COLOR ATLASES

14TH EDITION

Harrison's

PRINCIPLES of INTERNAL MEDICINE

14TH EDITION

Harrison's

PRINCIPLES of INTERNAL MEDICINE

EDITORS

Anthony S. Fauci, MD
Chief, Laboratory of Immunoregulation; Director, National Institute of Allergy and Infectious Diseases, National Institutes of Health, Bethesda

Eugene Braunwald, AB, MD, MA (Hon), MD (Hon), ScD (Hon)
Distinguished Hersey Professor of Medicine, Faculty Dean for Academic Programs at Brigham and Women's Hospital and Massachusetts General Hospital, Harvard Medical School; Vice-President for Academic Programs, Partners HealthCare System, Boston

Kurt J. Isselbacher, AB, MD
Mallinckrodt Professor of Medicine, Harvard Medical School; Physician and Director, Massachusetts General Hospital Cancer Center, Boston

Jean D. Wilson, MD
Charles Cameron Sprague Distinguished Chair and Clinical Professor of Internal Medicine, The University of Texas Southwestern Medical Center, Dallas

Joseph B. Martin, MD, PhD, FRCP (C), MA (Hon)
Dean of the Faculty of Medicine; Caroline Shields Walker Professor of Neurobiology and Clinical Neuroscience, Harvard Medical School, Boston

Dennis L. Kasper, MD, MA (Hon)
William Ellery Channing Professor of Medicine, Harvard Medical School; Director, Channing Laboratory; Co-Director, Division of Infectious Diseases; Executive Vice-Chairman, Department of Medicine, Brigham and Women's Hospital, Boston

Stephen L. Hauser, MD
Chairman and Betty Anker Fife Professor, Department of Neurology, University of California San Francisco, San Francisco

Dan L. Longo, AB, MD, FACP
Scientific Director, National Institute on Aging, National Institutes of Health, Gerontology Research Center, Bethesda and Baltimore

McGraw-Hill
HEALTH PROFESSIONS DIVISION

New York   St. Louis   San Francisco   Auckland   Bogotá   Caracas   Lisbon   London   Madrid
Mexico City   Milan   Montreal   New Delhi   San Juan   Singapore   Sydney   Tokyo   Toronto

A Division of The McGraw·Hill Companies

> **Note:** Dr. Fauci and Dr. Longo's works as editors and authors were performed outside the scope of their employment as U.S. government employees. These works represent their personal and professional views and not necessarily those of the U.S. government.

Harrison's
PRINCIPLES OF INTERNAL MEDICINE
Fourteenth Edition

1234567890 DOWDOW 9987
ISBN 0-07-020291-5 (COMBO)
0-07-020292-3 (VOL 1)
0-07-020293-1 (VOL 2)
0-07-912013-X (SET)

FOREIGN LANGUAGE EDITIONS
Arabic (Thirteenth Edition)—McGraw-Hill Libri Italia srl (est. 1996)
Chinese (Twelfth Edition)—McGraw-Hill Book Company–Singapore © 1994
Croatian (Thirteenth Edition)—McGraw-Hill Libri Italia srl (est. 1996)
French (Thirteenth Edition)—McGraw-Hill Libri Italia srl © 1995
German (Thirteenth Edition)—McGraw-Hill Libri Italia srl © 1995
Greek (Twelfth Edition)—Parissianos © 1994
Italian (Thirteenth Edition)—McGraw-Hill Libri Italia srl © 1995
Japanese (Eleventh Edition)—Hirokawa © 1991
Portuguese (Thirteenth Edition)—McGraw-Hill/Nueva Editorial Interamericana © 1995
Spanish (Thirteenth Edition)—McGraw-Hill Interamericana de España © 1994
Turkish (Thirteenth Edition)—McGraw-Hill Libri Italia srl (est. 1996)

This book was set in Times Roman by Monotype Composition Company. The editors were J. Dereck Jeffers, Martin J. Wonsiewicz, and Mariapaz Ramos Englis; editorial assistants were Rose Derario and Daniel J. Green. The production director was Robert Laffler. The index was prepared by Irving Tullar. The text and cover designer was Marsha Cohen/Parallelogram Graphics.

R.R. Donnelley and Sons, Inc., was the printer and binder.

Library of Congress Cataloging-in-Publication Data

Harrison's principles of internal medicine.—14th. ed./editors,
   Anthony S. Fauci . . . [et al.]
        p.   cm.
   Includes bibliographical references and index.
   ISBN 0-07-020291-5 (1 vol. ed.).—ISBN 0-07-912013-X (2 vol. ed.
: set).—ISBN 0-07-020292-3 (2 vol. ed. : bk 1).—ISBN
0-07-020293-1 (2 vol. ed. : bk 2)
   1. Internal medicine.   I. Harrison, Tinsley Randolph.
II. Fauci, Anthony S.
   [DNLM: 1. Internal Medicine.   WB 115 H322 1998]
RC46.H333   1998
616—dc21
DNLM/DLC
for Library of Congress   97-14184

CONTENTS

1990

CONTRIBUTORS

Numbers in brackets refer to chapters written or co-written by the contributor.

ELIAS ABRUTYN, MD
Professor of Medicine and Public Health and Vice-Chairman, Medicine, Allegheny University of the Health Sciences, MCP Hahnemann School of Medicine, Philadelphia [146, 147]

MICHAEL J. AMINOFF, MD, FRCP
Professor of Neurology, University of California San Francisco, San Francisco [21, 361, 368]

KENNETH C. ANDERSON, MD
Associate Professor of Medicine, Harvard Medical School; Medical Director, Blood Component Laboratory, Dana-Farber Cancer Institute, Boston [115]

ELLIOTT M. ANTMAN, MD
Associate Professor of Medicine, Harvard Medical School; Director, Coronary Care Unit, Brigham and Women's Hospital, Boston [243]

GORDON LEE ARCHER, MD
Professor of Medicine and Microbiology/Immunology; Chairman, Division of Infectious Diseases, Department of Medicine, Medical College of Virginia, Virginia Commonwealth University, Richmond [140]

JAMES O. ARMITAGE, MD
Professor and Chairperson, Department of Internal Medicine, University of Nebraska Medical Center, Omaha [116]

ARTHUR K. ASBURY, MD
Van Meter Professor of Neurology; Vice-Dean for Faculty Affairs, University of Pennsylvania School of Medicine, Philadelphia [23, 381]

JOHN R. ASPLIN, MD
Assistant Professor of Medicine, Section of Nephrology, University of Chicago Pritzker School of Medicine, Chicago [278, 279]

JOHN C. ATHERTON, MRCP
Lecturer, Department of Medicine, Division of Gastroenterology and Institute of Infections and Immunity, University of Nottingham, Nottingham, England [156]

PAUL S. AUERBACH, MD, MS
Chief Executive Officer, American Medical Partners; Clinical Professor of Emergency Medicine, Stanford University School of Medicine, Stanford [392]

K. FRANK AUSTEN, MD
Theodore B. Bayles Professor of Medicine, Harvard Medical School; Director, Inflammation & Allergic Diseases Research Section, Division of Rheumatology and Immunology, Department of Medicine, Brigham and Women's Hospital, Boston [310]

BERNARD M. BABIOR, MD, PhD
Head, Division of Biochemistry, Department of Molecular and Experimental Medicine, The Scripps Research Institute; Professor and Staff Physician, Division of Hematology and Oncology, Department of Medicine, Scripps Clinic and Research Foundation, La Jolla [108]

KAMAL F. BADR, MD
Professor of Medicine and Director, Center for Glomerulonephritis, Renal Division, Emory University; Chief, Renal Section, Atlanta VA Medical Center; Attending Physician, Emory University Hospital, Atlanta [277]

DONALD S. BAIM, MD
Professor of Medicine, Harvard Medical School; Chief, Interventional Cardiology Section, Beth Israel Deaconess Medical Center, Boston [229, 245]

ANN SULLIVAN BAKER, MD*
Associate Professor of Medicine (Ophthalmology), Harvard Medical School; Director, Infectious Disease Service, Massachusetts Eye and Ear Infirmary; Physician, Massachusetts General Hospital, Boston [30]

KENNETH J. BART, MD, MPH, MSHPM
Associate Director, Office of International and Refugee Health, Department of Health and Human Services, Rockville [122]

M. FLINT BEAL, MD
Professor of Neurology, Harvard Medical School, Boston [372, 380]

* Deceased

ARTHUR L. BEAUDET, MD
Investigator, Howard Hughes Medical Institute; Professor, Departments of Molecular and Human Genetics, Pediatrics and Cell Biology, Institute for Molecular Genetics, Baylor College of Medicine, Houston [65]

ROBERT S. BENJAMIN, MD
Internist and Professor of Medicine, Chairman, Department of Melanoma/Sarcoma Medical Oncology; Medical Director, Multidisciplinary Sarcoma Center, The University of Texas M.D. Anderson Cancer Center, Houston [100]

JOHN E. BENNETT, MD
Head, Clinical Mycology Section, Laboratory of Clinical Investigation, Division of Intramural Research, National Institute of Allergy and Infectious Diseases, National Institutes of Health; Director, Infectious Diseases Training Program, NIAID, NIH, Bethesda [202–210]

ERNEST BEUTLER, MD
Member and Chairman, Department of Molecular and Experiment Medicine, The Scripps Research Institute; Clinical Professor of Medicine, University of California, San Diego, San Diego [107]

DAVID R. BICKERS, MD
Carl Truman Nelson Professor, Chairman, Department of Dermatology, College of Physicians and Surgeons, Columbia University, New York [58]

BEVERLY M.K. BILLER, MD
Assistant Professor of Medicine, Harvard Medical School, Massachusetts General Hospital, Boston [328]

THOMAS D. BIRD, MD
Professor of Neurology, University of Washington; Chief of Neurology, Veterans Affairs Medical Center, Seattle [26, 367]

NEIL R. BLACKLOW, MD
Richard M. Haidack Distinguished Professor of Medicine, Molecular Genetics and Microbiology, and Chairman, Department of Medicine, University of Massachusetts Medical School, Worcester [189]

MARTIN J. BLASER, MD
The Addison B. Scoville Professor of Medicine; Director, Division of Infectious Diseases and Professor of Microbiology and Immunology, Vanderbilt University School of Medicine and VA Medical Center, Nashville [156, 160]

CLARA D. BLOOMFIELD, MD
Professor and Director, Division of Hematology and Oncology, Department of Internal Medicine; Director, Comprehensive Cancer Center, Ohio State University, Columbus [112]

JEAN L. BOLOGNIA, MD
Associate Professor of Dermatology, Yale University School of Medicine, New Haven [57]

GEORGE J. BOSL, MD
Chairman, Department of Medicine, Memorial Sloan-Kettering Cancer Center; Professor of Medicine, Cornell University Medical College, New York [98]

RICHARD C. BOUCHER, JR., MD
Professor of Medicine and Director, CF/Pulmonary Research and Treatment Center and Chief, Division of Pulmonary Disease/Critical Care Medicine, University of North Carolina at Chapel Hill; University of North Carolina Hospitals, Chapel Hill [257]

DAVID S. BRADFORD, MD
Chairman and Professor, Department of Orthopaedic Surgery, University of California San Francisco, San Francisco [16]

KAREN D. BRADSHAW, MD
Associate Professor of Obstetrics and Gynecology, The University of Texas Southwestern Medical Center, Dallas [52, 337]

HUGH R. BRADY, MD, PhD, FRCPI
Professor of Medicine and Therapeutics, University College Dublin; Mater Misericordiae Hospital, Dublin, Ireland [270, 273–275]

KENNETH D. BRANDT, MD
Professor of Medicine; Head, Rheumatology Division; Director, Multipurpose Arthritis and Musculoskeletal Diseases Center, Indiana University School of Medicine, Indianapolis [322]

EUGENE BRAUNWALD, AB, MD, MA (Hon), MD (Hon),
ScD (Hon), FRCP
Distinguished Hersey Professor of Medicine; Faculty Dean for Academic Programs at Brigham and Women's Hospital and Massachusetts General Hospital, Harvard Medical School; Vice-President for Academic Programs, Partners HealthCare System, Boston [1, 32–34, 36, 37, 226, 227, 232, 233, 237–241, 243, 244]

IRWIN M. BRAVERMAN, MD
Professor of Dermatology, Yale University School of Medicine, New Haven [57]

OTIS W. BRAWLEY, MD
Director, Office of Special Populations, Office of the Director, National Cancer Institute, National Institutes of Health, Bethesda [82]

GEORGE A. BRAY, MD
Professor of Medicine/Executive Director, Pennington Biomedical Research Center, Louisiana State University, Baton Rouge [75]

JOEL G. BREMAN, MD, DTPH
Deputy Director, Division of International Training and Research, Fogarty International Center, National Institutes of Health, Bethesda [216]

BARRY M. BRENNER, MD, AM (Hon), DSc (Hon), DMSc (Hon)
Samuel A. Levine Professor of Medicine, Harvard Medical School; Senior Physician and Director, Renal Division, Brigham and Women's Hospital, Boston [47, 49, 268–271, 273–277, 280]

CLAIRE V. BROOME, MD
Deputy Director, Centers for Disease Control and Prevention, Atlanta [145]

PHILIPPE BROUQUI, MD, PhD
Professor of Medicine, Faculté de Médecine, Marseilles, France [179]

ROBERT H. BROWN, JR., DPhil, MD
Associate Neurologist, Massachusetts General Hospital; Associate Professor of Neurology, Harvard Medical School, Boston [103, 370]

H. FRANKLIN BUNN, MD
Professor of Medicine, Harvard Medical School; Physician, Brigham and Women's Hospital, Boston [108, 109]

JOAN R. BUTTERTON, MD, MPhil, DTMH
Instructor in Medicine, Harvard Medical School; Clinical Assistant, Infectious Disease Division, Massachusetts General Hospital, Boston [128]

ALFRED E. BUXTON, MD
Professor of Medicine and Cardiology; Associate Chief of Cardiology, Temple University School of Medicine, Philadelphia [230, 231]

STEPHEN B. CALDERWOOD, MD
Associate Professor of Medicine (Microbiology and Molecular Genetics); Physician and Chief, Infectious Disease Division, Massachusetts General Hospital, Boston [128]

GRANT L. CAMPBELL, MD, PhD
Chief, Epidemiology Section, Bacterial Zoonoses Branch, Division of Vector-Borne Infectious Diseases, National Center for Infectious Diseases, Centers for Disease Control and Prevention, Fort Collins [164, 177]

CHARLES B. CARPENTER, MD
Professor of Medicine, Harvard Medical School; Director, Laboratory of Immunogenetics and Transplantation, Brigham and Women's Hospital, Boston [272, 306]

BRUCE R. CARR, MD
Professor of Obstetrics and Gynecology and Director, Division of Reproductive Endocrinology, The University of Texas Southwestern Medical Center, Dallas [52, 337]

GAIL H. CASSELL, PhD
Charles H. McCauley Professor and Chairman, Department of Microbiology; Professor, Departments of Pediatrics and Comparative Medicine, University of Alabama at Birmingham, Birmingham [180]

AGUSTIN CASTELLANOS, MD
Professor of Medicine and Director, Clinical Electrophysiology, University of Miami School of Medicine, Miami [39]

HUGO CASTRO-MALASPINA, MD
Associate Professor of Medicine; Associate Member, Memorial Sloan-Kettering Cancer Center, New York [110]

YUAN-TSONG CHEN, MD, PhD
Professor of Pediatrics and Chief, Division of Medical Genetics, Department of Pediatrics, Duke University Medical Center, Durham [347]

JOHN S. CHILD, MD
Professor of Medicine, University of California, Los Angeles; Co-Chief, Clinical Cardiology, UCLA Medical Center, Los Angeles [235]

L. CHINSOO CHO, MD
Assistant Professor, Department of Radiation Oncology, University of Texas Southwestern Medical Center, Harold C. Simmons Comprehensive Cancer Center, Dallas [396]

FREDRIC L. COE, MD
Professor of Medicine and Physiology and Chief, Nephrology Program, University of Chicago Pritzker School of Medicine, Chicago [268, 278, 279]

ALAN S. COHEN, MD
Distinguished Professor of Medicine in Rheumatology, Boston University School of Medicine, Boston [309]

JEFFREY I. COHEN, MD
Head, Medical Virology Section, National Institute of Allergy and Infectious Diseases, National Institutes of Health, Bethesda [186, 195]

JOHN M. COLFORD, JR., MD, MPH
Adjunct Assistant Professor, Department of Epidemiology and Biostatistics, University of California San Francisco, San Francisco [4]

FRANCIS S. COLLINS, MD, PhD
Director, National Human Genome Research Institute, National Institutes of Health, Bethesda [84]

WILSON S. COLUCCI, MD, FACC
Professor of Medicine and Physiology, Boston University School of Medicine; Chief, Cardiovascular Division, Boston Medical Center, Boston [241]

MAUREEN T. CONNELLY, MD, MPH
Instructor in Medicine, Harvard Medical School; Harvard Pilgrim Health Care, Boston [10]

MAX D. COOPER, MD
Professor of Medicine, Pediatrics, and Microbiology; Howard Hughes Medical Institute Investigator, University of Alabama at Birmingham, Birmingham [307]

LAWRENCE COREY, MD
Professor of Laboratory Medicine and Medicine and Head, Virology Division, University of Washington; Head, Program in Infectious Diseases, Fred Hutchinson Cancer Research Center, Seattle [184, 199, 201]

ANN M. COULSTON, MS, RD
Senior Research Dietitian, Stanford University Medical Center, Stanford [77]

MARK A. CREAGER, MD
Associate Professor of Medicine, Harvard Medical School; Director, Vascular Center, Brigham and Women's Hospital, Boston [247, 248]

RONALD G. CRYSTAL, MD
Bruce Webster Professor of Internal Medicine, Professor of Physiology and Biophysics; Chief, Division of Pulmonary and Critical Care Medicine, Department of Medicine, The New York Hospital–Cornell Medical Center, New York [320]

JOHN J. CUSH, MD
Medical Director, Arthritis Consultation Center, Presbyterian Hospital of Dallas, Dallas [321]

CHARLES A. CZEISLER, PhD, MD
Director, Sleep Disorders and Circadian Medicine, Associate Professor of Medicine, Harvard Medical School; Brigham and Women's Hospital, Boston [27]

GILBERT H. DANIELS, MD
Associate Professor of Medicine, Harvard Medical School; Co-Director, Thyroid Associates, Massachusetts General Hospital, Boston [328]

ROBERT B. DAROFF, MD
Professor of Neurology and Associate Dean, Case Western Reserve University; Chief of Staff and Senior Vice-President of Medical Affairs, University Hospitals of Cleveland, Cleveland [20]

CHARLES E. DAVIS, MD
Professor of Pathology and Medicine, University of California, San Diego School of Medicine; Director Emeritus, Microbiology Laboratory, UCSD Medical Center, San Diego [213]

MARGO DENKE, MD
Associate Professor of Internal Medicine, Center for Human Nutrition, The University of Texas Southwestern Medical Center, Dallas [72–74]

BRADLEY M. DENKER, MD
Assistant Professor of Medicine, Harvard Medical School; Associate Physician, Brigham and Women's Hospital, Boston [47]

DAVID T. DENNIS, MD, MPH
Chief, Bacterial Zoonoses Branch, Division of Vector-Borne Infectious Diseases, National Center for Infectious Diseases, Centers for Disease Control and Prevention, Fort Collins [164, 177]

ROBERT L. DERESIEWICZ, MD
Assistant Professor of Medicine, Harvard Medical School; Associate Physician, Channing Laboratory and the Division of Infectious Diseases, Brigham and Women's Hospital, Boston [142, 161]

ROBERT J. DESNICK, PhD, MD
Arthur J and Nellie Z Cohen Professor of Pediatrics and Genetics; Chairman, Department of Human Genetics, Mount Sinai School of Medicine, New York [343]

JULES L. DIENSTAG, MD
Associate Professor of Medicine, Harvard Medical School; Physician, Massachusetts General Hospital, Boston [93, 295–297, 301]

WILLIAM P. DILLON, MD
Professor of Radiology, Neurology, and Neurosurgery; Chief, Diagnostic Neuroradiology, University of California San Francisco, San Francisco [362]

ALAN R. DIMICK, MD
Professor of Surgery, University of Alabama at Birmingham; Director, Burn Center, University of Alabama Hospital, Birmingham [395]

CHARLES A. DINARELLO, MD
Professor of Medicine, University of Colorado Health Sciences Center, Denver [17, 125]

ROBERT G. DLUHY, MD
Associate Professor of Medicine, Harvard Medical School, Brigham and Women's Hospital, Boston [332]

RAPHAEL DOLIN, MD
Charles A. Dewey Professor and Chair, Department of Medicine, University of Rochester School of Medicine and Dentistry, Rochester [183, 191, 193]

DANIEL B. DRACHMAN, MD
Professor of Neurology and Neurosciences; Director, Neuromuscular Unit, The Johns Hopkins University School of Medicine, Baltimore [382]

JEFFREY M. DRAZEN, MD
Parker B. Francis Professor of Medicine, Harvard Medical School; Chief, Pulmonary Division, Brigham and Women's Hospital, Boston [249–251, 266]

THOMAS D. DUBOSE, JR., MD
Professor of Medicine and Integrative Biology; Director, Division of Renal Diseases and Hypertension; Vice-Chairman, Department of Internal Medicine, The University of Texas–Houston Medical School; Medical Director, Nephrology Section, Herman Hospital; Medical Director, University Kidney Center, Houston [50]

MARLENE DURAND, MD
Instructor, Harvard Medical School; Assistant in Medicine, Massachusetts General Hospital, Boston [30]

JANICE P. DUTCHER, MD
Professor of Medicine, Albert Einstein College of Medicine, Albert Einstein Cancer Center, Montefiore Medical Center, New York [104]

VICTOR J. DZAU, MD
Hersey Professor of the Theory and Practice of Medicine, Harvard Medical School; Chairman, Department of Medicine and Director of Research, Brigham and Women's Hospital, Boston [247, 248]

JEFFREY S. DZIECZKOWSKI, MD
Assistant Professor, Departments of Pathology and Internal Medicine, Wayne State University School of Medicine, Detroit [115]

J. DONALD EASTON, MD
Professor and Chair, Department of Clinical Neurosciences, Brown University School of Medicine; Neurologist-in-Chief, Rhode Island Hospital, Providence [366]

BARRY I. EISENSTEIN, MD
Vice-President, Science and Technology, Beth Israel Deaconess Medical Center, Boston [155]

LOUIS J. ELSAS II, MD
Professor of Pediatrics and Director of the Division of Medical Genetics, Emory University School of Medicine, Atlanta [349, 350]

JOHN W. ENGSTROM, MD
Associate Professor of Clinical Neurology, University of California San Francisco, San Francisco [16, 371]

ALAN EPSTEIN, MD
Assistant Professor of Medicine, Brown University, Providence [44, 288]

VIRGINIA L. ERNSTER, PhD
Professor of Epidemiology and Biostatistics, Department of Epidemiology and Biostatistics, University of California San Francisco, San Francisco [4]

KENNETH H. FALCHUK, MD
Associate Professor of Medicine, Harvard Medical School, Brigham and Women's Hospital, Boston [80]

ANTHONY S. FAUCI, MD
Chief, Laboratory of Immunoregulation; Director, National Institute of Allergy and Infectious Diseases, National Institutes of Health, Bethesda [1, 192, 305, 308, 319]

MURRAY J. FAVUS, MD
Professor of Medicine, Sections of Endocrinology and Nephrology, Department of Medicine, University of Chicago Pritzker School of Medicine, Chicago [279]

ROBERT G. FENTON, MD, PhD
Senior Investigator, Medicine Branch, Division of Clinical Sciences, National Cancer Institute, National Institutes of Health, Frederick [83]

THOMAS F. FERRIS, MD
Nesbitt Professor and Chairman, Department of Medicine, University of Minnesota; University of Minnesota Hospital and Clinics, Minneapolis [7]

HOWARD FIELDS, MD, PhD
Professor of Neurology and Physiology, University of California San Francisco, San Francisco [12]

GREGORY A. FILICE, MD
Associate Professor of Medicine, University of Minnesota; Chief, Infectious Disease Section, Veterans Affairs Medical Center, Minneapolis [167]

ROBERT W. FINBERG, MD
Professor of Medicine, Harvard Medical School; Chief, Division of Infectious Diseases, Dana-Farber Cancer Institute, Boston [87, 136]

JOYCE D. FINGEROTH, MD
Assistant Professor of Medicine, Harvard Medical School; Physician, Dana-Farber Cancer Institute, Boston [136]

DANIEL W. FOSTER, MD
Chairman and Professor of Internal Medicine, The University of Texas Southwestern Medical Center, Dallas [43, 76, 334, 335, 352]

ARNOLD S. FREEDMAN, MD
Associate Professor of Medicine, Harvard Medical School; Associate Professor of Medicine, Dana-Farber Cancer Institute, Boston [113]

GERALD H. FRIEDLAND, MD
Professor of Medicine and Epidemiology and Public Health, and Director, AIDS Program, Yale University School of Medicine, Yale-New Haven Hospital, New Haven [134]

LAWRENCE S. FRIEDMAN, MD
Associate Professor of Medicine, Harvard Medical School; Associate Physician, Massachusetts General Hospital, Boston [41, 42, 284, 287]

WILLIAM F. FRIEDMAN, MD
J.H. Nicholson Professor of Pediatrics (Cardiology); Senior Advisor, Clinical Affairs, to the Provost and Dean, University of California, Los Angeles School of Medicine and UCLA Medical Center, Los Angeles [235]

ROBERT F. GAGEL, MD
Professor of Medicine and Chief of the Section of Endocrinology, University of Texas M.D. Anderson Cancer Center, Houston [340]

JOHN I. GALLIN, MD
Director, NIH Warren Grant Magnuson Clinical Center; Associate Director for Clinical Research, Chief, Laboratory of Host Defenses, National Institute of Allergy and Infectious Diseases, National Institutes of Health, Bethesda [62]

JEFFREY A. GELFAND, MD
Sheldon M. Wolff Professor and Chairman, Department of Medicine, Tufts University School of Medicine; Physician-in-Chief, New England Medical Center, Boston [17, 125]

JAMES L. GERMAN III, MD
Member, New York Blood Center, Laboratory of Human Genetics, New York [66]

ANNE A. GERSHON, MD
Professor of Pediatrics, Columbia University College of Physicians and Surgeons; Attending Physician, Presbyterian Hospital, New York [196–198]

BRUCE C. GILLILAND, MD
Professor of Medicine and Laboratory Medicine, Associate Dean for Clinical Affairs, University of Washington School of Medicine, Seattle [314, 326]

HENRY N. GINSBERG, MD
Herbert and Florence Irving Professor of Medicine; Head, Division of Preventive Medicine and Nutrition, Department of Medicine, Columbia University College of Physicians and Surgeons, New York [341]

ELI GLATSTEIN, MD
Vice-Chairman and Clinical Director, Radiation Oncology, University of Pennsylvania Medical Center, Philadelphia [396]

ROBERT M. GLICKMAN, MD
Herrman L. Blumgart Professor of Medicine, Harvard Medical School; Chairman, Department of Medicine, Beth Israel Hospital, Boston [46, 286]

IRA J. GOLDBERG, MD
Professor of Medicine, Division of Preventive Medicine and Nutrition, Department of Medicine, Columbia University College of Physicians and Surgeons, New York [341]

ARY L. GOLDBERGER, MD
Associate Professor of Medicine, Harvard Medical School; Director of Electrocardiography and Arrhythmia Monitoring Laboratories, Beth Israel Deaconess Medical Center, Boston [228]

SAMUEL Z. GOLDHABER, MD
Associate Professor of Medicine, Harvard Medical School; Physician, Brigham and Women's Hospital, Boston [261]

LEE GOLDMAN, MD
Julius R. Krevans Distinguished Professor and Chairman, Department of Medicine and Associate Dean for Clinical Affairs, University of California, San Francisco School of Medicine, San Francisco [3, 11, 13]

DONALD E. GOODKIN, MD
Associate Professor, Department of Neurology; Medical Director, UCSF/Mt. Zion Multiple Sclerosis Center, San Francisco [376]

RAJ K. GOYAL, MD
Mallinckrodt Professor of Medicine, Harvard Medical School; Associate Chief of Staff for Research and Development, Brockton/West Roxbury VA Medical Center, West Roxbury [40, 283]

GREGORY C. GRAY, MD, MPH
Naval Health Research Center, Clinical Epidemiology Division, San Diego [180]

HARRY B. GREENBERG, MD
Professor of Medicine, Microbiology and Immunology, Stanford University School of Medicine and the VA Palo Alto Health Care System, Stanford [194]

NORTON J. GREENBERGER, MD, MACP
Professor and Chairman, Department of Medicine, University of Kansas Medical Center, Kansas City [285, 302–304]

JOHN S. GREENSPAN, BSc, BDS, PhD, FRCPath
Professor and Chair, Department of Stomatology and Director, Oral AIDS Center, School of Dentistry; Professor, Department of Pathology, and Director, AIDS Clinical Research Center, School of Medicine, University of California San Francisco, San Francisco [31]

JAMES E. GRIFFIN III, MD
Professor of Internal Medicine, The University of Texas Southwestern Medical Center, Dallas [336, 339]

ROBERT C. GRIGGS, MD
Professor of Neurology, Medicine, Pathology, Laboratory Medicine, and Pediatrics; Edward A. and Alma Vollertsen Professor of Neurophysiology; Chair, Department of Neurology, University of Rochester School of Medicine & Dentistry, Rochester [22, 383]

WILLIAM GROSSMAN, MD
Professor of Medicine, University of California San Francisco; Chief of Cardiology, University of California San Francisco Medical Center, San Francisco [229, 245]

RASIM GUCALP, MD, FACP
Associate Professor of Medicine, Department of Oncology, Montefiore Medical Center, Albert Einstein College of Medicine, New York [104]

BEVRA HANNAHS HAHN, MD, FACP
Professor of Medicine, Chief of Rheumatology, University of California, Los Angeles, Los Angeles [312]

ROBERT I. HANDIN, MD
Professor of Medicine, Harvard Medical School; Director, Hematology Division, Brigham and Women's Hospital, Boston [60, 117–119]

H. HUNTER HANDSFIELD, MD
Professor of Medicine, University of Washington School of Medicine; Director, STD Control Program, Seattle-King County Department of Public Health, Seattle [129]

STEPHEN L. HAUSER, MD
Chairman and Betty Anker Fife Professor, Department of Neurology, University of California San Francisco, San Francisco [1, 360, 366, 373, 376]

BARTON FORD HAYNES, MD
Frederic M. Hanes Professor and Chair, Department of Medicine; Professor, Department of Immunology, Director, Duke University Arthritis Center, Durham [305]

PATRICK H. HENRY, MD
Chairman, Department of Medicine, St. John's Mercy Medical Center, St. Louis [61]

BARBARA L. HERWALDT, MD, MPH
Medical Epidemiologist, Centers for Disease Control and Prevention, Division of Parasitic Diseases, Atlanta [217]

ROBERT S. HILLMAN, MD
Professor of Medicine, University of Vermont College of Medicine; Chairman of Medicine, Maine Medical Center, Portland [59, 106]

RAYMOND L. HINTZ, MD
Professor of Pediatrics, Head of the Division of Pediatric Endocrinology, Stanford University School of Medicine, Stanford [329]

MARTIN S. HIRSCH, MD
Professor of Medicine, Harvard Medical School; Physician, Massachusetts General Hospital, Boston [187]

BERNARD HIRSCHEL, MD
Associate Professor of Medicine; Head, HIV/AIDS Section, Division of Infectious Diseases, University Hospital, Geneva [173]

GARY S. HOFFMAN, MD, MS
Chairman, Department of Rheumatic and Immunologic Diseases, Cleveland Clinic Foundation; Professor of Medicine, Ohio State University, Columbus [323]

JOHN H. HOLBROOK, MD
Professor of Medicine and Chief, Division of General Internal Medicine, University of Utah School of Medicine, Salt Lake City [389]

MICHAEL F. HOLICK, PhD, MD
Professor of Medicine, Physiology and Dermatology, Boston University School of Medicine, Boston [353, 355]

STEVEN M. HOLLAND, MD
NIAID Investigator, Laboratory of Host Defenses, National Institute of Allergy and Infectious Diseases, National Institutes of Health, Bethesda [62]

STEVEN M. HOLLENBERG, MD
Assistant Professor of Medicine, Sections of Cardiology and Critical Care Medicine, Rush Medical College, Chicago [38]

KING K. HOLMES, MD, PhD
Professor of Medicine and Director, Center for AIDS and STD, University of Washington, Seattle [129, 130, 150, 166, 174]

RANDALL K. HOLMES, MD, PhD
Professor and Chair, Department of Microbiology, University of Colorado Health Sciences Center, Denver [144]

ERIC G. HONIG, MD
Associate Professor of Medicine, Emory University School of Medicine, Atlanta [258, 265]

JONATHAN C. HORTON, MD, PhD
Associate Professor of Ophthalmology, Neurology, and Physiology, University of California San Francisco, San Francisco [28]

THOMAS H. HOSTETTER, MD
Professor of Medicine, University of Minnesota School of Medicine; Director, Division of Renal Disease, University Hospital, Minneapolis [276]

LYN HOWARD, MB, DCh, FRCP, FACP
Head, Division of Clinical Nutrition, Professor of Medicine and Associate Professor of Pediatrics, The Albany Medical College, Albany [78]

HOWARD HU, MD, MPH, ScD
Associate Professor of Occupational Medicine, Harvard School of Public Health; Assistant Professor of Medicine, Harvard Medical School; Associate Physician, Channing Laboratory, Brigham and Women's Hospital, Boston [5, 390, 397]

GARY W. HUNNINGHAKE, MD
Professor of Internal Medicine and Director, Pulmonary, Critical Care and Occupational Medicine, University of Iowa College of Medicine, Iowa City [253]

DANIEL C. IHDE, MD
Professor of Medicine and Chief, Medical Oncology, Washington University School of Medicine, St. Louis [63]

EDWARD P. INGENITO, MD, PhD
Assistant Professor of Medicine, Harvard Medical School; Director, Pulmonary Function Laboratory, Brigham and Women's Hospital, Boston [266]

ROLAND H. INGRAM, JR, MD
Martha West Looney Professor, Emory University School of Medicine; Director, Pulmonary and Critical Care Medicine, Chief of Medicine, Emory-Crawford Long Hospital, Atlanta [32, 258, 265]

THOMAS S. INUI, ScM, MD
Professor and Chairman, Department of Ambulatory Care and Prevention, Harvard Medical School; Harvard Pilgrim Health Care, Boston [10]

CHARLES E. IRWIN, JR, MD
Professor of Pediatrics, Director of the Division of Adolescent Medicine, University of California San Francisco, San Francisco [8]

MARK A. ISRAEL, MD
Professor, Departments of Neurological Surgery and Pediatrics; Director, Preuss Laboratory of Molecular Neuro-Oncology, University of California San Francisco, San Francisco [375]

KURT J. ISSELBACHER, MD
Mallinckrodt Professor of Medicine, Harvard Medical School; Physician and Director, Massachusetts General Hospital Cancer Center, Boston [1, 41, 42, 44–46, 93, 281, 285, 288, 291–300, 302, 304, 342, 351]

RICHARD F. JACOBS, MD
Horace C. Cabe Professor of Pediatrics and Chief, Pediatric Infectious Diseases, Arkansas Children's Hospital and the University of Arkansas for Medical Sciences, Little Rock [163]

BRUCE E. JOHNSON, MD
Head, Lung Cancer Biology Section, Medicine Branch, National Cancer Institute, National Institutes of Health, Bethesda [102]

MICHAEL P. JOSEPH, MD
Physician, Weber Medical Clinic, Ltd., Olney [30]

MARK E. JOSEPHSON, MD
Professor of Medicine, Harvard Medical School; Director, Harvard-Thorndike Electrophysiology Institute and Arrhythmia Service, Beth Israel Deaconess Medical Center, Boston [230, 231]

EDWARD L. KAPLAN, MD
Professor, Department of Pediatrics, University of Minnesota Medical School, Minneapolis [236]

LEE M. KAPLAN, MD, PhD
Assistant Professor of Medicine, Harvard Medical School; Associate Chief for Research, Gastrointestinal Unit, Massachusetts General Hospital, Boston [45, 95]

DENNIS L. KASPER, MD, MA (Hon)
William Ellery Channing Professor of Medicine, Harvard Medical School; Director, Channing Laboratory; Co-Director, Division of Infectious Diseases; Executive Vice-Chairman, Department of Medicine, Brigham and Women's Hospital, Boston [1, 120, 127, 148, 152, 169]

LLOYD H. KASPER, MD
Professor of Medicine (Neurology) and Microbiology, Dartmouth Medical School, Hanover [219]

DONALD KAYE, MD
Klinghoffer Professor of Medicine, MCP Hahnemann School of Medicine, Allegheny University of the Health Sciences; Executive Vice-President for Health Affairs, Allegheny University of the Health Sciences; President and CEO, Allegheny University Hospitals, Philadelphia [126]

ELAINE T. KAYE, MD
Clinical Instructor in Dermatology, Harvard Medical School; Assistant in Medicine, Department of Medicine, Children's Hospital Medical Center, Boston [18]

KENNETH M. KAYE, MD
Assistant Professor of Medicine, Harvard Medical School; Associate Physician, Division of Infectious Diseases, Brigham and Women's Hospital, Boston [18]

JONATHAN R. KELLER, PhD
Head, Hematology and Gene Therapy Section, SAIC, Inc.; Intramural Research and Support Program, National Cancer Institute-Frederick Cancer Research and Development Center, Frederick [105]

GERALD T. KEUSCH, MD
Professor of Medicine and Chief, Division of Geographic Medicine and Infectious Diseases, New England Medical Center Hospitals, Boston [122, 158, 159, 161]

JAY S. KEYSTONE, MD, FRCPC
Professor of Medicine, University of Toronto; Tropical Disease Unit, Division of Infectious Disease, The Toronto Hospital, Toronto [123]

ELLIOTT D. KIEFF, MD, PhD
Harriet Ryan Albee Professor of Medicine; Professor of Microbiology and Molecular Genetics; Chairman, Virology Program, Harvard Medical School; Co-Director, Division of Infectious Diseases, Brigham and Women's Hospital, Boston [182]

LOUIS V. KIRCHHOFF, MD, MPH
Professor, Department of Internal Medicine, University of Iowa; Staff Physician, Department of Veterans Affairs Medical Center, Iowa City [218]

JAMES P. KNOCHEL, MD
Clinical Professor of Internal Medicine, University of Texas Southwestern Medical Center; Chairman, Department of Internal Medicine, Presbyterian Hospital, Dallas [356, 357]

HOWARD K. KOH, MD, PhD
Professor of Dermatology, Medicine and Public Health, Boston University Schools of Medicine and Public Health; Co-Director, Skin Oncology Program, Director, Cancer Prevention and Control Center, Boston [88]

ELISE C. KOHN, MD
Senior Investigator, Chief, Signal Transduction and Prevention Unit, Laboratory of Pathology, National Cancer Institute, National Institutes of Health, Bethesda [85]

ANTHONY L. KOMAROFF, MD
Professor of Medicine, Harvard Medical School, Boston [6]

WALTER J. KOROSHETZ, MD
Associate Professor of Neurology and Medicine; Associate Director, Stroke and Clinical Neurology Services, Massachusetts General Hospital, Harvard Medical School, Boston [378]

WILLIAM J. KOVACS, MD
Associate Professor of Medicine, Division of Endocrinology, Vanderbilt University School of Medicine, Nashville [53]

PHYLLIS E. KOZARSKY, MD
Associate Professor of Medicine, Emory University School of Medicine; Chief of Infectious Diseases, Emory Crawford Long Hospital, Atlanta [123]

BARNETT S. KRAMER, MD, MPH
Associate Director, Early Detection and Community Oncology Program, Division of Cancer Prevention and Control, National Cancer Institute, National Institutes of Health, Bethesda [82]

STEPHEN M. KRANE, MD
Persis, Cyrus, and Marlow B. Harrison Professor of Medicine, Harvard Medical School, Massachusetts General Hospital, Boston [353, 355, 358, 359]

DONALD W. KUFE, MD
Professor of Medicine, Harvard Medical School; Chief, Division of Cancer Pharmacology, Department of Medicine, Dana-Farber Cancer Institute, Boston [86]

HELENA KUIVANIEMI, MD, PhD
Associate Professor, Center for Molecular Medicine and Genetics, and Department of Surgery, Wayne State University School of Medicine, Detroit [348]

LEWIS LANDSBERG, MD
Irving S. Cutter Professor and Chairman, Department of Medicine, Northwestern University Medical School; Physician-in-Chief, Northwestern Memorial Hospital, Chicago [70, 333]

H. CLIFFORD LANE, MD
Head, Clinical and Molecular Retrovirology Section, Laboratory of Immunoregulation; Clinical Director, National Institute of Allergy and Infectious Diseases, National Institutes of Health, Bethesda [308]

THOMAS J. LAWLEY, MD
Professor and Chairman, Department of Dermatology, Emory University School of Medicine, Atlanta [54, 55, 311]

ALEXANDER R. LAWTON III, MD
Edward C. Stahlman Professor in Pediatric, Physiology and Cell Metabolism; Professor of Pediatrics and Microbiology, Head, Division of Pediatric Immunology and Rheumatology, Vanderbilt University School of Medicine, Nashville [307]

J. MICHAEL LAZARUS, MD
Associate Professor of Medicine, Harvard Medical School; Director of Clinical Services, Nephrology Division, Brigham and Women's Hospital, Boston [271, 272]

MATTHEW E. LEVISON, MD
Professor of Medicine and Chief, Division of Infectious Diseases, Allegheny University of the Health Sciences, Philadelphia [255]

ELLIOTT LEVY, MD
Instructor in Medicine, Harvard Medical School; Associate Physician, Brigham and Women's Hospital, Boston [276]

PETER LIBBY, MD
Professor of Medicine, Harvard Medical School; Director, Vascular Medicine and Atherosclerosis Unit, Brigham and Women's Hospital, Boston [242]

RICHARD W. LIGHT, MD
Professor of Medicine, Vanderbilt University; Director, Pulmonary Diseases Program, Saint Thomas Hospital, Nashville [262]

CHRISTOPHER LINDEN, MD
Associate Professor of Emergency Medicine, Division of Toxicology, University of Massachusetts Medical Center, Worcester [391]

LANCE A. LIOTTA, MD, PhD
Chief, Laboratory of Pathology, National Cancer Institute, National Institutes of Health, Bethesda [85]

MARC E. LIPPMAN, MD
Director, Lombardi Cancer Center; Professor of Medicine and Pharmacology, Georgetown University Medical School, Washington, DC [64, 91]

PETER LIPSKY, MD
Professor of Internal Medicine and Microbiology; Director, Harold C. Simmons Arthritis Research Center, Department of Internal Medicine, University of Texas Southwestern Medical Center at Dallas, Dallas [313, 317, 321]

LEO X. LIU, MD, DTMH
Assistant Professor of Medicine, Harvard Medical School; Division of Infectious Diseases, Department of Medicine, Beth Israel Deaconess Medical Center, Boston [214, 221, 222]

BERNARD LO, MD
Professor of Medicine and Director, Program in Medical Ethics, University of California San Francisco, San Francisco [2]

DAN L. LONGO, MD, FACP
Scientific Director, National Institute on Aging, National Institutes of Health, Gerontology Research Center, Bethesda and Baltimore [1, 61, 63, 81, 83, 105, 114, 192]

FRANK M. LONGO, MD, PhD
Associate Professor of Neurology, University of California San Francisco; Chief of Neurology, Veterans Affairs Medical Center, Department of Neurology, San Francisco [363]

NICOLA LONGO, MD, PhD
Assistant Professor of Pediatrics, Emory University School of Medicine, Atlanta [349, 350]

JOSEPH LOSCALZO, MD
Wade Professor and Chairman, Department of Medicine, Boston University School of Medicine; Physician-in-Chief, Boston Medical Center; Director, Whitaker Cardiovascular Institute, Boston [71]

FREDERICK H. LOVEJOY, JR, MD
William Berenberg Professor of Pediatrics, Harvard Medical School; Chief and Vice-Chairman, Department of Pediatrics, Children's Hospital, Boston [391]

DANIEL H. LOWENSTEIN, MD
Associate Professor of Neurology, Anatomy, and Neurosurgery, Robert B. and Ellinor Aird Chair in Neurology; Director, Epilepsy Research Laboratory, University of California San Francisco, San Francisco [365]

SHEILA A. LUKEHART, PhD
Research Professor of Medicine and Infectious Diseases, University of Washington, Seattle [174]

RICHARD B. LYNN, MD
Assistant Professor of Medicine, Jefferson Medical College, Thomas Jefferson University, Philadelphia [287]

HARALD S. MACKENZIE, MB, ChB, MRCP (UK)
Assistant Professor of Medicine, Harvard Medical School; Associate Physician, Brigham and Women's Hospital, Boston [269]

M. MONIR MADKOUR, DM (Cairo), FRCP (London)
Consultant Physician, Military Hospital, Riyadh [162]

LAWRENCE C. MADOFF, MD
Assistant Professor of Medicine, Harvard Medical School; Channing Laboratory, Brigham and Women's Hospital; Division of Infectious Diseases, Beth Israel Deaconess Medical Center, Boston [120, 135]

JAMES H. MAGUIRE, MD
Associate Professor of Medicine, Harvard Medical School; Associate Professor in Tropical Public Health, Harvard School of Public Health, Boston [132, 324, 393]

FRANCIS E. MARCHLINSKI, MD
Professor of Medicine, Allegheny University of the Health Sciences; Section Chief, Electrophysiology, Allegheny University Hospitals, Philadelphia [230, 231]

THOMAS J. MARRIE, MD, FRCPC
Professor of Medicine, Dalhousie University, Halifax [179]

JOSEPH B. MARTIN, MD, PhD, FRCP (C), MA (Hon)
Dean of the Faculty of Medicine; Caroline Shields Walker Professor of Neurobiology and Clinical Neuroscience, Harvard Medical School, Boston; formerly Professor of Neurology and Chancellor, University of California San Francisco, San Francisco [1, 12, 20, 24, 29, 360, 363, 366, 371, 372, 380]

JANET MAURER, MD
Head, Section of Lung Transplantation, Department of Pulmonary and Critical Care Medicine, The Cleveland Clinic Foundation, Cleveland [267]

ROBERT J. MAYER, MD
Professor of Medicine, Harvard Medical School; Clinical Director, Department of Medicine, Dana-Farber Cancer Institute, Boston [92, 94]

JOHN D. McCONNELL, MD
Professor and Chairman, Department of Urology, The University of Texas Southwestern Medical Center, Dallas [48, 51]

EDWARD REGIS McFADDEN, JR., MD
Argyl J. Beams Professor of Medicine and Director, Pulmonary and Critical Care Medicine, Case Western Reserve University School of Medicine, Cleveland [252]

MARGARET McGOVERN, MD
Assistant Professor of Human Genetics and Pediatrics, Mount Sinai School of Medicine, New York [346]

NANCY K. MELLO, PhD
Professor of Psychology (Neuroscience), Alcohol and Drug Abuse Research Center, McLean Hospital, Belmont [388]

JERRY R. MENDELL, MD
Chairman and Professor of Neurology; Director, Neuromuscular Disease Center, The Ohio State University, Columbus [383]

JACK H. MENDELSON, MD
Professor of Psychiatry (Neuroscience), Alcohol and Drug Abuse Research Center, McLean Hospital, Belmont [388]

M.-MARSEL MESULAM, MD
Ruth and Evelyn Dunbar Professor of Neurology and Psychiatry; Director, Center for Behavioral and Cognitive Neurology; Director, Alzheimer's Program, Northwestern University Medical School, Chicago [25]

RICHARD A. MILLER, MD
Associate Professor of Medicine, University of Washington School of Medicine; Chief, Infectious Diseases Section, Veterans Affairs Puget Sound Health Care System, Seattle [172]

JOHN D. MINNA, MD
Professor, Internal Medicine and Pharmacology; Director, Hamon Center for Therapeutic Oncology Research, University of Texas Southwestern Medical Center, Dallas [90]

JEROME H. MODELL, MD
Professor of Anesthesiology; Executive Associate Dean, University of Florida College of Medicine, Gainesville [394]

STEPHEN A. MORSE, MSPH, PhD
Associate Director, Science Division AIDS/STDs and Tuberculosis Laboratory Research, National Center for Infectious Diseases, Centers for Disease Control and Prevention, Atlanta; Adjunct Professor of Microbiology and Immunology, Emory School of Medicine, Atlanta, and University of Alabama at Birmingham, Birmingham [150]

ARNOLD M. MOSES, MD, FACP
Professor of Medicine, State University of New York Health Science Center, Syracuse [330]

ROBERT J. MOTZER, MD
Associate Attending Physician, Memorial Sloan-Kettering Cancer Center; Associate Professor of Medicine, Cornell University Medical College, New York [96, 98]

HARALAMPOS M. MOUTSOPOULOS, MD
Professor and Director, Department of Pathophysiology, National University of Athens School of Medicine; Corresponding member, Academy of Athens; Athens, Greece [316, 318]

LÜTFIYE MÜLAZIMOGLU, MD
Associate Professor of Infectious Diseases and Clinical Microbiology, Section of Infectious Diseases, Marmara University, School of Medicine, Istanbul [153]

ROBERT S. MUNFORD, MD
Jan and Henri Bromberg Professor of Internal Medicine; Professor of Microbiology, The University of Texas Southwestern Medical Center, Dallas [124]

TIMOTHY F. MURPHY, MD
Professor of Medicine and Microbiology; Director, Division of Infectious Diseases, State University of New York at Buffalo, Buffalo [152]

DANIEL M. MUSHER, MD
Professor of Medicine and Professor of Microbiology and Immunology, Baylor College of Medicine; Chief, Infectious Diseases Section, Veterans Affairs Medical Center, Houston [141, 151]

ROBERT J. MYERBURG, MD
Professor of Medicine and Physiology and Director, Division of Cardiology, University of Miami School of Medicine, Miami [39]

LEE M. NADLER, MD
Chair, Department of Adult Oncology, Dana-Farber Cancer Institute; Chief, Division of Oncology, Brigham and Women's Hospital; Professor of Medicine, Harvard Medical School, Boston [113]

THEODORE ELLIOTT NASH, MD
Senior Scientist; Head, Gastrointestinal Parasite Section, Laboratory of Parasitic Disease, National Institute of Allergy and Infectious Diseases, National Institutes of Health, Bethesda [220, 224]

ROBERT L. NORRIS, MD, FACEP
Assistant Professor of Surgery, Department of Surgery, Division of Emergency Medicine, Stanford University, Stanford [392]

THOMAS B. NUTMAN, MD
Head, Helminth Immunology Section, Laboratory of Parasitic Diseases, National Institute of Allergy and Infectious Diseases, National Institutes of Health, Bethesda [223, 225]

RICHARD J. O'BRIEN, MD
Chief, Research and Evaluation Branch, Division of Tuberculosis Elimination, National Center for HIV, STD, and TB Prevention, Centers for Disease Control and Prevention, Atlanta [171]

PATRICK T. O'GARA, MD
Assistant Professor of Medicine, Harvard Medical School; Director, Clinical Cardiology, and Vice-Chairman for Clinical Programs, Department of Medicine, Brigham and Women's Hospital, Boston [34]

YVONNE M. O'MEARA, MD, MRCPI
College Lecturer, Department of Medicine and Therapeutics, University College Dublin; Consultant Physician, Mater Misericordiae Hospital, Dublin, Ireland [274, 275]

RICHARD J. O'REILLY, MD
Chairman, Department of Pediatrics; Chief, Bone Marrow Transplantation, Memorial Sloan-Kettering Cancer Center, New York [110]

ROBERT A. O'ROURKE, MD
Charles Conrad Brown Distinguished Professor in Cardiovascular Disease, The University of Texas Health Science Center at San Antonio, San Antonio [227]

JOHN A. OATES, MD
Professor and Chairman, Department of Medicine, Vanderbilt University School of Medicine; Physician-in-Chief, Vanderbilt University Hospital, Nashville [68]

RICHARD K. OLNEY, MD
Professor of Clinical Neurology, School of Medicine, University of California San Francisco, San Francisco [21]

ANDREW B. ONDERDONK, PhD
Associate Professor of Pathology, Harvard Medical School; Director, Clinical Microbiology Laboratory, Brigham and Women's Hospital, Boston [121]

SCOTT OSLUND, MD
Attending Physician, St. Francis Medical Center, Lynwood [392]

JOSEPH E. PARRILLO, MD
James B. Herrick Professor of Medicine, Rush Medical College; Chief, Sections of Cardiology and Critical Care Medicine; Medical Director, Rush Heart Institute, Rush–Presbyterian–St. Luke's Medical Center, Chicago [38]

JEFFREY PARSONNET, MD
Associate Professor of Medicine and of Microbiology, Dartmouth Medical School; Staff Physician, Infectious Disease Section, Dartmouth-Hitchcock Medical Center, Hanover [142]

SHREYASKUMAR R. PATEL, MD
Associate Professor of Medicine, Department of Melanoma/Sarcoma Medical Oncology, The University of Texas MD Anderson Cancer Center, Houston [100]

PETER L. PERINE, MD
Professor of Epidemiology, University of Washington, Seattle; Professor of Tropical Public Health and Medicine Emeritus, Uniformed Services University of the Health Sciences, Bethesda [175]

C.J. PETERS, MD
Chief, Special Pathogens Branch, Division of Viral and Rickettsial Diseases, National Center for Infectious Diseases, Centers for Disease Control and Prevention, Atlanta [200]

WALTER L. PETERSON, MD
Professor of Medicine, University of Texas Southwestern Medical School; Staff Physician, Dallas VA Medical Center, Dallas [284]

KEVIN J. PETTY, MD, PhD
Associate Director, Clinical Development, US Human Health, Merck & Company, Inc, Westpoint, Pennsylvania [19]

ELIOT A. PHILLIPSON, MD
Sir John and Lady Eaton Professor of Medicine and Chair, Department of Medicine, University of Toronto; Physician-in-Chief, Mount Sinai Hospital, Toronto [263, 264]

GERALD B. PIER, PhD
Associate Professor of Medicine, Harvard Medical School; Channing Laboratory, Brigham and Women's Hospital, Boston [139]

DANIEL K. PODOLSKY, MD
Professor of Medicine, Harvard Medical School; Chief, Gastrointestinal Unit, Massachusetts General Hospital, Boston [281, 291–293, 298–300]

RONALD E. POLK, PharmD
Professor of Pharmacy and Medicine, School of Pharmacy, Medical College of Virginia, Virginia Commonwealth University, Richmond [140]

MATTHEW POLLACK, MD
Professor of Medicine, Uniformed Services University of the Health Sciences, F. Edward Hébert School of Medicine, Bethesda [157]

JOHN T. POTTS, JR., MD
The Jackson Professor of Clinical Medicine, Massachusetts General Hospital, Harvard Medical School, Boston [353, 354]

LAWRIE W. POWELL, MD, PhD
Professor of Medicine, The University of Queensland; Director, Queensland Institute of Medical Research, The Bancroft Centre, Brisbane, Queensland, Australia [342]

DARWIN J. PROCKOP, MD, PhD
Professor and Director, Center for Gene Therapy MCP Hahnemann School of Medicine, Allegheny University of the Health Sciences, Philadelphia [348]

LOUIS J. PTÁČEK, MD
Associate Professor of Neurology and Human Genetics, The University of Utah School of Medicine, Salt Lake City [383]

DIDIER RAOULT, MD, PhD
Professor of Medicine and President of the University of Aix, Marseilles, France [179]

NEIL H. RASKIN, MD
Professor of Neurology, School of Medicine, University of California San Francisco, San Francisco [15, 364]

MARIO C. RAVIGLIONE, MD
Medical Officer, Tuberculosis Research and Surveillance Unit, Global Tuberculosis Programme, World Health Organization, Geneva [171]

SHARON L. REED, MD
Associate Professor of Medicine and Pathology and Director, Microbiology and Virology Laboratories, University of California, San Diego Medical Center, San Diego [215]

ANTONIO J. REGINATO, MD
Head, Division of Rheumatology; Professor of Medicine, Cooper Hospital/University Medical Center, University of Medicine and Dentistry of New Jersey/Robert Wood Johnson Medical School at Camden, Camden [323]

RICHARD C. REICHMAN, MD
Professor of Medicine, Microbiology and Immunology and Head, Infectious Disease Unit, University of Rochester School of Medicine and Dentistry, Rochester [190]

NEIL M. RESNICK, MD
Associate Professor of Medicine, Harvard Medical School; Chief, Division of Gerontology, Brigham and Women's Hospital; Geriatric Research Education and Clinical Center, Brockton-West Roxbury Veterans Administration Medical Center, Boston [9]

VICTOR I. REUS, MD
Professor of Psychiatry, University of California San Francisco; Medical Director, Langley Porter Hospital, San Francisco [385]

HERBERT Y. REYNOLDS, MD
J. Lloyd Huck Professor of Medicine, The Pennsylvania State University; Chairman, Department of Medicine, University Hospital, The Milton S. Hershey Medical Center, Hershey [259]

STUART RICH, MD
Professor of Medicine, Rush Medical College; Director, Rush Heart Institute Center for Pulmonary Heart Disease, Chicago [260]

GARY S. RICHARDSON, MD
Instructor in Medicine, Harvard Medical School; Director, Sleep Disorders Service, Brigham and Women's Hospital, Boston [27]

HAL B. RICHERSON, MD
Professor of Internal Medicine, Allergy-Immunology Division, University of Iowa College of Medicine; University of Iowa Hospitals and Clinics, Iowa City [253]

CELESTE ROBB-NICHOLSON, MD, MPH
Assistant Professor of Medicine, Harvard Medical School; Assistant Physician, Massachusetts General Hospital, Boston [6]

CHERYL L. ROCK, PhD, RD
Associate Professor of Family and Preventive Medicine, University of California, San Diego, San Diego [77]

ALLAN H. ROPPER, MD
Chief of Neurology, St. Elizabeth's Medical Center; Professor of Neurology, Tufts University School of Medicine, Boston [24, 374]

LEON E. ROSENBERG, MD
Senior Vice-President, Scientific Affairs, Bristol-Myers Squibb Pharmaceutical Research Institute, Princeton [349, 350]

ROGER N. ROSENBERG, MD
Zale Distinguished Chair in Neurology; Professor of Neurology and Physiology, University of Texas Southwestern Medical Center; Attending Neurologist, Parkland Hospital and Zale-Lipsky University Hospital, Dallas [369]

WENDELL F. ROSSE, MD
Florence Reynaud McAlister Professor of Medicine and Medical Research, Department of Medicine, Duke University Medical School, Durham [109]

ARTHUR H. RUBENSTEIN, MD
Lowell T. Coggeshall Professor and Chairman of Medicine, University of Chicago Pritzker School of Medicine, Chicago [335]

MACK T. RUFFIN IV, MD, MPH
Assistant Professor, Department of Family Practice, Assistant Research Scientist, Department of Epidemiology, University of Michigan, Ann Arbor [77]

FRANCIS W. RUSCETTI, PhD
Chief, Laboratory of Leukocyte Biology, Division of Basic Sciences, National Cancer Institute–Frederick Cancer Research and Development Center, National Institutes of Health, Frederick [105]

THOMAS A. RUSSO, MD, CM
Assistant Professor of Medicine, Division of Infectious Diseases, Department of Medicine, State University of New York at Buffalo, Buffalo [168]

ARTHUR I. SAGALOWSKY, MD
Professor of Urology and Chief of Urologic Oncology, Department of Urology, The University of Texas Southwestern Medical Center, Dallas [97]

STEPHEN M. SAGAR, MD
Professor of Neurology, Case Western Reserve School of Medicine, Cleveland [375]

MATTHEW H. SAMORE, MD
Assistant Professor of Medicine, Harvard Medical School; Division of Infectious Diseases, Beth Israel Deaconess Medical Center, Boston [154]

I. HERBERT SCHEINBERG, MD
Senior Lecturer in Medicine, College of Physicians and Surgeons, Columbia University, New York [345]

W. MICHAEL SCHELD, MD
Professor of Internal Medicine and Neurosurgery; Associate Chair for Residency Programs, University of Virginia School of Medicine, Charlottesville [377]

HOWARD I. SCHER, MD
Chief, Genitourinary Oncology Service, Associate Attending Physician, Division of Solid Tumor Oncology, Department of Medicine, Memorial Sloan-Kettering Cancer Center; Associate Professor Medicine, Cornell University Medical College, New York [96]

ALAN L. SCHILLER, MD
Irene Heinz Given and John LaPorte Given Professor and Chairman of Pathology, Mount Sinai School of Medicine; Chairman of Pathology, The Mount Sinai Hospital, New York [359]

JOHN SPEER SCHROEDER, MD
Professor of Medicine, Stanford University School of Medicine; Division of Cardiovascular Medicine, Stanford Hospital, Stanford [234]

ANNE SCHUCHAT, MD
Medical Epidemiologist, Division of Bacterial and Mycotic Diseases, National Center for Infectious Diseases, Centers for Disease Control and Prevention, Atlanta [145]

MARC A. SCHUCKIT, MD
Professor of Psychiatry, University of California, San Diego, and Veterans Affairs Medical Center, San Diego [386, 387]

PETER H. SCHUR, MD
Professor of Medicine, Harvard Medical School; Senior Physician, Brigham and Women's Hospital, Boston [325]

DAVID S. SEGAL, PhD
Professor of Psychiatry, University of California, San Diego, La Jolla [387]

JULIAN L. SEIFTER, MD
Associate Professor of Medicine, Harvard Medical School; Physician, Brigham and Women's Hospital, Boston [280]

ANDREW P. SELWYN, MD, MA (Hon), FRCP, FACC
Professor of Medicine, Harvard Medical School; Director of Cardiac Catheterization, Brigham and Women's Hospital, Boston [244]

PETER A. SELWYN, MD, MPH
Associate Professor of Medicine, Epidemiology, and Public Health and Associate Director, AIDS Program, Yale University School of Medicine, Yale–New Haven Hospital, New Haven [134]

MARY-ANN SHAFER, MD
Professor of Pediatrics, Associate Director of the Division of Adolescent Medicine, University of California San Francisco, San Francisco [8]

STEVEN I. SHERMAN, MD
Assistant Professor of Medicine, University of Texas MD Anderson Cancer Center, Houston [340]

GEORGE R. SIBER, MD
Associate Professor of Medicine, Harvard Medical School, Boston; Vice-President and Chief Scientific Officer, Wyeth Lederle Vaccines and Pediatrics, Pearl River [154]

WILLIAM SILEN, MD
Johnson & Johnson Distinguished Professor of Surgery, Harvard Medical School; Surgeon-in-Chief Emeritus, Department of Surgery, Beth Israel Hospital, Boston [14, 289, 290]

FRED E. SILVERSTEIN, MD
Clinical Professor of Medicine, University of Washington; Partner, Frazier and Company, Seattle [282]

GARY G. SINGER, MD
Assistant Professor of Medicine, Washington University School of Medicine; Associate Director, Transplant Nephrology, Barnes-Jewish Hospital, St. Louis [49]

JEAN D. SIPE, PhD
Professor, Department of Biochemistry, Boston University School of Medicine, Boston [309]

CHRISTOPHER A. SLAPAK, MD
Assistant Professor of Medicine, Harvard Medical School; Division of Cancer Pharmacology, Dana-Farber Cancer Institute, Boston [86]

JAMES B. SNOW, JR., MD
Director, National Institute on Deafness and Other Communication Disorders, National Institutes of Health, Gaithersburg [29]

ARTHUR J. SOBER, MD
Associate Professor of Dermatology, Harvard Medical School; Associate Chief of Dermatology, Massachusetts General Hospital, Boston [88]

CLAUS O. SOLBERG, MD, PhD
Professor of Medicine and Chairman, Medical Department, University of Bergen, Bergen, Norway [149]

PETER SPEELMAN, MD
Chief, Division of Infectious Diseases, Tropical Medicine and AIDS, Department of Medicine, Academic Medical Center, University of Amsterdam, Amsterdam [176]

FRANK E. SPEIZER, MD
Edward H. Kass Professor of Medicine, Harvard Medical School; Co-Director, Channing Laboratory, Brigham and Women's Hospital, Boston [5, 254, 390]

ANDREW SPIELMAN, ScD
Professor of Tropical Public Health, Harvard School of Public Health, Boston [393]

JERRY L. SPIVAK, MD
Professor of Medicine and Oncology, The Johns Hopkins University School of Medicine, Baltimore [111]

WALTER E. STAMM, MD
Professor of Medicine and Head, Division of Allergy and Infectious Diseases, University of Washington, Seattle [131, 181]

ALLEN C. STEERE, MD
Professor of Medicine and Chief, Rheumatology/Immunology, New England Medical Center and Tufts University School of Medicine, Boston [178]

ROBERT S. STERN, MD
Professor, Department of Dermatology, Beth Israel Hospital, Boston [56]

DENNIS L. STEVENS, MD, PhD
Professor of Medicine, University of Washington School of Medicine, Seattle; Chief, Infectious Diseases, VA Medical Center, Boise [133]

RICHARD M. STONE, MD
Assistant Professor of Medicine, Harvard Medical School, Boston [101]

STEPHEN E. STRAUS, MD
Chief, Laboratory of Clinical Investigation, National Institute of Allergy and Infectious Diseases, National Institutes of Health, Bethesda [384]

DAVID H. P. STREETEN, MB, DPhil, FRCP
Professor of Medicine Emeritus, Department of Medicine, State University of New York, Health Science Center, Syracuse [330]

MORTON N. SWARTZ, MD
Professor, Department of Medicine, Harvard Medical School; Chief, James Jackson Firm Medical Services, Massachusetts General Hospital, Boston [378]

ROBERT A. SWERLICK, MD
Associate Professor, Department of Dermatology, Emory University School of Medicine, Atlanta [55]

RUP TANDAN, MD, MRCP
Associate Professor of Neurology; Director, Neuromuscular Disorders Section; Attending Neurologist, Medical Center Hospital of Vermont, Fletcher Allen Health Care, University of Vermont College of Medicine, Burlington [315]

JOEL D. TAUROG, MD
Professor of Internal Medicine, Department of Internal Medicine, University of Texas Southwestern Medical Center at Dallas, Dallas [317]

SCOTT J. THALER, MD
Instructor in Medicine, Harvard Medical School; Infectious Disease Division, Brigham and Women's Hospital, Boston [324]

LUCY STUART TOMPKINS, MD, PhD
Professor, Departments of Medicine (Division of Infectious Diseases and Geographic Medicine) and Microbiology and Immunology, Stanford University School of Medicine; Director, Clinical Microbiology Laboratory; Director, Hospital Epidemiology, Stanford University Medical Center, Stanford [165]

PHILLIP P. TOSKES, MD
Professor of Medicine and Director, Division of Gastroenterology, Hepatology and Nutrition; Associate Chairman for Clinical Affairs, Department of Medicine, University of Florida, Gainesville [303, 304]

NHU-LINH T. TRAN, MD
Fellow, Department of Dermatology, Emory University School of Medicine, Atlanta [88]

JEFFREY M. TRENT, PhD
Chief, Laboratory of Cancer Genetics; Director, Division of Intramural Research, National Human Genome Research Institute, National Institutes of Health, Bethesda [84]

GERARD TROMP, PhD
Assistant Professor, Center for Molecular Medicine and Genetics, Wayne State University School of Medicine, Detroit [348]

KENNETH L. TYLER, MD
Professor of Neurology, Medicine and Microbiology and Immunology, University of Colorado Health Sciences Center; Chief, Neurology Service, Denver Veterans Affairs Medical Center, Denver [379]

DAVID L. VALLE, MD
Professor of Pediatrics and Molecular Biology and Genetics, The Johns Hopkins Hospital School of Medicine, Baltimore [67]

EVERETT E. VOKES, MD
Professor of Medicine and Radiation and Cellular Oncology, University of Chicago, Chicago [89]

K. B. WAITES, MD
Associate Professor, Departments of Pathology, Microbiology, and Rehabilitation Medicine; Director of Clinical Microbiology, University of Alabama Hospitals and Clinics, Birmingham [180]

DAVID H. WALKER, MD
Professor and Chairman, Department of Pathology; Director, WHO Collaborating Center for Tropical Diseases, University of Texas Medical Branch, Galveston [179]

RICHARD J. WALLACE, JR., MD
Chairman, Department of Microbiology; Acting Director of Center for Pulmonary Infectious Disease Control; Professor of Medicine; John Chapman Professorship in Microbiology, University of Texas Health Center, Tyler [170]

PETER D. WALZER, MD
Professor of Medicine, University of Cincinnati College of Medicine; Associate Chief of Staff for Research, Cincinnati VA Medical Center, Cincinnati [211]

FREDERICK C.S. WANG, MD
Assistant Professor of Medicine, Harvard Medical School, Boston [182, 188]

LEONARD WARTOFSKY, MD
Professor of Medicine and Physiology, Uniformed Services University; Clinical Professor of Medicine, Georgetown, George Washington, and Howard University Schools of Medicine; Chairman of Medicine Washington Hospital Center, Washington DC [331]

CARL V. WASHINGTON, JR, MD
Assistant Professor of Dermatology, Emory University School of Medicine; Director, Mohs Surgery Unit, The Emory Clinic, Atlanta [88]

VISH WATKINS, MD
Clinical Research Physician, Lilly Research Laboratories, Eli Lilly and Company, Indianapolis [155]

STEVEN E. WEINBERGER, MD
Professor of Medicine, Harvard Medical School; Chief, Pulmonary and Critical Care Division, Beth Israel Deaconess Medical Center, Boston [33, 249–251, 256]

ROBERT A. WEINSTEIN, MD
Professor of Medicine, Rush Medical College; Chairman, Division of Infectious Diseases, Cook County Hospital, Chicago [138]

PETER F. WELLER, MD
Professor of Medicine, Harvard Medical School; Co-Chief, Division of Infectious Diseases and Chief, Allergy and Inflammation Division, Department of Medicine, Beth Israel Deaconess Medical Center, Boston [212, 214, 220–223, 225]

MICHAEL R. WESSELS, MD
Associate Professor of Medicine, Harvard Medical School; Channing Laboratory, Brigham and Women's Hospital; Division of Infectious Diseases, Beth Israel Deaconess Medical Center, Boston [143]

MEIR WETZLER, MD
Assistant Professor of Medicine, State University of New York at Buffalo, Buffalo [112]

NICHOLAS J. WHITE, DSc, MD, FRCP
Director, Wellcome-Mahidol University, Oxford Tropical Medicine Research Programme, Faculty of Tropical Medicine, Mahidol University, Bangkok; Wellcome Trust Clinical Research Unit, Centre for Tropical Diseases, Cho Quan Hospital, Ho Chi Minh City [216]

RICHARD J. WHITLEY, MD
Loeb Eminent Scholar in Pediatrics and Professor of Pediatrics, Microbiology and Medicine, University of Alabama at Birmingham, Birmingham [185]

GRANT R. WILKINSON, PhD
Professor of Pharmacology, Vanderbilt University School of Medicine, Nashville [68]

GORDON H. WILLIAMS, MD
Professor of Medicine, Harvard Medical School; Chief, Endocrine-Hypertension Division, Brigham and Women's Hospital, Boston [35, 246, 332]

JEAN D. WILSON, MD
Charles Cameron Sprague Distinguished Chair and Clinical Professor of Internal Medicine, The University of Texas Southwestern Medical Center, Dallas [1, 51, 53, 72–74, 79, 97, 327, 336, 338, 339]

BRUCE U. WINTROUB, MD
Professor of Dermatology, Executive Vice-Dean, School of Medicine, University of California San Francisco, San Francisco [56]

BEVERLY WOO, MD
Assistant Professor of Medicine, Harvard Medical School; Physician, Brigham and Women's Hospital, Boston [6]

ALASTAIR J.J. WOOD, MBChB, FRCP (Edin), FRCP (Lond)
Professor of Medicine and Professor of Pharmacology, Vanderbilt University School of Medicine; Attending Physician, Vanderbilt University Hospital, Nashville [69]

ROBERT L. WORTMANN, MD
Professor and Chairman of Medicine, East Carolina University School of Medicine, Greenville [344]

PAUL W. WRIGHT, MD
Director of Predoctoral Education and Professor of Family Practice, University of Texas Health Center, Tyler [170]

JOSHUA WYNNE, MD
Professor of Medicine and Chief, Division of Cardiology, Wayne State University; Chief, Section of Cardiology, Harper Hospital, Detroit [239]

KIM B. YANCEY, MD
Senior Investigator, Dermatology Branch, National Cancer Institute, National Institutes of Health, Bethesda [54, 311]

JAMES B. YOUNG, MD
Professor of Medicine, Northwestern University Medical School; Attending Physician, Northwestern Memorial Hospital, Chicago [70, 333]

ROBERT C. YOUNG, MD
President, Fox Chase Cancer Center, Philadelphia [99]

VICTOR L. YU, MD
Professor of Medicine, University of Pittsburgh; Chief, Infectious Disease Section, Veterans Affairs Medical Center, Pittsburgh [153]

DORI F. ZALEZNIK, MD
Assistant Professor of Medicine, Harvard Medical School; Physician, Beth Israel Deaconess Medical Center; Channing Laboratory, Brigham and Women's Hospital, Boston [127, 137, 148]

PETER J. ZIMETBAUM, MD
Instructor in Medicine, Harvard Medical School; Cardiovascular Division, Beth Israel Deaconess Medical Center, Boston [230, 231]

PHILIPPE E. ZIMMERN
Associate Professor of Urology, The University of Texas Southwestern Medical School, Dallas [48]

The first edition of *Harrison's Principles of Internal Medicine* was published nearly 50 years ago, and subsequent editions have incorporated advances that have occurred in biomedical research and clinical practice in the interim. In the 14th edition, the text has been revised to reflect further understanding of the biology and pathophysiology of disease and at the same time to retain those facts that, while not new, remain clinically useful and important. Virtually every chapter in the 14th edition has been completely or substantially rewritten, and major new chapters have been added. In this preface, we cannot describe all of these changes; however, we would like to call to the reader's attention those that are particularly noteworthy.

Part One, "Introduction to Clinical Medicine," contains new chapters dealing with the influence of environmental and occupational hazards on health. Disease prevention is becoming more important in the current era, and both general principles of prevention and specific guidelines for primary care physicians are presented in a new chapter on preventive medicine. Chapters on medical ethics, women's and adolescent health, geriatric medicine, medical complications of pregnancy, and cost awareness and quantitative aspects of medicine have been revised and updated.

Part Two, "Cardinal Manifestations and Presentation of Diseases," serves as a comprehensive introduction to clinical medicine. Major symptoms are reviewed by organ system and are correlated with specific disease states—the basis of differential diagnosis. New chapters have been added on fever and rash; hypothermia; faintness, syncope, and dizziness; weakness, abnormal movements, and imbalance; coma and acute confusional states; aphasia and other focal cerebral disorders; memory loss and dementia; heart murmur; hypertension; voiding dysfunction, incontinence, and other common urologic complaints; manifestations of cancer; and breast masses in women and men. For the first time in *Harrison's*, a comprehensive approach to the diagnosis and treatment of common eye disorders is presented. The chapter on diarrhea and constipation has been extensively revised, with a focus not only on etiology but also on acute and chronic treatment. The chapter on gastrointestinal bleeding has been rewritten to focus on early diagnosis and the latest approaches to treatment.

Part Three, "Genetics and Disease," has been extensively updated and includes a new formulation of the role of classic and molecular genetics in health and disease and a major revision of the chapter on cytogenetics.

Part Four, "Clinical Pharmacology," contains a new chapter on nitric oxide. Nitric oxide or its inhibition may be important in the management of coronary insufficiency, septic shock, erectile impotence, primary pulmonary hypertension, and the adult respiratory distress syndrome.

Part Five, "Nutrition," covers nutritional considerations related to clinical medicine, including nutritional requirements, assessment of nutritional status, protein-energy malnutrition, and diet therapy.

The core of *Harrison's* encompasses the disorders of the organ systems and is contained in Parts Six through Fifteen. These sections include succinct accounts of the pathophysiology of the major systems and emphasize disease manifestations, diagnostic procedures, differential diagnosis, and treatment strategies. The treatment sections of virtually every chapter have been amplified, supplemented by the liberal use of algorithms, and clearly highlighted.

Part Six, "Oncology and Hematology," has been completely reorganized and extensively rewritten under the direction of our newest editor, Dr. Dan L. Longo, who brings to the textbook a wealth of experience at the bench and bedside in both hematology and oncology. He has called upon a distinguished group of contributors to reorganize this section. The oncology chapters that were distributed among several sections in previous editions have been brought together in a single section on neoplastic disorders (with the exception of tumors of the thyroid, central nervous system, and heart). There are eight new chapters, including those on the approach to the patient with cancer, cancer prevention and early detection, cancer cell biology, invasion and metastasis, sarcomas and bone tumors, and oncologic emergencies. Twenty-seven additional chapters have new authors. An effort was made to organize the chapters in a more uniform fashion and to include molecular and genetic mechanisms involved in tumors (and their clinical correlations) where that information is known. The chapter on lymphoid malignancies includes the novel classification scheme of the International Lymphoma Working Group. Where appropriate, diagnostic and management algorithms have been incorporated.

Changes in Part Seven, "Infectious Diseases," include a greater emphasis on the treatment of infections and infestations. Specific, current recommendations for therapy are made against a background of up-to-date information on the etiology, epidemiology, diagnosis, and prevention of infectious diseases. Special care has been taken to update and expand the information presented on the biology of microorganisms, microbial resistance to therapeutic agents, and emerging and reemerging infections, including mycobacterial infections, recently identified viral infections, and infections due to other newly recognized pathogens such as *Helicobacter pylori*. The revised chapter on the laboratory diagnosis of infectious diseases is complemented in this edition by the inclusion (as Appendix B) of comprehensive instructions for the collection and transport of specimens for culture. New and expanded chapters cover the health risks to travelers, the approach to patients with parasitic infections, and recommendations for the administration of standard and special-use vaccines. The chapter on the human retroviruses has been revised and expanded, as have the chapters on the biology of viruses and antiviral therapy. This edition's chapter on *Pneumocystis carinii* infection appears in Section 15, "Fungal Infections," reflecting the change in the classification of this pathogen from a protozoan to a fungus.

In Part Eight, "Disorders of the Cardiovascular System," a new chapter on atherosclerosis focuses not only on the importance of traditional risk factors but also on factors that influence plaque stability and instability. The current approach to the prevention of atherosclerosis is clearly delineated. An understanding of prevention of plaque instability is of critical importance, since it is now clear that plaque rupture can cause acute coronary syndromes (unstable angina and acute myocardial infarction) and sudden death.

Despite major advances in its diagnosis and therapy, acute myocardial infarction is the most common cause of death in industrialized nations. The new chapter on acute myocardial infarction provides important information on myocardial reperfusion therapy—thrombolysis and primary coronary angioplasty—and summarizes guidelines for acute coronary care and for risk stratification in the postinfarct patient.

Pulmonary thromboembolism is a major complication of the postoperative state and of a variety of illnesses. In Part Nine, "Disorders of the Respiratory System," major advances in prevention and therapy are presented in a new chapter that includes a useful algorithm for the work-up of patients with suspected pulmonary embolic disease. Enormous strides have been made in the use of lung transplantation for selected patients with end-stage, irreversible, pulmonary parenchymal and vascular disease, and a new chapter on this topic focuses on patient selection for this therapy.

In Part Ten, "Disorders of the Kidney and Urinary Tract," there has been considerable revision. In Part Eleven, "Disorders of the Gastrointestinal System," the new chapter on peptic ulcer and gastritis focuses on the role of *Helicobacter pylori*, with particular attention to its diagnosis and treatment. This chapter can be viewed as *the* definitive chapter on peptic ulcer and gastritis. The chapters on irritable bowel syndrome and diverticular diseases are also new, and the chapters on acute hepatitis and complications of cirrhosis have been extensively revised, the latter with a specific focus on the treatment of hepatic coma, ascites, and portal hypertension.

In Part Twelve, "Disorders of the Immune System, Connective Tissue, and Joints," the updating focuses on therapy. The chapter on "Introduction to the Immune System" has been completely rewritten and provides a comprehensive review of the human immune system. The chapter on HIV disease and AIDS is comprehensive and up-to-date and includes coverage of the natural history, epidemiology, and immunopathogenic mechanisms of HIV disease. In addition, the chapter contains both an organ system by organ system approach and a delineation of the major complications of HIV disease. The sections on therapy include a state-of-the-art discussion of the treatment of HIV infection with combinations of antiretroviral agents.

In Part Thirteen, "Endocrinology and Metabolism," there are new chapters on the hyperlipoproteinemias, lysosomal storage diseases, and glycogen storage disease. The chapter on diabetes mellitus includes a discussion of the impact of tight control on the development of diabetic complications.

As a new editor, Dr. Stephen L. Hauser, Chairman of the Department of Neurology at the University of California San Francisco, joins Dr. Joseph Martin in providing a comprehensive neurology section applicable to general internal medicine. Dr. Hauser's contributions to Part Fourteen, "Neurologic Disorders," have been substantial, including chapters on multiple sclerosis, disorders of the spinal cord, and stroke. The entire section on neurology has been extensively revised and updated. New or extensively rewritten chapters on neuroimaging, epilepsy, stroke, Alzheimer's disease, Parkinson's disease, ataxia, spinal cord disease, tumors, and chronic meningitis provide an up-to-date summary of this rapidly changing field. The traditional focus of *Harrison's* textbook—providing an in-depth review of the pathophysiologic basis of each neurologic disorder—has been retained, and important advances in molecular pathogenesis and treatment have been included. When possible, diagnostic and therapeutic algorithms have been prepared that standardize and simplify the approach to different neurologic problems. A major effort has been made to expand the neuroimaging figures throughout the section. The anatomic figures have also been expanded and improved.

Finally, Part Fifteen, "Environmental and Occupational Hazards," has been expanded and reorganized.

Beginning with the 12th edition of *Harrison's*, the editors decided to provide laboratory values expressed in two ways: according to the International System (SI) and according to the conventional laboratory terminology used by hospitals in the United States. We felt that this was important because, although the SI units are used in many scientific and medical journals in the United States and elsewhere and in hospitals in many parts of the world, there remains considerable resistance to their adoption from some hospitals and some medical journals. Thus, it is apparent that physicians in many parts of the world will have to live indefinitely with two systems of laboratory values—one for the practice of medicine and another for access to large parts of biomedical science. Consequently, in this edition we continue to list the SI units first and the conventional units in parentheses for all measurements except blood pressure, which is given only in millimeters of mercury, and for those measurements in which the values are the same in both systems, as in the case of serum sodium measurements (expressed in meq/L and mmol/L). In most instances, the interconversion between SI and conventional units is straightforward. However, it is imperative that readers consult their own laboratory for normal values. Perhaps the greatest potential danger inherent in the existence of the two systems is in the interpretation of plasma glucose and plasma calcium levels, but caution should be observed in the interpretation of all laboratory values.

In view of the requirements for continuing education for licensure and relicensure, as well as the emphasis on certification and recertification, a revision of the *Pre-Test Self-Assessment and Review* will be published with this edition. It consists of several hundred questions based on *Harrison's*, along with answers and explanations for the answers. The *Companion Handbook* that was pioneered as a supplement to the 11th edition of *Harrison's* has been updated and will appear shortly after the publication of this edition. The 13th edition of *Harrison's* has been available in a CD-ROM version. An expanded CD-ROM version of the 14th edition will be available and will be regularly updated.

We wish to express our appreciation to our many associates and colleagues, who, as experts in their fields, have helped us with constructive criticism and helpful suggestions. We acknowledge especially the contributions of Gary Abrams, David Acker, Robert Alpern, Donna Ambrosino, Joseph Antin, Karen Antman, James Armitage, Cameron Ashbaugh, Tamar Barlam, Arthur L. Beaudet, Richard Blumberg, Timothy Brewer, Bruce Chabner, Paul Choi, Hal Churchill, Jeffrey Cohen, Oren Cohen, George Curlin, Richard T. Davey, Jr., Margo A. Denke, Judith Falloon, Christopher Fanta, Mark Feinberg, Paul Fitzgerald, Lawrence Friedman, Joseph L. Goldstein, Daryl Gress, Rachel Haft, Helen H. Hobbs, Stephanie James, Clay Johnston, Keith Joiner, Stephen Kohl, Catherine Lachenauer, John LaMontagne, H. Clifford Lane, James Maguire, James Mastrianni, Carol Mendelsohn, Kirk Miller, James Murtagh, Thomas Nutman, Mario Ostrowski, David Ozonoff, Jeffrey Parsonnet, John Reilly, Elizabeth Robbins, David Rosenthal, John Rutherford, Richard Schwartzstein, Robert Seder, Ellen Seely, Julian Seifter, John Spengler, Ray Swanson, Jorge Tavel, Scott Thaler, Kenneth Tyler, Mark Udey, Sasha Vinogradov, C. Fordham von Reyn, Ronald Walls, Fred Wang, Arnold Weinberg, Michael Weinblatt, Scott Weiss, Peter Weller, Michael Wessels, and Stephen Zucker.

This book could not have been edited without the dedicated help of our co-workers in the editorial offices of the individual editors. We are especially indebted to Pat Duffey, Caroline Figoni, Christy K. Gonzales, Terry Jones, Leslie LaPiana, Julie McCoy, Pamela Oliver, Jaylyn Olivo, Kathryn Saxon, Marie Scurti, and Elin Woodger.

Finally, we continue to be indebted to three outstanding members of the McGraw-Hill organization: Mariapaz Ramos Englis, Managing Editor; J. Dereck Jeffers, Editor-in-Chief; and Martin J. Wonsiewicz, Editorial Director. They are an effective team who have given the editors constant encouragement and sage advice and have been of enormous help in bringing this edition to fruition in a timely manner.

The Editors

1   *The Editors*

THE PRACTICE OF MEDICINE

WHAT IS EXPECTED OF THE PHYSICIAN   The practice of medicine combines both science and art. The role of science in medicine is clear. Science-based technology is the foundation for the solution to many clinical problems; the dazzling advances in biochemical methodology and in biophysical imaging techniques that allow access to the remotest recesses of the body are the products of science. So too are the therapeutic maneuvers that increasingly are a major part of medical practice. Yet skill in the most sophisticated application of laboratory technology and in the use of the latest therapeutic modality alone does not make a good physician. The ability to extract from a mass of contradictory physical signs and from the crowded computer printouts of laboratory data those items that are of crucial significance, to know in a difficult case whether to "treat" or to "watch," to determine when a clinical clue is worth pursuing or when to dismiss it as a "red herring," and to estimate in any given patient whether a proposed treatment entails a greater risk than the disease are all involved in the decisions that the clinician, skilled in the practice of medicine, must make many times each day. This combination of medical knowledge, intuition, and judgment defines the *art of medicine*. It is as necessary to the practice of medicine as is a sound scientific base.

The editors of the first edition of this book articulated what is expected of the physician in words that, although they reflect the gender bias of that era, still ring true as a universal principle:

> No greater opportunity, responsibility, or obligation can fall to the lot of a human being than to become a physician. In the care of the suffering he needs technical skill, scientific knowledge, and human understanding. He who uses these with courage, with humility, and with wisdom will provide a unique service for his fellow man, and will build an enduring edifice of character within himself. The physician should ask of his destiny no more than this; he should be content with no less.

Tact, sympathy and understanding are expected of the physician, for the patient is no mere collection of symptoms, signs, disordered functions, damaged organs, and disturbed emotions. He is human, fearful, and hopeful, seeking relief, help and reassurance. To the physician, as to the anthropologist, nothing human is strange or repulsive. The misanthrope may become a smart diagnostician of organic disease, but he can scarcely hope to succeed as a physician. The true physician has a Shakespearean breadth of interest in the wise and the foolish, the proud and the humble, the stoic hero and the whining rogue. He cares for people.

THE PATIENT-PHYSICIAN RELATIONSHIP   It may be trite to emphasize that physicians need to approach patients not as "cases" or "diseases" but as individuals whose problems all too often transcend the complaints that bring them to the doctor. Most patients are anxious and frightened. Often they go to great ends to convince themselves that illness does not exist, or unconsciously they set up elaborate defenses to divert attention from the real problem that they perceive to be serious or life-threatening. Some patients use illness to gain attention or to serve as a crutch to extricate themselves from a stressful situation; some even feign physical illness. Whatever the patient's attitude, the physician needs to consider the setting in which an illness occurs—in terms not only of the patients themselves but also of their families and social backgrounds. Medical workups and records often fail to include essential information about the patient's origins, schooling, job, home and family, hopes and fears. Without this knowledge, it is difficult for the physician to gain rapport with the patient or to develop insight into the illness. The ideal physician-patient relationship is based on thorough knowledge of the patient, on mutual trust, and on the ability to communicate with one another.

The direct, one-to-one physician-patient relationship, which traditionally characterized the practice of medicine, is in jeopardy, primarily because of the changing setting in which medicine is being practiced. Often the management of the individual patient requires the participation of a variety of trained professional personnel and of several physicians and indeed may be a team effort. The patient can benefit greatly from such collaboration, but *it is the duty of the primary physician to guide the patient through an illness*. To carry out this difficult task, the physician must have some familiarity with the techniques, skills, and objectives of specialist physicians and of colleagues in the fields allied to medicine. In giving the patient an opportunity to receive all the benefits of the important advances of science, the primary physician must, in the last analysis, retain responsibility for the major decisions concerning diagnosis and treatment.

Furthermore, patients are increasingly cared for by groups of physicians, clinics, hospitals, or health-maintenance organizations (HMOs) rather than by individual, independent practitioners. Whatever the potential advantages of such organized medical groups, there are also drawbacks, the chief of which is the *loss of the concept of the physician who is primarily and continuously responsible*. Even in the group setting, it is essential that each patient have a physician who has an overview of the problems and who is familiar with the patient's reaction to the illness, to the drugs given, and to the challenges that the patient faces. Moreover, because a number of physicians may, at any one time, contribute to the care of a particular patient, accurate and detailed medical records are essential to patient care.

The practice of medicine in a "managed care" setting puts additional stress on the classic paradigm of the physician-patient relationship. Many physicians find themselves in an environment where they must deal with a patient within a restricted time frame, with limited access to specialists, and under organizational guidelines that may at times compromise their ability to exercise their optimal clinical judgment. These circumstances provide a unique challenge to the physician to deliver excellent medical care while complying with the guidelines of the organization within which he or she practices. As difficult as these restrictions may be, it is the ultimate responsibility of the physician to determine what is best for the patient; this responsibility cannot be relinquished in the name of compliance with organizational guidelines.

Satisfactory physician-patient relationships in the tertiary care setting require that the physician be well versed in etiquette and ethics as well as in medicine. The diagnostic and treatment dilemmas of referring physicians must be respected, although the treatment provided prior to admission may not have been up to the standards of the current hospital or care setting. Differences of opinion that arise about patient management are best resolved in private discussions away from the bedside. When students or residents are involved in the care of a patient, they must be supervised by a senior physician. On the other hand, physicians must never misuse their position of authority in any manner that potentially exploits patients, staff, or trainees.

The modern hospital constitutes an intimidating environment for most patients. Lying in a bed surrounded by air jets, buttons, and lights; invaded by tubes and wires; beset by the numerous members of the health care team—nurses, nurses' aides, physicians' assistants, social workers, technologists, physical therapists, medical students, house officers, attending and consulting physicians, and many others; transported to special laboratories and x-ray chambers replete with blinking lights and strange sounds, it is little wonder that patients lose their sense of reality. In fact, the physician is often the only tenuous link between the patient and the real world, and a strong personal relationship with the physician helps to sustain the patient in such a stressful situation.

Many trends in contemporary society tend to make medical care impersonal. Some of these have been mentioned already and include (1) vigorous efforts to reduce the escalating costs of health care; (2) the increasing reliance on technologic advances and computerization for many aspects of diagnosis and treatment; (3) the increased geographic mobility of both patients and physicians; (4) the growing number of HMOs, in which the patient may have little choice in selecting a physician; (5) the need for more than a single physician to be involved in the care of most patients who are seriously ill; and (6) an increasing tendency on the part of patients to express their disappointments with the health care system by legal means (i.e., by malpractice litigation). Given these changes in the medical care system, maintaining the humane aspects of medical care and the empathetic qualities of the physician is a major challenge. It is now more important than ever that the physician consider each patient to be a unique individual deserving of humane treatment, regardless of personal or financial circumstances.

The American Board of Internal Medicine has defined humanistic qualities as encompassing integrity, respect, and compassion. Availability, the expression of sincere concern, the willingness to take the time to explain all aspects of the illness, and an attitude of being nonjudgmental with patients who have lifestyles, attitudes, and values different from those of the physician and which he or she may in some instances even find repugnant are just a few of the characteristics of the humane physician. Every physician will, at times, be challenged by patients who evoke strongly negative (and occasionally strongly positive) emotional responses. Physicians should be alert to their own reactions to such patients and situations and should consciously monitor and control their behavior so that the patients' best interests remain the principal motivation for their actions at all times.

The famous statement of Dr. Francis Peabody is even more relevant today than when delivered more than a half century ago:

> The significance of the intimate personal relationship between physician and patient cannot be too strongly emphasized, for in an extraordinarily large number of cases both the diagnosis and treatment are directly dependent on it. One of the essential qualities of the clinician is interest in humanity, for the secret of the care of the patient is in caring for the patient.

CLINICAL SKILLS **History Taking** The written history of an illness should embody all the facts of medical significance in the life of the patient. If the history is recorded in chronologic order, recent events should be given the most attention. Likewise, if a problem-oriented approach is used, the problems that are clinically dominant should be listed first. Ideally, the narration of symptoms or problems should be in the patient's own words. However, few patients have sufficient powers of observation or recall to give a history without some guidance from the physician, who must be careful not to suggest the answers to the questions being posed. Often a symptom of concern to a patient has little significance, while a seemingly minor complaint may be of importance. Therefore, the physician must be alert to the possibility that any event related by the patient, however trivial or apparently remote, may be the key to the solution of the medical problem.

An informative history is more than an orderly listing of symptoms. Something is always gained by listening to patients and noting the way in which they describe their symptoms. Inflections of voice, facial expression, and attitude may betray important clues to the meaning of the symptoms to the patient. In listening to the history, the physician discovers not only something about the disease but also something about the patient.

With experience, the pitfalls of history taking become apparent. What patients relate for the most part consists of subjective phenomena colored by past experience; they differ widely in their responses to the same stimuli and in their coping mechanisms. Their attitudes are variably influenced by fear of disability and death and by concern over the consequences of their illness to their families. Sometimes the accuracy of the history is affected by language or sociologic barriers, by failing intellectual powers that interfere with recall, or by disorders of consciousness that make them unaware of their illness. It is not surprising, then, that even the most careful physician may at times despair of collecting factual data and be forced to proceed with evidence that represents little more than an approximation of the truth. It is in obtaining the history that the physician's skill, knowledge, and experience are most clearly in evidence.

The family history serves several functions. First, in rare single-gene defects a positive family history of a similarly affected individual or a history of consanguinity may have important diagnostic implications. Second, in diseases of multifactorial etiology with a familial aggregation, it may be possible to identify patients at risk for disease and to intervene before the development of overt manifestations. For example, recent weight gain may be a more ominous development in a woman who has a family history of diabetes than in one who does not. In certain situations the family history has major implications for preventive medicine. When a diagnosis of a hereditary condition known to predispose to cancer is made, it is the physician's obligation to follow up this possibility carefully in the patient, to survey the family, and to educate them about the need for long-term follow-up.

However accurate and complete, the medical history does much more than provide facts of critical importance. The very act of taking the history provides the physician with the opportunity to establish or enhance the unique bond that is the basis for the physician-patient relationship. An effort should be made to place the patient at ease, regardless of the circumstances. The patient should, at some point, have the opportunity to tell his or her own story of the illness without frequent interruption and, when appropriate, receive expressions of interest, encouragement, and empathy from the physician. It is helpful to develop an appreciation of the patient's perception of the illness, the patient's expectations of the physician and the medical care system, and the financial and social implications of the illness to the patient. The confidentiality of the physician-patient relationship should be emphasized, and the patient should be given the opportunity to identify any aspects of the history that should not be disclosed.

Physical Examination Physical signs are the objective indications of disease and represent solid, indisputable facts. Their significance is enhanced when they confirm a functional or structural change already suggested by the patient's history. At times, the physical signs may be the only evidence of disease, especially when the history is inconsistent, confused, or lacking altogether.

The physical examination should be performed methodically and thoroughly, with consideration for the patient's comfort and modesty. Although attention is often directed by the history to the diseased organ or part of the body, the examination of a new patient must extend from head to toe in an objective search for abnormalities. Unless the physical examination is systematic, important parts may be omitted, a common error even among skilled clinicians. The results of the examination, like the details of the history, should be recorded at the time they are elicited, not hours later when they are subject to the distortions of memory. Many inaccuracies stem from writing or dictating notes long after the examination has been concluded. Skill in physical diagnosis is acquired with experience, but it is not merely technique that determines success in eliciting signs. The detection of a few scattered petechiae, a faint diastolic murmur, or a small mass in the abdomen is not a question of keener eyes and ears or more sensitive fingers but of a mind alert to these findings. Skill in physical diagnosis reflects a way of thinking more than a way of doing. Physical findings are subject to change. Just because the examination is normal on one occasion does not guarantee that it will be normal on subsequent examinations. Likewise, abnormal findings may disappear during the course of illness. The physical examination should be repeated as frequently as the clinical situation warrants.

Laboratory Tests The increase in the number and availability of laboratory tests has increased our reliance on these studies for the solution of clinical problems. It is essential, however, to bear in mind the limitations of such procedures, which by virtue of their impersonal quality and complexity often gain an aura of authority regardless of the fallibility of the tests themselves, the instruments used in the tests, and the individuals performing or interpreting them. Moreover, the accumulation of laboratory data does not relieve the physician from the responsibility of careful observation and study of the patient. Physicians also must weigh the hazards and expense involved in the laboratory procedures they order. Moreover, laboratory tests are rarely ordered and reported singly. Rather, they are produced as "batteries" of multiple tests. The various combinations of laboratory tests are often useful. For example, they may provide the clue to such nonspecific symptoms as generalized weakness and increased fatigability by revealing abnormalities of hepatic function, suggesting the diagnosis of chronic liver disease. Sometimes a single abnormality, such as an elevated serum calcium level, points to a specific disease, such as hyperparathyroidism.

The thoughtful use of screening tests should not be confused with indiscriminate laboratory testing. The use of screening tests is based on the fact that a group of laboratory determinations can be carried out conveniently on a single specimen of blood at relatively low cost. Biochemical measurements, together with simple laboratory examinations such as blood count, urinalysis, and sedimentation rate, often provide the major clue to the presence of a pathologic process. At the same time, the physican must learn to evaluate occasional abnormalities among the screening tests that may not necessarily connote significant disease. An in-depth workup following a report of an isolated laboratory abnormality in a patient who is otherwise well is almost invariably wasteful and unproductive. Among the more than 40 tests that are performed on many patients, one or two are often slightly abnormal. If there is no suspicion of an underlying illness, these tests are ordinarily repeated to ensure that the abnormality does not represent a laboratory error. If an abnormality is confirmed, it is important to distinguish a minor one (less than two standard deviations) from a major one (more than two standard deviations). Even in the latter case, the decision of whether to proceed with further workup is left to the physician's clinical judgment.

Imaging Techniques The availability of ultrasonography, a variety of scans that employ isotopes to visualize organs heretofore inaccessible, computed tomography with its varying permutations, magnetic resonance imaging, and positron emission tomography has opened new diagnostic vistas, and has benefited patients because these new techniques have largely supplanted more invasive ones. While the enthusiasm for noninvasive technology is understandably justified, the expense entailed in performing these imaging tests is often substantial and is not always considered when ordering them. These examinations should be used judiciously.

Continued Learning The conscientious physician must be a perpetual student since the body of medical knowledge is constantly expanding and being refined. The profession of medicine should be inherently linked to a career-long thirst for new knowledge that can be used for the good of the patient. It is the responsibility of a physician to pursue continually the acquisition of new knowledge by reading, attending conferences and courses, and consulting with colleagues. This is often a difficult task under the circumstances of a busy practice; however, such a commitment to continued learning is such an integral part of being a physician that it should be given the highest priority.

Medicine on the Internet The explosion in use of the World-Wide Web, or Internet, through personal computers has had an important impact on many practicing physicians. The "Net" provides almost instantaneous availability of a wide range of information directly to the desk of a physician at any time of day or night and from anywhere in the world. It holds enormous potential for providing useful up-to-date practice guidelines, information on state-of-the-art conferences, journal contents, textbook chapters, and direct communication with other physicians and specialists, thereby expanding the depth and breadth of information available to the physician about the

diagnosis and care of patients. The potential benefit of this medium for the practicing physician is enormous, and it behooves physicians to become familiar with the use of the Internet. It is likely that most medical journals will ultimately be on-line. Yet, there is one important caveat. Certain authors post prepublication manuscripts on the Internet, and others supply unpublished data. In this regard, it is relatively easy to publish virtually anything on the Internet by using either a home page or a file server, thus circumventing the peer review process that is an essential feature of quality publication. Therefore, physicians who search the Internet for medical information must be aware of this potential for misinformation. Notwithstanding this limitation, appropriate use of the Internet is revolutionizing information access for physicians and will be a positive force in the practice of medicine.

THE DIAGNOSIS OF DISEASE Clinical diagnosis requires both aspects of logic—analysis and synthesis—and the more difficult the clinical problem, the more important is a logical approach to it. Such an approach requires that the physician list carefully each problem suggested by the symptoms and physical and laboratory findings and seek answers to each. Most physicians attempt consciously or unconsciously to fit a given problem into one of a series of syndromes. *The syndrome is a group of symptoms and signs of disordered function related to one another by means of some anatomic, physiologic, or biochemical peculiarity*. It embodies a hypothesis concerning the deranged function of an organ, organ system, or tissue. Congestive heart failure, Cushing's syndrome, and dementia are examples. In congestive heart failure, dyspnea, orthopnea, cyanosis, dependent edema, engorged neck veins, pleural effusion, rales, and hepatomegaly are connected by a single pathophysiologic mechanism—insufficiency of the cardiac pump mechanism. In Cushing's syndrome, moon facies, hypertension, diabetes mellitus, and osteoporosis are the consequence of excess glucocorticoids. In dementia, deterioration of memory, incoherent thinking, impaired language functions, visual-spatial disorientation, and faulty judgment are related to destruction of the association areas of the cerebrum.

A syndrome usually does not identify the precise cause of an illness, but it narrows the possibilities and may suggest certain special clinical and laboratory studies. The diagnosis is simplified greatly if a clinical problem conforms neatly to a well-defined syndrome, because only a few diseases need to be considered in the differential diagnosis. In contrast, the search for the cause of an illness that does not conform to a syndrome is more difficult because more diseases have to be considered. Even here an orderly approach that proceeds from symptom to sign to laboratory findings will usually result in the diagnosis.

CARING FOR THE PATIENT Patient care begins with the development of a personal relationship between the patient and the physician. In the absence of trust and confidence on the part of the patient, the effectiveness of most therapeutic measures is diminished. When there is confidence in the physician, reassurance may be the best treatment and all that is needed. Likewise, in those cases that do not lend themselves to easy solutions, a feeling by the patient that the physician is doing all that is possible is one of the most important benefits that can be provided. An important aspect of clinical decision making and patient care involves the "quality of life," a subjective assessment of what each patient values most. Such an assessment requires detailed, sometimes intimate knowledge of the patient, which can usually be obtained only through deliberate, unhurried, and often repeated conversation. As mentioned above, it is in these situations that the time constraints of a managed care setting may prove problematic. In situations where cure is impossible, enhancement of the quality of life is the major goal of therapy.

Assessing the Outcome of Treatments Clinicians generally use *objective* and readily measurable parameters to judge the outcomes of a therapeutic intervention. For example, findings on physical or laboratory examination—such as the level of blood pressure, the patency of a coronary artery on an angiogram, the size of a mass on a radiologic examination, or the titer of an antibody—can provide information of critical importance. However, patients usually seek medical attention for *subjective* reasons; they wish relief from pain, to preserve or regain function, and to enjoy life. Although these goals are often nebulous and differ among individuals, a patient's health status or quality of life can be separated into categories, such as bodily comfort, physical activity, social activity, personal and professional function, sexual function, cognitive function, sleep, vitality, and overall perception of health. Function in each of these important areas can be assessed by means of structured interviews or specially designed questionnaires. In a less formal way such assessments also provide useful parameters by which the physician can judge the patient's view of his or her disability and the response to treatment, particularly of chronic illness. The humane practice of medicine requires consideration and integration of both objective and subjective outcomes.

Drug Therapy   Many new drugs have only a marginal advantage over the agents they are aimed to replace. The barrage of new information with which practitioners are deluged does little to provide a clear picture of clinical pharmacology; on the contrary, to most physicians new drugs are confusing. With some exceptions, however, the approach to a new drug should be one of caution. Unless the new agent is established beyond doubt to be a real advance, it is wiser to use agents whose efficacy and safety are well established.

Care of the Elderly   Over the next several decades, the practice of medicine will be greatly influenced by the health care needs of the increasing numbers of the elderly. In the United States the population over age 65 will almost triple over the next 30 years, and it is essential that we understand and appreciate the physiologic processes associated with aging; the different responses of the elderly to common diseases; and disorders that occur commonly with aging such as depression, dementia, frailty, urinary incontinence, and fractures. The elderly have more adverse reactions to medications, in large part due to altered pharmacokinetics and pharmacodynamics. Commonly used drugs such as digoxin have prolonged half-lives, and tissues such as the central nervous system become more sensitive to certain drugs, such as the benzodiazepines and narcotics.

Diseases in Men versus Women   There are significant gender differences in diseases that afflict both men and women. These have not been clearly evident because in the past many epidemiologic and clinical studies were carried out only in adult men. In ischemic heart disease, mortality rates may be higher in women. Hypertension is more prevalent in African-American women than in their male counterparts; diseases involving the immune system such as lupus erythematosus, multiple sclerosis, and primary biliary cirrhosis occur more frequently in women; and women have a greater longevity than men. Recently, considerable attention has been paid to women's health issues, a subject that has regrettably not received sufficient attention in the past. Such consideration should enhance our understanding of the mechanisms of gender differences in the course and outcome of certain diseases.

Iatrogenic Disorders   An *iatrogenic disorder* occurs when the deleterious effects of a therapeutic or diagnostic regimen cause pathology independent of the condition for which the regimen is given. No matter what the clinical situation, it is the responsibility of the physician to use powerful therapeutic measures wisely, with due regard to their action, potential dangers, and cost. Every medical procedure, whether diagnostic or therapeutic, has the potential for harm, but it would be impossible to provide the benefits of modern scientific medicine if reasonable steps in diagnosis and therapy were withheld because of possible risks. *Reasonable* implies that the physician has weighed the pros and cons of a procedure and has concluded that it is advisable or essential for the relief of discomfort or the cure or amelioration of disease. For example, the use of glucocorticoids to arrest progressive systemic lupus erythematosus may produce Cushing's syndrome. In this instance, the benefits usually exceed the untoward side effects. However, much harm can result when the deleterious effects of a procedure or a drug exceed any possible advantages that might have been anticipated. Examples include the harmful and even fatal drug reactions that occasionally follow the use of antibiotics given for minor respiratory infections, the gastric hemorrhage or perforation caused by the administration of glucocorticoids for mild arthritis, and the development of fatal liver disease after needless transfusions of virus-contaminated blood or plasma.

However, the harm that a physician can do is not limited to the imprudent use of medication or procedures. Equally important are ill-considered or unjustified remarks. Many a patient has developed a cardiac neurosis because the physician ventured a grave prognosis on the basis of a misinterpreted finding of a heart murmur on auscultation. Not only the treatment itself but the physician's words and behavior are capable of causing injury.

The physician must never become so absorbed in the disease as to forget the patient who is its victim. As the science of medicine advances, it is all too easy to become so fascinated by the manifestations of disease that one disregards the ailing person's fears and concerns about suffering and death, job and family, the cost of medical care, and the specter of economic insecurity. Treatment of a patient consists of more than the dispassionate confrontation of a disease. It embodies also the expression of warmth, compassion, and understanding.

Informed Consent   Patients often require diagnostic and therapeutic procedures that are painful and that pose some risk, such as surgical procedures, including biopsies, endoscopy, radiographic maneuvers involving the insertion of catheters, and many others. In most hospitals and clinics, patients undergoing such procedures are required to sign a form consenting to them. More important, however, the patient must understand clearly the risk entailed in these procedures; this is the definition of *informed consent*. It is incumbent on the physician to explain to the patient, in a clearly understandable manner, the procedures he or she faces, and to ascertain that the patient understands both the procedure and the attendant risks. By doing this conscientiously, much of the dread of the unknown that is inherent in hospitalization will be mitigated.

Accountability   Throughout the world, physicians, once licensed to practice medicine, have not had to account for their actions except to their peers. In the United States, however, there have been increasing demands for physicians to account for the way in which they practice medicine by meeting certain standards prescribed by federal and state governments. The hospitalization of patients whose health care is reimbursed by the government (Medicare and Medicaid) and other third parties is subjected to utilization review. This means that the physician must defend the cause for and duration of a patient's hospitalization if it falls outside certain "average" standards. In some instances, a second opinion is necessary before a patient can have elective surgery. The purpose of these regulations is both to improve standards of health care and to contain spiraling health care costs. It is likely that this type of review will be extended to all phases of medical practice and will alter the practice of medicine profoundly.

Physicians also may be expected to give account of their continuing competence by mandatory continuing education, patient-record audit, recertification by examination (time-limited certification), or relicensing. While these measures probably enhance the physician's factual knowledge, there is no evidence that they have a similar effect on the quality of practice.

Practice Guidelines   Physicians are faced with a large, often bewildering array of potentially useful diagnostic techniques and therapeutic measures from which to choose as they deal with individual patients. The intelligent and cost-effective practice of medicine consists of selecting those most appropriate to a particular patient and clinical situation. To aid physicians and other care-givers in making these selections, professional organizations and government agencies are developing formal clinical practice guidelines. These guidelines may be viewed as double-edged swords. On the one hand, when they are current and properly applied, they can provide a useful framework for managing patients with particular diagnoses or symptoms. They also offer guidelines that protect patients—particularly those with inadequate health care benefits—from receiving substandard care. They can also protect conscientious caregivers from inappropriate charges of malpractice, and they can protect society from the excessive costs associated with the overuse of medical resources. However, clinical guidelines tend to oversimplify the complexities of medicine. Different groups with differing perspectives may develop divergent recommendations regarding issues as basic as the need for a periodic sigmoidoscopy in middle-aged persons. Furthermore, guidelines do not—and cannot be expected to—take into account the uniqueness of each individual and of his or her illness. The practice of medicine strictly according to guidelines carries with it the danger of transforming medicine from a learned profession rooted in the biologic and behavioral sciences to a technical vocation. The challenge for the physician is to accept and incorporate into clinical practice the useful recommendations offered by the experts who prepare clinical practice guidelines without accepting them blindly or being inappropriately constrained.

Evidence-Based Medicine The concept of evidence-based medicine means that clinical decisions are formally supported by data, particularly data derived from randomized, controlled clinical trials. There is a perception that many therapeutic decisions are made in the absence of a formal clinical trial that establishes efficacy. However, in a 1995 study at a university-affiliated hospital, it was concluded that 82 percent of primary treatments administered at that hospital were, in fact, evidence based. Evidence-based medicine was defined in the study as an intervention whose value had been established in one or more randomized controlled clinical trials or an intervention whose validity was so clear that randomized trials were unanimously judged to be unnecessary and would have been unethical if a placebo were involved. Eighteen percent of patients received symptomatic and supportive care without substantial evidence that it was superior to some other intervention, including no therapy. Nonetheless, there is a trend to require that therapy be scientifically validated. This approach will obviously have an impact on resource utilization.

Cost-Effectiveness in Medical Care As the cost of medical care continues to rise, it is necessary to establish priorities in the expenditure of money for health care. In some instances, preventive measures offer the greatest return for the expenditure; outstanding examples include vaccination, immunization, reduction in accidents and occupational hazards, improved environmental control, and biochemical and molecular biologic screening of newborns. For example, the detection of phenylketonuria by newborn screening may result in a net saving of many thousands of dollars.

As resources become increasingly constrained, it is necessary to weigh the justification of performing costly procedures that provide only a limited life expectancy against the pressing need for more primary care for those persons who do not have adequate access to medical services. At the level of the individual patient, it is important to reduce costly hospital admissions as much as possible if total health care is to be provided at a cost that most can afford. This, of course, implies and depends on a close cooperative effort between patients, their physicians, their employers, third-party carriers, and government. It is equally important for individual physicians to know the cost of medicines that they prescribe and to monitor both the cost and effectiveness of those drugs. In the last analysis, the medical profession should provide leadership and guidance to the public in matters of cost control, and physicians must take this responsibility seriously without being or seeming to be self-serving. It is important, however, that the socioeconomic aspects of health care delivery not interfere with the welfare of patients. The patient must be able to rely on the individual physician as his or her principal advocate in matters of health care.

Research and Teaching The title *doctor* is derived from the Latin *docere*, "to teach," and the physician should share information and medical knowledge with colleagues and with students of medicine and related professions. The practice of medicine is dependent on the sum total of medical knowledge, which in turn is based on an unending chain of scientific discovery, clinical observation, analysis, and interpretation. Advances in medicine depend on the acquisition of new information, i.e., on research, which must often involve patients; improved medical care requires the transmission of this information. As part of broader societal responsibilities, the physician should encourage patients to participate in ethical and properly approved clinical investigations if they do not impose undue hazard, discomfort, or inconvenience.

Incurability and Death No problem is more distressing than that presented by the patient with an incurable disease, particularly when premature death is inevitable. What should the patient and family be told, what measures should be taken to maintain life, and how is death to be defined?

Although some would argue otherwise, there is no ironclad rule that the patient must immediately be told "everything," even if the patient is an adult and the head of a family. How much the patient is told should depend on the individual's ability and capacity to deal with the possibility of imminent death; often this capacity grows with time, and whenever possible, gradual rather than abrupt disclosure is the best strategy. A wise and insightful physician is often guided by an understanding of what a patient wants to know and when he or she wants to know it. This decision also may take into consideration the patient's religious beliefs, financial and business status, and to some extent the wishes of the family. The patient must be given an opportunity to talk with the physician and ask questions. Patients may find it easier to share their feelings about death with their physician, who is likely to be more objective and less emotional than family members.

One thing is certain; it is not for you to don the black cap and, assuming the judicial function, take hope away from any patient . . . hope that comes to us all.

William Osler

Even when the patient directly inquires, "Doctor, am I dying?" the physician must attempt to determine whether this is a request for information, a demand for reassurance, or even an expression of hostility. Most would agree that only open communication between the patient and the physician can resolve these questions and guide the physician in what to say and how to say it.

The physician should provide or arrange for emotional, physical, and spiritual support and must be compassionate, unhurried, and open. There is much to be gained by the laying on of hands. Pain should be adequately controlled, human dignity maintained, and isolation from family avoided. The last two in particular tend to be overlooked in hospitals, where the intrusion of life-sustaining apparatuses can so easily detract from attention to the whole person and encourage concentration instead on the life-threatening disease. The physician also must prepare to deal with guilt feelings on the part of the family when a member becomes gravely or hopelessly ill. It is important for the doctor to be able to assure the family that everything possible has been done.

The President's Committee for the Study of Ethical Problems in Medicine defined death as (1) irreversible cessation of circulatory and respiratory function or (2) irreversible cessation of all functions of the entire brain, including the brainstem. Clinical and electroencephalographic criteria permit the reliable diagnosis of cerebral death. According to the criteria adopted by the staff of the Massachusetts General Hospital and the Harvard Committee on Brain Death, death occurs when all signs of receptivity and responsivity are absent, including all brainstem reflexes (pupillary reactions, ocular movement, blinking, swallowing, breathing), and the electroencephalogram is isoelectric. Occasionally, intoxications and metabolic disorders may simulate this state; hence the diagnosis requires expert evaluation. Under the aforementioned circumstances, to continue with heroic, highly costly supportive measures merely for the purpose of preserving cardiac function is against the best interests of patient, family, and society. In such instances, the dilemma of continuing care could be avoided if the medical profession, in accord with social sanction, can be brought to redefine life and death by these criteria.

The following guidelines are deserving of consideration:

1. The diagnosis of brain death, based on the preceding criteria, should be corroborated by another physician and confirmed by clinical examination and EEG, repeated one or more times.

2. The family should be informed of the irreversibility of loss of brain function but should not be requested to ratify the decision whether the medical treatment should be discontinued. An exception to this limited decision-making power of the family might apply where the patient has directed the family that he or she wishes them to make the decision.
3. The physician, after consultation with a professional colleague, may withdraw supportive measures, assuming that nothing more can be offered.
4. The possibility that such patients may become sources of organs for grafting should not enter into the aforementioned decisions, although prior to the cessation of heart action the family may be asked whether this would be their wish, or the family may suggest that organs be used for this purpose. In many states, laws now require physicians to request organ donations. A question arises when the patient has indicated in advance a wish to be an organ or tissue donor whether the family must be approached, since many believe the patient's prior wishes carry overriding weight. This issue is controversial.

"Do Not Resuscitate" Orders and Cessation of Therapy When carried out in a timely and expert manner, cardiopulmonary resuscitation is often useful in the prevention of sudden, unexpected death. However, unless there are reasons to the contrary, it should not be carried out when it merely prolongs life in a patient with terminal, incurable disease. The decision not to resuscitate a patient and decisions about the intensity of therapy and, indeed, whether or not treatment is to be delivered or continued to patients who are incurably and terminally ill must be reviewed frequently and must take into consideration any unexpected changes in the patient's condition. In this context the administration of fluids and food are considered therapies that may be withdrawn or withheld. These decisions also must take into account both the underlying medical condition and the wishes of the patient or, if these cannot be or have not been ascertained directly, those of a close relative or other surrogate who can be relied on to transmit the patient's feelings and to be guided by the patient's best interests and wishes. The patient's autonomy—whether the choice is to continue or discontinue treatment or to be resuscitated in the event of a cardiopulmonary arrest—is paramount. The courts have ruled that competent patients may be able to refuse therapy and that an incompetent patient's previously stated wishes regarding life support should be respected. The issues involving death and dying are among the most difficult in medicine. In approaching them rationally and consistently, the physician must combine both the art and the science of medicine.

BIBLIOGRAPHY

ELLIS J et al: Inpatient general medicine is evidence based. Lancet 346:407, 1996

LEWIN DI, SHURKIN JN: Scientific publishers rush journals into virtual print. J NIH Res 7:23, 1995

TAUBES G: Looking for the evidence in medicine. Science 272:22, 1996

| 2 | *Bernard Lo* |

ETHICAL ISSUES IN CLINICAL MEDICINE

Physicians frequently confront ethical issues in clinical practice that are perplexing, time-consuming, and emotionally draining. Experience, common sense, and simply being a good person do not guarantee that physicians can identify or resolve ethical dilemmas. Knowledge about common ethical dilemmas is also essential.

FUNDAMENTAL ETHICAL GUIDELINES

In patient care, physicians should follow two fundamental but frequently conflicting ethical guidelines: respecting patient autonomy and acting in the patient's best interests.

RESPECTING PATIENT AUTONOMY Competent, informed patients may exercise their self-determination and liberty by refusing recommended interventions and choosing among the available alternatives.

Informed Consent Informed consent requires physicians to discuss with the patient the nature of the proposed care, the alternatives, the risks and benefits of each, and the likely consequences and to obtain the patient's agreement to care. Informed consent involves more than obtaining patients' signatures on consent forms. Physicians need to educate patients, discuss options with them, answer questions, make recommendations, and help them deliberate. Patients can be overwhelmed with medical jargon, needlessly complicated explanations, or too much information at once.

Nondisclosure of Information Physicians may consider withholding a serious diagnosis, misrepresenting it, or limiting discussions of prognosis or risks out of fear that a patient will develop severe anxiety or depression or refuse needed care. Patients should not be forced to receive information against their will. Most people, however, want to know their diagnosis and prognosis, even if they are terminally ill. Generally, physicians should provide relevant information, while offering empathy and hope and helping patients cope with bad news.

Emergency Care Informed consent is not required when patients cannot give consent and delaying treatment would place their life or health in peril. People are presumed to want such emergency care, unless they have indicated otherwise.

Futile Interventions Autonomy does not entitle patients to insist on whatever care they want. Physicians are not obligated to provide futile interventions that have no physiologic rationale or when maximal treatment is failing. For example, cardiopulmonary resuscitation would be futile in a patient with multisystem failure that is worsening despite maximal therapy. But physicians should be wary of using the term "futile" in looser senses to justify withholding interventions when they believe that the probability of success is too low, no worthwhile goals can be achieved, the patient's quality of life is unacceptable, or the costs are too high. Such looser usages of the term are problematic because they may be inconsistent and mask hidden value judgments.

ACTING IN THE BEST INTERESTS OF PATIENTS The guideline of *beneficence* requires physicians to take actions for patients' benefit. Laypeople do not possess medical expertise and may be vulnerable because of their illness. They justifiably rely on physicians to provide sound advice and to promote their well-being. Physicians encourage such trust. For these reasons, physicians have a fiduciary duty to act in the best interests of their patients. Furthermore, the interests of the patient should take priority over physicians' self-interest or the interests of third parties, such as hospitals or insurers. These fiduciary obligations contrast sharply with the business world, where the goal is to maximize profits, not to act in the best interests of customers. The guideline of *"do no harm"* forbids physicians from providing ineffective interventions or acting without due care. This precept, while often cited, provides only limited guidance, because many beneficial interventions also have serious risks.

CONFLICTS BETWEEN BENEFICENCE AND AUTONOMY Patients' refusals of care may thwart their own goals or cause them serious harm. For example, a young man with asthma may refuse mechanical ventilation for reversible respiratory failure. Simply to accept such refusals, in the name of respecting autonomy, would fail to show caring. Physicians can elicit patients' expectations and concerns, correct misunderstandings, and try to persuade them to accept beneficial therapies. If disagreements persist after discussions, the patient's informed choices and view of his or her best interests should prevail. While refusing recommended care does not render a patient incompetent, it may lead the physician to probe further to ensure that the patient is able to make informed decisions.

Patients may not be able to make informed decisions because of unconsciousness, dementia, delirium, or other conditions. Physicians need to ask two questions regarding such patients: Who is the appropriate surrogate? What would the patient want done?

ASSESSING CAPACITY TO MAKE MEDICAL DECISIONS All adults are considered legally competent unless declared incompetent by a court. In practice, physicians usually determine that patients lack the capacity to make health care decisions and arrange for surrogates to make them, without involving the courts. By definition, competent patients can express a choice and appreciate the medical situation, the nature of the proposed care, the alternatives, and the risks, benefits, and consequences of each. Their choices should be consistent with their values and should not result from delusions or hallucinations. Psychiatrists may help in difficult cases because they are skilled at interviewing mentally impaired patients and can identify treatable depression or psychosis. When impairments are fluctuating or reversible, decisions should be postponed if possible until the patient recovers decision-making capacity.

CHOICE OF SURROGATE Physicians routinely ask family members to serve as surrogates for patients who lack decision-making capacity. Most patients want their family members to be surrogates, and family members generally know the patient's preferences and have the patient's best interests at heart. Patients may designate a particular individual to serve as proxy; such choices should be respected. Some states have established a prioritized list of which relative may serve as surrogate if the patient has not designated a proxy.

STANDARDS FOR SURROGATE DECISION MAKING

Advance Directives These are statements by competent patients to direct care if they lose decision-making capacity. They may indicate (1) what interventions they would refuse or accept or (2) who should serve as surrogate. Following the patient's advance directives respects his or her autonomy.

Oral conversations are the most frequent form of advance directives. While such conversations are customarily followed in clinical practice, casual or vague comments may not be trustworthy.

Living wills direct physicians to forego or provide life-sustaining interventions if the patient develops a terminal condition or persistent vegetative state. Generally patients may refuse only interventions that "merely prolong the process of dying."

A health care power of attorney allows patients to appoint a proxy to make health care decisions if they lose decision-making capacity. It is more flexible and comprehensive than the living will, applying whenever the patient is unable to make decisions.

Physicians can encourage patients to provide advance directives, to indicate both what they would want and who should be surrogate, and to discuss their preferences with surrogates. In discussions with patients, physicians can ensure that advance directives are informed, up-to-date, and address likely clinical scenarios. The federal Patient Self-Determination Act requires hospitals and health maintenance organizations to inform patients of their right to make health care decisions and to provide advance directives.

Substituted Judgment In the absence of clear advance directives, surrogates and physicians should try to decide as the patient would under the circumstances, using all information that they know about the patient. While such substituted judgments try to respect the patient's values, they may be speculative or inaccurate. A surrogate may be mistaken about the patient's preferences, particularly when they have not been discussed explicitly.

Best Interests When the patient's preferences are unclear or unknown, decisions should be based on the patient's best interests. Patients generally take into account the quality of life as well as the duration of life when making decisions for themselves. It is understandable that surrogates would also consider quality of life of patients who lack decision-making capacity. Judgments about quality of life are appropriate if they reflect the patient's own values. Bias or discrimination may occur, however, if others project their values onto the patient

or weigh the perceived social worth of the patient. Most patients with chronic illness rate their quality of life higher than their family members and physicians do.

Legal Issues Physicians need to know pertinent state laws regarding patients who lack decision-making capacity. A few state courts allow life-sustaining treatments to be withheld only if patients have provided written advance directives or very specific oral ones.

Disagreements Disagreements may occur among potential surrogates or between the physician and surrogate. Physicians can remind everyone to base decisions on what the patient would want, not what they would want for themselves. Consultation with the hospital ethics committee or with another physician often helps resolve disputes. Such consultation is also helpful when patients have no surrogate and no advance directives. The courts should be used only as a last resort when disagreements cannot be resolved in the clinical setting.

DECISIONS ABOUT
LIFE-SUSTAINING INTERVENTIONS

Although medical technology can save lives, it can also prolong the process of dying. Competent, informed patients may refuse life-sustaining interventions. Such interventions also may be withheld from patients who lack decision-making capacity on the basis of advance directives or decisions by appropriate surrogates. Courts have ruled that foregoing life-sustaining interventions is neither suicide nor murder.

MISLEADING DISTINCTIONS People commonly draw distinctions that are intuitively plausible but prove untenable on closer analysis.

Extraordinary and Ordinary Care Some physicians are willing to forego "extraordinary" or "heroic" interventions, such as surgery, mechanical ventilation or renal dialysis, but insist on providing "ordinary" ones, such as antibiotics, intravenous fluids, or feeding tubes. However, this is not a logical distinction because all medical interventions have both risks and benefits. Any intervention may be withheld, if the burdens for the individual patient outweigh the benefits.

Withdrawing and Withholding Interventions Many health care providers find it more difficult to discontinue interventions than to withhold them in the first place. Although such emotions need to be acknowledged, there is no logical distinction between the two acts. Justifications for withholding interventions, such as refusal by patients or surrogates, also are justifications for withdrawing them. In addition, an intervention may prove unsuccessful, or new information about the patient's preferences or condition may become available after the intervention is started. If interventions could not be discontinued, patients and surrogates might not even attempt treatments that might prove beneficial.

DO NOT RESUSCITATE (DNR) ORDERS When a patient suffers a cardiopulmonary arrest, cardiopulmonary resuscitation (CPR) is initiated unless a DNR order has been made. Although CPR can restore people to vigorous health, it can also disrupt a peaceful death. After CPR is attempted on a general hospital service, only 14 percent of patients survive to discharge, and even fewer in certain subgroups. DNR orders are appropriate if the patient or surrogate requests them or if CPR would be futile. To prevent misunderstandings, physicians should write DNR orders and the reasons for them in the medical record. "Slow" or "show" codes that merely appear to provide CPR are deceptive and therefore unacceptable. Although a DNR order signifies only that CPR will be withheld, DNR orders may lead to a reconsideration of the plans for care.

ASSISTED SUICIDE AND ACTIVE EUTHANASIA Proponents of these controversial acts believe that competent, terminally ill patients should have control over the end of life and that physicians should help them end their suffering. Opponents assert that such actions violate the sanctity of life, that suffering can generally be relieved, that abuses are inevitable, and that such actions are outside the physician's proper role. Whatever their personal views regarding these illegal acts, physicians need to respond to patients' inquiries with compassion and concern. Physicians need to elicit and address any underlying problems, such as unrelieved suffering, loss of control, or depression. Distress usually can be relieved more effectively, and after this is done patients generally withdraw their requests for these acts.

CARE OF DYING PATIENTS Patients often suffer unrelieved pain during their final days of life. Physicians may hesitate to order high doses of narcotics and sedatives, fearing they will hasten death. Relieving pain in terminal illness and alleviating dyspnea when patients forego mechanical ventilation enhances patient comfort and dignity. If lower doses of narcotics and sedatives have failed to relieve suffering, increasing the dose to levels that may suppress respiratory drive and hasten death is different from active euthanasia and is ethically appropriate. Physicians can also relieve suffering by spending time with dying patients, listening to them, and attending to their psychological distress.

CONFLICTS OF INTEREST

Acting in the patient's best interests may conflict with the physician's self-interest or the interests of third parties such as insurers or hospitals. The ethical ideal is to keep the patient's interests paramount. Even the appearance of a conflict of interest may undermine trust in the profession.

FINANCIAL INCENTIVES In managed care systems, physicians may serve as gatekeepers or bear financial risk for expenditures. Although such incentives are intended to reduce inefficiency and waste, the concern is that physicians may withhold beneficial care in order to control costs. In contrast, physicians have incentives to provide more care than indicated when they receive fee-for-service reimbursement or when they refer patients to medical facilities in which they have invested. Regardless of financial incentives, physicians should recommend available care that is in the patient's best interests—no more and no less.

DENIALS OF COVERAGE Utilization review programs designed to reduce unnecessary services may also deny coverage for care that the physician believes will benefit the patient. Physicians should inform patients when a plan is not covering standard care and act as patient advocates by appealing such denials of coverage. Patients may ask physicians to misrepresent their condition to help them obtain insurance coverage or disability. While physicians understandably want to help patients, such misrepresentation undermines physicians' credibility and violates their integrity.

GIFTS FROM PHARMACEUTICAL COMPANIES Physicians may be offered gifts ranging from pens and notepads to lavish entertainment. Critics worry that any gift from drug companies may impair objectivity, increase the cost of health care, and give the appearance of conflict of interest. A helpful rule of thumb is to consider whether patients would approve if they knew physicians had accepted such gifts.

OCCUPATIONAL RISKS Some health care workers, fearing fatal occupational infections, refuse to care for persons with human immunodeficiency virus (HIV) infection or multidrug-resistant tuberculosis. Such fears about personal safety need to be acknowledged, and institutions need to reduce occupational risk by providing proper training, equipment, and supervision. Physicians should provide appropriate care within their clinical expertise, despite personal risk.

MISTAKES Mistakes are inevitable in clinical medicine. They may cause serious harm to patients or require substantial changes in management. Physicians and students may fear that disclosing such mistakes could damage their careers. Without disclosure, however, patients cannot understand their clinical situation or make informed choices about subsequent care. Similarly, unless attending physicians are informed of trainees' mistakes, they cannot provide optimal care and help trainees learn from mistakes.

LEARNING CLINICAL SKILLS Learning clinical medicine, particularly how to perform invasive procedures, may present inconve-

nience or risk to patients. To ensure patient cooperation, students may be introduced as physicians, or patients may not be told that trainees will be performing procedures. Such misrepresentation undermines trust, may lead to more elaborate deception, and makes it difficult for patients to make informed choices about their care. Patients should be told who is providing care, what benefits and burdens can be attributed to trainees, and how trainees are supervised. Most patients, when informed, allow trainees to play an active role in their care.

IMPAIRED PHYSICIANS Physicians may hesitate to intervene when colleagues impaired by alcohol abuse, drug abuse, or psychiatric or medical illness place patients at risk. However, society relies on physicians to regulate themselves. If colleagues of an impaired physician do not take steps to protect patients, no one else may be in a position to do so.

CONFLICTS FOR TRAINEES Medical students and residents may fear that they will receive poor grades or evaluations if they act on the patient's behalf by disclosing mistakes, avoiding misrepresentation of their role, and reporting impaired colleagues. Discussing such dilemmas with more senior physicians can help trainees check their interpretation of the situation and obtain advice and assistance.

ADDITIONAL ETHICAL ISSUES

MAINTAINING CONFIDENTIALITY Maintaining the confidentiality of medical information respects patients' autonomy and privacy, encourages them to seek treatment and to discuss their problems candidly, and prevents discrimination. Physicians need to guard against inadvertent breaches of confidentiality, as when talking about patients in elevators. Maintaining confidentiality is not an absolute rule. The law may require physicians to override confidentiality in order to protect third parties, for example, reporting to government officials persons with specified infectious conditions, such as tuberculosis and syphilis, persons with gunshot wounds, and victims of elder abuse and domestic violence.

ALLOCATING RESOURCES JUSTLY Allocation of limited health care resources is unavoidable. Ideally, allocation decisions should be made as public policy, with physician input. At the bedside, physicians generally should act as patient advocates within constraints set by society and sound practice. *Ad hoc* rationing by the individual physician at the bedside may be inconsistent, discriminatory, and ineffective. In some cases, however, two patients may compete for the same limited resources, such as physician time or a bed in intensive care. When this occurs, physicians should ration their time and resources according to patients' medical needs and the probability of benefit.

ASSISTANCE WITH ETHICAL ISSUES Discussing perplexing ethical issues with other members of the health care team, colleagues, or the hospital ethics committee often clarifies ethical issues and suggests ways to improve communication and to deal with strong emotions. When struggling with difficult ethical issues, physicians may need to reevaluate their basic convictions, tolerate uncertainty, and maintain their integrity while respecting the opinions of others.

BIBLIOGRAPHY

AMERICAN COLLEGE OF PHYSICIANS: *American College of Physicians Ethics Manual.* Ann Intern Med, 117:947,1992

BEAUCHAMP TL, CHILDRESS JF: *Principles of Biomedical Ethics*, 4th ed. New York, Oxford University Press, 1994

DUNN PM et al: Medical ethics: An annotated bibliography. Ann Intern Med 121:627, 1994

EMANUEL LL: A professional response to demands for accountability: Practical recommendations regarding ethical aspects of patient care. Ann Intern Med 124:240, 1996

JONSEN AR et al: *Clinical Ethics*, 3d ed. New York, Macmillan, 1991

KASSIRER JP: Managed care and the morality of the marketplace. N Engl J Med 333:50, 1995

Lo B: *Resolving Ethical Dilemmas: A Guide for Clinicians.* Baltimore, Williams & Wilkins, 1995

MEISEL A: *The Right to Die*, 2d ed. New York, Wiley, 1995

PELLOGRINO ED: The metamorphosis of medical ethics—a 30-year retrospective. JAMA 269:1158, 1993

QUANTITATIVE ASPECTS OF CLINICAL REASONING

The process of clinical reasoning is poorly understood but is based on factors such as experience and learning, inductive and deductive reasoning, interpretation of evidence that itself varies in reproducibility and validity, and intuition that often is difficult to define. In an effort to improve clinical reasoning, a number of attempts have been made to analyze quantitatively the many factors involved, including defining the cognitive approaches that clinicians apply to difficult problems, devising computerized decision support systems that are designed to emulate certain features of decision making, and applying decision theory to understand how judgments should be reached. While each of these approaches has advanced the understanding of the diagnostic process, all have practical and/or theoretical problems that limit their direct applicability to the care of the individual patient.

Nevertheless, these preliminary attempts to apply the rigor and logic inherent in the quantitative method have provided significant insights into the process by which clinical reasoning is accomplished, have identified ways in which the process may be improved, and have made it possible to minimize certain features of the workup that are not cost-effective.

In a simplified model, quantitative clinical reasoning includes five phases. The *first* consists of an investigation of the chief complaint through key questions that are included in the history of the present illness (Table 3-1). These questions are supplemented by the past medical history and by a physical examination that emphasizes detailed investigation of potential key organ systems. In the *second* phase, the physician may select from an array of diagnostic tests, each with its own accuracy and usefulness for investigating the possibilities raised in the differential diagnosis. Since each test has its costs, and some entail risk and discomfort as well, the physician must ask whether the history and physical examination are sufficiently diagnostic before ordering tests. *Third*, the clinical data must be integrated with test results to estimate the likelihood of conditions in the differential diagnosis. *Fourth*, the comparative risks and benefits of further diagnostic and therapeutic options must be weighed to reach a recommendation for the patient. In the *fifth* and final phase, this recommendation is presented to the patient, and after appropriate discussion of the options, a therapeutic plan is initiated. Each of the five steps in this simplified model of the clinical reasoning process can be analyzed individually.

HISTORY AND PHYSICAL EXAMINATION It originally had been assumed that physicians begin investigating a patient's chief complaint by obtaining a comprehensive history, which includes many, if not most, of the questions included in a full review of systems, and by performing an all-inclusive physical examination. However, experienced clinicians begin to form hypotheses based on the chief complaint and on the responses to initial questioning, and they ask further questions in a sequence that allows them to evaluate the initial hypotheses and, if necessary, shorten or amend the list of possibilities. In such a way, high-priority questions are selected from the almost limitless number that might be asked, and these specific questions are incorporated into the history of the present illness. Often, a key re-

Table 3-1

Phases of Clinical Reasoning and Decision Making

---

1. Investigation of the complaint by means of clinical examination (history and physical examination)
2. Ordering of diagnostic tests, each with its own intrinsic accuracy and usefulness
3. Integration of clinical findings with test results to assess diagnostic probabilities
4. Weighing of comparative risks and benefits of alternative courses of action
5. Determination of patient's preferences and development of a therapeutic plan

sponse, such as a history of melena, will be selected, a list of potential explanations for it will be formulated, and this list will then be trimmed, based on the response to more probing questions, so that a principal diagnosis can be selected and then tested. This process, termed *iterative hypothesis testing*, is an efficient approach to diagnosis and is preferable to attempts to gather every conceivable piece of information prior to formulating a differential diagnosis.

Advocacy of iterative hypothesis testing does not argue against the need for a systematic, thorough, and complete history of the present illness, past medical history, review of systems, family history, social history, and physical examination. For example, if a patient presents with abdominal pain, the physician should gather information regarding its location and quality as well as the factors that precipitate and/or relieve it. The physician then asks questions relating to the diagnoses that may be suspected based on the response to the initial questions. If the pain is suggestive of pancreatitis, the clinician would ask about alcohol intake, the use of thiazide diuretics or glucocorticoids, symptoms suggestive of concomitant gallbladder disease, a family history of pancreatitis, and questions aimed at uncovering the possibility of a posterior penetrating ulcer. Alternatively, if the discomfort seems more typical of reflux esophagitis, a different sequence of questions would be triggered. The use of iterative hypothesis testing encourages the physician to elicit detailed information in high-yield areas, without forgoing a systematic and thorough approach to the patient. The careful use of clear and, when possible, precise questions can increase the reproducibility and validity of the medical history but still cannot eliminate all variability. Findings on the history and physical examination should influence each other. The history focuses the physical examination on certain organs, and findings on physical examination should encourage more detailed review of certain systems.

Despite limitations in the reproducibility and validity of the medical history and physical examination, their critical importance in clinical reasoning should not be undervalued. Rather, they emphasize that care and diligence are critical in the application of these skills, and that physicians must recognize their limitations. For example, the history and physical examination are of limited value in predicting whether back pain is caused by a serious underlying disease, but careful auscultation of the heart during various bedside maneuvers (see Chap. 227) has been shown to be remarkably accurate in determining the cause of systolic murmurs. Even in the latter case, however, confirmation echocardiography will often be helpful.

When physicians use the history and the physical examination to arrive at a diagnosis, they are rarely certain of it. Therefore, it would be better to assess the likelihood of the diagnosis in terms of probabilities. All too frequently this probability is not expressed as an actual percentage but rather in such terms as "nearly always," "commonly," "sometimes," or "rarely." Since different physicians may assign different probabilities to the same terms, these imprecise words can lead to major misunderstandings among physicians or between the physician and the patient. Physicians should be as rigorous and quantitative as possible in their assessments, and when feasible, a quantitative expression of probability should be used. For example, rather than saying that it is unlikely that a radiographic pattern is indicative of a carcinoma of the colon, it would be preferable, if possible, to provide a more precise indication of the probability of carcinoma with this radiographic pattern. A 10 to 15 percent probability of carcinoma may be interpreted as "unlikely" but from a clinical perspective usually warrants further evaluation because of the serious consequences of missing a potentially resectable tumor.

Although such quantitative estimates would be desirable, they usually are not available in practice. Even experienced physicians often are unable to estimate accurately the likelihood of particular conditions. There is a tendency to overestimate the likelihood of relatively uncommon conditions, and physicians are especially poor at quantifying probabilities that are very high or very low. For example, a physician may not know whether the probability of bacterial meningitis or of another disease that could be diagnosed by a lumbar puncture in a patient with a severe headache is 1 in 20 or 1 in 2000. In both situations, the probability is low, but the decision as to whether a lumbar puncture should be performed may depend on this estimate.

As was emphasized in Chap. 1, the history and physical examination have other important purposes. They allow the physician to evaluate the emotional status of the patient and to understand how the present problems fit into the context of the patient's social and family life, and they encourage the development in the patient of confidence in the physician, which is so necessary for reaching an agreement on the coming plan of action.

DIAGNOSTIC TESTS: INDICATIONS, ACCURACY, AND USEFULNESS A diagnostic test should be ordered for specified clinical indications, be sufficiently accurate to be efficacious for such indications, and be the least expensive and/or risky of the available efficacious tests. No diagnostic test is totally accurate, and physicians often have difficulty interpreting test results. It is therefore critical to understand several commonly used terms in test analysis and epidemiology, including prevalence, sensitivity, specificity, positive predictive value, and negative predictive value (Table 3-2).

Although reports of the accuracies of diagnostic tests are commonly expressed in terms of positive and negative predictive values, these calculated values are dependent on the prevalence of the disease in the population being studied (Table 3-3). A test with a particular sensitivity and specificity has different positive and negative predictive values when used in groups of patients that have different prevalences of disease. For example, a mildly abnormal alkaline phosphatase level in a young adult with a known lymphoma suggests hepatic involvement by the tumor (i.e., it is likely to be a *true positive*), while the same alkaline phosphatase level as part of a routine screening battery of blood tests in an asymptomatic person of the same age is unlikely to be due to tumor (i.e., in this setting it is more likely to be a *false positive*).

Although the sensitivity and specificity of a test do not depend on the prevalence (or percentage of patients being tested who have the disease), they do depend on the spectrum of patients in whom the test is being evaluated. For example, measurement of a prostate-specific antigen for diagnosing carcinoma of the prostate (see Chap. 97) will appear to have a nearly perfect sensitivity and specificity if

Table 3-2

Definitions of Commonly Used Terms in Epidemiology and Decision Making

Test Result	Disease State	
	Present	**Absent**
Positive	a (true positive)	b (false positive)
Negative	c (false negative)	d (true negative)
Prevalence (prior probability)	$= (a + c)/(a + b + c + d)$	= all patients with the disease/all patients tested
Sensitivity	$= a/(a + c)$	= true-positive test results/all patients with the disease
Specificity	$= d/(b + d)$	= true-negative test results/all patients without the disease
False-negative rate	$= c/(a + c)$	= false-negative test result/all patients with the disease
False-positive rate	$= b/(b + d)$	= false-positive test results/all patients without the disease
Positive predictive value	$= a/(a + b)$	= true-positive test results/all patients with positive test results
Negative predictive	$= d/(c + d)$	= true-negative test results/all patients with negative results
Overall accuracy	$= (a + d)/(a + b + c + d)$	= true-positive + true-negative test results/ all tests

the diseased population has a palpable prostate nodule and an elevated serum acid phosphatase level while the nondiseased population is composed of normal medical students. If, however, without changing the prevalence of disease in the population being tested, the spectrum of the diseased and nondiseased patients is altered by including patients with other characteristics (i.e., if the population of patients with carcinoma of the prostate were composed principally of those without palpable nodules and with stage 1 disease, while the population without carcinoma of the prostate included elderly men with marked benign

Table 3-3

How the Positive and Negative Predictive Values of the Same Test Vary Depending on the Prior Probability of Disease

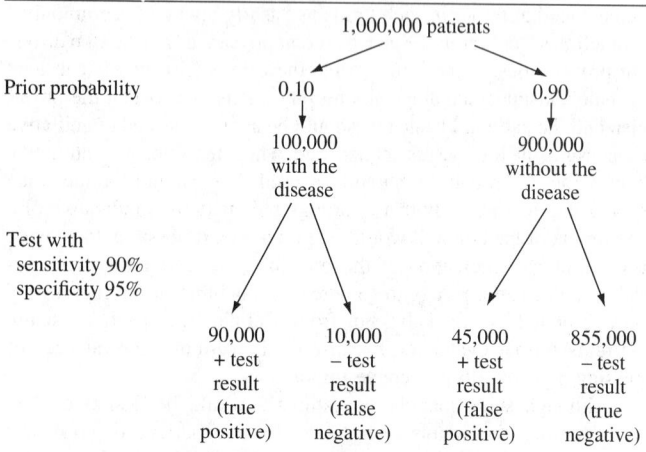

INTERPRETATION OF TEST RESULT WHEN 10% OF PATIENTS TESTED HAVE THE DISEASE (PRIOR PROBABILITY = 10%)

The probability of disease in a patient with a positive test result (positive predictive value) = 90,000/135,000 = 67%
The probability of no disease in a patient with a negative test result (negative predicative value) = 855,000/865,000 = 99%

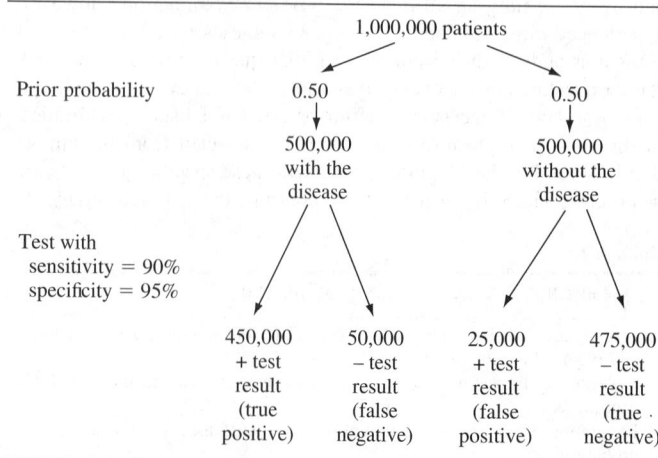

INTERPRETATION OF TEST RESULT WHEN 50% OF PATIENTS TESTED HAVE THE DISEASE (PRIOR PROBABILITY = 50%)

The probability of disease in a patient with a positive test result (positive predictive value) = 450,000/475,000 = 95%
The probability of no disease in a patient with a negative test result (negative predicative value) = 475,000/525,000 = 90%

prostate hypertrophy), the sensitivity and specificity of the test would change dramatically. In the latter situation, the sensitivity and specificity of the prostate-specific antigen are not only lower than in the first example, because the spectrum of diseased and nondiseased patients has been changed, but more important, they may not be high enough for even this relatively accurate test to be recommended as a routine screening procedure. This example also demonstrates the methodologic problems encountered when applying data from one study to a different type of patient or when pooling data from studies of different subsets of patients.

In some situations, uncertainty about the sensitivity and specificity of the test in the type of patient being assessed may limit its clinical value. Since the physician rarely knows (or can know) the population on which every test that is ordered has been standardized, the results provide information that is far less decisive than usually thought. Furthermore, it may be quite difficult to distinguish random laboratory errors from test results that might be falsely positive or negative because of coexistence of a process that can affect the test, such as the finding of an elevated level of CK (creatine kinase) in a patient who has undergone strenuous exercise and is being evaluated for chest pain.

Because no single value or cutoff point of an individual test can be expected to have both a perfect sensitivity and a perfect specificity, it is often necessary to determine which value or cutoff point is the most appropriate to guide decision making. A graph (Fig. 3-1) of the test's *receiver operating characteristic curve*, which displays the inevitable trade-off between emphasizing a high sensitivity, such as defining an exercise electrocardiogram as abnormal if it shows ≥0.5 mm of ST-segment depression, versus emphasizing a high specificity, such as defining an exercise electrocardiogram as abnormal only if it shows ≥2.0 mm of ST-segment depression, can help the clinician understand the implications of various definitions of a "positive" test result. Such a graph demonstrates that different definitions of normal versus abnormal may be appropriate depending on whether one wishes to rule in the disease via a positive result on a test that has a high specificity or to exclude the disease via a negative result on a test that has a high sensitivity. Different tests may have different sensitivities and specificities, and better tests may have both a higher sensitivity and a higher specificity than poorer tests.

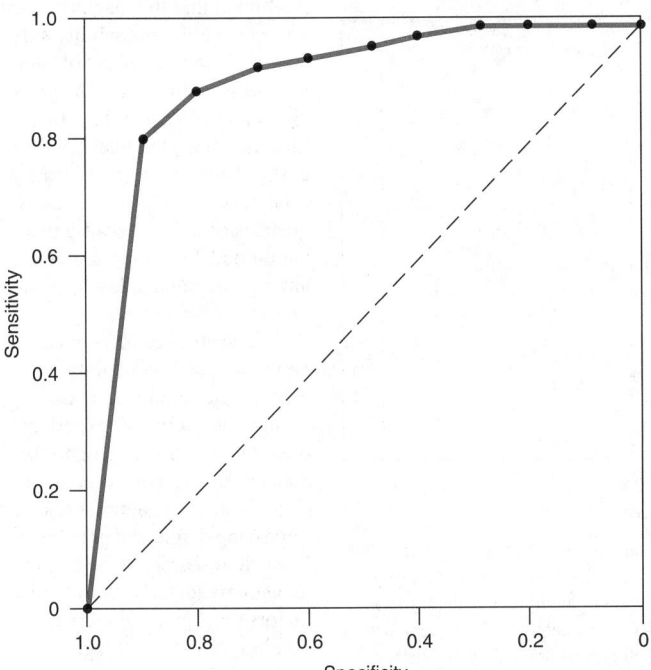

FIGURE 3-1 The inherent trade-off between sensitivity and specificity. For any diagnostic test, an increase in sensitivity will be associated with a decline in specificity. The closer this curve comes to the upper-left-hand corner, the more useful the test; the closer to the broken line, the less useful it is. When deciding on the cutoff between normal versus abnormal, one must determine what sensitivity and specificity are most useful clinically.

One example of a sensitive test is an enzyme-linked immunosorbent assay (ELISA) to test for the presence of antibodies to human immunodeficiency virus type 1 (HIV-1). This relatively inexpensive test has a high sensitivity for detecting HIV-1 antibodies but is not sufficiently specific to be used as the basis for making a firm diagnosis. Thus, if the ELISA assay is positive, it is commonly repeated. Confirmation of the diagnosis of HIV-1 antibody positivity requires a western blot, or an equivalently specific test, to exclude the possibility of a false-positive ELISA assay (see Chap. 308). A common example of a reasonably specific test would be an electrocardiogram to diagnose acute myocardial infarction. While the precise specificity depends on the spectrum of patients being tested, the presence of new ST-segment elevations exceeding 1.0 mm in two or more electrically contiguous leads in patients who present to an emergency department with prolonged acute chest pain consistent with myocardial ischemia is sufficiently specific, i.e., sufficiently unlikely to be a false-positive result, that admission to an intensive care unit and treatment with either intravenous thrombolysis or emergent percutaneous transluminal coronary angioplasty is virtually always recommended. However, this test is not sensitive, and if admission to the hospital were restricted to patients with this electrocardiographic finding, almost half of patients with myocardial infarctions presenting to hospital emergency departments would be missed.

INTEGRATION OF CLINICAL DATA AND TEST RESULTS Although, as we have seen, neither clinical data nor test results may be entirely accurate, the integration of the two can lead to better diagnostic predictions than either alone. By knowing the probability that the patient has a particular condition before a test is performed (the prior, or pretest, probability), and by knowing the sensitivity and the specificity of the test, the posttest probability can be calculated. A common mathematical technique for integrating clinical data and a test result is the odds-likelihood form of Bayesian analysis (Table 3-4). A pretest probability can be expressed as odds (as in a horse race, for example) and multiplied by the likelihood ratio (which is the sensitivity of the test divided by 1 minus the specificity of the test) to yield the posttest odds, which may be transformed back into a posttest probability. This approach can be employed in any situation in which the physician can use clinical findings to estimate a pretest diagnostic probability and integrate this with the result as well as the sensitivity and specificity of the diagnostic test. Many clinical situations may be so complex that it is not practical to estimate the prior probabilities of all likely diagnoses or to know the sensitivities and specificities of each of the tests that might be performed individually or in sequence. Nevertheless, attempts in this direction will stimulate critical thinking, expose uncertainties, and generate ideas for original investigations or a review of past experiences to facilitate the application of Bayesian analysis to the integration of clinical data and laboratory tests.

The results of Bayesian analyses often can be expressed in graphic form, such as the value of exercise electrocardiograms for predicting the presence of coronary artery disease (Fig. 3-2). This series of curves also demonstrates how to consider a test whose result may be in the "gray zone" rather than clearly positive or clearly negative.

One of the key assumptions inherent in most such analyses is that the correlation between the pretest probability and the test result is no greater than expected by chance. If the diagnostic test simply duplicates information that has already been obtained by the clinical examination, it will not have any additional benefit for predicting whether or not the disease is present. For example, in trying to determine whether or not a patient with carcinoma of the colon has hepatic metastases, the finding of jaundice on physical examination should be a strong predictor. The degree of hyperbilirubinemia also can be measured, but the bilirubin level in a patient with clinical jaundice does not add substantial *independent* information to that obtained by a careful physical examination. When integrating a diagnostic test with clinical information, the test is helpful only when it adds incremental

Table 3-4

Example of the Use of Bayesian Analysis to Integrate the Pretest Probability with the Test Result to Calculate a Posttest Probability

Example 1: Prior probability of disease = 25%; a test with a sensitivity (true-positive rate) of 90% and a specificity of 80% (which implies a false-positive rate of 20%) gives a positive result

Clinical data

↓

Prior probability → prior odds

25%   1:3

$$\frac{0.90}{0.20} \leftarrow \frac{\text{sensitivity*}}{(1-\text{specificity})^{\dagger}} \leftarrow \text{positive test}$$

Posttest odds

$(1:3) \times \dfrac{0.90}{0.20} = 4.5:3$

Posttest probability

$\dfrac{4.5}{7.5} = 60\%$

Example 2: Same pretest probability and test, but now the test gives a negative result. Here the true-negative rate would be 80% and the false-negative rate (which is 1 − sensitivity) would be 10%.

Clinical data

↓

Prior probability → prior odds

25%   1:3

$$\frac{0.10}{0.80} \leftarrow \frac{(1-\text{sensitivity})^{\ddagger}}{\text{specificity}^{\S}} \leftarrow \text{negative test}$$

Posttest odds

$(1:3) \times \dfrac{0.10}{0.80} = 0.125:3 = 1:24$

Posttest probability

$\dfrac{1}{25} = 4\%$

* Sensitivity = probability of a positive test result in a patient with the disease
† (1 − specificity) = probability of a positive test result in a patient without the disease

‡ (1 − sensitivity) = probability of a negative test result in a patient with the disease.
§ Specificity = probability of a negative test result in a patient without the disease.

information to what can be inferred based on the history and physical examination and on prior, less costly or less risky diagnostic tests. If a diagnostic test (such as a retrograde cholangiogram in a patient with hyperbilirubinemia) provides information that cannot be inferred directly, it is less likely that its results are associated with pretest probabilities to an extent greater than would be expected by chance.

A diagnostic test has an impact on the evaluation of a specific patient only if it changes the diagnostic probability to the extent that the new probability dictates a change in the diagnostic strategy or therapeutic plans or if the test serves as part of a sequence of tests that moves the probability across such a threshold. An example is a patient suspected of having a pulmonary embolism, with an estimated probability of 50 percent based on clinical data alone. The finding of a "low probability for pulmonary embolus" pulmonary ventilation-perfusion scan may reduce the probability of pulmonary embolism, but if the goal is to exclude pulmonary embolism with the highest possible degree of certainty, a pulmonary angiogram would be required (Chap. 261).

Because diagnostic tests often do not provide important new information even when their results are accurate, several questions should be considered in deciding when to order diagnostic tests. First, how likely is the disease in question? Second, what would be the clinical consequences if the diagnosis were missed or if the patient were mistakenly treated for a disease that is not present? Third, what is the likelihood that the diagnostic test will change the probability sufficiently to have an effect on either diagnosis or therapy? The physician should consider the probabilities, the risks, the likelihood and costs of obtaining new information, and the adverse consequences of delay, because observation and follow-up are always among the available diagnostic options.

Since the establishment of valid diagnostic probabilities is a cornerstone to clinical reasoning, accumulated clinical experience, often in the form of computerized data banks, has been used to generate statistical approaches for improving diagnostic predictions. In such research, it is common to begin by identifying individual factors that have a univariate correlation with the diagnosis in question. Then these univariate correlates may be included in a multivariate analysis to determine which of them are significant independent predictors of the diagnosis. Some analyses may identify the important predictive

FIGURE 3-2 How the exercise tolerance test affects the probability of coronary artery disease. The before-test probability of coronary artery disease (CAD) will be modified by the result of the exercise electrocardiogram to yield an after-test probability of CAD. Note that the finding of <1 mm of ST-segment depression will reduce the probability of CAD, whereas ≥1 mm of ST-segment depression will increase the probability. For example, if a patient with a before-test probability of CAD of 90 percent (about that of a middle-aged man with typical anginal symptoms) had 2 to 2.49 mm on ST-segment depression on exercise testing, the after-test probability of CAD would be 99.5 percent. In contrast, the same exercise test result in a patient with 30 percent before-test probability of CAD (about that of a patient with atypical anginal symptoms) would yield an after-test probability of about 90 percent. In an asymptomatic patient, with a before-test probability of about 5 percent, the same exercise test result would yield an after-test probability of about 50 percent. Thus the same test yields different after-test probabilities in patients with different before-test probabilities. (*Adapted, with permission of the New England Journal of Medicine, from RD Rifkin, WB Hood, Bayesian analysis of electrocardiographic exercise stress testing. N Engl J Med 297:684, 1977.*)

factors and then assign them "weights," which can be transformed to calculate a probability. Alternatively, the analysis may result in a limited number of categories of patients, each with a discrete probability of the diagnosis.

These quantitative approaches to the estimation of various diagnostic probabilities, which are often termed "prediction rules," are especially helpful if they are in a format that is readily usable by the clinician and if they have been validated prospectively on a sufficient number and spectrum of patients. For example, by carefully defining the key historical questions, findings on physical examination, and electrocardiographic abnormalities that might predict the probability of acute myocardial infarction among emergency department patients with chest pain, accurate guidelines can be developed for the triage of patients to settings ranging from intensive care to discharge home. For such prediction rules to be useful to the clinician, they must be derived from relevant patient populations and use tests that are reproducible and readily available so that the results can be extrapolated to local medical practice.

COMPARING RISKS AND BENEFITS: DECISION ANALYSIS Inherent in the concept that probabilities can guide decision making is the assumption that one can arrive at a reasonable threshold by knowing the relative risks (or costs) and benefits of various options and deciding at what probability this ratio changes to favor an alternative strategy. Decision analysis is an organized process for evaluating such situations and identifies the key issues and problems.

One problem with applying decision-analysis techniques to difficult clinical problems is that the decision analysis is no better than the data on which it is based. In some instances, an attempted decision analysis of a complex clinical problem may yield no more information than that the critical data required for the analysis are missing and that more research in the field needs to be performed. In addition, when clinicians are uncertain about diagnostic or therapeutic strategies, formal analyses may indicate that the differences in outcome among various strategies are very small. In such cases, the formal analysis may have such inherent error that it is not definitive. Even when decision analysis is potentially helpful, it may not be feasible to complete the detailed estimations and calculations within the time constraints of bedside decision making. Nevertheless, the value of the analytic approach to decision making is that it integrates available data, mandates rigorous thinking, and exposes areas of uncertainty or ignorance.

Decision analysis depicts graphically two types of issues in the decision-making process: first, the decisions (or choices) available to the physician and, second, the probabilities of all the events that may result from each decision. To illustrate how this process works, consider a very simplified decision analysis of whether to use an intravenous thrombolytic agent in a patient with a suspected acute myocardial infarction (see Chap. 243). Figure 3-3 depicts the simplified decision tree for this problem. The square box or "node" labeled A indicates a decision that the physician must make. The circular nodes, labeled B through O, indicate where different outcomes, each of which has an estimatable probability, could occur. In this analysis, the initial choices were to treat the patient with an intravenous thrombolytic agent or not to treat. The use of such an agent may or may not result in serious complications of therapy, especially bleeding and intracranial hemorrhage.

Each of the possible outcomes for a patient is typically assigned a "utility," which is the relative preference for the outcome, where 1.0 is a perfect outcome and 0 is the worst possible outcome. Each terminal branch of the decision tree is assigned the utility corresponding to its outcome, and the "expected value" of each terminal branch is calculated by multiplying its probability by its utility. To calculate the expected value of each of the two possible courses of action (see Fig. 3-3, node A), the expected values of each of the terminal branches that originate from it would be summed. The preferred course of action is the one which, when all possible outcomes are considered, including the risks and benefits of therapy, yields the highest expected value, which is the sum of the product of the probability multiplied by the utility for each of its possible outcomes.

In performing any decision analysis, the relevant probabilities must be known or estimated, a process that sometimes requires guess-

FIGURE 3-3 Simplified decision tree for the decision of whether or not to use an intravenous thrombolytic agent in a patient with a suspected acute myocardial infarction. The square node represents the decision point, and the round nodes denote chance events (see text for details).

work. Next, utilities could be assigned to each of these outcomes. A major practical limitation of decision analysis is the subjective judgment often required to estimate utilities. It is also difficult to adjust future years of life for their quality in any numerical fashion, e.g., in considering how treatment complications, such as an intracranial hemorrhage, or the advantages of treatment, such as congestive heart failure averted because an infarction was smaller, affect the quality of future years of life.

The results and usefulness of a decision analysis depend on the probabilities and utilities that are used in the calculation, and it is imperative for decision analyses to include a *sensitivity analysis*, in which various estimates for each probability are included in the analysis to determine if the conclusions would be changed. For example, in the analysis in Fig. 3-3, some range of probabilities must be assumed for the risk of serious bleeding complications and for the likelihood that any particular patient is having an acute myocardial infarction. If the conclusions of an analysis were altered by relatively minor changes in the assumptions on which it was based, the analysis would not be sufficiently reliable to become the basis for decision making. Because of the impressive benefit of thrombolysis for improving survival in patients with acute myocardial infarctions presenting early after the onset of symptoms, decision analyses have shown treatment to be the preferred option even when an acute myocardial infarction is not certain and even in most elderly patients.

Decision analysis sometimes demonstrates a clear and dramatic advantage with one particular option. In other circumstances, there may be little difference between two options; either option may be reasonable, or secondary issues that cannot be taken into account in the formal analysis, such as the patient's feelings about taking risks or the recent local experience with particular interventions, should be the final determinants in the decision. Physicians who perform a decision analysis therefore must determine the probabilities of each of the possible events by reviewing the pertinent patient experience at their own institution or practice or by reviewing the pertinent literature. Even when the outcome of the analysis seems clear, the physician or the patient may believe that the situation in question is an exception to the rule. Other reasonable alternatives, such as emergent percutaneous transluminal coronary angioplasty in this example, must also be considered. Furthermore, even the best analyses, like all clinical intuition, are based on assumptions that may be open to debate.

Decision analysis can indicate the preferred strategy in terms of outcome, but it does not routinely consider the costs at which such benefits might be achieved. In determining health policy, a formal cost-effectiveness analysis can be performed to determine how many dollars must be spent to achieve a unit of benefit, often defined as a life saved, a year of life saved, or a quality-adjusted year of life saved, in which the years are adjusted to take into account the quality of life during that time. For example, in 1997 dollars, 1 year of in-center hemodialysis can be estimated to cost about $35,000 to $45,000 per quality-adjusted year of life saved; this figure includes only the direct medical costs and not indirect costs related to issues such as time lost or travel or any benefits in terms of a patient's ability to work. In some situations, the ability of the patient to maintain gainful employment may offset some or all of the direct medical expenses. In other situations, such as with pneumococcal vaccine, the savings from episodes of pneumonia that are averted may more than offset the cost of the vaccine in high-risk persons.

ETHICS AND PATIENT INPUT   In both quantitative and non-quantitative clinical reasoning, the physician must consider ethical issues as well as the patient's values and preferences. While a detailed discussion of these issues is beyond the scope of this chapter, it is important to emphasize that patients' preferences for alternative therapies may not agree with the preferences that the physicians propose on the basis of their own clinical judgment or the results of a decision-analysis approach. For example, the preferred treatment for many patients with benign prostatic hypertrophy depends critically on how much the patient is bothered by urinary symptoms. It is imperative that physicians assess those characteristics of life which the patient prizes most (the elusive "quality of life") prior to basing controversial decisions solely on quantitative approaches, the physicians' own subjective impressions of the likely medical benefits, their own personal preferences, or their assumptions about the patient's preferences. While quantitative analyses may apply to groups of patients, judgment must be exercised when adapting them to the individual patient. Therefore, the final plan should reflect an agreement between a well-informed patient and a sympathetic physician who has detailed knowledge of the relevant medical issues and of the impact of the various possible outcomes on the specific patient.

BIBLIOGRAPHY

GASPOZ et al: Cost-effectiveness of a new short-stay unit to "rule out" acute myocardial infarction in low risk patients. J Am Coll Cardiol 24:1249, 1994

HULL RD et al: A non-invasive strategy for the treatment of patients with suspected pulmonary embolism. Arch Intern Med 154:289, 1994

KASSIRER JP: Teaching problem solving—how are we doing? N Engl J Med 332:1507, 1995

SACKETT DL et al: *Clinical Epidemiology: A Basic Science for Clinical Medicine*, 2d ed. Boston, Little, Brown, 1991

SLOAND EM et al: HIV testing: State of the art. JAMA 266:2861, 1991

SOX HC JR (ed): *Common Diagnostic Tests: Use and Interpretation*, 2d ed. Philadelphia, American College of Physicians, 1990

ST CLAIR EW et al: Assessing housestaff diagnostic skills using a cardiology patient simulator. Ann Intern Med 117:751, 1992

TORIBARA NW et al: Screening for colorectal cancer. N Engl J Med 332:861, 1995

VAN DEN HOOGEN HM et al: On the accuracy of the history, physical examination, and erythrocyte sedimentation rate in diagnosing low back pain in general practice. A criteria-based review of the literature. Spine 20:318, 1995

WASSON JH et al: A comparison of transurethral surgery with watchful waiting for moderate symptoms of benign prostatic hypertrophy. N Engl J Med 332:75, 1995

4   *Virginia L. Ernster, John M. Colford, Jr.*

HOST AND DISEASE: INFLUENCE OF DEMOGRAPHIC AND SOCIOECONOMIC FACTORS*

Marked variations in disease occurrence and survival exist among different subgroups of the U.S. population. Some of these are attributable to demographic and social factors such as age, gender, race/ethnicity, sexual orientation, geographic location, and socioeconomic status (SES). Although individual physicians have limited ability to influence these characteristics, it is important to recognize the role of these factors in determining environmental exposures, behavioral risk factors, access to health care, and compliance with recommended preventive and therapeutic regimens, all of which can influence disease etiology and prognosis. Although not reviewed here, other social factors including culture and acculturation, religion, and psychosocial factors (e.g., life events, social mobility, and social networks) also affect the impact of disease.

This chapter describes variations in measures of health across demographic and socioeconomic subgroups. Improvements in mortality and life expectancy have occurred during the twentieth century, but despite overall improvements, differences in morbidity, quality of survival, and mortality continue to exist across racial/ethnic groups. Individuals of lower SES experience greater morbidity and mortality, and differences in SES explain many of the variations in health status across racial/ethnic groups. Differences in behavioral risk factors explain many, but not all, of the differences in disease prevalence across sociodemographic groups. For the already advantaged segments of our population, future improvements in health status will likely result in only minor increases in average life expectancy but may lengthen the period of "healthy life."

DEMOGRAPHIC FACTORS   Age   The specialties of pediatrics, adolescent medicine, and geriatrics developed because the clinical expressions of disease differ across the age spectrum. The biologic, medical, and sociologic characteristics of persons in these age groups are discussed in other chapters. Within the adult range, mortality rates from the leading causes of death vary widely by age group. Additionally, the prevalence of health risk behaviors such as smoking and alcohol use varies by age.

Gender   Although most illnesses affect both men and women, there are notable exceptions. By definition, many disorders of the reproductive tract occur exclusively in one gender. Others, such as carcinoma of the breast, rarely occur in men, whereas recessive disorders linked to the X chromosome, such as hemophilia and Duchenne's muscular dystrophy, are more common in males. Other conditions occur regularly in both sexes but predominate or tend to be more severe in one or the other. Examples include diabetes mellitus, connective tissue diseases, iron deficiency anemia, and osteoporosis in women; coronary atherosclerosis in young and middle-aged men; and gout in men. Other aspects of women's health are discussed in Chap. 6.

Race/Ethnicity   Race and ethnicity also play an important role in the expression of disease. In addition to genetic factors, persons with similar ethnic backgrounds share cultural, nutritional, environmental, economic, and social characteristics that influence disease. There are numerous examples of differences in the risk, incidence, and expression of disease across ethnic groups: sickle cell anemia and other hemoglobinopathies are found almost exclusively in persons of African, Arabic, Indian, Greek, and Italian ancestry; the age-adjusted prevalence of hypertension in African-Americans is two to four times that of whites (with the highest rates in black women); the prevalence of non-insulin diabetes mellitus is approximately twice as high in African-Americans and Native Americans as in whites; the age-adjusted mortality rates for stroke and sudden death are higher in blacks than in whites; the rates for symptomatic coronary artery disease are higher in black than in white women; the prevalence and incidence of tubercu-

*This chapter includes the contributions of Eugene Braunwald and Jean Wilson from prior editions.

losis are approximately twice as high in blacks as in whites; osteoporosis and vertebral fractures occur more frequently in women than in men and in white than in black women; and ankylosing spondylitis and Reiter's syndrome are more common in whites.

Social class, racism, and other sociocultural factors affect health-related behaviors and outcomes across racial/ethnic groups. Even when income, health status, age, sex, and history of chronic disease are taken into account, blacks in the United States have fewer ambulatory visits and are less likely to see a physician, suggesting disadvantages in access to care.

Less is known about the mortality and morbidity data for racial/ethnic groups other than whites and blacks. Moreover, there are serious concerns about the accuracy of such data as do exist, given documented discrepancies in the coding of race/ethnicity among agencies that collect vital statistics. Broad categories such as "Hispanic," "Asian," or "Native American" include diverse populations with diverse disease risks. For example, Mexican-Americans appear to have a low risk of cerebrovascular disease, whereas Puerto Ricans have a high risk of stroke, which would make it difficult to interpret statistics for Hispanics based on the combined experience. More precise ethnic categories, particularly for Asians and Pacific Islanders, often have too few individuals for reliable calculation of cause-specific death rates. Furthermore, the increasing interracial admixture of the population makes traditional racial categories less meaningful over time.

Sexual Orientation The incidence of some diseases varies greatly in subgroups of the population defined by sexual orientation and practices. For example, the incidence of AIDS, gonorrhea, syphilis, and hepatitis B is higher among homosexual than among heterosexual men. Colitis due to parasites ("gay-bowel syndrome") and anal and oropharyngeal carcinomas also occur more frequently in homosexual men. The increased incidence of these conditions is related to the numbers of sexual partners and sexual practices and not to homosexuality itself. Among lesbians, rates of infection with syphilis, gonorrhea, chlamydia, herpesvirus, and human papillomavirus appear to be lower than among heterosexual women. Many lesbians are nulliparous, and nulliparous women are at increased risk for breast and ovarian cancer.

Geography Geography can influence disease incidence in several ways. Some diseases occur only in those who have resided for long periods in specific areas. Goiter caused by iodine deficiency occurs mainly in people who live in areas previously covered by glaciers; toxic waste syndromes usually require prolonged residence in an area exposed to toxins; pulmonary hypertension is more common in those living at high altitudes; sarcoidosis is more common in residents of the coniferous belt of the southern United States; multiple sclerosis is more common in temperate climates. Some infectious diseases (e.g., melioidosis, leprosy, leishmaniasis, Chagas' disease, and filariasis) tend to occur in people who live in specific locations for a long time. The advent of widespread airborne travel, refugee resettlement, and immigration requires that clinicians in the United States consider a broad differential diagnosis of disease encompassing conditions related to geographic exposure.

Health indicators and practice patterns differ among diverse geographic regions. In 1990 to 1992, the age-adjusted death rate for residents of large cities in the United States was 19 percent greater than in suburbs around large cities. One study found substantial regional variation in the use of cardiac medications and procedures for the management of acute myocardial infarction in the United States.

THE RELATIONSHIP OF AGE, GENDER, AND RACE/ETHNICITY TO MEASURES OF HEALTH Life Expectancy Since 1900, life expectancy in the United States increased by nearly 60 percent for whites and 100 percent for blacks. By 1992, average life expectancy at birth was 73.2 and 79.8 years, respectively, for white males and females and 65.0 and 73.9 years for black males and females (Table 4-1). These gains in life expectancy are the result of declines in age-adjusted mortality rates (Fig. 4-1). Nevertheless, there is a continuing gap in life expectancy between blacks and whites, a slowing of life expectancy gains in blacks beginning in the mid-1980s, and a persistent twofold excess in infant mortality among blacks.

The male-female gap in life expectancy widened and then narrowed during this century, consistent with the pattern of cigarette

Table 4-1

Life Expectancy at Birth for Whites and Blacks, by Gender: United States, 1900–1992

	White		Black	
	Male	**Female**	**Male**	**Female**
1900	46.6	48.7	32.5	33.5
1950	66.5	72.2	58.9	62.7
1960	67.4	74.1	60.7	65.9
1970	68.0	75.6	60.0	68.3
1980	70.7	78.1	63.8	72.5
1990	72.7	79.4	64.5	73.6
1991	72.9	79.6	64.6	73.8
1992	73.2	79.8	65.0	73.9

SOURCE: National Center for Health Statistics.

smoking, first by men and later by women. Life expectancy among whites was on average 2.1 years longer for women than men in 1900, 7.6 years longer in 1970, and 6.6 years longer in 1992.

Mortality Rates Since the mid-1960s, most of the decline in overall mortality rates in the United States is due to reductions in death from coronary heart disease (CHD) and stroke, affecting primarily the older age groups. Age-adjusted CHD death rates have declined by more than 40 percent since 1970; between 1980 and 1992 alone, age-adjusted heart disease mortality rates in the population aged 55 to 64 years declined 30 percent, from 494.1 to 346.5 per 100,000. For all of the leading causes of death (except diabetes mellitus) in the United States, there is a male excess in age-adjusted death rates; the excess is greater than twofold for deaths due to accidents, suicide, chronic liver disease and cirrhosis, homicide, and human immunodeficiency virus infection (Table 4-2). Data on disease rates among Hispanics,

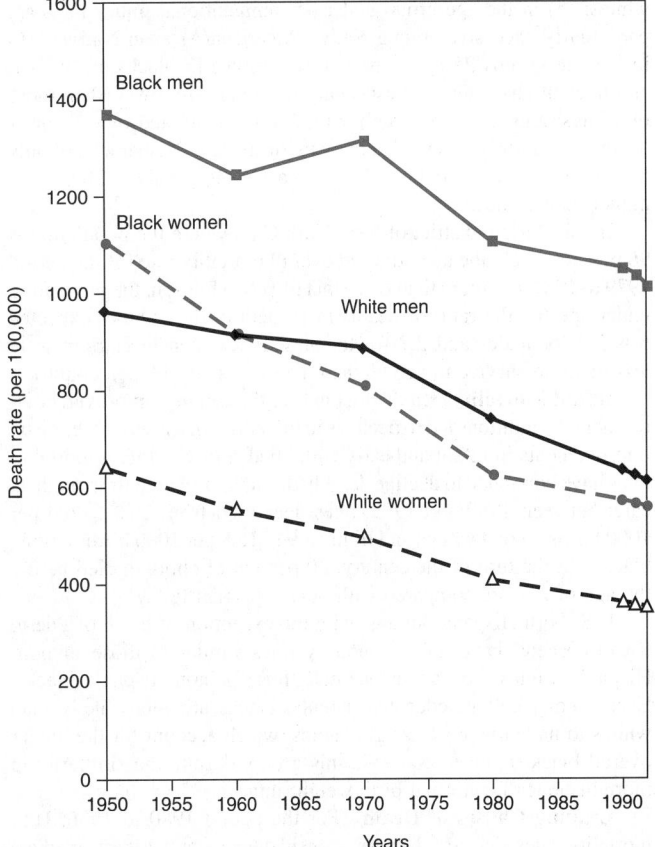

FIGURE 4-1 Age-adjusted death rates per 100,000, 1950–1992, for white and black males and females, age-adjusted to the 1940 U.S. population. (*After National Center for Health Statistics.*)

Table 4-2

Age-Adjusted Death Rates (per 100,000 Population) and Ratios for the Leading Causes of Death by Gender and Race: United States, 1992

Causes	White		Black		Ratio of white male rate to white female rate	Ratio of black male rate to black female rate	Ratio of black male rate to white male rate	Ratio of black female rate to white female rate
	Male	Female	Male	Female				
Heart disease	190.3	98.1	264.1	162.4	1.9	1.6	1.4	1.7
Malignant neoplasms	157.3	110.3	238.1	136.6	1.4	1.7	1.5	1.2
Cerebrovascular diseases	26.3	22.5	52.0	39.9	1.2	1.3	2.0	1.8
Chronic obstructive pulmonary diseases	26.8	16.1	24.8	11.2	1.7	2.2	0.9	0.7
Motor vehicle crashes	22.2	9.6	25.0	8.7	2.3	2.9	1.1	0.9
Pneumonia and influenza	15.8	9.7	25.0	12.2	1.6	2.0	1.6	1.3
Human immunodeficiency virus infection	18.1	1.6	61.8	14.3	11.3	4.3	3.4	8.9
Diabetes mellitus	11.6	9.6	24.2	25.8	1.2	0.9	2.1	2.7
Suicide	19.5	4.6	12.4	2.1	4.2	5.9	0.6	0.5
Homicide and legal intervention	9.3	2.8	68.1	13.0	3.3	5.2	7.3	4.6
Chronic liver disease and cirrhosis	11.1	4.6	17.2	6.9	2.4	2.5	1.5	1.5
Alcohol-induced causes	9.9	2.6	22.3	6.3	3.8	3.5	2.3	2.4
Drug-induced causes	5.5	2.7	10.6	3.6	2.0	2.9	1.9	1.3
All causes	620.9	359.9	1026.9	568.4	1.7	1.8	1.7	1.6

SOURCE: National Center for Health Statistics.

Asians/Pacific Islanders, and Native American/Alaskan Native populations, as well as blacks and whites, assembled by the National Center for Health Statistics, suggest the following: (1) for all age groups, overall death rates are lowest among Asians; (2) blacks have the highest overall death rates for all age groups except ages 15 to 24, when rates are slightly higher for Native American/Alaskan Natives; (3) in all age groups under 65, overall death rates among whites and Hispanics are intermediate between the low rates of Asians and the high rates of blacks; (4) in young people aged 15 to 24, blacks are seven times more likely, and Hispanics and Native Americans are three to four times more likely, to die of homicide than Asians and whites; (5) in the age group under 45, unintentional injury rates are particularly excessive among Native American/Alaskan Natives; (6) in the age groups 25 to 64, heart disease rates in blacks are higher, and rates in Hispanics and especially in Asians are lower, than those of whites; and (7) among the population 65 years and older, cancer death rates among Asians, Native Americans, and Hispanics are only half or less those of whites, whereas black rates are about 20 percent higher than whites.

In the Harlem district of New York City, where the population is 96 percent black, the age-adjusted overall mortality rate for the period 1979 to 1981 was more than twice that of U.S. whites; in the population under age 65, the ratio of deaths in Harlem to the number expected was 2.9 for males and 2.7 for females. Black men in Harlem were less likely to survive to age 65 than men in less-developed countries.

Infant Mortality   In the first half of the century, improved environmental conditions led to declines in infectious diseases and dramatic improvements in infant and early childhood survival. Infant mortality rates have continued to decline, largely due to improvements in medical care; between 1950 and 1992, rates decreased from 26.8 to 6.9 per 1000 births among whites and from 43.9 to 16.8 per 1000 births among blacks. At the turn of the century, 30 percent of children died before the age of 5 years compared with only 2 percent today.

U.S.-born Hispanic infants, with the exception of those of Puerto Rican descent, have infant mortality rates similar to those of non-Hispanic whites, i.e., about one-half those of non-Hispanic blacks. Even among college-educated parents, blacks are more likely than whites to have low birth weight babies, which account for the higher overall black infant mortality in this group, despite the similarity in mortality rates for normal birth weight infants.

Leading Causes of Death   For the period 1980 to 1986, U.S. mortality rates due to 12 causes considered preventable by medical intervention (tuberculosis, cervical cancer, Hodgkin's disease, rheumatic heart disease, hypertensive heart disease, acute respiratory disease, pneumonia and bronchitis, influenza, asthma, appendicitis, her-

nias, and cholecystitis) were 4.5 times higher in blacks than whites, with highest relative differences for tuberculosis, hypertensive heart disease, and asthma.

Morbidity   Morbidity data are consistent with the mortality data. In 1988, 16.3 percent of blacks and 12.8 percent of whites reported limitation of their activity due to chronic conditions. In a study in Manhattan (New York), incidence rates of Parkinson's disease were highest for black men. One population-based study reported hypertensive end-stage renal disease rates in blacks to be 4.5 times higher than in whites, adjusting for age, prevalence of hypertension, diabetes, and education level. On the other hand, malignant melanoma is more common in whites than in blacks.

Access to Care   In Massachusetts, black patients with ischemic heart disease undergo coronary angiography and coronary artery bypass grafting less often than whites, even controlling for age, sex, income, source of payment, primary diagnosis, and the number of secondary diagnoses. In Los Angeles County from 1986 through 1988, blacks and Latinos were less likely than whites and Asians to undergo bypass surgery. Among Medicare patients, sex- and age-adjusted rates for coronary artery bypass grafting among blacks were about one-third those among whites in 1986 and were not related to admission rates for acute myocardial infarction. Many of the residual differences may be due to inadequate control for SES, but the disparities exist nonetheless.

SOCIOECONOMIC STATUS   Socioeconomic status is measured in various ways, including education, income, occupation, population density, poverty area residence, and combined indices. Different measures of SES are not necessarily interchangeable; it is preferable to have more than one indicator. When a single SES indicator must suffice, education appears to provide the most valid measure. However measured, low SES has adverse health consequences and appears to be largely responsible for the differences in health status between whites and other racial/ethnic groups, especially blacks, in the United States (see below). Increasing attention is being given to understanding mediators of this impressive relationship of SES to disease.

RELATIONSHIP OF SOCIOECONOMIC STATUS TO MEASURES OF HEALTH   Mortality Data   In a study of 340,000 individuals who died in 1960, clear inverse gradients were found in mortality by education, income, and occupation for white and nonwhite males and females. The mortality of white females with 4 or more years of college education, for example, was only 71 percent of the overall rate for white females, whereas those with fewer than 5 years of education had a mortality ratio of 127 percent. Similarly, life expectancy for white women aged 25 with at least 1 year of college education was almost 10 years greater (56.4 years) than for those with fewer than 5 years of schooling. The decline in heart disease mortality among males between 1960 and 1971 to 1984 was sharpest for those with more years of education.

Mortality differentials by occupational status have been well documented, and social class differences in mortality in Britain may be widening. In the United States, a population-based 18-year follow-up study in Alameda County, California, found that death rates in individuals with inadequate family income were twice as high as in those with adequate income. The Western Collaborative Group Study of 3154 employed, middle-aged men showed an association between SES and mortality, even after adjustment was made for other causes of mortality.

Incidence of Disease When SES is controlled, black/white differences in the incidence of some cancers, including invasive cervical cancer and male lung cancer, are reduced or disappear. In fact, unadjusted for SES, overall cancer rates are higher in blacks compared with whites in the United States, but adjusted rates are higher in whites than in blacks. Differences in heart disease rates across occupational groups in the United States are greater than differences between blacks and whites. Even the onset of the decline in CHD rates among white women in the United States occurred first in geographic areas where average income, education, and occupational levels were highest.

Survival Black women have poorer survival from breast cancer than white women, but race is not significant if SES is controlled. Although infant mortality rates are twice as high among normal birth weight black babies compared with white babies in the general population, no differences are found in comparisons of normal birth weight infants born to black and white college-educated parents. In one study, those with annual household incomes of $40,000 or greater were about half as likely to die within 5 years as patients with lower incomes.

Morbidity Morbidity is also inversely related to income. In the United States in 1993, 26.0 percent of individuals whose family income was less than $14,000 reported limitation of activity due to chronic conditions, compared with only 9.2 percent of those whose income was $50,000 or greater (Table 4-3). Other analyses demonstrate that most preventable morbidity and functional limitation in the U.S. population before age 75 occurs in the lower SES strata. Even among children the average number of disability days in 1980 was 9.1 for those whose families had annual incomes of $5000, compared with 4 days for those from families with incomes of $25,000 or more. The incidence of lower respiratory illness is inversely related to educational level of the head of household, and in one study the lowest income group had a threefold increase in the odds of CHD compared with the highest income group. The pattern was similar in blacks and whites.

There are notable exceptions to the inverse gradient between SES and disease. For example, the incidence of breast cancer is higher in upper SES groups. However, the general validity of the inverse gradient of social class to so many seemingly unrelated causes of disease is impressive.

Differences in health status across SES and racial groups are partially due to differences in the distribution of known disease risk factors. Cigarette smoking, the leading cause of preventable death in the United States, shows a strong inverse relationship to SES. In the population 18 years of age and older, 37.3 percent of males and 27.1 percent of females with less than a high school education were current smokers in 1990, compared with 14.5 percent and 12.3 percent, respectively, of college graduates. The inverse relation of smoking prevalence

and educational status is seen for both white and black, males and females (Table 4-4). It is projected that by the year 2000 smoking prevalence among those with a high school education or less will be about 30 percent, whereas it will be less than 10 percent among college graduates. In California between 1984 and 1989, smoking, nonuse or infrequent use of seat belts, not exercising outside of work, being overweight, and hypertension among women were all more common in those with a high school education or less (Table 4-5). Nationwide data for 1987 to 1989 indicate that self-reports of mammographic screening and of having had a Pap smear within the previous year are positively associated with income level. Finally, the proportion of children in the United States who are vaccinated for measles, rubella, diphtheria/tetanus/pertussis (DTP), polio, and mumps is about 15 to 20 percent higher among white children compared with children of other racial groups (Table 4-6), which may largely reflect SES differences.

For many diseases, however, control for differences in known risk factors diminishes but does not eliminate differences across SES and racial groups. In British civil servants, about 40 percent of the differential in CHD mortality across different employment grades remained after controlling for serum cholesterol, systolic blood pressure, smoking, physical activity, body mass, and other factors. Similarly, adjustment for age and risk factors resulted in only modest reductions in the elevated relative risks of death from heart disease among the least educated men and women aged 45 to 74 in one survey. An examination of follow-up data from the same survey for adults aged 35 to 54 found that the ratio of black to white mortality rates decreased from 2.3 to 1.9 when adjusted for six risk factors (smoking, systolic blood pressure, cholesterol level, body-mass index, alcohol intake, and diabetes) and was further reduced

Table 4-4

Age-Adjusted Prevalence of Current Cigarette Smoking by Persons 25 Years of Age and Over, by Sex, Race, and Education: United States, 1993

Education, years	Male		Female	
	White	Black	White	Black
<12	39.7	47.2	31.7	29.8
12	29.7	36.4	27.6	23.9
13–15	26.9	30.1	21.9	22.7
>16	14.1	16.0*	12.5	13.3*
Total	26.3	36.0	23.1	22.2

* These age-adjusted percents should be considered unreliable because of small sample size.

SOURCE: National Center for Health Statistics.

Table 4-5

Prevalence of Behavioral Risk Factors by Education Level in California, Ages 35–44, 1984–1989

Risk Factor	Males		Females	
	≤ High School, %	> High School, %	≤ High School, %	> High School, %
Current smoking	40.7	25.6	30.1	19.1
Irregular, nonuse of seatbelts	29.6	17.8	20.9	10.9
No exercise outside of work	39.4	14.4	31.9	20.2
Overweight	33.1	19.6	21.6	14.1
Hypertension	13.1	20.0	15.9	10.9
Chronic drinking	13.9	12.8	4.0	2.5
Drinking and driving	6.7	5.2	1.1	1.3

SOURCE: Based on responses to telephone interviews conducted as part of the CDC's ongoing Behavioral Risk Factor Survey. n = 10,650 California participants during 1984–1989.

Table 4-3

Limitation of Activity due to Chronic Conditions by Family Income, United States, 1993

Family Income, $	Percent of Population
<14,000	26.0
14,000–24,999	17.3
25,000–34,999	13.4
35,000–49,999	11.1
50,000 or more	9.2

SOURCE: National Center for Health Statistics.

Table 4-6

Vaccination of White and Black Children Aged 19–35 Months for
Selected Diseases, by Race, United States, 1993

	White	Black
Measles	84.2	80.8
DTP*	88.3	78.0
Polio	74.7	67.4
Haemophilus b	64.4	46.5

* Diphtheria/tetanus/pertussis.
SOURCE: National Center for Health Statistics.

to 1.4 when adjustment for family income was included; 31 percent of the excess mortality in blacks was, therefore, due to the six risk factors, and 38 percent was due to family income, leaving 31 percent unexplained. On the other hand, lower cardiovascular disease mortality has been reported in Mexican-American compared to white males, despite higher levels of cardiovascular risk factors in the former.

One theme under consideration is the role of relative deprivation, as opposed to absolute levels of income or other measures of SES, in determining health status in developed countries. In Britain, for example, among individuals in nonmanual occupations who are homeowners, mortality is still lower in those with two cars compared to those with only one car. Across the 12 countries of the European Community, a strong correlation between income distribution and life expectancy has been reported.

Nevertheless, avoidable risk factors account for part of the differences in disease status in all SES groups, even among the elderly. Priority areas for health promotion (individual behaviors), health protection (environmental and regulatory measures), and preventive services (counseling, screening, immunization, or chemoprophylactic intervention in clinical settings) are extensively documented. Attempts to promote healthy lifestyles among the socially disadvantaged deserve high priority. In the face of the difficulties of daily life, however, such efforts may not be a high priority for the individuals who are in greatest need, and such education will have little impact unless coupled with adequate income, employment, and housing. It is disturbing that social class disparities, as measured by income, are widening, and it is important that the paucity of national disease data by social class be corrected.

THE FUTURE: IMPROVEMENTS IN YEARS OF HEALTHY LIFE VS. LENGTH OF LIFE It is not clear whether it is biologically possible to extend average life expectancy much beyond that presently attained by the most advantaged members of our society, i.e., around 85 years of age. If it is not possible, our major goal in health promotion should be the "compression of morbidity," i.e., postponement of debilitating illness until as close as possible to the time of death. Stated otherwise, we should focus on the morbidity and quality-of-life outcomes of our prevention efforts: "Add life to your years, not years to your life."

That said, it is important to acknowledge that sizable disadvantaged segments of our population have yet to approximate the purported maximum life span and that attempts to change established behavioral risk factors, while critically important, will not compress morbidity for the population as a whole. Improvements in SES and recognition of the continuing impact of racism on health outcomes are fundamental to achieving that goal.

BIBLIOGRAPHY

ADLER NE et al: Socioeconomic inequalities in health. No easy solution. JAMA 269:3140, 1993

BRAUNWALD E, WILSON JD: Host and disease: Influence of demographic factors, in *Harrison's Principles of Internal Medicine*, 13th ed, KJ Isselbacher et al (eds). New York, McGraw-Hill, 1994, pp 8–10

BUCHER HC et al: Socioeconomic indicators and mortality from coronary heart disease and cancer: A 22-year follow-up of middle-aged men. Am J Public Health 85:1231, 1995

CARLISLE DM et al: Racial and ethnic differences in the use of invasive cardiac procedures among cardiac patients in Los Angeles County, 1986 through 1988. Am J Public Health 85:352, 1995

DENENBERG R: Report on lesbian health. Womens Health Issues 5:81, 1995

DIEZ-ROUX AV et al: Social inequalities and atherosclerosis: The atherosclerosis risk in communities study. Am J Epidemiol 141:960, 1995

DOLL R: Health and the environment in the 1900s. Am J Public Health 82:933, 1992

HAHN RA: The state of federal health statistics on racial and ethnic groups. JAMA 267:268, 1992

KRIEGER N et al: Social class: The missing link in U.S. health data. Int J Health Serv 24:25, 1994

LEE PR et al: Measuring social inequalities in health. Report on the Conference of the National Institutes of Health. Public Health Rep 110:302, 1995

MAYEUX R et al: The frequency of idiopathic Parkinson's disease by age, ethnic group, and sex in northern Manhattan, 1988–1993. Am J Epidemiol 142:820, 1995

NATIONAL CENTER FOR HEALTH STATISTICS: *Health, United States, 1994.* DHHS publication No. (PHS) 95-1232, Hyattsville, MD, 1995

PILOTE L et al: Regional variation across the United States in the management of acute myocardial infarction. N Engl J Med 333:565, 1995

US DEPARTMENT OF HEALTH AND HUMAN SERVICES: *Healthy People 2000.* DHHS publication No. (PHS) 91-50213, Washington, DC, 1990

WHITE et al: Lesbian health care. What a primary care physician needs to know. Western J Med 162:463, 1995

WILKINSON RG: National mortality rates: The impact of inequality? Am J Public Health 82:1082, 1992

5

Howard Hu, Frank E. Speizer

INFLUENCE OF ENVIRONMENTAL AND OCCUPATIONAL HAZARDS ON DISEASE

Exposures to hazardous materials and processes in the home, the workplace, and the community can cause or exacerbate a multitude of diseases. Physicians commonly treat the sequelae of such diseases in the practice of medicine; however, unless the underlying connection with hazardous exposures is identified and mitigated, treatment of manifestations rather than the cause at best only ameliorates the condition. At worst, the neglect of hazardous exposures may lead to both failure of treatment and failure to recognize a public health problem with wide significance.

No existing surveillance or reporting system can estimate the total contribution of hazardous exposures to morbidity and mortality. However, careful histories have identified occupational factors as etiologic in more than 10 percent of all admissions to general internal medicine wards in hospitals, with even higher percentages when the primary illness is either respiratory or musculoskeletal. Estimates of the number of new cases of disease due to work in the United States range from 125,000 to 350,000 per year; these cases do not include 5.3 million work-related injuries.

Environmental exposures are increasingly associated with decrements in measures of health whose outcomes range from subclinical to clinically catastrophic. For example, exposure to lead at levels that are common in the general population has been associated with increased blood pressure and decreased creatinine clearance. Ambient air pollution with respect to levels of ozone and fine-particulate matter recently has been related to increased rates of hospital admissions for respiratory and cardiovascular diseases and to increased mortality, respectively. Indoor exposures to radon and passive environmental tobacco smoke have been linked with an increased risk of lung cancer. While such data are suggestive but not necessarily conclusive with respect to causation, there is pressure on clinicians to be aware of and act on this type of information.

Patients are becoming increasingly concerned about hazardous exposures. More than 15 percent of patients seen in one study conducted in a primary care clinic expressed the opinion that their health problems were work-related, and 75 percent of this subgroup of patients reported exposure to one or more recognized toxic agents. Patients often want answers to very specific questions, such as: Is the water in our town safe to drink? Could my breathing problem be related to the new roofing sealant used in my building at work? Physicians are consulted because they are the most trusted sources of information on health risks, including chemical risks. Unfortunately, few physicians have more than rudimentary training in environmental and occupational medicine. Therefore, it becomes important for primary care physicians to be able to recognize cases having these elements and either to manage them or to make appropriate referrals.

Many manifestations of exposure-related illnesses are nonspecific (e.g., dizziness, headache) or are commonly encountered in general internal medicine (e.g., myocardial infarction, cancer). The establishment of a connection with a hazard requires a high index of suspicion and the application of fundamental concepts of environmental/occupational medicine. Furthermore, early recognition by physicians of unusual patterns of illness or of evidence of asymptomatic exposure to toxins with low-level effects (e.g., an elevated blood lead level) can alert health officials to the need for control measures. Case reports either sent to local authorities or published in the literature often prompt follow-up studies that can lead to the identification of new hazards. In many states and countries, the reporting by physicians of occupational/environmental diseases is mandatory. For instance, beginning in 1992, physicians in Massachusetts were required to report cases of pneumoconiosis, occupational asthma, carpal tunnel syndrome, and carbon monoxide poisoning, among other conditions. Identification of an environmental/occupational etiology of an illness may have important economic ramifications for the patient (e.g., the awarding of worker's compensation, which covers medical bills as well as lost wages). Finally, physicians are frequently asked to provide expert medical testimony during litigation on the causal relationship between toxic exposures and disease. In this setting, the more knowledgeable the physician is about potential hazardous exposures, the better prepared he/she is to serve the patient.

THE ILL PATIENT
RECOGNIZING A CHEMICAL
OR OTHER ENVIRONMENTAL ETIOLOGY

DEFINITION OF ENVIRONMENTAL/OCCUPATIONAL HAZARDS The term *hazards* encompasses chemical factors as well as other risks posed by the physical environment (changes in temperature and in altitude and/or pressure, exposures to ionizing and nonionizing radiation) and by select natural phenomena (venoms and stings). A detailed discussion of specific hazards can be found in Part 15. Unless otherwise defined, the terms *toxins* and *toxic exposures* are synonymous with *hazards*. These hazards may exist in the general environment or in the workplace. Strictly speaking, smoking, alcohol ingestion, nutritional factors and infectious diseases can also be considered chemical or environmental hazards.

THE ENVIRONMENTAL/OCCUPATIONAL HISTORY For a physician, the most critical steps toward recognizing these disorders are remembering to consider them in the differential diagnosis and taking an appropriate environmental/occupational history as part of the medical workup. The level of detail that is called for depends on the clinical situation. *Information should always be obtained on current and major past occupations, and patients should be asked whether they think their health problem is related to their work or to any particular environmental exposure.* In the review of systems, patients should also be asked if they have been exposed to dusts, fumes, chemicals, radiation, loud noise. When patient and physician are confronted with an illness of uncertain etiology, these factors should be explored in more detail, with the environmental/occupational history as the point of departure. (A brief outline of a sample history is shown in Table 5-1.)

Table 5-1

Initial Clinical Approach to the Recognition of Illness Caused by Environmental or Occupational Hazards

A. Screening questions
  1. Chief symptom and history of present illness
     - What kind of work do you do?
     - Do you think your health problems are related to your work, home, or any other particular environment or exposures?
     - Does the timing of your symptoms have any relation to being at work or at home or to any other particular exposures or activities?
  2. Review of systems
     - Are you now or have you previously been exposed to dusts, fumes, chemicals, radiation, or loud noise?
B. Detailed questioning based on initial suspicion
  - Chronology of jobs: Job title, type of industry, dates of work, description of job, a typical day, potentially hazardous exposures, protective equipment used
  - Chronology of residences: Description of potentially hazardous exposures (e.g., furnaces, pesticide application, home hobbies involving chemicals)
  - Identification of other employees or household members who have similar health problems
  - Exploration in detail of the temporal link between potential exposures and the chief symptom
  - Clinical clues (suspicious scenarios; see text)

SOURCE: Adapted from Newman, 1995.

The identification of specific chemical exposures can be difficult. Household products must list chemical ingredients on their labels, and this information may prove useful. For workplace exposures, the U.S. Occupational Safety and Health Administration (OSHA) requires chemical suppliers to provide material safety data sheets with their products and requires employers to retain these sheets and make them available to employees. The data sheets can be obtained by the physician or employee by a telephoned or written request; failure of an employer to provide them within 30 days of such a request is a violation of OSHA regulations and is punishable by fines. In addition to providing information on chemical ingredients and percent composition, the material safety data sheets provide basic information on toxicity. This information is seldom adequate from a clinical perspective but may indicate the general type of toxicity to be anticipated.

EVALUATION OF POSSIBLE CHEMICAL OR ENVIRONMENTAL HAZARDS Given the wide variety of toxic exposures that may be uncovered during a workup, a clinician should routinely consult additional reference material to evaluate whether particular hazards may be associated with the illness at hand. Many sources of information exist. OSHA and some regional poison-control centers have extensive information on hazards and brief summary documents that can be transmitted by telephone or facsimile. Depending on the area, other resources may include county and state health departments; regional offices of the National Institute for Occupational Safety and Health and the Environmental Protection Agency; the Consumer Products Safety Commission in Washington, D.C.; academic institutions; and individual toxicologists, occupational/environmental medicine specialists, or industrial hygienists. Sophisticated computerized databases are also available, including detailed listings on CD-ROM information systems. MEDLARS, the electronic database maintained by the National Library of Medicine, is accessible by modem and is familiar to many physicians. Files other than MEDLINE, such as the Hazardous Substances Databank, provide specific toxicity information on chemicals and include toxicologic references not covered by MEDLINE. Many of these databases can also be accessed through the Internet.

As with any other illness, laboratory investigation may be crucial. For example, tests of carboxyhemoglobin level to document carbon monoxide exposure or of serum anticholinesterase level to document organophosphate pesticide absorption should be performed within hours of exposure. As in cases of acute drug overdose, it is useful to freeze samples of urine and serum from any patient suspected of having had an acute chemical exposure; such specimens can be analyzed at a later date by sensitive methods of detection. Use of other tests must rely on knowledge of the specific hazard or illness in question.

SUSPICIOUS SCENARIOS Some medical problems or clinical scenarios demand a particularly high degree of suspicion of occupational or environmental factors as causative or contributing agents.

Respiratory Disease The contribution of occupational/environmental factors to respiratory disease is generally underrecognized, particularly among patients who smoke and among the elderly (see Chap. 254). For instance, asthma related to chemical exposure may be treated without regard to cause or may be erroneously diagnosed as acute tracheobronchitis. Shortness of breath from asbestosis may be attributed to chronic obstructive pulmonary disease. Chemical pneumonitis may be misdiagnosed as a bacterial infection.

Cancer Many cancers are thought to be causally related to occupational and environmental factors in addition to tobacco. Some are particularly likely to have a chemical etiology or another environmental cause, including cancers of the skin (solar radiation, arsenic, coal tar, soot); lung (asbestos, arsenic, nickel, radon); pleura (almost exclusively asbestos); nasal cavity and sinuses (chromium, nickel, wood and leather dusts); liver (arsenic, vinyl chloride); bone marrow (benzene, ionizing radiation); and bladder (aromatic amines).

Coronary Disease Carbon monoxide exposure is common, particularly in homes with malfunctioning furnaces or in workplaces close to motor vehicle exhaust. By reducing oxygen transport by hemoglobin and inhibiting mitochondrial metabolism, carbon monoxide can aggravate coronary disease. Methylene chloride, a solvent used in paint stripping, is converted to carbon monoxide and thus poses the same risk. Exposure to carbon disulfide, a chemical used in the production of rayon, accelerates the rate of atherosclerotic plaque formation.

Hepatitis/Chronic Liver Disease In the absence of evidence that a virus infection, alcohol ingestion, or drug use is the main cause of hepatitis (see Chaps. 295, 296, and 297), the involvement of a toxin must be considered. Toxin-induced hepatic injury may be cytotoxic, cholestatic, or both. The list of hepatotoxic agents is long, including organic synthetic compounds such as carbon tetrachloride (used in solvents and cleaning fluids) and methylene diamine (a resin hardener); pesticides such as chlordecone (Kepone); metals, particularly arsenic (used in pesticides and paints and found in well water); and natural toxins such as the pyrrolidizine alkaloids.

Kidney Disease Many chemical and environmental factors can cause renal injury (see Chap. 270). The etiology of much chronic kidney disease, however, remains unknown. An increasing body of evidence now links chronic renal failure with hypertension to lead exposure. Some studies suggest that chronic exposure to hydrocarbons (e.g., gasoline, paints, solvents) may lead to various types of glomerulonephritis, including Goodpasture's syndrome.

Peripheral Neuropathy Organic solvents such as *n*-hexane, heavy metals such as lead and arsenic, and some organophosphate compounds can damage the axons of peripheral nerves. Dimethylaminopropionitrile, an industrial catalyst, causes bladder neuropathy. Nerve entrapment syndromes of the upper extremity, such as carpal tunnel syndrome, may be caused by jobs that involve repetitive motion, especially those requiring the maintenance of awkward positions.

Neuropsychiatric Symptoms Fatigue, memory loss, difficulty in concentration, and emotional lability have been linked to chronic exposure to solvents such as toluene and perchloroethylene. Painters, metal degreasers, plastics workers, and cleaners are commonly exposed to solvents and develop these symptoms at a high rate. Characteristic patterns on formal neurobehavioral testing and stabilization of symptoms with gradual improvement after discontinuation of the exposure are among the features that distinguish these patients. Other substances associated with neurobehavioral dysfunction include metals, particularly lead, mercury, arsenic, and manganese; pesticides, such as or-

ganophosphates and organochlorines; and gases such as carbon monoxide.

Teratogenesis and Reproductive Problems Toxins can impair successful reproduction at a variety of levels. Examples include insecticides and herbicides, PCBs (polychlorinated biphenyls) and PBBs (polybrominated biphenyls), ethylene oxide (a sterilizing gas used in hospitals), metals (lead, arsenic, cadmium, mercury), and solvents. Dibromochloropropane, a nematocide, suppresses spermatogenesis. Some toxins, such as PCBs, PBBs, and chlorinated pesticides, are concentrated in milk.

Immunosuppression, Autoimmunity, and Hypersensitivity Evidence is increasing that exposures to some chemical agents can compromise the immune system, thereby leading to a generalized increased incidence of tumors (e.g., exposure to PBBs) or infections (e.g., respiratory infections after exposure to common air pollutants). Mercury, dieldrin, and methylcholanthrene are known to elicit autoimmune responses. Some chemicals are potent allergic sensitizers that cause dermal and respiratory problems (see Chaps. 254 and 311).

BIOLOGICAL MARKERS An increasing number of methods are available for measuring and interpreting toxic exposure, including (1) the internal dose of specific toxins and (2) markers of the biological effects of toxins. Internal-dose markers are relevant for toxins that are sequestered in the human body, such as lead (in blood), arsenic (in hair), and other metals (see Chap. 397), and halogenated compounds (such as PCBs). Markers of the biological effects of toxins include depressed levels of acetylcholinesterase in serum after exposure to organophosphate pesticides and sister chromatid exchanges in peripheral lymphocytes after exposure to the carcinogen ethylene oxide.

MANAGING A HAZARD-RELATED ILLNESS

Once a chemical or another environmental hazard has been identified as an important contributor to an illness, the next step is to prevent further exposure. For chronic diseases such as cancer, this step is irrelevant; the illness remains when the exposure has come and gone. For others, the physician *must be willing to become an active advocate for the patient*. This advocacy may involve writing a letter stating that the patient should no longer be exposed to a hazard or should remain out of work. Alternatively, it may involve contacting appropriate officials in government, industry, or labor or other advocates who can deal with a hazardous exposure. Treatment is dependent on the specific hazard.

In few areas of medicine does a physician deal with more scientific uncertainty. Comprehensive information on toxicants is available for only a small percentage of chemicals. In general, the physician should take a conservative approach (i.e., advise the patient to avoid a hazard likely to have contributed to illness) and should use common sense and up-to-date information to evaluate causal relationships.

LOW-LEVEL EXPOSURES AND THEIR EFFECTS

The subclinical effects of toxins that are widespread in our environment and our workplaces are of increasing concern. Given the absence of any demonstrable effect threshold, low-level exposure to carcinogens should be avoided; not only carcinogenic but also noncarcinogenic effects of chronic low-level exposure to these substances are important.

Perhaps lead provides the most important example of low-level noncarcinogenic effects that constitute a major public health problem. Multiple pathways of exposure, including the combustion of leaded gasoline, the use of lead-based paints and solder, and the presence of lead in cans containing food, have contributed to exposure of the entire population. Such low-level exposures can impair neurobehavioral development in infants and children and can raise blood pressure in adults. Furthermore, absorbed lead is stored in the skeleton and may reenter the circulation at times of heightened bone turnover (e.g., pregnancy, lactation, osteoporosis, hyperthyroidism). Subclinical toxic effects can be prevented if chronic low-level exposure is detected early and curtailed. In the case of lead, such exposure is detected by tests of blood lead level, which should be performed regularly in young children living in old neighborhoods and as a precautionary measure in adults with a history of lead exposure.

BIBLIOGRAPHY

BALMES J et al: Hospital records as a data source for occupational disease surveillance: A feasibility study. Am J Ind Med 21:341, 1992

DOCKERY DW et al: An association between air pollution and mortality in six U.S. cities. N Engl J Med 329:1753, 1993

GENNART J-P et al: Importance of accurate employment histories of patients admitted to units of internal medicine. Scand J Work Environ Health 17:386, 1991

HIMMELSTEIN JS, FRUMKIN H: The right to know about toxic exposures: Implications for physicians. N Engl J Med 312:687, 1985

INSTITUTE OF MEDICINE: *Role of the Primary Care Physician in Occupational and Environmental Medicine.* Washington, DC, National Academy Press, 1988

————: *Environmental Medicine—Integrating a Missing Element into Medical Education,* AM Pope, DP Rall (eds). Washington, DC, National Academy Press, 1995

KNEIP TJ, CRABLE JV: *Methods for Biological Monitoring—A Manual for Assessing Human Exposure to Hazardous Substances.* Washington, DC, American Public Health Association, 1988

MORRIS RD et al: Ambient air pollution and hospitalization for congestive heart failure among elderly people in seven large U.S. cities. Am J Public Health 85:1361, 1995

MULLAN RJ, MURTHY LI: Occupational sentinel health events: An up-dated list for physician recognition and public health surveillance. Am J Ind Med 19:775, 1991

NEWMAN LS: Current concepts: Occupational illness. N Engl J Med 333:1128, 1995

PAUL M (ed): *Occupational/Environmental Hazards and Reproductive Health: A Guide for Clinicians.* Baltimore, Williams & Wilkins, 1992

ROSENSTOCK L, CULLEN MR (eds): *Textbook of Clinical Occupational and Environmental Medicine.* Philadelphia, WB Saunders, 1994

SULLIVAN JB JR, KRIEGER GR (eds): *Hazardous Materials Toxicology.* Baltimore, Williams & Wilkins, 1992

6

Anthony L. Komaroff, Celeste Robb-Nicholson, Beverly Woo

WOMEN'S HEALTH

In recent years, the medical problems and health care of women have received increasing attention. There are differences in morbidity and mortality between men and women. Most illnesses that can affect both men and women have not been as well studied in women. Many research studies of disease prevention and pathophysiology have included only male subjects. There are poorly understood differences in the expression of diseases in the two sexes. Finally, it appears that women receive different care than men for certain health problems that are common to both sexes.

MORBIDITY AND MORTALITY IN WOMEN   **Morbidity** Over and above obstetric and gynecologic conditions, women experience or report greater morbidity than men. Studies have found that women experience a 25 percent higher rate of restricted activity and a 40 percent higher rate of bed disability, adjusted across all ages. Women also make more visits to physicians, particularly for acute self-limited illnesses. It is unclear whether there are real differences in the prevalence of morbidity or differences in care-seeking behavior following the perception of symptoms.

Mortality In the developed nations, women live longer than men. In 1995, in the United States, the projected average life expectancy from birth is 79.7 years for females and 72.8 years

for males. Although more male fetuses are conceived than female fetuses, females have a survival advantage over males in all age groups. The longer life expectancy of women in developed countries, compared to men, is due in large part to the difference in mortality caused by ischemic heart disease (IHD).

As shown in Table 6-1, the leading causes of death among young women in the United States are accidents, homicide, and suicide. During the middle years, breast cancer is a slightly more common cause of death than IHD and lung cancer. In women between ages 65 and 74, IHD, lung cancer, and cerebrovascular disease overtake breast cancer as the leading causes of death. Among women of *all* ages, IHD is the leading cause of death, by a substantial margin, with a mortality rate five to sixfold higher than the rate for either lung or breast cancer. Nevertheless, a recent Gallup poll found that U.S. women believe breast cancer poses the greatest threat to their lives.

Social Factors Influencing Morbidity and Mortality Gender differences in morbidity and mortality may be explained in part by psychosocial factors such as socially defined gender roles, poverty, participation in the work force, health insurance, and life-style factors.

In the past 30 years in the United States, there has been a "feminization of poverty"—i.e., a rapid growth in the relative percentage of people in female-headed households who are living in poverty. One-third of families headed by women currently live in poverty, and the fraction is greater than one-half for African-American and Latina women. Almost a fifth of women over age 65 in the United States live below the poverty level. Women constitute a majority of the poor in all societies. People of lower socioeconomic status experience poorer health and a higher mortality rate than those in higher income groups. Although women of lower socioeconomic status have a smaller risk of breast cancer than women of higher socioeconomic status, they are less likely to be diagnosed at an early stage of the disease. The poor are more likely to smoke and less likely to use recommended preventive measures, including cancer screening. Lack of adequate health insurance is a major problem for many women, especially minority women, poor and low-income women, and women of reproductive age. Women in general are more likely than men to have low-paying, part-time, non-union jobs that do not provide health insurance. Women who are divorced or widowed may also lose health insurance that they had through their husbands.

Biological Factors Influencing Morbidity and Mortality Certain biological differences also contribute to the greater longevity of women. The most obvious is the exposure to estrogen that most women experience for about 40 years of their lives, which may provide some protection from IHD.

PREVENTION (See also Chap. 10) Primary prevention and screening are crucial elements in improving the health of women. Although there are few definitive clinical trials of preventive interventions in women, a growing number of large case-control and prospec-

Table 6-1

Death Rates (per 100,000) for the Leading Causes of Death in U.S. Women, 1990

Ages 24–34 Total: 74.2	Ages 45–54 Total: 342.7	Ages 65–74 Total: 1991.2	All Ages Total: 812.0
1. Motor vehicle accidents (11.5)	1. Breast cancer (45.4)	1. Ischemic heart disease (415.2)	1. Ischemic heart disease (185.6)
2. Homicide (7.2)	2. Ischemic heart disease (33.6)	2. Lung cancer* (181.7)	2. Cerebrovascular disease (68.6)
3. Suicide (5.6)	3. Lung cancer* (35.3)	3. Cerebrovascular disease (126.9)	3. Lung cancer* (40.4)
4. Non-motor vehicle accidents (4.6)	4. Cerebrovascular disease (17.0)	4. Breast cancer (111.7)	4. Breast cancer (34.0)

* Cancer of respiratory and intrathoracic organs, predominantly lung cancer.

SOURCE: Adapted from National Center for Health Statistics: *Vital Statistics of the United States, 1990,* vol II: *Mortality,* Part A. Washington, Public Health Service, 1994. DHHS Publication No. (PHS)95-1101, pp 40–52.

tive cohort observational studies (such as the Nurses' Health Study) have evaluated the prevention of disease in women. Based on available literature and experience, various authoritative organizations (e.g., the U.S. Preventive Services Task Force, Canadian Task Force, American College of Physicians, American Heart Association, American Cancer Society) have published guidelines on preventive practices in women.

While the annual comprehensive physical examination is no longer recommended, most physicians believe that a baseline history and physical examination is useful to set the stage for preventive measures appropriate to each patient. Most authorities recommend that blood pressure be measured every other year throughout life. Counseling on diet, smoking cessation, exercise, and use of seatbelts are of demonstrated value in the primary prevention of diseases and accidents. Counseling about safe sexual practices, alcohol abuse, and violence are recommended.

Screening for glaucoma is recommended for African-American women over age 40 and for Caucasian women over age 50. Yearly examinations to test visual acuity are recommended for women over age 70.

Regular screening for breast, cervical, and colorectal cancer is recommended, but how often tests should be performed and which tools to use are controversial. Most authorities recommend annual clinical breast examination in all women beginning at age 35 to 40. There is strong evidence to support the efficacy of annual mammography in women aged 50 to 59. For women aged 60 and older, the evidence for screening is less strong. Screening for women between the ages of 40 and 49 remains controversial.

Most authorities recommend Pap-smear screening beginning at age 18 or when a woman becomes sexually active. After two or three consecutive normal Pap smears, most groups recommend Pap smear testing every 3 years. If Pap smears have been normal for 10 years, they can be discontinued in women after age 65.

Recommendations for colorectal cancer screening vary, and there are no randomized controlled trials that have demonstrated a benefit. Rectal examination and fecal occult blood testing lack sensitivity and specificity. Randomized trials are underway to evaluate the benefit of flexible sigmoidoscopy.

One major risk factor, cigarette smoking, has been well studied in women. In 1990, 28 percent of men and 23 percent of women were regular smokers. Over the past 60 years there has been a sharp decline in smoking among men, but not among women. "Low-yield" cigarettes are marketed heavily to women; however, users of these cigarettes have the same risk of myocardial infarction as users of higher-yield brands. The Nurses' Health Study showed that one-third of the excess risk of IHD was eliminated two years after smoking cessation, and that all of the excess risk was eliminated by 10 to 14 years after smoking cessation.

Although reduction of serum cholesterol has been associated with a decreased risk of IHD in men, primary prevention studies have included far smaller numbers of women. It is likely that improvement of lipid profiles will decrease the risk of IHD in women, but that has not been proved. The National Cholesterol Education Program recommends that total cholesterol and high-density lipoprotein (HDL) levels be measured once. If both are normal, a repeat test after 5 years is recommended.

Postmenopausal estrogen therapy is associated with a 40 to 50 percent reduction in deaths due to IHD, a finding supported by several case-control studies. Calcium and estrogen replacement therapy have been shown to slow the development of osteoporosis and to reduce the frequency of hip and vertebral fracture in the postmenopausal woman.

Considerable research indicates that a relatively high dietary intake of various antioxidants (including vitamins C and E) is associated with lower rates of vascular disease and malignancies. Randomized trials of supplemental antioxidants are under way. Preliminary research indicates that regular aspirin use is associated with reduced rates of IHD and colorectal carcinoma.

GENDER DIFFERENCES IN DISEASE Obviously, some diseases and conditions occur exclusively (or nearly exclusively) in women—e.g., menopause and various breast and gynecologic disorders. These are discussed elsewhere in this book (Chaps. 48, 91, 337, 338). In this chapter, we seek primarily to highlight some gender differences in diseases that occur in both women and men.

Ischemic Heart Disease (See also Chap. 244) Many persons think of IHD as primarily a problem of men, perhaps because men have more than twice the total incidence of cardiovascular morbidity and mortality than women between the ages of 35 and 84. However, as stated earlier, in the United States IHD is the leading cause of death among women as well as men (Table 6-1), although the curve for mortality rate from IHD lags behind that for men by about a decade. Nearly 250,000 women die annually from IHD; after age 40, one in three women will die from heart disease. Although IHD mortality has been falling in the United States over the past 30 years, the rate of decline has been lower in women than in men.

Why are rates of IHD lower in women? Women have a more favorable risk profile in some respects: higher HDL cholesterol levels, lower triglyceride levels, and less upper-body obesity than men. But women also have a less favorable risk profile in other respects: more obesity, higher blood pressure, higher plasma cholesterol levels, higher fibrinogen levels, and more diabetes. The simplest explanation for the sex differential in IHD is a "cardioprotective" effect of estrogen, due to improvement of the lipid profile, a direct vasodilatory effect, and perhaps other factors. HDL cholesterol levels appear to be a particularly important risk factor for IHD in women. HDL levels are higher in all age groups in women compared to men, and are higher in premenopausal and estrogen-treated postmenopausal women than in non-estrogen-treated postmenopausal women. Smoking is the most important risk factor for IHD in women.

IHD presents differently in men and women. In the Framingham study, angina was the most frequent initial symptom of IHD in women, occurring in 47 percent of women. Myocardial infarction was the most frequent initial symptom in men, occurring in 46 percent of men. The exercise electrocardiogram appears to have a lower specificity for IHD in women than in men.

Women, particularly African-American women, have higher risks of morbidity and mortality than men following a myocardial infarction. Compared to men, women having coronary artery bypass graft surgery have more advanced disease, a higher perioperative mortality rate, less relief of angina, and less graft patency, but similar 5 and 10 year survival rates. Women undergoing percutaneous transluminal coronary angioplasty have lower rates of clinical and angiographic success than men, but also a lower rate of restenosis and a better long-term outcome. Women may benefit less and have more frequent serious bleeding complications from thrombolytic therapy than do men. Factors such as older age, more comorbid conditions, and more severe IHD in women at the time of events or procedures appear to account for at least part of the gender differences observed. As demonstrated in the CARE trial, women with IHD benefit at least as much as men, and perhaps more, from reductions in cholesterol level.

Hypertension (See also Chap. 246) Hypertension is more common in U.S. women than men, largely owing to the high prevalence of hypertension in older age groups and the longer survival of women. Renovascular hypertension from fibromuscular dysplasia occurs more often in women. Other causes of secondary hypertension occur with equal frequency in women and men. Both the effectiveness and the adverse effects of various antihypertensive drugs appear to be comparable in women and men. Benefits of treatment for severe hypertension have been dramatic in both women and men. However, in clinical trials of the treatment of mild to moderate hypertension, women have had a smaller decrease in morbidity and mortality than men, perhaps because women have a lower risk of myocardial infarction and stroke than men to begin with. Older women benefit at least as much as men from treatment, as demonstrated by the Systolic Hypertension in the Elderly study. When oral contraceptives were first introduced, many women had a small increase in blood pressure, with 5 percent showing an increase to above 140/90 over a 5-year period. The incidence of hypertension appears to be lower with the current low-dose oral contraceptives. Postmenopausal estrogen therapy is not associated with increases in blood pressure.

Immune-Mediated Diseases Several immune-mediated diseases—e.g., rheumatoid arthritis, systemic lupus erythematosus, multiple sclerosis, Graves' disease, and thyroiditis—occur much more frequently in women than in men. In animal models of rheumatoid arthritis, lupus, and multiple sclerosis, for example, it is females that are predominantly affected. On the other hand, animal studies indicate that females are less susceptible to infection.

In short, women and female animals appear to have more vigorous immune responses, with both beneficial and adverse consequences. Increasing evidence indicates that estrogens up-regulate both cellular and humoral immunity. Some immunocytes contain receptors for estrogen, progestin, and androgens, and the uterus produces a variety of cytokines. The reproductive and immune systems clearly interact in a complex way.

Osteoporosis Estrogen secretion also appears to play an important role in the control of bone density. While it is clear that the risk of osteoporosis in postmenopausal women is much greater than in men of the same age, and while postmenopausal estrogen supplementation is associated with a decreased incidence of osteoporosis, the mechanisms by which estrogen exerts its protective effects are not fully elucidated.

Psychological Disorders Depression, bulimia, and anorexia nervosa occur more often in women, as may anxiety disorders. Epidemiologic studies from both developed and developing nations consistently find major depression to be twice as common in women as in men, with the gender disparity becoming evident in early adolescence. The incidence of major depression in women diminishes after age 45. Interestingly, the incidence of depression does not increase with the onset of menopause, a time of symbolic and actual loss. Depression in women also appears to have a worse prognosis than in men: episodes of depression last longer, and there is a lower rate of spontaneous remission.

Depression occurs in 10 percent of women during pregnancy and in 10 to 15 percent of women during the first several months of the postpartum period. The treatment of depression during pregnancy or in the postpartum nursing mother is problematic: Relatively little is known about the possible teratogenic effects of many antidepressants, and it is uncertain whether the dosing of psychotropic drugs should be different in pregnancy.

Social factors may account for the greater prevalence of some disorders in women; the traditionally subordinate role of women in society may generate helplessness and frustration which, in turn, contribute to psychiatric illness. In addition, it is likely that biological factors, including hormonally influenced neurochemical changes, also play an important role. The limbic system and hypothalamus, areas of the brain thought to subserve appetite, satiety, and emotion, contain estradiol and testosterone receptors.

Alcohol Abuse One-third of Americans who suffer from alcoholism are women. Women alcoholics are less likely to be diagnosed than men. On average, alcoholic women drink less than alcoholic men but exhibit the same degree of impairment. Blood alcohol levels are higher in women than in men after drinking equivalent amounts of alcohol (adjusted for body weight). This greater bioavailability of alcohol in women is probably due to the higher proportion of body fat and to a lower gastric "first-pass metabolism" of alcohol, associated with lower activity of gastric alcohol dehydrogenase. In addition, alcoholic women are more likely than alcoholic men to abuse tranquilizers, sedatives, and amphetamines.

Women alcoholics have a higher mortality rate than both nonalcoholic women and alcoholic men. Compared to men, women also appear to develop alcoholic liver disease and other alcohol-related diseases with shorter drinking histories and lower levels of alcohol consumption. Alcohol abuse also poses special risks to a woman, adversely affecting fertility and the health of the baby (fetal alcohol syndrome).

Human Immunodeficiency Virus Infection (See also Chap. 308) In the United States, more than 20,000 women have developed AIDS, and an estimated 80,000 to 140,000 women have been infected with human immunodeficiency virus (HIV). In 1994, 18 percent of the reported cases of AIDS in persons over age 12 occurred in women, compared to 7 percent of the reported AIDS cases in 1985. The disease continues to affect women in racial/ethnic minorities and lower socioeconomic classes disproportionately. More than half of American women with AIDS are current or past users of intravenous drugs, compared to more than 70 percent of American men with AIDS. Heterosexual contact with an at-risk partner is the fastest-growing transmission category for women and is associated with most of the cases in non-intravenous drug users. About half of women who apparently were infected with HIV by heterosexual transmission did not know that they had been exposed to HIV.

Studies have not consistently demonstrated gender-related differences in the natural history of HIV infection. Compared with men, HIV-infected women more frequently suffer from esophageal candidiasis and less frequently develop Kaposi's sarcoma. Preventive and therapeutic measures appear to be comparably effective for HIV-infected women and men. Some studies have found that women have less access to care than do men.

Violence Against Women There has been a growing awareness of the enormous problem of violence against women, both rape and domestic violence. Rape has been redefined recently in many statutes as "nonconsensual sexual penetration of an adolescent or adult obtained by physical force, by threat of bodily harm, or when the victim is incapable of giving consent by virtue of mental illness, mental retardation, or intoxication." Epidemiologic studies in the United States suggest that at least 20 percent of adult women have experienced sexual assault during their lifetime. Nearly 100,000 cases of rape are reported annually in the United States, and this undoubtedly represents only a fraction of the actual number of cases. Adult women are much more likely to be raped by a spouse, ex-spouse, or acquaintance than by a stranger.

Domestic violence is an enormous problem in the United States. The American Medical Association guidelines define domestic violence as "an ongoing, debilitating experience of physical, psychologic, and/or sexual abuse in the home, associated with increasing isolation from the outside world and limited personal freedom and accessibility to resources." Every year in the United States, more than two million women (likely a low estimate, owing to underreporting) are severely injured and more than 1000 women are killed by their current or former male partner. Domestic violence is the most common cause of physical injury in women, exceeding the combined incidence of all other types of injury (such as from rape, mugging, and auto accidents). Surveys of women seeking medical care for any reason in internal medicine and emergency room practices have reported that the prevalence of domestic violence is an astonishing 15 to 30 percent. Domestic violence is a major health problem in women from all age, ethnic, and socioeconomic groups.

Women who have been raped or injured, as well as women who have been molested during childhood, frequently seek medical care for headaches, sleep and eating disorders, abdominal or pelvic pain, vaginal discharge, or musculoskeletal symptoms. They may also present to physicians with depression, suicidal ideation, and substance abuse. Given this indirect presentation of the consequences of violence, and the high prevalence of violence, clinicians should have a low threshold for pursuing the possibility of violence in female patients, particularly those with vague symptoms and psychological disorders.

The immediate treatment of rape and domestic violence is focused on assessing and treating physical injuries, on providing emotional support, on assessing and dealing with the risks of sexually transmitted infection and pregnancy, on evaluating the safety of the patient and other family members, and on documenting the patient's history and physical examination findings. In addition to dealing with the medical and psychological issues, appropriate care includes providing information about legal services, shelters and safe houses, hotlines, support groups, and counseling services.

RESEARCH IN WOMEN'S HEALTH Although women seek medical attention and use medications more frequently than men, historically relatively few women had been involved in studies of the prevention, pathophysiology, and treatment of diseases that involve both women and men. However, the growing recognition of the importance of women's health has spawned a number of research efforts. The U.S. National Institutes of Health (NIH) has introduced guidelines to mandate the inclusion of women in clinical studies.

Studies of Prevention The Framingham Study, an observational study of men and women under way since 1947, has been increasingly analyzing data specific to women. Since 1976, the Nurses' Health Study has been following more than 120,000 women, prospectively collecting data about their smoking, diet, physical activity, medications, prevention and screening behaviors, and some psychosocial factors. This study already has revealed information about how these factors contribute to the relative risk of developing a number of medical disorders, including breast cancer, ischemic heart disease, stroke, diabetes, and fracture, as well as to causes of mortality.

The Postmenopausal Estrogens/Progestins Intervention (PEPI) Trial was the first major trial testing the effects of postmenopausal hormone replacement therapy. It was a 3-year, multicenter, randomized, double-blind, placebo-control trial of the effects of three estrogen/progestin regimens on risk factors for cardiovascular disease, bone mineral density, and endometrial tissue. Thus far, the study has reported that estrogen alone or in combination with progestin increased serum levels of HDL and decreased low-density lipoprotein (LDL) and fibrinogen levels. While unopposed estrogen (without progestins) resulted in the most beneficial effects on lipids, it also was associated with an increased risk of endometrial hyperplasia.

In 1992, the NIH funded the Women's Health Initiative (WHI)—a study of the health of postmenopausal women. The WHI, the largest research study ever funded by the NIH, will involve 160,000 postmenopausal women at 45 clinical centers across the United States through the year 2002. The WHI includes both a prospective observational study and an interventional randomized trial designed to test strategies to prevent cardiovascular disease, breast cancer, and osteoporotic fractures—among the leading causes of death, disability, and diminished quality of life for older women. The clinical trial component of the WHI will involve 63,000 women in a randomized, controlled trial of the effects of a low-fat diet, hormone replacement therapy, and calcium and vitamin D supplementation on the risks for the illnesses cited above.

There are many other ongoing studies of the pathophysiology and prevention of diseases that affect women, and the next decade should be rich in data from this research.

Pharmacologic Treatment Over $30 billion worth of pharmaceuticals are sold each year in the United States, and the great majority are used by women. Women have been underrepresented in drug trials. In 1992, the U.S. Government Accounting Office reviewed pharmaceutical products that received Food and Drug Administration (FDA) approval between 1988 and 1991. The review concluded that 25 percent of the trials did not actively recruit women, that 30 percent included a smaller number of women than the FDA had recommended, and that in 60 percent of trials women were underrepresented relative to the gender distribution of the disease being treated. Two reasons are commonly given for conducting most clinical pharmacologic studies in men. First, cyclic hormonal changes in females could make experiments more difficult to control and interpret. Second, particularly with new drugs, concern about unsuspected pregnancy and subsequent teratogenic effects have discouraged the recruitment of female subjects.

The underrepresentation of women in drug trials is changing. The FDA now requires information on the safety and effectiveness of experimental drugs in women, on the effects of the menstrual cycle and menopause on a drug's pharmacokinetics, as well as on a drug's influence on the effectiveness of oral contraceptives. The increased emphasis on women in drug trials is likely to yield important information. Those studies that have included women indicate that there are clinically significant differences in the way women respond to a number of frequently prescribed pharmaceuticals, including sedative-hyp-

notics, antidepressants, antipsychotics, anticonvulsants, and beta-adrenoceptor blocking agents. The 1992 FDA Annual Adverse Experience Report found that women have a higher frequency of adverse drug reactions than men. Other studies suggest that the efficacy of many drugs may be different in women. For example, women require lower doses of neuroleptics to control schizophrenia than men do. The reasons for these differences are not clear. Estrogens may affect drug clearance via the cytochrome P450 oxidase system. In some instances, drug pharmacokinetics may change during the menstrual cycle. For example, there is reasonable evidence that some anticonvulsants and lithium may be metabolized more rapidly in the premenstrual period, resulting in an increased frequency of premenstrual ("catamenial") seizures and increased symptoms of bipolar disorder, respectively, in women treated with these drugs.

WOMEN AND HEALTH CARE REFORM The U.S. health care system is in the midst of major changes. Women, as the chief consumers of health care, and supported by an effective lay health movement, are having an increasing voice in this change. A number of women are seeking health care in multidisciplinary women's health units that combine expertise in gynecology, psychiatry, and internal or family medicine. Some internal medicine residency training programs are establishing tracks in women's health. The number of women physicians has grown by 300 percent between 1970 and 1990, and more than 40 percent of all U.S. medical students now are women. This infusion of women into the physician work force is likely to encourage the trend toward a greater recognition of the unique aspects of health and disease of women.

BIBLIOGRAPHY

BLUME SB: Women and alcohol. A review. JAMA 256:1467, 1986

BLUMENTHAL SJ et al: *Towards a Women's Health Research Agenda. Findings of the Scientific Advisory Meeting.* Washington, DC, Bass and Howes, 1991

BRAVEMAN P et al: Women without health insurance: Links between access, poverty, ethnicity, and health. West J Med 149:708, 1988

COLDITZ GA: The Nurses' Health Study: A cohort of U.S. women followed since 1976. JAMWA 50:40, 1995

COUNCIL ON SCIENTIFIC AFFAIRS, AMERICAN MEDICAL ASSOCIATION: Violence against women. Relevance for medical practitioners. JAMA 267:3184, 1992

GIJSBERS VAN WIJK CMT et al: Symptom sensitivity and sex differences in physical morbidity: A review of health surveys in the United States and the Netherlands. Women Health 17:91, 1991

KAPLAN NM: The treatment of hypertension in women. Arch Intern Med 185:563, 1995

MINKOFF HL, DEHOVITZ JA: Care of women infected with the human immunodeficiency virus. JAMA 266:2253, 1991

MURABITO JM: Women and cardiovascular disease: Contributions from the Framingham Heart Study. JAMWA 50:35, 1995

RICH-EDWARDS JW et al: The primary prevention of coronary heart disease in women. N Engl J Med 332:1758, 1995

RODIN J, ICKOVICS JR: Women's health. Review and research agenda as we approach the 21st century. Am Psychol 45:1018, 1990

THE WRITING GROUP FOR THE PEPI TRIAL: Effects of estrogen or estrogen/progestin regimens on heart disease risk factors in postmenopausal women: The Postmenopausal Estrogen/Progestin Interventions Trial. JAMA 273:199, 1995

VERBRUGGE LM, WINGARD DL: Sex differentials in health and mortality. Women Health 12:103, 1987

WEISSMAN MM, OLFSON M: Depression in women: Implications for health care research. Science 269:799, 1995

7

Thomas F. Ferris

MEDICAL DISORDERS DURING PREGNANCY

Pregnancy may be complicated by chronic disease or a new illness. In the past, many disorders were considered contraindications to pregnancy, but now, with appropriate care, excellent outcomes for both mother and child are the rule.

Systemic vascular resistance is reduced in pregnancy. In spite of a 40 percent increase in cardiac output during the second trimester, blood pressure falls (usually to 100/70 mmHg or lower). Although a modest rise may occur during the last month of normal pregnancy, an increase in systolic pressure of 30 mmHg or in diastolic pressure of 15 mmHg at any time during gestation is abnormal. Perinatal mortality increases with blood pressure levels that would be normal in nonpregnant women. For example, when mean arterial blood pressure (diastolic plus one-third of the pulse pressure) is 90 mmHg or higher during the second trimester, there is a greater risk for stillbirth, fetal growth retardation, and preeclampsia.

Hypertension during pregnancy usually has one of four causes: (1) preeclampsia (toxemia); (2) chronic essential hypertension; (3) gestational hypertension; and (4) renal disease.

PREECLAMPSIA (TOXEMIA)   Preeclampsia is a disease of late pregnancy in which hypertension is associated with hepatic, neurologic, hematologic, or renal involvement. Rapid development of edema, particularly of the face and hands, along with a rise in blood pressure, often signals the onset of this condition. Jaundice and abnormal liver function may be present. Hyperreflexia, visual disturbances, and headache indicate neurologic involvement and raise concern for the development of convulsions, termed "eclampsia." Hematologic manifestations of preeclampsia include thrombocytopenia with elevated levels of lactate dehydrogenase (LDH), microangiopathic hemolytic anemia, and thrombocytopenia. This condition is termed HELLP (*h*emolysis, *e*levated *l*iver function tests, *l*ow *p*latelets). In fulminant preeclampsia, disseminated intravascular coagulation may cause a reduction in plasma fibrinogen and elevated circulating fibrin degradation products (Chap. 119).

Proteinuria indicates renal involvement, and is one of the hallmarks of preeclampsia. Since the glomerular filtration rate (GFR) increases by about 50 percent in normal gestation, a reduction in GFR heralds the onset of preeclampsia even with normal levels of blood urea nitrogen (BUN) and serum creatinine. Indeed, a BUN of 6.4 mmol/L (18 mg/dL) or a creatinine level of 90 μmol/L (1 mg/dL) during pregnancy may reflect a 50 percent decline in GFR. In preeclampsia, urate clearance decreases, because of increased proximal tubular reabsorption of urate, which in turn is probably due to the reduction of vascular volume. Hyperuricemia usually precedes the rise in serum creatinine and BUN; in fact, a plasma uric acid level above 270 μmol/L (4.5 mg/dL) in a hypertensive pregnant woman suggests preeclampsia. Volume contraction is similar to that in some other hypertensive states in which venoconstriction causes capillary pressure to rise, with expansion of interstitial volume at the expense of intravascular volume, but a generalized increase in capillary permeability may contribute also.

Fibrin deposits in the glomeruli, with characteristic swelling of the glomerular endothelial cells, are evident in renal biopsies; peripheral necrosis with fibrin deposits in the sinusoids may be present in the liver. Tomographic scanning techniques [computed tomography (CT) or magnetic resonance imaging (MRI)] reveal hypodense areas consistent with small cerebral infarctions in approximately half of the women with eclampsia.

An abnormality in endothelial integrity has been proposed as the cause of the widespread fibrin deposits. Increased synthesis of two vasodilator prostaglandins—prostaglandin (PGE_2) and prostacyclin (PGI_2)—may explain the vasodilation and resistance to angiotensin II in normal pregnancy. In preeclampsia, the synthesis of PGI_2 decreases while sensitivity to angiotensin II increases, and the balance that normally exists between the platelet-aggregative and vasoconstrictor effects of thromboxane A_2 (produced by platelets) and the counteracting antiaggregative and vasodilating effects of PGI_2 (produced by endothelial cells) may be lost, contributing to hypertension and platelet aggregation. The incidence of preeclampsia may be reduced in high-risk women when low-dose aspirin (an inhibitor of thromboxane A_2 synthesis) is administered throughout pregnancy. However, no benefit from low-dose aspirin therapy has been demonstrated in low-risk women.

℞ **TREATMENT**

Once preeclampsia is diagnosed, hospitalization is indicated, since the disease can progress rapidly to multisystem involvement, including eclampsia, characterized by convulsions. The definitive treatment of preeclampsia and eclampsia is delivery of the conceptus, which should be carried out promptly if fetal size and maturity are adequate. If the fetus is immature, bed rest, restriction of sodium intake to 2 g/d or less, and antihypertensive therapy may be attempted. However, if clinical deterioration occurs in the mother or fetus despite these measures, the fetus should be delivered regardless of gestational age. Beta blockers, calcium antagonists, hydralazine, and central sympathetic antagonists are all useful agents. Angiotensin converting enzyme (ACE) inhibitors are *contraindicated in pregnancy* since they increase the risk for fetal loss.

If an immediate reduction in blood pressure is needed, as in other forms of severe, uncontrolled hypertension (Chap. 246), several agents are useful. These include intravenous hydralazine (10 mg every 15 min until the desired effect is maintained); 500 mg α-methyldopa given over 30 min; and labetalol (1 mg/kg given intravenously, followed by a continuous infusion of 20 mg/h). Intravenous magnesium sulfate is an anticonvulsant and vasodilator that increases the synthesis of PGI_2 by endothelial cells and is used to prevent the development or recurrence of eclampsia. Recently, magnesium sulfate has been shown to be superior to phenytoin or diazepam in this regard.

CHRONIC ESSENTIAL HYPERTENSION (Chap. 246) Like normal women, those with chronic essential hypertension experience a reduction in peripheral resistance during pregnancy. Indeed, a "normal" blood pressure may be obtained for the first time during pregnancy. Women with chronic hypertension are at higher risk for preeclampsia. Careful monitoring for proteinuria and of serum levels of creatinine and uric acid are important in detecting the onset of this complication. There is no evidence that pregnancy has an adverse effect on the course of chronic essential hypertension. Thus, antihypertensive medication (other than ACE inhibitors) should be continued throughout pregnancy in women with essential hypertension. α-Methyldopa has been used extensively in pregnancy, and children born to mothers who have taken this drug throughout pregnancy develop normally.

GESTATIONAL HYPERTENSION Hypertension that develops late in pregnancy (with no end-organ manifestations characteristic of preeclampsia) and disappears after delivery is termed *gestational hypertension*. Usually, women with this condition are overweight; others have a family history of hypertension, develop chronic essential hypertension later in life, and have a high incidence of recurrence during subsequent pregnancies. Attention must be directed toward detecting increases in urinary protein and serum levels of uric acid, creatinine, or BUN, since these remain normal in gestational hypertension and become elevated in preeclampsia. A beta blocker or α-methyldopa are usually effective in lowering blood pressure.

RENAL DISEASE

The increase in GFR during normal pregnancy is due to a rise in renal plasma flow without a concomitant elevation in glomerular pressure. However, in renal disease, any rise in GFR depends on an elevation in glomerular pressure, which can increase proteinuria and worsen the underlying disease. Hypertension becomes more severe during pregnancy in most women with chronic renal disease, and proteinuria increases in approximately 20 percent. Since autoregulation of renal blood flow may be impaired in renal disease, any increase in blood pressure is more apt to raise glomerular pressure. The development or worsening of hypertension during pregnancy in patients with renal disease may be due to preeclampsia superimposed on renal disease.

It is desirable to maintain blood pressure below 120/80 mmHg in pregnant women with chronic renal disease. The 24-h urine protein excretion should be assessed throughout pregnancy, and an increase in proteinuria with no clinical evidence of toxemia usually reflects elevated glomerular pressure. Antihypertensive drugs other than ACE inhibitors should be used.

Many women have had successful pregnancies after renal transplantation. Although these patients receive chronic immunosuppressive therapy throughout gestation, the incidence of congenital malformations does not appear to be increased.

If systemic lupus erythematosus (SLE) (Chap. 312) is quiescent for 12 to 18 months prior to conception, pregnancy does not appear to activate the disease. In nonpregnant women, flare-ups of lupus nephropathy are usually associated with extrarenal manifestations of the disease, i.e., arthritis, rash, and fever, accompanied by a reduction in serum complement and a rise in anti-DNA antibodies. In contrast, pregnant women with SLE may manifest an increase in blood pressure and proteinuria along with a reduction in renal function in the absence of extrarenal manifestations. The renal exacerbations may be due to superimposed preeclampsia or to the effect of hypertension on the nephropathy, since there is no clinical evidence of lupus activity and no increase in anti-DNA antibodies. This is an important distinction, because these women may be treated inappropriately with higher doses of glucocorticoids or immunosuppressive agents (which may exacerbate hypertension) when antihypertensive therapy or delivery (depending on gestational age and maternal condition) is indicated instead. Conversely, women with active SLE who could be treated with glucocorticoids are often delivered inappropriately early for the mistaken diagnosis of preeclampsia.

CARDIAC DISEASE

As noted above, pregnancy is associated with a reduction in systemic vascular resistance. Normally, increases occur in blood volume, stroke volume, heart rate, and cardiac output; these changes often produce systolic (flow) murmurs and third heart sounds. The rise in cardiac output exceeds the increase in oxygen consumption, so the arteriovenous oxygen difference falls. Marked fluctuations in cardiac output occur during normal labor and delivery, and the following four cardiac disorders are adversely affected by pregnancy: (1) valvular heart disease; (2) primary pulmonary hypertension; (3) the Eisenmenger syndrome; and (4) the Marfan syndrome. Delivery or pregnancy termination appear to be the times of greatest risk for these patients.

VALVULAR HEART DISEASE (See Chap. 237) The increased cardiac output associated with pregnancy may cause deterioration in women with *mitral stenosis*. If severe mitral stenosis is identified *prior* to pregnancy, valvulotomy should be carried out before conception, if possible. Asymptomatic pregnant women with mitral stenosis require close observation but not definitive therapy. However, if symptoms of pulmonary congestion develop, diuretics and restriction of activity are indicated. Atrial fibrillation should be treated with oral digoxin and/or a beta blocker to slow the ventricular rate. The latter type of agent may also be useful in patients with sinus rhythm and relatively rapid heart rates (>80 beats per minute). Thromboembolism associated with mitral stenosis necessitates anticoagulation with intravenous heparin; warfarin is *contraindicated* in pregnancy because of its teratogenic effects. A closed mitral valvulotomy (surgical or, preferably, by balloon mitral valvuloplasty) can be carried out during pregnancy when symptoms of mitral stenosis are severe; open-heart surgery is associated with an increase in fetal loss.

Mitral regurgitation is usually well tolerated during pregnancy, presumably because peripheral resistance is lower. Critical *aortic stenosis* is a contraindication for pregnancy until the lesion has been corrected. A maternal mortality rate of 15 percent has been reported in women with critical aortic stenosis.

Balloon flotation (Swan-Ganz) catheters allow precise hemodynamic assessment and control during labor and delivery and in the immediate postpartum period.

Artificial heart valves in pregnant women are associated with many problems. It is mandatory to continue full anticoagulation in patients with mechanical valvular prostheses. Warfarin is contraindicated because of its teratogenic effects; subcutaneous heparin is preferable but may cause bleeding and fetal loss. Tissue valves are less thrombogenic, but their limited durability in young adults is a serious disadvantage. Therefore, in women with serious valvular heart disease, every effort should be made to allow pregnancy to go to completion prior to valve replacement, and subsequent pregnancies should be avoided once a mechanical valve has been implanted.

In women with prosthetic valves, antibiotic prophylaxis with agents effective against genitourinary organisms is mandatory during the peripartum period.

PULMONARY HYPERTENSION AND EISENMENGER SYNDROME (See Chaps. 260 and 235) Pulmonary hypertension of all causes is a strong contraindication for pregnancy. If moderate or severe pulmonary hypertension (systolic pulmonary artery pressure >45 mmHg) is detected during the first trimester, termination of the pregnancy is advisable. In women with congenital heart disease, pulmonary hypertension, and a right-to-left shunt—i.e., the Eisenmenger syndrome, both maternal and fetal mortality are high, the latter increasing with the severity of maternal cyanosis. Bed rest may be required in severe cases. Systemic hypotension increases the right-to-left shunt in such patients and must be avoided.

MARFAN SYNDROME (See Chap. 348) Cardiovascular manifestations of the Marfan syndrome include mitral valve prolapse, mitral and aortic valve abnormalities, and aortic regurgitation due to enlargement of the aortic root. When the aortic root diameter as measured by echocardiography exceeds 40 mm, the risk of aortic dissection and rupture during pregnancy is increased. Women with the Marfan syndrome, especially those with a dilated aortic root, should avoid pregnancy; however, if such women become pregnant and refuse abortion, beta-adrenoceptor blocker therapy should be instituted to reduce the force of myocardial contraction and the resultant shear stress on the aorta.

OTHER FORMS OF CARDIAC DISEASE In the absence of pulmonary hypertension, atrial septal defect (p. 1303) is well tolerated by pregnant women, although the risk of fetal loss is increased. Patients with ventricular septal defect (p. 1304) without pulmonary hypertension also tolerate pregnancy well, but this lesion may be complicated by infective endocarditis, so antibiotic prophylaxis at the time of delivery is mandatory. Mitral valve prolapse (p. 1316), which is common among pregnant women, does not appear to complicate the pregnancy, nor does pregnancy complicate prolapse, although antibiotic prophylaxis is warranted. Women with hypertrophic cardiomyopathy (p. 1330) generally tolerate pregnancy well; indeed, the gestational hypervolemia may be associated with a reduction of the intraventricular pressure gradient and thus ameliorate symptoms. Because of its poor prognosis, chronic dilated cardiomyopathy (p. 1328) accompanied by heart failure is a contraindication to pregnancy.

Peripartum cardiomyopathy, a form of acute dilated cardiomyopathy that may be associated with a myocarditis, appears around the time of delivery (most frequently during the first 6 weeks postpartum), is sometimes associated with preeclampsia, and may actually be caused by pregnancy (p. 1330). Infant mortality is high if congestive heart failure ensues, and maternal mortality may be as high as 30 percent within the first few months. Treatment should include bed rest, digitalis, diuretics, and a vasodilator (other than an ACE inhibitor). About one-third of patients show functional recovery, but one-third have persistent severely impaired left ventricular function. Subsequent pregnancies should be avoided, since peripartum cardiomyopathy may recur.

Premature atrial or ventricular systoles occurring during pregnancy can be treated by the elimination of stimulants, avoidance of excessive fatigue, and reassurance. Drug therapy should be avoided, if possible, but cardioversion has been used safely for tachyarrhythmias during pregnancy.

PULMONARY EMBOLISM (See also Chap. 261)

In pregnancy, the levels of all of the coagulation factors (except factors XI and XIII) are increased, and the level of antithrombin III, a major inhibitor of coagulation, is reduced. Pulmonary embolism occurs about once per 750 pregnancies. Because of the immediate need to prevent embolism and the other long-term complications of deep vein thrombosis (DVT), it is important to recognize the latter condition. DVT may occur during pregnancy owing to compression of the iliac veins by the enlarged uterus as well as to changes in the coagulation and fibrinolytic systems that favor thrombosis. DVT also occurs at an increased incidence in the postpartum period. Impedance plethysmography and Doppler ultrasonography are noninvasive, nonradiologic techniques useful in documenting DVT. When pulmonary embolism is suspected, perfusion lung scanning can be accomplished with smaller quantities of isotope, and pulmonary angiography can be carried out if the abdomen is shielded. Despite the potential small hazard of fetal irradiation posed by the latter procedures, it is extremely important to diagnose pulmonary embolism.

℞ TREATMENT

Anticoagulant therapy is indicated in pregnant women with DVT, to prevent pulmonary embolism. Heparin, which does not cross the placenta, can be administered at a dose of 1000 U/h by continuous infusion until early during labor. Protamine can then be used to reverse the drug's effects, and heparin can be restarted within 2 h of delivery and continued for 3 to 4 days, after which subcutaneous heparin or oral warfarin therapy may be instituted for 6 months. When venous thrombosis or pulmonary embolism occurs in the early postpartum period, heparin treatment should be instituted for 7 to 10 days, followed by warfarin for about 3 months.

DIABETES MELLITUS (See also Chap. 334)

In pregnancy, there are two major opposing metabolic states: accelerated starvation and insulin resistance. Blood sugar and amino acids are low, while plasma free fatty acids, ketones, and triglycerides are increased. After an overnight fast, plasma glucose is lower by 0.8 to 1.1 mmol/L (15 to 20 mg/dL) than in nonpregnant women; when fasting lasts longer than 12 h, plasma glucose may fall to 2.2 to 2.5 mmol/L (40 to 45 mg/dL), while plasma hydroxybutyrate and acetoacetate rise to levels two to four times higher than in nonpregnant women. As a consequence, ketoacidosis develops in the absence of striking hyperglycemia in pregnant diabetics. Maternal insulin and glucagon do not cross the placenta, but acetoacetate and β-hydroxybutyrate cross readily and are oxidized by the fetal brain and liver.

In spite of the fetal demand for glucose, pregnancy is also a diabetogenic state by virtue of the development of insulin resistance. Elevation of several hormones in pregnancy may be responsible for insulin resistance, including progesterone, estrogen, prolactin, and human placental lactogen.

PREGNANCY IN INSULIN-DEPENDENT AND NON-INSULIN DEPENDENT DIABETES MELLITUS Pregnancy in diabetics is associated with a higher perinatal mortality (3 to 5 percent, vs. 1 to 2 percent in nondiabetic women) and a higher incidence of congenital anomalies (6 to 12 percent, vs. 2 to 3 percent in nondiabetics). Therapeutic control of blood glucose, particularly during organogenesis, reduces the incidence of congenital anomalies. Counseling should emphasize the importance of home monitoring of glucose levels and the need to adjust the insulin dose to maintain fasting blood sugar at a normal level and postprandial glucose no higher than 7.8 mmol/L (140 mg/dL), both prior to conception and throughout pregnancy. Glycosylated hemoglobin should also be monitored during pregnancy. Ultrasound evaluation of the fetus should be carried out during the second trimester, and alpha-fetoprotein levels should be assessed in the 20th week to detect neural tube defects.

Women with diabetic nephropathy have an excellent chance of a normal pregnancy, the rate of perinatal survival being approximately 90 percent. As with other renal diseases, hypertension can worsen late in pregnancy, with an increase in proteinuria and a decrease in creatinine clearance that represent either superimposed preeclampsia or a rise in glomerular pressure. There is no evidence that pregnancy worsens diabetic nephropathy, but care of pregnant women with diabetic nephropathy requires management by obstetricians skilled in high-risk pregnancies and by neonatologists, diabetologists, and nephrologists. Hypertension should be treated as described earlier in this chapter.

GESTATIONAL DIABETES The insulin resistance of normal pregnancy may also contribute to gestational diabetes in women in whom the capacity for insulin secretion is not sufficient to meet the increased insulin demands of pregnancy. The overall prevalence of gestational diabetes is between 1 and 3 percent. An important reason for recognizing the disorder early is that, because glucose crosses the placenta, the condition results in excessive fetal insulin secretion, which in turn can cause fetal macrosomia and increase the risk of birth trauma, need for cesarean section, and neonatal hypoglycemia.

There are no universally accepted criteria for the diagnosis or screening for gestational diabetes if the fasting glucose is normal. Some obstetricians recommend "universal" screening of all pregnant women with normal fasting blood sugar levels between the 24th and 28th weeks of gestation using a 50-g oral glucose load. If the 1-h glucose level exceeds 7.8 mmol/L (140 m/dL), a 100-g oral glucose test is performed after an overnight fast. A diagnosis of gestational diabetes is made if any two of the following values are reached: 1 h, >10.5 mmol/L (>190 ng/dL); 2 h, >9.2 mmol/L (>165 ng/dL); 3 h, >8.0 mmol/L (>145 ng/dL). In contrast, the American College of Obstetricians and Gynecologists recommends screening only for women at high risk, namely women over age 30; women with previous macrosomic, malformed, or stillborn infants; and those with obesity, hypertension, or glycosuria.

℞ TREATMENT

Gestational diabetes is treated first with dietary measures. If the fasting or postprandial glucose level remains elevated, insulin therapy should be started. Following delivery, carbohydrate tolerance may return to normal, but 30 percent or more of women with gestational diabetes develop diabetes mellitus within 5 years of the pregnancy.

THYROID DISEASE (See also Chap. 331)

The diagnosis of thyroid disease in pregnancy is complicated by the increases in thyroid size, radioactive iodine uptake, basal metabolic rate, and thyroxine-binding globulin level during normal pregnancy. Plasma T_3 and T_4 levels are elevated, but levels of free T_3, T_4, and thyroid-stimulating hormone (TSH) usually remain normal, while the T_3 resin uptake value is in the hypothyroid range. Maternal thyrotoxicosis occurs about once per 500 pregnancies, and the diagnosis may be difficult because the increase in cardiac output, tachycardia, skin warmth, and heat intolerance that are typical of pregnancy can mimic hyperthyroidism. Values of T_4 concentration above 154 mmol/L (12 μg/dL) with a resin T_3 uptake in the euthyroid range (25 to 35 percent) suggests hyperthyroidism in a pregnant woman. Pregnant women can tolerate mild degrees of hyperthyroidism without difficulty, and thyrotoxicosis does not increase fetal loss. Although hyperthyroidism may worsen in the first trimester, it is often more easily controlled in the third trimester. The treatment of gestational thyrotoxicosis involves a choice between antithyroid drugs and ablative surgery. Propylthiouracil is the drug of choice, since methimazole has been associated with aplasia cutis in the fetus. The goal should be to maintain the maternal T_4 concentration in the upper part of the normal range, because at that level fetal thyroid function is normal. The lowest possible dose of propylthiouracil should be used, because the drug crosses the placenta and inhibits fetal synthesis of thyroxine. If the mother is overtreated, fetal goiter occasionally develops owing to stimulation of fetal TSH. When surgery is planned for the treatment of thyrotoxicosis, propylthiouracil should be administered preoperatively to control the hyperthyroid state.

TREATMENT

Hypothyroidism during pregnancy should be treated with hormone replacement, with the knowledge that the dose requirement may increase. The increase in dose requirement has been shown to occur as early as 8 weeks of gestation. The reason for this increased requirement is unclear and may involve the increase in concentration of binding proteins, transplacental transfer of T_4, or placental metabolism of T_4.

DISORDERS OF CALCIUM METABOLISM (See also Chap. 354)

Although the serum calcium level normally falls in pregnancy because of the decrease in serum albumin, the concentration of ionized calcium remains unchanged. Earlier studies of parathyroid hormone (PTH) levels, which used assays that measure PTH fragments, suggested that PTH levels increase during pregnancy with no change in phosphate clearance. However, more recent studies using assays that measure intact PTH have demonstrated a fall in PTH levels in pregnancy. Urinary calcium excretion is approximately 7.5 mmol/d (300 mg/d), compared with 2.5 mmol/d (100 mg/d) in nonpregnant women, and urinary calculi develop in about one of 2000 pregnant women. It may be that the increase in 1,25-dihydroxyvitamin D (which has a placental contribution) is the primary event leading to increased calcium absorption, a fall in PTH, and hypercalciuria. When hyperparathyroidism with hypercalcemia occurs during pregnancy, the neonate may exhibit tetany because of the suppression of fetal PTH secretion.

HEMATOLOGIC DISORDERS

During pregnancy, plasma volume increases more than does red cell mass, so that a fall in hemoglobin concentration of 10 to 20 g/L (1 to 2 g/dL) is usual. Two potential causes of anemia during pregnancy are deficiencies of iron or folate. Since the developing fetus uses these substances in large amounts, these deficiencies may be prevented by providing iron and folate supplements. Pregnancy also results in a leukocytosis that can sometimes reach 18,000 μL.

Sickle cell anemia (Chap. 107) may be complicated by pregnancy, and vasoocclusive crises become more frequent, particularly during labor and the postpartum period. The risks of spontaneous abortion, prematurity, and neonatal death are high.

Thrombocytopenia in pregnancy is most often due to preeclampsia, although sepsis and idiopathic thrombocytopenic purpura may also be responsible. In the last-named condition, antiplatelet antibodies cross the placenta and can cause thrombocytopenia in the fetus as well. Cesarean section is indicated if the fetal platelet count obtained by percutaneous umbilical cord sampling performed at 36 to 37 weeks is less than 50,000/ml.

Stillbirth, often associated with placental venous thrombosis, occurs in women with the so-called lupus anticoagulant (Chap. 312), an immunoglobulin that binds to negatively charged phospholipids and interferes with vitamin K–dependent coagulation factors. The lupus anticoagulant is actually more apt to cause thrombosis than bleeding, and treatment with low-dose aspirin and prednisone throughout pregnancy may reduce the rate of fetal loss.

Disseminated intravascular coagulation may occur as a result of abruptio placentae, a retained dead fetus, amniotic fluid embolism, saline-induced abortion, or fulminant preeclampsia and can be cured by treating the underlying cause.

GASTROINTESTINAL AND LIVER DISEASES

Nausea and vomiting occur in approximately 90 percent of women between the 6th and 16th weeks of pregnancy. When severe, the problem can be treated with oral dimenhydrinate, 50 to 100 mg every 4 h, or D-oxylamine, 12.5 mg every 4 h. In its severe form, *hyperemesis gravidarum* can cause dehydration that requires parenteral feeding. Heartburn, which may be due to relaxation of the lower esophageal sphincter, is usually responsive to treatment with antacids and H_2 receptor blocking agents.

Pregnancy in women with inflammatory bowel disease may be uncomplicated, but it is difficult to anticipate the course in advance. Most patients do well, but in some the pregnancy may exacerbate the disease; rarely the pregnancy may need to be terminated. If the disease is active at the time of conception, the incidence of spontaneous abortion is higher than in normal pregnancy.

Although pregnancy is associated with supersaturation of the bile with cholesterol, the incidence of cholelithiasis in a first pregnancy does not appear to be increased. However, the risk for this complication increases with multiparity. The serum triglyceride and cholesterol levels are elevated during pregnancy; although serum bilirubin remains normal, there is a striking rise in the level of alkaline phosphatase (which originates from the placenta); this level may reach a peak two to four times normal at term.

Although total serum protein concentration declines by approximately 20 percent in midpregnancy because of a decrease in albumin, hepatic synthesis of other plasma proteins increases. In a normal pregnancy, the serum levels of γ-glutamyl transpeptidase and LDH are increased, whereas serum levels of aminotransferases and aspartate aminotransferase are normal.

Intrahepatic cholestasis of pregnancy usually appears in the third trimester and is manifested by pruritus, with bilirubin levels usually less than 100 μmol/L (6 mg/dL). Although bilirubin levels usually remain in the range of 34 to 86 μmol/L (2 to 5 mg/dL), there is a striking increase in the alkaline phosphatase level. The cholestasis and pruritus disappear promptly after delivery, but the syndrome may recur with subsequent pregnancies. Aside from pruritus, the mother does not suffer any adverse effect. However, there appears to be an increase in stillbirths, which is thought to be secondary to the toxicity of bile acids to the fetus. Therefore, fetal surveillance should be carried out once the diagnosis of intrahepatic cholestasis of pregnancy is established. Treatment of pruritus consists of antihistamines and of cholestyramine, 4 g four times a day.

Acute fatty liver of pregnancy, with histologic changes showing hepatocytes with increased microvesicular fat and fibrin deposits in the hepatic sinusoids, may occur late in pregnancy and may be associated with preeclampsia. The serum bilirubin level may exceed 170 μmol/L (10 mg/dL), and the levels of aspartate aminotransferase and alanine aminotransferase are in the range of 5 to 8 μkat/L (300 to 500 U/L). Prothrombin time may be prolonged, and disseminated intravascular coagulation may cause depressed fibrinogen levels, an increase in fibrin degradation products, and thrombocytopenia. Maternal deaths may occur, but this condition usually ameliorates following delivery.

Hepatitis B (Chap. 295) during pregnancy increases the rates of prematurity and fetal death, with a high risk of transmission to the infant, particularly in mothers who are positive for the HBe antigen at the time of delivery. Women who are positive for the HBs antigen and negative for the HBe antigen transmit the disease less frequently. Approximately 5 to 10 percent of infants infected with hepatitis B acquire the disease by the transplacental route. Infants born to mothers with hepatitis B should be treated with both hepatitis B immune globulin and hepatitis B vaccine.

The severity of viral hepatitis A is not altered by pregnancy, and the risk of transmission to the neonate is small.

INFECTIONS

Infectious diseases constitute a serious risk to both the pregnant woman and the fetus.

BACTERIAL INFECTIONS Urinary tract infections (see Chap. 131) are the most common type of bacterial infection in pregnancy. Asymptomatic bacteriuria occurs in up to 7 percent of pregnancies. Physiologic changes in pregnancy, such as hormone-induced dilation of the urinary tract, hydroureter, and vesicoureteral reflux predispose to asymptomatic bacteriuria, and one-third of patients with these conditions develop pyelonephritis, usually during the last trimester. Most cases of pyelonephritis developing late in pregnancy were preceded by asymptomatic bacteriuria early in the pregnancy. Therefore, over 75 percent of cases of pregnancy-associated acute pyelonephritis can be avoided by treating asymptomatic bacteriuria, and screening for bacteriuria at the first prenatal visit is recommended. *Escherichia coli* is the most commonly isolated organism, and treatment of asymptomatic bacteriuria for 3 days with ampicillin, cephalexin, nitrofurantoin, or sulfisoxazole is appropriate, although the latter drug should not be used during the final month of gestation because it may cause jaundice in the infant. In women with asymptomatic bacteriuria, urine cultures should be obtained at monthly intervals for the remainder of the pregnancy. Relapse requires retreatment.

Intrauterine infection occurs in up to 4 percent of pregnancies and is associated with increased rates of morbidity and mortality in the prenatal period. Intraamniotic infection is most common when ascending infection follows rupture of the membranes, but it is also seen with intact membranes, especially in cases of preterm labor. Infection is usually polymicrobial, involving *E. coli* anaerobes, genital mycoplasmas, *Gardnerella vaginalis*, and group B streptococci. Since early clinical signs may be subtle, diagnosis requires a high degree of suspicion. Clinical clues include fever, maternal or fetal tachycardia, uterine tenderness, uncommonly foul-smelling amniotic fluid, and leukocytosis. In addition to the clinical findings, the diagnosis is based on the results of Gram's staining of amniotic fluid and on the glucose concentration and leukocyte esterase activity of amniotic fluid. Delivery of the fetus is indicated. Antibiotic therapy should begin during labor, rather than afterward. Antibiotics with broad coverage, such as ampicillin and gentamicin, are indicated.

Postpartum infections remain the most common cause of maternal mortality in the United States. Most of these deaths are related to postpartum endometrial infections complicated by pelvic abscess, peritonitis, or pelvic thrombophlebitis. Rates of endometritis vary from 1 to 3 percent after vaginal delivery and from 6 to 18 percent after cesarean section. Endometritis should be suspected when a patient has a fever developing 1 to 2 days after delivery. Rupture of the membranes and cesarean delivery following onset of labor are important risk factors for postpartum endometritis. Few patients exhibit all of the classical manifestations, such as fever, abdominal pain, malaise, and purulent or foul-smelling lochia. The workup should include a complete blood count, blood cultures, and a genital tract culture. Postpartum endometritis is usually a polymicrobial infection. The most common bacterial pathogens responsible for the condition are group B streptococci, mixed anaerobic and aerobic organisms, *E. coli*, and enterococci. Group B streptococci are the most frequent blood culture isolates in patients with endometritis. Treatment depends on the organism cultured, but broad-spectrum antibiotics or combinations such as ampicillin, an aminoglycoside, and clindamycin are usually used.

Group B *Streptococcus* (Chap. 143) has become a major cause of postpartum bacteremia, accounting for 10 to 20 percent of blood culture isolates from women admitted to obstetrical services. The source of these infections is group B streptococci colonizing the female genital tract. Although most of these patients have an uncomplicated course following appropriate antibiotic therapy, complications such as pelvic abscesses, septic shock, and septic thrombophlebitis are occasionally seen. Most severe group B *Streptococcus* infections in pregnancy are associated with an identifiable source, such as endometritis or a urinary tract infection. Group B streptococci may be transmitted to the neonate during the perinatal period. The attack rate of serious group B streptococcal infections in newborns is 1.8 per 1000 live births.

Listeria monocytogenes (see Chap. 145) is another bacterial pathogen that can produce specific pregnancy-related morbidity. Infection can occur at any time during pregnancy, but it is most common during the third trimester. Symptoms are frequently suggestive of a urinary tract infection, but urine cultures are sterile. Diagnosis is made by a positive blood culture. The infection can range in clinical severity from a mild febrile illness to severe illness. This infection can precipitate labor and result in premature birth of a dead or infected infant. Treatment should be with ampicillin or penicillin.

Neisseria gonorrhoeae (see Chap. 150) can be transmitted from mother to infant in utero, during delivery, or in the postpartum period. The most common clinical problem caused by this transmission is gonococcal conjunctivitis of the newborn. Conjunctival instillation of a 1% aqueous solution of silver nitrate is effective in preventing blindness caused by this infection. Congenital syphilis (see Chap. 174) occurs by infection of the fetus in utero. Transmission of *Treponema pallidum* to the fetus, which is most common in the early stages of syphilis, can occur at any time during pregnancy. Infection of the fetus before the fourth month is rare. Syphilis can have severe effects on the offspring, including stillbirth, neonatal disease, or latent infection.

VIRAL INFECTIONS These are of major concern during pregnancy because of the consequences to the fetus. Since transplacental transmission may occur, maternal infections with cytomegalovirus (CMV), rubella, varicella zoster, and herpes simplex virus have the greatest teratogenic potential, particularly during the first trimester. Perinatal infection can result from transmission of the virus to the infant during passage through an infected uterine cervix.

CMV (see Chap. 187) is the most common cause of congenital viral infection. The virus is ubiquitous; 35 to 100 percent of the adult population have evidence of prior infection, with the highest prevalence among lower socioeconomic groups. CMV is usually acquired by the oral-respiratory route, through sexual contact, or by blood transfusion. CMV infection establishes a lifelong latent infection in the host, which can be reactivated later by immunosuppression. Rates of cervical infection with CMV increase in later stages of pregnancy. Although during pregnancy CMV can be shed with no evidence of clinical disease in the mother, high numbers of CMV in the cervix suggest that the neonate is at risk during birth. Approximately 1 to 2 percent of all newborn infants in the United States are infected with CMV in utero, but the vast majority of these infants are normal. Clinically apparent congenital infections are most common in the first infant of mothers with primary infection during pregnancy. CMV disease occurs in infants whose mothers are not immune. Cytomegalic inclusion disease is characterized by jaundice, hepatosplenomegaly, a petechial rash, and multiple system and organ involvement. Other manifestations range from subtle neurologic sequelae to severe microcephaly.

Rubella (see Chap. 197) can have severe outcomes in the fetus, including fetal death and premature delivery, if the mother is infected during early pregnancy. A variety of congenital defects are caused by rubella, including cataracts, cardiac abnormalities, deafness, and mental retardation. Fetal abnormalities are greatest when maternal rubella occurs during the first trimester, with 80 percent of children affected; the percentage falls to about 25 percent when infection occurs at the end of the second trimester. Congenital infection can be diagnosed prenatally by detecting rubella IgM antibody in fetal blood obtained under ultrasound guidance. In places where immunization programs have been widely used, the problem has been eliminated. The vaccine can be administered during pregnancy without harm to the fetus. Infection during pregnancy with varicella zoster virus (VZV) represents a health risk to the mother (see Chap. 185). There is nearly a 10 percent risk for severe pneumonia. Antiviral therapy should be instituted early if there is any suspicion of chickenpox-related pneumonia. Although most infants born to VZV-infected mothers are normal, there is a risk to the unborn child of developing congenital teratogenic infection.

Infection of the newborn with herpes simplex virus (HSV) can range from mild localized infection to fatal dissemination (see Chap. 184). Retrograde infection or birth through a maternal genital tract infected with HSV-2 can result in serious disseminated neonatal infection.

OTHER INFECTIONS OF PREGNANCY *Vulvovaginal candidiasis* (see Chap. 207) is more common in pregnant than nonpregnant women. High estrogen levels apparently encourage growth of this organism. Infection rates increase as the gestational period progresses, with up to 55 percent of third-trimester women being colonized and with symptomatic disease developing in most of those colonized.

Toxoplasmosis (see Chap. 219) causes symptoms in only 10 to 20 percent of women infected during pregnancy. Unfortunately, the fetus is at risk whether or not the mother is symptomatic. Transmission to the fetus can occur transplacentally or at birth. One-third of infants born to mothers infected during pregnancy become infected. The risk for congenital infection is greater when maternal infection occurs during the third trimester than the first, although the risk of spontaneous abortion is highest when infection is acquired in the first trimester. Infected infants may have no symptoms at birth but may develop symptoms, particularly chorioretinitis, by adolescence. Less common manifestations include strabismus, epilepsy, and psychomotor retardation. Toxoplasmosis does not cause fetal malformation. Treatment of acutely infected pregnant women decreases the incidence and attenuates the severity of fetal infections.

HUMAN IMMUNODEFICIENCY VIRUS INFECTION

Approximately 80 percent of women with AIDS are of childbearing age. The incidence of infection with human immunodeficiency virus (HIV) will increase in women in the United States during the 1990s (see also Chap. 308). Worldwide, particularly in developing countries, HIV infection is spread mainly heterosexually, with the male-to-female ratio in certain countries approaching 1. Currently, most of the women in the United States who have AIDS are either intravenous drug users (IVDUs) or the heterosexual partners of IVDUs. The geographic distribution of HIV infection among women closely parallels that among IVDUs, with the highest incidence in the Northeast and Southeast seaboard states and Puerto Rico.

EFFECT OF HIV INFECTION ON PREGNANCY Although earlier studies suggested that HIV-positive women were at a higher risk of an unfavorable outcome of pregnancy, at present the accumulating evidence indicates that HIV infection alone does not impose a significant negative effect on pregnancy, particularly when the infection is in the asymptomatic stage. An acceleration of HIV disease during pregnancy is uncommon and may be due to other factors associated with confounding issues present in the women most likely to be infected, such as intravenous drug use and inadequate access to prenatal care.

Primary infection is generally associated with a burst of viremia with or without an acute HIV syndrome, the latter occurring in approximately 50 to 70 percent of individuals following initial infection. It is unclear what effect this burst of viremia has on the pregnancy itself; however, given the strong association between high levels of viremia and transmission of infection to the fetus, it is highly likely that primary infection of the mother during pregnancy increases the chances of transmission of HIV to the fetus.

TRANSMISSION OF HIV TO THE FETUS/INFANT The rate of transmission of HIV from mother to fetus/infant averages approximately 30 percent, ranging from 13 percent in a European collaborative study to 45 percent in Central Africa (see Chap. 308). Higher rates of transmission have been associated with the symptomatic stage in the mother with high levels of plasma viremia in the mother, and with low maternal CD4+ T lymphocyte counts. Although infection of the fetus can occur throughout pregnancy, transmission is thought to occur most often during the perinatal period. Nonetheless, caesarean sections are not currently recommended unless there are other, obstetrical reasons for performing one. Postnatal transmission from mother to infant has been documented, and colostrum and breast milk have been clearly implicated.

In developed countries where other forms of nutrition are available to the infant, breast feeding by an infected mother is absolutely contraindicated.

 TREATMENT

In HIV-infected pregnant women, administration of zidovudine to the mother before and during delivery and to the newborn for 6 weeks reduced the risk of maternal-infant HIV transmission by approximately 66 percent.

NEOPLASTIC DISEASES

Transmission of leukemia or lymphoma to the fetus has not been reported, and there is no clear evidence that pregnancy adversely affects the course of any type of malignancy; however, it is possible that the high estrogen levels of pregnancy accelerate the course of breast cancer.

Deciding whether a pregnancy should be terminated in a woman with a neoplastic disease requires judgment about whether the pregnant state presents a significant obstacle to effective therapy and whether the fetus will be harmed as a result of such therapy. Although most antineoplastic agents are potentially teratogenic or cause fetal wastage, many healthy full-term infants have been born despite active maternal chemotherapy at the time of conception or during the first trimester. Thus, while it would be safer to avoid fetal exposure, the decision to terminate a pregnancy must take into account the parents' desire to have a child. Pregnant women with leukemia who are given the usual chemotherapy for this condition have done surprisingly well; in some studies, the maternal survival rate has been 100 percent, and the incidence of congenital abnormalities in the newborn is less than 10 percent.

BIBLIOGRAPHY

BRIGGS GG et al: *Drugs in Pregnancy and Lactation*, 3d ed. Baltimore, Williams & Wilkins, 1990

BURROW GN, FERRIS TF: *Medical Complications During Pregnancy*, 4th ed. Philadelphia, Saunders, 1994

CLASP (COLLABORATIVE LOW-DOSE ASPIRIN STUDY IN PREGNANCY) COLLABORATIVE GROUP: CLASP: A randomised trial of low-dose aspirin for the prevention and treatment of pre-eclampsia among 9364 pregnant women. Lancet 343:619, 1994

CONNOR EM et al: Reduction of maternal-infant transmission of HIV type 1 with zidovudine treatment. N Engl J Med 331:1173, 1994

LUCAS MJ et al: A comparison of magnesium sulfate with phenytoin for the prevention of eclampsia. N Engl J Med 333:201, 1995

MANDEL SJ et al: Increased need for thyroxine during pregnancy in women with primary hypothyroidism. N Engl J Med 323:91, 1990

8

Charles E. Irwin, Jr., Mary-Ann Shafer

ADOLESCENT HEALTH PROBLEMS

———— *Approach to the Patient* ————

Adolescence is the period between childhood and adulthood. This period is usually defined by the rapid onset of biological and psychological growth and development prior to or at the second decade of life and ending before age 20. Major social and environmental factors influence the onset, duration, and completion of adolescence. Over the next decade, the numbers of adolescents will increase, adolescents will include more ethnic and racial minorities than the general population, and the adolescent population will become more impoverished, thereby decreasing their access to health care. Currently, the adolescent population in the United States is the group least likely to have health insurance. Physicians need a careful understanding of the biological and psychosocial changes of adolescence, the associated environmental

Table 8-1

CHAPTER 8
Adolescent Health Problems

31

Sexual Maturity Ratings for Females

A Pubertal development in size of female breasts
Stage 1: Prepubertal. Elevation of the papilla only.
Stage 2: Breast bud stage. A small mound of breast tissue causes
elevation of the breast contour and papilla. Areolar diameter enlarges.
Stage 3: Further enlargement of breast and areola with no separation of
their contours.
Stage 4: Projection of the areola and papilla to form a secondary mound
above the level of the breast.
Stage 5: Adult. The breasts resemble those of a mature female. The
areola has recessed to become contiguous with the contour of the breast.

B Pubertal development of female pubic hair
Stage 1: Prepubertal. There is no pubic hair.
Stage 2: Sparse growth of long, slightly pigmented, downy hair, straight
or only slightly curled, primarily along the labia majora.
Stage 3: The hair becomes darker, coarser, and more curled and spreads
sparsely over the junction of the pubes.
Stage 4: The hair, now adult in type, covers a smaller area than in the
adult and does not extend onto the medial surface of the thighs.
Stage 5: Adult. The hair is adult in quantity and type, with extension
onto the thighs.

SOURCE: Modified from van Wieringen JC et al: *Growth Diagrams*. Gronigen, Neth.,
Woplter-Noorhoff Publishing, 1971.

changes, and the legal and ethical issues that affect the provision of
health care services to adolescents.

Biological Maturation PUBERTY *(See also Chaps. 336 and
337)* Puberty is defined as the sequential biological processes that
ultimately lead to reproductive capacity. The onset and tempo of
puberty vary by sex, population group, and individual. During puberty,
major alterations in the hormonal regulatory systems in the central
nervous system, gonads, and adrenals cause changes in skeletal growth
and body composition and the acquisition of secondary sexual characteristics. The mechanisms responsible for the initiation of puberty
through activation of the hypothalamic-pituitary-gonadal axis remain undefined.

The sexual maturity ratings (SMRs) of Marshall and Tanner are
helpful in monitoring the development of secondary sexual characteristics of pubertal maturation, which are the somatic manifestations of
adrenal and gonadal activity. These ratings correlate more closely with
bone age than chronologic age. The SMRs for girls are based upon
breast and pubic hair development, each in five stages (Table 8-1).

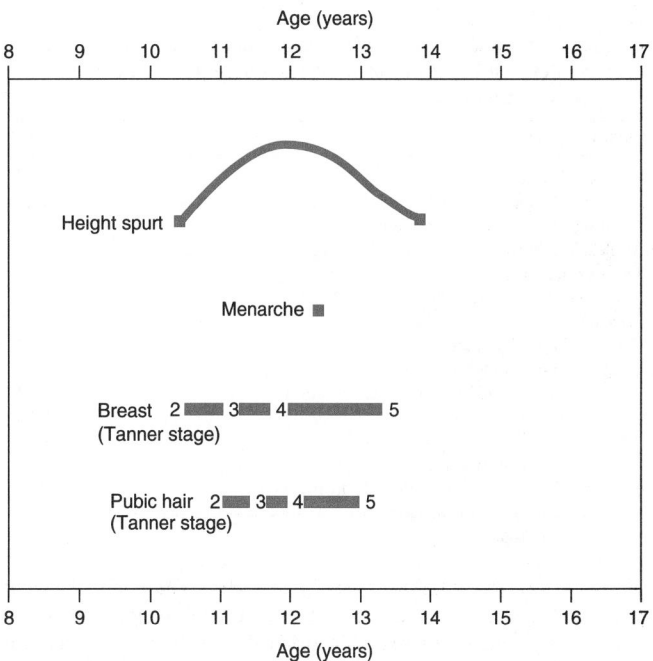

FIGURE 8-1 Pubertal events in females.

The ratings for boys are based upon genital and pubic hair development
(Table 8-2).

The mean age of onset of puberty for girls as defined by breast
budding is 11.2 ± 1.6 years, and the mean age of onset for boys as
defined by enlargement of testes is 11.6 ± 1.1 years. The mean age
of menarche in the United States is 13.3 ± 1.3 years, and the mean
age for spermarche is between 13.5 and 14.5 years. The average
duration of puberty for girls is 4 years, with a range of 1.5 to 8 years,
and for boys is 3 years, with a range of 2 to 5 years. Even though
the timing and duration of the events vary, each adolescent follows
an orderly sequence in somatic growth and development (Figs. 8-1
and 8-2). Monitoring these events by history and physical examination
is helpful in identifying disorders that become manifest during adolescence (Table 8-3).

Table 8-2

Sexual Maturity Ratings for Males

A Pubertal development in size of male genitalia
Stage 1: Prepubertal. Penis, testes, and scrotum are of childhood size.
Stage 2: The scrotum and testes enlarge with testicular measurement
greater than 2.5 cm in length (testicular volume, 4–7 mL). Penis usually
shows no growth. Scrotal skin reddens or darkens.
Stage 3: Further growth of testes (testicular volume, 8–10 mL) and
scrotum with enlargement of penis, mainly in length.
Stage 4: Continued growth of the testes (testicular volume, 10–15 mL)
and scrotum with increased size of the penis, especially in breadth.
Stage 5: Adult. The genitalia are adult in size (testicular volume, 20–25
mL) and shape.

B Pubertal development of male pubic hair
Stage 1: Prepubertal. Pubic hair is absent.
Stage 2: Sparse growth of long, slightly pigmented, downy hair, straight
or only slightly curled, primarily at the base of the penis.
Stage 3: The hair is considerably darker, coarser, and more curled. The
hair spreads sparsely over the junction of the pubes.
Stage 4: The hair, now adult in type, covers a smaller area than in the
adult and does not extend onto the medial surface of the thighs.
Stage 5: Adult. The hair is adult in quantity and type, with extension
onto the thighs.

SOURCE: Modified from van Wieringen JC et al: *Growth Diagrams*. Gronigen, Neth.
Woplter-Noorhoff Publishing, 1971.

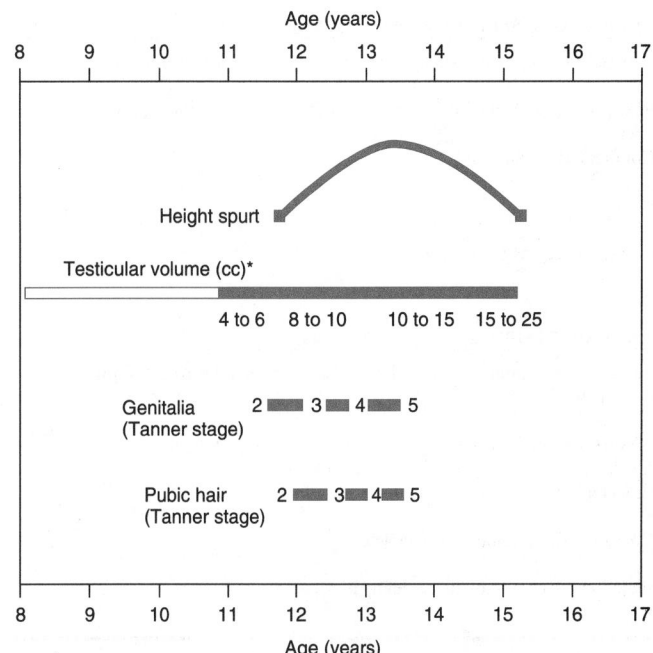

FIGURE 8-2 Pubertal events in males.

Table 8-3

Relation Between Development of Features of Maturation and Sexual Maturity Ratings (SMR)

Clinical Feature	SMR
Hematocrit rise (male)	2–5
Alkaline phosphatase peak (male)	3
Alkaline phosphatase peak (female)	2
Adolescent hormonal levels (rise in estrogen for females, testosterone for males)	2–5
Peak height velocity (male)	3–4
Peak height velocity (female)	2–3
Usual timing of menarche	3–4
Slipped capital femoral epiphysis	2–3
Acute worsening of idiopathic adolescent scoliosis	2–4
Osgood-Schlatter disease	3
Appearance of "normal" gynecomastia	2–3
Usual appearance of acne vulgaris	2–3
Increased levels of serum uric acid in males	2–5

SOURCE: After Daniel.

SKELETAL GROWTH (See also Chap. 329) The pubertal height spurt accounts for about 25 percent of final adult height and begins at an average age of 12 years for girls (SMR 2–3) and 14 years for boys (SMR 3–4). During this spurt, females gain 9.0 ± 1.03 cm/year and reach a final mean adult height of 163 cm at 16 years; males gain 10.3 ± 1.54 cm/year and reach a final mean adult height of 177 cm at 18 years. Assessment of skeletal growth during adolescence should be done through a height velocity curve with consideration of the sexual maturity rating. Bone age can be determined through the utilization of hand roentgenograms.

CHANGES IN BODY COMPOSITION Weight gain during the growth spurt accounts for 40 percent of ideal body weight. Lean body mass increases in boys from 80 to 90 percent and decreases in girls from 80 to 75 percent. In boys mean body fat increases from 4.3 to 11.2 percent by late puberty and is distributed primarily in the truncal area. In girls, mean body fat increases from 15.7 to 26.7 percent and is deposited in the pelvic, breast, upper back, and arm areas. Shortly after the growth spurt is completed, muscle mass peaks and is greater in boys than in girls.

CARDIORESPIRATORY CHANGES At puberty stroke volume, cardiac output, and blood pressure increase, and heart rate decreases. The lungs increase in size. The male larynx, under the influence of androgens, develops an acute 90-degree angle in the anterior thyroid cartilage; male vocal cords are three times the length of those in females. These changes account for the deepening of the voice.

Psychological Development Adolescence is often viewed as a tumultuous period (Table 8-4). However, most adolescents pass through puberty without disruption in their lives. The clinician must assess whether psychosocial development of the adolescent is normal. Adolescence involves a series of changes, which, if mastered, allow normal function as an adult. These changes include separation from the family, maturation of sexual identity, planning for education and career, and development of the capacity for intimacy. Adolescents also undergo cognitive changes with behavioral and social sequelae. The functional and cognitive changes do not necessarily correlate with physical maturation. The early adolescent (ages 10 to 13) tends to focus on the physical changes in his or her body and may have concerns about the maturation process.

Table 8-4

Biopsychosocial Development During Adolescence

Characteristics	Impact
EARLY ADOLESCENCE (Age 10 to 13 Years)	
Onset of puberty, becomes concerned with developing body	Major questions concerning normality of physical maturation; often concerned about the stages of sexual development and how the process relates to peers of same gender. Masturbation begins.
Begins to expand social radius beyond family and concentrate on relationships with peers	Encourage some external responsibilities alone in consultation with parents, i.e., visit with health care provider, contacts with school counselors.
Cognition is usually concrete	Concrete thinking requires dealing with most health situations in a simple, explicit manner using visual and verbal cues.
MIDDLE ADOLESCENCE (Age 14 to 16 Years)	
Pubertal development usually complete and sexual drives emerge	Explores ability to attract opposites. Sexual behavior and experimentation (same and opposite sex) begin. Masturbation increases.
Peer group sets behavioral standards, although some family values persist	Peer group affects compliance, and peers rather than parents offer key support.
Conflicts over independence	Increased assumption of independent action, together with continued need for parental support and guidance; able to discuss and negotiate changes in rules; ambivalence on part of adolescent in discussion and negotiation.
Cognition begins to be abstract	Begins to consider full range of possibilities with poor ability to integrate into real life because of immaturity and incomplete cognitive development.
LATE ADOLESCENCE (Age 17 to 21 Years)	
Physical maturation complete. Body image and gender role definition are secured	Begins to feel comfortable with relationships and decisions regarding sexuality and preference. Individual relationships become more important than peer group.
Narcissism declines; there is a process of giving and sharing	More open to specific questioning regarding behavior.
Idealistic	Idealism may lead to conflicts with family and other authority figures.
Emancipation is nearly secured	With emancipation, more awareness about consequences of personal actions.
Cognitive development is complete	Most are capable of understanding a full range of options for health issues.
Functional role begins to be defined	Often interested in significant discussion of life goals because this is the primary function of this stage.

SOURCE: After Shafer and Irwin.

Middle adolescence (ages 14 to 16 years) is the period of rapid cognitive growth when formal operational thinking emerges. Adolescents begin to understand abstract concepts and may question the judgment of adults. The individual then shifts from the egocentric world of the early adolescent to the sociocentric world of the middle and late adolescent and begins to modulate impulsive behavior.

Late adolescence (ages 17 to 21 years) is the period of establishment of personal identity and intimate relationships and the beginning of the assumption of a role in society. The late adolescent views life in a more sociocentric view, characteristic of adulthood. The late adolescent may be altruistic, and conflicts with the family and society may center on moral issues rather than egocentric considerations.

Families can facilitate adolescence by providing a graduated increase in independence and in responsibilities. Adolescents require both individuality and involvement with family and society to facilitate development of identity and of rational competence. Clinicians should support this process by encouraging adolescents to make their own appointments, assisting the chronically ill adolescent in assuming more responsibility for his or her health care, and encouraging parents to decrease their role in clinical management issues.

Psychological Changes Associated with Pubescence HORMONES AND BEHAVIOR Specific behavioral changes are associated with puberty and its timing. Androgens are involved in this process. During peak height velocity (stages 3 to 4), boys tend to have conflicts with their mothers, and as boys complete puberty mothers tend to defer more to their sons. Girls also tend to have more conflict with their mothers and to decrease interactions with their fathers. Other activities associated with changes in androgens include heterosocial and heterosexual behavior. Boys with rising levels of testosterone tend to initiate sexual intercourse and are reported to be more impatient, irritable, and aggressive. Rising levels of adrenal androgens correlate with increased masturbatory activity and heterosocial behavior in girls.

TIMING OF MATURATION Timing of puberty is associated with psychological and behavioral sequelae. Earlier physical maturation in girls is associated with more dissatisfaction with their bodies, lower self-esteem, and general unhappiness. Early-developing girls also receive less support from peer groups and may associate with older adolescents. The early-developing girl initiates sexual behavior before her age peers, experiences an early identity crisis, has greater interest in independence and decision-making, and tends to have more behavioral problems and less interest in academic activities. Early physical maturation in boys is associated with earlier initiation of sexual behavior, and late maturation in boys is more often associated with negative psychological sequelae. The late-maturing boy tends to have a negative self-concept and body image and an increased frequency of identity crises.

Environmental Changes SOCIAL ENVIRONMENT Changes in the social environment during the second decade may affect health status. The family tends to provide less supervision and allow more freedom in choices regarding free time, often providing the adolescent opportunity to engage in risky behaviors. Schools are transformed from supportive elementary schools to the large, impersonal, and less structured environments of middle/junior high schools, high schools, and colleges. Work environments provide even less supervision and on-the-job guidance for the adolescent. With the ongoing restructuring of social programs of the 1990s fewer nurturing programs are available for youth after school. Increased poverty has had a negative effect on the health status of children and adolescents.

LEGAL ENVIRONMENT The law in most states requires consent of a parent for medical care for children below age 18. The involvement of parents is usually not a barrier to the provision of health services, but some sensitive health issues (e.g., sexual behavior and substance use) may interfere with access to health care for adolescents. The Mature Minor Doctrine generally allows adolescents to seek health care independently if they are capable of understanding the risks and benefits of the proposed treatment and therefore capable of informed consent. There is usually little risk of liability in providing health care to the older mature minor (14 years or older) if the care is for the

individual's benefit or is an emergency. In many states adolescents can seek care without parental permission for sensitive issues such as sexually transmitted diseases, contraception, pregnancy, substance use, and some psychiatric problems. Adolescents may also be treated without parental permission if the condition is an emergency and a delay in treatment would be detrimental. Emancipated minors (adolescents who live away from home, are no longer subject to parental control, are economically self-supporting, are married, or are members of the military service) may also consent to their own health care.

MORBIDITY AND MORTALITY

The concept that adolescence is the healthiest period of life is based on measures of mortality and morbidity that do not include functional assessment of health status or the effects of behaviors initiated during adolescence on adult mortality and morbidity.

MORTALITY Mortality rates are low, but since 1985, there has been an increase in mortality for adolescents and young adults. Mortality (per 100,000) increases from 26 in 10 to 14 year olds to 88 in 15 to 19 year olds to 110 in 20 to 24 year olds. Most adolescent mortality is due to violence, particularly motor vehicle accidents, homicide, and suicide. In 1990 injuries accounted for most deaths between the ages of 10 and 24, and mortality rates for males are double those of females. Ethnic and racial groups differ in respect to the cause of death: black males of 15 to 19 years old have a ninefold greater rate of death from homicide than white males and the lowest life expectancy of all adolescents. In contrast, white male adolescents have higher death rates from suicide and motor vehicle accidents. Unintentional injuries account for more than half of deaths in the second decade. Risky driving habits account for half of fatal crashes, and adolescent and young adult (ages 15 to 24) drivers have the highest rates of motor vehicle fatalities. Alcohol is also implicated in fatal bicycle, boating, skateboard, and swimming accidents. Suicide is responsible for 13 percent of deaths between ages 15 and 24. Native American males have high rates, and black adolescents have low rates of suicide. Between ages 15 and 24 homicide accounts for 14 percent of deaths. Homicide is the leading cause of death in black male adolescents and young adults, accounting for 58 percent and 54 percent of the deaths, respectively. Adolescents in impoverished metropolitan areas are more likely to be victims of homicide. Cardiovascular diseases account for 1.4 to 4.1 deaths, and malignancies cause 3.1 to 5.5 deaths per 100,000 persons aged 10 to 24.

MORBIDITY Most morbidity during adolescence originates from substance abuse, sexual activity, and injuries. Additional causes include mental health problems and skeletal and reproductive disorders.

Skeletal System (See also Chap. 329) Rapid growth of the long bones and closure of the epiphyses are associated with several orthopedic problems. Slipped capital femoral epiphyses occur primarily at the time of rapid growth spurt and are more common in the obese. Osgood-Schlatter disease (osteochondrosis of the tibial tuberosity) and idiopathic scoliosis are disorders of adolescence, and neoplasms of osseous origins peak during adolescence. Fractures due to injuries are common throughout adolescence.

Female Reproductive Health Problems Reproductive problems are a common cause of morbidity in young women.

Anovulatory cycles (See also Chap. 337) Dysfunctional uterine bleeding (DUB) is characterized by frequent, irregular, painless menses. Primary DUB results from anovulatory cycles, i.e., oscillations of estrogen levels that lack the characteristic surge in luteinizing hormone and subsequent corpus luteum development, progesterone production, and endometrial maturation of a mature cycle. Without progesterone, the endometrial lining becomes thickened and fragile, resulting in intermittent sloughing and irregular, frequently excessive menstrual bleeding. The differential diagnosis includes pregnancy, stress, rapid weight change, chronic illness, substance abuse, disorders of coagulation, and disorders of the vagina, cervix, uterus, and ovary. Anovulatory cycles may persist for 5 years following menarche.

Dysmenorrhea Dysmenorrhea, both primary and secondary, is a major complaint of menstruating adolescents and a major cause of school absenteeism. Primary dysmenorrhea is due to prostaglandin-stimulated myometrial contractions during ovulatory cycles. Secondary dysmenorrhea is associated with pelvic infections, intrauterine and extrauterine pregnancy, intrauterine devices, and congenital anomalies. Primary dysmenorrhea is treated by suppressing production of the prostaglandins and/or inhibiting ovulation. If the subject fails to respond to oral contraceptives and prostaglandin inhibitors, further evaluation is required.

Sexually transmitted diseases (STD) (See also Chap. 129) Sexually active adolescents have the highest rates of STD of any age group in the United States. Complications include cervical intraepithelial neoplasia, pelvic inflammatory disease, ectopic pregnancy, infertility, genital cancers, neonatal infections, and AIDS. As of June 1995, 2184 cases of AIDS had been diagnosed in 13 to 19 year olds and 17,745 cases in the 20- to 24-year-old cohort. The extent of seroprevalence of human immunodeficiency virus in adolescents is not well defined. When one STD is diagnosed, the clinician must screen for other STDs and counsel the young patient about risks.

Male Reproductive Health Problems (See also Chap. 336) Testicular masses and varicoceles may become evident during puberty and are usually discovered during a routine physical examination. Surgical repair may be indicated to enhance fertility and in the following situations: genital discomfort, testicular volume loss, abnormal semen analysis, or abnormal luteinizing hormone–releasing hormone stimulation test. Testicular cancer is rare in adolescents, but teaching young men to perform self testicular examinations may increase early identification of tumors.

RISK-TAKING BEHAVIORS

SUBSTANCE USE AND ABUSE Since 1991 there has been a reversal in the downward trends of substance use that occurred in the 1980s. This increase in substance abuse has been accompanied by a decrease in the perception of harm by such behavior. In 1994 45.6 percent of high school seniors reported illicit substance use at some time. Rates of lifetime use of LSD and heroin among high school seniors increased to 10.5 and 1.2 percent respectively, and 3 percent of high school seniors reported use of crack cocaine. Lifetime alcohol and tobacco use approximated 87 percent and 62 percent, respectively, among high school seniors in 1994. Binge drinking (the consumption of at least five drinks or more in a row at least once in the previous 2 weeks) was reported by 31 percent of high school seniors and by 40 percent of college students. Initiation of substance abuse during adolescence has major negative health consequences in adulthood, including more common habituation. Girls consistently report greater use of cigarettes, whereas boys use alcohol more commonly. Approximately 19 percent of adolescents leave high school as smokers, and 21 percent of young adults are regular smokers. The lower rates of cigarette smoking in boys may be due to the increase in use of snuff and chewing tobacco.

Surveys may underestimate the true prevalence of substance use, but it is clear that patterns of substance use vary by region, age, gender, and ethnicity. Substance use generally increases with age. Native American adolescents have the highest prevalence rates for cigarettes, alcohol, and most illicit drugs, followed by rates for whites, Hispanics, African-Americans, and Asian-Americans.

UNINTENTIONAL INJURIES Injuries, particularly motor vehicle accidents, account for more than half of deaths in adolescents, and hospitalization for injury accounts for the largest number of hospital days. Alcohol, high speed, and reckless behavior play important roles in these injuries and are also implicated in injuries with bicycles,

skateboards, swimming, and boating. Males outnumber females by greater than 2 to 1 in all injury situations.

SEXUAL BEHAVIOR Adolescents now initiate heterosexual behavior earlier than cohorts of previous generations. By age 15, 26 percent of white females and males, 24 percent of black females, and 69 percent of black males experience coitus. By age 19 these figures increase to 76 percent of white females, 85 percent of white males, 83 percent of black females, and 96 percent of black males. White adolescent females report more frequent sexual intercourse and more partners than their age-related black cohorts. Adolescent females with earlier menarche begin to have intercourse earlier than those with a later menarche. Adolescents who initiate sexual behavior early tend to have more sexual partners and are more likely to acquire a sexually transmitted disease or become pregnant. Fewer than half of sexually active adolescents use condoms. Reported rates of unprotected heterosexual anal intercourse are from 12 percent to 26 percent. Reliable data on same-sex behavior during adolescence are not available, but rates may approximate 5 to 10 percent. Retrospective studies of adult homosexual and bisexual men indicate that half initiated same-sex sexual behavior by age 16.

Overall birth rates have declined over the past decade, but the number of births to unmarried adolescent girls has increased. Furthermore, there were an estimated 412,275 abortions in adolescents in 1992. Pregnancy, birth, and abortion rates vary by race and ethnicity.

COVARIATION OF RISK BEHAVIORS The practice of one risk behavior is associated with a greater likelihood for initiation of another in the near future. The association between alcohol abuse and injury is well established. Other activities that predispose to injury include reckless driving and failure to use seat belts and helmets.

The strongest evidence for covariation is in substance abuse, sexual activity, and delinquent behavior. The major risk for initiation of cigarette, alcohol, and marijuana use is by age 20 and for illicit substance use is by age 21. Young adults who have not used these substances are unlikely to do so thereafter. During early and middle adolescence, less serious substance use predicts subsequent use of more serious substances. Alcohol use precedes marijuana use, and marijuana use precedes other illicit drugs (including psychedelics, cocaine, heroin, and nonprescribed stimulants, sedatives, and tranquilizers). In girls, cigarette use is predictive of subsequent substance use. The influence of alcohol and tobacco use on subsequent marijuana use is independent of age. The earlier adolescents begin using marijuana the more likely the use of other illicit substances. Substance use is also correlated with delinquent behavior, violent behavior, suicide, homicide, early sexual debut, and less effective contraceptive use.

MENTAL HEALTH PROBLEMS

Approximately 10 percent of adolescents have symptoms of psychological distress. Psychiatric conditions that may begin in childhood include anxiety and panic disorders, personality disorders, schizophrenia, suicide, and eating disorders. Three common problems during adolescence are suicide, depression, and eating disorders.

SUICIDE Suicide is the fourth leading cause of death in early adolescence (10 to 14 years old) and the third leading cause in late adolescence and young adulthood. The greatest increase in suicide rates since 1970 is among men aged 15 to 24. Suicide is relatively uncommon before puberty and increases after age 16 with most occurring between ages 18 and 24, particularly in white and Native American late adolescent boys and young men. The relationship between male sex and substance abuse and conduct disorders may be responsible for this predominance. For every completed suicide, there may be 20 to 50 attempted suicides, with a female preponderance. Differences in methods may be responsible for the sex differences between fatal and attempted suicides. Methods for fatal suicide include firearms, hanging, and jumping from heights. Drug ingestion, which rarely causes fatality, is the most common method for suicide attempts in adolescents.

Etiology of Suicide Common factors in suicidal adolescents include a history of suicide in family members, alcohol and substance abuse, attention deficit disorder, conduct disorders, depression, anxiety states, and knowing someone who has committed or attempted suicide. Precipitating factors include acute stress, trouble with the law, trouble at school such as cheating or truancy, substance abuse, pregnancy or fear of pregnancy, hypochondriasis, social isolation, and anxiety. In occasional girls perfectionism and anxiety about academic performance (in the presence of average intelligence) or environmental change appear to be causal. Many suicide victims are intoxicated at the time of death.

Recognition of the At-Risk Suicidal Adolescent Recognition of the suicidal adolescent may be difficult. The most common underlying psychiatric factor in suicidal adolescents is depression, manifested by feelings of hopelessness, low self-esteem, despair, and somatic complaints. In the younger adolescent, depressive equivalents of school problems and acting-out behavior may include legal problems. The younger adolescent may also have difficulty in describing his or her feelings. In the older adolescent, substance abuse is more common. Injured adolescents should be queried about the cause of the injury to rule out suicidal behavior. Adolescents with a family history of suicide, a history of psychiatric disorders, or a past history of suicidal behavior need to be screened for suicide risk. The depressed adolescent contemplating suicide usually welcomes the opportunity to communicate his or her feelings.

Once a suicidal adolescent is identified, an extensive evaluation is required to assess the problem. Comprehensive workup should include evaluation of the adolescent, the family, and the family together with the adolescent. Confidentiality is immaterial in the face of potential suicide, and parents and/or guardians should be informed immediately about the suicidal behavior. Suicidal intent is as important as the lethality of the method. Many adolescents have little knowledge of lethality. Evaluation should focus on mental health disorders in the family, past history of mental health problems in the adolescent, sexual abuse, and sexual behavior including same-sex behavior, since homosexual adolescents appear to be at greater risk for suicide. All suicidal adolescents need evaluation by a psychiatrist as soon as possible.

In emergencies, the physician must decide if outpatient or inpatient care is appropriate. If immediate treatment is needed, psychiatric consultation is obtained when the patient is stable medically. If the patient is initially medically stable, the physician must decide whether he or she is at continuing risk for suicide. Some programs recommend hospitalization for all suicidal adolescents, and hospitalization is always advisable for the following groups: (1) those still intent on suicide; (2) those with previous suicide attempts; (3) all males; (4) all severely depressed patients; (5) those impaired by substance abuse; (6) those whose attempt was with a lethal method (e.g., firearm, hanging, or jumping from a high place); and (7) those without a supportive environment at home.

When the patient is discharged, the physician needs to monitor compliance with the mental health treatment program and to query the family about the availability of firearms at home. Adolescents who are depressed or suicidal are difficult to engage in treatment programs, and a follow-up appointment with the primary care physician is the best way to monitor compliance. If the adolescent fails to keep the appointment, the physician should telephone and reschedule it.

Depression (See also Chap. 385) Depression is the most common feature in patients who attempt suicide. The prevalance of major depressive disorders in adolescence is between 4 and 6 percent with a slight preponderance of females to males. The diagnostic criteria for depression during adolescence are the same as in adulthood (Table 8-5) and include changes in mood and relationships, cognitive functioning, and bodily functioning. Depressive equivalents in the adolescent include hypochondriasis, substance abuse, decrements in school functioning, problems with the law, and major family conflicts.

EATING DISORDERS (See also Chap. 76) Eating disorders generally have their onset in postpubertal adolescents, and adolescents may fulfill the DSM-IV criteria for anorexia nervosa or bulimia nervosa prior to the completion of puberty (See Tables 76-1 and 76-2). Adolescents with subclinical eating disorders may need the same treatment

Table 8-5

DSM-III-R Criteria for Diagnosis of Major Depression

Diagnosis requires symptom 1 or 2 and at least four other symptoms for a 2-week period

1. Depressed or irritable mood
2. Diminished interest or pleasure
3. Weight loss or weight gain
4. Insomnia or hypersomnia
5. Psychomotor agitation or retardation
6. Fatigue or loss of energy
7. Feelings of worthlessness or excessive guilt
8. Decreased concentration or indecisiveness
9. Thoughts of death, suicidal ideation, or suicide attempt

SOURCE: After American Psychiatric Association, p 217.

as adolescents with full-fledged disorders. While the eating patterns in many adolescents appear abnormal, and adolescent girls commonly have dissatisfaction with weight and shape and some fear of gaining weight, these feelings and fears are extreme in the adolescent with an eating disorder.

THE CLINICAL VISIT OF THE ADOLESCENT

TRANSITION INTERVIEW Establishing an effective doctor-patient relationship with the adolescent is a formidable task for the physician whose practice is primarily with adults. A transition interview for the adolescent and family helps to define the relationship between the physician and the emerging adult. Areas to be emphasized include the necessity for the physician to interview and examine the adolescent privately and the need for the patient to generate his or her own questions including initiating appointments. Normal adolescence and the continuing need for some decisions to be made with family guidance and support should be discussed. The payment mechanisms and responsibility for fees should be clarified. During this interview, the physician should inquire about the previous health care and request authorization to contact the former physician.

CONFIDENTIALITY Confidentiality is fundamental to any doctor-patient relationship. Adolescents need to be able to discuss all matters with the physician openly, honestly, and confidentially, and the physician must provide assurance of the confidential nature of all information. Prior to queries about sexual behavior or substance use, it may be useful to restate the confidential nature of the questioning. With life-threatening behaviors or diseases (e.g., suicidal behavior or management of chronic disease), the physician generally has the right to intervene including identification of a parent, guardian, or supportive adult to assist in the management.

OBTAINING THE HISTORY History taking should be guided by the developmental stage of the patient (Table 8-4). The adolescent may not disclose his or her primary concern until a secure and confidential relationship has been established. General screening should be undertaken for the major health-damaging behaviors of adolescence, including sexual activity, substance use, depression and its equivalents, and dietary changes suggestive of an eating disorder. Distinguishing between risk-taking behaviors that are temporary, though dangerous, and those that are pathologic is a challenge. This judgment requires assessing the effects of risky behavior on the health status and the motivation for engaging in them and determining whether normal psychosocial development is impaired. Figure 8-3 summarizes the biopsychosocial and environmental factors that increase vulnerability for initiating risky behaviors. Male sex, positive attitudes toward risky behaviors, lack of parental supervision, contact with peers engaging in the behavior, and multiple school transitions are associated with an increased propensity for risky behaviors. The physician should be

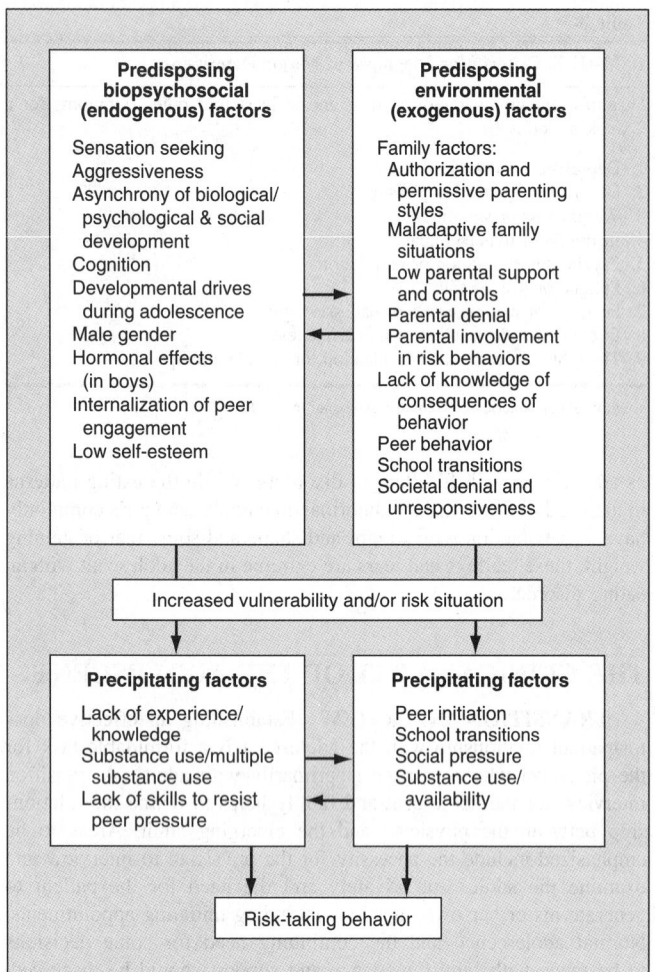

FIGURE 8-3 Principal factors in risk-taking behaviors. (Adapted from Irwin and Millstein.)

specific in questioning about individual risk behaviors, including their frequency and their intensity. One behavior may serve as a warning sign for another risky behavior. For example, early substance abuse correlates with early sexual activity. Guidelines have been developed to assist physicians in screening youth at risk, including *Bright Futures* (Green, 1995) and *Guidelines for Adolescent Preventive Services* (Elster and Kuznets, 1994) (see "Bibliography").

Frequently, adolescents do not want to disclose current behavior, and the physician may query instead about general risk taking and the behavior of peer groups. The physical signs and symptoms associated with risky behaviors are similar to those in adults, but the consequences of such behaviors may have a greater effect on the adolescent, including more family conflicts, impaired academic performance, unwise peer relationships and activities, and changes in extracurricular activities.

Immunization history needs to be reviewed. Previously immunized adolescents who received a complete series of immunizations prior to 5 years of age need to receive a second vaccination for measles alone or for measles, mumps, and rubella. Adolescents who have never been immunized or for whom the immunization history is not available should receive a three-dose primary series of immunizations for tetanus, diphtheria, and poliomyelitis and a two-dose primary series for measles, mumps, rubella, and hepatitis B. Hepatitis A vaccine should be given to sexually active adolescents.

The physical examination and laboratory assessment are guided by the general complaints and the associated physical stigmata of risky behaviors.

BIBLIOGRAPHY

ADAMS LB, SHAFER MA: Early manifestations of eating disorders in adolescents: Defining those at risk. J Nutr Ed 20:307, 1988

AMERICAN PSYCHIATRIC ASSOCIATION: *Diagnostic and Statistical Manual of Mental Disorders*, 4th ed. Washington, DC, The American Psychiatric Association, 1994

BACHMAN JAG et al: Racial/ethnic differences in smoking, drinking and illicit drug use among American high school seniors, 1976–89. Am J Public Health 81:372, 1991

BLUMENTHAL SJ, KUPFER DJ: *Suicide over the Life Cycle*. Washington, DC, American Psychiatric Press, 1990

CENTERS FOR DISEASE CONTROL: *HIV/AIDS Surveillance Report, 1995*, 7(No. 1). Atlanta, Centers for Disease Control and Prevention. 1995

———: Premarital sexual experience among adolescent women—United States, 1970–1988. MMWR 39:929, 1991

COPELAND KC et al: Assessment of pubertal development. Ross Laboratories PREP series. Columbus, Ross Laboratories, 1986

DANIEL WA: Growth at adolescence: Clinical correlates. Semin Adolesc Med 1:15, 1985

ELSTER AB, KUZNETS NJ: AMA Guidelines for Adolescent Preventive Services (GAPS): Recommendations and Rationale. Baltimore, Williams & Wilkins, 1994

ENGLISH A: Treating adolescents: Legal and ethical considerations. Med Clin North Am 74:1097, 1990

FELDMAN SS, ELLIOTT GR: *At the Threshold: The Developing Adolescent*. Cambridge, Harvard University, 1990

FRIEDMAN SB et al (eds): *Comprehensive Adolescent Health Care*. St. Louis, Quality Medical Publishing, 1992

GREEN M: Bright Futures. Arlington, VA, National Center for Education in Maternal and Child Health, 1995

GREULICH WW, PYLE SI: *Radiographic Atlas of Skeletal Development of the Hand and Wrist*, 2d ed. Stanford, Stanford University, 1959

IRWIN CE JR: The theoretical concept of at-risk adolescents. Adolesc Med: State Art Rev 1:1, 1990

———, MILLSTEIN SG: Biopsychosocial correlates of risk taking behavior during adolescence: Can the physician intervene? J Adolesc Health Care 7:82S, 1986

———, SHAFER MA: Adolescent sexuality: Negative outcomes of a normative behavior, in *Adolescents at Risk: Medical and Social Perspectives*, DE Rogers, E Ginzberg (eds). Boulder, Westview Press, 1992, pp 35–79

JOHNSTON LD et al: *National Survey Results on Drug Use from the Monitoring the Future Study, 1975–94*. Vol 1, *Secondary Students*. Rockville, MD, NIH Publication No. 95-4026, 1995

KASS EJ: Adolescent varicocele: Current concepts. Semin Urol 6:140, 1988

MARSHALL W, TANNER JM: Variation in the pattern of pubertal changes in boys. Arch Dis Child 45:13, 1970

———, ———: Variation in the pattern of pubertal changes in girls. Arch Dis Child 44:291, 1969

MCANARNEY ER et al: *Textbook of Adolescent Medicine*. Philadelphia, Saunders, 1992

MILLSTEIN SG et al: Health risk behaviors among young adolescents. Pediatrics 89:422, 1992

———: *Promoting the Health of Adolescents*. New York, Oxford University, 1994

NATIONAL CENTER FOR HEALTH STATISTICS: *Vital Statistics of the United States, 1990*, vol 2, *Mortality, part A*. DHHS publication no (PHS) 95-1101, 1994, pp 14–39

NEWACHECK PW et al: Health insurance coverage of adolescents: A current profile and assessment of trends. Pediatrics 90:589, 1992

NOTTELMANN ED et al: Developmental processes in early adolescence: Relations between adolescent adjustment problems and chronologic age, pubertal stage and puberty-related hormones. J Pediatr 110:473, 1987

SHAFER MAB, IRWIN CE JR: The adolescent patient, in *Rudolph's Pediatrics*, 20th ed, A Rudolph (ed). Norwalk, Appleton and Lange, 1995

SHAFFER D et al: Preventing teenage suicide: A critical review. J Am Acad Child Adolesc Psychiatry 27:675, 1988

SINGER MI et al: *Handbook for Screening Adolescents at Psychosocial Risk*. New York, Lexington Books, 1993

STYNE D, GRUMBACH MM: Disorders of puberty in males and females, in *Reproductive Endocrinology*, SS Yen, RB Jaffee (eds). Philadelphia, Saunders, 1991, pp 511–54

SUBSTANCE ABUSE AND MENTAL HEALTH SERVICES ADMINISTRATION, US DHHS: *Preliminary Estimates from the 1993 National Household Survey on Drug Abuse*, 1993

TANNER JM, DAVIES PSW: Clinical longitudinal standards for height and weight velocity for North American Children. J Pediatr 107:317, 1985

UDRY JR: Biological predispositions and social control in adolescent sexual behavior. Am Soc Rev 53:709, 1988

US Dept. of Health and Human Services (PHS), Division of STD Preven- tion: *Sexually Transmitted Disease Surveillance, 1994.* Atlanta, Centers for Disease Control and Prevention, 1995

US Office of Technology Assessment: *Adolescent Health*, vol III, *Cross- cutting Issues in the Delivery of Health and Related Services*, OTA-H- 467, Washington, DC, 1991

US Preventive Services Task Force: *Guide to Clinical Preventive Services: An Assessment of the Effectiveness of 169 Interventions.* Baltimore, Wil- liams & Wilkins, 1989

9 | *Neil M. Resnick*

GERIATRIC MEDICINE

Of all the people who have ever lived to age 65, more than half are now alive. This statistic has important demographic and economic implications, and its impact on medical care is also substantial.

BIOLOGY OF AGING

Numerous molecular concomitants of aging have been described. For instance, there is an increase in chromosome structural abnormalities, DNA cross-linking, and frequency of single-strand breaks, a decline in DNA methylation, and loss of DNA telomeric sequences. The primary structure of proteins is unaltered, but posttranslational changes, such as deamidation, oxidation, cross-linking, and nonenzy- matic glycation, increase. Mitochondrial structure also deteriorates, albeit not universally.

However, the biological changes are clearer than the mechanisms that mediate them. In fact, although the senescent phenotype appears to be ubiquitous, biologists disagree about whether senescence even exists beyond zoos and civilized societies and whether it occurs at all in many species. There is little evolutionary rationale for a process that happens after reproduction is complete, particularly one associated with such a long and complex course. In nature, senescence is most notable for its absence; nearly all animals die of predation, disease, or environmental hazards rather than aging. The argument that different species have different maximum lifespans can be explained without invoking a specific aging process: while growth and development are based on a genetic template, aging may reflect merely the accumulation of random damage rather than a specific mechanism.

If aging exists as a distinct process, there is consensus that the mechanisms are likely multifactorial and species-specific, if not organ-and cell-specific, making the paucity of available human data particularly problematic. As a result, there are nearly as many theories of aging as investigators. Most theories overlap or are not mutually exclusive, and none is completely compatible with the dearth of data. As a group, the theories can be divided into two broad categories, based on whether they attribute aging to a genetic program or to progressive and random damage to homeostatic systems. Of the genetic theories, "pleiotropic antagonism" is the only viable one compatible with the limited evolutionary selection pressure present following completion of reproduction. Proposed 35 years ago and still inadequately investigated, it suggests that aging may be caused by the late and deleterious effects of genes that are conserved because of their beneficial effects prior to reproduction. The "random damage" theories are based on the possibility that the balance between ongoing damage and repair is disrupted. The theories differ in the emphasis placed on increased damage (e.g., by free radicals, oxidation, or glycation) versus deficient repair and about the mechanisms that might mediate each. Although such theories are attractive, it remains unclear whether the described abnormalities are the cause or the result of senescence.

Many mechanisms previously postulated to mediate aging have not been borne out, including the somatic mutation theory (in which aging would result from cumulative spontaneous mutations), the error catastrophe theory (in which aging would result from errors in the synthesis of proteins critical to the synthesis of genetic material or protein-synthesizing machinery), and the intrinsic mutagenesis theory (in which aging is the result of ongoing intrinsic DNA rearrangements).

To date, the only intervention known to delay aging is caloric restriction. Its salutary effect has been documented in multiple species, from single-cell organisms to rodents. In rodents, it not only increases average life expectancy and maximum life span but also delays the onset of some typical age-associated diseases as well as deterioration of physiologic systems (e.g., immune responsiveness, glucose metabo- lism, muscle atrophy). The mechanism is still not determined, but it is specific to caloric restriction rather than to reduction of any dietary component (e.g., fat intake) or supplements with vitamins or antioxi- dants. Unfortunately, adequate data from primates are not yet available, and the impact of caloric restriction in humans is still unknown.

PRINCIPLES OF GERIATRIC MEDICINE

Despite the biological controversy, from a physiologic standpoint hu- man aging is characterized by progressive constriction of the homeo- static reserve of every organ system. This decline, often referred to as *homeostenosis*, is evident by the third decade and is gradual and progressive, although the rate and extent of decline vary. The decline of each organ system (Table 9-1) appears to occur independently of changes in other organ systems and is influenced by diet, environment, and personal habits as well as by genetic factors.

Several important principles follow from these facts: (1) Individu- als become more dissimilar as they age, belying any stereotype of aging; (2) an *abrupt* decline in any system or function is always due to disease and not to "normal aging"; (3) "normal aging" can be attenuated by modification of risk factors (e.g., increased blood pres- sure, smoking, sedentary lifestyle); and (4) "healthy old age" is not an oxymoron. In fact, *in the absence of disease, the decline in homeostatic reserve causes no symptoms and imposes few restrictions on activities of daily living regardless of age.*

Appreciation of these facts may make it easier to understand the striking increases that have occurred in life expectancy. Average life expectancy is now 17 years at age 65, 11 years at age 75, 6 years at age 85, 4 years at age 90, and 2 years at age 100. Moreover, the bulk of these years is characterized by a lack of significant impairment (Table 9-2)—only 35 percent of people over age 85 are impaired in any activity required for daily living, and only 20 percent reside in a nursing home. Yet, as individuals age they are more likely to suffer from disease, disability, and the side effects of drugs, all of which, when combined with the decrease in physiologic reserve, make the older person more vulnerable to environmental, pathologic, and phar- macologic challenges.

The following concepts underlie the remainder of the chapter:
1. The onset of a new disease in the elderly (usually defined as over age 75 to 80) generally affects the organ system made most vulnerable by prior physiologic and pathologic changes. Because this organ system often differs from the newly diseased organ system, disease presentation in the elderly is often atypical. For example, fewer than one-fourth of older patients with hyperthyroidism present with goiter, tremor, and exophthalmos; more likely are atrial fibrillation, confusion, depression, syncope, and weakness. Significantly, because the "weakest link" is so often the brain, the lower urinary tract, or the cardiovascular or musculoskeletal system, a limited number of presenting symptoms predominate—acute confusion, depression, in- continence, falling, and syncope—no matter what the underlying dis- ease. Thus for the most common geriatric syndromes, regardless of the presenting symptom, the differential diagnosis is often largely similar. The corollary is equally important: The organ system usually associated with a particular symptom is less likely to be the source of that symptom in older individuals than in younger ones. Compared with middle-aged individuals, for example, acute confusion in older patients is less often due to a new brain lesion, depression to a psychiat-

ric disorder, incontinence to bladder dysfunction, falling to a neuropathy, or syncope to heart disease.

2. Because of decreased physiologic reserve, older patients often develop symptoms at an earlier stage of their disease. For example, heart failure may be precipitated by mild hyperthyroidism, cognitive dysfunction by mild hyperparathyroidism, urinary retention by mild prostatic enlargement, and nonketotic hyperosmolar coma by mild glucose intolerance. Paradoxically, therefore, treatment of the underlying disease may be easier because it is frequently less advanced at the time of presentation. A corollary is that drug side effects can occur with drugs and drug doses unlikely to produce side effects in younger people (Chap. 69). For instance, an antihistamine may cause confusion,

diuretics may precipitate urinary incontinence, digoxin may induce depression even with normal serum levels, and over-the-counter sympathomimetics may precipitate urinary retention in men with mild prostatic obstruction.

Unfortunately, the predisposition to develop symptoms at an earlier stage of disease is often offset by the change in illness behavior that occurs with age. Raised at a time when symptoms and debility were accepted as normal consequences of aging, the elderly are less likely to seek attention until symptoms become disabling. Thus, any symptom, particularly those associated with a change in functional status, must be taken seriously and evaluated promptly.

3. Since many homeostatic mechanisms may be compromised concurrently, there are usually multiple abnormalities amenable to treatment, and small improvements in each may yield dramatic benefits overall. For instance, cognitive impairment in patients with Alz-

Table 9-1

Selected Age-Related Changes and Their Consequences

Organ/System	Age-Related Physiologic Change*	Consequences of Age-Related Physiologic Change	Consequences of Disease, not Age
General	↑Body fat	↑Volume of distribution for fat soluble drugs	Obesity
	↓Total body water	↓Volume of distribution for water soluble drugs	Anorexia
Eyes/ears	Presbyopia	↓Accommodation	
	Lens opacification	↑Susceptibility to glare	Blindness
		Need for increased illumination	
	↓High-frequency acuity	Difficulty discriminating words if background noise is present	Deafness
Endocrine	Impaired glucose homeostasis	↑Glucose level in response to acute illness	Diabetes mellitus
	↓Thyroxine clearance (and production)	↓T_4 dose required in hypothyroidism	Thyroid dysfunction
	↑ADH, ↓renin, and ↓aldosterone		↓Na^+, ↑K^+
	↓Testosterone		Impotence
	↓Vitamin D absorption and activation	Osteopenia	Osteomalacia, fracture
Respiratory	↓Lung elasticity and ↑chest wall stiffness	Ventilation/perfusion mismatch and ↓P_{O_2}	Dyspnea, hypoxia
Cardiovascular	↓Arterial compliance and ↑ systolic BP →LVH	Hypotensive response to ↑HR, volume depletion, or loss of atrial contraction	Syncope
	↓β-adrenergic responsiveness	↓Cardiac output and HR response to stress	Heart failure
	↓Baroreceptor sensitivity and ↓SA node automaticity	Impaired blood pressure response to standing, volume depletion	Heart block
Gastrointestinal	↓Hepatic function	Delayed metabolism of some drugs	Cirrhosis
	↓Gastric acidity	↓Ca^+ absorption on empty stomach	Osteoporosis, B_{12} deficiency
	↓Colonic motility	Constipation	Fecal impaction
	↓Anorectal function		Fecal incontinence
Hematologic/immune system	↓Bone marrow reserve(?)		Anemia
	↓T cell function	False-negative PPD response	
	↑Autoantibodies	False-positive rheumatoid factor, antinuclear antibody	Autoimmune disease
Renal	↓GFR	Impaired excretion of some drugs	↑Serum creatinine
	↓Urine concentration/dilution (see also "Endocrine")	Delayed response to salt or fluid restriction/overload; nocturia	↓↑Na^+
Genitourinary	Vaginal/urethral mucosal atrophy	Dyspareunia, bacteriuria	Symptomatic UTI
	Prostate enlargement	↑Residual urine volume	Urinary incontinence; urinary retention
Musculoskeletal	↓Lean body mass, muscle		Functional impairment
	↓Bone density	Osteopenia	Hip fracture
Nervous system	Brain atrophy	Benign senescent forgetfulness	Dementia, delirium
	↓Brain catechol synthesis		Depression
	↓Brain dopaminergic synthesis	Stiffer gait	Parkinson's disease
	↓Righting reflexes	↑Body sway	Falls
	↓Stage 4 sleep	Early wakening, insomnia	Sleep apnea

* Changes generally observed in healthy elderly subjects free of symptoms and detectable disease in the organ system studied. The changes are usually important only when the system is stressed or other factors are added (e.g., drugs, disease, or environmental challenge); they rarely result in symptoms otherwise. Abbreviations: T_4, thyroxine; BP, blood pressure; HR, heart rate; ADH, antidiuretic hormone; GFR, glomerular filtration rate.

Table 9-2

CHAPTER 9
Geriatric Medicine

39

Life Expectancy and Number of Remaining Years Free of Dependency
in Activities of Daily Living

	Life Expectancy*, av		Disability-Free Years Remaining	
Age	Men	Women	Men	Women
65–69	13	20	9	11
70–74	12	16	8	8
75–79	10	13	7	7
80–84	7	10	5	5
≥85	7	8	3	3

* For independent noninstitutionalized elderly men and women in Massachusetts. Longevity and disability-free longevity are surprisingly long and must be incorporated into treatment decisions. Av, average. All figures rounded to nearest year. See text for more recent data on longevity alone.

SOURCE: S Katz et al, N Engl J Med 309:1218, 1983.

heimer's disease may be exacerbated by hearing or visual impairment, depression, heart failure, and electrolyte imbalance. Similarly, urinary incontinence can be worsened by fecal impaction, medications, and excess urinary output. In each case, substantial functional improvement can result from treating the contributing factors even if—as in Alzheimer's disease—the disease itself is untreatable.

4. Many findings that are abnormal in younger patients are relatively common in older people—e.g., bacteriuria, premature ventricular contractions, low bone mineral density, impaired glucose tolerance, and uninhibited bladder contractions. However, they may not be responsible for a particular symptom but only be incidental findings that result in missed diagnoses and misdirected therapy. For instance, the finding of bacteriuria should not end the search for a source of fever in an acutely ill older patient, nor should an elevated random blood sugar—especially in an acutely ill patient—be incriminated as the cause of neuropathy. On the other hand, certain other abnormalities must not be dismissed as due to old age—e.g., there is no anemia, impotence, depression, or confusion of old age.

5. Because symptoms in older people are often due to multiple causes, the diagnostic "law of parsimony" often does not apply. For instance, fever, anemia, retinal embolus, and a heart murmur prompt almost a reflex diagnosis of infective endocarditis in a younger patient but may reflect aspirin-induced blood loss, a cholesterol embolus, insignificant aortic sclerosis, and a viral illness in an older patient.

6. Because the older patient is more likely to suffer the adverse consequences of disease, treatment—and even prevention—may be equally or even more effective. For instance, the benefits of thrombolysis and beta-blocker therapy after a myocardial infarction are as impressive in older patients as in younger ones; and treatment of hypertension and transient ischemic attacks, as well as immunization against influenza and pneumococcal pneumonia are more effective in older patients. In addition, prevention in older patients often must be seen in a broader context. For instance, although interventions to increase bone density may be limited in older patients, fracture still may be prevented by efforts to improve balance, strengthen legs, reduce peripheral edema, treat other contributing medical conditions, replete nutritional deficits, eliminate environmental hazards, and remove adverse medications—not so much those that affect bone metabolism, but rather those that induce orthostasis, confusion, and extrapyramidal stiffness.

HISTORY TAKING IN ELDERLY PATIENTS Most older patients are able to provide a reliable medical history; however, a multitude of complaints may make obtaining a history more difficult and adequate time must be allotted. If the patient is unable to comprehend or communicate, data should be sought from family, friends, and caregivers. The history also should include drug ingestion; a dietary history; and history of falling, of incontinence, and of depression and anxiety.

Advance Directives All older patients should be asked whether they have drafted advance health care directives, and, if they have, a copy should be placed in the record. Such directives may consist of a health care proxy or durable power of attorney for health care, in which patients designate a surrogate decision-maker who makes health care decisions if the patient cannot, and/or a living will or medical directive, in which patients specify their desires for treatment in specific situations if they cannot communicate at the critical time.

Whether or not the patient has formally drafted these directives, it is useful to indicate in the record who should make health care decisions if the patient is no longer able to do so. Patients should then be encouraged to discuss with the physician as well as the designated proxy their feelings about resuscitation, intubation, feeding tubes, hospitalization, etc., in their current state of health and possible future declining states of health. The early elicitation of a patient's preferences and values can often help both physicians and families in subsequent difficult decisions by giving surrogate decision-makers the sense that they are doing as the patient would have wanted.

PHYSICAL EXAMINATION Certain features of the examination should receive special attention, depending in part on clues from the history. Weight and postural blood pressure should be measured at each visit. Vision and hearing should be checked; if hearing is impaired, excess cerumen should be removed from the external auditory canals. Denture fit should be assessed, and the oral cavity should be inspected with the dentures removed. Although thyroid disease becomes more common with age, the sensitivity and specificity of related findings are substantially lower than in younger individuals; consequently, the physical examination can rarely corroborate or exclude thyroid dysfunction in older patients. The breasts should not be overlooked, since older women are more likely to have breast cancer and less likely to do breast self-examination. The systolic murmur of aortic sclerosis is common and may be difficult to differentiate from aortic stenosis, especially since the presence of a fourth heart sound in an elderly person does not imply significant cardiac disease, and the carotid upstroke normally increases owing to age-related arterial stiffening.

In inactive patients and those with fecal or urinary incontinence, one should check for fecal impaction. In patients with urinary incontinence—especially men—a distended bladder must be looked for, since it may be the only finding in urinary retention; perineal sensation and the bulbocavernosus reflex also should be tested. Patients who fall should be observed standing up from a chair, bending down, reaching up, walking 10 feet, turning, returning, and sitting again; abnormalities of gait and balance should be evaluated with the patient's eyes open and closed and in response to a sternal push. It should be appreciated that "frontal release signs" (e.g., "snout," "glabellar," or palmomental reflexes) and absent ankle jerks and vibratory sense in the feet may be normal in the elderly.

MENTAL STATUS EXAMINATION In addition to evaluating mood and affect, some form of cognitive testing is essential in all elderly patients, even if it involves only checking different components of the history for consistency. People with mild degrees of dementia usually retain their social graces and may mask intellectual impairment by a cheerful and cooperative manner. Thus, the examiner should always probe for content. For patients who follow the news, one can ask what stories they are particularly interested in and why; the same applies to reading, social events—even the soap operas on television.

If there is any suspicion of a cognitive deficit after this kind of conversational probing, further questioning is indicated. An examination that tests only orientation as to person, place, and time is insufficient to detect mild or moderate intellectual impairment. As a quick screen, simply assessing orientation and asking the patient to draw a clock with the hands at a set time (e.g., 10 min before 2:00) can be very informative regarding cognitive status, visuospatial deficits, ability to comprehend and execute instructions in logical sequence, and presence or absence of perseveration. For slightly more detailed examinations, many practical mental status tests are available. The most widely used is the Mini-Mental Status Examination of Folstein (Chap. 24), which provides a numerical score that can be obtained in 5 to 10 min. Regardless of the test employed, the total score is less useful diagnostically than is knowledge of the specific domain of the deficit. As a general rule, disproportionate difficulty with immediate recall (e.g., of a list of three items) suggests depression, while predominant difficulty with recalling the items 5 min later suggests dementia. For patients with deficits of attention—recognized by inability to spell simple words backwards, repeat five digits, or recite the months of the year backwards—delirium is probably present, and the accuracy of the remainder of the test is dubious. However, the test can be interpreted accurately only in the context of a comprehensive evaluation.

EVALUATION OF FUNCTIONAL CAPACITY A clear description of the patient's degree of functional incapacity based on both medical and psychosocial problems is essential. The functional assessment includes determination of the patient's ability to perform basic activities of daily life (ADL), which are those needed for personal self-care, as well as the ability to perform more complex tasks required for independent living, the instrumental activities of daily living (IADL). ADLs include bathing, dressing, toileting, feeding, getting in and out of chairs and bed, and walking. IADLs include shopping, cooking, money management, housework, using a telephone, and traveling outside the home. For frail patients, an assessment in the home by a trained observer may be required, but for most patients a questionnaire dealing with these activities can be completed by the family or patient. In either case, the physician must determine the cause of any impairment and whether it can be treated. The assessment should conclude with determination of the socioeconomic circumstances and social support systems.

Since disease can present atypically in the elderly, acute functional decline may represent the first sign of serious acute illness. Thus, *acute functional decline presenting as the onset or worsening of falls, confusion, depression, or incontinence should prompt immediate medical evaluation.*

MANAGEMENT OF COMMON GERIATRIC CONDITIONS

Diseases more common in the elderly are covered elsewhere in the text. The medical problems discussed below do not usually present as clear-cut organ-specific diagnoses and are most common in the frail elderly, especially those over 80 years of age.

INTELLECTUAL IMPAIRMENT The predominant causes of impaired mentation in older patients are delirium, dementia, and depression. Each condition is covered elsewhere in the text in detail (Chaps. 24 and 367), but their management in the elderly is discussed here.

Differentiating the causes of impaired mentation is important, but in older patients they frequently coexist. Thus, the most important first step is to search for and correct all factors that may contribute to cognitive impairment, even in patients with dementia. Evidence of dangerous behavior also should be sought (e.g., leaving the stove on, wandering, and getting lost) and plans should be devised to deal with it. Although there is no specific pharmacologic treatment for Alzheimer's disease and agents such as tacrine are of limited efficacy and tolerability, this does not mean that the physician has no further role in treating the patient and family. In addition to discontinuing all nonessential medications and treating new intercurrent illness, the physician should help the family and patient predict and deal with the disease; indeed, the family often needs the physician's support more than the patient does.

 TREATMENT
Community services should be suggested as needed, including a visiting nurse, a home health aid to assist with personal hygiene, a homemaker to assist with housework, meal delivery and transportation services, day health centers, and respite care to ease the burden on family members. Support groups such as the Alzheimer's Associ-

ation often are of value to the family and help them to anticipate problems. Signs of patient abuse by an overstressed caregiver should be watched for. Legal counsel should be recommended to help the patient and family devise plans for ongoing management and ultimate disposition of assets.

Finally, abrupt worsening of mentation or the onset of disruptive behavior should always prompt a search for new illness or medication. Exacerbation of cognitive dysfunction may occur with mild infections (e.g., subungual toe abscess, vaginitis, or pressure ulcer); with "therapeutic" levels of many drugs; with use of nonprescribed drugs or alcohol; with modest abnormalities of serum sodium, calcium, glucose, or thyroxine; with mild hypoxia; with borderline nutritional deficiencies; and with the development of fecal impaction, urinary retention, pain, or change in environment, particularly in frail older patients. However, if a cause is not found and behavior does not respond to environmental manipulation, low doses of an antipsychotic medication may be helpful (e.g., haloperidol 0.25 to 2 mg per day orally; see below).

DEPRESSION Depression of significant degree occurs in 5 to 10 percent of community-dwelling elderly but is often overlooked. At highest risk are individuals with recent medical illness (e.g., stroke), bereavement, lack of social supports, recent nursing home admission, or psychiatric history (including alcohol abuse). The diagnosis requires the presence of a depressed mood for at least two consecutive weeks plus at least four of the following eight signs: sleep disturbance, lack of interest, feelings of guilt, decreased energy, decreased concentration, decreased appetite, psychomotor agitation/retardation, and suicidal ideation. Also helpful diagnostically are a personal or family history of depression, anhedonia (loss of pleasure), and past response to an antidepressant. It is essential to bear in mind that depression in older patients is often caused or contributed to by drugs or a systemic illness.

 TREATMENT
For the hospitalized patient in whom acute depression delays recovery or rehabilitation—when correction of medical and pharmacologic contributing factors is ineffective and there is no prior history of mania or major depression—methylphenidate, 5 to 10 mg at 8 A.M. and noon (to avoid insomnia) is often very effective, with benefits discernible within a few days. For patients with major depression, there is no ideal antidepressant drug. All are about equally effective, but the side effects differ (see below and Chap. 385). Consequently, one should become familiar with one or two agents for patients with psychomotor retardation (e.g., desipramine, sertraline) and for those with agitation (e.g., nortriptyline or trazodone). Because of its potent anticholinergic and orthostatic side effects, amitriptyline should be avoided whenever possible in older patients. Initial low dosages should be increased slowly to avoid serious side effects; low doses of each medication (e.g., nortriptyline, 10 to 50 mg daily; desipramine, 25 to 75 mg daily; or sertraline 50 to 150 mg daily) are often effective in the elderly. Careful follow-up is required to anticipate and minimize anticholinergic side effects, orthostatic hypotension, sedating effects, confusion, bizarre mental symptoms, cardiovascular complications, and drug overdose with suicidal intent. Adverse drug reactions should not be assumed to be due to the aging process.

Cautious use of the monoamine oxidase inhibitors is sometimes of benefit when other antidepressants are ineffective. Monoamine oxidase inhibitors should not be used in combination with the cyclic compounds. Electroconvulsive therapy has been successful and is usually well tolerated by elderly patients who remain severely depressed despite drug treatment, particularly if they also have delusions.

URINARY INCONTINENCE **Transient Incontinence** (Table 9-3) Because urinary continence requires adequate mobility, mentation, motivation, and manual dexterity—in addition to integrated

Table 9-3

Classification of Incontinence

TRANSIENT

Delirium/confusional state
Infection—urinary (symptomatic)
Atrophic urethritis/vaginitis
Pharmaceuticals
Psychological, especially depression
Excessive urine output (e.g., CHF, hyperglycemia)
Restricted mobility
Stool impaction

ESTABLISHED

Detrusor overactivity
Detrusor underactivity
Urethral obstruction
Urethral incompetence

SOURCE: Adapted from NM Resnick, Medical Grand Rounds 3:281, 1984.

control of the lower urinary tract—problems outside the bladder can result in incontinence.

1. *Delirium.* A clouded sensorium impedes recognition of both the need to void and the location of the nearest toilet; once delirium clears, incontinence resolves.
2. *Infection.* Symptomatic urinary tract infection commonly causes or contributes to incontinence; asymptomatic infection does not.
3. *Atrophic urethritis/vaginitis.* Atrophic urethritis/vaginitis, characterized by the presence of vaginal telangiectasia, petechiae, erosions, erythema, or friability, commonly contributes to incontinence in women and responds to a short course of low-dose estrogen or vaginal estrogen creams.
4. *Pharmaceutical.* The drugs most commonly causing transient incontinence are listed in Table 9-4.
5. *Psychologic.* Depression and psychosis are uncommon but treatable causes.
6. *Excess urine output.* Excess urine output may overwhelm the ability to reach a toilet in time. Causes include diuretics, excess fluid intake, and metabolic abnormalities (e.g., hyperglycemia, hypercalcemia, diabetes insipidus); nocturnal incontinence may result from mobilization of peripheral edema.
7. *Restricted mobility.* If mobility cannot be improved, access to a urinal or commode may restore continence. (See "Immobility" below.)
8. *Stool impaction.* This is a common cause of urinary incontinence, especially in hospitalized or immobile patients. Although the mechanism is unknown, a clue to its presence is the coexistence of both urinary and fecal incontinence. Disimpaction restores continence.

Established Incontinence (Table 9-3)   The causes of established incontinence include irreversible functional deficits, such as *end-stage* Alzheimer's disease, and intrinsic lower urinary tract dysfunction. Lower urinary tract dysfunction should be sought after transient causes have been excluded.

Detrusor Overactivity   This disorder (involuntary bladder contraction) accounts for two-thirds of geriatric incontinence in both sexes, regardless of whether patients are demented. Detrusor overactivity can be diagnosed presumptively in a woman when leakage occurs in the absence of stress maneuvers or urinary retention and is preceded by the abrupt onset of an intense urge to urinate that cannot be forestalled. In men, the symptoms are similar, but since detrusor overactivity often coexists with urethral obstruction, urodynamic testing should be done if prescription of a bladder relaxant is planned. Because detrusor overactivity also may be due to bladder stones or tumor, the abrupt onset of otherwise unexplained urge incontinence—especially if accompanied by perineal/suprapubic discomfort or sterile hematuria—should prompt cystoscopy and cytologic examination.

Table 9-4

Commonly Used Medications That May Affect Continence

Type of Medication	Examples	Potential Effects on Continence
Sedatives/hypnotics	Long-acting benzodiazepines (e.g., diazepam, flurazepam)	Sedation, delirium, immobility
Alcohol		Polyuria, frequency, urgency, sedation, delirium, immobility
Anticholinergics	Dicyclomine, disopyramide, antihistamines	Urinary retention, overflow incontinence, delirium, impaction
Antipsychotics	Thioridazine, haloperidol	Anticholinergic actions, sedation, rigidity, immobility
Antidepressants	Amitriptyline, desipramine	Anticholinergic actions, sedation
Antiparkinsonians	Trihexyphenidyl, benztropine mesylate (not L-dopa/selegiline)	Anticholinergic actions, sedation
Narcotic analgesics	Opiates	Urinary retention, fecal impaction, sedation, delirium
Alpha-adrenergic antagonists	Prazosin, terazosin, doxazosin	Urethral relaxation may precipitate stress incontinence in women
Alpha-adrenergic agonists	Nasal decongestants	Urinary retention in men
Calcium channel blockers	All dihydropyridines*	Urinary retention; nocturnal diuresis due to fluid retention
Potent diuretics	Furosemide, bumetanide	Polyuria, frequency, urgency
Angiotensin-converting enzyme inhibitors	Captopril, enalapril, lisinopril	Drug-induced cough can precipitate stress incontinence in women and in some men with prior prostatectomy
Vincristine		Urinary retention

* Examples include nifedipine, nicardipine, israpidine, felodipine, nimodipine.
SOURCE: Adapted from NM Resnick, in Current Medical Diagnosis and Treatment, LT Tierney et al (eds), Norwalk, Appleton & Lange, 1993.

 TREATMENT

The cornerstone of treatment is behavioral therapy. Patients without dementia are instructed to void every 1 to 2 h (while awake only) and to suppress urgency in between; once daytime continence is restored, the interval between voiding can be progressively increased. Demented patients are "prompted" to void at similar intervals. When drugs are necessary, they should be added to these regimens and monitored to avoid inducing urinary retention. Effective drugs include anticholinergics (e.g., propantheline, 7.5 to 30 mg three to five times daily), oxybutynin (2.5 to 5 mg three or four times daily), dicyclomine (10 to 30 mg three times daily), and imipramine or doxepin (25 to 100 mg at bedtime).

Indwelling catheterization is rarely indicated for detrusor overactivity. If all measures fail, an external collection device or protective pad or undergarment may be required.

Stress incontinence This disorder, the second most common cause of established incontinence in older women (it is rare in men), is characterized by symptoms and evidence of *instantaneous* leakage of urine in response to stress. Leakage is worse or occurs only during the day unless another abnormality (e.g., detrusor overactivity) is also present. On examination, with the bladder full and the perineum relaxed, instantaneous leakage upon coughing strongly suggests stress incontinence, especially if it reproduces symptoms and if urinary retention has been excluded by a postvoiding residual determination; a several-second delay suggests that leakage is instead caused by an involuntary bladder contraction induced by coughing.

TREATMENT
Surgery is the most effective treatment with a cure rate of 75 to 85 percent. For women who can comply indefinitely, pelvic muscle exercises are an option for mild to moderate stress incontinence; if not contraindicated, an alpha-adrenergic agonist (e.g., phenylpropanolamine) is also helpful in such cases, especially if combined with estrogen. Occasionally, a pessary or even a tampon (for women with vaginal stenosis) provides some relief.

Urethral obstruction Rarely present in women, urethral obstruction (due to prostatic enlargement, urethral stricture, bladder neck contracture, or prostate cancer) is the second most common cause of established incontinence in older men. It can present as dribbling incontinence after voiding, urge incontinence due to detrusor overactivity (which coexists in two-thirds of cases), or overflow incontinence due to urinary retention. Renal ultrasound is recommended to exclude hydronephrosis in men whose postvoiding residual volume exceeds 100 to 200 mL; in older men for whom surgery is planned, urodynamic confirmation of obstruction is strongly advised.

TREATMENT
Surgical decompression is the most effective treatment for obstruction, especially if there is urinary retention. For a nonoperative candidate, intermittent or indwelling catheterization is used; a condom catheter is contraindicated when urinary retention is present. For a man with prostatic obstruction who is not in retention, treatment with an alpha-adrenergic antagonist (e.g., terazosin 5 to 10 mg daily) may lessen symptoms in a few weeks. The 5α-reductase inhibitor finasteride also may ameliorate symptoms in a third or more of patients, but its impact is modest and not apparent for many months. Combined treatment with both agents has proved no better than treatment with an alpha blocker alone.

Detrusor underactivity Whether idiopathic or due to sacral lower motor nerve dysfunction, this is the least common cause of incontinence (<10 percent of cases). When it causes incontinence, detrusor underactivity is associated with urinary frequency, nocturia, and frequent leakage of small amounts. The elevated postvoiding residual volume (generally over 450 mL) distinguishes it from detrusor overactivity and stress incontinence, but only urodynamic testing (rather than cystoscopy or intravenous urography) differentiates it from urethral obstruction in men; such testing usually is not required in women, in whom obstruction is rare.

TREATMENT
For the patient with a poorly contractile bladder, augmented voiding techniques (e.g., double voiding or applying suprapubic pressure) are often effective; pharmacologic agents (e.g., bethanechol) are rarely effective. If further emptying is needed or for the patient with an acontractile bladder, intermittent or indwelling catheterization is the only option. Antibiotics should be used for symptomatic upper tract infection, or as prophylaxis for recurrent symptomatic infections only in a patient using intermittent catheterization; they should not be used as prophylaxis with an indwelling catheter.

FALLS Falls are a major problem for elderly people, especially women. Thirty percent of community-dwelling elderly fall each year, and the proportion increases with age. Nonetheless, falling must *not* be viewed as accidental, inevitable, or untreatable.

Causes of Falls Balance and ambulation require a complex interplay of cognitive, neuromuscular, and cardiovascular function and the ability to adapt rapidly to an environmental challenge. Balance becomes impaired and sway increases with age. The resulting vulnerability predisposes the older person to fall when challenged by an additional insult to *any* of these systems. Thus, a seemingly minor fall may be due to a serious problem, such as pneumonia or a myocardial infarction.

Much more commonly, however, falls are due to the complex interaction between a variably impaired patient and an environmental challenge. While a warped floorboard may pose little problem for a vigorous, unmedicated, alert person, it may be sufficient to precipitate a fall and hip fracture in the patient with impaired vision, strength, balance, or cognition. Thus, falls in older people are rarely due to a single cause, and effective prevention entails a comprehensive assessment of the patient's intrinsic deficits (usually diseases and medications), the routine activities, and the environmental obstacles.

Intrinsic deficits are those that impair sensory input, judgment, blood pressure regulation, reaction time, and balance and gait (Table 9-5). Medications and alcohol use are among the most common, significant, and reversible causes of falling. Other treatable contributors include postprandial hypotension (which peaks 30 to 60 min after a meal), insomnia, urinary urgency, foot problems, and peripheral edema (which can burden impaired leg strength and gait with an additional 5 to 10 pounds).

Environmental obstacles are listed in Table 9-6. Since most falls occur in or around the home, a visit by a visiting nurse, physical therapist, or physician often reaps substantial dividends.

Complications of Falls and Treatment One out of four people who fall suffers serious injury. Five percent of falls result in fractures, and an equal proportion cause serious soft tissue damage. Falls are the sixth leading cause of death for older people and a contributing factor in 40 percent of admissions to nursing homes. Resultant hip problems and fear of falls are major causes of loss of independence.

Subdural hematoma is a treatable but easily overlooked complication of falls that must be considered in any elderly patient presenting with new neurologic signs, including confusion alone, even in the absence of a headache. Dehydration, electrolyte imbalance, pressure sores, and hypothermia also may occur and endanger the patient's life following a fall.

The risk of falling and consequent injury, disability, and potential institutionalization can be reduced by modifying where possible those factors outlined above and in Tables 9-5 and 9-6. Gait training by a physical therapist often alleviates fear of falling. Ensuring the availability of phones at floor level, a portable phone, or a lightweight radio call system is also important.

IMMOBILITY The main causes of immobility are weakness, stiffness, pain, imbalance, and psychological problems. Weakness may result from disuse of muscles, malnutrition, electrolyte disturbances, anemia, neurologic disorders, or myopathies. The most common cause of stiffness in the elderly is osteoarthritis; however, Parkinson's disease, rheumatoid arthritis, gout, pseudogout, and antipsychotic drugs such as haloperidol may also contribute. Pain, whether from bone (e.g., osteoporosis, osteomalacia, Paget's disease, metastatic bone cancer, trauma), joints (e.g., osteoarthritis, rheumatoid arthritis, gout), bursa, muscle (e.g., polymyalgia rheumatica, intermittent claudication, or "pseudoclaudication"), or foot problems may immobilize the patient.

Imbalance and fear of falling are major causes of immobilization. Imbalance may result from general debility, neurologic causes (e.g., stroke; loss of postural reflexes; peripheral neuropathy due to diabetes mellitus, alcohol, or malnutrition; and vestibulocerebellar abnormalities), orthostatic or postprandial hypotension, or drugs (e.g., diuretics, antihypertensives, neuroleptics, and antidepressants) or may occur following prolonged bed rest. Psychological conditions such as severe anxiety or depression also may contribute to immobilization.

Consequences In addition to thrombophlebitis and pulmonary embolus, there are multiple hazards of bed rest in the elderly. Deconditioning of the cardiovascular system occurs within days and involves fluid shifts, fluid loss, decreased cardiac output, decreased peak oxygen uptake, and increased resting heart rate. Striking changes also occur in skeletal muscle. At the cellular level, intracellular ATP and glycogen concentrations decrease, rates of protein degradation increase, and contractile velocity and strength decline, while at the whole-muscle level, atrophy, weakness, and shortening are seen. Pressure sores are another serious complication; mechanical pressure, moisture, friction, and shearing forces all predispose to their development. As a result, within days of being confined to bed, the risk of postural hypotension, falls, and skin breakdown rises. Moreover, these changes usually take weeks to months to reverse.

℞ TREATMENT

The most important step is preventive—to avoid bedrest whenever possible. When it cannot be avoided, several measures can be employed to minimize its consequences. Patients should be positioned as close to the upright position as possible several times daily. Range of motion exercises should begin immediately, and the skin over pressure points should be inspected frequently. Isometric and isotonic exercises should be performed while the patient is in bed, and whenever possible patients should assist their own positioning, transferring, and self-care. As mobility becomes feasible, graduated ambulation should begin. For individuals confined to a wheelchair, ring-shaped devices ("donuts") should not be used to prevent pressure ulcers since they cause venous congestion and edema and actually increase the risk.

If a pressure ulcer develops, therapy depends on its stage. Stage 1 ulcers are characterized by nonblanchable erythema of intact skin; stage 2 lesions involve an ulcer of the epidermis, dermis, or both; stage 3 ulcers extend to the subcutaneous tissue; and stage 4 lesions involve muscle, bone, and/or the supporting tissues. For stage 1 lesions, eliminating excess pressure and ensuring adequate nutrition and hygiene are sufficient. For the remaining types, the caregiver must also ensure that the wound stays clean and moist; thus, if saline dressings are used they should be changed when they are damp rather than dry. Synthetic dressings are more expensive than saline but are more effective because they require fewer changes (with less disruption of reepithelialization) and protect against contamination. Because bacterial colonization of pressure ulcers is universal, swab cultures should not be performed and topical treatment should be considered only for patients whose ulcers have not healed after 2 weeks of therapy. By contrast, associated cellulitis, osteomyelitis, or sepsis requires systemic therapy after cultures of blood and the wound border (by needle aspiration or biopsy) have been obtained. Surgical or enzymatic debridement is required for stage 3 and 4 lesions. In addition to a daily multivitamin, prescribing vitamin C (500 mg twice daily) is also useful. For debilitated patients, special mattresses are beneficial, including those that reduce pressure (e.g., static air mattress or foam) and those that relieve it (e.g., dynamic units that sequentially inflate and deflate).

In addition to treating all identified factors that contribute to immobility, consultation with a physical therapist should be sought. Installing handrails, lowering the bed, and providing chairs of proper height with arms and rubber skid guards may allow the patient to be safely mobile in the home. A properly fitted cane or walker may be helpful.

IATROGENIC DRUG REACTIONS For several reasons, older patients are two or three times more likely to have adverse drug reactions (Chap. 69). Drug clearance is often markedly reduced. This

Table 9-5

Intrinsic Risk Factors for Falling, and Possible Interventions

Risk Factor	Interventions	
	Medical	Rehabilitative or Environmental
Reduced visual acuity, dark adaptation, and perception	Refraction; cataract extraction	Home safety assessment
Reduced hearing	Removal of cerumen; audiologic evaluation	Hearing aid if appropriate (with training); reduction in background noise
Vestibular dysfunction	Avoidance of drugs affecting the vestibular system; neurologic or ear, nose, and throat evaluation, if indicated	Habituation exercises
Proprioceptive dysfunction, cervical degenerative disorders, and peripheral neuropathy	Screening for vitamin B_{12} deficiency and cervical spondylosis	Balance exercises; appropriate walking aid; correctly sized footwear with firm soles; home safety assessment
Dementia	Detection of reversible causes; avoidance of sedative or centrally acting drugs	Supervised exercise and ambulation; home safety assessment
Musculoskeletal disorders	Appropriate diagnostic evaluation	Balance-and-gait training; muscle-strengthening exercises; appropriate walking aid; home safety assessment
Foot disorders (calluses, bunions, deformities, edema)	Shaving of calluses; bunionectomy; treatment of edema	Trimming of nails; appropriate footwear
Postural hypotension	Assessment of medications; rehydration; possible alteration in situational factors (e.g., meals, change of position)	Dorsiflexion exercises; pressure-graded stockings; elevation of head of bed; use of tilt table if condition is severe
Use of medications (sedatives: benzodiazepines, phenothiazines, antidepressants; antihypertensives; others: antiarrhythmics, anticonvulsants, diuretics, alcohol)	Steps to be taken: 1. Attempted reduction in the total number of medications taken 2. Assessment of risks and benefits of each medication 3. Selection of medication, if needed, that is least centrally acting, least associated with postural hypotension, and has shortest action 4. Prescription of lowest effective dose 5. Frequent reassessment of risks and benefits	

SOURCE: After ME Tinetti and M Speechley, N Engl J Med 320:1055, 1989.

Table 9-6

Environmental Factors Affecting the Risk of Falling

Environmental Area or Factor	Objective and Recommendations
All areas	
Lighting	Adequacy of illumination (older people need twice as much as younger people); absence of glare and shadows; accessible switches at room entrances; night light in bedroom, hall, bathroom
Floors	Nonskid backing for throw rugs; carpet edges tacked down; carpets with shallow pile; nonskid wax on floors; cords out of walking path; small objects (e.g., clothes, shoes) off floor
Stairs	Lighting sufficient, with switches at top and bottom of stairs; securely fastened bilateral handrails that stand out from wall; top and bottom steps marked with bright, contrasting tape; stair rises of no more than 6 in; steps in good repair; no objects stored on steps
Kitchen	Items stored so that reaching up and bending over are not necessary; secure step stool available if climbing is necessary; firm, nonmovable table
Bathroom	Grab bars for tub, shower, and toilet; nonskid decals or rubber mat in tub or shower; shower chair with handheld shower; nonskid rugs; raised toilet seat; door locks removed to ensure access in an emergency
Yard and entrances	Repair of cracks in pavement, holes in lawn; removal of rocks, tools, and other tripping hazards; well-lit walkways, free of ice and wet leaves; stairs and steps as above
Institutions	All the above; bed at proper height (not too high or low); spills on floor cleaned up promptly; appropriate use of walking aids and wheelchairs
Footwear	Shoes with firm, nonskid, nonfriction soles; low heels (unless person is accustomed to high heels); avoidance of walking in stocking feet or loose slippers

SOURCE: After ME Tinetti and M Speechley, N Engl J Med 320:1055, 1989.

is due to a decrease in renal plasma flow and glomerular filtration rate and a reduced hepatic clearance. The last is due to a decrease in activity of the drug-metabolizing microsomal enzymes and an overall decline in blood flow to the liver with aging. The volume of distribution of drugs also is affected, since the elderly have a decrease in total body water and a relative increase in body fat. Thus, water-soluble drugs become more concentrated, and fat-soluble drugs have longer half-lives. In addition, serum albumin levels decline, particularly in sick patients, so that there is a decrease in protein binding of some drugs (e.g., warfarin, phenytoin), leaving more free (active) drug available.

In addition to impaired drug clearance, which alters pharmacokinetics, older patients have altered responses to similar serum drug levels, a phenomenon known as altered pharmacodynamics. They are more sensitive to some drugs (e.g., opiates, anticoagulants) and less sensitive to others (e.g., beta-adrenergic agents). Finally, the older patient with multiple chronic conditions is likely to be taking several drugs, including nonprescribed agents. Thus, adverse drug reactions and dosage errors are more likely to occur, especially if the patient has visual, hearing, or memory deficits.

Precautions to Avoid Drug Toxicity *Drug selection and administration* Before initiating treatment, the physician should first ensure that the symptom requiring treatment is not itself due to another drug. For example, antipsychotic agents can cause symptoms that mimic depression (flat affect, restlessness, and pacing); such symptoms should prompt lowering of the dose rather than initiation of an antidepressant. In addition, drug therapy should be employed only after nonpharmacologic means have been considered or tried and only when the benefit clearly outweighs the risk.

Once pharmacotherapy has been decided upon, it should begin at less than the usual adult dosage and the dose should be increased slowly. However, given the marked variability in pharmacokinetics and pharmacodynamics in the elderly, dose escalation should continue until either a successful endpoint is reached or an intolerable side effect is encountered. The final dosage schedule should be kept as simple as possible and the number of pills should be kept as low as possible. Serum drug levels are often useful in older patients, especially for monitoring drugs with narrow therapeutic indices such as phenytoin, theophylline, quinidine, aminoglycosides, lithium, and psychotropic agents such as nortriptyline. However, toxicity can occur even with "normal" therapeutic levels of some drugs (e.g., digoxin, phenytoin).

Over-the-counter agents Nearly three-quarters of the elderly regularly use nonprescribed drugs, many of which cause significant symptoms. Frequent offenders include nonprescribed agents for insomnia (all of which are anticholinergics), and nonsteroidal anti-inflammatory drugs (NSAIDs), which can hamper control of hypertension in addition to causing renal dysfunction, and gastrointestinal bleeding. Because older patients often consider such agents "nostrums" rather than drugs, the physician must ask about them directly.

Sedative-hypnotics If nonpharmacologic treatment of insomnia is unsuccessful, short-term use of an intermediate-acting agent whose metabolism is not affected by age (e.g., oxazepam, 10 to 30 mg/d) may be useful. Because of the increased risk of confusion and other adverse effects, benzodiazepines with either short (e.g., triazolam) or long duration of action (e.g., flurazepam and diazepam) should be avoided. An antidepressant should not be prescribed for insomnia unless the patient is depressed.

Antibiotics Serum creatinine is not a good index of renal function in old people; however, when it is elevated special care must be taken with the administration of drugs normally excreted by the kidneys. Concentrations of relevant antibiotics should be measured directly.

Cardiac drugs In older patients, digitalis, procainamide, and quinidine have prolonged half-lives and narrow therapeutic windows; toxicity is common at the usual dosages. For example, digoxin toxicity—especially anorexia, confusion, or depression—can occur even with therapeutic digoxin levels.

H_2 *receptor antagonists* Most of these agents interfere with hepatic metabolism of other drugs, and all can produce confusion in the elderly. Because they are renally excreted, lower doses should be used to minimize the risk of toxicity in older individuals.

Antidepressants and antipsychotics These drugs can produce anticholinergic side effects in old people (e.g., confusion, urinary retention, constipation, dry mouth). This can be minimized by switching to a nonanticholinergic agent (e.g., sertraline or trazodone) or one with less anticholinergic effect (e.g., desipramine). In general, the least potent agents for psychosis (e.g., chlorpromazine) have the most sedating and anticholinergic effects and are the most likely to induce postural hypotension. By contrast, the most potent antipsychotic agents (e.g., haloperidol) have the least sedating, anticholinergic, and hypotensive side effects but cause extrapyramidal side effects, including dystonia, akathisia, rigidity, and tardive dyskinesia. Thus all of these agents are potentially toxic. Moreover, since both depression and agitation often remit spontaneously, cautious discontinuation of these drugs should be considered periodically.

Glaucoma medications Both topical beta-blockers and carbonic anhydrase inhibitors can cause systemic side effects. The latter can cause malaise and anorexia independent of the induced metabolic acidosis.

Anticoagulants Elderly patients benefit from anticoagulation as much as do younger individuals but are more vulnerable to serious bleeding. Hence, more careful monitoring and less aggressive anticoagulation are advisable.

Avoid overtreatment Drugs are not necessarily indicated in some common clinical situations. For instance, antibiotics need not be given for asymptomatic bacteriuria unless obstructive uropathy, other anatomic abnormalities, or stones are also present. Ankle edema is often due to venous insufficiency, drugs such as NSAIDs or some calcium antagonists, or even inactivity or malnutrition in chairbound patients. Diuretics are usually not indicated unless edema is associated with heart failure. Fitted, pressure gradient stockings are often helpful. Regular exercise is much more useful for claudication than is pentoxyfylline. Finally, since older patients generally tolerate aspirin and other NSAIDs less well than do younger patients, localized pain should be treated when possible with local measures such as injection, physical therapy, heat, ultrasound, or transcutaneous electrical stimulation (see Chap. 12).

PREVENTION

Much can be done to prevent the progression and even the onset of disease in older people. Dietary inadequacies in the elderly should be corrected. Daily calcium intake should approximate 1500 mg, and most elderly people should take 400 to 800 IU of vitamin D daily (contained in one to two multivitamin tablets). Tobacco and alcohol use should be minimized, since the benefits of discontinuing these accrue even to individuals over age 65. The importance of reviewing all of a patient's medications and discontinuing them whenever feasible cannot be overemphasized.

The benefits of treating both isolated systolic hypertension and combined systolic and diastolic hypertension in ambulatory elderly have now been documented. Treatment reduces the risk of stroke and the risk of death due to cardiovascular causes in this age group. Conclusive results have been achieved using *low doses* of a thiazide-like diuretic (e.g., chlorthalidone, 12.5 to 25 mg/d) as the first step (alone effective in almost half of patients) and adding low-dose reserpine (0.05 to 0.1 mg/d) or atenolol (25 to 50 mg/d) only as needed. Benefits are dramatic, side effects are minimal, cost is trivial, and concerns about potential toxicity have not been borne out.

Because of the prevalence, functional impact, and ease of treatment, glaucoma should be screened for, and visual and auditory impairment should be corrected. Dentures should be assessed for their fit, and oral lesions beneath them should be detected.

Because thyroid dysfunction is more prevalent in the elderly, difficult to detect clinically, and treatable, serum levels of thyroid-stimulating hormone should be measured at least once in asymptomatic older people. Serum cholesterol is worth measuring in those with established coronary heart disease, but in those without apparent disease, screening for hypercholesterolemia is controversial. It seems reasonable to screen those who would be willing to comply with therapy, whose quality of life is good (from the patient's viewpoint), whose life expectancy exceeds several years (long enough to potentially benefit from therapy), and whose other risk factors—for which benefit of treatment has been definitely established—have already been addressed. A Papanicolaou test should be done in women who have not had one before, since the incidence of both preventable cervical carcinoma and associated death increases with age, especially in this group; it should be repeated triennially in all older women unless two previous tests have been normal. Immunizations for influenza, pneumococcal pneumonia, and tetanus should be current. PPD testing should be done on residents of chronic care facilities and on others at high risk of tuberculosis; those who have recently converted probably should be treated. Since responsiveness wanes with age, the test, if negative, should be repeated in a week to increase the chances of detecting all exposed patients. Because older women with breast cancer are more likely to die *of* it than *with* it, screening mammography is indicated every 1 to 2 years at least until age 75 and thereafter if a positive finding would result in therapeutic intervention. The relative risks and benefits of low-dose aspirin and (for women) estrogen replacement therapy have not yet been elucidated sufficiently in the elderly to warrant routine use, but they should be considered on an individual basis.

Exercise should be encouraged not only because of its beneficial effects on blood pressure, cardiovascular conditioning, glucose homeostasis, bone density, and functional status, but also because it may improve mood and social interaction, reduce insomnia and constipation, and prevent falls. Spinal flexion exercises should be avoided in patients with osteopenia; consultation with a physical therapist may be helpful.

Measures should be taken to prevent falling, as outlined in Tables 9-5 and 9-6. Counseling about driving is important, especially for patients with cognitive impairment. But perhaps the most valuable procedure for prevention of disease in old people is to take a careful history, focusing not only on the "chief complaint" but also on common and often hidden conditions such as falls, confusion, depression, sexual dysfunction, and incontinence. In addition, one should always identify the complications for which the specific patient is at risk and take steps to avert them. For instance, a patient with cognitive impairment who smokes is at risk not only for lung cancer but also for starting a fire, and a patient who requires narcotics is at risk for fecal impaction, delirium, urinary retention, and confusion. Community-dwelling patients who are at highest risk of rapid deterioration and institutionalization and who should be monitored more closely include those over age 80, those who live alone, those who are bereaved or depressed, and those who are intellectually impaired.

BIBLIOGRAPHY

BIOLOGY OF AGING

MASORO EJ (ed): *Handbook of Physiology.* Section 11: *Aging.* New York: Oxford Univ Press (for the American Physiological Society), 1995
RUSTING RL: Why do we age? Sci Am 12:130, 1992
VIJG J, WEI JY: Understanding the biology of aging: The key to prevention and therapy. J Am Geriatr Soc 43:426, 1995
WEINDRUCH R: Caloric restriction and aging. Sci Am 273(1):46, 1996

FUNCTIONAL ASSESSMENT

CORTI M-C et al: Serum albumin and physical disability as predictors of mortality in older persons. JAMA 272:1036, 1994
GURALNIK JM et al: Lower-extremity function in persons over the age of 70 years as a predictor of subsequent disability. N Engl J Med 332:556, 1995
IKEGAMI N: Functional assessment and its place in health care. N Engl J Med 332:598, 1995
LACHS MS et al: A simple procedure for general screening for functional disability in elderly patients. Ann Intern Med 112:699, 1990

DEMENTIA, DELIRIUM, DEPRESSION

CARLSON DL et al: Management of dementia-related behavioral disturbances: A nonpharmacologic approach. Mayo Clin Proc 70:1108, 1995
FLEMING KC, EVANS MD: Pharmacologic therapies in dementia. Mayo Clin Proc 70:1116, 1995
INOUYE SK: The dilemma of delirium: Clinical and research controversies regarding diagnosis and evaluation of delirium in hospitalized elderly medical patients. Am J Med 97:278, 1994
NIH CONSENSUS DEVELOPMENT PANEL: Diagnosis and treatment of depression in late life. JAMA 268:1018, 1992
RUMMANS TA et al: Delirium in elderly patients: Evaluation and management. Mayo Clin Proc 70:989, 1995

URINARY INCONTINENCE

OUSLANDER JG, SCHNELLE JF: Incontinence in the nursing home. Ann Intern Med 122:438, 1995
RESNICK NM: Urinary incontinence. Lancet 346:94, 1995

FALLS/IMMOBILITY/PRESSURE ULCERS

BERGSTROM N et al: *Treatment of Pressure Ulcers.* Clinical Practice Guideline, No. 15. Rockville, MD: US Department of Health and Human Services, Public Health Service, Agency for Health Care Policy and Research (AHCPR) publication NO. 95-0652. December 1994
RUBENSTEIN LZ et al: Falls in the nursing home. Ann Intern Med 121:442, 1994
TINETTI ME et al: A multifactorial intervention to reduce the risk of falling among elderly people living in the community. N Engl J Med 331:821, 1994

GERIATRIC PHARMACOLOGY

AVORN J, GURWITZ JH: Drug use in the nursing home. Ann Intern Med 123:195, 1995
NIH CONSENSUS CONFERENCE: Optimal calcium intake. JAMA 272:1942, 1994
ROCHON PA, GURWITZ JH: Drug therapy. Lancet 346:32, 1995

PREVENTION

DENKE MA, WINKER MA: Cholesterol and coronary heart disease in older adults: No easy answers. JAMA 274:575, 1995

FABACHER D et al: An in-home preventive assessment program for independent older adults: A randomized controlled trial. J Am Geriatr Soc 42:630, 1994

FIATARONE MA et al: Exercise training and nutritional supplementation for physical frailty in very old people. N Engl J Med 330:1769, 1994

FLAHERTY JH: Driving and older persons. Clin Geriat 3(3):44, 1995

KERLIKOWSKE K et al: Efficacy of screening mammography. A meta-analysis. JAMA 273:149, 1995

MARTINEZ R: Older drivers and physicians. JAMA 274:1060, 1995

MULROW CD et al: Hypertension in the elderly. JAMA 272:1932, 1994

US PREVENTIVE SERVICE TASK FORCE: Guide to Clinical Preventive Services, 2d ed. Baltimore, Williams & Wilkins, 1996

MISCELLANEOUS

HARRIS J: The treatment of cancer in an aging population. JAMA 268:96, 1992

JANSEN REMM, LIPSITZ LA: Postprandial hypotension: Epidemiology, pathophysiology, and clinical management. Ann Intern Med 122:286, 1995

LIBOW LS, STARER P: Care of the nursing home patient. N Engl J Med 321:93, 1989

WEBER DC et al: Rehabilitation of geriatric patients. Mayo Clin Proc 70:1198, 1995

---

10   *Maureen T. Connelly, Thomas S. Inui*

PRINCIPLES OF DISEASE PREVENTION

PERSPECTIVES ON PREVENTION

The primary goals of prevention in medicine are to prolong life, to decrease morbidity, and to improve quality of life—all with the available resources. Working in partnership with patients, physicians play critical roles as educators, managers of access to screening and intervention services, and interpreters of divergent recommendations for promoting health. Despite evidence of the effectiveness of many preventive services in prolonging healthy life and decreasing medical costs, physicians frequently do not integrate appropriate preventive practices into their care. Obstacles to providing optimal preventive care include lack of appropriate training, doubt about the effectiveness of preventive interventions, skepticism about patients' commitment to change, limited reimbursement and time, and conflicting professional recommendations. Success achieved for populations may not be visible to individuals, and physicians may not appreciate the cumulative benefit of their efforts. Despite considerable success in some areas, such as the reduction of smoking by U.S. adults from 40 percent to 25 percent in the last 30 years, effective behavior change in other domains is often elusive, challenging and frustrating physicians and patients alike.

DEFINITIONS   This chapter will be devoted to a discussion of *primary* and *secondary* prevention. Primary prevention, including various forms of health promotion and vaccination, is care intended to minimize risk factors and the subsequent incidence of disease. Secondary prevention is screening for detection of early disease, for example the use of mammography to detect preclinical breast cancer. While the term *secondary prevention* is also sometimes used for the prevention of recurrent episodes of an existing illness, most would consider this activity to be *tertiary prevention*, care intended to ameliorate the course of established disease.

Deciding what types of primary and secondary preventive care clinicians should offer to their patients is not a trivial matter. The United States Preventive Services Task Force (USPSTF), The Canadian Task Force on the Periodic Health Examination, and the American College of Physicians, among other organizations, have critically re-

viewed the strength of available evidence for preventive practices and have made recommendations. Adopting an evidence-based approach to the development of preventive practices policy is an essential step to assuaging provider concerns about the validity of particular recommendations, to identifying the specific basis of controversies in prevention, and to reassuring patients that certain interventions will do more good than harm.

PRIMARY PREVENTION

RISK MODIFICATION   Of the more than 2 million deaths that occur in the United States each year, as many as half may be due to preventable causes (Table 10-1). Life-style and behavior play a central role in the primary causes of morbidity and mortality for adults—coronary heart disease, cancer, and injuries.

Tobacco   Perhaps the largest potentially modifiable risk to health is the abuse of tobacco products. Responsible for more than 400,000 deaths each year and an estimated annual cost to society as high as $50 billion, tobacco abuse accounts for a substantial fraction of cardiovascular, cancer, and pulmonary morbidity and mortality. Recent evidence also suggests that passive exposure to tobacco smoke results in chronic pulmonary disease as well as lung cancer for some adults. Because of the addictive properties of nicotine, preventing the initiation of tobacco abuse is the tobacco control intervention of choice. Most adult smokers acquire their habit as teenagers, and primary efforts to discourage initial tobacco use must engage younger audiences.

Counseling regarding the health risks of tobacco and methods for quitting is advised by all prevention advisory panels. Particular attention should be paid to groups at highest risk for tobacco abuse, such as men, blacks, and those with only a high school education or less. Because 70 percent of smokers come into contact with health professionals each year, the medical encounter provides an opportunity to address the health implications of tobacco abuse. Ninety percent of successful quitters will stop smoking without the aid of programmatic interventions. A review of smoking habits, recommendation to stop, and support from a health care provider may generate the impetus for an individual to make an effort to stop smoking. Respect for patients' self-efficacy, reflected in questions such as "What do you understand about the health consequences of smoking?", "Are you ready to quit?", and "What would it take for you to stop smoking?" has been suggested as a means to engage patients in the process. Setting a date to quit, arranging follow-up visits or phone calls during the initial quitting period, providing literature, and considering the use of nicotine replacement systems for those who will completely desist from the use of other tobacco products are all interventions that may improve the quitting success rate.

Table 10-1

Actual Causes of Preventable Deaths in the United States in 1990

	Deaths	
Cause	**Estimated No.***	**Percentage of Total Deaths**
Tobacco	400,000	19
Diet/activity patterns	300,000	14
Alcohol	100,000	5
Microbial agents	90,000	4
Toxic agents	60,000	3
Firearms	35,000	2
Sexual behavior	30,000	1
Motor vehicles	25,000	1
Illicit use of drugs	20,000	<1
TOTAL	1,060,000	50

* Composite approximation drawn from studies that use different approaches to derive estimates, ranging from actual counts (e.g., firearms) to population attributable risk calculations (e.g., tobacco). Numbers over 100,000 are rounded to the nearest 100,000; those over 50,000 are rounded to the nearest 10,000; those below 50,000 are rounded to the nearest 5000.

SOURCE: McGinnis JM, Foege WH: Actual causes of death in the United States. JAMA 270:2207, 1993.

Alcohol and Drugs The use of alcohol and drugs accounts for more than 100,000 deaths annually. While the ability of health care providers to prevent the initiation of such behaviors has not been proven, screening for exposure and addiction could potentially direct medical effort to the prevention of alcohol and drug-associated problems such as injury, violence, and medical complications of drug abuse. Although instruments such as the CAGE questionnaire have proven to be valuable for detection of alcohol abuse, no comparable brief screening strategy is available for the routine identification of illicit drug abuse. Health care providers screen inadequately for both disorders, despite evidence for effective early treatment of addictions and their complications. Recent data suggesting that moderate alcohol intake may prevent heart disease for some individuals and the lack of a biologic "gold standard" criterion for alcoholism contribute to difficulties in diagnosing alcohol abuse. Legal implications of identifying illicit drug use may hinder detection of this problem. When screening for these disorders is feasible, interventions that have proven effective include brief counseling, referral to ambulatory and in-patient treatment programs, use of 12-step and other community organizations, and appropriate use of medications such as methadone for heroin abuse.

Diet Mounting evidence suggests that modification of caloric intake, both quantity and quality, can result in decreased morbidity and mortality from cardiovascular disease, cancer, and diabetes. Excess weight is an independent risk factor for coronary disease, in addition to its contribution to the incidence of diabetes, hyperlipidemia, and hypertension. Between 20 and 30 percent of Americans are overweight, defined as 20 percent above the acceptable body-mass index (kg/m^2), and more than 40 percent of certain subpopulations, such as black, Native American, and Mexican-American women, are overweight.

Americans derive excess calories from fats, particularly saturated fats, rather than from more beneficial sources such as complex carbohydrates and fiber. Since intake of saturated fat correlates with cholesterol level, and coronary heart disease is reduced by 2 to 3 percent for every 1 percent reduction in plasma cholesterol level, dietary modification will play a central role in decreasing the primary cause of mortality in America. Excess dietary fat intake has also been associated with breast, colon, prostate, and lung cancer in epidemiologic studies. Reducing calories from all fats to 30 percent and from saturated fat to 10 percent are widely accepted goals. Increasing the intake of dietary fiber, such as from plant, legume, and grain sources, may contribute specifically to a decrease in colon cancer incidence.

Dietary sodium restriction may benefit those who have salt-sensitive hypertension, although the need for such restriction in the general population is unclear. Calcium and vitamin D are protective against osteoporosis, particularly in young women prior to reaching menopause, and evidence suggests that females at all ages have an inadequate intake. Menstruating women are at risk for iron-deficiency anemia. To achieve the recommended daily intake of vitamins and minerals, a varied diet including fish, lean meats, dairy products, whole grains, and five to six servings of fruits and vegetables daily is recommended, rather than the use of vitamin supplements. While evidence supporting the use of antioxidants such as vitamins E and C is still incomplete, the recommended quantities of these micronutrients can be obtained from a balanced diet. Physicians play a critical role in effecting dietary change in their patients. The value of providing counseling and literature, referring patients to appropriate community groups and nutrition professionals, and helping patients set goals and limits for diet modification cannot be overemphasized. Despite concern about the risk of weight cycling, the health hazards of obesity appear to outweigh the potential harm of repeated weight loss and gain.

Physical Activity A key counterpart to decreased caloric intake is increased energy expenditure. Not only can increased physical activity decrease obesity, but avoiding a sedentary life-style can also decrease the incidence of cardiac disease, hypertension, diabetes, and osteoporosis. It is estimated that only 22 percent of U.S. adults engage in at least light to moderate physical activity, such as walking for 30 min three to five times per week. A full quarter of the population pursues no vigorous physical activity at all. The magnitude of benefit derived from physical activity may be as great as a 35 percent reduction in coronary heart disease, and even light exercise is preferable to no exercise. While the ultimate goal for optimal cardioprotective physical activity is 20 to 30 min of vigorous activity most days of the week, patients should be encouraged to approach this level gradually. A sudden onset of vigorous activity in the unfit may increase the risk for myocardial infarction and sudden death. Patients should be informed that, despite previous physical inactivity, the incremental adoption of a regular fitness program can decrease their risk of cardiovascular and other diseases to the level of those who have remained fit throughout their lives. Successful exercise programs are integrated into daily routines, self-directed, and injury-free.

Sexual Behavior Because of the substantial risks of infectious diseases and unwanted pregnancy from unprotected sexual activity, patients should be strongly advised to use barrier methods for all high-risk practices such as oral, anal, and vaginal intercourse as well as additional contraceptive methods when pregnancy would not be welcome.

Environment Physicians should adopt a broad construction of environmental risks to health, considering the physical, social, and occupational environments of their patients. Taking a complete exposure history, focusing on home, work, neighborhood, hobbies, and dietary habits can help direct interventions and recommendations. While local circumstances will dictate specific risks to which patients should be alerted, such as regional infectious diseases or particular toxic exposures produced by local industry, certain general recommendations should be adopted universally for health promotion.

Since skin cancers, the vast majority of them secondary to sun exposure, constitute the most common form of malignancy, all patients should be counseled to avoid sun overexposure and to use sunscreens. Patients should be encouraged to consider potential toxin exposures, such as those due to air pollution, household smoking, or carbon monoxide and radon gases, and be informed of the medical symptoms and consequences of such exposures. Proper food preparation and storage decrease the incidence of food-borne infectious disease.

Unintended injury constitutes a significant preventable burden of morbidity and mortality and is the leading cause of death for the general population under 40. Automobile accidents are the leading cause of unintentional injuries. The risk of being involved in a disabling traffic accident may be as high as 30 percent in the course of an individual's lifetime, and 50 percent of deaths from automobile accidents could be prevented with regular seatbelt use. Physicians should recommend seatbelt use, as well as helmet use for motorcycle and bicycle riders, since evidence supports a higher likelihood of use among patients who receive such advice. Clinicians should also recommend against operating a motor vehicle after drinking, since alcohol (and illicit drugs) is a clear-cut risk cofactor.

Smoke detectors are underused, being found in only 80 percent of homes. Since most deaths due to fire occur in the residential setting, patients should be encouraged to install at least one on each floor of their home.

Attention to health hazards in the workplace can identify those at risk and prevent long-term consequences of exposure. Evaluation of the work environment should include questions about exposure to metals, dusts, fibers, chemicals, fumes, radiation, loud noises, extreme temperatures, and biologic agents.

Community and family violence, particularly through the misuse of firearms, is the second leading cause of death from unintentional injury. Firearms, especially handguns, are far more likely to injure a family member than an intruder and are associated with increased rates of suicide and harm to children. Patients should be encouraged to remove their weapons from the home and should be informed of the risks associated with improper security and storage of firearms. While community and family violence are epidemic in the United States, interventions to curtail violent behavior are not well established. Screening for exposure to relationship violence, developing plans for safe havens, and referrals to appropriate community and government agencies can prevent continued abuse.

IMMUNIZATION As many as 70,000 deaths due to influenza, pneumococcal infections, and hepatitis B occur in the United States annually. Despite good availability and evidence for the cost-effectiveness of recommended vaccinations for adults, only 40 percent or fewer members of target populations are immunized. Factors explaining poor adherence to adult immunization guidelines include lack of confidence in vaccine efficacy among providers and patients, underestimation of the severity of the target diseases, incomplete reimbursement, lack of systems to identify and vaccinate high-risk populations, and the absence of an adult requirement for vaccination equivalent to our vaccination policies for school-age children. Table 10-2 lists recommended adult immunizations.

CHEMOPROPHYLAXIS There is significant supportive evidence for the use of certain medications in primary prevention. Therapy of this nature in the otherwise healthy person, however, is not risk-free. The use of aspirin for the prevention of cardiovascular disease or colorectal cancer, for example, is supported by evidence from cohort and, in the case of cardiovascular disease, randomized controlled trials. The potential for cerebral bleeds and gastrointestinal intolerance, however, must be balanced against a patient's individual risk for the target diseases. Although no randomized trials have measured the impact on mortality, postmenopausal hormone replacement therapy is another therapy given to healthy women for the prevention of future disease (coronary heart disease and osteoporosis), as well as to control menopausal symptoms. These benefits must be weighed against the risks of possible breast and endometrial carcinoma. Patient involvement in the decision-making process, perhaps even informed consent, is

recommended to ensure compliance, proper use of medication, and sustained monitoring for side effects.

SECONDARY PREVENTION

SCREENING Widespread screening for the presence of existing diseases should meet the following criteria:

1. The targeted disease must be sufficiently burdensome to the population that a screening program is warranted. Minor changes in relative risk should have a substantial impact on the absolute risk within the population.
2. The target disease must have a well-understood natural history with a long preclinical latent period.
3. The screening method must have acceptable technical performance parameters, detecting the disease at an earlier stage than would be possible without screening and minimizing false-positive and false-negative results.
4. Efficacious treatment for the target illness must be available.
5. Early detection must improve disease outcome.
6. Cost, feasibility, and acceptability of screening and early treatment should be established.

While physicians underprovide certain screening services that have met these criteria (for example, regular mammograms for women over age 50 years), it is also the case that some prevalent screening practices today are not solidly rooted in evidence. Screening tests such as measurement of prostate-specific antigen and mammography in women under 50 have been adopted for use by many clinicians despite lack of complete current evidence that these services will decrease the risk of morbidity or mortality or improve the quality of life. See Table 10-2 recommendations of the USPSTF for screening of adults who are at average risk for target conditions. Recommendations for special-risk and vulnerable populations are available in the USPSTF *Guide*.

COMMUNITY HEALTH ADVOCACY

In addition to the direct clinical provision of preventive and health-promoting services, physicians can bring their knowledge, expertise, clinical experience, and influence to bear at the community level to promote health. Whether arguing for the denormalization of tobacco use or providing data about the health risks of local incinerators, physicians are the important sources of information and support for improving health beyond the clinical office. Such activities are consistent with the overall objective of caring for patients and may have a substantial impact on decreasing the prevalence of the root causes of disease.

Table 10-2

Recommendations for Preventive Medical Care

Screening
 Blood pressure
 Height and weight
 Pap smear
 FOBT and/or sigmoidoscopy*
 Mammography ± breast exam†
 Assess for problem drinking
 Total blood cholesterol (men aged 35 to 64, women aged 45 to 64>
 Vision screening‡
 Assess for hearing impairment‡
Counseling
 Tobacco cessation
 Avoidance of alcohol and drugs when driving, swimming, boating
 Limitation of fat, cholesterol
 Maintenance of caloric balance
 Emphasis on grains, fruits, vegetables in diet
 Adequate calcium
 Physical activity
 Lap/shoulder belts
 Motorcycle and bicycle helmets
 Smoke detectors
 Storage or removal of firearms
 STD prevention
 Dental visits, fluoride, flossing
 Contraception
 Fall prevention‡
 CPR training for household‡
 Hot water heater at <120°‡
Immunization
 Tetanus-diphtheria (Td)
 Pneumococcal vaccine‡
 Influenza vaccine‡
Chemoprophylaxis
 Discussion of hormone replacement therapy with perimenopausal women

---

* After age 49
† After age 49; before age 70
‡ Ages 65+

SOURCE: Adapted from the U.S. Preventive Services Task Force *Guide to Clinical Preventive Services.* Consult full report for details and recommendations for high-risk individuals.

BIBLIOGRAPHY

AMERICAN COLLEGE OF PHYSICIANS: Preventing firearm violence: A public health imperative. Ann Intern Med 122:311, 1995

FEDSON DS: Adult immunization: Summary of the National Vaccine Advisory Committee Report. JAMA 272:1133, 1994

Healthy People 2000: National Health Promotion and Disease Prevention Objectives. Department of Health and Human Services Publication (PHS) 91-50213, 1991

HELZLSOUER KJ et al: Summary of the round table discussion on strategies for cancer prevention: Diet, food, additives, supplements, and drugs. Cancer Res 54:2044s, 1994

McCORMICK WC, INUI TS: Geriatric preventive care: Counseling techniques in practice settings. Clin Geriat Med 8:215, 1992

POPE AM, RALL DP (eds): *Environmental Medicine: Integrating a Missing Element into Medical Education.* Washington, DC, National Academy Press, 1995

SCHWARTZ JS et al: Internists' practices in health promotion and disease prevention. Ann Intern Med 114:46, 1991

SOX HC: Preventive health services in adults. N Engl J Med 330:1589, 1994

U.S. PREVENTIVE SERVICES TASK FORCE: *Guide to Clinical Preventive Services,* 2d ed. Baltimore, Williams & Wilkins, 1995

WILLIAMS GC et al: "The facts concerning the recent carnival of smoking in Connecticut" and elsewhere. Ann Intern Med 115:59, 1991

COST AWARENESS
IN MEDICINE

COSTS OF HEALTH CARE IN THE UNITED STATES

Through the 1980s and early 1990s, health care expenditures in the United States rose at a rate of more than 10 percent per year, which exceeded the rates of inflation and of growth in the gross national product (GNP). As a consequence, the percentage of the GNP that is spent on health care increased from about 7 percent in 1970 to 9 percent in 1980 and to more than 12 percent by the early 1990s. This escalation exceeded the increases in other western countries, such as the United Kingdom and Canada. Much of the difference between the United States and Canada is explained by higher physician fees rather than by a higher per capita use of services. The United States also spends substantially more on the administrative costs of health care than Canada or Great Britain.

The reasons for the increase in health care costs are multifactorial. The aging of the population and the availability of new diagnostic and therapeutic advances have increased the demand for health care. Furthermore, the supply of specialists has increased dramatically, providing Americans with easier access to advanced medical services but also suggesting than an oversupply of physicians contributed to an excessive escalation in costs. The costs of care are especially influenced by decisions regarding hospital admission and surgery and by decisions affecting the use of intensive care units, life-sustaining treatments, and long-term care facilities. Efforts at cost-containment have attempted to identify unnecessary services, such as routine preoperative electrocardiograms in healthy young patients, or situations in which extraordinary expenses occur, such as in the last 6 months of life. Attempts to reduce "fat" in the health care system may be counterbalanced, at least in part, by growth in the number and age of the population and by continued advances in technology.

Despite these rising costs, an estimated 40 million Americans, or about 15 percent of the population, do not have health care insurance of any kind, even though nearly half are in households in which someone is employed. This lack of insurance coverage and access to health care is often blamed for the fact that the United States, despite its high expenditures on health care, ranks about twentieth in the world in infant mortality and is not in the top ten in life expectancy.

HEALTH INSURANCE Traditional fee-for-service insurance reimburses the hospital and the physician for services rendered but frequently does not cover preventive care. Even when insurance provides coverage for a service, the patient may be responsible for an initial "deductible" and a copayment, which is usually a fixed percentage of the entire amount charged.

Patients who must pay such out-of-pocket charges for some of their medical care seek less care than those whose care is fully covered by insurance. In the working poor this may result in reduced utilization of services and in an increase in the prevalence of serious disease. When adults of all socioeconomic classes lose health insurance coverage, they may use fewer medical services; as a result, their health status tends to decline.

Most alternatives to traditional fee-for-service medical care require enrolled persons to prepay a fixed premium, which, except when a relatively small copayment is required, usually covers acute, chronic, and preventive medical services and sometimes covers medications and other health care needs. Prepaid plans have varying organizational and financial structures. Early on in their development, staff-model health maintenance organizations (HMOs) were among the most popular formats. In this model, groups of salaried physicians practiced physically together in one or a few central facilities to provide prepaid care. In recent years, independent practice associations (IPAs) have shown the most rapid growth. IPAs provide prepaid care to the patient by contracting with office-based practitioners who agree to see patients on a prenegotiated fee schedule or for a fixed monthly per-patient capitated payment. To balance the normal fee-for-service incentives and control utilization, IPAs employ various forms of administrative controls and review. The number of days of hospitalization have been markedly reduced among enrollees in HMOs, and HMOs have been among the leaders in attempts to reduce hospital costs and lengths of stay.

REIMBURSEMENT OF HOSPITALS AND PHYSICIANS In 1983, Medicare introduced a system of prospective reimbursement using diagnosis-related groups (DRGs), whereby hospitals were paid a predetermined sum based on the patient's principal diagnosis, procedures, complications, and comorbidities regardless of the costs or charges that were actually generated by the hospital stay. This reimbursement system was designed to reward hospitals for being more efficient, and hospitals could actually be paid more than their costs. While the prospective reimbursement system has undoubtedly stimulated efficiency, it also has raised concerns about the practice of discharging patients prematurely or transferring them to other institutions if the projected cost of caring for them exceeds the expected reimbursement.

Since the introduction of federal prospective reimbursement, the number of inpatient hospital days has decreased. This reduction has been accompanied by a marked increase in ambulatory services, including a shift to the outpatient arena of services that previously were delivered only on an inpatient basis. This shift should lower the cost of delivering an individual unit of service, such as the cost of a breast biopsy, but the overall cost of medical care will rise if, for example, the breast biopsy is performed on an ambulatory basis *and* the inpatient resources that the breast biopsy patient would have used are now consumed by new services such as the treatment of a breast cancer patient with bone marrow transplantation.

Methods of physician payment also have been revised. Physician reimbursement in the United States, whether by Medicare or by private insurers, traditionally was a direct payment based on the doctor's "usual and customary" fee. Medicare changed this approach when it adopted the *relative value scale*, which is based on the concept that payment rates for medical services should, as with other economic "goods," reflect the costs of producing those services. This change suggests that procedural tasks were being reimbursed at rates exceeding those of nonprocedural tasks that require comparable time, skill, and experience. Medicare's relative rates are similar to preexisting fee schedules in Canada.

CONTROL OF HEALTH CARE COSTS Two different approaches have been suggested to control health care costs: regulation and competition. Regulations, such as per diem rate setting, attempt to control costs by setting and enforcing practice or reimbursement standards. Other regulatory means of attempting to reduce costs include mandatory second opinions prior to elective hospitalization or surgery, but such programs usually do not save more than the costs of administration of the programs themselves.

The competitive approach encourages hospitals and providers to bid in a free-market atmosphere, in which consumers will presumably make rational choices based on the perceived cost and quality of the available alternatives. Insurance plans that utilize deductibles and copayments reflect this approach. It also has been proposed that physicians who practice inexpensively should be rewarded financially, but if physicians are paid to perform fewer services, the quality of care may suffer. In the absence of legislative reform, the U.S. health care system has been changing rapidly in response to competitive forces. In some parts of the country, employers have joined together to demand lower insurance premiums or to contract directly with hospitals and physicians. In other areas, hospitals, doctors, or doctors with their hospitals have contracted with insurance carriers to establish comprehensive systems that can deliver the full range of health services to a large population of individuals. For-profit insurers and hospitals often compete actively with more traditional not-for-profit entities.

Much of the new competition is in "managed care," by which physicians and institutions agree to provide services for a predetermined price. This price may be a discount of historic fee-for-service prices or it may be negotiated for a specific package of services on behalf of multiple providers, such as when physicians and their hospital agree to perform a kidney transplantation, as well as pre- and posttransplant services, for a specific price. In this arrangement, the various providers then divide the total reimbursement according to an internally negotiated formula. Increasingly, however, physicians, often in conjunction with their hospitals, are negotiating full-risk capitation contracts with employers and insurers. Under this arrangement, providers agree to deliver comprehensive medical services, commonly including preventive and long-term care, to a panel of subscribers for a negotiated reimbursement per member per month. The providers who take responsibility for the care of a panel of patients will not be paid more if their expenses exceed their contracted capitation price, but they are able to retain any prenegotiated payments that are in excess of the costs of the services they provide. In many capitated settings, risk-sharing arrangements are used to dissuade individual physicians from utilizing more tests or procedures than desired by the health care system. For example, a portion of the payment earned by a physician, either via a modified fee-for-service arrangement or as part of a monthly capitated fee, may be "withheld" until the overall financial performance of the system is known not to be in deficit. By 1995, about 20 percent of the U.S. population was in managed care plans, and in some parts of the United States the enrollment was above 50 percent. It is projected that 70 percent or more of the population will be in managed care plans by the end of the century.

Reimbursement mechanisms that give physicians incentives to ration services or that directly link the financial stability of the physician's employer to the ability to reduce costs create an inherent conflict of interest. Of course, a different type of conflict of interest exists under traditional fee-for-service reimbursement, by which a physician is paid more to do more.

In managed care systems, the utilization of health services, particularly specialty care, tends to decline. As a result, current forecasts suggest a substantial excess of specialty physicians and hospital beds. Primary care physicians are thought to be inequitably distributed nationwide but only slightly, if at all, insufficient in numbers.

In the presence of competition and an oversupply of hospital beds and specialist physicians, insurers can negotiate lower prices. As a result, insurance premiums are declining in many parts of the United States, even as the insurers keep an increasing percentage of the premium and distribute a smaller percentage to physicians and hospitals. Total reimbursements to all physicians and hospitals are projected to decline by as much as 25 percent in the coming years.

COSTS AND COST-EFFECTIVENESS

The costs of medical care include direct costs, such as the salaries of health personnel, and indirect costs, such as utilities, maintenance, and mortgage payments. Some costs are fixed (i.e., they do not vary with the volume of services provided), and other costs are variable (i.e., they depend on volume). For example, consider a situation in which a new instrument to perform a blood chemistry test costs $1000 and will last for 1 year. Also assume that each individual chemical analysis has an incremental cost of $10 in reagents, personnel time, and other resource inputs. If the laboratory utilizes the instrument to analyze 100 specimens in a year, the average cost per specimen is $20 ($10 each in fixed and variable costs), but if it analyzes 10,000 specimens, the average cost per specimen is $10.10 ($0.10 in fixed costs and $10.00 in variable costs) because the fixed costs are spread over more specimens.

The charges for medical services do not necessarily correspond to the true costs of providing the services. This occurs in part because the costs are difficult to measure and in part because charges are usually fixed regardless of volume, while costs vary with volume. Many analyses of cost and cost-effectiveness in medicine are based on charges rather than on true costs.

The net costs for a health care program include the costs of providing the program, costs that are generated by adverse side effects of treatment, and costs for treating disease that would not have occurred if the patient had not lived longer as a result of the original treatment. From these costs, the savings in health care, rehabilitation, or custodial costs due to prevention or alleviation of disease are subtracted to determine the net cost. For example, consider a program to perform mammography in women over age 40. The program would have its own direct costs related to advertising, screening, mammography, physician visits, breast biopsy, etc. Some women would have false-positive mammograms and would receive unnecessary breast biopsies. Other women would live longer as a result of early diagnosis and treatment of breast cancer, but they might develop other illnesses, such as coronary disease, in the interim. If they developed conditions such as Alzheimer's disease, the custodial costs might be substantial. However, these costs would be countered by savings from hospitalizations for advanced cancer and by a potential increase in productive wage-earning years.

In all analyses of costs, it is important to consider *when* the costs will be incurred and *when* the effects in health benefits may be realized. Present dollars or health benefits are considered to have greater worth than a promise of future dollars or health benefits for several reasons. Other events may intercede so that a projected future cost or benefit may never occur, and there is always the possibility that money spent now will not achieve the desired effect at some time in the future. Furthermore, another illness may intervene, or there might be better ways to spend the money in the future. The principle by which future dollars and benefits are less highly valued than known immediate costs and benefits is termed *discounting*. It is independent of monetary inflation. By this concept, it is preferable to spend $1000 today to prevent someone from dying today than it is to spend $1000 today in the expectation that someone will not die 10 years from now.

It is unusual for any program simultaneously to achieve the greatest possible benefit and have the lowest possible cost. Instead, one usually either determines the desired benefit and then finds the lowest cost needed to achieve it or determines the resources available and then finds the greatest possible benefit that can be achieved.

Analyses of cost-effectiveness commonly examine the ratio of cost to effectiveness, i.e., the number of dollars required to save a year of life or a quality-adjusted year of life, in which the analysis considers not only the quantity but also the patient-assessed quality of the health benefit. Such analyses are relevant to medicine because interventions only rarely both save lives and reduce costs. Hence it is important to estimate the tradeoff of costs for gains in health. Two strategies with the same ratio may have quite different absolute costs and absolute benefits. For example, a program that saves 100 lives for $100,000 has the same cost-effectiveness ratio as one that saves 1000 lives for $1 million, but the absolute costs and absolute benefits vary tenfold. The choice between these two programs may depend on how much money is available to spend. In assessing any program, it is important to measure incremental costs and effects rather than average costs and effects. For example, consider two programs to reduce death from lung cancer. If, on average, program A costs $100 million to save 100,000 years of life (average of $1000 per year of life) and program B costs $200 million to save 100,100 years of life (about $2000 per year of life), the *incremental* cost of program B versus program A is $1 million per year of life saved.

The cost-effectiveness of an intervention depends on its own cost, the costs it may avert or induce, and the patient's risks. The cost-effectiveness of an intervention will vary dramatically depending on the type of patient to whom it is applied (Table 11-1).

SOCIETAL ISSUES IN COSTS It is rare to find a medical intervention, such as measles vaccination programs, that both saves lives and reduces overall costs because the savings from disease prevention more than outweigh the expenses of the treatment itself. More commonly, medical practices that are truly of benefit also cause an associated increase in medical care costs. Among the more cost-effective examples is coronary artery bypass surgery in patients with left main coronary artery disease, which costs under $10,000 per year of life saved.

The shift of services from the inpatient to the outpatient setting or from the hospital to the home generally reduces the expense of delivery of that aspect of medical care. For example, home dialysis is less expensive than dialysis in an outpatient center, which in turn is less expensive than dialysis in a hospital. Similarly, the administration of parenteral nutrition and intravenous antibiotics at home and the home care for patients with AIDS have greatly reduced the need for hospitalization for conditions in which skilled nursing care is otherwise not required. However, a by-product of this strategy is an increased percentage of severely ill hospital inpatients who require more intensive and expensive care than the less sick patients who otherwise might have occupied hospital beds.

Even now, society has been reluctant to make ethical decisions regarding the amount of cost appropriate for any particular net benefit. Neither medicine nor society is accustomed to placing a dollar value on a life or a year of life. In many analyses, however, the projected annual costs of approximately $35,000 to $45,000 (in 1997 dollars) for renal dialysis for 1 year of useful life have been used as a benchmark of how much the United States is willing to spend to save a year of life, because such a program is supported with tax dollars and presumably is a reasonable reflection of national priorities.

HEALTH SCREENING   *Screening* refers to the performance of a medical evaluation and/or diagnostic tests in asymptomatic persons in the hope that early diagnosis may lead to improved outcome. This important subject is discussed in Chap. 10.

HEALTH PROMOTION AND DISEASE PREVENTION Health promotion and disease prevention require investment of time, energy, and resources in the hope that the yield in terms of improved health warrants this investment. Unfortunately, there is limited information on the effectiveness of health promotion and disease prevention efforts. Interventions that result in a specified *relative* reduction in adverse outcomes have a greater *absolute* effect in higher-risk populations. For example, the same relative reduction in serum cholesterol will be of greater absolute benefit in persons with higher serum cholesterol levels or other unfavorable risk factors. In general, interventions to alter risk factors have a diminishing effect as risk factors decrease in severity.

Both patients and society commonly expect physicians to play a leadership role in health promotion and disease prevention. Patients expect and desire their physicians to make recommendations regarding physical activity, diet, and other lifestyle issues, and physicians often fail in this regard. If physicians do not become involved, patients seek advice elsewhere, risking the possibility that fads or other erroneous sources may influence their choices.

When physicians become actively involved in health promotion, patients respond frequently and make appropriate behavior changes. For example, a physician's encouragement to increase physical activity, especially if combined with explicit suggestions, is likely to lead to changes in behavior so that the time spent by the physician appears to be cost-effective. Advice by a physician that a patient should lose weight or discontinue smoking is successful in only a small minority of cases, but it is an excellent first step toward health promotion and disease prevention (Chap. 389).

Physician-directed dietary interventions commonly lower the serum cholesterol level by as much as 8 percent. Drug treatment may be more effective but is more expensive. For example, treatment with lovastatin in men for the primary prevention of coronary heart disease costs more than $50,000 per year of life saved except in very high risk persons. Treatment strategies for hypertension are more cost-effective; the approximate cost of screening and treating hypertension, given the average medication compliance rates and treatment with a generic beta-adrenergic antagonist, ranges from a projection of about $15,000 per year of life saved for a patient with a diastolic blood pressure of 105 mmHg or higher to about $25,000 to $30,000 for a person with a diastolic blood pressure of 95 to 104 mmHg. Costs would be higher with more expensive medications, although the cost could be warranted if a reduction in side effects led to an improvement in an individual's quality of life.

Immunizations, including pneumococcal and influenza vaccination in elderly and high-risk patients, are effective ways to reduce disease and its associated costs (see Chap. 122).

DIAGNOSTIC TESTING   As detailed in Chap. 3, diagnostic tests are valuable only to the extent that they provide new, *incremental* information that cannot be obtained less expensively from the history, physical examination, or other less expensive tests. Although these tests may often be of psychological benefit in reassuring the patient or the physician, they commonly generate redundant information, often result in a needless expense, and may entail risk. For example, in the evaluation of left ventricular function, the physician must decide whether a two-dimensional echocardiogram is sufficient or the more precise but more expensive measurement by radionuclide ventriculog-

Table 11-1

Example of Costs, Effectiveness, and Cost-Effectiveness for a Hypothetical Intervention in 10,000 Patients for 5 Years* (High-Risk Patients Compared with Low-Risk Patients)

	High Risk		Low Risk	
	Untreated	**Treated**	**Untreated**	**Treated**
Annual death rate	10%	5%	1%	0.5%
Years of life saved[†]	0	5209	0	614
Cost of treatment (in $ millions) at $2000 per year	0	90.5	0	99.0
Annual CABG rate	6%	3%	0.6%	0.3%
Cost per CABG	$20,000	$20,000	$20,000	$20,000
Annual MI rate	4%	2%	0.4%	0.2%
Cost per MI	$10,000	$10,000	$10,000	$10,000
Annual rate of other events	4%	2%	0.4%	0.2%
Cost per other event	$5000	$5000	$5000	$5000
Medical costs (in $ millions)	70.0	39.7	8.8	4.4
Total cost (in $ millions)	70.0	130.2	8.8	103.4
Total cost difference (in $ millions)		60.2		94.8
Approximate cost per year of life saved		$11,500*		$155,000*

* Simplified so that the intervention reduces all risks by 50%, neither costs nor health effects are discounted, all patients are assumed to die at midyear, and the analysis considers only the first 5 years.
† By life-table analysis.
NOTE: CABG, coronary artery bypass grafting; MI, myocardial infarction.
SOURCE: Reprinted from L Goldman et al, J Am Coll Cardiol 27:1020, 1996.

raphy is worthwhile. The physician faces analogous choices when deciding whether to obtain both an abdominal ultrasound examination and an abdominal computed tomography (CT) scan or, in a different case, whether CT and magnetic resonance imaging of the head are both required.

Ideally, each test should be ordered in sequence only to the extent that it is expected to add to the data available. However, this iterative approach can be expensive in hospitalized patients, where the sequencing of tests may lead to delays in scheduling and performing them. In these situations, the expense of the additional days of waiting may more than offset the savings from possibly avoiding a particular test. Usually, careful consideration of the problem by a physician is one of the most cost-effective ways to evaluate the patient. Expert consultation may be more cost-effective and helpful than ordering more diagnostic tests. Although interventions designed to reduce utilization have met with variable success, those that have been successful have generally included educational components, full endorsement by locally respected leaders, frequent reinforcement and attempts to modify the system by which care is delivered.

TREATMENT CHOICES In choosing among various treatments, physicians try to enhance the likelihood of an optimal outcome. It is important to consider whether an equivalent outcome could be achieved at a lower cost. For example, generic medications may be substituted for more expensive brand-name counterparts. Similarly, outcome is not usually compromised by interventions designed to encourage the use of less expensive antibiotic regimens. Endorsement by the medical profession of restricted indications for procedures such as pacemaker implantation and tonsillectomy have led to decreased utilization without any detectable reduction in life expectancy or quality of life. Whenever possible, diagnostic and therapeutic options should be subjected to strict evaluation of both benefit and cost-effectiveness, and physicians have responsibility to assist in such evaluations and to learn from their results.

INDIVIDUALIZATION

The physician has a unique responsibility. On the one hand, the physician must serve as an advocate for the individual patient, within the limits set by society, and recommend the course of action most likely to be beneficial to the patient. The overriding nature of the patient-physician relationship is the cornerstone of humane medical care. On the other hand, physicians must understand the costs as well as the benefits of medical interventions so that they can choose from among the wide range of options. The physician must serve as the advocate for providing the best options to the individual patient and should know which options are of little or no value or are more likely to do harm than good. The physician must, with the assistance and consent of the patient and the family, set priorities for the patient's management within any limits or restrictions imposed by society; such limits may be expressed, for example, in a finite number of dollars available for the treatment of a specific illness.

In addition, physicians have a broad role in determining health costs. Individually and through various professional organizations, physicians have a responsibility to help set national priorities, based on their appreciation of the finite resources available for health care and their knowledge of the relative benefits and costs of various diagnostic and therapeutic options in particular types of patients. The financial incentives of capitation, by which physicians are paid a fixed amount per patient per month regardless of what services are delivered, presents a new series of ethical challenges for physicians to avoid incentives toward underutilization. These challenges are magnified by the pressures of insurers and health care systems to reduce costs. Inappropriate attempts to reduce costs, exemplified by limiting Medicaid payments for effective medications, are counterproductive in that they worsen health and ultimately lead to increased overall costs.

Special consideration revolves around the use of expensive procedures in medical care, such as liver, heart, lung, and bone marrow transplantation. In these situations, the limited availability of donors makes it necessary to choose the best possible recipients from among a wide range of potential candidates and to "ration." Although rationing is not pleasant, physicians have often responded well in situations with limited resources. For example, when faced with a reduction in intensive care unit availability, physicians are usually successful at maintaining normal admission rates for patients who most require intensive care so that little, if any, adverse effects occur in those excluded from intensive care.

There is marked variability in the rates at which various procedures are performed in different geographic areas, even though there are no obvious differences in the types or ages of patients. To date, relatively little difference in health care outcomes can be detected despite wide differences in the rates of various procedures, suggesting that lower utilization rates often do not adversely affect the quality of care. In some circumstances, however, lower rates of expensive and potentially risky procedures have been associated with poorer functional status, indicating that variations may in part be related to patients' preferences and in part to differing beliefs among physicians regarding optimal medical care choices. When the records of patients who have undergone such procedures are reviewed to determine how the indications for their procedure compared with the standards recommended by experts, a substantial proportion of procedures are deemed inappropriate. However, so far there is no close correlation between the percentage of cases deemed inappropriate and the rate at which the procedure is performed in a given location. There is no definitive evidence that high rates of performance can be equated with a high rate of unnecessary use.

The variations in rates of utilization, the proportion of cases in which some procedures seem not to be necessary, and the ability of physicians to respond to situations in which rationing is necessary suggest that in many situations the quality of medical care and the likelihood of a favorable outcome can be maintained while lowering costs. Society, with the input of physicians, must exercise this role without compromising the physician's responsibility to the individual patient and without restricting access on the basis of sex, socioeconomic status, or ethnic background.

BIBLIOGRAPHY

BARR DA: The effects of organizational structure on primary care outcomes under managed care. Ann Intern Med 122:353, 1995

COUNCIL ON ETHICAL AND JUDICIAL AFFAIRS, AMERICAN MEDICAL ASSOCIATION: Ethical issues in managed care. JAMA 273:330, 1995

EPSTEIN AM: US teaching hospitals in the evolving health care system. JAMA 273:1203, 1995

GOLBERG MA et al: The relation between universal health care insurance and cost control. N Engl J Med 332:742, 1995

GOLDMAN L: Cost-effective strategies in cardiology, in *Heart Disease*, 5th ed, E Braunwald (ed). Philadelphia, Saunders, 1997, pp 1741–1756

HYAMS AL et al: Practice guidelines and malpractice litigation: A two-way street. Ann Intern Med 122:450, 1995

IGLEHART JK: Recent changes for academic medical centers. N Engl J Med 332:407, 1995

KUPERSMITH J et al: Cost effectiveness analysis in heart disease. Part III: Ischemia, congestive heart failure, and arrhythmias. Prog Cardiovasc Dis 37:307, 1995

LINDFORS KK et al: The cost-effectiveness of mammographic screening strategies. JAMA 274:881, 1995

LUBITZ J et al: Longevity and medicare expenditures. N Engl J Med 332:999, 1995

MCGLYNN EA et al: Comparison of the appropriateness of coronary angiography and coronary artery bypass graft surgery between Canada and New York state. JAMA 272:934, 1994

PILOTE L et al: Regional variation across the United States in the management of acute myocardial infarction. N Engl J Med 333:565, 1995

RASELL ME: Cost-sharing in health insurance—a reexamination. N Engl J Med 332:1164, 1995

SCHROEDER SA: The latest forecast. Managed care collides with physician supply. JAMA 272:239, 1994

12

Howard L. Fields, Joseph B. Martin

PAIN: PATHOPHYSIOLOGY AND MANAGEMENT

The task of medicine is to preserve and restore health and to relieve suffering. Understanding pain is essential to both these goals. Because pain is universally understood as a signal of disease, it is the most common symptom that brings a patient to a physician's attention. The function of the pain sensory system is to detect, localize, and identify tissue-damaging processes. Since different diseases produce characteristic patterns of tissue damage, the quality, time course, and location of a patient's pain complaint and the location of tenderness provide important diagnostic clues and are used to evaluate the response to treatment.

THE PAIN SENSORY SYSTEM

Pain is an unpleasant sensation localized to a part of the body. It is often described in terms of a penetrating or tissue-destructive process (e.g., stabbing, burning, twisting, tearing, squeezing) and/or of a bodily or emotional reaction (e.g., terrifying, nauseating, sickening). Furthermore, any pain of moderate or higher intensity is accompanied by anxiety and the urge to escape or terminate the feeling. These properties illustrate the duality of pain: It is both sensation and emotion. When it is acute, pain is characteristically associated with behavioral arousal and a stress response consisting of increased blood pressure, heart rate, pupil diameter, and plasma cortisol levels. In addition, local muscle contraction (e.g., limb flexion, abdominal wall rigidity) is often seen.

THE PRIMARY AFFERENT NOCICEPTOR A peripheral nerve consists of the axons of three different types of neurons: primary sensory afferents, motor neurons, and sympathetic postganglionic neurons (Fig. 12-1). The cell bodies of primary afferents are located in the dorsal root ganglia in the vertebral foramina. The primary afferent axon bifurcates to send one process into the spinal cord and the other to innervate tissues. Primary afferents are classified by their diameter, degree of myelination, and conduction velocity. The largest-diameter fibers, A-beta, respond maximally to light touch and/or moving stimuli; they are present primarily in nerves that innervate the skin. In normal individuals, the activity of these fibers does not produce pain. There are two other classes of primary afferents: the small-diameter myelinated (A-delta) and the unmyelinated (C fiber) axons (see Fig. 12-1). These fibers are present in the nerves to the skin and to deep somatic and visceral structures. Some tissues, such as the cornea, are innervated only by A-delta and C afferents. Most A-delta and C afferents respond maximally only to intense (painful) stimuli and produce the subjective experience of pain when they are electrically stimulated; this de-

fines them as *primary afferent nociceptors (pain receptors)*. The ability to detect painful stimuli is completely abolished when A-delta and C axons are blocked.

Individual primary afferent nociceptors can respond to several different types of noxious stimuli. For example, most nociceptors respond to heating, intense mechanical stimuli such as a pinch, and application of irritating chemicals.

Sensitization When intense, repeated, or prolonged stimuli are applied in the presence of damaged tissue or inflammation, the threshold for activating primary afferent nociceptors is lowered and the frequency of firing is higher for all stimulus intensities. Inflammatory mediators such as bradykinin, some prostaglandins, and leukotrienes contribute to this process, which is called *sensitization*. In sensitized tissues normally innocuous stimuli can produce pain. Sensitization is a clinically important process that contributes to tenderness, soreness, and hyperalgesia. A striking example of sensitization is sunburned skin, in which severe pain can be produced by a gentle slap on the back or a warm shower.

Compared with superficial structures (e.g., skin, cornea), viscera are relatively insensitive to noxious stimuli under normal conditions. In contrast, when affected by a disease process with an inflammatory component, deep structures such as joints or hollow viscera characteristically become exquisitely sensitive to mechanical stimulation.

A large proportion of A-delta and C afferents innervating viscera are completely insensitive in normal noninjured, noninflamed tissue. That is, they cannot be activated by known mechanical or thermal stimuli and are not spontaneously active. However, in the presence of inflammatory mediators, these afferents become sensitive to mechanical stimuli. Such afferents have been termed *silent nociceptors*, and their characteristic properties may explain how under pathologic conditions the relatively insensitive deep structures can become the source of severe and debilitating pain and tenderness.

Nociceptor-Induced Inflammation One important concept to emerge in recent years is that afferent nociceptors also have a neuroeffector function. Most nociceptors contain polypeptide mediators that are released from their peripheral terminals when they are activated

FIGURE 12-1 Components of a typical cutaneous nerve. There are two distinct functional categories of axons: primary afferents with cell bodies in the dorsal root ganglion and sympathetic postganglionic fibers with cell bodies in the sympathetic ganglion. Primary afferents include those with large-diameter myelinated (A-β), small-diameter myelinated (A-δ), and unmyelinated (C) axons. All sympathetic postganglionic fibers are unmyelinated.

(Fig. 12-2). An example is substance P, an 11-amino-acid peptide. Substance P is released from primary afferent nociceptors and has multiple biologic activities. It is a potent vasodilator, degranulates mast cells, is a chemoattractant for leukocytes, and increases the production and release of inflammatory mediators. Interestingly, depletion of substance P from joints reduces the severity of experimental arthritis. Primary afferent nociceptors are not simply passive messengers of threats to tissue injury but also play an active role in tissue protection through these neuroeffector functions.

CENTRAL PATHWAYS FOR PAIN   The Spinal Cord and Referred Pain   The axons of primary afferent nociceptors enter the spinal cord via the dorsal root. They terminate in the dorsal horn of the spinal gray matter (Fig. 12-3). The terminals of primary afferent axons contact spinal neurons that transmit the pain signal to brain sites involved in pain perception. The axon of each primary afferent contacts many spinal neurons, and each spinal neuron receives convergent inputs from many primary afferents.

From a clinical standpoint, the convergence of many sensory inputs to a single spinal pain-transmission neuron is of great importance

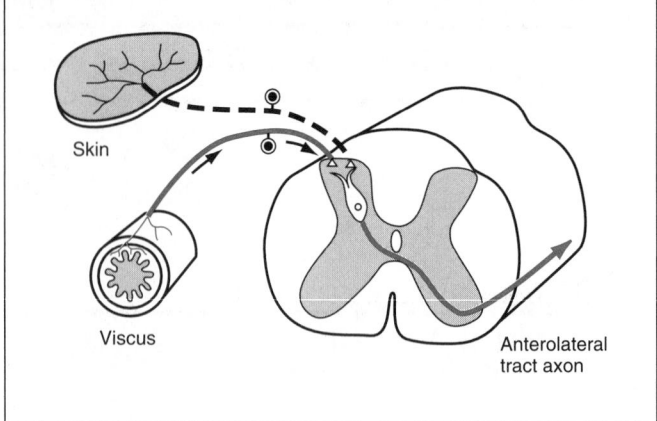

FIGURE 12-3   The convergence-projection hypothesis of referred pain. According to this hypothesis, visceral afferent nociceptors (S) converge on the same pain-projection neurons as the afferents from the somatic structures in which the pain is perceived. The brain has no way of knowing the actual source of input and mistakenly "projects" the sensation to the somatic structure.

because it underlies the phenomenon of referred pain. All spinal neurons that receive input from the viscera and deep musculoskeletal structures also receive input from the skin. The convergence patterns are determined by the spinal segment of the dorsal root ganglion that supplies the afferent innervation of a structure. For example, the afferents that supply the central diaphragm are derived from the third and fourth cervical dorsal root ganglia. Primary afferents with cell bodies in these same ganglia supply the skin of the shoulder and lower neck. Thus sensory inputs from both the shoulder skin and the central diaphragm converge on pain-transmission neurons in the third and fourth cervical spinal segments. *Because of this convergence and the fact that the spinal neurons are most often activated by inputs from the skin, activity evoked in spinal neurons by input from deep structures is mislocalized by the patient to a place that is roughly coextensive with the region of skin innervated by the same spinal segment.* Thus inflammation near the central diaphragm is usually reported as discomfort near the shoulder. This spatial displacement of pain sensation from the site of the injury that produces it is known as *referred pain*.

Ascending Pathways for Pain   A majority of spinal neurons contacted by primary afferent nociceptors send their axons to the contralateral thalamus. These axons form the contralateral spinothalamic tract which lies in the anterolateral white matter of the spinal cord, the lateral edge of the medulla, and the lateral pons and midbrain. The spinothalamic pathway is crucial for pain sensation in humans. Interruption of this pathway produces permanent deficits in pain and temperature discrimination.

Spinothalamic tract axons connect to thalamic neurons that project to somatosensory cortex (Fig. 12-4). This pathway from spinal cord to thalamus to somatosensory cortex appears to be particularly important for the sensory aspects of pain, i.e., its location, intensity, and quality. Spinothalamic tract axons also connect to thalamic and cortical regions linked to emotional responses, such as the cingulate gyrus and frontal lobe. This pathway is thought to subserve the affective or unpleasant emotional dimension of pain.

PAIN MODULATION   The pain produced by similar injuries is remarkably variable in different situations and in different people. For example, athletes have been known to sustain serious fractures with only minor pain, and Beecher's classic World War II survey revealed that many men were unbothered by battle injuries that would have produced agonizing pain in civilian patients. Furthermore, even the suggestion of relief can have a significant analgesic effect (placebo). On the other hand, many patients find even minor injuries (such as venipuncture) unbearable, and the expectation of pain has been demonstrated to induce pain *without a noxious stimulus*.

The powerful effect of expectation and other psychological variables on the perceived intensity of pain implies the existence of brain circuits that can modulate the activity of the pain-transmission path-

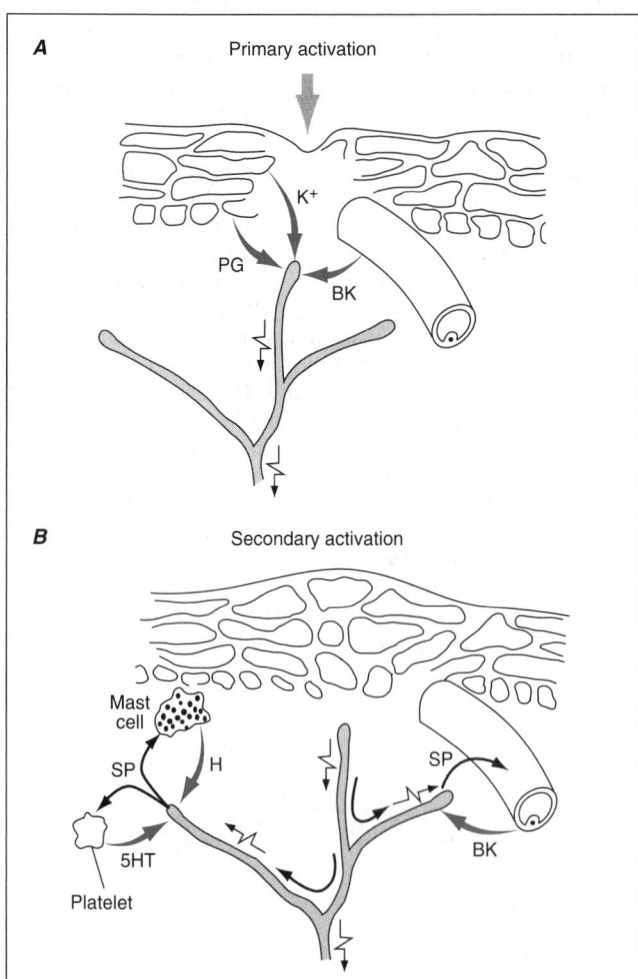

FIGURE 12-2   Events leading to activation, sensitization, and spread of sensitization of primary afferent nociceptor terminals. *A.* Direct activation by intense pressure and consequent cell damage. Cell damage leads to release of potassium (K^+) and to synthesis of prostaglandins (PG) and bradykinin (BK). Prostaglandins increase the sensitivity of the terminal to bradykinin and other pain-producing substances. *B.* Secondary activation. Impulses generated in the stimulated terminal propagate not only to the spinal cord but also into other terminal branches where they induce the release of peptides, including substance P (SP). Substance P causes vasodilation and neurogenic edema with further accumulation of bradykinin. Substance P also causes the release of histamine (H) from mast cells and serotonin (5HT) from platelets.

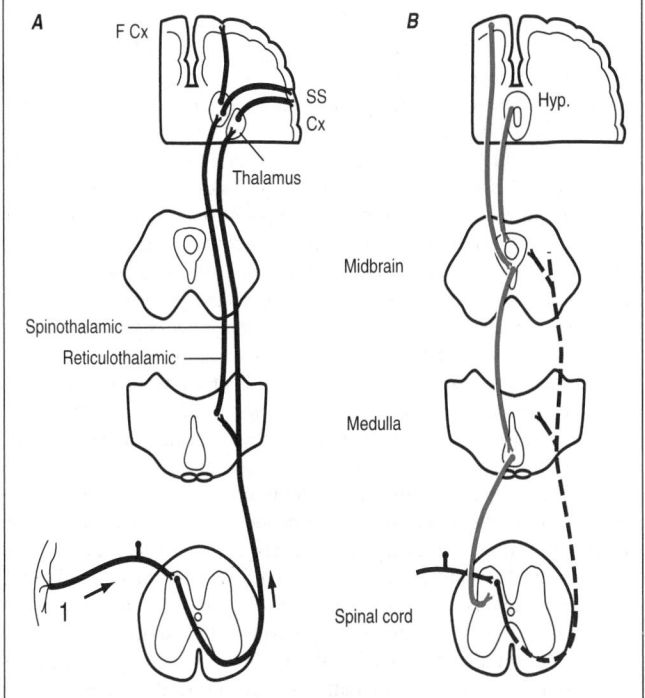

FIGURE 12-4 *A.* Transmission system for nociceptive messages. Noxious stimuli activate the sensitive peripheral ending of the primary afferent nociceptor by the process of transduction (1). The message is then transmitted over the peripheral nerve to the spinal cord, where it synapses with cells of origin of the two major ascending pain pathways, the spinothalamic and spinoreticulothalamic. The message is relayed in the thalamus to both the frontal (F Cx) and the somatosensory cortex (SS Cx). *B.* Pain-modulation network. Inputs from frontal cortex and hypothalamus (Hyp.) activate cells in the midbrain, that control spinal pain-transmission cells via cells in the medulla.

ways. Although there are probably several circuits that can modulate pain, only one has been studied extensively. This circuit has links in the hypothalamus, midbrain, and medulla, and it selectively controls spinal pain-transmission neurons through a descending pathway (see Fig. 12-4).

There is good evidence that this pain-modulating circuit contributes to the pain-relieving effect of narcotic analgesic medications. Each of the component structures of the pathway contains opioid receptors and is sensitive to the direct application of opioid drugs. Furthermore, lesions of the system reduce the analgesic effect of systemically administered opioids such as morphine. Along with the opioid receptor, the component nuclei of this pain-modulating circuit contain endogenous opioid peptides such as the enkephalins and beta-endorphin.

The most reliable way to activate this endogenous opioid-mediated modulating system is by prolonged pain and/or fear. There is evidence that pain-relieving endogenous opioids are released following operative procedures and in patients given a placebo for pain relief.

Pain modulation is bidirectional. Pain-modulating circuits not only produce analgesia but are also capable of increasing pain. Both pain-inhibiting and pain-facilitating neurons in the medulla project to and control spinal pain-transmission neurons. Since pain-transmission neurons can be activated by modulatory neurons, it is theoretically possible to generate a pain signal with no peripheral noxious stimulus. Some such mechanism could account for the finding that pain can be induced by suggestion alone and may provide a framework for understanding how psychological factors can contribute to chronic pain.

NEUROPATHIC PAIN   The normal nervous system transmits coded signals that result in pain. Thus lesions of the peripheral or central nervous system may result in a loss or impairment of pain sensation. Paradoxically, damage or dysfunction of the nervous system can produce pain. For example, damage to peripheral nerves, as occurs

in diabetic neuropathy, or to primary afferents, as in herpes zoster, can result in pain that is referred to the body region innervated by the damaged nerves. Though rare, pain also may be produced by damage to the central nervous system, particularly the spinothalamic pathway or thalamus. Such neuropathic pains are often severe and are notoriously intractable to standard treatments for pain.

Neuropathic pains typically have an unusual burning, tingling, or electric shock–like quality and may be triggered by very light touch. These features are rare in other types of pain. On examination, a sensory deficit is characteristically present in the area of the patient's pain.

A variety of mechanisms contribute to neuropathic pain. As with sensitized primary afferent nociceptors, damaged primary afferents, including nociceptors, become highly sensitive to mechanical stimulation and begin to generate impulses in the absence of stimulation. Damaged primary afferents also may develop sensitivity to norepinephrine. Interestingly, spinal pain-transmission neurons cut off from their normal input may become spontaneously active. Thus both central and peripheral nervous system changes may contribute to neuropathic pain.

Sympathetically Maintained Pain   A certain percentage of patients with peripheral nerve injury develop a severe burning pain (causalgia) in the region innervated by the nerve. The pain typically begins after a delay of hours to days or even weeks. The pain is accompanied by swelling of the extremity, periarticular osteoporosis, and arthritic changes in the distal joints. A similar syndrome called *reflex sympathetic dystrophy* can be produced without obvious nerve damage by a variety of injuries, including fractures of bone, soft tissue trauma, myocardial infarction, and stroke (see Chap. 371). Although the pathophysiology of this condition is poorly understood, the pain can be relieved within minutes by blocking the sympathetic nervous system. This implies that sympathetic activity activates nociceptors even if they are not obviously damaged. These results also suggest that the sympathetic nervous system can, under some circumstances, play an active role in inflammation.

Ⓡ TREATMENT

The ideal treatment for any pain is to remove the cause. Sometimes this is possible, but more often after diagnosis and initiation of appropriate treatments for the cause, there is a lag period before the pain subsides. Furthermore, some conditions are so painful that rapid and effective analgesia is essential (e.g., the postoperative state, burns, trauma, cancer, sickle cell crisis). Analgesic medications are a first line of treatment in these cases, and their use should be familiar to all practitioners.

Aspirin, Acetaminophen, and Nonsteroidal Anti-Inflammatory Agents (NSAIDS)   These drugs are considered together because they are used for similar problems and may have a similar mechanism of action (Table 12-1). All these compounds inhibit cyclooxygenase and, except for acetaminophen, all have anti-inflammatory actions, especially at higher dosages. They are particularly effective for mild to moderate headache and for pain of musculoskeletal origin.

Since they are effective for these common types of pains and are available without prescription, cyclooxygenase inhibitors are by far the most commonly used analgesics. They are absorbed well from the gastrointestinal tract and, with occasional use, side effects are minimal. With chronic use, gastric irritation is a common side effect of aspirin and NSAIDs and the problem that most frequently limits the dose that can be given. Gastric irritation is most severe with aspirin, which may cause erosion of the gastric mucosa, and because aspirin irreversibly acetylates platelets and interferes with coagulation of the blood, gastrointestinal bleeding is a risk. The NSAIDs are less problematic in this regard. Although toxic to the liver when taken in a high dose, acetaminophen rarely produces gastric irritation and does not interfere with platelet function. Table 12-1 lists the dosages and durations of action of the commonly used drugs of this class.

The introduction of a parenteral form of NSAID, ketorolac, extends the usefulness of this class of compounds in the management of acute severe pain. Ketorolac is sufficiently potent and rapid in onset to supplant opioids for many patients with acute severe headache and musculoskeletal pain.

Opioid Analgesics Opioids are the most potent pain-relieving drugs currently available. Furthermore, of all analgesics, they have the broadest range of efficacy, providing the most reliable method for rapidly relieving pain. Although side effects are common, except for respiratory depression, they are usually not serious and can be reversed rapidly with the narcotic antagonist naloxone. The physician should not hesitate to use opioid analgesics in patients with acute severe pain. Table 12-1 lists the most commonly used opioid analgesics.

Opioids produce analgesia by actions in the central nervous system. They activate pain-inhibitory neurons and directly inhibit pain-transmission neurons. Most of the commercially available opioid analgesics act at the same opiate receptor (mu receptor), differing mainly in potency, speed of onset, duration of action, and optimal route of administration. Although the dose-related side effects (sedation, respiratory depression, pruritus, constipation) are similar among the different opioids, some side effects are due to accumulation of nonopioid metabolites that are unique to individual drugs. One striking example of this is normeperidine, a metabolite of meperidine. Normeperidine produces hyperexcitability and seizures that are not reversible with naloxone. Normeperidine accumulation is much greater in patients with renal failure.

The most rapid relief with opioids is obtained by intravenous administration; relief with oral administration is significantly slower. Common acute side effects include nausea, vomiting, and sedation. These effects are dose-related, and there is great variability among patients in the doses that relieve pain and produce side effects. Because of this, initiation of therapy requires titration to optimal dose and interval. The most important principle is to provide adequate pain relief. This requires asking the patient whether the drug has relieved the pain and, if so, when the relief wears off. *The most common error made by physicians in managing severe pain with opioids is to prescribe an inadequate dose. Since many patients are reluctant to complain, this practice leads to needless suffering.* In the absence of sedation at the expected time of peak effect, a physician should not hesitate to repeat the initial dose to achieve satisfactory pain relief.

An innovative approach to the problem of achieving adequate pain relief is the use of patient-controlled analgesia (PCA). PCA requires a device that immediately delivers a pre-programmed dose of an opioid drug when the patient pushes a button. The device can be programmed to limit the total hourly dose so that overdosing is impossible. The patient can then titrate the dose to the optimal level. This approach is used most extensively for the management of postoperative pain, but there is no reason why it should not be used for any hospitalized patient with persistent severe pain. PCA is also used for home care of patients with intractable pain, such as metastatic cancer.

Table 12-1

Drugs for Relief of Pain

NONNARCOTIC ANALGESICS: USUAL DOSES AND INTERVALS

Generic Name	Dose, mg	Interval	Comments
Acetylsalicylic acid	650 PO	q 4 h	Enteric-coated preparations available
Acetaminophen	650 PO	q 4 h	Side effects uncommon
Ibuprofen	400 PO	q 4–6 h	Available without prescription
Naproxen	250–500 PO	q 12 h	Delayed effects may be due to long half-life
Fenoprofen	200 PO	q 4–6 h	pa
Indomethacin	25–50 PO	q 8 h	Gastrointestinal side effects common
Ketorolac	15–60 IM	q 4–6 h	Available for parenteral use (IM)

NARCOTIC ANALGESICS: USUAL DOSES AND INTERVALS

Generic Name	Parenteral Dose, mg	PO Dose, mg	Comments
Codeine	30–60 q 4 h	30–60 q 4 h	Nausea common
Oxycodone	—	5–10 q 4–6 h	Usually available with acetaminophen or aspirin
Morphine	10 q 4 h	60 q 4 h	
Morphine sustained release	pa	60–180 bid to tid	Oral slow-release preparation
Hydromorphone	1–2 q 4 h	2–4 q 4 h	Shorter acting than morphine sulfate
Levorphanol	2 q 6–8 h	4 q 6–8 h	Longer acting than morphine sulfate; absorbed well PO
Methadone	10 q 6–8 h	20 q 6–8 h	Delayed sedation due to long half-life
Meperidine	75–100 q 3–4 h	300 q 4 h	Poorly absorbed PO; normeperidine a toxic metabolite
Butorphanol	—	1–2 q 4 h	Intranasal spray
Fentanyl	—	—	Transdermal patch

ANTICONVULSANTS AND ANTIARRHYTHMICS

Generic Name	PO Dose, mg	Interval
Phenytoin	300	daily/qhs
Carbamazepine	200–300	q 6 h
Clonazepam	1	q 6 h
Mexiletine	150–300	q 6–12 h

TRICYCLIC ANTIDEPRESSANTS

Generic Name	Uptake Blockade		Sedative Potency	Anticholinergic Potency	Orthostatic Hypotension	Cardiac Arrhythmia	Average Dose, mg/day	Range, mg/day
	5HT	NE						
Doxepin	+ +	+	High	Moderate	Moderate	Less	200	75–400
Amitriptyline	+ + + +	+ +	High	Highest	Moderate	Yes	150	25–300
Imipramine	+ + + +	+ +	Moderate	Moderate	High	Yes	200	75–400
Nortriptyline	+ + +	+ +	Moderate	Moderate	Low	Yes	100	40–150
Desipramine	+ + +	+ + + +	Low	Low	Low	Yes	150	50–300

Many physicians, nurses, and patients have a certain trepidation about using opioids that is based on an exaggerated fear of patients becoming addicted. In fact, there is a vanishingly small chance of patients becoming addicted to narcotics as a result of their appropriate medical use.

The availability of new routes of administration has extended the usefulness of opioid analgesics. Most important is the availability of spinal administration. Opioids can be infused through a spinal catheter placed either intrathecally or epidurally. By applying opioids directly to the spinal cord, regional analgesia can be obtained using a relatively low total dose. In this way, such side effects as sedation, nausea, and respiratory depression can be minimized. This approach has been used extensively in obstetrical procedures and for lower-body postoperative pain. Opioids also can be given intranasally (butorphanol), rectally, and transdermally (fentanyl), thus avoiding the discomfort of frequent injections in patients who cannot be given oral medication.

OPOID AND CYCLOOXYGENASE INHIBITOR COMBINATIONS When used in combination, opioids and cyclooxygenase inhibitors have additive effects. Because a lower dose of each can be used to achieve the same degree of pain relief and their side effects are nonadditive, such combinations can be used to lower the severity of dose-related side effects. Fixed-ratio combinations of an opioid with acetaminophen carry a special risk. Dose escalation as a result of increased severity of pain or decreased opioid effect as a result of tolerance may lead to levels of acetaminophen that are toxic to the liver.

CHRONIC PAIN

PATIENT EVALUATION Managing patients with chronic pain is intellectually and emotionally challenging. The patient's problem is often difficult to diagnose: such patients are demanding of the physician's time and often appear emotionally distraught. The traditional medical approach of seeking an obscure organic pathology is usually unhelpful. On the other hand, psychological evaluation and behaviorally based treatment paradigms are frequently helpful, particularly in the setting of a multidisciplinary pain-management center.

There are several factors that can cause, perpetuate, or exacerbate chronic pain. First, of course, the patient may simply have a disease that is characteristically painful for which there is presently no cure. Arthritis, cancer, migraine headaches, fibromyalgia, and diabetic neuropathy are examples of this. Second, there may be secondary perpetuating factors that are initiated by a bodily disease and persist after that disease has resolved. Examples include damaged sensory nerves, sympathetic efferent activity, and painful reflex muscle contraction. Finally, a variety of psychological conditions can exacerbate or even cause pain.

There are certain areas to which special attention should be paid in the medical history. Because depression is the most common emotional disturbance in patients with chronic pain, they should be questioned about their mood, appetite, sleep patterns, and daily activity. A simple standardized questionnaire, such as the Beck Depression Inventory, can be a useful screening device. It is important to remember that major depression is a common, treatable, and potentially fatal illness.

Other clues that a significant emotional disturbance is contributing to a patient's chronic pain complaint include: pain occurs in multiple unrelated sites; a pattern of recurrent, but separate, pain problems beginning in childhood or adolescence; pain beginning at a time of emotional trauma, such as the loss of a parent or spouse; a history of physical or sexual abuse; and past or present substance abuse.

On examination, special attention should be paid to whether the patient guards the painful area and whether certain movements or postures are avoided because of pain. Discovering a mechanical component to the pain can be useful both diagnostically and therapeutically. Painful areas should be examined for deep tenderness, noting whether this is localized to muscle, ligamentous structures, or joints. Chronic myofascial pain is very common, and in these patients deep palpation may reveal highly localized trigger points that are firm bands or knots in muscle. If injection of local anesthetic into these trigger points

relieves the pain, it supports the diagnosis. A neuropathic component to the pain is indicated by evidence of nerve damage, such as sensory impairment, exquisitely sensitive skin, weakness and muscle atrophy, or loss of deep tendon reflexes. Evidence suggesting sympathetic nervous system involvement includes the presence of diffuse swelling, changes in skin color and temperature, and hypersensitive skin and joint tenderness compared with the normal side. Relief of the pain with a sympathetic block is diagnostic.

A guiding principle in evaluating patients with chronic pain is to assess both emotional and organic factors before initiating therapy. Addressing these issues together, rather than waiting to "rule out" organic causes of the pain, improves compliance in part because it assures patients that a psychological evaluation does not mean that the physician is questioning the validity of their complaint. Even when an organic cause for a patient's pain can be found, it is still wise to look for other factors. For example, cancer patients with painful bony metastases also may have pain due to nerve damage and significant depression. Optimal therapy requires that each of these factors be looked for and treated.

℞ **TREATMENT**

Once the evaluation process has been completed and the likely causative and exacerbating factors identified, an explicit treatment plan should be developed. An important part of this process is to identify specific and realistic functional goals for therapy, such as getting a good night's sleep, being able to go shopping, or returning to work. A multidisciplinary approach that utilizes medications, counseling, physical therapy, nerve blocks, and even surgery may be required to improve the patient's quality of life. This may require referral to a pain clinic; however, this is not necessary for all chronic pain patients. For some, pharmacologic management alone can provide significant help.

Antidepressant Medications The tricyclic antidepressants (see Table 12-1) are extremely useful for the management of patients with chronic pain. Although developed for the treatment of depression, the tricyclics have a spectrum of dose-related biologic activities that include the production of analgesia in a variety of clinical conditions. Although the mechanism is unknown, the analgesic effect of tricyclics has a more rapid onset of action and occurs at a lower dose than is typically required for the treatment of depression. Furthermore, patients with chronic pain who are not depressed obtain pain relief with antidepressants. There is evidence that tricyclic drugs potentiate opioid analgesia, so they are useful adjuncts for the treatment of severe persistent pain such as occurs with malignant tumors. Table 12-2 lists some of the painful conditions that respond to tricyclics. Tricyclics are of particular value in the management of neuropathic pains such as painful diabetic neuropathy and postherpetic neuralgia, for which there are few other therapeutic options.

The tricyclics that have been shown to relieve pain have significant side effects. Unfortunately, some of the newer antidepressants such as fluoxetine (Prozac) that have fewer and less serious side effects have not been shown to provide pain relief.

Table 12-2

Painful Conditions that Respond to Tricyclic Antidepressants

Postherpetic neuralgia*
Diabetic neuropathy*
Tension headache*
Migraine headache*
Rheumatoid arthritis*†
Chronic low back pain†
Cancer

* Controlled trials demonstrate analgesia.
† Controlled studies indicate benefit but not analgesia.
SOURCE: Fields, 1987, p 291.

Anticonvulsants and Antiarrhythmics (See Table 12-1) These drugs are useful primarily for patients with neuropathic pain. Phenytoin (Dilantin) and carbamazepine (Tegretol) were first shown to relieve the pain of trigeminal neuralgia. This pain has a characteristic brief, shooting, electric shock–like quality. In fact, anticonvulsants seem to be helpful largely for pains that have such a lancinating quality.

Antiarrhythmic drugs such as low-dose lidocaine and mexiletine (Mexitil) are also effective for neuropathic pains. These drugs block the spontaneous activity of primary afferent nociceptors that appears when they are damaged.

Chronic Opioid Medication The long-term use of opioids is accepted for patients with pain due to malignant disease. Although its use for chronic pain of nonmalignant origin is controversial, it is clear that for many such patients opioid analgesics are the only option available for obtaining effective relief. This is understandable since opioids are the most potent and have the broadest range of efficacy of any analgesic medications. Although addiction is rare in patients who first use opioids for pain relief, some degree of tolerance and physical dependence are likely to occur with long-term use. Therefore, before embarking on opioid therapy, other options should be explored, and the limitations and risks of opioids should be explained to the patient. It is also important to point out that some opioid analgesic medications have mixed agonist-antagonist properties (e.g., pentazocine and butorphanol). From a practical standpoint, this means that they may worsen pain by inducing an abstinence syndrome in patients who are physically dependent on other opioid analgesics.

With long-term outpatient use of orally administered opioids it is desirable to use long-acting compounds such as levorphanol, methadone, or sustained-release morphine (see Table 12-1). The pharmacokinetic profile of these drugs enables prolonged pain relief, minimizes side effects such as sedation that are associated with high peak plasma levels, and, perhaps, reduces the likelihood of rebound pain associated with a rapid fall in plasma opioid concentration. Constipation is a virtually universal side effect of opioid use and should be treated expectantly.

It is worth emphasizing, in conclusion, that many patients, especially those with chronic pain, seek medical attention primarily because they are suffering and because only physicians can provide the medications required for their relief. Clearly, it is a primary responsibility of all physicians to attempt to minimize the physical and emotional discomfort of their patients. Familiarity with pain mechanisms and analgesic medications is an important step toward accomplishing this aim.

BIBLIOGRAPHY

BASBAUM AI, FIELDS HL: Endogenous pain control systems: Brainstem spinal pathways and endorphin circuitry. Ann Rev Neurosci 7:309, 1984

FIELDS HL (ed): *Pain Syndromes in Neurology.* London, Butterworth, 1990

———: *Pain.* New York, McGraw-Hill, 1987

———, LIEBESKIND JC (eds): *Pharmacological Approaches to the Treatment of Chronic Pain: New Concepts and Critical Issues.* Seattle, IASP Press, 1994

GALER BS: Neuropathic pain of peripheral origin: Advances in pharmacologic treatment. Neurology 45:517, 1995

MELZACK R, CASEY KL: Sensory, motivational, and central control determinants of pain, in *International Symposium on the Skin Senses*, DR Kenshalo (ed). Springfield, Ill, Charles C Thomas, 1968, p 423

ROWBOTHAM MC: Chronic pain: From theory to practical management. Neurology 45:5, 1995

STEIN C: The control of pain in peripheral tissue by opioids. N Engl J Med 332:1685, 1995

WALL PD, MELZACK R (eds): *Textbook of Pain* 3d ed. New York, Churchill Livingstone, 1994

WILLIS WD (ed): *Hyperalgesia and Allodynia.* New York, Raven Press, 1992

———, COGGESHALL RE: *Sensory Mechanism of the Spinal Cord.* New York, Plenum Press, 1991

13   *Lee Goldman*

CHEST DISCOMFORT AND PALPITATION

CHEST DISCOMFORT

Chest discomfort is one of the most frequent complaints for which patients seek medical attention; the potential benefit (or harm) resulting from the proper (or improper) assessment and management of the patient with this complaint is enormous. Failure to recognize a serious disorder, such as ischemic heart disease, may result in the dangerous delay of much-needed treatment, while an incorrect diagnosis of a potentially hazardous condition such as angina pectoris is likely to have harmful psychological and economic consequences and may lead to unnecessary cardiac catheterization. There is little relation between the severity of chest discomfort and the gravity of its cause. Therefore, a frequent problem in patients who complain of chest discomfort or pain is distinguishing trivial complaints from coronary artery disease and other serious disorders (Table 13-1).

CAUSES OF CHEST DISCOMFORT **Discomfort due to Myocardial Ischemia** Discomfort due to myocardial ischemia occurs when the oxygen supply to the heart is deficient in relation to

Table 13-1

Some Causes of Chest Discomfort and the Types of Discomfort Associated with Them

Cause	New, Acute, Often Ongoing	Recurrent, Episodic	Persistent, Even for Days
CARDIAC			
Coronary artery disease	+	+	—
Aortic stenosis	—	+	—
Hypertropic cardiomyopathy	—	+	—
Pericarditis	+	+	+
VASCULAR			
Aortic dissection	+	—	—
Pulmonary embolism	+	+	—
Pulmonary hypertension	+	+	—
Right ventricular strain	+	+	—
PULMONARY			
Pleuritis or pneumonia	+	+	+
Tracheobronchitis	+	+	+
Pneumothorax	+	—	+
Tumor	—	—	+
Mediastinitis or mediastinal emphysema	+	—	+
GASTROINTESTINAL			
Esophageal reflux	+	+	+
Esophageal spasm	+	+	+
Mallory-Weiss tear	+	—	—
Peptic ulcer disease	+	+	—
Biliary disease	+	+	—
Pancreatitis		+	+
MUSCULOSKELETAL			
Cervical disk disease	—	+	+
Arthritis of the shoulder or spine	—	+	+
Costochondritis	+	+	+
Intercostal muscle cramps	+	+	+
Interscalene or hyperabduction syndromes	—	+	+
Subacromial bursitis	+	+	+
OTHER			
Disorders of the breast	—	+	+
Chest wall tumors	—	—	+
Herpes zoster	+	—	+
Emotional	+	+	+

the oxygen need. The blood flow through the coronary arteries is directly proportional to the pressure gradient between the aorta and the ventricular myocardium (during systole) or the ventricular cavity (during diastole). However, in the presence of critical stenosis, it is also proportional to the fourth power of the radius of the coronary arteries. A relatively slight alteration in coronary luminal diameter below a critical level can produce a large decrease in coronary flow, provided that other factors remain constant. Coronary blood flow occurs primarily during diastole, when it is unopposed by systolic myocardial compression of the coronary vessels.

When the epicardial coronary arteries are narrowed critically (>70 percent stenosis of the luminal diameter), the intramyocardial coronary arterioles dilate in an effort to maintain total flow at a level that will avert myocardial ischemia at rest. The further dilation that would normally occur during exercise is, therefore, not possible. Hence, any condition in which increased heart rate, arterial pressure, or myocardial contractility occurs in the presence of coronary obstruction tends to precipitate anginal attacks by increasing myocardial oxygen needs in the face of a fixed oxygen supply.

By far the most frequent underlying cause of myocardial ischemia is organic narrowing of the coronary arteries secondary to coronary atherosclerosis (see also Chap. 244). Acute thrombosis superimposed on an atherosclerotic plaque is frequently the cause of unstable angina and acute myocardial infarction (see Chaps. 243 and 244).

Aside from conditions that narrow the lumen of the coronary arteries, the only other frequent causes of myocardial ischemia are disorders such as valvular aortic stenosis (Chap. 237) or hypertrophic cardiomyopathy (Chap. 239), which cause a marked disproportion between the coronary perfusion pressure and the heart's oxygen requirements. Under such conditions, the rise in left ventricular systolic pressure is not, as in hypertensive states, balanced by a corresponding elevation of aortic perfusion pressure. Epidemiologic studies indicate that chest pain is no more common in patients with mitral valve prolapse than in those without it.

The chest discomfort of myocardial ischemia, most commonly from coronary artery disease but also occasionally from the other causes of ischemia noted above, is angina pectoris. Myocardial ischemia secondary to coronary atherosclerosis is more common in adults, especially the elderly who have hypercholesterolemia, diabetes mellitus, hypertension, obesity, or who smoke cigarettes (Chap. 242). Toxins, including cocaine ingestion or withdrawal of chronic exposure to nitroglycerin, can cause sufficient coronary vasoconstriction to result in myocardial ischemia, and cocaine also can cause myocardial infarction.

Angina pectoris   (See also Chap. 244)   Angina pectoris is usually described as a heaviness, pressure, squeezing, or sensation of strangling or constriction in the chest, but it also may be described as an aching or burning pain, or even as indigestion. Some patients steadfastly deny pain but will admit to a discomfort or unusual feeling or may complain of difficulty in breathing.

Typically, angina pectoris develops gradually during exertion, after heavy meals, and with anger, excitement, frustration, and other emotional states; it is not precipitated by coughing, respiratory movements, or other motion. When angina is induced by walking, it often forces the patient to stop or to reduce speed. Anginal pain typically resolves within 5 to 30 min. More prolonged myocardial ischemia often represents a myocardial infarction, while more prolonged pain without other evidence for myocardial ischemia suggests a noncoronary etiology.

The correct diagnosis of angina pectoris may be aided by noting that the pain disappears more rapidly (usually within 5 min) and more completely when sublingual nitroglycerin is used. The demonstration that the time required for a given exercise to produce pain is consistently and considerably longer when it is undertaken within a few minutes after a sublingual nitroglycerin pill than after a placebo may, in some instances, be powerful clinical evidence for the diagnosis of angina pectoris. Angina is rarely relieved within a few seconds of lying down. It is not precipitated by stooping forward or by chest palpation, deep breathing, or simple changes in position.

Angina occurs most typically in the substernal region, anteriorly

across the midthorax; it may radiate to or rarely occur alone in the intercapsular region, arms, shoulders, teeth, or abdomen. It rarely radiates to below the umbilicus, to the back of the neck, or to the occiput. Although the radiation of chest discomfort to the left arm increases the likelihood that myocardial ischemia or infarction is present, impulses from the skin and from visceral structures, such as the esophagus and heart, converge on a common pool of neurons in the posterior horn of the spinal cord, and their origin may be confused by the cerebral cortex.

An increase in heart rate is especially harmful in patients with coronary atherosclerosis or with aortic stenosis, because it both increases myocardial oxygen need and shortens diastole more than systole, thereby decreasing the total available perfusion time per minute. Tachycardia, a decline in arterial pressure, thyrotoxicosis, and diminution in arterial oxygen content (such as occurs in anemia or arterial hypoxia) are precipitating and aggravating factors rather than underlying causes of angina.

Patients with marked *right ventricular hypertension* may have exertional pain that is quite similar to that of angina. This discomfort probably results from relative ischemia of the right ventricle brought about by the increased oxygen needs and by the elevated intramural resistance, with reduction of the normally large systolic pressure gradient that perfuses this chamber.

Myocardial infarction   Myocardial infarction is usually associated with a discomfort that is similar in quality and distribution to that of angina but of longer duration (usually 30 min) and usually of greater intensity. In contrast to angina, the pain of myocardial infarction is not rapidly relieved by rest or by coronary dilator drugs and may require large doses of narcotics. It may be accompanied by diaphoresis, nausea, and hypotension (see Chap. 243).

Physical examination   The results of physical examination may be normal in patients with myocardial ischemia caused by coronary atherosclerosis. However, myocardial ischemia can cause a third or fourth heart sound because of an impairment of myocardial contraction or relaxation. Ischemic papillary muscle dysfunction can cause transient mitral regurgitation and its associated murmur. Myocardial infarction and, less commonly, severe and generalized ischemia can cause congestive heart failure.

The chest discomfort from myocardial ischemia that is caused by aortic stenosis, hypertrophic cardiomyopathy, and nonatherosclerotic causes of coronary artery disease is generally similar to that of angina pectoris from coronary atherosclerosis. However, in these conditions the physical examination will usually reveal classic findings of an aortic systolic murmur in patients with aortic stenosis (see Chap. 237) and will reveal dynamic outflow obstruction in many patients with hypertrophic cardiomyopathy (see Chap. 239).

Chest Pain due to Pericarditis   The visceral surface of the pericardium ordinarily is insensitive to pain, as is the parietal surface, except in its lower portion, which has a relatively small number of pain fibers carried in the phrenic nerves. The pain associated with pericarditis is believed to be due to inflammation of the adjacent parietal pleura. These observations explain why noninfectious pericarditis (e.g., that associated with uremia and with myocardial infarction) and cardiac tamponade with relatively mild inflammation are usually painless or accompanied by only mild pain, whereas infectious pericarditis, being nearly always more intense and spreading to the neighboring pleura, is usually associated with pain (Chap. 240).

Pericarditis can cause pain in several locations (see Chap. 240). Since the central part of the diaphragm receives its sensory supply from the phrenic nerve (which arises from the third to fifth cervical segments of the spinal cord), pain arising from the lower parietal pericardium and central tendon of the diaphragm is felt characteristically at the tip of the shoulder, the adjoining trapezius ridge, and the neck. Involvement of the more lateral part of the diaphragmatic pleura, supplied by branches from the sixth to ninth intercostal nerves, causes pain not only in the anterior part of the chest but also in the upper part of the abdomen or corresponding region of the back, sometimes simulating the pain of acute cholecystitis or pancreatitis.

Pericardial pain commonly has a pleuritic component; i.e., it is related to respiratory movements and aggravated by cough and/or deep inspiration, because of pleural irritation. It is sometimes brought on by swallowing, because the esophagus lies just behind the posterior portion of the heart, and is often altered by a change of body position, becoming sharper and more left-sided in the supine position and milder when the patient sits upright, leaning forward.

In some patients, however, pericardial pain may be described as a steady substernal discomfort that can mimic the pain of acute myocardial infarction. The mechanism of this steady substernal pain is not certain, but it may arise from marked inflammation of the relatively insensitive inner parietal surface of the pericardium or from irritated afferent cardiac nerve fibers lying in the periadventitial layers of the superficial coronary arteries. Occasionally, both pleuritic and steady pain may be present simultaneously.

Vascular Causes of Chest Pain   *Aortic dissection* develops as a result of a subintimal hematoma, which may start either because a tear has developed in the intima of the aorta or because of bleeding into the vasa vasorum. Antegrade movement of this hematoma can compromise major branches off the aorta, while retrograde spread can occlude a coronary artery, disrupt the aortic valve annulus, or rupture into the pericardial space.

The pain due to *acute dissection of the aorta* (Chap. 247) or to an expanding aortic aneurysm results from stimulation of nerve endings in the adventitia. The pain usually begins abruptly, reaches an extremely severe peak rapidly, is felt in the center of the chest and/or in the back depending on the site of the dissection, lasts for hours, and requires unusually large amounts of analgesics for relief. Patients commonly describe a true pain rather than the vague discomfort that is sometimes described with myocardial ischemia. The pain is not aggravated by changes in position or respiration.

Chest Pain due to Pulmonary Embolism   The acute pain from massive *pulmonary emboli* (Chap. 261) is thought to be related to pulmonary hypertension and to distention of the pulmonary artery. Infarction of a segment of the lung that is adjacent to the pleura commonly irritates the pleural surface and causes chest discomfort hours or even days later. The pain resulting from pulmonary embolism may resemble that of acute myocrdial infarction, and in cases of massive embolism it is located substernally. In patients with smaller emboli, the pain is caused by focal pulmonary infarction and is usually located more laterally, is pleuritic in nature, and sometimes is associated with hemoptysis.

Other Pulmonary Causes of Chest Discomfort   A variety of diseases of the lung can cause chest discomfort. Pleural pain, which is usually a brief, sharp, knifelike pain that is precipitated by inspiration or coughing, is very common and generally results from stretching of a parietal pleura that is inflamed by fibrinous pleurisy or any pneumonic process (see Chap. 262).

Gastrointestinal Causes of Chest Discomfort   *Esophageal pain* commonly presents as a deep thoracic burning discomfort, which is the hallmark of acid-induced pain. Ingestion of aspirin, alcohol, or certain foods typically exacerbates this burning discomfort, and the discomfort may be relieved promptly by antacids or even by one or two swallows of food or water. Patients may have accompanying dysphagia, regurgitation of undigested food, or weight loss. The symptoms of a hiatus hernia tend to be exacerbated by lying down, and all forms of acid-peptic disease may be worse in the early morning, when acidic secretions are not neutralized by food. Esophageal spasm, which may be induced by reflux of gastric acid into an esophagus in which the mucosa has been previously irritated, can cause a squeezing pain that may be indistinguishable from that of myocardial ischemia and that may even have a similar pattern of radiation. Pain resulting from injury of the esophagus, such as in the case of a Mallory-Weiss tear that is caused by severe vomiting, can cause severe acute chest pain (Chap. 283).

Occasionally, other gastrointestinal diseases, including *peptic ulcer disease, biliary disease*, and *pancreatitis*, may present with chest discomfort as well as abdominal discomfort. Pain resulting from gastric or duodenal ulcer (Chap. 284) is epigastric or substernal, usually commences about 1 to 1.5 h after meals, and is usually relieved in several minutes by antacids or milk.

The discomfort caused by acute cholecystitis is more commonly described as an ache, which may be epigastric or substernal. It most commonly occurs an hour or so after meals and not in relation to exertion. The presence of an abdominal disorder, such as a hiatus hernia or a duodenal ulcer, does not constitute proof that the patient's chest pain is related to it. Such disorders are frequently asymptomatic and are not at all uncommon in patients who also have myocardial ischemia.

Neuromusculoskeletal Causes of Chest Discomfort   Neuromusculoskeletal chest discomfort can be caused by *cervical disk disease* because of compression of nerve roots, by *arthritis of the shoulder or spine*, or by *costochondritis*, which is an inflammation of the costochondral junctions. Inflammation of the subacromial bursa or, less commonly, the supraspinatus or deltoid tendon may cause pain that radiates to the chest. *Intercostal muscle cramps* may occur throughout the chest. Anterior scalene and hyperabduction syndromes also can cause chest discomfort.

The *costochondral and chondrosternal articulations* are the most common sites of anterior musculoskeletal chest pain. Objective signs in the form of swelling (Tietze's syndrome), redness, and heat are rare, but sharply localized tenderness is common. The pain may be darting and last for only a few seconds or may be a dull ache enduring for hours or days. An associated feeling of tightness due to muscle spasm (see below) is frequent. *Pressure on the chondrosternal and costochondral junctions and on the pectoralis muscles is an essential part of the examination of every patient with chest pain* and will reproduce the pain arising from these tissues.

Emotional Causes of Chest Pain   Emotional disorders are commonly associated with chest pain. Usually, the discomfort is experienced as a sense of "tightness," sometimes called "aching," and occasionally it may be designated as a pain of considerable magnitude. Since the discomfort may be described as a tightness or constriction and is often localized at least in part beneath the sternum, it is not surprising that this type of discomfort is frequently confused with that of myocardial ischemia. Ordinarily, it lasts for a half hour or more, is unrelated to exertion, and fluctuates slowly in intensity. The association with fatigue or emotional strain is usually clear, although this may not be volunteered by the patient. Associated hyperventilation can cause innocent changes in the T waves and ST segments, which can be confused with coronary artery disease. Alternatively, chest pain associated with emotional disorders may be sharp and very brief and located near the left nipple.

DIFFERENTIAL DIAGNOGIS OF CHEST DISCOMFORT
The key issue in the evaluation of the patient with chest discomfort is to distinguish potentially life-threatening conditions such as coronary artery disease, aortic dissection, or pulmonary embolism from other causes of chest discomfort. Even patients who have brief episodes of pain and are otherwise in apparently excellent health may have intermittent myocardial ischemia or recurrent pulmonary emboli. One useful approach to the patient with chest pain is to determine whether the syndrome represents new, acute, and often ongoing pain; recurrent, episodic pain; or pain that is persistent, perhaps for days (Fig. 13-1). The various causes of chest pain (Table 13-1) can, in part, be distinguished by their likelihood to present in these three different ways.

New, Acute, often Ongoing Pain   In a patient who presents with this syndrome, the physician must immediately distinguish whether the pain represents a condition for which acute circulatory or respiratory insufficiency is a substantial risk (Fig. 13-2). Emergent stabilization and treatment must precede detailed diagnostic evaluation.

In the patient with acute chest discomfort, the diagnostic evaluation begins with a focused history and physical examination that is designed to evaluate the likelihood of conditions, such as acute myocardial

Determine type of syndrome

New, acute, often ongoing pain → See Fig. 13-2

Recurrent, episodic pain → See Fig. 13-4

Persistent (perhaps for days) pain → See Fig. 13-5

FIGURE 13-1 Approach to the patient with chest pain.

infarction, aortic dissection, or pulmonary embolism, that could be life-threatening even in a patient who currently appears to be stable. Accumulated data from large numbers of patients who have presented to emergency departments with acute chest pain can aid in the assessment of the probability that an individual is experiencing an acute myocardial infarction. In this setting, an emergent electrocardiogram is the single best diagnostic test (Fig. 13-3). In patients in whom the electrocardiogram shows Q waves of at least 0.04 s duration or ST-segment elevation that is not known to be old in two more leads, the probability of acute myocardial infarction is 75 percent. In patients in whom the electrocardiogram shows evidence of ST-segment depression of 1 mm or more or T-wave inversion that is not known to be old in two or more leads, the probability of acute myocardial infarction is about 20 percent. On the basis of substantial empirical data, patients with either of these electrocardiographic changes and a clinical syndrome suspicious for acute myocardial ischemia require urgent admission to an intensive care unit, partly for further evaluation but mainly because of the substantial short-term risk of developing life-threatening complications (see Chap. 243). For patients with ST-segment elevation, the likelihood of occlusion of an infarct-related artery mandates urgent reperfusion unless otherwise contraindicated or unless a diagnosis other than acute myocardial infarction is being considered very seriously. For patients with changes suggesting ischemia but without ST elevation, treatment is usually for presumed unstable angina (see Chap. 244).

For patients without electrocardiographic changes of new (or presumably new) ischemia or infarction, further observation with serial electrocardiograms and cardiac enzymes is useful if the clinical presentation nevertheless raises a reasonable likelihood of acute myocardial infarction or acute myocardial ischemia. In this assessment, multiple factors must be taken into account, especially in patients who do not have evident changes on the initial electrocardiogram. For example, a patient is more likely to be having acute myocardial ischemia if the pain is clearly similar to prior known angina pectoris but somehow worse in terms of intensity, duration, or failure to respond to usual measures. In patients wih no prior history of ischemic heart disease, multiple factors, including the patient's age and gender and the location and description of pain, influence whether further observation is required. New approaches to these patients include admission to chest pain observation units in which patients are

watched for up to 6 to 12 h with serial testing. After this observation period, further cardiac testing with a standard exercise electrocardiogram, a myocardial perfusion scintiscan, or a stress echocardiogram may aid in establishing the diagnosis. In patients in whom no myocardial cause is evident, a musculoskeletal and/or gastrointestinal evaluation may be helpful, but such testing can usually be performed on an outpatient basis.

Acute aortic dissection (Chap. 247) may be suggested by the sudden onset of symptoms, the finding of asymmetric pulses, and a history of hypertension or Marfan's syndrome. The routine chest radiograph may show a dilated aortic root to suggest or support this diagnosis, which may then be established by transesophageal echocardiography, computed tomography, or magnetic resonance imaging. Aortography has traditionally been the definitive test, but, because of its invasiveness, it is often now replaced by magnetic resonance imaging in hemodynamically stable patients and preceded by a screening transesophageal echocardiogram in unstable patients.

Acute pulmonary embolism (Chap. 261) may be suggested on the basis of respiratory symptoms, hemoptysis, pleuritic chest discomfort, or a history of deep venous thrombosis or coagulation abnormalities. The evaluation usually requires a lung scan and/or pulmonary arteriogram to evaluate pulmonary perfusion.

Of the various potential gastrointestinal causes of chest discomfort, the most worrisome include a Mallory-Weiss esophageal tear, acute cholecystitis, pancreatitis, and a perforating gastric or duodenal ulcer. For peptic ulcer disease, cholecystitis, and pancreatitis, the abdominal examination usually is critical to the diagnosis. Mallory-Weiss tears

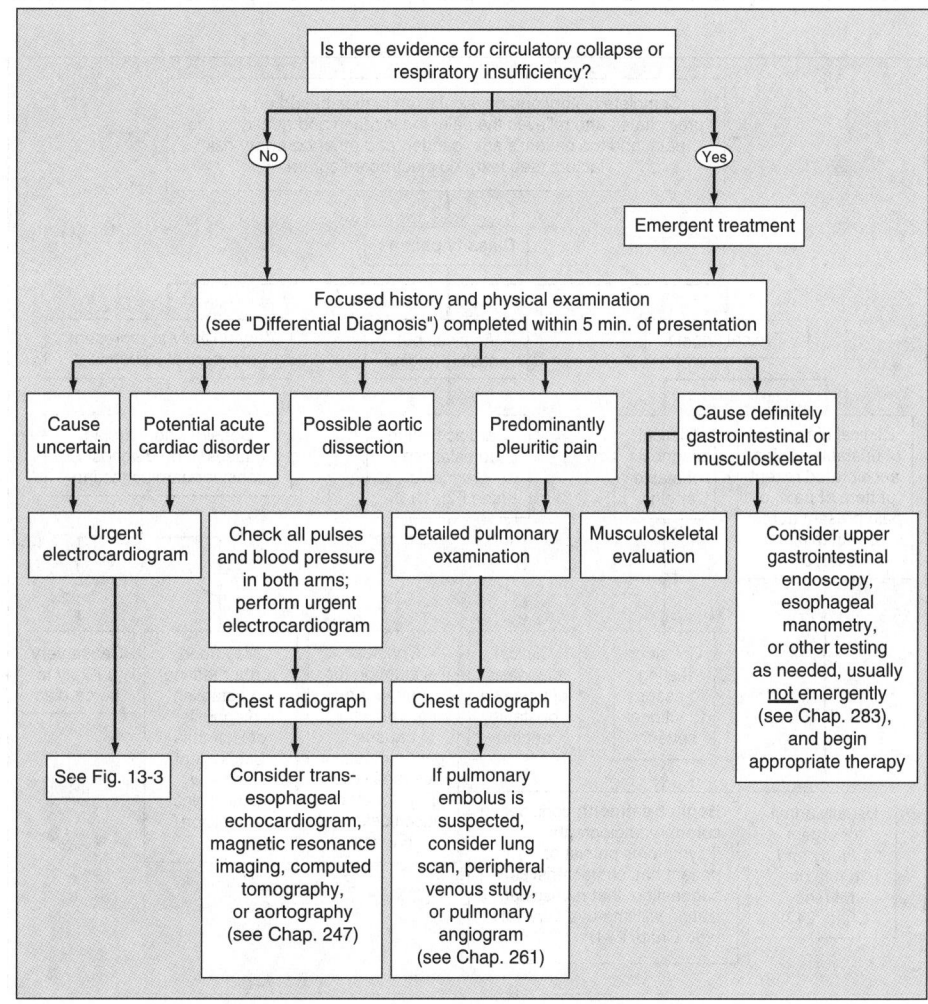

FIGURE 13-2 Approach to the patient with new, acute, often ongoing pain.

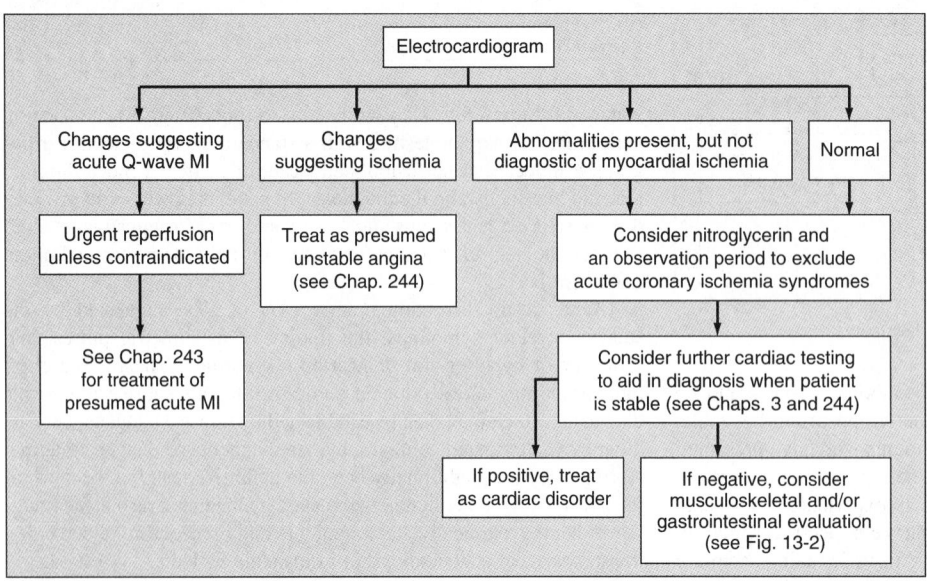

FIGURE 13-3 Approach to the patient with new, acute, often ongoing pain potentially of cardiac etiology or of uncertain cause. (MI, myocardial infarction.)

are commonly associated with hematemesis. In the acute setting, esophageal disease may be a diagnosis of exclusion in patients who have no evidence for cardiac, pulmonary, or vascular causes. Upper gastrointestinal endoscopy or an upper gastrointestinal roentgenogram can diagnose esophageal or peptic ulcer disease. Esophageal manometry and measurement of lower esophageal sphincter pressure are useful in identifying esophageal spasm. The Bernstein acid perfusion test, in which an attempt is made to reproduce the pain by infusion of

hydrochloric acid into the esophagus, can help establish acid reflux as the cause of chest pain (see Chap. 283).

Recurrent Episodic Pain In the patient with recurrent, episodic pain, the diagnostic and therapeutic tempo is different than in the patient with new, acute, and often ongoing pain. Although life-threatening conditions such as acute myocardial infarction, recurrent pulmonary emboli, or even aortic dissection can sometimes present in this way, patients with recurrent, episodic pain are more likely to have a variety of less critical diagnoses (Table 13-1).

In this setting, a detailed and meticulous history of the behavior of the pain is the cornerstone of the evaluation (Fig. 13-4). One useful approach is to divide recurrent, episodic pain into those syndromes that represent a high likelihood for angina, those that are atypical but possibly represent angina, and those that are very unlikely to be caused by angina or myocardial ischemia. The history, physical examination, and subsequent diagnostic testing can be guided by this approach.

The *history* should focus on the behavior of the pain as the cornerstone of the evaluation. The location, radiation, quality, intensity, and duration of the episodes are important. Even more so is the story of the aggravating and alleviating factors. A history of intense aggravation by breathing, coughing, or other respiratory movements will usually point toward the pleura and pericardium or mediastinum as the site, although chest wall pain is likewise affected by respiratory motion. Similarly, a pain that regularly appears on rapid walking, or with other exertion such as sexual activity, and vanishes a few minutes after stopping suggests the diagnosis of angina pectoris, although a similar story will occasionally be obtained from patients with skeletal disorders.

A thorough *physical examination* can provide important clues to the cause of chest discomfort. Blood pressure should be checked in both arms if aortic dissection is being considered. Examination of the skin may reveal cyanosis, which suggests hypoxemia from either diminished cardiac output or impaired respiratory function, or xanthelasthma, which would suggest hyperlipidemia and associated coronary disease. The finding of lymphadenopathy suggests a tumor. The examination of the chest wall should include both inspection and palpation to search for costochondritis and other musculoskeletal abnormalities. Lung examination may reveal a pleural rub, signs of pneumonic consolidation, or evidence of congestive heart failure. The physical examination may be totally normal in persons with severe myocardial ischemia, but it also may demonstrate abnormalities of vital signs, a third or fourth heart sound, or mitral regurgitation from papillary muscle dysfunction. Aortic stenosis will be accompanied by its typical murmur (Chap. 237). The cardiac examination also

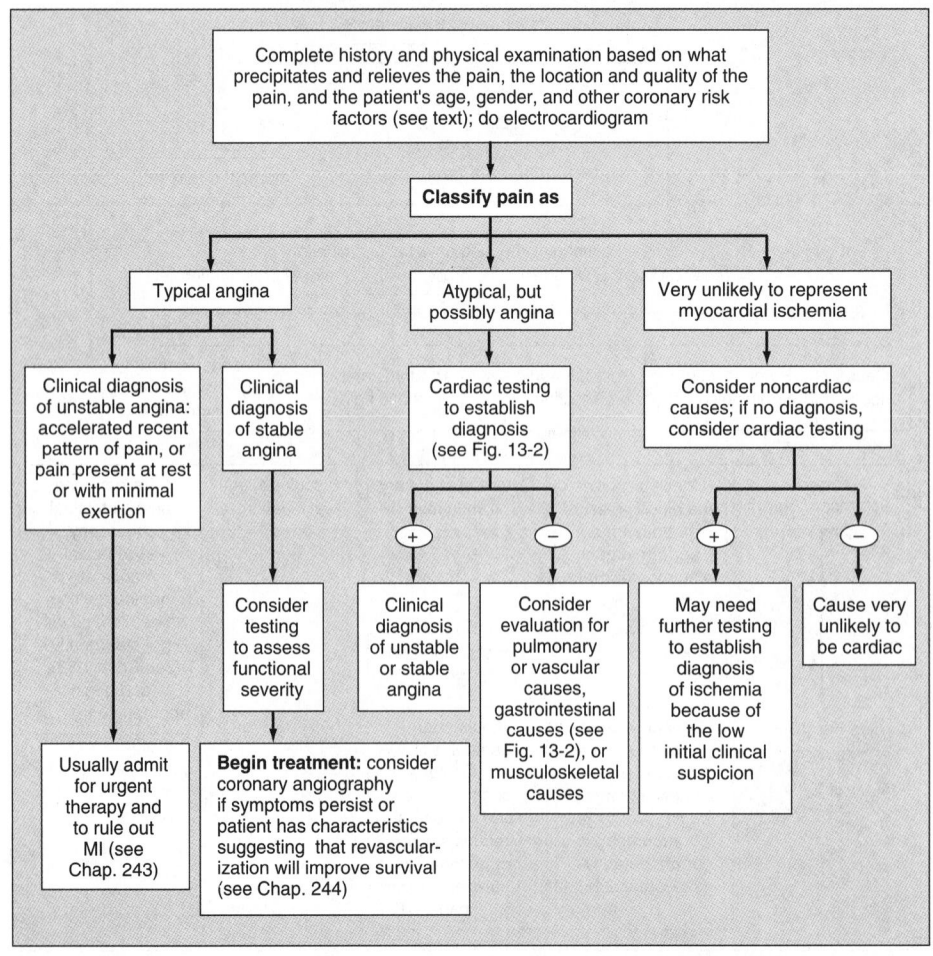

FIGURE 13-4 Approach to the patient with recurrent episodic pain. (MI, myocardial infarction.)

should search for an increased pulmonic second sound that may indicate elevated pulmonary artery pressure, such as is found in pulmonary embolism, and the pericardial friction rub that strongly suggests pericarditis. A careful upper abdominal examination may be the first clue to peptic ulcer disease or cholecystitis.

Critical information can often be obtained by attempts to produce or alleviate the pain, such as with nitroglycerin. Careful palpation of the chest wall, subacromial bursa, deltoid tendon, abdomen, and other structures may be very helpful if it reproduces the chest discomfort. Shoulder and arm motion commonly reproduces pain related to these structures. Evaluation of the patient at the time of a spontaneous episode, such as with an electrocardiogram during pain, is also extremely helpful.

Persistent Chest Discomfort Pain that persists unabated for many hours or days is more likely to represent a noncoronary cause, such as pericarditis, a musculoskeletal condition, a pulmonary abnormality, or one of several gastrointestinal conditions. Once again, a complete history and physical examination is mandatory, and further testing is guided by the findings (Table 13-2). If pericarditis is suspected, an electrocardiogram, chest radiograph, and echocardiogram may establish or exclude the diagnosis. Potential pulmonary conditions are commonly evaluated with a chest radiograph. Suspected musculoskeletal abnormalities may be confirmed, if necessary, by radiographic studies and/or the response to targeted therapies, including a local injection of lidocaine. Potential gastrointestinal causes may be evaluated with a variety of tests as described above. Although acute myocardial infarction, pulmonary embolism, and aortic dissection rarely present as persistent pain, these diagnoses must also be considered in patients in whom the more common causes of persistent pain are not found.

In considering diagnostic tests for all the various causes of chest discomfort, the clinician must remember that a useful test result is commonly one that moves the likelihood of a diagnostic possibility across a threshold, so the test result would lead to a change in management, either by influencing the decision to order additional tests or by causing a change in treatment. In the case of chest discomfort, the decisions cannot be based on a 50 percent threshold: Probabilities of coronary artery disease, pulmonary embolism, or aortic dissection that are well below 50 percent may still demand further evaluation because of the dire consequences of missing one of these important diagnoses. The physician must be prepared to embark on an appropriate evaluation when the history and physical examination do not exclude these diagnoses with a reasonable degree of certainty. The degree of certainty must be determined for the individual condition and patient at hand, typically after an appropriately full and frank discussion between the patient and the physician.

Weighing the Evidence The assessment of the probability of the various causes of chest pain requires the integration of multiple pieces of data, because no single clinical feature can be considered decisive. Each of the conditions that can cause chest discomfort can have varied presentations, and the diagnostic tests upon which physicians often rely can also have false-positive or false-negative results. Thus the principles of clinical reasoning (Chap. 3) should be applied to the evaluation of the patient with chest discomfort.

The information obtained from a careful medical history and physical examination can be used to develop a differential diagnosis of the causes of chest discomfort in an individual patient, to rank these diagnostic possibilities, and often to assign approximate percent probabilities to them. Although the various causes of chest discomfort have typical characteristics, these characteristics must be interpreted in light of the prior probability that a person with a given age and sex and with a particular past medical history would have such a cause of chest discomfort. For example, the possibility of angina pectoris as a cause of precordial or substernal discomfort must be seriously considered in a middle-aged man with coronary risk factors such as hypercholesterolemia and smoking, even if the description of the discomfort is not perfectly typical for angina pectoris. Conversely, when a 20-year-old woman describes the onset of new discomfort in a way that is seemingly classic for angina pectoris, such a diagnosis is relatively

unlikely because the prior probability of ischemic heart disease, given her age and sex, is so low.

Although it is not always possible to assign numerical probabilities to the various causes of chest discomfort in an individual patient, experienced clinicians either implicitly or explicitly assess the relative likelihoods of various potential explanations for any chest discomfort syndrome to help guide their future diagnostic evaluations and therapy. For example, a middle-aged or elderly man with typical characteristics for angina pectoris has about an 85 percent probability of having hemodynamically significant coronary artery disease. By comparison, the same man with a history of chest discomfort that has some characteristics that are typical for angina pectoris but other characteristics that are atypical has a probability of important coronary disease ranging from about 30 to 60 percent. Even persons with chest pain that is decidedly unlikely to represent coronary disease still have some finite possibility of coronary disease, with a likelihood ranging from exceedingly small in a young woman to somewhere in the 10 percent range in a middle-aged man with many coronary risk factors.

Diagnostic tests Although myocardial ischemia commonly is associated with electrocardiographic changes (Chap. 244), many patients have normal tracings between attacks, and in some the electrocardiogram may even be normal during an episode of pain. However, depression of the ST segments, caused by myocardial ischemia, typically occurs during exertion and is accompanied by anginal discomfort; moreover, electrocardiographic evidence of myocardial ischemia may occur at rest and with or without accompanying chest discomfort. The finding of flat or down-sloping ST-segment depressions of 0.1 mV or greater during an attack of pain substantially increases the likelihood that the pain is anginal in origin. Exercise electrocardiography will show ischemic changes in about 50 to 80 percent of persons with symptomatic coronary disease but also in about 10 to 15 percent of patients who do not have coronary disease. The accuracy of ambulatory ischemia monitoring in the general population is less clear.

Although exercise electrocardiography and exercise thallium scintigraphy are of value in distinguishing between cardiac and noncardiac causes of chest discomfort, the results must be interpreted in light of the prior probability of coronary artery disease, which is the probability that the patient has coronary disease based on the presenting clinical characteristics, age, and sex (see Fig. 3-2). Since exercise perfusion scintigraphy appears to provide information that is correlated with the standard exercise electrocardiogram no more than would be expected by chance, it can provide additional independent information (Chap. 3) and further change the probability of coronary artery disease (Fig. 13-1). If absolute diagnostic knowledge is required, cardiac catheterization with coronary angiography serves as the gold standard—i.e., the test that is considered definitive regarding the presence or absence of coronary disease—even though the presence of anatomic disease does not guarantee that the coronary stenoses are causing the chest discomfort.

A sequence of consistently negative cardiologic test results reduces the probability of coronary artery disease to below 10 percent in patients with atypical chest discomfort. However, even after a normal exercise electrocardiogram and exercise perfusion scintigram, the probability of coronary disease will still be about 30 percent in a

Table 13-2

Approach to the Patient with Persistent Pain (Lasting Perhaps for Days)

1. Complete history and physical examination
2. Testing guided by data may include:
    Electrocardiogram
    Chest radiograph
    Computed tomography of chest
    Gastrointestinal evaluation (see Fig. 13-2)
    Spine, shoulder, or rib radiographs
    Echocardiogram

middle-aged or elderly patient with a typical history of angina pectoris (Fig. 13-2). By recognizing the potential change in probabilities that can be obtained with positive and negative results of the diagnostic tests that are planned, the physician can decide whether these potential changes in probability are sufficient to warrant the test. For example, the physician should commonly decide that a patient with typical angina pectoris and a positive exercise electrocardiogram does not require an exercise thallium scintigram to *diagnose* coronary disease, although under some circumstances this examination might aid in the estimation of the patient's subsequent prognosis.

PALPITATIONS

Palpitations are a common, disagreeable symptom that may be defined as an awareness of the beating of the heart, an awareness most commonly brought about by a change in the heart's rhythm or rate or by an augmentation of its contractility. Palpitations are not pathognomonic of any particular group of disorders; indeed, often they signify not a primary physical disorder but rather a psychological disturbance. Even when they occur as a more or less prominent complaint, the diagnosis of the underlying disease is made largely on the basis of other associated symptoms and data. Nevertheless, palpitations are frequently of considerable importance in the minds of patients, who fear they may indicate heart disease. Concern is all the more pronounced in patients who have been told that they *may* have heart disease; to them palpitations may seem to be an omen of impending disaster. Since the resulting anxiety may be associated with increased activity of the autonomic nervous system, with consequent increases in the cardiac rate and rhythm and the vigor of contraction, the patient's awareness of these changes may then lead to a vicious cycle, which may ultimately be responsible for incapacitation.

Palpitations may be described by the patient in various terms, such as "pounding," "fluttering," "flopping," and "skipping," and in most cases it will be obvious that the complaint is of a sensation of disturbed heartbeat. The sensitivity to alterations in cardiac activity among different individuals varies widely. Some patients seem to be unaware of the most serious and chaotic dysrhythmias; others are seriously troubled by an occasional extrasystole. Patients with anxiety states often exhibit a lowered threshold at which disorders of rate and rhythm result in palpitation. The awareness of the heartbeat also tends to be more common at night and during introspective moments than during activity. Patients with organic heart disease and chronic disorders of cardiac rate, rhythm, or stroke volume tend to accommodate to these abnormalities and are often less sensitive than normal persons to such events. Persistent tachycardia and/or atrial fibrillation may not be accompanied by continuous palpitations, in contrast to a sudden, brief alteration in cardiac rate or rhythm, which often causes considerable subjective discomfort. Palpitations are particularly prominent when the precipitating cause for increased heart rate or contractility or arrhythmia is recent, transient, and episodic. Conversely, in emotionally well-adjusted individuals, palpitations commonly become progressively less disconcerting as they become more chronic.

DIFFERENTIAL DIAGNOSIS   The patient's description of palpitations represents the most important clue to their etiology (Fig. 13-5). Every effort should be made to ask the patient to check the radial pulse during episodes of palpitation to assist in the diagnosis. If the rhythm is steady and regular and the rate is normal, the patient may be aware of an abnormal stroke volume from a condition such as aortic regurgitation but more likely is reporting a heightened awareness of normal cardiac function, sometimes in response to routine stress. Conversely, if the rhythm is steady and regular but the rate is clearly increased, especially above 120 beats per minute at a time when activity or other stresses should not result in tachycardia, the papitations may well represent a supraventricular or sometimes even a ventricular tachycardia.

An irregular pulse noted during an episode of palpitation virtually

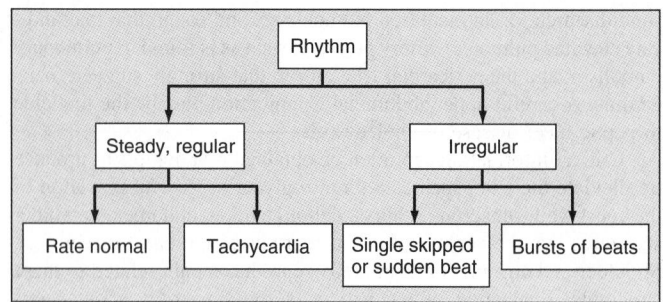

FIGURE 13-5   Flowchart for the description of palpitations.

always represents a true arrhythmia. The arryhthmia may be as simple as an occasional extrasystole. The premature contraction and post-premature beat after an extrasystole are often described as a "flopping," or the patient may say that it feels as if "the heart were turning over." The pause following the premature contraction may be felt as an actual cessation of the heart beat. The first ventricular contraction after the pause may be felt as an unusually vigorous beat and often be described as "pounding" or "thudding." By the patient's account alone, numerous extrasystoles may be difficult to distinguish from atrial fibrillation (Chap. 231). Bursts of beats may represent atrial fibrillation or brief episodes of a supraventricular or ventricular tachycardia.

Ectopic tachycardias commonly begin instantaneously and stop suddenly, sometimes followed by a pause before sinus rhythm resumes. Patients are usually acutely aware of both the onset and ending of the arrhythmia. A variety of vagal maneuvers (Chap. 231) may already have been used by the patient or may be suggested by the physician to aid in cessation of the ectopic arrhythmia.

All of the various arrhythmic causes of palpitations may be more common in the setting of thyrotoxicosis (Chap. 331), hypoglycemia (Chap. 335), pheochromocytoma (Chap. 333), fever (Chap. 17), and certain drugs. These arrhythmias may also be precipitated by tobacco, coffee, tea, alcohol, epinephrine, ephedrine, aminophylline, atropine, or thyroid medication. The physical examination should include a search for evidence of valvular heart disease, hyperthyroidism, and pulmonary disease.

ASSOCIATED SYMPTOMS   While palpitations are extremely common in healthy individuals, regardless of whether they are caused by a true arrhythmia or not, the presence of associated signs, symptoms, or other conditions helps to determine the potential seriousness of palpitations. Palpitations associated with symptoms of dizziness, shortness of breath, or chest discomfort, or occurring in a patient with an underlying history of cardiac disease, often require further evaluation. In such individuals, palpitations may be a manifestation of important arrhythmias that influence prognosis and, in some situations, require treatment (Chap. 231).

Approach to the Patient

The most common initial test for a patient with palpitations is a continuous (Holter) monitor, especially if the palpitations occur on a daily basis. For individuals with less frequent symptoms, a variety of loop recorders can be worn for days and activated by the patient at the time that the palpitations are experienced. It should be remembered that many patients have asymptomatic irregularities of the heart rhythm.

In addition to ambulatory electrocardiographic monitoring, exercise testing is sometimes of value in reassuring both the patient and the physician that vigorous exercise does not produce a worrisome arrhythmia. In general, arrhythmias that disappear with exercise are more likely to be more benign than those that are precipitated by it.

The management of palpitations focuses on the treatment of specifically diagnosed arrhythmias, on the elimination of precipitating factors (medications, tobacco, coffee, tea, alcohol), or on the recognition of associated syndromes, including hyperthyroidism, pheochromocytoma, hypoglycemia, menopausal symptoms, or an anxiety state.

As a rule, palpitations themselves often produce anxiety and fear out of proportion to the seriousness to the underlying condition. When the cause has been accurately determined and the significance is explained to the patient, concern is often ameliorated or eliminated. In patients with no important cause, evaluation and appropriate reassurance may be critical to helping the patient regain confidence and return to a normal quality of life.

BIBLIOGRAPHY

ACC/AHA Task Force: Guidelines for clinical use of cardiac radionuclide imaging. J Am Coll Cardiol 25:521, 1995

Barsky AJ et al: The clinical course of palpitations in medical outpatients. Arch Intern Med 155:1782, 1995

Gersh B et al: Chronic ischemic heart disease, in *Heart Disease*, 5th ed, E Braunwald (ed). Philadelphia, Saunders, 1997, pp 1289–1365

Lam HGT et al: Acute noncardiac chest pain in a coronary care unit: Evaluation by a 24-hour pressure and pH recording of the esophagus. Gastroenterology 102:453, 1992

Nienaber CA et al: The diagnosis of thoracic aortic dissection by noninvasive imaging procedures. N Engl J Med 328:1, 1993

Singh S et al: The contribution of gastroesophageal reflux to chest pain in patients with coronary artery disease. Ann Intern Med 117:824, 1992

Wolf MA: Palpitations and disturbances of cardiac rhythm, in *Office Practice of Medicine*, 3d ed, WT Branch Jr (ed). Philadelphia, Saunders, 1994

14 | *William Silen*

ABDOMINAL PAIN

The correct interpretation of acute abdominal pain is one of the most challenging demands made of any physician. Since proper therapy may require urgent action, the luxury of the leisurely approach suitable for the study of other conditions is sometimes denied. Few other clinical situations demand greater experience and judgment, because the most catastrophic of events may be forecast by the subtlest of symptoms and signs. Nowhere in medicine is a meticulously executed, detailed history and physical examination of greater importance. The etiologic classification in Table 14-1, although not complete, forms a useful frame of reference for the evaluation of patients with abdominal pain.

The diagnosis of "acute or surgical abdomen" so often heard in emergency wards is not an acceptable one because of its often misleading and erroneous connotation. The most obvious of "acute abdomens" may not require operative intervention, and the mildest of abdominal pains may herald the onset of an urgently correctable lesion. Any patient with abdominal pain of recent onset requires early and thorough evaluation with specific attempts at accurate diagnosis.

SOME MECHANISMS OF PAIN ORIGINATING IN THE ABDOMEN   Inflammation of the Parietal Peritoneum   The pain of parietal peritoneal inflammation is steady and aching in character and is located directly over the inflamed area, its exact reference being possible because it is transmitted by somatic nerves supplying the parietal peritoneum. The intensity of the pain is dependent on the type and amount of foreign substance to which the peritoneal surfaces are exposed in a given period of time. For example, the sudden release into the peritoneal cavity of a small quantity of *sterile* acid gastric juice causes much more pain than the same amount of grossly contaminated neutral fecal material. Enzymatically active pancreatic juice incites more pain and inflammation than does the same amount of sterile bile containing no potent enzymes. Blood and urine are often so bland as to go undetected if exposure of the peritoneum has not been sudden and massive. In the case of bacterial contamination, such as in pelvic inflammatory disease, the pain is frequently of low intensity early in the illness until bacterial multiplication has caused the elaboration of irritating substances.

So important is the rate at which the irritating material is applied to the peritoneum that cases of perforated peptic ulcer may be associated with entirely different clinical pictures dependent only on the rapidity with which the gastric juice enters the peritoneal cavity.

The pain of peritoneal inflammation is invariably accentuated by pressure or changes in tension of the peritoneum, whether produced by palpation or by movement, as in coughing or sneezing. The patient with peritonitis lies quietly in bed, preferring to avoid motion, in contrast to the patient with colic, who may writhe incessantly.

Another characteristic feature of peritoneal irritation is tonic reflex spasm of the abdominal musculature, localized to the involved body segment. The intensity of the tonic muscle spasm accompanying peritoneal inflammation is dependent on the location of the inflammatory process, the rate at which it develops, and the integrity of the nervous system. Spasm over a perforated retrocecal appendix or perforated ulcer into the lesser peritoneal sac may be minimal or absent because of the protective effect of overlying viscera. A slowly developing process also often greatly attenuates the degree of muscle spasm. Catastrophic abdominal emergencies such as a perforated ulcer have been repeatedly associated with minimal or occasionally no detectable pain or muscle spasm in obtunded, seriously ill, debilitated elderly patients or in psychotic patients.

Obstruction of Hollow Viscera   The pain of obstruction of hollow abdominal viscera is classically described as intermittent, or colicky. Yet the lack of a truly cramping character should not be misleading, because distention of a hollow viscus may produce steady pain with only very occasional exacerbations. Although not nearly as

Table 14-1

Some Important Causes of Abdominal Pain

PAIN ORIGINATING IN THE ABDOMEN

1. Parietal peritoneal inflammation
   a. Bacterial contamination, e.g., perforated appendix, pelvic inflammatory disease
   b. Chemical irritation, e.g., perforated ulcer, pancreatitis, mittelschmerz
2. Mechanical obstruction of hollow viscera
   a. Obstruction of the small or large intestine
   b. Obstruction of the biliary tree
   c. Obstruction of the ureter
3. Vascular disturbances
   a. Embolism or thrombosis
   b. Vascular rupture
   c. Pressure or torsional occlusion
   d. Sickle cell anemia
4. Abdominal wall
   a. Distortion or traction of mesentery
   b. Trauma or infection of muscles
5. Distention of visceral surfaces, e.g., hepatic or renal capsules

PAIN REFERRED FROM EXTRAABDOMINAL SOURCE

1. Thorax, e.g., pneumonia, referred pain from coronary occlusion
2. Spine, e.g., radiculitis from arthritis
3. Genitalia, e.g., torsion of the testicle

METABOLIC CAUSES

1. Exogenous
   a. Black widow spider bite
   b. Lead poisoning and others
2. Endogenous
   a. Uremia
   b. Diabetic ketoacidosis
   c. Porphyria
   d. Allergic factors (C'1 esterase inhibitor deficiency)

NEUROGENIC CAUSES

1. Organic
   a. Tabes dorsalis
   b. Herpes zoster
   c. Causalgia and others
2. Functional

well localized as the pain of parietal peritoneal inflammation, some useful generalities can be made concerning its distribution.

The colicky pain of obstruction of the small intestine is usually periumbilical or supraumbilical and is poorly localized. As the intestine becomes progressively dilated with loss of muscular tone, the colicky nature of the pain may become less apparent. With superimposed strangulating obstruction, pain may spread to the lower lumbar region if there is traction on the root of the mesentery. The colicky pain of colonic obstruction is of lesser intensity than that of the small intestine and is often located in the infraumbilical area. Lumbar radiation of pain is common in colonic obstruction.

Sudden distention of the biliary tree produces a steady rather than colicky type of pain; hence the term *biliary colic* is misleading. Acute distention of the gallbladder usually causes pain in the right upper quadrant with radiation to the right posterior region of the thorax or to the tip of the right scapula, and distention of the common bile duct is often associated with pain in the epigastrium radiating to the upper part of the lumbar region. Considerable variation is common, however, so that differentiation between these may be impossible. The typical subscapular pain or lumbar radiation is frequently absent. Gradual dilatation of the biliary tree, as in carcinoma of the head of the pancreas, may cause no pain or only a mild aching sensation in the epigastrium or right upper quadrant. The pain of distention of the pancreatic ducts is similar to that described for distention of the common bile duct but, in addition, is very frequently accentuated by recumbency and relieved by the upright position.

Obstruction of the urinary bladder results in dull suprapubic pain, usually low in intensity. Restlessness without specific complaint of pain may be the only sign of a distended bladder in an obtunded patient. In contrast, acute obstruction of the intravesicular portion of the ureter is characterized by severe suprapubic and flank pain which radiates to the penis, scrotum, or inner aspect of the upper region of the thigh. Obstruction of the ureteropelvic junction is felt as pain in the costovertebral angle, whereas obstruction of the remainder of the ureter is associated with flank pain that often extends into the corresponding side of the abdomen.

Vascular Disturbances A frequent misconception, despite abundant experience to the contrary, is that pain associated with intraabdominal vascular disturbances is sudden and catastrophic in nature. The pain of embolism or thrombosis of the superior mesenteric artery or that of impending rupture of an abdominal aortic aneurysm certainly may be severe and diffuse. Yet, just as frequently, the patient with occlusion of the superior mesenteric artery has only mild continuous diffuse pain for 2 or 3 days before vascular collapse or findings of peritoneal inflammation appear. The early, seemingly insignificant discomfort is caused by hyperperistalsis rather than peritoneal inflammation. Indeed, absence of tenderness and rigidity in the presence of continuous, diffuse pain in a patient likely to have vascular disease is quite characteristic of occlusion of the superior mesenteric artery. Abdominal pain with radiation to the sacral region, flank, or genitalia should always signal the possible presence of a rupturing abdominal aortic aneurysm. This pain may persist over a period of several days before rupture and collapse occur.

Abdominal Wall Pain arising from the abdominal wall is usually constant and aching. Movement, prolonged standing, and pressure accentuate the discomfort and muscle spasm. In the case of hematoma of the rectus sheath, now most frequently encountered in association with anticoagulant therapy, a mass may be present in the lower quadrants of the abdomen. Simultaneous involvement of muscles in other parts of the body usually serves to differentiate myositis of the abdominal wall from an intraabdominal process that might cause pain in the same region.

REFERRED PAIN IN ABDOMINAL DISEASES Pain referred to the abdomen from the thorax, spine, or genitalia may prove a vexing diagnostic problem, because diseases of the upper part of the abdominal cavity such as acute cholecystitis or perforated ulcer are frequently associated with intrathoracic complications. A most important, yet often forgotten dictum is that the possibility of intrathoracic disease must be considered in every patient with abdominal pain, especially if the pain is in the upper part of the abdomen. Systematic questioning and examination directed toward detecting the presence or absence of myocardial or pulmonary infarction, pneumonia, pericarditis, or esophageal disease (the intrathoracic diseases that most often masquerade as abdominal emergencies) will often provide sufficient clues to establish the proper diagnosis. Diaphragmatic pleuritis resulting from pneumonia or pulmonary infarction may cause pain in the right upper quadrant and pain in the supraclavicular area, the latter radiation to be sharply distinguished from the referred subscapular pain caused by acute distention of the extrahepatic biliary tree. The ultimate decision as to the origin of abdominal pain may require deliberate and planned observation over a period of several hours, during which time repeated questioning and examination will provide the proper explanation.

Referred pain of thoracic origin is often accompanied by splinting of the involved hemithorax with respiratory lag and decrease in excursion more marked than that seen in the presence of intraabdominal disease. In addition, apparent abdominal muscle spasm caused by referred pain will diminish during the inspiratory phase of respiration, whereas it is persistent throughout both respiratory phases if it is of abdominal origin. Palpation over the area of referred pain in the abdomen also does not usually accentuate the pain and in many instances actually seems to relieve it. The frequent coexistence of thoracic and abdominal disease may be misleading and confusing, so differentiation may be difficult or impossible. For example, the patient with known biliary tract disease often has epigastric pain during myocardial infarction, or biliary colic may be referred to the precordium or left shoulder in a patient who has suffered previously from angina pectoris. → *For an explanation of the radiation of pain to a previously diseased area, see Chap. 12.*

Referred pain from the spine, which usually involves compression or irritation of nerve roots, is characteristically intensified by certain motions such as cough, sneeze, or strain and is associated with hyperesthesia over the involved dermatomes. Pain referred to the abdomen from the testicles or seminal vesicles is generally accentuated by the slightest pressure on either of these organs. The abdominal discomfort is of dull aching character and is poorly localized.

METABOLIC ABDOMINAL CRISES Pain of metabolic origin may simulate almost any other type of intraabdominal disease. Here several mechanisms may be at work. In certain instances, such as hyperlipidemia, the metabolic disease itself may be accompanied by an intraabdominal process such as pancreatitis, which can lead to unnecessary laparotomy unless recognized. C'1 esterase deficiency associated with angioneurotic edema is also often associated with episodes of severe abdominal pain. Whenever the cause of abdominal pain is obscure, a metabolic origin always must be considered. Abdominal pain is also the hallmark of familial Mediterranean fever (Chap. 288).

The problem of differential diagnosis is often not readily resolved. The pain of porphyria and of lead colic usually is difficult to distinguish from that of intestinal obstruction, because severe hyperperistalsis is a prominent feature of both. The pain of uremia or diabetes is nonspecific, and the pain and tenderness frequently shift in location and intensity. Diabetic acidosis may be precipitated by acute appendicitis or intestinal obstruction, so if prompt resolution of the abdominal pain does not result from correction of the metabolic abnormalities, an underlying organic problem should be strongly suspected. Black widow spider bites produce intense pain and rigidity of the abdominal muscles and of the back, an area infrequently involved in disease of intraabdominal origin.

NEUROGENIC CAUSES Causalgic pain may occur in diseases that injure nerves of sensory type. It has a burning character and is usually limited to the distribution of a given peripheral nerve. Normal stimuli such as touch or change in temperature may be transformed into this type of pain, which is also frequently present in a patient at rest. A helpful finding is the demonstration that cutaneous pain spots are irregularly spaced, and this may be the only indication of an old nerve lesion underlying causalgic pain. Even though the pain may be precipitated by gentle palpation, rigidity of the abdominal muscles is absent, and the respirations are not disturbed. Distention of the abdomen is uncommon, and the pain has no relationship to the intake of food.

Pain arising from spinal nerves or roots comes and goes suddenly and is of a lancinating type (see Chap. 16). It may be caused by herpes zoster, impingement by arthritis, tumors, herniated nucleus pulposus, diabetes, or syphilis. Again, it is not associated with food intake, abdominal distention, or changes in respiration. Severe muscle spasm, as in the gastric crises of tabes dorsalis, is common but is either relieved or is not accentuated by abdominal palpation. The pain is made worse by movement of the spine and is usually confined to a few dermatome segments. Hyperesthesia is very common.

Psychogenic pain conforms to none of the aforementioned patterns of disease. Here the mechanism is hard to define. The most common problem is the hysterical adolescent or young person who develops abdominal pain and who frequently loses an appendix or other organs because of it. Ovulation or some other natural event that causes brief mild abdominal discomfort may sometimes be experienced as an abdominal catastrophe.

Psychogenic pain varies enormously in type and location but usually has no relation to meals. It is often at its onset markedly accentuated during the night. Nausea and vomiting are rarely observed, although occasionally the patient reports these symptoms. Spasm is seldom induced in the abdominal musculature and, if present, does not persist, especially if the attention of the patient can be distracted. Persistent localized tenderness is rare, and if found, the muscle spasm in the area is inconsistent and often absent. Restriction of the depth of respiration is the most common respiratory abnormality, but this is in the nature of a smothering or choking sensation and is part of an anxiety state. It occurs in the absence of thoracic splinting or change in the respiratory rate.

Approach to the Patient

There are few abdominal conditions that require such urgent operative intervention that an orderly approach need be abandoned, no matter how ill the patient. Only those patients with exsanguinating hemorrhage must be rushed to the operating room immediately, but in such instances, only a few minutes are required to assess the critical nature of the problem. Under these circumstances, all obstacles must be swept aside, adequate access for intravenous fluid replacement obtained, and the operation begun. Many patients of this type have died in the radiology department or the emergency room while awaiting such unnecessary examinations as electrocardiograms or films of the abdomen. *There are no contraindications to operation when massive hemorrhage is present.* Although exceedingly important, this situation fortunately is relatively rare.

Nothing will supplant an orderly, painstakingly *detailed history*, which is far more valuable than any laboratory or roentgenologic examination. This kind of history is laborious and time-consuming, making it not especially popular, even though a reasonably accurate diagnosis can be made on the basis of the history alone in the majority of cases. Recent studies of computer-aided diagnosis of abdominal pain indicate that this technique provides no advantage over clinical assessment alone. In cases of *acute* abdominal pain, a diagnosis is readily established in most instances, whereas success is not so frequently achieved in patients with *chronic* pain. Since the irritable bowel syndrome is one of the most common causes of abdominal pain, the possibility of this diagnosis must always be kept in mind (see Chap. 287). The *chronological sequence of events* in the patient's history is often more important than emphasis on the location of pain. If the examiner is sufficiently open-minded and unhurried, asks the proper questions, and listens, the patient will usually provide the diagnosis. Careful attention should be paid to the extraabdominal regions that may be responsible for abdominal pain. An accurate menstrual history in a female patient is essential. Narcotics or analgesics should be withheld until a definitive diagnosis or a definitive plan

has been formulated, because these agents often make it more difficult to secure and to interpret the history and physical findings.

In the examination, simple critical inspection of the patient, e.g., of facies, position in bed, and respiratory activity, may provide valuable clues. The amount of information to be gleaned is directly proportional to the *gentleness* and thoroughness of the examiner. Once a patient with peritoneal inflammation has been examined brusquely, accurate assessment by the next examiner becomes almost impossible. For example, eliciting rebound tenderness by sudden release of a deeply palpating hand in a patient with suspected peritonitis is cruel and unnecessary. The same information can be obtained by gentle percussion of the abdomen (rebound tenderness on a miniature scale), a maneuver that can be far more precise and localizing. Asking the patient to cough will elicit true rebound tenderness without the need for placing a hand on the abdomen. Furthermore, the forceful demonstration of rebound tenderness will startle and induce protective spasm in a nervous or worried patient in whom true rebound tenderness is not present. A palpable gallbladder will be missed if palpation is so brusque that voluntary muscle spasm becomes superimposed on involuntary muscular rigidity.

As in history taking, there is no substitute for sufficient time spent in the examination. It is important to remember that abdominal signs may be minimal but nevertheless, if accompanied by consistent symptoms, may be exceptionally meaningful. Signs may be virtually or actually totally absent in cases of pelvic peritonitis, so careful *pelvic and rectal examinations are mandatory in every patient with abdominal pain*. The presence of tenderness on pelvic or rectal examination in the absence of other abdominal signs must lead the examiner to consider such important operative indications as perforated appendicitis, diverticulitis, twisted ovarian cyst, and many others.

Much attention has been paid to the presence or absence of peristaltic sounds, their quality, and their frequency. Auscultation of the abdomen is probably one of the least rewarding aspects of the physical examination of a patient with abdominal pain. Severe catastrophes, such as strangulating small intestinal obstruction or perforated appendicitis, may occur in the presence of normal peristalsis. Conversely, when the proximal part of the intestine above an obstruction becomes markedly distended and edematous, peristaltic sounds may lose the characteristics of borborygmi and become weak or absent even when peritonitis is not present. It is usually the severe chemical peritonitis of sudden onset that is associated with the truly silent abdomen. Assessment of the patient's state of hydration is important. The hematocrit and urinalysis permit an accurate estimate of the severity of dehydration so that adequate replacement can be carried out.

Laboratory examinations may be of enormous value in assessment of the patient with abdominal pain, yet with but a few exceptions they rarely establish a diagnosis. Leukocytosis should never be the single deciding factor as to whether or not operation is indicated. A white blood cell count greater than $20,000/\mu L$ may be observed with perforation of a viscus, but pancreatitis, acute cholecystitis, pelvic inflammatory disease, and intestinal infarction may be associated with marked leukocytosis. A normal white blood cell count is by no means rare in cases of perforation of abdominal viscera. The diagnosis of anemia may be more helpful than the white blood cell count, especially when combined with the history.

The urinalysis is also of great value in indicating to some degree the state of hydration or to rule out severe renal disease, diabetes, or urinary infection. Determination of the blood urea nitrogen, blood sugar, and serum bilirubin levels also may be helpful. The serum amylase determination is overrated. Since many diseases other than pancreatitis, e.g., perforated ulcer, strangulating intestinal obstruction, and acute cholecystitis, may be associated with very marked increase in the serum amylase, great care must be exercised in denying an operation to a patient solely on the basis of an elevated serum amylase level. The determination of the serum lipase may have a somewhat greater accuracy than the serum amylase.

Plain and upright or lateral decubitus roentgenograms of the abdomen may be of the greatest value. They are usually unnecessary in patients with acute appendicitis or strangulated external hernias. However, in cases of intestinal obstruction, perforated ulcer, and a variety of other conditions, films may be diagnostic. In rare instances, barium or water-soluble medium examination of the upper part of the gastrointestinal tract may demonstrate partial intestinal obstruction that may elude diagnosis by other means. If there is any question of obstruction of the colon, oral administration of barium sulfate should be avoided. On the other hand, barium enema is of inestimable value in cases of colonic obstruction and should be used with greater frequency where the possibility of perforation does not exist.

Peritoneal lavage is a safe and effective diagnostic maneuver in patients with acute abdominal pain. It is of special value in patients with blunt trauma to the abdomen, in whom evaluation of the abdomen may be difficult because of other multiple injuries to the spine, pelvis, or ribs and in whom blood in the peritoneal cavity produces only a very mild peritoneal reaction. In the absence of trauma, peritoneal lavage has been replaced by ultrasound, computed tomography (CT), and laparoscopy. Ultrasonography has proved to be useful in detecting an enlarged gallbladder or pancreas, the presence of gallstones, an enlarged ovary, or a tubal pregnancy. Laparoscopy is especially helpful in diagnosing pelvic conditions, such as ovarian cysts, tubal pregnancies or salpingitis, and acute appendicitis. Radioisotopic scans (HIDA) may help differentiate acute cholecystitis from acute pancreatitis. A CT scan may demonstrate an enlarged pancreas, ruptured spleen, or thickened colonic wall and streaking of the mesocolon characteristic of diverticulitis.

Sometimes, even under the best of circumstances with all available auxiliary aids and with the greatest of clinical skill, a definitive diagnosis cannot be established at the time of the initial examination. Nevertheless, despite lack of a clear anatomic diagnosis, it may be abundantly clear to an experienced and thoughtful physician and surgeon that on clinical grounds alone operation is indicated. Should that decision be questionable, watchful waiting with repeated questioning and examination will often elucidate the true nature of the illness and indicate the proper course of action.

BIBLIOGRAPHY

ATTARD AR et al: Safety of early pain relief for acute abdominal pain. BMJ 305:554, 1992

BUGLIOSI TF et al: Acute abdominal pain in the elderly. Ann Emerg Med 19:1383, 1990

DAVIES AH et al: Ultrasonography in the acute abdomen. Br J Surg 78:1178, 1991

GATZEN C et al: Management of acute abdominal pain: Decision making in the accident and emergency department. J R Coll Surg Edinb 36:121, 1991

LEEK BF: Abdominal and pelvic visceral receptors. Br Med Bull 33:163, 1977

SCOTT HJ, ROSIN RD: The influence of diagnostic and therapeutic laparoscopy on patients presenting with an acute abdomen. J R Soc Med 86:699, 1993

TAOUREL P et al: Acute abdomen of unknown origin: Impact of CT on diagnosis and management. Gastrointest Radiol 17:287, 1992

15   *Neil H. Raskin*

HEADACHE

Few of us are spared the experience of head pain during our lifetimes; indeed, severe, disabling headache is reported to occur at least annually by 40 percent of individuals worldwide. This incidence occurs whether subjects live in large urban environments or in rural villages. In some individuals, stress and anxiety may trigger "benign" headaches, but emotional factors are not necessary for the symptom to occur. The more severe the headache, the more likely it is to be associated with

nausea and to be experienced as a pulsing or pounding discomfort; photophobia and hyperacusis are also more likely to be reported. Moreover, there does not appear to be any utility in having headache; most sufferers report the contrary. A useful classification of the many causes of headache, adapted from recommendations of the International Headache Society, is shown in Table 15-1.

Headache is usually a benign symptom, and only occasionally is it the manifestation of a serious illness such as brain tumor, subarachnoid hemorrhage, meningitis, or giant cell arteritis. Even in emergency settings, only 5 percent of patients who present with headache are found to have a serious underlying neurologic disorder. Nonetheless, it is imperative that these serious conditions be recognized and treated appropriately. Thus, the first issue to resolve in confronting the patient who complains of headache is to make the distinction between benign and more ominous etiologies.

GENERAL CONSIDERATIONS

The quality, location, duration, and time course of the headache and the conditions that produce, exacerbate, or relieve it should be carefully reviewed.

Ascertaining the *quality* of cephalic pain is occasionally helpful. Most headaches are dull, deeply located, and aching. Superimposed on such nondescript pain may be other types of pain that have greater diagnostic value. It is useful to identify *all* types of pain that have been experienced by the patient, regardless of their frequency or intensity. A throbbing quality and tight muscles about the head, neck, and shoulder girdle are common nonspecific accompaniments of headache. It was formerly believed that tight "hat-band" headaches indicated stress, anxiety, or depression, but investigations have not supported this view. Jabbing, brief, sharp cephalic pain, often occurring multifocally (ice pick-like pain), is the signature of a benign disorder.

Pain *intensity* seldom has diagnostic value—in the head or in any other somatic location. From the patient's perspective, it is, of course, the single aspect of pain that is most important. Physicians should be cautious about assessing pain intensity by visually inspecting a patient. People respond to pain in a variety of ways that range from overt histrionic behavior to stoicism. It is of more value to inquire as to how pain disturbs day-to-day function. *Response to placebo medication or procedures produces no useful information*—either diagnostic or therapeutic. It simply identifies a "placebo responder," about 30 percent of the population. There is no evidence that placebo responders have lower pain levels than nonresponders or do not really have pain. Patients entering emergency departments with the most severe headache of their lives usually have migraine. Meningitis, subarachnoid hemorrhage, and cluster headache also produce intense cranial pain. Contrary to common belief, the headache produced by a brain tumor is not usually distinctive or severe.

Data regarding *location* of headache may be informative. If the source is an extracranial structure, as in giant cell arteritis, the correspondence with the site of pain is fairly precise. Inflammation of an extracranial artery causes pain and exquisite tenderness localized to the site of the vessel. Lesions of paranasal sinuses, teeth, eyes, and upper cervical vertebrae induce less sharply localized pain, but pain that is still referred in a regional distribution. Intracranial lesions in the posterior fossa cause pain that is usually occipitonuchal, and supratentorial lesions most often induce frontotemporal pain.

Duration and *time-intensity* curves of headaches are diagnostically useful. A ruptured aneurysm results in head pain that peaks in an instant, thunderclap-like; much less often, unruptured aneurysms may signal their presence in the same way. Cluster headache attacks reach their peak over 3 to 5 min, remain at maximal levels for about 45 min, and then taper off. Migraine attacks build up over hours, are maintained for several hours to days, and are characteristically relieved by sleep. Sleep disruption is characteristic of headaches produced by brain tumors.

Recurrent headache may bear a relationship to certain biologic events or environmental exposures. The following exacerbating phenomena make a benign etiology highly probable: provocation by red wine, sustained exertion, organic odors, hunger, lack of sleep, weather change, and menses. The association of diarrhea with attacks and the amelioration of headache during pregnancy, especially the second and third trimesters, are pathognomonic of migraine. Patients with continuous benign headaches often observe a pain-free interlude of several minutes upon awakening before head pain commences. This phenomenon occurs with other pain syndromes, such as thalamic pain, but does not occur when inflammation (meningitis or giant cell arteritis) is the cause of pain. When attempts are made to elicit this information, patients commonly respond negatively to initial inquiries because the provocative stimuli or quality of the pain may be variable or inconsistent. Induction of pain by red wine and hunger, for example, is *always* inconsistent, for reasons that are unclear. It is important that patients understand that recollection of inciting factors for even some of their headaches may be of diagnostic value and may save unnecessary neuroimaging procedures.

A history of amenorrhea or galactorrhea should lead one to question whether the polycystic ovary syndrome or a prolactin-secreting pituitary adenoma is the source of headache. Headache arising de novo in a patient with known malignancy suggests either cerebral metastases and/or carcinomatous meningitis. When there is striking accentuation of pain with eye movement, a systemic infection and particularly meningitis should be seriously considered. Head pain appearing abruptly after bending, lifting, or coughing can be the clue to a posterior fossa mass or the Arnold-Chiari malformation. Orthostatic

headache occurs after lumbar puncture and also with subdural hematoma and benign intracranial hypertension. The eye itself is seldom the cause of acute orbital pain if the sclerae are white and not injected; a "red eye" is the sign of ophthalmic disease. In optic neuritis, pain is typically localized to the eye or supraorbital region and is exacerbated by eye movements. Similarly, acute sinusitis nearly always declares itself through a dark green, purulent nasal exudate.

The analysis of facial pain requires a different approach. Trigeminal and less commonly glossopharyngeal neuralgia are frequent causes of facial pain (see Chap. 372). "Neuralgias" are painful disorders characterized by paroxysmal, fleeting, often electric shock–like episodes that are often caused by demyelinating lesions of nerves (the trigeminal or glossopharyngeal nerves in cranial neuralgias). Certain maneuvers characteristically trigger paroxysms of pain. However, the most common cause of facial pain by far is dental; provocation by hot, cold, or sweet foods is typical. The application of a cold stimulus will repeatedly induce dental pain, whereas in neuralgic disorders a refractory period usually occurs after the initial response so that pain cannot be repeatedly induced. The presence of refractory periods can nearly always be elicited in the history so that patients need not be put through a painful experience.

The effect of eating on facial pain may provide insight into its

Table 15-1

The Classification of Headache

1. **Migraine**
   Migraine without aura
   Migraine with aura
   Ophthalmoplegic migraine
   Retinal migraine
   Childhood periodic syndromes that may be precursors to or
     associated with migraine
   Migrainous disorder not fulfilling above criteria

2. **Tension-type headache**
   Episodic tension-type headache
   Chronic tension-type headache

3. **Cluster headache and chronic paroxysmal hemicrania**
   Cluster headache
   Chronic paroxysmal hemicrania

4. **Miscellaneous headaches not associated with structural lesion**
   Idiopathic stabbing headache
   External compression headache
   Cold stimulus headache
   Benign cough headache
   Benign exertional headache
   Headache associated with sexual activity

5. **Headache associated with head trauma**
   Acute posttraumatic headache
   Chronic posttraumatic headache

6. **Headache associated with vascular disorders**
   Acute ischemic cerebrovascular disorder
   Intracranial hematoma
   Subarachnoid hemorrhage
   Unruptured vascular malformation
   Arteritis
   Carotid or vertebral artery pain
   Venous thrombosis
   Arterial hypertension
   Other vascular disorder

7. **Headache associated with nonvascular intracranial disorder**
   High CSF pressure
   Low CSF pressure
   Intracranial infection

7. **Headache associated with nonvascular intracranial disorder (cont.)**
   Sarcoidosis and other noninfectious inflammatory diseases
   Related to intrathecal injections
   Intracranial neoplasm
   Associated with other intracranial disorder

8. **Headache associated with substances or their withdrawal**
   Headache induced by acute substance use or exposure
   Headache induced by chronic substance use or exposure
   Headache from substance withdrawal (acute use)
   Headache from substance withdrawal (chronic use)

9. **Headache associated with noncephalic infection**
   Viral infection
   Bacterial infection
   Other infection

10. **Headache associated with metabolic disorder**
    Hypoxia
    Hypercapnia
    Mixed hypoxia and hypercapnia
    Hypoglycemia
    Dialysis
    Other metabolic abnormality

11. **Headache or facial pain associated with disorder of facial or cranial
    structures**
    Cranial bone
    Eyes
    Ears
    Nose and sinuses
    Teeth, jaws, and related structures
    Temporomandibular joint disease

12. **Cranial neuralgias, nerve trunk pain, and deafferentation pain**
    Persistent (in contrast to ticlike) pain of cranial nerve origin
    Trigeminal neuralgia
    Glossopharyngeal neuralgia
    Nervus intermedius neuralgia
    Superior laryngeal neuralgia
    Occipital neuralgia
    Central causes of head and facial pain other than tic douloureux

13. **Headache not classifiable**

SOURCE: After Olesen; and Dalessio.

cause. Is it the chewing, swallowing, or taste of the food that elicits pain? Chewing points toward trigeminal neuralgia, temporomandibular joint dysfunction, or giant cell arteritis ("jaw claudication"), whereas swallowing *and* taste provocation points toward glossopharyngeal neuralgia. Pain upon swallowing is common among patients with carotidynia (see Chap. 364) because the inflamed, tender carotid artery abuts the esophagus during deglutition.

Many patients with facial pain do not experience stereotypic neuralgias; the term *atypical facial pain* has been used in this setting. Vague, poorly localized, continuous facial pain is *characteristic* of nasopharyngeal carcinoma; a burning pain often develops as deafferentation occurs and evidence of cranial neuropathy appears. Burning facial pain may also occur with tumors of the fifth cranial nerve (meningioma or schwannoma) or with lesions of the pons that interrupt the dorsal root entry zone of the nerve (multiple sclerosis). In patients with facial pain, the finding of objective sensory loss is an important clue to a serious underlying disorder. Occasionally, the cause of a pain problem cannot be resolved promptly, necessitating periodic follow-up until further signs appear.

PAIN-SENSITIVE STRUCTURES OF THE HEAD

Pain is most commonly due to tissue injury resulting in stimulation of peripheral nociceptors in an intact nervous system, as in the pain of scalded skin or appendicitis. Pain can also result from damage to or anomalous activation of pain-sensitive pathways of the peripheral or central nervous system. Headache may originate from either mechanism. The following cranial structures are sensitive to mechanical stimulation: the scalp and aponeurotica, middle meningeal artery, dural sinuses, falx cerebri, and the proximal segments of the large pial arteries. The ventricular ependyma, choroid plexus, pial veins, and much of the brain parenchyma are pain-insensitive. Electrical stimulation of the midbrain in the region of the dorsal raphe has resulted in migraine-like headaches. Thus whereas most of the brain is insensitive to electrode probing, a site in the midbrain represents a possible source of headache generation.

Sensory stimuli from the head are conveyed to the central nervous system via the trigeminal nerves for structures above the tentorium in the anterior and middle fossae of the skull and via the first three cervical nerves for those in the posterior fossa and the inferior surface of the tentorium. The ninth and tenth cranial nerves supply part of the posterior fossa and refer pain to the ear and throat.

Headache can occur as the result of (1) distention, traction, or dilation of intracranial or extracranial arteries; (2) traction or displacement of large intracranial veins or their dural envelope; (3) compression, traction, or inflammation of cranial and spinal nerves; (4) spasm, inflammation, or trauma to cranial and cervical muscles; (5) meningeal irritation and raised intracranial pressure; and (6) possibly, perturbation of intracerebral serotonergic projections. By and large, intracranial masses cause headache when they deform, displace, or exert traction on vessels, dural structures, or cranial nerves at the base of the brain; this often happens long before intracranial pressure rises. Such mechanical displacement mechanisms do not explain the headaches resulting from cerebral ischemia or from benign intracranial hypertension after the pressure is reduced, nor the headaches that are so common in febrile illnesses and systemic lupus erythematosus. Perturbation of intracerebral serotonergic projections has been suggested as a possible mechanism for these phenomena.

PRINCIPAL CLINICAL VARIETIES OF HEADACHE

Normally there is little difficulty in diagnosing the headache of glaucoma, purulent sinusitis, bacterial meningitis, and brain tumor because of the clues provided by the associated symptoms and signs. The headache symptom alone is often nondescript. It is when headache is chronic, recurrent, and unattended by other important signs of disease that the physician faces a challenging but ultimately gratifying medical problem. The headache syndromes described below should be considered (see also Table 15-2).

MIGRAINE A useful definition of migraine is a benign and recurring syndrome of headache, nausea, vomiting, and/or other symptoms of neurologic dysfunction in varying admixtures. Migraine can often be recognized by its activators (red wine, menses, hunger, lack of sleep, glare, estrogen, worry, perfumes, let-down periods) and its deactivators (sleep, pregnancy, exhilaration, sumatriptan). → *Migraine, by far the most common cause of headache, is considered in detail in Chap. 364.*

CLUSTER HEADACHE The most common form of this syndrome is manifested by one to three short-lived daily attacks of periorbital pain over a 4- to 8-week interval followed by a pain-free interval that averages 1 year. The painful attacks are often associated with a homolateral red, tearing eye, nasal stuffiness, and ptosis. → *This subject is further discussed in Chap. 364.*

TENSION HEADACHE The term *tension headache* is still commonly used to describe a chronic head pain syndrome characterized by tight bandlike discomfort. Patients may report that the head feels as if it is in a vise or that the posterior neck muscles are tight. The pain typically builds slowly, fluctuates in severity, and may persist more or less continuously for many days. In some patients, anxiety or depression coexist with tension headache. Many investigators believe that periodic tension headache is biologically indistinguishable from migraine (Chap. 364).

LUMBAR PUNCTURE HEADACHE Headache following lumbar puncture (Chap. 360) usually begins within 48 h but may be delayed for up to 12 days. Its incidence is between 10 and 30 percent. Head pain is dramatically positional; it begins when the patient sits or stands upright; there is relief upon reclining or with abdominal compression. The longer the patient is upright, the longer the latency before head pain subsides. It is worsened by head shaking and jugular vein compression. The pain is usually a dull ache but may be throbbing; its location is occipitofrontal. Nausea and stiff neck often accompany headache, and occasional patients report blurred vision, photophobia, tinnitus, and vertigo. The symptoms resolve over a few days but may on occasion persist for weeks to months.

Loss of cerebrospinal fluid (CSF) volume decreases the brain's supportive cushion, so that when a patient is upright there is probably dilation and tension placed on the brain's anchoring structures, the pain-sensitive dural sinuses, resulting in pain. Intracranial hypotension often occurs, but severe lumbar puncture headache may be present even in patients who have normal CSF pressure.

Treatment with intravenous caffeine sodium benzoate given over a few minutes as a 500-mg dose will promptly terminate headache in 75 percent of patients; a second dose given in 1 h brings the total success rate to 85 percent. An epidural blood patch accomplished by injection of 15 mL of autologous whole blood rarely fails for those who do not respond to caffeine. The mechanism for these treatment effects is not straightforward. The blood patch has an *immediate* effect, making it unlikely that sealing off a dural hole with blood clot is its mechanism of action.

POSTCONCUSSION HEADACHES Following seemingly trivial head injuries and particularly after rear-end motor vehicle collisions, many patients report varying combinations of headache, dizziness, vertigo, and impaired memory. Anxiety, irritability and difficulty with concentration are other hallmarks of this syndrome. Symptoms may remit after several weeks or persist for months and even years after the injury. Postconcussion headaches may occur whether or not a person was rendered unconscious by head trauma. Typically, the neurologic examination is normal with the exception of the behavioral abnormalities, and computed tomography (CT) or magnetic resonance imaging (MRI) studies are unrevealing. Chronic subdural hematoma may on occasion mimic this disorder. Although the cause of postconcussive headache disorder is not known, it should not in general be viewed as a primary psychological disturbance. It often persists long after the settlement of pending lawsuits. The treatment is symptomatic support. Repeated encouragement that the syndrome eventually remits is important.

TEMPORAL ARTERITIS (See also Chaps. 28 and 319) Temporal (giant cell) arteritis is an inflammatory disorder of arteries that frequently involves the extracranial carotid circulation. This is a common disorder of the elderly; its average annual incidence is 77:100,000 in individuals aged 50 and older. The average age of onset is 70 years, and women account for 65 percent of cases. Fifty percent of patients with untreated temporal arteritis develop blindness due to involvement of the ophthalmic artery and its branches; indeed, the ischemic optic neuropathy induced by giant cell arteritis is the major cause of rapidly developing bilateral blindness in the patient over 60 years of age. Because treatment with glucocorticoids is effective in preventing this complication of temporal arteritis, prompt recognition of this disorder is important.

Typical presenting symptoms include headache, polymyalgia rheumatica (Chap. 319), jaw claudication, fever, and weight loss. Headache is the dominant symptom and often appears in association with malaise and muscle aches. Head pain may be unilateral or bilateral and is located temporally in 50 percent of patients but may involve any and all aspects of the cranium. Pain usually appears gradually over a few hours before peak intensity is reached; occasionally, it is explosive in onset. The quality of pain is only seldom throbbing; it is almost invariably described as dull and boring with superimposed episodic ice pick–like lancinating pains similar to the sharp pains that appear in migraine. Most patients can recognize that the origin of their head pain is superficial, external to the skull, rather than originating deep within the cranium (the pain site for migraineurs). Scalp tenderness is present, often to a marked degree; brushing the hair or resting the head on a pillow may be impossible because of pain. Headache is usually worse at night and is often aggravated by exposure to cold. Reddened, tender nodules or red streaking of the skin overlying the temporal arteries may be found in patients with headache, as is tenderness of the temporal, or less commonly, the occipital arteries.

The erythrocyte sedimentation rate (ESR) is often but not always elevated; a normal ESR does not exclude giant cell arteritis. A temporal artery biopsy and the initiation of prednisone at 80 mg daily for the first 4 to 6 weeks should be instituted when clinical suspicion is high. The prevalence of migraine among the elderly is substantial, considerably higher than that of giant cell arteritis. Migraineurs often report amelioration of their headaches with prednisone, so that one must be cautious about interpreting the therapeutic response.

COUGH HEADACHE A male-dominated (4:1) syndrome, cough headache is characterized by transient, severe head pain upon coughing, bending, lifting, sneezing, or stooping. Head pain persists for seconds to a few minutes. Many patients date the origins of the syndrome to a lower respiratory infection accompanied by severe coughing or to strenuous weight-lifting programs. Headache is usually diffuse but is lateralized in about one-third of patients. The incidence of serious intracranial structural anomalies causing this condition is about 25 percent; the Arnold-Chiari malformation (Chap. 373) is a common cause. Thus, MRI is indicated for most patients with cough headache. The benign disorder may persist for a few years; it responds dramatically to indomethacin at doses ranging from 50 to 200 mg daily. Approximately half of patients will also show a response to therapeutic lumbar puncture with removal of 40 mL of CSF.

Many patients with migraine note that attacks of headache may be provoked by *sustained* physical exertion, such as during the third mile of a 5-mile run. Such headaches build up over hours, in contrast to cough headache. The term *effort migraine* has been used for this syndrome to avoid the ambiguous term *exertional headache*.

Table 15-2

Common Types of Headaches

Type	Usual Site	Age and Sex	Clinical Features	Life Profile
Migraine, with or without aura	Frontotemporal, uni- or bilateral	All ages; highest incidence in children and young adults Female > male in adults Female = male in children	Onset after awakening; quelled by sleep Provoked by menses, odors, foods Stops after 2d trimester of pregnancy Duration: 6 h to 2 days	Cycles of several months to years Less frequent and less severe with aging
Cluster headache	Lateralized, orbital or temporal	All ages above 10; peaks at 30–50 Male preponderance (90%) Provoked by alcohol	Periodic attacks 1–2 attacks per day, commonly awakens from sleep Duration: 45 min Associated with red eye and stuffy nose homolaterally	Daily attacks for 6 weeks with annual recurrence of bout
Tension headache	Generalized	All ages; principally young adults Female preponderance	Nondescript, tight bandlike discomfort continuously Exacerbations provoked by factors similar to migraine	Cycles of several years
Brain tumor	Variable	All ages, both sexes	Interrupts sleep, unrelieved by sleep Exacerbated by orthostatic changes Steadily worsening pain; may be preceded by days to weeks of nausea and vomiting	Monophasic illness lasting weeks to months
Giant cell arteritis	Lateralized, temporal or occipital	Over 55 years, either sex	Marked scalp tenderness with superimposed jabbing and jolting pain Deep, intermittent throbbing Associated with malaise and morning stiffness and pain in shoulders and hips	Monophasic illness lasting weeks to months
Lumbar puncture headache	Bifrontal and/or bioccipital	Over 10 years, either sex	Orthostatic; head pain present with patient sitting or standing and disappears in prone or supine positions	Arises 1–2 days after lumbar puncture and persists for 3–4 days

COITAL HEADACHE This is another male-dominated (4:1) syndrome. Attacks occur periorgasmically, are very abrupt in onset, and subside in a few minutes if coitus is interrupted. These are nearly always benign events and usually occur sporadically; if they persist for hours or are accompanied by vomiting, subarachnoid hemorrhage must be excluded (Chap. 366).

BRAIN TUMOR HEADACHE About 30 percent of patients with brain tumors consider headache to be their chief complaint. The head pain syndrome is usually nondescript—an intermittent deep, dull aching of moderate intensity, which may worsen with exertion or change in position and may be associated with nausea and vomiting. This pattern of symptoms results from migraine far more often than from brain tumor. Headache of brain tumor disturbs sleep in about 10 percent of patients. Vomiting that precedes the appearance of headache by weeks is highly characteristic of posterior fossa brain tumors. → *A detailed discussion of brain tumors can be found in Chap. 375.*

PSEUDOTUMOR CEREBRI Headache, clinically resembling that of brain tumor, is a common presenting symptom of pseudotumor cerebri, an unusual disorder of raised intracranial pressure probably resulting from impaired CSF absorption by the arachnoid villi. Transient visual obscurations, and papilledema with enlarged blind spots and loss of peripheral visual fields, are additional manifestations. Most patients are young, female, and obese. → *Treatment of pseudotumor cerebri is discussed in Chap. 28.*

HEADACHE CAUSED BY SYSTEMIC ILLNESS There is hardly any illness that is never manifested by headache; however, some illnesses are *characteristically* associated with headache. These include infectious mononucleosis, systemic lupus erythematosus, chronic pulmonary failure with hypercapnia (early morning headaches), Hashimoto's thyroiditis, inflammatory bowel disease, many of the illnesses associated with human immunodeficiency virus, and the acute blood pressure elevations that occur in pheochromocytoma and in malignant hypertension. The last two examples are the exceptions to the generalization that hypertension per se is a very uncommon cause of headache; diastolic pressures of at least 120 mmHg are requisite for hypertension to cause headache. Some drugs and drug-withdrawal states, for example oral contraceptives, ovulation-promoting medications, and glucocorticoid withdrawal, are also associated with headache in some individuals.

Approach to the Patient

Entirely different diagnostic possibilities are raised by a patient who presents with the first severe headache ever and a patient who has had recurrent headache over many years. In the first instance, the probability of finding a potentially serious cause is considerably greater than in the second; some of the causes that should be considered include meningitis, subarachnoid hemorrhage, epidural or subdural hematoma, glaucoma, and purulent sinusitis. In general, acute, severe headache with stiff neck and fever suggests meningitis and without fever suggests subarachnoid hemorrhage; in the former case, lumbar puncture is mandatory, whereas in the latter case a neuroimaging procedure (CT) is the study of choice. Acute persistent headache and fever are often the manifestations of an acute systemic viral infection; if the neck is supple in such a patient, lumbar puncture may be deferred. There is always the possibility of a first attack of migraine, but fever would be a rare associated feature. Clinical features that indicate a possible serious underlying etiology to a headache are summarized in Table 15-3.

A complete neurologic examination is an essential first step in the evaluation of chronic headache. In most cases, an abnormal examination should be followed by a CT or MRI study. In patients with recurrent migraine headaches and a normal examination, neuroimaging procedures are not indicated. In other patterns of headache and a normal examination, imaging studies may be indicated, although their

Table 15-3

Headache Symptoms That Suggest a Serious Underlying Disorder

First severe headache ever
Subacute worsening over days or weeks
Disturbs sleep or present immediately upon awakening
Abnormal neurologic examination
Fever or other unexplained systemic signs
Vomiting precedes headache
Induced by bending, lifting, cough
Known systemic illness (e.g., cancer, collagen-vascular disease)
Onset age 55 or older

---

yield is low. As a screening procedure for intracranial pathology in this setting, CT and MRI methods appear to be equally sensitive.

A general evaluation of recurring headache should consider the investigation of cardiovascular and renal status by blood pressure monitoring and urine examination; eyes by fundoscopy, intraocular pressure measurement, and refraction; cranial arteries by palpation; cervical spine by the effect of passive movement of the head and imaging; and the psychological state of the patient.

The adolescent with chronic daily frontal or holocephalic headache represents a special type of problem. Extensive diagnostic batteries are most often unrevealing, including the psychiatric assessment. Fortunately, the headaches tend to stop after a few years, and symptomatic management with analgesics can enable these teenagers to move through secondary school and enter college. By the time they reach the late teens, the cycle has usually ended.

The relationship of head pain to depression is not straightforward. Many patients in chronic daily pain cycles become depressed, a not unreasonable sequence of events; moreover, there is a greater-than-chance coincidence of migraine with both bipolar (manic depressive) and unipolar major depressive disorders. Yet studies of large populations of depressed patients do not reveal headache prevalence rates that are different from the general population; the high prevalence of headache in the population at large may account for this apparent paradox. The physician should be cautious about assigning depression as the cause of recurring headache; drugs with antidepressant actions are also effective in migraine.

Finally, a note on recurring headache that may be pain-driven. Temporomandibular joint dysfunction is an example; in general, it produces preauricular pain that is associated with chewing food. The pain may radiate to the head but is not easily confused with headache per se. On the other hand, headache-prone patients may observe that headaches are more frequent and severe in the presence of a painful temporomandibular joint problem. Similarly, headache disorders may be activated by pain that follows otologic or endodontic surgical procedures. Treatment of the headache problem is largely ineffective until the cause of the primary pain problem is dealt with. Thus pain about the head as the result of diseased tissue or trauma may reawaken an otherwise quiescent migrainous syndrome.

BIBLIOGRAPHY

COUCH JR: Headache to worry about. Med Clin North Am 77:141, 1993
DALESSIO DJ: Diagnosing the severe headache. Neurology 44(Suppl 3): 56,1994
FRISHBERG BM: The utility of neuroimaging in the evaluation of headache in patients with normal examination. Neurology 44:1191, 1994
JOHNS D: Benign sexual headache within a family. Arch Neurol 43:1158, 1986
LANCE JW: *Mechanism and Management of Headache*, 5th ed. London, Butterworth Scientific, 1993
OLESEN J: Headache Classification Committee of the International Headache Society. Classification and diagnostic criteria for headache disorders, cranial neuralgia, and facial pain. Cephalalgia 8(Suppl 7): 1, 1988
PASCUAL J, IGLESIAS F, OTERINO A, VAZQUEZ-BARQUERO A, BERCIANO J: Cough, exertional, and sexual headaches: An analysis of 72 benign and symptomatic cases. Neurology 46:1520, 1996
RASKIN NH: Lumbar puncture headache: A review. Headache 30:197, 1990
————: The cough headache syndrome: Treatment. Neurology 45:1784, 1995
————: *Headache*, 2d ed. New York, Churchill Livingstone, 1988
RASMUSSEN BK, OLESEN J: Symptomatic and nonsymptomatic headaches in a general population. Neurology 42:1225, 1992

BACK AND NECK PAIN

The importance of back and neck pain in our society is underscored by the following: (1) the annual societal cost of back pain in the United States is estimated to be between $20 and $50 billion, (2) back symptoms are the most common cause of disability in patients under 45 years of age, (3) 50 percent of working adults, in one survey, admitted to having a back injury each year, and (4) approximately 1 percent of the U.S. population is chronically disabled because of back pain.

There is enormous economic pressure to provide rational and efficient care of patients with back pain. As a result, clinical practice guidelines (CPGs) for patients with back pain are evolving rapidly. CPGs are defined as evaluation or treatment algorithms based upon indications for tests or treatment at specific steps in patient care. CPGs for *acute back pain* are based upon incomplete evidence (see algorithms, Fig. 16-7) but reflect common medical practice. Major revisions in these CPGs can be anticipated in the future. Management of patients with *chronic low back pain* (CLBP) is complex and not amenable yet to a simple algorithmic approach.

A clear understanding of spine anatomy, pertinent features of history and examination, relevant laboratory studies, causes of back pain, and management will optimize patient care.

RELEVANT ANATOMY OF THE SPINE

The anterior portion of the spine consists of cylindrical vertebral bodies separated by intervertebral disks and held together by the anterior and posterior longitudinal ligaments. The intervertebral disks are composed of a central gelatinous nucleus pulposus surrounded by a tough cartilagenous ring, the annulus fibrosis; they are responsible for one-fourth of the length of the spinal column (Figs. 16-1 and 16-2). The disks are thickest in the cervical and lumbar regions where movements of the spine are greatest. The disks are elastic in youth and allow the bony vertebrae to move easily upon each other. Elasticity is lost with age. The function of the anterior spine is to absorb the shock of body movements that comprise motor activities of daily living (walking, running).

The posterior portion of the spine consists of the vertebral arches and seven processes. Each arch consists of paired cylindrical pedicles anteriorly and paired laminae posteriorly (Fig. 16-1). The vertebral arch gives rise to two transverse processes laterally, one spinous process posteriorly, and two superior and two inferior articular facets. The functions of the posterior spine are to protect the spinal cord and nerves within the spinal canal and to stabilize the spine by providing sites for the attachment of muscles and ligaments. The contraction of muscles attached to the spinous and transverse processes produces a system of pulleys and levers that results in flexion, extension, and lateral bending movements of the spine. Normal upright posture in humans places the center of gravity anterior to the spine. The graded contraction of well-developed paraspinal muscles attached to the laminae, transverse processes, and spinous processes is necessary to maintain normal upright posture.

Some anatomic features are of considerable clinical importance. The nerve roots exit at a level above their respective vertebral bodies in the cervical region (the C7 nerve root exits at the C6-C7 level) and below their respective vertebral bodies in the thoracic and lumbar regions (the L4 nerve root exits at the L4-L5 level). The spinal cord ends at the L1 or L2 level of the bony spine. As a consequence, the lumbar nerve roots follow a long course within the lumbar spinal canal and can be injured anywhere from the upper lumbar spine to their exit at the intervertebral foramen. For example, it is common for disk herniation at the L4-L5 level to produce compression of the S1 nerve root (Fig. 16-3). In contrast, cervical nerve roots follow a short intraspinal course and exit at the level of their respective spinal cord segments (upper cervical) or one segment below the corresponding levels (lower

FIGURE 16-1 Vertebral anatomy. (*From FH Netter, vol. 1, Part I, 1983, with permission.*)

cervical cord). Cervical spine pathology can result in spinal cord compression, but lumbar spine pathology cannot. Pain-sensitive structures in the spine include the vertebral body periosteum, dura, facets, annulus fibrosus of the intervertebral disk, epidural veins, and the posterior longitudinal ligament. Damage to these nonneural structures may be the source of referred pain. The nucleus pulposus of the intervertebral disk is not pain-sensitive. Pain sensation is provided by the sinuvertebral nerve that arises from the spinal nerve at each spine segment and reenters the spinal canal through the intervertebral foramen at the same level. Disease of these pain-sensitive spine structures may explain many cases of back pain without nerve root compression.

The lumbar and cervical spine possess the greatest potential for movement and injury.

GENERAL CLINICAL CONSIDERATIONS

TYPES OF LOW BACK PAIN   There are five types of low back pain: local pain, pain referred to the spine, pain of spine origin referred to the legs or buttocks, radicular pain, and muscular spasm. The history is of paramount importance to uncover risk factors for serious underlying disease that requires specific evaluation by physical examination or laboratory tests. Back pain quality varies considerably, but there are features that help to distinguish anatomic sources and etiologies of back pain.

Local pain is caused by processes that compress or irritate sensory nerve endings. They are usually due to fractures, tears, or stretching of pain-sensitive structures. The site of the pain is near the affected part of the spine. Local pain that does not vary with changes in position suggests spine tumor or infection.

Pain referred to the spine may arise from abdominal or pelvic viscera. The pain is usually described as abdominal or pelvic as well as spinal and is often unaffected by position of the spine. This type of pain may be described occasionally as back pain only.

Pain of spine origin may be referred to the buttocks and legs. Diseases affecting the upper lumbar spine may refer pain to the lumbar region, groin, or anterior thighs. Diseases affecting the lower lumbar spine may result in pain referred to the buttocks, posterior thighs, or rarely the calves or feet. Provocative injections into pain-sensitive structures of the spine (diskography) may produce leg pain that does not follow a dermatomal distribution. The exact pathogenesis of this "sclerotomal" pain is unclear.

Classic *radicular back pain* is usually sharp and radiates from the spine to the leg within the territory of a nerve root (see "Lumbar Disk Disease"). Coughing, sneezing, or voluntary contraction of abdominal muscles (lifting heavy objects or straining at stool) often elicits radiating pain. The patient notices increased pain in postures that stretch the nerves and nerve roots. Sitting stretches the sciatic nerve (L5 and S1 roots) because the nerve passes posterior to the hip. The femoral nerve (L2, L3, and L4 roots) passes anterior to the hip and is not stretched by sitting. The description of the pain alone usually fails to distinguish clearly between pain of bony spine origin and radiculopathy.

The *pain associated with muscle spasm*, although of obscure origin, is commonly associated with many spine disorders. The spasms are accompanied by abnormal posture, taut paraspinal muscles, and dull pain.

Back pain at rest or unassociated with posture should raise the index of suspicion for underlying spine tumor, fracture, infection, or referred pain from visceral structures. Leg pain initiated by ambulation or standing and relieved by the sitting or supine position is suggestive of spinal stenosis. Knowledge of the circumstances associated with back pain onset are important when weighing possible serious underlying causes for the pain. The diagnostic utility of back symptoms and signs suggestive of a serious underlying cause are discussed in the management section. Some patients involved in accidents or work injuries may exaggerate their pain for the purpose of compensation or for psychological reasons.

EXAMINATION OF THE LOW BACK   A general physical examination that includes the abdomen and rectum is advisable. Back pain referred from visceral organs may be reproduced during palpation of the abdomen (pancreatitis, abdominal aortic aneurysm) or percussion over the costovertebral angles (pyelonephritis, adrenal disease, L1-L2 transverse process fracture).

Inspection of the normal spine (Fig. 16-2) reveals a normal thoracic kyphosis, lumbar lordosis, and cervical lordosis. Exaggeration of these normal alignments may result in hyperkyphosis (lameback) or hyperlordosis (swayback) of the lumbar spine. Spasm of lumbar

SPINAL COLUMN

Anterior view   Left lateral view   Posterior view

Atlas (C1)
Axis (C2)
Atlas (C1)
Axis (C2)
C7
C7
T1
T1
T12
T12
L1
L1
L5
L5
Sacrum (S1-5)
Sacrum (S1-5)
Coccyx
Coccyx

FIGURE 16-2   Spinal column. (*From FH Netter, vol. 1, Part I, 1983, with permission.*)

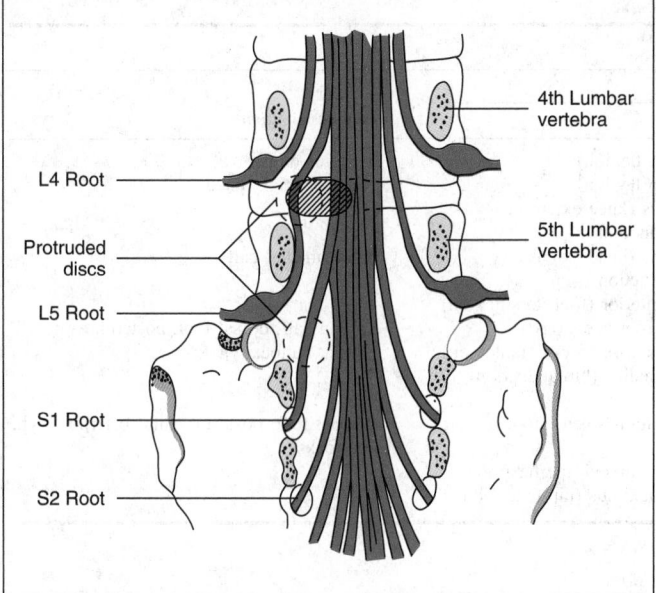

FIGURE 16-3 Locations of compression of lumbar and sacral roots by herniated disks. (*From RD Adams, M Victor, A Ropper, Prinicples of Neurology, 7th ed, New York, McGraw-Hill, 1997, with permission.*)

paraspinal muscles results in flattening of the usual lumbar lordosis. Inspection may reveal lateral curvature of the spine (scoliosis) or an asymmetry in the appearance of the paraspinal muscles, suggesting muscle spasm. Taut paraspinal muscles limit the motion of the lumbar spine in coronal and sagittal planes. Local back pain is often reproduced by palpation or percussion over the spinous process of the affected vertebrae.

Forward bending is frequently limited by paraspinal muscle spasm which accompanies disease of pain-sensitive spine structures. Flexion of the hips is normal in patients with lumbar spine disease (spondylosis), but flexion of the lumbar spine is limited and sometimes painful. Lateral bending to the side opposite the injured spinal element may stretch the damaged tissues, worsen pain, and result in limited motion. Hyperextension of the spine (with the patient prone or standing) is limited when nerve root compression or bony spine disease is present.

Pain from hip disease may mimic the pain of lumbar spine disease. The first movement to be limited is internal rotation of the hip. Manual internal and external rotation at the hip with the knee and hip in flexion may reproduce the pain, as may percussion of the patient's heel with the palm of the examiner's hand.

Passive flexion of the thigh on the abdomen while the knee is extended produces stretching of the L5 and S1 nerve roots and the sciatic nerve. The sciatic nerve passes posterior to the hip. Passive dorsiflexion of the foot during the maneuver adds to the stretch. Flexion to at least 80° is normally possible without causing pain, but tight hamstrings may limit motion. This *straight leg–raising* (SLR) *sign* is positive if the maneuver reproduces the patient's pain. The SLR sign may be elicited in the sitting position to determine if the finding is reproducible. The patient may describe pain in the low back, buttocks, posterior thigh, or lower leg. The *crossed SLR sign* is positive when performance of the maneuver on one leg reproduces the patient's pain symptoms in the opposite leg or buttocks. The nerve or nerve root lesion is always on the side of the pain. The *reverse SLR sign* is elicited by placing the patient in the prone position and passively extending the thigh. This maneuver stretches the L2-L4 nerve roots and the femoral nerve, which pass anterior to the hip. The reverse SLR test is positive if the maneuver reproduces the patient's pain.

The neurologic examination includes a search for weakness, atrophy, asymmetric or age-inappropriate absence of reflexes, diminished sensation in the legs, and signs of spinal cord injury. Examination findings that can be found with specific nerve root lesions are shown in Tables 16-1 and 16-2 and are discussed further in the sections on lumbar and cervical disk disease.

LABORATORY STUDIES "Routine" laboratory studies are rarely needed for the initial evaluation of acute (<3 months), nonspecific, low back pain. If risk factors for underlying serious disease are present (see "Treatment" and algorithms, Fig. 16-7), then laboratory studies (guided by the history and examination) may be helpful. Simple screening tests used in the setting of suspected malignancy or infection include a complete blood count, erythrocyte sedimentation rate, and urinalysis.

Plain films of the lumbar or cervical spine are helpful when risk factors for vertebral fracture (trauma, chronic steroid use) are present. *In the absence of risk factors, routine x-rays of the lumbar spine in the setting of acute, nonspecific, low back pain are expensive and not helpful.* Magnetic resonance imaging (MRI) and CT-myelography

Table 16-1

Cervical Radiculopathy—Neurologic Findings

| Cervical Nerve Roots | Changes | | | Pain Distribution |
	Reflex	Sensory	Motor	
C5	Biceps	Over deltoid +/− Thumb, index finger	Supraspinatus* (initial arm abduction) Infraspinatus* (arm external rotation) Deltoid* (arm abduction) Biceps (arm flexion)	Lateral arm, medial scapula
C6	Biceps	Thumb, index fingers Radial hand/forearm	Biceps (arm flexion) Pronator teres (internal forearm rotation)	Lateral forearm, thumb, index finger
C7	Triceps	Middle fingers Dorsum forearm	Triceps* (arm extension) Wrist extensors* Extensor digitorum* (finger extension) Pronator teres (internal forearm rotation)	Posterior arm, dorsal forearm, lateral hand
C8	Finger flexors	Little finger Medial hand and forearm	Abductor pollicis brevis (abduction D2) First dorsal interosseous (abduction D1) Abductor digit minimi (abduction D5)	4th and 5th fingers, medial forearm
T1	Finger flexors	Axilla and medial arm	Abductor pollicis brevis (abduction D2) First dorsal interosseous (abduction D1) Abductor digit minimi (abduction D5)	Medial arm, axilla, deep shoulder

* These muscles receive the majority of innervation from the root in the same horizontal row.

Table 16-2

Lumbosacral Radiculopathy—Neurologic Findings

Lumbosacral Nerve Roots	Changes			Pain Distribution
	Reflex	Sensory	Motor	
L2†	—	Upper anterior thigh	Psoas (hip flexion)	Anterior thigh
L3†	—	Lower anterior thigh Anterior knee	Psoas (hip flexion) Quadriceps (knee extension) Thigh adduction	Anterior thigh, knee
L4†	Quadriceps (knee)	Medial calf	Quadriceps (knee extension)* Thigh adduction Tibialis anterior (foot dorsiflexion)	Knee, medial calf
L5‡	—	Dorsal surface—foot Lateral calf	Peroneii (foot eversion)* Tibialis anterior (foot dorsiflexion) Gluteus medius (hip abduction) Toe dorsiflexors	Lateral calf, dorsal foot, posterolateral thigh, buttocks
S1‡	Gastrocnemius/soleus (ankle)	Plantar surface—foot Lateral aspect—foot	Gastrocnemius/soleus (foot plantar flexion)* Abductor hallucis (toe flexors)* Gluteus maximus (hip extension)	Bottom foot, posterior calf, posterior thigh, buttocks

* These muscles receive the majority of innervation from the root in the same horizontal row.
† Reverse straight-leg raising sign present—see examination of the spine.
‡ Straight-leg raising sign present—see examination of the spine.

have emerged as the radiologic texts of choice for evaluation of most spinal diseases; specific indications appear below.

CONDITIONS CAUSING DISABLING PAIN IN THE LOW BACK

CONGENITAL ANOMALIES OF THE LUMBAR SPINE *Spondylolysis* consists of a bony defect probably caused by a stress fracture to a congenitally abnormal segment in the pars interarticularis (a segment near the junction of the pedicle with the lamina) of the vertebra. The defect (usually bilateral) is best visualized on oblique projections in plain x-rays or by computed tomography (CT) scan and occurs in the setting of a single injury, repeated minor injuries, or growth. The vertebral body, pedicles, and superior articular facets may slip anteriorly and leave the posterior elements behind. This latter abnormality (*spondylolisthesis*) more often results in symptoms. The patient may complain of pain in the low back radiating into the legs, and tenderness may be elicited near the segment that has "slipped" forward (most often L5 on S1 or occasionally L4 on L5). A "step" may be present on deep palpation of the posterior elements of the segment above the spondylolisthetic joint. The trunk may be shortened and the abdomen protuberant as a result of extreme forward displacement of L5 on S1 in severe degrees of spondylolisthesis. In these cases, cauda equina syndrome may occur (Chap. 373).

TRAUMA TO THE LOW BACK AND NECK Trauma constitutes an important cause of acute low back and neck pain. These patients require careful initial evaluation. A patient complaining of back or neck pain and inability to move the legs may have a spine fracture. In acute injuries that may involve fracture or dislocation of the vertebral segments, the examining physician must be careful to avoid further damage to the spinal cord or nerve roots. The neck or back (depending on the location of the trauma) should be immobilized pending plain x-rays to exclude the presence of a fracture or dislocation.

Sprains and Strains The terms *lumbosacral sprain* and *strain* are used loosely by patients and physicians and do not clearly describe a specific anatomic lesion. The terms *low back strain*, *sprain*, or *mechanically induced muscle spasm* are used for minor, self-limited injuries associated with lifting a heavy object, a fall, or a sudden deceleration as occurs in an automobile accident. Patients with low back pain often assume unusual postures related to paraspinal muscle spasm. The pain is usually confined to the lower back, and there is no radiation to the buttocks or legs.

Vertebral Fractures Most traumatic fractures of the lumbar vertebral bodies result from compression or flexion injuries and consist of anterior wedging or compression. With more severe trauma, the patient may sustain a fracture dislocation or a "burst" fracture involving not only the vertebral body but posterior elements as well. Vertebral fractures are caused by falls from a height (a pars interarticularis fracture of the L5 vertebra is common), sudden deceleration in an automobile accident, or direct injury. Neurologic impairment is commonly associated with these injuries, and early treatment produces a more favorable outcome. When fractures occur with minimal or no trauma, the bone is presumed to be weakened by a pathologic process. The cause is usually postmenopausal (type 1) or senile (type 2) osteoporosis (see Chap. 355), but underlying systemic disorders such as osteomalacia, hyperparathyroidism, hyperthyroidism, multiple myeloma, metastatic carcinoma, or glucocorticoid use may also weaken the vertebral body. The clinical context (trauma, patient age, steroid use), examination findings (neurologic deficit, paraspinal muscle spasm), and x-ray appearance of the spine will establish the diagnosis.

Transverse process fractures are associated with severe injury to the paravertebral muscles—principally the psoas. Associated retroperitoneal hemorrhage may result in a low hematocrit or hypovolemic shock. Such injuries may produce deep tenderness at the injury site and limitation of all lumbar movements. CT or MRI scans establish the diagnosis.

Lumbar Disk Disease This disorder is a common cause of chronic or recurrent low back and leg pain. Disk disease is most likely to occur at the L4-L5 and L5-S1 levels, but upper lumbar levels are involved occasionally. The cause of the disk injury is often unknown. Degeneration of the nucleus pulposus and the annulus fibrosus, which increases with age, may have been asymptomatic or painful. A sneeze, cough, or trivial movement may cause the nucleus pulposus to prolapse, pushing the frayed and weakened annulus posteriorly. In severe disk disease, the nucleus may protrude through the annulus (herniation) or become extruded to lie as a free fragment in the vertebral canal.

The symptoms of a ruptured intervertebral disk consist of pain, abnormal posture, and limitation of spine motion (particularly flexion), or radicular pain. The pattern of radicular pain may suggest involvement of one or several nerve roots. A dermatomal pattern of sensory disturbance (paresthesia, hypersensitivity, or hyposensitivity) or asymmetric reduction or loss of a deep tendon reflex is more suggestive of a specific root lesion than the pain pattern. Motor abnormalities (focal weakness or fasciculations, muscle atrophy) occur less frequently, but a myotomal pattern of involvement can suggest specific nerve root involvement. Lumbar disk disease is usually unilateral (Fig. 16-4), but bilateral involvement can be seen with large

FIGURE 16-4 Lumbar herniated disk; left S1 radiculopathy. Sagittal T1-weighted image on the left with arrows outlining disk margins. Sagittal T2 image on the right reveals a protruding disk at the L5-S1 level (*arrows*) which displaces the central thecal sac.

central disk herniations that compress several nerve roots at the same level. Reflex, sensory, motor, and pain distribution findings pertinent to specific lumbosacral nerve root lesions are summarized in Table 16-2.

The examiner must be cautious to avoid overinterpretation of individual neurologic findings. The suggestion of a nerve root lesion by history and examination does not specify the underlying cause. Epidural abscesses or tumors may produce a syndrome similar to a herniated disk. Fever, constant pain uninfluenced by position, sphincter abnormalities, or signs of spinal cord disease suggest an etiology other than lumbar disk disease. Bilateral absence of ankle reflexes can be a normal finding in old age or a sign of bilateral S1 radiculopathy. An absent deep tendon reflex or focal sensory loss may reflect injury to a nerve root, but other sites of injury along the nerve must also be considered. For example, an absent knee reflex may be due to a femoral neuropathy rather than an L4 nerve root injury. A focal decrease in sensation over the foot and distal lateral calf may result from a peroneal neuropathy rather than an L5 nerve root injury. Paresthesia, when present, may be in the entire cutaneous distribution of the root or in only a portion of the distal nerve root territory. "Weakness" may be due to unsustained effort (breakaway weakness) associated with radicular pain, true weakness, or both. Electromyography (EMG) can often distinguish true weakness from breakaway weakness. Asymmetric muscle atrophy may reflect chronic motor axonal loss associated with nerve root injury, nerve injury, or disuse.

There are five indications for disk surgery: (1) progressive motor weakness from nerve root injury, (2) progressive impairment demonstrated by EMG and nerve conduction studies, (3) abnormal bowel or bladder function or other signs of spinal cord disease, (4) incapacitating nerve root pain despite conservative treatment for at least 4 weeks, and (5) recurrent incapacitating pain despite conservative treatment. The latter two criteria are more subjective and less well established than the first three indications.

Degeneration of the intervertebral disk without frank extrusion of disk tissue may give rise to low back pain with little or no leg pain or, occasionally, leg pain with little or no discomfort in the back. There are no signs of nerve root involvement, but the back pain may be referred to the thigh or leg. Lumbar disk syndromes are usually unilateral, but large central disk herniations (with or without extrusion of a large, free fragment into the spinal canal) can cause bilateral symptoms and signs. Large central disk herniations may result in

cauda equina syndrome with bilateral symptoms and signs from involvement of lumbosacral roots.

Diagnosis is straightforward when all the symptoms and signs indicative of disk disease with radiculopathy are present. When one symptom is present (particularly backache), a specific diagnosis can be difficult. Spine MR scans yield exquisite views of intraspinal and adjacent soft tissue anatomy and are more likely to establish a specific diagnosis or "road map" for surgical therapy than plain films or myelography. Occasional lateral recess or intervertebral foramen bony lesions may be seen with optimal clarity on CT-myelographic studies.

OTHER CAUSES OF LOW BACK PAIN Spinal stenosis, facet hypertrophy, lumbar adhesive arachnoiditis, and failed back syndrome are other sources of back pain.

Spinal stenosis is caused by a narrowed spinal canal. The symptoms include back and leg pain induced by walking or standing (pseudoclaudication) and relieved by the sitting or supine positions. Symptoms in the legs are usually bilateral. Focal weakness, sensory loss, or reflex changes may occur. Unlike vascular claudication, the symptoms are usually provoked by standing without walking. Unlike lumbar disk disease, the symptoms are usually relieved by sitting. Severe neurologic deficits, including paralysis and urinary incontinence, occur in a small minority of patients. Spinal stenosis usually results from acquired (75 percent), congenital, or mixed acquired/congenital factors. Congenital forms (achondroplasia, idiopathic) are characterized by short, thick pedicles that produce both anteroposterior (central) spinal canal stenosis and lateral recess stenosis. Acquired factors that may contribute to spinal stenosis include degenerative diseases (spondylosis, spondylolisthesis, scoliosis), trauma, spine psurgery (postlaminectomy, fusion), metabolic or endocrine disorders (epidural lipomatosis, osteoporosis, acromegaly, renal osteodystrophy, hypoparathyroidism), and Paget's disease. MRI or CT-myelography provide the best definition of the abnormal anatomy (Fig. 16-5).

Conservative treatment includes nonsteroidal anti-inflammatory drugs (NSAIDs), exercise programs, and symptomatic treatment of acute pain exacerbations. Surgical therapy is considered when medical therapy does not relieve pain sufficiently to allow for activities of daily living or when significant focal neurologic signs are present. Between 65 and 80 percent of patients treated surgically experience greater than 75 percent relief of back and leg pain. Up to 25 percent develop recurrent stenosis at the same spinal level or an adjacent level 5 years after the initial surgery; recurrent symptoms usually respond to a second surgical decompression.

FIGURE 16-5 Spinal stenosis; back pain and leg claudication induced by walking and relieved by sitting. Sagittal T2 fast spin echo MRI of a normal (left) and stenotic (right) lumbar spine, revealing multifocal narrowing of the CSF spaces surrounding the nerve roots within the thecal sac.

Unilateral *facet joint hypertrophy* can produce radicular pain that is exacerbated and relieved by many of the same factors that influence disk-related radiculopathies. Patients often exhibit back pain and a SLR sign. Focal motor weakness, hyporeflexia, and sensory loss may occur. MRI, CT-myelography, and surgical exploration reveal hypertrophic superior or inferior facets. Foraminotomy and facetectomy result in long-term relief of leg and back pain in 80 to 90 percent of patients.

Lumbar adhesive arachnoiditis with radiculopathy is the result of a fibrotic process following an inflammatory response to local tissue injury within the subarachnoid space. The fibrosis results in nerve root adhesions, producing back and leg pain associated with motor, sensory, and reflex deficits. The classic clinical setting is in patients who have had multiple lumbar operations or oil-based myelography (Pantopaque). Myelography-induced arachnoiditis has become rare with the abandonment of oil-based contrast and the maturation of noninvasive imaging techniques (CT and MRI). Other causes of arachnoiditis include chronic spinal infections, spinal cord injury, intrathecal hemorrhage, intrathecal injection of steroids and anesthetics, and foreign bodies. MRI is the method of choice to demonstrate arachnoiditis. The nerve roots may clump together centrally or adhere to the dura peripherally or loculations of cerebrospinal fluid (CSF) may form within the thecal sac that obscure visualization of the roots. Treatment is unsatisfactory. Microsurgical lysis of adhesions, dorsal rhizotomy, and dorsal root ganglionectomy have produced poor results. Dorsal column stimulation for pain relief has produced varying results. Epidural steroid injections have been of limited value.

The cause of the low back pain sometimes remains unclear. Some patients have had multiple operations for disk disease but have persistent pain and disability. The original indications for surgery may have been questionable with back pain only, no definite neurologic signs, and a minor disk bulge noted on CT or MRI. Scoring systems based upon neurologic signs, psychological factors, physiologic studies, and imaging studies have been devised to minimize the likelihood of unsuccessful surgical explorations and to avoid selection of patients with psychological profiles that predict poor functional outcomes.

Surgical treatment should be considered if the pain and/or neurologic findings do not disappear or substantially improve within 3 to 4 weeks and in patients with worsening symptoms. Surgery must be preceded by a lumbar CT or MRI to determine the location and type of pathology (disk herniation or, rarely, intra- or extradural tumor). The usual surgical procedure is a partial hemilaminectomy with excision of the involved prolapsed intervertebral disk. Arthrodesis of the involved segments is rarely indicated and should be considered only in the presence of significant spinal instability such as degenerative spondylolisthesis or isthmic spondylolysis. In the cervical spine, herniated disks are usually managed surgically through the anterior approach. Diskectomy is usually followed by an anterior interbody fusion.

ARTHRITIS   Arthritis of the spine is a major cause of back and neck pain.

Spondylosis   Osteoarthritic spine disease occurs in later life and primarily involves the cervical and lumbosacral spine. Patients often complain of pain centered in the spine that is increased by motion and associated with stiffness and limitation of motion. The relationship between clinical symptoms and radiologic findings is often not straightforward; pain may be prominent when x-ray findings are minimal and large osteophytes can be seen in asymptomatic patients in middle and later life. Hypertrophied facets and osteophytes may compress nerve roots in the lateral recess or intervertebral foramen. Osteophytes arising from the vertebral body may cause central spinal canal stenosis. Loss of intervertebral disk height reduces the vertical dimensions of the intervertebral foramen, causing the descending pedicle to compress the nerve root exiting at that level. Osteoarthritic changes in the lumbar spine may on occasion compress the cauda equina. Degenerative spondylolisthesis (slipping of a vertebral body over the vertebra below) occurs most often at the L5-S1 level and may further contribute to

root compression. Surgical procedures should be considered only after failure of conservative management.

Ankylosing Spondylitis (See also Chap. 317)   This distinctive form of arthritic spine disease typically presents with the insidious onset of low back and buttock pain in a man under the age of 40 years and is associated with morning back stiffness, nocturnal back pain, back pain unrelieved by rest, an elevated sedimentation rate, and the presence of histocompatibility antigen HLA-B27. The differential diagnosis in early stages includes tumor and infection, but the back pain of ankylosing spondylitis characteristically improves with exercise. Loss of the normal lumbar lordosis and exaggeration of thoracic kyphosis are seen as the disease progresses. Inflammation and erosion of the outer fibers of the annulus fibrosus at the point of contact with the vertebral body are followed by ossification and growth of bone. This bony growth (syndesmophyte) bridges adjacent vertebral bodies and results in reduced spine mobility for anterior flexion, lateral flexion, and extension. The radiologic hallmarks of the disease are periarticular destructive changes, subsequent sclerosis of the sacroiliac joints, and bridging of vertebral bodies by bone to produce the characteristic immobile and fused "bamboo spine." Similar patterns of restricted movement may accompany Reiter's syndrome, psoriatic arthritis, and chronic inflammatory bowel disease. Stress fractures through the spontaneously ankylosed posterior bony elements of the rigid, osteoporotic spine may result in focal spine pain and either spinal cord compression or cauda equina syndrome. Occasional atlantoaxial subluxation with spinal cord compression occurs. Bilateral ankylosis of the ribs to the spine and a decrease in the height of axial thoracic structures may cause marked impairment of respiratory function.

OTHER DESTRUCTIVE DISEASES   **Neoplasm** (See also Chap. 373)   Back pain was the most common neurologic symptom among patients with systemic cancer in one large series. One-third of the patients with undiagnosed back or neck pain and systemic cancer had epidural extension or metastasis, and one-third had pain associated with vertebral metasases alone. Eleven percent had back pain unrelated to metastatic disease. Metastatic carcinoma (breast, lung, prostate, thyroid, kidney, gastrointestinal tract), multiple myeloma, and non-Hodgkin's and Hodgkin's lymphomas are malignant tumors that frequently involve the spine. Back pain may be the presenting symptom because the primary tumor site may be overlooked or asymptomatic. The pain tends to be constant, dull, unrelieved by rest, and worse at night. In contrast, mechanical low back pain is usually improved with rest. Radiographic changes are manifest usually as destructive lesions in one or several vertebral bodies without involvement of the disk space. Disk space involvement increases the likelihood of an infectious process. MRI or CT-myelography are the studies of choice in the setting of suspected spinal metastasis. Debate over which test is preferred continues, but the trend of evidence favors the use of MRI. As a practical matter, the test most rapidly available is the procedure of choice because the patient may worsen during a diagnostic delay.

Infection   *Vertebral osteomyelitis* is usually caused by staphylococci, but other bacteria or the tubercle bacillus (Pott's disease) may be the responsible organisms. In 40 percent of patients a primary source of infection can be identified, most often from the urinary tract, skin, or lungs. Intravenous drug use is a well-recognized risk factor. Back pain exacerbated by motion and unrelieved by rest, spine tenderness over the involved spine segment, and an elevated erythrocyte sedimentation rate are the most common findings. Fever is present in only one-fourth, and an elevated white blood cell count in only one-third, of patients. Plain radiographs may show narrowing of a disk space with erosion and destruction of adjacent vertebrae, but these diagnostic changes may take weeks or even months to appear. MRI is highly sensitive and specific for osteomyelitis; definition of soft tissue detail is exquisite. CT scan is also sensitive and specific, and compared to MRI may be more readily available and better tolerated by some patients with severe back pain.

Spinal epidural abscess (discussed in Chap. 373) presents with back pain (aggravated by palpation or movement) and fever. The patient may have radicular complaints, often bilateral, which can progress to spinal cord compression with focal sensory loss, focal weakness, incontinence, and paraplegia. Spine MRI best defines the extent of this lesion, which may extend over multiple spinal levels.

Osteoporosis and Osteosclerosis   A considerable loss of bone substance may occur with or without symptoms in many medical disorders, including hyperparathyroidism, chronic steroid use, or immobilization. Compression fractures occur in up to half of patients with severe osteoporosis. The sole manifestation of a compression fracture may be a complaint of focal aching (often after a trivial injury) in the lumbar or thoracic spine, which is exacerbated by movement. Other patients may experience thoracic or upper lumbar radicular pain. Focal spine tenderness is common. When compression fractures are found, treatable risk factors for additional fractures and possible underlying causes should be considered carefully. Compression fractures above the midthoracic region are suggestive of malignancy. Paget's disease of the spine is readily identifiable as osteosclerosis on routine x-ray studies and may result in back pain (related to involvement of pain-sensitive structures or secondary anatomic distortion of these structures) or be painless. Spinal cord or nerve root compression may occur due to bony encroachment on the spinal canal or intervertebral foramina. Single dual-beam photon absorptiometry or quantitative CT can be used to detect small changes in bone mineral density. → *For further discussion of these bone disorders, see Chaps. 354, 355, and 358.*

REFERRED PAIN FROM VISCERAL DISEASE   Diseases of the pelvis, abdomen, or thorax may produce local pain or referred pain to the posterior portion of the spinal segment that innervates the diseased organ. Occasionally, back pain may be the first and only sign. In general, pelvic diseases refer pain to the sacral region, lower abdominal diseases to the lumbar region (around the second to fourth lumbar vertebrae), and upper abdominal diseases to the lower thoracic or upper lumbar spine (eighth thoracic to the first and second lumbar vertebrae). Local signs (pain with spine palpation, paraspinal muscle spasm) are absent, and little or no pain accompanies normal movements of the spine.

Low Thoracic and Upper Lumbar Pain in Abdominal Disease   Peptic ulcer or tumor of the posterior wall of the stomach or duodenum typically results in epigastric pain (see Chaps. 92 and 284), but spinal pain may be produced if there is retroperitoneal extension. The pain may be midline, paraspinal, or both. Other characteristics of the pain may provide clues to its origin. For example, back pain due to peptic ulcer may be induced after ingestion of an orange, alcohol, or coffee and relieved by food and antacids. Fatty foods are more likely to induce back pain associated with biliary disease. Diseases of the pancreas (pancreatitis, cyst, or tumor) may cause back pain to the right of the spine (if the head of the pancreas is involved) or to the left (if the body or tail are involved). Diseases of retroperitoneal structures (hemorrhage, tumors, pyelonephritis) may produce paraspinal pain with radiation to the lower abdomen, groin, or anterior thighs. A mass in the iliopsoas region often produces unilateral lumbar pain with radiation toward the groin, labia, or testicle. The sudden appearance of lumbar pain in a patient receiving anticoagulants should raise the suspicion of retroperitoneal hemorrhage.

Isolated low back pain occurs in 15 to 20 percent of patients with rupture of an abdominal aortic aneurysm. The classic triad of abdominal pain, shock, and back pain in an elderly man occurs in fewer than 20 percent of patients. Two of the three clinical features are present in two-thirds of patients; hypotension is present in half. This condition has a high mortality rate if untreated, thus it is essential to consider the possibility of a ruptured aneurysm in the appropriate clinical context. The diagnosis is initially missed in one-third of patients, in part because the symptoms and signs can be nonspecific. Common misdiagnoses include nonspecific back pain, diverticulitis, renal colic, sepsis, and myocardial infarction. A careful abdominal examination revealing a pulsatile mass (present in 50 to 75 percent of patients) is the most important physical finding.

Lumbar Pain with Lower Abdominal Diseases   Inflammatory bowel disorders (colitis, diverticulitis) or colonic neoplasms may cause lower abdominal pain (between the umbilicus and pubis) and/or pain in the midlumbar spine region. The pain may have a beltlike distribution around the body. A lesion in the transverse colon or first part of the descending colon may cause midline or left-sided pain referred to the L2-L3 level in the back. Sigmoid colon disease may refer pain to the upper sacral region, midline suprapubic region, or left lower quadrant of the abdomen.

Sacral Pain in Gynecologic and Urologic Disease   Pelvic organs are rarely the cause of low back pain, although gynecologic disorders that involve the uterosacral ligaments are an important source of chronic back pain. Endometriosis or carcinoma of the uterus (body or cervix) may invade the uterosacral ligaments, while malposition of the uterus may cause uterosacral ligament traction. The pain is referred to the sacral region. In endometriosis, the pain begins during the premenstrual phase and often continues until it merges with menstrual pain. Malposition of the uterus (retroversion, descensus, and prolapse) may lead to sacral pain after standing for several hours.

Menstrual pain may be felt in the sacral region. It is a poorly localized, cramping pain that can radiate down the legs. Other pelvic sources of low back pain include neoplastic invasion of pelvic nerves, radiation necrosis, and pregnancy. Pain due to neoplastic infiltration of nerves is typically continuous, progressive in severity, and unrelieved by rest at night. X-ray therapy of pelvic tumors may produce sacral pain from late radiation necrosis of tissue or nerves. Low back pain with radiation into one or both thighs is common in the last weeks of pregnancy.

Urologic sources of sacral back pain include chronic prostatitis, prostate carcinoma with spinal metastasis, and diseases of the kidney and ureter. Lesions of the bladder and testes do not usually produce back pain. The diagnosis of metastatic prostate carcinoma is established by rectal examination, spine imaging studies (MRI or CT), and measurement of prostate-specific antigen (PSA) (Chap. 97). Infectious, inflammatory, or neoplastic renal diseases may result in ipsilateral lumbar pain, as can renal artery or vein thrombosis. Ureteral obstruction due to renal stones may produce paraspinal lumbar pain.

Postural Back Pain   There is a group of patients with chronic, nonspecific low back pain in whom no anatomic or pathologic lesion can be found despite exhaustive investigation. Some of these individuals complain of vague, diffuse back pain with prolonged sitting or standing that is relieved by rest. The physical examination is unrevealing except for "poor posture." Imaging studies and laboratory evaluations are normal. Exercises to strengthen the paraspinal and abdominal muscles are sometimes therapeutic.

Psychiatric Disease   CLBP may be encountered in patients with compensation hysteria, malingering, substance abuse, chronic anxiety states, or depression. Many patients with CLBP managed medically or with unsuccessful spine surgery have a history of psychiatric illness (depression, anxiety, substance abuse) or childhood trauma (physical or sexual abuse) that antedates the onset of back pain. Preoperative psychological assessment has been used to exclude patients with marked psychological impairment who are at high risk for a poor surgical outcome. These considerations not withstanding, it is important to be certain that back pain in these patients does not represent serious spine or visceral pathology in addition to the impaired psychological state.

PAIN IN THE NECK AND SHOULDER

Neck pain commonly arises from diseases of the cervical spine and soft tissues of the neck. Neck and low back pain share many clinical features. Neck pain arising from the cervical spine may be precipitated by neck movements and accompanied by focal spine tenderness and limitation of motion. Pain arising from the brachial plexus, shoulder, or peripheral nerves can occasionally be confused with cervical spine disease, but the history and examination usually identify a more distal site of origin for the pain.

CERVICAL SPINE TRAUMA   Unlike injury to the low back, trauma to the cervical spine (fractures, subluxation) places the spinal cord at risk for compression. The resulting bladder dysfunction, quadriparesis, and respiratory failure (with upper cervical cord compression; see Chap. 373) can be devastating. Immobilization of the neck is a top priority to minimize further cord injury due to movement of unstable cervical spine segments. The patient may also exhibit combined spinal cord and nerve root findings (myeloradiculopathy).

Whiplash injury is due to trauma (usually in automobile accidents) causing cervical musculoligamental sprain or strain due to hyperflexion or hyperextension. This diagnosis excludes patients with fractures, disk herniation, head injury, or alteration of consciousness. A prospective study of patients with whiplash injury found that 18 percent had persistent injury-related symptoms 2 years after the car accident. Such patients were older, had a higher incidence of inclined or rotated head position at impact, greater intensity of initial neck and head pain, greater number of initial symptoms, and more osteoarthritic changes on cervical spine x-rays at baseline compared to patients in remission. Objective data on the pathology of the soft tissue injuries is lacking. In general, patients with severe initial injury are at increased risk for poor long-term outcome.

CERVICAL DISK DISEASE   Acute or subacute lower cervical disk herniation is a common cause of neck, shoulder, arm, and hand pain. Neck pain (worse with neck movement), stiffness, and limited range of motion are the rule. Nerve root compression may cause radiation of pain into the shoulder or arm. Extension and lateral rotation of the neck (Spurling's sign) may narrow the neural foramen and reproduce the radicular symptoms. Acute cervical nerve root compression from a ruptured disk is often due to trauma in young individuals and is less common than acute lumbar nerve root compression. Subacute radiculopathy is less likely to be related to a specific traumatic incident and may involve both disk disease and spondylosis. Cervical disk herniations are usually posterolateral near the lateral recess and intervertebral foramen. The usual patterns of reflex, sensory, and motor changes and pain distribution with common cervical nerve root lesions are listed in Table 16-2. Nerve root function normally varies somewhat from patient to patient, and overlap in function between nerve roots is common. The anatomic pattern of pain is the most variable of the clinical features. The distribution of symptoms and signs often occupies only part of the associated nerve root territory.

CERVICAL SPONDYLOSIS   Osteoarthritis of the cervical spine may cause neck pain that radiates into the back of the head, shoulders, or arms. Arthritic or other pathologic conditions of the upper cervical spine may be the source of headaches in the posterior occipital region (supplied by the C2-C4 nerve roots). Cervical spondylosis with osteophyte formation in the lateral recess or hypertrophic facet joints may result in a monoradiculopathy (Fig. 16-6). Narrowing of the spinal canal by osteophyte formation, ossification of the posterior longitudinal ligament, or herniation of a large central disk may result in spinal cord compression with bladder symptoms and motor, sensory, and reflex changes. An electrical sensation elicited by neck flexion and radiating down the spine (Lhermitte's symptom) indicates spinal cord involvement. When little or no neck pain accompanies the cord compression, the diagnosis may be confused with amyotrophic lateral sclerosis (Chap. 370), multiple sclerosis (Chap. 376), spinal cord tumors (Chap. 373), or syringomyelia (Chap. 373). The possibility of treatable cervical spinal cord disease must be considered even when the patient presents with complaints in the legs only. In some patients, a combination of spondylitic changes results in cervical spinal stenosis with myeloradiculopathy. Lumbar spinal stenosis may mask associated findings of coexistent cervical myelopathy. MRI or CT-myelography will reveal the full extent of the anatomic abnormalities in cervical spondylosis and cervical disk disease. EMG and nerve conduction studies are useful to quantify the severity and localize the levels of nerve root injury.

OTHER CAUSES OF NECK PAIN   *Rheumatoid arthritis* (RA) (see Chap. 313) of the cervical apophyseal joints results in neck pain, stiffness, and limitation of motion. The diagnosis of RA is straightforward in typical cases with symmetric inflammatory polyarthritis. In advanced RA, synovitis of the atlantoaxial joint (C1-C2; see Fig. 16-2) may damage the transverse ligament of the atlas, producing forward displacement of the atlas on the axis (atlantoaxial subluxation). Atlantoaxial subluxation occurs radiographically in 30 percent of patients with. RA, and the degree of subluxation correlates with the severity of erosive disease. When subluxation is present, neurologic examination and MR or CT scans are useful to assess the presence and clinical importance of any associated spinal cord compression. Occasional patients develop high spinal cord compression, leading to quadriparesis, respiratory insufficiency, and death. Although low back pain is common in RA patients, the frequency of facet disease, fracture, and spondylolisthesis is no greater than among age- and sex-matched controls with mechanical low back pain.

Ankylosing spondylitis can cause neck pain and occasional atlantoaxial subluxation with spinal cord compression. Herpes zoster may cause neck and posterior occipital pain in a C2-C3 distribution prior to the outbreak of vesicles. Neoplasms metastatic to the cervical spine, infections (osteomyelitis and epidural abscess), and metabolic bone

A

B

FIGURE 16-6   Cervical spondylosis; left C6 radiculopathy. *A.* Sagittal T2 fast spin echo MRI reveals a hypointense osteophyte which protrudes from the C5-C6 level into the thecal sac, displacing the spinal cord posteriorly (*white arrow*). *B.* Axial 2-mm section from a 3-D volume gradient echo sequence of the cervical spine. The high signal of the right C5-C6 intervertebral foramen contrasts with the narrow high signal of the left C5-C6 intervertebral foramen produced by osteophytic spurring (*arrows*).

diseases may also cause neck pain. Diagnostic considerations are similar to those described above for low back pain. Neck pain may be referred from the heart in coronary artery ischemia (cervical angina syndrome).

THORACIC OUTLET The thoracic outlet is an anatomic region containing the first rib, the subclavian artery and vein, the brachial plexus, the clavicle, and the lung apex. Injury to these structures may produce thoracic outlet syndrome (TOS), characterized by pain around the shoulder and supraclavicular region induced by certain tasks and positions. There are at least three subtypes of TOS. *True neurogenic thoracic outlet syndrome* results from compression of the lower trunk of the plexus by an anomalous band of tissue connecting an elongate transverse process at C7 with the first rib. Neurologic deficits include weakness of intrinsic muscles of the hand and diminished sensation on the palmar aspect of the 4th and 5th digits. EMG and nerve conduction studies confirm the diagnosis. The *arterial thoracic outlet syndrome* results from compression of the subclavian artery by a cervical rib; the compression results in poststenotic dilatation of the artery and thrombus formation. A reduced blood pressure in the affected limb may be accompanied by signs of emboli in the hand. Neurologic signs are absent. Noninvasive Doppler techniques confirm the diagnosis. The *disputed thoracic outlet syndrome* includes a large number of patients with chronic arm and shoulder pain of unclear cause. The lack of sensitive and specific changes on physical examination or laboratory markers for this condition frequently results in diagnostic uncertainty, and treatment of this form of TOS is often unsuccessful.

BRACHIAL PLEXUS AND NERVES Pain from injury to the brachial plexus or peripheral nerves can on occasion be confused with pain of neck origin. Infiltration of peripheral nerves by neoplasm may occur in the lower trunk of the brachial plexus and produce shoulder pain radiating down the arm, numbness of the fourth and fifth fingers, and weakness of intrinsic hand muscles innervated by the ulnar and median nerves. Postradiation fibrosis (breast carcinoma is the most common setting) or a Pancoast tumor of the lung (Chap. 90) may produce similar findings. A Horner's syndrome is present in two-thirds of patients with Pancoast tumor. Suprascapular neuropathy may produce severe shoulder pain, weakness, and wasting of the supraspinatus and infraspinatus muscles. Acute brachial neuritis is often confused with radiculopathy. The acute onset of severe shoulder or scapular pain is followed over days to weeks by weakness of the proximal arm and shoulder girdle corresponding to muscles innervated by the upper trunk of the plexus. Antecedent infection and immunization have been associated with acute brachial neuritis, but a causal link is circumstantial. Identification of this syndrome is important because slow, complete recovery occurs in 75 percent of patients after 2 years and in 89 percent after 3 years. Occasional cases of carpal tunnel syndrome produce pain and paresthesia extending into the forearm, arm, and shoulder resembling a C5 or C6 root lesion. Lesions of the radial or ulnar nerve can mimic a radiculopathy at C7 or C8, respectively. EMG and nerve conduction studies can accurately localize lesions to the nerve roots, brachial plexus, or nerves. Peripheral nerve disorders are discussed more fully in Chap. 381.

SHOULDER Pain in the shoulder region can be difficult to separate clearly from neck pain. If the symptoms and signs of radiculopathy are absent, then the differential diagnosis includes mechanical shoulder pain (tendonitis, bursitis, rotator cuff tear, partial cuff tear, adhesive capsulitis, and cuff impingement under the acromion) and referred pain (subdiaphragmatic irritation, angina, Pancoast tumor). Mechanical pain is often worse at night, associated with local shoulder tenderness, and aggravated by abduction, internal rotation, or extension of the arm. The pain of shoulder disease may at times radiate into the arm or hand, but the sensory, motor, and reflex changes that indicate disease of the nerve roots, plexus, or peripheral nerves are absent.

℞ **TREATMENT**

Acute Low Back Pain A practical approach to the management of low back pain is to consider acute and chronic presentations separately. Acute low back pain is defined as pain of less than 3 months' duration. Full recovery can be expected in 85 percent of

patients with acute low back pain unaccompanied by leg pain. Most of these patients exhibit "mechanical" symptoms—pain that is aggravated by motion and relieved by rest. Despite the staggering annual costs of back pain to society, there is a paucity of well-controlled clinical trials in this area.

Recent observational, population-based studies (North Carolina Back Pain Project) have been used to justify a minimalist approach to individual patient care. These studies share a number of limitations: (1) comparison of treatment groups often lacks a true placebo control group, (2) it is assumed that patients who consult different provider groups (generalists, orthopedists, neurologists) have similar etiologies for their back pain, (3) no information is provided about the details of treatment within each provider group or between provider groups, and (4) there is no attempt to tabulate serious causes of low back pain. The appropriateness of specific diagnostic procedures or therapeutic interventions for low back pain cannot be assessed from these studies.

Competitive pressures in the health care marketplace have encouraged the rapid development of CPGs for the treatment of back pain. In December 1994, the Agency for Health Care Policy and Research (AHCPR) published a summary guideline entitled "Acute Low Back Problems in Adults." The following characteristics of evidence were considered in developing the guidelines: the quality and amount of evidence for efficacy, the strength of an effect for the diagnostic/therapeutic method, the consistency of findings between studies when multiple studies were available, the clinical applicability of the evidence to adult patients, and evidence on complications or cost.

Entry into the AHCPR guideline begins with adults (patients > 18 years of age) who have less than 3 months of activity intolerance due to low back pain and/or back-related leg symptoms. The term *back problems* was defined as pain of sufficient magnitude to limit a return to functional activities. The next guideline phase focused on the use of the medical history and physical examination to divide patients into management subcategories. "Red flags" were used to identify features that raised the likelihood that a serious underlying disease requiring rapid evaluation and treatment was present. Findings on neurologic examination were heavily weighted in the initial screen. If the history, physical examination, and neurologic screening examination did not yield red flags, then patients were treated symptomatically. No diagnostic tests were deemed necessary. The common serious etiologies considered as red flags were cancer metastatic to spine, spine fracture, and spine infection.

The guidelines attempted to use available medical literature to create management recommendations and often quoted specific values for the sensitivity and specificity (SAS) of certain tests. However, the applicability of these values to common outpatient clinical settings is limited for numerous reasons: (1) many of the studies used to calculate SAS were retrospective series comprising patients who ultimately had surgery, and they excluded nonsurgical patients with abnormal findings on examination (e.g., SLR) who never underwent surgery; (2) patients were preselected by virtue of referral to orthopedic surgeons and thus may not have reflected a general medical population; (3) different entry criteria and protocols for evaluation were employed in different studies; (4) many studies were performed prior to the era of modern neuroimaging; (5) surgical outcome was assessed by anatomic endpoints (compression of nerve roots) and not by functional status; and (6) none of the studies documented the natural history of disk lesions associated with a focal neurologic deficit. These limitations emphasize the point that the use of current CPGs for the treatment of low back pain should not substitute for sound clinical judgment in specific circumstances.

The proposed algorithms (Fig. 16-7) for management of acute back pain draw considerably from published guidelines. The initial assessment must exclude serious causes of spine pathology that require urgent intervention, including infection, cancer, and trauma. Risks factors for a possible serious underlying cause of back pain include: age > 50 years, prior diagnosis of cancer or other serious medical illness, bed rest without relief, duration of pain > 1 month, urinary incontinence or recent nocturia, focal leg weakness or numbness, pain radiating into the leg(s) from the back, intravenous drug use, chronic infection (pulmonary or urinary), pain increasing with standing and relieved by sitting, history of spine trauma, and glucocorticoid use. Clinical signs associated with a possible serious etiology include unexplained fever, well-documented and unexplained weight loss, positive SLR sign, reverse SLR sign, crossed SLR sign, percussion tenderness over the spine or costovertebral angle, an abdominal mass (pulsatile or non-pulsatile), a rectal mass, focal sensory loss (saddle anesthesia or focal limb sensory loss), or leg weakness, spasticity, and asymmetric leg reflexes. Laboratory studies are unnecessary at this time unless a serious underlying cause is suspected based upon the symptoms and signs (Fig. 16-7, Algorithms

1 and 2). Plain spine films are rarely indicated in the first month of symptoms unless a spine fracture is suspected.

The roles of bed rest, early exercise, and traction in the treatment of acute low back pain among patients lacking clinical features to suggest a serious underlying cause have been the subject of recent studies. Clinical trials fail to demonstrate any benefit of prolonged (>2 days) bed rest. Theoretical advantages of early activity following the onset of acute low back pain include maintenance of cardiovascular conditioning, improved disk and cartilage nutrition, improved bone and muscle strength, and increased endorphin levels. A recent trial did not show benefit from an early *vigorous* exercise program, but the benefits of less vigorous exercise or other exercise programs remain unknown. The effect of bed rest on patients with sciatica or acute back pain and focal neurologic findings is also unknown. Early resumption of usual physical activity (without heavy manual labor) is beneficial. Well-designed clinical studies of traction, which include a sham traction group, fail to show a benefit of this treatment for acute low back pain. Despite this knowledge, a recent study of physician perceptions of treatment effectiveness identified strict bed rest for more than 3 days, trigger point injections (see below), and physical therapy as beneficial in over 50 percent of patients with acute low back pain. A highly variable perception of treatment effectiveness was present between physicians within a given specialty. In many instances, the behavior of treating physicians does not reflect the current medical literature.

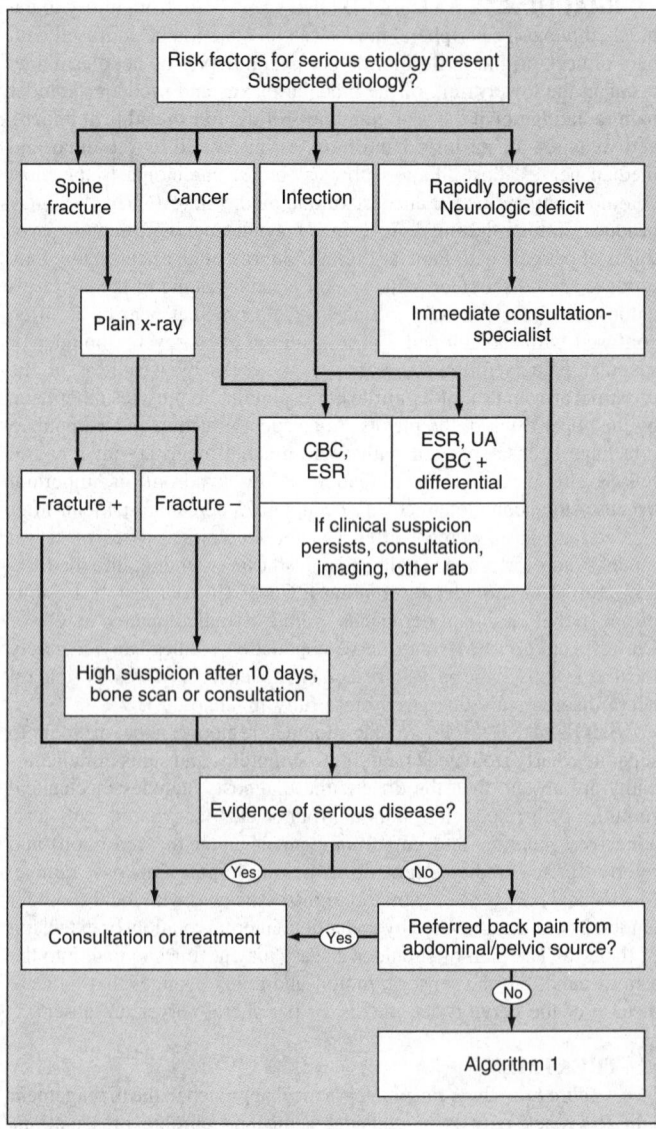

FIGURE 16-7 Algorithms for management of acute low back pain. Algorithm 1: First 4 weeks; ①, adults ≥18 years of age, symptoms <3 months; ②, see Algorithm 2; ③, excluding heavy manual labor.

FIGURE 16-7 *(continued)* Algorithm 2: Low back pain of possible serious etiology.

Proof is lacking to support the treatment of acute back and neck pain with acupuncture, transcutaneous electrical nerve stimulation, massage, ultrasound, diathermy, or electrical stimulation. Cervical collars can limit spontaneous and reflex neck movements that exacerbate pain, Evidence regarding the efficacy of self-application of ice and heat or use of shoe insoles is lacking. These interventions remain a therapeutic option given the lack of negative evidence, low cost, and low risk. Biofeedback has not been studied rigorously. Facet joint, trigger point, and ligament injections are not recommended in the treatment of acute low back pain.

A beneficial role of specific exercises or modification of posture has not been validated by rigorous clinical studies. As a practical

matter, temporary suspension of activity known to increase mechanical stress on the spine such as heavy lifting, prolonged sitting, bending or twisting, or straining at stool may be helpful.

Patient education is an important part of treatment. Clinical studies reveal that patient satisfaction and the likelihood of follow-up increases when patients are educated about prognosis, treatment methods, activity modifications, and strategies to prevent future exacerbations. In one study, patients who felt they did not receive an adequate explanation for their symptoms wanted more diagnostic tests. The evidence for the efficacy of structured education programs about low back pain ("back school") is inconclusive; in one controlled study, patients attending back school had a shorter duration of sick leave during the initial episode but not during subsequent episodes.

Medications used in the treatment of acute low back pain include NSAIDs, acetaminophen, muscle relaxants, and opioids. NSAIDs are superior to placebo for back pain relief. Acetaminophen is superior to placebo in the treatment of other types of pain but has not been compared against placebo for low back pain. Muscle relaxants provide short-term (4 to 7 days) benefit compared with placebo, but drowsiness often limits their use. The efficacy of muscle relaxants compared to NSAIDs or in combination with NSAIDs is unclear. Opioid analgesics have not been shown to be more effective than NSAIDs or acetaminophen for relief of acute low back pain or likelihood of return to work. Short-term use of opioids in selected patients unresponsive to or unable to take acetaminophen or NSAIDs may be helpful. There is no evidence to support the use of oral glucocorticoids or tricyclic antidepressants in treatment of acute low back pain. Equivocal data suggests that epidural steroids may occasionally produce short-term pain relief in patients with acute low back pain and radiculopathy, but proof is lacking for pain relief beyond 1 month. Epidural anesthetics, steroids, or opioids are not indicated as initial treatment for patients with acute low back pain unaccompanied by radiculopathy.

A short course of spinal manipulation for symptomatic relief of uncomplicated, acute low back pain is an option. A mild benefit of manipulation is seen only during the first 2 weeks after onset of treatment but may lessen pain and improve daily function in this situation. Treatment longer than 1 month or treatment of patients with radiculopathy is of unknown value and carries potential risk. The appropriate frequency or duration of spinal manipulation has not been adequately addressed.

CHRONIC LOW BACK PAIN CLBP is defined as pain lasting longer than 12 weeks. Patients with CLBP comprise 5 percent of all back pain patients but consume 50 percent of back pain costs. The initial approach to these patients is similar to that for acute low back pain. The differential diagnosis of CLBP includes most of the conditions described in this chapter. Treatment of this heterogeneous group of patients is based upon identification of the underlying cause.

Many diseases that result in CLBP can be defined by the combination of neuroimaging and electrophysiologic studies. MRI, CT, or CT-myelography are not indicated within the first month of back pain symptoms in the absence of risk factors for a serious underlying cause. Spine MRI or CT-myelography is the technique of choice; their sensitivity and specificity in the diagnosis of lumbar disk disease and lumbar spinal stenosis are equivalent, but MRI does not expose the patient to ionizing radiation and the definition of soft tissue structures by MRI is superior. Both techniques are noninvasive. CT-myelography provides optimal imaging of bony lesions in the region of the lateral recess and intervertebral foramen and is tolerated by claustrophobic patients. With rare exceptions, conventional myelography and bone scan are inferior to MRI and CT-myelography. The selection of diagnostic procedures for individual patients is often aided by appropriate neurologic, surgical, or medical consultation. Imaging studies should be performed only in circumstances where the results are likely to influence surgical or medical treatment.

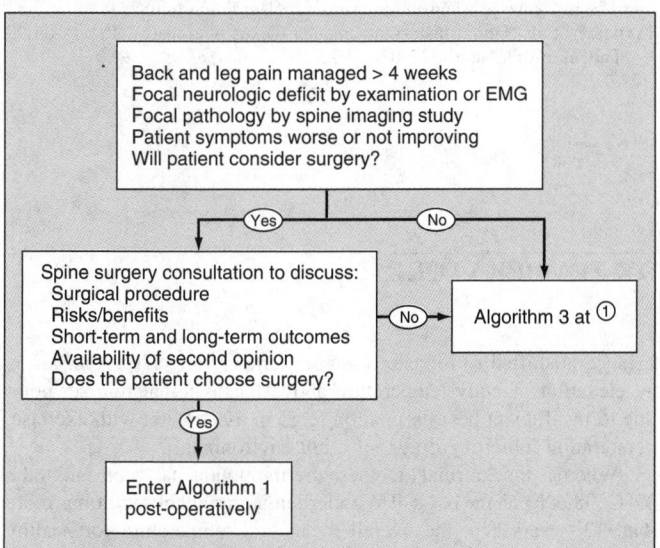

FIGURE 16-7 *(continued)* *Top.* Algorithm 3: Management for weeks 4 to 12; ①, entry point from Algorithm 4 postoperatively or if patient declines surgery. *Bottom.* Algorithm 4: Surgical options.

Diskography is of questionable value in the evaluation of back pain. No additional anatomic information is provided beyond what is available by MRI scan. Reproduction of the patient's typical pain with the injection provides evidence for a specific disk as a pain generator, but controversy exists regarding how to use this information to decide whether or not to operate. There is no proven role for thermography in the management of radiculopathy.

Sensory nerve conduction studies, motor nerve conduction studies, and needle EMG (Chap. 361) are used to assess the functional integrity of the peripheral nervous system in the setting of back pain. Sensory nerve conduction studies are normal when a circumscribed sensory loss is due to nerve root damage proximal to the dorsal root ganglion (DRG). The amplitude of motor nerve compound muscle action potentials (CMAP) may be reduced when there is significant loss of motor axons in a damaged nerve root. The diagnostic yield of needle EMG is higher than that of nerve conduction studies for radiculopathy. Denervation changes in a myotomal (segmental) distribution are detected by sampling multiple muscles supplied by different nerve roots and nerves; the pattern of muscle involvement indicates the nerve root(s) responsible for the injury. Needle EMG can also provide objective information about motor nerve fiber injury when the clinical evaluation of weakness is limited by pain or lack of patient effort. EMG and nerve conduction studies will be normal when only limb pain or sensory nerve root injury or irritation is present. Mixed nerve somatosensory evoked potentials and F-wave studies are of uncertain value in the evaluation of nerve root lesions.

The diagnosis of nerve root injury is most secure when the history and examination and results of imaging studies and EMG are concordant. The correlation between CT and EMG for localization of nerve root injury is between 65 and 73 percent. Up to 25 percent of asymptomatic individuals have a herniated disk detected by CT or MRI scans. Thus, surgical intervention based solely upon radiologic findings and pain increases the likelihood of an unsuccessful outcome.

CLBP can be treated with a variety of conservative measures. Acute and subacute exacerbations are managed with NSAIDs and comfort measures. Bed rest should not exceed 2 days. Activity tolerance is the primary goal, while pain relief is secondary. Exercise programs can reverse type II muscle fiber atrophy in paraspinal muscles and result in improved trunk extension strength. Supervised, intensive physical exercise or "work hardening" regimens (under the guidance of a physical therapist) have been effective in returning patients to work, improving walking distances, and diminishing pain. The benefit can be sustained among patients who follow home exercise regimens. Compliance with the exercise regimen strongly influences outcome. A reduction in sick leave days, long-term health care

utilization, and pension expenditures may offset the initial expense of multidisciplinary treatment programs. Hydrotherapy resulted in diminished duration and intensity of back pain, reduced analgesic drug consumption, improved spine mobility, and improved functional score in one study comparing 3 weeks of hydrotherapy versus routine ambulatory care. Functional score returned to baseline at the 9-month follow-up, but all other beneficial effects were sustained.

BIBLIOGRAPHY

AGENCY FOR HEALTH CARE POLICY AND RESEARCH (AHCPR): *Acute Low Back Problems in Adults*. U.S. Department of Health and Human Services. Public Health Service. ACHPR Publication No. 95-0642. Rockville, MD

AMINOFF MJ et al: Electrophysiologic evaluation of lumbosacral radiculopathies: Electromyography, late responses, and somatosensory evoked potentials. Neurology 35:1514, 1985

AMUNDSEN T et al: Lumbar spinal stenosis. Clinical and radiologic features. Spine 20:1178, 1995

BATEMAN JL, PEVZNER MM: Spinal osteomyelitis: A review of 10 years' experience. Orthopedics 18:561, 1995

BEURSKENS AJ et al: Efficacy of traction for non-specific low back pain: A randomised clinical trial. Lancet 346:1596, 1995

BODEN SD et al: Abnormal magnetic-resonance scans of the lumbar spine in asymptomatic subjects. J Bone Joint Surg 72A:403, 1990

CAPUTY AJ, LUESSENHOP AJ: Long-term evaluation of decompressive surgery for degenerative lumbar stenosis. J Neurosurg 77:669, 1992

CAREY TS et al: The outcomes and costs of care for acute low back pain among patients seen by primary care practitioners, chiropractors, and orthopedic surgeons. N Engl J Med 333:913, 1995

CLOUSTON PD et al: The spectrum of neurological disease in patients with systemic cancer. Ann Neurol 31:268, 1992

DAROUICHE RO et al: Bacterial spinal epidural abscess. Medicine 71:369, 1992

DEYO RA et al: How many days of bed rest for acute low back pain? A randomized clinical trial. N Engl J Med 315:1064, 1986

ELAM KC et al: How emergency physicians approach low back pain: Choosing costly options. J Emerg Med 13:143, 1995

FROST H et al: Randomised controlled trial for evaluation of fitness programme for patients with chronic low back pain. BMJ 310:151, 1995

HELLER JG: The syndromes of degenerative cervical disease. Orthop Clin North Am 23:381, 1992

KORI SH et al: Brachial plexus lesions in patients with cancer: 100 cases. Neurology 31:45, 1981

MALMIVAARA A et al: The treatment of acute low back pain—bed rest, exercises, or ordinary activity? N Engl J Med 332:351, 1995

MARSTON WA et al: Misdiagnosis of ruptured abdominal aortic aneurysms. J Vasc Surg 16:17, 1992

MARTIN RJ, YUAN HA: Neurosurgical care of spinal epidural, subdural, and intramedullary abscesses and arachnoiditis. Orthop Clin North Am 27:125, 1996

PEARSON SD et al: Critical pathways as a strategy for improving care: Problems and potential. Ann Intern Med 123:941, 1995

STURZENEGGER M et al: Presenting symptoms and signs after whiplash injury: The influence of accident mechanisms. Neurology 44:688, 1994

TSAIRIS P et al: Natural history of brachial plexus neuropathy: Report on 99 patients. Arch Neurol 27:109, 1972

SECTION 2

ALTERATIONS IN BODY TEMPERATURE

17

Jeffrey A. Gelfand, Charles A. Dinarello

FEVER AND HYPERTHERMIA

Fever is an elevation of body temperature above the normal circadian range as the result of a change in the thermoregulatory center located in the anterior hypothalamus. A normal body temperature is ordinarily maintained, despite environmental variations, through the ability of the thermoregulatory center to balance heat production by the tissues (notably, muscles and the liver) with heat dissipation. With fever, the balance is shifted to increase the core temperature. *Hyperthermia* is an elevation of body temperature above the hypothalamic set point due to insufficient heat dissipation (e.g., in association with exercise, perspiration-inhibiting drugs, or a hot environment).

Whereas the "normal" temperature in humans has been said to be 37°C (98.6°F) on the basis of Wunderlich's original observations more than 120 years ago, the overall mean oral temperature for healthy individuals aged 18 to 40 years is actually 36.8 ± 0.4°C (98.2 ± 0.7°F), with a nadir at 6 A.M. and a zenith at 4 to 6 P.M. The maximum normal oral temperature at 6 A.M. is 37.2°C (98.9°F), and the maximum normal oral temperature at 4 P.M. is 37.7°C (99.9°F)—both values defining the 99th percentile for healthy individuals. Given these criteria, *an A.M. temperature of greater than 37.2°C (98.9°F) or a P.M. temperature of greater than 37.7°C (99.9°F) would define a fever.* Rectal temperatures are generally 0.6°C (1°F) higher. Lower esophageal temperatures closely reflect core temperature. The temperature of a freshly passed urine specimen is close to rectal values. The normal 24-h circadian temperature rhythm is associated with temperatures varying typically by 0.5°C (0.9°F) but occasionally by as much as 1°C between the A.M. nadir and the P.M. peak. This morning-low and evening-high pattern is usually preserved in febrile diseases but not in hyperthermia. In menstruating women, the A.M. temperature is generally lower in the 2 weeks prior to ovulation, rising by about 0.6°C (1°F) with ovulation and remaining at that level until menses occur. In addition, there may be a seasonal variation in body temperature. Finally, such physiologic factors as postprandial state, pregnancy, endocrine alterations, and age may affect baseline temperatures.

PYROGENS Substances that cause fever are called *pyrogens* and may be either exogenous or endogenous. *Exogenous pyrogens* come from outside the host, whereas endogenous pyrogens are produced by the host, generally in response to initiating stimuli that are usually triggered by infection or inflammation. The majority of exogenous pyrogens are microorganisms, their products, or toxins. The best-characterized type of exogenous pyrogen consists of a heterogeneous group of molecules that is common to all gram-negative bacteria and is referred to as *endotoxin* (lipopolysaccharide, LPS). LPS, which is found in the outer membrane of all gram-negative bacteria, comprises lipid A and a polysaccharide core linked to an O-polysaccharide side chain composed of repeating units of sugars that vary with the gram-negative organism. Gram-positive organisms also are sources of potent pyrogens. These include cell wall–derived lipoteichoic acid and peptidoglycans. Several exotoxins and enterotoxins produced by pathologic strains of streptococci and staphylococci act as bacterial superantigens—polyclonal T-lymphocyte activators that bind to the variable region of the T-cell receptor rather than in the antigen-binding pocket of the receptor. This binding leads to the activation of cells of many specificities, with resultant mediator release and tissue damage. These toxins are thought to contribute to both staphylococcal and streptococcal toxic shock. In vivo, as little as 1 ng of LPS/kg is capable of producing fever in humans; although there are no in vivo data for humans, gram-positive cell-wall constituents generally require a 2- to 3-log larger amount of material by weight to induce the production of endogenous pyrogens in vitro.

In general, exogenous pyrogens act primarily by inducing the formation of endogenous pyrogens through stimulation of the host's cells—usually monocytes and macrophages. However, the distinction between exogenous and endogenous pyrogens is sometimes blurred. For example, LPS may act directly on endothelial cells in the brain to generate fever, whereas many exogenous products result in the release of endogenous pyrogens, thereby causing fever. Such endogenous substances include antigen-antibody complexes with complement, complement cleavage products, steroid hormone metabolites, bile acids, and some cytokines.

Endogenous pyrogens are polypeptides produced by a variety of host cells, particularly monocytes/macrophages. Endogenous pyrogens, produced either systemically or locally, gain entrance to the circulation and produce fever at the level of the thermoregulatory center of the hypothalamus.

It was originally thought that there was a single endogenous pyrogen. The standard experimental model utilized injection of leukocyte supernatants or sera from febrile rabbits into normal rabbits. It was then realized that there are two leukocyte endogenous pyrogens: interleukin (IL) 1α and IL-1β. These two interleukins have a common molecular weight of approximately 17.5 kDa, have only 26 percent amino acid sequence homology, and bind to the same receptors. Originally thought to be produced only by phagocytic cells, IL-1α or IL-1β is also produced by endothelial cells, B lymphocytes, natural killer cells, fibroblasts, smooth-muscle cells, keratinocytes, and glial cells. Because of the ubiquitous production of these and other interleukins, cell-derived inflammatory polypeptides, and growth-promoting

peptides, the more general term *cytokine* has been adopted to refer to these substances. Cytokines are regulatory polypeptides produced by a large variety of nucleated cells. Specifically, cytokines are produced by monocytes/macrophages, lymphocytes, endothelial cells, hepatocytes, epithelial cells, keratinocytes, and fibroblasts as well as other cells. Cytokines typically act locally, initiating autocrine (self-stimulating) or paracrine (nearby-stimulating) effects. When found in the circulation, cytokines are usually present in picogram-per-milliliter concentrations.

The major fever-inducing cytokines appear to be IL-1α, IL-1β, tumor necrosis factor α (TNFα), interferon (IFN) α, and IL-6. When any of these cytokines is administered intravenously to humans, chills and fever develop within 1 h. IL-1α and -1β are the most pyrogenic, with temperatures of 39°C developing in response to doses of 1 to 10 ng/kg of body weight. Doses of 100 ng/kg have caused higher fevers and rigors. TNFα produces chills and a temperature of 39°C at somewhat higher doses (50 to 100 ng/kg). IL-6 is the least pyrogenic of these cytokines, producing a temperature of 39°C at 10 μg/kg. IFNα and IFNγ have been administered primarily by the subcutaneous route; therefore, chills and fever develop after 3 to 4 h. On a weight basis, the interferons are less potent than IL-1 or TNFα and similar to IL-6. Moreover, the degree of fever elicited decreases with repeated injections of interferon. Studies with genetically altered mice have revealed that IL-1 and TNFα cause fever by inducing IL-6 in the brain.

HYPOTHALAMIC CONTROL OF TEMPERATURE Body temperature is controlled by the hypothalamus. Neurons in both the preoptic anterior hypothalamus and the posterior hypothalamus receive two kinds of signals—one from peripheral nerves that reflect receptors for warmth and cold and the other from the temperature of the blood bathing the region. These two signals are integrated by the thermoregulatory center of the hypothalamus to maintain normal temperature. In a neutral environment, the metabolic rate of humans consistently produces more heat than is necessary to maintain the core body temperature at 37°C. Therefore, the hypothalamus controls temperature by mechanisms of heat loss.

Clusters of neurons in the preoptic/anterior hypothalamus are supplied by a rich and permeable vascular network with limited blood-brain barrier function. The specialized vascular network is called the *organum vasculosum laminae terminalis*. It is likely that the endothelial cells of this network release arachidonic acid metabolites when exposed to endogenous pyrogenic cytokines from the circulation. The arachidonic acid metabolites—mainly prostaglandin E_2 (PGE$_2$)—then presumably diffuse into the preoptic/anterior hypothalamic region and initiate fever. It is also possible that PGE$_2$ or other arachidonic acid products induce a second messenger such as cyclic AMP, which in turn raises the thermoregulatory set point. PGE$_2$ is the most potent of the fever-producing arachidonic acid derivatives when injected directly into the hypothalamus and is believed to mediate the rise in the thermoregulatory set point. With the new, higher "thermostatic setting," signals go to various efferent nerves, particularly those sympathetic fibers innervating the peripheral blood vessels, which in turn initiate vasoconstriction and promote heat conservation. The thermoregulatory center also sends signals to the cerebral cortex, initiating behavioral changes such as seeking a warm environment, putting on more clothes, and special posturing. With the shunting of blood from the periphery and these behavioral changes, the body temperature usually rises by 2 to 3°C; if the hypothalamus calls for more heat, shivering (involuntary muscle contraction) is triggered to increase heat production. The combination of heat conservation and increased heat production continues until the temperature of the blood bathing the anterior hypothalamic neurons matches the new "setting." At that point, the hypothalamus maintains the new febrile temperature (Fig. 17-1).

The hypothalamic set point is reset downward by the disappearance of stimulating pyrogenic cytokines or by the inhibition of local prostaglandin synthesis by cyclooxygenase inhibitors such as aspirin and ibuprofen. The reduction of fever by acetaminophen involves the metabolism of the drug by brain cytochromes and the subsequent inhibition of brain cyclooxygenase by the metabolites. Vasodilation and sweating dissipate heat through radiation and conduction from the skin. Behavioral changes, such as the removal of insulating clothing or bedding, may be triggered. There are also endogenous antipyretic substances. These include arginine vasopressin, adrenocorticotropin, α-melanocyte-stimulating hormone, and corticotropin-releasing hormone, each of which appears to alter the ability of endogenous pyrogens to stimulate prostaglandin production.

Specific cytokine antagonists and inhibitory cytokines may play a role in modulating fever. The IL-1 receptor antagonist (IL-1Ra) is a 23- to 25-kDa protein that blocks the binding of IL-1 to its receptors. Whereas IL-1Ra blocks the hypotensive effects of IL-1 and gram-negative and gram-positive bacteremia in experimental animals, in volunteers it has failed to prevent fever in response to small doses of intravenous LPS. Peak molar concentrations of IL-1Ra may exceed those of IL-1β by 100-fold, but these levels tend to be reached 1 h after the IL-1β peak and may be part of the recovery process.

Endogenous binding proteins for TNFα are produced by cleavage of the extracellular domains of the two TNFα receptors. Circulating levels of these two soluble TNFα receptor fragments (type I and type II) are higher than circulating levels of TNFα. In addition, cytokines that inhibit the production of the major pyrogens IL-1 and TNFα include transforming growth factor β, IL-4, and IL-10. There is little information on the role of these cytokines in modulating the febrile response.

BIOLOGIC ACTIVITIES OF IL-1, TNFα, AND IL-6 It is important to distinguish between the critical physiologic roles of local IL-1 and TNFα and the high systemic blood levels of these cytokines that are often seen with severe and life-threatening diseases. IL-1 and TNFα mediate local phagocytic-cell emigration and activation as well as the release of lipid-derived mediators such as PGE₂, thromboxane,

and platelet-activating factor. IL-1 induces the synthesis of IL-8, which in turn is a potent neutrophil and monocyte chemotactic factor. IL-8 stimulates the release of enzymes from neutrophils, further enhancing the host's attack on invading microbes. Vasodilation, the induction of adhesive glycoproteins, the activation of T and B lymphocytes, and the enhancement of killing by phagocytic cells are directly or indirectly mediated by these pyrogenic cytokines. The acute-phase response is stimulated, resulting in changes in protein synthesis in the liver. Serum albumin levels decrease, and the production of acute-phase proteins, including antiproteases, complement components, fibrinogen, ceruloplasmin, ferritin, and haptoglobin, is increased. Levels of C-reactive protein, which binds to damaged and necrotic cells and to some microorganisms, may increase by 1000-fold. Concentrations of serum amyloid A protein also may increase markedly, with the protein deposited in various organs to cause secondary amyloidosis. Decreases in serum iron and zinc levels deprive invading microbes of these critical growth factors. Although IL-1 and TNFα can induce these hepatic changes, IL-6 is thought to be the prime mediator of the acute-phase response.

IL-1 and TNFα act synergistically to mediate local and systemic inflammatory effects. Amounts of each cytokine that cause little inflammation individually produce refractory hypotension and the failure of mutiple organ systems in combination. Suppression of either of these two cytokines may have a significant therapeutic effect by blocking this synergistic toxicity. Furthermore, IL-1–induced activation of T and B cells is greater at 39°C than at 37°C. Both IL-1 and TNFα increase the loss of mean body mass and cause anorexia, contributing to the cachexia of chronic febrile states. IL-1 and TNFα are found in the circulation only briefly but nevertheless induce IL-6. Levels of IL-6 correlate better with the degree of fever and other pathologic findings in a variety of infectious diseases than do levels of IL-1 or TNFα because of the persistence of IL-6 in the circulation. However, there is little or no evidence that IL-6 is—like IL-1 and TNFα—a lethal cytokine.

WHY FEVER? From an evolutionary perspective, the phenomenon of fever has been operative for hundreds of millions of years. Fish, amphibians, and reptiles develop fever. When fish are injected with bacterial endotoxin or gram-negative bacteria, they raise their body temperature by swimming to warmer water. When lizards are injected with bacteria or pyrogens, they generate fever by basking in the sun to raise their core temperature to "febrile" levels. In many situations, the elevation of body temperature increases chances for survival. The growth and virulence of several bacterial species are impaired at high temperatures; thus, for example, fever therapy was used in neurosyphilis before antibiotics became available. Type III pneumococci are particularly sensitive to high temperature and at 41°C grow poorly and may autolyze. Inhibition of fever in rabbits infected with type III pneumococci increases the mortality rate. Temperatures in the febrile range appear to increase the phagocytic and bactericidal activity of neutrophils and the cytotoxic effects of lymphocytes. Thus fever probably enhances the ability to survive infection. Redundancies among the pyrogens (IL-1β, IL-1α, TNFα, IL-6, interferons) suggest that it is beneficial to preserve a number of pathways for eliciting this response.

However, fever involves considerable "costs" to the host in addition to discomfort. For each elevation of body temperature by 1°C, there is an increase in O₂ consumption of 13 percent and an increase in caloric and fluid requirements. The increased metabolic demand may stress fetuses as well as patients with marginal cardiac or cerebral vascular supply. IL-1 and TNFα accelerate muscle catabolism, an effect leading to a loss of body weight and a negative nitrogen balance. Essentially, skeletal muscle is utilized as an energy source, with liberation of amino acids for gluconeogenesis and for the synthesis of acute-phase proteins and formation of clones of immune cells. Fever reduces mental acuity and can produce delirium and stupor. Children are prone to develop seizures with fevers, particularly if they have a history of seizures. A single episode of a temperature of ≥37.8°C (100°F) in the first trimester of pregnancy doubles the risk of neural tube defects in the fetus.

ACCOMPANIMENTS OF FEVER Not surprisingly, many features associated with fever, including back pain, generalized myal-

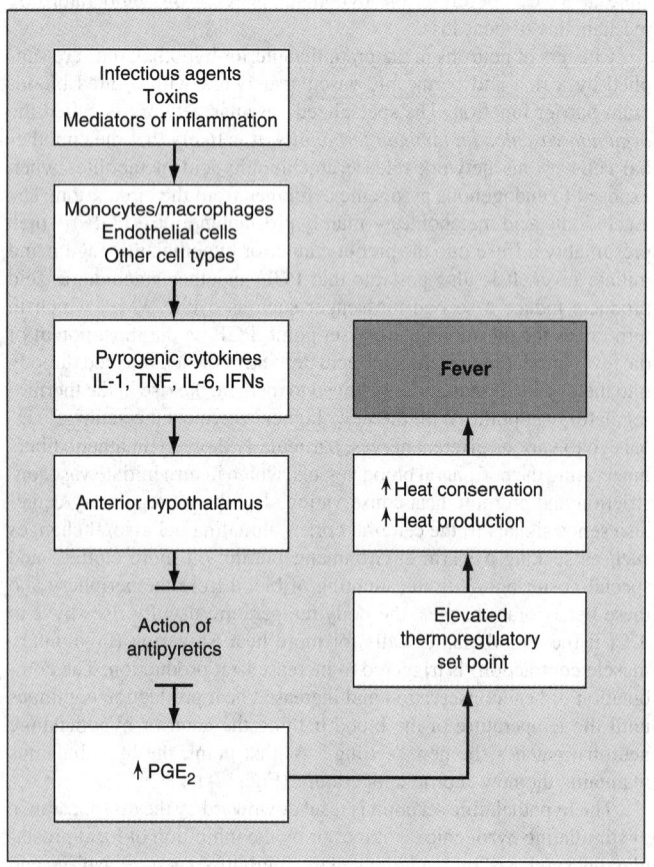

FIGURE 17-1 Chronology of events required for the induction of fever.

gias, arthralgias, anorexia, and somnolence, can be reproduced by infusions of purified cytokines. These symptoms may be reduced by cyclooxygenase inhibitors. *Chills*, a sensation of cold occurring in most fevers, are part of the central nervous system (CNS) response to the thermoregulatory set point's call for more heat. A *rigor*, a profound chill with piloerection ("goose flesh") accompanied by chattering of the teeth and severe shivering, is common in bacterial, rickettsial, and protozoal diseases and in influenza (but not in other viral diseases). Rigors can be produced by sepsis; by systemic infections such as leptospirosis, brucellosis, rat-bite fever, and endocarditis; by malaria; by the intermittent sepsis seen with abscesses; and by lymphoma, leukemia, renal cell carcinoma, and hepatoma. Rigors are also common with drug-induced fevers. *Sweats* occur with the activation of heat-loss mechanisms by antipyretic treatment, by attainment of a new "thermal ceiling," or by elimination of the febrile stimulus. The intermittent administration of antipyretics may exaggerate swings of temperature, thereby causing chilliness, discomfort, and exhaustion. Hypothalamic reflexes trigger sweating, which allows rapid dissipation of heat by evaporative loss.

Alterations of mental status and convulsions are common among the very young and the very old and among patients with dementia, hepatic failure, or chronic renal failure. A progression from irritability to delirium to frank obtundation usually clears with the abating of fever.

Convulsions typically develop in febrile infants and in febrile children less than 5 years old, being particularly common at the onset of febrile disease and at higher temperatures (>40°C). Febrile convulsions in children are not necessarily a sign of significant cerebral disease, but a CNS disorder must be excluded in these cases. Fever may precipitate seizures in epileptic adults as well.

_____ *Approach to the Patient* _____

History   It is in the diagnosis of a febrile illness that the science and art of medicine come together. In no other clinical situation is a meticulous history more important. Painstaking attention must be paid to the chronology of symptoms in relation to the use of drugs (including those taken without a physician's supervision) or treatments such as surgical or dental procedures. The exact nature of any prosthetic materials and/or implanted devices should be ascertained. A careful occupational history should include exposures to animals; toxic fumes; potential infectious agents; possible antigens; or other febrile or infected individuals in the home, workplace, or school. A history of the geographic areas in which the patient has lived and a travel history should include locations during military service. Information on unusual hobbies, dietary proclivities (such as raw or poorly cooked meat, raw fish, and unpasteurized milk or cheeses), and household pets should be elicited, as should that on sexual orientation and practices, including precautions taken or omitted. Attention should be directed to the use of tobacco, marijuana, intravenous drugs, or alcohol; trauma; animal bites; tick or other insect bites; and prior transfusions, immunizations, drug allergies, or hypersensitivities. A careful family history should include information on family members with tuberculosis, other febrile or infectious diseases, arthritis or collagen vascular disease, or unusual familial symptomatology such as deafness, urticaria, fevers and polyserositis, bone pain, or anemia. Ethnic origin may be critical. For example, blacks are more likely than persons in other groups to have hemoglobinopathies. Turks, Arabs, Armenians, and Sephardic Jews are especially likely to have familial Mediterranean fever.

Patterns of Fever   The widespread use of antipyretics, glucocorticoids, and antibiotics can alter the course of fever so that "classic" fever patterns are not seen. Some patterns are clinically informative, however. Whereas the circadian temperature pattern is preserved and in fact exaggerated in most fevers, it may be reversed in typhoid fever and disseminated tuberculosis. Temperature-pulse dissociation (relative bradycardia) is seen in typhoid fever as well as in brucellosis, leptospirosis, some drug-associated fevers, and many factitious fevers. Bradycardia in the presence of fever also may signify cardiac conduction abnormalities, as it does in acute rheumatic fever, Lyme disease, viral myocarditis, or valve-ring abscess complicating bacterial endocarditis.

Fever may be sustained, intermittent, remittent, or relapsing. A *sustained* fever is one in which temperature elevation is persistent, with minimal variation. With *intermittent* fever, there is an exaggeration of the normal circadian rhythm; when this variation is extremely large, the fever is termed *hectic* or *septic*. Intermittent, hectic, and septic patterns are common in deep-seated or systemic infections, malignancy, and drug fevers. When hectic fevers occur daily, they are sometimes termed *quotidian*.

Remittent fever, in which the temperature falls each day but not to normal, is typical for tuberculosis, viral diseases, many bacterial infections, and noninfectious conditions. It should be emphasized that newborns, the elderly, patients with chronic renal or hepatic failure, patients taking glucocorticoids, or patients with bacteremic shock may fail to generate fever altogether; in these individuals, *hypothermia* may be a sign of severe infection.

With *relapsing* fevers, febrile episodes are separated by intervals of normal temperature; when paroxysms occur on the first and third days, the fever is called *tertian*. *Plasmodium vivax* causes tertian fevers. *Quartan* fevers are associated with paroxysms on the first and fourth days and are seen with *Plasmodium malariae*. Other relapsing fevers are related to *Borrelia* infections and rat-bite fever, which are both associated with days of fever followed by a several-day afebrile period and then a relapse of days of fever. Pel-Ebstein fever, with fevers lasting 3 to 10 days followed by afebrile periods of 3 to 10 days, is classic for Hodgkin's disease and other lymphomas. Another characteristic fever is that of cyclic neutropenia, in which fevers occur every 21 days and accompany the neutropenia.

Physical Examination   A meticulous physical examination should be repeated on a regular basis. All the vital signs are relevant. The temperature may be taken orally or rectally, but the site used should be consistent. Axillary temperatures are notoriously unreliable, as are oral temperatures taken after recent consumption of hot or cold drinks, smoking, or hyperventilation.

In some cases, patients are thoroughly examined at the time of initial evaluation, but the diagnostic emphasis then shifts to laboratory data and other diagnostic procedures. Particular attention should be paid to daily (or sometimes more frequent) physical examination, which should continue until the diagnosis is certain and the anticipated response has been achieved. Special attention should be paid to the skin, lymph nodes, eyes, nail beds, cardiovascular system, chest, abdomen, musculoskeletal system, and nervous system. Rectal examination is imperative. The penis, prostate, scrotum, and testes should be examined carefully, and the foreskin, if present, retracted. Pelvic examination must be part of every complete physical examination of a woman.

Laboratory Tests   Few signs and symptoms in medicine have as many diagnostic possibilities as fever. If the history, epidemiologic situation, or physical examination suggests more than a simple viral illness or streptococcal pharyngitis, then laboratory testing is indicated. The tempo and complexity of the workup will depend on the pace of the illness, diagnostic considerations, and the immune status of the host. If findings are focal or if the history, epidemiologic setting, or physical examination suggests certain diagnoses, the laboratory examination can be focused. If fever is undifferentiated, the "diagnostic nets" must be cast farther, and certain guidelines are indicated, as follows.

CLINICAL PATHOLOGY   The workup should include a complete blood count; a differential count should be performed manually or with an instrument sensitive to the identification of eosinophils, juvenile or band forms, toxic granulations, and Döhle bodies, the last three of which are suggestive of bacterial infection. Neutropenia may be seen with some viral infections, particularly parvovirus B19 infection; drug reactions; systemic lupus erythematosus; typhoid; brucellosis; and infiltrative diseases of the bone marrow, including lymphoma, leukemia, tuberculosis, and histoplasmosis. Lymphocytosis may be seen with typhoid, brucellosis, tuberculosis, and viral disease. Atypical lymphocytes are documented in many viral diseases, including infection with

Epstein-Barr virus, cytomegalovirus, or human immunodeficiency virus; dengue; rubella; varicella; measles; and viral hepatitis. This abnormality also occurs in serum sickness and toxoplasmosis. Monocytosis is a feature of typhoid, tuberculosis, brucellosis, and lymphoma. Eosinophilia may be associated with hypersensitivity drug reactions, Hodgkin's disease, adrenal insufficiency, and certain metazoan infections. If the febrile illness appears to be severe or is prolonged, the smear should be examined carefully and the erythrocyte sedimentation rate should be determined. Urinalysis, with examination of urinary sediment, is indicated. It is axiomatic that any abnormal fluid accumulation (pleural, peritoneal, joint), even if previously sampled, merits reexamination in the presence of undiagnosed fever. Joint fluids should be examined for crystals. Bone marrow biopsy (not simple aspiration) for histopathologic studies (as well as culture) is indicated when marrow infiltration by pathogens or tumor cells is possible. Stool should be inspected for occult blood; an inspection for fecal leukocytes, ova, or parasites also may be indicated.

CHEMISTRY Electrolyte, glucose, blood urea nitrogen, and creatinine levels should be measured. Liver function tests are usually indicated if efforts to identify the cause of fever do not point to the involvement of another organ. Additional assessments (e.g., measurement of creatine phosphokinase) can be added as the workup progresses.

MICROBIOLOGY Smears and cultures of specimens from the throat, urethra, anus, cervix, and vagina should be assessed in appropriate situations. Sputum evaluation (Gram's staining, staining for acid-fast bacilli, culture) is indicated for any patient with fever and cough. Cultures of blood, abnormal fluid collections, and urine are indicated when fever is thought to indicate more than uncomplicated viral illness. Cerebrospinal fluid should be examined and cultured if meningismus, severe headache, or a change in mental status is noted.

RADIOLOGY A chest x-ray is usually part of the evaluation for any significant febrile illness.

Outcome of Diagnostic Efforts In most cases of fever, either the patient recovers spontaneously or the history, physical examination, and initial screening laboratory studies lead to a diagnosis. In the former case, a viral illness is usually considered to have been the source of the fever. When fever continues for 2 to 3 weeks, during which time repeat physical examinations and laboratory tests are unrevealing, the patient is provisionally diagnosed as having fever of unknown origin (see Chap. 125).

R_x TREATMENT

When to Treat Fever It is distressingly common in hospitals to find "routine," "standing," or "prn" orders for the use of antipyretics (such as acetaminophen) for a temperature above an arbitrary level; it is also common to find patients awake and alert but most uncomfortable, shivering on a cooling blanket. Such therapies have their appropriate application but are frequently used without therapeutic rationale. The first decision to make is whether an elevated temperature in fact reflects *fever* or *hyperthermia*.

Hyperthermia is an elevation of core temperature *without elevation of the hypothalamic set point*. Hyperthermia is most commonly due to inadequate heat dissipation, though more rarely the primary cause is excessive heat production with heat dissipation inadequate to compensate. The various syndromes of hyperthermia, as distinguished from true elevation of the hypothalamic set point, or fever, are listed in Table 17-1.

Heat stroke, caused by thermoregulatory failure in association with a warm environment, may be categorized as exertional or nonexertional. *Exertional heat stroke* typically occurs in younger individuals exercising at ambient temperatures and/or humidities that are higher than normal. Even in normal individuals, dehydration or the use of common medications (e.g., over-the-counter antihista-

mines with anticholinergic side effects) may help to precipitate exertional heat stroke.

Nonexertional or *classic heat stroke* typically occurs in elderly individuals, particularly during heat waves. For example, in Chicago in July 1995, a total of 465 deaths were certified as heat related. The elderly, the bedridden, persons taking anticholinergic or antiparkinsonian drugs or diuretics, and individuals confined to poorly ventilated and un-air-conditioned environments are most susceptible.

Drug-induced hyperthermia has become increasingly common as a result of the increased use of prescription psychotropic drugs and illicit drugs. Drug-induced hyperthermia may be caused by monoamine oxidase inhibitors, tricyclic antidepressants, and amphetamines and by the illicit use of phencyclidine, lysergic acid diethylamide (LSD), or cocaine.

Malignant hyperthermia is an inherited abnormality of skeletal-muscle sarcoplasmic reticulum that causes a rapid increase in intracellular calcium levels in response to halothane and other inhalational anesthetics or to succinylcholine. Elevated temperature, increased muscle metabolism, rigidity, rhabdomyolysis, acidosis, and cardiovascular instability develop rapidly. Cessation of anesthesia and administration of dantrolene sodium are the immediately indicated therapies. The *neuroleptic malignant syndrome* can occur with phenothiazines and other drugs such as haloperidol and is characterized by muscle rigidity, autonomic dysregulation, and hyperthermia. This disorder appears to be caused by the inhibition of central dopamine receptors in the hypothalamus, which results in increased heat generation and decreased heat dissipation. Thyrotoxicosis and pheochromocytoma can also cause increased thermogenesis.

A high core temperature in a patient likely to have hyperthermia (due to environmental exposure or treatment with anticholinergic or neuroleptic drugs, tricyclic antidepressants, succinylcholine, or halothane) along with appropriate clinical findings (dry skin, hallucinations, delirium, pupil dilation, muscle rigidity, and/or elevated levels of creatine phosphokinase) is characteristic of hyperthermia. The attempt to lower the already-normal hypothalamic set point is of little use. Physical cooling with sponging, fans, cooling blankets, and even ice baths should be initiated immediately in conjunction with the administration of intravenous fluids and appropriate pharmacologic agents (such as dantrolene for malignant hyperthermia and the neuroleptic malignant syndrome or physostigmine for tricyclic antidepressant overdose). If insufficient cooling is achieved by external means, internal cooling can be achieved by gastric or peritoneal lavage with iced saline. In extreme circumstances, hemodialysis or even cardiopulmonary bypass with cooling of blood may be performed.

Malignant hyperthermia should be treated immediately with intravenous dantrolene. The recommended dose of dantrolene is 1 to

Table 17-1

Causes of Hyperthermia Syndromes

Heat stroke
  Exertional: Exercise in higher-than-normal heat and/or humidity
  Nonexertional: Anticholinergics, including antihistamines; antiparkinsonian drugs; diuretics; phenothiazines

Drug-induced hyperthermia
  Amphetamines; monoamine oxidase inhibitors; cocaine; phencyclidine; tricyclic antidepressants; LSD

Neuroleptic malignant syndrome
  Phenothiazines; butyrophenones, including haloperidol and bromperidol; fluoxetine; loxapine; tricyclic dibenzodiazepines; metoclopramide; domperidone; thiothixene; molindone

Malignant hyperthermia
  Inhalational anesthetics; succinylcholine

Endocrinopathy
  Thyrotoxicosis
  Pheochromocytoma

SOURCE: After FJ Curley, RS Irwin.

2.5 mg/kg of body weight given intravenously every 6 h for at least 24 to 48 h—until oral dantrolene can be administered, if needed. Procainamide should also be administered to patients with malignant hyperthermia because of the likelihood of ventricular fibrillation in this syndrome. Dantrolene at similar doses is indicated in the neuroleptic malignant syndrome and drug-induced hyperthermia and may even be useful in the hyperthermia of thyrotoxicosis. The neuroleptic malignant syndrome may also be treated with bromocriptine, levodopa, amantadine, or nifedipine or by induction of muscle paralysis with curare and pancuronium.

With *hyperpyrexia* (temperature ≥41°C), treatment with antipyretics is clearly indicated, and physical cooling while "resetting" the hypothalamic set point with antipyretics will speed the process. Antipyretics also suppress the constitutional symptoms that accompany fever (myalgias, chills, headache.). However, there is little evidence that low-grade or moderate fever is harmful or that antipyretic therapy for such fever is beneficial, with the aforementioned exceptions—children with febrile seizures, pregnant women, and patients with impaired cardiac, pulmonary, or cerebral function. Temperature is often suppressed needlessly, and "routine" antipyretic orders may obscure the important clinical information to be gained by following the upward or downward course of a patient's temperature. Nonsteroidal anti-inflammatory drugs (NSAIDs) and glucocorticoids may mask the inflammatory features of a localized infection, thus preventing its detection and even encouraging its spread. In addition, the drugs themselves may cause adverse effects. The administration of aspirin to children with viral diseases is to be avoided because of the possibility of Reye's syndrome, which occurs in association with influenza and varicella and occasionally with enterovirus infection. The antiplatelet and even antiphagocytic effects of aspirin have led to the general use of acetaminophen. Acetaminophen is a poor cyclooxygenase inhibitor in peripheral tissue and thus lacks anti-inflammatory activity; in the CNS, the oxidation of acetaminophen converts it to an active cyclooxygenase inhibitor—an event explaining its antipyretic effect. Ibuprofen may be safe for children, with possibly more pronounced and more prolonged temperature reduction at doses similar to those of acetaminophen. Ibuprofen does not appear to pose a risk of Reye's syndrome, but the caveat about bacterial infections remains. Other NSAIDs, particularly indomethacin and naproxen, are also useful as antipyretics.

Glucocorticoids are potent antipyretics. They inhibit PGE_2 synthesis by inhibiting phospholipase A_2, and they block both mRNA transcription for IL-1 and TNFα and translation of these cytokines. The potent immunosuppressive and antiphagocytic effects of glucocorticoids limit their use as antipyretics to febrile states in which inflammation is a major pathogenic factor—such as bacterial meningitis, tuberculous pericarditis, and vasculitis. The severe rigors that accompany some fevers can be reduced with meperidine, morphine sulfate, prochlorperazine, or chlorpromazine. These two classes of agents combined have an additive suppressive effect on rigors; however, care must be taken to avoid hypotension when these agents are administered either singly or together.

Specific Therapy The advantages and disadvantages of antipyretic therapy have just been discussed. More specific therapy is based on the differential diagnosis for a given patient, including the relative probabilities of syndromes that are imminently life-threatening, the risks of not treating, and the risks of treatment itself. Sepsis of various etiologies is a leading consideration in determining the need for therapy.

Sepsis is defined as evidence of infection with a systemic response. *Sepsis syndrome* refers to a systemic response sufficient to produce organ dysfunction, and *septic shock* is the sepsis syndrome with documented hypotension. In a nonimmunocompromised adult with sepsis, gram-positive infection, gram-negative rod infection, and meningococcal infection can be "covered" by a variety of antibiotic combinations, including imipenem, ticarcillin/clavulanate, or a third-generation cephalosporin. The suspected involvement of a methicillin-resistant strain of *Staphylococcus aureus* dictates the addition of vancomycin to the regimen. If the patient has had a

splenectomy, therapy with ampicillin/sulbactam, ceftriaxone, cefotaxime, or cefuroxime is indicated. Suspicion of *Legionella* dictates the addition of erythromycin (possibly with rifampin) or, alternatively, of clarithromycin or azithromycin. In appropriate settings, the involvement of rickettsiae should be suspected, and the administration of either doxycycline or chloramphenicol is indicated. If a case of septic shock has no evident source, the differential diagnosis should include meningococcemia, staphylococcal and streptococcal toxic shock syndromes, and (rarely) gram-negative bacteremia. A combination of high-dose penicillin and penicillinase-resistant synthetic penicillins (nafcillin, oxacillin) will cover these cocci. Clindamycin and early fasciotomy of any putative soft-tissue lesion should be considered in cases of streptococcal toxic shock; tampons or wounds should be sought in staphylococcal toxic shock. A third-generation cephalosporin suffices to treat gram-negative bacteremia. Ticarcillin/clavulanate or piperacillin/tazobactam is an alternative. If a typhoidal syndrome is suspected, therapy with a fluoroquinolone such as ciprofloxacin or ofloxacin is indicated. Intravenous penicillin should be used if leptospirosis is suspected. In appropriate geographic areas, plague is a consideration; treatment with an aminoglycoside or chloramphenicol is indicated in this situation. Suspected endocarditis should be treated with a combination of penicillin, oxacillin/nafcillin, or vancomycin and gentamicin, depending on the type of patient and the suspected origin of infection. In intravenous drug users, the involvement of methicillin-sensitive or -resistant *S. aureus* and gram-negative bacilli should also be considered.

A febrile patient with headache, myalgia, cough, abdominal pain, nausea, or vomiting who develops interstitial infiltrates and/or respiratory distress may be infected with hantavirus. A controlled trial of intravenous ribavirin, performed in China with the Korean form of the disease, suggested benefit from therapy.

Consideration must also be given to acute febrile conditions in which the prevention of tissue damage requires immediate therapeutic intervention with agents other than anti-infectives. Examples include aspirin for acute rheumatic fever, intravenous gamma globulin for the Kawasaki syndrome, and glucocorticoids and/or cyclophosphamide for various forms of acute vasculitis.

Ultimately, the physician's task in dealing with these diverse diagnostic and therapeutic possibilities is to thoughtfully distill the data acquired by meticulous history-taking, physical examination, and laboratory studies; to narrow the possibilities; and to make a risk-benefit assessment regarding empirical therapy. In the "art" of medicine, this skill is known as "judgment." There is no formula for this type of judgment in any textbook.

BIBLIOGRAPHY

ATKINS E: Fever: Historical aspects, in *Interleukin-1, Inflammation, and Disease*, R Bomford, B Henderson (eds). New York, Elsevier Science Publishers, 1989, pp 3–15

CANNON JG et al: Circulating interleukin-1 and tumor necrosis factor in septic shock and experimental endotoxin fever. J Infect Dis 161:79, 1990

CENTERS FOR DISEASE CONTROL AND PREVENTION: Heat-related mortality—Chicago. MMWR 44:577, 1995

CURLEY FJ, IRWIN RS: Disorders of temperature control. Hyperthermia, in *Intensive Care Medicine*, 3d ed, JM Rippe et al (eds). Boston, Little, Brown, 1996, pp 859–873

DINARELLO CA: Interleukin-1 and interleukin-1 antagonism. Blood 77: 1627, 1991

———, WOLFF SM: Pathogenesis of fever, in *Principles and Practice of Infectious Diseases*, 3d ed, GL Mandell et al (eds). New York, Wiley, 1990, pp 462–467

——— et al: New concepts on the pathogenesis of fever. Rev Infect Dis 10:168, 1988

HECKER RB et al: Bayesian analysis of noninvasive versus oral temperature measurements to determine hypothermia in postoperative patients. South Med J 89:71, 1996

MACKOWIAK PA et al: A critical appraisal of 98.6°F, the upper limit of the normal body temperature, and other legacies of Carl Reinhold August Wunderlich. JAMA 268:1578, 1992

————: Carl Reinhold August Wunderlich and the evolution of clinical ther-
mometry. Clin Infect Dis 18:458, 1994

MILENO MD et al: Coagulation of whole blood stimulates interleukin-1β gene
expression. J Infect Dis 172:308, 1995

MILUNSKY A et al: Maternal heat exposure and neural tube defects. JAMA
268:882, 1992

STEINMETZ HT et al: Increase in interleukin-6 serum level preceding fever in
granulocytopenia and correlation with death from sepsis. J Infect Dis
171:225, 1995

18   *Elaine T. Kaye, Kenneth M. Kaye*

FEVER AND RASH

The acutely ill patient with fever and rash often presents a diagnostic
challenge for physicians. The distinctive appearance of an eruption in
concert with a clinical syndrome may facilitate a prompt diagnosis
and the institution of life-saving therapy or critical infection-control
interventions.

Approach to the Patient

A thorough history of patients with fever and rash includes the following relevant information: immune status, medications taken within the
previous month, specific travel history, immunization status, exposure
to domestic pets and other animals, history of animal or arthropod
bites, existence of cardiac abnormalities, presence of prosthetic material, recent exposure to ill individuals, and exposure to sexually transmitted diseases. The history should also include the site of onset of
the rash and its direction and rate of spread.

The acutely ill patient... A thorough physical examination entails close attention to the rash,
with an assessment and precise definition of its salient features. First, it
is critical to determine the *type* of lesions that make up the eruption.
Macules are flat lesions defined by an area of changed color (i.e., a
blanchable erythema). *Papules* are raised, solid lesions <5 mm in diameter; *plaques* are lesions >5 mm in diameter with a flat, plateau-like
surface; and *nodules* are lesions >5 mm in diameter with a more rounded
configuration. *Wheals* (urticaria, hives) are papules or plaques that are
pale pink and may appear annular (ringlike) as they enlarge; classic
(nonvasculitic) wheals are transient, lasting only 24 to 48 h in any defined area. *Vesicles* (<5 mm) and *bullae* (>5 mm) are circumscribed,
elevated lesions containing fluid. *Pustules* are raised lesions containing
purulent exudate; vesicular processes such as varicella or herpes simplex
may evolve to pustules. *Nonpalpable purpura* is a flat lesion that is due
to bleeding into the skin; if <3 mm in diameter, the purpuric lesions are
termed *petechiae*; if >3 mm, they are termed *ecchymoses*. *Palpable
purpura* is a raised lesion that is due to inflammation of the vessel wall
(vasculitis) with subsequent hemorrhage.

Other pertinent features of rashes include their *configuration* (i.e.,
annular or target), the *arrangement* of their lesions, and their *distribution* (i.e., central or peripheral). → *For further discussion, see Chaps.
54 and 57.*

CLASSIFICATION OF RASH This chapter reviews rashes
that reflect systemic disease but does not include localized skin eruptions (i.e., cellulitis, impetigo) that may also be associated with fever
(see Chap. 133). Rashes are classified herein on the basis of the
morphology and distribution of lesions. For practical purposes, this
classification system is based on the most typical disease presentations.
However, morphology may vary as rashes evolve, and the presentation
of diseases with rashes is subject to many variations (see Chap. 57).
For instance, the classic petechial rash of Rocky Mountain spotted
fever (RMSF) may initially consist of blanchable erythematous macules on the hands and feet; at times, the rash associated with RMSF
may not be predominantly acral, or a rash may not develop at all.

Diseases with fever and rash may be classified by type of eruption:
centrally distributed maculopapular, peripheral, confluent desquamative erythematous, vesiculobullous, urticarial, nodular, and purpuric
(Table 18-1). For a more detailed discussion of each disease associated
with a rash, the reader is referred to the chapter dealing with that
specific disease. (Reference chapters are cited in the text and listed
in Table 18-1.)

Centrally Distributed Maculopapular Eruptions Centrally
distributed rashes, in which lesions are primarily truncal, are the most
common type of eruption. The rash of *measles* (rubeola) starts at the
hairline 2 to 3 days into the illness and moves down the body, sparing
the palms and soles (see Chap. 196). It begins as discrete erythematous
lesions, which become confluent as the rash spreads. Koplik's spots
(1- to 2-mm white or bluish lesions with an erythematous halo on the
buccal mucosa) are pathognomonic for measles and are generally seen
during the first 2 days of symptoms. They should not be confused
with Fordyce's spots (ectopic sebaceous glands), which have no erythematous halos and are found in the mouth of healthy individuals.
Koplik's spots may briefly overlap with the measles exanthem.

German measles (rubella) also spreads from the hairline downward; unlike that of measles, however, the rash of rubella tends to
clear from originally affected areas as it migrates and may be pruritic
(see Chap. 197). Forchheimer spots (palatal petechiae) may develop
but are nonspecific since they also develop in mononucleosis (Chap.
186) and scarlet fever (Chap. 143). Postauricular and suboccipital
adenopathy and arthritis are common among adults with German measles. Exposure of pregnant women to ill individuals should be avoided,
as rubella causes severe congenital abnormalities. Numerous strains
of enteroviruses (Chap. 195), primarily echoviruses and coxsackieviruses, cause nonspecific syndromes of fever and eruptions that may
mimic rubella or measles. Both infectious mononucleosis caused
by Epstein-Barr virus and primary infection with human immunodeficiency virus (HIV; Chap. 308) may also include pharyngitis,
lymphadenopathy, and a nonspecific maculopapular exanthem.

The rash of *erythema infectiosum* (fifth disease), which is caused
by human parvovirus B19, primarily affects children 3 to 12 years
old; it develops after fever has resolved as a bright blanchable erythema
on the cheeks ("slapped cheeks") with perioral pallor (Chap. 189). A
more diffuse rash (often pruritic) appears the next day on the trunk
and extremities and then rapidly develops into a lacy reticular eruption
that may wax and wane (especially with temperature change) over 3
weeks. Adults with fifth disease often have arthritis, and fetal hydrops
can develop in association with this condition in pregnant women.

Exanthem subitum (roseola) is most common among children
under 3 years of age (Chap. 187). As in erythema infectiosum, the
rash usually appears after fever has subsided. It consists of 2- to
3-mm rose-pink macules and papules that rarely coalesce, occur initially on the trunk and sometimes on the extremities (sparing the face),
and fade within 2 days.

Though drug reactions have many manifestations, including urticaria, exanthematous *drug-induced eruptions* (Chap. 56) are most
common and are often difficult to distinguish from viral exanthems.
Eruptions elicited by drugs are usually more intensely erythematous
and pruritic than viral exanthems, but this distinction is not reliable.
A history of new medications and an absence of prostration may help
to distinguish a drug-related rash from an eruption of another etiology.
Rashes may persist for up to 2 weeks after administration of the
offending agent is discontinued. Certain populations are more prone
than others to drug rashes. Of HIV-infected patients, 50 to 60 percent
develop a rash in response to sulfa drugs; 50 to 100 percent of patients
with mononucleosis due to Epstein-Barr virus develop a rash when
given ampicillin.

Rickettsial illnesses (Chap. 179) should be considered in the evaluation of individuals with centrally distributed maculopapular eruptions.
The usual setting for *epidemic typhus* is a site of war or natural disaster
in which people are exposed to body lice. A diagnosis of recrudescent
typhus should be considered in European immigrants to the United
States. However, an indigenous form of typhus, presumably transmitted by flying squirrels, has been reported in the southeastern United

Table 18-1

Diseases Associated with Fever and Rash

Disease	Etiology	Description	Group Affected/ Epidemiological Factors	Clinical Syndrome	Chapter Reference
CENTRALLY DISTRIBUTED MACULOPAPULAR ERUPTIONS					
Measles (rubeola, first disease)	Paramyxovirus	Discrete lesions that become confluent as rash spreads from hairline downward, sparing palms and soles; lasts ≥3 d; Koplik's spots	Nonimmune individuals	Cough, conjunctivitis, coryza, severe prostration	196
German measles (rubella, third disease)	Togavirus	Spreads from hairline downward, clearing as it spreads; Forchheimer spots	Nonimmune individuals	Adenopathy, arthritis	197
Erythema infectiosum (fifth disease)	Human parvovirus B19	Bright-red "slapped-cheek" appearance followed by diffuse lacy reticular rash that waxes and wanes over 3 weeks	Most common in children aged 3–12 years; occurs in winter and spring	Mild fever; arthritis in adults	189
Exanthem subitum (roseola, sixth disease)	Human herpesvirus 6	Diffuse maculopapular eruption (sparing face); resolves within 2 d	Usually affects children <3 years old	Rash following resolution of fever; similar to Boston exanthem (echovirus 16)	187
Primary HIV infection	HIV	Nonspecific diffuse macules and papules; may be urticarial; palatal ulcers in some cases	Individuals recently infected with HIV	Pharyngitis, adenopathy, arthralgias	308
Infectious mononucleosis	Epstein-Barr virus	Diffuse maculopapular eruption (10–15% of cases; 90% if ampicillin is given); urticaria in some cases; periorbital edema (50%); palatal petechiae (25%)	Adolescents, young adults	Hepatosplenomegaly, pharyngitis, cervical lymphadenopathy, atypical lymphocytosis, heterophile antibody	186
Other viral exanthems	Echoviruses 2, 4, 9, 11, 16, 19, and 25; coxsackieviruses A9, B1, and B5	Skin findings mimicking rubella or measles	Affect children more commonly than adults	Nonspecific viral syndromes	195
Exanthematous drug-induced eruption	Drugs (antibiotics, anticonvulsants, diuretics, etc.)	Intensely pruritic, bright-red macules and papules, symmetric on trunk and extremities; may become confluent	Occurs 2–3 d after exposure in those previously sensitized; otherwise, after 2–3 weeks (but can occur anytime, even after drug is discontinued)	Variable findings: fever and eosinophilia	56
Epidemic typhus	*Rickettsia prowazekii*	Maculopapular eruption, usually sparing face, palms, soles; evolves from blanchable macules to confluent eruption with petechiae; rash evanescent in recrudescent typhus (Brill-Zinsser disease)	Exposure to body lice; occurrence of recrudescent typhus as relapse after 30–50 years	Headache, myalgias; 10–40% mortality if untreated; milder clinical presentation in recrudescent form	179
Endemic (murine) typhus	*Rickettsia typhi*	Maculopapular eruption, usually sparing palms, soles	Exposure to rat or cat fleas	Headache, myalgias	179
Scrub typhus	*Rickettsia tsutsugamushi*	Diffuse macular rash starting on trunk; eschar at site of mite bite	Endemic in South Pacific, Australia, Asia; transmitted by mites	Headache, myalgias, regional adenopathy, mortality up to 30% if untreated	179
Rickettsial spotted fevers	*Rickettsia conorii* (boutonneuse fever), *Rickettsia australis* (North Queensland tick typhus), *Rickettsia sibirica* (Siberian tick typhus)	Eschar at site of bite; maculopapular (rarely, vesicular and petechial) eruption on proximal extremities, spreading to trunk and face	Exposure to ticks; *R. conorii* in Mediterranean region, India, Africa; *R. australis* in Australia; *R. sibirica* in Siberia, Mongolia	Headache, myalgias, regional adenopathy	179
Ehrlichiosis	*Ehrlichia* species	Maculopapular eruption (40% of cases), sparing extremities, palms, soles; feature distinguishing from RMSF is central distribution with peripheral *sparing*	Tick-borne; most common in U.S. Southeast and southern Midwest	Headache, myalgias, leukopenia	179

(continued)

Table 18-1—*(Continued)*

Diseases Associated with Fever and Rash

Disease	Etiology	Description	Group Affected/ Epidemiological Factors	Clinical Syndrome	Chapter Reference
Leptospirosis	*Leptospira interrogans*	Maculopapular eruption; conjunctivitis; scleral hemorrhage in some cases	Exposure to water contaminated with animal urine	Myalgias; aseptic meningitis; *fulminant form:* icterohemorrhagic fever (Weil's disease)	176
Lyme disease	*Borrelia burgdorferi*	Papule expanding to erythematous annular lesion with central clearing (ECM; average diameter, 15 cm), sometimes with concentric rings, sometimes with indurated or vesicular center; multiple secondary ECM lesions in some cases	Bite of tick vector	Headache, myalgias, chills, photophobia occurring acutely; CNS disease, myocardial disease, arthritis weeks to months later in some cases	178
Typhoid fever	*Salmonella typhi*	Blanchable erythematous macules and papules, 2–4 mm, usually on trunk (rose spots)	Ingestion of contaminated food or water (rare in U.S.)	Variable abdominal pain and diarrhea; headache, myalgias, hepatosplenomegaly	158
Rat-bite fever (sodoku)	*Spirillum minus*	Eschar at site of bite; then blotchy violaceous or red-brown central rash	Rate bite; primarily found in Asia; rare in U.S.	Regional adenopathy, recurrent fevers if untreated	135
Relapsing fever	*Borrelia* species	Central rash at end of febrile episode; petechiae in some cases	Exposure to ticks or body lice	Recurrent fever, headache, myalgias, hepatosplenomegaly	177
Erythema marginatum (rheumatic fever)	Group A *Streptococcus*	Erythematous annular papules and plaques occurring as polycyclic lesions in waves over trunk, proximal extremities; evolving and resolving within hours	Patients with rheumatic fever	Pharyngitis preceding polyarthritis, carditis, subcutaneous nodules, chorea	236
Systemic lupus erythematosus	Autoimmune disease	Macular and papular erythema, often in sun-exposed areas; discoid lupus lesions (local atrophy, scale, pigmentary changes); periungual telangiectasis; malar rash; vasculitis sometimes causing urticaria, palpable purpura; oral erosions in some cases	Most common in young to middle-aged women; flares precipitated by sun exposure	Arthritis; cardiac, pulmonary, renal, hematologic, and vasculitic disease	312
Adult-onset Still's disease	Autoimmune disease	Transient 2- to 5-mm erythematous papules appearing at height of fever on trunk, proximal extremities; lesions evanescent	Young adults; more common in females	High spiking fever, polyarthritis, splenomegaly; erythrocyte sedimentation rate, >100 mm/h	326

PERIPHERAL ERUPTIONS

Disease	Etiology	Description	Group Affected/ Epidemiological Factors	Clinical Syndrome	Chapter Reference
Chronic meningococcemia, disseminated gonococcal infection*	—	—	—	—	149, 150
RMSF	*Rickettsia rickettsii*	Rash beginning on wrists and ankles and spreading centripetally; appears on palms and soles late in disease; lesion evolution from blanchable macules to petechiae	Tick vector; widespread but more common in southeastern and southwest-central U.S.	Headache, myalgias, abdominal pain; mortality up to 40% if untreated	179
Secondary syphilis	*Treponema pallidum*	Coincident primary chancre in 10% of cases; copper-colored, scaly papular eruption, diffuse but prominent on palms and soles; rash never vesicular in adults; condyloma latum, mucous patches, and alopecia in some cases	Sexually transmitted	Fever, constitutional symptoms	174

(continued)

Disease	Etiology	Description	Group Affected/ Epidemiological Factors	Clinical Syndrome	Chapter Reference
Atypical measles	Paramyxovirus	Maculopapular eruption beginning on distal extremities and spreading centripetally; may evolve into vesicles or petechiae; edema of extremities; Koplik's spots absent	Individuals contracting measles who received killed measles vaccine between 1963 and 1967 in U.S.	Headache, nodular pneumonia	196
Hand-foot-and-mouth disease	Coxsackievirus A16	Tender vesicles, erosions in mouth; 0.25-cm papules on hands and feet with rim of erythema evolving into tender vesicles	Summer and fall; primarily children under 10 years; multiple family members	Transient fever	195
Erythema multiforme	Drugs, infection, idiopathic causes	Target lesions (central erythema surrounded by area of clearing and another rim of erythema) up to 2 cm; symmetric on knees, elbows, palms, soles; may become diffuse; may involve mucosal surfaces	Drug intake (i.e., sulfa, phenytoin, penicillin); herpes simplex or *Mycoplasma pneumoniae* infection	Varies with predisposing factor	—†
Rat-bite fever (Haverhill fever)	*Streptobacillus moniliformis*	Maculopapular rash over palms, soles, extremities; may be purpuric; may desquamate	Rat bite	Myalgias; arthritis (50%); fever recurrence in some cases	135
Bacterial endocarditis	*Streptococcus, Staphylococcus,* etc.	*Subacute course:* Osler's nodes (tender pink nodules on finger or toe pads); petechiae on skin and mucosa; splinter hemorrhages. *Acute course (S. aureus):* Janeway lesions (painless erythematous or hemorrhagic macules on palms and soles)	Abnormal heart valve, intravenous drug use	New heart murmur	126

CONFLUENT DESQUAMATIVE ERYTHEMAS

Disease	Etiology	Description	Group Affected/ Epidemiological Factors	Clinical Syndrome	Chapter Reference
Scarlet fever (second disease)	Group A *Streptococcus* (pyrogenic exotoxins A, B, C)	Diffuse blanchable erythema beginning on face and spreading to trunk and extremities; circumoral pallor; "sandpaper" texture to skin; accentuation of linear erythema in skin folds (Pastia's lines); enanthem of white evolving into red "strawberry" tongue; desquamation in second week	Most common in children aged 2–10 years; usually follows group A streptococcal pharyngitis	Fever, pharyngitis, headache	143
Kawasaki disease	Idiopathic causes	Rash similar to scarlet fever (scarlatiniform) or erythema multiforme; fissuring of lips, strawberry tongue; conjunctivitis; edema of hands, feet; desquamation later in disease	Children under 8 years	Cervical adenopathy, pharyngitis, coronary artery vasculitis	57, 319
Streptococcal toxic shock syndrome	Group A *Streptococcus* (associated with pyrogenic exotoxin A or certain M types)	When present, rash often scarlatiniform	May occur in setting of severe group A streptococcal infections, such as necrotizing fasciitis, bacteremia, pneumonia	Multiorgan failure, hypotension; 30% mortality rate	143
Staphylococcal toxic shock syndrome	*S. aureus* (toxic shock syndrome toxin 1, enterotoxin B or C)	Diffuse erythema involving palms; pronounced erythema of mucosal surfaces, conjunctivitis; desquamation 7–10 d into illness	Colonization with toxin-producing *S. aureus*	Fever >39°C (102°F), hypotension, multiorgan dysfunction	142

(continued)

Table 18-1—*(Continued)*

Diseases Associated with Fever and Rash

Disease	Etiology	Description	Group Affected/ Epidemiological Factors	Clinical Syndrome	Chapter Reference
Staphylococcal scalded-skin syndrome	*S. aureus*, phage group II	Diffuse tender erythema, often with bullae and desquamation; Nikolsky's sign	Colonization with toxin-producing *S. aureus*; occurs in children under 10 (termed "Ritter's disease" in neonates) or adults with renal dysfunction	Irritability; nasal or conjunctival secretions	142
Exfoliative erythroderma syndrome	Underlying psoriasis, eczema, drug eruption, mycosis fungoides	Diffuse erythema (often scaling) interspersed with lesions of underlying condition	Usually occurs in adults over age 50; more common in men	Fever, chills (i.e., difficulty with thermoregulation); lymphadenopathy	55, 56
Toxic epidermal necrolysis	Drugs, other causes (infection, neoplasm, graft-vs.-host disease)	Diffuse erythema or target-like lesions progressing to bullae, with sloughing and necrosis of the entire epidermis; Nikolsky's sign	Uncommon in children; more common in patients with HIV infection or graft-vs.-host disease	Dehydration, sepsis sometimes resulting from lack of normal skin integrity; 25% mortality	56, 308

VESICULOBULLOUS ERUPTIONS

Disease	Etiology	Description	Group Affected/ Epidemiological Factors	Clinical Syndrome	Chapter Reference
Hand-foot-and-mouth syndrome‡; staphylococcal scalded-skin syndrome, toxic epidermal necrolysis§	—	—	—	—	—†
Varicella (chickenpox)	Varicella-zoster virus	Macules (2–3 mm) evolving into papules, then vesicles (sometimes umbilicated), on an erythematous base ("dewdrops on a rose petal"); pustules then forming and crusting; lesions appearing in crops; may involve scalp, mouth; intensely pruritic	Usually affects children; 10% of adults susceptible; most common in late winter and spring	Malaise; mild disease in healthy children; more severe disease with complications in adults and immunocompromised children	185
Rickettsialpox	*Rickettsia akari*	Eschar found at site of mite bite; diffuse rash involving face, trunk, extremities; 2- to 10-mm papules and plaques evolving into vesicles and then crusting	Seen in urban settings; transmitted by mouse mites	Headache, myalgias, regional adenopathy; mild disease	179
Disseminated *Vibrio vulnificus* infection	*V. vulnificus*	Erythematous lesions evolving into hemorrhagic bullae and then into necrotic ulcers	Patients with cirrhosis; exposure by ingestion of contaminated saltwater seafood	Hypotension; 50% mortality	161
Ecthyma gangrenosum	*Pseudomonas aeruginosa*, other gram-negative rods, fungi	Indurated plaque evolving into hemorrhagic bulla or pustule that sloughs, resulting in eschar formation; erythematous halo; most common in axillary, groin, perianal regions	Usually affects neutropenic patients; occurs in up to 28% of individuals with *Pseudomonas* bacteremia	Clinical signs of sepsis	157

URTICARIAL ERUPTIONS

Disease	Etiology	Description	Group Affected/ Epidemiological Factors	Clinical Syndrome	Chapter Reference
Urticarial vasculitis	Serum sickness, connective-tissue disease, infection, idiopathic causes	Erythematous, circumscribed areas of edema; occasionally indurated; pruritic or burning; lesions sometimes purpuric; individual lesions lasting up to 5 d	In serum sickness, occurs 8–14 d after antigen exposure in nonsensitized individuals; may occur within 36 h in sensitized individuals	Malaise, lymphadenopathy, myalgias, arthralgias	319†

(continued)

Disease	Etiology	Description	Group Affected/ Epidemiological Factors	Clinical Syndrome	Chapter Reference
NODULAR ERUPTIONS					
Disseminated infection	Fungi (e.g., candidiasis, histoplasmosis, cryptococcosis, sporotrichosis, coccidioidomycosis); mycobacteria	Subcutaneous nodules (up to 3 cm); fluctuance, draining common with mycobacteria; necrotic nodules (extremities, periorbital or nasal regions) common with *Aspergillus*, *Mucor*	Immunocompromised hosts (i.e., bone marrow transplant recipients, patients undergoing chemotherapy, HIV-infected patients, alcoholics)	Features vary with organism	—†
Erythema nodosum (septal panniculitis)	Infections (e.g., streptococcal, fungal, mycobacterial, yersinial); drugs (e.g., sulfas, penicillins, oral contraceptives); sarcoidosis; idiopathic causes	Large, violaceous, nonulcerative, subcutaneous nodules; exquisitely tender; usually on lower legs but also on upper extremities	More common in females aged 15–30	Arthralgias (50%); features vary with associated condition	—†
Sweet's syndrome (acute febrile neutrophilic dermatosis)	Yersinial infection; lymphoproliferative disorders; idiopathic causes	Tender edematous nodules giving impression of vesiculation; usually on face, neck, upper extremities; when on lower extremities, may mimic erythema nodosum	More common in women and in persons aged 30–60	Headache, arthralgias, leukocytosis	57
PURPURIC ERUPTIONS					
RMSF, rat-bite fever, endocarditis‡; epidemic typhus¶	—	—	—	—	—†
Acute meningococcemia	*Neisseria meningitidis*	Petechiae rapidly becoming numerous, sometimes enlarging and becoming vesicular; trunk, extremities most commonly involved; may appear on face, hands, feet; may include purpura fulminans reflecting DIC (see below)	Most common in children, individuals with asplenia or terminal complement component deficiency (C5-C8)	Hypotension, meningitis (sometimes preceded by upper respiratory infection)	149
Purpura fulminans	Severe DIC	Large ecchymoses with sharply irregular shapes evolving into hemorrhagic bullae and then into black necrotic lesions	Individuals with sepsis (e.g., involving *N. meningitidis*), malignancy, or massive trauma; asplenic patients at high risk for sepsis	Hypotension	124, 149
Chronic meningococcemia	*N. meningitidis*	Variety of recurrent eruptions, including pink maculopapular; nodular (usually on lower extremities); petechial (sometimes developing vesicular centers); purpuric areas with pale blue-gray centers	Individuals with complement deficiencies	Fevers, sometimes intermittent; arthritis, myalgias, headache	149
Disseminated gonococcal infection	*Neisseria gonorrhoeae*	Papules (1–5 mm) evolving over 1–2 d into hemorrhagic pustules with gray necrotic centers; hemorrhagic bullae occurring rarely; lesions (usually fewer than 40) distributed peripherally near joints (more commonly on upper extremities)	Sexually active individuals (more often females), some with complement deficiency	Low-grade fever, tenosynovitis, arthritis	150
Enteroviral petechial rash	Usually echovirus 9 or coxsackievirus A9	Disseminated petechial lesions (may also be maculopapular, vesicular, or urticarial)	Often occurs in outbreaks	Pharyngitis, headache; aseptic meningitis with echovirus 9	195

(continued)

Table 18-1—(Continued)

Diseases Associated with Fever and Rash

Disease	Etiology	Description	Group Affected/ Epidemiological Factors	Clinical Syndrome	Chapter Reference
Viral hemorrhagic fever	Arboviruses and arenaviruses	Petechial rash	Residence in or travel to endemic areas	Triad of fever, shock, hemorrhage from mucosa or gastrointestinal tract	200, 201
Thrombotic thrombocytopenic purpura	Idiopathic causes	Petechiae	Usually affects young adults; more common in women; hemolytic-uremic syndrome seen in children after gastroenteritis caused by *Escherichia coli* O157:H7	Fever, hemolytic anemia, thrombocytopenia, neurologic and renal dysfunction; coagulation studies normal	57, 109, 117

* See "Purpuric eruptions."
† See etiology-specific chapters.
‡ See "Peripheral eruptions."
§ See "Confluent desquamative erythemas."
¶ See "Centrally distributed maculopapular eruptions."
NOTE: DIC, disseminated intravascular coagulation; ECM, erythema chronicum migrans; HIV, human immunodeficiency virus; RMSF, Rocky Mountain spotted fever.

States. *Endemic typhus* or *leptospirosis* (caused by a spirochete; see Chap. 176) may be seen in urban environments where rodents proliferate. Outside the United States, other rickettsial diseases cause a spotted-fever syndrome and should be considered in residents of or travelers to endemic areas. Similarly, *typhoid fever*, a nonrickettsial disease caused by *Salmonella typhi* (Chap. 158), is usually acquired during travel outside the United States.

Some centrally distributed maculopapular eruptions have distinctive features. Erythema chronicum migrans (ECM), the rash of Lyme disease (Chap. 178), typically manifests as singular or multiple annular plaques. Untreated ECM lesions usually fade within a month but may persist for more than a year. *Erythema marginatum*, the rash of acute rheumatic fever (Chap. 236), has a distinctive pattern of enlarging and shifting transient annular lesions.

Collagen vascular diseases may cause fever and rash. Patients with *systemic lupus erythematosus* (Chap. 312) typically develop a sharply defined, erythematous eruption in a butterfly distribution on the cheeks (malar rash) as well as many other skin manifestations. *Still's disease* (Chap. 326) manifests as an evanescent salmon-colored rash on the trunk that coincides with fever spikes.

Peripheral Eruptions These rashes are alike in that they are most prominent peripherally or begin in peripheral (acral) areas before spreading centripetally. Early diagnosis and therapy are critical in RMSF (Chap. 179) because of its grave prognosis if untreated. Lesions evolve from macular to petechial, start on the wrists and ankles, spread centripetally, and appear on the palms and soles only later in the disease. The rash of *secondary syphilis* (Chap. 174), which may be diffuse but is prominent on the palms and soles, should be considered in the differential diagnosis of pityriasis rosea, especially in sexually active patients. *Atypical measles* (Chap. 196) is seen in individuals contracting measles who received the killed measles vaccine between 1963 and 1967 in the United States and who were not subsequently protected with the live vaccine. *Hand-foot-and-mouth disease* (Chap. 195) is distinguished by tender vesicles distributed peripherally and in the mouth; outbreaks commonly occur within families. The classic target lesions of *erythema multiforme* appear symmetrically on the elbows, knees, palms, and soles. In relatively severe cases, these lesions may spread diffusely and involve mucosal surfaces. Lesions may develop on the hands and feet in *endocarditis* (Chap. 126).

Confluent Desquamative Erythemas These eruptions consist of diffuse erythema, often followed by desquamation. The eruptions caused by group A *Streptococcus* or *Staphylococcus aureus* are toxin mediated. Certain disease features may provide diagnostic clues. *Scarlet fever* (Chap. 143) usually follows pharyngitis; patients have a facial flush, a "strawberry" tongue, and accentuated petechiae in body folds (Pastia's lines). *Kawasaki disease* (Chaps. 57 and 319) presents in the pediatric population as fissuring of the lips, a strawberry tongue, conjunctivitis, adenopathy, and sometimes cardiac abnormalities. *Streptococcal toxic shock syndrome* (Chap. 143) manifests with hypotension, multiorgan failure, and often a severe group A streptococcal infection (e.g., necrotizing fasciitis). *Staphylococcal toxic shock syndrome* (Chap. 142) also presents with hypotension and multiorgan failure, but usually only *S. aureus* colonization—not a severe *S. aureus* infection—is documented. *Staphylococcal scalded-skin syndrome* (Chap. 142) is seen primarily in children and in immunocompromised adults. Generalized erythema is often evident during the prodrome of fever and malaise; profound tenderness of the skin is distinctive. In the exfoliative stage, the skin can be induced to form bullae with light lateral pressure (Nikolsky's sign). In a mild form, a scarlatiniform eruption mimics scarlet fever, but the patient does not exhibit a strawberry tongue or circumoral pallor. In contrast to the staphylococcal scalded-skin syndrome, in which the cleavage plane is superficial in the epidermis, *toxic epidermal necrolysis* (Chap. 56) involves sloughing of the entire epidermis, resulting in severe disease. This condition is uncommon among children and relatively common among HIV-infected patients (Chap. 308). *Exfoliative erythroderma syndrome* (Chaps. 55 and 56) is a serious reaction associated with systemic toxicity that is often due to eczema, psoriasis, mycosis fungoides, or a severe drug reaction.

Vesiculobullous Eruptions *Varicella* (Chap. 185) is highly contagious, often occurring in winter or spring. At a given time within a given region of the body, varicella lesions are in different stages of development. In immunocompromised hosts, varicella vesicles may lack the characteristic erythematous base or may appear hemorrhagic. *Rickettsialpox* (Chap. 179) is often documented in urban settings and is characterized by vesicles and pustules. It can be distinguished from varicella by an eschar at the side of the mouse-mite bite. *Disseminated Vibrio vulnificus infection* (Chap. 161) or *ecthyma gangrenosum* due to *Pseudomonas aeruginosa* (Chap. 157) should be considered in immunosuppressed individuals with sepsis and hemorrhagic bullae.

Urticarial Eruptions Individuals with classic urticaria ("hives") usually have a hypersensitivity reaction without associated fever. In the presence of fever, urticarial eruptions are usually due to *urticarial vasculitis* (Chap. 319). Unlike individual lesions of classic urticaria, which last up to 48 h, these lesions may last up to 5 days. Etiologies include serum sickness (often induced by drugs such as penicillins, sulfas, salicylates, or barbiturates), connective-tissue disease (e.g., systemic lupus erythematosus or Sjögren's syndrome), and infection (e.g., with hepatitis B virus, coxsackievirus A9, or parasites). Malignancy may be associated with fever and chronic urticaria (Chap. 57).

Nodular Eruptions In immunocompromised hosts, nodular lesions often represent disseminated infection. Patients with disseminated *candidiasis* (often due to *Candida tropicalis*) may have a triad of fever, myalgias, and eruptive nodules (Chap. 207). Disseminated *cryptococcosis* lesions (Chap. 206) may resemble molluscum contagiosum. Necrosis of nodules should raise the suspicion of *aspergillosis* (Chap. 208) or *mucormycosis* (Chap. 209). *Erythema nodosum* presents with exquisitely tender nodules on the lower extremities. *Sweet's syndrome* (Chap. 57) should be considered in individuals with multiple nodules and plaques, often so edematous that they give the appearance of vesicles or bullae. Sweet's syndrome may affect either healthy individuals or persons with lymphoproliferative disease.

Purpuric Eruptions *Acute meningococcemia* (Chap. 149) classically presents in children as a petechial eruption, but initial lesions may appear as blanchable macules or urticaria. RMSF should be considered in the differential diagnosis of acute meningococcemia. *Echovirus 9 infection* (Chap. 195) may mimic acute meningococcemia; patients should be treated as if they have bacterial sepsis since prompt differentiation of these conditions may be impossible. Large ecchymotic areas of *purpura fulminans* reflect severe underlying disseminated intravascular coagulation, which may be due to infectious or noninfectious causes. The lesions of *chronic meningococcemia* (Chap. 149) may have a variety of morphologies, including petechial. Purpuric nodules may develop on the legs and resemble erythema nodosum but lack its exquisite tenderness. Lesions of *disseminated gonococcemia* (Chap. 150) are distinctive, sparse, countable hemorrhagic pustules, usually located near joints. The lesions of chronic meningococcemia and those of gonococcemia may be indistinguishable in terms of appearance and distribution. *Viral hemorrhagic fever* (Chaps. 200 and 201) should be considered in patients with an appropriate travel history and a petechial rash. *Thrombotic thrombocytopenic purpura* (Chaps. 57, 109, and 117) is a noninfectious cause of fever and petechiae.

BIBLIOGRAPHY

CHERRY JD: Contemporary infectious exanthems. Clin Infect Dis 16:199, 1993
————: Cutaneous manifestations of systemic infections, in *Textbook of Pediatric Infectious Diseases*, vol. 1, 3d ed, RD Feigin and JD Cherry (eds). Philadelphia, Saunders, 1992, pp 755–782
FITZPATRICK TB et al (eds): *Dermatology in General Medicine*, 4th ed. New York, McGraw-Hill, 1993
HURWITZ S (ed): *Clinical Pediatric Dermatology*. Philadelphia, Saunders, 1981
LEVIN S, GOODMAN LJ: An approach to acute fever and rash (AFR) in the adult. Curr Clin Top Infect Dis 15:19, 1995
WEBER DJ, COHEN MS: The acutely ill patient with fever and rash, in *Principles and Practice of Infectious Diseases*, vol 1, 4th ed, GL Mandell et al (eds). New York, Churchill Livingstone 1995, pp 549–561
WENNER HA: Virus diseases associated with cutaneous eruptions. Prog Med Virol 16:269, 1973

19 *Kevin J. Petty*

HYPOTHERMIA

Hypothermia is defined arbitrarily as a core body temperature of 35°C or below and is classified as mild (35 to 32°C), moderate (< 32 to 28°C), or severe (< 28°C). Hypothermia can have several causes and is usually multifactorial in origin. Precise estimates of the incidence are difficult to obtain because nonfatal hypothermia is often not detected or reported and fatal hypothermia is probably underreported. Between 1979 and 1991 approximately 770 deaths per year occurred in the United States due to environmental hypothermia. Among those deaths,

67 percent were men, 61 percent were white, and more than half were above 65 years of age. Most cases occur in the winter months in areas with cold climates, but hypothermia can occur in mild climates at any season. Risk factors include extremes of age (especially the elderly), homelessness, ethanol use, malnutrition, poverty, mental illness, use of neuroleptic medications, and hypothyroidism. A common setting is chronic indoor cold exposure in an impoverished elderly person with underlying illnesses and immobility. Homeless male alcoholics are at great risk.

THERMOREGULATION Heat is generated in most tissues of the body and is lost by radiation (55 percent), evaporation (5 percent from airways, 25 percent from skin), conduction (15 percent), and convection (5 percent). Immersion in water results in hypothermia more rapidly because the thermal conductivity of water is 20 to 30 times greater than that of air. The balance between heat production and heat loss in the body is regulated by the hypothalamus (preoptic and posterior regions). Exposure to cold activates cutaneous cold receptors that transmit the signal via the lateral spinothalamic tracts to the preoptic nuclei of the hypothalamus. The posterior hypothalamus activates the sympathetic nervous system to increase muscle tone and cause shivering, which in turn increases the metabolic rate from a normal level of 40 to 60 kcal/h to as high as 300 kcal/h. Even at maximum metabolic rates, heat loss from the body can exceed heat production. As the body temperature drops below 30°C, metabolic processes slow and shivering stops, thereby accelerating the development of hypothermia.

CAUSES Extreme environmental conditions can cause hypothermia in healthy individuals, but it rarely requires medical attention. Most severe hypothermia occurs in persons with underlying medical conditions that lead to excessive heat loss (usually involving environmental exposure) or inadequate heat production, and both processes are usually involved (Table 19-1). It is worthwhile keeping in mind that body temperature never falls below the environmental temperature.

Most environmental exposures are accidental. Iatrogenic hypothermia can occur when obtunded patients are left uncovered in hospital rooms or during surgical procedures when large body surface areas are exposed for long periods in the operating room. The shivering response is inhibited by anesthesia, enhancing the likelihood of hypothermia. Its only manifestation in this setting may be difficult in achieving hemostasis due to inactivation of clotting factors at low temperatures. Enhanced blood flow to the skin (burns, psoriasis) can also produce hypothermia in the presence of slight environmental challenge because heat conservation via peripheral vasoconstriction is impaired.

Decreased heat production can contribute to the development of hypothermia. Malnutrition and/or starvation deplete the stores of glycogen and fat necessary for effective heat production. Hypothermia occurs in more than 10 percent of patients with sepsis (usually bacterial) and is often associated with a poor prognosis. Approximately 40 percent of resting oxygen consumption is regulated by thyroid hormone, and hypothermia is common in severe hypothyroidism where the metabolic rate can be reduced to as much as 40 percent below normal. Hypothermia in hepatic failure is often due to a combination of hypoglycemia from inadequate hepatic gluconeogenesis and altered hypothalamic function (decreased shivering). Hypoglycemia from any cause (glucocorticoid deficiency, ethanol use, hyperinsulinism), uremia, and diabetic ketoacidosis also predispose to hypothermia.

Hypothalamic lesions (tumor, inflammation) can cause thermoregulatory instability and hypothermia. Spinal cord lesions at the first thoracic nerve root or above can lead to hypothermia by blocking shivering and interrupting cold-induced compensatory reflexes mediated by the lateral spinothalamic tracts. Episodic spontaneous hypothermia with hyperhidrosis is a rare disorder associated with excessive sweating in the absence of shivering; nearly half of these patients have agenesis of the corpus callosum (Shapiro's syndrome), suggesting a central nervous system (CNS) etiology.

Table 19-1

Causes of Hypothermia

I. Excessive heat loss
  A. Environmental exposure
    1. Accidental
    2. Iatrogenic
  B. Increased cutaneous blood flow—burns, psoriasis, toxic epidermal necrolysis
II. Inadequate heat production
  A. Decreased metabolism
    1. Malnutrition
    2. Hypothyroidism
    3. Adrenal insufficiency
    4. Hepatic failure
    5. Hypoglycemia
    6. Diabetic ketoacidosis
  B. Altered thermoregulation
    1. Sepsis
    2. Uremia
    3. Hypothalamic dysfunction
    4. Spinal cord injury—T1 or above
    5. Episodic spontaneous hypothermia with hyperhidrosis
  C. Drug-induced
    1. Phenothiazines
    2. Barbiturates
    3. Ethanol
    4. Opiates
    5. Clonidine
    6. Lithium
    7. Benzodiazepines

Several drugs can contribute to hypothermia. Phenothiazines, barbiturates, opiates, benzodiazepines, and ethanol inhibit shivering through their CNS effects. Ethanol inhibits shivering, impairs hepatic gluconeogenesis, and enhances heat loss by inducing peripheral vasodilatation. Clonidine inhibits central sympathetic outflow.

EFFECTS ON ORGAN SYSTEMS Acute cold exposure causes tachycardia, increased cardiac output, peripheral vasoconstriction, and increased peripheral vascular resistance secondary to sympathetic stimulation. As body temperature drops below 32°C, cardiac conduction becomes impaired, and heart rate and cardiac output decrease. Atrial fibrillation with slow ventricular response is common below 32°C, and ventricular fibrillation may occur below 28°C. Electrocardiographic changes include the characteristic Osborn (J) wave (a positive deflection occurring at the junction of the QRS complex and the ST segment).

Peripheral vasoconstriction shunts blood to the central circulation and increases central blood volume; a diuresis (cold diuresis) ensues, tending to lower intravascular volume in a compensatory fashion. With prolonged cold exposure the combination of cold diuresis, additional volume losses due to impaired sodium and water reabsorption by the kidneys (due to impaired function of epithelial transport mechanisms), and intravascular fluid shifts with intracellular and peripheral edema can cause severe volume depletion and hypotension. Volume depletion in turn leads to hemoconcentration and increased blood viscosity that predispose to thrombosis. Conversely, bleeding due to inefficient clotting at lower temperatures, thrombocytopenia, and disseminated intravascular coagulation can cause even minor trauma to result in significant blood loss.

The acid-base and electrolyte derangements depend on the duration of cold exposure. Lactic acidosis due to decreased peripheral tissue perfusion can lead to a compensatory respiratory alkalosis. In severe hypothermia depression of respiration can cause respiratory acidosis. Levels of serum electrolytes are usually normal, but movement of potassium into cells can cause hypokalemia in the absence of trauma or rhabdomyolysis.

Cold exposure can induce bronchorrhea and bronchospasm. Early tachypnea is followed by hypoventilation as hypothermia becomes more severe. Decreased mental status predisposes to aspiration because of loss of coughing and gag reflex, and pulmonary edema can occur. Shift of the oxygen dissociation curve of hemoglobin to the left at lower temperatures impairs oxygen delivery to hypothermic tissues, an impairment mitigated by decreased tissue oxygen requirements due to decreased metabolism.

The nervous system manifestations are diverse. Cerebral blood flow decreases, and nerve conduction velocity slows as neuronal metabolism declines. Manifestations include dysarthria, ataxia, amnesia, hallucinations, confusion, slow pupillary reflexes, and delayed deep tendon reflexes; the latter phenomenon may make it hard to recognize hypothyroidism in the presence of hypothermia. Chronic hypothermia can be a primary or contributing cause of altered mental status in the elderly. Hypothermic individuals may remove their clothing because of feeling warm ("paradoxical undressing"). In severe hypothermia coma can be associated with an isoelectric electroencephalogram (EEG); in this setting an isoelectric EEG is not indicative of brain death and may be reversible.

Enhanced secretion of hypothalamic-releasing hormones by acute cold exposure results in increased secretion of ACTH and thyroid-stimulating hormone (TSH). Levels of serum cortisol and catecholamines increase as with other acute stresses. The acute release of vasopressin by expansion of the central blood volume contributes to cold diuresis. Levels of serum thyroid hormones increase only slightly, and serum free thyroxine levels remain normal in euthyroid individuals. Moderate to severe hypothermia inhibits insulin action and leads to decreased glucose utilization and hyperglycemia except when hypoglycemia is a cause of the hypothermia. Severe hypothermia eventually inhibits the release and action of ACTH and steroid hormones.

Intestinal hypomotility is common in moderate hypothermia. Decreased hepatic metabolism can prolong the serum half-life of compounds normally cleared by the liver. Pancreatitis and hyperamylasemia occur in as many as half of patients after rewarming. It is unclear whether hypothermia per se causes pancreatitis because ethanol abuse, a common factor in hypothermia, is an independent cause of pancreatitis.

DIAGNOSIS Oral thermometers are often calibrated only down to 34.4°C. Accurate temperature measurement in the low range requires the use of a thermometer capable of reading down to 15°C or preferably a rectal thermocouple probe inserted at least 15 cm. The reliability of infrared tympanic thermography in this setting has not been established. Therefore, when an initial body temperature of 35°C or less is obtained, it is important to remeasure core temperature accurately.

Historical data, when available, are often helpful in determining the cause and duration of the hypothermia. Preexisting medical conditions, medications, home environment, and the length and severity of exposure should be ascertained. Due to vasoconstriction blood pressure may be difficult to obtain without the use of Doppler ultrasound. Pulse oximetry is of little value for the same reason. Evidence of trauma and of coexisting medical conditions should be carefully sought. The ingestion of alcohol (which may be detected on the breath) is a common contributing factor. Neurologic function can range from alertness to obtundation and correlates with the severity of hypothermia. Focal findings on neurologic examination should prompt a search for specific intracranial lesions.

Initial laboratory evaluation should include a complete biochemical profile [electrolytes, blood urea nitrogen (BUN), creatinine, calcium, phosphorous, magnesium, glucose, liver function], measurement of amylase levels, complete blood count, prothrombin/partial thromboplastin times (PT/PTT), electrocardiogram, chest x-ray, urinalysis, arterial blood gas analysis, and toxicologic screen. Blood and urine cultures should be obtained because of the relatively high prevalence of bacteremia and sepsis in hypothermic patients (nearly 40 percent in one urban hospital). Serum TSH should be measured in most, if not all, hypothermic patients to assess for hypothyroidism. Appropriate imaging studies (computed tomography, magnetic resonance imaging) should be obtained when trauma or head injury is suspected. Arterial blood gas is usually analyzed at 37°C and should not be corrected for the body temperature.

℞ TREATMENT

Rewarming techniques can be active or passive, internal or external. Passive external rewarming involves covering the patient with blankets and clothing in a warm environment to allow endogenous heat production to correct the hypothermia; it is important to keep the head covered because up to 30 percent of body heat can be lost from the head. This is the easiest and safest method and should be used first in most patients with mild hypothermia. Body temperature increases of 0.5 to 2.0°C/h can be expected.

Active external rewarming involves direct application of heat sources (heating blankets, heat lamps, warm water immersion) to external body surfaces. This procedure can worsen the condition in two ways if not performed properly. First, the direct application of heat to the skin can produce shock by relieving cold-induced vasoconstriction, thereby removing an important support for maintenance of blood pressure in the volume-depleted patient. Second, the relief of peripheral vasoconstriction allows cooler peripheral blood to enter the central circulation and can cause core temperature to drop even further (a phenomenon referred to as "afterdrop"). There is a risk of burn injury when heat sources are applied directly to the skin. Direct heat should be applied only to the thorax if active external rewarming is used.

Active internal rewarming can be achieved by several techniques. The simplest method is airway rewarming in which the patient inspires humidified oxygen heated to 42°C via face mask or endotracheal tube. Rewarming rates of 1 to 2°C/h can be achieved with airway rewarming. Intravenous fluids should be heated to 40°C, but their use has minimal effects on core rewarming. Lavage of the stomach, bladder, or colon with warmed fluids produces limited warming and generally is not used if rapid rewarming is needed. Peritoneal and pleural lavage induce warming rates of 2 to 4°C/h but should be used only in moderate to severe hypothermia where there is cardiovascular instability or when external rewarming is ineffective.

The most efficient rewarming technique is extracorporeal blood warming by hemodialysis or cardiopulmonary bypass. Both methods involve continuous removal of blood that is circulated and warmed externally before being reinfused. Cardiopulmonary bypass is the most efficient technique and can increase core temperature 1 to 2°C every 3 to 5 min. These procedures are reserved for the most severe cases of hypothermia (e.g., cardiac arrest) and when peritoneal and/or pleural lavage are ineffective.

The volume depletion should be corrected with isotonic fluids. Warmed normal saline (or 5% dextrose/normal saline) should be given intravenously. Lactated Ringer's solution should be avoided because lactate metabolism is impaired by hypothermia. Physical manipulation of the patient should be minimized, and central vein lines, nasogastric tubes, and endotracheal tubes should be inserted carefully because of the possibility of cardiac arrhythmia. Treatment of acidosis is usually not necessary since rewarming corrects most abnormalities, and drugs should be administered with caution because their effectiveness may be impaired at lower body temperatures and because their metabolic clearance is prolonged. If sepsis is a possibility, it is appropriate to administer empiric broad-spectrum antibiotics until the results of blood cultures are available (see Chap. 124).

Rewarming often corrects hyperglycemia. Insulin is inactive at body temperatures below 32°C, and excess insulin can produce late hypoglycemia when body temperature is raised. Furthermore, prolonged shivering can cause depletion of muscle glycogen and predispose to hypoglycemia. Therefore, insulin should not be administered until it is clear that hyperglycemia persists after rewarming. Hypokalemia may correct with rewarming alone as potassium shifts to the extracellular space, but serum potassium levels should be monitored during rewarming. Development of hyperkalemia during hypothermia suggests significant tissue necrosis (rhabdomyolysis) with or without renal failure.

Continuous cardiac monitoring is essential. Atrial arrhythmias are common and are usually reversible with rewarming alone. Antiarrhythmic or vasopressor drugs should not be administered until body temperature is normal. Ventricular arrhythmias in the hypothermic patient tend to be refractory to drugs and to defibrillation. Bretylium tosylate is the drug of choice for ventricular fibrillation. Only one attempt at electrical defibrillation should be made when the core temperature is <30°C. When cardiac arrest is present, active internal rewarming and cardiopulmonary resuscitation should be initiated simultaneously.

It is occasionally difficult to distinguish reversible from irreversible hypothermia. Apnea, asystole, and absence of brain activity are usually signs of death but can also be present in severe, reversible hypothermia, particularly in victims of immersion hypothermia and near-drowning. The lowest recorded body temperature in a patient who was resuscitated successfully was 15.2°C in a 23-day-old infant. Generally, cardiopulmonary resuscitation of hypothermic patients should continue until core body temperature has been raised at least to 32°C or until cardiovascular status has stabilized.

Once body temperature is corrected and the patient is stabilized, a search should be made for precipitating causes. Empiric broad-spectrum antibiotic therapy may be given because the usual manifestations of infection are masked. A careful neurologic examination should be performed. Coexisting medical conditions (myocardial infarction, diabetic ketoacidosis, renal failure, hepatic failure, gastrointestinal bleeding, pancreatitis, rhabdomyolysis, hypothyroidism) should be treated aggressively if present.

Preventive measures in high-risk individuals such as the elderly include use of layered clothing and headgear, adequate shelter, increased caloric intake, and avoidance of ethanol.

BIBLIOGRAPHY

DANZL DF, POZOS RS: Accidental hypothermia. N Engl J Med 331:1756, 1994

HARCHELROAD F: Acute thermoregulatory disorders. Clin Geriatr Med 9:621, 1993

JOLLY B, GHATS K: Accidental hypothermia. Emerg Med Clin North Am 10:311, 1992

KOLODZIK PW: Hypothermia, in *Presenting Signs and Symptoms in the Emergency Department*, GC Hamilton (ed). Baltimore, Williams & Wilkins, 1993, p 248

20

Robert B. Daroff, Joseph B. Martin

FAINTNESS, SYNCOPE, DIZZINESS, AND VERTIGO

Syncope is defined as transient loss of consciousness with postural collapse caused by an acute decrease in cerebral blood flow. Although often preceded by faintness or light-headedness (presyncope), it may not be when caused by cardiac asystole or ventricular tachycardia. Presyncope symptoms may be manifest as "dizziness," always without true vertigo, or may be mimicked by a warning (aura) prior to a seizure. The sequence of symptoms is reasonably stereotyped and includes increasing lightheadedness, visual blurring proceeding to blindness, diaphoresis, and heaviness in the lower limbs progressing to postural sway. These symptoms increase in severity until consciousness is lost or the ischemia is corrected, often by assuming the recumbent position. The differentiation of syncope from seizure is an important, sometimes difficult, diagnostic problem.

In this chapter syncope and dizziness are considered with particular reference to clinical manifestations, differential diagnosis, and treatment.

SYNCOPE

At the beginning of a syncopal attack, the patient is nearly always in the upright position, either sitting or standing. A cardiac etiology, such as a Stokes-Adams attack, is exceptional in this respect (see Chap. 230). The patient is warned of the impending faint by a sense of "feeling bad," of giddiness, and of movement or swaying of the floor or surrounding objects. The patient becomes confused and may yawn, visual spots and dimming may occur, and the ears may ring. Nausea and sometimes vomiting accompany these symptoms. There is a striking pallor or ashen gray color of the face, and generalized perspiration ensues. In some patients, a deliberate onset with presyncopal symptoms may allow time for protection against injury; in others, the syncope is sudden and without warning. The onset varies from instantaneous to 10 to 30 s, rarely longer.

The depth and duration of unconsciousness vary. Sometimes the patient remains partly aware of the surroundings, or there may be profound coma. The patient may remain in this state for seconds to minutes or even as long as half an hour. Usually the patient lies motionless with skeletal muscles relaxed, but a few clonic jerks of the limbs and face may occur shortly after the beginning of the unconsciousness. In some situations there may be a brief tonic-clonic seizure. Sphincter control is usually maintained. The pulse is feeble or apparently absent, the blood pressure may be low to undetectable, and breathing may be almost imperceptible. Once the patient is in a horizontal position, gravity no longer hinders the flow of blood to the brain. The strength of the pulse may then improve, color begins to return to the face, breathing becomes quicker and deeper, and consciousness is regained. There is usually an immediate recovery of consciousness. Some patients may, however, be keenly aware of physical weakness, and rising too soon may precipitate another faint. In other patients, particularly those with transient tachyarrhythmias, there may be no residual symptoms following the initial syncope. Headache and drowsiness, which, with mental confusion, are the usual sequelae of a convulsion, do not follow a syncopal attack.

ETIOLOGY The list of causes in Table 20-1 is based on established or assumed physiologic mechanisms. The more common types of faint are reducible to a few simple mechanisms. Syncope results from a sudden impairment of brain metabolism usually brought about by hypotension with reduction of cerebral blood flow.

Several mechanisms subserve circulatory adjustments to the upright posture. Approximately three-fourths of the systemic blood volume is contained in the venous bed, and any interference with venous

return may lead to a reduction in cardiac output. Cerebral blood flow may still be maintained, as long as systemic arterial vasoconstriction occurs, but when this adjustment fails, serious hypotension with resultant cerebral underperfusion to less than half normal results in syncope. Normally, the pooling of blood in the lower parts of the body is prevented by (1) pressor reflexes that induce constriction of peripheral arterioles and venules, (2) reflex acceleration of the heart by means of aortic and carotid reflexes, and (3) improvement of venous return to the heart by activity of the muscles of the limbs. Placing a normal person on a tilt table to relax the muscles and tilting upright slightly diminishes cardiac output and allows the blood to accumulate in the legs to a slight degree; this may then be followed by a slight transitory

Table 20-1

Causes of Faintness and Disturbances of Consciousness

I. Circulatory (reduced cerebral blood flow)
  A. Inadequate vasoconstrictor mechanisms
    1. Vasovagal (vasodepressor)
    2. Postural hypotension
    3. Primary autonomic insufficiency
    4. Sympathectomy (pharmacologic, due to antihypertensive medications such as methyldopa and hydralazine, or surgical)
    5. Diseases of central and peripheral nervous systems, including autonomic nerves (Chaps. 371 and 381)
    6. Carotid sinus syncope (see also "Bradyarrhythmias," below)
    7. Hyperbradykininemia
  B. Hypovolemia
    1. Blood loss—gastrointestinal hemorrhage
    2. Addison's disease
  C. Mechanical reduction of venous return
    1. Valsalva maneuver
    2. Cough
    3. Micturition
    4. Atrial myxoma, ball valve thrombus
  D. Reduced cardiac output
    1. Obstruction to left ventricular outflow: aortic stenosis, hypertrophic subaortic stenosis
    2. Obstruction to pulmonary flow: pulmonic stenosis, primary pulmonary hypertension, pulmonary embolism
    3. Myocardial: massive myocardial infarction with pump failure
    4. Pericardial: cardiac tamponade
  E. Arrhythmias (Chaps. 230 and 231)
    1. Bradyarrhythmias
      a. Atrioventricular (AV) block (second- and third-degree), with Stokes-Adams attacks
      b. Ventricular asystole
      c. Sinus bradycardia, sinoatrial block, sinus arrest, sick-sinus syndrome
      d. Carotid sinus syncope (see also inadequate vasoconstrictor mechanisms, above)
      e. Glossopharyngeal neuralgia (and other painful states)
    2. Tachyarrhythmias
      a. Episodic ventricular tachycardia with or without associated bradyarrhythmias
      b. Supraventricular tachycardia without AV block
II. Other causes of disturbances of consciousness
  A. Altered state of blood to the brain
    1. Hypoxia
    2. Anemia
    3. Diminished carbon dioxide due to hyperventilation (faintness common, syncope seldom occurs)
    4. Hypoglycemia (episodic weakness common, faintness occasional, syncope rare)
  B. Cerebral
    1. Cerebrovascular disturbances (cerebral ischemic attacks, see Chap. 366)
      a. Extracranial vascular insufficiency (vertebral-basilar, carotid)
      b. Diffuse spasm of cerebral arterioles (hypertensive encephalopathy)
    2. Emotional disturbances, anxiety attacks, and hysterical seizures

fall in systolic arterial pressure and, in patients with defective vasomotor reflexes, may produce faints.

TYPES OF SYNCOPE **Vasodepressor (Vasovagal) or Neurocardiogenic Syncope** This form of syncope is the common faint that may be experienced by normal persons and accounts for about 50 percent of all instances of syncope. It is frequently recurrent and commonly precipitated by emotional stress (especially in a warm, crowded room), fear (e.g., in a dentist's chair), extreme fatigue, injury, or pain. Many episodes, however, occur without obvious antecedent cause. In its classic form, vasodepressor syncope comprises a constellation of symptoms including hypotension, bradycardia, nausea, pallor, and diaphoresis. Syncope typically occurs in the setting of diminished venous return that leads to reduced stroke volume and a reflex increase in sympathetic activity. In susceptible individuals, this increase in sympathetic activity causes cardiac hypercontractility and excessive stimulation of ventricular mechanoreceptors (afferent vagal C fibers), which, in turn, leads to sympathetic withdrawal and activation of the parasympathetic nervous system via a centrally mediated vasomotor reflex. The net result is a vicious cycle of *inappropriate peripheral vasodilatation* and *relative bradycardia* leading to progressive hypotension and syncope that can be reversed by assumption of supine posture and elevation of the legs. Orthostatic stress induced by prolonged upright tilt testing at 60 to 80 degrees is a sensitive technique for reproducing syncope in many patients with this syndrome. The use of low-dose isoproterenol infusion enhances the sensitivity of upright tilt testing but leads to false-positive tests when used in high doses. Vasodepressor syncope may occur with sudden severe pain, particularly if it originates in the viscera, and may also rarely accompany a severe migraine headache.

Postural (Orthostatic) Hypotension with Syncope This type of syncope affects persons who have a chronic defect in, or variable instability of, vasomotor reflexes. The fall in blood pressure on assumption of upright posture is due to a loss of vasoconstriction reflexes in resistance and capacitance vessels of the lower extremities. Although the syncopal attack differs little from vasodepressor syncope, the effect of posture is critical. Sudden arising from a recumbent position or standing quietly are precipitating circumstances.

Postural syncope may occur in the following conditions:

1. In otherwise normal persons who have defective postural reflexes. In such individuals, fainting may occur when they are tilted on a table. Under such circumstances the blood pressure at first diminishes slightly and then stabilizes at a lower level. Shortly thereafter, the compensatory reflexes suddenly fail and the arterial pressure falls precipitously. The condition is often familial.
2. In *primary autonomic insufficiency* and in the *dysautonomias*. Three syndromes have been delineated:

Acute or subacute dysautonomia In this rare condition, an otherwise healthy adult or child develops, over a period of a few days or weeks, a partial or complete paralysis of the parasympathetic and sympathetic nervous systems. Pupillary reflexes are lost, and lacrimation, salivation, and sweating are absent or diminished. Impotence, paresis of bladder and bowel musculature, and orthostatic hypotension are present. The cerebrospinal fluid (CSF) protein is often increased. Sensory and motor nerves are intact, but unmyelinated autonomic nerves degenerate. The disease appears to represent a variant of Guillain-Barré syndrome, and recovery usually occurs within a few months.

Chronic postganglionic autonomic insufficiency This is a disease of the middle-aged and elderly who gradually develop chronic orthostatic hypotension, sometimes in conjunction with impotence and sphincter disturbances. Typically, after standing for 5 to 10 min, the blood pressure falls by at least 35 mmHg, the pulse pressure narrows, and there is no compensatory tachycardia, pallor, or nausea. Men are more often affected than women.

Chronic preganglionic autonomic insufficiency In this condition, orthostatic hypotension with anhidrosis, impotence, and sphincter disturbances is combined with a disorder of the central nervous system (CNS). These disorders, designated *multisystem atrophies*, include

syndromes characterized by (1) tremor, extrapyramidal rigidity, and akinesia (Shy-Drager syndrome); (2) progressive cerebellar degeneration, some instances of which are familial; and (3) a more variable extrapyramidal and cerebellar disorder (striatonigral degeneration). These syndromes lead to severe disability and often death within a few years (see Chaps. 368 and 371).

The differentiation of chronic peripheral postganglionic and central preganglionic insufficiency is based on pathologic and pharmacologic evidence. In the postganglionic type, neurons of the sympathetic ganglia degenerate, whereas in the central type, intermediolateral horn preganglionic cells of the thoracic spinal cord degenerate. In the postganglionic peripheral type, resting levels of norepinephrine are subnormal because of failure to release norepinephrine from postganglionic endings, and there is hypersensitivity to injected norepinephrine. In the central type, resting levels of norepinephrine are normal. On standing, unlike the reaction in the normal individual, there is little, if any, rise in norepinephrine levels in either type. And in both types, the levels of plasma dopamine β-hydroxylase (the enzyme that converts dopamine to norepinephrine) are subnormal.

Other causes of postural syncope (1) After physical deconditioning, e.g., after prolonged illness with recumbency, especially in elderly individuals with reduced muscle tone, or after prolonged weightlessness, as in space flight. (2) After a sympathectomy that has abolished vasopressor reflexes. (3) In diabetic, alcoholic, and other neuropathies. The most common neurogenic orthostatic hypotension accompanies diseases of the peripheral nervous system. Diabetic polyneuropathy, beriberi, amyloid polyneuropathy, and the Adie syndrome are examples. Usually the orthostatic hypotension is associated with disturbances in sweating, impotence, and sphincter difficulties. Presumably the lesion involves postganglionic, unmyelinated fibers in peripheral nerves. (4) In patients receiving antihypertensive and vasodilator drugs as well as those who may be hypovolemic because of diuretics, excessive sweating, or adrenal insufficiency.

Micturition syncope, a condition usually seen in elderly men during or after urination, particularly after arising from sleep, is probably a special type of vasodepressor syncope. Release of intravesicular pressure may trigger vasodilatation and vagally mediated bradycardia.

Cardiac Syncope Cardiac syncope results from a sudden reduction in cardiac output, caused most commonly by a cardiac arrhythmia. In normal individuals, slow ventricular rates, but above 35 to 40 beats per minute, and fast rates not exceeding 180 beats per minute do not reduce cerebral blood flow, especially if the person is in the supine position. However, changes in pulse rate outside these limits may impair cerebral circulation and function. Upright posture, cerebrovascular disease, anemia, and coronary, myocardial, or valvular disease all reduce the tolerance to alterations in rate.

Atrioventricular block High-degree atrioventricular block is commonly associated with fainting (*Stokes-Adams-Morgagni syndrome*; see Chap. 230). In patients with these attacks, the block may be persistent or intermittent. When the block is high-grade or complete and the pacemaker below the block fails to function, or functions at too slow a rate, syncope occurs. Stokes-Adams attacks occur precipitously, usually without warning symptoms. Should cardiac asystole persist more than 8 to 10 s, the patient turns pale, falls unconscious, and may exhibit a few clonic jerks. With longer periods of asystole, cyanosis ensues, breathing is irregular, and fixed pupils, incontinence, and bilateral Babinski signs may be present. While recovery following a Stokes-Adams attack is usually prompt and complete, prolonged confusion and neurologic signs due to cerebral ischemia may occur in some patients, and permanent impairment of mental function may occasionally result, although focal neurologic signs are rare. The patient usually does not recall presyncopal symptoms. Cardiac faints of this type may recur several times a day. Commonly the heart block is transitory, and the electrocardiogram (ECG) taken later may not show any arrhythmia. Ventricular tachycardia or fibrillation may follow a period of asystole, resulting in prolonged coma or sudden death.

Sinus node disorders Disorders of sinus node automaticity or sinoatrial conduction may result in asystole or bradycardia of sufficient severity to cause presyncope or syncope. This disorder is most frequently detected with ambulatory ECG monitoring. Findings consistent with a diagnosis of sinus node dysfunction include symptomatic sinus pauses (>3 s) resulting from sinus arrest or sinoatrial block and severe unexplained sinus bradycardia (<40 beats per minute). The *bradycardia-tachycardia syndrome* is a common form of sinus node dysfunction in which syncope generally occurs as a result of marked sinus pauses following termination of paroxysmal supraventricular tachycardia. Electrophysiologic testing is sometimes helpful in unmasking diagnostic abnormalities in patients with syncope and suspected sinus node dysfunction in whom the diagnosis is not established by ambulatory ECG recording.

Tachyarrythmias Recurrent paroxysmal tachyarrhythmias also may cause presyncope and syncope as a result of a sudden reduction in cardiac output. The magnitude of tachycardia-induced hypotension is dependent on the interaction of several variables, including the rate and mechanism of the tachycardia, the type and severity of underlying cardiac disease, the patient's posture and activity level at the onset of the tachycardia, the sensitivity of the tachycardia to endogenous catecholamines, and the integrity of compensatory autonomic reflexes. *Supraventricular tachyarrhythmias* are not commonly associated with syncope. However, even in the absence of structural heart disease, the extremely high heart rates may impair cardiac filling and output sufficiently to cause loss of consciousness. These tachycardias result most commonly from the occurrence of paroxysmal atrial flutter, atrial fibrillation, or reentry involving the atrioventricular (AV) node or accessory pathways that bypass part or all of the AV conduction system (see Chap. 230). Patients with the Wolff-Parkinson-White syndrome are susceptible to several forms of supraventricular tachycardia, the most dangerous of which is atrial fibrillation with rapid antegrade conduction to the ventricles over an accessory AV connection that may result in syncope and, in rare instances, sudden death. When abnormal conduction over an accessory AV connection or an AV nodal reentry rhythm is suspected as a cause of syncope, electrophysiologic testing is indicated to define the mechanism and pathway of the tachycardia and to facilitate the selection of an effective therapeutic intervention (see also Chap. 230).

Paroxysmal ventricular tachycardia is a relatively common cause of syncope, particularly in patients with structural heart disease. Typically, the tachycardias are rapid and associated with abrupt loss of consciousness without premonitory symptoms. Usually the patient is unaware of palpitations, and recovery following an episode is prompt and complete without residual neurologic or cardiac sequelae. Unexplained syncope in a patient with structural heart disease is a potentially ominous finding and merits careful evaluation. The presence of pathologic Q waves on the ECG, indicative of a prior transmural myocardial infarction, is strongly associated with ventricular tachycardia as a cause of syncope in patients with ischemic heart disease. Other forms of heart disease such as hypertrophic and dilated cardiomyopathy, right ventricular dysplasia, and the long-QT-interval syndromes are also frequently associated with paroxysmal ventricular tachycardia and syncope (see Chap. 231).

Reflexive heart block In another form of cardiac syncope, the heart block is reflexive and is due to irritation of the vagus nerves. Examples of this phenomenon have been observed in patients with esophageal diverticula, mediastinal tumors, gallbladder disease, carotid sinus disease, glossopharyngeal neuralgia, and pleural and pulmonary irritation. In these conditions, reflex bradycardia is more commonly of the sinoatrial than the atrioventricular type.

Other causes Cardiac syncope also may result from *acute massive myocardial infarction*, particularly when associated with cardiogenic shock. *Aortic stenosis* often sets the stage for exertional syncope, most commonly by limiting cardiac output in the face of peripheral vasodilatation, with resultant myocardial and cerebral ischemia and

occasionally arrhythmias. *Idiopathic hypertrophic subaortic stenosis* also may lead to exertional syncope because of intensified obstruction, ventricular arrhythmias, or both (Chap. 239). In *primary pulmonary hypertension*, a relatively fixed cardiac output and bouts of acute right ventricular failure may be associated with syncope (Chap. 238). However, vagal reflexes may be involved in this condition as well as in the syncope that occurs with *pulmonary embolism*. Ball-valve thrombus in the left atrium, left atrial myxoma, or thrombosis or malfunction of a prosthetic valve may produce sudden mechanical obstruction of the circulation and syncope. *Tetralogy of Fallot* is the congenital cardiac malformation most commonly responsible for syncope. In this condition, systemic vasodilatation, perhaps associated with infundibular spasm, greatly increases the right-to-left shunt and produces arterial hypoxia, which leads to syncope (Chap. 235).

Carotid Sinus Syncope The carotid sinus is normally sensitive to stretch and gives rise to sensory impulses carried via the nerve of Hering, a branch of the glossopharyngeal nerve, to the medulla oblongata. Massage of one or both of the carotid sinuses, particularly in elderly persons, causes (1) a reflex cardiac slowing (sinus bradycardia, sinus arrest, or even AV block), the so-called vagal type of response, and (2) a fall of arterial pressure without cardiac slowing, the so-called depressor type of response. Both types of carotid sinus response may coexist.

Syncope due to carotid sinus sensitivity is extremely uncommon and said to be initiated by turning of the head to one side, by a tight collar, or by shaving over the region of the sinus. In a patient displaying faintness on compression of one carotid sinus, it is important to distinguish between the benign disorder (carotid sinus hypersensitivity) and a much more serious condition such as carotid artery stenosis on the opposite side (see Chap. 366). Thus, carotid compression is a risky maneuver that may lead to cerebral ischemia.

Glossopharyngeal Neuralgia This painful disorder may induce reflex fainting. The sequence is always pain, followed by syncope. The pain is localized to the jaw, base of the tongue, pharynx or larynx, tonsillar area, and ear. The cardiovascular effects are attributable to excitation of the dorsal motor nucleus of the vagus via collateral fibers from the nucleus of the tractus solitarius. Treatment of the neuralgia with carbamazepine is often effective for the syncope, as well as for the pain.

Cough Syncope This is a rare condition that follows paroxysm of coughing, usually in chronic bronchitis. After forceful coughing, the patient suddenly becomes weak and loses consciousness momentarily. The coughing increases intrathoracic pressure and the elevated pressure is transmitted via the great veins to the intracranial compartment, causing increased intracranial pressure and secondarily decreased cerebral blood flow. At a critically low blood flow, syncope ensues.

Stretch Syncope This is a rare condition that occurs in otherwise normal adolescents. The provoking maneuver is simultaneous neck extension and upper limb stretching. The mechanism seems to be compression of the vertebral arteries in the neck.

DIFFERENTIAL DIAGNOSIS Anxiety Attacks and the Hyperventilation Syndrome Anxiety, such as occurs in panic attacks, is frequently interpreted as a feeling of faintness or dizziness without loss of consciousness. The symptoms are not accompanied by facial pallor and are not relieved by recumbency. The diagnosis is made on the basis of the associated symptoms, and the attack can be reproduced by hyperventilation. Hyperventilation results in hypocapnia, alkalosis, increased cerebrovascular resistance, and decreased cerebral blood flow. The release of epinephrine in anxiety states also contributes to the symptoms.

Hypoglycemia Severe hypoglycemia is usually traceable to a serious disease such as a tumor of the islets of Langerhans; advanced adrenal, pituitary, or hepatic disease; or to excessive administration of insulin; it leads to confusion or loss of consciousness. Mild hypoglycemia, often reactive type and occurring 2 to 5 h after eating, is not usually associated with a disturbance of consciousness.

Acute Hemorrhage Acute hemorrhage, usually within the gastrointestinal tract, is an occasional cause of syncope. In the absence of pain and hematemesis, the cause of the weakness, faintness, or even unconsciousness may remain obscure until the passage of a black stool.

Cerebral Transient Ischemic Attacks (TIAs) TIAs occur in patients with atherosclerotic narrowing, occlusion, or emboli to the major arteries of the brain. The symptoms are manifold (see Chap. 366). Sudden drop attacks may mimic syncope. Isolated loss of consciousness is rare.

Hysterical Fainting The attack is usually unattended by an outward display of anxiety. Lack of change in pulse and blood pressure or color of the skin and mucous membranes distinguishes it from the vasodepressor faint.

Approach to the Patient

Type of Onset (see Fig. 20-1) The timing and type of onset may assist in determining the cause. Syncope that begins over a period of a few seconds is most likely due to postural hypotension, sudden AV block, asystole, or ventricular tachycardia. When symptoms develop gradually during a period of several minutes, hyperventilation or hypoglycemia should be considered. Onset of syncope during or immediately after exertion suggests aortic stenosis, idiopathic hypertrophic subaortic stenosis or excessive bradycardia, and, in elderly subjects, postural hypotension. Exertional syncope is seen occasionally in persons with aortic insufficiency. In patients with ventricular standstill or ventricular fibrillation, loss of consciousness occurs 8 to 10 s later and then often by brief clonic muscle contractions.

Position at Onset of Attack Epilepsy and syncopal attacks due to hypoglycemia, hyperventilation, or heart block are likely to be independent of posture. Faintness associated with a drop in blood pressure and with ectopic tachycardia usually occurs only in the sitting or standing position, whereas faintness resulting from orthostatic hypotension is apt to begin shortly after change from the recumbent to the standing position.

Associated Symptoms Symptoms such as palpitation may be present when the attack is due to anxiety or hyperventilation, ectopic tachycardia, or hypoglycemia. Numbness and tingling in the hands and face are frequent accompaniments of hyperventilation. Genuine convulsions during the attack may occasionally occur with heart block, asystole, or ventricular tachycardia.

In patients with recurrent syncope an attempt to reproduce an attack may assist in diagnosis.

Symptoms induced by hyperventilation can be reproduced readily by having the subject breathe rapidly and deeply for 2 to 3 min. Anxiety attacks induced by hyperventilation tend to be lessened when the patient learns that the symptoms can be produced and alleviated at will simply by controlling breathing.

Other conditions in which the diagnosis is commonly clarified by reproducing the attacks are orthostatic hypotension and orthostatic tachycardia (observations of pulse rate, blood pressure, and symptoms in the recumbent and standing positions), and cough syncope (by inducing the Valsalva maneuver). In each instance, the crucial point is not whether symptoms are produced (the procedures mentioned frequently induce symptoms in healthy persons) but whether the exact pattern of symptoms that occurs in the spontaneous attacks is reproduced in the artificial ones. Continuous ambulatory ECG monitoring is essential to identify arrhythmias responsible for syncope, particularly in patients with frequently recurring symptoms. Monitoring is diagnostic if it shows episodes of asystole, extreme bradycardia, or tachyarrhythmia.

In cases of recurrent syncope of unknown cause in which ambulatory ECG monitoring is unrevealing and there is underlying heart disease, particularly ischemic and prior myocardial infarction, the use of intracardiac electrophysiologic techniques with programmed stimulation can be helpful in detecting cardiac rhythm abnormalities and in establishing effective treatment. During stimulation, up to two-thirds of such patients can be shown to have rapid ventricular tachycardia. Occasionally, intracardiac electrophysiologic studies are helpful in identifying significant His bundle conduction delays or sick-sinus syndrome. The diagnostic yield of intracardiac electrophysiologic test-

ing is lower in patients with nonischemic heart disease and in patients with structurally normal hearts than in patients with ischemic heart disease. Recently, the signal-averaged ECG has proved to be useful in identifying patients with unexplained syncope who are likely to have ventricular tachycardia induced by electrophysiologic study.

Head-up tilt testing is a useful provocative technique for the diagnosis of vasodepressor syncope. Upright tilt to a maximum of 60 to 70 degrees usually precipitates symptomatic hypotension or syncope within 10 to 30 min in patients with this syndrome. In normal subjects, passive tilting to 60 degrees causes a small decrease in systolic blood pressure and an increase in diastolic blood pressure and heart rate. Recently, tilt testing has been used in conjunction with electrophysiologic testing to assess the efficacy of prophylactic pacing in selected patients with vasodepressor syncope and to evaluate the impact of posture on the hemodynamic consequences of some tachyarrhythmias. Sublingual nitroglycerine administered during head-up tilt testing may unmask certain vasovagal-induced causes of syncope.

Syncope should be distinguished from disturbances of cerebral function caused by a seizure. A seizure may occur day or night, regardless of the position of the patient; syncope rarely appears when the patient is recumbent, the only common exception being the Stokes-Adams attack. The patient's color may not change in seizures, though there may be cyanosis; pallor is an early and invariable finding in all types of syncope, except chronic orthostatic hypotension and hysteria, and it precedes unconsciousness. Seizures are often heralded by an aura, which is caused by a focal seizure discharge and hence has brain-localizing significance. The aura is usually followed by rapid return to normal or by loss of consciousness. The onset of syncope is usually more deliberate and without aura. Injury from falling is frequent in a

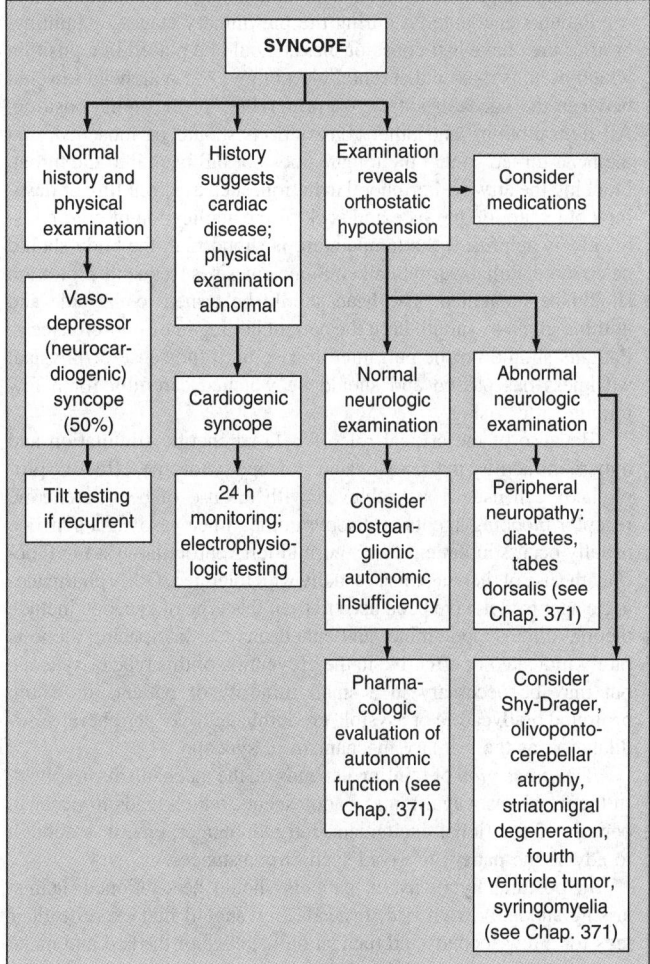

FIGURE 20-1 Approach to the patient with syncope.

seizure and rare in syncope for the reason that only in seizures are protective reflexes abolished instantaneously. Tonic-convulsive movements are a feature of seizures and usually do not occur with syncope, although, as stated above, brief tonic clonic seizurelike activity can accompany fainting episodes. Upward deviation of the eyes occurs with both conditions. The period of unconsciousness tends to be longer in seizures than in syncope. Urinary incontinence is frequent in seizures and rare in syncope. The return of consciousness is prompt in syncope, slow after a seizure. Mental confusion, headache, and drowsiness are common sequelae of seizures; physical weakness with a clear sensorium characterizes the postsyncopal state. Repeated spells of unconsciousness in a young person at a rate of several per day or month are more suggestive of epilepsy than of syncope.

The electroencephalogram (EEG) may be helpful in differentiating syncope from seizures. In the interval between epileptic seizures, it may show some degree of abnormality in up to 80 percent of patients. In the interval between syncopal attacks, the EEG should be normal.

℞ **TREATMENT**

The treatment of cardiac arrythmias is given in Chap. 230. In most instances, fainting is relatively benign. In dealing with patients who have fainted, the physician should think first of those causes of fainting that constitute a therapeutic emergency. Among them are massive internal hemorrhage and myocardial infarction, which may be painless, and cardiac arrhythmias. In elderly persons, a sudden faint, without obvious cause, should arouse the suspicion of complete heart block or a tachyarrhythmia, even though all findings are negative when the patient is seen.

Patients encountered during the preliminary stages of fainting, or after they have lost consciousness, should be placed in a position which permits maximal cerebral blood flow, i.e., with head lowered between the knees, if sitting, or, preferably, in the supine position. All tight clothing and other constrictions should be loosened, and the head turned so that the tongue does not fall back into the throat, blocking the airway. Peripheral irritation, such as sprinkling or dashing cold water on the face and neck or the application of cold moist towels, is helpful. If the temperature is subnormal, the body should be covered with a warm blanket. Since emesis is frequent, aspiration should be prevented. The head should be turned to the side and nothing given by mouth until the patient has regained consciousness. Patients should not be permitted to rise until the sense of physical weakness has passed and should be watched carefully for a few minutes after rising.

Because of the critical role of beta-adrenergic stimulation and hypercontractility in the vasovagal syncope syndrome, effective prophylaxis can usually be achieved with the use of beta-adrenergic receptor blocking agents or disopyramide. Since vasovagal syncope usually occurs in patients with normal left ventricular systolic function, the use of these agents is usually well tolerated. Other pharmacologic agents that have been used to treat this type of syncope include theophylline, scopolamine, and ephedrine. Cardiac pacing alone is rarely indicated or effective in the prevention of this type of syncope but may be necessary in a small minority of patients in whom profound bradycardia or asystole predominates over peripheral vasodilatation as the primary mechanism of syncope.

The *prevention* of fainting depends on the mechanisms involved. In the usual vasovagal faint of adolescents, which tends to occur in periods of emotional excitement, fatigue, hunger, etc., it is enough to advise the patient to avoid such circumstances.

In postural hypotension, patients should be cautioned against arising suddenly from bed. Instead, they should first exercise their legs for a few seconds and then sit on the edge of the bed and make certain they are not lightheaded or dizzy before starting to walk. Sleeping with the headposts of the bed elevated on wooden blocks 8 to 12 in. high and wearing a snug elastic abdominal binder and elastic stockings are often helpful. The distinction made between the various types of orthostatic hypotension has therapeutic significance. In the peripheral postganglionic type, the most effective treatment is 9α-fluorohydrocortisone (oral dose 0.1 to 0.2 mg/d) and salt loading to increase blood volume, supplemented by mechanical devices to prevent pooling of blood in the legs and lower trunk (g suit). However, salt together with mineralocorticoids may induce serious supine hypertension, and the dose of the drug must be adjusted for this. For the central preganglionic type, there has been greater success with use of a sympathomimetic amine such as tyramine (which releases norepinephrine from intact postganglionic endings) supplemented by a monoamine oxidase inhibitor (to prevent destruction of the amine) and possibly propranolol. Levodopa has been effective in some cases. In the postganglionic type, judicious use of phenylephrine or ephedrine may be beneficial if they do not cause insomnia. If there are no contraindications, a high intake of sodium chloride, which expands the extracellular fluid volume, may be tried.

The treatment of carotid sinus syncope involves first of all instructing the patient in measures that minimize the hazards of a fall (see below). Loose collars should be worn, and the patient should learn to turn the whole body, rather than the head alone, when looking to one side. Atropine or the ephedrine group of drugs should be used, respectively, in patients with pronounced bradycardia or hypotension during attacks. The treatment of the various cardiac arrhythmias that may induce syncope is discussed in Chap. 230. The treatment of hypoglycemia is found in Chap. 335.

The chief hazard of a faint in most elderly persons is not the underlying disease but fracture or other trauma due to the fall. Therefore, patients subject to recurrent syncope should cover the bathroom floor and bathtub with rubber mats and should have as much of their home carpeted as is feasible. Especially important is the floor space between the bed and the bathroom, because faints are common in elderly persons when walking from bed to toilet. Outdoor walking should be on soft ground rather than hard surfaces, and the patient should avoid standing still, which is more likely than walking to induce an attack.

DIZZINESS AND VERTIGO

Dizziness is a common and often vexing symptom. Patients use the term to encompass a variety of sensations, including those that seem semantically appropriate (e.g., lightheadedness, faintness, spinning, giddiness, etc.) and those that are misleadingly inappropriate, such as mental confusion, blurred vision, headache, tingling, or "walking on cotton." Moreover, some patients with gait disturbances and no abnormal cephalic sensations will describe their problem as "dizziness." A careful history is necessary to determine exactly what a patient who states, "Doctor, I'm dizzy," is experiencing.

After eliminating the misleading symptoms such as confusion, "dizziness" usually means either *faintness* (analogous to the feelings that precede syncope) or *vertigo* (an illusory or hallucinatory sense of environmental or self-movement). In other instances, neither of these terms accurately describes a patient's symptoms, and the explanation may only become apparent when the neurologic examination reveals spasticity, parkinsonism, or other ambulation disturbances as the cause of the complaint. Operationally, dizziness is classified into four categories: (1) faintness, (2) vertigo, (3) miscellaneous head sensations, and (4) gait disturbances.

FAINTNESS Fainting (syncope) is a loss of consciousness secondary to cerebral ischemia, more specifically ischemia to the brainstem. Prior to the actual faint, there are often prodromal symptoms (faintness) reflecting ischemia to a degree insufficient to impair consciousness (see above).

VERTIGO Vertigo is a hallucination of self- or environmental movement, most commonly a feeling of spinning, usually due to a disturbance in the vestibular system. The end organs of this system, situated in the bony labyrinths of the inner ears, consist of the three semicircular canals and the otolithic apparatus (utricle and saccule) on each side. The canals transduce angular acceleration, while the otoliths transduce linear acceleration and static gravitational forces, the latter providing a sense of head position in space. The neural output of the end organs is conveyed to the vestibular nuclei in the brainstem via the eighth cranial nerve. The principal projections from the vestibular nuclei are to the nuclei of cranial nerves III, IV, and VI, the spinal cord, the cerebral cortex, and the cerebellum. The vestibuloocular reflex (VOR) serves to maintain visual stability during head movement and depends on direct projections from the vestibular nuclei to the sixth cranial nerve (abducens) nuclei in the pons and, via the medial longitudinal fasciculus, to the third (oculomotor) and fourth (trochlear) cranial nerve nuclei in the midbrain. These connections account for the nystagmus (to-and-fro oscillation of the eyes) that is an almost invariable accompaniment of vestibular dysfunction. The vestibulospinal pathways assist in the maintenance of postural stability. Projections to the cerebral cortex, via the thalamus, provide conscious awareness of head position and movement. The vestibular nerves and nuclei project to areas of the cerebellum (primarily the flocculus and nodulus) that modulate the VOR.

The vestibular system is one of three sensory systems subserving spatial orientation and posture; the other two are the visual system (retina to occipital cortex) and the somatosensory system that conveys peripheral information from skin, joint, and muscle receptors. The three stabilizing systems overlap sufficiently to compensate (partially or completely) for each other's deficiencies. Vertigo may represent either physiologic stimulation or pathologic dysfunction in any of the three systems.

Physiologic Vertigo This occurs when (1) the brain is confronted with a mismatch among the three stabilizing sensory systems; (2) the vestibular system is subjected to unfamiliar head movements to which it has never adapted, such as in seasickness; or (3) unusual head/neck positions, such as the extreme extension when painting a ceiling. Intersensory mismatch explains carsickness, height vertigo, and the visual vertigo most commonly experienced during motion picture chase scenes; in the latter, the visual sensation of environmental movement is unaccompanied by concomitant vestibular and somatosensory movement cues. *Space sickness*, a frequent transient effect of active head movement in the weightless zero-gravity environment, is another example of physiologic vertigo.

Pathologic Vertigo This results from lesions of the visual, somatosensory, or vestibular systems. Visual vertigo is caused by new or incorrect spectacles or by the sudden onset of an extraocular muscle paresis with diplopia; in either instance, CNS compensation rapidly counteracts the vertigo. Somatosensory vertigo, rare in isolation, is usually due to a peripheral neuropathy that reduces the sensory input necessary for central compensation when there is dysfunction of the vestibular or visual systems.

The most common cause of pathologic vertigo is vestibular dysfunction. The vertigo is frequently accompanied by nausea, jerk nystagmus, postural unsteadiness, and gait ataxia. Since vertigo increases with rapid head movements, patients tend to hold their heads still.

Labyrinthine dysfunction This causes severe rotational or linear vertigo. When rotational, the hallucination of movement, whether of environment or self, is directed away from the side of the lesion. The fast phases of nystagmus beat away from the lesion side, and the tendency to fall is toward the side of the lesion.

When the head is straight and immobile, the vestibular end organs generate a tonic resting firing frequency that is equal from the two sides. With any rotational acceleration, the anatomic positions of the semicircular canals on each side necessitate an increased firing rate from one and a commensurate decrease from the other. This change in neural activity is ultimately projected to the cerebral cortex, where it is summed with inputs from the visual and somatosensory systems to produce the appropriate conscious sense of rotational movement. After cessation of movement, the firing frequencies of the two end organs reverse; the side with the initially increased rate decreases, and the other side increases. A sense of rotation in the opposite direction is experienced; since there is no actual head movement, this hallucinatory

sensation is *vertigo*. Any disease state that changes the firing frequency of an end organ, producing unequal neural input to the brainstem and ultimately the cerebral cortex, causes vertigo. The symptom can be conceptualized as the cortex inappropriately interpreting the abnormal neural input from the brainstem as indicating actual head rotation. Transient abnormalities produce short-lived symptoms. With a fixed unilateral deficit, central conpensatory mechanisms ultimately diminish the vertigo. Since compensation depends on the plasticity of connections between the vestibular nuclei and the cerebellum, patients with brainstem or cerebellar disease have diminished adaptive capacity, and symptoms may persist indefinitely. Compensation is always inadequate for severe fixed bilateral lesions despite normal cerebellar connections: these patients are permanently symptomatic.

Acute unilateral labyrinthine dysfunction is caused by infection, trauma, and ischemia. Often, no specific etiology is uncovered, and the nonspecific terms *acute labyrinthitis*, *acute peripheral vestibulopathy*, or *vestibular neuritis* are used to describe the event. It is impossible to predict whether a patient recovering from the first bout of vertigo will have recurrent episodes.

Acute bilateral labyrinthine dysfunction is usually the result of toxins such as drugs or alcohol. The most common offending drugs are the aminoglycoside antibiotics.

Schwannomas involving the eighth cranial nerve (*acoustic neuroma*) grow slowly and produce such a gradual reduction of labyrinthine output that central compensatory mechanisms can prevent or minimize the vertigo; auditory symptoms of hearing loss and tinnitus are the most common manifestations. While lesions of the brainstem or cerebellum can cause acute vertigo, associated signs and symptoms usually permit distinction from a labyrinthine etiology (Table 20-2). However, labyrinthine ischemia may be the sole manifestation of vertebrobasilar insufficiency. Occasionally, an acute lesion of the vestibulocerebellum may present with monosymptomatic vertigo indistinguishable from a labyrinthopathy.

Table 20-2

Differentiation of Peripheral and Central Vertigo

Sign or Symptom	Peripheral (Labyrinth)	Central (Brainstem or Cerebellum)
Direction of associated nystagmus	Unidirectional; fast phase opposite lesion*	Bidirectional or unidirectional
Purely horizontal nystagmus without torsional component	Uncommon	Common
Vertical or purely torsional nysagmus	Never present	May be present
Visual fixation	Inhibits nystagmus and vertigo	No inhibition
Severity of vertigo	Marked	Often mild
Direction of spin	Toward fast phase	Variable
Direction of fall	Toward slow phase	Variable
Duration of symptoms	Finite (minutes, days, weeks) but recurrent	May be chronic
Tinnitus and/or deafness	Often present	Usually absent
Associated central abnormalities	None	Extremely common
Common causes	Infection (labyrinthitis), Ménière's, neuronitis, ischemia, trauma, toxin	Vascular, demyelinating, neoplasm

* In Ménière's disease, the direction of the fast phase is variable.

Recurrent unilateral labyrinthine dysfunction, in association with signs and symptoms of cochlear disease (progressive hearing loss and tinnitus), is usually due to Ménière's disease. When auditory manifestations are absent, the term *vestibular neuronitis* denotes recurrent monosymptomatic vertigo. TIAs of the posterior cerebral circulation (vertebrobasilar insufficiency) very infrequently cause recurrent vertigo without concomitant motor, sensory, visual, cranial nerve, or cerebellar signs.

Positional vertigo is precipitated by a recumbent head position, either to the right or to the left. Benign paroxysmal positional (or positioning) vertigo (BPPV) is particularly common. Although the condition may be due to head trauma, usually no precipitating factors are identified. It generally abates spontaneously after weeks or months. The vertigo and accompanying nystagmus have a distinct pattern of latency, fatigability, and habituation that differs from the less common central positional vertigo (Table 20-3) due to lesions in and around the fourth ventricle. Moreover, the pattern of nystagmus in BPPV is distinctive. The lower eye displays a large-amplitude torsional nystagmus, and the upper eye has a lesser degree of torsion combined with upbeating nystagmus. If the eyes are directed to the upper ear, the vertical nystagmus in the upper eye increases in amplitude.

Vestibular epilepsy, vertigo secondary to temporal lobe epileptic activity, is rare and almost always intermixed with other epileptic manifestations.

Psychogenic vertigo, usually a concomitant of agoraphobia (fear of large open spaces, crowds, or leaving the safety of home), should be suspected in patients so "incapacitated" by their symptoms that they adopt a prolonged housebound status. Despite their discomfort, most patients with organic vertigo attempt to function. Organic vertigo is accompanied by nystagmus; a psychogenic etiology is almost certain when nystagmus is absent during a vertiginous episode.

Evaluation of patients with pathologic vestibular vertigo The evaluation depends on whether a central etiology is suspected (see Table 20-2). If so, magnetic resonance imaging of the head is mandatory. Such an examination is rarely helpful in cases of recurrent monosymptomatic vertigo with a normal neurologic examination. Typical BPPV requires no investigation after the diagnosis is made (see Table 20-3).

Vestibular function tests serve to (1) demonstrate an abnormality when the distinction between organic and psychogenic is uncertain, (2) establish the side of the abnormality, and (3) distinguish between peripheral and central etiologies. The standard test is electronystagmography, where warm and cold water (or air) are applied, in a prescribed fashion, to the tympanic membranes, and the slow-phase velocities of the resultant nystagmus from the right and left ears are compared. A velocity decrease from one side indicates hypofunction ("canal paresis"). An inability to induce nystagmus with ice water denotes a "dead labyrinth." Some institutions have the capability of quantitatively determining various aspects of the vestibuloocular reflex using computer-driven rotational chairs and precise oculographic recording of the eye movements.

 TREATMENT

Treatment of acute vertigo consists of bed rest and vestibular suppressant drugs such as antihistaminics (meclizine, dimenhydrinate, promethazine), centrally acting anticholinergics (scopolamine), or a tranquilizer with GABA-ergic effects (diazepam). If the vertigo persists beyond a few days, most authorities advise ambulation in an attempt to induce central compensatory mechanisms, despite the short-term discomfiture to the patient. Chronic vertigo of labyrinthine origin may be treated with a systematized exercise program to facilitate compensation.

Prophylactic measures to prevent recurrent vertigo are variably effective. Antihistamines are commonly utilized. Ménière's disease may respond to a very low salt diet (1 g/day). Persisting (beyond 4 to 6 weeks) BPPV responds dramatically to specific exercise programs.

There are a variety of inner ear surgical procedures for all forms of refractory chronic or recurrent vertigo, but these are only rarely necessary.

Miscellaneous Head Sensations This designation is used, primarily for purposes of initial classification, to describe dizziness that is neither faintness nor vertigo. Cephalic ischemia or vestibular dysfunction may be of such low intensity that the usual symptomatology is not clearly identified. For example, a small decrease in blood pressure or a slight vestibular imbalance may cause sensations different from distinct faintness or vertigo but that may be identified properly during provocative testing techniques. Other causes of dizziness in this category are hyperventilation syndrome, hypoglycemia, and the somatic symptoms of a clinical depression; these patients should have normal neurologic examinations and vestibular function tests.

Gait Disturbances Some individuals with gait disorders complain of dizziness despite the absence of vertigo or other abnormal cephalic sensations. The causes include peripheral neuropathy, myelopathy, spasticity, parkinsonian rigidity, and cerebellar ataxia. In this context, the term *dizziness* is being used to describe disturbed mobility. There may be mild associated lightheadedness, particularly with impaired sensation from the feet or poor vision; this is known as *multiple-sensory-defect dizziness* and occurs in elderly individuals who complain of dizziness only during ambulation. Decreased position sense (secondary to neuropathy or myelopathy) and poor vision (from cataracts or retinal degeneration) create an overreliance on the aging vestibular apparatus. A less precise, but sometimes comforting, designation is *benign dysequilibrium of aging*.

――――――― *Approach to the Patient* ―――――――

The most important diagnostic tool is a careful history focused on the meaning of "dizziness" to the patient. Is it faintness? Is there a sensation of spinning? If either of these is affirmed and the neurologic examination is normal, appropriate investigations for the multiple etiologies of cephalic ischemia or vestibular dysfunction are undertaken.

When the meaning of "dizziness" is uncertain, provocative tests may be helpful. These office procedures simulate either cephalic ischemia or vestibular dysfunction. Cephalic ischemia is obvious if the dizziness is duplicated during orthostatic hypotension. Further provocation involves the Valsalva maneuver, which decreases cerebral blood flow and should reproduce ischemic symptoms.

The simplest provocative test for vestibular dysfunction is rapid rotation and abrupt cessation of movement in a swivel chair. This always induces vertigo that the patients can compare with their symptomatic dizziness. The intense induced vertigo may be unlike the spontaneous symptoms, but shortly thereafter, when the vertigo has all but subsided, a lightheadedness supervenes that may be identified as "my dizziness." When this occurs, the dizzy patient, originally classified as suffering from "miscellaneous head sensations," is now properly diagnosed as having mild vertigo secondary to a vestibulopathy.

Table 20-3

Benign Paroxysmal Positional Vertigo (BPPV) and Central Positional Vertigo

Features	BPPV	Central
Latency*	3–40 s	None: immediate vertigo and nystagmus
Fatigability†	Yes	No
Habituation‡	Yes	No
Intensity of vertigo	Severe	Mild
Reproducibility§	Variable	Good

* Time between attaining head position and onset of symptoms.
† Disappearance of symptoms with maintenance of offending position.
‡ Lessening of symptoms with repeated trials.
§ Likelihood of symptom production during any examination session.

Patients with symptoms of positional vertigo should be appropriately tested (see Table 20-3); positional testing is more sensitive with special spectacles that preclude visual fixation (Frenzel lenses).

A final provocative test, requiring the use of Frenzel lenses, is vigorous head shaking in the horizontal plane for about 10 s. If nystagmus develops after the shaking stops, even in the absence of vertigo, vestibular dysfunction is demonstrated. The maneuver can then be repeated in the vertical plane. If the provocative tests establish the dizziness as a vestibular symptom, the previously described evaluation of vestibular vertigo is undertaken.

Hyperventilation is the cause of dizziness in many anxious individuals; tingling of the hands and face may be absent. Forced hyperventilation for 1 min is indicated for patients with enigmatic dizziness and normal neurologic examinations. Similarly, depressive symptoms (which patients usually insist are "secondary" to the dizziness) must alert the examiner to a clinical depression as the *cause*, rather than the effect, of the dizziness.

CNS disease can produce dizzy sensations of all types. Consequently, a neurologic examination is always required even if the history or provocative tests suggest a cardiac, peripheral vestibular, or psychogenic etiology. Any abnormality on the neurologic examination should prompt appropriate neurodiagnostic studies.

BIBLIOGRAPHY

BALOH RW: Approach to the evaluation of the dizzy patient. Otolaryngol Head Neck Surg 112:3, 1995

BRANDT T et al: Therapy for benign paroxysmal positioning vertigo, revisited. Neurology 44:796, 1994

BRIGNOLE M et al: Mechanisms of syncope caused by transient bradycardia and the diagnostic value of electrophysiologic testing and cardiovascular reflexivity maneuvers. Am J Cardiol 76:273, 1995

BRUNI J: Episodic impairment of consciousness, in *Neurology in Clinical Practice*, WG Bradley et al (eds). Boston, Butterworth-Heinemann, 1996, chap 2

CALKINS H et al: Clinical presentation and long-term follow-up of athletes with exercise-induced vasodepressor syncope. Am Heart J 129:1159, 1995
——— et al: The value of the clinical history in the differentiation of syncope due to ventricular tachycardia, atrioventricular block, and neurocardiogenic syncope. Am J Med 98:365, 1995

EVANS RW: Neurologic aspects of hyperventilation syndrome. Semin Neurol 15:115, 1995

FERRANTE L et al: Glossopharyngeal neuralgia with cardiac syncope. Neurosurgery 36:58, 1995

GOMEZ CR et al: Isolated vertigo as a manifestation of vertebrobasilar ischemia. Neurology 47:94, 1996

KLEIN GJ et al: Electrophysiological testing: The final court of appeal for diagnosis of syncope? Circulation 92:1332, 1995

KUSUMOTO FM, GOLDSCHLAGER N: Cardiac pacing. N Engl J Med 334:89, 1996

LANDAU WM: Neuroskepticism: Sovereign remedy for the carotid sinus syndrome. Neurology 44:1570, 1994
———, NELSON DA: Feinting science: Neurocardiogenic syncope and collateral vasovagal confusion. Neurology 46:609, 1996
——— et al: Benign positional vertigo: Recognition and treatment. BMJ 311:489 and 799, 1995

LEMPERT T et al: Syncope: A videometric analysis of 56 episodes of transient cerebral hypoxia. Ann Neurol 36:233, 1994
——— LEMPERT T et al: The eye movements of syncope. Neurology 46:1086, 1996

LIPPMAN N et al: Failure to decrease parasympathetic tone during upright tilt predicts a positive tilt-table test. Am J Cardiol 75:591, 1995

LOW PA: Update on the evaluation, pathogenesis, and management of neurogenic orthostatic hypotension. Neurology 45:suppl 5, 54–532, 1995

MATHIAS CJ: Disorders of the autonomic nervous system, in *Neurology in Clinical Practice*, WG Bradley et al (eds). Boston, Butterworth-Heinemann, 1996, chap 82

MATTLE HP et al: Transient cerebral circulatory arrest coincides with fainting in cough syncope. Neurology 45:498, 1995

NADOL JB: Vestibular neuritis. Otolaryngol Head Neck Surg 112:162, 1995

SHARPE JA: Neuro-ophthalmic implications of vestibular disorders, in *Neuro-Ophthalmological Disorders*, RJ Tusa, SA Newman (eds). New York, Dekker, 1995, chap 18

STURZENEGGER M et al: Transcranial Doppler and angiographic findings in adolescent stretch syncope. J Neurol Neurosurg Psychiatry 58:367, 1995

TROOST BT: Dizziness and vertigo, in *Neurology in Clinical Practice*, WG Bradley et al (eds). Boston, Butterworth-Heinemann, 1996, chap 18

| 21 | *Richard K. Olney, Michael J. Aminoff* |

WEAKNESS, ABNORMAL MOVEMENTS, AND IMBALANCE

Motor dysfunction may result from weakness, movement disorders, ataxia, imbalance, and other disturbances in the initiation or coordination of movement. In this chapter, we describe the normal anatomy and physiology of the neural structures that subserve these functions, review the manner in which this physiology is altered to produce symptoms, and present a clinical approach toward the diagnosis of these various types of motor dysfunction.

WEAKNESS

Weakness is a reduction in normal power of one or more muscles. Patients may use the term differently; thus one or more specific examples of weakness should be elicited during the history. Increased fatigability or limitation in function due to pain is often confused with weakness by patients. Increased fatigability is the inability to sustain the performance of an activity that should be normal for a person of the same age, gender, and size.

Weakness is commonly described by severity and distribution. Paralysis and the suffix "-plegia" indicate weakness that is so severe that it is complete or nearly complete. "Paresis" refers to weakness that is mild. The prefix "hemi-" refers to one half of the body, "para-" to both legs, and "quadri-" to all four limbs.

Recognition of altered tone is important in localizing the cause of weakness. *Tone* is the resistance of a muscle to passive stretch. Central nervous system abnormalities that cause weakness generally produce *spasticity*, an increase in tone due to upper motor neuron disease. Spasticity is velocity dependent, has a sudden release after reaching a maximum (the "clasp-knife" phenomenon), and predominantly affects antigravity muscles (i.e., upper limb flexors more than extensors and lower limb extensors more than flexors). Spasticity is distinct from rigidity and paratonia, two other types of increased tone. *Rigidity* is increased tone that is present throughout the range of motion (a "lead pipe" or "plastic" stiffness) and affects flexors and extensors equally. In some patients, rigidity has a cogwheel quality that is enhanced by voluntary movement of the contralateral limb (reinforcement). Rigidity occurs with certain extrapyramidal disorders. *Paratonia*, also referred to as *gegenhalten*, is increased tone that varies irregularly in a manner that may seem related to the degree of relaxation, is present throughout the range of motion, and affects flexors and extensors equally. Paratonia usually results from disease of the frontal lobes. Weakness with decreased tone (flaccidity) or normal tone occurs with disorders of the *motor unit*, that is, a single lower motor neuron and all of the muscle fibers it innervates.

Three basic patterns of weakness can usually be recognized based on the signs summarized in Table 21-1. One results from upper motor neuron pathology, and the other two from disorders of the motor unit (lower motor neuron and myopathic weakness). Fasciculations and the early presence of atrophy help to distinguish lower motor neuron (neurogenic) weakness from myopathic weakness. A *fasciculation* is a visible or palpable twitch within a single muscle due to the spontaneous discharge of one motor unit. Neurogenic weakness also produces more prominent hypotonia and greater depression of tendon reflexes than myopathic weakness.

PATHOGENESIS OF WEAKNESS Upper Motor Neuron Weakness This pattern of weakness results from disorders that affect the upper motor neurons or their axons in the cerebral cortex, subcortical white matter, internal capsule, brainstem, or spinal cord.

Upper motor neurons have their cell bodies in layer V of the cerebral cortex. Most are contained in the primary motor cortex (the precentral gyrus, or Brodmann's area 4) and in the premotor and

Table 21-1

Signs that Distinguish Patterns of Weakness

Sign	Upper Motor Neuron	Lower Motor Neuron	Myopathic
Atrophy	None	Severe	Mild
Fasciculations	None	Common	None
Tone	Spastic	Decreased	Normal/decreased
Distribution of weakness	Pyramidal/regional	Distal/segmental	Proximal
Tendon reflexes	Hyperactive	Hypoactive/absent	Normal/hypoactive
Babinski's sign	Present	Absent	Absent

supplemental motor cortex (area 6). A significant minority are in the primary sensory cortex (areas 3, 1, and 2) and the superior parietal lobule (areas 5 and 7). The upper motor neurons in the primary motor cortex are somatotopically organized. Those that activate facial muscles are at the lower end of the precentral gyrus, those that activate arm and hand muscles are higher in this gyrus, and those that activate the leg muscles are in the paracentral lobule over the medial surface of the cerebral hemisphere. Somatotopic organization of the upper motor neurons is also preserved in other cortical motor areas (e.g., premotor and supplemental motor cortices).

Axons of the upper motor neurons descend through the subcortical white matter and the posterior limb of the internal capsule. Those axons that comprise the *pyramidal* or *corticospinal system* descend through the brainstem in the cerebral peduncles of the midbrain, the basis pontis, and the medullary pyramids (Fig. 21-1). At the cervicomedullary junction, most pyramidal axons decussate into the contralateral corticospinal tract of the lateral spinal cord, but 10 to 30 percent remain ipsilateral in the anterior spinal cord. Pyramidal neurons include both the large corticomotoneurons and the smaller corticospinal neurons. The corticomotoneurons are glutamatergic and make direct monosynaptic connections with lower motor neurons. They innervate most densely the lower motor neurons of hand muscles and are involved in the execution of learned, fine movements. The corticospinal neurons are also glutamatergic, but they synapse on neurons in the dorsal horn and interneurons in the intermediate zone of the spinal cord to facilitate cortically initiated movements. Corticobulbar neurons are upper motor neurons that are similar to corticospinal neurons but innervate brainstem motor nuclei. Although analogous in function and often referred to as pyramidal in general contexts, corticobulbar neurons are not strictly part of the pyramidal system, as their axons never traverse the medullary pyramids.

Bulbospinal upper motor neurons influence strength and tone but are not part of the pyramidal system (Fig. 21-1). Corticorubral, corticoreticular, corticopontine, and other cortical-brainstem pathways contribute to lower motor neuron activity indirectly through these pathways. The cortical neurons influence the red nucleus and superior colliculus of the midbrain and the vestibular nuclei, the inferior olivary nucleus, and reticular formation of the pons and medulla. The descending *ventromedial bulbospinal pathways* originate in the tectum of the midbrain (tectospinal pathway), the lateral and medial vestibular nuclei (vestibulospinal pathway), and the reticular formation (reticulospinal pathway). These pathways influence axial and proximal muscles and are involved in the maintenance of posture and integrated movements of the limbs and trunk. The

descending *ventrolateral bulbospinal pathways*, which originate predominantly in the magnocellular portion of the red nucleus (rubrospinal pathway), facilitate distal limb muscles. The bulbospinal system is sometimes referred to as the *extrapyramidal upper motor neuron system*.

The pyramidal and bulbospinal pathways contribute to normal strength, tone, coordination, and gait. Clinical lesions generally affect both pyramidal and bulbospinal pathways and are rarely purely pyramidal. Purely pyramidal lesions in animals produce an acute flaccid contralateral hemiplegia that spares the face and is associated with an extensor plantar (Babinski) response; strength recovers over weeks to months, and spasticity and hyperreflexia do not develop. In upper motor neuron weakness in humans, the development of spasticity and hyperreflexia has been reported with the rare cases of pure bilateral pyramidal infarction.

Upper motor neuron lesions produce weakness through decreased activation of the lower motor neurons that innervate muscles in one or more regions of the body. Upper motor neuron weakness always affects more than one muscle group and uncommonly affects all muscles within a limb. In general, distal muscle groups are affected more severely than proximal ones, and axial movements are spared unless the lesion is severe and bilateral. With corticobulbar involvement, weakness is usually observed only in the lower face and tongue; extraocular, upper facial, pharyngeal, and jaw muscles are almost always spared. With bilateral corticobulbar lesions, *pseudobulbar palsy* often develops, in which dysarthria, dysphagia, dysphonia, and emotional lability accompany bilateral facial weakness. Spastic tone accompanies upper motor neuron weakness, unless it is acute. Acute

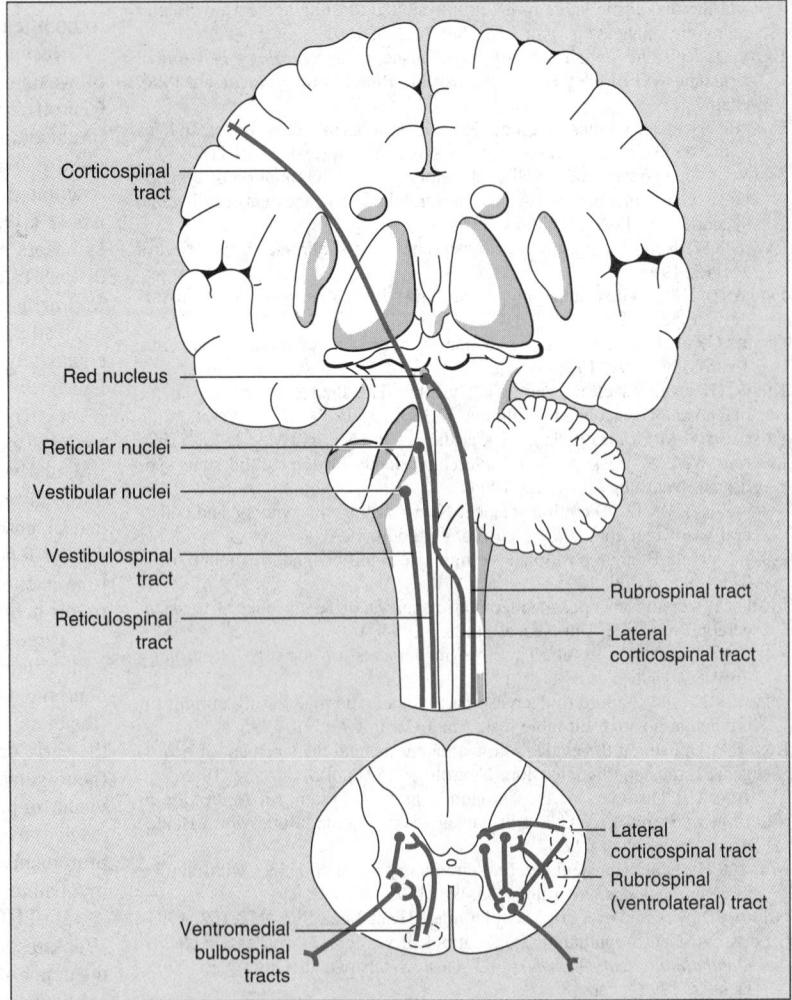

Corticospinal tract

Red nucleus

Reticular nuclei

Vestibular nuclei

Vestibulospinal tract

Reticulospinal tract

Rubrospinal tract

Lateral corticospinal tract

Lateral corticospinal tract

Rubrospinal (ventrolateral) tract

Ventromedial bulbospinal tracts

FIGURE 21-1 The corticospinal and bulbospinal upper motor neuron pathways. The axons of the bulbospinal neurons are contained in both ventromedial and ventrolateral tracts. In all figures, nerve cell bodies and axon terminals are shown, respectively, as closed circles and forks.

lesions below the foramen magnum usually produce *spinal shock* if weakness is severe. During spinal shock, tendon reflexes are absent and tone is flaccid. Spasticity subsequently develops over days to weeks.

Upper motor neuron lesions also cause incoordination that is manifest as slow, coarse movements for which normal rhythmicity is maintained. Finger-nose-finger and heel-knee-shin are performed slowly but adequately. The incoordination is more obvious with rapidly repeated movements, such as tapping the index finger on the thumb.

Lower Motor Neuron Weakness This pattern results from disorders of cell bodies of lower motor neurons in the brainstem motor nuclei and the anterior horn of the spinal cord, or from dysfunction of the axons of these neurons as they pass to skeletal muscle.

Lower motor neurons are divided into alpha and gamma types (Fig. 21-2). Gamma motor neurons are smaller than alpha motor neurons and innervate the intrafusal muscle fibers of the muscle spindle. Activation of the gamma motor neuron increases the tension on muscle spindles and facilitates stretch reflexes and other local reflex mechanisms that activate a muscle through the alpha motor neurons. Each muscle is innervated by many (usually several hundred) alpha motor neurons. Each alpha motor neuron activates many extrafusal muscle fibers, several hundred for limb and axial muscles or fewer than twenty for extraocular muscles, through release of acetylcholine.

Lower motor neuron axons exit the brainstem in certain cranial nerves and the spinal cord in the ventral roots. The ventral roots fuse with the dorsal roots at the intervertebral foramen to form spinal nerves. For innervation of limb muscles, several adjacent spinal nerves fuse to form plexuses before dividing into peripheral nerves. Most peripheral nerves branch one or more times as they innervate different muscles. Each alpha motor axon extensively arborizes just before reaching the many muscle fibers that it innervates.

The alpha motor neuron receives direct excitatory, glutamatergic input from corticomotoneurons and primary muscle spindle afferents. The alpha and gamma motor neurons also receive direct or indirect excitatory input from other descending upper motor neuron pathways, segmental sensory inputs, and interneurons. The alpha motor neurons in the spinal cord receive direct postsynaptic inhibition from Renshaw cell interneurons, which release glycine. Other interneurons produce presynaptic inhibition on dorsal horn neurons through release of gamma-aminobutyric acid (GABA); this indirectly inhibits the alpha and gamma motor neurons. Other descending upper motor neuron pathways and segmental sensory inputs also produce direct or indirect inhibition of the alpha and gamma motor neurons.

When the balance of descending upper motor neuron and segmental inputs is excitatory, the pool of lower motor neurons that innervates a muscle is activated in an orderly manner. The lower motor neurons with the smallest cell bodies are activated first. With increasing effort,

these motor units discharge more rapidly, and larger motor units are then gradually recruited. With maximum effort, the entire lower motor neuron pool is activated to produce maximum power.

Lower motor weakness is produced by a decrease in the number of motor units that can be activated, due to a loss of the alpha motor neurons or disruption of their connections to muscle. With a decreased number of motor units, fewer muscle fibers are activated with full effort and maximum power is reduced. Loss of gamma motor neurons does not cause weakness but decreases tension on the muscle spindles. Muscle tone and tendon reflexes depend on gamma motor neurons, muscle spindles, their afferent fibers, and the alpha motor neurons. A tap on a tendon stretches muscle spindles and activates the primary spindle afferent fibers. These monosynaptically stimulate the alpha motor neurons in the spinal cord through release of glutamate. The activated alpha motor neurons produce a brief muscle contraction, which is the familiar tendon reflex. Loss of the gamma motor neuron input to the intrafusal muscle fibers decreases both continuous discharge of spindle afferents (which increase muscle tone) and phasic discharge of spindle afferents in response to stretch (which produces the tendon reflex).

When a motor unit becomes diseased, especially in anterior horn cell diseases, it may spontaneously discharge, producing a fasciculation, without being recruited in the normal manner. These isolated small twitches may be seen or felt clinically or recorded by electromyography (EMG) (See Chap. 361). When alpha motor neurons or their axons degenerate, the denervated muscle fibers spontaneously discharge in a manner that cannot be seen or felt but can be recorded with EMG. These small single muscle fiber discharges are called *fibrillation potentials*. The recruitment of surviving motor units can be assessed with EMG. If significant lower motor neuron weakness is present, recruitment of motor units is delayed or reduced, meaning that fewer than normal are activated at a given discharge frequency. This contrasts with upper motor neuron weakness, in which a normal number of motor units are activated at a given frequency but in which the maximum discharge frequency is decreased.

Myopathic Weakness This pattern of weakness is produced by disorders within the motor unit that affect the muscle fibers or the neuromuscular junctions.

Two types of muscle fibers exist. Type I muscle fibers are rich in mitochondria and oxidative enzymes, produce relatively low force, but have low energy demands that can be supplied by ongoing aerobic metabolism. They produce sustained postural and nonforceful movements. Type II muscle fibers are rich in glycolytic enzymes, can produce relatively high force, but have high energy demands that cannot be supplied for long by ongoing aerobic metabolism. Thus, these units can be activated maximally for only brief periods of time to produce high-force movements.

For graded voluntary movements, type I muscle fibers are activated earliest in recruitment. For each muscle fiber, if the nerve terminal releases a normal number of acetylcholine molecules presynaptically and a sufficient number of postsynaptic acetylcholine receptors are opened, the end plate reaches threshold and thereby generates an action potential that spreads across the muscle fiber membrane and into the transverse tubular system. This electrical excitation activates intracellular events that produce an energy-dependent contraction of the muscle fiber (excitation–contraction coupling).

Myopathic weakness is produced by a decrease in the number or contractile force of muscle fibers activated within the motor unit. With muscular dystrophies, inflammatory myopathies, or myopathies with muscle fiber necrosis, decreased numbers of muscle fibers survive within many motor units. As demonstrated with EMG, the size of each motor unit action potential is decreased so that motor units must be recruited more rapidly than normal to produce the power necessary for a certain movement. Neuromuscular junction diseases produce weakness in a similar manner, although the loss of muscle fibers within the motor unit is functional rather than actual. Furthermore, the number

FIGURE 21-2 Alpha and gamma motor neurons and the primary spindle afferent neuron.

of muscle fibers activated can vary over time, depending on the state of rest of the neuromuscular junctions. Some myopathies produce weakness through loss of contractile force of muscle fibers. These may not affect the size of the motor unit action potentials and are detected by a discrepancy between the electrical activity and force of a muscle.

Nonparalytic Disorders of Movement Other disorders of movement occur that do not cause weakness. Those that are classified as movement disorders or as imbalance and ataxia will be discussed later in this chapter. Others are caused by disorders in initiation or integration of movement. Such disorders are produced by diseases that affect the cerebral hemispheres without causing obvious upper motor neuron weakness.

Most functional movements require the integrated coordination of many muscle groups. For example, consider a simple movement, such as grasping a ball. The primary movement is a flexion of the thumb and fingers of one hand, with opposition of the thumb and little finger. This requires the contraction of several muscles, including flexor digitorum superficialis, flexor digitorum profundus, flexor pollicis longus, flexor pollicis brevis, opponens pollicis, and opponens digiti minimi. These prime movers for this action are called *agonists*. In order for the grasping to be smooth and forceful, the thumb and finger extensors need to relax at the same rate as the flexors contract. The muscles that act in a directly opposing manner to the agonists are *antagonists*. A secondary action of the thumb and finger flexors is to flex the wrist; because wrist flexion tends to weaken finger flexion if both occur, activation of wrist extensors assists the grasping movement. Muscles that produce such complementary movements are *synergists*. Finally, the arm needs to be held in a stable position as the grasp occurs, so that the ball is not knocked away before it is secured. Muscles that stabilize the arm position are *fixators*.

The coordination of activity by agonists, antagonists, synergists, and fixators is regulated by a three-level hierarchy of motor control. The lowest level of control is mediated through segmental reflexes in the spinal cord. These reflexes facilitate agonists and reciprocally inhibit the antagonists. Spinal segments also control rhythmic patterns of movement that involve more than a single pair of agonists and antagonists. For example, the lumbosacral spinal cord contains the basic programming for cyclical stepping movements that involve the synergistic activation of different muscle groups over time. The intermediate level of control is mediated through the descending bulbospinal pathways, which integrate visual, proprioceptive, and vestibular feedback into the execution of an action (discussed later). For example, the locomotor center in the mesencephalon is required to modify the cyclical stepping movements in order that balance be maintained and forward movement occur. The highest level of control is mediated by the cerebral cortex. Superimposition of this highest level of control is necessary for activities, such as walking, to be goal-directed. Precise movements that are learned and improved through practice are also initiated and controlled by the motor cortex. Although only the agonists are directly activated, during the course of a complex sequence of actions, such as playing the piano, the sequential activation of different groups of agonists for each note or chord is a part of the learned motor program. Further, the execution of these actions also involves input from the basal ganglia and cerebellar hemispheres to facilitate agonists, synergists, and fixators and to inhibit undesired antagonists.

Apraxia is a disorder of initiating and planning movement (see also Chap. 25). Unilateral apraxia of the right hand may be due to a lesion of the left frontal lobe (especially anterior or inferior), the left temporoparietal region (especially the supramarginal gyrus), or their connections. Left body apraxia is produced by lesions of these regions in the right hemisphere or by lesions in the corpus callosum that disconnect the right temporoparietal or frontal regions from those on the left. Bilateral apraxia is often due to bilateral frontal lobe lesions or diffuse bilateral hemispheric disease.

DIAGNOSTIC APPROACH AND DIFFERENTIAL DIAGNOSIS FOR COMMON CLINICAL PRESENTATIONS OF WEAKNESS Clinical Assessment of Weakness
When there is a discrepancy between the history and physical findings, it is usually because the patient complains of weakness, whereas symptoms are actually due to other causes, such as incoordination. The proper approach to weakness requires that its mode of onset, distribution, and associated features be carefully defined in order to identify the responsible anatomic lesion and the likely etiology.

Power may be examined in a variety of ways. Direct testing is most often used to determine whether weakness is present and to assess its distribution. The patient is asked to push or pull in a specified direction against the resistance of the physician, and the strength in each muscle group is graded from 0 to 5 by the scale developed by the Medical Research Council (Table 21-2). A second method is indirect testing through observation of task performance such as holding the arms outstretched. This is especially useful in detecting mild, asymmetric upper motor neuron weakness through the observation of a downward drift with pronation of the forearm on one side. A third method is functional testing, which involves quantitation of activities. Common tests include counting the number of times a person can perform a deep-knee bend or step on a stool or chair, or timing the length of time the arms can be held abducted to 90 degrees. Functional testing for weakness is time-consuming and any weakness is difficult to localize to a specific muscle or group of muscles; however, it provides reproducible data for assessment of changes in the patient's status over time.

Other essential parts of the motor examination include appraisal of muscular bulk, inspection for fasciculations, and assessment of tone in all four limbs. The presence of fasciculations is most easily determined by observing relaxed limbs that are illuminated from behind. Fasciculations can also be palpated as irregular low-amplitude twitches within the muscle. Tone is assessed by passive movement of each limb at its various joints and at several different speeds. In the clinical context of weakness, tone may be spastic or decreased. The presence of cogwheel rigidity, lead-pipe rigidity, or paratonia suggests a nonparalytic disorder of movement.

Hemiparesis Hemiparesis results from an upper motor neuron lesion above the midcervical spinal cord; most lesions that produce hemiparesis are located above the foramen magnum. More precise localization of the lesion is aided by recognition of associated signs. Language disorders, cortical sensory disturbances, cognitive disorders, disorders of visual-spatial integration, apraxia, and seizures identify a cortical lesion. Homonymous visual field defects reflect either a cortical or a subcortical hemispheric lesion. A hemiparesis of the face, arm, and leg without associated signs indicates a small, discrete lesion in the posterior limb of the internal capsule, cerebral peduncle, or upper pons. Some brainstem lesions produce the classic findings of ipsilateral cranial nerve signs and contralateral hemiparesis. These "crossed paralyses" are discussed further in Chap. 366. The absence of cranial nerve signs or facial weakness suggests that a hemiparesis is due to a lesion in the high cervical spinal cord, especially if associated with ipsilateral loss of proprioception and contralateral loss of pain and temperature sense (the Brown-Séquard syndrome). However, most spinal cord lesions produce quadriparesis or paraparesis.

Table 21-2

Medical Research Council Grading of Strength

Grade	Definition
5	Normal strength
4	Active movement against gravity and resistance
3	Active movement against gravity (no resistance from physician)
2	Active movement with gravity eliminated (no resistance from physician)
1	Flicker or trace contraction
0	No visible or palpable contraction

Acute hemiparesis usually has a vascular pathogenesis (Chap. 366). Less commonly, hemorrhage may occur into primary or metastatic brain tumors (Chap. 375) or from rupture of normal vessels due to trauma (Chap. 374); the trauma may be trivial in patients who are anticoagulated or elderly. Less likely possibilities include a focal inflammatory lesion from multiple sclerosis or sarcoidosis (Chap. 376), or an acute bacterial abscess (Chap. 377). The diagnostic approach begins immediately with a computed tomography (CT) scan of the brain, and subsequent decisions are based upon the result (Fig. 21-3). If CT of the brain is normal and an ischemic stroke is unlikely, magnetic resonance imaging (MRI) of the brain or cervical spine may be required.

Subacute hemiparesis has a long differential diagnosis. Subacute subdural hematoma is a common cause of hemiparesis that develops over days to a few weeks; this readily treatable condition must always be considered, especially in elderly patients or those who are anticoagulated, even in the absence of a history of trauma (Chap. 374). Infectious possibilities include cerebral bacterial abscess (Chap. 377), fungal granuloma or meningitis (Chap. 378), and parasitic infection. Weakness from malignant primary and metastatic neoplasms may evolve over days to weeks (Chap. 375). AIDS (Chap. 308) may present with subacute hemiparesis due to toxoplasmosis or primary central nervous system lymphoma. Noninfectious inflammatory processes, such as multiple sclerosis (Chap. 376) or, less commonly, sarcoidosis, are further considerations. The diagnostic approach is summarized in Fig. 21-3; if the brain MRI is normal, MRI of the cervical spine may be required.

Chronic hemiparesis that develops over months (as opposed to one that develops acutely and then persists for months) is usually due to a histologically benign neoplasm (Chap. 375), an unruptured arteriovenous malformation (Chap. 366), a chronic subdural hematoma (Chap. 374), or a degenerative disease (Chaps. 368 to 371). The initial diagnostic test is often an MRI of the brain, especially if the clinical findings suggest brainstem pathology. If MRI of the brain is normal, less likely possibilities of a foramen magnum or high cervical spinal cord lesion should be considered (Fig. 21-3).

Paraparesis Paraparesis most commonly results from an intraspinal lesion at or below the upper thoracic spinal cord level. A sensory level over the trunk identifies the approximate level of the cord lesion. Other causes for paraparesis include other upper motor neuron lesions (parasagittal lesions and hydrocephalus) and lower motor neuron lesions (anterior horn cell disorders, cauda equina syndromes, and atypical peripheral neuropathies).

Acute paraparesis due to spinal cord disease may be difficult to distinguish from disorders affecting lower motor neurons or cerebral hemispheres. With paraparesis or paraplegia from acute spinal cord disease, the upper motor neuron deficit is usually associated with urinary and fecal incontinence and often lower limb numbness that extends rostrally to a level on the trunk; tone is typically flaccid, and tendon reflexes absent. With a sensory level and sphincter involvement, the diagnostic approach starts with an imaging study of the spinal cord (Fig. 21-3). The diagnostic possibilities include epidural metastasis, epidural hematoma, and spinal cord ischemia from a dural arteriovenous fistula or other vascular anomaly, each of which requires acute intervention. These need to be distinguished from transverse myelitis and lesions outside the spinal cord (Chap. 373). Diseases of the cerebral hemispheres that result in acute paraparesis include anterior cerebral artery ischemia, superior sagittal sinus thrombosis, cortical venous thrombosis, or acute hydrocephalus. If upper motor neuron signs are associated with drowsiness, confusion, seizures, or other cortical signs but not a sensory level over the trunk, the diagnostic approach starts with an MRI of the brain. Paraparesis is part of the cauda equina syndrome, which may result from trauma to the low back, a midline disk herniation, or lumbar intraspinal metastasis; although sphincters are affected, hip flexion is often spared as is sensation over the anterolateral thighs. Paraparesis is rarely caused by acute demyelinating polyneuropathy (the most common form of Guillain-Barré syndrome) or, rarely, a myopathy. In such cases, electrophysiologic studies are diagnostically helpful and refocus the subsequent evaluation (Chaps. 381 and 383).

Subacute or *chronic paraparesis* with spasticity is caused by upper motor neuron disease. When paraparesis develops over weeks or months with lower limb sensory loss and sphincter involvement, possible spinal cord disorders include multiple sclerosis, intraparenchymal tumor, chronic spinal cord compression from degenerative disease of the spine, subacute combined degeneration due to vitamin B_{12} deficiency, and hereditary diseases. Chronic progressive multiple sclerosis usually presents in the fourth or fifth decade with progressive paraparesis (Chap. 376). Primary spinal cord gliomas typically produce a progressive myelopathy that is painful (Chap. 375). The clinical approach begins with MRI or myelography to image the spinal cord. If the imaging study is normal and spasticity is present, MRI of the brain may also be indicated. If cortical signs are present, parasagittal meningioma or chronic hydrocephalus is likely and MRI of the brain is the initial test. Progression over months to years may also be due to degenerative disorders, such as primary lateral sclerosis (Chap. 370) or hereditary disorders, such as familial spastic paraparesis and adrenomyeloneuropathy (Chap. 373). In

FIGURE 21-3 An algorithm for the initial work-up of a patient with weakness. CT, computed tomography; EMG, electromyography; LMN, lower motor neuron; MRI, magnetic resonance imaging; NCS, nerve conduction studies; UMN, upper motor neuron.

the rare situations in which a chronic paraparesis is due to lower motor neuron or myopathic weakness, the localization is usually suspected on clinical grounds and confirmed by EMG and nerve conduction tests.

Quadriparesis Quadriparesis can result from upper motor neuron disease (localized to the upper cervical spinal cord or above), diffuse lower motor neuron disease, or a myopathy.

Acute quadriparesis The differential diagnosis for acute quadriparesis with onset over minutes includes many diseases of upper motor neurons (e.g., anoxia, hypotension, brainstem or cervical cord ischemia, trauma, and systemic metabolic abnormalities) and also rare forms of myopathic weakness (systemic toxins or periodic paralyses). Onset over hours to a few days may be due to upper motor neuron, lower motor neuron, or myopathic disorders. All three patterns of weakness are usually associated initially with hypotonia. If the acute quadriparesis is associated with stupor or coma, the evaluation begins with a CT scan of the brain. If upper motor neuron signs are present but the patient is alert, the initial test is usually an MRI of the cervical cord. If weakness is lower motor neuron, myopathic, or uncertain in origin, the clinical approach starts with an electrodiagnostic study. Acute demyelinating polyneuropathy (Chap. 381) is an important diagnostic possibility in this setting.

Subacute or chronic quadriparesis When quadriparesis due to upper motor neuron disease develops over weeks, months, or years, the distinction between disorders of the cerebral hemispheres, brainstem, and cervical spinal cord is usually possible by clinical criteria alone. The diagnostic approach begins with an MRI of the clinically suspected site of pathology. Lower motor neuron disease presents with weakness that is most profound distally, whereas myopathic weakness is typically proximal (Chaps. 381 and 383). The evaluation then begins with EMG and nerve conduction studies.

Monoparesis or Weakness within One Limb This is usually due to lower motor neuron disease, with or without associated sensory involvement. Upper motor neuron weakness occasionally presents with a monoparesis of distal and nonantigravity muscles. Myopathic weakness is rarely limited to one limb.

Acute monoparesis Distinguishing between upper and lower motor neuron disorders may be difficult with motor examination alone because tone and reflexes are frequently decreased in both at the time of acute presentation. If the weakness is predominantly in distal and nonantigravity muscles and not associated with sensory impairment or pain, focal cortical ischemia is likely (Chap. 366); in this setting, diagnostic possibilities are similar to those for acute hemiparesis. Acute lower motor neuron disease is usually accompanied by sensory loss and pain. The distribution of weakness is commonly localized to a single nerve root or peripheral nerve within one limb. If lower motor neuron weakness is suspected, or if the pattern of weakness is uncertain, the clinical approach begins with an EMG and nerve conduction study.

Subacute or chronic monoparesis or segmental weakness Weakness with atrophy of one limb that develops over weeks or months is almost always due to a localized disorder of lower motor neurons. If the weakness is associated with numbness, a peripheral nerve or spinal root origin is likely; uncommonly, the brachial or lumbosacral plexus is affected. If numbness is absent, segmental anterior horn cell disease is likely. In either case, an electrodiagnostic study is indicated. If upper rather than lower motor neuron signs are present, a tumor, vascular malformation, or other cortical lesion affecting the precentral gyrus may be responsible. Alternatively, if the leg is affected, a small thoracic cord lesion, often a tumor or demyelinative plaque, may be present. In these situations, the approach begins with an imaging study of the suspicious area.

Distal Weakness Involvement of two or four limbs distally suggests lower motor neuron or peripheral nerve disease. Acute distal lower limb weakness occurs occasionally from an acute toxic polyneuropathy or cauda equina syndrome. Distal symmetric weakness usually develops over weeks, months, or years and is due to metabolic, toxic,

hereditary, degenerative, or inflammatory diseases of peripheral nerves (Chap. 381). With peripheral nerve disease, weakness is usually less severe than numbness. Anterior horn cell disease may begin distally but is typically asymmetric and is not associated with numbness (Chap. 370). Rarely, myopathies also present with distal weakness without associated numbness (Chap. 383). The first step in evaluation is to obtain an electrodiagnostic study (Fig. 21-3).

Proximal Weakness Proximal weakness of two or four limbs suggests a disorder of muscle or, less commonly, neuromuscular junction or anterior horn cell. Proximal weakness that develops over weeks, months, or years is usually due to hereditary, inflammatory, metabolic, or endocrine disease. Myopathy often produces symmetric weakness of the pelvic or shoulder girdle muscles (Chap. 383). Diseases of the neuromuscular junction (such as myasthenia gravis) may present with symmetric proximal weakness (Chap. 382), often associated with ptosis, diplopia, or bulbar weakness and fluctuating in severity during the day. The proximal weakness of anterior horn cell disease is most often asymmetric, but may be symmetric if familial (Chap. 370). Numbness does not occur with any of these diseases. The evaluation usually begins with determination of the serum creatine kinase level and electrophysiologic studies.

MOVEMENT DISORDERS

Movement disorders are neurologic syndromes in which abnormal movements (or *dyskinesias*) occur due to a disturbance of fluency and speed of voluntary movement or the presence of unintended extra movements. Because they are so distinct from the pyramidal disorders that cause upper motor neuron weakness, movement disorders are often referred to as *extrapyramidal diseases*. Movement disorders are divided into hypokinetic and hyperkinetic types. *Hypokinetic movement disorders* are characterized by *akinesia* or *bradykinesia*, in which purposeful motor activity is absent or reduced. This is often described as "poverty of movement." *Hyperkinetic movement disorders* are those in which an excessive amount of spontaneous motor activity is seen or in which abnormal involuntary movements occur.

PATHOGENESIS OF MOVEMENT DISORDERS **Normal Functional Interconnections** Movement disorders result from disease of the basal ganglia, paired subcortical gray matter structures that form anatomically distinct nuclear groups. They consist of the caudate and the putamen (which together are called the striatum), the internal and external segments of the globus pallidus, the subthalamic nucleus, and the substantia nigra. The major interconnections and neurotransmitters involved in basal ganglia circuits are diagrammed in Fig. 21-4A. Cortically initiated movement is facilitated and competing movements are inhibited through the influence of the basal ganglia. The striatum receives somatotopically organized input from many areas of the cortex. These consist of multiple parallel segregated circuits that include input from the frontal, sensory, and motor cortex and from parietotemporooccipital association areas; however, only the precentral motor and postcentral somatosensory projections seem directly related to movement. These projections are glutamatergic and excitatory. The striatum has direct and indirect projections to the major outflow nuclei of the basal ganglia, the substantia nigra pars reticulata and the globus pallidus interna (also called the medial globus pallidus). These nuclei project in turn to the ventral anterior and ventral lateral nuclei of the thalamus via inhibitory GABA neurotransmission. The thalamic nuclei have glutamatergic, excitatory projections to cortical neurons. Thus, inhibition of the substantia nigra pars reticulata and the globus pallidus interna disinhibits thalamocortical projections that reinforce cortically initiated activity, and excitation of these outflow pathways inhibits thalamocortical projections for competing motor responses. The basal ganglia do not project directly to the spinal cord.

The direct pathway from the striatum to the substantia nigra pars reticulata and the globus pallidus interna is GABA-ergic and inhibitory. This direct pathway then functions to facilitate thalamocortical projections that reinforce cortically initiated movement. The indirect pathway is more complex and functions to inhibit thalamocortical projections to other areas of the motor cortex. The first connection of the indirect pathway is GABA-ergic; it inhibits activity in the globus pallidus externa (also called the lateral globus pallidus). The globus pallidus externa has GABA-ergic, inhibitory input on the subthalamic nucleus. The subthalamic nucleus has excitatory, glutamatergic feedback on the globus pallidus externa and excitatory, glutamatergic input on the substantia nigra pars reticulata and the globus pallidus interna. Thus, activation of the indirect pathway increases outflow from the substantia nigra pars reticulata and the globus pallidus interna, in contrast to the decreased outflow that is produced by activation of the direct pathway.

The direct and indirect pathways are influenced also by input from the substantia nigra pars compacta. This dopaminergic input on the striatum has a net inhibitory effect on direct pathway neurons that predominantly express D_1 dopamine receptors and has a net excitatory effect on indirect pathway neurons that predominantly express D_2 dopamine receptors. The striatum also has GABA-ergic, inhibitory feedback connections with the pars compacta. Striatal activity is further modulated by cholinergic interneurons within the striatum, which are functionally antagonistic to the dopaminergic projections.

Hypokinetic Movement Disorders   This model explains well the *hypokinetic movement disorders*. As diagrammed in Fig. 21-4*B*, the fundamental abnormality of Parkinson's disease consists of a loss of dopaminergic neurons in the substantia nigra pars compacta. This causes a loss of excitation of the D_1 striatal neurons in the direct pathway and a loss of inhibition of the D_2 striatal neurons in the indirect pathway. This combination of changes increases outflow from the substantia nigra pars reticulata and the globus pallidus interna, which increases inhibition of thalamocortical projections and results in loss of facilitation of cortically initiated movement. The resting tremor of Parkinson's disease is less readily explained by this model but may result from effects on cholinergic interneurons in the striatum.

Hyperkinetic Movement Disorders   As diagrammed in Fig. 21-4*C*, the pathogenesis of chorea in Huntington's disease is an initial loss of the striatal neurons that express D_2 receptors and normally project GABA-ergic inhibition through the indirect pathway. This disinhibits the globus pallidus externa, which in turn increases inhibition of the subthalamic nucleus. Because the glutamatergic input from the subthalamic nucleus is the primary source of excitation on the

substantia nigra pars reticulata and the globus pallidus interna, loss of this excitation reduces inhibition of the thalamus and cortically initiated movements are facilitated without normal feedback control. The pathogenesis of hemiballismus is similar but less complicated— a direct lesion of the glutamatergic neurons in the subthalamic nucleus leads to disinhibition of thalamocortical projections.

Some movement disorders, for example parkinsonism and chorea, may result from changes in discrete populations of neurons that use a specific neurotransmitter. Such selective vulnerability is commonly present in degenerative neurologic diseases, both hereditary and sporadic, and in toxic, nutritional, and inflammatory conditions. Structural disease that affects more than one cell type is common only in hemiballismus, in which a lesion of the subthalamic nucleus, usually a stroke, is almost always found.

DIAGNOSTIC APPROACH AND DIFFERENTIAL DIAGNOSIS FOR COMMON CLINICAL PRESENTATIONS OF MOVEMENT DISORDERS   An algorithm for the interpretation of abnormal movements is illustrated in Fig. 21-5. The initial step is to determine if the movement disorder is due to an excess or a poverty of movement (e.g., a hyperkinetic or a hypokinetic movement disorder).

Hyperkinetic Movement Disorders   Abnormal involuntary movements are divided into those that are rhythmical and those that are irregular. Those that are rhythmical are termed *tremors*. Tremors are divided into three types: rest tremor, postural tremor, and intention tremor. A *rest tremor* is maximal at rest and becomes less prominent with activity. It is characteristic of parkinsonism, a hypokinetic movement disorder, and is therefore commonly associated with bradykinesia and cogwheel rigidity. A rest tremor that develops acutely is usually due to toxins [such as exposure to 1-methyl-4-phenyl-1,2,3,6-tetrahydropyridine (MPTP)] or dopamine blocking drugs (such as phenothiazines). If insidious in onset, the diagnostic approach is the same as for Parkinson's disease (Chap. 368). A *postural tremor* is maximal while limb posture is actively maintained against gravity; it is lessened

FIGURE 21-4*A, B, C*   Diagram of the normal major functional connections and neurotransmitters involved in the basal ganglia circuits. *A.* The striatum receives glutamatergic afferents from the sensorimotor cortex and dopaminergic afferents from the substantia nigra pars compacta. The major output of the basal ganglia is GABA-ergic inhibition from the globus pallidus interna and the substantia nigra pars reticulata to the ventral anterior and ventral lateral nuclei of the thalamus. The striatum projects to the output nuclei by a direct and an indirect pathway. *B.* Parkinson's disease results from a loss of dopaminergic projections from the substantia nigra pars compacta to the striatum. Loss of

D_1 receptor stimulation results in disinhibition of the output nuclei by the direct pathway. Loss of D_2 receptor inhibition results in excitation of the output nuclei by the indirect pathway. Thus, inhibition of the thalamus is abnormally increased and cortically initiated movements are not facilitated. *C.* Huntington's chorea results from early loss of striatal neurons that express D_2 receptors and normally project GABA-ergic inhibition to the globus pallidus externa. This causes disinhibition of the thalamus and excess thalamocortical excitation of movements. GABA, gamma-aminobutyric acid; Glu, glutamate; ——➤, excitatory; --–➤, inhibitory.

by rest and is not markedly enhanced during voluntary movement toward a target. A postural tremor that develops acutely is usually due to toxic or metabolic factors (for example, hyperthyroidism) or stress. The insidious onset of a postural tremor suggests a benign or familial essential tremor (Chap. 368). An *intention tremor* is most prominent during voluntary movement toward a target and is not present during postural maintenance or at rest. It is a sign of cerebellar disease (Chap. 369). *Asterixis*, which may superficially resemble a tremor, is an intermittent inhibition of muscle contraction that occurs with metabolic encephalopathy. This leads, for example, to a momentary and repetitive partial flexion of the wrists during attempted sustained wrist extension (Chap. 380).

Abnormal involuntary movements that are irregular are characterized further by their speed and site of occurrence and by whether they can be suppressed voluntarily. The slowest are athetosis and dystonia. *Athetosis* is a slow writhing, sinuous movement that occurs nearly continuously in distal muscles. *Dystonia* is a slowly varying but nearly continuous deviation of posture about one or more joints; it may occur in a proximal or distal limb or in axial structures. Dystonia is a more sustained deviation of posture than athetosis, although these two phenomena overlap considerably. The further evaluation of athetosis and dystonia are discussed in Chap. 368.

Among the rapid irregular movements, *tics* are controlled with voluntary effort, while the others are not. Tics often occur repetitively in a single location but are sometimes multifocal (Chap. 368).

Chorea, hemiballismus, and myoclonus are rapid, irregular jerks that cannot be consciously suppressed. *Hemiballismus* is the most distinctive among them. It is manifest as a sudden and often violent flinging movement of a proximal limb, usually an arm (Chap. 368). Hemiballismus usually develops acutely due to infarction of the contralateral subthalamic nucleus but occasionally develops subacutely or chronically due to other lesions of this nucleus.

Chorea is a rapid, jerky, irregular movement that tends to occur in the distal limbs or face but may also occur in proximal limb and axial structures. Acute onset is usually toxic due to excess levodopa or dopamine-agonist therapy. In children, it may be associated with rheumatic fever and, in such cases, is referred to as *Sydenham's chorea*. The gradual onset of chorea is typical of degenerative neurologic diseases, such as Huntington's chorea (Chap. 367).

Myoclonus is a rapid, brief, irregular movement that is usually multifocal. Myoclonus can occur spontaneously at rest, in response to sensory stimuli, or with voluntary movements. It is a symptom that occurs in a wide variety of metabolic and neurologic disorders. Posthypoxic intention myoclonus is a special myoclonic syndrome that occurs as a sequel to transient cerebral anoxia. Myoclonus may result from lipid storage disease, encephalitis, Creutzfeldt-Jakob disease, or metabolic encephalopathies due to respiratory failure, chronic renal failure, hepatic failure, or electrolyte imbalance. Myoclonus is also a feature of certain types of epilepsy, as discussed in Chap. 365.

Hypokinetic Movement Disorders These syndromes are manifest as bradykinesia, with a masked expressionless facial appearance, loss of associated limb movements during walking, and rigid en bloc turning. If bradykinesia is associated only with a rest tremor, cogwheel rigidity, or impairment of postural reflexes (especially with a tendency to fall backwards), Parkinson's disease is likely (Chap. 368). If cognitive, language, upper motor neuron, sensory, or autonomic signs are also present, a multisystem *degenerative neurologic disease* is present. → *These disorders are discussed in Chaps. 368, 369, and 371.*

IMBALANCE AND DISORDERS OF GAIT

Imbalance is the impaired ability to maintain the intended orientation of the body in space. It is generally manifest as difficulty in maintaining an upright posture while standing or walking; a severe imbalance may also affect the ability to maintain posture while seated. Patients with imbalance commonly complain of a feeling of unsteadiness or dysequilibrium. Whereas imbalance and unsteadiness are synonymous, *dysequilibrium* implies the additional component of impaired spatial orientation even while lying down. Patients with dysequilibrium commonly also experience *vertigo*, defined as an hallucination of rotatory movement.

PATHOGENESIS OF IMBALANCE AND DISORDERS OF GAIT Imbalance Imbalance results from disorders of the spinocerebellar or vestibular sensory input, the integration of these inputs in the brainstem or cerebellum, or the motor output to the spinal neurons that control axial and proximal muscles.

The position of the head in space is normally detected by the inner ear. The utricle and saccule are sensitive to static head position and acceleration by sensing the direction of gravitational pull and changes in it. The semicircular canals are sensitive to rotatory motion. These sensations for static head position and movement are transmitted by the vestibular nerve to the vestibular nuclei in the lower pons and upper medulla (Fig. 21-6). Excitatory input from the vestibular nerve and nuclei is to the fastigial nucleus deep in the midline of the cerebellum and via glutamatergic mossy fibers to overlying ipsilateral granule cells of the flocculonodular cerebellar cortex.

The position of the head relative to the limbs and trunk is detected by receptors that respond to joint position, joint movement, and shortening or lengthening of muscle spindles in axial and proximal limb muscles. This sensory input is transmitted both along the posterior column and medial lemniscal pathways to the cerebrum and the spinocerebellar

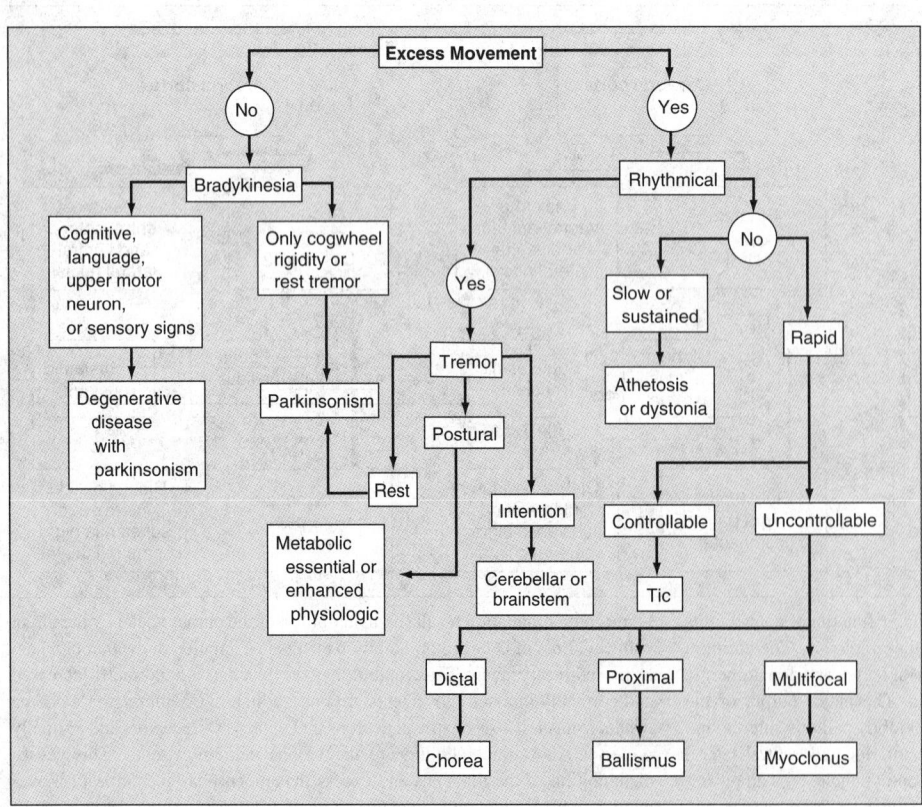

FIGURE 21-5 An algorithm for interpretation of abnormal movements.

pathways to the cerebellum. For the automatic maintenance of balance, proprioceptive sensory input ascends up the spinal cord in the ventral and dorsal spinocerebellar tracts and, for the head position, the cuneocerebellar tracts (Fig. 21-6). These enter the cerebellum as excitatory, glutamatergic mossy fiber inputs to the granule cells in the ipsilateral midline vermal cerebellar cortex and the ipsilateral fastigial nucleus. Visual input, by way of the tectum of the midbrain, is transmitted to the cerebellum through similar, excitatory mossy fibers.

The midline cerebellar cortex and nuclei are of paramount importance in the integration of these inputs and in control of appropriate motor responses required to maintain normal balance. In both midline and lateral cerebellar cortices, several neuronal cell types mediate these complex interactions. The Purkinje cells of the middle cortical layer are the principal outflow neurons of cerebellar cortical activity. They have inhibitory GABA-ergic projections to the deep cerebellar nuclei. The granule cells of the inner cellular layer project an extensive network of axons to the outer molecular layer as parallel fibers, which run parallel to the long axis of the folia. The parallel fibers produce a weak excitatory, glutamatergic influence on the dendrites of many Purkinje cells in the molecular layer and on the basket and stellate cells, which are the interneurons of the molecular layer. Both basket and stellate cells have inhibitory projections onto the Purkinje cells. Basket cell axons run perpendicular to the parallel fibers and produce GABA-ergic inhibition on Purkinje cell bodies just outside the band of parallel fiber excitation. Thus, basket cells provide center-surround antagonism in the cerebellar cortex. A third inhibitory neuron that acts in the cerebellar cortex is the Golgi cell, which is found at the outer border of the granular layer. Golgi dendrites project to the molecular layer, where they receive excitatory parallel fiber input. The Golgi cells exert GABA-ergic feedback inhibition to the granule cells. The major output of the cerebellar cortex is inhibition of the deep cerebellar nuclei by the Purkinje cells. The deep cerebellar nuclei receive excitatory input from mossy fibers.

The major cerebellar output for balance is from the fastigial nuclei to the vestibular nuclei and reticular formation and, to a lesser extent, directly from the midline Purkinje cells to the vestibular nuclei. Vestibular nuclei and reticular formation project descending vestibulospinal and reticulospinal output via the ventromedial pathways to control the axial and proximal muscles of the limbs and trunk (Fig. 21-1).

The speed, fluency, and integration of limb movements are also controlled by the cerebellum. Spinocerebellar proprioceptive feedback from the limbs projects onto the granule cells in the ipsilateral intermediate cerebellar cortex and the ipsilateral interposed (globose and emboliform) nuclei as excitatory, glutamatergic mossy fiber inputs (Fig. 21-7). The major output system from the interposed nuclei is to the magnocellular portion of the contralateral red nucleus and then to the descending rubrospinal pathway, which is the major ventrolateral bulbospinal pathway that facilitates limb movements, in part through activation of gamma motor neurons.

The lateral cerebellar hemispheres coordinate a complex feedback circuit that modulates cortically initiated limb movement. Cortical motor commands influence the cerebellar hemispheres indirectly through pontocerebellar mossy fibers and olivocerebellar climbing fibers (Fig. 21-8). Descending corticopontine fibers excite the ipsilateral pontine nuclei. The pontocerebellar fibers decussate in the pons, project to the cerebellum through the middle cerebellar peduncle, and excite the granule cells and the dentate nucleus of the contralateral cerebellar hemisphere. The inferior olivary nucleus of the medulla receives input from the cortex as collaterals from corticospinal axons and from the basal ganglia, red nucleus, and reticular formation. Excitatory, climbing fibers from the inferior olivary nuclei decussate, pass through the inferior cerebellar peduncle, and stimulate the Purkinje cells of the lateral cerebellar hemispheres and dentate nuclei. The excitatory climbing fibers use aspartate as a neurotransmitter. The output from the cerebellar hemispheres is predominantly via the dentate nuclei to the parvocellular component of the contralateral red nucleus, to the ventrolateral nucleus of the thalamus, and then to the motor and premotor cerebral cortex. Lesions along this circuit result in cerebellar limb ataxia.

Sensory ataxia is caused by lesions that affect the peripheral sensory fibers, dorsal root ganglia cells, posterior columns of the spinal cord, lemniscal system in the brainstem, thalamus, or parietal cortex; relevant anatomy is discussed in Chap. 23. Impairment of the proprioceptive sensory feedback to the cerebellum, basal ganglia, and cortex produces sensory ataxia. Sensory ataxia results in imbalance and disturbs the fluency and integration of movements that can be partially alleviated by visual feedback.

Disorders of Gait Walking is one of the most complicated and common motor activities of daily life. Essentially all structures discussed in this chapter participate in normal walking. Cyclical stepping movements produced by the lumbosacral spinal cord centers are modified by cortical, basal ganglionic, brainstem, and cerebellar influences based on proprioceptive, vestibular, and visual feedback.

FIGURE 21-6 Cerebellar control of balance. The vestibular and spinocerebellar mossy fiber afferents excite the granule cells in the flocculonodular and vermal cortex and the fastigial nuclei. The Purkinje cells of the cerebellar cortex inhibit the fastigial nuclei. The major efferent projections are from the fastigial nucleus to the vestibular nuclei and the reticular formation. The vermis is a central portion of the cerebellum that is not illustrated in the figure because it overlies the brainstem and fastigial nuclei.

Labels in figure: Fastigial nucleus; Purkinje fibers; Flocculo-nodular lobe; Vestibular nerve; Ventral and dorsal spinocerebellar tracts; Dorsal spinocerebellar tract; Ventral spinocerebellar tract; Tegmentum; Juxtarestiform body; Vestibular nuclei; Reticular nuclei

DIAGNOSTIC APPROACH AND DIFFERENTIAL DIAGNOSIS FOR COMMON CLINICAL PRESENTATIONS OF IMBALANCE AND ABNORMAL GAIT **Examination for Imbalance, Incoordination, and Abnormal Gait** Neurologic examination of coordination, balance, and gait is typically performed together. The patient performs several maneuvers with each limb while coordination is assessed. The finger-nose-finger and the heel-knee-shin maneuvers are observed for signs of incoordination in general and dysmetria in particular. *Dysmetria* consists of irregular errors in the distance and force of limb movements. This is accentuated near the target or point of intention and hence termed *intention tremor*. The patient is also asked to maintain the arms outstretched against a resistance that is suddenly removed; excessive rebound indicates cerebellar dysfunction. The ability of the patient to rapidly and repetitively tap the hands and feet is assessed for speed and rhythmicity. Slow, coarse, but rhythmical movements indicate upper motor neuron incoordination. Errors in rhythm and irregular rate indicate cerebellar disease; this is most readily demonstrated by asking the patient to perform rapidly alternating movements. During attempts to tap alternately the dorsal and palmar surfaces of the hand as rapidly as possible, the rate, rhythm, and regularity of force cannot be sustained, a sign called *dysdiadochokinesia*. The patient is asked to demonstrate how to comb the hair or brush the teeth to assess the ability to initiate and execute a simple sequence of activity. Balance is examined by having the patient stand stationary with the feet together. If this position can be maintained, the eyes are closed for 5 to 10 s. Accentuation of sway or actual loss of balance is assessed. If balance is momentarily lost, several trials may be necessary to determine if the loss is consistently in the same direction. Walking along an uncrowded space, such as a hallway, is observed for 20 m or more. Symmetry of arm swing and various phases of the gait cycle are observed. Walking is then performed for several steps on the heels, on the toes, and in tandem.

Imbalance An algorithm for the interpretation of imbalance is presented in Fig. 21-9.

Cerebellar ataxia results from disorders of the cerebellum or of its afferent inputs or efferent projections. The examination frequently assists in localizing the anatomic site responsible for the ataxia. Abnormalities of the midline cerebellar vermis or the flocculonodular lobe are usually revealed during the process of rising from a chair, assuming the upright stance with the feet together, or performing some other activity while standing. Once a desired position is reached, imbalance may be surprisingly mild. As walking begins, the imbalance recurs. Patients usually learn to lessen the imbalance by walking with the legs widely separated. The imbalance is usually not lateralized and may be accompanied by symmetric nystagmus if the flocculonodular lobe or its connections are affected. These abnormalities of the midline vermis characteristically produce truncal ataxia; dysmetria of the lower limbs with intention tremor may also be present.

Abnormalities of the intermediate and lateral portions of the cerebellum typically produce impaired limb movements rather than truncal ataxia. If involvement is asymmetric, lateralized imbalance is common and usually associated with asymmetric nystagmus. Clinical signs of cerebellar limb ataxia include dysmetria, intention tremor, dysdiadochokinesia, and abnormal rebound. Muscle tone is often modestly reduced; this contributes to the abnormal rebound due to decreased activation of segmental spinal cord reflexes and also to pendular reflexes, i.e., a tendency for a tendon reflex to produce multiple swings to and fro after a single tap. Cerebellar diseases are discussed in Chap. 369.

Imbalance with vestibular dysfunction is characterized by a consistent tendency to fall to one side. The patient commonly complains of vertigo rather than imbalance, especially if the onset is acute. Acute vertigo associated with lateralized imbalance but no other neurologic signs is often due to disorders of the semicircular canal (Chaps. 20 and 372); the presence of other neurologic signs suggests brainstem ischemia (Chap. 366) or demyelinating disease (Chap. 376). When the vestibular dysfunction is peripheral, positional nystagmus and vertigo tend to resolve if a provocative position is maintained (extinction) or repeated (habituation). Lateralized imbalance of gradual onset or persisting for more than 2 weeks, accompanied by nystagmus, may result from lesions of the semicircular canal or vestibular nerve (Chap. 372), brainstem, or cerebellum.

Imbalance with sensory ataxia is characterized by marked worsening when visual feedback is removed. The patient can often assume the upright stance with feet together cautiously with eyes open. With eye closure, balance is rapidly lost (positive Romberg sign) in various directions at random. Sensory examination reveals impairment of proprioception at the toes and ankles, usually associated with an even more prominent abnormality of vibratory perception. Prompt evaluation for vitamin B_{12} deficiency is important, as this disorder is reversible if recognized early (Chap. 380). Depression or absence of reflexes points to peripheral nerve disorders (Chap. 381). Spasticity with extensor plantar responses suggest posterior column and spinal cord disorders (Chap. 373). Rarely, sensory ataxia produces lateralized imbalance. In these cases, the disorder is usually in the parietal lobe or thalamus (Chap. 23), but may also be due to

FIGURE 21-7 The most direct cerebellar control of limb movements is mediated by the rubrospinal pathway. Spinocerebellar afferents excite the granule cells of the intermediate hemispheres and the interposed nuclei. The interposed nuclei excite the magnocellular portion of the contralateral red nucleus.

an asymmetric sensory neuropathy (Chap. 381) or posterior column disease (Chap. 373).

Sensory limb ataxia is similar to cerebellar limb ataxia but is markedly worse when the eyes are closed. Examination also reveals abnormal proprioception and vibratory perception. The approach focuses on localizing the proprioceptive impairment to the peripheral nerves (Chap. 381), the posterior columns of the spinal cord (Chap. 373), or rarely the parietal lobe.

Other forms of imbalance occur, but the fundamental problem is usually a primary disorder of strength, extrapyramidal function, or cortical initiation of movement.

Abnormal Gait Each of the disorders discussed in this chapter produces a characteristic gait disturbance. If the neurologic examination is normal, except for an abnormal gait, diagnosis may be difficult, even for the experienced clinician.

Hemiparetic gait characterizes spastic hemiparesis. In its most severe form, an abnormal posture of the limbs is produced by spasticity. The shoulder is adducted and internally rotated, with flexion of the elbow, wrist, and fingers and with extension of the hip, knee, and ankle. Forward swing of the spastic leg during walking requires abduction and circumduction at the hip, often with contralateral tilt of the trunk. In its mildest form, the affected arm is held in a normal position, but swings less than the normal arm. The affected leg is flexed less than the normal leg during its forward swing and is more externally rotated. A hemiparetic gait is a common residual sign of a stroke (Chap. 366).

Paraparetic gait is a walking pattern in which both legs are moved in a slow, stiff manner with circumduction, similar to the leg movement in an hemiparetic gait. In many patients, the legs tend to cross with each forward swing ("scissoring"). A paraparetic gait is a common sign of spinal cord disease (Chap. 373) and also occurs in cerebral palsy.

Steppage gait is produced by weakness of ankle dorsiflexion. Because of the partial or complete foot drop, the leg must be lifted higher than usual to avoid catching the toe on the floor during the forward swing of the leg. If unilateral, steppage gait is usually due to L5 radiculopathy, sciatic neuropathy, or peroneal neuropathy (Chap. 381). If bilateral, it is the common result of a distal polyneuropathy or lumbosacral polyradiculopathy (Chap. 381).

Waddling gait results from proximal lower limb weakness, most often from myopathy (Chap. 383) but occasionally from neuromuscular junction disease (Chap. 382) or a proximal symmetric spinal muscular atrophy (Chap. 370). With weakness of hip flexion, the trunk is tilted away from the leg that is being moved to lift the hip and provide extra distance between the foot and the floor, and the pelvis is rotated forward to assist with forward motion of the leg. Because pelvic girdle weakness is customarily bilateral, the pelvic lift and rotation alternates from side to side, giving the waddling appearance to the gait.

Parkinsonian gait is characterized by a forward stoop, with modest flexion at the hips and knees. The arms are flexed at the elbows and adducted at the shoulders, often with a 4- to 6-Hz resting pronation-supination tremor but little other movement, even during walking. Walking is initiated slowly by leaning forward and maintained with short rapid steps, during which the feet shuffle along the floor. The pace tends to accelerate (festinate) as the upper body gradually leans further ahead of the feet, whether movement is forwards (propulsion) or backwards (retropulsion). The postural instability leads to falls (Chap. 368).

Apraxic gait results from bilateral frontal lobe disease with impaired ability to plan and execute sequential movements. This gait superficially resembles that of parkinsonism, in that the posture is stooped and any steps taken are short and shuffling. However, initiation and maintenance of walking are impaired in a different manner. Each movement that is required for walking can usually be performed, if tested in isolation while sitting or lying. However, when asked to step forward while standing, a long pause often occurs before any attempt is made to flex at the hip and advance. Furthermore, once walking is initiated, it is not maintained, even in an abnormal festinating manner. Rather, after one or several steps are taken, walking is stopped for several seconds or longer. The process is then repeated. This gait is usually accompanied by dementia (Chap. 367).

Choreoathetotic gait is characterized by an intermittent, irregular movement that disrupts the smooth flow of a normal gait. Flexion or extension movements at the hip are common and unpredictable but readily observed as a pelvic lurch (Chap. 368).

Cerebellar ataxic gait is a broad-based gait disorder in which the speed and length of stride varies irregularly from step to step. With midline cerebellar disease, as in alcoholics (Chap. 380), posture is erect but the feet are separated; lower limb ataxia is commonly present as well. Assumption of a particular stance or a change in position may cause instability, yet balance can usually be maintained well with the eyes open or closed. Walking may be rapid but cadence is irregular. Although patients commonly lack confidence in the stability of their walking, minimal support is often required for reassurance. With disease of the cerebellar hemispheres, limb ataxia and nystagmus are commonly present as well (Chap. 369).

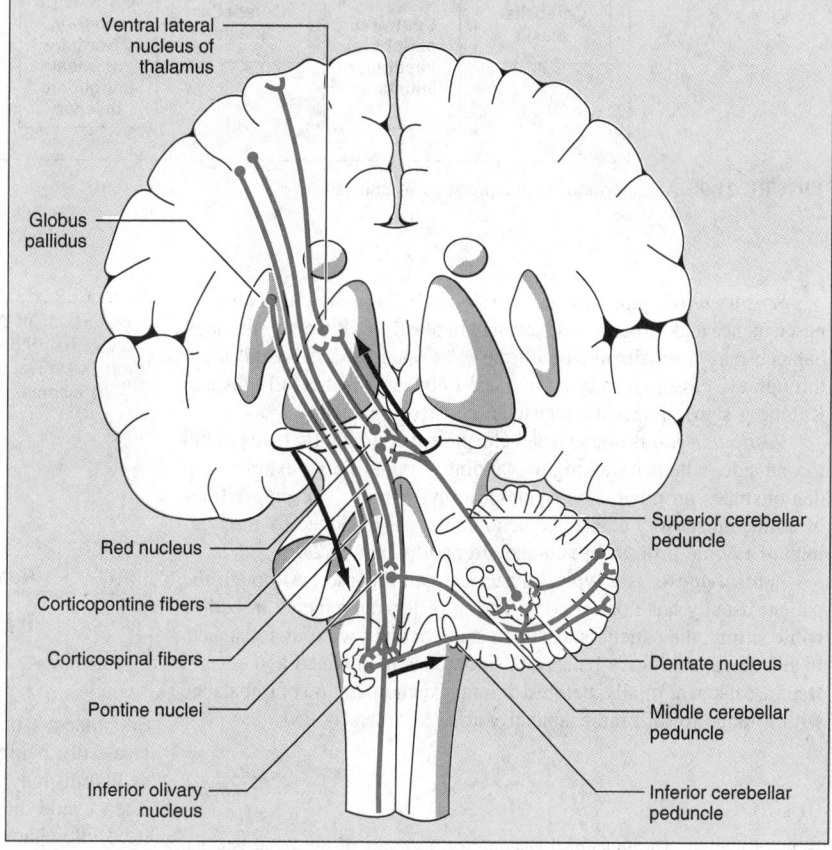

FIGURE 21-8 Cerebellar modulation of cortically initiated movement is mediated by a complex feedback circuit that involves the lateral cerebellar hemispheres. In response to stimulation by corticopontine fibers, pontocerebellar fibers decussate in the pons, project to the cerebellum through the middle cerebellar peduncle, and excite the granule cells and the dentate nucleus of the contralateral cerebellar hemisphere. The inferior olivary nucleus of the medulla projects excitatory, climbing fibers to the Purkinje cells of the contralateral lateral cerebellar hemispheres and dentate nuclei. The cerebellar output is predominantly to the contralateral red nucleus, to the ventrolateral nucleus of the thalamus, and from there to the motor and premotor cerebral cortex.

FIGURE 21-9 An algorithm for interpretation of imbalance.

Sensory ataxic gait may resemble a cerebellar gait, with its broad-based stance and difficulty with change in position. However, although balance may be maintained with the eyes open, loss of visual input through eye closure results in rapid loss of balance with a fall (positive Romberg sign), unless the physician assists the patient.

Vestibular gait is one in which the patient consistently tends to fall to one side, whether walking or standing. Cranial nerve examination demonstrates an obviously asymmetric nystagmus. The possibilities of unilateral sensory ataxia and hemiparesis are excluded by the findings of normal proprioception and strength (Chap. 372).

Astasia-abasia is a typical hysterical gait disorder. Although the patient usually has normal coordination of leg movements in bed or while sitting, the patient is unable to stand or walk without assistance. If distracted, stationary balance is sometimes maintained and several steps are taken normally, before a dramatic demonstration of imbalance with a lunge toward the examiner's arms or a nearby bed.

BIBLIOGRAPHY

ALBIN RL et al: The functional anatomy of disorders of the basal ganglia. Trends Neurosci 18:63, 1995

BRODAL A: *Neurological Anatomy in Relation to Clinical Medicine*, 3d ed. Oxford, Oxford University Press, 1981

COLES SK et al: The mesencephalic centre controlling locomotion in the rat. Neuroscience 28:149, 1989

HORE J et al: Cerebellar dysmetria at the elbow, wrist, and fingers. J Neurophysiol 65:563, 1991

JAGIELLA WM, SUNG JH: Bilateral infarction of the medullary pyramids in humans. Neurology 39:21, 1989

KANDEL ER et al: *Principles of Neural Science*, 3d ed. New York, Elsevier, 1991

ROSS CA et al: Messenger molecules in the cerebellum. Trends Neurosci 13:216, 1990

WICHMANN T et al: Parkinson's disease and the basal ganglia: Lessons from the laboratory and from neurosurgery. Neuroscientist 1:236, 1995

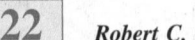

Robert C. Griggs

EPISODIC MUSCLE SPASMS, CRAMPS, AND WEAKNESS

Spontaneous or exercise-related discomfort from muscles or joints is usually benign and does not signal neuromuscular disease. Such symptoms may, however, provide clues to disabling disorders that too often evade diagnosis. The terms *pain*, *spasm*, and *cramp* are often used interchangeably by patients to describe symptoms referable to muscles. Other terms including *aching*, *heaviness*, and *stiffness* are also used and usually connote less certainty about the localization of the discomfort. In clinical terminology, *spasm* refers to a brief, unsustained contraction of a single or multiple muscles. *Cramp* is a paroxysmal, spontaneous, prolonged, and painful contraction of one or more muscles. Muscle pain may be associated with fatigue (asthenia) or weakness. This chapter discusses both fatigue and episodic weakness. The usual causes of weakness are considered in Chap. 21.

SPASMS Abnormal movements of muscle may arise from abnormal electrical activity of the central nervous system (CNS) mediated via the motor neuron or occur within the motor neuron or muscle fiber itself. It may be difficult on clinical grounds alone to determine the precise site of origin of the abnormal motor activity. In general, movements originating in the CNS affect the entire side of the body, an entire limb, or a group of muscles. Central disorders may be rhythmic or intermittent; those arising in the periphery are usually random. The electroencephalogram (EEG) may provide evidence for altered cortical activity in some conditions with a CNS etiology. The electromyogram (EMG) is less helpful because it reflects motor activity from any cause. EMG evidence of an underlying nerve or muscle disease may, however, be helpful in diagnosis (see Chap. 361).

Intermittent, nonrhythmic movements of an entire limb, of the trunk, or of a portion of the face may result from cerebral seizure activity (Chap. 361) or from myoclonus (Chap. 21). Flexor and extensor spasms of an entire side or of the lower limbs result from a loss of motor inhibition within the CNS (Chap. 21). *Segmental myoclonus* results from focal disease within the brainstem or spinal cord that causes an abnormal discharge of groups of motor neurons. Localized vascular disease, tumor, or another lesion may be implicated.

Abnormal Facial Movements *Hemifacial spasm* results from paroxysmal facial nerve activity, sometimes triggered by pressure from a tortuous blood vessel adjacent to the facial nerve as it leaves the brainstem. Hemifacial spasm commonly occurs in muscles about the eye but also may involve or spread to the entire side of the face. Symptoms are often intermittent and intensified when patients are using facial muscles in activities such as speaking. Hemifacial spasm is painless but embarrassing, especially to individuals dealing with the public. Since it is often intensified and more severe when the patient is in stressful situations, an erroneous diagnosis of tic is often made. Cerebellopontine angle lesions can occasionally produce a similar disorder. Neuroradiologic investigation is indicated in patients with hemifacial spasm. Injection of botulinum toxin into involved muscles alleviates spasm for up to 3 months; surgical exploration and shielding of the facial nerve from the adjacent vessel is often curative (Chap. 372).

Facial *tics* are stereotyped movements of the face such as eye blinking, head turning, or grimacing that are under voluntary control but may be suppressed only by effort and anxiety on the part of the subject (see Chap. 21). Some tics are so frequently encountered as to be considered mannerisms, analogous to excessive clearing of the throat. The repetitious elevation of the eyebrows by frontalis muscle contraction is an example. Certain hereditary movement disorders such as Gilles de la Tourette syndrome are characterized by multiple tics. Tics can often be controlled by neuroleptic agents (Chap. 21).

Synkinesias of the face result from aberrant regeneration of the facial nerve following facial paralysis from Bell's palsy or other facial nerve lesions. Nearly 50 percent of patients who recover from Bell's palsy display such movements; an example is *jaw winking*, where voluntary movements of the lower face elicit contraction of the orbicularis oculi muscle with unilateral eye closure (see Chap. 372).

Trigeminal neuralgia (tic douloureux) is characterized by brief, paroxysmal, lancinating pain in one side of the face (see Chap. 372). Although the portion of the nerve involved is almost exclusively sensory, the severity of the pain causes involuntary contraction of facial muscles, hence the name *tic*. Abnormal movements do not occur in the absence of pain.

Facial myokymia refers to a nearly continuous twitching of facial muscles. Although often benign, it may result from lesions of the pons such as a neoplasm or multiple sclerosis. Facial and limb myokymia occur in association with episodic ataxia in hereditary defects of nerve potassium ion channels. Similar movements occur in motor neuron diseases such as amyotrophic lateral sclerosis (see Chaps. 363 and 383).

Abnormal Limb Movements No movement should be visible in totally relaxed muscles. Diseases of motor neurons or their proximal axons are often associated with *fasciculations*, the spontaneous firing of an entire motor unit. Fasciculations are visible on inspection of muscle or perceived by the patient as a pulsation or quivering within

muscle. Fasciculations occur at times in most normal individuals, and unless weakness is present, they are seldom of any significance. Fasciculations are normal if observed in incompletely relaxed muscles and are frequently observed at rest in the calves of normal individuals. *Myokymia*, consisting of numerous, repetitive fasciculations, also may occur in limb muscles, giving a writhing appearance. Myokymia disappears with neuromuscular blockade, proving that the activity originates in anterior horn cells or in peripheral nerve. In patients with long-standing muscle denervation and reinnervation, motor unit size enlarges and fasciculations may be so large as to produce movement of the limbs, particularly of the fingers, a condition termed *minipoly-myoclonus*.

Certain conditions are characterized by a compulsion to move the extremities. *Akathisia*, or motor restlessness, occurs in Parkinson's disease and other disorders of the basal ganglia, including drug-induced movement disorders. The *restless legs syndrome* describes an uncomfortable sensation in muscles, usually in the legs and thighs, that occurs most commonly in middle-aged women. Patients feel they need to move their legs to relieve the abnormal sensation. The restless legs syndrome is frequent in uremia and may occur in other neuropathies, suggesting that the sensation is caused by an underlying neuropathy. It also may be familial, and detailed study of such patients has failed to demonstrate any evidence of neuropathy. The restless sensation may be accompanied by myoclonic jerks of muscle. These myoclonic jerks are similar to the myoclonus observed in normal individuals entering REM sleep (see Chap. 27).

These forms of muscle spasm and myoclonus are somewhat similar to a group of unusual *startle* syndromes or *hyperexplexias* characterized by sudden jerking of limbs or occasionally of trunk muscles. Sudden noise or touch may cause a patient to jump or to fling an extremity. Hyperexplexias result from mutations in the glycine receptor (see Chap. 363).

SUSTAINED MUSCLE CONTRACTIONS Distinguishing central from peripheral causes of sustained muscle contraction is often difficult. Abnormal muscle contractions with increased muscle tone usually result from CNS disease. Thus loss or disturbance of CNS inhibition may lead to abnormal muscle contraction characteristic of spasticity, rigidity, or "paratonic" rigidity. In most instances there is other evidence of CNS disorder (Chap. 21). Diseases of the basal ganglia, many of them hereditary, may lead to dystonia (see Chaps. 21 and 363).

Abnormal muscle contractions also may arise from repetitive depolarization of the component portions of the motor unit: the motor neuron, the peripheral axon of the neuron, the neuromuscular junction, or muscle fibers. Electrically inactive contractions may arise from disorders of the muscle contractile system.

Motor Neuron Disorders *Cramp* is a term often used by patients to refer to a painful, involuntary contraction of a single muscle or a muscle group. Muscle cramps can arise from spontaneous firing of groups of anterior horn cells followed by contraction of many motor units. EMG recordings indicate that motor units fire at a rate of up to 300 per second, much higher than occurs with voluntary contraction. Cramps occur frequently in the legs in elderly patients and, when severe, are followed by residual tenderness and evidence of muscle fiber necrosis, including elevation of serum creatine kinase. Cramps in the calf muscles are so common as to be considered normal, but more generalized cramps may be a sign of chronic disease of the motor neuron, such as amyotrophic lateral sclerosis. They may be particularly troublesome during pregnancy, in patients with electrolyte disturbances (hyponatremia), and in patients on hemodialysis. When recurrent and localized to one muscle group, they suggest nerve root disease. In many instances, however, it is impossible to determine the cause of cramps. Benign cramps, occurring commonly at night, may be relieved by quinine sulfate. Other causes of contractions arising from the motor neuron include *tetanus* (Chap. 146) and the *stiff-man syndrome*. In both disorders, a loss of inhibitory neuronal input to anterior horn cells may result in repeated firing of motor neurons, producing severe, painful muscle contraction. Antibodies to glutamic acid decarboxylase are often present in the stiff-man syndrome, and the disorder may respond to plasma exchange. A similar clinical picture may occur acutely with *strychnine poisoning*. Diazepam improves these spasms but may cause respiratory depression in doses sufficient to alleviate muscle contraction.

Peripheral Nerve Disorders *Tetany* is characterized by contractions of predominantly distal muscles, particularly in the hand (carpal spasm) and feet (pedal spasm). Laryngospasm also may occur. Tetany results from increased excitability of peripheral nerves. The muscle contractions are initially painless, but if sustained, they may cause muscle damage with pain. Severe tetany may involve spine musculature to produce opisthotonus. Tetany is usually caused by hypocalcemia, but it may occur with hypomagnesemia or severe respiratory alkalosis (see Chap. 354). Idiopathic normocalcemic tetany, *spasmophilia*, occurs in both hereditary and acquired forms. The acquired disorder is similar to Isaac's syndrome (neuromyotonia), in which hyperexcitability of peripheral nerve leads to muscle cramps and twitching. Such patients have responded to plasma exchange and it may be mediated by IgG autoantibodies to nerve membrane potassium channels.

Muscle Disorders *Myotonia* Repetitive depolarization of muscle cells can cause muscle contraction resulting in muscle stiffness and impaired relaxation. Myotonia is usually painless, but it may disable patients by interfering with fine hand movements or by slowing ambulation. Myotonic dystrophy is the most common disorder associated with myotonia, although other manifestations of the disease such as cataracts and muscle weakness are usually more symptomatic. A similar disorder, proximal myotonic myopathy (PROMM), is associated with muscle pain (see Chap. 383). Myotonia congenita and paramyotonia congenita are less common but more troublesome in terms of severity of myotonia. Myotonia is often worsened by cold and characteristically is attenuated by repeated muscle activity. *Myotonia congenita* has both autosomal dominant and recessive variants. Myotonia results from defects in chloride channel function and can also result from defects of sodium channel function. One such disorder is paramyotonia congenita, which is characterized by *paradoxical myotonia*: myotonia that worsens with repeated activity. These patients also suffer from episodic and cold-induced weakness (see Chap. 383). Myotonia can often be alleviated by quinine, phenytoin, or mexiletine.

Contracture Muscle contracture is a painful shortening of a muscle unassociated with muscle membrane depolarization. It occurs in disorders where a metabolic defect such as myophosphorylase deficiency limits the production of high-energy phosphates. Contractures are precipitated by exercise, are usually intensely painful, and result in muscle damage; widespread muscle contractures may cause sufficient myoglobinuria to precipitate renal failure. This use of the term *contracture* is confusing because the same word is used to describe the unrelated limitation of joint movement by shortening of muscle tendons seen in rheumatologic disorders, cerebral palsy, or chronic myopathies. Muscle rigidity from metabolic contracture can occur in the malignant hyperthermia syndrome, usually associated with general anesthesia. In the neuroleptic malignant syndrome, muscle rigidity arises from CNS overactivity, and intense electrical activity is present in muscle.

MUSCLE PAIN, ACHING, AND TENDERNESS Painful muscles do not always imply muscle disease. Joint and bone disease frequently produces complaints of muscle pain and may further confuse the anatomic localization of symptoms by resulting in disuse atrophy and moderate muscle weakness. Pain from disease of overlying subcutaneous tissue or fascia and of tendons also may be referred to muscle. Additionally, disease of major peripheral nerves or of their small intramuscular branches may produce both muscle pain and weakness. Muscle pain may be a major symptom in inflammatory, metabolic, endocrine, and toxic myopathies (see Chaps. 315 and 383).

Muscle Trauma Vigorous activity, even in conditioned athletes, may be associated with muscle and tendon tears, which lead to temporary acute muscle pain, swelling, and tenderness. Rupture of muscle tendons such as the biceps or gastrocnemius muscle may produce visible muscle shortening. Many such tears resolve without surgery but leave an abnormal appearance to the muscle belly.

The almost-pleasurable ache and fatigue of muscles after strenuous activity is separable only by degree from more severe, but still normal pain following severe, unaccustomed activity. Such symptoms are often associated with laboratory evidence of profound muscle damage, including a rise in serum enzymes (creatine kinase), focal edema on magnetic resonance imaging (MRI), and widespread muscle necrosis on biopsy. Myoglobinuria may occur. Particularly likely to produce muscle pain and necrosis are certain types of exercise: brief periods of contracting a muscle while it is lengthening (eccentric contractions) and prolonged exercise such as marathon running. The point at which such symptoms become abnormal is not clear. Many patients have pain with moderate activity. Such exertional muscle pain is also characteristic of metabolic disorders of muscle such as carnitine palmitoyl transferase deficiency; patients with partial defects in *dystrophin* may have recurrent exercise-induced myalgias. Complete deficiency of this protein causes Duchenne muscular dystrophy (see Chap. 383). Deficiencies of enzymes of glycolysis are more commonly associated with contractures (see Chap. 383). The majority of patients with exertional and postexertional muscle pain do not have a definable abnormality.

Diffuse Myalgias Muscle pain in the absence of muscle weakness can occur in acute infections caused by influenza virus and coxsackievirus. Fibrositis, fibromyalgia, and fibromyositis are synonyms for a disorder associated with pain and tenderness of muscle and adjacent connective tissue. Focal "trigger points" of tenderness can be identified, and systemic symptoms such as fatigue, insomnia, and depression are frequently present (see Chap. 315). Although patients often identify painful swellings, histologic evaluation discloses no abnormality of muscle or connective tissue. Symptoms may respond partially to amitriptyline or nonsteroidal anti-inflammatory agents, but the disorder tends to be chronic and unrelenting. A supportive program of physical reconditioning is sometimes helpful. Patients whose symptoms persist for months or years are often considered to be depressed; whether depression causes or results from symptoms is unclear.

Polymyalgia rheumatica occurs in patients over age 50 and is characterized by stiffness and pain in shoulder and hip musculature. Despite symptoms of pain localized to muscles, there is convincing evidence that the disease includes a proximal, inflammatory arthritis; joint effusions are often present in knees and other peripheral joints as well. Patients often develop profound disuse atrophy of muscles and complain of weakness, giving rise to a suspicion of polymyositis. However, creatine kinase levels are usually normal, and muscle biopsy shows atrophy without evidence of muscle necrosis or inflammation. The erythrocyte sedimentation rate is elevated in most patients, and temporal arteritis may be present (see Chap. 319). Treatment with nonsteroidal anti-inflammatory agents is advocated except in patients with temporal arteritis, for whom prednisone (40 to 60 mg/d) is recommended. Patients with polymyalgia rheumatica who fail to respond to nonsteroidal anti-inflammatory agents may require low-dose prednisone (10 to 20 mg/d). Myalgias are also frequent in other rheumatologic disorders, including rheumatoid arthritis, systemic lupus erythematosus, polyarteritis nodosa, scleroderma, and the mixed connective tissue syndrome. Patients with polymyositis and dermatomyositis may have myalgias, although in the majority muscles are not painful (see Chap. 315).

Diagnostic Algorithm Complaints of muscle pain and fatigue are among the most frequent symptoms offered by patients. The decision as to which patients require extensive diagnostic tests can usually be made by history, examination, and routine blood studies (Fig. 22-1).

EPISODIC WEAKNESS The term *weakness* is often used by a patient to describe a loss of stamina or decreased "energy." Even careful efforts at eliciting a history of true as opposed to subjective weakness may fail to distinguish the two conditions. The most helpful strategy is to ask the patient to identify whether a discrete loss of

FIGURE 22-1 Evaluation of muscle pain and fatigue. CBC, complete blood count; ESR, erythrocyte sedimentation rate; T$_4$, thyroxine; TSH, thyroid-stimulating hormone.

function has occurred and to elicit the circumstances in which symptoms are noted.

Weakness, whether true or perceived, may be due to disorders of the central or peripheral nervous system. Weakness from CNS disorders such as transient cerebral ischemia is usually associated with a change in level of consciousness or cognition, with increased muscle tone and muscle stretch reflexes, and often with alterations of sensation. Most neuromuscular causes of intermittent weakness are associated with normal mental function, diminished muscle tone, and muscle stretch reflexes. The major causes of intermittent weakness are listed in Table 22-1. Central causes are considered in Chaps. 21 and 366.

Episodic Asthenia Patients who describe intermittent "weakness" but actually have *fatigue*, suffer from asthenia, which can be separated from true weakness by the fact that patients do not lack the ability to do a task but rather the ability to perform it repetitively. Asthenia is a major problem in many patients with serious renal, hepatic, cardiac, or pulmonary disease. Examination of such patients usually confirms their ability to do all functional activities at least once, such as rising from a knee bend, climbing stairs, or rising from a chair. Fatigue is also characteristic of relatively selective damage to CNS descending motor tracts, in which signs of neurologic abnormality may be minimal. Fatigue that is worsened by activity is characteristic of *chronic fatigue syndrome* (see Chap. 384).

Intermittent weakness due to peripheral neuromuscular disease may result from abrupt changes in peripheral nerve function, intermittent destruction of muscle, alterations of electrophysiologic properties of muscle from abnormalities of blood electrolytes, genetic diseases of muscle ion channels, and intermittent failure of neuromuscular transmission.

Failure of Peripheral Nerve Conduction A number of uncommon peripheral neuropathies are associated with recurrent weakness. *Hereditary liability to pressure palsies*, often termed *tomaculous neuropathy* because of the sausage-like appearance of myelin on nerve biopsy, is characterized by abrupt paralysis following compression of a peripheral nerve. The disease is autosomal dominant and results in many families from an abnormality in peripheral myelin protein (PMP–22) (see Chap. 363). The paralysis is usually self-limited, lasting days to weeks. Other types of peripheral neuropathy also may predispose to the development of reversible, compressive neuropathies (see Chap. 381).

Disordered Neuromuscular Junction Transmission *Myasthenia gravis*, particularly in its initial manifestations, is characterized by transient weakness. Cranial muscles are usually affected first, caus-

ing double vision, ptosis, dysphagia, and dysarthria. Rarely, limb weakness may herald the onset of myasthenia gravis and in the absence of cranial muscle dysfunction may escape diagnosis for months. Diurnal variation in strength is typical, with weakness worsening as the day wears on. Other, less-common defects of the neuromuscular junction such as the Lambert-Eaton syndrome also may present with intermittent weakness (see Chap. 382).

Intermittent Alterations in Electrolytes Transient shifts in serum potassium are associated with profound alterations in muscle strength. Although the primary periodic paralyses (hypo- and hyperkalemic periodic paralysis) spring to mind in a patient with weakness and an abnormality in serum potassium, other causes of abnormal serum potassium are more frequently behind episodic weakness (see Chap. 383). Familial periodic paralysis seldom presents after age 30; other causes are usually present in older patients. Hypokalemic periodic paralysis may occur in patients with hyperthyroidism. Episodic weakness due to hypokalemia may occur with renal or gastrointestinal potassium loss (see Table 22-1).

Hyperkalemic weakness usually occurs in the setting of chronic renal or adrenal disease. Other electrolyte disturbances may produce intermittent weakness as the initial clinical manifestation of a severe metabolic abnormality (see Table 22-1). Correction of the metabolic derangement improves the weakness.

Metabolic Muscle Disease A number of uncommon defects in glycogen and lipid utilization are associated with impaired energy production by muscle and cause intermittent weakness, usually accompanied by muscle pain and evidence of muscle damage. Carnitine palmitoyl transferase deficiency is one such condition. Mitochondrial disorders such as cytochrome oxidase deficiency may produce severe exercise intolerance with fatigue and weakness associated with lactic acidosis. Muscle pain and destruction seldom occur. (See also Chap. 383.)

Other Disorders Recurrent attacks of a feeling of "weakness" often occur in patients with the *hyperventilation syndrome*; such patients are, however, of normal strength when tested. Similarly, *recurrent hypoglycemic episodes* are associated with subjective weakness, although hypoglycemia is uncommon as the cause of this symptom.

Table 22-1

Causes of Episodic Generalized Weakness

1. Electrolyte disturbances
   a. Hypokalemia: Primary aldosteronism (Conn's syndrome); barium poisoning; renal tubular acidosis; juxtaglomerular apparatus hyperplasia (Bartter's syndrome); villous adenoma of colon; alcoholism; diuretics; licorice; para-aminosalicylic acid; glucocorticoids
   b. Hyperkalemia: Addison's disease; chronic renal failure; hyporeninemic hypoaldosteronism
   c. Hypercalcemia
   d. Hypocalcemic tetany
   e. Hyponatremia
   f. Hypophosphatemia
   g. Hypermagnesemia
2. Neuromuscular junction disorders
   a. Myasthenia gravis
   b. Lambert-Eaton syndrome
3. Muscle disorders
   a. Sodium and chloride channelopathies: Periodic paralyses and myotonias
   b. Metabolic defects of muscle (impaired carbohydrate or fatty acid utilization)
4. Central nervous system causes
   a. Cataplexy and sleep paralysis associated with narcolepsy
   b. Multiple sclerosis
   c. Transient ischemic attacks
5. Disorders with only subjective weakness: Hyperventilation, hypoglycemia

Central nervous system disorders may cause generalized weakness without an associated alteration of consciousness. *Drop attacks* resulting from impaired blood supply to the motor pathways of the brainstem cause sudden paraparesis or quadriparesis, usually lasting only a few seconds. Patients with narcolepsy may have sudden loss of muscle strength and tone during episodes of *cataplexy*. A disorder of the reticular activating system is responsible for these episodes as well as for *sleep paralysis* that occurs as narcoleptic patients are falling asleep or awakening (see Chap. 27).

BIBLIOGRAPHY

ARGOV Z: Phosphorus magnetic resonance spectroscopy (^{31}P MRS) in neuromuscular disorders. Ann Neurol 30:90, 1991

BERTOLASI L et al: The influence of muscular lengthening on cramps. Ann Neurol 33:176, 1993

DEMIRKIRAN M, JANKOVIC J: Paroxysmal dyskinesias: Clinical features and classification. Ann Neurol 38:571, 1995

EDWARDS RHT et al: Muscle biochemistry and pathophysiology in postviral fatigue syndrome. Br Med Bull 47:826, 1991

GRIGGS RC et al: *Evaluation and Treatment of Myopathies*. Philadelphia, F.A. Davis, 1995

LAYZER RB: Muscle pain, cramps, and fatigue, in *Myology*, AG Engel, C Franzini-Armstrong (eds). New York, McGraw-Hill, 1994, pp 1754–1768

O'KEEFFE ST: Restless legs syndrome. Arch Intern Med 156:243, 1996

PTACEK LJ et al: Genetics and physiology of the myotonic muscle disorders. N Engl J Med 328:482, 1993

23 *Arthur K. Asbury*

NUMBNESS, TINGLING, AND SENSORY LOSS

Normal somatic sensation is a continuous process that commands considerable moment-to-moment nervous system activity. Little of the activity intrudes on consciousness or exacts notice. In contrast, disordered sensation, particularly pains and paresthesias, may be highly intrusive, alarming, tenacious, and may dominate attention. Abnormalities of sensation tend to make patients seek prompt medical attention. When abnormal sensations are perceived as painful, medical advice is sought even more quickly. For a consideration of pain, see Chap. 12. The physician must be able to assess abnormal sensations, estimate their likely site of origin, and recognize their implications.

POSITIVE AND NEGATIVE PHENOMENA All abnormal sensory phenomena may be divided into two categories, positive and negative. Positive phenomena include tingling, pins-and-needles, pricking, bandlike sensations, lightning-like shooting feelings (lancinations), aching, and knifelike, twisting, drawing, pulling, tightening, burning, searing, electrical, and raw sensations. These descriptors are frequently the actual words used by patients. Such sensations may or may not be experienced as painful. The basis for positive phenomena is thought to be ectopic generation of volleys of impulses at a site of lowered neural threshold along the sensory pathways, either in peripheral or central sensory fibers. Such trains of ectopically generated afferent impulses determine the nature of the abnormal sensation experienced, depending on the number, rate, and distribution of impulses and the type and function of nerve fibers in which they arise.

Positive phenomena represent heightened activity in sensory pathways; therefore, they are not necessarily associated with any sensory deficit upon examination.

Negative phenomena result from loss of sensory function and are characterized by diminution or absence of feeling, often experienced as numbness, in a particular distribution. Negative phenomena, in contrast to positive phenomena, are accompanied by abnormal findings on sensory examination. In disorders affecting peripheral sensation, it is estimated that at least half the afferent fibers innervating a given site must be lost or functionless in order for sensory deficit to be demonstrated. This estimate probably varies according to how rapidly sensory fibers have lost function. If the rate of loss is slow and chronic, lack of cutaneous feeling may be unnoticed by the patient and difficult to demonstrate on examination, even though few sensory fibers are functioning. Rapidly evolving sensory abnormality usually evokes positive phenomena of some type and is more readily recognized by patients than insidious deafferentation. Subclinical degrees of sensory dysfunction not demonstrable on clinical sensory examination may be revealed by sensory nerve conduction studies or somatosensory cerebral evoked potentials (see Chap. 361). Sensory symptoms may be either positive or negative, but sensory signs on examination are always negative phenomena.

Terminology Paresthesia and dysesthesia are terms used to denote positive phenomena (sensory symptoms). *Paresthesia* carries the implication that the abnormal sensation is perceived without an apparent stimulus, whereas *dysesthesia* is a more general term used to describe all types of positive sensations whether a stimulus is evident or not. Abnormalities on examination are denoted by *hypesthesia* or *hypoesthesia* (reduction of cutaneous sensation to a specific type of testing such as pressure, light touch, and warm or cold stimuli); *anesthesia* (complete absence of skin sensation to the same stimuli plus pinprick); and *hypalgesia* (referring to loss of pain perception, i.e., nociception, such as the pricking quality elicited by a pin). *Hyperesthesia* means exaggerated perception of sensations in response to mild stimuli (light touch or stroking of the skin). Similarly, *allodynia* describes the situation in which an ordinarily nonpainful stimulus, once perceived, is experienced as painful, even excruciating. An example is elicitation of a painful sensation by application of a vibrating tuning fork. *Hyperalgesia* denotes an exaggerated response to a noxious stimulus, and *hyperpathia*, a broad term, encompasses all the phenomena described by hyperesthesia, allodynia, and hyperalgesia.

Disorders of deep sensation, arising from muscle spindles, tendons, and joints, affect proprioception (position sense). Manifestations include imbalance, particularly with eyes closed or in the dark, clumsiness of precision movements, and unsteadiness of gait, which are referred to collectively as *sensory ataxia* (see Chap. 21). Other findings on examination include reduced or absent joint position and vibratory sensibility and absent deep tendon reflexes in the affected limbs. Romberg's sign is positive, which means that the patient sways or topples when asked to stand with feet close together and eyes closed.

In severe states of deafferentation involving deep sensation, the patient cannot walk or stand unaided or even sit unsupported. Continuous, sometimes wormlike involuntary movements, called *pseudoathetosis*, of the hands and arms occur, particularly with eyes closed. Such patients are severely disabled.

Normal Sensation Cutaneous afferent innervation is subserved by a rich variety of receptors, both naked endings (nociceptors and thermoreceptors) and encapsulated terminals (mechanoreceptors). Each has its own set of sensitivities to specific stimuli, size and distinctness of receptive fields, and adaptational qualities. Much of the knowledge about these receptors has come from the development of techniques to study single intact nerve fibers intraneurally in awake unanesthetized human subjects. It is possible not only to record from single nerve fibers, large or small, but also to stimulate single fibers in isolation. A single impulse, whether elicited by a natural stimulus or evoked by electrical microstimulation, in a large myelinated afferent fiber may be both perceived and localized.

Afferent fibers in peripheral nerve trunks traverse the dorsal roots and enter the dorsal horn of the spinal cord. From there the polysynaptic projections of the smaller fibers (unmyelinated and small myelinated), which in general subserve nociception and temperature sensibility, cross and ascend in the contralateral spinothalamic tract through spinal cord, through brainstem, to the ventral posterolateral nucleus (VPL) of the thalamus, and ultimately project to the postcentral gyrus of the parietal cortex (see Chap. 12). This is the *spinothalamic* pathway. The larger fibers that subserve tactile and position sense and kinesthesia project rostrally in the ipsilateral posterior column of the spinal cord and finally make their first synapse in the gracile or cuneate nuclei of the lower medulla (see Fig. 23-1). The second-order neuron decussates and ascends in the medial lemniscus located medially in the medulla and in the tegmentum of the pons and midbrain and synapses in the VPL. The third-order neuron projects to parietal cortex; this entire system is referred to as *lemniscal*.

Although the fiber types and functions that make up the spinothalamic and lemniscal systems are relatively well known, it has been found that many other fibers, particularly those associated with touch, pressure, and position sense, ascend in a diffusely distributed pattern both ipsilaterally and contralaterally in the anterolateral quadrants of the spinal cord. These anatomic facts explain why an individual with a known complete lesion of the posterior columns of the spinal cord may have little sensory deficit on examination.

EXAMINATION OF SENSATION   The initial step in examination of the somatosensory system is to conduct the tests of primary sensation, which by convention include the sense of pain, touch, vibration, joint position, and thermal sensation, both hot and cold (see Table 23-1).

Some general principles pertain. First, the examiner must depend on subjective patient response, which in turn depends on the level of alertness, motivation, and intelligence of the patient and also on the skill with which the examiner has made the task clear. In a stupefied or obtunded patient, sensory examination is reduced to observing the briskness of withdrawal and the complexity of defensive movements of the patient in response to a pinch or other noxious stimulus. In the alert but uncooperative patient, it is often possible to get some idea of proprioceptive function by noting covertly the patient's best performance of movements requiring balance and precision. Cutaneous sensation may be unexaminable.

Second, sensory examination should not be pressed if the patient is fatigued. An abbreviated survey will suffice until a more extensive examination can be carried out when the patient has rested. Third, sensory examination in a patient who has no neurologic complaints should be quite abbreviated and may consist of pin, touch, and vibration testing in the hands and feet plus evaluation of station and gait, including Romberg's maneuver, which also tests the integrity of motor and cerebellar systems. Fourth, patients should be tested with their eyes closed or covered during both primary sensation and cortical sensory function examination.

Primary Sensation   (See Table 23-1)   The sense of pain is usually tested with a pin, asking the patient to focus on the pricking or unpleasant quality of the stimulus and not just the pressure or touch sensation elicited. Areas of hypalgesia should be mapped by proceeding from the most hypalgesic zones to less affected ones (see Figs. 23-2 and 23-3).

Figure 23-1   Schematic diagram of lemniscal system, which subserves proprioception and discriminative touch.

Temperature sensation, both to hot and to cold, is probably best tested by touching the skin for a couple of seconds with a water flask filled with water of the desired temperature, using a thermometer to verify the temperature. For most purposes, it is satisfactory if a patient can identify as warm the flask that is 35 or 36°C and as cool the one that is 28 to 32°C. Between 28 and 32°C, most individuals can distinguish temperature differences in 1°C steps. Both cold and warm should be tested because different receptors respond to each.

Touch is usually tested with a wisp of cotton or a fine camel's hair brush. In general, it is better to avoid testing touch on hairy skin because of the profusion of sensory endings that surround each hair follicle. The patients, whose eyes are covered, should be asked to say

Table 23-1

Testing Primary Sensation

Sense	Test Device	Endings Activated	Fiber Size Mediating	Central Pathway*
Pain	Pinprick	Cutaneous nociceptors	Small	SpTh, also D
Temperature, heat	Flask with warm water	Cutaneous thermoreceptors for hot	Small	SpTh
Temperature, cold	Flask with cold water	Cutaneous thermoreceptors for cold	Small	SpTh
Touch	Cotton wisp, fine brush	Cutaneous mechanoreceptors, also naked endings	Large and small	Lem, also D and SpTh
Vibration	Tuning fork, 128 Hz	Mechanoreceptors, especially pacinian corpuscles	Large	Lem, also D
Joint position	Passive movement of specific joints	Joint capsule and tendon endings, muscle spindles	Large	Lem, also D

* D, diffuse ascending projections in ipsilateral and contralateral anterolateral columns; SpTh, spinothalamic projection, contralateral; Lem, posterior column and lemniscal projection, ipsilateral.

"now" each time they feel the stimulus. They also may be asked to point to the site where the stimulus was felt, although this tests not only the sense of touch but also touch localization (see "Cortical Sensation," below).

Joint position testing is a measure of proprioception, one of the most important functions of the sensory system. Joint position is usually tested first in the great toe and then in the fingers. Patients are asked to keep their eyes closed and to relax completely the part to be examined. In the case of the great toe, one starts with the toe in a neutral position and grasps it lightly between the thumb and the forefinger on either side of the toe (not top and bottom). The toe is moved a few degrees either in a dorsal or a plantar direction, and the patient is asked to say whether the movement was up or down. One must make sure that the patient understands that it is the direction of movement which is being tested and not the direction the toe is pointing when it stops. A patient with absence of position sense in the part being tested will have a 50 percent error rate because only two choices are available. Answers that are consistently greater than 50 percent in error should be viewed with skepticism. If errors are made in recognizing the direction of passive movements of the toe, then passive movements of the ankle or even of the knee should be undertaken in the same way. Similarly, position sense at the proximal interphalangeal joint of the index finger may be tested, and if abnormal, other finger joints and the wrist and elbow joints also should be tested. A test of proximal joint position sense, primarily at the shoulder, can be carried out by asking the patient to bring the two index fingers together with

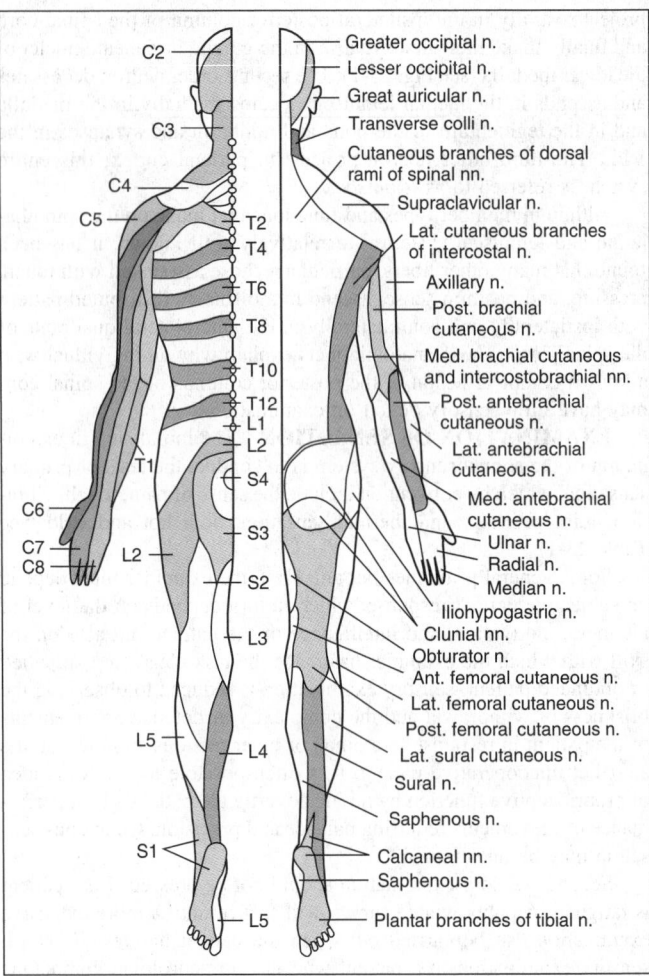

Figure 23-3 Posterior view of dermatomes *(left)* and cutaneous areas supplied by individual peripheral nerves *(right)*. *(Modified from MB Carpenter and J Sutin, in Human Neuroanatomy, 8th ed, Baltimore, Williams & Wilkins, 1983.)*

the arms extended and the eyes closed. Normal individuals should be able to do this quite accurately with errors of a centimeter or less.

The sense of vibration is tested with a tuning fork, preferably a large one that vibrates at 128 Hz. The decay of vibration using this fork is slow enough to be of quantitative use because it takes 15 to 20 s to decay below threshold. Vibration is usually tested at bony prominences, specifically the malleoli at the ankles, the patella, the anterior iliac spine, the spinous processes of the vertebral bodies, the metacarpal-phalangeal joints (knuckles), the styloid process of the ulna, the elbow, and the acromion of the shoulder. Control sites at which to test vibration are the sternum and the forehead. The examiner can compare the threshold at a given site in both patient and self. A crude approximation of degree of vibratory sense loss can be made by counting the seconds that the examiner can feel the sense of vibration longer than the patient. It must be clear to the patient that it is the sense of vibration and not just the pressure of the end of the tuning fork to which attention is directed.

Cortical Sensation Cortical sensory testing includes two-point discrimination, touch localization, stereognosis, graphesthesia, and bilateral simultaneous stimulation, to name the most commonly used methods. Abnormalities of these sensory tests, in the presence of normal primary sensation in an alert cooperative patient, signify a lesion of the parietal cortex or thalamocortical projections to the parietal lobe. If primary sensation is altered, it is not possible to test for these cortical discriminative functions.

Two-point discrimination is tested by special calipers whose points may be set from 2 mm to several centimeters apart and then applied simultaneously to the site to be tested. The pulp of the fingertips is a common site to test; a normal individual can distinguish about 3-mm

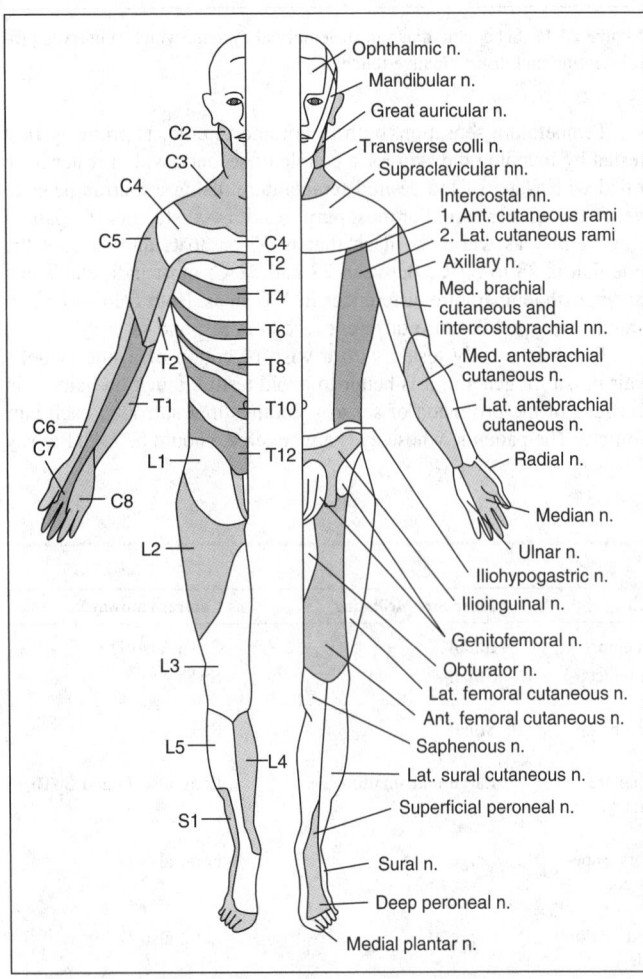

Figure 23-2 Anterior view of dermatomes *(left)* and cutaneous areas supplied by individual peripheral nerves *(right)*. *(Modified from MB Carpenter and J Sutin, in Human Neuroanatomy, 8th ed, Baltimore, Williams & Wilkins, 1983.)*

separation of points there. One can distinguish more closely set points on the tongue and lips, but the threshold for discriminating two points may be centimeters at other sites on the body. Comparisons should always be made between analogous sites on the two sides of the body, since the deficit, with a specific parietal lesion, is likely to be hemilateral. This point holds true for all cortical sensory testing.

Touch localization is usually carried out by light pressure with the examiner's fingertip, asking the patient, whose eyes are closed, to identify the site of touch. It is usual to ask the patient to touch the same site with a fingertip. Bilateral simultaneous stimulation at analogous sites (e.g., the dorsa of both hands) can be carried out to determine whether the perception of touch is extinguished consistently on one side or the other. The phenomenon is referred to as *extinction* on bilateral simultaneous stimulation.

Graphesthesia means the capacity to recognize with eyes closed letters or numbers drawn by the examiner's fingertip on various parts of the body. The usual comparison is the palm of one hand versus the palm of the other. Numbers should be drawn large enough to occupy most of the palm. Once again, the comparison of one side with the other is of prime importance. Failure to recognize numbers or letters is termed *agraphesthesia*.

Stereognosis refers to the ability to identify common objects by palpation, recognizing their shape, texture, and size. Common standard objects are the best test objects, such as a marble, a paper clip, a small rubber ball, or coins. Patients with normal stereognosis should be able to distinguish a dime from a penny and certainly a nickel from a quarter. Patients should only be allowed to feel the object with one hand at a time. If they are unable to identify it in one hand, it should be placed in the other for comparison. Individuals unable to identify common objects and coins in one hand who can do so in the other are said to have *astereognosis* of the abnormal hand. Note that the major comparison is one side of the body with the other.

Localization of Sensory Abnormalities Peripheral neuropathies are generally graded, distal, and symmetric in distribution of deficit. Although most peripheral neuropathies are pansensory and affect all modalities of sensation, selective sensory dysfunction according to nerve fiber size may occur. In small fiber neuropathies, the hallmark is burning, painful dysesthesias with reduced pinprick and thermal sensation but with sparing of proprioception, motor function, and even deep tendon jerks. Touch is variably involved, but when spared, the sensory pattern is referred to as *sensory dissociation* (see below). In contrast to small fiber neuropathies, large fiber neuropathies are characterized by position sense deficit, imbalance, absent tendon jerks, and variable motor dysfunction but preservation of most cutaneous sensation and few or no dysesthesias.

Paresthesias and dysesthesias may be of either peripheral nerve or spinal cord origin and probably can arise in the brainstem, but in every instance they are thought to represent abnormal showers of impulses generated from an ectopic focus or foci. By themselves, paresthesias may not be localizable, but when accompanied by other signs of neuropathy or of myelopathy, the correct site of origin may be deduced.

Dissociated sensory deficit patterns, in which pinprick and thermal sensation are lost but touch is spared, are usually a sign of spinothalamic tract involvement in the spinal cord, especially if the deficit is unilateral and has an upper level on the torso. Bilateral spinothalamic tract involvement occurs with lesions affecting the center of the spinal cord, such as happens with expansion of the central canal in syringomyelia. Sensory dissociation also may occur in peripheral neuropathies in which afferent cutaneous nerve fibers of small diameter are preferentially affected. Neuropathies in which sensory dissociation may occur include leprous neuritis, hereditary sensory neuropathy, and certain cases of amyloid and diabetic polyneuropathy (see Chap. 381).

Hemisensory disturbance with tingling numbness from head to foot is often thalamic in origin but can also be anterior parietal. If abrupt in onset, the lesion is likely to be due to a small stroke (lacunar infarction), particularly if localized to the thalamus. Occasionally, with lesions affecting the posterolateral thalamus (VPL) or adjacent white matter, a syndrome of thalamic pain, also called *Déjerine-Roussy*

syndrome, may ensue. This is a persistent unrelenting hemipainful state often described in dramatic terms such as "like the flesh is being torn from my limbs" or "as though that side is bathed in acid" (see Chap. 12). Harlequin patterns of sensory disturbance, in which one side of the face and the opposite side of the body are affected, localize to the lateral medulla, where a small lesion may damage both the ipsilateral descending trigeminal tract and ascending spinothalamic fibers (lateral lemniscus) subserving the opposite arm, leg, and hemitorso (see "Lateral Medullary Syndrome" in Fig. 366-7).

With lesions of the parietal lobe, either of the cortex or of subjacent white matter, the most prominent symptoms are contralateral hemineglect, hemi-inattention, and a tendency not to use the contralateral hand and arm. Tests of primary sensation may be normal or altered. Anterior parietal infarction may present as a pseudothalamic syndrome with hemilateral loss of primary sensation. Dysesthesias, or even a sense of numbness, also occur except in the special circumstance of focal sensory seizures. These are generally due to lesions in or near the postcentral gyrus. Symptoms of focal somatosensory seizures are usually combinations of numbness and tingling but frequently, additional, more complex sensations are present, such as a rushing feeling, a sense of warmth, a sense of movement without visible motion, or an unpleasantly dysesthetic quality. Duration of seizures is variable; they may be transient, lasting only seconds, or they may persist for hours. Focal motor features (clonic jerking) may supervene, and seizures can become generalized with loss of consciousness. Likely sites of symptoms are unilaterally in the lips, face, digits, or foot, and symptoms may spread as in a Jacksonian march. On occasion, symptoms may occur in a symmetric bilateral fashion, for instance, in both hands; this results from involvement of the second sensory area (unilaterally) located in the rolandic area at and just above the Sylvian fissure.

BIBLIOGRAPHY

BASSETTI C et al: Sensory syndromes in parietal stroke. Neurology 43:1942, 1993

LIGHT AR, PERL ER: Peripheral sensory systems, in *Peripheral Neuropathy*, PJ Dyck et al (eds). Philadelphia, Saunders, 1993, pp 149–165

OCHOA JL: Positive sensory symptoms in neuropathy: Mechanisms and aspects of treatment, in *Peripheral Nerve Disorders*, AK Asbury and PK Thomas (eds). Oxford, Butterworth-Heinemann, 1995, pp 44–58

24   *Allan H. Ropper, Joseph B. Martin*

ACUTE CONFUSIONAL STATES AND COMA

Confusional states and coma are among the most common problems in general medicine. It is estimated that over 5 percent of admissions to the emergency ward of large municipal hospitals are due to diseases that cause a disorder of consciousness. Because a clouding of consciousness (confusion) cannot easily be separated from a diminished level of consciousness (drowsiness, stupor, and coma) and the two are produced by many of the same medical disorders, these conditions are presented here.

Although the interpretation of consciousness is a psychological and philosophical matter, the distinction between *level* of consciousness, or wakefulness, and *content* of consciousness, or awareness, has neurologic significance. Wakefulness-alertness is maintained by a system of upper brainstem and thalamic neurons, the reticular activating system (RAS), and its broad connections to the cerebral hemispheres. Therefore, reduced wakefulness results from depression of the neuronal activity in either the cerebral hemispheres or in the RAS. *Awareness* and *thinking* are dependent on integrated and organized thoughts, subjective experiences, emotions, and mental processes, each of which resides to some extent in anatomically defined regions of the brain. Self-awareness requires that the organism senses this personal stream of thoughts and emotional experiences. The inability to maintain a coherent sequence of thoughts, accompanied usually by inattention and disorientation, is the best definition of *confusion* and is a disorder of the content of consciousness.

STATES OF REDUCED ALERTNESS The unnatural condition of reduced alertness and lessened responsiveness is a continuum that in extreme form characterizes the deep sleeplike state from which the patient cannot be aroused, called *coma*. *Drowsiness* is a disorder that simulates light sleep from which the patient can be easily aroused by touch or noise and can maintain alertness for some time. *Stupor* defines a state in which the patient can be awakened only by vigorous stimuli, and an effort to avoid uncomfortable or aggravating stimulation is displayed. As already indicated, both drowsiness and stupor are usually attended by some degree of mental confusion. Verbal responses in these states are therefore incorrect, slow, or absent during periods of arousal. *Coma* indicates a state from which the patient cannot be aroused by stimulation, and no purposeful attempt is made to avoid painful stimuli.

In clinical practice these terms must be supplemented by a narrative description of the behavioral state of the patient and of responses evoked by various stimuli precisely as they are observed at the bedside. Such descriptions are preferable to ambiguous summary terms such as semicoma or obtundation, the definitions of which differ between observers.

THE CONFUSIONAL STATE Confusion is a behavioral state of reduced mental clarity, coherence, comprehension, and reasoning. *Inattention and disorientation are the main early signs*; however, as an acute confusional state worsens there is deterioration in memory, perception, comprehension, problem solving, language, praxis, visuospatial function, and various aspects of emotional behavior that are each identified with particular regions of the brain. Early in the process it is difficult to know if these complex mental functions are reduced solely as a result of the pervasive defect in attention, but global cortical dysfunction is expected from the metabolic diseases and pharmacologic agents that are the most common sources of the acute confusional state. When there is in addition to confusion an element of drowsiness, the patient is said to have an *encephalopathy*.

Confusion may be a feature of a dementing illness, in which case the chronicity of the process and often a disproportionate effect on memory distinguish it from acute confusion. The confusional state may also derive from a single cortical deficit in higher mental function such as impaired language comprehension, loss of memory, or lack of appreciation of space, in which case each state is defined by the dominant behavioral change (namely, aphasia, dementia, agnosia) rather than characterizing the state as confusion (see Chap. 25).

The drowsiness caused by systemic metabolic changes or by brain lesions is typically accompanied by confusion (encephalopathy). In these instances the primary problem that is causing a diminished level of consciousness should be addressed. A difficult circumstance arises when a process that ultimately leads to drowsiness or stupor begins with confusion or delirium in a fully awake patient.

The confused patient is usually subdued, not inclined to speak, and is inactive physically. In certain cases confusion is accompanied by illusions (misperceptions of environmental sight, sound, or touch) or hallucinations (spontaneous endogenous perceptions). While psychiatrists use the term *delirium* interchangeably with confusion, neurologists prefer to reserve it as a description for an agitated, hypersympathotonic, hallucinatory state most often due to alcohol or drug withdrawal or to hallucinogenic drugs.

COMALIKE SYNDROMES AND RELATED STATES Coma is characterized by complete unarousability. Several other syndromes render patients apparently unresponsive or insensate but are considered separately because of their special significance. The *vege-* *tative state*, an unfortunate term, describes patients who were earlier comatose but whose eyelids have after a time opened, giving the appearance of wakefulness. There may be yawning, grunting, and random limb and head movements, but there is an absolute absence of response to commands and an inability to communicate—in essence, an "awake coma." There are accompanying signs of extensive damage to both cerebral hemispheres, i.e., Babinski signs, decerebrate or decorticate limb posturing, and absent response to visual stimuli. Autonomic nervous system functions such as cardiovascular, thermoregulatory, and neuroendocrine control are preserved and may be subject to periods of overactivity. The vegetative state results from global damage to the cerebral cortex, most often from cardiac arrest or head injury as discussed further in Chaps. 366 and 374. *Akinetic mutism* refers to a partially or fully awake patient who when unstimulated remains immobile and silent. The state may result from hydrocephalus, from masses in the region of the third ventricle, or from large bilateral lesions in the cingulate gyrus or other portions of both frontal lobes. Lesions in the periaqueductal or low diencephalic regions may cause a similar state. *Abulia* can be viewed as a mild form of akinetic mutism with the same anatomic origins. The abulic patient is hypokinetic and slow to respond but generally gives correct answers. It is typical to halt while reciting numbers or sequential calculations and, with a delay, to resume correctly. The *locked-in state* describes a pseudocoma in which patients are awake but deefferented, i.e., have no means of producing speech or limb, face, or pharyngeal movements. Infarction or hemorrhage of the ventral pons, which transects all descending corticospinal and corticobulbar pathways are the usual causes. The RAS arousal system, vertical eye movements, and lid elevation remain unimpaired. Such eye movements can be used by the patient to signal to the examiner. A similar awake state simulating unresponsiveness may occur as a result of total paralysis of limb, ocular, and oropharyngeal musculature in severe cases of acute Guillain-Barré syndrome (a peripheral nerve disease) (see Chap. 381). Unlike brainstem stroke, vertical eye movements are not selectively spared.

Certain psychiatric states can mimic coma by producing an apparent unresponsiveness. *Catatonia* is a peculiar hypomobile syndrome associated with major psychosis. In the typical form patients appear awake with eyes open but make no voluntary or responsive movements, although they blink spontaneously and may not appear distressed. It is characteristic but not invariable to have a "waxy flexibility," in which limbs maintain their posture when lifted by the examiner. Upon recovery, such patients have some memory of events that occurred during their catatonic stupor. Patients with *hysterical* or *conversion pseudocoma* show signs that indicate voluntary attempts to appear comatose, though it may take some ingenuity on the part of the examiner to demonstrate these. Eyelid elevation is actively resisted, blinking occurs to a visual threat when the lids are held open, and the eyes move concomitantly with head rotation, all signs belying brain damage.

ANATOMIC CORRELATES OF CONSCIOUSNESS A normal level of consciousness (wakefulness) depends upon activation of the cerebral hemispheres by neurons located in the brainstem RAS. Both of these components and the connections between them must be preserved for normal consciousness to be maintained. The principal causes of coma are therefore: (1) widespread damage in both hemispheres from ischemia, trauma, or other less common brain diseases; (2) suppression of cerebral function by extrinsic drugs, toxins, or hypoxia or by internal metabolic derangements such as hypoglycemia, azotemia, hepatic failure, or hypercalcemia; and (3) brainstem lesions that cause proximate damage to the RAS.

The RAS is a physiologic system contained within the rostral portion of the reticular formation; it consists of neurons located bilaterally in the medial tegmental gray matter of the brainstem that extends from the medulla to the diencephalon. Animal experiments and human clinicopathologic observations have established that the region of the reticular formation that is of critical importance for maintaining wakefulness extends from the rostral pons to the caudal diencephalon. A practical consideration follows: *Destructive lesions that produce coma also affect adjacent brainstem structures of the upper pons, midbrain, and diencephalon that are concerned with pupillary function and eye*

Abnormalities in these systems provide convenient, albeit indirect, evidence of direct brainstem damage as the source of coma. Lesions confined to the cerebral hemispheres do not immediately affect the brainstem RAS, although secondary dysfunction of the upper brainstem often results from compression by a mass in a cerebral hemisphere (see transtentorial herniation below).

Brainstem RAS neurons project rostrally to the cortex, primarily via thalamic relay nuclei that exert a tonic influence on the activity of the cerebral cortex. Experimental work in primates suggests that the brainstem RAS affects the level of consciousness by suppressing the activity of the nonspecific nuclei that, in turn, have a predominantly inhibitory effect on the cortex, but this is an oversimplification. It is believed that high-frequency (30 to 40 Hz) rhythms synchronize cortical and thalamic neurons during wakefulness. The basis of behavioral arousal by environmental stimuli (somesthetic, auditory, and visual) is related to the rich innervation that the RAS receives from these sensory systems.

The relays between the RAS and the thalamic and cortical areas are accomplished by neurotransmitters. Of these, the influences on arousal of acetylcholine and biogenic amines have been studied most extensively. Cholinergic fibers connect the midbrain to other areas of the upper brainstem, thalamus, and cortex. Serotonin and norepinephrine also subserve important functions in the regulation of the sleep-wake cycle (see Chap. 27). Their roles in arousal and coma have not been clearly established, although the alerting effects of amphetamines are likely to be mediated by catecholamine release.

A reduction in alertness is related in a semiquantitative way to the total mass of damaged cortex or RAS and is not focally represented in any region of the hemispheres, with the exception that large, acute, and purely unilateral hemispheral lesions, particularly on the left, may cause transient drowsiness even in the absence of damage to the opposite hemisphere or RAS. *Hemispheral lesions in most instances cause coma indirectly when a large mass in one or both hemispheres secondarily compresses the upper brainstem and diencephalic RAS.* This is most typical of cerebral hemorrhages and rapidly expanding tumors. The magnitude of decrease in alertness is also related to the rapidity of onset of the cortical dysfunction or RAS compression.

This secondary compressive effect has led to a concept of *transtentorial herniation* with progressive brainstem dysfunction to explain the neurologic signs that accompany coma from supratentorial mass lesions. Herniation refers to displacement of brain tissue away from a mass, past a less mobile structure such as the dura, and into a space that it normally does not occupy. The common herniations seen at postmortem examinations are transfalcial (displacement of the cingulate gyrus under the falx in the anterior midline), transtentorial (medial temporal lobe displacement into the tentorial opening), and foraminal (the cerebellar tonsils forced into the foramen magnum). Uncal transtentorial herniation, or impaction of the anterior medial temporal gyrus into the anterior portion of the tentorial opening, causes compression of the third nerve with pupillary dilation. Subsequent coma may be due to midbrain compression by the parahippocampal gyrus. Central transtentorial herniation denotes symmetric downward movement of the upper diencephalon (thalamic region) through the tentorial opening in the midline and is heralded by miotic pupils and drowsiness. These shifts in brain are thought to cause a progression of rostral to caudal brainstem compression of first the midbrain, then the pons, and finally the medulla, leading to the sequential appearance of neurologic signs corresponding to the level damaged and to progressively diminished alertness. However, many patients with supratentorial masses do not follow these stereotypic patterns; for example, an orderly progression of signs from midbrain to medulla is often bypassed in catastrophic lesions where all brainstem functions are lost almost simultaneously. Furthermore, drowsiness and stupor typically occur with moderate lateral shifts at the level of the diencephalon when there is only minimal vertical displacement of structures near the tentorial opening and well before downward herniation is evident on computed tomogaphy (CT) scan or magnetic resonance imaging (MRI).

PATHOPHYSIOLOGY OF COMA AND CONFUSION

Coma of metabolic origin is produced by interruption of energy substrate delivery (hypoxia, ischemia, hypoglycemia) or by alteration of the neurophysiologic responses of neuronal membranes (drug or alcohol intoxication, toxic endogenous metabolites, anesthesia, or epilepsy). These same metabolic abnormalites can cause widespread neuronal dysfunction in the cortex that reduces all aspects of mentation and results in an acute confusional state. In this way, acute confusion and coma can be viewed as a continuum in metabolic encephalopathy.

The neurons of the brain are dependent on cerebral blood flow (CBF), oxygen, and glucose. CBF is approximately 75 mL per 100 g/min in gray matter and 30 mL per 100 g/min in white matter (mean = 55 mL per 100 g/min). Oxygen consumption is 3.5 mL per 100 g/min, and glucose consumption is 5 mg per 100 g/min. Brain stores of glucose provide energy for approximately 2 min after blood flow is interrupted, and consciousness is lost within 8 to 10 s. Hypoxia and ischemia simultaneously exhaust glucose more rapidly. The EEG becomes diffusely slowed (typical of metabolic encephalopathies) when mean CBF is below 25 mL per 100 g/min; at 15 mL per 100 g/min, all recordable brain electrical activity ceases. If all other conditions such as temperature and arterial oxygenation remain normal, CBF less than 10 mL per 100 g/min causes irreversible brain damage. The rapidity of the development of ischemia and its duration are also important determinants of irreversible damage.

Confusion and coma due to hyponatremia, hyperosmolarity, hypercapnia, hypercalcemia, and the encephalopathies of hepatic and renal failure are associated with a variety of metabolic derangements of neurons and astrocytes. The reversible toxic effects of these conditions on the brain are not understood but may, in different cases, impair energy supplies, change ion fluxes across neuronal membranes, and cause neurotransmitter abnormalities. In some instances there are specific morphologic changes of nerve cells (see Chap. 380). For example, the high brain ammonia concentration associated with *hepatic coma* interferes with cerebral energy metabolism and the Na^+, K^+-ATPase pump, increases the number and size of astrocytes, causes increased concentrations of potentially toxic products of ammonia metabolism, and results in abnormalities of neurotransmitters, including possible "false" neurotransmitters, which may act competitively at receptor sites. Ammonia or other metabolites also may bind to benzodiazepine–gamma-aminobutyric acid receptors to cause central nervous system (CNS) depression by an endogenous mechanism. Furthermore, these changes are not mutually exclusive.

The mechanism of the encephalopathy of *renal failure* is also poorly understood. Unlike ammonia, urea itself does not produce CNS toxicity. A multifactorial cause has been proposed including an increased permeability of the blood-brain barrier to toxic substances such as organic acids and an increase in brain calcium or cerebrospinal fluid (CSF) phosphate content.

Abnormalities of *osmolarity* are involved in the coma and seizures caused by several systemic medical disorders, including diabetic ketoacidosis, the nonketotic hyperosmolar state, and hyponatremia. Brain water volume correlates best with level of consciousness in hyponatremic–hypoosmolar states, but other factors probably also play a role. Sodium levels below 125 mmol/L cause acute or subacute confusion and below 115 mmol/L are associated with coma and convulsions, depending on the rapidity with which the hyponatremia develops. Serum osmolarity is generally above 350 mosmol/L in hyperosmolar coma.

Hypercapnia produces a diminished level of consciousness proportional to the P_{CO_2} tension in the blood and to the rapidity of onset. A relationship between CSF acidosis and the severity of symptoms has been established. The pathophysiology of other metabolic encephalopathies such as hypercalcemia, hypothyroidism, vitamin B_{12} deficiency, and hypothermia are incompletely understood but must also reflect derangements of CNS biochemistry and membrane functioning.

The large group of *drugs* that depress the CNS, anesthetics, and some endogenous toxins appear to produce coma by suppression of both the RAS and the cerebral cortex. For this reason, combinations of cortical and brainstem signs occur in drug overdose and some other metabolic comas, which may lead to a specious diagnosis of structural brainstem damage.

Although all metabolic derangements alter neuronal electrophysiology, the only primary disturbance of brain electrical activity encountered in clinical practice is *epilepsy*. Continuous, generalized electrical discharges of the cortex (seizures) are associated with coma even in the absence of epileptic motor activity (convulsions). Coma following seizures, termed the *postictal state*, may be due to exhaustion of energy metabolites or be secondary to locally toxic molecules produced during the seizures. Recovery from postictal unresponsiveness occurs when neuronal metabolic balance is restored. The postictal state produces a pattern of continuous, generalized slowing of the background EEG activity similar to that of metabolic encephalopathy.

_____ *Approach to the Patient* _____

In Coma The diagnosis and acute management of coma depend on knowledge of its main causes in clinical practice, an interpretation of certain clinical signs, notably the brainstem reflexes, and the efficient use of diagnostic tests. It is common knowledge that acute respiratory and cardiovascular problems should be attended to prior to neurologic diagnosis. A complete medical evaluation, except for the vital signs, funduscopy, and examination for nuchal rigidity, may be deferred until the neurologic evaluation has established the severity and nature of coma.

HISTORY In many cases, the cause of coma is immediately evident (e.g., trauma, cardiac arrest, or known drug ingestion). In the remainder, historical information about the onset of coma is often sparse. The most useful historical points are (1) the circumstances and temporal profile of the onset of neurologic symptoms; (2) the precise details of preceding neurologic symptoms (confusion, weakness, headache, seizures, dizziness, diplopia, or vomiting); (3) the use of medications, illicit drugs, or alcohol; and (4) a history of liver, kidney, lung, heart, or other medical disease. Telephone calls to family and observers on the scene are an important part of the initial evaluation. Ambulance attendants often provide the best information in an enigmatic case.

PHYSICAL EXAMINATION AND GENERAL OBSERVATIONS The temperature, pulse, respiratory rate and pattern, and blood pressure should be measured. Fever suggests systemic infection, bacterial meningitis, encephalitis, or a brain lesion that has disturbed the temperature-regulating centers. High body temperature, 42° to 44°C, associated with dry skin should arouse the suspicion of heat stroke or anticholinergic drug intoxication. Hypothermia is observed with bodily exposure to lowered environmental temperature; alcoholic, barbiturate, sedative, or phenothiazine intoxication; hypoglycemia; peripheral circulatory failure; or hypothyroidism. Hypothermia itself causes coma only when the temperature is below 31°C. Aberrant respiratory patterns that may reflect brainstem disorders are discussed below. A change of pulse rate combined with hyperventilation and hypertension may signal an increase in intracranial pressure. Marked hypertension is a very helpful signature of hypertensive encephalopathy, cerebral hemorrhage, or hydrocephalus and occurs acutely, but to lesser degree, after head trauma. Hypotension is characteristic of coma from alcohol or barbiturate intoxication, internal hemorrhage, myocardial infarction, septicemia, and Addisonian crisis. The funduscopic examination is used to detect subarachnoid hemorrhage (subhyaloid hemorrhages), hypertensive encephalopathy (exudates, hemorrhages, vessel-crossing changes), and increased intracranial pressure (papilledema). Generalized cutaneous petechiae suggest thrombotic thrombocytopenic purpura or a bleeding diathesis associated with intracerebral hemorrhage.

GENERAL NEUROLOGIC ASSESSMENT An exact description of spontaneous and elicited movements is of great value in establishing the level of neurologic dysfunction. The patient's state should be observed first without examiner intervention. The nature of respirations and spontaneous movements are noted. Patients who toss about, reach up toward the face, cross their legs, yawn, swallow, cough, or moan are closest to being awake. The only sign of seizures may be small excursion twitching of a foot, finger, or facial muscle. An outturned leg at rest or lack of restless movements on one side suggests a hemiparesis.

The terms *decorticate* and *decerebrate rigidity*, or "posturing," describe stereotyped arm and leg movements occurring spontaneously or elicited by sensory stimulation. Flexion of the elbows and wrists and arm supination (decortication) suggest severe bilateral damage in the hemispheres above the midbrain, whereas extension of the elbows and wrists with pronation (decerebration) suggests damage to the corticospinal tracts in the midbrain or caudal diencephalon. Arm extension with minimal leg flexion or flaccid legs has been associated with lesions in the low pons. These terms, however, have been adapted from animal work and cannot be applied with the same precision to coma in humans. Acute lesions of any type frequently cause limb extension regardless of location, and almost all extensor posturing becomes flexion as time passes, so posturing alone cannot be utilized to make an anatomic localization. Metabolic coma, especially after acute hypoxia, also may produce vigorous spontaneous extensor (decerebrate) rigidity. Posturing may coexist with purposeful limb movements, usually reflecting subtotal damage to the motor system. Multifocal myoclonus is almost always an indication of a metabolic disorder, particularly azotemia, anoxia, or drug ingestion. In a drowsy and confused patient bilateral asterixis is a certain sign of metabolic encephalopathy or drug ingestion (see below).

ELICITED MOVEMENTS AND LEVEL OF AROUSAL If the patient is not aroused by conversational voice, a sequence of increasingly intense stimuli is used to determine the patient's best level of arousal and the optimal motor response of each limb. It should be recognized that the results of this testing may vary from minute to minute and that serial examinations are most useful. Nasal tickle with a cotton wisp is a strong arousal stimulus. Pressure on the knuckles or bony prominences is the preferred and humane form of noxious stimulus. Pinching the skin over the face, chest, or limbs causes unsightly ecchymoses and is not necessary.

Responses to noxious stimuli should be appraised critically. Abduction avoidance movement of a limb is usually purposeful and denotes an intact corticospinal system to that limb. Stereotyped posturing following stimulation of a limb indicates severe dysfunction of the corticospinal system. Adduction and flexion of the stimulated limbs may be reflex movements and imply corticospinal system damage. Brief clonic or twitching limb movements occur at the end of extensor posturing excursions and should not be mistaken for convulsions.

BRAINSTEM REFLEXES Brainstem signs are a key to localization of the lesion in coma (Fig. 24-1). As a rule, coma associated with normal brainstem function indicates widespread and bilateral hemispheral disease or dysfunction. The brainstem reflexes that allow convenient examination are pupillary light responses, eye movements, both spontaneous and elicited, and respiratory pattern.

Pupillary reaction is examined with a bright, diffuse light and, if the response is absent, confirmed with a magnifying lens. Light reaction in pupils smaller than 2 mm is often difficult to appreciate, and excessive room lighting mutes pupillary reactivity. Symmetrically reactive round pupils (2.5 to 5 mm in diameter) usually exclude midbrain damage as the cause of coma. One enlarged (greater than 5 mm) and unreactive or poorly reactive pupil results either from an intrinsic midbrain lesion (on the same side) or, far more commonly, is secondary to compression or stretching of the third nerve by the secondary effects of a mass. Unilateral pupillary enlargement usually denotes an ipsilateral mass, but this sign occasionally occurs contralaterally, possibly by compression of the midbrain or third nerve against the opposite tentorial margin. Oval and slightly eccentric pupils accompany early midbrain–third nerve compression. Bilaterally dilated and unreactive pupils indicate severe midbrain damage, usually from secondary compression by transtentorial herniation or from ingestion of drugs with anticholinergic activity. The use of mydriatic eye drops by a previous examiner, self-administration by the patient, or direct ocular trauma may cause misleading pupillary enlargement. Reactive and bilaterally small but not pinpoint pupils (1 to 2.5 mm) are most commonly seen in metabolic encephalopathy or after deep bilateral hemispheral lesions such as hydrocephalus or thalamic hemorrhage. This has been attributed to dysfunction of sympathetic nervous system efferents emerging from the posterior hypothalamus. Very small but reactive pupils (less than 1 mm) characterize narcotic or barbiturate overdose but also occur with acute, extensive bilateral pontine damage, usually from hemorrhage. The response to naloxone and the presence of reflex eye movements distinguish these. The unilaterally small pupil of a Horner's syndrome is detected by failure of the pupil to enlarge in the dark. It is rare in coma but may occur ipsilateral to a large cerebral hemorrhage that affects the thalamus. Lid tone, tested by lifting the eyelids, palpating resistance to opening, and speed of closure, is reduced progressively as coma deepens.

Eye movements are the second foundation of physical diagnosis in coma because their examination permits an analysis of a large portion of the brainstem. The eyes are first observed by elevating the lids and noting the resting position and spontaneous movements of the globes. Horizontal divergence of the eyes at rest is normally observed in drowsiness. As patients either awaken or coma deepens, the ocular axes become parallel again. An adducted eye at rest indicates lateral rectus paresis (weakness) due to a sixth nerve lesion, and when bilateral, it is often a sign of increased intracranial pressure. An abducted eye at rest, often accompanied by ipsilateral pupillary enlargement, indicates medial rectus paresis due to third nerve dysfunction. With few exceptions, vertical separation of the ocular axes, or *skew deviation*, results from pontine or cerebellar lesions.

Spontaneous eye movements in coma generally take the form of conjugate horizontal roving. This motion exonerates the midbrain and pons and has the same meaning as normal reflex eye movements (see below). Cyclic vertical downward movements are seen in specific

FIGURE 24-1 Brainstem reflexes in the coma examination. Midbrain and third nerve function are tested by pupillary reaction to light, pontine function by spontaneous and reflex eye movements and corneal responses, and medullary function by respiratory and pharyngeal responses.

Reflex conjugate, horizontal eye movements are dependent on the medial longitudinal fasciculus (MLF) interconnecting the sixth and contralateral third nerve nuclei. Eye movements are elicited by head rotation (oculocephalic reflex) or caloric stimulation of the labyrinths (oculovestibular reflex). These reflex movements are suppressed in the awake patient by the cerebral hemispheres via their connections to the brainstem.

circumstances. "Ocular bobbing" describes a brisk downward and slow upward movement of the globes associated with loss of horizontal eye movements and is diagnostic of bilateral pontine damage. "Ocular dipping" is a slower, arrhythmic downward movement followed by a faster upward movement in patients with normal reflex horizontal gaze and denotes diffuse anoxic damage to the cerebral cortex. The eyes may turn down and inward in thalamic and upper midbrain lesions.

"Doll's-eye," or *oculocephalic*, responses are reflex movements tested by moving the head from side to side or vertically, first slowly then briskly; eye movements are evoked in the opposite direction to head movement (see Fig. 24-1). These responses are generated by brainstem mechanisms originating in the labyrinths and cervical proprioceptors. They are normally suppressed by visual fixation mediated by the cerebral hemispheres in awake patients but appear as the hemispheres become suppressed or inactive. The neuronal pathways for reflex horizontal eye movements require integrity of the region surrounding the sixth nerve nucleus and are yoked to the contralateral third nerve via the medial longitudinal fasciculus (MLF) (see Fig. 24-1). Two disparate pieces of information are obtained from the reflex eye movements. First, in coma resulting from bihemispheral disease or metabolic or drug depression, the eyes move easily or "loosely" from side to side in a direction opposite to the direction of head turning. The ease with which the globes move toward the opposite side is a reflection of disinhibition of brainstem reflexes by damaged cerebral hemispheres. Second, conjugate oculocephalic movements demonstrate the integrity of brainstem pathways extending from the high cervical spinal cord and medulla, where vestibular and proprioceptive input from head turning originates, to the midbrain, at the level of the third nerve. Thus full and conjugate eye movements that are induced by the oculocephalic maneuver demonstrate the intactness of a large segment of brainstem and virtually exclude a primary lesion of the brainstem as the cause of coma.

Incomplete ocular adduction indicates an ipsilateral midbrain (third nerve) lesion or damage to the pathways mediating reflex eye movements in the MLF (i.e., internuclear ophthalmoplegia). Third nerve damage is usually associated with an enlarged pupil and horizontal ocular divergence at rest, whereas MLF lesions are unrelated to pupillary function and leave the globe in the primary position. Adduction of the globes is by nature more difficult to obtain than abduction, and subtle abnormalities in the doll's-eye maneuver should be interpreted with caution.

Caloric stimulation of the vestibular apparatus (*oculovestibular response*) is an adjunct to the oculocephalic test, acting as a stronger stimulus to reflex eye movements but giving fundamentally the same information. Irrigation of the external auditory canal with cool water causes convection currents in the endolymph of the labyrinths of the inner ear. An intact brainstem pathway from the labyrinths to the oculomotor nuclei of the midbrain is indicated, with brief latency, by tonic deviation of both eyes (lasting 30 to 120 s) to the side of cool-water irrigation. Bilateral conjugate eye movements therefore have similar significance as full oculocephalic responses. If the cerebral hemispheres are functioning properly, as in hysterical coma, an obligate rapid corrective movement is generated away from the side of tonic deviation. The absence of this nystagmus-like quick phase signifies that the cerebral hemispheres are damaged or suppressed.

Conjugate horizontal ocular deviation at rest or incomplete conjugate eye movements with head turning indicate damage in the pons on the side of the gaze paresis or frontal lobe damage on the opposite side. This phenomenon may be summarized by the following aphorism: *The eyes look toward a hemispheral lesion and away from a brainstem lesion.* It is usually possible to overcome the ocular deviation associated with frontal lobe damage by oculocephalic testing. Seizures also may cause aversive (opposite) eye deviation with rhythmic, jerky movements to the side of gaze. On rare occasions, the eyes may turn paradoxically away from the side of a deep hemispheral lesion ("wrong-way eyes"). In hydrocephalus with dilatation of the third ventricle, the globes frequently rest below the horizontal meridian. Two types of rapid rhythmic eye movements may occur in stupor or coma. *Ocular myoclonus* is a rapid horizontal oscillatory nystagmus usually associated with a similar movement of the palate and due to damage to the central tegmental fasciculus, a longitudinal tract in the brainstem. *Opsoclonus* is an irregular, jerky, saccadic movement varying in direction that results from cerebellar lesions.

A major pitfall in coma diagnosis may occur when reflex eye movements are suppressed by drugs. The eyes then move with the head as it is turned as if the globes locked in place, thus spuriously suggesting brainstem damage. Overdoses of phenytoin, tricyclic antidepressants, and barbiturates are commonly implicated as well as, on occasion, alcohol, phenothiazines, diazepam, and neuromuscular blockers such as pancuronium. The presence of normal pupillary size and light reaction will distinguish most drug-induced comas from brainstem damage. Small to midposition, 1- to 3-mm nonreactive pupils may occur with very high serum levels of barbiturates or secondary to hydrocephalus (see below).

Although the *corneal reflexes* are rarely useful alone, they may corroborate eye movement abnormalities because they also depend on the integrity of pontine pathways. By touching the cornea with a wisp of cotton, a response consisting of brief bilateral lid closure may be observed. The corneal response may be lost if the reflex connections between the fifth and seventh cranial nerves within the pons are damaged. The normal efferent response is bilateral, with closure of both eyelids. CNS depressant drugs diminish or eliminate the corneal responses soon after the reflex eye movements become paralyzed but before the pupils become unreactive to light.

RESPIRATION Respiratory patterns have received much attention in coma diagnosis but are of inconsistent localizing value. Shallow, slow, but well-timed regular breathing suggests metabolic or drug depression. Rapid, deep (Kussmaul) breathing usually implies metabolic acidosis but also may occur with pontomesencephalic lesions. Cheyne-Stokes respiration in its classic cyclic form, ending with a brief apneic period, signifies mild bihemispheral damage or metabolic suppression and commonly accompanies light coma. Agonal gasps reflect bilateral lower brainstem damage and are well known as the terminal respiratory pattern of severe brain damage. In brain-dead patients, shallow respiratory-like movements with irregular, nonrepetitive back arching may be produced by hypoxia and are probably generated by the surviving cervical spinal cord and lower medulla. Other cyclic breathing variations are not usually diagnostic of specific local lesions.

Approach to the Patient

With Acute Confusion Acute confusion is characterized by difficulty in maintaining a coherent stream of thinking and mental performance. This is manifested most obviously by inattention and disorientation, which in turn may generate difficulty with memory and all mental activities. Attention may be gauged by the clarity of and speed of response while the history is being taken but should also be examined by having the patient repeat strings of numbers (most adults easily retain seven digits forward and four backward) or perform serial calculations that require holding the result of one calculation in a working memory in order to pursue the next step—the serial 3-from-30 subtraction test is the usual paradigm. Orientation and memory are tested by asking the patient in a forthright manner the date, inclusive of month, day, year, and day of week; the precise place; and some items of generally acknowledged and universally known information (the name of the President, a recent national catastrophe, the state capital). Further probing may be necessary to reveal a defect—why is the patient in the hospital; what is his or her address, zip code, telephone number, social security number? Problems of increasing complexity may be pursued but they give little more practical information once a confusional state has been established.

Evidence of drug ingestion should be sought on general physical examination. Other salient neurologic findings are the level of alertness, which typically fluctuates in acute cases; indications of focal damage of the cerebrum such as hemiparesis, hemianopia, and particularly aphasia; adventitious movements of myoclonus; or convulsions. The most pertinent sign of a metabolic encephalopathy is *asterixis*, which is an arrhythmic flapping tremor that is typically elicited by asking the patient to hold the arm out straight with the wrist fully extended. After a few seconds, a large jerking lapse in the posture of the hand occurs and then a rapid return to the original position. The same can be appreciated in any tonically held posture, even of the tongue, and in extreme form the movements may intrude on voluntary limb motion. Bilateral asterixis always signifies a metabolic encephalopathy, for example, from hepatic failure or from drug ingestion, especially with anticonvulsants. Myoclonic jerking and tremor in an awake patient are typical of uremic encephalopathy or antipsychotic (butyrophone) drug ingestion.

The language of the confused patient may be disorganized and rambling, even to the extent of incorporating paraphasic words. These features, along with impaired comprehension that is due to inattention, may be mistaken for aphasia.

Distinguishing dementia from confusion is a great problem. The memory loss of dementia necessarily engenders a confusional state that varies in severity from hour to hour and day to day. Poor mental performance is derived mainly from incomplete recollection, inadequate access to names and ideas, and on the inability to retain new information, thus affecting orientation and factual knowledge; attention is preserved in the early stages of the process. Depending upon the nature of the dementing disease, there may be added specific deficits of language, praxis, visual-spatial performance, or a slowed frontal lobe state. Eventually dementia produces a chronic confusion with breakdown of all types of mental performance, and the distinction from confusion depends simply on the chronic nature of the condition.

LABORATORY EXAMINATION FOR ACUTE CONFUSION AND COMA Four laboratory tests are used most frequently in the diagnosis of confusion and coma: chemical-toxicologic analysis of blood and urine, CT or MRI, EEG, and CSF examination.

Chemical blood determinations are made routinely to investigate metabolic, toxic, or drug-induced encephalopathies. The major metabolic aberrations encountered in clinical practice are those of electrolytes, calcium, blood urea nitrogen (BUN), glucose, plasma osmolarity, and hepatic dysfunction (NH_3). Toxicologic analysis is of great value in any case of coma where the diagnosis is not immediately clear. However, the presence of exogenous drugs or toxins, especially alcohol, does not ensure that other factors, particularly head trauma, may not also contribute to the clinical state. Ethanol levels in nonhabituated patients of 200 mg/dL generally cause confusion and impaired mental activity and above 300 mg/dL are associated with stupor. The development of tolerance may allow the chronic alcoholic to remain awake at levels over 400 mg/dL.

The increased availability of CT and MRI has focused attention on causes of coma that are radiologically detectable (e.g., hemorrhages, tumors, or hydrocephalus). This approach, although at times expedient, is imprudent because most cases of confusion and coma are metabolic or toxic in origin. The notion that a normal CT scan excludes anatomic lesions as the cause of coma is also erroneous. Early bilateral hemisphere infarction, small brainstem lesions, encephalitis, meningitis, mechanical shearing of axons as a result of closed head trauma, absent cerebral perfusion associated with brain death, sagittal sinus thrombosis, and subdural hematomas that are isodense to adjacent brain are some of the lesions that may be overlooked by CT. Even MRI may fail to demonstrate these processes early in their evolution. Nevertheless, in coma of unknown etiology, a CT or MRI scan should be obtained. In those cases in which the etiology is clinically apparent, these provide verification and define the extent of the lesion (Fig. 24-2).

With acute mass lesions, 3 to 5 mm of horizontal displacement of the pineal body from the midline generally corresponds to drowsiness, 5 to 8 mm corresponds to stupor, and greater than 8 mm corresponds to coma. As a supratentorial mass enlarges, the opposite perimesencephalic cistern is first compressed from lateral movement of the brainstem, the ipsilateral cistern is widened, and finally, both are compressed from the lateral mass effect. The lateral ventricle opposite the mass becomes enlarged as the third ventricle is compressed. These radiologic features of tissue shifts near the tentorial opening are helpful in correlating the clinical state with the progress of a mass lesion on scans (Fig. 24-3). For technical reasons, MRI is difficult to perform in comatose patients, and it also does not demonstrate hemorrhages as well as CT (see Chap. 362).

The EEG is useful in metabolic or drug-induced confusional states but is rarely diagnostic in coma, with the exception of comas due to clinically unrecognized seizures, herpes virus encephalitis, and Creutzfeldt-Jakob disease. The amount of background slowing of the EEG is a useful gauge of the severity of any diffuse encephalopathy. Predominant high-voltage slowing (delta waves) in the frontal regions is typical of metabolic coma, as from hepatic failure and widespread fast (beta) activity implicates the effects of sedative drugs. A pattern of "alpha coma" is defined by widespread, invariant 8- to 12-Hz activity superficially resembling the normal alpha rhythm of waking but unresponsive to environmental stimuli. Alpha coma results from either high pontine or diffuse cortical damage and is associated with a poor prognosis. Coma due to persistent epileptic discharges that are not clinically manifested may be revealed by EEG recordings. Normal alpha activity on the EEG also may alert the clinician to the locked-in syndrome or a hysterical case. Computed on-line EEG analysis and evoked potential recordings (auditory and somatosensory) are useful additional methods for coma diagnosis and monitoring.

Lumbar puncture is now used more judiciously in cases of coma or confusion because the CT scan excludes intracerebral hemorrhages and most subarachnoid hemorrhages. The use of lumbar puncture in coma is limited to diagnosis of meningitis or encephalitis and instances of suspected subarachnoid hemorrhage in which the CT is normal. Lumbar puncture should not be deferred if meningitis is a strong clinical possibility. Xanthochromia is documented by spinning the CSF in a large tube and comparing the supernatant to water. This yellow coloration indicates preexisting blood in the CSF (or very high protein levels) and permits exclusion of a traumatic puncture. In addition, initial and final tubes should be inspected for a decrement in the number of erythrocytes, indicating traumatic puncture. Knowing the pressure within the subarachnoid space is of further help in interpreting abnormalities of the cell count and protein content of the CSF.

DIFFERENTIAL DIAGNOSIS OF CONFUSION AND COMA In most instances, confusion and coma are part of an obvious medical problem such as known drug ingestion, hypoxia, stroke, trauma, or liver or kidney failure. Attention is then appropriately focused on the primary illness. A complete listing of all diseases that cause confusion and coma would serve little purpose, since it would not aid diagnosis. Some general rules, however, are helpful. Illnesses that cause sudden or acute coma are due to drug ingestion or to one of the catastrophic brain lesions—hemorrhage, trauma, hypoxia, or, rarely, acute basilar artery occlusion. Coma that appears subacutely is usually related to preceding medical or neurologic problems, including the secondary brain swelling that surrounds a preexisting lesion. Coma diagnosis, therefore, requires familiarity with the common intracerebral catastrophes. These are described in more detail in Chap. 366 but may be summarized as follows: (1) basal ganglia and thalamic hemorrhage (acute but not instantaneous onset, vomiting, headache, hemiplegia, and characteristic eye signs); (2) subarachnoid hemorrhage (instantaneous onset, severe headache, neck stiffness, vomiting, third or sixth nerve lesions, transient loss of consciousness, or sudden coma with vigorous extensor posturing); (3) pontine hemorrhage (sudden onset, pinpoint pupils, loss of reflex eye movements and corneal responses, ocular bobbing, posturing, hyperventilation, and sweating); (4) cerebellar hemorrhage (occipital headache, vomiting, gaze paresis, and inability to stand); and (5) basilar artery thrombosis (neurologic prodrome or warning spells, diplopia, dysarthria, vomiting, eye movement and corneal response abnormalities, and asymmetric limb paresis). The most common stroke, namely, infarction in the territory of the middle cerebral artery, does not cause coma acutely. The syndrome of acute hydrocephalus causing coma may accompany many intracranial catastrophes, particularly subarachnoid hemorrhage. Acute symmetric enlargement of both lateral ventricles causes headache and sometimes vomiting followed by drowsiness that may progress quickly to coma, with extensor posturing of the limbs, bilateral Babinski signs, small nonreactive pupils, and impaired vertical oculocephalic movements.

A   B   C

FIGURE 24-2   Coma with right 3d nerve palsy due to stroke. *A.* T2-weighted fast spin echo MR image demonstrates a wedge-shaped area of abnormal signal intensity consistent with infarction within the midbrain extending from the aqueduct ventrally along the course of the 3d cranial nerve (arrows). *B.* T2-weighted image demonstrates bilateral thalamic infarctions (arrows). This area is perfused by the perforating arteries arising from the tip of the basilar artery. *C.* T2-weighted image with fluid attentuation (FLAIR). Note that the right thalamic infarction (*black arrow*) has abnormal high signal intensity while the left thalamic infarction (*white arrow*) has low signal intensity indicating a more chronic cavitated process. Also note the abnormal signal intensities along both trigones of the lateral ventricles consistent with small vessel ischemic disease. This patient suffered brainstem and bithalamic infarctions secondary to occlusion of the top of the basilar artery. (Prepared by William Dillon, M.D.)

A **B**

FIGURE 24-3 Unilateral intracranial mass lesion: coma, seizures, and right third nerve palsy. Axial post-contrast T$_1$-weighted MRI images through the suprasellar cistern (*A*) and third ventricle (*B*.) A heterogeneously enhancing mass in the right temporal lobe (*arrows*) compresses the right cerebral peduncle and midbrain (*white arrow*). This glioblastoma multiforme was resected and treated with a combination of radiation and chemotherapy. (Prepared by William Dillon, M.D.)

If the history and examination are not typical for any neurologic diagnosis and metabolic or drug causes are excluded, then information obtained from CT or MRI may be used as outlined in Table 24-1. The CT scan is useful to focus the differential diagnosis, and because of its accuracy and general availability, the diagnoses that it facilitates are listed in the table. As mentioned earlier, the majority of medical causes of coma are established without a CT or with the study being normal.

COMA AFTER HEAD TRAUMA Concussion is a common form of transient coma that results from torsion of the hemispheres about the midbrain-diencephalic junction with brief interruption of RAS function. Persistent coma after head trauma presents a more complex and serious problem (Chap. 374). The main causes are subdural or epidural hemorrhage, deep cerebral hemorrhage, bilateral frontotemporal contusions, and extensive white matter damage.

COMA WITH ISCHEMIC-ANOXIC BRAIN DAMAGE There are widespread and complex changes in the CNS following cardiac arrest, profound hypotension, or anoxia. Some of these are physiologic and mediated by alterations in electrical and neurotransmitter function, and others may result from endogenously released neurotoxins that ultimately lead to neuronal death. Several clinically recognizable patterns emerge that occur usually in pure form but that may coexist: (1) a deep coma with preserved brainstem function that evolves to the vegetative state or to a dementia, reflecting damage to neurons throughout the cortex—brainstem function may be suppressed in the first hours, thus emulating brain death, and the limbs may be either flaccid or show vigorous extensor posturing or myoclonic jerks; (2) syndromes of proximal bibrachial and paraparetic weakness or of cortical blindness that are due to bilateral infarctions of the watershed regions between major cortical vessel territories from diminished blood flow; (3) a Korsakoff-amnestic state that indicates the selective vulnerability of neurons in the hippocampal cortex; and infrequently (4) a cerebellar syndrome.

Brain Death Brain death is a state of total cessation of cerebral blood flow and global infarction of the brain at a time when respiration is preserved by artificial support and the heart continues to function. It is the only type of irrevocable loss of brain function currently recognized as equivalent to death. Many sets of roughly equivalent criteria have been advanced for the diagnosis of brain death, and it is essential to adhere to those endorsed as standard practice by the local medical community. Ideal criteria are simple, conducted at the bedside, and allow no chance of diagnostic error. There are three essential elements: (1) widespread cortical destruction shown by deep coma; (2) global brainstem damage demonstrated by absent pupillary light reaction, and absent oculovestibular and corneal reflexes; and (3) medullary destruction indicated by complete apnea. The pulse rate is also invariant and unresponsive to atropine. Most patients have diabetes insipidus, but in some it develops after the clinical signs of brain death. The pupils need not be enlarged but should not be constricted. The absence of deep tendon reflexes is not required because the spinal cord may remain functional.

The possibility of profound drug-induced or hypothermic CNS depression should always be excluded. Some period of observation, usually 6 to 24 h, is desirable during which this state is shown to be sustained. It is often advisable to delay clinical testing for up to 24 h if a cardiac arrest has caused brain death or if the inciting disease is not known.

Demonstration of apnea generally requires that the P$_{CO_2}$ be high enough to stimulate respiration. This can be accomplished safely in most patients by removal of the respirator and use of diffusion oxygenation sustained by a tracheal cannula connected to an oxygen supply. In brain-dead patients, CO_2 tension increases approximately 0.3 to 0.4 kPa/min (2 to 3 mmHg/min) during apnea. At the end of an appropriate interval, arterial P$_{CO_2}$ should be at least above 6.6 to 8.0 kPa (50 to 60 mmHg) for the test to be valid. Large posterior fossa lesions that compress the brainstem, CNS-depressant drugs, and profound hypothermia can simulate brain death, but adherence to recognized protocols for diagnosis will prevent these errors.

An isoelectric EEG is often used as a confirmatory test for total cortical damage, but it is not absolutely necessary. Radionuclide brain scanning, cerebral angiography, or transcranial Doppler measurements may also be used to demonstrate the absence of cerebral blood flow, but with the exception of the latter, they are cumbersome and have not been correlated extensively with pathologic material.

There is no explicit reason to make the diagnosis of brain death except when organ transplantation or difficult resource-allocation (intensive care) issues are involved. Although it is commonly accepted that the respirator can be disconnected from a brain-dead patient, most problems arise because of inadequate explanation and preparation of the family by the physician.

℞ **TREATMENT**

The immediate goal in acute coma is the prevention of further nervous system damage. Hypotension, hypoglycemia, hypercalcemia, hypoxia, hypercapnia, and hyperthermia should be corrected rapidly and assiduously. An oropharyngeal airway is adequate to keep the pharynx open in drowsy patients who are breathing normally. Tracheal intubation is indicated if there is apnea, upper airway obstruction, hypoventilation, or emesis, or if the patient is liable to aspirate. Mechanical ventilation is required if there is hypoventilation or if there is an intracranial mass and induced hypocapnia is necessary. Intravenous access is established, and naloxone and dextrose are administered if narcotic overdose or hypoglycemia are even remote possibilities. Thiamine is administered with glucose in order to avoid eliciting Wernicke's encephalopathy in malnourished patients. The veins of intravenous drug abusers may be difficult to cannulate; in such cases, naloxone can be injected sublingually through a small-guage needle. In cases of suspected basilar thrombosis with brainstem ischemia, intravenous heparin or a thrombolytic agent is administered after obtaining a CT scan, keeping in mind that cerebellar and pontine hemorrhages resemble the syndrome of basilar artery occlusion. Physostigmine, when used by experienced physicians with careful monitoring, may awaken patients with anticholinergic-type drug overdose, but many physicians believe that this is justified only to treat cardiac arrhythmias resulting from these overdoses. The use of benzodiazepine antagonists is promising for treatment of overdoses and has transient benefit in hepatic encephalopathy. Intravenous administration of water should be monitored carefully in any serious acute CNS illness because of the potential for exacerbating brain swelling. Neck injuries must not be overlooked, particularly prior to attempting intubation or eliciting oculocephalic responses. Headache accompanied by fever and meningismus indicates an urgent need for examination of the CSF to diagnose meningitis, and *lumbar puncture should not be delayed while awaiting a CT scan.*

Table 24-1

Approach to the Differential Diagnosis of Coma

NORMAL BRAINSTEM REFLEXES, NO LATERALIZING SIGNS

A. Bilateral hemispheral dysfunction without mass lesion (CT or MRI normal; primary test used for diagnosis is indicated in parentheses)
   1. Drug-toxin ingestion (toxicologic analysis)
   2. Endogenous metabolic encephalopathy (glucose, ammonia, calcium, osmolarity, P_{O_2}, P_{CO_2}, urea, sodium)
   3. Shock, hypertensive encephalopathy
   4. Meningitis (CSF analysis)
   5. Nonherpetic viral encephalitis (CSF analysis)
   6. Epilepsy (EEG)
   7. Reye's syndrome (ammonia, increased intracranial pressure)
   8. Fat embolism
   9. Subarachnoid hemorrhage with normal CT (CSF analysis)
   10. Creutzfeldt-Jakob disease (EEG)
   11. Hysterical coma or catatonia
B. Anatomic lesions of hemisphere found by CT or MRI
   1. Hydrocephalus
   2. Bilateral subdural hematomas
   3. Bilateral contusions, edema, or axonal shearing of hemispheres due to closed head trauma
   4. Subarachnoid hemorrhage
   5. Acute disseminated encephalomyelitis (CSF analysis)

NORMAL BRAINSTEM REFLEXES (WITH/WITHOUT UNILATERAL THIRD NERVE PALSY), LATERALIZING MOTOR SIGNS (CT OR MRI ABNORMAL)

A. Unilateral mass lesion
   1. Cerebral hemorrhage (basal ganglia, thalamus)
   2. Large infarction with surrounding brain edema
   3. Herpes virus encephalitis (temporal lobe lesion)
   4. Subdural or epidural hematoma
   5. Tumor with edema
   6. Brain abscess with edema
   7. Vasculitis with multiple infarctions
   8. Metabolic encephalopathy superimposed on preexisting focal lesions (i.e., stroke with hyperglycemia, hyponatremia, etc.)
   9. Pituitary apoplexy
B. Asymmetric signs accompanied by diffuse hemispheral dysfunction
   1. Metabolic encephalopathies with asymmetric signs (blood chemical determinations)
   2. Isodense subdural hematoma (MRI, CT with contrast)
   3. Thrombotic thrombocytopenic purpura (blood smear, platelet count)
   4. Epilepsy with focal seizures or postictal state (EEG)

MULTIPLE BRAINSTEM REFLEX ABNORMALITIES

A. Anatomic lesions in brainstem
   1. Pontine, midbrain hemorrhage
   2. Cerebellar hemorrhage, tumor, abscess
   3. Cerebellar infarction with brainstem compression
   4. Mass in hemisphere causing advanced upper brainstem compression
   5. Primary brainstem tumor, demyelination, or abscess
   6. Traumatic brainstem contusion-hemorrhage
B. Brainstem dysfunction without mass lesion
   1. Basilar artery thrombosis causing brainstem infarction (clinical signs, angiogram)
   2. Severe drug overdose (toxicologic analysis)
   3. Brainstem encephalitis
   4. Basilar artery migraine

Enlargement of one pupil usually indicates secondary midbrain compression by a hemispherical mass and demands immediate reduction of intracranial pressure (ICP) as discussed further in Chap. 374. Surgical evacuation of the mass may be appropriate. Medical management to reduce intracranial pressure consists of intravenous fluid normal saline (the safest fluid because it is slightly hyperosmolar in most patients). Therapeutic hyperventilation may be used to achieve an arterial P_{CO_2} of 3.7 to 4.2 kPa (28 to 32 mmHg), but its effects are brief. Hyperosmolar therapy with mannitol or an equivalent is the mainstay of ICP reduction. It may be used simultaneously with hyperventilation in critical cases. A ventricular puncture is necessary to decompress hydrocephalus if medical measures fail to improve alertness. The use of high-dose barbiturates and other neuronal sparing agents soon after cardiac arrest has not been shown in clinical studies to be beneficial and corticosteroids have no proven value except in cases of brain tumor.

PROGNOSIS OF COMA AND THE VEGETATIVE STATE Interest in predicting the outcome of coma is oriented toward allocating medical resources and limiting the support of hopeless cases. To date, no collection of clinical signs except those of brain death assuredly predicts outcome of coma, but certain constellations have prognostic value. Children and young adults may have ominous early clinical findings such as abnormal brainstem reflexes and yet recover. All schemes for prognosis should be taken as only approximate indicators, and medical judgments must be tempered by other factors such as age, underlying disease, and general medical condition. In an attempt to collect prognostic information from large numbers of patients with head injury, the Glasgow Coma Scale was devised; empirically it has predictive value in cases of brain trauma (see Chap. 374). Major points include a 95 percent death rate in patients whose pupillary reaction or reflex eye movements are absent 6 h after onset of coma, and a 91 percent death rate if the pupils are unreactive at 24 h (although roughly 5 percent make a good recovery).

Prognostication of nontraumatic coma is difficult because of the heterogeneity of contributing diseases. Metabolic coma generally has a more favorable prognosis than anoxic or traumatic coma. Unfavorable signs in the first hours after admission are the absence of any two of pupillary reaction, corneal reflex, or the oculovestibular response. One day after the onset of coma, the preceding signs, in addition to absence of eye opening and muscle tone, predict death or severe disability, and the same signs at 3 days strengthen the prediction of a poor outcome. In many patients, precise combinations of predictive signs do not occur, and coma scales lose their value. The use of evoked potentials aids prognostication in head-injured and post–cardiac arrest patients. Bilateral absence of cortical somatosensory evoked potentials is associated with death or a vegetative state in most cases. Medical practitioners are becoming less reluctant to withdraw support from non-brain-dead but severely neurologically injured patients as predictions become more reliable and resources more limited.

The prognosis for regaining full mental faculties once the vegetative state has supervened is almost nil. Most instances of dramatic recovery, when investigated carefully, yield to the usual rules for prognosis, but it must be acknowledged that rare instances of awakening to a condition of dementia or paralysis after months or years in this state have been documented.

BIBLIOGRAPHY

CELESIA GG et al: Persistent vegetative state—Report of the American Neurological Association Committee on Ethical Affairs. Ann Neurol 33:386, 1993

IVAN L, BRUCE D: *Coma.* Springfield, IL, Charles C Thomas, 1982

JENNET B et al: Prognosis of patients with severe head injury. Neurosurgery 4:283, 1979

LEVY D et al: Prognosis in non-traumatic coma. Ann Intern Med 94:229, 1981

PLUM F, POSNER J: *The Diagnosis of Stupor and Coma*, 3d ed. Philadelphia, Davis, 1980

ROPPER AH: Lateral displacement of the brain and level of consciousness in patients with an acute hemispheral mass. N Engl J Med 314:953, 1986

————: Coma and acutely raised intracranial pressure, in *Diseases of the Nervous System*, 2d ed, A Asbury et al (eds). Philadelphia, Saunders, 1992

————: *Neurological and Neurosurgical Intensive Care*, 3d ed. New York, Raven, 1992

YOUNG BY et al: *Coma and Impaired Consciousness*. New York, McGraw-Hill, 1997

25   *M.-Marsel Mesulam*

APHASIAS AND OTHER FOCAL CEREBRAL DISORDERS

The cerebral cortex is subdivided into five functional zones designated as (1) primary sensorimotor, (2) unimodal association, (3) heteromodal association, (4) paralimbic, and (5) limbic (Table 25-1, Fig. 25-1). The *primary sensorimotor zone*, devoted to elementary sensory and motor functions, takes up less than 10 percent of the cerebral cortex. The remaining four zones, collectively known as the *association cortex*, account for the vast majority of the cerebral cortex and sustain complex cognitive and behavioral functions. The conventional neurologic examination places a greater emphasis on testing of sensorimotor than cognitive function. Hence, detection of disease in the sensorimotor cortex and related pathways is more precise than detection of disease confined to the association cortex. A "normal" neurologic examination in a patient with a large frontal, parietal, or temporal lobe lesion is not uncommon in clinical experience. A systematic testing of cognitive function is necessary if the clinical assessment of the association cortex is to be guided by the same rational approach that guides the assessment of other components of the nervous system.

The interpretation of the traditional neurologic examination tends to be based on relatively invariant relationships between anatomy and function. Damage to the optic tract or striate cortex, for example, always leads to contralateral homonymous hemianopic visual field defects. The destruction of the sciatic nerve always leads to loss of the ankle jerk. The approach to higher cortical function was initially based on the expectation that analogous relationships would be uncovered in the association cortex; that it would be possible to identify centers for "hearing words," "perceiving space," or "storing memories"; and that it would consequently be possible to devise specific bedside tests for the precise localization of association cortex lesions. These expectations now need to be modified to incorporate more modern models of localization based on an understanding of *large-scale neural networks* and *selectively distributed processing*.

According to current thinking, cognitive and behavioral functions (domains) are coordinated by intersecting neural networks that contain interconnected cortical and subcortical components. The network approach to higher cortical function has at least four implications of clinical relevance: (1) a single domain such as language or memory can be disrupted by damage to any one of several areas, as long as

Table 25-1

Types of Cortical Areas and Their Corresponding Brodmann Numbers

PRIMARY SENSORY AND MOTOR CORTEX

Primary visual (area 17, striate cortex)
Primary auditory (areas 41, 42)
Primary somatosensory (areas 3, 1, 2 but mostly area 3b)
Primary motor (area 4)

UNIMODAL ASSOCIATION CORTEX

Unimodal visual [areas 18–19 (peristriate cortex, upstream visual association); 20–21, ?37 (downstream visual association)]
Unimodal auditory (area 22)
Unimodal somatosensory (area 5, rostral area 7)
Unimodal motor (areas 6, ?caudal 8, ?44, premotor cortex)

HETEROMODAL ASSOCIATION CORTEX

Heteromodal prefrontal (areas 9, 10, 45, 46, 47, rostral parts of areas 11, 12, 32)
Heteromodal parietotemporal (areas 39, 40, caudal parts of area 7, banks of superior temporal sulcus, ?area 36)

PARALIMBIC CORTEX

Insula (areas 14, 15), temporopolar cortex (area 38), caudal orbitofrontal cortex (caudal areas 11, 12), cingulate complex (areas 23, 24, ?31, 33, 25, 26, 29, caudal parts of area 32), parahippocampal cortex (areas 28, 34, 35, 30)

CORE LIMBIC AREAS

Corticoid formations (amygdala, substantia innominata, septal nuclei)
Allocortex (hippocampus, pyriform olfactory cortex)

FIGURE 25-1 Lateral (*top*) and medial (*bottom*) views of the cerebral hemispheres. The numbers refer to the Brodmann cytoarchitectonic designations. AG, angular gyrus; B, Broca's area; CC, corpus callosum; CG, cingulate cortex; DLPFC, dorsolateral prefrontal cortex; FEF, frontal eye fields (premotor cortex); FG, fusiform gyrus; IPL, inferior parietal lobule; ITG, inferior temporal gyrus; LG, lingual gyrus; MPFC, medial prefrontal cortex; MTG, middle temporal gyrus; OFC, orbitofrontal gyrus; PHG, parahippocampal gyrus; PPC, posterior parietal cortex; PSC, peristriate cortex; SC, striate cortex; SMG, supramarginal gyrus; SPL, superior parietal lobule; STG, superior temporal gyrus; STS, superior temporal sulcus; TP, temporopolar cortex; W, Wernicke's area.

these areas belong to the same network; (2) damage confined to a single area can give rise to multiple deficits, involving the functions of all networks that intersect in that region; (3) damage to a network component may give rise to minimal or transient deficits in the relevant domain if other parts of the network undergo compensatory reorganization; and (4) individual anatomic sites within a network display a relative (but not absolute) specialization for different behavioral aspects of the relevant function. Thus, damage to each anatomic component of a network may lead to impairments of the same domain but with different clinical patterns. Five anatomically defined large-scale networks are most relevant to clinical practice: a perisylvian network for language; a parietofrontal network for spatial orientation; an occipitotemporal network for object recognition; a limbic network for retentive memory; and a prefrontal network for attention and comportment (see Fig. 25-1).

THE LEFT PERISYLVIAN NETWORK FOR LANGUAGE: APHASIAS AND RELATED CONDITIONS **Definitions** Language allows the communication and reshaping of thoughts and experiences by linking them to arbitrary symbols known as words. The neural substrate of language is composed of a distributed network centered in the perisylvian region of the *left* hemisphere. The posterior pole of this network is known as *Wernicke's area* and includes the posterior third of the superior temporal gyrus and a surrounding rim of the inferior parietal lobule. An essential function of Wernicke's area is to transform sensory inputs into their neural word representations so that these can enter the distributed associations that lead to meaning. The anterior pole of the language network, known as *Broca's area*, includes the posterior part of the inferior frontal gyrus and a surrounding rim of prefrontal heteromodal cortex. An essential function of this area is to transform neural word representations into their articulatory sequences so that the words can be uttered in the form of spoken language. The sequencing function of Broca's area also appears to involve the ordering of words into sentences so that the resulting statement has a meaning-appropriate *syntax* (grammar). Wernicke's and Broca's areas are interconnected with each other and with additional perisylvian, temporal, prefrontal, and posterior parietal regions, making up a neural network subserving the various aspects of language function. Damage to any one of these components or to their interconnections can give rise to language disturbances (*aphasia*). Aphasia should be diagnosed only when there are deficits in the formal aspects of language such as naming, word choice, comprehension, spelling, and syntax. Dysarthria and mutism do not, by themselves, lead to a diagnosis of aphasia. The language network shows a left hemisphere dominance pattern in the vast majority of the population. In approximately 90 percent of right handers and 60 percent of left handers, aphasia occurs only after lesions of the left hemisphere. In some individuals no hemispheric dominance for language can be discerned, and in some others (including a small minority of right handers) there is a right hemisphere dominance for language. A language disturbance occurring after a right hemisphere lesion in a right hander is called *crossed aphasia*.

Clinical Examination The clinical examination of language should include the assessment of naming, spontaneous speech, comprehension, repetition, reading, and writing. A deficit of naming (*anomia*) is the single most common finding in aphasic patients. When asked to name common objects (pencil or wristwatch) or their parts (eraser, lead, stem, band), the patient may fail to come up with the appropriate word, may provide a circumlocutious description of the object ("the thing for writing"), or may come up with the wrong word (*paraphasia*). If the patient offers an incorrect but legitimate word ("pen" for "pencil"), the naming error is known as a *semantic paraphasia*; if the word approximates the correct answer but is phonetically inaccurate ("plentil" for "pencil") it is known as a *phonemic paraphasia*. Asking the patient to name body parts, geometric shapes, and component parts of objects (lapel of coat, cap of pen) can elicit mild forms of anomia in patients who can otherwise name common objects. In most anomias, the patient cannot retrieve the appropriate name when shown an object but can point to the appropriate object when the name is provided by the examiner. This is known as a one-way naming deficit. A two-way

naming deficit exists if the patient can neither provide nor recognize the correct name, a condition always associated with impairments of language comprehension. *Spontaneous speech* is described as "fluent" if it maintains appropriate phrase length and melody or as "nonfluent" if it is halting, dysarthric, and average phrase length is below four words. The examiner should also note if the speech is paraphasic or circumlocutious; if it shows a relative paucity of substantive nouns and action verbs versus function words (prepositions, conjunctions); and if word order, tenses, suffixes, prefixes, plurals, and possessives are appropriate. *Comprehension* can be tested by assessing the patient's ability to follow conversation, by asking yes-no questions ("Can a dog fly?", "Does it snow in summer?") or asking the patient to point to appropriate objects ("Where is the source of illumination in this room?"). Statements with embedded clauses or passive voice construction ("If a tiger is eaten by a lion, which animal stays alive?") help to assess the ability to comprehend complex syntactic structure. Commands to close or open the eyes, stand up, sit down, or roll over should not be used to assess overall comprehension since appropriate responses aimed at such axial movements are subserved by neural systems outside of the language network and can be preserved in patients who otherwise have profound comprehension deficits.

Repetition is assessed by asking the patient to repeat single words, short sentences, or strings of words such as "No ifs, ands, or buts". The testing of repetition with tongue-twisters such as "hippopotamus" or "Irish constabulary" provides a better assessment of dysarthria than aphasia. Aphasic patients may have little difficulty with tongue-twisters but have a particularly hard time repeating a string of function words. It is important to make sure that the number of words does not exceed the patient's attention span. Otherwise, the failure of repetition becomes a reflection of the narrowed attention span rather than an indication of an aphasic deficit. *Reading* should be assessed for deficits in reading aloud as well as comprehension. *Writing* is assessed for spelling errors, word order, and grammar. *Alexia* describes an inability to either read aloud or comprehend single words and simple sentences; *agraphia* (or *dysgraphia*) is used to describe an acquired deficit in the spelling or grammar of written language.

Each sector of the language network participates in several language functions but also displays local specializations. For example, Wernicke's area occupies the lexical-semantic pole of the language network, whereas Broca's area occupies its syntactic pole. This organization allows the classification of aphasic patients into specific clinical syndromes and helps to determine the most likely anatomic distribution of the underlying neurologic disease. It also has implications for etiology and prognosis (Table 25-2). The syndromes outlined below are idealizations; pure syndromes occur rarely. The correspondence between individual deficits of language function and lesion location does not display a rigid one-to-one relationship and should be conceptualized within the context of the distributed network model. With these considerations in mind, the aphasic syndromes can be divided into "central" syndromes, which result from damage to the two centers of the language network (Broca's and Wernicke's areas), and "disconnection" syndromes, which arise from lesions that interrupt the connections of these centers with each other and with the other components of the language network.

Wernicke's aphasia Comprehension is impaired for spoken and written language. Language output is fluent and maintains appropriate melody but is highly paraphasic and circumlocutious. The tendency for paraphasic errors may be so pronounced that it leads to strings of neologisms, which form the basis of what is known as "jargon aphasia." Speech contains large numbers of function words (e.g., prepositions, conjunctions) but few substantive nouns or verbs that refer to specific actions. The output is therefore voluminous but uninformative. For example, a 76-year-old man was brought to the emergency room because he started to talk "funny" while playing cards. In the following passage he is trying to describe how his wife accidentally threw away something important, perhaps his dentures: "We don't need it anymore, she says. And with it when that was downstairs was my teeth tick . . . a . . . den . . . dentith . . . my dentist. And they happened to be in that bag . . . see? How could this have happened? How could a thing like this happen . . . So she says we won't need it anymore . . . I didn't think we'd use it. And now if I have any problems anybody coming a month from now, four months from now, or six months from now, I have a new dentist. Where my two . . . two little pieces of dentist that I use . . . that I . . . all gone. If she throws the whole thing away . . . visit some friends of hers and she can't throw them away."

Gestures and pantomime do not improve communication. The patient does not seem to realize that his or her language is incomprehensible and may appear angry and impatient when the examiner fails to decipher the meaning of a severely paraphasic statement. In some patients this type of aphasia can be associated with severe agitation and paranoid behaviors. One area of comprehension that may be preserved is the ability to follow commands aimed at axial musculature. The dissociation between the failure to understand simple questions ("What is your name") in a patient who rapidly closes his or her eyes, sits up, or rolls over when asked to do so is characteristic of Wernicke's aphasia and helps to differentiate it from deafness, psychiatric disease, or malingering. Patients with Wernicke's aphasia cannot express their thoughts in meaning-appropriate words and cannot decode the meaning of words in any modality of input. This aphasia therefore has expressive as well as receptive components and should not be designated as a "sensory aphasia" or "receptive aphasia," two terms often used as synonyms for Wernicke's aphasia. In addition to the paraphasic speech and poor comprehension of spoken language, patients with Wernicke's aphasia also have impaired repetition, naming, reading, and writing.

The lesion site most commonly associated with Wernicke's aphasia is the posterior portion of the language network and tends to involve at least parts of Wernicke's area. An embolus to the inferior division of the middle cerebral artery, and to the posterior temporal or angular branches in particular, is the most common etiology (Chap. 366). Intracerebral hemorrhage, venous infarction, severe head trauma, or neoplasm are other causes. A coexisting right hemi- or superior quadrantanopia is common in patients with Wernicke's aphasia, and mild right nasolabial flattening may be found, but otherwise the examination is often unrevealing. The paraphasic, neologistic speech in an agitated patient with an otherwise uneventful neurologic examination may lead to the suspicion of a primary psychiatric disorder such as schizophrenia or mania, but the other components characteristic of acquired aphasia and the absence of prior psychiatric disease usually settle the issue. The prognosis for recovery is guarded in most cases; some patients with Wernicke's aphasia due to intracerebral hemorrhage or head trauma may improve as the hemorrhage or the injury heals.

Broca's aphasia Speech is nonfluent, labored, dysarthric, and interrupted by many word-finding pauses. It is impoverished in function words but enriched in meaning-appropriate nouns and verbs. Abnormal word order and the inappropriate deployment of *bound morphemes* (word endings used to denote tenses, possessives, or plurals) lead to a characteristic agrammatism. Speech is telegraphic and pithy but quite informative. In the following passage, a 45-year-old man with Broca's aphasia describes his medical history: "I see . . . the dotor, dotor sent me . . . Bosson. Go to hospital. Dotor . . . kept me beside. Two, tee days, doctor send me home."

Output may be reduced to a grunt or single word ("yes" or "no") which is emitted with different intonations in an attempt to express approval or disapproval. In addition to fluency, naming and repetition are also impaired. Comprehension of spoken language is intact, except for syntactically difficult sentences with passive voice structure or embedded clauses. Reading comprehension is also preserved, with the occasional exception of a specific inability to read small grammatical words such as conjunctions and pronouns. The last two features indicate that Broca's aphasia is not just an "expressive" or "motor" disorder and that it may also involve a comprehension deficit for function words and syntax. Patients with Broca's aphasia can be tearful, easily frustrated, and profoundly depressed. Insight into their condition is preserved, in contrast to Wernicke's aphasia. Even when spontaneous speech is severely dysarthric, the patient may be able to display a relatively normal articulation of words when singing. This dissociation has been used to develop specific therapeutic approaches (melodic intonation therapy) for treating patients with Broca's aphasia. Additional neurologic deficits that are usually encountered in these patients include right facial weakness, hemiparesis or hemiplegia, and a buccofacial apraxia characterized by an inability to carry out motor commands involving oropharyngeal and facial musculature (for example, show me how you would blow out a match, suck through a straw). Visual fields are intact. The cause is most often infarction of Broca's area (the inferior frontal convolution; see Fig. 25-1) and surrounding anterior perisylvian and insular cortex, due to occlusion of the superior division of the middle cerebral artery (Chap. 366). Mass lesions including tumor (either primary or metastatic), intracerebral or subdural hemorrhage, or abscess can also present as Broca's aphasia. Small lesions confined to the posterior part of Broca's area may lead to a nonaphasic and often reversible deficit of speech articulation. In these cases, the remaining parts of the language network appear sufficient for sustaining essential language functions. Patients frequently have limited motor deficits at presentation, for example, isolated facial weakness. By contrast, patients with dense hemiparesis or hemiplegia have larger lesions and less favorable prospects for recovery. When the cause is stroke, recovery of language function generally peaks within several months, after which time no further progress is made.

Global aphasia Speech output is nonfluent, and comprehension of spoken language is severely impaired. Naming, repetition, reading, and writing are also impaired. This syndrome represents the combined involvement of Broca's and Wernicke's areas and usually results from strokes that involve the entire middle cerebral artery distribution in the left hemisphere. Most patients are initially mute or say a few words, such as "hi" or "yes." Related signs include right hemiplegia, hemisensory loss, and homonomous hemianopia. Occasionally, a patient with a lesion in Wernicke's area will present with a global aphasia that soon resolves into Wernicke's aphasia. In this circumstance, the impaired fluency (which gives the initial impression of global aphasia) arises from a mechanism analogous to spinal shock or dias-

Table 25-2

Clinical Features of Aphasias and Related Conditions

	Comprehension	Repetition of Spoken Language	Naming	Fluency
Wernicke's	Impaired	Impaired	Impaired	Preserved or increased
Broca's	Preserved (except grammar)	Impaired	Impaired	Decreased
Global	Impaired	Impaired	Impaired	Decreased
Conduction	Preserved	Impaired	Impaired	Preserved
Nonfluent (motor) transcortical	Preserved	Preserved	Impaired	Impaired
Fluent (sensory) transcortical	Impaired	Preserved	Impaired	Preserved
Isolation	Impaired	Echolalia	Impaired	No purposeful speech
Anomic	Preserved	Preserved	Impaired	Preserved except for word-finding pauses
Pure word deafness	Impaired only for spoken language	Impaired	Preserved	Preserved
Pure alexia	Impaired only for reading	Preserved	Preserved	Preserved

chisis, where acute dysfunction in a network component leads to a remote and reversible dysfunction in other network components.

Conduction aphasia   Speech output is fluent but paraphasic; comprehension of spoken language is intact; repetition is severely impaired. Naming and writing are also impaired. Reading aloud is impaired, but reading comprehension is preserved. This type of aphasia represents a disconnection between the anterior and posterior poles of the language network. As a consequence of this disconnection, neural word representations formed in Wernicke's area and adjacent regions cannot be conveyed to Broca's area for assembly into corresponding articulatory patterns. The lesion sites spare Broca's and Wernicke's areas but involve projection paths that link the two or adjacent perisylvian regions such as the insula or supramarginal gyrus. Occasionally, a Wernicke's area lesion gives rise to a transient Wernicke's aphasia that rapidly resolves into a conduction aphasia. The paraphasic output in conduction aphasia interferes with the ability to express meaning, but this deficit is not nearly as severe as the one displayed by patients with Wernicke's aphasia. Associated neurologic signs in conduction aphasia vary according to the primary lesion site.

Nonfluent transcortical aphasia (transcortical motor aphasia)   The clinical features are somewhat similar to those of Broca's aphasia, but repetition is intact and the agrammatism may be less pronounced. The rest of the neurologic examination may be intact, but a right hemiparesis can also exist. The lesion site is one that leaves the core of the language network intact but that disconnects it from prefrontal areas of the brain. Characteristic lesion sites include the anterior half of the vascular watershed zone between anterior and middle cerebral artery territories or the supplementary motor cortex in the territory of the anterior cerebral artery.

Fluent transcortical aphasia (transcortical sensory aphasia)   Clinical features are similar to those of Wernicke's aphasia, but repetition is intact. The lesion site disconnects the intact core of the language network from other temporoparietal association areas. Associated neurologic findings may include hemianopia. Fluent transcortical aphasia can be associated with cerebrovascular lesions (e.g., infarctions in the posterior part of the watershed zone) or neoplasms that involve the temporoparietal cortex posterior to Wernicke's area.

Isolation aphasia   This rare syndrome represents a combination of the two transcortical aphasias. Comprehension is severely impaired, and there is no purposeful speech output. The patient may parrot fragments of heard conversations (*echolalia*), indicating that the neural mechanisms for repetition are relatively spared. This condition represents the pathologic function of the language network when it is isolated from other regions of the brain. Lesions are patchy and can be associated with anoxia, carbon monoxide poisoning, or complete watershed zone infarctions. Broca's and Wernicke's areas tend to be spared, but there is damage in surrounding frontal, parietal, and temporal cortex.

Anomic aphasia   This type of aphasia could be considered as the "minimal dysfunction" syndrome of the language network. Articulation, comprehension, and repetition are intact but confrontation naming, word finding, and spelling are impaired. Speech is enriched in function words but impoverished in substantive nouns and verbs denoting specific actions. Language output is fluent but paraphasic, circumlocutious, and uninformative. The lesion sites can be anywhere within the left hemisphere language network, including the middle and inferior temporal gyri. *Anomic aphasia is the single most common language disturbance seen in head trauma and metabolic encephalopathy.* This is also the most common aphasia seen in Alzheimer's disease. The language impairment of Alzheimer's disease almost always leads to fluent aphasias (e.g., anomic, Wernicke's, conduction, or fluent transcortical aphasia). The insidious onset and relentless progression of nonfluent language disturbances (Broca's or nonfluent transcortical aphasia) can be seen in patients with the syndrome of *primary progressive aphasia*, a degenerative disease that is most commonly associated with focal nonspecific neuronal loss or Pick's disease.

Pure word deafness   This is not a true aphasic syndrome because the language deficit is modality-specific. The most common lesions are either bilateral or left-sided in the superior temporal gyrus. The net effect of the underlying lesion is to interrupt the flow of information from the unimodal auditory association cortex to Wernicke's area. Patients with this syndrome have no difficulty understanding written language and can express themselves very well in spoken or written language. These patients are not deaf in the traditional sense and have no difficulty interpreting and reacting to environmental sounds since primary auditory cortex and subcortical auditory relays are intact. Since auditory information cannot be conveyed to the language network, however, it cannot be decoded into neural word representations and the patient reacts to speech as if it were in an alien tongue that cannot be deciphered. Patients with this syndrome cannot repeat spoken language but have no difficulty naming objects. In time, patients with pure word deafness teach themselves lip reading and may appear to have improved upon superficial bedside examination. There may be no additional neurologic findings, but agitated paranoid reactions are frequent. Cerebrovascular lesions are the most frequent causes of this syndrome.

Pure alexia without agraphia   This is the visual equivalent of pure word deafness. The lesions (usually a combination of damage to the left occipital cortex and to a posterior sector of the corpus callosum—the splenium) interrupt the flow of visual input into the language network. There is usually a right hemianopia, but the core language network remains unaffected. The patient can understand and produce spoken language, name objects in the left visual hemifield, repeat, and write. However, the patient acts as if he or she is completely illiterate when asked to read even the simplest sentence because the visual information from the written words (presented to the intact left visual hemifield) cannot reach the language network. According to Geschwind, objects in the left hemifield can be named accurately because they activate nonvisual associations in the right hemisphere, which, in turn, can access the language network through transcallosal pathways anterior to the splenium. Patients with this syndrome may also lose the ability to name colors, although they can match colors. This is known as a *color anomia*. The most common etiology of pure alexia is a cerebrovascular lesion in the distribution of the posterior cerebral artery or an infiltrating neoplasm in the left occipital cortex that involves the optic radiations as well as the crossing fibers of the splenium. Since the posterior cerebral artery also supplies medial temporal components of the limbic system, the patient with pure alexia may also experience an amnesia, but this is usually transient.

Aphemia   There is an acute onset of severely impaired fluency (often mutism) that resolves, in time, into a hoarse whisper. Writing, reading, and comprehension are intact, so this is not a true aphasic syndrome. Partial lesions of Broca's area or subcortical lesions that undercut its connections with other parts of the brain may be present. Occasionally, the lesion site is on the medial aspects of the frontal lobes and may involve the supplementary motor cortex of the left hemisphere.

Apraxia   Apraxia is a generic term that designates a complex motor deficit that cannot be attributed to pyramidal, extrapyramidal, cerebellar, or sensory dysfunction and that does not arise from the patient's failure to understand the nature of the task. The one form that is most frequently encountered in clinical practice is known as *ideomotor apraxia*. Commands to perform a specific motor act ("cough," "blow out a match") or to pantomime the use of a common tool (a comb, hammer, straw, or toothbrush) in the absence of the real object cannot be followed. The patient's ability to comprehend the command is ascertained by demonstrating multiple movements and establishing that the correct one can be recognized. Some patients with this type of apraxia can imitate the appropriate movement (when it is demonstrated by the examiner) and show no impairment when handed the real object, indicating that the sensorimotor mechanisms necessary for the movement are intact. Ideomotor apraxia represents a disconnection of the language network from pyramidal motor systems: commands to execute complex movements are understood but cannot be conveyed to the appropriate motor areas, even though the relevant motor mechanisms are intact. *Buccofacial apraxia* involves apraxic deficits in movements of the face and mouth. *Limb apraxia* encompasses apraxic deficits in movements of the arms and legs. Ideomotor apraxia is commonly associated with aphasic syndromes, especially Broca's aphasia and conduction aphasia. Its presence cannot be ascertained in patients with language comprehension deficits. As indicated above, the ability to follow commands aimed at axial musculature ("close the eyes," "stand up") is subserved by different pathways and may be intact in otherwise severely aphasic and apraxic patients. Patients with lesions of the anterior corpus callosum can display a special type of ideomotor apraxia confined to the left side of the body. Since the handling of real objects is not impaired, ideomotor apraxia, by itself, causes no limitation of daily living activities.

Two other types of apraxia are ideational apraxia and limb-kinetic apraxia. *Ideational apraxia* refers to a deficit in the execution of a goal-directed sequence of movements in patients who have no difficulty executing the individual components of the sequence. For example, when asked to pick up a pen and write, the sequence of uncapping the pen, placing the cap at the opposite end, turning the point towards the writing surface, and writing may be disrupted and the patient may be seen trying to write with the wrong end of the pen or even with the removed cap. These motor sequencing problems are usually seen in the context of confusional states and dementias rather than focal lesions associated with aphasic conditions. *Limb-kinetic apraxia* involves a clumsiness in the actual use of tools that cannot be attributed to sensory, pyramidal, extrapyramidal, or cerebellar dysfunction. This condition can emerge in the context of focal premotor cortex lesions or *corticobasal ganglionic degeneration.*

Gerstmann's syndrome The combination of *acalculia* (impairment of simple arithmetic), *dysgraphia* (impaired writing), *finger anomia* (an inability to name individual fingers such as the index or thumb), and *right-left confusion* (an inability to tell whether a hand, foot, or arm of the patient or examiner is on the right or left side of the body) is known as Gerstmann's syndrome. In making this diagnosis it is important to establish that the finger and left-right naming deficits are not part of a more generalized anomia and that the patient is not otherwise aphasic. When Gerstmann's syndrome is seen in isolation, it is commonly associated with damage to the inferior parietal lobule (especially the angular gyrus) in the left hemisphere.

Aprosodia Variations of melodic stress and intonation influence the meaning and impact of spoken language. For example, the two statements "He is clever." and "He is clever?" contain an identical word choice and syntax but convey vastly different messages because of differences in the intonation and stress with which the statements are uttered. This aspect of language is known as *prosody.* Damage to perisylvian areas in the right hemisphere can interfere with speech prosody and can lead to syndromes of aprosodia. Ross has pointed out that damage to right hemisphere regions corresponding to Wernicke's area yields a greater impairment in the decoding of speech prosody, whereas damage to right hemisphere regions corresponding to Broca's area yields a greater impairment in the ability to introduce meaning-appropriate prosody into spoken language. The latter deficit is the most common type of aprosodia identified in clinical practice— the patient produces grammatically correct language with accurate word choice but the statements are uttered in a monotone that interferes with the ability to convey the intended stress and affect. Patients with this type of aprosodia give the mistaken impression of being depressed or indifferent.

Subcortical aphasias The major aphasic syndromes in Table 25-2 are classified according to cortical lesion sites. However, damage to subcortical components of the language network (e.g., the head of the caudate and thalamus of the left hemisphere) can also lead to aphasia. The resulting syndromes contain combinations of deficits in the various aspects of language but rarely fit the specific patterns described in Table 25-2. An anomic aphasia accompanied by dysarthria

or a fluent aphasia with hemiparesis represents deviation from the major syndromes listed in Table 25-2 and should raise the suspicion of a subcortical lesion site.

THE PARIETOFRONTAL NETWORK FOR SPATIAL ORIENTATION: NEGLECT AND RELATED CONDITIONS

A number of clinical syndromes are recognizable with deficits in this network. They include hemispatial neglect, Balint's syndrome, simultanagnosia, dressing apraxia, and construction apraxia.

Hemispatial Neglect Adaptive orientation to significant events within the extrapersonal space is subserved by a large-scale network containing three major cortical components. The *cingulate cortex* provides access to a limbic-motivational mapping of the extrapersonal space, the *posterior parietal cortex* to a sensory-representational mapping, and the *frontal eye fields* in the frontal lobe to a motor-exploratory mapping. Subcortical components of this network include the striatum and the pulvinar nucleus of the thalamus. Contralesional hemispatial neglect represents one outcome of damage to any of the cortical or subcortical components of this network. *The traditional view that hemispatial neglect always denotes a parietal lobe lesion is inaccurate.* In keeping with this anatomic organization, the clinical manifestations of neglect display three behavioral components: sensory events (or their mental representations) within the neglected hemispace have a lesser impact on overall awareness; there is a paucity of exploratory and orienting acts directed toward the neglected hemispace; and the patient behaves as if the neglected hemispace was motivationally devalued.

The neural organization of spatial orientation displays a right hemisphere dominance pattern. The right hemisphere directs attention to the *entire* extrapersonal space, whereas the left hemisphere directs attention only to the contralateral right hemispace. Unilateral left hemisphere lesions do not give rise to contralesional neglect since the ipsiversive attentional mechanisms of the right hemisphere can compensate for the loss of the *contralaterally* directed attentional functions of the left hemisphere. Unilateral right hemisphere lesions, however, give rise to severe contralesional left hemispatial neglect because the unaffected left hemisphere does not contain ipsiversive attentional mechanisms. Contralesional neglect is consequently more common, severe, and lasting after damage to the right hemisphere than after damage to the left hemisphere. Severe neglect for the right hemispace is rare, even in left handers with left hemisphere lesions.

Patients with severe neglect may fail to dress, shave, or groom the left side of the body; may fail to eat food placed on the left side of the tray; and may fail to read the left half of sentences. When the examiner draws a large circle [12 to 16 cm (5 to 6 in.) in diameter] and asks the patient to place the numbers 1 to 12 as if the circle represented the face of a clock, there is a tendency to crowd the numbers on the right side and leave the left side empty. When asked to copy a simple line drawing, the patient fails to copy detail on the left; and when asked to write, there is a tendency to leave an unusually wide margin on the left.

Two bedside tests that are useful in assessing neglect are *simultaneous bilateral stimulation* and *visual target cancellation.* In the former, the examiner provides either unilateral or simultaneous bilateral stimulation in the visual, auditory, and tactile modalities. Following right hemisphere injury, patients who have no difficulty detecting unilateral stimuli on either side experience the bilaterally presented stimulus as coming only from the right. This phenomenon is known as *extinction* and is a manifestation of the sensory-representational aspect of hemispatial neglect. In the target detection task, targets (e.g., A's) are interspersed with foils (e.g., other letters of the alphabet) on a 21.5 $\times$ 28.0 cm (8.5 $\times$ 11 in.) sheet of paper and the patient is asked to circle all the targets. A failure to detect targets on the left is a manifestation of the exploratory deficit in hemispatial neglect. Hemianopia, by itself, does not interfere with performance in this task since the patient is free to turn the head and eyes to the left. The normal tendency in target detection tasks is to start from the left upper quadrant and move systematically in horizontal or vertical sweeps. Some patients show a tendency to start the process from the right and proceed in a haphazard fashion. This represents a subtle manifestation of left neglect, even if the patient eventually manages to detect all the appropriate targets. Some patients with neglect may also deny the existence of hemiparesis or hemihypesthesia and may even deny ownership of the paralyzed limb, a condition known as *anosognosia*.

The clinical manifestations of neglect are not identical in all patients. In general, lesions that are centered around the frontal component of the network for spatial orientation are likely to result in neglect syndromes with relatively more salient motor-exploratory deficits, whereas lesions centered around the parietal component are likely to result in neglect syndromes with more salient sensory-representational deficits. Cerebrovascular lesions and neoplasms in the right hemisphere are the most common causes of hemispatial neglect. Depending on the site of the lesion, the patient with neglect may also have hemiparesis, hemihypesthesia, and hemianopia on the left, but these are not invariant findings.

Balint's Syndrome, Simultanagnosia, Dressing Apraxia, and Construction Apraxia Bilateral involvement of the network for spatial orientation, especially its parietal components, leads to a state of severe spatial disorientation known as *Balint's syndrome*. Balint's syndrome involves deficits in the orderly visuomotor scanning of the environment (*oculomotor apraxia*) and in accurate manual reaching toward visual targets (*optic ataxia*). The third and most dramatic component of Balint's syndrome is known as *simultanagnosia* and reflects an inability to integrate visual information in the center of gaze with more peripheral information. The patient gets stuck on the detail that falls in the center of gaze without attempting to scan the visual environment for additional information. The patient with simultanagnosia "misses the forest for the trees." Complex visual scenes cannot be grasped in their entirety, leading to severe limitations in the visual identification of objects and scenes. For example, a patient who is shown a table lamp and asked to name the object may look at its circular base and call it an ash tray. Some patients with simultanagnosia report that objects they look at may suddenly vanish, probably indicating an inability to look back at the original point of gaze after brief saccadic displacements. Movement and distracting stimuli greatly exacerbate the difficulties of visual perception. Simultanagnosia can sometimes occur without the other two components of Balint's syndrome.

A modification of the letter cancellation task described above can be used for the bedside diagnosis of simultanagnosia. In this modification, some of the targets (e.g., A's) are made to be much larger than the others [7.5 to 10 cm vs. 2.5 cm (3 to 4 in. vs. 1 in.) in height], and all targets are embedded among foils. Patients with simultanagnosia display a counterintuitive but characteristic tendency to miss the larger targets (Fig. 25-2). This occurs because the information needed for the identification of the larger targets cannot be confined to the immediate line of gaze and requires the integration of visual information across a more extensive field of view. The greater difficulty in the detection of the larger targets also indicates that poor acuity is not responsible for the impairment of visual function and that the problem is central rather than peripheral. Balint's syndrome results from bilateral dorsal parietal lesions; common settings include watershed infarction between the middle and posterior cerebral artery territories, hypoglycemia, sagittal sinus thrombosis, or degenerative diseases such as Alzheimer's disease. In patients with Balint's syndrome due to stroke, bilateral visual field defects (usually inferior quadrantanopsias) are common.

Another manifestation of bilateral (or right sided) dorsal parietal lobe lesions is *dressing apraxia*. The patient with this condition is unable to align the body axis with the axis of the garment and can be seen struggling as he or she holds a coat from its bottom or extends his or her arm into a fold of the garment rather than into its sleeve. Lesions that involve the posterior parietal cortex in the right hemisphere also lead to severe difficulties in copying simple line drawings. This is known as a *construction apraxia*. In some patients, the drawing difficulties are confined to the left side of the figure and represent a manifestation of hemispatial neglect; in others, there is a more universal deficit in reproducing contours and three-dimensional perspective. Dressing apraxia and construction apraxia represent special instances of a more general disturbance in spatial orientation.

FIGURE 25-2 This 70-year-old woman with a 2-year history of degenerative dementia was asked to circle all the A's. She detects most of the small targets but ignores the larger ones. This is a manifestation of simultanagnosia.

THE OCCIPITOTEMPORAL NETWORK FOR OBJECT RECOGNITION: PROSOPAGNOSIA AND OBJECT AGNOSIA Perceptual information about faces and objects is initially encoded in primary (striate) visual cortex and adjacent (upstream) peristriate visual association areas. This information is subsequently relayed first to the downstream visual association areas of occipitotemporal cortex and then to other heteromodal and paralimbic areas of the cerebral cortex. Bilateral lesions in the fusiform and lingual gyri of occipitotemporal cortex disrupt this process and interfere with the ability of otherwise-intact perceptual information to activate the distributed multimodal associations that lead to the recognition of faces and objects. The resultant face and object recognition deficits are known as *prosopagnosia* and *visual object agnosia*.

The patient with prosopagnosia cannot recognize familiar faces, including, sometimes, the reflection of his or her own face in the mirror. This is not a perceptual deficit since prosopagnosic patients can easily tell if two faces are identical or not. Furthermore, a prosopagnosic patient who cannot recognize a familiar face by visual inspection alone can use auditory cues to reach appropriate recognition if allowed to listen to the person's voice. The deficit in prosopagnosia is therefore modality-specific and reflects the existence of a lesion that prevents the activation of otherwise intact multimodal templates by relevant visual input. Damasio has pointed out that the deficit in prosopagnosia is not limited to the recognition of faces but that it can also extend to the recognition of individual members of larger generic object groups. For example, prosopagnosic patients characteristically have no difficulty with the generic identification of a face as a face or of a car as a car, but they cannot recognize the identity of an individual face or the make of an individual car. This reflects a visual recognition deficit for proprietary features that characterize individual members of an object class. When recognition problems become more generalized and extend to the generic identification of common objects, the condition is known as visual object agnosia. In contrast to prosopagnosic patients, those with object agnosia cannot recognize a face as a face or a car as a car. It is important to distinguish visual object agnosia from anomia. The patient with anomia cannot name the object but can describe its use. In contrast, the patient with visual agnosia is unable either to name a visually presented object or to describe its use. The characteristic lesions in prosopagnosia and visual object agnosia consist of bilateral infarctions in the territory of the posterior cerebral arteries and involve the lingual and fusiform gyri. Associated deficits can include visual field defects (especially superior quadrantanopias) or a centrally based color blindness known as achromatopsia. Rarely, the responsible lesion is unilateral. In such cases, prosopagnosia is associated with lesions in the right hemisphere and object agnosia with lesions in the left.

As noted above, patients with Balint's syndrome also experience severe visual recognition difficulties based on abnormalities in the integration of visual percepts. The resulting face and object recognition deficits of Balint's syndrome are known as *apperceptive visual agnosias*, whereas the prosopagnosia and visual object agnosias described in this section are known as *associative agnosias* because they result from the failure of an intact percept to evoke the relevant multimodal associations.

THE LIMBIC NETWORK FOR MEMORY: AMNESIAS The core limbic and paralimbic areas listed in Table 25-1, the anterior and medial nuclei of the thalamus, the medial and basal parts of the striatum, and the hypothalamus collectively constitute a distributed network known as the *limbic system*. The behavioral affiliations of this network include the coordination of emotion, motivation, autonomic tone, and endocrine function. An additional area of specialization for the limbic network, and the one which is of most relevance to clinical practice, is that of declarative (conscious) memory for events and experiences. Damage to components of the limbic network can give rise to severe and global disturbances of retentive memory. This type of memory disturbance is known as an amnestic state. In the absence of deficits in motivation, attention, language, or visuospatial function, the clinical diagnosis of a persistent global amnestic state implies a primary disturbance in the core process of retentive memory and is always associated with bilateral lesions within the limbic network.

The memory disturbance in the amnestic state is multimodal and includes retrograde and anterograde components. The *retrograde amnesia* involves an inability to recall experiences that occurred before the onset of the amnestic state. Relatively recent events are more vulnerable to retrograde amnesia than more remote events. This is known as Ribot's gradient and explains why patients with even very severe retrograde amnesia rarely forget events of early childhood. A patient who comes to the emergency room complaining that he cannot remember his identity but who can remember the events of that day is almost certainly not suffering from a neurologic cause of memory disturbance. The second and most important component of the amnestic state is the *anterograde amnesia*, which indicates an inability to store, retain, and recall new knowledge. Patients with amnestic states are perfectly alert and motivated but cannot remember what they ate a few minutes ago or the details of an important event they may have experienced a few hours ago. In the acute stages, there may also be a tendency to fill in memory gaps with inaccurate, fabricated, and often implausible information. This is known as *confabulation*. Patients with the amnestic syndrome forget that they forget and tend to deny the existence of a memory problem when questioned.

The patient with an amnestic state is almost always disoriented, especially to time. Accurate temporal orientation and accurate knowledge of current news rule out a major amnestic state. Memory can be tested with a list of four to five words read aloud by the examiner up to five times or until the patient can immediately repeat the entire list without intervening delay. In the next phase of testing, no distraction is provided and the patient is allowed to concentrate on the words and to rehearse them internally for 1 min before being asked to recall them. Accurate performance in this phase indicates that the patient is motivated and sufficiently attentive to hold the words in consciousness for at least 1 min. The final phase of the testing involves a retention period of 5 to 10 min during which the patient is engaged in other tasks. Adequate recall at the end of this interval requires encoding, retention, and retrieval. Amnestic patients fail this phase of the task and may even forget that they were given a list of words to remember. Accurate recognition of the words by multiple choice in a patient who cannot recall them indicates a less severe memory disturbance that affects mostly the retrieval stage of memory.

Many neurologic diseases can give rise to an amnestic state. These include tumors (of the sphenoid wing, posterior corpus callosum, thalamus, or medial temporal lobe), infarctions (in the territories of the anterior or posterior cerebral arteries), head trauma, herpes simplex encephalitis, Wernicke-Korsakoff encephalopathy, paraneoplastic limbic encephalitis, and degenerative dementias such as Alzheimer's or Pick's disease. The one common denominator of all these diseases is that they lead to the bilateral involvement of one or more components in the limbic network. Occasionally, unilateral left sided lesions can give rise to an amnestic state, but the memory disorder tends to be transient. Depending on the nature and distribution of the underlying neurologic disease, the patient may also have visual field deficits, eye movement limitations, or cerebellar findings. In many patients there are no associated neurologic findings, and the differential diagnosis of psychiatric disease may occasionally be entertained. In this setting, the amnesia may remain undetected and lead to the inappropriate management of patients with head trauma or herpes simplex encephalitis.

Transient global amnesia is a distinctive syndrome usually seen in late middle age. Patients become acutely disoriented and repeatedly ask who they are, where they are, what they are doing. The spell is characterized by anterograde amnesia (inability to retain new information) and a retrograde amnesia for relatively recent events that occurred before the onset. The syndrome usually resolves within 24 to 48 h and is followed by the filling-in of the period affected by the retrograde amnesia, although there is persistent loss of memory for the events that occurred during the ictus. Recurrences are noted in approximately 20 percent of patients. Migraine, temporal lobe seizures, and transient ischemic events in the posterior cerebral territory (artery of Percheron; see Chap. 366) have been postulated as causes of transient global amnesia.

Although the limbic network is the site of damage for amnestic states, it is almost certainly not the storage site for memories. Memories are stored in widely distributed form throughout association cortex. The role attributed to the limbic network is to bind these distributed fragments into coherent events and experiences that can sustain conscious recall. Damage to the limbic network does not necessarily destroy memories but interferes with their conscious (declarative) recall in coherent form. The individual fragments of information remain preserved despite the limbic lesions and can sustain what is known as *implicit memory*. For example, patients with amnestic states can acquire new motor or perceptual skills, even though they may have no conscious knowledge of the experiences that led to the acquisition of these skills.

THE PREFRONTAL NETWORK FOR ATTENTION AND COMPORTMENT Approximately one-third of all the cerebral cortex in the human brain is located in the frontal lobes. The frontal lobes can be subdivided into motor-premotor, dorsolateral prefrontal, medial prefrontal, and orbitofrontal components. The terms *frontal lobe syndrome* and *prefrontal cortex* refer only to the last three of these four components. These are the parts of the cerebral cortex that show the greatest phylogenetic expansion in primates and especially in humans. The dorsolateral prefrontal, medial prefrontal, and orbitofrontal areas, and the subcortical structures with which they are interconnected (i.e., the head of the caudate and the dorsomedial nucleus of the thalamus), collectively make up a large-scale prefrontal network that coordinates exceedingly complex aspects of human cognition and comportment.

The orbitofrontal cortex provides a convergence site for neural inputs from association, paralimbic, and limbic cortices and constitutes a zone of intersection for the prefrontal and limbic networks. In keeping with this organization, the prefrontal network plays an important role in behaviors that require an integration of thought with emotion and motivation. There is no simple formula for summarizing the diverse functional affiliations of the prefrontal network. Its integrity appears important for the simultaneous (on-line) awareness of context, options, consequences, relevance, and perspectives so as to allow the formulation of adaptive inferences, decisions, and actions. Damage to this part of the brain impairs mental flexibility, foresight, judgment, and the ability to inhibit inappropriate responses. Behaviors impaired by prefrontal cortex lesions are often referred to as "executive functions."

Even very large bilateral prefrontal lesions may leave all sensory, motor, and basic cognitive functions intact while leading to isolated but dramatic alterations of personality and comportment. The associated impairments may emerge only in real-life situations when behavior is under minimal external control and may not be apparent within the structured environment of the medical office. The physician must therefore be prepared to make a diagnosis of frontal lobe disease on the basis of historical information alone even when the office examination of mental state may be quite intact. The most common clinical manifestations of damage to the prefrontal network take the form of two relatively distinct syndromes. In the *frontal abulic syndrome*, the patient shows a loss of initiative, creativity, and curiosity and displays a pervasive emotional blandness and apathy. In the *frontal disinhibition syndrome*, the patient becomes socially disinhibited and shows severe impairments of judgment, insight, and foresight. The dissociation between intact intellectual function and a total lack of even rudimentary common sense is striking. Despite the preservation of all essential memory functions, the patient cannot learn from experience and continues to display inappropriate behaviors without appearing to experience emotional pain, guilt, or regret when such behaviors repeatedly lead to disastrous consequences. Testing judgment by asking patients what they would do if they detected a fire in a theater or found a stamped and addressed envelope on the road is not very informative since patients who answer these questions wisely in the office may still do the wrong thing in the more complex real-life setting.

The abulic syndrome tends to be associated with damage to the dorsolateral prefrontal cortex, and the disinhibition syndrome with the medial prefrontal or orbitofrontal cortex. These syndromes tend to arise almost exclusively after bilateral lesions, most frequently in the setting of head trauma, stroke, ruptured aneurysms, hydrocephalus, or tumors (including metastases, glioblastoma, and falx or olfactory groove meningiomas). Unilateral lesions confined to the prefrontal cortex may remain silent until the pathology spreads to the other side. The emergence of developmentally primitive reflexes such as grasping, rooting, and sucking are also signs of frontal lobe disease. However, these reflexes are seen primarily in patients with large structural lesions that extend into the premotor components of the frontal lobes or in the context of metabolic encephalopathies. The vast majority of patients with prefrontal lesions and frontal lobe behavioral syndromes do not display these reflexes. Absent suck, root, and grasp reflexes therefore do not exclude a frontal lobe lesion.

Involvement of the prefrontal network impairs reasoning, abstract thinking, and hypothesis formation and leads to a stimulus-bound, concrete, and impulsive mode of mental functioning. Damage to this part of the brain also disrupts a variety of attention-related functions including concentration span, verbal fluency, the inhibition of immediate but inappropriate responses, and mental flexibility. Digit span (which should be seven forward and five reverse) is decreased; the recitation of the months of the year in reverse order (which should take less than 15 s) is slowed; and the number of words starting with a, f, or s that can be generated in 1 min (normally 12 or more per letter) is diminished even in nonaphasic patients. Characteristically, there is a progressive slowing of performance as the task proceeds; e.g., the patient asked to count backwards from 20 responds "20, 19, 18 . . . 17, ... 16," etc., and may not complete the task. In go–no go tasks (where the instruction is to raise the finger upon hearing one tap but to keep it still upon hearing two taps), the patient shows a characteristic inability to keep still in response to the "no go" stimulus; mental flexibility (tested by the ability to shift from one criterion to another in sorting or matching tasks) is impoverished; distractibility by irrelevant stimuli is increased; and there is a pronounced tendency for impersistence and perseveration. The effective scanning of internal information stores, the capacity for focusing on a trend of thought, and the ability to shift the focus of attention flexibly from one thought or stimulus to another are also impaired.

These attentional deficits contribute to the emergence of "working memory" impairments. The capacity for working memory refers to the amount of information that can be kept *on-line* at any given time. Working memory impairments interfere with the ability to maintain a coherent trend of thought and lead to confusion, especially in complex situations that require the simultaneous consideration of several variables. The attentional deficits disrupt the registration and retrieval of new information and lead to secondary memory deficits. These mem-

ory difficulties can be differentiated from those of the amnestic state by showing that they improve when the attentional load of the task is decreased. Working memory (also known as immediate memory) is an attentional function based on the temporary on-line holding of information. It is closely associated with the integrity of the prefrontal network and the ascending reticular activating system. Retentive memory, on the other hand, depends on the stable (off-line) storage of information and is associated with the integrity of the limbic network. The distinction of the underlying neural mechanisms is illustrated by the observation that severely amnestic patients who cannot remember events that occurred a few minutes ago may have intact if not superior working memory capacity as shown in tests of digit span. Working memory is closely related to the integrity of the dorsolateral prefrontal cortex, whereas other attentional functions such as the ability to inhibit inappropriate responses (as assessed by the go–no go task) depend primarily on the integrity of the medial prefrontal or orbitofrontal cortex.

The network approach postulates that the same cognitive domain can be impaired after damage to different parts of the brain as long as these parts belong to the same large-scale neural network. Accordingly, lesions in the caudate nucleus or in the dorsomedial nucleus of the thalamus (structures that can be considered as subcortical components of the prefrontal network) can also give rise to the clinical picture of a frontal lobe syndrome. This is one reason why the mental state changes associated with degenerative basal ganglia diseases, such as Parkinson's or Huntington's disease, may take the form of a frontal lobe syndrome. Because of its widespread connections with other regions of association cortex, one essential computational role of the prefrontal network is to function as an integrator or orchestrator for other networks. Bilateral multifocal lesions of the cerebral hemispheres, none of which are individually large enough to cause specific cognitive deficits such as aphasia or neglect, can collectively interfere with the connectivity and integrating function of prefrontal cortex. This is one reason why a frontal lobe syndrome is the single most common behavioral profile associated with a variety of bilateral multifocal brain diseases including metabolic encephalopathy, multiple sclerosis, Vitamin B_{12} deficiency, and others. In fact, the vast majority of patients with the clinical diagnosis of a frontal lobe syndrome tend to have lesions that do not involve prefrontal cortex but that involve either the subcortical components of the prefrontal network or its connections with other parts of the brain. In order to avoid the paradox of making a diagnosis of "frontal lobe syndrome" in a patient with no evidence of frontal cortex disease, it is advisable to use the diagnostic term *prefrontal network syndrome*, with the understanding that the responsible lesions can lie anywhere within this distributed network.

The patient with frontal lobe disease raises potential dilemmas in differential diagnosis: the abulia and blandness may be misinterpreted as depression, and the disinhibition as mania or acting-out. Appropriate intervention may be delayed while a treatable tumor keeps expanding. An informed approach to frontal lobe disease and its comportmental manifestations may help to avoid such errors.

CARING FOR THE PATIENT WITH DEFICITS OF HIGHER CORTICAL FUNCTION Some of the deficits described in this chapter are so complex that they may bewilder not only the patient and family but also the physician. It is imperative to carry out a systematic clinical evaluation in order to characterize the nature of the deficits and explain them in lay terms to the patient and family. Such an explanation can allay at least some of the anxieties, address the mistaken impression that the deficit (e.g., social disinhibition or inability to recognize family members) is psychologically motivated, and lead to practical suggestions for daily living activities. Patients with simultanagnosia, for example, should be given the counterintuitive instruction to stand back when they cannot find an item so that a greater search area falls within the immediate field of gaze. Physicians tend to place a great emphasis on signs that are elicited during the clinical examination. In some patients, however, the history may be more important and may conflict with the bedside examination. For example, patients with frontal lobe disease can be extremely irritable and abusive to spouses and yet display all the appropriate social graces during the visit to the medical office.

Reactive depression is common in patients with higher cortical dysfunction and should be treated. These patients may be sensitive to the usual doses of antidepressants or anxiolytics and deserve a careful titration of dosage. Brain damage may cause a dissociation between feeling states and their expression so that a patient who may superficially appear jocular could still be suffering from an underlying depression that deserves to be treated. In many cases, agitation may be controlled with reassurance. In other cases, treatment with benzodiazepines or sedating antidepressants may become necessary. The use of neuroleptics for the control of agitation should be reserved only for refractory cases since extrapyramidal side effects are frequent in patients with coexisting brain damage.

The assessment of higher cortical function can be as systematic as the rest of the neurologic examination but requires time and familiarity with specialized tests. The consultation of a skilled neuropsychologist may aid in the formulation of diagnosis and management. The availability of computed tomography, magnetic resonance imaging, positron emission tomography, and single-photon emission computed tomography does not obviate the need for careful clinical assessment since the complex results and implications of these diagnostic procedures can be interpreted fully only in the light of a thorough clinical evaluation.

Spontaneous improvement of cognitive deficits due to acute neurologic lesions is common. It is most rapid in the first few weeks but may continue for up to 2 years, especially in young individuals with single brain lesions. The mechanisms for this recovery are incompletely understood. Some of the initial deficits appear to arise from remote dysfunction (diaschisis) in parts of the brain that are interconnected with the site of initial injury. Improvement in these patients may reflect, at least in part, a normalization of the remote dysfunction. Other mechanisms may involve functional reorganization in surviving neurons adjacent to the injury or the compensatory use of homologous structures, for example, the right superior temporal gyrus with recovery from Wernicke's aphasia. Cognitive rehabilitation procedures have been used in the treatment of higher cortical deficits. There are few controlled studies, but some do show a benefit of rehabilitation in the recovery from hemispatial neglect and aphasia. In some of these patients, the recovery of cognitive deficits reflects the development of compensatory strategies. In other patients, recovery may involve a reorganization of the relevant neural networks. Some types of deficits may be more prone to recovery than others. For example, patients with nonfluent aphasias are more likely to benefit from speech therapy than patients with fluent aphasias and comprehension deficits. In general, lesions that lead to a denial of illness (e.g., anosognosia) are associated with cognitive deficits that are more resistant to rehabilitation. The recovery of higher cortical dysfunction is rarely complete. Periodic neuropsychological assessment is necessary for quantifying the pace of the improvement and for generating specific recommendations for cognitive rehabilitation, modifications in the home environment, and the time-table for returning to school or work.

BIBLIOGRAPHY

BENSON F: Aphasia and related disorders: A clinical approach, in *Principles of Behavioral Neurology*, M-M Mesulam (ed). Philadelphia, Davis, 1985, pp 193–238

DAFFNER KR et al: Dissociated neglect behavior following sequential strokes in the right hemisphere. Ann Neurol 28:97, 1990

DAMASIO AR: Disorders of complex visual processing: Agnosias, achromatopsia, Balint's syndrome, and related difficulties of orientation and construction, in *Principles of Behavioral Neurology*, M-M Mesulam (ed). Philadelphia, Davis, 1985, pp 259–288.

———: Aphasia. N Engl J Med 326:531, 1992

DEUEL RK, COLLINS RC: Recovery from unilateral neglect. Exp Neurol 81:733, 1983

GESCHWIND N: Disconnection syndromes in animals and man. Brain 88:237, 1965

GITELMAN DR et al: Functional imaging of human right hemispheric activation for exploratory movements. Ann Neurol 39:174, 1996

GRENSHAM GE et al: *Post-Stroke Rehabilitation*. In: U. S. Department of Health and Human Services Agency for Health Care Policy and Research, Publication No. 95-0662. Rockville, Maryland 1995

HEILMAN KM et al: Neglect and related disorders, in *Clinical Neuropsychology*, KM Heilman, E Valenstein (eds). New York, Oxford University Press, 1985, pp 279–336

MESULAM M-M: Patterns in behavioral neuroanatomy: Association areas, the limbic system, and hemispheric specialization, in *Principles of Behavioral Neurology*, M-M Mesulam (ed). Philadelphia, Davis, 1985, pp 1–70

———: Frontal cortex and behavior. Ann Neurol 19:320, 1986

———: Primary progressive aphasia—differentiation from Alzheimer's disease [editorial]. Ann Neurol 22:533, 1987

———: Large-scale neurocognitive networks and distributed processing for attention, language, and memory. Ann Neurol 28:597, 1990

———: Higher visual functions of the cerebral cortex and their disruption in clinical practice, in *Principles and Practice of Ophthalmology*, DM Albert, FA Jakobiec (eds). Philadelphia, Saunders, 1994, pp 2640–2653

MOHR JR et al: Broca's aphasia: Pathologic and clinical. Neurology 28:311, 1978

NAESER MA, HELM-ESTABROOKS N: CT scan lesion localization and response to melodic intonation therapy with nonfluent aphasia cases. Cortex 21:203, 1985

PRICE BH et al: Neuropsychological patterns and language deficits in 20 consecutive cases of autopsy-confirmed Alzheimer's disease. Arch Neurol 50:931, 1993

ROSS ED: Nonverbal aspects of language. Neurol Clin 11:9, 1993

SEECK M et al: Selectively distributed processing of visual object recognition in the temporal and frontal lobes of the human brain. Ann Neurol 37:538, 1995

SIGNORET J-L: Memory and amnesias, in *Principles of Behavioral Neurology*, M-M Mesulam (ed). Philadelphia, Davis, 1985, pp 169–192

TURNER RS et al: Clinical, neuroimaging, and pathologic features of progressive nonfluent aphasia. Ann Neurol 39:166, 1996

WEILLER C et al: Recovery from Wernicke's aphasia: A positron emission tomographic study. *Ann Neurol* 37:723, 1995

WEINTRAUB S, MESULAM M-M: The examination of mental state, in *Principles of Behavioral Neurology*, M-M Mesulam (ed). Philadelphia, Davis, 1985, pp 71–123

---

26 *Thomas D. Bird*

MEMORY LOSS AND DEMENTIA

DEFINITION Dementia is a serious and common problem that affects more than 4 million Americans and costs society more than $50 billion annually. Ten percent of persons over age 70 and 20 to 40 percent of individuals over age 85 have clinically identifiable memory loss. Dementia is a syndrome with many causes. A simple definition of dementia is a deterioration in cognitive abilities that impairs the previously successful performance of activities of daily living. Memory is the most common and most important cognitive ability that is lost. Other mental faculties may also be affected such as attention, judgment, comprehension, orientation, learning, calculation, problem solving, mood, and behavior. Agitation or withdrawal, hallucinations, delusions, insomnia, and loss of inhibitions are also common. Individuals with mental retardation and psychosis may become demented if a decline in intellectual function occurs. Many common forms of dementia are progressive, but some dementing illnesses are static and unchanging. Dementia is a chronic condition, whereas delirium is an acute confusional state associated with a change in level of consciousness (ranging from lethargy to agitation).

Memory is a complex function of the brain that has fascinated philosophers and scientists for centuries. Memory is currently viewed as a mental process using several storage buffers of differing capacity and duration (Table 26-1). Sensory memory lasts for about 250 ms in the visual mode (iconic memory) and 1 to 2 s in the auditory mode (echoic memory). Immediate (short-term or primary) memory has a duration of about half a minute and a limited capacity of approximately 5 to 10 items. Immediate memory is highly vulnerable to distraction, requiring attention and vigilance to maintain the content. It is often tested at the bedside by asking the patient to recall several digits forward and backward. Recent, or secondary, memory has been called both "short-term" and "long-term." It has a duration of minutes to weeks and exhibits a larger storage capacity than immediate memory. On entering this buffer, information undergoes a process of consolidation of variable duration. Recent memory is commonly tested in the clinical setting by asking a patient to recall three words after 3 to 5 min. Remote, or long-term, memory stores information lasting weeks to a lifetime and contains most of our personal experiences and knowledge. Some information appears to be stored accurately for an indefinite time, whereas other items fade or become distorted. Memory function includes registration (encoding or acquisition), retention (storage or consolidation), stabilization, and retrieval (decoding or recall). Registration and retrieval are conscious processes. Animal experiments have shown that long-term memory requires new protein synthesis, and the stabilization process probably involves physical changes at neuronal synapses.

Several additional classifications of memory are sometimes used by psychologists, particularly in reference to the content or use of the memory stores. Reference memory refers to a filing system that contains recent and remote information gained from previous experience. Working memory refers to an active process that is being updated continually by current experience. Episodic memory contains information about events occurring in a specific place and time. Semantic memory contains unchanging facts, principles, associations, and rules (for example, state capitals and the number of days in a week). Declarative (explicit) memory refers to facts about the world and past personal events that must be consciously retrieved to be remembered. Procedural (implicit) memory, in contrast, is involved in learning and retaining a skill or procedure such as how to ride a bicycle, get dressed, or drive a car. Abilities stored in procedural memory become automatic and do not require conscious implementation.

Finally, the term *executive function* refers to mental activity involved in planning, initiating, and regulating behavior. It is considered the central organizing function of the brain that results in systematic, goal-directed activity. Executive functions are active in nonroutine situations where reflex or automatic behavior is not adequate. The anatomic and physiologic substrates of executive function are presumed to involve the frontal lobes (see Chap. 25). Deficits in executive function occur frequently in patients with dementia.

FUNCTIONAL ANATOMY AND PATHOGENESIS Dementia results from disorders of cerebral neuronal circuits and is a result of the total quantity of neuronal loss combined with the specific location of such loss (Chap. 25). The anatomic basis of memory was initially clarified from study of the alcohol/thiamine deficiency syndrome of Korsakoff and the consequences of temporal lobe surgery performed for the treatment of epilepsy. In Korsakoff's syndrome lesions in the hypothalamus, mammillary bodies, and dorsomedial nuclei of the thalamus showed that these areas were important for learning, recall, and recognition. Unilateral temporal lobe surgery for epilepsy produced mild to moderate amnesia for either verbal or nonverbal material. Bilateral medial temporal lobe excision involving the hippocampal formation, the parahippocampal gyrus, and part of the amygdala produced a severe anterograde learning disorder, i.e., an inability to store new memories, often with retained ability to recall old ones. The components of the medial temporal lobe memory system include the hippocampus and adjacent cortex, including the entorhinal, perirhinal, and parahippocampal regions (Fig. 26-1). This includes a circular pathway of neurons from entorhinal cortex to dentate gyrus, CA3 and CA1 neurons of hippocampus to subiculum, and back to entorhinal cortex; this pathway is heavily damaged in Alzheimer's disease (AD). This system is fast, has limited capacity, and performs a crucial function at the time of learning and establishing declarative memory. Its role continues after learning during a lengthy period of reorganization and consolidation whereby memory stored in neocortex eventually becomes independent of the medial temporal lobe memory system. This process, by which the burden of long-term (permanent) memory storage is gradually assumed by neocortex, assures that the medial temporal lobe system is always available for the acquisition of new information. Recent functional brain imaging studies indicate that learning and memory involve many of the same regions of the cortex that process sensory information and control motor output. The forms of perceptual and motor learning that can occur without conscious recollections are mediated in part by contractions and expansions of representations in the sensory and motor cortex. One study, for example, has shown that the cortical representation of the fingers of the left hand of musical string players is larger than that in controls, suggesting that the representation of different parts of the body in the primary somatosensory cortex of humans depends on use and changes to conform to the current needs and experiences of the individual. Discrete cortical regions exist in which object knowledge (such as words related to color, animals, tools, or action) is organized as a distributed system in which the attributes of an object are stored close to the regions of the cortex that mediate perception of those attributes (Chap. 25). That is, brain regions active during object identification are partly dependent on the intrinsic properties of the object. Procedural (implicit) memory appears to involve centers outside the hippocampus such as amygdala, cerebellum, and sensory cortex.

Biochemically, the cholinergic system plays an important role in memory. Anticholinergic agents such as atropine and scopolamine interfere with memory. Choline acetyl transferase (the enzyme catalyzing the formation of acetylcholine) and nicotinic cholinergic receptors

---

Table 26-1

Classification of Memory

Type	Time Interval	Test/Example	Probable Cerebral Location
Sensory			
Iconic (visual)	<1 s	After image	Visual cortex
Echoic (auditory)	1–2 s	Cough/dog bark	Auditory cortex
Immediate (primary/working)	30 s	Digit span	Perisylvian cortex, frontal lobe
Recent (secondary/reference)	Minutes–weeks/months	Recall 3 words after 3–5 min	Hippocampus, mamillothalamic tract, dorsomedial thalamus
Declarative (explicit)			
Episodic		Recall trip last week	
Semantic		Recall names of months	
Procedural (implicit)		Ride a bike	Amygdala, cerebellum, association cortex, frontal lobe, ? other
		Get dressed	
Remote (reference)	Months–years	Recall high school graduation	Association cortex, ? other

SOURCE: Modified from Erickson.

are known to be deficient in the cortex of patients with AD. The brains of AD patients show severe neuronal loss in the nucleus basalis of Meynert, a major source of cholinergic input to the cerebral cortex. These findings form the basis for the use of tacrine (a cholinesterase inhibitor) in the treatment of AD, its modest benefit presumably arising from increased available levels of acetylcholine. Behavior and mood are modulated by noradrenergic, serotonergic, and dopaminergic pathways, and norepinephrine has been shown to be reduced in the brainstem locus coeruleus in AD. Neurotrophins are also postulated to play a role in memory in part by preserving cholinergic neurons.

Long-term potentiation (LTP), which refers to a long-lasting enhancement of synaptic transmission resulting from repetitive stimulation of excitatory synapses, is presumed to be involved in memory acquisition and storage. LTP occurs in hippocampus and is mediated by *N*-methyl-D-aspartate (NMDA) receptors. Gene knockout mouse models have been useful in the definition of secondary messenger systems that play a role in hippocampal LTP. For example, disruption of either calcium/calmodulin-dependent protein kinase or cytoplasmic tyrosine kinase (fyn) results in deficient hippocampal LTP and impaired spatial learning. On the other hand, mice in which a neuronal glycoprotein thy-1 has been inactivated show regionally selective impairment of LTP but intact spatial learning, suggesting that LTP in the entorhinal projection to the dentate gyrus of the hippocampus (Fig. 26-1) may not be necessary for some forms of spatial learning.

Most diseases causing dementia do not have highly restricted regions of pathology. Disorders such as AD appear to represent relatively diffuse neuronal deterioration throughout the cerebral cortex, whereas multi-infarct dementia associated with recurrent strokes causes more focal damage in a random patchwork of cortical regions. Diffuse white matter damage may disrupt intracerebral connections and cause dementia syndromes such as those associated with leukodystrophies, multiple sclerosis, and Binswanger's disease. Subcortical

structures such as the caudate, putamen, thalamus, and substantia nigra also modulate cognition and behavior in ways that are not yet well understood. Some investigators distinguish between cortical and subcortical types of dementia. Cortical dementia such as AD and Pick's disease primarily present as memory loss and are often associated with aphasia or other disturbance of language. Patients with subcortical dementia such as Huntington's disease (HD) are less likely to have memory and language problems and more likely to have difficulties with attention, judgment, and behavior. Both the clinical and anatomic characteristics of the cortical and subcortical dementias show considerable overlap, and the conditions are often not distinct.

Lesions of some relatively specific cortical-subcortical pathways may have significant effects on behavior (Chap. 25). The dorsolateral prefrontal cortex has connections with dorsolateral caudate, globus pallidus, and thalamus. Lesions of these pathways result in poor organization and planning, perseveration, and decreased cognitive flexibility with impaired judgment. The lateral orbital frontal cortex connects with the ventromedial caudate, globus pallidus, and thalamus. Lesions of these connections cause irritability, impulsiveness, and distractibility. The anterior cingulate cortex connects with the nucleus accumbens, globus pallidus, and thalamus. Interruption of these connections produces apathy and poverty of speech or even akinetic mutism.

The single strongest risk factor for dementia is increasing age. The prevalence of disabling memory loss increases with each decade over age 50 and is associated most often with the microscopic changes of AD at autopsy. Slow accumulation of mutations in neuronal mitochondria is hypothesized to contribute to the increasing prevalence of dementia with age. Yet many centenarians have intact memory function and no evidence of clinically significant dementia. Whether dementia is an inevitable consequence of normal human aging remains controversial.

DIFFERENTIAL DIAGNOSIS The many causes of dementia are listed in Table 26-2. The frequency of each condition depends on the age group under study, the country of origin, and perhaps racial or ethnic variations. AD is the most common cause of dementia in

FIGURE 26-1 The principal connections of the hippocampus. Afferent connections (*blue arrows*) from the cingulate gyrus (cortical association fibers) and amygdala converge on the entorhinal cortex (part of the parahippocampal gyrus) and connect with the hippocampus via a polysynaptic circuit (*black arrows*) from dentate to CA3, CA1, and subiculum neurons with output back to the entorhinal cortex. Efferent connections (*broken arrows*) are principally via the fornix to the anterior nucleus of the thalamus, septal nuclei, and mamillary body.

Vascular disease is the second most common cause of dementia in the United States, representing 20 to 25 percent, but is more common than AD in some Asian countries. Dementia associated with chronic alcoholism and Parkinson's disease (PD) represent the next two most common categories. Chronic intoxications including those resulting from prescription drugs are an important, potentially treatable cause of dementia. Other disorders listed in the table are uncommon but important because many are reversible. The classification of dementing illnesses into two broad groups of treatable and untreatable disorders is a useful approach to the differential diagnosis of dementia.

Subtle cumulative memory loss is a natural part of aging. This frustrating experience, often the source of jokes and humor, is referred to as *benign forgetfulness of the elderly*. Benign means that it is not so progressive or serious that it impairs reasonably successful and productive daily functioning, although the distinction between benign and more significant memory loss can be difficult to make. A proportion of persons with benign memory loss progress to frank dementia, usually caused by AD. It remains unclear why some individuals show progression and others do not. It was once assumed that a cumulative loss of hippocampal neurons with normal aging might underlie this forgetfulness, but recent quantitative neuronal counts indicate that this "natural" neuronal loss may not occur.

Alzheimer's disease is a slowly progressive dementing illness associated with diffuse cortical atrophy and specific neuropathologic hallmarks of amyloid plaques and neurofibrillary tangles. Although quite common in the elderly, it remains a diagnosis of exclusion to be confirmed definitively only at autopsy. The clinical diagnosis of AD established by experienced neurologists proves to be correct at autopsy approximately 85 to 90 percent of the time. → *This condition is described in greater detail in Chap. 367.*

Two major types of vascular dementia can be identified (Chap. 367). The first, often called multi-infarct dementia, results from an accumulation of discrete cerebral strokes that produce disabling deficits of memory, behavior, and other cognitive abilities. Such patients usually give a history of sudden, separate stroke episodes with stepwise deterioration. On examination, focal neurologic deficits such as hemiparesis, unilateral Babinski reflex, aphasia, or visual field defect are common. Brain imaging shows multiple areas of stroke, which may have been ischemic or hemorrhagic. A second, more subtle and insidious type of vascular dementia, Binswanger's disease, is a dementing illness associated with diffuse, subcortical white matter damage often occurring in patients with chronic hypertension and/or severe atherosclerosis. The white matter changes are dramatically visualized by magnetic resonance imaging (MRI). The pathogenesis of Binswanger's disease is unknown. Because AD and vascular dementia are common, occasional patients may have both conditions.

Dementia commonly accompanies *chronic alcoholism* (Chap. 380). This may be a result of associated malnutrition, especially of B vitamins and particularly thiamine. However, other as yet poorly defined aspects of chronic alcohol ingestion may also produce cerebral damage and atrophy. A rare idiopathic syndrome of dementia and seizures with degeneration of the corpus callosum has been reported primarily in male Italian drinkers of red wine (MarchiafavaBignami disease).

Thiamine (vitamin B_1) deficiency causes Wernicke's encephalopathy (Chap. 380). The clinical presentation is a malnourished individual (frequently but not necessarily alcoholic) with confusion, ataxia, and diplopia from ophthalmoplegia (Charcot's triad). Thiamine deficiency damages the thalamus, mammillary bodies, midline cerebellum, periaquaductal gray matter of the midbrain, and peripheral nerves. Damage to medial thalamic regions correlates most closely with memory loss. Prompt administration of parenteral thiamine (100 mg intravenously for 3 days followed by daily oral dosage) may reverse the disease if given in the first few days of symptom onset. However, prolonged untreated thiamine deficiency can result in an irreversible dementia/amnestic syndrome (Korsakoff's psychosis) or even death.

In *Korsakoff's syndrome*, the patient is unable to recall new information despite normal immediate memory, attention span, and level of consciousness. Memory for new events is seriously impaired, whereas memory of knowledge prior to the illness is relatively intact. Patients are easily confused, disoriented, and incapable of recalling new infor-

Table 26-2

Differential Diagnosis of Dementia

MOST COMMON CAUSES OF DEMENTIA

Alzheimer's disease	Alcoholism*
Vascular dementia	Parkinson's disease
Multi-infarct	Drug/medication intoxication*
Diffuse white matter disease (Binswanger's)	

LESS COMMON CAUSES OF DEMENTIA

Vitamin deficiencies	Toxic disorders
Thiamine (B_1): Wernicke's encephalopathy*	Drug, medication, and narcotic poisoning*
B_{12} (Pernicious anemia)*	Heavy metal intoxication*
Nicotinic acid (pellagra)*	Dialysis dementia (aluminum)
Endocrine and other organ failure	Organic toxins
Hypothyroidism*	Psychiatric
Adrenal insufficiency and Cushing's syndrome*	Depression (pseudodementia)*
Hypo- and hyperparathyroidism*	Schizophrenia*
Renal failure*	Conversion reaction*
Liver failure*	Degenerative disorders
Pulmonary failure*	Huntington's disease
Chronic infections	Pick's disease
HIV	Diffuse Lewy body disease
Neurosyphilis*	Progressive supranuclear palsy (Steel-Richardson syndrome)
Papovavirus (progressive multifocal leukoencephalopathy)	Multisystem degeneration (Shy-Drager syndrome)
Prion (Creutzfeldt-Jakob and Gerstmann-Sträussler-Scheinker diseases)	Hereditary ataxias (some forms)
Tuberculosis, fungal, and protozoal*	Motor neuron disease [amyotrophic lateral sclerosis (ALS); some forms]
Sarcoidosis*	Frontal lobe dementia
Whipple's disease*	Cortical basal degeneration
Head trauma and diffuse brain damage	Multiple sclerosis
Dementia pugilistica	Adult Down's syndrome with Alzheimer's
Chronic subdural hematoma*	ALS–Parkinson's–Dementia complex of Guam
Postanoxia	Miscellaneous
Postencephalitis	Vasculitis*
Normal-pressure hydrocephalus*	Acute intermittent porphyria*
Neoplastic	Recurrent nonconvulsive seizures*
Primary brain tumor*	Additional conditions in children or adolescents
Metastatic brain tumor*	Hallervorden-Spatz disease
Paraneoplastic limbic encephalitis	Subacute sclerosing panencephalitis
	Metabolic disorders (e.g., Wilson's and Leigh's diseases, leukodystrophies, lipid storage diseases, mitochondrial mutations)

* Potentially treatable dementia.

mation for more than a brief interval. Superficially, they may be conversant, entertaining, able to perform simple tasks, and follow immediate commands. Confabulation is common, although not always present, and may result in obviously erroneous statements and elaborations. There is no specific treatment because the previous thiamine deficiency has produced irreversible damage to the medial thalamic nuclei and mammillary bodies. Mammillary body atrophy may be visible on high-resolution MRI.

Vitamin B₁₂ deficiency, as can occur in pernicious anemia, causes a macrocytic anemia and may also damage the nervous system (Chaps. 373 and 380). Neurologically it most commonly produces a spinal cord syndrome (myelopathy) affecting the posterior columns (loss of position and vibratory sense) and the lateral corticospinal tracts (hyperactive tendon reflexes and Babinski responses); it also damages peripheral nerves, resulting in sensory loss with depressed tendon reflexes. Damage to cerebral myelinated fibers may also cause dementia. The mechanism of neurologic damage is unclear but may be related to a deficiency of *S*-adenosylmethionine (required for methylation of myelin phospholipids) due to reduced methionine synthase activity or accumulation of methylmalonate and propionate, providing abnormal substrates for fatty acid synthesis in myelin. The neurologic signs of vitamin B₁₂ deficiency are usually associated with macrocytic anemia, but on occasion may occur in its absence. Treatment with parenteral vitamin B₁₂ (1000 μg intramuscularly daily for a week, weekly for a month, and monthly for life for pernicious anemia) stops progression of the disease if instituted promptly, but reversal of advanced nervous system damage will not occur.

Deficiency of nicotinic acid (pellagra) is associated with sun-exposed skin rash, glossitis, and angular stomatitis (Chaps. 79 and 380). Severe dietary deficiency of nicotinic acid along with other B vitamins such as pyridoxine may result in spastic paraparesis, peripheral neuropathy, fatigue, irritability, and dementia. This syndrome has been seen in prisoner-of-war and concentration camps. Low serum folate levels appear to be a rough index of malnutrition, but isolated folate deficiency has not been proven to be a specific cause of dementia.

Approximately 20 percent of patients with PD (Chap. 368) eventually develop dementia. Treatment with L-dopa neither accelerates nor prevents this process. Some PD patients with dementia have cytoplasmic neuronal inclusions (Lewy bodies) or AD changes in cerebral cortex, but others have no specific identifiable cortical pathology.

Infections of the central nervous system (CNS) usually cause delirium and other acute neurologic syndromes. However, some chronic CNS infections such as tuberculosis or cryptococcosis may produce a dementing illness (Chap. 378). Between 20 and 30 percent of patients in the advanced stages of infection with human immunodeficiency virus (HIV) become demented (Chap. 308). Cardinal features include psychomotor retardation, apathy, and impaired memory. This may result from secondary opportunistic infections but can also be caused by direct involvement of CNS neurons with HIV, where there is a multinucleated giant cell encephalitis and diffuse pallor of white matter. The neuronal toxicity may be mediated by cytokines or the direct neurotoxic effect of the gp 120 envelope glycoprotein. In the absence of CNS opportunistic infection, elevated β2 microglobulin in CSF is a useful marker for HIV dementia. Herpes simplex encephalitis (Chap. 379) has a predilection for the inferior temporal lobes and may present as subacute confusion and disorientation but more often as an acute syndrome rather than a chronic dementia. Computed tomography (CT), MRI, and electroencephalogram (EEG) may all demonstrate the temporal lobe location of the lesions. Cerebrospinal fluid (CSF) usually shows increased protein and a lymphocytic pleocytosis. CNS syphilis (Chap. 174) was a common cause of dementia in the preantibiotic era; it is uncommon nowadays but can still be encountered in the population with multiple sex partners. Characteristic CSF changes consist of pleocytosis, increased protein, and positive VDRL test.

Prion disorders such as Creutzfeldt-Jakob disease (CJD) (Chap. 379) are very rare conditions (approximately 1 per million population) that commonly produce dementia. CJD is usually a rapidly progressive disease associated with dementia, rigidity, and myoclonus, causing death in less than 1 to 2 years. These clinical characteristics may also rarely be seen in AD, and the differential diagnosis usually depends on the slower progression of AD and the markedly abnormal periodic EEG discharges seen in CJD. Ataxia or cortical blindness may also accompany CJD. The transmissible agent, or prion, consists principally of an abnormal isoform of a host-encoded protein, the prion protein (PrP), which accumulates in affected brains. The abnormal disease-causing prion protein (PrP^SC) is derived from the normal prion protein (PrP^C) by a posttranslation mechanism that may represent a physical conformational change. PrP^SC apparently acts as a template that promotes the conversion of PrP^C to PrP^SC, and this cascading conformational change somehow produces neuronal damage and death. The disease is transmissible by tissue transplantation to animals or other humans and is occasionally inherited (familial CJD, or Gerstmann-Sträussler-Scheinker disease). The inherited variety has the unique characteristic of being both a genetic and a transmissible disorder. Sporadic cases are not inherited. CJD is not contagious by touch or airborne spread. Bovine spongiform encephalopathy in the United Kingdom is thought to have resulted from cattle feed containing sheep tissues contaminated with infectious prions (PrP scrapie). Possible transmission to the human population is under investigation. Immunoassay for a 14-3-3 brain protein in CSF may be a useful marker for transmissible spongiform encephalopathies in patients with dementia.

Primary and metastatic *neoplasms of the* CNS (Chap. 375) usually produce focal neurologic findings and seizures rather than dementia. However, if tumor growth begins in the frontal or temporal lobes, the initial manifestations may be memory loss or behavioral changes. A rare paraneoplastic syndrome of dementia associated with occult carcinoma (usually small cell lung cancer) has been termed *limbic encephalitis* (Chap. 103). In this syndrome, confusion, agitation, seizures, poor memory, and frank dementia may occur in association with sensory neuropathy. The CSF often shows an increase in cells and protein. There is neuronal loss and perivascular lymphocytic infiltration in the hippocampus, amygdala, and cingulate and frontal cortex. Circulating antineuronal nuclear antibodies may be present. There is no specific treatment.

The syndrome of *normal-pressure hydrocephalus* (Chap. 367) is frequently discussed but difficult to diagnose. Clinically, a triad of memory loss, gait disturbance, and bladder incontinence is typical. The gait abnormality is often the initial symptom, and the dementia is usually mild. On imaging studies, the lateral ventricles are enlarged but there is minimal or no cortical atrophy. Lumbar puncture shows a normal or slightly elevated opening pressure with normal CSF. The condition may be idiopathic or the result of previous meningitis or subarachnoid blood from a ruptured aneurysm or head trauma. The pathogenetic mechanism is presumably a block of normal CSF flow over the convexity and delayed absorption into the venous system, with resulting stretch and distortion of white matter tracts within the corona radiata. Some individuals improve with ventricular shunting but many do not. The condition is difficult to distinguish from AD (see Chap. 367).

A nonconvulsive *seizure disorder* may underlie a syndrome of confusion, clouding of consciousness, and garbled speech. Psychiatric disease is often suspected, but an EEG demonstrates the seizure discharges. If recurrent or persistent, the condition may be termed *complex partial status epilepticus*. The cognitive disturbance often responds to anticonvulsant therapy. The etiology may be previous small strokes or head trauma; some cases are idiopathic.

It is important to recognize systemic diseases that indirectly affect the brain and produce chronic confusion or dementia. Such conditions include dysthyroid states (especially hypothyroidism), vasculitis, and hepatic, renal, or pulmonary disease. Hepatic encephalopathy may begin with irritability and confusion and slowly progress to agitation, lethargy, and coma (Chap. 380).

Isolated angiitis of the CNS (CNS granulomatous angiitis) (Chaps. 319 and 366) occasionally causes a chronic encephalopathy associated with confusion, disorientation, and clouding of consciousness. Headache is common, and strokes and cranial neuropathies may occur. Brain imaging studies may be normal or nonspecifically abnormal. CSF studies reveal a mild pleocytosis or elevation in the protein level in half of the cases. Cerebral angiography often shows multifocal stenosis and narrowing of vessels. A few patients have only small-vessel disease that is not revealed on angiography. The angiographic appearance is not specific and may be mimicked by atherosclerosis, infection, or other causes of vascular disease. Brain or meningeal biopsy demonstrates abnormal arteries with endothelial cell proliferation and infiltrates of mononuclear cells. Autoantibodies and immune complexes are not present, and a cell-mediated process appears most likely. The prognosis is poor, but some patients respond to glucocorticoids or chemotherapy.

Chronic metal intoxications may also produce a dementing syndrome. The key to diagnosis is to elicit a history of exposure at work, home, or even as a consequence of a medical procedure such as dialysis. Lead poisoning has highly variable neurologic manifestations. Fatigue, depression, and confusion may be associated with episodic abdominal pain and peripheral neuropathy. Gray lead lines may appear in the gums. There is usually an associated anemia with basophilic stippling of red cells. The clinical presentation can resemble that of acute intermittent porphyria, including elevated levels of urine porphyrins as a result of the inhibition of δ-aminolevulinic acid dehydratase. Chronic lead poisoning from inadequately fired glazed pottery has been reported. The treatment is chelation therapy with agents such as EDTA. Chronic mercury poisoning may produce dementia, peripheral neuropathy, and a fine tremulousness that may progress to a cerebellar intention tremor or choreoathetosis. The confusion and memory loss of chronic arsenic intoxication is also associated with nausea, weight loss, peripheral neuropathy, pigmentation and scaling of the skin, and transverse white lines of the fingernails (Mee's lines). Treatment is chelation therapy with dimercaprol (BAL). Aluminum poisoning has been best documented with the dialysis dementia syndrome in which water used during renal dialysis was contaminated with excessive amounts of aluminum. This resulted in a progressive encephalopathy associated with confusion, memory loss, agitation, and, later, lethargy and stupor. Speech arrest and myoclonic jerking was common and associated with severe and generalized EEG changes. The condition was often fatal. There were no specific pathologic findings, but elevated brain aluminum content was documented. The condition has been eliminated by use of deionized water for dialysis. Although aluminum injected into experimental animals may produce neurofibrillary tangles, dialysis dementia patients had neither tangles nor amyloid plaques, and there has been no direct association of aluminum poisoning with AD.

Recurrent head trauma in professional boxers may lead to dementia, sometimes called the "punch drunk" syndrome or *dementia pugilistica*. The symptoms can be progressive and may begin late in a boxer's career or even long after retirement. The severity of the syndrome correlates with the length of the boxing career and the total number of bouts. Early in the condition there occurs a personality change associated with social instability and sometimes paranoia and delusions. Later, memory loss progresses to full dementia, often associated with parkinsonian signs and ataxia or intention tremor. At autopsy, the cerebral cortex may show changes similar to AD, although neurofibrillary tangles are usually more predominant than amyloid plaques (which are usually diffuse rather than neuritic). There may also be loss of neurons in the substantia nigra. Chronic subdural hematoma is also occasionally associated with dementia, often in the context of underlying cortical atrophy from conditions such as AD or HD. In these latter cases, evacuation of the subdural hematoma will not alter the underlying degenerative process.

Head injury (Chap. 374) may also be associated with temporary amnesia. The memory disturbance may include events that occurred both prior to the injury (retrograde amnesia) and during the postinjury period (posttraumatic or anterograde amnesia). Retrograde amnesia following severe head injury may extend back for hours or weeks prior to the injury; remote memory is usually intact. As patients recover, the extent of retrograde amnesia shrinks and may disappear. Often, retrograde amnesia causes permanent inability to recall the few minutes prior to the head injury, implying disruption of the immediate memory system and failure to register long-term memory. The length of posttraumatic amnesia generally corresponds to the length of the postconcussive confusional state but posttraumatic amnesia may persist even in the presence of normal immediate memory and digit span. The duration of posttraumatic amnesia indicates the severity of head injury; the ability to learn new material is often the last cognitive deficit to recover. There are reports of recovery from retrograde amnesia occurring months or years after the initial brain insult, the recovery sometimes stimulated by hypnosis, amobarbital interview, or electrical stimulation. One theory of such recovery envisions a resetting of distorted patterns of neuronal matrices subserving memory.

Transient global amnesia (TGA) is characterized by sudden onset of complete anterograde loss of memory and learning abilities, usually occurring in persons over age 50. Onset of memory loss may occur in the context of an emotional stimulus or physical exertion. During the attack the individual is alert and communicative, general cognition seems intact, and there are no other neurologic signs or symptoms. The patient may seem confused and repeatedly ask about present events. Ability to form new memories returns after a period of hours, and the individual returns to normal but has no recall for the period of the attack. Frequently no cause can be determined, but cerebrovascular disease, epilepsy (7 percent in one study), migraine, or cardiac arrhythmia are sometimes implicated. A Mayo Clinic review of 277 patients with TGA found a past history of migraine in 14 percent and cerebrovascular disease in 11 percent, but these conditions were not temporally related to the TGA episodes. About one-fourth of the patients had recurrent attacks, but they were not at increased risk for subsequent stroke. Rare instances of permanent memory loss after sudden onset have been reported.

Psychogenic amnesia for personally important memories is common, although whether this results from deliberate avoidance of unpleasant memories or from unconscious repression may be impossible to establish. The event-specific amnesia is particularly common after violent crimes such as homicide of a close relative or friend or sexual abuse. It also may occur with severe drug or alcohol intoxication and sometimes with schizophrenia. More prolonged psychogenic amnesia occurs in fugue states that also commonly follow severe emotional stress. The patient with a fugue state suffers from a sudden loss of personal identity and may be found wandering far from home. In contrast to organic amnesia, fugue states are associated with amnesia for personal identity and events closely associated with the personal past. At the same time, memory for other recent events and the ability to learn and use new information are preserved. The episodes usually last hours or days and occasionally weeks or months while the patient takes on a new identity. On recovery, there is a residual amnesic gap for the period of the fugue.

Psychiatric diseases may mimic dementia. Severely depressed individuals may appear demented, a phenomenon called *pseudodementia*. Unlike cortical dementias, memory and language are usually intact when carefully tested in depressed persons. The patients may feel confused and are unable to accomplish routine tasks. Vegetative symptoms are common, such as insomnia, lack of energy, poor appetite, and concern with bowel function. The psychosocial milieu may suggest prominent reasons for depression. The patients respond to antidepressant treatment. Schizophrenia is usually not difficult to distinguish from dementia but occasionally the distinction can be problematic. (Kraepelin's original term for schizophrenia was *dementia praecox*.) Schizophrenia usually has a much earlier age of onset (second and third decades) than most dementing illnesses, is associated with intact memory, and the delusions and hallucinations of schizophrenia are usually more complex and bizarre than those of dementia. Some chronic schizophrenics develop an unexplained progressive dementia late in life that is not related to AD. Memory loss may also be part of a conversion reaction. In this situation, patients commonly complain bitterly of memory loss but careful cognitive testing either does not confirm the deficits or demonstrates inconsistent or unusual patterns of cognitive problems. The patients' behavior and "wrong" answers to questions often indicate that they both understand the question and know the answer.

Clouding of cognition by chronic drug or medication use, often prescribed by physicians, is an important cause of dementia. Sedatives, tranquilizers, and analgesics used to treat insomnia, pain, anxiety, or agitation may cause confusion, memory loss, and lethargy, especially in the elderly. Discontinuation of such medication often improves mentation.

Approach to the Patient

The approach to the patient with dementia should always keep two major issues in the forefront: What is the most accurate diagnosis and is there a treatable condition? A broad overview of this approach is shown in Table 26-3.

History The history should concentrate on the onset, duration, and tempo of the memory loss. Acute or subacute confusion may represent delirium and suggests intoxication, infection, or metabolic derangement. An elderly person with slowly progressive memory loss over several years is likely to have AD. Initial symptoms often are difficulty with managing money, driving, shopping, following instructions, or finding one's way around town. A change in personality is also common. A history of sudden stroke with an irregular stepwise progression suggests multi-infarct dementia. Stroke is also commonly associated with a history of hypertension, atrial fibrillation, peripheral vascular disease, and diabetes. Rapid progression with rigidity and myoclonus suggests CJD. Seizures may indicate strokes or neoplasm. Trouble in walking may suggest PD or normal-pressure hydrocephalus, especially the latter when associated with bladder incontinence. Multiple sex partners or intravenous drug use may indicate CNS infection, especially with HIV. A history of recurrent head trauma could indicate chronic subdural hematoma, dementia pugilistica, or normal-pressure hydrocephalus. Alcoholism may suggest malnutrition and thiamine deficiency. A remote history of gastric surgery resulting in loss of intrinsic factor might indicate vitamin B_{12} deficiency. Certain occupations such as working in a battery or chemical factory might indicate heavy metal intoxication. Careful review of medication intake, especially of sedatives and tranquilizers, may raise the issue of chronic drug intoxication. A positive family history of dementia would be elicited in HD or familial AD. Recent death of a loved one, insomnia, or poor appetite suggest depression.

Physical Examination A careful examination is essential to document the dementia, look for other signs of nervous system involvement, and search for clues suggesting other systemic disease. Cognitive function should be assessed in terms of orientation, recent and remote memory, and calculation. Many of the simple, commonly used bedside tests of cognitive function (such as serial 7s, digits forward and backward) are most useful when they are performed normally; this makes the diagnosis of dementia unlikely. Mistakes on these simple tests are more difficult to interpret and are of less diagnostic importance. Drawing a clock and the trail-making test are frequently used tests of immediate memory and visual-spatial abilities. The mini-mental status exam (MMSE) is an easily administered 30-points test of cognitive function (Table 26-4). It is used to indicate a dementing process quickly, provide a rough assessment of its severity, and follow progression of the illness. The MMSE is influenced by culture and education and is less useful in the early and late stages of dementia. Language function should be tested by ability to read, write, comprehend, and name objects. Resting tremor, cogwheel rigidity, bradykinesia, and festinating gait indicates a parkinsonian syndrome. Gait ataxia or apraxia (inability to initiate and coordinate steps in a sequential fashion) suggests normal-pressure hydrocephalus. Confusion, sixth cranial nerve paresis, and ataxia suggests thiamine deficiency. Myoclonic jerks are present in CJD but also occur in AD. Hemiparesis or other focal neurologic deficits may occur in multi-infarct dementia or brain tumor. Bilateral hyperactive tendon reflexes, Babinski responses, and loss of vibration and position sensation suggest a myelopathy, such as occurs in vitamin B_{12} deficiency. Stocking-glove sensory loss and diminished tendon reflexes suggest a peripheral neuropathy, which could indicate underlying diabetes, vitamin deficiency, or heavy metal intoxication. Dry cool skin, hair loss, and bradycardia suggest hypothyroidism. Confusion associated with repetitive stereotyped movements may indicate ongoing seizure activity. Hearing impairment or visual loss may produce confusion and disorientation misinterpreted as dementia. Such sensory deficits are common in the elderly.

Laboratory Tests The use of multiple laboratory tests in the evaluation

Table 26-3

Evaluation of the Demented Patient

Routine Evaluation	Optional Focused Tests	Occasionally Helpful Tests
History	HIV	EEG
Physical examination	Chest x-ray	Parathyroid function
Laboratory tests	Lumbar puncture	Adrenal function
Thyroid function (TSH)	Liver function	Urine heavy metals
Vitamin B_{12}	Renal function	RBC sedimentation rate
Complete blood count	Urine toxin screen	Angiogram
Electrolytes	Psychometric testing	Brain biopsy
VDRL	Apolipoprotein E	
CT/MRI		

DIAGNOSTIC CATEGORIES

Treatable Causes	Untreatable/Degenerative Dementias	Psychiatric Disorders
Examples	Examples	Depression
Hypothyroidism	Alzheimer's	Schizophrenia
Thiamine deficiency	Pick's	Conversion reaction
Vitamin B_{12} deficiency	Huntington's	
Normal-pressure	Diffuse Lewy body disease	
hydrocephalus	Multi-infarct	
Chronic infection	Leukoencephalopathies	
Brain tumor	Parkinson's	
Drug intoxication		

Associated Treatable Conditions

Depression
Seizures
Insomnia
Agitation
Caregiver "burnout"
Drug side effects

of dementia is controversial. The physician does not want to miss a treatable cause, yet no single treatable cause stands out as common; thus a screen must employ multiple different tests, each of which has a low yield. Therefore, cost/benefit ratios are difficult to assess, and many laboratory screening algorithms for dementia discourage multiple tests. Nevertheless, even a test with only a 1 to 2 percent positive rate is probably worth undertaking if the alternative is missing a treatable cause of dementia. The algorithm in Table 26-3 lists most screening tests for dementia. Neuroimaging studies (CT and MRI) are especially controversial because of their costs. However, they are clearly of value to identify primary and secondary neoplasms, locate areas of infarction, or suggest normal-pressure hydrocephalus or diffuse white matter disease. They also lend support to the diagnosis of AD, especially if there is hippocampal atrophy in addition to diffuse cortical atrophy. On the other hand, attempts to relate cognition to neuroimaging measures of atrophy and white matter changes have only shown modest correlations. A diagnosis of AD is reached primarily by exclusion of other causes of dementia. (The indications for apolipoprotein E testing for AD are discussed in Chap. 367.) Serum levels of vitamin B_{12} and thyroid-stimulating hormone, complete blood count, electrolyte measurements, and VDRL are reasonable routine screening tests because they detect treatable conditions. Lumbar puncture need not be done routinely in the evaluation of dementia, but is indicated if CNS infection is a serious consideration, for example, in patients with delirium, fever, or nuchal rigidity. CSF levels of tau protein are increased, and $A\beta$ amyloid decreased, in some AD patients; however, the clinical utility of these changes is not yet clear. Formal psychometric testing is not necessary in every patient with dementia, but can be used to document the severity of dementia, suggest psychogenic causes, and provide a semiquantitative method for following the disease course. EEG is rarely helpful except to suggest CJD (repetitive bursts of diffuse high voltage sharp waves) or an underlying nonconvulsive seizure disorder (epileptiform discharges). Brain biopsy (including meninges) is not commonly advised except to diagnose vasculitis, potentially treatable neoplasms, unusual infections (such as sarcoid), or in young persons where the diagnosis is in doubt. Angiography is not likely to be of use except when multiple strokes or cerebral vasculitis is a possible cause of the dementia.

Table 26-4

The Mini-Mental Status Examination

	Points
Orientation	
Name: season/date/day/month/year	5 (1 for each name)
Name: hospital/floor/town/state/country	5 (1 for each name)
Registration	
Identify three objects by name and ask patient to repeat	3 (1 for each object)
Attention and calculation	
Serial 7s; subtract from 100 (e.g., 93–86–79–72–65)	5 (1 for each subtraction)
Recall	
Recall the three objects presented earlier	3 (1 for each object)
Language	
Name pencil and watch	2 (1 for each object)
Repeat "No ifs, ands, or buts"	1
Follow a 3-step command (e.g., "Take this paper, fold it in half, and place it on the table")	3 (1 for each command)
Write "close your eyes" and ask patient to obey written command	1
Ask patient to write a sentence	1
Ask patient to copy a design (e.g., intersecting pentagons)	1
TOTAL	**30**

The two major goals of management are, first, to treat any correctable cause of the dementia and, second, to provide comfort and support to the patient and caregivers. Treatment of underlying causes might include thyroid replacement for hypothyroidism, vitamin therapy for thiamine and B_{12} deficiency, antibiotics for opportunistic infections, ventricular shunting for normal-pressure hydrocephalus, and appropriate surgical, radiation, and/or chemotherapy for CNS neoplasms. Removal of sedating or cognition-impairing drugs and medications is often beneficial. If the patient is depressed rather than demented (pseudodementia), the depression should be vigorously treated. Patients with degenerative diseases such as AD and HD may also be depressed, and that portion of their condition may respond to antidepressant therapy. Antidepressants should be used with caution in demented patients because they may produce delirium. Antidepressants that are low in cognitive side effects, such as selective serotonin reuptake inhibitors, and tricyclic antidepressants with low anticholinergic activity, such as desipramine and nortriptyline, are advisable. Anticonvulsants are used to control seizures. Agitation, hallucinations, delusions, and confusion are difficult to treat. These behavioral problems represent major causes for nursing home placement and institutionalization. Drugs such as phenothiazines, haloperidol, and benzodiazepines may ameliorate the behavior problems but have untoward side effects such as sedation, rigidity, and dyskinesias. Medications that may calm agitation and insomnia without worsening dementia include low-dose haloperidol (0.5 to 2 mg), trazodone, buspirone, and propranolol. When patients do not respond it is usually a mistake to advance to higher doses or to use anticholinergics or sedatives (such as barbiturates or benzodiazepines).

Nondrug behavior therapy has an important place in the management of dementia. The primary goal is to make the demented patient's life comfortable, uncomplicated, and safe. Preparing lists, schedules, calendars, and labels can be helpful. It is also useful to stress familiar routines, short-term tasks, brief walks, and simple physical exercises. For many demented patients, the memory for facts is worse than that for routine activities, and they still may be able to take part in remembered physical activities such as walking, bowling, dancing, and golf. Demented patients usually object to losing control over familiar tasks such as driving, cooking, and handling finances. Attempts to help or take over may be greeted with complaints, depression, or anger. Hostile responses on the part of the caretaker are useless and sometimes harmful. Explanation, reassurance, distraction, and calm statements are more productive responses in this setting. Eventually, tasks such as finances and driving must be assumed by others, and the patient will conform and adjust. Safety is an important issue that includes not only driving but the environment of the kitchen, bathroom, and sleeping area. These areas need to be monitored, supervised, and made as safe as possible. A move to a retirement home, assisted-living center, or nursing home can initially increase confusion and agitation. Repeated reassurance, reorientation, and careful introduction to the new personnel will help to smooth the process. Provision of activities that are known to be enjoyable to the patient can be of considerable benefit. Attention should also be paid to frustration and depression in family members and caregivers. Caregiver guilt and burn-out are common. Family members often feel overwhelmed and helpless and may vent their frustrations on the patient, each other, and healthcare providers. Caregivers should be encouraged to take advantage of day-care facilities and respite breaks. Education and counseling about dementia are important. Local and national support groups can be of considerable help, such as the Alzheimer's Disease and Related Disorders Association.

BIBLIOGRAPHY

COREY-BLOOD J et al: Diagnosis and evaluation of dementia. Neurology 45:211, 1995

CUMMINGS JK: *Dementia: A Clinical Approach*, 2d ed. Boston, Butterworth-Heinemann, 1992

EBLY EM et al: Prevalence and types of dementia in the very old: Results from the Canadian Study of Health and Aging. Neurology 44:1593, 1994

ERICKSON K: Amnestic disorders. Pathophysiology and patterns of memory dysfunction. West J Med 152:159, 1990

FLEMING KC, EVANS JM: Pharmacologic therapies in dementia. Mayo Clin Proc 70:1116, 1995

HODGES JR, WARLOW CP: Syndromes of transient amnesia: Towards a classification. A study of 153 cases. J Neurol Neurosurg Psychiatry 53:834, 1990

MARTIN LM, FLEMING KC et al: Recognition and management of anxiety and depression in elderly patients. Mayo Clin Proc 70:999, 1995

SIU AL: Screening for dementia and investigating its causes. Ann Intern Med 115:122, 1991

WILLMER J et al: The usefulness of CT scanning in diagnosing dementia of the Alzheimer type. Can J Neurol Sci 20:210, 1993

27   *Charles A. Czeisler, Gary S. Richardson*

DISORDERS OF SLEEP AND CIRCADIAN RHYTHMS

Disturbed sleep is among the most frequent health complaints physicians encounter. One-third of adults in the United States experience occasional or persistent sleep disturbances. Sleep deprivation or disruption of the circadian timing system can lead to serious impairment of daytime functioning. Sleep disorders may either contribute to or result from related medical or psychiatric conditions. Twenty-five years ago, many such complaints were treated with hypnotic medications without further diagnostic evaluation. Since then, a distinct class of sleep and arousal disorders has been identified, and the field of sleep disorders is now an established clinical discipline. Two principal neurobiologic systems govern the sleep-wake cycle: one that actively generates sleep and sleep-related processes and another that times sleep within the 24-h day. Either intrinsic abnormalities in these systems or extrinsic disturbances (environmental, drug- or illness-related) can lead to sleep or circadian rhythm disorders.

PHYSIOLOGY OF SLEEP AND WAKEFULNESS

Most adults sleep 7 to 8 h per night, although the timing, duration, and internal structure of sleep vary among apparently healthy individuals and as a function of age. At the extremes, infants and the elderly have frequent interruptions of sleep. In the United States, adults of intermediate age tend to have one consolidated sleep episode per day, although in some cultures sleep may be divided into a midafternoon nap and a shortened night sleep. While there is a wide range of normal sleep lengths, epidemiologic studies suggest that adults with habitual sleep durations of fewer than 4 h or greater than 9 have increased mortality rates as compared to those who sleep 7 to 8 h per night.

STATES AND STAGES OF SLEEP   States and stages of human sleep are defined on the basis of characteristic patterns in the electroencephalogram (EEG), the electrooculogram (EOG—a measure of eye-movement activity), and the surface electromyogram (EMG).

The continuous recording of this array of electrophysiologic parameters to define sleep and wakefulness is termed *polysomnography.*

Polysomnographic profiles define two states of sleep: (1) rapid-eye-movement (REM) sleep, and (2) non-rapid-eye-movement (NREM) sleep. NREM sleep is in turn subdivided into four stages, characterized by increasing arousal threshold and slowing of the cortical EEG (Fig. 27-1). REM sleep is characterized by a low-amplitude, mixed-frequency EEG similar to that of NREM stage 1 (Fig. 27-1). The EOG shows bursts of REM similar to those seen during eyes-open wakefulness. EMG activity is absent, reflecting the complete brainstem-mediated muscle atonia that is characteristic of that state.

ORGANIZATION OF HUMAN SLEEP   Normal nocturnal sleep in adults displays a consistent organization from night to night (Fig. 27-2). After sleep onset, sleep usually progresses through NREM stages 1 to 4 within 45 to 60 min. Slow-wave sleep predominates in the first third of the night and comprises 15 to 25 percent of total nocturnal sleep time in young adults. The percentage of slow-wave sleep is influenced by several factors, most notably age (see below). Prior sleep deprivation increases the rapidity of sleep onset and both the intensity and amount of slow-wave sleep.

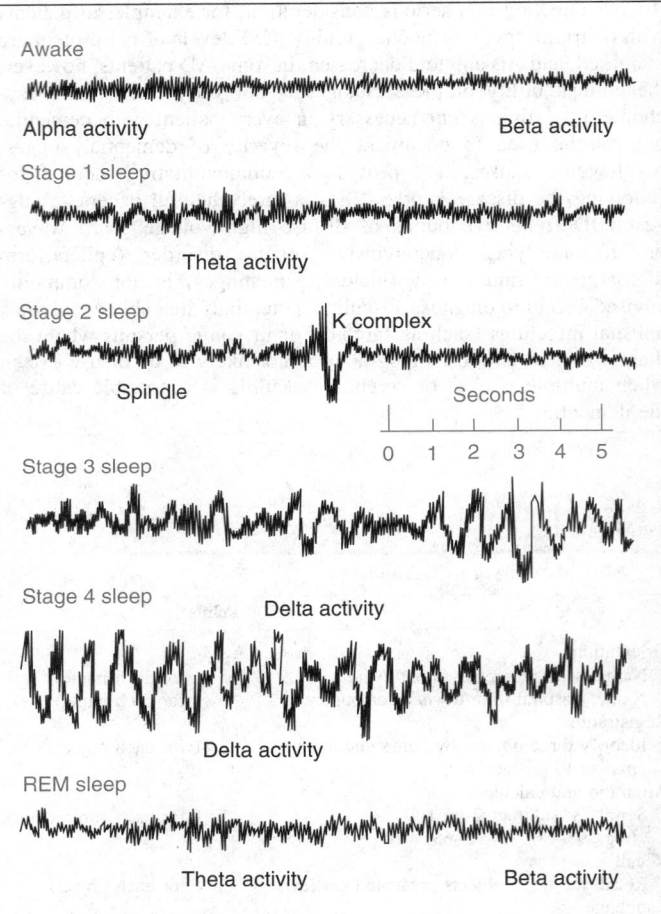

FIGURE 27-1   Electroencephalogram of human sleep stages. The first trace illustrates alpha activity seen in quiet wakefulness (eyes closed) and the beta activity of an alert subject. Stage 1 theta activity is seen in the second trace; stage 2 sleep (with associated sleep spindle and K complex) in the third. The fourth and fifth traces show slow-wave (stages 3 and 4) sleep, with prominent delta activity. This synchronous activity is absent in REM sleep (sixth trace), which resembles stage 1 EEG. However, REM sleep is accompanied by rapid eye movements and muscle paralysis. *(Reproduced from J Horne, Why We Sleep: The Functions of Sleep in Humans and Other Mammals. Oxford, Oxford University Press, 1988.)*

The first REM sleep episode usually occurs in the second hour of sleep. More rapid onset of REM sleep in a young adult may (particularly if less than 30 min) suggest pathology such as endogenous depression, narcolepsy, circadian rhythm disorders, or drug withdrawal. NREM and REM alternate through the night with an average period of 90 to 110 min (the "ultradian" cycle). Overall, REM sleep constitutes 20 to 25 percent of total sleep, and NREM stages (1 and 2) are 50 to 60 percent (increasing in elderly subjects).

Age has a large impact on sleep state organization (Fig. 27-2). Slow-wave sleep is most prominent during childhood, decreasing sharply at puberty and across the second and third decades of life. After age 30, there is a progressive, almost linear decline in the amount of slow-wave sleep, and the amplitude of delta EEG activity comprising slow-wave sleep is reduced. In the otherwise healthy elderly person, slow-wave sleep may be completely absent, particularly in males.

A different age profile exists for REM sleep. In infancy, REM sleep may comprise 50 percent of total sleep time, and the percentage is inversely proportional to developmental age. The amount of REM sleep falls off sharply over the first postnatal year as a mature REM-NREM cycle develops. During the rest of life into extreme old age, REM sleep occupies a more constant percentage of total sleep time than does slow-wave sleep.

BEHAVIORAL CORRELATES OF SLEEP STATES AND STAGES Polysomnographic staging of sleep correlates with behavioral changes during specific states and stages. Awakenings from REM sleep are associated with recall of vivid dream imagery more than 80 percent of the time. The reliability of dream recall increases with REM sleep episodes occurring later in the night. Imagery may also be reported after NREM sleep interruptions, though these typically lack the detail and vividness of REM sleep dreams. The incidence of NREM sleep dream recall can be increased by selective REM sleep deprivation, suggesting that REM sleep and dreaming per se are not inexorably linked. Sleep onset is associated with marked decrements in perception of both auditory and visual stimuli and lapses of consciousness. During stage 1 sleep, subjects may respond to faint auditory or visual signals without "awakening." Furthermore, memory incorporation is inhibited at the onset of NREM stage 1, and subjects aroused from that stage frequently deny having been asleep. At the same time, it is possible to continue performing routine and familiar motor tasks, such as driving an automobile, during the transitional state between wakefulness and sleep (stage 1 sleep) that often intrudes upon behavioral wakefulness in the sleepy individual. During such intrusions, typically lasting only seconds but known on occasion to persist for longer durations, visual and auditory perception are attenuated and reaction time is prolonged. Subsequently, the sleepy individual may be unaware that such an event has occurred. The dramatic perceptual and cognitive deficits associated with frequent brief intrusions of stage 1 sleep into behavioral wakefulness are a major component of the impaired psychomotor performance seen with sleepiness.

PHYSIOLOGIC CORRELATES OF SLEEP STATES AND STAGES All major physiologic systems are influenced by sleep. In some cases, concomitant behavior changes such as supine posture or inactivity are the proximal causes of altered physiologic function, but in most cases the sleep state itself appears to be responsible. Changes in cardiovascular function include a decrease in blood pressure and heart rate during NREM, and particularly during slow-wave, sleep. During REM sleep, phasic activity (bursts of eye movements) is associated with variability in both blood pressure and heart rate mediated principally by the vagus. Cardiac dysrhythmias may occur selectively during REM sleep. Respiratory function also changes (see Chap. 263). In comparison to relaxed wakefulness, respiratory rate becomes more regular during NREM sleep (especially slow-wave sleep) and tonic REM sleep and becomes very irregular during phasic REM sleep. Minute ventilation decreases in NREM sleep out of proportion to the decrease in metabolic rate at sleep onset, resulting in a higher P_{CO_2}. Multiple factors contribute to these sleep-related changes in breathing: (1) decreased upper airway patency and consequent increased upper airway resistance, likely the result of sleep-related relaxation of a subset of tonically active upper airway muscles that lack a clear pattern of respiratory activation; (2) change in responsiveness of the respiratory system to chemical stimuli, namely P_{CO_2} and P_{O_2}; (3) loss of respiratory responses to wakeful stimuli; and (4) decreased metabolic rate. In addition, the cough reflex is attenuated or absent during sleep. These changes in respiratory function may be relevant to the pathogenesis of obstructive sleep apnea and sudden infant death syndrome (see Chap. 263).

Endocrine function also varies with sleep. The most prominent changes are apparent in neuroendocrine parameters. Slow-wave sleep is associated with secretion of growth hormone, while sleep in general is associated with augmented secretion of prolactin. Sleep has a complex effect on the secretion of luteinizing hormone (LH); during puberty, sleep is associated with increased LH secretion, whereas sleep in the mature woman inhibits LH secretion in the early follicular phase of the menstrual cycle. Sleep onset (and probably slow-wave sleep)

FIGURE 27-2 Plots of the stages of REM sleep (solid bars), the four stages of NREM sleep and wakefulness over the course of the entire night for representative young (upper panel, age 23) and elderly (lower panel, age 68) adult men. The recording in the elderly subject illustrates the reduction of slow-wave sleep, frequent spontaneous awakenings, early sleep onset, and early morning awakening that are characteristic features of sleep in the aged, even in the absence of specific medical or psychiatric pathology. (*From the Circadian, Neuroendocrine, and Sleep Disorders Section, Endocrine Division, Brigham and Womens' Hospital.*)

is associated with inhibition of thyroid-stimulating hormone and of the adrenocorticotropic hormone–cortisol axis, an effect that is super-imposed on the circadian rhythms in the two systems. The pineal hormone melatonin is secreted predominantly at night, in both day- and night-active species, reflecting the direct modulation of pineal activity by the circadian pacemaker in the anterior hypothalamus (see below). Melatonin secretion is not dependent upon the occurrence of sleep, persisting in individuals kept awake at night. In addition, some recent data suggest that exogenous melatonin may increase sleepiness and potentiate sleep, particularly when administered during daylight hours when endogenous melatonin levels are low. However, further studies are required to verify and quantify putative sleep-promoting properties of melatonin.

Sleep is also associated with alterations of thermoregulatory function. NREM sleep is associated with an attenuation of thermoregulatory responses to either heat or cold stress, and animal studies of thermosensitive neurons in the hypothalamus document a NREM-sleep-dependent reduction of the thermoregulatory set-point. REM sleep is associated with complete absence of thermoregulatory responsiveness, effectively resulting in functional poikilothermy. However, the potential adverse impact of this failure of thermoregulation is blunted by inhibition of REM sleep by extreme ambient temperatures.

Neuroanatomy of Sleep Lesion studies in animals and neurologic diseases in humans have suggested distinct neuroanatomic sites in the generation of normal sleep and wakefulness. The studies of von Economo of patients with encephalitis lethargica suggested that the anterior hypothalamus contained a "sleep center" while the posterior hypothalamus contained a "wake center." Experimental studies in animals have variously implicated the medullary reticular formation, the thalamus, and the basal forebrain in the generation of sleep, while the brainstem reticular formation, the midbrain, the subthalamus, the thalamus, and the basal forebrain have all been suggested to play a role in the generation of wakefulness or EEG arousal (see also Chap. 24).

Despite many studies, there is little evidence for either a single, discrete "sleep center" or a single, discrete "wake center." Current hypotheses suggest that the capacity for sleep and wakefulness generation is distributed along an axial "core" of neurons extending from the brainstem rostrally to the basal forebrain. Complex commingling of neuronal groups occurs at many points along this brainstem-forebrain axis.

Nonetheless, the neuroanatomic correlates of REM sleep appear to be discretely localized. Specific regions in the pons are associated with each of the neurophysiologic correlates of REM sleep. Small lesions in the dorsal pons produce REM sleep without the descending muscle inhibition normally associated with that state; microinjections of carbachol into the pontine reticular formation appear to produce a state with all of the features of REM sleep. These experimental manipulations are mimicked by pathologic conditions in humans and animals. In narcolepsy, for example, abrupt, complete, or partial paralysis (cataplexy) occurs in response to a variety of stimuli. In dogs with this condition, physostigmine, a central cholinesterase inhibitor, increases the frequency of cataplectic attacks while atropine decreases their frequency. Conversely, in REM sleep behavior disorder (see below), patients suffer from incomplete motor inhibition during REM sleep, resulting in involuntary, occasionally violent movement during REM sleep.

Neurochemistry of Sleep Early experimental studies that focused on the raphe nuclei of the brainstem appeared to implicate serotonin as the primary sleep-promoting neurotransmitter, while catecholamines were considered to be responsible for wakefulness. Subsequent work has demonstrated that the raphe-serotonin system may facilitate sleep but is not necessary to its expression. The extensive pharmacology of sleep and wakefulness suggests roles for other neurotransmitters as well. Cholinergic neurotransmission is known to play a role in REM sleep generation. The alerting influence of caffeine

implicates adenosine, whereas the hypnotic effect of benzodiazepines and barbiturates suggests a role for endogenous ligands of the GABA-A receptor complex.

A variety of sleep-promoting substances have been identified. These include prostaglandin D_2, delta sleep–inducing peptide, muramyl dipeptide, interleukin 1, fatty acid primary amides, and melatonin (see above), and the hypnotic effect is commonly limited to NREM or slow-wave sleep, although peptides that increase REM sleep have also been reported. Many putative "sleep factors," including interleukin 1 and prostaglandin D_2, are immunologically active as well, suggesting a link between immune function and sleep-wake states.

PHYSIOLOGY OF CIRCADIAN RHYTHMICITY The sleep-wake cycle is the most evident of the many 24-h rhythms in humans. Prominent daily variations also occur in endocrine, thermoregulatory, cardiac, pulmonary, renal, gastrointestinal, and cognitive functions. However, in evaluating a daily variation, it is important to distinguish between those rhythmic components passively evoked by periodic environmental or behavioral changes (e.g., the increase in blood pressure and heart rate upon assumption of the upright posture), and those actively driven by an endogenous oscillatory process (e.g., the circadian variation in plasma cortisol that persists under a variety of environmental and behavioral conditions).

The suprachiasmatic nuclei (SCN) of the hypothalamus act as the central neural pacemakers driving endogenous circadian rhythms in mammals. Bilateral destruction of these nuclei results in a loss of endogenous circadian rhythmicity that can only be restored by transplantation of the same structure(s) from a donor animal. The period and phase of the endogenous neural oscillator are normally synchronized to the 24-h period of the environmental light-dark cycle. Entrainment of mammalian circadian rhythms by the light-dark cycle is mediated via the retinohypothalamic tract, a monosynaptic pathway that links the retina to the SCN.

The principal properties characterizing an endogenous circadian pacemaker are its *intrinsic period*, *entrained phase*, *amplitude*, and *resetting capacity*. In human subjects living in controlled laboratory environments free of time cues (*free-running*), the duration of the behavioral rest-activity cycle averages 25 h. However, the timing of the light-dark cycle has generally been uncontrolled in such free-running studies, with the subjects choosing to be exposed to light during their "subjective days" and to darkness during their "subjective nights." Recent work suggests that when the light-dark cycle is controlled, the observed period of the human circadian pacemaker is much closer to 24 h. Nonetheless, synchronization of the endogenous circadian pacemaker to the 24-h day requires that the pacemaker be reset each day, which is normally achieved by exposure to the environmental light-dark cycle.

Exposure to light can shift the phase of the endogenous circadian pacemaker, but both the magnitude and the direction of the phase shifts induced by light depend on the timing, duration, wavelength, and intensity of the light. Properly timed exposure to light of sufficient intensity can, within 2 to 3 d, reset the human circadian pacemaker (presumably the SCN) to any desired hour. Exposure to ordinary indoor room light also shifts circadian phase but not by as great a magnitude as brighter outdoor light.

The timing and internal architecture of sleep are directly coupled to the output of the endogenous pacemaker. Spontaneous sleep duration, sleepiness, REM sleep propensity, and both the ability and the tendency to sleep vary with circadian phase. Sleep tendency, sleepiness, and REM sleep propensity all peak just after the nadir of the endogenous circadian temperature cycle (approximately 1 to 3 h before awakening). In addition, 85 percent of all spontaneous awakenings of subjects living in constant environmental conditions occur on the rising slope of the temperature cycle. Furthermore, there are certain times (wake maintenance zones) when it is very difficult to fall asleep, even for subjects who are sleep-deprived. Misalignment of the output of the endogenous circadian pacemaker with the desired sleep-wake cycle is thought to be responsible for certain types of insomnia, as well as for the decrements of alertness and performance in night-shift workers and after jet lag.

DISORDERS OF SLEEP AND WAKEFULNESS

An international classification of sleep disorders (Table 27-1) divides these conditions into three major groups: dyssomnias, parasomnias, and medical psychiatric sleep disorders. A detailed description of each of these disorders may be found in the publication of the American Sleep Disorders Association.

Approach to the Patient

With a Sleep Complaint Patients may seek help from a physician because of: (1) an acute or chronic inability to sleep adequately at night; (2) chronic fatigue, sleepiness, or tiredness during the day; or (3) a behavioral manifestation associated with sleep itself. Disruption or disturbance of nocturnal sleep is directly related to decreased alertness and impairment of daytime cognitive and psychomotor performance, which is often of serious concern to the patient. Table 27-2 outlines the most common pathways encountered in the evaluation of the patient with a complaint of excessive daytime sleepiness.

Taking a careful history is critical in the evaluation of the patient with a sleep complaint. In particular, the duration, severity, and consistency of the complaint are important, along with the patient's esti-mate—in the case of an insomnia complaint—of the consequences of reported sleep loss on subsequent waking function. Information from a friend or family member can be an invaluable aid in assessing the severity of the complaint on daytime functioning, as some patients will underreport such potentially embarrassing symptoms as heavy snoring or falling asleep while driving.

Retrospective completion by the physician and patient of a day-by-day sleep-work-drug log in reverse chronologic order can help the physician better understand the nature of the complaint. Work times should be specified each day. Drug and alcohol use, including caffeine and hypnotics, should be noted each day. This log should be compared with a prospective sleep-work-drug log (including daytime naps and nocturnal awakenings) as recorded by the patient for at least 2 weeks. The sleep times should be plotted to facilitate recognition of circadian rhythm sleep disorders such as delayed sleep phase syndrome (see below).

Laboratory evaluation of objective sleep measures is necessary in the diagnosis of specific disorders such as narcolepsy and sleep apnea and may be of utility in other settings as well. In addition to the three electrophysiologic variables used to define sleep states and stages, the standard clinical polysomnogram includes measures of respiration (respiratory effort, air flow, and oxygen saturation), anterior tibialis EMG, and ECG. Evaluation of penile tumescence during nocturnal sleep also can be used to help determine whether the cause of erectile dysfunction in a patient is psychogenic or organic (see Chap. 51).

DAYTIME CONSEQUENCES OF SLEEP DISORDERS

While the experience of disrupted nocturnal sleep may be the most prominent symptom for patients with sleep disorders, particularly those with insomnia, the impact of this sleep disruption on daytime function is arguably the more important aspect from both clinical and public health perspectives. Sleepiness-related automobile accidents, for example, constitute an important health risk for the patient with disrupted sleep.

Daytime impairment due to sleep loss may be difficult to quantify in the clinical setting for several reasons. First, sleepiness is not necessarily proportional to subjectively assessed sleep deprivation. In obstructive sleep apnea, for example, the repeated brief interruptions of sleep associated with resumption of respiration at the end of apneic episodes result in significant waking impairment, despite the fact that the patient may be unaware of the sleep fragmentation. Second, subjective descriptions of waking impairment vary from patient to patient. Patients may describe themselves as "sleepy," "fatigued," or "tired" and may have a clear sense of the meaning of those terms, while others may use the same terms to describe a completely different condition. Third, sleepiness, particularly when profound, may affect judgment in a manner analogous to ethanol, such that subjective awareness of the condition and the consequent cognitive and motor impairments is reduced. Finally, patients may be reluctant to admit that sleepiness is a problem, both because they are generally unaware of what constitutes normal alertness and because sleepiness is generally viewed pejoratively, ascribed more often to a deficit in motivation than to an inadequately addressed physiologic need.

In assessing sleepiness in the clinical setting, specific questioning about the occurrence of sleep episodes during normal waking hours, both intentional and unintentional, can overcome the inconsistencies among subjective characterizations and will simultaneously provide an index of the adverse impact of sleepiness on daytime function. Specific areas to be addressed include the occurrence of inadvertent sleep episodes while driving or in other safety-related settings, sleepiness while at work or school (and the relationship of sleepiness to work and school performance), and the effect of sleepiness on social and family life. Evidence for significant daytime impairment (typically in association with the diagnosis of a primary sleep disorder such as narcolepsy or sleep apnea) raises the question of the physician's

---

Table 27-1

International Classification of Sleep Disorders

DYSSOMNIAS

Intrinsic sleep disorders	Extrinsic sleep disorders
Psychophysiologic insomnia	Inadequate sleep hygiene
Idiopathic insomnia	Environmental sleep disorder
Narcolepsy	Altitude insomnia
Recurrent or idiopathic hyper-somnia	Adjustment sleep disorder
Posttraumatic hypersomnia	Sleep-onset association disorder
Sleep apnea syndromes	Food allergy insomnia
Periodic limb movement disorder	Nocturnal eating (drinking) syn-drome
Restless legs syndrome	Drug- or alcohol-dependent sleep disorders
Circadian rhythm sleep disorders	
Time-zone change (jet lag) syn-drome	
Shift-work sleep disorder	
Delayed sleep phase syndrome	
Advanced sleep phase syndrome	
Non-24-h sleep-wake disorder	

PARASOMNIAS

Arousal disorders	Parasomnias usually associated with REM sleep
Confusional arousals	Nightmares
Sleepwalking	Sleep paralysis
Sleep terrors	Impaired sleep-related penile erections
Sleep-wake transition disorders	Sleep-related painful erections
Rhythmic movement disorder	REM sleep-related cardiac arrhythmias
Sleep talking	REM sleep behavior disorder
Nocturnal leg cramps	Other parasomnias
	Sleep bruxism
	Sleep enuresis
	Nocturnal paroxysmal dystonia

SLEEP DISORDERS ASSOCIATED WITH MEDICAL/PSYCHIATRIC DISORDERS

Associated with mental disorders	Associated with other medical dis-orders
Associated with neurologic dis-orders	Sleeping sickness
Cerebral degenerative disorders	Nocturnal cardiac ischemia
Parkinsonism	Chronic obstructive pulmonary disease
Fatal familial insomnia	Sleep-related asthma
Sleep-related epilepsy	Sleep-related gastroesophageal reflux
Sleep-related headaches	Peptic ulcer disease
	Fibrositis syndrome

SOURCE: Modified from the Diagnostic Classification Steering Committee.

responsibility to notify licensing authorities of the increased risk of sleepiness-related vehicle accidents. As with epilepsy, legal requirements vary from state to state, and existing legal precedents typically do not provide a consistent interpretation of the balance between the physician's responsibility and the patient's right to privacy. At a minimum, physicians should document discussions with the patient regarding the increased risk of operating a vehicle, as well as a recommendation that driving be suspended until successful treatment can be instituted.

Differentiation of sleepiness from fatigue can be difficult, particularly given the imprecise use of these terms by patients in describing subjective symptoms. The distinction can be useful in the differentiation of patients with complaints of fatigue or tiredness in the setting of disorders such as fibromyalgia, chronic fatigue syndrome (see Chap. 384), or endocrine deficiencies such as hypothyroidism or Addison's disease. While patients with these disorders can typically distinguish their daytime symptoms from the sleepiness that occurs with sleep deprivation, substantial overlap can occur. This is particularly true when the primary disorder also results in chronic sleep disruption (e.g., sleep apnea in hypothyroidism) or in abnormal sleep (e.g., fibromyalgia).

While clinical evaluation of the complaint of excessive sleepiness is usually adequate, objective quantification is sometimes necessary for diagnostic purposes or for the evaluation of treatment response. Assessment of daytime functioning as an index of the adequacy of sleep can be made with the multiple sleep latency test (MSLT), which involves repeated measurement of sleep latency (time to onset of sleep) under standardized conditions during a day following quantified nocturnal sleep. The average latency across four to six tests (administered every 2 h across the waking day) is taken as an objective measure of daytime sleep tendency. Disorders of sleep that result in pathologic daytime somnolence can be reliably distinguished with the MSLT. In addition, the multiple measurements of sleep onset may identify direct transitions from wakefulness to REM sleep that are suggestive of specific pathologic conditions (e.g., narcolepsy).

INSOMNIA Insomnia is the complaint of inadequate sleep; it can be classified according to the nature of sleep disruption and the duration of the complaint. The nature of the sleep disruption provides important information about the possible etiology of the insomnia and is also central to the selection of specific and appropriate treatment. Insomnia is subdivided into difficulty falling asleep (*sleep onset insomnia*), frequent or sustained awakenings (*sleep maintenance insomnia*), early morning awakenings (*sleep offset insomnia*), or persistent sleepiness despite sleep of adequate duration (*nonrestorative sleep*). Simi-

larly, the duration of the symptom is an important determinant of the nature of appropriate treatment. An insomnia complaint lasting one to several nights (within a single episode) is termed *transient insomnia*. Transient insomnia is typically the result of situational stress or a change in sleep schedule or environment (e.g., jet lag). *Short-term insomnia* lasts from a few days to 3 weeks. Disruption of this duration is usually associated with more protracted stress, such as recovery from surgery or short-term illness. *Long-term* or *chronic insomnia* lasts for months or years and commonly reflects perpetuating factors associated with a primary sleep disorder (see below). Chronic insomnia may present as recurrent episodes of insomnia, not necessarily associated with parallel variation in the underlying cause. Although some clinicians refer to this as recurrent insomnia, others suggest that this may be the typical pattern of all chronic insomniacs.

While an occasional night of poor sleep, typically in the setting of stress or excitement about external events, is both common and without lasting consequences, persistent insomnia can have important adverse consequences in the form of impaired daytime function, mood disturbances, and increased risk of injury due to accidents.

Psychophysiologic Insomnia Persistent psychophysiologic insomnia is a behavioral disorder in which patients are preoccupied with a perceived inability to sleep adequately at night. The sleep disturbance is often triggered by an emotionally stressful event; however, the poor sleep habits acquired during the stressful period persist long after the initial incident. Such patients become hyperaroused by their own persistent efforts to sleep and/or the sleep environment, and the insomnia is a conditioned or learned response. Patients with psychophysiologic insomnia fall asleep more easily at unscheduled times (when not trying) or outside the home environment. In these cases, polysomnographic recording reveals an objective sleep disturbance, often with an abnormally long sleep latency, frequent nocturnal awakenings, and an increased amount of stage 1 transitional sleep. Extrinsic factors may contribute to this condition (see below). Rigorous attention should be paid to sleep hygiene (see below) and correction of counterproductive, arousing behaviors before bedtime. Behavioral therapy (i.e., sleep hygiene, relaxation training, stimulus control therapy, sleep restriction therapy) is the treatment modality of choice for psychophysiologic insomnia, and such therapy appears best instituted without medication.

Extrinsic Insomnia A number of sleep disorders are the result of extrinsic factors that interfere with sleep. *Adjustment sleep disorder*, also called *transient situational insomnia*, can occur after a change in the sleeping environment (e.g., in an unfamiliar hotel or hospital bed) or before or after a significant life event, such as a change of occupation, loss of a loved one, illness, or anxiety over a deadline or examination. Increased sleep latency, frequent awakenings from sleep, and early morning awakening can all occur. Recovery generally occurs rapidly, certainly within 2 to 3 weeks. *Inadequate sleep hygiene* is characterized

Table 27-2

Evaluation of the Patient with the Complaint of Excessive Daytime Somnolence

Findings on History and Physical Examination	Diagnostic Evaluation	Diagnosis	Therapy
Obesity, snoring, hypertension	Polysomnography with respiratory monitoring	Obstructive sleep apnea	Continuous positive airway pressure; ENT surgery (e.g., uvulopalatopharyngoplasty); dental appliance; pharmacologic therapy (e.g., protriptyline); weight loss; (see Chap. 264)
Cataplexy, hypnogogic hallucinations, sleep paralysis, family history	Polysomnography with multiple sleep latency test	Narcolepsy-cataplexy syndrome	Stimulants (e.g., methylphenidate, pemoline); REM-suppressant antidepressants (e.g., protriptyline); genetic counseling
Restless legs syndrome, disturbed sleep, predisposing medical condition (e.g., anemia or renal failure)	Polysomnography with bilateral anterior tibialis EMG	Periodic limb movements of sleep	Treatment of predisposing condition, if possible; dopamine agonists (e.g., levodopa-carbidopa); benzodiazepines (e.g., clonazepam)
Disturbed sleep, predisposing medical conditions (e.g., asthma) and/or predisposing medical therapies (e.g., theophylline)	Sleep-wake diary	Insomnias (see text)	Treatment of predisposing condition and/or change in therapy, if possible; behavioral therapy; short-acting benzodiazepine receptor agonist (e.g., zolpidem)

NOTE: ENT, ears, nose, throat; REM, rapid eye movement; EMG, electromyogram.

by a behavior pattern prior to sleep and/or a bedroom environment that is not conducive to sleep. Noise and/or light in the bedroom can interfere with sleep, as can a bed partner with periodic limb movements during sleep or one who snores loudly. Luminous clocks can arouse the patient, heightening anxiety about the time it has taken to fall asleep. Drugs that act on the central nervous system, large meals, vigorous exercise, or hot showers just before sleep may interfere with sleep onset. In preference to hypnotic medications, patients should be counseled to develop a soporific bedtime ritual and to prepare and reserve the bedroom environment for sleeping. Consistent, regular rising times should be charted daily; total time in bed should be restricted to actual sleep time.

Altitude Insomnia   Sleep disturbance is a common consequence of exposure to high altitude. Periodic breathing of the Cheyne-Stokes type occurs during NREM sleep about half the time at altitude, with restoration of a regular breathing pattern during REM sleep. Central rather than obstructive sleep apnea appears to be responsible, characterized by regular respiratory pauses. Both hypoxia and hypocapnia are thought to be involved in the development of periodic breathing. Frequent awakenings and poor quality sleep characterize altitude insomnia, which is generally worst on the first few nights at high altitude but may persist. The duration of sleep is unchanged, but there are more arousals after sleep onset and less time in slow-wave (stages 3 and 4) sleep. Treatment with acetazolamide can decrease time spent in periodic breathing and substantially reduce hypoxia during sleep. Medroxyprogesterone acetate also reduces hypoxia but does not significantly reduce periodic breathing during sleep at altitude.

Drug- or Alcohol-Dependent Sleep Disorders   Disturbed sleep can result from ingestion of a wide variety of agents. Caffeine is perhaps the most common pharmacologic cause of insomnia in sensitive patients. It produces increased latency to sleep onset, more frequent arousals during sleep, and a reduction in total sleep time for up to 8 to 14 h after ingestion. Occasional patients are surprised to learn that their insomnia may be related to coffee consumption; a careful history will reveal that such patients may drink 15 to 20 cups per day. As few as 3 to 5 cups of coffee can significantly disturb sleep in some patients; therefore, a 1- to 2-month caffeine withdrawal period should be attempted in patients with these symptoms. Similarly, alcohol and nicotine can interfere with sleep, although many patients use them to relax and promote sleep. Although alcohol can increase drowsiness and shorten sleep latency, even moderate amounts of alcohol increase awakenings after sleep onset by interfering with the ability of the brain to maintain sleep. In addition, alcohol ingestion prior to sleep is contraindicated in patients with sleep apnea because of the inhibitory effects of alcohol on upper airway muscle tone. Acutely, amphetamines and cocaine suppress both REM sleep and total sleep time, which return to normal with chronic use. Withdrawal leads to a REM sleep rebound. Finally, rebound insomnia associated with the acute withdrawal of hypnotics can be severe, especially following the use of high doses of benzodiazepines with a short half-life. For this reason, hypnotics should rarely be prescribed for habitual use; doses should be low to moderate, the total duration of hypnotic therapy should be limited to 2 to 3 weeks, and drug dosage should be reduced prior to withdrawal.

NARCOLEPSY   Excessive daytime sleepiness with involuntary daytime sleep episodes, disturbed nocturnal sleep, and cataplexy (sudden weakness or loss of muscle tone without loss of consciousness that is elicited by emotion) are the most common symptoms of narcolepsy (see Table 27-3). Some patients also experience muscular paralysis and/or hallucinations at sleep onset or upon awakening. The severity varies. Patients may have two to three cataplectic attacks per day or per decade, and the extent and duration of an attack may vary from a transient sagging of the jaw lasting a few seconds to flaccid paralysis of the entire voluntary musculature for up to 20 to 30 min, in rare cases.

Narcolepsy affects about 1 in 4000 people in the United States and appears to have a genetic basis. Experiments in some canine models of narcolepsy suggest an autosomal recessive pattern of inheritance. First-degree relatives of narcoleptic patients have about a 1 percent incidence of narcolepsy, much higher than the general popula-

tion. In addition, nearly all narcoleptics are positive for the human leukocyte antigen DR15 (ordinarily found in 20 to 30 percent of the general population) (see Chap. 306). A high rate of discordance in identical twins indicates that one or more nonheritable factors contributes to its development.

Symptoms typically begin in the second decade, although the onset ranges from ages 5 to 50. Once established, the disease is chronic without remissions.

Diagnosis   Classically, the diagnosis of narcolepsy required the presence of the "narcolepsy tetrad," consisting of (1) excessive daytime somnolence, (2) cataplexy, (3) hypnogogic hallucinations (the occurrence of vivid hallucinatory dream imagery at sleep onset), and (4) sleep paralysis (an awareness that voluntary musculature is paralyzed coincident with the onset of sleep). The last three symptoms of the tetrad are all manifestations of the abnormal REM sleep regulation inherent in the syndrome. All patients with narcolepsy have objectively verifiable daytime somnolence, but the other three symptoms are variably present, and only cataplexy is unique to narcolepsy. At least half have cataplexy of some degree, and similar percentages report hypnogogic hallucinations and/or sleep paralysis. Other associated symptoms are useful but not specific. A history of "automatic behavior" during wakefulness (a trancelike state during which simple motor behaviors persist) serves principally to corroborate the presence of daytime somnolence but is not specific for mechanism. Patients with narcolepsy also commonly report severe disruption of nocturnal sleep.

A family history is important in the evaluation of the patient with excessive daytime somnolence. Careful observation of the children and siblings of known narcoleptics, particularly at the typical age of onset (second decade), can lead to early diagnosis. The diagnosis of narcolepsy in a patient with a suggestive history depends upon (1) objective verification of excessive daytime somnolence, typically using the MSLT after nocturnal sleep recording; (2) a history of unambiguous cataplexy; (3) documentation of abnormal REM sleep regulation as evidenced by REM sleep onset within 10 min of sleep onset, either during the nocturnal recording or on one or more of the MSLT determinations; and (4) exclusion of other disorders, such as sleep apnea, that cause excessive sleepiness.

 TREATMENT

The treatment of narcolepsy is symptomatic. Somnolence is treated with stimulants. Methylphenidate is considered the drug of choice by most. Pemoline, a common second choice, has a longer half-life and is associated with fewer side effects but may not be as effective. Dextroamphetamine and methamphetamine are also frequently used, particularly when methylphenidate and pemoline are inadequate.

Treatment of cataplexy, hypnogogic hallucinations, and sleep paralysis requires antidepressants, which are effective, in part, because of potent REM-suppressive effects. Protriptyline, imipramine, and clomipramine are commonly used in the United States. Efficacy is limited largely by anticholinergic side effects. Fluoxetine and other serotonin reuptake inhibitors are often effective for this condition.

Table 27-3

Prevalence of Symptoms in Narcolepsy

Symptom	Prevalence, %
Excessive daytime somnolence	100
Disturbed sleep	87
Cataplexy	76
Hypnagogic hallucinations	68
Sleep paralysis	64
Memory problems	50

SOURCE: Modified from TA Roth, L Merlotti in SA Burton et al (eds), *Narcolepsy 3rd International Symposium: Selected Symposium Proceedings*, Chicago, Matrix Communications, 1989.

SLEEP APNEA SYNDROMES Respiratory dysfunction during sleep is a common, serious cause of excessive daytime somnolence as well as of disturbed nocturnal sleep. An estimated 2 to 5 million people in the United States stop breathing for 10 to 150 s, from thirty to several hundred times every night during sleep. These cessations of breathing may be due to either an occlusion of the airway (*obstructive sleep apnea*), absence of respiratory effort (*central sleep apnea*), or a combination of these factors (*mixed sleep apnea*). Failure to recognize and appropriately treat these conditions may lead to serious cardiovascular complications and increased mortality. This problem is particularly prevalent in overweight men and in the elderly and is often associated with hypertension. Occult sleep-related breathing disorders may result in significant impairment of daytime alertness and functioning in otherwise healthy elderly persons. → *Readers are referred to Chap. 263 for a comprehensive review of the diagnosis and treatment of patients with these conditions.*

DYSSOMNIA ASSOCIATED WITH LIMB MOVEMENTS
Restless Legs Syndrome Patients with dyssomnia associated with the restless legs syndrome (RLS) report an irresistible urge to move their legs when awake and inactive, especially when lying in bed just prior to sleep. This interferes with the ability to fall asleep. They report a creeping or crawling sensation deep within the calves or thighs, or sometimes even in the upper limbs, that is only relieved briefly by movement, particularly walking. In contrast, paresthesia secondary to peripheral neuropathy persists with activity. The severity of this chronic, idiopathic disorder may wax and wane with time and can be exacerbated by caffeine and pregnancy. Iron- or folic acid-deficiency anemia and renal failure may actually cause RLS, which is then considered secondary RLS. Nearly all patients with restless legs also experience periodic limb movement disorder during sleep, although the reverse is not the case.

Periodic Limb Movement Disorder Periodic limb movement disorder, also known as *nocturnal myoclonus*, is the principal objective polysomnographic finding in 17 percent of patients with insomnia and 11 percent of those with excessive daytime somnolence. This condition can be documented in one-sixth of patients with insomnia seen at sleep disorders centers, although it is often thought to be an incidental finding rather than the cause of disturbed sleep. Stereotyped, rhythmic, 0.5- to 5.0-s extensions of the great toe and dorsiflexion of the foot recur every 20 to 40 s during NREM stages 1 and 2 sleep, in episodes lasting from minutes to hours. Most such episodes occur during the first half of the night. The disorder occurs in a wide variety of sleep disorders (including narcolepsy, sleep apnea, REM sleep behavior disorder, and various forms of insomnia) and is associated with frequent arousals and an increased number of sleep-stage transitions. However, it has not been demonstrated that these sleep disturbances always lead to insomnia. In fact, periodic limb movement may be secondary to chronic sleep-wake disturbance rather than the cause of it. The incidence increases with age; 44 percent of healthy subjects over age 65 without a sleep complaint and almost all patients with RLS have periodic limb movements. The pathophysiology is not well understood. Polysomnography with bilateral surface EMG recording of the anterior tibialis, extensor carpi radialis, triceps and/or biceps is used to establish the diagnosis. Treatment options are limited; some patients may respond to a combination of carbidopa and levodopa, clonazepam, or levodopa alone.

PARASOMNIAS The term *parasomnia* refers to behavioral disorders during sleep that are associated with brief or partial arousals but not with marked sleep disruption or impaired daytime alertness. The presenting complaint is usually related to the behavior itself. Most are more common in children but may persist into adulthood when their occurrence may have more pathologic significance.

Sleepwalking (Somnambulism) Patients affected by this disorder carry out automatic motor activities that range from minor to complex. Individuals may leave the bed, walk, urinate inappropriately, or exit from the house while remaining unconscious or uncommunica-

tive. Arousal is difficult, and untoward or even fatal activities can occur. Sleepwalking occurs in stage 3 or 4 NREM sleep. It is most common in children and adolescents. Episodes are usually isolated but may be recurrent in 1 to 6 percent of patients. The cause is unknown.

Sleep Terrors This disorder, also called *pavor nocturnus*, occurs primarily in young children during the first several hours after sleep onset, in stages 3 and 4 of NREM sleep. The child suddenly screams, exhibiting autonomic arousal with sweating, tachycardia, and hyperventilation. The individual may be difficult to arouse and rarely recalls the episode on awakening in the morning. Recurrent attacks are rare, and treatment is usually by way of reassurance of parents. Both sleep terrors and sleepwalking represent abnormalities of arousal. In contrast, *nightmares* (dream anxiety attacks) occur during REM sleep and cause full arousal, with memory for the dream-associated unpleasant episode.

REM Sleep Behavior Disorder This is a rare parasomnia arising from REM sleep instead of slow-wave sleep, as is characteristic of the other, more common parasomnias. It primarily afflicts men of middle age or older, many of whom have a history of prior neurologic disease (e.g., degenerative diseases, Guillain-Barré syndrome, dementia, subarachnoid hemorrhage, stroke). Presenting symptoms are of violent behavior during sleep, reported by a bed partner. In contrast to typical somnambulism, injury to patient or bystander is common, and, upon awakening, the patient reports vivid, often unpleasant dream imagery. The principal differential diagnosis is that of nocturnal seizures, which can be excluded with polysomnography. In REM sleep behavior disorder, seizure activity is absent, and the EEG/EOG REM sleep pattern exhibits a high-amplitude EMG. Complex, purposeful motor behavior occurs during REM sleep episodes. The pathogenesis is unclear, but the preexisting neurologic disease may have involved brainstem areas responsible for descending motor inhibition during REM sleep. In support of this hypothesis are the remarkable similarities between the REM sleep behavior disorder and the sleep of animals with bilateral lesions of the pontine tegmentum in areas controlling REM sleep motor inhibition. Treatment with clonazepam provides sustained improvement in almost all reported cases.

Sleep Bruxism Bruxism is an involuntary, forceful grinding of teeth during sleep that affects 10 to 20 percent of the population. The patient is usually unaware of the problem, and data on this parasomnia come from roommates and bed partners, alarmed by the loud grinding noise, and from dentists who see evidence of destruction of tooth enamel and dentum. The typical age of onset is 17 to 20 years, and spontaneous remission usually occurs by age 40. Sex distribution appears to be equal.

Hypotheses about the pathophysiology suggest contributory roles for dental abnormalities, e.g., malocclusion, and for central neural mechanisms. Psychological factors may also play a role in that stress exacerbates the disorder. Treatment is dictated by the risk of dental injury. In many cases, the diagnosis is made during dental examination, damage is minor, and no treatment is indicated. In more severe cases, treatment with a rubber tooth guard is necessary to prevent permanent and disfiguring tooth injury. Stress management or, in some cases, biofeedback can be useful when bruxism is a manifestation of severe stress. Useful pharmacologic therapy has not been described.

Sleep Enuresis Bedwetting, like sleepwalking and night terrors, is another parasomnia occurring during slow-wave sleep in the young. Before age 5 or 6, nocturnal enuresis should probably be considered a normal feature of development. The condition usually spontaneously improves at puberty, has a prevalence in late adolescence of 1 to 3 percent, and is rare in adulthood. The age threshold for initiation of treatment depends on parental and patient concern about the problem. Persistence of enuresis into adolescence or adulthood may reflect a variety of underlying conditions. In older patients with enuresis a distinction must be made between primary and secondary enuresis, the latter being defined as bedwetting in patients who have been fully continent for 6 to 12 months. Treatment of primary enuresis is reserved for patients of appropriate age (older than 5 or 6 years) and consists of bladder training exercises and behavioral therapy. Urologic abnormalities are more common in primary enuresis and must be assessed by urologic examination. Important causes of secondary enuresis include emotional disturbances, urinary tract malformations. In the patient for whom enuresis may be a source of significant stress, symptomatic pharmacotherapy may be appropriate while attention is also paid to underlying causes. This is usually accomplished with oxybutynin chloride or imipramine. Intranasal desmopressin has been used in some patients.

Miscellaneous Parasomnias Other clinical entities fulfill the definition of a parasomnia in that they occur selectively during sleep and are associated with some degree of sleep disruption. Examples include *jactatio capitis nocturna* (nocturnal headbanging), sleep talking, and nocturnal leg cramps.

SLEEP DISORDERS ASSOCIATED WITH MEDICAL/PSYCHIATRIC DISORDERS **Sleep Disorders Associated with Mental Disorders** Sleep architecture and physiology are disturbed in *schizophrenia* (with a decreased amount of stage 4 sleep and a lack of augmentation of REM sleep following REM sleep deprivation); chronic schizophrenics usually show day-night reversal, sleep fragmentation, and insomnia. Patients with other psychiatric disorders (anxiety disorders, affective illness, obsessive-compulsive disorders, and chronic alcoholism) also often sleep poorly. There is considerable heterogeneity, however, in the nature of the sleep disturbance both between conditions and among patients with the same condition.

Depression can be associated with sleep onset insomnia, sleep maintenance insomnia, and/or early morning wakefulness. However, hypersomnia occurs in some depressed patients, especially adolescents and those with either bipolar or seasonal (fall/winter) depression (see also Chap. 385). Indeed, sleep disturbance is an important vegetative sign of depression and may commence before any mood changes are perceived by the patient. Consistent polysomnographic findings in depression include decreased REM sleep latency, lengthened first REM sleep episode, and shortened first NREM sleep episode; however, these findings are not specific for depression, and the extent of these changes varies with age and symptomatology. Depressed patients also show decreased slow-wave sleep and reduced sleep continuity.

In *mania* and *hypomania*, sleep latency is increased and total sleep time can be reduced. Patients with *anxiety disorders* tend not to show the changes in REM sleep and slow-wave sleep seen in endogenously depressed patients. Finally, *chronic alcoholics* lack slow-wave sleep, have decreased amounts of REM sleep (as an acute response to alcohol), and have frequent arousals throughout the night. This is associated with impaired daytime alertness. The sleep of chronic alcoholics remains disturbed for years after discontinuance of alcohol usage.

Sleep Disorders Associated with Neurologic Disorders A variety of neurologic diseases result in sleep disruption through both indirect, nonspecific mechanisms (e.g., pain in cervical spondylosis or low back pain) or by impairment of central neural structures involved in the generation and control of sleep itself.

For example, the dementias have long been associated with disturbances in the timing of the sleep-wake cycle, often characterized by nocturnal wandering and an exacerbation of symptomatology at night (so-called sundowning). Such clinical observations are consistent with the neuropathologic report that 80 percent of the cells in the hypothalamic circadian pacemaker (the SCN) are lost in patients with senile dementia (Alzheimer's disease), though the report has not been replicated and a causal association remains unproven.

Epilepsy may rarely present as a sleep complaint (see also Chap. 365). Often the history is of abnormal behavior, at times with convulsive movements, during sleep, and the differential diagnosis includes REM sleep behavior disorder, sleep apnea syndrome, and periodic movements of sleep (see above). Diagnosis requires nocturnal EEG recording. Other neurologic diseases associated with abnormal movements, such as *Parkinson's disease*, *hemiballismus*, *Huntington's chorea*, and *Gilles de la Tourette syndrome*, are also associated with disrupted sleep, presumably through secondary mechanisms. Headache syndromes may show sleep-associated exacerbations (*migraine* or *cluster headache*) (see also Chaps. 15 and 364). The mechanism of association between sleep and headache is unknown.

Fatal familial insomnia is a rare hereditary disorder caused by bilateral degeneration of anterior and dorsomedial nuclei of the thalamus. Insomnia is a prominent early symptom. Progressively, the syndrome produces autonomic dysfunction, dysarthria, myoclonus, coma, and death. The pathogenesis of the thalamic destruction is unknown.

Sleep Disorders Associated with Other Medical Disorders A number of medical conditions are associated with disruptions of sleep. The association may be nonspecific, for example, that between sleep disruption and chronic pain from rheumatologic disorders. Attention to this association is important in that sleep-associated symptoms are the presenting complaint of many such patients. In addition, sleep disruption may stem from the appropriate use of drugs such as steroids or from the symptoms of another illness.

Among the most prominent associations is that between sleep disruption and *asthma*. In many asthmatics there is a prominent daily variation in airway resistance that results in marked increases in asthmatic symptoms at night, especially during sleep. In addition, treatment of asthma with theophylline-based compounds, adrenergic agonists, or glucocorticoids can independently disrupt sleep. When sleep disruption is a prominent side effect of asthma treatment, inhaled steroids (e.g., beclomethasone) that do not disrupt sleep may provide a useful alternative.

Cardiac ischemia may also be associated with sleep disruption. Variability in autonomic nervous system function during REM sleep may account for the association of sleep and angina, although this remains unproven. Patients may present with complaints of nightmares or vivid, disturbing dreams, with or without awareness of the more classical symptoms of angina. Recent work suggests that patients with nocturnal angina are likely to have obstructive sleep apnea, treatment of which may substantially improve the nocturnal angina symptoms. *Paroxysmal nocturnal dyspnea* can also occur as a consequence of sleep-associated cardiac ischemia that causes pulmonary congestion exacerbated by recumbent posture.

Chronic obstructive pulmonary disease is also associated with sleep disruption. Other conditions associated with sleep disruption include *cystic fibrosis*, *menopause*, *hyperthyroidism*, *gastroesophageal reflux*, *chronic renal failure*, and *liver failure*.

CIRCADIAN RHYTHM SLEEP DISORDERS

A subset of patients presenting with either insomnia or hypersomnia may have a disorder of sleep *timing* rather than sleep *generation*. Disorders of sleep timing can either be organic (i.e., due to an intrinsic defect in the circadian pacemaker or its input from entraining stimuli) or environmental (i.e., due to a disruption of exposure to entraining stimuli from the environment). Regardless of etiology, the symptoms reflect the influence of the underlying circadian pacemaker on sleep-wake function. Thus, effective therapeutic approaches should aim to entrain the oscillator at an appropriate phase.

RAPID TIME-ZONE CHANGE (JET LAG) SYNDROME More than 60 million people experience transmeridian air travel annually, which is often associated with excessive daytime sleepiness, sleep onset insomnia, and frequent arousals from sleep, particularly in the latter half of the night. Gastrointestinal discomfort is common. The syndrome is transient, typically lasting 2 to 14 d depending on the number of time zones crossed, the direction of travel, and the traveler's age and phase-shifting capacity. Travelers who spend more time outdoors reportedly adapt more quickly than those who remain in hotel rooms, presumably due to bright (outdoor) light exposure.

SHIFT-WORK SLEEP DISORDER About 7 million workers in the United States regularly work at night, either on a permanent or rotating schedule. In addition, each week millions of Americans elect to remain awake at night to meet deadlines, drive long distances, or participate in recreational activities, leading to an inversion of their sleep-wake cycle. Studies of regular night-shift workers indicate that the circadian timing system typically fails to adapt successfully to such inverted schedules. This leads to a misalignment between the desired work-rest schedule and the output of the pacemaker and in disturbed daytime sleep. Consequent sleep deprivation, increased length of time awake prior to work, and misalignment of circadian phase produce decreased alertness and performance and cause increased safety hazards among night workers. Routine tasks such as highway driving are particularly vulnerable to sleep-related accidents. There is a marked increase in the risk of fatal-to-the-driver road accidents between midnight and 6 A.M., even when alcohol is eliminated as a causal factor. In addition, chronic shift workers have higher rates of cardiac, gastrointestinal, and reproductive disorders.

Interventions should promote increased awareness of the hazards associated with night work and should be aimed at minimizing both circadian disruption and sleep deprivation. The work schedule should minimize: (1) exposure to night work; (2) the frequency of shift rotation so that shifts do not rotate more than once every 2 to 3 weeks; (3) the number of consecutive night shifts worked from seven (which is typical) to four or five; and (4) the duration of night shifts. In addition, strategic use of bright-light exposure can facilitate rapid adaptation to night-shift work, where feasible. These steps can lead to marked improvements in employee health and performance and to reduced accident rates among shift workers.

DELAYED SLEEP PHASE SYNDROME Delayed sleep phase syndrome is characterized by: (1) reported sleep onset and wake times intractably later than desired; (2) actual sleep times at nearly the same clock hours daily; and (3) essentially normal all-night polysomnography except for delayed sleep onset. Patients exhibit an abnormally delayed endogenous circadian phase, with the temperature minimum during the constant routine occurring later than normal. This delayed phase could be due to: (1) an abnormally long intrinsic period of the endogenous circadian pacemaker; (2) an abnormally reduced phase-advancing capacity of the pacemaker; or (3) an irregular prior sleep-wake schedule, characterized by frequent nights when the patient chooses to remain awake well past midnight (for social, school, or work reasons). In most cases, it is difficult to distinguish among these factors, since patients with an abnormally long intrinsic period are more likely to "choose" such late-night activities because they are unable to sleep at that time. Patients tend to be young adults. This self-perpetuating condition can persist for years and does not usually respond to attempts to reestablish normal bedtime hours.

Patients respond to a rescheduling regimen in which bedtimes are successively delayed by about 3 h/d until the desired (and earlier) bedtime is achieved. Treatment methods involving bright-light phototherapy during the morning hours also show promise in these patients.

ADVANCED SLEEP PHASE SYNDROME Advanced sleep phase syndrome is the converse of the delayed sleep phase syndrome and tends to occur in the elderly. Patients with this condition report excessive daytime sleepiness during the evening hours, when they have great difficulty remaining awake, even in social settings. The patients awaken from 3 to 5 A.M. each day, often several hours before their desired wake times. Although such patients have not been studied extensively, some of these patients may benefit from bright-light phototherapy during the evening hours, designed to reset the circadian pacemaker to a later hour.

NON-24-H SLEEP-WAKE DISORDER This condition can occur when the maximal phase-advancing capacity of the circadian pacemaker is not adequate to accommodate the difference between the 24-h geophysical day and the intrinsic period of the pacemaker in the patient. Alternatively, patients' self-selected exposure to artificial light may drive the circadian pacemaker to a longer than 24-h schedule. Patients affected are not able to maintain a stable phase relationship between the output of the pacemaker and the 24-h day. Such patients typically present with an incremental pattern of successive delays in sleep onsets and wake times, progressing in and out of phase with local time. When the patient's endogenous rhythms are out of phase

with the local environment, insomnia coexists with excessive daytime sleepiness. Conversely, when the endogenous rhythms are in phase with the local environment, symptoms remit. The intervals of alternation between symptomatic vs. asymptomatic intervals may last several weeks to several months. Blind individuals unable to perceive light are particularly susceptible to this disorder.

MEDICAL IMPLICATIONS OF CIRCADIAN RHYTHMICITY Understanding the role of circadian rhythmicity in the pathophysiology of illness may lead to improvements in diagnosis and treatment. For example, prominent circadian variations have been reported in the incidence of *acute myocardial infarction*, *sudden cardiac death*, and *stroke*, the leading causes of death in the United States. Platelet aggregability is increased after arising in the early morning hours, coincident with the peak incidence of these cardiovascular events. A better understanding of the possible role of circadian rhythmicity in the acute destabilization of a chronic condition such as atherosclerotic disease could improve the understanding of the pathophysiology.

Diagnostic and therapeutic procedures may also be affected by the time of day at which data are collected. Examples include blood pressure, body temperature, the dexamethasone suppression test, and plasma cortisol levels. The timing of chemotherapy administration has been reported to have an effect on the outcome of treatment. Few physicians realize the extent to which routine measures are affected by the time (or sleep/wake state) when the measurement is made.

In addition, both the toxicity and effectiveness of drugs can vary during the day. For example, more than a fivefold difference has been observed in mortality rates following administration of toxic agents to experimental animals at different times of day. Anesthetic agents are particularly sensitive to time-of-day effects.

Finally, it should be noted that the risk of errors and accidents due to inattention and/or sleepiness varies markedly with the time of day. Single-vehicle truck accidents, industrial errors and accidents, and lapses of attention all peak during a critical zone of vulnerability that typically occurs during the latter half of the night, coincident with maximal sleep drive within the brain. The physician must be increasingly aware of the public health risks associated with the ever-increasing demands made by the duty-rest-recreation schedules in our round-the-clock society.

BIBLIOGRAPHY

ALDRICH MS: Narcolepsy. Neurology 42 (Suppl 6):34, 1992

BECKER PM et al: Dopaminergic agents in restless legs syndrome and periodic limb movements of sleep: Response and complications of extended treatment in 49 cases. Sleep 16:713, 1993

BENCA RM et al: Sleep and psychiatric disorders. A meta-analysis. Arch Gen Psychiatry 49:651, 1992

BLIWISE DL: Sleep in normal aging and dementia. Sleep 16:40, 1993

CZEISLER CA et al: Exposure to bright light and darkness to treat physiologic maladaptation to night work. N Engl J Med 322:1253, 1990

———— et al: Association of sleep-wake habits in older people with changes in output of circadian pacemaker. Lancet 340:933, 1992

———— et al: Suppression of melatonin secretion in some blind patients by exposure to bright light. N Engl J Med 332:6, 1995

DIAGNOSTIC CLASSIFICATION STEERING COMMITTEE, THORPY MJ(chairman): *International Classification of Sleep Disorders: Diagnostic and Coding Manual.* Rochester, MN, American Sleep Disorders Association, 1990

DIJK D-J, CZEISLER CA: Contribution of the circadian pacemaker and the sleep homeostat to sleep propensity, sleep structure, electroencephalographic slow waves, and sleep spindle activity in humans. J Neurosci 15:3526, 1995

FARNEY RJ, WALKER JM: Office management of common sleep-wake disorders. Med Clin North Am 79:391, 1995

FINDLEY LJ et al: Drivers with untreated sleep apnea. A cause of death and serious injury. Arch Intern Med 151:1451, 1991

FRANKLIN KA et al: Sleep apnea and nocturnal angina. Lancet 345:1085, 1995

GUILLEMINAULT C et al: Nondrug treatment trials in psychophysiologic insomnia. Arch Intern Med 155:838, 1995

KRYGER MH et al (eds): *Principles and Practice of Sleep Medicine*, 2d ed. Philadelphia, Saunders, 1994

LYDIC R et al: Cholinergic reticular mechanisms influence state-dependent ventilatory response to hypercapnia. Am J Physiol 261:R738, 1991

POLO O et al: Management of obstructive sleep apnoea/hypopnoea syndrome. Lancet 344:656, 1994

RADECKI SF, BRUNTON SA: Management of insomnia in office-based practice: National prevalence and therapeutic patterns. Arch Fam Med 2:1129, 1993

SCHWARTZ WJ: A clinician's primer on the circadian clock: Its localization, function, and resetting. Adv Intern Med 38:81m, 1993

SHERIN JE et al: Activation of ventrolateral preoptic neurons during sleep. Science 271:216, 1996

TATEISHI J et al: First experimental transmission of fatal familial insomnia. Nature 376:434, 1995

U.S. CONGRESS, OFFICE OF TECHNOLOGY ASSESSMENT: *Biological Rhythms: Implications for the Worker*, OTA-BA-463. Washington, DC, U.S. Government Printing Office, September, 1991

SECTION 4

DISORDERS OF EYES, EARS, NOSE, AND THROAT

28 *Jonathan C. Horton*

DISORDERS OF THE EYE

THE HUMAN VISUAL SYSTEM

The visual system provides a supremely efficient means for the rapid assimilation of information from the environment to aid in the guidance of behavior. The act of seeing begins with the capture of images focused by the cornea and lens upon a light-sensitive membrane in the back of the eye, called the *retina*. The retina is actually part of the brain, banished to the periphery to serve as a transducer for the conversion of patterns of light energy into neuronal signals. Light is absorbed by photopigment in two classes of receptors: rods and cones. There are approximately 100 million rods and 5 million cones in the human retina. The rods are operative under scotopic, or dim, illumination. The cones, active under photopic, or daylight, conditions, are specialized for color perception and high spatial resolution. The majority of cones are located within the macula, the portion of the retina serving the central 10° of vision. In the middle of the macula a small pit termed the *fovea*, packed exclusively with cones, provides best visual acuity.

Photoreceptors hyperpolarize to light, activating bipolar, amacrine, and horizontal cells in the inner nuclear layer. After processing of the photoreceptor response by this complex retinal circuit, the flow of sensory information ultimately converges upon a final common pathway: the ganglion cells. These cells translate the visual image impinging upon the retina into a continuously varying barrage of action potentials that propagates along the primary optic pathway to visual centers within the brain. There are a million ganglion cells in each retina, and hence a million fibers in each optic nerve.

Ganglion cell axons sweep along the inner surface of the retina in the nerve fiber layer, exit the eye at the optic disc, and travel through the optic nerve, optic chiasm, and optic tract to reach targets in the brain. The majority of fibers synapse upon cells in the lateral geniculate body, a thalamic relay station. Cells in the lateral geniculate body project in turn to the primary visual cortex. This massive afferent retinogeniculocortical sensory pathway provides the neural substrate for visual perception. Although the lateral geniculate body is the main target of the retina, separate classes of ganglion cells project to other subcortical visual nuclei involved in different functions. The pupillary reflex is mediated by input to the pretectal olivary nuclei in the midbrain. These pretectal nuclei send their output to the ipsilateral and contralateral Edinger-Westphal nuclei of the oculomotor nuclear complex. Cells in the Edinger-Westphal nuclei provide parasympathetic innervation to the iris sphincter via an interneuron in the ciliary ganglion. Circadian rhythms are timed by a retinal projection to the suprachiasmatic nucleus. Visual orientation and eye movements are served by retinal input to the superior colliculus. Gaze stabilization and optokinetic reflexes are governed by a group of small retinal targets known collectively as the *brainstem accessory optic system*.

Finally, there is a sizeable retinal projection to the pulvinar, a large thalamic visual nucleus of obscure function.

The eyes must be rotated constantly within their orbits to place and maintain targets of visual interest upon the fovea. This activity, called *foveation*, or *looking*, is governed by an elaborate efferent motor system. Each eye is moved by six extraocular muscles, supplied by cranial nerves from the oculomotor (III), trochlear (IV), and abducens (VI) nuclei. Activity in these ocular motor nuclei is coordinated by pontine and midbrain mechanisms for smooth pursuit, saccades, and gaze stabilization during head and body movements. Large regions of the frontal and parietooccipital cortex control these brainstem eye movement centers by providing descending supranuclear input.

Visual function can be disturbed in myriad ways. The eyes are mounted in a prominent position on the head, where they are vulnerable to trauma, exposure, and infection. Vision can be damaged by diseases intrinsic to the eye, such as glaucoma, cataract, or retinal detachment. Many neurologic diseases produce ocular symptoms, because extensive areas of the cortex, thalamus, and brainstem are devoted to visual perception or to the execution of eye movements. In genetic disorders, eye manifestations are common and often help the clinician to recognize a rare syndrome. Finally, the eyes are affected frequently by acquired systemic diseases.

The eye is a specialized organ, requiring unique optical instruments for proper examination. The slit lamp and ophthalmoscope proffer a beautiful, magnified view of the transparent anatomy of the eye and afford the only opportunity for direct inspection of blood vessels in a living subject. Some physicians do not acquire sufficient facility with these instruments and consequently feel unable to care for patients with eye problems. Although it may be determined that a patient requires specialized eye care, the initial evaluation of ocular symptoms lies within the purview of all physicians, and the assessment of visual acuity, pupils, eye movements, visual fields, and the fundi remain part of any complete physical examination.

CLINICAL ASSESSMENT OF VISUAL FUNCTION

REFRACTIVE STATE In approaching the patient with reduced vision, the first step is to decide whether refractive error is responsible. In *emmetropia*, parallel rays from infinity are focused perfectly upon the retina. Sadly, this condition is enjoyed by only a minority of the population. In *myopia*, the globe is too long, and light rays come to a focal point in front of the retina. Near objects can be seen clearly, but distant objects require a diverging lens in front of the eye. In *hyperopia*, the globe is too short, and hence a converging lens is used to supplement the refractive power of the eye. In *astigmatism*, the corneal surface is not perfectly spherical, necessitating a cylindrical corrective lens. With the onset of middle age, *presbyopia* develops as the lens within the eye becomes unable to increase its refractive power to accommodate upon near objects. To compensate for presbyopia, the emmetropic patient must use reading glasses. The patient already wearing glasses for distance correction usually switches to bifocals. The only exception is the myope, who may achieve clear vision at near simply by removing glasses containing the distance prescription.

Refractive errors usually develop slowly and remain stable after adolescence, except in unusual circumstances. For example, the acute onset of diabetes mellitus can produce sudden myopia because of fluid imbibition and swelling of the lens induced by hyperglycemia. Testing vision through a pinhole aperture is a useful way to screen quickly for refractive error. If the visual acuity is better through a pinhole than with the unaided eye, the patient needs a formal refraction screening.

VISUAL ACUITY The Snellen chart is used to test acuity at a distance of 6 m (20 ft). For convenience, a scale version of the Snellen chart, called the Rosenbaum card, is held at 36 cm (14 in) from the patient (Fig. 28-1). All subjects should be able to read the 6/6 m (20/20 ft) line with each eye using the proper refractive correction. Patients who need reading glasses must wear them for accurate testing. If 6/6 (20/20) acuity is not present in each eye, the deficiency in vision must be explained. For acuity worse than 6/240 (20/800), the ability to count fingers, see hand motions, or perceive a bright light should be recorded. Legal blindness is defined by the Internal Revenue Service as a best corrected acuity of 6/60 (20/200) or less in the better eye, or a binocular visual field subtending 20° or less. For driving the laws vary by state, but most require a corrected acuity of 6/12 (20/40) in at least one eye. Patients with a homonymous hemianopia cannot drive.

PUPILS The pupils should be tested individually in dim light with the patient fixating upon a distant target. If they respond briskly to light, there is no need to check the near response, because isolated loss of constriction (miosis) to accommodation does not occur. For this reason, the ubiquitous abbreviation PERRLA (pupils equal, round, and reactive to light and accommodation) implies a wasted effort with the last step. However, it is important to test the near response if the light response is poor or absent. Light-near dissociation occurs with neurosyphilis (Argyll Robertson pupil), lesions of the dorsal midbrain (obstructive hydrocephalus, pineal region tumors), and after aberrant regeneration (oculomotor nerve palsy, Adie's tonic pupil).

An eye with no light perception has no pupillary response to direct light stimulation. If the retina or optic nerve is only partially injured, the direct pupillary response will be less than the consensual pupillary response evoked by shining a light into the other eye. This *relative afferent pupillary defect* (Marcus Gunn pupil) can be elicited with the swinging flashlight test (Fig. 28-2). It is an extremely useful sign in retrobulbar optic neuritis and other optic nerve diseases, where it may be the sole objective evidence for disease.

Subtle inequality in pupil size, up to 0.5 mm, is a fairly common finding in normal subjects. The diagnosis of essential or physiologic anisocoria is secure as long as the relative pupil asymmetry remains constant as ambient lighting varies. Anisocoria that increases in dim light indicates a sympathetic paresis of the iris dilator muscle. The triad of miosis with ipsilateral ptosis and anhidrosis constitutes Horner's syndrome, although anhidrosis is often absent. Brainstem stroke, carotid dissection, or neoplasm impinging upon the sympathetic chain are occasionally identified as the cause of Horner's syndrome, but the majority of cases are idiopathic.

Anisocoria that increases in bright light suggests a parasympathetic palsy. The first concern is an oculomotor nerve paresis. This possibility is excluded if the eye movements are full and the patient has no ptosis or diplopia. Acute pupillary dilation (mydriasis) can occur from damage to the ciliary ganglion in the orbit. Common mechanisms are infection (herpes zoster, influenza), trauma (blunt, penetrating, surgical), or ischemia (diabetes, temporal arteritis). After denervation of the iris sphincter the pupil does not respond well to light, but the response to near is often relatively intact. When the near stimulus is removed, the pupil redilates very slowly compared with the normal

pupil, hence the term *tonic pupil*. In Adie's syndrome, a tonic pupil occurs in conjunction with weak or absent tendon reflexes in the lower extremities. This benign disorder, which occurs predominantly in healthy young women, is assumed to represent a mild dysautonomia. Tonic pupils are also associated with Shy-Drager syndrome, segmental hypohidrosis, diabetes, and amyloidosis. Occasionally, a tonic pupil is discovered incidentally in an otherwise completely normal, asymptomatic individual. The diagnosis is confirmed by placing a drop of dilute (0.125%) pilocarpine into each eye. Denervation hypersensitivity produces pupillary constriction in a tonic pupil, whereas the normal pupil shows no response. Pharmacologic dilation from accidental or deliberate instillation of anticholinergic agents (atropine, scopolamine drops) into the eye can also produce pupillary mydriasis. In this situation, normal strength (1%) pilocarpine causes no constriction.

Both pupils are affected equally by systemic medications. They are small with narcotic use (morphine, heroin) and large with anticholinergics (scopolamine). Parasympathetic agents (pilocarpine, demecarium bromide) used to treat glaucoma produce miosis. In any patient with an unexplained pupillary abnormality, a slit-lamp examination

FIGURE 28-1 The Rosenbaum card is a miniature, scale version of the Snellen chart for testing visual acuity at near. When the visual acuity is recorded, the Snellen distance equivalent should bear a notation indicating that vision was tested at near, not at 6 m (20 ft), or else the Jaeger number system should be used to report the acuity.

FIGURE 28-2 Demonstration of a relative afferent pupil defect (Marcus Gunn pupil) in the left eye, done with the patient fixating upon a distant target. *A*. With dim background lighting, the pupils are equal and relatively large. *B*. Shining a flashlight into the right eye evokes equal, strong constriction of both pupils. *C*. Swinging the flashlight over to the damaged left eye causes dilation of both pupils, although they remain smaller than in *A*. Swinging the flashlight back over to the healthy right eye would result in symmetric constriction back to the appearance shown in *B*. Note that the pupils always remain equal; the damage to the left retina/optic nerve is revealed by weaker bilateral pupil constriction to a flashlight in the left eye compared with the right eye. (*From P Levatin, Arch Ophthalmol 62:768, 1959.*)

is helpful to exclude surgical trauma to the iris, an occult foreign body, perforating injury, intraocular inflammation, adhesions (synechia), angle-closure glaucoma, and iris sphincter rupture from blunt trauma.

EYE MOVEMENTS AND ALIGNMENT Eye movements are tested by asking the patient with both eyes open to pursue a small target such as a penlight into the cardinal fields of gaze. Normal ocular versions are smooth, symmetric, full, and maintained in all directions without nystagmus. Saccades, or quick refixation eye movements, are assessed by having the patient look back and forth between two stationary targets. The eyes should move rapidly and accurately in a single jump to their target. Ocular alignment can be judged by holding a penlight directly in front of the patient at about 1 m. If the eyes are straight, the corneal light reflex will be centered in the middle of each pupil. To test eye alignment more precisely, the cover test is useful. The patient is instructed to gaze upon a small fixation target in the distance. One eye is covered suddenly while observing the second eye. If the second eye shifts to fixate upon the target, it was misaligned. If it does not move, the first eye is uncovered and the test is repeated on the second eye. If neither eye moves, the eyes are aligned orthotropically. If the eyes are orthotropic in primary gaze but the patient complains of diplopia, the cover test should be performed with the head tilted or turned in whatever direction elicits the patient's diplopia. With practice the examiner can detect an ocular deviation (hetero-

tropia) as small as 1 to 2° with the cover test. Deviations can be measured by placing prisms in front of the misaligned eye to determine the power required to neutralize the fixation shift evoked by covering the other eye.

STEREOPSIS Stereoacuity is determined by presenting targets with retinal disparity separately to each eye using polarized images. The most popular office tests measure a range of thresholds from 800 to 40 seconds of arc. Normal stereoacuity is 40 seconds of arc. If a patient achieves this level of stereoacuity, one is assured that the eyes are aligned orthotropically and that vision is intact in each eye. Random dot stereograms have no monocular depth cues and provide an excellent screening test for strabismus and amblyopia in children.

COLOR VISION The retina contains three classes of cones, with visual pigments of differing peak spectral sensitivity: red (560 nm), green (530 nm), and blue (430 nm). The red and green cone pigments are encoded on the X chromosome; the blue cone pigment on chromosome 7. Mutations of the blue cone pigment are exceedingly rare. Mutations of the red and green pigments cause congenital X-linked color blindness in 8 percent of males. Affected individuals are not truly color blind, rather, they differ from normal subjects in how they perceive color and how they combine primary monochromatic lights to match a given color. Anomalous trichromats have three cone types, but a mutation in one cone pigment (usually red or green) causes a shift in peak spectral sensitivity, altering the proportion of primary colors required to achieve a color match. Dichromats have only two cone types and will therefore accept a color match based upon only two primary colors. Anomalous trichromats and dichromats have 6/6 (20/20) visual acuity, but their hue discrimination is impaired. Ishihara color plates can be used to detect red-green color blindness. The test plates contain a hidden number, visible only to subjects with color confusion from red-green color blindness. Because color blindness is almost exclusively X-linked, it is worth screening only male children.

The Ishihara plates are often used to test patients with acquired defects of color vision. Although they are not intended for this purpose, no other simple, convenient method for quantitative color vision testing is available for regular office use. Acquired defects in color vision frequently result from disease of the macula or optic nerve. For example, patients with a history of optic neuritis often complain of color desaturation long after their visual acuity has returned to normal. Color blindness can also occur from bilateral strokes involving the ventral portion of the occipital lobe (cerebral achromatopsia). Such patients can perceive only shades of gray and may also have difficulty recognizing faces (prosopagnosia). Infarcts of the dominant occipital lobe sometimes give rise to color anomia. Affected patients can discriminate colors, but they cannot name them.

VISUAL FIELDS Vision can be impaired by damage to the visual system anywhere from the eyes to the occipital lobes. One can localize the site of the lesion with considerable accuracy by mapping the visual field deficit by finger confrontation and then correlating it with the topographic anatomy of the visual pathway (Fig. 28-3). More quantitative data can be obtained by formal perimetric examination of the visual fields. In kinetic perimetry, the patient faces a tangent screen or a hemispheric bowl (Goldmann perimeter) while the examiner moves a small light target from the periphery towards the center. Such manual techniques largely have been supplanted by computer-driven perimeters (Humphrey, Octopus) that present a target of variable intensity at fixed positions in the visual field (Fig. 28-3A). By generating an automated printout of light thresholds, these static perimeters provide a sensitive means of detecting scotomas in the visual field. They are also useful for serial assessment of visual function in chronic diseases like glaucoma or pseudotumor cerebri.

The crux of visual field analysis is to decide whether a lesion is before, at, or behind the optic chiasm. If a scotoma is confined to one eye, it must be due to a lesion anterior to the chiasm, involving either the optic nerve or retina. Retinal lesions produce scotomas that correspond optically to their location in the fundus. For example, a superior-nasal retinal detachment results in an inferior-temporal field cut. Damage to the macula causes a central scotoma (Fig. 28-3*B*).

Optic nerve disease produces characteristic patterns of visual field loss. Glaucoma selectively destroys axons that enter the superotemporal or inferotemporal poles of the optic disc, resulting in arcuate scotomas shaped like a Turkish scimitar, which emanate from the blind spot and curve around fixation to end flat against the horizontal meridian (Fig. 28-3*C*). This type of field defect mirrors the arrangement of the nerve fiber layer in the temporal retina. The superb acuity of humans is achieved by thrusting aside all retinal elements at the fovea except photoreceptors, to minimize absorption and scattering of light. To avoid passing over the fovea, axons from cells in the temporal retina must follow an indirect course arching around the fovea to reach the optic disc. Arcuate or nerve fiber layer scotomas also occur from optic neuritis, ischemic optic neuropathy, optic disc drusen, and branch retinal artery occlusion.

Damage to the entire upper or lower pole of the optic disc causes an altitudinal field cut that follows the horizontal meridian (Fig. 28-3*D*). This pattern of visual field loss is typical of ischemic optic neuropathy but also occurs from retinal vascular occlusion, advanced glaucoma, and optic neuritis.

About half the fibers in the optic nerve originate from ganglion cells serving the macula. Damage to papillomacular fibers causes a cecocentral scotoma encompassing the blind spot and macula (Fig. 28-3*E*). If the damage is irreversible, pallor eventually appears in the temporal portion of the optic disc. Temporal pallor from a cecocentral scotoma may develop in optic neuritis, nutritional optic neuropathy, toxic optic neuropathy, Leber's hereditary optic neuropathy, and compressive optic neuropathy. It is worth mentioning that the temporal side of the optic disc is slightly more pale than the nasal side in most normal subjects. Therefore, it can sometimes be difficult to decide whether the temporal pallor visible on fundus examination represents a pathologic change. Pallor of the nasal rim of the optic disc is a less equivocal sign of optic atrophy.

At the optic chiasm, fibers from nasal ganglion cells decussate into the contralateral optic tract. For unknown reasons, crossed fibers are damaged more by compression than uncrossed fibers. As a result, mass lesions of the sellar region cause a temporal hemianopia in each eye. Tumors anterior to the optic chiasm, such as meningiomas of the tuberculum sella, produce a junctional scotoma characterized by an optic neuropathy in one eye and a superior temporal field cut in the other eye (Fig. 28-3*G*). More symmetric compression of the optic chiasm by a pituitary adenoma (Fig. 28-4), meningioma, craniopharyngioma, glioma, or aneurysm results in a bitemporal hemianopia (Fig. 28-3*H*). The insidious development of a bitemporal hemianopia often goes unnoticed by the patient and will escape detection by the physician unless each eye is tested separately.

It is difficult to localize a postchiasmal lesion accurately, because injury anywhere in the optic tract, lateral geniculate body, optic radiations, or visual cortex can produce a homonymous hemianopia, i.e., a temporal hemifield defect in the contralateral eye and a matching nasal hemifield defect in the ipsilateral eye (Fig. 28-3*I*). A unilateral postchiasmal lesion leaves the visual acuity in each eye unaffected, although the patient may read the letters on only the left or right half of the eye chart. Lesions of the optic radiations tend to cause poorly matched or incongruous field defects in each eye. Damage to the optic radiations in the temporal lobe (Meyer's loop) produces a superior quadrantic homonymous hemianopia (Fig. 28-3*J*), whereas injury to the optic radiations in the parietal lobe results in an inferior quadrantic homonymous hemianopia (Fig. 28-3*K*). Lesions of the primary visual cortex give rise to dense, congruous hemianopic field defects. Occlusion of the posterior cerebral artery supplying the occipital lobe is a frequent cause of total homonymous hemianopia. Some patients with hemianopia after occipital stroke have macular sparing, because the macular representation at the tip of the occipital lobe is supplied by collaterals from the middle cerebral artery (Fig. 28-3*L*). Destruction of both occipital lobes produces cortical blindness. This condition can be distinguished from bilateral prechiasmal visual loss by noting that the pupil responses and optic fundi remain normal.

Approach to the Patient

Red or Painful Eye *Corneal abrasions* are seen best by placing a drop of fluorescein in the eye and looking with the slit lamp using a cobalt-blue light. A penlight with a blue filter will suffice if no slit lamp is available. Damage to the corneal epithelium is revealed by yellow fluorescence of the exposed basement membrane underlying the epithelium. It is important to check for foreign bodies. To search the conjunctival fornices, the lower lid should be pulled down and the upper lid everted. A foreign body can be removed with a moistened cotton-tipped applicator after placing a drop of topical anesthetic, such as proparacaine, in the eye. Alternatively, it may be possible to flush the foreign body from the eye by irrigating copiously with saline or artificial tears. If the corneal epithelium has been abraded, antibiotic ointment and a patch should be applied to the eye. A drop of an intermediate-acting cycloplegic such as cyclopentolate hydrochloride 1%, helps to reduce pain by relaxing the ciliary body. The eye should be reexamined the next day. Minor abrasions may not require patching and cycloplegia.

Subconjunctival hemorrhage results from rupture of small vessels bridging the potential space between the episclera and conjunctiva. Blood dissecting into this space can produce a spectacular red eye, but vision is not affected and the hemorrhage resolves without treatment. Subconjunctival hemorrhage is usually spontaneous but can occur from blunt trauma, eye rubbing, or vigorous coughing. Occasionally it is a clue to an underlying bleeding disorder.

A *pinguecula* is a small, raised conjunctival nodule at the temporal or nasal limbus. In adults such lesions are extremely common and have little significance, unless they become inflamed (pingueculitis). A *pterygium* resembles a pinguecula but has crossed the limbus to encroach upon the corneal surface. Removal is justified when symptoms of irritation or blurring develop, but recurrence is a common problem.

Blepharitis refers to inflammation of the eyelids. The most common form occurs in association with acne rosacea or seborrheic dermatitis. The eyelid margins are usually colonized heavily by staphylococcus. Upon close inspection, they appear greasy, ulcerated, and crusted with scaling debris that clings to the lashes. Treatment consists of warm compresses, strict eyelid hygiene, and topical antibiotics such as erythromycin. An external *hordeolum* (sty) is caused by staphylococcal infection of the superficial accessory glands of Zeis or Moll located in the eyelid margins. An internal hordeolum occurs after suppurative infection of the oil-secreting meibomian glands within the tarsal plate of the eyelid. Systemic antibiotics, usually tetracyclines, are sometimes necessary for treatment of meibomian gland inflammation (meibomitis) or chronic, severe blepharitis. A *chalazion* is a painless, granulomatous inflammation of a meibomian gland that produces a pealike nodule within the eyelid. It can be incised and drained, or injected with glucocorticoids. Basal cell, squamous cell, or meibomian gland carcinoma should be suspected for any nonhealing, ulcerative lesion of the eyelids.

Dacrocystitis, or inflammation of the lacrimal drainage system, can produce epiphora (tearing) and ocular injection. Gentle pressure over the lacrimal sac evokes pain and reflux of mucus or pus from the tear puncta. Dacrocystitis usually occurs after obstruction of the lacrimal system. It is treated with topical and systemic antibiotics, followed by probing or surgery to reestablish patency. *Entropion* (inversion of the eyelid) or *ectropion* (sagging or eversion of the eyelid) can also lead to epiphora and ocular irritation.

Conjunctivitis is the most common cause of a red, painful eye. Pain is minimal, and the visual acuity is reduced only slightly. The most common viral etiology is adenovirus infection. It causes a watery discharge, mild foreign-body sensation, and photophobia. Bacterial infection tends to produce a more mucopurulent exudate. Mild cases

Monocular Pre-chiasmal Field Defects:

A 30° — blind spot — Normal Field Right Eye

B 30° — Central Scotoma

C 30° — Nerve-Fiber Bundle (Arcuate) Scotoma

D 30° — Altitudinal Scotoma

E 30° — Ceco-central Scotoma

F 30° — Enlarged Blind-Spot with Peripheral Constriction

Binocular Chiasmal or Post-chiasmal Field Defects:

(Left eye)   (Right eye)

G 30° — Junctional Scotoma

H 30° — Bitemporal Hemianopia

I 30° — Homonymous Hemianopia

J 30° — Superior Quadrantanopia

K 30° — Inferior Quadrantanopia

L 30° — Homonymous Hemianopia with Macular Sparing

100°   60°

Right   Left

Optic Nerve

Optic Chiasm

Optic Tract

Lateral Geniculate Body

Optic Radiations

Primary Visual Cortex

FIGURE 28-3 Ventral view of the brain, correlating patterns of visual field loss with the sites of lesions in the visual pathway. The visual fields overlap partially, creating 120° of central binocular field flanked by a 40° monocular crescent on either side. The visual field maps in this figure were done with a computer-driven perimeter (Humphrey Instruments, Carl Zeiss, Inc.). It plots the retinal sensitivity to light in the central 30° using a gray scale format. Areas of visual field loss are shown in black. The examples of common monocular, prechiasmal field defects are all shown for the right eye. By convention, the visual fields are always recorded with the left eye's field on the left, and the right eye's field on the right, just as the patient sees the world.

of infectious conjunctivitis usually are treated empirically with broad-spectrum topical ocular antibiotics, such as sulfacetamide 10%, poly-mixin-bacitracin-neomycin, or trimethoprim-polymixin combination. Smears and cultures are usually reserved for severe, resistant, or recurrent cases of conjunctivitis. To prevent contagion, patients should be admonished to wash their hands frequently, not to touch their eyes, and to avoid direct contact with others.

Allergic conjunctivitis is extremely common and often mistaken for infectious conjunctivitis. Three forms are recognized, with closely overlapping manifestations. *Hay fever conjunctivitis* has a seasonal incidence, related to the release of airborne antigens into the air by plants. IgE-mediated activation of mast cells in the conjunctiva causes itching, redness, and edema. *Vernal conjunctivitis* is also seasonal, becoming worse during warm months. It affects exclusively children or adolescents and is more common in boys. The cause is unknown, but airborne antigens are thought to trigger symptoms. Itching, photophobia, epiphora, and mucous discharge are typical. The palpebral conjunctiva may become hypertropic with giant excrescences called cobblestone papillae. Irritation from contact lenses or any chronic foreign body can also induce formation of cobblestone papillae. *Atopic conjunctivitis* occurs in subjects with atopic dermatitis or asthma. Symptoms caused by allergic conjunctivitis can be alleviated with cold compresses, topical vasoconstrictors, antihistamines, and mast-cell stablizers such as cromolyn sodium. Topical glucocorticoid solutions provide dramatic relief of immune-mediated forms of conjunctivitis, but their long-term use is ill-advised because of the complications of glaucoma, cataract, and secondary infection. Topical nonsteroidal anti-inflammatory agents (NSAIDs) like ketorolac tromethamine are a better alternative.

Keratoconjunctivitis sicca, or dry eye, produces burning, foreign-body sensation, injection, and photophobia. In mild cases the eye appears surprisingly normal, but tear production measured by wetting of a filter paper (Schirmer strip) is deficient. A variety of systemic drugs, including antihistaminic, anticholinergic, and psychotropic medications, result in dry eye by reducing lacrimal secretion. Disorders that involve the lacrimal gland directly, such as sarcoidosis or Sjögren's syndrome, also cause dry eye. Patients may develop dry eye after radiation therapy if the treatment field includes the orbits. Problems with ocular drying are also common after lesions affecting cranial nerves V or VII. Corneal anesthesia is particularly dangerous, because the absence of a normal blink reflex exposes the cornea to injury without pain to warn the patient. Dry eye is managed by frequent and liberal application of artificial tears and ocular lubricants. In severe cases the tear puncta can be plugged or cauterized to reduce lacrimal outflow.

Keratitis is a threat to vision because of the risk of corneal clouding, scarring, and perforation. Worldwide, the two leading causes of blindness from keratitis are trachoma from chlamydial infection and vitamin A deficiency related to malnutrition. In the United States, contact lenses play a major role in corneal infection and ulceration. They should not be worn by anyone with an active eye infection. In evaluating the cornea, it is important to differentiate between a superficial infection (*keratoconjunctivitis*) and a deeper, more serious ulcerative process. The latter is accompanied by greater visual loss, pain, photophobia, redness, and discharge. Slit-lamp examination shows disruption of the corneal epithelium, a cloudy infiltrate or abscess in the stroma, and an inflammatory cellular reaction in the anterior chamber. In severe cases, pus settles at the bottom of the anterior chamber, giving rise to a hypopyon. Immediate empiric antibiotic therapy should be initiated after corneal scrapings are obtained for Gram's stain, Giemsa stain, and cultures. Fortified topical antibiotics are most effective, supplemented with subconjunctival antibiotics as required. The most frequent bacterial pathogens are *Staphylococcus*, *Streptococcus* (particularly *S. pneumoniae*), *Pseudomonas*, Enterobacteriaceae, *Haemophilus*, and *Neisseria*. For *Neisseria*, systemic antibiotics should be given in addition to topical antibiotics to eliminate systemic infection. A fungal etiology should always be considered in the patient with keratitis. Fungal infection is common in warm humid climates, especially after penetration of the cornea by plant or vegetable material.

The *herpes viruses* are a major cause of blindness from keratitis. Most adults in the United States have serum antibodies to herpes simplex, indicating prior viral infection (Chap. 184). Primary ocular infection generally is caused by herpes simplex type 1, rather than type 2. It manifests as a unilateral follicular blepharoconjunctivitis, easily confused with adenoviral conjunctivitis, unless telltale vesicles appear on the periocular skin or conjunctiva. A dendritic pattern of corneal epithelial ulceration revealed by fluorescein staining is pathognomonic for herpes infection but is seen in only a minority of primary infections. Recurrent ocular infection arises from reactivation of the latent herpes virus. Viral eruption in the corneal epithelium may result in the characteristic herpes dendrite. Involvement of the corneal stroma produces edema, vascularization, and iridocyclitis. Herpes keratitis is

A　　　　　　　　　　　　　　　　　*B*

FIGURE 28-4　Pituitary adenoma: Coronal precontrast (*A*) and postcontrast (*B*) T1-weighted MRI through the sella turcica shows a large tumor (T) arising from the pituitary fossa. The optic chiasm (*black arrows*) is elevated and compressed, producing a visual field defect resembling that shown in Fig. 28-3H. There is peripheral enhancement around the mass due to displaced normal pituitary tissue (*white arrows*) and heterogeneous enhancement of the mass itself. The patient presented with decreased vision in both eyes of several years duration and optic pallor.

treated with topical antiviral agents, cycloplegics, and oral acyclovir. Topical glucocorticoids are effective in mitigating corneal scarring but must be used with extreme caution because of the danger of corneal melting and perforation. Topical steroids also carry the risk of prolonging infection and inducing glaucoma.

Herpes zoster from reactivation of latent varicella (chickenpox) virus causes a dermatomal pattern of painful vesicular dermatitis. Ocular symptoms can occur after zoster eruption in any branch of the trigeminal nerve but are particularly common when vesicles form on the nose, reflecting nasociliary (V1) nerve involvement (Hutchinson's sign). Herpes zoster ophthalmicus produces corneal dendrites, which can be difficult to distinguish from those seen in herpes simplex. Stromal keratitis, anterior uveitis, raised intraocular pressure, ocular motor nerve palsies, acute retinal necrosis, and postherpetic scarring and neuralgia are other common sequelae. Herpes zoster ophthalmicus is treated with antiviral agents and cycloplegics. In severe cases, steroids may be added to prevent permanent visual loss from corneal scarring.

Episcleritis is an inflammation of the episclera, a thin layer of connective tissue between the conjunctiva and sclera. Episcleritis resembles conjunctivitis but is a more localized process and discharge is absent. Most cases of episcleritis are idiopathic, but some occur in the setting of an autoimmune disease. *Scleritis* refers to a deeper, more severe inflammatory process, frequently associated with a connective tissue disease such as rheumatoid arthritis, lupus erythematosus, polyarteritis nodosa, Wegener's granulomatosis, or relapsing polychondritis. The inflammation and thickening of the sclera can be diffuse or nodular. In anterior forms of scleritis, the globe assumes a violet hue and the patient complains of severe ocular tenderness and pain. With posterior scleritis the pain and redness may be less marked, but there is often proptosis, choroidal effusion, reduced motility, and visual loss. Episcleritis and scleritis should be treated with NSAIDs. If these agents fail, topical or even systemic glucocorticoid therapy may be necessary, especially if an underlying autoimmune process is active.

Uveitis involving the anterior structures of the eye is called *iritis* or *iridocyclitis*. The diagnosis requires slit-lamp examination to identify inflammatory cells floating in the aqueous humor or deposited upon the corneal endothelium (keratic precipitates). Anterior uveitis develops in sarcoidosis, ankylosing spondylitis, juvenile rheumatoid arthritis, inflammatory bowel disease, psoriasis, Reiter's syndrome, and Behçet's disease. It is also associated with herpes infections, syphilis, Lyme disease, onchocerciasis, tuberculosis, and leprosy. Although anterior uveitis can occur in conjunction with many diseases, no cause is found to explain the majority of cases. For this reason, laboratory evaluation usually is reserved for patients with recurrent or severe anterior uveitis. Treatment is aimed at reducing inflammation and scarring by judicious use of topical steroids. Dilation of the pupil reduces pain and prevents the formation of synechiae.

Posterior uveitis is diagnosed by observing inflammation of the vitreous, retina, or choroid on fundus examination. It is more likely than anterior uveitis to be associated with an identifiable systemic disease. Some patients have panuveitis, or inflammation of both the anterior and posterior segments of the eye. Posterior uveitis is a manifestation of autoimmune diseases such as sarcoidosis, Behçet's disease, Vogt-Koyanagi-Harada syndrome, and inflammatory bowel disease. It also accompanies diseases such as toxoplasmosis, onchocerciasis, cysticercosis, coccidioidomycosis, toxocariasis, and histoplasmosis; infections caused by organisms such as *Candida*, *Pneumocystis carinii*, *Cryptococcus*, *Aspergillus*, herpes, and cytomegalovirus (**Plate III-1**); and other diseases such as syphilis, Lyme disease, tuberculosis, cat-scratch disease, Whipple's disease, and brucellosis. In multiple sclerosis, chronic inflammatory changes can develop in the extreme periphery of the retina (pars planitis or intermediate uveitis).

Acute angle-closure glaucoma is a rare and frequently misdiagnosed cause of a red, painful eye. Susceptible eyes have a shallow anterior chamber, either because the eye has a short axial length (hyperopia) or a lens enlarged by the gradual development of cataract.

When the pupil becomes mid-dilated, the peripheral iris blocks aqueous outflow via the anterior chamber angle and the intraocular pressure rises abruptly, producing pain, injection, corneal edema, obscurations, and blurred vision. In some patients, ocular symptoms are overshadowed by nausea, vomiting or headache, prompting a fruitless workup for abdominal or neurologic disease. The diagnosis is made by measuring the intraocular pressure during an acute attack or by performing gonioscopy to reveal the narrowed chamber angle by means of a specially mirrored contact lens. Acute angle closure is treated with oral or intravenous acetazolamide, topical beta blockers, and pilocarpine to induce miosis. If these measures fail, a laser can be used to create a hole in the peripheral iris to relieve pupillary block. Many physicians are reluctant to dilate patients routinely for fundus examination because they fear precipitating an angle-closure glaucoma. The risk is actually remote and more than outweighed by the potential benefit to patients of discovering a hidden fundus lesion visible only through a fully dilated pupil. Moreover, a single attack of angle closure after pharmacologic dilation rarely causes any permanent damage to the eye and serves as an inadvertent provocative test to identify patients with narrow angles who would benefit from prophylactic laser iridectomy.

Endophthalmitis occurs from bacterial, viral, fungal, or parasitic infection of the internal structures of the eye. It is usually acquired by hematogenous seeding from a remote site. Chronically ill, diabetic, or immunosuppressed patients, especially those with a history of indwelling intravenous catheters or positive blood cultures, are at greatest risk for endogenous endophthalmitis. Although most patients have ocular pain and injection, visual loss is sometimes the only symptom. Septic emboli, from a diseased heart valve or a dental abscess, that lodge in the retinal circulation can give rise to endophthalmitis. White-centered retinal hemorrhages (Roth's spots) are considered pathognomonic for subacute bacterial endocarditis, but they also appear in leukemia, diabetes, and many other conditions. Endophthalmitis also occurs as a complication of ocular surgery, occasionally months or even years after the operation. An occult penetrating foreign body or unrecognized trauma to the globe should be considered in any patient with unexplained intraocular infection or inflammation.

Transient or Sudden Visual Loss   Transient ischemic attack of the retina is called *amaurosis fugax*. Because neural tissue has a high rate of metabolism, interruption of blood flow to the retina for more than a few seconds results in *transient monocular blindness*, a term used interchangeably with amaurosis fugax. Patients describe a rapid fading of vision like a curtain descending, sometimes affecting only a portion of the visual field. Amaurosis fugax usually occurs from an embolus that becomes stuck within a retinal arteriole (**Plate III-2**). If the embolus breaks up or passes, flow is restored and vision returns quickly to normal without permanent damage. With prolonged interruption of blood flow, the inner retina suffers infarction. Ophthalmoscopy reveals zones of whitened, edematous retina following the distribution of branch retinal arterioles. Complete occlusion of the central retinal artery produces arrest of blood flow and a milky retina with a cherry-red fovea. Emboli are composed of either cholesterol (Hollenhorst plaque), calcium, or platelet-fibrin debris. The most common source is an atherosclerotic plaque in the carotid artery or aorta, although emboli can also arise from the heart, especially in patients with diseased valves, atrial fibrillation, or wall motion abnormalities.

In rare instances, amaurosis fugax occurs from low central retinal artery perfusion pressure in a patient with a critical stenosis of the ipsilateral carotid artery and poor collateral flow via the circle of Willis. In this situation, amaurosis fugax develops when there is a dip in systemic blood pressure or a slight worsening of the carotid stenosis. Sometimes there is contralateral motor or sensory loss, indicating concomitant hemispheric cerebral ischemia.

Amaurosis fugax warns of a patient at high risk for stroke. The carotid arteries should be studied by ultrasound. Endarterectomy for a stenosis of 60 percent or more, even in asymptomatic patients, has been shown to reduce the subsequent rate of ipsilateral stroke (Chap. 366). Therapy with aspirin, warfarin, or other anticoagulants is appropriate in selected patients. If no carotid lesion is found, cardiac ultrasound and ambulatory ECG monitoring should be undertaken.

Marked *systemic hypertension* causes sclerosis of retinal arterioles, splinter hemorrhages, focal infarcts of the nerve fiber layer (cotton-wool spots), and leakage of lipid and fluid (hard exudate) into the macula (**Plate III-3**). In hypertensive crisis, sudden visual loss can result from vasospasm of retinal arterioles and consequent retinal ischemia. In addition, acute hypertension may produce visual loss from ischemic swelling of the optic disc. Patients with acute hypertensive retinopathy should be treated by lowering the blood pressure. However, the blood pressure should not be reduced precipitously, because there is a danger of optic disc infarction from sudden hypoperfusion.

Impending *branch* or *central retinal vein occlusion* can produce prolonged visual obscurations that resemble those described by patients with amaurosis fugax. The veins appear engorged and phlebitic, with numerous retinal hemorrhages (**Plate III-4**). In some patients, venous blood flow recovers spontaneously, while others evolve a frank obstruction with extensive retinal bleeding ("blood and thunder" appearance), infarction, and visual loss. Venous occlusion of the retina is often idiopathic, but hypertension, diabetes, and glaucoma are prominent risk factors. The benefit of treatment with anticoagulants is unproven and carries the risk of hemorrhage into the vitreous. Polycythemia, thrombocythemia, or other factors leading to an underlying hypercoagulable state should be corrected.

Anterior ischemic optic neuropathy (AION) is caused by insufficient blood flow through the posterior ciliary arteries supplying the optic disc. It produces sudden, painless, monocular visual loss, although patients occasionally report premonitory obscurations. The optic disc appears swollen and surrounded by nerve fiber layer splinter hemorrhages (**Plate III-5**). AION is divided into two forms: arteritic and nonarteritic. The nonarteritic form of AION is most common. No specific cause can be identified, although diabetes and hypertension are frequent risk factors. No treatment is available. About 5 percent of patients, especially those over age 65, develop the arteritic form of AION in conjunction with giant cell (temporal) arteritis (Chap. 319). It is urgent to identify patients with arteritic AION so that glucocorticoid therapy can be instituted immediately to prevent blindness in the second eye. Symptoms of polymyalgia rheumatica may be present, and the sedimentation rate is usually elevated. In a patient with visual loss from suspected arteritic AION, temporal artery biopsy is helpful to confirm the diagnosis, but steroid treatment should be started without waiting for the biopsy to be completed. The diagnosis of arteritic AION is difficult to sustain in the face of a normal sedimentation rate and a negative temporal artery biopsy, but such cases do occur rarely.

Posterior ischemic optic neuropathy is an infrequent cause of acute visual loss. It is induced by the combination of severe anemia and hypotension, causing infarction of the retrobulbar optic nerve. Cases have been reported after major blood loss during surgery, exsanguinating trauma, gastrointestinal bleeding, and renal dialysis. The fundus usually appears normal, although optic disc swelling develops if the process extends far enough anteriorly. Vision can be salvaged in some patients by prompt blood transfusion and reversal of hypotension.

Optic neuritis is a common inflammatory disease of the optic nerve. In the recent Optic Neuritis Treatment Trial, the mean age of patients was 32 years, 77 percent were female, 92 percent had ocular pain (especially with eye movements), and 35 percent had optic disc swelling. In the majority of patients, the demyelinating event was retrobulbar and the ocular fundus appeared normal on initial examination (**Plate III-6**), although optic disc pallor slowly developed over subsequent months. Many patients with optic neuritis eventually develop multiple sclerosis, but for some patients optic neuritis remains an isolated event. Virtually all patients experience a gradual recovery of vision after a single episode of optic neuritis, even without treatment. This rule is so reliable that failure of vision to improve substantially after a first attack of optic neuritis casts doubt upon the original diagnosis.

Treatment of optic neuritis with glucocorticoids is controversial. The Optic Neuritis Treatment Trial showed that patients treated with a conventional dose of oral steroids (prednisone, 1 mg/kg per day for 14 days) did no better than patients treated with a placebo. Surprisingly, patients who received oral prednisone appeared to have an increased recurrence rate of optic neuritis. From these results, it is apparent that treatment of optic neuritis with oral glucocorticoids is of no help and may even heighten the risk of further attacks. High-dose intravenous methylprednisolone (250 mg every 6 h for 3 days) followed by oral prednisone (1 mg/kg per day for 11 days) led to a slightly faster recovery of visual function, but final acuity 6 months later was not significantly different in patients treated with a placebo. Remarkably, intravenous glucocorticoids were associated with a reduced rate of development of multiple sclerosis over a 2-year follow-up period, especially in the subgroup of patients with multiple foci of demyelination on their magnetic resonance (MR) scan. However, by the end of a 3-year follow-up period, patients treated with intravenous glucocorticoids versus placebo showed no difference in the rate of multiple sclerosis. Moreover, intravenous steroids did not reduce the likelihood of subsequent attacks of optic neuritis. To summarize: the study authors recommend an MR scan in patients with optic neuritis. If two or more foci of demyelination are found or visual loss is severe, they suggest treatment with intravenous steroids. The potential benefits of intravenous steroids are: (1) a slightly faster recovery of visual function, and (2) a potential reduction in the risk of subsequent neurologic events that would signify multiple sclerosis. Critics of the Optic Neuritis Treatment Trial have questioned these recommendations, pointing out that: (1) visual outcome is the same in the long run, (2) evidence indicating a reduced risk of eventual multiple sclerosis with intravenous steroid treatment is based upon follow-up data in a rather small number of patients, and (3) the protection against multiple sclerosis is transient, and no longer apparent 3 years later. In cases of unilateral optic neuritis, the decision whether to obtain an MR scan or to treat with intravenous steroids should be based upon clinical judgment and careful discussion with the patient. In cases of bilateral, simultaneous optic neuritis, the rationale for intravenous steroids is stronger.

Leber's hereditary optic neuropathy (Chap. 380) is a disease of young men, characterized by onset over a few weeks of painless, severe, central visual loss in one eye, followed weeks or months later by the same process in the other eye. Acutely, the optic disc appears mildly plethoric with surface capillary telangiectases, but no vascular leakage on fluorescein angiography. Eventually optic atrophy ensues. There is no treatment. Recently, Wallace discovered that Leber's optic neuropathy is caused by a point mutation at codon 11778 in the mitochondrial gene encoding nicotinamide adenine dinucleotide dehydrogenase (NADH) subunit 4. Subsequently, additional mutations responsible for the disease have been identified, most in mitochondrial genes encoding proteins involved in electron transport. Mitochrondrial mutations causing Leber's neuropathy are inherited from the mother by all her children, but usually only sons develop symptoms. This curious male predilection is a mystery.

Toxic optic neuropathy can result in acute visual loss with bilateral optic disc swelling and central or cecocentral scotomas. Such cases have been reported from ethambutol, methyl alcohol (moonshine), ethylene glycol (antifreeze), and carbon monoxide. In toxic optic neuropathy, visual loss can also develop gradually and produce optic atrophy without a phase of acute optic disc edema (**Plate III-7**). Many agents have been implicated as a cause of toxic optic neuropathy, but the evidence supporting the association for many is weak. The following is a partial list of potential offending drugs or toxins: disulfiram, ethchlorvynol, chloramphenicol, amiodarone, monoclonal anti-CD3 antibody, ciprofloxacin, digitalis, streptomycin, lead, arsenic, thallium, D-penicillamine, isoniazid, emetine, and sulfonamides. Deficiency states, induced either by starvation, malabsorption, or alcoholism, can lead to insidious visual loss. Thiamine, vitamin B_{12}, and folate levels should be checked in any patient with unexplained, bilateral central scotomas and optic pallor.

Papilledema connotes bilateral optic disc swelling from raised intracranial pressure **(Plate III-8)**. Headache is a frequent, but not invariable, accompaniment. All other forms of optic disc swelling, e.g., from optic neuritis or ischemic optic neuropathy, should be called "optic disc edema." This convention is arbitrary but serves to avoid confusion. Often it is difficult to differentiate papilledema from other forms of optic disc edema by fundus examination alone. Transient visual obscurations are a classic symptom of papilledema. They can occur in only one eye or simultaneously in both eyes. They usually last seconds but can persist for minutes if the papilledema is fulminant. Obscurations follow abrupt shifts in posture or happen spontaneously. When obscurations are prolonged or spontaneous, the papilledema is more threatening. Visual acuity is not affected by papilledema, unless the papilledema is severe, long-standing, or accompanied by macular edema and hemorrhage. Visual field testing shows enlarged blind spots and peripheral constriction (Fig. 28-3*F*). With unremitting papilledema, peripheral visual field loss progresses in an insidious fashion while the optic nerve develops atrophy. In this setting, reduction of optic disc swelling is an ominous sign of a dying nerve rather than an encouraging indication of resolving papilledema.

Evaluation of papilledema requires computed tomography (CT) or MR imaging to exclude a brain tumor. If none is found, MR angiography is appropriate in selected cases to investigate the possibility of a dural venous sinus occlusion or an arteriovenous shunt. If neuroradiologic studies are normal, the subarachnoid opening pressure should be measured by lumbar puncture to confirm that it is elevated. If it is elevated, without explanation, the diagnosis of *pseudotumor cerebri* (idiopathic intracranial hypertension) is made by exclusion. The majority of patients are young, female, and obese. Treatment with a carbonic anhydrase inhibitor such as acetazolamide lowers intracranial pressure by reducing the production of cerebrospinal fluid. Weight reduction is exceedingly important but often unsuccessful. If acetazolamide and weight loss fail, and visual field loss is progressive, lumboperitoneal shunting or optic nerve sheath fenestration should be undertaken without delay, when required, to prevent blindness.

Optic disc drusen are refractile deposits within the substance of the optic nerve head **(Plate III-9)**. They are unrelated to drusen of the retina, which occur in age-related macular degeneration. Optic disc drusen are most common in people of northern European descent, with an incidence of 3 to 4 per thousand. Their diagnosis is obvious when they are visible as glittering particles upon the surface of the optic disc. However, in many patients they are hidden beneath the surface, producing an elevated optic disc with blurred margins that is easily mistaken for papilledema. It is important to recognize pseudopapilledema due to optic disc drusen to avoid an unneccessary evaluation for papilledema. Ultrasound or CT scanning are sensitive for detection of buried optic disc drusen because they contain calcium. In most patients, optic disc drusen are an incidental, innocuous finding, but they can produce visual obscurations. On perimetry they give rise to enlarged blind spots and arcuate scotomas from damage to the optic disc. With increasing age, drusen tend to become more exposed on the disc surface as optic atrophy develops. Hemorrhage, choroidal neovascular membrane, and anterior ischemic optic neuropathy are more likely to occur in patients with optic disc drusen. No treatment for drusen is available.

Vitreous degeneration occurs in all individuals with advancing age, leading to chronic and acute visual symptoms. Opacities develop in the vitreous, casting annoying shadows upon the retina. As the eye moves, these distracting "floaters" move synchronously, with a slight lag caused by inertia of the vitreous gel. Vitreous traction upon the retina causes mechanical stimulation, resulting in perception of flashing lights. This photopsia is brief and confined to one eye, in contrast to the bilateral, prolonged scintillations of cortical migraine. Contraction of the vitreous can result in sudden separation from the retina, heralded by an alarming shower of floaters and photopsia. This process, known as *vitreous detachment*, is a frequent involutional event in the elderly. It is not harmful unless it damages the retina. A careful

examination of the dilated fundus is mandatory in any patient complaining of floaters or photopsia to search for peripheral tears or holes. If such a lesion is found, laser application or cryotherapy can forestall a retinal detachment. Occasionally a tear ruptures a retinal blood vessel, causing vitreous hemorrhage and sudden loss of vision. On attempted ophthalmoscopy the fundus is hidden by a dark red haze of blood. Ultrasound is required to examine the interior of the eye for a retinal tear or detachment. If the hemorrhage does not resolve spontaneously, the vitreous can be removed surgically. Vitreous hemorrhage also occurs from the fragile neovascular vessels that proliferate on the surface of the retina in diabetes, sickle cell anemia, and other ischemic ocular diseases.

Retinal detachment produces symptoms of floaters, flashing lights, and a scotoma in the peripheral visual field corresponding to the detachment **(Plate III-10)**. If the detachment includes the fovea, there is an afferent pupil defect and the visual acuity is reduced. In most eyes, retinal detachment starts with a hole, flap, or tear in the peripheral retina (rhegmatogenous retinal detachment). Patients with peripheral retinal thinning (lattice degeneration) are particularly vulnerable to this process. Once a break has developed in the retina, liquified vitreous is free to enter the subretinal space, separating the retina from the pigment epithelium. The combination of vitreous traction upon the retinal surface and passage of fluid behind the retina leads inexorably to detachment. Patients with a history of myopia, trauma, or prior cataract extraction are at greatest risk for retinal detachment. The diagnosis is confirmed by ophthalmoscopic examination of the dilated eye.

Classic migraine (Chap. 364) usually occurs with a visual aura lasting about 20 min. In a typical attack, a small central disturbance in the field of vision marches toward the periphery, leaving a transient scotoma in its wake. The expanding border of migraine scotoma has a scintillating, dancing, or zig-zag edge, resembling the bastions of a fortified city, hence the term "fortification spectra." Patients' descriptions of fortification spectra vary widely and can be confused with amaurosis fugax. Migraine patterns usually last longer and are perceived in both eyes, whereas amaurosis fugax is briefer and occurs in only one eye. Migraine phenomena also remain visible in the dark or with the eyes closed. Generally they are confined to either the right or left visual hemifield, but sometimes both fields are involved simultaneously. Patients often have a long history of stereotypic attacks. After the visual symptoms recede, headache develops in most patients.

Transient ischemic attacks from *vertebrobasilar insufficiency* result in acute homonymous visual symptoms. Many patients mistakenly describe symptoms in their left or right eye, when in fact they are occurring in the left or right hemifield of both eyes. Interruption of blood supply to the visual cortex causes a sudden fogging or graying of vision, occasionally with flashing lights or other positive phenomena that mimic migraine. Cortical ischemic attacks are briefer in duration than migraine, occur in older patients, and are not followed by headache. There may be associated signs of brainstem ischemia, such as diplopia, vertigo, numbness, weakness, or dysarthria.

Stroke occurs when interruption of blood supply from the posterior cerebral artery to the visual cortex is prolonged. The only finding on examination is a homonymous visual field defect that stops abruptly at the vertical meridian. Occipital lobe stroke is usually due to thrombotic occlusion of the vertebrobasilar system, embolus, or dissection. Lobar hemorrhage, tumor, abscess, and arteriovenous malformation are other common causes of hemianopic cortical visual loss.

Factitious (functional, nonorganic) *visual loss* is claimed by hysterics or malingerers. The latter comprise the vast majority, seeking sympathy, special treatment, or financial gain by feigning loss of sight. The diagnosis is suspected when the history is atypical, physical findings are lacking or contradictory, inconsistencies emerge on testing, and a secondary motive can be identified. In our litigious society, the fraudulent pursuit of recompense has spawned an epidemic of factitious visual loss.

Chronic Visual Loss *Cataract* is a clouding of the lens sufficient to reduce vision. Most cataracts develop slowly as a result of aging, leading to gradual impairment of vision. The formation of cataract occurs more rapidly in patients with a history of ocular trauma, uveitis, or diabetes mellitus. Cataracts are acquired in a variety of genetic diseases, such as myotonic dystrophy, neurofibromatosis type 2, and galactosemia. Radiation therapy and glucocorticoid treatment can induce cataract as a side effect. The cataracts associated with radiation or steroids have a typical posterior subcapsular location. Cataract can be detected by noting an impaired red reflex when viewing light reflected from the fundus with an ophthalmoscope or by examining the dilated eye at the slit lamp.

The only treatment for cataract is surgical extraction of the opacified lens. Over a million cataract operations are performed each year in the United States. The operation is generally done under local retrobulbar anesthesia on an outpatient basis. Remarkable technical innovations have made it possible to aspirate the cataract while leaving the lens capsule intact (extracapsular cataract extraction), rather than removing the entire lens with its capsule (intracapsular cataract extraction). A plastic or silicone intraocular lens is then placed within the empty lens capsule in the posterior chamber, substituting for the natural lens, and leading to rapid recovery of sight. More than 95 percent of patients who undergo cataract extraction can expect an improvement in vision. In many patients, the lens capsule remaining in the eye after cataract extraction eventually turns cloudy, causing a secondary loss of vision. A small opening is made in the lens capsule with a laser to restore clarity.

Glaucoma is a slowly progressive, insidious optic neuropathy, usually associated with chronic elevation of intraocular pressure. In Americans of African descent it is the leading cause of blindness. The mechanism whereby raised intraocular pressure injures the optic nerve is not understood. Axons entering the inferotemporal and superotemporal aspects of the optic disc are damaged first, producing typical nerve fiber bundle or arcuate scotomas on perimetric testing. As fibers are destroyed, the neural rim of the optic disc shrinks and the physiologic cup within the optic disc enlarges (**Plate III-11**). This process is referred to colloquially as pathologic "cupping." The cup-to-disc diameter is expressed as a ratio, e.g., 0.2/1. The cup-to-disc ratio ranges widely in normal subjects, making it difficult to diagnose glaucoma reliably simply by observing an unusually large or deep optic cup. Careful documentation of serial prospective examinations is helpful. In the patient with physiologic cupping, the large cup remains stable, whereas in the patient with glaucoma it expands relentlessly over the years. Detection of visual field loss on formal perimetry also contributes to the diagnosis of glaucoma. Finally, most patients with glaucoma have raised intraocular pressure. However, a surprising number of patients with typical glaucomatous cupping and visual field loss have an intraocular pressure that apparently never exceeds the normal limit of 20 mmHg (so-called low-tension glaucoma).

In acute angle-closure glaucoma, the eye is red and painful due to abrupt, severe elevation of intraocular pressure. Such cases account for only a handful of patients with glaucoma. Most patients with glaucoma have open, nonoccludable anterior chamber angles. In open-angle glaucoma the cause of the raised intraocular pressure is unknown. Because the elevation of intraocular pressure develops gradually and is less marked than in angle-closure glaucoma, there is no pain or ocular injection. The central visual field and foveal acuity are spared until end-stage disease is reached. For these reasons, severe and irreversible damage can occur before either the patient or physician recognizes the diagnosis. Screening of patients for glaucoma by noting the cup-to-disc ratio on ophthalmoscopy and by measuring intraocular pressure (using a Schiotz, Tonopen, or Goldmann tonometer) is vital. Glaucoma is treated with topical adrenergic agonists (epinephrine, dipivefrin, apraclonidine), cholinergic agonists (pilocarpine), and beta blockers (betaxolol, carteolol, levobunolol, metipranolol, and timolol). Occasionally, systemic absorption of beta blocker from an eye

drop can be sufficient to cause side effects of bradycardia, hypotension, heart block, bronchospasm, impotence, or depression. Topical or oral carbonic anhydrase inhibitors are used to lower intraocular pressure by reducing aqueous production. Laser treatment of the trabecular meshwork in the anterior chamber angle improves aqueous outflow from the eye. If medical or laser treatments fail to halt optic nerve damage from glaucoma, a filter must be constructed surgically (trabeculectomy) to release aqueous from the eye in a controlled fashion.

Macular degeneration is a major cause of gradual, painless, bilateral central visual loss in the elderly. The old term, "senile macular degeneration," misinterpreted by many patients as an unflattering reference, has been replaced with "age-related macular degeneration." It occurs in a nonexudative (dry) form and an exudative (wet) form. The nonexudative process begins with the accumulation of extracellular deposits, called drusen, underneath the retinal pigment epithelium. On ophthalmoscopy they are pleomorphic but generally appear as small discrete yellow lesions clustered in the macula (**Plate III-12**). With time they become larger, more numerous, and confluent. The retinal pigment epithelium becomes focally detached and atrophic, causing visual loss by interfering with photoreceptor function. There is currently no way to prevent the development of age-related macular degeneration. Concoctions of various vitamins (A, C, and E) and minerals (zinc, copper, and selenium) have been marketed, without good evidence that they retard the process of macular degeneration.

Exudative macular degeneration, which develops in only a minority of patients, occurs when neovascular vessels from the choroid grow through defects in Bruch's membrane into the potential space beneath the retinal pigment epithelium. Leakage from these vessels produces elevation of the retina and pigment epithelium, with distortion (metamorphopsia) and blurring of vision. Although onset of these symptoms is usually gradual, bleeding from subretinal choroidal neovascular membranes sometimes causes acute visual loss. The neovascular membranes can be difficult to see on fundus examination because they are beneath the retina. Fluorescein angiography is extremely useful for their detection. In some patients, prompt laser ablation of choroidal neovascular membranes seen on fluorescein angiography can halt the exudative process. However, the neovascular membranes frequently recur, requiring constant vigilance and repeated photocoagulation.

Major or repeated hemorrhage under the retina from neovascular membranes results in fibrosis, development of a round (disciform) macular scar, and permanent loss of central vision. Surgical attempts to remove subretinal membranes in age-related macular degeneration have not improved vision in most patients. However, outcomes have been more encouraging for patients with choroidal neovascular membranes from ocular histoplasmosis syndrome.

Central serous chorioretinopathy primarily affects males between the ages of 20 and 50. Leakage of serous fluid from the choroid causes small, localized detachment of the retinal pigment epithelium and the neurosensory retina. These detachments produce acute or chronic symptoms of metamorphopsia and blurred vision when the macula is involved. They are difficult to visualize with a direct ophthalmoscope because the detached retina is transparent and only slightly elevated. Diagnosis of central serous chorioretinopathy is made easily by fluorescein angiography, which shows dye streaming into the subretinal space. The cause of central serous chorioretinopathy is unknown. Symptoms may resolve spontaneously if the retina reattaches, but recurrent detachment is common. Laser photocoagulation has benefited some patients with this condition.

Diabetic retinopathy was a rare disease until 1921, when the discovery of insulin resulted in a dramatic improvement in life expectancy for patients with diabetes mellitus. It is now a leading cause of blindness in the United States. The retinopathy of diabetes takes years to develop but eventually appears in nearly all cases. Regular surveillance of the dilated fundus is crucial for any patient with diabetes. In advanced diabetic retinopathy, the proliferation of neovascular vessels leads to blindness from vitreous hemorrhage, retinal detachment, and glaucoma (**Plate III-13**). These complications can be avoided in most patients by administration of panretinal laser photocoagulation at the appropriate point in the evolution of the disease. → *The manifestations* and management of diabetic retinopathy are discussed further in Chap. 334.

Retinitis pigmentosa is a general term for a disparate group of rod and cone dystrophies characterized by progressive night blindness (nyctalopia), visual field constriction with a ring scotoma, loss of acuity, and an abnormal electroretinogram (ERG). It occurs sporadically or in an autosomal recessive, dominant, or X-linked pattern. Irregular black deposits of clumped pigment in the peripheral retina, called bone spicules because of their vague resemblance to the spicules of cancellous bone, give the disease its name (Plate III-14). The name is actually a misnomer because retinitis pigmentosa is not an inflammatory process. Most cases are due to a mutation in the gene for rhodopsin, the rod photopigment, or in the gene for peripherin, a glycoprotein located in photoreceptor outer segments. There is no effective treatment for retinitis pigmentosa. Vitamin A (15,000 IU/day) slightly retards the deterioration of the ERG but has no beneficial effect upon visual acuity or visual fields. Some forms of retinitis pigmentosa occur in association with rare, hereditary systemic diseases (olivopontocerebellar degeneration, Bassen-Kornzweig disease, Kearns-Sayre syndrome, Refsum's disease). Chronic treatment with chloroquine, hydroxychloroquine, and phenothiazines (especially thioridazine) can produce visual loss from a toxic retinopathy that resembles retinitis pigmentosa.

Epiretinal membrane refers to a fibrocellular tissue that grows across the inner surface of the retina, causing metamorphopsia and reduced visual acuity from distortion of the macula. With the ophthalmoscope one can see a crinkled, cellophane-like membrane on the retina. Epiretinal membrane is most common in patients over 50 years of age and is usually unilateral. Most cases are idiopathic, but some occur as a result of hypertensive retinopathy, diabetes, retinal detachment, or trauma. When visual acuity is reduced to the level of about 6/24 (20/80), vitrectomy and surgical peeling of the membrane to relieve macular puckering are recommended. Contraction of an epiretinal membrane sometimes gives rise to a *macular hole*. Most macular holes, however, are caused by local vitreous traction within the fovea. Vision is usually depressed to the level of 6/30 (20/100) or worse. Vitrectomy may improve visual acuity in some patients with macular hole. Fortunately, fewer than 10 percent of patients with macular hole develop a hole in their other eye.

Melanoma of the choroid is the most common primary tumor of the eye (Plate III-15). It causes photopsia, an enlarging scotoma, and loss of vision. A small melanoma is often difficult to differentiate from a benign choroidal nevus. Careful serial examinations are required to document a malignant pattern of growth. Treatment of melanoma is controversial. Options include enucleation, local resection, and irradiation. *Metastatic tumors* to the eye outnumber primary tumors of uveal origin. Breast and lung carcinoma have a special propensity to spread to the choroid or iris. Leukemia and lymphoma also commonly invade ocular tissues. Sometimes their only sign on eye examination is a cellular debris in the vitreous, which can masquerade as a chronic posterior uveitis. *Retrobulbar tumor* of the optic nerve (meningioma, glioma) or *chiasmal tumor* (pituitary adenoma, meningioma) produces gradual visual loss with few objective findings, except for optic disc pallor. Rarely, sudden expansion of a pituitary adenoma from infarction and bleeding (*pituitary apoplexy*) causes acute retrobulbar visual loss, with headache, nausea, and ocular motor nerve palsies. In any patient with visual field loss or optic atrophy, CT or MR scanning should be considered if the cause remains unknown after careful review of the history and thorough examination of the eye (Fig. 28-4).

Proptosis Proptosis is an abnormal forward protrusion of one or both eyes. It is measured using a Hertel exophthalmometer, a handheld instrument that records the position of the anterior corneal surface relative to the lateral orbital rim. If this instrument is not available, relative eye position can be judged by bending the patient's head forward and looking down upon the orbits. A proptosis of only 2 mm in one eye is detectable from this perspective. The development of proptosis implies a space-occupying lesion in the orbit. A CT or MR scan should be obtained in any patient with proptosis, unless the diagnosis of Graves' ophthalmopathy is certain.

Graves' ophthalmopathy is the leading cause of proptosis in adults (Chap. 331). Orbital inflammation and engorgement of the extraocular muscles, particularly the medial rectus and the inferior rectus, account for the protrusion of the globe. Corneal exposure, lid retraction, conjunctival injection, restriction of gaze, diplopia, and visual loss from optic nerve compression are cardinal symptoms. Optic nerve compression should be relieved promptly with radiation therapy or orbital decompression to prevent permanent visual loss.

Orbital pseudotumor is an idiopathic, inflammatory orbital syndrome, frequently confused with Graves' ophthalmopathy. Symptoms are pain, limited eye movements, proptosis, and congestion. Evaluation for sarcoidosis, Wegener's granulomatosis, and other types of orbital vasculitis or collagen-vascular disease is negative. Imaging often shows swollen eye muscles (orbital myositis) with enlarged tendons. By contrast, in Graves' ophthalmopathy the tendons of the eye muscles usually are spared. The Tolosa-Hunt syndrome may be regarded as an extension of orbital pseudotumor through the superior orbital fissure into the cavernous sinus. The diagnosis of orbital pseudotumor is difficult. Biopsy of the orbit frequently yields nonspecific evidence of fat infiltration by lymphocytes, plasma cells, and eosinophils. A dramatic response to a therapeutic trial of systemic glucocorticoids indirectly provides the best confirmation of the diagnosis.

Orbital cellulitis causes pain, lid erythema, proptosis, conjunctival chemosis, restricted motility, decreased acuity, afferent pupillary defect, fever, and leukocytosis. It often arises from a paranasal sinus, especially by contiguous spread of infection from the ethmoid sinus through the thin lamina papyracea of the medial orbit. A history of recent upper respiratory tract infection, chronic sinusitis, thick mucous secretions, or dental disease is significant in any patient with suspected orbital cellulitis. Blood cultures should be obtained, but they are usually negative. Most patients respond to empiric therapy with broad-spectrum intravenous antibiotics. Occasionally, orbital cellulitis follows an overwhelming course, with massive proptosis, blindness, septic cavernous sinus thrombosis, and meningitis. To avert this disaster, orbital cellulitis should be managed aggressively in the early stages, with immediate antibiotic therapy and imaging of the orbits. Prompt surgical drainage of an orbital abscess or paranasal sinusitis is indicated if optic nerve function deteriorates despite antibiotics.

Tumors of the orbit cause painless, progressive proptosis. The most common primary tumors are hemangioma, lymphangioma, neurofibroma, dermoid cyst, optic nerve glioma, optic nerve meningioma, and benign mixed tumor of the lacrimal gland. Metastatic tumor to the orbit occurs frequently in breast carcinoma, lung carcinoma, and lymphoma. Diagnosis by fine-needle aspiration followed by urgent radiation therapy can sometimes preserve vision.

Carotid cavernous fistulas with anterior drainage through the orbit produce proptosis, diplopia, glaucoma, and tortuous, red conjunctival vessels. Direct fistulas usually result from trauma. They are easily diagnosed because of the dramatic signs produced by high-flow, high-pressure shunting. Indirect fistulas, or dural arteriovenous malformations, are more likely to occur spontaneously, especially in older women. The signs are more subtle and the diagnosis is frequently missed. The combination of slight proptosis, diplopia, enlarged muscles, and an injected eye is often mistaken for thyroid ophthalmopathy. A bruit heard upon auscultation of the head, or reported by the patient, is a valuable diagnostic clue. Imaging shows an enlarged superior ophthalmic vein in the orbits. Carotid cavernous shunts can be eliminated by intravascular embolization.

Ptosis *Blepharoptosis* is an abnormal drooping of the eyelid. Unilateral or bilateral ptosis can be congenital, from dysgenesis of the levator palpebrae superioris, or from abnormal insertion of its aponeurosis into the eyelid. Acquired ptosis can develop so gradually that the patient is unaware of the problem. Inspection of old photographs is helpful in dating the onset. A history of prior trauma, eye surgery, contact lens use, diplopia, systemic symptoms (e.g., dysphagia or peripheral muscle weakness), or a family history of ptosis should be sought. Fluctuating ptosis that worsens late in the day is typical of myasthenia gravis. Examination should focus upon evidence for proptosis, eyelid masses or deformities, inflammation, pupil inequality, or limitation of motility. The width of the palpebral fissures is measured in primary gaze to quantitate the degree of ptosis. The ptosis will be underestimated if the patient is compensating by lifting the brow with the frontalis muscle.

Mechanical ptosis occurs in many elderly patients from stretching and redundancy of eyelid skin and subcutaneous fat (dermatochalasis). The extra weight of these sagging tissues causes the lid to droop. Enlargement or deformation of the eyelid from infection, tumor, trauma, or inflammation also results in ptosis on a purely mechanical basis.

Aponeurotic ptosis is an acquired dehiscence or stretching of the aponeurotic tendon, which connects the levator muscle to the tarsal plate of the eyelid. It occurs commonly in older patients, presumably from loss of connective tissue elasticity. Aponeurotic ptosis is also a frequent sequela of eyelid swelling from infection or blunt trauma to the orbit, cataract surgery, or hard contact lens usuage.

Myogenic ptosis includes myasthenia gravis (see Chap. 382) and a number of rare myopathies that manifest with ptosis. The term *chronic progressive external ophthalmoplegia* refers to a spectrum of systemic diseases caused by mutations of mitochrondrial DNA. As the name implies, the most prominent findings are symmetric, slowly progressive ptosis and limitation of eye movements. In general, diplopia is a late symptom because all eye movements are reduced equally. In the *Kearns-Sayre* variant, retinal pigmentary changes and abnormalities of cardiac conduction develop. Peripheral muscle biopsy shows characteristic "ragged-red fibers." *Oculopharyngeal dystrophy* is a distinct autosomal dominant disease with onset in middle age, characterized by ptosis, limited eye movements, and trouble swallowing. *Myotonic dystrophy*, another autosomal dominant disorder, causes ptosis, ophthalmoparesis, cataract, and pigmentary retinopathy. Patients have muscle wasting, myotonia, frontal balding, and cardiac abnormalities.

Neurogenic ptosis results from a lesion affecting the innervation to either of the two muscles that open the eyelid: Muller's muscle or the levator palpebrae superioris. Examination of the pupil helps to decide between these two possibilities. In Horner's syndrome, the eye with ptosis has a smaller pupil and the eye movements are full. In an oculomotor nerve palsy, the eye with the ptosis has a larger, or a normal, pupil. If the pupil is normal but there is limitation of adduction, elevation, and depression, a pupil-sparing oculomotor nerve palsy is likely (see next section). Rarely, a lesion affecting the small, central subnucleus of the oculomotor complex will cause bilateral ptosis with normal eye movements and pupils.

Double Vision   The first point to clarify is whether diplopia persists in either eye after covering the fellow eye. If it does, the diagnosis is monocular diplopia. The cause is usually intrinsic to the eye and therefore has no dire implications for the patient. Corneal aberrations (e.g., keratoconus, pterygium), uncorrected refractive error, cataract, or foveal traction may give rise to monocular diplopia. Occasionally it is a symptom of malingering or psychiatric disease. Diplopia alleviated by covering one eye is binocular diplopia and is caused by disruption of ocular alignment. Inquiry should be made into the nature of the double vision (purely side-by-side versus partial vertical displacement of images), mode of onset, duration, intermittency, diurnal variation, and associated neurologic or systemic symptoms. If the patient has diplopia while being examined, motility testing should reveal a deficiency corresponding to the patient's symptoms. However, subtle limitation of ocular excursions is often difficult to detect. For example, a patient with a slight left abducens nerve paresis may appear to have full eye movements, despite a complaint of horizontal diplopia upon looking to the left. In this situation, the cover test provides a more sensitive method for demonstrating the ocular malalignment. It should be conducted in primary gaze, and then with the head turned and tilted in each direction. In the above example, a cover test with

the head turned to the right will maximize the fixation shift evoked by the cover test.

Occasionally, a cover test performed in an asymptomatic patient during a routine examination will reveal an ocular deviation. If the eye movements are full and the ocular misalignment is equal in all directions of gaze (concomitant deviation) the diagnosis is strabismus. In this condition, which affects about 1 percent of the population, fusion is disrupted in infancy or early childhood. To avoid diplopia, vision is suppressed from the nonfixating eye. In some children, this leads to impaired vision (amblyopia, or "lazy" eye) in the deviated eye.

Binocular diplopia occurs from a wide range of processes: infectious, neoplastic, metabolic, degenerative, inflammatory, and vascular. One must decide if the diplopia is neurogenic in origin or due to restriction of globe rotation by local disease in the orbit. Orbital pseudotumor, myositis, infection, tumor, thyroid disease, and muscle entrapment (e.g., from a blowout fracture) cause restrictive diplopia. The diagnosis is confirmed by performing a forced duction test in the office. After applying topical anesthesia, the physician grasps the eye with forceps and pulls it toward the direction of deficient motion. If rotation of the globe is prevented by tethering, a restrictive process is at work. The utility of this test is limited by its unpopularity with patients; in practice, the diagnosis of restriction is made by recognizing other associated signs and symptoms of local orbital disease.

Myasthenia gravis (Chap. 382) is a major cause of diplopia. The diplopia is often intermittent, variable, and not confined to any single ocular motor nerve distribution. The pupils are always normal. Fluctuating ptosis may be present. Many patients have a purely ocular form of the disease, with no evidence of systemic muscular weakness. The diagnosis can be confirmed by an intravenous edrophonium injection or by an assay for antiacetylcholine receptor antibodies. Negative results from these tests do not exclude the diagnosis. *Botulism* from food or wound poisoning can mimic ocular myasthenia.

After restrictive orbital disease and myasthenia gravis are excluded, a lesion of a cranial nerve supplying innervation to the extraocular muscles is the most likely cause of binocular diplopia.

The *oculomotor nerve* (third cranial nerve) innervates the medial, inferior, and superior recti; inferior oblique; levator palpebrae superioris; and the iris sphincter. Total palsy of the oculomotor nerve lesion causes ptosis, a dilated pupil, and leaves the eye "down and out" because of the unopposed action of the lateral rectus and superior oblique. This combination of findings is obvious. More challenging is the diagnosis of an early or partial oculomotor nerve palsy. In this setting, any combination of ptosis, pupil dilation, and weakness of the eye muscles supplied by the oculomotor nerve may be encountered. Frequent serial examinations during the evolving phase of the palsy and a high index of suspicion help ensure that the diagnosis is not missed. The advent of an oculomotor nerve palsy with any degree of pupil involvement in an otherwise healthy patient, especially when accompanied by pain, raises the specter of a circle of Willis aneurysm. If an MR scan shows no compressive lesion, an arteriogram must be performed to rule out an aneurysm of either the posterior communicating artery or the basilar artery. If the pupil is entirely normal, with all other components of an oculomotor palsy present, aneurysm is so rare that an angiogram is seldom indicated.

A lesion of the oculomotor nucleus in the rostral midbrain produces signs that differ from those caused by a lesion of the nerve itself. There is bilateral ptosis because the levator muscle is innervated by a single central subnucleus. There is also weakness of the contralateral superior rectus, because it is supplied by the oculomotor nucleus on the other side. Occasionally both superior recti are weak. Isolated nuclear oculomotor palsy is quite rare. Usually neurologic examination reveals additional signs to suggest brainstem damage from infarction, hemorrhage, tumor, or infection.

Injury to structures surrounding fascicles of the oculomotor nerve descending through the midbrain has given rise to a number of classic eponymic designations. In *Nothnagel's syndrome*, injury to the superior cerebellar peduncle causes ipsilateral oculomotor palsy and contralateral cerebellar ataxia. In *Benedikt's syndrome*, injury to the red nucleus results in ipsilateral oculomotor palsy and contralateral tremor, chorea, and athetosis. *Claude's syndrome* incorporates features of both the aforementioned syndromes, by injury to both the red nucleus and the superior cerebellar peduncle. Finally, in *Weber's syndrome*, injury to the cerebral peduncle causes ipsilateral oculomotor palsy with contralateral hemiparesis.

In the subarachnoid space the oculomotor nerve is vulnerable to aneurysm, meningitis, tumor, infarction, and compression. In cerebral herniation the nerve becomes trapped between the edge of the tentorium and the uncus of the temporal lobe. Oculomotor palsy can also occur from midbrain torsion and hemorrhages during herniation. In the cavernous sinus, oculomotor palsy arises from carotid aneurysm, carotid cavernous fistula, cavernous sinus thrombosis, tumor (pituitary adenoma, meningioma, metastasis), herpes zoster infection, and the Tolosa-Hunt syndrome.

The etiology of an isolated, pupil-sparing oculomotor palsy often remains obscure, even after neuroimaging and extensive laboratory testing. Most cases are thought to result from microvascular infarction of the nerve, somewhere along its course from the brainstem to the orbit. Usually the patient complains of pain. Diabetes, hypertension, and vascular disease are major risk factors. Spontaneous recovery over a period of months is the rule. If this fails to occur, or if new findings develop, the diagnosis of microvascular oculomotor nerve palsy should be reconsidered. Aberrant regeneration is common when the oculomotor nerve is injured by trauma or compression (tumor, aneurysm). Miswiring of sprouting fibers to the levator muscle and the rectus muscles results in elevation of the eyelid upon downgaze or adduction. The pupil also constricts upon attempted adduction, elevation, or depression of the globe. Aberrant regeneration is not seen after oculomotor palsy from microvascular infarct and hence vitiates that diagnosis.

The *trochlear nucleus* (fourth cranial nerve) is located in the midbrain, just caudal to the oculomotor nerve complex. Its fibers exit the brainstem dorsally and cross to innervate the contralateral superior oblique. The principal actions of this muscle are to depress and to intort the globe. A palsy therefore results in hypertropia and excyclotorsion. The cyclotorsion is seldom noticed by patients. Instead, they complain of vertical diplopia, especially upon reading or looking down. The vertical diplopia also is exacerbated by tilting the head toward the side with the palsy, and alleviated by tilting it away. This "head tilt test" is a cardinal diagnostic feature.

Isolated trochlear nerve palsy occurs from all the causes listed above for the oculomotor nerve, except aneurysm. The trochlear nerve is particularly apt to suffer injury after closed head trauma. The mechanism is unknown, but the free edge of the tentorium may impinge upon the nerve during a concussive blow. Most isolated trochlear nerve palsies are idiopathic and hence diagnosed by exclusion as "microvascular." Spontaneous improvement occurs over a period of months in most patients. A base-down prism (conveniently applied to the patient's glasses as a stick-on Fresnel lens) may serve as a temporary measure to alleviate diplopia. If the palsy does not resolve, the eyes can be realigned by surgically adjusting other eye muscles.

The *abducens nerve* (sixth cranial nerve) innervates the lateral rectus muscle. A palsy produces horizontal diplopia, worse on gaze to the side of the lesion. A nuclear lesion has different consequences, because the abducens nucleus contains interneurons that project via the medial longitudinal fasciculus to the medial rectus subnucleus of the contralateral oculomotor complex. Therefore, an abducens nuclear lesion produces a complete lateral gaze palsy, from weakness of both the ipsilateral lateral rectus and the contralateral medial rectus. *Foville's syndrome* following dorsal pontine injury includes lateral gaze palsy, ipsilateral facial palsy, and contralateral hemiparesis incurred by damage to descending corticospinal fibers. *Millard-Gubler syndrome* from ventral pontine injury is similar, except for the eye findings. There is lateral rectus weakness only, instead of gaze palsy, because the abducens fascicle is injured rather than the nucleus. Infarct, tumor, hemorrhage, vascular malformation, and multiple sclerosis are the most common etiologies of brainstem abducens palsy.

After leaving the ventral pons, the abducens nerve runs forward along the clivus to pierce the dura at the petrous apex where it enters the cavernous sinus. Along its subarachnoid course it is susceptible to meningitis, tumor (meningioma, chordoma, carcinomatous meningitis), subarachnoid hemorrhage, trauma, and compression by aneurysm or dolichoectatic vessels. At the petrous apex, mastoiditis can produce deafness, pain, and ipsilateral abducens palsy (*Gradenigo's syndrome*). In the cavernous sinus, the nerve can be affected by carotid aneurysm, carotid cavernous fistula, tumor (pituitary adenoma, meningioma, nasopharyngeal carcinoma), herpes infection, and Tolosa-Hunt syndrome.

Unilateral or bilateral abducens palsy is a classic sign of raised intracranial pressure. The diagnosis can be confirmed if papilledema is observed on fundus examination. The mechanism is still debated but is probably related to rostral-caudal displacement of the brainstem. The same phenomenon accounts for abducens palsy from low intracranial pressure (e.g., after lumbar puncture, spinal anesthesia, or spontaneous dural cerebrospinal fluid leak).

Treatment of abducens palsy is aimed at prompt correction of the underlying cause. However, the cause remains obscure in many instances, despite diligent evaluation. As mentioned above for isolated trochlear or oculomotor palsy, most cases are assumed to represent microvascular infarcts because they often occur in the setting of diabetes or other vascular risk factors. Some cases may develop as a postinfectious mononeuritis (e.g., following a viral flu). Patching one eye or applying a temporary prism will provide relief of diplopia until the palsy resolves. If recovery is incomplete, eye muscle surgery can nearly always realign the eyes, at least in primary position. A patient with an abducens palsy that fails to improve should be reevaluated for an occult etiology (e.g., chordoma, carcinomatous meningitis, carotid cavernous fistula, myasthenia gravis).

Multiple ocular motor nerve palsies should not be attributed to spontaneous microvascular events affecting more than one cranial nerve at a time. This remarkable coincidence does occur, especially in diabetic patients, but the diagnosis is made only in retrospect after exhausting all other diagnostic alternatives. Neuroimaging should focus on the cavernous sinus, superior orbital fissure, and orbital apex, where all three ocular motor nerves are in close proximity. In the diabetic or compromised host, fungal infection (*Aspergillus*, Mucorales, *Cryptococcus*) is a frequent cause of multiple nerve palsies. In the patient with systemic malignancy, carcinomatous meningitis is a likely diagnosis. Cytologic examination may be negative despite repeated sampling of the cerebrospinal fluid. The cancer-associated Eaton-Lambert myasthenic syndrome can also produce ophthalmoplegia. Giant cell (temporal) arteritis occasionally manifests as diplopia from ischemic palsies of extraocular muscles. Fisher's syndrome, an ocular variant of Guillain-Barré, can produce ophthalmoplegia with areflexia and ataxia. Often the ataxia is mild, and the areflexia is overlooked because the physician's attention is focused upon the eyes.

Supranuclear disorders of gaze are often mistaken for multiple ocular motor nerve palsies. For example, Wernicke's encephalopathy can produce nystagmus and a partial deficit of horizontal and vertical gaze that mimics a combined abducens and oculomotor nerve palsy. The disorder occurs in malnourished or alcoholic patients and can be reversed by giving thiamine. Infarct, hemorrhage, tumor, multiple sclerosis, encephalitis, vasculitis, and Whipple's disease are other important causes of supranuclear gaze palsy.

The *frontal eye field* of the cerebral cortex is involved in generation of saccades to the contralateral side. After hemispheric stroke, the eyes usually deviate towards the lesioned side because of the unopposed action of the frontal eye field in the normal hemisphere. With time, this deficit resolves. Seizures generally have the opposite effect: the eyes deviate conjugately away from the irritative focus. *Parietal lesions* disrupt smooth pursuit of targets moving toward the side of the lesion. Bilateral parietal lesions produce Balint's syndrome, characterized by impaired eye-hand coordination (optic ataxia), difficulty initiating voluntary eye movements (ocular apraxia), and visuospatial disorientation (simultanagnosia).

Descending cortical inputs mediating *horizontal gaze* ultimately converge at the level of the pons. Neurons in the paramedian pontine reticular formation are responsible for controlling conjugate gaze toward the same side. They project directly to the ipsilateral abducens nucleus. A lesion of either the paramedian pontine reticular formation or the abducens nucleus causes an ipsilateral conjugate gaze palsy. Lesions at either locus produce nearly identical clinical syndromes, with the following exception: vestibular stimulation (oculocephalic maneuver or caloric) will succeed in driving the eyes conjugately to the side in a patient with a lesion of the paramedian pontine reticular formation, but not in a patient with a lesion of the abducens nucleus.

Internuclear ophthalmoplegia results from damage to the medial longitudinal fasciculus ascending from the abducens nucleus in the pons to the oculomotor nucleus in the midbrain (hence, "internuclear"). Damage to fibers carrying the conjugate signal from abducens interneurons to the contralateral medial rectus motoneurons results in a failure of adduction on attempted lateral gaze. For example, a patient with a left internuclear ophthalmoplegia will have slowed or absent adducting movements of the left eye. A patient with bilateral injury to the medial longitudinal fasciculus will have bilateral internuclear ophthalmoplegia. Multiple sclerosis is the most common cause, although tumor, stroke, trauma, or any brainstem process may be responsible. One-and-a half syndrome is due to a combined lesion of the medial longitudinal fasciculus and the abducens nucleus on the same side. The patient's only horizontal eye movement is abduction of the eye on the other side.

Vertical gaze is controlled at the level of the midbrain. The neuronal circuits affected in disorders of vertical gaze are not well elucidated, but lesions of the rostral interstitial nucleus of the medial longitudinal fasciculus and the interstitial nucleus of Cajal cause supranuclear paresis of upgaze, downgaze, or all vertical eye movements. Distal basilar artery ischemia is the most common etiology. *Skew deviation* refers to a vertical misalignment of the eyes, usually constant in all positions of gaze. The finding has poor localizing value because skew deviation has been reported after lesions in widespread regions of the brainstem and cerebellum.

Parinaud's syndrome (dorsal midbrain syndrome) is a distinct supranuclear vertical gaze disorder from damage to the posterior commissure. It is a classic sign of hydrocephalus from aqueductal stenosis. Pineal region tumors (germinoma, pineoblastoma), cysticercosis, and stroke also cause Parinaud's syndrome. Features include loss of upgaze (and sometimes downgaze), convergence-retraction nystagmus on attempted upgaze, downwards ocular deviation (setting sun sign), lid retraction (Collier's sign), skew deviation, pseudoabducens palsy, and light-near dissociation of the pupils. Disorders of vertical gaze, especially downwards saccades, are an early feature of progressive supranuclear palsy. Smooth pursuit is affected later in the course of the disease. Parkinson's disease, Huntington's chorea, and olivopontocerebellar degeneration can also affect vertical gaze.

Nystagmus is a rhythmical oscillation of the eyes, occurring normally from vestibular and optokinetic stimulation or abnormally in a wide variety of diseases. Blindness from anterior visual pathway disease in early life causes a complex, searching nystagmus with irregular pendular (sinusoidal) and jerk features. This nystagmus is commonly referred to as *congenital nystagmus*, a poor term, given that it is acquired often in early childhood. Sometimes it develops in a perfectly normal child.

Jerk nystagmus is characterized by a slow drift off the target, followed by a fast corrective saccade. By convention, the nystagmus is named after the quick phase. Jerk nystagmus can be downbeat, upbeat, horizontal (left or right), and torsional. The pattern of nystagmus may vary with gaze position. Some patients will be oblivious to their nystagmus. Others will complain of a subjective, to-and-fro movement of the environment (oscillopsia), corresponding to their nystagmus. Fine nystagmus may be difficult to see upon gross examination of the eyes. Observation of nystagmoid movements of the optic disc on ophthalmoscopy is a sensitive way to detect subtle degrees of nystagmus. The slit lamp is also useful.

Gaze-evoked nystagmus is the most common form of jerk nystagmus. When the eyes are held eccentrically in the orbits, they have a natural tendency to drift back to primary position. The subject compensates by making a corrective saccade to maintain the deviated eye position. Many normal patients have mild gaze-evoked nystagmus. Exaggerated gaze-evoked nystagmus can be induced by drugs (sedatives, anticonvulsants, alcohol), muscle paresis, myasthenia, demyelinating disease, and cerebellopontine angle, brainstem, and cerebellar lesions.

Vestibular nystagmus results from dysfunction of the labyrinth (Ménière's disease), vestibular nerve, or vestibular nucleus in the brainstem. Peripheral vestibular nystagmus often occurs in discrete attacks, with symptoms of nausea and vertigo. There may be associated tinnitus and hearing loss. Sudden shifts in head position may provoke or exacerbate symptoms.

Downbeat nystagmus occurs from lesions near the craniocervical junction (Chiari malformation, basilar invagination). It has also been reported in brainstem or cerebellar stroke, lithium or anticonvulsant intoxication, and multiple sclerosis. *Upbeat nystagmus* is associated with damage to the pontine tegmentum, from stroke, demyelination, or tumor.

Opsoclonus is a rare, dramatic disorder of eye movements consisting of bursts of consecutive saccades (saccadomania). When the saccades are confined to the horizontal plane, the term *ocular flutter* is preferred. It is a sign of neuroblastoma, encephalitis, trauma, or paraneoplastic syndrome. It has been reported as a benign, transient phenomenon in otherwise healthy patients, probably as a consequence of a mild, occult viral encephalitis.

BIBLIOGRAPHY

ALBERT DM, JAKOBIEC FA (eds): *Principles and Practice of Ophthalmology*. Philadelphia, Saunders, 1994

BECK RW et al: A randomized controlled trial of corticosteroids in the treatment of acute optic neuritis. N Engl J Med 326:581, 1992

——— et al: The effect of corticosteroids for acute optic neuritis on the subsequent development of multiple sclerosis. N Engl J Med 329:1764, 1993

BURDE RM et al: *Clinical Decisions in Neuro-ophthalmology*, 2d ed. St. Louis, Mosby, 1992

DUANE T (ed): *Clinical Ophthalmology*. Philadelphia, Lippincott, 1994

EXECUTIVE COMMITTEE FOR THE ASYMPTOMATIC CAROTID ATHEROSCLEROSIS STUDY: Endarterectomy for asymptomatic carotid artery stenosis. JAMA 273:1421, 1995

GASS JD: *Stereoscopic Atlas of Macular Diseases*, 4th ed. St. Louis, Mosby, 1996

GOLD DH, WEINGEIST TA (eds): *The Eye in Systemic Disease*. Philadelphia, Lippincott, 1990

LEIGH RJ, ZEE DS: *The Neurology of Eye Movements*, 2d ed. Philadelphia, Davis, 1991

MILLER NR: *Walsh and Hoyt's Clinical Neuroophthalmology*, 4th ed. Baltimore, Williams & Wilkins, 1995

NATHAN J et al: Molecular genetics of inherited variation in human color vision. Science 232:203, 1986

SINGH G: A mitochondrial DNA mutation as a cause of Leber's hereditary optic neuropathy. N Engl J Med 320:1300, 1989

SMOLIN G, THOFT RA (eds): *The Cornea*, 3d ed. Boston, Little, Brown, 1994

VAUGHN D et al: *General Ophthalmology*, 14th ed. Norwalk, Appleton & Lange, 1995

DISORDERS OF SMELL, TASTE, AND HEARING

SMELL

The sense of smell determines the flavor and palatability of food and drink. It serves along with the trigeminal system as a monitor of inhaled chemicals, including dangerous substances such as natural gas, smoke, and air pollutants. Although qualitative sensations of smell are subserved by the olfactory neuroepithelium, many substances are capable of producing somatic sensations of coolness, warmth, and irritation through the trigeminal, glossopharyngeal, and vagal afferents in the nose, oral cavity, tongue, pharynx, and larynx. The sense of smell should be considered as one of several chemosensory systems, since most chemical substances initiate olfactory, trigeminal, and taste perceptions.

The *olfactory neuroepithelium* is located in the superior part of the nasal cavities. It contains an orderly arrangement of bipolar olfactory receptor cells, microvillar cells, sustentacular cells, and basal cells. The dendritic process of the bipolar cell has a bulb-shaped knob or vesicle that projects into the mucous layer and bears six to eight cilia. The receptor sites for odorant molecules are located on the cilia. The microvillar cells are located adjacent to the receptor cells on the surface of the neuroepithelium. The sustentacular cells, unlike their counterparts in the respiratory epithelium, are not specialized to secrete mucus. Their function is unknown. The basal cells are progenitors of other cell types in the olfactory neuroepithelium, including the bipolar receptor cells. There is a regular turnover of the bipolar receptor cells, which function as the primary sensory neurons. In addition, with injury to the cell body or its axon, the receptor cell is replaced by a differentiated basal cell which reestablishes a central neural connection. *Hence these primary sensory neurons are unique among sensory systems in that they are regularly replaced and regenerate after injury.*

The unmyelinated axons of the receptor cells form the fila of the olfactory nerve, pass through the cribriform plate, and terminate within spherical masses of neuropil, termed *glomeruli*, in the olfactory bulb. The glomeruli are the focus of a high degree of convergence of information, since many more fibers enter than leave them. The main second-order neurons are the mitral cells. The primary dendrite of each mitral cell extends into a single glomerulus. Axons of the mitral cells project along with the axons of adjacent tufted cells to the limbic system, including the anterior olfactory nucleus, the prepiriform cortex, the periamygdaloid cortex, the olfactory tubercle, the nucleus of the lateral olfactory tract, and the corticomedial nucleus of the amygdala. Cognitive awareness of smell requires stimulation of the prepiriform cortex or the amygdaloid nuclei.

Odorants are absorbed into the mucus overlying the olfactory neuroepithelium, diffuse to the cilia, and reversibly bind to membrane receptor sites. The process causes conformational changes in the receptor proteins which induce a chain of biochemical events that results in generation of action potentials in the primary neurons. Transduction depends on the activation of G protein–coupled second messengers. Intensity appears to be coded by the amount of firing in the afferent neurons. Indeed, a clear relationship exists in humans between psychophysical measures of intensity and the magnitude of the evoked potential from the olfactory neuroepithelium. The discovery of a large family of receptor genes suggests that there may be specific receptors for each odorant. A single receptor neuron expresses only one receptor subtype of the multigene family. All receptor neurons expressing a given receptor subtype project their axons to one or two glomeruli in the olfactory bulb.

DISORDERS OF THE SENSE OF SMELL
Disorders of the sense of smell are caused by conditions that interfere with the access of the odorant to the olfactory neuroepithelium (transport loss), injure the receptor region (sensory loss), or damage central olfactory pathways (neural loss).

Transport olfactory loss can result from swollen nasal mucous membrane in acute viral upper respiratory infections, bacterial rhinitis and sinusitis, allergic rhinitis, and structural changes in the nasal cavity such as deviations of the nasal septum, polyps, and neoplasms. It is also likely that abnormalities of mucus secretion in which the olfactory cilia are immersed could result in a loss of olfactory sensitivity.

Sensory olfactory losses are caused by destruction of the olfactory neuroepithelium by viral infections, neoplasms, the inhalation of toxic chemicals, drugs that affect cell turnover, and radiation therapy to the head. *Neural olfactory losses* occur in head trauma, with or without fracture of the base of the anterior cranial fossa or cribriform plate area; Parkinson's disease, Alzheimer's disease, Korsakoff's psychosis, and vitamin B_{12} deficiency; neoplasms of the anterior cranial fossa; neurosurgical procedures; administration of neurotoxic agents (e.g., ethanol, amphetamines, topical cocaine, aminoglycosides, tetracycline, cigarette smoke); and in some congenital disorders such as Kallmann's syndrome. Other endocrine disorders, including Cushing's syndrome, hypothyroidism, and diabetes mellitus, can affect smell perception.

From the psychophysical point of view, disorders of the sense of smell may be categorized by either the patient's complaint or the objective sensory measurements as *total anosmia* (general anosmia)—inability to detect any qualitative olfactory sensations; *partial anosmia*—ability to detect some, but not all, qualitative olfactory sensations; *specific anosmia*—loss of ability to appreciate only one or a very limited number of odorants; *total hyposmia* (general hyposmia)—decreased sensitivity to all odorants; *partial hyposmia*—decreased sensitivity to some odorants; *dysosmia* (cacosmia or paraosmia)—distortion in the perception of an odor, i.e., the perception of an unpleasant odor when a pleasant odorant is being presented or the perception of an odor when there is no odorant in the environment; *total hyperosmia* (general hyperosmia)—increased sensitivity to all odorants; *partial hyperosmia*—increased sensitivity to some odorants; and *agnosia*—inability to classify, contrast, or identify odor sensations verbally, even though the ability to distinguish between odorants or to recognize them may be normal.

Clinical Evaluation
The history of the onset and development of the disorder of the sense of smell may be of paramount importance in making an etiologic diagnosis. Unilateral anosmia is rarely a complaint. Only by separate testing of smell in each nasal cavity can it be recognized. Bilateral anosmia, on the other hand, does bring patients to medical attention. Anosmic patients usually complain of a loss of the sense of taste even though their taste thresholds may be within normal limits. In actuality, they are complaining of a loss of flavor detection, which is mainly an olfactory function. Flavor appreciation depends on the olfactory detection of volatile substances in food and beverages as well as the sense of taste. The physical examination should include a complete examination of the ears, upper respiratory tract, and head and neck. A neurologic examination emphasizing the cranial nerves is essential. Computed tomography (CT) scans of the head with enhancement are required to rule out neoplasms of the anterior cranial fossa, unsuspected fractures of the anterior cranial fossa, paranasal sinusitis, and neoplasms of the nasal cavity and paranasal sinuses.

The sensory evaluation of olfactory function is necessary for corroboration of the patient's complaint, evaluation of the efficacy of treatment, and determination of the degree of permanent impairment. The first step in the sensory evaluation is to determine the degree to which qualitative sensations are present. For this assessment, a smell identification test is used that consists of a 40-item, forced choice, microencapsulated odor, scratch-and-sniff paradigm. For example, one of the items reads, "This odor smells most like (a) chocolate, (b) banana, (c) onion, or (d) fruit punch," and the patient is instructed to answer one of the alternatives. The test is highly reliable (short-term test-retest reliability $r = 0.95$) and is sensitive to age and sex differences (Fig. 29-1). It is an accurate quantitative determination of the relative degree of olfactory deficit. Persons with a total loss of smell function score in the range of 7 to 19 out of 40. The average score for total anosmics is slightly higher than that expected on the basis of chance because of the inclusion of some odorants that act by trigeminal stimulation.

The second step is to establish a detection threshold for the odorant phenyl ethyl alcohol, using a graduated stimulus. Sensitivity for each side of the nose is determined with a detection threshold for phenyl ethyl methyl ethyl carbinol. Nasal resistance is measured with anterior rhinomanometry for each side of the nose.

Techniques have been developed to biopsy the olfactory neuroepithelium, but in view of the widespread degeneration of the olfactory neuroepithelium and intercalation of respiratory epithelium in the olfactory area of adults with no apparent olfactory dysfunction, biopsy material must be interpreted cautiously.

Differential Diagnosis   At the present time, there are no psychophysical methods to differentiate sensory from neural olfactory losses. Fortunately, the history of the disease provides important clues to the cause. The leading causes of olfactory disorders are head trauma and viral infections. Head trauma is a more frequent cause of anosmia in children and young adults, and viral infections are more important causes of anosmia in older adults.

Cranial trauma is followed by uni- or bilateral impairment of smell in 5 to 10 percent of cases. Frontal injuries and fractures disrupt the cribriform plate and olfactory axons that perforate it. Sometimes there is an associated cerebrospinal fluid (CSF) rhinorrhea resulting from a tearing of the dura overlying the cribriform plate and paranasal sinuses. Anosmia also may follow blows to the occiput. Once traumatic anosmia develops, it is usually permanent; only about 10 percent of patients ever improve or recover. Perversion of the sense of smell may occur as a phase in the recovery process.

Viral infections destroy the olfactory neuroepithelium, and it is replaced by respiratory epithelium. Congenital anosmias are rare but important. Kallmann's syndrome is a neuronal migration defect for which the X-linked gene (KAL) has been cloned. It is characterized by congenital anosmia and hypogonadotropic hypogonadism (see Chap. 328). The hypothalamic and olfactory bulb defects result from failure of migration from the olfactory placode of olfactory receptor neurons and neurons synthesizing gonadotropin-releasing hormone. Anosmia also can occur in albinos. The receptor cells are present but are hypoplastic, lack cilia, and do not project above the surrounding supporting cells.

Meningioma of the inferior frontal region is the most frequent neoplastic cause of anosmia; rarely, anosmia can occur with glioma of the frontal lobe. Occasionally, pituitary adenomas, craniopharyngiomas, suprasellar meningiomas, and aneurysms of the anterior part of the circle of Willis extend forward and damage olfactory structures. These tumors and hamartomas also may induce seizures with olfactory hallucinations, indicating involvement of the uncus of the temporal lobe.

Dysosmia, subjective distortions of olfactory perception, may occur with intranasal disease that partially impairs smell or may represent a phase in the recovery from a neurogenic anosmia. Most dysosmic disorders consist of disagreeable or foul odors, and they may be accompanied by distortions of taste. Dysosmia is associated with depression.

℞ TREATMENT

Therapy for patients with transport olfactory losses due to allergic rhinitis, bacterial rhinitis and sinusitis, polyps, neoplasms, and structural abnormalities of the nasal cavities can be undertaken rationally and with a high chance of improvement. Allergy management, antibiotic therapy, topical and systemic glucocorticoid therapy, and operations for nasal polyps, deviation of the nasal septum, and chronic hyperplastic sinusitis are frequently effective in restoring the sense of smell.

There is no treatment with demonstrated efficacy for sensorineural olfactory losses. Fortunately, spontaneous recovery often occurs. Zinc and vitamin therapy are advocated by some. Profound zinc deficiency can undoubtedly result in losses and distortion of the sense of smell, but it is not a clinical problem except in very limited geographic areas. Vitamin therapy has mainly been in the form of vitamin A. The epithelial degeneration associated with vitamin A deficiency can cause anosmia, but vitamin A deficiency is not a common clinical problem in the United States.

TASTE

Many patients with a loss of olfactory sensitivity also complain of a loss of the sense of taste. On psychophysical testing, most of these patients have normal detection thresholds for taste. Disturbances of the sense of taste are far less frequent than disturbances of the sense of smell.

The taste receptor cells are located in the taste buds, spherical groups of cells arranged like the segments of a citrus fruit. At the surface, the taste bud has a pore into which microvilli of the receptor cells project. Taste buds have a similar appearance wherever they are located. Unlike the olfactory system, the receptor cell is not the primary neuron. Instead, gustatory afferent nerve fibers contact individual taste receptor cells. Transduction depends on activation of G protein–coupled second messengers but differs in details for each taste quality.

The sense of taste is mediated through the facial, glossopharyngeal, and vagal nerves. The gustatory system consists of at least five receptor populations. Taste buds are located in the foliate papillae along the lateral margin of the tongue, in the fungiform papillae throughout the dorsum of the tongue, in the circumvallate papillae at the junction of the dorsum and the base of the tongue, and in the palate, epiglottis, larynx, and esophagus. The chorda tympani branch of the facial nerve subserves taste from the anterior two-thirds of the tongue. The posterior third of the tongue is supplied by the lingual branch of the glossopharyngeal nerve. Afferents from the palate travel with the greater superficial petrosal nerve to the geniculate ganglion and thence via the facial nerve to the brainstem. The internal branch of the superior laryngeal nerve of the vagus nerve contains the taste afferents from the larynx including the epiglottis and esophagus.

The central connections of the nerves terminate in the brainstem in the nucleus of the tractus solitarius. The fibers of the chorda tympani and greater superficial petrosal nerves go to the cephalic portion of the nucleus. The glossopharyngeal gustatory fibers go to the middle, and the superior laryngeal nerve fibers go to the caudal portion of the nucleus. The central pathway from the nucleus of the tractus solitarius projects to the ipsilateral parabrachial nuclei of the pons. Two divergent pathways project from the parabrachial nuclei. One ascends to the gustatory relay in the dorsal thalamus, synapses, and continues to the

FIGURE 29-1   Smell identification test. Scores for a group of male and female subjects 5 to 99 years in age are shown. *(Reprinted with permission from RL Doty et al. Copyright 1984 by the AAAS.)*

cortex of the insula. There is also evidence for a direct pathway from the parabrachial nuclei to the cortex. (Olfaction and gustation appear to be unique among sensory systems in that at least some fibers bypass the thalamus.) The other pathway from the parabrachial nuclei goes to the ventral forebrain, including the lateral hypothalamus, substantia innominata, central nucleus of the amygdala, and the stria terminalis.

Tastants gain access to the receptor cells through the taste pore. Four classes of taste are recognized: sweet, salt, sour, and bitter. Individual gustatory afferent fibers almost always respond to a number of different chemicals. Response patterns of gustatory afferent axons can be grouped into classes based on the stimulus chemical that produces the largest response. For example, for sucrose–best response neurons, the second-best stimulus is almost always sodium chloride. The fact that individual gustatory afferent fibers respond to a large number of different chemicals led to the *across-fiber-pattern* theory of gustatory coding, while the best-stimulus analysis led to the concept of *labeled* afferents. It appears that labeled fibers are important for establishing gross quality, but the across-fiber pattern within a best-stimulus category, and perhaps among categories, is needed for discriminating chemicals within qualities. For example, sweetness may be carried by sucrose-best neurons, but the differentiation of sucrose and fructose may require a comparison of the relative activity among sucrose-best, salt-best, and quinine-best neurons. As with olfaction and other sensory systems, intensity appears to be encoded by the quantity of neural activity.

DISORDERS OF THE SENSE OF TASTE   Disorders of the sense of taste are caused by conditions that interfere with the access of the tastant to the receptor cells in the taste bud (transport loss), injure receptor cells (sensory loss), or damage gustatory afferent nerves and central gustatory pathways (neural loss).

Transport gustatory losses result from xerostomia due to many causes, including Sjögren's syndrome, heavy-metal intoxication, and bacterial colonization of the taste pore. The salivary milieu of the receptors may prove to be important to diverse causes of gustatory loss.

Sensory gustatory losses are caused by inflammatory and degenerative diseases in the oral cavity; a vast number of drugs, particularly those that interfere with cell turnover such as antithyroid and antineoplastic agents; radiation therapy to the oral cavity and pharynx; viral infections; endocrine disorders; neoplasms; and aging.

Neural gustatory losses occur with neoplasms, trauma, and operations in which the gustatory afferents are injured. Taste buds degenerate when their gustatory afferents are transected but remain when their somatosensory afferents are severed.

Clinical Manifestations   From the psychophysical point of view, disturbances of the sense of taste may be categorized by either the patient's complaint or the objective sensory measurements as *total ageusia*—inability to detect the qualities of sweet, salt, bitter, or sour; *partial ageusia*—ability to detect some of but not all the qualitative gustatory sensations; *specific ageusia*—inability to detect the taste quality of certain substances; *total hypogeusia*—decreased sensitivity to all tastants; *partial hypogeusia*—decreased sensitivity to some tastants; and *dysgeusia*—distortion in the perception of a tastant, i.e., the perception of the wrong quality when a tastant is presented or the perception of a taste when there has been no tastant ingested. Confusions of sour and bitter are common and, at times, may be semantic misunderstandings. Frequently, however, they have physiologic or pathophysiologic bases.

It may be possible to differentiate between the loss of flavor recognition in patients with olfactory losses who complain of a loss of taste as well as smell by asking if they are able to taste sweetness in sodas, saltiness in potato chips, etc.

Patients who complain of loss of taste should be evaluated psychophysically for gustatory function in addition to being evaluated for olfactory function. The first step is to perform suprathreshold whole-mouth taste testing for quality, intensity, and pleasantness perception with sucrose, citric acid, caffeine, and sodium chloride. In the quantification of the sense of taste, detection thresholds are obtained by applying graduated dilutions to the tongue quadrants or by whole-mouth sips. Finally, suprathreshold magnitude estimation may be used

to shed further light on the patient's complaint. Electric taste testing (*electrogustometry*) is used clinically to identify taste deficits in specific quadrants of the tongue.

Biopsy of the foliate or fungiform papillae for histopathologic study of taste buds remains experimental but holds promise of shedding light on the categorization of taste disorders.

Differential Diagnosis   As with olfaction, psychophysical methods for differentiating transport, sensory, and neural gustatory losses are not available. Once there is objective evidence of a disorder of taste, it is important to establish, as is done in other neurologic deficits, an anatomic diagnosis before proceeding to an etiologic diagnosis. The history of the disease often provides important clues to the cause. For example, absence of taste on the anterior two-thirds of the tongue associated with a facial paralysis indicates that the lesion is proximal to the point of junction of the chorda tympani branch with the facial nerve in the mastoid.

 TREATMENT

Therapy for gustatory losses remains limited. Artificial saliva benefits some patients with a disturbed salivary milieu. Treatment for bacterial and fungal infections of the oral cavity is appropriate and may be helpful. Withdrawal of drugs affecting cell turnover is usually helpful if the patient's general condition permits. Zinc and vitamin therapy for gustatory losses is advocated by some but lacks demonstrated efficacy. No therapeutic strategies exist for the sensorineural disorders of taste.

HEARING

Hearing occurs by air conduction and bone conduction. In air conduction, sound waves reach the ear by propagation in air, enter the external auditory canal, and set the tympanic membrane in motion, which in turn moves the malleus, incus, and stapes. Movement of the footplate of the stapes causes pressure changes in the fluid-filled inner ear eliciting a traveling wave in the basilar membrane of the cochlea. Hearing by bone conduction occurs when the sounding source, in contact with the head, results in vibration of the bones of the skull, including the temporal bone, producing a traveling wave in the basilar membrane. In either case, the traveling wave moves from the base to the apex of the cochlea. Hairs (stereocilia) of the hair cells of the organ of Corti, which rests on the basilar membrane, are in contact with the tectorial membrane and are deformed by the traveling wave. A point of maximal displacement of the basilar membrane determined by the frequency of the stimulating tone occurs with each traveling wave. High-frequency tones cause maximal displacement of the basilar membrane near the base of the cochlea. As the frequency of the stimulating tone decreases, the point of maximal displacement moves toward the apex of the cochlea.

The inner and outer hair cells of the organ of Corti have different innervation patterns, but both are mechanoreceptors. The afferent innervation relates principally to the inner hair cells, and the efferent innervation relates principally to outer hair cells. The outer hair cells have an internal organization that is in certain respects similar to muscle cells. Not only does the organ of Corti respond to acoustic stimulation, it also produces acoustic energy that can be detected in the external auditory canal with sensitive microphones. These otoacoustic emissions (OAE) occur spontaneously and can be evoked by acoustic stimulation. The sources of this acoustic energy are the outer hair cells.

Motility of outer hair cells occurs with mechanical (acoustical) and electrical stimulation, iontophoretically applied acetylcholine, and changes in their internal and external ionic milieu and is modulated by stimulation of the efferent olivocochlear bundle.

The outer hair cells are capable of slow and fast motility. Slow elongation and contraction occur with increased intracellular calcium in the presence of ATP, the application of acetylcholine, and changes in the ionic environment (increased potassium, which depolarizes the cell), while rapid motility occurs with mechanical (acoustic) and direct-current electrical stimulation. The electrokinetic membrane is located in the outer or lateral wall of the outer hair cell. Fast contractile activity occurs with changes in the membrane potential. The electromotility is driven by a novel and perhaps unique membrane-based force generator that can achieve audible frequencies.

The motility of the outer hair cells alters the micromechanics of the inner hair cells and thereby satisfies the long-sought cochlear amplifier required to explain the exquisite sensitivity and frequency selectivity of the cochlea.

A resting direct-current potential, the *endocochlear potential*, exists in the scala media and at the stereocilia end of the hair cells. It is generated by the stria vascularis. It is present whether there is acoustic stimulation or not. It has a magnitude of 80 mV, not unlike the intracellular potential, but its polarity is positive within the endolymph relative to the perilymph. It increases the potential differential at the stereocilia end of the hair cell, which undoubtedly is of importance in transduction.

As the traveling wave moves along the basilar membrane, the stereocilia are deformed and several receptor potentials are produced: the cochlear microphonic and the positive and negative summating potentials. It is thought that these receptor potentials arise at the apical end of the stereocilia. It may be that the summating potentials are generated largely by the inner hair cells and the cochlear microphonic potential is generated by the outer hair cells. The summating potential represents a direct-current shift that approximates the "envelope" of the acoustical stimulus. The cochlear microphonic potential is an alternating-current response that faithfully represents the frequency and intensity of the stimulating tone.

The current concept of cochlear transduction is that displacement of the tips of the stereocilia cause tip links between stereocilia to allow potassium to flow into the cell, resulting in its depolarization. The potassium causes calcium channels near the base to open and allow calcium to enter the cell. The calcium ions stimulate transmitter release. The action potential in the eighth nerve occurs 0.5 ms after the onset of the cochlear microphonic potential. The neurotransmitter at the hair cell and cochlear nerve dendrite interface is thought to be glutamate. Each of the cochlear nerve neurons can be activated at a frequency and intensity specific for that cell. This phenomenon of the characteristic or best frequency occurs at each point of the central auditory pathway: dorsal and ventral cochlear nuclei, trapezoid body, superior olivary complex, lateral lemniscus, inferior colliculus, medial geniculate body, and auditory cortex. At low frequencies, individual auditory nerve fibers can respond more or less synchronously with the stimulating tone. At higher frequencies, phase-locking occurs so that neurons take turns in responding to particular phases of the cycle of the sound wave. Intensity is encoded by the amount of neural activity in individual neurons, the number of neurons that are active, and the specific neurons that are activated.

DISORDERS OF THE SENSE OF HEARING A loss of hearing can result from lesions in the external auditory canal, middle ear, inner ear, or central auditory pathways. Lesions in the external auditory canal or middle ear cause conductive hearing losses, while lesions in the inner ear or eighth nerve cause sensorineural hearing losses.

Conductive hearing losses result from obstruction of the external auditory canal by cerumen, debris, and foreign bodies; swelling of the lining of the canal; stenosis and neoplasms of the canal; perforations of the tympanic membrane, as in chronic otitis media; disruption of the ossicular chain, as occurs with necrosis of the long process of the incus in trauma or infection; fixation of the ossicles, as in otosclerosis; and fluid, scarring, or neoplasms in the middle ear. *Sensory hearing losses* are due principally to damage to the hair cells of the organ of Corti caused by intense noise, viral infections, ototoxic drugs, fractures of the temporal bone, meningitis, cochlear otosclerosis, Ménière's disease, and aging. Neural hearing losses are due mainly to cerebellar

angle tumors such as vestibular schwannomas (acoustic neuromas) but also may result from any neoplastic, vascular, demyelinating, infectious, or degenerative disease or trauma affecting the central auditory pathways.

Clinical Evaluation of Hearing The physical examination should evaluate the external ear canal and tympanic membrane. Careful inspection of the nose, nasopharynx, and upper respiratory tract is indicated. The other cranial nerves should be carefully evaluated. Conductive and sensorineural hearing losses can be differentiated by comparing the threshold of hearing by air conduction with that elicited by bone conduction. Testing the hearing by air conduction is accomplished by presenting the stimulus in air. Hearing by air conduction is affected by the patency of the external auditory canal, the efficiency of the middle ear, and the integrity of the inner ear, eighth nerve, and central auditory pathways. Testing the hearing by bone conduction is accomplished by placing the stem of a vibrating tuning fork or an oscillator of an audiometer in contact with the head. Hearing by bone conduction bypasses the external auditory canal and middle ear and tests the integrity of the inner ear, eighth nerve, and central auditory pathways. If air-conduction thresholds are elevated and bone-conduction thresholds are in the normal range, the lesion causing hearing loss is in the external auditory canal or middle ear. If both air-conduction and bone-conduction thresholds are elevated, the lesion is in the inner ear, eighth nerve, or central auditory pathways. Of course, conductive and sensorineural hearing losses can coexist, in which case both the air-conduction and bone-conduction thresholds are elevated, but in this case, air-conduction thresholds are elevated more than bone-conduction thresholds.

The Weber and Rinne tuning fork tests are used to differentiate conductive from sensorineural hearing losses. The Weber tuning fork test may be performed with a 256- or 512-Hz fork. The Rinne tuning fork test is most sensitive in detecting mild conductive hearing losses if a 256-Hz fork is used. Weber's test is performed by placing the stem of a vibrating tuning fork on the head in the midline and asking the patient whether the tone is heard in both ears or better in one ear than in the other. With a unilateral conductive hearing loss, the tone is perceived in the affected ear. With a unilateral sensorineural hearing loss, the tone is perceived in the unaffected ear. Rinne's test compares the ability to hear by air conduction with the ability to hear by bone conduction. The tines of a vibrating tuning fork are held near the opening of the external auditory canal, and then the stem is placed on the mastoid process. The patient is asked to indicate whether the tone is louder by air conduction or bone conduction. Normally, a tone is heard louder by air conduction than by bone conduction. With a conductive hearing loss, the bone-conduction stimulus is perceived as louder than the air-conduction stimulus. With sensorineural hearing losses, both air-conduction and bone-conduction perceptions are reduced, but the air-conduction stimulus is perceived as louder, as it is in normal hearing. The combined information from the Weber and Rinne tests permits a tentative conclusion as to whether a conductive or sensorineural hearing loss is present.

Laboratory Assessment of Hearing Quantification of hearing loss is obtained with an audiometer, an electronic device that allows the presentation of specific frequencies at specific intensities to each ear by either air or bone conduction. The testing is done in a sound-attenuated chamber, and masking, usually with broad-spectrum noise, is presented to the nontest ear so that responses are based on perception from the ear under test. Frequencies from 250 to 8000 Hz are used in clinical testing. The responses are measured in decibels. A decibel (dB) is equal to 10 times the logarithm of the ratio of the acoustic power required to achieve threshold in the patient to the acoustic power required to achieve threshold in a normal hearing person. An *audiogram* is a plot of intensity in decibels required to achieve threshold versus frequency.

The audiometric pattern of hearing loss is often of diagnostic value. Conductive hearing losses usually have a fairly equal threshold elevation for each frequency. Conductive hearing losses with a large mass component, as is often seen in middle-ear effusions, have a greater elevation of thresholds in the higher frequencies. Conductive hearing losses with a large stiffness component, as in fixation of the footplate of the stapes in early otosclerosis, have a greater elevation of thresholds in the lower frequencies. In general, sensorineural hearing losses tend to have a greater threshold elevation at each higher frequency. Interesting exceptions to this generalization are noise-induced hearing loss, in which the loss at 4000 Hz is greater than it is at higher frequencies, and in Ménière's disease, particularly in the early stages of the disease, where thresholds are elevated more in lower than in higher frequencies.

Speech audiometry provides essential additional information. The *spondee threshold* is defined as the intensity at which speech is recognized as a meaningful symbol and is obtained by presenting through an audiometer two-syllable words with an equal accent on each syllable. The intensity at which the patient can repeat 50 percent of the words correctly is the spondee threshold and usually approximates the average threshold at the speech frequencies (500, 1000, and 2000 Hz). Once the spondee threshold is determined, the discrimination, or word-recognition ability, is tested by presenting one-syllable words at 25 to 40 dB above the spondee threshold. The words are phonetically balanced (PB) in that the phonemes (speech sounds) occur in the list of words at the same frequency that they occur in ordinary conversational English. An individual with normal hearing can repeat 90 to 100 percent of the PB words correctly. Likewise, individuals with a conductive hearing loss do well in discrimination testing. On the other hand, patients with a sensorineural hearing loss have a loss of discrimination attributable to the loss of peripheral analysis of sound in the inner ear or eighth nerve. With a lesion in the inner ear, the discrimination is moderately affected, usually in the 50 to 80 percent range, while with neural lesions, the discrimination is severely affected, often in the 0 to 50 percent range.

The discrimination testing may then be done at higher intensities than 25 to 40 dB above the spondee threshold to determine the performance-intensity function. A deterioration in discrimination ability at higher intensities suggests a lesion in the eighth nerve or central auditory pathways.

Tympanometry measures the impedance of the middle ear to sound. A sounding source and microphone are introduced into the ear canal with an airtight seal. The amount of sound that is absorbed through the middle ear or reflected from the middle ear is measured at the microphone. In conductive hearing losses, more sound is reflected than in the normal middle ear. The pressure in the ear canal can be increased or decreased from atmospheric pressure. Normally, the middle ear is most compliant at atmospheric pressure. With a negative pressure in the middle ear, as with eustachian tube obstruction, the point of maximal compliance occurs with negative pressure in the ear canal. With discontinuity of the ossicular chain, no point of maximal compliance can be obtained. Tympanometry is particularly useful in the identification and diagnosis of middle-ear effusions in children.

During tympanometry, an intense tone (80 dB above the hearing threshold) elicits contraction of the stapedius muscle. The change in compliance of the middle ear with contraction of the stapedius muscle can be detected. The presence or absence of this *acoustic reflex* is important in the anatomic localization of facial nerve paralysis. The presence or absence of *acoustic reflex decay* helps differentiate sensory from neural hearing losses. In neural hearing loss, the reflex adapts or decays with time.

In order to evaluate a patient with a loss of hearing, the minimum audiologic assessment should include the measurement of pure tone air-conduction and bone-conduction thresholds, spondee threshold, discrimination score, performance-intensity function, OAE, tympanometry, acoustic reflexes, and acoustic-reflex decay. This information provides a comprehensive screening evaluation of the whole auditory system and allows one to determine whether further differentiation of a sensory (cochlear) from a neural (retrocochlear) hearing loss is indicated.

In addition to these tests, testing for recruitment, the short increment sensitivity index, tone decay, Békésy audiometry, and auditory brainstem evoked responses (ABR) help differentiate sensory from neural hearing losses. Of these, ABR is the most powerful means of differentiating the site of sensorineural hearing loss (see Chap. 361). In response to sound, five distinct waves can be recorded with computer averaging from scalp surface electrodes. Poor or absent waveforms, abnormal latency of waves, and abnormal interwave latency are evidence of lesions in the eighth nerve and brainstem. In addition, ABR is valuable in situations in which patients cannot or will not give reliable voluntary thresholds. It is also used to measure auditory function in neonates and young children and to monitor the integrity of the auditory nerve and brainstem in various clinical situations, including intraoperatively and in determination of brain death.

Otoacoustic emissions can be measured with sensitive microphones inserted into the external auditory canal in infants, children, and adults. The emissions may be spontaneous or evoked with sound stimulation. The presence of OAE indicates that the outer hair cells are intact and can be used as important evidence in distinguishing sensory from neural hearing losses. Otoacoustic emissions are particularly robust in infants.

The measurement of OAE can be done rapidly and with limited technical expertise in newborns. It is uncertain whether this technique or automated ABR will become the preferred method of screening neonates for hearing impairment. One strategy is to screen all neonates with OAE and to confirm hearing impairment with ABR. High-risk factors include a family history of hearing impairment, prenatal infection, prematurity, low birth weight, neonatal anoxia, a low Apgar score, neonatal jaundice, and neonatal infection. Unfortunately, ABR fails to identify 50 percent of infants with profound hearing impairment among high-risk infants. In the United States, the average age of identification of profound hearing impairment is 2½ years.

The natural acquisition and development of oral speech and language depend on hearing language. The critical period for language acquisition is the first 2 years of life. Therefore, the early identification of hearing impairment in infants is of the greatest importance so that amplification with a hearing aid and special education can commence within the first several months of life.

In addition to the universal screening of infants for hearing impairment, hearing should be assessed in all children before the first formal educational experience (preschool or kindergarten). Hearing also should be measured in the late teenage period when otosclerosis and noise-induced hearing loss begin to appear and in the sixth decade of life when presbycusis makes its appearance. Known causes of hearing impairment in addition to the risk factors already mentioned are meningitis, cytomegalovirus infections, head trauma, middle-ear infections and effusions, administration of ototoxic drugs (e.g., salicylates, quinine and its synthetic analogues, aminoglycoside antibiotics, loop diuretics such as furosemide and ethacrynic acid, and cancer chemotherapeutic agents such as *cis*-platinum), and noise exposure. At any time in life when one of these hearing risks is encountered, an audiologic assessment should be carried out.

Ten million Americans have noise-induced hearing loss, and 20 million are exposed to hazardous noise in their employment. Noise-induced hearing loss results from recreational as well as occupational activities and begins in adolescence, particularly among boys as they begin to engage in high-risk activities, such as wood and metal working with electrical equipment and target practice and hunting with small firearms. All internal-combustion and electric engines, including snow and leaf blowers, snowmobiles, outboard motors, and chain saws, require protection of the user with hearing protectors such as ear plugs or fluid-filled ear muffs. Virtually all noise-induced hearing loss is preventable through education, which should begin before the teenage years.

Programs of industrial conservation of hearing are required when the exposure over an 8-h period averages 85 dB on the A scale. Workers in such noisy environments can be protected with preemployment audiologic assessment, the mandatory use of hearing protectors, and annual audiologic assessments.

_____ *Approach to the Patient* _____

Clinical Assessment of a Complaint of Hearing Loss   In evaluating patients who complain of loss of hearing, associated symptoms of tinnitus, vertigo, difficulty with balance, earache, otorrhea, and aural fullness should be sought along with a careful reconstruction of the history of evolution of the hearing deficit. A sudden onset of unilateral hearing loss, with or without tinnitus, may represent a viral infection in the inner ear. Gradual progression in a hearing deficit is common with otosclerosis, noise-induced hearing loss, vestibular schwannoma, or Ménière's disease. In the latter case, intermittent tinnitus and vertigo are usual. Hearing loss can occur with demyelinative lesions in the brainstem.

The genetic basis of hearing impairment is apparent in families in which hearing impairment occurs in multiple generations. Hearing impairment is also genetically predetermined in instances in which there are obvious environmental factors. For example, in certain Asian families the susceptibility to aminoglycoside ototoxicity is transmuted through a mitochondrial mutation. The variation in individual and familial susceptibility to noise-induced hearing loss and presbycusis is also probably genetically determined.

One in 1000 infants is born with profound hearing impairment. At least 50 percent of congenital deafness has a genetic basis. A larger number of individuals develop hereditary hearing impairment in childhood and later in life. Between 70 and 80 percent of hereditary hearing impairment is autosomal recessive, and between 15 and 20 percent is autosomal dominant. Less than 5 percent is X-linked. Hereditary hearing impairment also occurs in syndromes in which other organ systems are affected. Greater progress has been made in finding the genes for syndromes of hereditary deafness because of the ease of making the determination of the hereditary basis of the hearing impairment. The genes for Waardenburg's syndrome (failure of melanocytes to migrate from the neural crest, resulting in deafness and pigmentary and integumentary changes) have been mapped to chromosome 2 (type 1) and chromosome 3 (type 2), and the genes for Usher's syndrome (deafness, vestibular loss, and blindness due to retinitis pigmentosa) have been mapped to chromosome 1 (type 2) and chromosome 2 (type 1). The genes for one form of Alport's syndrome (deafness and glomerulonephritis leading to renal failure), albinism, and neurofibromatosis type 2 (bilateral acoustic neurinomas) have been found. The first nonsyndromic deafness gene was found in a Costa Rican kindred with an autosomal dominant hearing impairment on the long arm of chromosome 5. Several genes responsible for recessive nonsyndromic hereditary hearing impairment in isolated, consanguineous families have been located.

Between 30 and 35 percent of individuals over 65 years of age have a hearing loss that is sufficiently great to require a hearing aid. Presbycusis is characterized by a loss of discrimination for phonemes, recruitment (abnormal growth of loudness), and particular difficulty in understanding speech in noisy environments.

Tinnitus is defined as the perception of a sound when there is no sound in the environment. It may have a buzzing, roaring, or ringing quality and may be pulsatile (synchronous with the heartbeat). Tinnitus is usually associated with a conductive or sensorineural loss of hearing. The pathophysiology of tinnitus is not well understood. The cause of the tinnitus can usually be determined by finding the cause of the associated hearing loss. Tinnitus may be the first symptom of a serious condition such as a vestibular schwannoma. Pulsatile tinnitus requires evaluation of the vascular system of the head to exclude vascular tumors such as glomus jugulare tumors, aneurysms, and stenotic lesions.

Differential Diagnosis   Many patients with sensorineural hearing losses should have the vestibular system evaluated with electronystagmography and caloric testing (see Chap. 20). Most patients with conductive hearing losses should have CT of the temporal bones. Patients with unilateral or asymmetric sensorineural hearing losses should have magnetic resonance imaging of the head with gadolinium enhancement.

Prevention   Conductive hearing losses may be prevented by prompt and appropriate antibiotic therapy of adequate duration for acute otitis media and by reventilation of the middle ear with tympanostomy tubes in middle-ear effusions lasting 6 weeks or longer. Loss of vestibular function and deafness due to aminoglycoside antibiotics can largely be prevented by careful monitoring of serum peak and trough levels. Noise-induced hearing loss can be prevented by avoidance of exposure to loud noise or by regular use of ear plugs or fluid-filled muffs to attenuate intense sound. Vaccination of infants against type B *Haemophilus influenzae* meningitis will prevent a major cause of acquired deafness, as has immunization for measles, mumps, and rubella.

_____

℞ **TREATMENT**

Most patients with conductive hearing losses can have the middle ear reconstructed using procedures such as tympanoplasty after chronic otitis media and trauma and stapedectomy for otosclerosis. Tympanostomy tubes allow the prompt return of hearing to normal in children and adults with middle-ear effusions. Hearing aids are effective and well-tolerated for patients with conductive hearing losses. Patients with mild, moderate, and severe sensorineural hearing losses are regularly rehabilitated with hearing aids of varying configuration and strength. However, the problem of understanding conversation with a hearing aid in noise remains. Hearing aids have been improved to provide greater fidelity and have been miniaturized. High-frequency emphasis, needed for many sensorineural hearing losses, has been achieved principally by venting the ear mold and with filters. The augmentation of soft sounds and the nonamplification of intense sounds has been achieved. Digital hearing aids lend themselves to programming for the individual, and multiple and directional microphones at the ear level help some with difficulty of hearing with a hearing aid in noisy surroundings. Since all hearing aids amplify noise as well as speech, the only absolute solution to the problem found so far is to place the microphone closer to the speaker than the noise source. This arrangement is not possible with a self-contained, cosmetically acceptable device. It is cumbersome and requires a user-friendly environment.

In many situations, including lectures and the theater, hearing-impaired persons benefit from assistive devices that are based on the principle of having the speaker closer to the microphone than any source of noise. Assistive devices include infrared and FM transmission as well as an electromagnetic loop around the room for transmission to the individual's hearing aid. Hearing aids with telecoils also can be used with properly equipped telephones in the same way.

Cochlear implants are neural prostheses that convert sound energy to electrical energy and can be used to stimulate the auditory division of the eighth nerve directly. Cochlear implants consist of electrodes that are inserted into the cochlea, speech processors that extract acoustical elements of speech for conversion to electric currents, and a means of transmitting the electrical energy through the skin. Most commonly for this purpose an induction coil is held over an implanted induction coil with magnets in each coil. In most causes of profound hearing impairment, the auditory hair cells are lost, but the ganglionic cells of the auditory division of the eighth nerve are preserved. Cochlear implants are appropriate for children with congenital and acquired profound hearing impairment and adults with hearing impairment that is so severe that less than 30 percent of speech can be understood with a hearing aid in ideal listening circumstances. Worldwide, more than 14,000 deaf individuals, 2000 of whom are children, have had cochlear implants. They experience sound that helps with speech reading and allows some open-set word recognition. It is anticipated that improvements in the electrode design and speech processors will permit further improvement in understanding speech. The implant also allows the recipient to hear and identify environmental sounds and distinguish between men's and women's voices. It is also a help in modulating the person's own voice.

For individuals who have had both eighth nerves destroyed by trauma or bilateral vestibular schwannomas, a brainstem auditory implant has been placed near the cochlear nucleus on a limited, experimental basis. Recipients of the brainstem implant derive benefit similar to those with the cochlear implant.

The treatment of tinnitus is particularly problematic. The frequency range and intensity of tinnitus can often be matched with the use of an audiometer. Relief of the tinnitus may be obtained by masking it with background music. Hearing aids also are helpful in tinnitus suppression, as are tinnitus maskers, devices that present a sound to the affected ear that is more pleasant to listen to than the tinnitus. The use of a tinnitus masker is often followed by several hours of inhibition of the tinnitus.

Communicating with Hard-of-Hearing Individuals   First of all, unnecessary noise should be eliminated or reduced. The radio and television should be turned off. Persons with hearing impairment depend on speech reading. They should be allowed to see the face of the speaker at all times. Speaking directly into the ear is occasionally helpful, but usually more is lost in communication than gained when the speaker's face cannot be seen. The lighting of the face of the speaker should be considered. The hard-of-hearing person should sit with his or her back to the window so that the light will be on the speaker's face. Speech should be slow enough to make each word distinct, but overly slow speech is distracting and loses contextual and speech-reading benefits. Although speech should be in a loud, clear voice, one should be aware that in sensorineural hearing losses in general and in elderly hard-of-hearing persons in particular, recruitment (the ability to hear loud sounds normally loud) may be troublesome. Above all, optimal communication cannot take place without both parties giving it their full and undivided attention.

BIBLIOGRAPHY

Ballenger JJ, Snow JB (eds): *Otorhinolaryngology Head and Neck Surgery*, 15th ed. Baltimore, Williams & Wilkins, 1995

Doty RL et al: Smell identification ability: Changes with age. Science 226:1441, 1984

Firestein S, Shepherd GM: Interaction of anionic and cationic currents leads to a voltage dependence in the odor response of olfactory receptor neurons. J Neurophys 73:562, 1995

Franco B et al: A gene deleted in Kallmann's syndrome shares homology with neural cell adhesion and axonal path-finding molecules. Nature 353:529, 1991

Getchell TV et al: *Smell and Taste in Health and Disease*. New York, Raven Press, 1991

Kalinec F et al: A membrane-based force generation mechanism in auditory sensory cells. Proc Natl Acad Sci USA 89:8671, 1992

Prezant TR: Mitochondrial ribosomal RNA mutation associated with antibiotic-induced and nonsyndromic deafness. Nat Genet 4:288, 1993

Russler KJ et al: A zonal organization of odorant receptor gene expression in the olfactory epithelium. Cell 73:597, 1993

Warchol ME et al: Regenerative proliferation in inner ear sensory epithelia from adult guinea pigs and humans. Science 259:1619, 1993

| 30 | *Marlene Durand, Michael Joseph, Ann Sullivan Baker** |

INFECTIONS OF THE UPPER RESPIRATORY TRACT

Infections of the upper respiratory tract include some of the most common infectious diseases encountered by internists and other primary-care physicians. Pharyngitis, laryngitis, rhinitis, sinusitis, otitis externa, and otitis media account for millions of visits to physicians annually. Although these infections are usually mild enough to be

*Deceased.

treated on an outpatient basis, the primary-care physician must be able to recognize their serious complications, such as peritonsillar abscess from pharyngitis, subperiosteal abscess from frontal sinusitis, and temporal-bone osteomyelitis from invasive otitis externa. The physician must also identify potentially life-threatening infections of the head and neck, such as epiglottitis, Ludwig's angina, and rhinocerebral mucormycosis.

INFECTIONS OF THE NOSE AND FACE

Skin infections that commonly affect the nose and face include folliculitis, furunculosis, impetigo, and erysipelas. These are discussed in detail elsewhere (see Chap. 133, in particular Table 133-1).

Infection of the mucosal surface of the nose is most commonly due to respiratory viruses (e.g., rhinovirus) and presents as acute rhinitis. There are several rare, chronic intranasal infections. *Ozena*, or atrophic rhinitis, is characterized by atrophied mucosa overlaid by foul-smelling dry crusts (Greek *ozein*, "stench"). *Klebsiella ozaenae* is often isolated from nasal cultures, but whether it is a cause of illness or merely a colonizer is unclear. Intranasal irrigation with aminoglycosides (e.g., tobramycin ophthalmic solution) or oral administration of ciprofloxacin has resulted in clinical improvement in some cases. *Klebsiella rhinoscleromatis* causes *rhinoscleroma*, a chronic granulomatous disease of the upper respiratory tract mucosa that is seen in inhabitants of parts of Africa, Asia, and Latin America and was recently described in two patients positive for human immunodeficiency virus (HIV). Mikulicz cells (foamy histiocytes) are seen in the submucosa of biopsy specimens. Rhinoscleroma can be treated with streptomycin, trimethoprim-sulfamethoxazole, a quinolone, or tetracycline for 2 months. *Pseudomonas mallei* causes *glanders*, a respiratory disease of horses. Infection is rare in humans; nasal inoculation may produce a purulent nasal discharge followed by granulomatous intranasal lesions that ulcerate. Treatment with sulfadiazine is administered.

Neonatal congenital syphilis may present as rhinitis (snuffles), and the generalized osteochondritis that follows may result in a "saddle-nose" deformity. In *leprosy*, *Mycobacterium leprae* infiltrates the nasal mucosa and may cause chronic nasal congestion and nosebleeds. Involvement of the nasal cartilage may also result in a saddle nose.

Rhinosporidium seeberi is a fungus-like organism, not yet cultured, that causes *rhinosporidiosis*. Pedunculated nasal masses that grow over months or years cause obstruction and a foul odor and must be surgically excised. *Blastomyces dermatitidis*, a fungus prevalent in the Mississippi and Ohio River valleys, usually causes pulmonary disease but may cause chronic ulcerative lesions of the skin and nasal mucosa. *Mucormycosis*, a life-threatening fungal illness that occurs primarily in diabetic patients, may present as black eschars in the nasal cavity (see "Fungal Sinusitis").

SINUSITIS

The paranasal sinuses are aerated cavities in the bones of the face that develop as outpouches of the nasal cavity and communicate with this cavity throughout life. The maxillary and ethmoid sinuses are present at birth; the frontal and sphenoid sinuses develop after ages 2 and 7, respectively. Like the nose, the sinuses are lined with respiratory epithelium that includes mucus-producing goblet cells and ciliated cells. The mucous blanket is carried toward the sinus openings (ostia) at a speed of up to 1 cm/min by the beating of the cilia. The ostia are small; the ethmoid sinus ostia, for example, are only 1 to 2 mm in diameter. Delay in the mucociliary transport time or—more important—obstruction of the ostia may lead to retained secretions and sinusitis.

Sinusitis is a common problem. In the United States, this infection accounts for millions of office visits annually. The most common type, maxillary sinusitis, is followed in frequency by ethmoid, frontal, and sphenoid sinusitis. A viral infection of the upper respiratory tract is the most common precursor of sinusitis, although only about 0.5 percent of such infections are complicated by clinically evident acute bacterial sinusitis. Sinusitis develops primarily through ostial obstruction due to mucosal edema. Viral upper respiratory infections also increase the amount of mucus produced and may damage ciliated cells, thereby delaying mucus transport time. Allergic rhinitis is another common cause of ostial obstruction, either by mucosal edema or by polyps. Nasotracheal or nasogastric intubation can result in obstruction of the ostia and is a major risk factor for nosocomial sinusitis in intensive care units. Dental infections may cause 5 to 10 percent of all cases of maxillary sinusitis; the roots of the upper back teeth (second bicuspid, first and second molars) abut the floor of the maxillary sinus. Other causes of sinusitis include barotrauma from deep-sea diving or airplane travel, mucus abnormalities (e.g., cystic fibrosis), and chemical irritants. Foreign bodies, tumors (e.g., midline granuloma, intranasal lymphoma, or squamous cell carcinoma), and granulomatous diseases (e.g., Wegener's granulomatosis or rhinoscleroma) may all cause sinusitis secondary to obstruction.

ACUTE BACTERIAL SINUSITIS   Manifestations Symptoms of acute sinusitis include purulent nasal or postnasal drainage, nasal congestion, and sinus pain or pressure whose location depends on the sinus involved. Maxillary sinus pain is often perceived as being located in the cheek or upper teeth; ethmoid sinus pain, between the eyes or retroorbital; frontal sinus pain, above the eyebrow; and sphenoid sinus pain, in the upper half of the face or retroorbital with radiation to the occiput. Sinus pain is frequently worse when the patient bends over or is supine. Fever develops in about half of patients with acute maxillary sinusitis.

Diagnosis   The diagnosis of bacterial sinusitis may be difficult, as symptoms may resemble those of the inciting upper respiratory infection. The persistence of cold symptoms for 7 to 10 days (or longer than usual for a particular patient) is the most consistent clinical feature of bacterial sinusitis, according to some authors. Complete opacification of sinus, shown by transillumination of maxillary and frontal sinuses with a strong flashlight in a dark room, constitutes good evidence of sinusitis; normal light transmission correlates well with an absence of infection. Partial transmission (dullness) is not diagnostically helpful, as it indicates infection in only one-quarter of cases. Transillumination is not of diagnostic value in patients with increased sinus-bone thickness, including children under age 10 and patients with chronic sinusitis. Four-view sinus x-rays are helpful in the diagnosis of acute sinusitis: radiologic opacity, an air-fluid level, or 4 mm or more of sinus mucosal thickening correlates well with active bacterial infection. Computed tomography (CT) of the sinus is much more sensitive than routine radiography, particularly for ethmoid and sphenoid disease. Its use should be reserved for complicated cases and for cases in hospitalized patients, however. In light of the recent finding that sinus CT often shows reversible acute changes in patients with common colds, it is apparent that routine early use of CT would lead to overdiagnosis of bacterial sinusitis.

Etiology   The bacteriology of acute community-acquired maxillary sinusitis has been well defined by studies using direct sinus puncture and aspiration. In children and adults, *Streptococcus pneumoniae* and *Haemophilus influenzae* (not type b), the most common pathogens, cause about one-third and one-fourth of cases, respectively. In children, *Moraxella catarrhalis* is also important, accounting for 20 percent of cases. In adults, gram-negative bacilli play a role (9 percent of cases), and anaerobes (6 percent) are especially important in cases associated with dental infections. How often *Chlamydia pneumoniae* causes sinusitis is not known. Rhinoviruses as well as influenza and parainfluenza viruses are found alone or with bacteria in one-fifth of adult cases.

℞ **TREATMENT**
Empiric therapy for acute bacterial sinusitis should be directed against the common bacterial pathogens; sinus puncture is not indicated in routine cases, and cultures of nasal drainage are not very reliable. Amoxicillin or trimethoprim-sulfamethoxazole may be effective in the treatment of first-time cases. Other effective but more expensive antibiotics include amoxicillin/clavulanate, cefuroxime axetil, and loracarbef. Treatment should be given for 1 to 2 weeks. Intravenous administration of antibiotics may be necessary for the treatment of patients with severe disease who appear toxic. In nosocomial sinusitis, *Staphylococcus aureus* and gram-negative bacilli are most common, and sinus cultures are indicated as an aid in tailoring therapy. Initial broad-spectrum intravenous therapy (e.g., with nafcillin and ceftriaxone) should be adjusted on the basis of culture results. Surgery to widen the ostia and drain thick secretions may be essential in severe acute sinusitis, particularly when ethmoid, frontal, or sphenoid disease fails to respond to initial intravenous therapy.

CHRONIC BACTERIAL SINUSITIS   Manifestations Chronic sinusitis is characterized by symptoms of sinus inflammation lasting 3 months or more. Most experts believe that this condition is caused by dysfunction of the mucociliary blanket, usually as a result of repeated past infections, rather than by the persistence of bacterial infection. Patients complain of constant sinus pressure, nasal congestion, and postnasal drainage, especially in the morning. A temperature of $\geq38°C$ (100.5°F) is rare and may signify a superimposed acute bacterial infection. Many patients also note a change in nasal discharge (to thick and green) with acute exacerbations.

Diagnosis   Sinus CT should be used in all cases of chronic sinusitis to define the extent of disease and to help exclude other diagnoses, such as an obstructing tumor or a granulomatous process. Patients should also be evaluated for allergies and immunodeficiencies (e.g., hypogammaglobulinemia). Evaluation by an otolaryngologist is essential, as this specialist will be able to obtain additional information by an office nasal endoscopic examination. Surgery, now usually done endoscopically, may be necessary to correct blockage of the sinus ostia. This blockage occurs most often in the osteomeatal complex that drains the maxillary, frontal, and anterior ethmoid sinuses. Samples of sinus secretions obtained intraoperatively should be cultured for anaerobes, aerobes, and fungi. Fungal sinusitis may mimic chronic bacterial infection (see "Fungal Sinusitis").

Etiology   The bacteriology of chronic sinusitis is not well defined. Nearly all patients with chronic disease, especially those who have had prior sinus surgery, have sinus cultures positive for bacteria, which often represent colonization rather than infection. Patients who have received multiple courses of antibiotics may be colonized by *S. aureus* or by resistant species of gram-negative bacilli.

℞ **TREATMENT**
The need for antibiotic therapy must be assessed on an individual basis, with antibiotics chosen in light of recent culture results.

COMPLICATIONS OF BACTERIAL SINUSITIS   The most common complication of sinusitis is orbital cellulitis. This condition is usually secondary to ethmoid sinusitis, since the ethmoid is separated from the orbit by only a very thin bone (the lamina papyracea). Patients present with fever, periorbital edema and erythema, conjunctival injection and chemosis, and proptosis. CT or magnetic resonance imaging (MRI) should be used to rule out a drainable orbital abscess, especially in patients with decreased eye movement. Treatment with broad-spectrum antibiotics (e.g., nafcillin and ceftriaxone) should be started immediately. If there is no improvement within 24 h, the ethmoid sinus should be drained.

Another extracranial complication of sinusitis is frontal subperiosteal abscess (Pott's puffy tumor) from frontal sinusitis. Patients present with a tender doughy swelling over the forehead. Treatment consists of surgical drainage of the abscess and the frontal sinus and 6 weeks of intravenous antibiotic therapy.

Intracranial complications such as epidural abscess, subdural empyema, meningitis, cerebral abscess, and dural-vein thrombophlebitis may result from sinusitis, particularly from frontal or sphenoid infections. Because the sphenoid sinus sits between the two cavernous sinuses, sphenoid sinusitis is a major cause of cavernous sinus thrombophlebitis.

FUNGAL SINUSITIS Fungal sinusitis is categorized as non-invasive or invasive. *Noninvasive* disease is chronic and occurs in immunocompetent hosts. It has two forms that are analogous to the noninvasive pulmonary diseases of aspergilloma and allergic bronchopulmonary aspergillosis. A fungus ball (aspergilloma) inside a sinus may cause symptoms of obstruction without invading the mucosa. Typically, only one sinus (often maxillary) is affected, and patients have unilateral symptoms and opacification of only that sinus on CT. Treatment is surgical only, unless special fungal stains show tissue invasion on histopathology. Allergic fungal sinusitis was first described in 1983 and is seen mainly in patients with a history of nasal polyposis and asthma. It is characterized by extremely thick sinus mucus ("allergic mucin") that, on histopathologic examination, is found to contain numerous Charcot-Leyden crystals, eosinophils, and rare fungal hyphae. There is no evidence of tissue invasion. Surgical removal of the inspissated mucus may be curative, although some experts recommend the use of intranasal or systemic glucocorticoids to prevent recurrences.

Invasive fungal sinusitis presents differently in immunocompetent and immunocompromised hosts. In immunocompromised individuals, fungal disease has an acute presentation. Rhinocerebral mucormycosis is a life-threatening infection due to fungi of the order Mucorales (*Rhizopus, Mucor, Absidia*) that usually involves diabetic patients with ketoacidosis but may also involve leukemic patients with prolonged neutropenia as well as transplant recipients. The affected patients have facial pain, headache, and fever; there may be early signs of orbital cellulitis and altered mental status. Black eschars overlying necrotic tissue may be seen in the nasal passages and should be biopsied emergently. The finding of tissue invasion by broad-based, nonseptate hyphae necessitates extensive surgical debridement and intravenous therapy with amphotericin B. *Aspergillus* and other fungi may also cause invasive sinus disease.

Immunocompetent hosts with invasive fungal sinusitis, in contrast, have slowly progressive disease. Fungi in ethmoid and sphenoid sinuses may invade the orbital apex, causing proptosis, ptosis, limitation of eye movement, and decreased vision. Patients may mistakenly be treated with glucocorticoids for presumed optic neuritis or orbital pseudotumor until sinus disease is recognized and biopsies are undertaken. Treatment consists of surgical debridement of the sinuses involved and prolonged intravenous therapy with amphotericin B. In all cases of invasive fungal sinusitis, follow-up CT and MRI should be conducted frequently to evaluate the progression of disease.

Mortality from fungal sinusitis is high, even among immunocompetent hosts.

EAR AND MASTOID INFECTIONS

AURICULAR CELLULITIS AND PERICHONDRITIS
Auricular cellulitis usually presents as a swollen, erythematous, hot, mildly tender ear. The lobule is especially swollen and red. There may be a history of minor trauma to the ear (e.g., involving earrings, cotton swabs, or scratching). Treatment consists of warm compresses and intravenous administration of antibiotics active against *S. aureus* and streptococci.

Perichondritis, an infection of the perichondrium of the ear, is often accompanied by infection of the underlying cartilage of the pinna (chondritis). Associated interruption of the blood supply to the cartilage may lead to ear deformity. Patients present with a swollen, hot, red, and exquisitely tender pinna, usually with sparing of the lobule. The most common antecedents of the infection are burns or significant trauma to the ear (e.g., as a result of boxing). *Pseudomonas aeruginosa* and *S. aureus* are the most common pathogens. Perichondritis should be treated with antibiotics, such as intravenous ticarcillin/clavulanic acid or intravenous nafcillin plus oral ciprofloxacin, for at least 4 weeks. Incision and drainage may be helpful for culture and for resolu-

tion of infection, which is often slow. This infection must be distinguished from relapsing polychondritis, a rheumatologic condition (see Chap. 326).

OTITIS EXTERNA The external auditory canal is about 2.5 cm long and is lined by skin. Beneath this skin is cartilage in the lateral half of the canal, temporal bone in the medial half. The skin in the bony portion lacks a subcutaneous layer and is attached directly to the periosteum, an important feature in the pathogenesis of invasive otitis externa (see below). Cerumen, secreted by glands, acidifies the canal and suppresses bacterial growth. However, desquamated skin and retained moisture make the canal especially susceptible to the hydrophilic organism *P. aeruginosa*.

Acute otitis externa, or swimmer's ear, occurs mostly in the summer and may be due to a decrease in canal acidity and resulting bacterial overgrowth. The ear is pruritic and painful, and the canal appears swollen and red. The most common pathogens are *P. aeruginosa*, *S. aureus*, and streptococci. Treatment consists of cleansing of the ear with alcohol–acetic acid mixtures and the administration of topical antibiotic ear drops, such as polymyxin-neomycin (4 drops four times daily for 5 days). Herpes zoster in the external canal causes severe otalgia and is often accompanied by ipsilateral facial paralysis due to the involvement of the geniculate ganglion of cranial nerve VII (Ramsay Hunt syndrome). Recent reports suggest that treatment with intravenous acyclovir decreases the incidence of permanent facial-nerve palsy, but the results of relevant controlled trials have not yet been published.

Chronic otitis externa causes pruritus rather than ear pain and is often due to irritation from either repeated minor trauma to the canal (e.g., scratching or use of cotton swabs) or drainage of a chronic middle-ear infection. In the latter situation, treatment of chronic otitis media with oral antibiotics will also cover this condition.

Invasive ("malignant") otitis externa is a potentially life-threatening infection, usually due to *P. aeruginosa*, that slowly invades from the external canal into adjacent soft tissues, mastoid, and temporal bone and eventually spreads across the base of the skull. It occurs primarily in diabetic patients whose diabetes, unlike that of patients with mucormycosis, is usually under control. There is often a history of ear pain and drainage of several months' duration. Examination reveals an edematous canal, with granulation tissue in the posterior wall about halfway down the canal (the region of the cartilage-bone junction). Trismus or partial facial paralysis (cranial nerve VII) is evident in some instances. Cranial nerves IX, X, and XI are occasionally affected as well. Signs of intradural involvement, such as meningitis, temporal-lobe cerebritis, or brain abscess, are rare. Fever is rare in invasive otitis externa and when it does develop is usually low-grade.

Laboratory studies usually reveal a normal white blood cell count but a high sedimentation rate. CT and MRI studies are essential for defining the extent of bone and soft-tissue involvement and for helping the ear, nose, and throat surgeon decide on the optimal location for biopsy. Cultures of discharge from the external canal may be unreliable, and in nearly all cases antibiotics should be withheld until a deep-tissue specimen is obtained for culture and pathologic examination. Once this specimen has been collected, empiric therapy with intravenous antibiotics active against *Pseudomonas* (e.g., ticarcillin, pipericillin, or ceftazidime, plus an aminoglycoside) may be started intraoperatively. In more than 95 percent of cases, *P. aeruginosa* is the pathogen involved; in the remaining cases, the pathogens include *Staphylococcus epidermidis, Aspergillus, Fusobacterium,* and *Actinomyces*. Intravenous antibiotic treatment should be continued for 6 to 8 weeks in advanced cases; in early cases, oral ciprofloxacin alone (750 mg twice daily for 6 weeks) may follow the initial 2 weeks of combination intravenous therapy if intraoperative cultures reveal a *Pseudomonas* strain sensitive to this drug.

ACUTE OTITIS MEDIA The middle ear is connected to the nasopharynx via the eustachian tube. When this tube is blocked, fluid collects in the middle-ear and mastoid cavities, providing a culture medium for any bacteria present. Acute otitis media (AOM), or middle-ear infection, may result. Viral upper respiratory infections, which can cause edema of the eustachian tube mucosa, often precede or accompany episodes of AOM. Otitis media, like upper respiratory tract infections, is most common in fall, winter, and spring. The incidence of AOM declines with age. More than two-thirds of children under age 3 have had at least one episode of AOM; the prevalence among adults is only 0.25 percent.

Symptoms include ear pain, fever, and decreased hearing acuity. On examination, the tympanic membrane moves poorly with insufflation and is usually red, opaque, bulging, or retracted. Spontaneous perforations of the tympanic membrane and otorrhea are occasionally documented.

The bacteriology of AOM has been delineated for pediatric disease: *S. pneumoniae* (35 percent), *H. influenzae* (25 percent), and *M. catarrhalis* (15 percent) are the most common organisms in nonneonates; group B streptococci and gram-negative bacilli are important in neonates. Viruses, either alone or with bacteria, are found in one-quarter of pediatric cases. Small studies of AOM in adults have also found *S. pneumoniae* (21 percent) and *H. influenzae* (26 percent) to be the most common pathogens. About 90 percent of the *H. influenzae* infections are due to nontypable strains: those due to type b may be accompanied by bacteremia or meningitis.

℞ **TREATMENT**

Treatment of otitis media is empiric, as diagnostic tympanocentesis is indicated only for patients who appear toxic, who are immunocompromised, or whose infection is refractory to initial therapy. Although about one-third of *H. influenzae* strains and at least three-quarters of *M. catarrhalis* strains are β-lactamase producers, most authorities still find amoxicillin therapy to be successful in routine cases. Other drugs effective against most β-lactamase-positive strains include amoxicillin/clavulanate, trimethoprim-sulfamethoxazole, erythromycin-sulfisoxazole, clarithromycin, and second-generation oral cephalosporins (e.g., loracarbef, cefpodoxime proxetil, and cefuroxime axetil). Penicillin resistance in pneumococci, an increasing problem, is not mediated by β-lactamase. Resistant strains may respond to therapy with erythromycin or sulfa drugs; serious infections require treatment with intravenous vancomycin or a third-generation cephalosporin (e.g., ceftriaxone). Adjunctive treatment of AOM with antihistamines is of no proven benefit.

Recurrent episodes of AOM in children are due to the same pathogens that cause primary AOM (*S. pneumoniae*, *H. influenzae*, and *M. catarrhalis*). Most early recurrences (75 percent), however, are not relapses but are due to different organisms or to different strains of the organism that caused the initial episode. The pattern of recurrent AOM in adults is presumably similar but has not been well studied. Treatment for recurrent AOM should include drugs with activity against β-lactamase-positive strains. Patients with frequent recurrences (e.g., three episodes within 6 months) may benefit from antibiotic prophylaxis with once-daily amoxicillin or sulfisoxazole during the winter months, although this benefit must be weighed against the risk of selecting more antibiotic-resistant strains of bacteria.

SEROUS OTITIS MEDIA Otitis media with effusion, or serous otitis media, is characterized by the persistence of middle-ear fluid for several months without other signs of infection. This condition is associated with a 25-dB hearing loss in the affected ear. Cultures of middle-ear fluid are frequently negative, although effusions have resolved more quickly in antibiotic-treated children than in controls in several clinical trials. Adenoidectomy, myringotomy, or tympanostomy tubes have been shown to decrease the duration of effusion in some children.

CHRONIC SUPPURATIVE OTITIS MEDIA In chronic suppurative otitis media, patients discharge chronic purulent drainage from their ears through perforated tympanic membranes. Patients with chronic suppurative otitis media are divided into two groups: those with and those without cholesteatoma. Aerobic culture of draining fluid from both children and adults reveals a high percentage of *S. aureus*, *P. aeruginosa*, and enteric gram-negative bacilli (*Klebsiella*, *Escherichia coli*, *Proteus*). Anaerobes, including *Prevotella*, *Fusobacterium*, *Porphyromonas*, and some *Bacteroides* species, are found in 50 percent of cases, usually in mixed culture with aerobes. CT should be used to rule out a surgically treatable nidus of infection, such as an infected cholesteatoma or mastoid sequestrum. Surgical drainage of infected areas of the middle ear, followed by a prolonged course of topical antibiotic drops, has been the mainstay of therapy for chronic suppurative otitis media. Recent reports of nonsurgical cure of chronic suppurative otitis media in children without cholesteatoma by intravenous antibiotic therapy based on culture results are encouraging, however.

Tuberculous otitis media, a rare but frequently misdiagnosed cause of chronic suppurative otitis media, is characterized by a tympanic membrane with multiple perforations, extensive granulation tissue, and severe hearing loss. Antituberculous therapy should be administered.

MASTOIDITIS The mastoid is the portion of the temporal bone posterior to the ear that contains a honeycomb of air cells lined with respiratory epithelium. These air cells connect with the middle ear. Fluid in the middle ear, a prelude to otitis media, is almost always accompanied by fluid in the mastoid. True mastoiditis, however, has become rare in the antibiotic era, probably because of prompt treatment of otitis media.

Mastoiditis is characterized by erosion of the bony partitions between the mastoid air cells. Patients with acute mastoiditis present with pain, tenderness, and swelling over the mastoid. When there is an overlying subperiosteal abscess or cellulitis, the pinna is pushed out and forward. CT may show bony destruction or a drainable mastoid abscess.

The reported bacteriology of mastoiditis has varied. Some cases involve organisms similar to those implicated in AOM (*S. pneumoniae*, *H. influenzae*); others are attributable to *S. aureus* and gram-negative bacilli, including *Pseudomonas*. Ideally, therapy should be guided by the results of cultures of middle-ear fluid obtained by tympanocentesis. Initial broad-spectrum therapy, such as that with intravenous ticarcillin/clavulanate plus gentamicin, can later be narrowed.

COMPLICATIONS OF OTITIS MEDIA AND MASTOIDITIS Extracranial complications include hearing loss, labyrinthitis and resulting vertigo, and facial-nerve palsy. Additional complications from mastoiditis develop when infection tracks under the periosteum of the temporal bone to cause a subperiosteal abscess or breaks through the mastoid tip to cause a neck abscess deep to the sternocleidomastoid muscle (Bezold's abscess). Intracranial complications include epidural abscess, dural venous thrombophlebitis (usually sigmoid sinus), meningitis, and brain abscess.

INFECTIONS OF THE ORAL CAVITY AND PHARYNX

ORAL CAVITY INFECTIONS The oral cavity extends from the lips to the circumvallate papillae of the tongue and is heavily colonized with viridans streptococci and anaerobes. These organisms can cause several infections in this area. *Gingivitis* is an infection of the gums, the earliest form of periodontal disease. Anaerobes residing in the mouth, especially anaerobic gram-negative rods such as *Prevotella intermedia*, are the most common pathogens. Patients with *Vincent's angina*, also called *acute necrotizing ulcerative gingivitis* or *trench mouth*, have halitosis and ulcerations of the interdental papillae. Oral anaerobes are the cause, and therapy with oral penicillin plus metronidazole or with clindamycin alone is effective in both this condition and gingivitis.

Ludwig's angina is a rapidly spreading, life-threatening cellulitis of the sublingual and submandibular spaces that usually starts in an infected lower molar. Patients are febrile and may drool the secretions they cannot swallow. A brawny, boardlike edema in the sublingual area pushes the tongue up and back, sometimes causing airway obstruction. Treatment with intravenous antibiotics active against streptococci and oral anaerobes (e.g., ampicillin/sulbactam or high-dose penicillin plus metronidazole) and airway monitoring are essential. Intubation or tracheostomy may be necessary. Surgical opening of the infected tissue compartments is usually necessary.

Noma, or *cancrum oris*, is a fulminant gangrenous infection of the oral and facial tissues that occurs in severely malnourished and debilitated patients and is especially common among children. Beginning as a necrotic ulcer in the gingiva of the mandible, noma is caused by oral anaerobes, especially fusospirochetal organisms (e.g., *Fusobacterium nucleatum*). It is treated with high-dose penicillin, debridement, and correction of the underlying malnutrition.

Herpes simplex commonly causes cold sores of the lips but may also cause painful vesicles on the tongue and buccal mucosa. Primary infection may require intravenous hydration and should be treated with acyclovir. *Thrush*, a condition caused by an overgrowth of yeast (usually *Candida* species) that occurs in immunocompromised patients, is treated with topical antifungal solutions (e.g., nystatin) or with oral fluconazole.

PHARYNGITIS   Most cases of pharyngitis are thought to be viral. Many occur as part of common colds caused by rhinovirus, coronavirus, or parainfluenza virus. Patients have a scratchy or sore throat as well as coryza and cough. The pharynx is inflamed and edematous, but no exudate is evident. Influenza virus and adenovirus may cause a particularly severe sore throat, along with fever and myalgias. In infection with either of the latter viruses, there is pharyngeal erythema and edema; however, adenovirus infection also commonly causes an exudate, thus mimicking streptococcal pharyngitis. *Infectious mononucleosis* due to Epstein-Barr virus often causes a severe sore throat. Exudative pharyngitis or tonsillitis is documented in half of mononucleosis cases and may also mimic streptococcal infection. *Herpangina*, caused by coxsackievirus, is characterized by fever, sore throat, myalgias, and a vesicular enanthem on the soft palate between the uvula and the tonsils. There are usually only two to six lesions, which begin as small papules that vesiculate and then ulcerate. Fever and nonexudative pharyngitis are common symptoms of the acute retroviral syndrome that develops several weeks after infection with HIV.

The most important bacterial cause of pharyngitis is group A *Streptococcus* (*Streptococcus pyogenes*). This organism is responsible for about 15 percent of all cases of pharyngitis and can cause important complications, both suppurative (peritonsillar and retropharyngeal abscess) and nonsuppurative (scarlet fever, streptococcal toxic shock syndrome, rheumatic fever, acute poststreptococcal glomerulonephritis). Fever, severe sore throat, cervical adenopathy, and inflammation of the tonsils and pharynx (which are covered with exudate) are classic findings. However, many cases of streptococcal pharyngitis are mild, with minimal erythema and no exudate, and mimic the pharyngitis of the common cold. Although some patients may in fact have viral pharyngitis and may simply be colonized with group A streptococci, these individuals must nevertheless be treated for presumed streptococcal pharyngitis. Diagnosis is made by culture. Recently, rapid antigen tests have become available. These tests are specific but not very sensitive: a positive test may be considered equivalent to a positive culture, but a negative test requires culture confirmation. Ten days of treatment with oral penicillin (or with erythromycin in penicillin-allergic patients) are required; shorter courses do not eradicate the organism. A single dose of intramuscular benzathine penicillin is an alternative of equal efficacy. Other antibiotics active against streptococci may be used (e.g., cephalexin, amoxicillin, cefuroxime, or cefprozil), although studies of the prevention of rheumatic fever are available only for penicillin (see Chap. 236).

Other bacterial causes of pharyngitis include groups C and G *Streptococcus*, *Neisseria gonorrhoeae* (see Chap. 150), *Arcanobacterium haemolyticum*, *Yersinia enterocolitica*, and—very rarely—*Corynebacterium diphtheriae* (see Chap. 144). In addition, *Mycoplasma pneumoniae* (Chap. 180) and *C. pneumoniae* (Chap. 181) can cause pharyngitis.

A peritonsillar abscess (*quinsy*) may follow untreated streptococcal pharyngitis. Oral anaerobes also play a role in quinsy. Patients have a severe sore throat and speak with a "hot-potato" voice. Examination reveals pronounced unilateral peritonsillar swelling and erythema causing deviation of the uvula. Immediate aspiration by an otolaryngologist is required in conjunction with antibiotic therapy with penicillin plus metronidazole, clindamycin, or ampicillin/sulbactam.

LARYNGITIS, CROUP, AND EPIGLOTTITIS

LARYNGITIS   Laryngitis is characterized by hoarseness. Most cases of acute laryngitis are caused by viruses (rhinovirus, influenza virus, parainfluenza virus, coxsackievirus, adenovirus, or respiratory syncytial virus). Acute laryngitis may also be associated with group A *Streptococcus* and *M. catarrhalis*. Laryngitis must be differentiated from epiglottitis (see below). The goal of treatment is merely the relief of symptoms except when throat cultures are positive for group A *Streptococcus* (in which case penicillin should be used) or possibly for *M. catarrhalis* (in which case erythromycin should be used).

Chronic laryngitis due to infection is rare and must be distinguished from hoarseness of neoplastic etiology. *Tuberculous laryngitis* may be mistaken for laryngeal cancer when assessed by direct laryngoscopy. Laryngeal and supraglottic lesions include mucosal hyperemia and thickening, nodules, and ulcerations. In a recent study, a history of fever and night sweats was rare, and the most common chest radiographic finding was apical thickening and fibrosis. Biopsy reveals granulomas with acid-fast bacilli. Cultures should be performed to confirm the diagnosis and evaluate the sensitivities of the pathogen. Laryngeal tuberculosis is highly contagious and should be managed with the same precautions and therapy used for active pulmonary disease (see Chap. 171). Fungal infections causing laryngitis include histoplasmosis (Chap. 203), blastomycosis (Chap. 205), and candidiasis (Chap. 207). *Histoplasma* and *Blastomyces* may cause nodules on the larynx, with or without ulcerations. *Candida* may cause laryngitis, along with thrush, in immunosuppressed patients or in patients with chronic mucocutaneous candidiasis.

CROUP   Croup, or acute laryngotracheobronchitis, is an infection of the upper and lower respiratory tract that causes marked subglottic edema. It mainly affects 2- and 3-year-old children and usually follows the onset of upper respiratory tract infection by 1 to 2 days. Symptoms include fever, hoarseness, a "seal's bark" cough, and inspiratory stridor. The most common etiology is parainfluenza virus, although croup may also be caused by other respiratory viruses (e.g., influenza or respiratory syncytial virus) and by *M. pneumoniae*.

Croup must be differentiated from epiglottitis (see below). Epiglottitis usually progresses more rapidly and produces a more toxic appearance. Neck x-rays may be helpful but do not reliably exclude epiglottitis. In croup, the anterior-posterior neck x-ray shows subglottic edema (the "hourglass sign"); in epiglottitis, the lateral neck view shows a thick epiglottis.

Patients with severe croup should be hospitalized, monitored for hypoxemia through pulse oximetry, and watched for airway obstruction requiring intubation. Humidification is commonly prescribed, but few controlled trials have assessed its benefit. Nebulized epinephrine provides temporary (2-h) improvement in patients with marked stridor, but such patients must be observed for rebound edema. Glucocorticoid therapy is controversial.

EPIGLOTTITIS   Acute epiglottitis (supraglottitis) is a life-threatening, rapidly progressive cellulitis of the epiglottis that may cause complete airway obstruction. It begins as a cellulitis between the tongue base and the epiglottis that pushes the epiglottis posteriorly. The epiglottis itself then becomes swollen, threatening the airway. Epiglottitis is most common among children 2 to 4 years old but may also affect older children and adults. Since the advent of vaccination against *H. influenzae* type b in 1985, the overall incidence of epiglottitis among children has decreased.

The typical young child with epiglottitis has a several-hour history of fever, irritability, dysphonia, and dysphagia and presents sitting forward and drooling. Some adolescents and adults may have a less fulminant presentation, with symptoms (especially sore throat) of 1 or 2 days' duration. Adults may present with dyspnea (25 percent), drooling (15 percent), and stridor (10 percent). Epiglottitis constitutes a medical emergency, as airway occlusion may occur suddenly. Lateral neck films showing an enlarged epiglottis (the "thumb sign") are helpful if positive but may be falsely negative. The value of obtaining these films has also been questioned because doing so may cause a critical delay in securing the airway. Direct viewing of the pharynx by use of a tongue blade should not be attempted, as immediate laryngospasm and airway obstruction may result. Instead, a child with suspected epiglottitis should be transported—while sitting up—to the operating room for visualization of the epiglottis with a fiberoptic laryngoscope, with preparations made for immediate airway control. If the epiglottis is cherry-red, an uncuffed endotracheal tube should be placed. Diagnosis in adults is also made by direct viewing of the epiglottis with a flexible fiberoptic laryngoscope, again only after preparations are made to secure the airway.

All patients must be closely monitored in an intensive care unit and should be given antibiotics active against *H. influenzae*. This organism is responsible for nearly all pediatric cases and is isolated from the blood in almost 100 percent. In adults, blood cultures are positive in about 25 percent of cases, all of which are due to *H. influenzae*. Other pathogens isolated from the pharynx of adults with epiglottitis include *Haemophilus parainfluenzae*, *S. pneumoniae*, group A *Streptococcus*, and (rarely) *S. aureus*; the correlation between throat and epiglottis cultures is unclear, however. Children may be treated with intravenous cefuroxime, ceftriaxone, ampicillin/sulbactam, or trimethoprim-sulfamethoxazole. Adults may be treated with cefuroxime, ampicillin/sulbactam, or nafcillin plus ceftriaxone; those highly allergic to penicillin may be given clindamycin plus trimethoprim-sulfamethoxazole. If the patient with *H. influenzae* epiglottitis has household contacts that include an unvaccinated child under age 4, all members of the household and the patient should receive prophylactic rifampin to eradicate the carriage of *H. influenzae*.

DEEP NECK INFECTIONS

Deep neck infections may be life-threatening because of airway compromise, involvement of the carotid sheath, or spread into the mediastinum.

SUBMANDIBULAR SPACE INFECTIONS See *Ludwig's angina* above (under "Oral Cavity Infections").

LATERAL PHARYNGEAL SPACE INFECTIONS The lateral pharyngeal space, also called the parapharyngeal or pharyngomaxillary space, is in the superior lateral portion of the neck and extends from the hyoid bone to the base of the skull. It lies deep to the lateral wall of the pharynx and is lateral to the tonsil and carotid sheath and medial to the parotid gland. Infection in this space may follow tonsillitis, pharyngitis with adenoid involvement, parotitis, mastoiditis, or periodontal infection.

On presentation, most patients appear toxic and have fever, sore throat, pain on swallowing, and leukocytosis. Infection confined to the posterior (retrostyloid) portion of the lateral pharyngeal space causes swelling of the lateral pharyngeal wall, which may be missed because it is behind the palatopharyngeal arch. Involvement of the anterior portion of this space causes medial displacement of the tonsil, swelling over the parotid gland, and trismus. Rigidity of the neck or torticollis toward the opposite side may develop. Diagnosis is confirmed by CT with contrast.

Treatment includes securing of the airway, surgical drainage in the operating room, and administration of intravenous antibiotics active against streptococci and oral anaerobes (e.g., ampicillin/sulbactam). Major complications result from involvement of the carotid sheath and the vessels it contains. These complications are frequently fatal and include jugular vein thrombophlebitis, erosion into the carotid artery, and mediastinitis. Jugular vein thrombophlebitis is characterized by high fevers, chills, and neck tenderness at the angle of the mandible. Erosion into the carotid artery is usually heralded by repeated small bleeds into the mouth. The involvement of adjacent cranial nerves may result in ipsilateral Horner's syndrome, hoarseness, or unilateral tongue paresis. Extension of infection along the carotid sheath into the posterior mediastinum results in mediastinitis and a mortality of 50 percent. MRI is useful in delineating carotid and jugular involvement.

RETROPHARYNGEAL SPACE INFECTION The retropharyngeal space lies between the pharynx and the prevertebral fascia and extends from the base of the skull into the mediastinum. Infection in this space may result from the spread of lateral pharyngeal space infection or from the lymphatic spread of infection in more cephalad sites (posterior sinuses, adenoids, nasopharynx) to the retropharyngeal lymph nodes. Retropharyngeal abscess is most common among infants and young children, probably because the retropharyngeal nodes later involute. Retropharyngeal abscess may also follow trauma to the posterior pharynx (e.g., endoscopy in adults, lollipop-stick perforation in children) or may result from anterior extension of infection from cervical osteomyelitis.

Symptoms include fever, marked difficulty and pain with swallowing, and a "hot-potato" voice. Physical examination may document drooling, nuchal rigidity, and bulging of the posterior pharyngeal wall. Advanced cases include dyspnea and stridor. Diagnosis may be confirmed by a lateral neck soft-tissue x-ray or CT scan. Treatment requires securing of the airway and emergency surgical drainage. Intravenous antibiotics should be given; the agents chosen should be active against streptococci, oral anaerobes, *S. aureus*, and *H. influenzae* (e.g., ampicillin/sulbactam alone or clindamycin plus ceftriaxone). Potential complications include airway obstruction, intraoral rupture of the abscess causing aspiration pneumonia, and mediastinitis.

BIBLIOGRAPHY

BAKER AS, MONTGOMERY WW: Oropharyngeal space infections. Curr Clin Top Infect Dis 8:227, 1987

CHOW AW: Life-threatening infections of the head and neck. Clin Infect Dis 14:991, 1992

CODY DT II et al: Allergic fungal sinusitis: The Mayo Clinic experience. Laryngoscope 104:1074, 1994

DEL BECCARO MA et al: Bacteriology of acute otitis media: A new perspective. J Pediatr 120:81, 1992

DONALD PJ et al (eds): *The Sinuses*. New York, Raven Press, 1995

EVANS FO et al: Sinusitis of the maxillary antrum. N Engl J Med 293:735, 1974

GWALTNEY JM JR et al: Computed tomographic study of the common cold. N Engl J Med 330:25, 1994

HARRIS JP, DARROW DH: Complications of chronic otitis media, in *Surgery of the Ear and Temporal Bone*, JB Nadol Jr, HF Schuknecht (eds). New York, Raven Press, 1993, p 171

KLEIN JO: Otitis externa, otitis media, mastoiditis, in *Principles and Practice of Infectious Diseases*, 4th ed, GL Mandell et al (eds). New York, Churchill Livingstone, 1995, p 579

LIM DJ, BLUESTONE CD (eds): Recent advances in otitis media: Report of the Fifth Research Conference. Ann Otol Rhinol Laryngol 103(Suppl 164), 1994

PARADISE JL: Etiology and management of pharyngitis and pharyngotonsillitis in children: A current review. Ann Otol Rhinol Laryngol 155:51, 1992

SCHWARTZ LE, BROWN RB: Purulent otitis media in adults. Arch Intern Med 152:2301, 1992

SINAVE CP et al: The Lemierre syndrome: Suppurative thrombophlebitis of the internal jugular vein secondary to oropharyngeal infection. Medicine 68:85, 1989

WASHBURN RG et al: Chronic fungal sinusitis in apparently normal hosts. Medicine 67:231, 1988

ORAL MANIFESTATIONS
OF DISEASE

A thorough oral examination, to include the oral and pharyngeal soft tissues as well as the teeth, is an important part of the physical examination. The common oral diseases are due to infection by bacteria, fungi, or viruses. The complex development of the orofacial structures leads to close interposition of a wide range of tissues, most of which are prone to developmental anomalies, growth disturbances, and neoplasia.

DISEASES OF THE TEETH

DENTAL CARIES, PULPAL AND PERIAPICAL DISEASE, AND COMPLICATIONS Dental caries is a destructive disease of the hard tissues of the teeth due to infection with *Streptococcus mutans* and other bacteria. Formerly one of the most common human diseases, caries has shown marked changes in recent years. In the United States, fewer than half of those 17 years and younger now have carious lesions, although in many segments of the population and in developing countries this decrease has not occurred. Much of the decline is due to artificial fluoridation of drinking water to a level of 1 part per million, with additional effects due to fluoride-containing toothpastes and topical fluoride administration. Conversely, retention of teeth and the aging of the population have led to an increase in root caries. Increasing numbers of patients surviving with the consequences of cancer therapy and other special populations (diabetics and those with xerostomia due to Sjögren's syndrome or to medications) may experience severe caries unless appropriate topical fluoride prophylaxis is used. Treatment of caries involves removal of the softened and infected hard tissues, sealing of the exposed dentine, and restoration of the lost tooth structure with silver amalgam, composite plastic, gold, or porcelain.

If the carious lesion progresses, infection of the dental pulp may occur, causing *acute pulpitis*. The tooth may become sensitive to hot or cold, and then severe continuous throbbing pain ensues. At this stage, pulp damage is irreversible, and root canal therapy becomes necessary. The contents of the pulp chamber and root canals are removed, followed by thorough cleaning, antisepsis, and filling with an inert material. Alternatively, extraction of the tooth may be indicated.

If the pulpitis is not treated successfully, infection may spread beyond the tooth apex into the periodontal ligament. If the infection causes acute inflammation, pain on chewing or on percussion is present, and a *periapical abscess* may form, while chronic inflammation can produce a *periapical granuloma* within the alveolar bone. This may cause slight pain and tenderness or may be asymptomatic. Proliferation of epithelial cell rests may convert the granuloma into a *periapical cyst*. Both the granuloma and the cyst produce periapical radiolucencies, whereas the periapical abscess does not do so unless it forms as a complication of one of the other two lesions. The pus in the periapical abscess may track through the alveolar bone into soft tissues, causing cellulitis and bacteremia, or may discharge into the oral cavity (*parulis* or *gumboil*), into the maxillary sinus, or through the skin of the face or submandibular area. A severe form of cellulitis, *Ludwig's angina*, originates from an infected mandibular molar, involves the submandibular space, and extends throughout the floor of the mouth, with elevation of the tongue, dysphagia, and difficulty in breathing. Glottal edema may occur, necessitating emergency tracheotomy.

EFFECT OF SYSTEMIC FACTORS ON TEETH Systemic factors, occurring in utero or in infancy during the stages of crown formation, may influence the development and structure of the teeth. Enamel hypoplasia of the primary and/or permanent teeth, manifested by alterations ranging from white spots to gross defects in the surface structure of the crowns, may be caused by disturbances of calcium and phosphate metabolism such as are found in vitamin D–resistant rickets, hypoparathyroidism, gastroenteritis, and celiac disease. Prema-

ture birth or high fevers also may give rise to enamel hypoplasia. Tetracycline, when given during the second half of pregnancy, in infancy, and in childhood up to 8 years of age, causes both a permanent discoloration of the teeth and enamel hypoplasia. Daily ingestion of more than 1.5 mg fluoride can result in enamel discoloration (*mottling*). Prenatal factors appear to influence crown size. Larger teeth are associated with maternal diabetes, maternal hypothyroidism, and large birth size. Tooth size is reduced in Down's syndrome. Premature loss of the deciduous dentition is frequently the first symptom in juvenile hypophosphatasia. Systemic disease may give rise to pain that simulates pulpal disease. Maxillary sinusitis is frequently manifested as pain in the maxillary teeth, including sensitivity to thermal changes and percussion. Cardiac disease with angina pectoris may result in pain referred to the lower jaw, probably through the vagus nerve.

PERIODONTAL DISEASES

In adults, chronic destructive periodontal disease becomes responsible for more loss of teeth than caries, particularly in the aged. However, the prevalence and incidence of periodontal disease also appears to be declining in the United States. The most common form of periodontal disease starts as inflammation of the marginal gingiva (*gingivitis*) which is painless, although the gingiva may bleed on brushing. The disease spreads to involve the periodontal ligament and alveolar bone. As the latter is slowly resorbed, there is loss of periodontal ligament attachment between tooth and bone. The soft tissue separates from the tooth surface, causing "pocket" formation with bleeding on probing and during chewing. Acute inflammation may become superimposed on this chronic process, with the production of pus and the formation of a *periodontal abscess*. Ultimately, extreme bone loss, tooth mobility, and recurrent abscess formation lead to tooth exfoliation or may mandate tooth extraction.

Gingivitis and periodontitis are infections associated with the accumulation of *bacterial plaque*, which may become mineralized (*calculus*) and which can be prevented by appropriate *oral hygiene* measures, including tooth brushing, flossing, antibacterial mouth rinses, and the removal of impacted food debris. Poorly fabricated or deteriorated restorations may contribute through overextended or inadequate margins, while the role of occlusal trauma is unclear. Therapy is directed at the causative microflora and consists of removal of plaque and calculus, debridement of the pocket lining and superficial infected cementum, and elimination of other contributing factors.

Periodontal disease appears to be a group of conditions, including *adult periodontitis*, associated with *Porphyromonas gingivalis*, *Prevotella intermedia*, and other gram-negative organisms. *Localized juvenile periodontitis* (LJP) causes rapid, severe pocketing and bone loss and is associated with *Actinobacillus actinomycetemcomitans*, *Capnocytophaga*, *Eikenella corrodens*, and other anaerobes. *Acute necrotizing ulcerative gingivitis* (ANUG) involves sudden inflammation of the gingivae with necrosis, tissue loss, pain, bleeding, and halitosis and is associated with *P. intermedia* and spirochetes. ANUG and an aggressive and rapid form of periodontitis (*necrotizing ulcerative periodontitis*) are seen in association with human immunodeficiency virus (HIV) infection. Some of these cases progress to a destructive gangrene-like lesion of oral soft tissues and bone (*necrotizing stomatitis*) resembling the *noma* formerly seen in severely malnourished populations. Therapy involves local antibacterial measures, debridement, and, in severe cases, systemic antibiotics effective against gram-negative anaerobes.

Host factors may be involved in the pathogenesis of periodontal disease in other populations as well. Thus familial defects in neutrophil chemotaxis are found in LJP, and these may predispose to tissue destruction caused by the toxins of *A. actinomycetemcomitans*, including leucotoxin, collagenase, endotoxin, and a factor further inhibiting neutrophil chemotaxis. Patients with IgA deficiency and agammaglobulinemia probably have less periodontal disease than matched healthy individuals, whereas in *Down's syndrome* and *diabetes mellitus* severe periodontal disease may occur. During pregnancy there may be severe gingivitis and the formation of localized *pyogenic granulomas*. Certain drugs, notably the anticonvulsant *phenytoin* and the antiangina calcium channel blocker *nifedipine*, cause *fibrous hyperplasia* of the gingiva, which may cover the teeth, interfere with eating, and be unsightly. Similar clinical appearances can be due to *idiopathic familial gingival fibromatosis*. Surgical management is used for both conditions, although a change in medication may be appropriate for the drug-induced form.

Periapical and periodontal bacterial infections can cause transient bacteremia after tooth extraction and even routine dental prophylaxis. These can lead to bacterial endocarditis in patients with a history of rheumatic fever, other valvular disease, valvular graft, or heart or joint prostheses. Antibiotic coverage is appropriate in such cases.

DISEASES OF THE ORAL MUCOSA

INFECTIONS Most oral mucosal diseases involve microorganisms (see Table 31-1).

PIGMENTED LESIONS See Table 31-2

DERMATOLOGIC DISEASES See Tables 31-1, -2, and -3 and Chaps. 54 to 58

DISEASES OF THE TONGUE See Table 31-4

HALITOSIS See Table 31-5

HIV DISEASE AND AIDS (See Table 31-6 and Chaps. 192 and 308) Immunosuppression induced by HIV infection predisposes to numerous oral infections, neoplasms, and autoimmune and idiopathic lesions. Some of these, such as *oral candidiasis* (**Plate ID-42**) and *hairy leukoplakia* (**Plate ID-41**) [a benign epithelial hyperplasia associated with Epstein-Barr virus (EBV)], are common features of HIV disease and often precede or accompany full-blown AIDS. Some, such as oral Kaposi's sarcoma and lymphoma, are diagnostic of AIDS. Oral candidiasis is easily treated with topical or systemic antifungals. These include nystatin oral pastilles, clotrimazole oral troches, nystatin vaginal tablets used orally, fluconazole, and ketoconazole. While most oral lesions of HIV disease are also found in the general population, both hairy leukoplakia and necrotizing ulcerative periodontal disease are strongly associated with HIV infection and are seen only very rarely in other circumstances. Only small and variable amounts of HIV can be found in saliva, but blood, tissue fluid, and gingival crevicular exudate, found in the mouth as a result of lesions or of clinical manipulation, are certainly sources of other viruses, such as herpes simplex virus (HSV) and EBV, and the same may be true for HIV.

HEMATOLOGIC AND NUTRITIONAL DISEASE Gingival bleeding, necrotic ulcers, and enlargement due to malignant infiltrates are seen in all forms of leukemia, particularly *monocytic leukemia*. In *agranulocytosis* severe oral mucosal ulcers are seen, while in *thrombocytopenia* oral petechiae, ecchymoses, and gingival bleeding occur. In *Plummer-Vinson syndrome* (see Chap. 106), atrophy of oral mucosa, particularly the tongue papillae, causes redness and soreness as well as dysphagia. This is associated with increased susceptibility to oral cancer. A smooth tongue also can be seen in *pernicious anemia* (Chap. 108). Severe oral mucositis with ulcers, candidiasis, bacterial infections, and xerostomia complicate local radiotherapy for head and neck malignancies as well as chemotherapy for both local and other malignancies. Although now rarely seen in the United States, oral features of vitamin deficiency include oral mucositis and ulcers, glossitis, and burning sensations in the tongue (*B group vitamin deficiency*) and petechiae, gingival swelling, bleeding, and ulceration as well as loosening of teeth (*scurvy* of vitamin C deficiency).

DISEASES OF THE SALIVARY GLANDS

The major and minor salivary glands can be involved in mumps, sarcoidosis, tuberculosis, lymphoma, and Sjögren's syndrome (Chap.

316). The latter may cause dry eyes and dry mouth (*xerostomia*) and be associated with features of connective tissue diseases, including rheumatoid arthritis or systemic lupus erythematosus. Xerostomia also may be due to medications such as diuretics, antihistamines, or tricylic antidepressants as well as therapeutic irradiation for head and neck cancer. It may cause *cervical or incisal caries* and oral candidiasis. Management includes fluoride mouth rinses and topical applications, saliva substitutes, salivary stimulation with sugarless candies, and the avoidance of sugar-containing drinks or food. Candidiasis is treated with nystatin or other antifungals. Salivary stones (*sialolithiasis*), usually in the duct of a major salivary gland, cause *sialoadenitis* with pain and swelling, often on eating. Recurrent *parotitis* without apparent cause is seen in children.

The most common neoplasm of the salivary glands is the *pleomorphic adenoma*, which is benign but will recur unless fully enucleated; malignant tumors include *mucoepidermoid carcinoma, adenoid cystic carcinoma*, and *adenocarcinoma*. The pleomorphic adenoma causes a firm, slowly growing mass in the parotid, palate, or cheek, whereas malignant tumors grow faster and can cause ulceration and invade nerves, producing numbness or facial paralysis.

NEUROLOGIC DISTURBANCES AND OROFACIAL PAIN

The mouth and face may be the site of pain from a number of vascular, neurologic, muscle/connective tissue, or joint conditions. Interdisciplinary diagnosis and management programs involving neurologists, restorative dentists, oral surgeons, otorhinolaryngologists, and other specialists, together with new imaging techniques to diagnose or exclude organic lesions, have begun to clarify this complex field. *Temporal arteritis* causes pain in the face, jaws, and tongue and may mimic temporomandibular joint disease. Glucocorticoids may provide relief. *Myofascial pain* is a dull, constant ache with local tenderness in the muscles of the jaws and difficulty in opening the mouth. This may be related to clenching and grinding habits (*bruxism*). *Arthralgia* of the temporomandibular joint causes local pain, which may extend to the face and head. Both myofascial pain and arthralgia can be relieved with heat, rest, and anti-inflammatory agents. Displacement of the meniscus or condyle may cause pain, clenching, or locking of the mandible in the open position. The joint may become involved in *osteoarthritis* with minimal symptoms, whereas *rheumatoid arthritis* causes pain and swelling in the joint, limitation of movement, and, in the *juvenile* form, severe malocclusion in children. *Ankylosis* may occur, necessitating condylectomy (see Chap. 313).

Trigeminal neuralgia (tic douloureux) causes sudden, severe, unilateral lancinating pain initiated by touching a "trigger zone" or occurring spontaneously. Confusion with pulpal or periapical pain is common, leading to inappropriate endodontic or surgical therapy. Many cases respond to carbamazepine and phenytoin, but for a few, surgical intervention to decompress the trigeminal nerve is indicated. Similar symptoms in the distribution of the ninth cranial nerve (tongue, pharynx, soft palate) are due to *glossopharyngeal neuralgia*, which may be triggered by swallowing and may produce referred pain in the temporomandibular joint. *Postherpetic neuralgia* may follow trigeminal herpes zoster (see Chap. 372) and cause burning, aching, and long-lasting pain. *Facial palsy* is usually unilateral and may be due to trauma, surgical intervention, tumor, or infection of the seventh cranial nerve. *Bell's palsy* is a form with acute onset and unknown cause, possibly viral infection such as herpes zoster. The corner of the mouth droops, and there may be difficulty in speech, eating, and in closing the eye. The symptoms usually disappear spontaneously, but residual facial immobility and lip drooping may persist. Abnormal or reduced *taste sensation* may be due to xerostomia, disturbances of the facial and glossopharyngeal nerves or their central connections, aging, or the wearing of dentures. Disease involving the hypoglossal nerve may cause atrophy of the tongue muscles with protrusion, if bilateral, or deviation toward the affected side, if unilateral.

Table 31-1

Vesicular, Bullous, or Ulcerative Lesions of the Oral Mucosa

Condition	Usual Location	Clinical Features	Course
VIRAL DISEASES			
Primary acute herpetic gingivo-stomatitis (herpes simplex virus type 1, rarely type 2)	Lip and oral mucosa	Labial vesicles that rupture and crust, and intraoral vesicles that quickly ulcerate; extremely painful; acute gingivitis, fever, malaise, foul odor, and cervical lymphadenopathy; occurs primarily in infants, children, and young adults	Heals spontaneously in 10–14 days unless secondarily infected
Recurrent herpes labialis	Mucocutaneous junction of lip, perioral skin	Eruption of groups of vesicles that may coalesce then rupture and crust; painful to pressure or spicy foods	Lasts about 1 week, but condition may be prolonged if secondary infection occurs
Recurrent intraoral herpes simplex	Palate and gingiva	Small vesicles that rupture and coalesce; painful	Heal spontaneously in about 1 week
Chickenpox (varicella-zoster virus)	Gingiva and oral mucosa	Skin lesions may be accompanied by small vesicles on oral mucosa that rupture to form shallow ulcers; may coalesce to form large bullous lesions that ulcerate; mucosa may have generalized erythema	Lesions heal spontaneously within 2 weeks
Herpes zoster (reactivation of varicella-zoster virus)	Cheek, tongue, gingiva, or palate	Unilateral vesicular eruption and ulceration in linear pattern following sensory distribution of trigeminal nerve or one of its branches	Gradual healing without scarring; postherpetic neuralgia is common
Infectious mononucleosis (Epstein-Barr virus)	Oral mucosa	Fatigue, sore throat, malaise, low-grade fever, and enlarged cervical lymph nodes; numerous small ulcers usually appear several days before lymphadenopathy; gingival bleeding and multiple petechiae at junction of hard and soft palates	Oral lesions disappear during convalescence
Warts (papillomavirus)	Anywhere on skin and oral mucosa	Single or multiple papillary lesions, with thick, white keratinized surfaces containing many pointed projections; cauliflower lesions covered with normal-colored mucosa or multiple pink or pale bumps (focal epithelial hyperplasia)	Lesions grow rapidly and spread
Herpangina (coxsackievirus A; also possibly coxsackievirus B and echovirus)	Oral mucosa, pharynx, tongue	Sudden onset of fever, sore throat, and oropharyngeal vesicles, usually in children under 4 years, during summer months; diffuse pharyngeal congestion and vesicles (1–2 mm), grayish-white surrounded by red areola; vesicles enlarge and ulcerate	Incubation period 2–9 days; fever for 1–4 days; recovery uneventful
Hand, foot, and mouth disease (type A coxsackieviruses)	Oral mucosa, pharynx, palms, and soles	Fever, malaise, headache with oropharyngeal vesicles that become painful, shallow ulcers	Incubation period 2–18 days; lesions heal spontaneously in 2–4 weeks
Primary HIV infection	Gingiva, palate, and pharynx	Acute gingivitis and oropharyngeal ulceration, associated with febrile illness resembling mononucleosis and including lymphadenopathy	Followed by HIV seroconversion, asymptomatic HIV infection, and usually ultimately by HIV disease
BACTERIAL OR FUNGAL DISEASES			
Acute necrotizing ulcerative gingivitis ("trench mouth," Vincent's infection)	Gingiva	Painful, bleeding gingiva characterized by necrosis and ulceration of gingival papillae and margins plus lymphadenopathy and foul odor	Continued destruction of tissue followed by remission, but may recur
Prenatal (congenital) syphilis	Palate, jaws, tongue, and teeth	Gummatous involvement of palate, jaws, and facial bones; Hutchinson's incisors, mulberry molars, glossitis, mucous patches, and fissures of corners of mouth	Tooth deformities in permanent dentition irreversible
Primary syphilis (chancre)	Lesion appears where organism enters body; may occur on lips, tongue, or tonsillar area	Small papule developing rapidly into a large, painless ulcer with indurated border; unilateral lymphadenopathy; chancre and lymph nodes containing spirochetes; serologic tests positive by third to fourth weeks	Healing of chancre in 1–2 months, followed by secondary syphilis in 6–8 weeks
Secondary syphilis	Oral mucosa frequently involved with mucous patches, primarily on palate, also at commissures of mouth	Maculopapular lesions of oral mucosa, 5–10 mm in diameter with central ulceration covered by grayish membrane; eruptions occurring on various mucosal surfaces and skin accompanied by fever, malaise, and sore throat	Lesions may persist from several weeks to a year
Tertiary syphilis	Palate and tongue	Gummatous infiltration of palate or tongue followed by ulceration and fibrosis; atrophy of tongue papillae produces characteristic bald tongue and glossitis	Gumma may destroy palate, causing complete perforation

(*continued*)

Table 31-1—*(continued)*

Vesicular, Bullous, or Ulcerative Lesions of the Oral Mucosa

Condition	Usual Location	Clinical Features	Course
Gonorrhea	Lesions may occur in mouth at site of inoculation or secondarily by hematogenous spread from a primary focus elsewhere	Earliest symptoms are burning or itching sensation, dryness, or heat in mouth followed by acute pain on eating or speaking; tonsils and oropharynx most frequently involved; oral tissues may be diffusely inflamed or ulcerated; saliva develops increased viscosity and fetid odor; submaxillary lymphadenopathy with fever in severe cases	Lesions may resolve with appropriate antibiotic therapy
Tuberculosis	Tongue, tonsillar area, soft palate	A solitary, irregular ulcer covered by a persistent exudate; ulcer has an undermined, firm border	Lesions may persist
Cervicofacial actinomycosis	Swellings in region of face, neck, and floor of mouth	Infection may be associated with an extraction, jaw fracture, or eruption of molar tooth; in acute form resembles an acute pyogenic abscess, but contains yellow "sulfur granules" (gram-positive mycelia and their hyphae)	Acute form may last a few weeks; chronic form lasts months or years; prognosis excellent; actinomycetes respond to antibiotics (tetracyclines or penicillin) but not to antifungal drugs
Histoplasmosis	Any area in mouth, particularly tongue, gingiva, or palate	Numerous small nodules that may ulcerate; hoarseness and dysphagia may occur because of lesions in larynx, usually associated with fever and malaise	May be fatal
Candidiasis	Any area of oral mucosa	Pseudomembranous form has white patches that are easily wiped off leaving red, bleeding, sore surface; erythematous form is flat and red; rarely, candidal leukoplakia appears as white patch in tongue that does not rub off; angular cheilitis due to *Candida* involves sore cracks and redness at angle of mouth; *Candida* seen on KOH preparation in all forms	Responds to antifungals

DERMATOLOGIC DISEASES

Condition	Usual Location	Clinical Features	Course
Mucous membrane pemphigoid	Primarily mucous membranes of the oral cavity, but may also involve the eyes, urethra, vagina, and rectum	Painful, grayish-white collapsed vesicles or bullae with peripheral erythematous zone; gingival lesions desquamate, leaving ulcerated area	Protracted course with remissions and exacerbations; involvement of different sites occurs slowly; glucocorticoids may temporarily reduce symptoms but do not control the disease
Erythema multiforme (Stevens-Johnson syndrome)	Primarily the oral mucosa and skin of hands and feet	Intraoral ruptured bullae surrounded by an inflammatory area; lips may show hemorrhagic crusts; the "iris," or "target" lesion, on the skin is pathognomonic; patient may have severe signs of toxicity	Onset very rapid; condition may last 1–2 weeks; may be fatal; acute episodes respond to steroids
Pemphigus vulgaris	Oral mucosa and skin	Ruptured bullae and ulcerated oral areas; mostly in older adults	With repeated recurrence of bullae, toxicity may lead to cachexia, infection, and death within 2 years; often controllable with steroids
Lichen planus	Oral mucosa and skin	White striae in mouth; purplish nodules on skin at sites of friction; occasionally causes oral mucosal ulcers and erosive gingivitis	Protracted course, may respond to topical steroids

OTHER CONDITIONS

Condition	Usual Location	Clinical Features	Course
Recurrent aphthous ulcers	Anywhere on nonkeratinized oral mucosa (lips, tongue, buccal mucosa, floor of mouth, soft palate, oropharynx)	Single or clusters of painful ulcers with surrounding erythematous border; lesions may be 1–2 mm in diameter in crops (herpetiform), 1–5 mm (minor), or 5–15 mm (major)	Lesions heal in 1–2 weeks but may recur monthly or several times a year; topical steroids give symptomatic relief; systemic glucocorticoids may be needed in severe cases; a tetracycline oral suspension may decrease severity of herpetiform ulcers
Behçet's syndrome	Oral mucosa, eyes, genitalia, gut, and CNS	Multiple aphthous ulcers in mouth; inflammatory ocular changes, ulcerative lesions on genitalia; inflammatory bowel disease and CNS disease	Ulcers may persist for several weeks and heal without scarring
Traumatic ulcers	Anywhere on oral mucosa; dentures frequently responsible for ulcers in vestibule	Localized, discrete ulcerated lesion with red border; produced by accidental biting of mucosa, penetration by a foreign object, or chronic irritation by a denture	Lesions usually heal in 7–10 days when irritant is removed, unless secondarily infected

Table 31-2

Pigmented Lesions of the Oral Mucosa

Condition	Usual Location	Clinical Features	Course
Oral melanotic macule	Any area of the mouth	Discrete or diffuse localized, brown to black macule	Remains indefinitely
Diffuse melanin pigmentation	Any area of the mouth	Diffuse pale to dark-brown pigmentation; may be physiologic ("racial") or due to smoking	Remains indefinitely
Nevi	Any area of the mouth	Discrete, localized, brown to black pigmentation	Remains indefinitely
Malignant melanoma	Any area of the mouth	Can be flat and diffuse, painless, brown to black, or can be raised and nodular	Expands and invades early; metastasis leads to death
Addison's disease	Any area in mouth but mostly on buccal mucosa	Blotches or spots of bluish-black to dark-brown pigmentation occurring early in the disease, accompanied by diffuse pigmentation of skin; other symptoms of adrenal insufficiency	Condition controlled by steroid therapy
Peutz-Jeghers syndrome	Any area in mouth	Dark-brown spots on lips, buccal mucosa, with characteristic distribution of pigment around lips, nose, eyes, and on hands; concomitant intestinal polyposis	Pigmented lesions remain indefinitely; polyps may become malignant
Drug ingestion (tranquilizers, oral contraceptives, antimalarials)	Any area in mouth	Brown, black, or gray areas of pigmentation	Disappears following cessation of drug
Amalgam tattoo	Gingiva and mucobuccal fold	Small blue-black pigmented areas associated with embedded amalgam particles in soft tissues; these may show up on radiographs as radiopaque particles in some cases	Remains indefinitely
Heavy metal pigmentation (bismuth, mercury, lead)	Gingival margin	Thin blue-black pigmented line along gingival margin; due to prior treatment for syphilis with bismuth or mercury or to accidental absorption of lead	Long-lasting
Black hairy tongue	Dorsum of tongue	Elongation of filiform papillae of tongue, which take on a brown to black coloration	Long-lasting but may disappear spontaneously
Fordyce's "disease"	Buccal and labial mucosa	Aggregation of numerous small yellowish spots just beneath mucosal surface; no symptoms; due to hyperplasia of sebaceous glands	Remains without apparent change indefinitely

Table 31-3

White Lesions of Oral Mucosa

Condition	Usual Location	Clinical Features	Course
Lichen planus	Buccal mucosa, tongue, gingiva, and lips; skin	Striae, white plaques, red areas, ulcers in mouth; purplish papules on skin; may be asymptomatic, sore, or painful; lichenoid drug reactions may look similar	Protracted; responds to topical steroids
White sponge nevus	Oral mucosa, vagina, anal mucosa	Painless white thickening of epithelium; adolescent/early adult onset; familial	Benign and permanent
Smoker's leukoplakia and smokeless tobacco lesions	Any area of oral mucosa, sometimes related to location of habit	White patch that may become firm, rough, or red-fissured and ulcerated; may become sore and painful but usually painless	Occasionally premalignant; may or may not resolve on cessation of habit
Nicotinic stomatitis	Palate in pipe smokers	White nodular elevations on hard palate with central red areas	Benign; usually resolves on cessation of pipe smoking
Frictional keratosis	Any area in mouth	Elevated white lesion due to hyperkeratosis and thickening of the oral epithelium secondary to chronic irritation	Removal of irritant leads to healing in 2–3 weeks
Candidiasis ("candidosis," "moniliasis")	Any area in mouth	*Pseudomembranous type* ("thrush"): creamy white curdlike patches that reveal a raw, bleeding surface when scraped; found in sick infants, debilitated elderly patients receiving high doses of glucocorticoids or broad-spectrum antibiotics, or in patients with AIDS	Responds favorably to antifungal therapy and correction of predisposing causes where possible
		Erythematous type: flat, red, sometimes sore areas, same groups of patients	Course same as for pseudomembranous type
		Candidal leukoplakia: nonremovable white thickening of epithelium due to *Candida*	Responds to prolonged antifungals
		Angular cheilitis: sore fissures at corner of mouth	Responds to topical antifungals
Hairy leukoplakia	Usually lateral tongue, rarely elsewhere on oral mucosa	White areas ranging from small and flat to extensive and "hairy"; found in HIV carriers in all risk groups for AIDS; rarely causes discomfort	Due to EBV; many patients develop AIDS; responds to high dose acyclovir but recurs
Chemical burns	Any area in mouth	White slough due to necrosis of epithelium and underlying connective tissue caused by contact with agents (e.g., aspirin) applied locally or the use of undiluted sodium perborate or hydrogen peroxide as a mouthwash; removal of slough leaves a raw, painful surface	Lesion heals in several weeks if not secondarily infected

Table 31-4

Alterations of the Tongue

Type of Change	Clinical Features
SIZE OR MORPHOLOGY CHANGES	
Macroglossia	Enlarged tongue that may be part of a syndrome found in developmental conditions such as Down's syndrome; may be due to tumor (hemangioma or lymphangioma), metabolic disease (such as primary amyloidosis), or endocrine disturbance (such as acromegaly or cretinism)
Fissured ("scrotal") tongue	Dorsal surface and sides of tongue covered by painless shallow or deep fissures that may collect debris and become irritated
Median rhomboid glossitis	Congenital abnormality of tongue with ovoid, denuded area in median posterior portion of the tongue; may be associated with candidiasis and may respond to antifungals
COLOR CHANGES	
"Geographic" tongue (benign migratory glossitis)	Asymptomatic inflammatory condition of the tongue, with rapid loss and regrowth of filiform papillae, leading to appearance of denuded red patches "wandering" across the surface of the tongue
Hairy tongue	Elongation of filiform papillae of the medial dorsal surface area due to failure of keratin layer of the papillae to desquamate normally; brownish-black coloration may be due to staining by tobacco, food, or chromogenic organisms
"Strawberry" and "raspberry" tongue	Appearance of tongue during scarlet fever due to the hypertrophy of fungiform papillae plus changes in the filiform papillae
"Bald" tongue	Atrophy may be associated with xerostomia, pernicious anemia, iron-deficiency anemia, pellagra, or syphilis; may be accompanied by painful burning sensation; may be an expression of erythematous candidiasis and respond to antifungals

Table 31-5

Causes of Halitosis

1. Upper respiratory infection
   a. Bronchiectasis
   b. Lung abscess
2. Oral infection
   a. Acute primary herpetic gingivostomatitis
   b. Acute necrotizing ulcerative gingivitis
   c. Periodontal disease
   d. Caries
3. Smoking
4. Hepatic failure (fishy odor)
5. Azotemia (ammoniacal or urinary odor)
6. Diabetic ketoacidosis (sweet, fruity odor)

Table 31-6

Oral Lesions of HIV Disease and AIDS

  I. Fungal
   A. Candidiasis
     1. Pseudomembranous
     2. Erythematous
     3. Angular cheilitis
   B. Histoplasmosis
   C. Cryptococcosis
 II. Bacterial
   A. Acute necrotizing ulcerative gingivitis
   B. Necrotizing ulcerative periodontitis
   C. Necrotizing stomatitis
   D. *M. avium* complex and tuberculosis
   E. Stomatitis due to enteric organisms
III. Viral
   A. Herpes simplex
   B. Herpes zoster
   C. Hairy leukoplakia
   D. Warts
IV. Neoplastic
   A. Kaposi's sarcoma
   B. Lymphoma
 V. Other
   A. Recurrent aphthous ulcers
   B. Immune thrombocytopenic purpura
   C. Xerostomia
   D. Salivary gland enlargement

BIBLIOGRAPHY

BARKER FG et al: The long-term outcome of microvascular decompression for trigeminal neuralgia. N Engl J Med 334:1077, 1996

GENCO R et al: *Contemporary Periodontics.* St. Louis, Mosby, 1990

GREENSPAN D et al: *AIDS and the Mouth.* Chicago, Year Book, 1990

LYNCH MA et al: *Burket's Oral Medicine, Diagnosis and Treatment,* 8th ed. Philadelphia, Lippincott, 1994

NEWBRUN E: *Cariology,* 3d ed. Chicago, Quintessence, 1989

SECTION 5
ALTERATIONS IN CIRCULATORY AND RESPIRATORY FUNCTIONS

32

Roland H. Ingram, Jr., Eugene Braunwald

DYSPNEA AND PULMONARY EDEMA

DYSPNEA

The breathing pattern is controlled by a series of central and peripheral mechanisms that can adjust ventilation appropriate to increased metabolic demands during physical activity. It can also increase ventilation in excess of metabolic demands in conditions such as anxiety and fear. A normal resting person is unaware of the act of breathing, and while he or she may become conscious of breathing during mild to moderate exertion, no discomfort is experienced. However, during and following exhausting exertion, an individual may become unpleasantly aware of breathing yet feel reasonably assured that the sensation will be transitory and is appropriate to the level of exercise. Therefore, as a cardinal symptom of diseases affecting the cardiorespiratory system, *dyspnea* is defined as an *abnormally uncomfortable awareness of breathing*.

Although dyspnea is not painful in the usual sense of the word, it is, like pain, involved with both the perception of a sensation and the reaction to that perception. Patients experience a number of uncomfortable sensations related to breathing and use an even larger number of verbal expressions to describe these sensations, such as "cannot get enough air," "air does not go all the way down," "smothering feeling or tightness or tiredness in the chest," and a "choking sensation." It may be necessary, therefore, to review meticulously the patient's history in order to ascertain whether the more abstruse descriptions do, in fact, represent dyspnea. Once it is established that a patient does have dyspnea, it is of paramount importance to define the circumstances in which it occurs and to assess associated symptoms. There are situations in which breathing appears labored but in which dyspnea does not occur. For example, the hyperventilation associated with metabolic acidemia is rarely accompanied by dyspnea. On the other hand, patients with apparently normal breathing patterns may complain of shortness of breath.

QUANTITATION OF DYSPNEA The gradation of dyspnea may usefully be based on the amount of physical exertion required to produce the sensation. In assessing the severity of dyspnea, it is important to obtain a clear understanding of the patient's general physical condition, work history, and recreational habits. For example, the development of dyspnea in a trained runner upon running 2 mi may signify a much more serious disturbance than a similar degree of breathlessness in a sedentary person upon running a fraction of this distance. Interindividual variation in perception must also be considered. Some patients with severe disease may complain of only mild dyspnea; others with mild disease may experience more severe shortness of breath. Some patients with lung or heart disease may have such reduced capabilities due to other disease (e.g., peripheral vascular insufficiency or severe osteoarthritis of the hips or knees) that exertional dyspnea is precluded despite serious impairment of pulmonary or cardiac function.

Some patterns of dyspnea are not directly related to physical exertion. Sudden and unexpected dyspneic episodes at rest can be associated with pulmonary emboli, spontaneous pneumothorax, hypercapnea secondary to breath holding, or anxiety. Nocturnal episodes of severe paroxysmal dyspnea are characteristic of left ventricular failure. Dyspnea upon assuming the supine posture, *orthopnea* (see below), thought to be mainly characteristic of congestive heart failure, also may occur in some patients with asthma and chronic obstruction of the airways and is a regular finding in the rare occurrence of bilateral diaphragmatic paralysis. *Trepopnea* is used to describe the unusual circumstance in which dyspnea occurs only in a lateral decubitus position, most often in patients with heart disease, while *platypnea* is dyspnea that occurs only in the upright position. Positional alterations in ventilation-perfusion relationships (see Chap. 250) have been invoked to explain these patterns. Platypnea can also be seen with deficient abdominal musculature, a deficiency that results in loss of diaphragmatic support due to anterior protrusion of abdominal viscera in the upright posture. Upon lying down, the viscera resume support of the diaphragm, stretching it to its optimal operational length. This form of platypnea is alleviated by use of an abdominal binder.

MECHANISMS OF DYSPNEA (See Fig. 32-1) Physicians usually relate the symptom of dyspnea to a process such as obstruction of the airways or congestive heart failure and generally proceed with further diagnostic and/or therapeutic attempts, having satisfied themselves that they understand the mechanism of the dyspnea. In fact, elucidation of the *actual* mechanism(s) of dyspnea has eluded clinical investigators.

Dyspnea occurs whenever the work of breathing is excessive. Increased force generation is required of the respiratory muscles to produce a given volume change if the chest wall or lungs are less compliant or if resistance to airflow is increased. Increased work of breathing also occurs when the ventilation is excessive for the level of activity. Although an individual is more apt to become dyspneic when the work of breathing is increased, the work theory does not account for the perceptual difference between a deep breath with a normal mechanical load and a normal-sized breath with an increased mechanical load. The work might be the same with both breaths, but the normal one with the increased load will be associated with discomfort. In fact, with respiratory loading, such as adding a resistance at the mouth, there is an increase in respiratory center output that is disproportionate to the increase in the work of breathing. It has been postulated that whenever the force that muscles actually generate during breathing approaches some fraction of their maximal force-generating ability, which may vary among individuals, dyspnea ensues due to transduction of mechanical to neural stimuli. Such a theory would still not explain why patients who are completely paralyzed, either by cord transections or neuromuscular blockade, experience dyspnea although aided by a mechanical ventilator. It is probable, in these circumstances, that signals from the lungs and/or airways travel via the vagus nerve to the central nervous system to account for the sensation.

In all likelihood, several different mechanisms operate to different degrees in the various clinical situations in which dyspnea occurs. In some circumstances, dyspnea is evoked by stimulation of receptors in the upper respiratory tract; in others it may originate from receptors in the lungs, airways, respiratory muscles, chest wall, or some combination of these structures. In any event, dyspnea is characterized by an excessive or abnormal activation of the respiratory centers in the brainstem. This activation comes about from stimuli transmitted from

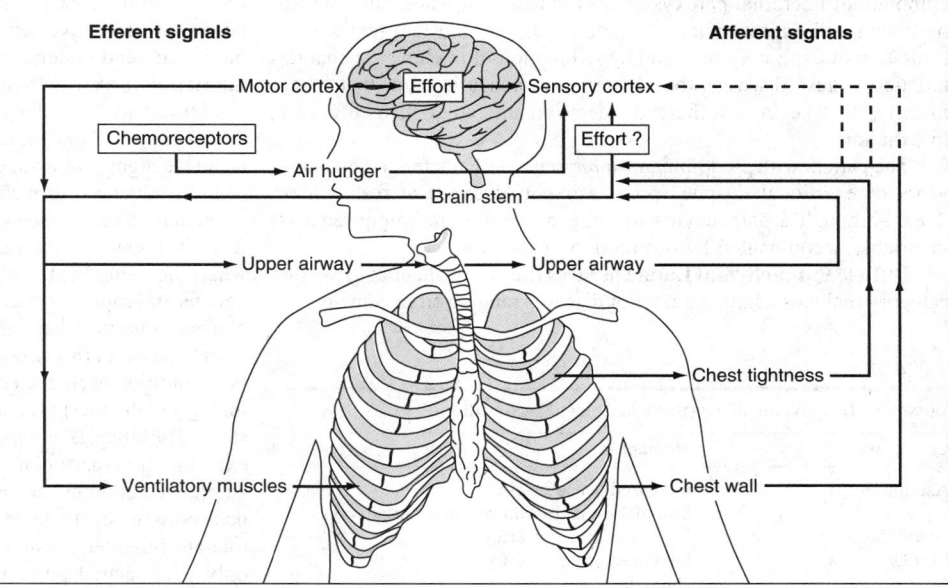

FIGURE 32-1 Efferent and afferent signals that contribute to the sensation of dyspnea. There is evidence that the sense of respiratory effort arises from a signal transmitted from the motor cortex to the sensory cortex simultaneously with the outgoing motor command to the ventilatory muscles. The motor output of the brainstem may also contribute to the sense of effort, as shown in the arrow from the brainstem to the sensory cortex. The sense of air hunger arises, in part, from increased respiratory activity within the brainstem, and the sensation of chest tightness probably results from stimulation of vagal-irritant receptors. While afferent information from airway, lung, and chest-wall receptors probably passes through the brainstem before reaching the sensory cortex, the dashed lines indicate uncertainty about whether some afferents bypass the brainstem and project directly to the sensory cortex. (*From Manning and Schwartzstein, with permission.*)

or through a variety of structures and pathways, including (1) intrathoracic receptors via the vagi; (2) afferent somatic nerves, particularly from the respiratory muscles and chest wall, but also from other skeletal muscles and joints; (3) chemoreceptors in the brain, aortic and carotid bodies, and elsewhere in the circulation; (4) higher (cortical) centers; and perhaps (5) afferent fibers in the phrenic nerves. In general, despite the interindividual variations described above, there is a reasonable correlation between the severity of dyspnea and the magnitude of disturbances of pulmonary or cardiac function that are responsible.

The mechanisms responsible for dyspnea may vary in different conditions (Table 32-1).

DIFFERENTIAL DIAGNOSIS **Obstructive Disease of Airways** (See also Chaps. 252 and 258)   Obstruction to airflow can be present anywhere from the extrathoracic airways out to the small airways in the periphery of the lung. Large extrathoracic airway obstruction can occur acutely, as with aspiration of food or a foreign body or with angioedema of the glottis. Circumstantial evidence or testimony from witnesses should cause the physician to suspect aspiration, and an allergic history together with a few scattered hives should raise the possibility of glottic edema. The acute form of upper airway obstruction is a medical emergency. More chronic forms can occur with tumors or with fibrotic stenosis following tracheostomy or prolonged endotracheal intubation. Whether acute or chronic, the cardinal symptom is dyspnea, and the characteristic signs are stridor and retraction of the supraclavicular fossae with *inspiration*.

Obstruction of intrathoracic airways can occur acutely and intermittently or can be present chronically with worsening during respiratory infections. Acute intermittent obstruction with wheezing is typical of *asthma* (Chap. 252). Chronic cough with expectoration is typical of *chronic bronchitis* (Chap. 258) and *bronchiectasis* (Chap. 256). Most often there is a prolongation of expiration and coarse rhonchi, which are generalized in chronic bronchitis and may be localized in the case of bronchiectasis. Intercurrent infection results in worsening of the cough, increased expectoration of purulent sputum, and more severe dyspnea. During such episodes, the patient may complain of nocturnal paroxysms of dyspnea with wheezing relieved by cough and expectoration of sputum. Despite the fact that severe limitation of expiratory flow and hyperinflation of the lung are characteristic of these diseases, the sensory experience is often that of an inability to take in a sufficiently deep breath rather than difficulty in exhaling.

The patient with predominant *emphysema* is characterized by many years of exertional dyspnea progressing to dyspnea at rest (Chap. 258). Although a parenchymal disease by definition, emphysema is invariably accompanied by obstruction of airways.

Diffuse Parenchymal Lung Diseases (See also Chap. 259)   This category includes a large number of diseases ranging from acute pneumonia to chronic disorders such as sarcoidosis and the various forms of *pneumoconiosis* (Chap. 254). History, physical findings, and radiographic abnormalities often provide clues to the diagnosis. The patients are often tachypneic with arterial P_{CO_2} and P_{O_2} values below normal. Exertion often further reduces the arterial P_{O_2}. Lung volumes are decreased, and the lungs are stiffer, i.e., less compliant than normal.

Pulmonary Vascular Occlusive Diseases (See also Chap. 261) Repeated episodes of dyspnea at rest often occur with recurrent pulmonary emboli. Evidence of a source for emboli, such as phlebitis of a lower extremity or the pelvis, is quite helpful in leading the physician to suspect the diagnosis. Arterial blood gases are most often abnormal, but lung volumes are frequently normal or only minimally abnormal.

Diseases of the Chest Wall or Respiratory Muscles (See also Chap. 263)   The physical examination establishes the presence of a chest wall disease such as severe kyphoscoliosis, pectus excavatum, or ankylosing spondylitis. Although all three of these deformities may be associated with dyspnea, only severe kyphoscoliosis regularly interferes with ventilation sufficiently to produce chronic cor pulmonale and respiratory failure.

Both weakness and paralysis of respiratory muscles can lead to respiratory failure and dyspnea (Chap. 263), but most often the signs and symptoms of the neurologic or muscular disorder are more prominently manifested in other systems.

Heart Disease   In patients with cardiac disease, exertional dyspnea occurs most commonly as a consequence of an elevated pulmonary capillary pressure, which in turn may be due to left ventricular dysfunction (Chaps. 232 and 233), reduced left ventricular compliance, and mitral stenosis. The elevation of hydrostatic pressure in the pulmonary vascular bed tends to upset the Starling equilibrium (see "Pulmonary Edema," below) with resulting transudation of liquid into the interstitial space, reducing the compliance of the lungs and stimulating J (juxtacapillary) receptors in the alveolar interstitial space. When it is prolonged, pulmonary venous hypertension results in thickening of the walls of small pulmonary vessels and an increase in perivascular cells and fibrous tissue, causing a further reduction in compliance. The competition for space among vessels, airways, and increased liquid within the interstitial space compromises the lumina of small airways, increasing the airways' resistance. Diminution in compliance and an increase in the airways' resistance increase the work of breathing. In advanced congestive heart failure, usually involving elevation of both pulmonary and systemic venous pressures, hydrothorax may develop, interfering further with pulmonary function and intensifying dyspnea.

Orthopnea, i.e., dyspnea in the recumbent position, and *paroxysmal nocturnal dyspnea*, i.e., attacks of shortness of breath that usually occur at night and awaken the patient from sleep, are characteristic of more advanced forms of heart failure associated with elevations of pulmonary venous and capillary pressures and are discussed in Chap. 233. Orthopnea is the result of the alteration of gravitational forces when the recumbent position is assumed, which elevates pulmonary venous and capillary pressures. These, in turn, increase the pulmonary closing volume (Chap. 250) and reduce the vital capacity.

Paroxysmal (nocturnal) dyspnea   Also known as *cardiac asthma*, this condition is characterized by attacks of severe shortness of breath that generally occur at night and usually awaken the patient from sleep. The attack is precipitated by stimuli that aggravate the previously existing pulmonary congestion; frequently, the total blood volume is augmented at night because of the reabsorption of edema from dependent portions of the body during recumbency. A sleeping patient can tolerate relatively severe pulmonary engorgement and may awaken only when actual pulmonary edema and bronchospasm have developed, with the feeling of suffocation and with wheezing respirations. Two other forms of nocturnal dyspnea must be distinguished from that due to heart failure. Chronic bronchitis is characterized by mucus hypersecretion and, after a few hours sleep, secretions can accumulate and produce dyspnea and wheezing, both of which are relieved by cough and expectoration of sputum. Asthma patients have circadian variations in their degree of airway obstruction. The obstruction becomes most severe between 1 A.M. and 2 A.M. and can be sufficiently severe that the patient awakens with a sense of suffocation, extreme

Table 32-1

Possible Mechanisms of Dyspnea in Selected Conditions

Condition	Mechanism
Asthma	Increased sense of effort
	Stimulation of irritant receptors in airways
Neuromuscular disease	Increased sense of effort
COPD	Increased sense of effort
	Hypoxia
	Hypercapnia
	Dynamic airway compression
Mechanical ventilation	Afferent mismatch
	Factors associated with the underlying condition
Pulmonary embolism	Stimulation of pressure receptors in pulmonary vasculature or right atrium (?)

NOTE: COPD, chronic obstructive pulmonary disease.
SOURCE: From Manning and Schwartzstein, with permission.

dyspnea, and wheezing. Although there is a prominent inflammatory component to nocturnal asthma, inhaled bronchodilators usually improve symptoms quickly.

Cheyne-Stokes respiration → See Chap. 233.

Diagnosis The diagnosis of cardiac dyspnea depends on the recognition of heart disease on the basis of the clinical examination supplemented by noninvasive testing. There may be a history of antecedent myocardial infarction, third and fourth heart sounds may be audible, and/or there may be evidence of left ventricular enlargement, jugular neck vein distention, and/or peripheral edema. Often there are radiographic signs of heart failure, with evidence of interstitial edema, pulmonary vascular redistribution, and accumulation of liquid in the septal planes and pleural cavity. Transthoracic echocardiography is particularly useful in establishing the diagnosis of structural heart disease, which can be responsible for dyspnea. Specifically, left atrial and/or left ventricular dilatation, left ventricular hypertrophy, a reduced left ventricular ejection fraction, and disorders of left ventricular wall motion may be clues to the presence of a cardiac etiology of otherwise unexplained dyspnea.

Differentiation between Cardiac and Pulmonary Dyspnea In most patients with dyspnea there is obvious clinical evidence of disease of the heart and/or lungs. Like patients with cardiac dyspnea, patients with chronic obstructive lung disease also may waken at night with dyspnea, but, as pointed out above, this is usually associated with sputum production; the dyspnea is relieved after these patients rid themselves of secretions. The difficulty in the distinction between cardiac and pulmonary dyspnea may be compounded by the coexistence of diseases involving both organ systems.

In patients in whom the etiology of dyspnea is not clear, it is desirable to carry out pulmonary function testing, for these tests may be helpful in determining whether dyspnea is produced by heart disease, lung disease, abnormalities of the chest wall, or anxiety (Chap. 250). In addition to the usual means of assessing patients for heart disease, determination of the ejection fraction at rest and during exercise by echocardiography or radionuclide ventriculography is helpful in the differential diagnosis of dyspnea. The left ventricular ejection fraction is depressed in left ventricular failure, while the right ventricular ejection fraction may be low at rest or may decline during exercise in patients with severe lung disease. Both left and right ventricular ejection fractions are normal at rest and during exercise in dyspnea due to anxiety or malingering. Careful observation during the performance of an exercise treadmill test will often help in the identification of the patient who is malingering or whose dyspnea is secondary to anxiety. Under these circumstances, the patient usually complains of severe shortness of breath but appears to be breathing either effortlessly or totally irregularly.

Anxiety Neurosis Dyspnea experienced by a patient with an anxiety neurosis is difficult to evaluate. The signs and symptoms of acute and chronic hyperventilation do not serve to distinguish between anxiety neurosis and other processes, such as recurrent pulmonary emboli. Another potentially confusing situation is seen when chest pain and electrocardiographic changes accompany the hyperventilation syndrome. When present and attributable to this condition, often referred to as *neurocirculatory asthenia* (Chap. 13), the chest pain is often sharp, fleeting, and in various loci, and the electrocardiographic changes are most often seen during repolarization. Frequent sighing respirations and an irregular breathing pattern point to a psychogenic origin of the dyspnea.

PULMONARY EDEMA See Table 32-2

CARDIOGENIC PULMONARY EDEMA (See Table 32-2, IA) An increase in pulmonary venous pressure, which results initially in engorgement of the pulmonary vasculature, is common in most instances of dyspnea in association with congestive heart failure. The lungs become less compliant, the resistance of small airways increases, and there is an increase in lymphatic flow that apparently serves to maintain a constant pulmonary extravascular liquid volume. Mild

tachypnea is present. If it is sufficient both in magnitude and duration, the increase in intravascular pressure results in a net gain of liquid in the extravascular space, i.e., *interstitial* edema develops. At this point symptoms worsen, tachypnea increases, gas exchange deteriorates further, and radiographic changes, such as Kerley B lines and loss of distinct vascular margins, are seen. At this stage, the capillary endothelial intercellular junctions have widened and allow passage of macromolecules into the interstices.

Further elevations in intravascular pressure result in disruption of the tight junctions between alveolar lining cells, and alveolar edema ensues with outpouring of liquid that contains both red blood cells and macromolecules. At this point *alveolar* edema is present. With yet more severe disruption of the alveolar-capillary membrane, edematous liquid floods the alveoli and airways. At this point, full-blown clinical pulmonary edema with bilateral wet rales and rhonchi occurs, and the chest radiograph may show diffuse haziness of the lung fields with greater density in the more proximal hilar regions. Typically, the patient is anxious and perspires freely, and the sputum is frothy and blood-tinged. Gas exchange is more severely compromised with worsening hypoxia. Without effective treatment (Chap. 233), progressive acidemia, hypercapnia, and respiratory arrest ensue.

Table 32-2

Classification of Pulmonary Edema Based on Initiating Mechanism

I. Imbalance of Starling forces
  A. Increased pulmonary capillary pressure
    1. Increased pulmonary venous pressure without left ventricular failure (e.g., mitral stenosis)
    2. Increased pulmonary venous pressure secondary to left ventricular failure
    3. Increased pulmonary capillary pressure secondary to increased pulmonary arterial pressure (so-called overperfusion pulmonary edema)
  B. Decreased plasma oncotic pressure
    1. Hypoalbuminemia
  C. Increased negativity of interstitial pressure
    1. Rapid removal of pneumothorax with large applied negative pressures (unilateral)
    2. Large negative pleural pressures due to acute airway obstruction alone with increased end-expiratory volumes (asthma)
II. Altered alveolar-capillary membrane permeability (acute respiratory distress syndrome)
  A. Infectious pneumonia—bacterial, viral, parasitic
  B. Inhaled toxins (e.g., phosgene, ozone, chlorine, Teflon fumes, nitrogen dioxide, smoke)
  C. Circulating foreign substances (e.g., snake venom, bacterial endotoxins)
  D. Aspiration of acidic gastric contents
  E. Acute radiation pneumonitis
  F. Endogenous vasoactive substances (e.g., histamine, kinins)
  G. Disseminated intravascular coagulation
  H. Immunologic—hypersensitivity pneumonitis, drugs (nitrofurantoin), leukoagglutinins
  I. Shock lung in association with nonthoracic trauma
  J. Acute hemorrhagic pancreatitis
III. Lymphatic insufficiency
  A. After lung transplant
  B. Lymphangitic carcinomatosis
  C. Fibrosing lymphangitis (e.g., silicosis)
IV. Unknown or incompletely understood
  A. High-altitude pulmonary edema
  B. Neurogenic pulmonary edema
  C. Narcotic overdose
  D. Pulmonary embolism
  E. Eclampsia
  F. After cardioversion
  G. After anesthesia
  H. After cardiopulmonary bypass

SOURCE: From Braunwald et al., with permission.

The earlier sequence of liquid accumulation described above follows the Starling law of capillary–interstitial liquid exchange:

$$\text{Liquid accumulation} = K[(P_c - P_{IF}) - \sigma(\pi_{pl} - \pi_{IF})] - Q_{lymph}$$

where K = hydraulic conductance (directly proportional to membrane surface area and inversely proportional to membrane thickness)
P_c = mean intracapillary pressure
π_{IF} = oncotic pressure of interstitial liquid
σ = reflection coefficient of macromolecules
P_{IF} = mean interstitial liquid pressure
π_{pl} = oncotic pressure of the plasma
Q_{lymph} = lymphatic flow

The pressures tending to move liquid out of the vessel are P_c and π_{IF}, which are normally more than offset by pressures tending to move liquid back into the vasculature, i.e., the algebraic sum of P_{IF} and π_{pl}. Implicit in the preceding equation is that lymphatic flow can increase in the case of imbalance of forces and result in no net accumulation of interstitial liquid. Further elevations in P_c not only increase the outward movement of liquid in each capillary region but also recruit more of the capillary bed, which increases K. These two effects lead to liquid filtration that exceeds clearance capability by the lymphatics, and liquid accumulates in the loose interstitial spaces of the lung. Even greater increases in P_c open first the loose endothelial intercellular junctions and later the tight alveolar intercellular junctions with an increase in permeability to macromolecules. This secondary disruption of both the function and structure of the alveolar-capillary membrane leads to alveolar flooding.

NONCARDIOGENIC PULMONARY EDEMA (See Table 32-2, IB, IC, II, III, and IV)   Several clinical conditions are associated with pulmonary edema based on an imbalance of Starling forces other than through primary elevations of pulmonary capillary pressure. Although diminished plasma oncotic pressure in hypoalbuminemic states (e.g., severe liver disease, nephrotic syndrome, protein-losing enteropathy) might be expected to lead to pulmonary edema, the balance of forces normally so strongly favors resorption that even in these conditions some elevation of capillary pressure is usually necessary before interstitial edema develops. Increased negativity of interstitial pressure has been implicated in the genesis of unilateral pulmonary edema following rapid evacuation of a large pneumothorax. In this situation, the findings may be apparent only by radiography, but occasionally the patient experiences dyspnea with physical findings localized to the edematous lung. It has been proposed that large negative intrapleural pressures during acute severe asthma may be associated with the development of interstitial edema. Lymphatic blockade secondary to fibrotic and inflammatory diseases or lymphangitic carcinomatosis may lead to interstitial edema. In such instances, both clinical and radiographic manifestations are dominated by the underlying disease process.

Other conditions characterized by increases in the interstitial liquid content of the lungs appear to be associated primarily with disruption of the alveolar-capillary membranes. Any number of spontaneously occurring or environmental toxic insults, including diffuse pulmonary infections, aspiration, and shock (particularly due to sepsis and hemorrhagic pancreatitis and following cardiopulmonary bypass), are associated with diffuse pulmonary edema that clearly does not have a hemodynamic origin. → *These conditions, which may lead to the acute respiratory distress syndrome, are discussed in Chap. 265.*

Other Forms of Pulmonary Edema   There are three forms of pulmonary edema that have not been clearly related to increased permeability, inadequate lymphatic flow, or an imbalance of Starling forces; hence their precise mechanism remains unexplained. *Narcotic overdose* is a well-recognized antecedent to pulmonary edema. Although illicit use of parenteral heroin is the most frequent cause, parenteral and oral overdoses of legitimate preparations of morphine, methadone, and dextropropoxyphene also have been associated with pulmonary edema. The earlier idea that injected impurities lead to the disorder is untenable. Available evidence suggests that there are alterations in the permeability of alveolar and capillary membranes rather than an elevation of pulmonary capillary pressure.

Exposure to high altitude in association with severe physical exertion is a well-recognized setting for pulmonary edema in unacclimatized yet otherwise healthy persons. Recent data show that acclimatized high-altitude natives also develop this syndrome upon return to high altitude after a relatively brief sojourn at low altitudes. The syndrome is far more common in persons under the age of 25 years. The mechanism for high-altitude pulmonary edema remains obscure, and studies have been conflicting, some suggesting pulmonary venous constriction and others indicating pulmonary arteriolar constriction as the prime mechanisms. A role for hypoxia at high altitude is suggested by the fact that patients respond to the administration of oxygen and/or return to lower altitudes. Hypoxia per se does not alter permeability of the alveolar-capillary membrane. Hence increased cardiac output and pulmonary arterial pressures with exercise combined with hypoxic pulmonary arteriolar constriction, which is more prominent in young persons, may combine to make this an example of prearteriolar, high-pressure pulmonary edema.

Neurogenic pulmonary edema has been described in patients with central nervous system disorders and without apparent preexisting left ventricular dysfunction. Although most experimental equivalents have implicated sympathetic nervous system activity, the mechanism whereby sympathetic efferent activity leads to pulmonary edema is a matter of speculation. It is known that a massive adrenergic nervous discharge leads to peripheral vasoconstriction with elevation of blood pressure and shifts of blood to the central circulation. In addition, it is probable that a reduction in left ventricular compliance also occurs, and both factors serve to increase left atrial pressures sufficiently to induce pulmonary edema on a hemodynamic basis. Some experimental evidence suggests that stimulation of adrenergic receptors increases capillary permeability directly, but this effect is relatively minor as compared with the imbalance of Starling forces.

TREATMENT OF PULMONARY EDEMA   → *See Chap. 233.*

BIBLIOGRAPHY

BRAUNWALD E et al: Clinical aspects of heart failure; High-output heart failure; Pulmonary edema, in *Heart Disease*, 5th ed, E Braunwald (ed). Philadelphia, Saunders, 1997, p 445
COLICE GL: Detecting the presence and cause of pulmonary edema. Postgrad Med 93:161, 169, 1993
ELLIOTT MW et al: The language of breathlessness: Use of verbal descriptors by patients with cardiopulmonary diseases. Am Rev Respir Dis 144:826, 1991
GILLESPIE DJ, STAATS BA: Unexplained dyspnea. Mayo Clin Proc 69:657, 1994
GROPPER MA et al: Acute cardiogenic pulmonary edema. Clin Chest Med 15:501, 1994
KILLIAN KJ, JONES NL: Mechanisms of exertional dyspnea. Clin Chest Med 15:247, 1994
MANNING HL, SCHWARTZSTEIN RM: Pathophysiology of dyspnea. N Engl J Med 333:1547, 1995

33   *Steven E. Weinberger, Eugene Braunwald*

COUGH AND HEMOPTYSIS

COUGH

Cough is an explosive expiration that provides a protective mechanism for clearing the tracheobronchial tree of secretions and foreign material. However, when excessive or bothersome, it is also one of the most common symptoms for which medical attention is sought. Reasons for the latter include discomfort from the cough itself, interference with normal lifestyle, and concern for the cause of the cough, especially fear of cancer or AIDS.

Coughing may be initiated either voluntarily or reflexively. As a defensive reflex it has both afferent and efferent pathways. The *afferent limb* includes receptors within the sensory distribution of the trigeminal, glossopharyngeal, superior laryngeal, and vagus nerves. The *efferent limb* includes the recurrent laryngeal nerve and the spinal nerves. The *sequence* of a cough starts with a deep inspiration and is followed by glottic closure, relaxation of the diaphragm, and muscle contraction against a closed glottis. The resulting markedly positive intrathoracic pressure causes narrowing of the trachea. Once the glottis opens, the large pressure differential between the airways and the atmosphere coupled with tracheal narrowing produces rapid flow rates through the trachea. The shearing forces that develop aid in the elimination of mucus and foreign materials.

ETIOLOGY As a protective mechanism against foreign or noxious material, cough can be initiated by a variety of airway irritants, which enter the tracheobronchial tree by inhalation (smoke, dust, fumes) or by aspiration (upper airway secretions, gastric contents, foreign bodies). When cough is due to irritation by upper airway secretions (as with postnasal drip) or gastric contents (as with gastroesophageal reflux), the initiating factor may go unrecognized and the cough can be persistent. Additionally, prolonged exposure to such irritants may initiate airway inflammation, which can itself trigger cough and sensitize the airway to other irritants.

Any disorder resulting in inflammation, constriction, infiltration, or compression of airways can be associated with cough. Inflammation commonly results from airway infections, ranging from viral or bacterial bronchitis to bronchiectasis. In viral bronchitis, airway inflammation sometimes persists long after resolution of the typical acute symptoms, thereby producing a prolonged cough, lasting for weeks. Pertussis infection is also a possible cause of persistent cough in adults; however, diagnosis is generally made on clinical grounds (see Chap. 154), and confirmation requires serologic testing for antibodies using an assay which is not readily available. Asthma, which is associated with airway inflammation as well as potentially reversible bronchoconstriction, is a common cause of cough. Although the clinical setting commonly suggests when a cough is secondary to asthma, some patients present with cough in the absence of wheezing or dyspnea, thus making the diagnosis more subtle ("cough variant asthma"). A neoplasm infiltrating the airway wall, such as bronchogenic carcinoma or a carcinoid tumor, is commonly associated with cough. Airway infiltration with granulomas may also trigger a cough, as seen with endobronchial sarcoidosis or tuberculosis. Compression of airways results from extrinsic masses, including lymph nodes, mediastinal tumors, and aortic aneurysms.

Examples of parenchymal lung disease potentially producing cough include interstitial lung disease, pneumonia, and lung abscess. Congestive heart failure may be associated with cough, probably as a consequence of interstitial as well as peribronchial edema. A nonproductive cough complicates the use of angiotensin-converting enzyme (ACE) inhibitors in 5 to 20 percent of patients taking these agents. Onset is usually within 1 week of starting the drug but can be delayed up to 6 months. Although the mechanism is not known with certainty, it may relate to accumulation of bradykinin or substance P, both of which are degraded by ACE.

_____ *Approach to the Patient* _____

A detailed history frequently provides the most valuable clues for etiology of the cough. Particularly important questions include:

1. Is the cough acute or chronic?
2. At its onset, were there associated symptoms suggestive of a respiratory infection?
3. Is it seasonal or associated with wheezing?
4. Is it associated with symptoms suggestive of postnasal drip (nasal discharge, frequent throat clearing) or gastroesophageal reflux (heartburn or sensation of regurgitation)?
5. Is it associated with fever or sputum? If sputum is present, what is its character?

6. Does the patient have any associated diseases or risk factors for disease (e.g., cigarette smoking, risk factors for infection with human immunodeficiency virus, environmental exposures)?
7. Is the patient taking an ACE inhibitor?

The general *physical examination* may point to a nonpulmonary cause of cough, such as heart failure, primary nonpulmonary neoplasm, or AIDS. Examination of the oropharynx may provide suggestive evidence for postnasal drip, including oropharyngeal mucus or erythema, or a "cobblestone" appearance to the mucosa. Auscultation of the chest may demonstrate inspiratory stridor (indicative of upper airway disease), rhonchi or expiratory wheezing (indicative of lower airway disease), or inspiratory crackles (suggestive of a process involving the pulmonary parenchyma, such as interstitial lung disease, pneumonia, or pulmonary edema).

Chest radiography may be particularly helpful in suggesting or confirming the cause of the cough. Important potential findings include the presence of an intrathoracic mass lesion, a localized pulmonary parenchymal infiltrate, or diffuse interstitial or alveolar disease. An area of honeycombing or cyst formation may suggest bronchiectasis, while symmetric bilateral hilar adenopathy may suggest sarcoidosis.

Pulmonary function testing (see Chap. 250) is useful for assessing the functional abnormalities that accompany certain disorders producing cough. Measurement of forced expiratory flow rates can demonstrate reversible airflow obstruction characteristic of asthma. When asthma is considered but flow rates are normal, bronchoprovocation testing with methacholine or cold-air inhalation can demonstrate hyperreactivity of the airways to a bronchoconstrictive stimulus. Measurement of lung volumes and diffusing capacity is useful primarily for demonstration of a restrictive pattern, often seen with any of the diffuse interstitial lung diseases.

If *sputum* is produced, gross and microscopic examination may provide useful information. Purulent sputum suggests chronic bronchitis, bronchiectasis, pneumonia, or lung abscess. Blood in the sputum may be seen in the same disorders, but its presence also raises the question of an endobronchial tumor. Gram and acid-fast stains and cultures may demonstrate a particular infectious pathogen, while sputum cytology may provide a diagnosis of a pulmonary malignancy.

More specialized studies are helpful in specific circumstances. *Fiberoptic bronchoscopy* is the procedure of choice for visualizing an endobronchial tumor and collecting cytologic and histologic specimens. Inspection of the tracheobronchial mucosa can demonstrate endobronchial granulomas often seen in sarcoidosis, and endobronchial biopsy of such lesions or transbronchial biopsy of the lung interstitium can confirm the diagnosis. Inspection of the airway mucosa by bronchoscopy can also demonstrate the characteristic appearance of endobronchial Kaposi's sarcoma in patients with AIDS. *High-resolution computed tomography* (HRCT) can confirm the presence of interstitial disease and can sometimes suggest a diagnosis based on the pattern of disease. It is the procedure of choice for demonstrating dilated airways and confirming the diagnosis of bronchiectasis.

A diagnostic algorithm for evaluation of chronic cough is presented in Fig. 33-1.

COMPLICATIONS Paroxysms of coughing may precipitate syncope (cough syncope; see Chap. 20), consequent to markedly positive intrathoracic and alveolar pressures, which diminish venous return, producing a decrease in cardiac output. Although cough fractures of the ribs may occur in otherwise normal patients, their occurrence should at least raise the possibility of pathologic fractures, which are seen with multiple myeloma, osteoporosis, and osteolytic metastases.

℞ **TREATMENT**
Definitive treatment of cough depends on determining the underlying cause and then initiating specific therapy. Elimination of an exogenous inciting agent (cigarette smoke, ACE inhibitors) or an endoge-

nous trigger (postnasal drip, gastroesophageal reflux) is usually effective when such a precipitant can be identified. Other important management considerations are treatment of specific respiratory tract infections, bronchodilators for potentially reversible airflow obstruction, chest physiotherapy to enhance clearance of secretions in patients with bronchiectasis, and treatment of endobronchial tumors or interstitial lung disease when such therapy is available and appropriate.

Symptomatic or nonspecific therapy of cough should be considered when: (1) the cause of the cough is not known or specific treatment is not possible, and (2) the cough performs no useful function or causes marked discomfort. An irritative, nonproductive cough may be suppressed by an antitussive agent, which increases the latency or threshold of the cough center. Such agents include codeine (15 mg qid) or nonnarcotics such as dextromethorphan (15 mg qid). These drugs provide symptomatic relief by interrupting prolonged, self-perpetuating paroxysms. However, a cough produc-

tive of significant quantities of sputum should usually not be suppressed, since retention of sputum in the tracheobronchial tree may interfere with the distribution of ventilation, alveolar aeration, and the ability of the lung to resist infection.

Other agents working by a variety of mechanisms have also been used to control cough, but objective information assessing their benefit is meager. The inhaled anticholinergic agent, ipratropium bromide (2 to 4 puffs qid), has been used with the rationale of inhibiting the efferent limb of the cough reflex. Inhaled glucocorticoids (e.g., beclomethasone or triamcinolone, 8 to 16 puffs per day divided over two to four doses) have been used for patients in whom airway inflammation is thought to be playing a role in the cough.

HEMOPTYSIS

Hemoptysis is defined as the expectoration of blood from the respiratory tract, a spectrum that varies from blood streaking of sputum to coughing up massive amounts of blood (i.e., >100 mL/24 h). Massive hemoptysis can represent an acutely life-threatening problem. Large amounts of blood can fill the airways and the alveolar spaces, not only seriously disturbing gas exchange but potentially causing the patient to suffocate. Expectoration of even relatively small amounts of blood is a frightening symptom, and quantitation by the patient may therefore be unreliable. It can be a marker for potentially serious disease, such as bronchogenic carcinoma.

ETIOLOGY Because blood originating from the nasopharynx or the gastrointestinal tract can mimic blood coming from the lower respiratory tract, it is important to determine initially that the blood is not coming from one of these alternative sites. Clues that the blood is originating from the gastrointestinal tract include a dark red appearance and an acidic pH, in contrast to the typical bright red appearance and alkaline pH of true hemoptysis.

The bronchial arteries, which are part of the high-pressure systemic circulation, originate either from the aorta or from intercostal arteries and are the source of bleeding in bronchitis or bronchiectasis or with endobronchial tumors.

An etiologic classification of hemoptysis can be based on the site of origin within the lungs (see Table 33-1). The most common site of bleeding is the airways, i.e., the tracheobronchial tree, which can be affected by inflammation (acute or chronic bronchitis, bronchiectasis) or by neoplasm (bronchogenic carcinoma, endobronchial metastatic carcinoma, or bronchial carcinoid tumor). Blood originating from the pulmonary parenchyma can be either from a localized source, such as an infection (pneumonia, lung abscess, tuberculosis), or from a process diffusely affecting the parenchyma (as with a coagulopathy or with an autoimmune process such as Goodpasture's syndrome). Disorders primarily affecting the pulmonary vasculature include pulmonary embolic disease and those conditions associated with elevated pulmonary venous and capillary pressures, such as mitral stenosis or left ventricular failure.

Although the relative frequency of the different etiologies of hemoptysis varies from series to series, most recent studies indicate

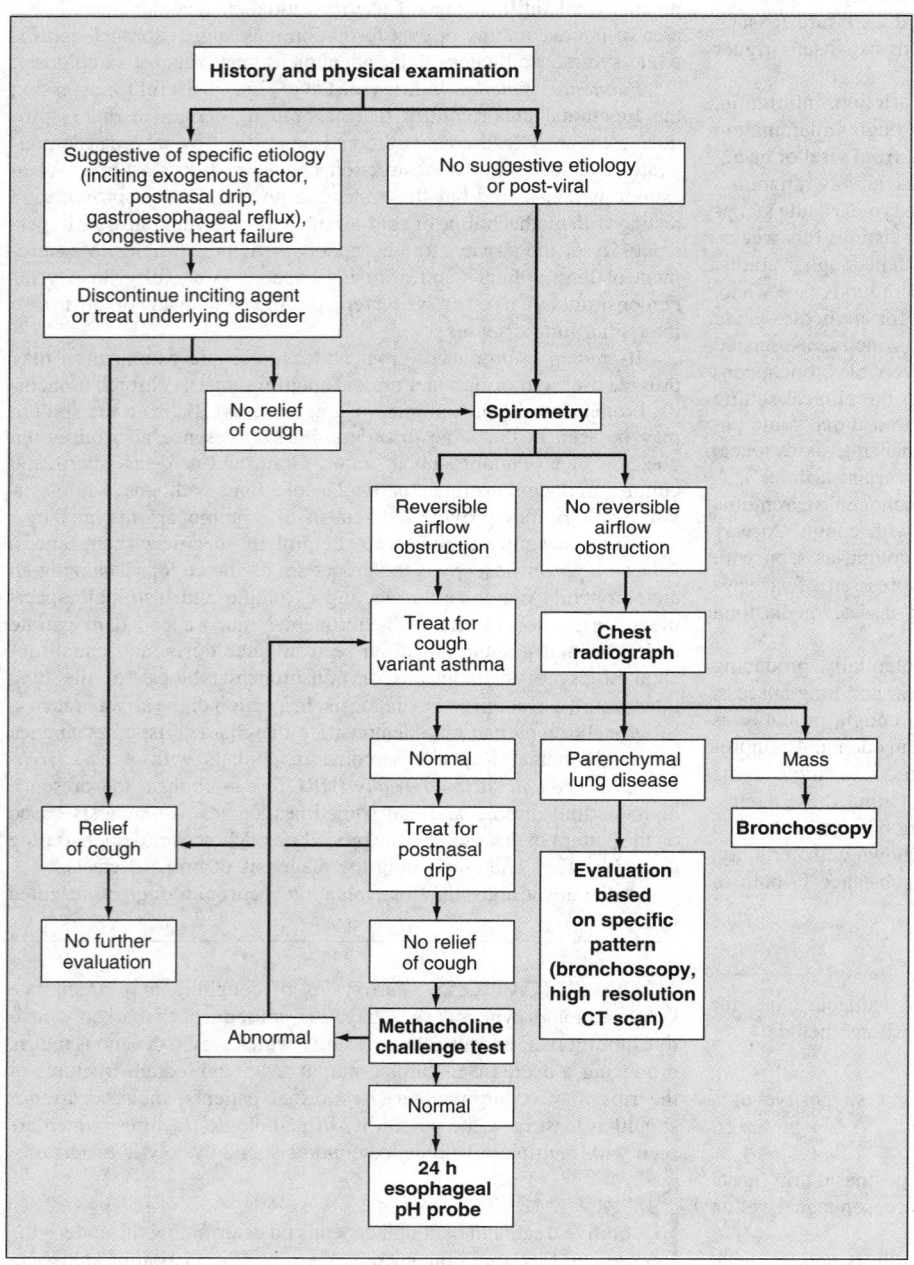

FIGURE 33-1 An algorithm for the evaluation of chronic cough.

that bronchitis and bronchogenic carcinoma are the two most common causes. Despite the lower frequency of tuberculosis and bronchiectasis seen in recent compared to older series, these two disorders still represent the most common causes of massive hemoptysis in several series. Even after extensive evaluation, a sizable proportion of patients (up to 30 percent in some series) have no identifiable etiology for their hemoptysis. These patients are classified as having idiopathic or cryptogenic hemoptysis, and subtle airway or parenchymal disease is presumably responsible for the bleeding.

Approach to the Patient

The history is extremely valuable. Hemoptysis that is described as blood-streaking of mucopurulent or purulent sputum often suggests bronchitis. Chronic production of sputum with a recent change in quantity or appearance favors an acute exacerbation of chronic bronchitis. Fever or chills accompanying blood-streaked purulent sputum suggests pneumonia, whereas a putrid smell to the sputum raises the possibility of lung abscess. When sputum production has been chronic and copious, the diagnosis of bronchiectasis should be considered, although the absence of chronic sputum production does not necessarily exclude a diagnosis of bronchiectasis (so-called dry bronchiectasis). Hemoptysis following the acute onset of pleuritic chest pain and dyspnea is suggestive of pulmonary embolism.

A history of previous or coexisting disorders should be sought, such as renal disease (seen with Goodpasture's syndrome or Wegener's granulomatosis), lupus erythematosus (with associated pulmonary hemorrhage from lupus pneumonitis), or a previous malignancy (either recurrent lung cancer or endobronchial metastasis from a nonpulmonary primary tumor). In a patient with AIDS, endobronchial or pulmonary parenchymal Kaposi's sarcoma should be considered. Risk factors for bronchogenic carcinoma, particularly smoking and asbestos exposure, should be sought. Patients should be questioned about previous bleeding disorders, treatment with anticoagulants, or use of drugs that can be associated with thrombocytopenia.

The *physical examination* may also provide helpful clues to the diagnosis. For example, examination of the lungs may demonstrate a

pleural friction rub (pulmonary embolism), localized or diffuse crackles (parenchymal bleeding or an underlying parenchymal process associated with bleeding), evidence of airflow obstruction (chronic bronchitis), or prominent rhonchi, with or without wheezing or crackles (bronchiectasis). Cardiac examination may demonstrate findings of pulmonary arterial hypertension, mitral stenosis, or heart failure. Skin examination may reveal Kaposi's sarcoma, arteriovenous malformations of Osler-Rendu-Weber disease, or lesions suggestive of systemic lupus erythematosus.

Diagnostic evaluation of hemoptysis starts with a chest radiograph to look for a mass lesion, findings suggestive of bronchiectasis (see Chap. 256), or focal or diffuse parenchymal disease (representing either focal or diffuse bleeding or a focal area of pneumonitis). Additional initial screening evaluation often includes a complete blood count, a coagulation profile, and assessment for renal disease with a urinalysis and measurement of blood urea nitrogen and creatinine levels. When sputum is present, examination by Gram and acid-fast stains (along with the corresponding cultures) is indicated.

Fiberoptic bronchoscopy is particularly useful for localizing the site of bleeding and for visualization of endobronchial lesions. When bleeding is massive, rigid bronchoscopy is often preferable to fiberoptic bronchoscopy because of better airway control and greater suction capability. In patients with suspected bronchiectasis, HRCT is now the diagnostic procedure of choice, having replaced bronchography.

A diagnostic algorithm for evaluation of nonmassive hemoptysis is presented in Fig. 33-2.

Rx TREATMENT

The rapidity of bleeding and its effect on gas exchange determine the urgency of management. When the bleeding is confined to either blood-streaking of sputum or production of small amounts of pure blood, gas exchange is usually preserved; establishing a diagnosis is the first priority. When hemoptysis is massive, maintaining adequate gas exchange, preventing blood from spilling into unaffected areas of lung, and avoiding asphyxiation are the highest priorities. Keeping the patient at rest and partially suppressing cough may help the bleeding to subside. If the origin of the blood is known and is limited to one lung, the bleeding lung should be placed in the dependent position, so that blood is not aspirated into the unaffected lung.

With massive bleeding, the need to control the airway and maintain adequate gas exchange may necessitate endotracheal intubation and mechanical ventilation. In patients in danger of flooding the lung contralateral to the side of hemorrhage despite proper positioning, isolation of the right and left mainstem bronchi from each other can be achieved with specially designed double-lumen endotracheal tubes. Another option involves inserting a balloon catheter through a bronchoscope by direct visualization and inflating the balloon to occlude the bronchus leading to the bleeding site. This technique not only prevents aspiration of blood into unaffected areas but also may promote tamponade of the bleeding site and cessation of bleeding.

Other available techniques for control of significant bleeding include laser phototherapy, embolotherapy, and surgical resection of the involved area of lung. With bleeding from an endobronchial tumor, the neodymium:yttrium-aluminum-garnet (Nd:YAG) laser can often achieve at least temporary hemostasis by coagulating the bleeding site. Embolotherapy involves an arteriographic procedure in which a vessel proximal to the bleeding site is cannulated, and a material such as Gelfoam is injected to occlude the bleeding vessel. Surgical resection is a therapeutic option either for the emergent therapy of life-threatening hemoptysis that fails to respond to other measures or for the elective but definitive management of localized disease subject to recurrent bleeding.

Table 33-1

Differential Diagnosis of Hemoptysis

Source other than the lower respiratory tract
    Upper airway (nasopharyngeal) bleeding
    Gastrointestinal bleeding

Tracheobronchial source
    Neoplasm (bronchogenic carcinoma, endobronchial metastatic tumor, bronchial carcinoid)
    Bronchitis (acute or chronic)
    Bronchiectasis
    Broncholithiasis
    Airway trauma
    Foreign body

Pulmonary parenchymal source
    Lung abscess
    Pneumonia
    Tuberculosis
    Mycetoma ("fungus ball")
    Goodpasture's syndrome
    Idiopathic pulmonary hemosiderosis
    Wegener's granulomatosis
    Lupus pneumonitis
    Lung contusion

Primary vascular disease
    Arteriovenous malformation
    Pulmonary embolism
    Elevated pulmonary venous pressure (esp. mitral stenosis)

Miscellaneous/rare causes
    Pulmonary endometriosis
    Systemic coagulopathy or use of anticoagulants

SOURCE: Adapted from SE Weinberger, Principles of Pulmonary Medicine, 2d ed, Philadelphia, Saunders, 1992

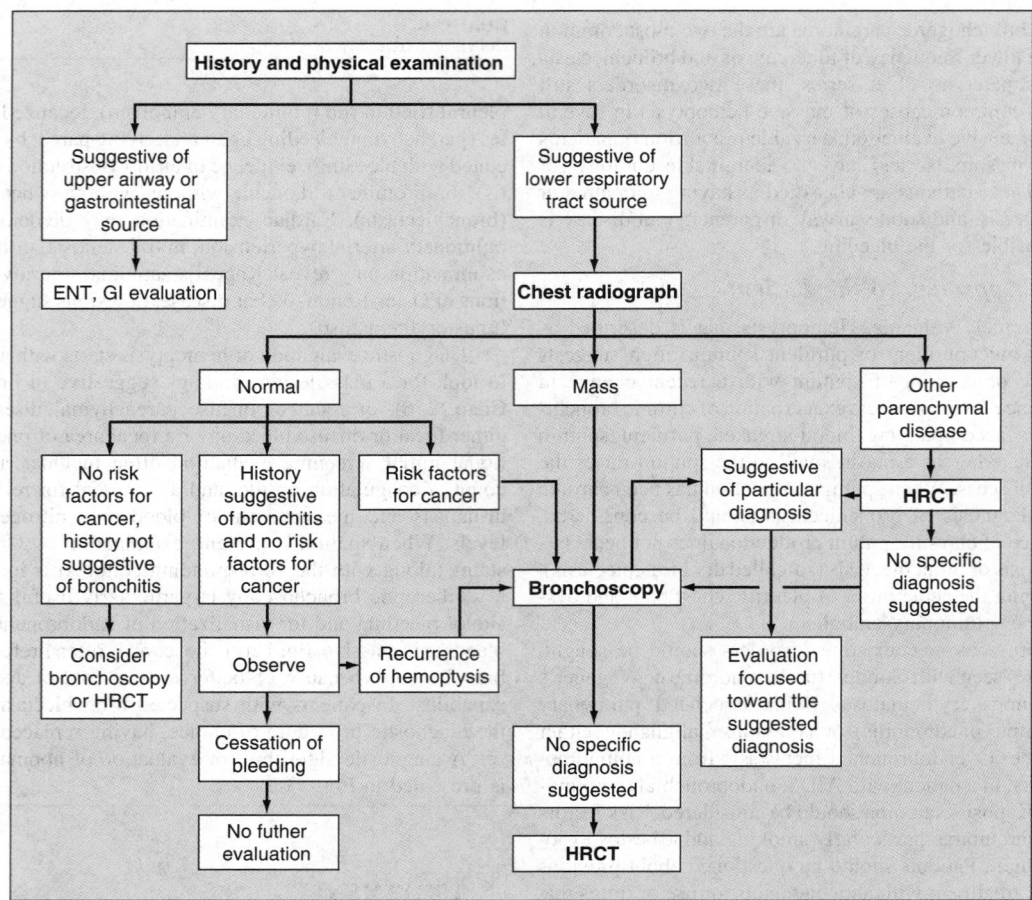

FIGURE 33-2 An algorithm for the evaluation of non-massive hemoptysis. HRCT, High resolution computer tomography.

BIBLIOGRAPHY

COUGH

ING AJ et al: Pathogenesis of chronic persistent cough associated with gastro-esophageal reflux. Am J Respir Crit Care Med 149:160, 1994

IRWIN RS et al: Appropriate use of antitussives and protussives. A practical review. Drugs 46:80, 1993

ISRAILI ZH, HALL WD: Cough and angioneurotic edema associated with angiotensin-converting enzyme inhibitor therapy. Ann Intern Med 117:234, 1992

PATRICK H, PATRICK F: Chronic cough. Med Clin North Am 79:361, 1995

PRATTER MR et al: An algorithmic approach to chronic cough. Ann Intern Med 119:977, 1993

WRIGHT SW et al: Pertussis infection in adults with persistent cough. JAMA 273:1044, 1995

HEMOPTYSIS

CAHILL BC, INGBAR DH: Massive hemoptysis: Assessment and management. Clin Chest Med 15:147, 1994

PRIMACK SL et al: Diffuse pulmonary hemorrhage: Clinical, pathologic, and imaging features. AJR 164:295, 1995

SANTIAGO S et al: A reappraisal of the causes of hemoptysis. Arch Intern Med 151:2449, 1991

THOMPSON AB et al: Pathogenesis evaluation, and therapy for massive hemoptysis. Clin Chest Med 13:69, 1992

34

Patrick T. O'Gara, Eugene Braunwald

APPROACH TO THE PATIENT WITH A HEART MURMUR

Auscultation of the heart constitutes the final step in the cardiovascular examination and for many patients with established or suspected cardiac disease represents the defining moment in the doctor-patient rela-tionship. The examiner must bring to this exercise an integrated approach that incorporates pertinent information simultaneously from several sources. The auscultatory findings must be interpreted in the context of the history and general physical examination and must be consonant with the observations made regarding the venous wave forms and major arterial pulses. In this way, abnormalities of the heart sounds, adventitious sounds, and murmurs can be placed in their proper perspective.

In many patients, a heart murmur is the only or the most conspicuous finding on physical examination. The recognition of a heart murmur commonly leads to additional testing, such as electrocardiography, chest radiography, and echocardiography, and may result in referral to a cardiologist. The differential diagnosis of a heart murmur should more properly begin with an unbiased and systemic evaluation of its major attributes: timing, duration, intensity, quality, frequency, configuration, location, radiation, and response to maneuvers (Table 227-1). Laboratory testing can be pursued thereafter to clarify any remaining ambiguity and to provide additional anatomic and physiologic information that will impact on patient management.

Heart murmurs are defined in terms of their timing within the cardiac cycle. *Systolic murmurs* begin with or after the first heart sound (S_1) and terminate at or before the component (A_2 or P_2) of the second heart sound (S_2) that corresponds to their side of origin (left or right). *Diastolic murmurs* begin with or after the associated component of S_2 and end at or before the subsequent S_1. *Continuous murmurs* are not confined to either phase of the cardiac cycle but rather begin in systole and proceed through S_2 into all or part of diastole.

The appropriate timing of heart murmurs is the first critical step in their identification. The distinction between S_1 and S_2, and, therefore, systole and diastole, is usually a straightforward process but can be difficult in the setting of a tachyarrhythmia, in which case the heart sounds can be distinguished by simultaneous palpation of the carotid arterial pulse. The upstroke should closely follow S_1. The principal causes of heart murmurs are shown in Table 34-1, and the critical importance of the timing of heart murmurs in the differential diagnosis is shown in Fig. 34-1.

SYSTOLIC HEART MURMURS

Systolic heart murmurs derive from the increased turbulence associated with (1) enhanced or accelerated flow across a normal semilunar valve

Table 34-1

Principal Causes of Heart Murmurs

ORGANIC SYSTOLIC MURMURS

Midsystolic (ejection)
  Aortic
    Obstructive
      Supravalvular—supraaortic stenosis, coarctation of the aorta
      Valvular—AS and sclerosis
      Subvalvular—discrete or HOCM
    Increased flow, hyperkinetic states, AR, complete heart block
    Dilatation of ascending aorta, atheroma, aortitis, aneurysm of aorta
  Pulmonary
    Obstructive
      Supravalvular—pulmonary arterial stenosis
      Valvular—pulmonic valve stenosis
      Subvalvular—infundibular stenosis
    Increased flow, hyperkinetic states, left-to-right shunt (e.g., ASD, VSD)
    Dilatation of pulmonary artery
Holosystolic (regurgitant)
  Atrioventricular valve regurgitation (MR, TR)
  Left-to-right shunt at ventricular level

EARLY DIASTOLIC MURMURS

Aortic regurgitation
  Valvular; rheumatic deformity; perforation, postendocarditis, posttraumatic, postvalvulotomy
  Dilatation of valve ring: aorta dissection, annuloectasia, cystic medial necrosis, hypertension
  Widening of commissures: syphilis
  Congenital: bicuspid valve, with VSD
Pulmonic regurgitation
  Valvular: postvalvulotomy, endocarditis, rheumatic fever, carcinoid
  Dilatation of valve ring: pulmonary hypertension; Marfan syndrome
  Congenital: isolated or associated with tetralogy of Fallot, VSD, pulmonic stenosis

MIDDIASTOLIC MURMURS

Mitral stenosis
Carey-Coombs murmur (middiastolic apical murmur in acute rheumatic fever)
Increased flow across nonstenotic mitral valve (e.g., MR, VSD, PDA, high-output states, and complete heart block)
Tricuspid stenosis
Increased flow across nonstenotic tricuspid valve (e.g., TR, ASD, and anomalous pulmonary venous return)
Left and right atrial tumors

CONTINUOUS MURMURS

Patent ductus arteriosus
Coronary AV fistula
Ruptured aneurysm of sinus of Valsalva
Aortic septal defect
Cervical venous hum
Anomalous left coronary artery
Proximal coronary artery stenosis
Mammary souffle
Pulmonary artery branch stenosis
Bronchial collateral circulation
Small (restrictive) ASD with MS
Intercostal AV fistula

NOTE: AR, aortic regurgitation; AS, aortic stenosis; ASD, atrial septal defect; AV, arteriovenous; HOCM, hypertrophic obstructive cardiomyopathy; MR, mitral regurgitation; MS, mitral stenosis; PDA, patent ductus arteriosus; TR, tricuspid regurgitation; VSD, ventricular septal defect.

SOURCE: E Braunwald, in Heart Disease, 4th ed, E. Braunwald (ed), Philadelphia, Saunders, 1992

or into a dilated great vessel, (2) flow across a structurally abnormal semilunar valve or through a narrowed ventricular outflow tract, (3) flow across an incompetent atrioventricular valve, and (4) flow across the interventricular septum. One approach to their differential diagnosis further subdivides these murmurs according to their time of onset and duration within the systolic phase of the cardiac cycle.

EARLY SYSTOLIC MURMURS Early systolic murmurs begin with S_1 and extend for a variable period of time, ending well before S_2. Their causes are relatively few in number. *Acute severe mitral regurgitation* into a normal-sized, relatively noncompliant left atrium results in an early and attenuated systolic murmur that is decrescendo in configuration and usually best heard at or just medial to the apical impulse (Chap. 237). These characteristics reflect the rapid rise in left atrial pressure caused by the sudden volume load into a nondilated chamber and contrast sharply with the auscultatory features of chronic mitral regurgitation. Clinical settings in which this occurs include: (1) papillary muscle rupture complicating acute myocardial infarction, (2) infective endocarditis, (3) rupture of chordae tendineae, and (4) blunt chest wall trauma.

FIGURE 34-1 Diagram depicting principal heart murmurs. *A.* Presystolic murmur of mitral or tricuspid stenosis. *B.* Pansystolic murmur of mitral or tricuspid incompetence or of ventricular septal defect. *C.* Aortic ejection murmur beginning with an ejection click and fading before the second heart sound. *D.* Systolic murmur in pulmonic stenosis spilling through the aortic second sound, pulmonic valve closure being delayed. *E.* Aortic or pulmonary diastolic murmur. *F.* Long diastolic murmur of mitral stenosis following the opening snap. *G.* Short middiastolic inflow murmur following a third heart sound. *H.* Continuous murmur of patent ductus arteriosus. *(Adapted from P Wood, Diseases of the Heart and Circulation, Philadelphia, Lippincott, 1968, with permission.)*

Acute mitral regurgitation from papillary muscle rupture usually accompanies an inferior, posterior, or lateral infarction. The murmur is associated with a precordial thrill in approximately one-half of cases and is to be distinguished from that associated with postinfarction ventricular septal rupture. The latter is more commonly (90 percent) accompanied by a thrill at the left sternal edge, is holosystolic, and complicates anterior infarctions as often as inferior-posterior events. The recognition of either of these mechanical defects mandates aggressive medical stabilization and emergent surgical intervention (Chap. 243).

The other potential causes of acute severe mitral regurgitation may be distinguished on the basis of associated findings. Spontaneous chordal rupture usually occurs on a substrate of myxomatous degeneration, such as that underlying most forms of mitral valve prolapse (Chap. 237). This lesion may be part of a more generalized process, as can occur with the Marfan or Ehlers-Danlos syndromes, or it may be an isolated phenomenon. Infectious endocarditis is associated with fever, peripheral embolic lesions, and positive blood cultures and most commonly occurs on a previously abnormal valvular apparatus (Chap. 126). Trauma is usually self-evident but may be disarmingly trivial (Chap. 241). It can result in papillary muscle contusion and rupture, chordal interruption, or leaflet avulsion or perforation.

Echocardiography should be performed in all cases of suspected acute severe mitral regurgitation to define the responsible mechanism, estimate the severity, and provide a preliminary assessment as to the feasibility of surgical repair (versus replacement).

Other causes of early systolic murmurs include congenital, small muscular ventricular septal defect. The duration of the murmur is attenuated by the closure of the defect during systolic contraction. The murmur is localized to the left sternal edge and is commonly of grade IV/VI or V/VI intensity. Signs of pulmonary hypertension or left ventricular volume overload are absent.

Tricuspid regurgitation with normal pulmonary artery pressures, such as that caused by infectious endocarditis in intravenous drug users, may produce an early systolic murmur. The murmur is soft, best heard at the lower left sternal edge, and may accentuate with inspiration (Carvallo's sign). Regurgitant $c-v$ waves may be visible in the jugular venous pulse.

MIDSYSTOLIC MURMURS Midsystolic murmurs begin at a short interval following S_1, end before S_2, and are usually crescendo-decrescendo in configuration (Fig. 34-1C). Semilunar valve stenosis is the classic prototype. With aortic valve stenosis the murmur is usually loudest in the second right intercostal space (aortic area) and radiates along the carotid arteries (Chap. 237). The intensity of the murmur varies directly with the cardiac output; aortic valve stenosis with severe heart failure may produce a misleadingly soft systolic murmur. With a normal cardiac output, a systolic thrill is usually indicative of severe stenosis with a peak gradient in excess of 50 to 60 mmHg. An accompanying early systolic ejection click may be audible in younger patients with a bicuspid valve; its presence localizes the obstruction to the valvular (as opposed to the sub- or supravalvular) level. The midsystolic murmur of aortic stenosis may be well transmitted to the apex, especially in older patients, where it becomes less harsh and slightly higher pitched (Gallavardin effect). The murmur of aortic stenosis should increase following a postpremature beat, whereas a mitral regurgitant murmur would not be expected to change in intensity.

Sclerosis of the aortic valve produces a murmur of similar location, radiation, and configuration, albeit without the usual signs of hemodynamic significance. The carotid upstroke is well preserved, the murmur peaks in midsystole and is not accompanied by a thrill, and only a modest gradient is estimated by Doppler echocardiography. Noncritical sclerodegenerative thickening of the aortic valve leaflets is perhaps the most common cause of a midsystolic murmur in an older adult. The similar midsystolic murmur of pulmonic valve stenosis, usually introduced by an ejection click, is best appreciated in the second and third left intercostal spaces (pulmonic area). The murmur lengthens and the intensity of P_2 diminishes with increasing degrees of stenosis. A midsystolic murmur in the aortic position of no functional significance can also be detected in hyperdynamic states (fever, thyrotoxicosis, pregnancy, anemia) and in the presence of isolated aortic regurgitation with the augmented flow into a dilated proximal aorta.

Crescendo-decrescendo midsystolic murmurs of grade II/VI or III/VI intensity heard in the pulmonic area may be innocent (Still's murmur), if unaccompanied by any other signs of cardiac disease in children or young adults, or they may reflect enhanced flow into a normal pulmonary artery in hyperkinetic states or augmented flow into a dilated pulmonary artery. The latter may occur with an atrial septal defect, in which case splitting of S_2 should be abnormal (fixed).

The midsystolic murmur of hypertrophic cardiomyopathy (Chap. 239) is usually loudest between the left sternal edge and apex, of grade II/VI to III/VI intensity, and crescendo-decrescendo in configuration. In contrast to aortic valve stenosis, the murmur does *not* radiate into the neck and the carotid upstrokes are brisk and full and may even be bifid. The intensity of the murmur associated with hypertrophic cardiomyopathy increases following maneuvers that decrease left ventricular volume (strain phase of the Valsalva maneuver, standing, amyl nitrite) or increase myocardial contractility (inotropic therapy). Conversely, the intensity of the systolic murmur decreases with maneuvers that increase ventricular volume (squatting, passive leg raising), impair contractility (beta-adrenoreceptor blockade), or raise preload and systemic afterload (squatting). Among these several maneuvers, auscultation in the standing and squatting positions, if possible, is perhaps the most sensitive technique to elicit a dynamic change in the intensity of the murmur associated with hypertrophic obstructive cardiomyopathy.

LATE SYSTOLIC MURMURS A late systolic murmur begins well after the onset of ejection and is usually best heard at the left ventricular apex or between the apex and the left sternal edge. When introduced by a nonejection click, it is usually indicative of systolic prolapse of the mitral valve leaflet(s) into the left atrium. The click and murmur move closer to S_1 following maneuvers that decrease left ventricular volume (standing, Valsalva) and move oppositely upon increases in volume (leg raising, squatting). The intensity of the murmur augments with increases in systemic afterload (squatting, pressor agents) and decrease with vasodilation (amyl nitrite). Isometric exercise, which also delays the onset of the murmur, accentuates the intensity.

HOLOSYSTOLIC MURMURS These murmurs, also termed *pansystolic murmurs*, begin with S_1 and continue through systole to S_2 (Fig. 34-1C). They are, with rare exception, indicative of atrioventricular valve regurgitation or of a ventricular septal defect; the differential diagnosis is shown in Fig. 34-2. The murmur of mitral regurgitation is loudest at the left ventricular apex. Its radiation reflects the direction of the regurgitant jet. With a flail posterior mitral leaflet due to ruptured chordae tendineae, for example, the jet is directed anterosuperiorly, and the murmur radiates prominently to the base of the heart where it might be confused with aortic valve stenosis unless the carotid upstrokes are carefully examined. Conversely, a flail anterior leaflet is associated with a posteriorly directed jet, which radiates into the axilla and the back. It may even strike the spine and be transmitted to the base of the neck. Severe mitral regurgitation is usually associated with a systolic thrill, a soft S_3, and a short diastolic rumbling murmur best appreciated in the left lateral decubitus position.

The holosystolic murmur of tricuspid regurgitation is generally softer (grades I to III/VI) than that of mitral regurgitation, is loudest at the left lower sternal edge, and increases in intensity upon inspiration. Associated signs include prominent "$c-v$" waves in the jugular venous pulse, systolic hepatic pulsations, and peripheral edema. Among the several causes of tricuspid regurgitation, annular dilatation from right ventricular enlargement in the setting of pulmonary artery hypertension is the most common.

Ventricular septal defect (Chap. 235) also produces a holosystolic murmur, the intensity of which varies inversely with the anatomic size of the defect. It is usually accompanied by a palpable thrill along the mid-left sternal border. The murmur of a ventricular septal defect is louder than that due to tricuspid regurgitation and does not share the latter's inspiratory increase in intensity or associated peripheral signs.

DIASTOLIC HEART MURMURS

Like systolic murmurs, diastolic murmurs also can be subcategorized according to their time of onset.

EARLY DIASTOLIC MURMURS (Fig. 34-1*E*) Early diastolic murmurs result from semilunar valve incompetence and begin at the valve closure sound (A_2 or P_2), which reflects their side of origin. They are generally high pitched and decrescendo in configuration, especially in states of chronic regurgitation, wherein their duration is a crude index of the severity of the lesion. The murmur of aortic regurgitation is generally, but not always, best heard in the second intercostal space at the left sternal edge. There is a tendency for the murmur associated with primary valvular pathology (e.g., rheumatic deformity, congenital bicuspid valve, endocarditis) to radiate more prominently along the *left* sternal border and to be well transmitted to the apex, while the murmur associated with primary aortic root pathology (e.g., annuloaortic ectasia, aortic dissection) radiates more often along the right sternal edge. It is occasionally necessary to examine the patient sitting forward in full expiration to appreciate the murmur, a maneuver that brings the aortic root closer to the anterior chest wall. Severe aortic regurgitation may be accompanied by a lower-pitched mid- to late-diastolic murmur at the apex (Austin Flint murmur), which is generally thought to reflect turbulence at the mitral inflow area from the mixing of the regurgitant (aortic) and forward (mitral) streams, and should be distinguished from mitral stenosis (see above). In the absence of significant heart failure, chronic severe aortic regurgitation is accompanied by several peripheral signs of significant diastolic runoff, including a wide systemic pulse pressure and water-hammer carotid upstrokes (Corrigan's pulse).

The murmur associated with *acute* aortic regurgitation is notably shorter in duration, lower pitched, and can be difficult to appreciate in the presence of tachycardia. Peripheral signs of significant diastolic runoff may be absent. These attributes reflect the abrupt rise in diastolic pressure within the noncompliant left ventricle, with a correspondingly rapid decline in the aortic diastolic–left ventricular pressure gradient.

The murmur of pulmonic valve regurgitation (Graham Steell murmur) begins with a loud (palpable) pulmonic closure sound (P_2) and is best heard in the pulmonic area with radiation along the left sternal border. Typically, it is high pitched, with a decrescendo quality, and is indicative of significant pulmonary artery hypertension with a diastolic pulmonary artery–right ventricular pressure gradient. Its increase in intensity upon inspiration is one means by which to distinguish it from aortic regurgitation. Signs of right ventricular pressure and volume overload are also usually present. With significant mitral stenosis, an early decrescendo diastolic murmur along the left sternal border is not uncommon and is almost always due to

aortic rather than pulmonic regurgitation, despite the coexistence of pulmonary artery hypertension.

Pulmonic valve regurgitation in the absence of pulmonary artery hypertension can occur on a congenital basis and rarely with infectious endocarditis. In these instances, the early diastolic murmur is softer and lower pitched than the classic Graham Steell murmur. It begins at or even after P_2, which should be easily separable from A_2 and thus produce appreciation of an early diastolic pause.

MIDDIASTOLIC MURMURS Middiastolic murmurs usually result from obstruction and/or augmented flow across the antrioventricular valves. The classic example is that of mitral stenosis due to rheumatic deformity (Fig. 34-1*F*). In the absence of extensive calcification, the first heart sound (S_1) is loud and the murmur begins after the opening snap; the time interval between S_2 and the opening snap is inversely related to the left atrial–left ventricular pressure gradient. The murmur is low pitched and best heard with the bell of the stethoscope over the apex, particularly in the left lateral decubitus position. While its intensity does not reflect the severity of the obstruction accurately, the duration of the murmur does provide some indication as to the magnitude of the obstruction. A longer murmur denotes persistence of a left atrioventricular pressure gradient over a greater proportion of the diastolic time interval. Presystolic accentuation of the murmur (Fig. 34-1*A*) is frequently appreciated in the presence of sinus rhythm and reflects a further increase in transmitral flow consequent to mechanical atrial systole.

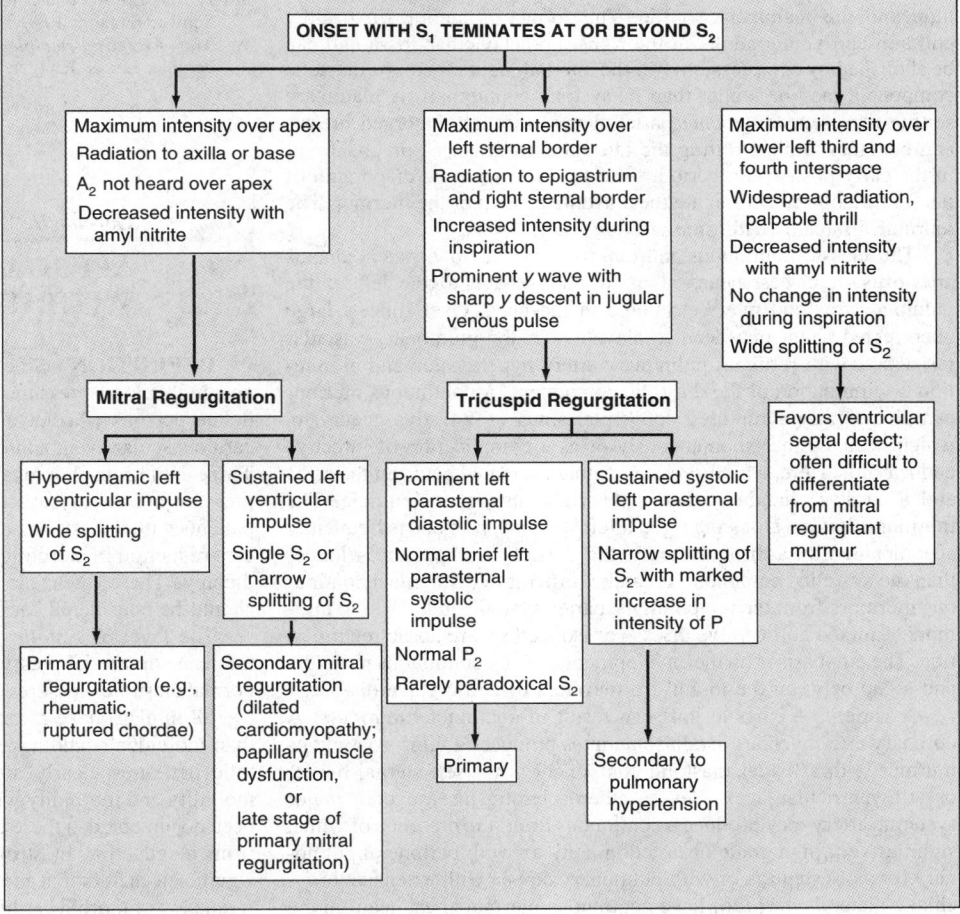

FIGURE 34-2 Differential diagnosis of pansystolic murmur (regurgitant). S_1, first heart sound; S_2, second heart sound; A_2, aortic component of the second heart sound; P_2, pulmonary component of the second heart sound (echo-Doppler evaluation should be considered for differential diagnosis). [*From C Chatterjee, in K Chatterjee et al (eds), Cardiology: An Illustrated Text/Reference, Philadelphia, Lippincott, 1991, with permission.*]

The murmur associated with tricuspid stenosis shares many of these features, but it is best heard at the lower left sternal border and, like most right-sided events, increases in intensity upon inspiration. The observant examiner may discern a prolonged *y* descent in the jugular venous pulse. Signs of right heart failure may predominate.

There are several other causes of mid-diastolic murmurs that are important to distinguish from mitral stenosis. *Left atrial myxomas* (Chap. 241) may masquerade as mitral stenosis, but the diastolic murmur is not accompanied by an opening snap or pre-systolic accentuation. Augmented flow across the mitral valve in diastole, such as occurs with severe mitral regurgitation or with large left to right intracardiac or great vessel shunts may produce a short, low pitched mid-diastolic apical murmur. The murmur usually follows a soft S_3 that is lower pitched and later in timing than the opening snap (Fig. 34-1*G*). Severe tricuspid regurgitation can also result in enhanced diastolic tricuspid flow and produce a right-sided filling complex similar to that which accompanies severe mitral regurgitation. The Austin Flint murmur of severe aortic regurgitation has been previously described and occurs in the presence of severe aortic regurgitation.

CONTINUOUS MURMURS

Continuous murmurs begin in systole, peak near S_2, and continue into all or part of diastole (Fig. 34-1*H*). Accordingly, they reflect the persistence of flow between two chambers during both phases of the cardiac cycle. The differential diagnosis of continuous murmurs is shown in Table 34-1. Two innocent variants are the cervical venous hum and the mammary souffle. The former is audible in healthy children and young adults in the right supraclavicular fossa and can be abolished by compression over the internal jugular vein. Its diastolic component may be louder than its systolic counterpart. A mammary souffle represents augmented arterial flow through engorged breasts and becomes audible during the late third trimester of pregnancy or in the early postpartum period. Firm pressure with the diaphragm of the stethoscope can eliminate the diastolic portion of the murmur. The murmur dissipates with time after delivery.

The classic continuous murmur is that due to a patent ductus arteriosus. It is best heard at or just above and to the left of the pulmonic area and may be audible in the back. Over time, a large uncorrected shunt may lead to elevation of the pulmonary vascular resistance, with resultant pulmonary artery hypertension and diminution or elimination of the diastolic component. A continuous murmur can also signify a ruptured congenital sinus of Valsalva aneurysm, which occurs either spontaneously or as a complication of infective endocarditis. Here, a high-pressure fistula is created between the aorta and a cardiac chamber, usually the right atrium or ventricle. The murmur is loudest along the right or left sternal border and is frequently accompanied by a thrill. Notably, the diastolic component is louder than the systolic component. It can be difficult to distinguish continuous murmurs from the temporally separate systolic and diastolic murmurs of mixed aortic valve disease or isolated severe aortic regurgitation. The emphasis is on the envelopment of S_2 by continuous murmurs and a gap between the to-and-fro murmurs of aortic valve disease.

A variety of other lesions can result in continuous murmurs. A coronary arteriovenous fistula sometimes produces a faint, continuous murmur with a louder diastolic component at the left sternal border or left ventricular apex. Severe atherosclerotic disease of a major systemic artery may produce a continuous bruit, the presence of which signifies very high grade obstruction. Patients with peripheral pulmonary (branch) stenosis or with pulmonary atresia with extensive bronchial collaterals may also have continuous murmurs best heard in the back or along the lateral thoracic cage. Similar findings are present in patients with severe aortic coarctation, a lesion that should be identifiable on the basis of weak and delayed lower extremity pulses and upper extremity hypertension. The continuous murmurs emanate from the enlarged collateral (intercostal) arteries.

In many patients the cause of a heart murmur can be readily elucidated from careful assessment of the murmur itself, as described in this chapter, when considered in the light of the history, general physical examination, and other features of the cardiac examination, as described in Chap. 227. When the diagnosis is in doubt, or when additional pathoanatomic and physiologic data are necessary in assessing the patient and planning treatment, a transthoracic echocardiogram with Droppler interrogation is of great value in identifying not only the etiology of the murmur but also the severity of the responsible lesion.

The majority of heart murmurs are midsystolic and soft (Grades I to II/VI). When such a murmur occurs in a child or young adult *without* other evidence of heart disease on clinical examination, it is usually benign and echocardiography is not generally required. On the other hand, echocardiographic examination is indicated in patients with loud systolic murmurs ($\geq$III/VI), especially those that are holosystolic, as well as in most patients with diastolic or continuous murmurs.

BIBLIOGRAPHY

GREWE K et al: Differentiation of cardiac murmurs by auscultation. Curr Prob Cardiol 13(10):669, 1988

LEMBO NJ et al: Bedside diagnosis of systolic murmurs. N Engl J Med 318(24):1572, 1988

PERLOFF JK: *The Clinical Recognition of Congenital Heart Disease,* 3d ed. Philadelphia, Saunders, 1987

———, BRAUNWALD E: Physical examination of the heart and circulation, in *Heart Disease,* 5th ed, E Braunwald (ed). Philadelphia, Saunders, 1997, pp 15–52

SAPIRA JD: *The Art and Science of Bedside Diagnosis.* Baltimore, Urban and Schwartzenberg, 1990

WEYMAN AE (ed): *Principles and Practice of Echocardiography,* 2d ed. Philadelphia, Lea & Febiger, 1994

---

35 *Gordon H. Williams*

APPROACH TO THE PATIENT WITH HYPERTENSION

DEFINITION Since there is no dividing line between normal and high blood pressure, arbitrary levels have been established to define persons who have an increased risk of developing a morbid cardiovascular event and/or will clearly benefit from medical therapy. These definitions should take into account not only the level of diastolic pressure but also systolic pressure, age, sex, and race. For example, patients with a diastolic pressure greater than 90 mmHg have a significant reduction in morbidity and mortality rate if they receive adequate therapy. These, then, are patients who have hypertension and who should be considered for treatment.

The level of *systolic* pressure is also important in assessing the influence of arterial pressure on cardiovascular morbidity. Males with normal diastolic pressures (<82 mmHg) but elevated systolic pressures (>158 mmHg) have a cardiovascular mortality rate 2.5 times higher than individuals who have similar diastolic pressures but whose systolic pressures clearly are normal (<130 mmHg). A reduction in mortality and morbidity with treatment, specifically in the elderly, has been documented in these patients. This beneficial effect results mainly from a reduction in strokes and occurs in women as well. Other significant factors that modify the influence of blood pressure on the frequency of morbid cardiovascular events are age, race, and sex, with young black males being most adversely affected by hypertension.

When hypertension is suspected, blood pressure should be measured at least twice during two separate examinations after the initial screening. In adults, a *diastolic* pressure below 85 mmHg is considered to be normal; one between 85 and 89 mmHg is high normal; one of

90 to 104 mmHg represents mild hypertension; one of 105 to 114 mmHg represents moderate hypertension; and one of 115 mmHg or greater represents severe hypertension. When the diastolic pressure is below 90 mmHg, a *systolic* pressure below 140 mmHg indicates normal blood pressure; one between 140 and 159 mmHg indicates borderline isolated systolic hypertension; and one of 160 mmHg or higher indicates isolated systolic hypertension. Increasing use of 12- or 24-h blood pressure monitoring may provide additional useful information in patients who are difficult to classify. However, normal values for this procedure and its usefulness in relation to therapeutic outcomes are not currently known. A useful classification of hypertension derived from the Joint Committee on Detection, Evaluation, and Treatment of High Blood Pressure is shown in Table 35-1.

Arterial pressure fluctuates in most persons, whether they are normotensive or hypertensive. Patients who are classified as having *labile hypertension* are those who sometimes, but not always, have arterial pressures in the hypertensive range. These patients are often considered to have borderline hypertension.

Sustained hypertension can become accelerated or enter a malignant phase, although that is unusual in treated patients. Though a patient with *malignant hypertension* often has a blood pressure above 200/140, the condition is defined by the presence of papilledema, usually accompanied by retinal hemorrhages and exudates, rather than by the absolute pressure level. *Accelerated hypertension* is defined as a significant recent increase over previous hypertensive levels associated with evidence of vascular damage on funduscopic examination but without papilledema.

PATIENT EVALUATION In evaluating patients with hypertension, the initial history, physical examination, and laboratory tests should be directed at (1) uncovering correctable secondary forms of hypertension (see Chap. 246), (2) establishing a pretreatment baseline, (3) assessing factors that may influence the type of therapy or be changed adversely by therapy, (4) determining if target organ damage is present, and (5) determining whether other risk factors for the development of arteriosclerotic cardiovascular disease are present (see Chap. 242). Ideally, this evaluation also would determine the underlying mechanism(s) in essential hypertension, particularly if such information leads to a more specific therapeutic program. Unfortunately, at present this aspect of the evaluation is limited by lack of knowledge of some of the underlying mechanisms, by uncertainty as to the correct treatment for a distinct subset even if the underlying mechanisms are known, or by the prohibitive cost of defining a subset of hypertensive patients even if specific therapy were available. However, with the accumulation of additional information, this sixth component of the evaluation of patients with hypertension may become increasingly important.

Table 35-1

Classification of Blood Pressure for Adults Aged 18 Years and Older

Category	Systolic Pressure, mmHg	Diastolic Pressure, mmHg
Normal*	<130	<85
High normal	130–139	85–89
Hypertension†		
Stage 1 (mild)	140–159	90–99
Stage 2 (moderate)	160–179	100–109
Stage 3 (severe)	180–209	110–119
Stage 4 (very severe)	≥210	≥120

* Optimal blood pressure with respect to cardiovascular risk is <120/80 mmHg. However, unusually low readings should be evaluated for clinical significance.

† Based on the average of ≥2 readings taken at each of two or more visits after an initial screening.

NOTE: Classification of blood pressure for adults aged 18 years and older not taking antihypertensive drugs and not acutely ill. When systolic and diastolic pressures fall into different categories, the higher category should be selected to classify the individual's blood pressure status.

SOURCE: From NK Hollenberg. Summary of the Joint National Committee (JNC)-V and WHO/International Society of Hypertension (ISH) Special Reports, in NK Hollenberg (ed): Hypertension: Mechanisms and therapy, in *Atlas of Heart Diseases*, vol. 1, E Braunwald (series ed). Philadelphia, Current Medicine, 1995, pp 13.1–13.16

Symptoms and Signs Most patients with hypertension have no specific symptoms referable to their blood pressure elevation and are identified only in the course of a physical examination. When symptoms do bring the patient to the physician, they fall into three categories. They are related to (1) the elevated pressure itself, (2) the hypertensive vascular disease, and (3) the underlying disease, in the case of secondary hypertension. Though popularly considered a symptom of elevated arterial pressure, headache is characteristic only of severe hypertension; most commonly such headaches are localized to the occipital region and are present when the patient awakens in the morning but subside spontaneously after several hours. Other complaints that may be related to elevated blood pressure include dizziness, palpitations, easy fatigability, and impotence. Complaints referable to vascular disease include epistaxis, hematuria, blurring of vision owing to retinal changes, episodes of weakness or dizziness due to transient cerebral ischemia, angina pectoris, and dyspnea due to cardiac failure. Pain due to dissection of the aorta or to a leaking aneurysm is an occasional presenting symptom.

Examples of symptoms related to the underlying disease in secondary hypertension are polyuria, polydipsia, and muscle weakness secondary to hypokalemia in patients with primary aldosteronism or weight gain, and emotional lability in patients with Cushing's syndrome. The patient with a pheochromocytoma may present with episodic headaches, palpitations, diaphoresis, and postural dizziness.

History A strong family history of hypertension, along with the reported finding of intermittent pressure elevation in the past, favors the diagnosis of essential hypertension. Secondary hypertension often develops before the age of 35 or after 55. A history of use of adrenal steroids or estrogens is of obvious significance. A history of repeated urinary tract infections suggests chronic pyelonephritis, although this condition may occur in the absence of symptoms; nocturia and polydipsia suggest renal or endocrine disease, while trauma to either flank or an episode of acute flank pain may be a clue to the presence of renal injury. A history of weight gain is compatible with Cushing's syndrome, and one of weight loss is compatible with pheochromocytoma. A number of aspects of the history aid in determining whether vascular disease has progressed to a dangerous stage. These include angina pectoris and symptoms of cerebrovascular insufficiency, congestive heart failure, and/or peripheral vascular insufficiency. Other risk factors that should be asked about include cigarette smoking, diabetes mellitus, lipid disorders, and a family history of early deaths due to cardiovascular disease. Finally, aspects of the patient's lifestyle that could contribute to the hypertension or affect its treatment should be assessed, including diet, physical activity, family status, work, and educational level.

Physical Examination The physical examination starts with the patient's general appearance. For instance, are the round face and truncal obesity of Cushing's syndrome present? Is muscular development in the upper extremities out of proportion to that in the lower extremities, suggesting coarctation of the aorta? The next step is to compare the blood pressures and pulses in the two upper extremities and in the supine and standing positions (for at least 2 min). A rise in diastolic pressure when the patient goes from the supine to the standing position is most compatible with essential hypertension; a fall, in the absence of antihypertensive medications, suggests secondary forms of hypertension. The patient's height and weight should be recorded. Detailed examination of the ocular fundi is mandatory, as funduscopic findings provide one of the best indications of the duration of hypertension and of prognosis. A useful guide is the Keith-Wagener-Barker classification of funduscopic changes (Table 35-2); the specific changes in each fundus should be recorded and a grade assigned. Palpation and auscultation of the carotid arteries for evidence of stenosis or occlusion are important; narrowing of a carotid artery may be a manifestation of hypertensive vascular disease, and it also may be a clue to the presence of a renal arterial lesion, since these two lesions may occur together. In examination of the heart and lungs, evidence of left ventricular hypertrophy and cardiac decompensation should be sought. Is there a left ventricular lift? Are third and fourth heart sounds present? Are there pulmonary rales? A third heart sound and pulmonary rales are unusual in uncomplicated hypertension. Their presence suggests ventricular dysfunction. Chest examination also includes a search for extracardiac murmurs and palpable collateral vessels that may result from coarctation of the aorta.

The most important part of the abdominal examination is auscultation for bruits originating in stenotic renal arteries. Bruits due to renal arterial narrowing nearly always have a diastolic component or may be continuous and are best heard just to the right or left of the midline above the umbilicus or in the flanks; they are present in many patients with renal artery stenosis due to fibrous dysplasia and in 40 to 50 percent of those with functionally significant stenosis due to arteriosclerosis. The abdomen also should be palpated for an abdominal aneurysm and for the enlarged kidneys of polycystic renal disease. The femoral pulses must be carefully felt, and, if they are decreased and/or delayed in comparison with the radial pulse, the blood pressure in the lower extremities must be measured. Even if the femoral pulse is normal to palpation, arterial pressure in the lower extremities should be recorded at least once in patients in whom hypertension is discovered before the age of 30 years. Finally, examination of the extremities for edema and a search for evidence of a previous cerebrovascular accident and/or other intracranial pathology should be performed.

Laboratory Investigation　　There is controversy as to what laboratory studies should be performed in patients presenting with hypertension. In general, the disagreement centers on how extensively the patient should be evaluated for secondary forms of hypertension or subsets of essential hypertension. The *basic* laboratory studies that should be performed in all patients with sustained hypertension are described below (Table 35-3). The *secondary studies* that should be added if (1) the initial evaluation indicates a form of secondary hypertension and/or (2) arterial pressure is not controlled after initial therapy as discussed in Chap. 246.

Renal status is evaluated by assessing the presence of protein, blood, and glucose in the urine and measuring serum creatinine and/or blood urea nitrogen. Microscopic examination of the urine is also helpful. The serum potassium level should be measured both as a screen for mineralocorticoid-induced hypertension and to provide a baseline before diuretic therapy is begun.

Other blood chemistry measurements also may be useful, particularly as they often can be ordered as a battery of automated tests at minimal cost to the patient. For example, a blood glucose determination is helpful both because diabetes mellitus may be associated with accelerated arteriosclerosis, renal vascular disease, and diabetic nephropathy in patients with hypertension and because primary aldosteronism, Cushing's syndrome, and pheochromocytoma all may be associated with hyperglycemia. Furthermore, since antihypertensive therapy with diuretics, for example, can raise the blood glucose level, it is important to establish a baseline. The possibility of hypercalcemia also may be investigated. Serum uric acid determination is useful because of the increased incidence of hyperuricemia in patients with renal and essential hypertension and because, as with blood glucose, the level may be raised subsequently by treatment with diuretics. Serum cholesterol, high density lipoprotein cholesterol, and triglycerides may be measured to identify other factors that predispose to the development of arteriosclerosis.

An electrocardiogram should be obtained in all cases to permit assessment of cardiac status, particularly if left ventricular hypertrophy

Table 35-3

Laboratory Tests for Evaluation of Hypertension

BASIC TESTS FOR INITIAL EVALUATION

A. Always included:
   1. Urine for protein, blood, and glucose
   2. Hematocrit
   3. Serum potassium
   4. Serum creatinine and/or blood urea nitrogen
   5. Electrocardiogram
B. Usually included, depending on cost and other factors:
   1. Microscopic urinalysis
   2. White blood cell count
   3. Plasma/blood glucose, cholesterol, HDL cholesterol, and triglycerides
   4. Serum calcium, phosphate, and uric acid
   5. Chest x-ray; echocardiogram

SPECIAL STUDIES TO SCREEN FOR SECONDARY HYPERTENSION

A. Renovascular disease: angiotensin converting enzyme inhibitor renogram, renal duplex ultrasound
B. Pheochromocytoma: 24-h urine assay for creatinine, metanephrines, and catecholamines or plasma catecholamines
C. Cushing's syndrome: overnight dexamethasone suppression test or 24-h urine cortisol

Table 35-2

Classification of Hypertensive and Arteriolosclerotic Retinopathy

| | **Hypertension** | | | | | **Arteriosclerosis** | |
| | **Arterioles** | | | | | | |
Degree	General Narrowing, AV ratio*	Focal Spasm†	Hemorrhages	Exudates	Papilledema	Arteriolar Light Reflex	AV Crossing Defects‡
Normal	3:4	1:1	0	0	0	Fine yellow line, red blood column	none
Grade I	1:2	1:1	0	0	0	Broadened yellow line, red blood column	Mild depression of vein
Grade II	1:3	2:3	0	0	0	Broad yellow line, "copper wire," blood column not visible	Depression or humping of vein
Grade III	1:4	1:3	+	+	0	Broad white line, "silver wire," blood column not visible	Right-angle deviation, tapering, and disappearance of vein under arteriole; distal dilation of vein
Grade IV	Fine, fibrous cords	Obliteration of distal flow	+	+	+	Fibrous cords, blood column not visible	Same as grade III

* Ratio of arteriolar to venous diameters.
† Ratio of diameters of region of spasm to proximal arteriole.
‡ Arteriolar length and tortuosity increase with severity.

is present, and to provide a baseline. The echocardiogram is more sensitive than either the electrocardiogram or physical examination in determining whether cardiac hypertrophy is present. Thus, in some circumstances, this modality may be a useful addition to the *baseline* evaluation of a hypertensive patient, particularly as left ventricular hypertrophy is an independent cardiovascular risk factor and its presence suggests the need for vigorous antihypertensive therapy. Furthermore, while a substantial increase in arterial pressure usually correlates with the presence of left ventricular hypertrophy, a mild increase may not. Thus, one cannot use the blood pressure as a surrogate marker for the presence or absence of left ventricular hypertrophy. On the other hand, because of the cost of an echocardiogram and the uncertainty as to whether the resultant information would modify therapy, it is unclear that routine *follow-up* echocardiograms during therapy are justified. The chest roentgenogram also may be helpful by providing the opportunity to identify aortic dilation or elongation and the rib notching that occurs in coarctation of the aorta.

Certain clues from the history, physical examination, and basic laboratory studies may suggest an unusual cause for the hypertension and dictate the need for special studies, which are outlined in Chap. 246.

℞ **TREATMENT**
See Chap. 246.

BIBLIOGRAPHY

GIFFORD RW et al: Office evaluation of hypertension: A statement for health professionals by a writing group of the Council for High Blood Pressure Research, American Heart Association. Circulation 79:721, 1989

GLYNN RJ et al: Evidence for a positive linear relation between blood pressure and mortality in elderly people. Lancet 345:825, 1995

JOINT NATIONAL COMMITTEE ON DETECTION, EVALUATION AND TREATMENT OF HIGH BLOOD PRESSURE: The fifth report. Arch Intern Med 153:154, 1993

KURTZ TW, SPENCE MA: Genetics of essential hypertension. Am J Med 94:77, 1993

LITTENBERG B et al: Screening for hypertension. Ann Intern Med 112:192, 1990

NATIONAL HIGH BLOOD PRESSURE EDUCATION PROGRAM WORKING GROUP: National High Blood Pressure Education Program Working Group report on hypertension in the elderly. Hypertension 23:145, 1994

SAGIE A et al: The natural history of borderline isolated systolic hypertension. N Engl J Med 329:1912, 1993

STAMLER J et al: Blood pressure, systolic and diastolic, and cardiovascular risks. US population data. Arch Intern Med 153:598, 1993

WEBER MA et al: Diagnosis of mild hypertension by ambulatory blood pressure monitoring. Circulation 90:2291, 1994

| **36** | *Eugene Braunwald* |

HYPOXIA, POLYCYTHEMIA, AND CYANOSIS

HYPOXIA

The fundamental purpose of the cardiorespiratory system is to deliver oxygen (and substrates) to the cells and to remove carbon dioxide (and other metabolic products) from them. Proper maintenance of this function depends on intact cardiovascular and respiratory systems and a supply of inspired gas containing adequate oxygen. Changes in oxygen and in carbon dioxide tension as well as changes in the intraerythrocytic concentration of certain *organic phosphate compounds*, especially 2,3-bisphosphoglyceric acid (2,3-BPG), cause shifts in the oxygen dissociation curve (see Fig. 107-1). When hypoxia occurs consequent to respiratory failure, Pa_{CO_2} usually rises (Chap. 250), and the oxygen dissociation curve is displaced to the right. Under these conditions or when the concentration of 2,3-BPG rises, the percentage saturation of the hemoglobin in the arterial blood at a given level of alveolar oxygen tension (Pa_{O_2}) declines. Thus arterial hypoxia and cyanosis are likely to be more marked in proportion to the degree of depression of Pa_{O_2} when such depression results from pulmonary dis-

ease than when the depression occurs as the result of a decline in the partial pressure of oxygen in the inspired air, in which case Pa_{CO_2} falls secondary to anoxia-induced hyperventilation and the oxygen dissociation curve is displaced to the left, limiting the decline in O_2 saturation of hemoglobin.

DIFFERENTIAL DIAGNOSIS Anemic Hypoxia Any decrease in hemoglobin concentration is attended by a corresponding decline in the oxygen-carrying capacity of the blood. The Pa_{O_2} remains normal, but the absolute amount of oxygen transported per unit volume of blood is diminished. As the anemic blood passes through the capillaries and the usual amount of oxygen is removed from it, the P_{O_2} in the venous blood declines to a greater degree than would normally be the case.

Carbon Monoxide Intoxication (Chap. 391)   The hemoglobin that is combined with carbon monoxide (carboxyhemoglobin) is unavailable for oxygen transport. In addition, the presence of carboxyhemoglobin shifts the hemoglobin dissociation curve to the left so that the oxygen can be unloaded only at lower tensions. By such formation of carboxyhemoglobin, a given degree of reduction in oxygen-carrying power produces a far greater degree of tissue hypoxia than the equivalent reduction in hemoglobin due to simple anemia.

Respiratory Hypoxia Arterial unsaturation is a common finding in advanced pulmonary disease. The most common cause of respiratory hypoxia is ventilation-perfusion mismatch, which results from perfusion of poorly ventilated alveoli. As discussed in Chap. 250, it may also be caused by hypoventilation, and it is then associated with an elevation of Pa_{CO_2}. These two forms of respiratory hypoxia are usually readily correctable by inspiring 100% O_2. A third cause is shunting of blood from right to left by perfusion of nonventilated portions of the lung, as in pulmonary atelectasis or through vascular abnormalities of the lung with arteriovenous connections. The low Pa_{O_2} in this situation is *not* correctable by inspiring 100% O_2.

Hypoxia Secondary to Right-to-Left Extrapulmonary Shunting From a physiologic viewpoint, this cause of hypoxia resembles intrapulmonary right-to-left shunting but is caused by congenital cardiac malformations such as tetralogy of Fallot, transposition of the great arteries, and Eisenmenger's complex (Chap. 235). As in pulmonary right-to-left shunting, the Pa_{O_2} cannot be brought to normal with inspiration of 100% O_2.

Circulatory Hypoxia As in anemic hypoxia, Pa_{O_2} is normal, but venous and tissue P_{O_2} values are reduced as a consequence of reduced tissue perfusion in the face of normal tissue oxygen consumption. Generalized circulatory hypoxia occurs in heart failure (Chap. 233) and in most forms of shock (Chap. 38).

Specific Organ Hypoxia Decreased circulation to a specific organ resulting in localized circulatory hypoxia may be due to organic arterial obstruction or may occur as a consequence of vasoconstriction (Chap. 248). The latter is seen in the upper extremities in Raynaud's phenomenon. In an attempt to maintain adequate perfusion to more vital organs, reduced circulation may occur in all limbs in patients with heart failure or hypovolemic shock. Ischemic hypoxia with accompanying pallor occurs in organic arterial obliterative disease. Localized hypoxia also may result from venous obstruction and the resultant congestion and reduced arterial inflow. Edema, which increases the distance through which oxygen diffuses before it reaches the cells, also can cause localized hypoxia.

Increased Oxygen Requirements If the oxygen consumption of the tissues is elevated without a corresponding increase in volume flow per unit of time, the P_{O_2} in venous blood (and hence capillary and tissue P_{O_2}) may be reduced. This will occur even if oxygen diffusion into blood perfusing the pulmonary capillary bed is normal and the hemoglobin is qualitatively and quantitatively normal. Such a situation may be encountered when fever or thyrotoxicosis occurs in patients in whom the cardiac output is fixed and cannot rise normally. Under these conditions, the circulation may be considered deficient relative to the metabolic requirements.

Ordinarily, the clinical picture of patients with hypoxia due to an elevated metabolic rate is quite different from that in other types of hypoxia; the skin is warm and flushed, owing to increased cutaneous blood flow which dissipates the excessive heat produced, and cyanosis is usually absent.

Exercise is a classic example of increased tissue oxygen requirements. These increased demands are normally met by several mechanisms operating simultaneously: (1) increasing the cardiac output and ventilation and thus oxygen delivery to the tissues; (2) preferentially directing the blood to the exercising muscles and away from resting muscles, skin, and viscera (by changing vascular resistances in various circulatory beds, directly and/or reflexly); (3) increasing oxygen extraction from the delivered blood and widening the arteriovenous oxygen differences; and (4) reducing the pH of the tissues and capillary blood, thereby unloading more oxygen from hemoglobin. If the capacity of these mechanisms is exceeded, then hypoxia, especially of the exercising muscles, will result.

Improper Oxygen Utilization Cyanide (Chap. 391) and several other similarly acting poisons cause a paradoxic state in which the tissues are unable to utilize oxygen, and as a consequence, the venous blood tends to have a high oxygen tension. This condition has been termed *histotoxic hypoxia.* Cyanide produces cellular hypoxia by paralyzing the electron-transfer function of cytochrome oxidase so that it cannot pass electrons to oxygen, whereas diphtheria toxin is believed to inhibit the synthesis of one of the cytochromes and thus interfere with oxygen consumption and energy production by the cells involved.

EFFECTS OF HYPOXIA Changes in the central nervous system, particularly the higher centers, are especially important. Acute hypoxia produces impaired judgment, motor incoordination, and a clinical picture closely resembling that of acute alcoholism. When hypoxia is long-standing, fatigue, drowsiness, apathy, inattentiveness, delayed reaction time, and reduced work capacity occur. As hypoxia becomes more severe, the centers of the brainstem are affected, and death usually results from respiratory failure. With reduction of Pa_{O_2}, cerebrovascular resistance decreases and cerebral blood flow increases, which tends to reduce the cerebral hypoxia. On the other hand, when the reduction of Pa_{O_2} is accompanied by hyperventilation and diminution of Pa_{CO_2}, cerebrovascular resistance rises, blood flow falls, and hypoxia is enhanced. Compared with the brain, the phylogenetically older spinal cord and peripheral nerves are relatively insensitive to hypoxia. Hypoxia also causes pulmonary arterial constriction, which serves the useful function of shunting blood away from poorly ventilated areas toward better-ventilated portions of the lung. However, it has the disadvantage of causing increased pulmonary vascular resistance and increased right ventricular afterload.

A complex disturbance of cellular functions results from the metabolic effects of severe acute hypoxia. In liver and muscles, the metabolism of the primary foodstuff, carbohydrate, normally proceeds anaerobically (i.e., without oxidation) to the stage of formation of pyruvic acid. The breakdown of pyruvate requires oxygen, and when this is deficient, increasing proportions of pyruvate are reduced to lactic acid, which cannot be broken down further. Hence there is an increase in the blood lactate, with decrease in bicarbonate and a corresponding metabolic acidosis. Under these circumstances, the total energy obtained from foodstuff breakdown is greatly reduced, and the amount of energy available for continuing resynthesis of energy-rich phosphate compounds becomes inadequate, leading to a complex disturbance of cellular function.

Most of the useful respiratory response to hypoxia originates in special chemosensitive cells in the carotid and aortic bodies, although the respiratory center in the brainstem is also stimulated directly by oxygen lack. The resultant increase in ventilation, with loss of carbon dioxide, leads to respiratory alkalosis. On the other hand, the diffusion of additional quantities of lactic acid from the tissues into the blood tends to produce metabolic acidosis. In either case, the total amount of bicarbonate, and hence the carbon dioxide–combining power, tends to be diminished (Chap. 50).

Diminished oxygen tension in any tissue results in local vasodilatation, and the diffuse vasodilatation that occurs in generalized hypoxia causes an elevation of total cardiac output. In patients with preexisting heart disease, the development of hypoxia and the requirements of the peripheral tissues for an increase of cardiac output may precipitate congestive heart failure. In patients with ischemic heart disease, a reduced Pa_{O_2} may intensify ischemia and further impair left ventricular function. Prolonged or severe hypoxia also may impair hepatic and renal function.

One of the important mechanisms of compensation for prolonged hypoxia is an increase in the hemoglobin concentration. This is due not to direct stimulation of the bone marrow but to the effect of erythropoietin. Assayable levels of erythropoietin are increased by hypoxia, and its production has been found to be regulated by the balance between tissue oxygen supply and demand.

POLYCYTHEMIA (See also Chap. 111)

The term *polycythemia* signifies an increase above normal in the number of red blood cells in the circulating blood. This elevation is usually, although not always, accompanied by a corresponding increase in the quantity of hemoglobin and in the hematocrit. The increase may or may not be associated with an elevation in the total quantity of red blood cells in the body. It is important to distinguish between *absolute* polycythemia (an increase in the total red cell mass) and *relative* (sometimes termed *spurious*), polycythemia, which occurs when, through loss of blood plasma, the *concentration* of the red cells in the circulating blood becomes greater than normal. This may be the consequence of abnormally lowered fluid intake, of the loss of plasma into the interstitial fluid, or of the marked loss of body fluids, such as occurs in persistent vomiting, severe diarrhea, copious sweating, or acidosis.

Because the term *polycythemia* is used loosely to refer to all varieties of increase in the number of red cells, the terms *erythrocytosis* and *erythremia* are preferred in referring to two forms of absolute polycythemia. Erythrocytosis denotes absolute polycythemia that occurs in response to some known stimulus, most commonly hypoxemia (secondary polycythemia); erythremia refers to the disease of unknown etiology—polycythemia vera. In secondary polycythemia, but not in polycythemia vera, the absolute increase in red cell mass is due to an increased production of erythropoietin. Erythrocytosis develops as a consequence of a variety of factors and represents a physiologic response to hypoxia. An approach to the differential diagnosis of erythrocytosis should begin with a consideration of its mechanisms (see Chap. 111).

Stress Erythrocytosis (Gaisböck's Syndrome) These terms have been applied to the polycythemia seen occasionally in active, hard-working, middle-aged white males who are typically hypertensive, overweight, and in a state of anxiety and who appear florid but have none of the other characteristic signs of polycythemia vera, i.e., no splenomegaly or leukocytosis with immature white blood cells. In such persons, the total red blood cell mass is normal, and the plasma volume is below normal. Thus they have a moderately elevated hematocrit, usually 50 to 60 percent, and *relative* polycythemia. *Smokers' polycythemia* is a closely related condition, but the high carboxyhemoglobin concentration may cause a small absolute increase in red cell mass which is often associated with a reduced plasma volume. Smoking should be discontinued.

SECONDARY POLYCYTHEMIA Sojourn at high altitudes leads to defective saturation of arterial blood with oxygen and stimulates the production of more red cells. The oxygen saturation, rather than oxygen tension, appears to be the more important determinant of the erythropoietic response to chronic hypoxia. A condition known as *chronic mountain sickness* or *soroche* (Monge's disease) may set in insidiously after several years of continued residence at high altitude. This condition appears to be caused by the development of alveolar hypoventilation superimposed on a lowered inspired O_2 concentration.

Prominent manifestations are a florid color that turns to cyanosis on mild exertion, impaired mental acuity, fatigue, and headache. Those affected are usually in the fourth to sixth decades. Return to sea level promptly relieves the symptoms. Living at high altitudes also evokes a number of compensatory reactions which act to increase oxygen delivery to the tissues. These include hyperventilation (which reduces the oxygen gradient between inspired and alveolar air), erythrocytosis, an augmentation of pulmonary capillary blood volume, an increase of pulmonary diffusing capacity, and an increase in cardiac output.

Any pulmonary disease that produces chronic hypoxia may lead to erythrocytosis. The increased blood viscosity secondary to the polycythemia elevates pulmonary arterial pressure and, combined with the elevation of pulmonary vascular resistance resulting from hypoxia, further elevates right ventricular pressure, contributing to the development or intensification of cor pulmonale (Chap. 238). The *abnormal ventilatory conditions* present in very obese individuals may cause alveolar hypoventilation and result in arterial unsaturation, erythrocytosis, hypercapnia, and somnolence (the Pickwickian syndrome; Chap. 263). This syndrome is also observed in nonobese persons (sleep-apnea syndrome) in whom decreased sensitivity of the respiratory center to CO_2 may play a role (Chap. 263).

The partial shunting of blood from the pulmonary circuit (right-to-left shunts), such as occurs in *congenital heart disease*, causes the most striking erythrocytosis resulting from abnormalities in the heart or lungs (Chap. 235). Erythrocyte counts as high as $12 \times 10^6/\mu L$, which are possible only when the red corpuscles are smaller than normal, have been observed in such patients, with a hematocrit as high as 86 percent. As the polycythemia develops, there is a progressive elevation of blood viscosity, which rises logarithmically when the volume of packed red blood cells exceeds 55 percent. The most common defects producing such polycythemia in the adult are tetralogy of Fallot and Eisenmenger syndrome. Other congenital cardiac malformations commonly responsible for polycythemia, but occurring more commonly in neonates, include transposition of the great arteries, tricuspid atresia, and persistent truncus arteriosus.

Rarely, patients with hepatic cirrhosis are hypoxemic secondary to intrapulmonary shunts or to right-to-left shunts from the portal to the pulmonary veins. The polycythemia of cyanotic congenital heart disease may lead to spontaneous thrombosis at any site, including the central nervous system.

The increase in hematocrit and the sharp increase in viscosity that occur when patients with congenital heart disease, large right-to-left shunts, and secondary polycythemia become dehydrated are particularly hazardous. Symptoms due to increased blood viscosity include reduced mentation, headache, fatigue, visual disturbance, and dizziness. This condition also may be accompanied by a variety of blood coagulation defects, including reduced fibrinogen and prothrombin concentrations, as well as thrombocytopenia. Reduction in red blood cell volume (phlebotomy with reinfusion of the plasma) is sometimes performed in severely symptomatic patients with extremely high hematocrit levels, usually exceeding 65 percent. It must be carried out slowly, with caution, and with the realization that the polycythemia is, in fact, an important compensatory mechanism. However, reduction of red blood cell volume may result in a reduction of the elevated blood viscosity which improves blood flow.

The excessive use of coal-tar derivatives and other forms of chronic poisoning, by producing abnormal hemoglobin pigments such as *methemoglobin* and *sulfhemoglobin* (Chap. 107), also may cause erythrocytosis. The production of erythropoietin and a secondary erythrocytosis *unassociated* with leukocytosis or thrombocytosis is stimulated in patients with abnormal hemoglobins that displace the oxygen dissociation curve to the left and interfere with oxygen unloading in the tissues (Chap. 107). Reductions in the synthesis of 2,3-bisphosphoglycerate also causes a shift to the left of the oxygen-hemoglobin dissociation curve.

Mild erythrocytosis is sometimes found in *Cushing's syndrome* and can be produced by the administration of large amounts of adrenocortical steroids and androgens. Especially intriguing are the instances of erythrocytosis observed in association with various *tumors* that

produce erythropoietin or an erythropoietin-like substance. These include vascular tumors (hemangioblastomas) in the posterior fossa, renal tumors (renal cell carcinoma, adenoma, and sarcoma), uterine myoma, hepatic carcinoma, and pheochromocytoma. Erythrocytosis also occurs occasionally in patients with solitary and polycystic disease of the kidneys, hydronephrosis, and renal artery stenosis. Plasma erythropoietin levels have been found to be elevated in a number of these patients with tumors and indeed all forms of secondary polycythemia. Erythropoietin-like activity has been demonstrated in tumor extracts and in renal cyst fluid, and erythrocytosis has disappeared after the associated tumor was removed.

CLINICAL FEATURES AND DIFFERENTIAL DIAGNOSIS Patients with polycythemia present with (in addition to the symptoms of the underlying condition) a characteristic "ruddy" cyanosis, dizziness, headache, epistaxes, and an increased incidence of thrombotic complications.

The *differential diagnosis* of absolute polycythemia is shown in Fig. 36-1 and is discussed further in Chap. 111. In polycythemia vera, erythropoietin levels are usually absent or below normal; leukocyte alkaline phosphatase, vitamin B_{12} binding capacity, vitamin B_{12} levels, and platelet and total white blood cell counts are usually elevated; and splenomegaly is common. Serum uric acid and lactate dehydrogenase (LDH) levels may be increased. The bone marrow shows hyperplasia of all elements. In secondary polycythemia with hypoxia, erythropoietin levels are elevated, while levels of leukocyte alkaline phosphatase and serum vitamin B_{12} and the platelet, total white blood cell, and differential counts are all normal. The liver and spleen are not enlarged, and the bone marrow shows only erythroid hyperplasia. In the absence of features of either polycythemia vera or polycythemia secondary to hypoxia or to a tumor, a hemoglobin with a high affinity for oxygen should be sought.

Workup of patients with polycythemia should include a chest roentgenogram, electrocardiogram, and arterial oxygen saturation determination to search for disease of the heart and lungs. In addition, imaging of the spleen should be carried out to assess its size and of the kidney to look for an erythropoietin-producing lesion (such as a renal cell carcinoma, hydronephrosis, or cyst). In patients who do not appear to have polycythemia vera or hypoxemia, the oxygen affinity of the patient's hemoglobin, i.e., the P_{O_2} at which 50 percent of the hemoglobin is deoxygenated (P_{50}) should be measured to detect hemoglobins which fail to release oxygen normally.

CYANOSIS

Cyanosis refers to a bluish color of the skin and mucous membranes resulting from an increased amount of reduced hemoglobin, or of hemoglobin derivatives, in the small blood vessels of those areas. It is usually most marked in the lips, nail beds, ears, and malar eminences. The florid skin characteristic of polycythemia vera (Chap. 111) must be distinguished from the true cyanosis discussed here. A cherry-colored flush, rather than cyanosis, is caused by carboxyhemoglobin (Chap. 391). The degree of cyanosis is modified by the quality of cutaneous pigment and the thickness of the skin, as well as by the state of the cutaneous capillaries. The accurate clinical detection of the presence and degree of cyanosis is difficult, as proved by oximetric studies. In some instances, central cyanosis can be detected reliably when the arterial saturation has fallen to 85 percent; in others, particularly in dark-skinned persons, it may not be detected until the saturation has declined to 75 percent.

The increase in the quantity of reduced hemoglobin in the cutaneous vessels that produces cyanosis may be brought about either by an increase in the quantity of venous blood in the skin as the result of dilatation of the venules and venous ends of the capillaries or by a reduction in the oxygen saturation in the capillary blood. In general, cyanosis becomes apparent when the mean capillary concentration of reduced hemoglobin exceeds 50 g/L (5 g/dL). It is the *absolute* rather than the *relative* quantity of reduced hemoglobin that is important in producing cyanosis. Thus, in a patient with severe anemia, the relative amount of reduced hemoglobin in the venous blood may be very large when considered in relation to the total amount of hemoglobin. However, since the concentration of the latter is markedly reduced, the *absolute* quantity of reduced hemoglobin may still be small, and therefore patients with severe anemia and even *marked* arterial desaturation do not display cyanosis. Conversely, the higher the total hemoglobin content, the greater is the tendency toward cyanosis; thus patients with marked polycythemia tend to be cyanotic at higher levels of arterial oxygen saturation than patients with normal hematocrit values. Likewise, local passive congestion, which causes an increase in the total amount of reduced hemoglobin in the vessels in a given area, may cause cyanosis. Cyanosis also is observed when nonfunctional hemoglobin such as methemoglobin or sulfhemoglobin (Chap. 107) is present in blood.

Cyanosis may be subdivided into central and peripheral types. In the *central* type, there is arterial blood unsaturation or an abnormal hemoglobin derivative, and the mucous membranes and skin are both affected. *Peripheral* cyanosis is due to a slowing of blood flow and abnormally great extraction of oxygen from normally saturated arterial blood. It results from vasoconstriction and diminished peripheral blood flow, such as occurs in cold exposure, shock, congestive failure, and peripheral vascular disease. Often in these conditions the mucous membranes of the oral cavity or those beneath the tongue may be spared. Clinical differentiation between central and peripheral cyanosis may not always be simple, and in conditions such as cardiogenic shock with pulmonary edema there may be a mixture of both types.

DIFFERENTIAL DIAGNOSIS **Central Cyanosis** (See Table 36-1) Decreased arterial oxygen saturation results from a marked reduction in the oxygen tension in the arterial blood. This may be brought about by a decline in the tension of oxygen in the inspired air without sufficient compensatory alveolar hyperventilation to maintain alveolar oxygen tension. Cyanosis does not occur to a significant degree in an ascent to an altitude of 2500 m (8000 ft) but is marked in a further ascent to 5000 m (16,000 ft). The reason for this becomes clear on studying the *S* shape of the oxygen dissociation curve (Fig. 107-1). At 2500 m (8000 ft) the tension of oxygen in the inspired air is about 120 mmHg, the alveolar tension is approximately 80 mmHg, and the hemoglobin is nearly completely saturated. However, at 5000 m (16,000 ft) the oxygen tensions in atmospheric air and alveolar air are about 85 and 50 mmHg, respectively, and the oxygen dissociation curve shows that the arterial blood is only about 75 percent saturated. This leaves 25 percent of the hemoglobin in the reduced form, an amount likely to be associated with cyanosis in the absence of anemia. Similarly, a mutant hemoglobin with a low affinity for oxygen (e.g., Hb Kansas) causes lowered arterial oxygen saturation and resultant central cyanosis (Chap. 107).

Seriously *impaired pulmonary function*, through alveolar hypoventilation or perfusion of unventilated or poorly ventilated areas of the lung, is a common cause of central cyanosis (Chap. 250). This may occur acutely, as in extensive pneumonia or pulmonary edema, or with chronic pulmonary diseases (e.g., emphysema). In the last situation polycythemia is generally present, and clubbing of the fingers may occur. However, in many types of chronic pulmonary disease with fibrosis and obliteration of the capillary vascular bed, cyanosis does not occur because there is relatively little perfusion of underventilated areas.

Another cause of decreased arterial oxygen saturation is *shunting of systemic venous blood into the arterial circuit*. Certain forms of congenital heart disease are associated with cyanosis (Chap. 235). Since blood flows from a higher-pressure to a lower-pressure region, in order for a cardiac defect to result in a right-to-left shunt, it must ordinarily be combined with an obstructive lesion distal to the defect or with elevated pulmonary vascular resistance. The most common congenital cardiac lesion associated with cyanosis in the adult is the combination of ventricular septal defect and pulmonary outflow tract obstruction (tetralogy of Fallot). The more severe the obstruction, the greater the degree of right-to-left shunting and resultant cyanosis. The mechanisms for the elevated pulmonary vascular resistance which may produce cyanosis in the presence of intra- and extracardiac communications without pulmonic stenosis (Eisenmenger syndrome) are discussed in Chap. 235. In patients with patent ductus arteriosus, pulmonary hypertension, and right-to-left shunt, *differential cyanosis* results; i.e., cyanosis occurs in the lower but not in the upper extremities.

Pulmonary arteriovenous fistulas may be congenital or acquired, solitary or multiple, microscopic or massive. The degree of cyanosis produced by these fistulas depends on their size and number. They occur with some frequency in hereditary hemorrhagic telangiectasia. Arterial oxygen unsaturation also occurs in some patients with cirrhosis, presum-

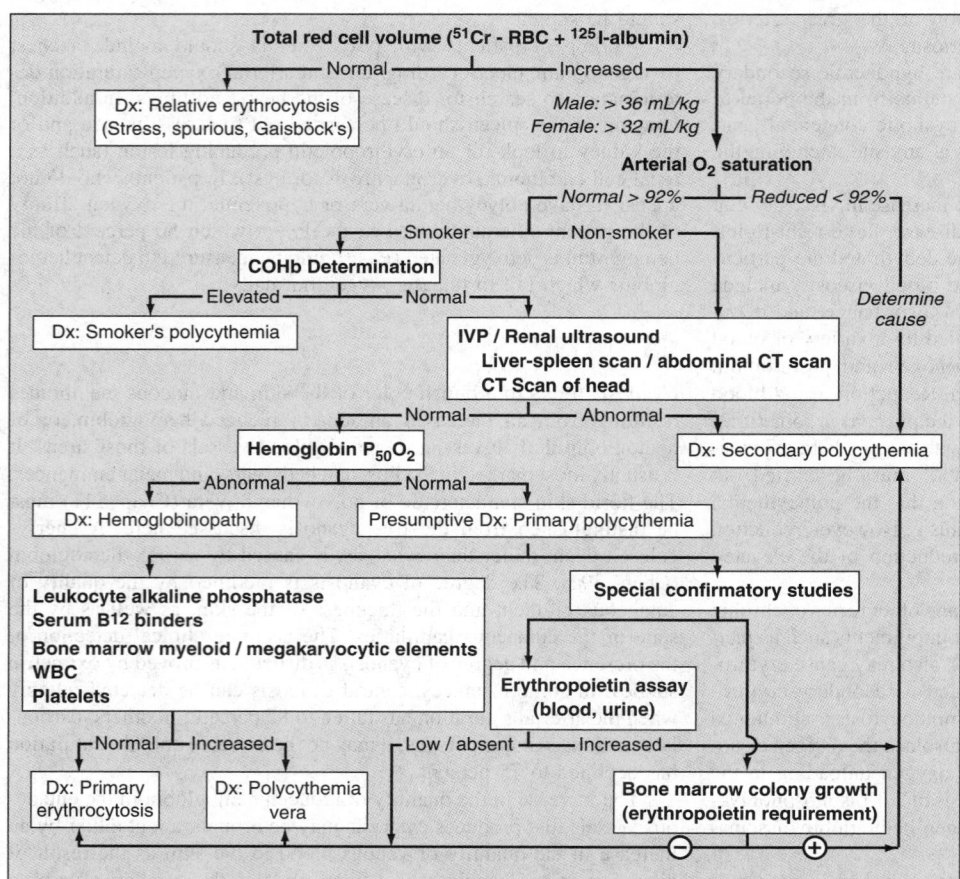

FIGURE 36-1 Algorithm for evaluation of an elevated hematocrit. COHb, carboxyhemoglobin; CT, computed tomography; IVP, intravenous pyelogram; $P_{50}O_2$, the P_{O_2} at which 50% of the hemoglobin is deoxygenated; RBC, red blood cells; WBC, white blood cells. *(From Fruchtman and Berk, with permission.)*

ably as a consequence of pulmonary arteriovenous fistulas or portal vein–pulmonary vein anastomoses.

In patients with cardiac or pulmonary right-to-left shunts, the presence and severity of cyanosis depend on the size of the shunt relative to the systemic flow as well as on the oxyhemoglobin saturation of the venous blood. In patients with central cyanosis due to arterial oxygen unsaturation, the severity of cyanosis increases with exercise. With increased extraction of oxygen from the blood by the exercising muscles, the venous blood returning to the right side of the heart is more unsaturated than at rest, and shunting of this blood or its passage through lungs incapable of normal oxygenation intensifies the cyanosis. Also, since the systemic vascular resistance normally decreases with exercise, the right-to-left shunt is augmented by exercise in patients with congenital heart disease and communications between the two sides of the heart. Secondary polycythemia occurs frequently in patients with arterial unsaturation and contributes to the cyanosis.

Cyanosis can be caused by small amounts of circulating methemoglobin and by even smaller amounts of sulfhemoglobin (Chap. 107). Although they are uncommon causes of cyanosis, these abnormal hemoglobin pigments should be sought by spectroscopy when cyanosis is not readily explained by malfunction of the circulatory or respiratory systems. Generally, clubbing does not occur with them. The diagnosis of methemoglobinemia can be suspected, if, on mixing the patient's blood in a test tube and exposing it to air, it remains brown.

Peripheral Cyanosis Probably the most common cause of peripheral cyanosis is generalized vasoconstriction resulting from exposure to cold air or water. This is a normal response. When cardiac output is low, as in severe congestive heart failure or shock, cutaneous vasoconstriction occurs as a compensatory mechanism, so blood is diverted from the skin to more vital areas such as the central nervous system and heart (Chap. 233), and intense cyanosis associated with cool extremities may result. Even though the arterial blood is normally saturated, the reduced volume flow through the skin and the reduced oxygen tension at the venous end of the capillary result in cyanosis.

Arterial obstruction to an extremity, as with an embolus, or arteriolar constriction, as in cold-induced vasospasm (Raynaud's phenomenon; Chap. 248), generally results in pallor and coldness, but there may be associated cyanosis. If there is venous obstruction and the extremity is congested, as with stagnation of blood flow, cyanosis is also present. Venous hypertension, which may be local (as in thrombophlebitis) or generalized (as in tricuspid valve disease or constrictive pericarditis), dilates the subpapillary venous plexuses and thereby intensifies cyanosis.

--- *Approach to the Patient* ---

Certain features are important in arriving at the proper cause of cyanosis:

1. The history, particularly the duration (cyanosis present since birth is usually due to congenital heart disease), and possible exposure to drugs or chemicals that may produce abnormal types of hemoglobin.
2. Clinical differentiation of central as opposed to peripheral cyanosis. Objective evidence by physical or radiographic examination of disorders of the respiratory or cardiovascular systems. Massage or gentle warming of a cyanotic extremity will increase peripheral blood flow and abolish peripheral but not central cyanosis.
3. The presence or absence of clubbing of the fingers (see below). Clubbing without cyanosis is frequent in patients with infective endocarditis and in association with ulcerative colitis; it may occasionally occur in healthy persons, and in some instances it may be occupational, e.g., in jackhammer operators. Slight cyanosis of the lips and cheeks, without clubbing of the fingers, is common in patients with mitral stenosis and is probably due to minimal arterial hypoxia resulting from fibrotic changes in the lungs secondary to long-standing congestion combined with reduction of cardiac output (Chap. 237). The combination of cyanosis and clubbing is frequent in patients with certain types of congenital cardiac disease and is seen occasionally in persons with pulmonary disease such as lung abscess or pulmonary arteriovenous shunts. On the other hand, peripheral cyanosis or acutely developing central cyanosis is not associated with clubbed fingers.
4. Determination of arterial blood oxygen tension or oxygen saturation, spectroscopic and other examinations of the blood for abnormal types of hemoglobin.

CLUBBING

The selective bullous enlargement of the distal segments of the fingers and toes due to proliferation of connective tissue, particularly on the dorsal surface, is termed *clubbing*; an increase occurs in the sponginess of the soft tissue at the base of the nail. Clubbing may be hereditary, idiopathic, or acquired and associated with a variety of disorders, including cyanotic congenital heart disease, infective endocarditis, and a variety of pulmonary conditions (among them primary and metastatic lung cancer, bronchiectasis, lung abscess, cystic fibrosis, and mesothelioma), as well as with some gastrointestinal diseases (including regional enteritis, chronic ulcerative colitis, and hepatic cirrhosis). Clubbing in patients with primary and metastatic lung cancer, mesothelioma, bronchiectasis, and hepatic cirrhosis may be associated with *hypertrophic osteoarthropathy*. In this condition, the subperiosteal formation of new bone in the distal diaphyses of the long bones of the extremities causes pain and symmetric arthritis-like changes in the shoulders, knees, ankles, wrists, and elbows. The diagnosis of hypertrophic osteoarthropathy may be confirmed by bone radiographs and scans. Although the mechanism of clubbing is unclear, it appears to be secondary to a (presumably humoral) substance which causes dilation of the vessels of the fingertip.

Table 36-1

Causes of Cyanosis

CENTRAL CYANOSIS

Decreased arterial oxygen saturation
 Decreased atmospheric pressure—high altitude
 Impaired pulmonary function
  Alveolar hypoventilation
  Uneven relationships between pulmonary ventilation and perfusion
   (perfusion of hypoventilated alveoli)
  Impaired oxygen diffusion
 Anatomic shunts
  Certain types of congenital heart disease
  Pulmonary arteriovenous fistulas
  Multiple small intrapulmonary shunts
 Hemoglobin with low affinity for oxygen
Hemoglobin abnormalities
 Methemoglobinemia—hereditary, acquired
 Sulfhemoglobinema—acquired
 Carboxyhemoglobinemia (not true cyanosis)

PERIPHERAL CYANOSIS

Reduced cardiac output
Cold exposure
Redistribution of blood flow from extremities
Arterial obstruction
Venous obstruction

BIBLIOGRAPHY

Doll DC, Greenberg BR: Cerebral thrombosis in smokers' polycythemia. Ann Intern Med 102:786, 1985

Fruchtman SM, Berk PD: Polycythemia vera and agnogenic myeloid multiplasia, in *Blood: Principles and Practice of Hematology,* RI Handin et al (eds). Philadelphia, Lippincott, 1995, pp 415–438

Hansen-Flaschen J, Nordberg J: Clubbing and hypertrophic osteoarthropathy. Clin Chest Med 8:287, 1987

HURTADO A: Some clinical aspects of life at high altitudes. Ann Intern Med 53:247, 1960

JANDL JH: Polycythemia: Erythrocytosis, in *Blood: Textbook of Hematology*, JH Jandl (ed). Boston, Little, Brown, 1996, pp 605–614

SCHWARCZ TH et al: Thromboembolic complications of polycythemia: Polycythemia vera vs. smokers' polycythemia. J Vasc Surg 17:518, 1993

SMITH JR, LANDAW SA: Smokers' polycythemia. N Engl J Med 298:6, 1978

SZIDON JP, FISHMAN AP: Cyanosis and clubbing, in *Pulmonary Diseases and Disorders*, 2d ed, A Fishman (ed). Philadelphia, Saunders, 1988, p 351

TERRITO MC, ROSOVE MH: Cyanotic congenital heart disease: Hematologic management. J Am Coll Cardiol 18:320, 1991

---

37 | *Eugene Braunwald*

EDEMA

Edema is defined as a clinically apparent increase in the interstitial fluid volume, which may expand by several liters before the abnormality is evident. Therefore, a weight gain of several kilograms usually precedes overt manifestations of edema, and a similar weight loss from diuresis can be induced in a slightly edematous patient before "dry weight" is achieved. *Ascites* (Chap. 46) and *hydrothorax* refer to accumulation of excess fluid in the peritoneal and pleural cavities, respectively, and are considered to be special forms of edema. *Anasarca* refers to gross, generalized edema.

Depending on its cause and mechanism, edema may be localized or have a generalized distribution; it is recognized in its generalized form by puffiness of the face, which is most readily apparent in the periorbital areas, and by the persistence of an indentation of the skin following pressure; this is known as "pitting" edema. In its more subtle form, it may be detected by noting that after the stethoscope is removed from the chest wall, the rim of the bell leaves an indentation on chest skin for a few minutes. When the ring on a finger fits more snugly than in the past or when a patient complains of difficulty in putting on shoes, particularly in the evening, edema may be present.

PATHOGENESIS About one-third of the total-body water is confined to the extracellular space. Approximately 25 percent of the latter, in turn, is composed of the plasma volume, and the remainder is interstitial fluid.

Starling Forces The forces that regulate the disposition of fluid between these two components of the extracellular compartment are frequently referred to as the *Starling forces* (see p. 194). The hydrostatic pressure within the vascular system and the colloid oncotic pressure in the interstitial fluid tend to promote movement of fluid from the vascular to the extravascular space. In contrast, the colloid oncotic pressure contributed by the plasma proteins and the hydrostatic pressure within the interstitial fluid, referred to as the *tissue tension*, promote the movement of fluid into the vascular compartment. Consequently there is a movement of water and diffusible solutes from the vascular space at the arteriolar end of the capillaries. Fluid is returned from the interstitial space into the vascular system at the venous end of the capillary and by way of the lymphatics, and unless these channels are obstructed, lymph flow tends to increase if there is net movement of fluid from the vascular compartment to the interstitium. These forces are usually balanced so that a steady state exists in the sizes of the intravascular and interstitial compartments, and yet a large exchange between them is permitted. However, should any one of the hydrostatic or oncotic forces be altered significantly, a net movement of fluid between the two components of the extracellular space will occur. The development of edema then depends on one or more alterations in the Starling forces so that there is a net movement of fluid from the vascular system into the interstitium or into a body cavity.

An increase in capillary pressure as a cause of edema may result from an elevation of venous pressure due to local obstruction in venous drainage. This increase in capillary pressure may be generalized, as occurs in congestive heart failure. The colloid oncotic pressure of the plasma may be reduced, owing to any factor that may induce severe hypoalbuminemia, such as malnutrition, liver disease, loss of protein into the urine or into the gastrointestinal tract, or a severe catabolic state.

Capillary Damage Edema may also result from damage to the capillary endothelium, which increases its permeability and permits the transfer of protein into the interstitial compartment. Injury to the capillary wall can result from chemical or bacterial agents as well as from thermal or mechanical trauma. Increased capillary permeability may also be a consequence of a hypersensitivity reaction and is characteristic of immune injury. Damage to the capillary endothelium is presumably responsible for inflammatory edema, which is usually nonpitting, localized, and accompanied by other signs of inflammation—redness, heat, and tenderness.

To formulate a hypothesis about the pathophysiology of an edematous state, it is important to discriminate between the *primary* events, such as venous or lymphatic obstruction, reduction of cardiac output, hypoalbuminemia, trapping of fluid in spaces such as the peritoneal cavity, or an increase in capillary permeability, and the predictable *secondary* consequences, which include the renal retention of salt and water in an attempt to restore the plasma volume. Both the primary event and the secondary consequences may contribute to the formation of edema.

Reduction of Effective Arterial Volume In many forms of edema the *effective arterial blood volume*, an as yet poorly defined parameter of the filling of the arterial tree, is reduced, and as a consequence a series of physiologic responses designed to restore it to normal are set into motion. A key element of these responses is the retention of an increment of salt and therefore of water, principally by the proximal tubule (Fig. 37-1), and in many instances this repairs the deficit of the effective arterial blood volume; often this occurs without the development of overt edema. If, however, the retention of salt and water is insufficient to restore and maintain the effective arterial blood volume, the stimuli are not dissipated, the retention of salt and water continues, and edema ultimately develops. This sequence of events is operative in dehydration and hemorrhage. Although in these conditions there is a reduction of effective arterial blood volume and activation of the entire sequence shown in the center of Fig. 37-2, including the diminished excretion of salt and water, edema does *not* occur because the net sodium and water balance is negative rather than positive. In most conditions that lead to edema the mechanisms responsible for maintaining a normal effective osmolality in the body fluids operate efficiently so that sodium retention promotes thirst and secretion of the antidiuretic hormone, which, in turn, lead to the ingestion and retention of approximately 1 L of water for each 140 mmol sodium retained. In edematous states, isotonic expansion of the extracellular fluid space may be massive, while the intracellular fluid volume is changed little or not at all.

Reduced Cardiac Output A reduction of cardiac output, whatever the cause, is associated with a reduction of the effective arterial blood volume as well as of renal blood flow, constriction of the efferent renal arterioles, and an elevation of the filtration fraction, i.e., the ratio of glomerular filtration rate to renal plasma flow. In severe heart failure there is a reduction in the glomerular filtration rate. Activation of the sympathetic nervous system and of the renin-angiotensin systems are responsible for renal vasoconstriction. The finding that alpha-adrenergic blocking agents and/or angiotensin-converting enzyme (ACE) inhibitors augment renal blood flow and induce diuresis supports the role of these two systems in elevating renal vascular resistance and salt and water retention.

Renal Factors Reduced cardiac output lowers effective arterial blood volume. There is increased reabsorption of glomerular filtrate in both the proximal (Fig. 37-1) and distal increases in sodium reabsorption in heart failure. Alterations in intrarenal hemodynamics appear to play a significant role. Heart failure, and other conditions such as nephrotic syndrome and cirrhosis that reduce effective arterial blood volume, cause renal efferent arteriolar constriction. This, in turn, reduces the hydrostatic pressure and raises the colloid osmotic pressure in the peritubular capillaries, thus enhancing salt and water reabsorption in the proximal tubule as well as in the ascending limb of the loop of Henle.

In addition, the diminished renal blood flow characteristic of states in which the effective arterial blood volume is reduced is translated by the renal juxtaglomerular cells into a signal for increased renin release (Chap. 332). The mechanisms responsible for this release include a baroreceptor response: reduced renal perfusion results in incomplete filling of the renal arterioles and diminished stretch of the juxtaglomerular cells, a signal that provides for the elaboration or release, or both, of renin. A second mechanism for renin release involves the macula densa; as a result of reduced glomerular filtration the sodium chloride load reaching the distal renal tubules is reduced. This is sensed by the macula densa, which signals the neighboring juxtaglomerular cells to secrete renin. A third mechanism involves the sympathetic nervous system and circulating catecholamines. Activation of the beta-adrenergic receptors in the juxtaglomerular cells stimulates renin release. These three mechanisms generally act in concert.

The Renin-Angiotensin-Aldosterone (RAA) System (See Chap. 332)   Renin, an enzyme with a molecular weight of about 40,000, acts on its substrate, angiotensinogen, an alpha$_2$ globulin synthesized by the liver, to release angiotensin I, a decapeptide, which is broken down to angiotensin II (AII), an octapeptide. This has generalized vasoconstrictor properties; it is especially active on the efferent arterioles, and independently increases Na$^+$ reabsorption in the proximal tubule. The RAA system has long been recognized as a hormone system. However, it also operates locally. Both circulating and intrarenally produced AII contribute to renal vasoconstriction and to salt and

water retention. These renal effects of AII are mediated by activation of AII type 1 receptors, which can be blocked by specific antagonists such as losartan. AII also enters the circulation and stimulates the production of aldosterone by the zona glomerulosa of the adrenal cortex. In patients with heart failure, not only is aldosterone secretion elevated but the biologic half-life of aldosterone is prolonged, which further increases the plasma level of the hormone. A depression of hepatic blood flow, particularly during exercise, secondary to a reduction in cardiac output, is responsible for the reduced hepatic catabolism of aldosterone. Aldosterone, in turn, enhances Na$^+$ reabsorption (and K$^+$ excretion) by the collecting tubule. The activation of the RAA system is most striking in the early phase of acute, severe heart failure and is less intense in patients with chronic, stable, compensated heart failure.

Although increased quantities of aldosterone are secreted in heart failure and in other edematous states and although blockade of the action of aldosterone by spironolactone (an aldosterone antagonist) or amiloride (a blocker of epithelial Na$^+$ channels) often induces a moderate diuresis in edematous states, persistent augmented levels of aldosterone (or other mineralocorticoids) alone do not always promote accumulation of edema, as witnessed by the lack of striking fluid retention in most instances of primary aldosteronism (Chap. 332). Furthermore, although normal individuals retain some salt and water under the influence of a potent mineralocorticoid, such as deoxycorticosterone acetate or fludrocortisone, this accumulation is self-limiting, despite continued exposure to the steroid, a phenomenon known as *mineralocorticoid escape*. The failure of normal individuals receiving large doses of mineralocorticoids to accumulate large quantities of extracellular fluid and to develop edema is probably a consequence of an increase in glomerular filtration rate (pressure natriuresis) and through the action of natriuretic substance(s) (see below). The continued secretion of aldosterone may be more important in the accumulation of fluid in edematous states because patients with edema are generally unable to repair the deficit in effective arterial blood volume. As a consequence they do not develop pressure natriuresis nor do they elaborate normal quantities of atrial natriuretic peptide.

Blockade of the RAA system, by blocking AII receptors or inhibiting the ACE reduces efferent arterial resistance and increases renal blood flow. This action (combined in patients with heart failure with a rise in cardiac output secondary to afterload reduction) as well as reduction in the secretion of aldosterone cause diuresis. However, in patients with moderate or severe impairment of renal function interference with the RAA system can cause paradoxical sodium retention due to intensification of renal failure.

Arginine Vasopressin (AVP) and Endothelin (See also Chap. 330)   The secretion of AVP occurs in response to increased intracellular osmolar concentration and by stimulating V$_2$ receptors increases the reabsorption of free water in the distal tubule, thereby increasing total-body water. Circulating AVP is elevated in many patients with heart failure secondary to an as yet unidentified nonosmotic stimulus, who fail to show the normal reduction of AVP with a reduction of osmolality, contributing to fluid retention and edema formation.

Endothelin   This is a potent peptide vasoconstrictor released by endothelial cells; its concentration is elevated in heart failure and contributes to renal vasoconstriction, Na$^+$ retention, and edema in heart failure.

Natriuretic Peptides   Atrial distention and/or a sodium load cause release into the circulation of atrial natriuretic peptide (ANP), a polypeptide; a high-molecular-weight precursor of ANP is stored in secretory granules within atrial myocytes. Release of ANP causes (1) excretion of sodium and water by augmenting glomerular filtration rate, inhibiting sodium reabsorption in the proximal tubule, and inhibiting release of renin and aldosterone; and (2) arteriolar and venous dilatation by antagonizing the vasoconstrictor actions of AII, AVP, and sympathetic stimulation. Thus, ANP has the capacity to oppose sodium retention and arterial pressure elevation in hypervolemic states.

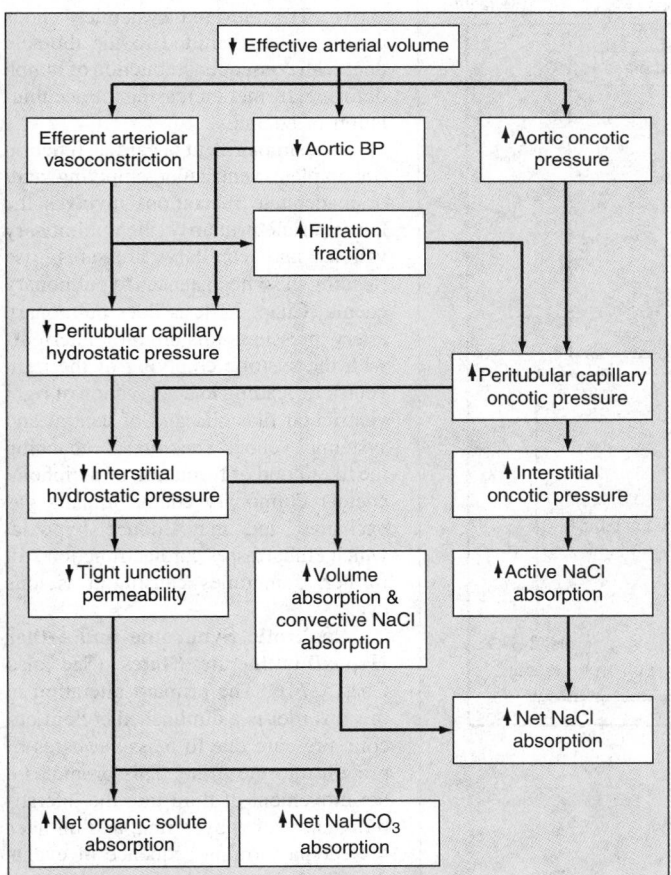

FIGURE 37-1   Effect of hemodynamic changes on proximal tubule solute transport: a summary. Hemodynamic mechanisms by which a reduction of effective arterial volume causes salt and water retention and thereby contributes to the formation of edema. *(From Seldin DW et al, Semin Nephrol 11:212, 1991, with permission.)*

The closely related brain natriuretic peptide (BNP) is stored primarily in cardiac ventricular myocardium and is released when ventricular diastolic pressure rises. Its actions are similar to ANP. Circulating levels of ANP and BNP are elevated in congestive heart failure but obviously not sufficient to prevent edema formation. In addition, in edematous states (particularly heart failure), there is abnormal resistance to the actions of natriuretic peptides.

CLINICAL CAUSES OF EDEMA **Obstruction of Venous (and Lymphatic) Drainage of a Limb** In this condition the hydrostatic pressure in the capillary bed upstream to the obstruction increases so that more fluid than normal is transferred from the vascular to the interstitial space. Since the alternative route (i.e., the lymphatic channels) may also be obstructed, this event causes an increased volume of interstitial fluid in the limb, i.e., a trapping of fluid in the extremity, at the expense of the blood volume in the remainder of the body, thereby reducing effective arterial blood volume and leading to the consequences shown in Fig. 37-2.

When venous and lymphatic drainage are obstructed in a limb, fluid accumulates in the interstitium at the expense of plasma volume. The latter stimulates the retention of salt and water until the deficit in plasma volume has been corrected. Tissue tension rises in the affected limb until it counterbalances the primary alterations in the Starling forces, at which time no further fluid accumulates. The net effect is a local increase in the volume of interstitial fluid. This same sequence occurs in ascites and hydrothorax, in which fluid is trapped or accumulates in the cavitary space, depleting the intravascular volume and leading to secondary salt and fluid retention, as already described.

Congestive Heart Failure (See also Chap. 233) In this disorder the defective systolic emptying of the chambers of the heart and/or the impairment of ventricular relaxation promotes an accumulation of blood in the heart and venous circulation at the expense of the arterial volume, and the aforementioned sequence of events (Fig. 37-2) is initiated. In mild heart failure, a small increment of total blood volume may repair the deficit of arterial volume and establish a new steady state because, through the operation of Starling's law of the heart, an increase in the volume of blood within the chambers of the heart promotes a more forceful contraction and may thereby increase the cardiac output (Fig. 233-1). However, if the cardiac disorder is more severe, retention of fluid cannot repair the deficit in effective arterial blood volume. The increment accumulates in the venous circulation, and the increase in capillary and lymphatic hydrostatic pressures promotes the formation of edema. In heart failure, a reduction occurs in baroreflex-mediated inhibition of the vasomotor center, which causes activation of renal vasoconstrictor nerves and the RAA system, causing sodium and water retention.

Incomplete ventricular emptying (systolic heart failure) and/or inadequate ventricular relaxation (diastolic heart failure) both lead to an elevation of ventricular diastolic pressure. If the impairment of cardiac function involves the right ventricle, pressures in the systemic veins and capillaries may rise, thereby augmenting the transudation of fluid into the interstitial space and enhancing the likelihood of peripheral edema in the presence of the accumulation of sodium and water, as described above. The elevated systemic venous pressure is transmitted to the thoracic duct with consequent reduction of lymph drainage, further increasing the accumulation of edema.

If the impairment of cardiac function (incomplete ventricular emptying and/or inadequate relaxation) involves the left ventricle primarily, then pulmonary venous and capillary pressures rise [leading in some instances to pulmonary edema (Chap. 32)], as does pulmonary artery pressure; this in turn interferes with the systolic emptying of the right ventricle, leading to an elevation of right ventricular diastolic and of central and systemic venous pressures, enhancing the likelihood of formation of peripheral edema. Pulmonary edema impairs gas exchange and may induce hypoxia, which embarrasses cardiac function still further, sometimes causing a vicious cycle.

Nephrotic Syndrome and Other Hypoalbuminemic States (See also Chap. 274) The primary alteration in this disorder is a diminished colloid oncotic pressure due to massive losses of protein into the urine. This promotes a net movement of fluid into the interstitium, causes hypovolemia, and initiates the edema-forming sequence of events described above, including activation of the RAA system. With severe hypoalbuminemia, the salt and water that are retained cannot be restrained within the vascular compartment, total and effective arterial blood volumes decline, and

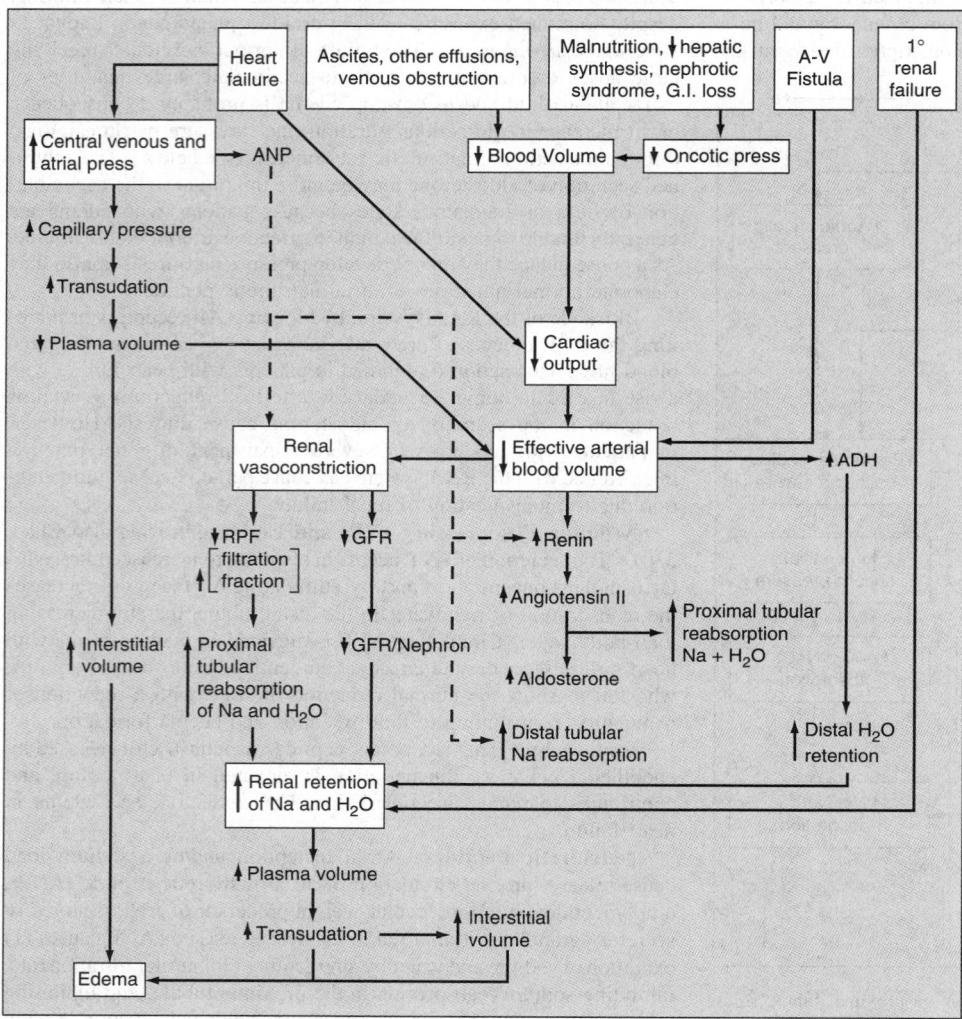

FIGURE 37-2 Sequence of events leading to the formation and retention of salt and water and the development of edema. ANP, atrial natriuretic peptide; RPF, renal plasma flow; GFR, glomerular filtration rate. Inhibitory influences are shown by broken lines. ADH, antidiuretic hormone

hence the stimuli to retain salt and water are not abated. A similar sequence of events occurs in other conditions that lead to *severe* hypoalbuminemia, including severe nutritional deficiency states, protein-losing enteropathy, congenital hypoalbuminemia, and severe, chronic liver disease. However, in the nephrotic syndrome, the impairment of renal function contributes to the retention of sodium.

Cirrhosis (See also Chaps. 46 and 298)   This condition is characterized by hepatic venous outflow blockade, which in turn causes expansion of the splanchnic blood volume and increased hepatic lymph formation. Intrahepatic hypertension acts as a potent stimulus for renal Na^+ retention and perhaps systemic vasodilation and a reduction of effective arterial blood volume as well. These alterations are frequently complicated by hypoalbuminemia secondary to reduced hepatic synthesis and reduce the effective arterial blood volume even further, leading to activation of the RAA system, of renal sympathetic nerves and other salt- and water-retaining mechanisms. The concentration of circulating aldosterone is elevated by the liver's failure to metabolize this hormone. Initially, the excess interstitial fluid is localized preferentially upstream to the congested portal venous system and obstructed hepatic lymphatics, i.e., in the peritoneal cavity. In later stages, particularly when there is severe hypoalbuminemia, peripheral edema may develop. The excess production of prostaglandins (PGE_2 and PGI_2) in cirrhosis attenuates renal Na^+ retention. When the synthesis of these substances is inhibited by nonsteroidal antiinflammatory agents, renal function deteriorates and Na^+ retention increases.

Idiopathic Edema   This syndrome, which occurs almost exclusively in women, is characterized by periodic episodes of edema (unrelated to the menstrual cycle), frequently accompanied by abdominal distention. Diurnal alterations in weight occur with orthostatic retention of sodium and water, so that the patient may weigh several pounds more after having been in the upright posture for several hours. Such large diurnal weight changes suggest an increase in capillary permeability which appears to fluctuate in severity and to be aggravated by hot weather. There is some evidence that a reduction in plasma volume occurs in this condition with secondary activation of the RAA system and impaired suppression of AVP release. Idiopathic edema should be distinguished from cyclical or premenstrual edema in which the sodium and water retention may be secondary to excessive estrogen stimulation. There are also some cases in which the edema appears to be "diuretic-induced." It has been postulated that in these patients, chronic diuretic administration leads to mild blood volume depletion, which causes chronic hyperreninemia and juxtaglomerular hyperplasia. Salt-retaining mechanisms appear to overcompensate for the direct effects of the diuretics. *Acute* withdrawal of diuretics can then leave the sodium-retaining forces unopposed, leading to fluid retention and edema. Decreased dopaminergic activity and reduced urinary kallikrein and kinin excretion have been reported in this condition and may also be of pathogenetic importance.

℞ **TREATMENT**

The treatment of idiopathic cyclic edema includes a reduction in salt intake, rest in the supine position for several hours each day, the wearing of elastic stockings (which are put on before arising in the morning), and an attempt to understand any underlying emotional problems. A variety of pharmacologic agents including ACE inhibitors, progesterone, the dopamine receptor agonist bromocriptine, and the sympathomimetic amine dextroamphetamine have all been reported to be useful when administered to patients who do not respond to simpler measures. Diuretics may be initially helpful but may lose their effectiveness with continuous administration; accordingly, they should be employed sparingly, if at all. Discontinuation of diuretics paradoxically leads to diuresis in "diuretic-induced" edema, described above.

DIFFERENTIAL DIAGNOSIS

Localized edema can usually be readily differentiated from generalized edema. The great majority of patients with generalized edema suffer from advanced cardiac, renal, hepatic, or nutritional disorders. Conse-

quently, the differential diagnosis of generalized edema should be directed toward identifying or excluding these several conditions.

LOCALIZED EDEMA (See also Chap. 248)   Edema originating from inflammation or hypersensitivity is usually readily identified. Localized edema due to venous or lymphatic obstruction may be caused by thrombophlebitis, chronic lymphangitis, resection of regional lymph nodes, filariasis, etc. Lymphedema is particularly intractable because restriction of lymphatic flow results in increased protein concentration in the interstitial fluid, a circumstance that aggravates retention of fluid.

EDEMA OF HEART FAILURE (See also Chap. 233)   The presence of heart disease, as manifested by cardiac enlargement and gallop rhythm, together with evidence of cardiac failure, such as dyspnea, basilar rales, venous distention, and hepatomegaly, usually provides an indication on clinical examination that edema results from heart failure. Noninvasive tests such as echocardiography and radionuclide angiography may be helpful in establishing the diagnosis of heart failure.

EDEMA OF THE NEPHROTIC SYNDROME (See also Chap. 274)   Marked proteinuria (>3.5 g/d), severe hypoalbuminemia (<2 g/dL), and in some instances hypercholesterolemia are present. This syndrome may occur during the course of a variety of kidney diseases, which include glomerulonephritis, diabetic glomerulosclerosis, and hypersensitivity reactions. A history of previous renal disease may or may not be elicited.

EDEMA OF ACUTE GLOMERULONEPHRITIS AND OTHER FORMS OF RENAL FAILURE   The edema occurring during the acute phases of glomerulonephritis is characteristically associated with hematuria, proteinuria, and hypertension. Although some evidence supports the view that the fluid retention is due to increased capillary permeability, in most instances the edema in this disease results from primary retention of sodium and water by the kidneys owing to renal insufficiency. This state differs from congestive heart failure in that it is characterized by a normal (or sometimes even increased) cardiac output and a normal arterial–mixed venous oxygen difference. Patients with edema due to renal failure commonly have evidence of pulmonary congestion on chest roentgenograms before cardiac enlargement is significant, but they usually do not develop orthopnea. Patients with chronic impairment of renal function may also develop edema due to primary renal retention of sodium and water.

EDEMA OF CIRRHOSIS (See also Chap. 298)   Ascites and biochemical and clinical evidence of hepatic disease (collateral venous channels, jaundice, and spider angiomas) characterize edema of hepatic origin. The ascites is frequently refractory to treatment because it collects as a result of a combination of obstruction of hepatic lymphatic drainage, portal hypertension, and hypoalbuminemia. Edema may also occur in other parts of the body in these patients as a result of hypoalbuminemia. Furthermore, the sizable accumulation of ascitic fluid may increase intraabdominal pressure and impede venous return from the lower extremities; hence, it tends to promote accumulation of edema in this region as well.

EDEMA OF NUTRITIONAL ORIGIN   A diet grossly deficient in protein over a prolonged period may produce hypoproteinemia and edema. The latter may be intensified by the development of beriberi heart disease, also of nutritional origin, in which multiple peripheral arteriovenous fistulas result in reduced effective systemic perfusion and effective arterial blood volume, thereby enhancing edema formation. Edema may actually become intensified when these famished subjects are first provided with an adequate diet. The ingestion of more food may increase the quantity of salt ingested, which is then retained along with water. So-called "refeeding edema" may also be linked to increased release of insulin, which directly increases tubular sodium reabsorption. In addition to hypoalbuminemia, hypokalemia and caloric deficits may be involved in the edema of starvation.

OTHER CAUSES OF EDEMA   These include hypothyroidism, in which the edema (myxedema) may be located typically in the pretibial region and which may also be associated with periorbital puffiness. Exogenous hyperadrenocortism, pregnancy, and administration of estrogens and vasodilators, particularly the calcium antagonist nifedipine, may also all cause edema.

DISTRIBUTION OF EDEMA   The distribution of edema is an important guide to the cause. Thus, edema limited to one leg or to one or both arms is usually the result of venous and/or lymphatic obstruction. Edema resulting from hypoproteinemia characteristically is generalized, but it is especially evident in the very soft tissues of the eyelids and face and tends to be most pronounced in the morning because of the recumbent posture assumed during the night. Less common causes of facial edema include trichinosis, allergic reactions, and myxedema. Edema associated with heart failure, on the other hand, tends to be more extensive in the legs and to be accentuated in the evening, a feature also determined largely by posture. When patients with heart failure have been confined to bed, edema may be most prominent in the presacral region. Unilateral edema occasionally results from lesions in the central nervous system affecting the vasomotor fibers on one side of the body; paralysis also reduces lymphatic and venous drainage on the affected side.

ADDITIONAL FACTORS IN DIAGNOSIS   The color, thickness, and sensitivity of the skin are significant. Local tenderness and increase in temperature suggest inflammation. Local cyanosis may signify a venous obstruction. In individuals who have had repeated episodes of prolonged edema, the skin over the involved areas may be thickened, indurated, and often red.

Measurement or estimation of the venous pressure is of importance in evaluating edema. Elevation in an isolated part of the body usually reflects localized venous obstruction. Generalized elevation of systemic venous pressure usually indicates the presence of congestive heart failure. Ordinarily, significant increase in venous pressure can be recognized by the level at which cervical veins collapse (Chap. 227). In patients with obstruction of the superior vena cava, edema is confined to the face, neck, and upper extremities, where the venous pressure is elevated compared with that in the lower extremities. Measurement of venous pressure in the upper extremities is also useful in patients with massive edema of the lower extremities and ascites; it is elevated when the edema is on a cardiac basis (e.g., constrictive pericarditis or tricuspid stenosis) but is normal when it is secondary to cirrhosis. Severe heart failure may cause ascites that may be distinguished from the ascites caused by hepatic cirrhosis by the jugular venous pressure, which usually is elevated in heart failure and normal in cirrhosis.

Determination of the concentration of serum albumin aids importantly in identifying those patients in whom edema is due, at least in part, to diminished intravascular colloid oncotic pressure. The presence of proteinuria also affords useful clues. The absence of protein in the urine is evidence against renal disease as a cause of edema. Slight to moderate proteinuria is the rule in patients with heart failure, whereas persistent massive proteinuria is characteristic of the nephrotic syndrome.

—————— Approach to the Patient ——————

An important first question is whether the edema is localized or generalized. If it is localized, those phenomena that may be responsible should be concentrated upon. Hydrothorax and ascites are forms of localized edema. Either may be a consequence of local venous or lymphatic obstruction, as in inflammatory or neoplastic disease.

If the edema is generalized, it should be determined, first, if there is serious hypoalbuminemia, e.g., serum albumin <2.5 g/dL. If so, the history, physical examination, urinalysis, and other laboratory data will help evaluate the question of cirrhosis, severe malnutrition, protein-losing gastroenteropathy, or the nephrotic syndrome as the underlying disorder. If hypoalbuminemia is not present, it should be determined if there is evidence of congestive heart failure of a severity to promote generalized edema. Finally, it should be determined whether the patient has an adequate urine output, or if there is significant oliguria or even anuria. These abnormalities are discussed in Chaps. 47, 270, and 271.

BIBLIOGRAPHY

ANAND IS et al: Studies of body water and sodium, renal function, hemodynamic indexes, and plasma hormones in untreated congestive heart failure. Circulation 80:299, 1989

ELLISON DH: Diuretic drugs and the treatment of edema: From clinic to bench and back again. Am J Kidney Dis 23:623, 1994

GOLDEN MHN: Protein deficiency, energy deficiency, and the oedema of malnutrition. Lancet 1:1261, 1982

GOLDSMITH SR: Control of arginine vasopressin and congestive heart failure. Am J Cardiol 71:629, 1993

LEIER C, BOUDOULAS H: Renal disorders and heart disease, in *Heart Disease,* 5th ed, E Braunwald (ed). Philadelphia, Saunders, 1997, pp 1914–1938

MARTIN PY, SCHRIER RW: Renal sodium excretion and edematous disorders. Endocrinol Metab Clin North Am 24:459, 1995

MILLER JA et al: Control of extracellular fluid volume and the pathophysiology of edema formation, in *The Kidney*, 5th ed, BM Brenner (ed). Philadelphia, Saunders, 1996, pp 817–872

PELOSI AJ et al: The role of diuretics in the aetiology of idiopathic oedema. Q J Med 88:49, 1995

STREETEN DH: Idiopathic edema. Pathogenesis, clinical features, and treatment. Endocrinol Metab Clin North Am 24:531, 1995

STRUTHERS AD: Ten years of natriuretic peptide research: A new dawn for their diagnostic and therapeutic use? BMJ 308:1615, 1994

38	*Steven M. Hollenberg, Joseph E. Parrillo*

SHOCK

Shock is the state in which failure of the circulatory system to maintain adequate cellular perfusion results in widespread reduction in delivery of oxygen and other nutrients to tissues. Circulatory insufficiency causes cellular and then organ dysfunction, which may become irreversible unless corrected promptly. Shock is a syndrome defined by a constellation of clinical signs that may arise from any of several causes. At the onset, the physiologic alterations accompanying shock reflect the nature of the initiating event. As the syndrome progresses, however, a common pattern emerges resulting from the consequences of inadequate tissue perfusion.

CONTROL OF ARTERIAL BLOOD PRESSURE

Maintenance of adequate perfusion of vital organs is critical for survival. Organ perfusion is dependent on arterial pressure, which is determined by two factors: cardiac output and vascular resistance. Hence, organ perfusion can be compromised by a decrease in cardiac output or by maldistribution of cardiac output. Within an organ, distribution of blood flow depends on perfusion pressure, vascular resistance, and patency of nutritional microvessels. Maldistribution of flow can aggravate organ dysfunction. Because the initiating factor in shock is inadequate tissue perfusion, it is important to understand the critical determinants of tissue perfusion. These determinants can be divided into cardiac, vascular, humoral, and microcirculatory factors.

CARDIAC FACTORS   Cardiac output is the product of stroke volume and heart rate. Stroke volume, in turn, is determined by three factors: preload, afterload, and myocardial contractility (Chap. 232).

VASCULAR FACTORS   Resistance to the flow of blood in a vessel is proportional to vessel length and viscosity of blood and inversely proportional to the fourth power of the vessel radius. Therefore, the cross-sectional area of a vessel is by far the most important determinant of the resistance to flow. Since the major site of resistance in the systemic vasculature is at the arteriolar level, and vascular smooth-muscle tone regulates the radius of the resistance arterioles, arteriolar smooth-muscle tone is the most important determinant of vascular resistance.

Arteriolar tone is regulated by extrinsic factors, which include neural and hormonal regulation, and intrinsic or local factors, which include the myogenic response, metabolic autoregulation, and endothelial-mediated regulation. Resistance arterioles receive a tonic vasoconstrictor stimulus from sympathetic nerves innervating the vascular smooth muscle; sympathetic tone is largely regulated by arterial and cardiopulmonary baroreceptors. Adrenal stimulation results in release of epinephrine and norepinephrine into the systemic circulation. Blood vessels can contract or relax in response to changes in transmural pressure so as to maintain a constant blood flow with changes in perfusion pressure; this *myogenic response* serves to maintain a constant arterial wall tension, ensuring local autoregulation of flow. Metabolic regulation results from release of vasodilators that increase tissue blood flow in response to increased metabolic activity; the most important of these are adenosine and vasodilator prostaglandins. Microvascular vesels also relax in the presence of low oxygen tensions, also due to release of prostaglandins. Vascular endothelial cells secrete a number of substances with local actions, including endothelium-derived relaxing factor (nitric oxide) (Chap. 71); the molecules derived from arachidonic acid, collectively termed *eicosanoids*; the vasoconstrictor peptides endothelin-1 and angiotensin II; and oxygen free radicals. The actions of and interactions among these mediators are important components of regulation of the local environment by endothelial cells.

HUMORAL FACTORS Circulating humoral substances play important roles in cardiovascular homeostasis. In shock, release of circulating mediators such as renin, vasopressin, prostaglandins, kinins, atrial natriuretic factor, and catecholamines is mediated both by central nervous system activation and by cellular effects of ischemia, toxins, and immunologic mechanisms.

MICROCIRCULATORY FACTORS Because shock results from microcirculatory failure, the most critical aspects of the pathogenesis of shock take place in the microcirculation. Normal blood delivery to an organ as a whole does not necessarily indicate that perfusion of all segments of that organ is commensurate with regional metabolic demand. Adhesion of leukocytes and platelets to activated or damaged vascular endothelial cells can cause sludging and occlusion of microvessels; activation of the coagulation system with fibrin deposition and accumulation of microthrombi can contribute to microvascular occlusion. Shunting can occur as a result of perfusion of vessels with inadequate capillary exchange. Decreased deformability of erythrocytes can also contribute to decreased microcirculatory flow and capillary exchange.

Microvascular flow is influenced by the balance between colloid osmotic pressure and capillary hydrostatic pressure, which in turn determines the balan...

vomiting, diarrhea, burns, or dehydration. Hypovolemic shock is the most common type of shock seen clinically; it has been well studied, because all gradations of hypovolemia can be reproducibly induced in animal models.

CARDIOGENIC SHOCK Cardiogenic shock (see also Chap. 243) results from severe depression of cardiac performance. Hemodynamically, it is characterized by a systolic blood pressure <80 mmHg, cardiac index $<1.8(L/min)/m^2$, and left ventricular filling pressure >18 mmHg; pulmonary edema is usually present. The most frequent cause is myocardial infarction with loss of substantial muscle mass (usually 40 percent or more of the left ventricular myocardium). Extensive right ventricular infarction can also precipitate cardiogenic shock. Pump failure can also result from acute myocarditis or from depression of myocardial contractility following cardiac arrest or prolonged cardiopulmonary bypass.

Cardiogenic shock can be caused by mechanical abnormalities. Severe valvular stenosis can decrease stroke volume and cardiac output. Acute, massive mitral or aortic regurgitation leads to a reduction in forward cardiac output that may result in pulmonary edema and cardiogenic shock. Acutely acquired ventricular septal defects, which usually occur in the setting of acute myocardial infarction, can also cause cardiogenic shock by reducing forward flow.

EXTRACARDIAC OBSTRUCTIVE SHOCK This form of shock is best exemplified by pericardial tamponade (Chap. 240). Increased pericardial pressure impairs ventricular diastolic filling, decreasing preload, stroke volume, and cardiac output. Tension pneumothorax can also impair cardiac filling by decreasing venous return to the heart. Massive pulmonary embolism is another form of extracardiac obstructive shock, although the mechanism is different (Chap. 261). When more than 50 to 60 percent of the pulmonary vascular bed is obstructed by thrombus, acute right ventricular failure can occur, and left ventricular filling is impaired.

Table 38-1

Classification of Forms of Shock

CARDIOGENIC SHOCK

...ic
...myocardial infarction
...cardiomyopathy
...dial depression in septic shock
...l
...egurgitation
...lar septal defect
...lar aneurysm
...ntricular outflow track obstruction (aortic stenosis, hypertrophic ...yopathy)

...RDIAC OBSTRUCTIVE SHOCK

...tamponade
...embolism (massive)
...nonary hypertension (primary or Eisenmenger)

...MIC SHOCK

...n

...E SHOCK

...(drug overdose)

...k
...hock

...rom SM Hollenberg and JE Parrillo, in Surgical Intensive Care, GT ...Barie (eds), New York, Little, Brown, 1993.

DISTRIBUTIVE SHOCK Distributive shock is caused by profound peripheral vasodilation; although cardiac output may be normal or high, organ and tissue perfusion pressures are inadequate. The prototype of distributive shock is septic shock, which is the most common cause of death in intensive care units in the United States; the pathogenesis of septic shock is considered in detail below. Other types of distributive shock include anaphylaxis, neurogenic shock, and adrenal insufficiency.

In the clinical setting, patients may demonstrate elements of more than one type of shock simultaneously. For example, during septic shock, elements of distributive and hypovolemic shock can be complicated by myocardial impairment. Traumatic shock can also be complicated by elements of both hypovolemic and distributive shock. In a given patient, the nature of the circulatory disturbance may change with time and with therapy.

PATHOGENESIS

Cellular dysunction in shock is the final outcome of a process with multiple stimuli. In early shock, compensatory mechanisms are activated in an attempt to restore pressure and flow to vital organs. When these compensatory mechanisms begin to fail, impairment of tissue perfusion is manifested as organ dysfunction. Excessive and prolonged reduction of tissue perfusion leads to damage to cellular membranes, leakage of lysosomal enzymes, and reduction in cellular energy stores and may result in cell death. Once a sufficiently large number of cells from vital organs have reached this stage, shock can become irreversible, and death can occur despite correction of the underlying cause. This concept of irreversibility is useful because it emphasizes the need to prevent the progression of shock.

Cellular dysfunction in shock occurs through three main mechanisms: cellular ischemia, inflammatory mediators and free radical injury. With cellular hypoperfusion, oxygen depletion leads to anaerobic glycolysis, which produces only 2 ATP molecules during the breakdown of 1 glucose molecule as opposed to the 36 ATP molecules produced by aerobic glycolysis. This results in depletion of ATP and intracellular energy reserves. Anaerobic glycolysis also causes accumulation of lactic acid, with resultant intracellular acidosis. Failure of energy-dependent ion transport pumps decreases transmembrane potential, causing accumulation of intracellular sodium and water. Normal gradients of potassium, chloride, and calcium cannot be maintained. Intracellular accumulation of calcium further exacerbates mitochondrial dysfunction. Cellular membrane dysfunction is manifested by changes in cellular structure. Initial pathologic changes include enlargement of the endoplasmic reticulum and formation of blebs at the cellular surface; progression leads to mitochondrial condensation. Swelling of the mitochondria heralds irreversible cell injury. Terminal events include accumulation of denatured proteins and chromatin in the cytoplasm, lysosomal breakdown, and fracture of the mitochondria, nuclear envelope, and plasma membrane.

SEPTIC SHOCK Disruption of cellular metabolism by the effects of inflammatory mediators plays a dominant role in the pathogenesis of septic shock and may be important in other forms of shock as well. Prominent among these mediators are cytokines such as tumor necrosis factor (TNF), interleukin (IL) 1, IL-2, interferon γ, eicosanoids, and platelet activating factor (PAF). TNF activates inflammatory cells, stimulates release of other inflammatory cytokines, promotes the expression of adhesion molecules on both endothelial cells and neutrophils, activates coagulation pathways, decreases transmembrane potential, causes arteriolar vasodilation, increases microvascular permeability, and can directly block intracellular pathways, leading to cellular dysfunction. IL-1 has similar effects and can potentiate the effects of TNF. Interferon γ promotes release of TNF and IL-1 and may act synergistically with these cytokines to produce cytotoxic activity. PAF also promotes release of TNF and eicosanoids and markedly increases microvascular permeability.

Free radicals are reactive oxygen intermediates that react with a variety of other molecules—inactivating proteins, damaging DNA, and, most importantly, inducing lipid peroxidation in the membrane. Massive production of free radicals can occur after ischemia and subsequent reperfusion. In shock, cellular ischemia and intracellular calcium accumulation can activate intracellular proteases and convert the enzyme xanthine dehydrogenase, which recycles ATP, to xanthine oxidase, which oxidizes purines with the formation of the highly toxic superoxide radical. When oxygen is reintroduced suddenly, large amounts of superoxide can be produced, and the cell's endogenous antioxidant defense systems can be overwhelmed. Lipid peroxidation is a self-sustaining process that severely impairs membrane integrity.

GENE EXPRESSION IN SHOCK Recent studies have suggested two common programs of gene expression in response to stress: the acute-phase response and the heat-shock response. The acute-phase response to adverse stimuli is involved in maintaining *systemic* homeostasis; specific cell types express different genes. This response is identifiable clinically by accumulation in the plasma of proteins collectively known as *acute-phase reactants*, which are synthesized and secreted by the liver. The heat-shock response is a generic cellular response involved in maintaining *intracellular* homeostasis; the proteins synthesized act within cells and cannot be measured in blood. Some heat-shock proteins function as "molecular chaperones," which play a role in folding, stabilizing, and translocating newly synthesized proteins. Other heat-shock proteins appear to be involved in the genetic program of cell death known as *apoptosis*, a physiologic mechanism that normally functions to remove senescent cells. Although induction of heat-shock proteins has been shown to make cells more resistant to subsequent stress, evidence is accumulating to suggest that overexpression of these proteins may be deleterious in shock. Induction of the heat-shock response can preempt expression of both acute-phase and other genes important in synthetic function. This execution of a genetic program of cellular defense by individual cells may not be beneficial for the organism as a whole. In addition to preempting vital programs of gene expression, heat-shock protein induction may also initiate programmed cell death.

TRANSITION TO IRREVERSIBLE DAMAGE Understanding the transition from reversible cellular dysfunction to irreversible cellular damage is important to an understanding of the pathogenesis of shock. This is thought to occur due to a self-amplifying and self-sustaining inflammatory process. Ordinarily, activation of the inflammatory system engenders counterregulatory anti-inflammatory mechanisms. If the inflammatory stimulus is sufficiently severe or prolonged, however, cellular autocrine and paracrine responses can lead to the development of positive feedback loops. Activation of endothelial cells ordinarily leads to expression of adhesion molecules and release of chemotactic factors and proinflammatory cytokines. In shock, these processes are excessive and unregulated. Adherent neutrophils and macrophages, in turn, become overactivated and release large quantities of inflammatory mediators. Similar self-sustaining mechanisms can be seen after free radical injury, in which lipid peroxidation leads to initiation of a cycle of autooxidation. Finally, accumulated injuries within a cell can reach a threshold at which self-destruction occurs.

ORGAN DYSFUNCTION

The clinical presentation of shock varies because each organ system is affected differently, depending on the severity of the perfusion deficit, the underlying cause of shock, and prior organ dysfunction. If circulatory failure persists and sufficient cellular dysfunction occurs, dysfunction of multiple organ systems results. Multiple organ failure may be fatal, even without massive cell death, if cellular dysfunction is severe enough to interfere with organ function in a manner incompatible with life.

HEART Cardiac dysfunction is frequent during circulatory shock. In cardiogenic shock, this dysfunction usually results from myocardial infarction or ischemia. Myocardial dysfunction, in turn, can exacerbate myocardial ischemia, setting up a vicious cycle. The increased ventricular diastolic pressures that result from heart failure reduce the pressure gradient for coronary perfusion, and the additional wall stress elevates myocardial oxygen requirements. Tachycardia reduces the time available for diastolic filling, further compromising coronary blood flow. Ischemia also decreases diastolic compliance, further increasing ventricular diastolic pressures.

In other forms of shock, most notably sepsis, ischemia is less important; myocardial dysfunction is associated with release of circulating myocardial depressant substances. Pulmonary hypertension and increased right ventricular afterload can cause right sided heart failure after pulmonary embolism and may contribute to limitation of cardiac output in sepsis. Decreased myocardial responsiveness to catecholamines and diastolic dysfunction may also contribute to myocardial dysfunction in sepsis.

BRAIN Most patients with circulatory failure have abnormalities of mental status, usually manifested as confusion. The etiology is multifactorial; hypoperfusion, hypoxemia, acid-base abnormalities, and electrolyte disturbances all contribute. Cerebral autoregulation compensates to an extent for hypoperfusion, but when mean arterial pressure is <60 mmHg, compensation begins to fail, and critical cerebral hypoperfusion can lead to ischemic injury.

LUNGS Pulmonary dysfunction occurs early in shock. Acute lung injury causes decreased compliance, impaired gas exchange, and shunting of blood through unventilated areas. The clinical consequence of this injury, severe hypoxemia with bilateral pulmonary infiltrates in the setting of normal filling pressures, constitutes the acute respiratory distress syndrome (ARDS) (see Chap. 265). Work of breathing increases, with increased respiratory muscle oxygen requirements in the setting of tissue hypoperfusion. Respiratory muscle fatigue and ventilatory failure can ensue, requiring mechanical ventilation. The pathologic hallmarks of early ARDS are neutrophil-fibrin aggregates within the pulmonary microvasculature. With progression, there is extension of inflammation into the interstitium and alveoli and exudation of proteinaceous fluid into the alveolar space. Consolidation and fibrosis are seen in the end stages.

KIDNEYS Renal perfusion is compromised by circulatory failure, in part because blood flow is directed preferentially toward the heart and brain and away from the kidney. Increased afferent arteriolar tone initially compensates for decreased renal blood flow and maintains glomerular perfusion. When this compensatory mechanism fails, reduction in renal cortical blood flow can lead to acute tubular necrosis and renal failure. Associated insults such as nephrotoxic drugs, intravenous contrast medium, or rhabdomyolysis can exacerbate renal injury in shock.

LIVER AND GASTROINTESTINAL TRACT Hepatic injury results from hypoperfusion, often complicated in septic and traumatic shock by activation of Kuppfer cells and release of cytokines. Derangements of metabolic function of the liver include impairment of both synthesis and detoxification. Phagocytic clearance within the hepatic reticuloendothelial system is also impaired. Increased serum levels of transaminases, lactic dehydrogenase, and bilirubin reflect hepatic parenchymal injury. Decreased levels of albumin and clotting factors indicate decreased synthetic capability. Dramatic increases in transaminases can be seen with profound hypoxemia or hypotension ("shock liver"); these are transient and resolve rapidly with reperfusion. Ischemic liver injury affects the center of the hepatic lobule (venous end) most prominently, with relative sparing of the portal (arterial) end; this is seen pathologically as central congestion and centrilobular necrosis. In septic shock, intrahepatic cholestasis can be present, with marked increases in bilirubin and only modest increases in transaminases; these changes may reflect dysfunction of bile canaliculi due to bacterial toxins.

Splanchnic blood flow is compromised in circulatory shock as blood flow is diverted elsewhere. Intestinal ischemia may occur, and injury may be further exacerbated by subsequent release of oxygen radicals during reperfusion following resuscitation. It has been hypothesized that ischemia/reperfusion injury may compromise the integrity of the intestinal mucosal barrier, leading to translocation of bacterial toxins, although this has not been demonstrated conclusively in patients. Splanchnic hypoperfusion can also lead to stress ulceration,

ileus, and malabsorption, and occasionally acalculous cholecystitis or pancreatitis may occur.

HEMATOLOGIC SYSTEM Abnormalities of coagulation are frequent in both septic and traumatic shock. Thrombocytopenia can result from hemodilution associated with volume repletion. Thrombocytopenia in sepsis is common, usually immunologically mediated, and often complicated by underlying illness and medications. Activation of the coagulation cascade within the microvasculature can lead to disseminated intravascular coagulation (Chap. 118), which leads to thrombocytopenia, microangiopathic hemolytic anemia, decreased fibrinogen, and circulating fibrin split products. Microvascular consumption of clotting factors can lead to their depletion, with subsequent hemorrhage.

PATHOGENESIS OF SPECIFIC FORMS OF SHOCK

The pathogenesis of different forms of shock is shown in Fig. 38-1. In hypovolemic, cardiogenic, and extracardiac obstructive shock, decreased tissue perfusion results from inadequate cardiac output. In distributive shock, decreased arterial pressure results from decreased systemic vascular resistance, and maldistribution of blood flow in the microcirculation is a major contributing factor to multiple organ system failure.

HYPOVOLEMIC SHOCK Hypovolemic shock has been studied extensively and its stages can be easily quantitated in experimental animals by the stepwise removal of blood from the intravascular space. Many of the lessons learned from these studies are applicable to other forms of shock with reduced cardiac output. With the loss of 10 percent of total blood volume, compensatory mechanisms are activated that maintain cardiac output despite decreased filling pressure and stroke volume. Increased adrenergic activity, resulting from both increased sympathetic discharge and adrenal release of catecholamines, leads to arterial vasoconstriction, venoconstriction with augmented venous return, and tachycardia. Reduction in hydrostatic pressure in the capillaries, along with precapillary arteriolar vasoconstriction, favors transudation of fluid from the extracellular space into the vessels. Intravas-

FIGURE 38-1 Pathogenesis of shock in humans. This schematic diagram depicts the present understanding of the pathogenetic relationships among the different types of shock and the cardiovascular abnormalities they usually produce.

cular volume contraction leads to activation of the renin-angiotensin system, increased release of antidiuretic hormone, and elevated levels of ACTH and aldosterone; renal sodium and water retention ensue. These adaptations may be sufficient to maintain arterial pressure, and orthostatic hypotension may be the only sign of early hypovolemia. However, if 20 to 25 percent of the blood volume is lost rapidly, the compensatory mechanisms begin to fail and the clinical shock syndrome ensues. Cardiac output declines, and there is hypotension despite generalized vasoconstriction. Reduced tissue perfusion leads to anaerobic metabolism, manifested by elevated lactate levels and metabolic acidosis. Reflex adrenergic discharge is intensified, and flow is redistributed to maintain perfusion to the brain and heart. This redistribution reflects the predominance of autoregulation of blood flow in the cerebral and coronary systems in contrast to the dependence of flow in other organs on sympathetic tone. Excessive vasoconstriction can reduce flow to the point that cellular damage occurs. Damage to the capillary endothelium leads to loss of fluid and proteins from the circulation, further exacerbating the hypovolemia. Ultimately end-organ damage and multiple organ system failure ensue.

CARDIOGENIC SHOCK (See also Chap. 243)   When myocardial function is depressed, several compensatory mechanisms are activated. Sympathetic stimulation increases heart rate and contractility, and renal fluid retention increases preload. If cardiac output cannot be maintained by these mechanisms, blood flow is redistributed to maintain cerebral and cardiac perfusion. In a failing heart, the compensatory mechanisms may ultimately become dysfunctional. Increased heart rate and contractility can raise myocardial oxygen demand and exacerbate ischemia. In addition, tachycardia decreases diastolic filling time, further compromising myocardial perfusion. Fluid retention may increase intravascular volume to the point where pulmonary congestion and hypoxemia occur. Ischemia also decreases ventricular diastolic compliance, further elevating left atrial pressures and worsening pulmonary congestion. Vasoconstriction to maintain blood pressure can compromise renal, splanchnic, and cutaneous perfusion. The increased systemic vascular resistance caused by this vasoconstriction increases myocardial afterload, further impairing cardiac performance and increasing myocardial oxygen demand. This increased demand, in the face of inadequate perfusion, leads to worsening ischemia and a vicious cycle that must be interrupted to prevent a downward spiral leading inexorably to the patient's demise.

PERICARDIAL TAMPONADE (See also Chap. 240)   Pericardial tamponade results from accumulation of fluid in the pericardium with resultant increases in intrapericardial pressure. This may be acute (e.g., hemopericardium associated with penetrating or closed chest trauma) or subacute (e.g., uremia, radiation, neoplasm, infection, or connective tissue disease). Tamponade can develop after cardiac surgery because of compression of the heart by a mediastinal hematoma or postpericardiotomy syndrome. The increase in pericardial pressure and consequent impairment of cardiac filling from a pericardial effusion depend on the rate of fluid accumulation, the volume of fluid, and the distensibility of the pericardium. As intrapericardial pressure increases, the gradient between peripheral venous and right atrial pressure is reduced and diastolic filling is compromised. When pericardial pressure impairs diastolic filling acutely, adrenergic stimulation leads to tachycardia, increased ejection fraction, and arterial vasoconstriction to maintain arterial pressure. Over a period of hours to days, fluid retention brings about elevated venous pressure, which enhances filling. Subacute, compensated tamponade presents with signs of systemic venous congestion with distended neck veins. Failure of compensation leads to shock, with tachycardia, tachypnea, low cardiac output, peripheral vasoconstriction, and hypotension.

DISTRIBUTIVE SHOCK   In this condition, tissue hypoperfusion results from abnormal shunting of a normal or increased cardiac output. Although the differential diagnosis includes anaphylaxis, drug overdose, neurogenic shock, and Addisonian crisis, the most important and prevalent etiology is septic shock (Chap. 124). In some forms of

distributive shock, organ blood flow appears adequate, but a mediator-induced "metabolic block" exists at the tissue level, preventing adequate utilization of oxygen and other nutrients. Lactate accumulates because cells are unable to use oxidative metabolic pathways normally. Thus, in some patients, blood flow through large vessels to tissues is adequate, but abnormalities of microvascular flow or an inability of cells to utilize nutrients leads to widespread cellular dysfunction and progressive shock.

Septic shock results when infectious agents or infection-induced mediators in the bloodstream induce cardiovascular decompensation. Septic shock is characterized at the onset by a high cardiac output and a low systemic vascular resistance. As shown in Fig. 38-2, septic shock usually begins with a nidus of infection that releases microorganisms into the bloodstream. Toxic effects can result from the organisms

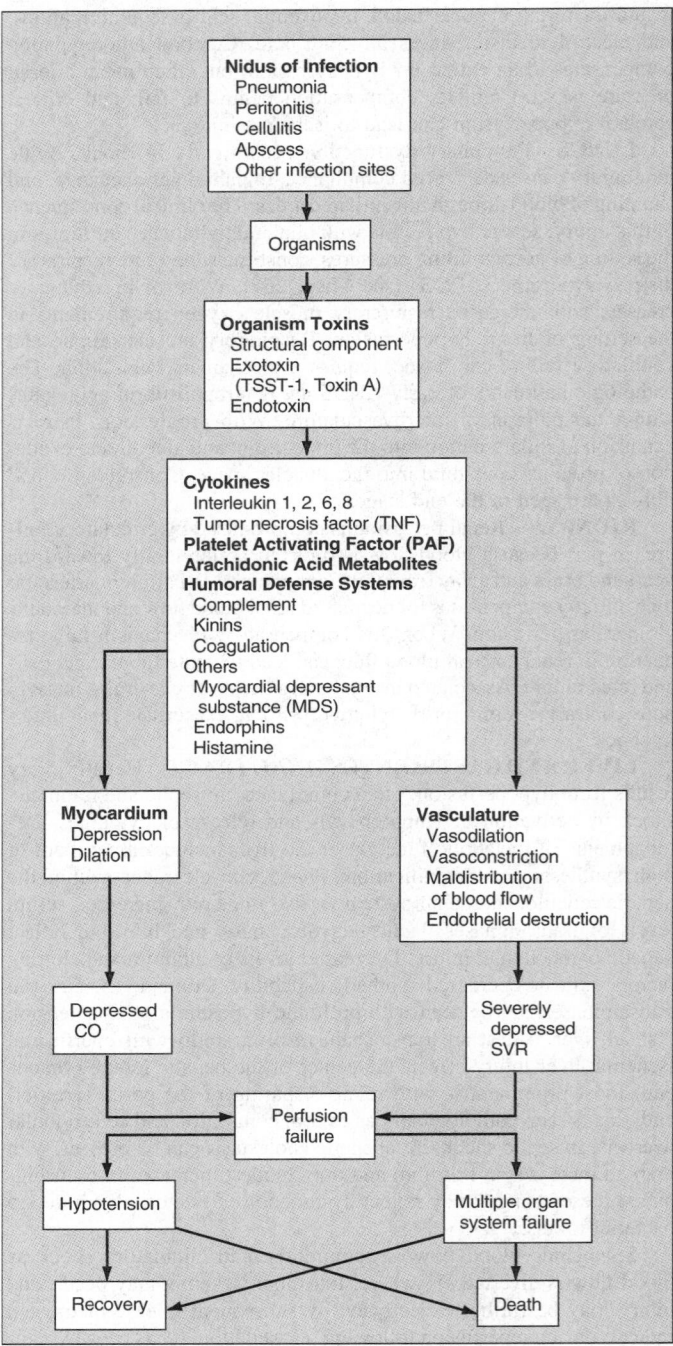

FIGURE 38-2 Pathogenesis of human septic shock. This schematic diagram represents the present understanding of the interrelationships in the pathogenesis of septic shock in humans. CO, cardiac output; SVR, systemic vascular resistance. (*Modified from Parrillo et al, 1990.*)

themselves; from components such as endotoxin, the lipopolysaccharide associated with the outer membrane of gram-negative bacteria; or from elaboration of exotoxins. The most important pathologic effects of these organisms and toxins may result from stimulation of the release of massive quantities of endogenous inflammatory mediators. Endotoxin is a potent trigger for release of cytokines, most notably the interleukins and TNF, which amplify the systemic response to endotoxin by stimulating neutrophils, endothelial cells, and platelets and by causing the release of other mediators, such as PAF, arachidonic acid metabolites, complement, kinins, histamine, and endorphins.

The effects of these mediators can be divided into two broad categories: effects on the peripheral vasculature and effects on the heart. Both exogenous and endogenous mediators have been shown to mediate peripheral vasodilation in sepsis. Administration of small doses of endotoxin to normal volunteers causes a decrease in arterial pressure, an increase in cardiac output, and a decrease in systemic vascular resistance similar to those seen in sepsis. Similar vasodilation with increased cardiac output occurs after administration of TNF, IL-1, or IL-2. A pivotal mediator of vasodilation in response to cytokines is nitric oxide, which is formed from arginine by the enzyme nitric oxide synthase (Chap. 71). Endotoxin, TNF, and interleukins can stimulate inducible nitric oxide synthase in macrophages and vascular smooth muscle cells, with release of large amounts of this vasodilatory molecule.

Endotoxin can also activate the intrinsic coagulation cascade along with the fibrinolytic system; this can lead to deposition of fibrin microaggregates in the microvasculature, obstructing flow and exacerbating tissue hypoxia. TNF and the interleukins activate both endothelial cells and neutrophils, leading to neutrophil aggregation and further microcirculatory insufficiency.

Although patients with septic shock have high cardiac outputs, left and right ventricular ejection fractions are reduced. Dilation of the ventricles allows normal stroke volumes to be maintained despite the depression of myocardial contractility, and tachycardia results in an elevated cardiac output. Septic patients also manifest a decreased ventricular stroke work response to volume infusion, further indicating depressed myocardial performance. The mechanisms responsible have not been completely clarified; it appears that cytokines, particularly TNF and IL-1, play an important role, possibly through generation of nitric oxide.

If septic shock persists, the combination of peripheral vascular abnormalities and myocardial depression results in a mortality of approximately 50 percent (Fig. 38-2). Death results from unrelenting hypotension and/or multiple organ system failure. The hypotension is associated with a severe and irreversible reduction in systemic vascular resistance. Occasionally (in about 10 percent of nonsurvivors) myocardial depression is so severe that cardiac output becomes low, exacerbating the hypotension.

CLINICAL MANIFESTATIONS

Some symptoms and signs are similar for all types of shock. The condition is almost always characterized by hypotension, which in adults generally refers to a mean arterial pressure below 60 mmHg. In interpreting any given level of arterial pressure, however, the chronic level of pressure must be considered; patients with severe chronic hypertension may be relatively hypotensive when their mean arterial pressure declines by 40 mmHg, even if it still exceeds 60 mmHg. Conversely, patients with chronically low arterial pressures may not exhibit clinical abnormalities until mean pressure falls below 50 mmHg. Common manifestations of shock include tachycardia, oliguria, a clouded sensorium, and cool, mottled extremities indicative of reduced blood flow to the skin. Metabolic acidosis, often due to elevated blood lactate levels, reflects prolonged inadequate blood flow to tissues.

Other clinical manifestations are specific to the type of shock. Patients with hypovolemic shock frequently have a history of gastrointestinal bleeding, hemorrhage from another site, or clear evidence of large volume losses via diarrhea and/or vomiting. Patients with

cardiogenic shock usually have symptoms and signs of heart disease, including elevated filling pressures, gallop rhythms, and other evidence of heart failure. Mechanical causes of cardiogenic shock frequently cause heart murmurs, such as those of mitral regurgitation, aortic stenosis, or ventricular septal defect. Patients with pericardial tamponade may demonstrate pulsus paradoxus and distant heart sounds. In patients with distributive shock due to sepsis, there may be evidence of localized infection as well as fever and chills. Patients with sepsis and neutropenia are less likely to have a clinically evident nidus of infection and may be septic from their own skin or bowel flora.

Approach to the Patient

Shock is an emergency. Optimal management entails balancing the need to initiate therapy before shock causes irreversible damage to vital organs against the need to perform the clinical assessment required to understand the cause of shock and target therapy to that cause. A practical approach is to make a rapid evaluation initially, based on a limited history and physical examination, and initiate specific diagnostic procedures directed toward determining the cause and severity of shock. Initial tests ordinarily include a chest x-ray, electrocardiogram, measurement of arterial blood gas and electrolyte levels, a complete blood count, and other tests directed as specific questions raised by the initial examination. Right heart catheterization with a balloon-tipped, flow-directed (Swan-Ganz) catheter is frequently useful. As this initial evaluation is in progress, therapy should be initiated. After stabilization, a more comprehensive diagnostic evaluation should be undertaken, and the response to the initial therapeutic interventions should be assessed.

USE OF RIGHT HEART CATHETERIZATION TO EVALUATE SHOCK
The different categories of shock (see Table 38-1) have different hemodynamic profiles (Table 38-2). Patients with mild hypovolemic shock may be treated successfully with simple fluid replacement. In patients with moderate or severe shock, however, right heart catheterization is often useful, not only for providing a diagnostic hemodynamic assessment but also for monitoring the response to therapy, because noninvasive evaluation is frequently incorrect in estimating filling pressures and cardiac output.

Table 38-2 summarizes the usual findings at right heart catheterization in patients with different forms of shock. Individual patients may present with hemodynamic features of more than one type of shock, but when these profiles are combined with clinical findings and the calculation of systemic vascular resistance, the etiology of most cases of shock can be categorized.

 TREATMENT

General Principles Whenever possible, patients should be treated in an intensive care unit. Continuous electrocardiographic monitoring should be performed for detection of rhythm disturbances, and an arterial line should be in place for beat-to-beat measurement of arterial pressures. Pulse oximetry is often useful to detect fluctuations in arterial oxygenation. In most case of shock that cannot be reversed rapidly, serial measurements of left and right ventricular filling pressures and cardiac output should be performed. Frequent measurements of arterial blood gases, serum electrolytes, complete blood counts, and coagulation parameters should be done to follow the patient's progress and to monitor the effects of therapy. Serum calcium, phosphorus and magnesium levels should be checked as well, because substantial reductions in these ions can be associated with depression of myocardial and respiratory muscle function. The frequency of measurements should be based on the clinical course and the perceived need to assess responses to therapy.

Guidelines for managing shock are listed in Table 38-3. In general, the goals of treating shock are to maintain mean arterial pressure and to ensure adequate perfusion and delivery of oxygen and other nutrients to the vital organs. Tissue hypoperfusion and

Table 38-2

Use of Right Heart Catheterization to Diagnose the Etiology of Shock

Diagnosis	Pulmonary Capillary Wedge Pressure	Cardiac output (CO)	Miscellaneous Comments
Cardiogenic shock			
Cardiogenic shock due to myocardial dysfunction	↑↑	↓↓	Usually occurs with evidence of extensive myocardial infarction (>40% of LV infarcted), severe cardiomyopathy, or myocarditis
Cardiogenic shock due to a mechanical defect			
Acute ventricular septal defect	↑	LVCO ↓↓ and RVCO > LVCO	Predominant shunt is left to right, pulmonary blood flow is greater than systemic blood flow: oxygen "step-up" occurs at RV level
Acute mitral regurgitation	↑↑	Forward CO ↓↓	V waves in pulmonary capillary wedge pressure tracing
Right ventricular infarction	Normal or ↓	↓↓	Elevated RA and RV filling pressures with low or normal pulmonary capillary wedge pressures
Extracardiac obstructive forms of shock			
Pericardial tamponade	↑	↓ or ↓↓	RA mean, RV end-diastolic pulmonary capillary wedge mean pressures are elevated and within 5 mmHg of one another
Massive pulmonary embolism	Normal or ↓	↓↓	Usual finding is elevated right-sided pressures
Hypovolemic shock	↓↓	↓↓	
Distributive forms of shock			
Septic shock	↓ or normal	↑ or normal, rarely ↓	
Anaphylactic shock	↓ or normal	↑ or normal	

↑↑ or ↓↓ designates a moderate to severe increase or decrease: ↑ or ↓ designates a mild to moderate increase or decrease; CO, cardiac output; RA, right atrium; RV, right ventricle; LV, left vetricle.

NOTE: Systemic vascular resistance is increased, initially, in all forms of shock except distributive shock, in which it is usually reduced.

SOURCE: Modified from SM Hollenberg and JE Parrillo, in Surgical Intensive Care, GT Shires, PL Barie (eds), New York, Little, Brown, 1993.

anaerobic metabolism can lead to formation and release of lactic acid into the bloodstream. A reduction of elevated serum lactate levels is one good indicator of successful resuscitation and is often used as a therapeutic goal. In addition to these general goals, specific forms of shock require therapy directed at the underlying processes.

Hypovolemic Shock Infusion of fluid is the fundamental treatment of acute hypovolemia. The challenge is to restore cardiac filling pressures to optimum levels promptly and adequately without inducing pulmonary edema and compromising oxygenation. A major increase in pulmonary microvascular pressure is the most important determinant of transudation of fluid into the pulmonary interstitium. The clinical implication of this observation is that monitoring of pulmonary hydrostatic pressure, by physical examination or measured hemodynamics, is critical during resuscitation. Regardless of the type and amount of fluid used for resuscitation, it is imperative to use physiologic endpoints to gauge the initial response to treatment and to adjust the therapy to meet the needs of the individual patient.

Crystalloids, either normal saline or Ringer's lactate, are usually used for initial resuscitation for most forms of hypovolemic shock. After the initial resuscitation, with up to several liters of crystalloid

Table 38-3

Guidelines for Managing Shock

Abnormality	Intervention*	Therapeutic Goal
Hypotension	ICU monitoring, volume expansion, vasopressor agents	Mean arterial pressure of at least 60 mmHg Pulmonary capillary wedge pressure between 14 and 18 mmHg
Tissue hypoperfusion	ICU monitoring, volume expansion, vasopressor agents, inotropic agents	Hemoglobin above 10 g/dL Oxygen saturation above 92% Cardiac index above 2.2(L/min)/m² Normal blood lactate concentration

Organ system dysfunction	ICU monitoring, volume expansion, vasopressors, inotropic agents	Normalize values or otherwise reverse evidence of dysfunction in the following systems:
		  Renal—blood urea nitrogen and creatinine levels, urine output
		  Hepatic—bilirubin level
		  Pulmonary—arterial P_{O_2} and alveolar-arterial gradient
		  Central nervous system—mental status

Infection	Appropriate antibiotics and surgical drainage, if necessary	Eradication of infection
Mediators producing toxic effects	Mediator inhibition†	Reversal of toxic effect

* ICU denotes intensive care unit.
† This therapy is still in the experimental phase.
SOURCE: Adapted from Parrillo, 1993

fluid, use of colloids, such as albumin or starch solutions, has been advocated as a more efficient and rapid method of fluid repletion that can help maintain colloid osmotic pressure. However, colloids are expensive, and despite numerous studies, a convincing benefit has not been demonstrated from administration of colloids rather than crystalloids for fluid repletion. Preliminary studies with hypertonic saline solutions suggest that effective resuscitation can be achieved using relatively small volumes of fluid; in some settings, such as burn resuscitation, such limitation of the volume of fluid administered may be important. In hemorrhagic shock, restoration of oxygen-carrying capacity is achieved through transfusion of packed red blood cells; the goal is to maintain a hemoglobin concentration of 10 g/dL.

Cardiogenic Shock In cardiogenic shock due to myocardial infarction (see also Chap. 243), therapy should be directed toward reducing myocardial ischemia and salvaging ischemic but reversibly damaged myocardium at the infarct border. Initial measures include supplemental oxygen and, when systolic blood pressure permits, administration of intravenous nitroglycerin. Insertion of an intraaortic balloon pump decreases ventricular afterload, improving myocardial performance and decreasing myocardial oxygen demand and improving coronary perfusion pressure by increasing aortic diastolic pressure. The possibility of acute mechanical abnormalities such as mitral regurgitation or ventricular septal defect should be excluded, with either echocardiography or right heart catheterization. Where possible, it is probably best to perform emergent coronary angiography to define the coronary anatomy and to attempt revascularization. Trials of revascularization with either angioplasty or bypass surgery for patients with cardiogenic shock have suggested improved survival compared to historical controls. Administration of thrombolytic agents is another alternative, although a mortality benefit for patients who present with myocardial infarction and cardiogenic shock has not been demonstrated in clinical trials.

Cardiogenic shock can also occur after prolonged cardiopulmonary bypass; the stunned myocardium may require hours or days to recover sufficiently to support the circulation. Treatment consists of cardiovascular support with the combination of inotropic agents such as dopamine, dobutamine, or amrinone and intraaortic balloon counterpulsation. Dopamine, which acts directly on myocardial beta$_1$-adrenergic receptors and indirectly by releasing norepinephrine, has both inotropic and vasopressor effects. Tachycardia and increased peripheral resistance with dopamine administration can potentially exacerbate myocardial ischemia. Dobutamine, a selective beta$_1$-adrenergic receptor agonist, can improve myocardial contractility and increase cardiac output without inducing marked changes in heart rate or systemic vascular resistance. Amrinone and milrinone are phosphodiesterase inhibitors with both positive inotropic and vasodilator actions. Amrinone and milrinone have longer half-lives than dobutamine and can cause hypotension, so they are often reserved for use when other agents have proven ineffective. Because they do not act directly through adrenergic receptors, they may be effective in situations in which beta-adrenergic receptors are diminished. The addition of amrinone or milrinone to dopamine or

dobutamine may be considered in patients who fail to respond to one class of agents alone.

Extracardiac Obstructive Shock Pericardial tamponade (Chap. 240) is the prototype of extracardiac obstructive shock and may be recognized by clinical manifestations (hypotension, jugular venous distention, pulsus paradoxus) and characteristic findings on echocardiography. Although intravascular volume expansion and sometimes vasopressor agents are useful temporizing measures, the only effective therapy is pericardial drainage via needle pericardiocentesis or surgery.

Pulmonary embolism (Chap. 261) is usually treated with systemic anticoagulation, but when massive pulmonary embolism causes right ventricular failure and shock, thrombolytic therapy should be strongly considered. In patients with contraindications to thrombolytic therapy, emergency surgical pulmonary embolectomy is an alternative, if there is sufficient time to make the diagnosis, mobilize the surgical team, and institute cardiopulmonary bypass.

Septic Shock (See also Chap. 124) Therapy of septic shock has three main components. First, the nidus of infection must be identified and eliminated, using surgical drainage, antibiotic therapy, or both. Rapid institution of appropriate antibiotic therapy leads to improved survival, but the specific organisms causing sepsis are usually not known when the patient presents. Accordingly, a broad-spectrum antibiotic regimen should be chosen initially that will be effective against all the likely causative microorganisms, given the patient's clinical presentation and the hospital's organism resistance patterns.

Second, while the source of sepsis is being eradicated, adequate organ system perfusion and function must be maintained, guided by cardiovascular monitoring. Since antibiotics usually require 48 h or more to sterilize a septic focus, maintenance of tissue oxygen delivery is crucial to a favorable outcome (Table 38-3). Since oxygen delivery is the product of blood hemoglobin concentration, oxygen saturation, and cardiac output, maintenance of a blood hemoglobin level greater than 10 g/dL, oxygen saturation higher than 92%, and adequate cardiac output are important therapeutic guidelines. Initial cardiovascular therapy should optimize preload by administering volume to attain a pulmonary artery wedge pressure of 14 to 18 mmHg. If the serum albumin level is low (<2 g/dL), concentrated albumin infusions may be used to increase intravascular oncotic pressure. Since tissue hypoperfusion in sepsis results in part from abnormal shunting of cardiac output, some clinicians advocate increasing cardiac output to very high, supranormal levels. However, use of inotropic agents to achieve such supranormal cardiac outputs has not been shown to be beneficial in controlled trials.

If fluid therapy alone fails to restore adequate arterial pressure and organ perfusion, therapy with vasopressor agents should be initiated (Table 38-4). For the persistently hypotensive patient, dopamine (Chap. 70) frequently raises arterial pressure and maintains or enhances blood flow to the renal and splanchnic circulations. Patients

Table 38-4

Commonly Used Vasopressor Agents (Relative Potency*)

Agent	Dose	Cardiac		Peripheral Vascular		
		Heart Rate	Contractility	Vasoconstriction	Vasodilation	Dopaminergic
Dopamine	1–4 (μ/kg)/min	1+	1+	0	1+	4+
	4–20 (μg/kg)/min	2+	2–3+	2–3+	0	2+
Norepinephrine	2–20 μg/min	1+	2+	4+	0	0
Dobutamine	2.5–15 (μg/kg)/min	1–2+	3–4+	0	2+	0
Isoproterenol	1–5 μg/min	4+	4+	0	4+	0
Epinephrine	1–20 μg/min	4+	4+	4+	3+	0
Phenylephrine	20–200 μg/min	0	0	3+	0	0

* The 1 to 4+ scoring system is an arbitrary system to allow a judgment of comparative potency among these vasopressor agents.
SOURCE: Adapted from JE Parrillo, Major Issues in Critical Care Medicine, JE Parrillo, SM Ayres (eds), Baltimore, Williams & Wilkins, 1984.

who remain hypotensive despite dopamine require norepinephrine, a more potent vasopressor. Once hypotension has been corrected, to optimize oxygen delivery to tissues, raising a low cardiac index with dobutamine can be useful.

The third therapeutic goal is to interrupt the pathogenic sequence leading to septic shock. Several multicenter trials have documented that early glucocorticoid therapy fails to improve either morbidity or mortality in septic shock. Newer therapies have focused on inhibiting potentially toxic mediators such as endotoxin, TNF, and IL-1. Trials of inhibitors of the mediators of sepsis, which include anti-endotoxin antibodies, anti-TNF antibodies, IL-1 receptor antagonists, and soluble TNF receptors, have not shown a significant reduction in mortality in septic patients to date. → *For further discussion, see also Chap. 124.*

BIBLIOGRAPHY

BUCHMAN TG et al: Molecular biology of circulatory shock. Part II. Expression of four groups of hepatic genes is enhanced after resuscitation from cardiogenic shock. Surgery 108:559, 1990

CIPOLLE MD et al: Secondary organ dysfunction. From clinical perspectives to molecular markers. Crit Care Clin 9:261, 1993

GATTINONI L et al: A trial of goal-oriented hemodynamic therapy in critically ill patients. N Engl J Med 333:1025, 1995

GOULD SA et al: Hypovolemic shock. Crit Care Clin 9:239, 1993

GUYTON AC: Cardiac output and circulatory shock, in *Human Physiology and Mechanisms of Disease*, 5th ed. Philadelphia, Saunders, 1991, pp 187–200

HOLLENBERG SM, CUNNIN RE: Endothelial and vascular smooth muscle function in sepsis. J Crit Care 9:262, 1994

MARTIN C et al: Norepinephrine or dopamine for the treatment of hyperdynamic septic shock. Chest 103:1826, 1993

MIMOZ O et al: Pulmonary artery catheterization in critically ill patients: A prospective analysis of outcome changes associated with catheter-prompted changes in therapy. Crit Care Med 22:573, 1994

PARRILLO JE: Pathogenetic mechanisms of septic shock. N Engl J Med 328:1471, 1993

———— et al: Septic shock in humans: Advances in the understanding of pathogenesis, cardiovascular dysfunction, and therapy. Ann Intern Med 113:227, 1990

SUFFREDINI AF: Current prospects for the treatment of clinical sepsis. Crit Care Med 22:S12, 1994

39 Robert J. Myerburg, Agustin Castellanos

CARDIOVASCULAR COLLAPSE, CARDIAC ARREST, AND SUDDEN CARDIAC DEATH

OVERVIEW AND DEFINITIONS

The vast majority of naturally occurring sudden deaths are caused by cardiac disorders. The magnitude of the problem of *cardiac* causes is highlighted by estimates that more than 300,000 sudden cardiac deaths (SCD) occur each year in the United States, as many as 50 percent of all cardiac deaths. SCD is a direct consequence of cardiac arrest, which is often reversible if responded to promptly. Since resuscitation techniques and emergency rescue systems are available to save patients who have out-of-hospital cardiac arrest, which was uniformly fatal in the past, understanding the SCD problem has practical importance.

SCD must be defined carefully. In the context of time, "sudden" is defined, for most clinical and epidemiologic purposes, as 1 h or less between the onset of the terminal clinical event and death. An exception is unwitnessed deaths in which pathologists may expand the definition of time to 24 h after the victim was last seen to be alive and stable.

Because of community-based interventions, victims may remain biologically alive for days or weeks after a cardiac arrest that has resulted in irreversible central nervous system damage. Confusion in terms can be avoided by adhering strictly to definitions of death, cardiac arrest, and cardiovascular collapse, as outlined in Table 39-1. Death is biologically, legally, and literally an absolute and irreversible event. Death may be delayed in a survivor of cardiac arrest, but "survival after sudden death" is contradictory. Currently, the accepted definition of SCD is *natural death due to cardiac causes*, heralded by abrupt loss of consciousness within *1 h* of the onset of acute symptoms, in an individual who may have known *preexisting* heart disease but in whom the *time* and *mode* of death are *unexpected*. When biologic death of the cardiac arrest victim is delayed because of interventions, the relevant pathophysiologic event remains the sudden and unexpected cardiac arrest that leads ultimately to death, even though delayed by artificial methods. The language used should reflect the fact that the index event was a cardiac arrest and that death was due to its delayed consequences.

ETIOLOGY, INITIATING EVENTS, AND CLINICAL EPIDEMIOLOGY

Extensive epidemiologic studies have identified populations at high risk for SCD. In addition, a large body of pathologic data provides information on the underlying *structural abnormalities* in victims of SCD, and clinical/physiologic studies have begun to identify a group of *transient functional factors* that may convert a long-standing underlying structural abnormality from a stable to an unstable state (Table 39-2). This information is developing into an understanding of the causes and mechanisms of SCD.

Cardiac disorders constitute the most common causes of sudden *natural* death. After an initial peak incidence of sudden death between birth and 6 months of age (the sudden infant death syndrome), the incidence of sudden death declines sharply and remains low through childhood and adolescence. The incidence begins to increase in young adults, reaching a second peak in the age range of 45 to 75 years. Increasing age in this range is a powerful risk factor for sudden *cardiac* death, and the proportion of cardiac causes among all sudden natural deaths increases dramatically with advancing years. From 1 to 13 years of age, only one of five sudden *natural* deaths is due to cardiac causes. Between 14 and 21 years of age, the proportion increases to 30 percent, and then to 88 percent in the middle-aged and elderly.

Young and middle-aged men and women have very different susceptibilities to SCD, but the gender differences decrease with advanc-

Table 39-1

Distinction Between Death, Cardiac Arrest, and Cardiovascular Collapse

Term	Definition	Qualifiers or Exceptions
Death	Irreversible cessation of all biologic functions	None
Cardiac arrest	Abrupt cessation of cardiac pump function which may be reversible by a prompt intervention but will lead to death in its absence	Rare spontaneous reversions; likelihood of successful interventions relates to mechanism of arrest and clinical setting
Cardiovascular collapse	A sudden loss of effective blood flow due to cardiac and/or peripheral vascular factors which may reverse spontaneously (e.g., neurocardiogenic syncope; vasovagal syncope) or only with interventions (e.g., cardiac arrest)	Nonspecific term which includes cardiac arrest and its consequences and also events which characteristically revert spontaneously

ing age. The overall male/female ratio is approximately 4:1, but in
the 45- to 64-year-old age group, the male SCD excess is nearly 7:1.
It falls to approximately 2:1 in the 65- to 74-year-old age group. The
difference in risk for SCD parallels the risks for other manifestations
of coronary heart disease in men and women. As the gap for other
manifestations of coronary heart disease closes in the seventh and
eighth decades of life, the excess risk of SCD also narrows. Despite
the lower incidence in women, the classic coronary risk factors still
operate in women—cigarette smoking, diabetes, hyperlipidemia, hypertension—and SCD remains an important clinical and epidemiologic problem.

Hereditary factors contribute to the risk of SCD, but largely in
a nonspecific manner: They represent expressions of the hereditary
predisposition to coronary heart disease. Except for a few specific
syndromes, such as the genetic hyperlipoproteinemias (Chap. 341),
congenital long QT interval syndromes (Chap. 231), and a number of
myopathic and dysplastic syndromes there are no *specific* hereditary
risk factors for SCD.

The major categories of structural causes of, and functional factors
contributing to, the SCD syndrome are listed in Table 39-2. Worldwide,
and especially in western cultures, coronary atherosclerotic heart disease is the most common structural abnormality associated with SCD.
Up to 80 percent of all SCDs in the United States are due to the
consequences of coronary atherosclerosis. The cardiomyopathies (di-

TABLE 39-2

Cardiac Arrest and Sudden Cardiac Death

STRUCTURAL CAUSES

I. Coronary heart disease
  A. Coronary artery abnormalities
    1. Chronic atherosclerotic lesions
    2. Acute (active) lesions
      (plaque fissuring, platelet aggregation, acute thrombosis)
    3. Anomalous coronary artery anatomy
  B. Myocardial infarction
    1. Healed
    2. Acute
II. Myocardial hypertrophy
  A. Secondary
  B. Hypertrophic cardiomyopathy
    1. Obstructive
    2. Nonobstructive
III. Dilated cardiomyopathy—primary muscle disease
IV. Inflammatory and infiltrative disorders
  A. Myocarditis
  B. Noninfectious inflammatory diseases
  C. Infiltrative diseases
V. Valvular heart disease
VI. Electrophysiologic abnormalities, structural
  A. Anomalous pathways in Wolff-Parkinson-White syndrome
  B. Conducting system disease
  C. Membrane channel structure (e.g., congenital long QT syndrome)

FUNCTIONAL CONTRIBUTING FACTORS

I. Alterations of coronary blood flow
  A. Transient ischemia
  B. Reperfusion after ischemia
II. Low cardiac output states
  A. Heart failure
    1. Chronic
    2. Acute decompensation
  B. Shock
III. Systemic metabolic abnormalities
  A. Electrolyte imbalance (e.g., hypokalemia)
  B. Hypoxemia, acidosis
IV. Neurophysiologic disturbances
  A. Autonomic fluctuations: central, neural, humoral
  B. Receptor function
V. Toxic responses
  A. Proarrhythmic drug effects
  B. Cardiac toxins (e.g., cocaine, digitalis intoxication)
  C. Drug interactions

lated and hypertrophic, collectively, Chap. 239) account for another
10 to 15 percent of SCDs, and all the remaining diverse etiologies
cause only 5 to 10 percent of these events. Transient ischemia in the
previously scarred or hypertrophied heart, hemodynamic and fluid and
electrolyte disturbances, fluctuations in autonomic nervous system
activity, and transient electrophysiologic changes caused by drugs
or other chemicals (e.g., proarrhythmia) have all been implicated as
mechanisms responsible for transition from electrophysiologic stability
to instability. In addition, spontaneous reperfusion of ischemic myocardium, caused by vasomotor changes in the coronary vasculature and/
or spontaneous thrombolysis, may cause transient electrophysiologic
instability and arrhythmias.

PATHOLOGY Data from postmortem examinations of SCD
victims parallel the clinical observations on the prevalence of coronary
heart disease as the major structural etiologic factor. More than 80
percent of SCD victims have pathologic findings of coronary heart
disease. The pathologic description often includes a combination of
long-standing, extensive atherosclerosis of the epicardial coronary
arteries and acute active coronary lesions, which include a combination
of fissured or ruptured plaques, platelet aggregates, hemorrhage, and
thombosis. In one study, chronic coronary atherosclerosis involving
two or more major vessels with ≥75 percent stenosis was observed
in 75 percent of the victims. In another study, atherosclerotic plaque
fissuring, platelet aggregates, and/or acute thrombosis were observed
in 95 of 100 individuals who had pathologic studies after SCD. Most of
these acute changes were superimposed on preexisting chronic lesions.

As many as 70 to 75 percent of males who die suddenly have
prior myocardial infarctions (MIs), but only 20 to 30 percent have
recent acute MIs. A high incidence of left ventricular (LV) hypertrophy
coexists with prior MIs.

**CLINICAL DEFINITION OF FORMS OF CARDIOVASCU-
LAR COLLAPSE** (Table 39-1) *Cardiovascular collapse* is a general term connoting loss of effective blood flow due to acute dysfunction of the heart and/or peripheral vasculature. Cardiovascular collapse
may be caused by vasodepressor syncope (vasovagal syncope, postural
hypotension with syncope, neurocardiogenic syncope—see Chap. 20),
a transient severe bradycardia, or cardiac arrest. The latter is distinguished from the transient forms of cardiovascular collapse in that it
usually requires an intervention to achieve resuscitation. In contrast,
vasodepressor syncope and many primary bradyarrhythmic syncopal
events are transient and non-life-threatening, and the patient will regain
consciousness spontaneously.

The most common electrical mechanism for true cardiac arrest is
ventricular fibrillation (VF), which is responsible for 65 to 80 percent
of cardiac arrests. Severe persistent bradyarrhythmias, asystole, and
pulseless electrical activity (an organized electrical activity without
mechanical response—formerly called electomechanical dissociation)
cause another 20 to 30 percent. Sustained ventricular tachycardia (VT)
with hypotension is a less common cause. Acute low cardiac output
states, having precipitous onset, also may present clinically as a cardiac
arrest. The causes include massive acute pulmonary emboli, internal
blood loss from ruptured aortic aneurysm, intense anaphylaxis, cardiac
rupture after myocardial infarction, and unexpected fatal arrhythmia
due to electrolyte disturbances.

CLINICAL CHARACTERISTICS OF
CARDIAC ARREST

PRODROME, ONSET, ARREST, DEATH SCD may be pres-
aged by days, weeks, or months of increasing angina, dyspnea, palpitations, easy fatigability, and other nonspecific complaints. However,
these *prodromal complaints* are generally predictive of any major
cardiac event; they are not specific for predicting SCD.

The *onset of the terminal event*, leading to cardiac arrest, is defined
as an acute change in cardiovascular status preceding cardiac arrest
by up to 1 h. When the onset is instantaneous or abrupt, the probability

that the arrest is cardiac in origin is >95 percent. Continuous ECG recordings, fortuitously obtained at the onset of a cardiac arrest, commonly demonstrate changes in cardiac electrical activity in the minutes or hours before the event. There is a tendency for the heart rate to increase and for advanced grades of premature ventricular contractions (PVCs) to evolve. Most cardiac arrests that occur by the mechanism of VF begin with a run of sustained or nonsustained VT, which then degenerates into VF.

Sudden unexpected loss of effective circulation may be separated into "arrhythmic events" and "circulatory failure." Arrhythmic events are characterized by a high likelihood of patients being awake and active immediately prior to the event, are dominated by VF as the electrical mechanism, and have a short duration of terminal illness (<1 h). In contrast, circulatory failure deaths occur in patients who are inactive or comatose, have a higher incidence of asystole than VF, have a tendency to a longer duration of terminal illness, and are dominated by noncardiac events preceding the terminal illness.

The onset of cardiac arrest may be characterized by typical symptoms of an acute cardiac event, such as prolonged angina or the pain of onset of MI, acute dyspnea or orthopnea, or the sudden onset of palpitations, sustained tachycardia, or light-headedness. However, in many patients, the onset is precipitous, without forewarning.

Cardiac arrest is, by definition, abrupt. Mentation may be impaired in patients with sustained VT during the onset of the terminal event. However, complete loss of consciousness is a *sine qua non* in cardiac arrest. Although rare spontaneous reversions occur, it is usual that cardiac arrest progresses to death within minutes (i.e., SCD has occurred) if active interventions are not undertaken promptly.

The ability to resuscitate the victim of cardiac arrest is related to the time from onset to institution of resuscitative efforts, the setting in which the event occurs, the mechanism (VF, VT, pulseless electrical activity, asystole), and the clinical status of the patient prior to the cardiac arrest. Those settings in which it is possible to institute prompt cardiopulmonary resuscitation (CPR) provide a better chance of a successful outcome. However, the outcome in intensive care units and other in-hospital environments is heavily influenced by the patient's preceding clinical status. The immediate outcome is good for cardiac arrest occurring in the intensive care unit in the presence of an acute cardiac event or transient metabolic disturbance, but the outcome for patients with far-advanced chronic cardiac disease or advanced noncardiac diseases (e.g., renal failure, pneumonia, sepsis, diabetes, cancer) is no more successful in hospital than in the out-of-hospital setting.

The success rate for initial resuscitation and ultimate survival from an out-of-hospital cardiac arrest depends in part on the mechanism of the event. When the mechanism is VT, the outcome is best (67 percent); VF is the next most successful (25 percent), and asystole and pulseless electrical activity generate dismal outcome statistics (Fig. 39-1). Advanced age also influences adversely the chances of successful resuscitation.

Progression to biologic death is a function of the mechanism of cardiac arrest and the length of the delay before interventions. VF or asystole, without CPR within the first 4 to 6 min, has a poor outcome, and there are few survivors among patients who had no life-support activities for the first 8 min after onset. Outcome statistics are improved considerably by lay bystander intervention (basic life support—see below) prior to definitive interventions (advanced life support—defibrillation) and by early defibrillation. Death during the hospitalization after a successfully resuscitated cardiac arrest relates closely to the severity of central nervous system injury. Anoxic encephalopathy and infections subsequent to prolonged respirator dependence account for 60 percent of the deaths. Another 30 percent occur as a consequence of low cardiac output states that fail to respond to interventions. Paradoxically, recurrent arrhythmias are the least common cause of death, accounting for only 10 percent of in-hospital deaths.

Among patients who have cardiac arrest in the setting of acute MI, it is important to distinguish between primary and secondary cardiac arrests. *Primary* cardiac arrests refer to those that occur in the absence of hemodynamic instability, and *secondary* cardiac arrests are those that occur in patients in whom abnormal hemodynamics dominate the clinical picture before cardiac arrest. The success rate for immediate resuscitation in primary cardiac arrest during acute MI in a monitored setting should approach 100 percent. In contrast, as many as 70 percent of patients with secondary cardiac arrest succumb immediately or during the same hospitalization.

IDENTIFICATION OF PATIENTS AT RISK FOR SUDDEN CARDIAC DEATH Primary prevention of cardiac arrest depends on the ability to identify individual patients at high risk. One must view the problem in the context of the total number of events and the population pools from which they are derived. In Fig. 39-2A, the inverted triangle demonstrates that the annual incidence of SCD among an unselected adult population is 1 to 2 per 1000 population, largely reflecting the prevalence of those coronary heart disease patients among whom SCD is the first clinically recognized manifestation (20 to 25 percent of first coronary events are SCD). The incidence (percent per year) increases progressively with addition of identified coronary risk factors to populations free of prior coronary events. The most powerful factors are age, elevated blood pressure, LV hypertrophy, cigarette smoking, elevated serum cholesterol level, obesity, and non-specific electrocardiographic abnormalities. These coronary risk factors are not specific for SCD but rather represent increasing risk for all coronary deaths. The proportion of coronary deaths that are sudden remains at approximately 50 percent in all risk categories. Despite the marked *relative* increased risk of SCD with addition of multiple risk factors (from 1 to 2 per 1000 population per year in an unselected population to as much as 50 to 60 per 1000 in subgroups having multiple risk factors for coronary artery disease), the *absolute* incidence remains relatively low when viewed as the relationship between the number of individuals who have a preventive intervention and the number of events that can be prevented. Specifically, a 50 percent reduction in annual SCD risk would be a huge *relative* decrease but would require an intervention in up to 200 unselected individuals to prevent one sudden death. These figures highlight the importance of primary prevention of coronary heart disease. Control of coronary risk factors may be the only practical method to prevent SCD in major segments of the population, because of the paradox that the majority of events occur in the large unselected subgroups rather than in the specific high-risk subgroups (compare "Events/Year" with "Percent/Year" in Fig. 39-2A). Under most conditions of higher level of risk,

	Ventricular fibrillation	Ventricular tachycardia	Asystole / Brady-arrhythmia	TOTAL
Out-of-hospital cardiac arrests	220	24	108	352
	↓(40%)	↓(88%)	↓(9%)	↓(33%)
Resuscitated and hospitalized	87	21	9	117
	↓(59%)	↓(76%)	↓(−)	↓(57%)
Discharged	51	16	0	67

FIGURE 39-1 Initial electrophysiologic mechanisms recorded during out-of-hospital cardiac arrest. The figures highlighted by the boxes indicate the number of patients in each of three mechanism categories (ventricular fibrillation, ventricular tachycardia, and bradyarrhythmia/asystole). In each category, the data indicate the number of prehospital cardiac arrests (*top*), the number of patients successfully resuscitated in the field and transferred to the hospital alive (*middle*), and the number of patients who survived to be discharged from hospital (*bottom*). The percentages in parentheses indicate survivals between each level of care for each category. (*Modified from RJ Myerburg et al: Clinical, electrophysiologic, and hemodynamic profile of patients resuscitated from prehospital cardiac arrest. Am J Med 68:568, 1980, with permission*).

particularly those indexed to a recent major cardiovascular event (e.g., MI, recent onset of heart failure, survival after out-of-hospital cardiac arrest), the highest risk of sudden death occurs within the initial 6 to 18 months and then decreases toward baseline risk of the underlying disease (Fig. 39-2B). Accordingly, preventive interventions are most likely to be effective when initiated early.

For patients with acute or prior clinical manifestations of coronary heart disease, high-risk subgroups having a much higher ratio of SCD risk to population base can be identified. The acute, convalescent, and chronic phases of MI provide large population subsets with more

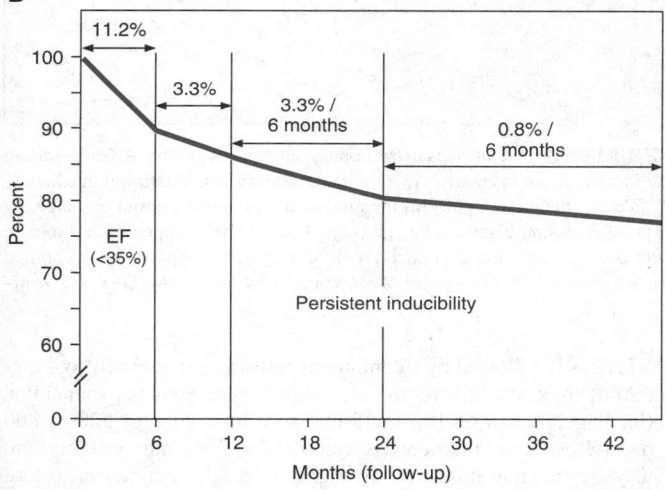

FIGURE 39-2 *A.* Incidence of sudden and nonsudden cardiac deaths in population subgroups, and the relation of total number of events per year to incidence figures. Approximations of subgroup incidence figures, and the related population pool from which they are derived, are presented. Approximately 50 percent of all cardiac deaths are sudden and unexpected. The incidence triangle on the left ("Percent/Year") indicates the approximate percentage of sudden and nonsudden deaths in each of the population subgroups indicated, ranging from the lowest percentage in unselected adult populations (0.1 to 2 percent per year) to the highest percentage in patients with VT or VF during convalescence after an MI (approximately 50 percent per year). The triangle on the right indicates the total number of events per year in each of these groups, to reflect incidence in context with the size of the population subgroups. The highest risk categories identify the smallest number of total annual events, and the lowest incidence category accounts for the largest number of events per year. (EF, ejection fraction; VT, ventricular tachycardia; VF, ventricular fibrillation; MI, myocardial infarction.) *B.* Time dependence of risk among survivors of out-of-hospital cardiac arrest. Recurrence risk is highest in the first 6 months of the index event. Survival is expressed as a percentage. High risk is best predicted initially by an ejection fraction ≤ 35 percent during the first 6 months, and subsequently persistent inducibility of VT during electrophysiologic testing becomes an added major risk. *n* = 101 at *t* = 0. [*After T Furukawa et al, in RJ Myerberg et al, Circulation 85(Suppl 1):2, 1992. Reproduced with permission of the American Heart Association.*]

highly focused risk (Chap. 243). The potential risk of cardiac arrest from the onset through the first 72 h after acute MI (the acute phase) may be as high as 15 to 20 percent. The highest risk of SCD in relation to MI is found in the subgroup that has experienced sustained VT or VF during the convalescent phase (3 days to 8 weeks) after MI. A greater than 50 percent mortality in 6 to 12 months has been observed among these patients, when managed with conservative medical therapy, and at least 50 percent of the deaths are sudden. Since the development of aggressive intervention techniques, the incidence appears to have fallen dramatically.

After the acute phase of MI, long-term risk for total mortality and SCD are predicted by a number of factors. The most important for both SCD and non-SCD is the extent of myocardial damage sustained during the acute event. This is measured by the degree of reduction in the ejection fraction (EF), functional capacity, and/or the occurrence of heart failure. Increasing *frequency* of postinfarction PVCs, with a plateau above the range of 10 to 30 PVCs per hour on 24-h ambulatory monitor recordings, also indicates increased risk, but advanced *forms* (salvos, nonsustained VT) are probably the more powerful predictor. PVCs interact strongly with decreased left ventricular EF. The combination of frequent PVCs, salvos or nonsustained VT, and an EF ≤ 30 percent identifies patients who have an annual risk of 20 percent. The risk falls off sharply with decreasing PVC frequency and the absence of advanced forms, as well as with higher EF. Despite the risk implications of postinfarction PVCs, improved outcome as a result of PVC suppression has not been demonstrated (Chap. 231).

The extent of underlying disease due to any cause and/or prior clinical expression of risk of SCD (i.e., survival after out-of-hospital cardiac arrest not associated with acute MI) identify patients at very high risk for subsequent (recurrent) cardiac arrest. Survival after out-of-hospital cardiac arrest predicts up to a 30 percent 1-year recurrent cardiac arrest rate in the absence of specific interventions (see below).

A general rule is that the risk of SCD is approximately one-half the total cardiovascular mortality rate. Thus, the SCD risk is approximately 20 percent per year for patients with advanced coronary heart disease or dilated cardiomyopathy severe enough to result in a 40 percent 1-year total mortality rate. As shown in Fig. 39-2A, the very high risk subgroups provide more focused population fractions ("Percent/Year") for predicting cardiac arrest or SCD; but the impact on the overall population, indicated by the absolute number of preventable events ("Events/Year"), is considerably smaller. The requirements for achieving a major population impact are effective prevention of the underlying diseases and/or new epidemiologic probes that will allow better resolution of subgroups within large general populations.

℞ TREATMENT

The individual who collapses suddenly is managed in four stages: (1) the initial response and basic life support, (2) advanced life support, (3) postresuscitation care, and (4) long-term management. The initial response and basic life support can be carried out by physicians, nurses, paramedical personnel, and trained lay persons. There is a requirement for increasing skills as the patient moves through the stages of advanced life support, postresuscitation care, and long-term management.

Initial Response and Basic Life Support   The initial response will confirm whether a sudden collapse is indeed due to a cardiac arrest. Observations for respiratory movements, skin color, and the presence or absence of pulses in the carotid or femoral arteries will promptly determine whether a life-threatening cardiac arrest has occurred. As soon as a cardiac arrest is suspected or confirmed, contacting an emergency rescue system (e.g., 911) should be the immediate priority.

Agonal respiratory movements may persist for a short time after the onset of cardiac arrest, but it is important to observe for severe stridor with a persistent pulse as a clue to aspiration of a foreign body or food. If this is suspected, a prompt Heimlich maneuver (see below) may dislodge the obstructing body. A precordial blow, or "thump," delivered firmly by the clenched fist to the junction of the middle and lower third of the sternum may occasionally revert VT or VF, but there is concern about converting VT *to* VF. Therefore, it has been recommended to use precordial thumps as an advanced life support technique when monitoring and defibrillation are available. This conservative application of the technique remains controversial.

The third action during the initial response is to clear the airway. The head is tilted back and chin lifted so that the oropharynx can be explored to clear the airway. Dentures or foreign bodies are removed, and the Heimlich maneuver is performed if there is reason to suspect that a foreign body is lodged in the oropharynx. If respiratory arrest precipitating cardiac arrest is suspected, a second precordial thump is delivered after the airway is cleared.

Basic life support, more popularly known as CPR, is intended to maintain organ perfusion until definitive interventions can be instituted. The elements of CPR are the establishment and maintenance of ventilation of the lungs and compression of the chest. Mouth-to-mouth respiration may be used if no specific rescue equipment is immediately available (e.g., plastic oropharyngeal airways, esophageal obturators, masked Ambu bag). Conventional ventilation techniques during CPR require the lungs to be inflated 10 to 12 times per minute, i.e., once every fifth chest compression when two persons are performing the resuscitation and twice in succession every 15 chest compressions when one person is carrying out both ventilation and chest wall compression.

Chest compression is based on the assumption that cardiac compression allows the heart to maintain a pump function by sequential filling and emptying of its chambers, with competent valves maintaining forward direction of flow. The technique is illustrated in Fig. 39-3. The palm of one hand is placed over the lower sternum, with the heel of the other resting on the dorsum of the lower hand. The sternum is depressed, with the arms remaining straight, at a rate of approximately 80 to 100 per minute. Sufficient force is applied to depress the sternum 3 to 5 cm, and relaxation is abrupt.

Advanced Life Support Advanced life support is intended to achieve adequate ventilation, control cardiac arrhythmias, stabilize the hemodynamic status (blood pressure and cardiac output), and restore organ perfusion. The activities carried out to achieve these goals include (1) intubation with an endotracheal tube, (2) defibrillation/cardioversion and/or pacing, and (3) insertion of an intravenous line. Ventilation with O_2 (room air if O_2 is not immediately available) may promptly reverse hypoxemia and acidosis. The speed with which defibrillation/cardioversion is carried out is an important element for successful resuscitation. When possible, immediate defibrillation should precede intubation and insertion of an intravenous line; CPR should be carried out while the defibrillator is being charged. As soon as a diagnosis of VT or VF is obtained, a 200-J shock should be delivered. Additional shocks at higher energies, up to a maximum of 360 J, are tried if the initial shock does not successfully abolish VT or VF. Epinephrine, 1 mg intravenously, is given after failed defibrillation, and attempts to defibrillate are repeated. The dose of epinephrine may be repeated after intervals of 3 to 5 min.

If the patient is less than fully conscious upon reversion, or if two or three attempts fail, prompt intubation, ventilation, and arterial blood gas analysis should be carried out. Intravenous $NaHCO_3$, which was formerly used in large quantities, is no longer considered routinely necessary and may be dangerous in larger quantities. However, the patient who is persistently acidotic after successful defibrillation and intubation should be given 1 meq/kg $NaHCO_3$ initially and an additional 50 percent of the dose repeated every 10 to 15 min.

After initial unsuccessful defibrillation attempts, or with persistent electrical instability, a bolus of 1 mg/kg lidocaine is given intravenously (Chap. 243), and the dose is repeated in 2 min in those patients who have persistent ventricular arrhythmias or remain in

FIGURE 39-3 Major steps in cardiopulmonary resuscitation. *A.* Make certain the victim has an open airway. *B.* Start respiratory resuscitation immediately. *C.* Feel for the carotid pulse in the groove alongside the thyroid cartilage. *D.* If pulse is absent, begin cardiac massage. Use 80–100 compressions a minute with one lung inflation after each group of five chest compressions. *(Modified from J Henderson, Emergency Medical Guide, 4th ed, New York, McGraw-Hill, 1978.)*

VF. This is followed by a continuous infusion at a rate of 1 to 4 mg/min. If lidocaine fails to provide control, intravenous procainamide (loading infusion of 100 mg/5 min to a total dose of 500 to 800 mg, followed by continuous infusion at 2 to 5 mg/min) or bretylium tosylate (loading dose 5 to 10 mg/kg in 5 min; maintenance dose 0.5 to 2 mg/min) may be tried. Intravenous calcium gluconate is no longer considered safe or necessary for routine administration. It is used only in patients in whom acute hyperkalemia is known to be the triggering event for resistant VF, in the presence of known hypocalcemia, or in patients who have received toxic doses of calcium channel antagonists.

Cardiac arrest secondary to bradyarrhythmias or asystole is managed differently. Once it is known that this type of rhythm is present, there is no role for external shock. The patient is promptly intubated, CPR is continued, and an attempt is made to control hypoxemia and acidosis. Epinephrine and/or atropine are given intravenously or by an intracardiac route. External pacing devices are now available to attempt to establish a regular rhythm, but the prognosis is generally very poor in this form of cardiac arrest. The one exception is bradyarrhythmic/asystolic cardiac arrest secondary to airway obstruction. This form of cardiac arrest may respond promptly to removal of foreign bodies by the Heimlich maneuver or, in hospitalized patients, by intubation and suctioning of obstructing secretions in the airway.

Postresuscitation Care This phase of management is determined by the clinical setting of the cardiac arrest. *Primary VF in acute MI* (Chap. 243) is generally very responsive to life-support techniques and easily controlled after the initial event. Patients are maintained on a lidocaine infusion at the rate of 2 to 4 mg/min for 24 to 72 h after the event. In the in-hospital setting, respirator support is usually not necessary or is needed for only a short time, and hemodynamics stabilize promptly after defibrillation or cardioversion. In *secondary VF in acute MI* (those events in which hemodynamic abnormalities predispose to the potentially fatal arrhythmia), resuscitative efforts are less often successful, and in those patients who are successfully resuscitated, the recurrence rate is high. The clinical picture is dominated by hemodynamic instability. In fact, the outcome is determined more by the ability to control hemodynamic dysfunction than by electrophysiologic abnormalities. Bradyarrhythmias, asystole, and pulseless electrical activity are commonly secondary events in hemodynamically unstable patients and are less responsive to interventions.

The outcome after in-hospital cardiac arrest associated with *noncardiac* diseases is poor, and in the few successfully resuscitated patients, the postresuscitation course is dominated by the nature of the underlying disease. Patients with cancer, renal failure, acute central nervous system disease, and uncontrolled infections, as a group, have a survival rate of less than 10 percent after in-hospital cardiac arrest. Some major exceptions are patients with transient airway obstruction, electrolyte disturbances, proarrhythmic effects of drugs, and severe metabolic abnormalities, most of whom may have an excellent chance of survival if they can be resuscitated promptly and maintained while the transient abnormalities are being corrected.

Long-Term Management After Survival of Out-of-Hospital Cardiac Arrest Patients who do not suffer irreversible injury of the central nervous system and who achieve hemodynamic stability should have extensive diagnostic and therapeutic testing to guide long-term management. This aggressive approach is driven by the fact that statistics from the 1970s indicated survival after out-of-hospital cardiac arrest was followed by a 30 percent recurrent cardiac arrest rate at 1 year, 45 percent at 2 years, and a total mortality rate of almost 60 percent at 2 years. Historical comparisons suggest that these dismal statistics may be significantly improved by newer interventions, but the magnitude of the improvement is unknown because of the lack of concurrently controlled intervention studies.

Among those patients in whom an acute transmural MI is the cause of out-of-hospital cardiac arrest, the management is the same as in any other patient who suffers cardiac arrest during the acute phase of a documented MI (see Chap. 243). For almost all other categories of patients, however, extensive diagnostic studies are carried out to determine etiology, functional impairment, and electrophysiologic instability as guides to future management. In general, patients who have out-of-hospital cardiac arrest due to chronic ischemic heart disease, without an acute MI, are evaluated to determine whether transient ischemia or chronic electrophysiologic instability was the more likely cause of the event. If there is reason to suspect an ischemic mechanism, coronary revascularization or drugs, most commonly beta blockers, are used to reduce ischemia. Electrophysiologic instability is best identified by the use of programmed electrical stimulation to determine whether sustained VT or VF can be induced (Chap. 231). If so, this information can be used as a baseline against which to evaluate drug efficacy for prevention of inducibility or to determine suitability for map-guided antiarrhythmic surgery, or whether an implantable cardioverter/defibrillator (ICD) might be the best strategy. Using this technique in patients with EF of 30 percent or more, the recurrent cardiac arrest rate is less than 10 percent during the first year of follow-up when inducibility is suppressed

by a drug. The outcome is not as good for patients with EF under 30 percent but may be still better than the apparent natural history of survival after cardiac arrest. For patients for whom successful drug therapy cannot be identified by this technique, insertion of an ICD, antiarrhythmic surgery (e.g., coronary bypass surgery, aneurysmectomy, cryoablation), or empiric amiodarone therapy can be considered options (Chap. 231). Primary surgical success, defined as surviving the procedure and reverting to a noninducible status without drug therapy, is better than 90 percent when patients are selecte for ability to be mapped in the operating room. However, only a small fraction of patients meet the criteria. In addition, VT/VF *cannot* be induced in a number of survivors of cardiac arrest (30 to 50 percent), and inducible arrhythmias can be suppressed by drugs in no more than 20 to 30 percent of those whose arrhythmias can be induced. Because of these limitations of drug therapy and surgical approaches, ICD therapy has evolved into the most commonly used strategy for cardiac arrest survivors. ICDs have very good success rates for sensing and reverting life-threatening arrhythmias, but improvement in long-term total survival outcomes remains ill defined.

The ESVEM study has suggested that ambulatory monitor-based suppression of ambient arrhythmias is equivalent to electrophysiologically guided testing in predicting long-term outcome. This conclusion has generated a debate which remains to be resolved.

BIBLIOGRAPHY

AKHTAR M et al: Implantable cardioverter-defibrillator therapy for prevention of sudden cardiac death. Cardiol Clin 11:97, 1993

CRANDALL BG et al: Implantable cardioverter-defibrillator therapy in survivors of out-of-hospital sudden cardiac death without inducible arrhythmias. J Am Coll Cardiol 21:1186, 1993

CUMMINS RO et al: Improving survival from sudden cardiac arrest: The "chain of survival" concept. Circulation 83:1832, 1991

ECHT DS et al: Mortality and morbidity in patients receiving encainide, flecainide, or placebo: The Cardiac Arrhythmia Suppression Trial. N Engl J Med 324:781, 1991

EMERGENCY CARDIAC CARE COMMITTEE AND SUBCOMMITTEES, AMERICAN HEART ASSOCIATION: Guidelines for cardiopulmonary resuscitation and emergency cardiac care. JAMA 268:2172, 1992

HEIMLICH HJ: A life-saving maneuver to prevent food choking. JAMA 234:398, 1975

JASTREMSKI MS: In-hospital cardiac arrest. Ann Emerg Med 22:113, 1993

JOSLYN et al: Survival from out-of-hospital cardiac arrest: Effects of patient age and presence of 911 Emergency Medical Services phone access. Am J Emerg Med 11:200, 1993

KANNEL WB, SCHATZKIN A: Sudden death: Lessons from subsets in population studies. J Am Coll Cardiol 5(suppl 6):141B, 1985

MASON JW, for the Electrophysiologic Study versus Electrocardiographic Monitoring Investigators: A comparison of electrophysiologic testing with Holter monitoring to predict antiarrhythmic drug efficacy for ventricular tachyarrhythmias. N Engl J Med 329:445, 1993

MYERBURG RJ, CASTELLANOS A: Cardiac arrest and sudden cardiac death, in *Heart Disease*, 5th ed, E Braunwald (ed). Philadelphia, Saunders, 1997, pp 742–779

——— et al: Epidemiology, transient risk, and intervention assessment. Ann Intern Med 119:1187, 1993

ORNATO JP: Use of adrenergic agonists during CPR in adults. Ann Emerg Med 22:411, 1993

WILBER DJ et al: Out-of-hospital cardiac arrest: Use of electrophysiologic testing in the prediction of long-term outcome. N Engl J Med 318:19, 1988

WILLICH SN et al: Sudden cardiac death. Support for a role of triggering in causation. Circulation 87:1442, 1993

40 Raj K. Goyal

DYSPHAGIA

Dysphagia is defined as a sensation of "sticking" or obstruction of the passage of food through the mouth, pharynx, or esophagus. It should be distinguished from other symptoms related to swallowing. *Aphagia* signifies complete esophageal obstruction, which is usually due to bolus impaction and represents a medical emergency. *Difficulty in initiating a swallow* occurs in disorders of the voluntary phase of swallowing. However, once initiated, swallowing is completed normally. *Odynophagia* means painful swallowing. Frequently, odynophagia and dysphagia occur together. *Globus pharyngeous* is the sensation of a lump lodged in the throat. However, no difficulty is encountered when swallowing is performed. *Misdirection of food*, resulting in nasal regurgitation and laryngeal and pulmonary aspiration of food during swallowing, is characteristic of oropharyngeal dysphagia. *Phagophobia*, meaning fear of swallowing, and *refusal to swallow* may occur in hysteria, rabies, tetanus, and pharyngeal paralysis due to fear of aspiration. Painful inflammatory lesions that cause odynophagia also may cause refusal to swallow. Some patients may feel the food as it goes down the esophagus. This esophageal sensitivity is not associated with the food sticking or obstruction, however. Similarly, the *feeling of fullness in the epigastrium* that occurs after a meal or after swallowing air should not be confused with dysphagia.

PHYSIOLOGY OF SWALLOWING The process of swallowing begins with a voluntary (oral) phase during which a bolus of food is pushed into the pharynx by the contraction of the tongue. The bolus then activates oropharyngeal sensory receptors that initiate the involuntary (pharyngeal and esophageal) phase, or deglutition reflex. The deglutition reflex is a complex series of events that serves both to propel food through the pharynx and the esophagus and to prevent its entry into the airway. When the bolus is propelled backward by the tongue, the larynx moves forward and the upper esophageal sphincter opens. As the bolus moves into the pharynx, contraction of the superior pharyngeal constrictor against the contracted soft palate initiates a peristaltic contraction that proceeds rapidly downward to move the bolus through the pharynx and the esophagus. The lower esophageal sphincter opens as the food enters the esophagus and remains open until the peristaltic contraction has swept the bolus into the stomach. Peristaltic contraction in response to a swallow involves inhibition followed by sequential contraction of muscles along the entire swallowing passage; this is called *primary peristalsis*. The inhibition that precedes the peristaltic contraction is called *deglutitive inhibition*. Local distention of the esophagus from food activates intramural reflexes in the smooth muscle and results in *secondary peristalsis*, limited to the thoracic esophagus. *Tertiary contractions* are nonperistaltic because they occur simultaneously over a long segment of the esophagus. Tertiary contractions may occur in response to a swallow or esophageal distention, or they may occur spontaneously.

PATHOPHYSIOLOGY OF DYSPHAGIA The normal transport of an ingested bolus through the swallowing passage depends on the size of the ingested bolus; the luminal diameter of the swallowing passage; the peristaltic contraction; and deglutitive inhibition, including normal relaxation of upper and lower esophageal sphincters during swallowing. Dysphagia caused by a large bolus or luminal narrowing is called *mechanical dysphagia*, whereas dysphagia due to incoordination or weakness of peristaltic contractions or to impaired deglutitive inhibition is called *motor dysphagia*.

Mechanical Dysphagia Mechanical dysphagia could be caused by a very large food bolus, intrinsic narrowing, or extrinsic compression of the lumen. In an adult, the esophageal lumen can distend up to a diameter of 4 cm because of the elasticity of the esophageal wall. When the esophagus cannot dilate beyond 2.5 cm in diameter, dysphagia to normal solid food can occur, but it is always present when it cannot distend beyond 1.3 cm. Circumferential lesions produce dysphagia more consistently than do lesions that involve only a portion of circumferences of the esophageal wall, as uninvolved segments retain their distensibility. The causes of mechanical dysphagia are listed in Table 40-1. Common causes include carcinoma, peptic and other benign strictures, and lower esophageal ring.

Motor Dysphagia Motor dysphagia may result from difficulty in initiating a swallow or from abnormalities in peristalsis and deglutitive inhibition due to diseases of the esophageal striated or smooth muscle.

Diseases of the striated muscle involve the pharynx, upper esophageal sphincter, and cervical esophagus. The striated muscle is innervated by a somatic component of the vagus with cell bodies of the lower motor neurons located in the nucleus ambiguus. These neurons are cholinergic and excitatory and are the sole determinant of the muscle activity. Peristalsis in the striated muscle segment is due to sequential central activation of neurons innervating muscles at different levels along the esophagus. Motor dysphagia of the pharynx results from neuromuscular disorders causing muscle paralysis, simultaneous nonperistaltic contraction, or loss of opening of the upper esophageal sphincter. Loss of opening of the upper sphincter is caused by paralysis of geniohyoid and other suprahyoid muscles or loss of deglutitive inhibition of the cricopharyngeus muscle. Because each side of the pharynx is innervated by ipsilateral nerves, a lesion of motor neurons occurring only on one side leads to unilateral pharyngeal paralysis. Although lesions of striated muscle also involve the cervical part of the esophagus, the clinical manifestations of pharyngeal dysfunction usually overshadow the manifestations due to esophageal involvement.

Diseases of the smooth muscle segment involve the thoracic part of the esophagus and the lower esophageal sphincter. The smooth muscle is innervated by the parasympathetic component of the vagal preganglionic fibers and postganglionic neurons in the myenteric ganglia. The vagal pathway consists of parallel excitatory and inhibitory pathways that use acetycholine and nitric oxide as neurotransmitters, respectively. The activation of inhibitory nerves causes inhibition that is followed by rebound contraction. These pathways are involved in the resting tone of the lower esophageal sphincter as well as swallow-induced lower esophageal sphincter opening and inhibition followed by peristaltic contractions in the esophageal body. Dysphagia results when the peristaltic contractions are weak or nonperistaltic or when the lower sphincter fails to open normally. Loss of contractile power occurs due to muscle weakness, as in scleroderma. The nonperistaltic contractions and impaired relaxation of the lower esophageal sphincter result from a defect in inhibitory vagal innervation and account for dysphagia in achalasia.

The causes of motor dysphagia are also listed in Table 40-1. The important causes are pharyngeal paralysis, cricopharyngeal achalasia, scleroderma of the esophagus, achalasia, and diffuse esophageal spasm and related motor disorders.

Approach to the Patient

History The history can provide a correct presumptive diagnosis in over 80 percent of patients. The type of food causing dysphagia provides useful information. Difficulty only with solids implies mechanical dysphagia with a lumen that is not severely narrowed. In advanced obstruction, dysphagia occurs with liquids as well as solids. In contrast, motor dysphagia due to achalasia and diffuse esophageal spasm is equally affected by solids and liquids from the very onset. Patients with scleroderma have dysphagia to solids that is unrelated to posture and to liquids in the recumbent but not in the upright posture. When peptic stricture develops in patients with scleroderma, dysphagia becomes more persistent.

The duration and course of dysphagia are helpful in diagnosis. Transient dysphagia of short duration may be due to an inflammatory process. Progressive dysphagia lasting a few weeks to a few months

Table 40-1

Causes of Dysphagia

MECHANICAL DYSPHAGIA	MOTOR (NEUROMUSCULAR) DYSPHAGIA

MECHANICAL DYSPHAGIA

I. Luminal
   A. Large bolus
   B. Foreign body
II. Intrinsic narrowing
   A. Inflammatory condition causing edema and swelling
      1. Stomatitis
      2. Pharyngitis, epiglottitis
      3. Esophagitis
         a. Viral (herpes simplex, varicella-zoster, cytomegalovirus)
         b. Bacterial
         c. Fungal (candidal)
         d. Mucocutaneous bullous diseases
         e. Caustic, chemical, thermal injury
   B. Webs and rings
      1. Pharyngeal (Plummer-Vinson syndrome)
      2. Esophageal (congenital, inflammatory)
      3. Lower esophageal mucosal ring (Schatzki ring)
   C. Benign strictures
      1. Peptic
      2. Caustic and pill-induced
      3. Inflammatory (Crohn's disease, candidal, mucocutaneous lesions)
      4. Ischemic
      5. Postoperative, postirradiation
      6. Congenital
   D. Malignant tumors
      1. Primary carcinoma
         a. Squamous cell carcinoma
         b. Adenocarcinoma
         c. Carcinosarcoma
         d. Pseudosarcoma
         e. Lymphoma
         f. Melanoma
         g. Kaposi's sarcoma
      2. Metastatic carcinoma
   E. Benign tumors
      1. Leiomyoma
      2. Lipoma
      3. Angioma
      4. Inflammatory fibroid polyp
      5. Epithelial papilloma
III. Extrinsic compression
   A. Cervical spondylitis
   B. Vertebral osteophytes
   C. Retropharyngeal abscess and masses
   D. Enlarged thyroid gland
   E. Zenker's diverticulum
   F. Vascular compression
      1. Aberrant right subclavian artery
      2. Right-sided aorta
      3. Left atrial enlargement
      4. Aortic aneurysm
   G. Posterior mediastinal masses
   H. Pancreatic tumor, pancreatitis
   I. Postvagotomy hematoma and fibrosis

MOTOR (NEUROMUSCULAR) DYSPHAGIA

I. Difficulty in initiating swallowing reflex
   A. Paralysis of the tongue
   B. Oropharyngeal anesthesia
   C. Lack of saliva (e.g., Sjögren's syndrome)
   D. Lesions of sensory components of vagus and glossopharyngeal nerves
   E. Lesions of swallowing center
II. Disorders of pharyngeal and esophageal striated muscle
   A. Muscle weakness
      1. Lower motor neuron lesion (bulbar paralysis)
         a. Cerebrovascular accident
         b. Motor neuron disease
         c. Poliomyelitis, postpolio syndrome
         d. Polyneuritis
         e. Amyotrophic lateral sclerosis
         f. Familial dysautonomia
      2. Neuromuscular
         a. Myasthenia gravis
      3. Muscle disorders
         a. Polymyositis
         b. Dermatomyositis
         c. Myopathies (myotonic dystrophy, oculopharyngeal myopathy)
   B. Nonperistaltic contractions or impaired deglutitive inhibition
      1. Pharynx and upper esophagus
         a. Rabies
         b. Tetanus
         c. Extrapyramidal tract disease
         d. Upper motor neuron lesions (pseudobulbar paralysis)
      2. Upper esophageal sphincter (UES)
         a. Paralysis of suprahyoid muscles (causes same as paralysis of pharyngeal musculature)
         b. Cricopharyngeal achalasia
III. Disorders of esophageal smooth muscle
   A. Paralysis of esophageal body causing weak contractions
      1. Scleroderma and related collagen-vascular diseases
      2. Hollow visceral myopathy
      3. Myotonic dystrophy
      4. Metabolic neuromyopathy (amyloid, alcohol?, diabetes?)
      5. Achalasia (classical)
   B. Nonperistaltic contractions or impaired deglutitive inhibition
      1. Esophageal body
         a. Diffuse esophageal spasm
         b. Achalasia (vigorous)
         c. Variants of diffuse esophageal spasm
      2. Lower esophageal sphincter
         a. Achalasia
            (1) Primary
            (2) Secondary
               (a) Chagas' disease
               (b) Carcinoma
               (c) Lymphoma
               (d) Neuropathic intestinal pseudoobstruction syndrome
               (e) Toxins and drugs
         b. Lower esophageal muscular (contractile) ring

is suggestive of carcinoma of the esophagus. Episodic dysphagia to solids lasting several years indicates a benign disease characteristic of a lower esophageal ring.

The localization of the site of dysphagia by the patient is helpful in determining the site of esophageal obstruction; the lesion is at or below the perceived location of dysphagia.

Associated symptoms provide important diagnostic clues. Nasal regurgitation and tracheobronchial aspiration with swallowing are hallmarks of pharyngeal paralysis or a tracheoesophageal fistula. Tracheobronchial aspiration unrelated to swallowing may be secondary to achalasia, a Zenker's diverticulum, or gastroesophageal reflux.

Severe weight loss that is out of proportion to the degree of dysphagia is highly suggestive of carcinoma. When hoarseness precedes dysphagia, the primary lesion is usually in the larynx. Hoarseness following dysphagia may suggest involvement of the recurrent laryngeal nerve by extension of esophageal carcinoma beyond the walls of

the esophagus. Sometimes hoarseness may be due to laryngitis secondary to gastroesophageal reflux. Association of laryngeal symptoms and dysphagia also occurs in various neuromuscular disorders. Hiccups suggest a lesion in the distal portion of the esophagus. Unilateral wheezing with dysphagia indicates a mediastinal mass involving the esophagus and a large bronchus.

Chest pain with dysphagia occurs in diffuse esophageal spasm and in related motor disorders. Chest pain resembling diffuse esophageal spasms also may occur in esophageal obstruction due to a large bolus. A prolonged history of heartburn and reflux preceding dysphagia indicates peptic stricture. Similarly, a history of prolonged nasogastric intubation, ingestion of caustic agents, ingestion of pills without water, previous radiation therapy, or associated mucocutaneous diseases may provide the cause of esophageal stricture. If odynophagia is present, candidal or herpes esophagitis or pill-induced esophagitis should be suspected.

In patients with AIDS or other immunodeficiency states, esophagitis due to opportunistic infections such as *Candida*, herpes simplex virus, or cytomegalovirus and tumors such as Kaposi's sarcoma and lymphoma should be suspected.

PHYSICAL EXAMINATION   Physical examination is important in motor dysphagia due to skeletal muscle, neurologic, and oropharyngeal diseases. Signs of bulbar or pseudobulbar palsy, including dysarthria, dysphonia, ptosis, tongue atrophy, and hyperactive jaw jerk, in addition to evidence of generalized neuromuscular disease, should be carefully searched for. The neck should be examined for thyromegaly or a spinal abnormality. A careful inspection of the mouth and pharynx should disclose lesions that may cause interference with passage of food from the mouth or esophagus because of pain or obstruction. Changes in the skin and extremities may suggest a diagnosis of scleroderma and other collagen-vascular diseases or mucocutaneous diseases such as pemphigoid or epidermolysis bullosa, which may involve the esophagus. Metastatic diseases to lymph nodes and liver may be evident. Pulmonary complications of acute aspiration pneumonia or chronic aspiration may be present.

DIAGNOSTIC PROCEDURES   All patients with dysphagia must be thoroughly investigated because the treatment depends on the underlying cause. If oropharyngeal dysphagia is suspected, videofluoroscopy of oropharyngeal swallowing should be obtained. If mechanical dysphagia is suspected on clinical history, barium swallow, esophagogastroscopy and endoscopic biopsies are the diagnostic procedures of choice. Barium swallow and esophageal motility studies are diagnostic tests for motor dysphagia. Esophagogastroscopy may be needed in patients with motor dysphagia to exclude an associated structural abnormality (see Chap. 283).

BIBLIOGRAPHY

CASTELL DO (ed): *The Esophagus.* Boston, Little, Brown, 2d ed, 1995
ENTERLINE H, THOMPSON J: *Pathology of the Esophagus.* New York, Springer-Verlag, 1984
GOYAL RK, PATERSON WG: Esophageal motility, in *Handbook of Physiology: Gastrointestinal System I.* Bethesda, MD, American Physiological Society, 1989, pp 865–908
GOYAL RK, HIRANO I: Mechanisms of disease: The enteric nervous system. N Engl J Med 334:110, 1996
HENDRIX TR: Art and science of history taking in patient with difficulty swallowing. Dysphagia 8:69, 1993
KOCH WM: Swallowing disorders. Diagnosis and therapy. Med Clin North Am 77:571, 1993
MORTON RE et al: Videofluoroscopy in the assessment of feeding disorders of children with neurological problems. J Dev Med Child Neurol 35:388, 1993
SHAKER R et al: Coordination of deglutition and phases of inspiration: Effect of aging, tachypnea, bolus volume, and chronic obstructive pulmonary disease. Am J Physiol 263:G750, 1992
YAMATO S et al: Role of nitric oxide in lower esophageal sphincter relaxation to swallowing. Life Sci 50:1263, 1992

41   *Lawrence S. Friedman, Kurt J. Isselbacher*

NAUSEA, VOMITING, AND INDIGESTION

NAUSEA AND VOMITING

Nausea and vomiting may occur independently of each other but generally are closely allied and are presumed to be mediated by the same neural pathways, so they may be considered together. *Nausea* denotes the feeling of an imminent desire to vomit, usually referred to the throat or epigastrium. *Vomiting* (or *emesis*) refers to the forceful oral expulsion of gastric contents. *Retching* denotes the labored rhythmic contraction of respiratory and abdominal musculature that frequently precedes or accompanies vomiting.

Nausea often precedes or accompanies vomiting. It is usually associated with diminished functional activity of the stomach (e.g., hypotonicity, hypoperistalsis, and hyposecretion) and altered small-intestinal motility (e.g., hypertonicity and reversed peristalsis of the duodenum). Often accompanying severe nausea is evidence of altered autonomic (especially parasympathetic) activity, such as skin pallor, increased perspiration, hypersalivation, defecation, and, occasionally, hypotension and bradycardia (vasovagal syndrome); anorexia is also usually present.

Nausea, retching, and hypersalivation frequently precede the act of vomiting, which is a highly integrated sequence of involuntary visceral and somatic motor events. The stomach plays a relatively passive role in the vomiting process, the major ejection force being provided by the abdominal musculature. With relaxation of the gastric fundus and gastroesophageal sphincter, a sharp increase in intraabdominal pressure is brought about by forceful contraction of the diaphragm and abdominal wall muscles. This, together with concomitant annular contraction of the gastric pylorus, results in the expulsion of gastric contents into the esophagus. Increased intrathoracic pressure results in the further movement of esophageal contents into the mouth. Reversal of the normal direction of esophageal peristalsis may play a role in this process. Reflex elevation of the soft palate during the vomiting act prevents the entry of the expelled material into the nasopharynx, whereas reflex closure of the glottis and inhibition of respiration help to prevent pulmonary aspiration.

Repeated emesis may have deleterious effects in a number of ways. The process of vomiting, if forceful, may lead to pressure rupture of the esophagus (Boerhaave's syndrome) or to linear mucosal (Mallory-Weiss) tears in the region of the cardioesophageal junction with resulting hematemesis. Prolonged vomiting may lead to dehydration, the loss of gastric secretions (especially hydrochloric acid) resulting in metabolic alkalosis with hypokalemia, malnutrition with various deficiency states, and dental caries. In states of central nervous system depression (e.g., coma), gastric contents may be aspirated into the lungs, with a resulting aspiration pneumonitis.

VOMITING MECHANISM   The act of vomiting is under the control of two functionally distinct medullary centers: the *vomiting center* in the dorsal portion of the lateral reticular formation and the *chemoreceptor trigger zone* in the area postrema of the floor of the fourth ventricle. The vomiting center controls and integrates the actual act of emesis. It receives afferent stimuli from the gastrointestinal tract and other parts of the body, from higher brainstem and cortical centers, especially the labyrinthine apparatus, and from the chemoreceptor trigger zone. Persons vary considerably in the threshold of their vomiting centers to different stimuli. The important efferent pathways in vomiting are the phrenic nerves (to the diaphragm), the spinal nerves (to the intercostal and abdominal musculature), and visceral efferent fibers in the vagus nerve (to the larynx, pharynx, esophagus, and stomach). The vomiting center is located near other medullary centers regulating respiratory, vasomotor, and autonomic functions that may be involved in the act of vomiting.

The chemoreceptor trigger zone by itself is incapable of mediating the act of vomiting; rather activation of this zone results in efferent impulses to the medullary vomiting center, which in turn initiates emesis. The chemoreceptor trigger zone is an emetic chemoreceptor that can be activated by a variety of stimuli or drugs, including apomorphine and other opiates, levodopa (after decarboxylation to dopamine), digitalis, bacterial toxins, radiation, and metabolic abnormalities as occur with uremia and hypoxia.

CLINICAL CLASSIFICATION   Nausea and vomiting are common manifestations of many organic and functional disorders. The precise mechanisms triggering vomiting in various clinical conditions are not well understood, making classification of mechanisms difficult.

Many *acute abdominal emergencies* that lead to the "surgical abdomen" are associated with nausea and vomiting. Vomiting may be seen with inflammation of a viscus, as in acute appendicitis or acute cholecystitis, intestinal obstruction, or acute peritonitis (see Chap. 288).

Other *disorders of the alimentary tract*, including those associated with chronic indigestion (see below), are frequently accompanied by nausea and vomiting. In peptic ulcer, emesis may be either spontaneous or self-induced and may lead to relief of symptoms, particularly if antral or pyloric edema has resulted in gastric outlet obstruction. Nausea and vomiting are also prominent in patients with disordered gastrointestinal motility, including postvagotomy, diabetic, or idiopathic gastroparesis (gastric atony); other gastric "dysrhythmias" resulting from abnormal myoelectric activity; and intestinal pseudoobstruction due to abnormal intestinal myogenic or neurogenic function. Gastroparesis may be demonstrated by gastric scanning after a radiolabeled meal or by radiography after ingestion of indigestible radiopaque solid markers. Experimentally, some patients with otherwise unexplained nausea and vomiting have been demonstrated to have accelerated ("tachygastria") or irregular ("gastric tachyarrhythmia") gastric electrical activity as measured by electrodes implanted surgically on the serosa of the stomach or placed on the abdominal surface ("electrogastrogram"). Typically, intestinal obstruction of any cause (e.g., adhesions, malignancy, hernia, volvulus) leads to vomiting, as do other disorders of the liver, pancreas, and biliary tract. Nausea and vomiting may accompany the distention and pain seen in the aerophagic syndromes (see below).

Viral, bacterial, and parasitic *infections of the intestinal tract* are typically associated with severe nausea and vomiting, often with diarrhea. *Acute systemic infections* with fever, especially in young children, are also frequently accompanied by vomiting and often by severe diarrhea. The mechanism whereby infections remote from the gastrointestinal tract produce these manifestations may relate to stimulation of the medullary chemoreceptor trigger zone by toxins or abnormal metabolites.

Central nervous system disorders that lead to increased intracranial pressure (e.g., neoplasms, encephalitis, hydrocephalus) may be accompanied by vomiting, which is often *projectile* (intensely forceful). Vertigo due to disorders of the labyrinthine apparatus, such as acute labyrinthitis and Ménière's disease, may be accompanied by vomiting with nausea and retching. Similarly, motion sickness is typically associated with anorexia, nausea, and vomiting as well as apathy, increased salivation, cold sweating, and headache. Additionally, migraine headaches, tabetic crises, acute meningitis, and the reactive phase of hypotension with syncope may be associated with nausea and vomiting.

Nausea and vomiting may be present in *acute myocardial infarction*, especially when posterior in location or transmural in extent, and in *congestive heart failure*, perhaps in relation to congestion of the liver. The possibility that these symptoms also may be due to drugs (e.g., opiates or digitalis) should always be borne in mind in patients with cardiac disease. Nausea and vomiting are common in cancer patients, especially those who are terminally ill.

Nausea and vomiting commonly accompany several *metabolic and endocrinologic disorders*, including uremia, diabetic ketoacidosis, hypo- and hyperparathyroidism, hyperthyroid crisis, and adrenal insufficiency, especially adrenal crisis. The morning sickness of early pregnancy is another instance of nausea and vomiting possibly related to hormonal changes; the term *hyperemesis gravidarum* is applied when fluid and electrolyte disturbances or nutritional deficiencies result.

The *side effects of many drugs and chemicals* include nausea and vomiting. In some cases, drugs have central emetic effects, as with digitalis, morphine, histamine, phenytoin, and some chemotherapeutic agents. In other cases, drug-induced gastric irritation leads to stimulation of the medullary vomiting center, as with salicylates, aminophylline, some antibiotics, and ipecac. The ingestion of a toxin (e.g., food poisoning) also may cause acute vomiting.

Psychogenic vomiting refers to chronic or recurrent vomiting that may result from an emotional or psychological disturbance. Often patients with emotional disorders and chronic vomiting maintain a relatively normal state of nutrition because only a relatively small amount of the ingested food is vomited. In some cases regurgitation rather than vomiting may predominate, and the degree of weight loss

may be out of proportion to the patient's description of the frequency and severity of vomiting. As discussed in Chap. 76, anorexia nervosa and bulimia are emotional disturbances that may be associated with vomiting and weight loss.

DIFFERENTIAL DIAGNOSIS Vomiting should be distinguished from *regurgitation*, which refers to the expulsion of food in the absence of nausea and without the abdominal diaphragmatic muscular contraction associated with vomiting. Regurgitation of esophageal contents may occur with esophageal strictures or diverticula. Regurgitation of gastric contents is generally seen in gastroesophageal reflux disease due to lower esophageal sphincter incompetence, in pyloric spasm or obstruction due to peptic ulcer, or in gastroparesis. *Hiccups* are a distinctive sound caused by contractions of the inspiratory muscles terminated abruptly by closure of the glottis. Brief episodes of hiccups may be caused by gastric distention, a sudden change in temperature, ingestion of alcohol, excess smoking, or excitement, whereas persistent hiccups may signify a serious underlying disease, such as a structural lesion or infection of the central nervous system, diaphragmatic irritation by a tumor or inflammatory process, metabolic derangement, vascular lesion, intraabdominal process, or systemic infection. In addition, a variety of drugs, including barbiturates and sedatives, general anesthesia, and psychogenic factors may lead to hiccups. *Rumination* is the effortless regurgitation of undigested food starting within minutes of a meal, presumably due to intraabdominal muscular contraction and simultaneous voluntary lower esophageal relaxation. It is rare in adults but more common in patients with bulimia nervosa and in infants, children, and mentally deficient persons.

The temporal relationship of vomiting to eating may be of help diagnostically. Vomiting that occurs predominantly in the morning is often seen early in pregnancy and in uremia. Alcoholic gastritis is also commonly accompanied by early-morning retching and emesis, the so-called dry heaves. Vomiting that occurs during or shortly after eating may suggest psychogenic vomiting or peptic ulcer with pylorospasm. Vomiting that occurs 4 to 6 h or longer after eating and involves the elimination of large quantities of undigested food often indicates gastric retention (e.g., pyloric obstruction, gastroparesis) or certain esophageal disorders (achalasia, Zenker's diverticulum). Vomiting that is projectile or without antecedent nausea suggests the possibility of a central nervous system lesion.

Associated symptoms also may provide diagnostic clues. For example, vertigo and tinnitus indicate the possibility of Ménière's disease. A long history of vomiting with little or no weight loss suggests psychogenic vomiting. Relief of abdominal pain with vomiting is typical of peptic ulcer. Early satiety is typical of gastroparesis.

The character of the vomitus also offers clues to the diagnosis. If the vomitus contains large amounts of free hydrochloric acid, gastric outlet obstruction due to an ulcer or a hypersecretory state such as Zollinger-Ellison syndrome should be considered. Absence of free hydrochloric acid is more compatible with gastric malignancy. A feculent or putrid odor reflects the results of bacterial action on the intestinal contents and may occur with distal intestinal obstruction, peritonitis, or gastrocolic fistula. Bile is commonly present in gastric contents whenever vomiting is prolonged; it has no significance unless constantly present in large quantities, when it may signify an obstructing lesion below the ampulla of Vater. The presence of blood in the gastric contents usually denotes bleeding from the esophagus, stomach, or duodenum.

Approach to the Patient

Every effort should be made to identify the underlying cause of nausea and vomiting. Evaluation should begin with a careful history taking, including a careful drug history; physical examination; and, if necessary, routine laboratory tests such as a complete blood count, erythrocyte sedimentation rate, electrolyte levels including blood urea nitrogen and creatinine, glucose levels, and liver function tests. Additional testing should be dictated by the age of the patient and clinical presentation, particularly when nausea and vomiting are chronic. In women of child-bearing age, a pregnancy test should be obtained. In selected cases urinalysis, cultures, a toxic screen, and tests of endocrine function (thyroid function tests, fasting morning cortisol level) may be indicated. The possibility of an underlying gastrointestinal or hepatobiliary disorder may be evaluated with plain and barium radiography, ultrasound, computed tomography (CT), and endoscopy. If neurologic disease is suspected, a CT scan of the head is indicated.

In over 50 percent of patients with chronic nausea and vomiting, the basic evaluation outlined above will be unrevealing, and in selected cases further specialized testing may be helpful, particularly if a gastrointestinal motility disorder is suspected. An array of tests may be considered, including esophageal motility and 24-h esophageal pH testing, gastric emptying and motility studies, and, if available, electrogastrography and small-intestinal motility testing. In occasional patients, a formal psychiatric consultation may prove to be revealing.

℞ TREATMENT

Effective therapy of nausea and vomiting usually depends on correction of the underlying cause. *Antiemetic agents* vary in their usefulness depending on the cause of the symptoms, responsiveness of the patient, and occurrence of side effects. *Antihistamines* such as dimenhydrinate, meclizine, and promethazine hydrochloride are effective for the control of nausea and vomiting due to motion sickness and other inner-ear disturbances and may be effective in pregnancy, uremia, and postoperative vomiting; they do not act on the chemoreceptor trigger zone and are of little value in other causes of vomiting. *Anticholinergics* such as scopolamine block central muscarinic receptors in afferent pathways of the vomiting reflex and are also effective in motion sickness. *Phenothiazine* derivatives such as prochlorperazine and the structurally related butyrophenone haloperidol inhibit cerebral dopamine receptors and act principally at the chemoreceptor trigger zone. They are often ineffective for severe nausea and vomiting and have the potential for causing sedation, hypotension, and Parkinson-like effects. *Metoclopramide* is the prototype of selective dopamine antagonists called *substituted benzamides*. Metoclopramide is useful in all types of vomiting except motion sickness and inner-ear dysfunction. In contrast to the phenothiazines, which have anticholinergic effects, metoclopramide has powerful peripheral cholinergic effects that enhance gastric emptying. Metoclopramide may be superior to phenothiazines in the treatment of severe nausea and vomiting and is particularly useful in the treatment of gastroparesis. The usual oral dosage is 5 to 20 mg four times daily, but intravenous doses up to 1 to 3 mg/kg, which also inhibit 5-hydroxytryptamine₃ receptors, may be effective as prophylaxis prior to potent chemotherapeutic agents (e.g., cisplatin). Unfortunately, neurologic side effects are frequent, including drowsiness, dystonic reactions, anxiety, insomnia, depression, parkinsonism, confusion, and a rise in prolactin level. Alternative newer agents such as *cisapride* and *domperidone* (the latter not yet licensed for use in the United States) exert peripheral antiemetic effects without the central nervous system side effects of metoclopramide. Cisapride has cholinomimetic effects but minimal antidopaminergic activity. The standard dose is 10 to 20 mg four times daily, generally before meals and at bedtime. *Glucocorticoids* are often combined with metoclopramide to control nausea and vomiting due to cancer chemotherapy; the mechanism of action may involve inhibition of prostaglandin formation. The sedative *lorazepam* may be added to this regimen. *Tetrahydrocannabinol*, the active ingredient of marijuana, is marketed as dronabinol for the prevention of nausea and vomiting after cancer chemotherapy; the mechanism of action is unknown. *Ondansetron* and *granisetron*, serotonin antagonists that bind to 5-hydroxytryptamine₃ receptors in the chemoreceptor trigger zone and

gut, are particularly effective in preventing chemotherapy-induced nausea and vomiting, especially when combined with intravenous dexamethasone. The recommended dose of ondansetron is 0.15 mg/kg infused intravenously over 15 min and given three times 4 h apart, beginning 30 min before the start of chemotherapy, although lower doses may be effective in some patients. The recommended dose of granisetron is 10 µg/kg intravenously infused over 5 min, beginning 30 min before the start of chemotherapy. The antibiotic *erythromycin*, which binds to motilin receptors in the gut, has been shown in doses as low as 125 mg four times daily to enhance gastric emptying in patients with gastroparesis; however, stimulation of antral contractility by erythromycin leads to abdominal cramps, nausea, and bloating and may limit its usefulness.

INDIGESTION

Indigestion is a term frequently used by patients to describe a variety of symptoms generally appreciated as upper abdominal distress and often associated with the intake of food. The term is nonspecific and may not have the same meaning for the patient and physician. Thus, in approaching the patient with indigestion, it is important for the physician first to elicit a precise description of this complaint. To some patients, indigestion refers to actual abdominal pain or pressure, which may be associated with postprandial fullness, early satiety, nausea, or bloating, and which is generally designated as *dyspepsia*. Others may use the term indigestion to describe either a vague feeling that digestion has not proceeded naturally or that intolerances to specific foods exist. Still others may use it to describe belching, a feeling of excessive gas, or flatulence. When heartburn is the predominant symptom, the patient can be presumed to have *gastroesophageal reflux disease* (see Chap. 283).

After having ascertained the patient's definition of indigestion, it is important to determine (1) the location and duration of the discomfort, (2) the temporal relation of the symptoms to the ingestion of food, and (3) the possible relation of the symptoms to the ingestion of specific types of food (e.g., milk, fatty foods) or drugs.

Indigestion may occur in association with diseases of the gastrointestinal tract or pathologic states in other organ systems. As a result of a systematic clinical and laboratory investigation, a definable pathophysiologic process sometimes can be shown to be responsible for the symptoms in a given case of indigestion. Frequently, however, a clear etiologic explanation for the patient's complaint of indigestion cannot be established, and descriptive designations are applied. For example, the term *nonulcer dyspepsia* is often used to describe ulcerlike symptoms when no ulcer is found. The term *flatulent dyspepsia* is used when belching, abdominal distention, and early satiety are prominent symptoms; the term *dysmotility-like dyspepsia* has been applied to the same constellation of symptoms. Unfortunately, these terms do not imply that the symptoms described are attributable to a particular pathogenic process. The term *functional dyspepsia* is used interchangeably with nonulcer dyspepsia when clinical evaluation fails to reveal an explanation for indigestion. In some cases of functional dyspepsia, sophisticated testing of gastrointestinal electrical activity and manometric studies may reveal disturbances of gastrointestinal motility, although the cause-and-effect relationship between such findings and the patient's symptoms may be difficult to prove. Indeed, some patients with functional dyspepsia also have features of the irritable bowel syndrome, suggesting a diffuse intestinal motility disturbance (see Chap. 287).

SYNDROMES COMMONLY DESCRIBED AS INDIGESTION **Pain** A careful elucidation of the pattern of pain may provide important diagnostic information. Visceral abdominal pain is mediated by visceral afferent nerves that accompany the abdominal sympathetic pathways (see Chap. 14). Visceral pain is described as dull and aching in nature, with a diffuse midline localization, or as fullness or pressure. The location of the discomfort generally corresponds to the segmental level of neural innervation of the affected organ. Abdominal visceral pain, which can be produced experimentally by artificially increasing pressure in a hollow viscus, results from distention or exaggerated muscular contraction of the viscus. Inflammation generally lowers the threshold for pain from such stimuli.

The visceral pain of indigestion should be distinguished from the sharp, localized pain patterns of many acute abdominal processes involving the peritoneum. In contrast to visceral pain, this somatic pain is mediated by cerebrospinal afferent nerves.

In view of the diffuse nature of visceral abdominal pain, the main clue to the cause comes from the *location* of the pain and the corresponding segmental level of neural innervation; however, in any given segmental region there is no way of determining which of several viscera is the source of the pain (Table 41-1). The following rules, already described in Chap. 14, are useful: *Substernal pain* of gastrointestinal origin usually arises from disorders of the esophagus or cardia of the stomach. Because pain in this area can emanate from the heart, cardiac disease must be carefully considered and excluded. *Epigastric pain* is generally of gastric, duodenal, biliary, or pancreatic origin. (The epigastrium is also a frequent location for "functional" pain.) As pathologic processes in the biliary tract or pancreas become more intense, pain may lateralize and localize, e.g., biliary pain to the right upper quadrant and tip of the scapula and pancreatic pain to the left upper quadrant and back. *Periumbilical pain* is generally associated with disease involving the small intestine. *Pain below the umbilicus* is often of appendiceal, colonic, or pelvic origin.

The unraveling of the *temporal relationships* of the patient's symptoms often provides additional diagnostic clues. It is important to ascertain whether the symptoms are *constant* (continually present over extended periods of time), as may occur with an infiltrating gastric carcinoma, or *intermittent*, as in acute gastritis or biliary colic. The symptoms may have a *diurnal* pattern, as in reflux esophagitis in which pain often occurs nocturnally and with recumbency. Pain that awakens the patient from a sound sleep may occur with duodenal ulcer. Occasionally symptoms are *seasonal*, as in peptic ulcer disease, in which some patients experience more discomfort in the spring and autumn than at other times.

Another helpful diagnostic feature is the relation of pain to *food ingestion*. Early postprandial symptoms may reflect esophageal disease, acute gastritis, or gastric carcinoma. Late postprandial indiges-

tion, i.e., occurring several hours after eating, may reflect failure of the stomach to empty adequately, as in gastric outlet obstruction, gastroparesis and other disorders of gastric motility, or duodenal ulcer, in which case pain results from exposure of ulcerated mucosa to acid secreted by the stomach and unbuffered by food. Conversely, the relief of pain following ingestion of food or antacids is characteristic of duodenal ulcer and is presumably due to the neutralization of acid. Late postprandial indigestion also may result from impaired digestive and absorptive processes, as in pancreatic insufficiency.

It is important to recognize that the pain patterns and relationships to the intake of food described above are generalizations, and many cases do not conform to classic "textbook" descriptions. For example, although pain limited to the right upper quadrant is often caused by gallbladder disease, about half of patients with this condition experience only epigastric pain. Similarly, there are some patients with duodenal ulcer whose pain is not relieved by food or antacids, while there are other patients with functional indigestion and even gastric carcinoma whose pain improves with food or antacids.

Nonulcer Dyspepsia Nonulcer dyspepsia refers to symptoms that suggest a diagnosis of peptic ulcer despite the documented absence of an ulcer by endoscopy or barium x-ray studies and the absence of any other demonstrable organic disorder (e.g., biliary tract disease) or evidence of the irritable bowel syndrome to account for the symptoms. Nonulcer dyspepsia is at least twice as common as peptic ulcer and may affect 20 to 30 percent of the population. Only 20 to 30 percent of patients with dyspepsia seek medical care. The pathogenesis of nonulcer dyspepsia is poorly understood; most patients have normal gastric acid secretion, and a relation between nonulcer dyspepsia and duodenitis or duodenal ulcer has not been demonstrated. Similarly, a role for *Helicobacter pylori* and associated chronic gastritis in causing dyspeptic symptoms in persons without peptic ulcer is unproven (see Chap. 284). Disordered gastroduodenal and small-intestinal motility appears to account for some cases of nonulcer dyspepsia. Between 25 and 50 percent of patients with nonulcer dyspepsia have postprandial antral hypomotility and delayed gastric emptying. Moreover, 50 percent experience abdominal discomfort in response to balloon distention at volumes lower than those that provoke pain in healthy controls, suggesting visceral hypersensitivity.

Heartburn Heartburn, or pyrosis, is a sensation of warmth or burning located substernally or high in the epigastrium with radiation into the neck and occasionally to the arms. Occasional heartburn is common in normal persons, but frequent and severe heartburn is generally a manifestation of esophageal dysfunction. Heartburn may result from abnormal motor activity or distention of the esophagus, sensitivity of the esophageal mucosa to refluxed acid or bile, or esophageal mucosal inflammation (esophagitis).

Heartburn is most often associated with gastroesophageal reflux (see Chap. 283). In this setting, heartburn typically occurs after a large meal, with stooping or bending, or when the patient is supine. It may be accompanied by the spontaneous appearance in the mouth of fluid which may be salty ("water brash"), sour (gastric contents), or bitter and green or yellow (bile). Heartburn may arise following the ingestion of certain foods (e.g., citrus fruit juices) or drugs (e.g., alcohol and aspirin). Characteristically, heartburn is alleviated promptly, even if only temporarily, by antacids.

Food Intolerance In some persons, specific foods or types of foods appear to be related to indigestion. Careful documentation of this relationship is sometimes of great help in arriving at an etiologic diagnosis.

Some foods may be poorly tolerated because of their consistency. Patients with esophageal stricture or carcinoma may tolerate liquids well but may experience discomfort, especially substernal distress, after ingesting solids (see Chaps. 40 and 283). Citrus fruits, perhaps because of their relatively low pH, and spicy foods often provoke symptoms in patients with peptic ulcer disease or peptic esophagitis. Certain foods may be tolerated poorly because of impaired intestinal

Table 41-1

Distribution of Visceral Pain and Examples of Disorders Frequently Involving the Specific Organ

Organ	Common Location of Pain	Examples of Disorders
Esophagus	Substernum, epigastrium	Peptic esophagitis, stricture, esophageal motility disorder, carcinoma
Stomach	Epigastrium	Gastric ulcer, gastritis, carcinoma
Duodenum (first and second portions)	Epigastrium	Duodenal ulcer
Small intestine (excluding first and second portions of duodenum)	Periumbilical region	Infectious gastroenteritis, Crohn's disease, lymphoma, intestinal obstruction
Gallbladder	Epigastrium, right upper quadrant, right upper back	Cholelithiasis, cholecystitis
Pancreas	Epigastrium, left upper quadrant, left side of back	Pancreatitis, pancreatic carcinoma
Liver	Right upper quadrant	Hepatitis, cirrhosis, passive congestion
Colon	Below umbilicus	Infectious colitis, ulcerative or Crohn's colitis, carcinoma, partial obstruction

digestion or absorption, as with the ingestion of fatty foods in patients with pancreatic or biliary tract disease.

Patients may have a congenital or acquired *deficiency of a specific enzyme* required for intestinal absorption of a certain nutrient. One example is the deficiency of lactase, the intestinal mucosal enzyme that catalyzes the hydrolysis of lactose. In persons who are lactase-deficient, the ingestion of milk (which contains lactose) results in abdominal cramps, distention, diarrhea, and flatulence (Chap. 285). Sucrose may lead to similar symptoms in persons with hereditary sucrase-isomaltase deficiency. Certain nutrients may lead to profound systemic effects because of *biochemical defects* in the patient that render the substances particularly hazardous, as in galactose intolerance in persons with galactosemia (see Chap. 351).

Some foods or food additives may initiate *allergic reactions*, which should be suspected when symptoms occur after ingestion of a specific food, recur on challenge testing, and are associated with other features of an allergic reaction, such as lip swelling, urticaria, angioedema, asthma, or, rarely, anaphylactic shock. Acute IgE-mediated reactions are most commonly associated with cow's milk (in infants), shellfish, wheat, eggs, nuts, and chocolate and may be confirmed by the radioallergosorbent test in some cases. Delayed hypersensitivity reactions also may occur; may be associated with less severe symptoms, including joint and muscle pain, fatigue, serous otitis, and altered spacial perception; and are more difficult to relate to specific foods. Some foods may exert *toxic effects* on the intestine in susceptible persons (e.g., gluten in patients with celiac sprue).

In many instances we do not understand the mechanism by which indigestion is associated with the ingestion of specific foods. Thus a history of fatty food intolerance or distress after eating spicy foods is commonly obtained from patients with indigestion; however, the mechanisms leading to these symptoms in these circumstances are often unclear.

Aerophagia In patients with a complaint of *chronic, repetitive eructation* (belching), each belch can often be observed to be preceded by a swallow of air, most of which passes only partway down the esophagus and is then regurgitated. Thus excessive eructation usually results from *aerophagia*, or air swallowing, not from excessive gas production in the stomach or the intestine. A degree of aerophagia occurs in normal persons, but some individuals gulp air excessively because of chronic anxiety, rapid eating, drinking carbonated beverages or any beverage through a straw, gum chewing, sucking on hard candy, smoking cigarettes, postnasal drip, poorly fitting dentures, or esophageal speech. Because eructation that follows aerophagia may provide temporary relief to the patient, a vicious cycle of aerophagia and eructation may ensue.

About 20 to 60 percent of intestinal gas represents swallowed air. Because nitrogen and oxygen are the only gases present in the atmosphere in appreciable concentrations, and because they are not produced in the gastrointestinal tract, their detection on chromatographic analysis of intestinal gas indicates that swallowed air is the source. Swallowed air that is not eructated passes into the stomach and intestine. Accumulation of swallowed air in the stomach may lead to postprandial fullness and pressure and the finding by x-ray of a large amount of air in the gastric fundus. This symptom complex, referred to as the *magenblase* (i.e., gastric bubble) *syndrome*, may occur when a patient lies supine after a large meal, thereby permitting gastric air to be "trapped" below the gastroesophageal junction by overlying fluid and unable to be eructated. Inability to eructate is also thought to underlie the "gas-bloat" syndrome observed after surgical repair of a hiatal hernia. Acute gastric distention by swallowed air can sometimes produce sharp pain, which may mimic angina pectoris. Swallowed air that successfully passes the stomach may either produce diffuse abdominal distention or become trapped in the splenic flexure of the colon. The latter condition, or *splenic flexure syndrome*, is characterized by a sensation of left upper quadrant fullness and pressure with radiation to the left side of the chest. Relief of pain often follows defecation or the expulsion of flatus. The diagnosis is suggested by the finding of increased tympany in the extreme left lateral portion of the upper abdomen on physical examination or of large amounts of air in the splenic flexure of the colon on a plain abdominal radiograph.

Gaseousness, Bloating, and Flatulence Despite the widely held belief that feelings of *diffuse abdominal pain and bloating* are often caused by excessive quantities of intestinal gas, studies employing an intestinal gas wash-out technique suggest that patients complaining of excessive gas actually have normal volumes of intestinal gas. In some cases, the primary abnormality causing functional bloating and pain appears to be a motility disturbance that causes the patient to perceive pain with an intestinal gas volume that is well tolerated by normal subjects. Alternatively, intestinal motility may be normal in such persons, but they may be excessively sensitive to normal impulses arising from the intestinal tract (visceral hypersensitivity).

A major source of intestinal gas is the fermentative action of intestinal bacteria on carbohydrates and proteins within the lumen. Normally such bacteria are limited to the colon, and the principal gases produced are carbon dioxide and hydrogen (in addition to minute quantities of odoriferous gases—indoles, skatols, and sulfur-containing compounds—which give flatus its characteristic odor). In the upper small bowel carbon dioxide is also produced when hydrochloric acid from the stomach or ingested fatty acids are neutralized by bicarbonate. (This may explain, in part, indigestion associated with fatty foods.) About one-third of adults produce appreciable quantities of methane in the colon; this appears to be a familial trait and unrelated to ingestion of specific foods.

An increase in intraluminal gas production resulting in *abdominal distention, bloating, and flatulence* occurs following the ingestion of certain foods, such as legumes and some grains, that contain significant quantities of nonabsorbable complex carbohydrates that pass into the colon, where they supply gas-forming substrates for colonic bacteria. The best-studied example of this is beans, which contain oligosaccharides (stachyose and raffinose) that cannot be split by intestinal mucosal enzymes but are metabolized by colonic bacteria. Less well appreciated is that fructose, a natural or added sweetener in fruit (particularly figs, dates, prunes, and grapes), fruit juices and soft drinks, and present in oligosaccharides in onions, asparagus, and wheat, may be incompletely absorbed in the small intestine and thereby contribute to abdominal distention, bloating, and flatulence. [In contrast, intestinal absorption of fructose is more likely to be complete when fructose is mixed with glucose or ingested as sucrose (glucose-fructose).] Intestinal malabsorption of sorbitol may underlie symptoms of abdominal distention, gaseousness, and diarrhea associated with certain fruits or when sorbitol is used as a sweetener in "sugar-free" gums and candies or as an "inert" ingredient in some medications. Increased intraluminal gas production also may result from abnormal bacterial colonization of the small intestine (bacterial overgrowth syndrome) or infection with *Giardia lamblia*.

Indigestion due to Extraintestinal Disease A number of extraintestinal diseases may lead to indigestion. Thus indigestion may be prominent in congestive heart failure, pulmonary tuberculosis, neoplastic disease, and uremia. Also, a variety of drugs such as aspirin, nonsteroidal anti-inflammatory agents, and glucocorticoids may cause indigestion because of their ulcerogenic properties.

Approach to the Patient

Indigestion represents a challenging and difficult diagnostic problem because of its nonspecific nature. It is essential to obtain a clear and detailed description of the specific symptoms, particularly the patient's definition of the term *indigestion*. The nature of the distress, its frequency and time of occurrence, its relationship to meals, and the special circumstances that lead to its exacerbation or relief should be elicited. Associated intestinal symptoms such as nausea and vomiting, abnormal bowel habits, diarrhea, steatorrhea, and melena should be sought, and an assessment of nutritional status, appetite, and changes in weight should be made. A careful history also should include an assessment of the patient's general health, including the possible presence of extraintestinal disorders that may produce indigestion. A careful dietary history is essential, and asking the patient to keep a diary of foods eaten may prove revealing. Similarly, the patient's medications should be reviewed, particularly for agents that may slow gut transit such as narcotics, anticholinergics, and calcium antagonists. Psychological factors may play an etiologic or contributory role, and the presence of anxiety, depressive symptoms, or hysteria should be noted.

Physical examination rarely establishes the specific diagnosis but may be useful in detecting diseases in other organ systems that can affect intestinal function (e.g., congestive heart failure). Stools should be examined for appearance and occult blood.

Whether further diagnostic studies are indicated depends on the specific nature of the patient's complaints and the patient's age (concern about the possibility of gastrointestinal malignancy being greater in older patients). Abdominal pain may be evaluated with radiologic and imaging studies of the esophagus, stomach, small intestine, colon, pancreas, and biliary tract. Esophagogastroscopy, endoscopic cholangiopancreatography, sigmoidoscopy, or colonoscopy may be considered depending on the specific symptoms. On the other hand, in patients under age 40 with epigastric pain typical of peptic ulcer, routine diagnostic studies are unlikely to disclose serious diseases (such as gastric carcinoma) and are often in fact negative; additional options in such patients include serologic testing for *H. pylori* and empiric treatment with "triple therapy" (a bismuth compound and two antibiotics) in persons who are seropositive or an empiric trial of antacids, H_2-receptor–blocking drugs, or sucralfate (see Chap. 284). In contrast to peptic ulcer, nonulcer dyspepsia improves inconsistently following antacids and other standard ulcer therapy. Esophagogastroscopy may be reserved for patients with symptoms that persist despite therapy or that recur soon after therapy is discontinued. However, in patients with *H. pylori* on endoscopic antral biopsy and no other explanation for indigestion (e.g., no ulcer), eradication of *H. pylori* has not been demonstrated in controlled trials to be of benefit. In fact, the cost-effective approach to the evaluation of dyspepsia, including the relative merits of initial endoscopy versus empiric therapy and the choice of empiric therapy, is still debated. In general, most authorities do not recommend treatment to eradicate *H. pylori* unless a peptic ulcer is confirmed (see Chap. 284). A suggested algorithm for the management of the patient with dyspepsia is shown in Fig. 41-1.

In individuals complaining of excessive eructation, the simple demonstration that aerophagia reproduces the symptoms may suffice to confirm the diagnosis and hopefully break the habit. Patients complaining of excessive gas, bloating, distention, and flatulence must be questioned carefully about dietary preferences and the relation of symptoms to ingestion of specific foods. In some cases, elimination of certain foods (e.g., milk, legumes) from the diet followed by rechallenge may be confirmatory. In other cases, a more detailed assessment, including stool examination for fat and muscle fibers and for parasites such as *G. lamblia*, breath tests to detect carbohydrate malabsorption or bacterial overgrowth, esophageal manometry and ambulatory pH monitoring, measurement of the rate of gastric emptying of a solid meal, and gastrointestinal motility studies, may be desirable. When no precise explanation for gaseousness can be identified, trials of activated charcoal to reduce gaseousness associated with carbohydrate malabsorption or simethicone to alter the elasticity of gas bubbles may be considered, although their value is uncertain.

In many cases of indigestion no clear explanation is obtained, even after careful diagnostic studies and therapeutic trials. Some cases represent gastrointestinal motility disturbances, perhaps due to subtle physiologic derangements not detectable by currently available methods. In some such instances, it may be beneficial to implement an empiric trial of a gastric prokinetic agent (e.g., cisapride, metoclopramide), which augments gastrointestinal motility. Other cases represent early stages of disease processes that may only be diagnosed by conventional methods at a later date. Still others are psychogenic and may respond to appropriate psychiatric measures. The ultimate evaluation of indigestion requires, therefore, the utmost in sensitivity, diligence, and concern on the part of the examining physician.

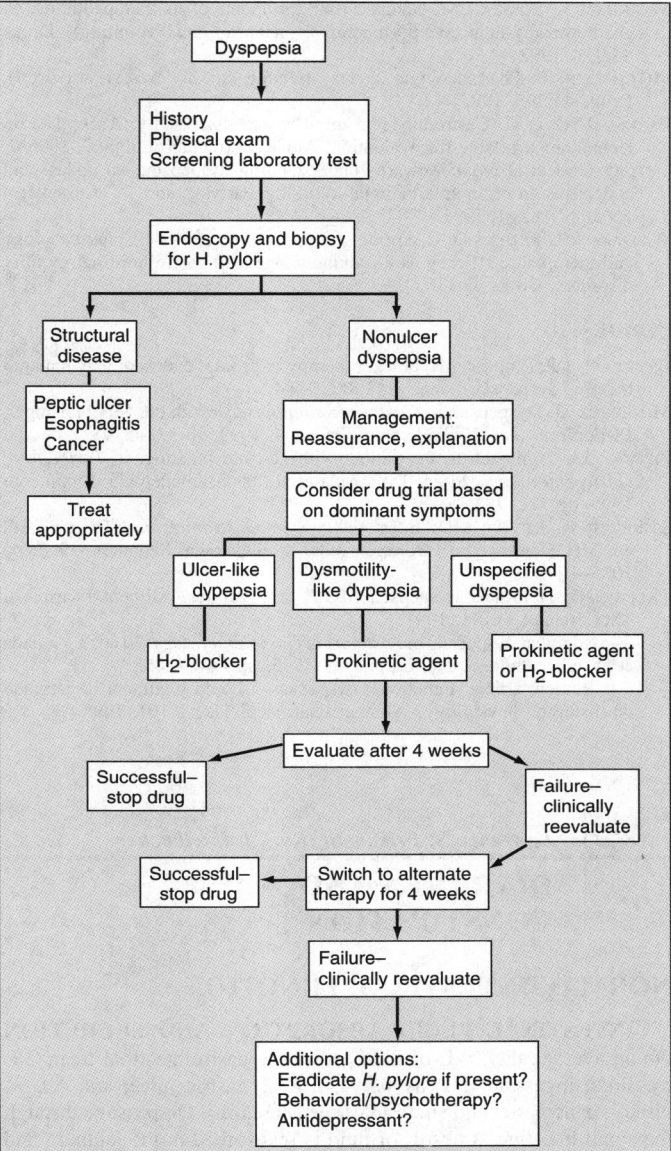

FIGURE 41-1   A suggested approach to the patent with dyspepsia. [Adapted from Talley NJ. Nonulcer dyspepsia, in *Textbook of Gastroenterology*, 2d ed, Yamada T et al (eds). Philadelphia, Lippincott, 1995, p. 1453.]

For further information, see Chap. 38 Agents affecting gastrointestinal water flux and motility, in Goodman and Gilman's The Pharmacological Basis of Therapeutics, *9th ed, New York, McGraw Hill, 1996.*

BIBLIOGRAPHY

NAUSEA AND VOMITING

GRUNBERG SM, HESKETH PJ: Control of chemotherapy-induced emesis. N Engl J Med 329:1790, 1993

KOCH KL: Approach to the patient with nausea and vomiting, in *Textbook of Gastroenterology*, 2d ed, T Yamada et al (eds). Philadelphia, Lippincott, 1995, pp 731–782

LEE M, FELDMAN M: Nausea and vomiting, in *Gastrointestinal Disease*, 5th ed, MH Sleisenger, JS Fordtran (eds). Philadelphia, Saunders, 1993, pp 509–523

MARKHAM A, SORKIN EM: Ondansetron: An update of its therapeutic use in chemotherapy-induced postoperative nausea and vomiting. Drugs 45:931, 1993

MITCHELSON F: Pharmacologic agents affecting emesis: A review (part I). Drugs 43:295, 1992

PARKMAN HP et al: Gastroduodenal motility and dysmotility: An update on techniques available for evaluation. Am J Gastroenterol 90:869, 1995

TYTGAT GNJ et al (eds): Towards understanding dyspepsia: An update and concensus from an International Working Party. Scand J Gastroenterol 26(suppl 182):1, 1991

WISEMAN LR, FAULDS D: Cisapride: An updated review of its pharmacology and therapeutic efficacy as a prokinetic agent in gastrointestinal motility disorders. Drugs 47:116, 1994

INDIGESTION

BYTZER P et al: Empirical H$_2$ blocker therapy or prompt endoscopy in management of dyspepsia. Lancet 343:811, 1994

MISIEWICZ JJ: Dyspepsia, in *Gastrointestinal Disease*, 5th ed, MH Sleisinger, JS Fordtran (eds). Philadelphia, Saunders, 1993, pp 572–579

PERMAN JA: Approach to the patient with gas and bloating, in *Textbook of Gastroenterology*, 2d ed, T Yamada et al (eds). Philadelphia, Lippincott, 1995, pp 772–782

STROCCHI A, LEVITT MD: Intestinal gas, in *Gastrointestinal Disease*, 5th ed, MH Sleisenger, JS Fordtran (eds). Philadelphia, Saunders, 1993, pp 1035–1042

TALLEY NJ: Non-ulcer dyspepsia: Myths and realities. Aliment Pharmacol Ther 5(suppl 1):145, 1991

————: Nonulcer dyspepsia, in *Textbook of Gastroenterology*, 2d ed, T Yamada et al (eds). Philadelphia, Lippincott, 1995, pp 1446–1455

————: Review article: Functional dyspepsia—should treatment be targeted on disturbed physiology? Aliment Pharmacol Ther 9:107, 1995

42   *Lawrence S. Friedman, Kurt J. Isselbacher*

DIARRHEA AND CONSTIPATION

NORMAL INTESTINAL FUNCTION

INTESTINAL FLUID ABSORPTION AND SECRETION

On an average day, 9 L of fluid enters the gastrointestinal tract: 2 L by direct ingestion, 1 L as saliva, 2 L as gastric juice, and 4 L as biliary, pancreatic, and small intestine secretions. On passage through the small intestine, 4 to 5 L of fluid is reabsorbed in the jejunum and 3 to 4 L in the ileum. Therefore, approximately 1 L of residual fluid enters the colon, where an additional 800 mL is reabsorbed before passage to the rectum and evacuation. Overall, the usual amount of fluid excreted in feces is approximately 200 mL/d.

In the intestine, water absorption follows active and passive sodium (Na$^+$) and nutrient absorption (Fig. 42-1). In the small intestine, Na$^+$ is cotransported with chloride (Cl$^-$) and nutrients such as glucose; in the terminal ileum, Na$^+$ is cotransported with bile salts; and in the colon, Na$^+$ is absorbed via Na$^+$ channels and by the electroneutral NaCl absorptive mechanism used in the small intestine. The cotransport mechanisms for Na$^+$ and nutrient absorption depend in part on Na$^+$ gradients across the apical membrane of intestinal epithelial cells created by the Na$^+$, K$^+$-ATPase pump of the basolateral membrane. The most important of these clinically is a Na$^+$-glucose cotransport carrier in the small intestine. Absorption of glucose by this mechanism results in accumulation of glucose in the epithelial cell, followed by its movement across the basolateral membrane by a facilitated transport mechanism, while Na$^+$ is actively pumped across the basolateral membrane by Na$^+$, K$^+$-ATPase. The absorption of Na$^+$ also promotes absorption of Cl$^-$ through a paracellular pathway. Water absorption follows passively to maintain isoosmolality in the intercellular space. Because the Na$^+$-glucose cotransport mechanism remains unaffected by most diarrheal diseases, administration of a glucose-salt solution

is useful clinically for the management of diarrhea and dehydration regardless of the cause.

Other cotransport mechanisms exist. A Na$^+$-Cl$^-$ cotransport mechanism is thought actually to be composed of an Na$^+$-H$^+$ exchange carrier and a Cl$^-$-HCO$_3^-$ exchange carrier. This mechanism permits entry of both Na$^+$ and Cl$^-$ into a cell in exchange for H$^+$ and HCO$_3^-$. Additional transport mechanisms have been identified for potassium (K$^+$), which may be absorbed in exchange for H$^+$, and for calcium (Ca^{2+}), the absorption of which is regulated by vitamin D and 1,25-dihydroxyvitamin D$_3$, parathyroid hormone, calcitonin, and a number of calcium-binding proteins.

In addition to its absorptive function, the intestine has a secretory function. Cl$^-$ can be secreted by intestinal crypt cells via an electrogenic mechanism, with Na$^+$, K$^+$, and water following passively through tight junctions. HCO$_3^-$ is secreted in the duodenum, other parts of the small intestine, and into the bile and pancreatic ducts. Because of the large acid load from the stomach, secreted HCO$_3^-$ is diluted and present in relatively low concentrations. However, in the distal gut, HCO$_3^-$ gradually becomes the predominant anion, permitting conservation of Cl$^-$, presumably via a Cl$^-$-HCO$_3^-$ exchange mechanism at the apical membrane of the epithelial cells. Intracellular cyclic nucleotides and ionized calcium (Ca^{2+}) initiate and regulate active Cl$^-$ secretion.

COLONIC FUNCTION   As in the small intestine, an Na$^+$ absorptive mechanism exists in the colon. Na$^+$ absorption is predominantly electrogenic in that the absorbed Na$^+$ ion is unaccompanied by cation exchange or anion cotransport. Na$^+$ enters colonic epithelial cells through channels in the apical membrane and is pumped out across the basolateral membrane by Na$^+$, K$^+$-ATPase.

A variety of neural and nonneural mediators regulate colonic ion transport and motility, but the precise mechanisms are not well understood. The colon and rectum are innervated by nerve fibers that release norepinephrine, acetylcholine, and other neurotransmitters. Parasympathetic nerves stimulate peristaltic contraction and electrolyte secretion, whereas adrenergic tone inhibits cholinergic stimulation and increases electrolyte absorption. Additional regulation is provided by local reflex arcs within the autonomous enteric nervous system and intrinsic contractile responses of the colonic smooth muscle.

DEFECATION   The defecatory reflex is initiated by acute distention of the rectum, which results in partial and transient relaxation of the internal anal sphincter via parasympathetic innervation. As sigmoid and rectal contractions increase the pressure within the rectum, the rectosigmoid angle created by tonic contraction of the puborectalis muscle, which forms a sling around the anorectal junction, is obliterated. Contraction of the external anal sphincter, which consists of at least three bundles of striated muscle surrounding the anal canal and innervated by the pudendal nerve, can delay defecation until a socially acceptable time. Concomitant relaxation of the internal and external anal sphincters then permits the evacuation of feces, which can be

FIGURE 42-1   Sodium, chloride, and glucose transport by intestinal epithelial cells. Passive and active transport mechanisms for sodium (Na$^+$), chloride (Cl$^-$), and sodium-glucose coupled uptake are shown. Na$^+$ is pumped out at basolateral border by the active ATPase pump; Cl$^-$ in part accompanies Na$^+$ but also is actively extruded by cyclic AMP. TJ, tight junction.

augmented by an increase in intraabdominal pressure created by the Valsalva maneuver.

DIARRHEA

DEFINITION   In developed countries, normal stool weight of an adult human is less than 200 g/d; stool water accounts for 60 to 85 percent of the weight. Normal bowel frequency ranges from three times a week to three times a day. Factors that influence stool weight, consistency, and frequency include the fiber content of the diet, gender (the average daily weight of stool in women is less than that of men), ingested medications, and possibly exercise and stress. *Diarrhea* is formally defined as an increase in daily stool weight above 200 g. Typically, the patient also may describe an abnormal increase in stool liquidity and frequency.

Diarrhea must be distinguished from *pseudodiarrhea* or *hyperdefecation*, which is an increased frequency of defecation without an increase in stool weight above normal, as occurs in patients with irritable bowel syndrome, proctitis, or hyperthyroidism. Diarrhea also must be distinguished from fecal *incontinence*, which is the involuntary release of rectal contents. Incontinence is more common when stool is liquid than solid and reflects abnormal function of the anorectum or pelvic muscles. Diarrhea is considered *acute* when lasting less than 7 to 14 days and *chronic* when lasting more than 2 to 3 weeks.

ACUTE DIARRHEA   The most common causes of acute diarrhea are infectious agents (Table 42-1). Acute diarrhea also may be caused by ingested drugs or toxins, the administration of chemotherapy, resumption of enteral feeding following a prolonged fast, fecal impaction (overflow diarrhea), or particular situations, such as marathon running. Additionally, acute diarrhea may represent the onset of a chronic diarrheal illness.

Table 42-1

Infectious Diarrhea: Pathophysiologic Mechanisms and Causes

Pathophysiologic Mechanism	Examples
Toxin production	
Preformed toxin	*Bacillus cereus*
	Clostridium perfringens
	Staphylococcus aureus
Enterotoxin	*Aeromonas* sp.
	Enterotoxigenic *E. coli*
	Vibrio cholerae
Cytotoxin	*Clostridium difficile*
	E. coli O157:H7
Enteroadherence	Cryptosporidiosis
	Cyclospora sp. (?)
	Enteroadherent and enteropathogenic *E. coli*
	Helminths
	Giardia
Mucosal invasion	
Minimal	Norwalk virus
	Rotavirus
	Other viruses (e.g., adenovirus, astrovirus, calicivirus, coronavirus, cytomegalovirus, herpes simplex virus)
Variable	*Aeromonas* sp.
	Campylobacter sp.
	Salmonella sp.
	Vibrio parahemolyticus
Severe	*Entamoeba histolytica*
	Enteroinvasive *E. coli*
	Shigella sp.
Systemic infection	Legionellosis
	Listeriosis
	Measles
	Psittacosis
	Rocky Mountain spotted fever
	Toxic shock syndrome
	Viral hepatitis

Infectious Diarrhea (see Chaps. 128, 142, 155, and 158 to 161)   Worldwide, acute infectious diarrhea accounts for more than 5 to 8 million deaths each year in children less than age 5, especially in developing nations, where acute infectious diarrhea is a major cause of protein-calorie malnutrition and dehydration. Contributing factors include inadequate sewage disposal and water supplies, lack of refrigeration, overcrowding and lack of personal hygiene, poverty, lack of access to health care, and lack of education. Even in the United States, significant economic loss results from acute infectious diarrhea, which accounts for 250,000 hospital admissions and nearly 8 million office visits to physicians each year.

Most infectious diarrheas are acquired by fecal-oral transmission by way of water or food contaminated by human waste as a result of poor sewage systems or by wild or domestic animal feces in inadequately purified water. Beef, pork, or poultry may be the source of infection (especially with *Escherichia coli* O157:H7) when improperly cooked. Food-preparing surfaces may be contaminated by organisms that are spread to uncooked food. Person-to-person transmission also may occur through aerosolization (Norwalk agent, rotavirus), contamination of hands (*Clostridium difficile*) or surfaces, or sexual activity.

In the United States, groups at particularly high risk of acute infectious diarrhea include travelers to or recently from developing nations, persons who ingest shellfish, male homosexuals (gay bowel syndrome), prostitutes, and intravenous drug users. Persons with AIDS in particular are at risk for a remarkable array of serious enteric infections (Table 42-2). Among children attending day-care centers, acute infectious diarrhea commonly results from person-to-person transmission. The most common organisms involved in day-care outbreaks of diarrhea are *Shigella*, *Giardia lamblia*, and *Cryptosporidium*. Secondary attack rates ranging between 10 and 20 percent represent an important source of infection for parents and siblings. Additional high-risk institutions for outbreaks of acute infectious diarrhea include residential homes for the mentally and developmentally handicapped, nursing homes, and hospitals.

Clinical Features   Patients with acute infectious diarrhea typically present with nausea, vomiting, abdominal pain, fever, and diarrhea, which may be watery, malabsorptive, or bloody, depending on the specific pathogen (see Table 42-1). Patients ingesting *toxins* or those with *toxigenic infection* typically have nausea and vomiting as prominent symptoms but rarely a high fever. Abdominal pain is mild, diffuse, and crampy and results from the high volumes of secreted fluid that stimulate peristalsis and cause watery diarrhea. Vomiting

Table 42-2

Possible Causes of Diarrhea in Patients with AIDS

Nonopportunistic pathogens
Shigella
Salmonella
Campylobacter
Entamoeba histolytica
Chlamydia
Neisseria gonorrhoeae
Treponema pallidum and other spirochetes
Giardia lamblia
Opportunistic infections
Protozoa
Cryptosporidium
Isospora belli
Microsporidia
Blastocystis hominis
Viruses
Cytomegalovirus
Herpes simplex
Adenovirus
Human immunodeficiency virus
Bacteria
Mycobacterium avium complex

that begins within several hours of ingesting a food should suggest food poisoning due to a preformed toxin. Parasites that do not invade the intestinal mucosa such as *Giardia lamblia* and *Cryptosporidium* usually cause only mild abdominal discomfort. *Giardia* also may be associated with mild steatorrhea, gaseousness, and bloating. *Invasive bacteria* such as *Campylobacter*, *Salmonella*, and *Shigella* and organisms that produce cytotoxins such as *C. difficile* and enterohemorrhagic *E. coli* (serotype O157:H7) cause severe intestinal inflammation, abdominal pain, and often a high fever; occasionally, peritoneal signs may suggest a surgical abdomen. *Yersinia* often infects the terminal ileum and cecum and presents with right lower quadrant pain and tenderness suggestive of acute appendicitis. Watery diarrhea is typical of organisms that invade the intestinal epithelium with *minimal inflammation*, such as enteric viruses, or organisms that *adhere* to but do not destroy the epithelium, such as enteropathogenic or enteroadherent *E. coli*, protozoa, and helminths. Some organisms such as *Campylobacter*, *Aeromonas*, *Shigella*, and *Vibrio* species (e.g., *Vibrio parahemolyticus* and *V. fulnifice*) both produce enterotoxins and invade the intestinal mucosa; patients therefore often present with watery diarrhea followed within hours or days by bloody diarrhea.

The presence of systemic symptoms may provide additional clues to the underlying cause of diarrhea. Both shigellosis and infection with enterohemorrhagic *E. coli* may be accompanied by the hemolytic-uremic syndrome, particularly in persons who are very young or very old. *Yersinia* infection and occasionally other enteric bacterial infections may be accompanied by Reiter's syndrome (arthritis, urethritis, and conjunctivitis), thyroiditis, pericarditis, or glomerulonephritis.

Differential Diagnosis Virtually any *medication* can cause diarrhea, and a careful drug history should be obtained in any patient with acute diarrhea (Table 42-3). Other ingested toxins also must be considered, including organophosphate insecticides, mushrooms, arsenic, and even caffeine. *Acute diverticulitis* occasionally may present with diarrhea accompanied by fever and abdominal pain (see Chap. 288). In patients with acute bloody diarrhea, diagnostic considerations may include *superior mesenteric arterial* or *venous thrombosis*, *ischemic* or *drug-induced colitis*, or *idiopathic inflammatory bowel disease* (ulcerative colitis or Crohn's disease) (see Chap. 286). In the elderly patient with acute colitis, differentiating an ischemic cause from enterohemorrhagic *E. coli* O157:H7 may be difficult because both diseases may be associated with submucosal hemorrhage that presents as "thumbprinting" on a plain abdominal radiograph. While colonoscopic and radiographic findings may be indistinguishable in infectious colitis and inflammatory bowel disease, histologic findings may be helpful

in suggesting one diagnosis or the other, since the inflammatory infiltrate in acute infectious diarrhea consists mainly of polymorphonuclear leukocytes rather than the chronic inflammatory infiltrate with crypt distortion typical of inflammatory bowel disease. The finding of pseudomembranes on colonoscopy points to *C. difficile* as the cause.

Laboratory Diagnosis Acute infectious diarrhea is usually self-limited, often resolving by the time the patient seeks medical attention. Because of the expense of stool cultures and other diagnostic tests, considerable judgment is required in deciding which patients with acute diarrhea should be evaluated and treated with antibiotics. For the patient presenting without high fever, bloody diarrhea, or dehydration, symptomatic therapy with oral fluids in the absence of specific diagnostic testing may suffice. On the other hand, a high fever, systemic toxicity, bloody diarrhea, and dehydration favor diagnostic testing, as do a known outbreak of food poisoning, recent overseas travel, immunocompromise, male homosexuality, or recent antibiotic use. In these situations, freshly collected stool should be examined for *occult blood* and *white blood cells*. The finding of primarily polymorphonuclear leukocytes on a Wright's or methylene blue stain suggests *Salmonella*, *Shigella*, invasive *E. coli*, *Yersinia*, or *Entamoeba histolytica*. Although it is common practice to obtain a qualitative fecal fat determination in patients with acute diarrhea, the presence of a small amount of fat in the stool is not uncommon in patients with acute diarrhea of any cause and provides no particular diagnostic information. The cornerstone of diagnosis in patients with severe and especially bloody diarrhea or a suggestive epidemiologic history is *bacterial culture* and *microscopic examination* of the stool for ova and parasites. Most laboratories routinely examine stool specimens sent for culture for *Salmonella*, *Shigella*, *Yersinia*, and *Campylobacter*, but special requests must be made to identify other organisms, including *C. difficile* (culture and toxin) and enterohemorrhagic *E. coli*. Special cultivation or staining techniques also may be required to identify organisms that cause watery diarrhea, including *Aeromonas*, *Cryptosporidium*, and *Vibrio* species. Certain organisms such as *Giardia* and *Strongyloides* as well as *Cryptosporidium* and *Isospora belli* may be difficult to detect in stool and are better diagnosed by *duodenal aspiration* or intestinal biopsy. Alternatively, a sensitive and specific enzyme-linked immunosorbent assay for *Giardia* antigen in stool may be used to confirm giardiasis. In patients with AIDS, electron microscopic examination of small intestinal biopsy specimens may facilitate detection of Microsporidia. *Sigmoidoscopy* and occasionally *colonoscopy* are generally reserved for patients with bloody diarrhea that does not improve within 10 days. As discussed above, mucosal changes may be nonspecific, although in some cases characteristic findings may be observed, such as pseudomembranes in *C. difficile*–induced colitis. *Barium radiographs* are also best deferred until the initial course of illness has been observed and appropriate stool specimens obtained. Even with the application of all available laboratory studies, between 20 and 40 percent of all acute infectious diarrheas remain undiagnosed.

Table 42-3

Drugs That Commonly Cause Diarrhea

Gastrointestinal drugs	Hypolipidemic agents
Magnesium-containing antacids	Clofibrate
Laxatives	Gemfibrozil
Misoprostol	Lovastatin
Olsalazine	Probucol
Cardiac drugs	Neuropsychiatric drugs
Digitalis	Lithium
Quinidine	Fluoxetine (Prozac)
Procainamide	Alprazolam (Xanax)
Hydralazine	Valproic acid
Beta blockers	Ethosuximide
Angiotensin-converting enzyme	L-Dopa
inhibitors	Others
Diuretics	Theophylline
Antibiotics	Thyroid hormones
Clindamycin	Colchicine
Ampicillin	Nonsteroidal anti-
Cephalosporins	inflammatory drugs
Erythromycin	
Chemotherapeutic agents	

℞ TREATMENT

General and nonspecific treatment of acute infectious diarrhea includes rest and fluid replacement. Because death in most instances of acute diarrhea results from dehydration, careful attention must be paid to correction of fluid and electrolyte deficits. Intravenous fluid therapy may be necessary in severely dehydrated individuals, especially infants and the elderly. Oral sugar-electrolyte solutions used in the treatment of patients with cholera can also be considered in patients with acute diarrhea due to other enterotoxin-producing bacteria. Antibiotic therapy in bacterial diarrheas is controversial and generally not necessary in patients with mild or resolving disease but should be considered in patients with shigellosis, traveler's diarrhea, pseudomembranous enterocolitis, cholera, and parasitic diseases. Regardless of the cause of infectious diarrhea, patients should be treated if they are immunocompromised, have a malignancy, have an abnormal heart valve or vascular or orthopedic prosthesis, have hemolytic anemia, or are extremely young or old. Anticholinergic drugs and opiates to control diarrhea should generally be avoided when an enteroinvasive organism is suspected because of the risk of prolonging colonization or causing ileus. However, loperamide and bismuth subsalicylate have been shown to be safe in patients with traveler's diarrhea who have neither a high fever nor blood or pus in the stool.

CHRONIC DIARRHEA Diarrhea that persists for weeks or months, whether constant or intermittent, requires evaluation. Although in the majority of cases the cause will prove to be irritable bowel syndrome, diarrhea may represent a manifestation of an underlying serious illness, and a careful search for disease should be undertaken. Chronic diarrhea can be categorized pathophysiologically as inflammatory, osmotic (malabsorption), secretory, due to intestinal dysmotility, or factitious (Table 42-4).

Inflammatory Diarrhea Inflammatory diarrheas are characterized generally by the presence of fever, abdominal tenderness, and blood or leukocytes in the stool, with inflammatory lesions on intestinal mucosal biopsy. In some cases, hypoalbuminemia, hypoglobulinemia, and protein-losing enteropathy may be present. In addition to inflammation, the mechanism of diarrhea may also be malabsorption or increased intestinal secretion.

In a patient who is not systemically ill, a liquid stool containing overt or occult blood raises the possibility of a *colonic neoplasm*. Patients with *ulcerative proctitis* also may present in this manner. In a patient who is systemically ill with chronic bloody diarrhea, the diagnosis of *inflammatory bowel disease* (either *ulcerative colitis* or *Crohn's disease*) is suggested. These disorders also should be suspected when chronic diarrhea is associated with prominent extraintestinal manifestations, including arthritis, skin lesions (such as erythema nodosum or pyoderma gangrenosum), uveitis, or vasculitis. Diarrhea in inflammatory bowel disease may result from damage to absorptive surface epithelium as well as the release into the circulation of secretagogues such as leukotrienes, prostaglandins, histamine, and other cytokines that stimulate intestinal secretion or the enteric nervous system.

Inflammatory diarrhea is seen in patients with *chronic radiation enterocolitis* as a result of pelvic irradiation for malignancies of the female urogenital tract or the male prostate. The segments usually involved are the terminal ileum, cecum, and rectosigmoid because they are fixed in the pelvis. The risk of radiation enterocolitis correlates with the radiation dose; the frequency is 1 to 5 percent with doses of 45 to 50 Gy (4500 to 5500 rad) and 35 percent with higher doses. Chronic radiation injury is characterized by progressive swelling of the endothelial cells in small arterioles of the submucosa leading to obliterative endarteritis and vascular thrombosis and resulting in ischemia with fibrosis, bowel wall thickening, ulceration, and fissuring of the mucosa. Colonoscopy may show luminal narrowing, ulceration, diffuse inflammatory changes, and characteristic mucosal telangiectases which may bleed severely. Diarrhea also may result from bile acid malabsorption because of ileal inflammation or bacterial overgrowth resulting from intestinal strictures or stasis.

Eosinophilic gastroenteritis is characterized by infiltration of any portion of the gastrointestinal tract with eosinophils. In addition to diarrhea, patients present with abdominal pain, nausea, vomiting, weight loss, and, in 75 percent of cases, peripheral eosinophilia; some patients may develop steatorrhea and protein-losing enteropathy. Severe *protein-losing enteropathy* is manifested by peripheral edema, ascites, and occasionally anasarca. It may occur in a variety of disease states, including infections (viral gastroenteritis, bacterial overgrowth, parasitic infestation, *C. difficile* enterocolitis, or Whipple's disease), inflammatory bowel disease, splanchnic congestion due to congestive heart failure, lymphoma, or other conditions associated with lymphatic obstruction, such as congenital intestinal lymphangiectasia, Ménétrier's disease, systemic lupus erythematosus, or milk allergy. Recently, an increasing number of infectious causes of chronic diarrhea have been associated with infection caused by the human immunodeficiency virus (HIV) or with AIDS (see Table 39-2 and Chap. 308). In many patients with AIDS and diarrhea, multiple potential pathogens may be present in the stool, although the exact cause of diarrhea may be uncertain because such pathogens may also be found in the stool of AIDS patients without diarrhea. HIV itself is also thought to cause diarrhea in some cases (AIDS enteropathy), but the mechanism is not understood.

Other miscellaneous diseases associated with inflammatory diarrhea include *Behçet's syndrome* and *graft-versus-host disease* following allogeneic bone marrow transplantation.

Osmotic Diarrhea (See Chap. 285) Osmotic diarrhea occurs when an orally ingested solute is not fully absorbed in the small intestine and thereby exerts an osmotic force that draws fluid into the intestinal lumen. The increased luminal fluid volume overwhelms the capacity of the colon for reabsorption. The nonabsorbed solute can be a maldigested or malabsorbed nutrient or drug. Clinical symptoms are usually recognized because of the malabsorption of *fat (steatorrhea)* or *carbohydrates*. Protein or *amino acid* malabsorption (*azotorrhea*) is generally not recognized clinically unless it is severe enough to cause malnutrition or the consequences of a specific deficiency in an amino acid. The various disorders associated with malabsorption and maldigestion are discussed in more detail in other chapters, specifically, mucosal malabsorptive disorders in Chap. 285 and pancreatic exocrine deficiency and related disorders in Chap. 304.

Table 42-4

Classification of Chronic Diarrhea

Mechanism	Clinical Features	Examples
INFLAMMATORY		
Mucosal and submucosal inflammation Damaged epithelium In some cases impaired intestinal absorption and excessive secretion	Fever, abdominal pain, blood and/or leukocytes in stool	Ulcerative colitis Crohn's disease Radiation enterocolitis Eosinophilic gastroenteritis Infections associated with AIDS
OSMOTIC		
Nonabsorbed or nondigested intraluminal solute	Improvement of diarrhea with fasting Bulky, greasy, foul-smelling stools; weight loss Nutrient deficiencies Osmotic gap in fecal water	Pancreatic insufficiency Bacterial overgrowth Celiac sprue Lactase deficiency Whipple's disease Abetalipoproteinemia Short bowel syndrome
SECRETORY		
Excessive secretion of electrolytes	Watery diarrhea, persists with fasting Dehydration Other systemic effects of hormones Absence of osmotic gap in fecal water	Carcinoid syndrome Zollinger-Ellison syndrome Vasoactive intestinal peptide-secreting pancreatic adenomas Medullary carcinoma of thyroid Villous adenoma of rectum Microscopic colitis Cholerrheic diarrhea
ALTERED INTESTINAL MOTILITY		
Rapid transit In some cases associated bacterial overgrowth	Alternating diarrhea and constipation Neurologic symptoms; bladder involvement	Irritable bowel syndrome Fecal impaction Neurologic diseases
FACTITIOUS		
Self-induced	Usually women Watery diarrhea with hypokalemia, weakness, edema	Laxative abuse

Intraluminal maldigestion may result from *pancreatic exocrine insufficiency*, which occurs when at least 90 percent of the secretory capacity of the pancreas is lost in patients with *chronic pancreatitis* or occasionally *pancreatic ductal obstruction*. Maldigestion and weight loss occur despite preserved appetite. In children, *cystic fibrosis* or *Shwachman's syndrome* may cause chronic pancreatic insufficiency. *Somatostatinoma* is a rare pancreatic islet tumor that leads to gallstones, diabetes, and steatorrhea thought to be caused by inhibition of pancreatic secretion. Intraluminal maldigestion also may result from *bile duct obstruction* as a result of cancer of the head of the pancreas or from severe liver disease with *cholestasis*. Deficiency of intraluminal bile salts usually results in only mild fat malabsorption. *Bacterial overgrowth* in a blind loop of intestine or a segment of stasis (e.g., due to enterocolonic fistula, jejunal diverticulosis, intestinal dysmotility due to scleroderma, diabetes, or chronic intestinal pseudo-obstruction) may result in steatorrhea due to deconjugation of the bile salts and impaired micelle formation; additional factors leading to diarrhea include brush border enzyme injury, mucosal inflammation, and hydroxylation of fat causing fatty acid diarrhea.

Osmotic diarrhea may result from the chronic ingestion of certain fruits or candy, gum, dietetic foods, and medications sweetened with unabsorbed carbohydrates such as sorbitol or fructose. Congenital absence of specific brush border carbohydrate hydrolases and transport proteins also may lead to chronic diarrhea; the most common of these is lactase deficiency resulting in lactose intolerance.

The classic example of *mucosal malabsorption* is *celiac sprue*, or gluten-sensitive enteropathy (see Chap. 285). In addition to presenting with typical symptoms and signs of malabsorption, patients with celiac sprue may have atypical presentations, including failure to thrive, muscle wasting, abdominal distention, and irritability in young children, and iron-deficiency anemia, growth retardation, and anorexia in adolescents or young adults. Later in life, patients may present with insidious nutritional deficiencies, infertility, and neuromuscular disease. Like celiac sprue, *tropical sprue* is characterized by malabsorption and histologic changes in the small bowel of villus atrophy, crypt hyperplasia, damaged surface epithelium, and a mononuclear infiltrate in the lamina propria. A disease affecting residents in certain tropical parts of the world, tropical sprue can occur even in visitors residing for as little as 1 to 3 months in an endemic area. The onset may be acute, suggesting an infectious etiology.

Intestinal malabsorption is typical of *Whipple's disease* due to *Tropheryma whippelii*, which usually affects middle-aged men but may present at any age and in patients of either sex. Additional manifestations include arthralgias, fever and chills, hypotension, lymphadenopathy, and involvement of the central nervous system (see Chap. 285). *Abetalipoproteinemia* is caused by the absence of Apo B resulting in defective chylomicron formation. Children with this disorder present with steatorrhea, acanthocytic red blood cells, ataxia, and retinitis pigmentosa (see Chap. 285). Steatorrhea also may result from infections with *Giardia*, *Isospora*, *Strongyloides*, and *Mycobacterium avium* complex. Ingestion of certain *drugs* may result in steatorrhea because of damage to enterocytes; examples include colchicine, neomycin, and *para*-aminosalicylic acid.

Intestinal lymphangiectasia (Chap. 285) causes protein-losing enteropathy with steatorrhea but preserved absorption of carbohydrates and is thus an example of *postmucosal obstruction of lymphatic channels*. The disease may be congenital or acquired as a result of trauma, lymphoma, carcinoma, or Whipple's disease.

Finally, extensive intestinal resection may result in the *short bowel syndrome*, in which steatorrhea results from an inadequate absorptive surface, decreased transit time, and a decreased bile salt pool. Other factors that may contribute to diarrhea in short bowel syndrome include the osmotic effect of nonabsorbed solutes, gastric hypersecretion, and in some cases bacterial overgrowth.

Secretory Diarrhea Secretory diarrhea is characterized by a large volume of fecal output caused by abnormal fluid and electrolyte transport not necessarily related to the ingestion of food. Therefore, diarrhea usually persists with fasting. The term *watery diarrhea* is often used synonymously with secretory diarrhea. Because there is no malabsorbed solute, fecal osmolality in secretory diarrheas can be accounted for by normal ionic constituents with no fecal osmotic gap (see below).

The classic examples of secretory diarrhea are those mediated by hormones (see Chaps. 95 and 284). Patients with metastatic *carcinoid tumors* of the gastrointestinal tract may have watery diarrhea as part of the carcinoid syndrome that includes episodic flushing, telangiectatic skin lesions, cyanosis, pellagra-like skin lesions, bronchospasm, and cardiac murmurs due to right-sided valvular lesions. The carcinoid syndrome results from secretion of a variety of vasoactive substances that are potent intestinal secretagogues, including serotonin, histamine, catecholamines, prostaglandin, and kinins. The *Zollinger-Ellison syndrome* is characterized by recurrent, refractory, and unusually located peptic ulcers due to a gastrinoma; diarrhea occurs in up to one-third of patients and may be the presenting symptom in 10 percent of cases. The diarrhea is due only in part to the high volumes of secreted hydrochloric acid but is also due to maldigestion of fat caused by inactivation of pancreatic lipase and precipitation of bile acids at low pH. *Non-beta cell pancreatic adenomas* may secrete a variety of peptides, including vasoactive intestinal polypeptide (VIP), pancreatic polypeptide, secretin, neurotensin, calcitonin, prostaglandins, and others. Those that secrete VIP may be associated with the *watery diarrhea/hypokalemia achlorhydria* (WDHA) *syndrome*, characterized by often massive secretory diarrhea, achlorhydria, hypokalemia, hypomagnesemia, hypercalcemia without hyperparathyroidism, and, in some cases flushing, myopathy, or nephropathy. Not all patients with WDHA syndrome have a *vipoma*, and in such cases, alternative mediators of intestinal secretion have been postulated. *Medullary carcinoma of the thyroid* (Chap. 331) may be sporadic or a feature of multiple endocrine neoplasia syndrome type IIa with pheochromocytomas and hyperparathyroidism. Watery diarrhea is thought to be mediated by calcitonin produced by the tumor, although in some cases other mediators may be found. The occurrence of diarrhea in medullary carcinoma of the thyroid is usually associated with metastases and a poor prognosis. *Systemic mastocytosis* (Chap. 285), which may be associated with the skin lesion urticaria pigmentosa, also may be associated with diarrhea that is secretory and mediated by histamine or malabsorptive and due to intestinal mucosal infiltration by mast cells.

Diarrhea associated with a *villous adenoma* (Chap. 92) of the rectum or rectosigmoid usually occurs with large tumors, often more than 3 to 4 cm in diameter. Hypokalemia due to potassium loss is common.

Microscopic or *lymphocytic colitis* and *collagenous colitis* (Chap. 286) may represent variants of the same disease. Their hallmarks are a characteristic histologic lesion, despite a normal mucosal appearance on colonoscopy, and diarrhea that is often secretory. In both disorders, histologic findings include infiltration of the lamina propria with inflammatory cells as well as intraepithelial lymphocytes, but only in collagenous colitis is there also a characteristic subepithelial collagen band.

Secretory diarrhea may result from *severe disease, resection*, or *bypass of the distal ileum* when less than 100 cm of the ileum is affected (Chap. 285). Presumably, diarrhea results from stimulation of colonic secretion by dihydroxy bile salts that escape absorption in the terminal ileum (cholerrheic diarrhea). By preventing gallbladder contraction and the delivery of large amounts of bile into the intestine, fasting eliminates this type of secretory diarrhea. When greater than 100 cm of terminal ileum is diseased or resected, hepatic synthesis cannot maintain an adequate intraluminal bile salt pool, and steatorrhea also ensues. Bile acid–induced diarrhea may occur following cholecystectomy because of the loss of the storage capacity of the gallbladder. Rarely, *primary (idiopathic) bile acid malabsorption* by the terminal ileum may account for otherwise unexplained secretory diarrhea. Rapid small intestinal transit resulting in increased delivery of bile acids to the colon also may account for *postvagotomy diarrhea*, which occurs in up to 30 percent of patients undergoing truncal vagotomy with a drainage procedure for peptic ulcer disease; diarrhea is much less common following proximal gastric vagotomy.

Altered Intestinal Motility Diarrhea may be associated with disorders that affect intestinal motility. The most common of these is *irritable bowel syndrome* (Chap. 287), in which diarrhea typically alternates with constipation and is associated with abdominal pain, the passage of mucus, and a sense of incomplete evacuation. However, in some patients, constipation alone with lower abdominal cramps is the predominant clinical manifestation, while others present only with painless diarrhea presumably due to disordered intestinal motility. Diarrhea may occasionally occur paradoxically as a result of *fecal impaction* or an obstructing tumor with the overflow of liquid colonic contents around the impacted stool or obstruction. A variety of *neurologic diseases* also may be associated with diarrhea because of altered autonomic control of bowel function. Profuse watery diarrhea, often with incontinence, may be seen in patients with *type 1 diabetes* and is often associated with severe neuropathy, nephropathy, and retinopathy. Additional contributing factors may include bacterial overgrowth secondary to intestinal dysmotility, pancreatic exocrine insufficiency, or, rarely, celiac sprue. Diarrhea also may occur in patients with *traumatic neuropathy*, the *Shy-Drager syndrome*, or *lesions of the cauda equina*.

Factitious Diarrhea Factitious diarrhea is self-induced by the patient and may result from intestinal infection, the addition of water or urine to the stool, or self-medication with laxatives. Patients are predominantly women with severe chronic watery diarrhea, abdominal pain, nausea and vomiting, weight loss, peripheral edema, and weakness resulting from hypokalemia. The diagnosis of factitious diarrhea should be suspected in a patient with a history of psychiatric disease or multiple previous negative evaluations for diarrhea. Additional diagnoses to consider in patients with chronic diarrhea of obscure origin are listed in Table 42-5.

Approach to the Patient

With Diarrhea A thorough history and physical examination are crucial initial steps in the evaluation of the patient with chronic diarrhea. The history in particular may direct the evaluation toward a general pathophysiologic mechanism or even a specific diagnosis and serves as a useful guide to the selection of a limited number of appropriate diagnostic studies.

Inflammatory diarrheas may be suggested by the presence of fever with abdominal pain, often localized to one of the lower quadrants. Extraintestinal manifestations such as arthritis, skin lesions, or ocular symptoms suggest idiopathic inflammatory bowel disease. The presence of peripheral edema, ascites, or anasarca is compatible with protein-losing enteropathy. Intestinal malabsorption is suggested by (1) bulky or greasy foul-smelling stools that are difficult to flush and leave oil in the bowl, (2) flatulence, and (3) weight loss. Malabsorption of specific essential nutrients may present as anemia, a bleeding tendency, osteopenia, amenorrhea, or infertility. Steatorrhea is typically more severe in pancreatic insufficiency than in intestinal mucosal disease, whereas flatulence and bloating are more typical of intestinal mucosal disease than pancreatic insufficiency because of associated carbohydrate malabsorption. Osmotic diarrhea of any cause often improves or resolves with fasting. In watery diarrheas, weight loss is

Table 42-5

Causes of Chronic Diarrhea of Obscure Origin

Drugs (see Table 42-3)
Laxative abuse
Microscopic or collagenous colitis
Bacterial overgrowth
Carbohydrate malabsorption
Bile acid malabsorption (including after cholecystectomy and
   ileal resection)
Diabetic diarrhea
Epidemic chronic diarrhea (? contaminated milk or water)
Chronic idiopathic secretory diarrhea
Fecal incontinence

unusual except in patients with advanced neuroendocrine tumors, which also may be suggested by characteristic systemic manifestations such as flushing. Symptoms of autonomic dysfunction such as postural hypotension, impotence, or disordered sweating are often found in patients with diabetic diarrhea. Diarrhea alternating with constipation is typical of the irritable bowel syndrome.

In addition to providing clues to the underlying cause of diarrhea, the physical examination is important in assessing the presence of volume depletion, as manifested by postural hypotension, tachycardia, absence of axillary sweat, decreased skin turgor, mental lethargy, and generalized weakness.

Laboratory studies may be employed in the evaluation of chronic diarrhea, but a "shotgun" approach should be avoided. In many patients it is helpful to start with routine blood studies such as a complete blood count and peripheral smear and serum electrolyte, calcium, phosphate, albumin, and quantitative immunoglobulin determinations.

Inflammatory diarrheas may be associated with leukocytosis, an elevated erythrocyte sedimentation rate, or hypoalbuminemia. The hallmark of inflammatory diarrheas is the presence of either *gross or occult blood and leukocytes* in the stool; leukocytes can be detected by a Wright's or methylene blue stain. Further evaluation usually involves *upper gastrointestinal endoscopy or colonoscopy* with diagnostic biopsies. An *upper gastrointestinal radiograph with a small bowel follow-through* also may be indicated to evaluate the small intestine. In rare instances, [111]*In-labeled white blood cell scans* may be used to detect bowel inflammation not apparent on endoscopy or conventional barium radiography. In patients with AIDS and chronic diarrhea, multiple stool specimens for culture and examination for ova and parasites should be obtained prior to more invasive diagnostic testing.

A wide array of tests may be helpful in evaluating the patient with an osmotic diarrhea. Decreased levels of iron, folate, vitamin B_{12}, and vitamin D may suggest malabsorption. The prothrombin time may be prolonged due to vitamin K deficiency, and serum carotene, cholesterol, and albumin levels may be decreased. A stool pH of less than 5.3 suggests carbohydrate malabsorption. The cornerstone of testing for intestinal malabsorption is the measurement of *fecal fat*, which is described in detail in Chap. 285.

The capacity of the small intestine to absorb simple sugars can be assessed by the D-*xylose absorption test*, in which 25 g of this five-carbon sugar is administered orally and urine is collected for the subsequent 5 h; normally, at least 25 percent of the administered dose is excreted in the urine. The sensitivity of this test may be increased by obtaining a blood sample following the oral dose; a blood level of greater than 30 mg/dL at 2 h is normal (see Chap. 285).

The definitive test for malabsorption due to intestinal mucosal disease is the *small-intestinal biopsy*, which may be performed via upper endoscopy with forceps biopsy of the distal duodenum or with a specialized small bowel biopsy instrument that reaches the jejunum. Small-intestinal biopsy is generally diagnostic in diseases characterized by diffuse involvement of the small intestine such as Whipple's disease, *M. avium complex* infection, or abetalipoproteinemia but may be falsely negative in diseases with a patchy distribution such as lymphoma, eosinophilic gastroenteritis, or amyloidosis. In celiac sprue, histologic findings may be suggestive, but the diagnosis can be confirmed only by demonstrating that the histologic lesion reverses following withdrawal of gluten from the diet. The diagnosis of celiac sprue is also suggested by detection of anti-endomysial and anti-gliadin antibodies in serum.

Protein-losing enteropathy is best confirmed by assaying for α_1-antitrypsin, an endogenous protein, on an aliquot of lyophilized stool (Chap. 285). One screening test of *pancreatic function* available in some countries is the *bentiromide test*, which depends on the ability of pancreatic chymotrypsin to cleave *para*-aminobenzoic acid (PABA) from the synthetic peptide *N*-benzoyl-L-tyrosyl *para*-aminobenzoic acid (bentiromide); the cleaved PABA is absorbed by the intestine, conjugated in the liver, and excreted in the urine. This and other tests of pancreatic function are discussed in Chap. 304.

The *Schilling test*, used in the evaluation of patients with suspected pernicious anemia, also can be used as a diagnostic test for pancreatic insufficiency, in which vitamin B_{12} absorption is impaired because gastric R-proteins are not cleaved from intrinsic factor as a result of diminished pancreatic proteolytic activity in the upper small intestine; vitamin B_{12} absorption improves when the test is repeated following oral administration of pancreatic enzymes.

Bacterial overgrowth may be detected by aspirating fluid from the upper small intestine through an endoscope or a small-intestinal tube placed under fluoroscopic guidance and finding a *bacterial colony count* of greater than 10^5 per mL. Alternatively, the diagnosis of bacterial overgrowth is suggested by an increase in exhaled $^{14}CO_2$ within 60 min of the ingestion of 1 g ^{14}C-D-xylose (*^{14}C-xylose breath test*) or after the ingestion of ^{14}[C]cholylglycine (*bile acid breath test*) or the detection of increased breath H_2 within the first 2 h after ingestion of either glucose or rice flour (*breath hydrogen test*) (see Chap. 285).

Radiologic tests may play a diagnostic role in patients with suspected malabsorption. An abdominal radiograph may demonstrate pancreatic calcification in patients with chronic pancreatitis. *Abdominal ultrasonography*, *computed tomography*, or *endoscopic retrograde cholangiopancreatography* also may be useful in the evaluation of suspected pancreatic disease. Standard *barium radiographs* of the gastrointestinal tract may suggest thickening of the valvulae conniventes due to infiltrative disease such as Whipple's disease, lymphoma, or amyloidosis or dilatation of the small bowel with flocculation of the barium in celiac sprue. Additional relevant findings may include a gastrocolic fistula, blind loop, stricture, or multiple diverticula.

Fecal osmolality measurements may be helpful in distinguishing osmotic from secretory diarrhea when the diarrhea is watery. Measured osmolality can be compared with the calculated fecal osmolality, which is the sum of the measured Na^+ and K^+ concentrations multiplied by 2 (to account for anions). The osmotic gap is the measured fecal osmolality minus the calculated fecal osmolality and corresponds approximately to the concentration of poorly absorbed solutes in fecal water. Measured fecal osmolality should approximate plasma osmolality, which, in general, is 290 mosmol/kg H_2O. (In fact, a measured fecal osmolality greater than 300 mosmol/kg H_2O indicates bacterial degradation of nonabsorbed carbohydrate in the collection jar or the addition of urine to the jar.) A fecal osmotic gap greater than 50 mosmol/kg H_2O is significant and suggests osmotic diarrhea due to a poorly absorbed carbohydrate or excessive ingestion of magnesium-containing laxatives. If the fecal osmolality is much lower than that of the plasma (290 mosmol/kg H_2O), fluid has been added to the stool.

In patients with watery diarrhea, blood levels of *serotonin*, *gastrin*, VIP, *calcitonin*, and other potential secretagogues should be obtained, in addition to a *urinary 5-hydroxyindole acetic acid* level. *Flexible sigmoidoscopy* or *colonoscopy* should be considered to exclude villous adenoma of the rectum or sigmoid as well as microscopic or collagenous colitis. Colonoscopy also may reveal melanosis coli due to abuse of anthraquinone laxatives. Ingestion of phenolphthalein laxatives may be detected by *alkalinizing the stool* with either NaOH or KOH, which results in a pink or purple color. When the index of suspicion for laxative abuse is high, a cautious room search may be diagnostic. In addition, spectrophotometry or thin-layer chromatography to detect bisacodyl, phenolphthalein, and anthraquinones can be performed on urine or stool water.

In cases of suspected ileal bile salt malabsorption, a ^{75}*selenahomotaurocholic acid* (^{75}*SeHCAT*) *test* may be available in some centers. ^{75}SeHCAT acid is an analogue of taurocholic acid and is thus absorbed in the terminal ileum; scanning with a gamma camera can be used to quantitate ileal absorption and increased bile acid loss. Alternatively, a therapeutic trial of the bile salt–binding resin *cholestyramine* may be administered.

R_x TREATMENT

While every effort should be made to identify and correct the specific cause of diarrhea, in many cases a cause that is specifically treatable may not be identifiable, and symptomatic therapy alone may be indicated. Psyllium and other hydrophilic agents absorb water and thereby enhance stool consistency. Most other available antidiarrheal agents act by altering intestinal motility; some also may have mild proabsorptive or antisecretory activity. *Opiate antidiarrheal agents* such as diphenoxylate and loperamide may be helpful in secretory diarrhea of mild to moderate severity. However, such antimotility agents may be contraindicated in diarrhea due to infectious agents because stasis may enhance tissue invasion by the organisms or delay their clearance from the bowel. In patients with severe inflammatory bowel disease, such drugs may contribute to the development of toxic megacolon and are contraindicated. *Octreotide*, a long-acting synthetic analogue of somatostatin, has a significant antisecretory effect in the carcinoid syndrome and other neuroendocrine tumors because of its specific inhibition of hormone secretion; it also may have some benefit in the short bowel syndrome. *Clonidine*, an alpha$_2$-adrenergic agonist, may be useful in the diarrhea of opiate withdrawal and diabetic diarrhea. *H^+, K^+-ATPase inhibitors*, such as omeprazole and lansoprazole, and *H_2-receptor antagonists* are useful in the diarrhea that results from gastric hypersecretion in the Zollinger-Ellison syndrome. Other drugs that may have some benefit in the treatment of neuroendocrine tumors or unexplained secretory diarrheas include *phenothiazines* and *calcium channel blockers*. *Indomethacin*, an inhibitor of prostaglandin synthesis and secretion, may have benefit in the diarrhea of medullary carcinoma of the thyroid and villous adenomas. A combination of H_1- and H_2-receptor antagonists may be helpful in treating the diarrhea of systemic mastocytosis. *Cholestyramine* is the drug of choice in diarrhea caused by ileal bile salt malabsorption.

CONSTIPATION

DEFINITION Constipation is a common complaint in clinical practice. Because of the wide range of normal bowel habits, constipation is difficult to define precisely. Most persons have at least three bowel movements per week, and *constipation* has been defined as a frequency of defecation of less than three times per week. However, stool frequency alone is not a sufficient criterion to use, because many constipated patients describe a normal frequency of defecation but subjective complaints of excessive straining, hard stools, lower abdominal fullness, and a sense of incomplete evacuation. Thus a combination of objective and subjective criteria must be used to define constipation.

CAUSES Pathophysiologically, constipation generally results from *disordered colonic transit or anorectal function* as a result of a primary motility disturbance, certain drugs, or in association with a large number of systemic diseases that affect the gastrointestinal tract. Constipation of any cause may be exacerbated by chronic illnesses that lead to physical or mental impairment and result in inactivity or physical immobility. Additional contributing factors may include a lack of fiber in the diet, generalized muscle weakness, and possibly stress and anxiety.

In the patient presenting with the recent onset of constipation, an *obstructing lesion* of the colon should be sought. In addition to a *colonic neoplasm*, other causes of colonic obstruction include *strictures* due to colonic ischemia, diverticular disease, or inflammatory bowel disease; *foreign bodies*; or *anal strictures*. Anal sphincter spasm due to painful *hemorrhoids* or *fissures* also may inhibit the desire to evacuate.

In the absence of an obstructing lesion of the colon, *disturbed colonic motility* may mimic colonic obstruction. Disruption of parasympathetic innervation to the colon as a result of injury or lesions of the lumbosacral spine or sacral nerves may produce constipation with hypomotility, colonic dilatation, decreased rectal tone and sensation, and impaired defecation. In patients with *multiple sclerosis*, constipation may be associated with neurogenic dysfunction of other organs. Similarly, constipation may be associated with *lesions of the central nervous system* caused by parkinsonism or a cerebrovascular accident. In South America, the parasitic infection *Chagas' disease* may result in constipation because of damage to myenteric plexus ganglion cells. *Hirschsprung's disease*, or aganglionosis, is characterized by absence of myenteric neurons in a segment of distal colon just proximal to the anal sphincter. This results in a segment of contracted bowel which produces obstruction and proximal dilatation. In addition, an absent rectosphincteric inhibitory reflex results in the failure of the internal anal sphincter to relax following rectal distention. Most patients with Hirschsprung's disease are diagnosed by 6 months of age, but in occasional cases symptoms are mild enough that the diagnosis may be delayed into adulthood (see Chap. 288).

Drugs that may lead to constipation include those with anticholinergic properties, such as antidepressants and antipsychotics, codeine and other narcotic analgesics, aluminum- or calcium-containing antacids, sucralfate, iron supplements, and calcium channel blockers. In patients with certain endocrinopathies such as *hypothyroidism* and *diabetes mellitus*, constipation is generally mild and responsive to therapy. Rarely, life-threatening megacolon occurs in patients with myxedema. Constipation is common during *pregnancy*, presumably as a result of altered progesterone and estrogen levels which decrease intestinal transit. *Collagen vascular diseases* may be associated with constipation, which may be a particularly prominent feature of *progressive systemic sclerosis*, in which delayed intestinal transit results from atrophy and fibrosis of colonic smooth muscle.

In the large majority of patients with severe constipation, no obvious cause can be identified. In *idiopathic childhood constipation*, both psychological and physiologic factors are thought to play a role. Affected children often have slow colonic transit localized to the distal colon and rectum, and voluntary withholding behavior or abnormal anorectal function has been suggested to play a role in this disorder. Young to middle-aged women may present with severe constipation characterized by infrequent defecation, excessive straining when defecating, and unresponsiveness to fiber supplements or mild laxatives. In 70 percent of such cases, slow colonic transit (colonic inertia) may be demonstrated by the delayed passage of radiopaque markers through the proximal colon. In 30 percent of cases colonic transit is normal, and abnormalities of anorectal sensory and motor function may be demonstrated. The terms *outlet obstruction* and *anismus* have been used to describe this form of constipation, which appears to result from failed relaxation or inappropriate contraction of the puborectalis and external anal sphincter muscles. Because relaxation of these muscles involves cortical inhibition of the spinal reflex during defecation and may be modified by biofeedback, it is speculated that such rectosphincteric dysfunction is an acquired or learned rather than an organic or neurogenic disease. Chronic straining at defecation itself may lead to descent of the perineal floor and stretching of the pudendal nerve, thus leading to an incompetent anal sphincter and fecal incontinence. *Rectal prolapse* may impair defecation as a result of rectal intussusception or chronic pudendal nerve injury. A *rectocele* is an anterior rectal herniation that may interfere with defecation by filling with feces preferentially during attempts at defecation.

Chronic idiopathic intestinal pseudoobstruction is a rare disorder in which episodes of intestinal obstruction are unaccompanied by evidence of mechanical blockage (see Chap. 288). This disorder may be familial as a result of a neuropathy or myopathy involving the bowel and in some cases the bladder. *Idiopathic megacolon* or *megarectum* is characterized by a dilated colon or rectum, respectively, with constipation and defecatory difficulties attributed to neurogenic dysfunction.

In young to middle-aged adults, constipation is most commonly attributable to the *irritable bowel syndrome*. Unlike some of the idiopathic constipation syndromes described above, irritable bowel syndrome is typically accompanied by abdominal pain, especially in the lower abdomen, as well as by the passage of small, hard stools with a sense of incomplete evacuation and excessive straining. Patients also may complain of flatulence, abdominal bloating, heartburn, nausea, dysphagia, back pain, and genitourinary symptoms. Colonic transit is usually normal in such patients, and the precise pathophysiologic basis for the symptoms is uncertain (see Chap. 287).

Approach to the Patient

With Constipation A precise description of symptoms and their duration should be obtained. A recent change in bowel habits always demands an evaluation for an obstructing neoplasm. A description of the frequency and nature of defecation should be obtained, including the presence of excessive straining, hard scybalous stools, or a sense of incomplete evacuation. The patient should be questioned about associated abdominal pain and bloating and upper gastrointestinal or genitourinary symptoms. It is especially important to obtain a history of prior laxative use and its duration. A gentle but careful assessment should be made for evidence of anxiety, emotional distress, or affective disorders and the use of mood-altering drugs.

Physical examination should be directed toward the detection of nongastrointestinal diseases that may contribute to constipation. Particular attention should be paid to the neurologic examination, including an assessment of autonomic function. The abdomen should be examined for evidence of prior surgery, bowel distention, or retained stool. A careful perineal and anorectal examination should be conducted for evidence of deformity, gluteal muscle atrophy, rectal prolapse, anal stenosis, anal fissure, rectal mass, or fecal impaction. The patient may need to strain to demonstrate evidence of a rectocele or rectal prolapse. A normal "anal wink" may be elicited by demonstrating reflex contraction of the anal canal following pinprick of the perineum. A variety of complications of constipation or its treatment also may be detected and may be the reason the patient seeks medical attention (Table 42-6).

Flexible sigmoidoscopy or *colonoscopy* may demonstrate melanosis coli as a brown-black discoloration of the bowel mucosa resulting from chronic use of anthraquinone laxatives. The absence of haustrations on endoscopy or barium enema suggests a "cathartic colon" due to laxative abuse. *Barium enema* also may demonstrate obstructing lesions of the colon, megacolon, or megarectum and in Hirschsprung's disease will show the characteristic denervated bowel segment with proximal dilatation of the colon. In such cases, rectal biopsies may be obtained to demonstrate the absence of neurons.

Studies of colonic and anorectal function should be reserved for patients with severe idiopathic constipation who fail to respond to simple therapeutic measures (see below). In patients with a complaint of infrequent defecation, *colonic transit studies* may demonstrate colonic inertia. Radiopaque markers are ingested and their transit is monitored by serial abdominal radiographs until at least 80 percent have passed or a defined period of time has elapsed. The upper limit of normal for most adults is approximately 70 h. In patients with suspected outlet obstruction, *anorectal motility studies* provide information about rectal sensation, viscoelasticity, relaxation of the internal anal sphincter, and defecation of air-filled balloons of various sizes inserted into the rectum. Whereas patients with constipation due to irritable bowel syndrome often have a low rectal compliance and tolerate rectal distention poorly, those with megarectum have a very high rectal compliance. The absence of internal anal sphincter relaxation suggests Hirschsprung's disease. In some centers, anorectal manometry is supplemented by *electromyogram studies* to record external anal sphincter function and *defecography*, in which thickened barium approximating the consistency of stool is introduced into the rectum

Table 42-6

Complications of Constipation or Its Treatment

Hemorrhoids	Ischemic colitis
Anal fissure	Colonic volvulus
Rectal prolapse	Colonic perforation
Stercoral ulcer	Fecal incontinence
Melanosis coli	Urinary retention
Cathartic colon	Cardiac and cerebrovascular dysfunction
Fecal impaction	(e.g., syncope, arrhythmias, angina)

and its evacuation monitored by fluoroscopy while the patient sits on a commode.

℞ TREATMENT

Treatment of constipation must be individualized, taking into account the duration and severity of constipation, potential contributing factors, the age of the patient, and the patient's expectations. Symptomatic therapy is quite empiric in that there is often little objective evidence to support a particular strategy. Initial therapy is usually dietary, with an emphasis on increasing dietary fiber intake. Although there is little evidence that constipated persons consume less dietary fiber than nonconstipated persons, many constipated persons respond to increases in dietary fiber to between 20 and 30 g/d. Fiber supplementation may increase stool weight and the frequency of defecation and decrease gastrointestinal transit time. Fiber supplementation is not appropriate for patients with obstructing lesions of the gastrointestinal tract or those with megacolon or megarectum.

Except for bulk laxatives, routine use of laxatives over long periods of time should be discouraged because of the risk of side effects such as lipid pneumonia due to mineral oil or damage to myenteric plexuses resulting in "cathartic colon" due to stimulant anthraquinone laxatives such as senna. *Bulk-forming laxatives* consist of natural (psyllium) or synthetic polysaccharides or cellulose derivatives that act in a manner similar to fiber. Fluid intake should be increased with the use of these preparations. *Emollient laxatives* include mineral oil, which when given orally or by enema penetrates and softens the stool, and docusate salts, which are anionic surfactants that lower the surface tension of stool to allow mixing of aqueous and fatty substances and thereby soften the stool. *Hyperosmolar agents* include mixed electrolyte solutions containing polyethylene glycol and nonabsorbable sugars such as lactulose and sorbitol, which act as osmotic agents and are used in bowel cleansing prior to colonoscopy. Lactulose may occasionally be prescribed for longterm use. *Saline laxatives* contain cations and anions that exert an osmotic effect to increase intraluminal water content; in elderly patients they may cause fluid retention. *Stimulant laxatives* include castor oil, anthraquinones such as senna, and diphenylmethanes such as phenolphthalein and bisacodyl. Castor oil is converted to ricinoleic acid, which stimulates intestinal secretion and increases intestinal motility. The anthraquinones increase fluid and electrolyte accumulation in the distal ileum and colon. Phenolphthalein and bisacodyl stimulate colonic motor activity and inhibit glucose and sodium absorption. Recently, the prokinetic agent cisapride has been shown to enhance intestinal transit through the proximal colon, but its role in the management of constipation is uncertain. A role for excessive endogenous opioids in constipation related to motility disorders has been hypothesized, and the benefit of opioid receptor antagonists in the treatment of constipation has been reported but requires further study. *Biofeedback* techniques have shown promise in the treatment of constipation resulting from inappropriate contraction of the pelvic floor muscles and external anal sphincter.

Surgical treatment for severe chronic constipation is generally controversial, except in Hirschsprung's disease, in which surgical resection of the aganglionic segment is the treatment of choice. In colonic inertia, subtotal colectomy with ileorectal anastomosis may be indicated in carefully selected patients in whom upper gastrointestinal motility is normal and anorectal dysmotility has been excluded. Surgery to reduce or resect a rectocele, intussusception, or prolapse should be undertaken with caution, because symptoms often are not alleviated.

BIBLIOGRAPHY

BOYCE TG et al: *Escherichia coli* O157:H7 and the hemolytic–uremic syndrome. N. Engl J Med 333:364, 1995

CAMILLERI M et al: Clinical management of intractable constipation. Ann Intern Med 121:520, 1994

DONOWITZ M et al: Evaluation of patients with chronic diarrhea. N Engl J Med 332:725, 1995

EHERER AJ, FORDTRAN JS: Fecal osmotic gap and pH in experimental diarrhea of various causes. Gastroenterology 103:545, 1992

FIELD M (ed): *Diarrheal Diseases*. New York, Elsevier, 1991

———— et al: Intestinal electrolyte transport and diarrheal disease. N Engl J Med 321:800, 1989

FINE KD, FORDTRAN JS: The effect of diarrhea on fecal fat excretion. Gastroenterology 102:1936, 1992

———— et al: Diarrhea, in *Gastrointestinal Disease: Pathophysiology, Diagnosis, Management*, 5th ed, MH Sleisenger, JS Fordtran (eds). Philadelphia, Saunders, 1993, pp 1043-1071

HEATON KW et al: Defecation frequency and timing, and stool form in the general population: A prospective study. Gut 33:818, 1992

PEMBERTON JH et al: Evaluation and surgical treatment of severe chronic constipation. Ann Surg 214:403, 1991

PHILLIPS S et al: Stool composition in factitial diarrhea: A 6-year experience with stool analysis. Ann Intern Med 123:97, 1995

POWELL DW: Approach to the patient with diarrhea, in *Textbook of Gastroenterology*, 2nd ed. T Yamada et al (eds). Philadelphia, Lippincott, 1995, pp 813-863

READ NW et al: Constipation and incontinence in the elderly. J Clin Gastroenterol 20:61, 1995

SCHILLER LR: Review article: Anti-diarrhoeal pharmacology and therapeutics. Aliment Pharmacol Ther 9:87, 1995

WALD A: Approach to the patient with constipation, in *Textbook of Gastroenterology*, 2nd ed, T Yamada et al (eds). Philadelphia, Lippincott, 1995, pp 864-880

WALD A: Colonic and anorectal motility testing in clinical practice. Am J Gastroenterol 89:2109, 1994

WENZL HH et al: Determinants of decreased fecal consistency in patients with diarrhea. Gastroenterology 108:1729, 1995

WISTROM J et al: Empiric treatment of acute diarrheal disease with norfloxacin. Ann Intern Med 117:202, 1992

43   *Daniel W. Foster*

GAIN AND LOSS IN WEIGHT

In normal persons weight is stable over long periods because food intake is matched to energy expenditure by neural activity in the hypothalamus that provides signals to eat or to stop eating. Because the system is usually effective, either weight gain or weight loss may bring a patient to the physician. No history is complete without ascertaining whether weight has been gained or lost and, if so, how much. In general, a change of 5 percent of body weight or 5 kg is considered significant. However, a 5-kg weight loss may not be of importance in a 130-kg man who is trying to lose weight, while a 2-kg weight loss may well be worrisome in a person weighing 40 kg.

WEIGHT GAIN

Weight gain is less likely to have a pathologic cause than weight loss. In most cases it is a consequence of overeating and inadequate exercise, and the diagnosis is usually simple obesity. Occasionally obesity may be the consequence of hypothyroidism, Cushing's syndrome, or hypothalamic disease such as craniopharyngioma (see Chap. 75). Workup for pathologic causes of weight gain is rarely indicated unless accompanying signs suggest an underlying cause. Sometimes weight gain is not fat but fluid, in which case the primary problems to be considered are congestive heart failure, renal failure, or cirrhosis with ascites.

There is an epidemic of obesity in the United States and some European countries such as Italy. The epidemic is almost certainly due to the availability of attractive, tasty food at low cost. Despite multiple studies suggesting altered metabolism or disturbed satiety signals as predisposing factors, one does not become fat without overeating. All obese patients have elevated, not depressed, absolute resting metabolic rates.

This is not to say that pathologic mechanisms may not play a role. Particular interest has focused on the presumed satiety signal, leptin, synthesized in and released from adipose tissue as the product of the *ob* gene. Leptin is believed to act in the hypothalamus to block the synthesis or release of neuropeptide Y, which appears to be a potent feeding signal. Although leptin deficiency is the cause of obesity in some strains of mice, mutations or deletions in the *ob* gene have not proven to be operative in humans. Resistance to leptin may be important in human obesity. However, at the time of this writing it is not documented that defects in leptin synthesis/action play any significant role in the obese state in humans.

Although rarely caused by disease, obesity predisposes to disease, especially diabetes mellitus but also to gall stones, degenerative joint disease, hyperlipidemia, atherosclerosis, hypertension, sleep apnea, and perhaps cancer.

WEIGHT LOSS

In all studies there are patients who lose weight without discernible cause, but significant involuntary weight loss is usually a marker of serious disease. *Even if no disease is found on initial evaluation, it should not be assumed that weight loss is idiopathic.* The patient should be followed at regular intervals with careful repeat examination since occult illness causing weight loss may not become manifest for long periods.

There are three general mechanisms of weight loss, but more than one may be operative in the same patient: increased energy expenditure, increased loss of energy in stool or urine, and decreased food intake. Decreased intake is by far the most common mechanism; it is usually due to loss of appetite but may result from obstruction in the esophagus or stomach secondary to stricture, compressive mass, or infiltrating malignancy. The only common causes of increased metabolism are hyperthyroidism, pheochromocytoma, and major exercise programs. Loss of ingested energy generally is due to either diabetes mellitus with glycosuria or intestinal malabsorption with steatorrhea. Chronic pancreatitis in alcoholics is the most common cause of steatorrhea, but malabsorption can occur with intestinal lymphoma, celiac sprue, islet cell tumors (such as somatostatinomas or gastrinomas), radiation injury, biliary tract obstruction, inflammatory bowel disease, and a variety of other disorders. If weight loss occurs with a history of increased food intake, the diagnosis is usually diabetes mellitus, hyperthyroidism, or malabsorption syndrome. Occasionally leukemias and lymphomas may present with weight loss in the absence of anorexia or even with increased food intake.

Large prospective studies of the causes of weight loss are not available, and the five retrospective studies published since 1981 involve relatively small numbers of patients, rendering all conclusions suspect. In young persons, the most likely diagnoses are diabetes mellitus, hyperthyroidism, anorexia nervosa, or infection, especially human immunodeficiency virus (HIV). In older persons, cancer is the most likely cause of significant weight loss, with psychiatric illness such as Alzheimer's disease and depression being a distant second.

Under most circumstances the diagnosis of the cause of weight loss is not difficult and is revealed by history, physical examination, and routine laboratory screening. The most common occult condition is cancer. Gastrointestinal, pancreatic, and hepatic malignancies are particularly prone to cause early weight loss. Infectious disease may occasionally be symptomatically silent. Weight loss may occur in HIV infection prior to AIDS-defining illness, and tuberculosis, fungal disease, bacterial endocarditis, or hepatitis may present as weight loss in the absence of defining symptoms. Eating disorders, early Alzheimer's disease, and depression may cause unexplained anorexia and weight loss. Uremia and hypercalcemia may be asymptomatic but are easily recognized through screening laboratory examination. Elevated calcium levels not only produce anorexia but sometimes induce nephrogenic diabetes insipidus, compounding the weight loss by volume depletion. Weight loss may or may not be a prominent feature of pheochromocytoma. Pernicious anemia may cause anorexia before hematologic changes occur, and early adrenal insufficiency

can cause weight loss in the absence of electrolyte changes, nausea, vomiting, or hypotension. Other causes of anorexic weight loss are chronic obstructive pulmonary disease/emphysema, congestive heart failure, chronic liver disease, and neurologic diseases such as Parkinsonism. For those returning from foreign countries, parasitic disease must always be considered.

A list of common causes of weight loss is given in Table 43-1.

DIAGNOSIS

Weight gain does not require much diagnostic expenditure since the vast majority of cases are simple obesity, as mentioned above. Three scenarios warrant laboratory testing: symptoms suggesting hypothyroidism [thyroid-stimulating hormone (TSH)]; central obesity, diabetes, and hypertension accompanied by quadriceps weakness and spontaneous bruising raising the possibility of Cushing syndrome (overnight dexamethasone suppression test, 24-h urinary free cortisol); and obesity accompanied by headache and endocrine dysfunction suggesting craniopharyngioma or pituitary tumor compressing or invading the hypothalamus [computed tomography (CT) or magnetic resonance imaging (MRI) of the head].

When weight loss is the chief complaint or cachexia is a major finding on physical examination, the diagnosis is often readily apparent on first evaluation. It is usually helpful to do a two-stage workup (Table 43-2). First-phase tests are done in every patient. The multiple chemistry panel will reveal diabetes mellitus, hypercalcemia, renal failure, liver disease, and electrolyte abnormalities that may suggest adrenal insufficiency or gastrointestinal illness. TSH should be assayed to rule out hyperthyroidism. HIV testing is indicated if risk factors are present. A chest x-ray must always be obtained. The stool should be checked for occult blood.

Second-phase testing is initiated if the cause of weight loss is still not apparent and in most instances begins with an abdominal CT scan. If hypercalcemia is present, measurements should be made of serum parathyroid hormone (PTH), human PTH-related peptide (a cancer marker), and 1,25-dihydroxyvitamin D and angiotensin-converting enzyme (markers for sarcoidosis). Mammography is indicated in women. Weakness, pigmentation, and hypoglycemia, with or without hyponatremia/hyperkalemia, require a short ACTH test to rule out adrenal insufficiency. Febrile weight loss makes it necessary to obtain blood cultures and, at times, bone marrow biopsy and culture. Iron deficiency anemia is an indication for colonoscopy and occasionally upper endoscopy. Weight loss with diarrhea may, in addition, require measure-

Table 43-1

Common Causes of Weight Loss

1. Increased energy expenditure
   a. Hyperthyroidism
   b. Pheochromocytoma
   c. Extensive exercise
2. Increased energy loss
   a. Diabetes mellitus
   b. Malabsorption syndromes
3. Diminished food intake*
   a. Cancer
   b. Infection (HIV, tuberculosis, endocarditis)
   c. Hypercalcemia (malignancy, hyperparathyroidism, sarcoidosis)
   d. Uremia
   e. Obstructive gastrointestinal disease
   f. Anorexia nervosa
   g. Adrenal insufficiency (primary or secondary)
   h. Pernicious anemia
   i. Alzheimer's disease
   j. Depression

* Many other diseases can be associated with anorexia, e.g., congestive heart failure, chronic obstructive pulmonary disease, chronic liver disease, neurologic disease, and inflammatory/autoimmune disease. The conditions listed above are emphasized because they have the capacity to be occult.

GASTROINTESTINAL BLEEDING

Table 43-2

Screening Tests for Involuntary Weight Loss

1. First-phase screen*
   a. CBC, erythrocyte sedimentation rate
   b. Urinalysis
   c. Multiphase chemical screen (SMA 20)
   d. TSH
   e. HIV test for persons at risk
   f. Chest x-ray
   g. Stool for occult blood
2. Second-phase screen
   a. Abdominal CT scan
   b. Mammography, serum protein electrophoresis, parathyroid hormone, human PTH-related peptide, angiotensin-converting enzyme, and 1, 25-dihydroxyvitamin D if hypercalcemia is present
   c. Colonoscopy if iron deficiency anemia or melena is found or inflammatory bowel disease is suspected
   d. Upper endoscopy for upper GI bleeding or dysphagia
   e. Short ACTH test for weakness, pigmentation, or hyponatremia/ hyperkalemia
   f. Blood cultures for fever of unknown origin with weight loss
   g. Bone marrow biopsy with culture for febrile weight loss with negative blood cultures
   h. 72-h stool fat for weight loss with chronic diarrhea
   i. Head CT or MRI for weight loss with headache, neurologic symptoms, or endocrine deficiency
   j. Spinal MRI if examination suggests paraspinal disease
   k. Vitamin B_{12}

---

* First-phase and second-phase screens are arbitrary definitions. The history and physical examination together with initial laboratory tests may move a second-phase test to an early time point. The suggested order is for true occult disease

ment of 72-h stool fat content or hormones such as gastrin, somatostatin, or glucagon. Even in the absence of anemia or macrocytosis, a vitamin B_{12} level should be measured in unexplained weight loss. New or severe headaches with or without neurologic symptoms are indications for CT examination, while back pain with fever and neurologic loss suggest the possibility of paraspinal or epidural abscess due to tuberculosis or staphylococci, especially in intravenous drug users.

SUMMARY

Weight loss is more often a diagnostic problem than a weight gain and is often a sign of serious organic illness. Diagnosis is usually quite straightforward. In cases where no ready explanation is available, persistence is essential. Initially the patient should be reexamined at monthly intervals with complete physical and laboratory examinations. If no cause is found by 6 months, the return intervals can be stretched.

BIBLIOGRAPHY

EZZELL C: Research in focus. Fat times for obesity research: Tons of new information, but how does it all fit together? J NIH Res 7:39, 1995

LEIBEL R et al: Changes in energy expenditure resulting from altered body weight. N Engl J Med 332:621, 1995

MACALLAN DC et al: Energy expenditure and wasting in human immunodeficiency virus and infection. N Engl J Med 333:83, 1995

OLEFSKY JM: Weighing in on the lean genes. J Clin Invest 95:2427, 1995

RABINOVITZ M et al: Unintentional weight loss: A retrospective analysis of 154 cases. Arch Intern Med 146:186, 1986

THOMPSON MP, MORRIS LK: Unexplained weight loss in the ambulatory elderly. J Am Geriatr Soc 39:497, 1991

WOLF-KLINE GP, SILVERSTONE FA: Weight loss and Alzheimer's disease: An international review of the literature. Int Psychogeriatr 6:135, 1994

Hematemesis is defined as the vomiting of blood, and *melena* as the passage of stools rendered black and tarry by the presence of blood. These clinical manifestations of gastrointestinal (GI) hemorrhage suggest a proximal source of bleeding. The color of vomited blood depends on the concentration of hydrochloric acid in the stomach and the duration of its contact with the blood. Thus, if vomiting occurs shortly after the onset of bleeding, the vomitus appears red, and later the appearance will be dark red, brown, or black. Precipitated blood clots and acid-degraded blood in the vomitus will produce a characteristic "coffee grounds" appearance when vomited. Hematemesis usually indicates bleeding proximal to the ligament of Treitz, because blood entering the GI tract below the duodenum rarely enters the stomach.

While bleeding sufficient to produce hematemesis usually results in melena, less than half of patients with melena have hematemesis. Melena usually denotes bleeding from the esophagus, stomach, or duodenum, but lesions in the jejunum, ileum, and even ascending colon may occasionally cause melena provided the gastrointestinal transit time is sufficiently prolonged. Approximately 60 mL of blood is required to produce a single black stool; acute blood loss greater than this may produce melena for as long as 7 days. After the stool color returns to normal, tests for occult blood may remain positive for over a week. The black color of melena results from contact of the blood with hydrochloric acid to produce hematin. Such stools are tarry ("sticky") and have a characteristic odor. This tarry consistency is in contrast to black or dark gray stools occurring after the ingestion of iron, bismuth, or licorice. GI bleeding, even if detected only by positive tests for occult blood, indicates potentially serious disease and must be further investigated.

Hematochezia, the passage of red blood per rectum, generally signifies bleeding from a source distal to the ligament of Treitz. However, brisk proximal bleeding can cause hematochezia due to rapid transit.

The clinical manifestations of GI bleeding depend on the extent and rate of hemorrhage and the presence of coincidental diseases. Blood loss of less than 500 mL is rarely associated with systemic signs; exceptions include bleeding in the elderly or in the anemic patient in whom smaller amounts of blood loss may produce hemodynamic alterations. Rapid hemorrhage of greater volume results in decreased venous return to the heart, decreased cardiac output, and increased peripheral resistance due to reflex vasoconstriction (see Chap. 38). Orthostatic hypotension greater than a change of 10 mmHg usually indicates a 20 percent or greater reduction in blood volume. Concomitant symptoms may include lightheadedness, syncope, nausea, sweating, and thirst. When blood loss is 25 to 40 percent of blood volume, shock frequently ensues with pronounced tachycardia and hypotension. Pallor is prominent, and the skin is cool. However, in the presence of beta-adrenergic and calcium channel blockers, these clinical signs may be blunted.

In the setting of rapid hemorrhage, the initial hematocrit may not accurately reflect the magnitude of blood loss, since equilibration with extravascular fluid and hemodilution often require over 8 h. Common laboratory findings include mild leukocytosis and thrombocytosis which develop within 6 h after the onset of bleeding. The blood urea nitrogen (BUN) may be elevated out of proportion to the creatinine, particularly in upper GI bleeding, due to breakdown of blood proteins to urea by intestinal bacteria as well as mild reduction in the glomerular filtration rate.

Occult bleeding, detected by card test for hemoglobin peroxidase (e.g., Hemocult), is an important means of finding colorectal neoplasia at earlier, potentially curable stages. Testing is advocated for patients over age 50 as a part of the yearly checkup. Multiple stools should be tested (usually two samples from three stools), and if any sample is positive, additional studies should be performed. A positive result can be due to physiologic blood loss, dietary peroxidases, undercooked meat, or any cause of upper or lower GI bleeding. The daily ingestion of over 500 mg of vitamin C may result in a false-negative test. To limit the confounding variables, patients should be tested on a high-fiber and low-meat diet with no ingestion of nonsteroidal anti-inflammatory agents (NSAIDs) or vitamin C, although the daily low dose of aspirin (80 to 325 mg) taken to prevent cardiovascular disease generally does not lead to false-positive results.

ETIOLOGY OF UPPER GI BLEEDING (See Table 44-1)   A careful history and physical examination of the oropharynx and nasal cavity should serve to exclude epistaxis or swallowed blood as a source of hematemesis or melena.

The most common causes of upper gastrointestinal hemorrhage are (1) erosive or hemorrhagic gastropathy, (2) duodenal ulcer, (3) gastric ulcer, (4) Mallory-Weiss tear, (5) varices or portal hypertensive gastropathy, and (6) arteriovenous malformations (AVMs). These entities account for over 90 percent of all cases of upper GI hemorrhage in which a specific source can be found.

Gastric erosions or *erosive, hemorrhagic gastropathy* are often associated with the ingestion of aspirin or other NSAIDs.

Peptic ulcers (either duodenal or gastric) caused by *Helicobacter pylori* are common causes of upper GI bleeding. Because hemorrhage may be the initial clinical manifestation of a peptic ulcer, the diagnosis should be considered even if a history characteristic of ulcer disease is not obtained. Concomitant use of NSAIDs increases the risk of peptic ulcer bleeding and the mortality associated with it.

Bleeding from *varices* or from *portal hypertensive gastropathy* is characteristically abrupt and massive. Bleeding from esophageal or gastric varices is usually the result of portal hypertension secondary to cirrhosis. Although alcoholic cirrhosis is the most prevalent cause in the United States, any condition producing portal hypertension may result in variceal bleeding. Further, while the presence of varices usually connotes long-standing portal hypertension, acute hepatitis or severe fatty infiltration of the liver may rarely produce varices that disappear once the hepatic abnormality resolves. Although upper GI bleeding in a patient with cirrhosis suggests a variceal source, up to one-quarter of those patients will be bleeding from another lesion, such as erosive gastropathy, peptic ulcer, gastritis, or Mallory-Weiss tear. Consequently, it is essential to determine the cause of bleeding promptly so that the appropriate treatment can be instituted.

Mallory-Weiss tears (esophagogastric mucosal tears) occur in the region of the esophagogastric junction and are often characterized historically by retching or nonbloody vomiting followed by hematemesis. However, a history of retching may be lacking in up to half of cases.

Esophagitis mostly due to gastroesophageal reflux may cause bleeding. Esophagitis associated with cancer or due to infections such as cytomegalovirus, herpes virus, or *Candida* rarely causes acute bleeding; however, it may cause chronic blood loss. Chronic blood loss may also result from linear mucosal tears in large sliding hiatal hernias as a result of the shearing effect caused by differences in intrathoracic and intragastric pressure.

Gastric carcinoma, lymphoma, polyps, and other tumors of the stomach and small bowel are uncommon causes of GI hemorrhage. Leiomyoma and leiomyosarcoma are uncommon, but they can lead to massive hemorrhage. Bleeding from duodenal or jejunal diverticula is an unusual cause of GI bleeding.

Rupture of arteriosclerotic aortic aneurysms into the small intestine is almost always fatal. Rupture usually occurs following arterial reconstructive surgery with fistula formation between the synthetic graft and bowel lumen. A small or "herald bleed" may precede a sudden massive hemorrhage from an aortoenteric fistula. Sudden bleeding also may occur from hemobilia following hepatic surgery or trauma.

Primary blood dyscrasias, vasculitis, hereditary hemorrhagic telangiectasia, and connective tissue disorders may result in significant GI bleeding. Uremia may produce gastrointestinal blood loss due to telangiectases throughout the GI tract. Pancreatic cancer may occasionally erode into the duodenum and produce upper GI bleeding.

ETIOLOGY OF LOWER GI BLEEDING (See Table 44-2)

Anal and Rectal Lesions   Small amounts of bright red blood on the surface of the stool and toilet tissue are often caused by hemorrhoids or anal fissures; such bleeding is generally precipitated by the strained passage of a hard stool. Proctitis is another source of rectal bleeding.

Colonic Lesions   Carcinoma of the colon as well as colonic polyps usually produce chronic occult blood loss but occasionally may produce brisk bleeding. Angiodysplasia, a mucosal vascular tuft, is a major source of acute or chronic bleeding in older patients. Bloody diarrhea may be the presenting symptom in patients with ulcerative colitis. Bleeding also may accompany diarrhea due to infections with *Shigella, Salmonella, Campylobacter jejuni, Clostridium difficile,* enterohemorrhagic toxigenic *Escherichia coli* O157:H7, ameba, and other parasites. In the elderly, diabetic patients, and patients with vascular disease, mesenteric ischemia may be a cause of bloody diarrhea.

Diverticula   Bleeding from colonic diverticula is a common cause of lower GI hemorrhage in persons over age 40. The usual presentation of a diverticular hemorrhage is that of the brisk painless passage of a maroon-colored stool. Meckel's diverticulum, a congenital anomaly most often in the distal ileum, is present in about 2 percent of the population and is an important cause of acute hemorrhage in children and young adults.

Approach to the Patient

With Acute Upper GI Bleeding   The approach to the bleeding patient depends on the site, extent, and rate of bleeding. The primary consideration in the care of the bleeding patient is maintaining adequate intravascular volume and hemodynamic stability. When first seen, the patient may be in shock. Prior to taking a history and performing a thorough physical examination, vital signs should be noted, blood sent for typing and cross-matching, and large-bore intravenous lines placed for infusion of saline or packed red blood cells.

HISTORY   A history or symptoms suggestive of peptic ulcer disease may provide a useful clue. Similarly, recent use of NSAIDs should make one suspect erosive gastropathy. If alcohol use has been long-standing and there are stigmata of chronic liver disease, esophageal varices may be a source of hemorrhage. Prior history of GI bleeding or a family history of intestinal disease or hemorrhagic diathesis may provide diagnostic clues. Recent retching followed by hematemesis should suggest the diagnosis of Mallory-Weiss tear.

PHYSICAL EXAMINATION   Following evaluation for orthostatic changes in pulse and blood pressure, clinical assessment of central

Table 44-1

Common Causes of Acute Upper GI Bleeding

1. Erosive, hemorrhagic gastropathy (aspirin, other NSAIDs)
2. Duodenal ulcer
3. Gastric ulcer
4. Mallory-Weiss tear
5. Varices / portal hypertensive gastropathy
6. Arteriovenous malformations

Table 44-2

Common Causes of Acute Lower GI Bleeding (in Order of Frequency)

Under Age 55	Over Age 55
1. Anorectal disease (hemorrhoids, fissures)	1. Anorectal disease (hemorrhoids, fissures)
2. Colitis (IBD,* infectious)	2. Diverticulosis
3. Diverticulosis	3. Angiodysplasia
4. Polyps, cancer (hyperplastic, hamartomas)	4. Polyps, cancer
5. Angiodysplasia	5. Enterocolitic (ischemic, infectious, IBD, radiation)

* IBD, inflammatory bowel disease.

venous pressure, and institution of volume repletion, the patient should be examined for clues to the underlying illness. A nonintestinal bleeding source should be excluded by careful examination of the oral cavity and nasopharynx. Dermatologic examination may disclose the characteristic telangiectatic lesions of Osler-Rendu-Weber disease (although these will not be visible if severe anemia is present). Stigmata of chronic liver disease such as spider angiomata, gynecomastia, testicular atrophy, jaundice, ascites, and hepatosplenomegaly suggest portal hypertension with bleeding from esophageal or gastric varices as an important potential source.

LABORATORY STUDIES Initial studies should include the hematocrit, hemoglobin, careful assessment of red blood cell morphologic features (hypochromic, microcytic red blood cells suggest that blood loss is chronic), white blood cell count, differential, and platelet count. Prothrombin time and partial thromboplastin time studies are needed to exclude primary or secondary clotting defects. An increase in BUN and the BUN to creatinine ratio may aid in suggesting upper GI bleeding. Abdominal films are rarely helpful in establishing a diagnosis unless a perforated or ischemic viscus is suspected or if intestinal obstruction is present. Although the initial studies are valuable and essential, repeated evaluation of the laboratory data is important as one follows the clinical course of the bleeding; a flow chart of data is desirable and should include the times that blood products and intravenous fluids were administered and their amounts.

DIAGNOSTIC AND THERAPEUTIC APPROACH (See Fig. 44-1) The diagnostic approach to the patient with GI hemorrhage must be individualized. When there is a history of melena or hematemesis or the suspicion of bleeding from the upper part of the GI tract, a nasogastric tube should be passed to empty the stomach and to determine whether the bleeding is proximal to the ligament of Treitz. If the initial nasogastric aspirate is clear or bilious, current active bleeding is unlikely and the tube may be removed.

If blood or "coffee grounds" material is aspirated from the nasogastric tube, water or saline lavage (at room temperature) should be initiated. Irrigation of the stomach serves two purposes: (1) it provides the clinician with an assessment of the rapidity of the bleeding, and (2) it clears the stomach of blood and blood clots prior to diagnostic endoscopy (EGD), which will improve the ability to view all mucosal surfaces. The pace of subsequent diagnostic evaluation will depend on the character of the nasogastric aspirate as well as on vital signs, transfusion requirements, and the number and color of stools.

Once the patient is hemodynamically stable, EGD should be performed to identify the source of bleeding (see Fig. 44-1). Early EGD also may provide prognostic information as to whether the patient is likely to rebleed and to permit endoscopic therapy. When there is evidence of persistent upper GI bleeding, based on continuing blood in the nasogastric tube drainage or failure of the patient to stabilize hemodynamically, the situation must be viewed as urgent, and EGD should commence as soon as possible. If the source of bleeding is found, the endoscopist needs to determine whether therapy via the endoscope may stop the bleeding. Bleeding from an ulcer may be controlled with injection of a vasoconstricting agent such as epinephrine or a sclerosing agent or by the use of electrocautery, most commonly performed with a bipolar or multipolar probe or a heater probe. Such therapy should be attempted when there is arterial spurting, which is unlikely to subside spontaneously, or when there is a "visible vessel," an exposed arteriole in the ulcer base that connotes a 50 percent bleeding risk. Erosive or hemorrhagic gastropathy (due to aspirin or other NSAIDs) is usually not amenable to endoscopic therapy. Fortunately, this condition often improves with cessation of the offending agent and the administration of H$_2$-receptor antagonists or proton pump inhibitors. AVMs, when bleeding, are frequently treated with bipolar electrocautery, but when detected they are usually not actively bleeding. Mallory-Weiss tears usually cease bleeding spontaneously but may require cautery or injection therapy if bleeding persists.

Esophageal variceal bleeding usually requires endoscopic intervention. The varices may be actively spurting or oozing blood or may show evidence of recent bleeding by "red wale" marks or cherry red spots. Until now, the most common approach to stop the bleeding has been sclerotherapy. This involves the injection of varices with sclerosing agents such as ethanolamine, sodium tetradecylsulfate, sodium morrhuate, or absolute ethanol. Esophageal variceal banding ligation (similar to rubber band ligation of hemorrhoids) is an increasingly used technique and is associated with a lower risk of esophageal stricture formation and systemic toxicity than sclerotherapy. Systemic infusion of vasopressin together with intravenous nitroglycerin lowers portal venous pressure and may be used adjunctively to control variceal bleeding. Similarly, systemic somatostatin or its analogues (e.g., octreotide) can lower portal pressure and help to control variceal bleeding without the peripheral vasoconstrictive side effects of vasopressin.

If endoscopic or pharmacologic measures fail to stop variceal bleeding, balloon tamponade with the Blakemore or Linton tube may be used to compress the varices directly and thereby stop bleeding temporarily until definitive therapy can be attempted. Another approach is the placement of a transjugular intrahepatic portosystemic

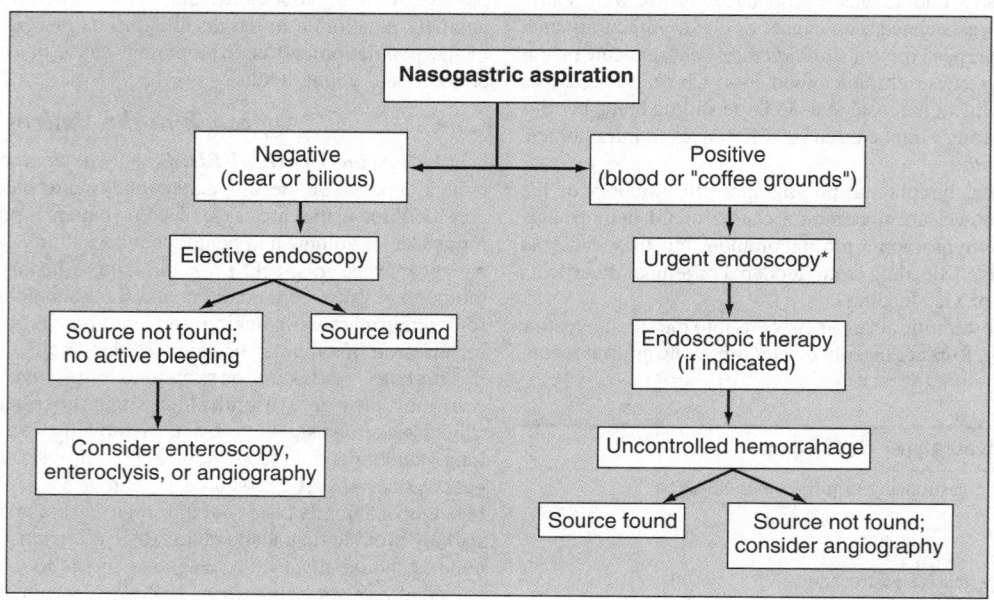

FIGURE 44-1 Approach to the patient with acute upper GI bleeding. (*Request surgical consultation early, in event operative intervention is required.)

shunt. This procedure involves placing an expandable metal stent through the liver to connect the portal and hepatic vein. Occasionally, upper GI bleeding is too brisk to visualize the bleeding site endoscopically; in such cases, angiography, such as selective mesenteric arteriography, may be appropriate. Bleeding of this magnitude usually requires surgical intervention once the bleeding site is localized, but on occasion intraarterial infusion of vasopressin or angiographic injection of Gelfoam or metallic coils may arrest the bleeding.

Approach to the Patient

With Acute Lower GI Bleeding The common causes of acute lower GI bleeding vary with age (see Table 44-2 and Fig. 44-2). In all instances, upper GI bleeding should be excluded, if necessary by nasogastric aspirate or even EGD, and there should be careful digital rectal examination and anoscopy to rule out anorectal pathology such as fissures and bleeding from internal hemorrhoids. A flexible sigmoidoscopic examination (after a gentle saline enema) should be performed to exclude rectosigmoid disease.

In the hemodynamically stable patient, elective colonoscopy should be performed after lavage with an oral polyethyleneglycol/electrolyte or phosphosoda solution. The therapeutic endoscopist may remove polyps, cauterize angiodysplastic lesions, and on occasion inject a bleeding diverticulum with epinephrine. If colonoscopy is negative but there is recurrent or intermittent lower GI bleeding, a tagged red blood scan may be considered. Images may be obtained for up to 48 h. If the scan shows a suspicious lesion, elective angiography helps to localize the site of bleeding more accurately. The patient with a torrential lower GI bleed usually cannot be prepped for colonoscopy nor wait for tagged red blood cell images; such a patient should promptly undergo mesenteric angiography after a nasogastric aspirate has ruled out brisk upper GI bleeding. Once the site of bleeding is localized by angiography, surgery is often required.

Acute upper and lower GI bleeding present a challenge both diagnostically and therapeutically. It requires optimal teamwork of emergency and intensive care room staff, internists, gastroenterologists, invasive radiologists and surgeons.

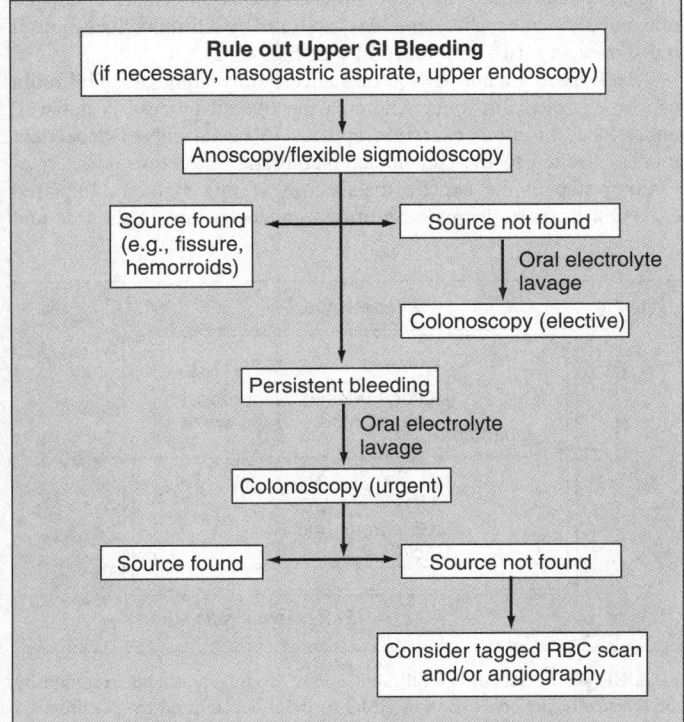

FIGURE 44-2 Approach to the patient with acute lower GI bleeding.

BIBLIOGRAPHY

CELLO JP et al: Endoscopic sclerotherapy versus portacaval shunt in patients with severe cirrhosis and acute variceal hemorrhage: Long-term follow-up. N Engl J Med 316:11, 1987

CHOJKIER M et al: A controlled comparison of continuous intraarterial and intravenous infusions of vasopressin in hemorrhage from esophageal varices. Gastroenterology 77:540, 1979

JENSEN DM, MACHICADO CA: Diagnosis and treatment of severe hemotochezia: The role of urgent colonoscopy after purge. Gastroenterology 95:1569, 1988

KANKARIA RG, FLEISHER DE: Critical management of nonvariceal upper gastrointestinal bleeding. Crit Care Clin 11:347, 1985

LAINE L: Multipolar electrocoagulation in the treatment of active upper gastrointestinal tract hemorrhage. N Engl J Med 316:1613, 1987

PETERSON WL et al: Routine early endoscopy in upper gastrointestinal tract bleeding: A randomized, controlled trial. N Engl J Med 304:925, 1981

REINUS JF, BRANDT LJ: Vascular ectasias and diverticulosis. Common causes of lower intestinal bleeding. Gastroenterol Clin North Am 23:1, 1988

RICHTER JM et al: Angiodysplasia: Clinical presentation and colonoscopic diagnosis. Dig Dis Sci 29:481, 1984

ROSEN RJ, SANCHEZ G: Angiographic diagnosis and management of gastrointestinal hemorrhage. Radiol Clin North Am 32:951, 1994

SUNG JJY et al: Prospective randomized study of the effects of octreotide on rebleeding from esophageal varices after endoscopic ligation. Lancet 346:1666, 1995

45   *Lee M. Kaplan, Kurt J. Isselbacher*

JAUNDICE

Accumulation of bilirubin in the bloodstream causes yellow pigmentation of the plasma, leading to discoloration of heavily perfused tissues. Serum bilirubin levels accumulate when its production from heme exceeds its metabolism and excretion. Imbalance between production and clearance may result either from excess release of bilirubin precursors into the bloodstream or from physiologic processes that impair the hepatic uptake, metabolism, or excretion of this metabolite (see Table 45-1). Clinically, hyperbilirubinemia appears as *jaundice* or *icterus*, yellow pigmentation of the skin and sclerae. Jaundice can usually be detected when the serum bilirubin level exceeds 34 to 43 μmol/L (2.0 to 2.5 mg/dL), or about twice the upper limit of the normal range, but may be detectable at lower bilirubin levels in patients with fair skin and profound anemia. Conversely, jaundice is frequently obscured in individuals with dark skin or edema. Scleral tissue is rich in elastin, which has a high affinity for bilirubin, so that scleral icterus is usually a more sensitive sign of hyperbilirubinemia than generalized jaundice. A similarly early sign of hyperbilirubinemia is darkening of the urine, which results from renal excretion of bilirubin in the form of bilirubin glucuronide. With pronounced jaundice, the skin may take

Table 45-1

Comparative Properties of Conjugated and Unconjugated Bilirubin

Properties and Reactions	Unconjugated	Conjugated
Water solubility	0	+
Affinity for lipids	+ +	±
Renal excretion	0	+
van den Bergh reaction	Indirect (total minus direct)	Direct
Binding to serum albumin (reversible)	+ + +	+
Formation of bilirubin-albumin complex (irreversible; delta bilirubin)	0	+ *

* Detectable in plasma under conditions of prolonged conjugated hyperbilirubinemia (see text).

on a greenish hue because of oxidation of some of the circulating bilirubin to biliverdin. This effect is seen more commonly with profound or long-standing *conjugated* hyperbilirubinemia such as in cirrhosis (see below). Other causes of yellowed skin include *carotenemia*, usually developing as a result of ingestion and absorption of large amounts of β-carotene and related pigmented compounds. Unlike hyperbilirubinemia, however, carotenemia does not cause scleral icterus.

PRODUCTION AND METABOLISM OF BILIRUBIN

Sources and Chemical Characterization of Serum Bilirubin

Normal serum bilirubin concentrations range from 5 to 17 μmol/L (0.3 to 1.0 mg/dL). More than 90 percent of serum bilirubin in normal individuals is in the unconjugated form, a nonpolar molecule circulating as an albumin-bound complex. The remainder is conjugated to a polar group (primarily glucuronide), rendering it water-soluble and thus able to be filtered and excreted by the kidney. When measured by routine clinical assays, the conjugated, or direct, fraction is frequently overestimated, leading to reported normal values of 1.7 to 8.5 μmol/L (0.1 to 0.5 mg/dL).

Approximately 80 percent of circulating bilirubin is derived from senescent red blood cells. When circulating erythrocytes reach the end of their normal life span of approximately 120 days, they are destroyed by reticuloendothelial cells (Fig. 45-1). Oxidation of the heme moiety dissociated from the hemoglobin within these cells generates biliverdin, which is then metabolized to bilirubin. Approximately 15 to 20 percent of circulating bilirubin is derived from other sources, including (1) ineffective erythropoiesis resulting from destruction of maturing erythroid cells in the bone marrow; and (2) the metabolism of other heme-containing proteins, most notably hepatic cytochromes, muscle myoglobin, and widely distributed heme-containing enzymes.

Unconjugated bilirubin liberated into the plasma is bound tightly, but noncovalently, to albumin. Certain organic anions, such as sulfonamides and salicylates, compete with bilirubin for binding sites on albumin, permitting the released pigment to enter tissues. Neonatal brain cells, especially those of the basal ganglia, have an affinity for unconjugated bilirubin facilitating its retention in the brain. This phenomenon may explain the neurotoxic effects of neonatal hyperbilirubinemia. Conjugated bilirubin is bound to albumin in two forms, reversible and irreversible. Reversible, noncovalent binding is similar to that of unconjugated bilirubin, although the complex is less stable. When present in serum for extended periods of time (e.g., with cholestasis, long-standing biliary obstruction, or chronic active hepatitis), conjugated bilirubin can form an irreversible, covalent complex with albumin referred to as *delta bilirubin* or *biliprotein*. Because of the irreversibility of binding, this complex is not excreted by the kidney. This delta bilirubin has a serum half-life similar to that of albumin (15 to 20 days) and thus remains detectable in serum for up to several weeks after relief of biliary obstruction or during recovery from hepatocellular disease.

Bilirubin is present in body fluids (joint effusions, ascites, pleural effusions, cysts, cerebrospinal fluid, etc.) in proportion to their albumin content and is absent from true secretions such as tears, saliva, and pancreatic juice. The appearance of jaundice is also influenced by blood flow and edema, with paralyzed extremities and edematous areas tending to remain uncolored.

Hepatic Metabolism of Bilirubin The liver has a central role in the metabolism of the bile pigments. This process can be divided into three distinct phases: (1) hepatic uptake, (2) conjugation, and (3) excretion into bile. Of these three phases, excretion appears to be the rate-limiting step and the one most susceptible to impairment when the liver cell is damaged.

Uptake Unconjugated bilirubin bound to albumin is presented to the liver cell, where the complex dissociates and the nonpolar bilirubin enters the hepatocyte by diffusion or transport across the plasma membrane. The uptake and subsequent hepatocyte storage of bilirubin involve binding of bilirubin to cytoplasmic anion-binding proteins, especially ligandin (glutathione-*S*-transferase B), that prevent efflux of bilirubin back into the plasma.

Conjugation Unconjugated bilirubin is water-insoluble unless complexed to an amphipathic molecule such as albumin. Since albumin is absent from bile, bilirubin must be converted to a water-soluble derivative before biliary excretion. This process is accomplished predominantly by conjugation of bilirubin to glucuronic acid, generating bilirubin glucuronide. The conjugation reaction occurs in the endoplasmic reticulum of hepatocytes and is catalyzed by bilirubin glucuronosyl transferase in a two-step reaction (see Fig. 45-2).

Excretion In normal circumstances, only conjugated bilirubin can be excreted into bile. Although the overall process is not well understood, bilirubin excretion appears to be an energy-dependent process limited to the canalicular membrane. Excretion is the rate-limiting step in the hepatic metabolism of this pigment. Impaired excretion leads to decreased bilirubin concentrations in the bile and

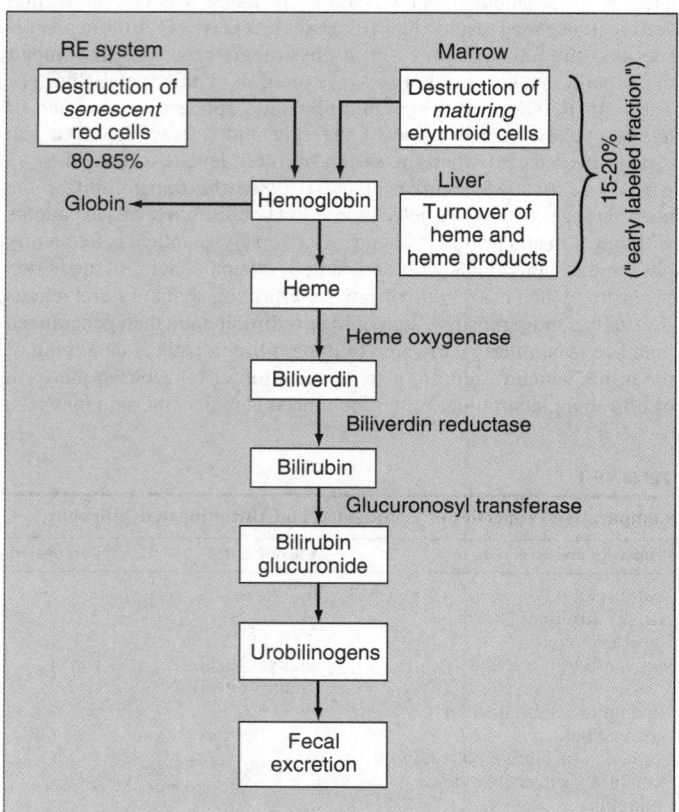

FIGURE 45-1 The sources and precursors of bilirubin and steps in its subsequent metabolism and excretion. RE, reticuloendothelial.

FIGURE 45-2 Scheme of bilirubin uptake, conjugation, and excretion by the liver cell. The conversion of BMG to BDG is catalyzed by glucuronosyl transferase of the endoplasmic reticulum. B, bilirubin; BMG, bilirubin monoglucuronide; BDG, bilirubin diglucuronide; UDP, uridine diphosphate.

concomitant efflux of *conjugated* bilirubin through the sinusoidal membrane of the hepatocyte into the bloodstream. The role of intracellular protein trafficking and membrane transport processes in normal and disordered bilirubin excretion are still incompletely understood.

Intestinal Phase of Bilirubin Metabolism After secretion into the bile, conjugated bilirubin is transported through the biliary ducts into the duodenum. Conjugated bilirubin is not reabsorbed by the intestinal mucosa. It is either excreted unchanged in the stool or metabolized by ileal and colonic bacteria to *urobilinogen* and related products. Urobilinogen can be reabsorbed from the small intestine and colon and enters the portal circulation. Some of the portal urobilinogen is taken up by the liver and reexcreted into the bile, and the remainder bypasses the liver and is excreted by the kidney. Under normal conditions, the daily urinary excretion of urobilinogen does not exceed 4 mg. When the hepatic uptake and excretion of urobilinogen is impaired (e.g., in hepatocellular disease) or the production of bilirubin is greatly increased (e.g., with hemolysis), daily urinary urobilinogen excretion may increase significantly. In contrast, cholestasis or extrahepatic biliary obstruction interferes with the intestinal phase of bilirubin metabolism and leads to markedly decreased production and urinary excretion of urobilinogen. Measurement of urinary urobilinogen can thus be a useful tool in distinguishing possible causes of hyperbilirubinemia.

Renal Excretion of Bilirubin The urine normally contains no detectable bilirubin by usual clinical assays, although traces may be detected by sensitive spectrophotometric procedures. Unconjugated bilirubin, being tightly bound into albumin, is not filtered by the renal glomeruli. Because there is no tubular secretory process for bilirubin, unconjugated bilirubin is not excreted in urine. In contrast, conjugated bilirubin is a polar molecule less tightly bound to albumin. A significant fraction circulates unbound, is filtered by the renal glomeruli, and appears in the urine. *The presence of bilirubin in the urine is evidence of conjugated hyperbilirubinemia* and can be a useful differentiating point early in the evaluation of jaundice. Bile salts enhance the glomerular filtration of conjugated bilirubin, and in conditions associated with increased circulating bile salts (e.g., cholestasis, extrahepatic biliary obstruction) renal bilirubin excretion is significantly enhanced. This increased renal excretion may explain the observation that serum conjugated bilirubin tends to plateau at levels below 510 to 680 μmol/L (30 to 40 mg/dL) in patients with *biliary tract obstruction*, while higher levels may occur in patients with severe hepatocellular injury. For additional information about the production, metabolism, and excretion of bilirubin, please refer to Chap. 294.

PATHOPHYSIOLOGIC CONSEQUENCES OF HYPER-BILIRUBINEMIA In most cases, hyperbilirubinemia itself has little pathophysiologic effect. Unlike circulating bile salts, whose levels are also elevated in cholestasis and biliary obstruction, bilirubin does not become deposited in cutaneous tissues and does not produce pruritus. However, unconjugated plasma bilirubin that is not bound to albumin can cross the blood-brain barrier. In conditions such as neonatal jaundice or type I or II Crigler-Najjar syndrome (see below), extremely high concentrations (>340 μmol/L or >20 mg/dL) of unconjugated bilirubin can accumulate, and the resulting diffusion of bilirubin into the central nervous system can cause encephalopathy (kernicterus) and permanent impairment of nervous function. The risk of kernicterus is increased by conditions that favor elevated circulating levels of *unbound*, unconjugated bilirubin, such as hemolysis, hypoalbuminemia, acidosis, and increased levels of compounds that compete for albumin binding such as free fatty acids and drugs. Circulating concentrations of unconjugated bilirubin can be decreased by removing these contributory factors and by facilitating the biliary excretion of unconjugated bilirubin. Exposure to blue light causes conformational changes in unconjugated bilirubin, rendering it more polar and water-soluble. These *photoisomers* are taken up and excreted by the liver and kidney, without need for conjugation. Intense treatment with blue light can provide sufficient isomerization of unconjugated bilirubin circulating through the skin to prevent kernicterus in patients with neonatal jaundice.

CHEMICAL TESTS FOR BILE PIGMENTS The most widely employed chemical test for bile pigments in serum is the van den Bergh reaction. The bilirubin pigments are exposed to sulfanilic acid to generate diazo conjugates, and the chromogenic products are measured colorimetrically. The van den Bergh reaction can be used to distinguish between unconjugated and conjugated bilirubin because of the different solubility properties of the pigments. When the reaction is performed in an aqueous medium, the water-soluble conjugated bilirubin reacts directly with sulfanilic acid, giving a positive *direct* van den Bergh reaction. When the reaction is performed in methanol, the intramolecular hydrogen bonds of unconjugated bilirubin are broken; thus, both conjugated and unconjugated pigments react, giving a measure of the *total* bilirubin level. The *indirect* value, representative of the unconjugated bilirubin fraction, is estimated by subtracting the direct-reacting fraction from the total measured bilirubin. The ability of the direct van den Bergh reaction to distinguish between conjugated and unconjugated bilirubin is dependent on the duration of the reaction. If the reaction is allowed to proceed longer than 1 min, a small amount of unconjugated pigment will react in the aqueous medium, giving a falsely high estimate of the direct-reacting (conjugated) fraction. This observation underscores the importance of considering these reactions as *approximations* rather than actual measurements of the conjugated and unconjugated fractions. More accurate measures of bilirubin fractions in biologic fluids reveal that normal serum contains predominantly (>96 percent) unconjugated bilirubin. This observation confirms the long-held suspicion that the small amount of direct-reacting bilirubin measured in normal serum by the van den Bergh method (2 to 5 μmol/L or 0.1 to 0.3 mg/dL) is an overestimate of the amount actually present. A summary of the key differences in the properties and reactions of the bilirubin pigments is shown in Table 45-1.

Qualitative determination of bilirubin in the urine may be accomplished by specific reaction with Ictotest tablets or dipstick. The foam test also is a simple qualitative test. When normal urine is shaken vigorously in a test tube, the foam is absolutely white. In urine containing bilirubin, the foam will be yellow. This difference may be subtle, becoming evident only after comparison with a similarly shaken specimen from a normal individual. Except for concentrated urine, the most common cause of a deep yellow-brown or dark urine is bilirubinuria. However, other causes of darkened urine need to be considered, including yellow or orange urine due to drugs (e.g., sulfasalazine, rifampin, thiamine), red urine due to porphyria, hemoglobinuria, myoglobinuria, or drugs (e.g., pyridium), and dark brown or black urine due to homogentisic acid (in ochronosis) or melanin (with melanoma).

ETIOLOGIC CONSIDERATIONS IN JAUNDICE Once jaundice is recognized clinically or chemically, it is important to determine whether it is predominantly due to unconjugated or conjugated hyperbilirubinemia (see Fig. 45-3). In the absence of available chemical determinations, a simple approach is to determine whether bilirubin is present in the urine. Its absence in the urine suggests unconjugated hyperbilirubinemia, since this pigment is not filtered by the renal glomeruli; its presence indicates conjugated hyperbilirubinemia. When chemical analysis (van den Bergh reaction) reveals 80 to 85 percent of the total serum bilirubin to be unconjugated, a patient is considered to have primarily *unconjugated hyperbilirubinemia*. A patient with more than 50 percent direct-reacting (conjugated) serum bilirubin is considered to have predominantly *conjugated hyperbilirubinemia*.

An approach to the classification of jaundice based on this important distinction is presented in Table 45-2. Derangements of bilirubin metabolism may occur through any of four mechanisms: (1) overproduction, (2) decreased hepatic uptake, (3) decreased hepatic conjugation, and (4) decreased excretion of bilirubin into bile (due either to intrahepatic dysfunction or extrahepatic mechanical obstruction). Jaundice may also be described on the basis of the pathogenic mechanisms or disease processes leading to increased bilirubin levels. Thus, the terms *hemolytic jaundice*, *hepatocellular jaundice*, and *obstructive* or *cholestatic jaundice* are often used. Though these classifications are helpful, in any one patient more than a single derangement in bilirubin metabolism may be operative, and more than a single "type" of jaundice may be present. For example, a patient with cirrhosis may have not only impaired hepatocyte function (and hence hepatocellular jaundice) but also hemolysis. Furthermore, as indicated above, obstructive jaundice or cholestasis may be due either to *mechanical* obstruction of the biliary radicles or to impaired *functional* hepatic excretion of bilirubin. This chapter presents a brief description of the major causes of jaundice. A more detailed discussion of individual diseases is found in Chap. 294.

Jaundice with Predominantly Unconjugated Bilirubinemia
Overproduction of bilirubin   An increased amount of hemoglobin released from senescent or hemolyzed red blood cells leads to increased bilirubin production. Erythrocyte destruction leading to hyperbilirubinemia most commonly results from intravascular hemolysis (e.g., autoimmune, microangiopathic, or hemoglobinopathy-associated) or resorption of a large hematoma. Excess bilirubin production is reflected in increased serum bilirubin levels of up to 51 to 68 μmol/L (3 to 4 mg/dL), with a predominance of unconjugated bilirubin. For further discussion of the causes of increased bilirubin production, refer to Chap. 294.

Impaired hepatic uptake of bilirubin   As indicated above, the uptake of bilirubin by hepatocytes requires dissociation of the nonpolar pigment molecule from albumin, transport across the cell membrane,

and binding to ligandin. In rare cases of drug-induced jaundice (e.g., from flavaspidic acid) and possibly in some patients with Gilbert's syndrome, there may be a disruption of this phase of bilirubin handling.

Impaired glucuronide conjugation   Deficiency in glucuronosyl transferase activity can occur as a result of both acquired and genetic defects. In the fetus and neonate, glucuronosyl transferase activity is normally low and the immature hepatocyte has an increased capacity for secretion of unconjugated bilirubin. Although transient, these alterations, together with increased neonatal intestinal absorption of unconjugated bilirubin, contribute to the development of *neonatal jaundice* that occurs between the second and fifth days of life. The significance of inherited deficiencies of glucuronosyl transferase depends on the level of residual enzyme activity. Gilbert's syndrome, associated with a *mild decrease* in activity, produces mild, asymptomatic, unconjugated hyperbilirubinemia. *Moderately decreased* activity occurs in Crigler-Najjar syndrome type II; this enzyme is *totally absent* in Crigler-Najjar syndrome type I, an autosomal recessive disorder associated with kernicterus and childhood mortality from central nervous system dysfunction. Acquired defects in glucuronosyl transferase activity may be induced by drugs (i.e., direct enzyme inhibition) or be associated with liver disease generally. However, in most hepatocellular disorders, bilirubin excretion is impaired to a greater extent than bilirubin conjugation, leading to primarily *conjugated* hyperbilirubinemia.

Jaundice with Predominantly Conjugated Bilirubinemia   *Impaired bilirubin excretion by hepatocytes*   Interference with the biliary excretion of conjugated bilirubin by hepatocytes leads to efflux

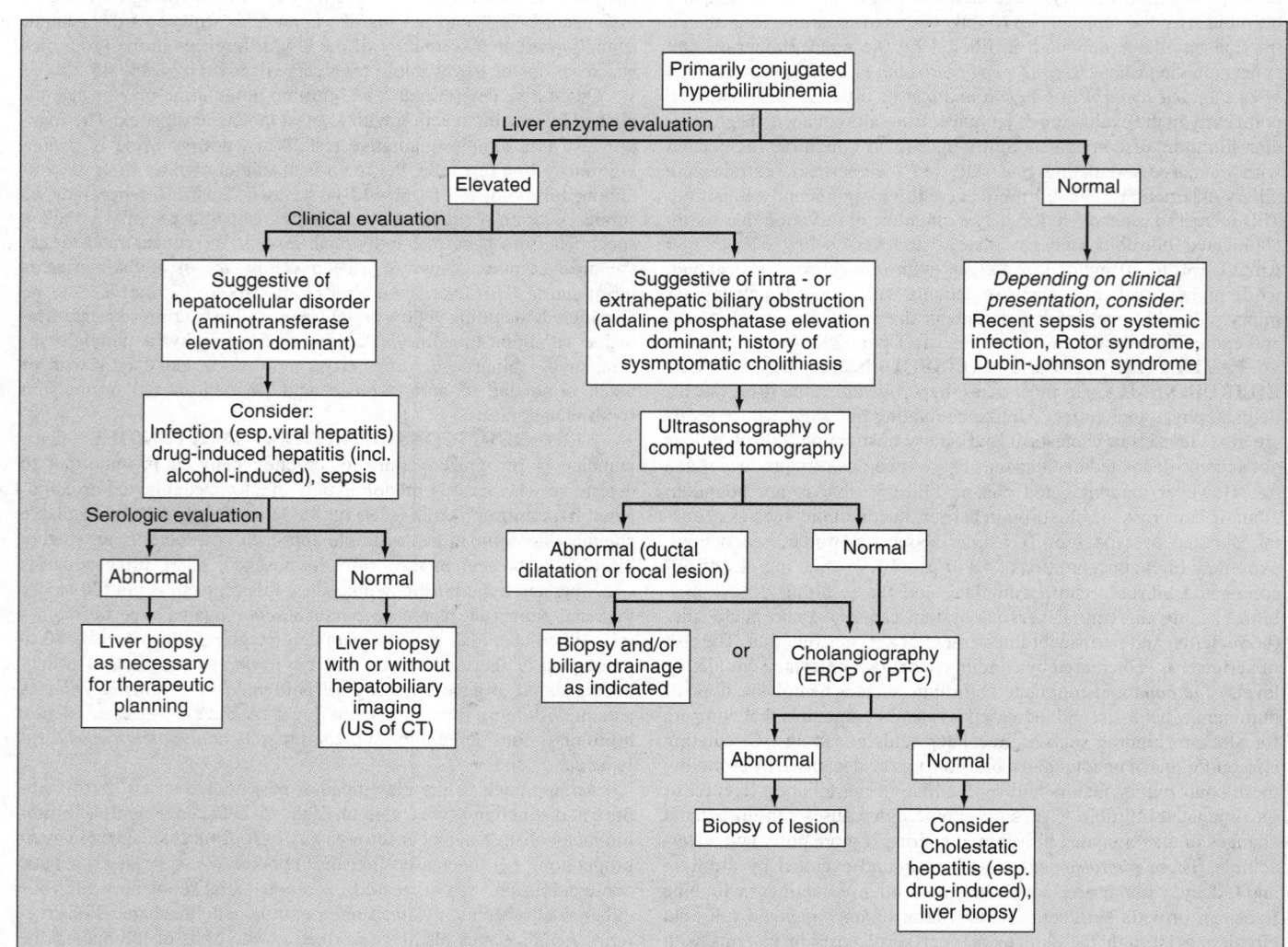

FIGURE 45-3   Algorithm for evaluation of conjugated hyperbilirubinemia. Abbreviations: CT, computed tomography, ERCP, endoscopic retrograde cholangiopancreatography; PTC, percutaneous transhepatic cholangiography; US, ultrasonography.

of this pigment into the systemic circulation, resulting in predominantly conjugated hyperbilirubinemia and consequent bilirubinuria. The mechanism for this efflux is unknown, although it is likely that impaired canalicular excretion leads to increased intracellular levels of conjugated bilirubin, which diffuses or is transported through the sinusoidal membrane into the blood. In addition, hepatocellular necrosis can promote rupture of the bile canaliculi, leading to direct reflux of bile into the hepatic sinusoids. Several mechanisms have been postulated to account for the decreased excretion of conjugated bilirubin in hepatocellular and cholestatic liver disease: (1) occlusion of the canaliculi by inspissated bile, (2) canalicular occlusion by swollen hepatocytes, (3) obstruction of the terminal intrahepatic bile ducts (cholangioles) by inflammatory cells, (4) altered hepatocyte permeability, allowing reuptake of excreted pigment, and (5) specific inhibition of membrane transport proteins.

Table 45-2

Classification of Jaundice Based on Underlying Derangement of Bilirubin Metabolism

PREDOMINANTLY *UNCONJUGATED* HYPERBILIRUBINEMIA

I. Overproduction
  A. Hemolysis (intra- and extravascular)
  B. Ineffective erythropoiesis
II. Decreased hepatic uptake
  A. Prolonged fasting
  B. Sepsis
III. Decreased bilrubin conjugation (decreased hepatic glucuronosyl transferase activity)
  A. Hereditary transferase deficiency
    1. Gilbert's syndrome (*mild* transferase deficiency)
    2. Crigler-Najjar type II (*moderate* transferase deficiency)
    3. Crigler-Najjar type I (*absence* of transferase)
  B. Neonatal jaundice (*transient* transferase deficiency; increased intestinal absorption of unconjugated bilirubin)
  C. Acquired transferase deficiency
    1. Drug inhibition (e.g., chloramphenicol, pregnanediol)
    2. Breast milk jaundice (transferase inhibition by pregnanediol and fatty acids in breast milk)
    3. Hepatocellular disease (hepatitis, cirrhosis)*
  D. Sepsis

PREDOMINANTLY *CONJUGATED* HYPERBILIRUBINEMIA

I. Impaired hepatic excretion (intrahepatic defects)
  A. Familial or hereditary disorders
    1. Dubin-Johnson syndrome
    2. Rotor syndrome
    3. Recurrent (benign) intrahepatic cholestasis
    4. Cholestatic jaundice of pregnancy
  B. Acquired disorders
    1. Hepatocellular disease (e.g., viral or drug-induced hepatitis, cirrhosis)*
    2. Drug-induced cholestasis (e.g., oral contraceptives, androgens, chlorpromazine)
    3. Alcoholic liver disease
    4. Sepsis
    5. Postoperative state
    6. Parenteral nutrition
    7. Biliary cirrhosis (primary or secondary)
II. Extrahepatic biliary obstruction
  A. Intraductal obstruction
    1. Gallstones
    2. Biliary malformation (e.g., stricture, atresia, choledochol cyst)
    3. Infection (e.g., *Clonorchis, Ascaris,* oriental cholangiohepatitis)
    4. Malignancy (cholangiocarcinoma, ampullary carcinoma)
    5. Hemobilia (trauma, tumor)
    6. Sclerosing cholangitis
  B. Compression of biliary ducts
    1. Malignancy (e.g., pancreatic carcinoma, lymphoma, metastases to portal lymph nodes)
    2. Inflammation (e.g., pancreatitis)

* In hepatocellular disease (hepatitis and cirrhosis) there is usually interference in the three major steps of bilirubin metabolism—uptake, conjugation, and excretion. However, excretion is the rate-limiting step and is usually impaired to the greatest extent. As a result, conjugated bilirubin predominates in serum.

Hepatocellular disorders in which jaundice may be associated with an obstructive, or cholestatic, phase include (1) drug reactions, especially those due to chlorpromazine or anabolic steroids, (2) alcoholic hepatitis and alcohol-induced fatty liver, (3) jaundice in the last trimester of pregnancy, (4) certain types of postoperative jaundice, (5) benign recurrent intrahepatic cholestasis, (6) Dubin-Johnson and Rotor syndromes, and (7) occasional cases of viral or autoimmune hepatitis. Impairment of bilirubin excretion is common in late-stage cirrhosis from any cause. It occurs much earlier in the course of primary biliary cirrhosis and in the rare cases of biliary cirrhosis occurring secondary to chronic, recurring choledocholithiasis or cholangitis.

Extrahepatic biliary obstruction *Complete obstruction* of the extrahepatic bile ducts leads to jaundice and predominantly conjugated hyperbilirubinemia associated with marked bilirubinuria and acholic stools. As noted above, the concentration of bilirubin rises progressively and plateaus at a level of 510 to 680 μmol/L (30 to 40 mg/dL). *Partial obstruction* of extrahepatic bile ducts also can lead to jaundice if the clearance of bilirubin into the duodenum is unable to match the level of pigment production. In such cases, intrabiliary pressure is usually increased (to levels approaching 250 mmHg). This increased pressure interferes with hepatocyte bilirubin secretion, further exaggerating the imbalance between bilirubin production and clearance. In partial biliary obstruction, the degree of jaundice and bilirubinuria depends on many factors, including the presence of concurrent hepatocellular disease or cholangitis, which can exacerbate the impairment of hepatocyte bilirubin excretion. The functional reserve of the liver is so great that occlusion of the intrahepatic bile ducts does not give rise to jaundice unless the drainage of bile from a large segment (>75 percent) of the parenchyma is interrupted. In most patients, either of the two major hepatic ducts or a large number of secondary radicles may be occluded without production of jaundice. In contrast, diffuse narrowing of the intrahepatic biliary ducts, even without complete obstruction, may produce jaundice in a manner analogous to partial obstruction of the extrahepatic ducts.

EVALUATION OF JAUNDICE The first task in the evaluation of jaundice is to consider whether the hyperbilirubinemia is due to hemolysis or hepatobiliary disease. This differentiation is most easily accomplished by measuring the direct and indirect bilirubin fractions. Predominantly unconjugated hyperbilirubinemia indicates a hemolytic disorder due to accelerated intravascular red blood cell destruction or resorption of a large hematoma. Exceptions to this rule are Gilbert's syndrome, the other, rare, hereditary disorders of glucuronosyl transferase, and end-stage hepatic failure. Further evaluation of the cause of hemolysis can then proceed as described in Chap. 108, "Megaloblastic Anemia," Chap. 107, "Hemoglobinopathies," and Chap. 109, "Anemias Due to Hemolysis and Acute Bood Loss."

Jaundice associated with predominantly (>50 percent) conjugated hyperbilirubinemia usually results from one of three groups of disorders: hepatocellular disease, intrahepatic biliary obstruction ("cholestasis"), and extrahepatic biliary obstruction. An early goal is the determination of which category of disease explains the patient's jaundice. Central to this determination is a careful *clinical* evaluation, including history, physical examination, basic tests of liver function, and a complete blood count. Using these simple tools, experienced clinicians can determine the overall nature of the jaundice in the majority of cases. Most importantly, however, the results of the clinical evaluation direct the physician to a logical progression of imaging studies, serologic tests, and pathologic evaluation. The initial clinical evaluation should focus on features of the patient's illness that distinguish between hepatocellular disease, intrahepatic cholestasis, and extrahepatic biliary obstruction. A general algorithm for the evaluation of jaundice due to conjugated hyperbilirubinemia is shown in Fig. 45-3.

History Historic evaluation should include determination of the length of symptoms, presence and character of abdominal pain, fever or other symptoms of active inflammation, and changes in appetite, weight, and bowel habits. Specific attention should be directed to a history of blood product transfusions, intravenous drug use, promiscuous sexual activity, and ethanol use. A history of medication use should be sought, particularly drugs known to cause either cholestasis, such as anabolic steroids and chlorpromazine, or hepatocellular necrosis, such as acetaminophen or isoniazid. A history of arthralgias may suggest acute viral hepatitis. Viral disease should also be considered in patients with a history of travel to developing countries endemic for enterally transmitted hepatitis E or East Asian countries, where the parenterally transmitted hepatitis B and C viruses are widespread. Pruritus is most commonly associated with chronic cholestasis, developing from either extrahepatic obstruction or cholestatic liver disease such as sclerosing cholangitis or primary biliary cirrhosis. In contrast, acholic stools develop more commonly in patients with extrahepatic biliary obstruction from tumor, choledocholithiasis, or secondary to a congenital biliary abnormality such as an inflamed choledochal cyst. The presence of acholic and heme-positive stool ("silver stools") should suggest a tumor of the distal biliary tract such as ampullary, periampullary, or cholangiocarcinoma. This combination may also be seen in patients with pancreatic carcinoma eroding into the biliary tract or duodenum. Jaundice, in the setting of previous biliary surgery, may suggest retained or recurrent stones, a biliary stricture, or recurrent obstruction from an enlarging tumor. Finally, a preexisting or underlying condition predisposing to hepatobiliary disease should be solicited. For example, inflammatory bowel disease, particularly ulcerative colitis, may be associated with sclerosing cholangitis. Pregnancy predisposes to cholestasis, steatosis, and acute liver failure. Right heart failure may result in hepatic congestion and cholestasis, and sepsis can cause selective disruption of bilirubin transport or generalized intrahepatic cholestasis.

Physical Examination The examination is also important for directing the subsequent evaluation. Excoriations suggest prolonged cholestasis or high grade biliary obstruction, and a greenish hue to the jaundice is associated with particularly severe or long-standing liver disease, such as biliary cirrhosis, sclerosing cholangitis, severe, chronic hepatitis, or long-standing malignant obstruction. Fever and epigastric or right upper quadrant tenderness are frequently associated with choledocholithiasis and cholangitis or cholecystitis. In contrast, malignant biliary obstruction commonly presents as painless jaundice. An enlarged, tender liver suggests acute hepatic inflammation or a rapidly enlarging hepatic tumor, while a palpable gallbladder suggests distal biliary obstruction from a malignant tumor. The presence of splenomegaly may provide a clue to the presence of portal hypertension, from chronic active hepatitis, severe alcoholic or acute viral hepatitis, or cirrhosis. Cirrhosis is also associated with a hyperestrogenic state that may be reflected in gynecomastia, testicular atrophy, or spider angiomata. Testicular atrophy may be particularly prominent in cirrhosis due to alcoholic liver disease or hemochromatosis. Palmar erythema, facial telangiectasia, and Dupuytren's contractures are also associated with cirrhosis, particularly as a result of chronic ethanol ingestion. Wasting or lymphadenopathy suggests malignancy, and in the presence of splenomegaly, these signs may direct consideration of a pancreatic tumor obstructing the splenic vein or a widely metastatic lymphoma. In patients whose history or examination suggests malignancy, particular attention should be directed toward physical findings suggestive of a primary tumor, including heme-positive stools, abdominal or breast masses, thyroid nodules, and supraclavicular lymphadenopathy. Physical findings associated with specific liver diseases include distended neck veins and hepatojugular reflux (right heart failure), xanthomata (primary biliary cirrhosis), and Kayser-Fleischer rings (Wilson's disease).

Laboratory Tests Initial laboratory evaluation should focus on serum bilirubin fractionation. Predominantly *unconjugated* (indirect) hyperbilirubinemia should prompt consideration of a hemolytic disorder, such as an autoimmune or microangiopathic hemolytic anemia, ineffective erythropoiesis, or resorption of a large hematoma. The most common cause of mild elevations in the unconjugated fraction, however, is Gilbert's syndrome, an inherited condition resulting from a mild deficiency in hepatic glucuronosyl transferase. Individuals with

Gilbert's syndrome experience variable elevations in circulating unconjugated bilirubin, especially in association with physical stress, fever, intercurrent infection or surgery, fasting, or heavy ethanol ingestion. This mild metabolic abnormality produces no symptoms other than jaundice, and is *not* associated with liver enzyme abnormalities or adverse long-term effects.

Conjugated (direct) hyperbilirubinemia usually results from hepatocellular or cholestatic liver disease or from extrahepatic biliary obstruction. Because hepatic glucuronosyl transferase activity is normally present in great abundance, adequate bilirubin glucuronide formation can occur even with severe liver disease. In patients with primarily conjugated hyperbilirubinemia, the presence and nature of liver enzyme abnormalities usually provide important clues about the nature of the underlying process. Conjugated hyperbilirubinemia without liver enzyme abnormalities is relatively uncommon but can be seen in pregnancy, sepsis, or after recent surgery. Isolated conjugated hyperbilirubinemia is the primary manifestation of two heritable disorders, Rotor and Dubin-Johnson syndromes, and can also be seen in some patients with the syndrome of recurrent benign intrahepatic cholestasis. As described more fully in Chap. 292, elevation of the aminotransferases out of proportion to other liver enzymes suggests hepatocellular damage, most commonly seen in toxic, viral, or ischemic hepatitis, while prominent elevations of the alkaline phosphatase, 5'-nucleotidase and/or gamma-glutamyl transpeptidase are more suggestive of intrahepatic cholestasis or extrahepatic obstruction. Although these patterns are not invariably diagnostic, they are helpful in directing the ensuing evaluation.

Patients with a clinical evaluation and laboratory findings suggestive of hepatocellular disease should be evaluated for evidence of viral hepatitis, drug toxicity, hepatic congestion, such as that produced by right ventricular failure or acute obstruction of the hepatic veins, or ischemic hepatitis. In the appropriate clinical setting, serologic studies are extremely helpful for establishing or excluding the diagnosis of hepatitis A; acute and chronic hepatitis B; hepatitis C, D, and E; and hepatitis from cytomegalovirus (CMV) or Epstein-Barr virus. Common causes of toxic hepatitis include acetaminophen, isoniazid, and halogenated anesthetic agents. Patients with alcoholic liver disease are particularly susceptible to acetaminophen toxicity, which may occur after therapeutic doses in these individuals. For patients with probable hepatocellular disease, liver biopsy can provide important diagnostic and prognostic information. The results of percutaneous, transjugular, or laparoscopic biopsy may also provide important information for optimal therapy. The role of hepatobiliary imaging in these patients is less clearly defined. In some cases, identification of focal lesions by computed tomography (CT), transabdominal ultrasonography (US), or magnetic resonance imaging (MRI) can increase the diagnostic accuracy of liver biopsy. These imaging techniques can also aid in diagnosis by suggesting the presence of hepatic fat deposition, cirrhosis, or the excessive hepatic iron deposition of hemochromatosis. Ultrasound is an exquisitely sensitive means of detecting ascites. Combined with Doppler flow analysis, it can also determine the patency and direction of flow in the portal and hepatic veins, frequently enabling noninvasive diagnosis of portal vein thrombosis and Budd-Chiari syndrome.

Hepatobiliary Imaging For patients whose clinical evaluation and liver chemistries suggest cholestasis or extrahepatic biliary obstruction, biliary imaging is an important early diagnostic tool to differentiate intrahepatic causes from extrahepatic obstruction. Both US and CT detect dilated extrahepatic biliary ducts with great sensitivity. In the absence of previous hepatobiliary surgery, the specificity of these tests for identifying dilated extrahepatic ducts is well above 90 percent. Both techniques are sensitive indicators of intrahepatic, portal, and pancreatic masses, and either can be effective in diagnosing biliary obstruction from tumors or impacted stones. In addition, US is an extremely effective means of detecting stones within the gallbladder and is somewhat more sensitive than CT. These imaging techniques are considerably less sensitive for detecting choledocholithiasis. Both fail to detect approximately 40 percent of intraductal stones, although selected studies suggest that CT is somewhat better at detecting stones within nondilated ducts.

In patients with clinical and radiographic evidence of extrahepatic biliary obstruction, further evaluation should be directed at determining the cause of the obstruction and providing rapid relief. Masses identified by transabdominal or endoscopic US, CT, or MRI are usually accessible to radiographically directed percutaneous or endoscopic biopsy. Further definition and relief of extrahepatic biliary obstruction can frequently be accomplished by *percutaneous* or *endoscopic cholangiography*. In the hands of experienced practitioners, dilated biliary ducts can be accessed percutaneously in more than 90 percent of patients, nondilated ducts in up to 70 percent. Percutaneous transhepatic cholangiography (PTC) may be particularly useful for imaging and drainage of patients with biliary obstruction well above the bifurcation of the common bile duct and in patients whose obstruction cannot be relieved during endoscopic cholangiography. Collection of bile for cytologic analysis may also allow identification of the obstructing lesion. Endoscopic retrograde cholangiopancreatography (ERCP) is frequently the preferred technique for diagnosing and treating distal biliary obstructions. In addition to cholangiography, ERCP provides the opportunity for inspection and biopsy of the ampulla of Vater and surrounding duodenum (common sites of tumors obstructing the bile ducts), visualization of the pancreatic ducts to detect evidence of pancreatic ductal stones or small pancreatic tumors, and direct biopsy of the bile duct epithelium and pancreatic head. Both PTC and ERCP can afford relief of malignant obstruction and dissolution or fragmenting of ductal stones. ERCP also provides the opportunity for long-term relief of stone disease via endoscopic papillotomy and is the preferred approach to intraductal stones remaining after surgical or laparoscopic cholecystectomy.

For patients with a clinical presentation of cholestasis who have ducts of *normal* caliber, attention should focus on intrahepatic cholestasis caused by primary biliary cirrhosis, drugs or toxins (including ethanol), and extrahepatic obstruction *without* ductal dilation, which can be caused by primary sclerosing cholangitis, primary biliary cirrhosis, or intrahepatic arterial chemotherapy and is occasionally seen in patients with cholangiocarcinoma. A related cholestatic process, termed *vanishing bile duct syndrome* (VBDS), can occur as a result of liver transplant rejection, AIDS, CMV infection, and radiation injury. VBDS is rarely associated with Hodgkin's disease and sarcoidosis and may develop after treatment with flucloxacillin, anticonvulsants, and other medications. If the clinical picture is more suggestive of cholestasis or biliary cirrhosis, liver biopsy may provide the most direct route to diagnosis. In contrast, cholangiography with cytologic analysis of the bile and/or biopsy of the ductal epithelium is indicated in patients whose presentation suggests extrahepatic obstruction, such as patients with jaundice and nondilated ducts in the setting of weight loss, lymphadenopathy, or inflammatory bowel disease.

BIBLIOGRAPHY

AONO S et al: Analysis of genes for UDP-glucuronosyl transferase in Gilbert's syndrome. Lancet 345:958, 1995

CHOWDHURY JR et al: Hereditary jaundice and disorders of bilirubin metabolism, in *The Metabolic Basis of Inherited Disease*, 7th ed. CR Scriver et al (eds). New York, McGraw-Hill, 1995, pp 2161–2208

FRANK BB et al: Clinical evaluation of jaundice: A guideline of the patient care committee of the American Gastroenterological Association. JAMA 262:3031, 1989

LAMONT JT, ISSELBACHER KJ: Postoperative jaundice, in *Wright's Liver and Biliary Disease*, 3d ed. GH Millward-Sadler et al (eds). Philadelphia, Saunders, 1992, pp 1372–1380

LESTER R (ed): The pathogenesis of cholestasis: Past and future trends. Semin Liver Dis 13:219, 1993

ROY-CHOWDHURY J et al: Bilirubin metabolism and its disorders, in *Hepatology*, 3d ed, D Zakim, T Boyer (eds). Philadelphia, Saunders, 1996, p 323

SHERLOCK S, DOOLEY J (eds): *Diseases of the Liver and Biliary System*, 9th ed. Oxford, Blackwell, 1993, pp 199–213

WEISS JS et al: The clinical importance of a protein-bound fraction of serum bilirubin in patients with hyperbilirubinemia. N Engl J Med 309:147, 1983

46   *Robert M. Glickman, Kurt J. Isselbacher*

ABDOMINAL SWELLING AND ASCITES

ABDOMINAL SWELLING   Abdominal swelling or distention is a common problem in clinical medicine and may be the initial manifestation of a systemic disease or of otherwise unsuspected abdominal disease. *Subjective* abdominal enlargement, often described as a sensation of fullness or bloating, is usually transient and is often related to a functional gastrointestinal disorder when it is not accompanied by objective physical findings of increased abdominal girth or local swelling. *Obesity* and lumbar lordosis, which may be associated with prominence of the abdomen, may usually be distinguished from true increases in the volume of the peritoneal cavity by history and careful physical examination.

Clinical History   Abdominal swelling may first be noticed by the patient because of a progressive increase in belt or clothing size, the appearance of abdominal or inguinal hernias, or the development of a localized swelling. Often, considerable abdominal enlargement has gone unnoticed for weeks or months, either because of coexistent obesity or because the ascites formation has been insidious, without pain or localizing symptoms. Progressive abdominal distention may be associated with a sensation of "pulling" or "stretching" of the flanks or groins and vague low back pain. Localized *pain* usually results from involvement of an abdominal organ (e.g., a passively congested liver, large spleen, or colonic tumor). Pain is uncommon in cirrhosis with ascites, and when it is present, pancreatitis, hepatocellular carcinoma, or peritonitis should be considered. Tense ascites or abdominal tumors may produce increased intraabdominal pressure, resulting in *indigestion* and *heartburn* due to gastroesophageal reflux or *dyspnea*, *orthopnea*, and *tachypnea* from elevation of the diaphragm. A coexistent pleural effusion, more commonly on the right, presumably due to leakage of ascitic fluid through lymphatic channels in the diaphragm, also may contribute to respiratory embarrassment. The patient with diffuse abdominal swelling should be questioned about increased alcohol intake, a prior episode of jaundice or hematuria, or a change in bowel habits. Such historical information may provide the clues that will lead one to suspect an occult cirrhosis, a colonic tumor with peritoneal seeding, congestive heart failure, or nephrosis.

Physical Examination   A carefully executed general physical examination can yield valuable clues concerning the etiology of abdominal swelling. Thus palmar erythema and spider angiomas suggest an underlying cirrhosis, while supraclavicular adenopathy (Virchow's node) should raise the question of an underlying gastrointestinal malignancy.

Inspection of the abdomen is important. By noting the abdominal contour, one may be able to distinguish localized from generalized swelling. The tensely distended abdomen with tightly stretched skin, bulging flanks, and everted umbilicus is characteristic of ascites. A prominent abdominal venous pattern with the direction of flow away from the umbilicus often is a reflection of portal hypertension; venous collaterals with flow from the lower part of the abdomen toward the umbilicus suggest obstruction of the inferior vena cava; flow downward toward the umbilicus suggests superior vena cava obstruction. "Doming" of the abdomen with visible ridges from underlying intestinal loops is usually due to intestinal obstruction or distention. An epigastric mass, with evident peristalsis proceeding from left to right, usually indicates underlying pyloric obstruction. A liver with metastatic deposits may be visible as a nodular right upper quadrant mass moving with respiration.

Auscultation may reveal the high-pitched, rushing sounds of early intestinal obstruction or a succussion sound due to increased fluid and gas in a dilated hollow viscus. Careful auscultation over an enlarged liver occasionally reveals the harsh bruit of a vascular tumor, especially a hepatocellular carcinoma, or the leathery friction rub of a surface nodule. A venous hum at the umbilicus may signify portal hypertension and an increased collateral blood flow around the liver. A fluid wave and flank dullness that shifts with change in position of the patient are important signs that indicate the presence of peritoneal fluid. In obese patients, small amounts of fluid may be difficult to demonstrate; on occasion, the fluid may be detected by abdominal percussion with patients on their hands and knees. Small amounts of ascites often can only be detected by ultrasound examination of the abdomen. Careful percussion should serve to distinguish generalized abdominal enlargement from localized swelling due to an enlarged uterus, ovarian cyst, or distended bladder. Percussion also can outline an abnormally small or large liver. Loss of normal liver dullness may result from massive hepatic necrosis; it also may be a clue to free gas in the peritoneal cavity, as from perforation of a hollow viscus.

Palpation is often difficult with massive ascites, and ballottement of overlying fluid may be the only method of palpating the liver or spleen. A slightly enlarged spleen in association with ascites may be the only evidence of an occult cirrhosis. When there is evidence of portal hypertension, a soft liver suggests that obstruction to portal flow is extrahepatic; a firm liver suggests cirrhosis as the likely cause of the portal hypertension. A very hard or nodular liver is a clue that the liver is infiltrated with tumor, and when accompanied by ascites, it suggests that the latter is due to peritoneal seeding. The presence of a hard periumbilical nodule (Sister Mary Joseph's nodule) suggests metastatic disease from a pelvic or gastrointestinal primary tumor. A pulsatile liver and ascites may be found in tricuspid insufficiency.

An attempt should be made to determine whether a mass is solid or cystic, smooth or irregular, and whether it moves with respiration. The liver, spleen, and gallbladder should descend with respiration unless they are fixed by adhesions or extension of tumor beyond the organ. A fixed mass not descending with respiration may indicate that it is retroperitoneal. Tenderness, especially if localized, may indicate an inflammatory process such as an abscess; it also may be due to stretching of the visceral peritoneum or tumor necrosis. Rectal and pelvic examinations are mandatory; they may reveal otherwise undetected masses due to tumor or infection.

Radiographic and laboratory examinations are essential for confirming or extending the impressions gained on physical examination.

Upright and recumbent films of the abdomen may demonstrate the dilated loops of intestine with fluid levels characteristic of intestinal obstruction or the diffuse abdominal haziness and loss of psoas margins suggestive of ascites. Ultrasonography is often of value in detecting ascites, determining the presence of a mass, or evaluating the size of the liver and spleen. Computed tomography (CT) scanning provides similar information. CT scanning is often necessary to visualize the retroperitoneum, pancreas, and lymph nodes. A plain film of the abdomen may reveal the distended colon of otherwise unsuspected ulcerative colitis and give valuable information as to the size of the liver and spleen. An irregular and elevated right side of the diaphragm may be a clue to a liver abscess or hepatocellular carcinoma. Studies of the gastrointestinal tract with barium or other contrast media are usually necessary in the search for a primary tumor.

ASCITES The evaluation of a patient with ascites requires that the *cause* of the ascites be established. In most cases ascites will appear as a part of a well-recognized illness, i.e., cirrhosis, congestive heart failure, nephrosis, or disseminated carcinomatosis. In these situations, the physician should determine that the development of ascites is indeed a consequence of the basic underlying disease and not due to the presence of a separate or related disease process. This distinction is necessary even when the cause of ascites seems obvious. For example, when the patient with compensated cirrhosis and minimal ascites develops progressive ascites that is increasingly difficult to control with sodium restriction or diuretics, the obvious temptation is to attribute the worsening of the clinical picture to progressive liver disease. However, an occult hepatocellular carcinoma, portal vein thrombosis, spontaneous bacterial peritonitis, or even tuberculosis may be responsible for the decompensation. The disappointingly low success in diagnosing tuberculous peritonitis or hepatocullar carcinoma in the patient with cirrhosis and ascites reflects the too-low index of suspicion for the development of such superimposed conditions. Similarly, the patient with congestive heart failure may develop ascites from a disseminated carcinoma with peritoneal seeding.

Diagnostic paracentesis (50 to 100 mL) should be part of the routine evaluation of the patient with ascites. The fluid should be examined for its gross appearance; protein content, cell count, and differential cell count should be determined, and Gram's and acid-fast stains and culture performed. Cytologic and cell-block examination may disclose an otherwise unsuspected carcinoma. Table 46-1

Table 46-1

Ascitic Fluid Characteristics in Various Disease States

Condition	Gross Appearance	Protein, g/dL	Serum-Ascites Albumin Gradient, g/dL	Cell Count		Other Tests
				Red Blood Cells, >10,000/μL	White Blood Cells, per μL	
Cirrhosis	Straw-colored or bile-stained	<25 (95%)	>1.1	1%	<250 (90%);* predominantly mesothelial	
Neoplasm	Straw-colored, hemorrhagic, mucinous, or chylous	>25 (75%)	<1.1	20%	>1000 (50%); variable cell types	Cytology, cell block, peritoneal biopsy
Tuberculous peritonitis	Clear, turbid, hemorrhagic, chylous	>25 (50%)	<1.1	7%	>1000 (70%); usually >70% lymphocytes	Peritoneal biopsy, stain and culture for acid-fast bacilli
Pyogenic peritonitis	Turbid or purulent	If purulent, >2.5	<1.1	Unusual	Predominantly polymorphonuclear leukocytes	+ Gram's stain, culture
Congestive heart failure	Straw-colored	Variable, 15–53	>1.1	10%	<1000 (90%); usually mesothelial, mononuclear	
Nephrosis	Straw-colored or chylous	<25 (100%)	>1.1	Unusual	<250; mesothelial, mononuclear	If chylous, ether extraction, Sudan staining
Pancreatic ascites (pancreatitis, pseudocyst)	Turbid, hemorrhagic, or chylous	Variable, often >25	<1.1	Variable, may be blood-stained	Variable	Increased amylase in ascitic fluid and serum

* Since the conditions of examining fluid and selecting patients were not identical in each series, the percentage figures (in parentheses) should be taken as an indication of the order of magnitude rather than as the precise incidence of any abnormal finding.

presents some of the features of ascitic fluid typically found in various disease states. In some disorders, such as cirrhosis, the fluid has the characteristics of a transudate (<25 g protein per liter and a specific gravity of <1.016); in others, such as peritonitis, the features are those of an exudate. Rather than the total protein content of ascites, some authors prefer the use of a *serum-ascites albumin gradient* (SAG) to characterize ascites. The gradient correlates directly with portal pressure. A gradient >1.1 g/dL is characteristic of uncomplicated cirrhotic ascites; a gradient <1.1 g/dL is seen in conditions characterized by exudative ascites. Although there is variability of the ascitic fluid in any given disease state, some features are sufficiently characteristic to suggest certain diagnostic possibilities. For example, blood-stained fluid with >25 g protein per liter is unusual in uncomplicated cirrhosis but is consistent with tuberculous peritonitis or neoplasm. Cloudy fluid with a predominance of polymorphonuclear cells and a positive Gram's stain are characteristic of bacterial peritonitis; if most cells are lymphocytes, tuberculosis should be suspected. The complete examination of each fluid is most important, for occasionally only *one* finding may be abnormal. For example, if the fluid is a typical transudate but contains more than 250 white blood cells per microliter, the finding should be recognized as atypical for cirrhosis and should warrant a search for tumor or infection. This is especially true in the evaluation of cirrhotic ascites where occult peritoneal infection may be present with only minor elevations in the white blood cell count of the peritoneal fluid (300 to 500 cells per microliter). Since Gram's stain of the fluid may be negative in a high proportion of such cases, careful culture of the peritoneal fluid is mandatory. Bedside innoculation of blood culture flasks with ascitic fluid results in a dramatically increased incidence of positive cultures when bacterial infection is present (90 versus 40 percent positivity with conventional cultures done by the laboratory). Direct visualization of the peritoneum (laparoscopy) may disclose peritoneal deposits of tumor, tuberculosis, or metastatic disease of the liver. Biopsies are taken under direct vision, often adding to the diagnostic accuracy of the procedure.

Chylous ascites refers to a turbid, milky, or creamy peritoneal fluid due to the presence of thoracic or intestinal lymph. Such a fluid shows Sudan-staining fat globules microscopically and an increased triglyceride content by chemical examination. Opaque milky fluid usually has a triglyceride concentration of >1000 mg/dL. A turbid fluid due to leukocytes or tumor cells may be confused with chylous fluid (pseudochylous), and it is often helpful to carry out alkalinization and ether extraction of the specimen. Alkali will tend to dissolve cellular proteins and thereby reduce turbidity; ether extraction will lead to clearing if the turbidity of the fluid is due to lipid. Chylous ascites is most often the result of lymphatic obstruction from trauma, tumor, tuberculosis, filariasis (see Chap. 223), or congenital abnormalities. It also may be seen in the nephrotic syndrome.

Rarely, ascitic fluid may be *mucinous* in character, suggesting either pseudomyxoma peritonei (Chap. 288) or rarely a colloid carcinoma of the stomach or colon with peritoneal implants.

On occasion, ascites may develop as a seemingly isolated finding in the absence of a clinically evident underlying disease. It is then that a careful analysis of ascitic fluid may indicate the direction the evaluation should take. A useful framework for the workup starts with an analysis of whether the fluid is an exudate or transudate. *Transudative ascites* of unclear etiology is most often due to occult cirrhosis, right-sided venous hypertension raising hepatic sinusoidal pressure, or hypoalbuminemic states such as nephrosis or protein-losing enteropathy. Cirrhosis with well-preserved liver function (normal albumin) resulting in ascites invariably is associated with signifi-

cant portal hypertension (see Chap. 298). Evaluation should include liver function tests, liver-spleen scan, or other hepatic imaging procedure (i.e., CT or ultrasound) to detect nodular changes in the liver or a colloid shift of isotope to suggest portal hypertension. On occasion, a wedged hepatic venous pressure can be useful to document portal hypertension. Finally, if clinically indicated, a liver biopsy will confirm the diagnosis of cirrhosis and perhaps suggest its etiology. Other etiologies may result in hepatic venous congestion and resultant ascites. Right-sided cardiac valvular disease and particularly constrictive pericarditis should raise a high index of suspicion and may require cardiac imaging and cardiac catheterization for definitive diagnosis. Hepatic vein thrombosis is evaluated by visualizing the hepatic veins using imaging techniques (Doppler ultrasound, angiography, CT scans, magnetic resonance imaging) to demonstrate obliteration, thrombosis, or obstruction by tumor. Uncommonly, transudative ascites may be associated with benign tumors of the ovary, particularly fibroma (Meigs' syndrome) with ascites and hydrothorax.

Exudative ascites should initiate an evaluation for primary peritoneal processes, most importantly infection and tumor. Routine bacteriologic culture of ascitic fluid often will yield a specific organism causing infectious peritonitis. Tuberculous peritonitis (see Table 46-1) is best diagnosed by peritoneal biopsy, either percutaneously or via laparoscopy. Histologic examination invariably shows granulomata that may contain acid-fast bacilli. Since cultures of peritoneal fluid and biopsies for tuberculosis may require 6 weeks, characteristic histology with appropriate stains allows antituberculosis therapy to be started promptly. Similarly, the diagnosis of peritoneal seeding by tumor can usually be made by cytologic analysis of peritoneal fluid or by peritoneal biopsy if cytology is negative. Appropriate diagnostic studies can then be undertaken to determine the nature and site of the primary tumor. Pancreatic ascites (see Table 46-1) is invariably associated with an extravasation of pancreatic fluid from the pancreatic ductal system, most commonly from a leaking pseudocyst. Ultrasound or CT examination of the pancreas followed by visualization of the pancreatic duct by direct cannulation (viz., endoscopic retrograde cholangiopancreatography, ERCP) will usually disclose the site of leakage and permit resective surgery to be carried out.

An analysis of the physiologic and metabolic factors involved in the production of ascites (see Chap. 298 for details), coupled with a complete evaluation of the nature of the ascitic fluid, will invariably disclose the etiology of the ascites and permit appropriate therapy to be instituted.

BIBLIOGRAPHY

EPSTEIN M: Treatment of refractory ascites. N Engl J Med 321:1675, 1989

HOEFS JC: Globulin correction of the albumin gradient: Correlation with measured ascites colloid osmotic pressure gradients. Hepatology 16:396, 1992

LIPSKY MS, STERNBACH MR: Evaluation and initial management of patients with ascites. Am Fam Physician 54:1327, 1996

PINTO PC et al: Large volume paracentesis in nonedematous patients with tense ascites: Its effect on intravascular volume. Hepatology 8:207, 1988

RECTOR WG JR, REYNOLDS TB: Superiority of the serum: ascites albumin difference over the ascites total protein concentration in separation of "transudative" and "exudative" ascites. Am J Med 77:83, 1988

RUNYON BA: Care of patients with ascites. N Engl J Med 330:337, 1994

——— et al: The serum-ascites albumin gradient in the differential diagnosis of ascites. Ann Intern Med 117:215, 1992

| 47 | *Bradley M. Denker, Barry M. Brenner* |

CARDINAL MANIFESTATIONS OF RENAL DISEASE

Renal diseases may present to the physician in several different ways depending upon the nature of the illness and the timing of presentation. Some patients with advanced renal disease have signs and symptoms of uremia with unremarkable urinalysis, while others have abnormalities of the urine but few, if any, disturbances in renal function. After a complete history and physical examination, the urinalysis and serum chemistries are essential aids in helping to distinguish among the various etiologies of renal disease. Urine characteristics including volume, specific gravity, electrolyte composition, and sediment (cells, casts, and crystals) can help define the specific process affecting the kidneys. This chapter focuses on the evaluation of patients with reduced glomerular filtration rate (GFR) and/or abnormalities of the urine.

AZOTEMIA

ASSESSMENT OF GLOMERULAR FILTRATION RATE

A reduced GFR leads to retention of nitrogenous waste products (azotemia) such as blood urea nitrogen (BUN) and creatinine. Azotemia may result from reduced renal perfusion, intrinsic renal disease, or postrenal processes (ureteral obstruction). Precise determination of GFR is problematic as commonly used markers (urea and creatinine) are partially handled by tubule transport. An ideal endogenous marker for GFR would be produced at a constant rate, freely filtered at the glomerulus, not protein-bound, and excreted without tubular modification (no reabsorption, secretion, or catabolism). BUN varies directly with protein intake, and urea is readily reabsorbed by the medullary collecting duct. The permeability of the tubule to urea is linked to water reabsorption; it is low in states of diuresis and low levels of arginine vasopressin (AVP) but is enhanced in states of decreased intravascular volume, low tubule fluid flow rate, and increased levels of AVP. Gastrointestinal bleeding, glucocorticoids, and tetracycline can also increase BUN, while reduced levels can be seen in patients with malnutrition and muscle wasting as seen in starvation or chronic liver disease. Urea clearance is generally an underestimate of GFR because of tubule urea reabsorption and may be as low as one-half of GFR measured by other techniques.

Creatinine is a small, freely filtered solute whose production varies little from day to day (since it is derived from metabolism of muscle creatine). However, serum creatinine can increase acutely from dietary ingestion of cooked meat. Creatinine can be secreted by the proximal tubule through an organic cation pathway that is saturable and can be blocked by some commonly used medications including cimetidine, trimethoprim, pyrimethamine, and dapsone. The secreted creatinine component confounds GFR measurements because it can vary within individuals over time; moreover, the proportion of secreted creatinine increases as GFR decreases. Extrarenal clearance of creatinine through gastrointestinal metabolism by bacterial flora can also affect GFR measurements when GFR is reduced. Most autoanalyzers of serum creatinine avoid contributions of noncreatinine chromogens, but high bilirubin levels can cause falsely low creatinine levels. Despite these shortcomings, creatinine clearance remains the most common clinical measure of GFR. The gradual loss of muscle from chronic illness, glucocorticoids, and malnutrition can mask significant changes in GFR through small or imperceptible changes in serum creatinine. More accurate determinations of GFR are available using inulin clearance or radionuclide-labeled markers such as ^{125}I-iothalamate or ^{51}Cr-ethylenediaminetetraacetic acid (EDTA).

Approach to the Patient

With Azotemia Once it has been established that GFR is reduced, the physician must decide if this represents acute or chronic renal failure. The clinical situation, history, and laboratory data often make this an easy distinction. Laboratory abnormalities characteristic of chronic renal failure include anemia, hypocalcemia, hyperphosphatemia, and radiographic evidence of renal osteodystrophy (Chap. 271). The urinalysis and renal ultrasound can also facilitate the distinction between acute and chronic renal failure. An approach to the evaluation of azotemic patients is shown in Fig. 47-1. Patients with advanced chronic renal failure often have some proteinuria, nonconcentrated urine (isosthenuria), and small kidneys on ultrasound, which is characterized by increased echogenicity and cortical thinning. Treatment should be directed toward slowing the progression of renal disease and providing symptomatic relief for edema, acidosis, anemia, and hyperphosphatemia, as discussed in Chap. 271. Acute renal failure can result from processes affecting renal blood flow (prerenal azotemia), intrinsic renal diseases (affecting vessels, glomeruli, or tubules), or postrenal processes (obstruction to urine flow in ureters, bladder, or urethra) (see Chap. 270).

PRERENAL FAILURE Decreased renal perfusion accounts for 40 to 80 percent of acute renal failure and, if appropriately treated, is readily reversible. The etiologies of prerenal azotemia include any cause of decreased circulating blood volume including volume loss (gastrointestinal hemorrhage, burns, diarrhea, diuretics), volume sequestration (pancreatitis, peritonitis, rhabdomyolysis), or decreased effective circulating volume (cardiogenic shock, sepsis). Renal perfusion can also be affected adversely by reductions in cardiac output from peripheral vasodilatation (sepsis, drugs) or profound renal vasoconstriction [severe heart failure, hepatorenal syndrome, drugs (e.g., nonsteroidal anti-inflammatory drugs, or NSAIDs)]. True, or "effective," hypovolemia leads to a fall in mean arterial pressure, which in turn triggers a series of neural and humoral responses that include activation of the sympathetic nervous system and renin-angiotensin-aldosterone system and AVP release. GFR is maintained by prostaglandin-mediated relaxation of afferent arterioles and angiotensin II–mediated constriction of efferent arterioles. Once the mean arterial pressure falls below 80 mmHg, there is a steep decline in GFR. Blockade of prostaglandin production by NSAIDs can result in severe vasoconstriction and acute renal failure in the presence of hypotension. Angiotensin-converting enzyme (ACE) inhibitors decrease efferent arteriolar tone and can thereby reduce glomerular capillary perfusion pressure. Patients on NSAIDs and/or ACE inhibitors are most susceptible to hemodynamically mediated acute renal failure when blood volume is reduced. Patients with renal artery stenosis are dependent upon efferent arteriolar vasoconstriction for maintenance of glomerular filtration pressure and are particularly susceptible to precipitous declines in GFR when given ACE inhibitors.

Prolonged renal hypoperfusion can lead to acute tubular necrosis (ATN), an intrinsic renal disease discussed below. The urinalysis and urinary electrolytes can be useful in distinguishing prerenal azotemia from ATN (Table 47-1). In prerenal failure the tubules are intact, leading to a concentrated urine (>500 mosmol/L), avid Na retention (urine Na concentration < 20 mmol/L; fractional excretion of Na < 1%), and urine/plasma creatinine ratio > 40 (Table 47-1). Urine sediment in prerenal failure is usually normal or has occasional hyaline and granular casts, while the sediment in ATN is usually filled with cellular debris and muddy brown granular casts.

INTRINSIC RENAL DISEASE When prerenal and postrenal azotemia have been excluded as etiologies of renal failure, an intrinsic parenchymal renal disease is present. Intrinsic renal disease can arise from processes involving large renal vessels, microvasculature and glomeruli, or tubular interstitium. Ischemic and toxic ATN account for about 90 percent of acute intrinsic renal failure. As outlined in Fig. 47-1, the clinical setting and urinalysis are helpful in separating the possible etiologies of acute intrinsic renal failure. Prerenal azotemia and ATN are part of a spectrum of renal hypoperfusion: evidence of structural tubule injury is present in ATN, whereas prompt reversibility occurs with prerenal azotemia upon restoration of adequate renal perfusion. Thus, ATN can often be distinguished from prerenal azotemia by urinalysis and urine electrolyte composition (Table 47-1 and Fig. 47-1). Ischemic ATN is observed most frequently in patients who have undergone major surgery, trauma, severe hypovolemia, overwhelming sepsis, or extensive burns. Nephrotoxic ATN complicates the administration of many common medications usually by inducing a combination of intrarenal vasoconstriction, direct tubule toxicity, and/or tubular obstruction. The kidney is vulnerable to toxic injury by virtue of its rich blood supply (25 percent of cardiac output) and its ability to concentrate and metabolize toxins. A diligent search for hypotension and nephrotoxins will usually uncover the specific etiology of ATN. → *An extensive list of potential drugs and toxins implicated in ATN can be found in Chap. 270.*

Processes that involve the tubules and interstitium can lead to acute renal failure. These include drug-induced interstitial nephritis (especially antibiotics, NSAIDs, and diuretics), severe infections (both bacterial and viral), systemic diseases (such as systemic lupus erythematosus), or infiltrative disorders (such as sarcoid, lymphoma, or leukemia) (see Chap. 276). The urinalysis usually shows mild to moderate proteinuria, hematuria, and pyuria and occasionally white blood cell casts. The finding of red blood cell casts in interstitial nephritis has been reported but should prompt a search for glomerular diseases. The finding of eosinophils in the urine is suggestive of allergic interstitial nephritis or atheroemboli.

Occlusion of large renal arteries and veins is an uncommon cause of acute renal failure. A significant reduction in GFR by this mechanism suggests bilateral processes or a unilateral process in a patient with a single functioning kidney. Renal arteries can be occluded with atheroemboli, thromboemboli, in situ thrombosis, aortic dissection, or vasculitis. Atheroembolic renal failure can occur spontaneously but is most often associated with recent aortic instrumentation. The emboli are cholesterol-rich and lodge in medium and small renal arteries, leading to an eosinophil-rich inflammatory reaction. The urinalysis in atheroembolic acute renal failure is usually normal but may contain eosinophils and casts. The diagnosis can be confirmed by renal biopsy, but this is often unnecessary when other stigmata of atheroemboli are present (livido reticularis, distal peripheral infarcts, eosinophilia). Renal artery thrombosis may lead to mild proteinuria and hematuria, whereas renal vein thrombosis usually induces heavy proteinuria and hematuria. → *These vascular catastrophes often require angiography for confirmation (Fig. 47-1) and are discussed in Chap. 277.*

Diseases of glomeruli (glomerulonephritis or vasculitis) and the renal microvasculature (hemolytic uremic syndromes, thrombotic thrombocytopenic purpura, or malignant hypertension) usually present with various manifestations of glomerular injury: proteinuria, hematuria, reduced GFR, and alterations of sodium excretion leading to hypertension, edema, and circulatory congestion (acute nephritic syndrome). These findings may occur as primary renal diseases or as renal manifestations of systemic diseases. The finding of red blood cell casts in the urine is an indication for early renal biopsy (Fig. 47-1) since the pathologic pattern has important implications for diagnosis, prognosis, and treatment. Hematuria without red blood cell casts can also be an indication of glomerular disease (Figs. 47-1 and 47-2). → *A detailed discussion of glomerulonephritis and diseases of the microvasculature is presented in Chap. 274.*

Table 47-1

Laboratory Findings in Acute Renal Failure

Index	Prerenal Azotemia	Oliguric Acute Renal Failure
BUN/P_{Cr} Ratio	>20:1	10–15:1
Urine sodium (U_{Na}), mEq/L	<20	>40
Urine osmolality, mOsm/L H_2O	>500	<350
Fractional excretion of sodium	<1%	>2%
$FE_{Na} = \dfrac{U_{Na} \times P_{Cr} \times 100}{P_{Na} \times U_{Cr}}$		
Urine/Plasma Creatinine (U_{Cr}/P_{Cr})	>40	<20

NOTE: BUN, Blood urea nitrogen; P_{Cr}, plasma creatinine; U_{Na}, urine sodium concentration; P_{Na}, plasma sodium concentration; U_{Cr}, urine creatinine concentration.

FIGURE 47-1 Approach to the patient with azotemia. (WBC, white blood cell; RBC, red blood cell; GBM, glomerular basement membrane.)

Postrenal azotemia Urinary tract obstruction accounts for fewer than 5 percent of cases of acute renal failure but is usually reversible and must be ruled out early in the evaluation (Fig. 47-1). Since a single kidney is capable of adequate clearance, acute renal failure from obstruction requires either obstruction at the urethra or bladder outlet, bilateral ureteral obstruction, or unilateral obstruction in a patient with a single functioning kidney. Obstruction is usually diagnosed by the presence of ureteral dilatation on renal ultrasound. However, early in the course of obstruction or if the ureters are unable to dilate (such as encasement by pelvic tumors), the ultrasound examination may be negative. → *The specific urologic conditions that cause obstruction are discussed in Chap. 280.*

Oliguria and anuria Oliguria refers to a 24-h urine output of <500 mL, and anuria is the complete absence of urine formation. Anuria can be caused by total urinary tract obstruction, total renal artery or vein occlusion, and shock (manifested by severe hypotension and intense renal vasoconstriction). Cortical necrosis, ATN, and rapidly progressive glomerulonephritis can occasionally cause anuria. Oliguria can accompany any cause of acute renal failure and carries a more serious prognosis for renal recovery in all conditions except prerenal azotemia. Nonoliguria refers to urine output >500 mL/d in patients with acute or chronic azotemia. With nonoliguric ATN, disturbances of potassium and hydrogen balance are less severe than in oliguric patients and recovery to normal renal function is usually more rapid.

ABNORMALITIES OF THE URINE

PROTEINURIA Large quantities of plasma proteins normally course through the glomerular capillaries but do not enter the urinary space. Both charge and size selectivity prevent virtually all of albumin, globulin, and other large-molecular-weight proteins from crossing the glomerular wall. Smaller proteins (<20 kDa) pass across the capillary wall but are readily reabsorbed by the proximal tubule. Most individuals excrete between 30 and 150 mg/d of total protein (normal upper limit 200 mg/d) and only about 30 mg/d of albumin. The remainder of the protein in the urine is secreted by the tubules (Tamm-Horsfall, IgA, and urokinase) or represents small amounts of filtered β_2-microglobulin, apoproteins, enzymes, and peptide hormones. Tubular proteinuria due to low-molecular-weight proteins occurs with diseases that damage tubules more than glomeruli (Chap. 276). The resulting proteinuria is usually between 1 and 3 g/d with only small amounts of albumin present. Current methods for measuring proteinuria vary significantly. The dipstick measurement detects mostly albumin and gives false-positive results when the pH > 7.0 and the urine is very concentrated or contaminated with blood. A very dilute urine may obscure significant proteinuria on dipstick. Tests to measure total urine concentration accurately rely on precipitation with sulfosalicylic or trichloracetic acids. Currently dipsticks are available to measure microalbuminuria (30 to 200 mg/L), an early marker of glomerular disease.

The normal glomerular endothelial cell forms a barrier (Fig. 47-2), penetrated by fenestrae of about 100 nm, that holds back cells and other particles but offers little impediment to passage of most proteins. The glomerular basement membranes traps most large proteins (>100 kDa), while the foot processes of epithelial cells (podocytes) cover the urinary side of the glomerular basement membrane and produce a series of narrow channels (slit diaphragms) to allow molecular passage of small solutes and water. The channels are coated with anionic glycoproteins that are rich in glutamate, aspartate, and sialic acid and that are negatively charged at physiologic pH. This negatively charged barrier impedes the passage of anionic molecules such as albumin. Glomerular disease can disrupt the basement membrane by immune complex deposition, allowing large-protein leakage. Several glomerular diseases affect primarily the epithelial cells and result in loss of foot processes with resulting albuminuria. When the

total daily excretion of protein (mostly albumin) exceeds 3.5 g, there is often associated hypoalbuminemia, hyperlipidemia, and edema (nephrotic syndrome). However, total urinary protein excretion greater than 3.5 g/d does occur without the other features of the nephrotic syndrome in some plasma cell dyscrasias (such as multiple myeloma). These diseases can be associated with large amounts of excreted light chains in the urine which may not be detected by dipstick, which detects mostly albumin. The light chains produced from these disorders are filtered by the glomerulus and overwhelm the reabsorptive capacity of the proximal tubule. A sulfosalicylic acid precipitate that is out of proportion to the dipstick estimate is suggestive of light chains (Bence Jones protein), and light chains typically redissolve upon warming of the precipitate. Renal failure from these disorders occurs through a variety of mechanisms including tubule obstruction (cast nephropathy) and light chain deposition (see Chap. 275).

Hypoalbuminemia in nephrotic syndrome occurs through excessive urinary losses, increased renal catabolism, and inadequate hepatic synthesis. The resulting decrease in plasma oncotic pressure contributes to edema formation by altering the Starling forces and favoring fluid movement from capillaries to interstitium. The resulting homeostatic mechanisms designed to correct the decrease in effective intravascular volume contribute to edema formation. These mechanisms include activation of the renin-angiotensin system, AVP, and the sympathetic nervous system, which contribute to excessive renal salt and water reabsorption and can contribute to unrelenting edema. The severity of edema correlates with the degree of hypoalbuminemia and is modified by other factors such as heart disease or peripheral vascular disease. The diminished plasma oncotic pressure and urinary losses of regulatory proteins appear to stimulate hepatic lipoprotein synthesis. The resulting hyperlipidemia results in lipid bodies (fatty casts, oval

FIGURE 47-2 *(Top)* Diagram showing normal structures separating the capillary lumen and urinary space in the glomerulus. In the process of glomerular filtration, an ultrafiltrate of plasma traverses the glomerular capillary wall through endothelial fenestrae, basement membrane, and slit diaphragms. Macromolecules in the plasma are believed to be restricted from entry into glomerular urine by each of these wall structures. In addition, circulating polyanions (e.g., albumin) are thought to be retarded by negatively charged glycosialoproteins, which, as shown by the shaded area in the upper panel, are distributed throughout the glomerular wall. *(Bottom)* A corresponding electron micrograph of the same structures. *(Drawing by NL Gahan from BM Brenner, R. Beeuwkes, Hosp. Pract., vol. 13, no. 7, 1978. Reproduced with permission.)*

fat bodies) in the urine. Other proteins are lost in the urine, leading to a variety of metabolic disturbances; these proteins include thyroxine-binding globulin, cholecalciferol-binding protein, transferrin, and metal-binding proteins. A hypercoagulable state frequently accompanies severe nephrotic syndrome due to urinary losses of antithrombin III, reduced serum levels of proteins S and C, hyperfibrinogenemia, and enhanced platelet aggregation. Some patients develop severe IgG deficiency with resulting defects in immunity.

HEMATURIA, PYURIA, AND CASTS Isolated hematuria without proteinuria, other cells, or casts is often indicative of bleeding from the urinary tract. Hematuria is defined as two to five red blood cells per high-power field and can be detected by dipstick. Common causes of isolated hematuria include stones, neoplasms, tuberculosis, trauma, and prostatitis. Gross hematuria with blood clots is almost never indicative of glomerular bleeding but rather suggests a postrenal source in the urinary collecting system. Evaluation of patients presenting with microscopic hematuria is outlined in Fig. 47-3. A single urinalysis with hematuria is common and can result from menstruation, viral illness, allergy, exercise, or mild trauma. However, persistent or significant hematuria (> three red blood cells per high-power field on three urinalyses, or single urinalysis with >100 red blood cells, or gross hematuria) identifies significant renal or urologic lesions. Even patients who are chronically anticoagulated should be investigated as outlined in Fig. 47-3.

Hematuria with pyuria and bacteriuria is typical of infection and should be treated with antibiotics after appropriate cultures. Acute cystitis or urethritis in women can cause gross hematuria. Hypercalciuria and hyperuricosuria are also risk factors for unexplained isolated hematuria in both children and adults. In some of these patients (50 to 60 percent), reducing calcium and uric acid excretion through

dietary interventions can eliminate the microscopic hematuria. → *Urologic etiologies of hematuria are discussed in more detail in Chap. 280.*

Isolated microscopic hematuria can be a manifestation of glomerular diseases. The red blood cells of glomerular origin are often dysmorphic when examined by phase-contrast microscopy. Irregular shapes of red blood cells may also occur due to pH and osmolarity changes in the distal tubule. There is, however, significant interobserver variability in detecting dysmorphic red blood cells, especially if a phase-contrast microscope is not available. The most common etiologies of isolated glomerular hematuria are IgA nephropathy (Chap. 275), hereditary nephritis, and thin basement membrane disease. IgA nephropathy and hereditary nephritis can have episodic gross hematuria. A family history of renal failure is often present in patients with hereditary nephritis, and patients with thin basement membrane disease often have other family members with microscopic hematuria. A renal biopsy is needed for the definitive diagnosis of these disorders, which are discussed in more detail in Chap. 275. Hematuria with dysmorphic red blood cells, red blood cell casts, and protein excretion >500 mg/d is virtually diagnostic of glomerulonephritis. Red blood cell casts form as red blood cells enter the tubular fluid, and become trapped in a cylindrical mold of gelled Tamm-Horsfall protein. Even in the absence of azotemia, these patients should undergo serologic evaluation and renal biopsy as outlined in Fig. 47-3.

Isolated pyuria is unusual since inflammatory reactions in the kidney or collecting system are also associated with hematuria. The presence of bacteria suggests infection, and white blood cell casts with bacteria are indicative of pyelonephritis. White blood cells and/or white blood cell casts may also be seen in tubulointerstitial processes such as interstitial nephritis, systemic lupus erythematosus, and transplant rejection. In chronic renal diseases, degenerated cellular casts called *waxy casts* can be seen in the urine. Broad casts are thought to arise in the dilated tubules of enlarged nephrons that have undergone compensatory hypertrophy in response to reduced renal mass (i.e., chronic renal failure). A mixture of broad casts together with cellular casts and red blood cells may be seen in smoldering processes such as chronic glomerulonephritis with persistent active glomerulitis.

ABNORMALITIES OF URINE VOLUME

The volume of urine produced varies depending upon the fluid intake, renal function, and physiologic demands of the individual. The causes of decreased (oliguria) or absent urine production (anuria) were discussed earlier in this chapter. → *The physiology of free water formation and renal water conservation are discussed in Chap. 269.*

POLYURIA From the history alone, it is often difficult to distinguish urinary frequency (often of small volumes) from polyuria; a 24-h urine collection is needed for evaluation (Fig. 47-4). It is necessary to determine if the polyuria represents a solute or water diuresis and if the diuresis is appropriate for the clinical circumstances. The average person excretes between 600 and 800 mosmol of solutes per day, primarily as urea and electrolytes. The urine osmolality can help distinguish a solute from a water diuresis. If the urine output is >3 L/d (arbitrarily defined as polyuria) and the urine is dilute (<250 mosmol/L), then total mosmol excretion is normal and a water diuresis is present. This circumstance could arise from polydipsia, inadequate secretion of AVP (central diabetes insipidus), or failure of renal tubules to respond to AVP (nephrogenic diabetes insipidus). If the urine volume is >3 L/d and urine osmolality is >300 mosmol/L, then a solute diuresis is clearly present and a search for the responsible solute(s) is mandatory.

Excessive filtration of a poorly reabsorbed solute such as glucose, mannitol, or urea can depress reabsorption of NaCl and water in the proximal tubule and lead to enhanced excretion in the urine. Poorly controlled diabetes mellitus is the most common cause of a solute diuresis, leading to volume depletion and serum hypertonicity. Since

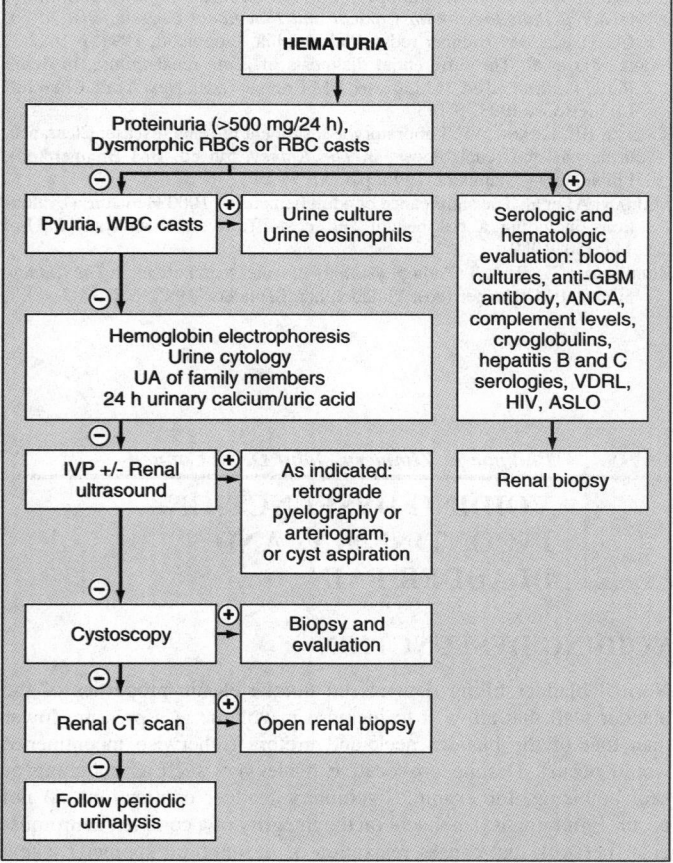

FIGURE 47-3 Approach to the patient with hematuria. (RBC, red blood cell; WBC, white blood cell; GBM, glomerular basement membrane; ANCA, antineutrophil cytoplasmic antibody; VDRL, venereal disease research laboratory; HIV, human immunodeficiency virus; ASLO, antistreptolysin O; UA, urinalysis; IVP, intravenous pyelography; CT, computed tomography.)

the urine Na concentration is less than that of blood, more water than Na is lost, causing hypernatremia and hypertonicity. Common iatrogenic solute diuresis occurs from mannitol administration, radiocontrast media, and high-protein feedings (enterally or parenterally), leading to increased urea production and excretion. Less commonly, excessive Na loss may occur from cystic renal diseases and Bartter's syndrome or during the course of a tubulointerstitial process (such as resolving acute tubular necrosis). In these so-called salt-wasting disorders, the tubule damage results in direct impairment of Na reabsorption and indirectly reduces the responsiveness of the tubule to aldosterone. Usually, the Na losses are mild, and the obligatory urine output is less than 2 L/d. (Resolving acute tubular necrosis and postobstructive diuresis are exceptions and may be associated with significant natriuresis and polyuria.)

Formation of large volumes of dilute urine represent polydipsic states or diabetes insipidus (Chaps. 276 and 330). Primary polydipsia can result from habit, psychiatric disorders, neurologic lesions, or medications. During deliberate polydipsia, extracellular fluid volume is normal or expanded and AVP levels are reduced because serum osmolality tends to be near the lower limits of normal. Reabsorption of water from the distal convoluted tubule and collecting duct is minimal with low AVP levels. The drive for water reabsorption is also reduced from washout of medullary hypertonicity gradients. The serum Na concentration may help to distinguish patients with primary polydipsia from those with diabetes insipidus; patients with polydipsia tend to have low-normal serum sodium concentrations, while patients with diabetes insipidus usually have normal to high-normal concentrations. A water deprivation test (see Chap. 330) may be needed to ascertain the exact diagnosis.

Central diabetes insipidus may be idiopathic in origin or secondary to a variety of hypothalamic conditions including posthypophysectomy, trauma and neoplastic, inflammatory, vascular, or infectious hypothalamic diseases. Idiopathic central diabetes insipidus is associated with selective destruction of the vasopressin-secreting neurons in the supraoptic and paraventricular nuclei and can be inherited as an autosomal dominant trait or occur spontaneously (Fig. 47-4), (see Chap. 330). Nephrogenic diabetes insipidus can occur in a variety of clinical situations as summarized in Fig. 47-4. Hypercalcemia and hypokalemia are reversible causes of nephrogenic diabetes insipidus, and familial conditions also exist. Usually nephrogenic diabetes insipidus is acquired from renal diseases or medications (Fig. 47-4). In both central and nephrogenic diabetes insipidus, water reabsorption is reduced along the distal nephron. Similar to the washout of medullary gradients seen with polydipsia, diabetes insipidus is also associated with dilution of the medullary solutes. Administering AVP can lead to formation of a more concentrated urine, but the maximal urine osmolality attained is often below normal (see Chap. 330).

Determination of the plasma AVP level is recommended as the best method for distinguishing between central and nephrogenic diabetes insipidus. Alternatively, a water deprivation test (Chap. 330) plus exogenous AVP may also distinguish primary polydipsia from central and nephrogenic diabetes insipidus.

BIBLIOGRAPHY

ANDERSON S et al: Renal and systemic manifestations of glomerular disease, in *The Kidney*, 5th ed, BM Brenner (ed). Philadelphia, Saunders, 1996, p 1981

ANDRES A et al: Isolated hematuria: Hypercalciuria and hyperuricosuria as risk factors. Kidney Int 36:96, 1989

BRADY HR et al: Acute renal failure, in *The Kidney*, 5th ed, BM Brenner (ed). Philadelphia, Saunders, 1996, p 1200

EDDY AA, MICHAEL AF: Immunopathogenic mechanisms of glomerular injury, in *Renal Pathology: With Clinical and Functional Correlations*, 2d ed, CC Tisher, BM Brenner (eds). Philadelphia, Lippincott, 1994, p 1622

FABER MD et al: The differential diagnosis of acute renal failure, in *Acute Renal Failure*, 3d ed, JM Lazarus, BM Brenner (eds). New York, Churchill Livingstone, 1993, p 133

KASISKE BL, KEANE WF: Laboratory assesssment of renal disease: Clearance, urinalysis and renal biopsy, in *The Kidney*, 5th ed, BM Brenner (ed). Philadelphia, Saunders, 1996, p 1137

MARIANI AJ et al: The signiicance of adult hematuria: 1000 Hematuria evaluations including a risk-benefit and cost-effectiveness analysis. J Urol 141:350, 1989

ROBERTSON GL, BERL T: Pathophysiology of water metabolism, in *The Kidney*, 5th ed, BM Brenner (ed). Philadelphia, Saunders, 1996, p 873

FIGURE 47-4 Approach to the patient with polyuria. (Osm, osmolality; ATN, acute tubular necrosis.)

48

Philippe E. Zimmern, John D. McConnell

VOIDING DYSFUNCTION, INCONTINENCE, AND BLADDER PAIN

VOIDING DYSFUNCTION

Normal bladder filling depends on unique elastic properties of the bladder wall that allow it to increase in volume at a pressure lower than that of the bladder neck and urethra (otherwise incontinence would occur). Despite provocative maneuvers such as coughing or heel bouncing, for example, voluntary bladder contractions do not occur. Emptying is dependent on the integrity of a complex neuromuscular network that causes relaxation of the urethral sphincter a few milliseconds before the onset of the detrusor (bladder muscle) contraction. With normal, sustained detrusor contraction, the bladder empties completely. A bladder that can fill and empty in this manner has a normal detrusor muscle and is described as *stable* according to conventional terminology.

Since the voluntary control of micturition depends on the neural connections between the cerebral cortex and the brainstem, disruption of these pathways (brain tumor, stroke, head trauma, Parkinson's disease) impairs the ability to suppress and control bladder contractions. A bladder contraction "without the owner's permission" (McGuire) characterizes an unstable bladder. Bladder or detrusor instability of neurologic origin is termed *detrusor hyperreflexia*. Conversely, the detrusor muscle that cannot contract during voiding is called *noncontractile* or *underactive*, and underactivity of the detrusor due to a lesion of the sacral cord or pelvic nerves is termed *detrusor areflexia*. These terms that characterize the function of the detrusor muscle and urethra have replaced terms such as atonic, hypotonic, autonomic, or flaccid, which refer to etiologies of dysfunction sometimes difficult to ascertain with certainty.

Contrary to common belief, the center that controls normal micturition is not in the spinal cord but in the brainstem. Proper coordination (synergia) between the detrusor and urethral sphincters requires an intact neural (autonomic and somatic nervous systems) communication between bladder and urethra. Injury to the upper spinal cord, for example, can cause dyssynergia between bladder and urethra that results in urge incontinence, residual urine retention, bladder wall changes (trabeculation and fibrosis), and possibly renal insufficiency.

A simple way to classify voiding dysfunction is to determine whether it is primarily a *storage failure* or an *emptying failure* by asking two questions:

Is the voiding dysfunction due to the bladder or outlet (bladder neck or urethra) (failure to store)?
Is the patient neurologically intact (failure to empty)?

Bladder storage and emptying problems may coexist in the same individual and can cause similar lower urinary tract symptoms (LUTS).

LOWER URINARY TRACT SYMPTOMS IN MEN The most common cause of LUTS in men of middle age and older is prostatic hyperplasia, which causes obstruction to urine flow by encroachment on the urethral lumen (see Chap. 97). Histologically, 50 to 80 percent of the prostatic volume is composed of stromal tissue (smooth muscle), while the remainder is glandular. The transitional zone, which is responsible for benign prostatic growth, comprises 10 to 15 percent of the prostate at the end of puberty but increases in volume after age 40. However, prostatic enlargement is not always accompanied by symptoms because the direction of growth can be outward, so that little change may occur in urine flow (at least up to a certain prostatic volume). Alternatively, men with early histologic evidence of prostatic hyperplasia can experience significant voiding symptoms. The reason for the latter phenomenon is believed to be an increased tone of the prostatic smooth muscle, possibly due to an increase in alpha-adrenergic receptors; in this circumstance enhanced prostatic tension within a nondistensible prostatic capsule can cause obstruction.

In response to obstruction, the bladder smooth muscle cells hypertrophy to generate the higher pressures necessary for voiding, and the increase in bladder muscle mass leads to reduced elasticity, or compliance, and decreased bladder capacity. Detrusor dysfunction from bladder outlet obstruction can cause any combination of the LUTS described above. When the obstruction progresses, infiltration of extracellular matrix between the smooth muscle bundles of the bladder wall can result in a hypocontractile or acontractile bladder (bladder failure).

Other complications such as urinary tract infections or bladder stones secondary to the large postvoid residuals (stasis) and upper tract damage (hydronephrosis, reflux) can develop during the course of the obstructive process. Although prostatic hyperplasia is the most common cause of bladder outlet obstruction in men, other sources of obstruction include prostate cancer, urethral stricture, and lack of proper sphincteric relaxation (neurologic cause). Nonobstructive causes of LUTS include diabetic neuropathy, which can affect the parasympathetic nerves of the bladder. Decreased sensation of bladder fullness leads to incomplete emptying and overdistention of the bladder and in turn to increased frequency and nocturia due to bladder overflow;

these symptoms are frequently made worse by the polydipsia/polyuria of diabetes mellitus. At times, storage symptoms can be caused by other neurologic causes such as stroke, multiple sclerosis, or Parkinson's disease.

The International Prostate Symptom Score (IPSS) is routinely employed to assess the severity of LUTS:

Decreased force of stream—over the past month how often have you had a weak urinary stream?
Intermittency—over the past month how often have you found you stopped and started again several times when urinating?
Incomplete emptying—over the past month how often have you had a sensation of not emptying your bladder completely after finishing urination?
Straining—over the past month how often have you had to push or strain to begin urination?

The IPSS also assesses the impact of storage symptoms:

Frequency—over the past month how often have you had to urinate again within 2 h after urinating?
Urgency—over the past month how often have you found it difficult to postpone urination?
Nocturia—over the past month how many times did you typically get up to urinate between going to bed and getting up in the morning? (Range: none to five or more times.)

Except for nocturia, the answers range from 0 (not at all) to 5 (almost always). A total score less than 8 indicates minimal voiding dysfunction; a total score of 13 or above is usually required to enroll patients in drug studies for the management of benign prostatic hyperplasia (BPH); and symptom scores above 23 suggest significant bladder outlet obstruction. Because similar symptoms can result from neurologic causes, the IPSS questionnaire cannot be used to make the diagnosis of prostatic hyperplasia but is only useful as an index of severity and of the response to treatment.

LOWER URINARY TRACT SYMPTOMS IN WOMEN Urethral obstruction is an uncommon cause of LUTS in women. A careful bimanual examination and passage of a urethral catheter are sufficient to exclude urethral stenosis, which is usually secondary to prior instrumentation or operative procedures, and urethral cancer. Urinary tract infection (cystitis) is more prevalent in women and must be excluded by urinalysis, and multiple sclerosis should be considered in middle-aged women presenting with frequency, urgency, or incontinence. In addition to many of the same disorders that produce voiding symptoms in men, estrogen deficiency, frequency-urgency syndrome, and interstitial cystitis (IC) with minimal pain must be considered. Cystocele and pelvic prolapse can cause urinary frequency secondary to impairment of bladder emptying.

EVALUATION Men and women with LUTS and concomitant neurologic disease should undergo a complete urodynamic evaluation. In the absence of neurologic disease, men with LUTS most commonly have prostatic hyperplasia. However, it is necessary to exclude prostate cancer, especially if there is a positive family history, an abnormal rectal examination, or an elevated level of prostate-specific antigen (PSA). In both sexes bladder cancer can also cause storage symptoms and is suggested by microscopic hematuria and/or abnormal urine cytology. Usually, a detailed genitourinary history, a symptom assessment, a careful neurologic examination including rectal examination and assessment of the bulbocavernosus reflex, measurements of urine flow and postvoid residual urine volume (by office bladder ultrasound), and limited laboratory evaluation (urinalysis, urine culture, PSA levels, urine cytology, urea/creatinine levels, as indicated) should be sufficient to direct therapy. More complex investigations of the lower urinary tract (cystoscopy, voiding cystography, urodynamics) and upper urinary tract (pyelogram or ultrasonography) are sometimes indicated.
→ *For therapy of BPH, see Chap. 97.*

INCONTINENCE

Incontinence is a condition where involuntary loss of urine is objectively demonstrated and is a social or hygienic problem. A common variant, *stress incontinence*, denotes involuntary loss of urine with physical exercise (coughing, sneezing, sports, sexual activity). *Urge incontinence* is an involuntary loss of urine associated with a strong desire to void, and *overflow incontinence* is an involuntary loss of urine when the elevation of intravesical pressure with bladder overfilling or distention exceeds the maximal urethral pressure. Loss of urine through channels other than the urethra is rare (ectopic ureter, fistulae) but causes total or continuous incontinence.

INCONTINENCE IN WOMEN Urinary incontinence affects approximately 20 million women in the United States. Among noninstitutionalized women 60 years of age and older, 25 to 30 percent have incontinence daily or weekly, and approximately half of the 1.5 million institutionalized women are incontinent more than once a day. The annual cost of caring for incontinent persons in the United States has been estimated at $10 billion.

Stress urinary incontinence (SUI) is secondary to urethral hypermobility or, less commonly (<10 percent), to intrinsic sphincteric deficiency (ISD). In the continent woman the bladder neck and proximal urethra are supported by the anterior vaginal wall and its lateral attachment to the levator muscles. Anterior vaginal wall relaxation causes urethral hypermobility, usually due to aging and/or estrogen deficiency or a prior traumatic delivery or pelvic surgery. Paradoxically, women can have clinical evidence of urethral hypermobility but no stress urinary incontinence.

Some women have an anatomically normal urethra and bladder neck but still have SUI due to damage to the internal sphincter (fixed, rigid, or "pipestem" urethra), due to prior anti-incontinence surgery, pelvic radiation or trauma, or neurologic disorders that cause denervation of the urethra. Urethral hypermobility and ISD can coexist in some patients and cause persistence (or rapid recurrence) of incontinence after a simple bladder neck suspension procedure that fixes the hypermobility but leaves the sphincter untreated.

Urge incontinence can be present alone or in association with SUI (mixed incontinence). The cause of the unsuppressible or uninhibited bladder contractions is usually idiopathic, but bacterial cystitis, bladder tumor, bladder outlet obstruction, and neurogenic bladder must be excluded. Overflow incontinence is due either to bladder outlet obstruction (rare in women), an acontractile bladder (diabetic neuropathy, multiple sclerosis), excessive smooth muscle relaxation from drugs (anticholinergic medications), or psychogenic retention.

INCONTINENCE IN MEN In men incontinence is less common than obstruction, but urgency and urge incontinence can occur as the result of bladder outlet obstruction (as from prostatic hyperplasia) that impairs detrusor smooth muscle function and leads to detrusor instability. Men with neurogenic bladders (diabetic neuropathy, multiple sclerosis, Parkinson's disease, stroke) can develop urge incontinence. Other causes such as bacterial cystitis or bladder tumor must be excluded. SUI in men is usually the result of distal sphincteric damage, for example, as the result of radical prostatectomy for prostate cancer.

INCONTINENCE IN THE ELDERLY Transient urinary incontinence is common in the elderly. A mnemonic devised by Resnick delineates its numerous causes, namely delirium, infection, atrophic urethritis, pharmacologic, psychological, excessive urine output (hyperglycemia, congestive heart failure), restricted mobility, and stool impaction (DIAPPERS). Urge incontinence is the next most common disorder in this age group and is attributed to the progressive loss of the modulating influence of the frontal lobes of the cortex on the micturition center in the brain stem.

EVALUATION The evaluation of urinary incontinence in women should include: history and quality-of-life assessment, voiding diary, physical examination including pelvic examination, urinalysis and urine culture, and measurement of postvoid residual urine volume. For patients with an unclear history or after prior pelvic or anti-incontinence procedures, evaluation may include cystoscopy, urodynamic evaluation, and imaging studies (lower and/or upper urinary tract). The history should define the onset, duration, evolution, and triggering events of leakage. Prior treatments with medications, frequent voiding schedules, and exercise regimens should be noted. Severity of incontinence is denoted by recording the type and number of pads used per day or at night and how the incontinence affects daily activities (incontinence-impact questionnaire). The amount and type of fluid consumed, sexual history (hormonal status, deliveries, venereal diseases), gastrointestinal function (fecal incontinence, constipation), and past urologic history (bed-wetting, surgeries) must also be documented. The physical examination should place special emphasis on the abdominal, genital, pelvic (associated prolapses), and neurologic systems. SUI must be demonstrated by asking the patient to cough, strain, or even stand or squat. While leakage during a cough confirms SUI, leakage after a cough is due to bladder instability (stress-induced instability). SUI in the absence of urethral hypermobility raises the suspicion of a sphincteric defect. More complex testing is needed to determine whether the urethral anatomy is normal (evaluation of urethral mobility, lateral view of the urethra on the voiding cystourethrogram, cystoscopy), whether urethral function is normal with adequate closure (leak point pressure, urethral profilometry, videourodynamics), or whether bladder function is normal (bladder volume based on home diary, filling cystometrogram).

℞ **TREATMENT**

Mild stress incontinence can be treated nonoperatively with medications, hormonal supplementation, or biofeedback techniques. Modalities such as urethral plugs and anterior vaginal wall prostheses are under investigation. Moderate to severe stress incontinence responds to surgical procedures aimed at supporting the anterior vaginal wall (vaginal, laparoscopic, or abdominal operations) or enhancing urethral closure when stress incontinence is secondary to internal sphincter deficiency (periurethral injection of teflon or collagen or insertion of an artificial urinary sphincter).

Urge incontinence responds to the management of its cause, for example, relief of outlet obstruction. When it is due to neurogenic or idiopathic causes, anticholinergic agents are partially effective, although side effects such as mouth dryness, blurring of vision, or constipation can limit their usefulness. Fluid restriction (which must be undertaken only with great caution) and bladder retraining with biofeedback may also be helpful. More aggressive intervention with bladder augmentation or urinary diversion are seldom necessary in the absence of neurologic disease.

BLADDER PAIN

Painful bladder disease is a general term for any bladder pathology that causes suprapubic, urethral, or pelvic pain. IC is the most common cause of bladder pain, but endometriosis, bacterial cystitis, and outlet obstruction that causes bladder instability can mimic the symptoms of IC.

INTERSTITIAL CYSTITIS IC is a severe, chronic bladder disorder that causes frequency, nocturia, and suprapubic pain. The disorder usually affects women and is rare in blacks. Routine urine culture is uniformly negative, and the symptoms do not respond to antibiotic therapy. The etiology is probably multifactorial (Table 48-1). Current hypotheses as to etiology include autoimmune reaction against bladder antigens, deficiency in the glycosaminoglycan layer of the bladder surface allowing presumed "toxins" to penetrate the mucosa, mast cell infiltration and activation leading to the histamine release, and local bladder wall damage from "cryptic" bacteria.

There are no universally accepted criteria to make the diagnosis, but the National Institutes of Health has established a series of criteria to define IC clinically (Table 48-2). The diagnosis is one of exclusion—infection, radiation cystitis, urethral diverticula, herpes simplex, and malignancy must be excluded. Cystoscopy under anesthesia may reveal

Table 48-1

Consensus Criteria for Diagnosis of Interstitial Cystitis

AUTOMATIC EXCLUSIONS

Less than 18 years old
Benign or malignant bladder tumors
Radiation cystitis
Bacterial cystitis
Vaginitis
Cyclophosphamide cystitis
Symptomatic urethral diverticulum
Uterine, cervical, vaginal, or urethral cancers
Active herpes
Bladder or lower urethral calculi
Waking frequency less than five times in 12 h
Nocturia less than twice nightly
Symptoms relieved by antibiotics, urinary antiseptics, urinary analgesics
  (e.g., phenazopyridine hydrochloride)
Duration less than 12 months
Involuntary bladder contractions (urodynamics)
Capacity greater than 400 mL, absence of sensory urgency

AUTOMATIC INCLUSIONS

Hunner's ulcer

POSITIVE FACTORS

Pain on bladder filling relieved by emptying
Pain (suprapubic, pelvic, urethral, vaginal, or perineal)
Glomerulations after hydrodistention on cystoscopy

---

glomerulations (submucosal vascular anomalies) or the infrequent Hunner's ulcer suggestive of IC; make it possible to estimate bladder capacity (an important guide to treatment); allow biopsy of the bladder wall when indicated; and, sometimes, provide therapeutic benefit with a reduction in pain level and urinary frequency up to 6 months, rarely longer.

EVALUATION Chronic urinary frequency and bladder pain affect the quality of life to an extreme degree, although most patients experience a waxing and waning evolution; only 10 percent of patients have a consistent progression in symptoms. Evaluation should include a detailed history; physical examination designed to exclude neurologic and gynecologic pathology; voiding cystogram to exclude urethral defects; and urodynamic testing to eliminate a neurogenic bladder, bladder instability, or outlet obstruction and to document sensory instability. Referral to specialists may be indicated to exclude adnexal pathology, endometriosis, or bowel dysfunction or to utilize modern pain management techniques to prevent drug addiction.

 TREATMENT

Empiric treatments that have been used include oral medications (amitriptyline, hydroxyzine) and intravesical agents (dimethyl sulfoxide, chlorpactin, heparin). These measures may improve the urinary symptoms and occasionally reduce pain but do not modify the long-term course. Surgical intervention (augmentation cystoplasty,

Table 48-2

Possible Causes of Interstitial Cystitis

Infection
  Fastidious bacteria
  Latent viruses
Dysfunctional bladder epithelium
  Defective glycosaminoglycan layer
  Abnormal intercellular junctions
Toxic substances in urine
Allergic/immune/autoimmune causes
Neurogenic disturbances
Bladder mastocytosis
Psychosomatic
Others
  Food intolerance
  Endocrine causes

---

urinary diversion) is indicated in fewer than 5 percent of cases because this is a non-life-threatening, chronic disease with occasional spontaneous remissions. "Last-resort" interventions such as removal of the bladder and urethra are not a guarantee of success because some patients continue to experience pelvic pain afterwards.

BIBLIOGRAPHY

Barry MJ et al: The American Urological Association symptom index for benign prostatic hyperplasia. The measurement committee of the American Urological Association. J Urol 148:1549, 1992

Berry SJ et al: The development of human benign prostatic hyperplasia with age. J Urol 132:474, 1984

Chai TB, Steers WD: Neurophysiology of micturition and continence. Urol Clin North Am 23:221, 1996

DuBeau CE: Interpreting the effect of common medical conditions on voiding dysfunction in the elderly. Urol Clin North Am 23:11, 1996

Gillenwater JY, Wein AJ: Summary of the National Institute of Arthritis, Diabetes, Digestive and Kidney Diseases Workshop on Interstitial Cystitis, National Institutes of Health, Bethesda, Maryland, August 28–29, 1987. J Urol 140:203, 1988

Hurst RE et al: Urinary glycosaminoglycan excretion as a laboratory marker in the diagnosis of interstitial cystitis. J Urol 149:31, 1993

Leach GE et al: Experience with 215 men with post-prostatectomy incontinence. J Urol 155:1256, 1996

McGuire EJ: Urodynamic evaluation of stress incontinence. Urol Clin North Am 22:551, 1995

Ratliff TL et al: The etiology of interstitial cystitis. Urol Clin North Am 21:21, 1994

Resnick N: Geriatric incontinence. Urol Clin North Am 23:55, 1996

Rivas DA, Chancellor MB: Neurogenic vesical dysfunction. Urol Clin North Am 22:579, 1995

Romanzi LJ et al: Preliminary assessment of the incontinent woman. Urol Clin North Am 22:513, 1995

Wein A: Neuromuscular dysfunction of the lower urinary tract, in *Campbell's Urology*, 6th ed, PC Walsh et al (eds). Philadelphia, Saunders, 1992, p 573

Gary G. Singer, Barry M. Brenner

FLUID AND ELECTROLYTE DISTURBANCES

SODIUM AND WATER

COMPOSITION OF BODY FLUIDS Water is the most abundant constituent in the body, comprising approximately 60 percent of body weight in men and 50 percent in women. This difference is attributable to differences in the relative proportions of adipose tissue in men and women. Total body water is distributed in two major compartments—55 to 75 percent is intracellular [intracellular fluid (ICF)], and 25 to 45 percent is extracellular [extracellular fluid (ECF)]. The ECF is further subdivided into intravascular (plasma water) and extravascular (interstitial) spaces in a ratio of 1:3.

The solute or particle concentration of a fluid is known as its osmolality and is expressed as milliosmoles per kilogram of water (mosmol/kg). Water crosses cell membranes to achieve osmotic equilibrium (ECF osmolality = ICF osmolality). The extracellular and intracellular solutes or osmoles are markedly different due to disparities in permeability, and the presence of transporters and active pumps. The major ECF particles are Na^+ and its accompanying anions Cl^- and HCO_3^-, whereas K^+ and organic phosphate esters (ATP, creatine phosphate, and phospholipids) are the predominant ICF osmoles. Solutes that are restricted to the ECF or the ICF determine the *effective osmolality* (or *tonicity*) of that compartment. Since Na^+ is largely restricted to the extracellular compartment, total body Na^+ content is a reflection of ECF volume. Likewise, K^+ and its attendant anions are predominantly limited to the ICF and are necessary for normal cell function. Therefore, the number of intracellular particles is relatively constant, and a change in ICF osmolality is usually due to a change in ICF water content. However, in certain situations, brain cells can vary the number of intracellular solutes in order to defend against large water shifts. This process of *osmotic adaptation* is important in the defense of cell volume and occurs in chronic hyponatremia and hypernatremia. This response is mediated initially by transcellular shifts of K^+ and Na^+, followed by synthesis, import, or export of organic solutes (so-called osmolytes) such as inositol, betaine, and glutamine. During chronic hyponatremia, brain cells lose solutes, thereby defending cell volume and diminishing neurologic symptoms. The converse occurs during chronic hypernatremia. Certain solutes, such as urea, do not contribute to water shift across cell membranes and are known as *ineffective osmoles*.

Fluid movement between the intravascular and interstitial spaces occurs across the capillary wall and is determined by the Starling forces—capillary hydraulic pressure and colloid osmotic pressure. The transcapillary hydraulic pressure gradient exceeds the corresponding oncotic pressure gradient, thereby favoring the movement of plasma ultrafiltrate into the extravascular space. The return of fluid into the intravascular compartment occurs via lymphatic flow.

WATER BALANCE (See also Chap. 269) The normal plasma osmolality is 275 to 290 mosmol/kg and is kept within a narrow range by mechanisms capable of sensing a 1 to 2 percent change in tonicity. To maintain a steady state, water intake must equal water excretion. Disorders of water homeostasis result in hypo- or hypernatremia. Normal individuals have an obligate water loss consisting of urine, stool, and evaporation from the skin and respiratory tract. Gastrointestinal excretion is usually a minor component of total water output, except in patients with vomiting, diarrhea, or high enterostomy output states. Evaporative or insensitive water losses are important in the regulation of core body temperature. Obligatory renal water loss is mandated by the minimum solute excretion required to maintain a steady state. Normally, about 600 mosmols must be excreted per day, and since the maximal urine osmolality is 1200 mosmol/kg a minimum urine output of 500 mL/d is required for neutral solute balance.

Water Intake The primary stimulus for water ingestion is *thirst*, mediated either by an increase in effective osmolality or a decrease in ECF volume or blood pressure. *Osmoreceptors*, located in the anterolateral *hypothalamus*, are stimulated by a rise in tonicity. Ineffective osmoles, such as urea and glucose, do not play a role in stimulating thirst. The average osmotic threshold for thirst is approximately 295 mosmol/kg and varies among individuals. Under normal circumstances, daily water intake exceeds physiologic requirements.

Water Excretion In contrast to the ingestion of water, its excretion is tightly regulated by physiologic factors. The principal determinant of renal water excretion is *arginine vasopressin* (AVP; formerly antidiuretic hormone), a polypeptide synthesized in the supraoptic and paraventricular nuclei of the hypothalamus and secreted by the posterior pituitary gland. The binding of AVP to V_2 receptors on the basolateral membrane of principal cells in the collecting duct activates adenylyl cyclase and initiates a sequence of events that leads to the insertion of water channels into the luminal membrane. These water channels that are specifically activated by AVP are encoded by the *aquaporin-2* gene (Chap. 330). The net effect is passive water reabsorption along an osmotic gradient from the lumen of the collecting duct to the hypertonic medullary interstitium. The major stimulus for AVP secretion is hypertonicity. Since the major ECF solutes are Na^+ salts, effective osmolality is primarily determined by the plasma Na^+ concentration. An increase or decrease in tonicity is sensed by hypothalamic osmoreceptors as a decrease or increase in cell volume, respectively, leading to enhancement or suppression of AVP secretion. The osmotic threshold for AVP release is 280 to 290 mosmol/kg, and the system is sufficiently sensitive that plasma osmolality varies by no more than 1 to 2 percent.

Nonosmotic factors that regulate AVP secretion include *effective circulating* (arterial) *volume*, nausea, pain, stress, hypoglycemia, pregnancy, and numerous drugs. The hemodynamic response is mediated by baroreceptors in the carotid sinus. The sensitivity of these receptors is significantly lower than that of the osmoreceptors. In fact, depletion of blood volume sufficient to result in a decreased mean arterial pressure is necessary to stimulate AVP release, whereas small changes in effective circulating volume have little effect. In the setting of hypovolemia, the osmotic regulation of AVP remains intact. However, the osmotic threshold, or set point, for AVP release is decreased, and the sensitivity is increased.

To maintain homeostasis and a normal plasma Na^+ concentration, the ingestion of solute-free water must eventually lead to the loss of the same volume of electrolyte-free water. Three steps are required for the kidney to excrete a water load: (1) filtration and delivery of water (and electrolytes) to the diluting sites of the nephron; (2) active reabsorption of Na^+ and Cl^- without water in the thick ascending limb of the loop of Henle and, to a lesser extent, in the distal nephron; and (3) maintenance of a dilute urine due to impermeability of the collecting duct to water in the absence of AVP. Abnormalities of any of these steps can result in impaired free water excretion, and eventual hyponatremia.

SODIUM BALANCE Sodium is actively pumped out of cells by the Na^+, K^+-ATPase pump. As a result, 85 to 90 percent of all Na^+ is extracellular, and the ECF volume is a reflection of total body Na^+ content. Normal volume regulatory mechanisms ensure that Na^+ loss balances Na^+ gain. If this does not occur, conditions of Na^+ excess or deficit ensue and are manifest as edematous or hypovolemic states, respectively. It is important to distinguish between disorders of osmoregulation and disorders of volume regulation since water and Na^+ balance are regulated independently. Changes in Na^+ concentration generally reflect disturbed water homeostasis, whereas alterations in Na^+ content are manifest as ECF volume contraction or expansion and imply abnormal Na^+ balance.

Sodium Intake Individuals eating a typical western diet consume approximately 150 mmol of NaCl daily. This normally exceeds basal requirements. As noted above, sodium is the principal extracellular cation. Therefore, dietary intake of Na^+ results in ECF volume expansion which, in turn, promotes enhanced renal Na^+ excretion to maintain steady state Na^+ balance.

Sodium Excretion (See also Chap. 269) The regulation of Na^+ excretion is multifactorial and is the major determinant of Na^+ balance. An Na^+ deficit or excess is manifest as a decreased or increased effective circulating volume, respectively. Changes in effective circulating volume tend to lead to parallel changes in glomerular filtration rate (GFR). However, tubule Na^+ reabsorption, and not GFR, is the major regulatory mechanism controlling Na^+ excretion. Almost two-thirds of filtered Na^+ is reabsorbed in the proximal convoluted tubule—this process is electroneutral and isoosmotic. Further reabsorption (25 to 30 percent) occurs in the thick ascending limb of the loop of Henle via the apical Na^+-K^+-$2Cl^-$ cotransporter—this is an active process and is also electroneutral. Distal convoluted tubule reabsorption of Na^+ (5 percent) is mediated by the *thiazide-sensitive Na^+-Cl^- cotransporter*. Final Na^+ reabsorption occurs in the cortical and medullary collecting ducts, the amount excreted being reasonably equivalent to the amount ingested per day (Chap. 269).

HYPOVOLEMIA

ETIOLOGY True volume depletion, or hypovolemia, generally refers to a state of combined salt and water loss exceeding intake, leading to ECF volume contraction. The loss of Na^+ may be renal or extrarenal (see Table 49-1).

Renal Many conditions are associated with excessive urinary NaCl and water losses, including diuretics. Pharmacologic diuretics inhibit specific pathways of Na^+ reabsorption along the nephron with a consequent increase in urinary Na^+ excretion. Enhanced filtration of non-reabsorbed solutes, such as glucose or urea, can also impair tubular reabsorption of Na^+ and water, leading to an osmotic or solute diuresis. This often occurs in poorly controlled diabetes mellitus and in patients receiving high-protein hyperalimentation. Mannitol is a diuretic that produces an osmotic diuresis because the renal tubule is impermeable to mannitol. Many tubule and interstitial renal disorders are associated with Na^+ wasting. Excessive renal losses of Na^+ and water may also occur during the diuretic phase of acute tubular necrosis (ATN) (Chap. 270) and following the relief of bilateral urinary tract obstruction. The natriuresis and water diuresis associated with these two conditions is often short-lived and an appropriate response to a state of ECF volume expansion that ensued as a result of prior oliguria. However, ongoing losses in the absence of adequate replacement fluids may eventually lead to a state of hypovolemia. Chronic renal insufficiency is associated with a diminished ability to regulate renal salt and water excretion appropriately (Chap. 271). Therefore, patients with a GFR of less than 25 mL/min have an obligatory renal Na^+ loss that may result in progressive ECF volume depletion if Na^+ intake is restricted. Finally, mineralocorticoid deficiency (hypoaldosteronism) causes salt wasting in the presence of normal intrinsic renal function.

Massive renal water excretion can also lead to hypovolemia. The ECF volume contraction is usually less severe since two-thirds of the volume lost is intracellular. Conditions associated with excessive urinary water loss include central and nephrogenic diabetes insipidus. These two disorders are due to impaired secretion of and renal unresponsiveness to AVP, respectively, and are discussed below.

Extrarenal Nonrenal causes of hypovolemia include fluid loss from the gastrointestinal tract, skin, and respiratory system and third space accumulations (burns, pancreatitis, peritonitis). Approximately 9 L of fluid enters the gastrointestinal tract daily, 2 L by ingestion and 7 L by secretion. Almost 98 percent of this volume is reabsorbed so that fecal fluid loss is only 100 to 200 mL/d. Impaired gastrointestinal reabsorption or enhanced secretion leads to volume depletion. Since gastric secretions have a low pH (high H^+ concentration), vomiting and diarrhea are often accompanied by metabolic alkalosis and acidosis, respectively.

Water evaporation from the skin and respiratory tract contributes to thermoregulation. These *insensible losses* amount to 500 mL/d. During febrile illnesses, prolonged heat exposure, or exercise, increased salt and water loss from skin, in the form of sweat, can be significant and lead to volume depletion. The Na^+ concentration of sweat is normally 20 to 50 mmol/L and decreases with profuse sweating due to the action of aldosterone. Since sweat is hypotonic, the loss of water exceeds that of Na^+. The water deficit is minimized by enhanced

thirst. Nevertheless, ongoing Na^+ loss is manifest as hypovolemia. Enhanced evaporative water loss from the respiratory tract may be associated with hyperventilation, especially in mechanically ventilated febrile patients.

Certain conditions lead to fluid sequestration in a *third space*. This compartment is extracellular but is not in equilibrium with either the ECF or the ICF. The fluid is effectively lost from the ECF and can result in hypovolemia. Examples include the bowel lumen in gastrointestinal obstruction, subcutaneous tissues in severe burns, retroperitoneal space in acute pancreatitis, and peritoneal cavity in peritonitis. Finally, severe hemorrhage from any source can result in volume depletion.

PATHOPHYSIOLOGY ECF volume contraction is manifest as a decreased plasma volume and hypotension. Hypotension is due to decreased venous return (preload) and diminished cardiac output; it triggers baroreceptors in the carotid sinus and aortic arch and leads to activation of the sympathetic nervous system and the renin-angiotensin system. The net effect is to maintain mean arterial pressure and cerebral and coronary perfusion. In contrast to the cardiovascular response, the renal response is aimed at restoring the ECF volume by decreasing the GFR and filtered load of Na^+ and, most importantly, by promoting tubular reabsorption of Na^+. Increased sympathetic tone increases proximal tubular Na^+ reabsorption and decreases GFR by causing preferential afferent arteriolar vasoconstriction. Sodium is also reabsorbed in the proximal convoluted tubule in response to increased angiotensin II and altered peritubular capillary hemodynamics (decreased hydraulic and increased oncotic pressure). Enhanced reabsorption of Na^+ by the collecting duct is an important component of the renal adaptation to ECF volume contraction. This occurs in response to increased *aldosterone* and AVP secretion, and suppressed *atrial natriuretic peptide* (ANP) secretion.

CLINICAL FEATURES A careful history is often helpful in determining the etiology of ECF volume contraction (e.g., vomiting, diarrhea, polyuria, diaphoresis). Most symptoms are nonspecific and secondary to electrolyte imbalances and tissue hypoperfusion and include fatigue, weakness, muscle cramps, thirst, and postural dizziness. More severe degrees of volume contraction can lead to end-organ ischemia manifest as oliguria, cyanosis, abdominal and chest pain, and confusion or obtundation. Diminished skin turgor and dry oral mucous membranes are poor markers of decreased interstitial fluid. Signs of intravascular volume contraction include decreased jugular venous pressure, postural hypotension, and postural tachycardia. Larger and more acute fluid losses lead to hypovolemic shock, manifest as hypotension, tachycardia, peripheral vasoconstriction, and hypoperfusion—cyanosis, cold and clammy extremities, oliguria, and altered mental status.

DIAGNOSIS A thorough history and physical examination are generally sufficient to diagnose the etiology of hypovolemia. Laboratory data usually confirm and support the clinical diagnosis. The blood urea nitrogen (BUN) and plasma creatinine concentrations tend to be elevated, reflecting a decreased GFR. Normally, the BUN:creatinine ratio is about 10:1. However, in *prerenal azotemia*, hypovolemia leads to increased urea reabsorption and a proportionately greater elevation in BUN than plasma creatinine, and a BUN:creatinine ratio of 20:1 or higher. An increased BUN (relative to creatinine) may also be due to increased urea production that occurs with hyperalimentation (high-protein), glucocorticoid therapy, and gastrointestinal bleeding.

Volume depletion may be associated with hyponatremia, hypernatremia, or a normal plasma Na^+ concentration, depending on the tonicity of the fluid lost, the presence of thirst, and the access to water. Hypokalemia is common in settings of increased renal or gastrointestinal K^+ loss, and hyperkalemia occurs in renal failure, adrenal insufficiency, and certain types of metabolic acidosis. Metabolic alkalosis occurs with diuretic-induced hypovolemia and in cases of vomiting or nasogastric suction. In contrast, metabolic acidosis is associated with renal failure, tubulointerstitial disorders, adrenal insufficiency, diarrhea, diabetic ketoacidosis, and lactic acid acidosis. Since albumin

Table 49-1

Causes of Hypovolemia

I. ECF volume contracted
  A. Extrarenal Na^+ loss
    1. Gastrointestinal
     (vomiting, nasogastric suction, drainage, fistula, diarrhea)
    2. Skin/respiratory
     (insensible losses, sweat, burns)
    3. Hemorrhage
  B. Renal Na^+ and water loss
    1. Diuretics
    2. Osmotic diuresis
    3. Hypoaldosteronism
    4. Salt-wasting nephropathies
  C. Renal water loss
    1. Diabetes insipidus (central or nephrogenic)
II. ECF volume normal or expanded
  A. Decreased cardiac output
    1. Myocardial, valvular, or pericardial disease
  B. Redistribution
    1. Hypoalbuminemia
     (hepatic cirrhosis, nephrotic syndrome)
    2. Capillary leak
     (acute pancreatitis, ischemic bowel, rhabdomyolysis)
  C. Increased venous capacitance
    1. Sepsis

and erythrocytes are confined to the intravascular compartment, ECF volume contraction often leads to a relative elevation in hematocrit (hemoconcentration) and plasma albumin concentration.

The appropriate response to hypovolemia is enhanced renal Na^+ and water reabsorption, which is reflected in the urine composition. Therefore, the urine Na^+ concentration should usually be less than 20 mmol/L except in conditions associated with impaired Na^+ reabsorption, as in acute tubular necrosis (Chap. 270). Another exception is hypovolemia due to vomiting since the associated metabolic alkalosis and increased filtered HCO_3^- impair proximal Na^+ reabsorption. In this case, the urine Cl^- is low (less than 20 mmol/L). The urine osmolality and specific gravity in hypovolemic subjects are generally greater than 450 mosmol/kg and 1.015, respectively, reflecting the presence of enhanced AVP secretion. However, in hypovolemia due to diabetes insipidus, urine osmolality and specific gravity are indicative of inappropriately dilute urine.

℞ TREATMENT

The therapeutic goals are to restore normovolemia with fluid similar in composition to that lost and to replace ongoing losses. Symptoms and signs, including weight loss, can help estimate the degree of volume contraction and should also be monitored to assess response to treatment. Mild volume contraction can usually be corrected via the oral route. More severe hypovolemia requires intravenous therapy. Isotonic or normal saline (0.9% NaCl or 154 mmol/L Na^+) is the solution of choice in normonatremic and mildly hyponatremic individuals and should be administered initially in patients with hypotension or shock. Severe hyponatremia may require hypertonic saline (3.0% NaCl or 513 mmol/L Na^+). Hypernatremia reflects a proportionally greater deficit of water than Na^+, and its correction will therefore require a hypotonic solution such as half-normal saline (0.45% NaCl or 77 mmol/L Na^+) or 5% dextrose in water. Patients with significant hemorrhage, anemia, or intravascular volume depletion may require blood transfusion or colloid-containing solutions (albumin, dextran). Hypokalemia may be present initially or may ensue as a result of increased urinary K^+ excretion; it should be corrected by adding appropriate amounts of KCl to replacement solutions.

HYPONATREMIA

ETIOLOGY A plasma Na^+ concentration less than 135 mmol/L usually reflects a hypotonic state. However, plasma osmolality may be normal or increased in some cases of hyponatremia, referred to as *pseudohyponatremia*. Plasma is 93 percent water, the remaining 7 percent consisting of plasma proteins and lipids. Since Na^+ ions are dissolved in plasma water, increasing the nonaqueous phase artificially lowers the Na^+ concentration measured per liter of plasma (except when Na^+-sensitive glass electrodes are used). The plasma osmolality and the Na^+ concentration remain normal. This type of hyponatremia has little clinical significance, except to ascertain the cause of the hyperproteinemia or hyperlipidemia. Isotonic or slightly hypotonic hyponatremia may complicate transurethral resection of the prostate or bladder because large volumes of isoosmotic (mannitol) or hypoosmotic (sorbital or glycine) bladder irrigation solution can be absorbed and result in a dilutional hyponatremia. The metabolism of sorbitol and glycine to CO_2 and water may lead to hypotonicity if the accumulated fluid and solutes are not rapidly excreted. Hypertonic hyponatremia is usually due to hyperglycemia or, occasionally, intravenous administration of mannitol. Relative insulin deficiency causes myocytes to become impermeable to glucose. Therefore, during poorly controlled diabetes mellitus, glucose is an effective osmole and draws water from muscle cells, resulting in hyponatremia. Plasma Na^+ concentration falls by 1.4 mmol/L for every 100 mg/dL rise in the plasma glucose concentration.

Most causes of hyponatremia are associated with a low plasma osmolality (Table 49-2). In general hypotonic hyponatremia is due

either to a primary water gain (and secondary Na^+ loss) or a primary Na^+ loss (and secondary water gain). Hyponatremia in the absence of water retention is usually associated with hypovolemic shock. Contraction of the ECF volume stimulates thirst and AVP secretion. The increased water ingestion and impaired renal excretion result in hyponatremia. It is important to note that *diuretic-induced hyponatremia* is almost always due to thiazide diuretics. Loop diuretics decrease the tonicity of the medullary interstitium and impair maximal urinary concentrating capacity. This limits the ability of AVP to promote water retention. In contrast, thiazide diuretics lead to Na^+ and K^+ depletion, and AVP-mediated water retention. In the presence of a large K^+ deficit, transcellular ion exchange (K^+ exits and Na^+ enters cells) may contribute to hyponatremia.

Hyponatremia in the setting of ECF volume expansion is usually associated with edematous states, such as congestive heart failure, hepatic cirrhosis, and the nephrotic syndrome. These disorders all have in common a decreased effective circulating arterial volume, leading to increased thirst and increased AVP levels. Additional factors impairing the excretion of solute-free water include a reduced GFR, decreased delivery of ultrafiltrate to the diluting site (due to increased proximal fractional reabsorption of Na^+ and water), and diuretic therapy. The degree of hyponatremia often correlates with the severity of the underlying condition and is an important prognostic factor. Oliguric acute and chronic renal failure may be associated with hyponatremia if water intake exceeds the ability to excrete equivalent volumes.

Hyponatremia in the absence of ECF volume contraction, decreased effective circulating arterial volume, or renal insufficiency is usually due to increased AVP secretion resulting in impaired water excretion. Ingestion or administration of water is also required since high levels of AVP alone are usually insufficient to produce hyponatremia. This disorder, commonly termed the *syndrome of inappropriate antidiuretic hormone (ADH) secretion* (SIADH), is the most common cause of normovolemic hyponatremia and is due to the nonphysiologic release of AVP from the posterior pituitary or an ectopic source (Chap. 330). Renal free water excretion is impaired while the regulation of Na^+ balance is unaffected. The most common causes of SIADH include neuropsychiatric and pulmonary diseases, malignant tumors, major surgery (postoperative pain), and pharmacologic agents. Severe pain and nausea are physiologic stimuli of AVP secretion; these stimuli are inappropriate in the absence of hypovolemia or hyperosmolality.

Table 49-2

Causes of Hyponatremia

I. Pseudohyponatremia
   A. Normal plasma osmolality
     1. Hyperlipidemia
     2. Hyperproteinemia
     3. Posttransurethral resection of prostate/bladder tumor
   B. Increased plasma osmolality
     1. Hyperglycemia
     2. Mannitol
II. Hypoosmolal hyponatremia
   A. Primary Na^+ loss (secondary water gain)
     1. Integumentary loss: sweating, burns
     2. Gastrointestinal loss: vomiting, tube drainage, fistula, obstruction, diarrhea
     3. Renal loss: diuretics, osmotic diuresis, hypoaldosteronism, salt-wasting nephropathy, postobstructive diuresis, nonoliguric acute tubular necrosis
   B. Primary water gain (secondary Na^+ loss)
     1. Primary polydipsia
     2. Decreased solute intake (e.g., beer potomania)
     3. AVP release due to pain, nausea, drugs
     4. Syndrome of inappropriate AVP secretion
     5. Glucocorticoid deficiency
     6. Hypothyroidism
     7. Chronic renal insufficiency
   C. Primary Na^+ gain (exceeded by secondary water gain)
     1. Heart failure
     2. Hepatic cirrhosis
     3. Nephrotic syndrome

A variety of central nervous system disorders may be associated with SIADH, such as meningitis, encephalitis, hemorrhage, stroke, psychosis, primary and metastatic tumors, and acute porphyria. Pneumonia, empyema, tuberculosis, and acute respiratory failure can be complicated by hyponatremia secondary to SIADH. Hypoxemia, hypercarbia, and positive-pressure ventilation are all nonosmotic stimuli for AVP release. Various tumors, notably oat cell carcinoma of the lung, have been demonstrated to secrete AVP ectopically. Many drugs either stimulate AVP release or potentiate its actions on the kidney. The pattern of AVP secretion can be used to classify SIADH into four subtypes: (1) erratic autonomous AVP secretion (ectopic production); (2) normal regulation of AVP release around a lower osmolality set point or *reset osmostat* (cachexia, malnutrition); (3) normal AVP response to hypertonicity with failure to suppress completely at low osmolality (incomplete pituitary stalk section); and (4) normal AVP secretion with increased sensitivity to its actions or secretion of some other antidiuretic factor (rare).

Hormonal excess or deficiency may cause hyponatremia. Adrenal insufficiency (Chap. 332) and hypothyroidism (Chap. 331) may present with hyponatremia and should not be confused with SIADH. Although decreased mineralocorticoids may contribute to the hyponatremia of adrenal insufficiency, it is the cortisol deficiency that leads to hypersecretion of AVP both indirectly (secondary to volume depletion) and directly (cosecreted with corticotropin-releasing factor). The mechanisms by which hypothyroidism leads to hyponatremia include decreased cardiac output and GFR and increased AVP secretion in response to hemodynamic stimuli.

Finally, hyponatremia may occur in the absence of AVP or renal failure if the kidney is unable to excrete the dietary water load. In psychogenic or *primary polydipsia*, compulsive water consumption may overwhelm the normally large renal excretory capacity of 12 L/d (Chap. 330). These patients often have psychiatric illnesses and may be taking medications, such as phenothiazines, that enhance the sensation of thirst by causing a dry mouth. The maximal urine output is a function of the minimum urine osmolality achievable and the mandatory solute excretion. Metabolism of a normal diet generates about 600 mosmol/d, and the minimum urine osmolality in humans is 50 mosmol/kg. Therefore, the maximum daily urine output will be about 12 L ($600 \div 50 = 12$). A solute excretion rate of greater than ~750 mosmol/d is, by definition, an *osmotic diuresis*. A low-protein diet may yield as few as 250 mosmol/d, which translates into a maximal urine output of 5 L/d at a minimum urine tonicity of 50 mosmol/kg. Beer drinkers typically have a poor dietary intake of protein and electrolytes and consume large volumes (of beer), which may exceed the renal excretory capacity and result in hyponatremia. This phenomenon is referred to as *beer potomania*.

CLINICAL FEATURES The clinical manifestations of hyponatremia are related to osmotic water shift leading to increased ICF volume, specifically brain cell swelling or cerebral edema. Therefore, the symptoms are primarily neurologic, and their severity is dependent on the rapidity of onset and absolute decrease in plasma Na^+ concentration. Patients may be asymptomatic, or complain of nausea and malaise. As the plasma Na^+ concentration falls, the symptoms progress to include headache, lethargy, confusion, and obtundation. Stupor, seizures, and coma do not usually occur unless the plasma Na^+ concentration falls acutely below 120 mmol/L or decreases rapidly. As described above, adaptive mechanisms designed to protect cell volume occur in chronic hyponatremia. Loss of Na^+ and K^+, followed by organic osmolytes, from brain cells decreases brain swelling due to secondary transcellular water shifts (from ICF to ECF). The net effect is to minimize cerebral edema and its symptoms.

DIAGNOSIS Hyponatremia is not a disease but a manifestation of a variety of disorders. The underlying cause can often be ascertained from an accurate history and physical examination, including an assessment of ECF volume status and effective circulating arterial volume. The differential diagnosis of hyponatremia, an expanded ECF volume, and decreased effective circulating volume includes congestive heart failure, hepatic cirrhosis, and the nephrotic syndrome. Hypothyroidism and adrenal insufficiency tend to present with a near-normal ECF

volume and decreased effective circulating arterial volume. All of these diseases have characteristic signs and symptoms. Patients with SIADH are usually euvolemic.

Four laboratory findings often provide useful information and can narrow the differential diagnosis of hyponatremia: (1) the plasma osmolality, (2) the urine osmolality, (3) the urine Na^+ concentration, and (4) the urine K^+ concentration. Since ECF tonicity is determined primarily by the Na^+ concentration, most patients with hyponatremia have a decreased plasma osmolality. If the plasma osmolality is not low, pseudohyponatremia must be ruled out. The appropriate renal response to hypoosmolality is to excrete the maximum volume of dilute urine, i.e., urine osmolality and specific gravity of less than 100 mosmol/kg and 1.003, respectively. This occurs in patients with primary polydipsia. If this is not present, it suggests impaired free water excretion due to the action of AVP on the kidney. The secretion of AVP may be a physiologic response to hemodynamic stimuli or it may be inappropriate in the presence of hyponatremia and euvolemia. Since Na^+ is the major ECF cation and is largely restricted to this compartment, ECF volume contraction represents a deficit in total body Na^+ content. Therefore, volume depletion in patients with normal underlying renal function results in enhanced tubule Na^+ reabsorption and a urine Na^+ concentration less than 20 mmol/L. The finding of a urine Na^+ concentration greater than 20 mmol/L in hypovolemic hyponatremia implies a salt-wasting nephropathy, diuretic therapy, hypoaldosteronism, or occasionally vomiting. Both the urine osmolality and the urine Na^+ concentration can be followed serially when assessing response to therapy.

SIADH is characterized by hypoosmotic hyponatremia in the setting of an inappropriately concentrated urine (urine osmolality greater than 100 mosmol/kg). Patients are typically normovolemic and have normal Na^+ balance. They tend to be mildly volume expanded secondary to water retention and have a urine Na^+ excretion rate equal to intake (urine Na^+ concentration usually greater than 40 mmol/L). By definition, they have normal renal, adrenal, and thyroid function and usually have normal K^+ and acid-base balance. SIADH is often associated with hypouricemia due to the uricosuric state induced by volume expansion. In contrast, hypovolemic patients tend to be hyperuricemic secondary to increased proximal urate reabsorption.

CLINICAL APPROACH See Fig. 49-1.

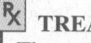 **TREATMENT**
The goals of therapy are twofold: (1) to raise the plasma Na^+ concentration by restricting water intake and promoting water loss; and (2) to correct the underlying disorder. → *For further discussion, see Chap. 330.*

HYPERNATREMIA

ETIOLOGY Hypernatremia is defined as a plasma Na^+ concentration greater than 145 mmol/L. Since Na^+ and its accompanying anions are the major effective ECF osmoles, hypernatremia is a state of hyperosmolality. As a result of the fixed number of ICF particles, maintenance of osmotic equilibrium in hypernatremia results in ICF volume contraction. Hypernatremia may be due to primary Na^+ gain or water deficit. The two components of an appropriate response to hypernatremia are increased water intake stimulated by thirst and the excretion of the minimum volume of maximally concentrated urine reflecting AVP secretion in response to an osmotic stimulus.

In practice, the majority of cases of hypernatremia result from the loss of water. Since water is distributed between the ICF and the ECF in a 2:1 ratio, a given amount of solute-free water loss will result in a twofold greater reduction in the ICF compartment than the ECF compartment. For example, consider three scenarios: the loss of 1 L of water, isotonic NaCl, or half-isotonic NaCl. If 1 L of water is lost, the ICF volume will decrease by 667 mL, whereas the ECF volume will fall by only 333 mL. Due to the fact that Na^+ is largely restricted to the ECF, this compartment will decrease by 1 L if the fluid lost is isoosmotic. One liter of half-isotonic NaCl is equivalent to 500 mL of water (one-third ECF, two-thirds ICF) plus 500 mL of isotonic saline (all ECF). Therefore, the loss of 1 L of half-isotonic saline decreases the ECF and ICF volumes by 667 mL and 333 mL, respectively.

The degree of hyperosmolality is typically mild unless the thirst mechanism is abnormal or access to water is limited. The latter occurs in infants, the physically handicapped, patients with impaired mental status, in the postoperative state, and in intubated patients in the intensive care unit. On rare occasions, impaired thirst may be due to *primary hypodipsia*. This usually occurs as a result of damage to the hypothalamic osmoreceptors that control thirst and tends to be associated with abnormal osmotic regulation of AVP secretion. Primary hypodipsia may be due to a variety of pathologic changes including granulomatous disease, vascular occlusion, and tumors. A subset of hypodipsic hypernatremia, referred to as *essential hypernatremia*, does not respond to forced water intake. This appears to be due to a specific osmoreceptor defect resulting in nonosmotic regulation of AVP release. Thus, the hemodynamic effects of water loading lead to AVP suppression and excretion of dilute urine.

The source of free water loss is either renal or extrarenal. Nonrenal loss of water may be due to evaporation from the skin and respiratory tract (insensible losses) or loss from the gastrointestinal tract. Insensible losses are increased with fever, exercise, heat exposure and severe burns and in mechanically ventilated patients. Furthermore, the Na^+ concentration of sweat decreases with profuse perspiration, thereby increasing solute-free water loss. Diarrhea is the most common gastrointestinal cause of hypernatremia. Specifically, osmotic diarrheas (induced by lactulose, sorbitol, or malabsorption of carbohydrate) and viral gastroenteritides result in water loss exceeding that of Na^+ and K^+. In contrast, secretory diarrheas (e.g., cholera, carcinoid, VIPoma) have a fecal osmolality (twice the sum of the concentrations of Na^+ and K^+) similar to that of plasma and present with ECF volume contraction and a normal plasma Na^+ concentration or hyponatremia.

Renal water loss is the most common cause of hypernatremia and is due to drug-induced or osmotic diuresis or diabetes insipidus (Chap. 330). Loop diuretics interfere with the countercurrent mechanism and produce an isoosmotic solute diuresis. This results in a decreased medullary interstitial tonicity and impaired renal concentrating ability. The presence of non-reabsorbed organic solutes in the tubule lumen impairs the osmotic reabsorption of water. This leads to water loss in excess of Na^+ and K^+, known as an osmotic diuresis. The most frequent cause of an osmotic diuresis is hyperglycemia and glucosuria in poorly controlled diabetes mellitus. Intravenous administration of mannitol and increased endogenous production of urea (high-protein diet) can also result in an osmotic diuresis. Hypernatremia secondary to nonosmotic urinary water loss is usually due to: (1) central or neurogenic diabetes insipidus characterized by impaired AVP secretion, or (2) nephrogenic diabetes insipidus resulting from end-organ (renal) resistance to the actions of AVP. The most common cause of *central diabetes insipidus* (CDI) is destruction of the neurohypophysis. This may occur as a result of trauma, neurosurgery, granulomatous disease, neoplasms, vascular accidents, or infection. In many cases, CDI is idiopathic and may occassionally be hereditary. The familial form of the disease is inherited in an autosomal dominant fashion and has been attributed to mutations in the propressophysin (AVP precursor) gene. *Nephrogenic diabetes insipidus* (NDI) may be either inherited or acquired. Congenital NDI is an X-linked recessive trait due to mutations in the V_2 receptor gene. Mutations in the autosomal aquaporin-2 gene may also result in NDI. The aquaporin-2 gene encodes the water channel protein whose membrane insertion is stimulated by AVP. The causes of sporadic NDI are numerous and include drugs (especially lithium), hypercalcemia, hypokalemia, and conditions that impair medullary hypertonicity (e.g., papillary necrosis or osmotic diuresis). Pregnant women, in the second or third trimester, may develop NDI as a result of excessive elaboration of vasopressinase by the placenta.

Finally, although infrequent, a primary Na^+ gain may cause hypernatremia. For example, inadvertent administration of hypertonic NaCl or $NaHCO_3$ or replacing sugar with salt in infant formula can produce this complication.

CLINICAL FEATURES   As a consequence of hypertonicity, water shifts out of cells, leading to a contracted ICF volume. A decreased brain cell volume is associated with an increased risk of subarachnoid or intracerebral hemorrhage. Hence, the major symptoms of hypernatremia are neurologic and include altered mental status, weakness, neuromuscular irritability, focal neurologic deficits, and occasionally coma or seizures. Patients may also complain of polyuria or thirst. For unknown reasons, patients with polydipsia from CDI tend to prefer ice-cold water. The signs and symptoms of volume depletion are often present in patients with a history of excessive sweating, diarrhea, or an osmotic diuresis. The mortality rate associated with a plasma Na^+ concentration greater than 180 mmol/L is very high. As with hyponatremia, the severity of the clinical manifestations is related to the acuity and magnitude of the rise in plasma Na^+ concentration. Chronic hypernatremia is generally less symptomatic as a result of adaptive mechanisms designed to defend cell volume. Brain cells initially take up Na^+ and K^+ salts, later followed by accumulation of organic osmolytes such as inositol. This serves to restore the brain ICF volume towards normal.

DIAGNOSIS   A complete history and physical examination will often provide clues as to the underlying cause of hypernatremia. Relevant symptoms and signs include the absence or presence of thirst, diaphoresis, diarrhea, polyuria, and the features of ECF volume contraction. The history should include a list of current and recent medications, and the physical examination is incomplete without a thorough mental status and neurologic assessment. Measurement of urine vol-

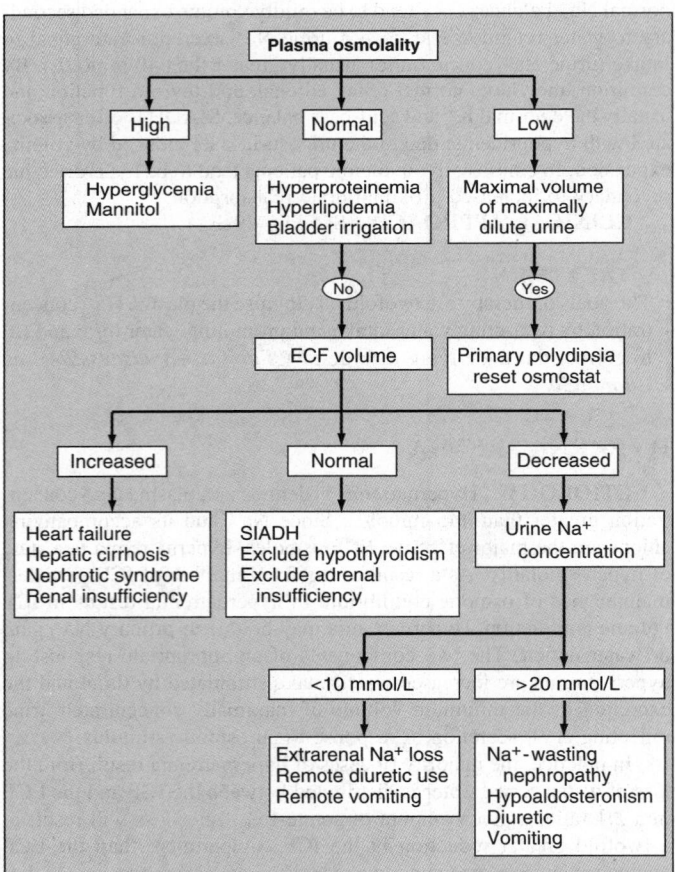

FIGURE 49-1   Algorithm depicting clinical approach to hyponatremia. ECF, extracellular fluid; SIADH, syndrome of inappropriate antidiuretic hormone secretion.

ume and osmolality are essential in the evaluation of hyperosmolality. The appropriate renal response to hypernatremia is the excretion of the minimum volume (500 mL/d) of maximally concentrated urine (urine osmolality greater than 800 mosmol/kg). These findings suggest extrarenal or remote renal water loss or administration of hypertonic Na^+ salt solutions. The presence of a primary Na^+ excess can be confirmed by the presence of ECF volume expansion and natriuresis (urine Na^+ concentration usually greater than 100 mmol/L). Many causes of hypernatremia are associated with polyuria and a submaximal urine osmolality. The product of the urine volume and osmolality, i.e., the solute excretion rate, is helpful in determining the basis of the polyuria (see above). To maintain a steady state, total solute excretion must equal solute production. As stated above, individuals eating a normal diet generate ~600 mosmol/d. Therefore, daily solute excretion in excess of 750 mosmol defines an osmotic diuresis. This can be confirmed by measuring the urine glucose and urea. In general, both CDI and NDI present with polyuria and hypotonic urine (urine osmolality less than 250 mosmol/kg). The degree of hypernatremia is usually mild unless there is an associated thirst abnormality. The clinical history, physical examination, and pertinent laboratory data can often rule out causes of acquired NDI. CDI and NDI can generally be distinguished by administering the AVP analogue desmopressin (10 µg intranasally) after careful water restriction. The urine osmolality should increase by at least 50 percent in CDI and will not change in NDI. Unfortunately, the diagnosis may sometimes be difficult due to partial defects in AVP secretion and action.

CLINICAL APPROACH   See Fig. 49-2.

 TREATMENT

The therapeutic goals are to stop ongoing water loss by treating the underlying cause and to correct the water deficit. The ECF volume should be restored in hypovolemic patients. The quantity of water required to correct the deficit can be calculated from the following equation:

$$\text{Water deficit} = \frac{\text{plasma } Na^+ \text{ concentration} - 140}{140} \times \text{total body water}$$

In hypernatremia due to water loss, total body water is approximately 50 and 40 percent of lean body weight in men and women,

respectively. For example, a 50-kg woman with a plasma Na^+ concentration of 160 mmol/L has an estimated free water deficit of 2.9 L [(160 − 140) ÷ 140 × (0.4 × 50)]. As in hyponatremia, rapid correction of hypernatremia is potentially dangerous. In this case, a sudden decrease in osmolality could potentially cause a rapid shift of water into cells that have undergone osmotic adaptation. This would result in swollen brain cells and increase the risk of seizures or permanent neurologic damage. Therefore, the water deficit should be corrected slowly over at least 48 to 72 h. When calculating the rate of water replacement, ongoing losses should be taken into account, and the plasma Na^+ concentration should be lowered by 0.5 mmol/L per hour and by no more than 12 mmol/L over the first 24 h. The safest route of administration of water is by mouth or via a nasogastric tube (or other feeding tube). Alternatively, 5% dextrose in water or half-isotonic saline can be given intravenously. The appropriate treatment of CDI consists of administering desmopressin intranasally (Chap. 330). Other options for decreasing urine output include a low-salt diet in combination with low-dose thiazide diuretic therapy. In some patients with partial CDI, drugs which either stimulate AVP secretion or enhance its action on the kidney have been useful. These include chlorpropamide, clofibrate, carbamazepine, and nonsteroidal anti-inflammatory drugs (NSAIDs). The concentrating defect in NDI may be reversible by treating the underlying disorder or eliminating the offending drug. Symptomatic polyuria due to NDI can be treated with a low-Na^+ diet and thiazide diuretics as described above. This induces mild volume depletion, which leads to enhanced proximal reabsorption of salt and water and decreased delivery to the site of action of AVP, the collecting duct. By impairing renal prostaglandin synthesis, NSAIDs potentiate AVP action and thereby increase urine osmolality and decrease urine volume. Amiloride may be useful in patients with NDI who need to be on lithium. The nephrotoxicity of lithium requires the drug to be taken up into collecting duct cells via the amiloride-sensitive Na^+ channel.

POTASSIUM

POTASSIUM BALANCE   Potassium is the major intracellular cation. The normal plasma K^+ concentration is 3.5 to 5.0 mmol/L, whereas that inside cells is about 150 mmol/L. Therefore, the amount of K^+ in the ECF (30 to 70 mmol) constitutes less than 2 percent of the total body K^+ content (2500 to 4500 mmol). The ratio of ICF to ECF K^+ concentration (normally 38:1) is the principal result of the resting membrane potential and is crucial for normal neuromuscular function. The basolateral Na^+,K^+-ATPase pump actively transports K^+ in and Na^+ out of the cell in a 2:3 ratio, and the passive outward diffusion of K^+ is quantitatively the most important factor that generates the resting membrane potential. The activity of the electrogenic Na^+,K^+-ATPase pump may be stimulated as a result of an increased intracellular Na^+ concentration and inhibited in the setting of digoxin toxicity of chronic illness such as heart failure or renal failure.

The distribution of K^+ is also affected by several other factors, including hormones, acid-base balance, osmolality, and cell turnover. Insulin increases Na^+,K^+-ATPase activity indirectly and independent of its effect on glucose transport, leading to K^+ shift into muscle and liver cells. Conversely, insulin deficiency results in K^+ movement from the ICF to the ECF compartment. Catecholamines have variable effects on K^+ distribution—beta$_2$-adrenergic agonists promote whereas alpha-adrenergic agonists impair K^+ uptake by cells. The Na^+,K^+-ATPase pump as well as insulin secretion are stimulated by beta$_2$-adrenergic agonists. In contrast, alpha-adrenergic agonists have the opposite effect. The major action of aldosterone is to increase K^+ excretion (see below). The role of extracellular pH in K^+ balance relates to the underlying acid-base disorder. In metabolic acidosis, 60 percent of the H^+ load is buffered inside cells. To maintain electroneutrality, the H^+ ion must either be accompanied by an anion or ex-

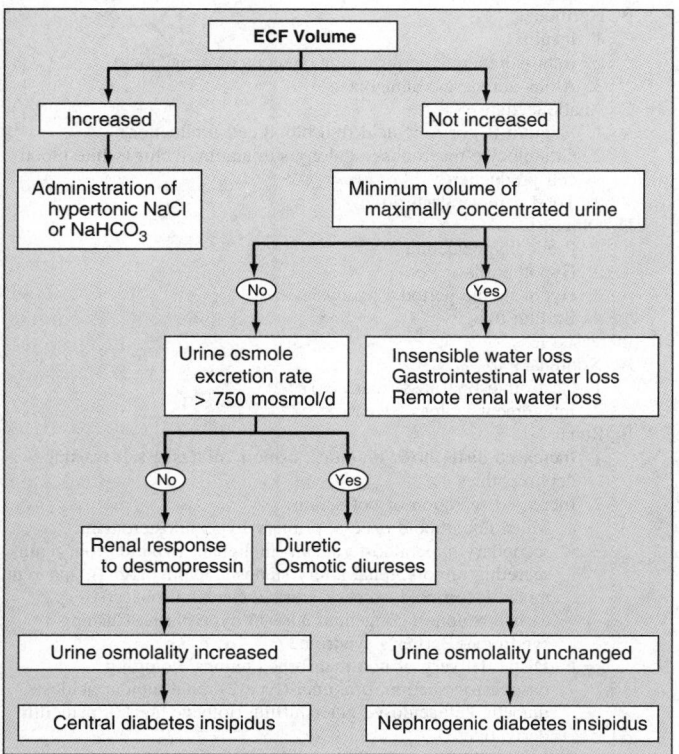

FIGURE 49-2   Algorithm depicting clinical approach to hypernatremia.

changed for intracellular K^+ (leading to hyperkalemia). Organic acidoses are not usually associated with a pH-related K^+ shift, since anions such as lactate and β-hydroxybutyrate can be readily taken up by the cell. The converse, movement of K^+ into cells, may be seen with metabolic alkalosis. However, this is less important due to diminished intracellular buffering. Primary respiratory disturbances in acid-base balance result in minimal transcellular K^+ shifts. In hyperosmolal states, K^+ diffuses out of cells along with water due to *solvent drag*. The concentration gradient favoring K^+ movement out of cells is also increased as a result of ICF water loss. Tissue destruction or breakdown results in the release of intracellular K^+, whereas the production of new cell shifts K^+ out of the ECF. Finally, moderate to severe exercise may be associatd with K^+ release from muscle, leading to glycogenolysis and local vasodilatation. This is usually transient but may affect the plasma K^+ concentration if patients repeatedly clench and unclench their fist prior to venipuncture.

The K^+ intake of individuals on an average western diet is 40 to 120 mmol/d or approximately 1 mmol/kg per day, 90 percent of which is absorbed by the gastrointestinal tract. Maintenance of the steady state necessitates matching K^+ ingestion with excretion. Initially, extrarenal adaptive mechanisms, followed later by urinary excretion, prevent a doubling of the plasma K^+ concentration that would occur if the dietary K^+ load remained in the ECF compartment. Immediately following a meal, most of the absorbed K^+ enters cells as a result of the initial elevation in the plasma K^+ concentration and facilitated by insulin release and basal catecholamine levels. Eventually, however, the excess K^+ is excreted in the urine (see below). The regulation of gastrointestinal K^+ handling is not well understood. The amount of K^+ lost in the stool can increase from 10 to 50 or 60 percent (of dietary intake) in chronic renal insufficiency. In addition, colonic secretion of K^+ is stimulated in patients with large volumes of diarrhea, resulting in potentially severe K^+ depletion.

POTASSIUM EXCRETION (See also Chap. 269) Renal excretion is the major route of elimination of dietary and other sources of excess K^+. The filtered load of K^+ (GFR × plasma K^+ concentration = 180 L/d × 4 mmol/L = 720 mmol/d is 10- to 20-fold greater than the ECF K^+ content. Ninety percent of filtered K^+ is reabsorbed by the proximal convoluted tubule and loop of Henle. Proximally, K^+ is reabsorbed passively with Na^+ and water, whereas the luminal Na^+-K^+-$2Cl^-$ cotransporter mediates K^+ uptake in the thick ascending limb of the loop of Henle. Therefore, K^+ delivery to the distal nephron (distal convoluted tubule and cortical collecting duct) approximates dietary intake. Net distal K^+ secretion or reabsorption occurs in the setting of K^+ excess or depletion, respectively. The cell responsible for K^+ secretion in the late distal convoluted tubule (or connecting tubule) and cortical collecting duct (CCD) is the principal cell. Virtually all regulation of renal K^+ excretion and total body K^+ balance occurs in the distal nephron. The driving force for K^+ secretion is a favorable electrochemical gradient across the luminal membrane of the principal cell. As a result of the action of the basolateral Na^+,K^+-ATPase pump, the intracellular K^+ concentration far exceeds that of the fluid in the lumen of the CCD. The electrical gradient is created by electrogenic Na^+ reabsorption leading to a lumen-negative transepithelial potential difference (TEPD), favoring K^+ secretion. The generation of a lumen-negative TEPD depends on the relative rates of reabsorption of Na^+ and its accompanying anion (primarily Cl^-). Equimolar reabsorption of Na^+ and Cl^- at equivalent rates is electroneutral, whereas reabsorption of Na^+ in excess of Cl^- is electrogenic. The cellular uptake of Na^+ by the principal cell occurs via an apical Na^+ channel and is driven by a low intracellular Na^+ concentration relative to that in the lumen of the CCD. The mechanism and regulation of distal nephron Cl^- transport is less clear. Obviously, factors that impact on either Na^+ or Cl^- reabsorption by the principal cell will influence the TEPD. Potassium secretion is regulated by two physiologic stimuli—aldosterone and hyperkalemia. Aldosterone is secreted by the zona glomerulosa cells of the adrenal cortex in response to high renin and angiotensin II or hyperkalemia. The actions of aldosterone on the principal cell include enhanced apical membrane Na^+ conductivity, stimulation of the basolateral Na^+,K^+-ATPase, and increased luminal K^+ channels. The plasma K^+ concentration, independent of aldosterone, can directly affect K^+ secretion. In addition to the K^+ concentration in the lumen of the CCD, renal K^+ loss depends on the urine flow rate, a function of daily solute excretion (see above). Since excretion is equal to the product of concentration and volume, increased distal flow rate can significantly enhance urinary K^+ output. Finally, in severe K^+ depletion, secretion of K^+ is reduced and reabsorption, via apical H^+,K^+-ATPase pumps in cortical and medullary collecting ducts, is upregulated.

HYPOKALEMIA

ETIOLOGY (See Table 49-3) Hypokalemia, defined as a plasma K^+ concentration less than 3.5 mmol/L, may result from one (or more) of the following: decreased net intake, shift into cells, or increased net loss. Diminished intake is seldom the sole cause of K^+ depletion since urinary excretion can be effectively decreased to less than 15 mmol/d as a result of net K^+ reabsorption in the distal nephron. With the exception of the urban poor and certain cultural groups, the amount of K^+ in the diet almost always exceeds that excreted in the urine. However, dietary K^+ restriction may exacerbate the hypokalemia secondary to increased gastrointestinal or renal loss. An unusual cause of decreased K^+ intake is ingestion of clay (geophagia), which binds dietary K^+ and iron. This custom was previously common among African-Americans in the American South.

Movement of K^+ into cells may transiently decrease the plasma K^+ concentration without altering total body K^+ content. For any

Table 49-3

Causes of Hypokalemia

I. Decreased intake
   A. Starvation
   B. Clay ingestion
II. Redistribution into cells
   A. Acid-base
      1. Metabolic alkalosis
   B. Hormonal
      1. Insulin
      2. Beta$_2$-adrenergic agonists (endogenous or exogenous)
      3. Alpha-adrenergic antagonists
   C. Anabolic state
      1. Vitamin B_{12} or folic acid (red blood cell production)
      2. Granulocyte-macrophage colony stimulating factor (white blood cell production)
      3. Total parenteral nutrition
   D. Other
      1. Pseudohypokalemia
      2. Hypothermia
      3. Hypokalemic periodic paralysis
      4. Barium toxicity
III. Increased loss
   A. Nonrenal
      1. Gastrointestinal loss (diarrhea)
      2. Integumentary loss (sweat)
   B. Renal
      1. Increased distal flow: diuretics, osmotic diuresis, salt-wasting nephropathies
      2. Increased secretion of potassium
         a. Mineralocorticoid excess: primary hyperaldosteronism, secondary hyperaldosteronism (malignant hypertension, renin-secreting tumors, renal artery stenosis, hypovolemia), apparent mineralocorticoid excess (licorice, chewing tobacco, carbenoxolone), congenital adrenal hyperplasia, Cushing's syndrome, Bartter's syndrome
         b. Distal delivery of non-reabsorbed anions: vomiting, nasogastric suction, proximal (type 2) renal tubular acidosis, diabetic ketoacidosis, glue-sniffing (toluene abuse), penicillin derivatives
         c. Other: amphotericin B, Liddle's syndrome, hypomagnesemia

given cause, the magnitude of the change is relatively small, often less than 1 mmol/L. However, a combination of factors may lead to a significant fall in the plasma K^+ concentration and may amplify the hypokalemia due to K^+ wasting. Alkalosis, especially that due to a primary increase in plasma HCO_3^- (metabolic alkalosis), is often associated with hypokalemia. This occurs as a result of K^+ redistribution as well as excessive renal or gastrointestinal K^+ loss. Treatment of diabetic ketoacidosis with insulin may lead to hypokalemia due to stimulation of the Na^+-H^+ antiporter and (secondarily) the Na^+,K^+-ATPase pump. Furthermore, uncontrolled hyperglycemia often leads to K^+ depletion from an osmotic diuresis (see below). Stress-induced catecholamine release and administration of beta$_2$-adrenergic agonists directly induce cellular uptake of K^+ and promote insulin secretion by pancreatic islet β cells. *Hypokalemic periodic paralysis* is a rare condition characterized by recurrent episodic weakness or paralysis (Chap. 383). Since K^+ is the major ICF cation, anabolic states can potentially result in hypokalemia due to a K^+ shift into cells. This may occur following rapid cell growth seen in patients with pernicious anemia treated with vitamin B_{12} or with neutropenia after treatment with granulocyte-macrophage colony stimulating factor. Massive transfusion with thawed washed red blood cells (RBCs) could cause hypokalemia since frozen RBCs lose up to half of their K^+ during storage.

Excessive sweating may result in K^+ depletion from increased integumentary and renal K^+ loss. Hyperaldosteronism, secondary to ECF volume contraction, enhances K^+ excretion in the urine (Chap. 332). Normally, K^+ lost in the stool amounts to 5 to 10 mmol/d in a volume of 100 to 200 mL. Hypokalemia subsequent to increased gastrointestinal loss can occur in patients with profuse diarrhea (usually secretory), villous adenomas, VIPomas, or laxative abuse. However, the loss of gastric secretions does not account for the moderate to severe K^+ depletion often associated with vomiting of nasogastric suction. Since the K^+ concentration of gastric fluid is 5 to 10 mmol/L, it would take 30 to 80 L of vomitus to achieve a K^+ deficit of 300 to 400 mmol typically seen in these patients. In fact, the hypokalemia is primarily due to increased renal K^+ excretion. Loss of gastric contents results in volume depletion and metabolic alkalosis, both of which promote kaliuresis. Hypovolemia stimulates aldosterone release, which augments K^+ secretion by the principal cells. In addition, the filtered load of HCO_3^- exceeds the reabsorptive capacity of the proximal convoluted tubule, thereby increasing distal delivery of $NaHCO_3$ which enhances the electrochemical gradient favoring K^+ loss in the urine.

In general, most cases of chronic hypokalemia are due to renal K^+ wasting. This may be due to factors that increase the K^+ concentration in the lumen of the CCD or augment distal flow rate. As described above, distal nephron K^+ secretion is driven by a lumen-negative TEPD, affected by aldosterone and the relative rates of reabsorption of Na^+ and its accompanying anion(s). Mineralocorticoid excess commonly results in hypokalemia (Chap. 332). *Primary hyperaldosteronism* is due to dysregulated aldosterone secretion by an adrenal adenoma (Conn's syndrome) or carcinoma or to adrenocortical hyperplasia. In a rare subset of patients, the disorder is familial (autosomal dominant) and aldosterone levels can be suppressed by administering low doses of exogenous glucocorticoid. The molecular defect responsible for *glucocorticoid-remediable hyperaldosteronism* is a rearranged gene (due to a chromosomal crossover), containing the 5′-regulatory region of the 11β-hydroxylase gene and the coding sequence of the aldosterone synthase gene. Consequently, mineralocorticoid is synthesized in the zona fasciculata and regulated by corticotropin. A number of conditions associated with hyperreninemia result in secondary hyperaldosteronism and renal K^+ wasting. High renin levels are commonly seen in both renovascular and malignant hypertension. Renin-secreting tumors of the juxtaglomerular apparatus are a rare cause of hypokalemia. Other tumors that have been reported to produce renin include renal cell carcinoma, ovarian carcinoma, and Wilms' tumor. Hyperreninemia may also occur secondary to decreased effective circulating arterial volume.

In the absence of elevated renin or aldosterone levels, enhanced distal nephron secretion of K^+ may result from increased production of

non-aldosterone mineralocorticoids in *congenital adrenal hyperplasia* (Chap. 332). Glucocorticoid-stimulated kaliuresis does not normally occur due to the conversion of cortisol to cortisone by 11β-hydroxysteroid dehydrogenase (11β-HSDH). Therefore, 11β-HSDH deficiency or suppression allows cortisol to bind to the aldosterone receptor and leads to the *syndrome of apparent mineralocorticoid excess*. Drugs that inhibit the activity of 11β-HSDH include glycyrrhetinic acid, present in licorice, chewing tobacco, and carbenoxolone. The presentation of Cushing's syndrome may include hypokalemia if the capacity of 11β-HSDH to inactivate cortisol is overwhelmed by persistently elevated glucocorticoid levels.

Liddle's Syndrome This is a rare familial (autosomal dominant) disease characterized by hypertension, hypokalemic metabolic alkalosis, renal K^+ wasting, and suppressed renin and aldosterone secretion (Chap. 332). This condition is caused by mutations in the β subunit of the principal cell apical Na^+ channel, resulting in increased conductivity. Appropriate therapy includes Na^+ restriction and treatment with amiloride, a specific inhibitor of the CCD luminal Na^+ channel. Increased distal delivery of Na^+ with a non-reabsorbable anion (not Cl^-) enhances the lumen-negative TEPD and K^+ secretion. Classically, this is seen with *proximal (type 2) renal tubular acidosis* (RTA) and vomiting, associated with bicarbonaturia. Diabetic ketoacidosis and toluene abuse (glue-sniffing) can lead to increased delivery of β-hydroxybutyrate and hippurate, respectively, to the CCD and to renal K^+ loss. High doses of penicillin derivatives administered to volume-depleted patients may likewise promote renal K^+ secretion as well as an osmotic diuresis. *Classic distal (type 1) RTA* is associated with hypokalemia due to increased renal K^+ loss, the mechanism of which is uncertain. Amphotericin B causes hypokalemia due to increased distal nephron permeability to Na^+ and K^+ and to renal K^+ wasting.

Bartter's Syndrome This is a disorder characterized by hypokalemia, metabolic alkalosis, hyperreninemic hyperaldosteronism secondary to ECF volume contraction, and juxtaglomerular apparatus hyperplasia (Chap. 332). The blood pressure is usually normal, and hypomagnesemia is often present as a result of renal Mg^{2+} wasting. The pathophysiology of Bartter's syndrome has yet to be elucidated. Proposed mechanisms include a defect in the Na^+-K^+-2Cl^- cotransporter of the thick ascending limb of the loop of Henle, impaired distal Cl^- reabsorption, and excessive renal prostaglandin synthesis. Hypokalemia refractory to K^+ repletion is suggestive of Mg^{2+} depletion. Although the pathogenesis is unclear, hypomagnesemia may stimulate aldosterone secretion or decrease distal Cl^- transport. Finally, diuretic use and abuse are common causes of K^+ depletion. Carbonic anhydrase inhibitors, loop diuretics, and thiazides are all kaliuretic. The degree of hypokalemia tends to be greater with long-acting agents and is dose-dependent. Increased renal K^+ excretion is due primarily to increased distal solute delivery and secondary hyperaldosteronism (due to volume depletion).

CLINICAL FEATURES The clinical manifestations of K^+ depletion vary greatly between individual patients, and their severity depends on the degree of hypokalemia. Symptoms seldom occur unless the plasma K^+ concentration is less than 3 mmol/L. Fatigue, myalgia, and muscular weakness of the lower extremities are common complaints and are due to a lower (more negative) resting membrane potential. More severe hypokalemia may lead to progressive weakness, hypoventilation (due to respiratory muscle involvement), and eventually complete paralysis. Impaired muscle metabolism and the blunted hyperemic response to exercise associated with profound K^+ depletion increase the risk of rhabdomyolysis. Smooth-muscle function may also be affected and manifest as paralytic ileus.

The electrocardiographic changes of hypokalemia (Fig. 228-19) are due to delayed ventricular repolarization and do not correlate well with the plasma K^+ concentration. Early changes include flattening or inversion of the T wave, a prominent U wave, ST-segment depression, and a prolonged QU interval. Severe K^+ depletion may result in a prolonged PR interval, decreased voltage and widening of the QRS complex, and an increased risk of ventricular arrhythmias, especially in patients with myocardial ischemia or left ventricular hypertrophy. Hypokalemia may also predispose to digitalis toxicity. Epidemiologic studies have linked a low-K^+ diet with an increased prevalence of hypertension, particularly among African-Americans. Furthermore, in patients with essential hypertension, systemic blood pressure may be lowered by K^+ supplementation. The mechanism of the hypertensive effect of K^+ depletion is not certain but may relate to enhanced distal NaCl reabsorption.

Hypokalemia is often associated with acid-base disturbances related to the underlying disorder. In addition, K^+ depletion results in intracellular acidification and an increase in net acid excretion or new HCO_3^- production. This is a consequence of enhanced proximal HCO_3^- reabsorption, increased renal ammoniagenesis, and increased distal H^+ secretion. This contributes to the generation of metabolic alkalosis frequently present in hypokalemic patients. Nephrogenic diabetes insipidus (see above) is not uncommonly seen in K^+ depletion and is manifest as polydipsia and polyuria. Glucose intolerance may also occur with hypokalemia and has been attributed to either impaired insulin secretion or peripheral insulin resistance.

DIAGNOSIS In most cases, the etiology of K^+ depletion can be determined by a careful history. Diuretic and laxative abuse as well as surreptitious vomiting may be difficult to identify but should be excluded. Rarely, patients with a marked leukocytosis (e.g., acute myeloid leukemia) and normokalemia may have a low measured plasma K^+ concentration due to white blood cell uptake of K^+ at room temperature. This *pseudohypokalemia* can be avoided by storing the blood sample on ice or rapidly separating the plasma (or serum) from the cells. After eliminating decreased intake and intracellular shift as potential causes of hypokalemia, examination of the renal response can help to clarify the source of K^+ loss. The appropriate response to K^+ depletion is to excrete less than 15 mmol/d of K^+ in the urine, due to increased reabsorption and decreased distal secretion. Hypokalemia with minimal renal K^+ excretion suggests that K^+ was lost via the skin or gastrointestinal tract or that there is a remote history of vomiting or diuretic use. As described above, renal K^+ wasting may be due to factors that either increase the K^+ concentration in the CCD or increase the distal flow rate (or both). The ECF volume status, blood pressure, and associated acid-base disorder may help to differentiate the causes of excessive renal K^+ loss. A rapid and simple test designed to evaluate the driving force for net K^+ secretion is the *transtubular K^+ concentration gradient* (TTKG). The TTKG is the ratio of the K^+ concentration in the lumen of the CCD ($[K^+]_{CCD}$) to that in peritubular capillaries or plasma ($[K^+]_P$). The validity of this measurement depends on three assumptions: (1) few solutes are reabsorbed in the medullary collecting duct (MCD), (2) K^+ is neither secreted nor reabsorbed in the MCD, and (3) the osmolality of the fluid in the terminal CCD is known. In most situations, reabsorption of Na^+ salts in the MCD will have a small effect on the TTKG. Significant reabsorption or secretion of K^+ in the MCD seldom occurs, except in profound K^+ depletion or excess, respectively. When AVP is acting, the osmolality in the terminal CCD is the same as that of plasma, and the K^+ concentration in the lumen of the distal nephron can be estimated by dividing the urine K^+ concentration ($[K^+]_U$) by the ratio of the urine to plasma osmolality (OSM_U/OSM_P):

$$[K^+]_{CCD} = [K^+]_U \div (OSM_U/OSM_P)$$

$$TTKG = [K^+]_{CCD} \div [K^+]_P = \frac{[K^+]_U \div (OSM_U/OSM_P)}{[K^+]_P}$$

The urine osmolality must exceed that of plasma in order to calculate the TTKG. There is no normal range of values for the TTKG since it is dependent on the state of total body K^+ balance. Hypokalemia with a TTKG greater than 4 suggests renal K^+ loss due to increased distal K^+ secretion. Plasma renin and aldosterone levels are often helpful in differentiating the various causes of hyperaldosteronism.

FIGURE 49-3 Algorithm depicting clinical approach to hypokalemia. RTA, renal tubular acidosis; TTKG, transtubular K^+ concentration gradient.

Bicarbonaturia and the presence of other non-reabsorbed anions also increase the TTKG and lead to renal K^+-wasting.

CLINICAL APPROACH See Fig. 49-3.

℞ TREATMENT

The therapeutic goals are to correct the K^+ deficit and to minimize ongoing losses. With the exception of periodic paralysis, hypokalemia resulting from transcellular shifts rarely requires intravenous K^+ supplementation, which can lead to rebound hyperkalemia. It is generally safer to correct hypokalemia via the oral route. The degree of K^+ depletion does not correlate well with the plasma K^+ concentration. A decrement of 1 mmol/L in the plasma K^+ concentration (from 4.0 to 3.0 mmol/L) may represent a total body K^+ deficit of 200 to 400 mmol, and patients with plasma levels under 3.0 mmol/L often require in excess of 600 mmol of K^+ to correct the deficit. Furthermore, factors promoting K^+ shift out of cells (e.g., insulin deficiency in diabetic ketoacidosis) may result in underestimation of the K^+ deficit. Therefore, the plasma K^+ concentration should be monitored frequently when assessing the response to treatment. Potassium chloride is usually the preparation of choice and will promote more rapid correction of hypokalemia and metabolic alkalosis. Potassium bicarbonate and citrate (metabolized to HCO_3^-) tend to alkalinize the patient and would be more appropriate for hypokalemia associated with chronic diarrhea or RTA.

Patients with severe hypokalemia or those unable to take anything by mouth require intravenous replacement therapy with KCl. The maximum concentration of administered K^+ should be no more than 40 mmol/L via a peripheral vein or 60 mmol/L via a central vein. The rate of infusion should not exceed 20 mmol/h unless paralysis or malignant ventricular arrhythmias are present. Ideally, KCl should be mixed in normal saline since dextrose solutions may initially exacerbate hypokalemia due to insulin-mediated movement of K^+ into cells. Rapid intravenous administration of K^+ should be used judiciously and requires close observation of the clinical manifestations of hypokalemia (electrocardiogram and neuromuscular examination).

HYPERKALEMIA

ETIOLOGY Hyperkalemia, defined as a plasma K^+ concentration greater than 5.0 mmol/L, occurs as a result of either K^+ release from cells or decreased renal loss. Increased K^+ intake is rarely the sole cause of hyperkalemia since the phenomenon of *potassium adaptation* ensures rapid K^+ excretion in response to increases in dietary consumption. Iatrogenic hyperkalemia may result from overzealous parenteral K^+ replacement or in patients with renal insufficiency. *Pseudohyperkalemia* represents an artificially elevated plasma K^+ concentration due to K^+ movement out of cells immediately prior to or following venipuncture. Contributing factors include prolonged use of a tourniquet with or without repeated fist clenching, hemolysis, and marked leukocytosis or thrombocytosis. The latter two result in an elevated serum K^+ concentration due to release of intracellular K^+ following clot formation. Pseudohyperkalemia should be suspected in an otherwise asymptomatic patient with no obvious underlying cause. If proper venipuncture technique is used and a plasma (not serum) K^+ concentration is measured, it should be normal. Intravascular hemolysis, tumor lysis syndrome, and rhabdomyolysis all lead to K^+ release from cells as a result of tissue breakdown. Metabolic acidoses, with the exception of those due to the accumulation of organic anions, can be associated with mild hyperkalemia resulting from intracellular buffering of H^+ (see above). As previously described (p. 271), insulin deficiency and hypertonicity (e.g., hyperglycemia) promote K^+ shift from the ICF to the ECF. The severity of exercise-induced hyperkalemia is related to the degree of exertion. It is due to release of K^+ from muscles and is usually rapidly reversible, often associated with rebound hypokalemia. Treatment with beta blockers rarely causes hyperkalemia but may contribute to the elevation in plasma K^+ concentration seen with other conditions. *Hyperkalemic periodic paralysis* (Chap. 383) is a rare autosomal dominant disorder characterized by episodic weakness or paralysis, precipitated by stimuli that normally lead to mild hyperkalemia (e.g., exercise). The genetic defect appears to be a single amino acid substitution due to a mutation in the gene for the skeletal muscle Na^+ channel. Hyperkalemia may occur with severe digitalis toxicity due to inhibition of the Na^+,K^+-ATPase pump. Depolarizing muscle relaxants such as succinylcholine can increase the plasma K^+ concentration, especially in patients with massive trauma, burns, or neuromuscular disease.

Chronic hyperkalemia is virtually always associated with decreased renal K^+ excretion due to either impaired secretion or diminished distal solute delivery (Table 49-4). The latter is seldom the only cause of impaired K^+ excretion but may significantly contribute to hyperkalemia in protein-malnourished (low urea excretion) and ECF

Table 49-4

Causes of Hyperkalemia

I. Renal failure
II. Decreased distal flow (i.e., decreased effective circulating arterial volume)
III. Decreased K^+ secretion
  A. Impaired Na^+ reabsorption
    1. Primary hypoaldosteronism: adrenal insufficiency, adrenal enzyme deficiency (21-hydroxylase, 3β-hydroxysteroid dehydrogenase, corticosterone methyl oxidase)
    2. Secondary hypoaldosteronism: hyporeninemia, drugs ACE inhibitors, NSAIDs, heparin)
    3. Resistance to aldosterone: pseudohypoaldosteronism, tubulointerstitial disease, drugs (K^+-sparing diuretics, trimethoprim, pentamidine)
  B. Enhanced Cl^- reabsorption (chloride shunt)
    1. Gordon's syndrome
    2. Cyclosporine

volume–contracted (decreased distal NaCl delivery) patients. Decreased K^+ secretion by the principal cells results from either impaired Na^+ reabsorption or increased Cl^- reabsorption, both of which give rise to a diminished (less lumen-negative) TEPD in the CCD. *Hyporeninemic hypoaldosteronism* is a syndrome characterized by euvolemia or ECF volume expansion and suppressed renin and aldosterone levels (Chaps. 332 and 334). This disorder is commonly seen in mild renal insufficiency, diabetic nephropathy, or chronic tubulointerstitial disease. Patients frequently have an impaired kaliuretic response to exogenous mineralocorticoid administration, suggesting that enhanced distal Cl^- reabsorption (electroneutral Na^+ reabsorption) may account for many of the findings of hyporeninemic hypoaldosteronism. NSAIDs inhibit renin secretion and the synthesis of vasodilatory renal prostaglandins. The resultant decrease in GFR and K^+ secretion is often manifest as hyperkalemia. As a rule, the degree of hyperkalemia due to hypoaldosteronism is mild in the absence of increased K^+ intake or renal dysfunction. Angiotensin-converting enzyme (ACE) inhibitors block the conversion of angiotensin I to angiotensin II, resulting in impaired aldosterone release. Patients at increased risk of ACE inhibitor–induced hyperkalemia include those with diabetes mellitus, renal insufficiency, decreased effective circulating arterial volume, bilateral renal artery stenosis, or concurrent use of K^+-sparing diuretics or NSAIDs.

Decreased aldosterone synthesis may be due to *primary adrenal insufficiency* (Addison's disease) or congenital adrenal enzyme deficiency (Chap. 332). Heparin (including low-molecular-weight heparin) inhibits production of aldosterone by the cells of the zona glomerulosa and can lead to severe hyperkalemia in a subset of patients with underlying renal disease; diabetes mellitus; or those receiving K^+-sparing diuretics, ACE inhibitors, or NSAIDs. *Pseudohypoaldosteronism* is a rare familial disorder characterized by hyperkalemia, metabolic acidosis, renal Na^+ wasting, hypotension, high renin and aldosterone levels, and end-organ resistance to aldosterone. The gene encoding the mineralocorticoid receptor is normal in these patients, and the electrolyte abnormalities can be reversed with suprapharmacologic doses of an exogenous mineralocorticoid (e.g., 9α-fludrocortisone) or an inhibitor of 11β-HSDH (e.g., carbenoxolone). The kaliuretic response to aldosterone is impaired by K^+-sparing diuretics. Spironolactone is a competitive mineralocorticoid antagonist, whereas amiloride and triamterene block the apical Na^+ channel of the principal cell. Two other drugs that impair K^+ secretion by blocking distal nephron Na^+ reabsorption are trimethoprim and pentamidine. These antimicrobial agents may contribute to the hyperkalemia often seen in patients infected with human immunodeficiency virus who are being treated for *Pneumocystis carinii* pneumonia.

Hyperkalemia frequently complicates acute oliguric renal failure due to increased K^+ release from cells (acidosis, catabolism) and decreased excretion. Increased distal flow rate and K^+ secretion per nephron compensate for decreased renal mass in chronic renal insufficiency. However, these adaptive mechanisms eventually fail to maintain K^+ balance when the GFR falls below 10 to 15 mL/min or oliguria ensues. Otherwise asymptomatic urinary tract obstruction is an often overlooked cause of hyperkalemia. Other nephropathies associated with impaired K^+ excretion include drug-induced interstitial nephritis, lupus nephritis, sickle cell disease, and diabetic nephropathy.

Gordon's Syndrome This is a rare condition characterized by hyperkalemia, metabolic acidosis, and a normal GFR. These patients are usually volume-expanded with suppressed renin and aldosterone levels as well as refractory to the kaliuretic effect of exogenous mineralocorticoids. It has been suggested that these findings could all be accounted for by increased distal Cl^- reabsorption (electroneutral Na^+ reabsorption), also referred to as a *Cl^- shunt*. A similar mechanism may be partially responsible for the hyperkalemia associated with cyclosporine nephrotoxicity. *Hyperkalemic distal (type 4) RTA* may be due to either hypoaldosteronism or a Cl^- shunt (aldosterone-resistant).

CLINICAL FEATURES Since the resting membrane potential is related to the ratio of the ICF to ECF K^+ concentration, hyperkalemia partially depolarizes the cell membrane. Prolonged depolarization impairs membrane excitability and is manifest as weakness, which may progress to flaccid paralysis and hypoventilation if the respiratory muscles are involved. Hyperkalemia also inhibits renal ammoniagenesis and reabsorption of NH_4^+ in the thick ascending limb of the loop of Henle. Thus, net acid excretion is impaired and results in metabolic acidosis, which may further exacerbate the hyperkalemia due to K^+ movement out of cells.

The most serious effect of hyperkalemia is cardiac toxicity, which does not correlate well with the plasma K^+ concentration. The earliest electrocardiographic changes include increased T-wave amplitude, or peaked T waves. More severe degrees of hyperkalemia result in a prolonged PR interval and QRS duration, atrioventricular conduction delay, and loss of P waves. Progressive widening of the QRS complex and merging with the T wave produces a sinewave pattern. The terminal event is usually ventricular fibrillation or asystole.

DIAGNOSIS With rare exceptions, chronic hyperkalemia is always due to impaired K^+ excretion. If the etiology is not readily apparent and the patient is asymptomatic, pseudohyperkalemia should be excluded, as described above. Oliguric acute renal failure and severe chronic renal insufficiency should also be ruled out. The history should focus on medications that impair K^+ handling and potential sources of K^+ intake. Evaluation of the ECF compartment, effective circulating volume, and urine output are essential components of the physical examination. The severity of hyperkalemia is determined by the symptoms, plasma K^+ concentration, and electrocardiographic abnormalities.

The appropriate renal response to hyperkalemia is to excrete at least 200 mmol of K^+ daily. In most cases, diminished renal K^+ loss is due to impaired K^+ secretion, which can be assessed by measuring the TTKG (see above). A TTKG of less than 10 implies a decreased driving force for K^+ secretion due to either hypoaldosteronism or

resistance to the renal effects of mineralocorticoid. This can be determined by evaluating the kaliuretic response to administration of mineralocorticoid (e.g., 9α-fludrocortisone). Primary adrenal insufficiency can be differentiated from hyporeninemic hypoaldosteronism by examining the renin-aldosterone axis. Renin and aldosterone levels should be measured in the supine and upright positions, following three days of Na^+ restriction (Na^+ intake less than 10 mmol/d) in combination with a loop diuretic to induce mild volume contraction. Aldosterone-resistant hyperkalemia can result from the various causes of impaired distal Na^+ reabsorption or from a Cl^- shunt. The former leads to salt wasting, ECF volume contraction, and high renin and aldosterone levels. In contrast, enhanced distal Cl^- reabsorption is associated with volume expansion and suppressed renin and aldosterone secretion. As mentioned above, hypoaldosteronism seldom causes severe hypokalemia in the absence of increased dietary K^+ intake, renal insufficiency, transcellular K^+ shifts, or antikaliuretic drugs.

CLINICAL APPROACH See Fig. 49-4.

℞ **TREATMENT**

The approach to therapy depends on the degree of hyperkalemia as determined by the plasma K^+ concentration, associated muscular weakness, and changes on the electrocardiogram. Potentially fatal hyperkalemia rarely occurs unless the plasma K^+ concentration exceeds 7.5 mmol/L and is usually associated with profound weakness and absent P waves, QRS widening, or ventricular arrhythmias on the electrocardiogram.

Severe hyperkalemia requires emergent treatment directed at minimizing membrane depolarization, shifting K^+ into cells, and promoting K^+ loss. In addition, exogenous K^+ intake and antikaliuretic drugs should be discontinued. Administration of calcium gluconate decreases membrane excitability. The usual dose is 10 mL of a 10% solution infused over 2 to 3 min. The effect begins within minutes but is short-lived (30 to 60 min), and the dose can be repeated if no change in the electrocardiogram is seen after 5 to 10 min. Insulin causes K^+ to shift into cells by mechanisms described previously and will temporarily lower the plasma K^+ concentration. Although glucose alone will stimulate insulin release from normal pancreatic β cells, a more rapid response generally occurs when exogenous insulin is administered (with glucose to prevent hypoglycemia). A commonly recommended combination is 10 to 20 units of regular insulin and 25 to 50 g of glucose. Obviously, hyperglycemic patients should not be given glucose. If effective, the plasma K^+ concentration will fall by 0.5 to 1.5 mmol/L in 15 to 30 min and the effect will last for several hours. Alkali therapy with intravenous $NaHCO_3$ can also shift K^+ into cells. This is safest when administered as an isotonic solution of 3 ampules per liter (134 mmol/L $NaHCO_3$) and ideally should be reserved for severe hyperkalemia associated with metabolic acidosis. Patients with end-stage renal disease seldom respond to this intervention and may not tolerate the Na^+ load and resultant volume expansion. When administered parenterally or in nebulized form, beta$_2$-adrenergic agonists promote cellular uptake of K^+ (see above). The onset of action is 30 min, lowering the plasma K^+ concentration by 0.5 to 1.5 mmol/L, and the effect lasts 2 to 4 h.

Removal of K^+ can be achieved using diuretics, cation-exchange resin, or dialysis. Loop and thiazide diuretics, often in combination, may enhance K^+ excretion if renal function is adequate. Sodium polystyrene sulfonate is a cation-exchange resin that promotes the exchange of Na^+ for K^+ in the gastrointestinal tract. Each gram binds 1 mmol of K^+ and releases 2 to 3 mmol of Na^+. When given by mouth, the usual dose is 25 to 50 g mixed with 100 mL of 20% sorbitol to prevent constipation. This will generally lower the plasma K^+ concentration by 0.5 to 1.0 mmol/L within 1 to 2 h and last for 4 to 6 h. Sodium polystyrene sulfonate can also be administered as a retention enema consisting of 50 g of resin and 50 mL of 70% sorbitol mixed in 150 mL of tap water. The sorbitol should be omitted from the enema in postoperative patients due to the increased incidence of sorbitol-induced colonic necrosis, especially following renal transplantation. The most rapid and effective way of lowering the plasma K^+ concentration is hemodialysis. This should be re-

FIGURE 49-4 Algorithm depicting clinical approach to hyperkalemia. NSAID, nonsteroidal antiinflammatory drug; ACE, angiotensin converting enzyme; RTA, renal tubular acidosis; TTKG, transtubular K concentration gradient.

served for patients with renal failure and those with severe life-threatening hyperkalemia unresponsive to more conservative measures. Peritoneal dialysis also removes K^+ but is only 15 to 20 percent as effective as hemodialysis. Finally, the underlying cause of the hyperkalemia should be treated. This may involve dietary modification, correction of metabolic acidosis, cautious volume expansion, and administration of exogenous mineralocorticoid.

BIBLIOGRAPHY

WATER AND SODIUM

ABRAHAM WT, SCHRIER RW: Body fluid volume regulation in health and disease. Adv Intern Med 39:23, 1994

FUJIWARA TM et al: Molecular biology of diabetes insipidus. Ann Rev Med 46:331, 1995

GINES P et al: Vasopressin in pathophysiological states. Semin Nephrol 14:384, 1994

GULLANS SR, VERBALIS JG: Control of brain volume during hyperosmolar and hypoosmolar conditions. Ann Rev Med 44:289, 1993

KOVACS L, ROBERTSON GL: Syndrome of inappropriate antidiuretics. Endocrinol Metabol Clin North Am 21:859, 1992

NARINS RG, RILEY LJ: Polyuria: Simple and mixed disorders. Am J Kidney Dis 17:237, 1991

ROBERTSON GL: Disorders of thirst in man, in *Thirst: Physiological and Psychological Aspects*, DJ Ramsay, DA Booth (eds). London, Springer-Verlag, 1991, p 453

———, BERL T: Pathophysiology of water metabolism, in *The Kidney*, 5th ed, BM Brenner (ed). Philadelphia, Saunders, 1996, pp 873–928

STERNS RH et al: Neurologic sequelae after treatment of severe hyponatremia: A multicenter perspective. J Am Soc Nephrol 4:1522, 1994

———: Hyponatremia: Pathophysiology, diagnosis, and therapy, in *Clinical Disorders of Fluid and Electrolyte Metabolism*, 5th ed, RG Narins (ed). New York, McGraw-Hill, 1994, pp 583–615

POTASSIUM

BROWN RS: Extrarenal potassium homeostasis. Kidney Int 30:116, 1986

DEFRONZO RA, SMITH JD: Clinical disorders of hyperkalemia, in *Clinical Disorders of Fluid and Electrolyte Metabolism*, 5th ed, RG Narins (ed). New York, McGraw-Hill, 1994, pp 697–754

FIELD MJ et al: Regulation of renal potassium metabolism, in *Clinical Disorders of Fluid and Electrolyte Metabolism*, 5th ed, RG Narins (ed). New York, McGraw-Hill, 1994, pp 147–174

KAMEL KS et al: Disorders of potassium homeostasis: An approach based on pathophysiology. Am J Kidney Dis 24:597, 1994

——— et al: Disorders of potassium balance, in *The Kidney*, 5th ed, BM Brenner (ed). Philadelphia, Saunders, 1996, pp 999–1037

KNOCHEL JP: Neuromuscular manifestations of electrolyte disorders. Am J Med 72:521, 1982

KUPIN WL, NARINS RG: The hyperkalemia of renal failure: Pathophysiology, diagnosis, and therapy. Contrib Nephrol 102:1, 1993

STEIN JH: The pathogenetic spectrum of Bartter's syndrome. Kidney Int 28:85, 1985

TANNEN RL: Diuretic-induced hypokalemia. Kidney Int 28:988, 1985

WHITE PC: Disorders of aldosterone biosynthesis and action. N Engl J Med 331:250, 1994

50   *Thomas D. DuBose, Jr.*

ACIDOSIS AND ALKALOSIS

NORMAL ACID-BASE HOMEOSTASIS

Systemic arterial pH is maintained between 7.35 and 7.45 by extracellular and intracellular chemical buffering together with respiratory and renal regulatory mechanisms. The control of arterial CO_2 tension (Pa_{CO_2}) by the central nervous system and respiratory systems and the control of the plasma bicarbonate by the kidneys stabilize the arterial pH by excretion or retention of acid or alkali. The metabolic and respiratory components that regulate systemic pH are described by the Henderson-Hasselbalch equation:

$$pH = 6.1 + \log \frac{[HCO_3{}^-]}{Pa_{CO_2} \times 0.0301}$$

Under most circumstances, CO_2 production and excretion are matched, and the usual steady-state Pa_{CO_2} is maintained at 40 mmHg. Underexcretion of CO_2 produces hypercapnia, and overexcretion causes hypocapnia. Nevertheless, production and excretion are again matched at a new steady-state Pa_{CO_2}. Therefore, the Pa_{CO_2} is regulated primarily by neural respiratory factors (Chap. 263) and is not subject to regulation by the rate of CO_2 production. Hypercapnia is usually the result of hypoventilation rather than of increased CO_2 production. Increases or decreases in Pa_{CO_2} represent derangements of neural respiratory control or are due to compensatory changes in response to a primary alteration in the plasma $[HCO_3{}^-]$.

Primary changes in Pa_{CO_2} can cause acidosis or alkalosis, depending on whether Pa_{CO_2} is above or below the normal value of 40 mmHg (respiratory acidosis or alkalosis, respectively). Primary alteration of Pa_{CO_2} evokes cellular buffering and renal adaptation, a slow process that becomes more efficient with time. A *primary* change in the plasma $[HCO_3{}^-]$ as a result of metabolic or renal factors results in compensatory changes in ventilation that blunt the changes in blood pH that would occur otherwise. Such respiratory alterations are referred to as *secondary*, or compensatory, changes, since they occur in response to primary metabolic changes.

The kidneys regulate plasma $[HCO_3{}^-]$ through three main processes: (1) "reabsorption" of filtered $HCO_3{}^-$, (2) formation of titratable acid, and (3) excretion of $NH_4{}^+$ in the urine. The kidney filters approximately 4000 mmol of $HCO_3{}^-$ per day. To reabsorb the filtered load of $HCO_3{}^-$, the renal tubules must therefore secrete 4000 mmol of hydrogen ions. Eighty to ninety percent of $HCO_3{}^-$ is reabsorbed in the proximal tubule. The distal nephron reabsorbs the remainder and secretes protons, as generated from metabolism, to defend systemic pH. While this quantity of protons, 40 to 60 mmol/d, is small, it must be secreted to prevent chronic positive H^+ balance and metabolic acidosis. This quantity of secreted protons is represented in the urine as titratable acid and $NH_4{}^+$. Metabolic acidosis in the face of normal renal function increases $NH_4{}^+$ production and excretion. $NH_4{}^+$ production and excretion are impaired in chronic renal failure, hyperkalemia, and renal tubular acidosis.

In sum, these regulatory responses, including chemical buffering, the regulation of Pa_{CO_2} by the respiratory system, and of $[HCO_3{}^-]$ by the kidneys, act in concert to maintain a systemic arterial pH between 7.35 and 7.45.

DIAGNOSIS OF GENERAL TYPES OF DISTURBANCES

The most common clinical disturbances are *simple* acid-base disorders, i.e., metabolic acidosis or alkalosis or respiratory acidosis or alkalosis. Since compensation is not complete, the pH is abnormal in simple disturbances. More complicated clinical situations can give rise to mixed acid-base disturbances.

SIMPLE ACID-BASE DISORDERS   Primary respiratory disturbances (primary changes in Pa_{CO_2}) invoke secondary metabolic responses (secondary changes in $[HCO_3{}^-]$), and primary metabolic disturbances elicit predictable respiratory responses. Physiologic compensation can be predicted from the relationships displayed in Table 50-1. Primary changes in Pa_{CO_2} or $[HCO_3{}^-]$ alter systemic pH and cause acidosis or alkalosis. To illustrate, metabolic acidosis due to an increase in endogenous acids (e.g., ketoacidosis) lowers extracellular fluid $[HCO_3{}^-]$ and decreases extracellular pH. As a result, the medullary chemoreceptors are stimulated to increase ventilation and to return the ratio of $[HCO_3{}^-]$ to Pa_{CO_2} and the subsequent pH toward normal. The degree of respiratory compensation expected in a simple form of metabolic acidosis can be predicted from the relationship: $Pa_{CO_2} = (1.5 \times [HCO_3{}^-]) + 8$, i.e., the Pa_{CO_2} is expected to decrease 1.25 mmHg for each mmol per liter decrease in $[HCO_3{}^-]$. Thus, a patient with metabolic acidosis and $[HCO_3{}^-]$ of 12 mmol/L would be expected to have a Pa_{CO_2} between 24 and 28 mmHg. Values for Pa_{CO_2} below 24

Table 50-1

Prediction of Compensatory Responses in Simple Acid-Base Disturbances

Disorder	Prediction of Compensation
Metabolic acidosis	$Pa_{CO_2} = (1.5 \times [HCO_3^-]) + 8$
	or
	Pa_{CO_2} will ↓ 1.25 mmHg per mmol/L ↓ in $[HCO_3^-]$
Metabolic alkalosis	Pa_{CO_2} will ↑ 0.75 mmHg per mmol/L ↑ in $[HCO_3^-]$
	or
	Pa_{CO_2} will ↑ 6 mmHg per 10-mmol/L ↑ in $[HCO_3^-]$
	or
	$Pa_{CO_2} = [HCO_3^-] + 15$
Respiratory alkalosis	
Acute	$[HCO_3^-]$ will ↓ 2 mmol/L per 10-mmHg ↓ in Pa_{CO_2}
Chronic	$[HCO_3^-]$ will ↓ 4 mmol/L per 10-mmHg ↓ in Pa_{CO_2}
Respiratory acidosis	
Acute	$[HCO_3^-]$ will ↑ 1 mmol/L per 10-mmHg ↑ in Pa_{CO_2}
Chronic	$[HCO_3^-]$ will ↑ 4 mmol/L per 10-mmHg ↑ in Pa_{CO_2}

or greater than 28 mmHg define a mixed disturbance (metabolic acidosis and respiratory alkalosis or metabolic acidosis and respiratory acidosis, respectively). Another way to judge the appropriateness of the response in $[HCO_3^-]$ or Pa_{CO_2} is to use an acid-base nomogram (Fig. 50-1). While the shaded areas of the nomogram show the 95 percent confidence limits for normal compensation in simple disturbances, finding acid-base values within the shaded area does not necessarily rule out a mixed disturbance. Imposition of one disorder over another may result in values lying

within the area of a third. Thus, the nomogram, while convenient, is not a substitute for the equations in Table 50-1.

MIXED ACID-BASE DISORDERS Mixed acid-base disorders—defined as independently coexisting disorders, not merely compensatory responses—are often seen in patients in critical care units. As with simple acid-base disorders, the differential diagnosis associated with each of the mixed disturbances should be considered in light of the clinical context. Mixed respiratory and metabolic acidosis or mixed respiratory and metabolic alkalosis can lead to dangerous extremes of pH. A patient with diabetic ketoacidosis (metabolic acidosis) may develop an independent respiratory problem leading to respiratory acidosis or alkalosis. Patients with underlying pulmonary disease may not respond to metabolic acidosis with an appropriate ventilatory response because of insufficient respiratory reserve. Such imposition of respiratory acidosis on metabolic acidosis can lead to severe acidemia and a poor outcome. When metabolic acidosis and metabolic alkalosis coexist in the same patient, the pH may be normal or near normal. When the pH is normal, an elevated anion gap (see below) denotes the presence of a metabolic acidosis. A diabetic patient with ketoacidosis may have renal dysfunction resulting in simultaneous metabolic acidosis. Patients who have ingested an overdose of drug combinations such as sedatives and salicylates may have mixed disturbances as a result of the acid-base response to the individual drugs (metabolic acidosis mixed with respiratory acidosis or respiratory alkalosis, respectively). Even more complex are triple acid-base disturbances. For example, patients with metabolic acidosis due to alcoholic ketoacidosis may develop metabolic alkalosis due to vomiting and superimposed respiratory alkalosis due to the hyperventilation of hepatic dysfunction or alcohol withdrawal.

DIAGNOSIS OF ACID-BASE DISORDERS Care should be taken when measuring blood gases to obtain the arterial blood sample without using excessive heparin. In the determination of arterial blood gases by the clinical laboratory, both pH and Pa_{CO_2} are measured, and the $[HCO_3^-]$ is calculated from the Henderson-Hasselbalch equation. This calculated value should be compared with the measured $[HCO_3^-]$ (total CO_2) on the electrolyte panel. These two values should agree within 2 mmol/L. If they do not, the values may not have been drawn simultaneously, a laboratory error may be present, or an error could have been made in calculating the $[HCO_3^-]$. After verifying the blood acid-base values, one can then identify the precise acid-base disorder.

The most common causes of acid-base disorders should be kept in mind while probing the history for clues about the etiology. For example, established chronic renal failure is expected to cause a metabolic acidosis, and chronic vomiting frequently causes metabolic alkalosis. Patients with pneumonia, sepsis, or cardiac failure frequently have respiratory alkalosis, and patients with chronic obstructive pulmonary disease or a sedative drug overdose often display a respiratory acidosis. The drug history is important since loop or thiazide diuretics may cause metabolic alkalosis, and the carbonic anhydrase inhibitor, acetazolamide, can result in metabolic acidosis.

Blood for electrolytes and arterial blood gases should be drawn simultaneously prior to therapy, since an increase

FIGURE 50-1 Acid-base nomogram. Shown are the 90 percent confidence limits of the normal respiratory and metabolic compensations for primary acid-base disturbances. [From TD DuBose et al: Acid-base disorders, in *The Kidney*, 5th ed, BM Brenner, FC Rector, Jr. (eds). Philadelphia, Saunders, 1996, pp. 929–998. Used with permission.]

in [HCO$_3$$^-$] occurs with metabolic alkalosis and respiratory acidosis. Conversely, a decrease in [HCO$_3$$^-$] occurs in metabolic acidosis and respiratory alkalosis.

Metabolic acidosis leads to hyperkalemia as a result of cellular shifts in which H$^+$ is exchanged for K$^+$ or Na$^+$. For each decrease in blood pH of 0.10, the plasma [K$^+$] should rise by 0.6 mmol/L. This relationship is not invariable. Diabetic ketoacidosis, lactic acidosis, diarrhea, and renal tubular acidosis are often associated with potassium depletion.

ANION GAP All evaluations of acid-base disorders should include a simple calculation of the anion gap (AG); it represents those unmeasured anions in plasma (normally 10 to 12 mmol/L) and is calculated as follows: AG = [Na$^+$] − ([Cl$^-$] + [HCO$_3$$^-$]). The unmeasured anions include anionic proteins, phosphate, sulfate, and organic anions. When acid anions, such as acetoacetate and lactate, accumulate in extracellular fluid, the AG increases, causing a high-AG acidosis. An *increase* in the AG may be due to a decrease in unmeasured cations (calcium, magnesium, potassium) or an increase in unmeasured anions. In addition, the AG may increase secondary to an increase in anionic albumin, either because of increased albumin concentration or alkalosis, which alters albumin charge. A *decrease* in the AG can be due to (1) an increase in unmeasured cations; (2) the addition to the blood of abnormal cations, such as lithium (lithium intoxication) or cationic immunoglobulins (plasma cell dyscrasias); (3) a reduction in the major plasma anion albumin concentration; (4) a decrease in the effective anionic charge on albumin by acidosis; or (5) hyperviscosity and severe hyperlipidemia, which can lead to an underestimation of sodium and chloride concentrations.

In the face of a normal serum albumin, a high AG is usually due to non-chloride-containing acids that contain inorganic (phosphate, sulfate), organic (ketoacids, lactate, uremic organic anions), exogenous (salicylate or ingested toxins with organic acid production), or unidentified anions. By definition, therefore, a *high-AG acidosis* has two identifying features: a low [HCO$_3$$^-$] and an elevated AG. The latter is present even if an additional acid-base disorder is superimposed to modify the [HCO$_3$$^-$] independently. Simultaneous metabolic acidosis of the high-AG variety plus either chronic respiratory acidosis or metabolic alkalosis represents such a situation in which [HCO$_3$$^-$] may be normal or even high. However, the AG is elevated, and [Cl$^-$] is depressed.

Similarly, normal values for [HCO$_3$$^-$], Pa$_{CO_2}$, and pH do not ensure the absence of an acid-base disturbance. For instance, an alcoholic who has been vomiting may develop a metabolic alkalosis with a pH of 7.55, Pa$_{CO_2}$ of 48 mmHg, [HCO$_3$$^-$] of 40 mmol/L, [Na$^+$] of 135, [Cl$^-$] of 80, and [K$^+$] of 2.8. If such a patient were then to develop a superimposed alcoholic ketoacidosis with a β-hydroxybutyrate concentration of 15 mM, arterial pH would fall to 7.40, [HCO$_3$$^-$] to 25 mmol/L, and the Pa$_{CO_2}$ to 40 mmHg. Although blood gases are normal, the AG is elevated at 26 mmol/L, indicating a mixed metabolic alkalosis and metabolic acidosis.

METABOLIC ACIDOSIS

Metabolic acidosis can occur because of an increase in endogenous acid production (such as lactate and ketoacids), loss of bicarbonate (as in diarrhea), or accumulation of endogenous acids (as in renal failure). Metabolic acidosis has profound effects on the respiratory, cardiac, and nervous systems. The fall in blood pH is accompanied by a characteristic increase in ventilation, especially tidal volume (Kussmaul respiration). Intrinsic cardiac contractility may be depressed, but inotropic function can be normal because of catecholamine release. Both peripheral arterial vasodilation and central venoconstriction can be present; the decrease in central and pulmonary vascular compliance predisposes to pulmonary edema with even minimal volume overload. Central nervous system function is depressed, with headache, lethargy, stupor, and, in some cases, even coma. Glucose intolerance may also occur.

 TREATMENT

It has been generally accepted that treatment of metabolic acidosis with alkali should be reserved for severe acidemia except when the patient has no "potential HCO$_3$$^-$" in plasma. Potential [HCO$_3$$^-$] can be estimated from the increment (Δ) in the anion gap (ΔAG = patient's AG − 10). It must be determined if the acid anion in plasma is metabolizable (i.e., β-hydroxybutyrate, acetoacetate, lactate) or nonmetabolizable (anions that accumulate in chronic renal failure and with toxin ingestion). The latter requires return of renal function to replenish the [HCO$_3$$^-$] deficit, a slow and often unpredictable process. Consequently, patients with no AG (hyperchloremic acidosis), a small AG (mixed hyperchloremic and AG acidosis), or an AG attributable to a nonmetabolizable anion in the face of renal failure should receive alkali therapy, either orally (NaHCO$_3$ or Shohl's solution) or intravenously (NaHCO$_3$), in an amount necessary to slowly increase the plasma [HCO$_3$$^-$] into the 20 to 22 mmol/L range.

Controversy exists, however, in regard to the use of alkali in patients with a pure AG acidosis owing to accumulation of a metabolizable organic acid anion (ketoacidosis or lactic acidosis). In general, severe acidosis (pH < 7.20) warrants the intravenous administration of 50 to 100 meq of NaHCO$_3$, over 30 to 45 min, during the initial 1 to 2 h of therapy. Provision of such modest quantities of alkali in this situation seems to provide an added measure of safety, but it is essential to monitor plasma electrolytes during the course of therapy, since the [K$^+$] may decline as pH rises.

As indicated above there are two major categories of clinical metabolic acidosis: (1) high-AG and (2) normal-AG, or hyperchloremic, acidosis (Tables 50-2 and 50-3).

HIGH-ANION-GAP ACIDOSES There are four principal causes of a high AG acidosis: (1) lactic acidosis, (2) ketoacidosis, (3) ingested toxins (Table 50-2), and (4) acute and chronic renal failure. Initial screening to differentiate the high AG acidoses should include: (1) a probe of the history for evidence of drug and toxin ingestion and measurement of arterial blood gas to detect coexistent respiratory alkalosis (salicylates); (2) determination of whether diabetes mellitus is present (diabetic ketoacidosis); (3) a search for evidence of alcoholism or increased levels of β-hydroxybutyrate (alcoholic ketoacidosis); (4) observation for clinical signs of uremia and determination of the blood urea nitrogen (BUN) and creatinine (uremic acidosis); (5) inspection of the urine for oxalate crystals (ethylene glycol); and (6) recognition of the numerous clinical settings in which lactate levels may be increased (hypotension, shock, cardiac failure, leukemia, cancer, and drug or toxin ingestion).

Lactic Acidosis Accumulation in plasma L-lactate may be secondary to obvious tissue hypoxia (type A)—circulatory insufficiency (shock, heart failure), severe anemia, cholera, mitochondrial enzyme defects, and inhibitors (carbon monoxide, cyanide)—or to more occult disorders (type B)—hypoglycemia (glycogen storage diseases), seizures, diabetes mellitus, ethanol, hepatic failure, malignancy, and

---

Table 50-2

Causes of High-Anion-Gap Metabolic Acidosis

Lactic acidosis (types A and B)
Ketoacidosis
    Diabetic
    Alcoholic
    Starvation
Toxins
    Ethylene glycol
    Methanol
    Salicylates
Renal failure (acute and chronic)

Table 50-3

Causes of Hyperchloremic Acidosis

  I. Gastrointestinal bicarbonate loss
    A. Diarrhea
    B. External pancreatic or small-bowel drainage
    C. Urterosigmoidostomy, jejunal loop, ileal loop
    D. Drugs
       1. Calcium chloride (acidifying agent)
       2. Magnesium sulfate (diarrhea)
       3. Cholestyramine (bile acid diarrhea)
 II. Renal acidosis
    A. Hypokalemia
       1. Proximal RTA (type II)
       2. Distal (classic) RTA (type I)
    B. Hyperkalemia
       1. Generalized distal nephron dysfunction (type IV RTA)
          a. Mineralocorticoid deficiency
          b. Mineralocorticoid resistance
          c. $\downarrow Na^+$ delivery to distal nephron
          d. Tubulointerstitial disease
          e. Ammonium excretion defect
    C. Normokalemia
       1. Early renal insufficiency
III. Drug-induced hyperkalemia (with renal insufficiency)
    A. Potassium-sparing diuretics (amiloride, triamterene, spironolactone)
    B. Trimethoprim
    C. Pentamidine
    D. Angiotensin-converting enzyme inhibitors
    E. Nonsteroidal anti-inflammatory drugs
    F. Cyclosporine
IV. Other
    A. Acid loads (ammonium chloride, hyperalimentation)
    B. Loss of potential bicarbonate: ketosis with ketone excretion
    C. Expansion acidosis (rapid saline administration)
    D. Hippurate
    E. Cation exchange resins

---

salicylates—in which overproduction and/or decreased hepatic removal of lactate can occur. Unrecognized bowel ischemia or infarction in a patient with severe atherosclerosis or cardiac decompensation receiving vasopressors is a common cause of lactic acidosis. D-Lactate acidosis, associated commonly with jejunoileal bypass or intestinal obstruction and due to formation by gut bacteria, may cause both an increased AG and hyperchloremia.

℞ **TREATMENT**

The underlying condition that disrupts lactate metabolism must first be corrected; tissue perfusion must be restored when it is inadequate. Vasoconstrictors should be avoided, if possible, since they may worsen tissue perfusion. Alkali therapy is generally advocated for acute, severe acidemia (pH < 7.1) to improve cardiac function and lactate utilization. However, $NaHCO_3$ therapy may paradoxically depress cardiac performance and exacerbate acidosis by enhancing lactate production (HCO_3^- stimulates phosphofructokinase). While the use of alkali in moderate lactic acidosis is controversial, it is generally agreed that attempts to return the pH or $[HCO_3^-]$ to normal by administration of exogenous $NaHCO_3$ are deleterious. A reasonable approach is to infuse sufficient $NaHCO_3$ to raise the arterial pH to no more than 7.2 over 30 to 40 min.

$NaHCO_3$ therapy can cause fluid overload and hypertension because the amount required can be massive when accumulation of lactic acid is relentless. Fluid administration is poorly tolerated because of central venoconstriction, especially in the oliguric patient. If the underlying cause of the lactic acidosis can be remedied, blood lactate will be converted to HCO_3^- and may result in an overshoot alkalosis.

Ketoacidosis *Diabetic ketoacidosis* (See also Chap. 334) This condition is caused by increased fatty acid metabolism and the accumu-

lation of ketoacids (acetoacetate and β-hydroxybutyrate). Diabetic ketoacidosis usually occurs in insulin-dependent diabetes mellitus in association with cessation of insulin or an intercurrent illness, such as an infection, gastroenteritis, pancreatitis, or myocardial infarction, which increases insulin requirements temporarily and acutely. The accumulation of ketoacids accounts for the increment in the AG and is accompanied most often by hyperglycemia [glucose > 17 mmol/L (300 mg/dL)]. The management of this condition is described in Chap. 234. Here it should be noted that since insulin prevents production of ketones, bicarbonate therapy is rarely needed except with extreme acidemia (pH < 7.1), and then in only limited amounts (as discussed above for correction of lactic acidosis).

Alcoholic ketoacidosis Chronic alcoholics can develop ketoacidosis when alcohol consumption is abruptly curtailed; it is usually associated with vomiting, abdominal pain, starvation, and volume depletion. The glucose concentration is low or normal, and acidosis may be severe because of elevated ketones, predominantly β-hydroxybutyrate. Mild lactic acidosis may coexist because of alteration in the redox state. The nitroprusside ketone reaction (Acetest) can detect acetoacetic acid but not β-hydroxybutyrate, so that the degree of ketosis and ketonuria can be underestimated. Typically, insulin levels are low, and concentrations of triglyceride, cortisol, glucagon, and growth hormone are increased.

℞ **TREATMENT**

This consists of intravenous volume repletion and glucose administration (5% dextrose in 0.9% NaCl). Hypophosphatemia, hypokalemia, and hypomagnesemia may coexist and should be corrected. Hypophosphatemia usually emerges 12 to 24 h after admission, may be exacerbated by glucose infusion, and, if severe, may induce rhabdomyolysis. Upper gastrointestinal hemorrhage, pancreatitis, and pneumonia may accompany this disorder.

Drug- and Toxin-Induced Acidosis *Salicylates* Salicylate intoxication in adults causes a high-AG metabolic acidosis, in which only a portion of the AG is due to the salicylates. Lactic acid production is also often increased, partly as a direct effect of the drug and partly as a result of the central stimulation of the respiratory center induced by salicylate causing a decrease in Pa_{CO_2} (respiratory alkalosis). Mixed acid-base disturbances (metabolic acidosis concomitant with respiratory alkalosis) from salicylates is common in adults.

℞ **TREATMENT**

This should begin with vigorous gastric lavage with isotonic saline (not $NaHCO_3$) followed by administration of activated charcoal. To facilitate removal of salicylate, intravenous $NaHCO_3$ is administered in amounts adequate to alkalinize the urine and to maintain urine output (urine pH > 7.5). While this form of therapy is straightforward in acidotic patients, a respiratory alkalosis may make this approach hazardous. Acetazolamide may be administered when an alkaline diuresis cannot be achieved, but this drug can cause systemic metabolic acidosis if $NaHCO_3$ is not given concomitantly. The hypokalemia, which may be severe, is a result of the alkaline diuresis from $NaHCO_3$ or acetazolamide or of the respiratory alkalosis and should be treated promptly and aggressively. Glucose-containing fluids should be administered because of the danger of hypoglycemia. Excessive insensible fluid losses may cause severe volume depletion and hypernatremia. If renal failure prevents rapid clearance of salicylate, hemodialysis can be performed against a bicarbonate dialysate.

Alcohols Under most physiologic conditions, sodium, urea, and glucose generate the osmotic pressure of blood. Plasma osmolality is calculated according to the following expression: $P_{osm} = 2Na^+ + Glu + BUN$ (all in mmol/L), or, using conventional laboratory values in which glucose and BUN are expressed in mg per dL: $P_{osm} = 2Na^+ + Glu/18 + BUN/2.8$. The calculated and determined osmolality should agree within 10 to 15 mmol/kg H_2O. When the measured osmolality exceeds the calculated osmolality by more than 15 to 20 mmol/kg H_2O, one of two circumstances prevails. Either the serum sodium is spuriously low, as with hyperlipidemia or hyperproteinemia (pseudohyponatremia), or osmolytes other than sodium salts, glucose, or urea have accumulated in plasma. Examples include mannitol, radiocontrast media, isopropyl alcohol, ethylene glycol, ethanol, methanol, and acetone. In this situation, the difference between the calculated osmolality and the measured osmolality (osmolar gap) is proportional to the concentration of the unmeasured solute. With an appropriate clinical history and index of suspicion, identification of an osmolar gap is helpful in identifying the presence of poison-associated AG acidosis.

Ethylene glycol Ingestion of ethylene glycol (commonly used in antifreeze) leads to a metabolic acidosis and severe damage to the central nervous system, heart, lungs, and kidneys. The increased AG and osmolar gap are attributable to ethylene glycol and its metabolites, oxalic acid, glycolic acid, and other organic acids. Lactic acid production increases secondary to inhibition of the tricarboxylic acid cycle and altered intracellular redox state. Diagnosis is facilitated by recognizing oxalate crystals in the urine.

℞ TREATMENT

This includes the prompt institution of a saline or osmotic diuresis, thiamine and pyridoxine supplements, ethanol, and dialysis. The administration of ethanol intravenously to achieve a level of 22 mmol/L (100 mg/dL) serves to lessen toxicity because it competes with ethylene glycol for metabolism by alcohol dehydrogenase and alters the cellular redox state.

Methanol The ingestion of methanol (wood alcohol) causes metabolic acidosis, and its metabolites formaldehyde and formic acid cause severe optic nerve and cental nervous system damage. Lactic acid, ketoacids, and other unidentified organic acids may contribute to the acidosis. Due to its low molecular weight (32 Da), an osmolar gap is usually present.

℞ TREATMENT

This is similar to that for ethylene glycol intoxication, including general supportive measures, ethanol administration, and hemodialysis.

Renal Failure (See also Chaps. 270 and 271) The hyperchloremic acidosis of moderate renal insufficiency is eventually converted to the high-AG acidosis of advanced renal failure. Poor filtration and reabsorption of organic anions contribute to the pathogenesis. As renal disease progresses, the number of functioning nephrons eventually becomes insufficient to keep pace with net acid production. Uremic acidosis is characterized, therefore, by a reduced rate of NH_4^+ production, primarily due to decreased renal mass. $[HCO_3^-]$ rarely falls below 15 mmol/L, and the AG rarely exceeds 20 mmol/L. The acid retained in chronic renal disease is buffered by alkaline salts from bone. Despite significant retention of acid (up to 20 mmol/d), the serum $[HCO_3^-]$ does not decrease further, indicating participation of buffers outside the extracellular compartment. Chronic metabolic acidosis results in significant loss of bone mass due to reduction in bone calcium carbonate. Chronic acidosis also increases urinary calcium excretion, proportional to cumulative acid retention.

℞ TREATMENT

Both uremic acidosis and the hyperchloremic acidosis of renal failure require oral alkali replacement to maintain the $[HCO_3^-]$ between 20 and 24 mmol/L. This can be accomplished with relatively modest amounts of alkali (1.0 to 1.5 mmol/kg body weight per day). It is assumed that alkali replacement prevents the harmful effects of H^+ balance on bone. Sodium citrate (Shohl's solution) or $NaHCO_3$ tablets are equally effective alkalinizing salts. Citrate enhances the absorption of aluminum from the gastrointestinal tract and should never be given together with aluminum-containing antacids because of the risk of aluminum intoxication. When hyperkalemia is present, furosemide (60 to 80 mg/d) should be added.

HYPERCHLOREMIC METABOLIC ACIDOSES Alkali can be lost from the gastrointestinal tract in diarrhea or from the kidneys (renal tubular acidosis). In these disorders (Table 50-3), reciprocal changes in $[Cl^-]$ and $[HCO_3^-]$ result in a *normal* AG. In pure hyperchloremic acidosis, therefore, the increase in $[Cl^-]$ above the normal value equals the decrease in $[HCO_3^-]$. The absence of such a relationship suggests a mixed disturbance.

Diarrhea causes the loss of large quantities of HCO_3^- and decomposed HCO_3^-. Since diarrheal stools contain a higher $[HCO_3^-]$ and decomposed HCO_3^- than plasma, metabolic acidosis develops along with volume depletion. Instead of an acid urine pH (as anticipated with systemic acidosis), urine pH is usually around 6 because metabolic acidosis and hypokalemia increase renal synthesis and excretion of NH_4^+, thus providing a urinary buffer that increases urine pH. Metabolic acidosis due to gastrointestinal losses with a high urine pH can be differentiated from renal tubular acidosis (RTA) (Chap. 278), because urinary NH_4^+ excretion is typically low in RTA and high with diarrhea. Urinary NH_4^+ levels can be estimated by calculating the urine net charge (UNC): $UNC = [Na^+ + K^+]_u - [Cl^-]_u$. When $[Cl^-]_u > [Na^+ + K^+]$, the urine ammonium level is appropriately increased, suggesting an extrarenal cause of the acidosis. In addition to diarrhea (HCO_3^- loss from the gastrointestinal tract), another extrarenal cause of hyperchloremic metabolic acidosis is parenteral hyperalimentation with the Cl^- salts of basic amino acids and insufficient alkali (acetate). However, if urine $[NH_4^+]$ is low, the cause is likely to be RTA. Caution is urged since ketonuria or the presence of drug anions in the urine invalidates the net negative charge estimate.

Loss of functioning renal parenchyma by progressive renal disease leads to hyperchloremic acidosis when the glomerular filtration rate (GFR) is between 20 and 50 mL/min and to uremic acidosis with a high AG when the GFR falls to below <20 mL/min. Such a progression occurs commonly with tubulointerstitial forms of renal disease, but hyperchloremic metabolic acidosis can persist with advanced glomerular disease. In advanced renal failure, ammoniagenesis is reduced in proportion to the loss of functional renal mass, and ammonium accumulation and trapping in the outer medullary collecting tubule may also be impaired. Because of adaptive increases in K^+ secretion by the collecting duct and colon, the acidosis of chronic renal insufficiency is typically normokalemic.

Most *proximal* RTA (type 2 RTA) is due to generalized proximal tubular dysfunction, with glycosuria, generalized aminoaciduria, and phosphaturia (*Fanconi syndrome*). The urine is appropriately acidified (pH < 5.5), and there is either a low plasma $[HCO_3^-]$ or a high fractional excretion of $[HCO_3^-]$ (>10 to 15 percent) with a near-normal serum HCO_3^- (>20 mmol/L). With proximal RTA, massive amounts of exogenous HCO_3^- are required, since HCO_3^- is not reabsorbed normally in the proximal tubule, resulting in enhanced renal potassium wasting and hypokalemia.

The typical findings in *classical distal* RTA (type 1 RTA) include hypokalemia, hyperchloremic acidosis, low urinary NH_4^- excretion (positive urine net charge), and inappropriately high urine pH (pH > 5.5). Such patients are unable to acidify the urine below pH = 5.5. These abnormalities suggest that one or both of the active proton pumps present in the collecting duct (the H^+-ATPase, or the H^+, K^+-ATPase) is defective. In addition, excretory rates of NH_4^+ are uniformly low when the degree of systemic acidosis is taken into account, indicating that the kidney is responsible for the metabolic acidosis. Ammonium excretion is low because of failure to trap NH_4^+ in the medullary collecting duct, as a result of higher than normal tubular fluid pH in this segment, and the urine pH is high because of impaired H^+ secretion. In amphotericin B poisoning, distal RTA is due to an inability to maintain a pH gradient across the collecting duct, whereas most other forms of distal RTA appear to be the result of deficient H^+ pump function or number.

Distal RTA usually occurs in association with a systemic illness, such as Sjögren's syndrome or multiple myeloma, and is referred to as "secondary" distal RTA. Conversely, distal RTA can occur as an inherited disorder unassociated with systemic disease. The RTA of renal transplantation can be either of the proximal or distal variety, but chronic rejection is usually associated with the distal type.

Although hyperchloremic metabolic acidosis and hyperkalemia occur with regularity in advanced renal insufficiency, in *type 4* RTA hyperkalemia is disproportionate to the reduction in GFR because of coexisting dysfunction of potassium and acid secretion. Urinary ammonium excretion is invariably depressed, and renal function may be compromised, for example, due to diabetic nephropathy, amyloidosis, or tubulointerstitial disease.

℞ TREATMENT

Chronic metabolic acidosis in classical distal RTA can usually be corrected by administration of sufficient oral alkali to neutralize the production of metabolic acids from the diet. In adult patients with distal RTA, this is usually equal to no more than 1 to 3 mmol/kg body weight per day in the form of Shohl's solution or $NaHCO_3$ tablets. Correction of acidosis reduces urinary potassium excretion, and hypokalemia and sodium depletion may resolve. Therefore, in most adult patients with distal RTA, potassium supplement is not necessary.

Hyporeninemic-Hypoaldosteronism (See also Chap. 332) This condition typically causes hyperchloremic metabolic acidosis, typically in older adults with diabetes mellitus or tubulointerstitial disease and renal insufficiency. Patients usually have mild to moderate renal insufficiency and acidosis with elevation in serum $[K^+]$ (5.2 to 6.0 mmol/L), concurrent hypertension, and congestive heart failure. Both the metabolic acidosis and the hyperkalemia are out of proportion to impairment in GFR. The nonsteroidal anti-inflammatory drugs also can cause hyperkalemia with hyperchloremic metabolic acidosis in patients with renal insufficiency. In hyporeninemic-hypoaldosteronism, plasma renin activity appears to be unresponsive to the usual physiologic stimuli, and aldosterone secretion is low as a result. Reduction in $[K^+]$ by administration of cation exchange resins may enhance renal ammoniagenesis and usually improves or corrects the metabolic acidosis and hyperkalemia. Mineralocorticoid replacement with fludrocortisone also improves net acid excretion but is contraindicated in the face of coexisting hypertension or congestive heart failure.

The combination of hyperchloremic metabolic acidosis, hyperkalemia, hypertension, undetectable plasma renin activity, and low aldosterone levels is termed *pseudohypoaldosteronism-type II*. This disorder is usually not associated with glomerular or tubulointerstitial disease. The acidosis is mild and can be accounted for by the hyperkalemia. Renin and aldosterone levels both increase if volume expansion is corrected by diuretics or salt restriction. Potassium excretion responds to sodium sulfate infusion. Mineralocorticoid resistance with salt wasting also causes hyperkalemic-hyperchloremic acidosis because of a decrease in mineralocorticoid effectiveness at the level of the cortical collecting tubule. Pseudohypoaldosteronism may occur with systemic lupus erythematosus, obstructive uropathy, sickle cell disease, drug-induced interstitial nephritis, cyclosporine therapy, or rejection of a kidney transplant.

℞ TREATMENT

Management of patients with metabolic acidosis and hyperkalemia with chronic renal insufficiency is not always necessary, and the decision to treat is often based on the severity of the hyperkalemia. Reduction in serum $[K^+]$ often improves the metabolic acidosis. Patients with hyporeninemic-hypoaldosteronism may respond to a cation-exchange resin (sodium polystyrene sulfonate), alkali therapy, or loop diuretics. Volume depletion should be avoided unless the patient is volume overexpanded or hypertensive. Supraphysiologic doses of mineralocorticoids may be necessary but should be administered in combination with a loop diuretic to avoid volume overexpan-

sion or aggravation of hypertension and to increase potassium excretion. Patients with pseudohypoaldosteronism-type II should receive thiazide diuretics coupled with dietary salt restriction.

METABOLIC ALKALOSIS

Metabolic alkalosis is manifested by an elevated arterial pH, an increase in the serum $[HCO_3^-]$, and an increase in Pa_{CO_2} as a result of compensatory alveolar hypoventilation. It is often accompanied by hypochloremia and hypokalemia. The patient with a high $[HCO_3^-]$ and a low $[Cl^-]$ has either metabolic alkalosis or chronic respiratory acidosis. As shown in Table 50-1, the Pa_{CO_2} increases 6 mmHg for each 10-mmol/L increase in the $[HCO_3^-]$ above normal. Stated differently, in the range of $[HCO_3^-]$ from 10 to 40 mmol/L, the predicted Pa_{CO_2} is approximately equal to the $[HCO_3^-]$ + 15. The arterial pH establishes the diagnosis, since it is increased in metabolic alkalosis and decreased or normal in respiratory acidosis. Metabolic alkalosis frequently occurs in association with other disorders such as respiratory acidosis or alkalosis or metabolic acidosis.

PATHOGENESIS Metabolic alkalosis occurs as a result of net gain of $[HCO_3^-]$ or loss of nonvolatile acid (usually HCl by vomiting) from the extracellular fluid. Since it is unusual for alkali to be added to the body, the disorder involves a *generative stage*, in which the loss of acid usually causes alkalosis, and a *maintenance stage*, in which the kidneys fail to compensate by excreting HCO_3^- because of volume contraction, a low GFR, or depletion of Cl^- or K^+.

Under normal circumstances, the kidneys have an impressive capacity to excrete HCO_3^-, and continuation of metabolic alkalosis represents a failure of the kidneys to eliminate HCO_3^- in the usual manner. For HCO_3^- to be added to the extracellular fluid, it must be administered exogenously or synthesized endogenously, in part or entirely by the kidneys. The kidneys will retain, rather than excrete, the excess alkali and maintain the alkalosis if one of two mechanisms is operative:

1. Cl^- deficiency (extracellular fluid contraction) existing concurrently with K^+ deficiency, reduced GFR, and/or enhanced proximal fraction HCO_3^- reabsorption. This combination of disorders evokes secondary hyperreninemic hyperaldosteronism and stimulates H^+ secretion by the collecting duct. The alkalosis is corrected by the administration of NaCl and KCl.
2. Hyperaldosteronism and hypokalemia are autonomous and unresponsive to increased extracellular fluid volume. The enhanced distal H^+ secretion is sufficient to reabsorb the increased filtered HCO_3^- load and to overcome the decreased proximal HCO_3^- reabsorption due to expansion of the extracellular fluid volume. To repair the alkalosis in this situation, it is necessary to inhibit the secretion or action of aldosterone or to surgically remove an aldosterone-secreting adrenal adenoma.

DIFFERENTIAL DIAGNOSIS To establish the cause of metabolic alkalosis (Table 50-4), it is necessary to assess the status of the extracellular volume (ECV), the recumbent and upright blood pressure, the serum K^+, and the renin-aldosterone system. For example, the presence of hypertension and hypokalemia in an alkalotic patient suggests either mineralocorticoid excess or a hypertensive patient receiving diuretics. Low plasma renin activity and normal urine $[Na^+]$ and $[Cl^-]$ in a patient who is not taking diuretics indicate a primary mineralocorticoid excess syndrome. The combination of hypokalemia and alkalosis in a normotensive, nonedematous patient can be due to Bartter's syndrome, magnesium deficiency, vomiting, exogenous alkali, or diuretic ingestion. Determination of urine electrolytes (especially the urine $[Cl^-]$) and screening of the urine for diuretics may be helpful. If the urine is alkaline, with elevated $[Na^+]$ and $[K^+]$ but low $[Cl^-]$, the diagnosis is usually either vomiting (overt or surreptitious) or alkali ingestion. If the urine is relatively acid and has low concentrations of Na^+, K^+, and Cl^-, the most likely possibilities are prior vomiting, the posthypercapnic state, or prior diuretic ingestion. If, on the other hand, neither the urine sodium, potassium, nor chloride concentrations are depressed, magnesium deficiency, Bartter's syndrome, or current diuretic ingestion should be considered.

Table 50-4

CHAPTER 50
Acidosis and Alkalosis

283

Causes of Metabolic Alkalosis

I. Exogenous HCO_3^- loads
  A. Acute alkali administration
  B. Milk-alkali syndrome
II. Effective ECFV contraction, normotension, K^+ deficiency, and secondary hyperreninemic hyperaldosteronism
  A. Gastrointestinal origin
    1. Vomiting
    2. Gastric aspiration
    3. Congenital chloridorrhea
    4. Villous adenoma
  B. Renal origin
    1. Diuretics
    2. Edematous states
    3. Posthypercapnic state
    4. Hypercalcemia/hypoparathyroidism
    5. Recovery from lactic acidosis or ketoacidosis
    6. Nonreabsorbable anions including penicillin, carbenicillin
    7. Mg^{2+} deficiency
    8. K^+ depletion
    9. Bartter's syndrome
  C. Gitelman's syndrome
III. ECFV expansion, hypertension, K^+ deficiency, and mineralocorticoid excess
  A. High renin
    1. Renal artery stenosis
    2. Accelerated hypertension
    3. Renin-secreting tumor
    4. Estrogen therapy
  B. Low renin
    1. Primary aldosteronism
      a. Adenoma
      b. Hyperplasia
      c. Carcinoma
    2. Adrenal enzyme defects
      a. 11β-Hydroxylase deficiency
      b. 17α-Hydroxylase deficiency
    3. Cushing's syndrome
      a. Ectopic corticotropin
      b. Adrenal adenoma
      c. Primary pituitary
    4. Other
      a. Licorice
      b. Carbenoxolone
      c. Chewer's tobacco
      d. Liddle's syndrome

NOTE: ECFV, extracellular fluid volume.

Alkali Administration Chronic administration of alkali to individuals with normal renal function results in minimal, if any, alkalosis. However, in patients with chronic renal insufficiency, alkalosis can develop following alkali administration when the normal capacity to excrete HCO_3^- is exceeded or when coexistent hemodynamic disturbances cause enhanced fractional reabsorption of HCO_3^-. Such patients include those who receive oral or intravenous HCO_3^-, acetate loads (parenteral hyperalimentation solutions), citrate loads (transfusions), or antacids plus cation-exchange resins (aluminum hydroxide and sodium polystyrene sulfonate). A rare cause is long-standing ingestion of excessive milk and antacids. Both hypercalcemia and vitamin D excess may increase renal HCO_3^- reabsorption and cause nephrocalcinosis, renal insufficiency, or metabolic alkalosis. Discontinuation of alkali ingestion or administration is usually sufficient to repair the alkalosis.

METABOLIC ALKALOSIS ASSOCIATED WITH ECFV CONTRACTION, K^+ DEPLETION, AND SECONDARY HYPERRENINEMIC HYPERALDOSTERONISM Gastrointestinal Origin *Vomiting and gastric aspiration* Gastrointestinal loss of H^+ results in retention of HCO_3^-. Increased H^+ loss through gastric secretions can be caused by vomiting, gastric aspiration, or a gastric fistula. The loss of fluid and NaCl in vomitus or nasogastric suction results in contraction of the extracellular fluid volume (ECFV) and an increase in the secretion of renin and aldosterone.

Volume contraction causes a reduction in GFR and an enhanced capacity of the renal tubule to reabsorb HCO_3^-. During active vomiting, there is continued addition of HCO_3^- to plasma in exchange for Cl^-, and the plasma $[HCO_3^-]$ exceeds the reabsorptive capacity of the proximal tubule. The excess $NaHCO_3$ reaches the distal tubule, where some Na^+ will be exchanged for K^+ by an aldosterone-mediated process. Because of contraction of the ECFV and hypochloremia, Cl^- is avidly conserved by the kidney. Upon cessation of vomiting, the plasma $[HCO_3^-]$ falls to the HCO_3^- threshold, which is elevated due to the combined effects of contraction of the ECFV, hypokalemia, and hyperaldosteronism. The alkalosis is less severe than during the phase of active vomiting, and the urine is relatively acidic with low concentrations of Na^+, Cl^-, and HCO_3^-. Correction of the contracted ECFV with NaCl may be sufficient to restore normal blood pH, even without repair of K^+ deficits. Good clinical practice, however, dictates K^+ repletion as well.

Villous adenoma Metabolic alkalosis has been described in cases of villous adenoma and is most likely the result of potassium depletion.

Renal Origin *Diuretics* (See also Chap. 233) Drugs that induce chloruresis without bicarbonaturia, such as thiazides and loop diuretics (furosemide, bumetanide, torsemide, and ethracrynic acid), *acutely* diminish the ECFV without altering the total body bicarbonate content. The serum $[HCO_3^-]$ increases. The Pa_{CO_2} does not increase commensurately, and a "contraction" alkalosis results. The degree of alkalosis is usually small, owing to cellular and non-HCO_3^- buffering. The chronic administration of diuretics tends to generate an alkalosis by increasing distal salt delivery, so that K^+ and H^+ secretion are stimulated. Diuretics, by blocking Cl^- reabsorption in the distal tubule or by increasing proton pump activity, may also stimulate distal H^+ secretion, as evidenced by an increase in net acid excretion. The alkalosis is maintained by persistence of the contraction of the ECFV, secondary hyperaldosteronism, K^+ deficiency, and the direct effect of the diuretic (as long as diuretic administration continues). Repair of the alkalosis is achieved by providing isotonic saline to correct the ECFV deficit.

Posthypercapnia Prolonged CO_2 retention with chronic respiratory acidosis enhances renal HCO_3^- absorption and the generation of new HCO_3^- (increased net acid excretion). If the Pa_{CO_2} is returned to normal, metabolic alkalosis results from the persistently elevated $[HCO_3^-]$. Alkalosis develops immediately if the elevated Pa_{CO_2} is abruptly returned toward normal by a change in mechanically controlled ventilation and the brisk bicarbonaturic response is proportional to the change in Pa_{CO_2}. The accompanying cation is predominantly K^+, especially if dietary K^+ is not limited, with natriuresis proportional to the salt intake. Secondary hyperaldosteronism in states of chronic hypercapnia may be responsible for this pattern of response. Associated ECFV contraction does not allow complete repair of the alkalosis by correction of the Pa_{CO_2} alone, and alkalosis persists until Cl^- supplementation is provided. Enhanced proximal acidification, the result of conditioning induced by the previous hypercapnic state, may also contribute to posthypercapnic alkalosis.

After treatment of lactic acidosis or ketoacidosis When an underlying stimulus for the generation of lactic acid or ketoacid is removed rapidly, as with repair of circulatory insufficiency or with insulin therapy, the lactate or ketones are metabolized to yield an equivalent amount of HCO_3^-; H^+ is consumed by metabolism of the organic anions, with the liberation of an equivalent quantity of HCO_3^-. This process will regenerate HCO_3^- if the organic acids are metabolized to HCO_3^- before their renal excretion. This is partly offset by urinary loss of organic ions. Other sources of new HCO_3^- are additive with the original amount generated by organic anion metabolism to create a surfeit of HCO_3^-. Such sources include (1) new HCO_3^- added to the blood by the kidneys as a result of enhanced acid excretion during the preexisting period of acidosis, and (2) alkali therapy during the treatment phase of the acidosis. Acidosis-induced contraction of the ECFV and K^+ deficiency act to sustain the alkalosis.

Nonreabsorbable anions and magnesium deficiency Administration of large quantities of nonreabsorbable anions, such as penicillin or carbenicillin, can enhance distal acidification and K^+ secretion by increasing the luminal potential difference. Mg^{2+} deficiency results in hypokalemic alkalosis by enhancing distal acidification through stimulation of renin and hence aldosterone secretion.

Potassium depletion Pure K^+ depletion causes a modest metabolic alkalosis. K^+ depletion increases urinary acid excretion as NH_4^+ and enhances HCO_3^- reabsorption. Alkalosis is mild because K^+ depletion also causes positive NaCl balance with or without mineralocorticoid administration. The salt retention, in turn, minimizes the alkalosis. When access to both NaCl and K^+ is restricted, alkalosis is more severe. Alkalosis associated with severe K^+ depletion is resistant to salt administration, whereas repair of the K^+ deficiency corrects the alkalosis.

Bartter's syndrome → *See Chap. 278.*

METABOLIC ALKALOSIS ASSOCIATED WITH ECFV EXPANSION, HYPERTENSION, AND HYPERALDOSTERONISM
Mineralocorticoid administration or excess production [primary aldosteronism of Cushing's syndrome and adrenal cortical enzyme defects (Chap. 332)] increases net acid excretion and may result in metabolic alkalosis, which may be worsened by associated K^+ deficiency. ECFV expansion from salt retention causes hypertension and antagonizes the reduction in GFR and/or increases tubule acidification induced by aldosterone and by K^+ deficiency. The kaliuresis persists and causes continued K^+ depletion with polydipsia, inability to concentrate the urine, and polyuria. Increased aldosterone levels may be the result of autonomous primary adrenal overproduction or of secondary aldosterone release due to renal overproduction of renin. In both situations, the normal feedback of ECFV on net aldosterone production is disrupted, and hypertension from volume retention can result.

Liddle's syndrome (Chap. 278) results from increased activity of collecting duct Na^+ channels and is a cause of volume expansion and hypokalemic alkalosis with normal aldosterone levels.

Symptoms These include changes in central and peripheral nervous system function similar to those of hypocalcemia; mental confusion, obtundation, and a predisposition to seizures, paresthesia, muscular cramping, tetany, aggravation of arrhythmias, and hypoxemia in chronic obstructive pulmonary disease. Related electrolyte abnormalities include hypokalemia and hypophosphatemia.

℞ TREATMENT

This is primarily directed at correcting the underlying stimulus for HCO_3^- generation. If primary aldosteronism is present, correction of the underlying cause will reverse the alkalosis. [H^+] loss by the stomach or kidneys can be mitigated by the use of H_2 blockers or the discontinuation of diuretics, respectively. The second aspect of treatment is to remove the factors that sustain HCO_3^- reabsorption, such as ECFV contraction or K^+ deficiency. Although K^+ deficits should be repaired, NaCl therapy is usually sufficient to reverse the alkalosis if ECFV contraction is present, as indicated by a low urine [Cl^-]. Unusual cases, termed *saline-resistant*, are associated with marked K^+ deficits (>1000 mmol), Mg^{2+} deficiency, Bartter's syndrome, or primary autonomous hypermineralocorticoid states. Therapy in these cases must be directed toward the underlying pathophysiologic problem.

If associated conditions preclude infusion of saline, renal HCO_3^- loss can be accelerated by administration of acetazolamide, a carbonic anhydrase inhibitor, which is usually effective in patients with adequate renal function but can worsen K^+ losses. Dilute hydrochloric acid (0.1 *N* HCl) is also effective but can cause hemolysis. Infusion of amino acids such as arginine hydrochloride is safer and as effective. Acidification can also be achieved with oral NH_4Cl, which should be avoided in the presence of liver disease. Finally, hemodialysis against a dialysate low in [HCO_3^-] and high in [Cl^-] can be effective when renal function is impaired.

RESPIRATORY ACIDOSIS

Respiratory acidosis can be due to severe pulmonary disease, respiratory muscle fatigue, or abnormalities in ventilatory control and is due to the increase in Pa_{CO_2} (Table 50-5). In acute respiratory acidosis, there is an immediate compensatory elevation (due to cellular buffering mechanisms) in HCO_3^-, which increases 1 mmol/L for every 10-mmHg increase in Pa_{CO_2}. In chronic respiratory acidosis (>24 h), renal adaptation occurs and the HCO_3^- increases by 4 mmol/L for every 10-mmHg increase in Pa_{CO_2}. The serum HCO_3^- usually does not increase above 38 mmol/L. Renal compensation (increased reabsorption of HCO_3^-) begins within 12 to 24 h and is not complete for about 5 days.

The clinical features vary according to the severity and duration of the respiratory acidosis, the underlying disease, and whether there is accompanying hypoxemia. A rapid increase in Pa_{CO_2} may cause anxiety, dyspnea, confusion, psychosis, and hallucinations and may progress to coma. Lesser degrees of dysfunction in chronic hypercapnia include sleep disturbances, loss of memory, daytime somnolence, personality changes, impairment of coordination, and motor disturbances such as tremor, myoclonic jerks, and asterixis. Headaches and other signs that mimic raised intracranial pressure, such as papilledema, abnormal reflexes, and focal muscle weakness, are due to vasoconstriction secondary to loss of the vasodilator effects of CO_2.

Depression of the respiratory center by a variety of drugs, injury, or disease can produce respiratory acidosis. This may occur acutely with general anesthetics, sedatives, and head trauma or chronically with sedatives, alcohol, intracranial tumors, and the syndromes of sleep-disordered breathing, including the primary alveolar and obesity-hypoventilation syndromes (Chaps. 263 and 264). Abnormalities or disease in the motor neurons, neuromuscular junction, and skeletal muscle can cause hypoventilation via respiratory muscle fatigue. Mechanical ventilation, when not properly adjusted and supervised, may result in respiratory acidosis, particularly if CO_2 production suddenly rises (because of fever, agitation, sepsis, or overfeeding) or alveolar ventilation falls because of worsening pulmonary function. High levels of positive end-expiratory pressure in the presence of reduced cardiac output may cause hypercapnia as a result of large increases in alveolar dead space (Chap. 266).

Table 50-5

Respiratory Acid-Base Disorders

I. Alkalosis
   A. Central nervous system lesions
   B. Pregnancy
   C. Endotoxemia
   D. Salicylates
   E. Hepatic failure
   F. Hypoxemia
   G. Anxiety
   H. Pain
II. Acidosis
   A. Central
      1. Drugs (anesthetics, morphine, sedatives)
      2. Stroke
      3. Infection
   B. Airway
      1. Obstruction
      2. Asthma
   C. Parenchyma
      1. Emphysema
      2. Pneumoconiosis
      3. Bronchitis
      4. Adult respiratory distress syndrome
      5. Barotrauma
   D. Neuromuscular
      1. Poliomyelitis
      2. Kyphoscoliosis
      3. Myasthenia
      4. Muscular dystrophies
   E. Miscellaneous
      1. Obesity
      2. Hypoventilation

Acute hypercapnia follows sudden occlusion of the upper airway or generalized bronchospasm as in severe asthma, anaphylaxis, inhalational burn, or toxin injury. Chronic hypercapnia and respiratory acidosis occur in end-stage obstructive lung disease. Restrictive disorders involving both the chest wall and the lungs can cause respiratory acidosis because the high metabolic cost of respiration causes ventilatory muscle fatigue. Advanced stages of intrapulmonary and extrapulmonary restrictive defects present as chronic respiratory acidosis.

The diagnosis of respiratory acidosis requires, by definition, the measurement of Pa_{CO_2} and arterial pH. A detailed history and physical examination often indicate the cause. Pulmonary function studies (Chap. 250), including spirometry, diffusion capacity for carbon monoxide, lung volumes, and arterial Pa_{CO_2}, and O_2 saturation usually make it possible to determine if respiratory acidosis is secondary to lung disease. The workup for nonpulmonary causes should include a detailed drug history, measurement of hematocrit, and assessment of upper airway, chest wall, pleura, and neuromuscular function.

TREATMENT

The management of respiratory acidosis depends on its severity and rate of onset. *Acute respiratory acidosis* can be life-threatening, and measures to reverse the underlying cause should be undertaken simultaneously with restoration of adequate alveolar ventilation. This may necessitate tracheal intubation and assisted mechanical ventilation. Oxygen administration should be titrated carefully in patients with severe obstructive pulmonary disease and chronic CO_2 retention who are breathing spontaneously (Chap. 258). When oxygen is used injudiciously, these patients may experience progression of the respiratory acidosis. Aggressive and rapid correction of hypercapnia should be avoided, because the falling Pa_{CO_2} may provoke the same complications noted with acute respiratory alkalosis (i.e., cardiac arrhythmias, reduced cerebral perfusion, and seizures). The Pa_{CO_2} should be lowered gradually in chronic respiratory acidosis, aiming to restore the Pa_{CO_2} to baseline levels and to provide sufficient Cl^- and K^+ to enhance the renal excretion of HCO_3^-.

Chronic respiratory acidosis is frequently difficult to correct, but measures aimed at improving lung function such as cessation of smoking, use of oxygen, bronchodilators, glucocorticoids, diuretics, and physiotherapy can help some patients and forestall further deterioration in most. The use of respiratory stimulants may be useful in selected patients, particularly if hypercapnia is out of proportion to the abnormality in lung function.

RESPIRATORY ALKALOSIS

Alveolar hyperventilation decreases Pa_{CO_2} and increases the HCO_3^-/Pa_{CO_2} ratio, thus increasing pH (Table 50-5). Nonbicarbonate cellular buffers respond by consuming HCO_3^-. Hypocapnia develops when a sufficiently strong ventilatory stimulus causes CO_2 output in the lungs to exceed its metabolic production by tissues. Plasma pH and $[HCO_3^-]$ appear to vary proportionately with Pa_{CO_2} over a range from 40 to 15 mmHg. The relationship between arterial hydrogen ion concentration and Pa_{CO_2} is about 0.7 mmol/L per mmHg (or 0.01 pH unit/mmHg), and that for plasma $[HCO_3^-]$ is 0.2 mmol/L per mmHg. Hypocapnia sustained longer than 2 to 6 h is further compensated by a decrease in renal ammonium and titratable acid excretion and a reduction in filtered HCO_3^- reabsorption. Full renal adaptation to respiratory alkalosis may take several days and requires normal volume status and renal function. The kidneys appear to respond directly to the lowered Pa_{CO_2} rather than to alkalosis per se. A 1-mmHg fall in Pa_{CO_2} causes a 0.4- to 0.5-mmol/L drop in HCO_3^- and a 0.3-mmol/L fall (or 0.003 rise in pH) in $[H^+]$.

The effects of respiratory alkalosis vary according to duration and severity but are primarily those of the underlying disease. Reduced cerebral blood flow as a consequence of a rapid decline in Pa_{CO_2} may cause dizziness, mental confusion, and seizures, even in the absence of hypoxemia. The cardiovascular effects of acute hypocapnia in the conscious human are generally minimal, but in the anesthetized or mechanically ventilated patient, cardiac output and blood pressure may fall because of the depressant effects of anesthesia and positive-pressure ventilation on heart rate, systemic resistance, and venous return. Cardiac arrhythmias may occur in patients with heart disease as a result of changes in oxygen unloading by blood from a left shift in the hemoglobin-oxygen dissociation curve (Bohr effect). Acute respiratory alkalosis causes intracellular shifts of Na^+, K^+, and PO_4^- and reduces free $[Ca^{2+}]$ by increasing the protein-bound fraction. Hypocapnia-induced hypokalemia is usually minor.

Respiratory alkalosis is the most common acid-base disturbance in critically ill patients and, when severe, portends a poor prognosis. Many cardiopulmonary disorders manifest respiratory alkalosis in their early to intermediate stages, and the finding of normocapnia and hypoxemia in a patient with hyperventilation may herald the onset of rapid respiratory failure and should prompt an assessment to determine if the patient is becoming fatigued. Respiratory alkalosis is common during mechanical ventilation.

The hyperventilation syndrome may be disabling. Paresthesia, circumoral numbness, chest wall tightness or pain, dizziness, inability to take an adequate breath, and, rarely, tetany may themselves be sufficiently stressful to perpetuate the disorder. Arterial blood-gas analysis demonstrates an acute or chronic respiratory alkalosis, often with hypocapnia in the range of 15 to 30 mmHg and no hypoxemia. Central nervous system diseases or injury can produce several patterns of hyperventilation and sustained Pa_{CO_2} levels of 20 to 30 mmHg. Hyperthyroidism, high caloric loads, and exercise raise the basal metabolic rate, but ventilation usually rises in proportion so that arterial blood gases are unchanged and respiratory alkalosis does not develop. Salicylates are the most common cause of drug-induced respiratory alkalosis as a result of direct stimulation of the medullary chemoreceptor. The methylxanthines, theophylline, and aminophylline stimulate ventilation and increase the ventilatory response to CO_2. Progesterone increases ventilation and lowers arterial Pa_{CO_2} by as much as 5 to 10 mmHg. Therefore, chronic respiratory alkalosis is a common feature of pregnancy. Respiratory alkalosis is also prominent in liver failure, and the severity correlates with the degree of hepatic insufficiency. Respiratory alkalosis is often an early finding in gram-negative septicemia, before fever, hypoxemia, or hypotension develop.

The diagnosis of respiratory alkalosis depends on measurement of arterial pH and Pa_{CO_2}. The plasma $[K^+]$ is often reduced, and the $[Cl^-]$ increased. In the acute phase, respiratory alkalosis is not associated with increased renal HCO_3^- excretion, but within hours net acid excretion is reduced. In general, the HCO_3^- concentration falls by 2.0 mmol/L for each 10-mmHg decrease in Pa_{CO_2}. Chronic hypocapnia reduces the serum $[HCO_3^-]$ by 5.0 mmol/L for each 10-mmHg decrease in Pa_{CO_2}. It is unusual to observe a plasma $HCO_3^- < 12$ mmol/L as a result of a pure respiratory alkalosis.

When a diagnosis of respiratory alkalosis is made, its cause should be investigated. The diagnosis of hyperventilation syndrome is made by exclusion. In difficult cases, it may be important to rule out other conditions such as pulmonary embolism, coronary artery disease, and hyperthyroidism.

TREATMENT

The management of respiratory alkalosis is directed toward alleviation of the underlying disorder. If respiratory alkalosis complicates ventilator management, changes in dead space, tidal volume, and frequency can minimize the hypocapnia. Patients with the hyperventilation syndrome may benefit from reassurance, rebreathing from a paper bag during symptomatic attacks, and attention to underlying psychological stress. Antidepressants and sedatives are not recommended, although beta-adrenergic blockers may ameliorate distressing peripheral manifestations of the hyperadrenergic state.

BIBLIOGRAPHY

ALPERN RJ et al: Metabolic alkalosis, in *The Kidney: Physiology and Pathophysiology*, 2d ed, DW Seldin, G Giebisch (eds). New York, Raven Press, 1992, pp 2733–2758

Molecular Bases of Inherited Disease, 7th ed, CR Scriver et al (eds). New York, McGraw-Hill, 1995, pp 3655–3690

——— et al: Acid-base disorders, in *The Kidney*, 5th ed, BM Brenner (ed). Philadelphia, Saunders, 1996, pp 929–998

EMMETT M et al: Metabolic acidosis, in *The Kidney: Physiology and Pathophysiology*, 2d ed, DW Seldin, G Giebisch (eds). New York, Raven Press, 1992, pp 2759–2836

MADIAS NE, COHEN JJ: Respiratory alkalosis and acidosis, in *The Kidney: Physiology and Pathophysiology*, 2d ed, DW Seldin, G Giebisch (eds). New York, Raven Press, 1992, pp 2837–2872

BIDANI A, DUBOSE TD JR: Cellular and whole body acid-base regulation, in *Fluid, Electrolyte, and Acid-Base Disorders*, 2d ed, AI Arieff, RA DeFronzo (eds). New York, Churchill Livingstone, 1995, pp 69–104

COGAN MG: Diagnosis of acid-base disorders, in *Fluid and Electrolytes*, MG Cogan (ed). Norwalk, Appleton & Lange, 1991, pp 198–202

DUBOSE TD JR, ALPERN RJ: Renal tubular acidosis, in *The Metabolic and*

SECTION 8
ALTERATIONS IN THE UROGENITAL TRACT

51 | *John D. McConnell, Jean D. Wilson*

IMPOTENCE

A variety of endocrine, vascular, neurologic, and psychiatric diseases disrupt normal sexual and reproductive function in men. Furthermore, sexual dysfunction may be the presenting symptom of systemic disease.

NORMAL SEXUAL FUNCTION

Penile erection is initiated by neuropsychologic stimuli that ultimately produce vasodilation of the sinusoidal spaces and arteries within the paired corpora cavernosa. Erection is normally preceded by sexual desire (or libido), which is regulated in part by androgen-dependent psychological factors. Although nocturnal and diurnal spontaneous erections are suppressed in men with androgen deficiency, erections may continue for long periods in response to erotic stimuli. Thus, continuing action of testicular androgens appears to be required for normal libido but not for the erectile mechanism itself.

The penis is innervated by sympathetic, parasympathetic, and somatic fibers. Somatic fibers in the dorsal nerve of the penis form the afferent limb of the erectile reflex by transmitting sensory impulses from the penile skin and glans to the S2–S4 dorsal root ganglia via the pudendal nerve. Unlike the corpuscular-type endings in the penile shaft skin, most afferents in the glans terminate in free nerve endings. The efferent limb begins with parasympathetic preganglionic fibers from S2–S4 that pass in the pelvic nerves to the pelvic plexus. Sympathetic fibers emerging from the intermediolateral gray areas of T11–L2 travel through the paravertebral sympathetic chain ganglia, superior hypogastric plexus, and hypogastric nerves to enter the pelvic plexus along with parasympathetic fibers. Somatic efferent fibers from S3–S4 that travel in the pudendal nerve to the ischiocavernosus and bulbocavernosus muscles and postganglionic sympathetic fibers that innervate the smooth muscle of the epididymis, vas deferens, seminal vesicle, and internal sphincter of the bladder mediate rhythmic contraction of these structures at the time of ejaculation.

Autonomic nerve impulses, integrated in the pelvic plexus, project to the penis through the cavernous nerves that course along the posterolateral aspect of the prostate before penetrating the pelvic floor muscles immediately lateral to the urethra. Distal to the membranous urethra, some fibers enter the corpus spongiosum, while the remainder enter the corpora cavernosa along with the terminal branches of the pudendal artery and exiting cavernous veins. If disruption of the cavernous nerves occurs following pelvic trauma or surgery, erectile impotence may ensue.

The brain exerts an important modulatory influence over spinal reflex pathways that control penile function. A variety of visual, auditory, olfactory, and imaginative stimuli elicit erectile responses that involve cortical, thalamic, rhinencephalic, and limbic input to the medial preoptic-anterior hypothalamic area, which acts as an integrating center. Other areas of the brain, such as the amygdaloid complex, may inhibit sexual function.

Although the parasympathetic nervous system is the primary effector of erection, the transformation of the penis to an erect organ is a vascular phenomenon. In the flaccid state the arteries, arterioles, and sinusoidal spaces within the corpora cavernosa are constricted due to sympathetic-mediated contraction of smooth muscle in the walls of these structures. The venules between the sinusoids and the dense tunica albuginea surrounding the cavernosa open freely to the emissary veins. Erection begins when relaxation of the sinusoidal smooth muscles leads to dilation of the sinusoids and a decrease in peripheral resistance, causing a rapid increase in arterial blood flow through internal pudendal and cavernosa arteries. Expansion of the sinusoidal system compresses the venules against the interior surface of the tunica albuginea, resulting in venous occlusion. The increase in intracorporeal pressure leads to rigidity; less than complete expansion of the sinusoidal spaces leads to less than complete rigidity.

Erection occurs when adrenergic-induced sinusoid tone is antagonized by sacral parasympathetic stimulation that produces sinusoidal relaxation primarily by synthesis and release of the nonadrenergic-noncholinergic (NANC) neurotransmitter nitric oxide (NO). The contribution of acetylcholine-dependent release of NO from the vascular endothelium is uncertain. In vitro electrical stimulation of isolated corpus cavernosum strips (with or without endothelium) produces sinusoidal relaxation by release of neurotransmitters within nerve terminals that is resistant to adrenergic and cholinergic blockers. Inhibitors of the synthesis of NO or of guanosine monophosphate (GMP), as well as nitric oxide scavengers, block sinusoidal relaxation. A variety of neuropeptides found in corporal tissues, including vasoactive intestinal peptide (VIP) and calcitonin gene–related peptide (CGRP), produce tumescence when injected into the penis but have uncertain physiologic roles. Norepinephrine plays an important role in the adrenergic mechanism of detumescence.

Seminal emission and ejaculation are under control of the sympathetic nervous system. Emission results from alpha-adrenergic–mediated contraction of the epididymis, vas deferens, seminal vesicles, and prostate which causes seminal fluid to enter the prostatic urethra. Concomitant closure of the bladder neck prevents retrograde flow of semen into the bladder, and antegrade ejaculation results from contraction of the muscles of the pelvic floor including the bulbocavernosus and ischiocavernosus muscles.

Orgasm is a psychosensory phenomenon in which the rhythmic contraction of the pelvic muscles is perceived as pleasurable. Orgasm can occur without either erection or ejaculation or in the presence of retrograde ejaculation.

Detumescence after orgasm and ejaculation is incompletely understood. Presumably, active tone in the vessels of the sinusoidal spaces is restored by contraction (probably adrenergic-mediated) of smooth muscles, which decreases the inflow of blood to the penis and promotes emptying of the erectile tissue. Following orgasm, there is a refractory period that varies in duration with age, physical condition, and psychic factors and during which erection and ejaculation are inhibited.

IMPOTENCE Simply defined, impotence is the failure to achieve erection, ejaculation, or both. Men with sexual dysfunction present with a variety of complaints, either singly, or in combination: loss of desire (libido), inability to initiate or maintain an erection, ejaculatory failure, premature ejaculation, or inability to achieve orgasm. Sexual dysfunction can be secondary to systemic disease or its treatment, to specific disorders of the urogenital or endocrine systems, or to psychological disturbance. It was previously thought that the majority of men with erectile impotency had a psychological etiology for the dysfunction, but it is now believed that most impotent men have a component of underlying organic disease. Since the selection and success of therapy depend upon the etiology, it is essential to evaluate all aspects of sexual function.

Loss of Desire A decrease in sexual desire, or libido, may be due to androgen deficiency (arising from either pituitary or testicular disease), psychological disturbance, or to some types of prescribed or habitually abused drugs. The possibility of androgen deficiency can be tested by measurement of plasma testosterone and gonadotropin. The minimal level of testosterone required for normal erectile function remains unknown. Hypogonadism may also result in the absence of emission, secondary to decreased secretion of ejaculate by the seminal vesicles and prostate.

Failure of Erection The organic causes of erectile impotence can be grouped into endocrine, drug, local, neurologic, and vascular causes (Table 51-1).

Decreased plasma testosterone secondary to testicular failure is an uncommon but easily recognized and treated disorder. A borderline decrease in plasma testosterone is not a cause of sexual dysfunction. However, hyperprolactinemia may cause impotence in some men with pituitary tumors and may not be obvious on physical examination; hyperprolactinemia suppresses the production of luteinizing hormone–releasing hormone (LHRH) and thus causes low or low-normal levels of plasma gonadotropin and testosterone. Bromocriptine, a dopamine agonist, may lower prolactin levels and reverse impotence in such patients.

Although many drugs are associated with impotence, antihypertensive agents, cimetidine, and monoamine oxidase inhibitors are more likely to lead to erectile dysfunction. Antihypertensive drugs with peripheral and central sympatholytic action or beta-adrenergic receptor blocking activity are the most frequently implicated. Angiotensin-converting enzyme inhibitors, calcium channel blockers, and peripheral vasodilators do not cause a significant incidence of sexual dysfunction. Histamine (H_2) receptor antagonists, such as cimetidine, have antiandrogenic properties in addition to increasing prolactin secretion. The 5α-reductase inhibitor, finasteride, used commonly for the treatment of benign prostatic hyperplasia, produces impotence, decreased libido, or impaired ejaculation in 10 to 12 percent of men. Monoamine oxidase inhibitors, antipsychotic drugs, and tricyclic depressants may impair sexual function via anticholinergic and sympatholytic actions.

Penile diseases including previous priapism, penile trauma, and Peyronie's disease can cause impotence due to fibrosis of the sinusoidal spaces of the corpora cavernosa, corporeal artery occlusion, or neurogenic mechanisms. Peyronie's disease is not rare; patients usually present with a painful plaque on the dorsum of the penis and may progress to development of penile curvature and decreased rigidity of erection.

Many types of neurologic disorders cause impotence, including lesions in the anterior temporal lobe, spinal cord disorders, insufficiency of sensory input as in tabes dorsalis, or damage to parasympathetic nerves, for example, following surgical procedures such as radical (total) prostatectomy or cystectomy. In contrast, transurethral prostatectomy does not cause organic impotence. Furthermore, the nerve supply to the penis (the cavernosal nerves) runs on the posterolateral surface of the prostate, and if the nerves are spared during radical prostate and bladder surgery, potency can be preserved in most men. If spinal cord injury is above the sacral region, reflex erections may occur, whereas diffuse injury of the sacral spinal cord results in total

Table 51-1

Some Organic Causes of Erectile Impotence in Men

I. Endocrine causes
  A. Testicular failure (primary or secondary)
  B. Hyperprolactinemia
II. Drugs
  A. Antiandrogens
    1. Histamine (H_2) blockers (e.g., cimetidine)
    2. Spironolactone
    3. Ketoconazole
    4. Finasteride
  B. Antihypertensives
    1. Central-acting sympatholytics (e.g., clonidine and methyldopa)
    2. Peripheral-acting sympatholytics (e.g., guanadrel)
    3. Beta blockers
    4. Thiazides
  C. Anticholinergics
  D. Antidepressants
    1. Monoamine oxidase inhibitors
    2. Tricyclic antidepressants
  E. Antipsychotics
  F. Central nervous system depressants
    1. Sedatives (e.g., barbiturates)
    2. Antianxiety drugs (e.g., diazepam)
  G. Drugs of habituation or addiction
    1. Alcohol
    2. Methadone
    3. Heroin
    4. Tobacco
III. Penile diseases
  A. Peyronie's disease
  B. Previous priapism
  C. Penile trauma
IV. Neurologic diseases
  A. Anterior temporal lobe lesions
  B. Diseases of the spinal cord
  C. Loss of sensory input
    1. Tabes dorsalis
    2. Disease of dorsal root ganglia
  D. Disease of nervi erigentes
    1. Radical prostatectomy and cystectomy
    2. Rectosigmoid operations
  E. Diabetic autonomic neuropathy and various polyneuropathies
V. Vascular disease
  A. Aortic occlusion (Leriche syndrome)
  B. Atherosclerotic occlusion or stenosis of the pudendal and/or cavernosa arteries
  C. Arterial damage from pelvic radiation
  D. Venous leak
  E. Disease of the sinusoidal spaces

impotence. As many as half of men with diabetes mellitus develop impotence within 6 years of the onset of diabetes, and impotence may be the first clinical manifestation of diabetic neuropathy. Vasculogenic dysfunction is a concomitant factor in most men with diabetic impotence. Several factors contribute to neuropathic impotence, including abnormalities in afferent sensory pathways, motor neuropathy in the cavernosa nerves (which carry the efferent pathways for vasodilation in the penis), and decreased level of neurotransmitters in the corpora cavernosa. In addition, denervation of the sinusoidal smooth muscle leads to a loss of contractile elements and fibrosis, which limits dilation of the spaces. Although the autonomic pathways in the penis can be tested by direct recording of electrical activity in the corporal smooth muscle, the test may not be necessary since most patients demonstrate other manifestations of autonomic neuropathy on careful examination. Many of the other polyneuropathies associated with impotence have similar effects.

Men with vasculogenic impotence may present with total erectile impotence, decreased penile rigidity, or loss of erection during intercourse. Vascular insufficiency may be due to aortic occlusion (Leriche syndrome) or to more distal atherosclerotic disease in the hypogastric, pudendal, and cavernosa arteries. The function of the sinusoidal tissue itself may be adversely affected by atherosclerosis and by the use of tobacco products, which contain a variety of vasocontractile agents. Significant disease in the pudendal and cavernosa arteries can occur in the absence of other clinical manifestations of peripheral vascular disease. The impotence commonly seen following pelvic radiation is probably due to vasculogenic causes. Together with neuropathy, vascular insufficiency contributes to the impotence in many men with diabetes mellitus.

Premature Ejaculation This disorder seldom has an organic cause. It is usually related to anxiety in the sexual situation, unreasonable expectations about performance, or emotional disorder. A variety of successful therapeutic modalities have been described, but behavioral therapy is most successful.

Absence of Emission This symptom may be produced by (1) retrograde ejaculation, (2) sympathetic denervation, (3) androgen deficiency, or (4) drugs. Retrograde ejaculation may occur following surgery on the bladder neck or develop spontaneously in diabetic men. Demonstration of sperm in a postcoital urine specimen establishes the diagnosis. Following sympathectomy or occasionally after extensive retroperitoneal surgery, the autonomic innervation of the prostate and seminal vesicles is lost, resulting in absence of smooth-muscle contraction at the time of ejaculation. Androgen deficiency results in a decrease in secretions of the prostate and seminal vesicles and in a decrease in the volume of ejaculate. Finally, drugs such as guanethidine, phenoxybenzamine, phentolamine, and sertraline primarily impair ejaculation rather than erection or libido.

Absence of Orgasm If libido and erectile function are normal, the absence of orgasm is almost always due to a psychiatric disorder.

Failure of Detumescence Priapism is a persistent painful erection, often unrelated to sexual activity. Priapism can be distinguished from a normal erection by the absence of tumescence of the glans penis. Priapism may be idiopathic but can be associated with sickle cell anemia, chronic granulocytic leukemia, spinal cord injury, or injection of vasodilator agents (such as alprostadil) into the penis. The disorder may be secondary to clotting of blood within the sinusoidal spaces of the penis or to abnormalities of the adrenergic-mediated mechanism for detumescence. Failure to treat priapism promptly usually results in fibrosis and subsequent loss of erectile function. In early phases, detumescence can sometimes be achieved by aspiration, irrigation of the corpora cavernosa, and injection of dilute vasoconstrictors. If this fails, surgical relief by shunting procedures may be necessary. In patients with priapism secondary to sickle cell anemia, conservative measures such as transfusion, oxygenation, and irrigation are generally preferred to shunting procedures.

EVALUATION OF IMPOTENCE The relative frequency of organic as opposed to psychogenic causes of erectile impotence is still debated. Nevertheless, anxiety and depressive states are common causes of impotence (see Chap. 385). Other psychological factors such as disinterest in the sexual partner, fear of sexual incompetence, marital discord, guilt about deviant sexual attitudes, worry, fatigue, and ill health often operate in various combinations to reduce sexual impulse. The central issue in the evaluation of impotence is to separate those instances due to psychological factors from those due to organic causes (Table 51-1). Often, the separation can be made on the basis of history. With the exception of severe depression, men with psychogenic impotence usually have normal nocturnal and early morning erections. From early childhood through the eighth decade, erections occur during normal sleep. This phenomenon, termed *nocturnal penile tumescence* (NPT), occurs during rapid eye movement sleep, and the total time of NPT averages 100 min per night. Consequently, if the impotent man gives a history of rigid erections under any circumstances (often when awakening in the morning), the efferent neurologic and circulatory systems that mediate erection are intact, and dysfunction is probably due to a psychiatric disorder. In these patients the workup should

be limited. (Occasional patients with early sensory neuropathy may have nocturnal erections.)

If the history of nocturnal erections is questionable, measurements of NPT can be made formally with the use of a strain gauge in a sleep laboratory, or informally attached to a recorder, by snap gauge or home monitor. Although false-negative and false-positive results are possible, this procedure helps to differentiate psychogenic and organic impotence. Patients with vasculogenic impotence may have some degree of penile tumescence without the development of adequate rigidity, which may result in a false-positive NPT test. An alternative to NTP testing is the visual sexual stimulation test, which utilizes videotaped erotic material in a laboratory setting to monitor erection by strain gauge. Other features in favor of organic impotence include a slow, insidious onset not associated with any particular psychiatric symptomatology, a previous uninterrupted period of normal erectile function, and persistent sexual desire.

Having deduced an organic cause, the fundamental problem is the differential diagnosis of the etiology (Table 51-1). The history should be probed for indications of diabetes mellitus, manifestations of peripheral neuropathy or bladder dysfunction, symptoms referable to the vascular system such as intermittent claudication, and symptoms of penile disease such as a history of priapism or penile curvature (Peyronie's disease). A thorough drug history should be obtained, and inquiry made concerning past surgery that may have produced neurologic damage. Smoking is not only a risk factor for atherosclerotic disease but may inhibit sinusoidal relaxation directly.

Physical examination should include a detailed genital examination to identify abnormalities of the penis, especially Peyronie's disease, usually easily felt as a fibrotic plaque on the dorsum of the penis. The testes should be palpated for size, symmetry, and abnormal masses; if the length is less than 3.5 cm, hypogonadism should be considered. Evidence of feminization, such as gynecomastia and abnormal body hair distribution, should be sought. All pulses should be palpated, and the presence of bruits should be sought. Often, the pulse in the dorsal penile artery can be felt. If there is an indication from either history or physical examination of a vascular etiology, direct measurement of penile blood flow may be indicated.

With the advent of minimally invasive treatment options, extensive diagnostic testing is infrequently indicated. An initial discussion of treatment options should precede invasive diagnostic procedures. If the patient prefers nonsurgical therapy, further testing beyond history, physical examination, and measurement of plasma testosterone is unlikely to change management.

Pudendal arteriography provides the most accurate assessment of penile arterial disease, but it is expensive and invasive. Moreover, distal arterial lesions may not be identified unless the procedure is performed under conditions of chemical erection (e.g., alprostadil injection). The penile/brachial index can be used to estimate penile blood flow by dividing the penile systolic blood pressure, as determined by Doppler technique, by the simultaneously determined supine brachial systolic pressure. An index of less than 0.6 suggests vasculogenic impotence. However, the test only evaluates flow through the dorsal penile artery, which is not directly involved in the erectile process. Significant disease may be present in the cavernosa arteries despite normal flow through the dorsal artery. Pulsed Doppler analysis and high-resolution ultrasonography can be used in conjunction with intracorporeal injection of alprostadil to assess blood flow in the cavernosal arteries. Alternatively, dynamic infusion cavernosography, in which pressure is measured directly within the corpora, can be utilized to assess arterial inflow. Abnormalities in the venous occlusive mechanism of the penis can cause impotence due to "venous leak" but are usually the result of abnormalities in sinusoidal smooth muscle function or impaired arterial inflow rather than venous abnormalities. Moreover, surgical attempts to eradicate venous leakage seldom restore erectile function in the long term. Therefore, testing to identify venous leak is rarely indicated.

The neurologic examination should measure anal sphincter tone, perineal sensation, and the bulbocavernosus reflex. This reflex is elicited by squeezing the glans penis and noting the degree of anal sphincter constriction. An examination for peripheral neuropathy should include assessment of distal muscle function; the tendon reflexes in the legs; and vibratory, position, tactile, and pain sensation. In the presence of peripheral neuropathy, tests to evaluate penile neuropathy are seldom necessary. In cases with an uncertain neurogenic component, electromyographic sacral signal tracing of the bulbocavernosus reflex or direct electrical recording of the corpora cavernosa by needle or surface electrodes may be helpful. A specific test to document abnormalities in the penile autonomic efferent pathways is not available.

In the absence of hypogonadism or feminization, the serum testosterone is usually normal. Hyperprolactinemia, however, may not be suspected on the basis of history and physical examination. Although endocrine causes of erectile dysfunction are uncommon, measurement of serum prolactin and pooled serum testosterone and luteinizing hormone (see Chap. 336) is appropriate since abnormalities of these parameters are treatable.

℞ TREATMENT

Medical therapy with androgens offers little more than placebo benefit except in hypogonadal men, and empirical therapy may actually delay identification of organic etiologies. If a prolactin-secreting pituitary tumor is present, however, either surgical removal or treatment with bromocriptine usually results in return of potency. Yohimbine, an alpha$_2$-adrenergic antagonist, is widely prescribed but works only in psychogenic impotence by placebo effect. Surgical therapy may be useful in the treatment of decreased potency related to aortic obstruction; however, potency can be lost rather than improved after aortic surgery if the autonomic nerve supply to the penis is damaged. Penile revascularization is appropriate only in young men with traumatic arterial disease. Very few men with venous leak impotence benefit from venous ligation.

The injection of a variety of vasoactive substances into the corpora cavernosa can produce erection. Self-injection with prostaglandin E$_2$ (alprostadil) produces erection in more than 90 percent of men with psychogenic, neurogenic, and mild-to-moderate vasculogenic impotency. Side effects include occasional pain on injection, priapism (1 percent), and penile fibrosis (2 percent). Commercially available mechanical devices that utilize a vacuum to produce an erection and a rubber band to restrict venous return at the base of the penis provide a successful nonsurgical alternative in many patients, including those with diabetes mellitus and severe vascular disease.

Penile prostheses are a therapeutic alternative in impotent patients refractory to other forms of therapy. Malleable plastic rods implanted into the penis provide the simplest system and the lowest complication rates; however, the cosmetic and functional performance of the device is not uniformly satisfactory. Multicomponent, hydraulically operated prostheses offer the advantage of more physiologic erection and greater increase in penile diameter, but these devices are subject to mechanical failure.

Even in patients with organic impotence, psychotherapy is often beneficial in alleviating concomitant psychogenic factors that limit the success of medical and surgical therapy.

BIBLIOGRAPHY

Abramowicz M et al: Drugs that cause sexual dysfunction. Med Let 29:65, 1987
Allen RP et al: Comparison of duplex ultrasonography and nocturnal penis tumescence in evaluation of impotence. J Urol 151:1525, 1994
Andersson KE: Pharmacology of lower urinary tract smooth muscles and penile erectile tissues. Pharmacol Rev 45:254, 1993
———, Wagner G: Physiology of penile erection. Physiol Rev 75:191, 1995
Burnett AL et al: Nitric oxide: A physiologic mediator of penile erection. Science 257:401, 1992
Fishman JF et al: Experience with inflatable penile prosthesis. Urology 23:86, 1984
Goldstein I et al: Radiation-associated impotence—a clinical study of its mechanism. JAMA 251:903, 1984
Kaiser FE, Korenman SG: Impotence in diabetic men. Am J Med 85(Suppl 5A):147, 1988
Kaplan HS: The combined use of sex therapy and intra penile injections in the treatment of impotence. J Sex Marital Ther 16:195, 1990
Kim N et al: A nitric-oxide like factor mediates nonadrenergic-noncholinergic neurogenic relaxation of penile corpus cavernosum smooth muscle. J Clin Invest 88:112, 1991
Knispel HH: Penile venous surgery in impotence: Results in highly selected cases. Urol Int 47:144, 1991
Kolodny RC et al: Sexual function in diabetic men. Diabetes 23:306, 1974
Krane RJ: Medical progress: Impotence. N Engl J Med 321:1648, 1989
Kwan M et al: The nature of androgen action on male sexuality: A combined laboratory–self-report study on hypogonadal men. J Clin Endocrinol Metab 57:557, 1983
Levine SB: Marital sexual dysfunction: Ejaculation disturbances. Ann Intern Med 84:575, 1976
Linet OL, Ogrinc FG: Efficacy and safety of intracavernosal alprostadil in men with erectile dysfunction. The Alprostadil Study Group. N Engl J Med 334(14):873, 1996
Lue TF et al: Vasculogenic impotence evaluated by high-resolution ultrasonography and pulsed Doppler spectrum analysis. Radiology 155:777, 1985
——— et al: Functional evaluation of penile veins by cavernosography in papaverine-induced erection. J Urol 135:479, 1986
Meuleman EJ, Diemont WL: Investigation of erectile dysfunction. Urol Clin North Am 22:803, 1995
Montague DK et al: Infusion pharmacocavernosometry and normal penile tumescence findings in men with erectile dysfunction. J Urol 145:768, 1991
Rajfer J: Nitric oxide as a mediator of relaxation in response to non-adrenergic, non-cholinergic neurotransmission. N Engl J Med 326:90, 1992
Saypol DC et al: Impotence. Are the newer diagnostic methods a necessity? J Urol 130:260, 1983
Tiefer L, Schuetz-Mueller D: Psychological issues in diagnosis and treatment of erectile disorders. Urol Clin North Am 22:767, 1995
Virag R et al: Intracavernous self-injection of vasoactive drugs in the treatment of impotence: 8-year experience with 615 cases. J Urol 145:287, 1991
Wabek AJ: Bulbocavernosus reflex testing in 100 consecutive cases of erectile dysfunction. Urology 25:495, 1985
Walsh PC et al: Impotence following radical prostatectomy: Insight into etiology and prevention. J Urol 128:492, 1982
Winter CC: Priapism. Urol Surv 28:163, 1978
Witherington R: Vacuum constriction device for management of erectile impotence. J Urol 141:320, 1989

52   *Bruce R. Carr, Karen D. Bradshaw*

DISTURBANCES OF MENSTRUATION AND OTHER COMMON GYNECOLOGIC COMPLAINTS IN WOMEN

Complaints related to the female reproductive tract can be categorized as disorders of menstruation, pelvic pain, disturbances in sexual function, or infertility. However, a single disorder, e.g., leiomyoma of the uterus, can present with symptoms referable to any one or more of these categories. Furthermore, sexual dysfunction can interdigitate with other problems in several ways. On the one hand, in women with complaints related to other reproductive tract functions, the underlying problem may actually be severe sexual dysfunction or marital conflict. Alternatively, women with severe organic disorders of the pelvis, e.g., pelvic inflammatory disease, may present with sexual dysfunction such as dyspareunia that in fact is only a minor manifestation of the underlying disease.

Since normal reproductive function depends on the integrated action of the central nervous system, the endocrine glands, and the reproductive organs, menstrual cycle abnormalities, sexual dysfunction, and infertility may be the result of systemic and psychological disorders as well as of primary defects in the endocrine and reproductive organs. The endocrine and physiologic control—normal and abnormal—of puberty, reproductive life, and menopause are discussed in Chap. 337. The focus of this chapter is on the initial evaluation of women with disturbances of the reproductive tract.

DISTURBANCES IN MENSTRUATION Disorders of menstruation can be divided into abnormal uterine bleeding and amenorrhea.

Abnormal Uterine Bleeding The menstrual cycle is defined as the interval between the onset of one bleeding episode and the onset of the next. In normal women the cycle averages 28 ± 3 days, the mean duration of menstrual flow is 4 ± 2 days, and the average blood loss is 40 to 100 mL. Between menarche and menopause most women experience one or more episodes of abnormal uterine bleeding, here defined as any bleeding pattern outside the normal ranges of frequency, duration, and/or amount of blood loss. The decision to evaluate a patient depends on the severity and frequency of the abnormal bleeding pattern.

When vaginal bleeding occurs, it should first be determined whether the blood is derived from the uterine endometrium. Rectal, bladder, cervical, and vaginal sources of bleeding must be excluded. Once the bleeding is established to be uterine in origin, a pregnancy-related disorder (such as threatened or incomplete abortion or ectopic pregnancy) must be ruled out by physical examination and appropriate laboratory tests. It should also be remembered that uterine bleeding also may be the initial or principal manifestation of a generalized bleeding diathesis. The remaining causes of abnormal uterine bleeding can be divided into those associated with ovulatory or anovulatory cycles.

Ovulatory cycles Menstrual bleeding with ovulatory cycles is spontaneous, regular in onset, predictable in duration and amount of flow, and frequently associated with discomfort; it is the consequence of progesterone withdrawal at the end of the luteal (postovulatory) phase and requires prior estrogen priming of the endometrium during the follicular (preovulatory) phase of the cycle. When deviations from an established pattern of menstrual flow occur but the cycles are still regular, the usual cause is disease of the outflow tract. For example, regular, prolonged, excessive bleeding episodes can result from abnormalities of the uterus such as submucous leiomyomas, adenomyosis, or endometrial polyps. On the other hand, cyclic, predictable menstruation characterized by spotting or light bleeding suggests obstruction of the outflow tract as with uterine synechiae or scarring of the cervix. Intermittent bleeding between cyclic ovulatory menses is often due to cervical or endometrial lesions.

Anovulatory cycles Uterine bleeding that is irregular in occurrence, unpredictable as to amount and duration of flow, and usually painless is called *dysfunctional or anovulatory uterine bleeding*. This type of bleeding is the result of a failure of normal follicular maturation with consequent anovulation and may be either transient or chronic. Transient disruption of ovulatory cycles occurs most often in the early menarcheal years, during the perimenopausal period, or as the consequence of a variety of stresses and intercurrent illnesses. Persistent dysfunctional uterine bleeding during the reproductive years can occur in several organic diseases that affect ovarian function and is most often due to estrogen breakthrough bleeding. Estrogen breakthrough bleeding occurs when estrogen stimulation of the endometrium is continuous and is not interrupted by cyclic progesterone withdrawal, as can occur in polycystic ovarian disease.

Amenorrhea *Amenorrhea* is defined either as failure of menarche by age 16, regardless of the presence or absence of secondary sexual characteristics, or as the absence of menstruation for 6 months in a woman with previous periodic menses. Amenorrhea in a woman who has never menstruated is termed *primary*; cessation of menses is termed *secondary amenorrhea*. Because some disorders can cause both primary and secondary amenorrhea, we prefer a functional classification based on the nature of the underlying defect, namely, anatomic defects of the outflow tract (uterus, cervix, or vagina), ovarian failure, and chronic anovulation.

Anatomic defects of the outflow tract include congenital defects of the vagina, imperforate hymen, transverse vaginal septa, cervical stenosis, intrauterine adhesions (synechiae), absence of the vagina or

uterus, and uterine maldevelopment. The diagnosis of an anatomic defect is usually made by physical examination and confirmed by demonstrating failure of bleeding following administration of estrogen plus a progestagen for 21 days. Pelvic ultrasonography, magnetic resonance imaging, hysterosalpingogram, or hysteroscopy may be helpful in defining the defect.

Causes of *ovarian failure* include gonadal dysgenesis, deficiency of $P450_{17\alpha}$, resistant ovary syndrome, and premature ovarian failure. Ovarian failure encompasses disorders in which the ovary is deficient in germ cells and those in which the germ cells are resistant to follicle-stimulating hormone (FSH). The diagnosis of ovarian failure as the cause of amenorrhea is confirmed by an elevated plasma FSH level.

Women with *chronic anovulation* fail to ovulate spontaneously but have the capability of ovulating with appropriate therapy. In some women with chronic anovulation, total estrogen production is adequate, but it is not secreted in a cyclic fashion. In others, estrogen production is deficient.

Women who have adequate estrogen production and demonstrate withdrawal bleeding after progestagen challenge usually have polycystic ovarian disease (see Fig. 337-8). Other causes include hormone-secreting ovarian and adrenal tumors. Women with deficient or absent estrogen production, and therefore with absence of withdrawal bleeding after progestagen administration, usually have hypogonadotropic hypogonadism due to organic or functional disorders of the pituitary or central nervous system such as brain tumors, pituitary tumors (especially prolactin-secreting adenomas), primary hypopituitarism, or Sheehan's syndrome.

PELVIC PAIN Pelvic pain may originate in the pelvis or be referred from another region of the body. A pelvic source is suggested by the history (e.g., dysmenorrhea and dyspareunia) and physical findings, but a high index of suspicion must be entertained for extrapelvic disorders that refer to the pelvis, such as appendicitis, cholecystitis, intestinal obstruction, and urinary tract infections (see Chap. 14).

"Physiologic" Pelvic Pain *Pain associated with ovulation ("mittelschmerz")* Many women experience low abdominal discomfort with ovulation, typically a dull aching pain at midcycle in one lower quadrant lasting from minutes to hours. It is rarely severe or incapacitating. The pain may result from peritoneal irritation by follicular fluid released into the peritoneal cavity at ovulation. The onset at midcycle and short duration of pain are often diagnostic.

Premenstrual or menstrual pain In normal ovulatory women, somatic symptoms during the few days prior to menses may be insignificant or disabling. Such symptoms include edema, breast engorgement, and abdominal bloating or discomfort. A symptom complex of cyclic irritability, depression, and lethargy is known as the *premenstrual syndrome* (PMS). The cause of PMS is unknown, and there is no consensus about therapy.

Severe or incapacitating uterine cramping during ovulatory menses and in the absence of demonstrable disorders of the pelvis is termed *primary dysmenorrhea*. Primary dysmenorrhea is caused by prostaglandin-induced uterine ischemia and is treated with prostaglandin synthetase inhibitors or oral contraceptive agents.

Pelvic Pain due to Organic Causes Severe dysmenorrhea associated with disease of the pelvis is termed *secondary dysmenorrhea*. Organic causes of pelvic pain can be classified as (1) uterine, (2) adnexal, (3) vulvar or vaginal, and (4) pregnancy-associated.

Uterine pain Pain of uterine etiology is often chronic and continuous and increases in intensity during menstruation and intercourse. Causes include leiomyomas of the uterus (particularly submucous and degenerating leiomyomas), adenomyosis, and cervical stenosis. Infections of the uterus associated with intrauterine manipulation following dilatation and curettage or with intrauterine devices also can cause pelvic pain (see Chap. 337). Pelvic pain due to endometrial or cervical cancer is usually a late manifestation (see Chap. 337).

Adnexal pain The most common cause of pain in the adnexae (fallopian tubes and ovaries) is infection (see Chap. 130). Acute salpingo-oophoritis presents as low abdominal pain, fever, and chills; begins a few days after a menstrual period; and is usually due to chlamydial or gonococcal disease with or without a superimposed pyogenic infection. Chronic pelvic inflammatory disease results from either a single episode or multiple episodes of infection and may present as infertility associated with chronic pelvic pain that increases in intensity with menses and intercourse. On physical examination, the adnexae are tender, and adnexal thickening and/or masses may be present. Pelvic inflammatory disease may become a surgical emergency if peritonitis results from rupture of a tuboovarian abscess. Ovarian cysts or neoplasms may cause pelvic pain that becomes more severe with torsion or rupture of the mass, and ectopic pregnancy must be considered in the differential diagnosis (see below). Endometriosis involving fallopian tubes, ovaries, or peritoneum may cause both chronic low abdominal pain and infertility; the magnitude of tissue involvement does not always correlate with the severity of symptoms. Endometriosis pain typically increases with menstruation and, if the posterior ligaments of the uterus are involved, with intercourse.

Vulvar or vaginal pain   Pain in these areas is most often due to infectious vaginitis caused by *Monilia*, *Trichomonas*, or bacteria and is characteristically associated with vaginal discharge and pruritus. Herpetic vulvitis, condyloma acuminatum, and cysts or abscesses of Bartholin's glands also may cause vulvar pain.

Pregnancy-associated disorders   Pregnancy must be considered in the differential diagnosis of pelvic pain during the reproductive years. Threatened abortion or incomplete abortion often presents with uterine cramping, bleeding, or passage of tissue following a period of amenorrhea. Ectopic pregnancy may be insidious in presentation or result in abrupt intraperitoneal hemorrhage and maternal death.

Evaluation of Pelvic Pain   The evaluation of pelvic pain requires a careful history and pelvic examination. This often leads to the correct diagnosis and institution of appropriate treatment. If the pain is severe and the diagnosis is unclear, the workup should follow that outlined for the acute abdomen (Chap. 14). A culdocentesis is indicated if a ruptured ectopic pregnancy is suspected. If there is a question of an adnexal mass or if the patient is so obese as to preclude a thorough pelvic examination, sonography may be useful. Serial human chorionic gonadotropin (hCG) measurements may help in establishing a diagnosis of tubal pregnancy. Finally, diagnostic laparoscopy and laparotomy may be indicated with pain of undetermined etiology.

SEXUAL DYSFUNCTION   Some women with sexual dysfunction describe minor complaints related to the reproductive tract as a means of bringing sexual problems to the attention of the physician. Alternatively, sexual dysfunction may be thought to be the cause of low abdominal discomfort or dyspareunia when the actual etiology is organic. However, more and more women seek medical advice because of sexual problems that interface in provenance between medicine and sociology.

The normal sexual response begins with sexual arousal, which causes genital vasocongestion that results in vaginal lubrication in preparation for intromission. The lubrication is due to the formation of a transudate in the vagina and in conjunction with genital congestion produces the so-called orgasmic platform prior to orgasm. Sexual stimuli (visual, tactile, auditory, and olfactory) as well as healthy vaginal tissue are prerequisites for genital vasocongestion and vaginal lubrication. During the second stage of the sexual response, involuntary contractions of the muscles of the pelvis result in a pleasurable cortical sensory phenomenon known as orgasm. Direct or indirect stimulation of the clitoris is important in the production of the female orgasm. In simple terms, sexual dysfunction can be due to interference with the arousal or orgasmic phases of the sexual response. Either disorder can be due to an organic or functional cause or both.

Illnesses that impair neurologic function such as diabetes mellitus or multiple sclerosis can prevent normal sexual arousal. Local pelvic diseases such as vaginitis, endometriosis, and salpingo-oophoritis may preclude normal sexual response because of resulting dyspareunia. Debilitating systemic diseases such as cancer and cardiovascular diseases may inhibit normal sexual response indirectly.

More commonly, failure of a normal sexual response is due to psychological factors that impair sexual arousal. Such problems include misinformation, e.g., the perception of sexual satisfaction as bad, or feelings of guilt about previous psychologically traumatic

events such as incest, rape, or unwanted pregnancy. In addition, women who have had previous hysterectomy or mastectomy may perceive themselves as "incomplete." Stresses such as anxiety, depression, fatigue, and marital or interpersonal conflicts may lead to failure of the vasocongestive response and prevent normal vaginal lubrication. Women with such experiences may be unable to achieve normal sexual response unless they receive professional counseling. Such problems are approached by attempting to identify and reduce the causative stresses.

Failure to achieve orgasm is a specific form of sexual dysfunction. In the absence of orgasm many women enjoy sexual encounters to variable degrees because of the pleasure derived from closeness in a cherished relationship, particularly with a loving partner. However, for other women sexual relations with rare or absent orgasms are frustrating and unsatisfying. In many instances, failure of orgasm is due to insufficient clitoral stimulation and may be rectified by appropriate counseling and patient education.

A specific entity, "vaginismus," painful, involuntary contractions of the musculature surrounding the entrance to the vagina, is a rare cause of dyspareunia. It is a conditioned response to a previous real or imagined frightening or traumatic sexual experience. Treatment is directed to elimination of the conditioned response by progressive vaginal dilation by the patient in conjunction with marital therapy.

REPRODUCTION   Infertility is discussed in detail in Chap. 337. The approach to infertile couples always involves evaluation of both the man and woman. The history should address the frequency of intercourse, the sexual responses of both, the use of contraceptives or lubricants, previous or past medical illnesses, and all medications taken.

Male-associated factors account for a third of infertility problems. Therefore, one of the first procedures in the workup of infertile couples should be a semen analysis (see Chap. 336). The initial evaluation of the woman includes documentation of normal ovulatory cycles. A history of regular, cyclic, predictable, spontaneous menses usually indicates ovulatory cycles, which may be confirmed by basal body temperature graphs, properly timed endometrial biopsies, or plasma progesterone measurements during the luteal phase of the cycle. Also, the diagnosis of luteal-phase dysfunction (low progesterone secretion during the luteal phase) can be established by these methods. Transvaginal ultrasonography is useful for evaluating follicular development. If the diagnosis is polycystic ovarian disease, attempts to induce ovulation can be undertaken by a variety of methods including administration of clomiphene, human menopausal gonadotropins, bromocriptine, or luteinizing hormone–releasing hormone (LHRH) agonists or by wedge resection of the ovaries (now usually done by laparoscopic cautery or laser drilling) (Chap. 337).

The most common cause of infertility in women is tubal disease, usually due to infection (pelvic inflammatory disease) or endometriosis. Tubal disease can be evaluated by obtaining a hysterosalpingogram or by diagnostic laparoscopy. Tubal diseases can usually be treated by laparoscopic tuboplasty and lysis of adhesions; in severe cases the infertility is treated by in vitro fertilization and embryo transfer.

A cervical factor as a cause of infertility is identified by a properly timed postcoital examination. During this examination, the sperm motility in cervical mucus is observed. Also, immunologic etiologies for infertility can be tested for by a variety of laboratory tests. The cause of infertility is unknown in 10 percent of couples. In many instances of infertility, it is now possible to use assisted reproductive technologies including in vitro fertilization and embryo transfer, gamete intrafallopian tube transfer, transfer of cryopreserved ova and embryos, and ovarian hyperstimulation with clomiphene citrate or gonadotropins followed by intrauterine insemination.

The desire for contraception is also a frequent cause for women to seek medical treatment or evaluation. The most widely used methods for fertility control include (1) rhythm and withdrawal techniques, (2) barrier methods, (3) intrauterine devices, (4) oral steroid contraceptives, (5) sterilization, and (6) abortion. These methods and their complications are discussed in Chap. 337.

BIBLIOGRAPHY

CARR BR, BLACKWELL RE: *Textbook of Reproductive Medicine*. Norwalk CT, Appleton & Lange, 1993

CUNNINGHAM FG et al: *Williams Obstetrics*, 19th ed. Norwalk, Appleton & Lange, 1993

HERBST AL et al: *Comprehensive Gynecology*, 2d ed. St. Louis, Mosby, 1992

FORDNEY DS: Dyspareunia and vaginismus. Clin Obstet Gynecol 21:205, 1978

HAMMOND DC: Screening for sexual dysfunction. Clin Obstet Gynecol 27:732, 1984

HATCHER RA et al: *Contraceptive Technology*, 16th ed. New York, Irvington, 1994

MASTERS W, JOHNSON V: *Human Sexual Response*. Boston, Little, Brown, 1966

ROSEN RJ et al: Prevention of sexual dysfunction in women. J Sex Med Ther 19:171, 1993

SPEROFF L et al: *Clinical Gynecologic Endocrinology and Infertility*, 4th ed. Baltimore, Williams & Wilkins, 1989

53   William J. Kovacs, Jean D. Wilson

HIRSUTISM AND VIRILIZATION

Hirsutism, male pattern hair growth in women, is a common and perplexing problem. The distribution and growth of hair in normal persons is under complex genetic and endocrine control so that there is considerable variability in hair growth among normal men and women. As a consequence, abnormal hair growth is difficult to define: Some patients may seek medical attention because of what the physician may consider an insignificant cosmetic defect. Others, because of personal or cultural factors, may be undisturbed by significant degrees of hirsutism. The central issue in dealing with such patients is the separation of those infrequent instances in which hirsutism is a manifestation of a serious and remediable underlying disorder from the majority of hirsute women in whom excess hair is fundamentally a cosmetic problem.

CONTROL OF NORMAL HAIR GROWTH AND DISTRIBUTION   Endocrine Control   Androgens are the major determinants of hair distribution in both sexes. There are three principal circulating androgens in women—dehydroepiandrosterone, derived from the adrenal; androstenedione, which is derived equally from adrenal and ovary; and testosterone, which is both secreted by the ovary and adrenal and formed in extraglandular tissue from circulating dehydroepiandrosterone and androstenedione. The production of adrenal androgen is regulated primarily by adrenocorticotropin, while ovarian androgen secretion is regulated by luteinizing hormone (LH). These various androgens must be converted to testosterone (or dihydrotestosterone) before they can bind to the androgen receptor of target cells and induce an androgenic response. Thus, adrenal androgens virilize only in so far as they serve as precursors for testosterone and dihydrotestosterone.

Several types of relationships can be defined between hair growth and androgens in normal individuals. Eyebrows, eyelashes, and vellus hairs are not dependent on androgens. Axillary and lower pubic hair are sensitive to small amounts of androgen; hair growth in these areas begins at the time of adrenarche under the control of adrenal androgens and is approximately equal in men and women. In some areas such as the face, upper pubic triangle, chest, and ears, hair growth is more typical of males and appears to require the greater androgen levels produced by the testes. Finally, scalp hair exhibits androgen-mediated regression. The reason different body regions respond differently to

the same or similar androgen is unknown. The metabolism of androgens might differ in the various sites. The hair follicle, like some other androgen targets, requires conversion of testosterone to dihydrotestosterone for expression of androgen action, and hair follicles from all regions of the body perform this conversion. Moreover, the same receptor that is essential for androgen action in other cells (Chap. 336) mediates the effects of dihydrotestosterone in the hair follicle. Genetic disorders with normal testosterone production but absent androgen receptor have deficient or absent axillary, pubic, facial, truncal, and limb hair (Chap. 339). Regional differences in androgen responsiveness of hair in normal individuals could also be the consequence of regional differences in the amount of androgen receptor in hair follicles.

Genetic Factors   Despite similar hormone levels, the distribution of hair varies among individuals and among different ethnic and racial groups. Dark-haired, darkly pigmented whites of either sex tend to be more hirsute than blond or fair-skinned persons. Asians, native Americans, and blacks on average are less hirsute than whites. Asians have scant facial and body hair except in the pubic and axillary regions, and native Americans, in addition, rarely develop baldness. Heterogeneity of hair patterns also exists within families. The inheritance of hair patterns is complex and probably polygenic in nature.

Other factors   Aging is a prerequisite for some types of hair development. For example, in men hair on the trunk and extremities frequently increases for several years after maximal levels of plasma androgens have been reached. Conversely, loss of androgen may not result in diminution of normal hair growth in men or complete reversal of hirsutism in women. Women in the first trimester of pregnancy commonly have increased hairiness of the face, extremities, and breasts. Menopause is often associated with the loss of hair in the pubic area, axillae, and extremities, whereas growth of hair on the face increases in postmenopausal women. These changes cannot be explained solely by changes in androgen levels.

PATHOLOGIC HAIR GROWTH AND DISTRIBUTION   A central consideration in the evaluation of women with hirsutism is whether evidence of virilization or defeminization is also present (Table 53-1) since such signs suggest profound androgen excess. In patients with overproduction of androgen, defeminizing signs, such as disturbances of menstruation, are more frequent than virilization. However, the presence or absence of overt virilization should be interpreted with caution for at least two reasons. First, signs of virilization (clitoromegaly, balding, coarsening of the hair, hirsutism) indicate androgen excess at some time in the patient's life but do not necessarily mean that active disease is present at the time of evaluation. It is necessary to measure plasma androgen levels and/or production rates to determine if androgen excess is ongoing. Second, severe overandrogenization may exist in the absence of marked virilization, i.e., at the same level of androgen production clitoromegaly may be present in one patient but not in another.

Diagnostic Considerations   *Drugs*   Excessive hair growth can be caused by drugs that exert their effects independent of androgens and do not produce defeminization or virilization. Such drugs include phenytoin, minoxidil, diazoxide, cyclosporine, and hexachlorobenzene; hair growth produced by these agents is usually vellus in character. Androgens produce hirsutism as well as virilization. Some synthetic progestagens have androgenic activity.

Table 53-1

Clinical Signs of Defeminization and Virilization

Signs of Defeminization	Signs of Virilization
Amenorrhea	Frontal balding
Decrease in breast size	Increase in size of shoulder
Loss of female body contours	girdle muscles
	Clitoromegaly
	Coarsening of the voice
	Acne

SOURCE: After L Karp, WL Herrmann, Diagnosis and treatment of hirsutism in women. Obstet Gynecol 41:283, 1973.

Tumors   The rapid onset of hair growth with or without accompanying signs of frank virilization suggests a neoplastic source of androgen. Such tumors include adenomas and carcinomas of the adrenal and ovarian tumors such as arrhenoblastoma, which secrete androgens directly, and Krukenberg tumors of the ovary, which stimulate the surrounding ovarian stromal tissue to produce excess androgen.

Polycystic ovarian disease   The most common cause of ovarian hyperandrogenism is polycystic ovarian disease. This disorder has a broad spectrum of manifestations that range from mild hirsutism to amenorrhea and virilization. The salient feature for the diagnosis is the pubertal onset of chronic anovulation and hirsutism. Enlarged cystic ovaries, obesity, and amenorrhea (i.e., the Stein-Leventhal syndrome) are present in half or fewer of women with this disorder and need not be present for the diagnosis (see Chap. 337). The fundamental abnormality in polycystic ovarian disease is not fully understood, but elevated levels of plasma LH cause enhanced androgen secretion by stromal and thecal cells of the ovary.

Attenuated forms of adrenal hyperplasia   The adrenal can be the source of excess androgen in the absence of tumor. Heritable defects in adrenal steroidogenesis (congenital adrenal hyperplasia) such as deficiencies of 21-hydroxylase (P450$_{C21}$), 11β-hydroxylase (P450$_{C11B}$), and 3β-hydroxysteroid dehydrogenase isomerase (3β-HSD) can produce virilization, and each can occur in a "late-onset" form in which hirsutism or virilization and menstrual irregularities appear at the time of expected puberty or in adulthood (see Chap. 339). The clinical features in these cases resemble those in polycystic ovarian disease. Late-onset 21-hydroxylase deficiency is the most common attenuated form of congenital adrenal hyperplasia and has been studied extensively; its incidence in the general population of hirsute, oligomenorrheic women is on the order of 1 to 5 percent. The presence of elevated plasma levels of adrenal androgens (such as dehydroepiandrosterone sulfate) or of dexamethasone-suppressible hyperandrogenism does not necessarily imply that the overandrogenization is due to a specific adrenal steroidogenic defect, but these findings may be useful as a guide to therapy.

Idiopathic hirsutism   In many women with hirsutism a specific diagnosis cannot be made. The term *idiopathic hirsutism* applies to those women with evidence of androgen excess but with normal menses, normal-sized ovaries, no evidence of tumors of the adrenal or ovary, and normal adrenal function. Slight elevations of plasma androstenedione and testosterone levels are common in such women, and testosterone production rates are increased, although to a lesser degree than in patients with polycystic ovarian disease.

Experience with the antiandrogens cyproterone acetate and flutamide indicates that this form of hirsutism is androgen-mediated, since therapy results in improvement. Women with idiopathic hirsutism might constitute the extreme end of a normal continuum of androgen production or represent a true pathologic subset. Some women with the tentative diagnosis of idiopathic hirsutism actually have mild or early polycystic ovarian disease, but in most, hirsutism is not accompanied by or followed by signs of ovarian dysfunction. If such women are merely extremes of the normal range of androgen production, then their hirsutism is fundamentally a cosmetic defect.

DIAGNOSTIC EVALUATION

The decision as to when to undertake a complex diagnostic evaluation depends on several factors. Such evaluation is appropriate in all women with hirsutism accompanied by virilization; whether it should be performed in women with iso-

lated hirsutism depends upon the severity, distribution, and rate of hair growth. An approach to the diagnostic evaluation of hirsute patients is shown in Fig. 53-1. The clinical history is taken with particular attention to drug ingestion and to the details of pubertal development and menstrual history and their relation to the onset of excessive hair growth. The physical examination is directed to the assessment of sites of growth of androgen-dependent hair (pubic, axillary, facial, truncal, and extremity) and evaluation for signs of virilization, which correlate with higher levels of androgen overproduction and raise the concern of androgen-producing neoplasms. Such signs include laryngeal enlargement (deepening of the voice), temporal balding, clitoromegaly, and increased muscle mass in the shoulder girdle. Signs of cortisol excess (plethora, centripetal obesity, striae, and enlarged dorsocervical and supraclavicular fat pads) should also be sought. Pelvic examination should include a search for palpable ovarian masses. Laboratory tests include measurement of serum androgens and, when indicated, radiologic imaging of ovaries and adrenal glands. Basal measurements of dehydroepiandrosterone sulfate greater than 22 μmol/L (8000 ng/mL) or of serum testosterone over 7 nmol/L (2 ng/mL) suggest neoplastic sources of androgen excess; plasma testosterone levels in the normal range are more difficult to interpret because total levels in women do not necessarily reflect the free or unbound levels of hormone under conditions when testosterone-binding globulin levels are either increased or decreased. Suspected Cushing's syndrome should be evaluated if a screening test (such as urinary free cortisol excretion or overnight dexamethasone suppression test) is abnormal. The diagnosis of polycystic ovarian disease is made from the history and clinical features in a woman with chronic anovulation. Women may be screened for delayed-onset adrenal hyperplasia by the short ACTH stimulation test and measurement of plasma 17-hydroxyprogesterone (see Chap. 332).

℞ **TREATMENT**

In the case of drug-induced hirsutism and neoplastic disease of the ovary or adrenals treatment is straightforward; administration of the drugs should be stopped, or the tumor should be removed. Adrenal steroidogenic defects are treated with glucocorticoids to suppress

FIGURE 53-1   Diagnostic approach to the hirsute patient. T, testosterone; DHEA-S, dehydroepiandrosterone sulfate.

excess ACTH and inhibit adrenal androgen secretion. In most instances (polycystic ovarian disease as well as idiopathic hirsutism) both cosmetic treatment and suppression of androgen production or antagonism of its action at the receptor level need to be employed.

Cosmetic therapy is directed at the concealment or removal of hair from exposed skin areas. Small amounts of hair can be bleached with hydrogen peroxide. Methods for removal of hair are classified as depilatory (removal of hair from the surface of the skin) or epilatory (removal of the intact hair with the root). Depilatory techniques include shaving and chemical methods. Shaving does not have an adverse effect on hair growth rate or coarseness (although the blunt ends may feel coarse), but shaving of areas other than axillae or legs is unacceptable to most women. Chemical depilatories are effective for limited areas of hair removal and are generally safe if used properly. Most available depilatories are substituted mercaptans, such as thioglycollic acid, which reduce the disulfide bonds in the peptide chains of keratin. The hair fiber swells and softens to a consistency that can be washed from the skin. Care must be taken to avoid skin irritation because of the alkalinity of these preparations. Temporary epilation can be achieved by plucking (useful only for isolated hairs), wax treatment, or the use of epilatory devices. The waxes are melted and applied to the skin. When the wax cools and sets, it is stripped off, removing hair with it. The procedure is uncomfortable, and best results can be obtained by salon treatments. Permanent epilation can be achieved only by electrolysis. The treatments are expensive and time-consuming, and success depends on the skill of the electrologist.

While cosmetic treatment is undertaken, attempts to suppress androgen overproduction may also be appropriate. Treatment with combination oral contraceptives suppresses ovarian androgen secretion when restoration of fertility is not an objective. To minimize side effects oral contraceptives should contain progestagens with the least androgenic side effects (such as desogestrel or norgestimate) and the lowest effective dosage of estrogen. Women over 35 years of age, smokers, and those with hypertension, a history of thromboembolic disease, impaired liver function, or suspected estrogen-dependent neoplasm should not be treated with oral contraceptives. The combination of oral contraceptives and luteinizing hormone–releasing hormone analogues does not offer any advantage over oral contraceptives alone. Suppression of adrenal androgen overproduc-

tion can be achieved with small doses of dexamethasone and is most useful in late-onset 21-hydroxylase deficiency.

Antagonism of the effects of androgens at the hair follicle is the basis for treatment with antiandrogens. Cyproterone acetate has been used with success but is available in the United States only for compassionate use. The androgen receptor antagonist flutamide is also effective, but it can cause hepatic failure and probably should not be used for this purpose. Spironolactone has a dual action of blocking the androgen receptor and of inhibiting androgen production and is a useful alternative therapy. Cimetidine also binds to the androgen receptor and acts as an androgen antagonist but is not of general benefit in the treatment of hirsutism. The 5α-reductase inhibitor finasteride has been used successfully for this purpose but can cause toxic effects if it crosses the placenta.

If pharmacologic therapy is undertaken, the patient should be prepared to make a commitment of 6 months for an adequate trial of efficacy. Even when treatment is long-term, dramatic reversal of established hair growth is unlikely to be achieved by interference with androgen synthesis or action. Such hormonal manipulations can arrest or slow the rate of hair growth, but established hair must be dealt with by use of cosmetic treatment.

BIBLIOGRAPHY

CARR BR et al: Oral contraceptive pills, gonadotropin-releasing hormone agonists, or use in combination for treatment of hirsutism: A clinical research center study. J Clin Endocrinol Metab 80:1169, 1995

CUSAN L et al: Treatment of hirsutism with the pure antiandrogen flutamide. J Am Acad Dermatol 23:462, 1990

DERKSEN J et al: Identification of virilizing adrenal tumors in hirsute women. N Engl J Med 331:968, 1994

EHRMAN DA, ROSENFIELD RL: An endocrinologic approach to the patient with hirutism. J Clin Endocrinol Metab 71:1, 1990

FRUZZETTI F et al: Effects of finasteride, a 5alpha-reductase inhibitor, on circulating androgens and gonadotropin secretion in hirsute women. J Clin Endocrinol Metab 79:1115, 1994

KILLEEN AA et al: Prevalence of nonclassical congenital adrenal hyperplasia among women self-referred for treatment of hirsutism. Am J Med Genet 42:197, 1992

MCKENNA TJ: Screening for sinister causes of hirsutism. N Engl J Med 331:1015, 1994

O'BRIEN RC et al: Comparison of sequential cyproterone acetate/estrogen versus spironolactone/oral contraceptive in the treatment of hirsutism. J Clin Endocrinol Metab 72:1008, 1991

RITTMASTER RS: Medical treatment of androgen-dependent hirsutism. J Clin Endocrinol Metab 80:2559, 1995

SECTION 9

ALTERATIONS IN THE SKIN

54

Thomas J. Lawley, Kim B. Yancey

APPROACH TO THE PATIENT WITH SKIN DISORDER

The challenge of examining the skin lies in distinguishing normal from abnormal and significant findings from trivial ones and in integrating pertinent signs and symptoms into an appropriate differential diagnosis. The fact that the largest organ in the body is visible is both an advantage and a disadvantage to those who examine it. It is advantageous because no special instrumentation, other than a magnifying glass, is necessary and because the skin can be biopsied with little morbidity. However, the casual observer can be overwhelmed by a variety of stimuli and overlook important, subtle signs of skin or

systemic disease. For instance, the sometimes minor differences in color and shape that distinguish a malignant melanoma from a benign pigmented nevus can be difficult to recognize. To aid in the interpretation of skin lesions, a variety of descriptive terms have been developed to characterize cutaneous lesions (Tables 54-1 and 54-2 and Fig. 54-1). Mastery of this terminology is important not only for categorizing the skin lesions of a particular case but also in formulating a differential diagnosis (Table 54-3). For instance, the finding of large numbers of scaling papules, usually indicative of a primary skin disease, places the patient in a different diagnostic category than would hemorrhagic papules, which may indicate vasculitis or sepsis. It is important to differentiate primary skin lesions from secondary skin changes. If the examiner focuses on linear erosions overlying an area of erythema and scaling, he or she may incorrectly assume that the erosion is the primary lesion and the redness and scale are secondary, while the correct interpretation

Table 54-1

CHAPTER 54
Approach to the Patient with Skin Disorder   **295**

Descriptions of Primary Skin Lesions

Macule: A flat, colored lesion, <2 cm in diameter, not raised above the surface of the surrounding skin. A "freckle," or ephelid, is a prototype pigmented macule.

Patch: A large (>2 cm), flat lesion with a color different from the surrounding skin. This differs from a macule only in size.

Papule: A small, solid lesion, <1 cm in diameter, raised above the surface of the surrounding skin and hence palpable (e.g., a closed comedone, or whitehead, in acne).

Nodule: A larger (1–5 cm), firm lesion raised above the surface of the surrounding skin. This differs from a papule only in size (e.g., dermal nevus).

Tumor: A solid, raised growth >5 cm in diameter.

Plaque: A large (>1 cm), flat-topped, raised lesion; edges may either be distinct (e.g., in psoriasis) or gradually blend with surrounding skin (e.g., in eczematous dermatitis).

Vesicle: A small, fluid-filled lesion, <1 cm in diameter, raised above the plane of surrounding skin. Fluid is often visible, and the lesions are often translucent [e.g., vesicles in allergic contact dermatitis caused by *Toxicodendron* (poison ivy)].

Pustule: A vesicle filled with leukocytes. Note: The presence of pustules does not necessarily signify the existence of an infection.

Bulla: A fluid-filled, raised, often translucent lesion >1 cm in diameter.

Cyst: A soft, raised, encapsulated lesion filled with semisolid or liquid contents.

Wheal: A raised, erythematous papule or plaque, usually representing short-lived dermal edema.

Telangiectasia: Dilated, superficial blood vessels.

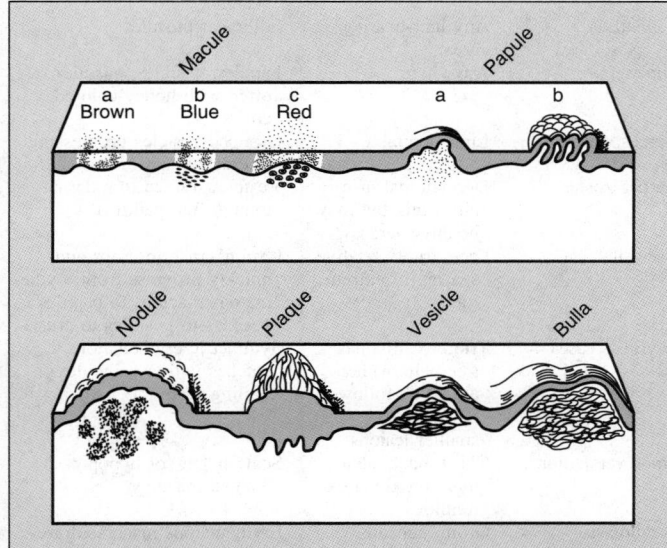

FIGURE 54-1   A schematic representation of several common primary skin lesions (see Table 54-1).

Table 54-2

Common Dermatologic Terms

Lichenification: A distinctive thickening of the skin that is characterized by accentuated skin-fold markings and that feels thick and firm on palpation.

Crust: Dried exudate of body fluids that may be either yellow (serous exudate) or red (hemorrhagic exudate).

Milia: Small, firm, white papules that are filled with keratin (and may in part resemble pustules).

Erosion: Epithelial deficit resulting in a superficial disruption of skin integrity.

Ulcer: Epithelial deficit resulting in a deep surface disruption.

Excoriations: Linear, angular erosions that may be covered by crust and are caused by scratching.

Atrophy: An acquired loss of substance. In the skin, this may appear as a depression with intact epidermis (i.e., loss of dermal or subcutaneous tissue) or as sites of shiny, delicate, wrinkled lesions (i.e., epidermal atrophy).

Scar: A change in the skin secondary to trauma or inflammation. Sites may be erythematous, hypopigmented, or hypertrophic depending on their age or character. Sites on hair-bearing areas may be characterized by destruction of hair follicles.

would be that the patient has a pruritic eczematous dermatitis and the erosions have been caused by scratching.

Approach to the Patient

In examining the skin it is usually advisable to assess the patient before taking a history. This way, the entire cutaneous surface is sure to be evaluated, and objective findings can be integrated with relevant historical data. Four basic features of any cutaneous lesion must be noted and considered in the examination of skin: the distribution of the eruption, the type(s) of primary lesion, the shape of individual lesions, and the arrangement of the lesions. In the initial examination it is important that the patient be disrobed as completely as possible. This will minimize chances of missing important individual skin lesions and make it possible to assess accurately the distribution of the eruption. The patient should first be viewed from a distance of about 1.5 to 2 m (4 to 6 ft) so that the general character of the skin and the distribution of lesions can be evaluated. Indeed, distribution of lesions often correlates highly with diagnosis (Fig. 54-2). For example, a hospitalized patient with a generalized erythematous exanthem is more likely to have a drug eruption than is a patient with a similar rash limited to the sun-exposed portions of the face. The presence or absence of lesions on mucosal surfaces also should be determined. Once the distribution of the lesions has been established, the nature of the primary lesion must be determined. Thus, when lesions are distributed on elbows, knees, and scalp, the most likely possibility based solely on distribution is psoriasis or dermatitis herpetiformis. The primary lesion in psoriasis is a scaly papule that soon forms erythematous plaques covered with a white scale, whereas that of dermatitis herpetiformis is an urticarial papule that quickly becomes a small vesicle. In this manner, identification of the primary lesion directs the examiner toward the proper diagnosis. Secondary changes in skin also can be quite helpful. For example, scale represents excessive epidermis, while crust is the result of an inadequate or inconsistent epithelial cell layer. Palpation of skin lesions also can yield insight into the character of an eruption. Thus red papules on the lower extremities that blanch with pressure can be a manifestation of many different diseases, but hemorrhagic red papules that do not blanch with pressure indicate palpable purpura characteristic of necrotizing vasculitis.

The shape of lesions is also an important feature. Flat, round, erythematous papules and plaques are common in many cutaneous diseases. However, target-shaped lesions that consist in part of erythematous plaques are specific for erythema multiforme. In the same way, the arrangement of individual lesions is important. Erythematous papules and vesicles can occur in many conditions, but their arrangement in a specific linear array suggests an external etiology such as allergic contact or primary irritant dermatitis. In contrast, lesions with a generalized arrangement are common and suggest a systemic etiology.

As in other branches of medicine, a complete history should be obtained to emphasize the following features:

1. Evolution of lesions
   a. Site of onset
   b. Manner in which eruption progressed or spread
   c. Duration
   d. Periods of resolution or improvement in chronic eruptions
2. Symptoms associated with the eruption
   a. Itching, burning, pain, numbness
   b. What, if anything, has relieved symptoms
   c. Time of day when symptoms are most severe
3. Current or recent medications (prescribed as well as over-the-counter)
4. Associated systemic symptoms (e.g., malaise, fever, arthralgias)
5. Ongoing or previous illnesses
6. History of allergies
7. Presence of photosensitivity
8. Review of systems

DIAGNOSTIC TECHNIQUES   Many skin diseases can be diagnosed on gross clinical appearance, but sometimes relatively simple diagnostic procedures can yield valuable information. In most instances, they can be performed at the bedside with a minimum of equipment.

Skin Biopsy   A skin biopsy is a straightforward minor surgical procedure; however, it is important to biopsy the anatomic site most likely to yield diagnostic findings. This decision may require expertise in skin diseases and knowledge of superficial anatomic structures in selected areas of the body. In this procedure, a small area of skin is anesthetized with 1% lidocaine with or without epinephrine. The skin lesion in question can be excised with a scalpel or removed by punch biopsy. In the latter technique, a punch is pressed against the surface of the skin and rotated with downward pressure until it penetrates to the subcutaneous tissue. The circular biopsy is then lifted with forceps, and the bottom is cut with iris scissors. Biopsy sites may or may not need suture closure depending on size and location.

KOH Preparation   A potassium hydroxide (KOH) preparation is performed on scaling skin lesions when a fungal etiology is suspected. The edge of such a lesion is scraped gently with a scalpel blade, and the removed scale is collected on a glass microscope slide and treated with 1 to 2 drops of a solution of 10 to 20% KOH. KOH dissolves keratin and allows easier visualization of fungal elements. Brief heating of the slide accelerates dissolution of keratin. When the preparation is viewed under the microscope, the refractile hyphae will be seen more easily when the light intensity is reduced. This technique can be utilized to identify hyphae in dermatophyte infections, pseudohyphae and budding yeast in *Candida* infections, and fragmented hyphae and spores in tinea versicolor. The same sampling technique can be used to obtain scale for culture of selected pathogenic organisms.

Table 54-3

Selected Common Dermatologic Conditions

Diagnosis	Common Distribution	Usual Morphology	Diagnosis	Common Distribution	Usual Morphology
Acne vulgaris	Face, upper back	Open and closed comedones, erythematous papules, pustules, cysts	Seborrheic keratosis	Trunk, face	Brown plaques with adherent, greasy scale; "stuck on" appearance
Rosacea	Blush area of cheeks, nose, forehead, chin	Erythema, telangiectasias, papules, pustules	Folliculitis	Any hair-bearing area	Follicular pustules
Seborrheic dermatitis	Scalp, eyebrows, perinasal	Erythema with greasy yellow-brown scale	Impetigo	Anywhere	Papules, vesicles, pustules, often with honey-colored crusts
Atopic dermatitis	Antecubital and popliteal fossae; may be widespread	Patches and plaques of erythema, scaling, and lichenification; pruritus	Herpes simplex	Lips, genitalia	Grouped vesicles progressing to crusted erosions
			Herpes zoster	Dermatomal, usually trunk but may be anywhere	Vesicles limited to a dermatome (often painful)
Stasis dermatitis	Ankles, lower legs	Patches of erythema and scaling on background of hyperpigmentation associated with signs of venous insufficiency	Varicella	Face, trunk, relative sparing of extremities	Lesions arise in crops and quickly progress from erythematous macules to papules to vesicles to pustules to crusts
Dyshidrotic eczema	Palms, soles, sides of fingers and toes	Deep vesicles	Pityriasis rosea	Trunk (Christmas tree pattern) herald patch followed by multiple smaller lesions	Symmetric erythematous patches with a collarette of trailing scale
Allergic contact dermatitis	Anywhere	Localized erythema, vesicles, scale, and pruritus, e.g., fingers, earlobes—nickel; dorsal aspect of foot—shoe dermatitis; exposed surfaces—poison ivy dermatitis; etc.	Tinea versicolor	Chest, back, abdomen, proximal extremities	Scaly hyper- or hypopigmented macules
Psoriasis	Elbows, knees, scalp, lower back, fingernails (may be generalized)	Papules and plaques covered with silvery scale; nails have pits	Candidiasis	Groin, beneath breasts, vagina, oral cavity	Erythematous macerated areas with satellite pustules; white, friable patches on mucous membranes
Lichen planus	Wrists, ankles, mouth (may be widespread)	Violaceous flat-topped papules and plaques	Dermatophytosis	Feet, groin, beard, or scalp	Varies with site, e.g., tinea corporis—scaly annular patch
Keratosis pilaris	Extensor surfaces of arms and thighs, buttocks	Keratotic follicular papules with surrounding erythema	Scabies	Groin, axillae, between fingers and toes, beneath breasts	Excoriated papules, burrows, pruritus
Melasma	Forehead, cheeks, temples, upper lip	Tan to brown patches	Insect bites	Anywhere	Erythematous papules with central puncta
Vitiligo	Periorificial, trunk, extensor surfaces of extremities, flexor wrists, axillae	Chalk-white macules	Cherry angioma	Trunk	Red, blood-filled papules
			Keloid	Anywhere (site of previous injury)	Firm tumor, pink, purple, or brown
			Dermatofibroma	Anywhere	Firm red to brown nodule that shows dimpling of overlying skin with lateral compression
Actinic keratosis	Sun-exposed areas	Skin-colored or red-brown macule or papule with dry, rough, adherent scale	Acrochordons (skin tags)	Groin, axilla, neck	Fleshy papules
Basal cell carcinoma	Face	Papule with pearly, telangiectatic border on sun-damaged skin	Urticaria	Anywhere	Wheals, sometimes with surrounding flare, pruritus
			Transient acantholytic dermatosis	Trunk, especially anterior chest	Erythematous papules
Squamous cell carcinoma	Face, especially lower lip, ears	Indurated and possibly hyperkaratotic lesions often showing ulceration and/or crusting	Xerosis	Extensor extremities, especially legs	Dry, erythematous, scaling patches, pruritus

Tzanck Smear A Tzanck smear, named after Arnault Tzanck, is a cytologic technique most often used in the diagnosis of herpesvirus infections (simplex or varicella-zoster). An early vesicle, not a pustule or crusted lesion, is unroofed, and the base of the lesion is scraped gently with a scalpel blade. The material is then placed on a glass slide, air-dried, and stained with Giemsa or Wright's stain. Multinucleated giant cells suggest the presence of herpes, but culture or immunofluorescence testing must be performed to identify the specific virus.

Diascopy Diascopy is designed to assess whether a skin lesion will blanch with pressure as, for example, in determining whether a red lesion is hemorrhagic or simply blood-filled. For instance, a hemangioma will blanch with pressure, whereas a purpuric lesion caused by necrotizing vasculitis will not. Diascopy is performed by pressing a microscope slide or magnifying lens against a specified lesion and noting the amount of blanching that occurs. Granulomas often have an "apple jelly" appearance on diascopy.

Wood's Light A Wood's lamp generates 360-nm ultraviolet (or "black") light that can be used to aid the evaluation of certain skin disorders. For example, a Wood's lamp will cause erythrasma (a superficial, intertriginous infection caused by *Corynebacterium minutissimum*) to show a characteristic coral red color, and wounds colo-

nized by *Pseudomonas* to appear pale blue. Tinea capitis caused by certain dermatophytes such as *Microsporum canis* or *M. audouini* exhibits a yellow fluorescence. Pigmented lesions of the epidermis such as freckles are accentuated, while dermal pigment such as post-inflammatory hyperpigmentation fades under a Wood's light. Vitiligo appears totally white under a Wood's lamp, and previously unsuspected areas of involvement often become apparent. A Wood's lamp also may aid in the demonstration of tinea versicolor and in recognition of ash leaf spots in patients with tuberous sclerosis.

Patch Tests Patch testing is designed to document sensitivity to a specific antigen. In this procedure, a battery of suspected allergens is applied to the patient's back under occlusive dressings and allowed to remain in contact with the skin for 48 h. The dressings are then removed, and the area is examined for evidence of delayed hypersensitivity reactions (e.g., erythema, edema, or papulovesicles). This test is best performed by physicians with special expertise in patch testing and is often helpful in the evaluation of patients with chronic dermatitis.

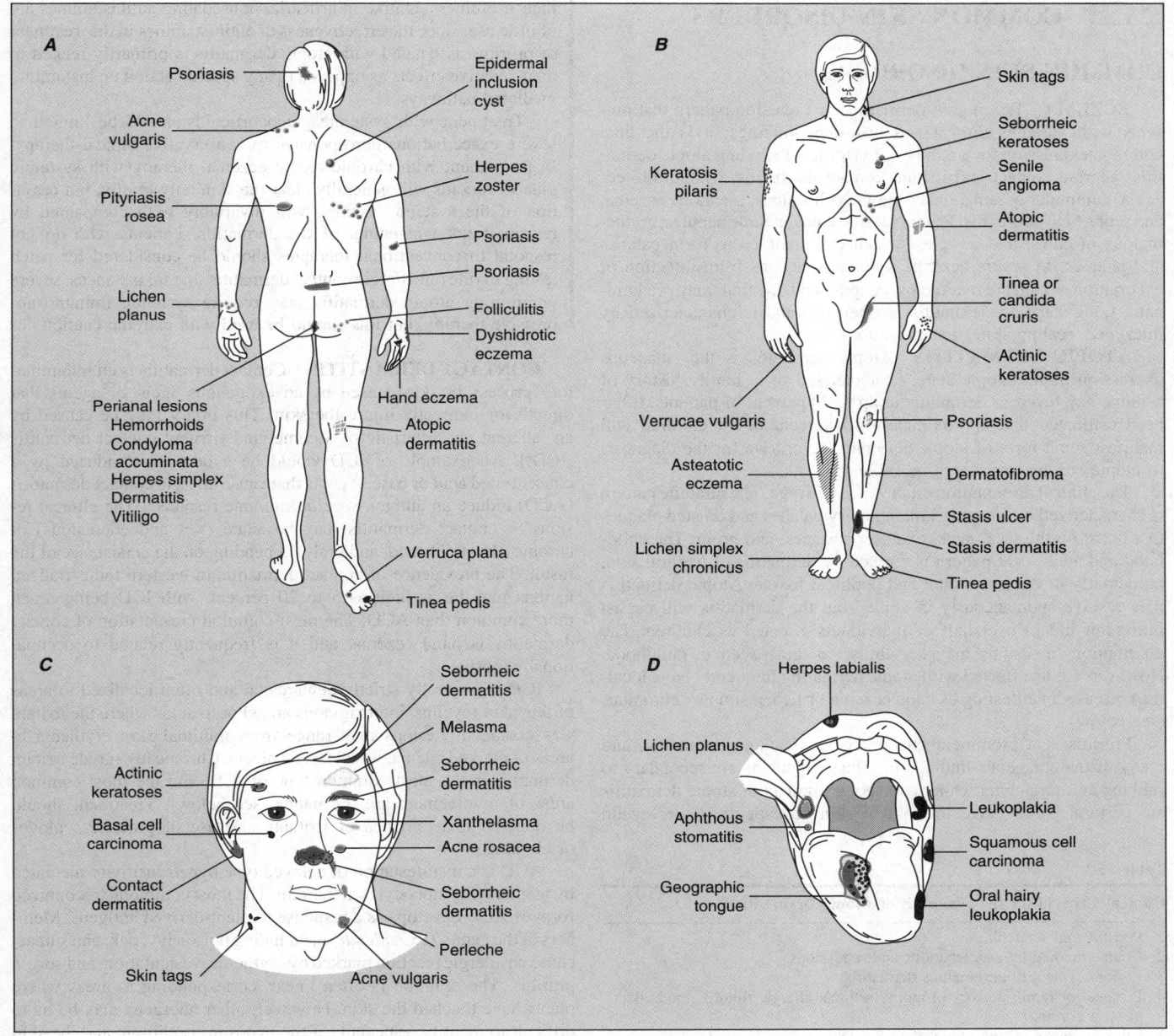

FIGURE 54-2 *A–D.* The distribution of some common dermatologic diseases and lesions.

BIBLIOGRAPHY

ARNDT KA et al (eds): *Cutaneous Medicine and Surgery, An Integrated Program in Dermatology*. Philadelphia, Saunders, 1996

ARNOLD HL et al (eds): *Andrew's Diseases of the Skin*, 8th ed. Philadelphia, Saunders, 1990

FITZPATRICK TB et al (eds): *Dermatology in General Medicine*, 4th ed. New York, McGraw-Hill, 1993

LOOKINGBILL DP, MARKS JG: *Principles of Dermatology*. Philadelphia, Saunders, 1986

ROOK A et al (eds): *Textbook of Dermatology*, 5th ed. Oxford, Blackwell Scientific, 1992

55	*Robert A. Swerlick, Thomas J. Lawley*

ECZEMA, PSORIASIS, CUTANEOUS INFECTIONS, ACNE, AND OTHER COMMON SKIN DISORDERS

COMMON SKIN DISORDERS

ECZEMA   Eczema, or dermatitis, is a reaction pattern that presents with variable clinical and histologic findings; it is the final common expression for a number of disorders including atopic dermatitis, allergic contact and irritant contact dermatitis, dyshidrotic eczema, nummular eczema, lichen simplex chronicus, asteatotic eczema, and seborrheic dermatitis. Primary lesions may include papules, erythematous macules, and vesicles, which can coalesce to form patches and plaques. In severe eczema, secondary lesions from infection or excoriation, which are marked by weeping and crusting, may predominate. Long-standing dermatitis is often dry and is characterized by thickened, scaling skin (lichenification).

ATOPIC DERMATITIS   Atopic dermatitis is the cutaneous expression of the atopic state, characterized by a family history of asthma, hay fever, or dermatitis in up to 70 percent of patients. It has been estimated that approximately 10 percent of all children will manifest some form of atopic eczema. The criteria for the diagnosis of atopic eczema are shown in Table 55-1.

The clinical presentation often varies with age. The infantile pattern is characterized by weeping inflammatory patches and crusted plaques that occur on the face, neck, extensor surfaces, and groin. The childhood and adolescent pattern is marked by dermatitis of flexural skin, particularly in the antecubital and popliteal fossae. Atopic dermatitis may resolve spontaneously in adults, but the dermatitis will persist into adult life in over half of individuals affected as children. The distribution of lesions may be similar to those seen in childhood. However, adults affected with atopic dermatitis frequently have localized disease, manifesting as hand eczema or lichen simplex chronicus (see below).

Pruritus is a prominent characteristic of atopic dermatitis, and many of the cutaneous findings in affected patients are secondary to rubbing and scratching. Other cutaneous stigmata of atopic dermatitis are perioral pallor, an extra fold of skin beneath the lower eyelid

Table 55-1

Clinical Criteria for the Diagnosis of Atopic Dermatitis

1. Pruritus and scratching
2. Course marked by exacerbations and remissions
3. Lesions typical of eczematous dermatitis
4. Personal or family history of atopy (asthma, allergic rhinitis, food allergies, or eczema)
5. Clinical course lasting longer than 6 weeks

(Dennie's line), increased palmar markings, and increased incidence of cutaneous infections, particularly with *Staphylococcus aureus*. Atopic individuals often have dry, itchy skin, abnormalities in cutaneous vascular responses, and in some instances, elevated levels of serum IgE.

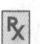 **TREATMENT**

Therapy of atopic dermatitis should be based on avoidance of cutaneous irritants, adequate cutaneous hydration, judicious use of low- or midpotency topical glucocorticoids, and prompt treatment of secondarily infected skin lesions. Patients should be instructed to bathe using warm, but not hot, water and to limit their use of soap. Immediately after bathing, the skin should be lubricated with a low- or midpotency topical glucocorticoid in a cream or ointment base. Crusted and weeping skin lesions should be treated with systemic antibiotics with activity against *Staph. aureus*, since secondary infection often exacerbates eczema. The role of dietary allergens in atopic dermatitis is controversial, but there is little evidence that they play any role outside of infancy.

Control of pruritus is essential for treatment, since atopic eczema often represents "an itch that rashes." Antihistamines are useful to control the pruritus that accompanies eczema, but sedation may limit their usefulness. Unlike in urticaria, nonsedating antihistamines are of little use, since the effectiveness of antihistamines in the treatment of pruritus associated with atopic dermatitis is primarily related to their sedative effects as opposed to any specific action on histamine-mediated pathways.

Treatment with systemic glucocorticoids should be limited to severe exacerbations unresponsive to conservative topical therapy. In the patient with chronic atopic eczema, therapy with systemic glucocorticoids will generally clear the skin only briefly, but cessation of the systemic therapy will invariably be accompanied by return, if not worsening, of the dermatitis. Patients who do not respond to conventional therapies should be considered for patch testing to rule out allergic contact dermatitis. In rare instances, severe unremitting atopic dermatitis may require systemic immunosuppressive therapy, but this should be used with extreme caution.

CONTACT DERMATITIS   Contact dermatitis is an inflammatory process in skin caused by an exogenous agent or agents that directly or indirectly injure the skin. This injury may be caused by an inherent characteristic of a compound [irritant contact dermatitis (ICD)]. An example of ICD would be a dermatitis induced by a concentrated acid or base. Agents that cause allergic contact dermatitis (ACD) induce an antigen-specific immune response. The clinical lesions of contact dermatitis may be acute (wet and edematous) or chronic (dry, thickened, and scaly) depending on the persistence of the insult. The prevalence of contact dermatitis in western industrialized nations may be as high as 5 to 20 percent, with ICD being much more common than ACD. The most common presentation of contact dermatitis is hand eczema, and it is frequently related to occupational exposures.

ICD is generally strictly demarcated and often localized to areas of thin skin (eyelids, intertriginous areas) or to areas where the irritant was occluded. Lesions may range from minimal skin erythema to areas of marked edema, vesicles, and ulcers. Chronic low-grade irritant dermatitis is the most common type of ICD, and the most common areas of involvement are the hands (see below). Treatment should be directed to avoidance of irritants and use of protective gloves or clothing.

ACD is a manifestation of delayed type hypersensitivity mediated by memory T lymphocytes in the skin. The most commonly recognized form of ACD develops as a response to plant-derived antigens. Members of the genus *Toxicodendron*, including poison ivy, oak, and sumac, cause an allergic reaction marked by erythema, vesiculation, and severe pruritus. The eruption is often linear, corresponding to areas where plants have touched the skin. However, other allergens may be more difficult to identify, especially if the exposure is chronic and the skin becomes thickened and scaly.

TREATMENT

If ACD is suspected and an offending agent is identified and removed, the eruption will resolve. Usually, treatment with a high-potency fluorinated topical glucocorticoid is enough to relieve symptoms while the ACD runs its course. Patients with particularly widespread disease, or disease involving the face or genitalia, may require treatment with oral glucocorticoids. Since the natural course of ACD is 2 to 3 weeks, therapy should be continued for that length of time. Treatment of ACD with very short, rapidly tapered courses of oral glucocorticoids is almost always accompanied by recurrence of skin lesions. Additionally, when systemic glucocorticoids are utilized, they are best given as single daily morning doses to limit potential side effects.

Identification of a contact allergen can be a difficult and time-consuming task. Patients with a dermatitis unresponsive to conventional therapy or with an unusual and patterned distribution should be suspected of having ACD. They should be questioned carefully regarding occupational exposures, topical medicaments, and oral medications. Common sensitizers include preservatives in topical preparations, nickel sulfate, potassium dichromate, neomycin sulfate, fragrances, formaldehyde, and rubber-curing agents. Patch testing is helpful in identifying these agents but should not be used on patients with widespread active dermatitis or on those taking systemic glucocorticoids.

HAND ECZEMA   Hand eczema is a very common, chronic skin disorder. It represents the overwhelming majority of occupation-associated skin disease, which is responsible for a significant proportion of occupation-associated injury and time lost from work. It may be associated with other cutaneous disorders such as atopic dermatitis or may occur by itself. As with other forms of dermatitis, both exogenous and endogenous factors play important roles in the expression of hand dermatitis. Chronic, excessive exposure to water and detergents may initiate or aggravate this disorder. It may present with dryness and cracking of the skin of the hands, as well as with variable amounts of erythema and edema. Often the dermatitis will begin under rings where water and irritants are trapped. A variant of hand dermatitis, dyshidrotic eczema, presents with multiple, intensely pruritic, small papules and vesicles occurring on the thenar and hypothenar eminences and the sides of the fingers. Lesions tend to occur in crops that slowly form crusts and heal.

The evaluation of a patient with hand eczema should include an assessment of potential occupation-associated exposures. Predominant involvement of the dorsal surface of the hands with sparing of the palmar surface should suggest a possible contact dermatitis. The history should be directed to identifying possible irritant or allergen exposures. The use of rubber gloves to protect dermatitic skin is sometimes associated with the development of delayed type hypersensitivity reactions to agents used for cross-linking rubber. These delayed type hypersensitivity reactions can be detected by patch testing. Less commonly, patients may manifest hand dermatitis as a consequence of developing immediate type hypersensitivity reactions to latex. These reactions are of particular concern since these patients are at risk for anaphylactic reactions. The most sensitive method of detection is the use of scratch testing with latex extract. However, this should be done with extreme caution only in a setting where an anaphylactic reaction can be treated. A latex radioallergosorbent test (RAST) is avialable, but it is only about 60 percent sensitive.

TREATMENT

Therapy of hand dermatitis is directed toward avoidance of irritants, identification of possible contact allergens, treatment of coexistent infection, and application of topical glucocorticoids. Whenever possible, the hands should be protected by gloves, preferably vinyl. Most patients can be treated with cool moist compresses (dressings) to dry and debride acute inflammatory lesions and to decrease swelling, followed by application of a mid- to high-potency topical glucocorticoid in a cream or ointment base. As with atopic dermatitis,

treatment of secondary infection from staphylococci or streptococci is essential for good control. Additionally, patients with hand dermatitis should be examined for dermatophyte infection by potassium hydroxide (KOH) preparation and culture (see below).

NUMMULAR ECZEMA   Nummular eczema is characterized by circular or oval "coinlike" lesions. Initially, this eruption consists of small edematous papules that become crusted and scaly. The most common locations are on the trunk or the extensor surfaces of the extremities, particularly on the pretibial areas or dorsum of the hands. It occurs more frequently in men and is most commonly seen in middle age. The etiology of nummular eczema is unknown. Whether nummular eczema represents a variant of atopic eczema is controversial. The treatment of nummular eczema is similar to that for other forms of dermatitis.

LICHEN SIMPLEX CHRONICUS   Lichen simplex chronicus may represent the end stage of a variety of pruritic and eczematous disorders. It consists of a well-circumscribed plaque or plaques with lichenified or thickened skin due to chronic scratching or rubbing. Common areas involved include the posterior nuchal region, dorsum of the feet, or ankles. Treatment of lichen simplex chronicus centers around breaking the cycle of chronic itching and scratching, which often occur during sleep. High-potency topical glucocorticoids are helpful in alleviating pruritus in most cases, but in recalcitrant cases, application of topical glucocorticoids under occlusion or intralesional injection of glucocorticoids may be required. Oral antihistamines are useful as antipruritics primarily due to their sedating action and are particularly useful at bedtime.

ASTEATOTIC ECZEMA   Asteatotic eczema, also known as xerotic eczema or "winter itch," is a mildly inflammatory variant of dermatitis that develops most commonly on the lower legs of elderly individuals during dry times of year. Fine cracks, with or without erythema, resembling cracks seen in china or porcelain characteristically develop on the anterior surface of the lower extremities. Pruritus is variable. Asteatotic eczema responds well to avoidance of irritants, rehydration of the skin, and application of topical emollients.

STASIS DERMATITIS AND STASIS ULCERATION   Stasis dermatitis develops on the lower extremities secondary to venous incompetence and chronic edema. Early findings in stasis dermatitis may consist of mild erythema and scaling associated with pruritus. The typical initial site of involvement is over the medial aspect of the ankle, often over a distended vein. As the disorder progresses, the dematitis becomes progressively pigmented, due to chronic erythrocyte extravasation leading to cutaneous hemosiderin deposition. As with other forms of dermatitis, stasis dermatitis may become acutely inflamed, with crusting and exudate. Chronic stasis dermatitis is often associated with dermal fibrosis that clinically is recognized as brawny edema of the skin. Stasis dermatitis is often complicated by secondary infection and contact dermatitis. Severe stasis dermatitis may precede the development of stasis ulcers.

TREATMENT

Avoidance of irritants and use of emollients and/or midpotency topical glucocorticoids are the cornerstones of therapy for stasis dermatitis. Control of chronic edema is important to prevent leg ulcers. Patients should be encouraged to elevate the affected extremity whenever sitting. A compression stocking with a gradient of at least 30 to 40 mmHg is most effective for edema control and is much more effective for preventing chronic edema than antiembolism hose.

Stasis ulcers are difficult to treat, and resolution of these lesions is slow even under the best of circumstances. It is extremely important to elevate the affected limb as much as possible. The ulcer should be kept clear of necrotic material by gentle debridement and covered with a semipermeable dressing under pressure. Glucocorticoids should not be applied to ulcers, since they may retard healing. Secondarily infected lesions should be treated with appropriate oral antibiotics, but it should be noted that all ulcers will become colonized with bacteria, and the purpose of antibiotic therapy should not be to clear all bacterial growth. Some ulcers may take months to heal or require skin grafting.

SEBORRHEIC DERMATITIS Seborrheic dermatitis is a common, chronic disorder characterized by greasy scales overlying erythematous patches or plaques. The most common location is in the scalp, where it may be recognized as severe dandruff. On the face, seborrheic dermatitis affects the eyebrows, eyelids, glabella, nasolabial fold, or ears. Scaling within the external ear is often mistaken for a chronic fungal infection (otomycosis), and postauricular dermatitis often becomes macerated and tender. Additionally, seborrheic dermatitis may develop in the central chest, axilla, groin, submammary folds, and gluteal cleft. Rarely, it may cause a widespread generalized dermatitis. Seborrheic dermatitis is usually symptomatic, with patients complaining of itching or burning.

Seborrheic dermatitis may be evident within the first few weeks of life, and within this context it occurs in the scalp ("cradle cap"), face, or groin. It is rarely seen in children beyond infancy but becomes evident again during adult life. Although it is frequently seen in patients with Parkinson's disease, in those who have had cerebrovascular accidents, and in those with human immunodeficiency virus (HIV) infection, the overwhelming majority of individuals with seborrheic dermatitis have no underlying disorder.

 TREATMENT

Treatment with low-potency topical glucocorticoids in conjunction with shampoos containing coal tar and/or salicylic acid is generally sufficient to control activity of this disorder. High potency topical glucocorticoid solutions (betamethasone or fluocinonide) are effective for control of scalp involvement. Fluorinated topical glucocorticoids should not be used on the face since this is often associated with the development of rebound worsening and steroid induced rosacea or atrophy.

PAPULOSQUAMOUS DISORDERS (Table 55-2)

PSORIASIS Psoriasis is one of the most common dermatologic diseases, affecting up to 1 to 2 percent of the world's population. It is a chronic inflammatory skin disorder clinically characterized by erythematous, sharply demarcated papules and rounded plaques, covered by silvery micaceous scale. The skin lesions of psoriasis are variably pruritic. Traumatized areas often develop lesions of psoriasis (Koebner or isomorphic phenomenon). Additionally, other external factors may exacerbate psoriasis including infections, stress, and medications (lithium, beta blockers, and antimalarials).

The most common variety of psoriasis is called *plaque type*. Patients with plaque-type psoriasis will have stable, slowly growing plaques, which remain basically unchanged for long periods of time. The most common areas for plaque psoriasis to occur are the elbows, knees, gluteal cleft, and the scalp. Involvement tends to be symmetrical. *Inverse psoriasis* affects the intertriginous regions including the axilla, groin, submammary region, and navel, and it also tends to affect the scalp, palms, and soles. The individual lesions are sharply demarcated plaques but may be moist due to their location. Plaque-type psoriasis generally develops slowly and runs an indolent course. It rarely spontaneously remits.

Eruptive psoriasis (guttate psoriasis) is most common in children and young adults. It develops acutely in individuals without psoriasis or in those with chronic plaque psoriasis. Patients present with many small erythematous, scaling papules, frequently after upper respiratory tract infection with beta-hemolytic streptococci. The differential diagnosis should include pityriasis rosea and secondary syphilis. Patients with psoriasis may also develop pustular lesions. These may be localized to the palms and soles or may be generalized and associated with fever, malaise, diarrhea, and arthralgias.

About half of all patients with psoriasis have fingernail involvement, appearing as punctate pitting, nail thickening, or subungual hyperkeratosis. About 5 to 10 percent of patients with psoriasis have associated joint complaints, and these are most often found in patients with fingernail involvement. Although some have the coincident occurrence of classic rheumatoid arthritis (see Chap. 313), many have joint disease that falls into one of five types associated with psoriasis: (1) disease limited to a single or a few small joints (70 percent of cases); (2) a seronegative rheumatoid arthritis–like disease; (3) involvement of the distal interphalangeal joints; (4) severe destructive arthritis with the development of "arthritis mutilans"; and (5) disease limited to the spine.

The etiology of psoriasis is still poorly understood, but there is clearly a genetic component. Over 50 percent of patients with psoriasis report a positive family history, and twin studies report a 65 to 72 percent concordance among monozygotic twins. Evidence has accumulated clearly indicating a role for T cells in the pathophysiology of psoriasis. Psoriasis may become particularly severe in individuals who are HIV-infected (see Chap. 308). Stimulation of immune function with cytokines such as interleukin 2 has been associated with abrupt worsening of preexisting psoriasis, and bone marrow transplantation has resulted in clearance of disease. In addition, agents that inhibit activated T cell function are often effective for the treatment of severe psoriasis.

 TREATMENT

Treatment of psoriasis depends on the type, location, and extent of disease. All patients should be instructed to avoid excess drying or irritation of their skin and to maintain adequate cutaneous hydration.

Table 55-2

Papulosquamous Disorders

	Clinical Features	Other Notable Features	Histologic Features
Psoriasis	Sharply demarcated, erythematous plaques with mica-like scale; predominantly elbows, knees, and scalp; atypical forms may localize to intertriginous areas; eruptive forms may be associated with infection (Reiter's syndrome)	May be aggravated by certain drugs, infection; severe forms seen associated with HIV	Acanthosis, vascular proliferation
Lichen planus	Purple polygonal papules marked by severe pruritus; lacy white markings, especially associated with mucous membrane lesions	Certain drugs may induce: thiazides, antimalarial drugs	Interface dermatitis
Pityriasis rosea	Rash often preceded by herald patch; oval to round plaques with trailing scale; most often affects the trunk, and eruption lines up in skin folds give a "fir tree"-like appearance; generally spares palms and soles	Variable pruritus; self-limited resolving in 2–8 weeks; may be imitated by secondary syphilis	Pathologic features often nonspecific
Dermatophytosis	Polymorphous appearance depending on dermatophyte, body site, and host response; sharply defined to ill-demarcated scaly plaques with or without inflammation; may be associated with hair loss	KOH preparation may show branching hyphae; culture helpful	Hyphae and neutrophils in stratum corneum

Most patients with localized plaque-type psoriasis can be managed with midpotency topical glucocorticoids, although their long-term use is often accompanied by loss of effectiveness (tachyphylaxis). Crude coal tar (1 to 5% in an ointment base) is an old but useful method of treatment in conjunction with ultraviolet light therapy. A topical vitamin D analogue (calcipitriol) is also efficacious in the treatment of psoriasis.

Ultraviolet light is an effective therapy for patients with widespread psoriasis. The ultraviolet B (UV-B) spectrum is effective alone or may be combined with coal tar (Goeckerman regimen) or anthralin (Ingram regimen). Natural sunlight or an artificial light source can be used. The combination of the UV-A spectrum and either oral or topical psoralens (PUVA) is also extremely effective for the treatment of psoriasis, but long-term use may be associated with an increased incidence of squamous cell cancer of the skin.

Various other agents can be used for widespread psoriatic disease. Methotrexate is an effective agent, especially in patients with associated psoriatic arthritis. Liver toxicity from long-term use limits its use to patients with widespread disease not responsive to less aggressive modalities. The synthetic retinoid, etretinate, has been shown to be effective in some patients with severe psoriasis, but it is a potent teratogen with an extremely long tissue half-life, thus precluding its use in women with childbearing potential.

LICHEN PLANUS Lichen planus (LP) is a papulosquamous disorder in which the primary lesions are pruritic, polygonal, flat-topped, violaceous papules. Close examination of the surface of these papules will often reveal a network of gray lines (Wickham's striae). The skin lesions may occur anywhere, but they have a predilection for the wrists, shins, lower back, and genitalia. Involvement of the scalp may lead to hair loss. LP commonly involves mucous membranes, particularly the buccal mucosa, where it can present as a white netlike eruption. Its etiology is unknown, but cutaneous eruptions clinically resembling LP have been observed after administration of numerous drugs, including diuretics, gold, antimalarials, penicillamine, and phenothiazines, and in patients with skin lesions of chronic graft-versus-host disease. Additionally, LP associated with abnormal liver function has been correlated with viral hepatitis, particularly hepatitis C infection. The course of LP is variable, but most patients have spontaneous remissions 6 months to 2 years after the onset of disease. Topical glucocorticoids are the mainstay of therapy.

PITYRIASIS ROSEA Pityriasis rosea (PR) is a papulosquamous eruption of unknown etiology that occurs more commonly in the spring and fall. Its first manifestation is the development of a 2- to 6-cm annular lesion (the herald patch). This is followed in a few days to a few weeks by the appearance of many smaller annular or papular lesions with a predilection to occur on the trunk. The lesions are generally oval with their long axis parallel to the skin fold lines. The individual lesions may range in color from red to brown and have a trailing scale. PR shares many clinical features with the eruption of

secondary syphilis, but palm and sole lesions are extremely rare in PR and common in secondary syphilis. The eruption tends to be moderately pruritic and lasts 3 to 8 weeks. Treatment is generally directed at alleviating pruritus and consists of oral antihistamines, midpotency topical glucocorticoids, and, in some cases, the use of UV-B phototherapy.

CUTANEOUS INFECTIONS (Table 55-3)

IMPETIGO AND ECTHYMA Impetigo is a common superficial bacterial infection of skin caused by group A beta-hemolytic streptococci (see Chap. 143) or *Staph. aureus* (see Chap. 142). The primary lesion is a superficial pustule that ruptures and forms a characteristic yellow-brown "honey-colored" crust. Lesions caused by staphylococci may be tense, clear bullae, and this less common form of the disease is called *bullous impetigo.* Lesions may occur on normal skin or in areas already affected by another skin disease. Ecthyma is a variant of impetigo that generally occurs on the lower extremities and causes punched-out ulcerative lesions. Treatment of both ecthyma and impetigo involves gentle debridement of adherent crusts, which is facilitated by the use of soaks and topical antibiotics, in conjunction with appropriate oral antibiotics.

ERYSIPELAS AND CELLULITIS (See Chap. 133)

DERMATOPHYTOSIS Dermatophytes are fungi that infect skin, hair, and nails and include members of the genera *Trichophyton*, *Microsporum*, and *Epidermophyton*. Infection of the foot (tinea pedis) is most common and is often chronic; it is characterized by variable erythema and edema, scaling, pruritus, and occasionally vesiculation. Involvement may be widespread or localized, but almost invariably the web space between the fourth and fifth toes is affected. Infection of the nails (tinea unguium) occurs in many patients with tinea pedis and is characterized by opacified, thickened nails and subungual debris. The groin is the next most commonly involved area (tinea cruris), with males affected much more often than females. It presents as a scaling erythematous eruption that spares the scrotum. Microscopic examination of either untreated tinea pedis or tinea cruris scale after digestion with KOH preparation will generally demonstrate hyphae.

Dermatophyte infection of the scalp (tinea capitis) has returned in epidemic proportions, particularly in inner city clinics. The predominant organism is *T. tonsurans*. This organism can produce an inflammatory or relatively noninflammatory infection that may present with either well-defined or irregular, diffuse areas of mild scaling and hair loss. Tinea corporis, or widespread infection on non-hair-bearing skin, may have a variable appearance, depending on the extent of the associated inflammatory reaction. It may have the typical annular appearance

Table 55-3

Common Skin Infections

	Clinical Features	Etiologic Agent	Treatment
Impetigo	Honey-colored crusted papules, plaques, or bullae	Group A *Streptococcus* and *Staphylococcus aureus*	Systemic or topical anti-staphylococcal antibiotics
Dermatophytosis	Inflammatory or noninflammatory annular scaly plaques; may have hair loss; groin involvement spares scrotum; hyphae on KOH preparation	*Trichophyton*, *Epidermophyton*, or *Microsporum* sp.	Topical azoles, systemic griseofulvin, or azoles
Candidiasis	Inflammatory papules and plaques with satellite pustules, frequently in intertiginous areas; may involve scrotum; pseudohyphae on KOH preparation	*Candida albicans* and other *Candida* species	Topical nystatin or azoles; systemic azoles for resistant disease
Tinea versicolor	Hyperpigmented or hypopigmented scaly patches on the trunk; characteristic mixture of hyphae and spores on KOH preparation ("spaghetti and meatballs")	KOH preparation may show branching hyphae; culture helpful	Topical selenium sulfide lotion or azoles

of "ringworm" or appear as deep inflammatory nodules (on the scalp known as a *kerion*) or granulomas. KOH examination of scale or hair from patients with tinea capitis or inflammatory tinea corporis often does not reveal hyphae, and diagnosis may require culture or biopsy.

℞ TREATMENT

Both topical and systemic therapies may be used to treat dermatophyte infection. Treatment depends on the site involved and the type of infection. Topical therapy is generally effective for uncomplicated tinea corporis, tinea cruris, and tinea pedis. It is not effective as monotherapy for tinea capitis or tinea ungium. Topical imidazoles (miconazole, ketoconazole, econazole, clotrimazole, oxiconazole, and sulconazole), triazoles (terconazole), and allylamines (terbinafine and naftifine) may all be effective topical therapies for dermatophyte infections. Haloprogin, undecylenic acid, ciclopirox olamine, and tolnaftate are also effective, but nystatin is not active against dermatophytes. Treatment should continue until the patient is clear of infection by clinical examination and culture. Tinea pedis often requires longer treatment courses and is associated with very high relapse rates.

Griseofulvin is the drug of choice for dermatophyte infections requiring systemic therapy. A daily dose of 500 mg of microsized or 350 mg of ultramicrosized griseofulvin administered with a fatty meal is an adequate dose for most dermatophyte infections. Unresponsive infections may respond to doubling the dose. The most common side effects of griseofulvin are gastrointestinal distress and headache. It is also rarely associated with blood and liver function abnormalities, and patients on long-term therapy should be monitored at regular intervals.

For chronic noninflammatory tinea pedis, topical agents are useful to limit the pruritus and scaling but are rarely curative. Treatment with oral griseofulvin is effective for tinea pedis, but it may require months of therapy for cure. Even then, it is associated with a high relapse rate, particularly if the nails are involved. The therapy of tinea corporis depends on the extent of disease. Localized infection is best treated with topical imidazoles, but widespread disease, particularly in patients with decreased cellular immunity, requires systemic antifungal therapy. Dermatophyte infection of hair-bearing areas (such as tinea capitis) requires systemic antifungal therapy, and treatment should be continued for 6 to 8 weeks. The adjunctive use of topical antifungal agents in addition to systemic therapy may be useful, but topical therapy alone is not adequate. Markedly inflammatory tinea capitis may result in scarring and hair loss, and systemic or topical glucocorticoids may be helpful in preventing this sequela.

Systemic azoles are now available for oral administration. Ketoconazole was the first oral broad-spectrum azole available in the United States. Its use has been limited by idiosyncratic hepatic toxicity that has been estimated to occur in 1 in 10,000 patients. Both fluconazole and itraconazole are now available for systemic fungal infections, and studies are now underway examining their effectiveness for dermatophyte infections, particularly of the nails. These agents may ultimately replace griseofulvin as first-line therapy for dermatophyte infection.

TINEA VERSICOLOR Tinea versicolor is caused by a nondermatophyte dimorphic fungus, which is a normal inhabitant of the skin. As the yeast form *Pityrosporum orbiculare*, it generally does not cause disease (except for folliculitis in certain individuals). However, in some individuals, it converts to the hyphal form and causes characteristic lesions. The expression of infection is promoted by heat and humidity. The typical lesions consist of oval scaly macules, papules, and patches concentrated on the chest, shoulders, and back, but only rarely on the face or distal extremities. On dark skin, they often appear as hypopigmented areas, while on light skin, they are slightly hyperpigmented. In some darkly pigmented individuals, they may only appear as scaling patches. A KOH preparation from scaling lesions will dem-

onstrate a confluence of short hyphae and round spores (so-called spaghetti and meatballs). Solutions containing sulfur, salicylic acid, or selenium sulfide will clear the infection if used daily for a week, and then intermittently thereafter. Topical imidazoles are also effective.

CANDIDIASIS Candidiasis is a fungal infection caused by a related group of yeasts, whose manifestations may be localized to the skin or rarely may be systemic and life-threatening. The causative organism is usually *Candida albicans* but may also be *C. tropicalis*, *C. parapsilosis*, or *C. krusei*. These organisms are normal saprophytic inhabitants of the gastrointestinal tract but may overgrow (usually due to broad-spectrum antibiotic therapy) and cause disease at a number of cutaneous sites. Other predisposing factors include diabetes mellitus, chronic intertrigo, oral contraceptive use, and cellular immune deficiency. Candidiasis is a very common infection in HIV-infected individuals (see Chap. 308). The oral cavity is commonly involved. Lesions may occur on the tongue or buccal mucosa (thrush) and appear as white plaques. Microscopic examination of scrapings will demonstrate both pseudohyphae and yeast forms. Fissured, macerated lesions at the corners of the mouth (perlèche) are often seen in individuals with poorly fitting dentures and may also be associated with candidal infection. Additionally, candidal infections have an affinity for sites that are chronically wet and macerated and may occur around nails (onycholysis and paronychia) and in intertriginous areas. Intertriginous lesions are characteristically edematous, erythematous, and scaly, with scattered "satellite pustules." In males there is often involvement of the penis and scrotum as well as the inner aspect of the thighs. In contrast to dermatophyte infections, candidal infections are frequently accompanied by a marked inflammatory response. Diagnosis of candidal infection is based upon the clinical pattern and demonstration of yeast on KOH preparation, or culture.

TREATMENT

Treatment routinely involves removing any predisposing factors such as antibiotic therapy or chronic wetness and the use of appropriate topical or systemic antifungal therapy. Effective topical agents include nystatin or topical azoles (miconazole, clotrimazole, econazole, or ketoconazole). These agents are generally effective in clearing mucous membrane or glabrous skin involvement in nonimmunosuppressed patients. The associated inflammatory response that often accompanies candidal infection on glabrous skin should be treated with a mild glucocorticoid lotion or cream (2.5% hydrocortisone) in a drying base. Systemic therapy is generally reserved for immunosuppressed patients or individuals with chronic or recurrent disease who fail to respond to or tolerate appropriate topical therpay. Vulvovaginal candidiasis may respond to treatment with a single dose of fluconazole (150 mg).

WARTS Warts are cutaneous neoplasms that are caused by papilloma viruses. Over 50 different human papilloma viruses (HPV) have been described, and this number will almost certainly continue to grow. Typical verruca vulgaris lesions are sessile, dome-shaped, usually about a centimeter in diameter, and their surface is made up of many small filamentous projections. The HPV that cause typical verruca vulgaris also cause typical plantar warts, flat warts (or verruca plana), and filiform warts in intertriginous areas. Plantar warts are endophytic and are covered by thick keratin. Paring of the wart will generally demonstrate a central core of keratinized debris and punctate bleeding points. Filiform warts are most commonly seen on the face, neck, and skin folds and present as papillomatous lesions on a narrow base. Flat warts are only slightly elevated and have a velvety, nonverrucous surface. They have a propensity for the face, arms, and legs and often are spread by shaving.

Multiple HPV types have been associated with genital tract lesions. They generally begin as small papillomas that may grow to form large fungating lesions. In women, they may involve either the labia, perineum, or perianal skin. Additionally, the mucosa of the vagina, urethra, and anus can be involved, as well as the cervical epithelium. In men, the lesions often occur initially in the coronal sulcus but may be seen on the shaft of the penis, the scrotum, perianal skin, or in the urethra.

Within the past decade, appreciable evidence has accumulated that suggests HPV plays a role in the development of neoplasia of the uterine cervix and external genitalia (see Chap. 99). HPV types 16 and 18 have been most intensely studied, while recent evidence also implicates other types. Lesions may initially appear as small, flat, velvety, hyperpigmented papules occurring on the genitalia or perianal skin. Histologic examination of biopsies from affected sites may reveal changes associated with typical warts and/or features typical of intraepidermal carcinoma (Bowen's disease). Squamous cell carcinomas associated with papilloma virus infections have also been observed in extragenital skin (see Chap. 88). This is most commonly seen in patients immunosuppressed after organ transplantation.

 TREATMENT

There are many modalities available to treat warts, but no single therapy is universally effective. Perhaps the most useful and convenient method for treating warts in almost any location is cryotherapy with liquid nitrogen. Equally effective, but requiring much more patient compliance, is the use of keratolytic agents such as salicylic acid plasters or combinations of lactic acid and salicylic acid. For genital warts, application of podophyllin solution is moderately effective but may be associated with marked local reactions in certain individuals. Other topical agents used include trichloracetic acid or cantharidin. Electrodessication and curettage or carbon dioxide laser excision are also effective therapies but require local anesthesia. Recurrence of warts appears to be common to all these modalities because viral genomic material is present in normal-appearing skin adjacent to the clinical lesions. Treatment of warts should be tempered by the observation that an overwhelming majority of warts in normal individuals resolve spontaneously within 1 to 2 years. Also, only an extremely small proportion of warts are associated with neoplasia, and those are almost exclusively located on the genitalia or perianal skin.

HERPES SIMPLEX   See Chap. 184
HERPES ZOSTER   See Chap. 185

ACNE

ACNE VULGARIS   Acne vulgaris is usually a self-limited disorder primarily of teenagers and young adults, although perhaps 10 to 20 percent of adults may continue to experience some form of the disorder. The permissive factor for the expression of the disease in adolescence is the increase in sebum release by sebaceous glands after puberty. Small cysts, called *comedones*, form in hair follicles due to blockage of the follicular orifice by retention of sebum and keratinous material. The activity of lipophilic yeast (*P. orbiculare*) and bacteria (*Proprionobacterium acnes*) within the comedones releases free fatty acids from sebum, causes inflammation within the cyst, and results in rupture of the cyst wall. An inflammatory foreign-body reaction develops as a result of extrusion of oily and keratinous debris from the cyst.

The clinical hallmark of acne vulgaris is the comedone, which may be closed (whitehead) or open (blackhead). Closed comedones appear as 1- to 2-mm pebbly white papules, which are accentuated when the skin is stretched. They are the precursors of inflammatory lesions of acne vulgaris. The contents of closed comedones are not easily expressed. Open comedones, which rarely result in inflammatory acne lesions, have a large dilated follicular orifice and are filled with easily expressible oxidized, darkened, oily debris. Comedones are usually accompanied by inflammatory lesions: papules, pustules, or nodules.

The earliest lesions seen in early adolescence are generally mildly inflamed or noninflammatory comedones on the forehead. Subsequently, more typical inflammatory lesions develop on the cheeks, nose, and chin. The most common location for acne is the face, but involvement of the chest and back is not uncommon. Most disease remains mild and does not lead to scarring. However, a small number of patients develop large inflammatory cysts and nodules, which may drain and result in significant scarring.

Exogenous and endogenous factors can alter the expression of acne vulgaris. Friction and trauma may rupture preexisting microcomedones and elicit inflammatory acne lesions. This is commonly seen with headbands or chin straps of athletic helmets. Application of comedogenic topical agents in cosmetics or hair preparations or chronic topical exposure to certain industrial compounds that are comedogenic may elicit or aggravate acne. Glucocorticoids, applied topically or administered systemically in high doses, may also elicit acne. Other systemic medications such as lithium, isoniazid, halogens, phenytoin, and phenobarbital may produce acneiform eruptions, or aggravate preexisting acne.

 TREATMENT

Treatment of acne vulgaris is directed toward elimination of comedones, decreasing the population of lipophilic bacteria and yeast, and decreasing inflammation. Although areas affected with acne should be kept clean, there is little evidence to suggest that removal of surface oils plays an important role in therapy. Overly vigorous scrubbing may aggravate acne due to mechanical rupture of comedones. Oral tetracycline or erythromycin in doses of 250 to 1000 mg daily will decrease follicular colonization with some of the lipophilic organisms. They also appear to have an anti-inflammatory effect independent of their antibacterial effect. Topical agents such as retinoic acid, benzoyl peroxide, or salicylic acid may alter the pattern of epidermal desquamation, preventing the formation of comedones and aiding in the resolution of preexisting cysts. Topical antibacterial agents such as benzoyl peroxide, topical erythromycin, clindamycin, or tetracycline are also useful adjuncts to therapy. Severe nodulocystic acne not responsive to oral antibiotics and topical therapy may be treated with the synthetic retinoid isotretinoin. It is used at doses of 0.5 to 2.0 mg/kg as a single daily dose for 15 to 20 weeks. The use of this drug is limited by its teratogenicity, and female patients must be screened for pregnancy prior to initiating therapy, maintain a method of birth control during therapy, and be screened for pregnancy during their treatment course. Patients receiving this medication develop extremely dry skin and cheilitis and must be followed for development of hypertriglyceridemia.

ACNE ROSACEA   Acne rosacea is an inflammatory disorder predominantly affecting the central face. It is seen almost exclusively in adults, only rarely affecting patients under 30 years of age. Rosacea is seen more often in women, but those most severely affected are men. It is characterized by the presence of erythema, telangiectases, and superficial pustules but is not associated with the presence of comedones. Rosacea only rarely involves the chest or back.

There is a relationship between the tendency for pronounced facial flushing and the subsequent development of acne rosacea. Often, individuals with rosacea initially demonstrate a pronounced flushing reaction. This may be in response to heat, emotional stimuli, alcohol, hot drinks, or spicy foods. As the disease progresses, the flush persists longer and longer and may eventually become permanent. Papules, pustules, and telangiectases can become superimposed on the persistent flush. Rosacea of very long standing may lead to connective tissue overgrowth, particularly of the nose (rhinophyma). Rosacea may also be complicated by various inflammatory disorders of the eye, including keratitis, blepharitis, iritis, and recurrent chalazion. These ocular problems are potentially sight-threatening and warrant ophthalmologic evaluation.

 TREATMENT

Acne rosacea can generally be effectively treated with oral tetracycline in doses ranging from 250 to 1000 mg/daily. Topical metronidazole has also been shown to be effective. In addition, the use of low-potency, nonfluorinated topical glucocorticoids, particularly after cool soaks, is helpful in alleviating facial erythema. Fluorinated topical glucocorticoids should be avoided since chronic use of these preparations may actually elicit rosacea. Topical therapy is not effective treatment for ocular disease.

BIBLIOGRAPHY

ARNDT KA et al (eds): *Cutaneous Medicine and Surgery: An Integrated Program in Dermatology.* Philadelphia, Saunders, 1996

BATA-CSORGO Z et al: Intralesional T-lymphocyte activation as a mediator of psoriatic epidermal hyperplasia. J Invest Dermatol 105:89S, 1995

FITZPATRICK TB et al (eds): *Dermatology in General Medicine,* 4th ed. New York, McGraw-Hill, 1993

GOTTLIEB SL et al: Response of psoriasis to a lymphocyte-selective toxin (DAB389 IL-2) suggests a primary immune, but not keratinocyte, pathogenic basis. Nat Med 1:442, 1995

HANAFIN JM et al: Recombinant interferon gamma therapy for atopic dermatitis. J Am Acad Dermatol 28:189, 1993

MARKS JG JR, DELEO VA: *Contact and Occupational Dermatitis.* St. Louis, Mosby Year Book, 1992

MURPHY GF (ed): *Dermatopathology: A Practical Guide to Common Disorders.* Philadelphia, Saunders, 1995

PETO R, ZUR HAUSEN H: *Viral Etiology of Cervical Cancer. Banbury Report.* Cold Spring Harbor, NY, Cold Spring Harbor Laboratory, 1986

PLEWIG G, KLIGMAN AM: *Acne: Morphogenesis and Treatment.* New York, Springer, 1975

SOWDEN JM et al: Double-blind, controlled, cross-over study of cyclosporin in adults with severe refractory atopic dermatitis. Lancet 338:137, 1991

56 *Bruce U. Wintroub, Robert S. Stern*

CUTANEOUS DRUG REACTIONS

Cutaneous reactions are among the most frequent adverse reactions to drugs. Early in drug-induced illness, prompt therapeutic intervention may limit toxicity. This chapter focuses on adverse cutaneous reactions to drugs other than topical agents and reviews the incidence, patterns, and pathogenesis of cutaneous reactions to drugs and therapeutic agents.

USE OF PRESCRIPTION DRUGS IN THE UNITED STATES More than 1.5 billion prescriptions for 60,000 drug products, which include approximately 2000 different active agents, are dispensed each year in the United States. Hospital inpatients alone receive annually about 120 million courses of drug therapy, and half of adult Americans receive prescription drugs on a regular outpatient basis. As much as 15 percent of hospital days are devoted to treatment for drug toxicity.

INCIDENCE OF CUTANEOUS REACTIONS Although adverse drug reactions are common, it is difficult to ascertain their incidence, seriousness, and ultimate health effects. The fact that comprehensive information on these reactions is inadequate in part reflects the difficulty in establishing a system for postmarketing surveillance that is both economically feasible and capable of generating clinically useful data. Available information comes from evaluations of hospitalized patients, epidemiologic surveys, premarketing studies, and voluntary reporting.

In one study about 2 percent of medical inpatients had skin reactions consisting of rash, urticaria, or pruritus during hospitalization, and the overall reaction rate per course of drug therapy was 3:1000. Penicillins, sulfonamides, and blood products accounted for two-thirds of cutaneous reactions. Specific algorithmic estimates of drug-specific quantitative reaction rates for drugs commonly used in inpatients were calculated. Reaction rates for selected commonly used drugs are summarized in Table 56-1. This study showed that most cutaneous reactions occur within 1 week of exposure to the drug. Exceptions were semisynthetic penicillins and ampicillin; about half the reactions to these drugs occurred more than 1 week after initial administration. The risk of allergic reactions was not related to age, diagnosis, or blood level of urea nitrogen on admission. Skin reactions were more frequent among women.

Table 56-1

Rates (per 1000 Recipients) of Skin Reactions to Selected Medications

Drug	Reaction Rate
Amoxicillin	51
Trimethoprim-sulfamethoxazole	34
Ampicillin	33
Other penicillins	20
Blood	21
Allopurinol	8
Gentamycin	5
Barbiturates	4

SOURCE: Adapted from Bigby et al.

The distribution of morphologic patterns of drug eruptions cared for within a Finnish hospital dermatology department with a special interest in fixed drug eruptions included exanthematous reactions (32 percent), urticaria and/or angioedema (20 percent), fixed drug eruptions (34 percent), erythema multiforme (2 percent), Stevens-Johnson syndrome (1 percent), exfoliative dermatitis (1 percent), and photosensitivity reactions (3 percent).

Documenting the risk of the most serious forms of drug eruptions associated with specific drugs remains an important challenge. Based on successful population-based retrospective case registries of toxic epidermal necrolysis (TEN) and Stevens-Johnson syndrome in Germany and France, there are now prospective registries that serve as the basis for case-control studies in these and other countries. These data, together with data from health-maintenance organizations and Medicaid, suggest that the risk of these reactions is from 1 to 10 per million person-years. The drugs most often associated with these reactions include the sulfonamide antibiotics, the aminopenicillins, phenytoin and structurally related antiseizure medications, and some nonsteroidal anti-inflammatory drugs.

PATHOGENESIS OF DRUG REACTIONS

Untoward cutaneous responses to drugs can arise as a result of immunologic or nonimmunologic mechanisms. Immunologic reactions require activation of host immunologic pathways and are designated *drug allergy.* Drug reactions occurring through nonimmunologic mechanisms may be due to activation of effector pathways, overdosage, cumulative toxicity, side effects, ecologic disturbance, interactions between drugs, metabolic alterations, exacerbation of preexisting dermatologic conditions, or inherited protein or enzyme deficiencies. Nonimmunologic cutaneous reactions to drugs are more common, and immunologic reactions are unpredictable when they do occur. It is often not possible to specify the responsible drug or pathogenic mechanism because the skin responds to a variety of stimuli through a limited number of reaction patterns. The mechanism of many drug reactions is unknown.

IMMUNOLOGIC DRUG REACTIONS Drugs frequently elicit an immune response, but only a small number of individuals experience clinical hypersensitivity reactions. For example, most patients exposed to penicillin develop demonstrable antibodies to penicillin but do not manifest drug reactions when exposed to penicillin. Multiple factors determine the capacity of a drug to elicit an immune response, including the *molecular characteristics* of the drug and *host effects.*

Increases in *molecular* size and complexity are associated with increased immunogenicity, and macromolecular drugs such as protein or peptide hormones are highly antigenic. Most drugs are small organic molecules less than 1000 daltons in size, and the capacity of such small molecules to elicit an immune response depends on their ability to act as haptens, i.e., to form stable, usually covalent, bonds with tissue macromolecules. Fortunately, most drugs have little or no ability to form covalent bonds with tissue components, and clinical sensitization results from minor contaminants or conversion of the drugs themselves to reactive metabolic products.

Route of administration of a drug or simple chemical can influence the nature of the *host* immune response. For example, topical application of antigens tends to induce delayed hypersensitivity, and exposure to antigens via oral or nasal cavities stimulates production of secretory immunoglobins, IgA and IgE, and occasionally IgM. Some agents, such as pentadecacatechol, sensitize readily if applied to the skin but do so poorly if ingested orally or applied to a mucosal surface. Frequency of sensitization through intravenous administration of drugs varies, but anaphylaxis is a more likely clinical consequence with this route of exposure.

The degree of drug exposure and individual variability in absorption and metabolism of a given agent may alter immunogenic load. The variable degree of in vivo acetylation of hydralazine provides a clinical example of this phenomenon. Hydralazine produces a lupus-like syndrome associated with antinuclear antibody formation more frequently in patients who acetylate the drug slowly. Frequent high-dose and interrupted courses of therapy are also important risk factors for development of drug allergy.

Pathogenesis of Allergic Drug Reactions   Allergic drug reactions are most commonly IgE-dependent or immune-complex–dependent. Cytotoxicity and delayed hypersensitivity have not been shown to cause systemic cutaneous drug reactions.

IgE-dependent reactions   IgE-dependent drug reactions are usually manifest in the skin and gastrointestinal, respiratory, and cardiovascular systems (see Chap. 310). Primary symptoms and signs include pruritus, urticaria, nausea, vomiting, cramps, bronchospasm, and laryngeal edema and, on occasion, anaphylactic shock with hypotension and death. Immediate reactions may occur within minutes of drug exposure, and accelerated reactions occur hours or days after drug administration. Accelerated reactions are usually urticarial and may include laryngeal edema. IgE-dependent reactions are usually due to penicillins; manifestations are caused by release from sensitized tissue mast cells or circulating basophilic leukocytes of chemical mediators such as histamine, adenosine, leukotrienes, prostaglandins, platelet-activating factor, enzymes, and proteoglycans. Release is triggered when polyvalent drug protein conjugates cross-link IgE molecules fixed to sensitized cells. The clinical manifestations are determined by interaction of the released chemical mediator with its target organ, i.e., skin, respiratory, gastrointestinal, and/or cardiovascular systems. Certain routes of administration favor different clinical patterns (i.e., oral route: gastrointestinal effects; intravenous route: circulating effects).

Immune-complex–dependent reactions   Serum sickness is produced by circulating immune complexes and is characterized by fever, arthritis, nephritis, neuritis, edema, and an urticarial, papular, or pruritic rash (see Chap. 319). The syndrome requires an antigen that remains in the circulation for prolonged periods so that when antibody is synthesized, circulating antigen-antibody complexes are formed. Serum sickness was first described following administration of foreign sera, but drugs are now the usual cause. Drugs that produce serum sickness include the penicillins, sulfonamides, thiouracils, cholecystographic dyes, phenytoin, aminosalicylic acid, streptomycin, heparin, and antilymphocyte globulin. Symptoms develop 6 days or more after exposure to a drug, the latent period representing the time needed to synthesize antibody. The antibodies responsible for immune-complex–dependent drug reactions are largely of the IgG or IgM class.

NONIMMUNOLOGIC DRUG REACTIONS   While nonimmunologic mechanisms are responsible for the majority of drug reactions, only the most important mechanisms will be discussed.

Nonimmunologic Activation of Effector Pathways   Drug reactions may result from nonimmunologic activation of effector pathways by three mechanisms: First, drugs may release mediators directly from mast cells and basophils and present as anaphylaxis or as urticaria and/or angioedema. Urticarial anaphylactic reactions induced by opiates, polymyxin B, tubocurarine, radiocontrast media, and dextrans may occur by this mechanism. Second, drugs may activate complement in the absence of antibody. This is an additional mechanism through which radiocontrast media may act. Third, drugs such as aspirin and other nonsteroidal anti-inflammatory agents may alter pathways of arachidonic acid metabolism; such drugs inhibit the cyclooxygenase

that catalyzes the generation of prostaglandins from arachidonic acid in vitro.

Phototoxicity   Phototoxic reactions may be drug-induced or may occur in metabolic disorders in which an appropriate photosensitizing chemical is overproduced. In each case the phototoxic reaction occurs when enough chromophore (drug or metabolic product) absorbs sufficient radiation in reactive tissue. Drug-induced phototoxic reactions can occur on first exposure, and the incidence of phototoxicity is a direct function of the concentration of sensitizer and amount of light. At least three distinct photochemical mechanisms have been described: First, the reaction between the excited state of a phototoxic molecule and a biologic target may cause formation of a covalent photoaddition product. Second, the phototoxic molecule may absorb protons to form stable photoproducts that are toxic to biologic substrates. Third, radiation of a phototoxic molecule may result in transfer of energy to oxygen molecules and cause formation of toxic oxygen species, such as singlet oxygen, superoxide anion, or hydroxyl radical. Interaction of these species with biologic targets produces photooxidized molecules. Serum protein–dependent systems and circulating effector cells play a role in acute in vivo phototoxic tissue damage due to exogenous agents; normal numbers of polymorphonuclear leukocytes and an intact complement system are required for the full development of demeclocycline-induced phototoxic lesions.

Exacerbation of Preexisting Diseases   A variety of agents can exacerbate preexisting diseases. For example, lithium can exacerbate acne and psoriasis in a dose-dependent manner. Beta-blocking agents and lithium may induce a psoriasiform dermatitis, and withdrawal of glucocorticoids can exacerbate psoriasis or atopic dermatitis. Exacerbations of cutaneous lupus have been noted in association with cimetidine use. Vasodilators may exacerbate rosacea.

Inherited Enzyme or Protein Deficiencies   Specific genetically determined defects in the ability of an individual to detoxify toxic reactive drug metabolites may predispose such individuals to the development of severe drug reactions, especially hypersensitivity syndrome and TEN associated with use of sulfonamides and anticonvulsants.

Alterations of Immunologic Status   Alterations in patients' immunologic status also may modify the risk of cutaneous reactions. Bone marrow transplant patients often experience cutaneous reactions to drugs. These reactions may be very difficult to differentiate from acute graft-versus-host reactions even when skin biopsy is obtained.

Persons infected with human immunodeficiency virus (HIV) are about 5- to 10-fold more likely to develop cutaneous eruptions, and this increased risk is not accounted for merely by the higher number of drugs utilized by these patients (see Chap. 308). The risk of these reactions increases as immunologic function deteriorates. Skin reactions to trimethoprim-sulfamethoxazole are seen in about a third of HIV-infected users of this drug. Dapsone, trimethoprim alone, and amoxicillin-clavulanate are also frequent causes of drug eruptions in these patients. Some drugs result in specific problems in HIV-infected persons. For example, foscarnet causes a painful penile ulcer in a substantial fraction of users. HIV-infected persons are at higher risk of the most serious types of reactions, including TEN and Stevens-Johnson syndrome.

CHARACTERISTIC FEATURES OF CUTANEOUS DRUG REACTIONS

Cutaneous disorders induced by drugs by known mechanisms include urticaria, photosensitivity, disturbances of pigmentation, vasculitis, phenytoin hypersensitivity syndrome, and warfarin necrosis of skin. Reactions of uncertain mechanism include morbilliform reactions, erythema multiforme, fixed drug reactions, erythema nodosum, lichenoid reactions, bullous drug reaction, and TEN.

REACTIONS OF KNOWN CAUSE   Urticaria   *Urticaria* is a skin reaction characterized by pruritic, red wheals. Lesions may vary from a small point to a large area. Individual lesions rarely last more than 24 h. When deep dermal and subcutaneous tissues are also swollen, this reaction is known as *angioedema*. Angioedema may involve mucous membranes and may be part of a life-threatening anaphylactic reaction. Urticarial lesions, along with pruritus and morbilliform (or maculopapular) eruptions, are among the most frequent types of cutaneous reactions to drugs.

Drug-induced urticaria may be caused by three mechanisms: an IgE-dependent mechanism, circulating immune complexes (serum sickness), and nonimmunologic activation of effector pathways. IgE-dependent urticarial reactions usually occur within 36 h but can occur within minutes. Reactions occurring within minutes to hours of drug exposure are termed *immediate reactions*, whereas those which occur 12 to 36 h after drug exposure are designated *accelerated reactions*. Immune-complex–induced urticaria associated with serum sickness may occur from 4 to 12 days after challenge. In this syndrome, the urticarial eruption may be accompanied by fever, hematuria, arthralgias, hepatic dysfunction, and neurologic symptoms.

Certain drugs, such as nonsteroidal anti-inflammatory agents, the angiotensin-converting enzyme (ACE) inhibitors, and radiographic dyes, may induce urticarial reactions, angioedema, and anaphylaxis in the absence of drug-specific antibody. Although aspirin, penicillin, and blood products are the most frequent causes of urticarial eruptions, urticaria has been observed in association with nearly all drugs.

Drugs also may cause chronic urticaria, which lasts more than 6 weeks. The mechanisms of chronic urticaria are unclear. Aspirin frequently exacerbates this problem.

The treatment of urticaria or angioedema depends on the severity of the reaction and the rate at which it is evolving. In addition to drug withdrawal, for patients with only cutaneous symptoms and without symptoms of angioedema or anaphylaxis, oral antihistamines are usually sufficient. For patients with anaphylaxis, systemic glucocorticoids, sometimes intravenously administered, are helpful. In cases with severe respiratory or cardiovascular compromise, epinephrine is useful.

Photosensitivity Eruptions Photosensitivity eruptions are usually most marked in sun-exposed areas but may extend to sun-protected areas. Phototoxic reactions are more common than photoallergic reactions. Phototoxic reactions usually resemble sunburn, can occur with the first exposure to a drug, and are dose-related. The action spectrum for phototoxicity is similar to the ultraviolet absorption spectrum of the drug. No single test system seems to be a successful predictor of the photosensitivity potential for a given compound.

The mechanism for photoallergy to systemic medications is not well defined. Drug, immune response, and light are required to produce clinical photoallergy, and photoallergic reactions may be delayed hypersensitivity responses. Eruptions range from lichenoid papules to eczematous changes.

Orally administered drugs that cause photoallergic or phototoxic reactions include chlorpromazine, tetracycline, thiazides, two nonsteroidal anti-inflammatory agents (benoxaprofen and piroxicam), and the quinalone antibiotics. Based on test systems, the majority of the common photosensitizers seem to have action spectrums in the long-wave ultraviolet A (UV-A) range and are usually phototoxic. This is fortunate, since phototoxic reactions will abate with removal of either the drug or ultraviolet radiation, but some photoallergic reactions may persist after the drug is withdrawn. Because UV-A and visible light which trigger these reactions are not easily absorbed by nonopaque sunscreens, these reactions may be difficult to block.

Photosensitivity reactions are treated by avoiding exposure to ultraviolet light (sunlight) and treating the reaction as one would a sunburn. It should be remembered that individuals who have severe photosensitive reactions may react for some weeks after avoidance of sunlight as the drug may persist in the skin for some time. Occasionally, individuals develop persistent sensitivity to light, necessitating long-term avoidance of sun exposure.

Pigmentation Changes Drugs may cause a variety of pigmentary changes in the skin. Some drugs stimulate melanocytic activity and increase pigmentation. Drug deposition also can lead to pigmentation; this phenomenon occurs with heavy metals. Phenothiazines may be deposited in the skin and cause a slate-gray color. Antimalarial drugs may cause a slate-gray or yellow pigmentation. Long term minocycline use may cause slate-gray hyperpigmentation, especially in areas of chronic inflammation. Inorganic arsenic, once used to treat psoriasis, is associated with diffuse macular pigmentation. Other heavy metals that cause pigmentary changes include silver, gold, bismuth, and mercury. Long-term use of phenytoin can produce a chloasma-like pigmentation in women. Certain cytostatic agents also can cause pigmentary changes. Histologic examination is often diagnostic for drug deposition diseases.

Zidovudine (AZT) is a frequent cause of pigmentation, especially of the nails. Clofazimine, an aminophenazine dye used in the treatment of leprosy, causes a red skin color that is so marked that some patients discontinue therapy. Methysergide produces a red color in the skin and an orange-peel-like texture. Nicotinic acid in large doses may cause brown pigmentation. Oral contraceptives may produce chloasma, and adrenocorticotropin may cause a hypermelanosis similar to that of primary adrenal insufficiency. In addition, amiodarone may cause violaceous hyperpigmentation that is increased in sun-exposed skin. Drugs such as heavy metals, copper, antimalarial and arsenical agents, and ACTH also may discolor oral mucosa.

Vasculitis Cutaneous necrotizing vasculitis often presents as palpable purpuric lesions that may be generalized or limited to the lower extremities or other dependent areas (see Chap. 319). Urticarial lesions, ulcers, and hemorrhagic blisters also occur. Vasculitis may involve other organs, including the liver, kidney, brain, and joints. Drugs are only one cause of vasculitis. Immune-complex–dependent mechanisms are probably responsible for drug-induced vasculitis and/or serum sickness. Propylthiouracil induces a cutaneous vasculitis that is accompanied by leukopenia and splenomegaly. Direct immunofluorescent changes in these lesions suggest immune-complex deposition. Drugs implicated in vasculitic eruptions include allopurinol, thiazides, penicillin, and phenytoin.

Phenytoin (Anticonvulsant) Hypersensitivity Reaction The phenytoin hypersensitivity reaction, one of many phenytoin-induced cutaneous reactions, is an erythematous eruption that eventually becomes purpuric and is accompanied by fever, facial and periorbital edema, tender generalized lymphadenopathy, leukocytosis (often with atypical lymphocytes and eosinophils), hepatitis, and sometimes nephritis. The cutaneous reaction usually begins 1 to 3 weeks after phenytoin is begun and resolves rapidly with drug cessation and treatment with systemic glucocorticoids. The eruption recurs with rechallenge, and cross-reactions with other aromatic anticonvulsants, including carbamazepine and barbiturates, are frequent. This syndrome apparently results from an inherited deficiency of epoxide hydrolase, an enzyme required for metabolism of a toxic intermediate arene oxide that is formed during metabolism of phenytoin by the cytochrome P450 system. Although controlled studies are unavailable, systemic glucocorticoids (prednisone, 0.5 to 1.0 mg/kg) will reduce symptoms, signs, and laboratory evidence of severe anticonvulsant hypersensitivity reactions.

Warfarin Necrosis of the Skin This rare reaction occurs usually between the third and tenth days of therapy with warfarin derivatives, usually in women. Lesions are sharply demarcated, erythematous, indurated, and purpuric and may resolve or progress to formation of large, irregular, hemorrhagic bullae with eventual necrosis and slow-healing eschar formation.

Development of the syndrome is unrelated to drug dose or underlying condition. Favored sites are breasts, thighs, and buttocks. The course is not altered by discontinuation of the drug after onset of the eruption. Similar reactions have been associated with heparin. Warfarin reactions are associated with protein C deficiency. Protein C is a vitamin K–dependent protein with a shorter half-life than other clotting proteins and is in part responsible for control of fibrinolysis. Since warfarin inhibits synthesis of vitamin K–dependent coagulation factors, warfarin anticoagulation in heterozygotes for protein C deficiency causes a precipitous fall in circulating levels of protein C, permitting hypercoagulability and thrombosis in the cutaneous microvasculature, with consequent areas of necrosis. Heparin-induced necrosis may have clinically similar features but is probably due to heparin-induced platelet aggregation with subsequent occlusion of blood vessels.

Warfarin-induced cutaneous necrosis is treated with vitamin K and heparin. Vitamin K reverses the effects of warfarin, and heparin acts as an anticoagulant. Treatment with protein C concentrates may also be helpful in individuals with deficiencies of protein C, the predisposing factor for development of these reactions.

REACTIONS OF UNCERTAIN CAUSE   Morbilliform Reactions   *Morbilliform* or *maculopapular eruptions* may be the most common of all drug-induced reactions, often start on the trunk or areas of pressure or trauma, and consist of erythematous macules and papules that are frequently symmetric and may become confluent. Involvement of mucous membranes, palms, and soles is variable; the eruption may be associated with moderate to severe pruritus and fever.

The pathogenesis is unclear. A hypersensitivity mechanism has been suggested, although these reactions do not always recur following drug rechallenge. Diagnosis is rarely assisted by laboratory tests; differentiation from viral exanthem is the principal differential diagnostic consideration. While these reactions usually require discontinuation of drug, eruptions occasionally may decrease or fade with continued use of the responsible drug.

Morbilliform reactions usually develop within 1 week of initiation of therapy and last 1 to 2 weeks; however, reactions to some drugs, especially penicillin, may begin more than 2 weeks after therapy has begun and last as long as 2 weeks after therapy has ceased. These eruptions are common in patients receiving ampicillin, amoxicillin, or allopurinol; trimethoprim-sulfamethoxazole causes frequent reactions in AIDS patients.

Morbilliform eruptions are usually treated symptomatically. Oral antihistamines and soothing baths are useful for treatment of pruritus. Topical antihistamines may also have some useful effect as do emollients. Short courses of potent topical glucocorticoids can reduce inflammation and symptoms and are probably helpful. The beneficial effect of systemic glucocorticoids relative to risk is less clear for morbilliform eruptions.

Fixed Drug Reactions   These reactions are characterized by one or more sharply demarcated, erythematous lesions in which hyperpigmentation results after resolution of the acute inflammation; with rechallenge, the lesion recurs in the same (i.e., "fixed") location. Lesions often involve the face, genitalia, and oral mucosa and cause burning. Fixed drug eruptions have been associated with phenolphthalein, sulfonamides, tetracycline, phenylbutazone, and barbiturates. Although cross-sensitivity appears to occur between different tetracycline compounds, cross-sensitivity was not elicited when different sulfonamide compounds were administered to patients as part of provocation testing.

Documentation of a characteristic papillary-dermal mononuclear cell infiltrate in close approximation to the dermoepidermal junction may confirm the clinical diagnosis. Extensive basal cell degeneration can lead to formation of bullae and pigment dispersion. Even when lesions are completely healed, melanin-laden macrophages are present in the dermis.

Erythema Nodosum   *Erythema nodosum* is a panniculitis characterized by tender, subcutaneous, erythematous nodules, usually on the anterior portion of the legs. Drug hypersensitivity, frequently involving oral contraceptives, is one cause of this reaction. The mechanism is unknown.

Lichenoid Drug Eruptions   A *lichenoid cutaneous reaction*, clinically and morphologically indistinguishable from lichen planus, is associated with a variety of drugs and chemicals. Eosinophils in lichen planus are more common when the reaction is drug-induced. Gold and antimalarials are most often associated with this eruption. Antihypertensive agents, including beta blockers and captopril, also have been reported to cause a lichenoid reaction.

Bullous Eruptions   Blisters accompany a wide variety of cutaneous reactions, especially the severe morbilliform eruptions, and may be an integral part of phototoxic reactions, Stevens-Johnson syndrome, TEN, and fixed drug eruptions. Nalidixic acid and furosemide cause blistering eruptions indistinguishable from the primary bullous diseases. Other examples are a pemphigus foliaceus–like eruption seen with penicillamine and cicatricial pemphigoid that has been seen with clonidine.

Pustular Eruptions   Active *pustular exanthemic eruptions* also are associated with exposure to drugs, most notably antibiotics. These eruptions can be distinguished from pustular psoriasis by more rapid onset of fever and pustulation and their rapid spontaneous resolution with drug withdrawal.

Erythema Multiforme   *Erythema multiforme* is an acute, self-limited inflammatory disorder of skin and mucous membranes characterized by distinctive iris or target lesions, usually acrally distributed and often associated with sore throat and malaise. Many drugs, including sulfonamides, penicillin, phenytoin, and phenylbutazone, have been reported to cause erythema multiforme; long-acting sulfonamides are the best-studied. Erythema multiforme most often has nondrug causes, most commonly herpes simplex infection.

Stevens-Johnson Syndrome   Stevens-Johnson syndrome (SJS) is a blistering disorder that is usually more severe than erythema multiforme. In addition to erosions of multiple mucous membranes, small blisters developing on dusky or purpuric macules or atypical target lesions characterize this eruption. Total percent of body surface area detachment is less than 10 percent. Overlap SJS/TEN shares characteristics of both SJS and TEN, with 10 to 30 percent of body surface area epidermal detachment. Fever and malaise also occur.

Toxic Epidermal Necrolysis   TEN is the most serious cutaneous drug reaction and may be fatal. Drugs are the most frequent cause of TEN in adults. Onset is generally acute and is characterized by epidermal necrosis involving >30 percent of body area. This reaction is most often associated with sulfonamides, aminopenicillins, anticonvulsants, the oxicam nonsteroidal anti-inflammatory agents, and allopurinol.

DRUGS OF SPECIAL INTEREST

PENICILLIN   The incidence of reactions to penicillin is about 1 percent. Not all adverse reactions are immunologic, as illustrated by ampicillin-induced morbilliform eruptions and central nervous system reactions to procaine penicillin.

IgG, IgM, and IgE antibodies can be produced; IgG and IgM antipenicillin antibodies play a role in the development of hemolytic anemia, whereas anaphylaxis and serum sickness appear to be due to IgE antibodies in serum.

Since penicillin reactions often occur in patients without a prior history of penicillin allergy, the utility of accurate and easily administered tests for sensitization is apparent. Current practice is to perform skin testing with a commercially available penicilloyl determinant preparation (Pre-pen, Kremers-Urban) and with fresh penicillin and, if possible, with another source of minor (nonpenicilloyl) determinants such as aged or base-treated penicillin. Antibodies to minor determinants are common in patients experiencing anaphylaxis. Testing with major determinants alone detects most patients at risk for anaphylaxis.

Twenty-seven percent (10 to 36 percent) of patients with a positive history of penicillin allergy also have a positive skin test, while 6 percent (3 to 10 percent) with a negative history demonstrate a positive skin response to penicillin. Administering penicillin to those patients with a positive skin test produces reactions in a high proportion (50 to 100 percent); conversely, only a few patients (about 0.5 percent) with negative skin tests react to the drug, and reactions tend to be mild and to occur late. Since a negative skin test may occur during or just after an acute reaction, testing should be performed either prospectively or several months after a suspected reaction. As many as 80 percent of patients lose anaphylactic sensitivity and IgE antibody after several years. Radioallergosorbent test (RAST) and other in vitro tests offer no advantage over properly performed skin testing.

Some cross-reactivity exists between penicillin and nonpenicillin β-lactam antibiotics (e.g., cephalosporins). About half of patients who react to penicillin skin testing also react to cephalosporin skin testing; anaphylaxis from cephalosporins has occurred in patients testing positive to penicillin. The benefit of skin testing with penicillin derivatives and cephalosporins in addition to penicillin is uncertain; in one study, none of 120 patients with negative results to penicillin skin tests reacted to semisynthetic penicillinase-resistant agents.

In the face of a positive clinical history of penicillin reaction, another drug should be chosen. If this is not feasible or prudent (e.g., in a pregnant patient with syphilis; with enterococcal endocarditis), skin testing with penicillin is warranted. If skin tests are negative, cautious administration of penicillin is acceptable, although some recommend desensitization of such patients. In those with positive skin tests, desensitization is mandatory if therapeutic use of β-lactam antibiotics is to be undertaken. Various protocols are available, including oral and parenteral approaches. Oral desensitization appears to carry a lesser risk of serious anaphylactic reactions during desensitization. However, desensitization carries the risk of anaphylaxis regardless of how it is performed. After desensitization, many patients experience non-life-threatening IgE-mediated untoward reactions to penicillin during their course of therapy. Desensitization is not effective in those with exfoliative dermatitis or morbilliform reactions due to penicillin.

NONSTEROIDAL ANTI-INFLAMMATORY DRUGS Nonsteroidal anti-inflammatory drugs (NSAIDs), including aspirin (but not salicylates in general) and indomethacin (indometacin), cause two broad categories of allergic-like symptoms in susceptible individuals: (1) approximately 1 percent of persons experience urticaria or angioedema, and (2) about half as many (0.5 percent) experience rhinosinusitis and asthma; however, about 10 percent of adult asthmatics and one-third of individuals with nasal polyposis and sinusitis may respond adversely to aspirin.

Urticaria/angioedema may be delayed up to 24 h and may occur at any age. The rhinosinusitis-asthma syndrome generally develops within 1 h of drug administration. In young people, the reaction pattern often begins as watery rhinorrhea, which can be complicated by nasal and sinus infection, and polyposis, bloody discharge, and nasal eosinophilia. In many individuals with this syndrome, asthma eventually ensues that can be life-threatening whenever NSAIDs are subsequently ingested, and symptoms may persist despite avoidance of these drugs. Proof of the association of symptoms and NSAID use requires either clear-cut history of symptoms following drug ingestion or an oral challenge. For the latter to be performed with relative safety, (1) asthma must be under good control, (2) the procedure must be conducted in a hospital setting by experienced personnel capable of recognizing and treating acute respiratory responses, and (3) the challenge should begin with very low doses (i.e., <30 mg) of aspirin and increase every 1 to 2 h in doubling doses as tolerated to 650 mg. In a study of 50 consecutive patients with a positive history of aspirin-induced bronchospasm, 84 percent developed pulmonary or naso-ocular symptoms with aspirin, but 16 percent did not react; moreover, when subjects who initially tested positive to a challenge were reexposed to aspirin, the clinical reaction pattern was identical in only 60 percent.

While cross-reactivity between NSAIDs is common, it is not immunologic, and patients who are sensitive to NSAIDs cannot be identified by assessment of IgE antibody to aspirin, lymphocyte sensitization, or in vitro immunologic testing. All cross-reacting drugs are cyclooxygenase inhibitors, although salicylates also inhibit cyclooxygenase but (except for aspirin) do not cause the response.

"Desensitization" to the adverse effects of NSAIDs can be accomplished by the challenge procedure above, although repeated challenge at the initial provocation dose may be required. Desensitization works by unknown mechanisms, renders the subject tolerant to all NSAIDs yet studied, persists for at least 24 and up to 96 h, and is probably universal but does not have a positive effect on the underlying disorder.

RADIOCONTRAST MEDIA Large numbers of patients are exposed to radiocontrast agents, and 5 to 10 percent of patients receiving them develop some reaction: urticaria in 1 percent, dyspnea in 0.25

percent, and death in 0.01 percent. Reactions consisting of urticaria and angioedema, asthma, and hypotension mimicking anaphylaxis occur in fewer than 1 percent of radiocontrast procedures. About one-third of those with mild reactions to previous exposure rereact on reexposure.

There is no proof of an immunologic mechanism for radiocontrast media reactions. Elevations in plasma histamine levels occur in those with and without reaction and may be due to the hypertonicity of these media. In addition, complement activation by both classic and alternative pathways occurs in normal and reactive individuals. In short, the mechanism for these reactions is not understood, and no test identifies patients at risk for a radiocontrast medium reaction. Because repeat reactions are common, obtaining a thorough history is the best available technique for identifying those most likely to experience an adverse reaction. Several pretreatment regimens are claimed to decrease the repeat reaction rate to about 10 percent. One such regimen consists of 50 mg prednisone at 13, 7, and 1 h before the procedure and 50 mg diphenhydramine 1 h before the procedure.

HYDANTOINS Phenytoin and other hydantoins cause morbilliform eruptions, erythema multiforme, and TEN, as well as a hypersensitivity reaction (described above) and the pseudolymphoma syndrome. In one study, 5 percent of children treated with phenytoin developed a mild dose-dependent, maculopapular eruption lasting 3 to 5 days and occurring within 2 weeks of starting treatment.

The pseudolymphoma syndrome, consisting of lymphadenopathy and histopathologic lymph node atypia, is a more chronic form of the phenytoin hypersensitivity syndrome, and the cutaneous changes are less marked in this syndrome.

Use of phenytoin is frequently associated with gingival hyperplasia and rarely with a syndrome similar to systemic lupus erythematosus, severe exfoliative dermatitis, and polyarteritis nodosa. Because many hydantoin side effects may be dose-related, drugs that interfere with its elimination (e.g., chloramphenicol) effectively prolong those effects. Sulfasalazine, other sulfonamides, and allopurinol cause reactions that are indistinguishable from the phenytoin hypersensitivity syndrome.

THIAZIDES AND SULFONAMIDES Thiazides are among the most common causes of drug-induced urticaria and morbilliform eruptions; they also cause erythema multiforme, drug-induced cutaneous vasculitis, and lichenoid and photosensitivity eruptions. Because they are substituted sulfonamides, antibodies to these diuretics may cross-react with sulfonamide antibiotics and sulfonamide-based hypoglycemic agents. The combination of sulfamethoxazole and trimethoprim causes two distinct cutaneous reactions: (1) an urticarial eruption beginning in the first few days of treatment and (2) a morbilliform eruption often occurring more than 1 week after therapy has begun. The morbilliform reaction is frequent in patients with AIDS and is associated with pancytopenia in some patients. The eruption may have an intensely purpuric character, independent of the presence of vasculitis. One patient developed TEN and pancytopenia following administration of sulfamethoxazole-trimethoprim.

AGENTS USED IN CANCER CHEMOTHERAPY Since many agents used in cancer chemotherapy inhibit cell division, rapidly proliferating elements of the skin, including hair, mucous membranes, and appendages, are sensitive to their effects; as a result, stomatitis and alopecia are among the most frequent dose-dependent side effects of chemotherapy. Onychodystrophy (dystrophic changes in nails) is also seen with bleomycin, hydroxyurea (hydroxycarbamide), and 5-fluorouracil. Sterile cellulitis and phlebitis and ulceration of pressure areas occur with many of these agents. Urticaria, angioedema, exfoliative dermatitis, and erythema of the palms and soles also have been seen, as has local and diffuse hyperpigmentation. Diagnosis and treatment of these reactions are especially difficult because of the underlying malignancy.

TETRACYCLINES While urticaria and morbilliform eruptions are unusual, tetracyclines sometimes cause other cutaneous side effects, including a photosensitivity reaction (as a result of drug-induced phototoxicity) and onycholysis (sometimes with no apparent cutaneous photosensitivity). These reactions occur with demeclocycline, doxycycline, minocycline, tetracycline, and oxytetracycline. Tetracyclines also cause fixed drug and lichenoid eruptions. An acne-like, gram-negative folliculitis with long-term use of tetracycline is due to overgrowth of resistant bacteria.

Several pigmentary abnormalities have been noted. If used during pregnancy or early childhood, tetracycline stains the teeth, sometimes permanently. Minocycline also has been associated with a flulike syndrome (accompanied by headaches, malaise, and eosinophilia) that recurred with rechallenge.

GLUCOCORTICOIDS Both systemic and topical glucocorticoids cause a variety of skin changes, including acneiform eruptions, atrophy, striae, and other stigmata of Cushing's syndrome, and in sufficiently high doses can retard wound healing. Patients using glucocorticoids are at higher risk for bacterial, yeast, and fungal skin infections that may be misinterpreted as drug eruptions but are in fact drug side effects instead.

ANTIMALARIAL AGENTS Antimalarial agents are used as therapy for several skin diseases, including the skin manifestations of lupus and polymorphous light eruption, but they also can induce cutaneous reactions. In patients with asymptomatic porphyria cutanea tarda, chloroquine increases porphyrin levels and may exacerbate the disease.

Pigmentation disturbances, including black pigmentation of the face, mucous membranes, and pretibial and subungual areas, occur with antimalarials, and quinacrine (mepacrine) causes generalized, cutaneous yellow discoloration. Antimalarial agents may exacerbate psoriasis, and exfoliative dermatitis, fixed drug eruptions, lichenoid dermatitis, and erythema annulare centrifugum have all been reported with their use.

GOLD Chrysotherapy has been associated with a variety of dose-related dermatologic reactions (including maculopapular eruptions) that can develop as long as 2 years after initiation of therapy and require months to resolve. Erythema nodosum, psoriasiform dermatitis, vaginal pruritus, eruptions similar to pityriasis rosea, hyperpigmentation, and lichenoid eruptions resembling those seen with antimalarial agents have been reported. After a cutaneous reaction, it is sometimes possible to reinstitute gold therapy at lower doses without recurrence of the dermatitis.

DIAGNOSIS OF DRUG REACTIONS

Possible causes of an adverse reaction can be assessed as definite, probable, possible, or unlikely based on six variables: (1) previous experience with the drug in the general population, (2) alternative etiologic candidates, (3) timing of events, (4) drug levels or evidence of overdose, (5) patient reaction to drug discontinuation, and (6) patient reaction to rechallenge.

PREVIOUS EXPERIENCE Tables of relative reaction rates are available and are useful to assess the likelihood that a given drug is responsible for a given cutaneous reaction. The specific morphologic pattern of a drug reaction, however, may modify these reaction rates by increasing or decreasing the likelihood that a given drug is responsible for a given reaction. For example, since fixed eruptions due to drug are more often seen with barbiturates than with penicillin, a fixed drug reaction in a patient taking both types of agents is more likely to be due to the barbiturate, even though penicillins have a higher overall drug reaction rate.

ALTERNATIVE ETIOLOGIC CANDIDATES A cutaneous eruption may be due to exacerbation of preexisting disease or to development of new disease unrelated to drugs. For example, a patient with psoriasis may have a flare-up of disease coincidental with administration of penicillin for streptococcal infection; in this case, infection is a more likely cause for the flare-up than drug reaction.

TIMING OF EVENTS Since most drug reactions of the skin occur within 1 to 2 weeks of initiation of therapy, reactions beginning after 2 weeks are less likely to be due to drugs.

DRUG LEVELS Some cutaneous reactions are dependent on dosage or cumulative toxicity. For example, lichenoid dermatoses due to gold administration appear more often in patients taking high doses.

DISCONTINUATION Most adverse cutaneous reactions to drugs remit with discontinuation of the suspected agent. A reaction

Table 56-2

Clinical and Laboratory Findings Associated with More Serious Drug-Induced Cutaneous Clinical Findings

Cutaneous
 Confluent erythema
 Facial edema or central facial involvement
 Skin pain
 Palpable purpura
 Skin necrosis
 Blisters or epidermal detachment
 Positive Nikolsky's sign
 Mucous membrane erosions
 Urticaria
 Swelling of tongue

General
 High fever [temperature >40°C (>104°F)]
 Enlarged lymph nodes
 Arthralgias or arthritis
 Shortness of breath, wheezing, hypotension

Laboratory results
 Eosinophil count >1000/μL
 Lymphocytosis with atypical lymphocytes
 Abnormal liver function tests

SOURCE: Adapted from Roujeau and Stern.

is unlikely to be drug-related if improvement occurs while the drug is continued or if a patient fails to improve after stopping the drug and appropriate therapy.

RECHALLENGE Rechallenge provides the most definitive information concerning adverse cutaneous reactions to drugs, since a reaction failing to recur on rechallenge with a drug is unlikely to be due to that agent. Rechallenge is frequently impractical, however, because the need to ensure patient safety and comfort outweighs the value of the possible information derived from rechallenge.

Of special importance is the rapid recognition of reactions that may become serious or life-threatening. Table 56-2 lists clinical and laboratory features that, if present, suggest the reaction may be serious. Table 56-3 provides key features of the most serious adverse cutaneous reactions.

DIAGNOSIS OF DRUG ALLERGY

Tests for IgE responses include in vivo and in vitro methods, but such tests are available only for a limited number of drugs, including penicillins and cephalosporins, some peptide and protein drugs (insulin, xenogeneic sera), and some agents used for general anesthesia. In vivo testing is accomplished by prick puncture and/or by intradermal skin testing. A wheal-and-flare response 2 × 2 mm greater than that seen with a saline control within 20 min is considered indicative of IgE-mediated mast cell degranulation, provided (1) the patient is not dermographic, (2) the drug does not nonspecifically degranulate mast cells, (3) the drug concentration is not high enough to be irritating, and (4) the buffer itself does not cause wheal-and-flare responses.

Skin testing with major and minor determinants of penicillins or cephalosporins has proved useful for identifying patients at risk of anaphylactic reactions to these agents. However, skin tests themselves carry a small risk of anaphylaxis. Negative skin tests do not rule out IgE-mediated reactivity, and the risk of anaphylaxis in response to penicillin administration in patients with negative skin tests is about 1 percent; about two-thirds of patients with a positive skin test and history of a previous adverse reaction to penicillin experience an allergic response on rechallenge. Skin tests may be negative in allergic patients receiving antihistamines or in those whose allergy is to determinants not present in the test reagent. Although less well studied, similar techniques can identify patients who are sensitive to protein

Table 56-3

Clinical Features of Selected Severe Cutaneous Reactions Often Induced by Drugs

Diagnosis	Mucosal Lesions	Typical Skin Lesions	Frequent Signs and Symptoms	Alternative Causes not Related to Drugs
Stevens-Johnson syndrome	Erosions usually at ≥two sites	Small blisters on dusky purpuric macules or atypical targets; rare areas of confluence; detachment ≤10% of body surface area	10–30% of cases involve fever, lesions of the respiratory and gastrointestinal tracts	Postinfectious erythema multiforme major (especially in the case of infection with herpes simplex or mycoplasma)
Toxic epidermal necrolysis	Erosions usually at ≥two sites	Individual lesions like those seen in Stevens-Johnson syndrome; confluent erythema; outer layer of epidermis separates readily from basal layer with lateral pressure; large sheet of necrotic epidermis; total detachment of >30% of body surface area	Nearly all cases involve fever, "acute skin failure," leukopenia, lesions of the respiratory and gastrointestinal tracts	
Hypersensitivity syndrome	Infrequent	Severe exanthematous rash (may become purpuric), exfoliative dermatitis	30–50% of cases involve fever, lymphadenopathy, hepatitis, nephritis, carditis, eosinophilia, atypical lymphocytes	Cutaneous lymphoma
Small-vessel vasculitis	Infrequent	Palpable purpura, most often on the legs; nodules, ulcerations; urticaria	30–50% of cases involve the gastrointestinal tract, neuritis, fever, glomerulonephritis	Infection, rheumatic diseases, lymphomas
Serum sickness or reactions resembling serum sickness	Absent	Morbilliform lesions, sometimes with urticaria	Fever, arthralgias	Infection
Anticoagulant-induced necrosis	Infrequent	Erythema then purpura and necrosis, especially of fatty areas	Pain in affected areas	Disseminated intravascular coagulopathy, septicemia
Angioedema	Often involved	Urticaria or swelling of central part of face	Respiratory distress, cardiovascular collapse	Insect stings, foods

SOURCE: Adapted from Roujeau and Stern.

drugs and to agents such as gallamine and succinylcholine. Most other drugs are small molecules, and skin testing with them is unreliable.

In vitro testing for IgE may be done by assessing the ability of serum to bind to antigen and then to bind radiolabeled antibody to IgE (RAST test) or by assessing the ability of the drug to cause histamine release from basophils from drug-sensitive individuals. The RAST test is sensitive and specific but is not available for most drugs; even in the case of penicillin it is available for major determinants only. Similarly, basophil histamine release is a research technique that is not generally available.

There are no generally available and reliable tests for sensitivity to NSAIDs, to agents that directly degranulate mast cells, or to drugs that cause manifestations via immune-complex–mediated complement activation. Although it is possible to screen for the absence of IgA antibody, the utility of this maneuver in preventing transfusion-associated anaphylaxis in IgA-deficient individuals has not been documented.

BIBLIOGRAPHY

ALANKO K et al: Cutaneous drug reactions: Clinical types and causative agents. Five-year survey of inpatients (1981–1985). Acta Derm Venereol (Stockh) 69:223, 1989

BASTUJI-GARIN S et al: Clinical classification of cases of toxic epidermal necrolysis, Stevens-Johnson syndrome, and erythema multiforme. Arch Dermatol 129(1):92, 1993

BIELORY L et al: Human serum sickness: A prospective analysis of 35 inpatients treated with equine anti-thymocyte globulin for bone marrow failure. Medicine 67:40, 1988

BIGBY M et al: Drug-induced cutaneous reactions: A report from the Boston Collaborative Drug Surveillance Program on 15,438 consecutive inpatients, 1975–1982. JAMA 256:3358, 1986

CHAN HL et al: The incidence of erythema multiforme, Stevens-Johnson syndrome, and toxic epidermal necrolysis: A population-based study with particular reference to reactions caused by drugs among outpatients. Arch Dermatol 126:43, 1990

COOPMAN SA et al: Cutaneous disease and drug reactions in HIV infection. N Engl J Med 328(23):1670, 1993

JUNG AC, PAAUW DS: Management of adverse reactions to trimethoprim-sulfamethoxazole in human immunodeficiency virus-infected patients. Arch Intern Med 154(21):2402, 1994

KAUFMANN D et al: Severe episode of high fever with rash, lymphadenopathy, neutropenia, and eosinophilia after minocycline therapy for acne. Arch Intern Med 154(17):1983, 1994

ROUJEAU JC, STERN RS: Severe adverse cutaneous reactions to drugs. N Engl J Med 331(19):1272, 1994

——— et al: Acute generalized exanthematous pustulosis: Analysis of 63 cases. Arch Dermatol 127:1333, 1991

57

Jean L. Bolognia, Irwin M. Braverman

SKIN MANIFESTATIONS OF INTERNAL DISEASE

It is now a generally accepted concept in medicine that the skin can show signs of internal disease. Therefore, in textbooks of medicine one finds a chapter describing in detail the major systemic disorders that can be identified by cutaneous signs. The underlying assumption of such a chapter is that the clinician has been able to identify the disorder in the patient and needs only to read about it in the textbook.

In reality, concise differential diagnoses and the identification of these disorders are actually difficult for the nondermatologist because he or she is not well versed in the recognition of cutaneous lesions or their spectrum of presentations. Therefore, the authors of this chapter have decided to cover this particular topic of cutaneous medicine not by discussing individual disorders but by describing and discussing the various presenting clinical signs and symptoms that indicate the presence of these disorders. Concise differential diagnoses will be generated in which the significant diseases will be briefly discussed and distinguished from the more common disorders that have no significance for internal diseases. The latter disorders are reviewed in table form and always need to be excluded when considering the former. For a detailed description of individual diseases, the reader should consult a dermatologic text. The categories of skin lesions that are discussed include papulosquamous lesions, erythroderma, alopecia, figurate lesions, acne, pustules, telangiectasias, hypopigmentation, hyperpigmentation, vesicles/bullae, exanthems, urticaria, papulonodular lesions, purpura, and ulcers. In an attempt to determine the appropriate category for a particular lesion, it is important to examine carefully its surface qualities, shape, and color in addition to the location and distribution (see Chap. 54).

PAPULOSQUAMOUS SKIN LESIONS (Table 57-1) When an eruption is characterized by elevated lesions, papules (<1 cm) or plaques (>1 cm), in association with scale, it is referred to as *papulosquamous*. The most common papulosquamous diseases—*psoriasis*, *tinea*, *pityriasis rosea*, and *lichen planus*—are primary cutaneous disorders (Table 57-2). When psoriatic lesions are accompanied by arthritis, the possibility of psoriatic arthritis or *Reiter's disease* should be considered. A history of oral ulcers, conjunctivitis, uveitis, and/or urethritis points to the latter diagnosis. In *guttate psoriasis* there is an acute onset of small, widely scattered, uniform lesions, often in association with a streptococcal infection. Lithium, beta blockers, human immunodeficiency virus (HIV) infection, and a rapid taper of systemic glucocorticoids are also known to exacerbate psoriasis. Epidermal hyperproliferation and incomplete maturation are responsible for the plaque formation and scale that is characteristic of psoriasis. The papulosquamous diseases are discussed in detail in Chap. 55.

Whenever the diagnosis of pityriasis rosea or lichen planus is made, it is important to review the patient's medications because the

Table 57-1

Selected Causes of Papulosquamous Skin Lesions

1. Primary cutaneous disorders
   a. Psoriasis*
   b. Tinea*
   c. Pityriasis rosea*
   d. Lichen planus*
   e. Parapsoriasis
   f. Bowen's disease (squamous cell carcinoma in situ)†
2. Drugs
3. Systemic diseases
   a. Lupus erythematosus‡
   b. Cutaneous T cell lymphoma
   c. Secondary syphilis
   d. Reiter's disease

* Discussed in detail in Chap. 55.
† Associated with chronic sun exposure and exposure to arsenic.
‡ See also "Red Lesions" in "Papulonodular Skin Lesions."

eruption can be treated by simply discontinuing the offending agent. Pityriasis rosea–like drug eruptions are seen most commonly with beta blockers, captopril, gold, and metronidazole, while the drugs that can produce a lichenoid eruption include gold, antimalarials, thiazides, quinidine, phenothiazines, sulfonylureas, beta blockers, and captopril. Lichen planus–like lesions are also observed in chronic graft-versus-host disease.

Parapsoriasis is an intermediate disease, for it can remain solely as a primary cutaneous disease or it can progress to cutaneous T cell lymphoma (CTCL) after a latency period of as long as 40 years. There are several forms of parapsoriasis, including small plaque (0.5 to 5 cm), large plaque (>6 cm), and retiform. The lesions of both small plaque and large plaque parapsoriasis are thin and salmon-pink in color with fine white scale. In small plaque forms, the lesions are commonly on the trunk but can be widely scattered. In large plaque forms, the most common location is the "girdle" area, and fine wrinkling secondary to epidermal atrophy is often seen. Retiform parapsori-

Table 57-2

Papulosquamous Skin Diseases (Primary Cutaneous Disorders)*

	Characteristic Lesion	Location	Other Findings	Diagnostic Aids	Treatment†
Psoriasis	Pink-red, silvery scale; sharply demarcated	Elbows, knees, scalp, presacral area	Nail dystrophy: pitting, onycholysis, yellow discoloration Arthritis: primarily small joints (hands and feet)	Skin biopsy Culture for beta-hemolytic streptococci	Discontinue possible offending agents; topical glucocorticoids, keratolytics, tars, and vitamin D; UV-B‡; PUVA§; methotrexate
Tinea	Pink-red; central clearing common; active, scaling border	Inner thigh (tinea cruris), palms, soles, any area of body	Invasion of stratum corneum by dermatophytes	KOH and/or fungal culture of scale	Topical or systemic antifungals, e.g., imidazoles, triazoles, allylamines, griseofulvin
Pityriasis rosea	Salmon-pink; oval shape; long axis follows lines of cleavage in the skin, peripheral collarette of scale	Trunk, proximal extremities	Herald patch: initial lesion and usually the largest in size Spontaneous resolution over 2–3 months	Skin biopsy, VDRL to exclude secondary syphilis	Discontinue possible offending agents; antihistamines; topical glucocorticoids; UV-B‡ if widespread
Lichen planus	Violet-colored; polygonal, flat-topped, traversed by thin white lines (Wickham's striae)	Flexor wrists, ankles, presacral area, glans penis	Oral mucosa: lacelike white plaques and/or erosions Pruritus Nail dystrophy: pterygium, longitudinal ridging	Skin biopsy	Discontinue possible offending agents; topical glucocorticoids; PUVA§; oral glucocorticoids

* Discussed in detail in Chap. 55.
† When multiple treatments are listed, the treatments for mild to moderate disease are listed first, followed by those for severe involvement.
‡ UV-B, ultraviolet B.
§ PUVA, psoralens + ultraviolet A irradiation.

asis forms a netlike pattern, and the individual papules are red-brown and flat-topped. The latter two forms of parapsoriasis, large plaque and retiform, can progress to CTCL.

A clue to the development of *CTCL* within lesions of large plaque or retiform parapsoriasis is an increase in the palpable component of the plaque (increased infiltration). In its early stages, CTCL may be confused with ezcema or psoriasis, but it often fails to respond to the appropriate therapy for those inflammatory diseases. The diagnosis of CTCL is established by skin biopsy in which collections of atypical T lymphocytes are found in the epidermis and dermis. As the disease progresses, cutaneous tumors and lymph node involvement may appear.

In *secondary syphilis* there are scattered red-brown papules with thin scale. The eruption often involves the palms and soles, and it can resemble pityriasis rosea. Associated findings are helpful in making the diagnosis, and they include annular plaques on the face, nonscarring alopecia, condyloma lata (broad-based and moist), and mucous patches as well as lymphadenopathy, malaise, fever, headache, and myalgias. The interval between the primary chancre and the secondary stage is usually 4 to 8 weeks, and spontaneous resolution without appropriate therapy is seen.

ERYTHRODERMA (Table 57-3)   *Erythroderma* is the term used when the majority of the skin surface is erythematous (red in color). There may be associated scale, erosions, or pustules as well as shedding of the hair and nails. Potential systemic manifestations include fever, chills, hypothermia, reactive lymphadenopathy, peripheral edema, hypoalbuminemia, and high-output cardiac failure. The major etiologies of erythroderma are (1) *cutaneous diseases* such as psoriasis and dermatitis (Table 57-4), (2) *drugs*, (3) *systemic diseases*, most commonly CTCL, and (4) *idiopathic*. In the first three groups, the location and description of the initial lesions, prior to the development of the erythroderma, aid in the diagnosis. For example, a history of red scaly plaques on the elbows and knees would point to psoriasis. It is also important to examine the skin carefully for a migration of the erythema and associated secondary changes such as pustules or erosions. Migratory waves of erythema studded with superficial pustules are seen in *pustular psoriasis*.

An erythroderma secondary to an underlying cutaneous disease is most commonly due to *psoriasis* or one of the various forms of *dermatitis* (eczema). Each type of dermatitis has its own distinguishing features, but they may be limited to the initial lesions (Table 57-4).

Drug-induced erythroderma (exfoliative dermatitis) may begin as a morbilliform eruption (Chap. 56), or it may arise as diffuse erythema. Fever and peripheral eosinophilia often accompany the eruption, and occasionally there is an associated allergic interstitial nephritis. A number of *drugs* can produce an erythroderma, including penicillins, sulfonamides, carbamazepine, phenytoin, gold, allopurinol, captopril, and granulocyte-macrophage colony stimulating factor. While reactions to anticonvulsants can lead to a pseudolymphoma syndrome, reactions to allopurinol may be accompanied by hepatitis, gastrointestinal bleeding, and nephropathy.

Table 57-3

Causes of Erythroderma

1. Primary cutaneous disorders
   a. Psoriasis*
   b. Dermatitis (atopic, stasis, contact, seborrheic)*
   c. Pityriasis rubra pilaris
2. Drugs
3. Systemic diseases
   a. Cutaneous T cell lymphoma
   b. Lymphoma
4. Idiopathic

* Discussed in detail in Chap. 55.

The most common malignancy that is associated with erythroderma is *CTCL*; in some series, up to 25 percent of the cases of erythroderma were due to CTCL. The patient may progress from isolated plaques and tumors, but more commonly the erythroderma is present throughout the course of the disease (Sézary syndrome). In the Sézary syndrome, there are circulating atypical T lymphocytes, pruritus, and lymphadenopathy. In cases of erythroderma where there is no apparent cause (idiopathic), longitudinal follow-up is mandatory to monitor for the possible development of CTCL. Other types of *lymphoma* can be associated with erythroderma, including Hodgkin's and non-Hodgkin's lymphoma, the former being more common. There also have been isolated case reports of erythroderma secondary to some solid tumors—lung, liver, prostate, thyroid, and colon—but it is usually in a late stage of the disease.

ALOPECIA (Table 57-5)   The two major forms of *alopecia* are scarring and nonscarring. In *scarring alopecia* there is associated fibrosis, inflammation, and loss of hair follicles. A smooth scalp with a decreased number of follicular openings is usually observed clinically, but in some cases the changes are seen only in biopsy specimens from the affected areas. In *nonscarring alopecia* the hair shafts are gone, but the hair follicles are preserved, explaining the reversible nature of nonscarring alopecia.

Primary cutaneous disorders are the most common causes of nonscarring alopecia and they include *telogen effluvium, androgenetic alopecia, alopecia areata, tinea capitis,* and *traumatic alopecia* (Table 57-6). In women with androgenetic alopecia, an elevation in circulating levels of androgens may be seen as a result of ovarian or adrenal gland dysfunction. When there are signs of virilization, such as a deepened voice and enlarged clitoris, the possibility of an ovarian or adrenal gland tumor should be considered.

Exposure to various *drugs* also can cause diffuse hair loss, usually by inducing a telogen effluvium. An exception is the anagen effluvium observed with antimitotic agents such as daunorubicin. Alopecia is a side effect of the following drugs: warfarin, heparin, propylthiouracil, carbimazole, vitamin A, isotretinoin, etretinate, lithium, beta blockers, colchicine, amphetamines, and thallium. Fortunately, spontaneous regrowth usually follows discontinuation of the offending agent.

Less commonly, nonscarring alopecia is associated with *lupus erythematosus* and *secondary syphilis*. In systemic lupus there are two forms of alopecia—one is scarring secondary to discoid lesions (see below) and the other is nonscarring. The latter form may be diffuse and involve the entire scalp, or it may localized to the frontal scalp in the form of multiple short hairs ("lupus hairs"). Scattered, poorly circumscribed patches of alopecia with a "moth-eaten" appearance are a manifestation of the secondary stage of syphilis (see "Papulosquamous Skin Lesions"). Diffuse thinning of the hair is also associated with hypothyroidism, hyperthyroidism, hypopituitarism, HIV infection, and deficiencies of protein, iron, biotin, and zinc.

Scarring alopecia is more frequently the result of a primary cutaneous disorder such as *lichen planus, folliculitis decalvans, cutaneous lupus,* or *linear scleroderma (morphea)* than it is a sign of systemic disease. Although the scarring lesions of *discoid lupus* can be seen in patients with systemic lupus, in the majority of cases the disease process is limited to the skin. Less common causes of scarring alopecia include *sarcoidosis* (see "Papulonodular Skin Lesions") and cutaneous *metastases*.

In the early phases of discoid lupus, lichen planus, and folliculitis decalvans, there are circumscribed areas of alopecia. Fibrosis and subsequent loss of follicles are observed primarily in the center of the individual lesions, while the inflammatory process is most prominent at the periphery. The areas of active inflammation in *discoid lupus* are erythematous with scale, whereas the areas of previous inflammation are often hypopigmented with a rim of hyperpigmentation. In *lichen planus* the peripheral perifollicular macules are violet-colored, and postinflammatory hyperpigmentation is a characteristic finding. Complete examination of the skin and oral mucosa combined with a biopsy and direct immunofluorescence microscopy will aid in distinguishing these two entities. The peripheral active lesions in *folliculitis decalvans* are perifollicular pustules that routinely grow *Staphylococ-*

Table 57-4

Erythroderma (Primary Cutaneous Disorders)

	Initial Lesions	Location of Initial Lesions	Other Findings	Diagnostic Aids	Treatment
Psoriasis*	Pink-red, silvery scale, sharply demarcated	Elbows, knees, scalp, presacral area	Nail dystrophy, arthritis, pustules	Skin biopsy	Etretinate ± PUVA†; methotrexate
Dermatitis:*					
Atopic	Acute: Erythema, fine scale, crust, indistinct borders. Chronic: Lichenification (increased skin markings)	Antecubital and popliteal fossae, neck, hands	Pruritus. Family history of atopy, including asthma, allergic rhinitis or conjunctivitis, and atopic dermatitis. Rule out secondary infection with *S. aureus*. Rule out superimposed irritant contact dermatitis	Skin biopsy	Topical glucocorticoids, tar, and antipruritics; oral antihistamines; open wet dressings; UV-B‡ + UV-A§; PUVA; oral/IM** glucocorticoids. Topical or oral antibiotics
Stasis	Erythema, crusting, excoriations	Lower extremities	Pruritus, lower extremity edema. History of venous ulcers, thrombophlebitis, and/or cellulitis. Rule out cellulitis. Rule out superimposed contact dermatitis, e.g., topical neomycin	Skin biopsy	Topical glucocorticoids; open wet dressings; leg elevation; pressure stockings
Contact	Local: Erythema, crusting, vesicles, and bullae	Depends on offending agent	Irritant—onset often within hours. Allergic—delayed-type hypersensitivity; lag time of 48 h	Patch testing	Remove irritant or allergen; topical glucocorticoids; oral antihistamines; oral/IM** glucocorticoids
Contact	Systemic: Erythema, fine scale, crust	Generalized	Patient has history of allergic contact dermatitis to topical agent and then receives systemic medication that is structurally related, e.g., ethylenediamine (topical) aminophylline (IV)	Patch testing	Same as local
Seborrheic	Pink-red, greasy scale	Scalp, nasolabial folds, eyebrows, intertriginous zones	Flares with stress, HIV infection. Associated with Parkinson's disease	Skin biopsy	Topical glucocorticoids and imidazoles
Pityriasis rubra pilaris	Orange-red, perifollicular, papules	Generalized, but characteristic "skip" areas of normal skin	Wax-like keratoderma. Rule out cutaneous T cell lymphoma	Skin biopsy	Isotretinoin or etretinate; methotrexate

* Discussed in detail in Chap. 55.
† PUVA, psoralens + ultraviolet A irradiation.
‡ UV-B, ultraviolet B.
§ UV-A, ultraviolet A.
** IM, intramuscular.

cus aureus or normal flora. These patients often have other forms of acne and folliculitis and can develop a reactive arthritis.

FIGURATE SKIN LESIONS (Table 57-7) In *figurate* eruptions, the lesions form rings and arcs that are usually erythematous but can be flesh-colored to brown. Most commonly, they are due to primary cutaneous diseases such as *tinea, urticaria, erythema annulare centrifugum,* and *granuloma annulare* (Table 57-8). An underlying systemic illness is found in a second, less common group of migratory annular erythemas. It includes *erythema gyratum repens, erythema migrans, erythema marginatum,* and *necrolytic migratory erythema.*

In *erythema gyratum repens,* one sees hundreds of mobile concentric arcs and wavefronts that resemble the grain in wood. A search for an underlying malignancy is mandatory in a patient with this eruption. *Erythema migrans* is the cutaneous manifestation of Lyme disease, which is caused by the spirochete *Borrelia burgdorferi.* In the initial stage (3 to 30 days after tick bite), a single annular lesion is usually seen, which can expand to ≥10 cm in diameter. Within several days, approximately half the patients develop multiple smaller erythematous lesions at sites distant from the bite. Associated symptoms include fever, headache, myalgias, photophobia, arthralgias, and malar rash. *Erythema marginatum* is seen in patients with rheumatic fever, primarily on the trunk. Lesions are pink-red in color, flat to mildly elevated, and transient.

There are additional cutaneous diseases that present as annular eruptions, but they lack an obvious migratory component. Examples include *CTCL, annular cutaneous lupus,* also referred to as *subacute*

lupus, secondary syphilis, and *sarcoidosis* (see "Papulonodular Skin Lesions").

ACNE (Table 57-9) *Acne vulgaris* and *acne rosacea* are the two major forms of acne (Table 57-10 and Chap. 55). Estrogens decrease sebaceous gland activity, whereas androgens enhance sebum production. Therefore, acne vulgaris in an adult, especially if it is of recent onset, may be a reflection of increased levels of circulating *androgens.* Dysfunction of the ovary or adrenal gland, e.g., polycystic ovary

Table 57-5

Causes of Alopecia

I. Nonscarring alopecia	II. Scarring alopecia
A. Primary cutaneous disorders	A. Primary cutaneous disorders
1. Telogen effluvium	1. Cutaneous lupus
2. Androgenetic alopecia	2. Lichen planus
3. Alopecia areata	3. Folliculitis decalvans
4. Tinea capitis	4. Linear scleroderma (morphea)
5. Traumatic alopecia	B. Systemic diseases
B. Drugs	1. Lupus erythematosus
C. Systemic diseases	2. Sarcoidosis
1. Lupus erythematosus	3. Cutaneous metastases
2. Secondary syphilis	
3. Hypothyroidism	
4. Hyperthyroidism	
5. Deficiencies of protein, iron, biotin, and zinc	
6. HIV infection	

Table 57-6

Nonscarring Alopecia (Primary Cutaneous Disorders)

	Clinical Characteristics	Pathogenesis	Treatment
Telogen effluvium	Diffuse shedding of normal hairs Follows either major stress (high fever, severe infection) or change in hormones (post partum) Reversible without treatment	Stress causes the normally asynchronous growth cycles of individual hairs to become synchronous; therefore, large numbers of growing (anagen) hairs simultaneously enter the dying (telogen) phase	Observation; discontinue any drugs that have alopecia as a side effect; check for underlying metabolic causes, e.g., hypothyroidism, hyperthyroidism
Androgenetic alopecia	Miniaturization of hairs along the midline of the scalp Recession of the anterior scalp line in men and some women	Increased sensitivity of affected hairs to the effects of testosterone Increased levels of circulating androgens (ovarian or adrenal source in women)	If no evidence of hyperandrogen state, then topical minoxidil ± tretinoin; hair transplant
Alopecia areata	Well-circumscribed, circular areas of hair loss, 2–5 cm in diameter In extensive cases, coalescence of lesions and/or involvement of other hair-bearing surfaces of the body Pitting of the nails	The germinative zones of the hair follicles are surrounded by T lymphocytes Occasional associated diseases: hyperthyroidism, hypothyroidism, vitiligo, Down's syndrome	Topical anthralin; intralesional glucocorticoids; topical contact sensitizers
Tinea	Varies from scaling with minimal hair loss to discrete patches with "black dots" (broken hairs) to boggy plaque with pustules (kerion)	Invasion of hairs by dermatophytes, most commonly *Trichophyton tonsurans*	Oral griseofulvin plus 2.5% selenium sulfide or ketoconazole shampoo; examine family members
Traumatic alopecia	Broken hairs Irregular outline	Traction with curlers, rubber bands, braiding Exposure to heat or chemicals Mechanical pulling (trichotillomania)	Discontinuation of offending hair style or chemical treatments; trichotillomania may require hair clipping and observation of shaved pila or biopsy for diagnosis followed by psychotherapy

Table 57-7

Causes of Figurate Skin Lesions

I. Primary cutaneous disorders
  A. Tinea
  B. Urticaria
  C. Erythema annulare centrifugum
  D. Granuloma annulare
II. Systemic diseases
  A. Migratory
    1. Erythema migrans
    2. Erythema gyratum repens
    3. Erythema marginatum
    4. Pustular psoriasis
    5. Necrolytic migratory erythema (glucagonoma syndrome)*
  B. Nonmigratory
    1. Sarcoidosis
    2. Subacute lupus erythematosus
    3. Secondary syphilis
    4. Cutaneous T cell lymphoma

* Migratory erythema with erosions; favors lower extremities and girdle area.

disease, Cushing's syndrome, or partial deficiency of the enzyme 21-hydroxylase, can lead to the hormonal imbalance. Examination of the patient for signs such as hirsutism, androgenetic alopecia, hypertension, and redistribution of subcutaneous fat will aid in the diagnosis.

Exacerbations of acne vulgaris follow the ingestion of several *drugs*, such as iodides, bromides, glucocorticoids, and lithium, as well as the application of oil-containing compounds. Acne-like lesions can be seen in patients with Behçet's disease (see "Ulcers"), and in immunocompromised hosts, disseminated *cryptococcosis* may present as an acneiform eruption.

Patients with the carcinoid syndrome have episodes of flushing of the head, neck, and sometimes the trunk. Resultant skin changes of the face, in particular telangiectasias, mimic the clinical appearance of acne rosacea. Suffusion of the face, as is seen in polycythemia vera, also can be confused with acne rosacea.

PUSTULAR LESIONS *Acneiform eruptions* (see "Acne") and *folliculitis* represent the most common pustular dermatoses. An important consideration in the evaluation of perifollicular pustules is a

Table 57-8

Figurate Eruptions (Primary Cutaneous Disorders)

	Clinical Characteristics	Pathogenesis	Treatment
Tinea	Active, scaling erythematous border with central clearing Expands slowly	Invasion of stratum corneum by dermatophytes	Topical or oral antifungals, e.g., imidazoles, allylamines
Urticaria	Central wheal with erythematous flare Transient and/or migratory Pruritic	Release of histamine from mast cells via immunologic (IgE, type 1 hypersensitivity) or nonimmunologic mechanisms (e.g., morphine)	Remove offending agent; antihistamines; if chronic, exclude urticarial vasculitis
Erythema annulare centrifugum	Enlarges slowly Erythematous, flat or slightly raised "Trailing scale"—scale on inner aspect of expanding ring Buttock, upper thighs	Not known Usually idiopathic Sometimes associated with tinea pedis, drug hypersensitivity Rarely, paraneoplastic	Observation; treat underlying fungal infection
Granuloma annulare	Border composed of flesh-colored to red-brown papules Extremities	Granulomatous process is limited to the skin Unknown etiology Disseminated form is associated with diabetes mellitus	Topical and intralesional glucocorticoids; niacinamide

Table 57-9

CHAPTER 57
Skin Manifestations of Internal Disease

315

Causes of Acneiform Eruptions

I. Primary cutaneous disorders
  A. Acne vulgaris
  B. Acne rosacea
II. Drugs
III. Systemic diseases
  A. Increased androgen production
    1. Adrenal origin, e.g., Cushing's disease, 21-hydroxylase
      deficiency
    2. Ovarian origin, e.g., polycystic ovary disease
  B. Cryptococcosis, disseminated
  C. Behçet's disease

determination of the associated pathogen, e.g., normal flora, *S. aureus*, *Pityrosperum*. Noninfectious forms of folliculitis include eosinophilic folliculitis and folliculitis secondary to drugs such as glucocorticoids and lithium. Eosinophilic folliculitis can be seen in HIV-infected individuals, and it is characterized by multiple pruritic lesions on the face and trunk. Administration of high-dose oral glucocorticoids can result in a widespread eruption of perifollicular pustules on the trunk, characterized by lesions in the same stage of development. With regard to underlying systemic diseases, pustules are a characteristic component of pustular psoriasis and can be seen in septic emboli of bacterial or fungal origin (see "Purpura"). For example, the cutaneous lesions of disseminated gonococcemia often have a halo of erythema surrounding a central pustule.

TELANGIECTASIAS (Table 57-11)   In order to distinguish the various types of telangiectasias, it is important to examine the shape and configuration of the dilated blood vessels. *Linear telangiectasias* are seen on the face of patients with *actinically damaged skin* and *acne rosacea* and are found on the legs of patients with *venous hypertension* and *essential telangiectasia* (Table 57-12). Patients with an unusual form of *mastocytosis* (telangiectasia macularis eruptiva perstans), the *carcinoid* syndrome (see "Acne"), and *ataxia-telangiectasia* also have linear telangiectasias. In ataxia-telangiectasia, linear telangiectasias appear on the bulbar conjunctiva during childhood. Eventually, there is involvement of the ears, eyelids, cheeks, and/or flexural areas such as the antecubital and popliteal fossae. Lastly, linear telangiectasias are found in areas of cutaneous inflammation. For example, lesions of discoid lupus frequently have telangiectasias within them.

Poikiloderma is a term used to describe a patch of skin with (1) reticulated hypo- and hyperpigmentation, (2) wrinkling secondary to epidermal atrophy, and (3) telangiectasias. Poikiloderma does not imply a single disease entity—it is seen in skin damaged by *ionizing radiation*, in the disorders *poikiloderma vasculare atrophicans* (PVA) and *xeroderma pigmentosum*, as well as in patients with connective-tissue diseases, primarily *dermatomyositis* (DM). PVA is a precursor lesion of CTCL, and the areas of poikiloderma usually begin in the flexural areas of the axillae and groin.

In *scleroderma*, the dilated blood vessels have a unique configuration and are known as *mat telangiectasias*. The lesions are broad

macules that usually measure 2 to 7 mm in diameter; occasionally, they are larger in size. Mats have a polygonal or oval shape, and their erythematous color may be uniform or the result of delicate telangiectasias. The most common locations for mat telangiectasias are the face, oral mucosa, and hands—peripheral sites that are prone to intermittent ischemia. The CREST (*c*alcinosis cutis, *R*aynaud's phenomenon, *e*sophageal dysmotility, *s*clerodactyly, and *t*elangiectasia) variant of scleroderma (see Chap. 314) is associated with a chronic course and anticentromere antibodies. Mat telangiectasias are an important clue to the diagnosis of the CREST syndrome as well as systemic scleroderma, for they may be the only cutaneous finding.

Periungual telangiectasias are pathognomonic signs of the three major connective tissue diseases—*lupus erythematosus, scleroderma,* and DM. They are easily visualized by the naked eye, and they occur in at least two-thirds of these patients. In both DM and lupus there is associated nailfold erythema, and in DM the erythema is often accompanied by "ragged" cuticles and fingertip tenderness. Under $10 \times$ magnification, the blood vessels in the nailfolds of lupus patients are tortuous and resemble "glomeruli," whereas in scleroderma and DM there is a loss of capillary loops and those that remain are markedly dilated.

In *hereditary hemorrhagic telangiectasia* (Osler-Rendu-Weber disease), the lesions usually appear during adulthood and are most commonly seen on the mucous membranes, face, and distal extremities, including under the nails. They represent arteriovenous (AV) malformations of the dermal microvasculature, are dark red in color, and are usually slightly elevated. When the skin is stretched over an individual lesion, an eccentric punctum with radiating legs is seen. Although the degree of systemic involvement varies in this autosomal dominant disease, the major symptoms are recurrent epistaxis and gastrointestinal bleeding. The fact that these mucosal telangiectasias are actually AV communications helps to explain their tendency to bleed.

HYPOPIGMENTATION (Table 57-13)   Disorders of hypopigmentation are classified as either diffuse or localized. The classic example of *diffuse* hypopigmentation is *oculocutaneous albinism* (OCA). The most common forms are due to mutations in the tyrosinase gene (type I) or the *P* gene (type II); some of the patients with type I OCA have a total lack of enzyme activity. At birth, different forms of OCA can appear similar—white hair, gray-blue eyes, and pink-white skin. However, the patients with no tyrosinase activity maintain this phenotype, whereas those with decreased activity or *P* gene mutations will acquire some pigmentation of the eyes, hair, and skin as they age. The degree of pigment formation is a function of their racial background, but a pigmentary dilution is readily apparent when they are compared to their first-degree relatives.

The ocular findings in OCA correlate with the degree of hypopigmentation and include decreased visual acuity, nystagmus, photophobia, and monocular vision. Generalized vitiligo, phenylketonuria, and homocystinuria are other unusual causes of diffuse pigmentary dilu-

Table 57-10

Acne (Primary Cutaneous Disorders)*

	Clinical Characteristics	Pathogenesis	Treatment
Acne vulgaris	Erythematous papules, pustules, open comedones (blackheads), closed comedones (whiteheads), and cysts	Epithelial hyperproliferation within the infundibulum of the hair follicle leads to comedone formation	Topical erythromycin, clindamycin, benzoyl peroxide, and tretinoin; oral antibiotics; if severe, isotretinoin
	Areas that contain sebaceous glands: face, neck, upper trunk	Additional factors: sebum-derived free fatty acids, *Propionibacterium acnes*	
Acne rosacea	Papules, pustules; central face	Unknown	Topical and oral antibiotics; topical metronidazole; avoidance of hot or spicy foods and alcohol
	Telangiectasias of nose and cheeks	No increased reactivity of cutaneous blood vessels to vasodilators	
	Facial erythema	Sebum production normal	
	Flushing reaction to hot foods and alcohol		
	Ocular involvement: conjunctivitis, blepharitis, keratitis		

* See Chap. 55.

Table 57-11

Causes of Telangiectasias

I. Primary cutaneous disorders
  A. Linear
    1. Acne rosacea
    2. Actinically damaged skin
    3. Venous hypertension
    4. Essential telangiectasia
  B. Poikiloderma
    1. Ionizing radiation
    2. Poikiloderma vasculare
      atrophicans
  C. Spider angioma
    1. Idiopathic
    1. Pregnancy

II. Systemic diseases
  A. Linear
    1. Carcinoid
    2. Ataxia-telangiectasia
    3. Mastocytosis
  B. Poikiloderma
    1. Dermatomyositis
    2. Xeroderma pigmentosum
    3. Cutaneous T cell
      lymphoma
  C. Mat
    1. Scleroderma
  D. Periungual
    1. Lupus erythematosus
    2. Scleroderma
    3. Dermatomyositis
  E. Papular
    1. Hereditary hermorrhagic
      telangiectasia
  F. Spider angioma
    1. Cirrhosis

Table 57-13

Causes of Hypopigmentation

I. Primary cutaneous disorders
  A. Diffuse
    1. Generalized vitiligo
  B. Localized
    1. Vitiligo
    2. Chemical leukoderma
    3. Piebaldism
    4. Nevus depigmentosus
    5. Postinflammatory
    6. Tinea versicolor

II. Systemic diseases
  A. Diffuse
    1. Oculocutaneous albinism
      a. Hermansky-Pudlak
        syndrome*
      b. Chédiak–Higashi
        syndrome†
  B. Localized
    1. Vogt-Koyanagi-Harada
    2. Scleroderma
    3. Melanoma-associated
      leukoderma
    4. Tuberous sclerosis
    5. Hypomelanosis of
      Ito/mosaicism
    6. Sarcoidosis
    7. Tuberculoid and indeterminate
      leprosy
    8. Cutaneous T cell lymphoma

* Platelet storage defect and restrictive lung disease secondary to deposits of ceroid-like material.
† Giant lysosomal granules and recurrent infections.

tion. In generalized vitiligo, melanocytes are not found in affected skin, whereas in OCA they are present but have decreased activity. Appropriate laboratory tests exclude the other disorders of metabolism.

The differential diagnosis of *localized* hypomelanosis includes the following primary cutaneous disorders: *vitiligo, chemical leukoderma, piebaldism, nevus depigmentosus* (see below), *postinflammatory hypomelanosis*, and *tinea versicolor* (Table 57-14). In this group of diseases, the areas of involvement are macules or patches with a decrease or absence of pigmentation, and in the first four disorders, secondary changes such as scale or crust are absent. Patients with vitiligo have an increased incidence of several autoimmune disorders, including hypothyroidism, Graves' disease, pernicious anemia, Addison's disease, uveitis, alopecia areata, chronic mucocutaneous candidiasis, and the polyglandular autoimmune syndromes (types I and II). Diseases of the thyroid gland are the most frequently associated disorders, occurring in up to 30 percent of patients with vitiligo. Circulating autoantibodies are often found, and the most common ones are antithyroglobulin, antimicrosomal, and antiparietal cell antibodies.

There are three systemic diseases that should be considered in a patient with skin findings suggestive of vitiligo—*Vogt-Koyanagi-Harada syndrome, scleroderma,* and *melanoma-associated leukoderma.* A history of aseptic meningitis, nontraumatic uveitis, tinnitus, hearing loss, and/or dysacousis points to the diagnosis of the Vogt-

Koyanagi-Harada syndrome. In these patients, the face and scalp are the most common locations of pigment loss. The vitiligo-like leukoderma seen in patients with scleroderma has a clinical resemblance to idiopathic vitiligo that has begun to repigment as a result of treatment; that is, perifollicular macules of normal pigmentation are seen within areas of depigmentation. The basis of this leukoderma is unknown; there is no evidence of inflammation in areas of involvement, but it can resolve if the underlying connective-tissue disease becomes inactive. In contrast to idiopathic vitiligo, melanoma-associated leukoderma often begins on the trunk, and its appearance should prompt a search for metastatic disease. The possibility exists that the destruction of normal melanocytes is the result of an immune response against malignant melanocytes.

There are two systemic disorders that may have the cutaneous findings of piebaldism (see Table 57-14). They are *Hirschsprung's disease* and *Waardenburg's syndrome.* A possible explanation for both disorders is an abnormal embryonic migration or survival of two neural crest–derived elements, one of them being melanocytes and the other myenteric ganglion cells (Hirschsprung's disease) or auditory nerve cells (Waardenburg's syndrome). The latter syndrome is characterized by congenital sensorineural hearing loss, dystopia canthorum (lateral displacement of the inner canthi but normal interpupillary distance), heterochromic irises, and a broad nasal root, in addition to the piebaldism. Patients with Waardenburg's syndrome have been shown to have mutations in two genes that encode DNA-binding proteins,

Table 57-12

Telangiectasias (Primary Cutaneous Disorders)

Type	Associated Disorder	Clinical Characteristics	Pathogenesis	Treatment
Linear: Simple red or blue line that disappears with diascopy (pressure)	Acne rosacea	Face Associated with flushing, erythema, papulopustules, and rhinophyma	Vasodilatation	Laser, pulsed dye
	Actinically damaged skin	Face, arms, upper trunk Associated with hypopigmentation, hyperpigmentation, and keratoses	Damage to supportive connective tissue	Laser, pulsed dye
	Essential telangiectasia	Netlike sheets Begins on lower extremities May be widespread More common in women	Unknown	?Sclerotherapy
Spider angioma: Central pulsating punctum with radiating legs	Idiopathic Pregnancy	Upper half of the body Halo of pallor secondary to local steal phenomenon	Proliferation of blood vessels in association with increased circulating estrogens	Laser, pulsed dye

PAX-3 and *MITF*, while some patients with Hirschsprung's disease and white spotting have a mutation in one of the two endothelin receptors.

In *tuberous sclerosis*, the earliest cutaneous sign is an ash leaf spot. These lesions are often present at birth and are usually multiple; however, detection may require Wood's lamp examination, especially in fair-skinned individuals. The pigment within them is reduced but not absent. The average size is 1 to 3 cm, and the common shapes are oval, polygonal, and lance-ovate, whereas the less common shapes are dermatomal and confettilike. Examination of the patient for additional cutaneous signs such as adenoma sebaceum (multiple angiofibromas of the face), ungual and gingival fibromas, fibrous plaques of the forehead, and connective-tissue nevi (shagreen patches) is recommended. It is important to remember that an ash leaf spot on the scalp will result in *poliosis*, which is a circumscribed patch of gray-white hair. Internal manifestations include seizures, mental retardation, central nervous system (CNS) and retinal hamartomas, renal angiomyoli-

pomas, and cardiac rhabdomyomas. The latter can be detected in up to 60 percent of children (<18 years) with tuberous sclerosis by echocardiography.

Nevus depigmentosus is a stable, well-circumscribed hypomelanosis that is present at birth. There is usually a single circular or rectangular lesion, but occasionally the nevus has a dermatomal or whorled pattern. It is important to distinguish this entity from ash leaf spots especially when there are multiple lesions. In *hypomelanosis of Ito* (incontinentia pigmenti achromians), swirls and streaks of hypopigmentation run parallel to one another in a pattern that resembles a marble cake. Lesions may progress or regress with time, and in at least a third of patients, associated abnormalities are found including in the musculoskeletal system (asymmetry), the CNS (seizures and mental retardation), and the eyes (strabismus and hypertelorism). Chro-

Table 57-14

Hypopigmentation (Primary Cutaneous Disorders, Localized)

	Clinical Characteristics	Wood's Lamp Examination (UV-A; Peak = 365 nm)	Skin Biopsy Specimen	Pathogenesis	Treatment
Vitiligo	Acquired; progressive Symmetric areas of complete pigment loss Periorifical—around mouth, nose, eyes, nipples, umbilicus, anus Other areas—flexor wrists, extensor distal extremities Segmental form is less common—unilateral, dermatomal-like	More apparent Chalk-white	Absence of melanocytes Minimal inflammation	Possible autoimmune phenomenon that results in destruction of melanocytes—humoral and/or cellular Alternative hypothesis is self-destruction of melanocytes and circulating antibodies against melanocytes as a secondary phenomenon	Topical glucocorticoids; PUVA*; transplants; depigmentation if widespread
Chemical leukoderma	Similar appearance to vitiligo Often begins on hands Satellite lesions in areas not exposed to chemicals	More apparent Chalk-white	Decreased number or absence of melanocytes	Exposure to chemicals that selectively destroy melanocytes, in particular, phenols and catechols (germicides; rubber products) Release of cellular antigens and activation of circulating lymphocytes may explain satellite phenomenon	Avoid exposure to offending agent, then treat as vitiligo
Piebaldism	Autosomal dominant Congenital, stable White forelock Areas of hypomelanosis contain normally pigmented and hyperpigmented macules of various sizes Symmetric involvement of central forehead, ventral trunk, and mid regions of upper and lower extremities	Enhancement of leukoderma and hyperpigmented macules	Hypomelanotic areas— few to no melanocytes	Defect in migration of melanoblasts from neural crest to ventral skin or failure of melanoblasts to survive or differentiate in these areas Mutations within the *c-kit* proto-oncogene that encodes the tyrosine kinase receptor for mast/stem cell growth factor	None; occasionally transplants
Postinflammatory	Hypopigmentation can develop within active lesions, as in subacute lupus, or after the lesion fades, as in dermatitis	Depends on particular disease Usually less enhancement than in vitiligo	Type of inflammatory infiltrate depends on specific disease	Block in transfer of melanin from melanocytes to keratinocytes could be secondary to edema or decrease in contact time Destruction of melanocytes if inflammatory cells attack basal layer	Treat underlying inflammatory disease
Tinea versicolor	Common disorder Upper trunk and neck Shawl-like distribution Young adults Macules have fine white scale when scratched	Golden fluorescence	Hyphae and budding yeast in stratum corneum	Invasion of stratum corneum by the yeast *Pityrosporum* Yeast is lipophilic and produces C_9 and C_{11} dicarboxylic acids which in vitro inhibit tyrosinase	Selenium sulfide 2.5%; topical imidazoles; oral imidazoles or triazoles

* PUVA = psoralens + ultraviolet A irradiation

mosomal mosaicism and diploid/triploid mixoploidy have been reported in these patients; this lends support to the hypothesis that the pattern is the result of the migration of two clones of primordial melanocytes, each with a different pigment potential.

Localized areas of decreased pigmentation are commonly seen as a result of cutaneous inflammation (see Table 57-14) and have been observed in the skin overlying active lesions of *sarcoidosis* (see "Papulonodular Skin Lesions") as well as in *CTCL*. Cutaneous infections also present as disorders of hypopigmentation, and in *tuberculoid leprosy* there are a few asymmetric patches of hypomelanosis that have associated anesthesia, anhidrosis, and alopecia. Biopsy specimens of the palpable border show dermal granulomas that lack *Mycobacterium leprae* organisms.

HYPERPIGMENTATION (Table 57-15) Disorders of hyperpigmentation are also divided into two groups—localized and diffuse. The *localized* forms are due to an epidermal alteration, a proliferation of melanocytes, or an increase in pigment production. Both *seborrheic keratoses* and *acanthosis nigricans* belong to the first group (Table 57-16). Seborrheic keratoses are common lesions, but in one clinical setting they are a sign of systemic disease, and that setting is the sudden appearance of multiple lesions, often with an inflammatory base and in association with acrochordons (skin tags) and acanthosis nigricans. This is termed the *sign of Leser-Trélat*, and it signifies an internal malignancy. *Acanthosis nigricans* also can be a reflection of an internal malignancy, most commonly of the gastrointestinal tract, and it appears as velvety hyperpigmentation (see Table 57-16). In the majority of patients, acanthosis nigricans is associated with obesity, but it may be a reflection of an endocrinopathy such as acromegaly, Cushing's syndrome, the Stein-Leventhal syndrome, or insulin-resistant diabetes mellitus (type A, type B, and lipoatrophic forms).

A proliferation of melanocytes results in the following pigmented lesions: *lentigo, melanocytic nevus,* and *melanoma* (see Table 57-16). In an adult, the majority of lentigines are related to sun exposure, which explains their distribution. However, in the Peutz-Jeghers and LEOPARD [*l*entigines; *E*CG abnormalities, primarily conduction defects; *o*cular hypertelorism; *p*ulmonary stenosis and subaortic valvular stenosis; *a*bnormal genitalia (cryptorchidism, hypospadias); *r*etardation of growth; and *d*eafness (sensorineural)] syndromes, lentigines do serve as a clue to systemic disease. In the multiple lentigines or *LEOPARD syndrome*, hundreds of lentigines develop during childhood and are scattered over the entire surface of the body. The lentigines in patients with *Peutz-Jeghers syndrome* are located primarily around the nose and mouth, on the hands and feet, and within the oral cavity. While the pigmented macules on the face may fade with age, the oral lesions persist. However, similar intraoral lesions are also seen in Addison's disease and as a normal finding in darkly pigmented individuals. Patients with this autosomal dominant syndrome have multiple benign polyps of the gastrointestinal tract, ovarian tumors, and an approximately 6 percent risk of developing a gastrointestinal malignancy when the polyps arise in the stomach, duodenum, or colon.

Lentigines are also seen in association with cardiac myxomas and have been described in two syndromes whose findings overlap: *LAMB* (*l*entigines, *a*trial myxomas, *m*ucocutaneous myxomas, and *b*lue nevi) *syndrome* and *NAME* [*n*evus, *a*trial myxoma, *m*yxoid neurofibroma, and *e*phelides (freckles)] *syndrome*. These patients also can have evidence of endocrine overactivity in the form of Cushing's syndrome, acromegaly, or sexual precocity.

The third type of localized hyperpigmentation is due to a local increase in pigment production, and it includes *ephelides* (see Table 57-16) and café au lait (CAL) spots. The latter are most commonly associated with two disorders—neurofibromatosis (NF) and Albright's syndrome. *CAL spots* are flat, uniformly light brown in color, and can vary in size from 0.5 to 12 cm. Approximately 80 percent of adult patients with *type I NF* will have six or more CAL spots measuring 1.5 cm or greater in diameter. Additional findings are discussed in the section on neurofibromas (see "Papulonodular Skin Lesions"). In

comparison with NF, the CAL spots in patients with *Albright's disease* [polyostotic fibrous dysplasia with precocious puberty in females due to mosaicism for a mutation in a G protein $(G_s\alpha)$] are usually larger, more irregular in outline, and respect the midline. CAL spots also have been associated with pulmonary stenosis (Watson syndrome), tuberous sclerosis, the LEOPARD syndrome, and ataxia telangiectasia, but a few such lesions can be found in normal individuals.

In incontinentia pigmenti, dyskeratosis congenita, and bleomycin pigmentation, the areas of localized hyperpigmentation form a pattern—swirled in the first, reticulated in the second, and flagellate in the third. Patients with the X-linked dominant disorder *incontinentia pigmenti* can have linear blisters and verrucous papules during infancy. During childhood, parallel swirls and streaks of hyperpigmentation appear on the trunk, and occasionally streaks of hypopigmentation appear on the extremities. Associated findings include seizures, mental retardation, strabismus, cataracts, and delayed or impaired dentition. Biopsy of the streaks will show pigment within dermal macrophages ("incontinent pigment"). In *dyskeratosis congenita*, atrophic reticulated hyperpigmentation is seen on the neck, thighs, and trunk, and it is accompanied by nail dystrophy, pancytopenia, and leukoplakia of the oral and anal mucosa. The latter often develops into squamous cell carcinoma. In addition to the flagellate pigmentation (linear

---

Table 57-15

Causes of Hyperpigmentation

I. Primary cutaneous disorders
  A. Localized
    1. Epidermal alteration
      a. Seborrheic keratosis
      b. Acanthosis nigricans (obesity)
      c. Pigmented actinic keratosis
    2. Proliferation of melanocytes
      a. Lentigo
      b. Nevus
      c. Melanoma
    3. Increased pigment production
      a. Ephelides (freckles)
      b. Café au lait spots
  B. Localized and diffuse
    1. Drugs
II. Systemic diseases
  A. Localized
    1. Epidermal alteration
      a. Seborrheic keratoses (sign of Leser-Trélat)
      b. Acanthosis nigricans (endocrine disorders, paraneoplastic)
    2. Proliferation of melanocytes
      a. Lentigines (Peutz-Jeghers, LEOPARD syndromes, xeroderma pigmentosum)
      b. Nevi [Carney complex (LAMB and NAME syndromes)]*
    3. Increased pigment production
      a. Café au lait spots (neurofibromatosis, Albright's syndrome)
      b. Urticaria pigmentosa (see "Papulonodular Skin Lesions")
    4. Dermal pigmentation
      a. Incontinentia pigmenti
      b. Dyskeratosis congenita
  B. Diffuse
    1. Endocrinopathies
      a. Addison's disease
      b. Nelson's syndrome
      c. Ectopic ACTH syndrome
    2. Metabolic
      a. Porphyria cutanea tarda
      b. Hemochromatosis
      c. Vitamin B_{12}, folate deficiency
      d. Pellagra
      e. Malabsorption, Whipple's disease
    3. Melanosis secondary to metastatic melanoma
    4. Autoimmune
      a. Biliary cirrhosis
      b. Scleroderma
      c. POEMS syndrome
      d. Eosinophilia-myalgia syndrome
    5. Drugs and metals

* Also lentigines.

streaks) on the trunk, patients receiving bleomycin often have hyperpigmentation on the elbows, knees, and small joints of the hand.

Localized hyperpigmentation is seen as a side effect of several other *systemic medications*, including those that produce fixed drug reactions (phenolphthalein, tetracyclines, sulfonamides, barbiturates, and analgesics) and those that can complex with melanin (antimalarials). Fixed drug eruptions recur in the same location as circular areas of erythema that can become bullous and then resolve as brown macules. The eruption usually appears within hours of administration of the offending agent, and common locations include the genitalia, extremities, and perioral region. Chloroquine and hydroxychloroquine produce gray-brown to blue-black discoloration of the shins, hard palate, and face, while blue macules can be seen on the lower extremities and in sites of inflammation with prolonged minocycline administration. Estrogen in oral contraceptives can induce melasma—symmetric brown patches on the face, especially the cheeks, upper lip, and forehead. Similar changes are seen in pregnancy, in patients receiving hydantoin, and in the adult form of Gaucher's disease. In the latter group there is also hyperpigmentation of the distal lower extremities.

In the *diffuse* forms of hyperpigmentation, the darkening of the skin may be of equal intensity over the entire body, or it may be accentuated in sun-exposed areas. The causes of diffuse hyperpigmentation can be divided into four groups—endocrine, metabolic, autoimmune, and drugs. The endocrinopathies that frequently have associated hyperpigmentation include *Addison's disease*, *Nelson's syndrome*, and *ectopic ACTH syndrome*. In these diseases, the increased pigmentation is diffuse, but it is accentuated in the palmar creases, sites of friction, scars, and the oral mucosa. An overproduction of any or all of the pituitary hormones α-MSH (melanocyte-stimulating hormone), ACTH, and β-lipotropin can lead to an increase in melanocyte activity. All these peptides are products of the proopiomelanocortin gene, and therefore, they exhibit homology; e.g., α-MSH and ACTH share 13 amino acids. A minority of the patients with Cushing's disease or hyperthyroidism have generalized hyperpigmentation.

The metabolic causes of hyperpigmentation include *porphyria cutanea tarda* (PCT), *hemochromatosis*, *vitamin B$_{12}$ deficiency*, *folic acid deficiency*, *pellagra*, *malabsorption*, and *Whipple's disease*. In patients with *PCT* (see "Vesicles/Bullae"), the skin darkening is seen in sun-exposed areas and is a reflection of the photoreactive properties of porphyrins. The increased level of iron in the skin of patients with *hemochromatosis* stimulates melanin pigment production and leads to the classic bronze color. Patients with *pellagra* have a brown discoloration of the skin, especially in sun-exposed areas, as a result of nicotinic acid (niacin) deficiency. In the areas of increased pigmentation, there is a thin varnishlike scale. These changes are also seen in patients who are vitamin B$_6$ deficient, have functioning carcinoid tumors (increased consumption of niacin), or take isoniazid. Approximately 50 percent of the patients with *Whipple's disease* have an associated generalized hyperpigmentation in association with diarrhea, weight loss, arthritis, and lymphadenopathy. A diffuse slate-blue color is seen in patients with melanosis secondary to *metastatic melanoma*. Although there is a debate as to whether the color is due to single-cell metastases in the dermis or to a widespread deposition of melanin resulting from the high concentration of circulating melanin precursors, there is more evidence to support the latter.

Of the autoimmune diseases associated with diffuse hyperpigmentation, *biliary cirrhosis* and *scleroderma* are the most common, and occasionally, both disorders are seen in the same patient. The skin is dark brown in color, especially in sun-exposed areas. In biliary cirrhosis the hyperpigmentation is accompanied by pruritus, jaundice, and xanthomas, whereas in scleroderma it is accompanied by sclerosis of the extremities, face, and, less commonly, the trunk. Additional clues to the diagnosis of scleroderma are telangiectasias, calcinosis cutis, Raynaud's phenomenon, and distal ulcerations (see "Telangiectasias"). The differential diagnosis of cutaneous sclerosis with hyperpigmentation includes the *POEMS syndrome* [polyneuropathy; organomegaly

Table 57-16

Hyperpigmentation (Primary Cutaneous Disorders, Localized)

	Clinical Characteristics	Histopathology	Treatment
Seborrheic keratosis	Tan to black papule Warty and/or greasy surface "Stuck on" appearance Trunk	Epidermal hyperplasia	Observation; if irritation or bleeding, removal
Acanthosis nigricans	Velvety surface Neck, axillae, groin Occasionally on dorsum of the hand, corners of mouth	Epidermal folds Increased pigment in basal layer	Topical tretinoin, α-hydroxy acids or keratolytics; weight loss if associated with obesity
Pigmented actinic keratosis	Brown macule, 3–10 mm Rough scale Sun-exposed areas, in particular face and dorsum of hand	Dysplasia of keratinocytes in lower third of epidermis Increased pigment in epidermis	Curettage or cryosurgery
Ephelides (freckles)	2–5-mm macule Tan color Sun-exposed surfaces Darkens following sun exposure	Increased pigment in epidermis	None
Lentigo	0.3–1.5 cm macule Tan to black Most commonly in sun-exposed areas Face, upper trunk, and extremities	Increased number of melanocytes in epidermis Increased pigment in epidermis	Observation; cryosurgery; lasers that target melanin
Nevus			
Junctional	Brown to black macule 2–6 mm	Nests of melanocytes at dermoepidermal junction	Observation for change
Compound	Tan to brown papule 2–8 mm	Nests of melanocytes in epidermis and dermis	Observation for change
Dermal	Flesh-colored papule	Nests of melanocytes in dermis	Observation
Melanoma	Variation in color—brown, black, blue, red, white Irregular outline and surface >5 mm in diameter Asymmetric	Malignant neoplasm of melanocytes	Excision, margins (0.5–2 + cm) dependent on Breslow depth*

* See Chap. 88.

(liver, spleen, lymph nodes); *endocrinopathies* (impotence, gynecomastia); *M*-protein; and *skin changes*]. The skin changes include hyperpigmentation, skin thickening, hypertrichosis, and angiomas.

Recently, an epidemic of the eosinophilia-myalgia syndrome was described that is presumably due to contaminated L-tryptophan preparations. In addition to maculopapular eruptions and alopecia, large areas of sclerodermalike induration are observed with overlying hyperpigmentation.

Diffuse hyperpigmentation that is due to *drugs* or *metals* can result from one of several mechanisms—induction of melanin pigment formation, complexing of the drug or its metabolites to melanin, and deposits of the drug in the dermis. Busulfan; cyclophosphamide; long-term, high-dose ACTH; and inorganic arsenic induce pigment production. Complexes containing melanin or hemosiderin plus the drug or its metabolites are seen in patients receiving chlorpromazine and minocycline. The sun-exposed skin as well as the conjunctivae of patients on long-term, high-dose chlorpromazine can become blue-gray in color. Patients taking minocycline may develop a diffuse blue-gray, muddy appearance in sun-exposed areas in addition to pigmentation of the mucous membranes, teeth, nails, bones, and thyroid. Administration of amiodarone can result in both a phototoxic eruption (exaggerated sunburn) and/or a brown or blue-gray discoloration of sun-exposed skin. Biopsy specimens of the latter show yellow-brown granules in dermal macrophages, which represent intralysosomal accumulations of lipids, amiodarone, and its metabolites. Actual deposits of a particular drug or metal in the skin are seen with silver (argyria), where the skin appears blue-gray in color; gold (chrysiasis), where the skin has a brown to blue-gray color; and clofazimine, where the skin appears reddish brown. The associated hyperpigmentation is accentuated in sun-exposed areas, and discoloration of the eye is seen with gold (sclerae) and clofazimine (conjunctivae).

VESICLES/BULLAE (Table 57-17) Depending on their size, cutaneous blisters are referred to as *vesicles* (<0.5 cm) or *bullae* (>0.5 cm). The primary blistering disorders include *pemphigus vulgaris, pemphigus foliaceus, pemphigus erythematosus, bullous pemphigoid, herpes gestationis, cicatricial pemphigoid, epidermolysis bullosa acquisita, linear IgA disease,* and *dermatitis herpetiformis* (see Chap. 311).

Vesicles and bullae are also seen in *contact dermatitis*, both allergic and irritant forms (see Chap. 55). When there is a linear arrangement of vesicular lesions, an exogenous cause should be suspected. Bullous disease secondary to the ingestion of drugs can take one of several forms, including phototoxic eruptions, isolated bullae, toxic epidermal necrolysis, and erythema multiforme (Chap. 56). Clinically, phototoxic eruptions resemble an exaggerated sunburn with diffuse erythema and bullae in sun-exposed areas. The most commonly associated drugs are thiazides, tetracyclines, sulfonamides, phenothiazines, nonsteroidal anti-inflammatory drugs (NSAIDs), and psoralens. The development of a phototoxic eruption is dependent on the doses of both the drug and UV-A irradiation.

Toxic epidermal necrolysis (TEN) is characterized by bullae that arise on widespread areas of erythema and then slough. This results in large areas of denuded skin. The associated morbidity, such as sepsis, and mortality are relatively high, and they are a function of the extent of epidermal necrosis. In addition, these patients also may have involvement of the mucous membranes and intestinal tract. Drugs are the primary cause of TEN, and the most common offenders are phenytoin, barbiturates, sulfonamides, penicillins, and NSAIDs. Severe acute graft-versus-host disease (grade 4) also can resemble TEN.

In *erythema multiforme* (EM), the primary lesions are pink-red macules and edematous papules, the centers of which may become vesicular. The clue to the diagnosis of EM rather than of a drug-induced morbilliform exanthem is the development of a "dusky" violet color or petechiae in the center of the lesions. Target or iris lesions are also characteristic of EM, and they arise as a result of active centers and borders in combination with centrifugal spread. However,

iris lesions need not be present to make the diagnosis of EM. Preferred sites of involvement include the hands, extensor forearms, palms, soles, and mucous membranes (oral, nasal, ocular, and genital). Hemorrhagic crusts of the lips are characteristic of EM as well as of two other blistering disorders—pemphigus vulgaris and TEN. Fever, malaise, myalgias, sore throat, and cough may precede or accompany the eruption. The lesions of EM usually resolve over 3 to 6 weeks, but they may be recurrent.

Drugs can induce EM, in particular sulfonamides, phenytoin, barbiturates, penicillins, and carbamazepine, but they do not cause the majority of cases, especially in young adults. Infections with herpes simplex are the most common cause of EM in this age group, and the lesions appear 7 to 12 days after the viral eruption. Other infectious agents associated with EM include *Mycoplasma pneumoniae, Histoplasma capsulatum, Coccidioides immitis, Yersinia enterocolitica,* and several viruses (echovirus, coxsackievirus, Epstein-Barr, and influenza). EM also can follow vaccinations with BCG, poliomyelitis, or vaccinia viruses; radiation therapy; and exposure to environmental toxins.

In addition to primary blistering disorders and hypersensitivity reactions, bacterial and viral infections can lead to vesicles and bullae. The most common infectious agents are herpes simplex (see Chap. 184), herpes varicella-zoster (see Chap. 185), and staphylococci (see Chap. 142).

Staphylococcal scalded-skin syndrome (SSSS) and *bullous impetigo* are two blistering disorders associated with staphylococcal (phage group II) infection. In SSSS, the initial findings are redness and tenderness of the central face, neck, trunk, and intertriginous zones. This is followed by short-lived flaccid bullae and a slough or exfoliation of the superficial epidermis. Crusted areas then develop, characteristically around the mouth. SSSS is distinguished from TEN by the following features: younger age group, more superficial site of blister formation, no oral lesions, shorter course, less morbidity and mortality, and an association with staphylococcal exfoliative toxin ("exfoliatin"), not drugs. A rapid diagnosis of SSSS versus TEN can be made by a frozen section of the blister roof or exfoliative cytology of the blister contents. In SSSS the site of staphylococcal infection is usually extracutaneous (conjunctivitis, rhinorrhea, otitis media, pharyngitis, tonsillitis), and the cutaneous lesions are sterile, whereas in *bullous impetigo* the skin lesions are the site of infection. Impetigo is more localized than SSSS, and it usually presents with honey-colored crusts. Occasionally, superficial purulent blisters also form. *Cutaneous emboli* from gram-negative infections may present as isolated bullae, but the base of the lesion is purpuric or necrotic, and it may develop into an ulcer (see "Purpura").

Table 57-17

Causes of Vesicles/Bullae

I. Primary cutaneous diseases	II. Systemic diseases
A. Primary blistering diseases (autoimmune)	A. Autoimmune
1. Pemphigus*	1. Paraneoplastic pemphigus
2. Bullous pemphigoid†	B. Infections
3. Herpes gestationis†	1. Cutaneous emboli†
4. Cicatricial pemphigoid†	C. Metabolic
5. Dermatitis herpetiformis†	1. Diabetic bullae*†
6. Linear IgA disease†	2. Porphyria cutanea tarda†
7. Epidermolysis bullosa acquisita†	3. Porphyria variegata†
. Secondary blistering diseases	4. Pseudoporphyria†
1. Contact*	5. Bullous dermatosis of hemodialysis†
2. Erythema multiforme*†	D. Ischemia
3. Toxic epidermal necrolysis*†	1. Coma bullae
C. Infections	
1. Varicella/zoster*‡	
2. Herpes simplex*‡	
3. Staphylococcal scalded-skin syndrome*	
4. Bullous impetigo*	

* Intraepidermal.   † Subepidermal.   ‡ Also systemic.

Several metabolic disorders are associated with blister formation, including diabetes mellitus, renal failure, and porphyria. Local hypoxia secondary to decreased cutaneous blood flow also can produce blisters, which explains the presence of bullae over pressure points in comatose patients (coma bullae). In *diabetes mellitus*, tense bullae with clear viscous fluid arise on normal skin. The lesions can be as large as 6 cm in diameter and are located on the distal extremities. There are several types of porphyria, but the most common form with cutaneous findings is *PCT*. In sun-exposed areas (primarily the face and hands), the skin is very fragile, and trauma leads to erosions and tense vesicles. These lesions then heal with scarring and formation of milia; the latter are firm, 2- to 3-mm white or yellow papules that represent epidermoid inclusion cysts. Associated findings can include hypertrichosis of the lateral malar region (males) or face (females) and, in sun-exposed areas, hyperpigmentation and firm sclerotic plaques. An elevated level of urinary uroporphyrins confirms the diagnosis and is due to a decrease in uroporphyrinogen decarboxylase activity. Precipitating agents include alcohol, iron, chlorinated hydrocarbons, and hepatitis C infection.

The differential diagnosis of PCT includes (1) *porphyria variegata*—the skin signs of PCT plus the systemic findings of acute intermittent porphyria; it has a diagnostic plasma porphyrin fluorescence emission at 626 nm; (2) *drug-induced bullous photosensitivity* (pseudoporphyria)—the clinical and histologic findings are similar to PCT, but porphyrins are normal; etiologic agents are furosemide, tetracycline, nalidixic acid, dapsone, naproxen, and pyridoxine; (3) *bullous dermatosis of hemodialysis*—the same appearance as PCT, but porphyrins are usually normal or occasionally borderline elevated; patients have chronic renal failure and are on hemodialysis; (4) PCT associated with hepatomas, hepatic carcinomas, and hemodialysis; and (5) *epidermolysis bullosa acquisita* (see Chap. 311).

EXANTHEMS (Table 57-18) Exanthems are characterized by an acute generalized eruption. The two most common presentations are erythematous macules and papules (morbilliform) and confluent blanching erythema (scarlatiniform). *Morbilliform* eruptions are usually due to either *drugs* or *viral infections*. For example, up to 5 percent of the patients receiving penicillins, sulfonamides, captopril, phenytoin, or gold will develop a maculopapular eruption. Accompanying signs may include pruritus, fever, eosinophilia, and transient lymphadenopathy. Similar maculopapular eruptions are seen in the classic childhood viral exanthems, including (1) *rubeola* (measles)—a prodrome of coryza, cough, and conjunctivitis followed by Koplik's spots on the buccal mucosa; the eruption begins behind the ears, at the hairline, and on the forehead and then spreads down the body, often becoming confluent; (2) *rubella*—it begins on the forehead and face and then spreads down the body; it resolves in the same order and is associated with retroauricular and suboccipital lymphadenopathy; and (3) *erythema infectiosum* (fifth disease)—erythema of the cheeks is followed by a reticulated pattern on extremities; it is secondary to a parvovirus infection, and an associated arthritis is seen in adults.

Both measles and rubella are seen in unvaccinated young adults, and an atypical form of measles is seen in adults immunized with either killed measles vaccine or killed vaccine followed in time by live vaccine. In contrast to classic measles, the eruption of atypical measles begins on the palms, soles, wrists, and knuckles, and the lesions may become purpuric. The patient with atypical measles can have pulmonary involvement and be quite ill. Rubelliform and roseoliform eruptions are also associated with *Epstein-Barr virus* (5 to 15 percent of patients), *echovirus, coxsackievirus*, and *adenovirus* infections. Detection of specific IgM antibodies or fourfold elevations in IgG antibodies allows the proper diagnosis. Occasionally, a maculopapular eruption is the result of a drug-viral interaction. For example, about 95 percent of the patients with infectious mononucleosis who are given ampicillin will develop a rash.

Of note, early in the course of infections with *Rickettsia* and *meningococcus*, prior to the development of purpura, the lesions may be erythematous macules and papules. This is also the case in chickenpox prior to the development of vesicles. Maculopapular eruptions

are associated with early *HIV infection*, early secondary *syphilis*, *typhoid fever*, and *acute graft-versus-host* disease. In the last, lesions frequently begin on the palms and soles; the macular rose spots of typhoid fever involve primarily the anterior trunk.

The prototypic *scarlatiniform* eruption is seen in *scarlet fever* and is due to an erythrotoxin produced by group A beta-hemolytic streptococcal infections, most commonly pharyngitis. This eruption is characterized by diffuse erythema, which begins on the neck and upper trunk, and red perifollicular puncta. Additional findings include a white strawberry tongue (white coating with red papillae) followed by a red strawberry tongue (red tongue with red papillae); petechiae of the palate; a facial flush with circumoral pallor; linear petechiae in the antecubital fossae; and desquamation of the involved skin, palms, and soles 5 to 20 days after onset of the eruption. A similar desquamation of the palms and soles is seen in toxic shock syndrome, Kawasaki's disease, and after severe febrile illnesses. Certain strains of staphylococci also produce an erythrotoxin that leads to the same clinical findings as in streptococcal scarlet fever, except that the antistreptolysin O titers are not elevated.

In *toxic shock syndrome* (TSS), staphylococcal (phage group I) infections produce an exotoxin (TSST-1) that causes the fever and rash, as well as enterotoxins. Initially, the majority of cases were reported in menstruating women who were using tampons. However, other sites of infection, including wounds and vaginitis, may produce TSS. The diagnosis of TSS is based on clinical criteria, and three of these involve mucocutaneous sites. The clinical criteria are (1) fever; (2) diffuse erythema of the skin; (3) desquamation of the palms and soles 1 to 2 weeks after onset of illness; (4) hypotension; and (5) involvement of three or more organ systems, including the gastrointestinal tract, muscles, kidney, liver, CNS, hematologic (thrombocytopenia), and mucous membranes. The latter is characterized as hyperemia of the vagina, oropharynx, or conjunctivae. Similar systemic findings have been described in *Streptococcal toxic shock–like syndrome* (Chap. 143), and although an exanthem is seen less often than in TSS due to a staphylococcal infection, the underlying infection is often in the soft tissue.

The cutaneous eruption in *Kawasaki's disease* (mucocutaneous lymph node syndrome) is polymorphous, but the two most common forms are morbilliform and scarlatiniform. The majority of cases are seen in children less than 5 years of age, but adult cases have been reported. The diagnosis is based on a fever lasting more than 5 days plus four of the five following criteria: (1) bilateral conjunctival injection; (2) exanthem; (3) cervical lymphadenopathy, usually unilateral; (4) erythema and edema of the hands and feet followed by desquamation; and (5) diffuse erythema of the oropharynx, red strawberry

Table 57-18

Causes of Exanthems

I. Morbilliform
   A. Drugs
   B. Viral
      1. Rubeola (measles)
      2. Rubella
      3. Erythema infectiosum
      4. Epstein-Barr, echovirus, coxsackievirus, and adenovirus
      5. Early HIV
   C Bacterial
      1. Typhoid fever
      2. Early secondary syphilis
      3. Early *Rickettsia*
      4. Early meningococcus
   D. Acute graft-versus-host disease
II. Scarlatiniform
   A. Scarlet fever
   B. Toxic shock syndrome
   C. Kawasaki's disease

tongue, and erosions with crusting on the lips. This clinical picture can resemble TSS and scarlet fever, but clues to the diagnosis of Kawasaki's disease are the cervical lymphadenopathy, lip erosions, and increased platelets. The most serious associated systemic finding in this disease is coronary aneurysm secondary to arteritis. Aneurysms may lead to sudden death, primarily within the first 30 days of the illness. Scarlatiniform eruptions are also seen in the early phase of SSSS (see "Vesicles/Bullae") and as reactions to drugs.

URTICARIA (Table 57-19) *Urticaria* (hives) are transient lesions that are composed of a central wheal surrounded by an erythematous halo. Individual lesions are round, oval, or figurate, and they are often pruritic. *Acute* and *chronic* urticaria have a wide variety of allergic etiologies. Less common systemic causes of urticaria are mastocytosis (urticaria pigmentosa), hyperthyroidism, malignancy, and juvenile rheumatoid arthritis (JRA). In JRA, the lesions coincide with the fever spike and are transient but not migratory as in erythema marginatum.

The common *physical urticarias* include *dermographism, solar urticaria, cold urticaria*, and *cholinergic urticaria*. Patients with dermographism exhibit linear wheals following minor pressure or scratching of the skin. It is a common disorder, affecting approximately 5 percent of the population. Solar urticaria characteristically occur within minutes of sun exposure and are a skin sign of one systemic disease—erythropoietic protoporphyria. In addition to the urticaria, these patients have subtle pitted scarring of the nose and hands. Cold urticaria are precipitated by exposure to the cold, and therefore, exposed areas are usually affected. In some cases, the disease is associated with abnormal circulating proteins—more commonly cryoglobulins and cold hemolysins and less commonly cryofibrinogens and cold agglutinins. Additional systemic symptoms include wheezing and syncope, thus explaining the need for these patients to avoid swimming in cold water. Cholinergic urticaria are precipitated by heat, exercise, or emotion and are characterized by small wheals with relatively large flares. They are occasionally associated with wheezing.

Whereas urticaria are the result of dermal edema, subcutaneous edema leads to the clinical picture of *angioedema*. Sites of involvement include the eyelids, lips, tongue, larynx, and gastrointestinal tract as well as the subcutaneous tissue. Angioedema occurs alone or in combination with urticaria, including urticarial vasculitis and the physical urticarias. Both acquired and hereditary (autosomal dominant) forms of angioedema occur (see Chap. 310), and in the latter, urticaria is rarely seen.

Urticarial vasculitis is an immune complex disease that may be confused with simple urticaria. In contrast to simple urticaria, individual lesions tend to last longer than 24 h, and they usually develop central petechiae that can be observed even after the urticarial phase has resolved. The patient also may complain of burning rather than pruritus. On biopsy, there is a leukocytoclastic vasculitis of the small blood vessels. Although many cases of urticarial vasculitis are idio-

pathic in origin, it can be a reflection of an underlying systemic illness such as lupus erythematosus, Sjögren's syndrome, or hereditary complement deficiency. There is a spectrum of urticarial vasculitis that ranges from purely cutaneous to multisystem involvement. The most common systemic signs and symptoms are arthralgias and/or arthritis, nephritis, and crampy abdominal pain, with asthma and chronic obstructive lung disease seen less often. Hypocomplementemia occurs in one- to two-thirds of patients, even in the idiopathic cases. Similar cutaneous, joint, and renal findings can be seen in the prodrome of *hepatitis B infection, serum sickness*, and *serum sickness–like illnesses*.

PAPULONODULAR SKIN LESIONS (Table 57-20) In the *papulonodular diseases*, the lesions are elevated above the surface of the skin and may coalesce to form plaques. The location, consistency, and color of the lesions are the keys to their diagnosis. This section is organized on the basis of color, and the color groups are white, flesh, pink, yellow, red, red-brown, blue, violaceous, purple, and brown-black.

White Lesions In *calcinosis cutis* there are firm white to white-yellow papules with an irregular surface. When the contents are discharged, a chalky white material is seen. *Dystrophic* calcification is seen at sites of previous inflammation or damage to the skin. It develops in acne scars as well as on the distal extremities of patients with scleroderma and in the subcutaneous tissue and intermuscular fascial planes in DM. The latter is more extensive and is more commonly seen in children. An elevated calcium phosphate product, as in secondary hyperparathyroidism, can lead to nodules of *metastatic* calcinosis cutis, which tend to be subcutaneous and periarticular. This form is often accompanied by calcification of muscular arteries and subsequent ischemic necrosis (calciphylaxis).

Flesh-Colored Lesions There are several types of flesh-colored lesions, including epidermoid inclusion cysts, lipomas, rheumatoid nodules, neurofibromas, angiofibromas, neuromas, and adnexal tumors such as tricholemmomas. Both *epidermoid inclusion cysts* and *lipomas* are very common mobile subcutaneous nodules—the former are rubbery and compressible, and they drain cheeselike material (sebum and keratin) if incised. Lipomas are firm and somewhat lobulated on palpation. When extensive facial epidermoid inclusion cysts develop in childhood or there is a family history of such lesions, the patient should be examined for other signs of Gardner's syndrome, including osteomas and desmoid tumors. *Rheumatoid nodules* are firm, 0.5- to 4-cm nodules that tend to localize around pressure points, especially the elbows. They are seen in approximately 20 percent of patients with rheumatoid arthritis and 6 percent of patients with Still's disease. Biopsies of the nodules show palisading granulomas. Similar lesions that are smaller and shorter-lived are seen in rheumatic fever.

Neurofibromas (benign Schwann cell tumors) are soft papules or nodules that exhibit the "button-hole" sign, that is, they invaginate into the skin with pressure in a manner similar to a hernia. Single lesions are seen in normal individuals, but multiple neurofibromas, usually in combination with six or more CAL spots measuring >1.5 cm (see "Hyperpigmentation") and multiple Lisch nodules, are seen in von Recklinghausen's disease (NF type I). Lisch nodules are 1-mm yellow-brown spots within the iris that are best observed with slit-lamp examination. Additional manifestations include axillary freckling and peripheral and CNS tumors (see Chap. 375). In some patients the neurofibromas are localized and unilateral, whereas in others they are limited to the CNS.

Angiofibromas are firm, pink to flesh-colored papules that measure from 3 mm to several centimeters in diameter. When they are located on the central cheeks (adenoma sebaceum) or multiple fibromas are seen around the nails, the patient has tuberous sclerosis. It is an autosomal disorder, and the associated findings are discussed in the section on ash leaf spots as well as in Chap. 375.

Neuromas (benign proliferation of nerve fibers) are also firm, flesh-colored papules. They are more commonly found at sites of amputation and as rudimentary supernumerary digits. However, when there are multiple neuromas on the eyelids, lips, distal tongue, and/or oral mucosa, the patient should be investigated for other signs of the multiple

Table 57-19

Causes of Urticaria

I. Primary cutaneous disorders
   A. Acute and chronic urticaria
   B. Physical urticaria
      1. Dermatographism
      2. Solar urticaria*
      3. Cold urticaria*
      4. Cholinergic urticaria*
   C. Angioedema (hereditary and acquired)*
II. Systemic diseases
   A. Urticarial vasculitis
   B. Hepatitis B infection
   C. Serum sickness
   D. Angioedema (hereditary and acquired)

* Also systemic.

Table 57-20

CHAPTER 57
Skin Manifestations of Internal Disease   **323**

Papulonodular Skin Lesions According to Color Groups

I. White
  A. Calcinosis cutis
II. Flesh
  A. Rheumatoid nodule
  B. Neurofibromas (von Recklinghausen's disease)
  C. Angiofibromas (tuberous sclerosis)
  D. Neuromas (multiple endocrine neoplasia syndrome, type 2b)
  E. Adnexal tumors
    1. Basal cell epitheliomas (basal cell nevus syndrome)
    2. Tricholemmomas (Cowden's disease)
  F. Primary cutaneous disorders
    1. Epidermal inclusion cysts
    2. Lipomas
III. Pink/translucent
  A. Amyloidosis
  B. Papular mucinosis
IV. Yellow
  A. Xanthomas
  B. Tophi
  C. Necrobiosis lipoidica
  D. Pseudoxanthoma elasticum
  E. Sebaceous adenomas (Torre's syndrome)
V. Red
  A. Papules
    1. Angiokeratomas (Fabry's disease)
    2. Bacillary angiomatosis (primarily in AIDS)
  B. Papules/plaques
    1. Cutaneous lupus
    2. Lymphoma cutis
    3. Leukemia cutis

  C. Nodules
    1. Panniculitis
    2. Cutaneous polyarteritis nodosa
    3. Systemic vasculitis
  D. Primary cutaneous disorders
    1. Arthropod bites
    2. Cherry hemangiomas
    3. Infections, e.g., erysipelas, sporotrichosis
    4. Polymorphous light eruption
    5. Lymphocytoma cutis (pseudolymphoma)
VI. Red-brown
  A. Sarcoidosis
  B. Sweet's syndrome
  C. Urticaria pigmentosa
  D. Erythema elevatum diutinum (chronic leukocytoclastic vasculitis)
  E. Lupus vulgaris
VII. Blue
  A. Venous malformations (blue rubber bleb syndrome)
  B. Primary cutaneous disorders
    1. Venous lake
    2. Blue nevus
VIII. Violaceous
  A. Lupus pernio (sarcoidosis)
  B. Lymphoma cutis
  C. Cutaneous lupus
IX. Purple
  A. Kaposi's sarcoma
  B. Angiosarcoma
  C. Palpable purpura
X. Brown-black
  See "Hyperpigmentation"
XI. Any color
  A. Metastases

endocrine neoplasia syndrome, type 2b. Associated findings include marfanoid habitus, protuberant lips, intestinal ganglioneuromas, and medullary thyroid carcinoma (>75 percent of patients) (see Chap. 340).

Adnexal tumors are derived from pluripotential cells of the epidermis that can differentiate toward hair, sebaceous, apocrine, or eccrine glands or remain undifferentiated. *Basal cell epitheliomas* (BCEs) are examples of adnexal tumors that have little or no evidence of differentiation. Clinically, they are translucent papules with rolled borders, telangiectasias, and central erosion. BCEs commonly arise in sun-damaged skin of the head and neck. When a patient has multiple BCEs, especially prior to age 30, the possibility of the basal cell nevus syndrome should be raised. It is inherited as an autosomal dominant trait and is associated with jaw cysts, palmar and plantar pits, frontal bossing, rib anomalies, and calcification of the falx cerebri and diaphragma sellae. *Tricholemmomas* are also flesh-colored adnexal tumors, but they differentiate toward hair follicles and can have a wartlike appearance. The presence of multiple tricholemmomas on the face and oral mucosa points to the diagnosis of Cowden's disease (multiple hamartoma syndrome). The oral tricholemmomas are found primarily on the tongue and gingiva and give these areas a cobblestone appearance. Internal organ involvement (in decreasing order of frequency) includes fibrocystic disease and carcinoma of the breast, adenomas and carcinomas of the thyroid, and gastrointestinal polyposis. Keratoses of the palms, soles, and dorsa of the hands are also seen.

Pink Lesions The cutaneous lesions associated with primary systemic *amyloidosis* are pink in color and translucent. Common locations are the face, especially the periorbital and perioral regions, and flexural areas. On biopsy, homogeneous deposits of amyloid are seen

in the dermis and in the walls of blood vessels; the latter lead to an increase in vessel wall fragility. As a result, petechiae and purpura develop in clinically normal skin as well as in lesional skin following minor trauma, hence the term "pinch purpura." Amyloid deposits are also seen in the striated muscle of the tongue and result in macroglossia.

Even though specific mucocutaneous lesions are rarely seen in secondary amyloidosis and are present in only about 30 percent of the patients with primary amyloidosis, a rapid diagnosis of systemic amyloidosis can be made by an examination of abdominal subcutaneous fat. By special staining, deposits are seen around blood vessels or individual fat cells in 40 to 50 percent of patients. There are also three forms of amyloidosis that are limited to the skin and that should not be construed as cutaneous lesions of systemic amyloidosis. They are macular amyloid (upper back), lichenoid amyloidosis (usually lower extremities), and nodular amyloidosis. In macular and lichenoid amyloidosis, the deposits are composed of altered epidermal keratin. Recently, macular and lichenoid amyloidosis have been associated with multiple endocrine neoplasia syndrome, type 2a.

Patients with *multicentric reticulohistiocytosis* also have pink-colored papules and nodules on the face and mucous membranes as well as on the extensor surface of the hands and forearms. They have a polyarthritis that can mimic rheumatoid arthritis clinically. On histologic examination, the papules have characteristic giant cells that are not seen in biopsies of rheumatoid nodules. Pink to flesh-colored papules that are firm, 2 to 5 mm in diameter, and often in a linear arrangement are seen in patients with *papular mucinosis*. This disease is also referred to as *lichen myxedematosus* or *scleromyxedema*. The latter name comes from the brawny induration of the face and extremities that may accompany the papular eruption. Biopsy specimens of the papules show localized mucin deposition, and serum protein electrophoresis demonstrates a monoclonal spike of IgG, usually with a λ light chain.

Yellow Lesions Several systemic disorders are characterized by yellow-colored cutaneous papules or plaques—hyperlipidemia (xanthomas), gout (tophi), diabetes (necrobiosis lipoidica), pseudoxanthoma elasticum, and Torre's syndrome (sebaceous tumors). Eruptive xanthomas are the most common form of *xanthomas*, and they are associated with hypertriglyceridemia (types I, III, IV, and V). Crops of yellow papules with erythematous halos occur primarily on the extensor surfaces of the extremities and the buttocks in association with elevations of the circulating triglycerides. They spontaneously involute with a fall in serum lipids. Increased β-lipoproteins (primarily types II and III) result in one or more of the following types of xanthoma: xanthelasma, tendon xanthomas, and plane xanthomas. Xanthelasma are found on the eyelids, whereas tendon xanthomas are frequently associated with the Achilles and extensor finger tendons; plane xanthomas are flat and favor the palmar creases, face, upper trunk, and scars. Tuberous xanthomas are frequently associated with hypertriglyceridemia, but they are also seen in patients with hypercholesterolemia (type II) and are found most frequently over the large joints or hand. Biopsy specimens of xanthomas show collections of lipid-containing macrophages (foam cells).

Patients with several disorders, including biliary cirrhosis, can have a secondary form of hyperlipidemia with associated tuberous and planar xanthomas. However, patients with myeloma have *normolipemic* flat xanthomas. This latter form of xanthoma may be ≥12 cm in diameter and is most frequently seen on the upper trunk or side of the neck. It is also important to note that the most common setting for eruptive xanthomas is uncontrolled diabetes mellitus. The least specific sign for hyperlipidemia is xanthelasma because at least 50 percent of the patients with this finding have normal lipid profiles.

In *tophaceous gout* there are deposits of monosodium urate in the skin around the joints, particularly those of the hands and feet. Additional sites of *tophi* formation include the helix of the ear and the olecranon and prepatellar bursae. The lesions are firm, yellow in color, and occasionally discharge a chalky material. Their size varies from

1 mm to 7 cm, and the diagnosis can be established by polarization of the aspirated contents of a lesion. Lesions of *necrobiosis lipoidica* are found primarily on the shins (90 percent), and the majority of patients have diabetes mellitus or develop it subsequently. Characteristic findings include a central yellow color, atrophy (transparency), telangiectasias, and an erythematous border. Ulcerations also can develop within the plaques. Biopsy specimens show necrobiosis of collagen, granulomatous inflammation, and obliterative endarteritis.

In *pseudoxanthoma elasticum* (PXE) there is an abnormal deposition of calcium on the elastic fibers of the skin, eye, and blood vessels. In the skin, the flexural areas such as the neck, axillae, antecubital fossae, and inguinal area are the primary sites of involvement. Yellow papules coalesce to form reticulated plaques that have an appearance similar to that of plucked chicken skin. In severely affected skin, hanging, redundant folds develop. Some patients have a more subtle macular form of the disease, and careful inspection is required. Biopsy specimens of involved skin show swollen and irregularly clumped elastic fibers with deposits of calcium. In the eye, the calcium deposits in Bruch's membrane lead to angioid streaks and choroiditis; in the arteries of the heart, kidney, gastrointestinal tract, and extremities, the deposits lead to angina, hypertension, gastrointestinal bleeding, and claudication, respectively. Long-term administration of D-penicillamine can lead to PXE-like skin changes as well as elastic fiber alterations in internal organs.

Adnexal tumors that have differentiated toward sebaceous glands include sebaceous adenoma, sebaceous epithelioma, sebaceous carcinoma, and sebaceous hyperplasia. Except for sebaceous hyperplasia, which is commonly seen on the face, these tumors are fairly rare. Patients with Torre's syndrome have *sebaceous adenomas*, and in the majority of cases there are multiple such tumors. These patients also can have sebaceous carcinomas and sebaceous hyperplasia as well as keratoacanthomas. The internal manifestations of Torre's syndrome include *multiple* carcinomas of the gastrointestinal tract (primarily colon) as well as cancers of the larynx, genitourinary tract, ovary, and endometrium. Some patients also have a strong family history of cancer.

Red Lesions   Cutaneous lesions that are red in color have a wide variety of etiologies, and in an attempt to simplify their identification, they will be subdivided into papules, papules/plaques, and subcutaneous nodules. Common red papules include *arthropod bites* and *cherry hemangiomas*; the latter are small, bright-red, dome-shaped papules that represent benign proliferation of capillaries. In patients with AIDS, the development of multiple red hemangioma-like lesions points to bacillary angiomatosis, and biopsy specimens show clusters of bacilli that stain positive with the Warthin-Starry stain; the pathogens have been identified as *Rochalimaea henselae* and *Bartanella quintana*. Disseminated visceral disease is seen primarily in immunocompromised hosts but can occur in immunocompetent individuals.

Multiple *angiokeratomas* are seen in Fabry's disease, an X-linked recessive lysosomal storage disease that is due to a deficiency of α-galactosidase A. The lesions are red to red-blue in color and can be quite small in size (1 to 3 mm), with the most common location being the lower trunk. Associated findings include chronic renal failure, peripheral neuropathy, and corneal opacities (cornea verticillata). Electron photomicrographs of angiokeratomas and clinically normal skin demonstrate lamellar lipid deposits in fibroblasts, pericytes, and endothelial cells that are diagnostic of this disease. Widespread acute eruptions of erythematous papules are discussed in the section on exanthems.

There are several infectious diseases that present as erythematous papules or nodules in a sporotrichoid pattern, that is, in a linear arrangement along the lymphatic channels. The two most common etiologies are *Sporothrix schenckii* (sporotrichosis) and *Mycobacterium marinum* (atypical mycobacteria). The organisms are introduced as a result of trauma, and a primary inoculation site is often seen in addition to the lymphatic nodules. Additional causes include *Nocardia, Leishmania,*

and other dimorphic fungi; culture of lesional tissue will aid in the diagnosis.

The diseases that are characterized by erythematous plaques with scale are reviewed in the papulosquamous section, and the various forms of dermatitis are discussed in the section on erythroderma. Additional disorders in the differential diagnosis of red papules/plaques include *erysipelas, polymorphous light eruption* (PMLE), *lymphocytoma cutis, cutaneous lupus, lymphoma cutis,* and *leukemia cutis*. The first three diseases represent primary cutaneous disorders. PMLE is characterized by erythematous papules and plaques in a primarily sun-exposed distribution—dorsum of the hand, extensor forearm, and face. Lesions follow exposure to both UV-B and UV-A, and in northern latitudes PMLE is most severe in the late spring and early summer. A process referred to as "hardening" occurs with continued UV exposure, and the eruption fades, but in temperate climates it will recur in the spring. PMLE must be differentiated from cutaneous lupus, and this is accomplished by histologic examination and direct immunofluorescence of the lesions. Lymphocytoma cutis (pseudolymphoma) is a *benign* proliferation of lymphocytes in the skin that presents as infiltrated pink-red to red-purple papules and plaques. It must be distinguished from cutaneous lupus and lymphoma cutis.

Several types of red plaques are seen in patients with systemic *lupus*, including (1) erythematous urticarial plaques across the cheeks and nose in the classic butterfly rash; (2) erythematous discoid lesions with fine or "carpet-tack" scale, telangiectasias, central hypopigmentation, peripheral hyperpigmentation, follicular plugging, and atrophy located on the face, scalp, external ears, arms, and upper trunk; and (3) psoriasiform or annular lesions of subacute lupus with hypopigmented centers located on the face, extensor arms, and upper trunk. Additional cutaneous findings include (1) a violaceous flush on the face and vee of the neck; (2) urticarial vasculitis (see "Urticaria"); (3) lupus panniculitis (see below); (4) diffuse alopecia; (5) alopecia secondary to discoid lesions; (6) periungual telangiectasias and erythema; (7) erythema multiforme–like lesions that may become bullous; and (8) distal ulcerations secondary to Raynaud's phenomenon, vasculitis, or livedoid vasculitis. Patients with only discoid lesions usually have the form of lupus that is limited to the skin. However, 2 to 10 percent of these patients eventually develop systemic lupus. Direct immunofluorescence of involved skin shows deposits of IgG or IgM and C3 in a granular distribution along the dermal-epidermal junction.

In *lymphoma cutis* there is a proliferation of malignant lymphocytes or histiocytes in the skin, and the clinical appearance resembles that of lymphocytoma cutis—infiltrated pink-red to red-purple papules and plaques. Lymphoma cutis can occur anywhere on the surface of the skin, whereas the sites of predilection for lymphocytomas are the malar ridge, tip of the nose, earlobes, forearms, and scrotum. Patients with non-Hodgkin's lymphomas have specific cutaneous lesions more often than those with Hodgkin's disease, and occasionally, the skin nodules precede the development of extracutaneous non-Hodgkin's lymphoma. Arcuate lesions are sometimes seen in lymphoma and lymphocytoma cutis as well as in CTCL. *Leukemia cutis* has the same appearance as lymphoma cutis, and specific lesions are seen more commonly in monocytic leukemias than in lymphocytic or granulocytic leukemias. Cutaneous chloromas (granulocytic sarcomas) may precede the appearance of circulating blasts in acute nonlymphocytic leukemia and, as such, represent a form of aleukemic leukemia cutis.

Common causes of erythematous subcutaneous nodules include inflamed epidermoid inclusion cysts, acne cysts, and furuncles. *Panniculitis*, an inflammation of the fat, also presents as subcutaneous nodules and is frequently a sign of systemic disease. There are several forms of panniculitis, including erythema nodosum, erythema induratum, lupus profundus, Weber-Christian disease, α_1-antitrypsin deficiency, factitial, and fat necrosis secondary to pancreatic disease. In all these disorders, except for erythema nodosum, the lesions may break down and ulcerate or heal with a scar. The shin is the most common location for the nodules of erythema nodosum, whereas the calf is the most common location for lesions of erythema induratum. In erythema nodosum the nodules are initially red but then develop a blue color as they resolve. Patients with erythema nodosum and no underlying systemic illness can still have fever, malaise, leukocytosis, arthralgias and/or arthritis. However, the possibility of an underlying illness should be excluded, and the most common associations are streptococcal infections, upper respiratory infections, sarcoidosis, and inflammatory bowel disease. The less common associations include tuberculosis, histoplasmosis, coccidioidomycosis, psittacosis, drugs (oral contraceptives, sulfonamides, aspartame, bromides, iodides), cat-scratch fever, and infections with *Yersinia*, *Salmonella*, and *Chlamydia*.

In many patients, erythema induratum/nodular vasculitis is an idiopathic disease; however, in approximately 25 to 50 percent of patients, polymerase chain reaction (PCR) analysis will demonstrate *Mycobacterium tuberculosis* complex DNA. The lesions of lupus profundus are found primarily on the face, upper arms, and buttocks (sites of abundant fat) and are seen in both the cutaneous and systemic forms of lupus. The overlying skin may be normal, erythematous, or have the changes of discoid lupus. The subcutaneous fat necrosis that is associated with pancreatic disease is presumably secondary to circulating lipases and is seen in patients with pancreatic carcinoma as well as in patients with acute and chronic pancreatitis. In this disorder and in Weber-Christian disease there may be an associated arthritis, fever, and inflammation of visceral fat. Histologic examination of deep incisional biopsy specimens will aid in the diagnosis of the particular type of panniculitis.

Subcutaneous erythematous nodules are also seen in *cutaneous polyarteritis nodosa* (PAN) and as a manifestation of *systemic vasculitis*, e.g., systemic PAN, allergic granulomatosis, or Wegener's granulomatosis. Cutaneous PAN presents with painful subcutaneous nodules and ulcers within a red-purple, netlike pattern of livedo reticularis. The latter is due to slowed blood flow through the superficial horizontal venous plexus. The majority of lesions are found on the lower extremity, and while arthralgias and myalgias may accompany cutaneous PAN, there is no evidence of systemic involvement. In both the cutaneous and systemic forms of vasculitis, skin biopsy specimens of the associated nodules will show the changes characteristic of a vasculitis; the size of the vessel involved will depend on the particular disease.

Red-Brown Lesions The cutaneous lesions in *sarcoidosis* are classically red to red-brown in color, and with diascopy (pressure with a glass slide) a yellow-brown residual color is observed that is secondary to the granulomatous infiltrate. The waxy papules and plaques may be found anywhere on the skin, but the face is the most common location. Usually there are no surface changes, but occasionally the lesions will have scale. Biopsy specimens of the papules show "naked" granulomas in the dermis, i.e., granulomas surrounded by a minimal number of lymphocytes. Other cutaneous findings in sarcoidosis include annular lesions with an atrophic or scaly center, papules within scars, hypopigmented macules and papules, alopecia, acquired ichthyosis, erythema nodosum, and lupus pernio (see below). Additional physical findings are peripheral lymphadenopathy and parotid and lacrimal gland enlargement. When there is cutaneous involvement of the hands, radiographs often will show lytic lesions in the underlying bone.

The differential diagnosis of sarcoidosis includes foreign-body granulomas produced by chemicals such as beryllium and zirconium, late secondary syphilis, and *lupus vulgaris*. Lupus vulgaris is a form of cutaneous tuberculosis that is seen in previously infected and sensitized individuals. There is often underlying active tuberculosis elsewhere, usually in the lungs or lymph nodes. At least 90 percent of the lesions occur in the head and neck area and are red-brown plaques with a yellow-brown color on diascopy. Secondary scarring and squamous cell carcinomas can develop within the plaques. Cultures or PCR analysis of the lesions should be done because it is rare for the acid-fast stain to show bacilli within the dermal granulomas.

Sweet's syndrome is characterized by red to red-brown plaques and nodules that are frequently painful and occur primarily on the head, neck, and upper extremities. The patients also have fever, neutrophilia, and a dense dermal infiltrate of neutrophils in the lesions. In approximately 10 percent of the patients there is an associated malignancy, most commonly acute nonlymphocytic leukemia. Sweet's syndrome also has been reported with lymphoma, chronic leukemia, myeloma, myelodysplastic syndromes, and solid tumors (primarily of the genitourinary tract). Extracutaneous sites of involvement include joints, muscles, eye, kidney (proteinuria, occasionally glomerulonephritis), and lung (neutrophilic infiltrates). The idiopathic form of Sweet's syndrome is seen more often in women, following a respiratory tract infection.

A generalized distribution of red-brown macules and papules is seen in the form of mastocytosis known as *urticaria pigmentosa* (see Chap. 310). Each lesion represents a collection of mast cells in the dermis, with hyperpigmentation of the overlying epidermis. Stimuli such as rubbing and heat cause these mast cells to degranulate, and this leads to the formation of localized urticaria (Darier's sign). Additional symptoms can result from mast cell degranulation and include headache, flushing, diarrhea, and pruritus. Mast cells also infiltrate various organs such as the liver, spleen, and gastrointestinal tract in up to 30 to 50 percent of patients with urticaria pigmentosa, and accumulations of mast cells in the bones may produce either osteosclerotic or osteolytic shadows on radiographs. In the majority of these patients, however, the internal involvement remains fairly static. A subtype of chronic leukocytoclastic vasculitis, *erythema elevatum diutinum* (EED), also presents with papules that are red-brown in color. The papules coalesce into plaques on the extensor surfaces of knees, elbows, and the small joints of the hand. Flares of EED have been associated with streptococcal infections.

Blue Lesions Lesions that are blue in color are the result of either vascular ectasias and tumors or melanin pigment in the dermis. *Venous lakes* (ectasias) are compressible dark blue lesions that are found commonly in the head and neck region. *Venous malformations* are also compressible blue papules and nodules that can occur anywhere on the body, including the oral mucosa. When they are multiple rather than single congenital lesions, the patient may have the blue rubber bleb syndrome or Mafucci's syndrome. Patients with the blue rubber bleb syndrome also have vascular anomalies of the gastrointestinal tract that may bleed, whereas patients with Mafucci's syndrome have associated dyschondroplasia and osteochondromas. In the case of single hemangiomas that are relatively large in size, there can be associated platelet consumption (Kasabach-Merritt syndrome). *Blue nevi* (moles) are seen when there are collections of pigment-producing nevus cells in the dermis. These benign papular lesions are dome-shaped and occur most commonly on the dorsum of the hand and arm.

Violaceous Lesions Violaceous papules and plaques are seen in *lupus pernio*, *lymphoma cutis*, and *cutaneous lupus*. Lupus pernio is a particular type of sarcoidosis that involves the tip of the nose and the earlobes, with lesions that are violaceous in color rather than red-brown. This form of sarcoidosis is associated with involvement of the upper respiratory tract. The plaques of lymphoma cutis and cutaneous lupus may be red or violaceous in color and were discussed above.

Purple Lesions Purple-colored papules and plaques are seen in vascular tumors, such as *Kaposi's sarcoma* (see Chap. 308) and *angiosarcoma*, and when there is extravasation of red blood cells into the skin in association with inflammation, as in *palpable purpura* (see "Purpura"). Patients with congenital or acquired arteriovenous fistulas and venous hypertension can develop purple papules on the lower extremities that can resemble Kaposi's sarcoma clinically and histologically, and this condition is referred to as pseudo-Kaposi sarcoma (acral angiodermatitis). *Angiosarcoma* is found most commonly on the scalp and face of elderly patients or within areas of chronic lymphedema and presents as purple papules and plaques. In the head and neck region the tumor often extends beyond the clinically defined borders and may be accompanied by facial edema.

Brown and Black Lesions Brown- and black-colored papules are reviewed in "Hyperpigmentation."

Cutaneous Metastases These are discussed last because they can have a wide range of colors. Most commonly they present as either firm, flesh-colored subcutaneous nodules or firm, red to red-brown papulonodules. The lesions of lymphoma cutis range from pink-red to plum in color, whereas metastatic melanoma can be pink, blue, or black in color. Cutaneous metastases develop from hematogenous or lymphatic spread and are most often due to the following primary carcinomas: in men, lung, colon, melanoma, and oral cavity; and in women, breast, colon, and lung. These metastatic lesions may be the initial presentation of the carcinoma, especially when the primary site is the lung, kidney, or ovary.

PURPURA (Table 57-21) *Purpura* are seen when there is an extravasation of red blood cells into the dermis, and as a result, the lesions do not blanch with pressure. This is in contrast to those erythematous or violet-colored lesions that are due to localized vasodilatation—they do blanch with pressure. Purpura ($\geq$3 mm) and petechiae ($\leq$2 mm) are divided into two major groups, palpable and nonpalpable. The most frequent causes of *nonpalpable* petechiae and purpura are primary cutaneous disorders such as *trauma, solar purpura,* and *capillaritis*. Less common causes are *steroid purpura* and *livedoid vasculitis* (see "Ulcers"). Solar purpura are seen primarily on the extensor forearm, while glucocorticoid purpura secondary to potent topical steroids or endogenous or exogenous Cushing's syndrome can be more widespread. In both cases there is alteration of the supporting connective tissue that surrounds the dermal blood vessels. In contrast, the petechiae that result from capillaritis are found primarily on the lower extremities. In capillaritis there is an extravasation of erythrocytes as a result of perivascular lymphocytic inflammation. The petechiae are bright red, 1 to 2 mm in size, and scattered within annular or coin-shaped yellow-brown macules. The yellow-brown color is caused by hemosiderin deposits within the dermis.

Systemic causes of nonpalpable purpura fall into several categories, and those secondary to clotting disturbances and vascular fragility will be discussed first. The former group includes *thrombocytopenia* (see Chap. 117), *abnormal platelet function* as is seen in uremia, and *clotting factor defects*. The initial site of presentation for thrombocytopenia-induced petechiae is the distal lower extremity. Capillary fragility leads to nonpalpable purpura in patients with systemic *amyloidosis* (see "Papulonodular Skin Lesions"), disorders of collagen production such as *Ehlers-Danlos syndrome*, and *scurvy*. In scurvy there are flattened corkscrew hairs with surrounding hemorrhage on the lower extremities, in addition to gingivitis. Vitamin C is a cofactor for lysyl hydroxylase, an enzyme involved in the posttranslational modification of procollagen that is necessary for cross-link formation.

In contrast to the previous group of disorders, in which either capillary fragility or a clotting abnormality is responsible for the nonpalpable purpura, the purpura seen in the following group of diseases are associated with thrombi formation within vessels. It is important to note that these thrombi are demonstrable in skin biopsy specimens. This group of disorders includes *disseminated intravascular coagulation* (DIC), *monoclonal cryoglobulinemia, thrombotic thrombocytopenic purpura,* and *reactions to warfarin*. DIC is triggered by several types of infection (gram-negative, gram-positive, viral, and rickettsial) as well as by tissue injury and neoplasms. Widespread purpura and hemorrhagic infarcts of the distal extremities are seen. Similar lesions are found in purpura fulminans, which is a form of DIC associated with fever and hypotension that occurs more commonly in children following an infectious illness such as varicella, scarlet fever, or an upper respiratory tract infection. In both disorders, hemorrhagic bullae can develop in involved skin.

Monoclonal cryoglobulinemia is associated with multiple myeloma, Waldenström's macroglobulinemia, lymphocytic leukemia, and lymphoma. Purpura, primarily of the lower extremities, and hemorrhagic infarcts of the fingers and toes are seen in these patients. Exacerbations of disease activity can follow cold exposure or an increase in serum viscosity. Biopsy specimens show precipitates of the cryoglobulin within dermal vessels. Similar deposits have been found in the lung, brain, and renal glomeruli. Patients with *thrombotic throm-*

bocytopenic purpura also can have hemorrhagic infarcts as a result of intravascular thromboses. Additional signs include thrombocytopenic purpura, fever, and microangiopathic hemolytic anemia (see Chap. 109).

Administration of *warfarin* can result in painful areas of erythema that become purpuric and then necrotic with an adherent black eschar. This reaction is seen more often in women and in areas with abundant subcutaneous fat—breasts, abdomen, buttocks, thighs, and calves. The erythema and purpura develop between the third and tenth day of therapy, most likely as a result of a transient imbalance in the levels of anticoagulant and procoagulant vitamin K–dependent factors. Continued therapy does not exacerbate preexisting lesions, and patients with an inherited or acquired deficiency of protein C are at increased risk for this particular reaction as well as for purpura fulminans.

Purpura secondary to *cholesterol emboli* are usually seen on the lower extremities of patients with atherosclerotic vascular disease. They often follow anticoagulant therapy or an invasive vascular procedure such as an arteriogram but also occur spontaneously from disintegration of atheromatous plaques. Associated findings include livedo reticularis, gangrene, cyanosis, subcutaneous nodules, and ischemic ulcerations. Multiple step sections of the biopsy specimen may be necessary to demonstrate the cholesterol clefts with the vessels. Petechiae are also an important sign of *fat embolism* and occur primarily on the upper body 2 to 3 days after a major injury. By using special fixatives, the emboli can be demonstrated in biopsy specimens of the petechiae. Emboli of tumor or thrombus are seen in patients with atrial myxomas and marantic endocarditis.

In the *Gardner-Diamond syndrome* (autoerythrocyte sensitivity), female patients develop large ecchymoses within areas of painful, warm erythema. An episode of significant trauma frequently precedes the onset of this syndrome. Intradermal injections of autologous erythrocytes or phosphatidyl serine derived from the red cell membrane can reproduce the lesions in some patients; however, there are instances where a reaction is seen at an injection site of the forearm but not in the midback region. The latter has led some observers to view Gardner-Diamond syndrome as a cutaneous manifestation of severe emotional stress. *Waldenström's hypergammaglobulinemic purpura* is a chronic disorder characterized by petechiae on the lower extremities. There are circulating complexes of IgG–anti-IgG molecules, and exacerbations are associated with prolonged standing or walking.

Palpable purpura are further subdivided into vasculitic and embolic. In the group of vasculitic disorders, *leukocytoclastic vasculitis*

Table 57-21

Causes of Purpura

I. Primary cutaneous disorders	c. Thrombotic thrombocytopenic purpura
A. Nonpalpable	d. Warfarin reaction
1. Trauma	4. Emboli
2. Solar purpura	a. Cholesterol
3. Steroid purpura	b. Fat
4. Capillaritis	5. Possible immune complex
5. Livedoid vasculitis*	a. Gardner-Diamond syndrome (autoerythrocyte sensitization)
II. Systemic diseases	b. Waldenström's hypergammaglobulinemic purpura
A. Nonpalpable	B. Palpable
1. Clotting disturbances	1. Vasculitis
a. Thrombocytopenia (including ITP)	a. Leukocytoclastic vasculitis
b. Abnormal platelet function	b. Polyarteritis nodosa
c. Clotting factor defects	2. Emboli
2. Vascular fragility	a. Acute meningococcemia
a. Amyloidosis	b. Disseminated gonococcal infection
b. Ehlers-Danlos syndrome	c. Rocky Mountain spotted fever
c. Scurvy	d. Ecthyma gangrenosum
3. Thrombi	
a. Disseminated intravascular coagulation	
b. Monoclonal cryoglobulinemia	

* Also systemic.

(LCV), also known as *allergic vasculitis*, is the one most commonly associated with palpable purpura (see Chap. 319). *Henoch-Schönlein purpura* is a subtype of acute LCV that is seen primarily in children and adolescents following an upper respiratory infection. The majority of lesions are found on the lower extremities and buttocks. Systemic manifestations include fever, arthralgias (primarily of the knees and ankles), abdominal pain, gastrointestinal bleeding, and nephritis. Direct immunofluorescence examination shows deposits of IgA within dermal blood vessel walls. In *polyarteritis nodosa*, specific cutaneous lesions result from a vasculitis of arterial vessels rather than postcapillary venules as in LCV. The arteritis leads to ischemia of the skin, and this explains the irregular outline of the purpura (see below).

Several types of infectious emboli can give rise to palpable purpura. These embolic lesions are usually *irregular* in outline as opposed to the lesions of leukocytoclastic vasculitis, which are *circular* in outline. The irregular outline is indicative of a cutaneous infarct, and the size corresponds to the area of skin that received its blood supply from that particular arteriole or artery. The palpable purpura in LCV are circular because the erythrocytes simply diffuse out evenly from the postcapillary venules as a result of inflammation. Infectious emboli are most commonly due to gram-negative cocci (meningococcus, gonococcus), gram-negative rods (Enterobacteriaceae), and gram-positive cocci (staphylococcus). Additional causes include *Rickettsia* and, in immunocompromised patients, *Candida* and *Aspergillus*.

The embolic lesions in *acute meningococcemia* are found primarily on the trunk, lower extremities, and sites of pressure, and a gunmetal-gray color often develops within them. Their size varies from 1 mm to several centimeters, and the organisms can be cultured from the lesions. Associated findings include a preceding upper respiratory tract infection, fever, meningitis, DIC, and, in some patients, a deficiency of the terminal components of complement. In *disseminated gonococcal infection* (arthritis-dermatitis syndrome), a small number of papules and vesicopustules with central purpura or hemorrhagic necrosis are found over the joints of the distal extremities. Additional symptoms include arthralgias, tenosynovitis, and fever. To establish the diagnosis, a Gram stain of these lesions should be performed. *Rocky mountain spotted fever* is a tick-borne disease that is caused by *Rickettsia rickettsii*. A several-day history of fever, chills, severe headache, and photophobia precedes the onset of the cutaneous eruption. The initial lesions are erythematous macules and papules on the wrists, ankles, palms, and soles. With time, the lesions spread centripetally and become purpuric.

Lesions of *ecthyma gangrenosum* begin as edematous, erythematous papules or plaques and then develop central purpura and necrosis. Bullae formation also occurs in these lesions, and they are frequently found in the girdle region. The organism that is classically associated with ecthyma gangrenosum is *Pseudomonas aeruginosa*, but other gram-negative rods such as *Klebsiella*, *Escherichia coli*, and *Serratia* can produce similar lesions. In immunocompromised hosts, the list of potential pathogens is expanded to include *Candida* and *Aspergillus*.

ULCERS (Table 57-22)   As an approach to the patient with a cutaneous ulcer, the etiologies are divided into two major groups: (1) primary cutaneous disorders and (2) underlying systemic diseases. Within the group of *primary cutaneous disorders*, there are three categories: vascular, tumor-associated, and infectious. The *peripheral vascular* group is the first to be discussed because it contains the most common cause of lower extremity ulcers in adults, *venous hypertension*. Stasis ulcers are characteristically painless and contain adequate granulation tissue. They are often found on the medial malleoli against a background of varicosities, stasis dermatitis, edema, and hemosiderin deposition (yellow-brown discoloration of the skin).

In contrast, lower extremity ulcers due to *arteriosclerosis obliterans* are often painful and are associated with cool, hairless, atrophic skin and dystrophic nails—all a reflection of a decrease in blood flow. The majority of patients are men, and they frequently have evidence of atherosclerosis in other large- and medium-sized arteries. *Thromboangiitis obliterans* (Buerger's disease) and *Mönckeberg's arteriosclerosis* are two less common arterial diseases that can lead to ulcers of the distal upper extremity as well as the lower extremity. The latter is found in patients with primary or secondary hyperparathyroidism,

and the calcification of the tunica media of involved muscular arteries is seen radiographically as a diffuse pipestem calcification. Buerger's disease occurs primarily in young men (ages 25 to 40) who smoke or have been smokers.

Livedoid vasculitis (atrophie blanche) represents a combination of a vasculopathy with intravascular thrombosis. Purpuric lesions and livedo reticularis are found in association with painful ulcerations of the lower extremities. These ulcers are often slow to heal, but when they do, irregularly shaped white scars are formed. The majority of cases are idiopathic in origin, but possible underlying illnesses include systemic lupus, the antiphospholipid syndrome, scleroderma, cryoglobulinemia, and cryofibrinogenemia. Patients with the antiphospholipid syndrome have anticardiolipin antibodies, biologic false-positive tests for syphilis, and prolonged activated partial thromboplastin times; the latter are due to a circulating lupus anticoagulant. These antiphospholipid antibodies are seen most commonly in patients with systemic lupus but are also associated with other connective tissue diseases. In addition to the lesions of livedoid vasculitis, patients with the antiphospholipid syndrome have recurrent venous thrombosis, arterial thrombosis (including cerebrovascular accidents), spontaneous abortions, and thrombocytopenia.

Several *carcinomas* can present as cutaneous ulcers, e.g., basal cell carcinoma, squamous cell carcinoma, and, less often, melanoma. When an ulcer on the lower extremity does not heal, despite appropriate treatment, it should be biopsied to rule out carcinoma, primarily squamous cell carcinoma. The same holds true for ulcers that develop within scars. Bacterial and viral *infections* also lead to cutaneous ulceration, and one of the more commonly isolated organisms is *Streptococcus*. The term *ecthyma* is used to describe the often widespread ulcerative lesions that are caused by this bacteria. Ecthyma is a primary cutaneous disorder and should not be confused with ecthyma gangrenosum, which is secondary to blood-borne emboli (see "Purpura"). In Meleney's ulcer, a gradually expanding ulcer begins at a site of trauma or surgery. The clinical appearance is similar to that of pyoderma gangrenosum, but the ulcer is due to a synergistic infection that usually includes anaerobic streptococci.

Table 57-22

Causes of Cutaneous Ulcers

I. Primary cutaneous disorders
   A. Peripheral vascular disease
      1. Venous
      2. Arterial
   B. Livedoid vasculitis*
   C. Squamous cell carcinoma, e.g., within scars
   D. Infections, e.g., ecthyma
II. Systemic diseases
   A. Legs
      1. Leukocytoclastic vasculitis
      2. Hemoglobinopathies
      3. Cryoglobulinemia, cryofibrinogenemia
      4. Cholesterol emboli
      5. Necrobiosis lipoidica
      6. Antiphospholipid syndrome
   B. Hands and feet
      1. Raynaud's phenomenon
   C. Generalized
      1. Pyoderma gangrenosum
      2. Infections, e.g., dimorphic fungi, chronic herpes varicella–zoster
      3. Lymphoma
   D. Mucosal
      1. Behçet's syndrome
      2. Erythema multiforme
      3. Primary blistering disorders
      4. Lupus erythematosus
      5. Inflammatory bowel disease

---

* Also systemic.

For one group of patients with cutaneous ulcers due to an underlying systemic disease, the lower extremity is the primary location for the lesions. In a young patient, ischemic cutaneous ulcers on the leg should raise the possibility of a *hemoglobinopathy* or *hereditary spherocytosis*. Intravascular thrombosis is the presumed cause of these ulcers as well as for the ulcers seen in patients with *monoclonal cryoglobulinemia* (see "Purpura"). Primary and secondary forms of *LCV* as well as *emboli of cholesterol* can result in cutaneous ulceration, again primarily on the lower extremities (see "Purpura"). For example, lower extremity ulcers in patients with rheumatoid arthritis are often due to vasculitis. In addition, the yellow atrophic plaques of *necrobiosis lipoidica* can break down centrally into an ulcer (see "Papulonodular Skin Lesions").

Vasospasm occurs in patients with *Raynaud's phenomenon* and can lead to ulcerations of the hands as well as the feet. Raynaud's phenomenon is defined as a triphasic reaction of pallor, cyanosis, and hyperemia in response to cold or emotional stress. Vasospasm is also seen in patients who receive systemic norepinephrine, vasopressin, ergot, and bleomycin. The patient with Raynaud's phenomenon and ulcerations on the tips of the digits should be examined carefully for periungual and mat telangiectasias, the subtle signs of scleroderma. Raynaud's phenomenon is also seen in patients with DM, systemic lupus, cryoglobulinemia, cervical rib and scalenus anticus syndromes, pneumatic hammer disease, and occupational acro-osteolysis (associated with the manufacture of polyvinyl chloride).

In *pyoderma gangrenosum*, the border of the ulcers has a characteristic appearance of an undermined necrotic bluish edge and a peripheral erythematous halo. The ulcers often begin as pustules that then expand rather rapidly to a size as large as 20 cm. Although these lesions are most commonly found on the lower extremities, they can arise anywhere on the surface of the body, including sites of trauma (pathergy). An estimated 30 to 50 percent of cases are idiopathic, and the most common associated disorders are ulcerative colitis and Crohn's disease. Less commonly, it is associated with chronic active hepatitis, seropositive rheumatoid arthritis, acute and chronic granulocytic leukemia, polycythemia vera, and myeloma. Additional findings in these patients, even those with idiopathic disease, are cutaneous anergy and a benign monoclonal gammopathy. Because the histology of pyoderma gangrenosum is nonspecific, the diagnosis is made clinically by excluding less common causes of similar-appearing ulcers such as necrotizing vasculitis, Meleney's ulcer (see above), dimorphic fungi, cutaneous amebiasis, spider bites, and factitial. In the myeloproliferative disorders, the ulcers may be more superficial with a pustulobullous border, and these lesions provide a connection between classic pyoderma gangrenosum and acute febrile neutrophilic dermatosis (Sweet's syndrome).

The clinical diagnosis of *Behçet's disease* (see Chap. 318) requires the presence of recurrent oral ulceration (at least three times in a 12-month period) in addition to two of the four following criteria: (1) recurrent genital ulcers, primarily of the vulva and scrotum; (2) eye lesions, either uveitis or retinal vasculitis; (3) skin lesions; and (4) a positive pathergy test. The oral ulcers are usually painful and well defined with an erythematous halo, whereas the genital ulcers tend to be deeper and heal with scarring. Erythema nodosum, "pseudofolliculitis," papulopustular lesions, *or* acneiform nodules in a postadolescent patient not on glucocorticoids are the entities included under the heading of skin lesions. The test for pathergy, which is defined as a reproduction of cutaneous lesions by trauma, is performed by injecting sterile saline into the dermis. Before the diagnosis of Behçet's disease can be made, the following disorders must be excluded: recurrent EM (see "Vesicles/Bullae"), herpes simplex, inflammatory bowel disease, systemic lupus, and primary blistering disorders.

FEVER AND RASH The major considerations in a patient with a fever and a rash are inflammatory diseases versus infectious diseases. In the hospital setting, the most common scenario is a patient who has a drug rash plus a fever secondary to an underlying infection.

However, it should be emphasized that a drug reaction can lead to both a cutaneous eruption and a fever ("drug fever"). Additional inflammatory diseases that are often associated with a fever include pustular psoriasis, erythroderma, and Sweet's syndrome. Lyme disease, secondary syphilis, and viral and bacterial exanthems (see "Exanthems") are examples of infectious diseases that produce a rash and a fever. Lastly, it is important to determine whether or not the cutaneous lesions represent septic emboli (see "Purpura"). Such lesions usually have evidence of ischemia in the form of purpura, necrosis, or impending necrosis (gunmetal-gray color). In the patient with thrombocytopenia, however, purpura can be seen in inflammatory reactions such as morbilliform drug eruptions and infectious lesions.

BIBLIOGRAPHY

ARNDT KA et al: *Cutaneous Medicine and Surgery*. Philadelphia, Saunders, 1995

BORK K: *Cutaneous Side Effects of Drugs*. Philadelphia, Saunders, 1988

BRAVERMAN IM: *Skin Signs of Systemic Disease*, 2d ed. Philadelphia, Saunders, 1981

CALLEN JP: *Dermatology Clinics*, vol 8, no 2: *Skin Signs of Internal Disease II*. Philadelphia, Saunders, 1990

———, JORIZZO JL: *Dermatology Clinics*, vol 7, no 3: *Skin Signs of Internal Disease*. Philadelphia, Saunders, 1989

CHAMPION RH et al (eds): *Textbook of Dermatology*, 5th ed. Oxford, Blackwell Scientific, 1992

LEVER WF, SCHAUMBURG-LEVER G: *Histopathology of the Skin*, 7th ed. Philadelphia, Lippincott, 1990

NOVICE FM et al: *Handbook of Genetic Skin Disorders*. Philadelphia, Saunders, 1994

ZURCHER K, KREBS A: *Cutaneous Drug Reactions*, 2d ed. Basel, Karger, 1992

58 *David R. Bickers*

PHOTOSENSITIVITY AND OTHER REACTIONS TO LIGHT

SOLAR RADIATION Sunlight is the most visible and obvious source of comfort in the environment. This natural proclivity for the sun has the beneficial results of warmth and vitamin D synthesis but also can produce pathologic consequences. Few effects of sun exposure beyond those on the skin have been identified, but cutaneous exposure to sunlight can evoke immunosuppressive responses and genetic changes that may be relevant to the pathogenesis of nonmelanoma skin cancer and perhaps infections such as herpes simplex.

The sun's energy encompasses a broad range from ultrashort ionizing radiation (10^{-2} μm) to ultralong radiowaves of very low photon energy (10^7 μm). Thus, the emission spectrum ranges over nine orders of magnitude, but that reaching the earth's surface is narrow and is limited to components of the ultraviolet (UV), visible light, and portions of the infrared. The cutoff at the short end of the UV is at approximately 290 nm, because stratospheric ozone is formed by ionizing radiation of wavelengths less than 100 nm and absorbs solar energy between 120 and 310 nm, thereby preventing penetration to the earth's surface of the shorter, more energetic, potentially more harmful wavelengths of solar radiation. Indeed, concern about destruction of the ozone layer by chlorofluorocarbons released into the atmosphere has led to international agreements to reduce production of these chemicals.

Measurements of solar flux indicate that there is a twentyfold regional variation in the amount of energy at 300 nm that reaches the earth's surface. This variability relates to seasonal effects, the path of sunlight transmission through ozone and air, the altitude (4 percent increase for each 300 m of elevation), the latitude (increasing intensity with decreasing latitude), and the amount of cloud cover, fog, and pollution.

The major components of the photobiologic action spectrum include the UV and visible wavelengths between 290 and 700 nm. In addition, the wavelengths beyond 700 nm in the infrared primarily evoke heat, but warming of the skin may enhance biologic responses to wavelengths in the UV and visible spectrum.

The UV spectrum is arbitrarily divided into three major segments: C, B, and A. This includes the wavelengths between 10 and 400 nm. Ultraviolet C (UV-C) consists of wavelengths between 10 and 290 nm and does not reach the earth because of its absorption by stratospheric ozone. These wavelengths are not a cause of photosensitivity except in occupational settings where artificial sources of this energy are employed, e.g., for germicidal effects. Ultraviolet B (UV-B) consists of wavelengths between 290 and 320 nm. This portion of the photobiologic action spectrum is the most efficient in producing redness or erythema in human skin and hence is sometimes known as the "sunburn spectrum." Ultraviolet A (UV-A) represents those wavelengths between 320 and 400 nm and is approximately 1000-fold less efficient in producing skin hyperemia than is UV-B. The UV-A has also been divided into two parts known as UV-A 1 (340 to 400 nm) and UV-A 2 (320 to 340 nm).

The visible wavelengths between 400 and 700 nm include the familiar white light which when directed through a prism can be shown to consist of various colors including violet, indigo, blue, green, yellow, orange, and red. The energy possessed by photons in the visible spectrum usually is not capable of damaging human skin in the absence of a photosensitizing chemical. The absorption of energy is critical to the development of photosensitivity. Thus the *absorption spectrum* of a molecule is defined as the range of wavelengths absorbed by it, whereas the *action spectrum* for an effect of incident radiation is defined as the range of wavelengths that evoke the response.

Photosensitivity occurs when a photon-absorbing chemical (chromophore) present in the skin absorbs incident energy, becomes excited, and transfers the absorbed energy to various structures or to oxygen. The absorbed energy must be dissipated by processes including heat, fluorescence, and phosphorescence. It is important to emphasize that absorption spectra and action spectra need not be superimposable, but there must be overlap at some point to produce photosensitization.

STRUCTURE AND FUNCTION OF SKIN The skin's exposure to sunlight permits the absorption of some wavelengths and the transmission of others. Essentially, human skin is a sandwich of two distinctive compartments, the epidermis and dermis, separated by a basement membrane. The outer epidermis is a stratified squamous epithelium comprising the surface stratum corneum (a protein- and lipid-rich compact membrane), the stratum granulosum, stratum spinosum, and the basal cell layer. The basal cell layer contains a heterogeneous population of cells, a subset of which migrate upward in the process of terminal differentiation that results in the expression of specific keratin genes and the formation of the stratum corneum. Epidermal cells include resident keratinocytes and melanocytes and immigrant cells, including the immunologically active Langerhans cells, lymphocytes, polymorphonuclear leukocytes, monocytes, and macrophages, making the epidermis a major component of the immune system. Branches of sensory nerve endings also reach into this compartment.

The second major component of skin is the dermis, which is relatively large and less densely populated with cells that include fibroblasts, endothelial cells within dermal vessels, and mast cells. Tissue macrophages and sparsely distributed inflammatory cells are also present. All these cells exist within an extracellular matrix of collagen, elastin, and glycosaminoglycans. In contrast to the epidermis, rich vascularization of the dermis allows it to play an important role in temperature regulation.

UV RADIATION (UVR) AND SKIN The epidermis and the dermis contain several chromophores capable of interacting with incident solar energy. These interactions include reflection, refraction, absorption, and transmission. The stratum corneum is a major impediment to the transmission of UV-B, and less than 10 percent of incident wavelengths in this region penetrate the basement membrane. Approximately 3 percent of radiation below 300 nm, 20 percent of radiation below 360 nm, and 33 percent of short visible radiation reaches the basal cell layer in untanned human skin. Proteins and nucleic acids absorb intensely in the short UV-B. In contrast, UV-A 1 and 2 penetrate

the epidermis efficiently to reach the dermis, where they likely produce changes in structural and matrix proteins that contribute to the aged appearance of chronically sun-exposed skin, particularly in individuals of light complexion.

One of the consequences of UV-B absorption by DNA is the production of pyrimidine dimers. These structural changes can be repaired by mechanisms that result in their recognition, excision, and the reestablishment of normal base sequences. The efficient repair of these structural aberrations is crucial, since individuals with defective DNA repair are at high risk for the development of cutaneous cancer. For example, patients with xeroderma pigmentosum, an autosomal recessive disorder, are characterized by variably decreased repair of UV-induced photoproducts, and their skin may develop the xerotic appearance of photoaging as well as basal cell and squamous cell carcinomas and melanoma in the first two decades of life. Studies in mice using knockout gene technology have verified the importance of genes regulating these repair pathways in preventing the development of UV-induced cancer.

Cutaneous Optics and Chromophores Chromophores are endogenous or exogenous chemical components that can absorb physical energy. Endogenous chromophores of skin are of two types: (1) chemicals that are normally present, including nucleic acids, proteins, lipids, and 7-dehydrocholesterol, the precursor of vitamin D; and (2) chemicals, such as porphyrins, synthesized elsewhere in the body that circulate in the bloodstream and diffuse into the skin. Normally, only trace amounts of porphyrins are present in the skin, but in the diseases known as the porphyrias, increased amounts are released into the circulation and are transported to the skin, where they absorb incident energy both in the Soret band around 400 nm (short visible) and to a lesser extent in the red portion of the visible spectrum (580 to 660 nm). This results in structural damage to the skin that may be manifest as erythema, edema, urticaria, or blister formation (see Chap. 343).

Acute Effects of Sun Exposure The immediate cutaneous consequences of sun exposure include sunburn and vitamin D synthesis.

Sunburn This very common affliction of human skin is caused by exposure to UVR. Generally speaking, the individual's ability to tolerate sunlight is inversely proportional to his or her melanin pigmentation. Melanin is a complex polymer of tyrosine that functions as an efficient neutral-density filter with broad absorbance within the UV portion of the solar spectrum. Melanin is synthesized in specialized epidermal dendritic cells termed *melanocytes* and is packaged into *melanosomes* that are transferred via dendritic processes into *keratinocytes*, where they provide photoprotection. Sun-induced melanogenesis is a consequence of increased tyrosinase activity in melanocytes that in turn may be due to a combination of eicosanoid and endothelin-1 release. Tolerance of sun exposure is a function of the efficiency of the epidermal-melanin unit and can usually be ascertained by asking an individual two questions: (1) Do you burn after sun exposure? and (2) Do you tan after sun exposure? By the answers to these questions, it is usually possible to divide the population into six skin types varying from type I (always burn, never tan) to type VI (never burn, always tan) (see Table 58-1).

There are two general theories about the pathogenesis of the sunburn response. First, the lag phase in time between skin exposure and

Table 58-1

Skin Type and Sunburn Sensitivity

Type	Description
I	Always burn, never tan
II	Always burn, sometimes tan
III	Sometimes burn, sometimes tan
IV	Sometimes burn, always tan
V	Never burn, sometimes tan
VI	Never burn, always tan

the development of visible redness (usually 4 to 12 h) suggests an epidermal chromophore that causes delayed production and/or release of vasoactive mediator(s), or cytokines, that diffuse to the dermal vasculature to evoke vasodilatation. Indeed UVR stimulates the release of numerous proinflammatory cytokines and nitric oxide by keratinocytes. Second, it is possible that the small amount of incident UV-B radiation (10 percent or less) that penetrates to the dermis can be absorbed directly by endothelial cells in the vasculature, thereby resulting in vasodilatation. The issue remains unresolved.

The action spectrum for sunburn erythema includes the UV-B and UV-A regions. Photons in the shorter UV-B are at least a 1000-fold more efficient than photons in the longer UV-B and the UV-A in evoking the response. However, UV-A may contribute to sunburn erythema at midday when much more UV-A than UV-B is present.

The mechanism of injury remains poorly defined, but the action spectrum for UV-B erythema closely resembles the absorption spectrum for DNA after adjusting for the absorbance of incident energy by the stratum corneum. Apoptotic keratinocytes (so-called sunburn cells) are visible histologically within an hour of exposure and are maximal within 24 h. UV-A is less effective than UV-B in producing sunburn cells. Mast cells may release inflammatory mediators after exposure to UV-B and UV-A. For example, erythema doses of both UV-B and UV-A increase histamine levels in suction blisters of human skin that return to normal after 24 h (before visible erythema has subsided). Prostaglandin E_2 increases to approximately 150 percent of control levels after 24 h and then diminishes. Since prostaglandins evoke both pain and redness when injected intradermally, their presence in suction blisters after UV-B exposure suggests a role in UV-B erythema. Age-related declines occur in the amount of inflammatory mediators detectable in human skin after UV-B irradiation. UV-A erythema results in few epidermal sunburn cells, but vascular endothelial injury is greater than with UV-B. In addition, there are increased levels of arachidonic acid and of prostaglandins D_2, E_2, and I_2 that peak within 5 to 9 h and then subside before peak redness occurs. Despite evidence for the role of prostaglandins in both UV-B- and UV-A-irradiated skin, administration of nonsteroidal anti-inflammatory drugs is more effective in reducing erythema evoked by UV-B than by UV-A. UV-B also induces cutaneous matrix-degrading metalloproteinases within hours of exposure.

Vitamin D photochemistry   Cutaneous exposure to UV-B causes photolysis of epidermal previtamin D_3 (7-dehydrocholesterol) to previtamin D_3, which then undergoes a temperature-dependent isomerization to form the stable hormone vitamin D_3. This compound then diffuses to the dermal vasculature and circulates systemically where it is converted to the functional hormone 1,25-dihydroxy vitamin D_3 [$1,25(OH)_2D_3$]. Vitamin D metabolites from the circulation or those produced in the skin itself can augment epidermal differentiation signaling. Aging substantially decreases the ability of human skin to produce vitamin D_3. This, coupled with the widespread use of sunscreens that filter out UV-B, has led to concern that vitamin D deficiency may become a significant clinical problem in the elderly. Indeed, studies have shown that the use of sunscreens can prevent the production of vitamin D_3 in human skin.

Chronic Effects of Sun Exposure: Nonmalignant   The clinical features of photodamaged sun-exposed skin consist of wrinkling, blotchiness, telangiectasia, and a roughened, irregular, "weatherbeaten" appearance. Whether these changes, which some refer to as *photoaging* or *dermatoheliosis*, represent accelerated chronologic aging or a separate and distinct process is not clear.

Within chronically sun-exposed epidermis there is thickening (acanthosis) and morphologic heterogeneity within the basal cell layer. Higher but irregular melanosome content may be present in some keratinocytes, indicating prolonged residence of the cells in the basal cell layer. These structural changes may help to explain the leathery texture and the blotchy discoloration of sun-damaged skin.

The dermis is the major site for sun-associated chronic damage, manifest as a massive increase in thickened irregular masses of tangled elastic fibers resulting from enhanced expression of elastin genes. Collagen fibers are also abnormally clumped in the deeper dermis. Fibroblasts are increased in number and show morphologic signs suggesting activation. Degraded mast cells may be present in the dermis, the relevance of which remains unclear.

These morphologic changes, both gross and microscopic, are features of chronically sun-exposed skin. The chromophore(s), the action spectra, and the specific biochemical events orchestrating these changes are unknown.

Chronic Effects of Sun Exposure: Malignant   One of the major known consequences of chronic skin exposure to sunlight is nonmelanoma skin cancer. The two types of nonmelanoma skin cancer are basal cell and squamous cell carcinoma (see Chap. 88). There are three major steps for cancer induction: initiation, promotion, and progression. Chronic exposure of animal skin to artificial light sources that mimic solar UVR results in *initiation*, a step whereby structural (mutagenic) changes in DNA evoke an irreversible alteration in the target cell (keratinocyte) that begins the tumorigenic process. Exposure to a tumor initiator is believed to be a necessary but not sufficient step in the malignant process, since initiated skin cells not exposed to tumor promoters do not generally develop tumors. The second stage in tumor development is *promotion*, a multistep process whereby initiated cells are exposed to chemical and physical agents that evoke epigenetic changes that culminate in the clonal expansion of initiated cells and cause the development, over a period of weeks to months, of benign growths known as *papillomas*. Again, using transgenic animals, the importance of UV effects on the expression of additional oncogenes such as *fos* and *jun* in developing papillomas has been demonstrated. UV-B is a *complete carcinogen*, meaning that it can function as both an initiator and a promoter, leading to tumor induction. *Incomplete carcinogens* can initiate tumorigenesis but require additional skin exposure to tumor promoters to elicit tumors. The prototype tumor promoter is the phorbol ester 12-*O*-tetradecanoyl phorbol-13-acetate. Tumor promotion usually requires multiple exposures over time to evoke a neoplasm.

The final step in the malignant process is the conversion of benign precursors into malignant lesions, a process thought to require additional genetic alterations in already transformed cells. Indeed *ras* gene mutations have been detected in a minority of human nonmelanoma skin cancers. Mutations of the tumor suppressor gene p53 also occur in sun-damaged human skin.

Sun exposure is believed to cause nonmelanoma and melanoma cancers of the skin, although the evidence is far more direct for its role in nonmelanoma (basal cell and squamous cell carcinoma) than in melanoma. Approximately 80 percent of nonmelanoma skin cancers develop on exposed body area, including the face, the neck, and the hands. Men of fair complexion who work outdoors are twice as likely as women to develop these types of cancers. Whites of darker complexions (e.g., Hispanics) have one-tenth the risk of developing such cancers as do light-skinned individuals. Blacks are at lowest risk for all forms of skin cancer. Between 600,000 and 800,000 individuals in the United States develop nonmelanoma skin cancer annually, and the lifetime risk for a white individual to develop such a neoplasm is estimated at approximately 15 percent. A consensus exists that the incidence of nonmelanoma skin cancer in the population is rising for reasons that are unclear.

The relationship of sun exposure to melanoma is less clear-cut, but suggestive evidence supports an association. Melanomas occasionally develop by the teenage years, indicating that the latent period for tumor growth is less than that of nonmelanomas. Melanomas are among the most rapidly increasing of all human malignancies. Epidemiologic studies of immigrants of similar ethnic stock indicate that individuals born in one area or who migrated to the same locale before age 10 have higher age-specific melanoma rates than individuals arriving later. It is thus reasonable to conclude that life in a sunny climate from birth or early childhood increases the risk of melanoma. In general, risk does not correlate with cumulative sun exposure but may relate to sequelae of sun exposure in childhood. Thus a blistering sunburn is associated with a doubling of melanoma risk at the site of the reaction.

Immunologic Effects Exposure to solar radiation influences both local and systemic immune responses. UV-B appears to be most efficient in altering immune responses, likely related to the capacity of such energy to affect antigen presentation in skin by interacting with epidermal Langerhans cells. These bone marrow–derived dendritic cells possess surface markers characteristic of monocytes and macrophages. Following skin exposure to erythema doses of UV-B, Langerhans cells undergo both morphologic and functional changes that result in decreased contact allergic responses when haptens are applied to the irradiated site. This diminished capacity for sensitization is due to the induction of antigen-specific suppressor T lymphocytes. Indeed, while the immunosuppressive effect of irradiation is limited to haptens applied to the irradiated site, the net result is systemic immune suppression to that antigen because of the induction of suppressor T cells.

Higher doses of radiation evoke diminished immunologic responses to antigens introduced either epicutaneously or intracutaneously at sites distant from the irradiated site. These suppressed responses are also associated with the induction of antigen-specific suppressor T lymphocytes and may be mediated by as yet undefined factors that are released from epidermal cells at the irradiated site. The implications of this generalized immune suppression in terms of altered susceptibility to cutaneous cancer or to infection remain to be defined.

It is known that UV-induced tumors in murine skin are antigenic and are rapidly rejected when transplanted into normal syngeneic animals. If the tumors are transplanted into animals previously exposed to subcarcinogenic doses of UV-B, they are not rejected and instead grow progressively in the recipients. This failure of irradiated animals to reject the transplanted tumors is due to the development of T suppressor cells that prevent the rejection response. While the mechanism of suppression of tumor rejection is unknown, such a response might be a critical determinant of cancer risk in human skin.

PHOTOSENSITIVITY DISEASES The diagnosis of photosensitivity requires a careful history to define the duration of the signs and symptoms, the length of time between exposure to sunlight and the development of subjective complaints, and visible changes in the skin. The age of onset also can be a helpful clue; for example, the acute photosensitivity of erythropoietic protoporphyria almost always begins in childhood, whereas the chronic photosensitivity of porphyria cutanea tarda typically begins in the fourth and fifth decades. A history of exposure to topical and systemic drugs and chemicals may provide important information. Many classes of drugs can cause photosensitivity on the basis of either phototoxicity or photoallergy. Fragrances such as musk ambrette contained in numerous cosmetic products are also potent photosensitizers.

Examination of the skin also may offer important clues. Anatomic areas that are naturally protected from direct sunlight such as the hairy scalp, the upper eyelids, the retroauricular areas, and the infranasal and submental regions may be spared, whereas exposed areas show characteristic features of the pathologic process. These anatomic localization patterns are often helpful but not infallible in making the diagnosis. For example, airborne contact sensitizers that are blown onto the skin may produce dermatitis that can be difficult to distinguish from photosensitivity, despite the fact that such material may trigger skin reactivity in areas shielded from direct sunlight.

Many dermatologic conditions may be caused or aggravated by light (Table 58-2). The role of light in evoking these responses may be dependent on genetic abnormalities ranging from well-described defects in DNA repair that occur in xeroderma pigmentosum to the inherited abnormalities in heme synthesis that characterize the porphyrias. In certain photosensitivity diseases, the chromophore has been identified, whereas in the majority, the energy-absorbing agent is unknown.

Polymorphous Light Eruption After sunburn, the most common type of photosensitivity disease is *polymorphous light eruption*, the mechanism of which is unknown. Many affected individuals never seek medical attention because the condition is often transient, becoming manifest each spring with initial sun exposure but then subsiding spontaneously with continuing exposure, a phenomenon known as "hardening." The major manifestations of polymorphous light eruption include pruritic (often intensely so) erythematous papules that may coalesce into plaques on exposed areas of the face and arms or other areas as well, making the distribution spotty and uneven.

The diagnosis can be confirmed by skin biopsy and by performing phototest procedures in which skin is exposed to multiple erythema doses of UV-A and UV-B. The action spectrum for polymorphous light eruption is usually within these portions of the solar spectrum.

Treatment of this disease includes the induction of hardening by the cautious administration of UV light, either alone or in combination with photosensitizers such as the psoralens (see below).

Phototoxicity and Photoallergy These photosensitivity disorders are related to the topical or systemic administration of drugs and other chemicals. Both reactions require the absorption of energy by a drug or chemical resulting in the production of an excited-state photosensitizer that can transfer its absorbed energy to a bystander molecule or to molecular oxygen, thereby generating tissue-destructive chemical species.

Phototoxicity is a nonimmunologic reaction caused by drugs and chemicals, a few of which are listed in Table 58-3. The usual clinical manifestations include erythema resembling a sunburn that quickly desquamates or "peels" within several days. In addition, edema, vesicles, and bullae may occur.

Table 58-2

Classification of Photosensitivity Diseases

Type	Disease
Genetic	Erythropoietic porphyria
	Erythropoietic protoporphyria
	Porphyria cutanea tarda—familial
	Variegate porphyria
	Hepatoerythropoietic porphyria
	Albinism
	Xeroderma pigmentosum
	Rothmund-Thompson disease
	Bloom's disease
	Cockayne's disease
	Phenylketonuria
Metabolic	Porphyria cutanea tarda—sporadic
	Hartnup disease
	Kwashiorkor
	Pellagra
	Carcinoid syndrome
	Pseudoporphyria
Phototoxic	
Internal	Drugs
External	Drugs, plants, food
Photoallergic	
Immediate	Solar urticaria
Delayed	Drug photoallergy
	Persistent light reaction/chronic actinic dermatitis
Neoplastic and degenerative	Photoaging
	Actinic keratoses
	Basal cell carcinoma
Idiopathic	Polymorphous light eruption
	Hydroa aestivale
	Actinic reticuloid
Photoaggravated	Lupus erythematosus
	Systemic
	Subacute cutaneous
	Dermatomyositis
	Pemphigus foliaceus
	Herpes simplex
	Lichen planus actinicus
	Acne vulgaris (aestivale)
	Transient acantholytic dermatosis

Photoallergy is distinct in that the immune system participates in the pathologic process. The excited-state photosensitizer may create highly unstable haptenic free radicals that bind covalently to macromolecules to form a functional antigen capable of evoking a delayed hypersensitivity response. Some of the drugs and chemicals that produce photoallergy are listed in Table 58-4. The clinical manifestations typically differ from those of phototoxicity in that an intensely pruritic eczematous dermatitis tends to predominate and evolves into lichenified, thickened, "leathery" changes in sun-exposed areas. A small subset (perhaps 5 to 10 percent) of patients with photoallergy may develop a persistent exquisite hypersensitivity to light even when the offending drug or chemical is identified and eliminated. Known as *persistent light reaction*, this may be incapacitating for years. Some have used the term *chronic actinic dermatitis* to encompass these chronic hyperresponsive states.

Diagnostic confirmation of phototoxicity and photoallergy often can be obtained using phototest procedures. In patients with suspected phototoxicity, determination of the minimal erythema dose (MED) while the patient is exposed to a suspected agent and then repeating the MED after discontinuation of the agent may provide a clue to the causative drug or chemical. Photopatch testing can be performed to confirm the diagnosis of photoallergy. This is a simple variant of ordinary patch testing in which a series of known photoallergens is applied to the skin in duplicate and one set is irradiated with a suberythema dose of UV-A. Development of eczematous changes at sites exposed to sensitizer and light is a positive result. The characteristic abnormality in patients with persistent light reaction is a diminished threshold to erythema evoked by UV-B. Patients with chronic actinic dermatitis may have a broad spectrum of UV hyperresponsiveness.

The management of drug photosensitivity is first and foremost to eliminate exposure to the chemical agents responsible for the reaction and to minimize sun exposure. The acute symptoms of phototoxicity may be ameliorated by cool, moist compresses, topical glucocorticoids, and systemically administered nonsteroidal anti-inflammatory agents. In severely affected individuals, a rapidly tapered course of systemic glucocorticoids may be useful. Judicious use of analgesics may be necessary.

Photoallergic reactions require similar management techniques. Furthermore, individuals suffering from persistent light reactivity must be meticulously protected against light exposure. In selected patients in whom chronic systemic high-dose glucocorticoids pose unacceptable risks, it may be necessary to employ cytotoxic agents such as azathioprine or cyclophosphamide.

Porphyria The porphyrias (see Chap. 343) are a group of diseases that have in common various derangements in the synthesis of heme. Heme is an iron-chelated tetrapyrrole or porphyrin, and the nonmetal chelated porphyrins are potent photosensitizers that absorb light intensely in both the short (400 to 410 nm) and the long (580 to 650 nm) portions of the visible spectrum.

Heme cannot be reutilized and must be continuously synthesized, and the two body compartments with the largest capacity for its production are the bone marrow and the liver. Accordingly, the porphyrias originate in one or the other of these organs, with the end result of excessive endogenous production of potent photosensitizing porphyrins. The porphyrins circulate in the bloodstream and diffuse into the skin, where they absorb solar energy, become photoexcited, and evoke cutaneous photosensitivity. The mechanism of porphyrin photosensitization is known to be photodynamic or oxygen-dependent and is mediated by reactive oxygen species such as superoxide anions.

Porphyria cutanea tarda is the most common type of human porphyria and is associated with decreased activity of the enzyme uroporphyrinogen decarboxylase associated with a number of gene mutations. There are two basic types of porphyria cutanea tarda: the sporadic or acquired type, generally seen in individuals ingesting ethanol or receiving estrogens, and the inherited type, in which there is autosomal dominant transmission of deficient enzyme activity. Both forms are associated with increased hepatic iron stores.

In both types of porphyria cutanea tarda, the predominant feature is a chronic photosensitivity characterized by increased fragility of sun-exposed skin, particularly areas subject to repeated trauma such as the dorsa of the hands, the forearms, the face, and the ears. The predominant skin lesions are vesicles and bullae that rupture, producing moist erosions often with a hemorrhagic base, and that heal slowly with crusting and purplish discoloration of the affected skin. Hypertrichosis,

Table 58-3

Phototoxic Drugs and Chemicals

	Topical	Systemic
COAL TAR DERIVATIVES		
Acridine	+	
Anthracene	+	
Phenanthrene	+	
DRUGS		
Amiodarone		+
Dacarbazine		+
Fluoroquinolones		+
5-Fluorouracil	+	+
Furosemide		+
Nalidixic acid		+
Phenothiazines		+
Psoralens	+	+
Retinoids	+	+
Sulfonamides		+
Sulfonylureas		+
Tetracyclines		+
Thiazides		+
Vinblastine		+
DYES		
Anthraquinone		+
Eosin		+
Methylene blue		+
Rose bengal		+

Table 58-4

Photoallergic Drugs and Chemicals

	Topical	Systemic
Antibiotics		
Sulfonamides		+
Antifungals		
Fenticlor	+	
Jadit	+	
Multifungin	+	
Diuretics		
Thiazides		+
Fragrances		
Musk ambrette	+	
6-Methylcoumarin	+	
Plant oleoresins	+	
Halogenated salicylanilides		
Bithionol	+	
Tetrachlorosalicylanilides	+	
Tribromosalicylanilide	+	
Nonsteroidal Anti-Inflammatory Agents		
Piroxicam	+	
Phenothiazines		
Chlorpromazine	+	
Promethazine	+	
Sulfonylureas		+
Sunscreens		
p-Aminobenzoic acid and esters	+	
Whitening Agents		
Stilbenes	+	

mottled pigmentary change, and scleroderma-like induration are associated features. Biochemical confirmation of the diagnosis can be obtained by measurement of urinary porphyrin excretion, plasma porphyrin assay, and by assay of uroporphyrinogen decarboxylase. Multiple mutations of the uroporphyrinogen decarboxylase gene have been identified in human populations including exon skipping and base substitutions.

Treatment consists of repeated phlebotomies to diminish the excessive hepatic iron stores and/or intermittent low doses of the antimalarial drugs chloroquine and hydroxychloroquine. Long-term remission of the disease can be achieved if the patient eliminates exposure to porphyrinogenic agents.

Erythropoietic protoporphyria originates in the bone marrow and is due to a decrease in the mitochondrial enzyme ferrochelatase secondary to a number of gene mutations. The major clinical features include an acute photosensitivity characterized by subjective burning and stinging of exposed skin that often develops during or just after exposure. There may be associated skin swelling and, after repeated episodes, a waxlike scarring.

The diagnosis is confirmed by demonstration of measurement of free elevated erythrocyte protoporphyrin. Detection of increased plasma protoporphyrin helps to differentiate lead poisoning and iron-deficiency anemia, in both of which elevated erythrocyte protoporphyrin occurs in the absence of cutaneous photosensitivity and of elevated plasma protoporphyrin.

Treatment consists of reducing sun exposure and the oral administration of the carotenoid β-carotene, which is an effective scavenger of free radicals. This drug increases tolerance to sun exposure in many affected individuals, although it has no effect on deficient ferrochelatase.

An algorithm for the approach to a patient with photosensitivity is illustrated in Fig. 58-1.

PHOTOPROTECTION Since photosensitivity of the skin results from exposure to sunlight, it follows that avoidance of the sun would eliminate these disorders. Unfortunately, social pressures make this an impractical alternative for most individuals, and this has led to a search for better approaches to photoprotection.

Natural photoprotection is provided by structural proteins in the epidermis, particularly keratins and melanin. The amount of melanin and its distribution in cells is genetically regulated, and individuals of darker complexion (skin types IV to VI) are at decreased risk for the development of cutaneous malignancy.

Other forms of photoprotection include clothing and sunscreens. Clothing constructed of tightly woven sun-protective fabrics, irrespective of color, affords substantial protection. Wide-brimmed hats, long sleeves, and trousers all reduce direct exposure. Sunscreens are of two major types—chemical and physical. Chemical sunscreens are chromophores that absorb energy in the UV-B and/or UV-A regions, thereby diminishing photon absorption by the skin (Table 58-5). Sunscreens are rated for their photoprotective effect by their *sun protective factor* (SPF). The SPF is simply a ratio of the time required to produce sunburn erythema with and without sunscreen application. SPF ratings of 15 or higher provide effective protection against UV-B and, to a lesser extent, UV-A. The major categories of chemical sunscreens include *p*-aminobenzoic acid and its esters, benzophenones, anthranilates, cinnamates, and salicylates. Physical sunscreens are light-opaque mixtures containing metal particles such as titanium oxide that scatter light, thereby reducing photon absorption by the skin.

In addition to light absorption, a critical determinant of the photoprotective effect of sunscreens is their ability to remain on the skin, a property known as *substantivity*. In general, the *p*-aminobenzoic acid esters formulated in moisturizing vehicles provide the greatest substantivity.

Photoprotection also can be achieved by limiting the time of exposure during the day. Since the majority of an individual's total lifetime sun exposure may occur by the age of 18, it is important to educate parents and young children about the hazards of sunlight. Simply eliminating exposure at midday will substantially reduce lifetime UV-B exposure.

PHOTOTHERAPY AND PHOTOCHEMOTHERAPY

UVR can also be used therapeutically. The administration of UV-B alone or in combination with topically applied agents can induce remissions of psoriasis and atopic dermatitis.

Photochemotherapy in which topically applied or systemically administered *psoralens* are combined with *UV-A* (PUVA) is also effective in treating psoriasis and in the early stages of cutaneous T cell lymphoma and vitiligo. Psoralens are tricyclic furocoumarins that, when intercalated into DNA and exposed to UV-A, form adducts with pyrimidine bases and eventually form DNA cross-links. These

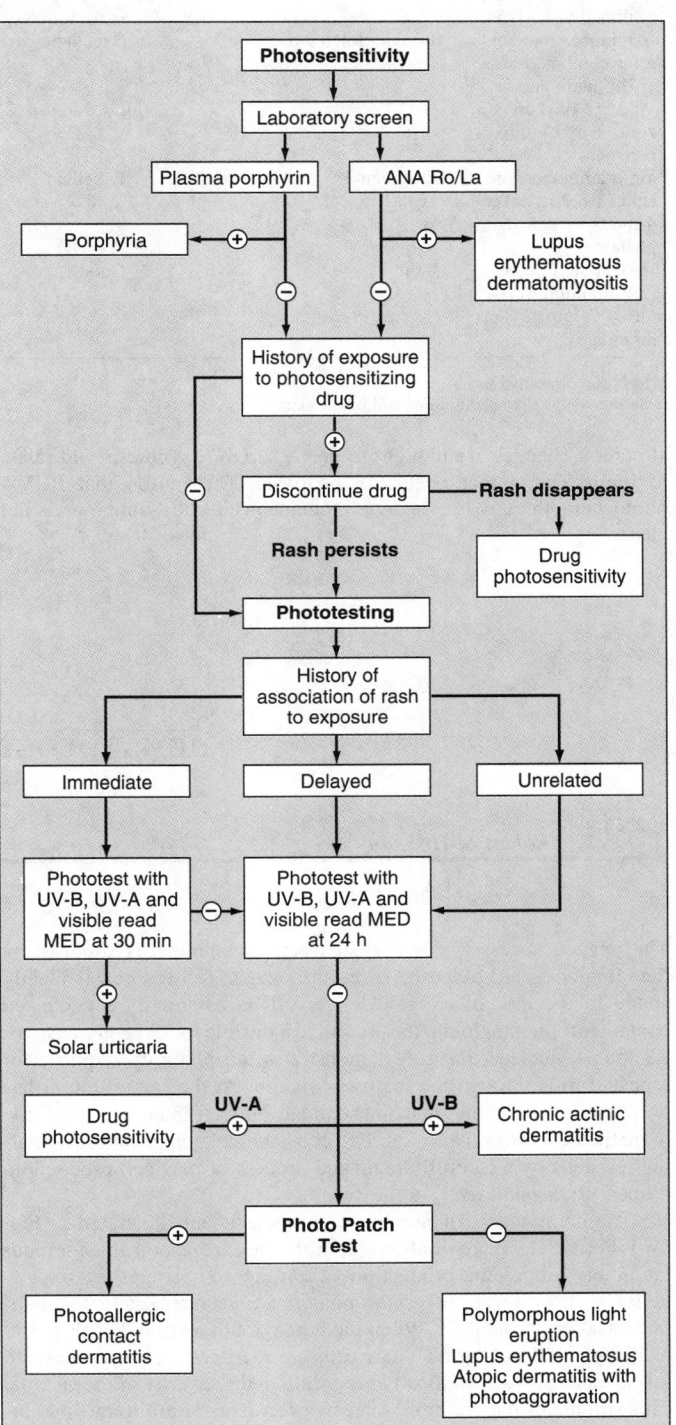

FIGURE 58-1 An algorithm for the diagnosis of a patient with photosensitivity.

Table 58-5

Properties of Selected Sunscreens

Ingredients	Trade Names	SPF* (Outdoors)	Substantivity†
p-Aminobenzoic acid (PABA) (5% in ethanol)	Pre-Sun-15	10–12	Excellent
p-Aminobenzoic acid esters (3.5% padimate A + 3.0% octyldimethyl PABA)	Original Eclipse	4–6	Fair
p-Aminobenzoic acid ester combinations (7.0% padimate O + 2.5% oxybenzone + 5.0% dioxybenzone)	Bain de Soleil	9	Excellent
Non-p-aminobenzoic acid (3% 2-hydroxy-4-methoxy benzophenone)	Ti-Screen-15	10–12	Excellent
Physical sunscreens (5% titanium dioxide + 5% methylanthranilate)	A-Fil	4–6	Good

* SPF, sun protective factor.
† Substantivity is the ability to remain on the skin.

structural changes are thought to decrease DNA synthesis and relate to improvement that occurs in psoriasis. The reason that PUVA photochemotherapy is effective in cutaneous T cell lymphoma is not clear.

In addition to its effects on DNA, PUVA photochemotherapy also stimulates melanin synthesis, and this provides the rationale for its use in the depigmenting disease vitiligo. Oral 8-methoxypsoralen and UV-A appear to be most effective in this regard, but as many as 100 treatments extending over 12 to 18 months may be required to promote satisfactory repigmentation.

The major side effects of UV-B phototherapy and PUVA photochemotherapy are due to the cumulative effects of photon absorption and include skin dryness, actinic keratoses, and an increased risk of nonmelanoma skin cancer. Despite these risks, the therapeutic index of these modalities is quite acceptable.

BIBLIOGRAPHY

FISHER GJ et al: Molecular basis of sun-induced premature skin aging and retinoid antagonism. Nature 379:335, 1996

GILCHREST BA et al: Mechanisms of ultraviolet light-induced pigmentation. Photochem Photobiol 63:1, 1996

GOULD JW et al: Cutaneous photosensitivity diseases induced by exogenous agents. J Am Acad Dermatol 33:551, 1995

HARBER LC, BICKERS DR: *Photosensitivity Diseases*, 2d ed. Toronto, Decker, 1989

HONIGSMANN H, STINGL G: *Therapeutic Photomedicine*. Basel, Karger, 1986

MAGNUS IA: *Dermatological Photobiology*. Oxford, Blackwell, 1976

PATHAK MA et al: Preventive treatment of sunburn, dermatoheliosis, and skin cancer with sun-protective agents, in *Dermatology in General Medicine*, 4th ed, TB Fitzpatrick et al (eds). New York, McGraw-Hill, 1993, Chap. 137

ZIEGLER A et al: Sunburn and p53 in the onset of skin cancer. Nature 372:773, 1994

SECTION 10
HEMATOLOGIC ALTERATIONS

59 *Robert S. Hillman*

ANEMIA

The oxygen necessary for normal tissue metabolism is supplied by the circulating red blood cells (erythrocytes). The red cell is ideally suited to the task of oxygen delivery. It is essentially a dedicated container for hemoglobin, the protein responsible for oxygen transport. Lacking a nucleus, the cell demonstrates the pliability required for repeated trips through the microcirculation. At the same time, it has only enough metabolic machinery to sustain cell integrity for a little more than 100 days. This requires a constant replenishment of circulating red cells by a carefully regulated process of new cell production, termed *erythropoiesis*.

The components of normal erythropoiesis are illustrated in Fig. 59-1. Peritubular interstitial cells of the kidney are responsible for regulating erythropoietin production according to changes in oxygen delivery. Low levels of erythropoietin are secreted daily to maintain basal erythropoiesis. When the hemoglobin level falls below 100 to 120 g/L (10 to 12 g/dL), new cells are recruited and erythropoietin levels increase logarithmically according to the severity of the anemia. This stimulates the erythroid marrow precursors to proliferate and increase red blood cell production severalfold. This functional capacity of the erythron requires normal renal function, a healthy marrow, and an adequate supply of key nutrients, especially iron. A defect in any

one or several of the key components in erythropoiesis will result in anemia.

By definition, a patient has an anemia whenever the hemoglobin level or the number of circulating red blood cells is significantly reduced. From a laboratory standpoint, the presence and severity of an anemia are easily described based on the deviation of the patient's hemoglobin/hematocrit from a standard set of normal values. From a clinical perspective, however, the diagnosis of an anemia is more complex. If it were feasible, the most sensitive indicator of anemia would be a direct measure of the level of oxygen delivered to peripheral tissues. Lacking this, a clinically significant anemia is best detected and defined from observed changes in the normal process of erythropoiesis. Measurements of red blood cell production, maturation, morphology, and iron supply are used to identify and initially classify an anemia as a defect in either marrow production, erythroid precursor maturation, or adult red blood cell survival. This functional classification of anemia then serves to guide the selection of a number of clinical and laboratory studies to complete the differential diagnosis of individual disease states.

CLINICAL PRESENTATION

The presence of an anemia may be suspected based on the nature of the patient's illness. Severe hemorrhage will produce an acute blood loss anemia, while chronic blood loss can be expected to result in iron deficiency. On the other hand, a patient with a collagen vascular disease is likely to present with an autoimmune hemolytic anemia. The clinical signs and symptoms of anemia will depend on how rapidly it appears, its severity, and the age of the patient. A mild anemia is easily compensated for by the inate ability of the hemoglobin–oxygen dissociation curve to maintain oxygen delivery to tissues as the hemoglobin level falls (Fig. 107-2). However, the shift in the curve will progressively reduce the capacity of the red cells to respond to situations of increased demand. Patients will report a loss in stamina, a rapid heart rate, and shortness of breath with exercise. When the hemoglobin falls below 70 to 80 g/L (7 to 8 g/dL), exercise capacity is markedly reduced; any exertion is associated with dyspnea, palpitations, a pounding headache, and rapid exhaustion. Older individuals who suffer from cardiovascular disease can develop worsening angina, claudication, and heart failure.

The ability to compensate also depends on the cause and rate of onset of the anemia. Acute blood loss involves a sudden reduction in both the blood volume and the red blood cell mass. While the hemoglobin–oxygen dissociation curve adjustment to release more oxygen to the tissues can make up for a reduced number of circulating red cells (see Chap. 107), even a modest fall in the total blood volume interferes with the cardiovascular response. A patient with severe hemorrhage will demonstrate signs and symptoms of both tissue hypoxia and vascular collapse. This is not true for patients who develop a more chronic anemia where the total blood volume remains normal and changes in cardiac output and regional blood flow help compensate for the loss in oxygen-carrying capacity.

Approach to the Patient

A detailed history and physical examination are essential to the diagnosis and management of an anemia. Clues to the etiology may appear in any part of the history, present illness, past medical history, family history, or review of systems. Symptoms of an acute or chronic illness, information as to transfusion history, past blood count measurements, nutritional habits, drug or alcohol intake, and family history of anemia can all be valuable. Racial background is important since many of the red blood cell metabolic defects follow ethnic lines. Certain complaints provide clues to specific types of anemia. For example, the sickle cell anemia patient will describe a lifelong history of periodic, severe bone and joint pain. Patients with severe iron deficiency often report a sore mouth and difficulty swallowing or have a craving for ice or dirt (pica or picophagia).

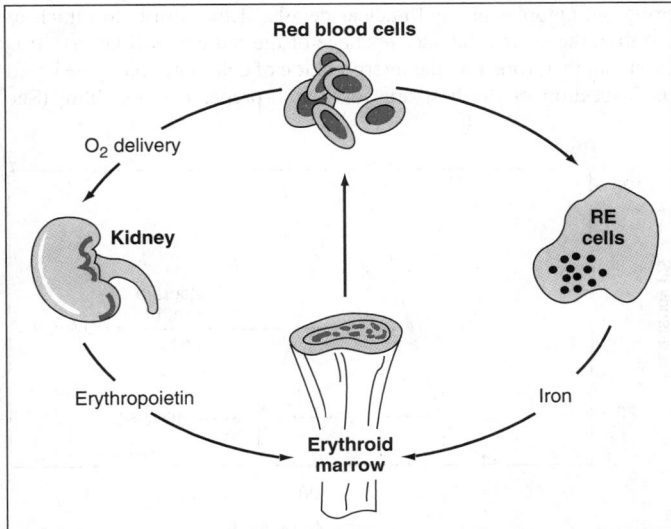

FIGURE 59-1 Components of normal erythropoiesis. The daily replacement of circulating red blood cells and the proliferative response to anemia is regulated by the kidney via release of erythropoietin. The response of the erythroid marrow to increasing levels of erythropoietin requires both a normal marrow and an adequate supply of iron from reticuloendothelial stores and oral intake.

The physical examination of a patient with anemia should emphasize the evaluation of tissue oxygen delivery. With acute blood loss, signs of hypovolemia and tissue hypoxia are the most reliable indicators of anemia severity. When more than 30 percent of the blood volume is suddenly lost, patients are unable to compensate with the usual mechanisms of venospasm and changes in regional blood flow. They will want to remain supine and will exhibit postural hypotension and tachycardia if mobilized. If the blood volume loss exceeds 40 percent (i.e., > 2000 mL in the average-sized adult), signs of hypovolemic shock including confusion, air hunger, diaphoresis, hypotension, and tachycardia will appear. Such patients are experiencing significant deficits in vital organ perfusion and require immediate volume replacement therapy.

When an anemia develops more gradually, hypovolemia is not a concern. In fact, a slight expansion of the blood volume and an increase in cardiac output are signs of effective compensation. The patient will exhibit a forceful apical impulse, strong peripheral pulses with a wide pulse pressure, and a mid- or holosystolic murmur secondary to increased blood flow and turbulence. Pallor of the skin and mucous membranes is another sign of severe anemia [a hemoglobin level < 80 to 100 g/L (8 to 10 g/dL)]. This is less reliable in patients with subcutaneous edema, marked reductions in skin blood flow, or deeply pigmented skin. Therefore, the examination should focus on areas where vessels are close to the surface, for example, the mucous membranes, nail beds, and palmar creases of the hand. When the palmar creases are lighter in color than the surrounding skin, the hemoglobin level is usually less than 80 g/L (8 g/dL).

Very mild anemias produce little in the way of clinical symptoms or signs. This is a tribute to the built-in mechanism of red cell compensation—the ability of the hemoglobin–oxygen dissociation curve to adjust oxygen delivery to tissues. Normally, only the topmost portion of the hemoglobin–oxygen dissociation curve is used, providing a considerable excess capacity for oxygen delivery for increased oxygen demands (see Fig. 107-2). In the case of acute anemia, slight changes in pH and CO_2 concentration at the periphery will instantaneously shift the curve to the right (Bohr effect), thereby increasing the release of oxygen to the tissues. With chronic anemia, the individual red cell maintains this shift by increasing the intracellular production of 2,3 bisphosphoglycerate. By itself, this mechanism of compensation is sufficient to maintain a normal delivery of oxygen to tissues despite hemoglobin falls of 20 to 30 g/L (2 to 3 g/dL). Because of this, a mild anemia is usually first detected from a screening measurement of hemoglobin or hematocrit, rather than from the history or physical examination.

Laboratory Evaluation The clinical laboratory provides a number of tests useful in the diagnosis of anemia (Table 59-1). The most important of these are the complete blood count (CBC), reticulocyte count, and measurements of iron supply, including the serum iron, total iron-binding capacity, and serum ferritin. In patients with severe anemia and abnormalities in red blood cell morphology, a bone marrow aspirate and biopsy are important diagnostic tools. Other assays of value in the diagnosis of specific anemias are discussed in chapters on specific disease states.

COMPLETE BLOOD COUNT Automated cell counters measure a number of parameters as a part of the CBC, including the hemoglobin, red blood cell count, red blood cell volume distribution, platelet count, and white blood cell count. The counter also calculates the hematocrit (based on the RBC count and volume), the mean cell volume (MCV) (based on volume distribution), mean cell hemoglobin (MCH) (hemoglobin divided by RBC count), mean cell hemoglobin concentration (MCHC) (hemoglobin divided by hematocrit), and the red cell distribution width (RDW). The red cell indices and RDW are used together with a direct inspection of the Wright-stained blood smear to evaluate red blood cell morphology.

The CBC provides a window into a number of the key components of erythropoiesis. The hemoglobin level and hematocrit are used inter-

Table 59-1

Laboratory Tests in Anemia Diagnosis

I. Complete blood count (CBC)
  A. Red blood cell count
    1. Hemoglobin
    2. Hematocrit
  B. Red blood cell indices
    1. Mean cell volume (MCV)
    2. Mean cell hemoglobin (MCH)
    3. Mean cell hemoglobin concentration (MCHC)
    4. Red cell distribution width (RDW)
  C. White blood cell count
    1. Cell differential
    2. Nuclear segmentation of neutrophils
  D. Platelet count
  E. Cell morphology
    1. Cell size
    2. Hemoglobin content
    3. Anisocytosis
    4. Poikilocytosis
    5. Polychromasia
II. Reticulocyte count
III. Iron supply studies
  A. Serum iron
  B. Total iron-binding capacity
  C. Serum ferritin, marrow iron stain
IV. Marrow examination
  A. Aspirate
    1. E/G ratio*
    2. Cell morphology
    3. Iron stain
  B. Biopsy
    1. Cellularity
    2. Morphology

* E/G ratio, ratio of erythroid to granulocytic precursors.

changeably to identify the presence and severity of an anemia according to a set of standard "normal" values (Table 59-2). Normal variations in the CBC with age are shown in the Appendix (Tables A-7 and A-8). Several physiologic and environmental factors can affect these normal values. The influences of age, sex, and pregnancy are recognized in Table 59-2. Higher normal values may be established for adult men and women who live at a high altitude or smoke more than 1 pack of cigarettes per day. This reflects a normal compensation for a decrease in arterial oxygen saturation. Heavy smokers can show an increase in the hemoglobin level of 5 to 10 g/L (0.5 to 1 g/dL) secondary to carbon monoxide binding to hemoglobin. It is also important to recognize that the range of normal values for the hemoglobin and hematocrit describe a Gaussian distribution around the normal mean. Therefore, the actual probability that a patient is anemic will depend on just how much lower the hemoglobin or hematocrit is from the reference value as well as the prevalence of various types of anemia in the population. A hemoglobin level < 100 g/L (< 10 g/dL) in an adult woman is definitely abnormal, while a value of 110 or 120 g/L (11 or 12 g/dL) may or may not indicate anemia.

Other components of the CBC can help in the detection and classification of an anemia. The red blood cell indices, especially the MCV,

Table 59-2

Normal Hemoglobin and Hematocrit Values

Age/Sex	Hemoglobin, g/L	Hematocrit, %
Adolescents	130	40
Adult men	160 (±20)*	47 (±6)*
Adult women	130 (±20)	40 (±6)
Adult women (postmenopausal)	140 (±20)	42 (±6)
Pregnancy (3rd trimester)	120 (±20)	37 (±6)

* ± 2 standard deviations.

Table 59-3

Normal Values for Red Cell Indices

Mean cell volume (MCV)	90 ± 9 fL
Mean cell hemoglobin (MCH)	32 ± 2 pg
Mean cell hemoglobin concentration (MCHC)	33 ± 3%
Red cell distribution width (RDW)	
RDW-CV	13 ± 1%
RDW-SD	42 ± 5 fL

will detect an increase (*macrocytosis*) or decrease (*microcytosis*) in red blood cell volume, while the MCH is sensitive to defects in hemoglobin production (*hypochromia*). The normal values for each of these measurements are listed in Table 59-3. Automated counters are quite precise in describing the red cell volume distribution (Fig. 59-2). The MCV that represents the peak of the distribution curve is not sensitive to the appearance of small populations of macrocytes or microcytes. Measurement errors can also be introduced by major distortions in red cell shape, red blood cell agglutination, or the presence of very high numbers of white blood cells. The technician or clinician can correct for these measurement errors by reviewing the actual red blood cell distribution curve produced by the counter and by direct inspection of the peripheral blood smear.

Automated counters also provide a numerical index of the distribution of red blood cell volumes, the RDW. As shown in Fig. 59-2, the RDW can be measured at two points on the red cell volume distribution curve. The RDW-CV is a ratio calculated as the width of the histogram at one standard deviation divided by the MCV, while the RDW-SD represents the width of the distribution curve at the 20 percent frequency level. Since it is a ratio, the RDW-CV will tend to magnify variations in cell size in patients with microcytic anemias. It is useful, therefore, in separating patients with early iron deficiency who have a mixed population of small and normal sized cells from the patient with thalassemia minor with more uniform microcytosis. At the same time, the RDW-CV is less sensitive to early macrocytosis. In contrast, the RDW-SD is very sensitive to the appearance of even small populations of microcytes or macrocytes.

PERIPHERAL BLOOD FILM Inspection of the peripheral blood film can provide important information as to the presence and nature of an erythropoietic defect. Careful preparation of the blood film is very important. Using glass slides or coverslips and a cytocentrifuge, a small drop of blood can be spread to create a monolayer of red blood cells. The well-dried blood film is then stained with Wright's stain to bring out cytoplasmic and nuclear details. If the film is too thick or too thin, the normal biconcave shape of the red cell will be lost. It is essential, therefore, that the interpretation of cell morphology be based on inspection of the best area of a well-prepared blood film. (**See**

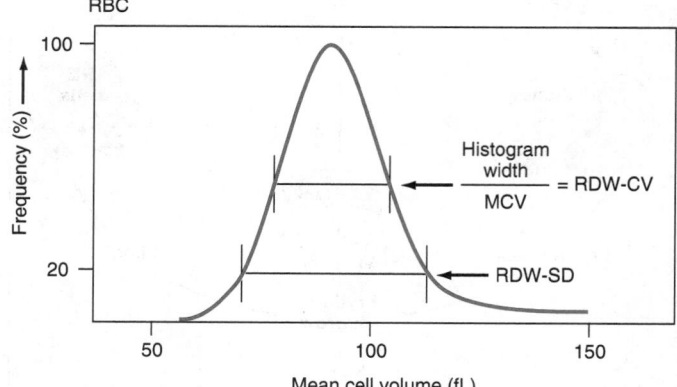

FIGURE 59-2 Automated cell counters display a distribution curve of the red blood cell volume and calculate two measurements of the width of the distribution curve. The RDW-CV is calculated as a ratio of the width of the curve at 1 standard deviation divided by the MCV. The RDW-SD is simply the width of the curve measured at the 20 percent frequency level (RDW, red cell distribution width). (From Hillman and Ault.)

Plate IV-1.) As a complement to the red cell indices, changes in individual cell diameter, shape, and hemoglobin content are looked for to identify microcytosis or macrocytosis even before there is a dramatic change in MCV, MCH, or RDW. The blood film is also important in describing variations in cell size (*anisocytosis*) and shape (*poikilocytosis*). The degree of anisocytosis usually correlates with increases in the RDW. Poikilocytosis suggests a defect in red blood cell precursor maturation or fragmentation hemolysis. The smear should also be inspected for *polychromasia*, that is, the presence of polychromatic macrocytes—cells that are slightly larger and grayish-blue in color. These are marrow reticulocytes containing residual amounts of RNA and ribosomes. They appear in the circulation in response to increased levels of erythropoietin stimulation and, therefore, can be used as a marker of the appropriateness of the erythropoietin response. Other individual cell abnormalities, including the appearance of nucleated red blood cells, Howell-Jolly bodies, targeting, sickle cells, etc., are clues to specific disease states.

RETICULOCYTE COUNT Like the CBC, an accurate measure of the reticulocyte count is key to the initial classification of any anemia. Reticulocytes are newborn red blood cells that contain sufficient residual RNA that they can be stained with a supravital dye and counted as a percent of the circulating red cell population. In the basal state, the normal reticulocyte count ranges from 1 to 2 percent according to the counting method. This correlates with the normal daily replacement of approximately 1 percent of the circulating red blood cell population. Increases in the reticulocyte count provide a reliable measure of the red blood cell production response to anemia.

To use the reticulocyte count as a production measure, it must first be corrected for changes in the patient's hematocrit and for the effect of erythropoietin on the early release of marrow reticulocytes into circulation. The hematocrit (Hct) correction converts the reticulocyte percentage to an absolute number:

$$\% \text{ Reticulocytes} \times \frac{\text{patient Hct}}{45\%} = \text{absolute \% reticulocytes}$$

The marrow reticulocyte ("shift") correction involves dividing the absolute percentage by a factor of 1.5 to 2.5 whenever there is prominent polychromasia on the peripheral blood smear (Fig. 59-3). The shift correction should always be applied to any patient with anemia and a very high reticulocyte count to provide a true index of effective red blood cell production. A normal patient will respond to a hematocrit less than 30 percent with a two- to threefold increase in the reticulocyte production index. Patients with severe, chronic hemolytic anemias can easily demonstrate a reticulocyte index of greater than five to six times normal. This measure alone, therefore, will confirm the fact that the patient has an appropriate erythropoietin response, a normal erythroid marrow, and sufficient iron supply to meet the challenge. When the reticulocyte index falls below 2, a defect in marrow proliferation or precursor maturation must be present.

TESTS OF IRON SUPPLY Standard measurements of iron supply include the serum iron, transferrin iron-binding capacity (TIBC), and the serum ferritin level. The normal serum iron ranges from 9 to 27 μmol/L (50 to 150 μg/dL), while the normal TIBC is 54 to 64 μmol/L (300 to 360 μg/dL). Therefore, in the basal state, only 30 to 50 percent of the transferrin in circulation is saturated with iron. Important information is provided by each measurement as well as the calculated percent saturation. The serum ferritin is used to evaluate body iron stores. Adult males have serum ferritin levels of between 50 and 150 μg/L, corresponding to iron stores of from 600 to 1000 mg. Adult females have lower serum ferritin levels (15 to 50 μg/L) and smaller iron stores (0 to 300 mg). Lower serum ferritin levels are observed as iron stores are depleted; levels below 15 μg/L indicate store exhaustion and iron deficiency. Iron overload (hemachromatosis and hemosiderosis) can produce levels in excess of 500 to 1000 μg/L.

BONE MARROW EXAMINATION A sample of bone marrow is readily obtained by needle aspirate or biopsy. It is of greatest value in patients who have a hypoproliferative anemia or a disorder of red blood cell maturation, providing valuable information as to marrow structure and cellularity, as well as precursor proliferation and maturation. The ratio of erythroid to granulocytic precursors (E/G ratio) is used to assess the proliferative capacity of erythroid precursors. A patient with a hypoproliferative anemia and a reticulocyte index < 2 will demonstrate an E/G ratio ≤ 1:3 or 1:2. In contrast, the hemolytic anemia patient with a production index ≥ 3 to 5 will have an E/G ratio > 1:1. Red cell precursor maturation defects are identified from the mismatch between the E/G ratio and reticulocyte production index. These individuals demonstrate an E/G ratio of greater than 1:1 together with a low reticulocyte index, typical of the ineffective erythropoiesis of a maturation disorder.

ADDITIONAL LABORATORY MEASUREMENTS There are a number of other laboratory tests that are of value in the diagnosis of specific disease states. Details as to the use of these tests are covered in the discussion of individual disorders. Normal values are listed in the "Appendix: Laboratory Values of Clinical Importance."

APPROACH TO ANEMIA DIAGNOSIS

The evaluation of anemia, whether a primary hematologic disorder or secondary to other illness, is common in clinical practice. Success will depend not only on the clinician's knowledge and understanding of causes of anemia but also on the speed and skill of the evaluation. As a rule, a significant anemia should be studied without delay, using a battery of laboratory tests so as to get a clear picture of the erythropoietic abnormality. This will help avoid the misinterpretation of a test because of a change in the patient's clinical status. For example, the ability to diagnose a nutritional anemia will be confounded as a patient changes diet or receives vitamin or mineral supplements. A blood transfusion given before the workup will, by reducing the erythropoietin response, change the red cell production measurements needed for diagnosis. It is also important never to assume a diagnostic relationship. Even when the cause of the anemia is suggested by the clinical presentation, a full laboratory evaluation is essential. Anemias are often the result of several contributing factors and not a single etiologic component.

INITIAL CLASSIFICATION OF ANEMIA The first step in anemia diagnosis is the classification according to the functional defect in erythropoiesis—whether there is a failure in red blood cell produc-

Hematocrit (%)	Marrow normoblasts and reticulocytes (days)	Peripheral blood reticulocytes (days)
45	3.5	1.0
35	3.0	1.5
25	2.5	2.0
15	1.5	2.5

"SHIFT" correction factor

FIGURE 59-3 Reticulocyte "shift" correction. As the level of erythropoietin stimulation increases with worsening anemia, marrow reticulocytes leave the marrow at an earlier point in their maturation. This effectively lengthens the maturation time in circulation and allows them to be counted for more than 1 day. This needs to be taken into account when interpreting the reticulocyte count. Whenever there is prominent polychromasia on the peripheral smear, the predicted delay in maturation of from 1.5 to 2.5 days should be used as a "shift" correction factor to calculate the true reticulocyte production index:

$$\frac{\text{Absolute \% reticulocytes}}{\text{"Shift" factor}} = \text{reticulocyte production index}$$

(From Hillman and Ault.)

tion, an abnormality in precursor maturation, or an increase in red blood cell destruction. In a patient with a moderate to severe anemia, the CBC and reticulocyte index are enough to make this distinction. As shown in Fig. 59-4, a defect in red cell production (hypoproliferative anemia) will show a low reticulocyte production index together with little or no change in red blood cell morphology, that is, a normocytic, normochromic anemia. Maturation disorders also demonstrate a low reticulocyte index but accompanied by either a macrocytic or microcytic morphology. Increased red blood cell destruction secondary to hemolysis or hemorrhage typically results in an increase in the reticulocyte index to levels greater than three times normal. Red blood cell morphology will depend on the specific disease state. The MCV is usually normal or slightly increased depending on the level of reticulocytosis. Inspection of the smear may reveal distinctive cell shapes that help make a specific diagnosis. Classifying an anemia according to the functional defect helps organize the subsequent use of laboratory studies.

HYPOPROLIFERATIVE ANEMIAS The majority of anemias seen in clinical practice are hypoproliferative, that is, they result from a failure in the appropriate erythroid marrow production response for the degree of anemia. As illustrated in Fig. 59-4, they can result from marrow damage (Chap. 110), iron deficiency, or a failure of the normal erythropoietin response to anemia (Chap. 106). The latter can reflect a suppression of erythropoietin release by inflammatory cytokines, a reduced metabolic need, or the permanent loss of peritubular interstitial cells as a part of end-stage renal disease. The laboratory measurements that help distinguish between these defects include the iron supply studies and bone marrow examination. Patients with the anemia of acute or chronic inflammation demonstrate a distinctive pattern of serum iron, TIBC, and serum ferritin. The same is true for iron loss leading to iron

deficiency. A primary failure in precursor proliferation due to marrow damage by a drug, leukemic change, or tumor infiltration can usually be diagnosed from the bone marrow morphology.

MATURATION DISORDERS Defects in erythroid precursor maturation are initially recognized from the combination of a low reticulocyte production index and a distinctive change in morphology. Patients present with either a macrocytic (MCV > 100 fL) or microcytic (MCV < 80 fL) anemia. The low reticulocyte index is a reflection of the ineffective erythropoiesis that results from the defect in precursor maturation. An examination of marrow morphology will show an increase in the E/G ratio to levels greater than 1:1, confirming the proliferation of the erythroid marrow. The reason for the failure in precursor development may also be apparent. A defect in nuclear maturation that produces a macrocytic anemia will demonstrate megaloblastic bone marrow morphology (Chap 108). Patients with cytoplasmic maturation defects will have poor hemoglobinization of the more mature erythroid precursors.

The most common causes of the nuclear and cytoplasmic maturation defects are listed in Fig. 59-4. Severe iron deficiency and the inherited defects in globin chain synthesis, the thalassemias, produce a moderate to marked microcytic, hypochromic anemia (Chap. 107). These disorders may be differentiated simply on the basis of blood smear morphology and the racial background of the patient. If not, measurements of iron supply will help make the diagnosis. Inherited or acquired abnormalities in mitochondrial function can result in either a microcytic or macrocytic anemia. Based on the distinctive finding of ringed sideroblasts on the marrow iron stain, they are initially classified as sideroblastic anemias (Chap. 106). Here again, iron supply studies are important to the differential diagnosis and management of the patient. Defects in nuclear maturation result from a deficiency in folic acid or vitamin B_{12}, exposure to a chemotherapeutic agent, and as a component of a myelodysplastic or preleukemic state (Chap. 110). As with the differential diagnosis of cytoplasmic defects, marrow morphology and iron studies are helpful in the differential diagnosis of the etiology of the disorder. Measurements of folic acid and vitamin B_{12} levels are of value in identifying a reversible vitamin deficiency.

INCREASED RED CELL DESTRUCTION This category of anemia is easily identified from the increase in the reticulocyte production index, together with normocytic or only slightly macrocytic red cell morphology (Fig. 59-4). This is a reflection of the capacity of the erythroid marrow to compensate for a blood loss or red cell hemolysis anemia with an increase in red blood cell production. The level of response will depend on both the severity of the anemia and the nature of the underlying disease process. Because the response to blood loss is limited by the availability of sources of iron supply, the initial reticulocyte response usually does not exceed three times the basal level and may be short-lived. In contrast, patients with acute or chronic hemolytic anemias will achieve much higher production levels and sustain them indefinitely.

While acute blood loss is usually clinically obvious, hemolytic anemias can present in different ways (Chap. 109). Some will appear suddenly as an acute, self-limited episode of intravascular or extravascular hemolysis. This pattern of presentation is often seen in patients with red blood cell metabolic defects or autoimmune hemolytic anemias. Patients with inherited defects of hemoglobin or membrane structure will generally describe a lifelong clinical history typical of the disease process. This is especially true for patients with a hemoglobinopathy such as sickle cell disease or combinations of sickle hemoglobin with other hemoglobinopathies (Chap. 107). Similarly, the patient with hereditary spherocytosis, a common membrane structural defect, will present with a complication stemming from their lifelong need to maintain a high level of red blood cell production, a hemolytic or aplastic crisis, symptomatic bilirubin gallstones, or significant splenomegaly (Chap. 109).

The differential diagnosis of the cause of an acute or chronic hemolytic anemia requires the careful integration of racial and family history data, the pattern of clinical presentation, and a number of targeted laboratory studies. Some of the more common congenital hemolytic anemias may be identified from the red blood cell morphol-

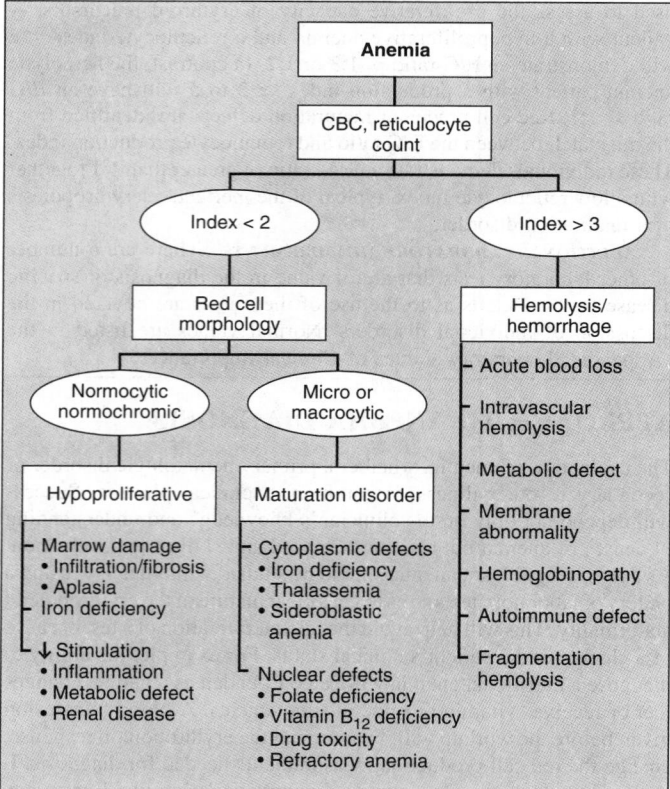

FIGURE 59-4 The classification of anemia. The complete blood count and reticulocyte index are used initially to classify an anemia as either hypoproliferative, a maturation disorder, or a hemolytic/hemorrhagic anemia. This provides a guide to the subsequent differential diagnosis of specific disease states within each category. The bone marrow examination and measurements of iron supply are very important in this differential.

ogy or a routine laboratory test such as the hemoglobin electrophoresis or an enzyme screening test. For example, the common β-chain hemoglobinopathies—sickle cell disease, hemoglobin SC disease, and sickle-thalassemia—have distinctive hemoglobin electrophoretic patterns. Glucose-6-phosphate dehydrogenase (G6PD) deficiency, a common red blood cell metabolic defect, can be easily screened for using a G6PD enzyme spot test. There are, however, a large number of other defects of red cell membrane, hemoglobin, and intracellular metabolism that can only be diagnosed with the help of an expert hematology reference laboratory.

℞ TREATMENT

The management of anemia begins at the time of evaluation. While it is important to perform a careful history, physical examination, and order a complete battery of laboratory tests without delay, it is equally important to quickly initiate any indicated treatment. When an anemia is so severe as to threaten the patient's survival, immediate steps must be taken to guarantee oxygen delivery to tissues. This will involve the appropriate infusion of electrolyte and colloid solutions to correct hypovolemia and red blood cell transfusions to guarantee tissue oxygen delivery. Administration of supplemental oxygen may be required. It may also involve the administration of an essential vitamin or chemotherapeutic drug(s) to address a specific disease process.

If the anemia is less severe, red cell transfusions and vitamin or mineral therapy should be withheld until the diagnosis is certain. "Shotgun" therapy where several vitamins and iron are administered simultaneously is never appropriate. The selection of the right therapy should be firmly based on the documented cause or causes of the anemia. Often, more than one etiologic component must be addressed in management. For example, a patient with the anemia of end-stage renal disease will require erythropoietin therapy to correct for the loss of erythropoietin-secreting cells. However, the effectiveness of recombinant erythropoietin will depend on the patient's iron status. If the patient lacks adequate reticuloendothelial iron stores, a failure in iron supply will prevent the erythroid marrow from proliferating in the face of erythropoietin therapy. It is important, therefore, to fully evaluate the patient's iron status before and during therapy.

The therapeutic options for the treatment of various anemias has expanded dramatically during the past two decades. Blood components are readily available and extremely safe. Effective therapies are now well established for the nutritional anemias, the hypoproliferative anemias associated with end-stage renal disease and chronic inflammation, severe aplastic anemia, and the hemolytic anemia associated with autoimmune diseases. Effective chemotherapy to help prevent sickle cell crises in sickle cell anemia patients has become available. In the future, it is anticipated that many of the congenital defects in hemoglobin structure and hemoglobin synthesis will be treated using the newer techniques of molecular engineering.

BIBLIOGRAPHY

BEUTLER E et al (eds): *Williams Hematology*, 5th ed. New York, McGraw-Hill, 1995, pp 3–22
HILLMAN RS, AULT KA: *Hematology in Clinical Practice*. New York, McGraw-Hill, 1995
———, FINCH CA: *Red Cell Manual*, 7th ed. Philadelphia, FA Davis, 1996

60 *Robert I. Handin*

BLEEDING AND THROMBOSIS

Hemorrhage, intravascular thrombosis, and embolism are common clinical manifestations of many diseases. The normal hemostatic system limits blood loss by precisely regulated interactions between components of the vessel wall, circulating blood platelets, and plasma proteins. However, when disease or trauma damage large arteries and veins, excessive bleeding may occur, despite a normal hemostatic system. Less frequently, hemorrhage is caused by an inherited or acquired disorder of the hemostatic machinery itself. A large number of such bleeding disorders have now been identified.

In addition, unregulated activation of the hemostatic system may cause thrombosis and embolism, which can reduce blood flow to critical organs like the brain and myocardium. Although we understand less about the pathophysiology of thrombosis than of hemostatic failure, certain patient groups have been identified that are particularly prone to thrombosis and embolism. These include patients who (1) are immobilized after surgery, (2) have chronic congestive heart failure, (3) have atherosclerotic vascular disease, (4) have a malignancy, or (5) are pregnant. Most of these "thrombosis-prone" patients have no identifiable hemostatic disorder. However, there are certain patient groups who have inherited or acquired a "hypercoagulable" or "prethrombotic" state which predisposes them to recurrent thrombosis.

The cardinal manifestations of disordered hemostasis which cause bleeding or thrombosis are discussed below, along with the clinical approach to diagnosis and evaluation of these patients. Certain information in the patient's history, such as the mode of onset and sites of bleeding, a family bleeding tendency, and a record of drug ingestion help establish the correct diagnosis. Physical examination can identify bleeding in the skin or joint deformities due to previous hemarthroses. Ultimately, however, bleeding disorders are diagnosed by laboratory tests. General screening tests are used first, to document a systemic disorder, and are then supplemented by specific tests of coagulation protein or platelet function to arrive at an accurate diagnosis.

The hypercoagulable or prethrombotic patient can also be identified by a careful history. There are three important clues to this diagnosis: (1) repeated episodes of thromboembolism without an obvious predisposing condition; (2) a family history of thrombosis; and (3) well-documented thromboembolism in adolescents and young adults. Although several tests are being evaluated, there are, as yet, no clinically useful screening tests for the prethrombotic state. However, several of the inherited prethrombotic disorders can be diagnosed with specific immunologic and functional assays.

NORMAL HEMOSTASIS

Accurate diagnosis and treatment of patients with either bleeding or thrombosis requires some knowledge of the pathophysiology of hemostasis. The process can be divided into primary and secondary components and is initiated when trauma, surgery, or disease disrupt the vascular endothelial lining and blood is exposed to subendothelial connective tissue. *Primary hemostasis* is the name given to the process of platelet plug formation at sites of injury. It occurs within seconds of injury and is of prime importance in stopping blood loss from capillaries, small arterioles, and venules (Fig. 60-1). *Secondary hemostasis* consists of the reactions of the plasma coagulation system that result in fibrin formation. It requires several minutes for completion. The fibrin strands that are produced strengthen the primary hemostatic plug. This reaction is particularly important in larger vessels and prevents recurrent bleeding from occurring hours or days after the initial injury. Although presented here as separate events, primary and secondary hemostasis are closely linked. For example, activated platelets accelerate plasma coagulation, and products of the plasma coagulation reaction, such as thrombin, induce platelet activation.

Effective primary hemostasis requires three critical events—platelet adhesion, granule release, and platelet aggregation. Within a few seconds of injury, platelets adhere to collagen fibrils in vascular subendothelium via a specific platelet collagen receptor, glycoprotein Ia/IIa, which is a member of the integrin family. As shown in Fig. 60-2, this interaction is stabilized by the von Willebrand factor, an adhesive glycoprotein which allows platelets to remain attached to the vessel wall despite the high shear forces generated within the vascular lumen. The von Willebrand factor accomplishes this task by

FIGURE 60-1 Schematic presentation of the major events in primary hemostasis. The first event is platelet adhesion, the interaction of platelets with a nonplatelet surface such as vascular subendothelium. This is followed by platelet activation and secretion. Some of the products secreted by platelets are depicted. Abbreviations: ADP, adenosine diphosphate; PDGF, platelet-derived growth factor; vWF, von Willebrand's factor. The final event is the binding of activated platelets to the adherent monolayer in the process of platelet aggregation.

forming a link between a platelet receptor site on glycoprotein Ib/IX and subendothelial collagen fibrils. The adherent platelets then release preformed granule constituents and generate de novo mediators like those depicted in Fig. 60-1.

As in other cells, platelet activation and secretion are regulated by changes in the level of cyclic nucleotides, the influx of calcium, hydrolysis of membrane phospholipids, and phosphorylation of critical intracellular proteins. The relevant pathways are depicted in Figs. 60-3 and 60-4. The binding of agonists such as epinephrine, collagen, or thrombin to platelet surface receptors activates two membrane enzymes—phospholipase C and phospholipase A$_2$. These enzymes catalyze the release of arachidonic acid from two of the major membrane phospholipids, phosphatidylinositol and phosphatidylcholine. Initially, a small quantity of the released arachidonic acid is converted to throm-

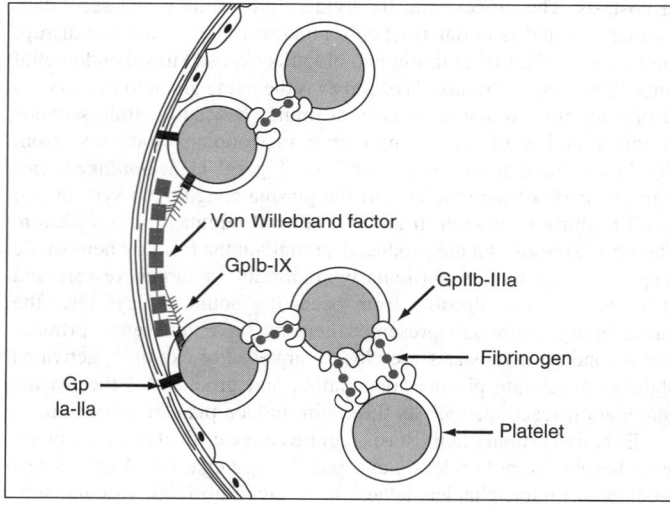

FIGURE 60-2 The molecular basis of platelet adhesion and aggregation. Adhesion of platelets to vascular subendothelium is facilitated by von Willebrand's factor, which forms a bridge between collagen fibrils in the vessel wall and receptors on platelet glycoprotein Ib/IX (GpIb–IX). In a similar manner, platelet aggregation is mediated by fibrinogen which links adjacent platelets via receptors on the platelet glycoprotein IIb and IIIa complex (GpIIb–IIIa).

FIGURE 60-3 Generation of thromboxane A$_2$ in platelets and prostacyclin (PGI$_2$) in endothelial cells.

boxane A$_2$ (TXA$_2$), which, in turn, can activate phospholipase C. The formation of TXA$_2$ from arachidonic acid is mediated by the enzyme cyclooxygenase (see Fig. 60-3). This enzyme is inhibited by aspirin and nonsteroidal anti-inflammatory drugs. Inhibition of TXA$_2$ synthesis is a cause of mild bleeding in some patients, as well as the basis for the action of some antithrombotic drugs.

Hydrolysis of the membrane phospholipid phosphatidylinositol 4,5-bisphosphate (PIP$_2$) produces diacylglycerol (DAG) and inositol triphosphate (IP$_3$), both of which play critical roles in platelet metabolism. IP$_3$ mediates the movement of calcium into the platelet cytosol and stimulates the phosphorylation of myosin light chains. The latter interact with actin to facilitate granule movement and platelet shape

FIGURE 60-4 The biochemical basis of platelet activation and secretion. Binding of agonists such as thrombin, epinephrine, or collagen sets in motion a chain of events which hydrolyzes membrane phospholipids, inhibits adenylate cyclase, mobilizes intracellular calcium, and phosphorylates critical intracellular proteins. The net result is shape change, movement of granules to the canalicular system, generation of mediators like thromboxane A$_2$, and granule secretion. Abbreviations: AC, adenylate cyclase; G, guanine nucleotide–binding protein; PIP$_2$, phosphatidylinositol 4,5-bisphosphate; PLC, phospholipase C; DAG, diacylglycerol; PLA$_2$, phospholipase A$_2$; PC, phosphatidylcholine; AA, arachidonic acid; CO, cyclooxygenase; O$_2$, oxygen; IP$_3$, inositol triphosphate; cAMP, cyclic AMP; Ca-CM, calcium calmodulin complex; MLCK, myosin light chain kinase.

change. DAG activates protein kinase C which, in turn, phosphorylates several substrates, including myosin light chain kinase and a 47,000-Da protein (plekstrin). Phosphorylation of these or other proteins may regulate platelet granule secretion.

A finely balanced mechanism controls the rate and extent of platelet activation, illustrated in Fig. 60-3. TXA$_2$, a platelet product of arachidonic acid, stimulates platelet activation and secretion. In contrast, prostacyclin (PGI$_2$), an endothelial cell product of arachidonic acid metabolism, inhibits platelet activation by raising intraplatelet levels of cyclic adenosine monophosphate (cyclic AMP). Similar pathways to regulate activation and secretion occur in other cells.

Following activation, platelets secrete their granule contents into plasma. Endoglycosidases and a heparin-cleaving enzyme are released from lysosomes; calcium, serotonin, and adenosine diphosphate (ADP) are released from the dense granules; and several proteins, including the von Willebrand factor, fibronectin, thrombospondin, the platelet-derived growth factor (PDGF), and a heparin-neutralizing protein (platelet factor 4) are released from alpha granules. Released ADP binds to a specific puringergic receptor which, when activated, changes the conformation of the glycoprotein IIb/IIIa complex so that it binds fibrinogen, linking adjacent platelets into a hemostatic plug (Fig. 60-2). Released PDGF stimulates the growth and migration of fibroblasts and smooth muscle cells within the vessel wall, which is an important part of the repair process.

As the primary hemostatic plug is being formed, plasma coagulation proteins are activated to initiate secondary hemostasis. An overall picture of the coagulation scheme, including the role of various inhibitors, is shown in Fig. 60-5. The coagulation pathway can be broken down into a series of reactions (outlined in Fig. 60-6) which culminate in the production of sufficient thrombin to convert a small portion of plasma fibrinogen to fibrin. Each of the reactions requires the formation of a surface-bound complex and the conversion of inactive precursor proteins into active proteases by limited proteolysis, and each is regulated by both plasma and cellular cofactors and calcium.

In *reaction 1*, the intrinsic or contact phase of coagulation, three plasma proteins, Hageman factor (factor XII), high-molecular-weight kininogen (HMWK), and prekallikrein (PK) form a complex on vascular subendothelial collagen. After binding to HMWK, factor XII is slowly converted to an active protease (XIIa), which then converts both PK to kallikrein and factor XI to its active form (XIa). Kallikrein (K) in turn accelerates the conversion of XII to XIIa, while XIa participates in subsequent coagulation reactions. Although these interactions are well characterized in vitro, an alternative mechanism for the activation of factor XI may exist, as patients who are deficient in either factor XII, HMWK, or PK have apparently normal hemostasis and no clinical bleeding.

Reaction 2 provides a second pathway to initiate coagulation by converting factor VII to an active protease. In this extrinsic or tissue-factor-dependent pathway, a complex is formed between factor VII, calcium, and tissue factor, a ubiquitous lipoprotein present in cellular membranes which is exposed following cellular injury. There is increasing evidence that the tissue factor–VII pathway is continuously active and makes a major contribution to basal coagulation. Factor VII and three other coagulation proteins—factors II (prothrombin), IX, and X—require calcium and vitamin K for biologic activity. These proteins are synthesized in the liver, where a vitamin K–dependent carboxylase catalyzes a unique posttranslational modification which adds a second carboxyl group to certain glutamic acid residues. Pairs of these di-γ-carboxyglutamic acid (Gla) residues bind calcium, which anchors these proteins to negatively charged phospholipid surfaces and confers biologic activity. Inhibition of this posttranslational modification by vitamin K antagonists (e.g., warfarin) is the basis of one of the most common forms of anticoagulant therapy.

In *reaction 3*, factor X is activated by the proteases generated in the two previous reactions. In one reaction, a calcium- and lipid-dependent complex is formed between factors VIII, IX, and X. Within this complex, factor IX is first converted to IXa by factor XIa that was generated within the intrinsic pathway (reaction 1). Factor X is then activated by factor IXa in concert with factor VIII. Alternatively, both factors IX and X can be activated more directly by factor VIIa, which has been generated via the extrinsic pathway (reaction 2). Activation of factors IX and X provides an important link between the intrinsic and extrinsic coagulation pathways (see Fig. 60-5).

Reaction 4, the final step, converts prothrombin to thrombin in the presence of factor V, calcium, and phospholipid. Although prothrombin conversion can take place on various natural and artificial phospholipid-rich surfaces, it proceeds several thousand times faster on the surface of activated platelets. Thrombin, the product of this reaction, has multiple functions in hemostasis. Although its principal role in hemostasis is the conversion of fibrinogen to fibrin, it also activates factors V, VIII, and XIII and stimulates platelet aggregation and secretion. Following the release of fibrinopeptides A and B from the α and β chains of fibrinogen, the modified molecule, now called fibrin monomer, polymerizes into an insoluble gel. The fibrin polymer is then stabilized by the cross-linking of individual chains by factor XIIIa, a plasma transglutaminase (Fig. 60-5).

Although the classic view of coagulation outlined above had clinical utility, it left several important questions unanswered. These included the following: (1) Why does factor XII deficiency produce a dramatically prolonged partial thromboplastin time (PTT) but not cause bleeding? (2) Why is there heterogeneity in the bleeding symptoms of patients with factor XI deficiency? (3) Why do deficiencies in factors VIII or IX produce such dramatic bleeding even though the "extrinsic" pathway remains intact? It is now thought that factors IX and X activation by the tissue factor–VIIa complex plays a major role in the initiation of hemostasis. Once coagulation is initiated by this interaction, a recently discovered protein, the tissue factor pathway inhibitor (TFPI), blocks the pathway, and elements of the intrinsic pathway, particularly factors VIII and IX, become the dominant regulators of thrombin generation. This new step in the pathway would help to explain why factor XIII–deficient patients are asymptomatic and

FIGURE 60-5 A schematic diagram of some of the clinically important coagulation reactions. The unactivated or precursor proteins are indicated by roman numerals, and the active form by the addition of a lowercase "a"—a standard convention. Other abbreviations: HMWK, high-molecular-weight kininogen; PK, prekallikrein; PL, phospholipid; TM, thrombomodulin; Ca^{2+}, calcium. There are two independent activation pathways, the contact system and the tissue factor–mediated or extrinsic system. They merge at the point of factor X activation and lead to the generation of thrombin, which converts fibrinogen into fibrin. These reactions are regulated by antithrombin, which forms complexes with all of the coagulation protein serine proteases except factor VII, and by the protein C–protein S system, which inactivates factors V and VIII.

why factor XI–deficient patients have a mild to moderate bleeding diathesis. This scheme is illustrated in Fig. 60-7.

Clot lysis and vessel repair begin immediately after the formation of the definitive hemostatic plug. There are three potential activators of the fibrinolytic system: Hageman factor fragments, urinary plasminogen activator (uPA) or urokinase (UK), and tissue plasminogen activator (tPA). The principal physiologic activators, tPA and uPA, diffuse from endothelial cells and convert plasminogen, adsorbed to the fibrin clot, into plasmin (Fig. 60-8). Plasmin then degrades fibrin polymer into small fragments, which are cleared by the monocyte-macrophage scavenger system. Although plasmin can also degrade fibrinogen, the reaction remains localized because (1) tPA and some forms of uPA activate plasminogen more effectively when it is adsorbed to fibrin clots, (2) any plasmin that enters the circulation is rapidly bound and neutralized by the α_2 plasmin inhibitor (the importance of this inhibitor is underscored by the fact that patients who lack it have unchecked fibrinolysis and bleed), and (3) endothelial cells release a plasminogen activator inhibitor (PAI-1), which directly blocks the action of tPA.

As noted above, the plasma coagulation system is tightly regulated so that only a small quantity of each coagulation enzyme is converted to its active form. As a consequence, the hemostatic plug does not propagate beyond the site of injury. Precise regulation is important, since there is enough clotting potential in a single milliliter of blood to clot all the fibrinogen in the body in 10 to 15 s. Blood fluidity is maintained by the flow of blood itself, which reduces the concentration of reactants; by the adsorption of coagulation factors to surfaces; and by the presence of multiple inhibitors in plasma. Antithrombin, proteins C and S, and TFPI are the most important inhibitors, collectively maintaining blood fluidity.

These inhibitors have distinct modes of action. Antithrombin forms complexes with all the serine protease coagulation factors except factor VII (see Fig. 60-5). Rates of complex formation are accelerated by heparin and heparin-like molecules on the surface of the endothelial cells. This ability of heparin to accelerate the activity of antithrombin is the basis for heparin's action as a potent anticoagulant. Protein C is converted to an active protease by thrombin after it is bound to an endothelial cell protein called thrombomodulin. Activated protein C

FIGURE 60-7 The contribution of the tissue factor–VIIa complex (TF-VIIa) and tissue factor pathway inhibitor (TFPI) to coagulation. Initial activation of factor IX by TF-VIIa compensates for deficiencies in the early factors, e.g. factors XII and XI. The subsequent inhibition of TF-VIIa by TFPI makes sustained activation of factor X by IXa and VIIIa critical for normal hemostasis. PL, phospholipid.

then inactivates the two plasma cofactors V and VIII by limited proteolysis, which slows down two critical coagulation reactions. Protein C may also stimulate the release of tissue plasminogen activator from endothelial cells. The inhibitory function of protein C is enhanced by protein S. As one might predict, reduced levels of antithrombin or proteins C and S, or dysfunctional forms of these molecules, result in a hypercoagulable or prethrombotic state. In addition, a particularly common heritable defect associated with a hypercoagulable state is the presence of a form of factor V (factor V Leiden) that is resistant to protein C inhibition. Twenty to fifty percent of patients with unexplained venous thromboembolism may have this defect.

The preceding description of blood coagulation implies that the process is uniform throughout the body. In fact, the process is not uniform, and the composition of the blood clot varies with the site of injury. Hemostatic plugs or thrombi that form in veins where blood flow is slow are rich in fibrin and trapped red blood cells and contain relatively few platelets. They are often called *red thrombi* because of their appearance in surgical and pathologic specimens. The friable ends of these red thrombi, which often form in leg veins, can break off and embolize to the pulmonary circulation. Conversely, clots that form in arteries under conditions of high flow are predominantly composed of platelets and have little fibrin. These *white thrombi* may readily dislodge from the arterial wall and embolize to distant sites, causing temporary or permanent ischemia. These clots are a particularly common cause of embolism in the cerebral and retinal circulation, where they may lead to transient neurologic dysfunction (transient ischemic attacks), including temporary monocular blindness (amaurosis fugax), or to strokes. In addition, most episodes of myocardial infarction are due to thrombi that form after the rupture of atherosclerotic plaques within diseased coronary arteries. It is important to remember that there is little difference between hemostatic plugs, which are a physiologic response to injury, and pathologic thrombi. To underscore the similarity, thrombosis has been described as coagulation occurring in the wrong place or at the wrong time.

FIGURE 60-6 The major coagulation reactions are subdivided and depicted in schematic form to emphasize their similarity. They all rely on the formation of surface-bound enzyme-cofactor complexes. Abbreviations: PK, prekallikrein; K, kallikrein; HMWK, high-molecular-weight kininogen; TF, tissue factor; Ca^{2+}, calcium; PT, prothrombin; Thr, thrombin. By convention, other coagulation factors are indicated by roman numerals, with a lowercase "a" appended to indicate their active form. The ∧∧∧ is used to indicate the Gla (di-γ-carboxyglutamic acid)–containing domains of factors VII, IX, X, Xa, and PT, which bind calcium and phospholipid. Hatching is used to indicate proteins that adhere to surfaces by hydrophobic interaction.

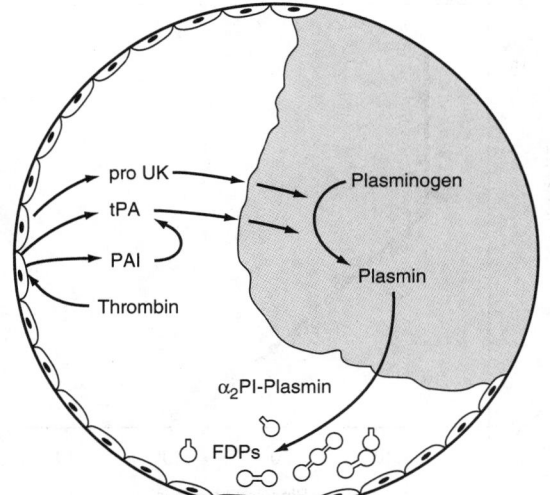

FIGURE 60-8 A schematic diagram of the fibrinolytic pathway. Tissue plasminogen activator (tPA) is released from endothelial cells, enters the fibrin clot, and activates plasminogen to plasmin. Any free plasmin is complexed with alpha$_2$ plasmin inhibitor (α_2PI). Fibrin is degraded to low-molecular-weight fragments, fibrin degradation products (FDPs).

CLINICAL EVALUATION

HISTORY Certain elements of the history are particularly useful in determining whether bleeding is caused by an underlying hemostatic disorder or by a local anatomic defect. One clue is a history of bleeding following common hemostatic stresses such as dental extraction, childbirth, or minor surgery. Bleeding that is sufficiently severe to require a blood transfusion merits special attention. A family history of bleeding and bleeding from multiple sites that cannot be linked to trauma or surgery also suggest a systemic disorder. Since bleeding can be mild, lack of a family history of bleeding does not exclude an inherited hemostatic disorder.

It may be possible to localize the defect to either the platelet or the plasma coagulation system (Table 60-1). Bleeding from a platelet disorder is usually localized to superficial sites such as the skin and mucous membranes, comes on immediately after trauma or surgery, and is readily controlled by local measures. In contrast, bleeding from secondary hemostatic or plasma coagulation defects occurs hours or days after injury and is unaffected by local therapy. Such bleeding most often occurs in deep subcutaneous tissues, muscles, joints, or body cavities. A careful and thorough history is probably the most important step in establishing the presence of a hemostatic disorder and in guiding initial laboratory testing.

Table 60-1

Differences in the Clinical Manifestations of Disorders of Primary and Secondary Hemostasis

Manifestations	Defects of Primary Hemostasis (Platelet Defects)	Defects of Secondary Hemostasis (Plasma Protein Defects)
Onset of bleeding after trauma	Immediate	Delayed—hours or days
Sites of bleeding	Superficial—skin, mucous membranes, nose, gastrointestinal and genitourinary tracts	Deep—joints, muscle, retroperitoneum
Physical findings	Petechiae, ecchymoses	Hematomas, hemarthroses
Family history	Autosomal dominant	Autosomal or X-linked recessive
Response to therapy	Immediate; local measures effective	Requires sustained systemic therapy

PHYSICAL EXAMINATION In conjunction with a careful history, physical examination can also be of help in evaluating patients with hemostatic disorders. The most common site to observe bleeding is in the skin and mucous membranes. Collections of blood in the skin are called *purpura* and may be subdivided on the basis of the site of bleeding in the skin. Small pinpoint hemorrhages into the dermis due to the leakage of red cells through capillaries are called *petechiae* and are characteristic of platelet disorders—in particular, severe thrombocytopenia. Larger subcutaneous collections of blood due to leakage of blood from small arterioles and venules are called *ecchymoses* (common bruises) or, if somewhat deeper and palpable, *hematomas*. They are also common in patients with platelet defects and result from minor trauma. There are other skin and mucous membrane lesions, like dilated capillaries or *telangiectasia*, that may cause bleeding without any hemostatic defect. In addition, the loss of connective tissue support for capillaries and small veins that accompanies aging increases the fragility of superficial vessels, such as those on the dorsum of the hand, leading to extravasation of blood into subcutaneous tissue—*senile purpura*. Menorrhagia is sometimes a serious problem in women with severe thrombocytopenia or platelet dysfunction. In addition, some patients with primary hemostatic defects, especially von Willebrand's disease, may have recurrent gastrointestinal hemorrhage.

As mentioned previously, bleeding into body cavities, the retroperitoneum, or joints is a common manifestation of plasma coagulation defects. Repeated joint bleeding may cause synovial thickening, chronic inflammation, and fluid collections and may erode articular cartilage and lead to chronic joint deformity and limited mobility. Such deformities are particularly common in deficiencies of factors VIII and IX, the two sex-linked coagulation disorders referred to as the *hemophilias*. For unclear reasons, hemarthroses are much less common in patients with other plasma coagulation defects. Blood collections in various body cavities or soft tissues can cause secondary necrosis of tissues or nerve compression. Retroperitoneal hematomas can cause femoral nerve compression, and large collections of poorly coagulated blood in soft tissues occasionally mimic malignant growths—the pseudotumor syndrome. Two of the most life-threatening sites of bleeding are in the oropharynx, where bleeding can compromise the airway, and in the central nervous system. Intracerebral hemorrhage is one of the leading causes of death in patients with severe coagulation disorders.

LABORATORY TESTS The most important screening tests of the primary hemostatic system are (1) a *bleeding time* (a sensitive measure of platelet function) and (2) a *platelet count*. The latter is particularly useful, as it is readily available and correlates well with the propensity to bleed. The normal platelet count is 150,000 to 450,000 platelets per microliter of blood. As long as the count is above 100,000/μL, however, patients usually are not symptomatic, and the bleeding time remains normal. Platelet counts of 50,000 to 100,000/μL cause mild prolongation of the bleeding time, so that bleeding occurs after severe trauma or other stress. Patients with platelet counts of less than 50,000/μL have easy bruising, which is manifested by skin purpura after minor trauma and bleeding after mucous membrane surgery. Patients with a platelet count below 20,000/μL have an appreciable incidence of spontaneous bleeding, usually have petechiae, and may have intracranial or other spontaneous internal bleeding. The major causes of thrombocytopenia are outlined in Table 60-2.

Patients with qualitative platelet abnormalities have a normal platelet count and a prolonged bleeding time (Table 60-3). The bleeding time is ascertained by making a small, superficial skin incision and timing the duration of blood flow from the wounded area. Although this is a rather crude "bioassay," by careful standardization it has become a reliable and sensitive test of platelet function. The most widely used technique uses a template or an automated scalpel to control the length and depth of the incision (usually 1 mm deep by 9 mm long) and a sphygmomanometer inflated to 40 mmHg to distend the capillary bed of the forearm uniformly. In order to be useful, the

Table 60-2

Causes of Thrombocytopenia

Decreased marrow production of megakaryocytes
  Marrow infiltration with tumor, fibrosis
  Marrow failure—aplastic, hypoplastic anemias, drug effects
Splenic sequestration of circulating platelets
  Splenic enlargement due to tumor infiltration
  Splenic congestion due to portal hypertension
Increased destruction of circulating platelets
  Nonimmune destruction
    Vascular prostheses, cardiac valves
    Disseminated intravascular coagulation
    Sepsis
    Vasculitis
  Immune destruction
    Autoantibodies to platelet antigens
    Drug-associated antibodies
    Circulating immune complexes (systemic lupus erythematosus, viral
      agents, bacterial sepsis)

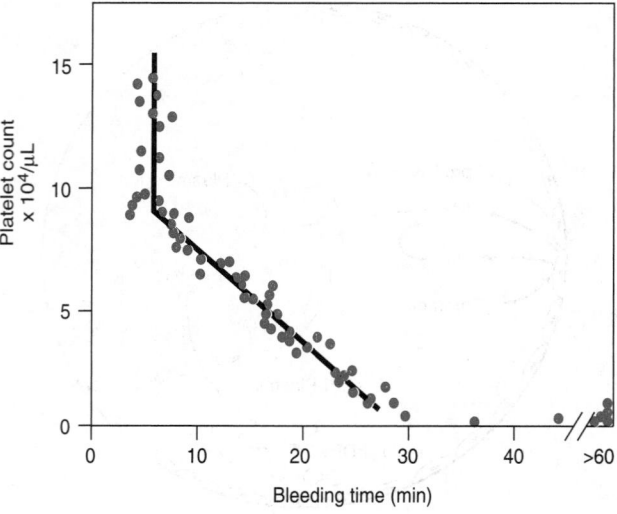

FIGURE 60-9 The relationship between the platelet count and the bleeding time. *(From LA Harker, Hemostasis Manual, 2d ed. Philadelphia, FA Davis Company, 1974.)*

bleeding time test must be performed by an experienced technician, as small differences in technique have a big effect on outcome. Although any patient with a bleeding time over 10 min has an increased risk of bleeding, the risk does not become great until the bleeding time exceeds 15 or 20 min. As shown in Fig. 60-9, there is a roughly linear relationship between the platelet count and the bleeding time. When a defect in primary hemostasis is uncovered, specialized testing is needed to determine the cause of the platelet dysfunction (Table 60-3). A precise diagnosis is important, since patients with bleeding due to a primary hemostatic disorder may need therapy with platelets, with one of several hormones (desmopressin, estrogen, glucocorticoids), or with plasma fractions, depending on the nature of the disorder. Occasional patients with a strong history of bleeding, particularly those with mild von Willebrand's disease, may have a normal bleeding time when initially tested, owing to cyclical variations in the level of the von Willebrand factor. Repeated testing may be necessary to establish an accurate diagnosis.

Plasma coagulation function is readily assessed with a few simple laboratory tests—the partial thromboplastin time (PTT), prothrombin time (PT), thrombin time (TT), and quantitative fibrinogen determination (Fig. 60-5, Table 60-4). The PTT screens the intrinsic limb of the coagulation system and tests for the adequacy of factors XII, HMWK, PK, XI, IX, and VIII. The PT screens the extrinsic or tissue factor–dependent pathway. Both tests also evaluate the common coagulation pathway involving all the reactions that occur after the activation of factor X. Prolongation of the PT and PTT that does not resolve

after the addition of normal plasma suggests a coagulation inhibitor. A specific test for the conversion of fibrinogen to fibrin is needed when both the PTT and PT are prolonged—either a TT or a clottable fibrinogen level can be employed. When abnormalities are noted in any of the screening tests, more specific coagulation factor assays can be ordered to determine the nature of the defect.

There are several rare coagulation abnormalities that may be missed as they do not perturb the results of the screening tests just discussed. They are factor XIII deficiency, α_2 plasmin inhibitor deficiency, PAI-1 deficiency (PAI-1 is the major inhibitor of plasminogen activators), and Scott's syndrome, a platelet coagulant defect. A test for factor XIII–dependent fibrin cross-linking, such as clot solubility in 5 M urea, should be ordered when the PT and PTT are both normal but there is a strong history of bleeding. The fibrinolytic system can be assessed by measuring the rate of clot lysis with the euglobulin lysis or whole blood clot lysis tests and by measuring the levels of α_2 plasmin inhibitor and PAI-1. Scott's syndrome can be detected by measuring the serum prothrombin time, which assesses the amount of residual prothrombin.

Table 60-3

Primary Hemostatic (Platelet) Disorders

Defects of platelet adhesion
  Von Willebrand's disease
  Bernard-Soulier syndrome (absence or dysfunction of GpIb/IX)
Defects of platelet aggregation
  Glanzmann's thrombasthenia (absence or dysfunction of GpIIb/IIIa)
Defects of platelet release
  Decreased cyclooxygenase activity
    Drug-induced—aspirin, nonsteroidal anti-inflammatory agents
    Congenital
  Granule storage pool defects
    Congenital
    Acquired
  Uremia
  Platelet coating (e.g., penicillin or paraproteins)
Defect of platelet coagulant activity
  Scott's syndrome

ABBREVIATION: Gp, glycoprotein.

Table 60-4

Relationship between Secondary Hemostatic Disorders and Coagulation Test Abnormalities

Prolonged partial thromboplastin time (PTT)
  No clinical bleeding—factors XII, HMWK, PK
  Mild or rare bleeding—factor XI
  Frequent, severe bleeding—factors VIII and IX
Prolonged prothrombin time (PT)
  Factor VII deficiency
  Vitamin K deficiency—early
  Warfarin anticoagulant ingestion
Prolonged PTT and PT
  Factor II, V, or X deficiency
  Vitamin K deficiency—late
  Warfarin anticoagulant ingestion
Prolonged thrombin time (TT)
  Mild or rare bleeding—afibrinogenemia
  Frequent, severe bleeding—dysfibrinogenemia
  Heparin-like inhibitors or heparin administration
Prolonged PT and/or PTT not corrected with normal plasma
  Specific or nonspecific inhibitor syndromes
Clot solubility in 5 M urea
  Factor XIII deficiency
  Inhibitors or defective cross-linking
Rapid clot lysis
  α_2 plasmin inhibitor

ABBREVIATIONS: HMWK, high-molecular-weight kininogen; PK, prekallikrein.

Table 60-5

CHAPTER 61
Enlargement of Lymph Nodes and Spleen

345

Thrombotic Disorders

Inherited
  Defective inhibition of coagulation factors
    factor V Leiden (resistant to inhibition by activated protein C)
    antithrombin III deficiency
    protein C deficiency
    protein S deficiency
  Impaired clot lysis
    dysfibrinogenemia
    plasminogen deficiency
    tPA deficiency
    PAI-1 excess
  Uncertain mechanism
    homocystinuria
Acquired
  Diseases or syndromes
    lupus anticoagulant
    malignancy
    myeloproliferative disorder
    thrombotic thrombocytopenic purpura
    estrogen treatment
    hyperlipidemia
    diabetes mellitus
    hyperviscosity
    nephrotic syndrome
    congestive heart failure
    paroxysmal nocturnal hemoglobinuria
  Physiologic states
    pregnancy (especially postpartum)
    obesity
    postoperative state
    immobilization
    old age

Conditions associated with thrombosis are listed in Table 60-5. There are as yet no useful tests to screen patients suspected of having hypercoagulable or prethrombotic disorders. Tests have been developed in research laboratories which measure small peptides or enzyme-inhibitor complexes generated during coagulation. For example, radioimmunoassays have been developed for fibrinopeptides A and B, for the thrombin-antithrombin complex, and for prothrombin cleavage fragments. Elevated levels of these products have been reported in patients with prethrombotic disorders and in patients with thromboembolism. These tests require meticulous phlebotomy, special anticoagulants, and special handling of the blood and are not in general clinical use. At present, patients suspected of having a hypercoagulable state on the basis of clinical information should be tested with specific assays to screen for the small number of known defects (Table 60-5). Currently available tests can identify 10 to 20 percent of the cases of familial thrombosis, a small fraction of the many patients who present to physicians with thromboembolism.

Inhibitor syndromes or circulating anticoagulants are usually due to antibodies that impair coagulation factor activity. They are an infrequent cause of bleeding and require specialized diagnostic testing. Inhibitors are likely when screening test abnormalities cannot be reversed by adding normal plasma to patient plasma. Antibodies against specific coagulation factors may develop in (1) postpartum women, (2) patients with autoimmune disorders such as systemic lupus erythematosus, (3) patients taking drugs such as penicillin and streptomycin, and (4) otherwise healthy elderly individuals. In addition, between 10 and 20 percent of patients with severe hemophilia who have received multiple plasma infusions develop inhibitor antibodies. Some patients, especially those with systemic lupus erythematosus, may also have a nonspecific form of anticoagulant antibody which interferes with phospholipid binding of coagulation factors and prolongs the PT and PTT but does not cause clinical bleeding. The presence of the lupus anticoagulant may increase the risk of thromboembolism and may cause placental infarction and recurrent midtrimester abortion. Occasionally, patients develop inhibitors that are not antibodies. For example, several patients with clinical bleeding have been found to have circulating mucopolysaccharides that have heparin-like activity.

BIBLIOGRAPHY

BROZE GJ: The role of tissue factor pathway inhibitor in a revised coagulation cascade. Blood 29:159, 1992

COLMAN RW et al (eds): *Hemostasis and Thrombosis: Basic Principles and Clinical Practice*, 4th ed. Philadelphia, Lippincott, 1996

HANDIN RI: Diseases of the platelet and vessel wall, in *Hematology of Infancy and Childhood*, 5th ed., DG Nathan et al (eds). Philadelphia, Saunders, 1997 (in press)

——— et al (eds): *Blood: Principles and Practice of Hematologic Oncology*, 4th ed. Philadelphia, Lippincott, 1994

LIND SE: The bleeding time does not predict surgical bleeding. Blood 77:2547, 1991

ROBERTS HR, LOZIER JN: New perspectives on the coagulation cascade. Hosp Pract Jan 1992, 97

61 *Patrick H. Henry, Dan L. Longo*

ENLARGEMENT OF LYMPH NODES AND SPLEEN

This chapter is intended to serve as a guide to the evaluation of patients who present with enlargement of the lymph nodes (*lymphadenopathy*) or the spleen (*splenomegaly*). Lymphadenopathy is a rather common clinical finding in primary care settings, whereas palpable splenomegaly is less so.

LYMPHADENOPATHY

Lymphadenopathy may be an incidental finding in patients being examined for various reasons or it may be a presenting sign or symptom of the patient's illness. The physician must eventually decide whether the lymphadenopathy is a normal finding or one that requires further study, up to and including biopsy. Soft, flat, submandibular nodes (<1 cm) are often palpable in healthy children and young adults, and healthy adults may have palpable inguinal nodes of up to 2 cm, which are considered normal. Further evaluation of these normal nodes is not warranted. In contrast, if the physician believes the node(s) to be abnormal, then pursuit of a more precise diagnosis is needed.

Approach to the Patient

Lymphadenopathy may be a primary or secondary manifestation of numerous disorders, as shown in Table 61-1. Many of these disorders are infrequent causes of lymphadenopathy. Analysis of lymphadenopathy in primary care practice has shown that more than two-thirds of patients have nonspecific causes or upper respiratory illnesses (viral or bacterial), and fewer than 1 percent have a malignancy. In one study, researchers reported that 186 of 220 patients (84 percent) referred for evaluation of lymphadenopathy had a "benign" diagnosis. The remaining 34 patients (16 percent) had a malignancy (lymphoma or metastatic adenocarcinoma). Sixty-three percent (112) of the 186 patients with benign lymphadenopathy had a nonspecific or reactive etiology (no causative agent found), and the remainder had a specific cause demonstrated, most commonly infectious mononucleosis, toxoplasmosis, or tuberculosis. Thus, the vast majority of patients with lymphadenopathy will have a nonspecific etiology requiring few diagnostic tests.

Clinical Assessment The physician will be aided in the pursuit of an explanation for the lymphadenopathy by a careful medical history, physical examination, selected laboratory tests, and perhaps an excisional lymph node biopsy.

The *medical history* should reveal the setting in which lymphadenopathy is occurring. Symptoms such as sore throat, cough, fever, night sweats, fatigue, weight loss, or pain in the nodes should be sought. The patient's age, sex, occupation, exposure to pets, sexual

Table 61-1

Diseases Associated with Lymphadenopathy

1. Infectious diseases
   a. Viral—infectious mononucleosis syndromes (EBV, CMV), infectious hepatitis, herpes simplex, herpesvirus-6, varicella-zoster virus, rubella, measles, adenovirus, HIV, epidemic keratoconjunctivitis, vaccinia
   b. Bacterial—streptococci, staphylococci, cat-scratch disease, brucellosis, tularemia, plague, chancroid, melioidosis, glanders, tuberculosis, atypical mycobacterial infection, primary and secondary syphilis, diphtheria, leprosy
   c. Fungal—histoplasmosis, coccidioidomycosis, paracoccidioidomycosis
   d. Chlamydial—lymphogranuloma venereum, trachoma
   e. Parasitic—toxoplasmosis, leishmaniasis, trypanosomiasis, filariasis
   f. Rickettsial—scrub typhus, rickettsialpox
2. Immunologic diseases
   a. Rheumatoid arthritis
   b. Juvenile rheumatoid arthritis
   c. Mixed connective tissue disease
   d. Systemic lupus erythematosus
   e. Dermatomyositis
   f. Sjögren's syndrome
   g. Serum sickness
   h. Drug hypersensitivity—diphenylhydantoin, hydralazine, allopurinol, primidone, gold, carbamazepine, etc.
   i. Angioimmunoblastic lymphadenopathy
   j. Primary biliary cirrhosis
   k. Graft-vs.-host disease
   l. Silicone-associated
3. Malignant diseases
   a. Hematologic—Hodgkin's disease, non-Hodgkin's lymphomas, acute or chronic lymphocytic leukemia, hairy cell leukemia, malignant histiocytosis, amyloidosis
   b. Metastatic—from numerous primary sites
4. Lipid storage diseases—Gaucher's, Niemann-Pick, Fabry, Tangier
5. Endocrine diseases—hyperthyroidism
6. Other disorders
   a. Castleman's disease (giant lymph node hyperplasia)
   b. Sarcoidosis
   c. Dermatopathic lymphadenitis
   d. Lymphomatoid granulomatosis
   e. Histiocytic necrotizing lymphadenitis (Kikuchi's disease)
   f. Sinus histiocytosis with massive lymphadenopathy (Rosai-Dorfman disease)
   g. Mucocutaneous lymph node syndrome (Kawasaki's disease)
   h. Histiocytosis X
   i. Familial mediterranean fever
   j. Severe hypertriglyceridemia
   k. Vascular transformation of sinuses
   l. Inflammatory pseudotumor of lymph node

behavior, and use of drugs such as diphenylhydantoin are other important historical points. For example, children and young adults usually have benign (i.e., nonmalignant) disorders, such as viral or bacterial upper respiratory infections, infectious mononucleosis, toxoplasmosis, and, in some countries, tuberculosis, which account for the observed lymphadenopathy. In contrast, after age 50 the incidence of malignant disorders increases and benign disorders decreases.

The *physical examination* can provide useful clues such as the extent of lymphadenopathy (localized or generalized), size of nodes, texture, presence or absence of nodal tenderness, signs of inflammation over the node, skin lesions, and splenomegaly. A thorough ear, nose, and throat (ENT) examination is indicated in adult patients with cervical adenopathy and a history of tobacco use. Localized or regional adenopathy implies involvement of a single anatomic area. Generalized adenopathy has been defined as involvement of three or more noncontiguous lymph node areas. Many of the causes of lymphadenopathy (Table 61-1) can produce localized *or* generalized adenopathy, so this distinction is of limited utility in the differential diagnosis. Nevertheless, generalized lymphadenopathy is frequently associated with non-

malignant disorders such as infectious mononucleosis [Epstein-Barr virus (EBV) or cytomegalovirus (CMV)], toxoplasmosis, AIDS, other viral infections, systemic lupus erythematosus (SLE), and mixed connective tissue disease. Acute and chronic lymphocytic leukemias and malignant lymphomas also produce generalized adenopathy in adults.

The site of localized or regional adenopathy may provide a useful clue about the cause. Occipital adenopathy often reflects an infection of the scalp, and preauricular adenopathy accompanies conjunctival infections and cat-scratch disease. The most frequent site of regional adenopathy is the neck, and most of the causes are benign—upper respiratory infections, oral and dental lesions, infectious mononucleosis, other viral illnesses. The chief malignant causes include metastatic cancer from head and neck, breast, lung, and thyroid primaries. Enlargement of supraclavicular and scalene nodes is always abnormal. Because these nodes drain regions of the lung and retroperitoneal space, they can reflect either lymphomas, other cancers, or infectious processes arising in these areas. Virchow's node is an enlarged left supraclavicular node infiltrated with metastatic cancer from a gastrointestinal primary. Metastases to supraclavicular nodes also occur from lung, breast, or genital cancers. Tuberculosis, sarcoidosis, and toxoplasmosis are (non-malignant) causes of supraclavicular adenopathy. Axillary adenopathy is usually due to injuries or localized infections of the ipsilateral upper extremity. Malignant causes include melanoma or lymphoma and, in women, breast cancer. Inguinal lymphadenopathy is usually secondary to infections or trauma of the lower extremities and may accompany sexually transmitted diseases such as lymphogranuloma venereum, primary syphilis, genital herpes, or chancroid. These nodes may also be involved by lymphomas and metastatic cancer from primary lesions of the rectum, genitalia, or lower extremities (melanoma).

The size and texture of the lymph node(s) and the presence of pain are useful parameters in evaluating a patient with lymphadenopathy. Nodes <1.0 cm² in area (1.0 × 1.0 cm or less) are almost always secondary to benign, nonspecific reactive causes. In one retrospective analysis of younger patients (9 to 25 years) who had a lymph node biopsy, a maximum diameter of >2 cm served as one discriminant for predicting that the biopsy would reveal malignant or granulomatous disease. Another study showed that a lymph node size of 2.25 cm² (1.5 cm × 1.5 cm) was the best discriminating limit for distinguishing malignant or granulomatous lymphadenopathy from other causes of lymphadenopathy. Patients with node(s) ≤1.0 cm² should be observed after excluding infectious mononucleosis and/or toxoplasmosis unless there are symptoms and signs of an underlying systemic illness.

The texture of lymph nodes may be described as soft, firm, rubbery, hard, discrete, matted, tender, movable, or fixed. Tenderness is found when the capsule is stretched during rapid enlargement, usually secondary to an inflammatory process. Some malignant diseases such as acute leukemia may produce rapid enlargement and pain in the nodes. Nodes involved by lymphoma tend to be large, discrete, symmetric, rubbery, firm, mobile, and nontender. Nodes containing metastatic cancer are often hard, nontender, and nonmovable because of fixation to surrounding tissues. The coexistence of splenomegaly in the patient with lymphadenopathy implies a systemic illness such as infectious mononucleosis, lymphoma, acute or chronic leukemia, SLE, sarcoidosis, toxoplasmosis, cat-scratch disease, or other less common hematologic disorders. The patient's story should provide helpful clues about the underlying systemic illness.

Nonsuperficial presentations (thoracic or abdominal) of adenopathy are usually detected as the result of a symptom-directed diagnostic workup. Thoracic adenopathy may be detected by routine chest roentgenography or during the workup for superficial adenopathy. It may also be found because the patient complains of a cough or wheezing from airway compression; hoarseness from recurrent laryngeal nerve involvement; dysphagia from esophageal compression; or swelling of the neck, face, or arms secondary to compression of the superior vena cava or subclavian vein. The differential diagnosis of mediastinal and hilar adenopathy includes primary lung disorders and systemic illnesses that characteristically involve mediastinal or hilar nodes. In the young, mediastinal adenopathy is associated with infectious mononucleosis and sarcoidosis. In endemic regions, histoplasmosis can cause unilateral paratracheal lymph node involvement that mimics lymphoma. Tuberculosis can also cause unilateral adenopathy. In older patients, the differential diagnosis includes primary lung cancer (especially among smokers), lymphomas, metastatic carcinoma (usually lung), tuberculosis, fungal infection, and sarcoidosis.

Enlarged intraabdominal or retroperitoneal nodes are usually malignant. Although tuberculosis may present as mesenteric lymphadenitis, these masses usually contain lymphomas or, in young men, germ cell tumors.

Laboratory Investigation The laboratory investigation of patients with lymphadenopathy must be tailored to elucidate the etiology suspected from the patient's story and physical findings. One study from a family practice clinic evaluated 249 younger patients with "enlarged lymph nodes, not infected" or "lymphadenitis." The author found that 51 percent had no laboratory studies. When studies were performed, the most common were a complete blood count (33 percent), throat culture (16 percent), chest x-ray (12 percent), or monospot test (10 percent). Only eight patients (3 percent) had a node biopsy, and half of those were normal or reactive. The complete blood count can provide useful data for the diagnosis of acute or chronic leukemias, EBV or CMV mononucleosis, lymphoma with a leukemic component, pyogenic infections, or immune cytopenias in illnesses such as SLE. Serologic studies may demonstrate antibodies specific to components of EBV, CMV, human immunodeficiency virus (HIV), and other viruses; *Toxoplasma gondii*; *Brucella*; etc. If SLE is suspected, then antinuclear and anti-DNA antibody studies are warranted.

The chest x-ray is usually negative, but the presence of a pulmonary infiltrate or mediastinal lymphadenopathy would suggest tuberculosis, histoplasmosis, sarcoidosis, lymphoma, primary lung cancer, or metastatic cancer and demands further investigation.

The indications for lymph node biopsy are imprecise, yet it is a valuable diagnostic tool. The decision to biopsy may be made early in a patient's evaluation or delayed until a sufficient period (approximately 2 weeks) of observation has occurred. Prompt biopsy should occur if the patient's history and physical findings suggest a malignancy; examples include a solitary, hard, nontender cervical node in an older patient who is a chronic user of tobacco; supraclavicular adenopathy; and solitary or generalized adenopathy that is firm, movable, and suggestive of lymphoma. If a primary head and neck cancer is suspected as the basis of a solitary, hard cervical node, then a careful ENT examination should be performed. Any mucosal lesion that is suspicious for a primary neoplastic process should be biopsied first. If no mucosal lesion is detected, an excisional biopsy of the largest node should be performed. Fine-needle aspiration should not be performed as the first diagnostic procedure. Most diagnoses require more tissue than such aspiration can provide and it often delays a definitive diagnosis. Fine-needle aspiration should be reserved for thyroid nodules and for confirmation of relapse in patients whose primary diagnosis is known. If the primary physician is uncertain about whether to proceed to biopsy, consultation with a hematologist or medical oncologist should be helpful. In primary care practices, fewer than 5 percent of lymphadenopathy patients will require a biopsy. That percentage will be considerably larger in referral practices, i.e., hematology, oncology, or otolaryngology (ENT).

Two groups have reported algorithms that they claim will identify more precisely those lymphadenopathy patients who should have a biopsy. Both reports were retrospective analyses in referral practices. The first study involved patients age 9 to 25 years of age who had a node biopsy performed. Three variables were identified that predicted those young patients with peripheral lymphadenopathy who should undergo biopsy; lymph node size >2 cm in diameter and abnormal chest x-ray had positive predictive values, whereas recent ENT symptoms had negative predictive values. The second study evaluated 220 lymphadenopathy patients in a hematology unit and identified five variables [lymph node size, location (supraclavicular or non-supraclavicular), age (>40 years or <40 years), texture (nonhard or hard), and tenderness] that were utilized in a mathematical model to identify those patients requiring a biopsy. Positive predictive value was found for age >40 years, supraclavicular location, node size >2.25 cm², hard texture, and lack of pain or tenderness. Negative predictive value was evident for age <40 years, node size <1.0 cm², nonhard texture, and tender or painful nodes. Ninety-one percent of those who required biopsy were correctly classified by this model. Since both of these studies were retrospective analyses and one was limited to young patients, it is not known how useful these models would be if applied prospectively in a primary care setting.

Most lymphadenopathy patients do not require a biopsy, and at least half require no laboratory studies. If the patient's history and physical findings point to a benign cause for lymphadenopathy, then careful follow-up at a 2- to 4-week interval can be employed. The patient should be instructed to return for reevaluation if the node(s) increase in size. Antibiotics are not indicated for lymphadenopathy unless there is strong evidence of a bacterial infection. Glucocorticoids should not be used to treat lymphadenopathy because their lympholytic effect obscures some diagnoses (lymphoma, leukemia, Castleman's disease) and they contribute to delayed healing or activation of underlying infections. An exception to this statement is the life-threatening pharyngeal obstruction by enlarged lymphoid tissue in Waldeyer's ring that is occasionally seen in infectious mononucleosis.

SPLENOMEGALY

STRUCTURE AND FUNCTION OF THE SPLEEN The spleen is a reticuloendothelial organ that has its embryologic origin in the dorsal mesogastrium at about 5 weeks' gestation. It arises in a series of hillocks, migrates to its normal adult location in the left upper quadrant, and is attached to the stomach via the gastrolienal ligament and to the kidney via the lienorenal ligament. When the hillocks fail to unify into a single tissue mass, accessory spleens may develop in around 20 percent of persons. The function of the spleen has been elusive. Galen believed it was the source of "black bile" or melancholia, and the word *hypochondria* (literally, beneath the ribs) and the idiom "to vent one's spleen" attest to the beliefs that the spleen had an important influence on the psyche and emotions. Some but not all of its secrets have yielded to scientific inquiry. In humans, its normal physiologic roles seem to be the following:

1. Maintenance of quality control over erythrocytes in the red pulp by removal of senescent and defective red blood cells. The spleen accomplishes this function through a unique organization of its parenchyma and vasculature (Fig. 61-1).
2. Synthesis of antibodies in the white pulp.
3. The removal of antibody-coated bacteria and antibody-coated blood cells from the circulation.

An increase in these normal functions may result in splenomegaly with or without hypersplenism.

The spleen is composed of red pulp and white pulp, which are Malpighi's terms for the red blood–filled sinuses and reticuloendothelial cell–lined cords and the white lymphoid follicles arrayed within the red pulp matrix. The spleen is in the portal circulation. The reason for this is unknown but may relate to the fact that lower blood pressure allows less rapid flow and minimizes damage to normal erythrocytes. Blood flows into the spleen at a rate of about 150 mL/min through the splenic artery, which ultimately ramifies into central arterioles. Some blood goes from the arterioles to capillaries and then to splenic veins and out of the spleen, but the majority of blood from central arterioles flows into the macrophage-lined sinuses and cords. The blood entering the sinuses reenters the circulation through the splenic venules, but the blood entering the cords is subjected to an inspection of sorts. In order to return to the circulation, the blood cells in the cords must squeeze through slits in the cord lining to enter the sinuses that lead to the venules. Old and damaged erythrocytes are less deformable and are retained in the cords, where they are destroyed and

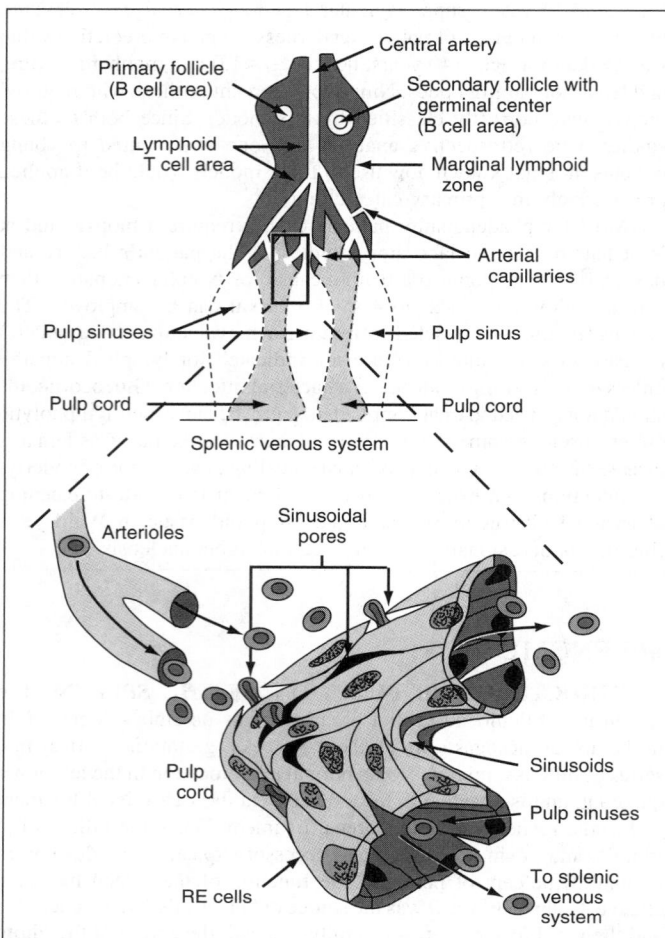

FIGURE 61-1 Schematic spleen structure. The spleen comprises many units of red and white pulp centered around small branches of the splenic artery, called central arteries. White pulp is lymphoid in nature and contains B cell follicles, a marginal zone around the follicles, and T cell–rich areas sheathing arterioles. The red pulp areas include pulp sinuses and pulp cords. The cords are dead ends. In order to regain access to the circulation, red blood cells must traverse tiny openings in the sinusoidal lining. Stiff, damaged, or old red cells cannot enter the sinuses. *(Bottom portion of figure from RS Hillman, KA Ault: Hematology in Clinical Practice. New York, McGraw-Hill, 1995.)*

their components recycled. Red cell inclusion bodies such as parasites, nuclear residua (Howell-Jolly bodies), or denatured hemoglobin (Heinz bodies) are pinched off in the process of passing through the slits, a process called *pitting*. The culling of dead and damaged cells and the pitting of cells with inclusions appear to occur without significant delay since the blood transit time through the spleen is only slightly slower than in other organs.

The spleen is also capable of assisting the host in adapting to its hostile environment. It has at least three adaptational functions: (1) clearance of bacteria and particulates from the blood, (2) the generation of immune responses to certain invading pathogens, and (3) the generation of cellular components of the blood under circumstances in which the marrow is unable to meet the needs (i.e., extramedullary hematopoiesis). The latter adaptation is a recapitulation of the blood-forming function the spleen plays during gestation. In some animals, the spleen also serves a role in the vascular adaptation to stress because it stores red blood cells (often hemoconcentrated to higher hematocrits than normal) under normal circumstances and contracts under the influence of beta-adrenergic stimulation to provide the animal with an autotransfusion and improved oxygen-carrying capacity. However, the normal human spleen does not sequester or store red blood cells and does not contract in response to sympathetic stimuli. The normal human spleen contains approximately one-third of the total body platelets and a significant number of marginated neutrophils. These sequestered cells are available when needed to respond to bleeding or infection.

Approach to the Patient

Clinical Assessment The most common *symptoms* produced by diseases involving the spleen are pain and a heavy sensation in the left upper quadrant. Pain may result from acute swelling of the spleen with stretching of the capsule, infarction, or inflammation of the capsule. For many years, it was believed that splenic infarction was clinically silent, which at times is true. However, Soma Weiss, in his classic 1942 report of the self-observations by a Harvard medical student on the clinical course of subacute bacterial endocarditis, documented that severe left upper quadrant and pleuritic chest pain may accompany thromboembolic occlusion of splenic blood flow. Vascular occlusion, with infarction and pain, is commonly seen in children with sickle cell crises. Rupture of the spleen, either from trauma or infiltrative disease that breaks the capsule, may result in intraperitoneal bleeding, shock, and death. The rupture itself may be painless.

A palpable spleen is the major *physical sign* produced by diseases affecting the spleen and suggests enlargement of the organ. The normal spleen is said to weigh less than 250 g, decreases in size with age, normally lies entirely within the rib cage, has a maximum cephalocaudad diameter of 13 cm by ultrasonography or maximum length of 12 cm and/or width of 7 cm by radionuclide scan, and is usually not palpable. However, a palpable spleen was found in 3 percent of 2200 asymptomatic, male, freshman college students. Follow-up at 3 years revealed that 30 percent of those students still had a palpable spleen without any increase in disease prevalence. Ten-year follow-up found no evidence for lymphoid malignancies. Furthermore, in some tropical countries (e.g., New Guinea) the incidence of splenomegaly may reach 60 percent. Thus, the presence of a palpable spleen does not always equate with presence of disease. Even when disease is present, splenomegaly may not reflect the primary disease, but rather a reaction to it. For example, in patients with Hodgkin's disease, only two-thirds of the palpable spleens show involvement by the cancer.

Physical examination of the spleen utilizes primarily the techniques of palpation and percussion. Inspection may reveal a fullness in the left upper quadrant which descends on inspiration, a finding associated with a massively enlarged spleen. Auscultation may reveal a venous hum or a friction rub.

Palpation can be accomplished by bimanual palpation, ballotment, and palpation from above (Middleton maneuver). For bimanual palpation, which is at least as reliable as the other techniques, the patient is supine with flexed knees. The examiner's left hand is placed on the lower rib cage and pulls the skin toward the costal margin allowing the fingertips of the right hand to feel the tip of the spleen as it descends while the patient inspires slowly, smoothly, and deeply. Palpation is begun with the right hand in the left lower quadrant with gradual movement toward the left costal margin, thereby identifying the lower edge of a massively enlarged spleen. When the spleen tip is felt, the finding is recorded as centimeters below the left costal margin at some arbitrary point, i.e., 10 to 15 cm, from the midpoint of the umbilicus or the xiphisternal junction. This allows other examiners to compare findings or the initial examiner to determine changes in size over time. Bimanual palpation in the right lateral decubitus position adds nothing to the supine examination.

Percussion for splenic dullness is accomplished with any of three techniques described by Nixon, Castell, or Barkun:

1. *Nixon's method*: The patient is placed on the right side so that the spleen lies above the colon and stomach. Percussion begins at the lower level of pulmonary resonance in the posterior axillary line and proceeds diagonally along a perpendicular line toward the lower midanterior costal margin. The upper border of dullness is normally 6 to 8 cm above the costal margin. Dullness greater than 8 cm in an adult is presumed to indicate splenic enlargement.

2. *Castell's method*: With the patient supine, percussion in the lowest intercostal space in the anterior axillary line (8th or 9th) produces a resonant note if the spleen is normal in size. This is true during expiration or full inspiration. A dull percussion note on full inspiration suggests splenomegaly.

3. *Percussion of Traube's semilunar space*: The borders of Traube's space are the sixth rib superiorly, the left midaxillary line laterally, and the left costal margin inferiorly. The patient is supine with the left arm slightly abducted. During normal breathing, this space is percussed from medial to lateral margins, yielding a normal resonant sound. A dull percussion note suggests splenomegaly.

Studies comparing methods of percussion and palpation with a standard of ultrasonography or scintigraphy have revealed sensitivity of 56 to 71 percent for palpation and 59 to 82 percent for percussion. Reproducibility among examiners is better for palpation than percussion. Both techniques are less reliable in obese patients or patients who have just eaten. Thus, the physical examination techniques of palpation and percussion are imprecise at best. It has been suggested that the examiner perform percussion first and, if positive, proceed to palpation; if the spleen is palpable, then one can be reasonably confident that splenomegaly exists. However, not all left upper quadrant masses are enlarged spleens; gastric or colon tumors and pancreatic or renal cysts or tumors can mimic splenomegaly.

The presence of an enlarged spleen can be more precisely determined, if necessary, by liver-spleen radionuclide scan, computed tomography (CT), magnetic resonance imaging (MRI), or ultrasonography. The latter technique is the current procedure of choice for routine assessment of spleen size (normal = a maximum cephalocaudad diameter of 13 cm) because it has high sensitivity and specificity and is safe, noninvasive, quick, mobile, and less costly. Nuclear medicine scans are accurate, sensitive, and reliable but they are costly, require greater time to generate data, and utilize immobile equipment. They have the advantage of demonstrating accessory splenic tissue. CT and MRI provide accurate determination of spleen size, but the equipment is immobile and the procedures are expensive. MRI appears to offer no advantage over CT. Changes in spleen structure such as mass lesions, infarcts, inhomogeneous infiltrates, and cysts are more readily assessed by CT, MRI, or ultrasonography. None of these techniques is very reliable in the detection of patchy infiltration (e.g., Hodgkin's disease).

Differential Diagnosis Many of the diseases associated with splenomegaly are listed in Table 61-2. They are grouped according to the presumed basic mechanism responsible for organ enlargement:

1. Hyperplasia or hypertrophy related to a particular splenic function such as reticuloendothelial hyperplasia (work hypertrophy) in diseases such as hereditary spherocytosis or thalassemia syndromes that require removal of large numbers of defective red blood cells; immune hyperplasia in response to systemic infection (infectious mononucleosis, sub-

acute bacterial endocarditis) or to immunologic diseases (immune thrombocytopenia, SLE, Felty's syndrome).

2. Passive congestion due to decreased blood flow from the spleen in conditions that produce portal hypertension (cirrhosis, Budd-Chiari syndrome, congestive heart failure).

3. Infiltrative diseases of the spleen (lymphomas, metastatic cancer, amyloidosis, Gaucher's disease, myeloproliferative disorders with extramedullary hematopoiesis).

The differential diagnostic possibilities are much fewer when the spleen is "massively enlarged," that is, it is palpable more than 8 cm below the left costal margin or its drained weight is ≥1000 g (Table 61-3). The vast majority of such patients will have non-Hodgkin's lymphoma, chronic lymphocytic leukemia, hairy cell leukemia, chronic myelogenous leukemia, myelofibrosis with myeloid metaplasia, or polycythemia rubra vera.

Laboratory Assessment The major laboratory abnormalities accompanying splenomegaly are determined by the underlying systemic illness. Erythrocyte counts may be normal, decreased (thalassemia major syndromes, SLE, cirrhosis with portal hypertension), or increased (polycythemia rubra vera). Granulocyte counts may be normal, decreased (Felty's syndrome, congestive splenomegaly, leukemias),

Table 61-2

Diseases Associated with Splenomegaly Grouped by Pathogenic Mechanism

ENLARGEMENT DUE TO INCREASED DEMAND FOR SPLENIC FUNCTION	ENLARGEMENT DUE TO ABNORMAL SPLENIC OR PORTAL BLOOD FLOW
Reticuloendothelial system hyperplasia (for removal of defective erythrocytes)	Cirrhosis
Spherocytosis	Hepatic vein obstruction
Early sickle cell anemia	Portal vein obstruction, intrahepatic or extrahepatic
Ovalocytosis	Cavernous transformation of the portal vein
Thalassemia major	Splenic vein obstruction
Hemoglobinopathies	Splenic artery aneurysm
Paroxysmal nocturnal hemoglobinuria	Hepatic schistosomiasis
Nutritional anemias	Congestive heart failure
Immune hyperplasia	Hepatic echinococcosis
Response to infection (viral, bacterial, fungal, parasitic)	Portal hypertension (any cause including the above): "Banti's disease"
Infectious mononucleosis	
AIDS	**INFILTRATION OF THE SPLEEN**
Viral hepatitis	
Cytomegalovirus	*Intracellular or extracellular depositions*
Subacute bacterial endocarditis	Amyloidosis
Bacterial septicemia	Gaucher's disease
Congenital syphilis	Niemann-Pick disease
Splenic abscess	Tangier disease
Tuberculosis	Hurler's syndrome and other mucopolysaccharidoses
Histoplasmosis	Hyperlipidemias
Malaria	*Benign and malignant cellular infiltrations*
Leishmaniasis	Leukemias (acute, chronic, lymphoid, myeloid, monocytic)
Trypanosomiasis	Lymphomas
Disordered immunoregulation	Hodgkin's disease
Rheumatoid arthritis (Felty's syndrome)	Myeloproliferative syndromes (e.g., polycythemia vera)
Systemic lupus erythematosus	Angiosarcomas
Collagen vascular diseases	Metastatic tumors (melanoma is most common)
Serum sickness	Eosinophilic granuloma
Immune hemolytic anemias	Histiocytosis X
Immune thrombocytopenias	Hamartomas
Immune neutropenias	Hemangiomas, fibromas, lymphangiomas
Drug reactions	Splenic cysts
Angioimmunoblastic lymphadenopathy	
Sarcoidosis	**UNKNOWN ETIOLOGY**
Thyrotoxicosis (benign lymphoid hypertrophy)	
Extramedullary hematopoiesis	Idiopathic splenomegaly
Myelofibrosis	Berylliosis
Marrow damage by toxins, radiation, strontium	Iron-deficiency anemia
Marrow infiltration by tumors, leukemias, Gaucher's disease	

Table 61-3

Diseases Associated with Massive Splenomegaly*

Chronic myelogenous leukemia
Lymphomas
Hairy cell leukemia
Myelofibrosis with myeloid metaplasia
Polycythemia rubra vera
Gaucher's disease
Chronic lymphocytic leukemia
Sarcoidosis
Autoimmune hemolytic anemia
Diffuse splenic hemangiomatosis

* The spleen extends greater than 8 cm below left costal margin and/or weighs more
than 1000 g.

or increased (infections or inflammatory disease, myeloproliferative disorders). In a similar manner the platelet count may be normal, decreased when there is enhanced sequestration or destruction of platelets in an enlarged spleen (congestive splenomegaly, Gaucher's disease, immune thrombocytopenia), or increased in the myeloproliferative disorders such as polycythemia rubra vera.

The complete blood count may reveal cytopenia of one or more blood cell types, which should suggest *hypersplenism*. This condition is characterized by splenomegaly, cytopenia(s), normal or hyperplastic bone marrow, and a response to splenectomy. The latter characteristic is less precise because reversal of cytopenia, particularly granulocytopenia, is sometimes not sustained after splenectomy. The cytopenias result from increased destruction of the cellular elements secondary to reduced flow of blood through enlarged and congested cords (congestive splenomegaly) or to immune-mediated mechanisms. In hypersplenism, various cell types usually have normal morphology on the peripheral blood smear, although the red cells may be spherocytic due to loss of surface area during their longer transit through the enlarged spleen. The increased marrow production of red cells should be reflected as an increased reticulocyte production index, although the value may be less than expected due to increased sequestration of reticulocytes in the spleen.

As mentioned earlier, the size of the spleen can be confirmed, if necessary, by ultrasound, radionuclide scan, CT, or MRI. The need for additional laboratory studies is dictated by the differential diagnosis of the underlying illness of which splenomegaly is merely a manifestation.

SPLENECTOMY Splenectomy is infrequently performed for diagnostic purposes, especially in the absence of clinical illness or other diagnostic tests that suggest underlying disease. More often splenectomy is performed for staging the extent of disease in patients with Hodgkin's disease, for symptom control in patients with massive splenomegaly, for disease control in patients with hairy cell leukemia or prolymphocytic leukemia, for bleeding control in patients with traumatic splenic rupture, or for correction of cytopenias in patients with hypersplenism or immune-mediated destruction of one or more cellular blood elements. Splenectomy is necessary for routine staging of patients with Hodgkin's disease only in patients with clinical stage I or II disease in whom radiation therapy is contemplated as the treatment. Noninvasive staging of the spleen in Hodgkin's disease is not a sufficiently reliable basis for treatment decisions because one-third of normal-sized spleens will be involved with Hodgkin's disease and one-third of enlarged spleens will be tumor-free. Although it has been clearly shown that splenectomy in chronic myelogenous leukemia does not affect the natural history of disease, removal of the massive spleen usually makes patients significantly more comfortable and simplifies their management by significantly reducing transfusion requirements. Splenectomy is an effective treatment for two chronic B cell leukemias, hairy cell leukemia and prolymphocytic leukemia, and for

the very rare splenic marginal zone lymphoma. Splenectomy in these diseases is associated with significant tumor regression in bone marrow and other sites of disease. Similar regressions of systemic disease have been noted after splenic irradiation in some types of lymphoproliferative disease, especially chronic lymphocytic leukemia. This has been termed the *abscopal effect*. Such systemic tumor responses to local therapy directed at the spleen suggest that there may be some hormone or growth factor produced by the spleen that affects tumor cell proliferation, but this conjecture is not yet substantiated. The most common indication for splenectomy is traumatic or iatrogenic splenic rupture. In a fraction of patients with splenic rupture, peritoneal seeding of splenic fragments can lead to splenosis—the presence of multiple rests of spleen tissue not connected to the portal circulation. This ectopic spleen tissue may cause pain or gastrointestinal obstruction, as in endometriosis. A large number of hematologic, immunologic, and congestive causes of splenomegaly can lead to destruction of one or more cellular blood elements. In the majority of such cases, splenectomy can correct the cytopenias, particularly anemia and thrombocytopenia. Perhaps the only contraindication to splenectomy is the presence of marrow failure, in which the enlarged spleen is the only source of hematopoietic tissue.

The absence of the spleen has minimal long-term effects on the hematologic profile. In the immediate postsplenectomy period, there may be some leukocytosis (up to 25,000/μL) and thrombocytosis (up to $1 \times 10^6/\mu$L), but within 2 to 3 weeks, blood cell counts and survival of each cell lineage are usually normal. The chronic manifestations of splenectomy are marked variation in size and shape of erythrocytes (anisocytosis, poikilocytosis) and the presence of Howell-Jolly bodies (nuclear remnants), Heinz bodies (denatured hemoglobin), basophilic stippling, and an occasional nucleated erythrocyte in the peripheral blood. When such erythrocyte abnormalities appear in a patient whose spleen has not been removed, one should suspect splenic infiltration by tumor that has interfered with its normal culling and pitting function.

The most serious consequence of splenectomy is increased susceptibility to bacterial infections, particularly those with capsules such as *Streptococcus pneumoniae*, *Haemophilus influenzae*, and some gram-negative enteric organisms. Patients under age 20 years are particularly susceptible to overwhelming sepsis with *S. pneumoniae*, and the overall actuarial risk of sepsis in patients who have had their spleens removed is about 7 percent in 10 years. About 25 percent of such patients will develop a serious infection at some time in their life. The frequency is highest within the first 3 years after splenectomy. About 15 percent of the infections are polymicrobial, and lung, skin, and blood are the most common sites. There appears to be no increased risk of viral infection in patients who have no spleen. The susceptibility to bacterial infections relates to the inability to remove opsonized bacteria from the bloodstream and a defect in making antibodies to T cell–independent antigens such as the polysaccharide components of bacterial capsules. Pneumococcal vaccine may be prophylactic if administered before splenectomy, but there are no data supporting its use after splenectomy. In fact, because patients cannot make antibody to pneumococcal polysaccharide after splenectomy, administration of the vaccine may actually lower the titer of specific pneumococcal antibodies and, theoretically, could make patients more susceptible to infection. The vaccine to *H. influenzae* should also be given to patients in whom elective splenectomy is planned. No other vaccines are routinely recommended in this setting. Once the spleen has been removed, vaccines to T cell–dependent antigens are not contraindicated but those to T cell–independent antigens are ineffective.

In addition to an increased susceptibility to bacterial infections, splenectomized patients are also more susceptible to the parasitic disease babesiosis. The splenectomized patient should avoid areas where the parasite *Babesia* is endemic (e.g., Cape Cod, MA).

Surgical removal of the spleen is an obvious cause of *hyposplenism*. Patients with sickle cell disease often suffer from autosplenectomy as a result of splenic destruction by the numerous infarcts associated with sickle cell crises during childhood. Indeed, the presence of a palpable spleen in a patient with sickle cell disease after age 5 suggests a coexisting hemoglobinopathy, e.g., thalassemia or hemoglobin C.

In addition, patients who receive splenic irradiation for a neoplastic or autoimmune disease are also functionally hyposplenic. The term *hyposplenism* is preferred to *asplenism* in referring to the physiologic consequences of splenectomy because asplenia is a rare, specific, and fatal congenital abnormality in which there is a failure of the left side of the coelomic cavity (which includes the splenic anlagen) to develop normally. Infants with asplenia have no spleens, but that is the least of their problems. The right side of the developing embryo is duplicated on the left so there is liver where the spleen should be, there are two right lungs, and the heart comprises two right atria and two right ventricles.

BIBLIOGRAPHY

BARKUN AN et al: Splenic enlargement and Traube's space: How useful in percussion? Am J Med 87:562, 1989

——— et al: The bedside assessment of splenic enlargement. Am J Med 91:512, 1991

CASTELL DO: The spleen percussion sign: A useful diagnostic technique. Ann Intern Med 67:1265, 1967

GRAVES SA et al: Does this patient have splenomegaly? JAMA 270:2218, 1993

KUBOTA T: The evaluation of peripheral adenopathy. Primary Care 7:461, 1980

MCINTYRE OR, EBAUGH FG JR: Palpable spleens: Ten year follow-up. Ann Intern Med 90:130, 1979

———, ———: Palpable spleens in college freshmen. Ann Intern Med 66:301, 1967

NIXON RK JR: The detection of splenomegaly by percussion. N Engl J Med 250:166, 1954

PANGALIS GA et al: Clinical approach to lymphadenopathy. Semin Oncol 20:570, 1993

SLAP GB et al: Validation of a model to identify young patients for lymph node biopsy. JAMA 255:2768, 1986

WEISS S: Self-observation and psychologic reactions of medical student A.S.R. to the onset and symptoms of subacute bacterial endocarditis. J Mt Sinai Hospital 8:1079, 1942

WILLIAMSON HA JR: Lymphadenopathy in a family practice: A descriptive study of 240 cases. J Fam Pract 20:449, 1985

ZUELZER W, KAPLAN J: The child with lymphadenopathy. Semin Hematol 12:323, 1975

62 Steven M. Holland, John I. Gallin

DISORDERS OF GRANULOCYTES AND MONOCYTES

Leukocytes are the major cellular components of inflammatory and immune responses and include neutrophils, T and B lymphocytes, natural killer (NK) cells, monocytes, eosinophils, and basophils. These cells have been assigned specific functions, such as antibody production by B lymphocytes or destruction of bacteria by neutrophils, but in no single infectious disease is the exact role of each of the cell types completely established. Thus, whereas neutrophils are classically thought to be critical to host defense against bacteria, there is increasing evidence that neutrophils play important roles in viral infections.

The blood is the most readily obtainable source of leukocytes and serves as the vehicle for their delivery to the various tissues from the bone marrow, where they are produced. Normal blood leukocyte counts are given in the Appendix (Tables A-7 and A-8). The various leukocytes are thought to derive from a common stem cell in the bone marrow. Three-fourths of the nucleated cells of bone marrow are committed to the production of leukocytes. Leukocyte maturation in the marrow is under the regulatory control of a number of different factors, known as colony stimulating factors and interleukins (see Chap. 105). Because an alteration in the number and type of leukocytes is a frequent association with disease processes, a total white blood count (WBC) (cells per microliter) and differential counts are obtained frequently. The lymphocytes and basophils are discussed in Chaps. 305 and 310, respectively. This chapter focuses on the neutrophils, monocytes, and eosinophils.

NEUTROPHILS

MATURATION Important events in the neutrophil life are summarized in Fig. 62-1. In normal humans, neutrophils are produced only in the bone marrow. Best estimates indicate that the appropriate number of stem cells necessary to support hematopoiesis is between 400 and 500. There is convincing evidence that human blood monocytes and tissue macrophages produce colony stimulating factors, hormones required for the growth of monocytes and neutrophils in the bone marrow. The hematopoietic system not only produces enough neutrophils (approximately 1.3×10^{11} cells per 80-kg person per day) to carry out physiologic functions but also has a large reserve stored in the marrow which can be mobilized in response to inflammation or infection. An increase in the number of blood neutrophils is called *neutrophilia*, and the presence of immature cells is termed a *shift to the left*. A diminution in the number of blood neutrophils is referred to as *neutropenia*.

Neutrophils and monocytes evolve from pluripotent stem cells under the influence of cytokines and colony stimulating factors (Fig. 62-2). The myeloblast is the first recognizable precursor cell and is followed by the *promyelocyte* (**Plate IV-15**). The promyelocyte evolves when the classic lysosomal granules, called the *primary* or *azurophil granules*, are produced. The primary granules contain hydrolases, elastase, myeloperoxidase, cationic proteins, and bactericidal/permeability-increasing (BPI) protein important for killing gram-negative bacteria. Azurophil granules also contain *defensins*, a family of cysteine-rich polypeptides with broad antimicrobial activity against bacteria, fungi, and certain enveloped viruses. The promyelocyte divides to produce the *myelocyte*, a cell responsible for the synthesis of the *specific* or *secondary granules* which contain unique (specific) constituents such as lactoferrin, vitamin B_{12}–binding proteins, membrane components of the nicotinamide-adenine dinucleotide phosphate (NADPH) oxidase required for hydrogen peroxide production, histaminase, and receptors for certain chemoattractants and adherence-promoting factors (CR3) as well as receptors for the connective tissue element laminin. The secondary granules do not contain acid hydrolases and therefore are not classic lysosomes. They are readily released extracellularly, and their mobilization is probably important in modulating inflammation. During the final stages of maturation there is no cell division, and the cell passes through the *metamyelocyte* stage and then to the *band* neutrophil with a sausage-shaped nucleus (**Plate IV-17**). As the band cell matures, the nucleus assumes a lobulated configuration. The nucleus of neutrophils normally contains up to four segments. Excessive segmentation (greater than five nuclear lobes) may be a manifestation of folate or vitamin B_{12} deficiency (**Plate IV-18**). The Pelger-Hüet anomaly (**Plate IV-19B**), an infrequent dominant benign inherited trait, results in neutrophils with distinctive bilobed nuclei that must be distinguished from band forms. The physiologic role of the multilobed nucleus of neutrophils is unknown, but it may allow great deformation of neutrophils during migration into tissues at sites of inflammation.

In settings of severe acute bacterial infection, prominent neutrophil cytoplasmic granules called *toxic granulations* are occasionally seen (**Plate IV-16**). Toxic granulations are thought to be immature or abnormally staining azurophil granules. Cytoplasmic inclusions, also called *Döhle bodies* (**Plate IV-17**), can be seen during infection and probably represent fragments of ribosome-rich endoplasmic reticulum. Large neutrophil vacuoles are often present in acute bacterial infection and probably represent pinocytosed (internalized) membrane.

Neutrophils have long been thought to be a homogeneous population of cells. However, studies of neutrophil function have suggested that they are heterogeneous. Recently, monoclonal antibodies have been developed that recognize only a subset of mature neutrophils. The meaning of neutrophil heterogeneity is not known.

MARROW RELEASE AND CIRCULATING COMPARTMENTS Specific signals, including interleukin (IL) 1, tumor necro-

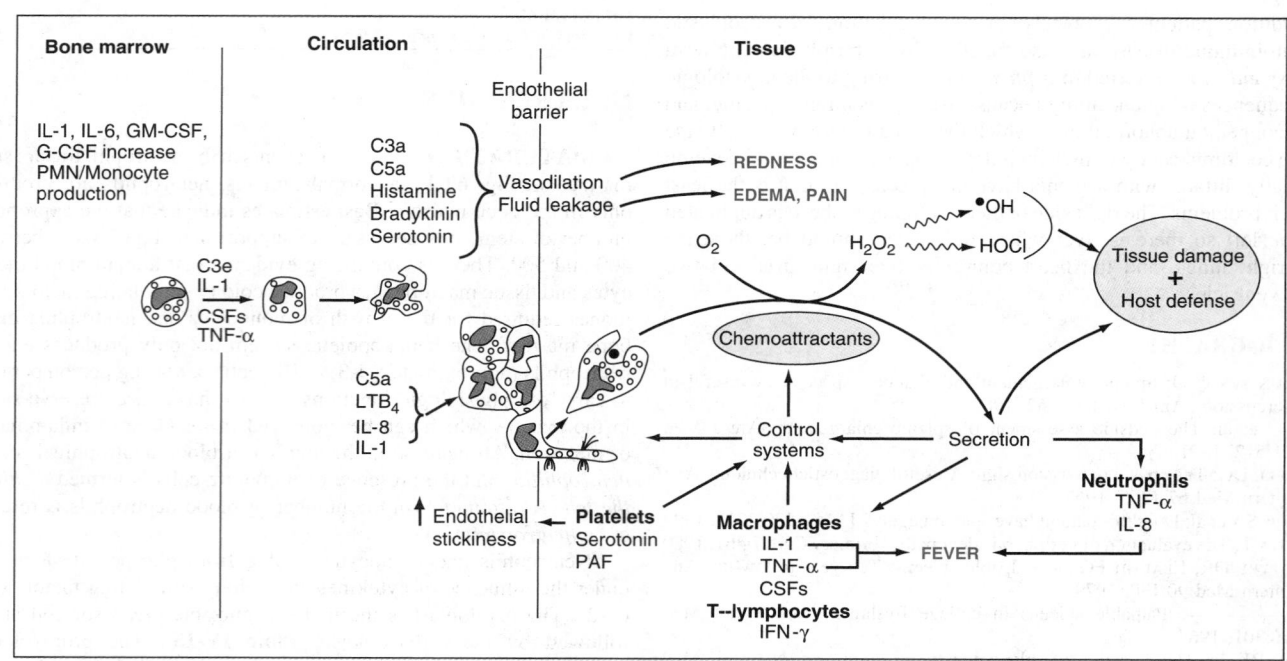

FIGURE 62-1 Events in inflammation. The four basic symptoms of inflammation are indicated by bold blue print.

Cell	Stage	Surface Markers*	Characteristics
	MYELOBLAST	CD33, CD13, CD15	Prominent Nucleoli
	PROMYELOCYTE	CD33, CD13, CD15	Large cell Primary granules appear
	MYELOCYTE	CD33, CD13, CD15, CD14, CD11b	Secondary granules appear
	METAMYELOCYTE	CD33, CD13, CD15, CD14, CD11b	Kidney–bean shaped nucleus
	BAND FORM	CD33, CD13, CD15, CD14, CD11b CD10, CD16	Condensed, band shaped nucleus
	NEUTROPHIL	CD33, CD13, CD15, CD14, CD11b, CD10, CD16	Condensed multilobed nucleus

* CD= Cluster Determinant; ⊘ Nucleolus; ● Primary granule; ○ Secondary granule.

FIGURE 62-2 Stages of neutrophil development are schematically shown. G-CSF and GM-CSF are critical to this process. Identifying cellular characteristics and specific cell-surface markers are listed for each maturational stage.

sis factor α (TNFα), the colony stimulating factors, the complement fragment C3e, and perhaps other cytokines mobilize leukocytes from the bone marrow and deliver them to the blood in an unstimulated state. Under normal conditions, about 90 percent of the neutrophil pool is in the bone marrow, 2 to 3 percent in the circulation, and the remainder in the tissues (Fig. 62-3).

The circulating pool exists in two dynamic compartments: freely flowing and marginated. The freely flowing pool is about one-half the neutrophils in the basal state and is composed of those cells that are in the blood and not in contact with the endothelium. Marginated leukocytes are those that are in close physical contact with the endothelium (Fig. 62-4). In the pulmonary circulation, where there is an extensive capillary bed (about 1000 capillaries per aleveolus), margination occurs because the capillaries are about the same size as a mature neutrophil. Therefore, neutrophil fluidity and deformability are necessary to make the transit through the pulmonary bed. Increased neutrophil rigidity and decreased deformability lead to augmented neutrophil trapping and margination in the lung. In contrast, in the systemic postcapillary venules, margination is mediated by the interaction of specific cell-surface molecules. *Selectins* are glycoproteins expressed on neutrophils and endothelial cells, among others, that cause a low-affinity interaction resulting in "rolling" of the neutrophil along the endothelial surface. On neutrophils, the molecule L-selectin [cluster determinant (CD) 62L] binds to glycosylated proteins on endothelial cells [e.g., glycosylation-dependent cell adhesion molecule (GlyCAM) 1 and CD34]. Glycoproteins on neutrophils, most importantly sialyl-Lewis^x (SLe^x, CD15s), are targets for binding of selectins expressed on endothelial cells [E-selectin (CD62E) and P-selectin (CD62P)] and other leukocytes. In response to

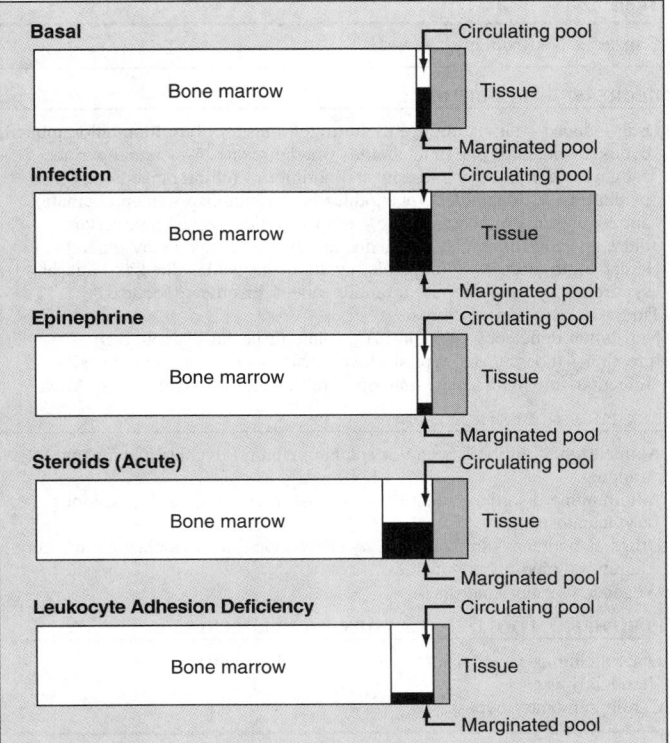

FIGURE 62-3 Schematic neutrophil distribution and kinetics between the different anatomic and functional pools.

chemotactic stimuli from injured tissues (e.g., the complement product C5a, the arachidonic acid derivative leukotriene B₄, the cytokine IL-8) or bacterial products [e.g., *N*-formylmethionylleucylphenylalanine (f-metleuphe)], neutrophil adhesiveness increases and they "stick" to the endothelium through *integrins*. The integrins are leukocyte glycoproteins that exist as complexes of a common CD18 β-chain with CD11a (LFA-1), CD11b (also called either Mac-1, CR3, or the C3bi receptor), and CD11c (p150,95). CD11a/CD18 and CD11b/CD18 mediate binding to specific endothelial receptors [intercellular adhesion molecules (ICAM)] 1 and 2.

Receptors for chemoattractants and opsonins are also mobilized; the phagocytes orient toward the chemoattractant source in the extravascular space, increase their motile activity (chemokinesis), and migrate with direction (chemotaxis) into tissues. The biochemistry and cell biology of these processes are rapidly unfolding (see "Bibliography"). The process of migration into tissues is called *diapedesis* and involves the crawling of neutrophils between postcapillary endothelial cells that open junctions between adjacent cells to permit leukocyte passage. Diapedesis involves platelet/endothelial cell adhesion molecule (PECAM) 1 (CD31), which is expressed on both the emigrating leukocyte and the endothelial cells. The endothelial responses (increased blood flow secondary to increased vasodilation and

permeability) are mediated by anaphylatoxins (e.g., complement products C3a and C5a) as well as vasodilators such as histamine, bradykinin, serotonin, and prostaglandins E and I. In the healthy adult, most neutrophils leave the body by migration through the mucous membrane of the gastrointestinal tract. Normally, neutrophils spend a relatively short time in the circulation, with a half-life of 6 to 7 h. Senescent neutrophils are cleared from the circulation by macrophages in the lung and spleen. Once in the tissues, neutrophils release enzymes such as collagenase and elastase, which may help establish abscess cavities. Neutrophils ingest (phagocytose) pathogenic materials that have been properly altered (opsonized) by substances such as IgG and the complement product C3b. Fibronectin and the tetrapeptide tuftsin facilitate the phagocytic process.

Concomitant with phagocytosis there is a burst of oxygen consumption and activation of the hexose-monophosphate shunt. A membrane-associated NADPH oxidase, consisting of membrane and cytosolic components, is assembled and catalyzes the reduction of oxygen to superoxide anion, which is then converted to hydrogen peroxide and other toxic oxygen products (e.g., hydrogen peroxide and hydroxyl radical). Hydrogen peroxide + chloride + neutrophil myeloperoxidase provide a particularly toxic system that generates hypochlorous acid (bleach), hypochlorite, and chlorine. These products oxidize and halogenate microorganisms and tumor cells and, when uncontrolled, can damage host tissue. Strongly cationic proteins and defensins also participate in microbial killing. Other enzymes, such as lysozyme and acid proteases, help digest microbial debris. After 1 to 4 days in tissues neutrophils die. Under certain conditions, such as in delayed-type hypersensitivity immunity, monocyte accumulation occurs within 6 to 12 h of initiation of inflammation. Neutrophils, monocytes, microorganisms in various states of digestion, and altered local tissue cells make up the inflammatory exudate, pus. Neutrophils shed their

FIGURE 62-4 Neutrophil travel through the pulmonary capillaries is dependent on neutrophil deformability. Neutrophil rigidity (e.g., caused by C5a) enhances pulmonary trapping and response to pulmonary pathogens in a way that is not so dependent upon cell-surface receptors. Intraalveolar chemotactic factors, such as those caused by certain bacteria (e.g., *Streptococcus pneumoniae*) lead to diapedesis of neutrophils from the pulmonary capillaries into the alveolar space. Neutrophil interaction with the endothelium of the systemic postcapillary venules is dependent on molecules of attachment. The neutrophil "rolls" along the endothelium using selectins: neutrophil CD15s (sialyl-Lewisˣ) binds to CD62E (E-selectin) and CD62P (P-selectin) on endothelial cells; CD62L (L-selectin) on neutrophils binds to CD34 and other molecules (e.g., GlyCAM-1) expressed on endothelium. Chemokines or other activation factors stimulate integrin-mediated "tight adhesion": CD11a/CD18 (LFA-1) and CD11b/CD18 (Mac-1, CR3) bind to CD54 (ICAM-1) and CD102 (ICAM-2) on the endothelium. Diapedesis occurs between endothelial cells: CD31 (PECAM-1) expressed by the emigrating neutrophil interacts with CD31 expressed at the endothelial cell-cell junction.

L-selectin molecules into the circulation upon entry into inflammatory sites. Myeloperoxidase (previously called verdoperoxidase) confers the characteristic green color to pus and may participate in turning off the inflammatory process by inactivating chemoattractants and immobilizing phagocytic cells.

Neutrophils react to certain cytokines [interferon γ (IFNγ), granulocyte-macrophage colony stimulating factor (GM-CSF), IL-8] and produce cytokines [TNFα, IL-8, macrophage inflammatory protein (MIP) 1α] that modulate the inflammatory response. An expanding class of proinflammatory peptides important for neutrophil and monocyte recruitment and activation are the *chemokines* (*chemo*attractant cyto*kines*). These small proteins are produced by many different cell types, including endothelial cells, fibroblasts, epithelial cells, neutrophils, and monocytes, and are necessary in the development of the inflammatory response. The chemokines transduce their signals through heterotrimeric G protein–linked receptors that have seven cell membrane–spanning domains, the same type of cell-surface receptor that mediates the response to the classical chemoattractants N-f-met-leuphe and C5a. There are two major structural and functional classes of chemokines: The α chemokines (e.g., IL-8) are mainly chemoattractant for neutrophils, whereas the β chemokines (e.g., MIP-1α) are more chemoattractant for monocytes and lymphocytes.

NEUTROPHIL ABNORMALITIES A defect anywhere in the neutrophil life cycle can lead to dysfunction and compromised host defenses. Inflammation is often depressed, and the clinical result is often recurrent and severe bacterial and fungal infections creating difficult management problems. Diagnosis of phagocytic cell disorders is suggested by clinical evaluation. Aphthous ulcers of mucous membranes (gray ulcers without pus) and gingivitis and periodontal disease are common. Patients with congenital phagocyte defects can have infections within the first few days of life. Skin, ear, upper and lower respiratory tract, and bone infections are common. Sepsis and meningitis are rare. In some disorders the frequency of infection is variable, and patients can go for months or even years without major infection. In the past it was unusual for persons with congenital defects to live beyond the age of 30 years. However, aggressive management of these diseases has extended the life span of patients.

Neutropenia The consequences of absent neutrophils are a dramatic demonstration of their importance in host defense. A large body of clinical data indicates that susceptibility to infectious diseases increases sharply when neutrophil levels fall below 1000 cells/μL. When the absolute neutrophil count (ANC; band forms and mature neutrophils combined) falls below 500 cells/μL, control of endogenous microbial flora (e.g., mouth, gut) is impaired; when there are fewer than 200 cells/μL, the inflammatory process is absent. The causes of neutropenia are related to depressed production, increased peripheral destruction, or excessive peripheral pooling. A falling neutrophil count or a significant decrease in neutrophils below steady state levels, together with a failure to increase neutrophil counts in the setting of infection or other challenge to the bone marrow reserve, requires investigation. Acute neutropenia, such as that caused by cancer chemotherapy, is more likely to be associated with increased risk of infection than neutropenia of long duration (months to years) that reverses in response to infection or carefully controlled administration of endotoxin (see "Laboratory Diagnosis," below).

Some causes of inherited and acquired neutropenia are listed in Table 62-1. The most common neutropenias are iatrogenic, resulting from the widespread use of cytotoxic or immunosuppressive therapies for malignancy or control of autoimmune disorders. These drugs cause neutropenia because they are toxic and result in decreased production of rapidly growing progenitor (stem) cells of the marrow. Cytotoxic chemotherapeutic agents fall into this category, but certain antibiotics such as chloramphenicol, trimethoprim-sulfamethoxazole, flucytosine, vidarabine, and the antiretroviral drug zidovudine may cause neutropenia by inhibiting proliferation of myeloid precursors. The marrow suppression is generally dose-related and dependent on continued

Table 62-1

Causes of Neutropenia

DECREASED PRODUCTION

Drug-induced—alkylating agents (nitrogen mustard, busulfan, chlorambucil, cyclophosphamide); antimetabolites (methotrexate, 6-mercaptopurine, 5-flucytosine); noncytotoxic agents [antibiotics (chloramphenicol, penicillins, sulfonamides), phenothiazines, tranquilizers (meprobamate), anticonvulsants (carbamazepine), antipsychotics (clozapine), certain diuretics, anti-inflammatory agents, antithyroid drugs, many others]
Hematologic diseases—idiopathic, cyclic neutropenia, Chédiak-Higashi syndrome, aplastic anemia, infantile genetic disorders (see text)
Tumor invasion, myelofibrosis
Nutritional deficiency—vitamin B$_{12}$, folate (especially alcoholics)
Infection—tuberculosis, typhoid fever, brucellosis, tularemia, measles, infectious mononucleosis, malaria, viral hepatitis, leishmaniasis, AIDS

PERIPHERAL DESTRUCTION

Antineutrophil antibodies and/or splenic or lung (alveolar macrophage) trapping
Autoimmune disorders—Felty's syndrome, rheumatoid arthritis, lupus erythematosus
Drugs as haptens—aminopyrine, α-methyl dopa, phenylbutazone, mercurial diuretics, some phenothiazines
Wegener's granulomatosis

PERIPHERAL POOLING (TRANSIENT NEUTROPENIA)

Overwhelming bacterial infection (acute endotoxemia)
Hemodialysis
Cardiopulmonary bypass

administration of the drug. Recombinant human granulocyte colony stimulating factor (G-CSF) is an important drug for reversing this form of neutropenia and is particularly useful in cancer chemotherapy.

Another important mechanism for iatrogenically induced neutropenia is the effect of drugs that serve as immune haptens and sensitize neutrophils or neutrophil precursors to immune-mediated peripheral destruction. This form of drug-induced neutropenia can be seen within 7 days of exposure to the drug; with previous drug exposure, resulting in preexisting antibodies, neutropenia may occur a few hours after administration of the drug. Although any drug can cause this form of neutropenia, the most frequent causes are commonly used antibiotics, such as sulfa-containing compounds, penicillins, and cephalosporins. Fever and eosinophilia also may be associated drug reactions, but often these signs are not present. Drug-induced neutropenia can be severe, but discontinuation of the sensitizing drug is sufficient for recovery, which is usually seen within 5 to 7 days and is complete by 10 days. Readministration of the sensitizing drug should be avoided, since abrupt neutropenia often will result. For this reason, diagnostic challenge should be avoided in most situations.

Autoimmune neutropenias caused by circulating antineutrophil antibodies are another form of acquired neutropenia that results in increased destruction of neutrophils. Acquired neutropenia also may be seen with viral infections, including those with the human immunodeficiency virus. Rarely, acquired neutropenia may be cyclic in nature, occurring at intervals of several weeks. Acquired cyclic neutropenia may be associated with increased natural NK cells and may be responsive to steroids.

Syndromes have been described in which expansion of large granular lymphocytes (LGL) is associated with neutropenia. Patients with LGL lymphocytosis may have moderate blood and bone marrow lymphocytosis, neutropenia, polyclonal hypergammaglobulinemia, splenomegaly, and absence of lymphadenopathy. Such patients may have a chronic and relatively stable course. Recurrent bacterial infections are frequent. There are both benign and malignant forms of this syndrome. In some patients, a spontaneous regression has occurred even after 11 years, suggesting an immunoregulatory defect as the basis for at least one form of the disorder.

Hereditary neutropenias are rare and may manifest in early childhood as a profound constant neutropenia or agranulocytosis. Examples of congenital forms of neutropenia include Kostmann's syndrome

Table 62-2

CHAPTER 62
Disorders of Granulocytes and Monocytes

355

Causes of Neutrophilia

INCREASED PRODUCTION

Idiopathic
Drug-induced—glucocorticoids
Infection—bacterial, fungal, rarely viral
Inflammation—thermal injury, tissue necrosis, myocardial and pulmonary infarction, hypersensitivity states, collagen vascular diseases
Myeloproliferative diseases—myelocytic leukemia, myeloid metaplasia, polycythemia vera

INCREASED MARROW MOBILIZATION

Glucocorticoids
Acute infection (endotoxin)
Inflammation—thermal injury

DEFECTIVE MARGINATION

Drugs—epinephrine, glucocorticoids, nonsteroidal anti-inflammatory agents
Stress, excitement, vigorous exercise
Leukocyte adhesion deficiency type 1 (integrin β chain, CD18), Leukocyte adhesion deficiency type 2 (selectin ligand, CD15s, sialyl-Lewis^x)

MISCELLANEOUS

Metabolic disorders—ketoacidosis, acute renal failure, eclampsia, acute poisoning
Drugs—lithium
Other—metastatic carcinoma, acute hemorrhage or hemolysis

(fewer than 100 neutrophils/μL), which is often fatal; more benign chronic idiopathic neutropenia (300 to 1500 neutrophils/μL); the hair-cartilage-hypoplasia syndrome; Shwachman syndrome associated with pancreatic insufficiency; and neutropenias associated with other immune defects (X-linked agammaglobulinemia, ataxia telangiectasia, IgA deficiency). Recently, forms of severe congenital neutropenia have been identified in which the G-CSF receptor encoded on chromosome 1 is mutated, leading to poor G-CSF responsiveness and apparently predisposing to development of myeloid malignancy. Hereditary cyclic neutropenia, an autosomal dominant trait, may occur in infancy and is characterized by a remarkably regular 3-week cycle. Hereditary cyclic neutropenia actually is cyclic hematopoiesis. Although the mechanism for hereditary cyclic neutropenia is not known, steroids and G-CSF blunt the cycling in some patients. Maternal factors can be associated with neutropenia in the newborn. Transplacental transfer of IgG directed against antigens on fetal neutrophils can result in peripheral destruction. Drugs (e.g., thiazide) ingested during pregnancy can cause neutropenia in the newborn by either depressed production or peripheral destruction.

The presence of immunoglobulin directed toward neutrophils is seen in Felty's syndrome (triad of rheumatoid arthritis, splenomegaly, and neutropenia; see Chap. 61). Patients with Felty's syndrome who respond to splenectomy with an increase in their neutrophil count also have lower postoperative serum neutrophil-binding IgG, a result suggesting that one beneficial effect of splenectomy is reduction in antibodies to neutrophils. Splenomegaly with peripheral trapping and destruction of neutrophils is also seen in lysosomal storage diseases and in portal hypertension.

Neutrophilia Neutrophilia results from increased neutrophil production, marrow release, or defective margination (Table 62-2). The most important acute cause of neutrophilia requiring prompt medical attention is infection. Neutrophilia from acute infection represents both increased production and increased marrow release. Increased production is also associated with chronic inflammation and certain myeloproliferative diseases. Increased marrow release and mobilization of the marginated leukocyte pool are induced by glucocorticoids. Release of epinephrine, as with vigorous exercise, excitement, or stress, will demarginate neutrophils in the spleen and lungs and double the neutrophil count. Leukocytosis with counts of 10,000 to 25,000 cells/μL occurs in response to infection and other forms of acute inflammation and results from both release of the marginated pool and mobilization of marrow reserves. Persistent neutrophilia of 30,000 to 50,000 cells/μL or greater is called a *leukemoid reaction*, a term often used to distinguish this degree of neutrophilia from leukemia. In a leukemoid reaction, the circulating neutrophils are usually mature and not clonally derived.

Abnormal Neutrophil Function The types of inherited and acquired abnormalities of phagocyte function are described in Table 62-3. The resulting diseases are best considered in terms of the functional defects of adherence, chemotaxis, and microbicidal activity. The distinguishing features of the important inherited disorders of phagocyte function are shown in Table 62-4, several of which are discussed below.

Two types of leukocyte adhesion deficiency (LAD) have been described: Both are autosomal recessive traits and result in the inability of neutrophils to exit the circulation to sites of infection, leading to constant leukocytosis and increased susceptibility to infection. Patients with LAD 1 have mutations in CD18, the common component of the integrins LFA-1, Mac-1, and p150,95, leading to a defect in tight adhesion between neutrophils and the endothelium. The heterodimer formed by CD18/CD11b (Mac-1) is also the receptor for the comple-

Table 62-3

Types of Granulocyte and Monocyte Disorders

Function	Cause of Indicated Dysfunction		
	Drug-Induced	**Acquired**	**Inherited**
Adherence-aggregation	Aspirin, colchicine, alcohol, glucocorticoids, ibuprofen, piroxicam	Neonatal state, hemodialysis	Leukoctye adhesion deficiency types 1 and 2
Deformability		Leukemia, neonatal state, diabetes mellitus, immature neutrophils	
Chemokinesis-chemotaxis	Glucocorticoids (high dose), auranofin, colchicine (weak effect), phenylbutazone, naproxen, indomethacin, interleukin 2	Thermal injury, malignancy, malnutrition, periodontal disease, neonatal state, systemic lupus erythematosus, rheumatoid arthritis, diabetes mellitus, sepsis, influenza virus infection, herpes simplex virus infection, acrodermatitis enteropathica, AIDS	Chédiak-Higashi syndrome, neutrophil-specific granule deficiency, hyper IgE–recurrent infection (Job's) syndrome (in some patients), Down syndrome, α-mannosidase deficiency, severe combined immunodeficiency, Wiskott-Aldrich syndrome
Microbicidal activity	Colchicine, cyclophosphamide, glucocorticoids (high dose)	Leukemia, aplastic anemia, certain neutropenias, tuftsin deficiency, thermal injury, sepsis, neonatal state, diabetes mellitus, malnutrition, AIDS	Chédiak-Higashi syndrome, neutrophil-specific granule deficiency, chronic granulomatous disease

ment-derived opsonin C3bi (CR3). The CD18 gene is located on distal chromosome 21q. Variable expression of the defect determines the magnitude of clinical disease. Complete lack of expression of the leukocyte adhesion proteins by resting neutrophils results in the severe phenotype in which inflammatory cytokines do not increase the expression of leukocyte adhesion proteins on neutrophils or activated T and B cells. The functional abnormalities are predictable because of the role these molecules play in normal leukocyte function. Neutrophils (and monocytes) from patients with LAD 1 adhere poorly to endothelial cells and protein-coated surfaces and exhibit defective spreading, aggregation, and chemotaxis. Patients with this syndrome have recurrent bacterial and fungal infections involving skin, oral and genital mucosa, and respiratory and intestinal tracts; persistent leukocytosis (15,000 to 20,000 neutrophils/μL) because cells do not marginate; and, in severe cases, a history of delayed separation of the umbilical stump. Infections, especially of the skin, tend to become necrotic with progressively enlarging borders, slow healing, and the development of dysplas-

tic scars. The most common bacteria are *Staphylococcus aureus* and enteric gram-negative bacteria. LAD 2 is caused by an abnormality of SLe^x (CD15s), the ligand on neutrophils that interacts with selectins on endothelial cells.

Abnormal neutrophil and monocyte chemotaxis occurs in the *hyper-immunoglobulin E–recurrent infection* (HIE) or *Job's syndrome*. The molecular basis for this syndrome is not known, but some cases appear to have autosomal dominant transmission. Patients with this syndrome have coarse facies; bone abnormalities including hyperostosis frontalis externa, hypertelorism, kyphoscoliosis, and osteoporosis; and eczema. They develop recurrent sinopulmonary and cutaneous infections that tend to be much less inflamed than appropriate for the degree of infection and have been referred to as "cold abscesses." A high degree of suspicion is required to diagnose infections in these patients, who may appear well despite extensive disease. For many years the cold abscesses were thought to be a reflection of impaired chemotaxis with too few phagocytes arriving too late, perhaps secondary to a lymphocyte factor inhibiting chemotaxis. However, it is now clear that the chemotactic defect in these patients is variable and the fundamental basis for the impaired defenses is complex and inadequately delineated.

Table 62-4

Inherited Disorders of Phagocyte Function: Differential Features

Clinical Manifestations	Cellular or Molecular Defects	Diagnosis
CHRONIC GRANULOMATOUS DISEASES OF CHILDHOOD (60% X-LINKED, 40% AUTOSOMAL RECESSIVE)		
Severe infections of skin, ears, lungs, liver, and bone with catalase-positive microorganisms such as *S. aureus*, *Burkholderia cepacia*, *Aspergillus* sp., *Chromobacterium violaceum*; often hard to culture organism; excessive inflammation with granulomas, frequent lymph node suppuration; granulomas can obstruct GI or GU tracts; gingivitis, aphthous ulcers, seborrheic dermatitis	Absent respiratory burst due to the lack of one of four NADPH oxidase subunits in neutrophils, monocytes, and eosinophils	NBT test; absent superoxide and H_2O_2 production by neutrophils; absent chemiluminescence; immunoblot for NADPH oxidase components
CHÉDIAK-HIGASHI SYNDROME (AUTOSOMAL RECESSIVE)		
Recurrent pyogenic infections, especially with *S. aureus*; many patients get lymphomatous-like illness during adolescence; periodontal disease; partial oculocutaneous albinism, nystagmus, progressive peripheral neuropathy, mental retardation in some patients	Reduced chemotaxis and phagolysosome fusion, increased respiratory burst activity, defective egress from marrow, abnormal skin window	Giant primary granules in neutrophils and other granule-bearing cells (Wright's stain)
SPECIFIC GRANULE DEFICIENCY (AUTOSOMAL RECESSIVE?)		
Recurrent infections of skin, ears, and sinopulmonary tract; delayed wound healing; decreased inflammation; bleeding diathesis	Abnormal chemotaxis, impaired respiratory burst and bacterial killing, failure to upregulate chemotactic and adhesion receptors with stimulation, defect in transcription of granule proteins	Lack of secondary (specific) granules in neutrophils (Wright's stain), absent neutrophil-specific granule contents (i.e., lactoferrin), absent defensins, platelet alpha granule abnormality
MYELOPEROXIDASE DEFICIENCY (AUTOSOMAL RECESSIVE)		
Clinically normal except in patients with underlying disease such as diabetes mellitus; then candidiasis or other fungal infections	Absent myeloperoxidase due to pre- and posttranslational defects	Absent peroxidase in neutrophils
LEUKOCYTE ADHESION DEFICIENCY (AUTOSOMAL RECESSIVE)		
Type 1 Delayed separation of umbilical cord, sustained granulocytosis, recurrent infections of skin and mucosa, gingivitis, periodontal disease	Impaired phagocyte adherence, aggregation, spreading, chemotaxis, phagocytosis of C3bi-coated particles; defective production of CD18 subunit common to leukocyte integrins	Reduced phagocyte surface expression of the CD18-containing integrins using monoclonal antibodies against LFA-1 (CD18/CD11a), Mac-1 or CR3 (CD18/CD11b), p150,95 (CD18/CD11c)
Type 2 Severe mental retardation, short stature, Bombay (hh) blood phenotype, recurrent infections, granulocytosis	Impaired phagocyte rolling along endothelium	Reduced phagocyte surface expression of Sialyl-Lewis^x, using monoclonal antibodies against CD15s
HYPER IgE–RECURRENT INFECTION SYNDROME (AUTOSOMAL) (JOB'S SYNDROME)		
Eczematoid or pruritic dermatitis, "cold" skin abscesses, recurrent pneumonias with *S. aureus* with bronchopleural fistulas and cyst formation, mild eosinophilia, mucocutaneous candidiasis, atopy, coarse facies, restrictive lung disease, scoliosis	Reduced chemotaxis in some patients, reduced suppressor T cell activity	Clinical features, serum IgE > 2000 IU/mL, high serum anti-*S. aureus* IgE, low or absent serum and salivary anti-*S. aureus* IgA

The most common neutrophil defect is *myeloperoxidase deficiency*, which is inherited as an autosomal recessive trait and may have an incidence as high as about 1 in 2000 persons. Isolated myeloperoxidase deficiency is not associated with clinically compromised defenses, because other defense systems such as hydrogen peroxide generation are accelerated. Microbicidal activity of neutrophils is delayed but not absent. However, if another underlying defect in host defense, such as poorly controlled diabetes mellitus, accompanies myeloperoxidase deficiency, then host defenses are likely to be significantly compromised. An acquired form of myeloperoxidase deficiency occurs in myelomonocytic leukemia and acute myeloblastic leukemia.

Chédiak-Higashi syndrome (CHS) is a rare disease with autosomal recessive inheritance. Neutrophils and all cells containing lysosomes from patients with CHS characteristically have large granules (**Plate IV-19A**). CHS patients have increased infections due to a multitude of infectious agents. CHS neutrophils and monocytes have impaired chemotaxis and abnormal rates of microbial killing due to slow rates of fusion of the lysosomal granules with phagosomes. Natural killer cell function is also impaired.

Chronic granulomatous disease (CGD) represents a group of disorders of granulocyte and monocyte oxidative metabolism. Although CGD is rare, currently estimated to occur once in 250,000 individuals, it is an important model of defective neutrophil oxidative metabolism. Most often CGD is inherited as an X-linked recessive pattern, although in about 40 percent of patients the disease is inherited with an autosomal recessive pattern. Mutations of four genes corresponding to four proteins that assemble at the plasma membrane account for all patients with CGD. Two proteins (a 91-kDa protein, abnormal in X-linked CGD, and a 22-kDa protein, absent in one form of autosomal recessive CGD) form the heterodimer cytochrome b-558 in the plasma membrane. Two other proteins (47 and 67 kDa, abnormal in the other autosomal recessive forms of CGD) are cytoplasmic in origin and interact with the cytochrome following cell activation to form NADPH oxidase, required for hydrogen peroxide production. Leukocytes from patients with CGD have severely diminished hydrogen peroxide production. The genes involved in each of the defects have been cloned and sequenced and the chromosome locations identified. Patients with CGD characteristically have increased infection with catalase-positive microorganisms (organisms that destroy their own hydrogen peroxide). When patients with CGD become infected, they often have extensive inflammatory reactions, and lymph node suppuration is common despite the administration of appropriate antibiotics. Aphthous ulcers and chronic inflammation of the nares are usually present. Granulomas are frequent and can obstruct the gastrointestinal or genitourinary tracts. The excessive inflammatory reactions probably reflect abnormal turnoff of inflammation by failure to degrade chemoattractants and failure to degrade antigens that cause persistent neutrophil accumulation. Impaired killing of intracellular microorganisms by macrophages may lead to persistent cell-mediated immunity and granuloma formation.

MONONUCLEAR PHAGOCYTES

The mononuclear phagocyte system is defined as a continuum linking monoblasts, promonocytes, and monocytes with the structurally diverse tissue macrophages that make up what was previously referred to as the reticuloendothelial system. Macrophages are long-lived phagocytic cells capable of many of the functions of neutrophils. In addition, they are important secretory cells that, through their receptors and secretory products, participate in many complex immunologic and inflammatory processes not attributed to neutrophils. Monocytes leave the circulation by diapedesis more slowly than neutrophils and have a half-life in the blood of 12 to 24 h.

After blood monocytes arrive in the tissues, they differentiate into macrophages ("big eaters") with specialized functions suited for specific anatomic locations. Macrophages are particularly abundant in capillary walls of the lung, spleen, liver, and bone marrow, where they function to remove microorganisms and other noxious elements from the blood. Alveolar macrophages, liver Kupffer cells, splenic macrophages, peritoneal macrophages, bone marrow macrophages, lymphatic macrophages, brain microglial cells, and dendritic macrophages all have specialized functions. Macrophage-secreted products include lysozyme, neutral proteases, acid hydrolases, arginase, numerous complement components, enzyme inhibitors (plasmin, α_2 macroglobulin), binding proteins (transferrin, fibronectin, transcobalamin II), nucleosides, and cytokines (TNFα, IL-1, -8, -12). Interleukin 1 (see Chaps. 17 and 305) has many important functions, including stimulating the hypothalamus to initiate fever, mobilizing leukocytes from the bone marrow, as well as activating lymphocytes and neutrophils. Tumor necrosis factor α (also called *cachectin*) is a pyrogen that duplicates many of the actions of IL-1 and plays an important role in the pathogenesis of gram-negative shock (see Chap. 124). It can stimulate vigorous production of hydrogen peroxide and related toxic oxygen species by macrophages and neutrophils. In addition, TNFα induces the catabolic responses of chronic inflammation, which contribute to the profound wasting (cachexia) associated with many chronic diseases.

Other macrophage-secreted products include reactive oxygen metabolites, bioactive lipids (arachidonate metabolites and platelet-activating factors), chemokines, bone marrow colony stimulating factors, and factors stimulating fibroblast and microvasculature proliferation. Macrophages help regulate the replication of lymphocytes and participate in the killing of tumors, viruses, and certain bacteria (*Mycobacterium tuberculosis* and *Listeria monocytogenes*). Macrophages are key effector cells in the elimination of intracellular microorganisms. Their ability to fuse to form giant cells that coalesce into granulomas in response to some inflammatory stimuli is important in the elimination of intracellular microbes and may be under the control of IFNγ.

Macrophages play an important role in the immune response (see Chap. 305). They process and present antigen to lymphocytes and secrete cytokines that modulate and direct lymphocyte development and function. Macrophages participate in autoimmune phenomena by removing immune complexes and other immunologically active substances from the circulation. Furthermore, they play a role in wound healing, in the disposal of senescent cells, and in the development of atheromas.

DISORDERS OF THE MONONUCLEAR PHAGOCYTE SYSTEM Many disorders of neutrophils extend to mononuclear phagocytes. Thus drugs that suppress neutrophil production in the bone marrow usually lead to monocytopenia. Transient monocytopenia also can be seen after stress or glucocorticoid administration. Monocytosis is associated with certain infections such as tuberculosis, brucellosis, subacute bacterial endocarditis, Rocky Mountain spotted fever, malaria, and visceral leishmaniasis (kala azar). Monocytosis is also seen in malignancies, leukemias, myeloproliferative syndromes, hemolytic anemias, chronic idiopathic neutropenias, and granulomatous diseases such as sarcoidosis, regional enteritis, and some collagen vascular diseases. Patients with LAD, HIE (Job's) syndrome, CHS, and chronic granulomatous diseases all have defects in the mononuclear phagocyte system. Impaired monocyte cytokine production has been found in some patients with disseminated nontuberculous mycobacterial infection who are not infected with the human immunodeficiency virus (HIV).

Certain viral infections impair mononuclear phagocyte function. For example, influenza virus infection is associated with abnormal monocyte chemotaxis. Mononuclear phagocytes can be infected by the HIV, and abnormal monocyte chemotaxis and abnormal clearance of IgG-coated erythrocytes (discussed below) by macrophages is also seen in AIDS (see Chap. 308). It is likely that the defects of the monocyte-macrophage system in AIDS contribute to the disordered immunoregulation and increased susceptibility to opportunistic infection due to intracellular microorganisms such as *Pneumocystis carinii* and *M. avium* complex. T lymphocytes produce IFNγ, which induces Fc-receptor expression and phagocytosis and stimulates hydrogen peroxide production by mononuclear phagocytes and neutrophils. In certain diseases, such as AIDS, IFNγ production may be deficient, while in other diseases, such as T cell lymphomas, excessive release of IFNγ is thought to cause erythrophagocytosis by splenic macrophages.

Specific defects of mononuclear phagocytes have been described in certain autoimmune diseases. Removal of IgG-coated radiolabeled autologous erythrocytes, presumably via the Fc receptor of splenic macrophages, is profoundly abnormal in patients with active systemic lupus erythematosus. Patients with other autoimmune diseases characterized by tissue deposition of immune complexes, as seen in Sjögren's syndrome, mixed cryoglobulinemia, dermatitis herpetiformis, and chronic progressive multiple sclerosis, also have defects in Fc-receptor function as judged by clearance of IgG-coated erythrocytes (see Chap. 311). Clinically, normal subjects with genetic haplotypes commonly associated with autoimmune disease (i.e., HLA-B8/DRw3) also have an increased incidence of defective Fc-receptor–specific functional activity, suggesting that this defect may predispose individuals with this genetic profile to immune-complex disease.

Monocytopenia occurs with acute infections, with stress, and following administration of glucocorticoids. Monocytopenia also occurs in aplastic anemia, hairy cell leukemia, and acute myelogenous leukemia and as a direct result of myelotoxic and immunosuppressive drugs.

EOSINOPHILS

Eosinophils and neutrophils share similar morphology, many lysosomal constituents, phagocytic capacity, and oxidative metabolism. Eosinophils express a specific chemoattractant receptor and respond to a specific chemokine, eotaxin. However, there are major differences between the two cell types, and little is known about the natural function of eosinophils. Eosinophils are much longer lived than neutrophils, and unlike neutrophils, tissue eosinophils can recirculate. During most infections, eosinophils do not appear to have any important function. However, in invasive helminthic infections, such as hookworm, schistosomiasis, strongyloidiasis, toxocariasis, trichinosis, filariasis, echinococcosis, and cysticercosis, the eosinophil likely plays a central role in host defense. Eosinophils are also associated with bronchial asthma, cutaneous allergic reactions, and other hypersensitivity states.

The characteristic red-staining eosinophil granules (Wright's stain) contain a number of unique constituents. The distinctive feature of the eosinophil granule is its crystalline core consisting of an arginine-rich protein (major basic protein) with histaminase activity, which is probably important in host defense against parasites. Eosinophil granules also contain a unique eosinophil peroxidase that catalyzes the oxidation of many substances by hydrogen peroxide and may facilitate killing of microorganisms.

Eosinophil peroxidase, in the presence of hydrogen peroxide and halide, initiates mast cell secretion in vitro and thereby may contribute to inflammation. Other substances found in eosinophils include cationic proteins, some of which bind to heparin and reduce its anticoagulant activity. Eosinophil cytoplasm contains Charcot-Leyden crystal protein, a hexagonal bipyramidal crystal first described in leukemia and then in sputum from asthma patients, which is lysophospholipase and may function to restrict the toxicity of certain lysophospholipids. Eosinophils also contain a powerful neurotoxin. Patients with hypereosinophilic syndrome and cerebral spinal fluid eosinophilia exhibit varied neurologic abnormalities.

Several factors enhance the eosinophil's function in host defense. For example, stimulated T cell–derived factors enhance the ability of eosinophils to kill parasites. Mast cell–derived eosinophil chemotactic factor of anaphylaxis (ECFa) increases the number of eosinophil complement receptors and enhances eosinophil killing of parasites. In addition, eosinophil colony stimulating factors (e.g., IL-5) produced by macrophages may not only increase eosinophil production in the bone marrow but also may activate eosinophils to kill parasites.

EOSINOPHILIA Eosinophilia is the presence of more than 500 eosinophils/μL of blood and is common in many settings besides parasite infection. Significant tissue eosinophilia can occur without an elevated blood count. The most common cause of eosinophilia is probably allergic reactions to drugs such as iodides, aspirin, sulfonamides, nitrofurantoin, penicillins, and cephalosporins. Allergies such as hay fever, asthma, eczema, serum sickness, allergic vasculitis, and pemphigus commonly are associated with eosinophilia. Eosinophilia is also seen in collagen vascular diseases (e.g., rheumatoid arthritis, eosinophilic fasciitis, allergic angiitis, and periarteritis nodosa) and malignancies (e.g., Hodgkin's disease, mycosis fungoides, chronic myelogenous leukemia, and cancer of the lung, stomach, pancreas, ovary, or uterus), as well as in rare diseases such as Job's syndrome and CGD; the mechanisms for the eosinophilia in these diseases are not known. Eosinophilia is commonly seen in the helminthic infections. Therapeutic administration of the cytokines IL-2 and GM-CSF frequently leads to transient eosinophilia. The most dramatic hypereosinophilic syndromes are Loeffler's syndrome, Loeffler's endocarditis, eosinophilic leukemia, and idiopathic hypereosinophilic syndrome (with counts as high as 50,000 to 100,000/μL).

The idiopathic hypereosinophilic syndrome represents a heterogeneous group of disorders with the common feature of prolonged eosinophilia of unknown cause and associated organ system dysfunction, including the heart, central nervous system, kidneys, lungs, gastrointestinal tract, and skin. The bone marrow is involved in all subjects, but the most severe complications involve the heart and central nervous system. Eosinophils are found in the involved tissues and are thought to cause tissue damage by local deposition of toxic eosinophil proteins such as eosinophil cationic protein and eosinophil major basic protein. In the heart, the pathologic changes lead to thrombosis, which may result in endocardial fibrosis and restrictive endomyocardiopathy. Similar pathologic changes are thought to contribute to the damage of tissues in other organ systems. Although the mechanism for the hypereosinophilia is not known, it has been shown that chemotherapy with glucocorticoids usually induces remission. In patients unresponsive to glucocorticoids, a cytotoxic agent such as hydroxyurea has been used successfully to lower the peripheral blood eosinophil counts and to improve markedly the prognosis. Interferon α also is effective in some patients, including those unresponsive to hydroxyurea. Aggressive medical and surgical approaches are employed for management of patients with cardiovascular complications.

The *eosinophilia-myalgia syndrome* is a multisystem disease with prominent cutaneous, hematologic, and visceral manifestations that frequently evolves into a chronic course and can occasionally be fatal. The syndrome is characterized by eosinophilia (greater than 1000 eosinophils/μL) and generalized disabling myalgias without other recognized causes. Eosinophil fasciitis, pneumonitis and myocarditis, neuropathy culminating in respiratory failure, and encephalopathy have been described. The association of the disease with ingestion of L-tryptophan–containing products originating from a single source has led to the identification and characterization of putative etiologic agents present as contaminants in these preparations. Although the accumulation of eosinophils, lymphocytes, macrophages, and fibroblasts in the affected tissues suggests that these cells play important roles in the pathogenesis of the eosinophilia-myalgia syndrome, the precise mechanism of their involvement has not been established. Several studies have demonstrated the activation of eosinophils and the deposition of eosinophil-derived toxic proteins in affected tissues. Fibroblast activation and increased expression of genes coding for various connective tissue molecules have been demonstrated. Furthermore, IL-5 and transforming growth factor β have been implicated as potential mediators. Treatment has included withdrawal of L-tryptophan–containing products and the administration of glucocorticoids. Most patients recover fully, remain stable, or show slow recovery, but in some patients (up to 5 percent) the disease can be fatal. This disease emphasizes the importance of chemical and environmental factors in the development of systemic disorders characterized by chronic inflammation and fibrosis.

EOSINOPENIA This occurs with stress, such as acute bacterial infection, and following administration of glucocorticoids. The mechanism of eosinopenia of acute bacterial infection is unknown but is independent of endogenous glucocorticoids, since it occurs in animals following total adrenalectomy. There is no known adverse effect of eosinopenia.

LABORATORY DIAGNOSIS AND MANAGEMENT

Initial studies of WBC and differential and often a bone marrow examination are followed by assessment of bone marrow reserves (steroid challenge test), marginated circulating pool of cells (epinephrine challenge test), and marginating ability (endotoxin challenge test) (see Fig. 62-3). In vivo assessment of inflammation is possible with a Rebuck skin window test or an in vivo blister assay, which measures the ability of leukocytes and inflammatory mediators to accumulate locally within the skin. In vivo clearance of IgG-coated erythrocytes provides a useful way to monitor the mononuclear phagocyte system. In vitro tests of phagocyte aggregation, adherence, chemotaxis, phagocytosis, degranulation, and microbicidal activity (for *Staph. aureus*) help pinpoint cellular or humoral lesions that can then be further characterized at the molecular level. Deficiencies of oxidative metabolism are screened with the nitroblue tetrazolium (NBT) dye test, which is based on the ability of products of oxidative metabolism to reduce yellow, soluble NBT to blue-black formazan, an insoluble material that precipitates intracellularly and can be seen microscopically. Further aspects of neutrophil oxidative metabolism are defined by studies of superoxide and hydrogen peroxide production.

The most important aspect of patient management is to appreciate that patients with leukopenias or leukocyte dysfunction often have delayed inflammatory responses. Therefore, clinical manifestations may be minimal despite overwhelming infection, and unusual infections must always be suspected. Early signs of infection demand prompt, aggressive culturing for microorganisms and use of antibiotics and surgical drainage of abscesses. Prolonged antibiotics are often required. Daily white blood cell transfusions (enriched for neutrophils) are controversial. In patients with CGD, prophylactic antibiotics trimethoprim-sulfamethoxazole) diminish the frequency of life-threatening infections. Surgery is required for thorough drainage of abscesses in lung, liver, and bones. Short courses of glucocorticoids have had dramatic effects in the management of the granulomas of CGD. For example, obstruction of the gastrointestinal or genitourinary tract in CGD can be diminished with a short course of steroids followed by a long one of a nonsteroidal anti-inflammatory agent. Recombinant human IFNγ, which nonspecifically stimulates phagocytic cell function, reduces the frequency of infections in CGD patients by 70 percent and reduces the severity of infection (hospital days for infection) as well. This effect of IFNγ in CGD is additive to the effect of prophylactic antibiotics. Interferon γ has been approved by the U.S. Food and Drug Administration for use in CGD at a recommended dose of 50 μL/m² of body surface area, subcutaneously three times weekly. Interferon γ also has been used successfully in the treatment of leprosy, nontuberculous mycobacteria, and visceral leishmaniasis.

Rigorous oral hygiene reduces but does not eliminate the discomfort of gingivitis, periodontal disease, and aphthous ulcers; chlorhexidine mouthwash and tooth brushing with a hydrogen peroxide–sodium bicarbonate paste helps many patients. Ketoconazole has caused dramatic improvement of mucocutaneous candidiasis in patients with Job's syndrome. Treatment to restore myelopoiesis in patients with neutropenia due to impaired production has included use of androgens, glucocorticoids, lithium, and immunosuppressive therapy. Recombinant G-CSF is useful in the management of certain forms of neutropenia due to depressed production, especially that related to cancer chemotherapy. Patients with chronic neutropenia with evidence of a good bone marrow reserve should not receive prophylactic antibiotics.

Patients with constant or cyclic neutrophil counts below 500 cells/μL may benefit from prophylactic antibiotics and G-CSF during periods of neutropenia. Oral trimethoprim-sulfamethoxazole (160/800 mg) twice daily is commonly used to prevent infection, although concerns about its predisposing to fungal infections have been raised. Increased fungal infection is not seen in CGD patients on this regimen. Oral quinolones such as norfloxacin and ciprofloxacin have been suggested alternatives.

In the setting of cytotoxic chemotherapy with severe, persistent neutropenia, the proven effectiveness of trimethoprim-sulfamethoxazole in preventing *P. carinii* pneumonia may offer another incentive to use this form of prophylaxis. These patients, and patients with phagocytic cell dysfunction, should avoid heavy exposure to airborne soil, dust, or decaying matter (mulch, manure), which are often rich in spores of *Aspergillus* or other fungi. Restriction of activities or social contact probably makes little difference in risk of infection.

Cure of some congenital phagocyte defects is theoretically possible by bone marrow transplantation (see Chap. 116). However, complications of bone marrow transplantation are still serious, and with rigorous medical care many patients with phagocytic disorders can go for years without a life-threatening infection. The identification of specific gene defects in patients with LAD 1 and CGD has led to in vitro correction of B cells from these patients by gene transfer. Gene correction has been performed on peripheral blood progenitor cells from patients with CGD. This approach has been successful in vitro, leading to restoration of a functional NADPH oxidase. Initial experiments also have been carried out in humans, making gene therapy for CGD and other genetic disorders a likely emerging reality.

BIBLIOGRAPHY

Cassatella MA: The production of cytokines by polymorphonuclear neutrophils. Immunol Today 16:21, 1995

Dong F et al: Mutations in the gene for the granulocyte colony-stimulating factor receptor in patients with acute myeloid leukemia preceded by severe congenital neutropenia. New Engl J Med 333:487, 1995

Gallin JI et al: Interferon-γ in the management of infectious diseases. Ann Intern Med 123:216, 1995

Hogg JC, Doerschuk CM: Leukocyte traffic in the lung. Annu Rev Physiol 57:97, 1995

Holland SM, Gallin JI: Neutrophil disorders, in *Samter's Immunologic Diseases*, MM Frank et al (eds). Boston, Little, Brown, 1995, p 529

Kuhns DB et al: Increased circulating cytokines, cytokine antagonists, and E-selectin after intravenous administration of endotoxin in humans. J Infect Dis 171:145, 1995

Leto TL et al: Assembly of the phagocyte NADPH oxidase:binding of Src homology 3 domains to proline-rich targets. Proc Natl Acad Sci USA 91:10650, 1994

Lieschke GJ, Burgess AW: Granulocyte colony-stimulating factor and granulocyte-macrophage colony-stimulating factor. N Engl J Med 327:28, 99, 1992

Springer TA: Traffic signals for lymphocyte recirculation and leukocyte emigration: The multistep paradigm. Cell 76:301, 1994

Varga J et al: The cause and pathogenesis of the eosinophil-myalgia syndrome. Ann Intern Med 116:140, 1992

63   *Daniel C. Ihde, Dan L. Longo*

PRESENTATIONS OF THE PATIENT WITH CANCER: SOLID TUMORS IN ADULTS

THE MAGNITUDE OF THE PROBLEM

Cancer is a major cause of morbidity in the United States. In 1996, the American Cancer Society estimated that 1,359,150 people were diagnosed with a malignant neoplasm and 554,740 died from one of these diseases. Cancer is responsible for 23.9 percent of all American deaths and is exceeded only by heart disease as a cause of mortality (33.0 percent of deaths). Unfortunately, cancer mortality is increasing, while that from cardiac disease is declining, and sometime early in the next century cancer is expected to become the leading cause of death in this country, as it already is in Japan.

All cancers share the characteristic of disordered normal control over cell division, growth, and differentiation. Their initial clinical manifestations are extremely heterogeneous, however, since over 70 types of cancer arising in virtually every organ or tissue in the body are recognized. They may be entirely asymptomatic until late in the disease course. Symptoms related to cancerous cell growth generally fall into one of three categories: (1) local—pain or swelling that may be painful or painless in a site of tumor cell expansion; (2) regional—dysfunction in the organ of origin or in adjacent or distant organs, related to the local or metastatic growth of the tumor; and (3) systemic—remote effects of tumor related to production of hormones or cytokines by the tumor or the host reaction to the tumor (see Table 63-1). In addition to problems related to the tumor itself, there are also psychosocial manifestations related to the *diagnosis* of cancer. Psychological distress, anxiety, and depression may occur out of proportion to the prognosis in response to the diagnosis of cancer. → *The problems associated with the diagnosis of cancer are discussed in Chap. 81.*

Local effects may include pain without a mass or a painful or painless mass or swelling. Regional effects may include edema or effusion from obstruction of lymphatic drainage; organ dysfunction (e.g., liver function abnormality or myelophthisic anemia); obstruction of flow of air, blood, urine, cerebrospinal fluid, bile, stool, or lymph; nerve dysfunction from compression (e.g., hoarseness from laryngeal nerve compression); and breach of structural integrity (e.g., bone fracture, blood vessel rupture, or viscus perforation). → *The paraneoplastic effects of cancer are numerous and are discussed in greater detail in Chaps. 102 and 103.*

Nearly every cardinal manifestation of disease discussed in this book may be associated with cancer. However, certain manifestations are more likely to be found in the more common tumors. This chapter is therefore confined to discussing the more frequent presenting symptoms or findings that lead to the diagnosis of a malignant neoplasm in patients with the 10 most common solid tumors of both men and women, which are quantitatively by far the major causes of death from cancer. → *A similar discussion of diagnostic considerations in the evaluation of patients with hematopoietic neoplasia (leukemias and lymphomas) may be found in Chaps. 61 and 62.*

Table 63-2 illustrates that there is considerable overlap among the specific types of solid tumors that are most frequently diagnosed in men and women. Six of these cancers—those of the lung, colon and rectum, bladder, kidney, and pancreas and cutaneous melanoma—are among the 10 most common tumors in both genders. Four of the common cancers are gender-specific—endometrium, ovary, and cervix in women and prostate in men—and a fifth, breast cancer, occurs in women over 99 percent of the time. The remaining three, oropharyngeal/laryngeal, stomach, and brain, are among the 10 most common

cancers of men but are not rare in women. It is noteworthy that the number of cases of newly diagnosed cancer within the categories of the 10 most common solid tumors in each gender totals 1,090,100 individuals, 80.2 percent of all cancer patients diagnosed in 1996. Thus, knowledge of common symptoms and presentations in individuals who develop one of the 10 most common cancers in either men or women will be applicable to a substantial majority of all cancer patients.

CANCERS GROUPED BY ORGAN SYSTEM

UPPER AERODIGESTIVE TRACT CANCERS Oropharyngeal/Laryngeal Asymptomatic and symptomatic oral neoplasms, both precancerous and cancerous, are often first noted during dental examination. Leukoplakia, a whitish patch in the mouth that cannot be wiped away, and erythroplakia, a reddish, sometimes raised or velvety painless lesion, are sometimes precancerous lesions, especially when associated with dysplasia on biopsy. Squamous carcinoma is the most common persisting ulceration in the oral cavity. These lesions are often painless and exhibit both infiltrative (crater-like with raised borders) and whitish exophytic growth patterns. Unexplained oral ulcers that do not heal after several weeks should be biopsied.

Oropharyngeal, hypopharyngeal, and laryngeal tumors often present with nodal metastasis in the neck; excisional biopsy should always be considered for a persisting noninflammatory neck mass. Hoarseness is associated with laryngeal and oropharyngeal cancers, difficulty in swallowing with oropharyngeal lesions, and otalgia with hypopharyngeal tumors. These symptoms are often associated with more advanced disease. Malodorous breath and hemoptysis may also occur.

Lung A myriad of symptoms or signs can raise the first suspicion of lung cancer. Symptoms arising from the primary tumor include

Table 63-1

Manifestations of Malignant Disease

Local
  Pain
  Swelling
Regional and distant
  Pain
  Swelling
  Edema
  Organ dysfunction
  Obstruction of flow (air, blood, urine, CSF, bile, stool)
  Compression of nerves
  Weakening or breach of structural integrity (bone, blood vessels, bowel)
Paraneoplastic syndromes (see Chap. 102)
  Metabolic disorders
    Hypercalcemia
    Cachexia
    Fever
    Hyponatremia
  Ectopic hormone production
    ACTH
  Neuropathy and CNS abnormalities (see Chap. 103)
  Dermatologic conditions (see Chap. 57)
  Hematologic abnormalities, including clotting and bleeding
  Immunosuppression or autoimmunity
Psychosocial effects
  Anxiety
  Depression
  Loss of autonomy
  Fear of death and dying
  Fear of pain and altered body image
  Alienation

NOTE: CSF, cerebrospinal fluid; ACTH, adrenocorticotropic hormone; CNS, central nervous system.

postobstructive pneumonia, stridor, dyspnea from intrinsic or extrinsic tumor or a pleural effusion, hemoptysis, and cough. Regional intrathoracic symptoms vary and may include superior vena cava syndrome, diaphragmatic paralysis from phrenic nerve compression, hoarseness from recurrent laryngeal nerve compression by mediastinal nodes, dysphagia from esophageal compression, severe pain radiating down the arm from brachial nerve compression in Pancoast tumors, and pericardial tamponade.

The patient may first come to attention because of a distant tumor metastasis resulting in a seizure from brain or pain from bone or liver involvement. Paraneoplastic syndromes may include hypercalcemia or hypertrophic pulmonary osteoarthropathy in non-small cell lung cancer and Eaton-Lambert syndrome, inappropriate secretion of antidiuretic hormone, and ectopic Cushing's syndrome in small cell tumors. Decreased appetite and weight loss are not uncommon and are probably manifestations of a poorly characterized paraneoplastic syndrome. Among patients presenting with a carcinoma of unknown primary site, lung cancers are one of two tumors most often identified later. Discovery of a lung mass in an asymptomatic patient for whom a chest radiograph is ordered for another reason is not uncommon; these patients usually have a better prognosis.

BREAST CANCER Over the past decade, breast cancer is being diagnosed much earlier in the course of its natural history. The majority of patients now present with stage I disease (no evidence of lymph node involvement) or carcinoma in situ. Thus, a mammographic abnormality detected during a screening examination or a lump in the breast now constitute the most common presentations. → *A detailed discussion of evaluation of breast abnormalities is presented in Chap. 64.*

GASTROINTESTINAL CANCERS Stomach Cancer Few symptoms are associated with early gastric cancer, and most patients are diagnosed only after the disease is more advanced. The epigastric discomfort, anorexia, and minor weight loss that sometimes occur are relatively nonspecific. Unexplained anemia may lead to endoscopic evaluation and a diagnosis, but gastrointestinal bleeding infrequently occurs in more treatable early stage disease. Grave symptoms and signs such as early satiety from a diffusely infiltrating tumor, vomiting from pyloric obstruction, palpation of a left supraclavicular node or a rectal mass (Blumer's shelf), and ovarian metastases usually indicate incurable disease.

Pancreatic Cancer Most patients are incurable at the time of diagnosis. Severe pain radiating to the back, probably due to splanchnic nerve invasion, and weight loss are hallmarks of the disease. Obstructive jaundice, especially when not accompanied by pain and weight loss, is associated with tumors of the pancreatic head, which are more often surgically resectable. Tumors of the body do not cause obstruction and are usually not resectable when diagnosed. Gastric or duodenal obstruction by tumor is associated with disordered intestinal motility, possibly from infiltration of the splanchnic nerves.

Colorectal Cancer Colorectal cancer can be diagnosed in a patient with symptoms or as a result of a screening program with fecal occult blood tests or endoscopic examination. Patients with early, resectable disease are often asymptomatic or have only nonspecific symptoms; individuals shown not to have colorectal neoplasms also sometimes note changes in bowel habits, abdominal pain, and rectal bleeding.

Symptomatic patients with colorectal cancer usually have abdominal pain or nausea and vomiting due to obstruction; bleeding from the tumor, sometimes accompanied by anemia; or chronic or acute bowel perforation. In more advanced disease, hyperbilirubinemia or other biochemical abnormalities from liver metastases may be present.

Right colon tumors are more insidious and less likely to cause obstruction, because the bowel lumen is more ample and the stool more liquid. Malignant obstruction usually occurs in left-sided lesions, where the lumen diameter is smaller and the stool more solid. Rectal tumors more often present with hematochezia and tenesmus.

GYNECOLOGIC CANCERS Ovarian Cancer Some patients with ovarian cancer have nonspecific symptoms of nausea, dyspepsia, or a sensation of swelling or discomfort in the lower abdomen; others have no complaints at all. More striking symptoms, such as abdominal pain, distention or masses, and vaginal bleeding, are usually manifestations of advanced disease. At diagnosis, cancer has spread beyond the ovaries in 75 percent of patients and beyond the pelvis in 60 percent. All perimenopausal or postmenopausal women with pelvic or abdominal symptoms should have a pelvic and general physical examination. An adnexal mass in a postmenopausal woman should usually prompt exploratory laparotomy, since functional ovarian cysts should not occur in nonmenstruating women.

Endometrial Cancer Almost all women with carcinoma of the endometrium develop vaginal bleeding, either a serosanguinous discharge or frank bleeding. In the three-fourths of patients who are postmenopausal, this should be readily detectable. However, only about one-fifth of women with postmenopausal bleeding have endometrial cancer. Pelvic examination and endometrial biopsy should be obtained. Pyometria in a postmenopausal woman should also prompt pelvic examination and endometrial biopsy. Pain, vaginal discharge, weight loss, and urinary or gastrointestinal complaints usually occur only in the setting of more advanced disease.

Cervical Cancer Carcinoma in situ of the uterine cervix can be detected by Pap smear but is not associated with any symptoms. Early invasive cancer can be associated with vaginal discharge or bleeding, especially postcoital spotting. In more aggressive invasive cancer, serosanguinous or purulent vaginal discharge progressively increases. Intermenstrual bleeding becomes more pronounced. Pelvic pain and urinary and rectal symptoms can be associated with tumor necrosis or chronic inflammation. Low back or leg pain may indicate compression of lumbosacral nerves or ureteral obstruction. Urinary frequency or urgency, rectal tenesmus, and bleeding are consequences of direct bladder or rectal invasion.

Pap smears should be obtained during the pelvic examination of any woman but especially those with pelvic symptoms described above. Any visually abnormal findings should be followed up with colposcopy, endocervical curretage, and colposcopically directed cervical biopsies. If this examination reveals a positive endocervical curretage, unsatisfactory colposcopic visualization, or microinvasion or other abnormalities, a diagnostic cone biopsy is performed, which removes a conical portion of the cervix including the entire transformation zone and some of the endocervix.

Table 63-2

Ten Most Common Solid Tumors in Men and Women, 1996

	Men			Women	
Rank	Type	New Cases		Type	New Cases
1.	Prostate	317,100		Breast	184,300
2.	Lung	98,900		Lung	78,100
3.	Colorectal	67,600		Colorectal	65,900
4.	Bladder	38,300		Endometrial	34,000
5.	Oropharyngeal/laryngeal	29,300		Ovary	26,700
6.	Cutaneous melanoma	21,800		Cutaneous melanoma	16,500
7.	Kidney/upper urinary track	18,500		Cervix	15,700
8.	Stomach	14,000		Bladder	14,600
9.	Pancreas	12,400		Pancreas	13,900
10.	Brain/CNS	10,400		Kidney/upper urinary tract	12,100
	Total	628,300		Total	461,800

NOTE: CNS, central nervous system.

SOURCE: After Parker et al, with permission.

GENITOURINARY CANCERS   Renal/Upper Urinary Tract Cancer   The classic triad of pain, hematuria, and a flank mass occurs in fewer than 20 percent of patients with adenocarcinoma of the kidney (hypernephroma). About one-third of patients present with metastatic disease, one-quarter with locally advanced disease, and 45 percent with localized tumor. Systemic manifestations of disease include hypochromic anemia, fever, weight loss, and nonmetastatic abnormalities of liver function; the latter are associated with a poor prognosis but may be reversible if the primary tumor is removed. Up to 5 percent of patients have polycythemia or hypercalcemia.

Transitional cell carcinomas of both the renal pelvis and ureters are associated with cigarette abuse. These tumors are manifestations of a field defect in which patients with larger tumors and carcinoma in situ are at high risk of multifocal recurrences. Hematuria is the presenting symptom in most cases.

Bladder Cancer   Gross or microscopic hematuria, usually painless, is by far the most common presentation in patients with bladder cancer, occurring in approximately 75 percent. Intermittent microscopic hematuria may be the initial manifestation of cancer. Vesical irritation is present in about 30 percent of patients and is associated with carcinoma in situ. In patients with advanced bladder cancer, pelvic pain from an enlarging tumor mass or nerve root compression may be present. Flank pain is a prominent symptom in patients with ureteral obstruction. Lower extremity edema due to lymphatic or venous obstruction can also occur.

Prostate Cancer   Localized prostate cancer is often asymptomatic but can be detected by palpation of one or more nodules on digital rectal examination. Of the more than half of patients who present with locally advanced tumor or distant metastases, symptoms of urinary outlet obstruction or bone pain frequently occur. In the minority who present with more advanced disease, spinal cord compression, weight loss, anemia, and renal failure due to ureteral obstruction are sometimes observed.

More recently, early detection of prostate cancer by screening for elevated levels of prostate-specific antigen (PSA) in the serum has been achieved. Many patients who are diagnosed by this test have no palpable prostatic nodules, and cancer is documented by means of ultrasound-guided or blind biopsies. Such patients more frequently have lower stage disease, with tumors more often pathologically confined to the prostate, than patients whose tumors are detected because of clinical findings. Whether this earlier detection will result in reduced mortality from prostate cancer requires the results of controlled clinical trials of PSA-based screening programs and further follow-up.

CUTANEOUS MELANOMA   Malignant melanomas are deeply pigmented tumors of the skin, which may arise in any part of the body but are more common on women's legs and men's trunks. Variation in color, an irregular border with indentations, an irregular raised surface, and ulcerations on the surface of the lesions are typical features that lead to biopsy and diagnosis. Since melanomas can evolve into a variety of appearances, any pigmented lesion that changes in appearance should be biopsied.

People at greater risk of developing cutaneous melanoma include those with a tendency to severe sunburns, red or blond hair, fair skin, and more than 20 pigmented nevi. Individuals with dysplastic nevi or familial melanoma are at greatly increased risk and should have their entire skin surface examined frequently.

BRAIN TUMORS   Neoplasms of the brain in adults are more often metastases from cancer in other organs than from tumors that originate in the brain itself. The most common primary brain tumors in adults are astrocytomas, which comprise over half of all such tumors and arise from glial or supporting cells. They exhibit heterogeneous clinical behaviors, ranging from indolent growth rates in low-grade gliomas to a markedly aggressive course in glioblastoma multiforme. Headache, usually most prominent upon arising in the morning, is the most common presenting symptom of gliomas and usually results from increased intracranial pressure due to tumor mass. Seizures are the second most common manifestation of primary brain tumors in adults. Numerous symptoms are specific to the portion of the brain in which the tumor arises, for example, homonymous hemianopsia in occipital lobe lesions. Thorough neurologic examination and magnetic resonance imaging of the brain are indicated when a primary brain tumor is suspected.

CANCER'S SEVEN WARNING SIGNS

For many years, the American Cancer Society has publicized a list of seven warning signs of possible cancer to the general public. The presence of any of these signs should prompt examination by a physician.

1. Change in bowel or bladder habits. Development of diarrhea, constipation, difficulty passing the stool, and gray or black stools may indicate jaundice or gastrointestinal bleeding. Blood or pus in the urine, frequent painful urination, and sudden development of nocturia may indicate urinary tract bleeding or prostatic or other obstruction.
2. A sore on the skin that does not heal may indicate a skin cancer.
3. Unusual bleeding or discharge from the nose, mouth, skin, nipple, or vagina, although more often a sign of infection, may also be a manifestation of cancer.
4. A thickening or lump in the breast or elsewhere may be the first indication of a breast cancer or a sarcoma of the soft tissues.
5. Indigestion or difficulty in swallowing, although overwhelmingly due to benign causes such as a hiatal hernia, may be due to a tumor in the esophagus or stomach. If these symptoms persist or worsen, they should be brought to the attention of a physician.
6. Obvious changes in a wart or mole, such as increasing size, change in color, or change in shape, may be a sign of malignant melanoma. Medical attention should be sought.
7. Nagging cough, particularly if associated with expectoration of blood, and hoarseness, which may be due to compression of a nerve innervating the vocal cord, may both be signs of lung cancer, particularly if these symptoms occur in a cigarette smoker.

BIBLIOGRAPHY

BEATTIE EJ: Seven warning signs of cancer: A fuller explanation for patients. Prim Care Cancer September: 45, 1989
CONN RB (ed): *Current Diagnosis*, 8th ed. Philadelphia, Saunders, 1991
DEVITA VT et al (eds): *Cancer: Principles and Practice of Oncology*, 5th ed. Philadelphia, Lippincott, 1997
PARKER SL et al: Cancer statistics, 1996. CA Cancer J Clin 46:5, 1996

64   *Marc E. Lippman*

EVALUATION OF BREAST MASSES IN MEN AND WOMEN

Because the breasts are a common site of fatal disease in women and because they frequently provide clues to underlying systemic disease in both men and women, examination of the breasts is an essential part of the physical examination. Unfortunately, internists frequently do not examine the breasts in men and, in women, they are apt to refer this evaluation to gynecologists. Because of the association between early detection and improved outcome, it is the duty of every physician to distinguish breast abnormalities at the earliest possible stage and to institute a definitive diagnostic workup whenever appropriate. It is for this reason that all women should be trained in self-examination of the breasts. Although breast cancer in men is unusual, unilateral lesions should be evaluated in the same manner as in women, with the recognition that gynecomastia in men can sometimes begin unilaterally and is often asymmetric. Nevertheless, about as many suspicious breast lesions are now detected by screening mammography as by physical examination.

Virtually all breast cancer is diagnosed by biopsy of a nodule detected either on a mammogram or by palpation. A series of algorithms have been developed to enhance the likelihood of diagnosing breast cancer and to reduce the frequency of unnecessary biopsy.

THE PALPABLE BREAST MASS   Women should be strongly encouraged to self-examine the breasts monthly. The minimum benefit of this practice is the greater likelihood of detecting a mass at a smaller size, when it can be treated with limited surgery. Breast examination by the physician should be performed in good light so as to see retractions and other skin changes. The nipple and areolae should be inspected, and an attempt should be made to elicit nipple discharge. All areas where regional lymph nodes are present should be examined, and any lesions should be measured. While lesions with certain features are more likely to be cancerous (hard, irregular, tethered or fixed, or painless lesions), physical examination alone cannot exclude malignancy. Furthermore, a negative mammogram in the presence of a persistent lump in the breast does not exclude malignancy.

In premenopausal women, lesions that are either equivocal or nonsuspicious on physical examination should be reexamined in 2 to 4 weeks, during the the follicular phase of the menstrual cycle. Days 5 to 7 of the cycle are the best time for breast examination. A dominant mass in a postmenopausal woman or a dominant mass that persists through a menstrual cycle in a premenopausal woman should be aspirated by fine needle biopsy or referred to a surgeon. If nonbloody fluid is aspirated and the lesion is thereby cured permanently, then diagnosis, therapy, and reassurance have all been accomplished at once. Solid lesions and persistent, recurrent, complex, or bloody cysts require mammography and biopsy, although in selected patients triple diagnostic techniques can be used to avoid biopsy (Figs. 64-1 to 64-3). Ultrasound can be used in place of fine needle aspiration to distinguish cysts from solid lesions. Not all solid masses are detected by ultrasound, however, so a palpable mass that is not visualized on ultrasound must be presumed to be solid.

Several points are essential in pursuing these management decision trees. First, risk factor analysis is not part of the decision process. Second, fine needle aspiration should be used only in centers that have proven skill in obtaining such specimens *and* analyzing them cytopathologically. Although the likelihood of cancer is low in the setting of a "triple negative" (benign-feeling lump, negative mammo-

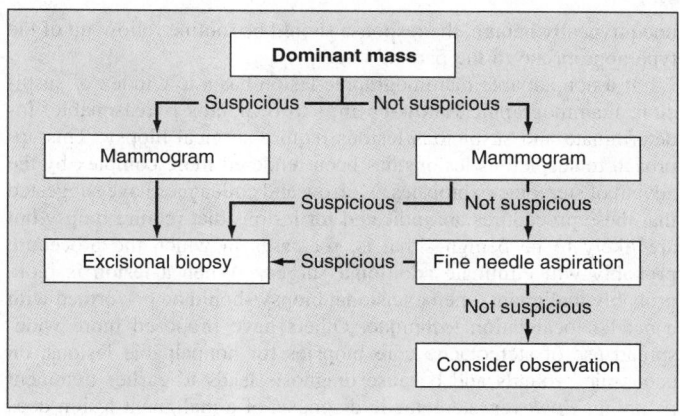

FIGURE 64-2   The "triple diagnosis technique."

gram, and negative fine-needle aspiration), it is not zero, and the patient and physician should be willing to assume about a 1 percent risk of false negativity. Third, additional technologies such as magnetic resonance imaging, ultrasound, and Sestamibi imaging cannot be used to exclude the need for biopsy, although in unusual circumstances they may provoke a biopsy.

THE ABNORMAL MAMMOGRAM   Screening mammography has reduced the lethality of breast cancer by promoting detection at an earlier stage. The procedure is justified on an annual basis for women over age 50, and a meta-analysis suggests a benefit for women over age 40, but this is controversial.

Screening mammography should not be confused with diagnostic mammography which is performed after a palpable abnormality has been detected. Diagnostic mammography generally is aimed at evaluating the rest of the breast before biopsy is performed, or, occasionally, is part of the "triple test" strategy to exclude immediate biopsy.

Subtle abnormalities that are first detected by screening mammography should be evaluated carefully almost invariably by compression or magnified views. These abnormalities include clustered microcalcifications, densities (especially if spiculated), and new or enlarging architectural distortion. For some nonpalpable lesions, ultrasound may be helpful either to identify cysts or to guide biopsy. In general, the management of patients with findings of this type is straightforward. If there is no palpable lesion and detailed mammographic studies are

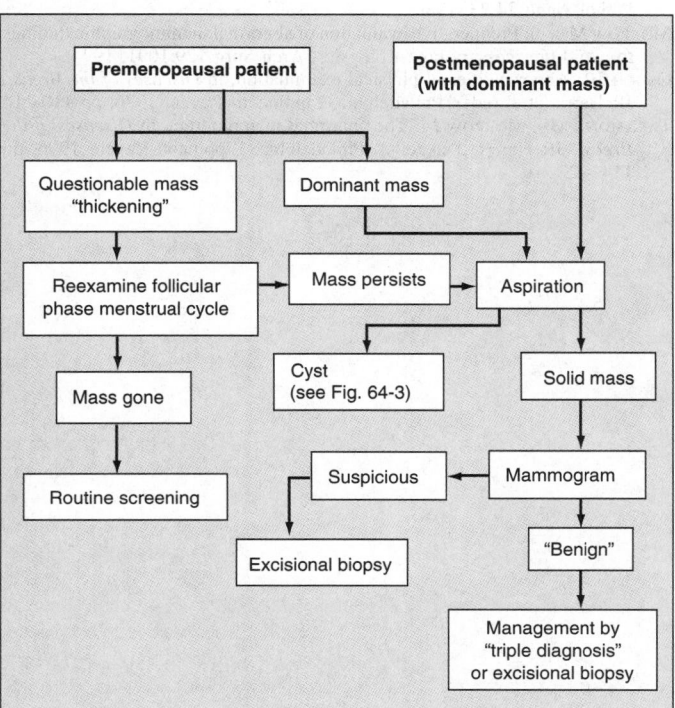

FIGURE 64-1   Approach to a palpable breast mass.

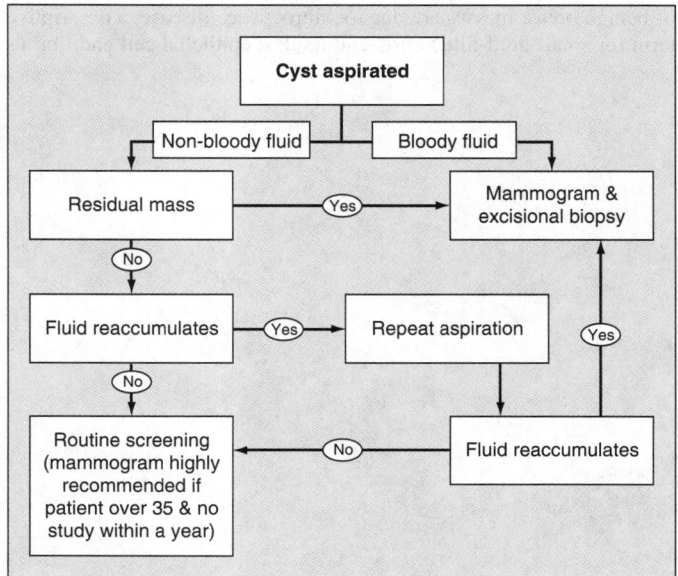

FIGURE 64-3   Management of a breast cyst.

unequivocally benign, the response should be routine follow-up of the type appropriate to the patient's age.

If a nonpalpable mammographic lesion has a low index of suspicion, mammographic follow-up in 3 to 6 months is reasonable. Indeterminate and suspicious lesions require surgical biopsy. This approach to suspicious lesions has been rendered more complex by the advent of stereotactic biopsies. Morrow and colleagues have suggested that these procedures are indicated for lesions that require biopsy but are likely to be benign—that is, for cases in which the procedure probably will eliminate additional surgery. When a lesion is more probably malignant, open excisional biopsy should be performed with a needle localization technique. Others have proposed more widespread use of stereotactic core biopsies for nonpalpable lesions, on economic grounds and because diagnosis leads to earlier treatment planning. However, stereotactic diagnosis of a malignant lesion does not eliminate the need for definitive surgical procedures, particularly if breast conservation is attempted. For example, after a breast biopsy with needle localization (i.e., local excision) of a stereotactically diagnosed malignancy, reexcision may still be necessary to remove the cancer with negative margins. To some extent, these issues are decided on the basis of referral pattern and the availability of the resources for stereotactic core biopsies. A reasonable approach is shown in Fig. 64-4.

Careful attention to these guidelines will greatly reduce the chance of failing to diagnose breast cancer.

BREAST MASSES IN THE PREGNANT OR LACTATING WOMAN During pregnancy, the breast grows under the influence of estrogen, progesterone, prolactin, and human placental lactogen. Lactation is suppressed by estrogen and progesterone, which block the effects of prolactin. After delivery, lactation is promoted by the fall in estrogen and progesterone levels, which leaves the effects of prolactin unopposed. The development of a dominant mass during pregnancy or lactation should never be attributed to the hormonal changes, and biopsy should be performed under local anesthesia. Breast cancer develops in one in every 3000 to 4000 pregnancies. Stage for stage, breast cancer in pregnant patients is no different from premenopausal breast cancer in nonpregnant patients. However, pregnant women often have more advanced disease because a breast mass was ignored.

BENIGN BREAST MASSES Only about one in every 5 to 10 patients who undergo a biopsy has a diagnosis of cancer, although the rate of positive biopsies varies in different countries. (These differences may be related to interpretation of mammograms.) The vast majority of benign breast masses are due to "fibrocystic" disease, a descriptive term for small fluid-filled cysts and modest epithelial cell and fibrous

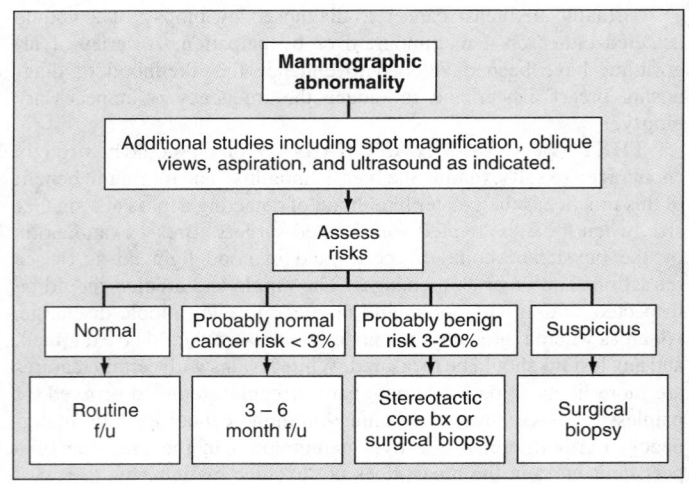

FIGURE 64-4   Approaches to abnormalities detected by mammogram.

tissue hyperplasia. However, fibrocystic disease is a histologic, not a clinical diagnosis, and women who have had a biopsy with benign findings are at a greater risk of developing breast cancer than those who have not had a biopsy. Indeed, the subset of women with ductal or lobular cell proliferation (about 30 percent of patients), particularly the small fraction (3 percent) with atypical hyperplasia, have a fourfold greater risk of developing breast cancer than unbiopsied women, and the increase in risk is about ninefold for women in this category who also have an affected first-degree relative. Thus, careful follow-up of these patients is required. By contrast, patients with a benign biopsy without atypical hyperplasia are at little risk and may be followed routinely.

→*The approach to the patient presenting with a nipple discharge or mastalgia is discussed in Chap. 338.*

BIBLIOGRAPHY

DONEGAN WL: Evaluation of a palpable breast mass. N Engl J Med 327:937, 1992

KERLIKOWSKE K et al: Efficacy of screening mammography. A meta-analysis. JAMA 273:149, 1995

LAYFIELD LJ et al: Fine needle aspiration in the management of breast masses. Pathol Annu 24:23, 1989

MORROW M et al: Preoperative evaluation of abnormal mammographic findings to avoid unnecessary breast biopsies. Arch Surg 129:1091, 1994

OSUCH JR: Abnormalities in physical examination, in *Diseases of the Breast*, JR Harris et al (eds). Philadelphia, Lippincott–Raven, 1996, pp 110-114

TALAMONT MS, MORROW M: The abnormal mammogram, in *Diseases of the Breast*, JR Harris et al (eds). Philadelphia, Lippincott-Raven, 1996, pp 114–122

65 Arthur L. Beaudet

GENETICS AND DISEASE

GENOMIC MEDICINE

Genomic medicine can be defined as the use of genotypic analysis (DNA testing) to enhance the quality of medical care, including presymptomatic identification of predisposition to disease, preventive intervention, selection of pharmacotherapy, and individual design of medical care based on genotype. The progress of the human genome project and research in molecular medicine have made genomic medicine an important strategy. Genotype can be deduced by analysis of protein (e.g., hemoglobin or α_1-antitrypsin), RNA, or DNA, but analysis of DNA is the usual method. It can be argued that there are no new principles or concepts involved in genomic medicine but that it will change the way medicine is practiced, particularly in regard to intervention for common diseases. Testing for predisposition to disease does have the potential for harm because it opens the possibility of various forms of discrimination, but it also has the potential of extraordinary benefits. Primary care physicians are in a pivotal position to provide the benefits and minimize the harm. Genotypic analysis is standard practice for diseases in which a single gene plays a prominent role, but the role of genetic testing in complex disease traits—where multiple genes and nongenetic factors are implicated—is less established. Nevertheless, genomic medicine has the potential of reducing the burden of these disorders. Genotypic information has two broad applications: first, to modify the medical care provided to the individual; and second, to make possible reproductive counseling to couples who wish to have children. It is important to distinguish those genotypic results that provide potential for benefit and/or intervention (e.g., hemochromatosis) as compared to those situations where no clear intervention is available (e.g., Alzheimer's or Huntington's disease), but most disorders fall in an intermediate category where opportunity for treatment or prevention is significant but limited.

The concept that it is good medical practice to screen the population to identify individuals with risks and to intervene to prevent disease processes in such persons is well established. For example, blood pressure and cholesterol are measured for screening purposes to identify individuals who are asymptomatic but have a predisposition to cardiovascular disease, and attempts are made to intervene in such individuals through pharmacology and changes in lifestyle. Although treatment is not always effective, there is frequent benefit to individuals and to society. Likewise, in perinatal medicine, population-based screening is used to identify individuals with particular genotypes who can benefit from prompt intervention, as exemplified by phenylketonuria. The rationales for routine mammography, screening for blood in the stool, measurement of prostate-specific antigen, and glaucoma screening are based on similar principles that early diagnosis can lead to beneficial intervention. Although some of these procedures test for disease rather than for predisposition to disease, all such strategies are based on the concept that early intervention can provide a medical benefit. The boundary between predisposition to disease and presymptomatic disease is not a clear one. Is hypertension a disease or a predisposition to a symptomatic event such as a stroke? Is a mutation in the breast and ovarian cancer gene BRCA1 a predisposition to breast cancer or an early phase of the disease process? As with any medical strategy, intervention based on genotypic information is valid only if the benefit to the individual outweighs the potential harm of genotypic analysis (see "Discrimination and Ethical Concerns," below). An example in which opportunities for genomic medicine have

been largely unutilized is population-based screening to identify individuals with predisposition to emphysema because of α_1-antitrypsin deficiency; such individuals can be identified by analysis of protein or DNA and should be counseled regarding the certainty of injury from smoking. The application and follow-up of widespread screening of this type may require major reorganization of medical care and its financing.

Recombinant DNA methods, the polymerase chain reaction (PCR), the human genome project, new technologies for analyzing DNA, and research in molecular medicine make it possible to obtain large amounts of genotypic information at very low cost using current and developing technologies but does not provide insight into which genotypic information can be used in a beneficial manner. As DNA information becomes routine, it should be incorporated into medical practice and into the medical record in the same way that blood pressure, cholesterol, and hemoglobin measurements are currently utilized. Proposals that DNA information be treated differently than other aspects of medical information reflect an exaggerated view of the predictive power of most DNA information. Indeed, many relatively public pieces of information such as obesity, alcohol intake, smoking, past medical conditions, and parental health history are likely to have greater predictive implications than most DNA analyses.

SINGLE-GENE DISORDERS   Genotypic analysis is available for the diagnosis, counseling, and management of many so-called single-gene disorders in which one gene plays a predominant role in determining disease. The relevant genes have been cloned, and mutations have been identified for most common genetic disorders, including neurofibromatosis, Marfan's syndrome, familial hypercholesterolemia, osteogenesis imperfecta, myotonic dystrophy, achondroplasia, familial polyposis of the colon, Huntington's disease, adult polycystic kidney disease, cystic fibrosis, and globin disorders. For these disorders, genotypic analysis can confirm the diagnosis, determine the status of relatives at risk, sometimes predict severity, provide the option of presymptomatic diagnosis, and provide the basis for genetic counseling. An excellent example of the benefits of genotypic analysis is in multiple endocrine neoplasia type 2, where mutation analysis can eliminate the need for burdensome, expensive, and imprecise endocrine screening for large numbers of family members not carrying the mutation and makes possible improved preventive and therapeutic strategies for individuals found to have the mutant gene. Similar benefits attributable to precise diagnosis are now available for many genetic disorders. Single-gene mutations also can influence pharmacogenetic susceptibilities where administration of a particular drug may result in catastrophic side effects among a subgroup of patients with a susceptible genotype. Examples include glucose-6-phosphate dehydrogenase deficiency, suxamethonium sensitivity, malignant hyperthermia, 5-fluorouracil sensitivity, 6-mercaptopurine sensitivity, and others (see "Pharmacogenetics," below).

COMPLEX DISEASE TRAITS AND HETEROGENEITY   In complex disease traits, also known as multifactorial diseases, multiple genes and nongenetic factors interact to contribute to the presence or absence of disease in a single individual. One example of a complex disease trait is type 1, or insulin-dependent, diabetes mellitus where familial clustering is believed to involve at least 10 genes, including the HLA region and the insulin gene. No one gene appears to contribute the major effect for type 1 diabetes. The situation where single genes have a predominant effect but in which the gene involved can vary from family to family is termed *genetic heterogeneity*. Examples of genetic heterogeneity include maturity onset diabetes of youth (MODY), where the causative gene may be the glucokinase gene or genes mapped to other chromosomes; hereditary breast cancer, which can be due to mutations in the BRCA1 gene on chromosome 17 or the BRCA2 gene on chromosome 13; and colon cancer, which can be caused by mutations in the gene for hereditary polyposis of the colon on chromosome 5 or by mutations in other genes that cause hereditary nonpolyposis colon cancer. Coronary artery disease (and perhaps most other common adult disorders) may involve either complex disease traits or genetic heterogeneity. Some individuals may have early onset coronary artery disease primarily due to mutations at a single locus, as for familial hypercholesterolemia or apolipoprotein E abnormalities, while most instances are thought to be due to interactions of nongenetic factors (e.g., smoking and diet) with variations in multiple genes, including apolipoprotein (a), apolipoprotein B, other apolipoproteins, lipoprotein receptors, lipoprotein lipase, angiotensin-converting enzyme, genes affecting homocysteine levels, genes affecting the clotting system, leukocyte and endothelial cell adhesion genes, and many others. Even when a single gene has a predominant effect, as in heterozygous familial hypercholesterolemia, other genes have secondary or modifier effects. The fact that there may be both major and minor effects in an individual disorder blurs the boundary between the concepts of complex disease traits and genetic heterogeneity.

Genetic heterogeneity is well documented for hypertension, with major single-gene effects involving the β or γ subunit of the renal amiloride-sensitive sodium channel, the enzyme 11β-hydroxysteroid dehydrogenase, dysregulated fusion genes (aldosterone synthase/11β-hydroxylase) leading to aldosterone synthesis under the control of ACTH, the renal thiazide-sensitive Na-Cl cotransporter, and many other loci. These disorders demonstrate dominant effects in some cases and recessive in others, considerable variation in findings even within a single family, and the need for different therapeutic intervention based on the specific defect. The extensive discoveries in the genetic basis of hypertension are shrinking the concept of "essential hypertension" and illustrate the potential for the practice of genomic medicine.

DISCRIMINATION AND ETHICAL CONCERNS There are widespread fears that discrimination in regard to employment, health care, and insurance underwriting will be based on the results of genetic testing. Such concerns are analogous to those related to other medical information including hypertension, hypercholesterolemia, family history of a specific genetic disorder such as Huntington's disease, or strong family history of breast cancer or coronary artery disease. It is imperative that individuals not be discriminated against based on genotype, and it is a challenge for society and for the medical profession to procure the benefits of genomic medicine and to prevent discrimination. Societal, governmental, and legal steps should be taken as needed to prohibit such discrimination (particularly based on genotype or predisposition) in the case of employment and health care. Many societies guarantee universal access to health care, and it is possible that genetic testing may increase the impetus in the United States for universal access to health care at standardized costs. The issues involved in this problem are complex, are not unique to genetics, and will continue to be debated. Anonymous genetic testing has been suggested as one option if individuals wish to obtain predictive information and minimize the risk of breach of confidentiality (e.g., anonymous testing for Huntington's disease or cancer susceptibility). Anonymous testing creates difficulties in assuring that individuals with burdensome results will be provided with proper interpretation, supportive counseling, and medical care, but there are some parallels to the experience with anonymous testing for human immunodeficiency virus.

MOLECULAR BASIS OF GENE EXPRESSION

The human genome is estimated to contain 50,000 to 100,000 genes, each of which is composed of a linear polymer of DNA. The genes are assembled into lengthy linear strands that, together with the proteins of chromatin, form the *chromosomes*. All normal nucleated human cells other than sperm or ova contain 46 chromosomes, arrayed in 23 pairs, one of each pair derived from each of the individual's parents.

The discovery that genes are not contiguous sequences of DNA but consist of coding sequences (exons) interrupted by intervening sequences (introns) led to a more complex view of gene expression.

Some approximations regarding the magnitude and organization of the human genome are presented in Fig. 65-1. The estimated 50,000 to 100,000 genes are encoded within the 3 billion base pairs (bp) of DNA that comprise a haploid genome. DNA length is ordinarily quantitated in kilobase (kb) units of 1000 bp or megabase (Mb) units of 1 million bp. Linkage studies indicate that the human genome is composed of approximately 3000 centimorgans (cM) in recombination distance. A centimorgan (1/100 of a Morgan) is a measure of genetic distance that reflects the probability of a crossover between two loci during meiosis. One centimorgan approximates a 1 percent chance of a crossover during meiosis. Thus, an average chromosome contains 2000 to 5000 genes within 130 million bp of DNA and is equivalent to about 130 cM of genetic material. A typical microband on a chromosome (stained at the 800 band level of resolution) should contain 3 to 5 million bp and 60 to 120 genes. This formulation oversimplifies many issues. Estimates of the total number of genes are imprecise, and although the average recombination distance is approximately 1 cM per million bp of DNA, there is wide variation in this rate over shorter distances and differences in recombination distance with sex. Genes range in size from small (1.5 kb for a globin gene) to large (about 2000 kb for the Duchenne muscular dystrophy locus). *Cis*-acting regulatory elements (i.e., on the contiguous DNA strand) may be a considerable distance from the coding region, e.g., 50 kb 5′ and 20 kb 3′ to the β-globin gene, thus extending the functional domains of genes and complicating the definition of boundaries. The human genome also contains numerous highly reiterated sequences of unknown function.

If one were to print *one copy* of *one strand* of the haploid human genome, it would fill a text 170 times the size of *Harrison's*. The analogy of the human genome to a large text can be carried further. The text can be envisioned as being bound into 23 separate volumes of various sizes, each the equivalent of one chromosome. Individuals would inherit one paternal set of 23 volumes and one maternal set of 23 volumes. The mutation that causes sickle cell anemia would be the equivalent of changing a single letter on one page of one volume

FIGURE 65-1 Perspectives on the amount of DNA, number of genes, and genetic distance in the human genome. The arrows in the lowest panel indicate hypothetical transcripts, with vertical lines indicating exons within genes. (*From Scriver et al, with permission.*)

from each of the sets, while deletion of the α-globin gene cluster in α-thalassemia would be equivalent to the loss of one or two pages of text in each set. This text can also be envisioned as having been copied over and over again for thousands of generations, with multiple errors or alterations (mutations) being introduced and passed to the progeny copies. Finally, to carry this analogy to the concept of crossing-over and linkage, each volume of each set can exchange parts with its corresponding partner at one to six sites per volume, so that a unique 23-volume text comprising mixed portions of the two available sets is passed to the next generation. This results in the unique genotype that is the basis of our genetic individuality.

THE MOLECULAR FLOW OF INFORMATION Much is known about how living organisms store, transmit, and utilize genetic information. Two excellent textbooks by Alberts et al. and by Darnell et al. provide a more systematic and comprehensive treatment of cellular and molecular biology, and the texts by Watson et al., 1987, and by Lewin provide a detailed view of molecular genetics.

The genetic information carried on chromosomes is transmitted to daughter cells under two different sets of circumstances. *Mitosis* occurs each time a somatic cell (i.e., a nongerm cell) divides and functions to transmit two identical copies of each gene to each daughter cell, thus maintaining a uniform genetic composition in all cells of a single organism. The other set of circumstances, *meiosis*, prevails when genetic information is to be transmitted from one individual to an offspring. In meiosis, the 46 chromosomes of an immature germ cell arrange themselves in 23 pairs at the center of the nucleus, each pair being composed of one chromosome derived from the mother and its homologous chromosome derived from the father. During the meiotic process, the two partner chromosomes separate, only one of each pair going into each gamete. Thus, meiosis reduces the number of chromosomes from 46 to 23, each gamete receiving one chromosome from each of the 23 pairs. The assortment of each pair of chromosomes is random, so that each gamete receives a different combination of maternal and paternal chromosomes. Fusion at fertilization of ovum and sperm cell, each of which has 23 chromosomes, produces an individual with 46 chromosomes.

The independent assortment of chromosomes into gametes during meiosis produces an enormous diversity among the possible genotypes of the progeny. For each 23 pairs of chromosomes, there are 2^{23} different combinations of chromosomes that could occur in a gamete, and the likelihood that one set of parents will produce two offspring with the identical complement of chromosomes is one in 2^{23} or one in 8.4 million (excepting monozygotic twins). Adding even further to the enormous genetic diversity in humans is the phenomenon of *genetic recombination* (see "The Genetic Map and the Principle of Genetic Linkage," below).

THE STRUCTURE OF DNA Most organisms store their genetic information in *deoxyribonucleic acid* (DNA). DNA is a linear polymer of four different monomeric units, collectively called *deoxyribonucleotides* or simply *nucleotides*, that are linked together in a chain by phosphodiester bonds. A typical DNA molecule consists of two interwound polynucleotide chains, each containing many thousand to several million bp. Each nucleotide in one chain is specifically linked by hydrogen bonds to a nucleotide in the other chain. Only two nucleotide pairings are found in DNA: deoxyadenosine monophosphate with thymidine monophosphate (A-T pairs) and deoxyguanosine monophosphate with deoxycytidine monophosphate (G-C pairs). Thus, the sequence of nucleotides of one chain fixes the sequence of the other, and the two chains are therefore said to be *complementary* to each other.

The sequence of the four nucleotides along a polynucleotide chain varies among the DNAs of unrelated organisms and indeed is the molecular basis of their genetic diversity. Because most genetic characteristics are stably transmitted from parent to progeny, the sequence of nucleotides in DNA must be faithfully copied or replicated as the organism reproduces itself. This occurs by unwinding of the two chains and polymerization of two daughter chains along the separated parental strands. The nucleotide sequence and the genetic information are conserved during this process because each nucleotide in the daughter

chains is paired specifically with its complement in the parental or template chains before polymerization occurs.

The actual replication process is mechanically complex but conceptually simple. The two strands of DNA separate, and each is copied by a series of enzymes that inserts a complementary base opposite each base on the original strand of DNA. Thus, two identical double helices are generated from one.

THE GENETIC CODE The sequence of bases in a gene ultimately dictates the sequence of amino acids in a specific protein (Fig. 65-2). This colinearity between the DNA molecule and the protein sequence is achieved by means of the *genetic code*. The four types of bases in DNA are arranged in groups of three, each triplet forming a code word, or *codon*, that ultimately signifies a single amino acid. Triplet codons exist for each of the 20 amino acids that occur in proteins (Fig. 65-3); there are slight differences in the genetic code in mitochondria. Since 64 different triplets can be generated from the four bases and only 20 amino acids exist, the genetic code is said to be *degenerate*. That is, most amino acids are specified by more than one codon, each of which is completely specific. Thus, the double-stranded sequence adenine-adenine-adenine (or AAA) in the antisense [complementary to messenger RNA (mRNA)] strand and thymine-thymine-thymine (or TTT) in the sense (same sequence as mRNA) strand of DNA code for uridine-uridine-uridine (or UUU) in mRNA, which is translated to phenylalanine in protein (Fig. 65-2).

DNA → RNA → PROTEIN To translate its genetic information into a protein, a segment of DNA is first transcribed into mRNA. The mRNA contains a sequence of purine and pyrimidine bases that is complementary to the bases of the antisense strand of the DNA. By this mechanism each adenine of DNA becomes a uridine of RNA, each cytosine of DNA becomes a guanine of RNA, each thymine of DNA becomes an adenine of RNA, and each guanine of DNA becomes a cytosine of RNA. Thus, each DNA triplet codon is translated into a corresponding RNA triplet codon.

The mRNA for each gene is processed extensively within the cell nucleus including splicing to remove intronic sequences. It then crosses the nuclear membrane and enters the cytoplasm, where it serves as a template for the synthesis of a specific protein. To translate the mRNA

FIGURE 65-2 Prototypical eukaryotic gene. In schematic form, a cellular gene is depicted in which exons or coding regions (boxes) are separated by intervening sequences (introns). Introns begin with a dinucleotide GT and end with AG. A short motif of AATAA (or modified versions) direct endonucleolytic cleavage and polyadenylation of nascent RNAs. Promoter elements, shown as empty parentheses, lie upstream from the start of the gene and are often multiple in nature. Common promoter elements include motifs such as TATA and CCAAT (TATA and CAT boxes) GGCGGG (the Spl nuclear factor binding site). Additional sequences, known as enhancers, augment transcription and can lie either before, within, or downstream from the gene. After transcription, the RNA is processed to yield mature mRNA, which is translated to yield protein. (*From Scriver et al, with permission.*)

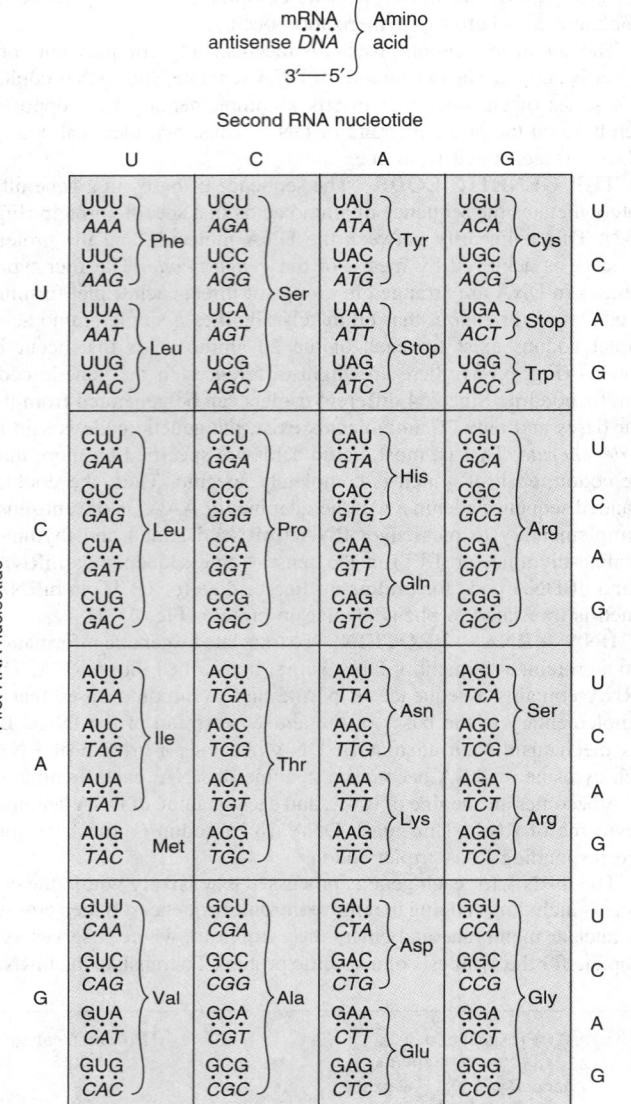

5′—— 3′
mRNA } Amino
antisense *DNA* } acid
3′—— 5′

Second RNA nucleotide

FIGURE 65-3 The genetic code. The RNA codons appear in boldface type; the complementary DNA codons are in italics. A, adenine; C, cystosine; G, guanine; T, thymine; U, uridine (replaces thymine in RNA). In RNA, adenine is complementary to thymine of DNA; uridine is complementary to adenine of DNA; cytosine is complementary to guanine and vice versa. "Stop" is punctuation. The three-letter and single-letter abbreviations for the amino acids are as follows: Ala (A), alanine; Arg (R), arginine; Asn (N), asparagine; Asp (D), aspartic acid; Cys (C), cysteine; Gln (Q), glutamine; Glu (E), glutamic acid; Gly (G), glycine; His (H), histidine; Ile (I), isoleucine; Leu (L), leucine; Lys (K), lysine; Met (M), methionine; Phe (F), phenylalanine; Pro (P), proline; Ser (S), serine; Thr (T), threonine; Trp (W), tryptophan; Tyr (Y), tyrosine; Val (V), valine. *(From Scriver et al, with permission.)*

code into a protein, the mRNA binds to a complex structure called a *ribosome*, which is composed of a different type of RNA [ribosomal RNA (rRNA)] and a large number of proteins. In order to be inserted into its proper place in the protein sequence, each of the 20 amino acids is attached in the cytoplasm to an additional type of RNA [transfer RNA (tRNA)]. Each tRNA contains an anticodon loop, which includes a sequence of three bases that is complementary to a specific codon in the corresponding mRNA. For example, phenylalanine is attached to a tRNA whose anticodon loop contains the sequence AAA, which is complementary to the mRNA codon UUU, which codes for phenylalanine.

Under the influence of cytoplasmic factors (initiation, elongation, and termination factors), peptide bonds are formed between the various amino acids that are aligned along the mRNA. Eventually, a terminator codon is reached, and the completed polypeptide is released from the ribosome. Since the primary sequence of bases in the coding regions of the DNA determines the sequence of amino acids in the protein, the gene and its protein are said to be *colinear*. This means that any alteration of the sequence of bases in the gene causes an alteration of the protein at a specific point in its sequence.

CONTROL OF GENE EXPRESSION The control of gene expression at a transcriptional level is complex. *Cis*-acting regulatory DNA sequences are part of the same duplex DNA molecule as the coding sequence, and *trans*-acting factors (usually proteins) are encoded by other genes. The *trans*-acting factors interact with the *cis* sequences to control the process of transcription. Many *cis*-acting transcriptional control elements are short distances upstream from the initiation site for transcription, but some occur at great distances (e.g., 5 to 50 kb) upstream and downstream from the initiation site for transcription.

The first described family of transcription factors was the helix-turn-helix proteins, and the homeodomain proteins contain a type of helix-turn-helix motif. Complex clusters of homeotic genes have been characterized in mouse and human; a number of these genes have been mutated in the mouse using gene-targeting methodology and an increasing number of human mutations are known. Another group of transcription factors contains "zinc finger" motifs such as the steroid receptors. Other families of transcription factors include proteins with "leucine zipper" motifs or helix-loop-helix motifs. Leucine zippers are characterized by heptad repeats of leucines, which promote dimer formation. The leucine zipper proteins can form various heterodimers that can activate or repress transcription. The helix-loop-helix proteins also appear to form dimers that can have positive or negative regulatory effects.

Regulation of gene expression also occurs at a posttranscriptional level, including regulation of export of mRNA from nucleus to cytoplasm, alternative splicing of transcripts, polyadenylation of transcripts, translation of mRNA, and stabilization of mRNA. There are numerous examples where gene function is regulated through alternative splicing, including control of immunoglobulin secretion, production of calcitonin or calcitonin gene–related peptide, and modulation of the structure and function of troponin-T.

MUTATION AS THE ORIGIN OF NORMAL VARIATION AND GENETIC DISEASE

Mutation was traditionally defined as a stable, heritable change in DNA, a definition that does not depend on the functional significance of the change. This definition implies a change in primary nucleotide sequence, and other changes such as those involving methylation are usually referred to as *epigenetic events*. Mutations in somatic cells may be relevant to cancer or aging and otherwise may be of less phenotypic significance. Mutations in germ cells have their impact on offspring of an individual. The concept that mutations are stable changes remains generally true, but the discovery of expanding triplet repeat mutations emphasizes that some mutations can be unstable either in somatic or in germ cells. Some mutations are genetically lethal and cannot be passed from one generation to the next, while others are less deleterious and are tolerated in the descendants. From the viewpoint of evolution, mutations provide sufficient genetic diversity to permit species to adapt to environmental changes through the mechanism of natural selection.

Mutations are quite diverse (Table 65-1) and can involve gross alterations (millions of base pairs) in the structure of a chromosome; these include duplications, deletions, and translocations of a portion of one chromosome to another (see Chap. 66). Mutations can even involve the entire genome (3 billion bp) as in triploidy, where there is a third copy of the whole chromosome constitution. On the other hand, mutations can be minute, involving deletion, insertion, or replacement of a single base. Single-base or very small mutations are

Table 65-1

CHAPTER 65
Genetics and Disease

369

Common Mechanisms of Mutation

Type	Usual Effect	Examples
LARGE MUTATION		
Deletions	Null*	Duchenne's dystrophy
Insertions	Null	Contiguous gene Hemophilia A/LINE repeat
Duplications	Null, gene disrupted	Duchenne's dystrophy
	Dosage, gene intact	Charcot-Marie-Tooth
Inversions	Null	Hemophilia A
Expanding triplet	Null	Fragile X
	?Gain of function	Huntington's disease
POINT MUTATION		
Silent (in or out of coding)	None	Cystic fibrosis
Missense or in-frame deletion	Null, hypomorphic, altered function, gain of function, benign	Globin Cystic fibrosis
Nonsense	Null	Cystic fibrosis
Frameshift	Null	Cystic fibrosis
Splicing (ag/gt)†	Null	Globin
Splicing (outside ag/gt)†	Hypomorphic	Globin
Regulatory (TATA, other)	Hypomorphic	Globin
Regulatory (poly A site)	Hypomorphic	Globin

* "Null" indicates no functional gene product.

† "ag/gt" indicates mutations in the almost absolutely canonical first two and last two base pairs of each intron, while "outside ag/gt" indicates splicing mutations in less canonical sequences of introns or exons.

called *point mutations.* If deletions or insertions of one or two bases occur in a coding region, they give rise to *frameshift mutations*, because they alter the reading frame of the triplet genetic code in the mRNA so that every codon distal to the mutation in the same gene is read in the wrong frame. Frameshift mutations alter the protein sequence and usually result in premature termination of the peptide chain because of the occurrence of a termination codon in the altered reading frame. Small deletions or insertions can also affect transcription, splicing, or RNA processing depending on their location.

When one base is replaced by another in the coding region, the point mutations may be of three types: (1) a *synonymous* or *silent mutation* (comprising about 23 percent of random base substitutions in coding regions), in which the base replacement does not lead to a change in the amino acid but only to the substitution of a different codon for the same amino acid (e.g., a replacement of a single base pair in the DNA so that a RNA codon for phenylalanine will be

transcribed into RNA not as UUU but as UUC, which still codes for phenylalanine); (2) a *missense mutation* (about 73 percent of base substitutions in coding regions), in which the base replacement changes the codon for one amino acid to another (e.g., the replacement of a base pair in DNA in the codon for phenylalanine such that it will be transcribed into RNA not as UUU but as UUA, which would change the codon to leucine); and (3) a *nonsense mutation* (about 4 percent of base substitutions in coding regions), in which the base replacement changes the codon to one of the termination codons (e.g., the replacement of a base pair in the codon for tyrosine such that it is transcribed into RNA not as UAU but as the stop codon UAA). Occasionally a base substitution in the coding region will alter RNA splicing either by creating a cryptic splice site or by interfering with function of a normal splice site. For missense mutations, the single letter amino acid code is often used to indicate substitutions, such that R560T indicates replacement of arginine (R) at position 560 in the protein by threonine (T).

Larger deletions may affect a portion of a gene, an entire gene, or a set of contiguous genes. Contiguous gene syndromes are discussed in Scriver et al. Such deletion mutations may interrupt or remove the coding region of a gene, causing the absence of its protein product. Alternatively, a deletion can bridge between the coding regions of two genes and produce a fusion, resulting in the production of a hybrid protein containing the initial sequence of one protein followed by the terminal sequence of another protein. This latter type of mutation may occur particularly by unequal crossing over between tandemly repeated homologous genes such as the globin genes. The range of mutations seen at the human β-globin locus provides a good perspective on the heterogeneity of possible mutations. More than 200 missense mutations cause amino acid substitutions in the β-globin locus, and various δβ and βδ fusions can occur. Numerous transcriptional, splicing, and RNA processing mutations cause β-thalassemia as depicted in Fig. 65-4. The reciprocal products of deletions caused by unequal crossover are duplications, and such duplications are the most common form of mutation causing type IA Charcot-Marie-Tooth disease. Insertions in genomic DNA also occur by retrotransposition as exemplified by the appearance of a repeat sequence in the factor VIII gene as a cause of hemophilia A. Inversion affecting the factor VIII gene is a common cause of severe hemophilia A.

Expanding triplet repeat mutations are known to cause fragile X mental retardation, myotonic dystrophy, spinobulbar muscular atrophy, Huntington's disease, spinocerebellar ataxia type I, and other disorders. These triplet repeat sequences can occur in the 5' untranslated, coding, intronic, or 3' untranslated regions. Longer repeat sequences are generally associated with a more severe and/or earlier onset phenotype, and repeat sequences slightly longer than normal

FIGURE 65-4 Point mutations in β thalassemia. The β-globin gene is shown with numbered hatched areas representing the coding regions of exons. Boxed open areas between the exons are introns, and boxed open areas at the 5' and 3' ends of the gene are untranslated regions that appear in the messenger RNA. The various types of mutations are depicted by different symbols. *(From HH Kazazian, Jr., CD Boehm, Blood 72:1107, 1988, with permission.)*

may function as premutations in asymptomatic individuals. The premutant and mutant expanded triplet repeats are unstable and may become more unstable when transmitted from females, as in the case of fragile X syndrome and myotonic dystrophy, or when transmitted from males as in Huntington's disease and spinocerebellar ataxia. For many of the neurodegenerative disorders (Huntington's disease, spinobulbar muscular atrophy, and spinocerebellar ataxia type I, and others), the expanded triplet repeat encodes a polyglutamine tract in the protein, but the mechanism by which this repeat causes neurodegeneration is not known. Expanding triplet repeat mutations are one mechanism underlying the phenomenon of *anticipation*, in which the phenotype of a disease may worsen over successive generations within a family.

The type and frequency of human mutations are complex topics (see Scriver et al.). Mutations that cause chromosomal aneuploidy occur at increasing frequency with advancing age of the mother. Some classes of mutations occur with increased frequency with advancing age of the father. Some loci such as those for Duchenne's muscular dystrophy and achondroplasia are subject to high rates of new mutation. In Duchenne's muscular dystrophy, this may be related in part to the unusually large size of the gene. The structure of a gene, its position within the genome, and the constraints on the gene product may contribute to the frequency of new mutations. The occurrence of 5-methylcytosine at the sites of CG base pairs provides sites of increased mutational frequency due to spontaneous deamination of 5-methylcytosine to yield a thymine base. This propensity leads to increased frequency of polymorphisms at CG sites in the genome and accounts for certain mutational hot spots; in achondroplasia one specific C-to-T base change is remarkably frequent, but similar alterations also occur for hemophilia A and B and many other disorders. The availability of recombinant DNA techniques makes possible the definition of the exact nature of mutations, determination of whether they arose from a maternal or paternal gamete, and analysis of whether the mutation is of recent or ancient origin. Mutations that are widespread in the population but are descended from a single event can be recognized by the occurrence of specific haplotypes of DNA polymorphisms surrounding the mutations; this has been well studied for thalassemia, phenylketonuria, and cystic fibrosis. A *haplotype* is a group of genetic markers linked together on a single chromosome, such as a group of close DNA polymorphisms or a group of human leukocyte antigen (HLA) alleles.

When mutations occur in germ cells, the altered expression of the mutant gene does not affect the phenotype of the individual in whom the mutation occurs but is manifest in subsequent generations. Usually such *new mutations* are sporadic events in human populations, but a mutation that occurs in somatic cells at an early developmental stage may affect the individual harboring the mutation and may or may not be passed to subsequent generations. The individual harboring such a somatic cell mutation is said to be a *mosaic* because two populations of cells are present: normal cells and cells harboring the mutant gene. Mutations occurring in an early germ line cell can give rise to gonadal mosaicism so that numerous mutant gametes may be descended from a single event. Gonadal mosaicism is documented in osteogenesis imperfecta and in Duchenne's muscular dystrophy and presumably occurs for many other genes. The reason for the more frequent occurrence of gonadal mosaicism for osteogenesis imperfecta compared to its rarity for disorders such as achondroplasia is unknown, but mutations arising at meiosis (e.g., unequal crossing-over) or later in life should not show gonadal mosaicism. Mutations associated with advanced paternal age (e.g., achondroplasia) are unlikely to involve gonadal mosaicism.

In the clinical context, human mutations fall into two general categories. Some mutations are relatively ancient, and the same mutation is found in thousands or millions of individuals as in the case of sickle cell anemia, the Z allele for α_1-antitrypsin deficiency, and the common mutation for cystic fibrosis. These ancient mutations either tend to be recessive so that the mutant allele persists in the population

through heterozygotes or are sufficiently benign as to permit reproduction. The presence of the same mutant allele in large numbers of individuals has implications for strategies in DNA diagnosis and screening (see "Analysis of Mutations," below). If genetic predisposition to common adult disorders were associated with ancient mutations, population screening with molecular methods would be feasible. Other human mutations are either recent or new to the first case diagnosed in a family. This circumstance is most common for autosomal dominant, deleterious mutations and for X-linked mutations that impair or prevent reproduction in males. These mutations tend to be heterogeneous with a different mutation in each family studied, with only rare recurrence of identical mutations. This scenario is typical for disorders such as Duchenne's muscular dystrophy, neurofibromatosis, retinoblastoma, and many other disorders that have an effect on reproductive fitness. New mutations are discussed further below (see "Dominant New Mutations" and "X-Linked New Mutations").

GENETIC DIVERSITY IN HUMANS: GARROD'S CHEMICAL INDIVIDUALITY AND THE CONCEPT OF POLYMORPHISM

In 1902, Garrod recognized that the aberrant metabolism seen in a condition such as alkaptonuria might imply far more extensive chemical individuality, and his concept of chemical individuality has found its explanation with the realization that the gene for a given protein frequently exists in different forms in different normal individuals and with the recognition that even more extensive variation exists in the DNA sequence of genomes among individuals. The widespread nature of genetic diversity was first apparent when it became possible to study enzymes by electrophoresis of cell extracts and thereby to detect structurally variant forms of enzymes without the necessity of purification. With the use of this technique, it was demonstrated that many proteins exist in two or more forms in the population. These multiple forms are due to the existence in the population of multiple variations of a gene (called *alleles*) at the same genetic locus coding for the same protein. For most loci, each individual possesses two alleles, one derived from each parent. If the two alleles are identical, the individual is said to be *homozygous*; if they differ, the individual is *heterozygous*. The various alleles have been derived from a single precursor allele by mutations during the evolution of the species; in general, they differ from each other only in the substitution of one base for another (missense mutations). In most cases, the proteins produced by both alleles at a given locus are equally functional, i.e., the amino acid difference is "neutral" or nearly so from the standpoint of natural selection.

At the level of protein sequence, many genetic loci (such as that for the β chain of hemoglobin) have a standard sequence/allele that accounts for the majority of alleles in the population, whereas the other alleles are rare. At other genetic loci, no single allele occurs with sufficient frequency to be designated as standard or normal. Variations in the α chain of haptoglobin and in apolipoprotein(a) represent examples of such extreme genetic polymorphism. A polymorphic locus (or nucleotide site) is one at which the most common allele has a frequency of less than 0.99. Note that this definition is concerned only with the frequency of variants at a locus and not with the functional consequences of the variant.

The recognition of polymorphism has been extended by the discovery of extraordinary variation at the DNA sequence level. Between 1 in 100 and 1 in 200 bp in the human genome is polymorphic; this is consistent with heterozygosity at 1 in 250 to 1 in 500 bp. It is possible to detect single-base DNA polymorphisms that represent synonymous differences or amino acid polymorphisms in coding regions, and DNA polymorphisms occur with even greater frequency outside of coding regions in parts of the genome that have little or no effect on gene expression. DNA polymorphisms include, in addition to single-base differences, insertions, deletions, and variation in numbers of tandemly repeated sequences. The latter are termed *variable number tandem repeats* (VNTR) if the repeats are long or *short tandem repeats* (STR) if the repeats are very short, e.g., tetra-, tri-, di-, or mononucleotide repeats.

With the recognition of the extent of DNA polymorphism (millions of nucleotide differences between two random haploid genomes), it is clear that the DNA of each individual contains millions of differences compared to the DNA of another individual, except in the case of identical twins. These DNA differences can be divided into four broad categories: (1) those with no phenotypic effect (e.g., DNA polymorphisms used for identity testing); (2) those causing phenotypic differences without affecting disease susceptibility (e.g., differences in height, hair color); (3) those making minor or modest contributions to disease processes (e.g., as for complex disease traits); and (4) those having a major role in causing a disease phenotype (e.g., as for single gene disorders).

METHODS FOR ANALYSIS OF HUMAN DNA

Molecular analyses of clinical relevance rely on multiple features and strategies, including: (1) the ability to clone genes and DNA fragments using recombinant methods, (2) determination of the sequence of DNA fragments, (3) the specificity of nucleic acid hybridization, (4) the specificity of recognition sites of restriction endonucleases, (5) the power of DNA amplification using the PCR, and (6) the ability to transcribe and translate DNA in vitro for analysis of the protein product. Various combinations of these approaches are used for diagnostic procedures, and some methods utilize mRNA rather than DNA as the starting material.

MOLECULAR CLONING AND SEQUENCING   The size, complexity, and variability of the human genome constitute barriers to the analysis of individual traits and genes. The feasibility for such analysis was greatly enhanced by the development of recombinant DNA technology, which allows for isolation of small DNA fragments and production of unlimited amounts of the cloned material. Hundreds of human genes have been cloned, including the genes for cystic fibrosis, Marfan's syndrome, polyposis of the colon, neurofibromatosis, myotonic dystrophy, fragile X mental retardation, Huntington's disease, breast cancer (BRCA1), hereditary nonpolyposis colon cancer, and many other disorders. Once cloned, the various genes and gene products can be utilized for studies of gene structure and function in normal and disease states, with diagnostic, therapeutic, counseling, and research implications.

The cloning of DNA involves isolation of DNA fragments and their insertion into the nucleic acid from another biologic source (vector) for manipulation and propagation. These vectors can accommodate DNA fragments of tens to hundreds of kilobases in size. Various methods for DNA cloning are described in Watson et al., 1992.

Most genes are divided into coding exons and intervening introns in the genomic DNA. The mRNA from a gene is spliced to link the coding segments, and mRNA can be copied in vitro to synthesize cDNA (DNA complementary to mRNA) for analysis and cloning. Genomic DNA and cDNA clones have been isolated for hundreds of human genes, and for thousands of gene fragments and *anonymous* sequences. The anonymous genomic DNA regions represent unique sites in the genome and often are associated with polymorphic markers that map to that site. Complete cDNA clones or even fragments thereof can be deduced to encode protein sequences which may be homologous to known proteins. Radioactive, biotinylated, or otherwise modified copies of DNA can be prepared from any cloned fragment and can serve as a specific molecular *probe*. Radioactive probes can be detected by autoradiography, whereas biotinylated probes can be detected using avidin and secondary nonradioactive detection methods. Some of the fruits of molecular cloning are the availability of probes for analytical procedures, the availability of DNA sequence data both to deduce protein sequence and to allow for DNA amplification (see "Polymerase Chain Reaction," below), and the ability to analyze for disease mutations.

NUCLEIC ACID HYBRIDIZATION   Many of the steps in recombinant DNA analysis take advantage of the complementary nature of nucleic acid interaction, which is so essential for the synthesis of DNA and RNA. Linear pieces of double-stranded (native) DNA can be treated with heat or alkali to dissociate the two strands to yield single-stranded (denatured) DNA. The denatured DNA can be incubated under conditions that allow for nucleic acid hybridization, i.e., the recognition of two complementary strands and reformation of double-stranded molecules by base pairing. Nucleic acid hybridization is so sensitive that a single-stranded DNA molecule can be hybridized specifically to a complementary strand of RNA or DNA and detected if present at about 1 part in 10,000. It is possible to identify and distinguish fully homologous and partially homologous sequences. The specificity of nucleic acid hybridization, often in combination with fractionation or amplification procedures, allows detection of a single gene among tens of thousands or of nucleic acid from an infectious organism, which may be present at a frequency of less than one copy per human cell. The majority of hybridization probes have been prepared in radioactive form, but the use of nonradioactive detection methods is increasing.

A particularly useful variation of nucleic acid hybridization involves the use of allele-specific oligonucleotides (ASO). The ASO probe is a synthetic, single-stranded oligonucleotide, usually 15 to 20 bases in length. Two probes are synthesized usually differing at the mutation site by a single base, one perfectly matching the normal sequence and one perfectly matching the mutant sequence, with the variable nucleotide in the midportion of the oligonucleotide. Hybridization conditions are adjusted so that the oligonucleotide detects a perfectly matched sequence but fails to hybridize if there is a single base mismatch. ASO can be used in combination with Southern blotting but are now more widely used in combination with DNA amplification.

RESTRICTION ENDONUCLEASES   The discovery in microorganisms of restriction endonucleases, commonly known as restriction enzymes, facilitated recombinant DNA manipulations. Each enzyme recognizes a specific short sequence in double-stranded DNA, typically 4 to 8 bp, and cleaves the DNA at this site. Hundreds of enzymes are known, each recognizing a unique DNA sequence (Fig. 65-5). For example, one enzyme (*Hae*III) that recognizes sequences only 4 bp in length cleaves the sequence 5′-GGCC-3′. The sequence specificity of restriction enzymes is a powerful tool in dissection of large genomes. When human DNA is digested with a particular restriction enzyme, hundreds of thousands of DNA fragments are reproducibly generated that vary from a few base pairs to several thousand base pairs in length, depending on the enzyme used. Restriction enzymes that recognize a sequence only 4 bp long cleave the DNA into smaller fragments than enzymes that recognize longer sequences, since shorter recognition sites occur more often. With the use of multiple restriction enzymes, it is possible to define a detailed map of restriction endonuclease cleavage sites for a particular segment of DNA. Such a map can span a region of from several hundred to tens of thousands of base pairs of DNA. Enzymes that cut the DNA infrequently can be used to prepare DNA maps over megabase dis-

FIGURE 65-5   DNA sequence specificity and nuclease activity for three restriction endonucleases. *Hae*III leaves a blunt end, while the other enzymes leave single-stranded ends.

tances. As described below, variations in the sequences of cleavage sites may reveal polymorphisms or mutations in the human genome.

SOUTHERN BLOTTING Many analyses of the human genome utilize the blotting procedure developed by E. M. Southern, which involves hybridizing DNA in solution to DNA fixed on a membrane support. For clinical analysis, *Southern blotting* (Fig. 65-6) begins with the isolation of genomic DNA from sources such as peripheral leukocytes or fetal cells. The sensitivity of Southern blotting is achieved by cleaving the DNA into small segments, fractionating the fragments by electrophoresis on agarose gels, and applying a sensitive detection method to identify specific fragments (nucleic acid hybridization). Overall, this method can detect unique genomic DNA fragments that typically represent about 1 part in 1 million in the genome. The clinical power of Southern blotting resides in the capacity to analyze a specific small portion of the primary structure of human genomic DNA from an individual. The procedure is useful for detecting gross rearrangements in DNA and some point mutations, but most point mutations are not detected by routine Southern blotting.

An analogous procedure starting with RNA for analysis has been termed *northern blotting*—in contrast to Southern blotting. In this procedure, the presence or absence and approximate size of a particular mRNA can be determined. The term *immunoblotting*, or *western blot-*

ting, describes a procedure designed to analyze protein antigens. Proteins are separated by electrophoresis and transferred to a solid membrane through a blotting procedure. The membrane is analyzed by incubation with antibodies followed by a second step for enzymatic or radioactive detection of bound antibody. Thus, Southern blotting, northern blotting, and immunoblotting or western blotting each combines a fractionation and a detection method to provide a sensitive technique for the analysis of DNA, RNA, and protein, respectively (Table 65-2).

POLYMERASE CHAIN REACTION The technique of PCR for DNA amplification has had a revolutionary impact on molecular diagnosis. The technique is based on knowing the nucleic acid sequence for a region that, for a diagnostic application, is to be analyzed repeatedly from different individuals. Oligonucleotide primers are prepared that are complementary to opposite strands of the DNA and are separated by up to a few hundred base pairs (Fig. 65-7). The oligonucleotide primers are incubated with the target DNA to be amplified and with a DNA polymerase that synthesizes a complementary strand in a 5′-to-3′ direction. Considerable specificity is provided by the requirement that primers must lead to convergent synthesis for amplification to be effective. The reaction is subjected to a series of temperature variations including a denaturing temperature where double-stranded DNA is dissociated to single-stranded DNA, an annealing temperature where oligonucleotide primers hybridize to target DNA, and a polymerization temperature for the synthetic step. The reaction is usually carried out using a thermostable polymerase so that the polymerase remains active during the temperature cycles (usually ranging from 50 to 95°C). After a number of such cycles, typically 20 to 30 or more, hundreds of thousands of copies of the original target sequence are synthesized as depicted in Fig. 65-7. The bulk of the product is a double-stranded DNA fragment of specific length. The technique is so sensitive that it can be used to amplify and analyze DNA from a single human sperm that contains one duplex target DNA molecule. PCR is easily performed with minimal preparation of crude and even degraded samples, allowing analysis from whole blood, dried blood filters, mouthwash, old tissue sections, and other sources. PCR can be performed starting with genomic DNA as the template; alternatively, RNA can be reverse transcribed to yield cDNA for use as a template, a procedure known as reverse transcription-PCR (RT-PCR). Molecular diagnosis with PCR can include: (1) determining the presence or the absence of an amplified product, (2) digesting the amplified product with a restriction enzyme, (3) hybridizing the PCR product with allele-specific oligonucleotides, (4) direct sequencing of the PCR product, (5) analyzing the ratio of RNA from two alleles using RT-PCR, and (6) analysis for expression in vitro to search for truncation mutations. Variations and modifications include synthesis of single-stranded DNA by altering the ratio of the oligonucleotide primers, preparation of recombinant DNA constructs, mutagenesis of cloned DNA, detection of rare nucleotide sequences, and detection of nucleotide sequences of infectious agents. The PCR method offers extremely rapid analysis (single day), ease of automation, relative economy, and extraordinary specificity.

PROTEIN TRUNCATION TESTS Protein truncation tests (PTT) can be used to detect any mutation that results in premature termination of the peptide during protein synthesis; these are primarily nonsense, frameshift, and some splicing mutations (Fig. 65-8). In PTT,

FIGURE 65-6 Southern blotting analysis of genomic DNA. RFLP, restriction fragment length polymorphism.

Table 65-2

Analytical Blotting Procedures

Blot Method	Material Analyzed	Fractionation	Detection
Southern	DNA	Electrophoresis	Nucleic acid hybridization
Northern	RNA	Electrophoresis	Nucleic acid hybridization
Western or immunoblot	Protein	Electrophoresis	Immunologic

FIGURE 65-7   Polymerase chain reaction for amplification of DNA. The target DNA is shown as a solid line in cycle 1. Newly synthesized DNA is indicated by dotted lines in each cycle. Primer oligonucleotides are indicated by solid rectangles. Each DNA strand is marked with an arrow indicating 5′-to-3′ orientation.

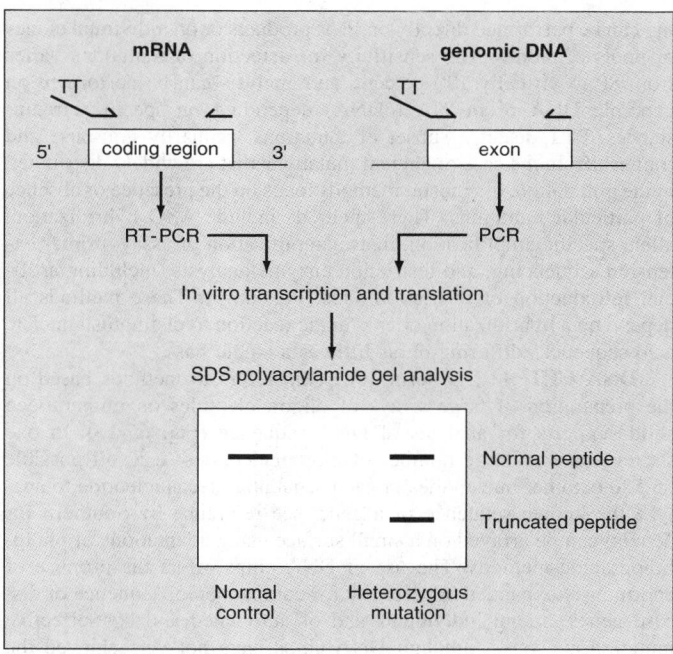

FIGURE 65-8   Protein truncation testing. Polymerase chain reaction (PCR) is performed starting with genomic DNA or reverse transcription-PCR (RT-PCR) is performed utilizing mRNA. Sequences for transcription and translation (TT) are introduced at the 5′ end of the coding segments. Mutations leading to truncation of a protein are detected by gel analysis.

fication, chemical cleavage of mismatches, single-strand conformation polymorphism analysis, heteroduplex analysis, and sequencing of DNA (Fig. 65-9). These methods involve chemical or enzymatic recognition of mismatches in nucleic acid duplexes, electrophoretic separation of single- or double-stranded DNA, or sequencing. DNA sequenc-

the amplified genomic DNA encoding an exon or amplified cDNA is transcribed and translated in vitro, and the protein products are analyzed using gel electrophoresis to detect truncated proteins. PTT have been used mostly to detect heterozygous mutations in autosomal dominant disorders, but the method is generally applicable and is particularly suited for detection of loss-of-function mutations.

ANALYSIS OF MUTATIONS   The challenge of detecting unknown mutations is different from diagnostic testing for the presence of known mutations. Large mutations are more easily detected, using Southern blotting or PCR to detect expansions of triplet repeats, deletions, insertions, and other rearrangements. RT-PCR is useful to detect absence of or major reduction in mRNA from a mutant allele; first, common polymorphisms are used to identify heterozygosity within an exon of genomic DNA, followed by analysis of the ratio of mRNA from the two alleles. This strategy will detect any mutation that profoundly reduces the level of mRNA. More discriminating methods are required for detection of point mutations. The best characterized methods for detection of unknown mutations include ribonuclease cleavage, denaturing gradient-gel electrophoresis, carbodiimide modi-

Method	Normal	Mutant	Principle
Carbodiimide (CDI) modification			CDI conjugate slower in gel or blocks primer extension
Denaturing gradient gel electrophoresis (DGGE)			Mutant slower in gel
Single-strand conformational polymorphism (SSCP)			Mutation changes shape and mobility in gel
Heteroduplex analysis			Bubble makes mutant duplex slower in gel
RNAse or chemical cleavage method			Mismatch cleaved in mutant
Allele-specific oligonucleotide			No binding of oligonucleotide to mutant
Ligation detection			No ligation of mutant
Allele-specific amplification			No PCR product of mutant
Single base primer extension			Different base in extension in mutant
Artificial introduction of restriction sites			Mutant has enzyme cut site engineered

FIGURE 65-9   Methods for detection of mutations. The asterisk represents the position of the mutation. PCR, polymerase chain reaction. (*Modified from Cotton, Hum Mutat 285:125, 1993, with permission.*)

ing can be performed directly on PCR products or on individual clones or pools of clones. The sensitivity for detection of mutations varies from 80 to virtually 100 percent, and analysis can be performed on genomic DNA or mRNA (cDNA) depending on specific circumstances. PTT detect a subset of mutations, primarily nonsense and frameshift. In the case of ancient mutations that are widely distributed in the population, diagnostic methods focus on the presence or absence of particular mutations. These methods include ASO hybridization, allele-specific amplification, ligase amplification or assay, primer extension sequencing, and restriction enzyme analysis (including artificial introduction of restriction sites; Fig. 65-9). These methods all depend on a hybridization or enzymatic reaction to distinguish nucleic acid sequences differing by as little as a single base.

DNA CHIPS The term *DNA chip* refers to methods based on the preparation of large arrays of oligonucleotides on miniaturized solid supports for analysis of DNA sequence (Fig. 65-10). In one strategy, a very large number of oligonucleotides (e.g., all possible 65,536 octomer nucleotides or each sequential decanucleotide to analyze the known sequence of a gene; see reference by Southern for details) can be arrayed on a small surface using adaptations of photolithographic methods. The use of DNA chips offers the promise of enormously expanded opportunity for comparison of sequence of disease genes among individuals and of automated and cost-effective mutation analysis. Although DNA chips have not yet achieved the status of practical application, these devices may become a key component of medical diagnosis in the future.

ANALYZING THE HUMAN GENOME

The topographic map of our genomic DNA can be divided into regions corresponding to the chromosomal bands visually identified by standard cytogenetic analysis of the 24 chromosomes (22 autosomes

FIGURE 65-10 Use of DNA chips for molecular analysis. Large numbers of unique oligonucleotides are arrayed on a solid support and analyzed as indicated. See reference by Southern for detailed discussion.

and X and Y). As of early 1996, about 3700 loci were assigned to specific positions on the human genetic map according to *Online Mendelian Inheritance in Man* (electronic address: http://www3.ncbi.nlm.nih.gov/omin/). Two kinds of maps describing the relative order and distance of genetic markers and their position within a defined region have been developed—the genetic and the physical maps; the first is an indirect statistical analysis based on genetic recombination, whereas the second hinges on direct measurement of the length of DNA.

THE GENETIC MAP AND THE PRINCIPLE OF GENETIC LINKAGE Genetic linkage is essential for preparation of the map of the human genome and is used routinely for molecular diagnosis. Genetic distance, which is expressed in centimorgans, is a measure of the likelihood of crossover between two loci. Two loci are 1 cM apart if there is a 1 percent probability of a crossover between them at meiosis. There are on average 30 to 35 crossovers during meiosis in males, and perhaps twice as many during meiosis in females.

The feasibility of human linkage analysis was revolutionized by the demonstration of genetic variation in the size of fragments generated by digestion of normal human DNA with restriction endonucleases. These restriction fragment length polymorphisms (RFLPs) are the consequence of the DNA sequence polymorphisms and are inherited according to Mendelian principles (Fig. 65-11). Restriction enzyme digestion and Southern blotting make it possible to utilize these polymorphisms as genetic markers for sites within the genome. If one of the base pairs in the recognition sequence for a restriction enzyme differs between individual copies of the genome or if there is a length variation in the DNA, there will be variation in the size of DNA fragments generated by the restriction enzyme digestion.

A particularly informative subset of RFLPs is the result of VNTR. These are sites of length variation in which a DNA sequence is variably and tandemly repeated on different chromosomes so that many different sizes of DNA fragments can be regarded as different alleles at a VNTR site. The repeat unit in VNTRs can be tens or hundreds of bases in length, with variation arising through unequal crossing-over. In the case of the gene for the apolipoprotein (a), a VNTR repeat unit includes two exons and gives rise to polymorphism in both the length of the gene and the protein. STRs are repeats of tetra-, tri-, di-, and mononucleotides in the genome in which variation has arisen through "slippage" of the DNA polymerase at replication to increase or decrease the number of repeat units on a chromosome. STRs are highly polymorphic, easily analyzed, and widely distributed in the genome (Fig. 65-12). An essential feature of linkage analysis, whether for construction of the human gene map or for clinical diagnosis, is that DNA markers have different alleles at the marker locus of interest so that the two chromosomes of the individual can be distinguished.

Genetic linkage can be assessed between any group of markers, one of which may represent a mutation that causes a disease phenotype. For autosomal genes, each individual inherits one copy of each chro-

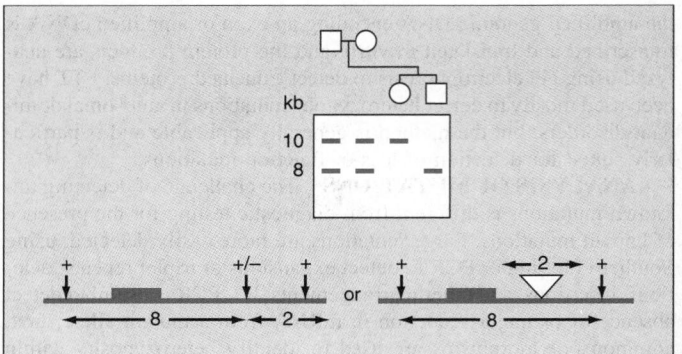

FIGURE 65-11 Example of restriction fragment length polymorphism (RFLP) in human DNA using Southern blotting. The solid blocks indicate segments of DNA used as probe. Parents are heterozygous and children are homozygous for the RFLP. Symbols above the arrows indicate cutting (+) or noncutting (−) by the restriction endonuclease. Numbers indicate DNA length in kilobases.

FIGURE 65-12 Depiction of a short tandem repeat polymorphism for a dinucleotide $(GT)_n$ repeat. Each repeat is separated by a vertical line. Sites for two primers for polymerase chain reaction (PCR) are indicated by arrows. Four alleles of 24, 21, 18, and 15 GT repeats are indicated. Inheritance of the alleles in a family as detected by PCR is shown below.

abundant DNA markers and the identification and cloning of the genes in a region.

Major strategies for physical mapping of the human genome include in situ hybridization, deletion mapping, long-range restriction mapping, and isolation of yeast artificial chromosome (YAC) or other large insert clones. With in situ hybridization, the direct hybridization of a DNA marker to a chromosome allows the assignment of the marker to a specific chromosomal band. With the advent of fluorescent in situ hybridization (FISH), it is now possible to use different colored probes for simultaneous mapping of more than one DNA marker, and hybridization to interphase nuclei allows determination of the order of markers within a particular chromosomal region. This technique is also very effective for the identification of chromosomal abnormalities (see Chap. 66).

Deletion mapping is based on the presence or absence of a particular region or locus in the DNA from patients with chromosomal abnormalities or from human/rodent somatic cell hybrids that contain defined segments of the human chromosomes. Deletion mapping is particularly useful for mapping of the X chromosome, because deletions of the X

mosome from each parent. Panel A of Fig. 65-13 depicts one pair of chromosomes ready to enter meiosis with one normal copy of a gene (open square) and one defective copy of the same gene (solid square). Four DNA markers, typically dinucleotide repeat polymorphisms, with A/B, F/G, K/L, and R/S alleles are depicted at 0, 1, 10, and >50 cM from the disease gene. After meiosis and three crossover events, gametes are formed containing one chromosome with various segments of the original chromosomes. Alleles A and F are at DNA markers within (A) or close to (F), the gene of interest, and remain on the chromosome with the normal copy of the gene. DNA markers further away have a greater probability to undergo crossing-over, and the L allele of one DNA marker is now on the chromosome with the normal copy of the defective copy of the gene. The greater the distance between markers and genes, the greater the probability of crossovers. Alleles for a gene and markers on different chromosomes are inherited in a completely independent fashion.

Panel B of Fig. 65-13 depicts the analysis of DNA markers in a family with an autosomal dominant disorder such as Huntington's disease. Data are shown for the K/L DNA marker that is 10 cM from the disease gene and for a Y/Z DNA marker on a different chromosome. A researcher trying to map a disease gene is likely to study many DNA markers, like the Y/Z marker, that show no correlation between which allele of the marker gene is inherited and whether the disease phenotype is inherited. Eventually a marker is discovered, such as K/L, that is close to the disease gene. Analysis of additional families can provide conclusive statistical evidence that a polymorphic DNA marker is near a disease gene and makes possible immediate application of the marker for diagnosis within a family such as that shown in Fig. 65-13 (see "Diagnosis by Linkage Analysis," below) and opens the way for positional cloning of the disease gene (see "Cloning and Identifying Human Disease Genes," below). The frequency of crossovers as shown for the last offspring in Fig. 65-13 is a measure of the genetic distance between the DNA marker and the disease gene. Once a linked DNA marker is found, closer DNA markers can be identified rapidly.

THE PHYSICAL MAP The physical map is based on direct DNA analysis and is not influenced by regional differences in recombination frequency. A physical map facilitates both the isolation of

FIGURE 65-13 Depiction of meiotic crossing-over and linkage analysis. *A.* Two copies of one chromosome (one in solid line and one in dashed line) from an individual before (above) and after (below) meiotic crossing-over. The individual is heterozygous for a disease locus with a normal allele (open square) and a disease allele (solid square) and is heterozygous for four DNA markers with alleles A/B, F/G, K/L, and R/S at 0, 1, 10, and >50 cM from the disease locus, respectively. *B.* Analysis in a family for an autosomal dominant disorder. The DNA marker with K/L alleles at 10 cM from the disease locus on chromosome 4 and another marker with Y/Z alleles on chromosome 7 are depicted. The chromosomes 4 and 7 for each parent are shown, and the genotypes given for each family member. The disease phenotype is inherited from the father with the L allele for the DNA marker, except for the last child who represents a crossover of the type shown in *A.* See text for discussion.

chromosome frequently result in a disease phenotype in males and because the nullisomic regions can be defined without having to separate the abnormal chromosome in somatic cell hybrids. Deletion mapping is also useful in establishing relative orders of sets of markers in the genome, although it does not provide precise information as to the distance involved.

Information about physical distance is provided by long-range restriction mapping. In this technique, high-molecular-weight DNA is cut into large fragments (from 100 kb up to 4 Mb), using restriction enzymes that cut very rarely in the genome, and these fragments are separated by pulsed-field gel electrophoresis (PFGE) and hybridized to several DNA markers using Southern blotting procedures. If, for example, two DNA probes hybridize to the same 200-kb restriction fragment, it can be concluded that the maximum distance between the two loci is 200 kb.

Another strategy in physical mapping utilizes YAC clones, which carry large fragments of genomic DNA (from 50 kb to 1 or 2 Mb in length). These YAC vectors contain yeast telomeres and centromeres, and the clones are actually propagated as separate chromosomes in a yeast host.

THE HUMAN GENOME PROJECT   The human genome project is an international effort, started in the mid 1980s, aimed at the complete characterization of human genomic DNA. Specific goals include: (1) development of detailed physical and genetic maps, (2) cloning of the entire genome in overlapping YACs or other large insert vectors, (3) identification and characterization of all genes, (4) sequencing of all the haploid human genome, and (5) biologic interpretation of the information encrypted in the nucleotide sequence. This project will almost certainly enhance knowledge both in basic biology and in medicine. In the latter field, an important goal is the identification of genes involved in genetic predisposition to cancer and to complex diseases such as hypertension and atherosclerosis.

As of 1996, a detailed map of the human genome was available with the analysis of 5264 highly informative, short tandem dinucleotide repeat polymorphisms; 2032 of these markers could be ordered with strong confidence, providing an average interval between markers of 1.6 cM. Sequencing has been performed for thousands of fragments of cDNA (expressed sequence tags), and this sequence information makes it possible to perform computerized searches of DNA and to deduce protein sequences. Numerous electronic databases are available to access the information accumulating from the human genome project.

CLONING AND IDENTIFYING HUMAN DISEASE GENES   There are four general strategies for cloning human disease genes: (1) starting with knowledge and availability of the protein; (2) using the ability to select for function of the gene; (3) determining the precise genetic location (positional cloning); and (4) some combination of information regarding the phenotype, the genetic map location of the gene in question, and the genetic map location of relevant genes (a positional candidate gene approach). Many of the early gene cloning successes relied on purification of a protein, determination of partial amino acid sequence, preparation of antibodies, and development of enzymatic or other assays. Using this information, cDNA clones were isolated using approaches such as mRNA purification, hybridization screening with oligonucleotides based on available amino acid sequence, PCR amplification based on similar oligonucleotides, immunologic screening of expression cDNA libraries, and other related approaches. Currently, expressed DNA sequences can often be found in databases if minimal amino acid sequence is available. In some instances genes have been cloned based on a functional property, without knowing the protein or the genetic map location. For example, various genes involved in DNA repair disorders have been isolated using selection in tissue culture to identify clones that correct the cellular phenotype of defective DNA repair.

Positional cloning is the isolation of a disease gene based on its location in the genome with no knowledge of its function. This strategy depends on the analysis of DNA samples from affected families to find a DNA marker that is located close to the disease locus, as discussed above and illustrated Fig. 65-13B. Having localized the disease gene in a general way, it is possible to isolate the DNA of the relevant region in overlapping clones, identify genes in the region, and eventually prove which is the disease gene, often by identifying small mutations within one of the genes (Fig. 65-14). This strategy is facilitated if chromosomal translocations are available to assist in mapping and identifying the disease gene. This approach has yielded landmark successes as in the identification of the genes for Duchenne's muscular dystrophy, cystic fibrosis, retinoblastoma, polyposis of the colon, neurofibromatosis, Huntington's disease, and breast cancer (BRCA1 and BRCA2).

As more genes are described, the positional candidate-gene approach has become very productive for identifying disease genes. A pure candidate-gene strategy occasionally involves deducing the disease gene from among known proteins based on the disease phenotype, but more often the candidate-gene approach requires an approximate genetic mapping, but much less than would be adequate for a strictly positional cloning effort. Based on the limited mapping information, on knowledge about relevant genes mapping to the same region, and perhaps taking into account information from other species such as the mouse, one can formulate and test the hypothesis that a particular gene is mutated in a specific disease by amplification and/or cloning of the gene in question from affected patients to search for mutations. Such an approach led to the identification of mutations in the cardiac myosin heavy chain genes that cause familial hypertrophic cardiomyopathy, in the fibrillin gene in Marfan's syndrome, in the *RET* protooncogene in multiple endocrine neoplasia type 2, and in various mismatch DNA repair genes in hereditary nonpolyposis colon cancer. Use of information from the mouse led to the recognition that the *PAX3* gene is mutated in Waardenburg's syndrome. One variation on the candidate-gene approach involves the production of mice with targeted mutations and identifying candidate genes based on phenotypes in the mice that resemble a human phenotype. The map locations for many disorders are shown in Fig. 65-15, and the majority of these genes are cloned.

TRANSGENIC AND MUTANT MICE   Gene structure and function are usually similar in mouse and human, and studies in the mouse can often be of value in understanding human disease (Fig. 65-16). After microinjection of cloned DNA sequences into the male pronucleus of fertilized mouse eggs, the injected DNA becomes integrated into the mouse chromosomal DNA in a fraction of the injected cells, including the germ cells, so that a series of descendant animals will express the transgene. Each site of integration of foreign DNA behaves as a single Mendelian trait, and heterozygous and homozygous animals can be bred. This strategy can be used to produce mouse models of human disease in the case of dominant negative or gain-of-function alleles, as has been done for osteogenesis imperfecta and spinocerebellar ataxia type 1.

Transgenic animals are particularly useful for the evaluation of *cis*-acting regulatory DNA sequences that control tissue-specific and temporal aspects of gene expression. Putative regulatory sequences are linked to a reporter gene that encodes an easily detectable product. Using this strategy, it has been shown that short DNA sequences provide exquisite tissue specificity for genes such as insulin and elas-

FIGURE 65-14   A positional cloning strategy. DNA markers at sites A and B are found to flank a disease gene. Overlapping DNA clones are isolated for the region, and the disease gene is identified within the region.

tase and that more complex and distant regulatory sequences control the expression of globin genes. The transgenic method has also been utilized to introduce viral or cellular oncogenes in animals to induce tumors, opening up approaches for the study of tumor biology. For example, a tissue-specific regulatory sequence linked to the SV40 T antigen produces tumors in specific cell types. Another transgenic mouse strategy involves linking of regulatory sequences to a toxin that will selectively kill cells that express the sequence. As an example, linking of insulin regulatory sequences to diphtheria toxin can generate mice with selective absence of pancreatic β cells. In yet another application, larger transgenic animals can be used for production of pharmaceuticals to be harvested from milk or blood.

It is also possible to induce mutations in mice, and treatment of male animals with ethylnitrosourea is quite effective in inducing small mutations. Since integration of transgenic DNA is relatively random, such insertions can on occasion interrupt normal mouse genes. Retroviruses can also be used to infect mouse embryonic cells to produce random insertional mutagenesis, and mutant phenotypes can then be ascertained in the resulting heterozygous or homozygous mice, including identification of defects that are benign in heterozygotes but are embryonic lethals in the homozygous state. Because the retrovirus inserts at the site of the affected gene, it is possible to identify many new mutations and to clone the relevant genes.

Homologous recombination with mouse embryonic stem (ES) cells provides additional opportunities. ES cells are totipotent cells that can be manipulated in culture and then reintroduced into mouse embryos. Using homologous recombination in ES cells, it is possible to target a specific gene for subtle mutation or inactivation ("knockout"). Altered ES cells are injected into recipient blastocysts and give rise to chimeric animals composed partially of mutant cells derived from the ES cell culture. The genetically altered cells are often represented in the sperm of the resulting chimeric animals, and mutant mice can be obtained and bred to study the gene in heterozygotes and homozygotes. The technique has allowed the production of mouse models of retinoblastoma, p53 oncogene deficiency (Li-Fraumeni familial cancer syndrome), cystic fibrosis, the Lesch-Nyhan syndrome, Gaucher's disease, apolipoprotein E deficiency, and others. In some instances there are phenotypic differences for the same mutation in mice and humans, providing an opportunity for important biologic insights, and in others, the phenotype in mice and humans is very similar, so that the animals are valuable for studies of pathogenesis and for therapeutic trials. Mutant mice of these types will be useful for unraveling the genetic factors in complex disease processes such as atherosclerosis and for analysis of neurologic functions. The ability to obtain mouse mutants for virtually any cloned gene provides an opportunity for analyzing the function of cloned genes whose biologic roles are not delineated.

CATEGORIES OF GENETIC DISORDERS

Genetic diseases generally fall into one of three categories: (1) *Chromosomal disorders* involve the lack, excess, or abnormal arrangement of one or more chromosomes, producing large amounts of excessive or deficient genetic material and affecting many genes. (2) *Mendelian or monogenic disorders* are determined primarily by a single mutant gene. These disorders display simple (Mendelian) inheritance patterns that can be classified into autosomal dominant, autosomal recessive, or X-linked types. (3) *Complex disease traits* are caused by an interaction of multiple genes and multiple exogenous or environmental factors. Although many of these complex traits, such as diabetes mellitus, gout, and cleft lip and palate, exhibit familial clustering, the inheritance pattern is complex, and the risk to relatives is less than in the single-gene disorders. Each of these categories of genetic disease presents different problems with respect to pathogenesis, prevention, diagnosis, genetic counseling, and treatment. Furthermore, this classification is in fact an oversimplification. For example, small chromosomal deletions can cause the simultaneous presence of multiple Mendelian or monogenic disorders, as exemplified by males with cytogenetically visible deletions in the short arm of the X chromosome in association

with Duchenne's muscular dystrophy, chronic granulomatous disease, retinitis pigmentosa, and the McLeod phenotype. Deletions of the retinoblastoma locus on chromosome 13 may be visible or submicroscopic and may extend to nearby loci such as esterase D. Thus, these defects bridge the gap between chromosomal and monogenic disorders. The phenotype caused by chromosomal disorders obviously is due to the altered expression of single genes, within the abnormal region. Chromosomal translocations may interrupt single genes, as exemplified by some women with Duchenne's muscular dystrophy due to X/autosome translocations.

The phenotypes of many monogenic disorders are modified by the genes at other loci and by environmental factors. Indeed, a single locus *entirely* determines the disease phenotype in relatively few monogenic disorders. Examples of effects of nongenetic factors that influence monogenic disorders include drug exposure for glucose-6-phosphate dehydrogenase deficiency and acute intermittent porphyria, iron intake and blood loss for hemochromatosis, smoking for α_1-antitrypsin deficiency, and diet for lipoprotein lipase deficiency. Similarly, genes at other loci can modify the phenotype, as exemplified by the effect of the genotype at the α-globin cluster on sickle cell anemia. The border between monogenic disorders and complex traits is not a sharp one, since other genes frequently modify the phenotype of monogenic disorders and major genes often play a role in complex traits (e.g., HLA genotype and type 1 diabetes mellitus). Although monogenic disorders provide an excellent starting point for the study of human genetic disease, an even greater challenge is to understand the more common complex disease traits.

FREQUENCY OF GENETIC DISEASE In studies in Montreal, Baltimore, and Newcastle, 6 to 8 percent of diseases among hospitalized children were attributable to single-gene defects, and 0.4 to 2.5 percent were due to chromosomal abnormalities; another 22 to 31 percent were considered to be gene influenced. The overall frequency of monogenic disorders is about 1 percent, and about 5.3 percent of individuals below age 25 will have a disease with an important genetic component (single gene, chromosomal, or complex traits). If complex traits of late onset are included, about 60 percent of individuals have genetically influenced diseases at some time. Genetic factors contribute in a significant way to an even larger fraction of diseases in a population when common infectious disorders are controlled.

CHROMOSOMAL DISORDERS Chromosomal disorders involve the largest changes in DNA and can include an entire extra copy of the genome (triploidy), an extra chromosome (trisomy), deletions or duplications of portions of a chromosome, and other defects. Chromosomal abnormalities are frequent causes of spontaneous abortion, malformations, mental retardation, and tumors (Table 65-3). Chromosomal disorders are discussed in greater detail in Chap. 66.

MONOGENIC DISORDERS Although few phenotypes are entirely determined by a single locus, the concept of *monogenic disorders* is still valuable. Such disorders ordinarily exhibit one of three patterns of inheritance: (1) autosomal dominant, (2) autosomal recessive, or (3) X-linked. The overall population frequency of monogenic disorders is about 10 per 1000 live births, comprising about 7 in 1000 dominant, about 2.5 in 1000 recessive, and about 0.4 in 1000 X-linked conditions (excluding color blindness). Table 65-4 lists some of the more common Mendelian disorders in adults.

If a particular disease shows one of the three Mendelian patterns of inheritance, its pathogenesis, no matter how complex, must be due to an abnormality at a single site in the genome usually involving a single protein. For example, in sickle cell anemia, the entire clinical syndrome, including such seemingly unrelated disturbances as anemia, pain crises, nephropathy, and predisposition to pneumococcal infections, is the physiologic consequence of having a single base change at a specific site in the gene that codes for the β chain of hemoglobin, producing a substitution of a valine for a glutamic acid in the sixth amino acid position in the protein sequence. The mutant gene and

FIGURE 65-15 Morbid anatomy of the human genome adapted to emphasize disorders discussed in *Harrison's*.
(Courtesy of Joanna S. Amberger and Victor A. McKusick, M.D.)

FIGURE 65-15 *(Continued)*

FIGURE 65-16   Various strategies for producing transgenic and mutant mice. DNA can be injected into the male pronucleus of fertilized mouse eggs followed by implantation in pseudopregnant mothers. Mouse embryos can be infected with retroviruses in vivo or in vitro. Transgenic mice may be mosaic, but the transgene can be recovered in nonmosaic form in the offspring of these mice. These strategies are depicted on the left. On the right, cultured embryonic stem (ES) cells can be modified by homologous or nonhomologous recombination or by retroviral infection. The modified cells can be selected and injected into a mouse blastocyst to produce a chimeric mouse, with subsequent recovery of the mutation in the germline of the offspring of the chimeric mouse.

protein for many common Mendelian disorders are known, even when the full pathogenesis of a disorder is not known.

The basic biochemical lesions in monogenic disorders involve defects in a wide variety of proteins, including enzymes, receptors, transport proteins, peptide hormones, immunoglobulins, collagens, transcription factors, and coagulation factors. Defects in genes that do not encode proteins (e.g., defects in genes for tRNA in the mitochondrial genome) are rare.

SIGNIFICANCE OF DOMINANCE OR RECESSIVENESS

Unless otherwise specified, the terms *dominant* and *recessive* refer to the clinical phenotype associated with a particular allele. This distinction is useful for clinical diagnosis, for linkage analysis, and for genetic counseling, but there are a number of complexities inherent in the use of these terms. The circumstance is relatively simple if the heterozygous individual is indistinguishable from one or the other homozygote. In this case, the dominant trait (disease) or allele (mutation) is the one that prevails in the heterozygote. In true recessive

Frequency of Chromosomal Disorders Among Liveborn Infants

Disorders	Frequency
Autosomal abnormalities	
Trisomy 21 (Down's syndrome)	1 in 600
Trisomy 18	1 in 5000
Trisomy 13	1 in 15,000
Sex chromosome abnormalities	
Klinefelter syndrome (47,XXY)	1 in 700 males
XYY syndrome (47,XYY)	1 in 800 males
Triple-X syndrome (47,XXX)	1 in 1000 females
Turner syndrome (45,X or 45X/46XX or 45X/46,XY or isochromosome Xq)	1 in 1500 females

Table 65-4

Some Relatively Frequent Mendelian Disorders Affecting Adults

AUTOSOMAL DOMINANT DISORDERS

Familial hypercholesterolemia
Hereditary nonpolyposis colon cancer
Polyposis of the colon
BRCA1 and BRCA2 breast cancer
Hereditary hemorrhagic telangiectasia
Marfan's syndrome
Hereditary spherocytosis
Adult polycystic kidney disease
Huntington's chorea
Acute intermittent porphyria
Osteogenesis imperfecta tarda
von Willebrand's disease
Myotonic dystrophy
Familial hypertrophic cardiomyopathy
Neurofibromatosis
Tuberous sclerosis

AUTOSOMAL RECESSIVE DISORDERS

Deafness
Albinism
Wilson's disease
Hemochromatosis
Sickle cell anemia
β Thalassemia
Cystic fibrosis
Hereditary emphysema (α_1-antitrypsin deficiency)
Homocystinuria
Friedreich's ataxia
Phenylketonuria

X-LINKED DISORDERS

Hemophilia A
Glucose-6-phosphate dehydrogenase deficiency
Duchenne/Becker muscular dystrophy
Fabry's disease
Ocular albinism
Testicular feminization
Chronic granulomatous disease
Hypophosphatemic rickets
Fragile-X
Color blindness

disorders, the phenotype in heterozygotes is indistinguishable from normal, and in true dominant disorders, heterozygous individuals have a disease phenotype that is indistinguishable from homozygous affected individuals. Although many recessive medical disorders appear on the surface to qualify as true recessives, heterozygotes for many of these conditions exhibit subtle differences in phenotype that may be enhanced by environmental factors. Such subtle phenotypic consequences may be advantageous or disadvantageous. Even when clinically "normal," individuals who are heterozygous for recessive loss-of-function alleles often have demonstrable metabolic differences and always have demonstrable differences at the protein level. These complexities are exemplified by sickle cell anemia, which is clinically a recessive disorder in that heterozygotes are usually normal healthy individuals. Nevertheless, heterozygotes exhibit a selective advantage for resistance to malaria and have subtle physiologic abnormalities in renal concentrating ability and in cardiopulmonary function at high altitude. Subtle phenotypic effects in heterozygotes for recessive disorders may be more common than is generally recognized and may contribute to phenotypes usually considered to be complex disease traits. For example, heterozygotes for ataxia telangiectasia and other DNA repair disorders may be at increased risk of malignancy, heterozygosity for homocystinuria is probably a risk factor in vascular disease, and heterozygosity for α_1-antitrypsin deficiency may predispose to pulmonary disease. Heterozygosity for known recessive disorders makes a major contribution to biochemical and medical individuality.

The situation is different for dominant phenotypes; very few conditions qualify as true dominants, such as may be the case for Huntington's disease. Homozygotes for most dominant disorders are ascertained rarely, and, when recognized, the disease is usually more severe than in heterozygotes, indicating that most such disorders are actually semidominant (incompletely or partially dominant) traits (e.g., familial hypercholesterolemia and achondroplasia). The term *codominant* has relatively little clinical applicability and describes a situation such as the A and B blood group alleles in which the presence of one antigenic determinant does not affect the presence or absence of the other.

Additional complexities arise from the fact that the phenotypic consequences of heterozygosity may be inconsistent and cause uncertainty as to whether the disorder is dominant or recessive. Heterozygotes may display symptoms in only a very small fraction of cases, or heterozygotes may have subtle and mild symptoms that do not qualify as a disease diagnosis. Homozygotes for these traits typically have clear-cut disease manifestation. From a clinical and counseling vantage point, most medical disorders fall into the dominant or recessive category despite the fact that this classification is an arbitrary division of a continuum rather than a true biologic demarcation.

Although there is a tendency for a given disease locus to be considered as typically involving dominant or recessive mutations, the classification of a mutation or trait as dominant or recessive must be made on an allele-by-allele basis and not on a locus-by-locus basis, as in the case of osteogenesis imperfecta where different mutations in the same gene can have dominant or recessive effects. When two different mutant alleles are present at the same locus, patients are referred to as *compound heterozygotes* or *genetic compounds*. This is distinct from a double-heterozygote individual who is heterozygous at two different loci. Most compound heterozygous genotypes involve different recessive alleles at a locus, but phenotypic homozygotes for dominant traits (such as familial hypercholesterolemia) may be compound heterozygotes at a molecular level as well. Alternatively, compound heterozygotes may have one recessive allele and one dominant allele such that heterozygotes for the recessive allele are phenotypically normal, heterozygotes for the dominant allele have a disease process, and the compound heterozygote individuals have a disease process that is distinct (usually more severe) from the disease in heterozygotes for the dominant allele. Such instances are likely for osteogenesis imperfecta.

Mutant alleles may cause a total or partial loss of function (referred to as *null alleles* or *hypomorphic alleles*, respectively), may exhibit altered function, or may gain a novel function. In general, most loss-of-function alleles tend to be recessive, as in the case of the majority of enzyme deficiencies in humans and most null mutations produced in mice. However, some null alleles have phenotypic effects and cause human disease if a half-normal level of the encoded protein is insufficient for normal physiology. Whether a mutation generates a dominant or recessive disorder is determined by two factors: (1) the effect of the mutation on the function of the gene product, and (2) the tolerance of the biologic system to perturbation of that particular gene product. Mutations in tolerant systems tend to result in recessive phenotypes; mutations in less tolerant systems tend to result in dominant phenotypes. Loci that encode enzymes usually result in recessive phenotypes because of the catalytic nature of enzymes and because enzymes are usually present in excess of the quantity required to maintain relatively normal levels of substrates and products, so that a large change in enzyme activity can have a negligible effect on flux in many pathways. Examples where a heterozygous loss-of-function mutation causes a disease phenotype include several forms of porphyria, familial hypercholesterolemia, and osteogenesis imperfecta. In the case of recessive disorders, the presence of protein with residual function can result in mild forms of disorders, including disorders of amino acid metabolism and lysosomal storage diseases.

The term *dominant negative* is applied to mutant alleles in which a mutant protein interferes in one way or another with the function of normal protein being produced from the normal allele in a heterozygote. Dominant negative alleles occur when proteins are involved in subunit structures or when proteins interact with other proteins or nucleic acids. A dominant negative mechanism is often involved when a mutant allele causes a more severe phenotype in heterozygotes than

that caused by a null allele because of some adverse effect of the abnormal product on the function of the normal product. For example, in osteogenesis imperfecta, missense mutations can interfere with collagen fiber assembly and cause lethal osteogenesis imperfecta in heterozygotes, whereas null alleles cause a milder disease. In other instances, mutant alleles generate a novel biologic effect that cannot be described in terms of increased or decreased function of the normal allele; these are referred to as *gain-of-function alleles* or *neomorphic alleles*. In amyloidosis, the abnormal folding properties of the mutant protein lead to a harmful, extracellular deposition of material that appears unrelated to the normal function of the protein. The expanded polyglutamine tracts in the mutant alleles for Huntington's disease, spinocerebellar ataxia, and spinobulbar muscular atrophy may represent gain-of-function alleles, but the pathogenesis is not yet understood.

EXCEPTIONS TO THE RULES (UNSTABLE MUTATIONS, UNIPARENTAL DISOMY, IMPRINTED GENES, AND TRANSMISSION RATIO DISTORTION) The traditional formulation of single-gene disorders involved assumptions that are generally correct, including the stability of mutations, the inheritance of one allele from each parent for an autosomal locus, the equal expression of both alleles at an autosomal locus, and the random transmission of either allele to an offspring. Genetic counseling, linkage analysis, and interpretation of genetic data are based on these assumptions. However, examples of exceptions to these rules now abound.

As mentioned above, the clearest examples of unstable mutations involve the expanding triplet repeats that cause fragile X syndrome, myotonic dystrophy, Huntington's disease, spinobulbar muscular atrophy, spinocerebellar ataxia type 1, and other disorders. Previously, the significance of *anticipation* (defined as the worsening of a disease phenotype over generations within a family) was uncertain, and molecular documentation was lacking for the concept of premutation. Expanding triplet mutations have demonstrated that premutations can exist as modest expansions of triplet repeats (perhaps including minor sequence differences from stable alleles). These premutations do not themselves cause clear phenotypic effects but are prone to further expansion and causation of disease. The phenomenon of anticipation is due to increasing size of repeats, which causes earlier onset of disease or a more severe phenotype.

Recognition that individuals can inherit two copies of part or all of a chromosome from one parent and no copy from the other parent is also a rare departure from Mendelian inheritance. This phenomenon of *uniparental disomy* is relatively rare but contributes to the occurrence of the Prader-Willi and Angelman syndromes. The significance of uniparental disomy is in large part due to the existence of *imprinting*, whereby the maternal copy of a gene and the paternal copy of a gene are differentially expressed. The copies of the genes for insulin-like growth factor 2 (*IFG2*) and small nuclear ribonucleopolypeptide N (*SNRPN*) that are inherited from the father are expressed, while the copies inherited from the mother are repressed in mouse and human; in contrast, the maternal copy of the H19 gene is expressed, and the paternal copy is repressed in mouse and human. The gene(s) causing the Prader-Willi syndrome appear to be expressed from the paternal copy, while that causing Angelman's syndrome is expressed from the maternal copy. Patterns of inheritance for diseases involving mutations in imprinted genes deviate from usual Mendelian patterns (see "Disorders of Imprinted Genes," below).

Further deviations from simple Mendelian rules probably exist. *Transmission ratio distortion* (or meiotic drive) describes the circumstance where there is preferential transmission of an allele to the offspring from a heterozygous parent. This phenomenon is well documented for various alleles at the *T* locus in the mouse and may occur in humans.

AUTOSOMAL DOMINANT DISORDERS Dominant diseases are manifest in the heterozygous state, i.e., when only one abnormal gene (*mutant allele*) is present and the corresponding allele on the homologous chromosome is normal. By definition, the gene responsible for an autosomal dominant disorder must be located on one of the 22 autosomes; hence, both males and females can be affected. Since alleles segregate independently at meiosis, there is a 1 in 2 chance that the offspring of an affected heterozygote will inherit the mutant allele.

Figure 65-17 shows typical pedigrees involving an autosomal dominant trait: (1) each affected individual has an affected parent (unless the condition arose by a new mutation in the sperm or ovum that formed the individual or unless the mutant allele is present but without phenotypic effect in the affected parent as discussed under "Penetrance and Expressivity," below); (2) an affected individual has a 50 percent probability of passing the trait to each offspring; (3) normal children of an affected individual have only normal offspring; (4) males and females are affected in equal proportions except in sex-limited disorders; (5) each sex is equally likely to transmit the condition to male and female offspring, including male-to-male transmission; and (6) vertical transmission of the condition through successive generations occurs, when the trait does not impair reproductive capacity. Autosomal dominant disorders can be inherited in a sex-limited or sex-modified pattern, as exemplified by breast/ovarian cancer in women and by familial male precocious puberty in boys.

Dominant New Mutations For autosomal dominant diseases, a certain proportion of cases are due to new mutations rather than to inherited mutations. Since a rough estimate of the frequency of mutation is 5×10^{-6} mutations per gene per generation and since there are two copies of each autosomal gene, one would expect that about 1 in 100,000 newborn persons possess a new mutation at any given genetic locus. Many of these mutations either do not impair the function of the gene product or involve a recessive effect, so that the mutation is clinically silent. Others, however, give rise to dominant traits. The parent in whose germ cells the mutation arose is clinically normal, and the sibs of the affected individual are usually normal since the mutation affects one or only a few germ cells. Given the nature of germ-cell proliferation, mutations are most likely to occur at one of the later cell divisions, but multiple mutant gametes may be descended from a single mutational event in some cases (gonadal mosaicism). Given these factors, and since humans have few offspring, the probability of a recurrence of the disorder among the siblings of an individual with a new mutation generally is quite low. The presence of the identical mutation in siblings when neither parent has the mutation in somatic cells can occur through gonadal mosaicism and will cause a higher recurrence risk in siblings, as has been well documented for osteogenesis imperfecta and Duchenne's muscular dystrophy. It is possible to assess the proportion of gonadal mosaicism by molecular analysis of sperm in some cases. Individuals affected with new dominant mutations are able to transmit the disease, and each offspring is at 50 percent risk for the condition.

The proportion of dominant disorders due to new mutations is inversely proportional to the effect on biologic fitness (Table 65-5).

A

B

New mutant

■ , ● Affected male, female

□ , ○ Unaffected male, female

FIGURE 65-17 Pedigree pattern for an autosomal dominant trait. Note the *vertical* pattern of inheritance; compare new mutation and inherited pedigrees.

Table 65-5

Approximate Percentage of Patients Affected by New Germline Mutations in Some Autosomal Dominant Disorders

Disorder	Percentage
Achondroplasia	80
Tuberous sclerosis	80
Neurofibromatosis	40
Marfan's syndrome	30
Polyposis of the colon	30
Myotonic dystrophy	Anticipation*
Huntington's disease	Anticipation*
Adult polycystic kidney disease	1
Familial hypercholesterolemia	Very low
BRCA1 breast cancer	Very low

* Anticipation is intended to indicate a multistep process from wild type to premutation to mutation. A very high percentage of cases are inherited.

The term *biologic fitness* refers to the ability of an individual to produce children who survive to adult life and reproduce. In the extreme case, if a dominant mutation causes infertility, then all observed cases, of necessity, represent new mutations, and there would be no evidence of familial transmission. Thanatophoric dysplasia represents such a disorder. In moderately severe disorders, as in tuberous sclerosis, biologic fitness is about 20 percent of normal, and about 80 percent of cases are due to new mutations. In disorders such as familial hypercholesterolemia, in which there is little, if any, reduction in biologic fitness, almost all affected persons have a pedigree showing classic vertical transmission. The incidence of a dominant disorder is dependent both on the biologic fitness and on the mutation frequency for the locus, which is widely variable. Although the proportion of cases due to new mutation is directly related to biologic fitness, genetic counseling and reproductive planning now can alter this proportion.

Many new mutations occur in the germ cells of fathers who are of advanced age. For example, in Marfan's syndrome, the average age of fathers of sporadic or "new mutation" cases (37 years) is in excess of the age of fathers who transmit the disease as an inherited mutation (30 years). The paternal age effect is also prominent in achondroplasia. There is evidence that the mutations associated with advanced paternal age are frequently point mutations, often C to T transitions at CG dinucleotides. Differences in mutation rates for male and female gametes are discussed below under "X-linked New Mutations and Heterozygote Detection."

Before one concludes that a dominant disorder in a patient with unaffected parents is the result of a new mutation, it is important to consider two other possibilities: (1) the gene may be carried by one parent, in whom the mutant allele is not penetrant; and (2) nonpaternity may have occurred (i.e., the father is someone other than the putative father), as happens in 3 to 5 percent of randomly studied children in many cultures.

Penetrance and Expressivity These terms are frequently the subject of confusion and slight variations in usage. In the medical context, *penetrance* is the proportion of individuals with a given genotype who present with *any* phenotypic features of the disorder (i.e., it is an all-or-none phenomenon). Although in one sense penetrance may vary with age, as in the case of Huntington's disease, variation in age of onset is most often considered as an aspect of variable expression. In some cases, penetrance depends on environmental exposure, as in glucose-6-phosphate dehydrogenase deficiency. In the autosomal dominant context, it is instructive to consider the concept of penetrance from a counseling perspective and in terms of molecular diagnosis. Penetrance is the question at issue when the apparently unaffected offspring of an individual with a dominant disorder wish to know if they carry the mutant gene and if they are at risk of having affected offspring. The mutant gene is not penetrant if an individual carrying the mutant gene shows absolutely no phenotypic effects. In molecular terms, the presence or absence of the mutant gene can be determined with appropriate diagnostic tests, and a person without the mutant gene can be distinguished from one carrying the impenetrant mutant gene. Clinically, definition of penetrance often depends on the quality of clinical methodologies; for example, magnetic resonance imaging might demonstrate findings not previously recognizable. In the medical context, the gene is usually considered penetrant if diagnostic abnormalities can be demonstrated even if the individual is asymptomatic. In the biologic context, the gene can be considered penetrant if it affects the function of the individual.

Expressivity, or *variability in clinical expression*, describes the range of phenotypic effects in individuals carrying a given mutation. This variability can include the type and severity of symptoms and the age of onset of symptoms. Variability in clinical expression is illustrated dramatically in multiple endocrine neoplasia, type 1. Patients in the same family with the same abnormal gene may have hyperplasia or neoplasia of one or all of a wide variety of endocrine tissues, including the pancreas, parathyroid glands, pituitary gland, or adipose tissue. The resulting manifestations are extremely diverse; different members of the same family may develop peptic ulcers, hypoglycemia, kidney stones, or pituitary tumors. In the case of some dominant disorders characterized by tumor formation, random second mutations in tumor suppressor genes may explain some of the clinical variability.

Variation in age of onset is seen in disorders such as Huntington's disease and adult polycystic kidney disease. These disorders often do not become symptomatic until adult life, even though the mutant gene is present throughout life. Whether variation in age of onset is considered as a form of variation in expression is somewhat arbitrary. In one sense, it cannot be said that the mutant gene was impenetrant in an individual until the person has had a complete evaluation and has died from other causes. Lack of penetrance can be considered as the absolute mildest end of the spectrum of expression so that no phenotypic effects are observed. In the counseling context, variation in expression, as distinct from penetrance, is the point in question when an individual with a dominant disorder wishes to know whether an offspring who carries the mutation would have mild or severe symptoms. In molecular terms, analysis of the single gene locus will not answer this question (i.e., predict variation in expression within a family) but can determine whether the mutant gene is present and not penetrant.

At least three factors underlie lack of penetrance and variability in expression: (1) the effects of genes at the same or other loci, (2) exogenous or environmental factors, and (3) stochastic factors. Effects within the same gene locus can be seen with mutations in α-spectrin, where a polymorphism in the level of gene expression affects the phenotype. The low-expression allele moderates the phenotype of hereditary elliptocytosis when in *cis* with the mutation but worsens the phenotype when in *trans* in a heterozygote for the mutation. In the case of cystic fibrosis, the phenotypic severity of the R117H mutation varies through a *cis* effect on the level of functional mRNA due to a splice junction polymorphism that influences skipping of an exon. The genotype at the α-globin locus that affects the sickle cell anemia phenotype and various loci that affect the monogenic hyperlipidemias are examples of effects by genes at other loci. The phenotypes in the monogenic hyperlipidemias, the porphyrias, and hemochromatosis can be affected by diet, alcohol use, smoking, and exercise. The effects of stochastic factors are exemplified by variability in the severity and distribution of lesions among identical twins with retinoblastoma, neurofibromatosis, or tuberous sclerosis. Other examples of stochastic events that can affect phenotypes are differences in random X chromosome inactivation among identical twin female heterozygotes for an X-linked disorder and somatic rearrangements and mutations associated with expression of immunoglobulins and T cell receptors. Although the issues of penetrance and expressivity are often defined in the context of autosomal dominant disorders, these principles are relevant to chromosomal disorders, autosomal recessive and X-linked disorders, and complex disease traits as well.

Biochemical Basis of Dominant Alleles The biochemical and/or molecular defects causing dominant disorders such as familial hypercholesterolemia, amyloidosis, hereditary spherocytosis, osteogenesis imperfecta, hereditary retinoblastoma, neurofibromatosis, Marfan's syndrome, and Huntington's disease have been determined. A number

of mechanisms can account for an abnormal phenotype in the presence of one mutant gene. One mechanism is *haploinsufficiency*—meaning that a half-normal amount of gene product is insufficient to maintain a normal phenotype (i.e., the process is sensitive to reduced dosage). This is true, for example, when gene products regulate complex metabolic pathways, such as membrane receptors and rate-limiting enzymes in biosynthetic pathways under feedback control (e.g., familial hypercholesterolemia and dominant porphyrias). In other cases a dosage effect due to gene duplication can cause a dominant phenotype, as in the case of the common mutation in type 1A Charcot-Marie-Tooth disease where triploid dosage for the *PMP22* gene causes the condition. This means the organism is sensitive to 150 percent of the normal level of gene product. Another mechanism involves abnormalities of structural proteins where a complex network of direct protein interactions is involved (e.g., collagens in osteogenesis imperfecta and erythrocyte cytoskeleton proteins in spherocytosis and elliptocytosis). Dominant negative mutations are instances where the molecules of mutant gene product interfere with the function of the normal gene products. Many mutations involving structural proteins have a dominant negative component, and some missense mutations may be more deleterious than null mutations, as in the case of osteogenesis imperfecta. Dominant phenotypic effects can also occur when the remaining normal copy of a gene is mutated at a single-cell level so that both copies of the locus are inactivated (e.g., hereditary retinoblastoma). These defects may be considered dominant at the pedigree level and recessive at the single-cell level. Conceptually, it is useful to distinguish dominant mutations that generate products with new or neomorphic biologic properties and cause a harmful effect (e.g., amyloidosis) from those due to deficiency of normal gene product (e.g., familial hypercholesterolemia and porphyrias). In the former group, restoration of a normal level of gene product does not negate the effect of the mutant gene.

Disorders of Imprinted Genes If an autosomal locus is imprinted such that it is expressed from one allele and repressed from the other, there is no question of a dominant or recessive effect since the gene is functionally hemizygous. The familial pattern is more similar to dominant pedigrees since the disorder may occur over multiple generations (i.e., show vertical transmission; Fig. 65-18). There are good examples of large pedigrees with inherited phenotypes involving imprinted genes. Hereditary paragangliomas is a disorder in which the phenotype is expressed only when the mutant allele is inherited from the father (Fig. 65-18). In contrast, Angelman's syndrome is expressed only when the mutant allele is inherited from the mother (Fig. 65-18).

AUTOSOMAL RECESSIVE DISORDERS Autosomal recessive conditions are clinically apparent only in the homozygous or compound heterozygous state, i.e., when both alleles at a particular genetic locus are mutant. It is useful to distinguish phenotypic "homozygotes" (perhaps better referred to as affected individuals), in whom both copies of the gene are defective, from molecular homozygotes, in whom DNA analysis reveals identical mutations in both copies of the gene. By definition, the gene responsible for an autosomal recessive disorder must be located on one of the 22 autosomes so that both males and females can be affected.

Figure 65-19 shows two pedigrees for families with an autosomal recessive trait. Monoplex families (Fig. 65-19A) are the most common, but families with multiple affected individuals occur. The following features are characteristic: (1) the parents are clinically normal; (2) only sibs are affected, and vertical transmission usually does not occur; (3) males and females are affected in equal proportions, except for sex-limited effects; and (4) consanguinity can be a contributing factor.

The variety of recessive alleles and the requirement for two abnormal copies for clinical expression create special conditions for autosomal recessive inheritance: (1) the more infrequent the mutant gene in the population, the stronger the likelihood that affected individuals are the product of consanguineous matings (see "Consanguinity," below); (2) if both parents are carriers for the same autosomal recessive

FIGURE 65-18 Idealized pedigrees for disorders involving imprinted genes. Filled symbols indicate individuals carrying the mutation and affected by the disorder. Symbols with a solid dot in the center indicate individuals who are asymptomatic but carry the mutation on the silenced allele. Open symbols indicate individuals who do not carry the mutation and are asymptomatic. The upper pedigree depicts a maternally expressed gene as in the case of Angelman's syndrome, while the lower pedigree depicts a paternally expressed gene as in the case of hereditary paragangliomas. *(Adapted from Sapienza and Hall, in Scriver et al, with permission.)*

gene, the probability for disease in offspring is 0.25, for a heterozygote (carrier) it is 0.50, and for a normal (noncarrier) offspring it is 0.25; (3) if an affected individual mates with a heterozygote, there is a 50 percent probability of disease for each child, and a pedigree simulating dominant inheritance may result; and (4) if two individuals with the same recessive disease mate, all the children will be affected.

The clinical features of autosomal recessive disorders tend to be more uniform than those of dominant diseases, and recessive disorders are more commonly diagnosed in children. Many autosomal recessive disorders present or cause major morbidity in adulthood, including hemochromatosis (see Chap. 342), α_1-antitrypsin deficiency, hemoglobinopathies, some forms of hyperlipidemia (see Chap. 341), and late-onset lysosomal storage diseases (see Chap. 346).

Since the probability is that only one in four individuals in a sibship will be affected, most cases of autosomal recessive disease may occur as isolated individuals, particularly when small families are common. Consider, for example, 16 families in which both parents are heterozygous for the same recessive disorder, such as cystic fibrosis. If each family has 2 children, the probability is that 9 of the 16 families will have no affected children, 6 will have 1 affected and 1 normal child, and only 1 of the 16 families will have 2 affected children. Because of the tendency toward small families, physicians usually see isolated cases of a recessive disease without an affected sib to alert them to the possibility of a genetic disorder. Fortunately, because of the relatively uniform manifestations of recessive disorders and because many conditions can be diagnosed directly by biochemical or molecular tests, the diagnosis of a genetic disease can frequently be made even when no other members of a family are clinically affected. Autosomal recessive disorders can be inherited in a sex-limited manner as exemplified by steroid 5α-reductase 2 deficiency, where only 46,XY males are phenotypically abnormal.

Biochemical Basis of Recessive Alleles The biochemical defects underlying many autosomal recessive disorders have been identified. Most alleles are complete or partial loss-of-function mutations, often involving enzymatic proteins. In these conditions, recessive inheritance occurs because a mutation that impairs the catalytic activity of an enzyme usually does not impair the health of a heterozygote. Regulatory mechanisms function to avert clinical consequences of this 50 percent deficiency, and so heterozygotes for enzyme defects usually are clinically normal as discussed above. On the other hand, when an individual inherits abnormal alleles at both loci specifying an enzyme, a disease results.

Many of the enzyme deficiencies in recessive diseases involve enzymes in catabolic pathways, frequently enzymes that degrade organic molecules in the diet, such as galactose (galactosemia, see Chap. 349), phenylalanine (phenylketonuria, see Chap. 349), and phytanic acid (Refsum's syndrome). When deficiency affects an acid hydrolase (*lysosomal storage disorders*), the substrate, usually a complex lipid or polysaccharide, accumulates within swollen lysosomes. Examples of such lysosomal diseases include the mucopolysaccharidoses such as Hurler's syndrome (α-iduronidase deficiency) and the sphingolipidoses such as Gaucher's disease (glucocerebrosidase deficiency).

Population Genetics of Recessive Alleles In general, recessive diseases are rare because the reduced biologic fitness of homozygotes serves to remove the mutant gene from the population. A few lethal recessive disorders, such as cystic fibrosis, thalassemia, and sickle cell anemia are common. To explain this paradox, it has been postulated that the biologic fitness of heterozygotes is greater than that of noncarriers for these genes. In such a case, the frequency of the gene in the population depends on the balance between the increased fitness of the relatively numerous heterozygotes and the reduced fitness of the less common homozygotes. A small selective advantage of the heterozygote in terms of reproductive advantage results in a high gene frequency and hence a high birth frequency of homozygotes, even when the disease is lethal. Thus, about 1 in 25 Caucasians is heterozygous (a carrier) for the genetically lethal disease cystic fibrosis, and the disease occurs in about 1 in 2500 Caucasian births. To maintain such a high gene frequency, heterozygotes for cystic fibrosis may have a selective advantage over noncarriers, and this advantage may involve protection against death from childhood diarrhea. Alternatively, there could be a slight transmission ratio distortion (meiotic drive), i.e., gametes carrying the mutant gene could have a slightly greater probability of achieving fertilization compared to gametes with the normal gene, or disorders might achieve a high frequency without a selective advantage, i.e., by chance. Haplotype data indicate that chromosomes carrying the common ΔF508 allele for cystic fibrosis are descended from a single mutational event, but this does not explain why the mutant gene is so frequent. In sickle cell anemia, another recessive disorder with high frequency among certain populations, heterozygotes have increased resistance to falciparum malaria.

FIGURE 65-19 Pedigree pattern for an autosomal recessive trait. Note the *horizontal* pattern of inheritance and consanguinity in the multiplex pedigree (B) in comparison to the more common monoplex pedigree (A). *(From Scriver et al, with permission.)*

Consanguinity By definition, a recessive disease requires the inheritance of a mutant allele at the same genetic locus from each parent. When the genes are rare, the likelihood of unrelated parents being carriers for the same defect is small. If the parents have a common ancestor who carried a recessive gene, the likelihood that two of the descendants inherited the same allele is enhanced. The less frequent the recessive gene, the stronger the likelihood that an affected individual is the product of a consanguineous mating. On the other hand, when recessive genes are common in the population, the likelihood of two unrelated parents being carriers is great enough to minimize the role of consanguinity. For common traits such as sickle cell anemia, phenylketonuria, cystic fibrosis, and Tay-Sachs disease consanguinity is uncommon in the parents.

Recessive New Mutations New mutations for recessive disorders can rarely be identified because such mutations usually generate asymptomatic heterozygotes. Only generations later will the descendants of individuals with that mutation mate with other heterozygotes with a mutation at the same locus. The selective pressure to eliminate deleterious recessive traits from the population is low because these traits are easily passed on in heterozygous form. Most recessive diseases appear to be due to mutations that occurred many generations earlier, as indicated from haplotype analysis of mutations causing phenylketonuria, β-thalassemia, sickle cell anemia, Tay Sachs disease, cystic fibrosis, and other disorders.

X-LINKED DISORDERS The genes responsible for X-linked disorders are located on the X chromosome, and the clinical risks are different for the two sexes. Since a female has two X chromosomes, she may be either heterozygous or homozygous for a mutant gene, and the mutant allele may demonstrate either recessive or dominant expression. Expression in females is often variable and influenced by random X-chromosome inactivation. Males, on the other hand, have only one X chromosome, so they are more likely to display the full phenotype, regardless of whether the mutation produces a recessive or dominant allele in the female. Thus, the terms *X-linked dominant* or *X-linked recessive* refer only to the expression of the mutations in women.

The distinction of dominant and recessive X-linked disorders is complicated by the effect of X-chromosome inactivation. In both ornithine transcarbamoylase deficiency, often described as X-linked dominant, and Fabry's disease, often described as X-linked recessive, phenotypic abnormalities are relatively frequent in heterozygotes. Since there is no clear convention, it may be best to consider such disorders as simply X-linked without a dominant or recessive designation. The recessive or dominant descriptors are more useful for X-linked disorders in which heterozygotes are consistently asymptomatic (e.g., X-linked recessive Hunter's mucopolysaccharidosis) or consistently symptomatic in a manner similar to hemizygous males (e.g., X-linked dominant hypophosphatemic rickets).

An important feature of all X-linked inheritance is the absence of male-to-male (i.e., father-to-son) transmission of the trait. This follows because a male contributes his Y chromosome to his son and does not contribute an X chromosome. On the other hand, since a male contributes his sole X chromosome to each daughter, all daughters of a male with an X-linked disorder will inherit the mutant allele.

The pedigrees in Fig. 65-20 illustrate some of the characteristic features of X-linked inheritance. (1) In contrast to the vertical distribution in dominant traits (parents and children affected) and the horizontal distribution in autosomal recessive traits (sibs affected), the pedigree pattern in X-linked recessive traits tends to be oblique; that is, the trait occurs in the maternal uncles of affected males and in male cousins who are descended from the mother's sisters who are carriers (Fig. 65-20A). (2) Male offspring of carrier females have a 50 percent chance of being affected. (3) All female offspring of affected males are carriers, and affected males do not transmit the disease to their sons. (4) Unaffected males do not transmit the trait to any offspring. (5) Affected homozygous females occur only when an affected male mates with a carrier female.

Examples of X-linked recessive disorders in humans include the Lesch-Nyhan syndrome, glucose-6-phosphate dehydrogenase deficiency, testicular feminization, and Hunter's mucopolysaccharidosis.

Affected hemizygous male
Asymptomatic heterozygous female
Symptomatic heterozygous female
Unaffected male
Noncarrier female

FIGURE 65-20 Pedigree pattern for an X-linked trait. *A*. Note the *oblique* pattern of inheritance. *B*. Note the occurrence of symptomatic and asymptomatic heterozygous females in the same pedigree. Heterozygotes are consistently asymptomatic in some disorders (recessive) and are variably symptomatic in other disorders (see text). *C*. New mutations can give rise to either affected males or heterozygous females. (*From Scriver et al, with permission.*)

Color blindness is a frequent X-linked recessive trait (occurring in about 8 percent of white males), so that the occurrence of homozygous color-blind females is no rarity. A pedigree for an X-linked disorder with variable symptomatology in females is depicted in Fig. 65-20*B*, and X-linked disease on the basis of new mutation is shown by the pedigrees in Fig. 65-20*C* (see "X-linked New Mutations and Heterozygote Detection," below).

X-linked dominant inheritance is illustrated by the pedigree in Fig. 65-21. (1) Females are affected about twice as often as males, (2) an affected female has a 50 percent probability of transmitting the disorder to her sons or daughters, (3) an affected male transmits the disorder to all of his daughters and to none of his sons, and (4) the phenotype may be more variable and less severe in heterozygous affected females than in hemizygous affected males. One common trait, the Xg (a+) blood group, is inherited as an X-linked dominant trait, as are a few diseases, such as hypophosphatemic rickets.

Some rare conditions may be inherited as X-linked dominant traits in which there is lethality in the hemizygous male (Fig. 65-22). (1) The disorder occurs only in females who are heterozygous for the mutant gene; (2) an affected mother has a 50 percent probability of transmitting the trait to her daughters; (3) an increased frequency of spontaneous abortions occurs in affected women, the abortions representing affected male fetuses. An example of a condition that is transmitted by this mode of inheritance is incontinentia pigmenti. Some X-linked disorders are lethal in utero in males and impair reproduction in females so that a condition occurs primarily or exclusively

Affected hemizygous male
Affected heterozygous female
Unaffected male, female

FIGURE 65-21 Pedigree pattern of an X-linked dominant trait. (*From Scriver et al, with permission.*)

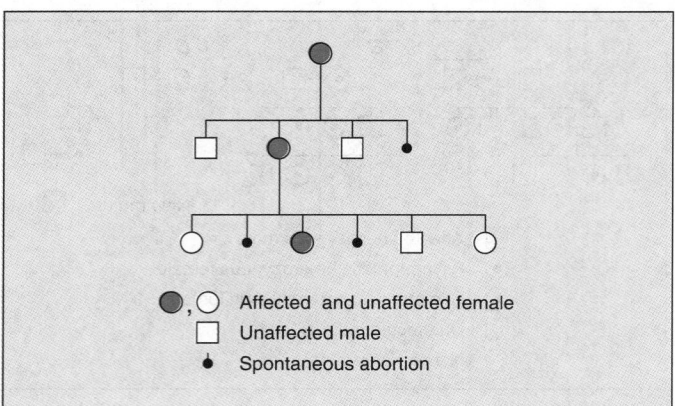

FIGURE 65-22 Pedigree pattern of an X-linked dominant trait lethal in the hemizygous male. *(From Scriver et al, with permission.)*

as a sporadic disorder in females due to new mutation. Aicardi's syndrome, Goltz's syndrome, and Rett's syndrome may represent such examples.

Genes in the pseudoautosomal region of the X chromosome have a homologous copy on the Y chromosome, and the pattern of inheritance of these genes is indistinguishable from autosomal circumstances, as the term implies.

X Inactivation   Phenotypic expression of X-linked traits in females is greatly influenced by the phenomenon of random X-chromosome inactivation. Early in embryonic development, one of the two X chromosomes in each somatic cell of a female is randomly inactivated so that for each cell there is an equal probability that the paternal or maternal X chromosome will be inactivated. The inactivation is stable so that all progeny of the initial cell inherit the same active and inactive X chromosomes. Thus, each female is a mosaic; on the average, half of the cells express the X chromosome of the father, and half express the X chromosome of the mother. If a mutation in a gene is carried on one of the X chromosomes, about one-half of the cells in each tissue will be normal and the other half will manifest the mutant phenotype. Chance or preferential survival of one clone of cells may alter these proportions in any given individual. Depending on the proportions of mutant and normal X chromosomes that are active in each tissue, a genetically heterozygous female may be clinically normal or have mild or severe manifestations of disease.

In each female cell the nonfunctional X chromosome can be identified as a condensed clump of chromatin—the Barr body. The inactive X chromosome is late replicating, and its DNA is more highly methylated. Methylation of DNA is thought to play a role in maintenance of X inactivation. The XIST gene [for X (inactive) specific transcripts] is transcribed exclusively from inactive X chromosomes and is required for X inactivation, but the molecular mechanism of X inactivation is not understood.

Random X inactivation is the most important determinant of expression in females for many X-linked disorders. Many individuals are asymptomatic, some have mild symptoms, and others have severe manifestations. The frequency of detectable phenotypic alterations depends on how carefully heterozygotes are examined and, in some instances, on the age at examination. Ornithine transcarbamylase deficiency exhibits variable phenotypic expression in heterozygotes. Many heterozygotes are asymptomatic; some have minimal protein intolerance; and others experience intermittent hyperammonemic coma, occasionally with fatal outcome. Hemizygous affected males are more consistently and more seriously symptomatic than are heterozygous females. Other examples in which clinical expression may occur in females include Duchenne's muscular dystrophy, hemophilia A, and Fabry's disease. In some cases the biochemical defect behaves in a cell autonomous fashion resulting in a mosaic tissue pattern, as

in choroideremia and certain forms of X-linked ocular albinism. If the defect involves a product that is secreted by cells, the phenotypic effect is an average for the relevant somatic tissues, as for factor VIII levels in hemophilia A. As already discussed under "X-Linked Disorders," it is preferable to describe these conditions as X-linked without applying the dominant or recessive descriptor since the literature is inconsistent.

X-Linked New Mutations and Heterozygote Detection   Identification of new mutations in X-linked genes is an important counseling issue in families ascertained because of an isolated affected male (monoplex families, Fig. 65-20C). In these families, the mother may be a noncarrier and may have contributed an egg with a new mutation. The father cannot contribute the new mutation, since he contributes a Y chromosome. Alternatively, the mother may be a carrier who received a gamete with a preexisting mutation from her mother or with a new mutation from either her father or her mother. If the new mutation rate for male gametes is greater than for female gametes, as is established in some instances, then a larger fraction of mothers of isolated male cases will be carriers. As formulated by Haldane, assuming that affected males do not reproduce, approximately two-thirds of mothers of isolated male cases are expected to be carriers, if the mutation rates for male and female gametes are identical. This proportion increases if the mutation rate for male gametes exceeds that for female gametes, a fact that is often ignored. Mutation rates for male and female gametes are similar for Duchenne's muscular dystrophy (a disorder predominantly due to large deletions), and the mutation rates for male gametes are higher for hemophilia A and B (disorders largely due to point mutations). Thus, a larger proportion of mothers of isolated hemophilia cases are carriers than are mothers of isolated Duchenne's muscular dystrophy cases.

Heterozygous females can sometimes be detected using biochemical methods, as in the Lesch-Nyhan syndrome, Fabry's disease, Hunter's syndrome, hemophilia A, hemophilia B, ornithine transcarbamylase deficiency, and Duchenne's muscular dystrophy. These biochemical methods are rarely completely accurate because random X inactivation may lead to a relatively normal biochemical result. Accuracy may be increased by sampling relatively clonal cells such as hair roots or cloned skin fibroblasts. Molecular methods can circumvent the problems of biochemical analysis of the gene product when the mutation can be detected directly.

Y-LINKED DISORDERS   Only a few genes are known on the Y chromosome, the gene encoding the sex-region determining Y (SRY) factor (also called the testis determining factor, TDF) being the most salient. Translocations between X and Y chromosomes can result in XY females where the Y chromosome is missing the SRY gene. The reciprocal situation exists in which XX males possess an X chromosome that carries a copy of the SRY gene. Point mutations that impair the function of the SRY factor can also result in XY females. For Y-linked genes, fathers pass the trait to all sons and to no daughters. The male phenotype is the most obvious Y-linked trait. The number of Y-linked disorders is likely to remain limited because of the small number of genes on the Y chromosome, but as many as 18 percent of men with severe oligospermia/azoospermia have microdeletions of the long arm of the Y chromosome that involve the azoospermia factor (AZF) gene.

MITOCHONDRIAL INHERITANCE   There are many genetic disorders affecting mitochondrial function. Mitochondria contain a 16.6-kb circular DNA genome that encodes the ribososomal RNAs and transfer RNAs for the distinct mitochondrial protein synthesis. This genome also encodes some of the proteins essential for oxidative phosphorylation, but many of the mitochondrial proteins are encoded in the nuclear genome, synthesized in the cytoplasm, and transported into mitochondria. Genetic disorders affecting mitochondria can be divided into two classes: mutations in the nuclear genome and those in the mitochondrial genome. For mutations in the nuclear genome, the inheritance is as for other nuclear genes, but mutations in the mitochondrial genome display a distinct pattern of inheritance.

There is wide variation in the number of mitochondria per cell and in the number of mitochondrial DNA genomes per mitochondrion (typically 2 to 10) so that each cell contains thousands of copies of mitochondrial DNA. Mitochondrial DNA is maternally inherited, with 200,000 to 300,000 copies per egg and insignificant contributions from sperm. This means that all individuals inherit their mitochondrial genome from their mothers. If a pathologic mutation is present in the mitochondrial genome, this typically affects some proportion of the mitochondrial genomes per cell, and this heterogeneity of mitochondrial DNA within a single cell and within an individual is referred to as *heteroplasmy*. If a woman carries a mutation in the mitochondrial genome, she will potentially transmit this mutation to all of her children, while a man with such a mutation will not transmit the trait to any of his children. This can give rise to a typical pattern of inheritance, with vertical transmission and the disease trait being passed to most or all of the offspring of affected women. The proportion of mutant to wild-type mitochondria may vary among individuals in a pedigree, leading to phenotypic heterogeneity. Disorders of the mitochondrial genome include chronic progressive external ophthalmoplegia, the Kearns-Sayre syndrome, Leber's hereditary optic neuropathy, myoclonic epilepsy, several forms of mitochondral myopathy, and other disorders (see Scriver et al.).

GENETIC HETEROGENEITY

Genetic heterogeneity can result from different mutations at a single locus (*allelic heterogeneity*) or from mutations at different genetic loci (*nonallelic* or *locus heterogeneity*). For example, Charcot-Marie-Tooth neurogenic atrophy, congenital sensorineural deafness, and retinitis pigmentosa all have autosomal dominant, autosomal recessive, and X-linked forms. Nonallelic heterogeneity is responsible in many cases, but allelic mutation also can account for dominant and recessive variation at a single locus. A similar bleeding disorder can be caused by mutations at either of two loci on the X chromosome, one causing deficiency of factor VIII (classic hemophilia, hemophilia A) and the other a deficiency of factor IX (Christmas disease, hemophilia B). Hereditary methemoglobinemia, once regarded as a homogeneous clinical entity, is the result of at least 10 different mutations at three distinct gene loci: two at the locus coding for the α chain of hemoglobin, three at the locus that encodes the β chain of hemoglobin, and at least five at the NADH dehydrogenase locus. Most hereditary diseases are genetically heterogeneous.

The extent of allelic heterogeneity is particularly impressive. Indeed, a large number of mutations have been characterized as causing hemoglobinopathies and thalassemias, cystic fibrosis, familial hypercholesterolemia, phenylketonuria, and breast cancer via the BRCA1 locus. A great deal of clinical heterogeneity is due to different mutations at a single locus. With detailed molecular characterization, many patients with autosomal recessive disorders are compound heterozygotes at a molecular level. Compound heterozygotes have different mutations in the mutant alleles, as exemplified by SC hemoglobinopathy or cystic fibrosis due to a ΔF508/G542X genotype. Exceptions to this generalization occur when a patient is the product of a consanguineous mating and when particular mutant alleles are present in high frequency in the population, e.g., sickle cell anemia with SS genotype or cystic fibrosis with a ΔF508/ΔF508 genotype.

Variation in manifestations due to allelic heterogeneity is particularly important. For example, Hurler's and Scheie's mucopolysaccharidoses were thought to be different genetic conditions based on the severe, lethal phenotype in Hurler's disease and the milder phenotype of bone and joint disease in Scheie's disease. In fact, these conditions are both due to deficiency of L-iduronidase. Similarly, the severe Duchenne's muscular dystrophy and milder Becker's muscular dystrophy are allelic disorders, each of which can be caused by gene deletions, most often out of frame for Duchenne's and in frame for Becker's. The classic and attenuated forms of adenomatous polyposis coli have about 15 years' difference in the age of onset, so that the attenuated disorder has minimal impact on reproduction, and unrecognized alleles of this type may be a significant contributor to the risk of colon cancer. Additional examples of different clinical manifestations due to allelic heterogeneity are found throughout genetics. In many instances a

classic phenotype occurs when no functional gene product is produced, and there is frequently a continuum of milder expression arising from mutations that partially impair the function of the gene product. Compound heterozygotes contribute to the complexity of the clinical continuum. At the mild end of the continuum, mutant alleles encode a product that leads to a nearly normal clinical phenotype or to a phenotype that is normal under most environmental circumstances. This continuum includes detectable biochemical variation that is ordinarily not associated with clinical effect. Obviously the amount of functional gene product required to prevent clinical symptoms depends on other genetic and environmental factors. As an example, an individual with "benign" methylmalonic acidemia is at risk during major catabolic disorders, so that the benign designation is merely conditional. This type of genetic heterogeneity forms a part of the border between monogenic disorders and multifactorial diseases.

COMPLEX DISEASE TRAITS

The common chronic diseases of adults (such as essential hypertension, gout, coronary heart disease, diabetes mellitus, peptic ulcer disease, and schizophrenia) and the common birth defects (such as cleft lip and palate, spina bifida, and congenital heart disease) have long been known to "run in families," indicating a genetic contribution to etiology. These disorders are *complex disease traits* or *multifactorial genetic diseases*. It is useful to recognize the heterogeneity of etiology of such disorders. For cleft lip and palate, some cases are due to single gene defects, some are due to chromosome abnormalities, and most appear to be due to multiple genetic and environmental factors. The concept of complex disease traits implies that in most instances multiple factors enter into the cause of a *single case*. Similarly, the etiology of coronary artery disease is heterogeneous; a small proportion of cases result from single gene defects (e.g., familial hypercholesterolemia), whereas most are multifactorial (i.e., multiple factors contribute to the etiology of individual cases). Complex disease traits imply the interaction of multiple genes and multiple environmental factors in the etiology of individual cases to cause familial aggregation without a simple Mendelian pattern of inheritance.

In complex disease traits, *constitutional (polygenic) components* consist of multiple genes at independent loci whose effects interact in a cumulative fashion. An individual who inherits a particular combination of these genes has a relative risk that may combine with an *environmental component* to cross a "threshold" of biologic significance so that the individual is affected with a disease. For another individual in the same family to express the same syndrome, a similar combination of genes would present similar risks. Since sibs share half of their genes, the probability of a sib inheriting the same combination of genes is $(1/2)^n$, where n is the number of genes required to express the trait (assuming that none of the genes is linked).

The number of genes responsible for polygenic traits is unknown, and risk estimates are based on empiric risk figures (i.e., a direct tally of the proportion of affected relatives in previously reported families). In contrast to the monogenic disorders, in which 25 or 50 percent of the first-degree relatives of an affected proband are at genetic risk, complex disease traits usually affect no more than 5 to 10 percent of first-degree relatives. Moreover, the recurrence risk for these conditions varies from family to family and is influenced by two factors: The greater number of affected relatives and the more severe their disease, the higher the risk to other relatives. For example, the risk of cleft lip in the sibs of a child with unilateral cleft lip is about 2.5 percent, but if the lesion in the index case is bilateral, the risk in the sibs rises to 6 percent.

Multifactorial etiology is thought to be important for many diseases that develop after adolescence, and diseases with later age of onset have decreased heritability on average. For example, in nine multifactorial diseases a decline in the impact of the genes on disease was evident with increasing age.

The hypothesis of a polygenic component in the inheritance of multifactorial diseases is supported by the findings that at least 28 percent of all gene loci harbor polymorphic alleles. This variation in normal genes provides a substrate for variations in response to environmental factors. At present, the genetic loci most strikingly associated with predisposition to specific diseases are those that constitute the major histocompatibility or HLA gene complex located on the short arm of chromosome 6 and consisting of multiple closely linked but distinct loci (A, B, DR, DQ, and DP). The products of these genes are proteins on the surface of cells involved in cellular immune recognition. Each HLA locus in the population consists of multiple alleles, each of which produces an immunologically distinct protein. For example, an individual may inherit any 2 of more than 36 alleles at the HLA-B locus. The inheritance of certain alleles predisposes to the development of certain diseases when the individual is exposed to an environmental challenge (see Chap. 306).

Complex disease traits are heterogeneous in etiology in the sense that the relative contribution of genetic ("risk genes") and environmental factors varies from patient to patient. As discussed above, among common phenotypes that are largely multifactorial, some cases may be due to monogenic or chromosomal abnormalities. For example, although coronary heart disease is usually of complex etiology, about 5 percent of patients with premature myocardial infarctions are heterozygotes for familial hypercholesterolemia, a single-gene disorder that produces atherosclerosis in the absence of an extraordinary environmental factor (see Chap. 341). However, even in a single-gene disorder such as familial hypercholesterolemia, other loci [e.g., the genes for apolipoprotein B, apolipoprotein (a), lipoprotein lipase, and apolipoprotein E] and nongenetic factors (diet and smoking) can influence the phenotype. The complexity of the etiology for coronary artery disease is detailed further in Chap. 242. Multiple genetic and nongenetic factors affect the risk. An appreciation of this etiologic heterogeneity and careful investigation of each patient are necessary prerequisites for counseling families at risk for these disorders.

Methods for unraveling the molecular basis of multifactorial etiology include the analysis of candidate genes using association studies, sib-pair analysis, and other complex strategies. The advantages of focusing on molecular variations that are important in gene function has been emphasized. The complexity of these approaches is daunting, but major loci have been identified for a number of multifactorial diseases, including hypertension (see "Complex Disease Traits," above) and insulin-dependent diabetes mellitus, in which several loci in addition to HLA are involved.

INTERACTION BETWEEN SINGLE GENETIC AND ENVIRONMENTAL FACTORS; PHARMACOGENETICS

In addition to polygenic states, many single-gene mutations can cause abnormal responses to environmental factors, as illustrated by disorders that produce major, often life-threatening idiosyncratic responses to drugs (Table 65-6). There is significant genetic variation is response to drugs such as isoniazid, some beta-adrenergic blockers, and tricyclic antidepressants. Other important interactions between genotype and drugs include glucose-6-phosphate dehydrogenase deficiency, acute intermittent porphyria, hemochromatosis, and muscle diseases with susceptibility to malignant hyperthermia.

Misinterpretation of adverse drug reactions can cause serious harm to patients, and unusual or idiosyncratic reactions should be considered to be genetically determined until proven otherwise. Fortunately, the pharmacogenetic disorders are a group of diseases for which therapy is straightforward: avoidance of the noxious drug by the patient and relatives at risk.

In addition to drugs, environmental factors may aggravate specific genetic traits. Cigarette smoke is particularly deleterious to persons homozygous (and possibly heterozygous) for α_1-antitrypsin deficiency, who are predisposed to the development of emphysema. Patients with xeroderma pigmentosum are sensitive to the ultraviolet exposure of sunlight. Avoidance of milk at an early age prevents the life-threatening complications of galactosemia, and diet is an important variable for most forms of hyperlipidemia. Unfortunately, a modern society is also subjected to an endless array of novel environmental exposures. The current widespread utilization of aspartame is an example of a special risk for persons with phenylketonuria.

TAKING THE FAMILY HISTORY

Recording a *family history* should be a routine part of primary care (Fig. 65-23) and should be performed with special care in patients with a likely genetic disorder. The first step is to obtain certain information on the *proband* or *index case* and on each of the *first-degree relatives* (i.e., the parents, siblings, and offspring of the proband). This information includes the given name, surname, maiden name, birth date

Table 65-6

Examples of Inherited Disorders Involving an Abnormal Response to Drugs

Disorder	Molecular Abnormality	Mode of Inheritance	Frequency	Clinical Effect	Drugs Producing Abnormal Response
Slow inactivation of isoniazid	Isoniazid acetylase in liver	Autosomal recessive	50% of U.S. population	Polyneuritis	Isoniazid, sulfamethazine, sulfamaprine, phenelzine, dapsone, hydralazine
Suxamethonium sensitivity	Pseudocholinesterase in plasma	Autosomal recessive	Several mutant alleles; most common affects 1 in 2500	Apnea	Suxamethonium, succinylcholine
Malignant hyperthermia	Ryanodine receptor	Autosomal dominant	1 in 20,000 anesthetized patients	Severe, hyperpyrexia, muscle rigidity, death	Such anesthetics as halothane, succinylcholine, methoxyflurane, ether, cyclopropane
Debrisoquine sensitivity	Cytochrome P450, CYP2D6	Autosomal recessive	5–10%; range 0–18% in ethnic groups	Toxicity of drugs, e.g., postural hypotension	Antiarrhythmics, beta blockers, neuroleptics, tricyclic antidepressants
Glucose-6-phosphate dehydrogenase deficiency	Glucose-6-phosphate dehydrogenase in erythrocytes	X-linked recessive	$\sim 1 \times 10^8$ affected persons in world; common in persons of African, Mediterranean, Asiatic origin; multiple mutant alleles	Hemolysis	Analgesics, sulfonamides, antimalarials, nitrofurantoin, other drugs

FIGURE 65-23 Suggested style for routine recording of family history. Individual II-2 is intended to represent a healthy individual (the patient) in a primary care setting.

Table 65-7

Examples of Simply Inherited Disorders that Occur with Increased Frequency in Specific Ethnic Groups

Ethnic Group	Simply Inherited Disorder
African blacks	Hemoglobinopathies, especially Hb S, Hb C, persistent Hb F, α and β thalassemia
	Glucose-6-phosphate dehydrogenase deficiency
Armenians	Familial Mediterranean fever
Ashkenazi Jews	Abetalipoproteinemia
	Bloom's syndrome
	Dystonia musculorum deformans (recessive form)
	Gaucher's disease (adult form)
	Tay-Sachs disease
	Breast ovarian cancer BRCA1 (specific mutation)
Chinese	α Thalassemia
	Glucose-6-phosphate dehydrogenase deficiency
	Adult lactase deficiency
Eskimos (Inuit)	Pseudocholinesterase deficiency
	Congenital adrenal hyperplasia
Finns	Congenital nephrosis
	Aspartylglucosaminuria
French Canadians	Tyrosinemia
	Familial hypercholesterolemia
Japanese	Acatalasemia
Lebanese	Familial hypercholesterolemia
Mediterranean peoples (Italians, Greeks, Sephardic Jews)	β Thalassemia
	Glucose-6-phosphate dehydrogenase deficiency
	Familial Mediterranean fever
	Glycogen storage disease, type III
Europeans	Cystic fibrosis
Scandinavians	α$_1$-antitrypsin deficiency
	LCAT (lecithin:cholesterol acyltransferase) deficiency
South African whites	Porphyria variegata
	Familial hypercholesterolemia

or current age, age at death, cause of death, and name or description of any disease or defect. Similar information should be recorded on reproductive partners where appropriate. More distant relatives should be included for autosomal dominant disorders, X-linked disorders, and chromosomal translocations. For reproductive counseling, the reproductive plans for a couple should be recorded, including use of contraception or previous sterilization procedure. It is important to ask specifically about spontaneous abortions, stillbirths, and childhood deaths, since these are frequently omitted and may provide information of great relevance. Pedigrees should be drawn in a manner that distinguishes siblings and half siblings.

Direct inquiry regarding possible consanguinity should be a routine part of recording the family history and is of particular relevance to the occurrence of autosomal recessive disorders. Reproductive couples can be asked whether they may be related in any way, and this information should be supplemented by inquiries regarding surnames, ethnic status, and geographic origin of families. Cousin marriages are common in many societies and in isolated areas. Incest is an extreme form of consanguinity and may occur in the context of sexual abuse of children and teenagers. The risk of autosomal recessive disorders, including mental retardation, is high for incestuous matings.

Interpretation of the family history is aided by understanding the variation in expression in specific genetic disorders. Assuming that the family history is focused on the presence of a specific disorder within the family, meticulous questioning regarding possible manifestations in relatives is important. In addition to recording the general health status of all first-degree relatives, inquiry should be made about other genetically determined conditions in the family. This is often best done by asking whether any relatives have experienced genetic diseases, rare conditions, mental retardation, birth defects, childhood deaths, or occurrence of common adult disorders at a young age. The philosophy of the physician should be to identify any genetic issues of potential importance for all family members and to urge appropriate evaluation, education, counseling, and intervention as appropriate.

Ethnic and geographic origin of family members can be an important part of the family history, because monogenic and complex disease traits occur at different frequencies in different populations (Table 65-7). Screening for diabetes mellitus, hypertension, and hyperlipidemia is particularly important in high-risk populations (e.g., the high incidence of diabetes mellitus in some native North American populations), and different options for reproductive screening are offered to different ethnic groups (e.g., Tay Sachs testing for Ashkenazi Jews, thalassemia testing for Mediterranean populations, sickle cell testing for populations of African descent, and perhaps cystic fibrosis testing for populations of European descent).

MOLECULAR STRATEGIES FOR ANALYSIS OF MENDELIAN DISORDERS

As for any form of clinical diagnosis, a detailed history, including family history, and clinical examination is the appropriate starting point. In some cases, the phenotype of the patient may be characteristic of a specific genetic disease, and the diagnostic information may be supplemented by the family history or by specific biochemical tests. A general scheme for utilization of molecular methods for diagnosis is depicted in Fig. 65-24. Although such techniques are powerful and provide precise information, the studies are often performed by research, academic, and commercial laboratories with variable levels of experience and attention to quality assurance. One report found 34 errors in a total of 360 tests analyzing for cystic fibrosis mutations in 40 laboratories. It is essential that clinicians be familiar with the quality of work in diagnostic laboratories and interpret data cautiously in the full context of the medical circumstance.

DEFINITE CLINICAL AND/OR BIOCHEMICAL GENETIC DIAGNOSIS In many cases, DNA analysis is undertaken to confirm a diagnosis already considered to be established. The goals in such cases may include genotype/phenotype correlation, i.e., predicting the severity of the disease based on the mutations. For example, some mutations cause nonneuronopathic Gaucher's disease, and others cause neuronopathic disease (see Chap. 346). Predicting the phenotype, future risks, and complications from the genotype is complex. Extensive studies are necessary, and great caution must be exercised to avoid overinterpretation or misinterpretation of molecular data. In principle, important therapeutic decisions can be based on genotypic data (e.g., α$_1$-antitrypsin deficiency or familial hypercholesterolemia), but exact predictions for individuals may be hazardous, due to variation in expression even when detailed molecular knowledge is available

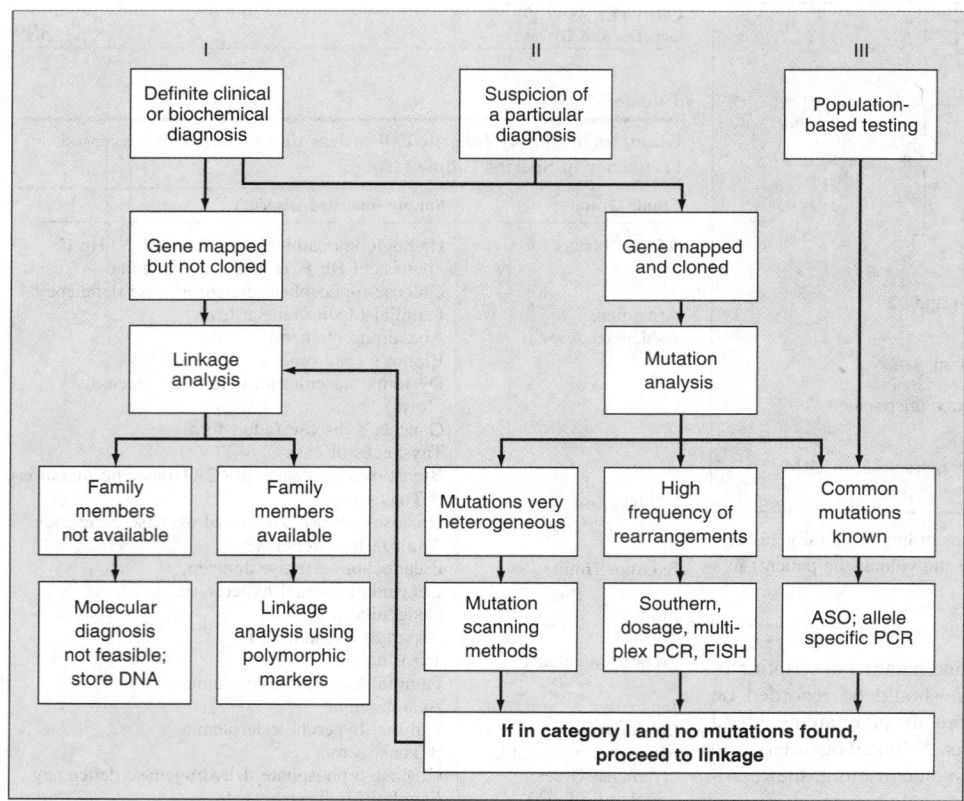

FIGURE 65-24   A scheme for utilization of DNA analysis for genetic diagnosis.

ular methods of population screening such as newborn screening; cholesterol measurements; mammography; prostate-specific antigen testing; carrier screening for Tay-Sachs, sickle-cell, or thalassemia; and screening for maternal serum alpha fetoprotein. As with established screening methods, DNA testing could be applied for (1) presymptomatic detection of disease susceptibility with plans for intervention, (2) carrier screening to offer reproductive counseling, or (3) prenatal testing. Many forms of genotypic analysis based on protein methods (e.g., sickle cell, α_1-antitrypsin, and Tay-Sachs testing) might be performed more specifically or economically in the future using DNA methods. Whether screening by DNA analysis for carriers of cystic fibrosis mutations should be offered routinely is being debated. With DNA variation of known or likely disease significance in apolipoprotein E, apolipoprotein(a), angiotensinogen, angiotensin-converting enzyme, α_1-antitrypsin, and many other genes, population-based DNA screening might become a powerful preventive approach by making possible pharmacologic and life-style interventions for individuals with high-risk genotypes. There is debate as to the appropriateness of population-based screening for disorders in which the definition of risk and potential for intervention are not fully known, as exemplified by BRCA1 mutations or mutations causing hereditary nonpolyposis colon cancer. Testing for disorders where specificity is low and/or there is no potential for intervention is generally discouraged (e.g., apolipoprotein E genotype and Alzheimer risk).

EXAMPLES OF MUTATION DETECTION   As indicated in the section designated "Gene Mapped and Cloned" in Fig. 65-24, different methods of analysis will be employed for molecular diagnosis depending on the most common type of mutation for a particular disorder, whether the mutations are large rearrangements or point mutations, and whether the mutations are of predictable type from ancient origins or are more heterogeneous and more recent in origin (Table 65-8).

Examples of large molecular defects that can be detected by Southern blotting include α thalassemia, some forms of β thalassemia, and hereditary persistence of fetal hemoglobin (Fig. 65-25). For Duchenne/Becker muscular dystrophy, 60 to 70 percent of cases involve large deletions that are easily detected by Southern blotting (Fig. 65-26). If one considers Fig. 65-26 in the context of carrier detection for family members, a case such as lane 1 with a novel, junctional DNA fragment is optimal since the presence of this fragment will be absolutely diagnostic for carrier status for females in this family. For cases such as lane 3, heterozygote detection would depend on dosage analysis with one copy of the deleted fragments in carrier females, and two copies of the nondeleted fragments. Dosage analysis is more difficult and requires meticulous quantitation and attention to internal controls. For families of the type depicted in lane 2, where Southern blotting is normal and does not detect a presumed point mutation in the gene, this analysis would not be useful for carrier detection. Deletions such as those seen in Duchenne/Becker dystrophy can also be detected using PCR to test for the presence or absence of various regions in the gene (Fig. 65-27). Deleted segments are identified by the absence of particular PCR products in a multiplex reaction testing for the presence of various sites along the length of the gene.

Expanding triplet repeat mutations are the cause of myotonic dystrophy, fragile X mental retardation, Huntington's disease, X-linked

(i.e., triplet repeat length in Huntington's disease). Extensive studies are in progress for Marfan's syndrome and breast cancer due to BRCA1 mutations, but the power and the limitations of genotype/phenotype correlations have not been defined for many disorders. Genotype/phenotype correlation and confirmation of diagnosis rely on mutation analysis and generally cannot be based on linkage analysis. Additional applications of molecular diagnosis include heterozygote detection, presymptomatic diagnosis, and prenatal diagnosis. Family studies should be performed using mutation analysis if possible, reserving linkage analysis as a secondary option.

CLARIFICATION OF A POSSIBLE GENETIC DIAGNOSIS   In some cases, there may be a suspicion of a particular genetic disease, but the findings may be inconclusive because it is too early in the clinical course or the findings are atypical in some way. This frequently occurs when it is possible to detect some mutations causing a disease, but when it is impractical to rule out the possibility of an undetected mutation. In the case of dominant disorders or X-linked diseases in males, a diagnosis may be established by demonstration of deletion, frameshift, or nonsense mutation; expanded triplet repeat; or unspecified truncation mutation. Failure to find a mutation does not rule out the diagnosis but makes it less likely if analysis is known to detect most disease mutations. Molecular analysis is particularly useful in the differential diagnosis of triplet repeat disorders, since virtually all clinically important expansions can be identified. Likewise, protein truncation testing can be helpful in evaluating possible cases of neurofibromatosis or hereditary breast cancer but will not detect all mutations. For autosomal recessive disorders, the situation may be complex (e.g., a phenotype of bronchiectasis possibly related to cystic fibrosis). Identification of pathologic mutations in both copies of the gene establishes a diagnosis, whereas identification of a pathologic mutation in one allele only increases the probability but does not prove that the suspect phenotype is related to mutation at this locus. Failure to identify any pathologic mutations lessens the likelihood that the disease is related to mutation at this locus but does not eliminate that possibility, since mutations can occur outside the coding sequence.

POPULATION-BASED DNA TESTING   Utilization of DNA testing as a population-based screening method is similar to nonmolecspinobulbar muscular atrophy, and other neurodegenerative disorders. With fragile X mental retardation and myotonic dystrophy, severity of the disease increases as premutation progresses to mutation and mild mutation progresses to severe mutation, the phenomenon of anticipation. Depending on the size of the expanded triplet repeat, these mutations can be detected by Southern blotting and/or PCR analysis. An example of an expanded triplet repeat mutation with more severe disease in later generations is depicted in Fig. 65-28. Although the size of a triplet repeat expansion has potential information for genotype/phenotype correlations, experience and caution are needed to make phenotypic predictions.

For many disorders, typically including any autosomal recessive disorders and autosomal dominant and X-linked disorders with minimal effect on reproduction, mutations of ancient origin may be present in many people in the population, but even when common mutations exist, there may still be extensive molecular heterogeneity, as for β thalassemia (Fig. 65-4). Likewise in cystic fibrosis, the common ΔF508 mutation accounts for about 70 percent of mutations in most populations, but hundreds of different mutations have been identified among the remaining 30 percent of mutant chromosomes. Common mutations of this type are usually best tested using some allele-specific method such as hybridization with allele-specific oligonucleotides. Typically, such analysis for a single disease may require testing for only a few alleles as in α_1-antitrypsin deficiency or for 10 to 30 mutations in the case of β thalassemia or cystic fibrosis (Figs. 65-29 and 65-30).

In some cases, mutation analysis is difficult because most patients

Table 65-8

Examples of the Role of Molecular Analysis for Diagnosis of Genetic Disease

Disease	Mutation Detection*	Linkage Analysis	Comments
Sickle cell anemia	+ + + +		PCR with ASO
Other globin disorders	+ + + +	+	PCR with ASO
Hemophilia A & B	+ + +	+ +	Mutation scanning and sequencing
Phenylketonuria	+	+ +	PCR with ASO
α_1-Antitrypsin ZZ	+ + + +		PCR with ASO
Familial hypercholesterolemia	+ +	+ +	Mutation scanning and sequencing
Lesch-Nyhan syndrome	+ + + +	+	PCR and direct sequencing
Tay-Sachs disease	+ + +	+	PCR with ASO in Ashkenazim
Duchenne's muscular dystrophy	+ + +		Multiplex PCR, Southern
Retinoblastoma	+ + +	+	Mutation scanning and sequencing
Huntington's disease	+ + + +		Southern and PCR for expanding triplet
Myotonic dystrophy	+ + + +		Southern and PCR for expanding triplet
Adult polycystic kidney disease	+ +	+ +	Mutation scanning and sequencing
Fragile X syndrome	+ + + +		Southern and PCR for expanding triplet
Cystic fibrosis	+ + +	+	PCR with ASO
Neurofibromatosis 1	+ +	+ +	Mutation scanning and sequencing, PTT
BRCA1 breast cancer	+ + +	+	ASO for some and PTT
Polyposis of colon	+ +	+ +	Mutation scanning and sequencing, PTT
Marfan's syndrome	+ +	+ +	Mutation scanning and sequencing
Gaucher's disease	+ + + +	+	PCR with ASO in Ashkenazim
Glycogen storage disease, Ia	+ + +	+	PCR with ASO
Familial hypertrophic cardiomyopathy	+ + + +	+	Southern and mutation sequencing
Spinal muscular atrophy	+ + +	+	Southern and PCR for deletions
Charcot-Marie-Tooth disease IA	+ + + +	+	PFGE or FISH for duplication
Prader-Willi syndrome	+ + + +		FISH for deletion and STR for uniparental disomy
DiGeorge/Velo-Cardio-Facial syndromes	+ + + +		FISH for deletion

* Symbols of + to + + + + indicate relative importance of an approach as of 1996; the status for disorders could change rapidly.

NOTE: PCR, polymerase chain reactions; ASO, allele-specific oligonucleotide; PFGE, pulsed-field gel electrophoresis; STR, short tandem repeat; FISH, fluorescence in situ hybridization; PTT, protein truncation test.

carry heterogeneous point mutations, including autosomal dominant disorders that impair reproductive fitness and X-linked disorders that limit reproduction in males. The factors influencing the proportion of cases of autosomal dominant disorders due to new mutation are discussed above. In these cases of heterogeneous mutations, some method for analyzing the entire gene is needed. Sequencing all of the exons of a gene is feasible in a few cases if the coding region of the gene is small, and this approach is used for a few genes. However, full-length sequencing is expensive and impractical for most genes with current technology, and identification of mutations depends on a variety of procedures designed to detect small mutations in DNA as discussed above (see "Analysis of Mutations"). Protein truncation testing is useful for detecting certain classes of mutations and is quite useful for polyposis of the colon (Fig. 65-31) and breast cancer due to BRCA1 mutations. In many cases, searching for mutations is an activity for research laboratories and beyond the capacity of routine clinical service.

DIAGNOSIS BY LINKAGE ANALYSIS When a gene is cloned but it is not practical to identify the mutation or mutations in a given family, it is sometimes possible to perform molecular diagnosis using linkage analysis. In other cases, mutation analysis is impossible because the disease gene is not cloned, but informative DNA markers may be available. In such cases, linkage diagnosis can be performed with a negligible possibility of crossovers (see Fig. 65-13). For linkage analysis, some genetic marker near the disease locus must be *informative*, namely, key individuals in the pedigree must have two different alleles at the marker locus. Linkage analysis is appropriate when an individual carries one mutant gene and one normal gene and when the goal is to determine which has been transmitted to the next generation. Many such analyses are informative because highly polymorphic STR polymorphisms are frequently present within and near genes causing diseases.

A second requirement for linkage analysis is that of *phase* information between the marker locus and the disease locus for genetic analy-

FIGURE 65-25 Depiction of Southern blot analysis of human globin genes. Above, DNA was isolated from a normal individual and from patients with homozygous hereditary persistence of fetal hemoglobin (HPFH) or homozygous α thalassemia. DNA was digested with the enzyme *Eco*RI. A mixed DNA probe was prepared by reverse transcription of reticulocyte globin mRNA. Below, arrows indicate *Eco*RI cut sites in the α- and β-globin regions, and numbers indicate DNA fragment sizes in kilobases. *(Adapted from YW Kan, AM Dozy, Proc Natl Acad Sci USA 75:5631, 1978, with permission.)*

FIGURE 65-26 Detection of deletions in the DNA isolated from Duchenne's muscular dystrophy patients using a dystrophin cDNA probe. Southern blot analysis detects deletions (absence of fragments) in five of eight patients (arrows). A junction fragment is clearly demonstrated in patients 1 and 6. *(From M Koenig et al, Cell 50:509, 1987, with permission.)*

sis. If an individual is heterozygous for a marker that is tightly linked to a mutation, it must be determined which allele for the marker is on the chromosome with the disease allele and which is on the homologous chromosome with the normal allele. When the genetic marker is informative and the phase is known, genetic diagnosis can include heterozygote detection, presymptomatic diagnosis, detection of lack of penetrance, and prenatal diagnosis. When the DNA probe or marker is within the mutant gene, crossing-over between the genetic marker and the disease causing mutation usually is negligible. Duchenne's muscular dystrophy is an exception, since the responsible gene is extremely large, and crossing-over occurs at a detectable frequency within the gene.

FIGURE 65-27 Multiplex amplification of DNA using polymerase chain reaction to detect deletions in the dystrophin gene. Nine amplifications detecting fragments of nine different exons are performed in a single tube and analyzed on an agarose gel. Deletions can be seen as missing fragments for the Duchenne's dystrophy patients shown in lanes b, d, e, g, and h, while no deletion is detected in lanes a, c, f, and i. φX indicates DNA markers. *(Used by permission, Multicenter Study Group, JAMA 267:2609, 1992.)*

FIGURE 65-28 Diagramatic representation of Southern blot analysis revealing an expanding triplet mutation in a myotonic dystrophy family. A grandmother and mother with the adult form of the disease and a child with the infantile form of the disease are shown. The normal size genomic DNA fragment (lowest band) is present in homozygous form in the unaffected individuals and in heterozygous form in the affected family members. The larger mutant fragment is present in all affected individuals, with increasing size from grandmother, to mother, to child.

Examples of molecular diagnosis by linkage, when there is negligible recombination between the loci, are shown in Fig. 65-32. Genetic marker data are presented as letters that might represent simple marker alleles or haplotypes of markers. A *haplotype* is a cluster of tightly linked specific alleles on a chromosome. Phase can usually be determined from a single index case for autosomal recessive disorders (Fig. 65-32A). Fetuses of AC genotype are predicted to be affected in Fig. 65-32A, while fetuses of AA or BC genotype are predicted to be carriers and those of AB genotype to be noncarriers. In Fig. 65-32B, carrier detection is sought for the aunt and uncle of the affected. The data on the maternal side require analysis of the grandparents and predict that the aunt is a noncarrier. Although the paternal grandparents are deceased, it is still possible to conclude that the uncle is a noncarrier since he does not inherit the C haplotype that is linked to disease allele on the paternal side. For autosomal dominant disorders, linkage phase usually cannot be determined from a single affected individual (Fig. 65-32C). Exceptions occur in retinoblastoma, when analysis of tumor DNA may distinguish the allele on the abnormal chromosome

FIGURE 65-29 Genotype analysis of polymerase chain reaction amplified genomic DNA using allele-specific oligonucleotide (ASO) probes. DNA was extracted from the blood of individuals of β-globin genotypes AA, AS, SS, SC, CC, and AC and homozygous deletion (XX). The DNA was applied to replicate filters for hybridization with ASO as follows: β^A probe (19A), β^S probe (19S) or β^C probe (19C). *(From K Mullis et al, Cold Spring Harbor Symp Quant Biol 51:263, 1986, with permission.)*

FIGURE 65-30 Reverse dot allele-specific oligonucleotide (ASO) analysis for various point mutations causing cystic fibrosis. For each mutation, the polymerase chain reaction product is hybridized to an ASO dot on the left for the normal allele and on the right for the mutant allele. The positions for each ASO are indicated as follows: F and Δ for the ΔF508 mutation, G and X for the G542X mutation, G and D for the G551D mutation, R and X for the R553X mutation, N and K for the N1303K mutation, and 10 or 11 or 21 under control for the ASO to detect the amplification of exons of those numbers. Mutations are designated by single-letter amino acid code (X, nonsense) with the normal amino acid followed by the position number followed by the substituted amino acid. Thus G551D is substitution of aspartic acid (D) for glycine (G) at position 551. ΔF508 is deletion of phenylalanine (F) at position 508. Letters at the right margin identify individuals of the following genotypes: A, no mutation; B, ΔF508/G542X compound heterozygote; C, ΔF508/R553X compound heterozygote; D, G542X heterozygote; E, G551D heterozygote; F, R553X heterozygote; G, N1303K heterozygote. *(Provided by H Erlich, Roche Molecular Systems.)*

(often retained in the tumor) from the allele on the normal chromosome (often lost in the tumor). Linkage phase for autosomal dominant disorders can be determined from two appropriate individuals, and it is not essential that both be affected if penetrance is complete. Fetuses of AA and AC genotype are predicted to be affected in Fig. 65-32*D*, while fetuses of AB and BC genotype are predicted to be affected in Fig. 65-32*E*. For X-linked disorders, phase information can be obtained from a single affected male individual (Fig. 65-32*F*). In general, although linkage information can predict the genotype of offspring of individuals of known genotype, it cannot be used consistently to determine the genotype of antecedents of individuals of known genotypes because of the possibility of new mutation from one generation to the next. This is exemplified by an X-linked disorder, where linkage information will not clarify whether or not the mother of an isolated affected male is a heterozygote (Fig. 65-32*G*). This limitation is an important difference between direct detection of a mutation and linkage analysis, but occasionally, linkage analysis can suggest the genotype of an antecedent. Note in Fig. 65-32*G* that the mutation arose on the chromosome from the unaffected maternal grandfather; it can be predicted that the maternal grandmother and the maternal aunt of the index case do not carry the mutation and that either the mother or the index case is the recipient of the new mutation. The situation is similar in Fig. 65-32*H*, except that the mutation is on the chromosome from the maternal grandmother, and the new mutation could go back further in the family. Still by linkage analysis, the maternal aunt is not a carrier of the mutation. The genotype of an antecedent also can be inferred when a woman has two sons with the same DNA marker, one son being affected and one son being unaffected with the X-linked disorder (Fig. 65-32*I*). In this instance, the mother is not a heterozygote for the X-linked disorder, although the possibility of gonadal mosaicism (i.e., some proportion of the maternal germ cells have the new mutation) is not eliminated.

Linkage analysis also can be performed with DNA markers that show detectable recombination with a disease locus, but this introduces probabilities of misdiagnosis due to recombination. Problems with recombination in linkage diagnosis become less common as innumerable highly informative markers are identified.

DIAGNOSIS AND PREVENTION OF GENETIC DISEASE

In the practice of medicine, it is important to recognize that many disease processes have a major contribution from a single gene. These single-gene disorders often go undiagnosed, or the genetic contribution to a disease process goes unrecognized unless the physician is well informed and has a high index of suspicion. Furthermore, partial genetic contribution to complex disease may be even more common. Primary care physicians should recognize the genetic contributions to disease and pursue the implications in regard to intervention and counseling. In many situations, genetic advice can be given by the primary physician once the relatively simple principles of medical genetics and genetic counseling are mastered. In other situations, the complexities may make referral to a genetic specialist necessary.

GENETIC COUNSELING WITH AN INDEX CASE The diagnosis of a single-gene disorder in an individual or family obliges the physician to provide appropriate genetic information and counseling. The first step is to establish the *correct diagnosis* with the maximum certainty, utilizing biochemical and/or molecular testing where possible. The certainty of the diagnosis is crucial for proper interpretation of the mode of genetic transmission and for calculating the risk of disease among relatives. Issues of new mutation, lack of penetrance, variation in expression, and genotype/phenotype correlations are frequently important. Family members should be counseled regarding

FIGURE 65-31 Protein assay for the detection of known truncating mutations causing familial polyposis. Representative samples of sporadic colorectal tumors (T1 through T8), known to have truncating mutations from sequence analysis, demonstrate the expected truncated APC (adenomatous polyposis coli) proteins. A substantial amount of normal, full-length APC protein is noted in the remaining normal alleles. A sample of normal tissue (N) is also shown. The numbers to the right of the horizontal bars indicate the predicted size of the truncated APC protein. *(From Powell et al, with permission.)*

options such as presymptomatic diagnosis, carrier testing, and availability of prenatal diagnosis.

REPRODUCTIVE COUNSELING, PRENATAL DIAGNOSIS, AND CARRIER SCREENING Prenatal diagnosis can be offered to couples with the known presence of a genetic disease in the family and in some routine pregnancies, as exemplified by cytogenetic testing in cases of advanced maternal age. Fetal samples obtained by amniocentesis or chorionic villus sampling (CVS) can be used for cytogenetic, biochemical, and molecular studies. Virtually all cytogenetic disorders can be detected using standard methods: fluorescent in situ hybridization can be used to detect subtle cytogenetic defects, most inborn errors of metabolism are detectable by biochemical methods, molecular methods can be used in many circumstances, and ultrasound methodology allows for detailed anatomic studies of the fetus.

Screening for genetic disorders and birth defects is a routine part of prenatal care, including analysis of maternal serum for alpha fetoprotein, human chorionic gonadotropin, and unconjugated estrol to screen for neural tube defects, trisomy, and other fetal pathology. Carrier testing for autosomal recessive disorders is an option for Tay Sachs disease and hemoglobinopathies in appropriate populations and may be used for disorders such as cystic fibrosis. Screening for serious X-linked disorders such as Duchenne's dystrophy and fragile X mental retardation is not routine at present.

POPULATION-BASED GENETIC SCREENING As discussed under "Genomic Medicine" at the beginning of this chapter, it may become practical to screen for genotypes that predispose to common adult diseases (hypertension, atherosclerosis, emphysema, hemochromatosis and various forms of cancer), although the pace at which such testing will become routine is difficult to predict. The usefulness of such testing is a function of the potential for medical intervention. Newborn screening for phenylketonuria is an example in which population-based screening for genetic disease in developed countries has provided extraordinary medical benefit. The future is likely to bring greater opportunity for medical benefit from population-based genetic testing.

ACKNOWLEDGMENTS This chapter represents the evolution of the cumulative contributions to chapters that have appeared in *Harrison's Principles of Internal Medicine* and in the *Metabolic and Molecular Bases of Inherited Disease*. Past contributors have included John B. Stanbury, James B. Wyngaarden, Donald S. Fredrickson, Joseph L. Goldstein, Michael S. Brown, Charles R. Scriver, William S. Sly, David Valle, and Andrea Ballabio. The author gratefully acknowledges the contributions of these predecessors and colleagues.

FIGURE 65-32 Examples of molecular diagnosis by genetic linkage with negligible recombination between the DNA probe and the disease locus. Letters below pedigree symbols indicate alleles for a DNA marker. Families *A* and *B* depict autosomal recessive disorders; *C* through *E* depict autosomal dominant disorders; and *F* through *I* depict X-linked disorders. Complete penetrance is assumed. See text for discussion.

BIBLIOGRAPHY

ALBERTS B et al: *Molecular Biology of the Cell*, 3d ed. New York, Garland Publishing, 1994

COLLINS FS: Positional cloning moves from perditional to traditional. Nat Genet 9:347, 1995

DARNELL J et al: *Molecular Cell Biology*, 3d ed. New York, Scientific American Books, 1995

HARPER PS: *Practical Genetic Counselling*, 4th ed. Stoneham, MA, Butterworth-Heinemann, 1993

LEWIN B: *Genes V.* New York, Oxford University Press, 1994

LIFTON RP: Molecular genetics of human blood pressure variation. Science 272:676, 1996

PATTERSON M, TODD JA: A complex issue. Trends Genet 11:592, 1995

POWELL SM et al: Molecular diagnosis of familial adenomatous polyposis. N Engl J Med 329:1982, 1993

RIMOIN DL et al: *Emery and Rimoin's Principles and Practice of Medical Genetics*, 3d ed. New York, Churchill and Livingstone, 1996

SCRIVER CR et al: *The Metabolic and Molecular Bases of Inherited Disease*, 7th ed. New York, McGraw-Hill, 1995

SIMPSON JL, ELIAS S: *Essentials of Prenatal Diagnosis*, vol I. New York, Churchill Livingstone, 1993

SOUTHERN EM: DNA chips: Analysing sequence by hybridization to oligonucleotides on a large scale. Trends Genet 12:110, 1996

THOMPSON MW et al: *Genetics in Medicine*, Philadephia, Saunders, 1993

VOGEL F, MOTULSKY AG: *Human Genetics: Problems and Approaches*, 3d ed. Berlin, Springer-Verlag, 1996

WATSON JD: *Molecular Biology of the Gene*, vols I and II, 4th ed. Menlo Park, CA, Benjamin/Cummings, 1987

———— et al: *Recombinant DNA*. New York, Freeman, 1992

66 *James German*

CYTOGENETIC ASPECTS OF HUMAN DISEASE

The chromosome complement is guarded carefully against change; most chromosome mutations, either structural or numerical, are deleterious. Only rarely is a structural rearrangement that results in neither deficiency nor duplication of chromosome segments introduced into the population and transmitted from generation to generation. As a rule, an abnormal number of autosomes results in early death, except for trisomy of the shortest chromosome. In contrast, an abnormal number of sex chromosomes is often tolerated reasonably well, although reproduction is usually impaired. Among human embryos, abnormalities in chromosome structure and number are the main known cause of fetal wastage. Not every fetus with an abnormal chromosome complement is aborted, however, and those that survive become the material of medical cytogenetics. Chromosome imbalances cause various features, including abnormal anatomic development, mental deficiency, behavioral disorders, and disturbances in growth and sexual development. Sometimes, apparently normal persons with abnormal chromosome complements are detected because of infertility, repeated abortion, or the birth of malformed children.

The chromosomal abnormalities just referred to affect tissues throughout the body. In addition, a change in the chromosome complement can occur in a single somatic tissue cell. Such a mutant cell may have a proliferative advantage over normal cells if the mutation affects certain growth-controlling loci, in which case a clone bearing the abnormal chromosome complement can develop among otherwise normal cells. Although many such mutant clones are clinically insignificant, some are of importance in the etiology of cancer.

This chapter addresses the aspects of normal chromosome structure and function that constitute the basis for understanding the important chromosome alterations that have been or will be discovered. Only a few such alterations and their consequences will be mentioned as examples.

CHROMOSOME STRUCTURE AND FUNCTION   The human autosomes are numbered 1 through 22, and the sex chromosomes are denoted X and Y. (Figure 66-1 shows the normal human chromosomes as seen in metaphase and defines several terms used in human cytogenetics.) Only seven of the chromosomes can be identified microscopically by their relative lengths and centromere positions (autosomes 1 through 3 and 16 through 18 and the Y chromosome), but unique staining characteristics—banding patterns—make possible the identification of all.

A mammalian chromosome consists of one double-stranded helix of DNA that extends from one end through the centromere to the other

end. The paternally and maternally derived autosomes that compose a pair, and the pair of X chromosomes in females are genetically homologous, their differences being qualitative, that is, dependent on the alleles received from each parent at polymorphic loci. In contrast, the X and Y chromosomes in males are almost completely different, with the exception of their *pseudoautosomal regions*, short homologous segments at the ends of the short arms, which in effect constitute a 24th pair of autosomes. The two homologues of each autosomal pair synapse and exchange chromatid segments at meiosis, as do the pseudoautosomal regions. In germ line cells in the ovary, the two Xs pair at meiosis and undergo *recombination* just as the autosomes do; in the male, pairing and recombination of the X and Y chromosomes normally is limited to the pseudoautosomal regions. In somatic cells of the female, except in early embryonic life, one X is extensively inactivated, thereby giving the male and female approximately equivalent numbers of active X-linked genes.

Cell-Division Cycle   Chromosomes must duplicate before cell division can occur. This duplication occurs prior to the onset of mitosis or meiosis, in a phase of the cell cycle termed *S*, for synthesis of DNA (Fig. 66-2). Thus, from the completion of S to the completion of metaphase, each chromosome contains two identical double-stranded

FIGURE 66-1   Normal human lymphocyte chromosomes arrested in metaphase and stained for G bands (G standing for Giemsa). The inset shows the arrangement of chromosomes in an intact cell, and the remainder of the figure shows them arranged into a karyotype. By the time mitosis begins, each chromosome consists of two identical parts called sister chromatids and is identified by its relative length, the location of its centromere (*short horizontal lines*), and a distinctive sequence of bands of varying lengths and depth of staining. The number of bands visible microscopically varies from cell to cell, depending on the degree of chromosome condensation. Approximately 500 bands can be seen in this cell, and with other techniques many of these bands could be resolved into subbands. Normally, the banding patterns of the two chromosomes of a homologous pair are alike, except in certain polymorphic regions. Examples of the latter are (1) the dark juxtacentromeric G band in chromosome 9 (located on the short arm in the chromosome on the right and in the usual position on the long arm in the chromosome on the left) and (2) the variant C bands shown in Fig. 66-3.

The centromere divides a chromosome into a short arm (p) and a long arm (q). Chromosomes 13 to 15, 21, 22, and Y are called *acrocentric* because of the nearly terminal position of their centromeres. The minute p arm of each acrocentric autosome bears a nucleolus-organizing region that often causes a secondary constriction in the metaphase chromosome (the primary constriction being the one at the centromere).

By standard nomenclature, the karyotype shown here is described as 46,XY, indicating that its chromosome number is 46 and its sex chromosomes are an X and a Y. The autosomes (the chromosomes other than the X and Y) number 44. The following examples show the general use of this nomenclature. A normal female karyotype is described as 46,XX. A female cell with an extra chromosome 18 (trisomic for 18) would be described as 47,XX, + 18. A cell with only one sex chromosome, an X, and with a deletion in the short arm of chromosome 5 would be described as 45,X,5p − . A male cell with a translocation between chromosomes 2 and 3, with breakpoints in band 13 of 2p and band 22 of 3p, would be described as 46,XY,t(2;3)(p13;p22). (See also footnote to Table 66-2.)

Figure 66-2 (graph)

Mitosis   Meiosis

Amount of DNA, c

4 — G₂ — I — (M)
3 — S
2 — G₁ — II
1
0

Time

FIGURE 66-2 Schematic representation of the mitotic and meiotic cell-division cycles, as described in the text. G_1 and G_2 = time gaps before and after S, the period in which DNA replicates. Each of these intervals is several hours in duration; together they constitute interphase. M = mitosis; I and II = the two divisions of meiosis. The DNA content of the cycling cells is indicated on the vertical axis: $1c$ = the content in a gamete; $2c$ = that in either an egg immediately after fertilization or a somatic cell emerging from mitosis; $4c$ = the amount in a cell which has completed chromosome duplication and is ready to enter mitosis or meiosis.

DNA helices, and the nucleus contains four times as much DNA as a spermatozoon or ovum. During mitosis, chromosomes are condensed, and the two sister chromatids can be visualized by late prophase or early metaphase (Fig. 66-1). (Metaphase is the stage in the cell-division cycle ordinarily employed for cytogenetic analysis.)

At the onset of anaphase, the centromeric regions of each chromosome separate, and the two chromatids move quickly to opposite poles of the mitotic spindle. When the poles receive their full complements of chromatids (now called chromosomes), nuclear membranes assemble about each cluster to form the nuclei of the two sister cells that will emerge from mitosis. (The nuclear membrane is disassembled late in prophase.) The sister cells emerge in what is called the G_1 phase of the cell cycle, where they remain unreplicated unless another division is to be prepared for, in which case they enter S. Cells engaged in a differentiated function ordinarily remain unreplicated, in which case G_1 can be referred to as G_0.

Most normal cells in the human body are diploid; that is, they have twice the *haploid* number of chromosomes (the number in a gamete; in humans, the haploid number is 23, and the diploid number is 46). In the germ-cell lineage, the cells devoted to gamete formation, and destined eventually to differentiate into spermatozoa or ova, undergo mitotic cell cycling until they enter *meiosis*, a series of two specialized divisions unique to this lineage. In meiosis, homologous chromosomes pair up (the paternally derived chromosome 1 with the maternally derived chromosome 1, etc.), and genetic recombination occurs by a process called *crossing over*, an exchange of entire segments between paternal and maternal chromosomes by which the genetic constitution of each is altered qualitatively (see Chap. 65). In the first meiotic division, homologous chromosomes are segregated, and the diploid chromosome number is reduced to the haploid; that is, each daughter cell then contains one of each of the 22 (duplicated) autosomes plus one (duplicated) sex chromosome. No S phase takes place between the first and second meiotic divisions (Fig. 66-2, *right*), so that, at the second division, in which sister chromatids separate, the emerging cells maintain the haploid number of chromosomes but have reduced their DNA content to half that of diploid G_1 cells of somatic tissues. With fertilization, both the chromosome constitution and the DNA content of the zygote are restored to that of a G_1 somatic cell. An S period in the zygote then prepares the way for the regular cell-division cycles characteristic of somatic cells.

Chromosome Differentiation Chromosomes are differentiated along their length, and some aspects of this differentiation are resolv-

able microscopically. The DNA is complexed with a number of proteins in a highly specific way. The DNA-protein complex, together with some associated RNA, is called *chromatin*. The fine structure of chromatin, the manner in which the DNA is compacted and interacts with proteins, and the organization of chromatin in the interphase nucleus are thought to be involved in the control of RNA production and DNA replication and perhaps of cellular differentiation as well.

The sequences of DNA nucleotide bases that constitute the genes and can be transcribed into messenger RNA are distributed throughout the length of the various chromosomes. (These sequences are too short to be resolved microscopically.) Approximately 3000 genes have been assigned to specific chromosomes, in many cases to specific bands of a chromosome, where the order in which they are *linked* also has been determined.

Certain visible segments of at least 12 chromosomes vary in length among individuals. These can be delineated by their staining characteristics (for example, see Fig. 66-3). These variable segments consist of nontranscribed, highly repetitive nucleotide sequences of DNA and, like genes, are transmitted from parent to child in a straightforward Mendelian fashion. The techniques of molecular genetics also make possible the identification and molecular definition of innumerable heritable polymorphic segments of DNA that, like genes themselves, are submicroscopic. These noncoding segments are referred to as *restriction fragment length polymorphisms* (RFLPs), *variable number of tandem repeats* (VNTRs), or *polymorphic short tandem repeats of di- or tetranucleotides*. These normal variations in both microscopically visible and invisible segments usually are not associated with a detectable phenotypic effect. However, they serve as useful genetic markers in prenatal diagnosis when they are tightly linked to disease-associated loci (e.g., in Duchenne's muscular dystrophy) and in the determination of the zygosity of twins, paternity, and the survival of transplants. Also, these DNA markers, especially the short tandem repeats, which are highly polymorphic and are widely dispersed throughout the genome, are invaluable in the effort to map the human genome. In this undertaking, loci of importance in normal development and differentiated cell function, including those that, when mutant, result in human disease, are being assigned their correct order and interrelationships along the chromosomes.

FIGURE 66-3 Metaphase chromosomes stained for C bands (C standing for centromeric or constitutive heterochromatin), showing inherited variation in lengths of the C bands in the chromosome 1 homologues (arrows).

Microscopically recognizable segments in the short arms of the acrocentric autosomes (see the legend to Fig. 66-1) are devoted to the production of ribosomal RNA and nucleoli. As mitosis progresses, these nucleolus-organizer regions remain relatively uncondensed. Consequently, at metaphase, they appear understained and demarcate condensed segments of chromatin distal to them on the chromosome arms—*satellites*. (The DNA of satellites contains no genes; they are examples of the polymorphic segments just mentioned.) Several other regions that remain relatively uncondensed at metaphase are recognizable in a low percentage of cells and are called *fragile sites* because they may undergo outright disruption ("breakage") in metaphase preparations. The only such region known to be of significance in relation to a human trait—the clinical condition called the *fragile X syndrome*—is one located near the distal end (the end away from the centromere) of the long arm of the X chromosome (see "Sex Chromosome Imbalance," below). Other examples of segmental specialization along the chromosome include *telomeres* and *centromeres*. Telomeres, the distal termini of each arm, have a relationship with the nuclear membrane and probably are important in the maintenance of order in the interphase nucleus and in the accurate pairing of homologues in meiosis; centromeric regions are sites of microtubule attachment at metaphase.

A further example of chromosome differentiation is the sequence by which various segments replicate during S; certain segments replicate early, others late. In general, late replication of a chromosome segment correlates with genetic inertness. This correlation is exemplified by one of the two X chromosomes in female cells; in one (either) X the entire chromosome, except for its terminal pseudoautosomal region and a few additional loci, is inactivated by a phenomenon referred to as the *Lyon effect* (see Chap. 65). The inactivated X is almost entirely late-replicating. During interphase it is tightly condensed and can be visualized microscopically as *sex chromatin* or the *Barr body*. The asynchrony of homologue replication that is best exemplified by the X chromosomes also occurs in short segments of some autosomes; its significance in autosomes is unknown but may be related to genomic imprinting (see below).

A little-understood type of chromatin is referred to as *heterochromatin*. It is tightly condensed, not just at metaphase but throughout interphase. Such condensation of chromatin correlates with genetic inactivity and also with late replication. Some regions are condensed and inactive in all cells (constitutive heterochromatin), while others, such as the X chromosome, may be either condensed and inactive or decondensed and active (facultative heterochromatin). The activity of genes can sometimes be altered, even abolished, if they are positioned aberrantly near regions of heterochromatin, as can occur with chromosome breakage and rearrangement. Therefore, in a chromosome imbalance, both the specific genetic loci and the particular types of chromatin deleted or duplicated are important. Many chromosome imbalances that permit viability beyond intrauterine life involve chromosome segments that are rich in this apparently inactive, or inactivatable, type of chromatin. This is true of the chromosomes that can be trisomic in live-born individuals or, in the case of the X, monosomic. Also, the significance of a chromosome rearrangement probably depends on the new and abnormal positioning of structural and regulatory genes in relation to each other and to heterochromatin.

Fortunately for the cytogeneticist, several differentiated features of the chromosome correlate with reproducible cytologic features that can be produced and visualized in the laboratory. A number of techniques are now in use to display the constant pattern of bands of various lengths and staining characteristics already mentioned (Figs. 66-1 and 66-3). These patterns are identical in each chromosome 1, each chromosome 2, etc., varying only in the inert polymorphic regions mentioned above, so that they can be used in clinical cytogenetics to identify chromosomes and to detect and define structural rearrangements.

Sources of Error   A large number of genetic loci must be active to produce and regulate the enzymes and structural proteins required

to initiate and complete a cell-division cycle. Precision and accuracy are demanded over and over in matters such as the passage of a cell from G₁ into S, the orderly progression of replication, the assembly of the mitotic spindle, the cohesion and then disjunction of the chromatids, and the spindle action that segregates chromatids at mitosis. In the germ line, additional loci are activated to undergo meiosis, which involves the pairing of homologous chromosomes, genetic recombination, and then the separation of recombined homologous chromosomes at anaphase of the first division. These mechanisms and processes are subject to errors, some spontaneous, others promoted by unfavorable environmental influences (Fig. 66-4) or by mutations that affect the cell cycle. Furthermore, the genetic material itself is subject to damage, and certain types of unrepaired or erroneously repaired lesions in DNA predispose to mutation, including chromosome rearrangement. Errors at many of these steps or errors introduced during the repair of damaged DNA must underlie chromosome imbalance. Chromosome mutations that arise in germ cells, during fertilization, or in early postfertilization divisions are important causes of embryonic maldevelopment and infertility; mutations in somatic cells are important causes of neoplasia.

CHROMOSOME ABNORMALITIES   Mutations of a single base in a gene and deletions and duplications of chromosome segments involving even hundreds of base pairs are not visible microscopically. In fact, for the normal chromosome banding pattern to be detectably disturbed, a long segment of DNA, perhaps more than 3 million base pairs, must be deleted, duplicated, or transposed. However, the same environmental agents that produce point mutations (mutagens in the usual sense) also act as chromosome-breaking agents (clastogens), and vice versa. Thus, mutations form a spectrum extending from those visible to the cytogeneticist to mutations that must be defined by nucleotide sequencing. Visible mutations ordinarily exert a more widespread effect on development than do point mutations; ordinary genes—often many of them—as well as other specialized types of chromatin of unknown function and significance are involved in cytologically visible mutations.

If an entire chromosome is affected in an imbalance, the genome is said to be either *trisomic* or *monosomic* for the chromosome (e.g., trisomy 13, monosomy X). Genes and chromatin carried on the affected chromosome then are present in a triple or a single dose, respectively, rather than in the normal double—*disomic*—dose. An abnormal dosage affecting less than an entire chromosome (the result of chromosome breakage and rearrangement) is often termed *partial trisomy* or *partial*

FIGURE 66-4   Breaks and rearrangements (*arrows*) in metaphase chromosomes of a blood lymphocyte that received ionizing irradiation before being stimulated by phytohemagglutinin to enter S and divide.

monosomy, to indicate that segments rather than entire chromosomes are involved (e.g., partial trisomy 13q, partial monosomy 4p). Some of the clinically important recurring chromosome imbalances, both numerical and structural, are listed in Table 66-1.

Uniparental disomy is the situation in which both chromosomes of a pair, or perhaps one of them plus a segment of the other, are erroneously inherited from a single parent. In such cases, the presence of a homozygous chromosome segment can have unfavorable effects on development. *Genomic imprinting* has critical effects on development (see "Autosome imbalance," below). In addition, the fact that the affected individual is homozygous at all the loci on the disomic chromosome (or segment) means that almost any deleterious recessive alleles that are present there may cause disease. The parent contributing the disomy would probably have been heterozygous at these loci and therefore healthy. (See also Chap. 65.)

Incidence The frequency with which chromosome imbalances are detectable depends on the population studied. At least 1 in 10 human conceptions has a chromosome abnormality, and chromosome imbalance is present in 5 to 6 percent of recognized pregnancies. In spontaneously aborted human embryos and fetuses, the incidence of chromosome imbalance peaks at 8 to 11 weeks of gestation. The contribution of chromosome imbalances to late abortion and stillbirth is also significant. Surveys of more than 65,000 live-born babies examined in different laboratories found an incidence of approximately 1 in 200 for significant chromosome abnormalities, either numerical or structural. In such studies, at least 1 in 700 infants is trisomic for one of the autosomes 21, 18, or 13; about 1 in 350 newborn boys has the complement 47,XXY or 47,XYY. One in every several thousand newborns has monosomy X. One in 500 has some structural rearrangement, most of which are genetically balanced. Samplings of the general adult population reveal an occasional inherited balanced structural rearrangement as well as the expected number of XXY, XYY, and XXX complements; the inherited, apparently innocuous segmental polymorphisms (e.g., the chromosome 9 polymorphism shown in Fig. 66-1 and the C-band polymorphisms in Fig. 66-3) are found in abundance.

Of individuals with mental deficiency, 10 to 15 percent have a significant chromosome abnormality; the proportion is greater among individuals who also have anatomic malformations. In some groups of men with behavioral disorders or infertility, an increased incidence of individuals with an extra X or Y chromosome is found. Infertile

Table 66-1

Some Recurring Chromosome Imbalances that Result in Distinct Syndromes*

Class of Imbalance	Chromosome Affected	Karyotypes†	Clinical Features‡
Monosomy	X	45,X	Turner syndrome
Segmental deficiency ("partial monosomy")	X	46,X,Xp−; 46,X,Xq−; 46,X,r(X); 46,X,iso(Xp); 46,X,iso(Xq)	Turner syndrome or some features of it
	Y	46,X,Yp−; 46,X,Yq−; 46,X,r(Y); 46,X,iso(Yp); 46,X,iso(Yq)	Turner syndrome, or some features of it, sometimes with "mixed gonadal dysgenesis" when a 45,X cell line coexists (mosaicism)
	4	46,XY,4p−	Gr, Cf, Mi, Ey, Sk, Ge, Ht, Co, Me
	5	46,XY,5p−	5p− syndrome: Cr, Mi, Cf, Me
	8	46,XY,del(8)(q22q24)	Langer-Gideon syndrome
	11	46,XY,11p− or del(11)(p13)	WT, Ge, Me
	13	46,XY,13q−	RB, Cf, Me
	15	46,XY,15q− or del(15)(q11q13)	Prader-Willi or Angelman syndrome
	17	46,XY,del(17)(p13)	Miller-Dieker syndrome
	18	46,XY,18p−	Gr, Cf, Ea, Te, Po, Sk, Ht, Me
	18	46,XY,18q−	Cf, Hy, Sk, Ey
	21	46,XY,r(21)	Cf, Hp, Ea, Me
Trisomy	X	47,XXX	Se, Me (mild), Ps
	X	47,XXY	Klinefelter syndrome
	Y	47,XYY	Ta, Ac, Su, B; but often normal
	8	46,XY/47,XY,+8	Cf, Sk, Me (moderate)
	13	47,XY,+13	Trisomy 13 syndrome: Cp, Ey, Pd, Po, Ht, D, V, Sc, F, Ar, Me
	18	47,XY,+18	Trisomy 18 syndrome: Cf, Ea, V, F, Gr, D, He, Me
	21	47,XY,+21	Trisomy 21 (Down syndrome)
Segmental duplication ("partial trisomy")	Y	46,X,t(X;Y)§	XX male
	9	9p+†	Cf
	21	21q+(distal q)	Trisomy 21 syndrome
	22	22q+¶	Gr, Cf, Ea, Cp, Hy, Co
Chimerism	Entire complement	46,XY/46,XX	Pseudo- or true hermaphroditism; dimorphism of blood-cell-surface antigens
Triploidy	Entire complement	69,XXY	Hc, Me, Sy, Ht, Ge, D

* For complete listing, consult DeGrouchy and Turleau.
† The sex chromosome constitution might be either XY or XX, but in the example karyotypes given, XY arbitrarily is used in most.
‡ The clinical features given include only some of the more constant ones. Deficiency of one segment often is accompanied by duplication of another, and the phenotypic effect is the consequence of the combined imbalance. Abbreviations are defined below.
§ Translocation onto an X of a segment of the Y bearing the locus responsible for testicular differentiation.
¶ Brought about through any of several rearrangements.

Abbreviations: −, absence of a chromosome if placed in front of a number, or deletion from or of the chromosome arm indicated in placed after it; +, the opposite of the minus sign; Ac, acne; Ar, arrhinencephaly; B, behavior disorder; Cr, characteristically abnormal cry; Cf, characteristic craniofacial dysmorphism; Co, convulsions; Cp, cleft lip–palate; D, early death; del, deletion; Ea, characteristically abnormal ears; Ey, eye anomaly; F, characteristically flared, overlapping fingers; Ge, abnormality of external genitalia; Gr, severe growth deficiency; Hc, hydrocephaly; Hp, hypertonia; Ht, cardiac malformation; Hy, infantile hypotonia; iso, isochromosome of the chromosome arm indicated in round brackets; Me, intellectual deficit; Mi, microcephaly; Om, omphalocele; p, short arm of a chromosome; Po, characteristically abnormal posture; Pd, polydactyly; Ps, psychotic predisposition; q, long arm of a chromosome; r, a ring chromosome; RB, retinoblastoma; Sc, scalp defect; Se, secondary amenorrhea; Sk, skeletal anomalies; Su, subfertility; Sy, syndactyly; t, translocation of the chromosome placed in round brackets; Ta, tallness; Te, characteristically abnormal teeth; V, visceral anomalies; WT, Wilms's tumor with aniridia.

and subfertile women also include many individuals with missing or abnormal sex chromosomes. Approximately one-fourth of women with primary amenorrhea have some abnormality of the X chromosome. An appreciable number of infertile men and women have structural chromosome rearrangements.

Numerical Abnormalities Trisomy (47 chromosomes) is the most common chromosome imbalance in early spontaneous abortuses, followed by monosomy (45 chromosomes) and triploidy (69 chromosomes). The extra or missing chromosomes can be either paternal or maternal in origin, and the error in segregation of chromosomes can occur in the germ line, in the fertilized egg, or in the early embryo. Trisomy of every chromosome except chromosome 1 has been observed in spontaneous abortions, trisomy 16 being the most frequent. Most trisomic chromosomes are maternal in origin, and the incidence increases with maternal age. Triploidy is usually the result of dispermy (simultaneous fertilization of an egg by two sperms.)

Sex chromosome trisomies (XXY, XYY, and XXX) are compatible with intrauterine survival, whereas autosomal trisomies rarely permit survival to term. However, a small proportion of infants with autosomal trisomies are born alive. For practical purposes, the viable trisomies are those involving chromosome 21, 18, or 13, in order of decreasing frequency. Trisomies 18 and 13 usually cause death during infancy. Therefore, the only trisomies of significance in adults are trisomies 21, XXY, XXX, and XYY. A few other autosomal trisomies, such as trisomy 8, occur rarely, usually in mosaicism with a normal cellular component. (*Mosaicism* is the coexistence in one individual of multiple, genetically different populations of cells, all of which are derived from a single zygote.)

Autosomal monosomy is rare even in abortion material, whereas monosomy X (45,X) occurs in approximately 1.5 percent of conceptions. It is present in approximately 10 percent of spontaneously aborted human embryos and in one in every several thousand live-born babies. The reason for the failure of 45,X embryos and fetuses to survive is unknown, although cardiovascular and renal anomalies are common in the few that do survive. The cause of the lethality may be hemizygosity for some vital locus or loci of which normal individuals have two copies (the second copy being located on the Y chromosome in males and, in females, on one of the parts of the X chromosome that is not inactivated by the Lyon effect, such as the pseudoautosomal region). Occasional 45,X individuals may survive because of occult mosaicism—that is, mosaicism in which the normal cells, perhaps limited just to a few tissues, go undetected. In monosomy X, the missing sex chromosome can have been either a Y or an X and, if an X, either paternal or maternal in origin. Often the second sex chromosome is not completely absent but is replaced by a structurally rearranged Y or X. Mosaicism is often demonstrable in live-born infants with monosomy X; the nonmonosomic cells may have either a normal 46,XY or 46,XX complement or a complement in which the second sex chromosome is rearranged in some way.

The phenotypic effects of the autosomal trisomies, of 47,XXY, and of monosomy X (45,X) are characteristic and well defined, so their diagnosis usually is not difficult (see Chap. 339). The effects of the 47,XYY and 47,XXX constitutions are less striking, and these complements are underdiagnosed. In mosaicism, the phenotype may be indistinguishable from normal.

The mechanisms responsible for the numerical abnormalities are undefined and may be multiple. The extra chromosome is maternal in 95 percent of trisomy 21 cases and usually resulted from nonsegregation at the first meiotic division. There is a maternal age effect in trisomies 21, 18, 13, XXY, and XXX. Over a third of babies with trisomy 21 are born to women over 35, whereas only about a tenth of all births occur in this group. The frequency of trisomy 21 rises from 0.5 to 0.7 per 1000 live births between ages 21 and 23 to 3 per 1000 at age 35, 10 per 1000 at age 40, and 34 per 1000 at age 45. After a child with trisomy 21 is born, the risk of recurrence in future pregnancies is about 1 percent. As to the cause of monosomy X, the

frequent association of the 45,X complement in mosaicism with normal cells and with cells with structural rearrangements of the X and Y suggests that it is due to a chromosome-breaking event in the zygote or very early embryo that only secondarily causes chromosome loss, rather than to a nondisjunctional event during meiosis as occurs in the trisomies.

Structural Abnormalities Some structural chromosome rearrangements are inherited, and others represent new mutations. The cause of the new rearrangements is unknown, although they are assumed to be partly spontaneous and partly the effect of environmental agents such as mutagenic chemicals or ionizing radiation (Fig. 66-4) acting on the germ line, zygote, or early embryo. Most de novo rearrangements are in paternally derived chromosomes.

Many chromosome rearrangements have been detected only once or a few times. Others are detected repeatedly in unrelated individuals and within families. For example, the most common translocation, which can either be inherited or arise by a de novo mutation, affects one chromosome 13 and one 14 at or near their centromeres. In this translocation, only inert chromatin or functional chromatin that is represented elsewhere in the genome—the nucleolus-organizing regions and satellites referred to earlier—is lost from the short arms. A similar recurring translocation affects chromosomes 14 and 21. The normal carriers of these abnormalities (so called Robertsonian translocations) have 45 rather than 46 chromosomes.

Chromosome complements bearing rearrangements can be genetically balanced—at least effectively so—and impart no unfavorable effect to their bearers; about two-thirds of rearrangements detected during surveys of live-born babies are balanced. Alternatively, the complement can be unbalanced and impair development, the usual case when rearrangements are detected in spontaneous abortuses or in individuals with multiple anomalies and mental deficiency.

Some balanced chromosome rearrangements are transmitted through multiple generations without producing clinical effects. In other cases, they cause the conception of embryos with unbalanced genomes. For example, inherited translocations involving chromosome 21 increase the chance of offspring with the trisomy 21 syndrome. Approximately 5 percent of live-born infants with that syndrome have a translocation, and in about a fifth of those it is detectable in one of the parents. Because most babies with trisomy 21 due to translocation are born to women under 30, a search should be made for a translocation when an affected child is born to young parents. Different translocations confer different risks of having offspring with unbalanced rearrangements (partial trisomies or partial monosomies). These risks frequently cannot be predicted on theoretical grounds. Empirical risk figures have been accumulated for the common translocations. In the case of the Robertsonian 14;21 translocation, for example, the risk of having a child with the trisomy 21 syndrome is 2 percent for a balanced male carrier and more than 10 percent for a female carrier.

Genetically Determined Chromosome Instability Many gene products interact with the chromosome in the course of DNA replication, transcription, recombination, and repair, including polymerases, helicases, topoisomerases, ligases, and deoxyribonucleases as well as gene products that regulate the cell cycle. Mutations in the genes that encode these proteins can have profound effects, including interference with the integrity of the chromosomes, as in DNA-repair defects, such as the one causing xeroderma pigmentosum, and chromosome breakage syndromes, such as Bloom's syndrome, ataxia-telangiectasia, Fanconi's anemia, and Werner's syndrome (see also Chap. 84). The chromosome breakage syndromes share two important features: a predisposition to cancer, and increased numbers of chromosome breaks and/or rearrangements in somatic cells. Bloom's syndrome is characterized by small body size, immunodeficiency, light-sensitive facial erythema, and a major predisposition to cancer. Ataxia-telangiectasia is associated with increased numbers of translocations, particularly involving the T cell receptor loci. Fanconi's anemia causes increased numbers of chromatid gaps and breaks, and Werner's syndrome is associated with translocations at various sites. As the genes mutated in these rare syndromes have been identified, the normal alleles of these genes have been found to play critical roles in genomic stability.

For example, the gene that is mutated in Bloom's syndrome codes for a DNA helicase that normally functions to guarantee the fidelity of chromosome replication. These rare syndromes are important models for the study of somatic mutational disorders.

Genomic imprinting can profoundly influence the developmental consequences of chromosome mutations. A few genetic loci are known to be subject to functional modulation that occurs presumably during passage through the germ line. The modulation differs depending on whether the genome passed through spermatogenesis or oogenesis. The parental source of a chromosome mutation that affects such an imprintable locus or loci can determine whether a developmental defect will arise and the nature of the defect. An example of imprinting concerns deletion of chromosome band 15q12; deletion of the region on the paternal chromosome (no paternal contribution) causes Prader-Willi syndrome, whereas deletion on the maternal chromosome causes the Angelman syndrome (Table 66-1). Because the disorders are due to lack of a contribution from a particular parent, uniparental disomy for chromosome 15 can also be responsible. For example, about one-fourth of Prader-Willi cases are due to maternal uniparental disomy; a smaller proportion of Angelman syndrome cases are due to paternal uniparental disomy. Chromosomes 7, 11, and 14 are also known to exert clinical effects by a uniparental disomy mechanism.

DISEASE ASSOCIATIONS Various combinations of abnormalities in malformed and mentally defective individuals suggest chromosome abnormalities.

Autosome Imbalance Of the three common autosomal trisomies found in live-born babies, only trisomy 21 is compatible with survival past infancy. The phenotype produced by an extra chromosome 21, formerly known as *mongolism* but now called the *Down syndrome* or *trisomy 21 syndrome*, is characteristic and easily diagnosed. Cardiac malformations lead to death in infancy in one-third of individuals, and other malformations may also cause early death. However, subjects who survive infancy often reach adulthood, and many reach old age. Early-onset Alzheimer's disease is common in adults with trisomy 21. Affected women occasionally become pregnant, and approximately half their children have trisomy 21.

Mosaicism of trisomy 21 with normal cells (46,XY/47,XY,+21) may occur in normal individuals or people with modified features of the trisomy 21 syndrome. Children of persons with such a mosaicism have a higher than normal risk of having trisomy 21. Unfortunately, however, the abnormal cell population is usually detected only after the birth of an affected child.

Partial trisomy, partial monosomy, or a combination of the two affecting any of numerous chromosomal segments throughout the genome causes many instances of multiple developmental defects combined with mental deficiency. Sometimes a balanced autosomal translocation is detected in a normally developed adult who has repeated spontaneous abortions or subnormal fertility, with or without abnormal live-born children.

Although the phenotypic effects of many segmental chromosome imbalances are varied and nonspecific, the anomalies sometimes constitute recognizable clinical syndromes. Two examples are as follows. (1) Partial trisomy of the distal band of the long arm of chromosome 21 causes development of the full Down syndrome. (A triple dose of other segments of the long arm of chromosome 21 also produces adverse effects, but not the Down syndrome.) (2) Partial monosomy of a short segment in the short arm of chromosome 5 causes mental deficiency, a characteristic facies, and a characteristic cry during infancy. This group of signs is known as the *5p−*, or *cri-du-chat syndrome*.

Some additional syndromes produced by imbalance of chromosome segments are listed in Table 66-1, e.g., the 4p−, 9p partial trisomy, 13q−, and 18q− syndromes, to name a few. Furthermore, the application of high-resolution banding techniques and fluorescence in situ hybridization (FISH) (described below in the section "Technical Considerations") make possible identification of the exact band(s) that are deficient or duplicated. Molecular analysis employing a battery of techniques shows that unbalanced translocations and deletions too short to be detected by microscopy nevertheless can cause develop-

mental defects and mental deficiency. Additional rearrangements and their corresponding clinical syndromes still are being recognized. These syndromes may either be due to de novo chromosome rearrangement or to formation of a genetically unbalanced gamete in a developmentally normal person carrying a rearrangement affecting the relevant segment in a balanced state.

Many individuals with a chromosome imbalance, regardless of the segments affected, exhibit a degree of phenotypic similarity. These recurring, nonspecific features include mental deficiency; growth deficiency; dysmorphic ears, nose, and mouth; cardiac malformations of standard types; abnormalities of dermal ridges and creases; and dysmorphic digits. (As a rule, autosomal imbalance need not be considered in the etiology of anatomic defects not accompanied by mental deficiency.) Why similar abnormalities occur with so many different segmental imbalances is unknown, but when several such features are present, they constitute a valuable indication for cytogenetic analysis. Imbalances affecting certain segments also causes specific phenotypic changes, examples being the 5p− syndrome, retinoblastoma [mutation of a particular band of chromosome 13 (band 13q14.2)], the WAGR syndrome (Wilms's tumor, aniridia, genital anomalies, and mental deficiency) caused by deletion of band 11p13, and the Prader-Willi syndrome, which is often the consequence of deletion of a specific band near the centromere of chromosome 15 (band 15q12). Whereas the nonspecific changes serve to call attention to the possibility of some chromosome imbalance, the specific features or constellation of features can suggest the exact segment of the genome affected.

Certain constellations of features are referred to as *contiguous gene-deletion syndromes*. The WAGR syndrome mentioned above is an example; another is caused by deletions of segments of Xp that result in the loss of contiguous loci that, individually, are responsible for Duchenne's muscular dystrophy, chronic granulomatous disease, retinitis pigmentosa, and the MacLeod phenotype.

Apparently balanced translocations are also found at higher frequency in mentally subnormal persons. In these cases, the abnormalities presumably are due to small imbalances not detectable at the ordinary level of microscopic resolution or to alterations in gene positioning. The discovery of such a new translocation in prenatal diagnostic studies presents a difficult counseling issue; limited data suggest that such translocations impart a risk of about 7 percent for abnormality.

Sex Chromosome Imbalance (See also Chap. 339) In contrast to autosomal trisomy, an extra sex chromosome causes relatively mild phenotypic effects. This is because X chromosomes beyond one in somatic cells are usually almost totally inactivated, because the pseudoautosomal region is much shorter than any of the autosomes, and because the strictly sex-linked portions of the Y bear few genes. X-linked loci (in contrast to autosomal loci) function normally in a single dose. Females are functionally hemizygous for most loci on the X through the Lyon effect; males, with only one X chromosome, are hemizygous for X-linked genes, with the exception of loci clustered in the pseudoautosomal segment and a few scattered in the proximal Yp and Yq. The addition of an extra sex chromosome has a phenotypic effect, but not one that interferes with intrauterine survival. Since major anatomic defects are usually absent, men with the complements 47,XXY and 47,XYY and 47,XXX females often go unrecognized.

The *Klinefelter syndrome* (Chap. 339) typically consists of small testes, infertility, gynecomastia, and a variable degree of underandrogenization, sometimes with mild mental deficiency, antisocial behavior, or both. It is caused by the addition of an extra X to the male complement (47,XXY). The extra X interferes with the survival of germ cells and causes atrophy of the spermatogenic tubules and azoospermia. Sometimes the phenotypic effects are mild, with testicular atrophy being the noteworthy feature in an otherwise healthy man. 46,XY/47,XXY mosaicism sometimes occurs and may ameliorate the phenotypic effect of the extra X. More extreme phenotypic effects and mental deficiency result when more than one extra X chromosome is added to the normal male complement (48,XXXY or 49,XXXXY).

The phenotypic effect of 47,XYY is less well defined; although increased height, behavioral difficulties, and infertility are common, the extra Y is sometimes found in otherwise normal men. The rare complement 48,XXYY results in infertility. The phenotype associated with 47,XXX is also poorly defined; women with this complement may have mild mental deficiency, psychosis, and menstrual abnormalities or may be normal.

Loss of the Y or of the second X has drastic effects on development. If it does not cause abortion (as already discussed), it may be recognizable in the newborn girl because of the presence of loose nuchal skin folds and edema of the hands and feet with or without renal or cardiovascular anomalies. The *Turner syndrome* (gonadal dysgenesis) is the manifestation in subsequent life (Chap. 339): short stature, infantilism of the female external and internal genitalia, germ-cell-free gonads (referred to as *gonadal streaks*), and variable renal, cardiovascular, skeletal, and ectodermal anomalies.

The Turner syndrome is associated with several chromosome constitutions besides 45,X. Mosaicism and structural abnormalities of the second sex chromosome, either a Y or an X, cause a spectrum of disorders at both the clinical and cytogenetic levels. Common abnormalities of the Y and X include isochromosome formation (one arm deleted and the other duplicated) or deletion of part or all of one arm. Thus, all cells may have 46 chromosomes, but the sex chromosomes may consist of one normal X plus an abnormal Y or X; an example is 46,XXp−, in which there is deletion of a segment of the short arm of one of the X chromosomes. In other cases, a second or third cellular component is present as well, for example, 45,X/46,XX/46,XXp−. Various combinations of these karyotypes can cause the Turner phenotype if one of them is either monosomic or partially monosomic for the X. However, when Y-bearing cells coexist with the 45,X cells, for example, 45,X/46,XY, genital ambiguity often develops, and gonadal morphology ranges from streaks to functional testes (the syndrome of *mixed gonadal dysgenesis*); when a Y cell line is present, the risk of gonadal neoplasia is significant. When 46,XX cells coexist with 45,X cells, varying degrees of ovarian function may be maintained, including ovulation. Thus, the phenotype associated with monosomy X and structural abnormality of the Y or X ranges from male through the Turner syndrome to female.

X-Linked Mental Deficiency In the general population, more males than females are mentally deficient, and familial mental deficiency affects males preferentially. In some kindreds, mental deficiency segregates as an X-linked trait, and several such syndromes are now recognized. The most common of these, the *fragile X syndrome*, is characterized by mental deficiency, a characteristic facies, and macroorchia. The condition can be recognized by cytogenetic techniques. In a variable but usually small proportion of metaphases from affected persons, the abnormal X chromosome exhibits a so-called fragile site near the distal end of Xq. This site is responsible for the decondensed appearance of the region at metaphase, and its fragility is due to excess amplification of the trinucleotide sequence CGG. This base sequence is normally repeated 2 to 50 times at the fragile-X locus, whereas in affected individuals the number of repeats is expanded to more than 200. This amplification is believed to affect the normal functioning of neighboring genetic determinants and thereby to cause the abnormal phenotype. This disorder is now diagnosed by molecular techniques.

Chromosome Changes in Cancer Most human cancers have chromosome complements that are altered in a microscopically detectable way. Indeed, the cytogenetic findings in leukemias and solid tumors were some of the first evidence of the clonal nature of human cancer. Table 66-2 lists some of the alterations found with regularity in human malignancies. In the leukemias, lymphomas, and certain myeloproliferative disorders, the alterations are less extensive than in solid tumors and, therefore, easier to define. As examples, chromosome 14 is often found to have undergone structural rearrangement in certain lymphomas, with the breakpoint near or in the immunoglobulin heavy chain locus; the rearrangement translocates the *c-myc* locus from its

Table 66-2

Some Recurring Chromosome Abnormalities Encountered in Human Neoplasms*

Neoplasm	Aberration	Chromosome Region Affected
Leukemia		
Chronic granulocytic	Translocation	9q34 and 22q11
Acute nonlymphocytic		
M1	Translocation	9q34 and 22q11
M2	Translocation	8q22 and 21q22
M3	Translocation	15q22 and 17q11
Chronic lymphocytic	Trisomy	12
Acute lymphocytic		
L1–L2	Translocation	9q34 and 22q11
L3	Translocation	4q21 and 11q23
	Translocation	8q24 and 14q32
Lymphoma		
Burkitt's	Translocation	8q24 and 14q32
Follicular	Translocation	14q32 and 18q21
Solid tumors		
Benign		
Meningioma	Deletion or monosomy	22q
Leiomyoma, uterus	Translocation	2q13–15 and 14q23–24
Adenomas, salivary gland	Translocation	3p25 and 8q12
Malignant		
Ewing's sarcoma	Translocation	11q24 and 22q12
Rhabdomyosarcoma, alveolar	Translocation	2q35–37 and 13q14
Germ cell tumors, testis	Isochromosome	12p
Lung, small cell carcinoma	Deletion	3p13–23
Liposarcoma, myxoid	Translocation	12q13 and 16p11
Sarcoma, synovial	Translocation	Xp11 and 18q11
Neuroblastoma	Deletion	1p31 to 3p36
Ovary, cystadenocarcinoma	Translocation	6q21 and 14q24
Retinoblastoma	Deletion	13q14
Wilms's tumor	Deletion	11p13

* For more complete listing, see Solomon.

NOTE: The FAB (French-American-British) classification of leukemias is employed above. The chromosome breakpoint and band nomenclature is that of the Paris Conference (Birth Defects: Original Articles Series VIII (7):1–46, 1971). The chromosome and chromosome-arm designation (e.g., 9q means the long arm of chromosome 9) appears first and is followed by the chromosome region and band on that arm (e.g., 9q34 means the fourth band in the third region of the long arm of chromosome 9).

normal position on chromosome 8 to chromosome 14. Also, in over 95 percent of cases of chronic granulocytic leukemia, a translocation affecting chromosomes 9 and 22 (already mentioned) is detected, resulting in the Philadelphia (Ph¹) chromosome, an abnormally short chromosome 22. If this leukemia progresses into a "blastic" phase, the already mutated karyotype evolves; certain new chromosome changes are added stepwise in a nonrandom sequence. In this and certain other leukemias, the chromosome changes, demonstrable either by conventional cytogenetic techniques and microscopy or by microscopy supplemented by molecular techniques, may have diagnostic utility as well as some value in prognosis and choice of therapy. Common carcinomas, such as those of the lung, breast, and colon, although more difficult to study by conventional cytogenetic techniques, also have specific chromosome mutations.

The chromosome mutations found with regularity in human neoplasms (Table 66–2) often affect loci that regulate growth in normal cells. In some cases, the chromosome breakpoints affect known cellular oncogenes, but analysis of cancer-associated breakpoints also has resulted in the identification of previously unrecognized important genes, including genes coding for factors that regulate transcription and loci concerned with the regulation of normal development. In some of the lymphoma examples given, *c-myc* in its new position on chromosome 14 is brought under the influence of the activating elements of the transcribing immunoglobulin locus in cells differentiated to synthesize antibodies. In follicular lymphoma, the translocation t(14;18)(q32;q21) results in activation of a locus that suppresses apoptosis and causes prolonged survival of lymphocytes. In the Ph¹ chromosome, the cellular oncogene *abl* is translocated from its normal position on chromosome 9 into a specific region on chromosome 22, thereby creating what is called a *fusion gene*; in myeloid cells, this mutant locus is transcribed, and the mRNA is translated into a novel protein that presumably helps to cause the growth of the neoplastic cell lineage that is recognized clinically as chronic granulocytic leukemia. Thus, chromosome mutations can cause activation of or de novo creation of growth-controlling genes.

Another process that appears to be important in the progression of some tumors is *gene amplification*. One particular chromosome segment is replicated selectively, sometimes to such a degree that the normal banding pattern at the chromosome region affected is visibly disturbed, a *homogeneously staining region* (HSR) appearing at the site. Sometimes the region amplified, rather than producing an HSR, is released from the chromosome, and multiple tiny centromereless bodies of DNA, known as *double minutes* (DMs), accumulate in the nucleus and can be seen at metaphase. Presumably, in both HSRs and DMs, amplification of the DNA of some particular locus is of selective value to the neoplastic cell, enhancing the neoplastic clone's progression or perhaps its resistance to chemotherapeutic agents.

Loss of a gene essential for the normal suppression of growth can also contribute to the initiation and progression of neoplasia. Such loss can occur from gene deletion or from disruption of a gene by a translocation breakpoint. Several such mutations are now recognized; they are considered to be recessive because the presence of a single wild type allele is sufficient to provide normal growth control. Such mutations can be inherited or arise de novo as new mutations; the chromosomal mechanisms by which normal genes can be lost in somatic cells include chromatid nondisjunction with loss of an entire chromosome, segmental deletion of a portion of a chromosome, and crossing over.

The consequence of hemi- or homozygosity at such a mutant locus is loss of normal growth control, that is, the acquisition of autonomous growth by the affected cell and its progeny. Such mutations were first recognized in the rare neoplasms retinoblastoma and Wilms's tumor, where the loci affected are on chromosomes 13 and 11, respectively. In some cases of retinoblastoma the original (recessive) mutation consisted of outright deletion of the locus; then, when somatic crossing-over occurred, homozygosity of the affected chromosome arm distal to the point of exchange was the consequence, and a cell and its progeny became *nullisomic* for the retinoblastoma locus. Transmission through the germ line of occult recessive mutations at such growth-suppressor loci explains why, in familial instances of those neoplasms, the pedigrees suggest dominant inheritance.

Thus, chromosome mutations of at least four types can serve as crucial steps in the initiation and progression of malignant neoplasia: (1) translocations that disturb the regulation of loci concerned with growth or that produce novel genes affecting growth; (2) deletion or mutation of recessive growth-controlling loci, such as the retinoblastoma locus just referred to (these mutations can either be inherited through the germ line or occur de novo in a somatic cell); (3) recombination yielding homozygosity for preexisting mutations affecting the last-mentioned type of locus; and (4) amplification of a locus that facilitates expansion of the neoplastic population. These mutations and their oncogenic consequences are the subject of intensive investigation. In turn, the breakpoints found in neoplasms help in identifying genetic determinants that regulate cellular proliferation and tissue growth.

TECHNICAL CONSIDERATIONS Human metaphase chromosomes can be examined by light microscopy in any tissue in which sufficient cells are cycling. Preparations can therefore be made from almost any embryonic tissue and from adult bone marrow, lymphoid tissue, and malignant tissues. To identify mosaicism and chimerism, multiple tissues usually have to be studied. Some tissues unlikely to contain metaphase cells can be placed in culture, and chromosome preparations can be made from cells that reach mitosis in vitro. Blood T lymphocytes stimulated to enter cell division cycles by phytohemagglutinin are the standard material for diagnosing constitutional chromosome imbalances. In some myeloproliferative disorders and leukemias,

unstimulated circulating blood cells divide spontaneously after a few hours in culture. Amniotic fluid cells, which are fetal in origin, are widely used in the prenatal diagnosis of chromosome imbalances. Metaphase preparations also can be made from chorionic villus cells obtained by biopsy during the first trimester of pregnancy or from aborted fetal tissue. Fibroblasts can be cultured from minute skin biopsy samples or from fragments of many other tissues, although it takes longer to obtain cytogenetic preparations from this source. Meiotic chromosome preparations from testicular biopsy samples are sometimes useful in obscure cases of infertility, for identification of translocations and genetically determined disturbances of meiotic pairing.

Combining conventional techniques with recombinant DNA technology and fluorescence microscopy makes it possible to detect abnormalities such as trisomy, translocation, and segmental duplication or deficiency. Molecular probes for many specific marker loci whose map positions are known and that together blanket the genome can be used to identify rearrangements not detectable by banding techniques alone. By FISH, molecular probes specific for each chromosome can be used to "paint" a chromosome differentially throughout its length, revealing, for example, whether part of one chromosome has been translocated to another or whether a chromosome or chromosome segment is trisomic. FISH also makes possible the chromosomal localization of known DNA sequences, including specific genes, and the determination of their order. For certain questions, study of interphase nuclei using either painting (chromosome-specific) probes or cloned gene sequences circumvents the need to bring cells into metaphase for identification of mutations. The use of FISH along with microscopy, Southern blotting, and the polymerase chain reaction can provide minute definition of chromosome rearrangements, whether constitutional or occurring in a neoplastic clone.

Sometimes, metaphase or anaphase chromosomes are analyzed to determine whether damage to the genetic material has been induced by some environmental agent (radiation, a chemical, a virus) or to identify constitutional genomic instability. Cells that have proliferated in vivo and then been incubated briefly in vitro may be used in searching for evidence of damage to the genetic material of a person or population (see Fig. 66-4).

BIBLIOGRAPHY

Cohen MM et al: Human cytogenetics: A current overview. Am J Dis Child 147:1159, 1993

De Grouchy J, Turleau C: *Clinical Atlas of Human Chromosomes*, 2d ed. New York, Wiley, 1984

Gardner RJM, Sutherland GR: *Chromosome Abnormalities and Genetic Counseling*, 2nd ed. New York, Oxford University Press, 1996

German JL: Studying human chromosomes today. Am Sci 58:182, 1970

———: Bloom syndrome: A Mendelian prototype of somatic mutational disease. Medicine 72:393, 1993

Grumbach MM, Conte FA: Disorders of sex differentiation, in *Williams Textbook of Endocrinology*, 8th ed, JD Wilson, DW Foster (eds). Philadelphia, Saunders, 1992, pp 853–951

Schizel A: *Catalogue of Unbalanced Chromosome Aberrations*. Berlin, Walter de Gruyter, 1983

Solomon E et al: Chromosome aberrations and cancer. Science 254:1153, 1991

David Valle

TREATMENT AND PREVENTION OF GENETIC DISEASE

Normal development and physiologic homeostasis depend on the coordinated interactions of the products of many genes working together in metabolic systems. These systems are adaptable within limits, allowing normal homeostasis to be maintained over a range of environmental conditions. For instance, the products of some 30 to 40 genes participate in blood glucose regulation; in concert they maintain a relatively constant blood glucose concentration despite intermittent and highly variable ingestion of glucose precursors. On a larger scale, developmental and homeostatic interactions of 10,000 or so gene products are believed to be necessary for normal development and function of the central nervous system. Mutations that reduce the adaptive capacity of these systems result in abnormalities that we recognize as genetic disease. The mutant gene may so compromise a particular developmental or homeostatic system that the system functions poorly or not at all under any circumstance, thereby producing a monogenic disorder. Alternatively, the mutant gene may have modest effects under ordinary conditions but in certain environments contribute to maldevelopment or dyshomeostasis that we recognize as a multifactorial disorder. Thus the role of the genes in health and disease is both central and complex. Consequently, treatment of genetic disease is both difficult and often less than completely effective.

℞ TREATMENT

Effective treatment of genetic disorders requires accurate diagnosis, early intervention prior to development of irreversible tissue damage, and an understanding of the abnormal biochemistry or metabolic pathophysiology. Progress in delineating the molecular basis of genetic disease has improved our capability for accurate diagnosis of monogenic disorders. Understanding of the metabolic pathophysiology is increasing at a slower rate, mainly because progress in this area often requires elucidation of integrative physiology by study of the intact organism. The development of noninvasive metabolic monitoring techniques such as positron emission tomography and topical magnetic resonance spectrometry, as well as new genetic technologies for the production of animal models of human genetic disease, offer great promise for progress in this area.

Approaches to treatment of genetic disease can be organized proceeding from the clinical phenotype through the abnormal metabolites and dysfunctional protein to the level of the defective gene (Table 67-1).

Treatment of the Clinical Phenotype Treatment of the clinical phenotype includes conventional medical practices such as patient education, pharmacologic interventions, and surgical procedures. It depends on a thorough understanding of the natural history of the particular disorder so that potential complications can be avoided or addressed early in the course to minimize the consequences. Although therapy at this level is not aimed at correcting the primary defect, it can markedly improve the quality of life. Examples include instruction to patients with albinism or xeroderma to limit sun exposure or to patients with glucose-6-phosphate dehydrogenase deficiency to avoid the offending drugs; administration of beta blockers to Marfan's syndrome patients to prevent or slow dilatation of the aortic root, anticonvulsants to patients with neurogenic disorders, or antihypertensive agents to patients with secondary hypertension; and a host of surgical interventions for patients with genetic malformations, skeletal dysplasias, and malignancies.

Treatment of the Metabolic Phenotype Treatment at the metabolite level involves nutritional or pharmacologic approaches and is dependent on understanding the biochemical pathophysiology (Fig. 67-1). Deficient function of a mutant protein may result in a disease phenotype for the following reasons: (1) a substrate accumulates to toxic levels (precursor toxicity); (2) the product of an alternative pathway is produced in excessive amounts (alternative pathway overflow); (3) formation of the reaction product or some downstream metabolite is reduced (product deficiency); or (4) there is some combination of these possibilities. Although this paradigm is most easily visualized for enzymes in a metabolic pathway, it holds for virtually all proteins. The pathophysiology may be *local* within the cell or tissue normally expressing the mutant protein, or it may

Table 67-1

Some Treatments for Monogenic Disorders

Level of Treatment and Method	Disorder(s)
CLINICAL PHENOTYPE	
Patient education	
Avoidance of aggravating agents (high carbohydrate diet, exposure to cold)	Periodic paralysis syndromes
Avoidance of certain drugs	Pharmacogenetic disorders, acute intermittent porphyria
Avoidance of sun exposure	Xeroderma pigmentosa, albinism
Avoidance of certain physical activity	Chondrodystrophies
Notify physician for rapid increase in size of mass or tinnitus	Neurofibromatosis
Pharmacologic	
Beta blockers	Marfan's syndrome
Anticonvulsants	Neurodegenerative disorders
Surgical	
Orthopedic reconstruction	Chondrodystrophies
Colectomy	Familial polyposis coli
Plastic reconstruction of facial malformations	Treacher-Collins syndrome, several monogenic cleft lip and/or palate syndromes
METABOLIC PHENOTYPE	
Metabolite alteration	
Substrate restriction	
Phenylalanine	Phenylketonuria
Branched-chain amino acids	Maple syrup urine disease
Galactose	Galactosemia
Fructose	Hereditary fructose intolerance
Lactose	Lactase deficiency
Phytanic acid	Refsum's disease
Alternative pathway utilization	
Benzoate and phenylacetate	Urea cycle disorders
Glycine	Isovaleric acidemia
Carnitine	Organic acidosis
Cysteamine	Cystinosis
Penicillamine	Wilson's disease
Metabolic inhibition	
Allopurinol	Gout
Mevinolin	Familial hypercholesterolemia
Replacement of deficient products	
Glucose polymers (cornstarch)	Glycogen storage disease, types I and III
Uridine	Hereditary orotic aciduria
Glucocorticoids	Congenital adrenal hyperplasia
Thyroxine	Familial goiter
Biotin	Biotinidase deficiency
Protein alteration	
Activation of the mutant protein	
Pyridoxine (vitamin B_6)	Homocystinuria
Thiamine	Maple syrup urine disease
Hydroxycobalamin (vitamin B_{12})	Some forms of methylmalonic acidemia
Replacement of the mutant protein	
Growth hormone	Growth hormone deficiency
Factor VIII	Classic hemophilia
α_1-Antitrypsin	α_1-Antitrypsin deficiency
Polyethylene glycol-adenosine deaminase	Adenosine deaminase deficiency
Mannose-terminated glucocerebrosidase	Gaucher's disease
Organ transplantation	
As a source for a specific protein	
Allogeneic bone marrow	Lysosomal storage diseases, β thalassemia
Liver	Glycogen storage disease, type I, familial hypercholesterolemia, ornithine transcarbamylase deficiency
As a protein source and replacement of damaged organ	
Liver	α_1-Antitrypsin deficiency, hepatorenal tyrosinemia
Kidney	Cystinosis

FIGURE 67-1 Pathophysiologic consequences of a genetic defect in a metabolic pathway. Substrate A is converted via a series of intermediates to a final product, D. The enzymes catalyzing these reactions are indicated by the horizontal arrows. A also is converted to F in an alternative pathway. Genetic deficiency of the enzyme converting A to B (indicated by the hatched rectangle) may have pathophysiologic consequences related to accumulation of A (precursor toxicity), overflow to F (alternative pathway overflow), reduced formation of D (product deficiency), or some combination of these possibilities.

involve *distant* biochemical effects as a consequence of perturbations of metabolite concentrations in the extracellular fluid. For example, the neurologic phenotype of Tay Sachs disease results from destruction of neurons caused by local deficiency of hexosaminidase A, whereas the mental retardation of untreated phenylketonuria due to deficiency of hepatic phenylalanine hydroxylase is a distant consequence of the systemic accumulation of phenylalanine.

PRECURSOR TOXICITY Correction of precursor toxicity frequently involves dietary restriction of a substrate whose major source is nutritional. Inborn errors of amino acid and carbohydrate metabolism are examples of this approach. A diet restricted in the branched-chain amino acids (leucine, isoleucine, valine) is effective in preventing the mental retardation associated with maple syrup urine disease caused by deficiency of branched-chain ketoacid decarboxylase (see Chap. 349). Such diets should be started soon after birth, continued for life, and monitored so that intake of these essential amino acids is just sufficient for normal growth. Illnesses that cause protein catabolism (e.g., those associated with intercurrent infections or trauma) periodically complicate this therapy by releasing large amounts of the offending amino acids from the breakdown of endogenous protein. These episodes may require hospitalization for administration of intravenous fluids or dialysis. Similarly, lifetime restriction of dietary galactose in patients with galactosemia due to deficiency of galactose-1-phosphate uridyl transferase corrects growth failure, prevents cataracts, and improves intellectual outcome (see Chap. 351).

ALTERNATIVE PATHWAY UTILIZATION For some disorders, alternative metabolic pathways may be utilized to remove toxic metabolites. The effectiveness of this approach is limited by the capacity of the alternative pathway and often must be combined with dietary restriction of the offending substrate. Administration of benzoate and phenylacetate to patients with inborn errors of urea metabolism is a good example of this approach. These compounds are conjugated with endogenous glycine and glutamine, forming hippurate and phenylacetylglutamine, respectively. When used in conjunction with restriction of dietary protein, this therapy reduces the accumulation of ammonia in patients with inborn errors of the urea cycle and organic acid metabolism. Similar approaches include the administration of carnitine, which conjugates with a variety of accumulated coenzyme A (CoA) esters, to patients with defects of organic acid metabolism; cysteamine, which helps to eliminate excess cystine in cystinosis; and penicillamine to reduce excessive stores of copper in Wilson's disease and iron in hemochromatosis.

INHIBITION OF AN OVERACTIVE PATHWAY For other disorders, particularly those in which alternative pathway overflow produces a toxic level of a particular metabolite, it may be possible to prevent the accumulation by inhibiting an enzyme in the affected pathway. This approach may lead to accumulation of upstream substrates that must be well tolerated if the treatment is to be successful. For instance, in gout and other disorders in which excessive purine degradation leads to uric acid accumulation, inhibition of xanthine oxidase by allopurinol reduces uric acid production and lowers the

incidence of uric acid nephropathy and gouty arthritis. Xanthine, which accumulates as a consequence, has greater aqueous solubility than uric acid and usually is well tolerated. In a similar fashion, hypercholesterolemic patients heterozygous for mutations of the low-density lipoprotein (LDL) receptor exhibit significant reductions in plasma cholesterol when treated with lovastatin, a drug that acts in part to inhibit hydroxymethylglutaryl CoA reductase that catalyzes an early, rate-limiting step in the synthesis of cholesterol (see Chap. 341).

PRODUCT DEFICIT For disorders in which the pathophysiology involves product deficit, nutritional or pharmacologic approaches to replenishing the product can be effective if the administered material reaches the appropriate physiologic compartment. For example, many of the inborn errors in hormone biosynthesis such as the various forms of congenital adrenal hyperplasia and hereditary defects in thyroid hormone biosynthesis respond well to pharmacologic replacement of the deficient hormones. By contrast, the administration of melanin to patients with albinism would not correct the pigment deficit in melanocytes.

Treatment Directed to the Protein Phenotype Therapy at the level of dysfunctional protein involves either activation or replacement of the mutant protein.

ACTIVATION OF THE MUTANT PROTEIN Activation may be possible if the protein requires a vitamin cofactor and the vitamin is one that is well tolerated in pharmacologic doses. Obviously, not all mutations of a gene encoding a vitamin-dependent protein will respond. Those that do are likely to be missense mutations that either decrease the affinity of an enzyme for its cofactor or destabilize a protein in a way that can be partially overcome by substantial increments in cofactor concentration. About one-third of the cases of homocystinuria due to deficiency of the pyridoxal phosphate–requiring enzyme cystathione-β-synthase exhibit a significant increment in the activity when treated with pharmacologic doses (50 to 500 mg/d) of pyridoxine (vitamin B_6). The actual increase in enzyme activity may be small, but it suffices to improve metabolic flux in the impaired pathway. Since activation of residual activity both reduces precursor accumulation and increases product formation, knowledge of the pathophysiologic mechanism is less critical for this form of treatment.

PROTEIN REPLACEMENT THERAPIES An alternative approach involves replacement with an exogenous supply of the protein. To be efficacious, the protein must be administered directly into or reach the appropriate physiologic compartment. Thus blood proteins or proteins that traverse the vascular compartment (e.g., peptide hormones) are candidates for this approach. Other considerations include the availability, stability, and immunogenicity of the protein. In some instances, the administered protein may be modified to enhance stability and/or targeting to the appropriate cell or tissue. For example, linkage of adenosine deaminase to polyethylene glycol increases stability, and partial deglycosylation of glucocerebrosidase exposes mannose residues on the surface of the protein that target it to macrophages via the mannose receptor. Recombinant DNA technology can frequently be utilized to supply sufficient amounts of the pure protein (e.g., human growth hormone, α_1-antitrypsin, and glucocerebrosidase). This advance ensures an adequate supply and avoids the risk of transmission of pathologic viruses contaminating protein purified from natural sources.

Organ Transplantation Organ transplantation is on the borderline between therapy at the level of the dysfunctional protein and gene therapy. On the one hand, a transplanted organ supplies a deficient protein; on the other, the transplant tissue also brings new genetic information which, in contrast to standard models of gene therapy, is not integrated into the recipient's genome. Kidney, liver, and bone marrow transplantation are utilized for a variety of genetic diseases. The development of more effective and specific immunosuppressants (cyclosporine and tacrolimus) and the inadequacy of many less invasive therapies account, in part, for the increased utilization of this form of treatment. In some instances, the goal of transplantation is to supply a tissue that can replace a mutant protein (e.g., liver transplant for deficiency of LDL receptor or one of the urea cycle enzymes). For other disorders (e.g., α_1-antitrypsin deficiency or hepatorenal tyrosinemia), the transplant both provides the protein and replaces a damaged organ. The pathophysiologic mechanism of the disease is relevant; the physician must consider if the newly supplied protein will only be used locally or, if not, will gain access to the involved tissue(s). The long-term efficacy and consequences of organ transplantation as treatment for genetic disorders remain to be determined.

Prospects for Gene Therapy Several methods are now available for introducing new genetic material into mammalian cells. These methods allow consideration of a more direct approach to treatment of genetic disease, namely, gene therapy or introduction of a functional gene to replace or supplement the activity of a resident defective gene. Typically, two strategies have been considered, germ-line and somatic cell gene therapy, which differ in the nature of the recipient cells. In the germ-line model, foreign DNA is introduced into the zygote or early embryo with the expectation that the newly introduced material will contribute to the germ line of the recipient, i.e., be passed on to the next generation. By contrast, in somatic gene therapy models, genetic material is introduced only into somatic cells and is not transmitted to the germ cells. A third approach to gene therapy involves activation of endogenous genes to augment or circumvent a defective gene. The use of hydroxyurea to increase fetal globulin synthesis for treatment of patients with β-hemoglobulinopathies is an excellent example of this strategy.

Much of the technology for germ-line gene therapy has been developed in transgenic mice. Fertilized mouse eggs are harvested from a superovulated female, microinjected with DNA molecules, and reimplanted in a pseudopregnant female. Several murine genetic diseases, including deficiency of growth hormone, myelin basic protein, and β-globin, have been "treated" in this fashion with the general result that the disease phenotype is markedly ameliorated.

These experiments have provided considerable information on the regulation of gene expression and the pathogenesis of genetic disease. However, the method is inefficient: Only 15 to 20 percent of injected eggs produce transgenic animals, and of these, only 20 to 30 percent actually express the introduced gene. Furthermore, there are appreciable risks, including damage to a resident gene by the random insertion of the foreign DNA (insertional mutagenesis), resulting in loss of function or aberrant regulation that can lead to cancer. For clinical medicine, availability of the molecular reagents necessary for attempting germ-line gene therapy would also make it possible to do prenatal diagnosis. The certainty of having an unaffected child as established by prenatal diagnosis is preferable to the uncertainty and risks of the transgenic approach. Thus, germ-line gene therapy is not applicable to human genetic disease.

In contrast, trials of somatic gene therapy for human genetic disease are underway. The methods for introducing the genetic material and the recipient cells vary, depending, in part, on the disease to be treated. The repertoire of delivery systems includes viral vectors (replication-deficient retrovirus, adenovirus, adeno-associated virus, herpes virus, and others) and nonviral systems such as liposomes, DNA-protein conjugates, and DNA-protein-defective virus conjugates. Delivery of the genetic material can be done ex vivo by introducing the genetic material into cultured cells that are then administered to the recipient. Alternatively, delivery can be done in vivo by transferring the gene and its vector directly to cells in the individual (Fig. 67-2). The latter method avoids problems of reintroducing adequate numbers of cells to a congenial and effective site in the patient. The former is still attractive for strategies that involve delivery to bone marrow stem cells and other cells that can be cultured ex vivo in large numbers. For both ex vivo and in vivo approaches it is important to consider the quantitative aspects of gene therapy. How much expression is required to ameliorate or correct the disease phenotype, and will the expression per transduced cell and number of transduced cells be adequate to achieve a therapeutic effect?

Viral vectors are being utilized for most trials of somatic gene therapy. Each has advantages and disadvantages. Replication-deficient retroviral vectors provide efficient integration of foreign DNA and permanent alteration of the recipient cell. However, they target

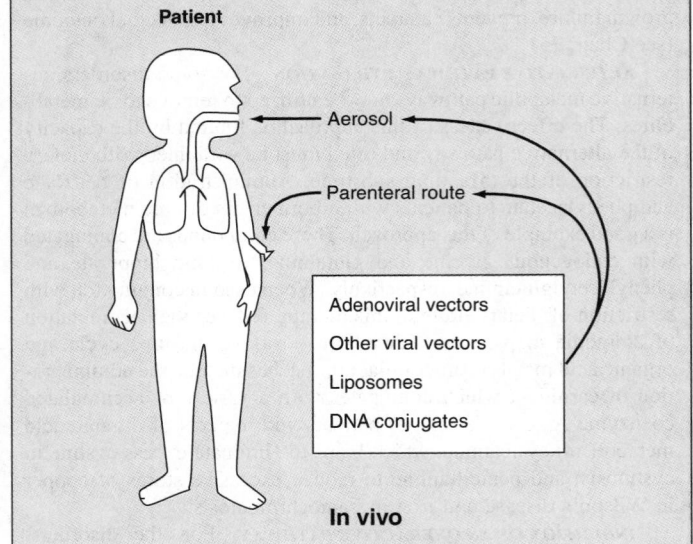

FIGURE 67-2 Comparison of ex vivo and in vivo strategies for somatic gene therapy. A procedure for ex vivo retroviral infection of bone marrow stem cells is shown on the left. On the right, this is compared to delivery by inhalation of aerosol for a disease such as cystic fibrosis or parenteral injection for targeting to organs such as liver or muscle using a variety of vectors or delivery systems. (*Courtesy of Arthur Beaudet, MD.*)

only dividing cells, have the risk of producing insertional mutations, and yield relatively low titers of recombinant virus, and the expression of the delivered gene often declines to unmeasurable levels over several months. Adenoviral vectors efficiently transfer genes to both dividing and nondividing cells, do not integrate and yield high titers of recombinant vector and high levels of expression of the introduced gene(s). However, the adenovirus vectors currently in use invoke nonspecific inflammation and antiviral cellular immunity responses, which limit expression to weeks or months. Thus, the viral vectors currently in use have major drawbacks. Considerable improvements in these and other vector systems will be necessary to make somatic gene therapy effective.

The number of candidate disorders for somatic gene therapy is expanding. The lessons learned from experience with conventional therapies will apply to gene therapy and should be considered for each candidate disorder. The importance of early intervention before the development of irreversible damage, consideration of the pathophysiologic mechanisms, and the need for regulated interactions of the product of the introduced gene with other members of the involved homeostatic system are all relevant. In addition to monogenic disorders, trials of somatic gene therapy are in progress for cancer, AIDS, and other disorders. The strategies under investigation for cancer include (1) alteration of cancer cells or other host cells to produce cytokines or other molecules to alter the host response to the malignancy; (2) expression of antigens (e.g., allogenic HLA proteins) on cancer cells to induce a host immune response; (3) insertion of tumor suppressor gene sequences or other sequences to slow cell growth; and (4) introduction of drug resistance genes into normal cells (e.g., bone marrow) to facilitate more aggressive chemotherapy. The first two immunomodulatory approaches are the basis of several current research protocols.

The ultimate contribution of somatic gene therapy to treatment of genetic disease and other disorders is unclear. After a detailed review of the field, it was concluded that the method has great promise but that considerable additional research is required to make gene therapy effective.

EVALUATION OF THERAPY FOR GENETIC DISEASE

Two general questions should be posed in an evaluation of therapy for a genetic disease. First, does the treatment provide therapeutic benefit? Second, does the treatment restore the patient to normality? These questions can be asked of any disease treatment but have special significance for genetic disorders that are predictable and preventable. In 1983 Costa, Scriver, and Childs evaluated the effect of therapy of 351 representative monogenic disorders on three basic variables: life span, reproductive capacity, and social adaptation; in their study, available therapies returned life span to normal in 15 percent, allowed reproductive capability in 11 percent, and improved social adaptation in 6 percent of the disorders. Slightly better outcomes were found with a subset of 65 diseases in which the basic defect is known. In a reexamination of the effect of treatment for the same 65 genetic diseases 10 years later, Treacy et al. found that therapy corrected all manifestations in 12 percent, was partially effective in 57 percent, and had no effect in 31 percent. Thus, the ability to treat genetic disease has improved but is still poor. It is hoped that increased understanding of the pathophysiology of specific diseases, in particular from study of disease models in "knockout" mice, and continued advances in gene therapy will result in substantial progress to treat genetic diseases in the future. Nevertheless, the slow rate of progress to date and recognition of the complexity of the problem make it clear that preventive measures for genetic disease should have high priority.

PREVENTION OF GENETIC DISEASE

Recognition of the limitation of therapy in genetic disease plus the predictability of the pattern of transmission of genes from one generation to the next have focused attention on prevention as the most reliable and effective means of dealing with hereditary disorders. The preventive approach includes genetic screening, counseling, and prenatal diagnosis.

GENETIC SCREENING   There are two types of genetic screening programs for autosomal recessive disorders: Homozygote screening programs search for individuals who have the disorder; by contrast, heterozygote screening programs search for individuals who are carriers of a mutant gene and thus are at risk of having offspring with a particular disorder. Successful homozygote screening programs require an inexpensive and reliable test, the recognition of some benefit (treatment, counseling) of early diagnosis, and education of the individuals and/or families screened so that they understand the significance of the results. The best example of such programs are the newborn screening programs. The diseases screened vary from state to state but include phenylketonuria, homocystinuria, maple syrup urine disease, galactosemia, cystic fibrosis, hypothyroidism, and sickle cell disease. In each instance, the screening test allows early detection and the opportunity to initiate appropriate therapy prior to the onset of irreversible damage. Also, the parents of an affected individual are made aware of the risk to future offspring and have the option of prenatal diagnosis. Heterozygote screening programs are best exemplified by the program to detect carriers of Tay Sachs disease, a fatal autosomal recessive lysosomal storage disease for which there is no effective treatment. Heterozygote screening of defined subpopulations with an increased carrier frequency (e.g., Ashkenazi Jews, in whom the carrier frequency is approximately 1/25 as compared with approximately 1/200 in Anglo Saxons) identifies couples at risk in which both potential parents are heterozygotes with a 25 percent chance of having an affected child. Prenatal diagnosis is possible, and the procedure provides a means for the couple to have unaffected children.

GENETIC COUNSELING   With the rapid growth in the general appreciation of the role of genes in disease, the demand for genetic counseling has increased. Individuals concerned about their own risk for a genetic disorder or about the risk of genetic disease in their offspring come to the physician with questions. Thus, all physicians should be familiar with the principles of medical genetics and use this knowledge to counsel patients. This effort may involve other professionals such as genetic counselors and medical geneticists who may perform the initial counseling with subsequent reinforcement and review provided by the personal physician.

Couples may be identified as being at increased risk for having a child with a genetic disease because of a previously affected child or other close relative. Alternatively, one or both parents may belong to a known high-risk group (e.g., identified as a carrier in a heterozygote screening test), or there may be advanced maternal age (35 years or greater at the time of delivery) with increased risk for an autosomal trisomy.

One aspect of genetic counseling involves determination of the risk for having an affected child and communication of this risk to the prospective parents so that they can make informed reproductive decisions. If a family member is affected with a genetic disease, the initial step is to assess the reliability of the diagnosis. This usually requires critical examination of existing medical data and/or additional evaluation of affected family member(s). The information is then assembled in the format of the family pedigree to determine the pattern of transmission within the family and to compare it with that expected for the diagnosed condition. Depending on the type of disease (monogenic, multifactorial, or chromosomal) and the reliability of the diagnosis, the risk to subsequent offspring may be predicted with a degree of certainty ranging from a rough estimate to nearly perfect. The reliability of the diagnosis will be influenced by whether multiple etiologies exist for a particular phenotype and the availability of specific diagnostic tests. Molecular tests that directly and unambiguously determine the parental genotype are sometimes available and allow precise prediction of the risk of recurrence and prenatal diagnosis for some monogenic disorders (see Chap. 65). For autosomal recessive and

X-linked disorders in which a primary biochemical defect is known, reliable diagnosis is possible by a functional test of the gene product (e.g., assay of enzyme activity). For many autosomal dominant disorders, the primary biochemical defect is not known, and the parental diagnosis is uncertain because of variable expressivity. Availability of linked molecular markers, e.g., restriction fragment length polymorphisms, and identification of the responsible genes greatly improves the reliability and precision of counseling for these conditions.

Counseling for many common multifactorial disorders (e.g., diabetes mellitus, hypertension, atherosclerosis, congenital malformations, and psychiatric disorders) is imperfect and will be so until we have a better understanding of the interactions of the various genes and environmental factors that produce these diseases. In some families the etiology may involve a major contribution of a single gene, and in others a mix of multiple genes and environmental factors is the cause. In the former the risk may be predicted by a monogenic model, while in the latter no simple model suffices. In these instances, the counselor must resort to empiric risk estimates derived from retrospectively assembled data based on the average outcome in many different families.

The risk, the prognosis, and the treatment of the disorder should be discussed, and the availability of prenatal diagnosis and carrier testing should be presented. Finally, the counselor must be sensitive to the emotional impact this information may have on those counseled.

During the counseling session, effective communication of the information depends on expressing the essentials in language understandable to those being counseled. Written notes and diagrams frequently are helpful and can be handed over at the end of the session. Finally, summary letters and reviews at subsequent visits help correct misconceptions and increase retention of the information. In this regard, the referring physician who has an established relationship with the family can reinforce information presented by a counselor who meets with the subjects on only one or two occasions.

PRENATAL DIAGNOSIS Following genetic counseling, the couple at risk for having a child with a genetic disease has several options depending, in part, on the type of disorder. They may feel reassured and proceed, despite the risk, without any subsequent monitoring. Or they may view the risks as too high and choose to have no additional children or to adopt. Alternatively, when both parents are heterozygous for an autosomal recessive disorder, they may choose to reduce the risk by utilizing artificial insemination by donor or donor eggs. The magnitude of the decrease in the risk provided by this option will depend on the carrier frequency for the particular disorder in the general population. For a couple with a 1 in 4, or 25 percent, chance of having a child with phenylketonuria, the risk with donor insemination will drop to 1 in 260 ($1 \times \frac{1}{65} \times \frac{1}{4}$), because the carrier frequency in the general population is 1 in 65. When mutant alleles for the gene in question are preferentially associated with particular linked markers (linkage disequilibrium) or if there is a prevalent mutant allele(s) in the population, it is possible to reduce the risk by prescreening the donors.

Finally, if the disorder can be detected antenatally, the couple may decide to proceed with reproduction and utilize prenatal diagnosis with elective abortion of affected fetuses. Because the risk of having an affected fetus ranges from a maximum of 50 percent for heterozygotes with autosomal dominant disorders to less than 10 percent for nearly all chromosomal and multifactorial disorders, the majority of pregnancies monitored by prenatal diagnosis have an unaffected fetus. This relatively low frequency of affected fetuses, together with an increase in reproductive activity which often results from the reassurance provided by the availability of prenatal diagnosis, leads to significant increases in the family size of at-risk couples. Thus, in contrast to some public misconceptions, availability of prenatal diagnosis actually results in increased numbers of offspring. Prenatal diagnosis is indicated when the risk of having an affected child is greater than the risk of the procedure (Table 67-2).

Table 67-2

Major Indications for Prenatal Diagnosis

Indication	Risk for Affected Fetus, %	Method of Detection
CHROMOSOMAL DISORDERS		
Advanced maternal age (≥ 35 y)	1–10 depending on maternal age	Chromosomal analysis of cells obtained by CVS* or amniocentesis
Parent with a balanced translocation	3–20 depending on the translocation	
Previous child with chromosomal abnormality	~1	
MONOGENIC DISORDERS		
Couple at risk for having a child with an autosomal recessive inborn error of metabolism	25	Biochemical and/or molecular analysis of cells obtained by CVS or amniocentesis
Couple at risk for having a child with a monogenic disorder for which molecular markers are available	25–50	Molecular analysis of DNA obtained from cells obtained by CVS or by amniocentesis
Couple at risk for having a child with a monogenic malformation syndrome without biochemical or molecular markers	25–50	Fetal imaging by ultrasound
MALFORMATION DISORDERS		
Couples at risk for having a child with a neural tube defect (anencephaly or meningomyelocele) or other multifactorial malformation syndrome	1–10	Fetal imaging by ultrasound and, for neural tube defects, measurement of alpha fetoprotein and other fetal markers in amniotic fluid obtained by amniocentesis

* CVS, chorionic villus sampling

Several methods for prenatal diagnosis are available (Table 67-3). Choice of a method depends on the disorder in question and on family preferences. Measurement of alpha fetoprotein (AFP) and other proteins in maternal serum is noninvasive and can be used to screen pregnancies for neural tube defects (increased maternal serum AFP) and for fetal aneuploidies (decreased maternal serum AFP). Ultrasonography can be used to visualize many fetal malformations and growth abnormalities and to monitor invasive fetal sampling techniques, with attendant reduction in the risks of the procedures. Second-trimester (15 to 16 weeks of gestation) fetal sampling by amniocentesis is widely used for obtaining fetal cells, and early amniocentesis at 12 to 14 weeks of gestation is available at some centers. Transcervical and transabdominal chorionic villus sampling (CVS) also provides fetal cells and can be performed at 10 to 12 weeks of gestation. CVS has the advantage of allowing the diagnosis to be made earlier, and if an abortion is chosen, it will take place at a stage of pregnancy when maternal-fetal bonding is less. Elective abortion at 12 weeks of gestation is a 2- to 3-h outpatient procedure, whereas a second-trimester elective abortion requires a 1- to 3-day hospitalization. The risks of CVS in experienced hands appear to compare well with those of amniocentesis, although in many centers the rate of miscarriages is slightly increased. The tissue obtained at CVS is fetal trophoblastic tissue, expresses nearly all enzymes found in amniocytes, and provides an excellent source of fetal DNA. Preimplantation prenatal diagnosis by molecular methods applied to a single cell removed from an 8-cell embryo produced by in vitro fertilization has been used successfully for a small number of monogenic disorders including cystic fibrosis and Tay Sachs disease. This method has the advantage that affected

Table 67-3

Methods of Prenatal Diagnosis

Method	Stage of Gestation, Weeks	Sample	Fetal Disorders	Risks
Maternal serum sampling	15–18	Alpha fetoprotein and other fetal proteins	Neural tube defects, aneuploidies	Negligible
Fetal ultrasonography	6–40	Image	Fetal dating, morphologic abnormalities, skeletal dysplasis	Negligible
Fetal sampling				
Chorionic villus sampling	9–12	Fetal trophoblastic tissue	Cytogenetic, biochemical, molecular	1–2% fetal loss
Amniocentesis	15–18	Amniotic fluid and cells	Cytogenetic, biochemical, molecular, neural tube defects	0.2–0.5% fetal loss
Fetal biopsy	18–20	Fetal skin	Dermatologic	~2% fetal loss
		Fetal liver	Liver-specific, enzyme deficiencies	2–5% fetal loss
		Umbilical cord, blood	Blood disorders	~2% fetal loss

embryos are not returned to the mother, obviating the need for abortion. However, the technique requires induction of ovulation and collection of eggs for in vitro fertilization and return of the normal embryos to the mother's uterus. These techniques are expensive and inefficient and require additional study to determine their reliability and risk.

BIBLIOGRAPHY

CHARACHE S et al: Effect of hydroxyurea on the frequency of painful crises in sickle cell anemia. N Engl J Med 332:1317, 1995

COSTA T et al: The effect of mendelian disease on human health: A measurement. Am J Hum Genet 21:231, 1985

CRYSTAL RG: Transfer of genes to humans: Early lessons and obstacles to success. Science 270:404, 1995

HARRISON MR et al: *The Unborn Patient: Prenatal Diagnosis and Treatment*, 2d ed. Philadelphia, Saunders, 1991

MARSHALL E: Gene therapy's growing pains. Science 269:1050, 1995

SCRIVER CR et al (eds): *The Metabolic and Molecular Bases of Inherited Disease*, 7th ed. New York, McGraw-Hill, 1995

TREACY E et al: Response to treatment in hereditary metabolic disease: 1993 survey and 10-year comparison. Am J Hum Genet 56:359, 1995

68   *John A. Oates, Grant R. Wilkinson*

PRINCIPLES OF DRUG THERAPY

QUANTITATIVE DETERMINANTS OF DRUG ACTION

Safe and effective drug therapy requires that drugs be delivered to their target tissues in concentrations within the range that yields efficacy without toxicity. Optimal precision in achieving concentrations of drug within this therapeutic "window" can be achieved with regimens that are based on the kinetics of the drug's availability to target sites. This chapter deals with the principles of drug elimination and distribution that form the basis for loading and maintenance regimens for the average patient and considers instances in which elimination of the drug is impaired (e.g., renal failure). The basis for optimal utilization of plasma level data is also discussed.

PLASMA LEVELS AFTER A SINGLE DOSE The levels of lidocaine in plasma following intravenous administration decline in two phases, as illustrated in Fig. 68-1; such a biphasic decline is typical for many drugs. Immediately after rapid injection, essentially all of the drug is in the plasma or central compartment, and the high initial plasma level (Cp_0) reflects the confinement of the drug to this small volume. The drug is then transferred into an extravascular or peripheral compartment during a period called the *distribution phase*. For lidocaine, the distribution phase is virtually complete within 30 min. A phase of slower decline, the *equilibrium phase* or *elimination phase*, then occurs. During this phase, the drug levels in the plasma and in tissues change in parallel. Although this disposition profile is common to many drugs given intravenously, the characteristic parameters vary among drugs.

Distribution Phase The pharmacologic events during the distribution phase depend on whether the level of drug at the receptor site is similar to that in the plasma. If that is the case, the pharmacologic effects, whether favorable or adverse, may be intense during this period because of the high initial levels in the plasma. For example, after a small bolus dose (50 mg) of lidocaine, antiarrhythmic effects may be evident during the early distribution phase, but they will disappear as levels fall below those which are minimally effective, even before equilibrium between plasma and tissue is reached. Thus, a larger single

FIGURE 68-1 Concentrations of lidocaine in plasma following the administration of 50 mg intravenously. The half-life ($t_{1/2}$) of 108 min is computed as the time required for levels to fall from any given value during the equilibrium phase ($Cp_{initial}$) to one-half that level. Cp_0 is the hypothetical concentration of lidocaine in plasma at time zero if equilibrium had been achieved instantly.

dose or multiple small doses must be administered to achieve an effect that is sustained into the equilibrium phase. Toxicity resulting from high levels of some drugs during the distribution phase precludes administration of a single intravenous loading dose that will yield therapeutic levels during the equilibrium phase. For example, the administration of the entire loading dose of phenytoin as a single intravenous bolus can cause cardiovascular collapse due to the high levels during the distribution phase. If a loading dose of phenytoin is administered intravenously, it must be given in fractions at intervals sufficient to permit substantial distribution between doses (e.g., 100 mg every 3 to 5 min). For similar reasons, the intravenous loading dose of many potent drugs that equilibrate rapidly with their receptors either is divided into fractional doses given at intervals or administered by infusion over a similar period.

A dose given orally results in lower plasma levels during the initial period than an intravenous bolus dose that delivers the same amount of drug to the systemic circulation. Because the drug is not absorbed instantly after oral administration and is delivered into the systemic circulation more slowly, much of it has been distributed by the time absorption is complete. Thus, procainamide, which is almost totally absorbed after oral administration, can be given orally as a single 750-mg loading dose with little risk of hypotension; in contrast, loading of this drug by the intravenous route is more safely accomplished by giving the dose in fractions of about 100 mg at 5-min intervals or by slow infusion to avoid hypotension during the distribution phase.

In contrast, some drugs are distributed slowly to their sites of action during the distribution phase. For example, the level of digoxin at the receptor site (and the drug's pharmacologic effect) do not reflect plasma levels during the distribution phase. Digoxin is transported (or bound) to its cardiac receptors slowly by a process that proceeds throughout distribution. Thus, over the distribution phase of several hours, plasma levels fall while the level at the site of action and the pharmacologic effect increase. Only at the end of the distribution phase, when the drug has reached equilibrium with the receptor, does the concentration of digoxin in plasma reflect pharmacologic effect. For this reason, there should be a 6- to 8-h wait after administration before plasma levels of digoxin are measured as a guide to therapy.

Equilibrium Phase After the concentration of drug in plasma has reached a dynamic equilibrium with that in the tissues, the levels in plasma and tissues fall in parallel as the drug is eliminated from the body. Thus, the *equilibrium phase* is also called the *elimination phase*. During this phase, drug concentrations measured in plasma provide the best index of drug levels in tissues.

Most drugs are eliminated as a first-order process. This means that the time required for the plasma level of the drug to fall to one-half the original value (the half-life, $t_{1/2}$) is the same regardless of the point on the plasma level curve at which measurement begins. Another characteristic of the first-order process is that a semilogarithmic plot of plasma concentration versus time is linear. From such a plot (Fig. 68-1), it can be seen that the half-life of lidocaine is 108 min.

If the half-life is known, one can calculate the amount of a dose remaining in the body at any time following administration. Table 68-1 shows how this amount changes over five successive half-lives.

From a clinical standpoint, elimination is essentially complete when it has reached about 90 percent. Therefore, for practical purposes, *a first-order elimination process reaches completion after three to four half-lives.*

DRUG ACCUMULATION—LOADING AND MAINTENANCE DOSES If a drug is given repeatedly at intervals shorter than the time required to eliminate a dose, both the amount of drug in the body and its pharmacologic effect increase with successive doses until they reach a plateau. Figure 68-2 shows the accumulation

Table 68-1

Amount of a Drug Dose Remaining in Body over Successive Half-Lives

No. of Elapsed Half-Lives	Amount of Dose Remaining in Body, %	Amount of Dose Eliminated, %
1	50	50
2	25	75
3	12.5	87.5
4	6.25	93.75
5	3.125	96.875

of digoxin administered in repeated maintenance doses (without a loading dose). Since the half-life of digoxin is about 1.6 days in a patient with normal renal function, 65 percent of a digoxin dose remains in the body at the end of 1 day. Thus, the second dose will raise the amount of digoxin in the body (and the average plasma level) to 165 percent of the level produced by the first dose. Each subsequent dose causes a further increase until a *steady state* is achieved. At that point, the drug intake per unit of time is the same as the rate of elimination, with the fluctuation between peak and trough plasma levels remaining constant. If the rate of drug delivery is then altered, a new steady state will be attained. Continuous infusion of a drug at constant rate also results in progressive accumulation to a predictable steady state (Fig. 68-3). In this case, the steady state plasma level (Cp_{ss}) is intermediate between the peak and trough levels produced by intermittent administration of the same amount of drug over the same period. For *all* drugs with first-order kinetics, the time required to achieve steady state levels can be predicted from the half-life, because accumulation is a first-order process with a half-life identical to that for elimination. Thus, accumulation reaches 90 percent of steady state levels at the end of three to four half-lives. This is true for either intermittent or continuous dosing (Fig. 68-3).

The time required to reach the steady state may be shortened by the administration of a *loading dose*—an amount of drug that will bring the equilibrium plasma concentration rapidly to the steady state level. The loading dose can be estimated if both the desired plasma level (Cp_{ss}) and the extent of the drug's extravascular distribution at equilibrium (the apparent volume of distribution V_d) are known:

$$\text{Loading dose} = \text{desired plasma level}$$
$$\times \text{ volume of distribution at steady state}$$
$$= Cp_{ss} \times V_d$$

Loading may be accomplished by the administration of a single loading dose or, if that would create a risk of toxicity, by the administration

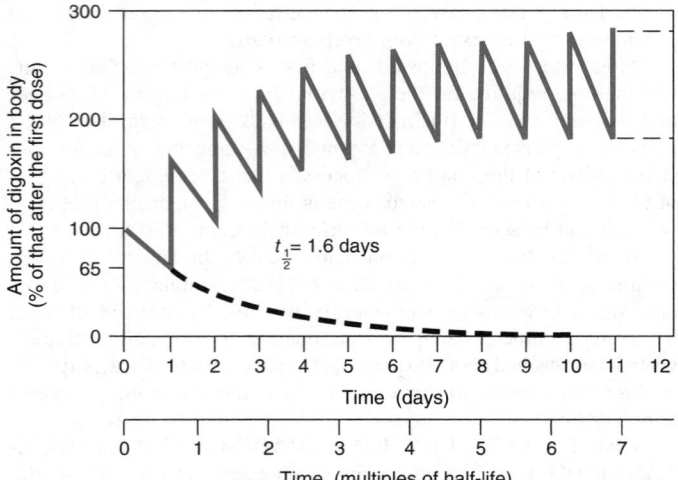

FIGURE 68-2 The time course of digoxin accumulation when a single daily maintenance dose is given without a loading dose. Note that accumulation is more than 90 percent complete by the end of four half-lives.

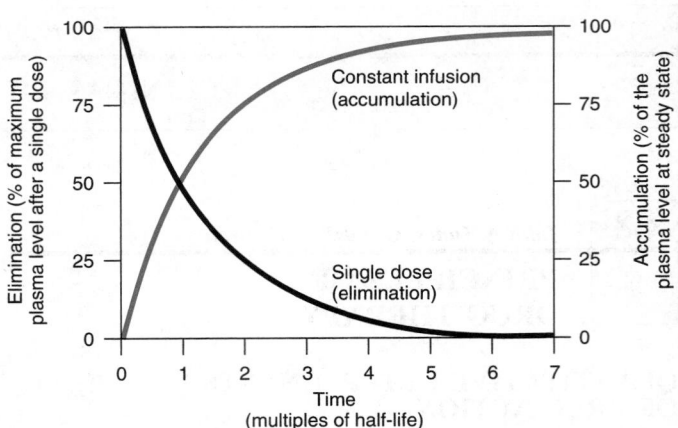

FIGURE 68-3 The time course of plasma levels of a drug following a single intravenous dose compared with those during a constant intravenous infusion. This relationship applies to all drugs that rapidly achieve equilibrium between plasma and tissues.

of the loading amount in a series of fractions. The latter approach is appropriate for most drugs that have a low therapeutic index. (The *therapeutic index* is the ratio of the toxic dose to the therapeutic dose.) This approach permits better individualization of the loading amount and minimizes adverse effects.

The loading amount required to achieve steady state plasma levels also can be determined from the fraction of drug eliminated during the dosing interval and the maintenance dose (in the case of intermittent drug administration). For example, if the fraction of digoxin eliminated daily is 35 percent and the planned maintenance dose is 0.25 mg daily, then the loading dose to achieve steady state levels should be 100/35 times the maintenance dose, or approximately 0.75 mg. Thus,

$$\text{Loading dose} = \frac{100}{\substack{\text{\% of drug eliminated} \\ \text{per dosage interval}}} \times \text{maintenance dose}$$

The fraction of drug eliminated during any dosing interval can be determined from a semilogarithmic graph in which the total amount in the body at time zero is set at 100 percent and the fraction remaining at the end of one half-life is 50 percent.[1]

To calculate a loading dose that will achieve the steady state plasma concentration of a known infusion rate,

$$\text{Loading dose} = \frac{\text{infusion rate}}{k}$$

where k is the fractional elimination constant that describes the rate of drug elimination.[1]

Regardless of the size of the loading dose, *after maintenance therapy has been given for three to four half-lives, the amount of drug in the body is determined by the maintenance dose.* The independence of the steady state plasma levels from the loading dose is illustrated in Fig. 68-3, which shows that the elimination of the loading dose would be practically complete after three to four half-lives.

DETERMINANTS OF PLASMA LEVELS DURING THE EQUILIBRIUM PHASE An important determinant of the level of drug in plasma during the equilibrium phase after a single dose is the extent to which the drug is distributed outside the plasma compartment. For example, if the distribution of a 3-mg dose of a large macromolecule is confined to a plasma volume of 3 L, then the concentration in plasma will be 1 mg/L. However, if a different drug is distributed so that 90 percent of it leaves the plasma compartment, then only 0.3

---

[1] Alternatively, the fraction of drug lost from the body during a dosage interval can be determined nongraphically from the following equation:

$$\text{Fraction of drug lost from body} = 1 - e^{-kt}$$

Values for e^{-kt} can be obtained from a table of natural exponential functions or by a calculator, where $k = (0.693/t_{1/2})$ is the fractional elimination constant (described in the next section) and t is the time interval after drug administration.

mg will remain in the 3-L plasma volume, and the concentration in plasma will be only 0.1 mg/L. The *apparent volume of distribution* V_d expresses the relationship between the amount of drug in the body and the plasma concentration at equilibrium:

$$V_d = \frac{\text{amount of drug in body}}{\text{plasma concentration}}$$

The amount of drug in the body is expressed as mass (e.g., milligrams), and the plasma concentration is expressed as mass per volume (e.g., milligrams per liter). Thus, V_d is a hypothetical volume into which a quantity of drug would distribute if its concentration in the entire volume were the same as that in plasma. Although it is not a real volume, it is an important concept because it determines the fraction of total drug in the plasma (central) compartment and therefore the fraction available to the organs of elimination. An approximation of V_d in the equilibrium phase can be obtained by estimating the concentration of drug in plasma at time zero (Cp_0) by back-extrapolation of the equilibrium-phase plot to zero time, as illustrated in Fig. 68-1. Then, after intravenous administration, when the amount in the body at time zero is the dose, we have

$$V_d = \text{dose}/Cp_0$$

For the administration of the large macromolecule mentioned above, the measured Cp_0 of 1 mg/L after a 3-mg dose indicates a V_d that is a real volume, the plasma volume. This is the exception, however, for the V_d of most drugs is larger than plasma volume; many drugs are so extensively taken up by cells that tissue levels exceed those in plasma. For such drugs, the hypothetical V_d is large, even greater than the volume of body water. For example, Fig. 68-1 indicates that the Cp_0 obtained by extrapolation after administration of 50 mg of lidocaine is 0.42 mg/L, yielding a V_d of 119 L.

Since elimination is performed largely by the kidneys and liver, it is useful to consider the elimination of drugs according to the *clearance* concept. For example, in the kidney, regardless of the extent to which removal of drug is determined by filtration, secretion, or reabsorption, the net result is a reduction of the concentration of drug in plasma as it passes through the organ. The extent of this reduction is expressed as the *extraction ratio*, E, which is constant as long as first-order elimination occurs.

$$E = C_a - C_v$$

where C_a = arterial plasma concentration and C_v = venous plasma concentration. If the extraction is complete, $E = 1$. If the total plasma flow to the kidneys is Q (mL/min), the total volume of plasma from which drug is completely removed in a unit of time (clearance, CL) is determined as

$$CL_{renal} = QE$$

If the renal extraction ratio of penicillin is 0.5 and renal plasma flow is 680 mL/min, then penicillin's renal clearance is 340 mL/min. If the extraction ratio is high, as is the case for renal extraction of aminohippurate or hepatic extraction of propranolol, then clearance is a function of organ blood flow.[2]

Clearance from the body (CL) is the sum of clearance from all organs of elimination and is the best measure of the efficiency of the elimination processes. If a drug is removed by both the kidney and liver, then

$$CL = CL_{renal} + CL_{hepatic}$$

Thus, if penicillin is eliminated by both renal clearance (340 mL/min) and hepatic clearance (36 mL/min) in a normal individual, the total clearance is 376 mL/min. If renal clearance is reduced by half, the total clearance is 170 + 36 or 206 mL/min. In anuria, total clearance equals hepatic clearance.

Only the drug in the vascular compartment can be cleared during each passage through an organ. To ascertain the effect of a given plasma clearance by one or more organs on the rate of removal of drug from the body, the clearance must be related to the volume of "plasma equivalents" to be cleared, that is, the volume of distribution.

If the volume of distribution is 10 L and clearance is 1 L/min, then one-tenth of the drug in the body is eliminated per minute. This fraction, CL/V_d, is known as a *fractional elimination constant* and is designated k:

$$k = CL/V_d$$

If the fraction k is multiplied by the total amount of drug in the body, the actual rate of elimination at any given time can be determined:

$$\text{Rate of elimination} = k \times \text{amount in body} = CL \cdot C_p$$

This is the general equation for all first-order processes and expresses the fact that rate is proportional to the declining quantity in a first-order process.

Since half-life is a temporal expression of the exponential first-order process, half-life ($t_{1/2}$) can be related to k as follows:

$$t_{1/2} = 0.693/k$$

Because

$$k = CL/V_d$$

then

$$t_{1/2} = 0.693V_d/CL$$

As shown in the section on drug dosage in renal failure ("Effects of Renal Disease," below), the linear relationship of k or CL to creatinine clearance makes k a useful parameter for the estimation of changes in drug elimination with reduction in creatinine clearance in renal insufficiency. By contrast, half-life is not linearly related to clearance.

The important relationship

$$t_{1/2} = 0.693V_d/CL$$

indicates clearly the dependence of half-life—a measure of rate of elimination—on the two physiologically independent variables of volume of distribution and clearance, the latter expressing the efficiency of elimination. For example, half-life is shortened when phenobarbital induces the enzymes responsible for hepatic clearance of a drug, and half-life is lengthened when a drug's renal clearance is attenuated in renal failure. Also, the half-life of some drugs is shortened when their volume of distribution is reduced. In treating patients after an overdose, the effects of hemodialysis on a drug's elimination depend on the drug's volume of distribution. When the volume of distribution is large, as with tricyclic antidepressants (the V_d of desipramine equals more than 1500 L), the removal of drug, even with a high-clearance dialyzer, proceeds slowly.

The extent to which a drug is bound to plasma proteins also determines the fraction extracted by the organ(s) of elimination. Altered binding changes the extraction ratio significantly, but only when elimination is limited to the unbound (free) drug in plasma. The extent to which binding influences elimination depends on the relative affinities of the drug for plasma binding and for the extraction process. The high affinity of the renal tubular anion transport system for many drugs leads to extraction of bound and unbound drug, and the efficient process by which the liver removes propranolol extracts most of this highly bound drug from blood. However, for drugs with low organ extraction ratios, only unbound drug is available for elimination.

STEADY STATE With a constant infusion of drug, the infusion rate equals elimination rate at steady state. Therefore,

$$\begin{array}{ccc} \text{Infusion rate} & = & Cp_{ss} \times & CL \\ \text{(amt/unit time)} & & \text{(amt/vol)} & \text{(vol/unit time)} \end{array}$$

when the units for amount, volume, and time are consistent.

Thus, if clearance (CL) is known, the infusion rate to achieve a given steady state plasma level can be calculated. Estimation of drug clearance is discussed in the section on renal disease.

When the dose is given intermittently instead of by infusion, the above relationship between plasma concentration and the dose administered at each dosage interval can be expressed as

$$\text{Dose} = Cp_{av} \times CL \times \text{dosage interval}$$

---

[2] When drug is present in the formed elements of blood and rapidly equilibrates with that in plasma, then it is more physiologically meaningful to calculate extraction and clearance from blood than from the plasma.

Because Cp_{av} is an average value, the actual plasma concentrations will be higher and lower at various points during the dosing interval, as shown in Fig. 68-2.

When a drug is given orally, the fraction F of the administered dose that reaches the systemic circulation is an expression of the drug's *bioavailability*. A reduction in bioavailability may reflect a poorly formulated dosage form that fails to disintegrate or dissolve in the gastrointestinal fluids. Regulatory standards have reduced the extent of this problem. Drug interactions also can impair absorption after oral dosing. Bioavailability also may be reduced by metabolism of the drug in the gastrointestinal tract and/or the liver during the absorption process, the *first-pass effect*. This is a particular problem for drugs that are extracted extensively by these organs, and there often is considerable interpatient variability in bioavailability. Lidocaine for the control of arrhythmias is not administered orally because of the first-pass effect. Drugs that are injected intramuscularly also may have low bioavailability, an example being phenytoin. An unexpected drug response should lead to consideration of bioavailability as a possible factor. The calculation of a dosage regimen may need to involve a correction for bioavailability:

$$\text{Oral dose} = \frac{Cp_{av} \times \text{CL} \times \text{dosage interval}}{F}$$

Localization of Drug Action Direct intraarterial administration of selected drugs may be considered as a means of achieving a pharmacologic effect that is targeted to a specific organ. For such a strategy to be beneficial, the drug must exert an efficacy in the target organ that is greater than oral or intravenous administration without increasing systemic adverse effects (i.e., a higher therapeutic ratio). To obtain a higher therapeutic ratio from intraarterial administration, a drug should be highly extracted by the organ during the first pass through its circulation. Furthermore, the local pharmacologic effect should be sustained for the duration required to achieve the therapeutic goal.

The intracoronary administration of nitroglycerin fulfills these criteria. Nitroglycerin is highly extracted during a single pass through an organ; it is a prodrug and its metabolism by the arterial wall to nitric oxide localizes its vasodilator action to the site of this metabolic activation. Experimentally, liposomes are being investigated as a means of targeted delivery of drugs, as they are highly extracted during the first circulatory passage through an organ. Evidence that a drug meets the criteria for achieving a higher therapeutic ratio by intraarterial administration should be strong enough to justify the risk of the required invasive procedure.

DRUG ELIMINATION THAT IS NOT FIRST-ORDER The elimination of some drugs, such as phenytoin, salicylate, propafenone, and theophylline, does not follow first-order kinetics when the amount of drug in the body is in the therapeutic range. For these drugs, the clearance changes as levels in the body fall during elimination or change after alterations in dose. This pattern of elimination is called *dose-dependent*. Accordingly, the time for the concentration to fall to one-half becomes less as plasma levels fall. (This halving time is not truly a half-life, because the term *half-life* applies to first-order kinetics and is a constant.) When a drug is eliminated by first-order kinetics, the plasma level at steady state is directly related to the amount of the maintenance dose, and a doubling of the dose should lead to doubling of the steady state plasma level. However, for drugs with dose-dependent kinetics, an increase in the dose may be accompanied by a disproportionate increase in the plasma level. Moreover, the magnitude of the increase is not predictable because of interpatient variability, in the extent to which elimination deviates from first order. Changes in dosage regimens for drugs with dose-dependent kinetics, such as phenytoin, theophylline, salicylates, and ethanol, should always be accompanied by surveillance for adverse effects and by measurement of the concentration of the drug in plasma after enough time has passed for a new steady state to be established. The mechanisms involved in dose-dependent kinetics may include the saturation of the rate-limiting step in metabolism or a feedback inhibition of the rate-limiting enzyme by a product of the reaction.

Optimal drug therapy requires administration of just the right amount of drug for the particular patient—too little and the drug is likely to be ineffective; too much and there is an increased risk of undesirable effects. When the desired response is a readily determined clinical effect, such as an alteration in blood pressure or coagulation time, then the optimal dosage can be achieved empirically. For potentially toxic drugs, however, changes in dosage should be modest (usually ≤50 percent of the existing dose) and should be made no more frequently than every two to three half-lives. In most cases, however, drug therapy must be guided by the concept of a "therapeutic window" in which drug concentrations must be maintained. If this therapeutic window is large—that is, if there is little dose-related toxicity—then maximal efficacy, should it be desired and achievable, may be obtained by administering a supraeffective dose. Such a strategy is often used for penicillins and many beta-adrenoceptor blocking agents. It is also possible to use this strategy to extend the duration of action of a drug, especially one that is eliminated rapidly from the body. Thus, 75 mg of captopril will result in reduced blood pressure for up to 12 h, even though the elimination half-life of this angiotensin converting enzyme inhibitor is about 2 h. The therapeutic window for most drugs, however, is much narrower, and in certain instances (see Table 68-5), as little as a twofold difference distinguishes the dose (concentration) of drug that produces the desired response from one that elicits an adverse effect. In these cases, the application of pharmacokinetic principles is critical to achieving the therapeutic objective.

During long-term therapy, the most important pharmacokinetic factor is the drug's clearance, since that determines the steady state plasma concentration. Thus, after an oral dose, and assuming that clearance is constant regardless of the dose (i.e., assuming first-order elimination),

$$Cp_{av} = \frac{\text{dosage rate}}{\text{clearance}} = \frac{F \times \text{oral dose}}{\text{CL} \times \text{dosage interval}}$$

Accordingly, steady state drug levels and, therefore, the intensity of response can be adjusted by modifying the dosing rate. In most cases, this is best achieved by changing the drug dose but not the dosing interval, for example, by giving 250 mg every 8 h instead of 200 mg every 8 h. A change of this type will cause a proportionate change in the average steady state drug level but will not alter the relative fluctuation between the maximum ($Cp_{max,SS}$) and minimum ($Cp_{min,SS}$) values. However, this approach is only acceptable if the resulting peak concentration is not toxic and the trough value does not fall below the minimum effective concentration for an undesirable length of time. Alternatively, the steady state may be changed by altering the frequency of intermittent dosing but not the size of each dose. In this case, the magnitude of the fluctuation around the average steady state level will change—the shorter the dosing interval, the smaller the difference between the peak and trough levels (Fig. 68-4).

EFFECTS OF RENAL DISEASE When urinary excretion is an important route of elimination, renal failure decreases the drug clearance and therefore slows the removal of the drug from the body, so that a given dosing schedule will produce a greater accumulation of drug in the body and thus an increased likelihood of toxicity. The goal in such cases is to modify the dosing schedule so that the profile of plasma drug concentration over time is as similar to the desired one as possible and so that the steady state is reached in about the same amount of time as in a patient with normal renal function. Careful modification of the dosing schedule is especially important for drugs with long half-lives and narrow therapeutic indexes (e.g., digoxin). Since

$$Cp_{av} = \frac{\text{dose}}{\text{dose interval}} \times \frac{F}{\text{CL}} = \frac{\text{dose}}{\text{dose interval}} \times \frac{F}{k\, V_d},$$

the Cp_{av} expected for a patient with normal renal function can be produced in a patient with renal impairment (and thus a decreased CL) by giving smaller doses, by lengthening the dosing interval, or by doing both. The modification factor for the dosing regimen depends on the ratio of the drug's clearance or rate of elimination in renal failure to that in uncompromised patients.

If the dose size alone is to be modified, then it is necessary to calculate the *fraction of the normal dose* to be given (at the usual dosing interval). This fraction can be determined from either the drug clearance (CL) or the fractional rate constant k, because both of these quantities are proportional to creatinine clearance (CL_{cr}). Creatinine clearance is best determined directly. However, serum creatinine (C_{cr}) may be used to estimate the value by the following equation (applicable to men):

$$CL_{cr} = \frac{(140 - age) \times weight\ (kg)}{72 \times C_{cr}\ (mg/dL)}\ (mL/min)$$

For women, the correct estimate is 85 percent of the value produced by this equation. This approach is not valid for patients with severe renal insufficiency ($C_{cr} > 5$ mg/dL) or when renal function is changing rapidly.

The Clearance Approach The most accurate basis for calculating drug dosage is the clearance of the drug. From data on the clearance of a drug, the dose in renal insufficiency ($Dose_{ri}$) may be calculated as follows:

$$Dose_{ri} = dose \times \frac{CL_{ri}}{CL}$$

where ri = renal insufficiency; CL = clearance from the whole body with normal renal function; CL_{ri} = clearance from the whole body with renal insufficiency; and Dose = maintenance dose with normal renal function ($CL_{cr} \approx 100$ mL/min).

The normal clearance and the clearance in renal impairment can be obtained by using the data in Table 68-2 in the following equations:

$$CL = CL_{renal} + CL_{nonrenal}$$

$$CL_{ri} = CL_{renal} \times \frac{measured\ CL_{cr}}{100\ mL/min} + CL_{nonrenal}$$

The CL_{renal} values in Table 68-2 are those found with $CL_{cr} = 100$ mL/min, and the renal clearance of drug in renal insufficiency is obtained by multiplying CL_{renal} by the ratio of measured CL_{cr} (in milliliters per minute) to 100 mL/min.

For gentamicin, which has a normal CL_{renal} of 78 mL/min and a $CL_{nonrenal}$ of 3 mL/min, the normal CL is 81 mL/min. Therefore, if the measured CL_{cr} in a patient with renal insufficiency is 12 mL/min, $CL_{ri} = 78 \times (12/100) + 3 = 12.4$ mL/min. If the dose of gentamicin for a given infection should be 4.5 mg/kg per day in the presence of normal renal function, and the dosing interval selected is 24 h, then

$$Dose_{ri} = \frac{4.5\ mg/kg}{24\ h} \times \frac{12.4\ mL/min}{81\ mL/min}$$
$$= 0.69\ mg/kg/24\ h$$

FIGURE 68-4 Plasma concentrations of a drug with an elimination half-life of 12 h during chronic therapy using different dosage regimens for a period sufficient to reach steady state. Proportionally reducing or increasing both the size of the maintenance dose and the interval between dosage changes the magnitude of the fluctuations in plasma levels but has no effect on the average steady state (Cp_{av}) value, since this depends on the ratio between D and τ.

Table 68-2

Clearance of Drugs

Drug	Renal Clearance,* mL/min	Nonrenal Clearance, mL/min
Ampicillin†	340	12
Carbenicillin	68	10
Digoxin†	110	36
Gentamicin	78	3
Kanamycin	60	0
Penicillin G‡	340	36

* The "normal" renal clearances are those associated with a clearance of creatinine of 100 mL/min.
† The fraction of digoxin absorbed after an oral dose (F) is approximately 0.75, and F for ampicillin is 0.5.
‡ One microgram of penicillin G = 1.6 units.

For a given dosing interval, the dose yielded by this calculation will produce the same average plasma level in the patient with renal insufficiency as the normal dose would produce in a patient with normal renal function. However, the difference between peak and trough levels will be smaller, the peak value could be below the therapeutic level and the trough level higher. To partially compensate for this flattening of the plasma concentration curve, the dosing interval for gentamicin in renal failure usually is adjusted, e.g., every 12 h for $CL_{cr} > 50$, every 24 h for $CL_{cr} = 10$ to 49 and every 48 h for $CL_{cr} < 10$ mL/min; the formula above would therefore be based on the appropriate dose for that dosing interval in a patient with normal renal function.

For some drugs, it is considered appropriate to modify only the dosing interval in renal failure, maintaining the same dose as with normal renal function:

$$Dosing\ interval \times \frac{CL}{CL_{ri}} = Dosing\ interval_{ri}$$

With this strategy, the potential that the plasma levels could be subtherapeutic for a deleterious period of time should be evaluated.

In some instances, it is desirable to calculate a dose that will yield a certain plasma level at steady state. This approach is most appropriate for constant intravenous infusions in which 100 percent of the dose is delivered to the systemic circulation. When the clearance of a drug in a patient with renal insufficiency is calculated as above, then

$$\begin{array}{ccc} Dose_{ri} & = & CL_{ri} \times Cp \\ (amt/unit\ time) & (vol/unit\ time) & (amt/vol) \end{array}$$

where the time, amount, and volume terms are uniform.

If a plasma concentration of carbenicillin of 100 μg/mL is the therapeutic objective in a patient with a creatinine clearance of 25 mL/min, the infusion rate is calculated as follows. Carbenicillin clearance is

$$CL_{ri} = \left(68 \times \frac{25}{100}\right) + 10 = 27\ mL/min$$

Therefore, carbenicillin should be infused at a rate of 2700 μg/min.

The Fractional Rate Constant (k) Approach For many drugs, clearance data in renal failure are not available. In these cases, the fraction of the normal dose that is required in a patient with renal failure can be approximated from the ratio of the fractional rate constant for elimination from the body in renal failure (k_{ri}) to that for normal renal function (k). This approach assumes that the distribution of the drug (V_d) is not affected by renal disease. The approach is the same as that employed with clearance data:

$$Dose_{ri} = dose \times \frac{k_{ri}}{k}$$

Since the ratio k_{ri}/k is the fraction of the usual dose employed in a given degree of renal insufficiency, it is termed the *dose fraction* and may be estimated from the information in Table 68-3 and the nomogram shown in Fig. 68-5. Table 68-3 gives the fraction of the usual

Table 68-3

Information for Estimation of Dose for Use in Patients with Renal Insufficiency

Drug	Dose fraction$_0$*	k (per hour)†
ANTIBIOTICS		
Amikacin	0.05	0.4
Amoxicillin	0.15	0.7
Ampicillin	0.1	0.6
Aztreonam	0.25	0.4
Carbenicillin	0.1	0.6
Cefazolin	0.06	0.35
Cefotaxime	0.3	0.7
Cefoxitin	0.1	0.8
Ceftazidime	0.1	0.4
Ceftriaxone‡	0.5	0.09
Cephalexin	0.04	0.7
Cephalothin	0.02	1.4
Chloramphenicol	0.8	0.3
Ciprofloxacin	0.33	0.2
Clindamycin	0.8	0.2
Cloxacillin	0.25	1.2
Dicloxacillin	0.5	1.2
Doxycycline	0.8	0.03
Erythromycin	0.7	0.5
Gentamicin	0.05	0.3
Imipenem	0.25	0.7
Isoniazid:		
Fast inactivators	0.8	0.5
Slow inactivators	0.5	0.25
Methicillin	0.12	1.4
Minocycline	0.9	0.06
Nafcillin	0.4	1.2
Norfloxacin	0.5	0.2
Ofloxacin	0.22	0.1
Oxacillin	0.25	1.4
Penicillin G	0.1	1.4
Piperacillin	0.33	0.5
Rifampin	1.0	0.25
Streptomycin	0.05	0.25
Sulfadiazine	0.45	0.7
Sulfamethoxazole	0.85	0.07
Tetracycline	0.12	0.08
Ticarcillin	0.1	0.6
Tobramycin	0.05	0.35
Trimethoprim	0.45	0.06
Vancomycin	0.03	0.12
MISCELLANEOUS DRUGS		
Chlorpropamide	0.4	0.02
Lidocaine	0.9	0.4
Sulfinpyrazone	0.55	0.3

CARDIAC GLYCOSIDES		
		k (per day)
Digitoxin	0.7	0.1
Digoxin	0.3	0.45

* Dose fraction$_0$, dose fraction for a patient with a creatinine clearance of zero.
† k, average overall fractional elimination rate constant for a patient with normal renal function.
‡ Extrarenal clearance also may be reduced in patients with renal failure who are uremic and/or ill.

dose of a drug required at a creatinine clearance of zero (dose fraction$_0$). The nomogram presents the dose fraction as a linear function of creatinine clearance.

To calculate the dose fraction$_{ri}$, the dose fraction$_0$ is obtained from Table 68-3, plotted on the left ordinate of the nomogram, and connected by a straight line to the upper right-hand corner of the nomogram. This line describes the dose fraction over a range of creatinine clearances from 0 to 100 mL/min. The point of intersection between the

FIGURE 68-5 Nomogram for estimation of the dose fraction in patients with renal insufficiency. Cr, creatinine; CL$_{cr}$, creatinine clearance. (*From Dettli L: Drug dosage in renal disease. Clin Pharmacokinet 1:126, 1976.*)

measured creatinine clearance (on the lower abscissa) and this dose-fraction line is a coordinate for which the dose fraction (on the left ordinate) corresponds to the particular creatinine clearance.

The elimination of many drugs is sufficiently rapid in patients with normal renal function that the time required to reach steady state is not significant, and usually no loading dose is used. In renal failure, however, the prolonged half-life may cause this accumulation period to become unacceptably long. In these cases, a loading dose may be indicated; the size of the loading dose would be the same as in patients with normal renal function (see "Drug Accumulation—Loading and Maintenance Doses," above).

General Considerations for Determining Dosage in Renal Insufficiency Because of the differences between patients in volumes of distribution and rates of metabolism, calculations of drug dose in renal failure must be viewed as valuable approximations that prevent the use of doses that are grossly excessive or inadequate for most patients. However, *maintenance dosages are most accurate when plasma-level data are used to adjust the dose as necessary.*

Active or toxic metabolites of drugs also may accumulate in renal failure. Meperidine, for example, is cleared largely by metabolism, and its concentration in plasma is little altered by renal insufficiency. However, the plasma concentration of one of its metabolites, normeperidine, is increased when its renal elimination is impaired. Since normeperidine has a stronger convulsant activity than meperidine, its accumulation probably accounts for the signs of central nervous system excitation, such as irritability, twitching, and seizures, that appear when multiple doses of meperidine are administered to patients with renal insufficiency.

EFFECTS OF LIVER DISEASE In contrast to the predictable decline in renal clearance of drugs when glomerular filtration is reduced, it is not possible to make a general prediction of the effect of liver disease on hepatic biotransformation of drugs (see Chap. 291). Rather, the possible effects of hepatitis or cirrhosis range from impaired to increased drug clearance. Even in advanced hepatocellular disease, drug clearance usually is impaired only about two- to fivefold. The extent of such changes, however, cannot be predicted by the common tests of liver function. Consequently, even when it is suspected that drug elimination is altered in liver disease, there is no quantitative basis on which to adjust the dosage regimen other than assessment of clinical response and the concentration of the drug in plasma.

Under conditions of decreased tissue perfusion, the cardiac output is redistributed to preserve blood flow to the heart and brain at the expense of other tissues (Chap. 38). As a result, the drug is distributed into a smaller volume of distribution, higher drug concentrations are present in the plasma and the tissues that are best perfused will be exposed to these higher concentrations. If either the brain or heart is sensitive to the drug, an alteration in response will occur.

Furthermore, the decreased perfusion of the kidney and liver may impair drug clearance by these organs directly or indirectly. Thus, in severe congestive heart failure, in hemorrhagic shock, and in cardiogenic shock, the response to the usual dose of drug may be excessive, and dosage modification may be necessary. For example, the clearance of lidocaine is reduced by about 50 percent in cardiac failure, and therapeutic plasma levels are achieved at infusion rates only about half those usually required. The volume of distribution of lidocaine also is reduced, meaning that the correct loading dose will be smaller than usual. Similar situations are thought to exist for procainamide, theophylline, and possibly quinidine. Unfortunately, predictors of these types of pharmacokinetic alterations are unavailable. Therefore, loading doses should be conservative, and continued therapy should be monitored closely, following clinical indicators of toxicity and plasma levels.

DISEASE-INDUCED CHANGES IN PLASMA BINDING Many drugs circulate in the plasma partly bound to plasma proteins. Since only the unbound (free) drug can distribute to the site of pharmacologic action, the therapeutic response should be related to the free rather than the total circulating plasma drug concentration. In most cases, the degree of binding is fairly constant across the therapeutic concentration range, so that the total drug levels in plasma can be used as a basis for adjusting dosage without resulting in significant error. However, conditions such as hypoalbuminemia, liver disease, and renal disease can decrease the extent of drug binding, particularly of acidic and neutral drugs, so that at any total plasma level there is a greater concentration of free drug than usual and thus a risk of increased response and toxicity. By contrast, conditions that lead to an increased plasma concentration of the acute-phase reactant alpha$_1$-acid glycoprotein—such as myocardial infarction, surgery, neoplastic disease, rheumatoid arthritis, and burns—cause an increase in drug binding for the basic drugs that bind to this macromolecule, resulting in an opposite set of effects. The drugs for which changes in binding are important are those that are normally highly bound in the plasma (>90 percent), because a small alteration in the extent of binding produces a large change in the amount of unbound drug.

The consequences of these binding changes, particularly with respect to total drug levels, depend on whether clearance is determined only by the unbound drug or by both forms of drug. For many drugs, elimination and distribution are restricted largely to the unbound fraction, and, therefore, a decrease in binding leads to an increase in the clearance and distribution of the drug. The relative magnitudes of these changes are such that the net effect is a shortened half-life.

In the case of drugs bound to alpha$_1$-acid glycoprotein, a disease-induced increase in binding has the opposite effects, reducing the clearance and distribution of the total drug. For example, a constant-rate infusion of lidocaine to control arrhythmias after myocardial infarction will lead to a greater accumulation of total drug.

VARIABLE ACTIONS OF DRUGS CAUSED BY GENETIC DIFFERENCES IN DRUG METABOLISM

ACETYLATION Isoniazid, hydralazine, procainamide, and a number of other drugs are metabolized by acetylation of a hydrazino or amino group. This reaction is catalyzed by *N*-acetyl transferase-2, an enzyme in the liver cytosol that transfers an acetyl group from acetyl coenzyme A to the drug. Individuals differ markedly in the rate at which drugs are acetylated, and there is a bimodal distribution of the population into "rapid acetylators" and "slow acetylators." The

rate of acetylation is under genetic control; slow acetylation is an autosomal recessive trait.

Acetylation phenotype can be determined by measuring the ratio of acetylated to nonacetylated dapsone or sulfamethazine in plasma or urine following administration of a test dose of these acetylation substrates. The ratio of monoacetyldapsone to dapsone in plasma at 6 h after dapsone administration is less than 0.30 for slow acetylators and more than 0.35 for rapid acetylators. At 6 h after the administration of sulfamethazine, the fraction of the drug in plasma that is in the acetylated form is <25 percent in slow acetylators and >25 percent in rapid acetylators; in the urine collected in the 5- to 6-h interval after administration, the fraction of drug in the acetylated form is <70 percent in slow acetylators and >70 percent in rapid acetylators. More recently, the acetylation of a metabolite of caffeine, possibly the most widely consumed drug in the world because of its presence in a variety of foods, has been used as an indicator of acetylator phenotype. In this procedure, the urinary molar ratio of 5-acetylamino-6-amino-3-methyluracil to methylxanthine after ingestion of a drink of coffee or cola is determined. Antimodes of about 1.8 and 6.6 separate slow, intermediate, and rapid acetylators; moreover, these three groups appear to correspond to the expected genotypes. The molecular bases of impaired *N*-acetyltransferase activity have now been established at the level of the gene, and several *NAT-2* alleles have been characterized. As a result, it is now possible to identify a slow acetylator by genotyping, using genomic DNA obtained from peripheral leukocytes.

METABOLISM BY MIXED-FUNCTION OXIDASES In healthy individuals taking no other medications, the major determinant of the rate of metabolism of drugs by the hepatic mixed-function oxidases is genetic. Hepatic endoplasmic reticulum contains a family of cytochrome P450 (CYP) isoforms with different substrate specificities. Many drugs undergo oxidative metabolism by more than one isoform, and the steady state concentrations of such drugs in the plasma is a function of the sum of the activities of these and other metabolizing enzymes. When a drug is metabolized by multiple pathways, the catalytic activities of the participating enzymes are regulated by a number of genes, so that the clearance rates and steady state concentrations of the drug tend to distribute unimodally within the population. The range of activity may differ markedly (tenfold or more) between different individuals, as is the case for chlorpromazine, and there is no way to predict the rate before beginning therapy.

Certain metabolic pathways show a bimodal distribution of activity, suggesting control by a single gene, and several polymorphisms have been identified. In these cases, two phenotypic populations are usually present, as for *N*-acetylation (see above). Most individuals are extensive metabolizers (the EM phenotype); a smaller group have a lower ability to metabolize the drug (or no ability at all) and are called poor metabolizers (the PM phenotype).

The cytochrome P450 isoform CYP2D6 is polymorphically distributed in the population, and about 8 to 10 percent of whites are deficient in this enzyme. CYP2D6 represents the main metabolic pathway for a number of drugs, including antiarrhythmic agents (propafenone, flecainide), beta-adrenoceptor blockers (timolol, metoprolol, and alprenolol), tricyclic antidepressants (nortriptyline, desipramine, imipramine, clomipramine), neuroleptic drugs (perphenazine, thioridazine, and possibly haloperidol), selective serotonin reuptake inhibitors (fluoxetine and paroxetine), and certain opiates, such as codeine and dextromethorphan. Thus, codeine has a much lower analgesic effect in PM patients because of impaired production of the active metabolite, morphine. Similarly, patients with the PM phenotype experience more pronounced systemic beta-adrenoceptor blockade after the administration of timolol ophthalmic solution. The catalytic activity of CYP2D6 in humans may be assessed by using a test drug, debrisoquin, which is eliminated almost entirely via hydroxylation by CYP2D6. A similar situation occurs with the oxidative polymorphism that involves the metabolism of mephenytoin by a different isoform, CYP2C19. This enzyme is also involved in the metabolism of omeprazole, proguanil, diazepam, and citalopram. The situation is further complicated by racial differences in the frequency of the polymorphisms. For example, impaired hydroxylation of mephenytoin is present in only 3 to 5 percent of whites, but the incidence is about 20 percent in individuals of Japanese and Chinese descent; likewise, the frequency of the PM phenotype for debrisoquin hydroxylation appears to decrease as one moves from Western (8 to 10 percent) to Eastern (0 to 1 percent) population groups.

Polymorphisms in drug-metabolizing ability may be associated with large differences in the disposition of a drug among individuals, especially when the involved pathway makes a major contribution to the elimination of the drug. For example, the clearance of mephenytoin given orally differs 100- to 200-fold between individuals of the EM and PM phenotypes. As a result, the peak plasma concentrations and bioavailability after oral administration may be much higher, and the rate of drug elimination much lower, in PM than in EM individuals. In PM individuals, the result is excessive drug accumulation and exaggerated pharmacologic responses, including toxicity, when usual drug dosages are administered. Inhibitory drug interactions involving compounds that are metabolized by CYP2D6 (e.g., certain selective serotonin reuptake inhibitors) or that noncompetitively inhibit the activity of the enzyme (e.g., quinidine), may be of considerable clinical importance in patients with the EM phenotype, as the concomitant administration of such agents often leads to impaired drug handling like that in the PM phenotype. Individualization of drug therapy is especially critical for drugs that exhibit polymorphic drug metabolism. As with the *NAT-2* polymorphism, the increasing availability of laboratory methods to identify the PM phenotype for CYP2D6 and CYP2C19 by genotyping should be useful for this purpose.

DRUG USE IN THE ELDERLY (See also Chap. 9)   The elderly (>65 years old) constitute about 12 percent of the U.S. population, and this fraction will increase to about 20 percent (50 to 60 million individuals) over the next 20 years. These patients use a disproportionate amount of prescription medications (30 percent). Also, 70 percent of the elderly regularly use over-the-counter drugs, compared with only 10 percent of the general adult population. Aging results in changes in organ function, especially of the organs involved in drug disposition, as well as alterations in body size and composition. Not surprisingly, therefore, pharmacokinetics are often different in elderly individuals than in younger adults. Unfortunately, few generalizations seem to be possible on the probable type, magnitude, or clinical importance of these age-related changes in an individual patient. Elderly patients often have multiple diseases and may therefore be taking a large number of drugs. Consequently, drug interactions as well as an increased vulnerability to morbidity and mortality, contribute to the higher incidence of adverse drug reactions in elderly patients. Increased sensitivity of target organs and impairment of physiologic control systems, such as those involved in the regulation of the circulation, also may be a factor. Accordingly, optimization of drug therapy in the elderly, particularly in frail patients, is often difficult, as a variety of factors (often poorly defined) accentuate the usual interindividual variability in drug response.

Although many individuals preserve good renal function into old age, elderly patients as a group have an increased likelihood of impaired renal excretion of drugs. Even in the absence of kidney disease, renal clearance is generally reduced by about 35 to 50 percent in elderly patients. Dosage adjustments analogous to those in patients with kidney dysfunction (see above) are therefore necessary for drugs that are eliminated mainly by the kidneys, such as digoxin, aminoglycosides, lithium, and other drugs listed in Table 68-3. In this regard, it is important to recognize that the reduced muscle mass of older individuals results in a reduced rate of creatinine production; thus, a normal serum creatinine concentration can be present even though creatinine clearance is impaired.

Aging also results in a decrease in the size of and blood flow to the liver and possibly in the activity of hepatic drug-metabolizing enzymes; accordingly, the hepatic clearance of some drugs is impaired

in the elderly. Unfortunately, no consistent pattern of clinical application appears to be present. Moreover, the changes are often modest relative to the interindividual variability in these patients. However, even a small reduction in hepatic extraction may significantly increase the oral bioavailability of drugs with a high first-pass effect, such as propranolol and labetalol.

Impaired clearance and/or increased distribution may cause the elimination half-life of a drug to increase with aging. Thus, if a dosage modification in an elderly patient is required, it is often possible to accomplish it by decreasing the frequency of drug administration, possibly along with a reduction in dose.

Even if the pharmacokinetics of a drug are not altered, an elderly patient may require a smaller dosage because of an increase in pharmacodynamic sensitivity. Examples include increased analgesic effects of opioids, increased sedation from benzodiazepines and other central nervous system depressants, and increased risk of bleeding while receiving anticoagulant therapy, even when clotting parameters are well controlled. Exaggerated responses to cardiovascular drugs are also common because of the impaired responsiveness of normal homeostatic mechanisms. Such age-related changes require close monitoring of the patient's clinical response and appropriate dosage titration.

In general, when administering drug therapy to an elderly patient, one should be alert to the possibility of moderate reductions in drug clearance and the chance of exaggerated pharmacodynamic responsiveness.

INTERACTIONS BETWEEN DRUGS

The effect of some drugs can be altered markedly by the administration of other agents. Such interactions can sabotage therapy by adversely increasing or decreasing the action of a drug. Drug interactions must be considered in the differential diagnosis of unexpected responses to drugs, and it should be recognized that patients often come to the physician with a legacy of drugs acquired during previous medical experiences. A meticulous drug history will minimize such unknown elements. It should include examination of the patient's medications and, if necessary, calls to the pharmacist to identify prescriptions.

There are two principal types of interactions between drugs. In *pharmacokinetic interactions*, the delivery of a drug to its site of action is altered, whereas in *pharmacodynamic interactions*, the responsiveness of the target organ or system is modified.

An index of the drug interactions discussed in this chapter is provided in Table 68-4. The table includes interactions that have verified significance in patients, plus a few that are so potentially dangerous that cognizance should be taken of the experimental data or case reports suggesting they occur.

I.   PHARMACOKINETIC INTERACTIONS CAUSING DIMINISHED DRUG DELIVERY

A.   Impaired Gastrointestinal Absorption   Cholestyramine, an ion-exchange resin, binds thyroxine, triiodothyronine, and the cardiac glycosides sufficiently strongly to impair their absorption from the gastrointestinal tract. This resin probably also interferes with the absorption of other drugs, and it is safest not to give it within 2 h of their administration. Aluminum ions, present in antacids, form insoluble chelates with the tetracyclines, preventing absorption of these drugs. Ferrous ions similarly block tetracycline absorption. Kaolin-pectin suspensions bind digoxin, and when these substances are administered together, digoxin absorption is reduced by about one-half. However, when kaolin-pectin is administered 2 h after digoxin, digoxin absorption is unaffected.

Ketoconazole is a weak base that dissolves well only at acidic pH. Histamine H_2 receptor antagonists, such as ranitidine and cimetidine, reduce gastric acidity and thus impair the dissolution and absorption of ketoconazole. By contrast, the absorption of fluconazole is not impaired by an increase in gastric pH. Oral administration of aminosalicylate interferes with the absorption of rifampin by an unknown mechanism.

B.   Induction of Hepatic Drug-Metabolizing Enzymes   When a drug is eliminated largely by metabolism, an increase in the rate of its metabolism reduces its availability to sites of action. Most drugs

Drug	Section of Chapter Describing Interaction
Allopurinol	IIA
p-Aminosalicylate	IA
Amiloride	III
Amiodarone	IIA, IIC
Amphetamine	IC
Antidepressants, tricyclic (desipramine, nortriptyline, imipramine, doxepin, protriptyline, amitriptyline)	IC
Aspirin	IIB, III
Astemizole	IIA
Azathioprine	IIA
Barbiturates (class)	IB
Carbamazepine	IB, IIA
Chlorpromazine	IC, IIA
Cholestyramine	IA
Cimetidine	IA, IIA, IIB
Cisapride	IIA
Clofibrate	IIA
Clonidine	IC
Codeine	IIA
Cotrimoxazole	IIA
Cyclosporine	IB, IIA
Dexamethasone	IB
Digoxin	IA, IIC
Diltiazem	IIA
Diuretics	III
Erythromycin	IIA
Ephedrine	IC
Ethanol	IIA
Fluconazole	IIA
Fluoxetine	IIA
Guanadrel	IC
Guanethidine	IC
Haloperidol	IIA
Indomethacin	III
Isoniazid	IIA
Itraconazole	IB, IIA
Kaolin-pectin	IA
Ketoconazole	IA, IB, IIA
Lidocaine	IIA
Lovastatin	IIA
6-Mercaptopurine	IIA
Methadone	IB
Methotrexate	IIB
Methylprednisolone	IB, IIA
Metronidazole	IB, IIA
Metyrapone	IB
Mexiletine	IB
Nicardipine	IIA
Nifedipine	IIA
Nonsteroidal antiinflammatory drugs	III
Oral contraceptive steroids	IB
Phenobarbital	IB
Phenylbutazone	IIA, IIB
Phenytoin (diphenylhydantoin)	IB, IIA
Piroxicam	III
Potassium	III
Prednisone	IB
Probenecid	IIB
Procainamide	IIB
Propranolol	III
Quinidine	IB, IIA, IIC, III
Ranitidine	IA, IIA
Rifampin	IA, IB
Salicylate	IIB
Spironolactone	III
Terfenadine	IIA
Tetracycline	IA
Theophylline	IIA
Thiazide diuretics	III
Tolbutamide	IIA
Triamterene	III
Triazolam	IIA
Verapamil	IB, IIA, IIC
Warfarin	IB, IIA, III

are metabolized largely in the liver because of this organ's large mass, high blood flow, and high concentration of drug-metabolizing enzymes. The first step in the metabolism of many drugs is catalyzed by a group of cytochrome P450 mixed-function oxidases located in the endoplasmic reticulum (see "Metabolism by Mixed-Function Oxidases," above). These enzyme systems oxidize drug molecules by a variety of reactions, including aromatic hydroxylations, N-demethylations, O-demethylations, and sulfoxidations. The products of these reactions are usually more polar than the parent compound (and more readily excreted by the kidney).

The expression of some of the mixed-function oxidase (CYP) isoforms is regulated, and their content in the liver can be increased by a number of drugs. Phenobarbital is the prototype of these inducers, and all the barbiturates in clinical use increase CYP enzyme activity. Induction with phenobarbital can occur with doses of as little as 60 mg daily. Mixed-function oxidases also are induced by rifampin, carbamazepine, phenytoin, and glutethimide, and by smoking, exposure to chlorinated insecticides such as DDT, and chronic alcohol ingestion.

Phenobarbital, rifampin, and other inducers lower plasma levels of many drugs, including warfarin, quinidine, mexiletine, verapamil, ketoconazole, itraconazole, cyclosporine, dexamethasone, methylprednisolone, prednisolone (the active metabolite of prednisone), oral contraceptive steroids, methadone, metronidazole, and metyrapone. These interactions all have obvious clinical significance. In the case of the coumarin anticoagulants, the patient is placed at major risk if the appropriate level of anticoagulation is achieved when an inducer is also being administered and the inducer is later discontinued (for example, at discharge from the hospital). The plasma levels of the coumarin anticoagulant will rise as the induction effect wears off, leading to excessive anticoagulation.

There is considerable variation among individuals in the extent to which drug metabolism can be induced. In some patients, phenobarbital leads to marked acceleration in the rate of drug metabolism, whereas little induction is seen in others.

In addition to inducing certain of the CYP isoforms, phenobarbital has other effects on hepatic function. It increases liver blood flow, bile flow, and the hepatocellular transport of organic anions. The conjugation of drugs and bilirubin also may be enhanced by inducing agents.

C. Inhibition of Cellular Uptake or Binding The guanidinium antihypertensive agents guanethidine and guanadrel are transported to their site of action in adrenergic neurons by an energy-requiring membrane transport system for biogenic monoamines. Although the physiologic function of the transport system is reuptake of the adrenergic neurotransmitter, it also transports a variety of ring-substituted bases, including guanethidine and related guanidiniums, which it can import against a concentration gradient. Inhibitors of norepinephrine uptake prevent the uptake of the guanidinium antihypertensive agents into adrenergic neurons and thereby block their pharmacologic effects. The tricyclic antidepressants are potent inhibitors of norepinephrine uptake. Consequently, concomitant administration of clinical doses of tricyclic antidepressants, including desipramine, protriptyline, nortriptyline, and amitriptyline, almost totally abolishes the antihypertensive effects of guanethidine and guanadrel. Although they are less potent inhibitors of norepinephrine uptake, doxepin and chlorpromazine produce dose-related antagonism of the action of the guanidinium antihypertensives. Ephedrine, a component of many drug combinations used in asthma, also antagonizes the effect of guanethidine. In patients with severe hypertension, the loss of control of blood pressure from these drug interactions can lead to stroke and malignant hypertension.

The antihypertensive effect of clonidine is partially antagonized by tricyclic antidepressants. Clonidine lowers arterial pressure by reducing sympathetic outflow from the blood pressure–regulating centers in the hindbrain (Chap. 246). This central hypotensive action is antagonized by the tricyclic antidepressants.

II. PHARMACOKINETIC INTERACTIONS CAUSING INCREASED DRUG DELIVERY

A. Inhibition of Drug Metabolism If the active form of a drug is eliminated largely by biotransformation, inhibition of its metabolism leads to reduced clearance, prolonged half-life, and accumulation of the drug during maintenance therapy. Excessive accumulation due to inhibited metabolism can lead to adverse effects.

Cimetidine is a potent inhibitor of the oxidative metabolism of many drugs, including warfarin, quinidine, nifedipine, lidocaine, theophylline, and phenytoin. Adverse reactions, many of them severe, have resulted from the administration of these drugs in conjunction with cimetidine. Cimetidine is a more potent inhibitor of mixed-function oxidases than ranitidine, whereas ranitidine is more potent as a histamine H_2 receptor antagonist. Thus, ranitidine, when administered in doses of 150 mg twice daily, does not inhibit the oxidative metabolism of most drugs; where reduced drug elimination has been observed, the effects of ranitidine have been less than those of cimetidine and have not had appreciable pharmacodynamic consequences. Doses of ranitidine higher than 150 mg, however, may produce greater inhibition of drug oxidation. Famotidine and nizatidine are not known to produce clinically appreciable inhibition of drug metabolism.

Knowledge of the CYP isoforms that catalyze the main pathway of metabolism of a drug provides a basis for predicting and understanding drug interactions. For example, the CYP3A subfamily of isoforms catalyze the metabolism of many drugs for which blockage of metabolism results in toxicity. Drugs that depend on CYP3A as a major route of metabolism include cyclosporine, quinidine, lovastatin, warfarin, nifedipine, lidocaine, terfenadine, astemizole, cisapride, erythromycin, methylprednisolone, carbamazepine, midazolam, and triazolam.

Erythromycin, ketoconazole, and itraconazole are potent inhibitors of enzymes in the CYP3A family. When fluconazole levels are elevated as a result of higher doses and/or renal insufficiency, this drug also can inhibit CYP3A. Some of the calcium antagonists, diltiazem, nicardipine, and verapamil also can inhibit CYP3A, as can some of its other substrates, such as cyclosporine. Thus, cyclosporine can cause serious toxicity when its metabolism is inhibited by erythromycin, ketoconazole, diltiazem, nicardipine, or verapamil. Lovastatin causes severe myopathy with rhabdomyolysis when administered together with erythromycin or cyclosporine, and it is highly probable that other of the known inhibitors of CYP3A also can inhibit the disposition of lovastatin. Terfenadine, astemizole, and cisapride can cause polymorphic ventricular tachycardia (torsade de pointes) when their metabolism is blocked by inhibitors of CYP3A, such as ketoconazole, itraconazole, and erythromycin.

Whenever erythromycin, ketoconazole, or itraconazole is administered to a patient, the physician should be alert to the possibility of serious interactions with drugs that are metabolized by CYP3A.

The CYP2D6 isoform that catalyzes the polymorphic metabolism of debrisoquin is markedly inhibited by quinidine and also is blocked by a number of neuroleptic drugs, such as chlorpromazine and haloperidol, and by fluoxetine. The analgesic effect of codeine depends on its metabolism to morphine via CYP2D6 in individuals with the extensive metabolizer phenotype. Thus, quinidine reduces the analgesic efficacy of codeine in extensive metabolizers. Since desipramine is cleared largely by metabolism via CYP2D6 in extensive metabolizers, its levels are increased substantially by concurrent administration of quinidine, fluoxetine, or the neuroleptic drugs that inhibit CYP2D6.

Some drugs are inactivated by mechanisms other than the hepatic drug-metabolizing enzymes. Azathioprine is converted in the body to an active metabolite, 6-mercaptopurine, which in turn is oxidized by xanthine oxidase to 6-thiouric acid. When allopurinol, a potent inhibitor of xanthine oxidase, is administered concurrently with standard doses of azathioprine or 6-mercaptopurine, life-threatening toxicity (bone marrow suppression) can result.

Other drugs that inhibit biotransformation of pharmacologic compounds (with examples of drugs whose metabolism is blocked by the inhibitor listed in parenthesis) include:

- Amiodarone (warfarin, quinidine)
- Clofibrate (phenytoin, tolbutamide)
- Excessive ingestion of ethanol (warfarin)
- Isoniazid (phenytoin)
- Metronidazole, cotrimoxazole (warfarin)
- Phenylbutazone (warfarin, phenytoin, tolbutamide)

B. Inhibition of Renal Elimination A number of drugs are secreted by the renal tubular transport systems for organic anions. Inhibition of this tubular transport system can cause excessive accumulation of a drug. Phenylbutazone, probenecid, and salicylates competitively inhibit this transport system. Salicylate, for example, reduces the renal clearance of methotrexate, an interaction that may lead to methotrexate toxicity. Renal tubular secretion contributes substantially to the elimination of penicillin, which can be inhibited by probenecid.

Inhibition of the tubular cation transport system by cimetidine impedes the renal clearance of procainamide and its active metabolite *N*-acetylprocainamide.

C. Inhibition of Clearance at Multiple Sites The concentrations of digoxin in plasma are elevated by quinidine, owing largely to inhibition of renal elimination and in part to inhibition of biliary secretion. An increase in cardiac arrhythmia may occur when quinidine is given in conjunction with a cardiac glycoside.

Amiodarone, cyclosporine, itraconazole, and verapamil also inhibit the clearance of digoxin and increase the concentration of digoxin in plasma.

III. PHARMACODYNAMIC AND OTHER INTERACTIONS BETWEEN DRUGS

Therapeutically useful interactions occur in which the effect of two drugs in combination is greater than the sum of their effects when used individually. Favorable drug combinations are described in specific therapeutic sections in this text, and this section focuses on interactions that create unwanted effects. Two drugs may act on separate components of a common process to yield effects greater than either has alone. For example, although small doses of aspirin (less than 1 g daily) do not alter the prothrombin time appreciably in patients who are receiving warfarin therapy, aspirin nevertheless increases the risk of bleeding in these patients because it inhibits platelet aggregation. Thus the combination of impaired functions of platelets and the clotting system increases the potential for hemorrhagic complications in patients receiving warfarin therapy.

Nonsteroidal antiinflammatory drugs cause gastric and duodenal ulcers, and, in patients treated with warfarin, the risk of bleeding from a peptic ulcer is increased almost threefold by concomitant use of a nonsteroidal antiinflammatory drug. This clearly is a serious drug interaction.

Indomethacin, piroxicam, and probably other nonsteroidal antiinflammatory drugs antagonize the antihypertensive effects of beta-adrenergic receptor blockers, diuretics, converting-enzyme inhibitors, and other drugs. The resulting elevation in blood pressure ranges from trivial to severe. Aspirin and sulindac, however, do not elevate the blood pressure in treated hypertensive patients.

Polymorphic ventricular tachycardia (torsade de pointes) during quinidine administration occurs much more frequently in patients receiving diuretics, probably owing to potassium and/or magnesium depletion.

The administration of supplemental potassium leads to more frequent and more severe hyperkalemia when potassium elimination is reduced by concurrent treatment with angiotensin-converting enzyme inhibitors, spironolactone, amiloride, or triamterene.

CONCENTRATION OF DRUGS IN PLASMA AS A GUIDE TO THERAPY

In many cases, the plasma concentration of a drug is measured as a guide in the individualization of therapy. Genetic variation in elimination rates, interactions with other drugs, disease-induced alterations in elimination and distribution, and other factors combine to yield a wide range of plasma levels in patients given the same dose. Furthermore, the problem of noncompliance with prescribed regimens during continuing therapy is an endemic and elusive cause of therapeutic failure (see below). Clinical indicators assist in the titration of some drugs into the desired range, and no chemical determination is a substitute for careful observations of the response to treatment. However, the therapeutic and adverse effects are not precisely quantifiable for all drugs, and, in complex clinical situations, estimates of the action of a drug may be misleading. For example, previously existing neurologic disease may obscure the neurologic consequences of intoxication with phenytoin. Because clearance, half-life, accumulation, and steady state plasma levels are difficult to predict, the measurement of plasma levels is often useful as a guide to the optimal dose. This is particularly true when there is a narrow range between the plasma levels yielding therapeutic and adverse effects. For drugs having such characteristics—e.g., digoxin, theophylline, lidocaine, aminoglycosides, and anticonvulsants—dose optimization should involve modification of the standard dose on the basis of the pharmacokinetic principles described above. In certain instances, predictive nomograms and algorithms have been developed to facilitate the necessary modifications. However, the most flexible and accurate method for individualizing drug dosage appears to be a feedback approach using a small number of previously obtained plasma levels and Bayesian forecasting. In controlled studies, this type of computer-assisted dosing has been shown to improve patient care. However, the overall cost/benefit ratio of such methods in routine management still remains to be concusively demonstrated.

For drugs with a narrow therapeutic window that exhibit first-order elimination, then, dosage adjustments may be made on the assumption that the average, maximum, and minimum steady state concentrations are related linearly to the dosing rate. Accordingly, the dose may be adjusted on the basis of the ratio between the desired and measured concentrations:

$$\frac{Cp_{SS} \text{ (desired)}}{Cp_{SS} \text{ (measured)}} = \frac{\text{dose (new)}}{\text{dose (previous)}}$$

For drugs that have dose-dependent kinetics (e.g., phenytoin and theophylline), plasma concentrations change disproportionately more than the alteration in the dosing rate. Not only should changes in dose be small to minimize the degree of unpredictability, but plasma concentration monitoring also is critical to ensure appropriate modification.

The variability among individual responses to given plasma levels must be recognized. This is illustrated by a hypothetical population concentration-response curve (Fig. 68-6) and its relationship to the

Table 68-5

Concentrations of Drugs in Plasma: Relation to Efficacy and Adverse Effects

Drug	Efficacy*	Adverse Effects†
Amikacin (peak)	20 μg/mL	40 μg/mL
Carbenicillin	100 μg/mL‡	300 μg/mL
Carbamazepine	3 μg/mL	10 μg/mL
Digitoxin	12 ng/mL	25–30 ng/mL
Digoxin	0.8 ng/mL	2.0 ng/mL
Ethosuximide	40 μg/mL	100 μg/mL
Gentamicin (peak)	5 μg/mL	10 μg/mL
Gentamicin (predose)		2.0 μg/mL
Lidocaine	1.5 μg/mL	5 μg/mL
Lithium	0.5 mEq/L	1.3 mEq/L
Penicillin G	1–25 μg/mL§	
Phenytoin (diphenylhydantoin)	10 μg/mL	20 μg/mL
Procainamide	4 μg/mL	10 μg/mL
Quinidine	2.5 μg/mL	6 μg/mL
Theophylline	8 μg/mL	20 μg/mL

* The therapeutic effect is infrequent or slight at levels below these.
† The frequency of adverse effects increases sharply when these levels are exceeded.
‡ Minimal inhibitory concentration (MIC) for most strains of *Pseudomonas aeruginosa*. MIC for other, more sensitive, organisms is less.
§ There is a wide range of MIC of penicillin for various organisms, and the MIC of all those for which penicillin is used is <20. "Massive" penicillin therapy with 20 million units daily achieves levels of 20 to 25 μg/mL in patients with clearance of creatinine of 100 mL/min.

therapeutic range or therapeutic window of desired plasma levels. The defined therapeutic window should include the levels at which the intended pharmacologic effect is achieved in most patients. However, a few persons, who are sensitive to the therapeutic effects, respond to lower levels, whereas others are refractory enough to require levels that may cause adverse effects. For example, a few patients with strong seizure foci require plasma levels of phenytoin exceeding 20 μg/mL to control seizures. Dosages to achieve this effect may be appropriate.

As also illustrated in Fig. 68-6, some patients are prone to adverse effects at levels that are tolerated by most of the population. Therefore, raising the plasma concentration of a drug to a level that has a high probability of being therapeutically effective may bring on unwanted actions in an occasional patient. Table 68-5 presents for a number of drugs the plasma concentrations that are associated with adverse and therapeutic effects in most patients. Use of this information according to the guidelines discussed should permit more effective and safer therapy for those patients who are not "average."

EFFECTIVE PARTICIPATION OF THE PATIENT IN THERAPY Measurement of the concentration of a drug in plasma is the most effective way to detect failure to take a drug. Such "noncompliance" is a frequent problem in the long-term treatment of diseases such as hypertension and epilepsy, occurring in 25 percent or more of patients in therapeutic environments in which no special effort is made to involve patients in the responsibility for their own health. Occasionally, noncompliance can be uncovered by sympathetic, nonincriminating questioning, but more often it is recognized only after determining that the concentration of drug in plasma is nil or is recurrently low. Because other factors can cause plasma levels to be lower than expected, comparison with levels obtained during inpatient treatment may be required to confirm that noncompliance has occurred. Once the physician is certain of noncompliance, a nonaccusatory discussion of the problem with the patient may clarify the reason for the noncompliance and serve as a basis for more effective cooperation on the part of the patient. Many approaches have been tried to make patients exercise more responsibility for their own treatment, most based on better communication regarding the nature of the disease and the chances of success or failure of the treatment. The patient is given a chance to discuss problems associated with treatment. The process may be improved by the involvement of nurses and other

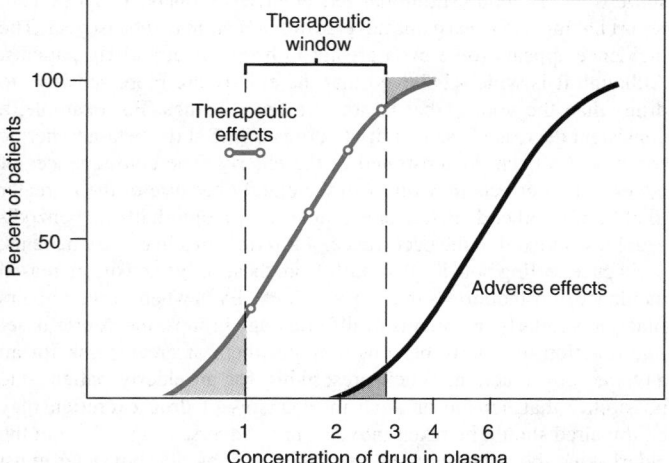

FIGURE 68-6 The cumulative percentage of patients responding to increasing levels of drug in plasma with both therapeutic and adverse effects. The therapeutic window defines the range of concentrations of drug that will achieve therapeutic effects in most patients with adverse effects in only a small percentage.

paramedical personnel. Minimizing the complexity of the regimen is helpful in terms of both the number of drugs and the frequency of administration. Educating patients to assume the principal role in their own health care requires a blend of the art and science of medicine.

BIBLIOGRAPHY

BENET LZ et al: Design and optimization of dosage regimens: Pharmacokinetic data, in *Goodman and Gilman's The Pharmacological Basis of Therapeutics*, 9th ed, JG Hardman et al (eds). New York, McGraw-Hill, 1995, Appendix II, p 1707

BENNETT WM et al: *Drug Prescribing in Renal Failure: Dosing Guidelines for Adults*, 2d ed. Philadelphia, American College of Physicians, 1991

BROWN GR et al: Drug concentration monitoring. An approach to rational use. Clin Pharmacokinet 24:187, 1993

MEYER UA: Drugs in special patient groups: Clinical importance of genetics in drug effects, in *Clinical Pharmacology: Basic Principles in Therapeutics*, 3d ed, KL Melmon et al (eds). New York, McGraw-Hill, 1992, p 875

NEBERT DW et al: The P450 superfamily: Update on new sequences, gene mapping, accession numbers and nomenclature. Pharmacogenetics 6:1, 1996

REYNOLDS DJ, ARONSON JK: ABCs of monitoring drug therapy. Making the most of plasma drug concentration measurements. BMJ 306:48, 1993

TUKEY RH, JOHNSON EF: Molecular aspects of regulation and structure of drug metabolizing enzymes, in *Principles of Drug Action: The Basis of Pharmacology*, 3d ed, WB Pratt, P Taylor (eds). New York, Churchill Livingstone, 1990, p 423

69 Alastair J. J. Wood

ADVERSE REACTIONS TO DRUGS*

The beneficial effects of drugs are coupled with the inescapable risk of untoward effects. The morbidity and mortality from these untoward effects often present diagnostic problems because they can involve every organ and system of the body and are frequently mistaken for signs of underlying disease. Major advances in the investigation, development, and regulation of drugs ensure in most instances that they are uniform, effective, and relatively safe and that their recognized hazards are publicized. However, the large number and variety of drugs available over the counter (OTC) or by prescription make it impossible for patient or physician to obtain or retain the knowledge necessary to use all drugs well. It is understandable, therefore, that many OTC drugs are used unwisely by the public and that restricted drugs may be prescribed incorrectly by physicians.

Most physicians use no more than 50 drug products in their practice, gaining familiarity with their effectiveness and safety. Most patients probably use only a limited number of OTC drugs. Nevertheless, many patients receive care and drug prescriptions from more than one physician, and in any 30-day period, many patients consume more than three different OTC drug products containing nine or more different chemical agents.

Twenty-five to fifty percent of patients make errors in self-administration of prescribed medicines, and these errors can be responsible for adverse drug effects. Elderly patients are the group most likely to commit such errors, perhaps in part because they consume more medicines. One-third or more of patients also may not take their prescribed medications. Similarly, patients commit errors in taking OTC drugs by not reading or following the directions on the containers. Physicians must recognize that providing directions with prescriptions does not always guarantee compliance.

* John A. Oates was coauthor in the 12th edition, and this chapter represents a revision of that work.

Every drug can produce untoward consequences, even when used according to standard or recommended methods of administration. When used incorrectly, the effectiveness may be reduced, and adverse reactions can be expected to occur more frequently. Also, the administration of several drugs concurrently may result in adverse drug interactions (see Chap. 68). In the hospital, all drugs a patient is given should be under the control of a physician, and patient compliance is, in general, ensured. Errors may occur nevertheless—the wrong drug or dose may be given, or the drug may be given to the wrong patient—although improved drug distribution and administration systems have reduced this problem. On the other hand, there are no means for controlling how ambulatory patients take prescription or OTC drugs.

EPIDEMIOLOGY Epidemiologic studies of adverse drug reactions have been helpful in evaluating the magnitude of the overall problem, in calculating the rate of reactions to individual drugs, and in characterizing some of the determinants of adverse drug effects.

Patients receive, on average, 10 different drugs during each hospitalization. The sicker the patient, the more drugs are given, and there is a corresponding increase in the likelihood of adverse drug reactions. When fewer than 6 different drugs are given to hospitalized patients, the probability of an adverse reaction is about 5 percent, but if more than 15 drugs are given, the probability is over 40 percent. Retrospective analyses of ambulatory patients have revealed adverse drug effects in 20 percent.

Thus, the magnitude of drug-induced disease is large. Of patients admitted to the medical and pediatric services of general hospitals, 2 to 5 percent are admitted because of illnesses attributed to drugs. The case/fatality ratio from drug-induced disease in hospitalized patients varies from 2 to 12 percent. Furthermore, some fetal or neonatal abnormalities are due to medicines taken by the mother during pregnancy or parturition.

A small group of widely used drugs accounts for a disproportionate number of reactions. Aspirin and other analgesics, digoxin, anticoagulants, diuretics, antimicrobials, steroids, antineoplastics, and hypoglycemic agents account for 90 percent of reactions, although the drugs involved differ between ambulatory and hospitalized patients. Estimates of the cost of drug-related morbidity and mortality in the ambulatory setting range from $30 billion to $130 billion.

ADVERSE DRUG REACTIONS IN THE ELDERLY (See also Chap. 9) The elderly as a group have a greater burden of disease and receive a greater number of medications than other persons. Thus, it is not surprising that adverse drug reactions occur frequently in elderly patients. The issue of whether an elderly individual is more likely to develop an adverse drug reaction than a young person with a similar number of concurrent diseases and taking the same number of drugs has not been answered unequivocally. However, in population surveys of the noninstitutionalized elderly, as many as 10 percent report having had at least one adverse drug reaction in the last year. The incidence appears to be even greater in hospitalized elderly patients. Although it is widely believed that the elderly are more sensitive to drugs than the young, that is not true for all drugs. For example, a consistent decrease in sensitivity to drugs acting at the beta-adrenergic receptor has been demonstrated in the elderly. The consequences of adverse drug effects may differ in the elderly because of their greater likelihood of other disease. For example, use of long–half-life benzodiazepines is linked to the occurrence of hip fractures in elderly patients, perhaps reflecting both a risk of falls from these drugs and the increased incidence of osteoporosis in elderly patients. Even when a drug impairs function similarly in patients of different age groups, the poorer baseline function in elderly persons may put them at greater risk for an adverse drug reaction. When prescribing for an elderly patient, the possibility that hepatic or renal mechanisms of drug excretion may be impaired should be taken into account. Adverse drug effects in the elderly may be subtle and, as in all populations, the physician must be alert to the possibility that a patient's signs and symptoms reflect an adverse effect of medication.

ETIOLOGY Most adverse drug reactions are preventable, and recent studies using a systems analysis approach suggest that the most common system failure associated with an adverse drug reaction is the failure to disseminate knowledge about drugs to individuals involved in prescribing and administering them. Most adverse reactions can be classified into two groups. The most frequent ones result from an exaggeration of a predicted pharmacologic action of the drug. Other adverse reactions ensue from toxic effects unrelated to the intended pharmacologic actions. The latter effects often are unpredictable, frequently are severe, and result from recognized as well as undiscovered mechanisms. Some mechanisms unrelated to the drug's primary pharmacologic activity include direct cytotoxicity, initiation of abnormal immune responses, and perturbation of metabolic processes in individuals with genetic enzymatic defects. Further understanding of interindividual differences in the expression of the enzymes responsible for drug metabolism has contributed to the understanding of adverse drug reactions that previously were thought to be idiosyncratic. For example, the hemotoxicity of dapsone, which includes hemolysis in patients with glucose-6-phosphate dehydrogenase (G6PD) deficiency as well as agranulocytosis, is thought to be due to the metabolism of dapsone to its hydroxylamine metabolite by specific cytochrome P450 enzymes. The extent to which dapsone is converted to this toxic metabolite depends on the activity of these cytochrome P450 enzymes in the individual, which thus determines the individual's susceptibility to the adverse effect. Conversely, an understanding of the enzymes responsible for producing the toxic metabolite may make it possible to coadminister specific enzyme inhibitors that will prevent the toxic effect. Prior consideration of the factors known to modify drug action often make it possible to prevent adverse reactions of this type.

An abnormally high drug concentration at the receptor site (site of action) owing to pharmacokinetic variability is the usual cause of these reactions (see Chap. 68). For example, a reduction in the volume of distribution, in the rate of metabolism, or in the rate of excretion all result in higher than expected concentration of drug at the receptor site, with a consequent increase in the pharmacologic effect.

Recently, the specific cytochrome P450s involved in drug metabolism have been identified. Recognition of the polymorphic distribution of some of these enzyme activities within the population provides an explanation for interindividual variability in drug clearance. Also, as simple tests are developed to characterize an individual's specific cytochrome P450 activity, it should become possible to identify in advance individuals at particular risk for concentration-related adverse effects. For enzymes whose activity is polymorphically distributed a proportion of the population has little or no enzyme activity. In these individuals, the concentration of drugs achieved will be higher than normal and may produce toxicity. Conversely, where toxicity or efficacy is produced by a metabolite, poor metabolizers will have limited toxicity or efficacy. The polymorphic distribution of drug-metabolizing enzymes may explain some adverse drug effects previously labeled as idiosyncratic.

Alteration in the dose-response curve due to increased receptor sensitivity results in an increase in drug effect at a given drug concentration. An example is the excessive response of elderly persons to the anticoagulant warfarin at normal or lower than normal blood levels.

The shape of the dose-response curve also determines the likelihood of adverse drug reactions. Drugs with a steep dose-response curve or a narrow therapeutic index (see Chap. 68) are more likely to cause dose-related toxicity because a small increase in dose produces a large change in pharmacologic effect. An increase in the dose of drugs that exhibit nonlinear kinetics, such as phenytoin (see Chap. 68), may produce a proportionately greater increase in the blood level, resulting in toxicity.

Concurrent administration of other drugs may affect pharmacokinetics or pharmacodynamics. Pharmacokinetics may be affected by alterations in bioavailability, protein binding, or the rate of metabolism or excretion. Pharmacodynamics may be altered by another drug that competes for the same receptor sites, that prevents the drug from reaching its site of action, or that antagonizes or enhances the drug's pharmacologic effect. Inhibition of the metabolism of one drug by another may occur when both drugs bind to the same cytochrome P450. Therefore, as the specific cytochrome P450s responsible for the metabolism of individual drugs becomes known, prediction of drug

interactions is put on a more rational scientific basis. An important recent example of such a mechanism is the inhibition of terfenadine's metabolism by inhibitors of Cyp3A, such as erythromycin and systemic antimycotics. Such inhibition has resulted in torsade de pointes and lethal cardiac arrhythmia (see Chap. 68).

TOXICITY UNRELATED TO A DRUG'S PRIMARY PHARMACOLOGIC ACTIVITY   Cytotoxic Reactions   The understanding of so-called idiosyncratic reactions has greatly improved with the recognition that many of them are due to irreversible binding of a drug or its metabolites to tissue macromolecules by covalent bonds. Some chemical carcinogens, such as the alkylating agents, combine directly with DNA. Usually, it is only after metabolic activation of a drug to reactive metabolites that covalent binding occurs. This activation usually occurs in the microsomal mixed-function oxidase system, the hepatic enzyme system responsible for the metabolism of many drugs (see Chap. 68). During the course of drug metabolism, reactive metabolites may covalently bind to tissue macromolecules, causing tissue damage. Because of the reactive nature of these metabolites, covalent binding often occurs close to the site of production. Typically that is the liver, but the mixed-function oxidase system is found in other tissues as well.

An example of this type of adverse drug reaction is the hepatotoxicity associated with isoniazid. This drug is metabolized principally by acetylation to acetylisoniazid, which is then hydrolyzed to acetylhydrazine. The further metabolism of acetylhydrazine by the mixed-function oxidase system liberates reactive metabolites that covalently bind to hepatic macromolecules, causing hepatic necrosis. The administration of drugs known to increase the activity of the mixed-function oxidase system, such as phenobarbital or rifampin, together with isoniazid results in the production of increased amounts of reactive metabolites, increased covalent binding, and a greater risk of hepatic damage.

The hepatic necrosis produced by overdosage of acetaminophen is also caused by reactive metabolites. Normally these metabolites are detoxified by combining with hepatic glutathione. When glutathione becomes exhausted, the metabolites bind instead to hepatic protein, with resultant hepatocyte damage. The hepatic necrosis produced by the ingestion of acetaminophen can be prevented, or at least attenuated, by the administration of substances such as *N*-acetylcysteine that reduce the binding of electrophilic metabolites to hepatic proteins. The risk of hepatic necrosis is increased in patients receiving drugs such as phenobarbital that increase the rate of drug metabolism and the rate of production of toxic metabolite(s).

It is likely, though as yet not proven, that other idiosyncratic reactions are caused by the covalent binding of reactive metabolites to tissue macromolecules, resulting either in direct cytotoxicity or in the initiation of an immune response.

Immunologic Mechanisms   Most pharmacologic agents are poor immunogens because they are small molecules with molecular weights of less than 2000. Stimulation of antibody synthesis or sensitization of lymphocytes by a drug or one of its metabolites usually requires in vivo activation and covalent linkage to protein, carbohydrate, or nucleic acid.

Drug stimulation of antibody production may mediate tissue injury by one of several mechanisms. The antibody may attack the drug when the drug is covalently attached to a cell, and thereby destroy the cell. This mechanism occurs in penicillin-induced hemolytic anemia. Antibody-drug-antigen complexes may be passively adsorbed by a bystander cell, which is then destroyed by activation of complement; this occurs in quinine- and quinidine-induced thrombocytopenia. Drugs or their reactive metabolites may alter a host tissue, rendering it antigenic and eliciting autoantibodies. For example, hydralazine and procainamide can chemically alter nuclear material, stimulating the formation of anti-nuclear antibodies and occasionally causing lupus erythematosus. Autoantibodies can be elicited by drugs that neither interact with the host antigen nor have any chemical similarity to the host tissue; for example, α-methyldopa frequently stimulates the formation of antibodies to host erythrocytes, yet the drug neither attaches to the erythrocyte nor shares any chemical similarities with the antigenic determinants on the erythrocyte.

Drug-induced *pure red cell aplasia* (Chap. 110) is due to an immune-based drug reaction. Red cell formation in bone marrow cultures can be inhibited by phenytoin and purified IgG obtained from a patient with pure red cell aplasia associated with phenytoin.

Serum sickness (Chap. 310) results from the deposition of circulating drug-antibody complexes on endothelial surfaces. Complement activation occurs, chemotactic factors are generated locally, and an inflammatory response develops at the site of complex entrapment. Arthralgias, urticaria, lymphadenopathy, glomerulonephritis, or cerebritis may result. Penicillin is the most common cause of serum sickness today. Many drugs, particularly antimicrobial agents, induce production of IgE, which binds to mast cell membranes. Contact with a drug antigen initiates a series of biochemical events in the mast cell and results in the release of mediators that can produce the urticaria, wheezing, flushing, rhinorrhea, and (occasionally) hypotension characteristic of anaphylaxis.

Drugs also may excite cell-mediated immune responses. Topically administered substances may interact with sulfhydryl or amino groups in the skin and react with sensitized lymphocytes to produce the rash characteristic of contact dermatitis. Other types of rashes also may result from the interaction of serum factors, drugs, and sensitized lymphocytes. The role of drug-activated lymphocytes in the immune mechanisms governing destruction of visceral tissue is unknown.

Toxicity Associated with Genetically Determined Enzymatic Defects In the porphyrias, drugs that increase the activity of enzymes proximal to the deficient enzyme in the biosynthetic pathway of porphyrins can increase the quantity of porphyrin precursors that accumulate proximal to the deficient enzyme (Chap. 343). These drugs are listed in Table 69-1.

Patients with a deficiency of G6PD develop hemolytic anemia in response to primaquine and a number of other drugs (Table 69-1) that do not cause hemolysis in patients with adequate quantities of this enzyme (Chap. 109).

DIAGNOSIS The manifestations of drug-induced diseases frequently resemble those of other diseases, and a given set of manifestations may be produced by different and dissimilar drugs. Recognition of the role of a drug or drugs in an illness depends on appreciation of the possible adverse reactions to drugs in any disease, on identification of the temporal relationship between drug administration and development of the illness, and on familiarity with the common manifestations of the drugs. Many associations between particular drugs and specific reactions have been described, but there is always a "first time" for a novel association, and any drug should be suspected of causing an adverse effect if the clinical setting is appropriate.

Illness related to a drug's pharmacologic action often is more easily recognized than illness attributable to immune or other mechanisms. For example, side effects such as cardiac arrhythmias in patients receiving digitalis, hypoglycemia in patients given insulin, and bleeding in patients receiving anticoagulants are more readily related to a

Table 69-1

Clinical Manifestations of Adverse Reactions to Drugs

I. MULTISYSTEM MANIFESTATIONS

Anaphylaxis	Drug-induced lupus erythematosus	Fever	Serum sickness
ACE* inhibitors and dialysis	Acebutolol	Aminosalicylic acid	Aspirin
Cephalosporins	Asparaginase	Amphotericin B	β-lactams
Demeclocycline	Barbiturates	Antihistamines	Penicillins
Dextran	Bleomycin	Carbenicillin	Propylthiouracil
Insulin	Cephalosporins	Intravenous immune globulin	Streptokinase
Intravenous immune globulin	Hydralazine	Novobiocin	Streptomycin
Iodinated drugs or contrast media	Iodides	Pamidronate	Sulfonamides
Iron dextran	Isoniazid	Penicillins	Vasculitis
Lidocaine	Methyldopa	Streptokinase	Allopurinol
Penicillins	Phenolphthalein	Hyperpyrexia	Aminopenicillins
Procaine	Phenytoin	Antipsychotics	Hydantoins
Streptomycin	Procainamide	Neuroleptic malignant syndrome	Penicillin
Sulfobromophthalein	Quinidine	Antipsychotics	Propylthiouracil
Angioedema	Sulfonamides	Antidopaminergics	Sulfonamides
ACE* inhibitors	Thiouracil		Thiazides
Penicillin			

II. ENDOCRINE MANIFESTATIONS

Addisonian-like syndrome	Gynecomastia (*cont.*)	Sexual dysfunction	Thyroid dysfunction (*cont.*)
Busulfan	Isoniazid	Decreased libido and impotence	Colestipol and nicotinic acid
Etomidate	Methyldopa	(*cont.*)	Dimercaprol
Ketoconazole	Phenytoin	Methyldopa	Gold salts
Galactorrhea (may also cause	Reserpine	Oral contraceptives	Iodides
amenorrhea)	Spironolactone	Sedatives	Lithium
Domperidone	Testosterone	Impairment of spermatogenesis or	Oral contraceptives
Methyldopa	Sexual dysfunction	oogenesis	Phenindione
Metoclopramide	Impaired ejaculation	Cytotoxic agents	Phenothiazines (long-term)
Phenothiazines	Bethanidine	Priapism	Phenylbutazone
Reserpine	Debrisoquin	Trazodone	Phenytoin
Tricyclic antidepressants	Guanethidine	Thyroid dysfunction (disorders	Sulfonamides
Gynecomastia	Thioridazine	causing abnormal results on	Tolbutamide
Calcium channel antagonists	Decreased libido and impotence	thyroid function tests)	Vaginal carcinoma
Clomiphene	Beta blockers	Acetazolamide	Diethylstilbestrol (given to
Digitalis	Clonidine	Amiodarone	mother)
Estrogens	Diuretics	Bromsulfophthalein	
Ethionamide	Lithium	Chlorpropamide	
Griseofulvin	Major tranquilizers	Clofibrate	

(*continued*)

Table 69-1—*(continued)*

Clinical Manifestations of Adverse Reactions to Drugs

III. METABOLIC MANIFESTATIONS

Hyperbilirubinemia
  Novobiocin
  Rifampin
Hypercalcemia
  Antacids with absorbable alkali
  Calcitonin
  Thiazides
  Vitamin D
Hyperglycemia
  Asparaginase
  Chlorthalidone
  Diazoxide
  Encainide
  Ethacrynic acid
  Furosemide
  Glucocorticoids
  Growth hormone
  Niacin
  Oral contraceptives
  Phenytoin
  Pentamidine
  Thiazides
Hypoglycemia
  Insulin
  Octreotide
  Oral hypoglycemics
  Pentamidine
  Quinine

Hyperkalemia
  ACE* inhibitors
  Amiloride
  Cyclosporine
  Cytotoxics
  Digitalis overdose
  Heparin
  Lithium
  NSAIDs†
  Pentamidine
  Potassium preparations
    including salt substitute
  Potassium salts of drugs
  Spironolactone
  Succinylcholine
  Triamterene
  Trimethoprin
Hypokalemia
  Alkali-induced alkalosis
  Amphotericin B
  Carbenoxolone
  Corticosteroids
  Diuretics
  Gentamicin
  Insulin
  Laxatives (abused)
  Mineralocorticoids, some
    glucocorticoids

Hypokalemia *(cont.)*
  Osmotic diuretics
  Sympathomimetic agents
  Tetracycline (degraded)
  Theophylline
  Vitamin B$_{12}$
Hyperuricemia
  Aspirin (low dose)
  Chlorthalidone
  Cyclosporine
  Cytotoxics
  Ethacrynic acid
  Fructose (IV)
  Furosemide
  Hyperalimentation
  Pyrazinamide
  Thiazides
Hyponatremia
  Dilutional:
    Antipsychotics
    Carbamazepine
    Chlorpropamide
    Cyclophosphamide
    Desmopressin
    Diuretics
    Intravenous immune globulin
    Octreotide
    Vincristine

Hyponatremia *(cont.)*
  Salt-wasting:
    Diuretics
    Enemas
    Mannitol
Metabolic acidosis
  Acetazolamide
  Metformin
  Paraldehyde (degraded)
  Phenformin
  Salicylates
  Spironolactone
Porphyria exacerbation
  Barbiturates
  Chlordiazepoxide
  Chlorpropamide
  Estrogens
  Glutethimide
  Griseofulvin
  Meprobamate
  Oral contraceptives
  Phenytoin
  Rifampin
  Sulfonamides

IV. DERMATOLOGIC MANIFESTATIONS

Acne
  Anabolic and androgenic steroids
  Bromides
  Glucocorticoids
  Iodides
  Isoniazid
  Oral contraceptives
  Troxidone
Alopecia
  Beta blockers
  Colchicine
  Cytotoxics
  Ethionamide
  Fluconazole
  Heparin
  Interferon
  Lithium
  Oral contraceptives (withdrawal)
  Retinoids
Eczema
  Captopril
  Cream and lotion preservatives
  Lanolin
  Topical antihistamines
  Topical antimicrobials
  Topical local anesthetics
Erythema multiforme or Steven-
  Johnson syndrome/toxic epidermal
  necrolysis
  Allopurinol
  Aminopenicillins
  Barbiturates
  Carbamazepine
  Cephalosporins
  Chlorpropamide
  Codeine
  Ethosuximide

Erythema multiforme *(cont.)*
  Imidazoles
  Iodides
  Lamotrigine
  Nalidixic acid
  Penicillins
  Phenolphthalein
  Phenylbutazone
  Phenytoin
  Piroxicam
  Quinolones
  Salicylates
  Sulfonamides
  Sulfones
  Tetracyclines
  Thiazides
  Tocainide
  Valproic acid
Erythema nodosum
  Oral contraceptives
  Penicillins
  Sulfonamides
Exfoliative dermatitis
  Barbiturates
  Gold salts
  Penicillins
  Phenylbutazone
  Phenytoin
  Quinidine
  Sulfonamides
Fixed drug eruptions
  Barbiturates
  Captopril
  Foscarnet (penile ulceration)
  Phenolphthalein
  Phenylbutazone
  Quinine

Fixed drug eruptions *(cont.)*
  Salicylates
  Sulfonamides
Hyperpigmentation
  Bleomycin
  Busulfan
  Chloroquine and other
    antimalarials
  Corticotropin
  Cyclophosphamide
  Gold salts
  Oral contraceptives
  Phenothiazines
  Vitamin A (hypervitaminosis A)
Hypertrichosis
  Cyclosporin
  Minoxidil
  Phenytoin
Lichenoid eruptions
  Aminosalicylic acid
  Antimalarials
  Chlorpropamide
  Gold salts
  Methyldopa
  Phenothiazines
Nail changes
  Penicillamine
  Retinoids
  Tetracyclines
Photodermatitis
  Captopril
  Chlordiazepoxide
  Furosemide
  Griseofulvin
  Nalidixic acid
  NSAIDs†
  Oral contraceptives

Photodermatitis *(cont.)*
  Phenothiazines
  Sulfonamides
  Sulfonylureas
  Tetracyclines, particularly
    demeclocycline
  Thiazides
Purpura (see also
  thrombocytopenia)
  Aspirin
  Glucocorticoids
  Rashes (nonspecific)
  Allopurinol
  Ampicillin
  Barbiturates
  Indapamide
  Methyldopa
  Phenytoin
Raynaud's disease or digital
  necrosis
  Beta blockers
  Bleomycin
  Ergot alkaloids
Skin necrosis
  Warfarin
Urticaria
  Aspirin
  Barbiturates
  Captopril
  Enalapril
  Intravenous immune
    globulin
  Penicillins
  Sulfonamides

(continued)

Table 69-1—*(continued)*

Clinical Manifestations of Adverse Reactions to Drugs

V. HEMATOLOGIC MANIFESTATIONS

Agranulocytosis (see also
  pancytopenia)
  Aprindine
  Captopril
  Carbimazole
  Cefotaxime
  Chloramphenicol
  Clozapine
  Co-trimoxazole
  Cytotoxics
  Gold salts
  Indomethacin
  Methimazole
  Oxyphenbutazone
  Phenothiazines
  Phenylbutazone
  Propylthiouracil
  Sulfonamides
  Ticlopidine
  Tolbutamide
  Tricyclic antidepressants
Clotting and bleeding abnormalities/
  hypothrombinemia
  Cefamandole
  Cefoperazone
  Ketorolac
  Mezlocillin
  Moxalactam
  Piperacillin
  Valproic acid
Eosinophilia
  Aminosalicylic acid
  Chlorpropamide
  Erythromycin estolate
  Imipramine
  L-Tryptophan

Eosinophilia (*cont.*)
  Methotrexate
  Nitrofurantoin
  Procarbazine
  Sulfonamides
Hemolytic anemia
  Aminosalicylic acid
  Cephalosporins
  Chlorpromazine
  Dapsone
  Insulin
  Isoniazid
  Levodopa
  Mefenamic acid
  Melphalan
  Methyldopa
  Penicillins
  Phenacetin
  Procainamide
  Quinidine
  Rifampin
  Sulfonamides
Hemolytic anemia (in G6PD
  deficiency)
  Aminosalicylic acid
  Antimalarials, e.g., primaquine
  Aspirin
  Chloramphenicol
  Co-trimoxazole
  Dapsone
  Nalidixic acid
  Nitrofurantoin
  Phenacetin
  Probenecid
  Procainamide
  Quinidine

Hemolytic anemia (*cont.*)
  Sulfonamides
  Vitamin C
  Vitamin K
Leukocytosis
  Glucocorticoids
  Lithium
Lymphadenopathy
  Phenytoin
  Primidone
Megaloblastic anemia
  Co-trimoxazole
  Folate antagonists
  Nitrous oxide (repeated or
    prolonged exposure)
  Oral contraceptives
  Phenobarbital
  Phenytoin
  Primidone
  Triamterene
  Trimethoprim
Pancytopenia (aplastic anemia)
  Carbamazepine
  Carbimazole
  Chloramphenicol
  Cytotoxics
  Felbamate
  Gold salts
  Mepacrine
  Mephenytoin
  Oxyphenbutazone
  Phenylbutazone
  Phenytoin
  Potassium perchlorate
  Quinacrine
  Sulfonamides

Pancytopenia (*cont.*)
  Thiouracils
  Trimethadione
  Zidovudine (AZT)
Pure red cell aplasia
  Azathioprine
  Chlorpropamide
  Isoniazid
  Phenytoin
Thrombocytopenia (see also
  pancytopenia)
  Acetazolamine
  Aspirin
  Carbamazepine
  Carbenicillin
  Chlorpropamide
  Chlorthalidone
  Co-trimoxazole
  Digitoxin
  Furosemide
  Gold salts
  Heparin
  Indomethacin
  Isoniazid
  Methyldopa
  Moxalactam
  Novobiocin
  Oxyphenbutazone
  Phenylbutazone
  Phenytoin and other
    hydantoins
  Quinidine
  Quinine
  Thiazides
  Ticarcillin

VI. CARDIOVASCULAR MANIFESTATIONS

Acute chest pain (nonischemic)
  Bleomycin
Angina exacerbation
  Alpha blockers
  Beta-blocker withdrawal
  Ergotamine
  Excessive thyroxine
  Hydralazine
  Methysergide
  Minoxidil
  Nifedipine
  Oxytocin
  Sumatriptan
  Vasopressin
Arrhythmias
  Adriamycin
  Antiarrhythmic drugs
  Astemizole
  Atropine
  Anticholinesterases
  Beta blockers
  Cisapride
  Daunorubicin
  Digitalis
  Emetine
  Erythromycin
  Guanethidine

Arrhythmias (*cont.*)
  Ketanserin
  Lithium
  Papaverine
  Pentamidine
  Phenothiazines, particularly
    thioridazine
  Probucol
  Sympathomimetics
  Terfenadine
  Theophylline
  Thyroid hormone
  Tricyclic antidepressants
  Verapamil
AV block
  Clonidine
  Methyldopa
  Verapamil
Cardiomyopathy
  Adriamycin
  Daunorubicin
  Emetine
  Lithium
  Phenothiazines
  Sulfonamides
  Sympathomimetics

Fluid retention/congestive heart
  failure/edema
  Beta blockers
  Calcium blockers
  Carbenoxolone
  Diazoxide
  Estrogens
  Indomethacin
  Mannitol
  Minoxidil
  Phenylbutazone
  Steroids
  Verapamil
Hypotension (see also arrhythmias)
  Amiodarone (perioperative)
  Calcium channel blockers, e.g.,
    nifedipine
  Citrated blood
  Diuretics
  Interleukin 2
  Levodopa
  Morphine
  Nitroglycerin
  Phenothiazines
  Protamine
  Quinidine

Hypertension
  Clonidine withdrawal
  Corticotropin
  Cyclosporine
  Glucocorticoids
  Monoamine oxidase
    inhibitors with
    sympathomimetics
  NSAIDs (some)
  Oral contraceptives
  Sympathomimetics
  Tricyclic antidepressants
    with sympathomimetics
Pericarditis
  Emetine
  Hydralazine
  Methysergide
  Procainamide
Pericardial effusion
  Minoxidil
Thromboembolism
  Oral contraceptives

(continued)

VII. RESPIRATORY MANIFESTATIONS

Airway obstruction (bronchospasm, asthma; see also anaphylaxis)
  Adenosine
  Beta blockers
  Cephalosporins
  Cholinergic drugs
  NSAIDs, e.g., aspirin, indomethacin
  Penicillins
  Pentazocine
  Streptomycin
  Tartrazine (drugs with yellow dye)

Cough
  ACE inhibitors
Nasal congestion
  Decongestant abuse
  Guanethidine
  Isoproterenol
  Oral contraceptives
  Reserpine
Pulmonary edema
  Contrast media
  Heroin
  Hydrochlorthiazide
  Interleukin 2
  Methadone
  Propoxyphene

Pulmonary hypertension
  Fenfluramine
Pulmonary infiltrates
  Acyclovir
  Amiodarone
  Azothioprine
  Bleomycin
  Busulfan
  Carmustine (BCNU)
  Chlorambucil
  Cyclophosphamide
  Gold
  Melphalan
  Methotrexate

Pulmonary infiltrates *(cont.)*
  Methysergide
  Mitomycin C
  Nitrofurantoin
  Procarbazine
  Sulfonamides
Respiratory depression
  Aminoglycosides
  Hypnotics
  Opiates
  Polymyxins
  Sedatives
  Trimethaphan

VIII. GASTROINTESTINAL MANIFESTATIONS

Cholestatic hepatitis
  Acetohexamide
  Anabolic steroids
  Androgens
  Chlorpropamide
  Clavulanic acid/amoxicillin
  Cyclosporine
  Erythromycin estolate
  Flucloxacillin
  Gold salts
  Methimazole
  Nitrofurantoin
  Oral contraceptives
  Phenothiazines
Constipation or ileus
  Aluminum hydroxide
  Barium sulfate
  Calcium carbonate
  Ferrous sulfate
  Ganglionic blockers
  Ion exchange resins
  Opiates
  Phenothiazines
  Tricyclic antidepressants
  Verapamil
Diarrhea or colitis
  Antibiotics (broad-spectrum)
  Clindamycin
  Cocaine
  Colchicine
  Digitalis
  Guanethidine
  Lactose excipients
  Lincomycin
  Magnesium in antacids
  Methyldopa
  Misoprostol
  Oral contraceptives
  Purgatives
  Reserpine
  Ticlopidine

Diffuse hepatocellular damage
  Acetaminophen (paracetamol)
  Acebutolol
  Allopurinol
  Aminosalicylic acid
  Amiodarone
  Aprindine
  Carbenicillin
  Cyclophosphamide
  Dapsone
  Diclofenac
  Erythromycin estolate
  Ethionamide
  Felbamate
  Glyburide
  Halothane
  Isoniazid
  Ketoconazole
  Labetalol
  Lovastatin
  Methimazole
  Methotrexate
  Methoxyflurane
  Methyldopa
  Monoamine oxidase inhibitors
  Niacin
  Nifedipine
  Nitrofurantoin
  Oxyphenisatin
  Phenytoin and other hydantoins
  Propoxyphene
  Propylthiouracil
  Pyridium
  Quinidine
  Rifampin
  Salicylates
  Sodium valproate
  Sulfonamides
  Tacrine
  Tetracyclines
  Trazodone
  Verapamil
  Zidovudine (AZT)

Gallstones/biliary pseudolithiasis
  Ceftriaxone
Intestinal ulceration
  Solid KCl preparations
Malabsorption
  Aminosalicylic acid
  Antibiotics (broad-spectrum)
  Cholestyramine
  Colchicine
  Colestipol
  Cytotoxic agents
  Neomycin
  Phenobarbital
  Phenytoin
  Primidone
Nausea or vomiting
  Digitalis
  Estrogens
  Ferrous sulfate
  Levodopa
  Opiates
  Potassium chloride
  Tetracyclines
  Theophylline
Oral conditions
  Dental discoloration:
    Tetracycline
  Dry mouth:
    Anticholinergics
    Clonidine
    Levodopa
    Methyldopa
    Tricyclic antidepressants
  Gingival hyperplasia:
    Calcium antagonists
    Cyclosporine
    Phenytoin
  Salivary gland swelling:
    Bethanidine
    Bretylium
    Clonidine

Oral conditions
  Salivary gland swelling *(cont.)*
    Guanethidine
    Iodides
    Phenylbutazone
  Taste disturbances:
    Acetazolamide
    Biguanides
    Captopril
    Griseofulvin
    Lithium
    Metronidazole
    Penicillamine
    Rifampin
  Ulceration:
    Aspirin
    Cytotoxic agents
    Gentian violet
    Isoproterenol (sublingual)
  Pancreatin
Pancreatitis
  Asparaginase
  Azathioprine
  Didanosine
  Estrogens
  Ethacrynic acid
  Furosemide
  Glucocorticoids
  Mercaptopurine
  Opiates
  Oral contraceptives
  Pentamidine
  Sulfonamides
  Thiazides
  Valproic acid
Peptic ulceration or hemorrhage
  Aspirin
  Ethacrynic acid
  Glucocorticoids
  NSAIDs†
  Reserpine (large doses)

(continued)

Table 69-1—*(continued)*

Clinical Manifestations of Adverse Reactions to Drugs

IX. RENAL MANIFESTATIONS

Bladder dysfunction/incontinence
  Anticholinergics
  Disopyramide
  Monoamine oxidase inhibitors
  Prazosin
  Terazosin
  Tricyclic antidepressants
Calculi
  Acetazolamide
  Vitamin D
Concentrating defect with polyuria
  (or nephrogenic diabetes insipidus)
  Demeclocycline
  Lithium
  Methoxyflurane
  Vitamin D
Hemorrhage cystitis
  Cyclophosphamide

Interstitial nephritis
  Cephalosporins
  Ciprofloxacin
  Allopurinol
  Furosemide
  NSAIDs†
  Penicillins, esp. methicillin
  Phenindione
  Rifampin
  Sulfonamides
  Thiazides
Nephropathies
  Analgesics (e.g., phenacetin)
Nephrotic syndrome
  Captopril
  Gold salts
  Ketoprofen

Nephrotic syndrome *(cont.)*
  Penicillamine
  Phenindione
  Probenecid
Obstructive uropathy
  Extrarenal: methysergide
Intrarenal:
  Acyclovir
  Cytotoxic agents
  Methotrexate
  Metyrosine
Renal dysfunction
  ACE inhibitors
  Cyclosporine
  NSAIDs
  Pentamidine
  Triamterene

Renal tubular acidosis
  Acetazolamide
  Amphotericin B
  Degraded tetracycline
Tubular necrosis
  Aminoglycosides
  Amphotericin B
  Cephaloridine
  Colistin
  Cyclosporine
  Intravenous immune
    globulin
  Methoxyflurane
  Polymyxins
  Radioiodinated contrast
    medium
  Sulfonamides
  Tetracyclines

X. NEUROLOGIC MANIFESTATIONS

Aseptic meningitis
  Intravenous immune globulin
CNS/vasculitis/cerebral hemorrhage
  Phenylpropanolamine
Exacerbation of myasthenia
  Aminoglycosides
  D-Penicillamine
  Polymyxins
Extrapyramidal effects
  Butyrophenones, e.g., haloperidol
  Levodopa
  Methyldopa
  Metoclopramide
  Oral contraceptives
  Phenothiazines
  Reserpine
  Tricyclic antidepressants
Headache
  Bromides
  Ergotamine (withdrawal)
  Glyceryl trinitrate
  Hydralazine

Headache *(cont.)*
  Indomethacin
  Intravenous immune globulin
Peripheral neuropathy
  Amiodarone
  Chloramphenicol
  Chloroquine
  Chlorpropamide
  Cisplatin
  Clioquinol
  Clofibrate
  Demeclocycline
  Disopyramide
  Ethambutol
  Ethionamide
  Glutethimide
  Hydralazine
  Isoniazid
  Methysergide
  Metronidazole
  Mustine
  Nalidixic acid

Peripheral neuropathy *(cont.)*
  Nitrofurantoin
  Perhexiline
  Phenelzine
  Phenytoin
  Polymyxin, colistin
  Procarbazine
  Streptomycin
  Tolbutamide
  Tricyclic antidepressants
  Vincristine
Pseudotumor cerebri (or intracranial
  hypertension)
  Amiodarone
  Glucocorticoids,
    mineralocorticoids
  Vitamin A (hypervitaminosis A)
  Oral contraceptives
  Tetracyclines
Seizures
  Amphetamines
  Analeptics

Seizures *(cont.)*
  Imipenem
  Isoniazid
  Lidocaine
  Lithium
  Nalidixic acid
  Meperidine
  Penicillins
  Phenothiazines
  Physostigmine
  Theophylline
  Tricyclic antidepressants
  Vincristine
Sleep disorders
  Lovastatin
Stroke
  Cocaine
  Oral contraceptives
Tremor
  Beta-adrenergic agonists

XI. OCULAR MANIFESTATIONS

Cataracts
  Busulfan
  Chlorambucil
  Glucocorticoids
  Phenothiazines
Color vision alteration
  Barbiturates
  Digitalis
  Methaqualone
  Streptomycin
  Sulfonamides

Color vision alteration *(cont.)*
  Thiazides
  Troxidone
Corneal edema
  Oral contraceptives
Corneal opacities
  Chloroquine
  Indomethacin
  Mepacrine
  Vitamin D

Eye pain
  Nifedipine
Glaucoma
  Ipratropium bromide
  Mydriatics
  Sympathomimetics
Optic neuritis
  Aminosalicylic acid
  Chloramphenicol
  Clioquinol
  Ethambutol

Optic neuritis *(cont.)*
  Isoniazid
  Penicillamine
  Phenothiazines
  Phenylbutazone
  Quinine
  Streptomycin
Retinopathy
  Chloroquine
  Phenothiazines

XII. EAR MANIFESTATIONS

Deafness
  Aminoglycosides
  Aspirin
  Bleomycin
  Chloroquine
  Cisplatin
  Deferoxamine
  Erythromycin

Deafness *(cont.)*
  Ethacrynic acid
  Furosemide
  Interferon
  Mustine
  Nortriptyline
  Quinine

Vestibular disorders
  Aminoglycosides
  Mustine
  Quinine

(continued)

Table 69-1—(continued)

Clinical Manifestations of Adverse Reactions to Drugs

XIII. MUSCULOSKELETAL MANIFESTATIONS

Bone disorders	Myopathy or myalgia	Rhabdomyolysis
Osteoporosis:	Amphotericin B	Gemfibrozil
Glucocorticoids	Carbenoxolone	Lovastatin
Heparin	Chloroquine	Tendon rupture
Gout: see Hyperuricemia	Cimetidine	Quinolones
Osteomalacia:	Clofibrate	
Aluminum hydroxide	Glucocorticoids	
Anticonvulsants	Oral contraceptives	
Glutethimide	Zidovudine	

XIV. PSYCHIATRIC MANIFESTATIONS

Delirious or confusional states	Depression	Hallucinatory states	Memory loss
Amantadine	Amphetamine withdrawal	Amantadine	Triazolam
Aminophylline	Beta blockers	Beta blockers	Schizophrenic-like or paranoid
Anticholinergics	Centrally acting antihypertensives	Levodopa	reactions
Antidepressants	(reserpine, methyldopa,	Meperidine	Amphetamines
Bromides	clonidine)	Narcotics	Bromides
Cimetidine	Glucocorticoids	Pentazocine	Glucocorticoids
Digitalis	Levodopa	Tricyclic antidepressants	Levodopa
Glucocorticoids	Drowsiness	Hypomania, mania, or excited	Lysergic acid
Isoniazid	Antihistamines	reactions	Monoamine oxidase
Levodopa	Anxiolytic drugs	Glucocorticoids	inhibitors
Methyldopa	Clonidine	Levodopa	Tricyclic antidepressants
Penicillins	Major tranquilizers	MAO inhibitors	Sleep disturbances
Phenothiazines	Methyldopa	Sympathomimetics	Anorexiants
Ranitidine	Reserpine	Tricyclic antidepressants	Levodopa
Sedatives and hypnotics	Tricyclic antidepressants	Hypersexuality	Monoamine oxidase
Vigabatrin		Antiparkinsonian agents	inhibitors
			Sympathomimetics

* ACE, angiotensin converting enzyme
† NSAID, non–steroidal anti–inflammatory drug

specific drug than are symptoms such as fever or rash, which may be caused by many drugs or by other factors.

Once an adverse reaction is suspected, discontinuance of the suspected drug followed by disappearance of the reaction is presumptive evidence of a drug-induced illness. Confirming evidence may be sought by cautiously reintroducing the drug and seeing if the reaction reappears. However, that should be done only if confirmation would be useful in the future management of the patient and if the attempt would not entail undue risk. With concentration-dependent adverse reactions, lowering the dosage may cause the reaction to disappear, and raising it may cause the reaction to reappear. When the reaction is thought to be allergic, however, readministration of the drug may be hazardous, since anaphylactic shock may develop. Readministration is unwise under these conditions unless no alternative drugs are available and treatment is necessary.

If the patient is receiving many drugs when an adverse reaction is suspected, the drugs likeliest to be responsible can usually be identified. All drugs may be discontinued at once, or, if that is not practical, they should be discontinued one at a time, starting with the one that is most suspect, and the patient observed for signs of improvement. The time needed for a concentration-dependent adverse effect to disappear depends on the time required for the concentration to fall below the range associated with the adverse effect, and that, in turn, depends on the initial blood level and on the rate of elimination or metabolism of the drug. Adverse effects of drugs with long half-lives, such as phenobarbital, take a considerable time to disappear.

Drugs recognized as producing a number of reactions are listed in Table 69-1. This table includes both well-documented and some less well-documented reactions, focusing on those that are sufficiently devastating to require consideration. This information should be used to suggest the drug likely to be causing a reaction; the absence of a drug from the table does not mean that it cannot be responsible for the reaction, however.

Serum antibody has been demonstrated in some persons with drug allergies involving cellular blood elements, as in agranulocytosis, hemolytic anemia, and thrombocytopenia. For example, both quinine and quinidine can produce platelet agglutination in vitro in the presence of complement and the serum from a patient who has developed thrombocytopenia following use of this drug.

Eliciting a drug history from patients is important for diagnosis. Attention must be directed to OTC as well as prescription drugs. Each type can be responsible for adverse drug effects, and adverse interactions may occur between OTC drugs and prescribed drugs. In addition, it is common for patients to be cared for by several physicians, and duplicative, additive, counteractive, or synergistic drug combinations may therefore be administered if the physicians are not aware of the patients' drug histories. Every physician should determine what drugs a patient has been taking, at least during the preceding 30 days, before prescribing any medications. A frequently overlooked source of additional drug exposure is topical therapy; for example, a patient complaining of bronchospasm may not mention that an ophthalmic beta blocker is being used unless specifically asked. A history of previous adverse drug effects in patients is common. Since these patients have shown a predisposition to drug-induced illnesses, such a history should dictate added caution in prescribing drugs.

Patients with biochemical abnormalities such as erythrocyte G6PD deficiency can be identified. Most patients with the G6PD defect are blacks or of Mediterranean descent. Drug-induced hemolytic crisis can be avoided by testing for the enzyme defect before administering drugs that could cause the reaction. Similarly, persons with an abnormal serum pseudocholinesterase level may have abnormally prolonged apnea when given succinylcholine.

GENERAL COMMENTS No drug is completely without side effects, and a side effect in one patient may be the desired pharmacologic effect in another. Current drug regulations allow physicians to have considerable confidence in the purity, bioavailability, and effectiveness of the drugs they prescribe. However, physicians have to weigh potential toxicity against possible benefits. Toxicity that would be acceptable for an effective antineoplastic agent would not be permitted in an oral contraceptive, for example. Because of the necessarily small number of patients treated in premarketing studies, rare adverse reactions may not be identified, so the first responsibility for identifying and reporting these effects must rest with the practicing clinician through the use of the various national adverse reaction reporting systems, such as those operated by the Food and Drug Administration in the United States and the Committee on Safety of Medicines in Great Britain. The publication of a newly recognized adverse reaction can in a short time stimulate many similar such reports of reactions that previously had gone unrecognized.

The prevention of adverse drug reactions first involves a high index of suspicion that the development of a new symptom or sign may be drug-related. Reduction of the dose or discontinuation of the suspected agent usually clarifies the issue in concentration-dependent toxic reactions. Physicians should be familiar with the common adverse effects of the drugs they use and, when in doubt, should consult the literature.

BIBLIOGRAPHY

BRENNAN TA et al: Incidence of adverse events and negligence in hospitalized patients: Results of the Harvard Medical Practice Study I. N Engl J Med 324:370, 1991

DAVIES DM: *Textbook of Adverse Drug Reactions*, 4th ed. New York, Oxford University Press, 1991

FELDMANN U: Design and analysis of drug safety studies, with special reference to sporadic drug use and acute adverse reactions. J Clin Epidemiol 46:237, 1993

HALLAS J et al: Drug related admissions to medical wards: A population based survey. Br J Clin Pharmacol 33:61, 1992

HOIGNÉ R et al: Risk factors for adverse drug reactions: Epidemiological approaches. Eur J Clin Pharmacol 39:321, 1990

JOHNSON JA, BOOTMAN JL: Drug-related morbidity and mortality: A cost-of-illness model. Arch Intern Med 155:1949, 1995

LEAPE LL et al: The nature of adverse events in hospitalized patients. Results of the Harvard Medical Practice Study II. N Engl J Med 324:377, 1991

ROUJEAU J-C et al: Medication use and the risk of Stevens-Johnson syndrome or toxic epidermal necrolysis. N Engl J Med 333:1600, 1995

———, STERN RS: Severe adverse cutaneous reactions to drugs. N Engl J Med 331:1272, 1994

WALLER PC: Measuring the frequency of adverse drug reactions. Br J Clin Pharmacol 33:249, 1992

70   *Lewis Landsberg, James B. Young*

PHYSIOLOGY AND PHARMACOLOGY OF THE AUTONOMIC NERVOUS SYSTEM

FUNCTIONAL ORGANIZATION OF THE AUTONOMIC NERVOUS SYSTEM

The autonomic nervous system innervates vascular and visceral smooth muscle, exocrine and endocrine glands, and parenchymal cells throughout the various organ systems. Functioning below the conscious level, the autonomic nervous system responds rapidly and continuously to perturbations that threaten the constancy of the internal environment. The many functions governed by this system include the distribution of blood flow and the maintenance of tissue perfusion, the regulation of blood pressure, the regulation of the volume and composition of the extracellular fluid, the expenditure of metabolic energy and supply of substrate, and the control of visceral smooth muscle and glands.

ANATOMIC ORGANIZATION The autonomic neurons, located in ganglia outside the central nervous system, give rise to the postganglionic autonomic nerves that innervate organs and tissues throughout the body (Fig. 70-1). The activity of autonomic nerves is regulated by central neurons responsive to diverse afferent inputs. After central integration of afferent information, autonomic outflow is adjusted to permit the functioning of the major organ systems in accordance with the needs of the organism as a whole. Connections between the cerebral cortex and the autonomic centers in the brainstem coordinate autonomic outflow with higher mental functions.

The Sympathetic and Parasympathetic Divisions The preganglionic neurons of the parasympathetic nervous system leave the central nervous system in the third, seventh, ninth, and tenth cranial nerves and in the second and third sacral nerves, while the preganglionic neurons of the sympathetic nervous system exit the spinal cord between the first thoracic and the second lumbar segments (Fig. 70-1). Responses to sympathetic and parasympathetic stimulation are frequently antagonistic, as exemplified by their opposing effects on heart rate and gut motility. This antagonism reflects highly coordinated interactions within the central nervous system; the resultant changes in parasympathetic and sympathetic activity, often reciprocal, provide more precise control of autonomic responses than could be achieved by the modulation of a single system.

Neurotransmitters *Acetylcholine* (ACh) is the preganglionic neurotransmitter for both divisions of the autonomic nervous system as well as the postganglionic neurotransmitter of the parasympathetic

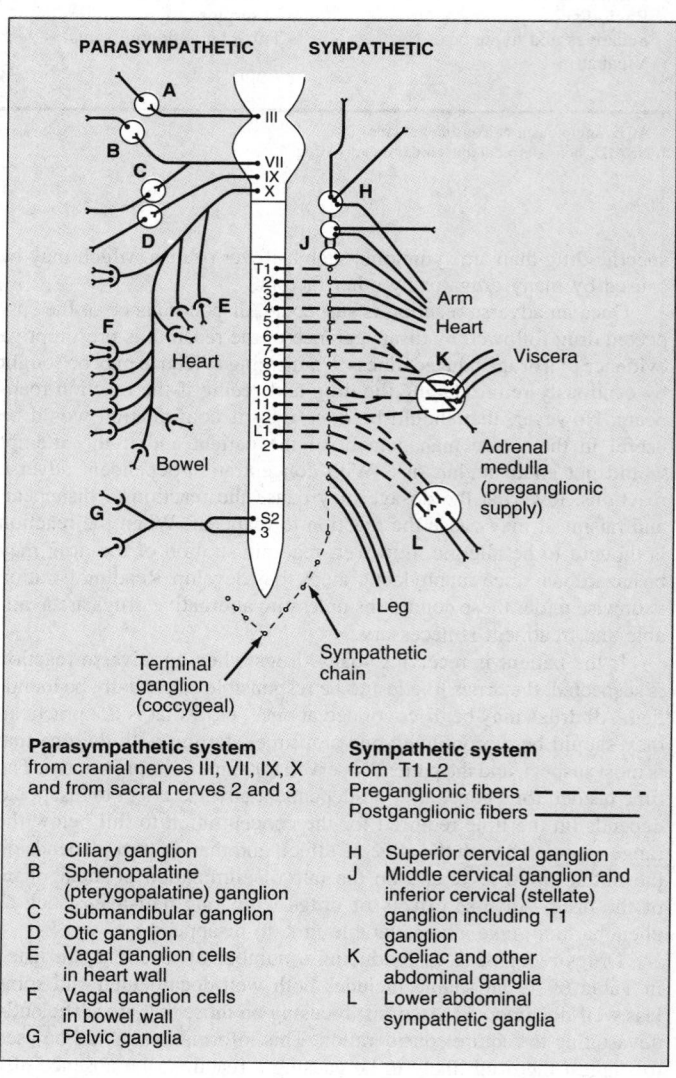

Parasympathetic system	Sympathetic system
from cranial nerves III, VII, IX, X and from sacral nerves 2 and 3	from T1 L2 Preganglionic fibers – – – – – Postganglionic fibers ————

A	Ciliary ganglion	H	Superior cervical ganglion
B	Sphenopalatine (pterygopalatine) ganglion	J	Middle cervical ganglion and inferior cervical (stellate) ganglion including T1 ganglion
C	Submandibular ganglion		
D	Otic ganglion		
E	Vagal ganglion cells in heart wall	K	Coeliac and other abdominal ganglia
F	Vagal ganglion cells in bowel wall		
G	Pelvic ganglia	L	Lower abdominal sympathetic ganglia

FIGURE 70-1 Schematic representation of the autonomic nervous system. *(From Moskowitz M. Clin Endocrinol Metab 6:77, 1977.)*

neurons. Nerves that release ACh are said to be cholinergic. *Norepinephrine* (NE) is the neurotransmitter of the postganglionic sympathetic neurons; these nerves are said to be adrenergic. Within the sympathetic outflow, postganglionic neurons innervating the eccrine sweat glands (and perhaps some blood vessels supplying skeletal muscle) are of the cholinergic type.

THE SYMPATHETIC NERVOUS SYSTEM AND THE ADRENAL MEDULLA

CATECHOLAMINES All three of the naturally occurring catecholamines, NE, *epinephrine* (E), and *dopamine*, function as neurotransmitters within the central nervous system. NE, the neurotransmitter of postganglionic sympathetic nerve endings, exerts its effects locally, in the immediate vicinity of its release. E, the circulating hormone of the adrenal medulla, influences processes throughout the body. A peripheral dopaminergic system also exists but has not been characterized in detail.

Biosynthesis (Fig. 70-2) Catecholamines are synthesized from the amino acid tyrosine, which is sequentially hydroxylated to form dihydroxyphenylalanine (dopa), decarboxylated to form dopamine, and hydroxylated on the beta position of the side chain to form NE. The initial step, the hydroxylation of tyrosine, is rate-limiting and is regulated so that synthesis of dopa is coupled to NE release. This regulation is achieved by alterations in both the activity and the amount of tyrosine hydroxylase. In the adrenal medulla and in those central neurons utilizing E as neurotransmitter, NE is *N*-methylated to E by the enzyme phenylethanolamine-*N*-methyltransferase (PNMT).

Catecholamine Metabolism The major metabolic transformations of catecholamines involve *O*-methylation at the meta-hydroxyl group and oxidative deamination. *O*-Methylation is catalyzed by the enzyme catechol-*O*-methyltransferase (COMT), and oxidative deamination is promoted by monoamine oxidase (MAO). COMT in liver and kidney is important in the metabolism of circulating catecholamines. MAO, a mitochondrial enzyme present in most tissues, including nerve endings, has a lesser role in the metabolism of circulating catecholamines but is important in regulating the catecholamine stores within the peripheral sympathetic nerve endings. The metanephrines and 4-hydroxy-3-methoxymandelic acid (VMA) are the major end products of E and NE metabolism. Homovanillic acid (HVA) is the end product of dopamine metabolism.

STORAGE AND RELEASE OF CATECHOLAMINES In both the adrenal medulla and sympathetic nerve endings catecholamines are stored in subcellular granules and released by exocytosis. The large stores of catecholamines in these tissues provide an important physiologic reserve that maintains an adequate supply of catecholamines in the face of intense stimulation. A variety of substances may be stored along with catecholamines in sympathetic nerve endings and adrenal medulla and released with catecholamines during exocytosis. These substances, which may function as cotransmitters or neuromodulators, include peptides such as neuropeptide Y, substance P, and enkephalins; purines such as ATP and adenosine; and other amines such as serotonin. At the neuroeffector junction, coreleased neuromodulators modify the response to NE, while cotransmitters exert physiologic effects independent of those induced by NE.

Adrenal Medulla The adrenal medullary chromaffin tissue in a pair of normal human adrenal glands weighs about 1 g and contains approximately 6 mg catecholamines, 85 percent of which is E.

Catecholamine secretion, stimulated by ACh from the preganglionic sympathetic nerves, occurs after calcium influx triggers fusion of the chromaffin granule membrane and cell membrane; obliteration of the cell membrane at the point of fusion and extrusion of the entire soluble contents of the granule into the extracellular space complete the process of exocytosis (Fig. 70-2). Although the molecular mechanisms involved in the exocytotic process are only partially understood, evidence has accumulated that specific calcium-binding proteins are involved. Once bound, calcium induces a conformational change in these proteins that induces fusion of granules and docking of granules at the cell membrane.

Peripheral Sympathetic Nerve Endings The peripheral sympathetic nerve endings form a reticulum or ground plexus that brings the terminal fibers into close contact with effector cells. All the NE in peripheral tissues is in the sympathetic nerve endings, and heavily innervated tissues contain as much as 1 to 2 μg/g of tissue. NE stored in the nerve endings is in discrete subcellular particles analogous to the adrenal medullary chromaffin granules. MAO in the mitochondria of the nerve endings plays an important role in regulating the local concentration of NE (Fig. 70-2). Amines in storage vesicles are protected from oxidative deamination; amines within the cytoplasm, however, are deaminated to inactive metabolites. Release from the nerve ending occurs in response to action potentials propagated in terminal sympathetic fibers.

THE PERIPHERAL ADRENERGIC NEUROEFFECTOR JUNCTION The peripheral sympathetic nerve endings possess an amine transport system that actively takes up amines from the extracellular fluid. Neuronal uptake or recapture of locally released NE terminates the action of the transmitter and contributes to the constancy of the NE stores.

A variety of factors alter the relationship between neuronal impulse traffic and NE release. Diminished temperature and acidosis, for example, both decrease the amount of NE released in response to sympathetic impulses. Several chemical mediators operate at the peripheral sympathetic nerve ending (referred to as *prejunctional* or *presynaptic sites*) to modify sympathetic neurotransmission by influencing the amount of NE released in response to nerve impulses. Prejunctional modulation may be either inhibitory or facilitatory.

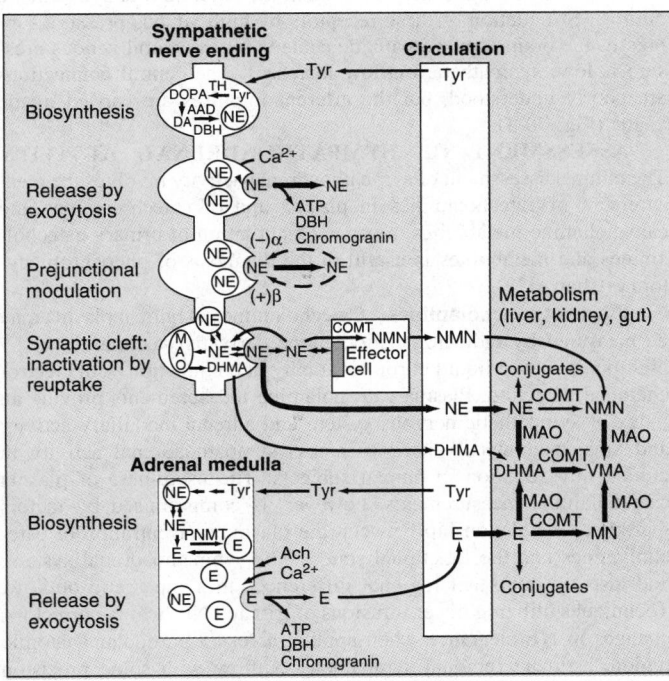

FIGURE 70-2 Catecholamine biosynthesis, release, and metabolism. Schematic representation of a peripheral sympathetic nerve ending is shown at the top; the bulbous areas on the terminal fiber represent varicosities identified by histochemical fluorescence techniques as areas of high neurotransmitter concentration. The processes of biosynthesis, release, modulation, and reuptake are shown sequentially for demonstration purposes only; in vivo they proceed concurrently. Adrenal medullary chromaffin cells are shown at the bottom of the diagram. (TH, tyrosine hydroxylase; AAD, aromatic-l-amino acid decarboxylase; DA, dopamine; DBH, dopamine-β-hydroxylase; NE, norepinephrine; PNMT, phenylethanolamine-*N*-methyltransferase; E, epinephrine; COMT, catechol-*O*-methyltransferase; NMN, normetanephrine; MAO, monoamine oxidase; DHMA, 3,4-dihydroxymandelic acid; VMA, 3-methoxy-4-hydroxymandelic acid.)

Certain modulators, such as catecholamines and ACh, may either inhibit or facilitate NE release, antagonistic effects that are mediated by different adrenergic or cholinergic receptors, respectively. Those compounds exerting an *inhibitory* effect on NE release at the prejunctional nerve ending include the following: catecholamines (alpha$_2$ receptor), ACh (muscarinic receptor), dopamine (D$_2$ receptor), histamine (H$_2$ receptor), serotonin, adenosine, enkephalins, and prostaglandins.

Catecholamines reduce NE release via prejunctional alpha receptors in a classic negative-feedback system. Feedback regulation is complicated by the fact that beta-receptor activation facilitates NE release.

Though both inhibitory and facilitatory effects of ACh on NE release have been described, the inhibitory effect of ACh, mediated by the muscarinic cholinergic receptor, occurs at lower ACh concentrations and is probably of greater physiologic significance.

CENTRAL REGULATION OF SYMPATHOADRENAL OUTFLOW Brainstem Sympathetic Centers

Sympathetic outflow is initiated from the reticular formation of the medulla oblongata and pons and from centers in the hypothalamus. The rostral ventral portion of the medulla, particularly the area designated the rostral ventrolateral medulla (RVLM), appears to contain especially important sympathoexcitatory areas. Descending fibers originating from these centers synapse in the intermediolateral cell column of the spinal cord with the preganglionic sympathetic neurons. Changes in the physical and chemical properties of the extracellular fluid, including the circulating levels of hormones and substrates, also affect sympathetic nervous system outflow. The area postrema, in the floor of the fourth ventricle, along with other circumventricular organs lie outside the blood-brain barrier and may play an important role in this regard. Although the hallmark of intense sympathoadrenal stimulation is a global response (the fight-or-flight reaction of Cannon), discrete changes in sympathetic outflow to different organ systems continuously regulate many autonomic functions.

Relationship between the sympathetic nervous system and the adrenal medulla Sympathetic nervous system activity and adrenal medullary secretion are coordinated but not always congruent. During periods of intense sympathetic stimulation, such as cold exposure and exhaustive exercise, the adrenal medulla is progressively recruited, and circulating E reinforces the physiologic effects of sympathetic stimulation. In other situations, the sympathetic nervous system and the adrenal medulla are stimulated independently. The response to upright posture, for example, involves predominantly the sympathetic nervous system, while hypoglycemia stimulates only the adrenal medulla.

Sympathetic Regulation of the Cardiovascular System

Stretch receptors in the systemic and pulmonary arteries and veins continuously monitor intravascular pressures; the resulting afferent impulses, after relay and integration in the brainstem, alter sympathetic activity in defense of blood pressure and blood flow to critical areas (Fig. 70-3).

Arterial baroreceptors An increase in blood pressure stimulates receptors in the carotid sinus and aortic arch. The ensuing afferent impulses, after relay within the nucleus of the solitary tract (NTS) in the brainstem, suppress the brainstem sympathetic centers (Fig. 70-3). This baroreceptor reflex arc forms a negative-feedback loop in which a rise in arterial pressure results in the inhibition of central sympathetic outflow. A brainstem noradrenergic pathway interacts with the NTS to participate in suppression of sympathetic outflow. This noradrenergic inhibitory pathway is stimulated by centrally acting alpha-adrenergic agonists and may be involved in the action of certain antihypertensive drugs, such as clonidine, that potentiate the baroreceptor-mediated vasodepressor response (Chap. 246). In the opposite manner, when the blood pressure falls, decreased afferent impulses diminish central inhibition, resulting in an increase in sympathetic outflow and a rise in arterial pressure.

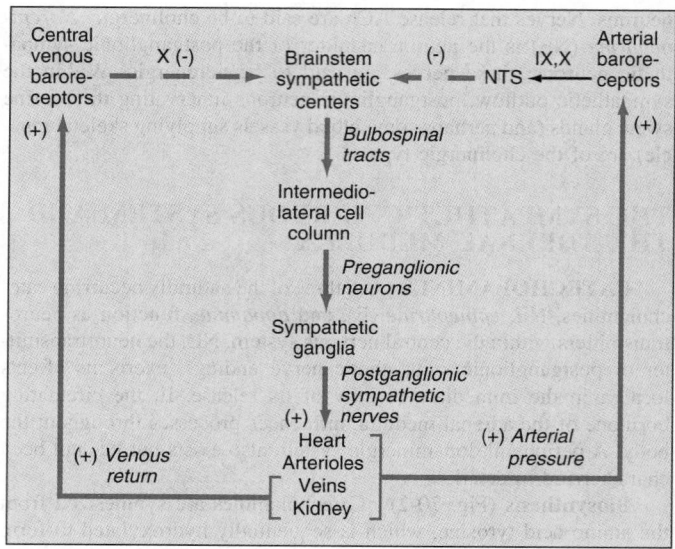

FIGURE 70-3 Sympathetic regulation of the circulation. Receptors in the venous and arterial circulations are stimulated by stretch, caused by an increase in pressure; afferent impulses from these receptors are carried to the central nervous system by the ninth (*IX*) and tenth (*X*) cranial nerves. The net result of these afferent impulses, after relay in the brainstem, is to inhibit central sympathetic outflow. The arterial baroreceptor reflex involves a relay in the nucleus of the tractus solitarius. (+, stimulation; −, inhibition.)

Central venous pressure Receptors in the walls of the great veins and within the atria are also involved in the regulation of sympathetic outflow. Stimulation of these receptors by high venous pressure suppresses the brainstem sympathetic centers; when central venous pressure is low, sympathetic outflow increases. The central connections are poorly understood, but the afferent impulses are carried in the vagus (Fig. 70-3).

ASSESSMENT OF SYMPATHOADRENAL ACTIVITY

The clinical assessment of sympathoadrenal activity involves the measurement of catecholamines in plasma and of catecholamines and catecholamine metabolites in urine. Quantitation of urinary catecholamines and metabolites is useful in the diagnosis of pheochromocytoma (Chap. 333).

Plasma Catecholamines Catecholamines in human plasma may be measured by radioenzymatic isotope derivative techniques or by high-performance liquid chromatography in conjunction with electrochemical detection. Plasma catecholamine measurements provide an index of sympathetic nervous system and adrenal medullary activity and have been widely used to assess sympathoadrenal activity in clinical investigation in human subjects. The usefulness of plasma catecholamine measurements, however, is compromised by factors that alter the relationship between the plasma concentration of catecholamines and the functional state of the sympathoadrenal system, and also by important regional differences in sympathetic outflow. Techniques utilizing tracer infusions of tritiated NE, which correct for changes in NE clearance when applied across a particular anatomic region, estimate regional sympathetic outflow with some precision and have helped to define differentiated sympathetic nervous system activity in the investigational setting. The clinical usefulness of plasma catecholamine levels remains limited to the evaluation of patients with autonomic insufficiency and, on occasion, patients with suspected pheochromocytoma (Chap. 333).

Basal plasma NE concentrations are in the range of 0.09 to 1.8 nmol/L (150 to 350 pg/mL); basal E levels are about 135 to 270 pmol/L (25 to 50 pg/mL). The half-time of disappearance of NE from the circulation is approximately 2 min. The plasma NE level is markedly affected by a variety of factors, including posture; accordingly, the conditions under which blood is obtained for assay must be controlled. By convention, basal plasma NE levels are those obtained through an indwelling intravenous line after the patient has rested supine in a relaxed environment for 30 min.

Plasma NE response to upright posture   The predictable increase in circulating NE concentration during upright posture provides a convenient test of sympathetic nervous system function. Five minutes of quiet standing results in a two- to threefold increase in plasma NE level. A normal response requires an intact afferent system, appropriate central nervous system relays, and an intact peripheral sympathetic nervous system; a defect of any of these components reduces the increment in circulating NE.

Plasma E levels are also dependent on the physical and mental state of the subject. Change in plasma E with upright posture is usually small. Hypoglycemia, strenuous exercise, and various types of mental stress, however, can cause large increases in the plasma E level.

PERIPHERAL DOPAMINERGIC SYSTEM

In addition to its role as neurotransmitter in the central nervous system, dopamine functions as an inhibitory transmitter in the carotid body and the sympathetic ganglia. A distinct peripheral dopaminergic system is also believed to exist. Dopamine elicits a variety of responses not attributable to stimulation of classic adrenergic receptors; it relaxes the lower esophageal sphincter, delays gastric emptying, causes vasodilation in the renal and mesenteric arterial circulation, suppresses aldosterone secretion, directly stimulates renal sodium excretion, and suppresses NE release at sympathetic nerve terminals by a presynaptic inhibitory mechanism. The mediation of these dopaminergic effects in vivo is poorly understood. Dopamine does not appear to be a circulating hormone.

ADRENERGIC RECEPTORS

Catecholamines influence effector cells by interacting with specific *receptors* on the cell surface. When stimulated by catecholamines, the adrenergic receptor initiates a series of membrane changes followed by a cascade of intracellular events that culminates in a measurable response.

Two major categories of response to catecholamines reflect the activation of two populations of adrenergic receptors, designated alpha and beta. Both alpha and beta receptors have been further divided into subtypes that serve different functions and are susceptible to differential stimulation and blockade.

ALPHA-ADRENERGIC RECEPTORS   Alpha-adrenergic receptors mediate vasoconstriction, intestinal relaxation, and pupillary dilatation. E and NE are approximately equipotent as alpha-receptor agonists. Distinct $alpha_1$- and $alpha_2$-receptor subtypes are also recognized. Originally the postsynaptic or postjunctional alpha-adrenergic receptors on effector cells were designated $alpha_1$, while the prejunctional alpha-adrenergic receptors on the sympathetic nerve endings were designated $alpha_2$. It is now recognized that nonneuronal (postsynaptic) processes are mediated by the $alpha_2$ receptor as well. The $alpha_1$ receptor mediates the classic alpha effects, including vasoconstriction; phenylephrine and methoxamine are selective $alpha_1$ agonists, and prazosin is a selective $alpha_1$ antagonist. The $alpha_2$ receptor mediates presynaptic inhibition of NE release from adrenergic nerves and other responses, including inhibition of ACh release from cholinergic nerves, inhibition of lipolysis in adipocytes, inhibition of insulin secretion, stimulation of platelet aggregation, and vasoconstriction in some vascular beds. Specific $alpha_2$ agonists include clonidine and α-methylnorepinephrine; these agents, the latter derived from α-methyldopa in vivo, exert an antihypertensive effect by interacting with $alpha_2$ receptors within the brainstem sympathetic centers that regulate blood pressure. Yohimbine is a specific $alpha_2$ antagonist.

BETA-ADRENERGIC RECEPTORS   Physiologic events associated with beta-adrenergic receptor responses include stimulation of heart rate and contractility, vasodilation, bronchodilation, and lipolysis. Beta-receptor responses also can be divided into two types. The $beta_1$ receptor responds equally to E and NE and mediates cardiac stimulation

and lipolysis. The $beta_2$ receptor is more responsive to E than to NE and mediates responses such as vasodilation and bronchodilation. Isoproterenol stimulates and propranolol blocks both $beta_1$ and $beta_2$ receptors. Other agonists and antagonists that have partial selectivity for the $beta_1$ or $beta_2$ receptors have been used therapeutically where the desired response involves predominantly one of the two subtypes.

Both pharmacologic and molecular genetic studies have demonstrated an additional distinct $beta_3$-adrenergic receptor that subserves lipolysis in white and brown adipose tissue as well as the stimulation of heat production in brown adipose tissue. The human $beta_3$-adrenergic receptor has been cloned, and a distinct polymorphism noted that may be associated with weight gain, insulin resistance, and type 2 diabetes mellitus. The $beta_3$-adrenergic receptor has a much greater affinity for NE than E and, unlike the $beta_1$ and $beta_2$ receptors, does not undergo desensitization. Synthetic agonists for the $beta_3$ receptor, currently under development, have a potential role in the treatment of obesity by increasing metabolic rate.

DOPAMINERGIC RECEPTORS   Specific dopaminergic receptors, distinct from the classic alpha- and beta-adrenergic receptors, are present in the central and peripheral nervous system and in several nonneural tissues. Two types of dopaminergic receptors serve different functions and have different second messengers. Dopamine is a potent agonist of both types of receptors; the action of dopamine is antagonized by phenothiazines and thioxanthenes. The D_1 receptor mediates vasodilation in the renal, mesenteric, coronary, and cerebral vascular beds. Fenoldopam is an investigational agonist selective for the D_1 receptor. The D_2 receptor inhibits transmission in the sympathetic ganglia, inhibits NE release from sympathetic nerve endings by an effect on the presynaptic membrane (Fig. 70-2), inhibits prolactin release from the pituitary, and causes vomiting. Selective agonists of the D_2 receptor include bromocriptine, lergotrile, and apomorphine, while butyrophenones such as haloperidol (active within the central nervous system), domperidone (does not cross blood-brain barrier readily), and the benzamide sulpiride are relatively selective D_2 antagonists.

STRUCTURE AND FUNCTION OF ADRENERGIC RECEPTORS   Adrenergic receptors belong to a superfamily of related membrane proteins, including the visual protein rhodopsin and the muscarinic acetylcholine receptors, that interacts with G proteins. These proteins share significant sequence homologies and, as deduced from the properties of the constituent amino acids, a similar topographic structure in the cell membrane. The postulated structure of this family of receptor proteins is shown schematically in Fig. 70-4. The characteristic features include seven membrane-spanning hydrophobic domains containing 20 to 28 amino acids each. The membrane-spanning domains, particularly M-7 (Fig. 70-4), appear to be important in determining the characteristic agonist binding.

Coupling of Receptor Occupancy with Cellular Response   The major mediators of adrenergic (as well as many other) cellular responses are a family of regulatory proteins termed *G proteins* that, when activated, bind the nucleotide guanosine triphosphate (GTP). The best-characterized G proteins are those that stimulate or inhibit adenylyl cyclase, designated G_s or G_i, respectively (Fig. 70-5). The $beta_1$, $beta_2$, and D_1 receptors are coupled to G_s; receptor occupancy is therefore associated with stimulation of adenylyl cyclase and results in an increase in intracellular cyclic adenosine monophosphate (AMP), which in turn results in activation of protein kinase A and other cyclic AMP–dependent protein kinases. The resultant protein phosphorylation alters the activity of enzymes and the function of other proteins, culminating in a cellular response that is characteristic of the tissue being stimulated. The $alpha_2$, M_2 subtype of the muscarinic acetylcholine receptor and the D_2 receptor are coupled to G_i, resulting in diminished adenylyl cyclase activity and a fall in cyclic AMP. The subsequent alterations in enzyme activity and function of other proteins produce an alternate, frequently opposite, series of cellular responses. Although many

FIGURE 70-4 Proposed structure of adrenergic receptors as deduced from primary amino acid sequences. The single protein chain contains a hydrophilic N terminus (extracellular) and C terminus (intracellular) connected by seven lipophilic membrane-spanning regions (M-1 to M-7) which are interconnected by three extracellular loops (E-I to E-III) and three cytoplasmic loops (C-I to C-III). The beta$_1$-, beta$_2$-, alpha$_1$-, and alpha$_2$-adrenergic receptors have appreciable sequence homologies and are believed to fit the general structural model represented. Specificity of agonist binding may be conferred by the tertiary structure of several of the membrane-spanning domains while specificity of intracellular response may be related to the length and tertiary structure of the cytoplasmic loops and C terminus. The top portion of the figure is a longitudinal representation of the receptor protein in the cell membrane; shown below is a hypothetical, more compact arrangement seen from the membrane surface. (ECF, extracellular fluid; ICF, intracellular fluid.) (*From Landsberg and Young, 1992, with permission.*)

alpha$_2$ responses can be explained by inhibition of adenylyl cyclase, other mechanisms may be involved as well.

The alpha$_1$-adrenergic receptor (as well as the M$_1$ subtype of the acetylcholine receptor) appears to be coupled to a different G protein that activates phospholipase C; this G protein has not been as well characterized but is sometimes designated G$_q$. Receptor occupancy in this system stimulates phospholipase C, which catalyzes the breakdown of membrane-bound phospholipids, particularly phosphatidyl-inositol-4,5-bisphosphate (PIP$_2$) with the production of inositol-1,4,5-trisphosphate (IP$_3$) and 1,2-diacylglycerol (DAG), both of which act as second messengers (Fig. 70-5). IP$_3$ rapidly mobilizes calcium from intracellular stores within the endoplasmic reticulum, producing an

increase in free cytoplasmic calcium which by itself and via calcium-calmodulin–dependent protein kinases influences cellular processes appropriate to the stimulated cell. The transient rise in calcium induced by IP$_3$ from the intracellular stores is reinforced in the presence of continued agonist stimulation by alterations in membrane calcium flux that result eventually in net calcium uptake from the extracellular fluid by mechanisms that have been incompletely defined.

DAG, the other second messenger produced by the action of phospholipase C on PIP$_2$ (as well as other membrane phospholipids), remains associated with the cell membrane and activates protein kinase C, which has different substrates than the calcium-calmodulin kinases stimulated by IP$_3$. Protein phosphorylation stimulated by protein kinase C contributes to the tissue-specific response in ways that remain poorly understood. Increases in intracellular calcium also potentiate the activation of protein kinase C (Fig. 70-5).

REGULATION OF ADRENERGIC RECEPTORS Prolonged exposure to alpha- or beta-adrenergic agonists decreases the number of corresponding adrenergic receptors on effector cells. Although the biochemical mechanisms involved are obscure, internalization of the beta-adrenergic receptor within the cell occurs during agonist exposure in some systems, suggesting that internal translocation contributes to the decrease in receptor number under these circumstances.

Alteration in agonist concentration also may affect the affinity of the receptor for the agonist. Adrenergic receptors that utilize adenylyl cyclase for the second messenger (beta receptors, alpha$_2$ receptors) exist in high and low affinity states; exposure to agonist diminishes the proportion of receptors in the high-affinity state. Such alterations in adrenergic receptors induced by adrenergic agonists are termed *homologous regulation*. Agonist-induced alterations in adrenergic-receptor density and affinity are believed to contribute to the diminished physiologic response that occurs after prolonged exposure of an effector tissue to adrenergic agonist, a phenomenon known as *tachyphylaxis* or *desensitization*.

Adrenergic receptors are also influenced by factors other than adrenergic agonists, so-called *heterologous regulation*. Enhanced alpha-adrenergic-receptor affinity, for example, may underlie the potentiation of alpha-adrenergic responses that occur in response to lowered environmental temperatures. Thyroid hormones potentiate beta-receptor responses by alterations in beta-receptor number and in the efficiency of coupling receptor occupancy with physiologic response. Estrogen and progesterone alter the sensitivity of the myometrium to catecholamines by effects on alpha-adrenergic receptors. Glucocorticoids may influence adrenergic function by antagonizing agonist-induced decreases in adrenergic receptors, thereby counteracting tachyphylaxis in response to intense adrenergic stimulation.

Alterations in sensitivity to catecholamines also occur as a consequence of postreceptor changes, although the latter remain poorly characterized.

FIGURE 70-5 Interaction of autonomic agonists with membrane-bound regulatory proteins and cellular effector systems. The designations α and β refer to adrenergic receptors, DA refers to dopaminergic receptors, and M, to muscarinic receptors. G designates the GTP-associated regulatory protein which may have a stimulatory (s) or inhibitory (i) effect on adenylyl cyclase or may stimulate phospholipase C (q). [(+) designates stimulation; (−) designates inhibition; PIP$_2$, phosphatidylinositol-4,5-bisphosphate; DAG, 1,2-diacylglycerol; IP$_3$, inositol-1,4,5-trisphosphate. See text for details.]

Catecholamines influence all of the major organ systems. The effects take place in seconds and may occur in anticipation of physiologic requirement. An increase in sympathoadrenal activity prior to strenuous exercise, for example, lessens the impact of exercise on the internal environment.

DIRECT EFFECTS OF CATECHOLAMINES **Cardiovascular system** Catecholamines stimulate vasoconstriction in the subcutaneous, mucosal, splanchnic, and renal vascular beds by alpha-receptor–mediated mechanisms. Although vasoconstriction was originally considered an alpha$_1$-receptor response, vascular tone appears to be more complexly regulated and, in many areas, involves alpha$_2$-mediated responses as well. The venous portion of the circulation, in particular, is endowed with alpha$_2$ receptors. Differential regulation of the two types of alpha receptors, under certain circumstances, contributes to an integrated physiologic response. Since vasoconstriction in the coronary and cerebral circulations is minimal, flow to these areas is maintained during sympathetic stimulation. Skeletal muscle vasculature contains beta receptors sensitive to low circulating levels of E so that skeletal muscle blood flow is augmented during adrenal medullary activation.

The effects of catecholamines on the heart are mediated by beta$_1$ receptors and include increase in heart rate, enhancement of cardiac contractility, and increase in conduction velocity. The increase in myocardial contractility is illustrated by a leftward and upward shift of the ventricular function curve (Fig. 232-6) that relates cardiac work to ventricular diastolic fiber length; at any initial fiber length, catecholamines increase cardiac work. Catecholamines also enhance cardiac output by stimulating venoconstriction, enhancing venous return, and increasing the force of atrial contraction, thereby augmenting diastolic volume and hence fiber length. The acceleration of conduction in the junctional tissues results in a more synchronous, and hence more effective, ventricular contraction. Cardiac stimulation increases myocardial oxygen consumption, a major factor in the pathogenesis and treatment of myocardial ischemia.

Metabolism Catecholamines increase metabolic rate. In small mammals, mitochondrial respiration in brown adipose tissue is functionally uncoupled by NE. In a reaction unique to brown adipose tissue, NE stimulates the beta$_3$-adrenergic receptor that activates a specific mitochondrial uncoupling protein that dissipates the proton gradient between the inner mitochondrial matrix and the cytoplasm, thereby uncoupling substrate utilization and ATP synthesis. In humans, a functional role for brown adipose tissue has not been established with certainty, but increasing evidence suggests a potential role for this tissue in catecholamine-stimulated heat production in human beings.

Substrate mobilization In a variety of tissues, catecholamines stimulate the breakdown of stored fuel with the production of substrate for local consumption; glycogenolysis in the heart, for example, provides substrate for immediate metabolism by the myocardium. Catecholamines also accelerate fuel mobilization in liver, adipose tissue, and skeletal muscle, liberating substrates (glucose, free fatty acids, lactate) into the circulation for use throughout the body.

Fluids and Electrolytes By a direct action on the renal tubule, NE stimulates sodium reabsorption, thereby defending extracellular fluid volume. Dopamine, in contrast, promotes sodium excretion. NE and E also promote cellular uptake of potassium, thereby defending against the development of hyperkalemia.

Viscera Catecholamines affect visceral function by actions on smooth muscle and glandular epithelium. Urinary bladder and intestinal smooth muscle are relaxed while the corresponding sphincters are stimulated. Gallbladder emptying also involves sympathetic mechanisms. Catecholamine-mediated smooth-muscle contraction in the female aids ovulation and ovum transport along the fallopian tubes, and in the male provides propulsive force for the seminal fluid during ejaculation. Inhibitory alpha$_2$ receptors on cholinergic neurons within the gut contribute to intestinal relaxation. Catecholamines induce bronchodilation by a beta$_2$-receptor mechanism.

INDIRECT EFFECTS OF CATECHOLAMINES The ultimate physiologic response induced by catecholamines involves changes in hormone secretion and in blood flow distribution, both of which support and amplify the direct effects of catecholamines.

Endocrine System Catecholamines influence the secretion of renin, insulin, glucagon, calcitonin, parathormone, thyroxine, gastrin, erythropoietin, progesterone, and, possibly, testosterone. Secretion of each of these hormones is governed by complex feedback loops. With the exception of thyroxine and the gonadal steroids, each is a polypeptide not under the direct control of the pituitary gland. Sympathoadrenal input into the secretion of these hormones provides a mechanism for regulation by the central nervous system and ensures a coordinated hormonal response in accord with the homeostatic needs of the organism.

Renin (See also Chap. 246) Sympathetic stimulation increases renin release by a direct beta-receptor effect independent of vascular changes within the kidney. The renin response to volume depletion is sympathetically mediated and is initiated by a fall in central venous pressure. Since renin secretion activates the angiotensin-aldosterone system, angiotensin-induced vasoconstriction supports the direct effects of catecholamines on blood vessels, while aldosterone-mediated sodium reabsorption complements the direct increase in sodium reabsorption induced by sympathetic stimulation. Beta-receptor blocking agents suppress renin secretion.

Insulin and glucagon Stimulation of pancreatic sympathetic nerves or an elevation in circulating catecholamines suppresses insulin and increases glucagon release. Inhibition of insulin secretion is mediated by the alpha$_2$ receptor, and stimulation of glucagon is mediated by the beta receptor. This combination of effects supports substrate mobilization, reinforcing the direct effects of catecholamines on hepatic glucose output and lipolysis. Although alpha-receptor–mediated suppression of insulin release usually predominates, a beta-receptor mechanism may augment insulin secretion under some circumstances.

SYMPATHOADRENAL FUNCTION IN SELECTED PHYSIOLOGIC AND PATHOPHYSIOLOGIC STATES **Support of the Circulation** The sympathetic nervous system functions to maintain an adequate circulation. During upright posture and volume depletion, reduction of afferent venous and arterial baroreceptor impulse traffic diminishes an inhibitory input to the vasomotor center, thereby increasing sympathetic activity (Fig. 70-3) and reducing efferent vagal tone. As a result, heart rate is increased, and cardiac output is diverted from the skin, subcutaneous tissues, mucosa, and viscera. Sympathetic stimulation of the kidney increases sodium reabsorption, and sympathetically mediated venoconstriction enhances venous return (Fig. 70-6). With pronounced hypotension, the adrenal medulla is recruited and E reinforces the effects of the sympathetic nervous system.

The intense sympathoadrenal stimulation that accompanies severe volume depletion may contribute to the development of ketoacidosis in alcoholics as well as to the ketoacidosis sometimes seen in association with hyperemesis gravidarum. Catecholamine-mediated suppression of insulin and stimulation of glucagon markedly potentiate ketogenesis in these disease states. Volume resuscitation and provision of adequate glucose promptly reverse the ketoacidosis in most cases.

Congestive heart failure The sympathetic nervous system also provides circulatory support during congestive heart failure (Chap. 233). Venoconstriction and sympathetic stimulation of the heart increase cardiac output while peripheral vasoconstriction directs blood flow to the heart and brain. The afferent signals are less clear than in simple volume depletion because the venous pressure is usually elevated. In severe heart failure, depletion of cardiac NE may impair the effectiveness of sympathetic circulatory support. On the other hand, the possibility has been raised that intense sympathetic stimulation may further impair cardiac function, suggesting possible benefit from beta-adrenergic blockade. The use of beta blockers in the treatment of congestive heart failure, however, should be considered experimental and undertaken only with great caution.

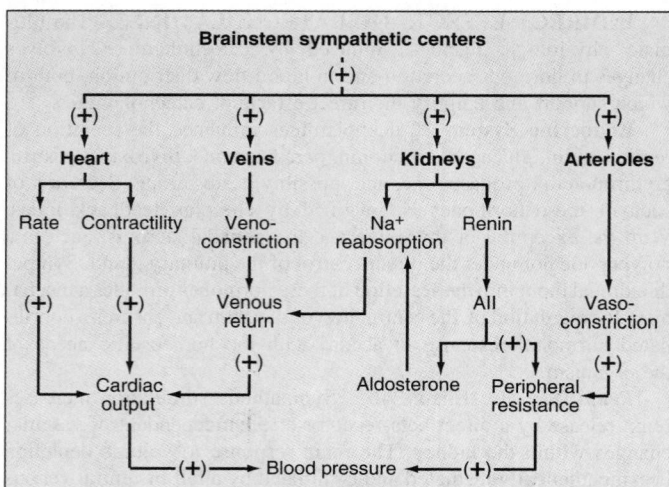

FIGURE 70-6 Sympathetic nervous system effects on blood pressure. Sympathetic stimulation (+) increases blood pressure by effects on the heart, the veins, the kidneys, and the arterioles. The net result of sympathetic stimulation is an increase in both cardiac output and peripheral resistance. AII = angiotensin II. [From JB Young, L Landsberg, in P Sleight et al (eds), Scientific Foundations of Cardiology, London, Heinemann, 1981.]

Trauma and shock In acute traumatic injury or shock, adrenal catecholamines support the circulation and mobilize substrates. In the chronic, reparative phase following injury, catecholamines also contribute to substrate mobilization and to the elevation in metabolic rate.

Exercise Sympathetic activation during exercise increases cardiac output and ensures sufficient substrate to meet the increased metabolic needs. Central neural factors, such as anticipation, and circulatory factors, such as fall in venous pressure, trigger the sympathetic response. Mild degrees of exercise stimulate the sympathetic nervous system alone; during more severe exertion the adrenal medulla is activated as well. Conditioning is associated with a decrease in sympathetic nervous system activity both at rest and during exercise, in comparison with the untrained state.

Hypoglycemia (See also Chap. 335) Hypoglycemia causes a marked increase in adrenal medullary E secretion. When glucose concentrations fall below overnight fasting levels, regulatory glucose-sensitive neurons in the central nervous system initiate a prompt increase in adrenal medullary secretion. The increase is especially intense at plasma glucose levels below 2.8 mmol/L (50 mg/dL), when plasma E levels increase 25 to 50 times above baseline, thereby increasing hepatic glucose output, providing alternative substrate in the form of free fatty acids, suppressing endogenous insulin release, and inhibiting insulin-mediated glucose utilization in muscle. Many clinical manifestations of hypoglycemia, such as tachycardia, palpitations, nervousness, tremor, and widened pulse pressure, are secondary to increased E secretion. These manifestations of E secretion constitute an "early warning" system in insulin-requiring diabetics. In patients with long-standing diabetes mellitus, however, the E response to hypoglycemia may be diminished or absent, leaving affected patients at greater risk to develop severe hypoglycemia.

Cold Exposure The sympathetic nervous system plays a critical role in the maintenance of normal body temperature during exposure to a cold environment. Receptors in the skin and central nervous system respond to a fall in temperature by activating hypothalamic and brainstem centers that increase sympathetic activity. Sympathetic stimulation leads to vasoconstriction in the superficial vascular beds, thereby diminishing heat loss. The sympathetic response involves a complex interaction between lowered environmental temperatures and alpha$_2$-adrenergic receptors. Acclimatization during chronic cold expo-

sure increases the capacity for metabolic heat production in response to sympathetic stimulation.

Dietary Intake Fasting suppresses and overfeeding stimulates the sympathetic nervous system. The reduction in sympathetic activity during fasting or starvation contributes to the decrease in metabolic rate, bradycardia, and hypotension in these states. Enhanced sympathetic activity during periods of increased caloric intake contributes to the elevation in metabolic rate associated with a chronic increase in dietary intake.

Hypoxia Chronic hypoxia is associated with stimulation of the sympathoadrenal system, and some of the cardiovascular changes attendant to hypoxia are dependent on catecholamines.

Orthostatic Hypotension The maintenance of arterial pressure during upright posture depends on an adequate blood volume, an unimpaired venous return, and an intact sympathetic nervous system. Significant postural hypotension, therefore, often reflects extracellular fluid volume depletion or dysfunction of the circulatory reflexes. Diseases of the nervous system, such as tabes dorsalis, syringomyelia, or diabetes mellitus, may disrupt these sympathetic reflexes with resultant orthostatic hypotension. Although any antiadrenergic agent may impair the postural sympathetic response, orthostatic hypotension is most prominent with drugs that block neurotransmission within the ganglia or adrenergic neurons.

The term *idiopathic orthostatic hypotension* refers to a group of degenerative diseases involving either the pre- or postganglionic sympathetic neurons (Chaps. 20 and 370).

Treatment of orthostatic hypotension is usually unsatisfactory except in the mildest cases. There is no way of reestablishing the normal relationship between fall in venous return and sympathetic neuronal activation. Volume expansion with fludrocortisone and a liberal salt diet in conjunction with fitted stockings to the waist, as well as elevation of the head of the bed to avoid recumbency, will maintain plasma volume and venous return and frequently provide symptomatic improvement.

PHARMACOLOGY OF THE SYMPATHOADRENAL SYSTEM

A variety of therapeutic agents affect sympathetic nervous system function or interact with adrenergic receptors, making it possible to stimulate or suppress effects mediated by catecholamines with some degree of specificity (Table 70-1).

SYMPATHOMIMETIC AMINES Sympathomimetic amines may directly activate adrenergic receptors (direct acting) or release NE from the sympathetic nerve endings (indirect acting). Many agents have both direct and indirect effects.

Epinephrine and Norepinephrine The naturally occurring catecholamines act predominantly by the direct stimulation of adrenergic receptors. NE is employed to support the circulation and elevate the blood pressure in hypotensive states (Chap. 38). Peripheral vasoconstriction is the major effect, although cardiac stimulation occurs as well. E, also employed as a pressor, has special usefulness in the treatment of allergic reactions, especially those associated with anaphylaxis. E antagonizes the effects of histamine and other mediators on vascular and visceral smooth muscle and is useful in the treatment of bronchospasm.

Dopamine *Dopamine* is used in treating hypotension, shock (Chap. 38), and certain forms of heart failure (Chap. 233). At low infusion rates it exerts a positive inotropic effect both by a direct action on the cardiac beta$_1$ receptors and by the indirect release of NE from sympathetic nerve endings in the heart. At low doses direct stimulation of dopaminergic receptors in the renal and mesenteric vasculature also results in vasodilation in the gut and kidney and facilitates sodium excretion. At higher infusion rates interaction with alpha-adrenergic receptors results in vasoconstriction, an increase in peripheral resistance, and an elevation of blood pressure.

Beta-Receptor Agonists *Isoproterenol*, a direct-acting beta-receptor agonist, stimulates the heart, decreases peripheral resistance, and relaxes bronchial smooth muscle. It raises the cardiac output and

Table 70-1

Some Commonly Used Autonomic Drugs[a,b,c]

Agent	Indication	Dose and Route	Comment
ADRENERGIC AGONISTS[d]			
Epinephrine	Anaphylaxis	300–500 μg SC or IM (0.3–0.5 mL of 1/1000 solution of hydrochloride salt); 25–50 μg IV (slowly) every 5–15 min; titrate as needed	Nonselective alpha and beta agonist; increases BP, heart rate Bronchodilation
Norepinephrine	Shock Hypotension	2–4 μg of NE base/min IV; titrate as needed	Alpha and beta$_1$ agonist Vasoconstriction predominates Extravasation causes tissue necrosis; infuse through IV cannula
Isoproterenol	Cardiogenic shock Bradyarrhythmias AV block Asthma	0.5–5.0 μg/min IV; titrate as needed Inhalation	Nonselective beta agonist Increases cardiac rate and contractility (beta$_1$) Tachycardia limits usefulness Dilates bronchi (beta$_2$); cardiac stimulation also occurs
Dobutamine	Refractory CHF Cardiogenic shock	2.5–25 (μg/kg)/min IV	Selective beta$_1$ agonist with greater effect on contractility than heart rate; a congener of dopamine but not a dopaminergic agonist
Phenylephrine	Hypotension	2–5 mg SC or IM 0.1–0.5 mg IV	Selective alpha$_1$ agonist; useful in antagonizing hypotension of spinal anesthesia
	Supraventricular tachycardia	150–800 μg slow IV push	Pressor effect induces vagotonic response; do not exceed 160 mmHg systolic BP
Terbutaline	Asthma	2.5–5.0 mg PO tid; 0.25–0.5 mg SC; inhalation every 4–5 h	Selective beta$_2$ agonist; beta$_1$ (cardiac) effects at higher doses (inhalation preferred route)
Bitolterol	Asthma	Inhalation every 4–6 h	Selective beta$_2$ agonist
Salmeterol	Asthma	Inhalation bid	Selective beta$_2$ agonist; long-acting agent for maintenance therapy
Albuterol	Asthma	2.0–4.0 mg PO tid or qid; 0.2 mg inhalation every 4–6 h	Selective beta$_2$ agonist; beta$_1$ effects (cardiac) at higher doses (inhalation preferred route)
Isoetharine	Asthma	Inhalation every 2–4 h	Selective beta$_2$ agonist; some beta$_1$ effects
Metaproterenol	Asthma	10–20 mg PO tid or qid; inhalation every 3–4 h	Selective beta$_2$ agonist; some beta$_1$ effects (inhalation preferred route)
Pirbuterol	Asthma	Inhalation every 4–6 h	Selective beta$_2$ agonist; some beta$_1$ effects
Ritodrine	Premature labor	50–350 μg/min IV	Selective beta$_2$ agonist; hypokalemia, hyperglycemia, hypotension, cardiac stimulation may occur Neonatal hypoglycemia, hypocalcemia reported
DOPAMINERGIC AGONISTS			
Dopamine	Shock	2–5 (μg/kg)/min IV (dopaminergic range) 5–10 (μg/kg)/min IV (dopaminergic and beta range) 10–20 (μg/kg)/min IV (beta range) 20–50 (μg/kg)/min IV (alpha range)	Pharmacologic effects are dose dependent: renal and mesenteric vasodilation predominate at lower doses; cardiac stimulation and vasoconstriction develop as the dose is increased
Bromocriptine	Amenorrhea-galactorrhea	2.5 mg PO bid or tid	Selective agonist of D$_2$ receptor; inhibits prolactin secretion
	Acromegaly	5–15 mg PO tid or qid	Lowers growth hormone in a minority of patients with acromegaly
INHIBITORS OF CENTRAL SYMPATHETIC OUTFLOW			
Clonidine	Hypertension	0.1–0.6 mg PO bid	Selective alpha$_2$ agonist; potentiates central baroreceptor depressor reflex Abrupt discontinuation may result in withdrawal syndrome with rebound hypertension
Methyldopa	Hypertension	250–500 mg PO every 6–8 h	Metabolized by decarboxylation and beta hydroxylation to α-methylnorepinephrine, a centrally active selective alpha$_2$ agonist
ADRENERGIC NEURON BLOCKING AGENTS			
Guanethidine	Hypertension	10–100 mg PO qd	Concentrated in sympathetic nerve endings; blocks release of NE in response to nerve impulses and depletes NE stores; prominent orthostatic hypotension
Bretylium	Ventricular fibrillation and tachycardia	150–300 mg IV 1–4 mg/min IV	In addition to blocking NE release, has direct effect on electrical properties of cardiac muscle

(continued)

Table 70-1—(continued)

Some Commonly Used Autonomic Drugs[a,b,c]

Agent	Indication	Dose and Route	Comment
BETA BLOCKING AGENTS[c]			
Propranolol	Hypertension	40–160 mg PO bid (or higher)	Lipophilic, nonselective Dosage highly variable
	Angina	10–40 mg PO tid or qid	
	Myocardial infarction	60–80 mg PO tid	Prolongs survival post MI
	Arrhythmias	10–30 mg PO tid or qid; 1–3 mg IV	
	Hypertrophic cardiomyopathy	20–40 mg PO tid or qid	
	Pheochromocytoma	10–20 mg PO tid or qid; 0.5–2.0 mg IV	After alpha blockade initiated
	Essential tremor	20–80 mg PO tid	
	Migraine	20–80 mg PO bid or tid	
	Hyperthyroidism	10–60 mg PO tid or qid	
Metoprolol	Hypertension	50–200 mg PO bid	Selective beta$_1$ (cardiac), lipophilic
	Myocardial infarction	100 mg PO bid	Prolongs survival post MI
Nadolol	Hypertension	80–320 mg PO qd	Hydrophilic, nonselective; lengthen dosage interval with renal failure
	Angina	80–240 mg PO qd	
Timolol	Hypertension	10–30 mg PO bid	Lipophilic, nonselective
	Myocardial infarction	10 mg PO bid	Prolongs survival post MI
Atenolol	Hypertension	50–100 mg PO qd	Selective beta$_1$, hydrophilic; lengthen dosage interval with renal failure
Pindolol	Hypertension	5–30 mg PO bid	Nonselective, lipophilic with partial agonist activity
	Angina	10 mg PO qid	
Acebutolol	Hypertension	200–800 mg qid	Selective beta$_1$, hydrophilic, partial agonist activity
	Arrhythmias	200–600 mg bid	
Penbutolol	Hypertension	20–40 mg PO qd	Nonselective
Betaxolol	Hypertension	15–20 mg PO qd	Selective β$_1$, hydrophilic
Carteolol	Hypertension	2.5–10 mg PO qd	Nonselective, partial agonist activity, hydrophilic; lengthen dosage interval with renal failure
Esmolol	Supraventricular tachycardia	50–200 (μg/kg)/min IV after loading dose of 500 μg/kg/min for 1 min	Selective beta$_1$, very short duration of action
Sotalol	Arrythmias	80–320 mg bid	Nonselective, hydrophilic
Bisoprolol	Hypertension	5–20 mg qd	Selective beta$_1$, lipophilic
ALPHA BLOCKING AGENTS			
Phenoxybenzamine	Pheochromocytoma	10–60 mg PO bid; titrate as needed	Noncompetitive, nonselective alpha blockade
Phentolamine	Pheochromocytoma	5 mg IV (after test dose of 0.5 mg)	Competitive, nonselective alpha blockade
Prazosin	Hypertension	1–5 mg PO bid or tid	Competitive, selective alpha$_1$ blockade
	CHF	2–7 mg PO qid	
Doxazosin	Hypertension Prostatism	1–16 mg PO qd	Competitive selective alpha$_1$ blockade, long duration of action
Terazosin	Hypertension Prostatism	1–5 mg PO qd	Competitive, selective alpha$_1$ blockade, long duration of action
COMBINED ALPHA-BETA BLOCKING AGENT			
Labetalol	Hypertension	100–1200 mg PO bid; titrate slowly as needed; 20–80 mg IV (by increments up to 300 mg); 2 mg/min by IV infusion	Competitive alpha and beta antagonist with relatively more activity against beta receptors
DOPAMINERGIC ANTAGONIST[f]			
Metoclopramide	Diabetic gastroparesis	10–15 mg PO qid	Competitive dopaminergic antagonist with prominent cholinergic agonist activity
	Gastroesophageal reflex	10–15 mg PO qid	
	Antiemetic (cancer chemotherapy)	10 mg IV	
GANGLIONIC BLOCKING AGENT			
Trimethaphan	Hypertensive crisis (aortic dissection)	0.5–5 mg/min IV	Competitive ganglionic blocker; some direct vasodilating effects; inhibits parasympathetic as well as sympathetic nervous system
CHOLINERGIC AGENT			
Bethanechol	Urinary retention (nonobstructive)	10–20 mg PO tid or qid; 2.5 mg SC	M$_2$ receptor agonist

Table 70-1—(continued)

Some Commonly Used Autonomic Drugs[a,b,c]

Agent	Indication	Dose and Route	Comment
ANTICHOLINESTERASE AGENTS[g]			
Physostigmine	Central cholinergic blockade	1–2 mg IV (slow)	Tertiary amine; penetrates CNS well; may cause seizures; used to reverse central anticholinergic effects produced by overdose of atropine or tricyclic antidepressants
Edrophonium	Paroxysmal supraventricular tachycardia	5 mg IV (after 1.0-mg test dose)	Induces vagotonic response; rapid onset, short duration of action; effects reversed by atropine
CHOLINERGIC BLOCKING AGENTS[h]			
Atropine	Bradycardia and hypotension	0.4–1.0 mg IV every 1–2 h	Competitive inhibition of M_1 and M_2 receptor; blocks hemodynamic changes associated with increased vagal tone
Ipratropium	Asthma Chronic obstructive pulmonary disease	500 mg by inhalation (nebulizer) tid or qid	Anticholinergic bronchodilator

[a] Consult complete prescribing information.   [b] Doses for children are not given.   [c] Only the more common indications and routes of administration are listed.
[d] Dopaminergic agonists are listed separately although dopamine, at high doses, is an adrenergic agonist as well.
[e] Clinical efficacy of most beta blockers appears similar for major indications. Not all beta blockers are FDA approved for all indications listed in the table. When beta-blocking agents are discontinued, gradual dosage reduction is recommended. Both beta₁ selective and nonselective agents have cardioprotective effects after myocardial infarction.
[f] Neuroleptic and antipsychotic agents are also dopaminergic antagonists; these are not included in the table.
[g] A major use of cholinesterase inhibitors is in myasthenia gravis (Chap. 382). These agents, quaternary amines that do not penetrate the CNS, are not included here.
[h] A wide variety of synthetic atropine derivatives are available for the purpose of (1) diminishing GI tract motility and secretion and (2) increasing urinary bladder capacity. Their usefulness is limited by anticholinergic side effects. Some may be useful as adjuncts in the treatment of peptic ulcer disease.

accelerates atrioventricular conduction while increasing the automaticity of ventricular pacemakers. Isoproterenol is used in the treatment of heart block and bronchoconstriction. *Dobutamine*, a congener of dopamine with relative selectivity for the beta₁ receptor and with a greater effect on myocardial contractility than on heart rate, is also used in the treatment of congestive heart failure, often in combination with vasodilators (Chap. 233). In conjunction with radionuclide imaging or echocardiographic assessment of wall motion, dobutamine, as well as other investigational congeners that have a relatively greater effect on heart rate, is used in the diagnosis of demand-induced myocardial ischemia.

Selective beta₂-receptor agonists The cardiac stimulation caused by nonselective beta agonists, such as isoproterenol or epinephrine, is occasionally dangerous when these agents are used in the treatment of bronchoconstriction (see Chap. 252). Selective beta₂ agonists, administered by inhalation for bronchoconstriction, include agents with an intermediate duration of action (*metaproterenol, albuterol, terbutaline, pirbuterol, isoetharine,* and *bitolterol*) and the newer long-acting agents (*salmeterol* and *formoterol*); these drugs improve the therapeutic ratio by achieving bronchial dilatation with less activation of the cardiovascular system (see Chaps. 252 and 258). Although selectivity is relative and cardiac stimulation may occur with these agents at higher dose levels, inhaled agonists at the usual doses result in relatively little cardiac stimulation. Oral administration, which is no longer preferred, is associated with more systemic beta-agonist effects. *Ritodrine*, another selective beta₂ agonist, is used as a tocolytic agent (as is *terbutaline*) to relax the uterus and antagonize premature labor.

Alpha-Adrenergic Agonists *Phenylephrine* and *methoxamine* are direct-acting alpha agonists that elevate blood pressure by increasing peripheral vasoconstriction. They are used primarily in the treatment of hypotension and paroxysmal supraventricular tachycardia (Chap. 231), in the latter case by increasing cardiac vagal tone through reflex baroreceptor stimulation. Phenylephrine and a related proprietary compound, *phenylpropanolamine*, are common constituents of decongestant medications (often combined with antihistamines) for the treatment of allergic rhinitis and upper respiratory infections.

Miscellaneous Sympathomimetic Amines with Mixed Actions *Ephedrine* has both direct beta-receptor agonist properties and an indirect effect on sympathetic nerve endings, from which it releases NE, and is used primarily as a bronchodilator. *Sudephedrine*, a conge-

ner of ephedrine, is less potent at dilating bronchi and serves as a nasal decongestant. *Metaraminol* has both direct and indirect effects on sympathetic nerve endings and is employed in the treatment of hypotensive states.

Dopaminergic Agonists The D_2-receptor agonist *bromocriptine* is used to suppress prolactin secretion (Chap. 328). *Apomorphine*, another D_2-receptor agonist, is used to induce emesis.

ANTIADRENERGIC OR SYMPATHOLYTIC AGENTS (See also Chap. 246) **Agents Inhibiting Central Sympathetic Outflow** The antihypertensive agents *methyldopa, clonidine, guanabenz,* and *guanfacine* diminish central sympathetic outflow by stimulating a central alpha-adrenergic pathway (alpha₂ receptor) that diminishes vasomotor outflow. Central nervous system side effects such as sedation are common. When administration of clonidine is stopped abruptly, a withdrawal syndrome characterized by rebound hyperactivity of the sympathetic nervous system can produce a state resembling the crises of patients with pheochromocytoma. *Opiates* also may exert a central sympatholytic effect; the sympathetic excitation of morphine withdrawal responds to clonidine and vice versa. *Propranolol* and *reserpine* may exert some sympatholytic effects at the level of the central nervous system.

Ganglionic Blocking Agents Ganglionic transmission may be antagonized by drugs that block the (nicotinic) cholinergic synapse between the preganglionic and postganglionic autonomic nerves. These agents inhibit the parasympathetic as well as the sympathetic nervous system. Only *trimethaphan* is in general clinical use; its major application is in the treatment of hypertensive crises, particularly aortic dissection, when controlled hypotension and decreased myocardial contractility are desirable (Chap. 246).

Agents Acting at the Peripheral Sympathetic Nerve Endings Adrenergic neuron-blocking agents depress the function of the peripheral sympathetic nerves by decreasing the amount of neurotransmitter released. *Guanethidine*, the prototype of this class of drugs, is concentrated in the sympathetic nerve endings by the amine-uptake mechanism. Within the terminal it blocks the release of NE in response to nerve impulses and eventually depletes the nerve of NE by displacing it from the intraneuronal storage granules. The drug is occasionally useful in the management of severe hypertension, although orthostatic hypotension is a limiting side effect. *Bretylium*, an agent whose effects are similar to those of guanethidine, is employed in the treatment of ventricular fibrillation (Chap. 231). Both guanethidine and bretylium are antagonized by agents that affect the amine-uptake transport process such as sympathomimetic amines, tricyclic antidepressants, phenoxybenzamine, and phenothiazines. The antihypertensive action of guanethidine may be rapidly reversed by these drugs.

Reserpine depletes catecholamines from the peripheral sympathetic nerve endings, the brain, and the adrenal medulla. Its antihypertensive effect in humans is usually attributed to depletion of peripheral NE stores within sympathetic nerve endings. The sedation and occasionally morbid depression attending its use result from NE depletion within the central nervous system.

Adrenergic-Receptor Blocking Agents Adrenergic blocking agents antagonize the effects of catecholamines at the level of the peripheral tissue.

Alpha-adrenergic-receptor blocking agents *Phenoxybenzamine* and *phentolamine* are utilized principally in treating pheochromocytoma (Chap. 333). Phenoxybenzamine produces prolonged, noncompetitive alpha blockade, while phentolamine leads to reversible, competitive blockade. Because of its rapid action and short duration, phentolamine is commonly used in the treatment of acute hypertensive paroxysms secondary to catecholamine excess, such as occur with pheochromocytoma. Both phentolamine and phenoxybenzamine antagonize alpha$_1$ and alpha$_2$ receptors, although phenoxybenzamine is more potent at the alpha$_1$ receptor site. *Prazosin*, an alpha-adrenergic blocking agent with selectivity for the alpha$_1$ receptor, possesses properties that resemble those of primary vasodilators and has been used in the treatment of essential hypertension and as an afterload-reducing agent in congestive heart failure. *Doxazosin* and *terazosin*, long-acting selective alpha$_1$ blockers, are more useful in the treatment of essential hypertension because of better dosing schedule and less orthostatic hypotension. These agents also lower triglyceride levels and raise high-density lipoprotein (HDL) cholesterol levels. Selective alpha$_1$ blockers are potentially useful in the symptomatic treatment of urinary outflow track obstruction and prostatism because they antagonize contraction of the sphincter at the bladder trigone.

Beta-adrenergic-receptor blocking agents These drugs antagonize the effects of catecholamines on the heart and are useful in the treatment of angina pectoris, hypertension, and cardiac arrhythmias. The benefit of beta blockade in angina derives from the decrease in myocardial oxygen consumption following reduction in heart rate and myocardial contractility (Chap. 244). The hypotensive effect of beta blockade is not clearly understood (Chap. 246). Diminished cardiac output, decreased NE release at postganglionic sympathetic nerve endings, reduced renin secretion, and suppressed central sympathetic outflow are possible mechanisms. The efficacy of beta-blocking agents in the treatment of arrhythmias depends on reduction of the rate of spontaneous depolarization of pacemaker cells in the sinus node and junctional pacemakers and on slowing conduction within the atria and atrioventricular node. Beta blockade is also effective in the symptomatic management of hyperthyroidism and the control of tachycardia and arrhythmias in patients with pheochromocytoma. Beta-adrenergic blocking agents are also useful in the treatment of migraine, essential tremor, idiopathic hypertrophic subaortic stenosis, and aortic dissection. Several trials have demonstrated that beta-receptor blocking agents, administered long-term, diminish mortality following acute myocardial infarction. The mechanism of this cardioprotective effect may involve antiarrhythmic action, prevention of reinfarction, and reduction in infarct size (Chap. 243).

Pharmacologic properties of beta-receptor blocking agents Thirteen beta-blocking agents (atenolol, acebutolol, betaxolol, bisoprolol, carteolol, esmolol, metoprolol, nadolol, pindolol, penbutolol, propranolol, sotalol, and timolol) are available for use in the United States. Other agents (alprenolol, bevantolol, dilevalol, oxprenolol, etc.) are in use in other countries and investigational within the United States. The utility of these agents is derived predominantly from blockade of

beta-adrenergic receptors. In general, the various agents have similar clinical efficacy.

Although much has been written about other pharmacologic properties, including cardioselectivity, membrane-stabilizing (local anesthetic) effects, intrinsic sympathomimetic (partial-agonist) activity, and lipid solubility, the clinical significance of these additional properties is small. Local anesthetic properties are most prominent with propranolol; however, membrane stabilization probably does not contribute substantially to the clinical utility. The various beta blockers do differ in their water and lipid solubility. The lipophilic agents (propranolol, metoprolol, oxprenolol, bisoprolol) are readily absorbed from the gastrointestinal tract, metabolized by the liver, have large volumes of distribution, and penetrate the central nervous system well; the hydrophilic agents (acebutolol, atenolol, betaxolol, carteolol, nadolol, sotalol) are less readily absorbed, not extensively metabolized, and have relatively long plasma half-lives. As a consequence, the hydrophilic agents may be administered once per day. Hepatic failure may prolong the plasma half-life of the lipophilic agents, whereas renal failure may prolong the action of the hydrophilic group. The degree of lipid solubility, therefore, provides a basis for choice of a particular agent in patients with hepatic or renal insufficiency. Although the hydrophilic agents penetrate the central nervous system less well, central nervous system side effects (sedation, depression, hallucinations) are well described with the hydrophilic as well as with the lipophilic agents.

Some beta-adrenergic blocking agents possess beta-agonist activity. This has been referred to as "intrinsic sympathomimetic activity" (ISA). Agents with partial agonist activity (pindolol, alprenolol, acebutolol, carteolol, dilevalol, oxprenolol) cause little or no depression of resting heart rate (partial agonist effect) while blocking the increase in heart rate that occurs in response to exercise or the administration of a beta agonist such as isoproterenol. The presence of partial agonist activity may be useful when bradycardia limits treatment in patients with slow resting heart rates. Pindolol also produces mild vasodilation, perhaps in part related to peripheral beta$_2$ stimulation. Agents with partial agonist activity cause less change in blood lipid levels than agents without agonist properties. On theoretical grounds, intrinsic sympathomimetic activity would be undesirable in the treatment of thyrotoxicosis, idiopathic hypertrophic subaortic stenosis, aortic dissection, and tachyarrhythmias.

Cardioselective (beta$_1$) adrenergic-receptor blocking agents Propranolol, the prototype of the nonselective beta-adrenergic blocking agent, induces a competitive blockade of both beta$_1$ and beta$_2$ receptors. Other nonselective beta-blocking agents include alprenolol, carteolol, dilevalol, nadolol, oxprenolol, penbutolol, pindolol, sotalol, and timolol. Metoprolol, esmolol, acebutolol, atenolol, and betaxolol possess relative selectivity for the beta$_1$ receptor. Although beta$_1$-(cardio-) selective agents have the theoretical advantage of producing less bronchoconstriction and less peripheral vasoconstriction, a clear-cut clinical advantage of the cardioselective agents has not been decisively demonstrated, since the beta$_1$ selectivity is only relative. Bronchoconstriction may occur when beta$_1$-selective agents are administered in full therapeutic doses.

Adverse effects of beta-receptor blocking agents Aside from the effects on the central nervous system, most adverse reactions to beta-blocking agents are consequences of beta-adrenergic blockade. These include the precipitation of heart failure in patients in whom cardiac compensation depends on enhanced sympathetic drive; the aggravation of bronchospasm in patients with asthma; predisposition to the development of hypoglycemia in insulin-requiring diabetics (blockade of catecholamine-mediated counterregulation and antagonism of the adrenergic warning signs of hypoglycemia); the development of hyperkalemia in diabetic or uremic patients with impaired potassium tolerance; the enhancement of coronary or peripheral arterial vasospasm; and elevation in triglycerides and depression of HDL levels. The lipid (and perhaps the peripheral vascular) effects are less (or absent) in agents with partial (beta$_2$) agonist activity.

Miscellaneous adrenergic blocking agents Labetalol, approved for use in the United States as an antihypertensive agent, is a competitive antagonist of both alpha- and beta-adrenergic receptors. Although labetalol induces relatively more beta- than alpha-receptor blockade, fall in peripheral resistance may be marked following acute administration of the drug. Vasodilation may be mediated in part by a partial agonist effect on the beta$_2$-adrenergic receptor; labetalol does not possess partial agonist activity for the beta$_1$ (cardiac) receptor.

Metoclopramide is a dopaminergic antagonist with cholinergic agonist properties. It enhances gastric emptying, increases the tone of the lower esophageal sphincter, increases prolactin and aldosterone secretion, and antagonizes emesis induced by apomorphine. It is useful clinically in enhancing gastric emptying (in the absence of organic obstruction such as in diabetic gastroparesis), in antagonizing gastroesophageal reflux, and as an antiemetic during cancer chemotherapy.

THE PARASYMPATHETIC NERVOUS SYSTEM

ACETYLCHOLINE ACh serves as the neurotransmitter at all autonomic ganglia, at the postganglionic parasympathetic nerve endings, at the postganglionic sympathetic nerve endings innervating the eccrine sweat glands, and at the skeletal muscle end plate (neuromuscular junction). The enzyme choline acetyltransferase catalyzes the synthesis of ACh from acetyl coenzyme A (CoA) produced within the nerve ending and from choline, actively taken up from the extracellular fluid. Within the cholinergic nerve endings, ACh is stored in discrete synaptic vesicles and released in response to nerve impulses that depolarize the nerve terminals and increase calcium influx.

Cholinergic Receptors Different receptors for ACh exist on the postganglionic neurons within the autonomic ganglia and at the postjunctional autonomic effector sites. Those within the autonomic ganglia and adrenal medulla are stimulated predominantly by nicotine (*nicotinic receptors*) and those on autonomic effector cells by the alkaloid muscarine (*muscarinic receptors*). Ganglionic blocking agents antagonize the nicotinic receptors, while atropine blocks the muscarinic receptors. The muscarinic (M) receptor, furthermore, has been recently subdivided into additional types. The M$_1$ receptor is localized to the central nervous system and perhaps parasympathetic ganglia; the M$_2$ receptor is the nonneuronal muscarinic receptor on smooth muscle, cardiac muscle, and glandular epithelium. Bethanechol is a selective agonist of the M$_2$ receptor; pirenzepine, an investigational agent, is a selective antagonist of the M$_1$ receptor that markedly reduces gastric acid secretion. The M$_2$ receptor inhibits adenylyl cyclase and utilizes the regulatory G$_i$ protein; the M$_1$ receptor interacts with G$_q$ and stimulates phospholipase C (Fig. 70-5). The M$_3$ receptor, present on smooth muscle and secretory glands, is antagonized by atropine and utilizes phospholipase C, IP$_3$, and DAG as second messengers. Other subtypes have been identified by molecular biologic techniques but have not yet been fully characterized.

Acetylcholinesterase Hydrolysis of ACh by acetylcholinesterase inactivates the neurotransmitter at cholinergic synapses. This enzyme (also known as specific or true cholinesterase) is present within neurons and is distinct from butyrocholinesterase (serum cholinesterase or pseudocholinesterase). The latter enzyme is present in plasma and nonneuronal tissues and is not primarily involved in the termination of the effects of ACh at autonomic effector sites. The pharmacologic effects of anticholinesterase agents are due to inhibition of neuronal (true) acetylcholinesterase.

PHYSIOLOGY OF THE PARASYMPATHETIC NERVOUS SYSTEM The parasympathetic nervous system participates in the regulation of the cardiovascular system, the gastrointestinal tract, and the genitourinary system. Tissues such as liver, kidney, pancreas, and thyroid also receive parasympathetic innervation, suggesting a role for the parasympathetic nervous system in metabolic regulation as well, although cholinergic effects on metabolism are not well characterized.

Cardiovascular System Parasympathetic effects on the heart are mediated by the vagus nerve. ACh reduces the rate of spontaneous depolarization of the sinoatrial node and decreases heart rate. ACh also delays impulse conduction within the atrial musculature while shortening the effective refractory period, a combination of factors that may initiate or perpetuate atrial arrhythmias. At the atrioventricular

node, ACh reduces conduction velocity, increases the effective refractory period, and thus diminishes the ventricular response during atrial flutter or fibrillation (Chap. 231). The decrease in inotropy induced by ACh is related to a prejunctional inhibitory effect on sympathetic nerve endings as well as to a direct inhibitory effect on the atrial myocardium. The ventricular myocardium is not much affected since innervation by cholinergic fibers is minimal. A direct cholinergic contribution to the regulation of peripheral resistance appears unlikely since parasympathetic innervation of the vasculature is not extensive. The parasympathetic nervous system, however, may influence peripheral resistance indirectly by inhibiting NE release from sympathetic nerves.

Gastrointestinal Tract Parasympathetic innervation of the gut is via the vagus nerve and the pelvic sacral nerves. The parasympathetic nervous system increases the tone of gastrointestinal smooth muscle, enhances peristaltic activity, and relaxes the gastrointestinal sphincters. ACh stimulates exocrine secretion from the glandular epithelium and enhances the secretion of gastrin, secretin, and insulin.

Genitourinary and Respiratory Systems Sacral parasympathetic nerves supply the urinary bladder and genitalia. ACh increases ureteral peristalsis, contracts the urinary detrusor muscle, and relaxes the trigone and sphincter, thereby playing a critical role in the coordination of urination. The respiratory tract is innervated with parasympathetic fibers derived from the vagus nerve. ACh increases tracheobronchial secretions and stimulates bronchial constriction.

PHARMACOLOGY OF THE PARASYMPATHETIC NERVOUS SYSTEM **Cholinergic Agonists** ACh itself has no therapeutic role because of its widespread effects and short duration of action. Congeners of ACh are less susceptible to hydrolysis by cholinesterase and have a narrower range of physiologic effects. Bethanechol, the only systemic cholinergic agonist in general use, stimulates gastrointestinal and genitourinary smooth muscle with minimal effect on the cardiovascular system. It is used in the treatment of urinary retention in the absence of outflow tract obstruction and, less commonly, in gastrointestinal disorders such as postvagotomy gastric atony. Pilocarpine and carbachol are topical cholinergic agonists used in the treatment of glaucoma.

Acetylcholinesterase Inhibitors Cholinesterase inhibitors enhance the effects of parasympathetic stimulation by diminishing the inactivation of ACh. The therapeutic application of reversible cholinesterase inhibitors depends on the role of ACh as neurotransmitter at the skeletal muscle neuroeffector junction and within the central nervous system and includes the treatment of myasthenia gravis (Chap. 382), the termination of neuromuscular blockade following general anesthesia, and the reversal of intoxication by agents with a central anticholinergic action. Physostigmine, a tertiary amine, penetrates the central nervous system well, while related quaternary amines (neostigmine, pyridostigmine, ambenonium, and edrophonium) do not. Organophosphorous cholinesterase inhibitors produce irreversible cholinesterase blockade; these agents are used principally as insecticides and are primarily of toxicologic interest. With regard to the autonomic nervous system, cholinesterase inhibitors are of limited use in the treatment of intestinal and bladder smooth-muscle dysfunction such as occurs in paralytic ileus and atonic urinary bladder. Cholinesterase inhibitors induce a vagotonic response in the heart and may be useful in terminating attacks of paroxysmal supraventricular tachycardia (Chap. 231).

Cholinergic-Receptor Blocking Agents *Atropine* blocks muscarinic cholinergic receptors, with little effect on cholinergic transmission at the autonomic ganglia and the neuromuscular junctions. Many of the central nervous system actions of atropine and atropine-like drugs are attributable to blockade of central muscarinic synapses. The related alkaloid, *scopolamine*, is similar to atropine but causes drowsiness, euphoria, and amnesia, effects that make it suitable as a preanesthetic medication.

Atropine increases heart rate and enhances atrioventricular conduction, actions that may be useful in combating the bradycardia or heart block associated with heightened vagal tone. In addition, atropine reverses cholinergically mediated bronchoconstriction and diminishes respiratory tract secretions. These effects contribute to its utility as a preanesthetic medication.

Atropine also decreases gastrointestinal tract motility and secretion. Although various derivatives and congeners of atropine (such as *propantheline, isopropamide*, and *glycopyrrolate*) have been advocated in patients with peptic ulcer or with diarrheal syndromes, the chronic use of such agents is limited by other manifestations of parasympathetic inhibition such as dry mouth and urinary retention. The investigational selective M_1 inhibitor pirenzepine inhibits gastric secretion at doses that have minimal anticholinergic effects at other sites; this agent may be useful in the treatment of peptic ulcer. Atropine and its congener *ipratropium*, when given by inhalation, cause bronchodilation and have been used experimentally in the treatment of asthma.

BIBLIOGRAPHY

ARNER P: The β_3-adrenergic receptor—a cause and cure of obesity? N Engl J Med 333:382, 1995

CARON MG, LEFKOWITZ RJ: Catecholamine receptors: Structure, function and regulation. Recent Prog Horm Res 48:277, 1993

CHALMERS J, PILOWSKY P: Brainstem and bulbospinal neurotransmitter systems in the control of blood pressure. J Hypertens 9:675, 1991

CLÉMENT K et al: Genetic variation in the β_3-adrenergic receptor and an increased capacity to gain weight in patients with morbid obesity. N Engl J Med 333:352, 1995

ESLER M et al: Overflow of catecholamine neurotransmitters to the circulation: Source, fate, and functions. Physiol Rev 70:963, 1990

KUPFERMANN I: Functional studies of cotransmission. Physiol Rev 71(3):683, 1991

LANDSBERG L, YOUNG JB: Catecholamines and the adrenal medulla, in *Williams' Textbook of Endocrinology*, 8th ed, DW Foster, JD Wilson (eds). Philadelphia, Saunders, 1992, p 621

LOKHANDWALA MF, AMENTA F: Anatomical distribution and function of dopamine receptors in the kidney. FASEB J 5:3023, 1991

LOW PA: Autonomic nervous system function. J Clin Neurophysiol 10:14, 1993

MEISTER B, APERIA A: Molecular mechanisms involved in catecholamine regulation of sodium transport. Semin Nephrol 13:41, 1993

NELSON H: β-Andrenergic bronchodilators. N Engl J Med 333:499, 1995

PACHOLCZYK T et al: Expression cloning of a cocaine- and antidepressant-sensitive human noradrenaline transporter. Nature 350:350, 1991

RUFFOLO RR et al: Structure and function of α-adrenoceptors. Pharmacol Rev 43:475, 1991

VAN ZWIETEN PA et al: The parasympathetic system and its muscarinic receptors in hypertensive disease. J Hypertens 13:1079, 1995

WIDÉN E et al: Association of a polymorphism in the β_3-adrenergic-receptor gene with features of the insulin resistance syndrome in Finns. N Engl J Med 333:348, 1995

WILLIAMS JL et al: Area postrema: A unique regulator of cardiovascular function. News Physiol Sci 7:30, 1992

71 | *Joseph Loscalzo*

NITRIC OXIDE: BIOLOGIC AND MEDICAL IMPLICATIONS

Nitric oxide (NO•) is a simple, heterodiatomic molecule with broad and diverse effects in human biology that have been recognized only recently. In 1980, Furchgott and Zawadzki reported that a product of the endothelial cell causes vasorelaxation, and this endothelium-derived relaxing factor (EDRF) was eventually shown to be NO•. NO• is now known to be produced by many cell types and to exert a wide range of biologic effects.

NO• is synthesized by a family of enzymes known as the nitric oxide synthases (NOSs) (Fig. 71-1). Three distinct isoforms have been identified, of which two are named after the cell types from which

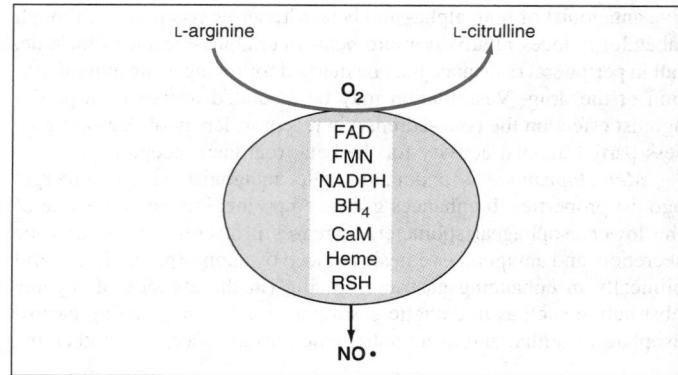

FIGURE 71-1 Nitric oxide synthases catalyze the five-electron oxidation of L-arginine to L-citrulline and nitric oxide. Cofactor requirements include flavin adenine dinucleotide (FAD), flavin mononucleotide (FMN), reduced β-nicotinamide adenine dinucleotide phosphate (NADPH), tetrahydrobiopterin (BH₄), calcium-calmodulin (CaM), a heme complex, and a thiol equivalent (RSH). (Adapted, with permission, from the Annual Review of Pharmacology and Toxicology, vol. 35, 1995, by Annual Reviews, Inc.)

they were first cloned: neuronal NOS (*nNOS, Nos1* gene product); inducible NOS (*iNOS, Nos2* gene product), present in monocytes/macrophages, smooth muscle cells, microvascular endothelial cells, fibroblasts, cardiomyocytes, hepatocytes, and megakaryocytes; and endothelial NOS (*eNOS, Nos3* gene product). As a free radical, NO• readily undergoes addition, substitution, redox, and chain-terminating reactions, which serve as the molecular basis for its biologic effects. NO• reacts with heme-bound iron to form a nitrosylated adduct. Reaction with the prosthetic heme group of guanylyl cyclase activates the enzyme; reaction with the heme group of hemoglobin traps NO•, making it biologically inactive and converting ferrous to ferric hemoglobin; reaction with the prosthetic heme groups of cytochromes uncouples oxidative phosphorylation.

PHYSIOLOGIC ACTIONS NO• is implicated in a wide variety of physiologic effects. The reaction of NO• with the heme group of guanylyl cyclase is the principal effector reaction of NO• in the cardiovascular system. This reaction leads to activation of guanylyl cyclase. In smooth muscle cells, the increase in cyclic guanosine 5'-monophosphate (cyclic GMP) leads to activation of cyclic GMP–dependent protein kinase, which, in turn, phosphorylates myosin light chain kinase. Phosphorylated myosin light chain kinase has a reduced affinity for the calcium-calmodulin complex and is less efficient at phosphorylating myosin light chain. Failure to phosphorylate the regulatory light chains of myosin stabilizes the inactive form of the enzyme and reduces smooth muscle contraction, thereby reducing vascular tone. Agonist–mediated increases in endothelial cell calcium activate *eNOS*. In addition, flow-mediated vasodilation with exercise depends in part on the flow-sensitive increase in endothelial cell calcium, which leads to an increase in *eNOS* activity.

Similar effects are exerted by NO• in smooth muscle cells of other organ systems. NO• relaxes gastrointestinal smooth muscle and leads to reduced motility, relaxation of the sphincter of Oddi, and relaxation of the lower esophageal sphincter. Relaxation of bronchial smooth muscle can be provoked by inhaled NO•, and endogenously produced NO• may contribute to the maintenance of basal bronchial and basal pulmonary arterial tone, as well.

Other effects of *eNOS* include maintenance of vascular integrity, impairment of leukocyte adhesion to the endothelium, and inhibition of smooth muscle migration and proliferation. Endothelial NO• also plays a critical role in hemostasis, making an important contribution to the normal inhibition of platelet function. Basal production of NO• by *eNOS* inhibits both adhesion and aggregation of platelets in the vasculature. Inhibition of platelet adhesion is a property of NO• not shared by the other principal antiplatelet product of the endothelium, prostacyclin.

Endothelial NO• is an important determinant of cerebral blood flow. *nNOS* in neuronal and glial cells contributes to the regulation of cerebrovascular tone and to memory and learning through its involvement in long-term potentiation in the central nervous system. NO• is a likely transmitter of nonadrenergic, noncholinergic neurons and may thereby participate in the regulation of myocardial contractility, heart rate, gastrointestinal motility, bronchial tone, and penile erection.

The production of NO• by *iNOS* in macrophages, lymphocytes, and neutrophils is an important determinant of immune and inflammatory responses. The bactericidal, fungicidal, viricidal, parasiticidal, and tumoricidal activities of macrophages are determined in part by the robust elaboration of NO• by *iNOS*. NO• also limits lymphocyte proliferation and attenuates the allogeneic immune response. Given the broad range of non-immune cell types shown to express *iNOS*, some investigators believe that NO• produced by this isoform is involved in nonspecific immunity, especially in the lung and liver. By a similar mechanism, NO• produced by *iNOS* may also be involved in apoptotic responses in a variety of cell types.

PATHOPHYSIOLOGIC EFFECTS OF NITRIC OXIDE
Both a deficiency and an excess of NO• are believed to be involved in several pathophysiologic states. NO• is a critical determinant of basal vascular tone, and a deficiency of NO• is associated with *hypertension*, as illustrated by recent observations in a murine model of *Nos3* gene inactivation by homologous recombination. Nevertheless, genetic linkage studies have thus far failed to suggest an association between the *Nos3* locus and essential hypertension. However, Deng and Rapp have demonstrated a clear linkage between the *Nos2* locus and salt-sensitive hypertension in the Dahl S rat. Also, the provision of L-arginine in the diet of these animals corrects the hypertensive response to dietary sodium chloride. In chronic renal failure, the plasma concentration of dimethylarginine, a naturally occurring derivative of L-arginine, is increased and competitively inhibits nitric oxide synthase activity, possibly contributing to the hypertension of chronic renal failure.

Common disorders that promote atherosclerosis, such as hypertension, hyperlipidemia, smoking, and diabetes, are all associated with abnormal endothelial function, one manifestation of which is a comparative deficiency of bioactive NO•. This deficiency, which represents either a true deficiency of the molecule or inactivation of it by reactive, oxygen-derived free radicals, is accompanied by increased vascular tone, reduced antithrombotic activity, decreased antiproliferative action, increased endothelial permeability, and enhanced susceptibility of low-density lipoprotein to oxidation. These many interrelated actions may promote atherosclerosis and its complications.

Expression of *iNOS* occurs in several disease states, the most prominent being *bacterial sepsis*. Induction of *Nos2* is induced by endotoxin and cytokines, and the elaboration of NO• in this setting accounts for the hypotension of septic shock states and contributes to the hemorrhagic diathesis of sepsis by profoundly inhibiting platelet function. The myocardial depression associated with septic shock may be explained in part by the inhibition of myocardial contractility by NO•. The cytokine-rich milieu that accompanies ischemia-reperfusion injury may also contribute to increased elaboration of NO• through increased expression of *iNOS* and the accompanying myocardial depression that follows successful coronary thrombolysis or revascularization.

A deficiency of NO•-producing neurons in the gastrointestinal tract is believed to be responsible for certain abnormalities in gastrointestinal motility, such as *Hirschsprung's disease, achalasia*, and *chronic intestinal pseudo-obstruction*. NO• is also believed to play an important role in gastric cytoprotection, possibly by way of increased mucosal blood flow and the modulation of gastric epithelial function.

Increased NO• production owing to the induction of *Nos2* in hepatocytes, fibroblasts, and endothelial cells is believed to underlie the hyperdynamic circulatory state of Laennec's cirrhosis. Also, NO• produced by hepatocyte *iNOS* plays a role in protection of these cells against a variety of hepatic toxins, including ethanol and acetaminophen. NO• inhibits protein synthesis in the hepatocyte at the posttranslational level and inhibits several mitochondrial enzymes involved in electron transport, including *cis*-aconitase, NADH-ubiquinone oxidoreductase, and succinate-ubiquinone oxidoreductase. NO• also inhibits glyceraldehyde-3-phosphate dehydrogenase activity in hepatocytes, thereby influencing glucose metabolism. On exposure to an oxidizing hepatic toxin, NO• prevents the consumption of cell reducing equivalents (reduced glutathione). These several effects of NO• on hepatic function suggest that hepatoprotection results from a reduction in the metabolic activity of the cell, which conserves the cell's energy stores.

Cytotoxicity by NO• also appears to be important in the central nervous system. Following neuronal injury, large amounts of L-glutamate are released and elicit neurotoxicity by activation of *N*-methyl-D-asparate receptors. Activation of these receptors augments *nNOS* activity. While *nNOS*-containing neurons are resistant to the cytotoxic effects of receptor stimulation, NO• released from them is responsible for cytotoxicity in adjacent neurons. Interestingly, NO• may also be cytoprotective in the central nervous system, an effect that depends on the molecule's redox state: NO^+ reacts with the *N*-methyl-D-aspartate receptor and thereby limits entry of excessive Ca^{2+} into the cell cytosol; NO•, by contrast, promotes Ca^{2+} entry into the cell and thus cytotoxicity.

Impairment of NO• production by endothelial cells in disorders of endothelial dysfunction or following percutaneous angioplasty may help to facilitate smooth muscle proliferative responses in these settings. In addition, elevated NO• may contribute to cytotoxic mechanisms in *graft-versus-host disease* and in *transplant rejection*. The cytoprotective and cytotoxic effects of NO• are important and contrasting; the balance between them is determined by the local concentration of NO• in a given organ, the availability of other free radicals that can react with NO• to form other oxidative compounds (such as $O_2•$, which reacts with NO• to form $OONO^-$), and the susceptibility of the cell or organ to the toxic effects of oxidant stress.

THERAPEUTIC IMPLICATIONS
Therapeutic manipulation of NO• levels—by providing the compound or by inhibiting its production—has profound effects in many clinical settings. For over 100 years, congeners of NO•, the nitrovasodilators, have been used to provide exogenous NO• to dysfunctional coronary arteries. These agents, including nitroglycerin, isosorbide mononitrate and dinitrate, and nitroprusside, promote vasodilation and platelet inhibition and are metabolized to NO• (or NO^+) to achieve these effects. Inhibition of *iNOS* can be used to restore normal arterial pressures in the setting of *septic shock*; however, the risk of intravascular platelet thrombosis is increased by this approach in animals. Interestingly, glucocorticoids inhibit *Nos2* transcription, which may account for part of their protective effect in septic syndromes. Owing to the importance of NO• in penile erection, NO• donors may be useful for the treatment of *erectile impotence*.

Given the relative pulmonary selectivity of inhaled NO•, this gas may be useful at concentration of 10 to 40 ppm for the treatment of *persistent pulmonary hypertension of the newborn*, the pulmonary vasoconstriction that accompanies congenital diaphragmatic hernia, *primary pulmonary hypertension*, and *adult respiratory distress syndrome*. Higher concentration of inhaled NO• may be toxic, owing to the reaction of NO• with oxygen to produce NO_2.

NO• may also be useful in the inhibition of proliferative responses following vascular injury. Local delivery of a long-acting NO^+ donor or gene therapy with *Nos3* limits vascular smooth muscle proliferation following denuding endothelial injury, which suggests potentially useful therapies for limiting restenosis following angioplasty.

The simplicity of the NO• molecule belies its wide range of complex biologic, pathobiologic, and therapeutic effects. Our understanding of the biologic roles of this molecule and its potential therapeutic uses are in their infancy. With a clearer understanding of the organ-specific effects of NO•, its toxic and therapeutic potential in specific organ systems, and the mechanisms by which its actions may be inhibited or promoted, the full potential of this molecule as a therapeutic agent may be realized.

BIBLIOGRAPHY

IGNARRO LJ: Signal transduction mechanisms involving nitric oxide. Biochem Pharmacol 41:485, 1991

LOSCALZO J: Nitric oxide and vascular disease. N Engl J Med 333:251, 1995

———, WELCH G: Nitric oxide and its role in the cardiovascular system. Prog Cardiovasc Dis 38:87, 1995

MONCADA S, HIGGS EA: The L-arginine:nitric oxide pathway. N Engl J Med 329:2002, 1993

NATHAN C: Nitric oxide as a secretory product of mammalian cells. FASEB J 6:3051, 1992

STAMLER JS et al: Biochemistry of nitric oxide and its redox-activated forms. Science 258:1898, 1992

ZHANG J, SYNDER SH: Nitric oxide in the nervous system. Annu Rev Pharmacol Toxicol 35:213, 1995

72 | Margo Denke, Jean D. Wilson

NUTRITION AND NUTRITIONAL REQUIREMENTS

Adequate nutrition is essential for health and for the management of disease. Eating is intermittent, whereas energy needs are continuous. For example, it is essential to maintain a steady fuel supply to the brain, which requires about 5 g/h of glucose in both the fed and fasted states. To meet these needs, metabolic and hormonal controls promote the storage of nutrients during the absorptive state, largely in the form of glycogen and adipose tissue, and their retrieval in the postabsorptive period and during prolonged fasting. The stability of body weight requires that energy intake and expenditure be balanced over time. The internal signals that balance caloric intake with energy needs are poorly understood, but they do not operate on a meal-to-meal basis but rather over a period of days to make compensatory changes in the volume of food eaten. Long-term aberrations in these control factors can cause obesity on the one hand and anorexia on the other.

NUTRITIONAL REQUIREMENTS, ALLOWANCES, AND TOLERANCES The body contains thousands of types of molecules but requires for health the intake of only a small number of organic compounds—9 essential amino acids, 1 fatty acid, and 13 vitamins—in addition to sufficient energy, water, and minerals. The majority of organic compounds in food, although metabolized and assimilated by the body, are nonessential in the sense that their deletion from the diet does not cause illness. The simplicity of the nutritional requirements of the healthy individual, in contrast to the chemical complexity of the body, is the result of the remarkable capacity for endogenous synthesis of a vast number of organic molecules. The body tends to preserve its composition, and dietary factors modify body composition only to a limited degree; the vast majority of compounds ingested in food, including complex lipids, carbohydrates, waxes, and proteins, are broken down to their component parts, which are used for the de novo synthesis of fuels and body constituents.

In contrast, most inorganic molecules in food are nutritionally essential: calcium, phosphorus, potassium, sodium, chloride, and magnesium are major constituents of the body; moderate amounts of iron and zinc are required; and fluoride, copper, chromium, iodine, manganese, molybdenum, and selenium are required in trace amounts (less than 1 mg/d).

The requirement of an essential nutrient is defined as the smallest amount that maintains normal body mass, chemical composition, morphology, and physiologic function and prevents any clinical or chemical sign of the corresponding deficiency state. For most essential nutrients this value is exceedingly difficult to define even for healthy adults, and requirements may differ at different periods, as in the developing embryo, the growing child, and the lactating or pregnant women. Minimal requirements differ among normal individuals due to a variety of environmental, genetic, hormonal, and physiologic variables.

Consequently, at the clinical level the concept that nutritional standards should be based on absolute nutritional requirements has been replaced by that of the recommended dietary allowances (RDA), namely, the levels of intake of essential nutrients that, on the basis of scientific knowledge, are judged by the Food and Nutrition Board of the National Research Council to be adequate to meet the nutrient needs of healthy persons (Table 72-1). The RDAs have had a major impact on nutrition policy and on nutrition education; they are based on many types of evidence that vary in completeness and accuracy, including replacement studies in persons with nutrient deficiency, nutrient balance studies, biochemical assessments of function in relation to nutrient intake, the nutrient intakes of healthy people, epidemiologic studies of the relation between nutrient status and nutrient intake, and, in some cases, extrapolation of data from animal experiments. When data are insufficient for formulating a RDA, the category of *safe and adequate* is utilized by the Food and Nutrition Board, as in the case of biotin, copper, manganese, and molybdenum (Table 72-2). In principle, in formulating both the RDAs and the safe-and-adequate category, the minimal physiologic requirement is adjusted to encompass the variations in requirement and different efficiencies of utilization among individuals and differing bioavailability in different food sources. The aim of these recommendations (Tables 72-1 and 72-2) is to provide a safety factor appropriate to each nutrient by exceeding the actual requirements of most individuals. However, neither the RDA nor the safe-and-adequate category defines the level of a nutrient necessary for the optimal health of an individual.

Just as intake of any essential nutrient below a critical level causes disease, intake of many nutrients above a specific level disturbs body structure or function. Intake higher than the maximal daily tolerance can cause acute, progressive, or permanent disability. Obesity, fluorosis, atherosclerosis, hypervitaminosis A, and hypervitaminosis D are examples of the long-term consequences of excessive ingestion of nutrients; acute manifestations of dietary intolerances include nausea, abdominal cramps, vomiting, and diarrhea (excess food intake); arrhythmias (potassium intoxication); and hyponatremia (water intoxication). A healthy diet provides levels of nutrient intake between the two thresholds of minimal requirement and maximal tolerance. Recognition that tolerance for a nutrient can be exceeded is particularly important for parenteral nutrition, when the gastrointestinal mechanisms (fullness, emesis, incomplete absorption, diarrhea) that ordinarily help protect from the ill consequences of excess nutrient intake are bypassed. The maximal tolerance for many nutrients is uncertain. For example, it is not known whether very high intake of protein and/or amino acids by athletes and by food faddists is safe.

ALTERATIONS OF NUTRITIONAL REQUIREMENTS Both the RDA and maximal tolerance for each nutrient are influenced by a variety of factors: age, rate of growth, exercise, pregnancy and lactation, composition of the diet, concomitant diseases, and drugs. As the differences between requirement and tolerance narrow, the design of appropriate intake becomes more difficult, as in the appropriate protein intake for a cachectic patient with cirrhosis of the liver and hepatic encephalopathy.

Physiologic Factors Growth, strenuous exercise, pregnancy, and lactation (Tables 72-1 and 72-2) increase the requirements for energy and most essential nutrients. Under climatic extremes, nutritional requirements may either increase or decrease, depending on energy expenditure. In the elderly requirements for nutrients and energy per unit of lean body mass are the same as in younger individuals. However, because of decreased lean body mass and reduced activity in the very elderly, energy requirements usually decrease with age; for both social and medical reasons the elderly are particularly prone to the development of protein-energy malnutrition and to the deficiency of micronutrients such as ascorbic acid and folic acid.

Composition of the Diet Given diets with identical contents of nutrients, the biologic availability of the nutrients can vary. For example, all proteins do not have equal biologic value in terms of optimal amino acid content and the ability to support maximal linear growth in children; in particular, tryptophan content can vary widely among proteins. Protein in milk, eggs, and meat has high biologic value, whereas the proteins of corn (maize), soy flour, and wheat gluten have lower biologic value. Even when diets are adequate, individual factors

Table 72-1

Recommended Dietary Allowances[a]

Category	Age, years, or Condition	Weight[b], kg	(lb)	Height[b], cm	(in)	Protein (g)	Fat-Soluble Vitamins			
							Vitamin A, μg RE[c]	Vitamin D, μg[d]	Vitamin E, mg α-TE[e]	Vitamin K, μg
Infants	0.0–0.5	6	(13)	60	(24)	13	375	7.5	3	5
	0.5–1.0	9	(20)	71	(28)	14	375	10	4	10
Children	1–3	13	(29)	90	(35)	16	400	10	6	15
	4–6	20	(44)	112	(44)	24	500	10	7	20
	7–10	28	(62)	132	(52)	28	700	10	7	30
Males	11–14	45	(99)	157	(62)	45	1000	10	10	45
	15–18	66	(145)	176	(69)	59	1000	10	10	65
	19–24	72	(160)	177	(70)	58	1000	10	10	70
	25–50	79	(174)	176	(69)	63	1000	5	10	80
	51+	77	(170)	173	(68)	63	1000	5	10	80
Females	11–14	46	(101)	157	(62)	46	800	10	8	45
	15–18	55	(120)	163	(64)	44	800	10	8	55
	19–24	58	(128)	164	(65)	46	800	10	8	60
	25–50	63	(138)	163	(64)	50	800	5	8	65
	51+	65	(143)	160	(63)	50	800	5	8	65
Pregnant						60	800	10	10	65
Lactating	1st 6 months					65	1300	10	12	65
	2nd 6 months					62	1200	10	11	65

[a]The allowances, expressed as average daily intakes over time, are intended to provide for individual variations among most normal persons as they live in the United States under usual environmental stresses. Diets should be based on a variety of common foods in order to provide other nutrients for which human requirements have been less well defined.
[b]Weights and heights of Reference Adults are actual medians for the U.S. population of the designated age, as reported by National Health and Nutrition Examination Survey (NHANES) II.
[c]Retinol equivalents, 1 retinol equivalent = 1 μg retinol or 6 μg β-carotene.

can influence bioavailability, e.g., the absorption of calcium and magnesium may be impaired by phytates in the diet, and the absorption of nonheme iron is reduced in meals containing low amounts of ascorbic acid.

Route of Administration The nutrient recommendations in Tables 72-1 and 72-2 apply to food intake through the gastrointestinal tract. The absorption of ingested amino acids, carbohydrates, fats, sodium, chloride, and potassium is so efficient that the RDAs are the same for people on parenteral nutrition and on oral intake. However, for most minerals net absorption is only 50 percent or less, and the mineral requirements for parenteral nutrition are less than the oral requirements. Timing of administration can also be important. For example, since excess amino acids are not stored but are converted to fuel, all essential amino acids must be supplied simultaneously to support maximal protein synthesis.

Disease Disease can alter nutritional requirements and tolerances by a variety of mechanisms, including induction of anorexia (cancer, AIDS, gastrointestinal obstruction), increased utilization of nutrients (fever, infection, trauma, hemolysis, cancer, recovery from malnutrition), malabsorption (cystic fibrosis, sprue), impaired metabolism of nutrients (kidney and liver disease), nutrient wastage (burns, blood loss, nasogastric suction, diarrhea), hyperabsorption (hyperabsorptive hypercalciuria, hemochromatosis), impaired excretion (uremia), and drug therapy (cholestyramine, colestipol).

THE ESSENTIAL NUTRIENTS **Water** For practical purposes, 1 mL of water per kcal energy expenditure is appropriate for adults under average conditions. However, the risk of water intoxication is so remote that the suggested intake is often increased to 1.5 mL/kcal energy expenditure to allow for variations in activity level, sweating, and solute load. Normally, 50 to 100 mL/d of water is excreted in the feces, 500 to 1000 mL is lost by evaporation or exhalation, and 1000 mL or more is lost in urine. Water intake must equal these amounts to avoid under- or overhydration, particularly when external losses increase. Fecal losses may approach 5 L/d in severe diarrhea, and each degree Celsius of fever causes a daily loss of about 200 mL water. Provided renal function is normal and solute intake is adequate, most normal adults can safely excrete up to 18 L of urine per day because of the large capacity of the kidney to excrete free water.

Special attention must be given to the water needs of the elderly whose thirst sensation may be blunted. The increased water needs of

pregnancy only amount to about 30 mL/d, but during the first 6 months of lactation the additional water requirement approximates 1000 mL/d. Water requirements are increased in infants because of their larger surface area, the limited capacity of their kidneys to handle solute loads, and the limited ability to communicate their thirst.

Energy To maintain stable weight energy intake must equal energy output, namely, the energy expenditure required for basal energy expenditure (BEE), metabolism of food (specific dynamic action), and physical activity. The Harris-Benedict equations take into account weight (w, kg), height (h, cm), and age (a, years) in estimating BEE:

$$BEE_{women} = 655 + (9.5 \times w) + (1.8 \times h) - (4.7 \times a)$$
$$BEE_{men} = 66 + (13.7 \times w) + (5.0 \times h) - (6.8 \times a)$$

To this basal expenditure 30, 50, or 100 percent is added for sedentary, moderate, or strenuous activity. Nonstressed hospitalized patients usually require 120 percent of BEE, whereas catabolic patients require 150 to 200 percent of BEE to prevent tissue breakdown or allow anabolism. Energy expenditure is increased by fever (13 percent for each degree Celsius above normal), burns (40 to 100 percent), trauma (40 to 100 percent), and hyperthyroidism (10 to 100 percent). Patients with malabsorption may absorb as few as 25 percent of ingested calories, and it may be impossible to supply the increased energy needs of the sick by mouth if increased nutrient intake causes diarrhea. In such circumstances parenteral nutrition may be required to prevent progressive malnutrition. In hypometabolic states such as hypothyroidism or adrenal insufficiency, energy requirements are decreased. The hospitalized patient should be weighed daily, and energy intake should be adjusted appropriately.

Protein Dietary protein is a source of energy and supplies the mixture of amino acids for protein synthesis. Healthy adults require nine essential amino acids (threonine, valine, isoleucine, leucine, lysine, tryptophan, methionine-cystine, phenylalanine-tyrosine, and histidine) in amounts that vary from 250 to 1100 mg/d each. The requirement of dietary protein depends on the biologic value of the protein (determined primarily by the essential amino acid content). The biologic value of the major protein foods follows the general sequence: animal products > legumes > cereals (rice, wheat, corn) > roots. The adult RDA for protein (Table 72-1), about 0.6 g/kg body weight, assumes a high biologic value characteristic of animal protein; the lower the biologic value, the higher the protein requirement. The

Water-Soluble Vitamins							Minerals						
Vitamin C, mg	Thiamin, mg	Riboflavin, mg	Niacin, mg NE^f	Vitamin B$_6$, mg	Folate, μg	Vitamin B$_{12}$, μg	Calcium, mg	Phosphorus, mg	Magnesium, mg	Iron, mg	Zinc, mg	Iodine, μg	Selenium, μg
30	0.3	0.4	5	0.3	25	0.3	400	300	40	6	5	40	10
35	0.4	0.5	6	0.6	35	0.5	600	500	60	10	5	50	15
40	0.7	0.8	9	1.0	50	0.7	800	800	80	10	10	70	20
45	0.9	1.1	12	1.1	75	1.0	800	800	120	10	10	90	20
45	1.0	1.2	13	1.4	100	1.4	800	800	170	10	10	120	30
50	1.3	1.5	17	1.7	150	2.0	1200	1200	270	12	15	150	40
60	1.5	1.8	20	2.0	200	2.0	1200	1200	400	12	15	150	50
60	1.5	1.7	19	2.0	200	2.0	1200	1200	350	10	15	150	70
60	1.5	1.7	19	2.0	200	2.0	800	800	350	10	15	150	70
60	1.2	1.4	15	2.0	200	2.0	800	800	350	10	15	150	70
50	1.1	1.3	15	1.4	150	2.0	1200	1200	280	15	12	150	45
60	1.1	1.3	15	1.5	180	2.0	1200	1200	300	15	12	150	50
60	1.1	1.3	15	1.6	180	2.0	1200	1200	280	15	12	150	55
60	1.1	1.3	15	1.6	180	2.0	800	800	280	15	12	150	55
60	1.0	1.2	13	1.6	180	2.0	800	800	280	10	12	150	55
70	1.5	1.6	17	2.2	400	2.2	1200	1200	320	30	15	175	65
95	1.6	1.8	20	2.1	280	2.6	1200	1200	355	15	19	200	75
90	1.6	1.7	20	2.1	260	2.6	1200	1200	340	15	16	200	75

^d As cholecalciferol. 10 μg cholecalciferol = 400 IU of vitamin D.
^e α-Tocopherol equivalents. 1 mg d-α tocopherol = 1 α-TE.
^f 1 NE (niacin equivalent) is equal to 1 mg of niacin or 60 mg of dietary tryptophan.
SOURCE: Recommended Dietary Allowances, 10th edition, National Academy Press, 1989.

Table 72-2

Estimated Safe and Adequate Daily Dietary Intakes of Selected Vitamins and Minerals

Category		Trace Elements*					Vitamins	
	Age, years	Copper, mg	Manganese, mg	Fluoride, mg	Chromium, μg	Molybdenum, μg	Biotin, μg	Pantothenic Acid, mg
Infants	0–0.5	0.4–0.6	0.3–0.6	0.1–0.5	10–40	15–30	10	2
	0.5–1	0.6–0.7	0.6–1.0	0.2–1.0	20–60	20–40	15	3
Children and adolescents	1–3	0.7–1.0	1.0–1.5	0.5–1.5	20–80	25–50	20	3
	4–6	1.0–1.5	1.5–2.0	1.0–2.5	30–120	30–75	25	3–4
	7–10	1.0–2.0	2.0–3.0	1.5–2.5	50–200	50–150	30	4–5
	11+	1.5–2.5	2.0–5.0	1.5–2.5	50–200	75–250	30–100	4–7
Adults		1.5–3.0	2.0–5.0	1.5–4.0	50–200	75–250	30–100	4–7

* Since the toxic levels for many trace elements may be only several times usual intakes, the upper levels for the trace elements given in this table should not be habitually exceeded.
SOURCE: Recommended Dietary Allowances, 10th edition, National Academy Press, 1989.

requirement for protein is also influenced by energy intake; when the energy requirement is met by nonprotein calories, ingested amino acids can be used for protein synthesis, but when energy intake is deficient, ingested amino acids tend to be diverted into the pathways of glucose synthesis and oxidation. Thus, energy undernutrition makes the individual more vulnerable to protein starvation, a phenomenon that accounts for the high prevalence of combined protein-energy malnutrition (see Chap. 74).

Protein requirements are increased by growth, pregnancy, lactation, and repletion after malnutrition and are decreased in liver failure and renal insufficiency. The decreased requirement in liver failure occurs because the catabolism of essential and nonessential amino acids is slowed and in renal failure is due to the fact that ammonia can be reutilized for the synthesis of nonessential amino acids. In both renal failure and liver disease, the tolerance for dietary protein is also decreased, and normal protein intake can precipitate encephalopathy in patients with cirrhosis of the liver and worsen the uremic state in those with renal failure.

Fat The absolute requirement for fat is only 1 g/d of linoleic acid (polyunsaturated fat) for prostaglandin synthesis. The typical American diet contains about 35 percent of the calories from fat, but to minimize the development of atherosclerosis it is recommended that no more than 30 percent of the calories should be from fat and that no more than a third of the fat intake should be saturated fat. In general carbohydrate is the nutrient that replaces fat. Diets devoid of fat are less palatable and may result in protein-energy malnutrition if food selections are not made carefully.

Minerals and Vitamins The RDAs and safe daily intakes of the vitamins and minerals are listed in Tables 72-1 and 72-2, and the clinical disorders that result from their deficiencies are described in Chaps. 79, 80, and 354 to 357. It is critical to remember that the excessive intake of fat-soluble vitamins (Chap. 79), minerals (Chaps. 80, 354, 356, and 357), and electrolytes (fluorosis, hypertension, potassium toxicity) is particularly dangerous.

BIBLIOGRAPHY

ASKEW EW: Environmental and physical stress and nutrient requirements. Am J Clin Nutr 61(Suppl 3):631S, 1995

BEATON GH: Uses and limits of the use of the Recommended Dietary Allowances for evaluating dietary intake data. Am J Clin Nutr 41:155, 1985

ELIA M: Changing concepts of nutrient requirements in disease: Implications for artificial nutrition support. Lancet 345:1279, 1995

FOOD AND NUTRITION BOARD, COMMISSION ON LIFE SCIENCES, NATIONAL RESEARCH COUNCIL: Recommended Dietary Allowances, 10th ed. Washington DC, National Academy Press, 1989

KENDRICK ZV et al: Metabolic and nutritional considerations for exercising older adults. Compr Ther 20:558, 1994

REEDS PJ, HUTCHENS TW: Protein requirements: From nitrogen balance to functional impact. J Nutr 124(Suppl 9):1754S, 1994

ROSENBERG IH: Nutrient requirements for optimal health: What does that mean? J Nutr 124(Suppl 9):1777S, 1994

73 | Margo Denke, Jean D. Wilson

ASSESSMENT OF NUTRITIONAL STATUS

Nutritional deficiency is rare among healthy people who live in industrialized nations. High-quality dietary protein and other foods are abundant, virtually eliminating kwashiorkor and marasmus. Improved food preservation, packaging, and distribution have reduced seasonal variations in micronutrient intake. Fortification of foodstuffs with vitamins and essential minerals, such as iodine in salt, vitamin D in milk, and iron and B-complex vitamins in flour, has nearly eliminated once-common deficiency states such as iodine-deficient goiter, rickets, and folic acid deficiency. Indeed, in industrialized nations the prevalent nutritional disorder is obesity (see Chap. 75).

The success of these public health programs in preventing common dietary deficiencies has in some minds made the routine assessment of nutritional status obsolete, and nutritional diagnoses rarely appear in charts in workups or in progress notes. However, undernutrition makes a major contribution to morbidity and to mortality. Such deficiencies are often attributed to the underlying disease, but in many instances the compromise in nutritional status predates the development of disease, contributes to mortality, and impairs recovery. Routine assessment of the nutritional status is necessary to identify those situations in which nutritional intervention is essential for recovery.

The nutritional assessment is designed to evaluate three aspects of overall nutrition—energy, protein, and micronutrient balance—and has three components: the nutritional history, appropriate physical examination with simple anthropometric measurements, and laboratory studies.

THE NUTRITIONAL HISTORY Nutritional assessment should begin with a chronologic record of body weight and changes in body weight (Table 72-1). Inquiry as to the individual's weight at life milestones such as graduation from high school, college, or marriage can facilitate this assessment. Significant changes in weight should be investigated carefully. Did the weight change follow changes in physical activity, alterations in dietary intake, or changes in health status? Hip fracture is often preceded by weight loss, and hypertension, hyperlipidemia, and insulin resistance are often associated with weight gain. It should be kept in mind that change in weight can sometimes be ambiguous, particularly in the presence of edema. Furthermore, an initially obese individual can lose 15 kg because of a wasting illness and present with a normal body weight, despite shrinkage of lean body mass. In such circumstances estimation of muscle mass should be made by balance techniques as described below.

A healthy person consuming a variety of foods is unlikely to have a dietary deficiency, but not all individuals consume a varied diet. To evaluate dietary intake, the patient should be asked to list everything eaten in the past 24 h (breakfast, lunch, dinner, and snacks), and this information can be used to determine the variety and adequacy of food consumed (Table 73-1). In a typical day, does the patient consume several servings of different fruits and vegetables and calcium-containing foods? What food groups are missing? Is the portion size adequate, too large, or too small? Are meals prepared by the patient or someone else? Do social, medical, or dental problems restrict food choices?

Illness can affect weight by several mechanisms, including reduced dietary intake from anorexia or because energy intake does not increase sufficiently to meet the increased demands from fever, infection, or trauma. The diagnostic workup itself may contribute to weight loss by requiring fasting for testing or diagnostic procedures. Drug therapy may alter taste or reduce appetite, leading to weight loss. Not all illnesses cause weight loss; when the major effect on energy balance

is a reduction in physical activity, weight gain can occur if energy intake remains unchanged or increases.

Acute and chronic illnesses increase the demands for energy, protein, and micronutrients. Protein requirements may triple in severe illnesses. Patients whose intake is restricted for any reason are at higher risk for nutritional deficiencies. When the initial assessment suggests dietary inadequacy, a formal assessment by a registered dietician is indicated.

In chronic illness, the duration, severity, and time course of weight loss or weight gain—steady, progressively worsening, waxing and waning—can provide a chronologic account of the course of the illness and of concomitant changes in appetite and physical activity. The nutritional history should encompass previous attempts to improve body weight and the presumed reasons for the success or failure of the attempts.

Nutrient Processing. Perhaps the most overlooked aspect of the nutritional history is the complex process by which nutrients and energy are absorbed (Table 73-2). The processing of food begins with appetite. Either anorexia or nausea can compromise the ability to maintain adequate intake. Do foods taste metallic or unpleasant? Are there mechanical difficulties with chewing such as poorly fitting dentures? Is there any difficulty swallowing? Is early satiety or a lack of satiety present? Is eating associated with gastrointestinal discomfort such as vomiting or diarrhea? Have there been changes in consistency, odor, and frequency of bowel movements? Queries regarding nutrient processing can uncover social problems, eating disorders, mechanical barriers to food ingestion, and malabsorption, any of which can alter nutritional status.

Associated Conditions That Increase Nutritional Demands Pregnancy, lactation, and, in children, periods of rapid growth increase metabolic demands and the requirements for specific nutrients. A series of acute illnesses, each in themselves self-limiting, can cumulatively compromise nutrition if adjustments are not made in food intake. A catalogue of these events and their duration and impact on general health status may help identify patients at risk.

Nutrient Supplements and Medication History Listing the amount and frequency of nutritional supplements together with both prescription and over-the-counter medications will provide insight as to whether intake of specific vitamins is excessive. Some medications alter nutrient bioavailability (see examples, Table 73-3), and use of these drugs should prompt inquiries regarding the intake of the nutrient affected.

PHYSICAL EXAMINATION Weight should be recorded at every outpatient visit. The presence and severity of edema or ascites should be noted, since these findings alter the interpretation of weight. Absolute body weight and changes in body weight have prognostic implications. Illness-associated weight loss of 10 to 20 percent over a period of 6 months or less can cause functional impairment of multiple organ systems. If weight loss exceeds 20 percent during illness, protein-energy malnutrition may be present.

Weight should be measured daily in the hospitalized patient. Total starvation causes a loss of approximately 0.4 kg/d of body weight; semi-starvation causes lesser degrees of weight loss. Most weight loss with starvation is initially from stored adipose tissue and then from catabolism of skeletal muscle protein and liver protein; other organ proteins are spared until wasting is extreme. Rapid increases in weight in the hospital setting are rarely due to increases in lean or fat mass. Hydration rapidly increases total body water and sodium, and renal compensation may be delayed. Rapid weight gain may occur when a starving patient is refed carbohydrate, replenishing glycogen stores and increasing hepatic water content.

Height should be measured annually and on every hospital admission. This measurement is of particular importance for detecting loss of height in subjects with metabolic bone disease and should be made with the patient standing straight and looking straight ahead. When loss in height is suspected and for individuals who cannot stand unassisted, maximal height can be estimated using knee height. Knee height is the distance between the sole of the foot to the anterior surface of the compressed thigh above the condyles of the femur and just proximal to the patella. It is measured with the patient in a sitting or recumbent position. Knee height is affected little by age or by changes in weight and can be calculated as follows:

$$\text{Height in men (cm)} = 64.19 - (0.04 \times \text{age}) + [2.2 \times \text{knee height (cm)}]$$

$$\text{Height in women (cm)} = 84.88 - (0.24 \times \text{age}) + [1.83 \times \text{knee height (cm)}]$$

Determination of *body mass index* (BMI) or *weight-for-frame size* provides insight as to whether the current weight is appropriate for the individual.

Body Mass Index   Assessment of BMI (weight in kg divided by height in m²) has the advantage of simplicity and is useful for

Table 73-1

Nutritional Assessment

Ambulatory Patients	Acute Illness	Chronic Illness
ENERGY REQUIREMENTS		
Body weight and weight for height are indices of energy balance. Imbalance between energy intake and expenditure causes weight loss or weight gain. Track weight at life milestones (graduation, marriage, etc.). Are changes in weight voluntary or involuntary?	Acute illness affects both components of energy balance. Illness can reduce appetite and energy intake and increase energy demands because of fever, infection, and trauma or decrease energy demands because of reduced physical activity.	Chronic illness requires a long-term adaptation to changes in energy balance. The duration of compromise and previous attempts to correct energy balance may provide insight into the disturbances in energy balance.
PROTEIN REQUIREMENTS		
Most patients meet their protein requirements from a combination of foods and not a single food. For example, 0.5% by weight of cooked vegetables, 4% of milk, 23% of meat, and 10% of uncooked pasta is protein. 40 g of protein (sufficient for 50-kg person) is contained in any of the following: 200 g fish, poultry, red meat; 150 g tree nuts; 130 g peanuts or peanut butter; 200 g brick cheese; 7 eggs or 12 egg whites; 400 g cooked rice plus 470 g cooked beans; 500 g tofu; 1000 g milk. Normal daily protein requirements: 0.8–1.0 g/kg	Illness may increase protein demands through: 1. Higher metabolic rates 2. Protein losses from skin (burns, exfoliation), gastrointestinal tract (protein losing enteropathy), or kidney (proteinuria) Daily protein requirements 1. Moderately stressed: 1.0–2.0 g/kg (infection, fractures, surgery) 2. Severely stressed: 2.0–2.5 g/kg (burns, multiple fractures)	Chronic illness may increase the demand for dietary protein: Nephrotic syndrome: dietary protein intake must be increased to compensate for protein loss or protein depletion can occur Chronic infection: increased catabolism of protein for energy; protein requirements typically double to maintain adequate pool of amino acids for synthesis of new protein Hyperthyroidism: increased metabolic rate, leading to a higher rate of catabolism of protein for energy; protein requirements may double Psoriasis: increased protein loss from skin; dietary protein requirements increase proportional to losses
MICRONUTRIENT REQUIREMENTS		
By assessing the variety of intake, risk for vitamin deficiency can be assessed. This assessment is particularly important for patients with a fixed income or who live alone.	Acute illness is self-limited; micronutrients most likely to be affected are rapid-turn over B vitamins.	Chronic illness may alter absorption of micronutrients: Gastric resection: impairs calcium and iron absorption if duodenum is bypassed Resection of proximal small intestine: impairs absorption of calcium, folic acid, water-soluble vitamins Resection of distal small intestine: impairs absorption of B_{12} and bile salts

Vitamin A — Meat, milk, egg, leafy green and deep yellow vegetables
Thiamine — Meat, milk, egg, enriched flour
Riboflavin — Meat, milk, egg
Niacin — Meat, starchy vegetables and grains
Vitamin B_6 — Meat, starchy vegetables
Vitamin B_{12} — Milk, meat, egg
Folic acid, pantothenic acid — Ubiquitous
Vitamin C — Vegetables, fruit, milk
Vitamin D — Fortified milk, meat
Vitamin E — Leafy green and deep yellow vegetables, meat, egg, fruit, milk
Iron — Meat, spinach, raisins, enriched flour, lentils
Calcium — Dairy products

Drugs may also alter micronutrient needs:
Chloroquine, levodopa, theophylline may induce a loss of appetite; propylthiouracil, rifampin change taste
Hydroxyzine, imipramine increase appetite
Ethanol excess may lead to a malabsorption of thiamine, B_{12}, and folate
Phenytoin, phenobarbital, primidone may reduce levels of folate, vitamin B_6, and vitamin B_{12} and increase vitamin D requirements
Methotrexate lowers folate levels by promoting folate excretion
Antimalarials (pyrimethamine and sulfadiazine) and the antibiotics (penicillins, sulfonamides) can reduce folate levels
Sodium bicarbonate may reduce folate absorption due to decreased jejunal pH
Salicylate may increase vitamin C and folate excretion and cause iron deficiency if gastrointestinal blood loss occurs
H_2 blockers impair B_{12} absorption, probably by reduced acid and pepsin production
Nonsteroidal anti-inflammatory agents may cause iron deficiency from gastrointestinal blood loss
Glucocorticoids increase calcium loss from bone

assessing both over- and undernutrition. A normal BMI is defined as 18.5 to 24.9 kg/m². Overweight is a BMI of 25.0 to 29.9 kg/m², obesity is a BMI of 30.0 to 39.9 kg/m², and morbid obesity is a BMI > 40 kg/m². Conversely, the risk for protein-energy malnutrition can be graded as mild: BMI = 17.0 to 18.4 kg/m²; moderate: BMI = 16.0 to 16.9 kg/m²; and severe: BMI < 16.0 kg/m². A BMI of 13 to 15 kg/m² suggests that the total body fat content is less than 5 percent of weight. The BMI is simple and is a widely used means of estimating energy balance, but it does not take into account differences in frame size.

Weight-for-Frame Size Frame size is conventionally divided into three categories—small, medium, and large. Large skeletons require greater muscle mass for locomotion. Actuarial tables such as those of the Metropolitan Life Insurance Company classify ranges of weight associated with lower mortality in terms of frame size. Whereas some databases use wrist circumference as a measure of frame size, the breadth of the epicondyle of the humerus is a more accurate index of frame size (Table 73-4) because its measurement is less influenced by subcutaneous fat. On the basis of frame size, height, and gender, valuable insight can be obtained as to appropriate ideal weights for the individual and how far the actual weight deviates from this norm (Table 73-5). In patients with amputations, adjustments for the missing extremity should be made before this value can be interpreted. For example, 7.1 percent of body weight should be subtracted from the reference weight for an above-the-knee amputation, and 18.6 percent should be subtracted if the entire leg is amputated. Such tables have to be interpreted with caution in pregnant women, for whom special tables must be used.

In addition to weight, which provides assessment of overall energy balance, it is often useful to have insight into specific aspects of *body composition*, particularly into fat and muscle (protein or nitrogen) mass. Caliper measurements of skin-fold thickness provide a useful index of *fat mass*. The triceps skin thickness differs with frame size and height (Table 73-6). This assessment does not provide much information beyond the measurement of BMI or weight-for-frame size in evaluating the obese but is particularly useful in identifying those individuals whose fat stores are dangerously depleted. More direct techniques to measure percent body fat such as underwater weighing, x-ray absorptiometry, and nuclear magnetic resonance imaging can also be employed under some circumstances.

Muscle mass can either be assessed as a part of the laboratory evaluation or measured directly as part of the physical examination. Midarm circumference is a function of muscle mass, skin, subcutaneous fat,

Table 73-3

Body Mass Index* (kg/m²) by Gender for Blacks and Whites, Ages 18 to 50

Percentile	Blacks		Whites	
	Men	**Women**	**Men**	**Women**
5th	18.8	18.4	19.6	18.4
50th	22.2	25.8	25.0	22.9

* Based on data from the National Health and Nutrition Examination Survey I.

Table 73-4

Frame Size Defined by Elbow Breadth* (cm)

Age	Men			Women		
	Small†	**Medium**	**Large†**	**Small**	**Medium**	**Large**
18–24	≤ 6.6	6.6 to 7.7	≥ 7.7	≤ 5.6	5.6 to 6.5	≥ 6.5
25–34	≤ 6.7	6.7 to 7.9	≥ 7.9	≤ 5.7	5.7 to 6.8	≥ 6.8
35–44	≤ 6.7	6.7 to 8.0	≥ 8.0	≤ 5.7	5.7 to 7.1	≥ 7.1
45–54	≤ 6.7	6.7 to 8.1	≥ 8.1	≤ 5.7	5.7 to 7.2	≥ 7.2
55–64	≤ 6.7	6.7 to 8.1	≥ 8.1	≤ 5.8	5.8 to 7.2	≥ 7.2
65–74	≤ 6.7	6.7 to 8.1	≥ 8.1	≤ 5.8	5.8 to 7.2	≥ 7.2

* Based on data from the combined National Health and Nutrition Examination Surveys I and II.
† By definition, small frame and large frame each account for 15% of U.S. population.
SOURCE: AR Frisancho, Am J Clin Nutr 40:808, 1984.

bone, and the neurovascular bundle of the arm, and of these parameters the amounts of muscle, skin, and fat are determined by nutritional state. Skin and subcutaneous fat are corrected for by subtracting the triscapular skin-fold before calculating the area of muscle mass:

Midarm muscle area

$$= \frac{[\text{Arm circumference} - (\pi \times \text{triscapular skin fold})]^2}{4\pi}$$

where all measurements are in centimeters. This assessment is a valuable means of identifying protein malnutrition, a particular problem in the elderly. Table 73-7 contains midarm muscle values from the National Health and Nutrition Examination Surveys (NHANES) I and II. In comparing the observed with the controlled values, certain caveats should be noted. The midarm muscle circumference also measures the humerus and neurovascular structures, which do not decrease in size with weight loss, and in some tables the bone mass in the arm is corrected for by subtracting 10 cm² for men or 6.5 cm² for women as an estimate of the size of the humerus; since these values are constants this subtraction is clinically unimportant. Atrophic muscle has more water, total lipid, and collagen than normal muscle, and, as a consequence, the mass of functional muscle in deconditioned or cachectic patients is probably overestimated by this technique.

LABORATORY ASSESSMENT
Routine laboratory measurements do not provide a sensitive index of the level of nutrition because changes in the levels of serum proteins occur late in the course of malnutrition but can, under some circumstances, be useful for assessing the effectiveness of nutritional intervention. For the ambulatory patient, laboratory assessment should be focused on potential deficiencies identified by history and physical examination. However, insufficient dietary protein and energy intake is not the only cause of low serum protein levels in illness because serum protein levels can be influenced by many factors.

Table 73-2

Nutrient Processing

Ambulatory Patients	Acute Illness	Chronic Illness
All patients should be queried about the process of nutrient assimilation: Appetite Mastication Swallowing Bite size Meal size Meal frequency Satiety Heartburn Dyspepsia Belching Bloating Diarrhea Constipation Foul-smelling stools Light/dark-colored stools Flatulence	Are changes in nutrient processing: 1. Temporally related to disease? 2. Temporally related to treatment?	Same as acutely ill patient, *plus* ascertain previous attempts to address problems such as: 1. Reducing drug dosages that alter appetite 2. Improving denture fitting 3. Trial of special meals such as pureed foods, high-fiber diets, low-acid foods 4. Improved meal planning and delivery 5. Controlling gastrointestinal symptoms after eating

Table 73-5

CHAPTER 73
Assessment of Nutritional Statuss   451

5th and 50th Percentiles of Weight for Frame Size, Height, and Gender,* Ages 25 to 74

| Height in cm (in Foam Slippers) | Weight in kg (in Examination Clothing) | | | | | |
| | Small | | Medium | | Large | |
	5th	50th	5th	50th	5th	50th
MEN						
157	46	64	51	68	57	82
160	48	61	52	71	58	83
163	49	66	54	71	59	84
165	52	66	59	74	60	79
168	56	67	58	75	60	84
170	56	71	62	77	62	84
173	56	71	60	78	63	86
175	57	74	63	78	68	89
178	59	75	64	81	68	87
180	60	76	62	81	73	91
183	62	74	68	84	73	91
185	63	79	70	85	72	93
188	65	80	68	88	69	92
WOMEN						
147	37	52	41	60	56	86
150	42	53	47	66	56	78
152	42	53	47	60	55	87
155	44	54	47	61	54	81
157	44	55	49	61	59	81
160	46	55	49	62	58	83
163	49	57	50	62	59	79
165	50	60	52	63	59	81
168	46	58	52	63	55	75
170	47	59	54	65	58	80
173	48	62	58	67	51	76
175	49	63	49	68	50	79
178	50	64	50	70	50	76

* Based on data from the combined National Health and Nutrition Examination Surveys I and II.

This problem is illustrated by *serum albumin*. Dehydration can lead to concentration of all plasma components and cause apparent increase in albumin levels. Shifts from intra- to extravascular spaces with surgery or burn injuries lower serum albumin levels, whereas semi-starvation shifts albumin to the intravascular space and may increase albumin levels more than total protein levels. Albumin synthesis can decline during acute illness, as synthesis of acute phase reactants increases, and physiologic stress can increase albumin catabolism. Albumin concentrations can also fall as a result of accelerated losses from skin, kidney, or gastrointestinal tract. Whereas dehydration and shifts between the intra- and extravascular spaces cause early alterations in serum albumin levels, changes in synthesis and catabolism do not alter serum albumin concentrations for several days because the half-life of serum albumin is normally 18 to 20 days. Serum albumin concentrations usually reach a nadir 5 to 7 days after the onset of a self-limiting illness, and it is common for serum albumin to fall 5 g/L after elective surgery. Measurement of serum proteins with shorter half-lives can provide a more accurate assessment of protein status. *Transferrin* has a half-life of 8 to 9 days, and *prealbumin*

Table 73-6

Assessment of Body Fat as Indicated by the 5th and 50th Percentiles of Triceps Skin Fold Thickness by Frame Size and Gender, Ages 25 to 74

| | Triceps Skin Fold, mm | | | | | |
| | Small Frame | | Medium Frame | | Large Frame | |
	5th	50th	5th	50th	5th	50th
Men	5	10	5	12	6	14
Women	10	20	12	24	16	32

* Based on data from the combined National Health and Nutrition Examination Surveys I and II.

Table 73-7

Assessment of Muscle Mass as Indicated by the 5th and 50th Percentiles of Midarm Muscle Area by Frame Size and Gender*

| | Midarm Muscle Area, cm² | | | | | |
| | Small Frame | | Medium Frame | | Large Frame | |
Age	5th	50th	5th	50th	5th	50th
MEN						
25–54	42	55	49	65	56	72
55–74	37	55	46	62	51	66
WOMEN						
25–54	26	33	28	37	32	46
55–74	26	35	29	40	35	50

* Based on data from the combined National Health and Nutrition Examination Surveys I and II.

has a half-life of 2 to 3 days. Unfortunately, the levels of these proteins in serum are affected by the same factors that influence albumin level. Measurement of serum proteins can be helpful in predicting prognosis. Low serum albumin in the chronically ill is associated with longer hospital stays, frequent readmissions for poor wound healing and infection, and increased mortality. Laboratory assessment can also help monitor intervention. If dietary protein is responsible for low serum protein levels, serum prealbumin levels rapidly increase in response to increased dietary protein.

Measurement of 24-h urinary creatinine can provide a simple estimate of *lean body mass* by the following equation:

Lean body mass (kg) = 7.138 + 0.02908 × urine creatinine (mg)

The ratio of 24-h urinary creatinine (mg) to height (cm) is another widely used index of muscle mass. In normal men ratios average 10.5 mg/cm, and ratios from 8.4 to 9.5 mg/cm, 7.4 to 8.4 mg/cm, and <7.4 mg/cm signify mild, moderate, and severe degrees of protein malnutrition, respectively. The usefulness of this measurement is tempered by the fact that urinary creatinine is impaired by renal failure and can be influenced by dietary protein intake, exercise, emotional stress, infection, fever, and trauma. As an index of response to replenishment regimens, a bedside estimate of daily nitrogen balance can be made as follows using daily measurements of protein intake and of 24-h urine urea nitrogen:

$$\text{N balance (g)} = \frac{\text{protein intake (g)}}{6.25} - \text{urine urea nitrogen (g)} + 2.5 \text{ g}$$

where 2.5 g is the approximate amount of fecal, integumental, and urinary nonurea nitrogen loss per day. This value provides an estimate of the change in protein mass during the period of observation but does not assess protein mass at the beginning or end of the intervention.

Regarding micronutrient adequacy, vitamin levels do not reflect vitamin stores with the exception of vitamin B_{12} (see Chap. 108), folate (see Chap. 108), and vitamin D (see Chaps. 354 and 355), and the diagnosis of vitamin deficiency is usually made on the basis of a high index of suspicion and documenting the response to specific replacement (see Chap. 79). Assessment of mineral status, particularly measurements of phosphorus, magnesium, calcium, potassium, and iron, is more useful clinically, although serum levels do not always change in parallel with body stores.

OVERALL ASSESSMENT The assessment of nutritional status is an important component of the history, physical examination, and laboratory evaluation. The intensity of the evaluation should match the severity of the illness and the degree of suspected malnutrition. For the ambulatory patient with adequate nutritional status, the focus should be on identifying potential factors that could produce future nutritional compromise, including change in weight, and guarding against impairment of nutrient processing.

For the hospitalized patient with acute or chronic illness, the most pressing issue is to identify that subset of patients with such severe nutritional compromise (fifth percentile or lower) that nutritional intervention is an essential component of acute management. For example, in a patient who cannot swallow because of a stroke it is appropriate to delay parenteral nutrition or assisted enteral nutrition for a week or 10 days if nutritional status is adequate, whereas delay of nutritional support might be disastrous in a cachectic individual. In most acute, self-limited disease, the focus should be on defining the interaction between the acute illness and the underlying nutritional state (weight, variety of dietary intake, and nutrient processing). The goal is to detect reversible factors that could influence the course of the disease and the risks for future complications. In chronic illness, the aim is to identify factors that contribute to nutritional compromise and to evaluate the effect of the nutritional compromise on the course of the illness. Anthropometric and laboratory measurements can be useful in this regard, but the basis of nutritional assessment rests on history and physical examination.

BIBLIOGRAPHY

GRANT A, DEHOOG S: Nutritional Assessment and Support, 1991. Anne Grant/Susan DeHoog, P.O. Box 75057 Northgate Station, Seattle, WA 98125

KERSTETTER JE et al: Malnutrition in the institutionalized older adult. *J Am Diet Assoc* 92:1109, 1992

LIPKIN EW, BELL S: Assessment of nutritional status. The clinician's perspective. *Clin Lab Med* 13:329, 1993

MANNING EM, SHENKIN A: Nutritional assessment in the critically ill. *Crit Care Clin* 11:603, 1995

MOWE M et al: Reduced nutritional status in an elderly population (>70 y) is probable before disease and possibly contributes to the development of disease. *Am J Clin Nutr* 59:317, 1994

OTTERY FD: Supportive nutrition to prevent cachexia and improve quality of life. *Semin Oncol* 22:98, 1995

SCHWENK A et al: Clinical risk factors for malnutrition in HIV-1-infected patients. *AIDS* 7:1213, 1993

SUITOR CW: Nutritional assessment of the pregnant woman. *Clin Obstet Gynecol* 37:501, 1994

74	*Margo Denke, Jean D. Wilson*

PROTEIN AND ENERGY MALNUTRITION

Insufficient consumption of protein and energy causes loss of both body mass and adipose tissue, although one or the other loss may predominate in a given individual. Protein-energy malnutrition (PEM) occurs primarily under two circumstances: in developing nations it may be present in endemic form, and under famine conditions the prevalence may approach 25 percent. The primary disorder occurs when socioeconomic factors limit the quantity and quality of food; it is a particular problem when vegetable proteins of low biologic value are major components of the diet and when the incidence of infectious diseases is high. The problem is accentuated when energy intake is insufficient so that dietary proteins are oxidized as fuel rather than utilized for the synthesis of body protein. In children of developing nations two syndromes of PEM have been distinguished: (1) *marasmus*, manifested by stunted growth, loss of adipose tissue, generalized wasting of protein mass, and no edema, is thought to be due to the combined effects of protein and energy malnutrition; and (2) *kwashiorkor*, manifested by growth failure, edema, hypoalbuminemia, fatty liver, and preservation of subcutaneous fat, is thought to be due to selective protein malnutrition. Mixed forms are common in both children and adults, and the distinction between pure protein malnutrition and PEM has little clinical significance.

In developed nations PEM occurs most commonly as a secondary disorder in people who were previously well nourished who develop the disorder in association with subacute or chronic illness. Predisposing features include anorexia, hypermetabolism, malabsorption, and drug and alcohol abuse, and, in the aged, depression, isolation, and low income may play a role. As many as half of the hospitalized elderly are malnourished at admission or develop nutritional deficits during hospitalization. Synergism between primary and secondary causes is common in that those individuals with scanty reserves of protein and energy develop clinical PEM more rapidly than well-nourished subjects when challenged by hypermetabolism, the anorexia of infection, or other catabolic illness.

EPIDEMIOLOGY The prevalence among a given population can be assessed by measuring subcutaneous fat, midarm muscle area, or the ratio of 24-h urine creatinine to height (Chap. 73). The magnitude of the problem worldwide is immense. In 1983 the World Health Organization estimated that 300 million children had growth retardation secondary to malnutrition; the consequences for mortality, cognitive function, social organization, and economic development are dire but impossible to quantify. Preschool children in developing countries are particularly susceptible, because of their dependence on others for food, their higher protein and energy requirements, and their enhanced susceptibility to infection, especially under nonhygienic conditions. Gastrointestinal infections frequently precipitate clinical PEM because of the associated diarrhea, associated anorexia, vomiting, increased metabolic needs, and decreased intestinal absorption; parasitic infections play a major role in the problem in many parts of the world.

In the United States protein deficiency in adults tends to be mild and subclinical, but poor nutrition is not limited to the adult poor. In one survey that focused on low-income areas of the United States, 22 to 35 percent of children 2 to 6 years old were below the 15th percentile for weight, and in another survey 11 percent of low-income children had height-for-age measurements below the 5th percentile. In hospitalized patients, severe as well as mild deficiencies are even more common. Moreover, the nutritional status of patients frequently declines during hospitalization, and the occurrence of postoperative infections, time required for the healing of surgical wounds, and duration of hospitalization are increased in such individuals, a disturbing phenomenon since malnutrition is both preventable and reversible.

PATHOPHYSIOLOGY When energy intake falls below the minimal requirements, the body responds with an orderly physiologic adaptation (Chap. 335), involving the hormones of energy metabolism, that causes mobilization of free fatty acids from adipose tissue and of amino acids from muscle to provide energy for the oxidative needs of the body and in particular of the brain. As amino acids are diverted into gluconeogenesis and oxidation, protein synthesis is curtailed, the metabolic rate declines, and lean body mass and adipose tissue contract. During the first week of starvation, 4 to 5 kg of body weight is lost, consisting of about 25 percent adipose tissue, 35 percent extracellular fluid, and 40 percent protein. During ensuing weeks, losses continue but at a slower pace. Different compartments contract at different rates: skeletal muscle faster than cardiac muscle; gastrointestinal tract and liver faster than kidney. Mobilization of amino acids from muscle supports the synthesis of some albumin so that hypoalbuminemia develops late.

The intake of protein can be more limiting than that of energy when proteins of low biologic value (chiefly vegetable proteins) are the major proteins of the diet or when glucose is the sole organic nutrient in the intravenous feeding of patients who cannot eat. The consequence in either case is to enhance insulin secretion, which in turn retards lipolysis of adipose tissue, preserves adipose tissue mass, and inhibits the mobilization of amino acids from muscle. Amino acid levels decline, and the synthesis of albumin and other proteins is impaired; hypoalbuminemia and edema are characteristic features, and fatty infiltration of the liver ensues. As stated above, these findings are typical of kwashiorkor.

Depletion of body minerals is in part due to contraction of body mass and extracellular fluid, but potassium and magnesium may be lost out of proportion to body mass due to shifts from intracellular stores. Deficiency of mineral intake (as in the patient in whom intravenous glucose is the sole energy source) and enhanced losses (diuresis, diarrhea, fistulas, etc.) may worsen mineral deficits.

Simple starvation, as described above, does not quickly lead to death but induces a gradual metabolic adaptation that involves the shift of the metabolism of the central nervous system to the oxidation of fatty acids and ketone bodies for energy and a profound reduction in the metabolic rate that conserves the residual protein stores. Starvation in the context of physical stress is considerably more deleterious. The extent to which the effects of stress are due to the direct metabolic consequences of inflammation, infection, fever, and wound healing as compared to the indirect consequences of the release of inflammatory cytokines such as tumor necrosis factor α, interleukin 2, and interleukin 6 is not clear, but the addition of stress to starvation increases the metabolic rate and accelerates the loss of weight and of nitrogen and micronutrients. It is for these reasons that severe PEM develops when both malnutrition and stress are present. It is of particular interest in this regard that PEM is a prominent feature of AIDS, where it is thought to be the consequence of anorexia (and diminished intake), fever, and diarrhea.

CLINICAL MANIFESTATIONS **Mild to Moderate PEM** Children fail to gain height and weight; adults generally lose weight, although edema may mask weight loss. Alternatively, if the individual was previously obese, loss of protoplasm can be hidden by a residue of fat. Triceps skin-fold thickness and midarm muscle area are reduced (see Tables 73-6 and 73-7). In the absence of renal disease the ratio of 24-h urine creatinine to height is a sensitive indicator of protein malnutrition and should be measured at weekly intervals. Levels of albumin, transferrin, and prealbumin in serum may be low. Serum triiodothyronine is decreased, the level of reverse triiodothyronine is increased, and the metabolic rate is low. Peripheral lymphopenia may be present, and glucose tolerance may be impaired. The heart size tends to be small.

Severe PEM Severe PEM is characterized by more profound abnormalities in body composition and in laboratory findings. Decrease in muscle mass is evident on physical examination, as indicated by excavation of the intercostal spaces and wasting of the temporal muscles and extremities, and subcutaneous adipose tissue is decreased or absent. Listlessness, easy fatigability, sensation of coldness, dry cracked skin, drawn facies, and dyspigmentation of the skin and hair are common. Decubiti and skin ulcers occur in advanced stages. Blood pressure is low, the pulse is decreased, and temperature may be low. There is a global impairment of organ system function.

Cardiovascular/renal/pulmonary The ventilatory response to hypoxia is blunted. During the course of malnutrition the heart and kidneys lose mass in proportion to the loss of lean body mass and the fall in metabolic rate, so that cardiac output and glomerular filtration rate are appropriate for body size and the metabolic state. However, congestive heart failure can occur during vigorous nutritional and volume repletion, with infection, and during other physical stresses.

Blood Blood volume, hematocrit, serum albumin, transferrin, and lymphocyte count are decreased. The anemia is normocytic and normochromic and is usually due to decreased red blood cell production, thought to reflect the general decrease in protein biosynthesis. Deficiencies of iron, folate, and pyridoxine may contribute to the anemia.

Metabolic rate In the absence of fever, basal metabolic rate falls and hypothermia is common, possibly the consequence of diminished levels of triiodothyronine and of the loss of the insulating protection of subcutaneous fat. Hypoglycemia may be a terminal event.

Gastrointestinal tract and pancreas Atrophy of the gastrointestinal tract involves the intestinal villi and both the exocrine and endocrine functions of the pancreas, and bacterial overgrowth may occur in the small intestine. Malabsorption and lactose intolerance may be present. The gastrointestinal manifestations may result, at least in part, from decreased oral feeding rather than starvation, since similar changes occur in individuals fully nourished by parenteral feeding.

Immune system Cell-mediated immunity is impaired, as indicated by all standard tests, whereas antibody responses are generally intact. Common infections and opportunistic infections can lead to increased morbidity and mortality. Pneumonia is common.

FIGURE 74-1 Hypothetical course of a typical patient with protein-energy malnutrition.

Wound healing All wounds and incisions heal more slowly in PEM. Wound dehiscence is common.

Reproduction Nearly every aspect of reproduction is impaired in the woman with PEM, including implantation, fetal growth, lactation, and parturition, and the infants are stunted in size and may have cognitive impairment if they survive.

COURSE A hypothetical course is illustrated in Fig. 74-1. In children slowing of growth is usually the first manifestation. Anemia, hypoalbuminemia, and amenorrhea follow, and loss of cell-mediated immunity predisposes to infection. The hypermetabolism and anorexia of infection accelerate the cachexia. In advanced PEM midarm fat below the fifth percentile and creatinine/height ratio less than 60 percent of the normal are associated with terminal infections.

RELATION TO OTHER DEFICIENCY STATES PEM rarely occurs as an isolated phenomenon. Common coexisting nutritional deficiencies include those for folic acid, thiamine, riboflavin, nicotinic acid, pyridoxine, and vitamin A; in children with PEM deficiency of vitamin A is a particular hazard. As PEM worsens and protoplasmic protein is consumed, the intracellular minerals potassium, phosphorous, and magnesium are excreted in parallel with nitrogen so that total-body deficits may become apparent upon refeeding.

℞ TREATMENT

In the case of mild to moderate PEM, any precipitating events must be addressed, and the intake of protein and energy (based on ideal weight) should be increased sufficiently to allow replenishment of deficits. It is appropriate to administer multivitamins to all such patients. It is also essential during repletion that the availability of all minerals and trace elements be adequate to prevent life-threatening hypokalemia, hypomagnesemia, hypophosphatemia, etc. from developing. Provided the patient can eat and swallow, most patients can be treated orally. However, if anorexia is a major problem or if the individual is edentulous, the diet may have to be supplemented with liquid formulas (Chap. 77) either by mouth or by assisted enteral feeding (Chap. 78).

Management of severe PEM is more emergent and more complicated for several reasons.

1. Precipitating illnesses tend to be more severe and difficult to manage, and it may not be possible to restore nitrogen balance until infection and fever are brought under control.

2. The degree of malnutrition itself may hamper recovery from associated life-threatening illness so that early intervention with

assisted enteral feeding or parenteral nutrition (Chap. 78) may be urgently required.

3. Introduction of nutrients in the gastrointestinal tract may itself cause diarrhea because of the atrophy of the intestinal mucosa and decrease in intestinal and pancreatic enzymes, and total parenteral nutrition may be necessary.

4. Associated deficiency states are common, and care must be taken to provide multivitamins, trace metals, and all essential minerals in sufficient amounts for replenishment of body stores.

Recovery in adults may be slow and limited, but children tend to recover within 3 to 4 months. Comprehensive programs of nutrition education, psychosocial stimulation, and rehabilitation should be instituted in all cases.

BIBLIOGRAPHY

ABBASI AA, RUDMAN D: Undernutrition in the nursing home: Prevalence, consequences, causes, and prevention. Nutr Rev 52:113, 1994

ALLEYNE GAO et al: *Protein-Energy Malnutrition.* London, Butler & Tanner, 1997

BECKER DJ: The endocrine responses to protein calorie malnutrition. Ann Rev Nutr 3:187, 1983

CAHILL GF: Starvation in man. N Engl J Med 200:220, 1970

HARDIN TC: Cytokine mediators of malnutrition: Clinical implications. Nutr Clin Pract 8:55, 1993

HEYMSFIELD SB et al: Nutritional assessment by anthropomorphic and biochemical methods, in *Modern Nutrition in Health and Disease,* 8th ed, ME Shils et al (eds). Philadelphia, Lea & Febiger, 1994, p 812

HOFFER LJ: Starvation, in *Modern Nutrition in Health and Disease,* 8th ed, ME Shils et al (eds). Philadelphia, Lea & Febiger, 1994, p 927

JAMES WP: The challenge of adult chronic energy deficiency. Eur J Clin Nutr 48(Suppl 3):S1, 1994

PARNES HL, AISNER J: Protein calorie malnutrition and cancer therapy. Drug Safety 7:404, 1992

POLLITT E: Functional significance of the covariance between protein energy malnutrition and iron deficiency anemia. J Nutr 125(Suppl 8):2272S, 1995

SULLIVAN DH: The role of nutrition in increased morbidity and mortality. Clin Geriatr Med 11:661, 1995

TORUM B, CHEW F: Protein-energy malnutrition, in *Modern Nutrition in Health and Disease,* 8th ed, ME Shils et al (eds). Philadelphia, Lea & Febiger, 1994, p 950

75 *George A. Bray*

OBESITY

Obesity is a chronic disease that is increasing in prevalence and that poses a serious risk for the development of diabetes mellitus, hypertension, heart disease, gall bladder disease, and certain forms of cancer. Obesity can be viewed as a consequence of the interaction between environmental forces and the individual genetic substrate, in particular with susceptibility genes. These genes enhance the storage of fat when food is limited and cause an increased risk of obesity when food is abundant and energy expenditure is reduced. The prevalence of obesity in the United States increased slowly after World War II and has increased 30 percent in the past decade. Against this environmental and genetic background, this chapter will define the problem, describe methods for measuring obesity, review the etiology and pathogenesis, consider the impact of differences in regional fatness as predictors of health risk, and summarize the available treatment options.

DEFINITION AND MEASUREMENT Both obesity and fat distribution are useful predictors of excess mortality and of the risks of diabetes mellitus, heart disease, hypertension, and gall bladder disease. *Obesity,* an increase in total body fat, is frequently used synonymously with *overweight* because the degree of overweight can readily be related

to the risks assigned to obesity and direct measures of body fat are expensive. Regional fat distribution, or fat topography, also has a profound influence on health risks. For example, increased deposits of visceral or abdominal fat correlate with the risks for heart disease, diabetes mellitus, high blood pressure, gall bladder disease, and breast cancer.

Of the techniques for estimating or measuring total body fat (Table 75-1), height and weight can be measured with accuracy and reliability and provide valuable information. Dual energy x-ray absorptiometry, which was developed to evaluate bone density, provides the best assessment of total body fat. Regional fat can be measured accurately by magnetic resonance imaging or computed tomography scanning; for practical purposes, waist circumference or the sagittal diameter is the most useful parameter. The ratio of waist circumference to hip circumference is widely used to estimate regional fat but is not accurate.

Overweight can be defined from tables of height and weight and from estimates of percent overweight or relative weight (ratio of actual to desirable weight). However, the most widely used formula for relating height and weight is the body mass index (BMI), which is weight/(height)^2, where weight is in kilograms and height is in meters. A nomogram for estimating BMI is shown in Fig. 75-1. A BMI between 20 and 25 kg/m^2 is usually considered a good weight for most individuals. Overweight is defined as a BMI above 27 kg/m^2, and obesity is defined as a body mass index above 30 kg/m^2. Weight gain may confer increased health risks even if the BMI does not exceed 25 kg/m^2. In women a weight gain of more than 5 kg (11 lb) is associated with increased risks of diabetes and heart disease, and in men any weight gain after age 25 appears to carry increased health risks. At the practical level, determination of the BMI, estimation of abdominal girth (see below), and assessment of the presence of heart disease, diabetes mellitus, gall bladder disease, or hypertension in the family provide valuable information for evaluating the obese patient. Based on these considerations, a table of good weights for men and women has been developed (Table 75-2).

Body fat and fat distribution are affected by gender, age, degree of physical activity, and a number of drugs. In both men and women body fat increases with age. In lean young men, body fat is less than 20 percent and may rise in older men to more than 25 percent. In young women, body fat stores may be below 30 percent and increase gradually to more than 35 percent in older women. At all ages after puberty women are fatter than men.

Table 75-1

Methods of Estimating Body Fat and Its Distribution

Method	Cost	Ease of Use	Accuracy	Measures Regional Fat
Height and weight	$	Easy	High	No
Skin folds	$	Easy	Low	Yes
Circumferences	$	Easy	Moderate	Yes
Ultrasound	$$	Moderate	Moderate	Yes
Density				
Immersion	$	Moderate	High	No
Plethysmograph	$$$	Difficult	High	No
Heavy water				
Tritiated	$$	Moderate	High	No
Deuterium oxide, or heavy oxygen	$$$	Moderate	High	No
Potassium isotope (^{40}K)	$$$$	Difficult	High	No
Total-body electrical conductivity	$$$	Moderate	High	No
Bioelectric impedance	$$	Easy	High	No
Fat-soluble gas	$$	Difficult	High	No
Absorptiometry (dual energy x-ray absorptiometry;				
dual photon absorptiometry)	$$$	Easy	High	No
Computed tomography	$$$$	Difficult	High	Yes
Magnetic resonance imaging	$$$$	Difficult	High	Yes
Neutron activation	$$$$	Difficult	High	No

NOTE: $, low cost; $$, moderate cost; $$$, high cost; $$$$, very high cost.

PREVALENCE The prevalence of obesity depends upon the criteria for diagnosis. In most European countries obesity is defined as a BMI above 30 kg/m², and overweight is frequently defined as a BMI between 25 and 30 kg/m² or between 27 and 30 kg/m². The National Center for Health Statistics in the United States defines overweight as weights above the 85th percentile in men and women age 20 to 29 years. There has been a slow increase in the prevalence in both genders since surveys began more than 40 years ago, and between 1988 and 1991 there was an increase of more than 30 percent both in the United States and abroad (Fig. 75-2).

PATHOGENESIS **Genetic Susceptibility** Genetic determinants can either play a major role in the pathogenesis of obesity or enhance susceptibility to its development. The dysmorphic forms of human obesity in which genetics play a major role include the Prader-Willi syndrome, Ahlstrom's syndrome, the Laurence-Moon-Biedl syndrome, Cohen's syndrome, and Carpenter's syndrome (Table 75-3).

Four genes have been cloned in which mutations cause obesity in animals, and some of them appear to be important in human biology (Table 75-4). The leptin gene is expressed only in adipose tissue, and in the recessively inherited ob/ob obesity in mice, both copies of the gene are defective because of the presence of a stop codon that truncates the protein at amino acid 105. The leptin protein is normally secreted from fat cells, and the levels of leptin mRNA in fat cells and the circulating level of leptin are both increased in animal and human obesities. Treatment of obese mice with leptin reduces food intake and body fat. Splicing defects in the leptin receptor are responsible for the obesity in the db/db mouse, which is phenotypically similar to the ob/ob mouse. The gene defect called *tub* results from a defective phosphatase and causes retinitis pigmentosa and obesity in mice, making it similar to the Lawrence-Moon-Biedl syndrome in humans. Additional genes, including those for the beta₃-adrenergic receptor, tumor necrosis factor α, and lipoprotein lipase, have been implicated in the development of human obesity, but their contribution to the overall disorder is small.

Genetic susceptibility to obesity has been studied extensively, and between 30 and 50 percent of the variability in total-body fat stores is believed to be genetically determined. In animals that become obese when fed a high-fat diet, at least 12 chromosomal loci play an important role in the expression of this susceptibility, and the basis for genetic susceptibility to obesity in human beings is likely to be equally complex.

The Fat Cell and Obesity In addition to its role in fat storage, the fat cell is an important secretory organ. It produces lipoprotein lipase, which is involved in hydrolyzing the triglycerides of very low density lipoproteins (VLDL) and chylomicrons, and complements D (adipsin) and C3b. The adipocyte also produces cytokines such as tumor necrosis factor α, angiotensinogen, and leptin. The fat cell generates large quantities of lactate and metabolizes glucose to provide glycerol-3-phosphate for triglyceride synthesis. Under conditions of dietary surfeit, human fat cells synthesize long chain fatty acids.

Most forms of obesity are associated with enlarged fat cells and higher rates of basal lipolysis. Fat cells also serve as a reservoir for storage of fatty acids released during the clearance of chylomicrons and can in turn release these stored fatty acids by the intracellular hormone-sensitive lipase. In many forms of severe childhood-onset obesity, the total number of fat cells is increased.

Environmental Factors Environmental factors interact with genetic susceptibility in the pathogenesis of obesity. For example, hypothalamic injury from trauma or surgery and destructive lesions in the region of the ventromedial or the paraventricular nucleus in the hypothalamus can produce obesity. The two major factors in hypothalamic obesity are hyperphagia and a disturbance in the autonomic nervous system consisting of increased parasympathetic and reduced sympathetic nervous system activity. One explanation for this sequence of events may be altered secretion of neuropeptide Y (NPY). NPY is produced in the arcuate nucleus and acts in the hypothalamus to stimulate eating; it can also impair reproductive function, decrease sympathetic activity, and increase parasympathetic activity—other key features of hypothalamic obesity.

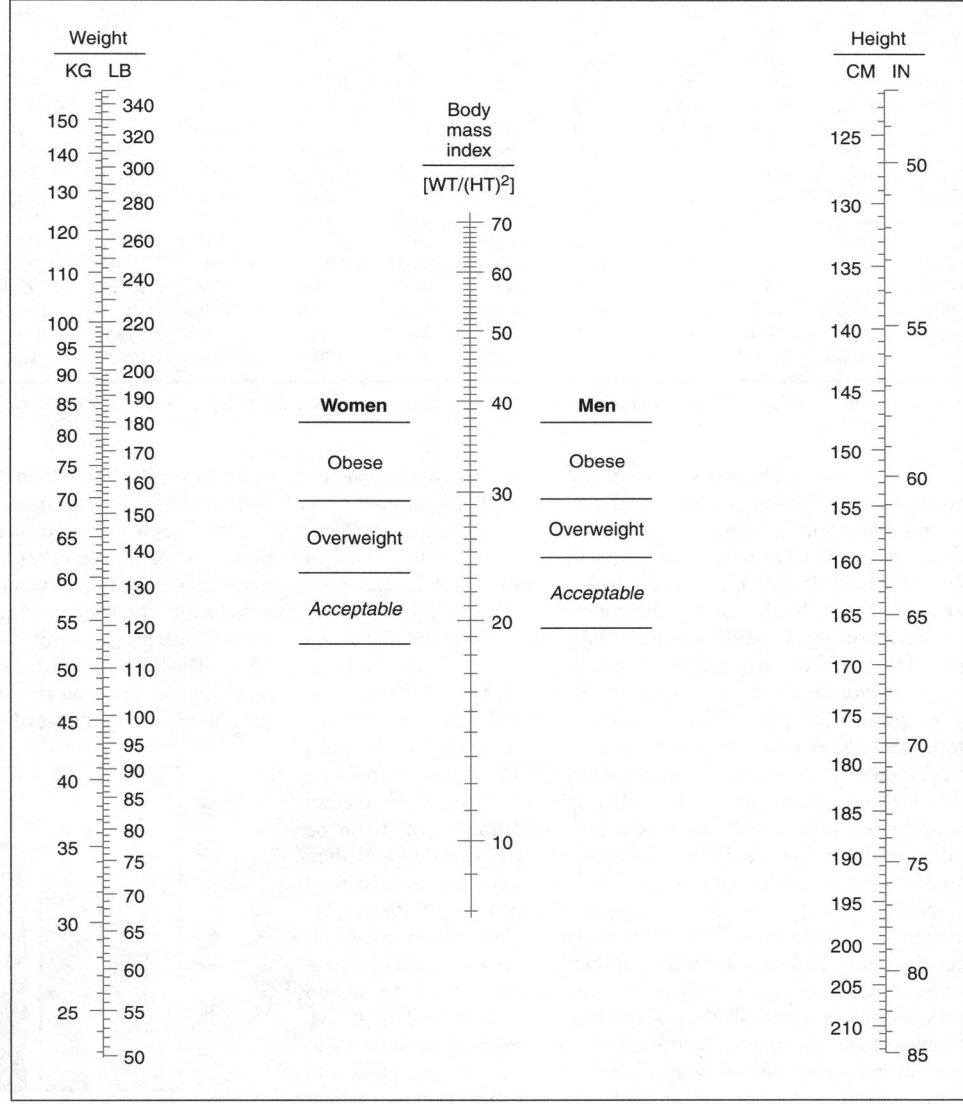

FIGURE 75-1 Nomogram for determining body mass index. To use this nomogram, place a ruler or other straight edge between the body weight (without clothes) in kilograms or pounds located on the left-hand line and the height (without shoes) in centimeters or in inches located on the right-hand line. The body mass index is read from the middle of the scale and is in metric units. (*Copyright 1978, George A. Bray. Used by permission.*)

Table 75-2

Chart to Find Body Mass Index (BMI) from Height and Weight, and Classification of Weight (Health Risk) According to BMI

Height	Weight													
			Good BMI				Borderline BMI				Increasing Risk BMI			
	19	20	21	22	23	24	25	26	27	28	29	30	35	40

Find your height on the left then move across the row to the weight which is closest to yours. Your BMI level is listed along the top.

HEIGHT IN CENTIMETERS, WEIGHT IN KILOGRAMS

Height	19	20	21	22	23	24	25	26	27	28	29	30	35	40
140.0	37.2	39.2	41.2	43.1	45.1	47.0	49.0	51.0	52.9	54.9	56.8	58.8	68.6	78.4
142.0	38.3	40.3	42.3	44.4	46.4	48.4	50.4	52.4	54.4	56.5	59.5	60.5	70.6	80.7
144.0	39.4	41.5	43.5	45.6	47.7	49.8	51.8	53.9	56.0	58.1	60.1	62.2	72.6	82.9
146.0	40.5	42.6	44.8	46.9	49.0	51.2	53.3	55.4	57.6	59.7	61.8	63.9	74.6	85.3
148.0	41.6	43.8	46.0	48.2	50.4	52.6	54.8	57.0	59.1	61.3	63.5	65.7	76.7	87.6
150.0	42.8	45.0	47.3	49.5	51.8	54.0	56.3	58.5	60.8	63.0	65.3	67.5	78.8	90.0
152.0	43.9	46.2	48.5	50.8	53.1	55.4	57.8	60.1	62.4	64.7	67.0	69.3	80.9	92.4
154.0	45.1	47.4	49.8	52.2	54.5	56.9	59.3	61.7	64.0	66.4	68.8	71.1	83.0	94.9
156.0	46.2	48.7	51.1	53.5	56.0	58.4	60.8	63.3	65.7	68.1	70.6	73.0	85.2	97.3
158.0	47.4	49.9	52.4	54.9	57.4	59.9	62.4	64.9	67.4	69.9	72.4	74.9	87.4	99.9
160.0	48.6	51.2	53.8	56.3	58.9	61.4	64.0	66.6	69.1	71.7	74.2	76.8	89.6	102.4
162.0	49.9	52.5	55.1	57.7	60.4	63.0	65.6	68.2	70.9	73.5	76.1	78.7	91.9	105.0
164.0	51.1	53.8	56.5	59.2	61.9	64.6	67.2	69.9	72.6	75.3	78.0	80.7	94.1	107.6
166.0	52.4	55.1	57.9	60.6	63.4	66.1	68.9	71.6	74.4	77.2	79.9	82.7	96.4	110.2
168.0	53.6	56.4	59.3	62.1	64.9	67.7	70.6	73.4	76.2	79.0	81.8	84.7	98.8	112.9
170.0	54.9	57.8	60.7	63.6	66.5	69.4	72.3	75.1	78.0	80.9	83.8	86.7	101.2	115.6
172.0	56.2	59.2	62.1	65.1	68.0	71.0	74.0	76.9	79.9	82.8	85.8	88.8	103.5	118.3
174.0	57.5	60.6	63.6	66.6	69.6	72.7	75.7	78.7	81.7	84.8	87.8	90.8	106.0	121.1
176.0	58.9	62.0	65.0	68.1	71.2	74.3	77.4	80.5	83.6	86.7	89.8	92.9	108.4	123.9
178.0	60.2	63.4	66.5	69.7	72.9	76.0	79.2	82.4	85.5	88.7	91.9	95.1	110.9	126.7
180.0	61.6	64.8	68.0	71.3	74.5	77.8	81.0	84.2	87.5	90.7	94.0	97.2	113.4	129.6
182.0	62.9	66.2	69.6	72.9	76.2	79.5	82.8	86.1	89.4	92.7	96.1	99.4	115.9	132.5
184.0	64.3	67.7	71.1	74.5	77.9	81.3	84.6	88.0	91.4	94.8	98.2	101.6	118.5	135.4
186.0	65.7	69.2	72.7	76.1	79.6	83.0	86.5	89.9	93.4	96.9	100.3	103.8	121.1	138.4
188.0	67.2	70.7	74.2	77.8	81.3	84.8	88.4	91.9	95.4	99.0	102.5	106.0	123.7	141.4
190.0	68.6	72.2	75.8	79.4	83.0	86.6	90.3	93.9	97.5	101.1	104.7	108.3	126.4	144.4
192.0	70.0	73.7	77.4	81.1	84.8	88.5	92.2	95.8	99.5	103.2	106.9	110.6	129.0	147.5
194.0	71.5	75.3	79.0	82.8	86.6	90.3	94.1	97.9	101.6	105.4	109.1	112.9	131.7	150.5
196.0	73.0	76.8	80.7	84.5	88.4	92.2	96.0	99.9	103.7	107.6	111.4	115.2	134.5	153.7
198.0	74.5	78.4	82.3	86.2	90.2	94.1	98.0	101.9	105.9	109.8	113.7	117.6	137.2	156.8
200.0	76.0	80.0	84.0	88.0	92.0	96.0	100.0	104.0	108.0	112.0	116.0	120.0	140.0	160.0

NOTE: The health risk from any level of BMI is increased if you have gained more than 5 kg (11 lb) since age 25 or if you have a waist circumference above 40 in (100 cm) due to central fatness.

The syndrome of hypothalamic obesity is at one end of the genetic-environmental continuum. At the same end of this continuum are several endocrine diseases associated with obesity, including Cushing's disease and the polycystic ovary syndrome, and drug-induced obesity (Table 75-5). One of the drugs, megestrol acetate, has been used to increase food intake in the anorexia of cancer cachexia.

Nutrition Intake and Substrate Oxidation To maintain normal body fat stores dietary nutrients must be oxidized in the body in the proportion in which they occur in the diet. A typical distribution of macronutrients in a 2000-kcal diet and the fraction of body stores that these nutrients represent are shown in Fig. 75-3. Since daily intake of carbohydrate nearly equals body stores of glucose, carbohydrate stores are more vulnerable to changes in dietary carbohydrate than either fat or proteins. Oxidation of food can be estimated from the respiratory quotient (RQ) (the ratio of carbon dioxide produced to oxygen used). The corresponding ratio in food is referred to as the food quotient. As the percent of dietary fat increases, the RQ must decline if weight is to remain stable. If RQ does not decline, the body continues to oxidize carbohydrate stores and must replace these by eating more food to obtain carbohydrate or synthesize endogenous glucose from protein stores. Whether this adjustment occurs efficiently and readily appears to have strong genetic determinants. Physiologically, the adaptation to a high-fat, western-type diet requires a decrease in carbohydrate oxidation to preserve carbohydrate stores. If carbohydrate oxidation is reduced, the oxidation of fat increases to provide for nutrient needs and lower the RQ. If the body is unable to reduce carbohydrate oxidation, the compensatory mechanism is increased food intake to provide needed carbohydrate with increasing fat storage until a point is reached at which the oxidation of fatty acids increases to meet average dietary intake.

Whether measured from room calorimeters or doubly labeled water, there is a positive correlation between energy expenditure and fat-free mass or body weight. To maintain body weight, therefore, heavier individuals must on average ingest more food to provide the necessary energy. Obese persons tend to underreport food intake significantly (Fig. 75-4). Thus, a patient who says 'Doctor, I hardly eat anything' is not recording or reporting food intake accurately. Because of almost uniform unreliability, dietary histories should probably be abandoned for

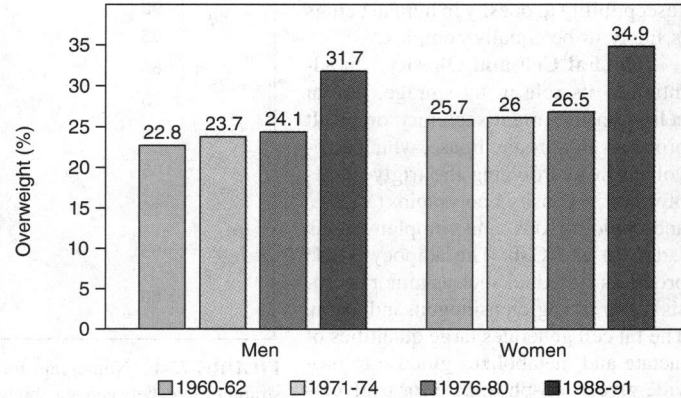

FIGURE 75-2 Prevalence of overweight status in four surveys. Data from the National Center for Health Statistics show the rise in prevalence of obesity over the past 30 years, particularly the past 10 years. (After Kuczmarski et al.)

Table 75-3

A Comparison of Syndromes of Obesity—Hypogonadism and Mental Retardation

Feature	Syndrome				
	Prader-Willi	Laurence-Moon-Biedl	Ahlstrom	Cohen	Carpenter
Inheritance	Sporadic; two-thirds have defect	Autosomal recessive	Autosomal recessive	Probably autosomal recessive	Autosomal recessive
Stature	Short	Normal; infrequently short	Normal; infrequently short	Short or tall	Normal
Obesity	Generalized Moderate to severe Onset 1–3 yrs	Generalized Early onset, 1–2 yrs	Truncal Early onset, 2–5 years	Truncal Mid-childhood, age 5	Truncal, gluteal
Cranofacies	Narrow bifrontal diameter Almond-shaped eyes Strabismus V-shaped mouth High arched palate	Not distinctive	Not distinctive	High nasal bridge Arched palate Open mouth Short philtrum	Acrocephaly Flat nasal bridge High arched palate
Limbs	Small hands and feet Hypotonia	Polydactyly	No abnormalities	Hypotonia Narrow hands and feet	Polydactyly Syndactyly Genu valgum
Reproductive status	1° Hypogonadism	1° Hypogonadism	Hypogonadism in males but not in females	Normal gonadal function or hypogonadotrophic hypogonadism	2° Hypogonadism
Other features	Enamel hypoplasia Hyperphagia Temper tantrums Nasal speech			Dysplastic ears Delayed puberty	
Mental retardation	Mild to moderate		Normal intelligence	Mild	Slight

Table 75-4

Molecular Biology of Obesity

	Gene Symbol	Chromosome	Gene Defect	Mechanism
ANIMALS				
Yellow mouse	A^y; A^{vy}; A^{iy}	2	Overexpression of 133-amino-acid Agouti protein	Agouti protein competes with MSH receptors
Obese mouse	ob	6	1. Stop codon at 105 in the 167-amino-acid leptin protein 2. Nonsense mutation in the leptin protein	Absence of leptin (ob protein), which appears to modulate steroid superfamily expression
Diabetes	db	4	Splicing defects in leptin receptor	Receptor for leptin absent
Fatty rat (syntenic to db locus)	fa	5	Not identified	Receptor for leptin probably absent
Tub		7	Not identified	?
Fat		8	Carboxypeptidase E	Failure of cleavage for many peptides
HUMANS				
Prader Willi		15q 1.2		
Laurence-Moon-Biedl		3 and 16		

estimating energy needs. In our clinic, a reasonable guideline for energy expenditure (kcal) in the obese is to multiply body weight by 10. An alternative method (Table 75-6) takes into account height, weight, and age to estimate of basal energy expenditure.

Table 75-5

Drugs Associated with Increased Body Weight

Phenothiazines (chlorpromazine > thioridazine ≥ trifluoperazine > mesoridazine > promazine ≥ mepazine ≥ perphenazine ≥ prochlorperazine haloperidol ≥ loxapine)
Antidepressants (amitriptyline > imipramine = doxepin = phenelzine > amoxapine = desipramine = trazodone = tranylcypromine)
Antiepileptics (valproate; carbamazepine)
Steroids (glucocorticoids; megestrol acetate)
Antihypertensives (terazosin)

There are three known predictors of future weight gain: a low metabolic rate; a high RQ, indicating carbohydrate oxidation and the need to eat to replace carbohydrate; and insulin resistance. The regulation of nutrient intake can be viewed as a feedback system with afferent and efferent signals (Fig. 75-5). Factors that increase hunger include a decrease in blood glucose, which precedes 60 percent or more of meals in animals and humans, and an increase in gastric contractions or abdominal uneasiness. These peripheral signals are integrated by neurotransmitters in the central nervous system to regulate food intake. Several neurotransmitters increase and a larger number decrease food intake. In addition, some neurotransmitters are specific modulators of the intake of one or another macronutrient (fat, carbohydrate, or protein). Thus, an increase or decrease in the intake of fat, carbohydrate, or protein can occur as major responses to specific neurotransmitters. These peptides and their monoamine substrates pro-

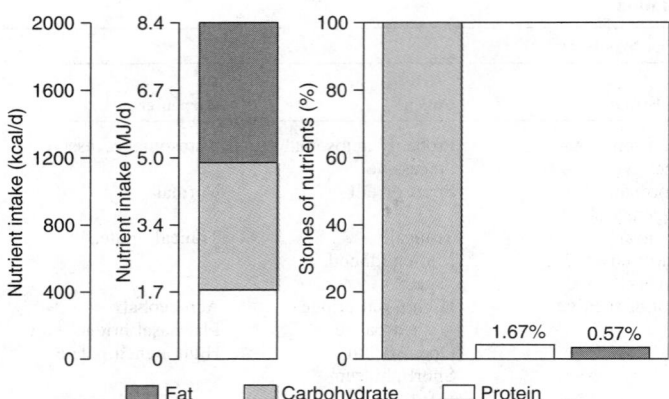

FIGURE 75-3 Nutrient intake versus stores. The daily intake of carbohydrate approximates body stores of carbohydrate. Intake of fat and protein are only a small fraction of the stored quantities of these nutrients.

FIGURE 75-4 Comparison of energy expenditure and reported food intake in obese subjects. Total energy expenditure was determined by using doubly labeled water ($^2H^{18}O_2$). Food intake was determined from reported dietary intakes. The obese subjects consistently reported eating less than half the calories that were needed to maintain body weight.

Table 75-6

Estimating Energy Needs

EQUATIONS FOR ESTIMATING BASAL METABOLIC RATE (BMR)*

Men

18–30 years = (0.0630 × actual weight in kg + 2.8957) × 240 kcal/day

31–60 years = (0.0484 × actual weight in kg + 3.6534) × 240 kcal/day

Women

18–30 years = (0.0621 × actual weight in kg + 2.0357) × 240 kcal/day

31–60 years = (0.0342 × actual weight in kg + 3.5377) × 240 kcal/day

ESTIMATED TOTAL ENERGY NEEDS

Energy expenditure = BMR × activity factor

Activity level	Activity factor
Low (sedentary)	1.3
Intermediate (some regular exercise)	1.5
High (regular activity or demanding job)	1.7

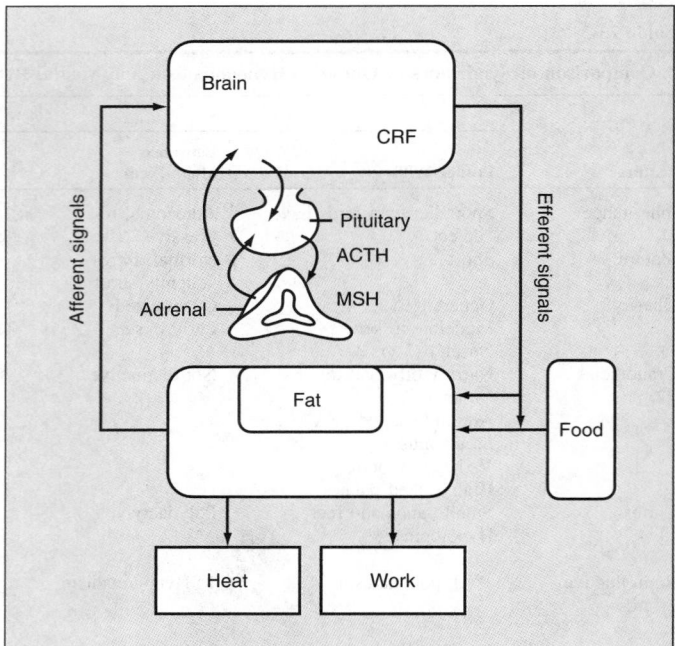

FIGURE 75-5 Model of a nutrient balance regulatory system for food intake. The afferent signals tell the brain about the state of nutrient stores and metabolism. This information is integrated in the central nervous system, which uses efferent endocrine and neural signals to modulate food intake and metabolism in the controlled system that digests, absorbs, metabolizes, or stores the ingested food.

vide a robust system for controlling the quantity and quality of food intake.

At least four processes are involved in the regulation of food intake: (1) olfactory and gustatory factors—these can stimulate intake when food is appetizing or inhibit intake when it is not; (2) gastrointestinal distention; (3) release of gastrointestinal hormones such as cholecystokinin and gastrin-releasing peptide; and (4) activation of a thermogenic component of the efferent sympathetic nervous system. These factors work together after food ingestion to induce satiety until the next glucose dip and increased gastric contractions produce a new arousal for seeking food.

OBESITY AND ITS ASSOCIATED RISKS The increased mortality associated with obesity results primarily from increased risks

FIGURE 75-6 Mortality ratio and body mass index. Data from the American Cancer Society study are plotted for men and women to show relationship of body mass index (BMI) to overall mortality. At BMI < 20 kg/m² and > 25 kg/m² there is an increase in relative mortality. The major causes for this increased mortality are listed along with a division of BMI groupings into various levels of risk. (*Copyright 1987, George A. Bray. Used with permission.*)

for cardiovascular disease, high blood pressure, diabetes mellitus, and, possibly, some types of cancer (Fig. 75-6).

Cardiovascular System   In addition to the increased work load on the heart, obesity is also associated with an increased risk of sudden death, probably due to cardiac arrhythmias, and with an increased risk of atherosclerosis, probably a reflection of an abnormal lipid profile including decreased levels of high-density lipoprotein (HDL) cholesterol and increased levels of low-density lipoprotein cholesterol, particularly when these are in the form of small dense VLDL particles (B pattern). The prevalence of hypertension is also increased, the mechanism being unclear. One hypothesis suggests that hyperinsulinemia and insulin resistance enhance sodium reabsorption by the renal tubule and increase sympathetic outflow to promote arterial constriction.

Diabetes Mellitus   Type 2 diabetes mellitus [non-insulin-dependent diabetes mellitus (NIDDM)] is almost nonexistent in individuals with a BMI below 22 kg/m². In the Pima Indians the increased risk of diabetes with obesity has a strong familial tendency; when one or both Pima Indian parents is diabetic, 100 percent of the offspring will develop diabetes if they become sufficiently obese. If neither parent has diabetes, fewer than 20 percent of the obese offspring develop diabetes. In nonhuman primates that develop diabetes mellitus, obesity precedes the onset of diabetes by months to years. Among the earliest predictors of subsequent diabetes in obese monkeys is the development of insulin resistance. As with human beings, prevention of obesity in nonhuman primates prevents diabetes.

Cancer   The incidence of endometrial and postmenopausal breast cancers in women, prostate cancer in men, and colonorectal cancer in men and women is related to the degree of obesity. Visceral obesity increases the risk of postmenopausal breast cancer independent of the degree of obesity. One explanation for susceptibility to endometrial and breast cancer in obese women is the increased production of estrogen from the aromatization of circulating androstenedione in adipose tissue.

Gall Bladder Disease   Gall bladder disease increases with obesity and age, possibly related to increased excretion of biliary cholesterol. The amount of cholesterol synthesized by the body each day increases by about 20 mg for each kilogram of adipose tissue, so that a 10-kg increase in adipose tissue mass increases daily cholesterol production and excretion by an amount comparable to the cholesterol in one egg. Disturbances in nidation factors in the bile and alterations in the level of bile acids and phospholipids may promote precipitation of cholesterol stones.

Pulmonary Function   Moderate obesity in the absence of underlying pulmonary disease has little effect on respiratory function. Sleep apnea, however, can occur in severely obese individuals and poses a potentially serious problem. Obstructive sleep apnea is believed to occur because of local fat accumulation in the tracheopharyngeal area. The obstructive episodes of sleep apnea produce interrupted sleep associated with hypoxia and hypercapnia. If not corrected, this condition can lead to right heart failure. Continuous positive airway pressure can be administered at night to reduce or eliminate the episodes of sleep apnea. Weight loss is of particular value in remediating this problem.

Joint and Skin Problems   The increased incidence of osteoarthritis is no doubt partly due to the added trauma of increased weight bearing, but the fact that osteoarthritis also occurs in non-weight-bearing joints in such patients suggests that additional factors are involved. The prevalence of gout is also increased and may reflect impairment in urate clearance. Ketone bodies compete at the renal tubule for reabsorption of urate, and increased production of ketones from fat metabolism may increase urate levels.

Among the skin problems associated with obesity are acanthosis nigricans, manifested by darkening of the skinfolds on the neck, elbows, and dorsal interphalangeal spaces. Acanthosis nigricans is also associated with insulin resistance and NIDDM. Skin turgor and friability may also be increased in obesity, enhancing the risk of fungal and yeast infections in skinfolds. Finally, venous stasis is increased in the obese.

Endocrine System   Insulin resistance leading to hyperinsulinemia is a uniform feature and is directly related to the degree of obesity. Growth hormone secretion is reduced, but insulin-like growth

factor I levels are normal, suggesting that the level of growth hormone is sufficient to stimulate production of this important hormone.

Testosterone levels are decreased in men, but levels of free testosterone decline only with massive obesity. Obesity leads to an earlier onset of menarche, to a greater frequency of irregular and anovulatory cycles, and to earlier menopause. Distribution of body fat influences steroid metabolism in women. Women with central or visceral fat have a higher production of androgens such as testosterone, and women with gluteofemoral obesity have increased levels of estrone due to peripheral aromatization of circulating androgens.

Changes in thyroid hormone and its metabolism occur with changes in the level of nutrient intake. Triiodothyronine (T_3) can be increased by overfeeding and decreased by starvation. T_3 levels are also increased by high-carbohydrate diets and lowered by low-carbohydrate diets. In contrast, levels of thyroxine and thyrotropin (TSH) are unaffected by diet.

Obesity can sometimes be mistaken for Cushing's syndrome. The normal pattern of diurnal variation in plasma cortisol and the concentration of urinary free cortisol are normal in obesity but abnormal in Cushing's disease. If these patterns are equivocal, dynamic tests of adrenal function may be indicated.

Fat Topography   Regional distributions of body fat play an important role in the risk factors of obesity. To assess the distribution of body fat, the ratio of the circumference of the waist to the circumference of the hips has been a valuable tool for epidemiologic studies. For the individual patient, however, this ratio is not as useful as waist circumference itself. A waist circumference above 100 cm in men and above 90 cm in women is associated with increased levels of triglyceride and reduced levels of HDL cholesterol. Quantitative estimates of central fat distribution can be obtained from magnetic resonance imaging or computed tomographic scans of the abdomen (see Table 75-1).

Weight Cycling and Intentional Weight Loss   Regaining body weight after dieting is common and is referred to as *weight cycling*. Review of the literature concerning weight cycling does not reveal any convincing detrimental effects. To the contrary, intentional weight loss reduces health risks. Among 28,000 women aged 40 to 64 who had never smoked and who had no other health problems, a 9.1-kg (20-lb) intentional weight loss in the previous year resulted in a 25 percent reduction in all-cause, cardiovascular, and cancer mortality. In 15,069 women of the same age with coexisting health problems, any amount of intentional weight loss resulted in a 10 percent decrease in cardiovascular disease, a 20 percent reduction in all-cause mortality, a 30 to 40 percent decrease in mortality related to diabetes mellitus, and a 40 to 50 percent reduction in mortality from cancers of the breast and colon.

℞ TREATMENT

Treatment of obesity should be undertaken with a clear understanding of the realities of the problem and its outcome. First, obesity is a chronic disease that is increasing in prevalence. Second, the etiology is usually unknown, making a cure unlikely and palliation the therapeutic goal. Third, both obesity and increased visceral fat increase health risks even when total-body weight and fat are not markedly elevated. Fourth, obesity is a stigmatized condition in which the overweight subject is frequently viewed as responsible for the condition. Fifth, treatment of obesity with medication suffers from the negative "amphetamine halo." The introduction of amphetamines for the treatment of obesity more than 50 years ago was soon followed by a spate of addictions and gave a bad name to the use of drugs of this type. The various drugs of this class, called β-phenethylamines, work through diverse mechanisms. Amphetamine releases norepinephrine and dopamine, whereas other drugs in this class either affect serotonin metabolism, norepinephrine metabolism, or both without influencing dopamine metabolism. Sixth, recidivism, i.e., weight regain, is common in obesity. Seventh, drugs and other treatments for obesity do not work unless they are used; when

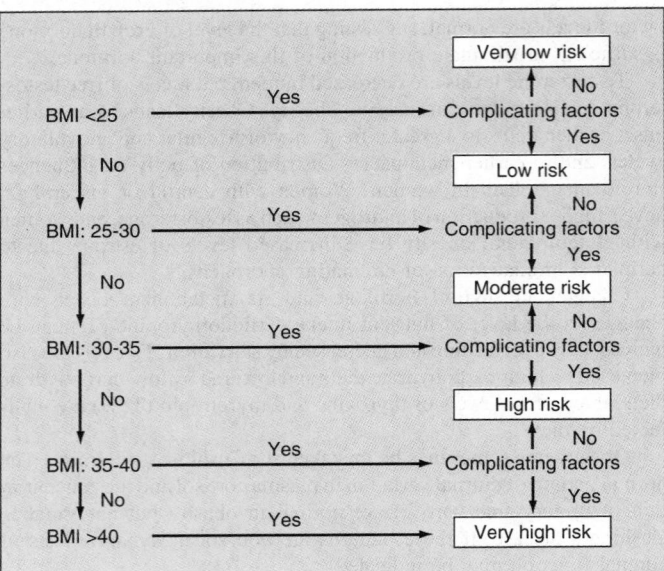

FIGURE 75-7 Risk classification algorithm. The patient is first placed into a category based on body mass index. The presence or absence of complicating factors determines the degree of health risk. Complicating factors include elevated abdominal-gluteal ratio (male: 0.95, female: 0.85), diabetes mellitus, hypertension, hyperlipidemia, male sex, and age < 40. (*Copyright 1987, George A. Bray. Used with permission.*)

reduction. The basic principles are those of operant conditioning and cognitive restructuring. Eating behavior is analyzed into its antecedents, the act of eating, and the consequences of eating by asking the patient to monitor and record these activities. The settings in which eating occurs, the eating event itself, and the use of rewards designed to change maladaptive behaviors are all monitored. Attempts are made to change thinking patterns from negative ones such as "I have just eaten that piece of cake, I am a bad person" into "I have just eaten a piece of cake, and now I need to go exercise" or other positive ways of solving the problem. Features of behavior modification of proven value in people who are successful in maintaining weight loss over an extended period of time include: (1) continued monitoring of food-related behaviors, (2) adoption of a low-fat diet, and (3) increased levels of physical activity.

Diet It is possible that increased dietary fat intake may be associated with increased risk of developing obesity in genetically susceptible subjects, and the prudent person should adopt a lower fat intake; the question is how low should this low-fat diet be? Extrapolation from experimental data suggests that a diet with fewer than 25 percent fat calories is a reasonable goal.

For anyone considering a weight-reducing diet, the quantity of food intake and the avoidance of settings in which excess quantities of high-fat food are eaten are equally important. Cafeterias and buffet meals are especially difficult. Controlling food intake is easier if the use of alcoholic beverages is reduced or eliminated, particularly since alcohol tends to blunt the ability to maintain other dietary controls. Increasing the frequency of eating is also a useful strategy. People who eat breakfast have a lower risk of developing obesity than individuals who do not. Ingestion of frequent small meals with relatively high carbohydrate and high fiber content is a way of decreasing fat intake and providing continued gastrointestinal fill.

Exercise Exercise is not good as a primary strategy for weight loss but is crucial in maintaining weight loss. Figure 75-8 illustrates the effect of adding exercise to a dietary program; of a group of men who completed an initial 8-week program, those who maintained an exercise program maintained the weight loss, whereas those who did not regained weight. This is clear demonstration of the importance of maintaining physical activity if body weight is to remain under control.

Use of Medication in the Management of Obesity Appetite-suppressing drugs may be useful but should be reserved for individuals with a BMI above 30 kg/m² or above 27 kg/m² if associated weight-related comorbid conditions are present. The options for pharmacologic intervention for obesity include several appetite-

appetite suppressing drugs are discontinued, patients regain weight, in keeping with the concept that the drugs do not cure obesity but only relieve its symptoms.

Selection of treatments can be made using the BMI as a guide and assessing the risks associated with obesity and central fat distribution (Fig. 75-7). Complicating factors include age; gender; comorbid conditions such as diabetes mellitus, hypertension, and hyperlipidemia; and a family history of hypertension, diabetes mellitus, or coronary heart disease. In young individuals under 40, especially men who have these risk factors or a positive family history, the need for treatment is more urgent.

Behavior Modification The principles of behavior modification provide the underpinnings for many current programs of weight

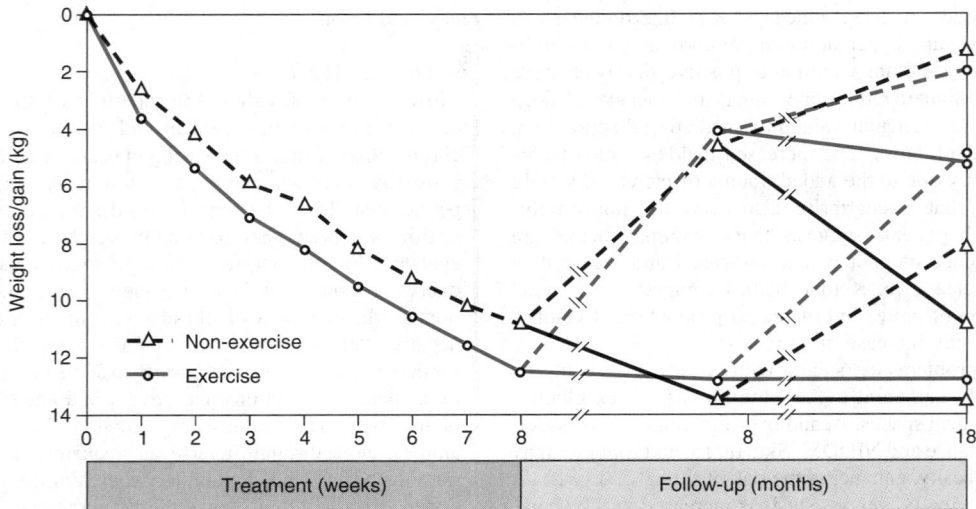

FIGURE 75-8 Weight loss and exercise. During the first 8 weeks, subjects were divided into two groups, one treated with diet and the other with diet plus exercise, with no difference in weight loss. Thereafter the subjects who exercised maintained better weight loss than those that did not. (*After Pavlou et al.*)

Table 75-7

Approved Appetite-Suppressing Drugs

	DEA Schedule	$t_{1/2}$, h	Tablet Size and Timing	Daily Dose Range, mg
NORADRENERGIC AGENTS				
Benzphetamine	III	6–12	25 or 50 mg before breakfast	25–50
Phendimetrazine	III	5–12	35 mg before meals or 105 mg (slow release) daily	17.5–105
Diethylpropion	IV	4–6	25 mg before meals; 75 mg in A.M. (slow release)	25–75 75
Mazindol	IV	10	1 or 2 mg at noon	1–2
Phentermine HCl	IV	7–24	8 mg before meals 15 or 37.5 mg before breakfast	15–37.5
Phentermine resin	IV		15 or 30 mg resin before breakfast	15–30
Phenylpropanolamine	Not scheduled (OTC)		25 mg before meals 75 mg (slow release) daily	25–75
SEROTONERGIC AGENTS				
Dexfenfluramine	IV	11–30	15 mg bid	30
Fenfluramine	IV	11–30	20 mg before meals	60–120

NOTE: DEA, Drug Enforcement Agency; OTC, over the counter.

suppressing drugs. The drugs shown in Table 75-7 increase extraneuronal norepinephrine by enhancing its release (benzphetamine, phendimetrazine, phentermine, mazindol, and diethylpropion), or by blocking its uptake, by inhibiting alpha$_1$-adrenergic receptors (phenylpropanolamine), or by releasing serotonin and blocking its reuptake (fenfluramine). Data from the first 34 weeks of a 210-week trial of placebo versus a combination of fenfluramine and phentermine are shown in Fig. 75-9. The patients on the drug combination lost more than 15 percent of their initial body weight and maintained the loss for the first year of the study. Those initially on placebo who were switched to a drug at the end of 34 weeks also showed a drop in body weight. In some individuals weight did not decrease, indicating that some patients do not respond to this therapy.

Amphetamine is classified by the U.S. Drug Enforcement Agency as an abusable drug. All other appetite suppressant drugs are similarly classified, but the risks of abuse for most of these agents are small. In the case of fenfluramine, there is no evidence of abuse potential, and the U.S. Food and Drug Administration's Drug Abuse Advisory Committee has recommended descheduling fenfluramine and its metabolites. Nevertheless, in considering the use of drugs for weight loss, it is necessary to understand the pharmacology of the specific agent and to provide a full disclosure of risks and benefits to the patient.

Surgery For individuals with a BMI above 35 kg/m² who have high risks for diabetes or family histories of early heart attacks and for individuals without these problems but with BMI above 40 kg/m², surgical manipulation of the gastrointestinal tract may be useful. A number of operative interventions have been used (Fig. 75-10). Data comparing different procedures suggest that the best long-term weight loss occurs with the gastric bypass operation in which a small upper pouch is attached by a Roux-en-Y anastomosis to the jejunum. Operative mortality is in the range of 0.1 to 0.5 percent. Weight regain and other problems are minimal with the Roux-en-Y operation and the vertically banded gastroplasty, the two recommended procedures.

FIGURE 75-9 Double-blind randomized control comparison of placebo and combination drug therapy in treatment of obesity. During the first 6 weeks, both groups were given similar programs in behavior modification, diet, and exercise. At the end of this period, the double-blind period of drug treatment was begun. At the end of 34 weeks, the patients treated with the combination of fenfluramine (F) and phentermine (Ph) had lost significantly more weight than the placebo-treated controls. (*Weintraub M et al, reproduced with permission*).

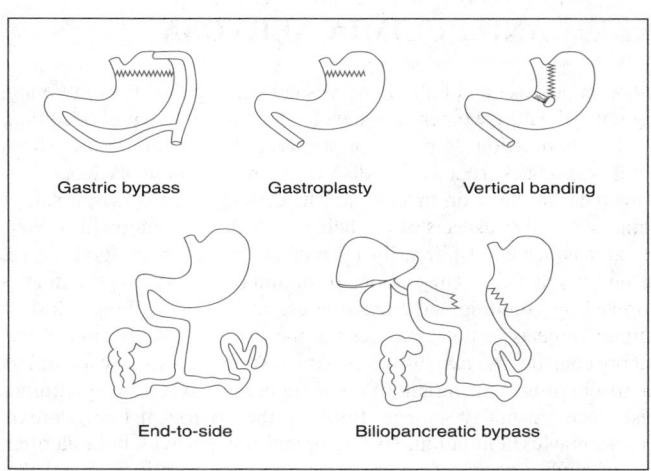

FIGURE 75-10 Examples of operative interventions used for surgical manipulation of the gastrointestinal tract.

BIBLIOGRAPHY

ANGEL A, BRAY GA: Synthesis of fatty acids and cholesterol by liver, adipose tissue and intestinal mucosa from obese and control patients. Eur J Clin Invest 9:355, 1979

ATKINSON RL et al: Weight cycling. JAMA 272:1196, 1994.

BALLOR DL, KEESEY RE: A meta-analysis of the factors affecting exercise-induced changes in body-mass, fat mass and fat-free mass in males and females. Int J Obes 15:717, 1991

BOUCHARD C (ed): *The Genetics of Obesity.* Boca Raton, FL, CRC Press, 1993

BRAY GA: Obesity, a disorder of nutrient partitioning: The MONA LISA hypothesis. J Nutr 121:1146, 1991

————: Evaluation of drugs for treating obesity. Obes Res 3:425S,1995

CAMPFIELD LA et al: Mouse OB protein: Evidence for a peripheral signal linking adiposity and central neural networks. Science 269:546, 1995

FOREYT JP et al: Psychological correlates of weight fluctuation. Int J Eating Dis 17:263, 1995

HALAAS JL et al: Weight-reducing effects of the plasma protein encoded by the obese gene. Science 269:543, 1995

KUCZMARSKI RJ et al: Increasing prevalence of overweight among US adults: The National Health and Nutrition Examination Surveys, 1960 to 1991. JAMA 272:205, 1994

LICHTMAN SW et al: Discrepancy between self-reported and actual caloric intake and exercise in obese subjects. N Engl J Med 327:1893, 1992

LISSNER L, HEITMANN BL: Dietary fat and obesity: Evidence from epidemiology. Eur J Clin Nutr 49:79, 1995

PAVLOU KN et al: Exercise as an adjunct to weight loss and maintenance in moderately obese subjects. Am J Clin Nutr 49:1115, 1989

PELLEYMOUNTER MA et al: Effects of the obese gene product on body weight regulation in ob/ob mice. Science 269:540, 1995

PORIES WJ et al: Surgical treatment of obesity and its effect on diabetes: 10-y follow-up. Am J Clin Nutr 55:S582, 1992

SCHAPIRA DV et al: Upper-body fat distribution and endometrial cancer risk. JAMA 266:1808, 1991

SJOSTROM LV: Morbidity of severely obese subjects. Am J Clin Nutr 55:508S, 1992

————: Mortality of severely obese subjects. Am J Clin Nutr 55(Suppl 2):516S, 1992

WEINTRAUB M et al: Long term weight control study I (weeks 0–34). Clin Pharmacol Ther 31:486, 1992

WEST DB et al: Dietary obesity linked to genetic-loci on chromosome-9 and chromosome-15 in a polygenic mouse model. J Clin Invest 94:1410, 1994

WILLETT WC et al: Weight, weight change and coronary heart disease in women: Risk within the normal weight range. JAMA 273:461, 1995

WILLIAMSON DF et al: Prospective study of intentional weight-loss and mortality in never-smoking overweight US white women aged 40–64 years. Am J Epidemiol 141:1128, 1995

76	*Daniel W. Foster*

ANOREXIA NERVOSA AND BULIMIA NERVOSA

Anorexia nervosa and bulimia nervosa are eating disorders in young, previously healthy women who develop a paralyzing fear of becoming fat. The population at risk consists largely of white women from middle-class backgrounds. The disorders rarely occur in black or oriental women, in the poor, or in men. The driving force is the pursuit of thinness, all other aspects of life being secondary. In anorexia nervosa this aim is achieved primarily by radical restriction of food intake, the end result being emaciation. In bulimia massive binge eating is followed by vomiting and excessive use of laxatives. Weight loss in bulimic subjects is not great despite the obsession with food. Some authors consider the two disorders to be distinct illnesses, while others classify bulimia as a variant of anorexia nervosa. Overlap syndromes exist since emaciated patients fulfilling the criteria of true anorexia nervosa may exhibit bulimic behavior and subjects with bulimia often pass through a phase of anorexia. In this chapter it is assumed that the two disorders are different expressions of a psychological obsession with body weight.

PREVALENCE/INCIDENCE The true prevalence and incidence of anorexia nervosa are not known. In high-risk populations, such as 16- to 18-year-old girls in private schools, the prevalence may be 1 percent, whereas public school girls of the same age have a prevalence of about 0.1 percent. In a study in Rochester, Minnesota, the prevalence was 0.2 percent in women and 0.02 percent in men. The probable prevalence is 0.2 to 1 percent in women and about one-tenth this level in men. The incidence rate (new case appearance), age- and sex-adjusted, was 7.3 per 100,000 population per year in the Rochester study.

The data for bulimia nervosa are even less satisfactory. A study in Ontario, Canada, suggested a lifetime prevalence in women of 1.1 percent and in men of 0.1 percent. All estimates of incidence are influenced by the cohort studied. For example, vomiting after eating occurs in up to 18 percent of women college students, a group in which incidence rates are high. Bulimia may now be more common than anorexia.

DIAGNOSIS The diagnosis of both disorders is made on clinical grounds. The standards of the American Psychiatric Association have "softened" so that the diagnoses are now made more frequently. Criteria of the 1994 *Diagnostic and Statistical Manual of Mental Disorders* (DSM-IV) are given in Tables 76-1 and 76-2. The weight criterion for diagnosis is 85 percent or less than expected ideal weight. Although DSM-IV does not use the body mass index [weight in kg/(height)^2 in m], a body mass index of less than 18 is considered the threshold level for diagnosis. Amenorrhea is an invariable feature. Anorexia nervosa is thus the only psychiatric illness including a mandatory endocrine component. An expressed intense fear of gaining weight or becoming fat, even when underweight, and a disturbance of body image (the way the body is perceived by the patient) complete the diagnostic tetrad. Two subtypes of anorexia nervosa are specified: restricting and binge eating/purging. In the former, bulimic behavior is absent, while in the latter gorging and purging are components.

Diagnostic criteria for bulimia nervosa require that an amount of food be ingested that is greater than most people would eat in a similar period of time. The binge episodes must be accompanied by a feeling that eating is out of control and must occur at least twice a week for 3 months, and there must be evidence of compensatory behavior to keep weight down. Bulimic symptoms must not occur exclusively in the presence of anorexia nervosa, i.e., the patient is assigned to anorexia nervosa rather than bulimia nervosa if weight reduction is sustained. Finally, as in anorexia, distortion of body image is an essential feature. The two subtypes of bulimia nervosa are purging and nonpurging. Obsessive/compulsive behavior, self-mutilation, and antisocial behavior are not essential criteria although they occur more frequently in bulimia than in anorexia nervosa and in control populations.

Table 76-1

Diagnostic Criteria for Anorexia Nervosa

1. Refusal to maintain body weight at or above a minimally normal weight for age and height (e.g., weight loss leading to maintenance of body weight less than 85% of that expected; or failure to make expected weight gain during period of growth, leading to body weight less than 85% of that expected).
2. Intense fear of gaining weight or becoming fat, even though underweight.
3. Disturbance in the way in which one's body weight or shape is experienced, undue influence of body weight or shape on self-evaluation, or denial of the seriousness of the current body weight.
4. In postmenarchal females, amenorrhea, i.e., the absence of at least three consecutive menstrual cycles. [a woman is considered to have amenorrhea if her periods occur only following hormone (e.g., estrogen) administration.]

Specify type:
   Restricting type: During the episode of anorexia nervosa the person does not regularly engage in binge-eating or purging behavior (i.e., self-induced vomiting or the misuse of laxatives, diuretics or enemas).
   Binge eating/purging type: During the episode of anorexia nervosa, the person regularly engages in binge-eating or purging behavior (i.e., self-induced vomiting or the misuse of laxatives, diuretics or enemas).

SOURCE: From Diagnostic and Statistical Manual of Mental Disorders, 4th ed, Washington, DC, American Psychiatric Association, 1994.

Table 76-2

CHAPTER 76
Anorexia Nervosa and Bulimia Nervosa **463**

Diagnostic Criteria for Bulimia Nervosa

1. Recurrent episodes of binge eating. An episode of binge eating is characterized by both of the following:
   a. Eating, in a discrete period of time (e.g., within any 2-h period), an amount of food that is definitely larger than most people would eat during a similar period of time and under similar circumstances.
   b. A sense of lack of control over eating during the episode (e.g., a feeling that one cannot stop eating or control what or how much one is eating).
2. Recurrent inappropriate compensatory behavior to prevent weight gain, such as self-induced vomiting, misuse of laxatives, diuretics, or other medications; fasting; or excessive exercise.
3. The binge eating and inappropriate compensatory behaviors both occur, on average, at least twice a week for 3 months.
4. Self-evaluation is unduly influenced by body shape and weight.
5. The disturbance does not occur exclusively during episodes of anorexia nervosa.

Specify type:
   Purging type: the person regularly engages in self-induced vomiting or the misuse of laxatives or diuretics.
   Nonpurging type: the person uses other inappropriate compensatory behaviors, such as fasting or excessive exercise, but does not regularly engage in self-induced vomiting or the misuse of laxatives or diuretics.

SOURCE: From Diagnostic and Statistical Manual of Mental Disorders, 4th ed, Washington, DC, American Psychiatric Association, 1994.

The diagnostic value of a disturbed perception of body image in patients with eating disorders has been questioned because many normal women evidence the same perceptual distortion. In practice a presumptive diagnosis of anorexia nervosa is justified if the following elements are present: (1) major weight loss; (2) absence of organic disease to account for weight loss; (3) absence of primary psychiatric illness that might account for failure to eat; (4) extreme restriction of food intake, with or without intermittent vomiting; (5) ritualized exercise; and (6) denial of hunger, fatigue, or emaciation. Late-onset disease is also now recognized, although usually symptoms begin in the teen years or early adulthood. While there is an emphasis on the absence of organic disease to cause weight loss, anorexia nervosa may coexist with other conditions that can cause loss of weight such as insulin-dependent diabetes mellitus.

The diagnosis of bulimia nervosa is secure if there is: (1) binge eating without major weight loss; (2) evidence of induced vomiting or regular use of laxatives or diuretics; (3) obsessive/compulsive behavior, antisocial activity or self-mutilation.

ETIOLOGY The cause of the eating disorders is unknown. Although primary dysfunction of the hypothalamus has been postulated, the recognized hypothalamic abnormalities revert to normal with weight gain and thus are secondary.

A psychiatric etiology is likely, but its nature is unclear. One view holds that the disorders begin in response to inadequate or destructive interpersonal relationships in families that are goal-oriented and highly achieving. Despite an outward normal appearance, interpersonal communications within such families tend to be inadequate, frequently following a pattern in which the father seeks success in work and the mother turns to the children for fulfillment and in the process becomes overdirective. Such families are said to be *enmeshed*, meaning that generational boundaries are blurred and that parents and children are deeply involved in each other's lives. Some investigators have suggested that sexual abuse plays a role, but this is controversial. Psychoanalytic interpretation tends to focus on anorexia as the mechanism whereby the patient reestablishes control of her own life independent of parental direction. It is not clear how this sequence might cause the intense fear of being fat that is central to both anorexia and bulimia. It is usually presumed that bulimia is a "backup" response in subjects at risk for anorexia but whose restrictive control fails.

The absence of serious psychiatric disease was previously required for the diagnosis of eating disorders, but depression and obsessive/compulsive behavior frequently accompany the disorders, especially bulimia. These abnormalities may be secondary or preexistent states that predispose to development of the eating disorder.

Some studies have suggested that a genetic component may be involved in the pathogenesis (e.g., increased prevalence of eating disorders in first-degree relatives of probands). Such a genetic component, if it exists, must be minor.

Cultural issues are important. The quest for health and slimness is a powerful force in modern society and may reinforce the fear of fatness in patients with an eating disorder or tip the borderline case into overt disease. Occupation may play a role. Dancers have a prevalence of anorexia nervosa 10 times that of the general population, and athletes, particularly runners, often seek to decrease body fat to very low levels (5 to 7 percent of body weight).

The defects that cause eating disorders remain obscure. There is some evidence of dysfunction in serotonin-mediated neurotransmission, thought to be a component of the satiety-signaling system. The peptide *leptin* (a product of the *ob* gene) is released into blood from adipose tissue and inhibits formation or release in the hypothalamus of neuropeptide Y, a powerful feeding signal. Serotonin may function as a neurotransmitter linking leptin and neuropeptide Y inhibition. Serotonin uptake inhibitors may be helpful in anorexia nervosa and in bulimia nervosa (see "Treatment"). Leptin levels have not been measured in either anorexia or bulimia.

CLINICAL FEATURES (Table 76-3). **Anorexia Nervosa** Anorexia nervosa usually begins before or shortly after puberty but may appear later (usually by the middle twenties). Many patients were overweight in childhood. Emaciation is similar to that in the concentration camp victims of World War II. Despite profound weight loss patients deny hunger, thinness, or fatigue. They are often physically active, and ritualized exercise is common. Frenzied calisthenics or running may follow food intake. There is preoccupation with food, and elaborate meals may be prepared for others. If social circumstances or binge eating causes more intake than usual, vomiting is induced as soon as possible, often in a public restroom. Constipation is common. Amenorrhea usually accompanies or follows weight loss but may appear prior to any physical change. Cold intolerance is presumably due to a defect in regulatory thermogenesis secondary to hypothalamic dysfunction.

In advanced cases bradycardia, hypothermia, and hypotension are present. Body fat is undetectable, and the bones protrude through the skin. Interestingly, breast tissue is often preserved. The skin may be

Table 76-3

The Eating Disorders

	Anorexia Nervosa	Bulimia
Predominant sex	Female	Female
Method of weight control	Restriction of intake	Vomiting
Binge eating	Uncommon	Invariant
Weight at diagnosis	Markedly decreased	Near normal
Ritualized exercise	Usual	Rare
Amenorrhea	100%	50%
Other endocrine changes	Common	Uncommon
Antisocial behavior	Rare	Frequent
Cardiovascular changes (bradycardia, hypotension)	Common	Uncommon
Skin changes (hirsutism, dryness, carotenemia)	Usual	Rare
Hypothermia	Usual	Rare
Edema	+/-	+/-
Medical complications	Hypokalemia, cardiac arrhythmias	Hypokalemia, cardiac arrhythmias, aspiration of gastric contents, esophageal or gastric rupture

NOTE: These features are characteristic of pure anorexia nervosa and pure bulimia. Overlap syndromes occur, and anorexia may evolve to bulimia. The bulimia→anorexia transformation is rare (see text).

dry and scaly and is often yellow due to carotenemia (particularly visible in the palms). Body hair is often increased and is usually of fine, lanugo quality, but frank hirsutism may occur. Parotid glands may be enlarged as in other forms of starvation. Mitral valve prolapse is due to valve–ventricular volume mismatch secondary to starvation-induced decrease in left ventricular volume. Edema in the absence of hypoalbuminemia is thought to be due to failure of extracellular fluid volume to contract proportionately with body mass during weight loss. Because of edema in the legs and parotid enlargement, which gives a fullness to the face, the true state of emaciation may be masked when the patient is dressed.

Laboratory abnormalities include anemia and leukopenia (with hypocellularity of the bone marrow), hypokalemia, and hypoalbuminemia. Serum β-carotene levels tend to be elevated. Vomiting and/or laxative use may cause prerenal azotemia with blood urea nitrogen levels as high as 21 to 25 mmol/L (60 to 70 mg/dL). Renal concentrating ability is impaired, possibly due to blunted responsiveness to vasopressin or diminished release of vasopressin in response to osmotic stimuli. Basal atrial natriuretic peptide levels are high and do not increase with saline infusion. Plasma cholesterol is occasionally high, but triglyceride levels are normal. Glucose tolerance is abnormal as in other forms of starvation. Additional abnormalities include low levels of IgG, IgM, and a variety of complement proteins. Despite these findings, immune function is generally preserved and serious infection is rare. Plasma iron and ceruloplasmin levels are normal, but iron-binding capacity is decreased. Serum zinc and copper are decreased, but levels of these metals are normal in hair. Serum amylase may be increased in the absence of pancreatitis.

Basal levels of luteinizing hormone (LH) and follicle stimulating hormone (FSH) are low when weight loss is severe, and the LH response to luteinizing hormone–releasing hormone (LHRH) is impaired. FSH response to LHRH is normal, although time to peak increase may be delayed. Studies of the 24-h circadian pattern of LH secretion show regression of the mature stage to the pattern characteristic of prepubertal or early pubertal girls, i.e., episodic LH release is missing or occurs only during sleep. These findings presumably account for the amenorrhea. Menses return with weight gain, although the weight required for reinitiation of menstruation may be somewhat higher (about 10 percent) than that needed for the original induction of menarche. Ovulatory menses may be induced in subjects with anorexia nervosa by appropriate treatment with LHRH agonists, suggesting that pituitary gonadotropin release is impaired because of hypothalamic dysfunction. Prolactin levels are normal. Plasma estradiol levels are low. Plasma testosterone is normal in women and low in men with anorexia nervosa.

Growth hormone (GH) may be normal or elevated in the basal state. A rise in GH occurs after injection of thyrotropin releasing hormone (TRH), as in other states with elevated basal levels of GH such as acromegaly, uremia, and protein-calorie malnutrition. Levels of insulin-like growth factor I are low and may contribute to growth hormone elevation via diminished negative feedback. Plasma cortisol levels are high due to increased secretion of corticotropin-releasing hormone from the hypothalamus because of impairment of negative feedback by cortisol. The suppression of plasma cortisol by dexamethasone and the stimulation of GH release by dexamethasone are both abnormal in many patients.

Levels of total thyroxine (T_4) and free T_4 are normal. Triiodothyronine (T_3) concentrations are reduced, while reverse T_3 (rT_3) levels are increased. Basal levels of thyroid stimulating hormone (TSH) and TSH response to TRH are normal. The primary defect in thyroid hormone metabolism is decreased activity of the $5'$-deiodinase that converts T_4 to T_3 and converts rT_3 to diiodothyronine in nonthyroidal tissues; these changes are characteristic of wasting diseases and are not specific for anorexia nervosa. Bone density is decreased; the mechanism has been thought to be estrogen deficiency, but estrogen replacement therapy does not restore bone density. Cortisol excess may contribute to bone loss. Plasma norepinephrine levels are decreased.

Bulimia Nervosa Bulimia, which means "ox-hunger," refers to the episodic, compulsive ingestion of large amounts of food, coupled with awareness that the eating is abnormal, a fear that eating cannot be stopped voluntarily, and feelings of depression at completion of the act. Bulimic patients have a morbid fear of becoming fat. While binge eating may occur in several types of emotional disorders, bulimic patients frequently give a history of overt or cryptic anorexia nervosa, suggesting that bulimia is a variant response to the same factors that cause anorexia nervosa. Episodes of binge eating are followed by induced vomiting, with or without the subsequent ingestion of laxatives. Initially vomiting is induced by placing a toothbrush or fingers in the throat or by ingestion of ipecac, but most patients learn to vomit reflexly. Bloating, flatulence, constipation, abdominal pain, borborygmi, and nausea are common.

Binge eating generally occurs daily; in one study the mean number of episodes per week was 12, ranging from 1 to 46, and the duration of the eating periods averaged 1.2 h but could last as long as 8 h. The amount of food ingested may be enormous, up to 200,000 kJ (50,000 kcal). High-carbohydrate foods are favored, and more than one food is usually eaten. The order of frequency in one report was: ice cream→bread→candy→doughnuts→soft drinks. The term *dietary chaos* describes the eating pattern. Because of the high-carbohydrate content of the diet, dental caries are frequent.

Secrecy about the eating-vomiting sequence is characteristic so that family and friends are often unaware. Stealing is common, and food is the item most often taken. There is a high rate of alcohol and drug abuse. Self-mutilation is not unusual and may be a manifestation of obsessive/compulsive disorder. Depression tends to be more severe than in anorexia nervosa, making suicide a definite risk. Hysterical behavior may occur. Families of patients with bulimia have a higher incidence of affective disorders, alcoholism, and illicit drug use than families of patients with anorexia nervosa.

Despite the close relationship with anorexia nervosa, a number of differences are noted. While many patients with bulimia are thin, weight is usually within 15 percent of the normal range as defined by ideal weight tables. Fluctuating weight is common, with cyclical gains and losses. Some patients are modestly overweight. In contrast to anorexia nervosa, many patients continue to menstruate and may become pregnant. Persistent menstruation probably reflects the absence of extreme weight loss. Sexual activity is greater in bulimic subjects than in those with anorexia.

The physical findings in bulimia nervosa are usually minimal. Scars from self-mutilation may be present and should be looked for in every patient.

The most common laboratory abnormality is hypokalemia secondary to vomiting and laxative use. Metabolic alkalosis may occur if potassium loss is significant. Endocrine changes are less prominent than in anorexia nervosa and may be absent. Some patients have deficient secretion of serotonin and cholecystokinin, the significance of which is unknown. Dexamethasone suppression of plasma cortisol is frequently abnormal. Unlike anorexia nervosa patients, some women with bulimia have low basal prolactin levels and an exaggerated prolactin response to TRH. Serum amylase may be elevated in the absence of pancreatitis in bulimia, as in anorexia nervosa.

COMPLICATIONS Patients with anorexia nervosa are vulnerable to sudden death from ventricular tachyarrhythmias. Electrocardiograms show prolonged QT intervals. The risk of death becomes high when weight declines 35 percent below ideal, probably because of protein deficiency. Complications of bulimia include aspiration, esophageal or gastric rupture, pneumomediastinum, hypokalemia with cardiac arrhythmias, pancreatitis, and ipecac-induced myopathy and/or cardiomyopathy.

PROGNOSIS The course of anorexia nervosa is variable. In long-term follow-up about half of patients achieve normal weight, 20 percent improve but remain underweight, 20 percent continue anorexic, 5 percent become obese, and 6 percent die. Even when weight gain occurs, binge eating, vomiting, and laxative use persist in up to two-thirds of patients. Death is usually due to starvation (cardiac arrhythmias primarily) or suicide. Poor prognostic signs include older age of onset, long duration of illness, bulimia or vomiting, extreme weight loss, and significant depression. Few long-term follow-up reports are available for bulimia. Because the psychiatric disturbance tends to be more severe (suicide occurs at high rates) and because of the medical dangers of gorging, prognosis is worse in bulimia than in anorexia. As many as 40 percent of treated patients remain bulimic after 18 months of treatment; relapse occurs in about two-thirds within a year of recovery. One study reported that about half of patients with bulimia still had an eating disorder after 5 years.

℞ TREATMENT

There is no specific treatment for anorexia nervosa or bulimia. The intense fear of becoming fat and the perceptual disturbance that causes overestimation of body size result in powerful resistance to therapy. The benefits of psychiatric intervention, behavior modification techniques, and group and family therapy are marginal. Supportive care by an understanding physician may accomplish as much as formal psychotherapy. The patient should be seen regularly for a review of weight change, diet, and exercise patterns. It is useful to establish a mutually agreeable explicit contract; for example, if the patient weighs 30 kg and ideal body weight is 52 kg, a goal of 40 kg might be set as a first stage. At every visit the patient should be reassured by the physician that "we will not let you get fat." A calm but realistic review of the dangers of starvation, including sudden death, should be given, coupled with statements like "my job is to help you deal with this illness so that you can have a normal life expectancy with reasonable happiness." The physician must be perceived not as an enemy or a parental surrogate but as an advisor and partner in the struggle.

A similar approach should also be used with bulimic patients. Even if the gorging-regurgitation cycle cannot be stopped, the lesser goals of limiting the load of food ingested (to minimize the chance of aspiration or gastric rupture) and decreasing the frequency of events may be achieved. Because depression and antisocial behavior are more common in bulimia, psychiatric therapy is sometimes required.

The issue of drug therapy is not settled. There is a general belief that antidepressants are helpful in bulimia nervosa but not anorexia nervosa. The serotonin uptake inhibitor fluoxetine may have an advantage over other antidepressants, and some reports suggest it is useful in anorexia as well. If used, a dose of 60 mg/d is suggested in adults instead of the usual dosages recommended for depression. Potassium supplementation may be necessary in vomiters or laxative users. Treatment of endocrine abnormalities is ordinarily not required since all revert if weight gain is achieved.

Hospitalization may be a lifesaving measure with severe anorexia nervosa. As noted above, sudden death may occur at weights more than 35 percent below ideal, particularly if weight loss has been rapid. Hypokalemia, hypotension, and prerenal azotemia due to volume depletion are other indications for hospitalization. A nasogastric tube may be required, but it is better to persuade the patient to eat. Total parenteral nutrition is rarely indicated. During initial hospitalization the patient should not be allowed to eat alone. Instruction about nutrition, occupational therapy, group therapy with the family, and individual psychotherapy may be useful. The "safety" of eating and assurances that obesity will not result should be emphasized repeatedly. Some specialists feel that all seriously affected anorexia patients benefit from initial hospitalization, but this view is not universal. Hospitalization for bulimic subjects is normally required only for medical complications (e.g., aspiration).

Treatment of the anorexia-bulimia syndromes is a long-term proposition, rife with failure, and requires perseverance by the patient, family, and physician.

BIBLIOGRAPHY

FOSTER DW: Eating disorders: Obesity, anorexia nervosa and bulimia nervosa in *Williams Textbook of Endocrinology*, 8th ed, JD Wilson, DW Foster (eds). Philadelphia, Saunders, 1992, p 1335

GARFINKEL PE et al: Bulimia nervosa in a Canadian community sample: Prevalence and comparison of subgroups. Am J Psychiatry 152:1052, 1995
HERZOG DB, COPELAND PM: Eating disorders. N Engl J Med 313:295, 1985
——— et al: Outcome in anorexia nervosa and bulimia nervosa. A review of the literature. J Nerv Ment Dis 176:131, 1988
ISNER JM et al: Anorexia nervosa and sudden death. Ann Intern Med 102:49, 1985
KAYE WH, WELTZIN TE: Neurochemistry of bulimia nervosa. J Clin Psychiatry Suppl 52:21, 1991
LEVY AB: Neuroendocrine profile in bulimia nervosa. Biol Psychiatry 25:98, 1989
LOVE L, GOLD PW: The hypothalamic-pituitary-adrenal axis in anorexia nervosa and bulimia nervosa: Pathophysiologic implications. Adv Pediatr 38:287, 1991
LUCAS ARE et al: Anorexia nervosa in Rochester, Minnesota: A 45-year study. Mayo Clin Proc 63:433, 1988
MITCHELL JE et al: Medical complications and medical management of bulimia. Ann Intern Med 107:71, 1987
NEWMAN MM, HALMI KA: The endocrinology of anorexia nervosa and bulimia nervosa. Endocrin Metab Clin North Am 7:195, 1988
SULLIVAN PF: Mortality in anorexia nervosa. Am J Pychiatry 152:1073, 1995
THIEL A et al: Obsessive-compulsive disorder among patients with anorexia nervosa and bulimia nervosa. Am J Psychiatry 152:72, 1995
WOODSIDE DB: A review of anorexia nervosa and bulimia nervosa. Curr Probl Pediatr 25:67, 1995

77 *Cheryl L. Rock, Ann M. Coulston, Mack T. Ruffin IV*

DIET THERAPY

Diet is an important component of health. Nutrition education and good eating patterns are essential for good health, nutritional problems contribute substantially to preventable illness and premature death, and alteration in food intake or dietary pattern is often an essential part of disease management. Nutritional requirements may be modified by disease, and dietary problems have an impact on the quality of life and the outcome of both acute and chronic diseases. For example, diet therapy plays a role both in the prevention of atherosclerosis and in the management of advanced coronary artery disease. Furthermore, major nutritional consequences can result from the treatment of disease, but nitrition and diet therapy are often of concern to the patient and the family, even when there is no solid evidence to support such therapy. In general, the usefulness of both new and traditional therapeutic diets deserves additional scientific scrutiny. As is true with all components of care, diet therapy should be soundly based and should be monitored to assess its impact on nutrition and health.

The first concept in diet therapy is that dietary intake or nutritional requirements may be altered as a result of disease or by the treatment (see Chap. 73), and the altered needs must be met by dietary modifications to prevent malnutrition. The second concept is that nutritional intervention can be critical for prevention, management, or treatment of disease. A complicating factor is that people eat food, rather than nutrients, so that the practical and psychosocial aspects of diet modification must be considered in making recommendations. Diet therapy is rarely an innocuous intervention, and adverse physical and psychological effects can result from inappropriate or ill-advised modification of the diet.

The aims of this chapter are to summarize the basic principles of diet therapy, to describe its application in common conditions, and to outline strategies for enhancing adherence to dietary recommendations.

BASIC DIETARY RECOMMENDATIONS

Variety, balance, and moderation are the basic components of dietary adequacy. The food guidance system developed by the U.S. Department of Agriculture and the Department of Health and Human Services is based on the "Dietary Guidelines for Americans," which emphasizes eating more grain products, vegetables, and fruits; eating less fat, saturated fat, and cholesterol; and choosing a diet moderate in sugars and sodium. By grouping foods into categories based on nutrient content, these guidelines can be translated into dietary prescriptions that meet nutritional requirements at different levels of energy intake (Table 77-1). The lower level of energy intake is usually appropriate for sedentary women and many older adults; the moderate level is for teenage girls, active women, and sedentary men; and the higher level is for teenage boys, many active men, and very active women. Alcohol contributes energy but little else nutritionally, and consumption should be no more than one to two drinks per day in adults who choose to drink.

Table 77-1

Sample Diets to Meet Daily Nutrient Requirements
and Dietary Guidelines

Food Group Category	Level of Energy Intake		
	Low, 1600 kcal/d	Moderate, 2200 kcal/d	High, 2800 kcal/d
Bread/starch group servings 1 slice bread, 1 ounce ready-to-eat cereal, 1/2 cup cooked rice or pasta	6	9	11
Vegetable group servings 1 cup raw leafy vegetables, 1/2 cup other vegetables, cooked or chopped raw	3	4	5
Fruit group servings 1 medium piece, 1/2 cup chopped, cooked, or canned fruit	2	3	4
Milk group servings 1 cup milk or yogurt	2–3*	2–3*	2–3*
Meat or meat substitute group† (ounces)	5	6	7
Total fat‡ (grams)	53	73	93
Total added sugars§ (teaspoons)	6	12	18

* Women who are pregnant or breast feeding, teenagers, and young adults to age 24 need 3 servings.
† Meat group amounts are in total ounces. One egg, 1/2 cup cooked dry beans, or 2 tablespoons peanut butter are equivalent to 1 ounce cooked lean meat, poultry, or fish.
‡ Fats are mainly contributed by choices within the milk and meat groups and from added fats (1 teaspoon, considered one serving, provides 5 g fat).
§ Sugars are mainly contributed by choices within the bread, fruit, and milk groups and from added sugars.
SOURCE: Adapted from Human Nutrition Information Service, US Department of Agriculture, *The Food Guide Pyramid*, Hyattsville, MD US Dept of Agriculture, 1992

Table 77-2

Average Nutrient Values per Serving

Food Group	Energy, kcal	Carbohydrate, g	Protein, g	Fat, g
Bread/starch	80	15	3	1 or less
Vegetable	25	5	2	—
Fruit	60	15	—	—
Milk				
Skim	90	12	8	0–3
Low-fat	120	12	8	5
Whole	150	12	8	8
Meat and meat substitutes				
Very lean	35	—	7	0–1
Lean	55	—	7	3
Medium-fat	75	—	7	5
High-fat	100	—	7	8
Fat	45	—	—	5

SOURCE: Adapted from The American Diabetes Association, Inc, The American Dietetic Association, *Exchange Lists for Weight Management*, Chicago, American Dietetic Association, 1995

This food group system can also form the basis of meal planning in diet therapy because energy and macronutrient content can be estimated on the basis of standardized serving sizes (Table 77-2).

SPECIFIC DIET THERAPIES

CARDIOVASCULAR DISEASE (See also Chaps. 242 and 341) Atherosclerotic cardiovascular disease (CVD) has multiple etiologies and involves a variety of risk factors. Modifiable risk factors include smoking, hypertension, hyperlipidemia, glucose intolerance, obesity, and physical inactivity. Elevation of plasma cholesterol, especially of low-density lipoprotein (LDL) cholesterol, is a major risk factor that can be at least partially modified by dietary intervention. The National Cholesterol Education Program (NCEP) has identified low risk as a total serum cholesterol concentration <5.2 mmol/L (200 mg/dL), moderate risk as 5.2 to 6.2 mmol/L (200 to 239 mg/dL), and high risk as >6.2 mmol/L (240 mg/dL). Hypertriglyceridemia and low levels of high-density lipoprotein (HDL) cholesterol are also risk factors. The basic diet therapy for patients with elevations of LDL cholesterol involves reduction in the intake of total and saturated fat to <30 percent and <10 percent of total calories, respectively. Sources of saturated fat include animal fats (fatty meat, poultry skin, butterfat) and some vegetable fats (coconut oil, cocoa butter, and palm oil). Cholesterol, found only in foods of animal origin, is not as important a determinant of plasma cholesterol as is saturated fat. Nevertheless, dietary intake of cholesterol should be <300 mg/d. In patients whose serum cholesterol does not respond to this degree of diet modification, the NCEP step 2 diets, which involve a greater restriction of saturated fat and cholesterol intake, should be prescribed (Table 77-3).

Obesity is also a risk factor for CVD (see also Chap. 75). For every excess kilogram of body weight, endogenous cholesterol synthesis is increased by 20 mg/d, so that with 10 kg of excess weight, 200 mg of additional cholesterol enters the body pool daily to be catabolized, excreted, or stored. Obesity is also associated with hypertriglyceridemia, decreased HDL-cholesterol, increased production of LDL from very low density lipoproteins (VLDL), and increased hepatic synthesis of VLDL. The insulin resistance associated with obesity and the resulting hyperinsulinemia improve with even modest (5 to 10 kg) weight reduction.

In some patients restriction of total dietary fat lowers HDL cholesterol and raises serum triglyceride concentrations. A decrease in HDL cholesterol is a cause for concern, especially when the baseline level is low [<0.9 mmol/L (35 mg/dL)]; the phenomenon appears to be related primarily to increased intake of carbohydrate and possibly to increased polyunsaturated fats. Monounsaturated oils (e.g., canola, olive, peanut) maintain HDL cholesterol and lower LDL cholesterol concentration, and when saturated fat is reduced to <10 percent of calories and monounsaturated fats make up the remainder of fat, a significant reduction in total cholesterol can be achieved without decreasing the total fat intake or increasing the proportion of calories

Table 77-3

Dietary Modifications for Hypercholesterolemia

Dietary Component	Step 1 Diet	Step 2 Diet
Total fat	<30% of kcal	<30% of kcal
Saturated fat	8–10% of kcal	<7% of kcal
Polyunsaturated fat	<10% of kcal	<10% of kcal
Monounsaturated fat	10–15% of kcal	10–15% of kcal
Carbohydrate	50–60% of kcal	50–60% of kcal
Protein	10–20% of kcal	10–20% of kcal
Cholesterol	<300 mg/d	<200 mg/d
Total energy intake	To achieve and maintain desirable weight	To achieve and maintain desirable weight

SOURCE: Adapted from US Department of Health and Human Services, *Step by Step: Eating to Lower Your High Blood Cholesterol*, publication no. 94-2920, Bethesda, MD, National Heart, Lung, and Blood Institute, 1994 from carbohydrate. These patients should be advised to substitute monounsaturated for saturated fat.

It has been suggested that trans-fatty acids are a risk factor for CVD. Trans-fatty acids are formed when vegetable oils are hydrogenated to be solid at room temperature. Margarine is the most significant source of trans-fatty acids in the U.S. diet. Consumption of trans-fatty acids in amounts >7 percent of calories may cause a significant increase in total and LDL cholesterol levels and a decrease in HDL cholesterol. However, the effect is a graded one, and intakes typical of the United States (≤4 percent of calories as trans-fatty acids) do not appear to have a deleterious effect. Consequently, patients need not be concerned about this issue at present.

Fish oils with polyunsaturated fats of the omega-3 type have potent triglyceride-lowering effects but do not lower LDL cholesterol. Any antiatherogenic effects of fish and fish oil consumption are probably mediated through the antithrombotic and anti-inflammatory actions of omega-3 fatty acids. Omega-3 fatty acids are sometimes useful in the treatment of hypertriglyceridemia (see Chap. 341).

Effective diet therapy for CVD should not rely on a "good food versus bad food" approach but should aim to modify the eating habits to attain desirable body weight and to reduce intake of saturated fatty acids. There are approaches to fit most lifestyles and to enhance compliance to life-long dietary changes necessary to the achieve this goal. To prevent cardiovascular disease, diet therapy is the first line of intervention, and pharmacologic agents are only adjunctive therapy.

Hypertension (See also Chap. 246) Elevated blood pressure increases the risk for CVD and stroke. Although not all hypertensive patients are salt-sensitive, dietary sodium should be reduced to 2000 mg/d routinely. Even modest amounts of weight reduction in the obese may reduce elevated blood pressure.

Congestive Heart Failure (See also Chap. 233) Cardiac cachexia is a type of malnutrition that occurs in patients with congestive heart failure and is due to reduced cardiac output, small bowel changes that lead to malabsorption, anorexia, and hypermetabolism secondary to increased work of breathing. Dietary intake is limited because of fatigue and early satiety with eating. Diet therapy involves the provision of adequate calories, protein, and other nutrients and the restriction of fluid (to 1 to 1.5 L/d) and sodium (to 1000 to 2000 mg/d).

CANCER Dietary factors influence survival rates in patients with certain malignancies, such as breast cancer. A possible link between diet and the risk for cancer has also been suggested but has been difficult to prove for cancers of the breast, colon, and prostate. For example, dietary factors that may increase risk for cancer, such as fat, tend to vary inversely with potentially protective factors, such as carotenoids. In addition, people on high-fat diets usually eat fewer vegetables and fruits and thus consume less of the protective factors contributed by those foods. As another example, dietary fat appears to increase and fiber appears to decrease the risk for colon cancer, and these usually have inverse concentrations in foods. Table 77-4 summarizes dietary practices that may reduce risk for some cancers.

Weight loss with cancer has many causes. The metabolic and

energy requirements of the tumor may promote weight loss by the host. Circulating factors (e.g., cytokines) originating either in the host or tumor are also probably involved in weight loss, but decreased food intake, frequently associated with anorexia, plays a major role in most patients. Indeed, many cancer patients have manifestations of malnutrition at the time of initial diagnosis, as evidenced by weight loss, weakness, anemia, and abnormalities in protein, lipid, and carbohydrate metabolism. However, in some cancers (breast and prostate cancer, melanoma) weight loss occurs late in the course.

The effects of chemotherapy, immunotherapy, and radiotherapy on dietary intake and nutritional status include nausea and vomiting, diarrhea, constipation, change in taste, sore or dry mouth, and dental problems. Surgical interventions may cause difficulties in chewing and swallowing, dumping syndrome, or malabsorption. Anorexia is the most common problem in the cancer patient, and agents such as megestrol acetate, glucocorticoids, hydrazine sulfate, and dronabinol may enhance appetite to some degree. Individual patients sometimes have distinct circadian patterns of appetite and anorexia that are identifiable by careful evaluation of food preferences and eating patterns. Dietary strategies to increase appetite or intake include providing salty foods, nutrient-dense beverages such as fruit juice, and easy-to-eat snacks. Attractive meals and snacks should be provided when appetite is good, and liquid food supplements can be administered when appetite is poor.

Nausea and vomiting in cancer patients may be related to the primary tumor (i.e., obstruction), to metastatic disease (i.e., central nervous system involvement), or to chemotherapy. In patients with reduced capacity of the stomach, small frequent feedings may circumvent early satiety and improve nutrition. One strategy that reduces both food aversions and nausea during chemotherapy is the ingestion of a diet composed primarily of low-stimuli (i.e., odorless, colorless) foods served cold or at room temperature. Mucositis and stomatitis in patients with head and neck cancers may be managed with diets that minimize oral irritation and ease swallowing difficulties. Diarrhea can also be minimized with dietary modifications (discussed below).

Criteria for instituting nutrition support (see Chap. 78) in cancer patients are progressive weight loss or the threat of serious weight loss. Although some features of cancer cachexia may be improved by parenteral or enteral feeding, few studies document improvement in body composition or disease outcome. One exception may be in patients undergoing surgery for cancer because the risks for complications of surgery are increased in the malnourished.

DIABETES MELLITUS (See also Chap. 334) Diabetes mellitus results from an absolute or relative lack of insulin, which regulates key aspects of carbohydrate, protein, and lipid metabolism, and diabetes is associated with accelerated atherogenesis and a high incidence of CVD. About 10 percent of patients have type 1 diabetes, manifested by a profound deficiency of endogenous insulin, and most of the rest have type 2 diabetes, in which endogenous insulin is synthesized but is insufficient to overcome peripheral insulin resistance. All patients with diabetes require diet therapy in conjunction with medication and exercise to achieve optimal control of blood glucose and blood lipids. The aim of therapy is to prevent acute complications (primarily hypoglycemia and hyperglycemia) and reduce the risk of long-term complications such as ophthalmopathy, renal failure, cardiovascular disease, and neuropathy. The major nutritional issues are (1) the distribution of the calorie-containing nutrients, carbohydrate, protein, and fat; (2) the impact of dietary carbohydrate and fat on plasma glucose and lipid concentrations; and (3) achievement of a healthful body weight (which means weight reduction for many patients).

Diabetes control improves with even modest weight loss (4 to 9 kg) in patients who are overweight (body mass index >30 kg/m^2). A moderate calorie restriction (250 to 500 kcal less than the daily energy requirement), coupled with an increase in physical activity, appears to be the best strategy. The improved metabolic control with such a regimen is probably due to a combination of decreased food intake,

Table 77-4

Dietary Recommendations that may Reduce Cancer Risk

1. Eat plenty of vegetables and fruits, especially cabbage family (cruciferous) vegetables, deeply pigmented fruits and vegetables containing β-carotene and other carotenoids, and fruits and vegetables rich in vitamin C. Aim for at least 5 servings of vegetables and fruits per day.
2. Eat plenty of high-fiber foods, such as whole grains, fruits, and vegetables, aiming for a daily fiber intake of 20–30 g/d.
3. Avoid obesity and aim for weight control through exercise and lower energy intake.
4. Decrease fat intake to 30% or less of total energy consumed.
5. Minimize consumption of salt-cured, smoked, and nitrite-cured foods, such as bacon, ham, and hot dogs.
6. Limit or eliminate alcohol intake.

SOURCE: Adapted from RR Butrum et al, Am J Clin Nutr 48:888, 1988; and Department of Health and Human Services, publication no. 95-3862, Bethesda, MD, National Cancer Institute, 1995 increased insulin sensitivity, and return of hepatic glucose production to normal, even when optimal body weight is not achieved.

For patients with diabetes, 10 to 20 percent of energy intake should consist of protein to ensure normal growth and development in children and maintain normal protein stores in adults. This intake is similar to the average protein intake in the United States of 14 to 18 percent of energy intake and is in accordance with the "recommended dietary allowance" of 0.8 g/kg body weight for adults. The intake of protein may accelerate the rate of renal failure, but a protein intake of 10 percent of caloric intake is tolerated by most diabetic patients. When nephropathy has progressed to end-stage renal disease, lower protein intakes (e.g., 0.6 g/kg body weight) may be necessary if patients are not on chronic dialysis (discussed below).

Carbohydrate and fat make up the remainder of the energy intake. Patients with diabetes have a dyslipidemia characterized by elevated total triglycerides and reduced HDL cholesterol concentrations. The hypertriglyceridemia is due to an increased hepatic production of triglyceride-rich VLDL and may be associated with increased circulating levels of small dense LDL. Because of the association of CVD with diabetes mellitus, dietary recommendations traditionally emphasized a low-fat (especially low saturated fat), high-carbohydrate intake, a diet that may enhance hypertriglyceridemia and lower HDL cholesterol. An alternative program is to replace saturated fat with monounsaturated fat, rather than with carbohydrate. This approach aims at adjusting dietary carbohydrate and fat to achieve the desired blood glucose and lipid concentrations, rather than to use a uniform, preconceived intake as a goal. Sugars and starches have the same effect on blood glucose, and the diet should contain both types of carbohydrate. Finally, diet therapy for patients with diabetes should be individualized according to lifestyle, cultural eating habits, and patient motivation (Table 77-5).

CHRONIC RENAL FAILURE (See also Chap. 271) Diet therapy plays an essential role in the management of all stages of renal failure but is of particular importance in end-stage renal disease. Patients with chronic renal failure are particularly susceptible to malnutrition due to inadequate intake and altered nutrient metabolism. Without intervention, vitamin D deficiency may cause decreased calcium absorption, hyperparathyroidism, and osteodystrophy. Dialysis itself depletes nutrients, and dialysis patients are at risk for deficiencies of vitamin B_6, vitamin C, and folate; elevated plasma vitamin A levels and increased or decreased body stores of vitamin A; and abnormalities in carnitine metabolism.

Excess protein intake increases glomerular filtration and can accelerate loss of renal function; conversely, dietary protein restriction may retard the progression of renal disease. Energy intake must be adequate

(35 kcal/kg per day) to spare the protein that is consumed and minimize endogenous protein catabolism and to reduce the risk of developing malnutrition. Patients with progressive renal failure may benefit from a diet providing 0.55 to 0.60 g protein/kg per day, including 0.35 g/kg per day of high-biological-value protein (animal proteins such as meat, eggs, and fish). If very low protein diets (0.28 g/kg per day of protein) are tried in patients with advanced renal failure, it is necessary to supplement them with amino acids or keto acids to prevent malnutrition. Reduced dietary phosphorus (5 to 10 mg/kg per day of phosphorus) is an inherent feature of a low-protein diet. More rigid dietary phosphorus restriction is necessary only if the serum phosphorus level is elevated. Restriction of dietary potassium is usually unnecessary for predialysis patients (unless hyperkalemia is present). Restriction of sodium intake to 1000 to 3000 mg/d is usually sufficient to control edema and hypertension of renal failure. Both nondialyzed and dialyzed patients with chronic renal failure often have elevated blood lipid levels. It is prudent to restrict dietary fat (<30 percent of energy), saturated fat (<10 percent energy), and cholesterol (<300 mg/d), although evidence that this strategy reduces lipid levels or mortality is limited.

Patients with end-stage renal disease on dialysis should be given increased dietary protein (1.0 to 1.4 g/kg per day for hemodialysis and 1.2 to 1.4 g/kg per day for peritoneal dialysis patients), along with adequate energy intake (approximately 35 kcal/kg per day) to compensate for the catabolic effects of dialysis. Indeed, hemodialysis patients consuming higher protein intakes (0.93 to 1.29 g/kg per day) may have lower mortality rates than those with lower intake (0.63 g/kg per day or less). Patients treated with continuous ambulatory or cycling peritoneal dialysis lose large amounts of protein in the dialysate, and glucose is absorbed from the peritoneal dialysate and must be included in calculations of energy intake.

Phosphorus retention with hyperphosphatemia occurs in end-stage renal disease, and management of patients on hemodialysis or peritoneal dialysis usually requires both phosphorus restriction (≤17 mg/kg per day) and administration of phosphorus-binding compounds. To maintain calcium balance, patients undergoing dialysis require 1400 to 1600 mg/d of calcium from the diet plus supplementation. To prevent hyperkalemia, potassium intake usually must be limited to 1500 to 2700 mg/d in patients treated with hemodialysis. Patients receiving peritoneal dialysis generally do not have elevated serum potassium levels, so that dietary potassium restriction is rarely necessary. Restrictions of sodium (1000 to 1500 mg/d) and fluids (700 to 1500 mL/d) are generally necessary for hemodialysis patients because they are usually oliguric or anuric, but achieving this degree of restriction is difficult for most patients. Higher intake of sodium and fluid (up to 6000 to 8000 mg/d of sodium and 3000 mL/d of fluids) is permitted for patients on peritoneal dialysis because the dialysate can be adjusted to remove the excess. Finally, supplementation with water-soluble vitamins and the active metabolite of vitamin D is necessary in end-stage renal disease, because of the likelihood of deficiency due to a restricted diet, excess losses, and metabolic abnormalities. Table 77-6 summarizes modifications of protein and minerals in the dietary management of chronic renal failure.

Table 77-5

Diet Therapy for Diabetes Mellitus

1. Maintain as near-normal levels of blood glucose as possible by balancing food intake with medications (insulin or oral agents) and activity.
2. Achieve optimal serum lipid levels.
3. Provide calories to maintain or achieve reasonable weight for adults or to promote recovery from catabolic illness. Promote weight loss in obese patients.
4. Aim for protein intake of 10–20% and saturated fat of <10% of daily calories.
5. Distribute the remaining 60–70% of daily calories between carbohydrate and fat based on treatment goals for blood glucose and lipid levels. Emphasize monounsaturated fats over polyunsaturated fats.
6. Sucrose and other "simple sugars" may be substituted for other carbohydrates.
7. As in the general population, aim for 20–35 g/d of dietary fiber.
8. If hypertension is present, limit sodium to <2400 mg/d.
9. Limit alcoholic beverages to <2/d.
10. Vitamin and mineral supplementation is unnecessary for most patients.

SOURCE: Adapted from The American Diabetes Association, Inc, The American Dietetic Association, J Am Diet Assoc 94:504, 1994

Table 77-6

Dietary Modifications for Chronic Renal Failure

Dietary Factor	Predialysis	Hemodialysis	Peritoneal Dialysis
Protein	0.55–0.60 g/kg per day (0.35 g/kg per day high biological value)	1.0–1.4 g/kg per day	1.2–1.4 g/kg per day
Calcium	1400–1600 mg/d	1400–1600 mg/d	1400–1600 mg/d
Phosphorus	5–10 mg/kg per day	≤17 mg/kg per day	≤17 mg/kg per day
Sodium	1000–3000 mg/d	1000–1500 mg/d	Remove excess with the dialysate
Potassium	Unnecessary unless hyperkalemic	1500–2700 mg/d	Rarely necessary

GASTROINTESTINAL DISORDERS Gastrointestinal disorders are nearly always associated with altered nutrient intake or utilization.

Lactose Intolerance (See also Chap. 285) About 25 percent of adults in the United States have lactose intolerance, as manifested by abdominal distention, flatulence, and diarrhea after the consumption of moderate to large amounts of lactose-containing foods. The disorder is managed by restricting the ingestion of these foods. Dairy products are the primary source of dietary lactose, but aged cheese (because of very low lactose content), yogurt with active cultures, and dairy products with added lactose-cleaving microbial enzymes are tolerated by most affected individuals. Indeed, most lactose-tolerant individuals have negligible symptoms when intake is limited to the equivalent of one cup of milk (approximately 12 g lactase) or less per day.

Diarrhea The symptomatic management of diarrhea involves volume repletion with isotonic saline, lactose restriction ($<$5 g per meal), and reduced intake of fat ($<$40 g/d) and fiber. Very restrictive diets, such as diets limited to bananas, rice, applesauce, and tea or toast, are not recommended because extreme dietary restriction may compromise recovery of gut mucosa. A cycle of malabsorption and diarrhea can result, especially in the immunologically compromised subject.

Constipation High-fiber diets, especially those with whole grain breads and cereals and bran products, are useful in the prevention and management of constipation. The typical U.S. diet provides $<$12 g/d of fiber, whereas a high-fiber diet provides 20 to 35 g/d of fiber from whole grain bread products, fruits, and vegetables. Very high intake of dietary fiber from supplements ($>$35 g/d) can cause gaseous distention, increase the risk for bowel obstruction, and cause malabsorption of micronutrients.

Gastroesophageal Reflux Dietary modifications may be useful in the management of gastroesophageal reflux. Because they decrease lower esophageal sphincter pressure, chocolate, fatty foods, and carminatives (e.g., spearmint, peppermint) should be avoided. Orange juice, tomato juice, and coffee should also be avoided because they are direct mucosal irritants. Weight loss for the obese, the use of drugs such as omeprozole (see Chap. 284), and allowing 3 h between meal ingestion and recumbency are other helpful strategies.

Irritable Bowel Syndrome Excessive intake of foods or beverages sweetened with fructose or sorbitol or of lactose-containing foods can produce symptoms suggestive of irritable bowel syndrome and may aggravate the syndrome if present. If constipation is present, a high-fiber diet may be useful, although studies evaluating the therapeutic effects of fiber (from the diet or from supplements) have yielded inconsistent results. Careful patient records of food intake in relation to symptoms make it possible to design individual diet therapy to control symptoms and ensure adequacy of nutrient intake (see Chap. 287).

Inflammatory Bowel Disease Weight loss is significant in 65 to 75 percent of patients with Crohn's disease and in 18 to 62 percent of patients with ulcerative colitis. Reduced dietary intake is a major cause of weight loss and is due to anorexia and pain with eating. Individual diet counseling may result in improved nutrition in these patients.

Protein-losing enteropathy and malabsorption of fat, fat-soluble vitamins, vitamin B_{12}, and minerals occur rarely in this disorder, but intestinal losses of nutrients (such as zinc with diarrhea and iron with blood loss) are more common. Food-drug interactions are also of importance: for example, sulfasalazine is a competitive inhibitor of folate absorption, and glucocorticoids decrease calcium absorption, cause osteopenia, and promote protein catabolism.

Dietary modifications useful in the management of these disorders include reduced intake of lactose (if intolerance is suggested by history) and fat ($<$70 g/d or adjusted to patient tolerance, particularly if steatorrhea is present) and sufficient intake of energy and protein to promote tissue healing. Dietary fiber should not be restricted unless partial bowel obstruction is present. Formula diets that have been useful in patients with inflammatory bowel disease (see Chap. 78) contain proteins that have been predigested to amino acids, carbohydrates, and

essential nutrients. The rationale is to reduce the exposure of the damaged gut wall to intact proteins that would promote a secondary immune response and at the same time provide adequate energy and nutrients. In practice, the liquid diets that have been evaluated in these disorders include those containing short-chain peptides and moderate amounts of lipids, and blenderized foods may have some usefulness. Although a reduction in symptoms has been observed in some studies, enteral nutrition support is inferior to glucocorticoids in inducing remission in active Crohn's disease. Intolerance to the formulas, especially when delivered orally, further limits their usefulness in some patients.

LIVER DISEASE The liver plays a central role in carbohydrate, lipid, and protein metabolism. Liver failure causes both decreased protein synthesis and enhanced protein breakdown, which, together with anorexia and reduced food intake, can lead to severe protein-energy malnutrition and limit the capacity for regeneration and functional recovery of the liver. Generally, the more severe the malnutrition, the worse the prognosis. In patients with massive hepatic necrosis or portal hypertension, a large load of protein nitrogen in the diet may promote or exacerbate hepatic encephalopathy, but severe dietary restriction of protein intake should not be imposed unnecessarily.

Patients with stable disease or in early hepatic failure benefit by receiving at least 1 g/kg per day of protein with adequate energy for efficient use of protein sources (at least 30 kcal/kg per day). Diet counseling should be provided to patients with stable chronic liver disease so as to maintain adequate dietary intake and prevent nutritional depletion. With progression of liver failure, modification in dietary protein intake may be necessary because of encephalopathy. Plant proteins tend to be better tolerated than animal proteins, possibly because plants contain less nonprotein nitrogen. Studies of the effects of specialized formula diets enriched in branched-chain amino acids on amino acid and ammonia levels and on hepatic encephalopathy have yielded inconsistent results. When prescribing dietary protein, the best approach is to determine patient tolerance by monitoring neurologic status, using 1 g/kg per day of protein as a goal for intake. As a minimum, 0.50 to 0.75 g/kg per day of protein, or approximately 40 g/d, is suggested; more severe protein restriction may promote the catabolism of body protein (see Chaps. 298 and 299).

In some patients with liver disease, dietary fat restriction ($<$30 g/d) may also be necessary, because of malabsorption and steatorrhea. To improve energy intake, restriction of long-chain fatty acids can be combined with the use of medium-chain triglyceride preparations, which can be absorbed without bile salts. Water-miscible forms of fat-soluble vitamins and other essential micronutrients should be given. Sodium restriction ($<$2 g/d) is usually necessary due to edema and ascites, but very low levels ($<$1 g/d) are not well tolerated and limit food choices, thus increasing the risk of malnutrition. Regular bread products, dairy products, and all processed foods (unless special low-sodium products) must be severely restricted to achieve $<$1000 mg/d of sodium.

CHRONIC NEUROLOGIC DISORDERS **Parkinson's Disease** Patients with Parkinson's disease are at risk of nutritional problems because of the effects of this disease on the gastrointestinal tract. Varying degrees of dysphagia, with or without aspiration, and constipation contribute to nutritional depletion in these patients. Diet counseling is recommended to ensure that the diet is adequate in the early stages of the disease.

The decrease in clinical efficacy of levodopa, which occurs commonly in the course of Parkinson's disease and which results in motor fluctuations and increased disability, may be improved by changing the timing of protein intake. The interaction between protein intake and clinical response appears to be due to inhibition by neutral amino acids in plasma of the uptake of levodopa into the central nervous system. Therefore, daytime restriction of dietary protein ($<$7 g protein intake prior to the evening meal) reduces unpredictable motor-response fluctuations during the active and productive periods of the day. At the evening meal, increased amounts of protein-rich foods can supply the daily requirements. Motivated individuals who adhere to this regimen usually improve and have no adverse effects on nutrition status, but this strategy increases the risk of malnutrition when regular diets are only marginally adequate.

Alzheimer's Disease Patients with Alzheimer's disease have more risk factors and more indications of poor nutritional status than elderly control populations. Diminished olfactory function causes poor eating habits and increases the risk of eating spoiled food, and choking and food refusal are common. Agitation and wandering increase energy requirements. Use of semi-solid or other nutritional supplements is one means of increasing nutrient intake in these patients. During the later stages patients often become unable to feed themselves and require assistance in eating. Throughout the course, monitoring of dietary intake is necessary to prevent weight loss and worsening of cognitive and physiologic function due to malnutrition and to prevent dehydration, aspiration, and increased risk of infectious illness.

PULMONARY DISEASE Malnutrition is common in patients with chronic obstructive pulmonary disease (COPD). Diaphragmatic muscle mass and area are reduced in association with weight loss in malnourished COPD patients when compared with patients with COPD who are of normal weight. The reduced tidal volume, carbon dioxide production, and oxygen consumption of malnourished individuals may predispose to pulmonary infections. Patients with COPD and weight loss have a shorter survival than patients with stable weight. Limited evidence suggests that improved nutrition improves respiratory muscle strength and endurance, even over the short term.

Patients with COPD have a >10 percent increase in basal energy requirements, associated with the increased work of breathing due to both increased pulmonary resistance and reduced efficiency of respiratory muscles. However, inadvertent provision of excessive energy intake can result in more harm than good. Increased carbon dioxide production resulting from overfeeding with excess energy (1.5 to 2.25 times the resting energy expenditure), especially carbohydrate loads, can cause respiratory distress. The prescription of low-carbohydrate, high-fat diets and energy-dense enteral formulas (containing 2 kcal/L) has been useful. These diets, which provide 50 to 55 percent of energy from fat and 25 to 35 percent of energy from carbohydrate, promote improvement in pulmonary function as compared to high-carbohydrate, low-fat diets (e.g., 74 percent of energy from carbohydrate, 9 percent of energy from fat). A diet containing 1.2 times the estimated resting energy expenditure is a beginning point in the provision of adequate calories, with protein at a level of 1.2 to 1.5 g/kg per day. However, individual diet therapy is necessary to avoid under- or overfeeding of these patients.

TRANSITIONAL AND OTHER DIETS Modifications in the consistency and texture of the diet can be important (see Table 77-7), especially for the hospitalized patient. A *clear liquid diet* provides an oral source of fluids, energy, and nutrients; leaves minimal residue in the gastrointestinal tract; and is used to prepare for diagnostic procedures, as an initial feeding following surgery or intravenous feeding, or during acute gastrointestinal dysfunction. These diets are not nutritionally adequate without nutritional supplements and should not be used for more than 3 days. A *full liquid diet* is liquid or semiliquid at room temperature and is prescribed for patients with chewing difficulties or as an intermediate progression to solid foods after surgery or intravenous feeding; it also may not be nutritionally adequate without enteral nutritional supplements. A *pureed diet*, which includes strained, pureed, and liquid foods, is useful for patients who are edentulous or have other problems that limit the ability to chew foods. A *soft diet* consists of foods that can be chewed more easily than those in a regular diet and includes tender meat and soft solids, while omitting raw fruits and vegetables and coarse breads and cereals. Pureed and soft diets are nutritionally adequate provided a sufficient quantity and variety of the foods are consumed.

Diets that eliminate specific dietary constituents, such as oxalates (for management of hyperoxaluria), galactose (for management of galactosemia), and gluten (for management of celiac disease), have also been described. For more details of these and other specific diet therapies the reader is referred to the diet manuals listed in the Bibliography.

Drug-Nutrient Interactions Diet modifications may be necessary because of drug-nutrient interactions. Certain foods or meal patterns can alter drug effectiveness, and conversely, drugs can alter nutrient requirements. Drug absorption is generally slower when administered with food. The metabolism of drugs, especially those that are substrates for cytochrome P450 enzymes, can be affected by changes in protein intake and micronutrient status. Table 77-8 lists examples of important drug-nutrient interactions. Drugs can also enhance or reduce appetite and dietary intake by central and/or peripheral effects.

Table 77-7

Diets Modified in Consistency

Diet	Examples of Foods Included
Clear liquid diet	Fat-free broth, bouillon, coffee, tea, carbonated beverages, clear fruit juice, gelatin, residue-free liquid nutritional supplements
Full liquid diet	Cream soups, coffee, tea, carbonated beverages, milk, yogurt, strained cooked cereal, vegetable and fruit juice, gelatin, sherbet, ice cream, custard, liquid nutritional supplements
Pureed diet	All soups, all beverages, strained or pureed meat or poultry, blended cottage cheese, gravy, milk, yogurt, mashed potatoes, strained or pureed vegetables and fruits, ice cream, custard
Soft diet	All beverages, cooked cereal, canned fruit, tender meat, cooked vegetables, milk, potatoes, rice, bread or rolls, ice cream, pudding

Table 77-8

Examples of Drug-Nutrient Interactions

Effects of Diet on Drugs	Compound
Absorption reduced by food	Atenolol
	Captopril
	Cephalexin
	Penicillin and derivatives
	Tetracycline
Absorption delayed by food	Digoxin
	Glipizide
	Phenytoin
	Piroxicam
	Theophylline
Absorption increased by food	Diazepam
	Griseofulvin
	Lithium
	Propranolol
	Thiazide diuretics

Effects of Drugs on Nutrients	Drug (Nutrient Affected)
Reduced absorption	Cimetidine (vitamin B_{12})
	Cholestyramine (fat-soluble vitamins)
	Glucocorticoids (calcium)
	Phenytoin (calcium)
	Sulfasalazine (folate)
Impaired utilization	Coumarin anticoagulants (vitamin K)
	Isoniazid (vitamin B_6)
	Methotrexate (folate)
	Nitrous oxide (vitamin B_{12})
	Oral contraceptives (folate)
Increased losses	Gentamicin (magnesium)
	Aspirin and nonsteroidal anti-inflammatory drugs (iron)
	Loop diuretics (thiamin)
	Penicillamine (zinc)
	Thiazide diuretics (potassium)

ALTERNATIVE DIET THERAPIES

New or alternative diet therapies are promoted by the popular nutrition literature, which is produced by an array of practitioners who devise and recommend various diet therapies based on different rationales and varying supportive data. In addition, both practitioners and patients can have beliefs and attitudes classified as food faddism, food cultism, or food quackery. Food faddism is an exaggerated belief in the effects of specific aspects of nutrition on health and disease. Food cultism implies beliefs about food that contain a religious or philosophical component, often with the involvement of a charismatic authority figure. Food quackery carries the implication of fraud but also refers to people who are sincere in their beliefs but misguided in the promotion of questionable diet therapies.

Popular diets often focus on limiting or regulating specific foods, using either speculative information or half-truths to explain the rationale. Unusual foods, food combinations, or other rituals for eating may also be prescribed. Table 77-9 lists examples of popular diets in a few general categories. Unproven diet therapies exist for the treatment of chronic fatigue syndrome, premenstrual syndrome, arthritis, multiple sclerosis, and numerous other medical problems. Vegetarian diets are sometimes considered alternative diets, although nutritional needs can be met quite easily by adults who consume dairy products but avoid meat, poultry, and fish. A vegan diet, which means that all animal products are eliminated, can also be nutritionally adequate, although more thoughtful food choices and supplementation with fortified foods and vitamin B_{12} may be necessary.

Although a randomized clinical trial is the ultimate test of efficacy, popular theories about diet and disease are often derived from epidemiologic studies such as ecologic, case-control, and cohort studies. Such studies are useful for generating hypotheses, but the apparent associations between diets and disease may be confounded by uncontrolled factors and other potential determinants of health and disease. As in any other medical therapy, the use of diet therapies should be based on a scientific rationale and sound data, not on anecdotal experience.

Feelings of medical abandonment or a need or desire to exert some control over the management of illness can motivate patients to adopt fad or popular diets. Such diets may have particular appeal to those with chronic illness. Awareness of alternative diet therapies being promoted, exploring with patients the issues surrounding nutrition and diet in a noncritical manner, and addressing concerns with reassurance are strategies to mimimize the chance of fad diets becoming health risks.

A few general questions are central to the evaluation of popular or alternative diets. Is the diet nutritionally adequate and appropriate for the patient? Comparing the diet composition with the guidelines for nutritional adequacy addresses this concern. Is the rationale for the diet scientifically sound? A basic understanding of nutritional requirements (see Chap. 72) makes it possible to assess the safety of the diet. Will physical or psychological risks or hazards result from the diet therapy? Even if the diet appears to involve health risk, some patients will still choose such a regimen, and the patient's decision must be respected. Suggesting that the therapy be tried for a limited time only and that the patient then return for reassessment can be helpful. Continued monitoring for adverse effects, along with support and follow-up, reduce the likelihood that conventional treatment will be completely abandoned.

PROMOTING ADHERENCE TO DIET THERAPY

No diet therapy can be effective if it is not followed or is followed incorrectly. Many factors, such as the complexity and cost of the diet, environmental and social circumstances, the nature and quality of the patient-clinician interaction, and the techniques used to counsel and teach the patient, will influence adherence. Compliance with medical therapies of all types, including prescription medications and diets, is universally poor. Traditional approaches, such as providing the patient a set menu plan or a list of foods to avoid, are usually unsuccessful. Similarly, interacting in a manner that creates a power struggle between the physician and the patient is doomed to failure.

Large-scale clinical trials have demonstrated that adherence can be improved, even when the diet is complex, when diet therapy includes specific educational and behavioral strategies. Such strategies are based on contemporary behavioral theory and a self-management approach, particularly when dietary changes must be maintained throughout the paient's life and when the degree of modification may be extensive. A self-management approach means that the physician or diet counselor and the patient are partners in the process: for long-term adherence, patients need to learn problem-solving skills and to believe in their own capabilities.

A basic strategy to enhance adherence is to focus on positive behavior and appropriate food choices rather than on food restrictions. One technique is to begin with the baseline diet as described by the patient and to identify changes that the patient is willing and able to make. Building on achievable goals, patients can practice and develop skills through continued support from a guiding expert. Frequent contact with the physician or diet counselor, who encourages the patient and reinforces progress, also increases adherence and promotes sustained motivation. For almost all patients, the involvement and assistance of family members and social support are mandatory if diet therapy is to succeed. Individualized and tailored education and communication are also necessary, taking into consideration the sociocultural influences on food choices and eating patterns.

Success of diet therapy is enhanced by working with a health care practitioner trained in nutrition. To obtain credentials as a registered dietitian involves completing an approved program of academic training that includes both didactic and supervised practice components. Dietitians provide nutritional care in the hospital and in ambulatory clinics, physician practice groups, community-based programs, and public health departments. A dietitian can function as the guiding and supportive expert, translating nutritional and metabolic needs into specific food choices and developing strategies that enable patients to effect changes in dietary habits.

BIBLIOGRAPHY

AMERICAN DIETETIC ASSOCIATION: *Manual of Clinical Dietetics*, 2d ed. Chicago, American Dietetic Association, 1992

COMMITTEE ON DIET AND HEALTH, FOOD AND NUTRITION BOARD, NATIONAL RESEARCH COUNCIL: *Diet and Health: Implications for Reducing Chronic Disease Risk*. Washington, DC, National Academy Press, 1989

COUNCIL ON SCIENTIFIC AFFAIRS, AMERICAN MEDICAL ASSOCIATION: Report of the Council on Scientific Affairs. Diet and cancer: Where do matters stand? JAMA 153:50, 1993

Eating Hints for Cancer Patients, Publication No. 94-2079. Bethesda, MD, National Cancer Institute, 1994

EXPERT PANEL ON DETECTION, EVALUATION, AND TREATMENT OF HIGH BLOOD CHOLESTEROL IN ADULTS: Summary of the Second Report of the National Cholestrol Education Program (NCEP) Expert Panel on Detection, Evaluation, and Treatment of High Blood Cholesterol in Adults (Adult Treatment Panel II). JAMA 269:3015, 1993

Table 77-9

Examples of Popular Diets

Diet Type	Characteristics	Examples
Low carbohydrate	Causes ketosis if <100 g/d	Atkin's diet Scarsdale diet Stillman's diet The Zone diet
Very low fat	Limited bioavailability of micronutrients; provides limited protein and energy	Macrobiotic diet McDougall diet Pritikin diet Rice-fruit diet
Novel diets	Unusual food combinations; unscientific rationale	Fit for Life diet Beverly Hills diet Yeast-free diet for allergies

FRANZ MJ et al: Nutrition principles for the management of diabetes and related complications. Diabetes Care 17:490, 1994

KLAHR S et al: The effects of dietary protein restriction and blood-pressure control on the progression of chronic renal disease. N Engl J Med 330:877, 1994

NELSON JK et al (eds): *Mayo Clinic Diet Manual*, 7th ed. St. Louis, Mosby 1994

PENNINGTON JA: *Bowes & Church's Food Values of Portions Commonly Used*, 16th ed. Philadelphia, Lippincott, 1994

SHILS ME et al (eds): *Modern Nutrition in Health and Disease*, 8th ed. Philadelphia, Lea & Febiger, 1994

78 Lyn Howard

ENTERAL AND PARENTERAL NUTRITION THERAPY

Parenteral and enteral nutrition provide life-sustaining therapy for patients who cannot take adequate food by mouth and who consequently are at risk for malnutrition and its effects, including susceptibility to infection and weakness and immobility, which predispose in turn to aspiration pneumonia, pulmonary embolism, and pressure sores, all of which delay recovery from illness and increase mortality.

The term *enteral* refers to feeding via the gut and hence includes normal eating, but in the present context the term implies the infusion of formulas via a tube into the upper gastrointestinal tract. *Parenteral* refers to the infusion of nutrient solutions into the bloodstream. While these are different approaches to nutritional support, their goals are by and large the same. Where feasible, enteral nutrition is the preferred route because it sustains the digestive, absorptive, and immunologic barrier functions of the gastrointestinal tract. The cost of enteral tube feeding is about one-tenth the cost of parenteral feeding.

Several developments have made tube feeding easier and more acceptable to patients. Small-bore pliable tubes have largely replaced large-bore rubber tubes, and double-bore tubes are now available with a gastric suction arm and jejunal feeding arm for use when there is concern about gastric retention and aspiration. Enteral tubes can be inserted into the stomach or jejunum through the nose or, for long-term use, directly through the abdominal wall, using endoscopic, radiologic, or surgical techniques. Once the enterocutaneous tract is established, the protruding tube can be replaced by a "button" entry port flush with the abdominal wall.

Complete nutrition by vein with sufficient calories, amino acids, minerals, and vitamins to permit wound healing, restoration of normal body composition of a cachectic patient, or growth in children became feasible in the 1960s with the development of high-flow central vein catheters and is now available in all large hospitals and for some patients at home. Adequate calories and other nutrients can be delivered in the form of high-energy, isotonic intravenous fat solutions via a peripheral vein. However, peripheral veins usually cannot sustain such infusions indefinitely, and long-term support requires central venous access.

THE DECISION PROCESS FOR USING PARENTERAL OR ENTERAL NUTRITION The decision to use specialized nutrition support should be based on the likelihood that averting or redressing malnutrition will improve the quality of life or the ability to recover from a serious illness. Approximately 15 to 20 percent of hospitalized patients have evidence of malnutrition. Some malnourished patients benefit from specialized nutrition support, but for others wasting is an inevitable component of a terminal disease. Distinguishing between these possibilities requires knowledge of the potential benefits and risks of nutritional support, and the physician must inform the patient and family of these benefits and risks with awareness of the legal issues involved. Figure 78-1 is a flow diagram of the steps involved in deciding whether specialized nutrition support should be undertaken and if so, how. Like all life-support measures, these therapies are difficult to withdraw once started.

The first step requires consideration of the nutritional implications of the disease process. Is the condition or its treatment likely to impair appetite or food ingestion and absorption for a prolonged period of time? Since prevention of malnutrition is easier than treatment, this issue must be considered in the initial evaluation. The second step is to determine whether the patient is already sufficiently malnourished that lean body mass is decreased and critical functions such as healing and ventilation will be impaired. The presence or absence of metabolic stress should be noted, since injury or infection can evoke the secretion of hormonal and cytokine factors that reduce the efficiency of nutrition repletion. The assessment of the nutritional status of patients is discussed in Chap. 73. Weight loss without physiologic impairment is probably of no consequence. Physiologic impairment usually becomes important when more that 20 percent of body protein is lost and is more likely if the relevant organ system is directly affected by disease. Once it is recognized that the patient is malnourished or at major risk, the question is whether specialized nutritional support will impact positively on the response to the disease and improve the quality of life. This issue involves risk-versus-benefit and ethical considerations. While the provision of food and water is part of basic medical care, nutrition support by enteral or parenteral means is associated with some risk and discomfort and should be recommended only when potential benefit exceeds risk and undertaken only with the consent of the patient.

If it is decided that preventing or treating malnutrition with specialized nutrition support would improve the prognosis and quality of life, the nutritional requirements must be determined and the route of nutrient delivery must be selected.

RISKS AND BENEFITS OF NUTRITION SUPPORT The risks are chiefly determined by the route required to deliver nutrition support. Providing nutritional requirements by special attention to oral intake of food or by adding oral liquid supplements together with monitoring food intake with frequent calorie counts is the best approach. It is also the most efficient metabolically because normal eating initiates the cephalic phase of digestion. Tube-fed infants grow better if the cephalic phase is stimulated by having the infant suck on a pacifier.

Anorexia, impairment of swallowing, or bowel disease may limit oral intake or the absorption of oral nutrients, in which case tube enteral nutrition is the next consideration. The bowel and its associated digestive organs derive 70 percent of their required nutrients directly from food in the lumen. In addition, glutamine, short-chain fatty acids, and nucleotides may have particular importance in maintaining gut integrity. Enteral feeding also supports gut function by stimulating splanchnic blood flow, neuronal activity, IgA antibody release, and secretion of gastrointestinal hormones such as epidermal growth factor that stimulate gut trophic activity. All these factors support the gut as an immunologic barrier against enteric pathogens.

For these reasons, some enteral nutrition should always be provided if possible, even when parenteral nutrition is required to provide most of the support. In the past, bowel rest through parenteral nutrition was thought to be the cornerstone of treatment of several severe gastrointestinal disorders, but the value of some enteral nutrition is now widely accepted and strict bowel rest is rarely advocated. Parenteral nutrition alone is still appropriate in the early phase of the extreme short bowel syndrome, severe hemorrhagic pancreatitis, necrotizing enterocolitis, prolonged ileus, and distal bowel obstruction.

Specialized nutrition support is expensive, accounting for over 1 percent of all health care dollars in 1992 (Table 78-1). Consequently, hard clinical endpoints such as rate of mortality, incidence of major complications, and duration of hospital stay are required of risk-benefit studies. Softer endpoints, such as better nitrogen balance, increased levels of serum albumin, and improved delayed hypersensitivity, are no longer acceptable.

Perioperative Nutrition While there is a clear-cut association between preoperative malnutrition and poor surgical outcome, it has

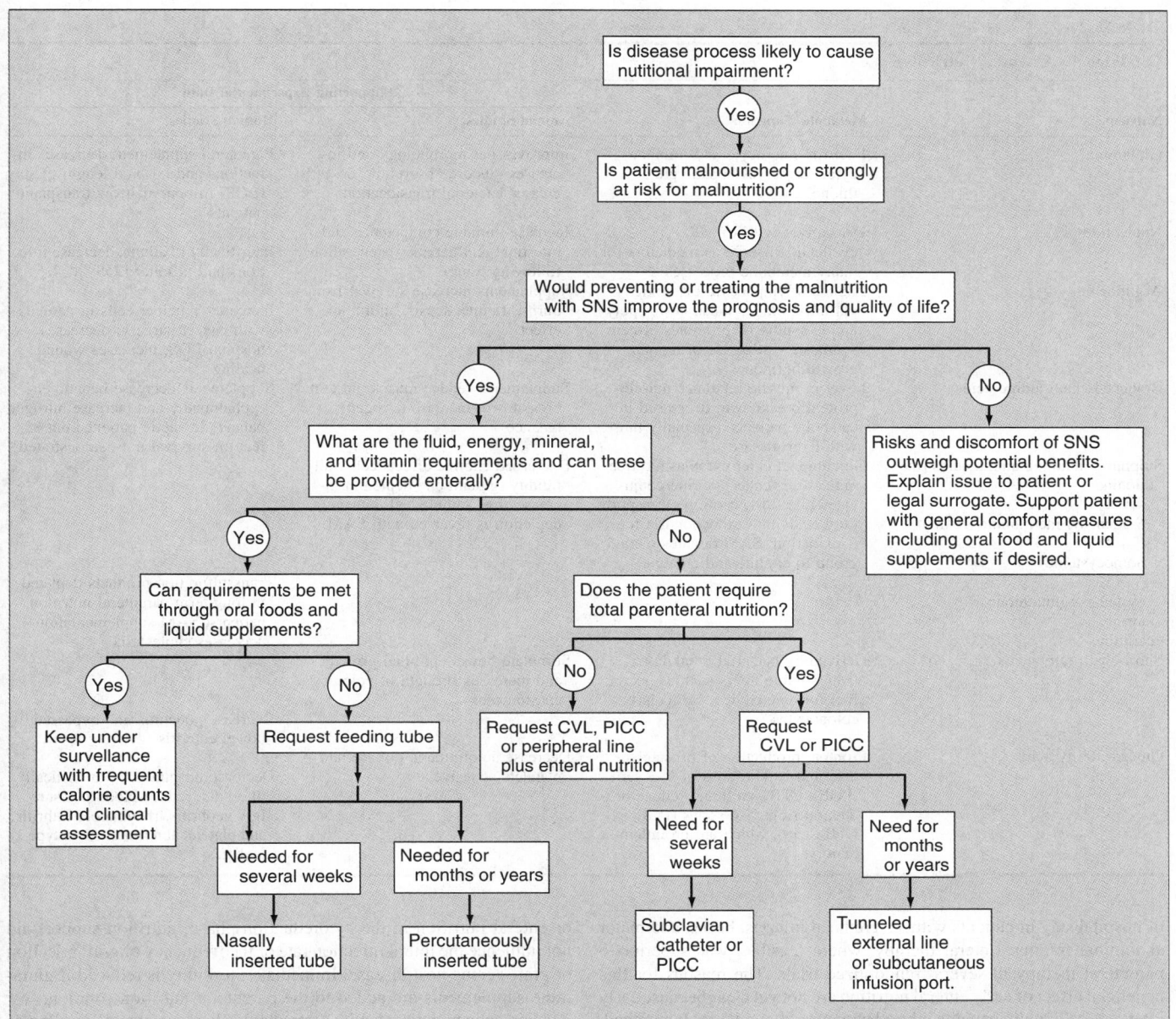

FIGURE 78-1 Should specialized nutrition support (SNS) be undertaken and if so, how? An algorithm. (PICC, Peripherally inserted, usually antecubital vein, central catheter; CVL, central venous line.)

been difficult to demonstrate the benefit of preoperative parenteral nutrition on the outcome of surgery in malnourished patients. However, a meta-analysis of 18 small studies and a large cooperative Veterans Administration study indicate that preoperative parenteral nutrition does improve the outcome of severely malnourished surgical patients.

Table 78-1

Estimate of Cost and Number of Persons Receiving Parenteral and Tube Enteral Nutrition in 1992 in the United States

Clinical Setting	Cost, $ Millions		Persons, Thousands	
	Parenteral	Enteral	Parenteral	Enteral
Hospital	6000	1200	500	1000
Home	780	357	40	152
Nursing home	6	410	<1	177
Dialysis center	20	<1	3	<1

SOURCE: Hospital estimate based on Anderson and Steinberg (data using quoted growth rates); nonhospital estimate based on Howard et al. (Medicare data and North American HPEN Registry information).

In treated patients, noninfectious complications (e.g., pulmonary emboli and delayed wound healing) are reduced in the postoperative period. In surgical patients with mild or moderate malnutrition, the risks of infection from preoperative parenteral therapy outweigh the benefits. These risks include line sepsis and infectious complications not directly related to the central line, such as pneumonia and wound infection. Effective preoperative restoration of nutrition by the parenteral route requires at least 7 to 14 days. Preoperative enteral nutrition, where feasible, is safe and more economical, especially if provided at home.

Immediate postoperative nutritional support is appropriate for patients who received preoperative support and for patients unlikely to resume oral feeding within 10 days. Commonly the parenteral route is used because of postoperative ileus or concern about disrupting a new bowel anastomosis. However, cautious jejunal feeding is often equally well tolerated. Specialized enteral formulas supplemented with a variety of conditionally essential nutrients may be particularly beneficial in debilitated and immunosuppressed postoperative patients (Table 78-2).

Critical Illness Very early nutrition support (within the first 48 h) improves survival, reduces infections, and reduces the length

Table 78-2

Conditionally Essential Nutrients

Nutrient	Metabolic Function	Supporting Experimental Data	
		Animal Studies	Human Studies
Glutamine	Fuel for enterocyte and immunocytes; preserves hepatic glutathione	Improves gut morphology and increases glucose absorption; decreases bacterial translocation	Parenteral supplement decreases infections and hospital length of stay (LOS) in bone marrow transplant patients
Nucleotides	Derivatives (cyclicAMP, cyclicGMP) serve as mediators for many metabolic processes	Increase immune competence and intestinal and hepatic regeneration following injury	In critically ill adults, decrease infections and hospital LOS
Arginine	Enhances lymphocyte cytotoxicity via nitric oxide; substrate for polyamine synthesis; promotes protein synthesis via release of human growth hormone	Supplements increase survival from burns, trauma, sepsis; antitumor effect	Increases T helper cells in patients with cancer surgery; decreases hospital LOS; increases wound healing
Branched-chain amino acids	Level in muscle regulates muscle-protein breakdown; decreased in catabolic patients, especially those with liver disease	Supplements reduce muscle protein breakdown, increase nitrogen balance	Supplements decrease hepatic encephalopathy and increase nitrogen balance in septic patients, but effect on survival not demonstrated
Sulphur-containing amino acids [methionine ↓ S-adenosyl methionine (SAM) ↓ homocysteine ↓ cysteine→glutathione taurine carnitine]	Glutathione, chief cytoplasmic free radical scavenger; taurine conjugates bile salts; carnitine transports fatty acids into mitochondria for β-oxidation; SAM donates methyl group to choline and creatine	Decreased choline affects cell-wall fluidity; glutathione depletion increases free radicle cell damage; depletion is reversed with SAM	Transsulfuration products depleted in long-term parenteral nutrition patients; SAM supplementation decreases cholestasis
Short-chain fatty acids	Derived by bacterial breakdown from soluble fibers such as pectin; fuel for enterocytes, particularly colonocytes	Stimulate bowel epithilial growth and increases strength of colonic anastomoses	Decrease pouchitis and bypassed bowel enteritis
Omega-3 fatty acids	Promote production of prostaglandins and leukotrienes of N-3 series (PGE$_3$, LTB$_5$, etc.) and reduce production from N-6 series (PGE$_2$, LTB$_4$, etc.), which are proinflammatory	Decrease autoimmune disease and platelets adhesiveness	Decrease hospital LOS in critically ill adults; reduce blood pressure, IgA nephritis, rheumatoid arthritis, and platelet abnormalities in type 1 diabetes

of hospital stay in patients with severe head injuries, burns, and major abdominal trauma. Enteral therapy, where feasible, was superior to parenteral therapy in several randomized trials. The reasons for this beneficial effect of early enteral nutrition are not yet clear because early intervention equally benefits injured patients not overtly malnourished. Animal studies suggest that enteral feeding results in decreased systemic infections from gut bacteria and in reduction of the systemic catabolic response. These phenomena have not been substantiated in humans, but early enteral feeding may prevent bacterial overgrowth and decrease aspiration pneumonia.

The practical issue is obtaining jejunal access in a critically ill patient, who is not easily transferred for endoscopic or radiologic placement. Sometimes a nasal or percutaneous combined gastric suction and jejunal feeding tube can be inserted at the bedside. When a surgical laparatomy is indicated, a feeding tube can be placed simultaneously.

Most studies of enteral feeding in critically ill patients used either a general polymeric formula or one with hydrolyzed protein. Parenteral formulas enriched with large amounts of branched-chain amino acids (BCAA) improve nitrogen balance but do appear to affect clinical outcome.

Cancer Cachexia Early nonrandomized studies suggested that patients with cancer cachexia benefit from parenteral nutrition, but randomized trials demonstrated more risk than benefit for patients receiving chemotherapy or radiation. Severely malnourished cancer patients undergoing surgery do appear to benefit from preoperative parenteral nutrition, as do other malnourished patients.

In two randomized, prospective trials, patients undergoing bone marrow transplantation had better long-term survival after parenteral or enteral nutrition in the cytoreduction phase; nutrition support did not influence the initial infection rate or the frequency of graft rejection or graft-versus-host disease. Immediate morbidity is reduced if glutamine supplements are added to the parenteral nutrition solution.

For cancer patients with untreatable disease, enteral feeding is usually justified if it is desired by the patient and family. Parenteral feeding should be provided only if clinical improvement can be expected and when quality survival at home for several months is predicted.

Liver Failure Malnutrition is common in advanced liver disease. Patients with acute or chronic liver failure have decreased levels of BCAA and elevated levels of aromatic amino acids (AAA) in plasma and cerebrospinal fluid. Randomized, prospective trials with parenteral and enteral formulas high in BCAA and low in AAA have demonstrated better nitrogen balance and less risk of encephalopathy. One large multicenter study also reported improved survival. The BCAA-enriched formulas are expensive and should be used only in patients who have encephalopathy or who develop encephalopathy when fed a standard protein formula providing 0.8 g protein/kg per day.

Renal Failure Since renal failure is associated with impaired nitrogen excretion, it is rational to assume that protein restriction might benefit patients with chronic renal failure and that more complete protein restriction might improve the course of acute renal failure. However, the progression of renal impairment in patients on chronic dialysis is not slowed by low-protein oral diets. Patients with acute renal failure given parenteral calories and amino acids have fewer infectious complications and a better chance of leaving the hospital than similar patients given only calories. An early randomized study showed benefit when essential amino acids were the sole source of nitrogen, but in other studies standard solutions supplying both essential and nonessential amino acids provide similar advantage. Thus, the benefit of using expensive formulas containing only essential amino acids or their keto analogues is not established.

Fifteen to twenty percent of patients with chronic renal failure on dialysis have significant nutritional impairment, usually due to profound anorexia. The anorexia sometimes improves with stepped-up dialysis or treatment of gastritis but usually persists. The resulting growth impairment in younger patients has been treated with supplemental tube enteral nutrition. This approach has not been widely used in older patients, but parenteral nutrition that provides some extra calories and amino acids can be administered in the last 90 min of hemodialysis treatment and is said to improve appetite, serum protein levels, and body weight. No randomized studies have documented better survival, so that the appropriateness of this regimen is not established. Standard continuous ambulatory peritoneal dialysis uses glucose to provide an osmotic load, and some glucose calories are absorbed. Amino acids can be substituted for glucose and are also partly absorbed, offsetting the loss of endogenous amino acids into the dialysate. This approach also awaits a randomized study.

Pancreatitis Parenteral nutrition does not improve the outcome of patients with mild or moderate pancreatitis. However, in severe pancreatitis survival decreases as malnutrition becomes more severe. When parenteral nutrition support was delayed beyond 72 h, patients with severe pancreatitis had a threefold higher complication and mortality rate, compared to similar patients treated earlier. In the absence of severe hyperlipidemia or thrombocytopenia, intravenous lipids appear safe and are especially useful if glucose intolerance is present. Several studies report successful enteral jejunal feeding in acute pancreatitis.

Inflammatory Bowel Disease (IBD) Evidence of nutritional deficiencies such as weight loss, growth failure, anemia, and hypoalbuminenia are common in IBD, more so in Crohn's disease than in ulcerative colitis (see Chap. 286). Nutrition support plays a role in correcting these nutritional deficiencies, particularly prior to elective surgery. Since IBD often improves with diversion of the fecal stream, the question is whether bowel rest and parenteral nutrition have a role as primary treatment. However, randomized, prospective studies have shown no special benefit from bowel rest. Elemental diets can be used in place of steroids for inducing remission in acute Crohn's disease, but relapse is common when a regular diet is resumed. In controlled studies remissions are prolonged if the Crohn's patient does not return to a regular diet but instead eliminates from the diet those foods that induce gastrointestinal symptoms. For the majority of Crohn's patients this leads to avoidance of cereals, dairy products, and yeast.

Because of the possibility that diets high in omega 3 fatty acids have a beneficial effect in immune disorders by altering prostaglandin synthesis, their value in IBD is under investigation. Some studies suggest that high-fiber diets benefit IBD patients, but fiber can also cause obstruction in patients with bowel strictures.

Short Bowel Syndrome Before the advent of parenteral nutrition, patients with acute short bowel syndrome from mesenteric vascular infarction or surgical resection seldom survived. Parenteral nutrition has allowed many patients to survive indefinitely with only a foot or two of small intestine. In some, the remaining bowel eventually adapts and allows the absorption of adequate calories and protein. However, fluid and electrolyte imbalance may persist so that some parenteral fluid and electrolyte support are required. Gradual increase of overnight tube enteral nutrition or constant sipping of an electrolyte solution may allow discontinuation of all parenteral support.

Pulmonary Disease Weight loss in patients with advanced pulmonary disease is due to increased work of breathing and poor food intake. Patients with chronic pulmonary disease who are less than 90% percent of their ideal weight have a greater 5-year mortality, independent of pulmonary status. The recommended energy intake for these patients is 1.7 times their resting energy expenditure. In cystic fibrosis, malnutrition may hasten pulmonary deterioration, and enteral feeding via gastrostomy tubes enhances growth and stabilizes or improves pulmonary function, particularly in young children. The criteria for selection of patients and the psychological costs of such treatment

have not been defined. The use of a low-carbohydrate formula is beneficial in the weaning of patients from ventilators, but the superiority of such formulas in ambulatory patients with chronic lung disease is not established.

Human Immunodeficiency Virus (HIV) Disease The role of specialized nutritional support in weight loss associated with HIV disease is not established. Studies by Kotler have shown that parenteral nutrition repletes lean body mass when weight loss is due to inadequate oral intake, either because of oral problems or esophageal disease or because of inadequate absorption due to small-bowel disease. However, wasting associated with systemic infection and increased cytokine secretion is not effectively repaired by parenteral nutrition. In patients with systemic infections, any weight gain reflects increased fat and body water rather than protein mass. Slow tube enteral infusion is often tolerated, and its role in the early phase of HIV-related weight loss is under investigation.

Pregnancy Severe hyperemesis gravidarum can make any oral or tube enteral nutrition impossible, and profound weight loss and ketosis may harm the developing fetus. The underlying mechanism of the disorder is not understood, but it is cured by abortion or delivery. Temporary parenteral nutrition usually results in a successful outcome in pregnancy complicated by severe hyperemesis, but nausea and vomiting tend to persist, despite bowel rest.

Home Parenteral and Enteral Nutrition Some patients require long-term nutrition support and this can be administered at home. Table 78-3 summarizes the outcome for patients with severe intestinal disorders, 11 treated parenterally and 2 treated enterally. Nutritional support is not appropriate in terminal patients, but it is an option if a patient can be expected to survive for several months. Such therapy must make sense to the patient, and sufficient help must be available so that the treatment can be given at home without undue hazard. Both home therapies are relatively safe, with less than a 5 percent mortality.

THE DESIGN OF INDIVIDUAL REGIMENS **Fluid Requirements** These can be estimated by adding the normal daily requirement (120 mL/kg of body weight for infants, 35 mL/kg of body weight for adults) to any abnormal loss. If the patient is on parenteral therapy, any enteral intake should be subtracted from the estimate (see Table 78-4.) Since abnormal loss of enteric fluid implies significant mineral losses, extra amounts of these nutrients (Table 78-5) must be added to any standard parenteral formula.

Energy Requirements These can be determined as outlined in Chap. 72. In the long run energy expenditure dictates energy requirements, but in the early phase of nutrition repletion, requirements may not reflect expenditure. For example, malnourished patients are hypometabolic and may expend only 85 kJ/kg (20 kcal/kg) per day, but more calories are needed for nutritional repletion because with refeeding the metabolic rate increases and extra calories are needed for tissue repair. Conversely, a highly stressed patient (burns, trauma) may expend 165 kJ/kg (40 kcal/kg) per day with a significant proportion of the calories coming from protein breakdown and gluconeogenesis and from catecholamine-induced lipolysis. Oxidation of exogenous glucose plateaus at 100 kJ/kg (25 kcal/kg) per day, and administering additional glucose induces hepatic steatosis. Furthermore, providing such patients with additional calories as exogenous fat does not suppress endogenous lipolysis. This is because the artificial chylomicrons of parenteral fat solutions, which are vegetable oils (soybean, safflower) emulsified with egg phospholipid, lack apoproteins and are are not metabolized like lipoproteins. For these reasons, modest hypocaloric glucose feeding with minimal parenteral fat is safer in the acutely stressed subject.

Parenteral lipid solutions are available as 10% or 20% isotonic solutions and can be infused separately from amino acids and glucose or as "three in one," obviating the need for an extra pump. However, three-in-one solutions are not as stable as the glucose and amino acid mix, and destabilized fat particles have the potential of coalescing into larger droplets and becoming fat emboli. To be safe, three-in-one solutions must be mixed by a pharmacist knowledgeable about the

Table 78-3

Summary of Outcome for Patients on Home Parenteral and Enteral Nutrition (HPEN)

Diagnosis	Number in Group	Age in Years	% Survival* on Therapy	Therapy Status, % at 1 year†‡ Full Oral Nutrition	Continued on HPEN Rx	Died	Rehabilitation‡§ Status, % in 1st year C	P	M	Complications¶ per Patient-Year HPEN‡	NonHPEN‡
HOME PARENTERAL NUTRITION											
Crohn's disease	562	36	96	70	25	2	60	38	2	0.9	1.1
Ischemic bowel disease	331	49	87	27	48	19	53	41	6	1.4	1.1
Motility disorder	299	45	87	31	44	21	49	39	12	1.3	1.1
Congenital bowel defect	172	5	94	42	47	9	63	27	11	2.1	1.0
Hyperemesis gravidarum	112	28	100	100	0	0	83	16	1	1.5	3.5
Chronic pancreatitis	156	42	90	82	10	5	60	38	2	1.2	2.5
Radiation enteritis	145	58	87	28	49	22	42	49	9	0.8	1.1
Chronic adhesive obstructions	120	53	83	47	34	13	23	68	10	1.7	1.4
Cystic fibrosis	51	17	50	38	13	36	24	66	16	0.8	3.7
Cancer	2122	44	20	26	8	63	29	57	14	1.1	3.3
AIDS	280	33	10	13	6	73	8	63	29	1.6	3.3
HOME ENTERAL NUTRITION											
Neurologic disorders of swallowing	1134	65	55	19	25	48	5	24	71	0.3	0.9
Cancer	1644	61	30	30	6	59	21	59	21	0.4	2.7

* Survival rates on therapy are values at 1 year, calculated by the life table method. This will differ from the percentage listed as died under Therapy Status, since all patients with known end points are considered in this latter measure. The ratio of observed versus expected deaths is equivalent to a Standard Mortality Ratio.
† Not shown are those patients who were back in hospital or who had changed therapy type by 12 months.
‡ Chi-square test, P < .05
§ Rehabilitation is designated complete (C), partial (P), or minimal (M), relative to the patient's ability to sustain normal age-related activity.
¶ Complications refer only to those complications that resulted in rehospitalization.
SOURCE: Derived from North American HPEN Registry.

appropriate mixing sequence of the ingredients and the amounts of divalent cations and trace elements that can be added. Patients who require parenteral iron and zinc must get these in non-lipid-containing parenteral solutions.

Polyunsaturated vegetable oils are used in most enteral formulas because they are better absorbed by the compromised gastrointestinal tract. The fat in parenteral and enteral formulas must supply the essential fatty acid requirement (1 to 4 percent of energy from linoleic and linolenic acid) (Table 78-6). In relatively stable patients the provision of 30 percent of energy as fat may reduce the problems that arise from providing glucose calories predominantly (e.g.,

hepatic steatosis). Substituting omega 3 polyunsaturated fish oils for ordinary polyunsaturated vegetable fats may reduce the catabolic response to burn injury, trauma, and radiation by reducing the synthesis of prostaglandins that enhance the inflammatory response (see Table 78-2).

Protein or Amino Acid Requirements The recommended dietary protein allowance of 0.8 g/kg per day is adequate for nonstressed patients, for example, a starved patient with a high-grade esophageal stricture. Catabolic patients, in contrast, may require up to 1.5 g/kg per day of protein to induce positive nitrogen balance and reconstitute normal body mass. Some studies suggest that nitrogen balance may be improved by giving human growth hormone, but it is not clear whether growth hormone increases muscle mass or enhances tissue healing. In a stable patient the adequacy of protein support can be assessed by analyzing protein balance:

Protein balance
= protein intake − protein loss

where protein loss = [(24-h urine urea nitrogen (g) + 4) × 6.25]. Over a long period, protein balance is assessed by documenting wound healing, restoration of normal body composition, or resumption of longitudinal growth.

In states of disturbed protein utilization (e.g., renal and hepatic failure), azotemia and abnormal plasma amino acid patterns develop. The benefit of special enteral and parenteral solutions that correct these aberrations is only established in hepatic encephalopathy (see "Risks and Benefits of Nutrition Support").

Table 78-4

Estimation of Daily Fluid Requirements

NORMAL 70-kg MAN

Intake
Normal requirement: 35 × 70 = ~2500 ml/d (derived from oral liquids of 1200 mL, or 5 glasses/cups per day and solid food providing 1300 mL, 1000 mL from water in food, 300 mL from water generated by metabolism of foods)

Output
Urine: 1600 mL/d
Insensible loss: 800 mL/d
Stool: 100 mL/d
[sweat loss can be up to 2 L/d; each degree of fever (C) = 200 mL/d]

TUBE ENTERAL PATIENT

58-kg woman recovering from total gastrectomy for gastric cancer and supported by jejunostomy feedings, taking nothing by mouth or intravenously but experiencing 600 mL of diarrheal losses/day:
Normal requirement 35 × 58 = ~2000 mL/d
Abnormal gastrointestinal loss 600 − 100 = 500 mL/d
Total per tube requirement = 2500 mL/d

PARENTERAL PATIENT

66-kg man with a high jejunostomy following massive bowel resection for Crohn's disease with oral intake of 2000 mL/day and jejunostomy loss of 4000 mL/day:
Normal requirement 35 × 66 = 2300 mL/d
Abnormal gastrointestinal loss (4000 − 100) minus oral intake (2000) = 1900 mL/d
Total parenteral requirement = 4200 mL/d

Table 78-5

CHAPTER 78
Enteral and Parenteral Nutrition Therapy   **477**

Enteric Fluid Volumes and Their Sodium, Potassium, Chloride, and Bicarbonate Content*

	L/d†	Na mmol/L	K‡ mmol/L	Cl mmol/L	HCO₃§ mmol/L
Oral intake	2–3				
Enteric secretions					
Saliva	1–2	10	30	10	30
Gastric juice	2	60	9	90	0
Bile	2–3	150	10	90	70
Small bowel	1	100	5	100	20
Colon	Variable	40	100	15	60

* Enteric secretions are also rich in divalent cations (Ca, Mg, Zn, Cu), and their loss is increased by steatorrhea, a high bowel fistula, or prolonged suction.

† Of the 9 L/d of oral and enteric fluid presented to the upper small bowel, normally 50 percent is absorbed in the jejunum, 40 percent in the ileum, and 10 percent in the colon. In short bowel patients, the colon can absorb greater amounts, up to 3 L/d.

‡ Potassium losses are small except in secretions distal to the ileocecal valve. The colon ion exchange is partly controlled by aldosterone, and therefore, Na⁺ depletion increases K⁺ loss in the stool.

§ Bicarbonate losses must be replaced in parenteral solutions as acetane or lactate because of potential precipitation of bicarbonate with ingredients such as calcium.

Certain organic compounds that can normally be synthesized endogenously become essential in severely ill patients when endogenous production or salvage pathways are impaired. This is true of glutamine, nucleotides, and the products of methionine metabolism (see Table 78-2). Glutamine, an important fuel for the enterocyte and lymphocyte, is fairly insoluble and is absent from standard parenteral formulas and present in low concentrations in most enteral formulas. Soluble glutamine-containing dipeptides are under investigation.

Nucleotides and their related metabolic products have beneficial effects on the immune system, growth of the small intestine, lipid metabolism, and hepatic function. Nucleotides can be synthesized de

Table 78-6

Daily Enteral (EN) and Parenteral (PN) Requirements of Essential Fatty Acids, Minerals, and Vitamins

Nutrient	Daily requirement, adult range	
	EN	PN
Essential fatty acids, % kcal	1–2	2–4
Calcium, g	0.8–1.2	0.2–0.4
Phosphorus, g	0.8–1.2	0.4–0.8
Potassium, g	2–5	3–4
Sodium, g	1–3	1–3
Chloride, g	2–5	3–4*
Magnesium, g	0.3	0.3
Iron, mg	10	1–2
Zinc, mg	15	3–12
Copper, mg	2–3	0.3–0.5
Iodine, mg	0.15	0.15
Manganese, mg	2–5	2–5
Chromium, μg	50–200	15–30
Molybdenum, μg	150–300	20–120
Selenium, μg	50–200	50–100
Ascorbic acid, mg	60	100
Thiamine, mg	1.4	3.0
Riboflavin, mg	1.6	3.6
Niacin, mg	18	40
Biotin, μg	60	60
Pantothenic acid, mg	5	15
Pyridoxine, mg	2.0	4.0
Folic acid, μg	400	400
Cobalamin, μg	3.0	5
Vitamin A, μg	1000	1000
Vitamin D, μg	10	5–10
Vitamin E, mg	8–10	10–15
Vitamin K, μg	70–140	200

* In addition to chloride anions there is a parenteral requirement for bicarbonate equivalents to protect normal acid-base balance. These are provided as 90 mmol or more per day of acetate or lactate because of potential precipitation of bicarbonate with ingredients such as calcium.

novo in all cells only in small amounts, and the body therefore depends on dietary nucleotides or on salvage pathways that recycle nucleotides from purine and pyrimidine turnover. Nutritionally depleted patients benefit from formulas enriched in nucleotides.

When amino acids are infused systemically rather than via the more physiologic portal vein, methionine, the only sulfur-containing amino acid in most parenteral solutions, is transaminated in peripheral tissues rather than transulfurated in the liver. As a result, downstream sulfur products such as carnitine, taurine, and glutathione become relatively deficient. Preliminary studies suggest that the addition of an intermediate compound, *S*-adenosyl methionine, to parenteral solutions results in less cholestasis.

Mineral and Vitamin Requirements Parenteral and enteral mineral and vitamin requirements are summarized in Table 78-6. Electrolyte modifications are necessary if the patient has significant gastrointestinal losses (Table 78-5) or renal failure. Requirements of some minerals and vitamins may be higher when they are administered parenterally for several reasons. First, the micronutrients are delivered into the systemic rather than the portal circulation, partially bypassing the liver and being excreted into the urine. Second, patients with bowel disease may have enteric loss of sodium, potassium, chloride, and bicarbonate and malabsorption of divalent cations, fat soluble vitamins, and vitamin B₁₂. Third, nutrients may adhere to the tubing and delivery bags, and exposure to oxygen and light may destroy vitamins (particularly vitamin A).

PARENTERAL NUTRITION   Infusion Technique and Patient Monitoring Partial and short-term total parenteral nutrition can be provided via a peripheral vein if the majority of the energy is supplied by isotonic fat solutions; long-term total parenteral nutrition using glucose as the chief energy source requires administration via a central vein catheter so that the hypertonic solution can be rapidly diluted in a high-flow system. The preferred site for central vein infusion is the superior vena cava, and the access and catheter choices are summarized in Table 78-7. Peripherally inserted central catheters are the most economical option for short-term parenteral nutrition. In one randomized study the number of catheter-related infections was the same with peripherally and centrally inserted catheters. Tunneled and implanted subcutaneous ports require operating room insertion and are more stable for long-term use. Central catheters should be changed when clinically indicated; routine changes are costly and hazardous. Chlorhexidine solution is a more effective local antiseptic than iodophor or alcohol. Although transparent dressings are helpful in stabilizing catheters and allow easy observation of the skin site, the incidence of catheter-related sepsis is higher than with traditional dry gauze dressings; newer transparent dressings that trap less moisture are under investigation. Catheters made from silastic material or polyurethane are associated with lower complications than polyvinylchloride catheters. Several types of needleless systems use hub valves; contamination rates for these devices are not yet known. Appropriate clinical and laboratory monitoring for patients on parenteral nutrition is summarized in Table 78-8.

Complications (See Table 78-9) *Mechanical* The insertion of a central venous catheter should be done only by trained personnel under aseptic techniques. Major mechanical complications include pneumothorax; hemothorax from laceration of the subclavian artery or vein; brachial plexus injury; and malpositioning of the catheter in a cerebral vein, the azygos vein, or the right ventricle. The correct catheter position must be confirmed by x-ray before hypertonic nutrient solution is infused. Catheters can subsequently back out of the vein, develop leaks, or become detached from the hub and embolize into the heart or pulmonary artery. Catheter thrombosis may occur, especially if the catheter is used for withdrawing blood samples, and extension of the thrombosis to the central vein is frequently coincident with infection. Thrombosed catheters can sometimes be unblocked by urokinase treatment. The addition of low-dose heparin (1000 units per liter) to limit thrombosis in parenteral catheters is controversial; no randomized, controlled studies dem-

Table 78-7

Central Venous Access for Parenteral Nutrition (PN)

Type of Catheters	Advantages	Disadvantages
Peripherally inserted central catheter (PICC) Single lumen Double lumen	Insertion cost low, can be done at bedside or by vascular radiology; especially advantageous for patients with neck wounds such as tracheostomies	High incidence of skin site irritation; tendency to break at hub; patient requires assistance with weekly dressing change
Centrally inserted externalized catheters (subclavian, jugular, femoral) Single lumen Triple lumen	Can be inserted at bedside; relatively low cost; can be changed over a guidewire if clinically indicated; catheter sepsis rate within subclavian < jugular < femoral vein	10% incidence of mechanical complication with insertion, higher if physician inexperienced; need dedicated PN line; multiple-lumen catheters have increased sepsis rate
Tunneled central catheters or subcutaneous ports	More stable for long-term use; when needle out, patients with ports have less disturbance of body image and can shower and swim without risk	More expensive device requiring operating room insertion; ports require needle stick.

onstrate benefit, and heparin can contribute to loss of bone mineral, which is already a problem with long-term parenteral nutrition.

Metabolic Fluid overload can cause congestive heart failure, particularly in elderly and debilitated patients. Glucose overload can cause an osmotic diuresis or stimulate insulin secretion, which in turn promotes extracellular to intracellular shifts of potassium and phosphorous. Such shifts are most dangerous in cachectic patients with depletion of potassium and phosphorus stores and can cause arrhythmias, cardiopulmonary dysfunction, and neurologic symptoms. To avoid these problems, parenteral nutrition should be started slowly and monitored carefully. Glucose content is increased gradually as the patient demonstrates tolerance of the high glucose load.

Late metabolic complications include cholestatic liver disease with bile sludging and gallstone formation. The exact cause of the liver disease is not understood, but lack of enteral stimulation of bile flow and defective sulfur amino acid metabolism appear to play a role. Cholestasis is less likely to occur if some enteral feeding is maintained. Parenteral nutrition induces hypercalcinuria, which can result in negative calcium balance and osteopenia. Hypercalcinuria may have several causes, including the high fixed-acid load of infused amino acids and the bisulfite preservative in the solutions. Earlier protein hydrolysates were contami-

nated with aluminum, which blocked bone mineralization, and aluminum is still a contaminant of some additives such as calcium gluconate. Once patients on long-term parenteral nutrition move from catabolic breakdown to sustained anabolism, deficiencies of micronutrients such as essential fatty acids, trace minerals, and vitamins may develop unless they are supplied in adequate amounts (see Table 78-6).

Infectious Infection of the access line rarely occurs in the first 72 h, and fever during this period is usually due to infection elsewhere or some other cause. Infection of the access line is likely if the fever defervesces when the infusion of the parenteral formula is tapered. Positive central line cultures suggests catheter sepsis, especially if no other infectious source is identified and if the organism is *Staphylococcus* or *Candida*. While removal of the central catheter may allow fungemia to clear spontaneously, antibiotic therapy is recommended for bacterial infections and the more invasive fungi. Catheter sepsis is equally likely with peripherally inserted central catheters, tunneled catheters, and single-lumen catheters dedicated exclusively to parenteral nutrition; multiple-lumen catheters are associated with a greater incidence of sepsis. While there is no evidence to support the use of prophylactic antibiotics, recurrent catheter sepsis may be avoided if cuffs are used around the catheter exit site or small amounts of an antibiotic solution are left in the line along with a heparin lock.

ENTERAL NUTRITION   Tube Placement and Patient Monitoring   The types of enteral feeding tubes, methods of insertion, their clinical uses, and potential complications are outlined in Table 78-10, and the various types of enteral formulas are listed in Table 78-11.

Table 78-8

Monitoring the Patient on Total Parenteral Nutrition

CLINICAL DATA MONITORED DAILY

Sense of well-being: symptoms suggesting fluid overload, high or low blood glucose, electrolyte imbalance, etc.
Strength as judged by graded activity: getting out of bed, walking, stair climbing.
Vital signs: temperature, blood pressure, pulse rate, and respiratory rate.
Fluid balance: weight; fluid input (intravenous +/− enteral) versus fluid output (urine, stool, gastric suction, etc.).
Delivery equipment for parenteral nutrition: composition of nutrient solution, tubing, pump, filter, catheter, dressing (skin checked for local infection at time of dressing change).

LABORATORY DATA

Plasma glucose	Four times daily until patient stable
Blood glucose Na^+, K^+, Cl^-, HCO_3^- Blood urea nitrogen	Daily until glucose infusion load and patient stable, then twice weekly
Serum albumin, transferrin (or TIBC) Liver function studies Serum creatinine Ca^{2+}, PO_4^{2+}, Mg^{2+} Hb/Hct, WBC	Baseline, then twice weekly
Prothrombin time, partial thromboplastin time Micronutrient tests as indicated	Baseline, then weekly

Table 78-9

Complications of Total Parenteral Nutrition (TPN)

First 48 h	First 2 Weeks	3 Months Onward
MECHANICAL		

Complications from catheter insertion:
  Cephalad displacement
  Pneumothorax
  Hemothorax
Detachment of line at catheter hub with blood loss or air embolism
	Catheter coming out of vein, more common if Silastic
	Detachment of line at catheter hub with blood loss or air embolism
		Detachment of line at catheter hub with blood loss or air embolism
		Fractures or tears in catheter

METABOLIC		
Fluid overload Hyperglycemia Hypophosphatemia Hypokalemia	Cardiopulmonary failure Hyperosmolar nonketotic hyperglycemic coma Acid-base imbalance Electrolyte imbalance	Essentially fatty acid deficiency Zinc, copper, chromium, selenium, molybdenum deficiency Iron deficiency Vitamin deficiencies Refeeding edema TPN metabolic bone disease TPN liver disease
INFECTIOUS		
	Catheter-induced sepsis Exit site infection	Catheter-induced sepsis Tunnel infections Exit site infection

Table 78-10

Enteral Feeding Tubes

Type/Insertion Technique	Clinical Uses	Potential Complications
NASOGASTRIC TUBE		
External measurement, nostril, ear, xiphisternum; tube stiffened by ice water or stylet; position verified by injecting air and auscultating, aspirating gastric acid, or by x-ray	Short-term clinical situation (weeks) or longer periods with intermittent insertion; bolus feeding simpler, but continuous drip with pump better tolerated	Aspiration; ulceration of nasal and esophageal tissues, leading to stricture
NASOJEJUNAL TUBE		
External measurement: nostril, ear, anterior superior iliac spine (medical malleolus in infants); tube stiffened by stylet and passed through pylorus under fluoscopy or with endoscopic loop	Short-term clinical situations where gastric emptying impaired or proximal leak suspected; requires continuous drip with pump	Spontaneous pulling back into stomach (position reverified by aspirating content pH > 6); diarrhea common, fiber-containing formula may help
GASTROSTOMY TUBE		
Percutaneous placement endoscopically, radiologically, or surgically: after tract established, can be converted to a gastric "button"	Long-term clinical situations, swallowing disorders, or impaired small-bowel absorption requiring continuous drip	Aspiration; irritation around tube exit site; peritoneal leak; balloon migration and obstruction of pylorus
JEJUNOSTOMY TUBE		
Percutaneous placement endoscopically or radiologically via pylorus or surgically into jejunum sutured to abdominal wall using fine-bore tube or larger tube	Long-term clinical situations where gastric emptying impaired; requires continuous drip with pump	Clogging or displacement of tube; jejunal fistula if large-bore tube used; diarrhea
COMBINED GASTROJEJUNOSTOMY TUBE		
Percutaneous placement endoscopically, radiologically, or surgically; intragastric arm for continuous or intermittent gastric suction; jejunal arm for enteral feeding	Used for patients with impaired gastric emptying and at high risk for aspiration or patients with acute pancreatitis or proximal leaks	Clogging; irritation around tube exit site

Table 78-11

Enteral Formulas

Composition Characteristics	Clinical Indication
STANDARD ENTERAL FORMULA	
1. Complete dietary products (+)*	Suitable for most patients requiring tube feeding; flavors available for oral use
a. Caloric density 1 kcal/mL	
b. Protein ~14% cals, caseinates, soy, lactalbumin	
c. Fat ~30% cals, corn, soy, safflower oils	
d. CHO ~60% cals, hydrolysed corn starch, maltodextrin, sucrose	
e. Recommended daily intake of all minerals and vitamins in ≥ 1500 kcal/d	
f. Osmolality (mosm/kg) ~300	
MODIFIED ENTERAL FORMULAS	
1. Caloric density 1.5–2 kcal/mL (+)	Fluid-restricted patients
2.	
a. High protein ~20% cals (+)	Protein malnutrition and ↓ wound healing
b. Hydrolysed protein to small peptides (+ +)	↓ Protein digestion/absorption or allergy
c. ↑ Glutamine, arginine, S-containing amino acids, nucleotides (+ + +)	Severely immunocompromised patients
d. ↑ Branch-chain amino acids, ↓ aromatic amino acids (+ + +)	Liver failure patients intolerant of 0.8 g/kg per day of regular protein
e. ↓ Protein, ↓ K, Mg, and P diets (+ +)	Renal failure patients
f. ↓ Protein, ↑ essential amino acids, ↓ minerals and vitamins (+ + +)	Renal failure patients not on dialysis
3.	
a. Low fat, partial MCT substitution (+)	Fat malabsorption
b. ↑ Fat >40% cals (+ +)	Pulmonary failure with ↑ P_{CO_2} on standard formulas
c. ↑ Fat from MUFA (+ +)	Poorly controlled diabetes mellitus
d. Fat ↑ in ω3 (fish oil) and ↓ ω6 (+ + +)	Immunocompromised and autoimmune disorder
4.	
a. Fiber provided as soy poly saccharide (+)	Diarrhea/constipation
b. Fiber provided as blenderized fruits and vegetables (+ +)	↓ Binding of dilantin
5. ↑ Minerals (Zn) and vitamins (A and C) (+ +)	Decubitus ulcers

* Cost: + inexpensive; + + moderately expensive; + + + very expensive.

NOTE: CHO, carbohydrate; MCT, medium chain triglyceride; MUFA, monunsaturated fatty acid, ω3 or ω6 polyunsatuated fat with first double bond at carbon 3 (fish oils) or carbon

Patients on enteral feeding are at risk for many of the same metabolic complications as those receiving parenteral nutrition and should be monitored in the same way (Table 78-8). Since small-bore tubes are easily displaced, tube position should be checked at intervals by aspirating and measuring the pH of the gut fluid (<4 in stomach, >6 in jejunum).

Complications *Aspiration* The debilitated patient with poor gastric emptying and impairment of the swallowing and cough mechanisms is at risk for aspiration; this is particularly so for those on respirators because tracheal suctioning induces coughing and gastric regurgitation and because the cuffs on the endotracheal tube or tracheostomy seldom provide protection against aspiration. Under these circumstances, it may be safer to use a large-bore feeding tube to allow for temporary removal of gastric contents during tracheal suction or to use jejunal feeding.

Constant gastric infusion of an enteral formula is better tolerated in sick patients than is intermittent bolus feeding. A continuous infusion is best achieved with a pump, especially when using fine-bore tubes that have a greater potential to clog. If long-term feeding is anticipated, endoscopic, radiologic, or surgical placement of a gastric tube is preferred by most patients. For long-term ambulatory patients, a gastrostomy tube can be converted to a gastric "button," an access device that is flush with the skin.

A nasojejunal tube reduces the risk of aspiration. However, fluoroscopic placement of fine bore tubes through the pylorus is time-consuming, and such tubes frequently pull back into the stomach. A large percutaneous gastric-suction and jejunal-feeding tube is more reliable. This can be placed radiologically, endoscopically, or surgically.

Diarrhea Enteral feeding often causes diarrhea, especially if bowel function is compromised by bowel disease or drugs. The diarrhea may be controlled by the use of continuous drip feeding or by the addition of bulking agents, such as psyllium hydrophilic mucilogs, or an anticholinergic medication in the formula. Diarrhea of enteral feeding does not necessarily imply inadequate absorption of nutrients, other than water and electrolytes. Furthermore, since luminal nutrients exert trophic effects on the gut mucosa and enhance the enteric immunologic barrier, it may be appropriate to persist, despite the diarrhea, even when this necessitates temporary supplemental parenteral fluid support.

THE COST OF NUTRITION SUPPORT As many as 25 percent of patients entering tertiary care hospitals have central catheters placed, and 20 to 30 percent of these catheters are used for parenteral nutrition. The incidence of catheter-related infection reflects the severity of the underlying medical conditions and varies from 2 to 30 per thousand catheter days, depending on the type of patients involved. In critically ill patients, catheter sepsis is associated with a 35 percent mortality rate and an attributable cost of about $40,000 per survivor. Most catheter-related complications derive from faulty insertion and management of the catheter rather than defects in the device. In large tertiary care hospitals, the insertion and management of these lines by specially trained teams can reduce complications by 80 percent, impacting significantly on outcome and costs.

The shift of focus of nutritional support of hospitalized patients from parenteral to enteral feeding also promises significant cost savings. Home parenteral nutrition costs approximately half as much as similar treatment in the hospital, and the cost of home enteral nutrition is one-tenth the cost of home parentral therapy.

BIBLIOGRAPHY

AMERICAN COLLEGE OF PHYSICIANS: Position paper: Parenteral nutrition in patients receiving cancer chemotherapy: A meta-analysis. Ann Intern Med 110:734, 1989

ANDERSON GF, STEINBERG EP: DRGs and specialized nutritional support: The need for reform. J Parenter Enter Nutr 10:3, 1986

BOWER RH et al: Early enteral administration of a formula (Impact) supplemented with arginine, nucleotides and fish oil in intensive care unit patients. Results of a multicenter, prospective, randomized, clinical trial. Crit Care Med 23:436, 1995

DALY JM et al: Enteral nutrition with supplemental arginine, RNA, and omega 3 fatty acids in patients after operation: Immunologic, metabolic and clinical outcome. Surgery 112:56, 1992

DETSKY AS et al: Perioperative parenteral nutrition: A meta-analysis. Ann Intern Med 107:195, 1987

FLYNN MB, LEIGHTTY FF: Preoperative outpatient nutritional support of patients with squamous cancer of the upper aerodigestive tract. Am J Surg 154:359, 1987

FREZZA M et al: Oral *S* adenosyl methionine in symptomatic treatment of intrahepatic cholestasis. Gastroenterology 99:211, 1990

GIAFFER MH et al: Controlled trial of polymeric versus elemental diet in treatment of active Crohn's disease. Lancet 335:816, 1990

GRAHM TW et al: The benefits of early jejunal hyperalimentation in the head-injured patient. Neurosurgery 25(5):729, 1989

GREENBERG GR et al: Controlled trial of bowel rest and nutritional support in the management of Crohn's disease. Gut 29:1309, 1988

HERNDON DN et al: Increased mortality with intravenous supplemental feeding in severely burned patients. J Burn Care Rehab 10:309, 1989

HILL GL: Body composition research: Implications for the practice of clinical nutrition. J Parenter Enter Nutr 16:197, 1992

HOWARD L et al: Current use and clinical outcome of home parenteral and enteral nutrition therapies in the United States. Gastroenterology 109:335, 1995

KALFARENTZOS FE et al: Total parenteral nutrition in severe acute pancreatitis. J Am Col Nutr 10(2):156, 1991

KUDSK KA et al: Enteral versus parenteral feeding: Effect on septic morbidity following blunt and penetrating trauma. Ann Surg 215(5):503, 1992

LIPMAN TO: Clinical trials of nutrition support in cancer. Hematol Oncol Clin North Am 5:91, 1991

MCCANN RM et al: Comfort care for terminally ill patients. JAMA 272:1263, 1994

MOORE FA et al: TEN vs. TPN following major abdominal trauma—reduced septic morbidity. J Trauma 29:916, 1989

——— et al: Clinical benefits of an immune-enhancing diet for early post injury enteral feeding. J Trauma 37:607, 1994

NAYLOR CD et al: Parenteral nutrition with branched-chain amino acids in hepatic encephalopathy: A meta-analysis. Gastroenterology 97:1033, 1989

Perioperative total parenteral nutrition in surgical patients: Veterans Administration total parenteral nutrition cooperative study. N Engl J Med 325:525, 1991

RAAD II et al: Infectious complications of indwelling vascular catheters. Clin Infect Dis 15:197, 1992

RIORDAN AM et al: Treatment of active Crohn's disease by exclusion diet: East Anglian Multicenter Controlled Trial. Lancet 342:1131, 1993

SITZMANN JV et al: Statement on guidelines for total parenteral nutrition. Dig Dis Sci 34:489, 1989

WEINSIER RL et al: Cost containment: A contribution of aggressive nutrition support in burn patients. J Burn Care Rehabil 6:436, 1985

WEISDORF S et al: Influence of prophylactic total parenteral nutrition on long-term outcome of bone marrow transplantation. Transplantation 43:833, 1987

WOLFSON M: Use of nutritional supplements in dialysis patients. Semin Dialysis 5:285, 1992

ZIEGLER TR et al: Clinical and metabolic efficacy of glutamine-supplemented parenteral nutrition after bone marrow transplantation. Ann Intern Med 116:821, 1992

79

Jean D. Wilson

VITAMIN DEFICIENCY AND EXCESS

Vitamins play several roles in human disease. Deficiencies of single vitamins are now rarely endemic, even in developing nations, and are more likely to occur either as a component of general malnutrition, as a result of food faddism, as a complication of another disease such as malabsorption or alcoholism, as a consequence of therapy such as hemodialysis or total parenteral nutrition, or as the result of an inborn error of metabolism. Indeed, disorders of vitamin excess may now be

In considering vitamin physiology, several points are worth emphasis: (1) The fact that organic compounds cannot be synthesized within the body and are required constituents of the diet is the result of mutations, and the provision of vitamins in the diet is a form of therapy for an inborn error of metabolism. In some instances, such as the limited ability to synthesize thiamine, the requirement is common to many, if not all, animals, and the defect must have arisen early in evolution; in others, such as the single-gene defect that prevents ascorbic acid synthesis, humans share the defect with only a few species, such as the guinea pig. (2) Only small amounts of vitamins are required in the diet in contrast to the relatively large amounts of essential amino acids and essential fatty acids. This is a consequence of the fact that vitamins function not as building blocks of tissue mass or as substrates for energy production but as prosthetic groups for quantitatively minor tissue constituents or as catalytic cofactors for biologic reactions; like most catalysts, they are required only in small amounts. (3) Deficiency of some vitamins (e.g., pantothenic acid) has never been described in humans, implying that these vitamins either are so ubiquitous in food sources or are conserved so efficiently by the body that deficiency can become manifest, if at all, only in the context of a mixed nutritional and vitamin deficiency. (4) The fact that many vitamin deficiencies develop on the background of alcoholism is the consequence of several interlocking factors, including diminished vitamin intake, impairment of absorption and storage of vitamins, and, in some cases, predisposing genetic factors. (5) Biochemical means of proving vitamin deficiency, once suspected, are limited, and the role of vitamin deficiency in disease states is frequently not recognized because nonspecific vitamin therapy is a common part of standard supportive care. As a consequence, knowledge of the manifestations of vitamin deficiency and a high index of suspicion in the appropriate setting are essential for considering the diagnosis, and demonstration of a response to replacement therapy may be the most accurate way to confirm a diagnosis. (6) Excessive amounts of vitamins can be consumed either as the indirect consequence of dietary practice or, more commonly, as the result of deliberate ingestion. Syndromes of excess for the fat-soluble vitamins A and D are well characterized, whereas the toxicity syndromes produced by the water-soluble vitamins are inconsistent and less well understood.

DEFICIENCY STATES

NIACIN (PELLAGRA) **Biochemistry** *Niacin* is the generic term for nicotinic acid (pyridine-3-carboxylic acid) and derivatives that exhibit the nutritional activity of nicotinic acid (Fig. 79-1). In one sense, niacin is not a vitamin, since it can be formed from the essential amino acid tryptophan. In the human, an average of about 1 mg of niacin is formed from 60 mg of dietary tryptophan. Accordingly, estimates of the adequacy of dietary intake must take into account the content of both tryptophan and niacin. Many foodstuffs, especially cereals, contain bound forms of niacin from which the vitamin is not nutritionally available.

The vitamin is absorbed rapidly from the intestine by both active and passive transport mechanisms. The capacity to absorb niacin is approximately 3 to 4 g/d in the human. Approximately one-fifth of the vitamin is decarboxylated to nicotinuric acid, and the remainder is excreted in the urine as methylated products, largely *N*-methylnicotinamide (NMN) and *N*-methyl-2-pyridone-5-carboxamide.

Mechanism of Action Niacin is an essential component of nicotinamide adenine dinucleotide (NAD) and nicotinamide adenine dinucleotide phosphate (NADP), coenzymes for many oxidation-reduction reactions.

Requirements The requirements and recommended daily allowances for niacin and tryptophan are listed in Table 72-1. In contrast to most vitamins, the requirement for niacin does not appear to be increased during pregnancy.

Experimental Depletion After the institution of a diet deficient in niacin and tryptophan, the urinary excretion of niacin metabolites reaches minimal values (<1.5 mg/d) after 1 to 2 months. Clinical deficiency develops shortly thereafter and consists of dermatitis, glossitis, stomatitis, diarrhea, proctitis, mental depression, abdominal pain, vaginitis, dysphagia, and amenorrhea, findings similar to those in pellagra.

Clinical Deficiency Pellagra was previously an endemic disease in the American South and in many other parts of the world. The endemic disease is usually associated with a high intake of maize (American corn) or of millet (sorghum, jowar) and can be cured by the administration of niacin; nevertheless, the fact that large populations of people exist on a diet in which maize is the major source of protein but are free of endemic pellagra indicates that the relation between maize intake and the development of the disease is not straightforward. The niacin equivalent (available niacin and tryptophan) of maize, although low, is no lower than that of some cereals that are unassociated with endemic pellagra. As a consequence, the concept of the pathogenesis of pellagra has evolved from that of a pure vitamin deficiency or a mixed deficiency of tryptophan and available niacin in the diet to a more complicated etiology. The disorder may be due to an imbalance in dietary amino acids or to a complex deficiency state. Alternatively, the milling of maize influences the bioavailability of the niacin in the cereal. Treatment of maize with alkali in the preparation of foods in Latin America may serve to hydrolyze bound nicotinic acid and inactivate toxins that accumulate in stored grain contaminated with molds. In contrast, degermination of the cereal during the common milling process in the United States may inhibit the liberation of bound niacin. The effect of these treatments, respectively, would be to prevent or to predispose to the development of pellagra when maize is a major element of the diet.

Whatever the cause, endemic pellagra disappeared coincident with the improvement of nutritional education and the widespread supplementation of grain cereals with niacin but still occurs on occasion in epidemic form, for example, among refugees. Pellagra is also a rare manifestation of the carcinoid syndrome, in which up to 60 percent of tryptophan is catabolized by what is ordinarily a minor pathway (see Chap. 95), and Hartnup disease (see Chap. 349), an inherited disorder in which several amino acids including tryptophan are absorbed poorly from the diet. In both conditions, pellagra is due to diminished availability of effective niacin equivalents and can be cured by the administration of large amounts of the vitamin.

Pellagra is a chronic wasting disease typically associated with dermatitis, dementia, and diarrhea. The dermatitis is bilateral, symmetric, and present in sites exposed to sunlight and is due to photosensitivity. The mental changes are less discrete; fatigue, insomnia, and apathy may precede the development of an encephalopathy characterized by confusion, disorientation, hallucination, loss of memory, and eventually, organic psychosis. Paresthesias and polyneuritis may be the result of coexisting deficiencies of other vitamins. Diarrhea, when present, results from widespread inflammation of the mucous surfaces; other mucosal abnormalities include achlorhydria, glossitis, stomatitis, and vaginitis. The skin lesions are characterized by hyperkeratosis, hyperpigmentation, and desquamation. The course is progressive over a several-year period, and death is usually due to secondary complications. The relation between the coenzyme functions of NAD and NADP and the symptoms has not been defined. The mental changes in pellagra may be due to diminished conversion of tryptophan to serotonin.

No biochemical test is of diagnostic value, and diagnosis must be based on suspicion and response to replacement therapy. As predicted, urinary excretion of the metabolites of nicotinic acid and tryptophan is low but not lower than in patients with generalized malnutrition. Plasma tryptophan and erythrocyte NAD and NADP levels are also low.

The administration of small amounts of niacin (10 mg/d) in the face of adequate amounts of dietary tryptophan is sufficient to cure

Vitamin	Active derivative or cofactor form	Principal function
Niacin	Nicotinamide adenine dinucleotide phosphate (NADP) and nicotine adenine dinucleotide (NAD)	Coenzymes for oxidations and reductions
Thiamine	Thiamine diphosphate	Coenzyme for cleavage of carbon-carbon bonds
Pyridoxine	Pyridoxal phosphate	Cofactor for enzymes of amino acid metabolism
Riboflavin	Flavin mononucleotide (FMN) and flavin adenine dinucleotide (FAD)	Cofactor for oxidation-reduction reactions and covalently attached prosthetic groups for some enzymes
Ascorbic acid	Ascorbic acid and dehydroascorbic acid	Participation as a redox ion in many biological oxidation reactions
Biotin	Biotin	Apoenzyme for carboxylase enzymes
Vitamin A	Retinol, retinal, and retinoic acid	Formation of carotenoid proteins (vision) and glycoproteins (epithelial cell function)
Vitamin E	Tocopherol	Antioxidant
Vitamin K	Menaquinone	Cofactor for post-translational carboxylation of many proteins including essential clotting factors

FIGURE 79-1 The structure and principal functions of some of the vitamins associated with human disorders.

endemic pellagra. Large amounts of niacin (40 to 200 mg/d) may be required in Hartnup disease and in the carcinoid syndrome.

THIAMINE (BERIBERI) Biochemistry Thiamine contains pyrimidine and thiazole moieties linked by a methylene bridge (see Fig. 79-1). The vitamin is synthesized by a variety of plants and microorganisms but not ordinarily by animals. However, rats and pigeons fed a thiamine-free diet can be protected from deficiency by large quantities of the pyrimidine and thiazole moieties, suggesting a small capacity to couple the subunits together. Small amounts may be synthesized by microorganisms in the gastrointestinal tract. Thiamine is absorbed both by an active-transport process and by passive diffusion. The capacity to absorb the vitamin in the human intestine is about 5 mg/d. Approximately 25 to 30 mg are stored in the body, 80 percent as thiamine diphosphate (pyrophosphate), 10 percent as thiamine triphosphate, and the remainder as thiamine monophosphate. Large amounts are present in skeletal muscles, heart, liver, kidneys, and brain. A number of thiaminase enzymes inactivate thiamine by splitting the vitamin into its two component parts. Several metabolites are excreted in the urine, principally thiamine itself (which is secreted by the renal tubules), an acetylated derivative, and derivatives of thiazole acetate and pyrimidine carboxylate.

Mechanism of Action Thiamine diphosphate acts as a coenzyme for several reactions that cleave carbon-carbon bonds—the oxidative decarboxylation of α-keto acids (pyruvate and α-ketoglutarate) and keto analogues of leucine, isoleucine, and valine and the transketolase reaction in the pentose phosphate pathway. Many features of thiamine deficiency are the result of inhibition of these enzymatic reactions and/or the accumulation of the proximal metabolites. Thiamine also may have a specific role in neurons independent of its function in general metabolism; thiamine and its esters are present in axonal membranes, and electrical stimulation of nerves effects the hydrolysis and release of thiamine diphosphate and triphosphate.

Requirements The recommended daily allowances for thiamine are given in Table 72-1. The vitamin has a widespread distribution in food and is absent only from oils, fats, cassava, and refined sugar. In vegetable products, the vitamin is largely in the form of thiamine. The outer layers of cereal grains are especially rich in the vitamin; hence machine-milled rice is a poor source. In animal tissues, thiamine is present largely in the form of phosphate esters. The esters are dephosphorylated by phosphatases in the intestine, and only the free vitamin is absorbed. A substantial loss of the vitamin takes place during cooking above 100°C.

Several factors influence the absorption and metabolism of the vitamin (and hence alter daily requirements). One is the presence of thiaminases in foods such as fresh fish, clams, shrimp, mussels, and some raw animal tissues and in microorganisms in the colon. Two, daily needs decrease when fat forms a large part of the diet and increase as carbohydrate intake increases. Requirements are increased by pregnancy, lactation, thyrotoxicosis, and fever. Accelerated loss of thiamine may occur with diuretic therapy, hemodialysis, peritoneal dialysis, and diarrhea. Defective absorption can occur in malabsorption states, alcoholism, chronic malnutrition, and folate deficiency.

Experimental Depletion Following the institution of a thiamine-free diet in control subjects, urinary thiamine excretion decreases to 5 percent of the control value after a week and is undetectable after 2 weeks. However, the excretion of the pyrimidine and thiazole catabolites remains unchanged for as long as a month, indicating that the body pool is slowly utilized when intake is low.

Within a week after the institution of a deficient diet, subjects develop a resting tachycardia, followed by the onset of weakness, decreased deep tendon reflexes, and (in some) sensory neuropathy. Symptoms include generalized malaise, headache, nausea, and aching of the muscles. Appearance of these symptoms is paralleled by a fall in red blood cell transketolase activity. Within a week of thiamine repletion (2 mg/d), all abnormal physical findings disappear, and the subjective symptoms clear after 2 weeks. (Experimental depletion in humans has not been carried to the point of development of severe manifestations.)

Clinical Deficiency In developed nations, thiamine deficiency occurs in alcoholics or food faddists and in special clinical situations, such as chronic peritoneal dialysis, hemodialysis, refeeding after starvation, after the administration of glucose to asymptomatic but thiamine-depleted patients, and in some studies in patients given large doses of diuretics chronically for congestive heart failure. In developing countries, the disorder is commonly due to the consumption of milled rice or foods containing thiaminases or (possibly) other antithiamine factors.

Development of thiamine deficiency in chronic alcoholics is due to low thiamine intake, impaired thiamine absorption and storage, accelerated destruction of thiamine diphosphate, and varying degrees of energy expenditure. However, clinical manifestations develop in only a fraction of alcoholics and other chronically malnourished persons. Genetic factors may be involved in susceptibility.

The two major manifestations of thiamine deficiency involve the cardiovascular (wet beriberi) and nervous systems (dry beriberi and the Wernicke-Korsakoff syndrome). The typical patient has mixed symptoms involving both the cardiovascular and nervous systems, but pure cardiovascular, neuropathic, and cerebral forms also occur. The relative preponderance of these manifestations is related in part to the duration and severity of deficiency, the degree of physical exertion, and the caloric intake. Severe physical exertion, high carbohydrate intake, and a moderate degree of chronic deficiency favor wet beriberi with little or no peripheral neuritis, whereas an equal deficiency with caloric restriction and relative inactivity favors the development of dry beriberi.

Beriberi heart disease comprises three major physiologic derangements: (1) peripheral vasodilatation leading to a high-output state, (2) retention of sodium and water leading to edema, and (3) biventricular myocardial failure. In the chronic form, peripheral vasodilatation leads to increased arteriovenous shunting of blood, rapid circulation time, tachycardia, increased cardiac output, and a venous congestive state characterized by elevated peripheral venous pressure, elevated right ventricular end-diastolic pressure, decreased arteriovenous extraction of oxygen, sodium retention, and edema. Decreased cerebral and renal blood flow and increased flow to muscles are common. Cardiac output increases so that notwithstanding the lowered peripheral vascular resistance, ventricular work, arterial blood pressure, and pulmonary wedge pressure tend to be elevated. Temporary appearance or worsening of hypertension may occur during thiamine repletion, presumably due to closing of arteriovenous shunts and temporary volume overload.

In acute fulminant cardiovascular (shoshin) beriberi, the myocardial lesion is the central feature of a course in which dyspnea, restlessness, and anxiety eventuate in acute cardiovascular collapse and death within hours to days. Physical findings include stocking-glove cyanosis, tachycardia, marked cardiomegaly, hepatomegaly, arterial bruits, and neck vein distention. The venous pressure is high, and the circulation time is rapid. Because of the fulminant course, edema may be minimal or absent. Administration of thiamine rapidly restores peripheral vascular resistance, but improvement in myocardial function may be delayed so that low-output failure supervenes during treatment.

Three types of nervous system involvement occur: peripheral neuropathy, Wernicke's encephalopathy (cerebral beriberi), and the Korsakoff syndrome. The neuropathy may or may not be painful and is characterized by a symmetric impairment of sensory, motor, and reflex function that affects predominantly the distal segments of limbs. The histologic lesion is a noninflammatory degeneration of myelin sheaths. No meaningful distinction can be made between this disorder and so-called alcoholic neuropathy on the basis of clinical criteria.

Wernicke's encephalopathy ordinarily develops in an orderly sequence and consists of vomiting, nystagmus (horizontal more commonly than vertical), palsies of the rectus muscles leading to unilateral or bilateral ophthalmoplegia (and decrease in the nystagmus), fever, ataxia, and progressive mental deterioration that eventuates in a global confusional state and may progress to coma and death. Improvement occurs after thiamine replacement, although Korsakoff's syndrome may

supervene. Thus the eye palsies are corrected, the nystagmus improves in one-half, the ataxia improves or disappears in two-thirds, and the global confusional state disappears to be replaced by Korsakoff's syndrome. The latter consists of retrograde amnesia, impaired ability to learn, and (usually) confabulation. The patient is typically alert and responsive and exhibits no serious defect in behavior. Recovery (complete or partial) from Korsakoff's syndrome occurs only in one-half.

In summary, Wernicke's encephalopathy and the amnesic psychosis of Korsakoff's syndrome are not separate clinical events; instead, the changing ocular and ataxic signs, the transformation of the global confusional state into the amnesic-confabulatory syndrome, and the development of a nonconfabulatory amnesic state are successive stages in the recovery from a single process. → *Cerebral beriberi is discussed further in Chap. 380.*

Biochemical tests to detect thiamine deficiency include the measurement of blood thiamine, pyruvate, α-ketoglutarate, lactate, and glyoxylate; measurement of the urinary excretion of thiamine and thiamine metabolites; the thiamine-loading test; and measurement of urinary methylglyoxal. The most reliable is the measurement of whole-blood or erythrocyte transketolase activity. Any enhancement in enzymatic activity resulting from added thiamine diphosphate (TPP) is referred to as the *TPP effect* (expressed in percent). If the activity of the enzyme is increased more than 15 percent by the added thiamine diphosphate, then a deficiency state is probably present. Measurement of isolated transketolase levels is not useful, but demonstration of an increase in activity after treatment, coupled with a positive TPP test prior to treatment, suggests thiamine deficiency.

Another criterion for the diagnosis is the assessment of clinical response to thiamine administration. Clinical improvement may be dramatic in cardiovascular beriberi, with an increase in blood pressure and a decrease in heart rate within 12 h after start of therapy and diuresis and reduction in heart size within 1 to 2 days.

Prompt administration of thiamine is indicated when beriberi is diagnosed or suspected. Fifty milligrams per day should be given intramuscularly for several days, after which 2.5 to 5 mg/d can be administered by mouth. Larger amounts are usually not absorbed. All patients also should receive other water-soluble vitamins in therapeutic quantities.

Thiamine-Responsive Inborn Errors of Metabolism Thiamine-responsive inborn errors of metabolism, in which patients may respond to pharmacologic doses of thiamine, include thiamine-responsive megaloblastic anemia, which is due to decreased cellular transport of thiamine; thiamine-responsive lactic acidosis, which is due to low activity of the pyruvate dehydrogenase complex; thiamine-responsive branched-chain ketoaciduria, which is due to low activity of a branched chain α-keto acid dehydrogenase; and a subset of subjects with Leigh's encephalomyelopathy due to abnormality of the E1 alpha subunit of pyruvate dehydrogenase.

PYRIDOXINE (VITAMIN B$_6$) **Biochemistry** The biologic activity of the vitamin B$_6$ group is displayed by pyridoxine, pyridoxal, and pyridoxamine and their 5-phosphate esters (see Fig. 79-1). The coenzyme form is pyridoxal-5-phosphate, and the other compounds owe their activity to conversion to pyridoxal-5-phosphate. The vitamin is widely and uniformly distributed in all foods; muscle meats, liver, vegetables, and whole-grain cereals are among the best sources.

Mechanism of Action Pyridoxal phosphate acts as a cofactor for many enzymes involved in amino acid metabolism, including transaminases, synthetases, and hydroxylases. In humans, the vitamin is of particular importance in the metabolism of tryptophan, glycine, serine, glutamate, and the sulfur-containing amino acids. Pyridoxal phosphate is also required for the synthesis of the heme precursor δ-aminolevulinic acid. A large portion of body stores is in muscle phosphorylase, where it functions to stabilize the enzyme rather than as a catalyst. It also plays a poorly understood role in neuronal excitability, possibly as a result of its function in transsulfuration reactions or in γ-aminobutyric acid (GABA) metabolism.

Requirements The recommended daily allowances are given in Table 72-1. Even more than for most vitamins, the requirement is increased in pregnancy and by the administration of estrogens. Estrogens appear to inhibit the role of pyridoxal phosphate in tryptophan metabolism. Pyridoxine requirement also may be increased by high protein intake and by either chronic hemodialysis or peritoneal dialysis. The ethanol metabolite acetaldehyde displaces pyridoxal phosphate from proteins and thus enhances its degradation.

Experimental Depletion The feeding of pyridoxine-deficient diets leads to chemical evidence of deficiency (increased xanthurenic acid and decreased pyridoxine in urine) within a week. Electroencephalographic abnormalities occur within 3 weeks, and some subjects have grand mal seizures. Deficiency induced with the pyridoxine antagonist deoxypyridoxine causes, in addition, seborrheic dermatitis, cheilosis, glossitis, nausea, vomiting, weakness, and dizziness.

Clinical Deficiency The widespread occurrence of the vitamin in food is probably the reason that pure pyridoxine deficiency is rare except when the pyridoxine content of food is destroyed during processing, as has happened in some infant formulas. It is a paradox, therefore, that pyridoxine deficiency is now common because many drugs act as pyridoxine antagonists. Isoniazid, cycloserine, penicillamine, and carbonyl reagents in general form complexes with the aldehyde moiety of the vitamin and inhibit its function as a coenzyme. In each case abnormal tryptophan metabolism and convulsions can be prevented by supplementation with the vitamin.

Estimates of vitamin deficiency have been based on the correction of clinical signs of deficiency following administration of the vitamin, measurement of the excretion of tryptophan metabolites after tryptophan-loading tests, measurement of various amino acid transaminase activities in blood, and measurement of the excretion of pyridoxine or its metabolites or of oxalate in urine. One index is the measurement of urinary tryptophan metabolites, particularly xanthurenic acid, following tryptophan loading. Alternatively, cystathionine can be assayed after administration of a methionine load. In vitro measurement of red blood cell glutamic pyruvic transaminase in the presence and absence of pyridoxal phosphate may be a better indicator of pyridoxine status than either loading test.

The appropriate management is prevention of deficiency. Supplementation of the diet with 30 mg pyridoxine returns tryptophan metabolism to normal in pregnancy, in users of oral contraceptives, and in patients taking isoniazid. Doses as high as 100 mg/d may be required in subjects taking penicillamine.

Pyridoxine-Responsive Diseases Several genetic disorders cause abnormalities in vitamin B_6 metabolism. In one group, infants develop convulsions and brain damage and die if not provided with large daily supplements of pyridoxine; the apoenzyme for glutamic acid decarboxylase in this disorder has a decreased binding affinity for pyridoxal phosphate. Consequently, these infants do not form normal amounts of GABA, a physiologic inhibitor of neurotransmission. Another group has pyridoxine-responsive sideroblastic anemia due to mutation in an erythrocyte-specific δ-aminolevulinate synthase; pyridoxine supplementation results in hematologic improvement but does not correct the morphologic abnormality in the erythrocytes.

The synthesis of cystathionine from homocystine and serine and its cleavage to cysteine and homoserine are catalyzed by two pyridoxal phosphate enzymes. Some patients with vitamin B_6–responsive xanthurenic aciduria or cystathioninuria have mutant apoenzymes that interact abnormally with pyridoxal phosphate, a defect that can be largely corrected by elevated concentrations of the cofactor. In contrast, the vitamin B_6 response in patients with homocystinuria due to cystathionine synthetase deficiency results from enhancement of the activity of the residual amount of normal enzyme present rather than from a restoration of the affected enzyme levels to normal.

RIBOFLAVIN Riboflavin in the form of the coenzymes flavin mononucleotide (FMN) and flavin adenine dinucleotide (FAD) (see Fig. 79-1) participates in a variety of oxidation-reduction reactions.

In addition, covalently attached flavins are essential to the structure of such enzymes as succinate dehydrogenase and monoamine oxidase. The vitamin is absorbed from the gastrointestinal tract either as free riboflavin or the 5′-phosphate by an active transport process. The recommended daily allowance is listed in Table 72-1. Covalently linked vitamin accounts for less than one-tenth of the tissue pool. The vitamin is excreted in urine predominantly in the free form, although a small fraction of the daily turnover is the result of catabolism by microorganisms in the gastrointestinal tract.

Riboflavin deficiency can be induced by feeding a riboflavin-deficient diet or by the administration of riboflavin antagonists such as galactoflavin. Deficiency is characterized by sore throat, hyperemia and edema of the oral mucous membranes, cheilosis, angular stomatitis, glossitis, seborrheic dermatitis, and normochromic, normocytic anemia due to red cell hypoplasia of the bone marrow. These features can be reversed by riboflavin administration. Thyroid hormones and adrenal steroids enhance FMN and FAD synthesis; phenothiazines and tricyclic antidepressants competitively inhibit flavin coenzyme biosynthesis, but these agents alone do not induce deficiency. Instead, riboflavin deficiency almost invariably occurs in combination with deficiencies of other water-soluble vitamins. Riboflavin requirements are increased in subjects on chronic hemodialysis or peritoneal dialysis.

VITAMIN C (SCURVY) Biochemistry In most animals, ascorbic acid (vitamin C) can be synthesized from glucose. However, humans, other primates, and the guinea pig are unable to synthesize L-ascorbic acid and require vitamin C in the diet (Fig 79-1). These species can perform the various reactions required for the biosynthesis of the vitamin from D-glucose except for one step, the conversion of L-gluconogammalactone to L-abscorbic acid. The enzyme that catalyzes this reaction (L-gluconolactone oxidase) is defective because of a mutation; thus the need for vitamin C in the diet is the result of an inborn error in carbohydrate metabolism.

Mechanism of Action L-Ascorbic acid readily undergoes reversible oxidation and reduction as follows:

$$\text{L-ascorbic acid} \rightleftharpoons \text{dehydro-L-ascorbic acid} + 2H^+ + 2e$$

This property of the vitamin is the key to understanding its role as a redox agent for biologic oxidation. However, ascorbic acid does not act as a conventional cofactor because its requirement can usually be replaced by other compounds with similar redox properties. The vitamin reduces the prosthetic metal ions in many enzymes and performs other antioxidant functions by removing free radicals. The best understood function is in the synthesis of collagen; absence of the vitamin leads to impairment of peptidyl hydroxylation of procollagen; nonhydroxylated collagen cannot form the triple helix required for normal tissue structure. In addition, the synthesis of both proteoglycan and collagen is decreased in ascorbic acid deficiency, possibly due to inhibition of insulin-like growth factor I. Many features of scurvy result from these defects in collagen synthesis, including the capillary fragility that underlies the hemorrhagic features, the poor healing of wounds, and (in part) the bony abnormalities of children. Collagens with the highest content of hydroxyproline are most severely affected, accounting for the early disruption of the adventitia, media, and basal laminae of blood vessels. Ascorbic acid also prevents oxidation of tetrahydrofolate and thus protects the active folic acid pool and regulates iron distribution and storage, probably by influencing the valence of stored iron and maintaining a normal ratio of ferritin to hemosiderin. Scorbutic patients excrete incompletely oxidized products of tyrosine metabolism, but the significance is not clear.

Requirements The recommended daily allowance for vitamin C is described in Table 72-1. The vitamin is present in milk and some meats (kidney, liver, fish) and is widely distributed in fruits and vegetables. A portion is lost after prolonged storage of unprocessed fruits and vegetables (e.g., potatoes), but it is partially preserved (half or greater) by most means of food processing (boiling, steaming, pressure cooking, preserving jams and jellies, freezing, dehydration, and canning). As a consequence, the recommended daily allowances can be met with even a modest intake of fruits and vegetables. Utilization of the vitamin is increased during pregnancy and lactation and in thyrotoxicosis, and absorption is decreased in diarrheal states and in achlorhydria.

Experimental Depletion The total-body pool of vitamin C varies from 1.5 to 3 g. When a deficient diet is instituted, the pool is depleted at a rate that approximates 4 percent per day. In monkeys, the major catabolic pathway involves oxidation of the alcohol at carbon 6 to an aldehyde and then to an acid. Because of differences in initial pool size and rates of turnover, differences in the completeness of deficiency in various experimental diets, and variation among normal subjects at the cellular or enzymatic level, the time required for development of symptoms ranges from 1 to 3 months in different studies. Manifestations of deficiency correlate better with the total pool size than with plasma or blood levels. The first symptoms (petechial hemorrhages and ecchymoses) develop when the pool size is less than 0.5 g; with further depletion (pool size 0.1 to 0.5 g), manifestations include gum involvement, hyperkeratosis, congested hair follicles, arthralgias, coiled hairs, and joint effusions. When depletion is extreme (pool size <0.1 g), dyspnea, edema, oliguria, and neuropathy supervene. Progress of the disease may then be rapid.

Symptoms do not improve until the pool is repleted, and the larger the therapeutic dose, the more rapid is the repletion. However, with doses as small as 6.5 mg/d the body pool eventually returns to normal, and amelioration of symptoms follows.

Clinical Deficiency Scurvy now occurs for the most part in areas of urban poverty. An increased incidence occurs at 6 to 12 months of age in infants whose processed milk formulas are unsupplemented with citrus fruit or vegetables as a result of maternal error or neglect. Another peak occurs in middle and old age; edentulous men who live alone and cook for themselves are particularly prone. Clinical scurvy is more severe than the experimental disease, doubtlessly because affected individuals usually have deficiencies of other dietary constituents as well and because the groups at risk (infants and the elderly) are especially vulnerable.

In adults, the features include perifollicular hyperkeratotic papules in which hairs become fragmented and buried; perifollicular hemorrhages; purpura beginning on the backs of the lower extremities coalescing to become ecchymoses (Fig. 79-2); hemorrhage into the muscles of the arms and legs with secondary phlebothromboses; hemorrhages into joints; splinter hemorrhages in the nail beds; gum involvement (only in people with teeth) that includes swelling, friability, bleeding, secondary infection, and loosening of the teeth; poor wound healing and breakdown of recently healed wounds; petechial hemorrhages in the viscera; and emotional changes. Symptoms resembling those of Sjögren's syndrome may occur. Terminally, icterus, edema, and fever are common, and convulsions, hypotension, and death may occur abruptly.

In infancy and childhood, hemorrhage into the periosteum of long bones causes painful swellings and may result in epiphyseal separation. The sternum may sink inward, leaving a sharp elevation at the rib margins (scorbutic rosary). Purpura and ecchymoses may develop in the skin, and gum lesions occur if the teeth have erupted. Retrobulbar, subarachnoid, and intracerebral hemorrhages rapidly culminate in death if treatment is delayed.

Normochromic, normocytic anemia is common and is due to bleeding into tissues. Anemia also may be macrocytic and/or megaloblastic (one-fifth of patients in one series). Many foods that contain vitamin C also contain folate, and diets that cause scurvy also may cause folate deficiency. However, ascorbic acid deficiency also results in an increased oxidation of formyl tetrahydrofolic acid to inactive folate metabolites and may cause a decrease in the active folate pool. Whether changes in iron distribution and storage are involved in the pathogenesis of the anemia is unclear. The anemia is corrected with replenishment of vitamin C and institution of a balanced diet.

In some hospitals, platelet ascorbic acid levels are useful in diagnosing scurvy and are usually less than one-fourth of the normal value. Plasma levels of the vitamin correlate less well with the clinical state. In infants, x-ray changes of the bones may be diagnostic. Bilirubin is frequently elevated. Capillary fragility is abnormal.

Scurvy is potentially fatal; if the diagnosis is suspected, blood

FIGURE 79-2 Hemorrhages and ecchymoses in a patient with scurvy. *(Photograph courtesy of Leonard L. Madison.)*

should be obtained, and ascorbic acid therapy should be instituted promptly. The usual dose in adults is 100 mg three to five times a day by mouth until 4 g has been administered, then 100 mg/d. In infants and children, administration of 10 to 25 mg three times a day is adequate. A diet rich in vitamin C should be initiated simultaneously. Spontaneous bleeding usually ceases within 24 h, muscle and bone pains subside quickly, and the gums begin to heal within 2 to 3 days. Even large ecchymoses and hematomas resolve in 10 to 12 days, although pigmentary changes in areas of hemorrhage may persist for months. Serum bilirubin becomes normal within 3 to 5 days, and the anemia is ordinarily corrected within 2 to 4 weeks.

BIOTIN Biotin (see Fig. 79-1) functions as a cofactor in mammalian carboxylases. The vitamin is largely ingested in a form bound to protein, hydrolyzed by pancreatic biotinidase, and absorbed by what is probably an active transport process. The recommended daily allowance is given in Table 72-1. In cells, biotin is covalently attached to apocarboxylases to form four haloenzymes that catalyze the incorporation of bicarbonate into substrate, acetyl-CoA carboxylase, pyruvate carboxylase, methylcrotonyl CoA carboxylase, and propionyl CoA carboxylase. Biotin deficiency in the human occurs under at least four conditions: following the prolonged consumption of raw egg white (which binds biotin in the gut and prevents its absorption), after parenteral nutrition without biotin supplementation in patients with malabsorption, as a component of protein-energy malnutrition, and in subjects with multiple carboxylase deficiency due to abnormalities in holocarboxylase synthetase or biotinidase. In all these conditions the common manifestations of biotin deficiency resemble those of essential fatty acid deficiency and include perioral dermatitis, conjunctivitis, alopecia, ataxia, and, in children, developmental delay. In addition, serious neurologic defects and organic aciduria may occur in multiple carboxylase deficiency.

The diagnosis can be established by documenting reduced urinary excretion of biotin or by demonstrating resolution of the deficiency in response to supplementation with 100 μg/d.

VITAMIN A   Biochemistry   Vitamin A (retinol) can either be ingested or synthesized within the body from plant carotenes (see Fig. 79-1). The best sources of preformed vitamin A are liver, milk, and kidney, where it occurs largely in the form of fatty acid esters. The esters are hydrolyzed during digestion, absorbed in the free form, reesterified with fatty acids within the intestinal mucosa, and enter the circulation with lymph chylomicrons. The carotene substrates for synthesis of vitamin A, mainly β-carotenes, are widely distributed in plants. β-Carotene can either be absorbed intact or cleaved in the intestinal tract to form two molecules of retinaldehyde. Retinaldehyde is subsequently reduced by an aldehyde reductase to retinol. Retinol from whatever source is stored as retinyl esters in the liver. The normal body pool is 300 to 900 mg.

Prior to release from the liver, retinyl esters are hydrolyzed, and the free alcohol is bound to a specific transport protein, retinol-binding protein (RBP), for transport to peripheral tissues. In vitamin A deficiency, the release of RBP from the liver is inhibited, and the protein accumulates in liver; with repletion, RBP is rapidly released from preformed stores. Approximately equal amounts of retinol are excreted in the bile and urine.

Mechanism of Action   The best-defined function of vitamin A is its role in vision; in the retina vitamin A constitutes the prosthetic group of carotenoid proteins that provide the molecular basis for visual excitation. In addition, vitamin A is required for growth, reproduction, and the maintenance of life. Retinol-phosphate-mannose glycolipid is present in a variety of cell membranes, and the vitamin plays a primary role in the synthesis of glycoproteins. The importance of glycoprotein to every cell implies that this is an equally important function of the vitamin. In all its functions, the vitamin is believed to act by binding to a transcription regulatory protein that controls gene expression (see Chap. 327).

Requirements   The recommended daily allowance for vitamin A is listed in Table 72-1. The assumed utilization efficiency for the conversion of β-carotene to vitamin A in the human is one-sixth (0.167). Other carotenoids with provitamin A activity have, on average, about half the activity of β-carotene. Pregnancy and disease states that cause impaired absorption or storage, excessive utilization, or increased excretion of vitamin A may lead to increased requirements.

Experimental Depletion   When experimental subjects are fed a diet deficient in both retinol and carotene, plasma levels fall, and the body pool shrinks to less than half the control value. Deficiency is manifested by follicular hyperkeratosis, impaired dark adaptation, and abnormalities of the electroretinogram. These changes are corrected after supplementation with 150 μg retinol or 300 μg β-carotene per day.

Clinical Deficiency   Endemic deficiency results from inadequate amounts of the vitamin and provitamins in the diet and occurs in conjunction with deficiency of other nutrients or complicating diseases. In some developing countries, vitamin A deficiency is a major cause of blindness in the young as a consequence of failure to incorporate green leafy vegetables or other sources of the provitamin or vitamin into the diet. Vitamin A–deficient children appear to be particularly susceptible to the complications of measles. Vitamin A deficiency also may be a component of protein-calorie malnutrition. In developed countries, vitamin A deficiency is usually due either to intestinal malabsorption (as in sprue or after intestinal bypass surgery), abnormal storage (liver disease), or enhanced destruction or excretion of the vitamin (proteinuria). Vitamin A deficiency also has occurred in patients receiving total parenteral nutrition because of loss of vitamin A after prolonged storage of intravenous fluid.

Night blindness is the earliest symptom of deficiency, followed by degenerative changes in the retina. The bulbar conjunctiva becomes dry (xerosis), and small gray plaques with foamy surfaces develop (Bitôt's spots). These early lesions are reversible with administration of vitamin A. The more serious effects of deficiency are ulceration and necrosis of the cornea (keratomalacia), leading to perforation, endophthalmitis, and blindness. Dryness and hyperkeratosis of the skin may be present.

Vitamin A levels in plasma are not reliable for the assessment of stores in individual cases. Measurements of dark adaptation, rod scotometry, and electroretinography are useful indicators of vitamin A stores but require trained personnel and expensive equipment; consequently, the diagnosis is usually based on a high index of suspicion in malnourished children or in patients with predisposing factors for its development.

Night blindness and the milder conjunctival changes respond well to 30,000 IU of vitamin A daily for a week. Corneal damage constitutes a therapeutic emergency, and the usual treatment is 20,000 IU/kg of body weight per day for 5 days. Children who are at risk for vitamin A deficiency and who develop measles should be given 200,000 IU orally each day for 2 days.

VITAMIN E   Biochemistry   Eight naturally occurring tocopherols possess vitamin E activity. The structure of alpha tocopherol, the most widely distributed and most active of the tocopherols, is shown in Fig. 79-1. The vitamin is absorbed from the gastrointestinal tract and enters the circulation via the lymph, associated first with chylomicrons and then with plasma β-lipoproteins. Indeed, plasma levels correlate with plasma lipid levels. The vitamin is stored in all tissues, and the tissue stores can protect against vitamin deficiency for long periods. Approximately three-fourths of the vitamin is excreted in bile, and the balance is excreted as glucuronides in urine. Metabolites with quinone structures (including one similar to ubiquinone) are present in tissues.

Mechanism of Action   The vitamin probably acts as an antioxidant rather than as a specific cofactor. In so acting it presumably inhibits oxidation of essential cellular constituents and prevents the formation of toxic oxidation products. Other antioxidants such as selenium, sulfur-containing amino acids, and the ubiquinone group can reverse the symptoms of vitamin E deficiency in animals.

Requirements   The recommended daily requirement is 10 to 30 mg/d (see Table 72-1). Diets containing large amounts of polyunsaturated fatty acids increase and diets containing antioxidants decrease the requirement. The vitamin is widely distributed in food, so a primary deficiency state has never been recognized in otherwise healthy children or adults. Newborn infants have plasma concentrations about one-fifth that of maternal levels, implying poor placental transfer, but human milk (in contrast to cow's milk) has sufficient levels to meet the requirements in infants.

Experimental Depletion   In long-term studies, vitamin E concentrations in plasma declined significantly only after months on a deficient diet. No manifestations of the depletion were detected in normal volunteers, making it difficult to establish that tocopherol is a human vitamin.

Clinical Deficiency   Nevertheless, vitamin E deficiency may be associated with a discrete syndrome, as when deficiency is due to a selective malabsorption of the vitamin or when an autosomal recessive mutation causes vitamin E deficiency and ataxia. More commonly, intestinal fat malabsorption can cause deficiency of all fat-soluble vitamins including vitamin E, and children with abetalipoproteinemia or chronic cholestatic liver disease appear to be particularly susceptible. Measurement of the ratio of serum vitamin E to total-serum lipid is the preferred index for assessing vitamin E status. The manifestations of deficiency include areflexia, gait disturbance, decreased proprioceptive and vibratory sensation, and paresis of gaze and are associated with degeneration of the posterior columns of the spinal cord, selective loss of large-caliber, myelinated axons in peripheral nerves, and appearance of spheroids in the gracile and cuneate nuclei of the brain. Treatment (50 to 100 IU/d by mouth) is most effective when initiated early in the course of the disease.

VITAMIN K Vitamin K consists of a quinone ring attached to a side chain (labeled R in Fig. 79-1) that varies depending on the source of the vitamin. Vitamin K_1 (phylloquinone) is present in most edible vegetables, particularly in green leaves. Vitamin K_2 is produced by intestinal bacteria but not in sufficient amounts to supply daily requirements. The many compounds with vitamin K activity are structurally related to the simpler compound, 2-methyl-1,4-naphthoquinone (menadione). Menadione is formed in the gut by the removal of the side chain from the vitamin by intestinal bacteria. After absorption, menadione is converted in the body to the active menaquinone. The vitamin is a component of a specialized microsomal enzyme system that effects the posttranslational γ carboxylation of glutamic acid in proteins of the plasma, bone, kidney, and urine, including clotting factors II, VII, IX, and X, and the coagulation inhibitors proteins C and S. Death from hemorrhage in deficiency states ensues before deficiency of the other carboxylated proteins becomes manifest. The warfarin anticoagulant drugs induce hypoprothrombinemia by inhibiting the γ carboxylation of the precursor protein.

Under ordinary circumstances, about 80 percent of vitamin K is absorbed from the small bowel into the intestinal lymph. Deficiency can occur in association with diseases that interfere with fat absorption. In addition, long-term treatment with oral antibiotics may temporarily eliminate intestinal bacteria as a source for vitamin K and promote deficiency when the diet is marginal.

Newborn infants tend to be deficient in vitamin K and have low plasma levels of several coagulation factors in the prothrombin complex. Such deficiencies result from minimal stores of vitamin K at birth, lack of an established intestinal flora, and a limited dietary intake of the vitamin, but it is not clear whether all infants should be supplemented routinely.

Determination of prothrombin should be performed prior to surgical procedures or delivery. Subjects with levels below 70 percent of normal should receive therapy with vitamin K. Vitamin K deficiency can be separated from hypoprothrombinemia of liver disease by demonstration of the noncarboxylated prothrombin precursor that accumulates in plasma in the vitamin deficiency.

VITAMIN EXCESS

According to the National Health Interview Survey, more than 50 percent of adults in the United States use vitamin and/or mineral supplements, and in many instances ingestion is within a potentially toxic range. Multivitamins are the usual type ingested by children, whereas single vitamins are consumed commonly by adults. Supplement use is higher with the level of education and income and in those whose health is good.

Fat-soluble vitamins are stored to a variable extent in the body and hence are more likely to cause adverse effects when taken in excess; excess states for vitamins D (see Chap. 354) and A are well characterized. Water-soluble vitamins are readily excreted in the urine and stored only to a limited extent. Consequently, toxicity states for these vitamins only occur when very large amounts are taken.

VITAMIN A AND CAROTENES Carotenemia Carotenemia results from excessive intake of vitamin A precursors in foods, principally carrots. Excess carotene is not injurious apart from the cosmetic effect; the fact that carotenemia does not cause hypervitaminosis A indicates that the conversion of carotene to vitamin A must be regulated. Carotenemia is manifested by yellowing of the skin with greatest intensity on the palms and soles and by a corresponding yellowness of serum. The yellowing of the skin differs from jaundice in that the sclerae remain white. Hypothyroid patients are particularly susceptible. The omission of carrots from the diet leads to the rapid disappearance of the pigmentation. Discoloration of the skin also can result from the consumption of large amounts of other colored fruits and vegetables.

Vitamin A Toxicity Hypervitaminosis A can result from accidental overingestion by hunters or explorers (polar bear liver), as the result of food faddism (usually caused by overly solicitous parents),

or as a side effect of inappropriate therapy. Acute toxicity from a single massive dose consists of abdominal pain, nausea, vomiting, headache, dizziness, sluggishness, papilledema, and in infants a bulging fontanel followed within a few days by generalized desquamation of the skin and recovery. Chronic toxicity occurs after ingestion of 25,000 units or more daily for protracted periods and is characterized by bone and joint pain, hyperostoses, hair loss, dryness and fissures of the lips, anorexia, benign intracranial hypertension, low-grade fever, pruritus, weight loss, and hepatosplenomegaly. The only diagnostic laboratory finding is elevation of the vitamin in serum, chiefly in the form of retinyl esters. The concentration of retinol-binding protein is normal, and the excess vitamin A circulates in association with lipoprotein. Relief is usually prompt on discontinuation of the vitamin, but cirrhosis of the liver can develop as a late complication of overdosage.

VITAMIN E Relatively large doses of vitamin E have been taken by some for extended periods without apparent harm. In others, malaise, gastrointestinal complaint, headaches, and possibly hypertension have occurred. However, true toxicity appears to occur in two situations—in subjects receiving oral anticoagulants and in premature infants. In large amounts, vitamin E can antagonize vitamin K and prolong the prothrombin time; this phenomenon results in a potentiation of oral anticoagulants. Premature infants given parenteral vitamin E have developed ascites associated with hepatosplenomegaly, cholestatic jaundice, azotemia, and thrombocytopenia.

VITAMIN K Large amounts of vitamin K can block the effects of oral anticoagulants and when given to pregnant women can cause jaundice in the newborn.

PYRIDOXINE Most adults can consume up to 10 times the recommended daily allowance of 2 mg pyridoxine per day without adverse effects. However, severe peripheral neuropathies have developed after ingestion of several grams per day for prolonged periods; symptoms include ataxia, perioral numbness, and clumsiness of the hands and feet, and the findings include loss of position and vibration sense without impairment of reflexes or sensory function. Recovery is slow after ingestion ceases. Lower doses (25 mg/d) can antagonize the effects of levodopa in Parkinson's disease and decrease the anticonvulsant effects of phenytoin and barbiturates.

In women who consume vitamin supplements, the median dose of pyridoxine approaches the level of 120 mg/d found to cause paresthesia and muscle weakness in normal volunteers who consumed the vitamin for 6 months or greater.

VITAMIN C Vitamin C is consumed by 85 percent of all vitamin users because of the belief that large amounts of the vitamin (a gram or greater per day) prevent or minimize the symptoms of the common cold. However, in controlled studies, no significant differences in occurrence, severity, or duration of colds have been demonstrated in subjects treated with the vitamin. Use of the vitamin in this way is unwarranted and probably unwise. The long-term use of ascorbic acid in these doses can interfere with the absorption of vitamin B_{12}, enhance blood levels of estrogens in women on exogenous estrogens, cause uricosuria, and predispose to formation of oxalate kidney stones. In addition, large doses enhance the development of metabolizing enzymes in the fetus and may cause rebound scurvy in the offspring of mothers who have ingested large amounts of the vitamin during pregnancy. However, pharmacologic doses (200 mg daily) may correct leukocyte abnormalities in patients with the Chédiak-Higashi syndrome (see Chap. 62).

NIACIN Large doses of niacin are used for treatment of hypercholesterolemia (see Chap. 341) and occasionally for other purposes. The vitamin causes release of histamine, which in turn can cause severe flushing, pruritus, and gastrointestinal disturbances and may aggravate asthma. Acanthosis nigricans may occur. In doses of 3 g/d niacin can cause elevation of serum uric acid and of glucose. Large doses can also cause hepatic toxicity including cholestatic jaundice.

For further information, see Chap. 62, Water-soluble vitamins, and Chap. 63, Fat-soluble vitamins, in Goodman & Gilman's The Pharmacological Basis of Therepeutics, *9th ed. New York, McGraw-Hill, 1996.*

BIBLIOGRAPHY

GENERAL

Bates CJ: Vitamin undernutrition. Proc Nutr Soc 52:143, 1993

Brown ML: *Present Knowledge in Nutrition.* Washington, International Life Science Institute, 1990

Combs GF Jr: *The Vitamins.* San Diego, Academic, 1992

Elsas LJ, McCormick DB: Genetic defects in vitamin utilization. Part I: General aspects and fat-soluble vitamins. Vitam Horm 43:103, 1986

Hoyumpa AM: Mechanisms of vitamin deficiencies in alcoholism. Alcohol Clin Exp Res 10:573, 1986

Linden MC: *Nutritional Biochemistry and Metabolism.* New York, Elsevier, 1991

Mudd SH: Inborn errors of metabolism. Vitamin-responsive genetic disease. J Clin Pathol 27(Suppl) 8:38, 1974

Rudman D, Williams PJ: Nutrient deficiencies during total parenteral nutrition. Nutr Rev 43:1, 1984

NIACIN DEFICIENCY

Carpenter KJ: The relationship of pellagra to corn and the low availability of niacin in cereals. Experientia(Suppl) 44:197, 1983

———, Lewin WJ: A reexamination of the composition of diets associated with pellagra. J Nutr 115:543, 1985

Castiello RJ, Lynch PJ: Pellagra and the carcinoid syndrome. Arch Dermatol 105:574, 1972

Fu CS et al: Biochemical markers for assessment of niacin status in young men. J Nutr 119:1949, 1989

Goldsmith GA: Experimental niacin deficiency. J Am Diet Assoc 32:312, 1956

Henderson LM: Niacin. Annu Rev Nutr 3:289, 1983

Jukes TH et al: The conquest of pellagra. Fed Proc 40:1519, 1980

Levy HL: Hartnup disorder, in *The Metabolic Basis of Inherited Disease,* 7th ed, CR Scriver et al (eds). New York, McGraw-Hill, 1995, p 3629

Malfait P et al: An outbreak of pellagra related to changes in dietary niacin among Mozambican refugees in Malawi. Int J Epidemiol 22:504, 1993

Oakley A, Wallace J: Hartnup disease presenting in an adult. Clin Exp Dermatol 19:407, 1994

THIAMINE DEFICIENCY

Bettendorff L: Thiamine in excitable tissues: Reflections on a non-cofactor role. Metab Brain Dis 9:183, 1994

Brady JA, et al: Thiamine status, diuretic medications, and the management of congestive heart failure. J Am Diet Assoc 95:541, 1995

De Meirleir L et al: Aberrant splicing of exon 6 in the pyruvate dehydrogenase-E1 alpha mRNA linked to a silent mutation in a large family with Leigh's encephalomyelopathy. Pediatr Res 36:707, 1994

Duran M, Wadman SK: Thiamine-responsive inborn errors of metabolism. J Inherit Metab Dis 8(Suppl 1):70, 1985

Dyckner T et al: Aggravation of thiamine deficiency by magnesium depletion. Acta Med Scand 218:129, 1985

Ellerine NP et al: Thiamin-responsive maple syrup urine disease in a patient antigenically missing dihydrolipoamide acyltransferase. Biochem Med Met Biol 49:363, 1993

Fineglas PM: Thiamin. Int J Vit Nutr Res 63:270, 1993

Haas RH: Thiamin and the brain. Annu Rev Nutr 8:483, 1988

Harper CG et al: Clinical signs in the Wernicke-Korsakoff complex: A retrospective analysis of 131 cases diagnosed at necropsy. J Neurol Neurosurg Psychiatry 49:341, 1986

Hoyumpa AM: Mechanisms of thiamine deficiency in chronic alcoholism. Am J Clin Nutr 33:2750, 1980

Kawai C et al: Reappearance of beriberi heart disease in Japan. Am J Med 69:383, 1980

Kozam RL et al: Cardiovascular beriberi. Am J Cardiol 30:418, 1972

Kuriyama M et al: Blood vitamin B_1, transketolase, and thiamine pyrophosphate (TPP) effect in beriberi patients. Clin Chim Acta 108:159, 1980

Naito E et al: Molecular analysis of abnormal pyruvate dehydrogenase in a patient with thiamine-responsive congenital lactic acidemia. Pediatr Res 36:340, 1994

Rindi G et al: Further studies on erythrocyte thiamin transport and phosphorylation in seven patients with thiamin-responsive megaloblastic anaemia. J Inherit Metab Dis 17:667, 1994

Shimon I et al: Improved left ventricular function after thiamine supplementa-

tion in patients with congestive heart failure receiving long term furosemide therapy. Am J Med 98:485, 1995

Victor M: Alcoholic dementia. Can J Neurol Sci 21:88, 1994

Ziporin ZZ et al: Excretion of thiamine and its metabolites in the urine of young adult males receiving restricted intakes of the vitamin. J Nutr 85:287, 1965

PYRIDOXINE DEFICIENCY

Bassier KH: Megavitamin therapy with pyridoxine. Int J Vitam Nutr Res 58:105, 1988

Bender DA: Novel functions of vitamin B_6. Proc Nutr Soc 53:625, 1994

Bhagavan HN, Brin M: Drug–vitamin B_6 interaction. Curr Concepts Nutr 12:1, 1983

Bitsch R: Vitamin B_6. Int J Vit Nutr Res 63:278, 1993

Cox TC et al: X-linked pyridoxine-responsive sideroblastic anemia due to a Thr388-to-Ser substitution in erythroid Δ-aminolevulinate synthase. N Engl J Med 330:675, 1994

Gershoff SN: Vitamin B_6, in *Nutrition Reviews' Present Knowledge in Nutrition,* 4th ed, DM Hegsted et al (eds). Washington, The Nutrition Foundation, 1976, p 149

Gospe SM Jr et al: Reduced GABA synthesis in pyridoxine-dependent seizures. Lancet 343:1133, 1994

Guilarte TR: Vitamin B_6 and cognitive development: Recent research findings from human and animal studies. Nutr Rev 51:193, 1993

Hu FL et al: Molecular basis of cystathionine beta-synthase deficiency in pyridoxine responsive and nonresponsive homocystinuria. Hum Mol Genet 2:1857, 1993

Kraus JP, Kozich V: Pyridoxine responsive and unresponsive homocystinuria. J Nutr Sci Vit Spec No: 589, 1992

Kretsch MJ et al: Electroencephalographic changes and periodontal status during short-term vitamin B_6 depletion of young nonpregnant women. Am J Clin Nutr 53:1266, 1991

Luhby AL et al: Vitamin B_6 metabolism in users of oral contraceptive agents: I. Abnormal urinary xanthurenic acid excretion and its correction by pyridoxine. Am J Clin Nutr 24:684, 1971

Mydlik M et al: Vitamin B_6 requirements in chronic renal failure. Int Urol Nephrol 24:453, 1992

Young RC, Bass JP: Iatrogenic nutritional deficiencies. Annu Rev Nutr 2:201, 1982

RIBOFLAVIN DEFICIENCY

Bates CJ: Human riboflavin requirements, and metabolic consequences of deficiency in man and animals. World Rev Nutr Diet 50:215, 1987

Merrill AH Jr et al: Formation and mode of action of flavoproteins. Annu Rev Nutr 1:281, 1981

Pinto JT, Rivlin RS: Drugs that promote renal excretion of riboflavin. Drug Nutr Interact 5:143, 1987

——— et al: Mechanisms underlying the differential effects of ethanol on the bioavailability of riboflavin and flavin adenine dinucleotide. J Clin Invest 79:1343, 1987

Roe DA: Riboflavin deficiency: Mucocutaneous signs of acute and chronic deficiency. Semin Dermatol 10:293, 1991

Ross NS, Hansen TP: Riboflavin deficiency is associated with selective preservation of critical flavoenzyme-dependent metabolic pathways. Biofactors 3:185, 1992

ASCORBIC ACID DEFICIENCY

Adelman HM et al: Scurvy resembling cutaneous vasculitis. Cutis 54:111, 1994

Barness LA: Nutritional aspects of vegetarianism, health foods, and fad diets. Nutr Rev 59:153, 1977

Boxer LA et al: Correction of leucocyte function in Chédiak-Higashi syndrome by ascorbate. N Engl J Med 295:1041, 1971

Burns JJ et al: *Third Conference on Vitamin C.* Ann NY Acad Sci Ser 498, 1987

England S, Seifter S: The biochemical functions of ascorbic acid. Annu Rev Nutr 6:365, 1986

Franceschi RT: The role of ascorbic acid in mesenchymal differentiation. Nutr Rev 50:65, 1992

Hodges RE et al: Clinical manifestations of ascorbic acid deficiency in man. Am J Clin Nutr 24:432, 1971

Levine M: New concepts in the biology and biochemistry of ascorbic acid. N Engl J Med 314:892, 1986

Padh H: Vitamin C: Newer insights into its biochemical functions. Nutr Rev 49:65, 1991

Peterkofsky B: Ascorbate requirement for hydroxylation and secretion of procollagen: Relationship to inhibition of collagen synthesis in scurvy. Am J Clin Nutr 54(Suppl 6):1135S, 1991

Reuler JB et al: Adult scurvy. JAMA 253:805, 1985

Sato P, Undenfriend S: Studies on ascorbic acid related to the genetic basis of scurvy, in *Vitamins and Hormones,* vol 36, P Munson et al (eds). New York, Academic, 1978, p 33

Tolbert BM et al: New information on synthesis and metabolism of ascorbic acid. Nutr Rev 35:22, 1977

Vilter RW: Effects of ascorbic acid deficiency in man, in *The Vitamins*, WH Sebrell Jr et al (eds). New York, Academic, 1967, vol 1, p 457

Wallerstein RO, Wallerstein RO Jr: Scurvy. Semin Hematol 13:211, 1976

BIOTIN

Marshall MM: The nutritional importance of biotin—an update. Nutr Today 22:26, 1987

Mock DM: Skin manifestations of biotin deficiency. Semin Dermatol 10:296, 1991

Sweetman L, Nyhan WL: Inheritable biotin-treatable disorders and associated phenomena. Annu Rev Nutr 6:317, 1986

Velazquez A et al: Biotin supplementation affects lymphocyte carboxylases and plasma biotin in severe protein-energy malnutrition. Am J Clin Nutr 61:385, 1995

Wolf B: Disorders of biotin metabolism, *The Metabolic and Molecular Basis of Inherited Disease*, 7th ed, in Scriver CR et al (eds). New York, McGraw-Hill, 1995, p 3151

VITAMIN A DEFICIENCY

Bates CJ: Vitamin A. Lancet 345:31, 1995

DeLuca LM: The direct involvement of vitamin A in glycosyl transfer reactions of mammalian membranes, in *Vitamins and Hormones*, vol 35, PL Munson et al (eds). New York, Academic, 1977, p 1

Fawzi WW et al: Vitamin A supplementation and child mortality. A meta-analysis. JAMA 269:898, 1993

Giguere V et al: Identification of a receptor for the morphogen retinoic acid. Nature 330:624, 1987

Goodman DS: Vitamin A and retinoids in health and disease. N Engl J Med 310:1023, 1984

Howard L et al: Vitamin A deficiency from long-term parenteral nutrition. Ann Intern Med 93:576, 1980

Olson JA: Hypovitaminosis A: Contemporary scientific issues. J Nutr 124(Suppl 8):1461S, 1994

Sauberlich HE et al: Vitamin A metabolism and requirements in the human studied with the use of labeled retinol, in *Vitamins and Hormones*, vol 32, RS Harris et al (eds). New York, Academic, 1974

Smith FR, Goodman DS: Vitamin A transport in human vitamin A toxicity. N Engl J Med 294:805, 1976

Sommer A: New imperatives for an old vitamin (A). J Nutr 119:96, 1989

Tee ES: Carotenoids and retinoids in human nutrition. Crit Rev Food Sci Nutr 31:103, 1992

Tielsch JM, Sommer A: The epidemiology of vitamin A deficiency and xerophthalmia. Annu Rev Nutr 4:183, 1974

Underwood BA: The role of vitamin A in child growth, development and survival. Adv Exp Med Biol 352:201, 1994

Vahlquist A: Clinical use of vitamin A and its derivatives—physiological and pharmacological aspects. Clin Exp Dermatol 10:133, 1985

Wald G: Molecular basis of visual excitation. Science 162:230, 1968

VITAMIN E DEFICIENCY

Bieri JG et al: Medical uses of vitamin E. N Engl J Med 308:1063, 1983

Doerflinger N et al: Ataxia with vitamin E deficiency: Refinement of genetic localization and analysis of linkage disequilibrium by using new markers in 14 families. Am J Hum Genet 56:1116, 1995

Kayden HJ: The neurologic syndrome of vitamin E deficiency: A significant cause of ataxia. Neurology 43:2167, 1993

———, Traber MG: Absorption, lipoprotein transport, and regulation of plasma concentrations of vitamin E in humans. J Lipid Res 34:343, 1993

Lloyd JK: The importance of vitamin E in human nutrition. Acta Paediatr Scand 79:6, 1990

Meydani M: Vitamin E. Lancet 345:170, 1995

Morrissey PA et al: Vitamin E. Int J Vitam Nutr Res 63:260, 1993

Sitrin MD et al: Vitamin E deficiency and neurologic disease in adults with cystic fibrosis. Ann Intern Med 107:51, 1987

Sokol RJ et al: Isolated vitamin E deficiency in the absence of fat malabsorption—familial and sporadic cases: Characterization and investigation of causes. J Lab Clin Med 111:548, 1988

——— et al: Intestinal malabsorption of vitamin E in primary biliary cirrhosis. Gastroenterology 96:479, 1989

——— et al: Multicenter trial of D-alpha-tocopheryl polyethylene glycol 1000 succinate for treatment of vitamin E deficiency in children with chronic cholestasis. Gastroenterology 104:1717, 1993

Traber MG et al: Lack of tocopherol in peripheral nerves of vitamin E–deficient patients with peripheral neuropathy. N Engl J Med 317:262, 1987

VITAMIN K DEFICIENCY

Bertina RM et al: New method for the rapid detection of vitamin K deficiency. Clin Chim Acta 105:93, 1980

Huysman MW, Sauer PJ: The vitamin K controversy. Curr Opin Pediatr 6:129, 1994

Iber FL et al: Vitamin K deficiency in chronic alcoholic males. Alcohol Clin Exp Res 10:679, 1986

Lipsky JJ: Nutritional sources of vitamin K. Mayo Clin Proc 69:462, 1994

Olson RE, Suttie JW: Vitamin K and γ-carboxyglutamate biosynthesis, in *Vitamins and Hormones*, vol 35, PL Munson et al (eds). New York, Academic, 1977, p 59

Shearer MJ: Vitamin K. Lancet 345:229, 1995

Suttie JW: Vitamin K and human nutrition. J Am Diet Assoc 92:585, 1992

——— et al: Vitamin K deficiency from dietary vitamin K restriction in humans. Am J Clin Nutr 47:475, 1988

VITAMIN EXCESS

Alhadeff L: Toxic effects of water-soluble vitamins. Nutr Rev 42:33, 1984

Chalmers TC: Effects of ascorbic acid on the common cold. Am J Med 58:532, 1975

Corrigan JJ Jr: The effect of vitamin E on warfarin-induced vitamin K deficiency. Ann NY Acad Sci 82:361, 1982

Dalton K, Dalton MJT: Characteristics of pyridoxine overdose neuropathy syndrome. Acta Neurol Scand 76:8, 1987

Geubel AP et al: Liver damage caused by therapeutic vitamin A administration: Estimate of dose-related toxicity in 41 cases. Gastroenterology 100:1701, 1991

Jorens PG et al: Vitamin A abuse: Development of cirrhosis despite cessation of vitamin A. A six-year clinical and histopathologic followup. Liver 12:381, 1992

Lemons JA, Maisels MJ: Vitamin E—how much is too much? Pediatrics 76:625, 1985

Lombaert A, Carton H: Benign intracranial hypertension due to A-hypervitaminosis in adults and adolescents. Eur Neurol 14:340, 1976

Lorch V et al: Unusual syndrome with fatalities among premature infants: Association with a new intravenous vitamin E product. Morb Mort Week Rep 33:198, 1984

Moss AJ et al: Use of vitamin and mineral supplements in the United States. Advance Data No. 174. Hyattsville, Md: National Center for Health Statistics, 1989

Roe DA: Assessment of risk factors for carotenodermia and cutaneous signs of hypervitaminosis A in college-aged populations. Semin Dermatol 10:303, 1991

Schaumburg H et al: Sensory neuropathy from pyridoxine abuse: A new megavitamin syndrome. N Engl J Med 309:445, 1983

Shin HB et al: Ascorbic acid–induced uricosuria: A consequence of megavitamin therapy. Ann Intern Med 84:385, 1976

Toxic effects of vitamin overdosage. Med Lett Drugs Ther 26:73, 1984

Woolliscroft JO: Megavitamins: Fact and fancy. Dis Mon 24:1, 1983

80 *Kenneth H. Falchuk*

DISTURBANCES IN TRACE ELEMENTS

CLASSIFICATION AND FUNCTIONS The *trace elements* comprise metals in biological fluids at concentrations <1 μg/g wet weight. Most are essential nutrients for humans (Table 80-1). Others (As, Ni, Sn, V, Si) are essential for some species and may be required by humans. The functions of trace elements and of more abundant metals (Na, K, Ca, Mg) are determined, in part, by their charges, mobilities, and binding constants to biological ligands. Some elements (Na, K) bind weakly to negatively charged ligands and cross cellular membranes without major impediment. They are used by living systems as charge carriers to conduct electric impulses along nerves, etc. Other elements (Mg, Ca) form moderately stable complexes with enzymes, nucleic acids, and other ligands. They act as "triggers," altering and/or controlling biological functions; for example, Ca affects muscle contraction and relaxation (Chap. 383). Those in a third group include Fe, Zn, Cu, and others that form strong static complexes with and become integral components of proteins and enzymes (Table 80-1).

METAL DEFICIENCY OR TOXICITY Metals can cause disease through deficiency, imbalance, or toxicity. Deficiency usually results when dietary intake is inadequate or when intake is adequate but other conditioning factors come into play. Conditioned deficiencies can be caused by metal malabsorption in chronic diarrheal diseases, surgical resection of the small intestine, or formation within the gastrointestinal tract of metal complexes that are not readily absorbed, for example, between phytates and Zn. Deficiency can also result from increased losses through urine, pancreatic juice, or other exocrine secretions or from metabolic imbalances produced by antagonistic or synergistic interactions between metals. Large amounts of Ca, for example, decrease the absorption of Zn. Zinc supplements in excess of 10 times the recommended daily allowance cause a conditioned deficiency of copper including anemia. Similarly, Mo and Cu compete so that excessive Mo in cattle leads to Cu deficiency characterized by diarrhea and wasting. Trace element deficiencies in humans were previously rare but have been recognized more frequently with the use of total parenteral nutrition (TPN) (Chap. 78). Criteria for the recognition of deficiency states include decreases in metal content of whole blood, serum, hair, and/or other accessible fluids and tissues; changes in the activities of metalloenzymes, and characteristic signs and symptoms (Table 80-2).

Toxic effects depend on the chemical form, the amount ingested, the route of entry into the body, the biological ligands bound by the metal, the tissue distribution, the concentration achieved, and the excretion rate. Mechanisms of toxicity include inhibition of enzyme activity by binding to essential amino acid residues, alterations in nucleic acid function and structure, impairment of protein synthesis, altered membrane permeability, and impairment of phosphorylation, among others. Metal toxicity in patients undergoing chronic hemodial-

ysis can be severe and can involve several elements, e.g., Al, Zn, Cu, Ni, and Sn (Chap. 272). For example, even when present only in trace amounts in dialysis fluids, Al is readily absorbed into blood and accumulates in brain, bone, and erythroid tissues and can cause disabling neurologic, skeletal, and hematologic manifestations including malaise, memory loss, asterixis, dementia, twitches, and other manifestations of metabolic encephalopathy, including seizures and death. Osteomalacia unresponsive to vitamin D, fractures, muscular pain, weakness, and anemia may occur. The diagnosis is made by documenting increase in plasma Al concentration following deferoxamine administration.

DISORDERS OF METABOLISM OF SPECIFIC METALS
Zinc The daily Zn requirement varies with age and growth state (Table 80-1); it is approximately 800 μg/day at 1 month of age, 3 to 10 mg/day between 1 and 10 years of age, and 10 to 15 mg/day in normal adults. During pregnancy, needs increase to 20 to 25 mg/day to provide Zn for the growing fetus. Absorption of Zn in the small intestine is decreased by fibers, phytate, phosphate, Ca, and Cu and increased by glucose, amino acids, peptides, iodoquinol, and other chelating agents. About 2 to 5 mg of Zn are excreted each day through secretions of the pancreas and intestine. Losses also occur through the renal proximal tubule (~500 to 800 μg/day) and from sweat glands (~500μg/day). Nearly 99 percent of total-body Zn (Table 80-1) is inside cells, the remainder is in plasma and extracellular fluids. The bplasma Zn concentration is approximately 100 μg/100 mL, 70 percent of which is bound to albumin and most of the rest is associated with α_2-macroglobulin, although a small amount is bound to uncharacterized proteins. Plasma Zn is the source of metal for cellular needs and its levels are fairly constant, with small diurnal variations. More significant changes take place under some circumstances. Plasma Zn levels are decreased in pregnancy and with the use of oral contraceptives, when intake or absorption is reduced (e.g., in regional enteritis), and when urinary losses are increased (e.g., in hypoalbuminemic states; with the administration of penicillamine or other chelating agents; in catabolic states such as trauma, burns, or surgery; and in hemolytic anemias and sickle cell disease). Plasma Zn levels also decrease with acute myocardial infarction, infections, malignancies, hepatitis, and

Table 80-1

Requirements and Functions of Trace Elements in Humans

Element	Requirements, mg/d*	Total, g/70 kg Body Wt	Serum μmol/L	Serum μ/dL	Selected Biochemical Functions	Enzyme and Protein Classes	Enzyme and Protein Examples
Fe	10–20	4.0	18	100	Oxygen transport	Oxidoreductases	Cytochrome oxidase
Zn	15–20	3.0	15	100	Nucleic acid and protein synthesis and degradation, alcohol metabolism	Transferases, hydrolases, lyases, isomerases, ligases, oxidoreductases, transcription factors	RNA polymerases, alcohol dehydrogenases, glucocorticoid receptor
Cu	2–6	0.25	16	100	Hemoglobin synthesis, connective tissue metabolism bone development	Oxidoreductases	Superoxide dismutase, ferroxidase (ceruloplasmin)
Co	0.0001	1.1	0.0001	0.0007	Methionine metabolism	Transferases	Homocysteine methyltransferase
Mn	2–5	0.02	0.001	0.06	Oxidative phosphorylation; fatty acid, mucopolysaccharide, and cholesterol metabolism	Oxidoreductases, hydrolases, ligases	Diamine oxidase, pyruvate carboxylase
Mo	0.15–0.5	0.07	0.007	0.07	Xanthine metabolism	Oxidoreductases	Xanthine oxidase
Se	0.05–0.2	(–)	1.6	13	Antioxidant	Oxidoreductases, transferases	Glutathione peroxidase
Ni	(–)	(–)	0.02	0.01	?Stabilizing RNA structure	Oxidoreductases, hydrolases	Urease
Cr	0.005–0.2	0.0006	0.004	0.02	?Binding of insulin to cells, glucose metabolism		

* Requirements may differ for different age groups and physiologic states, e.g., pregnancy.
† Reported normal values vary owing to differences in sample preparation, analytical instruments, and small quantities present in biologic materials.
NOTE: (–), Reported values variable or not available.

Table 80-2

CHAPTER 80
Disturbances in Trace Elements **491**

Disorders of Metal Metabolism in Humans

Element	Deficiency	Toxicity*
Fe	Anemia	Hepatic failure, diabetes, testicular atrophy, arthritis, cardiomyopathy, peripheral neuropathy, hyperpigmentation
Zn	Growth retardation, alopecia, dermatitis, diarrhea, immunologic dysfunction, failure to thrive, psychological disturbances, gonadal atrophy, impaired spermatogenesis, congenital malformations	Gastric ulcer, pancreatitis, lethargy, anemia, fever, nausea, vomiting, respiratory distress, pulmonary fibrosis
Cu	Anemia, growth retardation, defective keratinization and pigmentation of hair, hypothermia, degenerative changes in aortic elastin, mental deterioration, scurvy-like changes in skeleton	Hepatitis, cirrhosis, tremor, mental deterioration, *Kayser-Fleischer rings,* hemolytic anemia, renal dysfunction (*Fanconi-like* syndrome)
Mn	Bleeding disorder (increased prothrombin time)	Encephalitis-like syndrome, Parkinson-like syndrome, psychosis, pneumoconiosis
Co	Anemia (B_{12} deficiency)	Cardiomyopathy, goiter
Mo	?Esophageal cancer	?Hyperuricemia
Cr	?Impairment of glucose tolerance	Renal failure, dermatitis (occupational), pulmonary cancer
Se	Cardiomyopathy, congestive heart failure, striated muscle degeneration	Alopecia, abnormal nails, emotional lability, lassitude, garlic odor to breath
Ni	?	Dermatitis (occupational), lung and nasal carcinomas, liver necrosis, pulmonary inflammation
Si	?Impaired early bone development	Pulmonary inflammation, granuloma, fibrosis
F	?Impaired bone and dental structure	Mottled dental enamel, nausea, abdominal pain, vomiting, diarrhea, tetany, cardiovascular collapse

* Symptoms are dependent on route of entry and tissue distribution (see text).

many other diseases. The decreases may be due to redistribution from plasma to tissues such as liver and are probably mediated by corticotropin, cortisol, and/or interleukins 2 and 6. Liver uptake is associated with concomitant entry of amino acids, iron, and other metal ions.

The functions of Zn in cells and tissues depend on those of the metalloproteins and enzymes with which it is associated (Table 80-1); systems influenced by Zn include the reproductive, neurologic, immune, dermatologic, and gastrointestinal systems. Testicular Zn is critical for normal spermatogenesis and for sperm physiology; it preserves genomic integrity in the sperm and stabilizes attachment of sperm head to tail. The function of Zn in mammalian eggs is poorly understood, but Zn is essential for normal embryoic development. Deficiency results in malformations of the brain, eyes, bones, heart, and other organs. The survival of the embryo is placed at risk when Zn intake is reduced even for a period of days, particularly in the first trimester. Steroid hormone action is zinc-dependent in that the receptors require Zn to bind to the genes they activate.

In the brain the highest amounts of Zn are in the hippocampus and cerebral cortex, particularly the giant boutons of the mossy fiber system. Zinc may function in these areas to inhibit binding of peptides and other ligands to their neuroreceptors (opioid, muscarinic, acetylcholine, γ-aminobutyric acid, N-methyl-D-aspartate) and to influence neurotransmission.

Zinc is essential for the formation and function of the immune system. With Zn deprivation, the thymus atrophies, and viable thymocytes are not formed. The functions of macrophages and T cells are impaired. The result is an inability to respond to antigens or defend the organism against infection. Zn also may play a role in the sense of taste and in wound healing.

Human Zn deficiency (Table 80-2) was reported first in adolescents who consumed a diet rich in phytic acid and devoid of any animal protein and who also ate dirt; it was described subsequently in patients who received TPN without supplemental Zn (see Chap. 78) and in patients with Wilson's disease after treatment with penicillamine. Some patients with chronic diarrheal disease and malabsorption, including cystic fibrosis, regional enteritis, celiac sprue, and disaccharide malabsorption, exhibit signs and symptoms of Zn deficiency (Table 80-2). In the autosomal recessive defect *acrodermatitis enteropathica*, Zn deficiency may be the consequence of a defect in Zn absorption; symptoms often begin when an affected infant is weaned from human to cow's milk and include psoriasiform dermatitis with epidermal hyperplasia, parakeratosis, edema, and focal necrosis; flattening of intestinal villi and mucosal ulcerations; ovoid or rhomboid lysosomal-like inclusion bodies within Paneth cells; and a hypoplastic thymus with decreased or absent germinal centers in lymph nodes and spleen and immature plasma cells in paracortical areas.

Zinc-deficient cells fail to divide and differentiate, with consequent growth impairment; tissues with a high rate of cellular turnover, including skin, gastrointestinal mucosa, chondrocytes, spermatogonia, and thymocytes, are affected (Table 80-2). Dermatologic manifestations include hyperkeratosis, parakeratosis, acrodermatitis, and *alopecia*. Keratotic lesions usually occur in areas that are readily traumatized (elbows, knees) but can develop in other areas as well. The keratotic lesions can become pustular or crusting, red, scaly plaques. Immunologic defects of T cell function impair the ability to mount an immunologic response to parasites and may cause superinfections with either fungi or bacteria.

Toxicity follows inhalation of Zn fumes (by welders), oral ingestion, or intravenous administration. Inhalation of zinc oxide fumes leads to *metal-fume fever* or *brass chills*, manifested by fever, chills, excessive salivation, headaches, cough, and leukocytosis. Dialysis fluids can be contaminated with Zn from the adhesive on the dialysis coils or from galvanized pipes. Toxicity with hemodialysis is characterized by anemia, fever, and central nervous system disturbances (Table 80-2) and may be due to impaired chemotaxis, phagocytosis, pinocytosis, and platelet aggregation.

Copper The liver, kidney, heart, and brain contain the highest amounts of Cu. Over 90 percent of plasma Cu is associated with ceruloplasmin, and 60 percent of that in red blood cells is bound to superoxide dismutase. The major excretory pathway is through the bile. Serum Cu levels are normally constant. Increases in patients with acute myocardial infarction, leukemia, solid tumors, infections, cirrhosis of the liver, hemochromatosis, thyrotoxicosis, and connective tissue disorders are of uncertain significance. Decreases occur in the nephrotic syndrome, *kwashiorkor*, the hepatolenticular degeneration of *Wilson's disease* (see Chap. 345), severe diarrheal diseases with malabsorption, and conditions associated with increased excretion or decreased synthesis of ceruloplasmin. Premature infants fed diets deficient in Cu develop decreased serum ceruloplasmin and Cu levels, anemia, osteopenia, skin and hair depigmentation, and psychomotor retardation. Cu deficiency in subjects receiving TPN is associated with anemia and neutropenia.

A complex disorder of Cu metabolism occurs in *Menkes' disease*, an X-linked recessive disorder (see also Chap. 350). Intestinal Cu uptake is normal. Cu levels are normal or high in intestine, kidney, and skin (fibroblast) cells and low in serum, liver, brain, and (likely) vascular cells. Ceruloplasmin content and the activities of some Cu enzymes (e.g., connective tissue amine oxidases) are decreased. The clinical picture is similar to that of Cu deficiency in animals except that anemia does not occur (Table 80-2). The patients have kinky hair, and decreased amounts of mature collagen and elastin cause dissecting aneurysms, sudden cardiac rupture, emphysema, and osteoporosis. Death usually occurs in the first 5 years of life.

Excessive oral intake of Cu or hemodialysis with water contaminated with Cu causes toxicity manifested by hemolytic anemia, nausea, vomiting, and diarrhea. The renal and hepatic failure and the central nervous system disorders that eventually develop (Table 80-2) are typical of the manifestations of Cu toxicity in Wilson's disease (see Chap. 345).

Cobalt Co is a component of vitamin B_{12}, and deficiency syndromes are those associated with deficiency of the vitamin (see Chap. 108). Pharmacologic amounts of Co induce *erythropoiesis* and block iodine uptake by the thyroid, resulting in development of goiter.

Cardiomyopathy, congestive heart failure with pericardial effusions, polycythemia, thyroid enlargement, and neurologic abnormalities are manifestations of Co toxicity that occurred in drinkers of beer to which the metal had been added as a foam stabilizer. In the heart Co forms a complex with lipoic acid and interferes with decarboxylation reactions in pyruvate and fatty acid metabolism.

Manganese Mn acts as an activator of enzymes and as a component of metalloenzymes (Table 80-1). Mn deficiency in animals causes skeletal, central nervous, and gonadal manifestations. Mn deficiency in humans is rare; increases in prothrombin time, unresponsive to vitamin K, have been noted. In serum, Mn is bound to transmanganin, and it is excreted primarily in bile and pancreatic secretions.

Serum Mn increases following myocardial infarction and is decreased in children with convulsive disorders. Miners who inhale large quantities of Mn dust over long periods of time develop asthenia, anorexia, apathy, headache, impotence, leg cramps, speech disturbances, and occasionally even more severe symptoms (Table 80-2).

Selenium Se plays a critical role as a component of glutathione peroxidase in the control of oxygen metabolism, particularly in catalyzing the breakdown of H_2O_2. The metal is required for the growth of cells in tissue culture. Furthermore, Se cures or prevents *Keshan disease*, a syndrome characterized by multifocal myocardial necrosis and reduced serum Se content. The disorder is endemic to the Keshan Province in China, where the soil may be deficient in the metal. Manifestations vary from severe arrhythmias and cardiogenic shock to asymptomatic cardiac enlargement. Muscle degeneration causes peripheral myopathies (Table 80-2). Children and women of childbearing age are particularly susceptible. Se protects animals from a number of carcinogenic chemicals and viruses. Se binds Cd, Hg, and other metals and mitigates their toxic effects, even when tissue levels of the metals remain elevated. Se poisoning can occur after ingestion of water containing large amounts of the metal.

Other Trace Elements *Silicon* is present in bone and skin and may play a role in the cross-linkage of collagen. Deficiency in animals results in decreased growth, abnormal bone development, and decreased hexosamine content of epiphyses and epiphyseal plates. Deficiency has not been described in humans. Inhalation of fine particles of SiO_2 causes granuloma formation and fibrosis (*silicosis*) of the lungs (see Chap. 254).

Fluoride is a constituent of teeth and bone. In appropriate doses it prevents dental caries and increases bone density in patients with osteoporosis (see Chap. 355). Complications of long-term toxicity include calcification of bony ligaments and tendons and fluorosis, characterized by weakness, weight loss, anemia, brittle bones, and mottling of teeth (if taken during stages of enamel formation). Acute ingestion of toxic amounts, as found in some insect poisons, causes severe abdominal pain, nausea, vomiting, diarrhea, hypocalcemia, tetany, and on occasion cardiorespiratory arrest occur.

Deficiencies of *arsenic, nickel, tin,* or *vanadium* cause pathologic manifestations in plants and some vertebrates. Their roles in human health are undefined.

BIBLIOGRAPHY

ALFREY AC: Aluminum toxicity in patients with chronic renal failure. Ther Drug Monit 15:593, 1993

BEDWARL RS, BAKUGUNA A: Zinc, copper, and selenium in reproduction. Experentia 50:626, 1994

FALCHUK KH: Effect of acute disease and ACTH on serum zinc proteins. N Engl J Med 296:1129, 1977

GE K, YANG C: The epidmiology selenium deficiency in the etiological study of endemic diseases in China. Am J Clin Nutr 47(2 Suppl):2595, 1993

KLEIN GL: Aluminum in parenteral solutions revisited: Again. Am J Clin Nutr 61:449, 1995

NIELSEN FH: Nutritional refinement for boron, vanadium, nickel and arsenic: Current knowledge and speculations. FASEB J 56:2661, 1991

SEGHIZZI P et al: Cobalt cardiomyopathy: A critical review of literature. Sci Total Environ 150:105, 1994

TING-KAI L, VALLEE BL: The biochemical and nutritional roles of other trace elements, in *Modern Nutrition in Health and Disease*, RS Goodhart and ME Shills (eds). Philadelphia, Lea and Febiger, 6th ed, 1980, p 408

TZAMALOUKAS AH: Diagnosis and management of bone disorders in chronic renal failure and dialyzed-patients. Med Clin North Am 74:961, 1990

VALLEE BL, FALCHUK KH: The biochemical and pathological basis of zinc physiology. Physiol Rev 73:79, 1993

YARZE JL et al: Wilson's disease: Current status. Am J Med 92:643, 1992

YOKEE RA: Aluminum chelation: Chemistry, clinical and experimental studies and the search for alternatives to desferroxamine. J Toxicol Environ Health 41:131, 1994

ZLOTKIN SH et al: Trace elements in nutrition for premature infants. Clin Perinatol 22:223, 1995

81   *Dan L. Longo*

APPROACH TO THE PATIENT WITH CANCER

The application of current treatment techniques (surgery, radiation therapy, chemotherapy, and biological therapy) results in the cure of over 50 percent of patients diagnosed with cancer. Nevertheless, patients experience the diagnosis of cancer as one of the most traumatic and revolutionary events that has ever happened to them. Independent of prognosis, the diagnosis brings with it a change in a person's self-image and in his or her role in the home and workplace. The prognosis of a person who has just been found to have pancreatic cancer is the same as the prognosis of the person with aortic stenosis who develops the first symptoms of congestive heart failure (median survival, about 8 months). However, the patient with heart disease may remain functional and maintain a view of himself or herself as a fully intact person with just a malfunctioning part, a diseased organ ("a bum ticker"). By contrast, the patient with pancreatic cancer has a completely altered self-image and is viewed differently by family and anyone who knows the diagnosis. He or she is being attacked and invaded by a disease that could be anywhere in the body. Every ache or pain takes on desperate significance. Cancer is an exception to the coordinated interaction among cells and organs. In general, the cells of a multicellular organism are programmed for collaboration. Many diseases occur because the specialized cells fail to perform their assigned task. Cancer takes this malfunction one step further. Not only is there a failure of the cancer cell to maintain the specialized function of its tissue of origin, but also the cancer cell strikes out on its own; the cancer cell competes to survive using natural mutability and natural selection to seek advantage over normal cells in a recapitulation of evolution. One consequence of the traitorous behavior of cancer cells is that the patient feels betrayed by his or her body. The cancer patient feels that he or she, and not just a body part, is diseased.

THE MAGNITUDE OF THE PROBLEM

There is no nationwide cancer registry; therefore, the incidence of cancer is estimated on the basis of the National Cancer Institute's Surveillance, Epidemiology, and End Results (SEER) database, which tabulates cancer incidence and death figures from nine sites accounting for about 10 percent of the U.S. population and from population data from the Bureau of the Census. In 1996, 1.36 million new cases of invasive cancer (765,000 men, 595,000 women) were diagnosed and 555,000 people (292,000 men, 263,000 women) died from cancer. The percent distribution of new cancer cases and cancer deaths by site for men and women are shown in Fig. 81-1.

The most significant risk factor for cancer overall is age; two-thirds of all cases were in people over age 65 years. Cancer incidence increases as the third, fourth, or fifth power of age in different sites. Thus, the probability of a person developing cancer is age-dependent: For the interval between birth and age 39 years, 1 in 58 men and 1 in 52 women will develop cancer; for the interval between ages 40 and 59 years, 1 in 13 men and 1 in 11 women will develop cancer; and for the interval between ages 60 and 79 years, 1 in 3 men and 1 in 4 women will develop cancer.

Cancer is the second leading cause of death behind heart disease. However, deaths from heart disease have declined 45 percent in the United States since 1950 and continue to decline, while cancer deaths are increasing (Fig. 81-2). Early in the next century, cancer is projected to be the leading cause of death. The five leading causes of cancer deaths are shown for various populations in Table 81-1. Along with the increase in incidence has come an increase in survival for cancer patients. The 5-year survival for white patients was 39 percent in 1960–1963 and 58 percent in 1986–1991. Cancers are more often deadly in blacks; the 5-year survival was 42 percent for the 1986–1991 interval. The basis for these racial differences in survival is unclear.

PATIENT MANAGEMENT

Important information is obtained from every portion of the routine history and physical examination. The duration of symptoms may reveal the chronicity of disease. The past medical history may alert the physician to the presence of underlying diseases that may affect the choice of therapy or the side effects of treatment. The social history

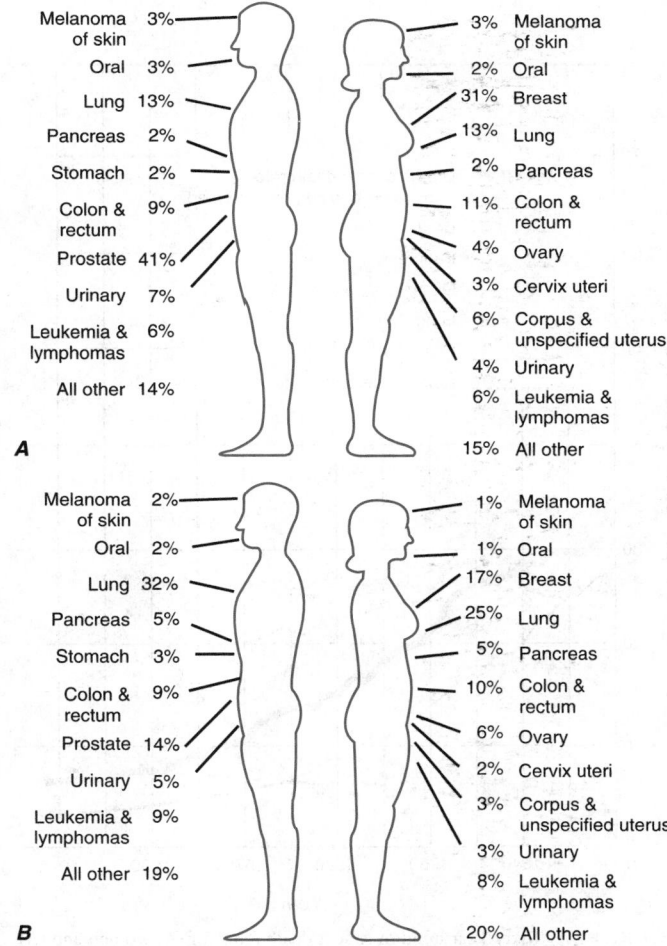

Melanoma of skin	3%		3%	Melanoma of skin
Oral	3%		2%	Oral
Lung	13%		31%	Breast
Pancreas	2%		13%	Lung
Stomach	2%		2%	Pancreas
Colon & rectum	9%		11%	Colon & rectum
Prostate	41%		4%	Ovary
Urinary	7%		3%	Cervix uteri
Leukemia & lymphomas	6%		6%	Corpus & unspecified uterus
			4%	Urinary
All other	14%		6%	Leukemia & lymphomas
A			15%	All other

Melanoma of skin	2%		1%	Melanoma of skin
Oral	2%		1%	Oral
Lung	32%		17%	Breast
Pancreas	5%		25%	Lung
Stomach	3%		5%	Pancreas
Colon & rectum	9%		10%	Colon & rectum
Prostate	14%		6%	Ovary
Urinary	5%		2%	Cervix uteri
Leukemia & lymphomas	9%		3%	Corpus & unspecified uterus
			3%	Urinary
All other	19%		8%	Leukemia & lymphomas
B			20%	All other

FIGURE 81-1 Distribution of (*A*) cancer incidence and (*B*) cancer deaths by sex for 1996. Data exclude basal and squamous cell skin cancers and carcinoma in situ except bladder. (*From Parker SL et al, CA Cancer J Clin 46:5, 1996.*)

may reveal occupational exposure to carcinogens, or habits, such as smoking or alcohol consumption, that may influence the course of disease and its treatment. The family history may suggest an underlying familial cancer predisposition and point out the need to begin surveillance or other preventive therapy for unaffected siblings of the patient. The review of systems may suggest early symptoms of metastatic disease or a paraneoplastic syndrome.

DIAGNOSIS The diagnosis of cancer relies most heavily on invasive tissue biopsy. The diagnosis should never be made without obtaining tissue; no noninvasive diagnostic test is sufficient to define a disease process as cancer. Although there are rare clinical settings (for example, thyroid nodules) where fine needle aspiration is an acceptable diagnostic procedure, in general, the diagnosis depends on removing from the patient adequate tissue to permit careful evaluation of the histology of the tumor, its grade, and its invasiveness and to yield further molecular diagnostic information, such as the expression of cell-surface markers or intracellular proteins that typify a particular cancer, or the presence of a molecular marker such as the t(8;14) translocation of Burkitt's lymphoma. Increasing evidence implicates the expression of certain genes with the prognosis and response to therapy (see Chaps. 83 and 84).

Occasionally a patient will present with a metastatic disease process that is defined as cancer on biopsy but has no apparent primary site of disease. Efforts should be made to define the primary site based on age, sex, sites of involvement, histology and tumor markers, and personal and family history. Particular attention should be focused on ruling out the most treatable causes (see Chap. 101).

Once the diagnosis of cancer is made, the management of the patient is best undertaken as a multidisciplinary collaboration among the primary care physician, medical oncologists, surgical oncologists, radiation oncologists, oncology nurse specialists, pharmacists, social workers, rehabilitation medicine specialists, and a number of other consulting professionals working closely with each other and with the patient and family.

DEFINING THE EXTENT OF DISEASE AND THE PROGNOSIS The first priority in patient management after the diagnosis of cancer is established and shared with the patient is to determine the extent of disease. The curability of a tumor usually is inversely proportional to the tumor burden. Ideally, the tumor will be diagnosed before symptoms develop (see Chaps. 63 and 64) or as a consequence of screening efforts (see Chap. 82). A very high proportion of such patients can be cured. However, most patients with cancer present with symptoms related to the cancer, caused either by mass effects of the tumor or by alterations associated with the production of cytokines or hormones from the tumor.

For most cancers, the extent of disease is evaluated by a variety of noninvasive and invasive diagnostic tests and procedures. This process is called *staging*. There are two types. *Clinical staging* is based on physical examination, radiographs, isotopic scans, computed tomography, and other imaging procedures; *pathologic staging* takes into account information obtained during a surgical procedure, which might include intraoperative palpation, resection of regional lymph nodes and/or tissue adjacent to the tumor, and inspection and biopsy of organs commonly involved in disease spread. Pathologic staging includes histologic examination of all tissues removed during the surgical procedure. Surgical procedures performed may include a simple lymph node biopsy or more extensive procedures such as thoracot-

FIGURE 81-2 Sixty-year trend in cancer death rates for (*A*) women and (*B*) men, by site in the United States, 1930–1992. Rates are per 100,000 age-adjusted to the 1970 U.S. standard population. Note: Due to changes in the ICD coding, numerator information has changed over time. Rates for cancer of the liver are particularly affected by these coding changes. Denominator information for the years 1930–1967 and 1991–1992 is based on intercensal population estimates, while denominator information for the years 1968–1990 is based on postcensal recalculation of estimates. (*From Parker SL et al, CA Cancer J Clin 46:5, 1996.*)

Table 81-1

The Five Leading Primary Tumor Sites for Patients Dying of Cancer Based on Age, Sex, and Race

Rank	All Ages	Age					Race	
		Under 15	15–34	35–54	55–74	75+	White	Black
1	M: lung (94,400; 30-yr trend, +85%) F: lung (64,300; 30-yr trend, +438%)	M and F: leukemia	M: leukemia F: breast	M: lung F: breast	M and F: lung	M and F: lung	Lung	Lung
2	M: prostate (41,400; 30-yr trend, +29%) F: breast (44,300; 30-yr trend, +4%)	M and F: brain and CNS	M: lymphoma F: leukemia	M: colon, rectum F: lung	M: colon, rectum F: breast	M: prostate F: colon, rectum	Colon, rectum	Colon, rectum
3	M: colon, rectum (27,400; 30-yr trend, −9%) F: colon, rectum (27,500; 30-yr trend, −31%)	M and F: endocrine	M: brain and CNS F: cervix	M: lymphoma F: colon, rectum	M: prostate F: colon, rectum	M: colon, rectum F: breast	Breast	Prostate
4	M: pancreas (13,600; 30-yr trend, −5%) F: ovary (14,800; 30-yr trend, −8%)	M: lymphoma F: bone	M: skin F: brain and CNS	M: brain and CNS F: ovary	M: pancreas F: ovary	M and F: pancreas	Prostate	Breast
5	M: lymphoma (12,400; 30-yr trend, +30%) F: pancreas (14,200; 30-yr trend, +12%)	M and F: sarcoma	M: Hodgkin's F: lymphoma	M: pancreas F: cervix	M: lymphoma F: pancreas	M: leukemia F: ovary	Pancreas	Pancreas

ABBREVIATIONS: F, female; M, male.

omy, mediastinoscopy, or laparotomy. Surgical staging may occur in a separate procedure or may be done at the time of definitive surgical resection of the primary tumor.

Knowledge of the predilection of particular tumors for spread to adjacent or distant organs helps direct the staging evaluation. The sites of metastatic disease for common tumors are given in Table 85-1.

Information obtained from staging is used to define the extent of disease either as localized, as exhibiting spread outside of the organ of origin to regional but not distant sites, or as metastatic to distant sites. The most widely used system of staging is the TNM (tumor, node, metastasis) system codified by the International Union Against Cancer and the American Joint Committee on Cancer (AJCC).* The TNM classification is an anatomically based system that categorizes the tumor on the basis of the size of the primary tumor lesion (T1–4, where a higher value of the subscript indicates a tumor of larger size), the presence of nodal involvement (usually N0 and N1 for the absence and presence, respectively, of involved nodes, although some tumors have more elaborate systems of nodal grading), and the presence of metastatic disease (M0 and M1 for the absence and presence, respectively, of metastases). The various permutations of T, N, and M scores are then broken into stages, usually designated by the roman numerals I through IV. Tumor burden increases and curability decreases with increasing stage. Other anatomic staging systems are used for some tumors, for example, the Dukes classification for colorectal cancers, the International Federation of Gynecologists and Obstetricians (FIGO) classification for gynecologic cancers, and the Ann Arbor classification for Hodgkin's disease.

Certain tumors cannot be grouped appropriately on the basis of anatomic considerations. For example, hematopoietic tumors such as leukemia, myeloma, and lymphoma are often disseminated at presentation and do not spread in the fashion typical of solid tumors. For these tumors, other prognostic factors have been identified (see Chaps. 112, 113, and 114).

In addition to tumor burden, a second major determinant of treatment outcome is the physiologic reserve of the patient. Patients who are bedridden before developing cancer are likely to fare worse, stage for stage, than fully active patients. Physiologic reserve is a determinant of how a patient is likely to cope with the physiologic stresses imposed by the cancer and its treatment. This factor is difficult to assess directly. Instead, surrogate markers for physiologic reserve are used, such as

the patient's age or Karnofsky performance status (Table 81-2). Older patients and those with a Karnofsky performance status of less than 70 have a poor prognosis unless the poor performance is a reversible consequence of the tumor.

Increasingly, biologic features of the tumor are being related to prognosis. The expression of particular oncogenes, drug resistance genes, apoptosis-related genes, and genes involved in metastasis are being found to influence response to therapy and prognosis. The presence of selected cytogenetic abnormalities may influence survival. Tumors with higher growth fractions, as assessed by expression of proliferation-related markers such as proliferating cell nuclear antigen (PCNA), behave more aggressively than tumors with lower growth fractions. Information obtained from studying the tumor itself will increasingly be used to influence treatment decisions.

MAKING A TREATMENT PLAN From information on the extent of disease and the prognosis and in conjunction with the patient's wishes, it is possible to determine whether the treatment approach should be curative or palliative in intent. Cooperation among the various professionals involved in cancer treatment is of the utmost importance in treatment planning. For some cancers, chemotherapy or chemotherapy plus radiation therapy delivered before the use of

Table 81-2

Karnofsky Performance Index

Performance Status	Functional Capability of the Patient
100	Normal; no complaints; no evidence of disease
90	Able to carry on normal activity; minor signs or symptoms of disease
80	Normal activity with effort; some signs or symptoms of disease
70	Cares for self; unable to carry on normal activity or do active work
60	Requires occasional assistance but is able to care for most needs
50	Requires considerable assistance and frequent medical care
40	Disabled; requires special care and assistance
30	Severely disabled; hospitalization is indicated although death is not imminent
20	Very sick; hospitalization necessary; active supportive treatment is necessary
10	Moribund, fatal processes progressing rapidly
0	Dead

* The AJCC *Manual for Staging Cancer* can be obtained from the AJCC at 55 East Erie Street, Chicago, IL, 60611.

definitive surgical treatment (so-called neoadjuvant therapy) may improve the outcome, as seems to be the case for locally advanced breast cancer and head and neck cancers. In certain settings in which combined modality therapy is intended, coordination among the medical oncologist, radiation oncologist, and surgeon is crucial to achieving optimal results. Sometimes the chemotherapy and radiation therapy need to be delivered sequentially, and other times concurrently. Surgical procedures may precede or follow other treatment approaches. It is best for the treatment plan either to follow precisely a standard protocol or else to be part of an ongoing clinical research protocol evaluating new treatments. Ad hoc modifications of standard protocols are likely to compromise treatment results.

The choice of treatment approaches was formerly dominated by the local culture in both the university and the practice settings. However, it is now possible to gain access electronically to standard treatment protocols and to every approved clinical research study in North America through a personal computer interface with the Internet.*

The skilled physician also has much to offer the patient for whom curative therapy is no longer an option. Often a combination of guilt and frustration over the inability to cure the patient and the pressure of a busy schedule greatly limit the time a physician spends with a patient who is receiving only palliative care. Resist these forces. In addition to the medicines administered to alleviate symptoms (see below), it is important to remember the comfort that is provided by holding the patient's hand, continuing regular examinations, and taking time to talk.

MANAGEMENT OF DISEASE AND TREATMENT COMPLICATIONS Because cancer therapies are toxic (see Chap. 86), patient management involves addressing complications of both the disease and its treatment as well as the complex psychosocial problems associated with cancer. In the short term during a course of curative therapy, the patient's functional status may decline. Treatment-induced toxicity is less acceptable if the goal of therapy is palliation. The most common side effects of treatment are nausea and vomiting (see below), febrile neutropenia (see Chap. 87), and myelosuppression (see Chap. 105). Therapeutic tools are now available to minimize the acute toxicity of cancer treatment.

New symptoms developing in the course of cancer treatment should always be assumed to be reversible until proven otherwise. The fatalistic attribution of anorexia, weight loss, and jaundice to recurrent or progressive tumor could result in a patient dying from a reversible intercurrent cholecystitis. Intestinal obstruction may be due to reversible adhesions rather than progressive tumor. Systemic infections, sometimes with unusual pathogens, may be a consequence of the immunosuppression associated with cancer therapy. Some drugs used to treat cancer or its complications (e.g., nausea) may produce central nervous system symptoms that look like metastatic disease or may mimic paraneoplastic syndromes such as the syndrome of inappropriate antidiuretic hormone. A definitive diagnosis should be pursued and may even require a repeat biopsy.

A critical component of cancer management is assessing the response to treatment. In addition to a careful physical examination in which all sites of disease are physically measured and recorded in a flow chart by date, response assessment usually requires periodic repeating of imaging tests that were abnormal at the time of staging. If imaging tests have become normal, repeat biopsy of previously involved tissue is performed to document complete response by pathol-

ogy criteria. Biopsies are not usually required if there is macroscopic residual disease. Responses are graded as complete, if there has been disappearance of all evidence of disease, and partial, if there has been greater than 50 percent reduction in the sum of the products of the perpendicular diameters of all measureable lesions. Progressive disease is defined as the appearance of any new lesion or an increase of greater than 25 percent in the sum of the products of the perpendicular diameters of all measurable lesions. Tumor shrinkage or growth that does not meet any of these criteria is considered stable disease. Some sites of involvement (e.g., bone) or patterns of involvement (e.g., lymphangitic lung or diffuse pulmonary infiltrates) are considered unmeasurable. No response is complete without biopsy documentation of their resolution but partial responses may exclude their assessment unless clear objective (though unmeasurable) progression has occurred.

Tumor markers may be useful in patient management in certain tumors. Response to therapy may be difficult to gauge with certainty. However, some tumors produce or elicit the production of markers that can be measured in the serum or urine and, in a particular patient, rising and falling levels of the marker are usually associated with increasing or decreasing tumor burden, respectively. Some clinically useful tumor markers are shown in Table 81-3. Tumor markers are not in themselves specific enough to permit a diagnosis of malignancy to be made, but once a malignancy has been diagnosed and shown to be associated with elevated levels of a tumor marker, the marker can be used to assess response to treatment.

The recognition and treatment of depression is an important component of management. The incidence of depression in cancer patients is about 25 percent overall and may be greater in patients with greater debility. This diagnosis is likely in a patient with a depressed mood (dysphoria) and/or a loss of interest in pleasure (anhedonia) for at least 2 weeks. In addition, three or more of the following symptoms are usually present: appetite change, sleep problems, psychomotor retardation or agitation, fatigue, feelings of guilt or worthlessness, inability to concentrate, and suicidal ideation. Patients with these symptoms should receive therapy. Medical therapy with a serotonin reuptake inhibitor such as fluoxetine (10 to 20 mg/d), sertraline (50 to 150 mg/d), or paroxetine (10 to 20 mg/d) or a tricyclic antidepressant such as amitriptyline (50 to 100 mg/d) or desipramine (75 to 150 mg/d) should be tried allowing 4 to 6 weeks for response. Effective therapy should be continued at least 6 months after resolution of symptoms. If therapy is unsuccessful, other classes of antidepressants may be used. In addition to medication, psychosocial interventions such as support groups, psychotherapy, and guided imagery may be of benefit.

Many patients opt for unproven or unsound approaches to treatment when it appears that conventional medicine is unlikely to be curative. Those seeking such alternatives are often well educated and may be early in the course of their disease. Unsound approaches are usually hawked on the basis of unsubstantiated anecdotes and not only cannot help the patient but may be harmful. Physicians should strive to keep communications open and nonjudgmental, so that patients are more likely to discuss with the physician what they are actually doing. The appearance of unexpected toxicity may be an indication that a supplemental therapy is being taken.*

LONG-TERM FOLLOW-UP/LATE COMPLICATIONS At the completion of treatment, sites originally involved with tumor are reassessed, usually by radiography or imaging techniques, and any persistent abnormality is biopsied. If disease persists, the multidisciplinary team discusses a new salvage treatment plan. If the patient has been rendered disease-free by the original treatment, the patient is followed regularly for disease recurrence. The optimal guidelines for follow-up care are not known. For many years, a routine practice has been to follow the patient monthly for 6 to 12 months, then every other month for a year, every 3 months for a year, every 4 months

---

* The National Cancer Institute maintains a database called PDQ (Physician Data Query) that is accessible on the Internet under the name CancerNet at wwwicic.nci.nih.gov/health.htm. Information can be obtained through a facsimile machine using CancerFax by dialing 301-402-5874. Patient information is also provided by the National Cancer Institute in at least three formats: on the Internet via CancerNet at wwwicic.nci.nih.gov/patient.htm, through the CancerFax number listed above, or by calling 1-800-4-CANCER. The quality control for the information provided through these services is rigorous.

* Information about unsound methods may be obtained from the National Council Against Health Fraud, Box 1276, Loma Linda, CA 92354, or from the Center for Medical Consumers and Health Care Information, 237 Thompson Street, New York, NY 10012.

for a year, every 6 months for a year, and then annually. At each visit, a battery of laboratory and radiographic and imaging tests were obtained on the assumption that it is best to detect recurrent disease before it becomes symptomatic. However, where follow-up procedures have been examined, this assumption has been found to be untrue. Studies of breast cancer, melanoma, lung cancer, colon cancer, and lymphoma have all failed to support the notion that asymptomatic relapses are more readily cured by salvage therapy than symptomatic relapses. In view of the enormous cost of a full battery of diagnostic tests and their manifest lack of impact on survival, new guidelines are emerging for less frequent follow-up visits during which the history and physical examination are the major investigations performed.

As time passes, the likelihood of recurrence of the primary cancer diminishes. For many types of cancer, survival for 5 years without recurrence is tantamount to cure. However, there are important medical problems that occur in patients treated for cancer that must be examined. For some tumor types, such as breast cancer and head and neck cancer, second primary tumors are a feature of the disease. Secondary tumors may also be a consequence of the treatment approach. For example, chronic administration of alkylating agents is associated with secondary acute leukemia. Radiation therapy is associated with the occurrence of second solid tumors in the treatment field. The risk of a second tumor from radiation therapy is about 0.5 to 1 percent per year; second tumors involving some organs, such as the thyroid or breast, may not appear until 20 years or more after the initial treatment. Mediastinal irradiation may produce accelerated coronary atherosclerosis. Abdominal or pelvic surgery or irradiation may lead to adhesions and bowel obstruction. Radiation of the neck usually leads to thyroid insufficiency and can result in the loss of salivary secretion and poor dentition. Chemotherapy that includes alkylating agents usually leads to infertility. Other sexual problems may be very slow to resolve after cancer treatment. Pulmonary complications also may occur after both radiation therapy and chemotherapy. Endocrine ablation is a goal of therapy in some tumors, and its long-term consequences must be managed. There are many medical conditions that the alert physician should anticipate in a patient who has undergone curative cancer therapy.

Despite these concerns, most patients who are cured of cancer return to normal lives.

SUPPORTIVE CARE In many ways, the success of cancer therapy depends on the success of the supportive care. Failure to control the symptoms of cancer and its treatment may lead patients to abandon curative therapy. Of equal importance, supportive care is a major determinant of quality of life. Even when life cannot be prolonged, the physician must strive to preserve its quality. Quality of life measurements have become common end-points of clinical research studies. Furthermore, palliative care has been shown to be cost-effective when approached in an organized fashion. A credo for oncology could be to cure sometimes, to extend life often, and to comfort always.

Pain Pain occurs with variable frequency in the cancer patient: 25 to 50 percent of patients present with pain at diagnosis, 33 percent have pain associated with treatment, and 75 percent have pain with progressive disease. The pain may have several causes. In about 70 percent of cases, pain is caused by the tumor itself—by invasion of bone, nerves, blood vessels, or mucous mem-

branes or obstruction of a hollow viscus or duct. In about 20 percent of cases, pain is related to a surgical or invasive medical procedure, to radiation injury (mucositis, enteritis, or plexus or spinal cord injury), or to chemotherapy injury (mucositis, peripheral neuropathy, phlebitis, steroid-induced aseptic necrosis of the femoral head). In 10 percent of cases, pain is unrelated to cancer or its treatment.

Assessment of pain requires the methodical investigation of the history of the pain, its location, character, temporal features, provocative and palliative factors, and intensity (see Chap. 12); a review of the oncologic history and past medical history as well as personal and social history; and a thorough physical examination. The patient should be given a 10-division visual analogue scale on which to indicate the severity of the pain. The clinical condition is often dynamic, making it necessary to reassess the patient frequently. Pain therapy should not be withheld while the cause of pain is being sought.

A variety of tools are available with which to address cancer pain. About 85 percent of patients will have pain relief from pharmacologic intervention. However, other modalities, including antitumor therapy (such as surgical relief of obstruction, radiation therapy, and strontium-89 treatment for bone pain), neurostimulatory techniques, regional analgesia, or neuroablative procedures are effective in an additional 12 percent or so. Thus, very few patients will have inadequate pain relief if appropriate measures are taken.

The World Health Organization (WHO) has devised a simple and effective method for the rational titration of oral analgesia, called the WHO ladder. The ladder has the following three steps. (1) For mild to moderate pain, one begins with acetaminophen (650 mg every 4 h or 975 mg every 6 h), aspirin (650 mg every 4 h or 975 mg every 6 h), or a nonsteroidal anti-inflammatory agent (NSAID; for example, ketoprofen, 25 to 60 mg every 6 h) with or without an adjuvant such as a glucocorticoid (dexamethasone) or an antidepressant (amitripty-

Table 81-3

Tumor Markers

Tumor Markers	Cancer	Non-Neoplastic Conditions
HORMONES		
Human chorionic gonadotropin	Gestational trophoblastic disease, gonadal germ cell tumor	Pregnancy
Calcitonin	Medullary cancer of the thyroid	
Catecholamines	Pheochromocytoma	
ONCOFETAL ANTIGENS		
Alphafetoprotein	Hepatocellular carcinoma, gonadal germ cell tumor	Cirrhosis, hepatitis
Carcinoembryonic antigen	Adenocarcinomas of the colon, pancreas, lung, breast, ovary	Pancreatitis, hepatitis, inflammatory bowel disease, smoking
ENZYMES		
Prostatic acid phosphatase	Prostate cancer	Prostatitis, prostatic hypertrophy
Neuron-specific enolase	Small cell cancer of the lung, neuroblastoma	
Lactate dehydrogenase	Lymphoma, Ewing's sarcoma	Hepatitis, hemolytic anemia, many others
TUMOR-ASSOCIATED PROTEINS		
Prostate-specific antigen	Prostate cancer	Prostatitis, prostatic hypertrophy
Monoclonal immunoglobulin	Myeloma	Infection, MGUS*
CA-125	Ovarian cancer, some lymphomas	Menstruation, peritonitis, pregnancy
CA 19-9	Colon, pancreatic, breast cancer	Pancreatitis, ulcerative colitis
CD30	Hodgkin's disease, anaplastic large cell lymphoma	—
CD25	Hairy cell leukemia, adult T-cell leukemia/lymphoma	—

* MGUS, monoclonal gammopathy of uncertain significance.

line). (2) When pain persists or increases, an opioid such as codeine or hydrocodone (30 mg every 3 to 4 h is roughly equivalent to 10 mg of intravenous morphine) should be added (not substituted); fixed combinations such as oxycodone/acetaminophen (Percocet) or oxycodone/aspirin (Percodan) are worth testing. (3) Pain that is persistent or that is moderate to severe at the outset should be treated by increasing the potency of the opioid or using higher dosages (for example, morphine, 15 to 30 mg every 3 to 4 h, or controlled-release morphine, 90 to 120 mg bid), and fixed opioid/NSAID combinations should be abandoned. Adjuvants may be used at all steps. The critical features of this approach are that the treatment is oral, should be given around the clock with supplemental doses as needed to control pain, and is tailored to the individual patient. Records of pain control should be a prominent component of the medical record. When opioids are used, the patient should be placed on a prophylactic regimen to prevent constipation.

Nausea Emesis in the cancer patient is usually caused by chemotherapy (see Chap. 86). Its severity can be predicted from the drugs used to treat the cancer. Three forms of emesis are recognized on the basis of their timing with regard to the noxious insult. *Acute emesis*, the most common variety, occurs within 24 h of treatment. *Delayed emesis* occurs 1 to 7 days after treatment; it is rare, but, when present, usually follows cisplatin administration. *Anticipatory emesis* occurs before administration of chemotherapy and represents a conditioned response to visual and olfactory stimuli previously associated with chemotherapy delivery.

Acute emesis is the best understood form. Stimuli that activate signals in the chemoreceptor trigger zone in the medulla, the cerebral cortex, and peripherally in the intestinal tract lead to stimulation of the vomiting center in the medulla, the motor center responsible for coordinating the secretory and muscle contraction activity that leads to emesis. Diverse receptor types participate in the process, including dopamine, serotonin, histamine, opioid, and acetylcholine receptors. The serotonin receptor antagonists ondansetron and granisetron are the most effective drugs against highly emetogenic agents, but they are expensive.

As with the analgesia ladder, emesis therapy should be tailored to the situation. For mildly and moderately emetogenic agents, prochlorperazine, 5 to 10 mg orally or 25 mg rectally, is effective. Its efficacy may be enhanced by administering the drug before the chemotherapy is delivered. Dexamethasone, 10 to 20 mg intravenously, is also effective and may enhance the efficacy of prochlorperazine. For highly emetogenic agents such as cisplatin, mechlorethamine, dacarbazine, and streptozocin, combinations of agents work best, and administration should begin 6 to 24 h before treatment. Ondansetron 8 mg orally every 6 h the day before therapy and intravenously on the day of therapy plus dexamethasone 20 mg intravenously before treatment is an effective regimen. Like pain, emesis is easier to prevent than to alleviate.

Delayed emesis may be related to bowel inflammation from the therapy and can be controlled with oral dexamethasone and oral metoclopramide, a dopamine receptor antagonist that also blocks serotonin receptors at high dosages. The best strategy for preventing anticipatory emesis is to control emesis in the early cycles of therapy to prevent the conditioning from taking place. If this is unsuccessful, prophylactic antiemetics the day before treatment may help. Experimental studies are evaluating behavior modification.

Effusions Fluid may accumulate abnormally in the pleural cavity, pericardium, or peritoneum. Asymptomatic malignant effusions may not require treatment. Symptomatic effusions occurring in tumors responsive to systemic therapy usually do not require local treatment but respond to the treatment for the underlying tumor. Symptomatic effusions occurring in tumors unresponsive to systemic therapy may require local treatment in patients with a life expectancy of at least 6 months.

Pleural effusions due to tumors may or may not contain malignant cells. Lung cancer, breast cancer, and lymphomas account for about 75 percent of malignant pleural effusions. Their exudative nature is usually gauged by an effusion/serum protein ratio of 0.5 or an effusion/serum lactate dehydrogenase ratio of 0.6. When the condition is symptomatic, thoracentesis is usually performed first. In most cases, symptomatic improvement occurs for less than 1 month. Chest tube drainage is required if symptoms recur within 2 weeks. Fluid is aspirated until the flow rate is less than 100 mL in 24 h. Then either 60 units of bleomycin or 1 g of doxycycline is infused into the chest tube in 50 mL of 5% dextrose in water; the tube is clamped; the patient is rotated on four sides, spending 15 min in each position; and, after 1 to 2 h, the tube is again attached to suction for another 24 h. The tube is then disconnected from suction and allowed to drain by gravity. If less than 100 mL drains over the next 24 h, the chest tube is pulled, and a radiograph taken 24 h later. If the chest tube continues to drain fluid at an unacceptably high rate, sclerosis can be repeated. Bleomycin may be somewhat more effective than doxycycline, but it is very expensive. Doxycycline is usually the drug of first choice. If neither doxycycline nor bleomycin is effective, talc can be used.

Symptomatic pericardial effusions are usually treated by creating a pericardial window or by stripping. If the patient's condition does not permit a surgical procedure, sclerosis can be attempted with doxycycline and/or bleomycin.

Malignant ascites is usually treated with repeated paracentesis of small volumes of fluid. If the underlying malignancy is unresponsive to systemic therapy, peritoneovenous shunts may be inserted. Despite the fear of disseminating tumor cells into the circulation, widespread metastases are an unusual complication. The major complications are occlusion, leakage, and fluid overload. Patients with severe liver disease may develop disseminated intravascular coagulation.

Nutrition Cancer and its treatment may lead to a decrease in nutrient intake of sufficient magnitude to cause weight loss and alteration of intermediary metabolism. The prevalence of this problem is difficult to estimate because of variations in the definition of cancer cachexia, but most patients with advanced cancer experience weight loss and decreased appetite. A variety of both tumor-derived factors (for example, bombesin, adrenocorticotropic hormone) and host-derived factors (for example, tumor necrosis factor, interleukins 1 and 6, growth hormone) contribute to the altered metabolism, and a vicious cycle is established in which protein catabolism, glucose intolerance, and lipolysis cannot be reversed by the provision of calories.

It remains controversial how to assess nutritional status and when and how to intervene. Efforts to make the assessment objective have included the use of a prognostic nutritional index based on albumin levels, triceps skin fold thickness, transferrin levels, and delayed-type hypersensitivity skin testing. However, a simpler approach has been to define the threshold for nutritional intervention as greater than 10 percent unexplained body weight loss, serum transferrin level less than 150 mg/dL, and serum albumin less than 3.4 g/dL.

The decision is important, because it appears that cancer therapy is substantially more toxic and less effective in the face of malnutrition. Nevertheless, it remains unclear whether nutritional intervention can alter the natural history. Unless there is some pathology affecting the absorptive function of the gastrointestinal tract, enteral nutrition provided orally or by tube feeding is preferred over parenteral supplementation. However, the risks associated with the tube may outweigh the benefits. Megestrol acetate, a progestational agent, has been advocated as a pharmacologic intervention to improve nutritional status. Research in this area may provide more tools in the future as cytokine-mediated mechanisms are further elucidated.

Psychosocial Support The psychosocial needs of patients vary with their situation. Patients undergoing treatment experience fear, anxiety, and depression. Self-image is often seriously compromised by deforming surgery and loss of hair. Women who receive cosmetic advice that enables them to look better also feel better. Loss of control over how one spends time can contribute to the sense of vulnerability. Juggling the demands of work and family with the demands of treatment may create enormous stresses. Sexual dysfunction is highly prevalent and needs to be discussed overtly with the patient. An empathetic health care team is sensitive to the individual patient's needs and permits negotiation where such flexibility will not adversely affect the course of treatment.

Cancer survivors have other sets of difficulties. Patients may have fears associated with the termination of a treatment they associate with their continued survival. Adjustments are required to physical losses and handicaps, real and perceived. Patients may be preoccupied with minor physical problems. They perceive a decline in their job mobility and view themselves as less desirable workers. They may be victims of job and/or insurance discrimination. Patients may experience difficulty reentering their normal past life. They may feel guilty for having survived and may carry a sense of vulnerability to colds and other illnesses. Perhaps the most pervasive and threatening concern is the ever-present fear of relapse (the Damocles syndrome).

Patients in whom therapy has been unsuccessful have other problems related to the end of life.

Death and Dying The most common causes of death in patients with cancer are infection (leading to circulatory failure), respiratory failure, hepatic failure, and renal failure. Intestinal blockage may lead to inanition and starvation. Central nervous system disease may lead to seizures, coma, and central hypoventilation. About 70 percent of patients develop dyspnea preterminally. However, many months usually pass between the diagnosis of cancer and the occurrence of these complications, and during this period the patient is severely affected by the possibility of death. The path of unsuccessful cancer treatment usually occurs in three phases. First, there is optimism at the hope of cure; when the tumor recurs, there is the acknowledgment of an incurable disease, and the goal of palliative therapy is embraced in the hope of being able to live with disease; finally, at the disclosure of imminent death, another adjustment in outlook takes place. The patient imagines the worst in preparation for the end of life and may go through stages of adjustment to the diagnosis. These stages include denial, isolation, anger, bargaining, depression, acceptance, and hope. Of course, patients do not all progress through all the stages or proceed through them in the same order or at the same rate. Nevertheless, developing an understanding of how the patient has been affected by the diagnosis and is coping with it is an important goal of patient management.

It is best to speak frankly with the patient and the family regarding the likely course of disease. These discussions can be difficult for the physician as well as for the patient and family. The critical features of the interaction are to reassure the patient and family that everything that can be done to provide comfort will be done. They will not be abandoned. Many patients prefer to be cared for in their homes or in a hospice setting rather than a hospital. The American College of Physicians has published a book called *Home Care Guide for Cancer: How to Care for Family and Friends at Home* that teaches an approach to successful problem solving in home care. With appropriate planning, it should be possible to provide the patient with the necessary medical care as well as the psychological and spiritual support that will prevent the isolation and depersonalization that can attend in-hospital death.

The care of dying patients may take a toll on the physician. A "burnout" syndrome has been described that is characterized by fatigue, disengagement from patients and colleagues, and a loss of self-fulfillment. Efforts at stress reduction, maintenance of a balanced life, and setting realistic goals may combat this disorder.

End-of-Life Decisions Unfortunately, a smooth transition in treatment goals from curative to palliative may not be possible in all cases because of the occurrence of serious treatment-related complications or rapid disease progression. Vigorous and invasive medical support for a reversible disease or treatment complication is assumed to be justified. However, if the reversibility of the condition is in doubt, the patient's wishes determine the level of medical care. These wishes should be elicited before the terminal phase of illness and reviewed periodically. This information can guide the physician should the patient be unable to speak for himself. The family cannot be expected to make such decisions without guidance from the patient and support from the physician when surrogate decisions are required. Advance directives such as the living will or the durable power of attorney for health care provide guidance for the health care team and

the family regarding the patient's wishes and may protect the patient's assets from depletion on expensive but unwanted care.

Only about 15 percent of the population has implemented an advance directive. Physicians should take the initiative to speak with patients and family members about advance directives.*

BIBLIOGRAPHY

Clinical Practice Guideline Number 9, Management of Cancer Pain. U.S. Department of Health and Human Services, Agency for Health Care Policy and Research publication no. 94-0592, 1994

GRUNBERG SM, HESKETH PJ: Control of chemotherapy-induced emesis. N Engl J Med 329:1790, 1993

HOLLAND JC, ROWLAND JH (eds): *Handbook of Psycho-oncology: Psychological Care of the Patient with Cancer.* New York, Oxford University Press, 1989.

LEVY MH: Pharmacologic treatment of cancer pain. N Engl J Med 335:1124, 1996

PARKER SL et al: Cancer statistics, 1996. CA Cancer J Clin 46:5, 1996

* Information about them can be obtained from the American Association of Retired Persons, 601 E Street, N.W., Washington, DC 20049, 202-434-2277 or Choice in Dying, 250 West 57th Street, New York, NY 10107, 212-366-5540.

---

82 *Otis W. Brawley, Barnett S. Kramer*

PREVENTION AND EARLY DETECTION OF CANCER

The prevention and control of cancer is a burgeoning field because of advances in the understanding of the biology of carcinogenesis. The field has expanded beyond the identification and avoidance of carcinogens to include studies of specific interventions to lower cancer risk, as well as screening for early detection of cancer.

Central to the prevention and control of cancer is the concept that carcinogenesis is not an event but a process, a series of discrete cellular changes that result in progressively more autonomous cellular processes. *Primary prevention* consists in the identification and manipulation of the genetic, biologic, and environmental factors in the causal pathway. Smoking cessation, diet modification, and chemoprevention are primary prevention activities. *Secondary prevention* consists in the identification of asymptomatic neoplastic lesions combined with effective therapy. Screening is a form of secondary prevention.

EDUCATION AND HEALTHFUL HABITS Public education on the avoidance of identified risk factors for cancer and the encouraging of healthy habits were among early efforts in cancer prevention and control. Many educational messages have come to the public through commercials in the print and electronic media and through school health courses. The physician is a potentially powerful messenger in this education campaign about the hazards of smoking, the benefits of a healthful diet, and sun avoidance.

Smoking Cessation Cigarette smoking is the most avoidable risk factor for cardiovascular disease and cancer. There are clear correlations between lung cancer mortality rates and the number of cigarettes smoked per day as well as the degree of inhalation of cigarette smoke. Also, those who stop smoking have a lower lung cancer mortality rate than those who continue smoking. In addition to lung cancer, cigarette smoking has been associated as a causative agent in cancers of the larynx, oropharynx, esophagus, and bladder. Cessation and avoidance of smoking have the potential to save and extend more lives than any other public health activity. It is estimated that 400,000 Americans die prematurely every year because of cigarette smoking. A smoker has a one in three lifetime risk of dying of a cancer, cardiovascular, or pulmonary disease caused by cigarette smoking. Indeed, more human lives are lost owing to cardiovascular disease caused by smoking than from smoking-related cancer. The risk of tobacco smoke is not necessarily limited to the smoker. Epidemiologic studies suggest that environmental tobacco smoke may cause lung cancer and other pulmonary diseases in nonsmokers.

Nonsmoking persons should be encouraged not to start smoking, and persons who smoke should be encouraged to stop. In one sense, tobacco-related disease is a pediatric issue. Surveys show that over 80 percent of American smokers begin smoking before the age of 18. Indeed, nearly 20 percent of Americans aged 12 to 18 have smoked a cigarette in the past month. Counseling of adolescents and young adults is critical to prevention of smoking. Studies show that a physician's simple advice to not start smoking or to quit smoking can be of benefit.

Current approaches to smoking cessation recognize that smoking is an addiction (see Chap. 389). The smoker who is quitting goes through a process with identifiable stages that include contemplation of quitting, an action phase in which the smoker quits, and a maintenance phase. Smokers who quit completely are more likely to be successful than those who gradually reduce the number of cigarettes smoked or change to cigarettes lower in tar or nicotine. More than 90 percent of the Americans who have successfully quit smoking did so on their own without participation in an organized cessation program, but cessation programs are helpful for some smokers. The Community Intervention Trial for Smoking Cessation (COMMIT) was a community-based 4-year program sponsored by the National Cancer Institute and completed in 1994. One community of each of 11 matched community pairs was randomly assigned to intervention. The intervention included public education through the media and community-wide events, health care providers, worksites and other organizations, and cessation resources. COMMIT demonstrated that light smokers can benefit from simple cessation messages and cessation programs. The quit rate (fraction of the cohorts followed who achieved and maintained cessation at the end of the trial) was 30.6 percent in the intervention communities and 27.5 percent in the control communities. This finding is statistically significant, but it also shows that there was a trend toward a decrease in smoking even in the control communities. The COMMIT interventions were not successful for heavy smokers (>25 cigarettes per day). Experts believe heavy smokers generally need an intensive, broad-based cessation program that includes counseling, behavioral strategies, and pharmacologic adjuncts such as nicotine gum and nicotine patches.

Smokeless tobacco is the fastest growing part of the tobacco industry and represents a significant health risk. Chewing tobacco is a carcinogen linked to dental caries, gingivitis, oral leukoplakia, and oral cancer. The systemic effects of smokeless tobacco may increase risks for other cancers. Nitrosamines found in smokeless tobacco cause lung cancer in laboratory animals.

Diet Modification Dietary modification may have significant potential for lowering cancer risk in Western culture. Studies of international dietary patterns and animal studies suggest that diets high in fat increase the risk for cancers of the breast, colon, prostate, and endometrium. These cancers have their highest incidence and mortalities in Western countries, where fat makes up an average of 40 to 45 percent of the total calories consumed. In populations at low risk for these cancers, fat accounts for less than 20 percent of dietary calories.

Nonetheless, dietary fat has not been accepted by all as important in the etiology of cancers. Case-control and cohort epidemiologic studies give conflicting results. Some have argued that the relatively homogeneous fat intake levels in many of these studies could mask an effect. In addition, diet involves a complex exposure to many nutrients and chemicals. The protection against cancer apparently afforded by low-fat diets may in part reflect exposure to anticarcinogens found in vegetables, fruits, legumes, nuts, and grains. Substances found in these foods that may be protective include phenols, sulfur-containing compounds, flavones, and fiber.

Dietary fiber appears to afford protection against colonic polyps and invasive cancer of the colon. The mechanisms involved are complex and speculative. They include binding of oxidized bile acids, a decrease in bowel transit time, and generation of soluble fiber products, such as butyrate, that may have differentiating properties. The fiber in high-fiber diets may also protect against breast and prostate cancer by absorbing and inactivating dietary compounds that serve as cancer promoters through estrogenic and androgenic activity.

A simple way for an individual to decrease dietary fat and increase dietary fiber is to consume at least five to nine servings of fruits and vegetables per day. Although the effects of such a diet have not been fully assessed, it is likely to decrease the risk of colon cancer and possibly lower the risk for cancers of the breast, endometrium, and prostate. Such a diet may also lower the risk of cardiac disease.

The U.S. National Institutes of Health (NIH) Women's Health Initiative, launched in 1994, is a long-term clinical trial enrolling more than 100,000 women aged 45 to 69. It studies the potential cancer-preventing effects of a low-fat diet and vitamin supplementation. It must be stressed that the scientific evidence does not currently establish the anticarcinogenic value of vitamin, mineral, or nutritional supplements in amounts greater than that provided by a good diet.

Sun Avoidance Epidemiologic studies suggest that nonmelanoma skin cancers (basal cell and squamous cell) are induced by cumulative exposure to ultraviolet radiation. Intermittent acute sun exposure and sun damage have also been linked to melanoma. Sunburns, especially in childhood and adolescence, are associated with an increased risk of melanoma in adulthood. Reduction of sun exposure through use of protective clothing and changes in the pattern of outdoor activities has been advocated as a way of reducing skin cancer risk. Sunscreens may provide some protection, but how much has not been established.

Educational interventions to help persons accurately assess their risk of developing skin cancer have some impact. Self-examination for skin pigment characteristics associated with melanoma, such as freckling, may be useful in helping high-risk individuals identify themselves. Persons who recognize themselves as being at risk tend to comply better with sun-avoidance recommendations. Possible risk factors for melanoma include a propensity to sunburn, a large number of benign melanocytic nevi, and atypical nevi.

CANCER CHEMOPREVENTION Chemoprevention of cancer is a relatively new concept. It involves the use of specific natural or synthetic chemical agents to reverse, suppress, or prevent carcinogenesis before the development of invasive malignancy. While the concept that pharmacologic agents can prevent a cancer is relatively new, the idea that a compound can prevent chronic disease is not. Clinicians routinely prevent heart disease, kidney disease, and stroke by treating hypertension with pharmacologic agents. Lipid-lowering drugs are used to prevent coronary artery disease.

Improved understanding of the biology of cancer makes chemoprevention a real possibility. Cancer develops through an accumulation of genetic changes, which are potential points of intervention for preventing cancer. The initial genetic changes are termed *initiation*. Alterations of this type can be inherited or can be acquired through the action of physical, viral, or chemical carcinogens. Like most human diseases, cancer arises through an interaction between genetics and environmental exposures (Table 82-1). Influences that cause the initiated cell to progress through the carcinogenic process and to change phenotypically are termed *promoters*. Examples of promoters are hormones such as androgens, linked to prostate cancer, and estrogen, linked to breast and endometrial cancer. The distinction between an initiator and a promoter is sometimes arbitrary; some components of cigarette smoke are so-called complete carcinogens, acting as both initiators and promoters. Cancer can be prevented or controlled through interference with the factors that cause initiation, promotion, or progression. Compounds of interest in chemoprevention often have antimutagenic, antioxidant, or antiproliferative activity.

Cancer chemoprevention is not yet established in clinical practice, although it has attracted great interest. Before a chemoprevention strategy can become standard practice, evidence of benefit must be gathered from clinical trials. These trials are usually large, long-term, randomized, placebo-controlled, and double-blinded. They often allow for the study of drugs for prevention of multiple cancers and the study of end-points other than cancer, such as other chronic diseases. Several large clinical trials have been completed, and a number will be continuing into the twenty-first century.

Multiple Cancer Site Prevention Trials The Physicians' Health Trial is a study that began in 1982. It involves 22,071 American male physicians. Participants were randomly assigned to receive β-carotene, aspirin, and/or placebo in a 2×2 factorial design and followed. All major medical events were recorded. In 1988, the aspirin arm was unblinded after the trial demonstrated that aspirin therapy causes a significant reduction in cardiovascular mortality. The β-carotene arm of the study will continue until 1998, when an analysis for cancer end-points is planned.

The Women's Health Study, launched in 1992, is an 8-year trial involving 44,000 female nurses. Subjects are randomly assigned to β-carotene, alpha tocopherol, aspirin, and/or placebo in a factorial design yielding eight different treatment groups. The end-points being studied are total epithelial cancers, breast cancer, lung cancer, colon cancer, and vascular disease.

The Women's Health Initiative, described earlier, uses a partial factorial design that places women in 22 intervention groups. Participants can receive calcium and vitamin D supplementation, hormone replacement therapy, and counseling to increase exercise and cease smoking. This study promises to render findings about prevention of a number of cancers, cardiovascular disease, osteoporosis, and other diseases.

Prevention of Hormonally Driven Cancers Hormonal manipulation is being tested in the primary prevention of breast and prostate cancer. Tamoxifen is an antiestrogen that has partial estrogen agonistic activity in some tissues, such as endometrium and bone. One of its actions is to up-regulate transforming growth factor β, which decreases breast cell proliferation. In randomized placebo-controlled trials to assess tamoxifen as an adjuvant in breast cancer treatment, this drug reduced the number of new breast cancers in the uninvolved breast by more than a third. The primary prevention capabilities of tamoxifen are being tested further in a decade-long trial involving 16,000 women at high risk of developing breast cancer.

Finasteride is a 5α-reductase inhibitor. It inhibits the conversion of testosterone to dihydrotestosterone, which is a more potent stimulator of prostate cell proliferation than testosterone. In an F344 rat model of carcinogen-induced prostate cancer, finasteride has been shown to decrease the incidence of cancers. Finasteride is being tested as a preventive agent for prostate cancer in a 10-year study involving 18,000 men age 55 and older.

Chemoprevention of Cancers of the Upper Aerodigestive Tract Smoking causes diffuse epithelial injury in the head, neck, esophagus, and lung. Patients cured of squamous cell cancers of the lung, esophagus, head, and neck are at high risk of developing a second malignancy (a risk as high as 5 percent per year of a second cancer of the upper aerodigestive tract). Cessation of cigarette smoking does not markedly decrease the cured cancer patient's risk of second malignancy, even though it does lower the cancer risk in those who have never developed a malignancy. Smoking cessation may halt the early stages of the carcinogenic process (such as metaplasia), but it may have no effect on late

stages of carcinogenesis. This "field carcinogenesis" hypothesis for cancer of the upper aerodigestive tract has made "cured" patients an important population for chemoprevention of second malignancies. A randomized, placebo-controlled clinical trial has demonstrated that adjuvant isoretinoin (13 *cis*-retinoic acid) can reduce the incidence of second primary tumors in patients treated with local therapy for head and neck cancer.

Oral leukoplakia, a premalignant lesion commonly found in smokers, has been used as an intermediate marker allowing the demonstration of chemopreventive activity in smaller, shorter-duration, randomized, placebo-controlled trials. Response was associated with up-regulation of retinoic acid receptor β. Therapy with isoretinoin causes regression of oral leukoplakia. However, the lesions recur when the agent is withdrawn, suggesting the need for chronic administration of retinoids. Premalignant lesions in the oropharyngeal area have also responded to β-carotene, retinol, alpha tocopherol (vitamin E), and selenium. Further study to better define the activity of these drugs is ongoing. The ability of isoretinoin to prevent second malignancies in patients cured of low-stage non–small cell lung cancer is also being assessed.

Several large-scale trials have been launched to assess agents in the chemoprevention of lung cancer in patients at high risk. In the Alpha-Tocopherol/Beta-Carotene (ATBC) Lung Cancer Prevention Trial, participants were male smokers, aged 50 to 69 at entry. At entry, participants had smoked an average of one pack of cigarettes per day for 35.9 years. Participants received alpha tocopherol, β-carotene, and/or placebo in a randomized, 2×2 factorial design. Surprisingly, after a median follow-up of 6.1 years, there was a statistically significant *increase* in lung cancer incidence and mortality in those receiving β-carotene. Alpha tocopherol had no significant impact on lung cancer mortality, and there was no evidence of interaction between the two drugs. Patients receiving alpha tocopherol had a higher incidence of hemorrhagic stroke. The Beta-Carotene and Retinol Efficacy Trial (CARET) involved 17,000 American smokers and workers with asbestos exposure. Entrants were randomly assigned to one of four arms and received β-carotene, retinol, and/or placebo in a 2×2 factorial

Table 82-1

Carcinogens and Associated Cancers or Neoplasms

Carcinogens*	Associated Cancer or Neoplasm
Alkylating agents	Acute myelocytic leukemia, bladder cancer
Androgens	Prostate cancer
Aromatic amines (dyes)	Bladder cancer
Arsenic	Cancer of the lung, skin
Asbestos	Cancer of the lung, pleura, peritoneum
Benzene	Acute myelocytic leukemia
Chromium	Lung cancer
Diethylstilbestrol (Prenatal)	Vaginal cancer (clear cell)
Epstein-Barr virus	Burkitt's lymphoma, nasal T-cell lymphoma
Estrogens	Cancer of the endometrium, liver
Ethyl alcohol	Cancer of the liver, esophagus, head and neck
Helicobacter pylori	Gastric cancer
Hepatitis B or C virus	Liver cancer
Human immunodeficiency virus	Non-Hodgkin's lymphoma, Kaposi's sarcoma, squamous cell carcinoma
Human T-cell lymphotropic virus type I (HTLV-I)	Adult T-cell leukemia/lymphoma
Immunosuppressive agents (azathioprine, cyclosporine, corticosteriods)	Non-Hodgkin's lymphoma
Nitrogen mustard gas	Cancer of the lung, head and neck, nasal sinuses
Nickel dust	Cancer of the lung, nasal sinuses
Phenacetin	Cancer of the renal pelvis and bladder
Polycyclic hydrocarbons	Cancer of the lung, skin (especially squamous cell carcinoma of scrotal skin)
Schistosomiasis	Bladder cancer (squamous cell)
Sunlight (ultraviolet)	Skin cancer (squamous cell and melanoma)
Tobacco (including smokeless)	Cancer of the upper aerodigestive tract, bladder
Vinyl chloride	Liver cancer (angiosarcoma)

* Agents that are thought to act as cancer initiators and/or promoters.

design. This trial demonstrated a lung cancer rate of 5 per 1000 subjects per year for those taking placebo and of 6 per 1000 subjects per year for those taking β-carotene.

These ATBC and CARET results demonstrate the importance of testing chemoprevention hypotheses before implementing them widely, because the results stand in contrast to a number of observational epidemiologic studies. In the ATBC, participants taking alpha tocopherol had a one-third reduction in the incidence of prostate cancer, compared to those not taking alpha tocopherol. Investigation of this surprising trial result continues.

Chemoprevention of Colon Cancer Many of the current colon cancer prevention trials are based on the premise that most colorectal cancers develop from adenomatous polyps. These trials use adenoma recurrence or disappearance as a surrogate end-point to assess colon cancer prevention. Early clinical trial results suggest that nonsteroidal antiinflammatory drugs (NSAIDs), such as piroxicam, sulindac, and aspirin, may prevent adenoma formation or cause regression of adenomatous polyps. The mechanism of the antiproliferative action of NSAIDs is unknown, but they are presumed to work through the cyclooxygenase pathway. In the Physicians' Health Trial, described above, aspirin had no effect on colon cancer incidence, although the 6-year assessment period was not long enough to definitively evaluate this end-point.

Epidemiologic studies suggest that diets high in calcium lower colon cancer risk. Calcium binds bile and fatty acids, which cause hyperproliferation of colonic epithelium. It is hypothesized that this effect reduces intraluminal exposure to these compounds. Cancer chemoprevention trials using calcium-containing compounds and NSAIDs are under way.

Vaccines and Cancer Prevention A number of infectious agents have been linked to the development of cancer, leading to interest in development of vaccines to protect against these agents. The hepatitis B vaccine is quite effective in preventing hepatitis and, presumably, also hepatomas due to chronic hepatitis B infection. Public health officials are encouraging widespread administration of this vaccine, especially in Asia, where the disease is epidemic. In the future, human papilloma virus vaccines could be developed to prevent cervical cancer, and *Helicobacter pylori* vaccines may be developed to prevent gastric cancer.

CANCER SCREENING Screening is best defined as a means of detecting disease early, in asymptomatic individuals, with the goal of decreasing morbidity and mortality. Screening for cancer is intuitively appealing and has attracted great public interest as technology has generated a number of diagnostic tests and procedures that are safe, quick, and inexpensive. While screening can potentially save lives, and has been shown clearly to do so in the case of breast, cervical, and colon cancer, it is also subject to a number of biases, which can suggest a benefit when actually there is none, or even mask a net harm. Early detection does not in itself confer benefit. To be of value, screening must detect disease earlier, and treatment of earlier disease must yield a better outcome than treatment at the onset of symptoms.

Because screening is done on asymptomatic, healthy persons, it should offer substantial likelihood of benefit. A critical approach to screening is necessary to ensure that this condition is met. Screening tests and their appropriate use should be carefully evaluated before their use is widely encouraged in screening programs as a matter of public policy.

Generally, screening examinations, tests, or procedures are not diagnostic of cancer but instead indicate that a cancer may be present. The diagnosis is then made following a workup that generally includes a biopsy and pathologic confirmation.

A number of genes have been identified as predisposing the bearer to a disease, and many more will be identified in the near future. Testing for these genes can define a high-risk population. The ability to predict the development of a particular cancer may some day present therapeutic options as well as ethical dilemmas. It may eventually allow for early

Table 82-2

Definition of Terms

Term	Definition
Sensitivity	The proportion of persons with the condition who test positive: $a/(a + c)$
Specificity	The proportion of persons without the condition who test negative: $d/(b + d)$
Positive predictive value	The proportion of persons with a positive test who have the condition: $a/(a + b)$
Negative predictive value	The proportion of persons with a negative test who do not have the condition: $d/(c + d)$

		Condition present	Condition absent
a = true positive			
b = false positive	Positive test	a	b
c = false negative			
d = true negative	Negative test	c	d

intervention to prevent a cancer or limit its severity. People at high risk will be ideal candidates for chemoprevention and screening; however, the efficacy of these interventions in the high-risk population should be investigated. Currently, persons at high risk for a particular cancer can engage in intensive screening. While this course is clinically prudent, it is not known if it saves lives in these populations.

The Accuracy of Screening Four indices are used to describe the accuracy, or ability to discriminate disease, of a screening test: sensitivity, specificity, positive predictive value, and negative predictive value (Table 82-2). *Sensitivity* is the proportion of people with the disease who test positive in the screen (i.e., the ability of the test to detect disease when it is present). *Specificity* is the proportion of people who do not have the disease and test negative in the screening test (i.e., the ability of a test to tell that the disease is not present). The *positive predictive value* is the proportion of persons who test positive and have the disease. Similarly, *negative predictive value* is the proportion who test negative and do not have the disease. The sensitivity and specificity of a test are relatively independent of the underlying prevalence (or risk) of the disease in the population screened, but the predictive values depend strongly on the prevalence of the disease (Table 82-3).

Table 82-3

Predictive Value Relationships*

Positive predictive value (PPV) is a function of sensitivity, specificity, and prevalence:

$$PPV = \frac{Prevalence \times Sensitivity}{(Prevalence \times Sensitivity) + (1 - Prevalence)(1 - Sensitivity)}$$

PPV values for a prevalence of 5 per 1000:

	PPV for a Sensitivity of	
Specificity	0.8	0.95
0.95	7%	9%
0.999	80%	83%

PPV values for a prevalence of 1 per 10,000:

	PPV for a Sensitivity of	
Specificity	0.8	0.95
0.95	0.2%	0.2%
0.999	7%	9%

* The positive predictive value is expressed as a percentage. It is influenced by the sensitivity and specificity of the screening test and the prevalence of the disease being screened for. As shown here, for relatively uncommon diseases, such as cancer, the positive predictive value is influenced particularly strongly by the specificity of the screening test at a given prevalence.

Screening is most beneficial, efficient, and economical when the target disease is common in the population being screened. To be valuable, the screening test should have a high specificity; sensitivity need not be very high, as demonstrated in Table 82-3.

Potential Biases of Screening Tests The common biases of screening are lead-time, length, and selection biases. These biases can make a screening test seem beneficial when actually it is not (or even causes net harm). Whether beneficial or not, screening can create the false impression of an epidemic by increasing the number of cancers diagnosed. It can also give the appearance of a shift in stage, thus improving survival statistics without reducing mortality (i.e., the number of deaths from a given cancer relative to the number of people at risk for the cancer). In such a case, the *apparent* duration of survival increases without lives being saved or life expectancy changing.

Lead-time bias occurs when a test does not lead to any change in the natural history of the disease; the patient is merely diagnosed at an earlier date. When lead time bias occurs, survival *appears* increased, but life is not really prolonged. The screening test only prolongs the time the subject is aware of the disease, which for cancer is not a benefit.

Length bias occurs when slow-growing, less aggressive, cancers are detected during screening. Cancers diagnosed owing to the onset of symptoms between scheduled screenings are on average more aggressive, and treatment outcomes are not as favorable. An extreme form of length bias is termed *overdiagnosis*, the detection of "pseudo-disease." The reservoir of some undetected slow-growing tumors is large. Many of these tumors fulfill the histologic criteria of cancer but will never become clinically significant or cause death. This problem is compounded by the fact that the most common cancers appear most frequently at ages when competing causes of death are more frequent.

Selection bias must be considered in assessing the results of any screening effort. The population most likely to seek screening may differ from the general population to which the screening test might be applied. The individuals screened may have volunteered because of a particular risk factor not found in the general population, such as a strong family history. In general, volunteers for studies may be more health conscious, and thus likely to have a better prognosis or lower mortality rate irrespective of the screening result. This is termed the "healthy volunteer effect."

Potential Drawbacks of Screening There are often risks associated with screening, including the risks of harm caused by the screening intervention itself, harm due to the further investigation of persons with positive test results (both true and false), and harm incident on the treatment of persons with a true-positive result, even if life is extended by treatment. The diagnosis and treatment of cancers that would never have caused medical problems can lead to the harm of unnecessary treatment and give patients the anxiety of a cancer diagnosis. The psychosocial impact of cancer screening, for persons with both positive and negative results, can also be substantial when applied to the entire population.

Assessment of Screening Tests Good clinical trial design can offset some biases of screening and demonstrate the relative risks and benefits of a screening test. A randomized, controlled screening trial with cause-specific mortality as the end-point provides the strongest support for a screening intervention. In a randomized trial, two like populations are randomly established. One is given the medical standard of care (which may be no screening at all), and the other receives the screening intervention being assessed. The two populations are compared over time. The efficacy of the test for the population studied is established when the group receiving the screening test has a better cause-specific mortality rate than the control group. Studies showing a reduction in the incidence of advanced-stage disease, an improved survival, or a stage shift are weaker evidence of benefit. These latter criteria are necessary but not sufficient to establish the value of a screening test.

Although a randomized, controlled screening trial provides the strongest evidence to support the usefulness of a screening test, it is not perfect. Unless the trial is population-based, it does not remove the issue of generalizability to the target population. Screening trials generally involve thousands of persons and last for years. Less defini-

tive study designs are therefore often used to estimate the effectiveness of screening practices. After a randomized controlled clinical trial, in descending order of strength, evidence may be derived from:

- The findings of internally controlled trials using intervention allocation methods other than randomization (e.g. allocation determined by birth date, date of clinic visit, etc.);
- The findings of cohort or case-control analytic observational studies;
- The results of multiple time series studies with or without the intervention;
- The opinions of respected authorities based on clinical experience, descriptive studies, or consensus reports of experts

The last of these forms of evidence is the weakest, because even experts can be misled by the biases described above.

Screening for Specific Cancers Studies have shown that widespread screening for breast, cervical, and colon cancer is beneficial for certain age groups. Special surveillance of those at high risk for a specific cancer because of a family history or a genetic risk factor may be prudent, but few studies have been carried out to assess the impact of this practice on mortality in specific high-risk populations. A number of organizations have considered whether or not to endorse routine use of certain screening tests. Because these groups have not used the same criteria to judge whether a screening test should be endorsed, they have arrived at different recommendations. The screening guidelines of the U.S. Preventive Services Task Force and those of the American Cancer Society are often quoted and show a range of recommendations (Table 82-4).

Breast cancer Breast self-examination, clinical breast examination by a care giver, and mammography have been advocated as useful screening tools. Only screening mammography alone and screening mammography with clinical exam have been evaluated in randomized controlled trials. In addition, there is an ongoing Canadian trial evaluating clinical breast exam with or without mammography in women aged 50 to 65, but final results have not yet been reported. A number of well-designed trials have demonstrated that annual or biennial screening with mammography or mammography plus clinical breast examination in women over the age of 50 saves lives. In these trials, the breast cancer mortality rate is decreased by about a third. These trials do not have enough statistical power to indicate definitively whether such screening is useful in normal-risk women younger than 50. Experts therefore disagree on whether average-risk women aged 40 to 49 should receive regular screening (see Table 82-4). An analysis of eight large randomized trials showed no benefit from mammographic screening for women aged 40 to 49 who were assessed 5 to 7 years after trial entry. However there may be a small benefit for women in these trials 10 to 12 years after study entry. What proportion of this possible benefit would be due to screening after these women turned 50 is not known but is an active area of study. While no study has shown breast self-examination to decrease mortality, it is recommended as prudent by many organizations.

Cervical cancer Cohort and case-control studies have shown that screening with Papanicolaou smears decreases cervical cancer mortality. The cervical cancer mortality rate has fallen significantly since the widespread use of the Pap smear, although this trend actually began earlier. Most screening guidelines recommend regular Pap testing for all women who are or have been sexually active or have reached the age of 18. With the onset of sexual activity comes the risk of sexual transmission of human papilloma virus, the most common etiologic factor for cervical cancer. The recommended interval for Pap screening varies from one to three years. It is not known whether there is an upper age limit at which screening ceases to be effective.

Colorectal cancer Fecal occult blood testing, rigid and flexible sigmoidoscopy, radiographic barium contrast studies, and colonoscopy have been considered for colorectal cancer screening. One randomized study indicates that annual fecal occult blood testing using hydrated specimens could reduce colorectal cancer mortality by a third. The sensitivity for fecal occult blood is increased if specimens are rehydrated before testing, but at the cost of lower specificity. The false-positive rate for rehydrated fecal occult blood testing is high; 1 to 5 percent of persons tested have a positive result. Approximately 10 percent of those with occult blood in the stool have cancer, and 20 to 30 percent have adenomas.

Two case-control studies suggest that regular screening of people over 50 with sigmoidoscopy decreases mortality. A quarter to a third of polyps can be discovered with the rigid sigmoidoscope; approximately half are found with a 35-cm flexible scope, and two-thirds to three-quarters are found with a 60-cm scope. Diagnosis of polyposis by sigmoidoscopy should lead to evaluation of the entire colon with colonoscopy and/or barium enema. The most efficient interval for screening sigmoidoscopy is unknown. Case-control studies suggest that testing at intervals of up to 9 years may confer benefit. Most authorities feel that full colonoscopy is too cumbersome and invasive for widespread use as a screening tool in standard-risk populations. It may be suitable for subjects at extremely high risk, however, such as members of families with a genetic predisposition to colorectal cancer. Likewise, barium contrast studies are often thought to be unsuitable for large-scale screening efforts.

Lung cancer   Screening chest radiographs and sputum cytology have been evaluated as methods for lung cancer screening. No significant reduction in lung cancer mortality has been found in these studies, although all the controlled trials performed have had low statistical power. Even screening of high-risk subjects (smokers) has not been proved to be beneficial.

Ovarian cancer   Adnexal palpation, transvaginal ultrasound, and serum CA-125 determination have been considered as methods for ovarian cancer screening. Adnexal palpation is considered by most to be far too insensitive to detect ovarian cancer at an early enough stage to substantially affect mortality. Neither transvaginal ultrasound nor CA-125 screening has been tested in a completed randomized prospective trial. Ovarian cancer screening can lead to an invasive diagnostic workup, which may include laparotomy. In a clinical study, 0.6 percent of 900 adult women had a serum CA-125 level greater than 35 U/ml. Thus, if 100,000 adult women were screened, 600 would be identified as having a high CA-125. The prevalence of ovarian cancer in the female adult population is approximately 20 per 100,000. Thus, the screening test would identify 600 women who would undergo further evaluation to identify 20 cases of ovarian cancer. Some of these 600

would only be inconvenienced by an ultrasound examination. Others would undergo an exploratory laparotomy. It should be noted that a large proportion of the 20 women identified as having ovarian cancer would have advanced, incurable disease and thus not benefit from screening. An NIH consensus conference in 1994 concluded that routine screening for ovarian cancer was not indicated for standard-risk women or for women with a single affected family member, but that it might be worthwhile in families with genetic ovarian cancer syndromes.

Prostate cancer   The most common prostate cancer screening modalities are digital rectal examination and assays for serum prostate-specific antigen (PSA). Newer serum tests, such as measurement of the ratio of bound to free serum PSA, have yet to be fully evaluated. An emphasis on PSA screening has caused prostate cancer to become the most common nonskin cancer diagnosed in American males. Screening for this disease is very prone to lead time bias, length bias, and overdiagnosis, and there is substantial debate among experts as to whether it is effective. Some experts are concerned that prostate cancer screening, more than screening for other cancers, may cause net harm. Prostate cancer screening clearly detects many asymptomatic cancers, but the ability to distinguish tumors that are lethal but still curable from those that pose little or no threat to health is limited. Men over age 50 have a very high prevalence of indolent, clinically insignificant prostate cancers. No well-designed trial has been completed to test the true benefit of prostate cancer screening and treatment, but trials are in progress.

The effectiveness of radical prostatectomy, radiation therapy, and other treatments for low-stage prostate cancer is also under study in randomized trials. Definitive treatment of cancers detected by screening may cause morbidity for some men, such as impotence and urinary incontinence, and carries a low but finite risk of death. Pending the completion of ongoing randomized trials comparing usual care to prostate screening and comparing definitive therapy to "watchful waiting," organizations have provided conflicting recommendations on prostate cancer screening (Table 82-4). All agree, however, that a man should have a life expectancy of at least 10 years to be eligible for screening.

Skin cancer   Visual examination of all skin surfaces by the patient or by a health care provider is used in screening for basal and squamous cell cancers and melanoma. No prospective randomized study has been performed to look for a mortality decrease. Observational epidemiologic evidence from Scotland and Australia suggest that screening programs have caused a stage shift in melanomas diagnosed. Screening may reinforce sun-avoidance and other skin cancer prevention behaviors.

Table 82-4

Screening Recommendations for Asymptomatic Subjects at Normal Risk*

Test or Procedure	USPSTF Recommendations	ACS Recommendations
Sigmoidoscopy	Over age 50: periodically Under age 50: not recommended	Ages 50 and over: every 3–5 years
Fecal occult blood testing	Ages 50 and over: every year	Ages 50 and over: every year
Digital rectal examination	No recommendation	Ages 40 and over: every year
Prostate-specific antigen determination	Recommended against	Men aged 50 and over: every year
Papanicolaou test	Women aged 18–65: every 1–3 years	Women over age 18: once yearly for 3 years; thereafter at physician's discretion
Pelvic examination	Not recommended; adnexal palpation should be performed during examination for other reasons	Women aged 18–40: every 1–3 years with Pap test; over age 40: every year
Endometrial tissue sampling	Not considered	At menopause if patient is obese or has a history of unopposed estrogen use
Breast self-examination	No recommendation	Women aged 20 and over: monthly
Clinical breast examination	Women over age 50: every year	Women aged 20–40: every 3 years; over age 40: yearly
Mammography	Women aged 50–75: every 1–2 years	Women aged 40–49: every 1–2 years; ages 50 and over: every year
Complete skin examination	Not recommended	Ages 20–39: every 3 years

* The above is a summary of the screening procedures recommended for the general population by the U.S. Preventive Services Task Force (USPSTF) and the American Cancer Society (ACS). These recommendations refer to asymptomatic persons who have no risk factors other than age or gender for the targeted condition.

BIBLIOGRAPHY

BLOCK G et al: Fruit, vegetables, and cancer prevention: A review of the epidemiological evidence. Nutr Cancer 18:1, 1992

DOLL R, PETO R: The cause of cancer: Quantitative estimates of avoidable risks of cancer in the United States today. J Natl Cancer Inst 66:1191, 1981

FLETCHER SW et al: Report of the International Workshop on Screening for Breast Cancer. J Natl Cancer Inst 85:1644, 1993

GREENWALD P et al: Chemoprevention. CA Cancer J Clin 45:31, 1995

———— et al: Cancer Prevention and Control. New York, Marcel Dekker, 1995

LIPPMAN SM et al: Cancer chemoprevention. J Clin Oncol 12:851, 1994

SOX HC: Preventive health services in adults. N Engl J Med 330:1589, 1995

THE ALPHA-TOCOPHEROL, BETA CAROTENE CANCER PREVENTION STUDY GROUP: The effect of vitamin E and beta carotene on the incidence of lung cancer and other cancers in male smokers. N Engl J Med 330:1029, 1994

THE COMMIT RESEARCH GROUP: Community intervention trial for smoking cessation (COMMIT): I. Cohort results from a four-year community intervention. Am J Public Health 85:183, 1995

————: Community intervention trial for smoking cessation (COMMIT): II. Changes in adult cigarette smoking prevalence. Am J Public Health 85:193, 1995

U.S. PREVENTIVE SERVICES TASK FORCE: Guide to Clinical Preventive Services, 2nd ed: Washington D.C., Government Printing Office, 1996

WOOLF SH: Screening for prostate cancer with prostate-specific antigen. N Engl J Med 333:1401, 1995

---

83 | Robert G. Fenton, Dan L. Longo

CELL BIOLOGY OF CANCER

Two characteristic features define a cancer: cell growth not regulated by external signals (i.e., autonomous) and the capacity to invade tissues and metastasize to and colonize distant sites (see Chap. 85). The first of these features, the uncontrolled growth of abnormal cells, is a property of all neoplasms, or new growths. A neoplasm may be benign or malignant. If invasion, the second cardinal feature of cancer, is present, the neoplasm is malignant. Cancer is a synonym for *malignant neoplasm*. Cancers of epithelial tissues are called *carcinomas*; cancers of nonepithelial (mesenchymal) tissues are called *sarcomas*.

Cancer is a genetic disease, but the level of its expression is the single cell. Although some forms of cancer are heritable, most mutations occur in somatic cells and are caused by intrinsic errors in DNA replication or are induced by carcinogen exposure. A single genetic lesion is usually not sufficient to induce neoplastic transformation of a cell. The malignant phenotype is acquired only after several (5 to 10) mutations (usually developing over many years) lead to derangements in a variety of gene products. Each genetic alteration may cause phenotypic changes typified by the progression in epithelial tissues from hyperplasia to adenoma to dysplasia to carcinoma in situ to invasive carcinoma. Resistance to neoplastic transformation is due to levels of control at every phase of cell function. Abnormalities in the function of one protein may be compensated by other proteins and pathways. An analogy can be drawn between the complex behavior of interacting signaling cascades and computer-based neural networks that can be adapted or trained to recognize patterns of complex inputs and respond to each pattern with a specific pattern of output.

The more than 200 discrete cell types in the body are not equally susceptible to developing cancer. Some cells, such as cardiac myocytes, sensory receptor cells for light and sound, and lens fibers, persist throughout life without dividing or being replaced. Neoplasia in such tissues is exceedingly rare. Most differentiated tissues undergo turnover characterized by cell death and replacement. When natural turnover rates are slow, fully differentiated cells may be induced to proliferate and produce fully differentiated daughter cells. For example, hepatocytes are capable of dividing to replace senescent, damaged, or surgically removed liver tissue.

In tissues with rapid turnover, such as skin, bone marrow, and gut, the differentiated function and the replacement function are carried out by different cell types. Under normal circumstances, an individual cell is on one of two largely mutually exclusive paths: division or differentiation. Cells capable of dividing are undifferentiated (stem cells), whereas terminally differentiated cells are unable to divide. Stem cells produce daughter cells that can either become new stem cells (thus replenishing the stem cell compartment) or undergo terminal differentiation, depending on the circumstances and the environmental signals. Stem cells are distinguished from differentiating cells by different patterns of gene expression. Gene expression is the product of the tissue-specific programming of gene expression interacting with environmental factors such as cell-to-cell contact; interactions with extracellular matrix; endocrine hormones; paracrine growth and differentiation factors; and stresses such as heat, oxidation, irradiation, and physical distortion or traction.

Cancer is most common in tissues with rapid turnover, especially those exposed to environmental carcinogens and whose proliferation is regulated by hormones. The most common genetic changes involve the activation of proto-oncogenes or the inactivation of tumor suppressor genes (see Chap. 84). Although genetic damage is nearly universal in human cancer, cells with neoplastic features can be generated in vitro without genetic damage. Removal and in vitro culture of cells from the epiblast of a murine embryo lead to the uncontrolled proliferation of the cells and the generation of a teratocarcinoma cell line capable of producing tumors when inoculated into animals. The removal of these normal embryonic cells from their normal environment leads to uncontrolled growth. However, if the teratocarcinoma cells are reinjected into an early embryo, under the inductive influence of their normal neighbors they can differentiate into normal organs and tissues appropriate for the location where they are injected.

Thus, environmental factors exert potent effects on the gene expression of target cells. The panoply of signals received by a particular cell leads to the activation of particular sets of transcription factors. The pattern of expression of transcription factors determines whether a cell will divide, differentiate, or die.

PRINCIPLES OF CELL CYCLE REGULATION

The mechanism of cell division is substantially the same in all dividing cells and has been conserved throughout evolution. The process assures that the cell accurately duplicates its contents, especially its chromosomes. The cell cycle is divided into four phases. During M phase, the replicated chromosomes are separated and packaged into two new nuclei by mitosis and the cytoplasm is divided between the two daughter cells by cytokinesis. The other three phases of the cell cycle are called *interphase*: G1 (gap 1), a period of growth during which the cell determines its readiness to commit to DNA synthesis; S (DNA synthesis), during which the genetic material is replicated and no re-replication is permitted; and G2 (gap 2), during which the fidelity of DNA replication is determined and errors are corrected.

During S phase, DNA synthesis begins with the unfolding of chromatin from the DNA and the addition of DNA helicase and single-strand binding proteins that help open the double helix. Replication origins are spaced roughly 100,000 nucleotide pairs apart throughout the genome. DNA polymerase and DNA primase attach to these sites and catalyze the polymerization of the DNA at a rate of about 50 nucleotides per second. Topoisomerases break and reseal DNA strands to prevent tangling. Although this system for replication is efficient and accurate, occasional mistakes are made, and these mistakes in the replicated sequences are repaired by a variety of mechanisms. In some cancers, the mismatch repair mechanisms are defective and errors are routinely passed along to daughter cells, increasing the development of new mutations. Once a DNA segment is replicated and the replication units reassembled, chromatin binds to the nascent DNA chain, assuring that each region is replicated only once. DNA polymerase is unable to replicate the end of a DNA chain completely. This problem has been solved by the addition of tandem repeats of a six-nucleotide sequence (GGGTTA) to the ends of each chromosome. These repeated sequences are called *telomeres* and are replicated through an RNA-dependent DNA polymerase called *telomerase*. Normal somatic cells do not express telomerase, presumably because they do not replicate or have a finite replication ability. Germ cells do express telomerase. The expression of telomerase in cancer cells is thought to be a component of the neoplastic process, assuring that the cell will be able to undergo many divisions without losing the information encoded near the ends of its chromosomes. Inhibition of telomerase activity in cancer cells could have antitumor effects.

The transitions between G1 and S and between G2 and M are tightly regulated to minimize errors in the replication process. Checkpoints in G1 and G2 that determine whether to enter S and M are regulated by protein kinases (cyclin-dependent kinases, or cdk) and kinase-associated proteins called *cyclins*. The enzymatic activity of the cdk is determined by their association with a cyclin and their phosphorylation state. There are at least seven cdk family members, each of which associates with a distinct cyclin molecule. The resulting complexes have characteristic substrate specificities, and are expressed in different phases of the cycle. Cyclin expression varies with the cell cycle, and the synthesis of these complexes is transcriptionally regulated and their degradation is mediated by ubiquitin-conjugation and destruction in proteasomes.

The cyclin B/cdc2 complex (also called *mitosis promoting factor*, or MPF) is the primary regulator of transition from G2 to M phase. It is activated by a cdk activating kinase (CAK) and a phosphatase (cdc25) that removes inhibitory phosphates. Some of the substrates of cyclinB/cdc2 are defined; its phosphorylation of histone H1, nuclear lamins, and microtubule-associated proteins facilitates chromosome condensation, nuclear membrane breakdown, and spindle formation, respectively.

The checkpoint regulating transition from G1 to S is frequently disrupted in cancer. The mechanism of the regulation is complex. Two cyclin/cdk complexes, cyclin D/cdk4 or -6 and cyclin E/cdk2, phosphorylate the retinoblastoma gene product, Rb, on 10 different sites and alter the ability of Rb to associate with cellular proteins. One such protein is E2F, a transcription factor that heterodimerizes with other transcription factors, such as DP1, and activates several genes required for S progression, including dihydrofolate reductase, thymidine kinase, DNA polymerase α, c-*myc*, c-*myb*, and cdc2 (Fig. 83-1). In addition to its role in promoting growth, Rb promotes differentiation through its association with transcription factors such as MyoD and activated transcription factor (ATF)/cyclic AMP response element binding (CREB) protein family members. Rb is the target of a number of transforming viruses including SV40 large T antigen, adenovirus E1A, and human papilloma virus E7.

The activity of cdk is also regulated by cdk inhibitors (cdki). These low-molecular-weight proteins either inhibit cdk activity broadly (p21$^{Cip1/Waf1}$, p27^{Kip1}, p57^{Kip2}) or selectively inhibit cyclin D/cdk4 or -6 complexes (p16^{INK4a}, p15^{INK4b}, p18). The first member of this family to be identified was p21, which inhibits both cdk and proliferating cell nuclear antigen (PCNA), a subunit of DNA polymerase δ. p21 is induced by DNA damage through transcriptional activation by p53 (see below) and inhibits cell cycle progression at several points, including G1 and S phases, and permits DNA repair to take place. If DNA damage is too great, a cell suicide pathway is induced to eliminate cells that may be dysfunctional (see below).

Cdki can be induced by growth inhibitors such as transforming growth factor (TGF) β and can be inhibited by positive growth factors such as interleukin (IL) 2. Genetic alterations in cdki, especially p16 and p15, occur with high frequency in certain tumors. Alterations at the p16 locus on chromosome 9p21 have been detected in 75 percent of pancreatic cancers; 40 to 70 percent of glioblastomas; 50 percent of esophageal cancers; and about 20 percent of non-small cell lung cancers, soft tissue sarcomas, and bladder cancers. Mutations in cdki often accompany cyclin D1 overexpression with the t(11;14) translocation in mantle cell lymphoma. Some tumors fail to express cdki because

FIGURE 83-1 The retinoblastoma gene product, pRb, regulates cell cycle progression at the restriction point by sequestering the E2F transcription factor. Hypophosphorylated pRb forms an inactive complex with E2F preventing its association with DP-1, or by repressing the interaction of E2F/DP-1 with the basal transcription machinery. The kinase activities of *cdk*4/cyclin D and *cdk*2/cyclin E convert pRb to the hyperphosphorylated state with loss of binding pocket activity. G1 cdk activity is positively regulated by growth factors and inhibited by a variety of physiologic signals from the cell microenvironment. E2F is released and forms transcriptionally active complexes with DP-1, which initiate transcription from promoters containing E2F binding sites. Many of these genes are necessary for S phase progression.

the genes are methylated, an epigenetic mechanism for blocking transcription. Table 83-1 summarizes some of the changes in cell cycle regulators detected in human cancers.

Whereas Rb, cyclin D, cdk4, and p16 are commonly altered in cancer, E2F overexpression or p21 mutations have not yet been seen. Additional study may reveal why some components of the system are susceptible to alterations and other components are not.

p53 is known as the "guardian of the genome" and the "guardian of the G1 checkpoint." It is not usually called upon to act in the course of normal replication. However, with DNA damage, p53 influences transcription to either halt cell cycle progression (e.g., through induction of p21 expression to inhibit cdk kinase activity) to permit repair of the DNA or, if the damage is too great, to initiate cell suicide (*apoptosis*). p53 is the target of many tumor-causing viruses: human

Table 83-1

Cell Cycle Regulators in Human Cancers

Gene	Functional or Genetic Change*	Tumors
Retinoblastoma	Deletion Point mutation	Retinoblastomas, osteosarcoma, soft tissue sarcoma, small cell lung carcinoma, bladder and breast carcinomas
Cyclin D	Chromosome translocation Gene amplification	Parathyroid adenomas, mantle cell lymphomas; breast, head and neck, esophageal, and hepatocellular carcinomas
cdk4	Amplification Point mutation	Glioblastoma, sarcoma; melanoma
p16^{INK4a} (p15^{INK4b})	Deletion Point mutations Methylation	Pancreatic, esophageal, non-small cell lung carcinomas; glioblastoma, sarcoma, familial melanoma, familial pancreatic cancer

* Each of these genetic lesions results in loss of physiologic regulation of the phosphorylation state of pRb late in G1 at a checkpoint called the restriction point. Aberrant regulation of the restriction point permits dysregulated entry into S phase, and is thought to occur as an early step in the genesis of most, if not all, tumors. By understanding the pathophysiology of these molecular defects, therapies can be devised that reestablish normal restriction point control.

papillomavirus E6 protein decreases p53 half-life, and adenovirus E1B proteins and SV40 large T antigen interfere with p53 function, for example. Mutations in p53 are the most common genetic alteration found in human cancer (>50 percent). Usually one p53 allele on chromosome 17p is deleted and the other is mutated. The mutations often involve the region between codons 120 and 290, the portion of the gene specifying the site of p53 involved in transcription. Some environmental agents cause mutations at specific sites. In 81 percent of hepatomas from developing countries, codon 249 is mutated due to exposure to the carcinogen, aflatoxin. Codon 249 mutations occur in only 11 percent of hepatomas from industrialized countries where aflatoxin exposure is low.

Regardless of the pathogenesis of the tumor, most have some mechanism(s) to bypass the G1 checkpoint, avoid activation of cell suicide pathways, and propagate cells with damaged DNA. An overview of cell cycle regulation is shown in Fig. 83-2.

SIGNALING FROM OUTSIDE THE CELL TO THE NUCLEUS

The behavior of every cell in the body is tightly regulated by environmental signals. The ability of a cell to respond to a specific set of signals determines whether the cell will live or die, differentiate, proliferate, or remain quiescent. In normal cells and tissues, coordinated action such as wound healing or the inflammatory response is regulated by signaling pathways that convert extracellular signals into the performance of specialized action in the responding cells. In cancer cells, the process of invading and metastasizing is influenced by signal transduction pathways activated by paracrine and autocrine factors.

The coupling of extracellular signals to cell response varies for different receptor and signaling systems, but the binding of a growth factor [e.g., epidermal growth factor (EGF)] to its receptor on the cell surface produces measurable changes in the cell within seconds and elicits a sequence of events that may last for days. Important mechanisms have evolved for preventing overstimulation of cells. The growth factors and local mediators are produced in minute quantities and usually act over short distances. When the growth factor or local mediator binds to its receptor, it is usually internalized rapidly and destroyed rather than released to stimulate other cells. In addition, receptor desensitization to the stimulus can occur by several mechanisms, including downregulation of receptors such that fewer receptors are on the cell and the likelihood of activation is reduced, and biochemical desensitization of the receptor through phosphorylations or methylations that alter the affinity for the ligand or prevent receptor coupling to downstream substrates.

Glucocorticoids, thyroid hormone, and retinoids all induce signals by binding to a family of cytoplasmic receptors (intracellular receptor or steroid hormone receptor superfamily; see Chap. 327) that, in the presence of ligand, move to the nucleus and bind to specific DNA sequence motifs, known as *response elements*, located within transcriptional promoter or enhancer regions. These response elements are located in proximity to the genes under the control of the hormones, usually upstream of the TATA box (a short thymidine- and adenine-rich double helical DNA sequence) that signals transcription initiation. For most other families of transcription factors, there are many interme-

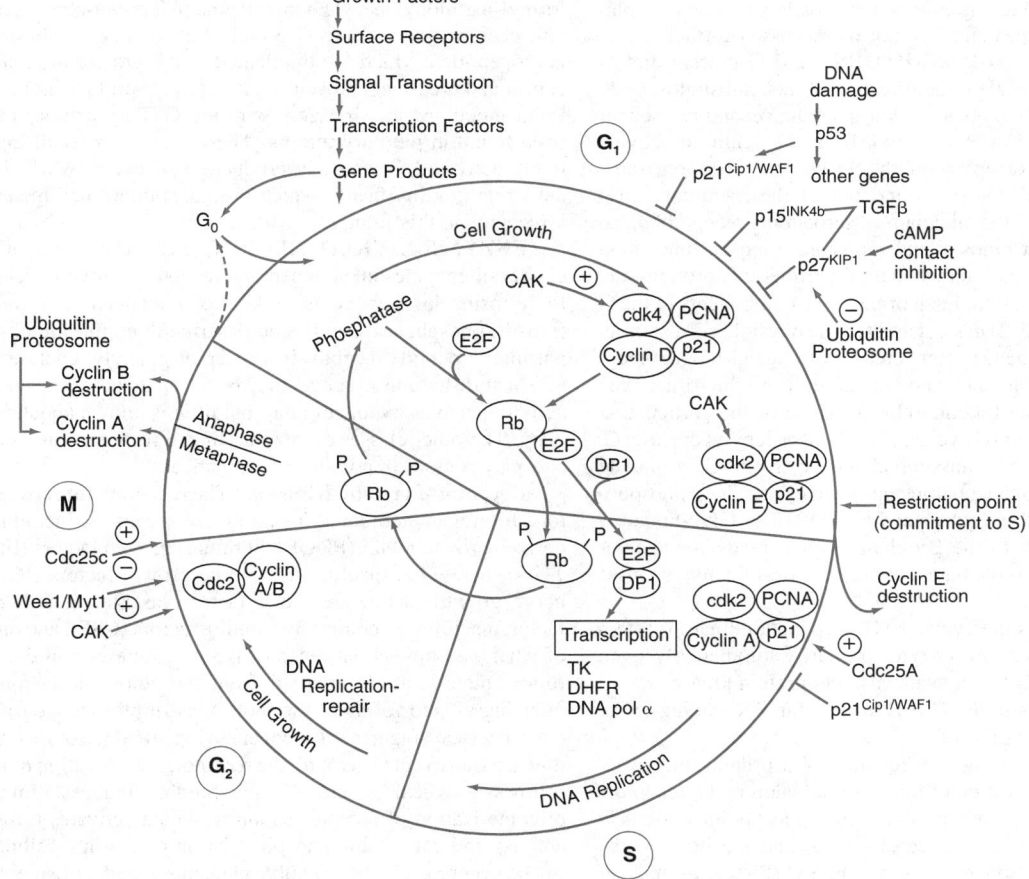

FIGURE 83-2 Integration of external stimuli with the mammalian cell cycle engine. Important checkpoint control mechanisms occur late in G1 near the restriction point and at the G2/M border. The phosphorylation of pRb by G1 cdk/cyclins releases E2F, which dimerizes with the transcription factor DP-1 and activates genes required for DNA synthesis. The cdk inhibitors p21, p15, and p27, induced in response to a variety of stimuli, block progression before the restriction point. External factors that positively or negatively influence the cycle are shown as impinging on the cycle. Cells in G1 may receive signals to halt proliferation and enter the G0 state, as occurs during differentiation, or continue cycling if growth factors and other stimulatory signals are present.

diate biochemical steps between the signaling molecule and the transcription factors it activates.

Derangements in steroid hormone receptors occur in some human cancers. For example, the t(15;17) translocation in acute promyelocytic leukemia generates a chimeric retinoic acid receptor α that has an abnormal cellular distribution and is associated with a differentiation arrest of tumor cells at the promyelocytic stage of development. However, administration of pharmacologic doses of tretinoin (all-*trans* retinoic acid), a ligand for retinoic acid receptor α, results in normal nuclear localization of the receptor and induces terminal differentiation of the tumor cells.

Some differentiated cells such as endothelial cells and macrophages respond to specific environmental signals by the production of nitric oxide (NO) gas through the enzymatic breakdown of arginine. NO serves as a signaling molecule; it diffuses into the cell and stimulates guanylyl cyclase to produce cyclic GMP, which can activate a class of ion channels important in membrane depolarization. NO mediates a variety of physiologic responses, including blood vessel relaxation, and may serve as a neurotransmitter in the central nervous system (see Chap. 71). NO may be responsible for some of the toxic effects associated with the use of biologic agents such as IL-2 and interferon γ.

Many signaling molecules are hydrophilic and act on specific cell surface membrane receptors to initiate a signal transduction cascade that leads to transcription factor activation. There are three families of cell surface receptors: ion channel–linked receptors, G protein–linked receptors, and enzyme-linked receptors. Although ion channel–linked receptors are a component of growth-related activation in many cell types, they are primarily involved in neurotransmitter signal transduction and are somewhat less important in the pathogenesis of neoplasia than the other two types and will not be discussed further.

G PROTEIN–LINKED RECEPTORS   The G protein–linked receptors do not induce covalent modification of their substrates, as do enzyme-linked receptors (see below), but generate second messenger molecules such as cyclic AMP, cyclic GMP, and calcium to activate downstream processes. Receptors of this class contain seven transmembrane segments that course in and out of the membrane in a serpentine fashion (thus, the nickname "serpentine receptors"), an extracellular domain that binds signal molecules, and an inner loop at the carboxyl terminal that interacts with the trimeric G proteins and regulates receptor sensitization. Each of the three components of the G protein complex (Table 83-2) has a characteristic physiologic response.

After association of the G protein complex to ligand-bound receptor, the Gα subunit binds to GTP and is released from the trimer. The GTP-α subunit mediates a function characteristic of the particular α subunit (G_s stimulates adenylyl cyclase; G_i inhibits adenylyl cyclase; G_s and G_o regulate calcium and potassium channels; G_q and G_{16} stimulate phospholipase Cβ; G_t couples photoreceptors to cyclic GMP phosphodiesterase) until the GTP is hydrolyzed to GDP. The GDP-bound α chain then reassociates with the βγ chains and is ready for another response. βγ Subunits also mediate a variety of physiologic responses (Table 83-2).

Cyclic AMP activates the cyclic AMP–dependent kinase (protein kinase A). The substrates of this enzyme primarily stimulate glycogen breakdown and inhibit glycogen synthesis, and protein kinase A activates transcription factors in the CREB protein family, leading to the transcription of a number of genes.

Perhaps the most important consequence of G protein–linked receptor activation is the elevation of intracellular calcium. G_q receptors activate phospholipase Cβ, which hydrolyses phosphoinositide 4,5-bisphosphate (PIP2) into diacylglycerol (DAG) and inositol triphosphate (IP3). DAG then activates protein kinase C (PKC), a family of serine threonine kinases that occur in a number of different forms with different substrates in different cell types. In many cells, PKC activates the MAP kinase cascade (see below) and phosphorylates IκB, an inhibitor molecule that keeps transcription factors of the *rel* family in the cytoplasm. A consequence of the activation of the MAP

kinase cascade is the generation of AP-1 transcription factor family members (usually heterodimeric proteins that include *fos* and *jun* family members). Phosphorylation of IκB leads to its release of *rel*/NFκB heterodimers and their translocation to the nucleus. The IP3 produced as a consequence of phospholipase C activity acts to release intracellular calcium stores, and the increase in intracellular calcium leads to the activation of a number of enzymes such as calcium/calmodulin-dependent protein kinases (CaM kinases).

The receptors for epinephrine, serotonin, chemotactic cytokines or chemokines (such as IL-8 and RANTES; see Chap. 305), and formyl-methionyl leucyl phenylalanine (f-met-leu-phe; a major neutrophil chemoattractant) are G protein linked. The bombesin family of neuropeptides, which are implicated in the growth of small cell lung cancer and breast and prostate cancers, use G protein–linked receptors. Point mutations that interfere with the GTPase activity of $G_s\alpha$ have been found in pituitary tumors. These mutations result in a constitutively activated G_s and overproduction of cyclic AMP. In addition, autocrine motility factor, which promotes tumor cell metastasis, uses a receptor in this family.

ENZYME-LINKED RECEPTORS   There are at least five classes of enzyme-linked receptors: receptor guanylyl cyclases, receptor tyrosine kinases, tyrosine kinase–associated receptors, receptor tyrosine phosphatases, and receptor serine/threonine kinases. The atrial natriuretic peptide receptor is a receptor guanylyl cyclase. Some disease manifestations in cancer may be related to atrial natriuretic peptide activity (such as hyponatremia), but little is known about this receptor class. The other classes of enzyme-linked receptors are better defined and play a more important role in cancer.

Receptor Tyrosine Kinases   The receptors for most growth factors are transmembrane tyrosine kinase receptors, including platelet-derived growth factor (PDGF), fibroblast growth factors (FGFs), EGF, TGFα, heregulin, insulin, insulin-like growth factors (IGF) I and II, nerve growth factor, stem cell factor, vascular endothelial growth factor, macrophage colony stimulating factors (CSF), and others. Much of what we know about receptor tyrosine kinases and the events that follow their ligation emerged from the study of the proliferation-inducing altered forms of the molecules (proto-oncogenes) that were the cancer-causing genes (oncogenes) in animal retroviruses. Although downstream events vary with the receptor, the activation of the receptor follows a typical pattern. Ligand binding induces dimerization or oligomerization of receptor subunits, which activates tyrosine kinase activity and causes autophosphorylation of the intracellular domains of the receptor chains. Finally, phosphorylated tyrosine residues on the receptors or on associated adaptor proteins form docking sights for other signal transduction molecules that contain one or more *src-homology region 2*, or SH2, domains, named because the sequence was first identified in the *src* nonreceptor tyrosine kinase. These associations via SH2 domains trigger subsequent events (Fig. 83-3).

Table 83-2

Heterotrimeric G Proteins

Subunits*	Effectors Regulated by α or βγ Subunits
Gα (16 genes, >20 proteins	
α_s (α_s, α_{olf})	Stimulates or inhibits adenylycyclase
(choleratoxin-sensitive)	Regulates calcium and potassium channels
α_i (α_i 1–3, α_o, α_t, α_{gust}, α_Z)	Activates cyclic AMP phosphodiesterase
(pertussis toxin–sensitive)	Activates PLCβ
α_q (α_q, α_{11}, α_{14}, α_{15}, α_{16})	Regulates sodium/potassium exchanger
α_{12} (α_{12}, α_{13})	
Gβ (5 isoforms)	Stimulates or inhibits adenylycyclase
Gγ (6 isoforms)	Activates potassium channels
	Stimulates PLCβ
	Activates βARK
	Activates *ras*-MAP kinase pathway

* Multiple Gα and Gβγ subunits mediate a variety of physiologic responses. Cells often express multiple types of G proteins, so integration of signaling information is a complex task. Both Gα and Gβγ subunits mediate these signaling events.

NOTE: PLCβ, phospholipase Cβ; βARK, β-adrenergic receptor kinase; MAP, mitogen-activated protein.

FIGURE 83-3 *A.* Structures of receptor tyrosine kinases activated by ligand-induced dimerization. Conserved extracellular domains, a single transmembrane spanning region, and a cytoplasmic domain encoding the tyrosine kinase characterize these receptors. The insulin and IGF-I receptors are disulfide-linked heterotetramers of α and β chains that undergo allosteric changes upon ligand binding. In the other cases shown, ligand binding induces homo- or heterodimerization within the subfamily followed by receptor autophosphorylation on tyrosine residues. Some kinase domains contain a kinase insert (KI). Flt-1 and Flk-1 are endothelial cell–specific receptors for vascular endothelial growth factor (VEGF) and are required for embryonic blood vessel differentiation and angiogenesis in the adult. Other members of the receptor tyrosine kinase family are not shown but share structural similarities. *B.* Multiple tyrosine autophosphorylation sites on activated PDGF receptor β chains serve as docking sites for signal transduction molecules. These include enzymes that activate downstream substrates and docking proteins to provide SH2 or P-Tyr binding sites for other proteins. These interactions lead to the formation of a signal transduction complex whose structure determines the nature of the signal transduction pathways activated by a particular ligand. SH2, SH3, pleckstrin homology (PH), proline-rich (Pro), phospholipase C (PLC), phosphoinositol 3′ kinase (PI3K), GTPase activating protein (GAP), and protein tyrosine phosphatase (PTPase) domains are shown.

The docking mechanisms of intracellular signaling molecules determine the specificity and kinetics of protein-protein interactions, and determine how a particular stimulus will lead to a characteristic response. The most common docking mechanisms are based on recog-

nition of particular protein sequences; the SH2 domains dock with phosphotyrosine-containing (P-Tyr) sequences, the SH3 domains dock with proline-rich sequences, and the pleckstrin homology domains (pleckstrin is a major PKC substrate in platelets) lead to associations by a mechanism not yet fully defined. Some molecules that do not have docking domains are brought into association with the receptors through the activity of adaptor proteins that are composed of docking domains only. Thus, the *ras* nucleotide exchange factor son of sevenless (SOS; named for its role in *Drosophila* eye development) is brought close to the membrane to activate *ras* through its association with the adaptor protein grb2 (identified because it "grabbed" phosphotyrosine-containing proteins).

Receptor tyrosine kinases in turn activate many signaling pathways including phospholipase C-γ, which stimulates calcium-dependent kinases and PKC; phosphoinositol 3′-kinase (PI3K), which activates protein kinase B and ribosomal S6 kinase (thus enhancing the efficiency of translation); and *src* family kinases, which leads to c-*myc* activation. Another consequence of receptor tyrosine kinase activation is stimulation of the *ras*/MAP kinase pathway that leads to activation of transcription factors in the *fos/jun*/AP-1 family. This pathway is frequently implicated in cancer cells.

ras is a 21-kDa member of a large family of proteins, including *rho*, *rac*, *rab*, and others, that regulate cytoskeletal changes, vesicular and nuclear transport, and proliferation and that share sequence homology with the Gα subunit of G protein–linked receptors. *ras* is attached to the inner cell membrane through an isoprenyl lipid group added by the enzyme farnesyl transferase. If the lipid group is not added, *ras* does not localize to the membrane and cannot function normally. In unstimulated cells, *ras* is bound to GDP and is inactive. Following activation of the receptor tyrosine kinase by its ligand, the guanine nucleotide exchange factor SOS is brought to the membrane by its association with grb2. SOS removes GDP from *ras* and adds GTP. GTP-bound *ras* then activates a cascade ending with MAP kinase, which migrates to the nucleus and phosphorylates (activates) a number of transcription factors (see Fig. 83-4).

About 30 percent of human cancers have mutated *ras*. The mutations usually involve codons 12, 13, or 61 and result in a *ras* that will not give up its GTP and is thus constitutively active. In the hereditary disorder, neurofibromatosis, a mutation in the gene that encodes neurofibromin, a GTPase activating protein (GAP), inhibits its ability to inactivate *ras* by converting the GTP to GDP. Some epithelial cancers overexpress one or more members of the receptor tyrosine kinase family. EGF receptors, IGF-I receptors, and HER-2/*neu* are overexpressed in lung, bladder, breast, head and neck, and ovarian cancers. Autocrine and paracrine sources of the relevant growth factors have been noted in some cases.

Tyrosine Kinase–Associated Receptors The receptors for growth hormone, prolactin, erythropoietin, IL-2, IL-3, IL-4, IL-6, IL-7, granulocyte CSF, granulocyte-macrophage CSF, interferon α, interferon γ, ciliary neurotrophic factor, and many other cytokines are members of the tyrosine kinase–associated receptor family. The receptors are often multisubunit receptors with each chain associating with a distinct set of signaling molecules via the docking mechanisms described above; however, the receptors themselves do not have tyrosine kinase activity. Three families of kinases are known to be associated with this class of receptors: *src* family (*src, yes, fgr, fyn, lck, lyn, hck, blk,* and counting), *syk* family (*syk,* ZAP-70), and Janus family (JAK1, JAK2, JAK3, Tyk2). The *src* family kinases can associate with receptor tyrosine kinases as well as tyrosine kinase–associated receptors, and, not surprisingly, signal transduction through either receptor class leads to the activation of similar signaling cascades. *myc* is one of the transcription factors activated as a consequence of *src* family activation. The *syk* family usually activates the *src* family member in the receptor complex. The Janus family leads to the phosphorylation and activation of a family of transcription factors called STATs (signal transduction and activation of transcription).

These receptors are often overexpressed on tumors of hematopoietic origin, and, similar to receptor tyrosine kinases, autocrine or paracrine stimulation may contribute to the neoplastic state of the tumor cell.

Serine/Threonine Kinase Receptors These receptors recognize TGFβ, bone morphogenetic factors, and other activins as ligands. Ligand binding leads to activation of the receptor kinase activity, but downstream events are not well defined. Bone morphogenetic factors are important in bone formation and in determining ventral vs. dorsal orientation in the developing embryo. TGFβ induces fibroblast proliferation but inhibits the proliferation of most cell types, probably through the induction of cdki. Loss of expression or loss of function of TGFβ receptors occurs in several tumor types including colon cancer and lymphomas.

Tyrosine Phosphatase Receptors The prototypical tyrosine phosphatase receptor is CD45; its ligand is unknown. CD45 plays a crucial role in T cell activation through its removal of phosphate from a negative regulatory site on the *src* family kinase, *lck*. This activates *lck* and permits signal transduction through the T cell antigen receptor. A role for CD45 in neoplasia has not been defined.

In addition to these known classes of receptors for soluble mediators and growth factors, some receptors bind and are triggered by components of the extracellular matrix (particular protein constituents or glycosaminoglycans) or by cell-cell adhesion. Integrins are the principal receptors involved in such interactions, and they influence the cytoskeleton of the cell through activation of kinases, such as focal adhesion kinase, and induce remodeling of actin filaments modulated through the *ras* family proteins, *rho* and *rac*. The intracellular pathway activated by these interactions is not well characterized.

CYTOSKELETON AND CELL ADHESION

The cytoskeleton, which controls the spatial organization of cells, is made up of three major types of fibers: microtubules, actin filaments, and intermediate filaments. Microtubules are polymers of tubulin that originate in the centrosome and terminate variably in the cytoplasm. Motor proteins use microtubules as "railways" to position organelles properly and transport some proteins to the nucleus. Actin filaments control the shape and movement of the cell; through directional polymerization and depolymerization, cell surface protrusions direct cell migration. Actin bundles are the main components of adhesion belts (special areas of interaction between adjacent cells, called *adherens junctions*) and focal contacts (adherens junctions with matrix rather than other cells). Intermediate filaments in different cells contain different proteins: epithelial cells use keratin, fibroblasts use vimentin, muscle cells use desmin, and so on. Intermediate filaments give the cell tensile strength and are components of the cell junctions that interface with neighboring cells (*desmosomes*) and with basal laminae (*hemidesmosomes*).

Cells of a particular tissue type maintain cell-cell contact through a calcium-dependent process involving cadherins that mediate interactions between the actin and intermediate filaments of the cells they join. Cells involved in host defense often maintain cell-cell contact between different cell types using one of a family of calcium-dependent carbohydrate-binding proteins called *selectins*. In some cell types, calcium-independent cell-cell interactions are mediated by intercellular adhesion molecules (ICAMs), members of the immunoglobulin supergene family.

In cancer, these highly organized mechanisms of intercellular interaction often become disrupted or are subsumed for the purpose of metastasizing (see Chap. 85). Individual cells no longer respond to signals from their neighbors, actin filaments are highly disorganized, and adherens junctions are lost. Although much less is known about how the cytoskeleton is disrupted than about the alterations in signal transduction, at least one example of a gene involved in cell adhesion is known to be involved in the etiology of a cancer. The adenomatous polyposis coli (APC) gene on chromosome 5 is defective in familial polyposis and is involved in the development of colon cancer. The *wnt* protein is a matrix-bound ligand that leads to the phosphorylation of the APC gene product. Phosphorylated APC binds to β-catenin and keeps levels of the protein low. The defective gene product cannot bind to β-catenin, and the free β-catenin disrupts adherens junctions and causes other cytoskeletal changes. Disruption of cell-cell communication is one of the many components of a multistep process leading to neoplastic transformation.

Drugs that attack the cytoskeleton, particularly tubulin (such as the vinca alkaloids and taxanes; see Chap. 86), are effective in a wide range of cancers.

REGULATION OF CELL DEATH

The homeostasis of adult organisms requires a balance between the generation of new cells and the death of old cells. Some cells die when their telomeres no longer protect the integrity of DNA replication. Some cells die when they have sustained sufficient hypoxic, heat, oxidative, or ultraviolet irradiation damage that cannot be repaired. A cell can be killed if it becomes infected with a virus or

FIGURE 83-4 The MAP kinase cascades. MAP kinase signal transduction cascades link *ras* activation with the nucleus. The overall framework of the MAP kinase cascades is shown in the box at the left. A series of sequential serine/threonine kinase events results in the activation of MAP kinase which has cytoplasmic and nuclear targets. The nuclear targets of MAP kinase are transcription factors bound to their DNA recognition sites that require phosphorylation to induce transactivating functions. ERKs (extracellular signal response kinases) target the ternary complex factor (TCF), while JNK/SAPK targets c-*jun* and ATF-2. Transcription factors associated with other promoters also serve as targets for MAP kinases. Other MAP kinase cascades exist in the cell. Each pathway is activated by different stimuli and the pattern of gene expression induced by each pathway is characteristic of that pathway. Interactions between pathways permit an integrated response to diverse signals.

other intracellular pathogen that destroys the cell or is recognized by the host's lymphocytes, which kill the infected cell. Multicellular organisms are a model of cellular cooperation; some cells die to preserve the rest of the organism.

Apoptosis is a form of cell death initiated by extracellular or intracellular signals in which enzymes are activated to degrade nuclear DNA by making intranucleosomal cuts, causing the cell to shrink and finally break up. Extracellular signals through the tumor necrosis factor (TNF) receptor or a related receptor (called *fas*) or intracellular signals related to p53 detection of irreparable DNA damage lead to the activation of a series of cellular proteases in the IL-1-converting enzyme (ICE) family (IL-1 must be processed by this enzyme to be released from cells). Activated ICE family proteases cleave specific proteins at asparagine residues and activate the cell death pathway. In the immune system, this process is activated to delete autoreactive lymphocytes.

The *bcl2* family of genes was originally noted when *bcl2* was cloned from the chromosome 18q contribution to the t(14;18) translocation in follicular lymphoma. The gene did not transform cells but prolonged the life of cells destined to die in the lymphoid follicle. Members of the *bcl2* family fall into two groups: *bcl2* and *bcl*-X_L prevent cell death, whereas *bax*, *bad*, *bak*, and others promote cell death. *bcl2* family members associate as homodimers or heterodimers; the combinatorial effects of the various dimers allow a fine level of control over cell survival. When any of the death promoters exist as homo- or heterodimers, the cell dies by apoptosis. When a death promoter heterodimerizes with either *bcl2* or *bcl*-X_L, cell death is prevented. Thus, the relative amounts of different *bcl2* family members determine whether a cell will survive potentially damaging insults. Furthermore, phosphorylation of *bcl2* family members by cellular kinases can alter the biologic activity of individual members, altering the balance in favor of death or survival.

In addition to its presumed role in the etiology of follicular lymphoma, *bcl2* is expressed in a number of cancers. It prevents the normal p53-mediated destruction of cells with damaged DNA and also appears to prevent the death of cells severely damaged by cancer chemotherapy. *bcl2* mediates drug resistance and contributes to neoplasia in a novel way, preventing the death that would normally eliminate the damaged cell, rather than promoting aberrant cell growth. Strategies to overcome *bcl2* function might well make available therapies more effective.

REGULATION OF GENE TRANSCRIPTION

Factors that regulate gene transcription recognize short stretches of double-helical DNA of a defined nucleotide sequence 6 to 12 bases in length. These recognition sites may be upstream or downstream of the transcription start site [the TATA box where the first subunit of the transcription machinery, transcription factor IID (TFIID) binds]. Transcription factors may affect transcription at sites remote from the start site by looping out large intervening DNA sequences.

Transcription factors contain specific amino acid sequences capable of recognizing the DNA sequence and usually form one of several structural motifs: helix-turn-helix, homeodomain, zinc finger, leucine zipper, and helix-loop-helix are all used as DNA-binding motifs or mediate dimerization of factors required for DNA binding. Transcription factors function in one or more of several ways. They can physically bend the DNA to permit the ordered addition of the components of the transcription machinery. They can facilitate the addition of those components. They can inhibit transcription by blocking binding of a positive transcription factor or preventing the assembly of a transcription complex. The complex interaction between positive and negative transcription factors dictates the level of gene transcription. Individual genes may have 20 or more sites for transcription factor binding.

Some growth factors and combinations of growth factors mediate different effects on different cell types. The receptors may be connected to a different combination of signaling pathways. Different combinations of transcription factors may be activated. Distinct patterns of chromatin condensation may make different regions of the genome available or unavailable for transcription. Some genes may be turned off in particular cell types by methylation of cytosine residues in critical cytosine- and guanosine-rich regions of the gene that prevent transcription. Most genes are regulated at multiple levels, though transcription initiation is the dominant control point. The von Hippel–Lindau gene on chromosome 3p (a tumor suppressor gene involved in the pathogenesis of renal cell cancer) appears to act by inhibiting the elongation of an RNA chain after transcription initiation. A message may be spliced alternatively and encode different proteins in different cells. Transport of the message from the nucleus to the cytoplasm may be altered. Messenger RNA turnover may be accelerated. Some proteins, such as apoferritin and thymidylate synthase, regulate the translation of their own messages (and perhaps other messages) by binding to mRNA and preventing initiation of protein synthesis. Thus, there are many levels at which gene expression may be influenced.

Some transcription factors were identified because of their transforming effects when their genes, usually in mutated form, were incorporated into animal retroviral genomes. *myc*, *rel*, *fos*, *jun*, and others are examples of proto-oncogene transcription factors that are overexpressed in certain cancers and that contribute to the malignant phenotype of tumor cells.

CELL BIOLOGY AND CANCER

For a cancer to arise, mutations must occur that affect a variety of pathways. Often the G1 cell cycle checkpoint is affected. The expression of telomerase is a common feature in cancers. Overexpression of growth factors and their receptors is frequently detected. Activation of the *ras* proto-oncogene or other changes leading to a constitutively active MAP kinase cascade are common. Changes in cytoskeleton and responsiveness to contact-mediated growth inhibition are frequent in cancer cells. Failure to induce expression of gene products required for apoptosis may be a component of the pathophysiology. Usually when a mutation occurs in one component of a signaling pathway, other mutations are seen in other pathways rather than in another component of the same pathway. The high level of mutability of cancer cells facilitates adaptation to the environment, including the development of resistance to anticancer drugs. As tumors progress, they acquire the ability to secrete proteases that aid in the escape from local barriers so that they may metastasize (see Chap. 85). Discrete steps in tumor progression lead to the production of factors by the tumor cells that permit neovascularization to supply nutrients to the growing tumor. Other mutations allow the tumor to escape immune surveillance mechanisms; for example, some tumors downregulate expression of class I major histocompatibility complex antigens so that they become invisible to T cells. The wide range of changes that must occur in a single cell to permit the behavior associated with a malignant neoplasm makes it clear why carcinogenesis is a multistep process and why human cancers may have 10 or more genetic lesions that account for the biology.

The characteristic of cancer cells that has dominated clinical thinking is their uncontrolled proliferation. However, the growth fraction of most human cancers is usually not higher than the growth fraction of normal gut epithelia or normal bone marrow, and most human tumor explants are difficult to propagate for long periods of time in culture. Cancer cell lines immortal in vitro may have additional genetic lesions that permit their growth in vitro. Naturally occurring tumors growing in vivo show a Gompertzian or exponential decline in their growth fraction because the daughter cells of a division are not uniformly capable of further division. The accumulation of genetic damage, poor oxygen or nutrient supply, and other unknown factors contribute to the senescence of some tumor cells, so that by the time a tumor becomes clinically apparent at a tumor burden of 10^8 to 10^9 cells, most of the proliferative capability of the tumor is finished. Often by this time, more malignant and highly selected clonal derivatives of the tumor have metastasized to other sites where new tumor deposits with more aggressive characteristics are formed. Thus, cancer cells can be viewed as having lost the altruism that usually characterizes cell behavior in multicellular organisms. Cancer cells operate under natural selection imposed by a hostile environment. Ironically, the more successful they are at achieving independence from environmental influences, the more assured is the destruction of their host and ultimately themselves.

Many potential therapeutic agents are in clinical development based on our concepts of tumor cell biology. They include the development of growth factor and growth factor receptor antagonists; inhibitors of phosphoryl transfer to block key kinases; selective inhibitors of PKC, phosphoinositol 3′ kinase, phospholipase C, and other targets; farnesyl transferase inhibitors that block the insertion of *ras* into the membrane; mutant versions of proteins such as *ras* and p53 that may make the cell vulnerable to immunologic attack if employed as a vaccine; inhibitors of angiogenesis or the steps in metastasis that may limit tumor growth and prevent its spread. However, it seems unlikely that a single target will be the highly sought after point of vulnerability. More likely, combinations of inhibitors will be required to improve antitumor effects. For example, the combination of chemotherapy and antibody to EGF receptors appears to produce greater antitumor effects than the sum of the effects produced individually.

BIBLIOGRAPHY

ALBERTS B et al: *Molecular Biology of the Cell*, 3d ed. New York, Garland, 1994
AMATI B, LAND H: Myc-Max, Mad: A transcription factor network controlling cell cycle progression, differentiation and death. Curr Opin Genet Dev 4:102, 1994
BERRIDGE MJ: Calcium signalling and cell proliferation. Bioessays 17:491, 1995
CANO E, MAHADEVAN LC: Parallel signal processing among mammalian MAP kinases. Trends Biochem Sci 20:117, 1995
COX LS, LANE DP: Tumor suppressors, kinases and clamps: How p53 regulates the cell cycle in response to DNA damage. Bioessays 17:501, 1995
HELDIN C-H: Dimerization of cell surface receptors in signal transduction. Cell 80:213, 1995
HILL CS, TREISMAN R: Transcriptional regulation by extracellular signals: Mechanisms and specificity. Cell 80:199, 1995
IHLE JN: Cytokine receptor signalling. Nature 377:591, 1995
WEINBERG RA: The retinoblastoma protein and cell cycle control. Cell 81:323, 1995

| 84 | *Francis S. Collins, Jeffrey M. Trent* |

CANCER GENETICS

THE CLONAL NATURE OF CANCER A critical feature of nearly all cancers is that they originate from a single cell. While multiple cumulative events are invariably required to move a cell from normal to the transformed phenotype (see below and Chap. 83), the origin of tumors from a single clone of cells is a critical discriminating feature between neoplasia and hyperplasia.

CANCER IS A GENETIC DISEASE Cancer arises because of alterations in DNA that result in unrestrained cellular proliferation. Most of these alterations involve actual sequence changes in the DNA (i.e., mutation). They may arise as a consequence of random replication errors, exposure to carcinogens (e.g., radiation), or faulty DNA repair processes.

While virtually all cancer is genetic, most cancer is not inherited. Certain individuals with cancer have inherited a germline mutation that predisposed them to the cancer, but even in that situation additional somatic mutations are required for a tumor to develop. In a truly sporadic cancer, *all* of the mutations responsible for the malignant

phenotype arise somatically. Such a cancer is caused by genetic alterations but has no hereditary implications.

RNA AND DNA TUMOR VIRUSES Many malignancies in animals are transmissible, and the etiologic agent is frequently a retrovirus, which possesses a single-stranded RNA genome. During the life cycle of the virus, the single-stranded RNA is converted to double-stranded DNA and is inserted at random into the host chromosome. On rare occasions, the virus can be remobilized, carrying along with it an adjacent segment of host DNA. Should this host DNA contain a growth-promoting gene, then the retrovirus is potentially transforming. Although efforts to identify retroviruses in human malignancies have mostly been fruitless, retroviruses are implicated in at least one human malignancy. Human T cell lymphotropic virus (HTLV) type I causes adult T cell lymphoma/leukemia, particularly in Japan and the Caribbean (see Chap. 192). Unlike animal retroviruses that induce neoplasia, HTLV-I does not contain a growth-promoting transforming oncogene. The tax protein, a 40-kDa molecule encoded in the pX region of the viral genome, induces the activation of a number of genes (including some promoting growth) through interactions with *rel* family and CREB (cyclic AMP response element binding protein) family transcription factors.

DNA tumor viruses are more commonly involved in human malignancy. Human papilloma viruses (especially types 16 and 18) cause cervical cancer (see Chap. 190), and both hepatitis B and hepatitis C viruses have been implicated in hepatocellular carcinoma (see Chap. 297). In addition, the Epstein-Barr virus, a herpesvirus that causes a mild illness in children but infectious mononucleosis in nonimmune adolescents and adults, causes Burkitt's lymphoma in Africa, nasopharyngeal carcinoma in the Orient, and lymphomas in the setting of immune deficiency (see Chap. 186).

GENERAL CLASSES OF CANCER GENES In 1914, Boveri hypothesized that cells become malignant either because of overactivation of a gene that promotes cell division or because of loss of function of a gene that normally restrains growth. This hypothesis is largely correct, although defects in DNA repair genes are also involved. Genes that promote normal cell growth are referred to as *proto-oncogenes*, and activation of such genes by point mutation, amplification, or dysregulation converts them to *oncogenes*.

Genes that normally restrain growth are called *tumor suppressors* (use of the alternative designation of anti-oncogenes is to be discouraged), and unregulated cell growth arises if their function is lost. The diploid nature of mammalian cells allows certain predictions about the consequences of somatic mutations of tumor suppressor genes. Loss of one allele is unlikely to have significant consequences in most instances, as the remaining normal allele is usually sufficient for normal function. Thus, most cells of an individual with an inherited loss of function of one tumor suppressor allele are functionally normal. Only the rare cell that loses or develops a mutation in the remaining normal copy will exhibit uncontrolled growth. This model correctly predicts that the inheritance pattern of cancer in a family with a tumor suppressor gene mutation will be expressed as an autosomal dominant trait, though the cellular mechanism is recessive.

The third category of genes that contribute to malignancy consists of the DNA repair genes. Every cell division involves the copying of 6 billion base pairs (bp) of DNA. DNA polymerase has a finite error rate, and many environmental influences can damage DNA; as a consequence, repair systems are essential to protect the integrity of the genome. When the repair systems themselves are faulty, either on the basis of inherited or acquired mutation, the rate of accumulation of mutations throughout the genome rises as cell divisions occur. To the extent that these mutations involve oncogenes and tumor suppressor genes, the likelihood of developing malignancy increases.

MENDELIAN CANCER SYNDROMES Roughly 100 syndromes of familial cancer have been reported, though many are rare. The majority are inherited as autosomal dominant traits, although some of those associated with DNA repair abnormalities (xeroderma pigmentosum, Fanconi anemia, ataxia telangiectasia) are autosomal recessives. Most of the genes responsible for the dominantly inherited cancer syndromes are tumor suppressor genes (Table 84-1). The hall-

Table 84-1

Selected Tumor Suppressor Genes Responsible for Familial Cancer Syndromes

Syndrome	Gene	Chromosome Location	Tumors
Basal cell nevus	*PTC*	9q22.3	Basal cell cancer, jaw cysts, medulloblastoma
Familial breast/ovarian cancer	*BRCA1*	17q21	Breast, ovarian, colon, prostate cancer
Familial breast cancer	*BRCA2*	13q12-13	Breast cancer, male breast cancer
Familial melanoma	p16	9p21	Melanoma, pancreatic cancer
Familial polyposis coli	*APC*	5q21	Intestinal polyposis, colorectal cancer
Familial retinoblastoma	*RB*	13q24	Retinoblastoma, osteosarcoma
Familial Wilms' tumor	*WT1*	11p13	Wilms' tumor, WAGR*
Hereditary multiple exostoses	*EXT1*	11p11-13	Exostoses, chondrosarcoma
Li-Fraumeni	p53	17q13	Sarcomas, breast cancer
Neurofibromatosis type 1	*NF1*	17q11.2	Neurofibroma, neurofibrosarcoma, brain tumor
Neurofibromatosis type 2	*NF2*	22q12	Acoustic neuroma, meningioma
Tuberous sclerosis	*TSC2*	16p13.3	Angiofibroma, renal angiomyolipoma
Von Hippel–Lindau	*VHL*	3p25-26	Renal cell cancer, pheochromocytoma, retinal angioma, hemangioblastoma

* WAGR, Wilms' tumor, aniridia, genitourinary abnormalities, and mental retardation.

marks of a tumor suppressor gene are as follows: (1) the germline mutation that affects one allele generally causes a loss of function, (2) tumors also show loss of the second normal allele as a result of a somatic mutation, and (3) often the *normal* function of the gene is to suppress unrestrained cellular growth or to promote differentiation.

The retinoblastoma (*RB*) gene is a paradigm of such a tumor suppressor gene. In a pedigree showing dominant inheritance of susceptibility to retinoblastoma, there is a loss-of-function germline mutation of one allele of the *RB* gene on chromosome 13. Analysis of the DNA from the tumors invariably shows that the wild-type allele has also been lost, by one of several possible mechanisms (Fig. 84-1). However, not all retinoblastoma tumors arise in the context of a strong family history. Sporadic retinoblastoma, which is usually unilateral and on average occurs at a slightly older age than familial retinoblastoma, is usually a consequence of somatic mutation in both alleles of the *RB* gene without any germline predisposition at all.

Another tumor suppressor gene is the p53 gene on chromosome 17p, which is frequently altered in solid tumors. p53 is somewhat unusual for a tumor suppressor gene in that missense mutations that produce a dominant negative protein product may also be growth promoting, so that not all alterations obliterate function. Given the role of p53 in a variety of tumors (mutations in p53 are found in nearly half of human tumors), it is not surprising that germline mutations in p53 have dramatic consequences, resulting in a phenotype known as the *Li-Fraumeni syndrome*, where affected individuals may develop a variety of sarcomas, brain tumors, and leukemia. Figure 84-2 illustrates a typical pedigree of this devastating disorder.

In many instances, the discovery of genes responsible for familial cancer syndromes has provided insight into the normal control of cell growth. For instance, in type I neurofibromatosis—one of the more common dominant disorders of humans—positional cloning efforts uncovered a previously unknown gene on chromosome 17q that, when mutated, produces a clinical phenotype of café au lait spots, neurofibromas, Lisch nodules of the iris, and a predisposition to neurofibrosarcoma and glioma. The responsible gene, which (like many of the genes in Table 84-1) has a close homo-

logue in yeast, is neurofibromin (*NF1*), a critical participant in the regulation of the proto-oncogene *ras*. As shown in Fig. 84-3, the NF1 protein is a GTPase-activating protein (GAP) that normally acts to convert *ras* from its active, growth-promoting, GTP-bound form to its inactive, GDP-bound form. Loss of both copies of *NF1* (one copy by inheritance, one by somatic mutation) thus renders a cell vulnerable to overgrowth, since *ras* is left in the "on" position.

While most autosomal dominant inherited cancer syndromes are due to mutations in tumor suppressor genes, there are a few interesting exceptions. Multiple endocrine neoplasia type II, a dominant disorder characterized by pituitary adenomas, medullary carcinoma of the thyroid, and (in some pedigrees) pheochromocytoma, is due to gain-of-function mutations in the proto-oncogene *ret* on chromosome 10. Interestingly, loss-of-function mutations in *ret* cause a totally different phenotype, namely Hirschsprung's disease (aganglionic megacolon) (see Chaps. 340 and 288).

Dominantly inherited colon cancer is sometimes associated with familial polyposis, which is usually due to mutations in the adenoma-

FIGURE 84-1 Diagram of possible mechanisms for tumor formation in an individual with familial retinoblastoma. On the left is shown the pedigree of an affected individual who has inherited the abnormal (RB) allele from her affected mother. The four chromosomes of her two parents are drawn to indicate their origin. Just below the retinoblastoma locus a polymorphic marker is also analyzed in this family. The patient is AB at this locus, like her mother, whereas her father is AA. Thus the B allele must be on the chromosome carrying the retinoblastoma disease gene. Tumor formation results when the normal allele (N), which this patient inherited from her father, is inactivated. On the right are shown four possible ways in which this could occur. In each case, the resulting chromosome 13 arrangement is shown, as well as the results of a Southern blot comparing normal tissue with tumor tissue. Note that in the first three situations the normal allele (A) has been lost in the tumor tissue, which is referred to as loss of heterozygosity. (*From TD Gelehrter and FS Collins, in Principles of Medical Genetics, Baltimore, Williams & Wilkins, 1990, with permission.*)

FIGURE 84-2 Pedigree of a family with the Li-Fraumeni syndrome. The affected individuals have developed sarcomas, brain tumors, leukemia, and breast cancer at an early age. All of the affected individuals were found to have a germline mutation in codon 252 of the p53 gene. *(After D Malkin, et al, Science 250:1233, 1990, with permission.)*

FIGURE 84-3 The *ras* pathway. The active form of the *ras* protein binds GTP and promotes cell division. The conversion to the inactive form, which binds GDP, is catalyzed by a number of proteins including the protein product of the neurofibromatosis type I (*NF1*) gene. Thus, loss of function of NF1 has the effect of leaving *ras* in the "on" position. Alternatively, mutations in the *ras* protein that block its inactivation also predispose to cancer.

tous polyposis coli (*APC*) tumor suppressor gene on chromosome 5 (Table 84-1). However, in most colon cancer families, affected individuals do not have familial polyposis, but instead the cancer arises from normal-appearing epithelium. Hereditary nonpolyposis colon cancer (HNPCC, or Lynch's syndrome) is commonly defined as the occurrence of colon cancer in at least three individuals over at least two generations and with at least one individual diagnosed under the age of 50. As many as 1 in 200 individuals in the general population may have HNPCC, although this number is somewhat controversial. Most HNPCC is due to mutations in one of four DNA mismatch repair genes (Table 84-2). All four of these genes are components of a repair system that is normally responsible for correcting errors in freshly copied DNA. Tumors in patients with HNPCC are characterized by profound genomic instability, especially for short repeated sequences called *microsatellites*. Figure 84-4 shows an example of the instability in allele sizes for dinucleotide repeats in the cancers in HNPCC. The unstable phenotype [sometimes referred to as the "mutator" phenotype, or the "RER$^+$" (replication error) phenotype] probably requires loss of both copies of the particular mismatch repair gene (one inherited, one somatic), so that the mechanism is similar to that typical of a tumor suppressor gene.

MORE COMPLEX INHERITED FORMS OF CANCER While the Mendelian forms of cancer described above have taught us much about mechanisms of cellular growth control, most forms of cancer do not follow such simple patterns of inheritance. In many instances (e.g., lung cancer), a strong environmental contribution is at work, but even in such circumstances some individuals may be genetically more susceptible to developing cancer given the appropriate exposure.

In the case of breast and ovarian cancer, circumstantial evidence indicates that a subset of affected individuals (perhaps 5 to 10 percent) might be accounted for by dominantly inherited high-penetrance susceptibility genes, and two of these genes have been identified by positional cloning. *BRCA1*, located on chromosome 17, is capable

Table 84-2

Genetic Alterations in Kindreds With Hereditary Nonpolyposis Colon Cancer (HNPCC)

Gene	Percent of Cases
MSH2	31
MLH1	33
PMS1	2
PMS2	4

SOURCE: Liu B et al, Nature Med 2:169, 1996

when mutated of producing a high risk (perhaps as high as 85 percent lifelong) of breast cancer and also of ovarian cancer (perhaps 50 percent lifelong risk). Roughly 1 in 500 women carries a germline *BRCA1* mutation, often giving rise to a strong family history. Men with *BRCA1* mutations may have a modestly increased risk of prostate cancer. There is an array of mutational heterogeneity described for *BRCA1* (Fig. 84-5), as is often the case for genetic disorders. An

FIGURE 84-4 Demonstration of microsatellite instability in normal and tumor tissue from HNPCC (hereditary nonpolyposis colon cancer) patients. In each case the lane marked T contains DNA from a tumor, and the lane marked N contains DNA from normal tissue of the same patient. The marker (*D2S123*, located on chromosome 2) is a microsatellite composed of a tandem repeat of the dinucleotide CA, which varies in length from chromosome to chromosome. Normally, however, the length of the repeat is stable in somatic tissues. In this example, a polymerase chain reaction analysis has been applied to genomic DNA, and new alleles for the marker are apparent in tumors 1, 2, 5, and 7. Because the tumor tissue is defective in DNA mismatch repair, clonal abnormalities in copying of the CA repeat have arisen. Errors are also occurring in functional genes, eventually resulting in the malignant phenotype. *(From LA Aaltonen et al, Clues to the pathogenesis of familial colorectal cancer. Science 260:812, 1993, with permission.)*

exception is the Ashkenazi Jewish population, where 1 in 100 individuals carries a particular 2-bp deletion (denoted 185delAG) of *BRCA1*, apparently as a consequence of descent from a common ancestor.

Mutations in another gene on chromosome 13, *BRCA2*, also confer a high risk of breast cancer (and a somewhat lower risk of ovarian cancer), and men with *BRCA2* mutations are also prone to develop breast cancer. The frequency of *BRCA2* mutations is estimated to be about half that of *BRCA1*. About 1 percent of Ashkenazi Jews again have a common mutation: 6174delT.

What then of the 90 to 95 percent of breast cancers that arise in individuals without germline alterations in *BRCA1* or *BRCA2*? Hereditary factors may still contribute to a significant fraction of these, but those factors must be weaker and therefore more difficult to discern. One such factor may be the heterozygous state for mutations in the ataxia telangiectasia gene at 11q22. Such individuals have as much as a four- to fivefold increased risk of breast cancer and are likely to represent about 1 percent of the population.

GENETIC TESTING AND COUNSELING FOR CANCER SUSCEPTIBILITY

The discovery of genes like *RB*, p53, *NF1*, *ret*, the HNPCC mismatch repair genes, *BRCA1*, and *BRCA2* raises the possibility of DNA analysis to predict risk of cancer. There are many complexities associated with such testing. First, one must know the sensitivity and specificity of the test; the mutational heterogeneity for each of these genes constitutes a considerable technical challenge, as it is often necessary to sample every nucleotide of the coding region, the splice junctions, and the promoter to identify most mutations. False-positive results, i.e., sequence alterations that turn out to be benign polymorphic variants (allelic variations) rather than disease-causing mutations, can present a thorny problem. Unless proven interventions are available and the test is sensitive, specific, and relatively inexpensive, it will be inappropriate to offer such tests to the general population, as the number of false-positive tests will exceed the number of true positives and a great deal of anxiety and expense will be incurred evaluating persons who are not at an increased risk. Generally, therefore, such testing is not considered except for individuals of higher-than-normal risk, usually on the basis of their family history. In deciding whether to offer such testing, it is critical to determine whether evidence exists for effective interventions to reduce the risk of cancer in those found to be at high risk. If such interventions do not exist (as is the case for Li-Fraumeni syndrome), then the value of the information is limited, and the major negative psychological consequences of this information must be seriously considered. For conditions such as colon and breast cancer, prophylactic measures exist (total colectomy and bilateral mastectomy, respectively), but these prophylactic measures are more radical and potentially disfiguring than the surgical procedures that would be used to treat the patient if the malignancies actually occurred (segmental bowel resection and lumpectomy, respectively). Other potential negative consequences of a positive genetic test include insurance and employment discrimination. One can still argue, of course, that a close relative of an individual known to carry a mutation in a cancer-causing gene is already sensitized to their personal risk of cancer, and that a test that establishes that an individual at risk does *not* harbor the mutation can be quite useful. Testing should never be undertaken, however, without a full consideration of how the individual will handle a positive as well as a negative result.

Despite these caveats, there are some cancer syndromes for which genetic testing already appears to have greater benefits than risks, and in those situations it is reasonable to offer testing to individuals at high risk. This would include conditions such as multiple endocrine neoplasia type 2 (see Chap. 340) and von Hippel–Lindau disease (see Chap. 375). More in the gray zone, although potentially applicable to much larger numbers of individuals, are tests for *BRCA1*, *BRCA2*, and the HNPCC genes. More research is urgently needed in those situations to determine the effectiveness of various interventions (lifestyle, diet, surveillance, or surgery). Until those answers are available, such testing should be offered only as part of a research protocol. As more susceptibility genes are identified, better answers become available about the effectiveness of interventions, and health insurance discrimination is legislatively prohibited, genetic testing will move into the mainstream of medicine. Every physician of the future will need to have the skills of a genetic counselor.

ACQUIRED MUTATIONS IN CANCER

The identification of mutations in the germline of patients with heritable cancers means that the alteration is present in every cell of the body. However, in most cancers, a normal cell becomes a malignant cell by a series of mutations that do not arise in the germline but in somatic cells. Usually mutations must occur in several genes to give rise to neoplasia. The underlying questions are "how many mutations cause a cancer?" and "what specific genes are affected?" rather than whether or not mutational events cause cancer.

While answers to these questions are not available for every human malignancy, advances in molecular and cellular biology and epidemiologic analyses of human and experimental cancers are providing insights in cancer causation. Table 84-3 summarizes evidence from several lines of investigation pointing to a mutational basis for cancer causation. One particularly striking feature is the fact that the overall incidence of cancer increases as the fourth to sixth power of age for most malignancies (Fig. 84-6A). For some tumors, the shape of the age-incidence curve suggests heterogeneity in molecular mechanisms. For example, Hodgkin's disease has a bimodal age distribution, sug-

FIGURE 84-5 Germline mutations that have been reported in the *BRCA1* gene, primarily found in families with a high incidence of breast cancer, ovarian cancer, or both. The numbers refer to the exons of the gene; there is no exon 4. *(Information is provided courtesy of the Breast Cancer Information Core data base, which is accessible on the World Wide Web at http://www.nchgr.nih.gov/dir/lab_transfer/bic/.)*

Table 84-3

Evidence That Mutations Cause Cancer

Malignant tumors are clonal in nature
Some cancers show a Mendelian pattern of inheritance
DNA from malignant cells can in some instances transform normal cells to
  a malignant phenotype
Most tumors contain somatic mutations in oncogenes and/or tumor
  suppressor genes
Recurring sites of chromosome change are observed in cancers at the sites
  of genes involved in cellular growth control
Most carcinogens are mutagens
Defects in DNA repair systems increase the probability of cancer

A

B

FIGURE 84-6 Relationship between age and cancer incidence. *A*. Age-specific incidence of skin, colon, and pancreas cancers in Canadian males. The curves appear as straight lines when plotted using logarithmic axes, fitting the multihit model of cancer (see text). *B*. For some tumor types (e.g., Hodgkin's disease), a bimodal age distribution is seen, perhaps indicative of a differing mutational basis (see text). (*From Tannock and Hall, with permission.*)

gesting that two etiologically (and therefore mutationally) distinct forms of this disease may exist (Fig. 84-6*B*).

MULTISTEP BASIS OF CANCER   From 5 to 10 accumulated mutations are thought to be necessary for a cell to move from the normal to the fully malignant phenotype. At each step, the mutated cell may gain a slight growth advantage, so that it is increased in its representation relative to its neighbors. Figure 84-7, a representation of a lineage diagram hypothesized by Peter Nowell, illustrates how a single cell, afflicted with progressive alterations in tumor suppressor genes and proto-oncogenes, can develop into a clonal malignancy.

We are beginning to understand the precise nature of the genetic alterations responsible for some malignancies and to get a sense of the order in which they occur. Perhaps the best studied example is colon cancer, where an analysis of DNA from tissues extending from normal epithelium through adenoma to carcinoma have identified some of the genes mutated along the way (Fig. 84-8). However, the order of mutational events is far from uniform, and the diagram in Fig. 84-8 should be considered a generalization and not a rigorous depiction. Similar data are being accumulated for other malignancies.

MECHANISMS OF SOMATIC MUTATION OF ONCO-GENES IN MALIGNANCY   Cellular proto-oncogenes, their necessity and importance in normal cell growth, and their responsibility for transformation-associated change after removal of normal growth controls are discussed in Chap. 83. Mechanisms that upregulate (or activate) cellular proto-oncogenes can be grouped into three broad areas: point mutations, DNA amplification, and chromosome rearrangements.

Point Mutation   A proto-oncogene that is commonly activated in solid tumors by point mutation is a member of the *ras* family of oncogenes; these were initially cloned from human bladder carcinoma cells and are critical regulators of normal and aberrant cell growth (Fig. 84-3). Mutations in one of the *ras* genes (H-*ras*, K-*ras*, or N-*ras*) are present in up to 15 percent of all human cancers. In studies of K-*ras* (particularly in lung and colon cancer), the mutational spectrum of this gene has been identified. Remarkably, and in contrast to the diversity of mutations observed in the *BRCA1* gene (Fig. 84-5), most of these activated genes contain point mutations in codons 12 or 61 (which convey resistance to the inactivating action of GAP). The specificity of this pattern of mutation means that it has potential value in diagnostic or prognostic studies of cancer. For K-*ras*, mutations may be a useful prognostic marker in lung cancer, but for most other cancers (including pancreas and colon cancer) no prognostic utility has been demonstrated. This is in part because *ras* mutations occur early in colon cancer (Fig. 84-8), being common in precancerous lesions of the bowel.

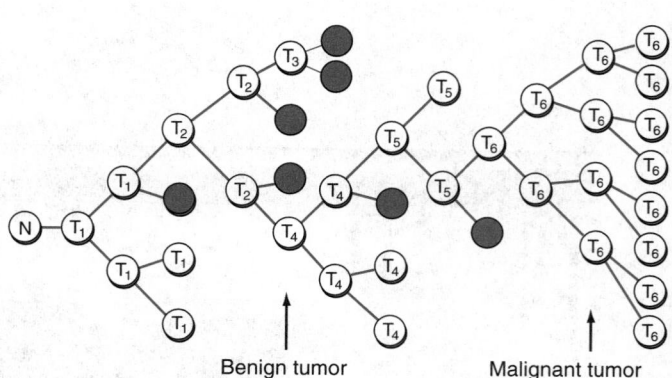

FIGURE 84-7 Multistep clonal development of malignancy. In this diagram, a series of five cumulative mutations (T1, T2, T4, T5, T6), each with a modest growth advantage acting alone, eventually results in a malignant tumor. Note that not all such alterations result in progression; for example, the T3 clone is a dead end. The actual number of cumulative mutations necessary to transform from the normal to the malignant state is unknown in most tumors. (*After P Nowell, Science 194:23, 1976, with permission.*)

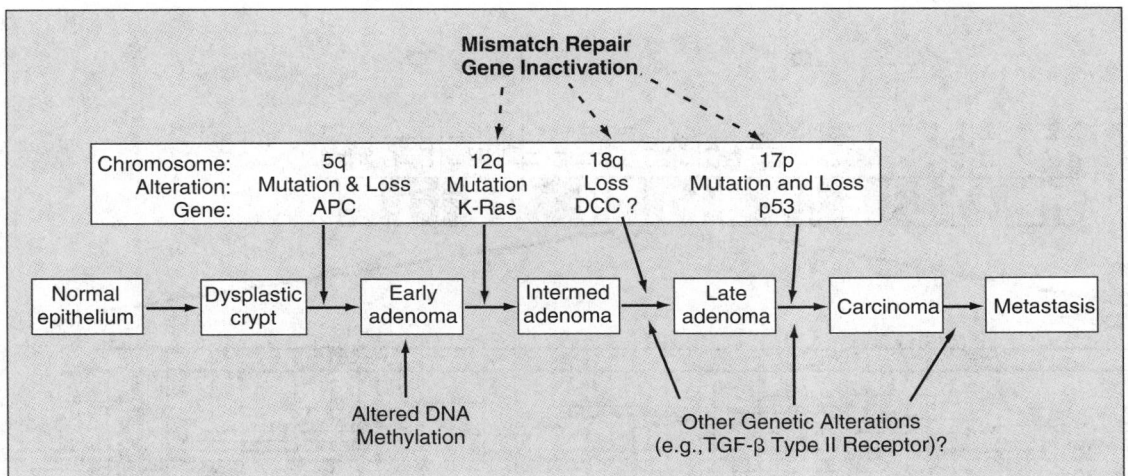

FIGURE 84-8 Progressive somatic mutational steps in the development of colon carcinoma. The accumulation of alterations in a number of different genes results in the progression from normal epithelium through early adenoma to full blown carcinoma. While the steps shown here do not always occur in this order, it is clear that an accumulation of somatic mutations is required before cancer develops. Patients with familial polyposis are already one step into this pathway, since they inherit a germline alteration of the *APC* gene.

DNA Amplification The second mechanism for activation of oncogene overexpression is DNA sequence amplification. This increase in DNA sequence copy number may cause cytologically recognizable chromosome alterations referred to as *homogeneous staining regions* (HSRs), if integrated within chromosomes, or *double minutes* (dmins), if extrachromosomal in nature (Fig. 84-9).

The recognition of DNA amplification was greatly facilitated by the development of a procedure based upon dual-color fluorescence in situ hybridization (FISH) called *comparative genomic hybridization* (CGH). DNA from tumor and normal cells is labeled with different fluorescent reporter molecules and then hybridized to normal metaphase chromosomes. Regions of duplications and deletions within tumor DNA are then demonstrated as quantifiable alterations in signal intensity at particular sites. With this technique, the entire genome can be surveyed for gains and losses of DNA sequences, thus pinpointing chromosomal regions likely to contain genes important in the development or progression of cancer.

Numerous genes are known to be amplified in human malignancies. Several genes including N-*myc* were identified because they were present within the amplified DNA sequences of a tumor and had homology to known oncogenes. Because the region amplified often extends to hundreds of thousands of base pairs, more than one oncogene may be amplified in some cancers (particularly sarcomas). Figure 84-10 illustrates the complex pattern of amplification observed in human sarcomas for a gene-dense region on human chromosome 12; genes simultaneously amplified in many cases include *MDM2*, *GLI*, *CDK4*, *SAS*, and others implicated in cellular growth control. The clinical implications of gene amplification have been explored for some cancers (most notably *ERBB2* in breast cancer and N-*myc* in neuroblastoma), and demonstration of amplification of a cellular gene is usually a predictor of poor prognosis. Once a patient has been exposed to the selective effects of chemotherapy, gene amplification may lead to drug resistance. Amplification of the dihydrofolate reductase gene may follow clinical exposure to methotrexate, a drug that inhibits the activity of the enzyme.

Chromosomal Alterations in Human Cancer Chromosomal alterations provide important clues as to the genetic changes in cancers. To date, most chromosome analyses have been performed on hematopoietic cancers, although solid tumors may also have translocations. The breakpoints of several recurring chromosome abnormalities often occur at the sites of cellular proto-oncogenes. Translocations are particularly common in lymphoid tumors, probably because these cell types normally rearrange DNA to generate antigen receptors. Indeed, antigen receptor genes are commonly involved in the translocations, implying that an imperfect regulation of receptor gene rearrangement may be involved in the pathogenesis. An example is Burkitt's lymphoma,

a B cell tumor characterized by a reciprocal translocation between chromosomes 8 and 14. Molecular analysis of Burkitt's lymphomas demonstrated that the breakpoints occurred within or near the *myc* locus on chromosome 8 and within the immunoglobulin heavy chain locus on chromosome 14, resulting in the transcriptional activation of

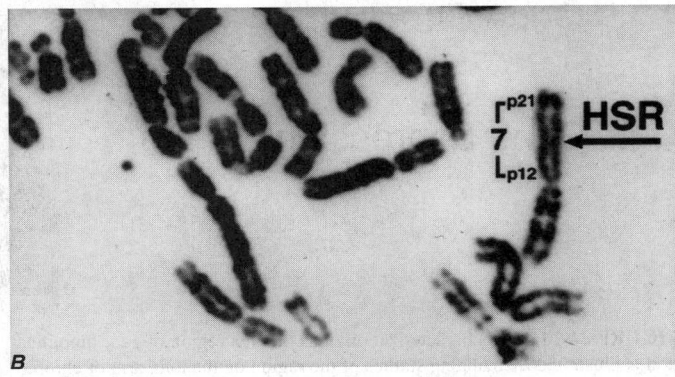

FIGURE 84-9 Representative examples of tumor cells containing cytogenetic evidence of gene amplification. *A*. Example of multiple copies of double minute (dmin) chromosomes from a patient with ovarian carcinoma. *B*. Example of a homogeneous staining region (HSR) on chromosome 7 from a patient with malignant melanoma.

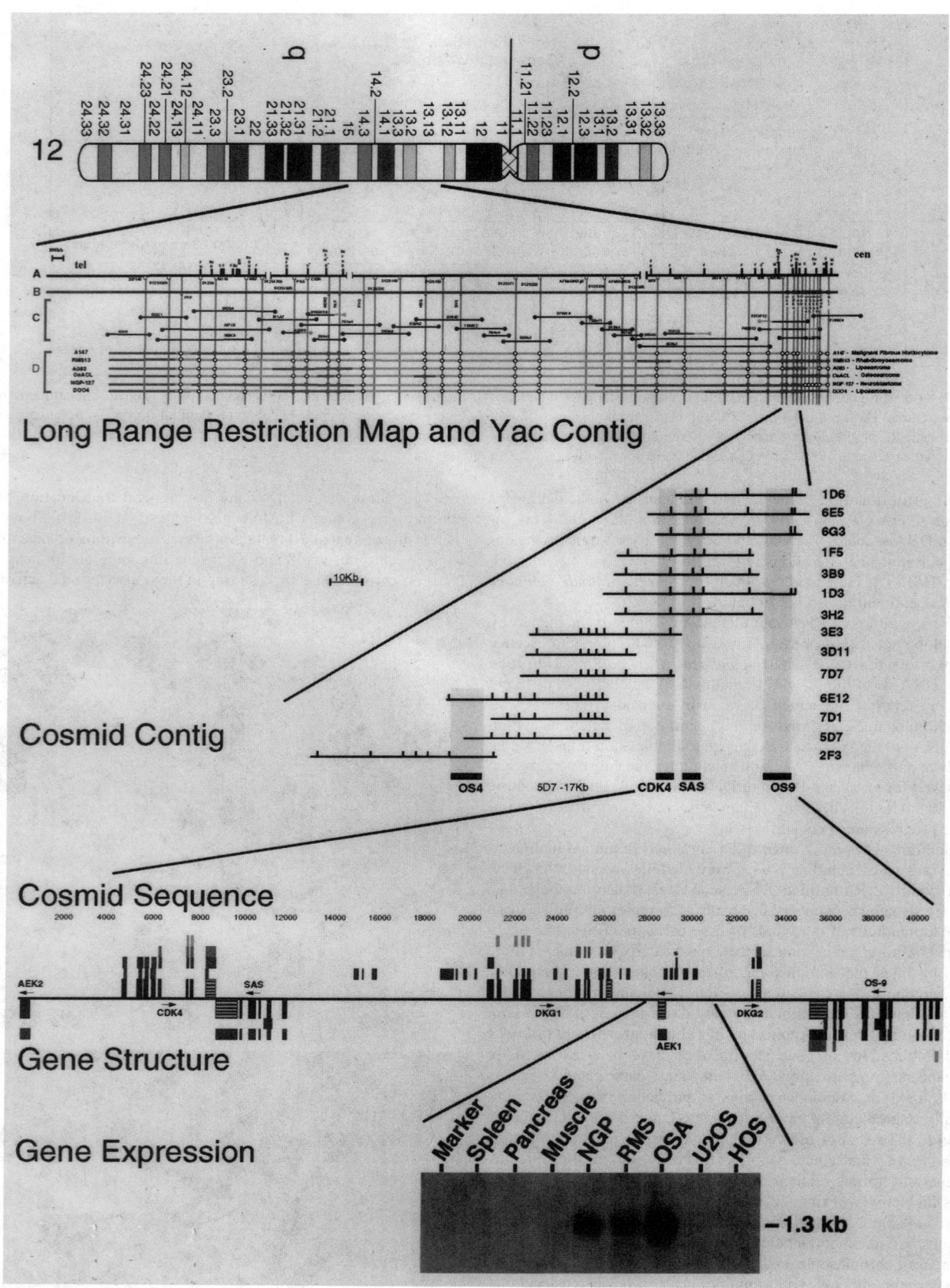

FIGURE 84-10 The characterization of a complex region of gene amplification is illustrated by mapping studies of the region on the long arm of chromosome 12 encoding the p53 regulator *MDM2* and the cyclin-dependent kinase *CDK4*. This region is frequently amplified in a subset of brain tumors and sarcomas. As shown at the top of the illustration, the amplicon is initially mapped at the relatively coarse level of the metaphase chromosome. Techniques of physical mapping are then used to define the segment(s) of the chromosome that contribute to the amplicon in various tumors. This defines the core region(s), which presumably contain the target gene(s). Higher resolution mapping and DNA sequencing are then applied to the core in order to localize genes within cosmids and their DNA sequence. Ultimately, the expression level of the genes identified in the amplification core is determined. *(Courtesy of AG Elkahloun and P Meltzer, NCHGR, NIH).*

Chromosome Translocation ⟶ **Chimeric Gene** ⟶ **Chimeric Protein**

Ph¹

BCR   ABL

Chr. 22q   Chr. 9q

BCR   ABL

9   22   9q+   22q-
t(9;22)(q34;q11)

Reciprocal translocation   Fusion of BCR and ABL   Chimeric BCR-ABL protein
generates Ph¹ chromosome   gene sequences

FIGURE 84-11 Specific translocation seen in chronic myelogenous leukemia (CML). The Philadelphia chromosome (Ph) is derived from a reciprocal translocation between chromosomes 9 and 22 with the breakpoint joining the sequences of the *ABL* oncogene with the *BCR* gene. The fusion of these DNA sequences allows the generation of an entirely novel fusion protein with modified function (see text). *(Courtesy of ER Fearon and KR Cho.)*

myc. Enhancer activation by translocation, although not universal, appears to play an important role in malignant progression.

Chromosome rearrangements can lead to the abnormal overexpression of a transcription factor that performs its normal function and turns on growth-related genes. The translocation may create a chimeric transcription factor that has altered function. For example, the t(15;17) of acute promyelocytic leukemia produces a retinoic acid receptor with an abnormal cell distribution that inhibits differentiation. Gene rearrangements most commonly involve transcription factors, but other components of signaling pathways may also be involved.

The first reproducible chromosome abnormality detected in human malignancy was the Philadelphia chromosome in chronic myelogenous leukemia (CML). This cytogenetic abnormality is generated by reciprocal translocation involving the *ABL* oncogene, a tyrosine kinase on chromosome 9 being placed in proximity to the *BCR* (breakpoint cluster region) on chromosome 22. Figure 84-11 illustrates the generation of the translocation and its protein product. The consequence of expression of the *BCR-ABL* gene product is the activation of signal transduction pathways, leading to cell growth independent of normal external growth factor signals.

In addition to transcription factors and signal transduction molecules, translocations may involve the overexpression of cell cycle regulatory proteins, such as cyclins, and of proteins that regulate cell death, such as bcl2. Table 84-4 lists representative examples of recurring chromosome alterations in malignancy and the associated gene(s) rearranged or dysregulated by the chromosomal change.

Technical obstacles have slowed the identification of recurring chromosome abnormalities in human solid tumors (particularly carcinomas) because of the complexity of chromosome alterations in such tumors, in contrast to the solitary, often reciprocal, nature of chromosome rearrangements in hematopoietic malignancies.

EPIGENETIC REGULATION OF GENE EXPRESSION AND CANCER The term *epigenetic* refers to mechanisms of gene regulation independent of DNA sequence. The inactivation of the second X chromosome in female cells is an example of an epigenetic mechanism that prevents gene expression from the inactivated chromosome. During embryologic development, entire regions of chromosomes from one parent are silenced and gene expression proceeds from the chromosome of the other parent. For most genes, expression occurs from both parental alleles or randomly from one parent or the other. The preferential expression of a particular gene exclusively from the allele contributed by one parent is called *parental imprinting* and is thought to be regulated by the methylation of the silenced allele.

The role of epigenetic control mechanisms in the development of human cancer is unclear. However, a general decrease in the level of DNA methylation has been noted as a common change in cancers. In addition, the loss of imprinting of the normally silent maternal allele

Table 84-4

Representative Oncogenes at Chromosomal Translocations

Gene (Chromosome)	Translocation	Malignancy
ABL (9q34.1) *BCR* (22q11)	(9;22)(q34;q11)	Chronic myelogenous leukemia
AML1 (21q22) *EAP* (3q26) *EVI1* (3q26)	(3;21)(q26;q22)	Acute myelogenous leukemia, myelodysplasia
ATF1 (12q13) *EWS* (22q12)	(12;22)(q13;q12)	Malignant melanoma of soft parts (MMSP)
BCL1 (11q13.3) *IgH* (14q32)	(11;14)(q13;q32)	Mantle cell lymphoma
BCL2 (18q21.3) *IgH* (14q32)	(14;18)(q32;q21)	Follicular lymphoma
BCL3 (19q13.1) *IgH* (14q32)	(14;19)(q32;q13)	B cell chronic lymphocytic leukemia
ERG (21q22.3) *EWS* (22q12)	(22;21)(q12;q22)	Ewing's sarcoma
FLI1 (11q24) *EWS* (22q12)	(11;22)(q24;q12)	Ewing's sarcoma
LCK (1p34) *TCRB* (7q35)	(1;7)(p34;q35)	T cell acute lymphocytic leukemia (ALL)
MLL/ALL1/HRX (11q23)	(4;11)(q21;q23)	ALL
myc (8q24)	(8;14)(q24;q32)	Burkitt's lymphoma, B cell ALL
TAN1 (9q34) deletion	(7;9)(q34;q34)	T cell ALL
WT1 (11p13) *EWS* (22q12)	(11;22)(p13;q12)	Desmoplastic small round cell tumor (DSRCT)
TLS/FUS (16p11) *CHOP* (12q13)	(12;16)(q13;p11)	Myxoid liposarcoma
PAX3 (2q35) *FKHR/ALV*(13q14)	(2;13)(q35;q14)	Alveolar rhabdomyosarcoma
PAX7 (1p36) *KHR/ALV*(13q14)	(1;13)(p36;q14)	Alveolar rhabdomyosarcoma
ret (10q11.2)	(10;17)(q11.2;q23)	Papillary thyroid carcinomas

SOURCE: After Hesketh.

519

of the insulin-like growth factor II gene at chromosome 11p15.5 has been implicated in some cases of the rare pediatric malignancy, Wilms' tumor. The loss of imprinting may result in the overexpression of the growth factor and a predisposition to malignant transformation.

THE FUTURE The real challenge in oncology is to convert the growing molecular understanding of cancer into clinical advances, particularly the development of new therapies. One can anticipate in the coming years that the molecular analysis of mutations in tumors will allow stratification of malignancies into more precise subgroups than is currently possible by histologic classification, including subgroups with particularly good or bad prognoses or that have a lower or higher likelihood of responding to a particular therapy. Some of this information is already accumulating, but usually only one or two genes are assessed; the promise of the future is to obtain a detailed molecular "fingerprint" of every tumor in order to provide the maximum information about its biology and response to therapy.

Genetics will also influence cancer prevention and early detection. The ability to identify cancer susceptibility genes presages a new era of cancer prevention, if the potential risks of such testing can be surmounted. Currently, most cancer early detection strategies (such as mammography, stool occult blood testing, or digital rectal examination) are applied to population groups. The ability to identify the individuals at highest risk and to focus preventive medicine efforts accordingly may be both better received by patients and more cost effective. Early detection strategies will be even more effective if we can develop the ability to identify very small numbers of malignant or premalignant cells at a time when the risk of metastasis is still very low.

More importantly, detailed molecular information about the regulation of the cell cycle and the interplay of tumor suppressor genes and proto-oncogenes that control it may lead to new effective therapies, based on pathophysiology rather than empiricism. Whether such strategies will rely on drugs of the traditional types or will be based on more novel strategies such as gene therapy or immunotherapy is hard to predict.

BIBLIOGRAPHY

COLLINS FS: BRCA1—lots of mutations, lots of dilemmas. N Engl J Med 334:186, 1996

ELKAHLOUN AG et al: Molecular cytogenetic characterization and physical mapping of 12q13-15 amplification in human cancers. Genes Chromosomes Cancer 17:205, 1996

FEARON ER, CHO KR: The molecular biology of cancer, in *Principles and Practice of Medical Genetics*, AE Emery, DL Rimoin (eds). New York, Churchill Livingstone, 1996, chap 20.

HEIM S, MITELMAN F: *Cancer Cytogenetics*, 2d ed. New York, Wiley, 1995

HESKETH R: *The Oncogene Facts Book*. San Diego, Academic Press, 1995

PARK M: Oncogenes: Genetic abnormalities of cell growth, in *The Metabolic and Molecular Bases of Inherited Disease*, 7th ed, CR Scriver et al (eds). New York, McGraw-Hill, 1995, chap 10

TANNOCK I, HALL R: *The Basic Science of Oncology*, 2d ed. New York, McGraw-Hill, 1992

VOGELSTEIN B, KINZLER KW: The multistep nature of cancer. Trends Genet 9:138, 1993

85

Elise C. Kohn, Lance A. Liotta

INVASION AND METASTASIS

Unregulated cellular proliferation may produce a neoplastic growth, but the defining features of malignancy are invasion and metastasis. A malignant neoplasm is a new growth with the potential to invade locally and/or to metastasize to distant sites in the body. Malignant neoplasms are the second most common cause of death in the industrialized world, leading to more than 500,000 deaths in the United States

yearly, with metastatic dissemination primarily responsible for most treatment failures and deaths. Metastasis is present in an occult or overt form in more than two-thirds of patients at the time of initial diagnosis and is often multifocal, making localized surgery, radiation, or chemotherapy ineffective.

Invasion is necessary for metastasis. The critical pathologic turning point for the patient is the initiation of local invasion and neovascularization leading to the dissemination of tumor cells. Tumor-induced angiogenesis provides a vascular entry portal that may precede primary tumor outgrowth by many years (Fig. 85-1A). Circulation of tumor cells is necessary but not sufficient, as circulating tumor cells may be detected in patients who never develop metastases. This clinical observation is supported by experimental studies indicating that metastasis initiation from circulating tumor cells is a low probability event, with fewer than 0.05 percent of circulating tumor cells successfully developing metastatic foci. Metastasis, like tumorigenesis, occurs only after a sufficient number of tumor cells with the requisite genotypic and phenotypic changes enter the circulation.

Invasion is the active translocation of neoplastic cells across tissue barriers and through host cellular and extracellular matrix barriers. It is not simply due to growth pressure but requires additional genetic and signaling dysregulation over that which caused malignant transformation. Invasion results from an imbalance and dysregulation of otherwise normal stimulatory and inhibitory events. Tightly controlled invasion occurs in many normal physiologic events, such as organ maintenance or remodeling, pregnancy and development, and wound healing. In cancer, this regulation is absent or attenuated so that malignant cells may not respond to signals originating from their environment and may rely on their own autocrine stimulation. In addition to invasion, metastasis requires angiogenesis and malignant cell proliferation. Successful metastasis requires that cells reach the secondary location, that they form colonies successfully at the secondary site, and that they avoid local and systemic host defenses. Thus, the process of invasion is a relatively individual process whereby the cell must be able to execute each of the required steps.

Historically, the changes occurring in the organization and integrity of the epithelial basement membrane have been considered by pathologists as the histologic markers of the transition from carcinoma in situ to invasive cancer (Fig. 85-1B). An early step that can be detected by simple histopathology is the interruption of basement membrane barriers in epithelial tumors. The basement membrane is a dense, acellular structure onto which epithelial or endothelial cells attach. It provides an infrastructure to support organ architecture or the vascular network. It is composed of a variety of glycoproteins and carbohydrates organized into a formidable barrier. The degradation of local basement membrane and surrounding interstitial stroma is necessary for invasion but is not sufficient for distant dissemination of malignant cells. The human breast provides an example of the progressive change from benign to malignant and invasive. Benign proliferative disorders of the human breast such as fibroadenoma, intraductal hyperplasia, and fibrocystic disease are all characterized by a continuous basement membrane separating the breast epithelium from its stroma. In contrast, multiple defects are found in the basement membrane of infiltrating malignancy. Defects in the basement membrane may also be observed adjacent or proximal to malignant cells in lymph nodes or at the site of parenchymal organ metastases.

Invasion and neovascularization may be very early events in cancer, frequently occurring even years before clinical detection. Invasion is required for advancement from in situ disease, and new blood vessel formation for adequate nutritional support for the growing tumors and as conduits for escape. Figure 85-1 shows a hypothetical time scale for the development of breast cancer. Note that invasion and angiogenesis occur several years before diagnosis, and that occult or overt metastases are present at the time of diagnosis. This is consistent with the data that in situ carcinoma of the breast is very infrequent.

Carcinomas can spread by both lymphatic and hematogenous routes, and metastases are found most commonly in organs fed by the downstream lymphatic and blood flow (Table 85-1). Sarcomas disseminate predominantly by vascular spread. In some cases, unusual

FIGURE 85-1 Cancer progression. *A.* Time course of cancer development and dissemination. This hypothetical time course shows the early initiation of angiogenesis and invasion in tumor progression. Diagnosis and treatment of cancer usually occur late in the disease course, when a high proportion of patients already have established occult or overt metastases. In contrast, progression through dysplasia to carcinoma in situ and the acquisition of the invasive and angiogenic phenotype may extend back over a period of years. This may define a window for therapeutic intervention before onset of metastasis. *B.* Progression to metastasis and associated genetic changes. Phenotypic progression from normal to hyperplastic, through carcinoma in situ to the initiation

of invasion and angiogenesis, leads to metastatic dissemination. Through new techniques in molecular diagnostics, gene loss through mutation and deletion and increased expression through amplification can now be more readily defined. The processes of invasion, angiogenesis, and metastasis are associated with both metastasis-suppressor genes, such as *nm*23 and E-cadherin, and metastasis-promoting genes, such as matrix metalloproteinases and autotaxin. Chromosomal mapping and microdissection of tumor cells with their adjacent normal cells will allow for a more detailed analysis of the genetic changes involved in metastasis and lead to new targets for diagnostics and therapeutics.

sites of metastases have been documented and may be explained by a permissive environment.

ANGIOGENESIS Angiogenesis is the process of blood vessel formation. Under normal conditions in the adult, neovascularization is limited to menstruation, pregnancy, and wound healing. During angiogenesis, normally quiescent endothelial cells acquire an invasive phenotype, breaching their own basement membrane to invade into interstitial stroma during the development of new capillary buds. These cells return to a quiescent and noninvasive phenotype when the angiogenic stimulus ceases. These angiogenic stimuli may include tumor-derived growth factors, extracellular matrix components, and endothelial cell–derived factors. The development of new vessels has been found to be a critical component of tumor development, benign and malignant; it is required for nutrient delivery and is necessary for metastatic dissemination. Subpopulations of highly metastatic tumor cells may exist at a very early stage in the development of primary tumors. It has been calculated that metastases from breast carcinomas,

for example, may be initiated as early as the point at which the primary tumor becomes vascularized, at a size of less than 0.125 cm². Tumor dormancy, a phenomenon where late or delayed tumor dissemination is observed, may arise as a consequence of inadequate vascular supply.

The clinical importance of vascular development has been demonstrated in several ways. Assessment of tumor vessel number is correlated positively with risk and degree of dissemination in breast cancer (both lymph node–positive and –negative disease), prostate cancer, and ovarian cancer. In addition, several endothelial cell–derived cytokines that stimulate endothelial cell proliferation and migration have also been found to stimulate proliferation of malignant cells and in some cases to be secreted by malignant cells as autocrine and paracrine factors.

Normally endothelial cells are quiescent; however, they can show a 100-fold increase in proliferation during neovascularization. Several antiangiogenic agents have been identified where the primary or secondary targets are the endothelial cells or the process of neovascularization.

Table 85-1

Patterns of Metastasis: Most Common Sites of Spread

	Metastatic Site (% Involvement)							
Primary	Adrenal	Brain	Bone	Skin	Kidney	Lung	Liver	Nodes Local/Distant
Breast	31	23	62	20	17	66	40–60	60–80
Bladder	35	7	26	5	19			
Cervix	31	9	21	3	26			
Colorectum	31	11	27	5	13	16	44	53
Kidney	20	19	10	5	21	72	44	
Lung	35	37	56		16	8	73	83/29
Melanoma	48	48	48	44	27	60	63	58
Ovary	20	3	12	5	6	34	48	48/58
Prostate	17	2	67	3	11	49	36	68

SOURCE: Adapted from Weiss, L: Clin Exp Metastasis 10:191–199, 1992, references inclusive.

INVASION Cellular adhesion, local proteolysis, and locomotion constitute the triad of invasion. While each is necessary for successful metastasis, none is sufficient individually. The cells at the invasive front undergo a dynamic cycling through the steps of invasion, in which they reach out and attach anew to the basement membrane or interstitial stroma. By secretion of proteinases or induction of proteinase secretion by stromal cells, tumor cells create local access through which to migrate into the vasculature or secondary organ sites. The basement membrane may also be a storage depot for latent proteinases or cytokines, released and/or activated during invasion and to which tumor cells or endothelial cells may respond.

Adhesion The interaction of cells with their scaffolding, the extracellular matrix and basement membrane, involves adhesion through specific receptors. Several classes of adhesion molecules have been shown to have critical roles in tumorigenesis. There are several predominant classes of adhesion receptors. These include the extracellular matrix protein receptors, the integrins; transmembrane cell adhesion molecules, the CAMs; and cadherins, extracellular adhesion molecules. The presence of selected adhesion receptors, such as particular integrin subunits, has shown a positive correlation with invasive potential and metastatic dissemination.

There are several members of the cadherin family. Genetic and biochemical analysis has demonstrated marked similarities between family members despite anatomic segregation. E-cadherin, or epithelial cadherin, forms extracellular homotypic interactions creating a functional bond between epithelial cells. Special intracellular proteins, the catenins, are required to link the extracellular cell-cell bond with the cell cytoskeleton. The interaction is regulated at several levels through protein-protein interactions, tyrosine phosphorylation, and cell-cell communication. Mutation or loss at several points along this cell adhesion pathway has been shown to occur naturally in tumors including breast, bladder, endometrial, and lung cancers. Furthermore, mutation or reduced expression has been associated with a more metastatic phenotype. Intact cadherins and catenins suppress metastasis.

The integrin family of cell surface extracellular matrix protein receptors consists of heterodimeric proteins, many of which have promiscuous binding preferences for the glycoproteins of the basement membrane and extracellular matrix. This family of receptors contains members where loss (in cancers such as breast, prostate, and colon) or increased expression (in melanoma and squamous cell cancer of the head and neck) has been associated with a more aggressive phenotype. Integrin occupation and cell surface clustering are critical components of basement membrane remodeling during angiogenesis. Integrin stimulation is necessary to provide a survival stimulus in several settings. For example, ligation of integrin $\alpha v \beta 3$ by melanoma cells is required for survival in collagen matrices. Alternatively, loss of stimulation of integrins has been shown to stimulate apoptosis. Thus, the same signaling pathways necessary for cellular processing of integrin information for adhesion, migration, and metastasis can also, in a different setting, cause cell death. This suggests that integrins may function as a 'go–no go' switch to trigger such diverse functions as metastatic spread or programmed cell death. While adhesion alone may not be sufficient for invasion and distant dissemination, loss of normally signaled adhesion functions may result in more aggressive invasion or loss of metastatic potential.

Proteolysis Degradation of local basement membrane and surrounding interstitial stroma is necessary for invasion, but it alone, like adhesion and motility, is not sufficient for distant dissemination of malignant cells. Important structural components of the basement membrane and interstitial stroma are the collagens, triple helical proteins that help form the latticework of the acellular matrix architecture. The major barrier to invasion is collagen. The interstitial or stromal collagens are generally composed of type I and III collagen, whereas types IV and V are the predominant collagens in the basement membrane. Enzymatic cleavage of the collagens, necessary to provide an escape route for tumor cells, is carried out by matrix metalloproteinases

with substrate selectivity. As with adhesion and angiogenesis, collagen production and collagenolytic degradation are functions of normal cells as well as malignant cells. The collagenases, neutral metal-binding proteases, are a well-studied family of enzymes whose function in metastatic dissemination has been used for prognostic assessment; they are now targets for therapeutic intervention. Collagenases are regulated by endogenous inhibitors, the tissue inhibitors of metalloproteinases (TIMP).

Several members of the metalloproteinase family have been shown to be overexpressed during the physiologic invasion of implantation of a fertilized ovum and during menstruation. These same enzymes have been shown to be overexpressed in the milieu of metastatic dissemination, whether in the interstitial stroma secreted by fibroblasts stimulated by local malignant cells or by the cancer cells themselves. Increased expression of a type IV collagenase (MMP-2, gelatinase A) is associated with increased metastatic progression in breast cancer, lung cancer, and colon cancer, among others. Increased circulating type IV collagenase in the blood of patients with bladder cancer correlates with their tumor burden. Similarly, TIMP expression has been shown to correlate with the invasive process. Overexpression of TIMP-2 or increased exogenous expression results in reduction in invasive phenotype in vitro and in vivo, whereas loss of TIMP-2 results in increased invasion, implying that TIMP-2 functions as a metastasis-suppressor gene. There is a critical balance between proteolysis (e.g., collagenases) and physiologic inhibition (TIMP). In invasive cancer, there is frequently an immediate local imbalance in protease and inhibitor that may not be evident when one studies the organ or individual as a whole. Collagenase excess permits a cell to invade and cross membrane barriers.

Motility The ability to translocate through local rents in the body's structural barriers requires that individual cells have a capacity for locomotion. There is a precedent in normal, physiologic invasion for migration. The movement of endothelial cells during vessel formation requires that a leading cell migrate into the stroma to initiate vascular bud formation. In infection, circulating monocytes must migrate into the stroma to initiate vascular bud formation. Tumor cells, likewise, must be able to migrate from the primary mass to reach a vascular conduit, intravasate, be carried by blood flow to a distant capillary bed, extravasate, and migrate some distance to initiate colony formation. Tumor cell migration can be directed by soluble factors emanating from target host tissues or by factors bound to the extracellular matrix. Soluble factors include cytokines such as hepatocyte growth factor, produced by stromal cells, and autocrine motility stimulatory enzymes such as autotaxin, produced by the tumor cells themselves. The receptor for hepatocyte growth factor is the oncogene, *met*, a tyrosine kinase–containing transmembrane receptor. Overexpression of *met* induces a tumorigenic and metastatic phenotype. Activation of *met* results in induction of an invasive phenotype with increased collagenase production, increased invasive potential in vitro, and metastasis production in vivo. Autotaxin, an exokinase secreted and tethered on the extracellular side of the tumor cell, is an autocrine motility factor. Autotaxin can be clipped near its transmembrane domain to yield the soluble motility-stimulating factor component. Its receptor has autophosphorylation, phosphatase, and phosphodiesterase activity.

Solid-phase migration factors include components of the extracellular matrix and basement membrane. Matrix glycoproteins and collagens can stimulate migration in vitro both as solid-phase attractants and in solution. Fragments of matrix proteins have also been demonstrated to be strong attractants to tumor cells and to cells involved in wound healing, endothelial cells, and fibroblasts. These fragments are produced physiologically by local proteolytic cleavage by invasion-associated proteinases, such as the matrix metalloproteinases that cleave basement membrane and interstitial stromal collagens. Hence, motility, like adhesion and proteolysis, requires interaction with the local environment and is the net balance of the production and secretion of stimulatory factors, such as hepatocyte growth factor and autotaxin; the activation of receptors, such as phosphorylation of *met*; and the response of the tumor and stromal cells.

DIAGNOSTICS, THERAPEUTICS, AND PATIENT MANAGEMENT Other genes have been identified that are specifically related to the invasive and metastatic phenotype. Loss of *nm*23 expression is correlated with increased aggressiveness of breast cancer, both node-positive and -negative. Expression of *nm*23 has also been associated with reduced aggressiveness of ovarian cancer. Experimental reexpression of *nm*23 caused a reduction in metastatic potential and reduced locomotion in vitro. The data define *nm*23 as a metastasis-suppressor gene.

Since invasion and angiogenesis are very early events in the time line of cancer progression leading to metastatic dissemination (Fig. 85-1), they provide novel targets for anticancer drug design. Batimastat (BB-94) is an agent that inhibits the proteolytic activity of type IV collagenase. Intraperitoneal administration of batimastat to animals bearing human ovarian cancer xenografts resulted in marked reduction in the cellularity and quantity of ascites formed, with some reduction in the tumor mass. It has had minimal toxicity in early clinical trials. Endothelial cell replication or invasion has been targeted because of the rare neovascularization occurring under physiologic conditions in adults. New antiangiogenic agents in development include derivatives of the fungal product fumagillin, such as TNP-470, that also have direct antiproliferative effects on cancer cells in vitro and in xenograft models.

Select signal transduction pathways have also been targeted. While dysregulation is not unique to invasion and metastasis of cancer and may be found in many pathologic states, normal cells appear to have better ability to accommodate alteration in their signaling pathways. Signal transduction agents under study include inhibitors of calcium influx, protein kinase C activity, *ras* farnesylation, and tyrosine phosphorylation. Most inhibitors of angiogenesis, metastasis, and signaling have been predominantly cytostatic agents, and many have shown selective anti-invasive and antiangiogenic activity. The cytostatic activity and minimal toxicity observed with these classes of compounds make them ideal candidates as chemopreventive agents against the early development of angiogenesis and invasion.

CONCLUSIONS The process of tumor invasion and metastasis is a complex cascade of biochemical and genetic events that are mediated by multiple signal transduction pathways and molecular systems. Simultaneously with an improved understanding of invasion and metastasis, new discoveries have yielded insight into the role of tumor heterogeneity, genetic progression, and the molecular events that modulate metastasis. Cellular and biochemical properties that are lost or augmented in metastatic cells will continue to be elucidated as research in this exciting field advances. In the future this knowledge will help identify new targets for diagnostic, therapeutic, and preventive modalities.

BIBLIOGRAPHY

Aaronson SA: Growth factors and cancer. Science 254:1146, 1991

Barsky SH et al: Loss of basement membrane components by invasive tumors but not their benign counterparts. Lab Invest 49:140, 1983

Folkman J: Seminars in medicine of the Beth Israel Hospital, Boston. Clinical applications of research on angiogenesis. N Engl J Med 333:1757, 1995

Kohn EC, Liotta LA: Molecular insights into cancer invasion: Strategies for prevention and intervention. Cancer Res 55:1856, 1995

Liotta LA et al: Quantitative relationships of intravascular tumor cells: Tumor vessels and pulmonary metastases following tumor implantation. Cancer Res 34:997, 1974

———— et al. Cancer metastasis and angiogenesis: An imbalance of positive and negative regulation. Cell 64:327, 1991

Montgomery AMP et al: Integrin alpha v-beta 3 rescues melanoma cells from apoptosis in three-dimensional dermal collagen. Proc Natl Acad Sci USA 91:8856, 1994

Stossel TP: On the crawling of cells. Science 260:1086, 1993

---

86 *Christopher A. Slapak, Donald W. Kufe*

PRINCIPLES OF CANCER THERAPY

The development of effective cancer therapy is a major focus of biomedical research. As a result of fundamental and applied research, certain previously lethal malignancies have become curable. Although progress in treating the most common epithelial-derived solid tumors has been slow, advances are leading to improvements in even these recalcitrant diseases. A further understanding of the process of malignant transformation has resulted in the identification of unique targets for therapeutic intervention. The discovery of biologic agents of potential clinical importance continues at a rapid pace. Tumor vaccine and gene transfer strategies are emerging from the laboratory and preclinical testing. New chemotherapeutic drugs, many with novel mechanisms of action, have entered clinical trials. The first differentiating agent effective in the treatment of a malignant disease has recently been approved for clinical use.

Cancer therapy is distributed among three interacting subspecialties. The role of the surgeon, the radiation oncologist, and the medical oncologist will continue to evolve as new agents become clinically available and a multimodality approach to cancer becomes the rule. The primary care physician will remain at the forefront of prevention and early detection of cancer. The further definition of cancer risk factors and the availability of more sensitive and specific screening procedures ensures that the internist will influence cancer morbidity and mortality. The approach to cancer therapy, whether it involves experimental therapeutics or standard therapy, must begin with an adequate data base. Each patient requires a proper histologic diagnosis of cancer. Every patient needs adequate staging and an appropriate plan of management.

DIAGNOSIS The histologic diagnosis of cancer and the proper categorization of the tumor type are pivotal in planning further workup and in deciding among treatment options. Although a histologic diagnosis may frequently appear straightforward, the clinician must realize its limitations. Histologic subtyping with biochemical and immunologic tissue characterization has resulted in a level of distinction among diagnoses not previously possible. In addition to substantiating the diagnosis of malignancy, this subtyping provides information essential in guiding therapy. The distinction between histologically similar tumors is important, as therapeutic options may differ. For example, when histologic subtyping is not possible, the decision to obtain additional tissue must be made in consultation with an experienced oncologist to determine whether it could alter the approach to treatment.

STAGING The extent of malignant disease is a prime determinant in planning appropriate therapy. Staging not only guides the selection of therapy but also provides important prognostic information and may help the clinician minimize morbid complications. The importance of staging has resulted in international attempts to adopt uniform criteria (see Chap. 81). No routine set of tests is appropriate for all patients. Understanding the natural history of the primary tumor, the pattern of spread to regional lymph nodes, and the possible sites of distant metastasis assists in the selection of tests. The risks to the patient from any study must be balanced against the benefits gained by having additional staging information.

MANAGEMENT A plan of management must be developed after diagnosis and staging. The plan must reflect the biology and natural history of the tumor, the available treatment options and their appropriateness to the patient's clinical situation, and the patient's wishes. The clinician must establish the goals of any treatment plan, and these goals should be explicitly communicated to the patient. Treatment with curative intent is clearly most desirable. The level of aggressiveness frequently required, often with attendant serious complications, requires the physician to evaluate realistically the potential for disease eradication. Treatment to improve longevity without long-term disease-free survival requires that the physician consider carefully the risk-to-benefit ratios of each therapeutic option. The expected gain in survival must be weighed against hospitalization time, potential complications, and side effects of therapy. Finally, treatment for palliation should not subject the patient to any unwarranted side effects, unnecessary complications, or other additional discomforts. The goals of palliation—relief of symptoms, prevention of complications, and maximization of quality of life—must always be kept in mind.

PRINCIPLES OF SURGICAL THERAPY

Surgery was the first modality used successfully in the treatment of cancer. After the development of ether anesthesia in the 1840s and of the principles of antisepsis in the 1860s, advances in cancer surgery were pioneered by Billroth, Halsted, and others. During the first part of this century, surgery was the only cancer treatment widely available. It is still the only curative therapy for many common solid tumors. Advances in surgical techniques, as well as improved multimodality therapy, have dramatically altered the surgical approach to many cancers. Limited surgical resections that do not affect the outcome but minimize loss of normal organ function are now feasible for some tumor types. Surgery has a primary role in the diagnosis, staging, and treatment of many tumors; surgical oncologists play an integral part in the multimodality approach to cancer therapy. Surgery is also effective in cancer prevention.

DIAGNOSIS A significant role of surgery in the treatment of patients with cancer is in the obtaining of adequate tissue samples for a histologic diagnosis. Accurate diagnosis is a critical first step in planning cancer therapy. Once the diagnosis of cancer is entertained, it is essential to involve a surgeon experienced in the principles of oncologic diagnosis. An improperly performed biopsy may compromise subsequent surgical management and, ultimately, the outcome for the patient.

Several techniques are available for obtaining tissue specimens. An *aspiration biopsy* is generally performed by inserting a fine needle into the tissue of interest and aspirating material for cytologic examination. The availability of an experienced cytologist is essential for a proper interpretation. Superficial lesions are amenable to aspiration, as are internal sites when the aspiration is guided by sonography or computed tomography (CT). A definitive diagnosis of cancer may not be possible by cytology alone, however. A *needle biopsy* obtains a core of tissue using a specially designed cutting needle. Radiologic guidance may permit a percutaneous approach to internal structures, such as the lung, liver, pancreas, and kidney. However, with some tumors, particularly lymphomas and sarcomas, a larger amount of tissue is usually required for a definitive diagnosis. With either aspiration or needle biopsy, sampling errors are a significant problem, and a negative result usually does not eliminate malignancy from the differential diagnosis. *Incisional biopsy*—the removal of a section or wedge of tissue from a larger tumor—is performed when removal of the entire tumor is impossible, as during an endoscopic examination. It is often performed before major surgical extirpation, as may be necessary for a soft tissue or bony sarcoma. Sampling errors are still a problem, as the resected portion may not be representative of the tumor as a whole. An *excisional biopsy* removes the entire lesion with little margin of normal tissue and, when possible, is to be preferred to incisional biopsy. Excising the entire lesion ensures sufficient tissue for pathologic examination, lessens the risk of tumor dissemination, and eliminates sampling problems. The choice of the appropriate procedure is dictated by anatomic considerations, the biology of the presumed tumor type, and the requirements of the pathologist. For some tumors, obtaining sufficient tissue for specialized studies such as immunophenotyping, cytogenetics, electron microscopy, or estrogen receptor status, requires specialized handling and close interaction with the pathologist.

STAGING Surgery is a principal means in the staging of many neoplastic diseases. Exploratory laparotomy to detect intraabdominal

spread of Hodgkin's disease is often indicated when conservative therapy is planned. Axillary lymph node sampling in breast carcinoma provides important prognostic information that may guide further therapy. Intraoperative staging by the sampling of celiac lymph nodes will help establish the appropriateness of an esophagectomy in a patient with esophageal carcinoma.

THERAPY Surgery is an effective way to cure patients whose tumors are confined to particular anatomic sites. However, at presentation, fewer than half of patients have tumors that are amenable to surgical treatment alone. The challenge is to identify the subset of patients that can be successfully treated by surgery alone, thus avoiding unnecessary surgical morbidity in the majority who will ultimately relapse. The most important determinants of a successful surgical intervention are the absence of distant metastases and little or no local tumor infiltration. For most solid tumors, the spread of disease beyond local confines prohibits a curative resection.

Understanding the typical patterns of cancer dissemination guides the preoperative assessment of patients. Cancer spreads by four routes: (1) by direct extension to adjacent structures; (2) through lymphatics to regional lymph nodes; (3) via hematogenous dissemination after entering the vascular system by direct vessel invasion; and (4) along serous cavities after growth through the wall of an organ. An individual tumor often uses more than one mode of dissemination. Careful clinical staging after the history, physical examination, and laboratory and imaging studies have been done is a requisite for deciding on the appropriateness of surgery.

Once the decision to treat by surgery has been made, it is essential to have an experienced oncologic surgeon; the best and usually only chance for curative resection is the first operation. Standard oncologic surgical practices are directed toward minimizing the risk of local tumor seeding and preventing dissemination at the time of the procedure. Such techniques include strict isolation of the tumor with avoidance of contamination to the operating field, minimal manipulation of the tumor, and early ligation of the vascular pedicle.

Removal of most solid tumors requires en bloc resections of the tumor plus a wide margin of normal tissue. The tumor type is the main factor determining how wide an adequate margin must be. The initial resection plan may have to be altered during the procedure as the full extent of the tumor becomes evident. Microscopic invasion of surrounding normal tissue by tumor that is imperceptible to the surgeon may necessitate examination of multiple frozen biopsy samples to establish tumor-free margins. Resection or sampling of regional lymph nodes is usually indicated; however, extended resection of several involved nodal groups is generally not warranted, as this approach has not resulted in improved survival.

Surgical resection of metastatic disease with the intent to cure may be appropriate in special circumstances. Generally, this approach is reserved for patients with slowly growing tumors who have a localized metastasis occurring well after resection of the primary disease. The metastasis should be the only evidence of distant disease found by imaging and laboratory studies, and it should be resectable with low morbidity. Examples include pulmonary metastases in patients with osteogenic sarcoma and solitary liver metastases in patients with colorectal carcinoma. In a minority of patients, resection of these lesions can lead to long-term disease-free survival.

Surgery may be used for palliation in patients for whom cure is not possible. The selection of patients who will benefit from this approach requires considerable judgment and skill. Appropriate, judicious use of surgery in patients with metastatic disease may alleviate symptoms and improve the quality of life. Surgery may be indicated to relieve pain, stop hemorrhage, or alleviate obstruction. For example, the excision of an occluding colon carcinoma when metastatic disease is present may greatly palliate symptoms. However, overly aggressive surgical intervention in a palliative setting may lead to prolonged hospitalizations, unnecessary discomfort, and an additional financial burden on the patient or family.

Modern surgical oncology is one component of combined-modality therapy, the goals of which are to improve outcome and allow a decrease in the extent of surgery. The surgeon, the medical oncologist, and the radiation therapist develop an integrated plan to deliver the most effective coordinated treatment. Combined-modality approaches have led to the successful development of adjuvant therapies. Adjuvant therapy, usually chemotherapy, is administered after definitive surgical resection to a patient who has no clinical, radiologic, or pathologic evidence of residual malignant disease. Adjuvant therapy is used in this setting to eliminate undetectable micrometastatic disease. The term *neoadjuvant treatment* refers to the administration of chemotherapy before definitive surgery. A patient who responds to neoadjuvant chemotherapy may benefit from more conservative local therapy. An example of multimodality therapy is the treatment of early-stage breast carcinoma. Mastectomy with axillary lymph node dissection can often be replaced by lumpectomy with lymph node sampling together with local radiotherapy and, when indicated, systemic adjuvant chemotherapy.

The use of surgery to achieve cytoreduction when complete excision is not possible has a role in some diseases, if combined with other therapeutic modalities. This approach has been most successful in childhood tumors, as in the surgical debulking of Wilms's tumor before administration of chemotherapy. In adults, this approach has a limited role in the treatment of ovarian carcinoma or Burkitt's lymphoma. A consideration of tumor cell biology demonstrates the difficulties of this approach: Debulking a mass 10 cm in diameter, containing approximately 1×10^{12} tumor cells, to a mass with a 1 cm diameter reduces the tumor burden by three orders of magnitude, leaving 1×10^9 tumor cells remaining.

Reconstructive surgery after a definitive resection can improve function and appearance and be of significant psychological benefit to the patient. The use of myocutaneous flaps and improvements in microvascular anastomotic techniques has had a profound effect on the ability to restore new tissue to a previous surgical area. Reconstruction after primary radiation therapy has also helped to restore function to damaged tissues. Stabilization of weight-bearing bones weakened by metastatic tumor may avert significant problems.

PREVENTION Surgery has a growing role in the prevention of cancer. Patients with conditions that predispose them to certain cancers or with genetic traits associated with cancer can have a normal life span with prophylactic surgery. Colectomy may be life-saving for patients with familial polyposis, nonpolyposis familial colon cancer, or ulcerative colitis. Women with multiple risk factors for breast cancer may benefit from prophylactic mastectomy. In light of the fact that the operation done for prophylaxis is more extensive than the operation done for control of the disease, most physicians would not recommend mastectomy unless the risk was more than 20 percent in 5 years. Oophorectomy is recommended for patients with familial ovarian cancer, and orchiectomy can prevent testicular cancer in men with undescended testes that have not been corrected before puberty. Orchiopexy can be preventive if performed early. Families with multiple endocrine neoplasia type II are at risk of developing medullary thyroid cancers. Thyroidectomy is prophylactic in this setting. Removal of premalignant skin lesions, such as dysplastic nevi and actinic keratoses, is the most common prophylactic surgery.

PRINCIPLES OF RADIATION THERAPY

Radiation therapy, like surgery, is a local modality used in the treatment of cancer. Its success depends on the inherent difference in radiosensitivity between the tumor and the adjacent normal tissues. Ideally, radiation therapy should destroy cancerous tissue while causing minimal disruption to surrounding normal structures. Other considerations are the ability of normal tissues to sustain and repair radiation-induced damage and for the patient to function adequately even if normal organ function is diminished.

PHYSICAL CHARACTERISTICS Radiation therapy for most solid tumors involves the administration of ionizing radiation in the form of x-rays or gamma rays to a tumor site. The term *x-ray* denotes high-energy electromagnetic radiation (4 to 25 MeV) produced by electron-level transitions within the atom. X-rays are generated by instruments such as linear accelerators. *Gamma rays* are also high-

energy radiation but are produced by radioactive isotope decay, typically from cobalt-60, cesium–137, or radium–226. Although there is no difference in the physical characteristics or biologic effects of x-rays and gamma rays, linear accelerators are more widely used and produce a more focused beam with a smaller penumbra. Megavoltage x-rays are commonly used to irradiate internal, deep-seated lesions, since high-energy, penetrating beams deliver a less intense superficial dose and spare the skin. Orthovoltage x-rays are of lesser energy and deliver a higher dose to superficial tissues; they can be used to treat skin cancers.

External beam therapy, or *teletherapy*, is radiation delivered from a source outside the body. Radiation delivered by sealed radioactive materials inserted in the body near or at the tumor site is called *brachytherapy*. Owing to the proximity of the radiation source to the tumor, the dose is more localized than with external beam therapy. Brachytherapy may consist of intracavitary inserts, used in the treatment of gynecologic malignancies such as cervical or vaginal carcinomas, or interstitial implants, such as those used for prostate carcinoma. Brachytherapy may also be used in conjunction with external beam therapy, for example in head and neck carcinoma, where the implants provide a high-intensity boost to the tumor bed.

Particle beam therapy, using neutron or proton beams, is available in specialized centers. This therapy has the advantage of more precise localization of energy release. The depth of particle penetration can be accurately controlled, with a resultant sparing of normal tissues. Electron beam therapy can be used to treat superficial tumors, such as skin cancers. The energy from these beams is rapidly absorbed, and, therefore, the dose to adjacent normal tissues is diminished.

BIOLOGIC CHARACTERISTICS Radiation therapy is a means of imparting energy to tissues that ultimately results in biological damage. Radiation dose, measured in gray (Gy), is defined as an amount of absorbed energy: 1 Gy is the absorption of 1 J of energy per kilogram of tissue. The previously used unit, the rad, equals 0.01 Gy (1 Gy equals 100 rad). A given dose of radiation kills a constant percentage of cells, not a constant number. At high doses of radiation, cell survival decreases with first-order kinetics in proportion to increasing radiation dose. At lower radiation doses, a shoulder in the curve results from a decreased rate of cell death and may represent the presence of cellular repair mechanisms (see Chap. 396).

DNA is the primary target for radiation-induced cell death. Ionizing radiation generates free radicals and reactive oxygen intermediates that damage local cellular constituents, especially DNA. DNA double-stranded breaks appear to be the critical lesion that results in cell death. Cellular demise associated with DNA breaks may occur within several hours or may become apparent only after cellular division, a process called *mitotic cell death*. In either instance, the process of *programmed cell death*, or *apoptosis*, may ensue after radiation-induced cellular damage in normal and tumor cells. Apoptosis is a genetically encoded program that involves the activation of endogenous nucleases and results in fragmentation of genomic DNA, nuclear condensation, and subsequent loss of cellular membrane integrity. The tumor suppressor gene *p53* is a key regulator of apoptosis. In a high percentage of tumors, mutation or deletion of *p53* may affect the ability of tumor cells to undergo programmed cell death in response to ionizing radiation. Cells that do not undergo apoptosis may succumb to *necrosis*, a process whereby cellular membrane integrity is lost before DNA degradation.

Rapidly proliferating normal tissues such as intestinal mucosa, bone marrow, and skin are particularly susceptible to ionizing radiation and readily show evidence of cytotoxicity. With slowly proliferating tissues, radiation-induced damage may not be apparent until much later or may occur only after stress to the normal tissues. For example, an irradiated long bone may not cause symptoms, except during prolonged healing following a fracture.

The capacity and extent of cellular repair mechanisms determine in part the radiosensitivity of a given tumor or normal tissue. Cellular repair in normal tissues is usually complete within 4 to 6 h after radiation exposure. Oxygen concentration is also an important determinant of radiation sensitivity. Oxygen is important for generating and sustaining the free radicals produced by radiation. Hypoxic tissues are relatively resistant to the effects of radiation; it takes a dose of radiation two to three times higher to kill anoxic cells as oxygenated ones. Poorly vascularized central areas of larger tumor masses are likely to exhibit relative insensitivity to radiation.

THERAPY Radiation therapy is planned and performed by a team of nurses, dosimetrists, physicists, and radiation oncologists. Achieving the goal of radiation therapy—to uniformly irradiate the entire tumor volume while sparing adjacent normal tissues—depends on appropriate treatment planning, in which extensive use should be made of imaging studies, particularly CT and magnetic resonance imaging (MRI) scans. A course of radiation therapy is preceded by a simulation session in which low-energy beams are used to produce radiographic images that indicate the exact beam location. The positioning of the patient used in the simulation must be reproduced exactly for each treatment to ensure maximal tumor killing with minimal complications.

Radiation therapy is usually delivered in fractionated doses, such as 180 to 300 cGy per day, five times a week for a total course of 5 to 8 weeks. Clinical experience has demonstrated that fractional treatment schedules improve the therapeutic index and result in better tumor control. This better outcome may be related to several factors, including cellular repair of normal tissues, repopulation of destroyed tissues, and reoxygenation of relatively hypoxic tumor sites. Accelerated fractionation schedules increase the daily dose and reduce the overall treatment time. Although this approach may produce more acute toxicity, it may benefit patients with tumors that have a rapid doubling time, such as some head and neck tumors. Hyperfractionation delivers smaller individual doses several times a day and thereby increases the total number of treatments. In theory, hyperfractionation improves the therapeutic index for some tumors.

Radiation therapy is delivered from multiple external sites or fields which together focus on the tumor. This approach distributes the radiotherapy and lessens its toxicity to the normal tissues by minimizing the dose to vital structures. Increasing the number of fields may cause a larger volume of normal tissue to receive irradiation, but at more moderate doses.

Radiation therapy with curative intent as the sole treatment modality is employed in limited-stage Hodgkin's disease, some non-Hodgkin's lymphomas, certain head and neck carcinomas, limited-stage prostate carcinoma, gynecologic tumors, central nervous system neoplasms, and some skin cancers. Radiation therapy also is often an integral part of curative multimodality approaches. For example, radiation therapy combined with chemotherapy has largely replaced surgery as a curative treatment for squamous cell carcinoma of the anus. Radiation therapy is a central component of breast conservation in the multimodality treatment of breast carcinoma.

Radiation therapy is also used in the palliative management of many tumors. Irradiation of bony metastases may alleviate pain and stabilize weight-bearing structures in an attempt to prevent pathologic fractures. Brain metastases are often irradiated to provide symptomatic relief and prevent further neurologic complications. Palliative radiation therapy can also be employed to treat significant bleeding, refractory visceral pain, and vital organ obstruction. In general, the doses employed for palliative management are lower than those used for curative therapy and result in less acute toxicity and discomfort to the patient.

Radiation therapy may be required on an urgent basis for the treatment of complications of malignant disease. Impending spinal cord compression in a patient with metastatic carcinoma is usually best treated with radiotherapy to the involved area. Alleviation of an obstructed airway or superior vena cava is generally treated effectively by radiotherapy.

COMPLICATIONS Radiation therapy is associated with both acute toxicity and long-term sequelae. Acute reactions occur during or immediately after therapy and represent interruption of the repopulation of rapidly dividing tissues. They are self-limited and usually do not limit the amount of radiation therapy that can be administered. Common manifestations include systemic symptoms, such as fatigue, and local skin reactions that range from erythema to moist desquamation. Gastrointestinal toxicity, with nausea, vomiting, dysphagia, or diarrhea, is associated with treatment to the abdomen or pelvis. Irradiation of the head and neck results in oropharyngeal mucositis and xerostomia. Significant myelosuppression, with leukopenia, thrombocytopenia, or anemia, is unusual but can occur if large amounts of the proliferative bone marrow are irradiated. If symptoms become problematic during therapy, treatment may need to be temporarily halted to allow normal tissue repair.

Long-term sequelae are dose-limiting and occur many months or years after the completion of therapy. The frequency of long-term complications increases as normal tissue tolerances are approached. These complications tend to be progressive rather than self-limited. Their occurrence does not correlate with the appearance or severity of acute reactions. The mechanism of late complications is believed to be the disruption of vascular endothelium or the depletion of normal tissue stem cells. Table 86-1 lists the tissue tolerances of some common structures that exhibit late complications. The normal tissue tolerance is defined as the dose at which no more than 5 percent of patients will have the stated complication within 5 years.

Radiation therapy is known to be mutagenic, carcinogenic, and teratogenic and is associated with an increased risk of developing both secondary leukemias and solid tumors. The most complete data for these complications come from studies of patients who are long-term survivors after therapy for Hodgkin's disease. Although secondary leukemias may appear within the first few years after therapy, the median time to appearance of secondary solid tumors is greater than 10 years. The relative risk for developing secondary tumors in Hodgkin's disease is related to extent of treatment, age, use of combined-modality therapy, and sex. The risk is higher for women than for men owing to the development of secondary breast cancers in young patients who received mantle radiation.

RADIONUCLIDES For decades, radionuclides have been used systemically to treat malignant disorders. They are administered by specialists in nuclear medicine or radiation therapy.

Radioactive iodine in the form of ^{131}I is effective therapy for well-differentiated thyroid carcinomas. Iodine is selectively metabolized by thyroid tissue; other tissues are spared the detrimental effects of ^{131}I. In practice, uptake of ^{131}I by tumors is variable and is less than that of normal thyroid tissue.

Strontium-89 is used for the treatment of bony metastases. Strontium is an alkaline earth element in the same family as calcium and is metabolized by the same biochemical pathways as calcium. Strontium is accumulated in sites of active osteogenesis and becomes localized in bone mineral. ^{89}Sr will selectively irradiate blastic sites of primary and metastatic bone involvement and spare normal tissues. It is used in a palliative manner to relieve pain; its major toxic effect is myelosuppression.

Table 86-1

Tolerance of Normal Tissues for Radiation Therapy

Tissue	Dose (cGy)	Complications
Brain	6000	Necrosis
Spinal cord	4500	Myelitis
Heart	4500	Pericarditis, myocardial damage
Intestine	4500	Stenosis, perforation
Liver	3000	Hepatitis, hepatic vein thrombosis
Lung	2000	Pneumonitis, fibrosis
Kidney	2000	Nephropathy, renal failure
Bone marrow	250	Aplasia
Ovary	200	Sterilization
Testes	100	Sterilization

PRINCIPLES OF CHEMOTHERAPY

BACKGROUND Systemic chemotherapy is the main treatment available for disseminated malignant disease. Progress in drug therapy has resulted in the development of curative chemotherapy regimens for several tumors (Table 86-2). Chemotherapy also has a significant role in palliation, often with improved survival, in a variety of other tumors (Table 86-2). However, chemotherapy has only minor activity in several common solid tumors. One of the most important and still evolving roles for systemic chemotherapy is its use in the adjuvant setting. Table 86-2 lists tumors that can be treated effectively with adjuvant chemotherapy.

Chemotherapy, whether given with curative or palliative intent, usually requires multiple cycles of treatment. It is often desirable to assess the therapeutic efficacy of the treatment before completing the entire course. The discontinuation of an ineffective treatment may allow a different salvage regimen to be instituted or, at least, will spare the patient unnecessary toxicity. Response to therapy can be measured directly by palpating superficial tumor masses or by imaging internal lesions. Indirect measurements can be used but generally are less desirable in the evaluation of tumor response.

Uniform criteria for describing a response to therapy are widely accepted and make it possible to compare the efficacy of alternative treatments. A *complete response* (*complete remission*) is the disappearance of all detectable malignant disease. A *partial response* is a decrease by more than 50 percent in the sum of the products of the perpendicular diameters of all measurable lesions; also, there can be no increase in size of any lesion nor the appearance of any new lesions. *Stable disease* means that there is no change in measurable tumor dimensions. *Progressive disease* means an increase by at least 25 percent in the sum of the products of the perpendicular diameters of measurable lesions, or the appearance of new lesions.

The modern era of chemotherapy treatment for malignant disease began after the observation in World War II that exposure to mustard gas led to bone marrow and lymph node hypoplasia. The clinical use of nitrogen mustard was pioneered by Gilman at Yale in the 1940s in the treatment of lymphoma. Farber at Harvard, also in the 1940s, first induced remissions in childhood leukemia using aminopterin, a folate antagonist. In 1955, chemotherapy was first used to cure a solid tumor, gestational trophoblastic carcinoma. The subsequent development of multidrug regimens for childhood acute leukemia and Hodgkin's disease in the 1960s demonstrated that chemotherapy could consistently cure a high percentage of patients with certain chemoresponsive diseases. To appreciate more fully the development and application of modern chemotherapeutic regimens in the treatment of neoplastic diseases, it is necessary to understand the principles of cytokinetics and pharmacodynamics.

CYTOKINETICS A primary determinant of malignant transformation is uncontrolled growth. All somatic cells, whether normal or malignant, multiply by cell division through the mitotic cell cycle (see Chap. 83). Many chemotherapeutic agents, such as the antimetabolites and the alkylating agents, are cell-cycle–active; that is, they are cytotoxic mainly to actively cycling cells. In addition, some cycle-active agents are phase-specific; that is, they are cytotoxic to cells in a particular phase of the cell cycle. Other agents are capable of exerting cytotoxicity at any phase of cell cycle, including G0/G1, and are not considered cycle-active.

A model elucidating the effectiveness of chemotherapy in eliminating a tumor mass was proposed by Skipper and coworkers in the 1960s and is called the *log cell kill model*. According to this model, tumor growth is exponential with first-order kinetics and progresses at that rate until a lethal tumor burden is reached (Fig. 86-1A). The time required for a tumor to increase from 10^6 cells to 10^9 cells (a three-log or 1000-fold increase) is the same as the time for the tumor to increase from 10^9 to 10^{12} cells. A given chemotherapy dose will destroy a constant percentage of cells, not a constant number, regardless of the tumor burden. Thus, if a given dose kills 99 percent of the tumor cells (a two-log reduction) a tumor mass of 10^{11} cells will be reduced to 10^9 cells (Fig. 86-1B). Assuming no tumor regrowth, an additional cycle of chemotherapy will reduce the tumor to 10^7 cells, at which point it would no longer be clinically detectable, and the patient would have achieved a complete response. However, an additional four cycles of chemotherapy will be required to reduce the tumor burden to less than 1 cell to achieve a cure.

Most human solid tumors do not grow with a constant doubling rate. Instead, the rate of growth slows progressively with increasing tumor size, a pattern called *Gompertzian growth* (Fig. 86-2). As tumors enlarge, the growth rate slows, the growth fraction decreases, and tumor volume begins to plateau. Patients with large tumors often respond poorly to chemotherapy, primarily because of unfavorable tumor cytokinetics. Chemotherapy is usually most effective on a small tumor burden for which the growth fraction is maximal, as in the adjuvant setting, in which tumor size and cytokinetics favor a response.

PHARMOCODYNAMICS Chemotherapeutic agents exhibit a dose-response effect (Fig. 86-3). At sufficiently low concentrations, no cytotoxicity is observed. At increasing concentrations, cell kill is proportional to drug exposure. At high concentrations, the effect reaches a plateau. Normal cells also are susceptible to the cytotoxic effects of chemotherapeutic drugs and exhibit a dose-response effect, but the response curve is shifted relative to that of malignant cells (Fig. 86-3). This difference represents the therapeutic index; the usefulness of many chemotherapeutic drugs is limited by the fact that they have a narrow therapeutic index. The toxicity to normal tissue that limits further dose escalation is the *dose-limiting toxicity*. The dose just below this point is the *maximum tolerated dose*. Proliferative normal tissues such as the bone marrow and gastrointestinal mucosa are generally the most susceptible to chemotherapy-induced toxicity.

The concentration range over which the dose-response curve remains linear for a particular drug is an important consideration in designing dose-intensive regimens. Drugs such as the alkylating agents characteristically have steep dose-response curves: An increase in the drug concentration by an order of magnitude or more results in a proportional increase in tumor cell kill. By contrast, the dose-response curve of phase-specific agents, such as the antimetabolites, typically

Table 86-2

Response of Tumors to Chemotherapy

CURABLE BY CHEMOTHERAPY

Acute lymphoblastic leukemia	Non-Hodgkin's lymphoma
Acute myeloid leukemia	Burkitt's lymphoma
Ewing's sarcoma	Diffuse large cell lymphoma
Gestational trophoblastic carcinoma	Follicular mixed lymphoma
Hodgkin's disease	Lymphoblastic lymphoma
	Rhabdomyosarcoma
	Testicular carcinoma
	Wilms's tumor

CHEMOTHERAPY HAS SIGNIFICANT ACTIVITY

Anal carcinoma	Head and neck carcinoma
Bladder carcinoma	Lung (small cell) carcinoma
Breast carcinoma	Multiple myeloma
Chronic lymphocytic leukemia	Non-Hodgkin's lymphoma
Chronic myelogenous leukemia	Follicular lymphoma
Hairy cell leukemia	Ovarian carcinoma

CHEMOTHERAPY HAS MINOR ACTIVITY

Brain tumors (astrocytoma)	Lung (non-small-cell) carcinoma
Cervical carcinoma	Melanoma
Colorectal carcinoma	Pancreatic carcinoma
Hepatocellular carcinoma	Prostate carcinoma
Kaposi's sarcoma	Soft tissue sarcoma

ADJUVANT CHEMOTHERAPY IS EFFECTIVE

Breast carcinoma	Ovarian carcinoma (stage III)
Colorectal carcinoma (stage III)	Testicular carcinoma
Osteogenic sarcoma	

FIGURE 86-1   Model of logarithmic cell growth and cell killing. *A.* Tumor cell growth proceeds with first-order kinetics from a clinically undetectable mass to a lethal tumor burden. *B.* Tumor regression in response to chemotherapy also follows first-order kinetics. A given dose of chemotherapy kills a constant percentage of cells regardless of tumor size. In the case shown here, two cycles of chemotherapy will render the tumor clinically undetectable, but six cycles will be required for total tumor eradication.

is linear over only a narrow range. These agents are less suitable for dose escalation. However, increased tumor cell kill is observed after prolonged exposure to these agents. Increasing the exposure time means that a larger percentage of the tumor cells will enter the cell cycle and thus become susceptible to the cytotoxic effects of the drugs. These agents are often referred to as *schedule-dependent.*

The ability of chemotherapy to eradicate tumor cells without causing lethal host toxicity depends on drug selectivity. The basis for anticancer drug selectivity remains incompletely understood. Although cytokinetics are important, other differences between normal and tumor cells in cellular processes, such as metabolic pathways and susceptibility to programmed cell death, also contribute.

Most chemotherapeutic agents are inducers of programmed cell death. Drugs such as the alkylating agents, the purine/pyrimidine analogs, and the topoisomerase inhibitors result in DNA damage (see below). In response to genotoxic damage, cells can arrest at two identified checkpoints: the G1/S and G2/M boundaries. G1 arrest is mediated in part by the tumor suppressor p53 via activation of the expression of the cyclin-dependent kinase inhibitor p21. G1 arrest may allow the cell to repair damage before DNA replication, and G2 arrest permits repair prior to mitosis. If the DNA damage is irreparable, apoptosis may occur via p53-dependent or -independent pathways.

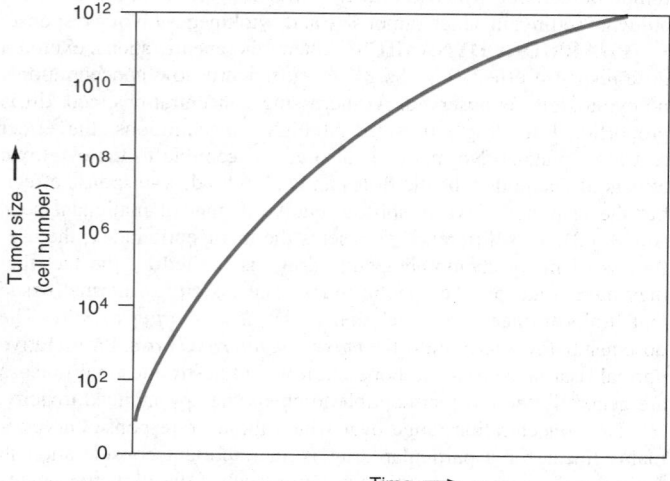

FIGURE 86-2   Model of Gompertzian growth. In Gompertzian growth, as the tumor size increases the growth rate slows and begins to plateau. Large tumors will be relatively insensitive to chemotherapy, owing primarily to unfavorable cytokinetics.

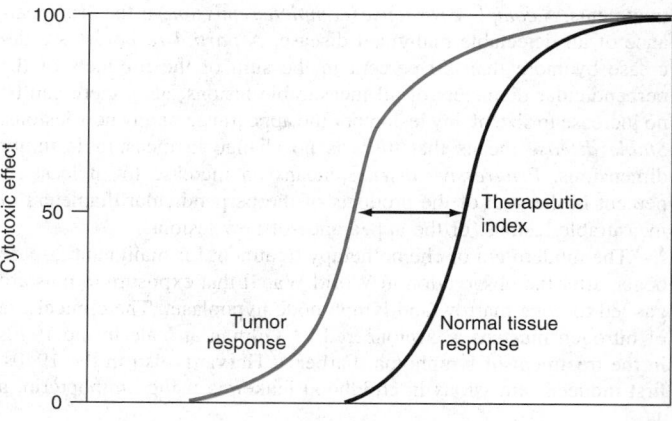

FIGURE 86-3   Dose-response effect. All cells, whether normal or malignant, demonstrate a dose-response effect when exposed to chemotherapeutic agents. The difference between the responses of the tumor and of normal tissue represents the therapeutic index.

CANCER CHEMOTHERAPY   Most of the commonly used cytotoxic antitumor agents are discussed below. They should be administered only by physicians experienced in their use and expert at handling potentially serious side effects. The dose of most chemotherapeutic agents is based on a patient's body surface area (in square meters) calculated according to height and weight. The major diseases for which individual agents are commonly used are listed in Table 86-3.

Antimetabolites   The antimetabolites induce cytotoxicity by serving as false substrates in biochemical pathways. They are cell-cycle–active and are specific mainly for the S phase. Many are nucleoside analogues that are incorporated into DNA or RNA and thereby inhibit nucleic acid synthesis. Other agents in this class inhibit enzymes involved in nucleotide biosynthesis.

Pyrimidine-Analogue Antimetabolites   The fluorinated pyrimidine, *fluorouracil* (5-fluorouracil; 5FU), is activated intracellularly to one of several metabolites. Fluorodeoxyuridine monophosphate (FdUMP) is a potent inhibitor of thymidylate synthase, an enzyme necessary for the synthesis of dTTP and ultimately DNA; fluorouridine triphosphate (FUTP) is incorporated into RNA and interferes with its processing and function. Fluorodeoxyuridine triphosphate (FdUTP) is incorporated into DNA and eventually leads to DNA strand breakage. The interference of FdUMP with thymidylate synthesis requires the presence of reduced folates. Leucovorin, a folate analogue, has been administered with fluorouracil in an attempt to increase antitumor activity. Extensive first-pass hepatic metabolism for fluorouracil has led to direct hepatic artery infusions for the treatment of hepatic metastases. The fluorouracil analogue *floxuridine*, (FUDR) is also available for intrahepatic infusion.

Fluorouracil toxicity is schedule-dependent. With bolus infusion, bone marrow suppression predominates, whereas with continuous infusion, gastrointestinal toxicity may be more limiting. Fluorouracil has been associated infrequently with a myocardial ischemic syndrome. Neurologic symptoms, usually reversible, include headaches, cerebellar ataxia, and somnolence. Dermatologic complaints, such as dermatitis, hyperpigmentation, and skin atrophy, are not uncommon.

Cytarabine (ara-C) is the 2' epimer of cytidine. After carrier-mediated uptake by the deoxycytidine transport system, this substance is phosphorylated sequentially to its active metabolite, ara-CTP, with deoxycytidine kinase activity being rate-limiting. Ara-CTP is incorporated into DNA and inhibits replication by acting as a chain terminator. Cytarabine can be degraded intracellularly to an inactive compound (ara-U) by cytidine deaminase. The net effects of cellular accumulation and of the balance between the activities of deoxycytidine kinase and cytidine deaminase ultimately determine the cellular toxicity of cytarabine.

Cytarabine is usually administered by continuous infusion and causes profound myelosuppression. Gastrointestinal toxicity, including oral mucositis, is frequently observed. High-dose regimens are associated with a syndrome of cholestatic jaundice, as well as cerebellar and cerebral toxicity. Patients with abnormal renal function, a greater than twofold elevation of alkaline phosphatase levels, or age greater than 40 are at increased risk for neurotoxicity. Conjunctivitis, preventable by ophthalmic corticosteroids, is common with high-dose regimens.

Gemcitabine is a difluorinated analogue of deoxycytidine. In a manner similar to cytarabine, it acts as a DNA chain terminator after carrier-mediated uptake and intracellular phosphorylation. However, gemcitabine appears to have better membrane permeability and greater affinity for deoxycytidine kinase. Once incorporated into DNA, it is more resistant to exonuclease excision than cytarabine. In addition, gemcitabine inhibits the enzyme ribonucleotide reductase and thereby leads to diminished pools of the competing natural compound, deoxycytidine. Myelosuppression is dose-limiting with gemcitabine. Other toxicities include lethargy and malaise.

Table 86-3

Antitumor Activities of Chemotherapeutic Agents

Agent	Tumors against which Agent Shows Activity*
ANTIMETABOLITES	
Pyrimidine analogs	
Cytarabine	Acute lymphoblastic leukemia, acute myeloid leukemia, non-Hodgkin's lymphoma
Fluorouracil (5FU)	Breast Ca, colorectal Ca, esophageal Ca, gastric Ca
Gemcitabine	Bladder Ca, non-small-cell lung Ca, pancreatic Ca
Purine analogues	
Cladribine	Hairy cell leukemia, follicular lymphoma
Fludarabine	Chronic lymphocytic leukemia, follicular lymphoma
Pentostatin	Hairy cell leukemia
Other	
Hydroxyurea	Chronic myelogenous leukemia, essential thrombocytosis
Methotrexate	Acute lymphoblastic leukemia, bladder Ca, breast Ca, gestational trophoblastic Ca, head/neck Ca, non-Hodgkin's lymphoma, osteogenic sarcoma
PLANT ALKALOIDS	
Taxanes	
Docetaxel	Breast Ca, ovarian Ca
Paclitaxel	Breast Ca, lung Ca, ovarian Ca
Vincas	
Vinblastine	Bladder Ca, breast Ca, Hodgkin's disease, lung Ca, non-Hodgkin's lymphoma, testicular Ca
Vincristine	Acute lymphoblastic leukemia, Hodgkin's disease, non-Hodgkin's lymphoma
Vinorelbine	Breast Ca, lung Ca
TOPOISOMERASE INHIBITORS	
Anthracyclines	
Daunorubicin	Acute lymphoblastic leukemia, acute myeloid leukemia
Doxorubicin	Bladder Ca, breast Ca, gastric Ca, hepatocellular Ca, Hodgkin's disease, lung Ca, non-Hodgkin's lymphoma, osteogenic sarcoma, soft tissue sarcoma
Idarubicin	Acute myeloid leukemia, non-Hodgkin's lymphoma
Epipodophyllotoxins	
Etoposide	Acute myeloid leukemia, lung Ca, non-Hodgkin's lymphoma, ovarian Ca, testicular Ca
Teniposide	Acute lymphoblastic leukemia, non-Hodgkin's lymphoma
Other	
Dactinomycin	Gestational trophoblastic Ca
Mitoxantrone	Acute myeloid leukemia, breast Ca, non-Hodgkin's lymphoma
ALKYLATING AGENTS	
Classic	
Busulfan	Chronic myelogenous leukemia
Chlorambucil	Chronic lymphocytic leukemia, Hodgkin's disease, non-Hodgkin's lymphoma
Cyclophosphamide	Bladder Ca, breast Ca, chronic lymphocytic leukemia, lung Ca, non-Hodgkin's lymphoma, ovarian Ca, soft tissue sarcoma
Ifosfamide	Breast Ca, non-Hodgkin's lymphoma, osteogenic sarcoma, testicular Ca
Mechlorethamine	Hodgkin's disease
Melphalan	Breast Ca, multiple myeloma, ovarian Ca
Thiotepa	Breast Ca, ovarian Ca
Nitrosoureas	
Carmustine	Astrocytoma, Hodgkin's disease, non-Hodgkin's lymphoma
Lomustine	Astrocytoma, Hodgkin's disease, non-Hodgkin's lymphoma
Platinum compounds	
Carboplatin	Bladder Ca, head/neck Ca, ovarian Ca
Cisplatin	Bladder Ca, esophageal Ca, head/neck Ca, lung Ca, osteogenic sarcoma, ovarian Ca, testicular Ca
ANTITUMOR ANTIBIOTICS	
Bleomycin	Hodgkin's disease, non-Hodgkin's lymphoma, testicular Ca
Mitomycin C	Breast Ca, colorectal Ca
MISCELLANEOUS AGENTS	
Dacarbazine	Hodgkin's disease, melanoma, soft tissue sarcoma
L-Asparaginase	Acute lymphoblastic leukemia
Procarbazine	Astrocytoma, Hodgkin's disease

* Ca, carcinoma.

Purine-Analogue Antimetabolites Three adenosine analogues have recently entered clinical practice. *Fludarabine* is a fluorinated derivative of the antiviral agent vidarabine (ara-A). Unlike vidarabine, it is resistant to intracellular deamination. Fludarabine is phosphorylated by deoxycytidine kinase before being incorporated into DNA and inhibiting DNA synthesis. A significant number (up to 20 percent) of patients experience mild, reversible neurotoxicity, although instances of severe, irreversible toxicity, including coma, have been reported. In addition to myelosuppression, fludarabine causes immunosuppression and episodes of opportunistic infection in some patients. *Cladribine* (chlorodeoxyadenosine) is also phosphorylated by deoxycytidine kinase before being incorporated into DNA and inhibiting DNA replication. Cladribine is myelosuppressive and immunosuppressive; other toxicities, such as gastrointestinal toxicity, are mild. *Pentostatin* (2'-deoxycoformycin) is an irreversible inhibitor of the enzyme adenosine deaminase, causing the toxic accumulation of deoxyadenosine nucleotides, particularly in lymphocytes. Pentostatin causes immunosuppression, especially of T-cell–mediated immunity. Myelosuppression, renal function impairment, central nervous system toxicity, and hepatoxicity have been attributed to treatment with this agent.

The thiopurine analogues *6-mercaptopurine* (6MP) and *6-thioguanine* (6TG) require modification by the enzyme hypoxanthine-guanine phosphoribosyltransferase (HGPRT) before they can inhibit purine biosynthesis. Patients receiving allopurinol require a 75 percent decrease in mercaptopurine dose size because elimination depends on the enzyme xanthine oxidase, the target for allopurinol inhibition. Cholestatic jaundice has been observed with both agents, although it is more common with 6MP. Both 6MP and 6TG produce myelosuppression and gastrointestinal toxicity, although the latter is usually mild.

Other Antimetabolites The antifolate *methotrexate* inhibits the enzyme dihydrofolate reductase. Dihydrofolate reductase activity is necessary to maintain intracellular pools of reduced tetrahydrofolates, which are required for the synthesis of purine nucleotides and thymidylate. After carrier-mediated cellular uptake, methotrexate is converted to a polyglutamate derivative that is more active than the parent drug. Administration of a reduced folate, such as leucovorin, bypasses the block created by methotrexate and can prevent severe gastrointestinal toxicity or marked bone marrow hypoplasia. It is generally used after administration of methotrexate at doses >100 mg/m^2. The accumulation of methotrexate in third-space fluids, such as pleural effusion or ascites, and the subsequent prolonged release of the agent can prolong drug elimination and lead to unusually severe toxicities.

Use of very high-dose methotrexate (>1000 mg/m^2) requires the monitoring of serum methotrexate levels to adjust the dose and schedule of leucovorin rescue. Methotrexate is cleared mainly by renal excretion, and patients with impaired renal function require dosage adjustments. High-dose regimens have been associated with acute renal injury, which may be prevented by vigorous hydration and alkalinization of the urine. In the absence of normal renal function, there are no satisfactory methods (including hemodialysis) to eliminate methotrexate. Acute or chronic administration of methotrexate has been associated with hepatoxicity and an idiosyncratic pneumonitis.

Hydroxyurea inhibits the enzyme ribonucleotide reductase, which converts ribonucleotides to deoxyribonucleotides. Hydroxyurea produces a predictable leukopenia that is usually reversible within days of discontinuing therapy. Gastrointestinal toxicity is usually mild. Patients receiving long-term hydroxyurea therapy may develop mild dermatologic changes.

Plant Alkaloids The vinca alkaloids *vincristine* and *vinblastine* were originally isolated from the periwinkle plant, *Catharanthus roseus*. *Vinorelbine* is a newer semisynthetic derivative. The vinca alkaloids inhibit microtubule assembly by binding to tubulin and thus are cytotoxic predominately during the M phase of the cell cycle. *Paclitaxel* and *docetaxel* are members of the taxane family. Paclitaxel is isolated from the Pacific yew (*Taxus brevifolia*), whereas docetaxel

is synthesized from a noncytotoxic precursor isolated from the more readily accessible European yew (*Taxus baccata*). They function by stabilizing microtubules and preventing their disassembly.

Neurotoxicity is dose-limiting with vincristine and is manifested as peripheral sensory neuropathy and/or an autonomic neuropathy. With continued use of the agent, a motor neuropathy may develop. Mild neuropathy generally improves with discontinuation of treatment. Vincristine has been associated with inappropriate secretion of antidiuretic hormone. Although vincristine is essentially nonmyelosuppressive, bone marrow hypoplasia is dose-limiting with vinblastine and vinorelbine. Major neurotoxicity is less commonly observed with vinblastine and vinorelbine.

Paclitaxel and docetaxel infusions are associated with hypersensitivity reactions. The vehicle in which they are dissolved, cremophor EL or Tween 80, may contribute. Bradyarrhythmias (especially atrioventricular block), atypical chest pain, and, rarely, more severe cardiac problems have also been associated with paclitaxel. Myelosuppression is dose-limiting for both agents. Peripheral neuropathy and severe alopecia are also common with both. Glucocorticoids may prevent the hypersensitivity.

Topoisomerase Inhibitors During transcription and replication, DNA acquires conformational and topologic changes that must be relieved. The enzymes topoisomerase I and topoisomerase II perform this function by introducing and then repairing single- or double-stranded DNA breaks. Agents that interfere with this process have been found to have antitumor activity. *Camptothecin*, derived from the tree *Camptotheca accuminata*, is the prototypical inhibitor of topoisomerase I. The camptothecin analogues *9-aminocamptothecin*, *topotecan*, and *irinotecan* (CPT-11) are in clinical trials.

By contrast, topoisomerase II inhibitors, such the epipodophyllotoxins and anthracyclines, include some of the most widely used antitumor agents. These agents inhibit the DNA-rejoining activity of topoisomerase II, leading to DNA fragmentation and ultimately cell death. A serious complication first reported for the epipodophyllotoxins and now also recognized for the anthracyclines is the development of secondary leukemias. Epipodophyllotoxin-related acute myeloid leukemia appears to evolve within 3 years of treatment with the drug and has been associated with cytogenetic abnormalities involving chromosome 11q23. The incidence may exceed 5 percent and appears to be dose- and schedule-dependent. The incidence of secondary leukemia induced by anthracyclines is much lower.

The epipodophyllotoxins *etoposide* and *teniposide* are semisynthetic derivatives of the natural product podophyllotoxin, which is derived from the mandrake plant, *Podophyllum peltatum*. Leukopenia is the dose-limiting toxicity for etoposide and teniposide, with white cell counts reaching their nadir at approximately 14 days. Intravenous administration of either drug is associated with fever, hypotension, bronchospasm, and, rarely, anaphylaxis. The incidence of these symptoms can be minimized by administering the drugs over 1 h.

The anthracyclines include *doxorubicin*, *daunorubicin*, and *idarubicin*. In addition, *epirubicin* is available for clinical use outside the United States. Although the anthracyclines are topoisomerase II inhibitors, they also undergo one- and two-electron reductions with the generation of intracellular free radicals, particularly hydroxyl radicals, which are highly cytotoxic. The anthracyclines are myelosuppressive and cause gastrointestinal toxicity. They are severe vesicants, and extravasation during infusion may lead to local tissue necrosis. In extreme cases, skin grafting may be required. The anthracyclines are metabolized by the liver, and patients with elevations of serum bilirubin require dosage modifications. Long-term administration is limited by cumulative dose-dependent cardiotoxicity. Irreversible cardiomyopathy is a significant risk in patients who have received doses in excess of 500 to 550 mg/m^2 of doxorubicin or daunorubicin. Previous chest radiotherapy or concomitant cyclophosphamide therapy may lower the tolerable cumulative dose. *Dexrazoxane* is a chelating agent that may prevent anthracycline-induced cardiomyopathy. Although data are not yet definitive, it appears that dexrazoxane does not significantly decrease tumor response rates. It is recommended for patients who have already received 300 mg/m^2 of anthracycline.

Mitoxantrone, an anthracenedione, is structurally related to the anthracyclines. Although the incidence of cardiomyopathy with this agent is lower than for doxorubicin, patients are still at risk who have received lifetime doses greater than 125 mg/m^2. Mitoxantrone also causes marked myelosuppression. *Dactinomycin* currently has limited clinical use. It causes myelosuppression and gastrointestinal toxicity.

Alkylating Agents The alkylating agents are among the most widely used antitumor agents. Most alkylating agents are bifunctional and are efficient at cross-linking DNA, leading to strand breakage and ultimately cell death. Alkyl groups are preferentially added to N-7 or O-6 of guanine, as well as at other nitrogen or oxygen positions in adenine and cytidine. Although alkylation of DNA can occur at any phase of the cell cycle, cytotoxicity is greatest in cells that are progressing through the cell cycle. These agents are best regarded as cell-cycle–active but non-phase-specific. The covalent alkylation of DNA is mutagenic and carcinogenic and results in long-term serious complications, including detrimental effects on spermatogenesis and oogenesis as well as the development of secondary leukemias.

Azoospermia resulting from treatment with alkylating agents has been found in men receiving therapy for lymphoma and may be permanent. The severity of gonadal injury appears to be dose-dependent and in some men is reversible. Women who have received alkylating agents may experience amenorrhea and ovarian atrophy. The likelihood that normal menstrual cycles will resume is inversely related to the age of the patient and the cumulative dose received.

Another serious long-term complication of alkylating agent chemotherapy is the development of secondary leukemias. In patients who have received an alkylating agent as part of combination chemotherapy for Hodgkin's or non-Hodgkin's lymphoma, the incidence of secondary acute myeloid leukemia is about 2 percent. The incidence is augmented by the addition of radiation therapy. Secondary leukemias have also followed the use of alkylating agent therapy for multiple myeloma and ovarian carcinoma. Not all the alkylating agents are equally leukemogenic. Melphalan appears to be associated with a higher incidence of secondary acute leukemia than cyclophosphamide when used in the treatment of ovarian carcinoma.

The most common dose-limiting toxicity of the alkylating agents is myelosuppression. The severity and duration varies with the individual drugs. Most of the alkylating agents are quite emetogenic and require extensive premedication. Gastrointestinal epithelial damage, however, is not prominent.

Cyclophosphamide is one of the most widely used broad-spectrum antitumor agents. It is activated by microsomal liver metabolism to 4-hydroxycyclophosphamide and is further metabolized in peripheral tissues to phosphoramide mustard and to acrolein. Cyclophosphamide therapy may be complicated by hemorrhagic cystitis. This complication is due to the metabolite acrolein, which is excreted unchanged in the urine. Adequate hydration with standard-dose therapy, and administration of the bladder protectant *mesna* with high-dose therapy, can help prevent this complication. Chronic bladder inflammation as a result of cyclophosphamide therapy has been associated with the development of malignant bladder tumors. Cyclophosphamide administration is associated with a syndrome of inappropriate antidiuresis due to a distal renal tubular effect. Cyclophosphamide is also a potent immunosuppressive agent. In very high doses it has been associated rarely with acute myocardial necrosis.

Ifosfamide is an analogue of cyclophosphamide that is less myelosuppressive but more urotoxic. It is usually administered with the uroprotectant agent mesna. A reversible neurotoxicity, manifested primarily as altered mental status, has been observed with ifosfamide. *Melphalan* is a derivative of the amino acid phenylalanine, does not require hepatic activation, and does not cause hemorrhagic cystitis. Melphalan appears to be one of the most leukemogenic alkylating agents and has been associated rarely with the development of pulmonary fibrosis. *Busulfan* is toxic to myeloid stem cells and can cause prolonged bone marrow hypoplasia. Busulfan therapy is also associated rarely with interstitial pneumonitis and progressive pulmonary fibrosis. *Mechlorethamine* (nitrogen mustard), the first alkylating agent to be used widely, currently has limited use. Mechlorethamine is highly

reactive in aqueous solution and is a severe vesicant. *Chlorambucil* is structurally related to mechlorethamine and is generally well tolerated. *Thiotepa* is a trivalent alkylating agent that currently has a limited clinical role.

Nitrosoureas The nitrosoureas *carmustine* (BCNU) and *lomustine* (CCNU) are a class of alkylating agents distinguished by high lipid solubility with excellent penetration into the central nervous system. The nitrosoureas produce a delayed myelosuppression lasting 4 to 6 weeks and appear to have a cumulative effect on the bone marrow. Moderate but reversible elevation of hepatic enzyme levels is common. A pulmonary fibrosis syndrome, similar to that seen with busulfan, has been reported. Prolonged treatment with the nitrosoureas can result in progressive renal insufficiency, even after cessation of therapy. Nitrosoureas are leukemogenic.

Platinum compounds The platinum compounds *cisplatin* and *carboplatin* are the only heavy metal compounds approved for use as antitumor agents. Although they are not true alkylating agents, they lead to the covalent cross-linking of DNA. Cisplatin is toxic to both proximal and distal renal tubule epithelial cells. Adequate intravenous hydration with saline diuresis, accompanied by administration of furosemide or mannitol, can decrease the incidence of nephrotoxicity. Nausea and vomiting are at times severe. Sensory neuropathy and high-frequency hearing loss after several cycles of therapy are not uncommon. Cisplatin produces modest myelosuppression. Carboplatin, a cisplatin analogue, is less nephrotoxic, less emetogenic, and less ototoxic, but more myelosuppressive.

Antitumor Antibiotics The antitumor antibiotics are isolated primarily from soil microorganisms. *Bleomycin* is a mixture of cytotoxic glycopeptides that interact with the ferrous iron ion (Fe^{2+}) and DNA simultaneously. This agent induces single- and double-stranded DNA breaks through free radical generation. It is cytotoxic mainly during the G2 and M phases of the cell cycle. Bleomycin has little myelosuppressive effect. Pulmonary toxicity manifested as a chronic interstitial pneumonitis is the most serious toxicity. The lifetime cumulative bleomycin dose should not exceed 200 U/m^2, and should be even less in patients with underlying pulmonary disease, previous chest radiotherapy, or advanced age. A test dose is often administered, because bleomycin infusion may be associated with hypersensitivity reactions.

Mitomycin C is activated intracellularly and then cross-links DNA. Mitomycin C exhibits delayed myelosuppression, with leukocyte and platelet counts reaching their nadir at 4 to 6 weeks. This agent can also precipitate progressive renal failure in association with a microangiopathic anemia (hemolytic-uremic syndrome).

Other Agents *Dacarbazine* appears to induce cytotoxicity by acting as an alkylating agent and damaging DNA after activation by hepatic microsomal enzymes. This agent produces moderate myelosuppression. Nausea and vomiting are often severe. *Procarbazine* is a monoamine oxidase inhibitor that, after oxidation by hepatic enzymes, functions like an alkylating agent, with methylation of nucleic acids. Procarbazine produces neurotoxicity manifested by peripheral sensory neuropathy and changes in mood and mental status. Nausea and vomiting may also be severe.

L-Asparaginase, the only enzyme used as an antitumor agent, results in depletion of extracellular pools of asparagine. Lymphocytes have a limited ability to synthesize the amino acid L-asparagine and are dependent on circulating pools. Asparaginase is associated with hypersensitivity reactions, and anaphylaxis may occur with the first dose. Hepatotoxicity, pancreatitis, and thromboses are occasionally observed.

COMBINATION CHEMOTHERAPY Most cancers are treated with multiagent chemotherapy. Although many regimens have been derived empirically, the principles that underlie most combinations of antitumor drugs can be summarized as follows. (1) Each of the agents in a regimen should have an independent activity against the specific tumor. Although unanticipated synergy may occur, adding an agent that by itself produces no response is likely to add toxicity without benefit. (2) Each drug should have a different mechanism of action. It is advantageous to target different steps along a biochemical pathway. Drugs that either inhibit the same enzyme or act by the same mechanism are less likely to have additive antitumor activity. (3) There should be no cross resistance among the agents used. A resistant tumor subpopulation selected by one drug is not likely to be cross-resistant to an agent that produces cytotoxicity through a different mechanism. (4) Each of the drugs should have a different dose-limiting toxicity. Administering two agents with the same toxicity profile at the maximum tolerated dose of each can produce unacceptable toxicity. Unfortunately, these principles are difficult to fulfill prospectively.

Bone marrow transplantation has been used to overcome severe myelosuppression after high-dose chemotherapy or chemoradiotherapy. The drugs most useful when transplantation is intended are generally the alkylating agents, such as busulfan and cyclophosphamide, which exhibit a linear response between drug dose and cell kill in vitro. Administering these drugs in myeloablative combination regimens results in higher tumor cytotoxicity. In autologous transplantation, the patient's bone marrow or peripheral blood stem cells are collected, cryopreserved, and then reinfused after delivery of systemic high-dose therapy. In allogeneic transplantation, bone marrow from a suitable donor is used to reconstitute the patient's hematopoietic system. Substantial evidence indicates that, in addition to the high-dose preparative regimens, immune effector mechanisms contribute to control of malignant disease after allogeneic bone marrow transplantation. The precise mediators of the so-called graft-versus-tumor effect remain to be elucidated. Transplantation has been most effective in treating tumors that are initially chemoresponsive, such as acute leukemia, Hodgkin's and non-Hodgkin's lymphoma, and testicular carcinoma. This approach has been ineffective, however, in treating common epithelial-derived malignancies, such as non-small cell lung carcinoma and colorectal carcinoma.

COMPLICATIONS Every chemotherapeutic regimen administered in adequate doses will have some deleterious side effect on normal tissues. Many complications can be anticipated, and considerable expertise has been gained in treating and preventing them. Myelosuppression, nausea and vomiting, stomatitis, and alopecia are the most frequently observed side effects.

Myelosuppression Chemotherapy-induced bone marrow suppression, manifested as leukopenia, thrombocytopenia, and anemia, is the most common dose-limiting toxicity. Blood counts usually reach their nadir between 10 and 14 days after treatment, with recovery noted by day 21 and a return to normal by day 28. Thus, most regimens are administered in cycles of 21 to 28 days. However, some agents, such as the nitrosoureas, involve a longer period of recovery and are usually administered every 6 weeks.

Neutropenia increases the risk of infectious complications. Fever is the hallmark of infection. Any patient with an absolute neutrophil count below 1.0×10^9/L and fever requires a prompt medical evaluation and subsequent administration of empirical, broad-spectrum parenteral antibiotics. Treatment with recombinant hematopoietic growth factors, particularly granulocyte colony stimulating factor and granulocyte-macrophage colony stimulating factor, can shorten the length of neutropenia associated with chemotherapy (see "Biologic Therapy," below).

Thrombocytopenia may occur in patients receiving chemotherapy but is less often dose-limiting than leukopenia. An increase in the bleeding time can be detected when the platelet count falls below 100×10^9/L, but most patients with platelet counts over 50×10^9/L are asymptomatic. The risk for a severe hemorrhagic complication, such as spontaneous intracranial bleeding, begins to increase when the platelet count falls below 20×10^9/L in patients with acute leukemia, or below 10×10^9/L in patients with solid tumors. Thrombocytopenia of this degree is usually observed only with very intense chemotherapeutic regimens, such as those used in the treatment of acute leukemia.

Some degree of anemia is to be anticipated with chemotherapy. However, except with dose-intensive regimens, transfusions usually are not required. In addition, there is no single hemoglobin level below which all patients should receive transfusions for chemotherapy-induced anemia. Rather, transfusions should be administered only after considering the long-term goals of therapy and weighing the risk-to-benefit ratio for each patient.

Nausea and Vomiting Nausea and vomiting are major side effects of cancer chemotherapy. Progress in preventing and treating chemotherapy-induced nausea and vomiting has resulted from the development of newer and more effective antiemetics, the completion of prospective clinical trials that addressed the problem, and the education of physicians regarding prevention and management.

Chemotherapy appears to induce nausea and vomiting through several pathways. Vomiting is controlled by two medullary centers, the vomiting center and the chemoreceptor trigger zone. The chemoreceptor trigger zone is stimulated directly by various toxins or drugs to release neurotransmitters, such as dopamine, which then interact with the vomiting center. The vomiting center coordinates the process of vomiting through multiple efferent tracts. Cerebral input, especially from visual or olfactory stimuli, can also stimulate the vomiting center.

Chemotherapeutic agents are not all equally emetogenic. Cisplatin consistently causes the most severe side effects. Dacarbazine, doxorubicin, and mechlorethamine are also highly emetogenic agents. However, many antimetabolites, such as methotrexate and fluorouracil, cause only minimal nausea and vomiting.

Prevention of nausea and vomiting should be a primary goal. Antiemetic regimens always should be given on a routine schedule, preferably beginning 24 h before chemotherapy administration. Treatment on an as-needed basis is generally inappropriate. Antiemetic regimens should err on the side of being too aggressive rather than insufficient, particularly for patients receiving chemotherapy for the first time. The treatment regimen should be commensurate with the emetogenic potential of the particular chemotherapy program.

The phenothiazines, such as *prochlorperazine* and *chlorpromazine*, are the most widely used antiemetic agents and appear to exert this effect through their antidopaminergic and antiserotoninergic activities. They are available in several formulations, making them useful for outpatient regimens. As single agents they are effective only for mildly emetogenic drugs, such as fluorouracil.

The benzamide *metoclopramide* appears to antagonize dopamine activity peripherally and centrally. When used parenterally in high doses (1 to 2 mg/kg every 2 to 4 h), it can effectively reduce the nausea and vomiting associated with the most emetogenic chemotherapeutic drugs. Metoclopramide used in high doses may cause extrapyramidal side effects and thus is often administered with an antihistamine (such as diphenhydramine) or a benzodiazepine (such as lorazepam).

The serotonin antagonists *ondansetron* and *granisetron* are the newest and among the most effective antiemetic agents. They selectively block the serotonin receptor 5-HT$_3$, which is present peripherally on the vagus nerve and centrally in the chemoreceptor trigger zone. They are effective in the treatment of nausea and vomiting due to cisplatin but are without the dystonic reactions that may accompany metoclopramide.

The cannabinoid *dronabinol* (Marinol) contains the principal psychoactive agent in marijuana, Δ-9-THC. It is available only in oral formulation and appears to be most effective against mild or moderately emetogenic chemotherapeutic regimens. It produces significant mood alterations, including dysphoria in some patients.

Other agents are frequently employed in combination antiemetic regimens. High-dose glucocorticoids, such as dexamethasone, may be used for brief intervals, particularly with metoclopramide. Benzodiazepines are useful as sedatives for patients with anticipatory nausea and vomiting and as amnestic agents. Antihistamines have modest antinausea properties but are useful to prevent dystonic reactions associated with phenothiazines or metoclopramide.

Stomatitis Stomatitis, an inflammation of the oral mucosa, is a major complication of cancer chemotherapy. Early signs of stomatitis are erythema and edema, which may progress to frank, painful ulcerations that persist for from several days to a week or longer. The painful ulcers result in poor oral intake with subsequent dehydration and malnutrition. They also may become secondarily infected and further complicate patient management. Virtually all chemotherapeutic agents will cause stomatitis if given at a sufficient dose intensity. With the antimetabolites, the duration of exposure is probably a greater risk factor for developing stomatitis than the peak drug level.

Currently, there are no means to prevent stomatitis except to modify the doses of the offending chemotherapeutic agents. Meticulous oral hygiene will help to diminish pathogenic oral flora and decrease the risk of secondary infections. Treatment with topical oral anesthetics, such as viscous xylocaine, can relieve pain and help to maintain adequate oral intake. Capsaicin may help in symptom control.

Alopecia Chemotherapy-induced hair loss is one of the most distressing aspects of cancer treatment for some patients. It is due to the cytotoxic effects of antineoplastic agents on the hair follicle. The hair loss tends to be patchy and most severe on the scalp, and it is usually noticeable 1 to 2 weeks after the beginning of therapy. After the cessation of chemotherapy, the hair should eventually return to pretreatment levels, although it may be different in texture and color. Cyclophosphamide, dactinomycin, doxorubicin, paclitaxel, and vincristine generally cause the most profound alopecia. Scalp-cooling devices, which apparently decrease scalp perfusion, have been employed with mixed results.

DRUG RESISTANCE Tumor cell resistance to chemotherapeutic agents is a central problem in medical oncology. With improvements in supportive care, including a new generation of antimicrobials, treatment with multicomponent blood products and hematopoietic growth factors, specialized oncology nursing, and high-technology intensive care units, drug resistance is probably the single most important obstacle to achieving higher cure rates.

The problem of drug resistance can be divided into two types: de novo resistance and acquired resistance. In de novo resistance, tumor cells are unresponsive to chemotherapy from the start. Unfortunately, many of the most common solid tumors show de novo resistance. In acquired drug resistance, tumors that are initially responsive to chemotherapy develop resistance with continued therapy. Acquired resistance is a primary reason why only a small percentage of the many tumors that respond to chemotherapy can be cured with chemotherapy alone.

The appearance of resistant clones within a larger population of cells was addressed initially by Delbruck and Luria in studies on bacteria and later by Law and then Goldie and Coldman in tumor cells. Delbruck and Luria observed that populations of bacteria exhibited varying degrees of resistance to bacteriophage infection. They showed that resistant cells were present in the population owing to spontaneous mutations that existed before exposure to the phage. Development of resistance depended on mutation frequency and population size.

The Delbruck-Luria principles were extended to tumor cell biology and treatment. An important property of tumor cells is genomic instability. As a tumor grows from a single transformed cell to a clinically detectable 1-cm^3 mass consisting of 10^9 cells, spontaneous mutations will give rise to a heterogeneous population of cells, some of which have mutated to a drug-resistant phenotype purely by chance. Treatment with chemotherapy will eliminate the most sensitive cells and leave the resistant subclones to grow. Clinically, this situation occurs in patients whose tumor has responded to therapy and entered a complete or partial remission, only to relapse and progress later in a drug-refractory form.

These concepts suggest important principles for maximizing the effectiveness of chemotherapy. Tumors are most likely to be responsive to chemotherapy when small in size, before multiple resistant subclones have developed. Regimens that are not effective against bulky tumors may be curative when used in the adjuvant setting. Effective treatment should consist of combination chemotherapy containing non-cross-resistant agents. The likelihood that a cell will undergo two simultaneous mutations affording resistance to two different classes of drugs is low (i.e., the product of two independent probabilities). Thus, the greater the number of non-cross-resistant drugs administered at full dose, the greater the chance of eliminating the entire tumor population.

Although the principle of combination chemotherapy is useful, limitations exist. Many antitumor agents, such as the alkylating agents, the anthracyclines, and the epipodophyllotoxins, are mutagenic and thus can actively promote the appearance of drug-resistant mutant clones. Furthermore, resistance to certain antitumor drugs can be associated with cross-resistance to other agents that are structurally and mechanistically distinct.

Mechanisms of Single-Agent Drug Resistance Much of what is known about drug resistance is a result of in vitro studies. Cell lines have been selected for resistance to various chemotherapeutic agents by exposing them to gradually increasing concentrations of the drug. Comparison of resistant sublines to the parental cell lines can reveal the resistance mechanisms. Determining the clinical importance of these in vitro mechanisms has been difficult. Examples of specific resistance mechanisms for various agents are given in Table 86-4.

Mechanisms of Multiple Drug Resistance Clinical refractoriness to chemotherapy is often characterized by resistance to multiple drugs. The phenomenon of in vitro multiple drug resistance was first described in the 1970s by Biedler and by Ling. In multiple drug resistance, cells selected for resistance to one drug show cross-resistance to other, structurally and functionally unrelated compounds. The drugs that constitute the multidrug-resistance family broadly include the anthracyclines, the vinca alkaloids, the epipodophyllotoxins, and the taxanes. Multidrug-resistant cells demonstrate an energy-dependent outward efflux of cytotoxic drugs. The resistant cell lines overexpress a membrane glycoprotein of 170 kDa termed *P-glycoprotein* or a 190 kDa membrane protein termed the *multidrug resistance protein* (MRP). Both belong to the family of ATP-binding cassette proteins.

Efflux mediated by P-glycoprotein can be blocked and multiple drug resistance circumvented by various modulating agents. Existing modulating agents, such as verapamil, quinine, and cyclosporine, have produced unacceptable toxicity when used at doses required to inhibit P-glycoprotein activity. Newer analogues, such as *dexverapamil* and *PSC 833* (a cyclosporine derivative), have entered clinical trials attempting to overcome multiple drug resistance. Agents that modulate MRP activity have to date been more difficult to identify. Although P-glycoprotein and MRP expression are well-defined mechanisms of in vitro multiple drug resistance, their role in clinical drug resistance has yet to be defined fully. In a few tumors, particularly adult acute myeloid leukemia and childhood neuroblastoma, P-glycoprotein expression at presentation portends a worse prognosis.

Altered activity and/or expression of the enzyme topoisomerase II is associated with resistance to the anthracyclines and epipodophyllo-

Table 86-4

Mechanisms of Single-Agent Drug Resistance

Mechanism	Drugs	Target
Defective transport	Methotrexate	Folate transporter
	Cytarabine	Nucleoside transporter
	Mechlorethamine	Choline transporter
Decreased activating enzyme	Cytarabine	Deoxycytidine kinase
	Mercaptopurine	Hypoxanthine-guanine phosphoribosyl transferase
	Methotrexate	Folyl-polyglutamylate synthetase
Increased drug inactivation	Bleomycin	Bleomycin hydrolase
	Cyclophosphamide	Aldehyde dehydrogenase
	Cytarabine	Cytidine deaminase
Increased target enzyme	Fluorouracil	Thymidylate synthase
	Methotrexate	Dihydrofolate reductase
	Pentostatin	Adenosine deaminase
Alteration in target	Fluorouracil	Thymidylate synthase
	Hydroxyurea	Ribonucleotide reductase
	Vincristine	Tubulin

toxins. Altered topoisomerase activity may also exist in cells that simultaneously exhibit more than one mechanism of multiple drug resistance. The clinical significance of topoisomerase II–mediated resistance is unknown.

An enhanced reducing environment with increased activity of glutathione detoxification pathways and elevated cellular pools of reduced glutathione has been described. Resistance to alkylating agents, including the nitrogen mustard derivatives and the nitrosoureas as well as the anthracyclines, has been associated with increased glutathione detoxification. *Buthionine sulfoximine*, an agent that depletes cellular glutathione levels, has entered clinical trials as a chemosensitizing agent.

Failure to undergo programmed cell death in response to genotoxic stress may contribute to insensitivity to both chemotherapy and ionizing radiation. The Bcl-2 protein is a key modulator of apoptosis and can prevent p53-dependent and -independent pathways of apoptosis. Other homologous proteins, Bcl-X and Bax, are also involved in the regulation of apoptosis. Bcl-X is expressed in two forms by differential RNA splicing. Bcl-X_L acts like Bcl-2 in preventing apoptosis. However, Bcl-X_S and Bax appear to promote cell death unless their function is blocked by heterodimerization with Bcl-2. The clinical importance of this family of proteins in chemotherapy insensitivity is an area of active investigation.

NEW DRUG DEVELOPMENT After the discovery in the 1940s of drugs with antitumor efficacy, the National Cancer Institute began a large-scale screening program. New compounds are tested against a panel of about 60 human cancer cell lines representing common solid tumors. Agents demonstrating in vitro antitumor activity are then tested against a panel of human tumor xenografts in nude mice. Compounds that are still promising then undergo further toxicology screening and formulation testing before beginning clinical trials. Antitumor agents proceed through a series of clinical trials marked by three distinct phases before they are accepted into widespread clinical use. It may take 10 years or longer for a compound to proceed from initial screening to approval by the Food and Drug Administration for a specific indication.

Phase I trials are performed to determine drug toxicity in humans. To be eligible, patients must have a cancer not responsive to available therapies. An initial dose is chosen on the basis of animal studies. Generally, small cohorts of patients are treated at a given dose before dose escalation, which proceeds sequentially until a dose-limiting toxicity is reached and the maximum tolerated dose is defined. Because phase I trials often involve a relatively small number of previously treated patients with diverse tumor types, lack of tumor response does not rule out ultimate clinical usefulness for the agent.

Phase II trials are designed to determine if a drug has activity for a particular tumor type. Generally, small groups of patients with advanced malignancies are treated according to a dose schedule determined from the phase I study. Patients must have measurable tumors, so that the efficacy of therapy can be assessed. A given compound may undergo several phase II studies against a broad array of tumor types. After the completion of phase II trials, a decision is made to proceed to phase III or to abandon further testing. Generally, compounds that induce responses in 20 percent or fewer of patients in phase II testing are not developed further.

Phase III studies are designed to test an agent against the standard existing therapy for a particular tumor. This testing usually requires a randomized, two-arm study. Patients generally have not received prior therapy at the time of treatment. Phase III trials require large numbers of patients and frequently are multi-institutional.

DIFFERENTIATING AGENTS Models of malignant transformation include the concept of maturation arrest. The clinical observation of residual differentiated masses after treatment of germ cell tumors or neuroblastoma with cytotoxic chemotherapy suggested that therapy aimed at promoting tumor cell differentiation may be effective. Studies in vitro have demonstrated that a variety of compounds could induce tumor cells to differentiate and to display characteristics of a more mature phenotype. Agents such as retinoids, vitamin D, phorbol esters, and polar/planar compounds (such as dimethyl sulfoxide) have been extensively characterized for their effects on tumor cell lines.

Retinoids stimulate the growth of normal myeloid and erythroid progenitors in culture and the differentiation of myeloid leukemia cell lines in vitro. Clinical trials showed that all-*trans*-retinoic acid (ATRA; *tretinoin*) induced remissions in a high percentage of patients with acute promyelocytic leukemia, although the duration of remission was on average short (<6 months). Tretinoin commonly produces headache and dermatologic toxicity. A minority of patients, however, will experience a syndrome of fever, pulmonary infiltrates, and respiratory distress. Prompt treatment with glucocorticoids may prevent worsening of the capillary leak syndrome. Clinical evaluation of tretinoin, as well as other retinoids and differentiating agents, continues.

ENDOCRINE THERAPY Endocrine therapy for hormone-responsive malignancies depends on the existence of underlying cellular growth control mechanisms derived from those of the normal tissues from which the tumor arose. For example, the presence of estrogen and progesterone receptors in breast carcinoma is predictive of a response to endocrine therapy. Many hormonal antitumor agents are functional agonists or antagonists of the steroid hormone family. Steroid hormones bind to specific intracellular receptors and induce a conformational change. The hormone-receptor complex interacts with DNA and functions as a transcription factor regulating gene expression.

Adrenocorticosteroids Because the toxicities of glucocorticoids do not overlap with those of many chemotherapeutic agents, and in particular do not include myelosuppression, glucocorticoids are frequently used in combination regimens for the treatment of lymphocytic leukemias and lymphomas. They function by binding to glucocorticoid-specific receptors present in lymphoid cells and initiating programmed cell death. Although several synthetic glucocorticoids are available, the agents most often used in cancer therapy are *prednisone*, *methylprednisolone*, and *dexamethasone*.

Antiandrogens The antiandrogen *flutamide* effectively blocks the binding of androgen to its receptor in peripheral tissues. Although serum testosterone levels may rise, levels in the target tissues are decreased. Flutamide is used in the treatment of disseminated prostate carcinoma and is often used with leuprolide. It has predictable antiandrogen side effects in men, including gynecomastia, decreased libido, and impotence. Elevation of hepatic transaminase levels has also been reported.

Estrogens Estrogen therapy was once a mainstay in the palliative treatment of disseminated prostate carcinoma, where it appears to function as a potent antiandrogen. Estrogens are occasionally used in the palliative treatment of breast carcinoma. Two commonly used preparations are *diethylstilbesterol* (DES) and *ethinyl estradiol*. Estrogen therapy can exacerbate underlying ischemic heart disease, may predispose to thromboembolic phenomena, and may lead to fluid retention. Gynecomastia and impotence in men is common.

Antiestrogens The antiestrogen *tamoxifen* is widely used in the therapy of breast carcinoma. It is employed in the adjuvant setting in postmenopausal women and as palliative therapy for metastatic disease in both premenopausal and postmenopausal women. Tamoxifen binds directly to the estrogen receptor and appears to function as a weak agonist/antagonist. It has a long plasma half-life and requires 4 weeks or longer to achieve steady state levels. Tamoxifen can cause amenorrhea, hot flashes, and, rarely, nausea and vomiting. It has been reported to modestly increase the risk of thromboembolic phenomenon. Chronic use is associated with a slightly increased risk of endometrial cancer. On the other hand, tamoxifen lowers the risk of death from cardiovascular disease and prevents osteoporosis.

Progestins Progestational agents such as *medroxyprogesterone* and *megestrol acetate* are used in the treatment of endometrial carcinoma and breast carcinoma. Studies suggest they may disrupt the hypothalamic-pituitary-gonadal axis, alter expression of estrogen receptors, or have androgenic effects. Progestins frequently cause menstrual irregularities. Fluid retention, elevated levels of hepatic enzymes, and thromboembolic events have all been reported.

Aromatase Inhibitor *Aminoglutethimide* inhibits the enzymatic pathway responsible for the conversion of androgens to estrogens in the peripheral tissues. It also inhibits the conversion of cholesterol to pregnenolone, a key step in steroid hormone biosynthesis. Aminoglutethimide treatment functions as a medical adrenalectomy, and patients receiving relatively high doses may need maintenance hydrocortisone and/or mineralocorticoid. It is used in the palliative treatment of metastatic breast carcinoma. Toxicity includes mild neurologic and dermatologic symptoms. On rare occasions, reversible leukopenia and thrombocytopenia have been observed.

Gonadotropin-Releasing Hormone Agonists The gonadotropin-releasing hormone (GnRH) agonist *leuprolide* is used in the treatment of disseminated prostate carcinoma. Continuous stimulation of the pituitary by GnRH—as opposed to the normal pulsatile control—leads to eventual downregulation of luteinizing hormone (LH) and follicle-stimulating hormone (FSH) secretion, with subsequent diminution of androgen levels. During the first weeks of therapy, increased LH and FSH release may precipitate a worsening of symptoms, which may be avoided by instituting antiandrogen treatment. Antiandrogen effects, including gynecomastia, impotence, and hot flashes, are seen to a varying degree.

Somatostatin Analogues The somatostatin analogue *octreotide* is used in the symptomatic treatment of patients with metastatic carcinoid or vasoactive intestinal peptide–secreting tumors. Somatostatin analogues suppress the release of gastric and pancreatic peptides in addition to suppressing growth hormone release. Patients with functional endocrine tumors who are receiving octreotide experience a dramatic decrease in endocrine-related symptoms. The drug must be injected subcutaneously two or three times daily to maintain adequate relief of symptoms. Because somatostatin inhibits insulin secretion, patients must be monitored for hyperglycemia.

BIOLOGIC THERAPY

Most biologic agents act as *biologic response modifiers*, meaning that they function by altering the host response to cancer; however, some cause direct cytotoxicity. Assessing the clinical usefulness of these agents is at times difficult because the paradigms for cytotoxic chemotherapy may be inappropriate for biologic agents. Biologic agents usually demonstrate peak activity within a narrow concentration range; higher or lower concentrations may result in a suboptimal effect. Thus, the optimal clinical dose is the one that produces the maximum desired effect, which may not be the highest dose tolerated without unacceptable toxicity.

IMMUNOTHERAPY Manipulation of the host immune response to cancer is a major goal of biologic therapy. Animal studies have conclusively shown that the immune system can recognize and eliminate malignant tumors in vivo. Rejection of tumor cells in several animal models appears to be mediated primarily by cytotoxic lymphocytes, including cytotoxic T lymphocytes and natural killer cells. Other effector cells, such as helper T cells, B cells, and macrophages, may also participate. However, antitumor immune responses have been difficult to demonstrate in patients with cancer. Furthermore, immune recognition of malignant cells can occur without resulting in tumor rejection. Cancer immunotherapy seeks to evoke effective immune responses to human tumors. Approaches have included administration of monoclonal antibodies, immunomodulatory cytokines, autologous or allogeneic immunocompetent cells, and tumor vaccines.

Monoclonal Antibodies The ability to produce monoclonal antibodies to a specific antigenic determinant led to high expectations for their widespread use in cancer therapy. Although monoclonal antibodies are important tools in cancer diagnosis, their use in cancer therapy has remained investigational. Trials of unconjugated monoclonal antibodies as cytotoxic therapy have generally proved disappointing. Obstacles have included difficulty in defining tumor-specific antigens serologically, antigenic modulation by tumor cells, and the development of human anti-mouse antibodies. Efforts to improve the efficacy of this approach have led to ongoing trials of antibodies conjugated to drugs, radioisotopes, or toxins. Clinical studies are evaluating the use of monoclonal antibodies in purging harvested bone marrow of tumor cells before autologous transplantation.

The immunophenotyping of leukemias and lymphomas using monoclonal antibodies directed primarily against myeloid and lymphoid differentiation antigens has improved our understanding of the pathogenesis of these diseases and has facilitated diagnosis. It is now common to analyze the immunophenotype of all lymphoid and myeloid specimens. Monoclonal antibody–based serum assays are commonly used for monitoring disease progress in solid tumors. CA-125 can be used to monitor ovarian carcinoma, and the prostate-specific antigen (PSA) to monitor prostate cancer, although widespread use of PSA as a tool for screening is controversial.

Immunomodulatory Cytokines Cytokines are intercellular messenger proteins. They include the interferons and interleukins. Interferons α and β share a common cellular receptor and are referred to as type I interferons. *Interferon* α is the product of a multigene family of at least 20 members, whereas *interferon* β is the product of a single gene. Type I interferons have immunoregulatory and antiproliferative effects. Recombinant interferon α is approved for use in the treatment of chronic myeloid leukemia, hairy cell leukemia, and AIDS-related Kaposi's sarcoma; it is an effective adjuvant therapy for high-risk melanoma. In addition, interferon α has activity in low-grade non-Hodgkin's lymphoma, multiple myeloma, and renal cell carcinoma. *Interferon* γ, produced by lymphocytes, is referred to as type II interferon and has immunomodulatory properties distinct from those of type I interferons. It appears to have less single-agent antitumor activity than type I interferons. It is used in the treatment of chronic granulomatous disease but remains investigational as an antitumor agent. All interferons can produce a flu-like syndrome with fever, malaise, myalgias, and fatigue. Modest leukopenia is also common, and elevations in hepatic transaminase levels can be seen.

The interleukins are cytokines that function predominantly as leukocyte messengers. At least 17 interleukins have been identified, and several have entered clinical trials, but only recombinant *interleukin 2* is an approved anticancer agent. Interleukin (IL)-2, previously known as T-cell growth factor, is a key regulatory hormone in cell-mediated immunity. It stimulates the proliferation and cytolytic activity of T cells and natural killer cells. High-dose IL-2 therapy produces a response in a minority of patients with metastatic renal cell carcinoma and melanoma. A small percentage (5 to 10 percent) of patients achieve a complete response associated with long-term disease-free survival. However, cardiovascular complications, largely due to a vascular leak syndrome, may necessitate intensive care unit management. Other toxicities, which can involve virtually every organ system (particularly renal, hepatic, pulmonary, neurologic, hematopoietic, and dermatologic toxicities), are seen but are generally reversible. Trials of outpatient therapy using reduced doses, often administered by continuous infusion, have resulted in less acute toxicity. The optimal dose and schedule of IL-2 therapy have not been defined.

The other interleukins remain investigational agents for cancer therapy. *Interleukin 4* is produced primarily by T cells and mast cells and has diverse immunohematopoietic effects. Several phase I/II trials of IL-4 alone or in combination with IL-2 have been completed. Although IL-4 can be safely administered with only moderate toxicity, the low rates of tumor response have diminished enthusiasm for its ultimate role as an antitumor agent. *Interleukin 6* is a pleiotropic cytokine that has direct antiproliferative activity in a variety of tumor model systems, in addition to immunohematopoietic activity that directly affects B cells, T cells, and megakaryocytes. Clinical trials have begun to assess IL-6 as an antitumor agent and as a thrombopoietic agent. *Interleukin 12* stimulates the function of both T cells and natural killer cells. Phase I trials of IL-12 in patients with cancer and AIDS have been conducted, and additional clinical studies are in progress.

Tumor necrosis factor (TNF) plays a central role in the inflammatory response. TNF administration produces impressive antitumor responses in animal models. However, pronounced toxicity (mainly cardiovascular) in humans after systemic administration, combined with low tumor response rates, has limited its clinical development. The use of TNF for local and regional therapy, as in isolated limb perfusion, is under investigation.

Cellular Therapy Adoptive cellular therapy consists of transferring either autologous or allogeneic immune effector cells to a tumor-bearing host. Autologous effectors generally are activated and expanded ex vivo before administration. Lymphokine-activated killer (LAK) cells, generated by culturing peripheral blood lymphocytes with IL-2, can directly lyse freshly isolated solid tumor cells. However, administration of LAK cells generated ex vivo together with IL-2 does not appear to be better than administration of IL-2 alone. Tumor-infiltrating lymphocytes (TIL), isolated directly from solid tumors, can also be expanded ex vivo with IL-2. In experimental systems, TIL demonstrate significantly more antitumor efficacy than LAK cells. Although early clinical trials in patients with metastatic melanoma are promising, it is not known whether administration of TIL is more effective than IL-2 alone. Allogeneic immune effector cells have been used to treat patients who have relapsed after bone marrow transplantation. Clinical, cytogenetic, and molecular complete remissions have been induced in patients with chronic myeloid leukemia after infusion of donor-derived buffy coats. Complications have included graft-versus-host disease and myelosuppression (See Chap. 116).

Tumor Vaccines The search for cancer vaccines effective in humans was stimulated by animal models that demonstrated protection from tumor challenges after immunization with syngeneic tumors or their derivatives. However, rejection of previously established solid tumors in experimental systems has been generally possible only when combined with a reduction in tumor burden, as by surgery. Thus, tumor vaccines may prove most effective in humans when used as adjuvants or in a setting of minimal disease. The question of which are the optimal immunogens remains unresolved. The injection of autologous whole tumor cells (unmodified, modified, or with an adjuvant) has resulted in modest objective tumor responses in some patients with melanoma. However, the generally low response rates and short remission duration have prompted further investigations. Gene transfer techniques to induce the expression of immunomodulatory molecules, such as B7, IL-12, or granulocyte-macrophage colony stimulating factor (GM-CSF), may increase the immunogenicity of the autologous tumor.

HEMATOPOIETIC GROWTH FACTORS Hematopoietic growth and differentiation are under the regulation of cytokines known as colony stimulating factors (CSFs). These agents were initially defined by their ability to stimulate and support hematopoietic colony formation in vitro using a semisolid culture system. Thus, the classification of a cytokine as a CSF or an interleukin is primarily a historical artifact. The isolation and subsequent clinical development of hematopoietic growth factors has substantially changed the clinical care of patients receiving myelosuppressive chemotherapy. In particular, the two agents that support neutrophil maturation, *granulocyte-macrophage CSF* (GM-CSF) and *granulocyte CSF* (G-CSF), have received widespread acceptance despite the fact that their optimal clinical use is not defined. To better guide clinicians, both the American Society of Clinical Oncology (ASCO) and the European Consensus Conference assembled expert panels to review the clinical data and to issue guidelines for the use of colony stimulating factors. The ASCO guidelines are summarized in Table 86-5 (see also Chap. 105).

GM-CSF promotes the differentiation of committed myeloid progenitors into mature granulocytes, monocytes, and eosinophils. It also stimulates growth of the multilineage hematopoietic precursors. Recombinant GM-CSF hastens myeloid reconstitution after autologous bone marrow transplantation. GM-CSF administration is associated with constitutional symptoms (fevers, chills, myalgias, anorexia, lethargy) and bone pain. G-CSF stimulates the growth and differentiation of committed neutrophilic progenitor cells. Administration of G-CSF to patients can shorten the period of neutropenia associated with

Table 86-5

Use of Colony Stimulating Factors in Patients with Cancer

Circumstance	Recommendation
Primary administration (beginning with first cycle of chemotherapy)	Not recommended for routine use (unless febrile neutropenia is expected in $\geq$40% of patients or patient has a preexisting risk factor)
Secondary administration (after an episode of febrile neutropenia)	May be used, although reduction in chemotherapy dose should be considered as an alternative unless dose intensity is important
In afebrile neutropenic patients	Not recommended for routine use
In febrile neutropenic patients	May be used if factors predictive of deterioration are present (such as pneumonia, hypotension, sepsis, fungal infection)
To make possible an increase in the dose intensity of chemoterapy	Not recommended for routine use
To shorten the duration of neutropenia after bone marrow transplantation	May be routinely recommended to mobilize peripheral blood progenitor cells and to speed hematopoietic reconstitution
In patients with acute myeloid leukemia	May be used after induction chemotherapy in patients $\geq$55 years
In patients with myelodysplasia	May be used intermittently (if neutropenia and recurrent infection are present)

chemotherapy-induced myeloid suppression. Clinical experience suggests that G-CSF may be better tolerated than GM-CSF, but randomized studies comparing the two cytokines have not been reported. Bone pain is the most common side effect of G-CSF.

Interleukin 3 stimulates the growth and differentiation of multipotent hematopoietic progenitors as well as committed erythroid, myeloid, and megakaryocytic precursors. Clinical trial results have been disappointing.

Erythropoietin, the primary regulator of erythropoiesis, induces erythroid maturation in committed progenitor cells and increases the release of reticulocytes from the bone marrow. Erythropoietin is produced by the kidney and liver in response to hypoxia. Recombinant erythropoietin is clearly beneficial in treating deficiency states such as the anemia of chronic renal failure. Patients receiving myelosuppressive chemotherapy experience anemia to varying degrees, and clinical trials have demonstrated that erythropoietin is modestly effective in ameliorating this form of anemia after at least 2 months of use. However, many patients with cancer suffer from the anemia of chronic disease, which is associated with a blunted response to erythropoietin, and they are thus less likely to benefit from its use.

Thrombopoietin (previously known as the Mpl ligand) has been identified. It has been shown to support megakaryocyte maturation and platelet production and has entered clinical trials.

Cytokines that appear to be responsible for maintenance of the multipotent hematopoietic stem cell have also been identified. The *Flk2/Flt3 ligand* and *stem-cell* or *Steel factor* activate specific tyrosine kinase receptors that appear to be restricted to the earliest stem cells. They act synergistically with later-acting hematopoietic growth factors, such as IL-3 or GM-CSF, to cause proliferation and expansion of hematopoietic progenitors. They are just beginning to be tested in humans.

See Chap. 51, Thyroid and antithyroid drugs, in Goodman & Gilman's The Pharmacological Basis of Therapeutics, *9th ed, JG Hardman, LE Zimbrid (eds), New York, McGraw-Hill, 1996.*

BIBLIOGRAPHY

AMERICAN SOCIETY OF CLINICAL ONCOLOGY UPDATE OF RECOMMENDATIONS FOR USE OF HEMATOPOIETIC COLONY-STIMULATING FACTORS: Evidence-based, clinical practice guidelines. J Clin Oncol 14:1957, 1996

BOOGAERTS M et al: Granulocyte growth factors: Achieving a consensus. Ann Oncol 6:237, 1995

CHABNER BA, LONGO DL: *Cancer Chemotherapy and Biotherapy: Principles and Practice*. Philadelphia, Lippincott, 1996

DEVITA VT et al (eds): *Biologic Therapy of Cancer*, 2d ed. Philadelphia, Lippincott, 1995

DRUGS OF CHOICE FOR CANCER CHEMOTHERAPY. Med Let 37:25, 1995

FISHER DE: Apoptosis in cancer therapy: Crossing the threshold. Cell 78:539, 1994

HOLLAND JF et al (eds): *Cancer Medicine*, 4th ed. Philadelphia, Lea & Febiger, 1996

PIZZO PH: Management of fever in patients with cancer and treatment-induced neutropenia. N Engl J Med 328:1323, 1993

87 *Robert Finberg*

INFECTIONS IN PATIENTS WITH CANCER

Infections are a common cause of death and an even more common cause of morbidity in patients with a wide variety of neoplasms. Autopsy studies show that most deaths from acute leukemia and half of deaths from lymphoma are caused directly by infection. With more intensive chemotherapy, patients with solid tumors have become more likely to die of infection rather than their underlying disease.

A physical predisposition to infection (Table 87-1) can be a result of the neoplasm's production of a break in the skin; for example, a squamous cell carcinoma may cause local invasion of the epidermis, which allows bacteria to gain access to the subcutaneous tissue and permits the development of cellulitis. The artificial closing of a normally patent orifice can also predispose to infection: Obstruction of a ureter by a tumor can cause urinary tract infection, and obstruction of the bile duct can cause cholangitis. Part of the host's normal defense against infection depends on the continuous emptying of a viscus; without emptying, a few bacteria present as a result of bacteremia or local transit can multiply and cause disease.

A similar problem can affect patients whose lymph node integrity has been disrupted by radical surgery, particularly patients who have had radical node dissections. A common clinical problem following radical mastectomy is the development of cellulitis (usually caused by streptococci or staphylococci) because of lymphedema and/or inadequate lymph drainage. In most cases, this problem can be addressed by local measures designed to prevent fluid accumulation and breaks in the skin, but antibiotic prophylaxis has been necessary in refractory cases.

A life-threatening problem common to many cancer patients is the loss of the reticuloendothelial capacity to clear microorganisms after splenectomy. Splenectomy is common in patients with Hodgkin's disease and in the management of hairy-cell leukemia, chronic lymphocytic leukemia (CLL), and refractory idiopathic thrombocytopenic purpura. Even after curative therapy for the underlying disease, the lack of a spleen predisposes such patients to rapidly fatal infections. The loss of the spleen through trauma similarly predisposes the normal host to overwhelming infection as long as 25 years after splenectomy. The splenectomized patient should be counseled about the risks of infection with certain organisms, such as the protozoan *Babesia* (Chap. 216) and *Capnocytophaga canimorsus* (formerly, dysgonic fermenter 2 or DF-2), a bacterium carried in the mouths of animals (Chap. 135). Since encapsulated bacteria (*Streptococcus pneumoniae, Haemophilus influenzae,* and *Neisseria meningitidis*) are the organisms most commonly associated with postsplenectomy sepsis, splenectomized persons should be vaccinated (and revaccinated; see Table 87-2) against the capsular polysaccharides of these organisms. Many clinicians recommend giving splenectomized patients a small supply of antibiotics effective against *S. pneumoniae, N. meningitidis,* and *H. influenzae* to avert rapid, overwhelming sepsis in the event that they cannot present for medical attention immediately after the onset of fever or other symptoms of bacterial infection.

The level of suspicion of infections with certain organisms should depend on the type of cancer diagnosed (Table 87-3). Diagnosis of multiple myeloma or CLL should prompt the measurement of immunoglobulin levels and the consideration of either antibody replacement or antibiotic prophylaxis. (In the case of CLL, antibiotic prophylaxis for likely pathogens has proven a cost-effective preventive measure.) Similarly, patients with acute lymphocytic leukemia (ALL), patients with non-Hodgkin's lymphoma, and all cancer patients treated with high-dose steroids (or steroid-containing chemotherapy regimens)

Table 87-1

Normal Barriers to Infections

Type of Defense	Specific Lesion	Cells Involved	Organisms	Cancer Association	Disease
Physical barrier	Breaks in skin	Skin epithelial cells	Staphylococci, streptococci	Head and neck, squamous cell carcinoma	Cellulitis, extensive skin infection
Emptying of fluid collections	Occlusion of orifices: ureters, bile duct, colon	Luminal epithelial cells	Gram-negative bacilli	Renal, ovarian, biliary tree, metastatic diseases of many cancers	Rapid, overwhelming bacteremia, urinary tract infection
Lymphatic disease	Node dissection	Lymph nodes	Staphylococci, streptococci	Breast cancer surgery	Cellulitis
Splenic clearance of microorganisms	Splenectomy	Splenic reticuloendothelial cells	*Streptococcus pneumoniae, Haemophilus influenzae, Neisseria meningitidis, Babesia, Capnocytophaga canimorsus*	Hodgkin's disease, leukemia, idiopathic thrombocytopenic purpura	Rapid, overwhelming sepsis
Phagocytosis	Lack of granulocytes	Granulocytes (neutrophils)	Staphylococci, streptococci, enteric organisms	Hairy-cell, acute myelocytic, and acute lymphocytic leukemias	Bacteremia
Humoral immunity	Lack of antibody	B cells	*S. pneumoniae, H. influenzae, N. meningitidis*	Chronic lymphocytic leukemia	Infections with encapsulated organisms, sinusitis, pneumonia
Cellular immunity	Lack of T cells	T cells and macrophages	*Mycobacterium tuberculosis, Listeria,* herpesviruses, fungi, other intracellular parasites	Hodgkin's disease, leukemia, T cell lymphoma	Infections with intracellular bacteria, fungi, parasites

should receive antibiotic prophylaxis for *Pneumocystis carinii* infection (Table 87-3).

In addition to their susceptibility to certain infectious organisms, patients with cancer are likely to manifest their infections in characteristic ways.

SYSTEM-SPECIFIC SYNDROMES

SKIN-SPECIFIC SYNDROMES (Plate ID-57) Skin lesions are common in cancer patients, and their appearance may permit the diagnosis of systemic bacterial or fungal infection. While cellulitis caused by skin organisms such as *Streptococcus* or *Staphylococcus* is common, neutropenic patients and those with impaired blood or lymphatic drainage may develop infections with unusual organisms. Innocent-looking macules or papules may be the first sign of bacterial or fungal sepsis in immunocompromised patients. In the neutropenic host, a macule progresses rapidly to ecthyma gangrenosum, a usually painless, round, necrotic lesion consisting of a central black or gray-black eschar with surrounding erythema. Ecthyma gangrenosum is located in nonpressure areas (as distinguished from necrotic lesions associated with lack of circulation) and is often associated with *Pseudomonas aeruginosa* bacteremia (Chap. 157) but may be caused by other bacteria.

Candidemia (Chap. 207) is also associated with a variety of skin conditions and commonly presents as a maculopapular rash. Punch biopsy of the skin may be the best method for diagnosis.

Cellulitis, an acute spreading inflammation of the skin, is most often caused by infection with group A *Streptococcus* or *Staphylococcus aureus*, virulent organisms normally found on the skin (Chap. 133). Although cellulitis tends to be circumscribed in normal hosts, it may spread rapidly in neutropenic patients [those with fewer than 500 functional polymorphonuclear leukocytes (PMNs) per cubic millimeter]. A tiny break in the skin may lead to spreading cellulitis, which is characterized by pain and erythema; in such patients, signs of infection (e.g., purulence) are often lacking. What might be a furuncle in a normal host may require amputation because of uncontrolled infection in a patient presenting with leukemia. A dramatic response to an infection that might be trivial in a normal host can mark the first sign of leukemia. Fortu-

nately, granulocytopenic patients are likely to be infected with certain types of organisms (Table 87-4); thus the selection of an antibiotic regimen is somewhat easier than it might otherwise be. (See discussion on the selection of antibiotics for use in neutropenic patients, below.) It is essential to recognize cellulitis early and to treat it aggressively. Patients who are neutropenic or have previously received antibiotics for other reasons may develop cellulitis with unusual organisms (e.g., *Escherichia coli*, *Pseudomonas*, or fungi). Early treatment, even of innocent-looking lesions, is essential to prevent necrosis and loss of tissue. Debridement to prevent spread may sometimes be necessary early in the course of disease, but it can often be performed after chemotherapy, when the PMN count increases.

Sweet's syndrome, or *febrile neutrophilic dermatosis*, was originally described in women with elevated white blood cell counts. The disease is characterized by the presence of leukocytes in the lower dermis, with edema of the papillary body. Ironically, this disease now is usually seen in patients with neutropenic cancer, most often in association with acute leukemia but also in association with a variety of other malignancies. Sweet's syndrome usually presents as red or bluish-red papules or nodules that may coalesce and form sharply bordered plaques. The edema may suggest vesicles, but on palpation the lesions are solid, and vesicles probably never arise in this disease. The lesions are most common on the face, neck, and arms. On the legs, they may be confused with erythema nodosum. The development of lesions is often accompanied by high fevers and an elevated erythrocyte sedimentation rate. Both the lesions and the temperature elevation respond dramatically to steroids. Treatment begins with high doses of steroids (60 mg of prednisone per day) followed by tapered doses over the next 2 to 3 weeks.

Recent data indicate that *erythema multiforme* with mucous membrane involvement is often associated with herpes simplex virus (HSV) infection and is distinct from Stevens-Johnson syndrome, which is associated with drugs and tends to have a more widespread distribution. Since cancer patients are both immunosuppressed (and therefore susceptible to herpes infections) and heavily treated with drugs (and therefore subject to Stevens-Johnson syndrome), both of these conditions are common in this population.

Cytokines, which are used as adjuvants or primary treatments for cancer, can themselves cause characteristic rashes, further complicating the differential diagnosis. This phenomenon is a particular problem in bone marrow transplant recipients (Chap. 136), who, in addition to having the usual chemotherapy-, antibiotic-, and cytokine-induced rashes, are plagued by graft-versus-host disease.

CATHETER-RELATED INFECTIONS Because intravenous catheters are commonly used in cancer chemotherapy and are prone to infection (Chap. 137), they pose a major problem in the care of patients with cancer. Recent reviews have emphasized that some infected catheters can be treated with antibiotics while others must be removed. If the patient has a "tunneled" catheter (which consists of an entrance site, a subcutaneous tunnel, and an exit site), a red streak over the subcutaneous part of the line (the tunnel) is grounds for immediate removal of the catheter. Failure to remove catheters under these circumstances may result in extensive cellulitis and tissue necrosis.

More common than tunnel infections are exit-site infections, often with erythema around the area where the line penetrates the skin. Most authorities (Chap. 142) recommend treatment (usually with vancomycin) for an exit-site

Table 87-2

Vaccination of Cancer Patients Receiving Chemotherapy

| Vaccine | Use in Indicated Patients | | |
	Intensive Chemotherapy	Hodgkin's Disease	Bone Marrow Transplantation
Diphtheria-tetanus (diphtheria, pertussis, tetanus; DPT) for children <7 years old	Primary series and boosters as necessary	No special recommendation	12 and 24 months after transplantation
Poliomyelitis*	Complete primary series and boosters	No special recommendation	12 and 24 months after transplantation
Haemophilus influenzae type b	Primary series and booster for children	Immunization before treatment and booster 2 years afterward	12 and 24 months after transplantation
23-Valent pneumococcal	Every 6 years	Immunization before treatment and booster 2 years afterward	12 and 24 months after transplantation
4-Valent meningococcal	Every 6 years	Immunization before treatment and booster 2 years afterward	12 and 24 months after transplantation
Influenza	Seasonal immunization	Seasonal immunization	Seasonal immunization
Measles/mumps/rubella	Contraindicated	Contraindicated	After 24 months in patients without graft-versus-host disease
Varicella-zoster virus	Contraindicated†	Contraindicated	Contraindicated

* Live virus vaccine is contraindicated; inactivated vaccine should be used.
† Contact the manufacturer for more information on use in children with acute lymphocytic leukemia.

infection caused by a coagulase-negative *Staphylococcus*. Treatment of coagulase-positive staphylococcal infection is associated with a poorer outcome, and it is advisable to remove the catheter. Similarly, many clinicians remove catheters associated with infections due to *P. aeruginosa* and *Candida* species, since such infections are difficult to treat, and bloodstream infections with these organisms are likely to be deadly.

GASTROINTESTINAL TRACT–SPECIFIC SYNDROMES
Upper Gastrointestinal Tract Disease The oral cavity is rich in aerobic and anaerobic bacteria (Chap. 169) that normally live in a commensal relationship with the host. The antimetabolic effects of chemotherapy cause a breakdown of host defenses, leading to ulceration of the mouth and the potential for invasion by resident bacteria. Mouth ulcerations afflict most patients receiving chemotherapy and have been associated with viridans streptococcal bacteremia. A variety of topical rinses and elixirs have been proposed to treat these ulcerations. Although some may have a local anesthetic effect, the efficacy of any of these therapies in the prevention of disease is unproven. Similarly, the efficacy of mouthwashes in the prevention of esophagitis or invasive candidiasis is doubtful. Fluconazole, on the other hand, is clearly effective in the treatment of both local infections (thrush) and systemic infections (esophagitis) due to *Candida albicans*.

Noma (or *cancrum oris*), commonly seen in malnourished children, is a penetrating disease of the soft and hard tissues of the mouth and adjacent sites, with resulting necrosis and gangrene. It has a counterpart in immunocompromised patients and is thought to be due to invasion of the tissues by *Bacteroides*, *Fusobacterium*, and other normal inhabitants of the mouth. It is associated with debility, poor oral hygiene, and immunosuppression.

Viruses, particularly HSV, are a prominent cause of morbidity in immunocompromised patients, in whom they are associated with severe mucositis. The use of acyclovir, either prophylactically or therapeutically, is of value.

The differential diagnosis of esophagitis (usually presenting as substernal chest pain upon swallowing) includes herpes simplex and candidiasis, both of which are readily treatable.

Lower Gastrointestinal Tract Disease Hepatic candidiasis (Chap. 207) results from seeding of the liver (usually from a gastrointestinal source) in neutropenic patients. It is most common in patients being treated for acute leukemia and usually develops around the time the neutropenia resolves. The characteristic picture is that of persistent fever unresponsive to antibiotics; abdominal pain and tenderness or nausea; and elevated serum levels of alkaline phosphatase in a patient with hematologic malignancy who has recently recovered from neutropenia. The diagnosis of this disease (which may present in an indolent manner and persist for several months) is based on the finding of yeasts or pseudohyphae in granulomatous lesions. Hepatic ultrasound or computed tomography (CT) may reveal bull's-eye lesions. In some cases, magnetic resonance imaging (MRI) reveals small lesions not visible by other imaging modalities. The pathology (a granulomatous response) and the timing (with resolution of neutropenia and an elevation in granulocyte count) suggest that the host response to *Candida* is an important component of the manifestations of disease. In many cases, although organisms are visible, cultures of biopsied material may be negative. The designation *hepatosplenic candidiasis* or *hepatic candidiasis* is a misnomer because the disease often involves the kidneys and other tissues; the term *chronic disseminated candidiasis* may be more appropriate. Because of the risk of bleeding with liver biopsy, diagnosis is often based on radiographic abnormalities.

Amphotericin B is traditionally used for therapy (often for several months, until all manifestations of disease have disappeared), but fluconazole may be useful for outpatient therapy.

Typhlitis *Typhlitis*, sometimes referred to as necrotizing colitis, neutropenic colitis, necrotizing enteropathy, ileocecal syndrome, or cecitis, is a clinical syndrome of fever and right-lower-quadrant tenderness in an immunosuppressed host. This syndrome is almost always seen in neutropenic patients after chemotherapy with cytotoxic drugs. It may be more common among children than among adults and appears to be much more common among patients with acute myelocytic leukemia (AML) or ALL. Physical examination reveals right-lower-quadrant tenderness, with or without rebound tenderness. Associated diarrhea (often bloody) is common, and the diagnosis can be confirmed by the finding of a thickened cecal wall on CT or ultrasonography. Plain films may reveal a right-lower-quadrant mass, but CT with contrast or MRI is a much more sensitive means of making the diagnosis. Although surgery is sometimes attempted to avoid perforation from ischemia, most cases resolve with medical therapy alone. The disease is sometimes associated with positive blood cultures (usually for aerobic gram-negative bacilli), and therapy is recommended for a broad spectrum of bacteria (particularly gram-negative bacilli, likely bowel flora). Recurrence is rare, and most patients recover uneventfully.

***Clostridium difficile*–Induced Diarrhea** Cancer patients seem to be predisposed to the development of *C. difficile* diarrhea (Chap. 148) as a consequence of chemotherapy alone. Thus, they may have positive toxin tests before receiving antibiotics. Obviously, such patients are also subject to *C. difficile*–induced diarrhea as a result of antibiotic pressure. It is worth noting that toxins other than *C. difficile* may be associated with diarrhea; therefore, the detection of nonspecific toxins in the stool—without a specific neutralization test—does not prove that *C. difficile* infection is present. → *The treatment of* C. difficile *infection is discussed in Chap. 148.*

CENTRAL NERVOUS SYSTEM–SPECIFIC SYNDROMES
Meningitis While meningitis in immunocompetent adults is likely to be caused by *S. pneumoniae*, the same is not true in immunocompromised patients. As noted previously, splenectomized patients are susceptible to rapid overwhelming infection with encapsulated bacteria (including *S. pneumoniae*, *H. influenzae*, and *N. meningitidis*). Similarly, patients who are antibody deficient (such as patients with CLL, those who have received intensive chemotherapy, or those who have undergone bone marrow transplantation) are likely to have infections with these bacteria. Other cancer patients, however, because of their defective cellular immunity, are likely to be infected with other patho-

Table 87-3

Infections and Cancer

Cancer	Underlying Immune Abnormality	Organisms Causing Infection
Multiple myeloma	Hypogammaglobulinemia	*Streptococcus pneumoniae*, *Haemophilus influenzae*, *Neisseria meningitidis*
Chronic lymphocytic leukemia	Hypogammaglobulinemia	*S. pneumoniae*, *H. influenzae*, *N. meningitidis*
Acute myelocytic or lymphocytic leukemia	Granulocytopenia, skin and mucous-membrane lesions	Extracellular gram-positive and gram-negative bacteria, fungi
Hodgkin's disease	Abnormal T-cell function	Intracellular pathogens (*Mycobacterium tuberculosis*, *Listeria*, *Salmonella*, *Cryptococcus*, *Mycobacterium avium*)
Non-Hodgkin's lymphoma and acute lymphocytic leukemia	Steroid chemotherapy, T- and B-cell dysfunction	*Pneumocystis carinii*
Colon and rectal tumors	Local abnormalities*	*Streptococcus bovis* (bacteremia)
Hairy-cell leukemia	Abnormal T-cell function	Intracellular pathogens (*M. tuberculosis*, *Listeria*, *Cryptococcus*, *M. avium*)

* The reason for this association is not well defined.

Table 87-4

Organisms Likely to Cause Infections in Granulocytopenic Patients

Gram-positive cocci	*Enterobacter* species
Staphylococcus epidermidis	*Serratia* species
Staphylococcus aureus	*Acinetobacter* species*
Viridans *Streptococcus*	*Citrobacter* species
Enterococcus faecalis	Gram-positive bacilli
Streptococcus pneumoniae	Diphtheroids
Gram-negative bacilli	JK bacillus*
Escherichia coli	Fungi
Klebsiella species	*Candida* species
Pseudomonas aeruginosa	*Aspergillus* species
Non-*aeruginosa Pseudomonas* species*	

* Often associated with intravenous catheters.

gens (see Table 87-3). The presentation of meningitis in patients with lymphoma, patients receiving chemotherapy (particularly with steroids) for solid tumors, and patients who have received bone marrow transplants suggests a diagnosis of cryptococcal or listerial infection.

Encephalitis The spectrum of disease resulting from viral encephalitis is expanded in immunocompromised patients. Infection with varicella-zoster virus (VZV) has been associated with encephalitis that may be caused by VZV-related vasculitis. The slow viruses (e.g., Creutzfeldt-Jakob agent) may also be associated with dementia and encephalitic presentations, and a diagnosis of progressive multifocal leukoencephalopathy should be considered when a patient who has received chemotherapy presents with dementia. Other abnormalities of the central nervous system (CNS) that may be confused with infection include normal-pressure hydrocephalus and vasculitis resulting from CNS irradiation. It may be possible to differentiate these conditions by MRI.

Brain Abscess Brain abscesses in immunocompromised patients are likely to be due to *Cryptococcus* (particularly in patients with lymphoma or those receiving steroids), *Nocardia*, or *Aspergillus*. *Aspergillus* may enter via the lungs or—like *Mucor*—may invade the hard and soft palates to cause pneumonia (see below) with or without brain abscesses.

PULMONARY INFECTIONS Pneumonia (Chap. 255) in immunocompromised patients may be difficult to diagnose because conventional methods of diagnosis depend on the presence of neutrophils. Bacterial pneumonia in neutropenic patients may present without purulent sputum—or, in fact, without any sputum at all—and may not produce physical findings suggestive of chest consolidation (rales or egophony).

In granulocytopenic patients with persistent or recurrent fever, the chest x-ray pattern may help to localize an infection and thus to determine which investigative tests and procedures should be undertaken and which therapeutic options should be considered (Table 87-5). The difficulties encountered in the management of pulmonary infiltrates relate in part to the difficulties of performing diagnostic procedures on the patients involved. When platelet counts can be increased to adequate levels by transfusion, microscopic and microbiologic evaluation of the fluid obtained by endoscopic bronchial lavage is often diagnostic. Lavage fluid should be cultured for *Mycoplasma*, *Chlamydia*, *Legionella*, *Nocardia*, fungi, and more common bacterial pathogens. In addition, the possibility of *P. carinii* pneumonia should be considered, especially in patients with ALL or lymphoma who have not received prophylactic trimethoprim-sulfamethoxazole. The characteristics of the infiltrate may be helpful in decisions about further diagnostic and therapeutic maneuvers. Nodular infiltrates suggest fungal pneumonia (e.g., that caused by *Aspergillus* or *Mucor*).

Aspergillus species (Chap. 208) can colonize the skin and respiratory tract or cause fatal systemic illness. Although *Aspergillus* may cause aspergillomas in a previously existing cavity or may produce allergic bronchopulmonary aspergillosis, the major problem posed by this genus in neutropenic patients is invasive disease due to *Aspergillus*

fumigatus or *Aspergillus flavus*. The organisms enter the host through colonization of the respiratory tract, with subsequent invasion of the blood vessels. The disease is likely to present as a thrombotic or embolic event because of the ability of the organisms to invade blood vessels. The risk of infection with *Aspergillus* correlates directly with the duration of neutropenia. In prolonged neutropenia, positive surveillance cultures for colonization of the nasopharynx with *Aspergillus* may predict the development of disease.

Patients with *Aspergillus* infection often present with pleuritic chest pain and fever, which are sometimes accompanied by cough. Hemoptysis may be an ominous sign. Chest x-rays may reveal new focal infiltrates or nodules (Table 87-5). Chest CT may reveal a characteristic halo consisting of a mass-like infiltrate surrounded by an area of low attenuation. The presence of a "crescent sign" on a chest x-ray or a chest CT scan, in which the mass progresses to central cavitation, is characteristic of invasive *Aspergillus* infection but may develop only with the resolution of the lesions.

In addition to causing pulmonary presentations, *Aspergillus* may invade through the nose or palate, with deep sinus penetration. The appearance of a discolored area in the nasal passages or on the hard palate should prompt a search for invasive *Aspergillus*. This situation is likely to require surgical debridement. Treatment (Chap. 208) with high doses of amphotericin B has been successful in curing granulocytopenic patients of invasive *Aspergillus* infection after the return of granulocytes. Catheter infections with *Aspergillus* usually require both removal of the catheter and antifungal therapy.

Diffuse interstitial infiltrates suggest viral or parasitic pneumonia. If the patient has a diffuse interstitial pattern on chest x-ray, it may be reasonable to institute empirical treatment with trimethoprim-sulfamethoxazole (for *Pneumocystis*) and erythromycin (for *Chlamydia*, *Mycoplasma*, and *Legionella*) while considering invasive diagnostic procedures. Noninvasive procedures, such as staining of sputum smears for *Pneumocystis* and serum cryptococcal antigen tests, may be helpful on occasion. In transplant recipients who are seropositive for cytomegalovirus (CMV), culture of a nonpulmonary site for CMV may be worthwhile. Infections with viruses that cause only upper respiratory symptoms in immunocompetent hosts, such as respiratory syncytial, influenza, and parainfluenza viruses, may be associated with fatal pneumonitis in immunocompromised hosts. An attempt at early diagnosis by nasopharyngeal aspiration should be considered so that appropriate treatment can be instituted.

While bleomycin is the most common cause of chemotherapy-induced lung disease, other causes include alkylating agents (such as cyclophosphamide, chlorambucil, and melphalan), nitrosoureas [carmustine (BCNU), lomustine (CCNU), and methyl-CCNU], busulfan, procarbazine, methotrexate, and hydroxyurea. Both infectious and noninfectious (drug- and/or radiation-induced) pneumonitis can cause fever and abnormalities on chest x-ray; thus, the differential diagnosis of an infiltrate in a patient receiving chemotherapy encompasses a

Table 87-5

Differential Diagnosis of Chest Infiltrates in Immunocompromised Patients

	Cause of Pneumonia	
Infiltrate	Infectious	Noninfectious
Localized	Common bacterial pulmonary pathogens, *Legionella*, mycobacteria	Local hemorrhage or embolism, tumor
Nodular	Fungi (e.g., *Aspergillus* or *Mucor*), *Nocardia*	Recurrent tumor
Diffuse	Viruses (especially CMV), *Chlamydia*, *Pneumocystis carinii*, *Toxoplasma gondii*, mycobacteria	Congestive heart failure, radiation pneumonitis, drug-induced lung injury, diffuse alveolar hemorrhage (described after BMT)

ABBREVIATIONS: CMV, cytomegalovirus; BMT, bone marrow transplantation.

broad range of conditions (Table 87-5). Since the treatment of radiation pneumonitis (which may respond dramatically to glucocorticoids) or drug-induced pneumonitis is different from that of infectious pneumonia, a biopsy may be important in the diagnosis. Unfortunately, no definitive diagnosis can be made in approximately 30 percent of cases, even after bronchoscopy.

Open lung biopsy is the gold standard of diagnostic techniques. Biopsy via a visualized thoracostomy can replace an open procedure in many cases. When a biopsy cannot be performed, empirical treatment can be undertaken with erythromycin and trimethoprim-sulfamethoxazole (in the case of diffuse infiltrates) or with amphotericin B (in the case of nodular infiltrates). The risks should be weighed carefully in these cases. If inappropriate drugs are administered, empirical treatment may prove toxic or ineffective; either of these outcomes may be riskier than biopsy.

CARDIOVASCULAR INFECTIONS Patients with Hodgkin's disease are prone to persistent infections by *Salmonella*, sometimes (and particularly often in elderly patients) affecting a vascular site. The use of intravenous catheters deliberately lodged in the right atrium is associated with a high incidence of bacterial endocarditis (presumably related to valve damage followed by bacteremia). Nonbacterial thrombotic endocarditis has been described in association with a variety of malignancies (most often solid tumors) and reportedly follows bone marrow transplantation as well. The presentation of an embolic event with a new cardiac murmur suggests this diagnosis. Blood cultures are negative in this disease of unknown pathogenesis.

ENDOCRINE SYNDROMES In addition to infections of the skin, gastrointestinal tract, and pulmonary system, infections of the endocrine system have been described in immunocompromised patients. *Candida* infection of the thyroid during neutropenia can be defined by indium-labeled white-cell scans or gallium scans after neutrophil counts increase. CMV infection can cause adrenalitis with or without resulting adrenal insufficiency. The presentation of a sudden endocrine anomaly in an immunocompromised patient may be a sign of infection in the involved end organ.

MUSCULOSKELETAL INFECTIONS Infection that is a result of vascular compromise (resulting in gangrene) can occur when a tumor compromises the blood supply to muscles, bones, or joints. The process of diagnosis and treatment of such infection is similar to that in normal hosts, with the following caveats: (1) In terms of diagnosis, a lack of physical findings resulting from a lack of granulocytes in the granulocytopenic patient should make the clinician more aggressive in obtaining tissue rather than relying on physical signs. (2) In terms of therapy, aggressive debridement of infected tissues may be required, but it is usually difficult to operate on patients who have recently received chemotherapy, both because of a lack of platelets (which results in bleeding complications) and because of a lack of white blood cells (which may lead to secondary infection). A blood culture positive for *Clostridium perfringens* (an organism commonly associated with gas gangrene) can have a number of meanings (Chap. 148). Bloodstream infections with intestinal organisms like *Streptococcus bovis* and *C. perfringens* may arise spontaneously from lower gastrointestinal lesions (tumor or polyps); alternatively, these lesions may be harbingers of invasive disease. The clinical setting must be considered in order to define the appropriate treatment for each case.

RENAL AND URETERAL INFECTIONS Infections of the urinary tract are common among patients whose ureteral excretion is compromised (Table 87-1). *Candida*, which has a predilection for the kidney, can invade either from the bloodstream or in a retrograde manner (via the ureters or bladder) in immunocompromised patients. The presence of "fungus balls" or persistent candiduria suggests invasive disease. Persistent funguria (with *Aspergillus* as well as *Candida*) should prompt a search for a nidus of infection in the kidney.

Certain viruses are typically seen only in immunosuppression. BK virus (polyomavirus hominis 1) has been documented in the urine of bone marrow transplant recipients and, like adenovirus, may be associated with hemorrhagic cystitis. BK-induced cystitis usually re-

mits with decreasing immunosuppression. Anecdotal reports have described the treatment of adenovirus with ribavirin in cases of severe hemorrhagic cystitis in immunocompromised patients.

ABNORMALITIES THAT PREDISPOSE TO INFECTION

THE LYMPHOID SYSTEM It is beyond the scope of this chapter to detail how all the immunologic abnormalities that result from cancer or from chemotherapy for cancer lead to infections. Disorders of the immune system are discussed in other sections of this book. As has been noted, patients with antibody deficiency are predisposed to overwhelming infection with encapsulated bacteria (including *S. pneumoniae*, *H. influenzae*, and *N. meningitidis*). Infections that result from the lack of a functional cellular immune system are described in the chapter on AIDS (Chap. 308). It is worth mentioning, however, that patients undergoing intensive chemotherapy for any form of cancer will have not only defects due to granulocytopenia but also lymphocyte dysfunction, which may be profound. Thus, these patients—especially those receiving steroid-containing regimens—should be given prophylaxis for *P. carinii* pneumonia.

THE HEMATOPOIETIC SYSTEM Initial studies in the 1960s revealed a dramatic increase in the incidence of infections (fatal and nonfatal) among cancer patients with a granulocyte count of <500/mm³. Recent studies have cited a figure of 48.3 infections per 100 neutropenic patients (<1000 granulocytes per cubic millimeter) with hematologic malignancies and solid tumors, or 46.3 infections per 1000 days at risk.

Neutropenic patients are unusually susceptible to infection with a wide variety of bacteria; thus, antibiotic therapy should be initiated promptly to cover likely pathogens if infection is suspected. Indeed, early initiation of antibacterial agents is mandatory to prevent deaths. These patients are susceptible to gram-positive and gram-negative organisms found commonly on the skin and in the bowel (Table 87-4). Because treatment with narrow-spectrum agents leads to infection with organisms not covered by the antibiotics used, the initial regimen should target pathogens likely to be initial causes of bacterial infection in neutropenic hosts (Fig. 87-1).

FIGURE 87-1 Diagnosis and treatment of febrile neutropenic patients: an algorithm.

℞ TREATMENT

Antibacterial Therapy Hundreds of antibacterial regimens have been tested for use in neutropenic patients with cancer. Many of the relevant studies involved small populations in which the outcomes were generally good, and most lacked the statistical power to detect differences among the regimens studied. Each febrile neutropenic patient should be approached as a unique problem, with particular attention given to previous infections and recent exposures to antibiotics. Several general guidelines are useful in the initial treatment of neutropenic patients with fever (Fig. 87-1):

1. It is necessary to use antibiotics active against both gram-negative and gram-positive bacteria (see Table 87-4) in the initial regimen.
2. An aminoglycoside or a quinolone (e.g., ciprofloxacin) alone is not adequate in this setting.
3. The agents used should reflect both the epidemiology and the antibiotic resistance pattern of the hospital. For example, in hospitals where there is gentamicin resistance, amikacin-containing regimens should be considered; in hospitals with frequent *P. aeruginosa* infections, a regimen with the highest level of activity against this pathogen (such as tobramycin plus a semisynthetic penicillin) would be reasonable for initial therapy.
4. A single third-generation cephalosporin constitutes an appropriate initial regimen in many hospitals (if the pattern of resistance justifies its use).
5. Most standard regimens are designed for patients who have not previously received prophylactic antibiotics. The development of fever in a patient receiving antibiotics affects the choice of subsequent therapy (which should target resistant organisms and organisms known to cause infections in patients being treated with the antibiotics already administered).

The initial antibacterial regimen should be refined on the basis of culture results (Fig. 87-1). Blood cultures are the most relevant cultures on which to base therapy; surface cultures of skin and mucous membranes may be misleading. In the case of gram-positive bacteremia or another gram-positive infection, it is important that the antibiotic be optimal for the organism isolated. If the infection is caused by certain gram-negative pathogens (such as *P. aeruginosa*), a synergistic combination of antibiotics (usually a semisynthetic penicillin, such as piperacillin, plus an aminoglycoside) may be appropriate. Although it is not desirable to leave the patient unprotected, the addition of more and more antibacterial agents to the regimen is not appropriate unless there is a clinical or microbiological reason to do so. *Planned progressive therapy* (the serial, empirical addition of one drug after another without culture data) is not efficacious in most settings and may have unfortunate consequences. Cephalosporins can cause bone marrow suppression, and vancomycin is associated with neutropenia in some healthy people (Chap. 140). Furthermore, the addition of multiple cephalosporins may induce β-lactamase production by some organisms; cephalosporins and double β-lactam combinations should probably be avoided altogether in *Enterobacter* infections.

Antifungal Therapy Fungal infections in cancer patients are most often associated with neutropenia. Neutropenic patients are predisposed to the development of invasive fungal infections, most commonly those due to *Candida* and *Aspergillus* species and occasionally those caused by *Fusarium*, *Trichosporon*, and *Bipolaris*. Cryptococcal infection, which is common among patients taking immunosuppressive agents, is uncommon among neutropenic patients receiving chemotherapy for AML. Invasive candidal disease is usually caused by *C. albicans* or *Candida tropicalis* but can be caused by *Candida krusei*, *Candida parapsilosis*, and *Candida glabrata*.

Most clinicians add amphotericin B to antifungal regimens if a neutropenic patient remains febrile despite 4 to 7 days of treatment with antibacterial agents. The rationale for the empirical addition of amphotericin B is that it is difficult to culture fungi before they cause disseminated disease and that mortality from disseminated fungal infections in granulocytopenic patients is high. The imidazoles (especially fluconazole) may have prophylactic efficacy in this regard, but their spectrum of activity is narrower than that of amphotericin B. Amphotericin B is the mainstay of therapy for disseminated *Candida* or *Aspergillus* infection in the neutropenic patient. The combined use of an imidazole and amphotericin B is controversial because of the theoretical antagonistic effects of these agents. The insolubility of amphotericin B has resulted in the marketing of several amphotericin B–lipid formulations. Most of these formulations appear to be less toxic than amphotericin B alone, but their therapeutic superiority has not yet been clearly proven in head-to-head trials. Thus, recommendations for their use as first-line therapy are problematic.

Other Therapeutic Modalities Another way to address the problems of the febrile neutropenic patient is to replenish the neutrophil population. Although granulocyte transfusions are efficacious in the treatment of refractory gram-negative bacteremia, they do not have a documented role in prophylaxis. Because of the expense, the risk of leukoagglutinin reactions (although this risk has probably been decreased by improved cell-separation procedures), and the risk of transmission of CMV from unscreened donors, granulocyte transfusion is reserved for patients unresponsive to antibiotics. This modality is efficacious for documented gram-negative bacteremia refractory to antibiotics, particularly in situations where granulocyte numbers will be depressed for only a short period.

A variety of cytokines, including granulocyte colony-stimulating factor and granulocyte-macrophage colony-stimulating factor, enhance granulocyte recovery after chemotherapy and consequently shorten the period of maximal vulnerability to fatal infections. The role of these cytokines in routine practice is still a matter of some debate. Most authorities recommend their use only when neutropenia is both severe and prolonged. The cytokines themselves may have adverse effects, including fever, hypoxemia, and pleural effusions or serositis in other areas. Since there is little evidence that their routine administration lessens the risk of death and since they are still expensive, the cytokines have not become the standard of care in all centers. The role of other cytokines (such as macrophage colony-stimulating factor for monocytes or interferon-γ) in preventing or treating infections in granulocytopenic patients is under investigation.

Once neutropenia has resolved, patients are not at high risk of infection. However, depending on what drugs they receive, patients who continue on chemotherapeutic protocols continue to be at high risk for certain diseases. Any patient receiving more than a maintenance dose of glucocorticoids (including many treatment regimens for diffuse lymphoma) should also receive prophylactic trimethoprim-sulfamethoxazole because of the risk of *P. carinii* infection; those with ALL should receive such prophylaxis for the duration of chemotherapy.

PREVENTION OF INFECTION IN CANCER PATIENTS

EFFECT OF THE ENVIRONMENT Outbreaks of fatal *Aspergillus* infection have been associated with construction and construction materials in several hospitals. The association between spore counts and risk of infection suggests the need for a high-efficiency air-handling system in hospitals that care for large numbers of neutropenic patients. The use of laminar-flow rooms and prophylactic antibiotics has decreased the number of infectious episodes in severely neutropenic patients. However, because of the expense of such a program and the failure to show that it dramatically affects mortality, most centers do not routinely use laminar flow to care for neutropenic patients. Some centers use "reverse isolation," in which health care providers and visitors to a patient who is neutropenic are dressed in

gowns and gloves. Since most of the infections these patients develop are due to organisms that colonize the patients' own skin and bowel, the validity of such schemes is dubious, and limited clinical data do not support their use. Hand washing by all staff caring for neutropenic patients should be required to prevent the spread of resistant organisms.

The presence of large numbers of bacteria (particularly *P. aeruginosa*) in certain foods, especially fresh vegetables, has led some authorities to recommend a special "low-bacteria" diet. A diet consisting of cooked and canned food is satisfactory to most neutropenic patients and does not involve elaborate disinfection or sterilization protocols.

PHYSICAL MEASURES Although few studies address this issue, patients with cancer are predisposed to infections resulting from anatomic compromise (e.g., lymphedema resulting from node dissections after radical mastectomy). Surgeons who specialize in cancer surgery can provide specific guidelines for the care of such patients, and patients benefit from common-sense advice about how to prevent infections in vulnerable areas.

ANTIBIOTIC PROPHYLAXIS There is no consensus on the use of prophylactic antibiotics in neutropenic patients. The incidence of infection is lower among patients who receive broad-spectrum antibiotic prophylaxis than among those who do not. Because of the prolongation of neutropenia associated with the use of trimethoprim-sulfamethoxazole, some clinicians use broad-spectrum agents such as quinolones (e.g., ciprofloxacin). Either regimen can be given orally, and both have the advantage of inactivity against anaerobic organisms; thus, neither is unlikely to disrupt the bowel flora and permit colonization with new aerobes or *Candida*. However, both regimens have adverse effects and can lead to the selection of resistant organisms in a hospital. For these reasons, many clinicians reserve their use for patients with the longest periods of neutropenia (e.g., bone marrow transplant recipients). The same issues apply to the use of antifungal agents. While agents such as fluconazole may prevent infections with susceptible organisms (e.g., *C. albicans*), they can cause a concomitant increase in infections due to resistant fungi (e.g., *C. krusei*). Thus, the decision to use antifungal prophylaxis may vary with the fungi endemic in a given hospital. Prophylaxis for *P. carinii* is mandatory for patients with ALL and for all cancer patients receiving steroid-containing chemotherapy regimens.

VACCINATION OF CANCER PATIENTS In general, patients undergoing chemotherapy respond less well to vaccines than normal hosts. Their greater need for vaccines thus leads to a dilemma in their management. Purified proteins and inactivated vaccines are almost never contraindicated and should be given to patients even during chemotherapy. For example, all adults should receive diphtheria-tetanus toxoid boosters at the indicated times, as well as seasonal influenza vaccine. However, if possible, vaccination should not be undertaken concurrent with chemotherapy. If patients are expected to be receiving chemotherapy for several months and vaccination is indicated (for example, influenza vaccination in the fall), the vaccine should be given midcycle—as far as possible from the antimetabolic agents that will prevent an immune response. The meningococcal and pneumococcal polysaccharide vaccines should be given to patients before splenectomy, if possible. The Advisory Committee on Immunization Practices recommends reimmunization every 6 years for the pneumococcal vaccine; although no official stand has been taken, this recommendation seems reasonable for the meningococcal vaccine as well. The *H. influenzae* type b conjugate vaccine should be administered to all splenectomized patients; there is no current recommendation for reimmunization, but immunity appears to be much longer-lasting than that induced by polysaccharide vaccines.

In general, live virus (or live bacterial) vaccines should not be given to patients during intensive chemotherapy because of the risk of disseminated infection. Recommendations on vaccination are summarized in Table 87-2.

BIBLIOGRAPHY

AMBROSINO DM, MOLRINE DC: Critical appraisal of immunization strategies for prevention of infection in the compromised host. Hematol Oncol Clin North Am 7:1027, 1993

AMERICAN SOCIETY OF CLINICAL ONCOLOGY: Recommendations for the use of hematopoietic colony-stimulating factors: Evidence-based, clinical practice guidelines. J Clin Oncol 12:2471, 1994

CARLISLE PS et al: Nosocomial infections in neutropenic cancer patients. Infect Control Hosp Epidemiol 14:320, 1993

GREENE JN: Catheter-related complications of cancer therapy. Infect Dis Clin North Am 10:255, 1996

LEW MA et al: Ciprofloxacin versus trimethoprim/sulfamethoxazole for prophylaxis of bacterial infections in bone marrow transplant recipients: A randomized, controlled trial. J Clin Oncol 13:239, 1995

MAYORDOMO JI et al: Improving treatment of chemotherapy-induced neutropenic fever by administration of colony-stimulating factors. J Natl Cancer Inst 87:803, 1995

MOONEY BR et al: Infection control and bone marrow transplantation. Am J Infect Control 21:131, 1993

SEPKOWITZ KA et al: *Pneumocystis carinii* pneumonia among patients without AIDS at a cancer hospital. JAMA 267:832, 1992

SICKLES EA et al: Clinical presentation of infection in granulocytopenic patients. Arch Intern Med 135:715, 1975

88 | *Arthur J. Sober, Howard K. Koh, Nhu-Linh T. Tran, Carl V. Washington, Jr.*

MELANOMA AND OTHER SKIN CANCERS

Pigmented skin lesions are among the most common findings on physical examination. The challenge is to distinguish cutaneous melanomas, which may be lethal, from the remainder, which with rare exceptions are benign. Cutaneous neoplasms are depicted in Section IB **(Plate IB-18 to 25)** of the Color Atlas; benign and malignant pigmented lesions are in Section IC **(Plate IC-26 to 31)**.

MELANOMA

Melanomas originate from melanocytes, pigment cells present normally in the epidermis and sometimes in the dermis. This tumor affects approximately 38,300 individuals per year in the United States, resulting in 7300 deaths. The tumor can affect adults of all ages, even young individuals (starting in the mid-teens); it has distinct clinical features that make it detectable at a time when cure by surgical excision is possible; and it is located on the skin surface, where it is visible. The incidence has increased dramatically (a 300 percent increase in the past 40 years). If the incidence continues to increase at the present rate, within a decade, lifetime risk of melanoma will approximate 1 percent or higher.

The reason for the increase in melanoma incidence is uncertain but may involve increased recreational sun exposure, especially early in life. Individuals of similar ethnic background who immigrate after childhood to areas of high sun exposure (e.g., Israel and Australia) have lower melanoma rates than individuals of similar age who were either born in those countries or immigrated before age 10. The individuals most susceptible to development of melanoma are those with fair complexions, red or blond hair, blue eyes, and freckles and who tan poorly and sunburn easily. In one literature survey, 9 of 11 studies linked increased melanoma risk to history of sunburn. Other factors associated with increased risk include a family history of melanoma (approximately 1 in 10 melanoma patients have a family member with melanoma); the presence of a clinically atypical mole (dysplastic nevus), a giant congenital melanocytic nevus, or a small to medium-sized congenital melanocytic nevus (see below); the presence of a higher than average number of ordinary melanocytic nevi; and immunosuppression (Table 88-1). A 64-fold increased risk for individuals with 50 or more moles ≥2 mm in size has been reported. About 30 percent of melanomas arise in a nevus. Melanoma is relatively rare in heavily pigmented peoples. Dark-skinned populations (such as those

Table 88-1

Risk Factors for Cutaneous Melanoma

High risk (>50-fold increase in risk)
  Persistently changing mole
  Clinically atypical moles in patient with two family members with melanoma
  Adulthood (vs. childhood)
  >50 nevi ≥2 mm in diameter
Intermediate risk (~10-fold increase in risk)
  Family history of melanoma
  Sporadic clinically atypical moles
  Congenital nevi (?)
  White ethnicity (vs. black or East Asian ethnicity)
  Personal history of prior melanoma
Low risk (2- to 4-fold increase in risk)
  Immunosuppression
  Sun sensitivity or excess exposure to sun

SOURCE: Adapted from Rhodes et al.

of India and Puerto Rico), blacks, and East Asians have rates 10 to 20 times lower than lighter-skinned whites. In keeping with the role of sun exposure, the incidence is inversely correlated with the latitude of residence; at any latitude, however, darker-skinned persons have the lowest incidence.

CLINICAL CHARACTERISTICS There are four types of cutaneous melanoma (Table 88-2). In three of these—superficial spreading melanoma, lentigo maligna melanoma, and acral lentiginous melanoma—the lesion has a period of superficial (so-called radial) growth during which it increases in size but does not penetrate deeply. It is during this period that the melanoma is most capable of being cured by surgical excision. The fourth type—nodular melanoma—does not have a recognizable radial growth phase and usually presents as a deeply invasive lesion, capable of early metastasis. When tumors begin to penetrate deeply into the skin, they are in the so-called vertical growth phase. Melanomas with a radial growth phase are characterized by irregular and sometimes notched borders, variation in pigment pattern, and variation in color. An increase in size or change in color is noted by the patient in 70 percent of early lesions. Bleeding, ulceration, and pain are late signs and are of little help in early recognition. Nodular melanomas are dark brown-black to blue-black nodules. Mela-nomas occasionally are amelanotic, in which case the diagnosis is established histologically after biopsy of a new or changing skin nodule. Lentigo maligna melanoma is usually confined to chronically sun-damaged, sun-exposed sites (face, neck, back of hands) in older individuals. Acral lentiginous melanoma occurs on the palms, soles, nail beds, and mucous membranes. While this type occurs in whites, it is most frequent (along with nodular melanoma) in blacks and East Asians. Superficial spreading melanoma is most frequent in whites. Melanomas arising in dysplastic nevi (see below) are usually of this type. The back is the most common site for melanoma in men. In women, the back and the lower leg (from knee to ankle) are frequent sites.

PROGNOSTIC FACTORS The most important prognostic factor is the stage at the time of presentation [see the discussion of revised American Joint Cancer Commission (AJCC) staging categories, below]. Five-year survival for clinical stages I and II (primary tumor; no clinical evidence of disease elsewhere) is about 85 percent. For clinical stage III (clinically palpable regional nodes that contain tumor), the 5-year survival is about 50 percent when only one node is involved and about 15 to 20 percent when four or more nodes are involved. The 5-year survival for clinical stage IV (disseminated disease) is less than 5 percent. Fortunately, most melanomas are diagnosed in clinical stages I and II. Within these stages, the prognosis depends on the thickness of the primary tumor (Table 88-3). This system is based on the rationale that the likelihood of metastasis should correlate with tumor volume, with thickness being the best single index of tumor volume. Melanomas less than 0.76 mm thick are usually cured by surgical removal (with 5-year survival rates of 96 to 99 percent). Approximately 40 percent of primary melanomas now fall in a low-risk category (thickness <1 mm). In low-risk patients who develop metastases, the primary tumors often exhibit either extensive microscopic features of regression or a vertical growth phase. Approximately 60 percent of individuals with melanomas ≥3.65 mm thick will develop metastatic disease and die of their melanoma. These thick tumors almost always are raised substantially above the plane of the skin. Two intermediate categories of thickness exist (Table 88-3). Certain anatomic sites affect the prognosis. The favorable sites appear to be the forearm and leg (excluding feet), while unfavorable sites include scalp, hands, feet, and mucous membranes. In general, women with stage I or II disease have a better survival than men, perhaps in part because of earlier diagnosis; women frequently have melanomas on the lower leg, where self-recognition is more likely and prognosis is better. Older individuals, in general, have poorer prognoses. This

Table 88-2

Clinical Features of Malignant Melanoma

Type	Site	Average Age at Diagnosis, Years	Duration of Known Existence, Years	Color
Lentigo maligna melanoma	Sun-exposed surfaces, particularly malar region of cheek and temple	70	5–20* or longer	In flat portions, shades of brown and tan predominant, but whitish gray occasionally present; in nodules, shades of reddish brown, bluish gray, bluish black
Superficial spreading melanoma	Any site (more common on upper back and, in women, on lower legs)	40–50	1–7	Shades of brown mixed with bluish red (violaceous), bluish black, reddish brown, and often whitish pink, and the border of lesion is at least in part visibly and/or palpably elevated
Nodular melanoma	Any site	40–50	Months to less than 5 years	Reddish blue (purple) or bluish black; either uniform in color or mixed with brown or black
Acral lentiginous melanoma	Palm, sole, nail bed, mucous membrane	60	1–10	In flat portions, dark brown predominantly; in raised lesions (plaques) brown-black or blue-black predominantly

* During much of this time, the precursor stage, lentigo maligna, is confined to the epidermis.

SOURCE: Adapted from AJ Sober, in *Pathophysiology of Dermatologic Diseases*, NA Soter, HP Baden (eds). New York, McGraw-Hill, 1984.

Table 88-3

CHAPTER 88
Melanoma and Other Skin Cancers **545**

Prognosis of Melanoma by Thickness (Breslow) and AJCC Stages: 5-Year Survival Rates

AJCC Stage	Thickness Range, mm	% Overall Survival
IA (localized)	≤0.75	96
IB (localized)	0.76–1.50	87
IIA (localized)	1.5–2.49	75
	2.50–3.99	66
IIB (localized)	≥4.00	47
III (metastatic to regional nodes)		45 (one node)
		<20 (two nodes)
IV (metastatic to distant sites)		8–10*

* One-year survival

finding has been explained in part by a tendency toward later diagnosis (and thus thicker tumors) in men and by a higher proportion in men of acral melanomas (palmar-plantar), which have a poorer prognosis. Melanoma may recur after many years. About 10 to 15 percent of first-time recurrences develop more than 5 years after treatment of the original lesion. The time to recurrence varies inversely with tumor thickness. Other prognostic factors for stages I and II melanoma include the presence of an ulcer in the primary tumor, the mitotic rate, and the presence of microscopic tumor satellites (foci of tumor ≥0.05 mm in diameter in the reticular dermis or subcutaneous fat, distinct from the main body of the tumor). The presence of microscopic satellites is also predictive of microscopic metastases to the regional lymph nodes. An alternate prognostic scheme for clinical stages I and II melanoma, proposed by Clark, is based on the anatomic level of invasion in the skin. Level I is intraepidermal (in situ); level II penetrates the papillary dermis; level III spans the papillary dermis; level IV penetrates the reticular dermis; and level V penetrates into the subcutaneous fat. The 5-year survival for these stages averages 100, 95, 82, 71, and 49 percent, respectively.

NATURAL HISTORY Melanomas may spread by the lymphatic channels or the bloodstream. The earliest metastases are often to regional lymph nodes. Surgical lymphadenectomy usually controls regional disease. Liver, lung, bone, and brain are common sites of hematogenous spread, but unusual sites, such as the anterior chamber of the eye, also may be involved. Once widespread metastatic disease is established, the likelihood of cure is low.

MANAGEMENT The entire cutaneous surface, including the scalp and mucous membranes, should be examined in each patient. Bright room illumination is important, and a 7× to 10× hand lens is helpful for evaluating variation in pigment pattern. A history of relevant risk factors should be elicited. Any suspicious lesions should be biopsied, evaluated by a specialist, or recorded by chart and/or photography for follow-up. Examination of the lymph nodes and palpation of the abdominal viscera are part of the staging examination for suspected melanoma. The patient should be advised to have other family members screened if either melanoma or clinically atypical moles (dysplastic nevi) are present. The detection of early melanoma in relatives on screening has been reported. Melanoma prevention is based on protection from the sun. Routine use of a sunblock of SPF ≥15, use of protective clothing, and avoiding intense midday ultraviolet exposure should be recommended. The patient should be educated in the clinical features of melanoma and advised to report any growth or other change in a pigmented lesion. Patient education brochures are available from the American Cancer Society, the American Academy of Dermatology, the National Cancer Institute, and the Skin Cancer Foundation. Self-examination at 6- to 8-week intervals may enhance the likelihood of detecting change between follow-up visits. The importance of routine follow-up visits for melanoma patients and patients with clinically atypical moles (dysplastic nevi) should be emphasized, as these visits may facilitate early detection of new tumors.

Precursor Lesions Clinically atypical moles, also termed *dysplastic nevi*, occur in certain families affected by melanoma. In some families, melanomas occur nearly exclusively in the individuals with dysplastic nevi. These nevi appear to be transmitted as an autosomal dominant trait that involves chromosome 9p16. In other families, the nevi may not be present in all individuals with an increased risk of melanoma. The melanomas may arise in clinically atypical moles or in normal skin; (in the latter situation the mole acts as a marker of increased risk). Individuals with clinically atypical moles and two family members with melanoma have been reported to have a greater than 50 percent lifetime risk for developing melanoma. Table 88-4 lists the features that are characteristic of clinically atypical moles and that differentiate them from benign acquired nevi. The number of clinically atypical moles may vary from one to several hundred. Clinically atypical moles usually differ from each other in appearance. The borders are often hazy and indistinct, and the pigment pattern is more highly varied than that in benign acquired nevi. Of the 90 percent of melanoma patients whose disease is regarded as sporadic (i.e., who lack a family history of melanoma), about 40 percent have clinically atypical moles, as compared with an estimated 5 to 10 percent of the population at large. Further studies to determine the background frequency of clinically atypical moles are required, once greater unanimity exists regarding their clinical and histopathologic features. The observation that at least 20 percent of sporadic melanomas arise in association with a clinically atypical mole makes this nevus the most important precursor for melanoma.

Less frequent precursors include the giant congenital melanocytic nevus and the small congenital melanocytic nevus (although the latter relationship is disputed by some). Congenital melanocytic nevi are present at birth or appear in the neonatal period (tardive form). The giant melanocytic nevus, also called the bathing trunk, cape, or garment nevus, is a rare malformation that affects perhaps 1 in 30,000 to 1 in 100,000 individuals. These nevi are usually greater than 20 cm in diameter and may cover more than half the body surface. Giant nevi often occur in association with multiple small congenital nevi. The borders are sharp, and hair may be present. The lesions are usually dark brown and may have darker and lighter areas. Pigment is haphazardly

Table 88-4

Clinical Features Distinguishing Atypical Moles from Benign Acquired Nevi

Clinical Feature	Clinically Atypical Moles	Benign Acquired Nevi
Color	Variable mixtures of tan, brown, black, or red/pink within a single nevus; nevi may look very different from each other	Uniformly tan or brown
Shape	Irregular borders; pigment may fade off into surrounding skin; macular portion at the edge of the nevus	Round; sharp, clear-cut borders between the nevus and the surrounding skin; may be flat or elevated
Size	Usually more than 6 mm in diameter; may be more than 10 mm; occasionally smaller than 6 mm	Usually less than 6 mm in diameter
Number	Often very many (more than 100), but occasionally may be only one	In a typical adult, 10 to 40 are scattered over the body; perhaps 15% of patients have no nevi
Location	Sun-exposed areas; the back is the most common site, but dysplastic nevi may also be seen on the scalp, breasts, and buttocks	Generally on the sun-exposed surfaces of the skin above the waist; the scalp, breasts, and buttocks are rarely involved

SOURCE: Modified from Friedman et al, 1991b.

displayed. The surface is smooth to rugose or cerebriform and may vary from one portion of the lesion to another. A lifetime risk of melanoma development of 6 percent has been estimated. The risk is greatest before age 5 and next greatest between ages 5 and 10. Early detection of melanoma is difficult in these lesions because of the deep dermal or subcutaneous origin of primary melanoma and because of the large and varied surface of the nevus. Prophylactic excision early in life can be accomplished by staged removal with coverage by split-thickness skin grafts. The use of cultured keratinocytes for coverage appears promising. At present, there are no uniform management guidelines for giant congenital nevi.

The small- to medium-sized congenital melanocytic nevus, which affects approximately 1 percent of persons, presents usually as a raised dark- to medium-brown lesion with a smooth or papillomatous surface. The border is sharp, and lesions may be oriented along lines of skin cleavage. Follicular hyper- and hypopigmentation may coexist in a salt-and-pepper configuration. The lesion may have an excess of thick, coarse hairs. The risk of melanoma developing in these lesions is not known; however, melanomas can arise in these lesions. Considerations of body surface area suggest that the incidence of melanomas arising in small congenital melanocytic nevi is probably higher than would be expected by chance. The remnants of a nevus with histopathologic features of a congenital nevus have been observed in 2 to 6 percent of melanomas. The management of small- to medium-sized congenital melanocytic nevi remains controversial; prophylactic removal under local anesthesia in the early teen years is appropriate. Melanomas in small congenital melanocytic nevi appear to occur after this period of life.

Differential Diagnosis The aim of differential diagnosis is to distinguish benign pigmented lesions from melanoma and its precursors. If melanoma is a consideration, then biopsy is appropriate. Some benign look-alikes may be removed in the process of trying to detect authentic melanoma. Table 88-5 summarizes the distinguishing features of benign lesions that may be confused with melanoma. Early detection of melanoma may be facilitated by applying the "ABCD rules": A—asymmetry, benign lesions are usually symmetric; B—border irregularity, most nevi have clear-cut borders; C—color variegation, benign lesions usually have uniform light or dark pigment; D—diameter >6 mm (the size of a pencil eraser).

Biopsy Any pigmented cutaneous lesion that has changed in size or shape or has other features suggestive of malignant melanoma is a candidate for biopsy. The recommended technique is a full-thickness excisional biopsy, as that facilitates pathologic assessment of the lesion, permits accurate measurement of thickness if the lesion is melanoma, and constitutes treatment if the lesion is benign. Shave biopsy or curettage of a suspected melanoma is contraindicated. For large lesions or lesions on anatomic sites where excisional biopsy may not be feasible (such as the face, hands, or feet), an incisional biopsy through the most nodular or darkest area of the lesion is acceptable; this should include the vertical growth phase of the primary tumor, if present. Data from prospective studies do not indicate that an incisional biopsy facilitates the spread of melanoma.

Staging Once the diagnosis of malignant melanoma has been confirmed, the tumor must be staged to determine prognosis and treatment. The history should probe for evidence of metastatic disease, such as malaise, weight loss, headaches, visual difficulty, or bone pain. The physical examination should be directed especially to the skin, regional draining lymph nodes, central nervous system, liver, and spleen. In the absence of signs or symptoms of metastasis, few laboratory or radiologic tests are indicated for staging purposes. Aside from a chest radiograph and, possibly, liver function tests, no other tests or scans are routinely indicated unless the history or physical examination suggests metastasis to a specific organ. Specifically, liver-spleen scans and computed tomography have a low yield and are not cost-effective. However, once signs of metastasis exist, favored sites of spread, such as the liver, lungs, bone, and brain, should be scanned.

Pigmented Lesions That Must Be Distinguished from Cutaneous Melanoma and Its Precursors

Lesion	Description
Blue nevus	Gunmetal or cerulean blue, blue-gray. Stable over time. One-half occur on dorsa of hand and feet. Lesions are usually single, small, 3 mm to <1 cm. Must be distinguished from nodular melanoma.
Compound nevus	Round or oval shape, well-demarcated, smooth-bordered. May be dome-shaped or papillomatous; colors range from flesh colored to very dark brown, with individual nevi being relatively homogeneous in color.
Hemangioma	Dome-shaped reddish, purple, blue nodule. Compression with a glass microscope slide may result in blanching. Must be distinguished from nodular melanoma.
Junctional nevus	Flat to barely raised brown lesion. Sharp border. Fine pigmentary stippling visible, especially upon magnification.

Lentigo
  Juvenile
  Solar
	Flat, uniformly medium or dark brown lesion with sharp border. Solar lentigines are acquired lesions on sites of chronic solar exposure (face and backs of hands). Lesions are 2 mm to ≥1 cm. Solar lentigines have reticulate pigmentation upon magnification.

Pigmented basal cell carcinoma	Papular border. May have central ulceration. Usually on a sun-exposed surface in an older patient. Patient usually has dark brown eyes and dark brown or black hair.
Pigmented dermatofibroma	Lesion is not well demarcated visually, is firm, and dimples downward when compressed laterally. Usually on extremities. Usually <6 mm.
Seborrheic keratosis	Rough, sharp-bordered lesions that feel waxy and "stuck on"; range in color from flesh to tan, to dark brown. Presence of keratin plugs in surface is helpful for discriminating especially dark lesions from melanoma.
Subungual hematoma	Maroon (red-brown) coloration. As lesion grows out from nail fold, a curving clear area is seen.
Tattoo (medical or traumatic)	In medical tattoo, lesions are small pigmentary dots, often blue or green, which make a regular pattern (rectangle). Traumatic tattoos are irregular, and pigmentation may appear black.

Appropriate evaluations place patients into four clinical stages (see Table 88-3).

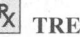 **TREATMENT**

Surgical Management For a newly diagnosed cutaneous melanoma, wide surgical excision of the lesion with a margin of normal skin is necessary to remove all malignant cells and minimize local recurrence. The appropriate width of the margin is a source of controversy. A World Health Organization trial prospectively randomized between 1- and 3-cm margins in 612 patients with thin malignant melanomas (≤2 mm thick) reported that the narrower margin resulted in higher rates of local recurrence but no difference in rates of nodal or distant metastases, disease-free survival, or overall survival after 7.5 years of follow-up. Another large randomized trial comparing 2- or 4-cm surgical margins for intermediate-thickness lesions (1 to 4 mm thick) also found no significant differences in overall survival. The following margins can be recommended for primary melanoma: in situ: 0.5 cm; invasive up to 1 mm thick: 1.0 cm; 1 to 4 mm thick: 2.0 cm; >4 mm thick: 2.5 to 3.0 cm. For lesions on the face, hands, and feet, strict adherence to these margins must give way to individual considerations about the constraints of surgery and minimization of morbidity. In all instances, however, inclusion of subcutaneous fat in the surgical specimen facilitates adequate thickness measurement and assessment of surgical margins by the pathologist.

Elective Regional Node Dissection   Elective regional node dissection in AJCC stage II disease (without palpable adenopathy) has been advocated, based on the hypothesis that melanoma metastasizes in an orderly fashion from the skin to regional lymph nodes and finally to distant sites. If that is the case, surgical excision of nodal micrometastases could theoretically provide definitive treatment at a time of relatively low tumor burden and perhaps improve survival. The efficacy of this procedure remains controversial; while some retrospective series suggest a survival benefit, two randomized studies examining this question in patients with limb melanomas and clinical stage I disease showed no survival advantage for wide local excision followed by immediate elective regional node dissection compared with wide local excision followed by delayed dissection (only if nodes became palpable). Furthermore, the procedure has associated morbidity, and some lesions, especially those on the trunk, have ambiguous nodal draining sites, making it difficult to decide which area to dissect. Results of biopsy of the first drainage node—the so-called sentinel node—predicts the likelihood of metastases in higher nodes. Sentinel nodes can be identified by injecting a blue dye or radioactive isotope around the primary tumor site. A negative biopsy result appears to obviate the need for elective regional nodal dissection. Patients with lesions <0.75 mm thick have an excellent prognosis and need no node dissection; at the other extreme, patients with lesions >3.50 mm thick have such a high risk for distant metastases that elective node dissection may not alter the ultimate clinical outcome. A subset of patients with AJCC stage II lesions of intermediate thickness may benefit from elective regional node dissection, but there is no consensus about which patients should undergo this procedure. An ongoing randomized surgical trial may resolve this issue.

Adjuvant Therapy   For patients who are free of disease but at high risk for metastases, adjuvant therapy that complements surgery is needed to destroy occult micrometastases, prolong disease-free survival, and improve the cure rate. Many strategies have been tried unsuccessfully. However, adjuvant interferon α (either 2a or 2b) is capable of improving disease-free and overall survival significantly, particularly in patients with nodal metastases (stage III disease). The FDA has recently approved a high dose interferon adjuvant protocol consisting of 20 million units per square meter intravenously 5 days a week for 4 weeks followed by 10 million units per square meter subcutaneously three times a week for 11 months. Ongoing studies are attempting to define the minimal effective dose, because, in nearly half of patients, these doses of interferon are associated with severe toxicity, including flu-like illness and decline in performance status. The toxicity reverses promptly with lower doses and when therapy is stopped.

Treatment of Metastatic Disease   Melanoma can metastasize to any organ, the brain being a particularly common site. Metastatic melanoma generally is incurable, with survival in patients with visceral metastases generally less than 1 year. Thus, the goal of treatment is usually palliation. Patients with soft-tissue and node metastases fare better than those with liver and brain metastases. Metastases limited to regional nodes (AJCC stage III disease) warrant a therapeutic lymph node dissection. Surgical excision of a single metastasis to the lung or to a surgically accessible brain site can prolong survival. Trials of stereotactic radiosurgery will determine its future role in the treatment of brain metastases. More often, however, patients have multiple brain metastases that require radiation therapy and glucocorticoids. Radiation therapy can provide local palliation for recurrent tumors or metastases. Patients who have advanced regional disease limited to a limb may benefit from hyperthermic limb perfusion with melphalan and tumor necrosis factor. Complete response rates greater than 90 percent have been reported; responses are associated with significant palliation of symptoms.

A number of drugs and biologicals have minimal antitumor activity (15 to 20 percent partial response rates) in metastatic melanoma, including dacarbazine (DTIC), the nitrosoureas carmustine (BCNU), lomustine (CCNU), and semustine (methyl-CCNU), platinum analogues such as cisplatin and carboplatin, vinca alkyloids such as vincristine, vinblastine, and vindesine, the taxanes paclitaxel (taxol) and docetaxel, interferon α, and interleukin 2 (IL-2). Single-agent dacarbazine is considered the standard treatment. This agent has been given at a number of different doses and schedules; 250 mg/m^2 intravenously every day for 5 days every 3 weeks is a standard schedule. There is increasing evidence that dacarbazine-based combination regimens are probably more effective. Ongoing trials are attempting to define superior combinations. Interferon and IL-2 produce response rates similar to those seen with cytotoxic agents; however, at active doses, they usually cause greater toxicity than chemotherapy.

Considerable evidence suggests that melanomas can express cell surface antigens that may be recognized by host immune cells. A number of melanoma-associated antigens have been discovered. Melanoma antigens (MAGEs)-1, -2, and -3 (endogenous proteins controlled by genes on the X chromosome; there may be up to 12 of these genes), and tyrosinase, an enzyme involved in melanin synthesis, are antigens that are processed into peptides and presented to T cells via HLA-A antigens on the tumor, particularly the HLA-A1 and A2 alleles, which are expressed in about 85 percent of patients with melanoma. In addition, there is a melanoma antigen called MART that is recognized in the context of class II MHC antigens. These melanoma-associated antigens alone or in combination may make it possible to develop vaccination strategies against melanoma. Such strategies include the use of purified proteins as immunogens and the use of genetically altered tumor cells to elicit a T-cell response. Alternative experimental approaches include efforts to expand tumor-specific T cells (obtained either from the tumor as tumor-infiltrating lymphocytes or harvested from the peripheral blood after vaccination) in vitro and transfer them into patients in large numbers. In addition, monoclonal antibodies to tumor antigens are being tested, with some early indication of efficacy in around 15 percent of patients. All of these experimental approaches will need considerable further development before being applicable on a wide scale. However, once an approach that appears to be active in metastatic disease is found, it is possible that it will prove most useful when administered as an adjuvant.

The absence of curative therapy for patients with metastatic melanoma underscores the importance of early detection and prevention as strategies to decrease melanoma mortality.

NONMELANOMA SKIN CANCER

Nonmelanoma skin cancer is the most common cancer in the United States, with an estimated annual incidence of more than 800,000 cases. Basal cell carcinomas (BCCs) account for 70 to 80 percent of nonmelanoma skin cancers. Squamous cell carcinomas (SCCs), while representing only about 20 percent of nonmelanoma skin cancers, are more significant because of their ability to metastasize; they account for most of the 2300 deaths annually. Incidence rates have risen dramatically over the past decade.

ETIOLOGY   The cause of BCC and SCC is multifactorial. Cumulative exposure to sunlight, principally the ultraviolet B (UV-B) spectrum, is the most significant factor. Other factors associated with a higher incidence of skin cancer are male sex, older age, Celtic descent, a fair complexion, a tendency to sunburn easily, and an outdoor occupation. The incidence of these tumors increases with decreasing latitude. Most tumors develop on sun-exposed areas of the head and neck. Tumors are more common on the left side of the body in the United States but on the right side in England, presumably owing to asymmetric exposure during driving. As the earth's protective ozone shield continues to thin, further increases in the incidence of skin cancer can be anticipated. In certain geographic areas, exposure to arsenic in well water or from industrial sources may significantly increase the risk of BCC and SCC. Skin cancer in affected individuals may be seen with or without other cutaneous markers of chronic arsenism (e.g., arsenical keratoses). Less common is exposure to the cyclic aromatic hydrocarbons in tar, soot, or shale. The risk of lip or oral SCC is increased with cigarette smoking. Human papillomaviruses and UV-B light may act as cocarcinogens.

Host factors associated with a high risk of skin cancer include immunosuppression induced by disease or drugs. Transplant recipients receiving chronic immunosuppressive therapy are particularly prone to SCC. The frequency of skin cancer is proportional to the duration of immunosuppression and the extent of sun exposure. Skin cancer is a not uncommon finding in patients infected with the human immunodeficiency virus (HIV), and it may be more aggressive in this setting. As the life span of HIV-infected persons increases, skin cancer may become a greater problem. Other factors include ionizing radiation, thermal burns, and certain scars and chronic ulcerations. Several heritable conditions have been associated with skin cancer (e.g., albinism, xeroderma pigmentosum, and BCC nevus syndrome).

CLINICAL PRESENTATION   Nonmelanoma skin cancers are often asymptomatic, but nonhealing ulceration, bleeding, or pain can occur.

Basal Cell Carcinoma   BCC is a malignancy arising from epidermal basal cells. There are several clinical types of BCC. The most common is *noduloulcerative BCC*, which begins as a small, pearly nodule, often with small telangiectatic vessels on its surface. The nodule grows slowly and may undergo central ulceration. Various amounts of melanin may be present in the tumor; tumors with a heavier accumulation are referred to as *pigmented BCC*. While clinically no more aggressive than the noduloulcerative variant, the latter may be mistaken for malignant melanoma. *Superficial BCC* consists of one or several erythematous, scaling plaques that slowly enlarge. Although they are more commonly found on the trunk and extremities, the head and neck also can be affected. The lesions may be confused with benign inflammatory dermatoses, especially nummular eczema and psoriasis. *Morpheaform (fibrosing) BCC* manifests itself as a solitary, flat or slightly depressed, indurated, whitish or yellowish plaque. Borders are typically indistinct, a feature associated with a greater potential for extensive subclinical spread.

Squamous Cell Carcinoma   Primary cutaneous SCC is a malignant neoplasm of keratinizing epidermal cells. Unlike BCC, which has a very low metastatic potential, SCC can metastasize and grow rapidly. The clinical features of SCC vary widely. Commonly, SCC appears as an ulcerated nodule or a superficial erosion on the skin or lower lip, but it may present as a verrucous papule or plaque. Unlike BCC, overlying telangiectasias are uncommon. The margins of this tumor may be ill-defined, and fixation to underlying structures may occur. Cutaneous SCC may develop anywhere on the body, but it usually arises on sun-damaged skin. A related neoplasm, keratoacanthoma, typically appears as a dome-shaped papule with a central keratotic crater, expands rapidly, and commonly regresses without therapy. This lesion can be difficult to differentiate from SCC.

SCC has several premalignant forms (actinic keratosis, actinic cheilitis, and some cutaneous horns) and in situ forms (e.g., Bowen's disease) that are confined to the epidermis. Actinic keratoses and cheilitis are hyperkeratotic papules and plaques that occur on sun-exposed areas. While the potential for malignant degeneration is low in any individual lesion, the risk of SCC increases with larger numbers of lesions. Bowen's disease presents as a scaling, erythematous plaque, which may develop into invasive SCC in up to 20 percent of cases. Controversy exists regarding the association of Bowen's disease with internal malignancy; however, recent evidence suggests that there is no significant relationship when other predisposing factors (e.g., arse-

nic) are absent. Treatment of premalignant and in situ lesions reduces the subsequent risk of invasive disease.

NATURAL HISTORY   **Basal Cell Carcinoma**   The natural history of BCC is that of a slowly enlarging, locally invasive neoplasm. The degree of local destruction and risk of recurrence vary with the size, duration, and location of the tumor, the histologic subtype, the presence of recurrent disease, and various patient characteristics. Location on the central face (e.g., the nose, the nasolabial fold, or the periorbital or perioral area), the ears, or the scalp may portend a higher risk. Small nodular, pigmented, cystic, or superficial BCCs respond well to most treatments. Large nodular, noduloulcerative, and especially morpheaform BCCs are usually more aggressive. The metastatic potential of BCC has been estimated to be 0.0028 to 0.1 percent. Persons with either BCC or SCC have an increased risk of developing subsequent skin cancers.

Squamous Cell Carcinoma   The natural history of SCC depends on both tumor and host characteristics. Tumors arising on actinically damaged skin have a lower metastatic potential than those on protected surfaces. The metastatic frequency of cutaneous SCC, reported at 0.3 to 3.7 percent, is lower than that of mucosal SCC. Tumors occurring on the lower lip and ear have metastatic potential approaching 13 and 11 percent, respectively. The metastatic potential of SCC arising in burn scars, chronic ulcerations, or the genitalia is higher. The overall metastatic rate for recurrent tumors may approach 30 percent. Poorly differentiated, deep tumors with perineural or lymphatic invasion often behave aggressively. Multiple tumors with rapid growth and aggressive behavior can be a therapeutic challenge in immunosuppressed patients. Regional lymph nodes are the most common site of metastasis. In patients with metastatic disease, the 5-year survival rate may be low.

℞ TREATMENT

Basal Cell Carcinoma   The treatment modalities used for BCC include electrodesiccation and curettage (ED&C), excision, cryosurgery, radiation therapy, Mohs micrographic surgery (MMS), and others. The mode of therapy chosen depends on tumor characteristics, on the age, medical status, and preferences of the patient, and on other factors. ED&C remains the method most commonly employed by dermatologists. This method is selected for low-risk tumors (e.g., a small primary tumor of a less aggressive subtype in a favorable location). Excision, which offers the advantage of histologic control, is usually selected for more aggressive tumors or those in high-risk locations, or, in many instances, for aesthetic reasons. Cryosurgery using liquid nitrogen may be used in certain low-risk tumors, but it requires specialized equipment (cryoprobes) to be effective for advanced neoplasms. Radiation therapy, while not employed as often as surgical modalities, offers an excellent chance for cure in many cases of BCC. It is useful in patients not considered surgical candidates and as a surgical adjunct in high-risk tumors. Younger patients may not be good candidates for radiation therapy because of the risks of long-term carcinogenesis and radiodermatitis. MMS is a specialized type of surgical excision which permits the ultimate in histologic control and preservation of uninvolved tissue. It is preferred for lesions that are recurrent, in a high-risk location, or large and ill-defined, and where maximal tissue conservation is critical (e.g., the eyelids). Topical chemotherapy with 5-fluorouracil (5FU) cream has limited usefulness in the management of BCC and should be used only for treating superficial BCC. Intralesional 5FU is being investigated as a treatment modality for BCC. Intralesional interferon is effective in certain primary tumors. Photodynamic therapy, which employs selective activation of a photoactive drug by visible light, may be useful in patients with numerous tumors, but further investigation is needed. Lasers also have been used for the treatment of skin cancer.

Squamous Cell Carcinoma   The therapy of cutaneous SCC should be based on an analysis of risk factors influencing the biologic behavior of the tumor. These include the size, location, and degree of histologic differentiation of the tumor and the age and physical condition of the patient. Surgical excision, MMS, and radiation are standard methods of treatment. Cryosurgery and ED&C have been used successfully for small primary tumors. Metastases are treated with lymph node dissection, irradiation, or both. 13-*Cis*-retinoic acid (1 mg orally every day) plus interferon α (3 million units subcutaneously or intramuscularly every day) may produce a partial response in most patients. Systemic chemotherapy combinations that include cisplatin may also be palliative in some patients.

PREVENTION   Since the vast majority of skin cancers are related to chronic UV-B exposure, patient and physician education could dramatically reduce their incidence. Emphasis should be placed on preventive measures beginning early in life. Patients must understand that damage from UV-B begins early, despite the fact that cancers develop years later. Regular use of sunscreens and protective clothing should be encouraged. Avoidance of tanning salons and sun exposure during midday (10 A.M. to 2 P.M.) is recommended. Precancerous and in situ lesions should be treated early. Early detection of small tumors affords simpler treatment modalities with higher cure rates and lower morbidity. In patients with a history of skin cancer, long-term follow-up for the detection of recurrence, metastasis, and new skin cancers should be emphasized. Chemoprophylaxis using synthetic retinoids is useful in controlling new lesions in some patients with multiple tumors.

OTHER TYPES OF CUTANEOUS CANCER

Neoplasms of cutaneous adnexa, and sarcomas of fibrous, mesenchymal, fatty, and vascular tissues make up 1 to 2 percent of nonmelanoma skin cancers. The recent rapid rise in the incidence of Kaposi's sarcoma is attributed to HIV infection and immunosuppressive therapy. Epidemiologic patterns suggest infectious agents as possible etiologic factors. A novel herpesvirus, human herpesvirus 8, is a potential cause of several types of Kaposi's sarcoma. Current therapy is palliative and depends on the symptoms and sites of involvement. Treatment modalities include cryosurgery, intralesional vinblastine, excision, radiation, interferon α, and systemic combination chemotherapy. As further etiologic factors are identified, safer and more effective therapy may be devised (see Chap. 308).

BIBLIOGRAPHY

ALBERT L et al: Dysplastic melanocytic nevi and cutaneous melanoma: Markers of increased melanoma risk for affected individuals and blood relatives. J Am Acad Dermatol 7:69, 1990
ARMSTRONG BK: Epidemiology of malignant melanoma: Intermittent or total accumulated exposure to the sun. J Dermatol Surg Oncol 14:835, 1988
BALCH CM et al (eds): *Cutaneous Melanoma: Clinical Management and Treatment Results Worldwide*, 2d ed. Philadelphia, Lippincott, 1992
——— et al: Efficacy of 2-cm surgical margins for intermediate-thickness melanomas (1–4 mm). Ann Surg 218:262, 1993
BOON T: Tumor antigens recognized by cytolytic T lymphocytes present perspectives for specific immunotherapy. Int J Cancer 54:177, 1993
CLARK WH JR et al: The histogenesis and biologic behavior of primary human malignant melanoma of the skin. Cancer Res 29:705, 1969
CREAGAN ET et al: Randomized surgical adjuvant clinical trial of recombinant interferon-alfa-2a in selected patients with malignant melanoma. J Clin Oncol 13:2776, 1995
DRAKE LA et al: Guidelines of care of basal cell carcinoma. J Am Acad Dermatol 26:117, 1992
——— et al: Guidelines of care for cutaneous squamous cell carcinoma. J Am Acad Dermatol 28:628, 1993
FRIEDMAN RJ et al: Malignant melanoma in the 1990s: The continued importance of early detection and the role of physician examination and self-examination of the skin. CA 41:201, 1991
——— et al (eds): *Cancer of the Skin*. Philadelphia, Saunders, 1991, pp 27–94
JOHNSON TM et al: Current therapy for cutaneous melanoma. J Am Acad Dermatol 32:689, 1995
KWA RE: Biology of cutaneous squamous cell carcinoma. J Am Acad Dermatol 26:1, 1992
KOH HK: Cutaneous melanoma. N Engl J Med 325:171, 1991
MARKS R: An overview of skin cancers. Incidence and causation. Cancer 75(Suppl):607, 1995
PRESTON DS et al: Nonmelanoma cancer of the skin. N Engl J Med 327:1649, 1992

LIPPMAN SM et al: 13cis-retinoic acid and interferon-α2a: Effective combination therapy for advanced squamous cell carcinoma of the skin. J Natl Cancer Inst 84:235, 1992
RHODES AR: Neoplasms: Benign neoplasias, hyperplasias, and dysplasias of melanocytes, in *Dermatology in General Medicine*, 4th ed, TB Fitzpatrick et al (eds). New York, McGraw-Hill, 1993, pp 996–1097
——— et al: Risk factors for cutaneous melanoma. JAMA 258:3146, 1987
RIGEL DS et al: Dysplastic nevi. Markers for increased risk for melanoma. Cancer 63:386, 1989
ROSENBERG SA: The immunotherapy and gene therapy of cancer. J Clin Oncol 10:180, 1992
VERONESI U et al: Delayed regional lymph node dissection in stage 1 melanoma of the skin of the lower extremities. Cancer 49:2420, 1982
———, CASCINELLI N: Narrow excision (1 cm margin), a safe procedure for thin cutaneous melanoma. Arch Surg 126:438, 1991

89   *Everett E. Vokes*

HEAD AND NECK CANCER

Epithelial carcinomas of the head and neck arise from the mucosal surfaces in the head and neck area and typically are squamous-cell in origin. This category includes tumors of the paranasal sinuses, the oral cavity, and the nasopharynx, oropharynx, hypopharynx, and larynx. Tumors of the salivary glands are discussed also in this chapter, although they differ from the more common carcinomas of the head and neck in etiology, histopathology, clinical presentation, and therapy. → *Thyroid malignancies are described in Chap. 331.*

INCIDENCE AND EPIDEMIOLOGY   The annual number of new cases of head and neck cancers in the United States is approximately 40,000, accounting for about 5 percent of adult malignancies. Head and neck cancers are more common in some other countries, and the worldwide incidence probably exceeds half a million cases annually. In North America and Europe, the tumors usually arise from the oral cavity, oropharynx, or larynx, whereas nasopharyngeal cancer is more common in the Mediterranean countries and in the Far East.

ETIOLOGY AND GENETICS   Alcohol and tobacco use are the most common risk factors for head and neck carcinogenesis in the United States, and the combination of alcohol and tobacco exposure is the most potent carcinogen. Even smokeless tobacco may be an etiologic agent for oral cancers. Other potential carcinogens include marijuana and occupational exposures such as nickel refining, exposure to textile fibers, and woodworking.

Dietary factors may contribute. There may be an inverse association between the consumption of fruits and vegetables and the incidence of head and neck cancer. Certain vitamins, including dietary carotenoids, may be protective; this relationship may provide a strategy for the prevention of head and neck cancers.

Some head and neck cancers may have a viral etiology. The DNA of human papilloma virus has been detected in the tissue of larynx and tonsil cancers, and there is an association with Epstein-Barr virus (EBV) infection and nasopharyngeal cancer. EBV DNA is present in nasopharyngeal cancers, and elevated antibody titers are present in most patients with nasopharyngeal cancer. The DNA of EBV has also been detected in premalignant lesions of the nasopharynx, further supporting a role for EBV in the pathogenesis. Nasopharyngeal cancer occurs endemically in some countries of the Mediterranean and Far East, where EBV antibody titers can be measured to screen high-risk populations. Nasopharyngeal cancer has also been associated with other environmental factors, such as consumption of salted fish.

No specific risk factors or environmental carcinogens have been identified for salivary gland tumors. Radiation exposure in early life is a risk factor for thyroid malignancies.

HISTOPATHOLOGY, CARCINOGENESIS, AND MOLECULAR BIOLOGY   The head and neck carcinomas of squamous cell origin can be divided into well-differentiated, moderately well-differentiated, and poorly differentiated categories. Patients with poorly differentiated tumors are believed to have a worse prognosis than those with well-differentiated tumors. In Mediterranean countries and the Far East, the less common differentiated squamous cell carcinoma is distinguished from nonkeratinizing and undifferentiated carcinoma (lymphoepithelioma) that contains infiltrating (bystander) lymphocytes.

Salivary gland tumors can arise from the major (parotid, submandibular, sublingual) or minor salivary glands (the latter located in the submucosa of the upper aerodigestive tract). Most parotid tumors are benign, but half of submandibular and sublingual gland tumors, and most minor salivary gland tumors, are malignant. Malignant tumors include mucoepidermoid and adenoidcystic carcinomas and adenocarcinomas.

The mucosal surface of the entire pharynx is exposed to alcohol and tobacco-related carcinogens and is at risk for the development of a premalignant or malignant lesion, such as erythroplakia or leukoplakia (hyperplasia, dysplasia), that can progress to invasive carcinoma. Alternatively, multiple synchronous or metachronous cancers can develop. In fact, patients with early-stage head and neck cancer are at greater risk of dying of a second malignancy than of dying from a recurrence of the primary disease.

Unlike the second malignancies that develop after combined-modality therapy for malignant lymphomas, second head and neck malignancies are not therapy-induced but, instead, reflect the exposure of the upper aerodigestive mucosa to the same carcinogens that caused the first cancer. These second primaries can develop in the head and neck area, the lung, or the esophagus.

Chromosomal deletions and other alterations, most frequently involving chromosomes 3p, 9p, 17p, and 13q, have been identified in both premalignant and malignant head and neck lesions as have been mutations in tumor suppressor genes, commonly the *p53* gene. Amplification of oncogenes is less common, but overexpression of PRAD-1/bcl-1 (cyclin D1) and the epidermal growth factor receptor have been described. The latter finding correlates positively with tumor size and poor outcome.

Attempts have been made to use this information in therapy. Resected tumor specimens with histopathologically negative margins ("complete resection") can have histopathologically undetectable residual tumor cells with persistent *p53* mutations at the margins. Thus, a tumor-specific *p53* mutation can be detected in some phenotypically "normal" surgical margins, indicating residual disease. Early data suggest that patients with such submicroscopic marginal involvement have a worse prognosis than patients with negative margins. It may also prove possible to use molecular techniques for the early diagnosis or screening of malignant or premalignant lesions in high-risk populations (smokers and drinkers).

CLINICAL PRESENTATION AND DIFFERENTIAL DIAGNOSIS Most head and neck cancers occur after age 50, although these cancers can appear in younger patients, including those without known risk factors. The manifestations vary according to the stage and primary site of the tumor. A high index of suspicion is warranted for patients with nonspecific signs and symptoms in the head and neck area, particularly if the symptoms persist longer than 2 to 4 weeks.

Cancer of the nasopharynx typically does not cause early symptoms. However, on occasion it may cause unilateral serous otitis media due to obstruction of the eustachian tube, unilateral or bilateral nasal obstruction, or epistaxis. Advanced nasopharyngeal carcinoma causes neuropathies of the cranial nerves.

Carcinomas of the oral cavity present as nonhealing ulcers, changes in the fit of dentures, or painful lesions. Tumors of the tongue base or oropharynx can cause decreased tongue mobility and alterations in speech. Cancers of the oropharynx or hypopharynx rarely cause early symptoms, but they may cause sore throat and/or otalgia.

Hoarseness may be an early symptom of laryngeal cancer, and persistent hoarseness requires referral to an otorhinolaryngologist for indirect laryngoscopy and/or radiographic studies. If a head and neck lesion treated initially with antibiotics does not resolve in a short period, further workup is indicated; to simply continue the antibiotic treatment may be to lose the chance of early diagnosis of a malignancy.

Advanced head and neck cancers in any location can cause severe pain, otalgia, airway obstruction, cranial neuropathies, trismus, odynophagia, dysphagia, decreased tongue mobility, fistulas, skin involvement, and massive cervical lymphadenopathy, which may be unilateral or bilateral. Some patients have enlarged lymph nodes even though no primary lesion can be detected by endoscopy or biopsy; these patients are considered to have carcinoma of unknown primary. If the enlarged nodes are located in the upper neck and the tumor cells are of squamous cell histology, the malignancy probably arose from a mucosal surface in the head and neck. Tumor cells in supraclavicular lymph nodes may also arise from a primary site in the chest or abdomen, however.

The physical examination should include scrutiny of all visible mucosal surfaces and palpation of the floor of mouth and tongue and of the neck. In addition to tumors themselves, leukoplakia—a white mucosal patch—or erythroplakia—a red mucosal patch—may be observed; these "premalignant" lesions can represent hyperplasia, dysplasia, or carcinoma in situ. Biopsy of all visible lesions is recommended. Further examination should be performed by the otorhinolaryngologist. Additional staging procedures include computed tomography of the head and neck to identify the extent of the disease. Patients with lymph node involvement should also undergo screening for distant metastases, including chest radiography and a bone scan. The definitive staging procedure is an endoscopic examination under anesthesia, which may include laryngoscopy, esophagoscopy, and bronchoscopy; during this procedure, multiple biopsy samples are obtained to establish a primary diagnosis, to define the extent of primary disease, and to identify any additional premalignant lesions or second primaries.

Head and neck tumors are classified according to the TNM system of the American Joint Committee on Cancer. This classification varies according to the specific anatomic subsite (Table 89-1); generally, T1 through T3 describe the size of the primary lesion, and T4 indicates involvement of a vital structure in the head and neck, such as the tongue base, a cranial nerve, or the thyroid cartilage. The lymph nodes are staged uniformly for head and neck cancers of all sites (Table 89-1). Distant metastases are found in less than 10 percent of patients at initial diagnosis, but in autopsy series, microscopic involvement of the lungs, bones, or liver is more common, particularly in patients with advanced neck lymph node disease.

In patients with lymph node involvement and no visible primary, the diagnosis should be made by lymph node excision. If the results indicate squamous cell carcinoma, a panendoscopy should be performed, with biopsy of all suspicious-appearing areas and directed biopsies of common primary sites, such as the nasopharynx, tonsil, tongue base, and pyriform sinus.

℞ TREATMENT

Generally, patients with head and neck cancer can be categorized into three clinical groups: those with localized disease, those with locally or regionally advanced disease, and those with recurrent and/or metastatic disease.

Localized Disease Approximately one-third of patients have localized disease; that is, T1 or T2 (stage I or stage II) lesions without detectable lymph node involvement or distant metastases. These lesions are treated with curative intent by surgery or radiation. The choice of modality differs according to institutional expertise. Generally, radiation therapy is preferred for laryngeal cancer to preserve voice function, and surgery is preferred for small lesions in the oral cavity to avoid the long-term complications of radiation, such as xerostomia and dental decay.

Locally Advanced Disease Locally or regionally advanced disease—that is, disease with a large primary tumor and/or lymph node metastases—can also be treated with curative intent. This treatment usually consists of extensive surgery followed by postoperative radiation therapy. However, unresectable lesions, such as cancers of the nasopharynx or tongue base, are treated solely with radiotherapy. Even with the use of this two-modality approach, most cancers recur in the head and neck region, usually within 2 years of therapy, and cause death. This fact reflects the inability of surgery and radiation to eliminate all microscopic disease. To improve the outcome, chemotherapy has been added, along two major investigational lines referred to as induction chemotherapy and concomitant chemoradiotherapy.

INDUCTION CHEMOTHERAPY In this strategy, patients with advanced disease receive chemotherapy before surgery and radiotherapy. The most common combination is cisplatin and fluorouracil (5FU). Most patients who receive three cycles of this combination show tumor reduction, and the response is clinically complete in up to half of these patients. It is not clear whether this "sequential" multimodality therapy cures more patients than surgery plus radiation therapy alone. Large, randomized studies comparing surgery and radiotherapy with chemotherapy followed by surgery and radiotherapy suggest that there is no benefit in terms of survival.

Nevertheless, induction chemotherapy allows for organ preservation. For example, one study comparing surgery and radiation therapy with chemotherapy and radiation therapy found no difference in survival (50 percent at 2 years) for patients with advanced larynx cancer; however, the use of chemotherapy allowed the preservation of the larynx in two-thirds of patients. Another study found similar results for patients with hypopharyngeal cancer. Thus, chemotherapy plus radiotherapy should be considered in this group of patients in place of laryngectomy plus radiotherapy.

Induction chemotherapy has also been studied in patients with nasopharyngeal cancer (who frequently present with advanced lymph node involvement). Preliminary results indicate a longer time to recurrence for chemotherapy and radiation therapy than for radiation therapy alone. Chemotherapy may also improve survival.

CONCOMITANT CHEMORADIOTHERAPY With the concomitant strategy, chemotherapy and radiation therapy are given simultaneously rather than sequentially. Because most patients with head and neck cancer develop recurrent disease in the head and neck area, this approach is aimed at killing radiation-resistant cancer cells with chemotherapy. Indeed, some chemotherapy agents appear to increase the cytotoxicity of radiation. Three studies in patients with unresectable disease have suggested that radiation therapy plus concomitant 5FU gives better survival than radiation therapy alone. However, because the survival benefit in all three studies was small and because toxicity (mucositis) was increased with concomitant chemoradiotherapy, this treatment is not widely used. The use of radiation therapy together with cisplatin has produced markedly improved survival in patients with nasopharyngeal cancer.

Recurrent and/or Metastatic Disease Patients with recurrent and/or metastatic disease are, with few exceptions, treated with palliative intent. Some patients may require local or regional radiotherapy for pain control, but most are given chemotherapy. Response rates to chemotherapy average only 30 to 50 percent, the duration of response averages only 3 months, and the median survival time is 6 months. Therefore, chemotherapy provides transient symptomatic

Table 89-1

TNM Classification for Head and Neck Cancer

T Grade	Lip	Oral Cavity	Oropharynx	Hypopharynx	Nasopharynx	Larynx
			Primary Tumor Site			
TX			Primary tumor cannot be assessed			
T0			No evidence of primary tumor			
Tis			Carcinoma in situ			
T1	0–2 cm	0–2 cm	0–2 cm	1 site	1 site	1 site or limited to vocal cords
T2	2.1–4 cm	2.1–4 cm	2.1–4 cm	>1 site, no vocal cord fixation	>1 site	>1 site or impaired cord mobility
T3	>4 cm	>4 cm	>4 cm	vocal cord paralysis	Extension to nasal cavity or oropharynx	Vocal cord paralysis
T4	>4 cm with massive invasion		Massive soft tissue, bone, or cartilage invasion			

REGIONAL LYMPH NODES (N)

NX	Regional lymph nodes cannot be assessed
N0	No regional lymph node metastasis
N1	Metastasis in a single ipsilateral lymph node, 3 cm or less in greatest dimension
N2	Metastasis in a single ipsilateral lymph node, more than 3 cm but not more than 6 cm in greatest dimension; or in multiple ipsilateral lymph nodes, none more than 6 cm in greatest dimension; or in bilateral or contralateral lymph nodes, none more than 6 cm in greatest dimension
N2a	Metastasis in single ipsilateral lymph node more than 3 cm but more than 6 cm in greatest dimension
N2b	Metastasis in multiple ipsilateral lymph nodes, none more than 6 cm in greatest dimension
N2c	Metastasis in bilateral or contralateral lymph nodes, none more than 6 cm in greatest dimension
N3	Metastasis in a lymph node more than 6 cm in greatest dimension

DISTANT METASTASIS (M)

MX	Presence of distant metastasis cannot be assessed
M0	No distant metastasis
M1	Distant metastasis

STAGE GROUPING

Stage 0	Tis	N0	M0	Stage IV	T4	N0	M0
Stage I	T1	N0	M0		T4	N1	M0
Stage II	T2	N0	M0		Any T	N2	M0
Stage III	T3	N0	M0		Any T	N3	M0
	T1	N1	M0		Any T	Any N	M1
	T2	N1	M0				
	T3	N1	M0				

benefit. Drugs with single-agent activity in this setting include methotrexate, 5FU, cisplatin, and paclitaxel. Combinations of cisplatin and 5FU, carboplatin and 5FU, and cisplatin and paclitaxel are also used.

CHEMOPREVENTION Another line of clinical research is aimed at preventing the transformation of premalignant disease into invasive carcinoma. β-Carotene and *cis*-retinoic acid can lead to the regression of leukoplakia. In addition, the use of *cis*-retinoic acid may reduce the incidence of second primaries. Large confirmatory randomized studies are under way to determine the effectiveness of this approach.

TREATMENT COMPLICATIONS Complications of the treatment of head and neck cancer are usually related to the extent of surgery. Several attempts have been made to limit the extent of surgery or to replace it with chemotherapy and radiation therapy. Acute complications of radiation include mucositis and dysphagia, and long-term complications include xerostomia, loss of taste, decreased tongue mobility, second malignancies, and dysphagia and neck fibrosis. The complications of chemotherapy vary with the regimen used but usually include myelosuppression, mucositis, nausea and vomiting, and nephrotoxicity (with cisplatin).

SALIVARY GLAND TUMORS Most benign salivary gland tumors are treated with surgical excision, and patients with invasive salivary gland tumors are treated with surgery and radiation. Neutron radiation may be particularly effective. These tumors may recur regionally; adenoidcystic carcinoma has a tendency to recur along the nerve tracks. Distant metastases may occur as late as 10 to 20 years after the initial diagnosis. For metastatic disease, therapy is given with palliative intent, usually chemotherapy with doxorubicin and/or cisplatin.

BIBLIOGRAPHY

ADELSTEIN DJ: The community approach to salvage therapy for advanced head and neck cancer. Semin Oncol 21(Suppl 7):52, 1994

BRENNAN JA et al: Molecular assessment of histopathological staging in squamous-cell carcinoma of the head and neck. N Engl J Med 332:429, 1995

BROWMAN GP, CRONIN L: Standard chemotherapy in squamous cell head and neck cancer: What we have learned from randomized trials. Semin Oncol 21:311, 1994

—— et al: Placebo-controlled randomized trial of infusional fluorouracil during standard radiotherapy in locally advanced head and neck cancer. J Clin Oncol 12:2648, 1994

FANDI A, et al: Nasopharyngeal cancer: Epidemiology, staging, and treatment. Semin Oncol 21:382, 1994

LIPPMAN SM, et al: Comparison of low-dose isotretinoin with beta carotene to prevent oral carcinogenesis. N Engl J Med 328:15, 1993

THE DEPARTMENT OF VETERANS AFFAIRS LARYNGEAL CANCER STUDY GROUP: Induction chemotherapy plus radiation compared with surgery plus radiation in patients with advanced laryngeal cancer. N Engl J Med 324:1685, 1991

VOKES EE, ATHANASIADIS I: Chemotherapy for squamous cell carcinoma of head and neck: The future is now. Ann Oncol 7:15, 1996

——, WEICHSELBAUM RR: Concomitant chemoradiotherapy: Rationale and clinical experience in patients with solid tumors. J Clin Oncol 8:911, 1990

—— et al: Head and neck cancer. N Engl J Med 328:184, 1993

| 90 | *John D. Minna* |

NEOPLASMS OF THE LUNG

Each year, primary carcinoma of the lung affects 99,000 males and 78,000 females in the United States, 86 percent of whom die within 5 years of diagnosis, making it the leading cause of cancer death in both men and women. The incidence of lung cancer peaks between ages 55 and 65 years. Lung cancer accounts for 32 percent of all cancer deaths in men and for 25 percent of all cancer deaths in women.

The effects of smoking cessation efforts begun 20 years ago have finally started to be seen in a slowing of the rate of age-adjusted cancer death from lung cancer in white males (57 per 100,000 male population), while, unfortunately, the rate in females is still increasing (26 per 100,000 female population). Lung cancer is the leading cancer killer in all racial groups in the United States. At the time of diagnosis, only 15 percent of all lung cancer patients will have local disease, while ~25 percent will have disease spread to regional lymph nodes, and >55 percent will have distant metastatic cancer. Even in the patients with localized disease, the 5-year survival is only 48 percent, while survival is 18 percent for patients with regional disease and 14 percent overall. Of clinical significance, the 5-year overall lung cancer survival rate has increased steadily from 8 percent in the 1960s to 14 percent in the 1990s. These increases have been seen in both whites and African Americans. The main cause of these changes appears to be advances in combined-modality treatment with surgery, radiotherapy, and chemotherapy. Thus, primary carcinoma of the lung is a major health problem with a generally grim prognosis. However, an orderly approach to diagnosis, staging, and treatment based on knowledge of the clinical behavior of lung cancer allows selection of the best therapy for either potential cure or optimal palliation of individual patients. This approach should be multidisciplinary, involving interaction of internists, chest physicians, medical, radiation, and surgical oncologists, pathologists, and supportive care personnel.

PATHOLOGY

The histologic classification of primary lung neoplasms recommended by the World Health Organization in 1981 should be used. The term *lung cancer* is usually reserved for tumors arising from the respiratory epithelium (bronchi, bronchioles, and alveoli). Mesotheliomas, lymphomas, and stromal tumors (sarcomas) usually are given a pathologic diagnosis distinct from epithelial lung cancer. Four major cell types make up 88 percent of all primary lung neoplasms (Table 90-1). These are *squamous* or *epidermoid carcinoma*, *small cell* (also called *oat cell*) *carcinoma*, *adenocarcinoma* (including bronchioloalveolar), and *large cell* (also called *large cell anaplastic*) *carcinoma*. The remainder include undifferentiated carcinomas, carcinoids, bronchial gland tumors (including adenoid cystic carcinomas and mucoepidermoid tumors), and rarer tumor types. The various cell types have different natural histories and responses to therapy, and thus a correct histologic diagnosis by an experienced pathologist is the first step to correct treatment. In the past 20 years, for unknown reasons, adenocarcinoma has replaced squamous cell carcinoma as the most frequent histologic subtype for all sexes and races combined (Table 90-1).

Major treatment decisions are made on the basis of whether a tumor is classified histologically as a small cell carcinoma or as one of the non-small cell varieties (which include epidermoid, adenocarcinoma, large cell carcinoma, bronchioloalveolar carcinoma—a subtype of adenocarcinoma—and mixed versions of these). Some of these distinctions are summarized in Tables 90-1 and 90-2. In general, small cell carcinomas have already spread at the time of presentation beyond the bounds where surgery with curative intent could be undertaken, and they are managed primarily by chemotherapy with or without radiotherapy. In contrast, non-small cell cancers that are found to be localized at the time of presentation should be considered for curative treatment with either surgery or radiotherapy. Further, the response of non-small cell cancers to chemotherapy usually is not dramatic, making such therapy less important in metastatic disease than it is in cases of small cell lung cancer.

Ninety percent of patients with lung cancer of all histologic types are current or former cigarette smokers. Currently, ~50,000 of the annual 177,000 new cases of lung cancer develop in former smokers. With increased success in smoking cessation efforts, this number will grow, and such former smokers will be important candidates for future early detection and chemoprevention efforts. By far the most common form of lung cancer arising in lifetime nonsmokers, in women, and in young patients (<45 years old) is adenocarcinoma. However, in nonsmokers with adenocarcinoma involving the lung, the possibility of other primary sites should be considered. Epidermoid and small cell cancers usually present as central masses with endobronchial growth, while adenocarcinomas and large cell cancers tend to present as peripheral nodules or masses, frequently with pleural involvement. Epidermoid and large cell cancers cavitate in approximately 10 to 20 percent of cases. Bronchioloalveolar carcinoma, a special form of adenocarcinoma arising from peripheral airways, can present as a single mass, as a diffuse, multinodular lesion, or as a fluffy infiltrate.

ETIOLOGY

The large majority of lung cancers are caused by carcinogens and tumor promoters ingested via cigarette smoking. The prevalence of smoking in the United States is 28 percent for males and 25 percent for females, 18 years old or older. Overall, the relative risk of developing lung cancer is increased about 13-fold by active smoking and about 1.5-fold by long-term passive exposure to cigarette smoke. Probably there is a cocarcinogenic effect of smoking and industrial or environmental pollutants such as radon gas from natural sources in the ground. There is a dose-response relationship between the lung cancer death rate and the total amount (often expressed in "cigarette pack-years") of cigarettes smoked, such that the risk is increased 60- to 70-fold for a man smoking two packs a day for 20 years as compared with a nonsmoker. Conversely, the chance of developing lung cancer decreases with cessation of smoking but may never return to the nonsmoker level. The increase in lung cancer rate in women is also associated with a rise in cigarette smoking. However, of great importance, women with lung cancer are more likely to have never smoked than men. Also, the dose-response odds ratio of developing lung cancer over cumulative exposure to cigarette smoking was ~1.5 higher in women than men for all histologic types. This gender difference is likely due to a higher susceptibility to tobacco carcinogens in women. As a preventive measure, efforts to get persons to stop smoking are mandatory. However, smoking cessation is extremely difficult, because the smoking habit represents a powerful addiction to nicotine (see Chap. 389). Therefore, it is of vital importance to prevent people from starting to smoke. This goal requires new efforts targeted at children, since addiction to cigarettes usually has occurred by the late teen years.

The poor prognosis for most patients with lung cancer requires the continued performance of well-designed clinical trials—trials of combinations of chemotherapy with surgery or radiotherapy and of the relative effectiveness of using chemotherapy and radiotherapy in an adjuvant (after surgery) and a neoadjuvant (before surgery) fashion; tests of biologic response modifiers, oncopeptide vaccines, and gene therapy; prospective testing of tumor sensitivity in vitro to drugs, radiation therapy, and biologic response modifiers; and tests of the application of newer methods for early detection and chemoprevention. The key intervention remains prevention, and broad efforts to help persons to stop smoking and to prevent persons from starting smoking must continue. Initial reports suggest that retinoids have a significant ability to prevent the development of second aerodigestive tract malignancies. Work in this area will expand rapidly in the immediate future, particularly in relation to former smokers. The detection of genetic lesions predisposing to malignancy in airway epithelial cells would be a major step forward in focusing preventive efforts, providing intermediate end-points and molecular means of early diagnosis, and eventually targeting therapy at the products of the lesions that make lung cancer cells malignant.

While human lung cancer is not thought of as a genetic disease, a variety of molecular genetic studies have shown

that lung cancer cells have acquired a number of genetic lesions, including activation of dominant oncogenes and inactivation of tumor suppressor or recessive oncogenes (Chaps. 83 and 84). In fact, lung cancer cells may have to accumulate a large number (perhaps 10 or more) of such lesions. For the dominant oncogenes, these include point mutations in the coding regions of the *ras* family of oncogenes (particularly in the K-*ras* gene in adenocarcinoma of the lung); amplification, rearrangement, and/or loss of transcriptional control of *myc* family oncogenes (c-, N-, and L-*myc*; changes in c-*myc* are found in non-small cell cancers, while changes in all *myc* family members are found in small cell lung cancer); and overexpression of *bcl-2*, *Her-2/neu*, and the telomerase gene (Table 90-2). Tumor mutations in *ras* genes are associated with a poor prognosis in non-small cell lung cancer, while tumor amplification of c-*myc* is associated with a poor prognosis in small cell lung cancer.

For the recessive oncogenes (*tumor suppressor genes*), cytogenetic and allelotyping analyses have shown deletions (allele loss) involving chromosome regions 1p, 1q, 3p12-13, 3p14 (*FHIT* gene region), 3p21, 3p24-25, 3q, 5q, 8p, 9p (*p16/CDKN2, p15* gene cluster), 11p13, 11p15, 13q14 (retinoblastoma, *rb*, gene), 16q, and 17p13 (*p53* gene), as well as other sites. There appear to be several candidate recessive oncogenes on chromosome 3p that are involved in nearly all lung cancers. The *p53* and *rb* genes are both mutated in more than 90 percent of small cell lung cancers, while *p53* is mutated in more than 50 percent and *rb* in 20 percent of non-small cell lung cancers. *p16/CDKN2* is abnormal in ~10 percent of small cell and >50 percent of non-small cell lung cancers. Rb and *p16/CDKN2* appear to be part of the same G1-to-S cell cycle regulatory pathway. Either one or the other of these elements appears to be mutated or to have its expression turned off (e.g., by hypermethylation) in the large majority of lung cancers. The large number of genetic lesions in clinically evident cancer has prompted a search for these mutations in lung tissue before classic cytopathologic evidence of malignancy can be found, to provide for molecular early diagnosis and as intermediate end-points in prevention efforts, including chemoprevention treatment. Histologically identifiable preneoplastic lesions found in the respiratory epithelium of lung cancer patients and smokers include hyperplasia, dysplasia (progressively severe), and carcinoma in situ. 3p allele loss (hyperplasia) followed by 9p (*p16/CDKN2*) allele loss (hyperplasia) are the earliest events; 17p (*p53*) abnormalities and then *ras* mutations usually are only found in carcinoma in situ and invasive cancer. Thus, molecular changes involving allele loss and microsatellite alteration can be found in the earliest preneoplastic lesions and potentially even before any histologic changes are noted. Clinical trials of early diagnosis will be needed to prove the usefulness of these molecular

Table 90-1

Frequency, Age-Adjusted Incidence, and Survival Rates for Different Histologic Types of Lung Cancer (All Races, Both Sexes, and All Stages)*

Histologic Type of Thoracic Malignancy	Frequency, %	Age-Adjusted Rate	5-year Survival Rate (All Stages)
Adenocarcinoma (and all subtypes)	32	17	17
Bronchioloalveolar carcinoma	3	1.4	42
Squamous cell (epidermoid) carcinoma	29	15	15
Small cell carcinoma	18	9	5
Large cell carcinoma	9	5	11
Carcinoid	1.0	0.5	83
Mucoepidermoid carcinoma	0.1	<0.1	39
Adenoid cystic carcinoma	<0.1	<0.1	48
Sarcoma and other soft tissue tumors	0.1	0.1	30
All others and unspecified carcinomas	11.0	6	NA
Total	100	52	14

* Data on histology frequency and age-adjusted incidence rates per 100,000 U.S. population are from 60,514 cases of invasive lung cancer involving all races and both sexes obtained from the data for 1983–1987 of the Surveillance, Epidemiology, and End Results (SEER) Program of the National Cancer Institute; 5-year relative survival rates for all stages, all races, and both sexes are from the SEER data on 87,128 carcinomas, 1978–1986. NA, not available.

SOURCE: Summarized from Travis et al.

markers in the identification of very early lung cancer and in the monitoring of treatment and chemoprevention.

The large number of lesions shows that lung cancer, like other common epithelial malignancies, is a multistep process that is likely to involve both carcinogens and tumor promoters. Prevention can be directed at both processes. Cell-biologic studies have shown that lung cancer cells both produce a large number of peptide hormones and express receptors for these hormones, which thereby can act to stimulate tumor cell growth in an "autocrine" fashion. Nicotine may play a very central role in lung cancer pathogenesis. Highly carcinogenic derivatives of nicotine are formed in cigarette smoke. Smoking is tied to nicotine addiction, and nicotine gum and patches are now widely used to help persons to stop smoking. Lung cancer cells of all histologic types express receptors for nicotine that are very similar to nicotinic acetylcholine receptors. Thus, it is possible that nicotine itself could be directly involved in lung cancer pathogenesis.

While lung cancer does not have a clear pattern of Mendelian inheritance, there are several indications of a potential for familial association. These include inherited mutations in *rb* (patients with retinoblastomas living to adulthood) and *p53* (Li-Fraumeni syndrome)

genes; studies that show that first-degree relatives of lung cancer probands have a two- to threefold excess risk of lung cancer or other cancers, many of which are not smoking-related; and a strong risk of developing lung cancer linked with the development of chronic obstructive pulmonary disease. Finally, genetic epidemiologic studies have proposed an association between the P450 enzyme or chromosome fragility (*mutagen sensitivity*) genotypes and the development of lung cancer. The genetic identification of persons at very high risk of developing lung cancer would be very important in early detection and prevention efforts.

CLINICAL MANIFESTATIONS AND MODE OF PRESENTATION

Lung cancer gives rise to signs and symptoms caused by local tumor growth, invasion or obstruction of adjacent structures, growth in regional nodes via lymphatic spread, growth in distant metastatic sites after hematogenous dissemination, or remote effects (paraneoplastic syndrome). The latter usually result from peptide hormone secretion by the tumor or immunologic cross-reaction between tumor and normal tissue antigens (Chap. 102).

Although 5 to 15 percent of patients are detected while asymptomatic, usually on a routine chest radiograph, the vast majority of patients

Table 90-2

Comparison Between Small Cell and Non-Small Cell Lung Cancers

	Small Cell	Non-Small Cell
Histology	Scant cytoplasm; small, hyperchromatic nuclei with fine chromatin pattern; nucleoli indistinct; diffuse sheets of cells	Abundant cytoplasm; pleomorphic nuclei with coarse chromatin pattern; nucleoli often prominent; glandular or squamous architecture
General neuroendocrine properties		
Dense-core granules	Present	Absent*
L-Dopa decarboxylase activity	High	Absent
Chromogranin	Present	Absent
Synaptophysin	Present	Absent
Neuron-specific enolase	High	Low
Creatine kinase BB isozyme	High	Low
CD56 and CD57 antigens	Present	Absent
Peptide hormone production		
Gastrin-releasing peptide gene products	Present	Absent
Other neuropeptides	ACTH, AVP, calcitonin, ANF	PTH
Other markers		
HLA, β₂-microglobulin	Absent/low	Present
Intermediate filament pattern	"SCLC"	"Non-SCLC"
Neurofilaments	Present	Absent
Opioid receptors	Present	Present
Nicotine receptors	Present	Present
EGF receptors	Low or absent	Present
Mucin	Absent	Present in adenocarcinomas
Surfactant-associated proteins	Absent	Often present
Carcinoembryonic antigen	Present	Present
Recessive oncogene (tumor suppressor gene) and allelotype abnormalities		
3p deletions	>90%	>80%
rb mutations	~90%	~20%
p16/CDKN2 mutations	~10%	~50%
p53 mutations	>90%	>50%
5q, 8p, 11p and other allele losses	Present	Present
Microsatellite alterations	Present	Present
Dominant oncogene abnormalities		
ras mutations	<1%	~30%
myc family overexpression	>50%	>50%
bcl-2 overexpression	>75%	>50%
Her-2/neu overexpression	<10%	~30%
Telomerase overexpression	>90%	>90%
Response to radiotherapy	Objective shrinkage in 80–90%; often complete response	Objective shrinkage in 30–50%; response uncommonly complete
Response to combination chemotherapy		
Overall regression rate	90%	30–40%
Rate of complete regression	50%	5%

* Ten percent of non-small cell lung cancers have populations of cells expressing neuroendocrine markers, and these are best demonstrated by immunohistochemical stains.

Abbreviations: ACTH, adrenocorticotropic hormone; ANF, atrial natriuretic factor; AVP, arginine vasopressin; CD56, neural cell adhesion molecule (NCAM)-1; CD57, Leu-7 or HNK-1; HLA, human leukocyte antigen; PTH, parathormone; SCLC, small cell lung cancer.

present with some sign or symptom. Signs and symptoms secondary to central or endobronchial growth of the primary tumor include cough, hemoptysis, wheeze and stridor, dyspnea, and postobstructive pneumonitis (fever and productive cough). Signs and symptoms secondary to the peripheral growth of the primary tumor include pain from pleural or chest wall involvement, cough, dyspnea on a restrictive basis, and symptoms of lung abscess resulting from tumor cavitation. Signs and symptoms related to the regional spread of tumor in the thorax (by contiguous growth or by metastasis to regional lymph nodes) include tracheal obstruction, esophageal compression with dysphagia, recurrent laryngeal nerve paralysis with hoarseness, phrenic nerve paralysis with elevation of the hemidiaphragm and dyspnea, and sympathetic nerve paralysis with Horner's syndrome (enophthalmos, ptosis, miosis, and ipsilateral loss of sweating). *Pancoast's* (or *superior sulcus tumor*) *syndrome* results from local extension of a tumor (usually epidermoid) growing in the apex of the lung with involvement of the eighth cervical and first and second thoracic nerves, with shoulder pain which characteristically radiates in the ulnar distribution of the arm, often with radiologic destruction of the first and second ribs. Often Horner's syndrome and Pancoast's syndrome coexist. Other problems of regional spread include *superior vena cava syndrome* from vascular obstruction; pericardial and cardiac extension with resultant tamponade, arrhythmia, or cardiac failure; lymphatic obstruction with resultant pleural effusion; and lymphangitic spread through the lungs with hypoxemia and dyspnea. In addition, bronchioloalveolar carcinoma can spread transbronchially, producing tumor growing along multiple alveolar surfaces with resultant impairment of oxygen transfer, respiratory insufficiency, dyspnea, hypoxemia, and production of large amounts of sputum.

Extrathoracic metastatic disease is found at autopsy in over 50 percent of patients with epidermoid carcinoma, 80 percent of patients with adenocarcinoma and large cell carcinoma, and over 95 percent of patients with small cell cancer. These autopsy studies have found lung cancer metastases in virtually every organ system. Thus, the majority of lung cancer patients eventually need therapy to palliate symptoms. Common clinical problems related to metastatic lung cancer include brain metastases with neurologic deficits; bone metastases with pain and pathologic fractures; bone marrow invasion with cytopenias or leukoerythroblastosis; liver metastases causing biochemical liver dysfunction, biliary obstruction, and pain; lymph node metastases in the supraclavicular region and occasionally in the axilla and groin; and spinal cord compression syndromes from epidural or bone metastases.

Paraneoplastic syndromes are common in lung cancer patients and may be the presenting finding or first sign of recurrence. In addition, paraneoplastic syndromes may mimic metastatic disease and, unless detected, lead to inappropriate palliative rather than curative treatment. Often the paraneoplastic syndrome may be relieved with successful treatment of the tumor, and tumor treatment is the basis for correcting such syndromes. In some cases, the pathophysiology of the paraneoplastic syndrome is known, particularly when a hormone with biologic activity is secreted by a tumor (Chap. 102). However, in many cases the pathophysiology is unknown. *Systemic symptoms* of anorexia, cachexia, weight loss (seen in 30 percent of patients), fever, and suppressed immunity are paraneoplastic syndromes of unknown etiology. *Endocrine syndromes* are seen in 12 percent of patients and have the best understood pathophysiology, including hypercalcemia and hypophosphatemia resulting from the ectopic production by epidermoid tumors of parathyroid hormone (PTH) or PTH-related peptide production, hyponatremia with the syndrome of inappropriate secretion of antidiuretic hormone or possibly atrial natriuretic factor by small cell cancer, and ectopic secretion by small cell cancer of adrenocorticotropic hormone (ACTH). ACTH secretion usually results in additional electrolyte disturbances, especially hypokalemia, rather than in the changes in body habitus seen in Cushing's syndrome from a pituitary adenoma.

Skeletal–connective tissue syndromes include clubbing in 30 percent of cases (usually non-small cell carcinomas) and hypertrophic pulmonary osteoarthropathy in 1 to 10 percent of cases (usually adenocarcinomas) with periostitis and clubbing giving pain, tenderness, and swelling over the affected bones and a positive bone scan. *Neurologic-*

myopathic syndromes are seen in only 1 percent of patients but are dramatic and include the myasthenic *Eaton-Lambert syndrome* and retinal blindness with small cell cancer, while peripheral neuropathies, subacute cerebellar degeneration, cortical degeneration, and polymyositis are seen with all lung cancer types. Many of these are caused by autoimmune responses such as the development of anti-voltage-gated calcium channel antibodies in the Eaton-Lambert syndrome (Chap. 103). *Coagulation, thrombotic, or other hematologic manifestations* occur in 1 to 8 percent of patients and include migratory venous thrombophlebitis (*Trousseau's syndrome*), nonbacterial thrombotic (marantic) endocarditis with arterial emboli, disseminated intravascular coagulation with hemorrhage, and anemia, granulocytosis, and leukoerythroblastosis. *Cutaneous manifestations* such as dermatomyositis and acanthosis nigricans are uncommon (1 percent or less), as are the *renal manifestations* of nephrotic syndrome or glomerulonephritis (1 percent or less).

DIAGNOSIS AND STAGING

EARLY DIAGNOSIS The screening of asymptomatic persons at high risk (men over 45 years of age who smoke 40 or more cigarettes per day) for lung cancer by means of sputum cytology and chest radiographs has not been proved effective. Studies using these screening procedures found a prevalence of lung cancer of 4 to 8 cases per 1000 persons. With follow-up screening every 4 months, four new cases of lung cancer are found per 1000 persons followed per year. These lung cancers are detected 72 percent of the time by radiographs alone and 20 percent by cytology alone, while 6 percent are detected by both methods. In contrast to nonscreened patients, 90 percent of these screened patients who develop lung cancer are asymptomatic, 62 percent have resectable lung cancer, and 53 percent of all the new cases are postoperative stage I (see below) with a 5-year survival probability of 45 percent. However, there was no difference in the survival rate between the screened and nonscreened groups of smoking males 45 years of age or older. The reason for this poor survival was the development of clinically silent and undetected metastases in the majority of patients even when primary tumors were detected at a very early stage. Newer screening methods involving fluorescent bronchoscopy and molecular analysis will be analyzed in clinical trials in the hope of improving the detection of lung cancer before metastases develop.

ESTABLISHING A TISSUE DIAGNOSIS OF LUNG CANCER Once signs, symptoms, or screening studies suggest lung cancer, it is necessary to establish a tissue diagnosis of malignancy, to determine the histologic cell type, and to stage the patient for appropriate treatment. In the initial evaluation of each patient, tumor tissue should be obtained so that a histologic diagnosis of cancer and tumor cell type can be made. Tumor tissue can be obtained by a bronchial or transbronchial biopsy during fiberoptic bronchoscopy; by node biopsy during mediastinoscopy; from the operative specimen at the time of definitive surgical resection; by percutaneous biopsy of an enlarged lymph node, soft tissue mass, lytic bone lesion, bone marrow, or pleural lesion; by fine-needle aspiration of thoracic or extrathoracic tumor masses using computed tomography (CT) guidance; or from an adequate cell block obtained from a malignant pleural effusion. In the vast majority of cases, the pathologist should be able to definitely make a diagnosis of epithelial malignancy and make the crucial distinction of small cell from non-small cell lung cancer.

STAGING PATIENTS WITH LUNG CANCER Lung cancer staging consists of two parts: first, a determination of the location of tumor (anatomic staging) and, second, an assessment of a patient's ability to withstand various antitumor treatments (physiologic staging). For example, in a patient with non-small cell lung cancer, it is crucial to determine both whether the tumor could be resected by a standard surgical procedure such as a lobectomy or pneumonectomy (determination of *resectability*), which depends on the anatomic stage of the tumor, and whether the patient could tolerate such a surgical procedure (determination of *operability*), which depends on the cardiopulmonary condition of the patient.

Non-Small Cell Lung Cancer The TNM international staging system (ISS), which was developed by the American Joint Committee (AJC) on End Results Reporting and modified by an international commission, should be used for cases of non-small cell lung cancer, particularly in preparing patients for curative attempts with surgery or radiotherapy (Table 90-3). The various T (tumor size), N (regional node involvement), and M (presence or absence of distant metastasis) factors are combined to form different stage groups (stages I, II, IIIA, IIIB, and IV) (Table 90-3). At presentation, approximately one-third of patients will have disease localized enough for a curative attempt with surgery or radiotherapy (patients with stage I or II disease and some with stage IIIA disease), one-third will have distant metastatic disease (stage IV disease), and the remaining one-third will have local or regional disease that may or may not be amenable to a curative attempt (some patients with stage IIIA disease and patients with stage IIIB disease) (see below). This staging system provides useful prognostic information.

Small Cell Lung Cancer A simple two-stage system is used. In this system, *limited-stage disease* (representing about 30 percent of all small cell cancer patients) is defined as disease confined to one hemithorax and regional lymph nodes (including mediastinal, contralateral hilar, and usually ipsilateral supraclavicular nodes), while *extensive-stage disease* (representing about 70 percent of all patients) is defined as disease exceeding those boundaries. Employed in staging are clinical studies such as physical examination, x-rays, scans, and bone marrow examination. In part, the definition of limited-stage disease relates to whether the known tumor can be encompassed within a tolerable radiation therapy port. Thus, contralateral supraclavicular nodes, recurrent laryngeal nerve involvement, and superior vena caval obstruction can all be part of limited-stage disease. However, cardiac tamponade, malignant pleural effusion, and bilateral pulmonary parenchymal involvement generally qualify disease as extensive-stage because of the size of the radiation therapy port required to cover all known disease.

GENERAL STAGING PROCEDURES (See Table 90-4) All lung cancer patients should have a complete history and physical examination, with evaluation of all other medical problems and a determination of performance status and weight loss, both of which have great prognostic value. An ear, nose, and throat examination is also necessary because of the frequent occurrence of second cancers in this area. While not done in every patient, fiberoptic bronchoscopy remains a cornerstone of lung cancer staging and follow-up, providing material for pathologic examination as well as information on tumor size, location, degree of bronchial obstruction, and recurrence.

Table 90-4

Pretreatment Staging Procedures for Lung Cancer Patients

ALL PATIENTS

Complete history & physical examination
    Determination of performance status and weight loss
    Ear, nose, and throat examination
Complete blood count with platelet determination
Measurement of serum electrolytes, glucose, calcium, and phosphorus; renal and liver function tests
Electrocardiogram
Skin test for tuberculosis
Chest x-ray
Computed tomography scan of brain, chest, and abdomen, and radionuclide scan of bone if any of the above studies suggest the presence of tumor metastasis in these organs
X-rays of suspicious bony lesions detected by scan or symptom
Barium-swallow radiographic examination if esophageal symptoms exist
Pulmonary function studies and arterial blood gas measurements if signs or symptoms of respiratory insufficiency are present
Biopsy of accessible lesions suspicious for cancer if a histologic diagnosis is not yet made or if treatment or staging decisions would be based on whether or not a lesion contained cancer

PATIENTS WITH NON-SMALL CELL LUNG CANCER WHO HAVE NO OBVIOUS CONTRAINDICATION TO CURATIVE SURGERY OR RADIOTHERAPY

All the above procedures, plus the following:
    Fiberoptic bronchoscopy with washings, brushings, and biopsy of suspicious areas
    Pulmonary function tests and arterial blood gas measurements
    Coagulation tests
    Computed tomographic scans of brain, chest, and abdomen
    If surgical resection is planned: surgical evaluation of the mediastinum at mediastinoscopy or at thoracotomy
    If the patient is a poor surgical risk or a candidate for curative radiotherapy: transthoracic fine-needle aspiration biopsy or transbronchial forceps biopsy of peripheral lesions if material from routine fiberoptic bronchoscopy is negative

PATIENTS PRESENTING WITH SMALL CELL OR NON-SMALL CELL LUNG CANCER THAT IS NOT CURABLE BY EITHER SURGERY OR RADIOTHERAPY ALONE*

For proven small cell lung cancer, all the procedures under "All Patients," plus the following:
    Fiberoptic bronchoscopy with washings and biopsy
    Chest, abdomen, and brain CT scans
    Bone marrow aspiration and biopsy
For non-small cell lung cancer or cancer of unknown histology, all the procedures under "All Patients," plus the following:
    Fiberoptic bronchoscopy if indicated by hemoptysis, obstruction, pneumonitis, or no histologic diagnosis of cancer
    Biopsy of accessible lesions suspicious for tumor to obtain a histologic diagnosis or if therapy would be altered by finding of tumor
    Transthoracic fine-needle aspiration biopsy or transbronchial forceps biopsy of peripheral lesions if fiberoptic bronchoscopy is negative and no other material exists for a histologic diagnosis
    Diagnostic and therapeutic thoracentesis if a pleural effusion is present

* Patients with non-small cell lung cancer and extrathoracic metastatic disease, malignant pleural effusion, or intrathoracic disease beyond the bounds of a tolerable radiotherapy port.

Table 90-3

International TNM (Tumor, Node, Metastasis) Staging System for Lung Cancer

Stage	TNM Descriptors	5-Year Survival (%)
I	T1–T2 N0 M0	60–80
II	T1–T2 N1 M0	25–50
IIIA	T3 N0–1 M0	25–40
	T1–3 N2 M0	10–30
IIIB	Any T4 or any N3 M0	<5
IV	Any M1	<5

TUMOR (T) STATUS DESCRIPTOR

T0   No evidence of a primary tumor
TX   Malignant cells found by cytologic examination but no lesion seen on x-ray or fiberoptic bronchoscopy
TIS   Carcinoma in situ
T1   Tumor <3 cm diameter
T2   Tumor >3 cm diameter or has distal atelectasis extending to hilum
T3   Tumor extends directly into pleura, chest wall, diaphragm, or pericardium, is <2 cm from carina, or causes total atelectasis
T4   Tumor invades mediastinum (heart, great vessels, trachea, esophagus, vertebral body, carina), or malignant pleural effusion is present

LYMPH NODE (N) INVOLVEMENT DESCRIPTOR

N0   No lymph node involvement
N1   Metastasis in bronchopulmonary or ipsilateral hilar lymph nodes
N2   Metastasis in ipsilateral mediastinal or subcarinal lymph nodes
N3   Metastasis to contralateral mediastinal or hilar lymph nodes or to any scalene or supraclavicular lymph nodes

DISTANT METASTASIS (M) DESCRIPTOR

M0   No known distant metastasis
M1   Distant metastasis present with site specified (e.g., brain)

SOURCE: Adapted from CF Mountain et al, Chest 96:475, 1989, and from Ginsberg et al.

Chest radiographs are needed to evaluate tumor size and nodal involvement, and it is very useful to obtain old x-ray films for comparison. CT scans are of use in the preoperative staging of non-small cell lung cancer to detect mediastinal nodes and pleural extension and occult abdominal disease (e.g., of the liver and adrenal glands), as well as in the planning of curative radiation therapy to allow the design of fields to encompass all the known tumor while avoiding as much normal tissue as possible. However, mediastinal nodal involvement should be documented histologically. Thus, sampling of lymph nodes via mediastinoscopy or thoracotomy to establish the presence or absence of N2 or N3 nodal involvement is of vital importance in considering or rejecting a curative surgical approach for non-small cell lung cancer patients with clinical stage I, II, or III disease. This is particularly true for patients with modest nodal abnormalities on chest CT scans. Likewise, unless the CT-detected abnormalities are unequivocal, malignancy of suspicious abdominal lesions should be confirmed by procedures such as fine-needle aspiration if the patient would otherwise be considered for curative treatment. In small cell lung cancer, CT scans are used in the planning of chest radiation treatment and in the assessment of the response to chemotherapy and radiation therapy. In following patients after surgery or radiotherapy—procedures that can make interpretation of conventional chest x-rays difficult—CT scans can provide good evidence of tumor recurrence.

If signs or symptoms suggest organ involvement by tumor, appropriate CT or radionuclide scans (e.g., of brain, liver, or bone) are performed, as well as radiography of any suspicious bony lesions. Any accessible lesions suspicious for cancer should be biopsied if a histologic diagnosis has not already been made or if treatment decisions would be based on whether or not the lesion contained cancer.

In patients presenting with a mass lesion on chest x-ray and no obvious contraindications to a curative approach with surgery or radiotherapy after the initial evaluation, the mediastinum must be investigated. Approaches vary between different centers and include performing chest CT scan and mediastinoscopy (for right-sided tumors) or lateral mediastinotomy (for left-sided lesions) on all patients and proceeding directly to thoracotomy for staging of the mediastinum. In patients presenting with disease that is confined to the chest but not resectable, and who thus are candidates for neoadjuvant chemotherapy plus surgery or for curative radiotherapy, other tests are done as indicated to evaluate specific symptoms. In patients presenting with non-small cell cancer that is not curable by surgery, radiotherapy, or a combination of either with chemotherapy, all the general staging procedures are done, plus fiberoptic bronchoscopy as indicated to evaluate hemoptysis, obstruction, or pneumonitis, as well as thoracentesis with cytologic examination (and chest tube drainage as indicated) if fluid is present. As a rule, a radiographic finding of an isolated lesion (such as an enlarged adrenal gland) should be confirmed as cancer by fine-needle aspiration before a curative attempt is rejected.

STAGING OF SMALL CELL LUNG CANCER Pretreatment staging for patients with histologically documented small cell lung cancer includes the initial general lung cancer evaluation as well as fiberoptic bronchoscopy with washings and biopsies to determine the tumor extent before therapy; brain CT scan, since 10 percent of patients have metastases; bone marrow biopsy and aspiration, since 20 to 30 percent of patients have tumor in the bone marrow; and CT (liver) and radionuclide scans (bone) if symptoms or other findings are suggestive of disease involvement in these areas. Chest and abdominal CT scans are very useful to evaluate and follow tumor response to therapy, and chest CT scans are helpful in planning chest radiotherapy ports.

If signs or symptoms of spinal cord compression or leptomeningitis develop at any time in lung cancer patients with disease of any histologic type, a CT scan or magnetic resonance scan and examination of the cerebrospinal fluid cytology are performed to determine the need for local therapy to the site of compression (usually with radiotherapy) and for intrathecal chemotherapy (usually with methotrexate) if malignant cells are detected. In addition, a brain CT scan is performed to search for brain metastases, which often are associated with spinal cord or leptomeningeal metastases.

DETERMINATION OF RESECTABILITY AND OPERABILITY In patients with non-small cell lung cancer, the following are major contraindications to curative surgery or radiotherapy alone: extrathoracic distant metastases; superior vena cava syndrome; vocal cord and, in most cases, phrenic nerve paralysis; malignant pleural effusion; cardiac tamponade; tumor within 2 cm of the carina (not curable by surgery but potentially curable by radiotherapy); metastasis to the contralateral lung; bilateral endobronchial tumor (potentially curable by radiotherapy); metastasis to the supraclavicular lymph nodes; lymph node metastasis in the contralateral mediastinum (potentially curable by radiotherapy); and involvement of the main stem pulmonary artery. While a histologic diagnosis of small cell lung cancer is usually highly correlated with other findings of unresectability, if all other findings suggest the potential for resection, that option should be considered. This situation is usually encountered in cases of small peripheral small cell lung cancer lesions (see below).

PHYSIOLOGIC STAGING Patients with lung cancer often have cardiopulmonary and other problems related to chronic obstructive pulmonary disease as well as other medical problems. To improve their preoperative condition, correctable problems (e.g., anemia, electrolyte and fluid disorders, infections, and arrhythmias) should be addressed, smoking stopped, and appropriate chest therapy instituted. Since it is not always possible to predict whether a lobectomy or pneumonectomy will be required until the time of operation, a conservative approach is to restrict resectional surgery to patients who could potentially tolerate a pneumonectomy. In addition to nonambulatory performance status, a myocardial infarction within the past 3 months is a contraindication to thoracic surgery because 20 percent of patients will die of reinfarction alone, while an infarction in the past 6 months is a relative contraindication. Other major contraindications include uncontrolled major arrhythmias, a maximum breathing capacity less than 40 percent of the predicted value, an FEV_1 (forced expiratory volume in 1 s) of less than 1 L, CO_2 retention (which is more serious than hypoxemia), and severe pulmonary hypertension. Recommending surgery when the FEV_1 is 1.1 to 2.4 L requires careful judgment, while an FEV_1 of over 2.5 L will usually permit a pneumonectomy. In patients with borderline pulmonary status or a question of pulmonary hypertension, split pulmonary function testing by ventilation-perfusion lung scans can define physiologic operability. The activity from quantitative scans is summed for each lung in the anterior and posterior views, and the ratio of the normal to total lung activity is multiplied by the FEV_1. Pneumonectomy usually is physiologically tolerable if this predicted value is greater than 1 L.

R̶x̶ **TREATMENT**

After a histologic diagnosis is obtained and appropriate anatomic and physiologic staging studies are completed, the overall treatment approach to patients with lung cancer may be formulated (Table 90-5). Even after the diagnosis is made, patients should be encouraged to stop smoking. Those who do fare better than those who continue to smoke.

Non-Small Cell Lung Cancer: Localized Disease SURGERY In patients with non-small cell lung cancer of stages I and II (see Table 90-3) who can tolerate operation, the treatment of choice is pulmonary resection. In stage IIIA cases where the patient's age and cardiopulmonary function and the anatomy are favorable, resection also should be considered. If a complete resection is possible, the 5-year survival rate for N1 disease is about 50 percent, while it is about 20 percent for N2 disease. However, only 20 percent of all cases of N2 disease are technically resectable, and most of these resectable cases are discovered to be N2 only at thoracotomy. Surgery for N2 disease is the most controversial area in the surgical management of lung cancer. In this regard, it is useful to divide N2 disease into "minimal" disease (involvement of only one node with microscopic foci, usually discovered at thoracotomy or mediastinoscopy); and the more common "advanced," bulky disease, clinically

Table 90-5

Summary of Treatment Approach to Lung Cancer Patients

NON-SMALL CELL LUNG CANCER

Stages I and II, some IIIA:
    Surgical resection for stages I, II
    Surgical resection with complete mediastinal lymph node dissection and
      consideration of neoadjuvant CT for stage IIIA disease with "minimal
      N2 involvement" (discovered at thoracotomy or mediastinoscopy)
    Postoperative RT for patients found to have N2 disease if no neoadjuvant
      therapy given
    Curative potential RT for "nonoperable" patients
Stage IIIA with selected types of stage T3 tumors:
    Tumors with chest wall invasion (T3): en bloc resection of tumor with in-
      volved chest wall and consideration of postoperative radiotherapy.
    Superior sulcus (Pancoast's) (T3) tumors: preoperative radiotherapy
      (3000–4500 cGy) followed by en bloc resection of involved lung and
      chest wall with consideration of postoperative radiotherapy or intraopera-
      tive brachytherapy.
    Proximal airway involvement (<2 cm from carina) without mediastinal
      nodes: sleeve resection if possible preserving distal normal lung or pneu-
      monectomy
Stages IIIA "advanced, bulky, clinically evident N2 disease" (discovered
  preoperatively) and IIIB disease that can be included in a tolerable radiotherapy port:
    Curative potential RT + CT if performance status is reasonable; other-
      wise, RT alone
    Consider neoadjuvant chemotherapy and surgical resection for IIIA dis-
      ease with advanced N2 involvement
Stage IIIB disease with carinal invasion (T4) but without N2 involvement:
  consider pneumonectomy with tracheal sleeve resection with direct reanastomosis to contralateral mainstem bronchus.
Stage IV and more advanced IIIB disease:
    RT to symptomatic local sites
    CT for patients with good performance status and evaluable lesions
    Chest tube drainage of large malignant pleural effusions
    Consider resection of primary tumor and metastasis for isolated brain or
      adrenal metastases

SMALL CELL LUNG CANCER

Limited stage (good performance status): combination chemotherapy +
  chest RT
Extensive stage (good performance status): combination chemotherapy
Complete tumor responders (all stages): prophylactic cranial RT
Poor-performance-status patients (all stages):
    Modified-dose combination chemotherapy
    Palliative RT

ALL PATIENTS

Radiotherapy for brain metastases, spinal cord compression, weight-bearing
  lytic bony lesions, symptomatic local lesions (nerve paralyses, obstructed
  airway, hemoptysis in non-small cell lung cancer and in small cell cancer
  not responding to chemotherapy)
Appropriate diagnosis and treatment of other medical problems and supportive care during chemotherapy
Encouragement to stop smoking
Entrance into clinical trial, if eligible

Abbreviations: CT, chemotherapy; RT, radiotherapy.

obvious on CT scans and discovered preoperatively. Patients with contralateral or bilateral positive mediastinal (N3) nodes, extracapsular nodal involvement, or fixed nodes are not considered resectable. New approaches that may make resection possible in situations where currently it is not include chest wall resection for direct extension of tumor, tracheal sleeve pneumonectomy, and sleeve lobectomy for lesions near the carina. Neoadjuvant (preoperative) chemotherapy gives tumor response rates of 50 to 60 percent and causes unresectable disease to become resectable in many responding patients. Video-assisted thoracic surgery (VATS) via thoracoscopy is being evaluated but is not a generally accepted approach for curative lung cancer resection.

The extent of resection is a matter of surgical judgment based on findings at exploration. In general, conservative resection that encompasses all known tumor gives survival equal to that obtained with more extensive procedures. However, lobectomy is superior to wedge resection in terms of reducing the rate of local recurrence. Thus, lobectomy is preferred to pneumonectomy and wedge resection, while wedge resection and segmentectomy are reserved for patients with poor pulmonary reserve and small peripheral lesions. Approximately 43 percent of all lung cancer patients will undergo thoracotomy. Of these, 76 percent will have a definitive resection, 12 percent will only be explored for disease extent, and 12 percent will have a palliative procedure with known disease left behind. The fraction of long-term survivors following definitive surgical therapy is remarkably consistent for all the major centers performing lung cancer surgery in the United States (Table 90-3). Approximately 30 percent of all patients treated with resection for cure survive 5 years, and 15 percent survive 10 years. The 30-day hospital mortality following pulmonary resection at major centers is also very consistent, being 3 percent for lobectomy and 6 percent for pneumonectomy. Thus, most patients who initially may be thought to have a "curative" resection ultimately die of metastatic disease (usually within 5 years of surgery).

MANAGEMENT OF OCCULT AND STAGE 0 CARCINOMAS In the uncommon situation where malignant cells are identified in a sputum or bronchial washing specimen but the chest radiograph appears normal (TX tumor stage), the lesion must be localized. Over 90 percent can be localized by meticulous examination of the bronchial tree with a fiberoptic bronchoscope under general anesthesia and collection of a series of differential brushings and biopsies. Often, carcinoma in situ or multicentric lesions are found in these patients. Current recommendations are for the most conservative surgical resection, allowing removal of the cancer and conservation of lung parenchyma, even if the bronchial margins are positive for carcinoma in situ. The 5-year overall survival for these occult cancers is approximately 60 percent. Close follow-up of these patients is indicated because of the high incidence of second primary lung cancers (approximately 5 percent per patient per year). A new approach to in situ or multicentric lesions uses systemically administered hematoporphyrin (which localizes to tumors and sensitizes them to light) followed by bronchoscopic phototherapy.

SOLITARY PULMONARY NODULE When a patient presents with an asymptomatic, solitary pulmonary nodule (defined as an x-ray density completely surrounded by normal aerated lung, with circumscribed margins, of any shape, usually 1 to 6 cm in greatest diameter, a decision to resect or follow the nodule must be made. Approximately 35 percent of all such lesions in adults will be malignant, most being primary lung cancer, while less than 1 percent are malignant in nonsmoking patients under 35 years of age. A complete history, including a smoking history, physical examination, routine laboratory tests, fiberoptic bronchoscopy, and old chest x-rays is obtained. If no diagnosis is immediately apparent, the following risk factors would all argue strongly in favor of proceeding with resection to establish a histologic diagnosis: a history of cigarette smoking; age 35 years or older; a relatively large lesion; lack of calcification; chest symptoms; associated atelectasis, pneumonitis, or adenopathy; and growth of the lesion revealed by comparison with old x-rays. At present, only two radiographic criteria are reliable predictors of the benign nature of a solitary pulmonary nodule: lack of growth over a period greater than 2 years and certain characteristic patterns of calcification. Calcification alone does not exclude malignancy. However, a dense central nidus, multiple punctate foci, and "bull's eye" (granuloma) and "popcorn ball" (hamartoma) calcifications are all highly suggestive of a benign lesion.

When old x-rays are not available and the characteristic calcification patterns are absent, the following approach is reasonable: Nonsmoking patients under 35 years can be followed with serial chest x-rays every 3 months for 1 year and then yearly. If any significant growth is found, a histologic diagnosis is needed. For patients over age 35 and all patients with a smoking history, a histologic diagnosis must be made. The sample for histologic diagnosis can be obtained either at the time of nodule resection or, if the patient is a poor operative risk, via transthoracic fine-needle biopsy. Some institutions would use preoperative fine-needle aspiration on all such lesions; however, all positive lesions will have to be resected, and negative cytologic findings will in most cases have to be confirmed by histology on a resected specimen. While much has been made of sparing patients an operation, the high probability of finding a malignancy (particularly in smokers over age 35) and the excellent chance for surgical cure when the tumor is small both suggest an aggressive approach to these lesions.

RADIOTHERAPY WITH CURATIVE INTENT   Patients with stage III disease, as well as patients with stage I or II disease who refuse surgery or appear not to be candidates for pulmonary resection for medical reasons, should be considered for radiation therapy with curative intent. The decision to administer high-dose and potentially curative radiotherapy is based on the extent of disease and the volume of the chest that requires irradiation. Patients with distant metastases, positive supraclavicular nodes, pleural effusion, or cardiac involvement are generally not considered for such curative radiation treatment. The median survival for patients with unresectable non-small cell lung cancer localized to the chest who undergo primary radiotherapy with curative intent is less than 1 year. However, 6 percent of these patients are alive at 5 years and are cured by radiotherapy alone. In addition to being potentially curative, radiotherapy, by controlling the primary tumor, may increase the quality and length of life of noncured patients. Treatment usually involves midplane doses of 55 to 60 Gy (5500 to 6000 rad), and the major concern is the amount of lung parenchyma and other organs in the thorax included in the treatment plan, including the spinal cord, heart, and esophagus. In patients with a major degree of underlying pulmonary disease, the treatment plan may have to be compromised because of the deleterious effect of radiation on pulmonary function. Recent studies suggest that continuous-fraction radiotherapy be given. The development of radiation pneumonitis is proportional to the dose of radiation and the volume of lung in the radiation field. The full clinical syndrome (dyspnea, fever, and radiographic infiltrate corresponding to the treatment port) occurs in 5 percent of cases. Acute radiation esophagitis occurs during treatment but usually is self-limited, while spinal cord injury should be avoided by careful treatment planning. Twice-daily fractionated chest radiotherapy may achieve high doses and avoid toxicity. This approach has been used primarily for small cell lung cancer. In addition, brachytherapy (local radiotherapy delivered by placing radioactive "seeds" in a catheter in the tumor bed) provides a way to give a high local dose while sparing surrounding normal tissue.

COMBINED-MODALITY THERAPY WITH CURATIVE INTENT   Many centers give high-dose postoperative radiation therapy if N1 or N2 nodal disease is found at operation, and postoperative radiation therapy currently is considered standard for N2 disease. However, a randomized trial of postoperative radiotherapy, while showing improved local tumor control, did not show a survival benefit.

As a special case, carcinomas of the superior pulmonary sulcus producing *Pancoast's syndrome* are usually treated with combined radiotherapy and surgery. These patients should have the usual preoperative staging procedures, including mediastinoscopy and CT scans to determine tumor extent and a neurologic examination (and sometimes nerve conduction studies) to document neurologic findings. Often a histologic diagnosis is not made, but the combination of tumor location and pain distribution permit a diagnostic accuracy for cancer of better than 90 percent. If mediastinoscopy is negative, two curative approaches may be used in treating a Pancoast's syndrome tumor. In the first, preoperative irradiation [30 Gy (3000 rad) in 10 treatments] is given to the area, followed by an en bloc resection of the tumor and involved chest wall 3 to 6 weeks later. At 3 years, survival figures of 42 percent for epidermoid and 21 percent for adeno- and large cell carcinomas have been reported. The second approach involves radiotherapy alone in curative doses and standard fractionation, which leads to survival rates similar to those from combined-modality therapy. Although small cell lung cancer responds to chemotherapy, this modality is not so effective for non-small cell lung cancer. While gratifying responses sometimes occur in patients with non-small cell lung cancer, substantial toxicities are associated with treatment and palliation, and survival benefits may be small. Because the toxicities, inconvenience, and expense of chemotherapy are borne alike by patients with responding and nonresponding disease and because the absolute survival benefits observed for chemotherapy of non-small cell lung cancer are relatively small, data from large numbers of patients participating in randomized clinical trials are needed to evaluate the clinical utility of chemotherapy in this setting.

A meta-analysis concerning the benefits of chemotherapy in non-small cell lung cancer was performed using updated data on 9,387 individual patients from 52 randomized trials, both published and unpublished, with the main outcome measure being survival. Overall, the results for modern regimens containing cisplatin favored chemotherapy in all comparisons. Trials in early-stage disease comparing surgery with surgery plus chemotherapy gave a hazard ratio of 0.87 (13 percent reduction in risk of death at 5 years) in favor of including chemotherapy. Trials in locally advanced disease comparing radical radiotherapy with radiotherapy plus chemotherapy also gave a hazard ratio of 0.87 (13 percent reduction in risk of death at 2 years) in favor of including chemotherapy.

While these results are statistically significant overall, the clinical benefits they show are only modest. This is particularly true for stage IV disease, where survival is increased by only a few months. The most clinically significant benefits were found when chemotherapy was added to radiotherapy for locally advanced disease (stage IIIB and some stage IIIA disease) and when chemotherapy was given preoperatively in a neoadjuvant fashion in stage IIIA disease. Thus, provided the risk:benefit ratio of using chemotherapy is discussed appropriately with patients, such therapy can be administered in a noninvestigational setting. While there are data supporting a benefit of chemotherapy as an adjuvant to surgery for early-stage disease, the confidence limits of these data are wide, and adjuvant chemotherapy cannot yet be recommended as standard therapy. In contrast to the beneficial results from trials using cisplatin, older trials using alkylating agents (not currently used for non-small cell lung cancer) tended to show a detrimental effect of chemotherapy. Randomized clinical trials also are needed to evaluate the usefulness of the new agents with activity against non-small cell lung cancer, including the taxanes (paclitaxel and docetaxel), vinorelbine, gemcitabine, and camptothecins (topotecan and CPT-11).

Disseminated Non-Small Cell Lung Cancer   The 70 percent of patients who have unresectable non-small cell cancer have a poor prognosis. For example, median survival times of 34, 25, 17, 8, and 4 weeks are seen for such patients with performance status scores of 0 (asymptomatic), 1 (symptomatic, fully ambulatory), 2 (in bed <50 percent of the time), 3 (in bed >50 percent of the time), and 4 (bedridden), respectively. Standard medical management, the judicious use of pain medications, and the appropriate use of radiotherapy form the cornerstone of management. Patients whose primary tumor is causing symptoms such as bronchial obstruction with pneumonitis, hemoptysis, or upper airway or superior vena cava (SVC) obstruction should, in general, have radiotherapy to the primary tumor. The case for prophylactic treatment of the asymptomatic patient is to prevent major symptoms from occurring within the thorax. However, if the patient can be followed closely, it is appropriate to defer treatment until symptoms develop. Usually a course of 30 to 40 Gy (3000 to 4000 rad) over 2 to 4 weeks is given to the tumor. Radiation therapy provides relief of intrathoracic symptoms with the following frequencies: hemoptysis, 84 percent; SVC syndrome, 80 percent; dyspnea, 60 percent; cough, 60 percent; atelectasis, 23 percent; and vocal cord paralysis, 6 percent. Other symptoms of metastatic disease treated with radiotherapy include cardiac-tamponade (treated with pericardiocentesis and radiation therapy to the entire cardiac silhouette), painful bony metastases (with relief in 66 percent of cases), brain or spinal cord compression, and brachial plexus involvement. Usually, with brain and cord compression, dexamethasone (25 to 100 mg per day in four divided doses) is also given and then rapidly tapered to the lowest dosage that relieves symptoms.

Brain metastases often are noted as isolated sites of relapse in patients with adenocarcinoma of the lung otherwise controlled by surgery or radiotherapy. However, there is no proven value for prophylactic cranial irradiation or for CT scans of the head in asymptomatic patients.

The key to effective palliation of lung cancer is to detect complications and begin radiotherapy as early as possible. Pleural effusions are common and are usually treated with thoracentesis as needed but not with radiotherapy. If they recur and are symptomatic, chest tube drainage with a sclerosing agent such as intrapleural doxycycline is used. First, the chest cavity is completely drained. Xylocaine 1% is instilled (15 mL), followed by 50 mL normal saline. Then 500 to 750 mg doxycycline HCl is dissolved in 100 mL normal saline, and this is injected via the chest tube. The chest tube is clamped for 4 h if tolerated, and the patient is rotated onto different sides to distribute the sclerosing agent. The chest tube is removed 24 to 48 h later, after drainage has become slight (usually less than 100 mL per 24 h). Recently, video-assisted thoracoscopy has been used to drain and treat large malignant effusions. Symptomatic endobronchial lesions that recur after surgery or radiotherapy or that develop in patients with severely compromised pulmonary function are difficult to treat with conventional therapy. There are several approaches to this problem. Neodynium-YAG (yttrium-aluminum-garnet) laser therapy administered via a flexible fiberoptic bronchoscope (usually under general anesthesia) can provide palliation in 80 to 90 percent of patients even when the tumor has relapsed after radiotherapy. Local radiotherapy delivered by brachytherapy, photodynamic therapy using a photosensitizing agent, and endobronchial stents are other measures that can relieve airway obstruction from tumor.

CHEMOTHERAPY The use of chemotherapy for non-small cell lung cancer requires careful judgment to balance potential benefits and toxicity. However, modest survival benefits (of 1 to 2 months) may accrue from such combination chemotherapy. From the large meta-analysis cited above, randomized trials in advanced disease comparing supportive care with supportive care plus chemotherapy gave a hazard ratio of 0.73 (27 percent reduction in risk of death at one year) in favor of including chemotherapy. Approximately 30 to 40 percent of patients will have objective tumor response to combination chemotherapy. However, a complete clinical regression of tumor (a *complete response*) occurs in less than 5 percent of cases. Those patients whose tumors respond to chemotherapy have significantly longer survival times (around 30 to 40 weeks median survival) than patients who do not respond to therapy (10 to 20 weeks median survival). The problem is that the responding patients also have better prognostic features (such as good performance status), and it is difficult to separate the effect of these features on survival from that of chemotherapy. However, in patients with good performance status, response to chemotherapy is also associated with prolonged survival and, in some cases, relief of symptoms. Thus, in patients with non-small cell lung cancer who desire chemotherapy, it is reasonable to give chemotherapy if the patient is fully ambulatory, has an evaluable tumor mass (so that the response to therapy can be followed), has not received prior chemotherapy, and is able to understand and accept the potential benefits and toxicities from such therapy. The chemotherapy should be delivered by a medical oncologist, who should use one of the published standard regimens, such as etoposide + cisplatin and also administer appropriate antiemetics and supportive care. New drugs with proven activity in non-small cell lung cancer include paclitaxel, vinorelbine, and gem-

citabine. Finally, all eligible patients should be encouraged to enter clinical studies that are designed to determine the benefits and toxicities of these new treatments.

Small Cell Lung Cancer Untreated patients with small cell lung cancer have median survivals of only 6 to 17 weeks, while patients treated with combination chemotherapy have median survivals of 40 to 70 weeks. Thus, the correct use of chemotherapy with or without radiotherapy or surgery is the cornerstone of the treatment of small cell cancer. The goal of treatment is to achieve a complete clinical regression of tumor documented by repeating the initial positive staging procedures, particularly fiberoptic bronchoscopy with washings and biopsy. The initial response, determined 6 to 12 weeks after the start of therapy, predicts both the median and long-term survival and the potential for cure. Patients who achieve a complete clinical regression survive longer than patients with only partial regression (shrinkage of the visible tumor by more than 50 percent with no sign of tumor progression elsewhere), who in turn survive longer than patients with no response. In addition, all long-term (>3-year) survivors come from the complete response group.

Following initial staging, patients are classified as having limited or extensive disease and as being physiologically able or not able to tolerate combination chemotherapy or combined-modality chemoradiotherapy. The overall mortality rate from initial combination chemotherapy even in these selected patients is about 5 percent at major centers. This figure is comparable with the operative mortality rate for pulmonary resection and indicates the need for physiologic staging of patients before chemotherapy. Such therapy should be reserved for ambulatory patients with no prior chemotherapy or radiotherapy, no other major medical problems, and adequate heart, liver, renal, and bone marrow function. The arterial P_{O_2} on room air should be above 6.6 kPa (50 mmHg), and there should be no CO_2 retention. For patients with limitations in any of these areas, the initial combined-modality therapy or chemotherapy must be modified to prevent undue toxicity. In all patients, these treatments must be coupled with supportive care for infectious, hemorrhagic, and other medical complications. This induction period is best supervised by a medical oncologist. Meticulous attention to the details of therapy and to the day-to-day management of the patient through the initial 6 to 12 weeks of treatment is essential if therapy-related mortality and morbidity are to be kept low.

CHEMOTHERAPY A variety of effective combination chemotherapy regimens have been reported for small cell lung cancer. At present, the combination most widely used is etoposide plus cisplatin, given every 3 weeks on an outpatient basis. Appropriate supportive care (antiemetic therapy, administration of fluid and saline boluses with cisplatin, monitoring of blood counts and blood chemistries, monitoring for signs of bleeding or infection, and, as required, administration of erythropoietin and granulocyte colony-stimulating factor) and adjustment of chemotherapy doses on the basis of nadir granulocyte counts are essential. The initial combination chemotherapy may result in moderate to severe granulocytopenia (e.g., granulocyte counts of less than 500 to 1500/μL) and thrombocytopenia (platelet counts of less than 50,000 to 100,000/μL). After the initial six to eight cycles of therapy, patients should be restaged to determine if they have entered a *complete clinical remission*, indicated by complete disappearance of all clinically evident lesions and paraneoplastic syndromes, or a *partial remission*, or have *no response* or tumor progression (seen in 10 percent or fewer of patients). Chemotherapy is then stopped in responding patients. More prolonged chemotherapy has not been shown to be of value. Patients whose tumors are progressing or not responding should be switched to a new chemotherapy regimen, preferably one involving a combination of agents that will not show cross-resistance with the previous combination, in an attempt to get an objective tumor response. Oral etoposide, as a single agent, has been shown to produce a clinical benefit in the initial treatment of patients who are elderly or have a very poor performance status.

RADIOTHERAPY High-dose [40 Gy (4000 rad)] radiotherapy to the whole brain should be given to patients with documented brain metastases. Prophylactic cranial irradiation (PCI) may be given to patients with complete responses, since it will significantly decrease the development of brain metastases (which occur in 60 to 80 percent of patients living 2 or more years who do not receive such prophylactic radiotherapy), but such prophylactic therapy has not been shown to prolong survival. Because some studies indicate possible deficits in cognitive ability that could be related to PCI, the long-term quality of life after PCI needs to be further studied. In the case of symptomatic, progressive lesions in the chest or at other critical sites, if radiotherapy has not yet been given to these areas, it may be administered in full doses [e.g., 40 Gy (4000 rad) to the chest tumor mass].

COMBINED-MODALITY THERAPY Most patients with limited-stage small cell lung cancer should receive combined-modality therapy with etoposide plus cisplatin and concurrent radiotherapy. There are definite toxicities of both an acute and chronic nature that should be expected with combined-modality chemoradiotherapy, particularly when the chemotherapy and radiotherapy are given concurrently. However, retrospective analyses of long-term survivors and analyses of local failures in the chest following chemotherapy alone suggest that chest radiotherapy is of benefit, and thus it is currently recommended for limited-stage patients. Patients should be selected (limited-stage disease and a performance status of 0 to 1 and initial good pulmonary function) such that radiotherapy can be given in full doses and in a manner that will not sacrifice too much lung function. The radiation oncologist must be prepared to deliver tailored radiotherapy with shaping of fields during treatment, much as is done for Hodgkin's disease. Several centers that give twice-daily radiotherapy concurrently with chemotherapy using etoposide plus cisplatin have reported improved local tumor control and acceptable toxicity. For extensive-stage disease, chest radiotherapy usually is not advocated. However, in favorable patients (e.g., those with a performance status of 0 to 1, good pulmonary function, and only one site of extensive disease), the addition of chest radiotherapy to chemotherapy can be considered. In all patients, if chemotherapy is inadequate to relieve local tumor symptoms, a course of radiotherapy can be added.

Several centers around the world have reported potential cure rates of 15 to 25 percent for limited-stage disease and of 1 to 5 percent for extensive-stage disease. Overall, approximately 50 percent of patients with limited-stage and 30 percent of patients with extensive-stage disease will enter a complete remission, and 90 to 95 percent of all patients will have some objective tumor shrinkage (complete or partial response). These responses increase the median survival to 10 to 12 months for patients with extensive-stage disease and 14 to 18 months for patients with limited-stage disease, as compared with 2 to 4 months for untreated patients. In addition, most patients have relief of their tumor-related symptoms and improvement of performance status. However, the maintenance of good performance status in a patient receiving outpatient chemotherapy requires judgment and skill on the part of the medical oncologist delivering the chemotherapy to avoid undue therapeutic toxicity. New treatments, such as new drug combinations, very intensive initial or "reinduction" therapy with autologous bone marrow infusion, and novel ways of combining chemotherapy, radiotherapy, and surgery, should all be given only in the context of an approved clinical protocol.

While surgical resection is not routinely recommended for small cell lung cancer, occasional patients with this cancer meet the usual requirements for resectability (stage I or II disease with negative mediastinal nodes). Also, in some patients, this histologic diagnosis is made only on review of the resected surgical specimen. Such patients have been reported to have high cure rates (above 25 percent) if adjuvant combination chemotherapy is used.

BENIGN LUNG NEOPLASMS

The benign neoplasms of the lung, representing less than 5 percent of all primary tumors, include bronchial adenomas and hamartomas (90 percent of such lesions) and a group of very uncommon neoplasms

(chondromas, fibromas, lipomas, hemangiomas, leiomyomas, teratomas, pseudolymphomas, and endometriosis). The diagnostic and primary-treatment approach is basically the same for all these neoplasms. They can present as central masses causing airway obstruction, cough, hemoptysis, and pneumonitis. The masses may or may not be visible on radiographs but usually are accessible to fiberoptic bronchoscopy. Alternatively, they can present without symptoms as solitary pulmonary nodules and thus will be evaluated as part of a solitary pulmonary nodule workup. In all cases, the extent of surgery must be determined at operation, and a conservative procedure with appropriate reconstructions is usually performed.

BRONCHIAL ADENOMAS Bronchial adenomas (80 percent of which are central) are slow-growing, endobronchial lesions; they represent 50 percent of all benign pulmonary neoplasms. A total of 80 to 90 percent are carcinoids, 10 to 15 percent are adenocystic tumors (or cylindromas), and 2 to 3 percent are mucoepidermoid tumors. Adenomas present in patients 15 to 60 years old (average age, 45) as endobronchial lesions and are often symptomatic for several years. Patients may have a chronic cough, recurrent hemoptysis, or obstruction with atelectasis, lobar collapse, or pneumonitis and abscess formation. Bronchial carcinoids, which usually follow a benign course, and small cell lung cancers, which are highly malignant, are both derived from the same normal bronchial epithelial component, the Kulchitsky cell. This cell is part of the amine precursor uptake and decarboxylation (APUD) system. Carcinoids, like small cell lung cancers, may secrete other hormones, such as ACTH or arginine vasopressin, and thus can cause paraneoplastic syndromes that resolve upon resection. In addition, bronchial carcinoid metastases (usually to the liver) may produce the carcinoid syndrome, with cutaneous flush, bronchoconstriction, diarrhea, and cardiac valvular lesions (see Chap. 95), which small cell lung cancer does not. Occasionally, pathologists may have difficulty in distinguishing carcinoids from small cell lung cancers. Carcinoid tumors that have an unusually aggressive histologic appearance (referred to as *atypical carcinoids*) metastasize in 70 percent of cases to regional nodes, liver, or bone, compared with only a 5 percent rate of metastasis for carcinoids with typical histology.

Bronchial adenomas of all types, because of their endobronchial and often central location, are usually visible by fiberoptic bronchoscopy, and tissue for histologic diagnosis is obtained in this manner. Because they are hypervascular, they can bleed profusely after bronchoscopic biopsy, and this problem should be anticipated. Bronchial adenomas must be dealt with as potentially malignant and thus require removal not only for symptom relief but also because they can be locally invasive or recurrent, potentially can metastasize, and may produce paraneoplastic syndromes. Surgical excision is the primary treatment for all types of bronchial adenomas. The extent of surgery is determined at operation and should be as conservative as possible. Often bronchotomy with local excision, sleeve resection, segmental resection, or lobectomy is sufficient. Five-year survival rates following surgical resection are 95 percent, decreasing to 70 percent if regional nodes are involved. The treatment of metastatic pulmonary carcinoids is currently unclear because they can either be indolent, growing slowly over several years, or behave more like small cell lung carcinoma. Assessment of the tempo and histology of the disease in the individual patient is necessary to determine if and when chemotherapy or radiotherapy is indicated.

HAMARTOMAS Pulmonary hamartomas have a peak incidence at age 60 and are more frequent in men than in women. Histologically, they contain normal pulmonary tissue components (smooth muscle and collagen) in a disorganized fashion. They are usually peripheral, clinically silent, and benign in their behavior. While it would be advantageous to avoid thoracotomy in these older patients, unless the radiographic findings are pathognomonic for hamartoma, with "popcorn" calcification, the lesions will usually have to be resected for diagnosis, particularly if the patient is a smoker.

METASTATIC PULMONARY TUMORS

The lung is a frequent site of metastases from primary cancers outside the lung. Usually such metastatic disease is considered incurable. However, two special situations should be borne in mind. The first is the development of a solitary pulmonary shadow on a chest x-ray in a patient known to have an extrathoracic neoplasm. This shadow may represent a metastasis or a new primary lung cancer. Because the natural history of lung cancer is worse than that of most other primary tumors, it is wise to approach a single pulmonary nodule in a patient with a known extrathoracic tumor as though the nodule is a primary lung cancer, particularly if the patient is over 35 years of age and a smoker. This means a vigorous evaluation looking for other sites of active cancer and, if none are found, surgical resection of the nodule. Second, in some cases, multiple pulmonary nodules can be resected with curative intent. This tactic is usually recommended if, after careful staging, it is decided that (1) the patient can tolerate the contemplated pulmonary resection, (2) the primary tumor has been definitively and successfully treated, and (3) all known metastatic disease can be encompassed by the projected pulmonary resection. The key is selection and screening of patients to exclude those with uncontrolled primary tumors and extrapulmonary metastases. Primary tumors whose pulmonary metastases have been successfully resected for cure include osteogenic and soft tissue sarcomas; colon, rectal, uterine, cervix, and corpus tumors; head and neck, breast, testis, and salivary gland cancer; melanoma; and bladder and kidney tumors. Five-year survival rates of 20 to 30 percent have been found in carefully selected patients, and the most dramatic results have been seen in osteogenic sarcomas, where resection of pulmonary metastases (sometimes requiring several thoracotomies) is becoming a standard curative treatment approach.

BIBLIOGRAPHY

BENOWITZ N: Pharmacologic aspects of cigarette smoking and nicotine addiction. N Engl J Med 319:1318, 1988

GAZDAR AF et al: Molecular genetic changes found in human lung cancer and its precursor lesions. Cold Spring Harbor Symp Quant Biol 59:565, 1994

GINSBERG RJ et al: Non-small cell lung cancer, in *Cancer: Principles and Practice of Oncology,* 5th ed, VT DeVita Jr et al (eds). Philadelphia, Lippincott-Raven, 1997, pp 858–911

IHDE DC et al: Small cell lung cancer, in *Cancer: Principles and Practice of Oncology,* 5th ed, VT DeVita Jr et al (eds). Philadelphia, Lippincott-Raven, 1997, pp 911–949

LIPPMAN SM et al: Epidemiology, biology, and chemoprevention of aerodigestive cancer. Cancer 74(Suppl 9):2719, 1994

MINNA JD et al: Molecular biology of lung cancer, in *Cancer: Principles and Practice of Oncology,* 5th ed, VT DeVita Jr et al (eds). Philadelphia, Lippincott-Raven, 1997, pp 849–857

MITCHELL JB et al: *Lung Cancer: Principles and Practice.* Philadelphia, Lippincott-Raven, 1996

NON-SMALL CELL LUNG CANCER COLLABORATIVE GROUP: Chemotherapy in non-small cell lung cancer: A meta-analysis using updated data on individual patients from 52 randomised clinical trials. BMJ 311:899, 1996

PARKER SL et al: Cancer statistics, 1996. CA Cancer J Clin 46(1):5, 1996

TRAVIS WD et al: Lung cancer. Cancer 75:191, 1995

ZANG EA, WYNDER EL: Differences in lung cancer risk between men and women: Examination of the evidence. J Natl Cancer Inst 88:183, 1996

91   *Marc E. Lippman*

BREAST CANCER

DEFINITION Breast cancer represents a malignant proliferation of epithelial cells lining the ducts or lobules of the breast. In 1996, there were approximately 185,000 cases of invasive breast cancer and 46,000 deaths in the United States. Breast cancer is the most common cancer in women (excluding skin cancer), although it is quite rare in men. This chapter will not consider rare malignancies of the breast, including sarcomas and lymphomas. Human breast cancer is a clonal disease. That is, a single transformed cell—the end result of a series of somatic (acquired) or germline (inherited) mutations—is able to express full malignant potential, in a series of events that occur in a sequential and stochastic manner. Thus, breast cancer may exist for a long period as either a noninvasive disease or an invasive but nonmetastatic disease. This fact makes the need for timely diagnosis and appropriate management more urgent.

GENETICS Probably only about 10 percent of human breast cancers can be linked directly to germline mutations. This area has undergone remarkable evolution with the identification of several genes responsible for the familial cases. The first to be identified were germline mutations in the tumor suppressor gene *p53*. In the disorder caused by these mutations—called the Li-Fraumeni syndrome—inherited mutations in *p53* lead to an increased incidence of breast cancer, osteogenic sarcomas, and other malignancies.

Another putative tumor suppressor gene, *BRCA-1*, has been identified at the chromosomal locus 17q21; this gene encodes a zinc finger protein, and the product therefore may function as a transcription factor. Women who inherit a mutated allele of this gene from either parent have an approximately 85 to 90 percent lifetime chance of developing breast cancer, as well as about a 33 percent chance of developing ovarian cancer. Men who carry a mutant allele of the gene have an increased incidence of prostate cancer but usually not of breast cancer. A third gene, termed *BRCA-2*, which has been localized to chromosome 11, is associated with an increased incidence of breast cancer in men and women.

The ataxia-telangiectasia gene is associated with remarkable radiation sensitivity even in the heterozygous state, which occurs in the population at a frequency of 1 to 2 percent. Because of their susceptibility to radiation-induced cancer, heterozygous carriers of this gene may be at risk from such procedures as screening mammography.

Even more important than the role these genes play in inherited forms of breast cancer susceptibility may be their role in sporadic breast cancer. For example, the *p53* mutation is present in approximately 40 percent of human breast cancers as an acquired defect. Thus far, evidence for *BRCA-1* mutation in primary breast cancer has not been reported. However, in a small series of sporadic breast cancers, decreased expression of BRCA-1 mRNA occurs. An abnormal cellular location of the BRCA-1 protein has also been found in some breast cancers, and BRCA-1 therefore may play a role in their pathogenesis. In addition, as evidenced by loss of heterozygosity, other types of tumor-suppressor activity appear to be lost in sporadic cases of human breast cancer. Finally, one dominant oncogene plays a role in about a quarter of human breast cancer cases. The product of this gene, a member of the EGF receptor superfamily called erbB2 (HER-2, neu), is overexpressed in these breast cancers owing to gene amplification, and this overexpression can transform human breast epithelium.

While restoration gene therapy is not a clinical reality yet, several approaches aimed at dealing with overexpressed genes are under clinical trial. The eventual hope for breast cancer is to alter the course of the disease by directly targeting the genes responsible for the malignant process.

EPIDEMIOLOGY Breast cancer is a hormone-dependent disease. Women without functioning ovaries who never receive estrogen replacement do not develop breast cancer. The female-to-male ratio for the disease is about 150 to 1. A host of findings indicate that hormones play a critical role as promoters of the disease. For most epithelial malignancies, a log-log plot of incidence versus age shows a straight-line increase with every year of life. A similar plot for breast cancer shows the same straight line increase, but with a decrease in slope beginning at the age of menopause. The three dates in a woman's life that have a major impact on breast cancer incidence are age of menarche, age at first full-term pregnancy, and age of menopause. Women who experience menarche at age 16 have only 50 to 60 percent of the lifetime breast cancer risk of women who experience menarche at age 12. Similarly, menopause occurring 10 years before the median age (52 years), whether natural or surgically induced, reduces lifetime breast cancer risk by about 35 percent. Compared with nulliparous women, women who have a first full-term pregnancy by age 18 have 30 to 40 percent the risk of breast cancer. Thus, length of menstrual life—particularly the fraction occurring before the first full-term pregnancy—is a substantial component of the total risk of breast cancer. This factor can account for 70 to 80 percent of the variation in breast cancer frequency in different countries.

International variation has provided some of the most important clues on hormonal carcinogenesis. A woman living to age 80 in North America has 1 chance in 9 of developing invasive breast cancer. Asian women have one-fifth to one-tenth the risk of breast cancer of women in North America or Western Europe. Asian women have substantially lower concentrations of estrogens and progesterone. These differences cannot be explained on a genetic basis, because Asian women living in a Western environment have a risk identical to that of their Western counterparts. These women also differ markedly in height and weight from Asian women in Asia; height and weight are critical regulators of age of menarche and have substantial effects on plasma concentrations of estrogens.

The role of diet in breast cancer etiology is controversial. While there are associative links between total caloric intake and breast cancer risk, the strongest link is with high dietary fat intake. However, within the range of dietary fat intake common in Western cultures, there is no convincing evidence that variations in dietary fat alter breast cancer risk. However, there is a risk associated with moderate alcohol intake; the mechanism is unknown. Recommendations favoring abstinence from alcohol must be weighed against other social pressures and the possible cardioprotective effect of moderate alcohol intake.

The potential role of exogenous hormones in breast cancer is of extraordinary importance, because millions of American women regularly use oral contraceptives. The most credible meta-analyses of oral contraceptive use suggest that these agents cause little if any increased risk of breast cancer. When the very substantial protective effect that oral contraceptives offer against ovarian epithelial tumors and endometrial cancers is considered, the data suggest that the use of oral contraceptives is highly protective against malignancy in general, with little impact on breast cancer. Far more controversial are the data surrounding hormone replacement therapy (HRT) in hypogonadal and/or menopausal women. First, HRT with estrogens alone, usually in the form of equine conjugated estrogens, provides less than the physiologic equivalent of premenopausal estrogens but is associated with an increased risk of endometrial cancer, a reduction in the symptoms of estrogen deprivation, a reduction in osteoporosis and resultant hip fractures, and a reduction by about one-third in the incidence of deaths due to cardiovascular disease. Meta-analyses suggest a small increase in breast cancer incidence, particularly with high dosages and a long duration of treatment. For the average woman, the negative effect on the breast is far outweighed by the protective effects on the bones and heart. Preliminary data suggest that there is a reduction in the risk of colon cancer as well.

The addition of progestogens to HRT regimens drastically reduces the risk of endometrial cancer. It is not clear whether the protective effects against cardiovascular and osteoporotic bone diseases are altered. However, progestogens are copromoters of breast cancer in model systems, and an increased risk of breast cancer is possible.

Whether a history of previous biopsy findings of atypical hyperplasia or in situ carcinoma or a strong family history of breast cancer alter the risk-to-benefit ratios for HRT is unknown. It is likely that the average woman benefits from HRT.

In addition to the other factors, radiation may be a risk factor in younger women. Women who have been exposed before age 30 to radiation in the form of multiple fluoroscopies (200 to 300 cGy) or treatment for Hodgkin's disease (>3600 cGy) have a substantially increased risk of breast cancer, whereas radiation exposure after age 30 appears to have a minimal carcinogenic effect on the breast.

DIAGNOSIS The diagnosis of breast cancer was described in Chap. 64. Suffice it to say that no combination of risk factors can be used to define a group of women who have no risk of breast cancer. However, identification of the *BRCA-1* gene makes it possible to identify women who face an 85 to 90 percent lifetime likelihood of

developing breast cancer (with a 70 percent risk of breast cancer by age 60). Breast cancer is virtually unique among epithelial tumors in adults in that screening (in the form of annual mammography) improves survival. Meta-analysis examining outcomes from every randomized trial of mammography conclusively shows a 25 to 30 percent reduction in the chance of dying from breast cancer with annual screening after age 50; the data for women between ages 40 and 50 are almost as positive. Although this remains an area of some controversy, it seems prudent to recommend annual mammography routinely for women past the age of 40. While the benefit of this practice may be debatable, for the vast majority of women it likely carries no risk. It should also be pointed out that no randomized study of breast self-examination has ever shown any improvement in survival. While breast self-examination should be encouraged, its major benefit appears to be identification of tumors appropriate for conservative local therapy, rather than a major increase in survival. It is hoped that better mammographic technology, including digitized radiography, routine use of magnified views, and greater skill in interpretation, combined with newer diagnostic techniques (magnetic resonance imaging, magnetic resonance spectroscopy, positron emission tomography, etc.) will make it possible to identify breast cancers yet more reliably and earlier.

STAGING Correct staging of breast cancer patients is of extraordinary importance. Not only does it permit an accurate prognosis, but in many cases therapeutic decision making is based largely on the TNM classification (Table 91-1). Comparison with historical series should be undertaken with caution, as the staging has changed in the past 10 years.

Table 91-1

Staging of Breast Cancer*

Primary Tumor (T)

T0	No evidence of primary tumor
Tis	Carcinoma in situ
T1	Tumor ≤2 cm
T2	Tumor >2 cm but ≤5 cm
T3	Tumor >5 cm
T4	Extension to chest wall, inflammation

Regional Lymph Nodes (N)

N0	No tumor in regional lymph nodes
N1	Metastasis to movable ipsilateral nodes
N2	Metastasis to matted or fixed ipsilateral nodes
N3	Metastasis to ipsilateral internal mammary nodes

Distant Metastasis (M)

M0	No distant metastasis
M1	Distant metastasis (includes spread to ipsilateral supraclavicular nodes)

Stage Grouping

Stage 0	TIS	N0	M0
Stage 1	T1	N0	M0
Stage IIA	T0	N1	M0
	T1	N1	M0
	T2	N0	M0
Stage IIB	T2	N1	M0
	T3	N0	M0
Stage IIIA	T0	N2	M0
	T1	N2	M0
	T2	N2	M0
	T3	N1, N2	M0
Stage IIIB	T4	Any N	M0
	Any T	N3	M0
Stage IV	Any T	Any N	M1

* Modified from the TNM classification proposed by the American Joint Committee on Cancer, 1992.

℞ TREATMENT

Primary Breast Cancer The management of breast cancer that is apparently localized to the breast or regional lymph nodes has changed since 1985. A series of randomized clinical trials both in the United States and abroad have shown that breast-conserving treatments, consisting of the removal of the primary tumor by some form of lumpectomy with or without irradiation to the breast, results in a survival that is as good as that after extensive procedures, such as mastectomy or modified radical mastectomy, with or without further irradiation. While breast conservation is associated with a possibility of recurrence in the breast, the 10-year survival is still as good as that after more radical surgery. Similarly, multiple studies have shown that the addition of radiotherapy to any form of mastectomy does not improve survival. However, radiation therapy can reduce the rate of local or regional recurrence, and, for women with high-risk primary tumors (i.e., T2 in size, positive margins, positive nodes), it may be considered following mastectomy. At present, approximately one-third of women with breast cancer in the United States are managed by lumpectomy. Breast-conserving surgery is not suitable for all patients, however. For example, it is not suitable for tumors larger than 7 cm (or for smaller tumors if the breast is small), for tumors involving the nipple areolar complex, for tumors with extensive intraductal disease involving multiple quadrants of the breast, for women with a history of collagen-vascular disease, and for women who either do not have the motivation for breast conservation or do not have convenient access to radiotherapy. However, these groups probably do not account for more than one-third of patients. The implication is that a great many women who undergo mastectomy could safely avoid this procedure.

An extensive intraductal component is a predictor of recurrence in the breast, and so are several clinical variables. Axillary lymph node involvement and involvement of vascular or lymphatic channels by metastatic tumor in the breast are associated with a higher risk of relapse in the breast but are not contraindications to breast-conserving treatment. When these patients are excluded, and when lumpectomy with negative tumor margins is achieved, breast conservation is associated with a recurrence rate in the breast of approximately 10 percent. The survival of patients who have recurrence in the breast is somewhat worse than that of women who do not. Thus, recurrence in the breast is a negative prognostic variable for long-term survival. However, recurrence in the breast is not the *cause* of distant metastasis. This conclusion is based on the fact that survival is the same for patients treated with breast-conserving therapy and patients treated with mastectomy. If recurrence in the breast caused metastatic disease, then women treated with lumpectomy, who have a higher rate of recurrence in the breast, should have a lower survival. Most patients should consult with a radiation oncologist before making a final decision concerning local therapy. However, a multimodality clinic approach in which the surgeon, radiation oncologist, medical oncologist, and other care givers cooperate to evaluate the patient and develop a treatment plan has gained widespread acceptance and is usually considered a major advantage by patients.

ADJUVANT THERAPY One of the significant advances in the treatment of solid tumors of adults has been the improved survival resulting from the use of systemic therapy after local management of breast cancer. While this therapy is imperfect in terms of effectiveness, toxicity, and patient selection, more than one-quarter of the women who would otherwise die of metastatic breast cancer remain disease-free when treated with the appropriate systemic regimen. In this section we will review patient selection, treatment regimens, and toxicities.

PROGNOSTIC VARIABLES At the time of local therapy, it is critical to identify patients at a substantial risk of eventual relapse. For patients likely to be cured by local therapy, systemic treatment offers no further benefit and involves a needless hazard. Furthermore, as therapies become increasingly specific, identification of variables associated with disease relapse may make it possible to choose the best therapy for the individual patient.

The most important prognostic variables are provided by *tumor staging*. The size of the tumor and the status of the axillary lymph nodes provide reasonably accurate information on the likelihood of tumor relapse. The relation of pathologic stage to 5-year survival is shown in Table 91-2. For most women, the need for adjuvant therapy can be readily defined on this basis alone. In the absence of lymph node involvement, involvement of microvessels (either capillaries or lymphatic channels) in tumors is considered by many as nearly equivalent to lymph node involvement. The greatest controversy concerns women with intermediate prognoses. Obviously, *there is no justification for adjuvant chemotherapy in women with tumors less than 1 cm in size whose axillary lymph nodes are negative*.

A large number of analyses have been performed to try to identify other significant prognostic variables. For each of these variables, differences in the methods of analysis and the populations studied, as well as the effects of chance, have resulted in discordant results. However, for several variables, the association with disease-free survival and overall survival seems clear. What is less clear is whether or not they add to the information from pathologic staging.

Estrogen and progesterone receptor status are of prognostic significance. Tumors that lack either or both of these receptors are more likely to recur than tumors that have them.

Several *measures of tumor growth rate* correlate with early relapse. S-phase analysis using flow cytometry is the most accurate measure, and indirect S-phase assessments using antigens associated with the cell cycle, such as PCNA and Ki67, are also valuable. Several studies suggest that tumors with a high proportion (more than the median) of cells in the S phase pose a greater risk of relapse and that chemotherapy offers the greatest survival benefit for these tumors. For this reason, some clinicians use S-phase assessment as a deciding factor for instituting adjuvant therapy when other pathologic features are unclear. Assessment of DNA content in the form of ploidy is of modest value, with nondiploid tumors having a somewhat worse prognosis.

Histologic classification of the tumor has also been used as a prognostic factor. Tumors with a poor nuclear grade have a higher degree of recurrence than tumors with a good nuclear grade. The reproducibility of this measurement is reasonable when semiquantitative measures such as Elston score are employed.

Molecular changes in the tumor are also useful. For example, tumors that overexpress the epidermal growth factor receptor erbB2 or that have a mutated *p53* gene have a bad prognosis. Particular interest has centered on erbB2 overexpression as measured by histochemistry. A cooperative group study suggests that tumors that overexpress erbB2 are more likely to respond to higher doses of doxorubicin-containing regimens. For this reason, erbB2 expression is usually worth measuring as a means of deciding on therapy.

To grow, a tumor must generate a neovasculature (see Chap. 85). On the basis of a semiquantitative scoring system, the presence of more microvessels in tumors has been shown by several groups to be associated with a worse prognosis.

Table 91-2

5-Year Survival Rate for Breast Cancer by Stage*

Stage	5-Year Survival (Percent of Patients)
0	99
I	92
IIA	82
IIB	65
IIIA	47
IIIB	44
IV	14

* Modified from data of the National Cancer Institute—Surveillance, Epidemiology, and End Results (SEER).

Other variables that have also been used to evaluate prognosis include proteins associated with invasiveness, such as type IV collagenase, cathepsin D, plasminogen activator, plasminogen activator receptor, and the metastasis suppressor gene *nm23*. None of these has been widely accepted as a prognostic variable for therapeutic decision-making.

One problem in interpreting these prognostic variables is that most of them have not been examined in a study using a substantial cohort of patients. For example, what should be done for a patient who has a 1-cm tumor with negative lymph nodes but has one or more bad prognostic variables? We aren't sure.

ADJUVANT REGIMENS Selection of appropriate adjuvant chemotherapy or hormone therapy regimens is a highly controversial issue in some situations. Meta-analyses have helped to define broad limits for therapy but do not help in choosing optimal regimens or in choosing a regimen for certain subgroups of patients. A general summary of recommendations is shown in Table 91-3. In general, premenopausal women for whom any form of adjuvant systemic therapy is indicated should receive chemotherapy. The effect on survival of adjuvant anti-estrogen (tamoxifen) therapy in premenopausal patients with any lymph node status is minimal, and this therapy should probably not be administered alone. The benefit of adding tamoxifen to chemotherapy in premenopausal women who are to be treated has not been well established, although it is common practice to follow chemotherapy with tamoxifen in premenopausal women whose tumors are positive for the estrogen receptor. Prophylactic castration may also be associated with a substantial survival benefit (primarily in estrogen receptor–positive patients), but this treatment has not been widely used in this country.

Data on postmenopausal women are also controversial. The impact of adjuvant chemotherapy is less clear-cut than in premenopausal patients, although some survival advantage has been shown. In general, the first decision is whether chemotherapy or tamoxifen should be used. While adjuvant tamoxifen improves survival regardless of axillary lymph node status, the improvement is modest for patients in whom multiple lymph nodes are involved. For this reason, it is usual to give chemotherapy to postmenopausal patients who have no medical contraindications and who have more than one positive lymph node; tamoxifen is commonly given simultaneously or subsequently. For postmenopausal women for whom systemic therapy is warranted but who have a more favorable prognosis, tamoxifen may be used as a single agent.

There is little agreement about optimal chemotherapy regimens. In fact, most comparisons of adjuvant chemotherapy regimens show little difference among them. However, dose-intensive doxorubicin-containing regimens appear to be better than lower-dose regimens of the same drugs. Whether this finding represents a threshold effect or a dose-response curve (in which case effectiveness would increase with even higher doses) is under examination. Combinations of very high drug doses and either stem cell or autologous bone marrow support for poor-prognosis stage II patients will be discussed in a separate section.

One approach—so-called neoadjuvant chemotherapy—involves the administration of adjuvant therapy before definitive surgery and radiation therapy. Because the objective response rates of patients with breast cancer to systemic therapy in this setting exceed 75 percent, many patients will be "down-staged" and may thus become candidates for breast-conserving therapy. Whether survival is improved by such approaches is unknown.

Other adjuvant treatments under trial include the use of new drugs, such as paclitaxel, and therapy based on alternative kinetic and biologic models. In such approaches, high doses of single agents are used separately in relatively dose-intensive cycling regimens. One randomized trial suggests that patients treated intensively with one drug combination followed by a second drug combination have better survival than patients given the same drugs in an alternating format. It would not be surprising if different uses of available drugs improved long-term survival. Regrettably, trials require a reasonably large number of homogeneous patients and prolonged follow-up.

Systemic Therapy for Metastatic Disease Unfortunately, after varying periods of disease-free survival, nearly half of patients treated for apparently localized breast cancer develop metastatic disease. Although some of these patients can be salvaged by combinations of systemic and local therapy, most eventually succumb. Soft tissue, bony, and visceral (lung and liver) metastases each account for approximately one-third of initial relapses. However, by the time of death, most patients will have bony involvement. Recurrences can appear at any time after primary therapy. In fact, half of all initial breast cancer recurrences occur more than 5 years after initial therapy.

Biopsy must be performed to demonstrate the presence of metastatic disease, because this diagnosis alters the outlook for the patient so drastically that it should not be made without certainty. Every oncologist has seen patients with tuberculosis, gallstones, primary hyperparathyroidism, or another nonmalignant disease misdiagnosed and treated as metastatic breast cancer. This is a catastrophic mistake and justifies biopsy for virtually every patient at the time of presentation of metastatic disease.

The choice of optimal therapy requires consideration of local therapy needs, of the overall medical condition of the patient, and of the hormone receptor status of the tumor, as well as the exercise of clinical judgment. Because therapy of systemic disease is palliative, the potential toxicities of therapies should be balanced against the response rates. Several variables influence the response to systemic therapy. For example, the presence of estrogen and progesterone receptors are strong indications for endocrine therapy, since the response rates for tumors that express both receptors may approach 70 percent. On the other hand, patients with short disease-free inter-

Table 91-3

Suggested Approaches to Adjuvant Therapy for Women

Age Group	Lymph Node Status*	Endocrine Receptor Status	Tumor	Recommendation	Comment
Premenopausal	Positive†	Any	Any	Multidrug chemotherapy	
Premenopausal	Negative	Any	>2 cm, or 1–2 cm with other poor prognostic variables	Multidrug chemotherapy	Role of tamoxifen not clear
Postmenopausal	Positive†	Negative	Any	Multidrug chemotherapy	
Postmenopausal	Positive†	Positive	Any	Tamoxifen with or without chemotherapy	
Postmenopausal	Negative	Positive	>2 cm, or 1–2 cm with other poor prognostic variables	Tamoxifen	
Postmenopausal	Negative	Negative	>2 cm, or 1–2 cm with other poor prognostic variables	Consider multidrug chemotherapy	

* As determined by pathologic examination.
† For patients with 6 or more positive nodes, consider enrollment in high dose chemotherapy trials.

vals, rapidly progressive visceral disease, lymphangitic pulmonary disease, or intracranial disease are unlikely to respond to endocrine therapy.

In many cases, systemic therapy can be withheld while the patient is treated with appropriate local therapy. The effectiveness of radiation therapy and occasionally of surgery for relieving the symptoms of metastatic disease, particularly when bony sites are involved, cannot be overemphasized. Many patients with bone-only or bone-dominant disease have a relatively indolent course. Under such circumstances, systemic chemotherapy has a modest effect, whereas radiation therapy may be effective for long periods. Other systemic treatments, such as strontium-89 and/or bisphosphonates, may provide a palliative benefit without inducing an objective response. Since the goal of therapy is to maintain well-being for as long as possible, emphasis should be placed on avoiding the most hazardous complications of metastatic disease, including pathologic fracture of the axial skeleton and spinal cord compression. New back pain in patients with cancer should be explored aggressively on an emergent basis; to wait for neurologic symptoms can be catastrophic. Also, metastatic involvement of endocrine organs can cause profound dysfunction, including adrenal insufficiency and hypopituitarism. Similarly, obstruction of the biliary tree or other impairment of organ function may be better managed with a local therapy than with a systemic approach.

ENDOCRINE THERAPY   Normal breast tissue is estrogen-dependent. Both primary breast cancer and metastatic breast cancer may retain this phenotype. The best means of ascertaining whether a breast cancer is hormone-dependent is through analyses of estrogen and progesterone receptor levels. Tumors that are positive for the estrogen receptor and negative for the progesterone receptor have a response rate of approximately 30 percent. Tumors that have both receptors have a response rate approaching 70 percent. If neither receptor is present, the objective response rates are less than 10 percent. In general, receptor analyses provide information as to the correct ordering of endocrine therapies. Because of the lack of toxicity and because some patients whose receptor analyses are reported as negative respond to endocrine therapy, an endocrine treatment should be attempted at some point in every patient with metastatic breast cancer. Potential endocrine therapies are summarized in Table 91-4. Little information suggests that any of these endocrine therapies is superior to another. The choice of endocrine therapy is usually determined by toxicity profile and availability. In most patients, the initial endocrine therapy is the antiestrogen tamoxifen. Newer antiestrogens that are free of agonist effects are in clinical trial. Cases in which tumors shrank in response to tamoxifen with-

Table 91-4

Endocrine Therapies for Breast Cancer

Therapy	Comments
Castration	For premenopausal women
Surgical	
LHRH agonists	
Antiestrogens	
Tamoxifen	Useful in pre- and postmenopausal women
"Pure" antiestrogens	Promising early clinical data
High-dose progestogens	Common second-line choice
Adrenalectomy	
Surgical	Rarely employed second-line choice
"Medical" adrenalectomy	Probably works to decrease the formation of estrogen precursors (aromatase inhibitor)
Aromatase inhibitors	Promising early clinical trials in postmenopausal women
Hypophysectomy	Rarely used
Additive androgens or estrogens	Plausible third-line therapies; potentially toxic

drawal (as well as withdrawal of pharmacologic doses of estrogens) have been reported. Endogenous estrogen formation may be blocked by aromatase inhibitors or analogues of luteinizing hormone–releasing hormone (LHRH). Additive endocrine therapies, including treatment with progestogens, estrogens, and androgens, may also be tried in patients who respond to initial endocrine therapy; the mechanism of action of these latter therapies is unknown. However, patients who respond to one endocrine therapy have at least a 50 percent chance of responding to a second endocrine therapy. It is not uncommon for patients to respond to two or three sequential endocrine therapies; however, combination endocrine therapies do not appear to be superior to individual agents, and combinations of chemotherapy with endocrine therapy are not useful. The median survival of patients with metastatic disease is approximately 2 years, and many patients, particularly older persons and those with hormone-dependent disease, respond to endocrine therapy for 3 to 5 years or longer.

CHEMOTHERAPY   Unlike other epithelial malignancies, breast cancer responds to several chemotherapeutic agents, including anthracyclines, alkylating agents, taxanes, and antimetabolites. Multiple combinations of these agents have been found to improve response rates somewhat, but they have had little impact on duration of response or survival. As previously mentioned, the median survival from diagnosis of metastatic disease to death is approximately 2 years. The choice among multidrug combinations frequently depends on whether adjuvant chemotherapy was administered and, if so, what type. While patients treated with adjuvant regimens of cyclophosphamide, methotrexate, and fluorouracil (CMF regimens) may subsequently respond to the same combination in the metastatic disease setting, most oncologists use drugs to which the patients have not been previously exposed. Once patients have progressed after combination drug therapy, it is most common to treat them with single agents. Given the significant toxicity of most drugs, the use of a single effective agent will minimize toxicity by sparing the patient exposure to drugs that would be of little value. Unfortunately, no form of in vitro drug sensitivity testing to select the drugs most efficacious for a given patient has been demonstrated to be useful.

Most oncologists use either an anthracycline or paclitaxel following failure with the initial regimen. However, the choice has to be balanced with individual needs.

HIGH-DOSE CHEMOTHERAPY INCLUDING AUTOLOGOUS BONE MARROW TRANSPLANTATION   Autologous bone marrow transplantation combined with high doses of single agents can produce improvement even in heavily pretreated patients. However, such responses are rarely, if ever, durable and are unlikely to substantially alter the clinical course for most patients with advanced metastatic disease. However, given the success of such regimens in chronic myelogenous leukemia and Hodgkin's disease, this approach has been tried in patients who have poor-prognosis breast cancer but a relatively small disease burden. These have included patients who have multiple axillary lymph node involvement at primary presentation, patients with stage III breast cancer, and patients with stage IV breast cancer who either have been rendered free of disease by localized therapy (that is, who had an apparently single metastasis and in whom surgical or radiation therapy resulted in disappearance of all objective disease) or showed a nearly complete response to conventional-dose systemic treatment. Several thousand patients in the United States have been treated with these regimens, but it is difficult to assess the success of the regimens because of the problem of comparing the results with historical controls. Nevertheless, the toxicity of these approaches has been reduced by the use of cytokine support and antibiotic prophylaxis, so that these therapies are more widely available. Some oncologists believe that this approach offers a significant advantage for patients.

Stage III Breast Cancer   Between 10 and 25 percent of patients have so-called locally advanced or stage III breast cancer at diagnosis. Many of these cancers are technically operable, whereas others, particularly cancers with chest wall involvement, inflammatory breast cancers, or cancers with large matted axillary lymph nodes, cannot be managed with surgery initially. Although no randomized trials have proved the efficacy of induction chemotherapy, this approach has gained widespread use. More than 90 percent of patients with locally advanced breast cancer show a partial or better response to multidrug chemotherapy regimens that include an anthracycline. Early administration of this treatment reduces the bulk of the disease and frequently makes the patient a suitable candidate for salvage surgery and/or radiation therapy. These patients should be managed in multimodality clinics if possible to coordinate surgery, radiationtherapy, and systemic chemotherapy. Most published series suggest that such approaches produce a long-term disease-free survival in about 30 to 50 percent of patients. It is difficult to make direct comparisons between the various reports because of differences in patient selection and drug regimens.

Breast Cancer Prevention The endocrine promotion of breast cancer has been reviewed in this chapter. Studies of hormone-dependent rodent models of breast cancer suggest that the endocrine milieu has a significant impact on the long-term risk of breast cancer.

Because tamoxifen is effective and relatively safe in both the advanced and adjuvant disease setting, the agent has been tried as a breast cancer preventive. Women who have one breast cancer are at risk of developing a contralateral breast cancer at a rate of approximately 0.5 percent per year. When adjuvant tamoxifen is administered to these patients, the rate of development of contralateral breast cancers is reduced. In other tissues of the body, tamoxifen has estrogen-like effects that are potentially beneficial. These include preservation of bone mineral density and long-term lowering of cholesterol. However, tamoxifen has estrogen-like effects on the uterus, leading to an increased risk of uterine cancer. Consequently, tamoxifen cannot at this time be regarded as a safe agent for prevention of breast cancer. Large-scale prevention trials are being carried out, however. Antiestrogens without estrogen-like effects are now in early clinical trials and may be even more effective in this regard.

Noninvasive Breast Cancer Breast cancer develops as a series of molecular changes in epithelial cells that lead to ever more malignant behavior. Increased use of mammography and better mammographic diagnosis have led to more frequent diagnosis of noninvasive breast cancer. These lesions fall into two groups: ductal carcinoma in situ (DCIS) and lobular carcinoma in situ (lobular neoplasia). The management of both entities is controversial, and careful consideration should be given to their treatment.

DUCTAL CARCINOMA IN SITU Proliferation of cytologically malignant breast epithelial cells within the ducts is termed DCIS. Significant pathologic disagreement can occur in differentiating atypical hyperplasia from DCIS. At least one-third of cases of untreated DCIS progress within 5 years to invasive breast cancer, and therefore appropriate therapy is warranted. For many years, the standard treatment for this disease was mastectomy. However, since treatment of this condition by lumpectomy and radiation therapy gives survival that is as good as the survival for invasive breast cancer treated by mastectomy, it appears paradoxical to recommend more aggressive therapy for a "less malignant" disease. Although both wide excision and wide excision plus radiation therapy are used for this disease in some centers, few randomized studies have compared different therapies; therefore, the optimal treatment is unclear. In one randomized trial, the combination of wide excision plus irradiation for DCIS caused a substantial reduction in the local recurrence rate as compared to wide excision alone with negative margins. Thus far, survival is identical in the two arms. Unfortunately, no studies have compared either of these regimens to mastectomy. Several prognostic features may help to identify patients at high risk for local recurrence after either lumpectomy alone or lumpectomy with radiation therapy. These include extensive disease, age less than 40, and cytologic features such as necrosis, poor nuclear grade, and comedo subtype with overexpression of erbB2. Some data suggest that adequate excision with careful determination of pathologically clear margins is associated with a low recurrence rate. When such surgery is combined with radiation therapy, recurrence (which is usually in the same quadrant) occurs with a frequency of 10 percent or less. Given the fact that half of these recurrences are invasive, about

5 percent will eventually develop into invasive breast cancer. A reasonable expectation of mortality for these patients is about 1 percent, a figure that approximates the mortality rate for DCIS managed by mastectomy. Although this train of reasoning has not formally been proved valid, it is reasonable at present to recommend that patients who desire breast preservation and in whom DCIS appears to be reasonably localized be managed by adequate surgery, with meticulous pathologic evaluation, followed by breast irradiation. The role of subsequent adjuvant tamoxifen in this setting is now being explored. For patients with localized DCIS, there is no need for axillary lymph node dissection. More controversial is the question of what management is optimal when there is any degree of invasion. Because of a significant likelihood (10 to 15 percent) of axillary lymph node involvement even when the primary lesion shows only microscopic invasion, it is prudent to do at least a level 1 and 2 axillary lymph node dissection for all patients with any degree of invasion. Management is dictated by the presence of nodal spread.

LOBULAR NEOPLASIA The management of patients with proliferation of cytologically malignant cells within the lobules (lobular neoplasia) is controversial. From historical data, it appears that approximately 30 percent of patients who have had adequate local excision of the lesion develop invasive breast cancer (usually infiltrating ductal cell carcinoma) over the next 15 to 20 years. Ipsilateral and contralateral disease are about equally common. Therefore, lobular neoplasia may be a premalignant lesion that suggests an elevated risk of subsequent breast cancer, rather than a form of malignancy itself, and aggressive local management seems unreasonable. Most patients should be followed with careful annual mammography and semiannual physical exams; whether they should receive tamoxifen is unknown. Additional molecular analysis of these lesions may make it possible to discriminate between patients who are at risk of further progression and require additional therapy and those in whom simple follow-up is adequate.

Breast Cancer in Men Breast cancer is about 1/150th as frequent in men as in women. It usually presents as a unilateral lump in the breast and is frequently not diagnosed promptly. Given the smaller amount of soft tissue and the unexpected nature of the problem, locally advanced presentations are somewhat more common. When male breast cancer is matched to female breast cancer by age and stage, its overall prognosis is identical. Although gynecomastia may initially be unilateral or asymmetrical, any unilateral mass in a man over the age of 40 should receive a careful workup all the way through biopsy. On the other hand, bilateral symmetrical breast development rarely represents breast cancer and is almost invariably due to endocrine disease or a drug effect. It should be kept in mind, nevertheless, that the risk of cancer is much greater in men with gynecomastia; in such men, gross asymmetry of the breasts should arouse suspicion of cancer. Male breast cancer is best managed by mastectomy and axillary lymph node dissection (modified radical mastectomy). Patients with locally advanced disease should also be treated with irradiation. Approximately 90 percent of male breast cancers have the estrogen receptor, and approximately 60 percent of cases with metastatic disease respond to endocrine therapy. There are no randomized studies exploring adjuvant therapy for male breast cancer. Two historical experiences suggest that the disease responds well to adjuvant systemic therapy, and, if not medically contraindicated, the same criteria for the use of adjuvant therapy in women should be applied to men.

The sites of relapse and spectrum of response to chemotherapeutic drugs are virtually identical for breast cancers in the two sexes.

Experimental Therapy Experimental approaches to the treatment of breast cancer include attempts to block the cell surface receptor erbB2, antiangiogenic therapies, and agents aimed at blocking cell-surface–receptor tyrosine kinases and other signal transduction pathways. An effort should be made to offer such experimental approaches to patients with breast cancer, given the relative lack of success of conventional therapies in prolonging the survival of patients with metastatic disease. Advances during the past 10 to 15 years have added to the quality of life for patients with breast cancer (breast-conserving surgery, more effective reconstructive surgery, the availability of cytokines to ameliorate toxicity, and less toxic endocrine therapies). It is hoped that the next generation of trials will have even greater impact on the long-term outlook for this disease.

BIBLIOGRAPHY

BYERS T: Nutritional risk factors for breast cancer. Cancer 74:288, 1994

DICKSON RB, LIPPMAN ME: Growth factors in breast cancer. Endocr Rev 16:559, 1995

EARLY BREAST CANCER TRIALISTS' COLLABORATIVE GROUP: Systemic treatment of early breast cancer by hormonal, cytotoxic, or immune therapy. Lancet 1:71, 1992

FISHER B et al: Ten-year results of a randomized clinical trial comparing radical mastectomy and total mastectomy with or without radiation. N Engl J Med 312:674, 1985

FRIEDMAN LS et al: The search for *BRCA1*. Cancer Res 54:6374, 1994

HARRIS J et al: Breast cancer: Recent trends and progress and future prospects. Parts I, II, III. N Engl J Med 327:319, 390, 473, 1992

────── et al (eds): *Diseases of the Breast*. Philadelphia, Lippincott-Raven, 1995

SANTEN RJ et al: Endocrine treatment of breast cancer in women. Endocr Rev 11:221, 1990

SHAPIRO S: Screening: Assessment of current studies. Cancer 74(Suppl):231, 1994

92 | Robert J. Mayer

GASTROINTESTINAL TRACT CANCER

After the prostate, the gastrointestinal tract is the second most common noncutaneous site for cancer in the United States. Cancer of the alimentary tract is the second major cause of cancer-related mortality in the American population, following respiratory tract cancer.

ESOPHAGEAL CANCER

INCIDENCE AND ETIOLOGY In the United States, cancer of the esophagus is a relatively uncommon but extremely lethal malignant condition. It is estimated that the diagnosis was made in 12,300 Americans in 1996, leading to 11,200 deaths. Worldwide, the incidence of esophageal cancer varies strikingly. It occurs frequently within a so-called Asian esophageal cancer belt extending from the southern shore of the Caspian Sea on the west to northern China on the east and encompassing parts of Iran, Central Asia, Afghanistan, Siberia, and Mongolia. High-incidence "pockets" of the disease also are present in such disparate locations as Finland, Iceland, Curaçao, southeastern Africa, and northwestern France. In North America and western Europe, the disease is far more common in blacks than whites, is more common in males than females, appears most often after age 50, and seems to be associated with a lower socioeconomic status.

A variety of causative factors have been implicated in the development of the disease (Table 92-1). In the United States, most esophageal cancer cases are believed to be attributable to excess consumption of alcohol and/or a long-standing history of cigarette smoking. The relative risk increases with the amount of tobacco smoked or alcohol consumed. The consumption of whiskey seems to be linked to a higher incidence than the consumption of wine or beer. The development of esophageal cancer has also been associated with the ingestion of other carcinogens such as nitrites, smoked opiates, and fungal toxins in pickled vegetables, as well as with mucosal damage caused by such

Table 92-1

Some Etiologic Factors Believed to Be Associated with Esophageal Cancer

Excess alcohol consumption
Cigarette smoking
Other ingested carcinogens
  Nitrates (converted to nitrites)
  Smoked opiates
  Fungal toxins in pickled vegetables
Mucosal damage from physical agents
  Hot tea
  Lye ingestion
  Radiation-induced strictures
  Chronic achalasia
Host susceptibility
  Esophageal web with glossitis and iron deficiency (i.e., Plummer-Vinson or Paterson-Kelly syndrome)
  Congenital hyperkeratosis and pitting of the palms and soles (i.e., tylosis palmaris et plantaris)
? Dietary deficiencies molybdenum, zinc, vitamin A
? Celiac sprue
Chronic gastric reflux (i.e., Barrett's esophagus) for adenocarcinoma

physical insults as long-term exposure to extremely hot tea, the ingestion of lye, radiation-induced strictures, and chronic achalasia. The presence of an esophageal web in association with glossitis and iron deficiency (i.e., Plummer-Vinson or Paterson-Kelly syndrome) and congenital hyperkeratosis and pitting of the palms and soles (i.e., tylosis palmaris et plantaris) have each been linked with esophageal cancer, as have dietary deficiencies of molybdenum, zinc, and vitamin A. The risk for esophageal cancer may be slightly greater in individuals with celiac sprue and is definitely increased in the presence of chronic gastric reflux (i.e., Barrett's esophagus). In contrast to other esophageal cancers, neoplasms arising from Barrett's esophagus afflict whites far more often than blacks.

CLINICAL FEATURES Approximately 15 percent of esophageal cancers occur in the upper third of the esophagus (cervical esophagus), 45 percent in the middle third, and 40 percent in the lower third. In the past, more than 75 percent of esophageal tumors were squamous cell carcinomas, arising from the squamous epithelium that lines the lumen of the esophagus. Adenocarcinomas, while less common, more often develop from columnar epithelium, which may appear dysplastic in the distal esophagus in association with chronic gastric reflux (i.e., Barrett's esophagus). Such dysplastic epithelium frequently contains cells with an abnormal DNA content (aneuploidy) and mutations in the *p53* tumor suppressor gene. These adenocarcinomas have the biologic behavior of gastric rather than esophageal cancers. The incidence of adenocarcinoma has risen steadily, while the number of cases of squamous cell carcinomas has remained relatively stable. Attempts at endoscopic and cytologic screening for carcinoma in patients with Barrett's esophagus, while effective as a means of detecting high-grade dysplasia, have not yet been shown to improve the prognosis in individuals found to have a carcinoma. Squamous cell carcinomas are more common in blacks than whites, while adenocarcinomas are more common in whites than blacks. Squamous cell carcinomas and adenocarcinomas of the esophagus cannot be distinguished radiographically or endoscopically.

Progressive dysphagia and weight loss of short duration are the initial symptoms in the vast majority of patients. Dysphagia initially occurs with solid foods and gradually progresses to include semisolids and liquids. By the time these symptoms develop, the disease is usually incurable, since difficulty in swallowing does not occur until 60 percent or more of the esophageal circumference is infiltrated with cancer. Dysphagia may be associated with pain on swallowing (odynophagia), pain radiating to the chest and/or back, regurgitation or vomiting, and aspiration pneumonia. The disease most commonly spreads to adjacent and supraclavicular lymph nodes, liver, lungs, and pleura. Tracheoesophageal fistulas may develop as the disease advances, leading to severe suffering. As with other squamous cell carcinomas, hypercalcemia occasionally may occur in the absence of osseous metastases. It is believed to result from parathormone-related peptide secreted by tumor cells (see Chap. 102).

DIAGNOSIS Routine contrast radiographs effectively identify esophageal lesions large enough to cause symptoms. In contrast to benign esophageal leiomyomas, which result in esophageal narrowing with preservation of a normal mucosal pattern, esophageal carcinomas characteristically cause ragged, ulcerating changes in the mucosa in association with deeper infiltration, producing a picture resembling achalasia. Smaller, potentially resectable tumors are often poorly visualized despite technically adequate esophagograms. Because of this, esophagoscopy should be performed in all patients suspected of having an esophageal abnormality, to visualize the tumor and to obtain histopathologic confirmation of the diagnosis. Because the population of persons at risk for squamous cell carcinoma of the esophagus (i.e., smokers and drinkers) also has a high rate of cancers of the lung and the head and neck region, endoscopic inspection of the larynx, trachea, and bronchi also should be done. A thorough examination of the fundus of the stomach (by retroflexing the endoscope) is imperative as well. Endoscopic biopsies of esophageal tumors fail to recover malignant tissue in one-third of cases because the biopsy forceps cannot penetrate deeply enough through normal mucosa pushed in front of the carcinoma. Cytologic examination of tumor brushings frequently complements standard biopsies and should be performed routinely. The extent of tumor spread to the mediastinum and paraaortic lymph nodes should also be assessed by computed tomography (CT) scans of the chest and abdomen.

℞ **TREATMENT**

The prognosis for patients with esophageal carcinoma is poor. Fewer than 5 percent of patients are alive 5 years after the initial diagnosis, leading many physicians to focus management efforts solely on symptomatic control. Surgical resection of all gross tumor (i.e., total resection) is feasible in only 40 percent of cases, with residual tumor cells frequently present at the resection margins. Such esophagectomies have been associated in the past with a postoperative mortality rate in excess of 20 percent due to anastomotic fistulas, subphrenic abscesses, and respiratory complications; more recent reports suggest far better tolerance and diminished morbidity from these surgical procedures. Fewer than 20 percent of patients who survive a total resection can be expected to be alive after 5 years. The therapeutic outcome following the administration of primary radiation therapy (5500 to 6000 cGy) is not dissimilar to that of radical surgery, sparing patients perioperative morbidity but often resulting in less satisfactory palliation of obstructive symptoms. The evaluation of chemotherapeutic agents in patients with esophageal carcinoma has been hampered by ambiguity in the definition of "response" (i.e., benefit) and the debilitated physical condition of many treated individuals. Nonetheless, significant reductions in the size of measurable tumor masses have been reported in 15 to 25 percent of patients given single-agent treatment and in 30 to 60 percent of patients treated with drug combinations that include cisplatin. Combination chemotherapy and radiation therapy as the initial therapeutic approach, either alone or followed by an attempt at operative resection, may be of benefit. When administered along with radiation therapy, chemotherapy produces a better survival outcome than radiation therapy alone. The use of preoperative chemotherapy and radiation therapy followed by esophageal resection appears to prolong survival as compared with historical controls and has been shown to be superior to surgery alone in at least one small randomized clinical trial.

For the incurable, surgically unresectable patient with esophageal cancer, dysphagia, malnutrition, and the management of tracheoesophageal fistulas loom as major issues. Approaches to palliation of these cancer-related complications include repeated endoscopic dilatation, the surgical placement of a gastrostomy or jejunostomy for hydration and feeding, and endoscopic placement of an expansive metal stent to bypass the tumor. Endoscopic fulguration of the obstructing tumor with lasers appears to be the most promising of these techniques.

TUMORS OF THE STOMACH

GASTRIC ADENOCARCINOMA **Incidence and Epidemiology** For unclear reasons, the incidence and mortality rates for gastric cancer have decreased markedly during the past 60 years. In 1930, gastric cancer was the leading cause of cancer-related deaths among American men by a factor of two, while in women the disease ranked just behind tumors of the uterine cervix and breast. During the ensuing years, the mortality rate from gastric cancer in the United States has dropped in men from 28 to 5.0 per 100,000 population, while in women, the rate has decreased from 27 to 2.3 per 100,000. Nonetheless, it was estimated in 1996 that 22,800 new cases of stomach cancer were diagnosed in the United States and that 14,000 Americans died of the disease. The decreased incidence in gastric cancer in the United States is also reflected worldwide. The incidence of gastric cancer varies widely among different countries, being comparatively high in Japan, China, Chile, and Ireland; however, a decrease in both incidence and mortality has occurred in these areas as well.

Epidemiologic surveys have suggested the risk of gastric cancer to be greater among lower socioeconomic classes. Furthermore, migrants from high- to low-incidence nations appear to maintain their susceptibility to gastric cancer, while the risk for their offspring more closely approximates that of the new homeland. These findings suggest that an environmental exposure, probably beginning early in life, is related to the development of gastric cancer, with dietary carcinogens considered the most likely factor(s).

Pathology Approximately 85 percent of stomach cancers are adenocarcinomas, with 15 percent due to non-Hodgkin's lymphomas and leiomyosarcomas. Gastric adenocarcinomas may be subdivided into two categories: a *diffuse type* in which cell cohesion is absent, so that individual cells infiltrate and thicken the stomach wall without forming a discrete mass; and an *intestinal type* characterized by cohesive neoplastic cells that form glandlike tubular structures. The diffuse carcinomas occur more often in younger patients, develop throughout the stomach, including the cardia, result in a loss of distensibility of the gastric wall (so-called linitis plastica or "leather bottle" appearance), and carry a far more ominous prognosis. Intestinal-type lesions are frequently ulcerative, more commonly appear in the antrum and lesser curvature of the stomach, and are often preceded by a prolonged precancerous process. While the incidence of diffuse carcinomas is similar in most populations, the intestinal type tends to predominate in the high-risk geographic regions mentioned earlier and is less likely to be found in areas where the frequency of gastric cancer is declining. Thus, different etiologic factor(s) may be involved in these two subtypes. In the United States, the distal stomach is the site of origin of about 30 percent of gastric cancers. Approximately 20 percent of these tumors arise in the midportion of the stomach, while upwards of 37 percent of gastric tumors now originate in the proximal third of the stomach. The remaining 13 percent of gastric carcinomas involve the entire stomach.

Etiology The relationship between dietary patterns and the development of gastric carcinoma has been investigated extensively. The long-term ingestion of high concentrations of nitrates in dried, smoked, and salted foods appears to be associated with a higher risk. The nitrates are thought to be converted to carcinogenic nitrites by bacteria (Table 92-2). Such bacteria may be introduced exogenously through the ingestion of partially decayed foods, which are consumed in abundance worldwide by the lower socioeconomic classes. Bacteria such as *Helicobacter pylori* may also contribute to this effect. Loss of gastric acidity may permit bacterial growth in the stomach. Loss of acidity may occur when acid-producing cells of the gastric antrum were removed surgically 15 to 20 years earlier in a partial gastrectomy performed to control benign peptic ulcer disease or when achlorhydria, atrophic gastritis, and even pernicious anemia develop in the elderly. Serial endoscopic examinations of the stomach in patients with atrophic gastritis have documented replacement of the usual gastric mucosa

Table 92-2

Nitrate-Converting Bacteria as a Factor in the Causation of Gastric Carcinoma*

Exogenous sources of nitrate-converting bacteria:
    Bacterially contaminated food (common in lower socioeconomic classes, who have a higher incidence of the disease; diminished by improved food preservation and refrigeration)
    ? *Helicobacter pylori* infection
Endogenous factors favoring growth of nitrate-converting bacteria in the stomach:
    Decreased gastric acidity
    Prior gastric surgery (antrectomy) (15 to 20 year latency period)
    Atrophic gastritis and/or pernicious anemia
    ? Prolonged exposure to histamine H_2-receptor antagonists

* Hypothesis: Dietary nitrates are converted to carcinogenic nitrites by bacteria.

by intestinal-type cells. This process of intestinal metaplasia may lead to cellular atypia and eventual neoplasia. Since the declining incidence of gastric cancer in the United States primarily reflects a decline in distal, ulcerating, intestinal-type lesions, it is conceivable that better food preservation and the availability of refrigeration to all socioeconomic classes have decreased the dietary ingestion of exogenous bacteria. It remains uncertain whether the iatrogenic achlorhydria induced by the widespread, prolonged use of histamine antagonists will result in a future increase in intestinal-type gastric cancer.

Several additional etiologic factors have been associated with gastric carcinoma. Gastric ulcers and adenomatous polyps have occasionally been so linked, but data regarding a cause-and-effect relationship are unconvincing. The inadequate clinical distinction between benign gastric ulcers and small ulcerating carcinomas may, in part, account for this presumed association. The presence of extreme hypertrophy of gastric rugal folds (i.e., Menetrier's disease), giving the impression of polypoid lesions, has been associated with a striking frequency of malignant transformation; such hypertrophy, however, does not represent the presence of true adenomatous polyps. Individuals with blood group A have been reported to have a higher incidence of gastric cancer than persons with blood group O; it is possible that this observation is related to differences in the mucous secretion of the various ABO blood groups, thereby leading to greater or lesser mucosal protection from carcinogens. No association has been identified between duodenal ulcers and gastric cancer.

Clinical Features Gastric cancers, when superficial and surgically curable, usually produce no symptoms. As the tumor becomes more extensive, patients may complain of an insidious upper abdominal discomfort varying in intensity from a vague, postprandial fullness to a severe, steady pain. Anorexia, often with slight nausea, is very common but is not the usual presenting complaint. Weight loss may eventually be observed, and nausea and vomiting are particularly prominent with tumors of the pylorus; dysphagia may be the major symptom caused by lesions of the cardia. There are no early physical signs of the disease, and the finding of a palpable abdominal mass generally indicates long-standing growth and regional extension.

Gastric carcinomas spread by direct extension through the gastric wall to the perigastric tissues, occasionally adhering to adjacent organs such as the pancreas, colon, or liver. The disease also spreads via lymphatics or by seeding of peritoneal surfaces. Metastases to intra-abdominal and supraclavicular lymph nodes occur frequently, as do metastatic nodules to the ovary (Krukenberg's tumor), periumbilical region ("Sister Mary Joseph node") or peritoneal cul-de-sac (Blumer's shelf palpable on rectal or vaginal exam); malignant ascites may also develop. The liver is the most common site for hematogenous spread of tumor.

The presence of iron-deficiency anemia in men and of occult blood in the stool in both sexes should mandate a search for an occult lesion in the gastrointestinal tract. Such a careful assessment is of particular

importance in patients having atrophic gastritis or pernicious anemia. Unusual clinical features associated with gastric adenocarcinomas include migratory thrombophlebitis, microangiopathic hemolytic anemia, and acanthosis nigricans.

Diagnosis A double-contrast radiographic examination is the simplest diagnostic procedure for the evaluation of a patient with epigastric complaints. The use of double-contrast techniques helps to detect small lesions by improving mucosal detail. The stomach should be distended at some time during every radiographic examination, since decreased distensibility may be the only indication of a diffuse infiltrative carcinoma. Although gastric ulcers can be detected fairly early, it may be impossible to distinguish benign from malignant lesions. The anatomic location of an ulcer is not in itself an indication of the presence or absence of a cancer.

Gastric ulcers that appear benign by radiography present special problems. Some physicians believe that gastroscopy is not mandatory if the radiographic features are typically benign, if complete healing can be visualized by x-ray within 6 weeks, and if a follow-up contrast radiograph obtained several months later shows a normal appearance. However, we recommend gastroscopic biopsy and brush cytology for all patients with a gastric ulcer in order to exclude a malignancy. It is crucial to identify malignant gastric ulcers before they penetrate into surrounding tissues, because the rate of cure of early lesions limited to the mucosa or submucosa is greater than 80 percent. Since gastric carcinomas are difficult to distinguish clinically or radiographically from gastric lymphomas, endoscopic biopsies should be made as deep as possible, due to the submucosal location of lymphoid tumors.

The staging system for gastric carcinoma is shown in Table 92-3.

℞ **TREATMENT**

Surgical removal of the complete tumor with resection of adjacent lymph nodes offers the only chance for cure. However, this is possible in fewer than one-third of patients. In general, a subtotal gastrectomy is the treatment of choice for patients with distal carcinomas, while total or near-total gastrectomies are required for more proximal tumors. The prognosis following complete surgical resection depends on the degree of tumor penetration into the stomach wall and is also adversely influenced by regional lymph node involvement, vascular invasion, and abnormal DNA content (i.e., aneuploidy), characteristics found in the vast majority of American patients. As a result, the probability of survival after 5 years for the 25 to 30 percent of patients in the United States able to undergo a complete resection of a gastric cancer is approximately 20 percent for distal tumors and less than 10 percent for proximal tumors, with recurrences continuing to occur for at least 8 years after surgery. In the absence of ascites or extensive hepatic or peritoneal metastases, however, even patients whose disease is believed to be incurable by surgery should be offered an attempt at resection of the primary lesion, since reduction of tumor bulk is the best form of palliation and may enhance the probability of benefit if chemotherapy and/or radiation therapy are administered.

Gastric adenocarcinoma is a relatively radioresistant tumor, and adequate control of the primary tumor requires doses of external beam irradiation that exceed the tolerance of surrounding structures, such as bowel mucosa and spinal cord. As a result, the major role of radiation therapy in patients with gastric cancer has been limited to palliation of pain. Radiation therapy alone after a complete resection does not prolong survival. In the setting of surgically unresectable disease limited to the epigastrium, patients treated with 3500 to 4000 cGy did not live longer than similar patients not receiving radiotherapy; however, survival was prolonged slightly when 5-fluorouracil (5-FU) was given in combination with radiation therapy. In this clinical setting, the 5-FU may well be functioning as a radiosensitizer.

The administration of combinations of cytotoxic drugs to patients with advanced gastric carcinoma has been associated with reductions of greater than 50 percent in measurable tumor mass ("partial responses") in 30 to 50 percent of cases, providing significant benefit to individuals who respond to treatment. Such drug combinations have generally included 5-FU and doxorubicin together with mitomycin-C, cisplatin, or high doses of methotrexate. Despite this encouraging response rate for a malignant condition once thought untreatable, complete disappearances of tumor masses remain uncommon; the partial responses are transient; and the overall impact of such multidrug therapy on survival has been a source of debate. The use of prophylactic (i.e., adjuvant) chemotherapy following the complete resection of a gastric cancer as a means of eradicating clinically undetectable micrometastases and improving the potential for cure has generally proven to be unsuccessful. The role of such adjuvant treatment as well as of preoperative ("neoadjuvant") chemotherapy should be considered investigational.

PRIMARY GASTRIC LYMPHOMA Primary lymphoma of the stomach is relatively uncommon, accounting for fewer than 15 percent of gastric malignancies and about 2 percent of all lymphomas. The stomach is, however, the most frequent extranodal location for lymphoma, and gastric lymphoma has appeared with increased frequency during the past 20 years. The disease is difficult to distinguish clinically from gastric adenocarcinoma; both tumors are most often detected during the sixth decade of life; present with epigastric pain, early satiety, and generalized fatigue; and are usually characterized by ulcerations with a ragged, thickened mucosal pattern demonstrated by contrast radiographs. The diagnosis of lymphoma of the stomach may occasionally be made through cytologic brushings of the gastric mucosa, but usually it requires a biopsy at the time of gastroscopy or laparotomy. Failure of gastroscopic biopsies to detect lymphoma in a given case should not be interpreted as being conclusive, since superficial biopsies may miss the deeper lymphoid infiltrate. The macroscopic pathology of gastric lymphoma may also mimic that of adenocarcinoma, consisting of either a bulky ulcerated lesion localized in the corpus or antrum or a diffuse process spreading throughout the entire gastric submucosa and even extending into the duodenum. Microscopically, the vast majority of gastric lymphoid tumors are non-Hodgkin's lymphomas of B cell origin; Hodgkin's disease involving the stomach is extremely uncommon. Histologically, these tumors may range from well-differentiated, superficial processes [mucosa-associated lymphoid tissue (MALT)] to high-grade, large cell lymphomas. Infection with *H. pylori*, the same bacterium associated with the development of gastric adenocarcinoma, appears to increase the risk for gastric lymphoma in general and MALT lymphomas in particular. Gastric lymphomas spread initially to regional lymph nodes (often to Waldeyer's ring) and may then disseminate. Gastric lymphomas are staged like other lymphomas (Chap. 113).

Previous concerns that the rapid destruction of lymphoma masses by chemotherapy might lead to life-threatening hemorrhage seem to have been eased by the results of clinical trials. Although radiation therapy to the abdomen has been employed in the past following surgical resection, this practice also has been questioned, because most recurrences develop at sites distant from the epigastrium and, consequently, outside the radiation treatment fields. If widespread disease is discovered at the time of laparotomy, combination chemotherapy should be used.

GASTRIC (NONLYMPHOID) SARCOMA Leiomyosarcomas are the most common of this group of gastric malignancies and make up approximately 1 to 3 percent of all gastric neoplasms. They most frequently involve the anterior and posterior walls of the gastric fundus and often ulcerate and bleed. Even those lesions that appear benign on histologic examination may behave in a malignant fashion. Leiomyosarcomas rarely invade adjacent viscera and characteristically do not metastasize to lymph nodes, but they may spread to the liver and lungs. The treatment of choice is surgical resection. Combination chemotherapy should be reserved for patients with metastatic disease.

COLORECTAL CANCER

INCIDENCE Cancer of the large bowel is second only to lung cancer as a cause of cancer death in the United States. Approximately 133,500 new cases occurred in 1996, resulting in 54,900 deaths. The incidence rate for this extremely common malignant condition has not changed substantially during the past 40 years, although, for some reason, the mortality rate has decreased in recent years, particularly in females. Colorectal cancer generally occurs in individuals 50 years of age or older.

POLYPS AND MOLECULAR PATHOGENESIS Most colorectal cancers, regardless of etiology, are believed to arise from adenomatous polyps. A polyp is a grossly visible protrusion from the mucosal surface and may be classified pathologically as a nonneoplastic hamartoma (*juvenile polyp*), a hyperplastic mucosal proliferation (*hyperplastic polyp*), or an adenomatous polyp. Only adenomas are clearly premalignant, and only a minority of such lesions ever develop into cancer. Population-screening studies and autopsy surveys have revealed that adenomatous polyps may be found in the colons of about 30 percent of middle-aged or elderly people. Based on this prevalence and the known incidence of colorectal cancers, it appears that fewer

℞ **TREATMENT**

Primary gastric lymphoma is a far more treatable disease than adenocarcinoma of the stomach, a fact that underscores the need for making the correct diagnosis. Antibiotic treatment to eradicate *H. pylori* infection has led to regression of about half of gastric MALT lymphomas and should be considered before surgery, radiation therapy, or chemotherapy are undertaken in patients having such tumors. Subtotal gastrectomy, usually followed by combination chemotherapy, has led to 5-year survival rates of 40 to 60 percent in patients with localized high-grade lymphomas. The need for this major surgical procedure has been questioned, particularly in patients with preoperative radiographic evidence of nodal involvement, for whom chemotherapy alone has been proposed as a substitution for resection.

Table 92-3

Staging System for Gastric Carcinoma

Stage	TNM	Features	Data from American College of Surgeons	
			Number of Cases, %	5-Year Survival, %
0	TisN0M0	Node negative; limited to mucosa	1	90
IA	T1N0M0	Node negative; invasion of lamina propria or submucosa	7	59
IB	T2N0M0	Node negative; invasion of muscularis propria	10	44
II	T1N2M0 T2N1M0	Node positive; invasion beyond mucosa but within wall		
		or	17	29
	T3N0M0	Node negative; extension through wall		
IIIA	T2N2M0 T3N1-2M0	Node positive; invasion of muscularis propria or through wall	21	15
IIIB	T4N0-1M0	Node negative; adherence to surrounding tissue	14	9
IV	T4N2M0	Node positive; adherence to surrounding tissue		
		or	30	3
	T1-4N0-2M1	Distant metastases		

than 1 percent of polyps ever become malignant. Most polyps produce no symptoms and remain clinically undetected. Occult blood in the stool may be found in fewer than 5 percent of patients with such lesions.

A number of molecular changes have been described in DNA obtained from adenomatous polyps, dysplastic lesions, and polyps containing microscopic foci of tumor cells (carcinoma in situ), which are thought to represent a multistep process in the evolution of normal colonic mucosa to life-threatening invasive carcinoma. These developmental steps towards carcinogenesis include point mutations in the K-*ras* proto-oncogene; hypomethylation of DNA, leading to gene activation; loss of DNA ("allelic loss") at the site of a tumor suppressor gene [the adenomatous polyposis coli (APC) gene] located on the long arm of chromosome 5 (5q21); allelic loss at the site of a tumor suppressor gene located on chromosome 18q [so-called the deleted in colorectal cancer (DCC) gene]; and allelic loss at chromosome 17p, associated with mutations in the *p53* tumor suppressor gene (see Chap. 84). Thus, the altered proliferative pattern of the colonic mucosa, which results in progression to a polyp and then to carcinoma, may involve the mutational activation of an oncogene followed by and coupled with the loss of genes that normally suppress tumorigenesis. While the present model includes five such molecular alterations, others are likely involved in the carcinogenic process. It remains uncertain whether the genetic aberrations always occur in a defined order. Based on this model, however, it is believed that neoplasia develops only in those polyps in which all of these mutational events take place.

Clinically, the probability of an adenomatous polyp becoming a cancer depends on the gross appearance of the lesion, its histologic features, and its size. Adenomatous polyps may be pedunculated (stalked) or sessile (flat-based). Cancers develop more frequently in sessile polyps. Histologically, adenomatous polyps may be tubular, villous (i.e., papillary), or tubulovillous. Villous adenomas, most of which are sessile, become malignant more than three times as often as tubular adenomas. The likelihood that any polypoid lesion in the large bowel contains invasive cancer is related to the size of the polyp, being negligible (<2 percent) in lesions smaller than 1.5 cm, intermediate (2 to 10 percent) in lesions 1.5 to 2.5 cm in size, and substantial (10 percent) in lesions larger than 2.5 cm.

Following the detection of an adenomatous polyp, the entire large bowel should be visualized endoscopically or radiographically, since synchronous lesions are present in approximately one-third of cases. Colonoscopy should then be repeated periodically, even in the absence of a previously documented malignancy, since such patients have a 30 to 50 percent probability of developing another adenoma and are at a higher-than-average risk for developing a colorectal carcinoma. Adenomatous polyps are thought to require more than 5 years of growth before becoming clinically significant; the results of a randomized trial conducted by the National Polyp Study have indicated that colonoscopy need not be carried out more frequently than every 3 years.

ETIOLOGY AND RISK FACTORS Risk factors for the development of colorectal cancer are listed in Table 92-4.

Diet The etiology for most cases of large-bowel cancer appears to be related to environmental factors. The disease occurs more often in upper socioeconomic populations who live in urban areas. Epidemiologic studies in various countries have documented a direct correlation between mortality from colorectal cancer and per capita consumption of calories, meat protein, and dietary fat and oil as well as elevations in the serum cholesterol concentration and mortality from coronary artery disease. Any geographic variations in incidence do not appear to be related to genetic differences, since migrant groups tend to assume the large-bowel cancer incidence rates of their adopted countries. Furthermore, population groups such as Mormons and Seventh Day Adventists, whose lifestyle and dietary habits differ somewhat from those of their neighbors, have incidence and mortality rates for colorectal cancer that are significantly lower than expected, while the appearance of colorectal cancer has increased in Japan since that nation

Table 92-4

Risk Factors for the Development of Colorectal Cancer

Diet
   Animal fat
   ? Fiber
Hereditary syndromes (autosomal dominant inheritance)
   Polyposis coli
   Nonpolyposis syndrome (Lynch syndrome)
Inflammatory bowel disease
Streptococcus bovis bacteremia
Ureterosigmoidostomy
? Tobacco use

has adopted a more "western" diet. It is therefore assumed that dietary patterns influence the development of colorectal cancer. At least two hypotheses have been proposed to explain this relationship, neither of which is fully satisfactory.

Animal fats Based on the association of colorectal cancer with hypercholesterolemia and coronary artery disease as well as the increased incidence of large-bowel tumors in geographic areas where meat is a dietary staple, it has been suggested that the ingestion of animal fats leads to an increased proportion of anaerobes in the gut microflora, resulting in the conversion of normal bile acids into carcinogens. This provocative hypothesis is supported by several reports of increased amounts of fecal anaerobes in the stools of patients with colorectal cancer. Moreover, prospective cohort and case control studies in large numbers of people have revealed a consistently enhanced risk for the development of colorectal adenomas and carcinomas in association with elevated serum cholesterol levels and diets high in animal (but not vegetable) fat.

Fiber The observation that South African Bantus ingest a diet far higher in roughage, produce more frequent, bulkier stools, and have a lower incidence of large-bowel cancer than their American and European counterparts led to the proposal that the higher rate of colorectal cancer in western society is in large part the result of a low intake of dietary fiber. This theory suggests that dietary fiber accelerates intestinal transit time, thereby reducing the exposure of colonic mucosa to potential carcinogens and diluting these carcinogens because of enhanced fecal bulk. Such a proposition appears somewhat simplistic when subjected to careful scrutiny. Although an enhanced fiber intake increases fecal bulk, there has been no consistent evidence that a higher fiber intake consistently shortens the transit time of stool. In addition, despite the generally higher fiber intake in low-incidence countries, the environmental differences between developing and industrialized nations are myriad and include such other important dietary variables as meat and fat consumption. Finally, a diet low in fiber may lead to chronic constipation and such associated conditions as diverticulosis. If a low-fiber diet alone were a significant factor in colorectal cancer, individuals having diverticulosis should be at higher risk for the development of large-bowel tumors; this does not appear to be the case.

Thus, the weight of epidemiologic evidence clearly implicates diet as being the major etiologic factor for colorectal cancer. The available data strongly associate a high intake of animal fat with the development of large-bowel cancer.

HEREDITARY FACTORS AND SYNDROMES As many as 25 percent of patients with colorectal cancer may have a family history of the disease, suggesting a hereditary predisposition. Such inherited large-bowel cancers can be divided into two main groups: the well-studied but uncommon polyposis syndromes and the increasingly well-defined, more common nonpolyposis syndromes (Table 92-5).

Polyposis Coli Polyposis coli (familial polyposis of the colon) is a rare condition characterized by the appearance of thousands of adenomatous polyps throughout the large bowel. It is transmitted in an autosomal dominant manner; the occasional patients with no family history are thought to have developed the condition due to a spontaneous mutation. Molecular studies have associated polyposis coli with a deletion in the long arm of chromosome 5 (including the APC gene) in both neoplastic (somatic mutation) and normal (germline mutation) cells. It has been hypothesized that the loss of this genetic material (i.e., allelic loss) results in the absence of tumor suppressor genes whose protein products would normally inhibit neoplastic growth. The presence of soft tissue and bony tumors and of ampullary cancers in addition to the colonic polyps characterizes a subset of polyposis coli known as *Gardner's syndrome*, while the appearance of malignant tumors of the central nervous system accompanying polyposis coli defines *Turcot's syndrome*. The colonic polyps in all these conditions are rarely present before puberty but are generally evident in affected individuals by age 25. If the polyposis is not treated surgically, colorectal cancer will develop in almost all patients before age 40. Polyposis coli has been studied intensively and appears to result from a defect in the colonic mucosa leading to an abnormal proliferative pattern and an impaired ability for cellular repair following exposure to radiation or ultraviolet light. Once the multiple polyps that constitute polyposis coli are detected, patients should undergo a total colectomy. In the past it was unclear whether the optimal operative approach in such a clinical setting was to resect the entire colon and rectum, leaving a young patient with a permanent ileostomy, or to perform an ileoproctostomy. While the latter procedure retained the distal rectum and anal sphincter, it placed the patient at continued risk for the development of cancer in the rectal remnant and necessitated semiannual or annual proctoscopic surveillance. The development of the ileoanal anastomotic technique allows removal of the entire bowel while retaining the anal sphincter; this appears to be the best treatment. Medical therapy with nonsteroidal anti-inflammatory drugs such as sulindac has been reported to decrease the number and size of polyps in patients with polyposis coli; however, this effect on polyps is only temporary. Colectomy remains the primary therapy for patients with polyposis coli. The offspring of patients with polyposis coli, who often are prepubertal when the diagnosis is made in the parent, have a 50 percent risk for the eventual development of this premalignant disorder and should be carefully screened by annual flexible sigmoidoscopy until age 35. Such proctosigmoidoscopy is a sufficient screening procedure because polyps tend to be evenly distributed from cecum to anus, making more invasive and expensive techniques such as colonoscopy or barium enema unnecessary. Testing for occult blood in the stool is an inadequate screening maneuver. An alternative and still experimental method for identifying carriers of this inherited trait is testing DNA from peripheral blood mononuclear cells for the presence of a mutated APC gene. The detection of such a germline mutation can lead to a definitive diagnosis before the development of polyps.

Hereditary Nonpolyposis Colon Cancer Hereditary nonpolyposis colon cancer (HNPCC), also known as Lynch syndrome, is another condition inherited in an autosomal dominant manner. It has the following characteristics: the presence of three or more relatives with histologically documented colorectal cancer, one of whom is a first-degree relative of the other two; one or more cases of colorectal cancer diagnosed before age 50 in the family; and colorectal cancer involving at least two generations. In contrast to polyposis coli, HNPCC is associated with an unusually high frequency of cancer arising in the proximal large bowel. The median age for the appearance of an adenocarcinoma is under 50 years, which is 10 to 15 years younger than the median age for the general population. Families with HNPCC often include individuals with multiple primary cancers; the association of colorectal cancer with either ovarian or endometrial carcinomas is especially strong in women. It has been recommended that members of such families undergo biennial colonoscopy beginning at age 25 years with in-

termittent pelvic ultrasonography and endometrial biopsy offered to potentially afflicted women; such a screening strategy has not yet been validated. HNPCC is associated with germline mutations of several genes, particularly *hMSH2* on chromosome 2 and *hMLH1* on chromosome 3. These mutations lead to errors in DNA replication and are thought to result in DNA instability because of defective repair of DNA mismatches, resulting in abnormal cell growth and tumor development.

INFLAMMATORY BOWEL DISEASE (See also Chap. 286) Large-bowel cancer represents a not infrequent complication in patients with long-standing inflammatory bowel disease. Neoplasms appear to develop more commonly in patients with ulcerative colitis than in those with granulomatous colitis, but this impression may result in part from the occasional difficulty of differentiating these two conditions. The risk of colorectal cancer in a patient with inflammatory bowel disease is relatively small during the initial 10 years of the disease, but then it appears to increase at a rate of approximately 0.5 to 1.0 percent per year. Actuarially derived cumulative cancer rates in such symptomatic patients have ranged from 8 to 30 percent after 25 years. The risk is generally considered to be higher in younger patients with pancolitis.

Cancer surveillance in patients with inflammatory bowel disease is unsatisfactory. Symptoms such as bloody diarrhea, abdominal cramping, and obstruction, which may signal the appearance of a tumor, are similar to the complaints caused by a flare-up of the underlying disease. In patients with a history of inflammatory bowel disease lasting 15 years or more who continue to experience exacerbations, the surgical removal of the colon can significantly reduce the risk for cancer and also eliminate the target organ for the underlying chronic gastrointestinal disorder. The value of such surveillance techniques as colonoscopy with mucosal biopsies and brushings for less symptomatic individuals with chronic inflammatory bowel disease is uncertain. The purpose of such procedures has been the identification of premalignant mucosal dysplasia, thereby justifying surgical intervention. The lack of uniformity regarding the pathologic criteria that characterize dysplasia and the absence of data that such surveillance reduces the development of lethal cancers, however, has made this costly practice an area of controversy.

OTHER HIGH-RISK CONDITIONS *Streptococcus bovis* **Bacteremia** For unknown reasons, individuals who develop endocarditis or septicemia from this fecal bacteria seem to have a high incidence of occult colorectal tumors and, possibly, upper gastrointestinal cancers as well. Endoscopic or radiographic screening appears advisable.

Table 92-5

Hereditable (Autosomal Dominant) Gastrointestinal Polyposis Syndromes

Syndrome	Distribution of Polyps	Histologic Type	Malignant Potential	Associated Lesions
Familial colonic polyposis	Large intestine	Adenoma	Common	None
Gardner's syndrome	Large and small intestine	Adenoma	Common	Osteomas, fibromas, lipomas, epidermoid cysts, ampullary cancers
Turcot's syndrome	Large intestine	Adenoma	Common	Brain tumors
Nonpolyposis syndrome (Lynch syndrome)	Large intestine (often proximal)	Adenoma	Common	Endometrial and ovarian tumors
Peutz-Jeghers syndrome	Small and large intestines, stomach	Hamartoma	Rare	Mucocutaneous pigmentation; tumors of the ovary, breast, pancreas, endometrium
Juvenile polyposis	Large and small intestines, stomach	Hamartoma, rarely progressing to adenoma	Rare	Various congenital abnormalities

Ureterosigmoidostomy There is a 5 to 10 percent incidence of colon cancer 15 to 30 years after ureterosigmoidostomy to correct congenital extrophy of the bladder. Neoplasms characteristically are found at a site distal to the ureteral implant where colonic mucosa is chronically exposed to both urine and feces.

Tobacco Use Prospective cohort studies have linked cigarette smoking to the development of colorectal adenomas, particularly after more than 35 years of tobacco use. No biologic explanation for this association has yet been proposed.

PRIMARY PREVENTION Several orally administered synthetic and naturally occurring materials have been assessed as possible inhibitors of colon cancer. The most effective class of these chemopreventive agents is aspirin and other nonsteroidal anti-inflammatory drugs, which are thought to suppress cell proliferation by inhibiting prostaglandin synthesis. Case-control studies have indicated that regular aspirin use reduces the risk for colonic adenomas and carcinomas as well as for death from large-bowel cancer; this inhibiting effect on colonic carcinogenesis appears to increase with the duration of drug use. While antioxidant vitamins such as ascorbic acid, tocopherols, and β-carotene are present in diets rich in fruits and vegetables, which have been associated with lower rates of colorectal cancer, they have been found to be ineffective in a prospectively randomized trial as a means of reducing the incidence of subsequent adenomas in patients who had undergone the removal of a colonic adenoma. Estrogen replacement therapy has been associated in prospective cohort studies with a reduction in the risk of colorectal cancer in women, conceivably by an effect on bile acid synthesis and composition. Possibly the otherwise unexplained reduction in colorectal cancer mortality in women may be a result of the widespread use of estrogen replacement in postmenopausal individuals. Oral calcium supplements have also been noted to inhibit colon epithelial cell proliferation, but efficacy in cancer prevention has not been proven.

SCREENING The rationale for colorectal cancer screening programs is that the earlier detection of localized, superficial neoplasms in asymptomatic individuals will increase the surgical cure rate. Such screening programs appear to be especially indicated for individuals having a family history of the disease in first-degree relatives. The relative risk for developing colorectal cancer increases to 1.75 in such people and may be even higher if the relative was afflicted before 60 years of age. Screening strategies have been based on the assumption that more than 60 percent of early lesions are located in the rectosigmoid, making them accessible to rigid proctosigmoidoscopy. For unexplained reasons, however, there has been a consistent decrease during the past several decades in the proportion of large-bowel cancers arising in the rectum, with a corresponding increase in the proportion of cancers in the more proximal descending colon. As such, the potential for rigid proctosigmoidoscopy to detect a sufficient number of occult neoplasms to make the procedure cost-effective has been questioned. Nonetheless, in support of periodic rigid proctosigmoidoscopic examination is a case-control study reporting a reduction in mortality from distal large bowel cancer in individuals who had undergone such screening. The availability of flexible, fiberoptic sigmoidoscopes, permitting trained operators to visualize the colon for up to 60 cm, should further enhance cancer detection and resolve this issue.

Most programs directed at the early detection of colorectal cancers have focused on digital rectal examinations and testing stool for the presence of occult blood. The digital examination should be part of any routine physical evaluation in adults older than age 40, serving as a screening test for prostate cancer in men, a component of the pelvic examination in women, and an inexpensive maneuver for the detection of masses in the rectum. The development of the Hemoccult test has greatly facilitated the detection of occult fecal blood. Unfortunately, even when performed optimally, the Hemoccult test has major limitations as a screening technique. Approximately 50 percent of patients with documented colorectal cancers have a negative fecal Hemoccult test, consistent with the intermittent bleeding pattern of

these tumors. When random cohorts of asymptomatic persons have been tested, 2 to 4 percent have Hemoccult-positive stools. Colorectal cancers have been found in only 5 to 10 percent of these "test-positive" cases, with benign polyps being detected in an additional 20 to 30 percent. Consequently, a colorectal neoplasm will not be found in most asymptomatic individuals with occult blood in their stool. Nonetheless, persons found to have Hemoccult-positive stool routinely undergo further medical evaluation, which includes sigmoidoscopy, barium enema, and/or colonoscopy—procedures that not only are uncomfortable and expensive but also are associated with a low but finite risk for significant complications. The added cost of these studies would appear justifiable if the small number of patients found to have occult neoplasms because of Hemoccult screening could be shown to have an improved prognosis and prolonged survival. Prospectively controlled trials addressing this issue are in progress. One of these studies, conducted at the University of Minnesota and involving more than 46,000 participants, reported a statistically significant reduction in mortality from colorectal cancer for individuals undergoing annual screening. However, this benefit only emerged after more than 13 years of follow-up and was extremely expensive to achieve, since all positive tests (most of which were false-positive) were followed by colonoscopy. Moreover, these colonoscopic examinations may have represented "chance selection" for more effective endoscopic screening and may also have provided the opportunity for cancer prevention through the removal of potentially premalignant adenomatous polyps.

Screening techniques for large-bowel cancer in asymptomatic persons remain unsatisfactory. Recommendations from governmental and private agencies are conflicting. At present, the American Cancer Society suggests annual digital rectal examinations beginning at age 40, annual fecal Hemoccult screening beginning at age 50, and sigmoidoscopy (preferably flexible) every 3 to 5 years beginning at age 50 for asymptomatic individuals having none of the high-risk factors for colorectal cancer. The use of colonscopy for screening has not yet been systematically examined. More effective techniques for screening are needed, perhaps taking advantage of the molecular changes that have been described in these tumors. An analysis for specific *ras* proto-oncogene mutations from DNA recovered from stool in patients with a history of colorectal cancer represents an initial step in this direction.

CLINICAL FEATURES **Presenting Symptoms** Symptoms vary with the anatomic location of the tumor.

Since stool is relatively liquid as it passes through the ileocecal valve into the right colon, neoplasms arising in the cecum and ascending colon may become quite large, significantly narrowing the bowel lumen, without resulting in any obstructive symptoms or noticeable alterations in bowel habits. Lesions of the right colon commonly ulcerate, leading to chronic, insidious blood loss without a change in the appearance of the stool. Consequently, patients with tumors of the ascending colon often present with symptoms such as fatigue, palpitations, and even angina pectoris and are found to have a hypochromic, microcytic anemia indicative of iron deficiency. Since the cancer may bleed intermittently, however, a random test for the presence of occult blood in the stool may be negative. As a result, the unexplained presence of iron-deficiency anemia in any adult (with the possible exception of a premenopausal, multiparous woman) mandates a thorough endoscopic and/or radiographic visualization of the entire large bowel (Fig. 92-1). For unknown reasons, blacks have a higher incidence of right colon lesions than do whites.

Since stool becomes more concentrated as it passes into the transverse and descending colon, tumors arising there tend to impede the passage of stool, resulting in the development of abdominal cramping, occasional obstruction, and even perforation. Radiographs of the abdomen often reveal characteristic annular, constricting lesions ("apple-core" or "napkin-ring") (Fig. 92-2).

Neoplasms arising in the rectosigmoid often are associated with hematochezia, tenesmus, and narrowing of the caliber of stool; nonetheless, anemia is an infrequent finding. While these symptoms may lead patients and their physicians to suspect the presence of hemorrhoids, the development of rectal bleeding and/or altered bowel habits

FIGURE 92-1 Double-contrast air-barium enema revealing a sessile tumor of the cecum in a patient with iron-deficiency anemia and guaiac-positive stool. The lesion at surgery was a stage B adenocarcinoma.

demands a prompt digital rectal examination and proctosigmoidoscopy.

Staging, Prognostic Factors, and Patterns of Spread The prognosis for individuals having colorectal cancer is closely related to the depth of tumor penetration into the bowel wall and the presence of both regional lymph node involvement and distant metastases. These variables are incorporated into the staging system introduced by Dukes and recently applied to a TNM classification method, in which T represents the depth of tumor penetration, N the presence of lymph node involvement, and M the presence or absence of distant metastases (Table 92-6). Patients with superficial lesions that do not penetrate into the muscularis or involve regional lymph nodes are designated as having *stage A* (T1N0M0) disease; patients whose tumors have penetrated more deeply but have not spread to lymph nodes have *stage B* disease [subclassified as *stage B₁* (T2N0M0) if lesions are restricted to the muscularis and as *stage B₂* (T3N0M0) if lesions involve or penetrate the serosa]; regional lymph node involvement defines *stage C* (TxN1M0) disease; and metastatic spread to sites such as liver, lung, or bone indicates *stage D* (TxNxM1) disease. Unless gross evidence of metastatic disease is present, it is impossible to accurately determine disease stage before surgical resection and pathologic analysis of the operative specimens.

Most recurrences after a surgical resection of a large-bowel cancer occur within the first 4 postoperative years, making the 5-year mark a fairly reliable indicator of cure. The likelihood for 5-year survival in patients with colorectal cancer is closely associated with their stage (Table 92-6). That likelihood has appeared to improve during the past several decades when similar surgical stages have been compared. The most plausible explanation for this improvement appears to be more thorough intraoperative and pathologic staging. In particular, more exacting attention to pathologic detail has revealed that the prognosis following the resection of a colorectal cancer is not related merely to the presence or absence of regional lymph node involvement but may be more precisely assessed by the number of involved lymph nodes (one to four lymph nodes versus five or more lymph nodes). Other predictors of a poor prognosis after a total surgical resection include tumor penetration through the bowel wall into pericolic fat, poorly differentiated histology, perforation and/or tumor adherence to adjacent organs (increasing the risk for an anatomically adjacent recurrence), and venous invasion by tumor (Table 92-7). Regardless of the clinicopathologic stage, a preoperative elevation of the plasma carcinoembryonic antigen (CEA) titer is suggestive of eventual tumor recurrence. The presence of an abnormal DNA content (i.e., aneuploidy) and specific chromosomal deletions, such as allelic loss in chromosome 18q (involving the DCC gene) in tumor cells, appears to predict a higher risk for metastatic spread, particularly in patients with stage B₂ (T3N0M0) disease. In contrast to most other carcinomas and sarcomas, the prognosis in individuals with colorectal cancer is not influenced by the size of the primary lesion when adjusted for nodal involvement and histologic differentiation.

Cancers of the large bowel generally spread to regional lymph nodes or to the liver via the portal venous circulation. The liver represents the most frequent visceral site of metastatic dissemination; it is the initial site of distant spread in one-third of recurring colorectal cancers and has become involved in more than two-thirds of such patients at the time of death. In general, colorectal cancer rarely metastasizes to the lungs, supraclavicular lymph nodes, bone, or brain without prior spread to the liver. A major exception to this rule occurs in

FIGURE 92-2 Annular, constricting adenocarcinoma of the descending colon. This radiographic appearance is referred to as an "apple-core" lesion and is always highly suggestive of malignancy.

Table 92-6

Staging of and Prognosis for Colorectal Cancer

Stage				Approximate 5-Year
Dukes	**TNM**	**Numerical**	**Pathologic Description**	**Survival, %**
A	T1N0M0	I	Cancer limited to mucosa and submucosa	>90
B₁	T2N0M0	II	Cancer extends into muscularis	85
B₂	T3N0M0	II	Cancer extends into or through serosa	70–80
C	TxN1M0	III	Cancer involves regional lymph nodes	35–65
D	TxNxM1	IV	Distant metastases (i.e. liver, lung, etc.)	5

Table 92-7

Predictors of Poor Outcome Following Total Surgical Resection
of Colorectal Cancer

Tumor spread to regional lymph nodes
Number of regional lymph nodes involved
Tumor penetration through the bowel wall
Poorly differentiated histology
Perforation
Tumor adherence to adjacent organs
Venous invasion
Preoperative elevation of CEA titer (>5.0 ng/mL)
Aneuploidy
Specific chromosomal deletion (e.g., allelic loss on chromosome 18q)

patients having primary tumors in the distal rectum, from which tumor cells may spread through the paravertebral venous plexus, escaping the portal venous system and thereby reaching the lungs or supraclavicular lymph nodes without hepatic involvement. The median survival after the detection of distant metastases may range from 6 to 9 months (hepatomegaly, liver abnormalities) to 24 to 30 months (small liver nodule initially identified by elevated CEA level and subsequent CT scan).

℞ **TREATMENT**

Total resection of tumor is the optimal treatment when a malignant lesion is detected endoscopically or radiographically in the large bowel. An evaluation for the presence of metastatic disease, including a thorough physical examination, a chest radiograph, biochemical assessment of liver function, and measurement of the plasma CEA level, should be performed before surgery. When possible, a colonoscopy of the entire large bowel should be performed to identify synchronous neoplasms and/or polyps. The detection of metastases should not preclude surgery in patients with tumor-related symptoms such as gastrointestinal bleeding or obstruction, but it often prompts the use of a less radical operative procedure. At the time of laparotomy, the entire peritoneal cavity should be examined, with thorough inspection of the liver, pelvis, and hemidiaphragm and careful palpation of the full length of the large bowel. Following recovery from a complete resection, patients should be observed carefully for 5 years by semiannual physical examinations and yearly blood chemistry measurements. If a complete colonoscopy was not performed preoperatively, it should be carried out within the first several postoperative months. Some authorities favor measuring plasma CEA levels at 3-month intervals because of the sensitivity of this test as a marker for otherwise undetectable tumor recurrence. Subsequent endoscopic or radiographic surveillance of the large bowel, probably at triennial intervals, is indicated, since patients who have been cured of one colorectal cancer have a 3 to 5 percent probability of developing an additional bowel cancer during their lifetime and a risk in excess of 15 percent for the development of adenomatous polyps. Anastomotic ("suture-line") recurrences are infrequent in colorectal cancer patients provided the surgical resection margins were adequate and free of tumor.

Radiation therapy to the pelvis is generally recommended for patients with rectal cancer because of the 30 to 40 percent probability of regional recurrences following complete surgical resection of stage B or C tumors, especially if they have penetrated through the serosa. This alarmingly high rate of local disease recurrence is believed to be due to the fact that the contained anatomic space within the pelvis limits the extent of the resection and because the rich lymphatic network of the pelvic side wall immediately adjacent to the rectum facilitates the early spread of malignant cells into surgically inaccessible tissue. The prophylactic use of radiation therapy, either pre- or postoperatively, reduces the likelihood of pelvic recurrences but does not appear to prolong survival. Preoperative radiotherapy is clearly indicated for patients with large, potentially unresectable rectal cancers, since such anatomically fixed lesions may shrink enough to permit subsequent surgical removal. Radiation therapy is not effective in the primary treatment of colon cancer.

Chemotherapy in patients with advanced colorectal cancer has proven to be of only marginal benefit. Since its introduction into clinical trials more than 30 years ago, 5-FU remains the most effective agent for this disease. It is as useful when given alone as when combined with other drugs, but its use has only a 15 to 20 percent likelihood of reducing measurable tumor mass by 50 percent or more (i.e., a partial response). While the probability of tumor response appears to be somewhat greater for patients with liver metastases when such chemotherapy is infused directly into the hepatic artery as compared to a peripheral vein, intraarterial treatment is costly and toxic and does not appear to prolong survival. The concomitant administration of folinic acid (also known as leucovorin or citrovorum factor) improves the efficacy of 5-FU in patients with advanced colorectal cancer, presumably by enhancing the binding of 5-FU to its target enzyme, thymidylate synthase, thereby increasing the suppression of DNA synthesis and accompanying cytotoxicity. A threefold improvement in the likelihood of partial response is noted when folinic acid is combined with 5-FU; however, the effect on survival appears to be marginal and the optimal dose schedule remains to be defined.

Patients with solitary hepatic metastases without clinical or radiographic evidence of additional tumor involvement should be considered for partial liver resection, because such procedures are associated with 5-year survival rates of 25 to 30 percent when performed on selected individuals by experienced surgeons.

The value of postoperative chemotherapy and/or radiation therapy has been assessed in patients with stage B or C cancers as a means of eradicating clinically undetectable micrometastases and thereby increasing the probability of cure. The administration of adjuvant 5-FU with the anthelmintic agent levamisole to patients with stage C cancers leads to a 40 percent decrease in the likelihood of recurrence and to a modest improvement in survival. No statistical benefit has been observed in patients with stage B_2 tumors. The levamisole is thought to act as a nonspecific immunomodulator. Comparisons of 5-FU and levamisole with 5-FU and folinic acid are in progress. In rectal cancer, postoperative radiation therapy, when combined with chemotherapy, appears to reduce the likelihood of regional recurrences and increase the chance of cure. The chemotherapy acts as a radiation sensitizer when given to individuals who have been operated on for rectal cancer, enhancing the biologic effect of the radiotherapy.

TUMORS OF THE SMALL INTESTINE

Small-bowel tumors make up only 3 to 6 percent of gastrointestinal neoplasms. Because of their rarity, a correct diagnosis is often delayed. Abdominal symptoms are usually vague and poorly defined, and conventional radiographic studies of the upper and lower intestinal tract often appear normal. Small-bowel tumors should be considered in the differential diagnosis in the following situations: (1) recurrent, unexplained episodes of crampy abdominal pain; (2) intermittent bouts of intestinal obstruction, especially in the absence of inflammatory bowel disease or prior abdominal surgery; (3) intussusception in the adult; and (4) evidence of chronic intestinal bleeding in the presence of negative conventional contrast radiographs. A careful small-bowel barium study is the diagnostic procedure of choice; the diagnostic accuracy may be improved by infusing barium through a nasogastric tube placed into the duodenum (enteroclysis).

BENIGN TUMORS In general, the histology of benign small-bowel tumors is difficult to predict on clinical and radiologic grounds alone. The symptomatology of benign tumors is not distinctive, with pain, obstruction, and hemorrhage being the most frequent symptoms. These tumors are usually discovered during the fifth and sixth decades of life, more often in the distal rather than the proximal small intestine.

The most common benign tumors are adenomas, leiomyomas, lipomas, and angiomas.

Adenomas These tumors include those of the islet cells and Brunner's glands as well as polypoid adenomas. *Islet cell adenomas* are occasionally located outside the pancreas; the associated syndromes are discussed in Chap. 95. *Brunner's gland adenomas* are not truly neoplastic but represent a hypertrophy or hyperplasia of submucosal duodenal glands. These appear as small nodules in the duodenal mucosa that secrete a highly viscous alkaline mucus. Most often, this is an incidental radiographic finding not associated with any specific clinical disorder.

Polypoid Adenomas Approximately 25 percent of benign small-bowel tumors are polypoid adenomas (see Table 92-5). They may present as single polypoid lesions or, less commonly, as papillary villous adenomas. As in the colon, the sessile or papillary form of the tumor is sometimes associated with a coexisting carcinoma. Occasionally, patients with Gardner's syndrome (a variant of polyposis coli) develop premalignant adenomas in the small bowel; such lesions are generally in the duodenum. Multiple polypoid tumors may occur throughout the small bowel (and occasionally the stomach and colorectum) in the Peutz-Jeghers syndrome. The polyps are usually hamartomas (juvenile polyps) having a low potential for malignant degeneration. Mucocutaneous melanin deposits as well as tumors of the ovary, breast, pancreas, and endometrium are also associated with this autosomal dominant condition.

Leiomyomas These neoplasms arise from smooth-muscle components of the intestine and are usually intramural, affecting the overlying mucosa. Ulceration of the mucosa may cause gastrointestinal hemorrhage of varying severity. Cramping, intermittent abdominal pain is frequently encountered.

Lipomas These tumors occur with greatest frequency in the distal ileum and at the ileocecal valve. They have a characteristic radiolucent appearance, are usually intramural and asymptomatic, but on occasion are associated with bleeding.

Angiomas While not true neoplasms, these lesions are important because they frequently cause intestinal bleeding. They may take the form of telangiectasia or hemangiomas. Multiple intestinal telangiectasias occur in a nonhereditary form confined to the gastrointestinal tract or as part of the hereditary Osler-Rendu-Weber syndrome. Vascular tumors may also take the form of isolated hemangiomas, most commonly in the jejunum. Angiography, especially during bleeding, is the procedure of choice in the evaluation of these lesions.

MALIGNANT TUMORS While rare, small-bowel malignancies occur in patients with long-standing regional enteritis and celiac sprue as well as in individuals with AIDS. In contrast to benign tumors, malignant tumors of the small bowel are frequently associated with fever, weight loss, anorexia, bleeding, and a palpable abdominal mass. After ampullary carcinomas (many of which arise from biliary or pancreatic ducts), the most frequently occurring small-bowel malignancies are adenocarcinomas, lymphomas, carcinoid tumors, and leiomyosarcomas.

Adenocarcinomas The most common primary cancers of the small bowel are adenocarcinomas, which account for about 50 percent of the malignant tumors. These neoplasms occur most often in the distal duodenum and proximal jejunum, where they tend to ulcerate and cause hemorrhage or obstruction. Radiologically, they may be confused with chronic duodenal ulcer disease or with Crohn's disease if the patient has long-standing regional enteritis. The diagnosis is best made by endoscopy and biopsy under direct vision. Surgical resection is the treatment of choice.

Lymphomas Lymphomatous involvement of the small bowel may be primary or secondary. A diagnosis of a primary intestinal lymphoma requires histologic confirmation in a clinical setting in which palpable adenopathy and hepatosplenomegaly are absent and there is no evidence of lymphoma on a chest radiograph, CT scan, or peripheral blood smear or on bone marrow aspiration and biopsy. In general, symptoms referable to the small bowel are present, usually accompanied by an anatomically discernible lesion. Secondary lymphoma of the small bowel consists of involvement of the intestine by

a lymphoid malignancy extending from involved retroperitoneal or mesenteric lymph nodes and hence is a manifestation of a generalized systemic neoplasm (see Chap. 113).

Primary intestinal lymphoma accounts for about 20 percent of malignancies of the small bowel. Essentially all these neoplasms are non-Hodgkin's lymphomas; they usually have a diffuse, large cell histology and usually are of T cell origin. Intestinal lymphoma involves the ileum more frequently than the jejunum, which, in turn, is more commonly affected than the duodenum, a pattern that mirrors the relative amount of normal lymphoid cells in these anatomic areas. The risk of small-bowel lymphoma is increased in patients with a prior history of malabsorptive conditions (e.g., celiac sprue), regional enteritis, and depressed immune function due to congenital immunodeficiency syndromes, prior organ transplantation, autoimmune disorders, or AIDS.

The development of localized or nodular masses that narrow the lumen results in periumbilical pain (made worse by eating) as well as weight loss, vomiting, and occasional intestinal obstruction. The diagnosis of small-bowel lymphoma may be suspected from the appearance on contrast radiographs of patterns such as infiltration and thickening of mucosal folds, mucosal nodules, areas of irregular ulceration, or stasis of contrast material. The diagnosis can be confirmed by surgical exploration and resection of involved segments. Intestinal lymphoma occasionally can be diagnosed by peroral intestinal mucosal biopsy, but since the disease mainly involves the lamina propria, full-thickness surgical biopsies are usually required.

Resection of the tumor constitutes the initial treatment modality. While postoperative radiation therapy has been given to some patients following such a total resection, most authorities favor short-term systemic treatment with combination chemotherapy. The frequent presence of widespread intraabdominal disease at the time of diagnosis and the occasional multicentricity of the tumor often make a total resection impossible. The probability of sustained remission or cure is approximately 75 percent in patients with localized disease but is 25 percent or less in individuals with unresectable lymphoma. In patients whose tumors are not resected, chemotherapy may lead to bowel perforation.

A unique form of small-bowel lymphoma, diffusely involving the entire intestine, was first described in oriental Jews and Arabs and is referred to as *immunoproliferative small intestinal disease* (IPSID), *Mediterranean lymphoma,* or α-*heavy chain disease*. This is a B cell tumor. The typical presentation includes chronic diarrhea and steatorrhea associated with vomiting and abdominal cramps; clubbing of the digits may be observed as well. A curious feature in many patients with IPSID is the presence in the blood and intestinal secretions of an abnormal IgA that contains a shortened α-heavy chain and is devoid of light chains. It is suspected that the abnormal α chains are produced by plasma cells infiltrating the small bowel. The clinical course of patients with IPSID is generally one of exacerbations and remissions, with death frequently resulting from either progressive malnutrition and wasting or the development of an aggressive lymphoma. The use of oral antibiotics such as tetracycline appears to be beneficial in the early phases of the disorder, suggesting a possible infectious etiology. Combination chemotherapy has been administered during later stages of the disease, with variable results. Results are better when antibiotics and chemotherapy are combined.

Carcinoid Tumors Among the more common epithelial tumors of the small intestine are carcinoid tumors. They arise from argentaffin cells of the crypts of Lieberkühn and are found from the distal duodenum to the ascending colon, areas embryologically derived from the midgut. More than 50 percent of intestinal carcinoids are found in the distal ileum, with most congregating close to the ileocecal valve. Most intestinal carcinoids are asymptomatic and of low malignant potential, but invasion and metastases may occur, leading to the carcinoid syndrome (Chap. 95).

Leiomyosarcomas Large, bulky tumors, leiomyosarcomas often are more than 5 cm in diameter and may be palpable on abdominal examination. Bleeding, obstruction, and perforation are common.

CANCERS OF THE ANUS

Cancers of the anus account for 1 to 2 percent of the malignant tumors of the large bowel. Most such lesions arise in the anal canal, which is defined as the anatomic area extending from the anorectal ring to a zone approximately halfway between the pectinate (or dentate) line and the anal verge. Carcinomas arising proximal to the pectinate line (i.e., in the transitional zone between the glandular mucosa of the rectum and the squamous epithelium of the distal anus) are known as basaloid, cuboidal, or cloacogenic tumors; approximately one-third of anal cancers have this histologic pattern. Malignancies arising distal to the pectinate line have a squamous cell histology, ulcerate more frequently, and constitute approximately 55 percent of anal cancers. The prognosis for patients with basaloid and squamous cell cancers of the anus is identical when corrected for tumor size and the presence or absence of nodal spread.

Anal cancers occur most commonly in individuals with a prior history of chronic anal irritation. Such irritation may result from condylomata accuminata (viral lesions thought to be caused by papillomavirus infection), perianal fissures and/or fistulas, chronic hemorrhoids, and leukoplakia. The risk for anal cancer appears to be increased among homosexual males, presumably relating to trauma from anal intercourse. The likelihood of developing anal cancers is also enhanced in both men and women with AIDS, possibly because their immunocompromised condition makes them more susceptible to papillomavirus infection. Anal cancers occur most commonly in middle-aged individuals, develop more frequently in women than men, and at the time of diagnosis are most often associated with bleeding, pain, the sensation of a perianal mass, and perianal pruritus.

Until recently, radical surgery (abdominal-perineal resection with lymph node sampling and a permanent colostomy) was the treatment of choice for this tumor type. The 5-year survival rate after such a procedure ranged from 55 to 70 percent in the absence of spread to regional lymph nodes and was less than 20 percent if nodal involvement was present. However, an alternative therapeutic approach combining external beam radiation therapy with concomitant chemotherapy has resulted in biopsy-proven disappearance of all tumor in more than 80 percent of patients whose initial lesion was less than 3 cm in size. Tumor has recurred in fewer than 10 percent of these patients. Thus, it appears that approximately 70 percent of patients with anal cancers can be cured with nonoperative treatment and that disfiguring surgery should be reserved for the minority of individuals who are found to have residual tumor after being managed initially with radiation therapy combined with chemotherapy.

BIBLIOGRAPHY

BLOT WJ: Esophageal cancer trends and risk factors. Semin Oncol 21:403, 1994

FLAM M et al: Role of mitomycin in combination with fluorouracil and radiotherapy, and of salvage chemoradiation in the definitive nonsurgical treatment of epidermoid carcinoma of the anal canal: Results of a phase III randomized intergroup study. J Clin Oncol 14:2527, 1996

FUCHS CS et al: A prospective study of family history and the risk of colorectal cancer. N Engl J Med 331:1669, 1994

————, MAYER RJ: Gastric carcinoma. N Engl J Med 333:32, 1995.

HAMILTON SR: The molecular genetics of colorectal neoplasia. Gastroenterology 105:3, 1993

HANSSON LE et al: The risk of stomach cancer in patients with gastric or duodenal ulcer disease. N Engl J Med 335:242, 1996

LYNCH HT, SMYRK T: Hereditary nonpolyposis colorectal cancer (Lynch syndrome). An updated review. Cancer 78:1149, 1996

MELBYE M et al: High incidence of anal cancer among AIDS patients. Lancet 343:636, 1994

MOERTEL CG et al: Fluorouracil plus levamisole as effective adjuvant therapy after resection of stage III colon carcinoma: A final report. Ann Intern Med 122:321, 1995

TORIBARA NW, SLEISENGER MH: Screening for colorectal cancer. N Engl J Med 332:861, 1995

WALSH TN et al: A comparison of multimodal therapy and surgery for esophageal carcinoma. N Engl J Med 335:462, 1996

WOTHERSPOON AC et al: Regression of primary low-grade B-cell gastric lymphoma of mucosa-associated lymphoid tissue after eradication of *Helicobacter pylori*. Lancet 342:575, 1993

---

93 | *Kurt J. Isselbacher, Jules L. Dienstag*

TUMORS OF THE LIVER AND BILIARY TRACT

BENIGN LIVER TUMORS

HEPATOCELLULAR ADENOMAS Hepatocellular adenomas are benign tumors of the liver found predominantly in women in their third and fourth decades. Their preponderance in women suggests a hormonal influence in their pathogenesis, and oral contraceptives have been implicated. There has been a striking increase in these adenomas since oral contraceptives were introduced, and most patients with those tumors have used these hormonal agents. Multiple hepatic adenomas have been associated with glycogen storage disease type I.

Hepatic adenomas occur predominantly in the right lobe of the liver, may be multiple, and are often quite large (>10 cm). Microscopically, they consist of normal or slightly atypical hepatocytes. These cells have an increased amount of glycogen, making them appear paler and larger than normal. Clinical features include pain and the presence of a palpable mass or features of intratumor hemorrhage (pain and circulatory collapse). The diagnosis is usually made by a combination of techniques: sonography, computed tomography (CT), magnetic resonance imaging (MRI), selective hepatic arteriography, and radionuclide scans. The angiographic appearance is typically hypervascular, but often also includes hypovascular regions. Technetium 99m scans usually show a defect, because phagocytosing Kupffer cells are absent. There is a risk of malignant change in the range of 10 percent; the risk is higher for large (>10 cm) and multiple adenomas.

As far as management is concerned, a patient taking oral contraceptives should stop doing so. If the lesion is large (8 to 10 cm), near the surface, and resectable, surgery is appropriate. Because of the risk of rupture, pregnancy should be avoided.

FOCAL NODULAR HYPERPLASIA Focal nodular hyperplasia is a benign tumor often identified incidentally on imaging studies or at laparoscopy done for other reasons. Like hepatic adenomas, it occurs predominantly in women; however, oral contraceptives do not appear to be implicated, and hemorrhage and necrosis are rare. The risk of hemorrhage, however, appears to be higher in women taking oral contraceptives. Typically, the lesion is a solid tumor, often in the right lobe, with a fibrous core and stellate projections. The fibrous projections contain atypical hepatocytes, biliary epithelium, Kupffer cells, and inflammatory cells. A radionuclide technetium scan will usually show a hot spot because of the presence of Kupffer cells. The lesion appears vascular on angiography, and septations may be detectable. If the lesion is asymptomatic, surgery is not indicated.

HEMANGIOMA AND OTHER BENIGN TUMORS *Hemangiomas* are probably the most common benign liver tumors, occurring predominantly in women and usually detected when abdominal imaging is done for unrelated symptoms, or unexpectedly at surgery. The prevalence in the general population is in the range of 0.5 to 7.0 percent. These vascular lesions are usually asymptomatic and can be identified by MRI, contrast-enhanced CT, labeled red blood cell nuclide scans, or hepatic angiography. They do not need to be removed unless they are large and are producing a mass effect. Hemorrhage is rare, and malignant change does not occur.

Nodular regenerative hyperplasia consists of multiple hepatic nodules resulting from periportal hepatocyte regeneration with surrounding atrophy. It may be associated with an underlying condition such as malignancy or connective tissue disease. Portal hypertension (in the absence of cirrhosis) is the most common clinical manifestation. Other, less common benign hepatic lesions include *bile duct adenomas* and *cystadenomas*. *Juvenile hemangioendotheliomas* occur in children in association with congestive heart failure and cutaneous hemangiomas.

CARCINOMAS OF THE LIVER

HEPATOCELLULAR CARCINOMA Epidemiology and Etiology Primary hepatocellular carcinoma is one of the most common tumors in the world. It is especially prevalent in regions of Asia and sub-Saharan Africa, where the annual incidence is up to 500 cases per 100,000 population. In the United States and western Europe, it is much less common, accounting for only 1 to 2 percent of malignant tumors at autopsy. Hepatocellular carcinoma is up to four times more common in men than in women and usually arises in a cirrhotic liver. The incidence peaks in the fifth to sixth decades of life in western countries but one to two decades earlier in regions of Asia and Africa with a high prevalence of liver carcinoma.

The principal reason for the high incidence of hepatocellular carcinoma in parts of Asia and Africa is the frequency of chronic infection with *hepatitis B virus* (HBV) and *hepatitis C virus* (HCV). These chronic infections frequently lead to cirrhosis, which itself is an important risk factor for hepatocellular carcinoma (the risk of liver cancer in a cirrhotic liver is ~3 percent per year); 60 to 90 percent of these tumors occur in patients with macronodular cirrhosis. The role of HBV as a factor has been fairly convincingly demonstrated. Studies in regions of Asia where hepatocellular carcinoma and HBV infection are prevalent have shown that the incidence over time of this cancer is about 100-fold higher in individuals with evidence of HBV infection than in noninfected controls. In China, the lifetime risk of developing hepatocellular carcinoma in patients with chronic hepatitis B approaches 40 percent. In patients with HBV infection and hepatocellular carcinoma, HBV DNA may be integrated into host genomic DNA, both in the tumor cells and in adjacent, uninvolved hepatocytes. In addition, there can be modifications of cellular gene expression by insertional mutagenesis, chromosomal rearrangements, or the transcriptional transactivating activity of the X and the pre-S2 regions of the HBV genome. These alterations probably occur during the process of liver cell injury and repair.

Since the discovery of hepatitis C virus as the agent responsible for most cases of non-A, non-B hepatitis, an increasing body of evidence has implicated HCV in hepatocellular carcinoma. In fact, in Europe and Japan HCV appears to be substantially more prevalent than HBV in cases of hepatocellular carcinoma. Both HBV and HCV can be demonstrated in some patients, but the clinical course of liver malignancy in these patients does not appear to differ from that when only one virus is implicated. One distinction in high-prevalence areas between hepatocellular carcinoma associated with HBV infection and with HCV infection is in the timing of onset. In Asia, HBV is acquired at birth via perinatal transmission, while HCV infection is acquired primarily during adulthood from transfused blood. Correspondingly, the onset of liver carcinoma occurs one to two decades earlier in those with lifelong hepatitis B than in persons with adult-acquired hepatitis C. Retrospective analysis indicates that hepatocellular carcinoma occurs on average approximately 30 years after HCV infection and almost exclusively in patients with cirrhosis.

Any agent or factor that contributes to chronic, low-grade liver cell damage and mitosis makes hepatocyte DNA more susceptible to genetic alterations. Thus, as indicated above, *chronic liver disease* of any type is a risk factor and predisposes to the development of liver cell carcinoma. These conditions include alcoholic liver disease, α_1-antitrypsin deficiency, hemochromatosis, and tyrosinemia. In Africa and southern China, *aflatoxin B1* is an important public health hazard. This mycotoxin appears to induce a very specific mutation at codon 249 in the tumor suppressor gene *p53*.

The loss, inactivation, or mutation of the *p53* gene has been implicated in tumorigenesis and is the most common genetic derangement present in human cancers. Thus HBV and aflatoxin B_1 have been implicated in the pathogenesis of hepatocellular carcinoma in regions of Africa and southern China where both agents are prevalent.

In view of the male predominance of liver cancer, hormonal factors also may play a role. Hepatocellular tumors may occur with long-term androgenic steroid administration, with exposure to thorium dioxide or vinyl chloride (see below), and possibly with exposure to estrogens in the form of oral contraceptives.

Clinical and Laboratory Features Cancers of the liver initially may escape clinical recognition because they often occur in patients with underlying cirrhosis, and the symptoms and signs may suggest progression of the underlying disease. The most common presenting features are abdominal *pain* with detection of an abdominal mass in the right upper quadrant. There may be a *friction rub* or *bruit* over the liver. Blood-tinged ascites occurs in about 20 percent of cases. Jaundice is rare, unless there is significant deterioration of liver function or mechanical obstruction of the bile ducts. Serum elevations of alkaline phosphatase and alpha fetoprotein (AFP) are common (see below). An abnormal type of prothrombin, des-γ-carboxy prothrombin, is also detectable and in general correlates with AFP elevations.

A small percentage of patients with hepatocellular carcinoma have evidence of *paraneoplastic syndrome*; erythrocytosis may result from erythropoietin-like activity produced by the tumor; hypercalcemia may result from secretion of a parathyroid-like hormone. Other manifestations may include hypercholesterolemia, hypoglycemia, acquired porphyria, dysfibrinogenemia, and cryofibrinogenemia.

Imaging procedures used to detect liver tumors include ultrasound, CT, MRI, hepatic artery angiography (see Chap. 281), and radionuclide scans with technetium 99m. Ultrasound is frequently used to screen high-risk populations and should be the first procedure if hepatocellular carcinoma is suspected; it is less costly than scanning procedures, is relatively sensitive, and can detect most tumors larger than 3 cm. MRI, however, is being used with increasing frequency.

AFP levels greater than 500 μg/L are found in about 70 to 80 percent of patients with hepatocellular carcinoma. Lower levels may be found in patients with large metastases from gastric or colonic tumors and in some patients with acute or chronic hepatitis. The presence and persistence of high levels of serum AFP (over 500 to 1000 μg/L) in an adult with liver disease and without an obvious gastrointestinal tumor strongly suggest hepatocellular carcinoma. A rising level suggests progression of the tumor or recurrence after hepatic resection or therapeutic approaches such as chemotherapy or chemoembolization (see below).

Percutaneous *liver biopsy* can be diagnostic if the sample is taken from an area localized by ultrasound or CT. Because these tumors tend to be vascular, percutaneous biopsies should be done with caution. Cytologic examination of ascitic fluid is invariably negative for tumor cells. Occasionally, *laparoscopy* or *minilaparotomy*, to permit liver biopsy under direct vision, may be used. This approach has the additional advantage of sometimes identifying patients who have a localized resectable tumor suitable for partial hepatectomy.

℞ **TREATMENT**
The course of clinically apparent disease is rapid; if untreated, most patients die within 3 to 6 months of diagnosis. When hepatocellular carcinoma is detected very early by serial screening of AFP and ultrasound, survival of 1 to 2 years is possible, as is resection. In selected cases, therapy may prolong life. *Surgical resection* offers the only chance for cure; however, few patients have a resectable tumor at the time of presentation, because of underlying cirrhosis, involvement of both hepatic lobes, or distant metastases (common sites are lung, brain, bone, and adrenal), and the 5-year survival is low. In patients at high risk for the development of hepatocellular carcinoma, such as patients positive for the hepatitis B surface anti-

gen (HBsAg) and patients with cirrhosis (including that caused by chronic hepatitis C), screening programs have been initiated to identify small tumors when they are still resectable. Because 20 to 30 percent of patients with early hepatocellular carcinoma do not have elevated levels of circulating AFP, ultrasonographic screening is recommended as well as AFP determination. In a study in the Far East, HBsAg-positive persons, with or without liver disease, were screened serially; a number of patients with small, subclinical tumors were identified, and surgical resection undertaken. Follow-up observation revealed a 5-year survival rate in this group of 70 percent and a 10-year survival rate of 50 percent. These Asian patients, however, were unusual in that they had minimal or no liver disease and their tumors tended to be unifocal or encapsulated. The findings are in contrast to a study in a large population of Italian patients with cirrhosis, associated in most cases with chronic HBV and/or HCV infections; screening every 3 to 12 months permitted the detection of a 3 percent annual incidence of cancer in this cohort, but in most cases failed to achieve the goal of early detection of surgically treatable disease.

Liver transplantation may be considered as a therapeutic option, but recurrence of tumor or metastases after transplantation have limited its usefulness (see Chap. 301). Other approaches include (1) hepatic artery embolization with chemotherapy (chemoembolization), (2) alcohol ablation via ultrasound-guided percutaneous injection, (3) ultrasound-guided cryoablation, (4) immunotherapy with monoclonal antibodies tagged with cytotoxic agents, and (5) gene therapy with retroviral vectors containing genes expressing cytotoxic agents.

Prevention is the preferred strategy. Hepatitis B vaccine can prevent infection and its sequelae. Treatment with interferon α lowers the risk of development of liver cancer in patients with hepatitis C–related chronic active hepatitis and cirrhosis (see Chap. 297).

OTHER MALIGNANT LIVER TUMORS

Fibrolamellar carcinoma differs from the typical hepatocellular carcinoma in that it tends to occur in young adults without underlying cirrhosis. This tumor is nonencapsulated but well circumscribed and contains fibrous lamellae; it grows slowly and is associated with a longer survival if treated. Surgical resection has resulted in 5-year survivals exceeding 50 percent; if the lesion is nonresectable, liver transplantation is an option, and the outcome far exceeds that observed in the nonfibrolamellar variety of liver cancer. *Hepatoblastoma* is a tumor of infancy that typically is associated with very high serum AFP levels. The lesions are usually solitary, may be resectable, and have a better 5-year survival than that of hepatocellular carcinoma. *Angiosarcoma* consists of vascular spaces lined by malignant endothelial cells. Etiologic factors include prior exposure to thorium dioxide (Thorotrast), polyvinyl chloride, arsenic, and androgenic anabolic steroids. *Epithelioid hemangioendothelioma* is of borderline malignancy; most cases are benign, but metastases occur. This tumor occurs in early adulthood, presents with right upper quadrant pain, is heterogeneous on sonography, hypodense on CT, and without neovascularity on angiography. Immunohistochemical staining reveals expression of factor VIII antigen. In the absence of extrahepatic metastases, these lesions can be treated by surgical resection or liver transplantation.

METASTATIC TUMORS Metastatic tumors of the liver are common, ranking second only to cirrhosis as a cause of fatal liver disease. In the United States, the incidence of clinically significant metastatic carcinoma is at least 20 times greater than that of primary carcinoma. At autopsy, hepatic metastases occur in 30 to 50 percent of patients dying from malignant disease.

Pathogenesis The liver is uniquely vulnerable to invasion by tumor cells. Its size, high rate of blood flow, double perfusion by the hepatic artery and portal vein, and its Kupffer cell filtration function combine to make it the next most common site of metastases after the lymph nodes. In addition, local tissue factors or endothelial membrane characteristics appear to enhance metastatic implants. Virtually all types of neoplasms except those primary in the brain may metastasize to the liver. The most common primary tumors are those of the gastrointestinal tract, lung, and breast, as well as melanomas. Less common are metastases from tumors of the thyroid, prostate, and skin.

Clinical Features Most patients with metastases to the liver present with symptoms referable only to the primary tumor, and the asymptomatic hepatic involvement is discovered in the course of clinical evaluation. Sometimes hepatic involvement is reflected by nonspecific symptoms of weakness, weight loss, fever, sweating, and loss of appetite. Rarely, features indicating active hepatic disease, especially abdominal pain, hepatomegaly, or ascites, are present. Patients with widespread metastatic liver involvement usually have suggestive clinical signs of cancer and hepatic enlargement. Some have localized induration or tenderness, and, occasionally, a friction rub may be found over tender areas of the liver.

Results of liver biochemical tests are often abnormal, but the elevations in marker levels often are only mild and nonspecific. These signs reflect the effects of fever and wasting as well as those of the infiltrating neoplastic process itself. An increase in serum alkaline phosphatase is the most common and frequently the only abnormality. Hypoalbuminemia, anemia, and occasionally a mild elevation of aminotransferase levels also may be found with more widespread disease. Substantially elevated serum levels of carcinoembryonic antigen are usually found when the metastases are from primary malignancies in the gastrointestinal tract, breast, or lung.

Diagnosis Evidence of metastatic invasion of the liver should be sought actively in any patient with a primary malignancy, especially of the lung, gastrointestinal tract, or breast, before resection of the primary lesion. An elevated level of alkaline phosphatase or a mass apparent on ultrasound, CT, or MRI examination of the liver may provide a presumptive diagnosis. Blind percutaneous needle biopsy of the liver will result in a positive diagnosis of metastatic disease in only 60 to 80 percent of cases with hepatomegaly and elevated alkaline phosphatase levels. Serial sectioning of specimens, two or three repeated biopsies, or cytologic examination of biopsy smears may increase the diagnostic yield by 10 to 15 percent. The yield is greatly increased when biopsies are directed by ultrasound or CT or obtained during laparoscopy.

℞ **TREATMENT**

Most metastatic carcinomas respond poorly to all forms of treatment, which is usually only palliative. On rare occasions, a single, large metastasis can be removed surgically. Systemic chemotherapy may slow tumor growth briefly and reduce symptoms, but it does not significantly alter the prognosis. Chemoembolization, intrahepatic chemotherapy, and alcohol ablation may provide palliation. It remains to be determined whether newer drugs, combination chemotherapy, or novel strategies (including immunologic targeting) will eventually prove to be more effective.

CHOLANGIOCARCINOMA Benign tumors of the extrahepatic bile ducts are extremely rare causes of mechanical biliary obstruction. Most of these are papillomas, adenomas, or cystadenomas and present with obstructive jaundice or hemobilia. Adenocarcinoma of the extrahepatic ducts is more common. There is a slight male preponderance (60 percent), and the incidence peaks in the fifth to seventh decades. Apparent predisposing factors include (1) some chronic hepatobiliary parasitic infestations, (2) congenital anomalies with ectatic ducts, (3) sclerosing cholangitis and chronic ulcerative colitis, and (4) occupational exposure to possible biliary tract carcinogens (employment in rubber or automotive plants). Cholelithiasis is not clearly a predisposing factor for cholangiocarcinoma. The lesions of cholangiocarcinoma may be diffuse or nodular; lesions of the latter type often arise at the bifurcation of the common bile duct (Klatskin tumors). This tumor is usually associated with a *collapsed gallbladder*, and that finding mandates that the proximal hepatic ducts be visualized by cholangiography.

Patients with cholangiocarcinoma usually present with biliary obstruction, painless jaundice, pruritus, weight loss, and acholic stools. A deep-seated, vaguely localized right upper quadrant pain may be an associated complaint. Hepatomegaly and a palpable, distended gallbladder (unless the lesion is high in the duct) are frequent accompanying signs. Fever is unusual unless associated with ascending cholangitis. Because the obstructing process is gradual, the cholangiocarcinoma is often far advanced by the time it presents clinically. The diagnosis is most frequently made by cholangiography following ultrasound demonstration of dilated intrahepatic bile ducts. Any focal strictures of the bile ducts should probably be considered malignant until proved otherwise. Survival of 1 to 2 years is possible in some cases with palliative drainage (stenting) of the biliary tree.

CARCINOMA OF THE PAPILLA OF VATER   The ampulla of Vater may be involved by extension of tumor arising elsewhere in the duodenum or may itself be the site of origin of a sarcoma, carcinoid tumor, or adenocarcinoma. Papillary adenocarcinomas are associated with slow growth and a more favorable clinical prognosis than diffuse, infiltrative cancers of the ampulla, which are more frequently widely invasive. The presenting clinical manifestation is usually obstructive jaundice. Endoscopic retrograde cannulation of the pancreatic duct (ERCP) is probably the preferred diagnostic technique when ampullary carcinoma is suspected, because it allows for direct endoscopic inspection and biopsy of the ampulla as well as for performance of pancreatography to exclude a diagnosis of pancreatic malignancy. Cancer of the papilla is usually treated by wide, often radical, surgical excision. Lymph node or other metastases are present at the time of surgery in approximately 20 percent of cases, and the 5-year survival rate following surgical therapy in this group is only 5 to 10 percent. In the absence of metastases, however, radical pancreaticoduodenectomy (the Whipple procedure) is associated with 5-year survival rates as high as 40 percent, and several long-term survivors have been reported.

CANCER OF THE GALLBLADDER   Most cancers of the gallbladder develop in conjunction with stones rather than polyps. In patients with gallstones, the risk for developing gallbladder cancer, while increased, is still quite low. In one study, gallbladder cancer developed in only 5 of 2583 patients with gallstones followed for a median of 13 years. In the United States, adenocarcinomas make up the vast majority of the estimated 6500 new cases of gallbladder cancer diagnosed each year. The female/male ratio is 4:1, and the mean age at diagnosis is approximately 70 years. The clinical presentation is most often one of unremitting right upper quadrant pain associated with weight loss, jaundice, and a palpable right upper quadrant mass. Cholangitis may supervene. The preoperative diagnosis of the condition has been facilitated by ultrasound and CT. CT is also useful in guiding fine needle aspiration and biopsy.

Once symptoms have appeared, spread of the tumor outside the gallbladder by direct extension or by lymphatic or hematogenous routes is almost invariable. Over 75 percent of gallbladder carcinomas are unresectable at the time of surgery, the exceptions being tumors discovered incidentally at laparotomy. The 1-year mortality rate for unresectable disease is approximately 95 percent, and only 5 percent of patients survive 5 years or more from the time of diagnosis. Radical operative resection does not appear to improve survival. Trials of radiation and chemotherapy in patients with primary gallbladder cancer also have been disappointing.

BIBLIOGRAPHY

DE BAC C et al: Pathogenic factors in cirrhosis with and without hepatocellular carcinoma: A multicenter Italian study. Hepatology 20:1225, 1994

FATTOVICH G et al: Occurrence of hepatocellular carcinoma and decompensation in western European patients with cirrhosis type B. Hepatology 21:77, 1995

GROUPE D'ETUDE ET DE TRAITMENT DU CARCINOMA HEPATOCELLULAIRE: A comparison of lipiodol chemoembolization and conservative treatment for unresectable hepatocellular carcinoma. N Engl J Med 332:1256, 1995

LIANG TJ et al: Viral pathogenesis of hepatocellular carcinoma in the United States. Hepatology 18:1326, 1993

OKA H et al: Prospective study of α-fetoprotein in cirrhotic patients monitored for development of hepatocellular carcinoma. Hepatology 19:61, 1994

OKUDA K: Hepatocellular carcinoma: Recent progress. Hepatology 15:948, 1992

SHEINER PA et al: Treatment of metastatic cancer to the liver. Semin Liver Dis 14:169, 1994

TAKANO S et al: Incidence of hepatocellular carcinoma in chronic hepatitis B and C: Prospective study of 251 patients. Hepatology 21:650, 1995

TAO LC: Oral contraceptive–associated liver cell adenoma and hepatocellular carcinoma: Cytomorphology and malignant transformation. Cancer 68:341, 1991

TSUKUMA H et al: Risk factors for hepatocellular carcinoma among patients with chronic liver disease. N Engl J Med 328:1797, 1993

VAUTHEY J-N et al: Recent advances in management of cholangiocarcinomas. Semin Liver Dis 14:109, 1994

WEITZ IC et al: Des-γ-carboxy (abnormal) prothrombin and hepatocellular carcinoma: A critical review. Hepatology 18:990, 1993

94   *Robert J. Mayer*

PANCREATIC CANCER

INCIDENCE AND ETIOLOGY   The incidence of pancreatic carcinoma in the United States has increased significantly as the median life expectancy of the American population has lengthened. The tumor results in the death of more than 98 percent of afflicted patients. Approximately 27,800 individuals died of pancreatic cancer in 1996, making it the fifth most common cause of cancer-related mortality. The disease appears to be somewhat more common in males than in females and in blacks than in whites. It rarely develops before the age of 50.

Little is known about the causes of pancreatic cancer. Cigarette smoking is the most consistently observed risk factor for the development of the tumor, with the disease being two to three times more common in heavy smokers than in nonsmokers. It is uncertain whether this apparent association reflects a direct carcinogenic effect of metabolites of cigarette smoking on the pancreas or whether an as yet undefined exposure that occurs more frequently in cigarette smokers is responsible for the enhanced risk. A large case-control study has correlated chronic pancreatitis with an increased risk of pancreatic cancer. A meta-analysis of 20 case-control and cohort studies has also shown a higher frequency of pancreatic cancer in persons with long-standing diabetes mellitus. There are no convincing data to link such epidemiologic factors as alcohol abuse or cholelithiasis with the development of pancreatic cancer. Furthermore, the weight of clinical data has failed to support any association between coffee consumption and pancreatic cancer. Mutations in K-*ras* genes have been found in more than 85 percent of specimens of human pancreatic cancer. The development of pancreatic cancer has also been associated with a mutation of the *p16^{INK4}* gene located on chromosome 9p21, a gene also implicated in the pathogenesis of cutaneous malignant melanoma.

CLINICAL FEATURES   More than 90 percent of pancreatic cancers are ductal adenocarcinomas, with islet cell tumors constituting the remaining 5 to 10 percent. Pancreatic cancers occur twice as frequently in the pancreatic head (about 70 percent of cases) as in the body (about 20 percent) or tail (about 10 percent) of the gland.

With the exception of jaundice, the initial symptoms associated with pancreatic cancer are often insidious and usually are present for more than 2 months before the cancer is diagnosed (Table 94-1). Pain and weight loss are present in more than 75 percent of patients. The pain typically has a gnawing, visceral quality, occasionally radiating from the epigastrium to the back. It generally is a more severe problem in lesions arising in the body or tail of the gland, as such tumors may become quite large before being detected. Characteristically, the pain improves somewhat when the patient bends forward.

Table 94-1

Presenting Signs and Symptoms of Pancreatic Carcinoma

Frequent
    Abdominal pain
    Weight loss
    Jaundice (lesions of pancreatic head only)
Infrequent
    Glucose intolerance
    Palpable gallbladder
    Migratory thrombophlebitis
    Gastrointestinal hemorrhage
    Splenomegaly

The development of significant pain is suggestive of retroperitoneal invasion and infiltration of the splanchnic nerves, indicating that the primary lesion is far advanced and is not surgically resectable. Rarely, such pain may be transient and associated with hyperamylasemia, indicative of acute pancreatitis caused by ductal obstruction by tumor. The weight loss observed in most patients having pancreatic carcinoma is primarily the result of anorexia, although in the initial period of the disease, subclinical malabsorption may also be a contributing factor.

Jaundice due to biliary obstruction is found in more than 80 percent of patients having tumors in the pancreatic head and is typically accompanied by darkening of urine, a claylike appearance of stool, and pruritus. In contrast to the "painless jaundice" sometimes observed in patients having carcinomas of the bile ducts, duodenum, or periampullary regions, most icteric individuals having ductal carcinomas of

the pancreatic head will complain of significant abdominal discomfort. Although the gallbladder is usually enlarged in patients with carcinoma of the head of the pancreas, it is palpable in less than 50 percent of cases (Courvoisier's sign). However, the presence of an enlarged gallbladder in a jaundiced patient without biliary colic should suggest malignant obstruction of the extrahepatic biliary tree.

Glucose intolerance, presumably a direct consequence of the tumor, often develops within 2 years of the clinical diagnosis. Other initial manifestations include venous thrombosis and migratory thrombophlebitis, gastrointestinal hemorrhage resulting from varices due to compression of the portal venous system by tumor, and splenomegaly caused by cancerous encasement of the splenic vein.

DIAGNOSTIC PROCEDURES (Fig. 94-1) Despite the availability of serologic tests for tumor-associated antigens, such as the carcinoembryonic antigen (CEA) and CA 19-9, and noninvasive imaging techniques, such as computed tomography (CT) and ultrasonography, the early diagnosis of a potentially resectable pancreatic carcinoma remains extremely difficult. The nonspecificity of the initial symptoms and the poor sensitivity of both serologic assays and noninvasive techniques have frustrated the development of effective screening procedures. When the disease is clinically suspected in a patient having vague, persistent abdominal complaints, ultrasound should be performed to visualize the gallbladder and the pancreas, as well as upper gastrointestinal contrast radiographs to rule out a hiatal hernia or a peptic ulcer. If these studies fail to provide an explanation for the symptoms, a CT scan should be considered. It should encompass not only the pancreas but also the liver, retroperitoneal lymph nodes, and pelvis, as pancreatic cancer frequently spreads within the abdomen. While more costly than ultrasonography, CT is technically simpler, more reproducible, provides better definition of the body and tail of the pancreas, and requires less interpretive skill. CT generally detects a malignant pancreatic lesion in over 80 percent of cases; in 5 to 15 percent of patients with proven pancreatic carcinoma, the CT scan shows only generalized pancreatic enlargement suggestive of pancreatitis rather than malignancy. False-positive results have also been reported in about 5 to 10 percent of cases where no tumor was found on laparotomy. Magnetic resonance imaging (MRI) has not been shown to be better than CT in the evaluation of pancreatic lesions. In selected situations in which clinical circumstances dictate additional diagnostic evaluation, endoscopic retrograde cholangiopancreatography (ERCP) may clarify the cause of ambiguous CT or ultrasound findings. The characteristic findings are stenosis or obstruction of either the pancreatic or the common bile duct; both duct systems are abnormal in over half the cases. It can be quite difficult to distinguish between carcinoma and chronic pancreatitis by ERCP, particularly if both diseases are present. False-negative results with ERCP are quite infrequent (less than 5 percent) and usually occur in the setting of islet cell, rather than ductal, carcinomas.

Selective and superselective angiography may be of value in some patients. Angiography is an effective means of detecting carcinomas in the body and tail of the pancreas by the demonstration of vascular narrowing, displacement, or occlusion by tumor. Angiography is also useful in assessing whether encasement of peripancreatic vessels is present; this

FIGURE 94-1 Carcinoma of the pancreas. *A.* Sonogram showing pancreatic carcinoma (P), dilated intrahepatic bile ducts (d), dilated portal vein (pv), and inferior vena cava (IVC). *B.* CT scan showing pancreatic carcinoma (*arrow*). *C.* ERCP showing abrupt cutoff of the duct of Wirsung (*arrow*). *D.* Arteriogram showing sheathing of splenic artery by tumor encasement (*arrow*).

assessment is of less importance in determining the potential for surgical resection.

Regardless of the results of the above diagnostic studies, a histologic confirmation of a presumed pancreatic cancer is mandatory to be absolutely certain that malignancy exists and to rule out the presence of such other neoplasms as islet cell tumor or lymphoma, for which the therapeutic approach and prognosis differ significantly from those for ductal carcinoma. Such tissue confirmation may be obtained through a percutaneous needle aspiration biopsy of the pancreas with CT or ultrasonographic guidance, thereby obviating surgical exploration.

Patients with carcinoma of the pancreas may undergo several months of investigation before a diagnosis is established. In the past, this period of diagnostic delay and accompanying emotional uncertainty led to the erroneous impression that the pain and weight loss might not have an organic cause, resulting in an association of pancreatic cancer and depression. The availability of CT scans has resulted in more prompt diagnosis and dispelled this incorrect notion. Unfortunately, however, even laparotomy may not provide a definitive diagnosis, because chronic pancreatitis may also produce a hard mass in the head of the pancreas indistinguishable from carcinoma by palpation. Furthermore, a superficial biopsy of such a mass may not show neoplastic tissue, revealing only evidence of pancreatitis, as the cancer is often surrounded by edematous, inflamed, and fibrotic tissue (i.e., chronic pancreatitis).

℞ TREATMENT

Complete surgical resection of pancreatic tumors offers the only effective treatment for this disease. Unfortunately, such "curative" operations are only possible in 10 to 15 percent of patients with pancreatic cancer, usually those individuals with a tumor in the pancreatic head in whom jaundice was the initial symptom. Patients considered for such a procedure should have no evidence of metastatic spread on a chest radiograph and abdominal-pelvic CT scan and should be operated on by an experienced surgeon, as mortality rates of greater than 15 percent have been associated with this procedure. Although the potential for cure in patients with pancreatic cancer is restricted to the few who are able to undergo a complete surgical resection, the 5-year survival rate following such operations is only 10 percent. Nonetheless, the procedure is worth attempting, particularly for lesions in the pancreatic head, since ductal carcinomas often cannot be distinguished preoperatively from ampullary, duodenal, and distal bile duct tumors or pancreatic cyst adenocarcinomas, all of which have far higher rates of resectability and cure. Furthermore, patients who undergo resection and eventually experience disease recurrence survive three to four times longer than those whose tumor is not excised, indicating that such operations have a palliative effect. The risk for tumor recurrence is not affected by the type of operative procedure—i.e., total pancreatectomy versus pancreaticoduodenectomy ("Whipple resection")—but it is increased by the presence of lymph node metastases or tumor invasion into adjacent viscera. As a rule, pancreaticoduodenectomy or distal pancreatectomy seems preferable to total pancreatectomy because of the retention of exocrine function and avoidance of brittle diabetes.

The median survival for patients whose pancreatic cancers are surgically unresectable is approximately 6 months. Management of such individuals should be directed at palliation of symptoms. Ambulatory patients having tumors in the pancreatic head should be considered for surgical diversion of the biliary system. If jaundice has already developed, therapeutic options include either nonoperative biliary decompression by endoscopic or percutaneous, transhepatic biliary drainage or surgical biliary bypass. External beam radiation in patients with unresectable tumors that have not spread beyond the pancreas does not appear to prolong survival, although a sufficient reduction in tumor size may lead to palliation of pain. However, the addition of chemotherapy with fluorouracil (5-FU) to external beam irradiation has increased the survival time for these patients, perhaps because 5-FU acts as a radiosensitizing agent. In a small patient population, a similar combination of radiation therapy and 5-FU appears to have prolonged the survival and increased the cure rate as compared to a prospectively randomized nontreatment control group of patients who had a complete surgical resection of their pancreatic cancer. This observation needs to be confirmed before it can be accepted. The possibility of administering such chemoradiation therapy at diagnosis and before surgery ("neoadjuvant" treatment), as a means of increasing the potential for resectability, is under investigation. Intraoperative radiation therapy has the potential to deliver higher doses of radiation to the tumor while sparing neighboring tissues. However, this strategy has not been shown to give better results than external beam treatment.

The experience of using chemotherapy in the management of patients with widely metastatic pancreatic cancer has been disappointing. Gemcitabine, a deoxycytidine analogue, has been shown to produce improvement in the quality of life for patients with advanced pancreatic cancer. However, duration of survival is only moderately improved. Newer forms of treatment, including therapies directed at specific molecular targets, such as K-*ras*, must be developed and should constitute the initial treatment for consenting, ambulatory patients. → *Pancreatic endocrine tumors are discussed in Chap. 95.*

BIBLIOGRAPHY

Cancer of the Pancreas Task Force: Staging of cancer of the pancreas. Cancer 47:1631, 1981

Connolly MM et al: Survival in 1001 patients with carcinoma of the pancreas. Ann Surg 206:366, 1987

Everhart J, Wright D: Diabetes mellitus as a risk factor for pancreatic cancer. A meta-analysis. JAMA 273:1605, 1995

Gastrointestinal Tumor Study Group: Pancreatic cancer. Adjuvant combined radiation and chemotherapy following curative resection. Arch Surg 120:899, 1985

Goldstein AM et al: Increased risk of pancreatic cancer in melanoma-prone kindreds with p16^INK4 mutations. N Engl J Med 333:970, 1995

Gullo L et al: Diabetes and the risk of pancreatic cancer. N Engl J Med 331:81, 1994

Janes RH Jr et al: National patterns of care for pancreatic cancer: Results of a survey by the Commission on Cancer. Ann Surg 223:261, 1996

Lin A, Feller ER: Pancreatic carcinoma as a cause of unexplained pancreatitis: Report of ten cases. Ann Intern Med 113:166, 1990

Lowenfels AB et al: Pancreatitis and the risk of pancreatic cancer. N Engl J Med 328:1433, 1993

Moertel CT et al: Therapy of locally unresectable pancreatic adenocarcinoma: A randomized comparison of high dose (6,000 rads) radiation alone, moderate dose radiation (4,000 rads) + 5-fluorouracil, and high dose radiation + 5-fluorouracil. The Gastrointestinal Tumor Study Group. Cancer 48:1705, 1981

Moore M et al: A randomized trial of gemcitabine (GEM) versus 5-FU as first-line therapy in advanced pancreatic cancer. Proc Am Soc Clin Oncol 14:199, 1995

Moossa AR, Levin B: The diagnosis of "early" pancreatic cancer: The University of Chicago experience. Cancer 47:1688, 1981

Schnall S, Macdonald JS: Chemotherapy of adenocarcinoma of the pancreas. Semin Oncol 23:220, 1996

Silverman DT et al: Cigarette smoking and pancreas cancer: A case-control study based on direct interview. J Natl Cancer Inst 86:1510, 1994

Speer AG et al: Randomized trial of endoscopic versus percutaneous stent insertion in malignant obstructive jaundice. Lancet 2:57, 1987

Steinberg WM et al: Comparison of the sensitivity and specificity of the CA 19-9 and carcinoembryonic antigen assays in detecting cancer of the pancreas. Gastroenterology 90:343, 1986

Wade TP et al: The Whipple resection for cancer in U.S. Department of Veterans Affairs hospitals. Ann Surg 221:241, 1995

Warshaw AL, Fernando-Del Castillo C: Pancreatic carcinoma. N Engl J Med 326:455, 1992

95 *Lee M. Kaplan*

ENDOCRINE TUMORS OF THE GASTROINTESTINAL TRACT AND PANCREAS

Tumors arising from neuroendocrine cells of the gastrointestinal tract and pancreas present special challenges in diagnosis and therapy. Unlike other gastrointestinal neoplasms, these tumors often cause symptoms from excess hormone secretion rather than from growth, invasion, or local anatomic effects. Frequently slow growing, they may nonetheless be life-threatening because of uncontrolled release of specific hormones and neurotransmitters. These neoplasms arise from within the gastrointestinal mucosa and pancreatic islets in cells that normally secrete regulatory monoamines and peptide hormones. For example, gastrin-secreting G cells within the gastric and duodenal mucosa regulate gastric acid secretion, and insulin-secreting β cells within the pancreatic islets have a crucial role in the homeostatic control of glucose metabolism. Overall, more than 30 distinct secretory products have been identified within neuroendocrine cells of the gut.

BIOLOGIC CONSIDERATIONS A striking feature of neuroendocrine tumors is the preservation of highly differentiated cell function. Tumor cells contain secretory granules and maintain the capacity for *a*mine *p*recursor *u*ptake and *d*ecarboxylation (APUD), a process essential for the production of monoamine neurotransmitters such as serotonin, dopamine, and histamine. This characteristic has fostered the term *APUDomas* for neoplasms derived from these cells, which can be located in the thyroid (C cells), adrenal medulla, lung (neuroendocrine cells), skin (melanocytes), and nervous system (glial cells and neuroblasts), as well as the gastrointestinal tract and pancreas. These cells also synthesize and secrete *peptide* hormones by a separate mechanism. Several of the known APUDomas are listed in Table 95-1. It was postulated that this specialized capability implies a common embryologic origin for these diverse cells, but in fact, cells of *varied* heritage can acquire the APUD phenotype during differentiation.

Studies of neuroendocrine cell physiology have revealed several important characteristics of secretory cells and the clinical syndromes caused by their humoral products:

1. Cellular phenotype does not predict the nature of the secreted product. Thus, neurons may secrete peptide "hormones" into the synaptic cleft, and endocrine cells may secrete monoamines previously classified as neurotransmitters. Individual cells have the capacity to synthesize and secrete both peptide and monoamine transmitters, which may coexist in individual secretory granules. Many symptoms of enterochromaffin cell tumors (carcinoid tumors) appear to arise from the combined actions of monoamine and peptide products.
2. Transmitter secretion by neuroendocrine cells is frequently episodic or pulsatile. Although the regulation of secretion is incompletely understood, the temporal pattern of hormone release may vary depending on the hormonal milieu, physiologic state, or stage of development. Thus, symptoms produced by abnormal secretion of hormones from neuroendocrine tumors may be intermittent, especially in early stages when tumor cells may behave more like their normal counterparts.
3. Individual cells have the *potential* to secrete a wide array of transmitters. This feature is particularly evident for the peptide hormones. Depending on the stage of development, cellular environment, and other as yet unidentified factors, neuroendocrine cells can change secretory profiles dramatically. For example, in cell culture, clonal populations may suddenly change from the secretion of insulin to secretion of cholecystokinin, gastrin, or even glucagon. Endocrine tumors may contain heterogeneous populations of cells, so that within individual tumors, a single cell type may predominate, or there may be multiple cell types in varying proportions. In addition, the secretory profile of a tumor may vary with time, producing a dramatic alteration of symptoms. Individual metastatic implants also can display different phenotypes from the primary tumor and from each other.
4. Individual hormones and transmitters secreted by neuroendocrine cells may regulate physiologic activity (e.g., secretion, absorption, or contractility), stimulate or inhibit growth, or affect the development of target cells. Thus, the humoral activity of gut neuroendocrine tumors can cause a wide variety of effects, including gastric acid hypersecretion, abnormal intestinal motility, gastric epithelial hyperplasia, gallstone formation, mesenteric and cardiac fibrosis, and necrosis of the skin.
5. Hormone production by neuroendocrine cells is tightly regulated at many levels, including RNA transcription, precursor peptide processing, and secretion. These cells, in addition, may be subject to control by neighboring secretory cells *(paracrine regulation)*. Thus, multiple cell types may act in concert to control the growth, secretory characteristics, and thus the clinical manifestations of individual tumors. Abnormal secretion by the tumors themselves may disrupt the normal regulated function of neighboring neuroendocrine cells, and neoplastic transformation may disturb hormone secretion by these cells. Cells may secrete partially processed hormone precursors, leading to unpredictable effects, or display altered susceptibility to regulation by exogenous stimuli. Occasionally, such characteristics can be exploited to permit specific diagnostic tests for individual tumors.

Neuroendocrine tumors of the gastrointestinal tract can be classified by cell type, major hormone secreted, and site of origin. These characteristics, alone or in combination, correlate well with the observed clinical syndromes. Table 95-2 lists the important tumors in this category, along with their clinical presentations, major secreted products, cells of origin, and biologic behavior.

DIAGNOSTIC CONSIDERATIONS Several distinct syndromes of hormone excess have been described in which symptoms may suggest the presence of an endocrine tumor of the gastrointestinal tract or pancreas. Moreover, these tumors may present as part of the type 1 multiple endocrine neoplasia (MEN 1) syndrome (see Chap. 340). MEN 1 patients frequently develop parathyroid and pituitary adenomas that may produce symptoms of hypercalcemia, hyperprolactinemia, hyperthyroidism, or growth hormone excess. Diagnosis is suggested by history, physical findings, elevated blood levels of the relevant peptide hormone(s), or elevated urinary levels of the major metabolites of monoamine transmitters. Further confirmation of hormone-producing tumors may be provided by provocative tests that reveal abnormalities in the regulation of hormone secretion. For example, tolbutamide may enhance somatostatin secretion from somatostatinoma cells. Normal somatostatin-secreting D cells do not show this effect. Other examples of *abnormal* regulation in tumor cells include enhancement by secretin of gastrin secretion in gastrinomas and pentagastrin stimulation of calcitonin secretion in medullary thyroid (C cell) tumors.

Anatomic definition for pancreatic tumors should be sought by computed tomography (CT) and/or endoscopic ultrasonography, and endoscopic visualization with ultrasonography or barium contrast studies should be obtained for suspected mucosal and submucosal tumors.

Table 95-1

Distribution of APUD Tumors

Origin	Tumors
Gastrointestinal tract	Carcinoid tumor
Pancreas	Islet cell carcinoma
Central nervous system	Ganglioneuroblastoma, neuroblastoma, chemodactoma, paraganglionoma
Thyroid	Medullary thyroid carcinoma
Skin	Melanoma
Adrenal medulla	Pheochromocytoma
Lung	Carcinoid tumor, small cell carcinoma

Table 95-2

Gastrointestinal Endocrine Tumor Syndromes

Syndrome	Cell Type	Clinical Features	Percentage Malignant	Major Products
Carcinoid syndrome	Enterochromaffin, enterochromaffin-like	Flushing, diarrhea, wheezing, hypotension	~100	Serotonin, histamine, miscellaneous peptides
Zollinger-Ellison, gastrinoma	Non-β islet cell, duodenal G cell	Peptic ulcers, diarrhea	~70	Gastrin
Insulinoma	Islet β cell	Hypoglycemia	~10	Insulin
VIPoma (Verner-Morrison, WDHA)	Islet D_1 cell	Diarrhea, hypokalemia, hypochlorhydria	~60	Vasoactive intestinal peptide
Glucagonoma	Islet A cell	Mild diabetes mellitus, erythema necrolytica migrans, glossitis	>75	Glucagon
Somatostatinoma	Islet D cell	Diabetes mellitus, diarrhea, steatorrhea, gallstones	~70	Somatostatin
GRFoma	Non-β islet cell	Acromegaly	—	Growth hormone–releasing hormone (GRF)
CRFoma	Non-β islet cell	Cushing's syndrome	—	Corticotropin-releasing hormone (CRF)
PPoma	Islet PP cell	Rare necrolytic erythema	—	Pancreatic polypeptide (PP)
Neurotensinoma	Non-β islet cell	Mild diarrhea	—	Neurotensin
Miscellaneous tumors	Non-β islet cell	Hypercalcemia, SIADH, hyperpigmentation	—	Parathyroid hormone, vasopressin, melanocyte-stimulating hormone

ABBREVIATION: SIADH, syndrome of inappropriate antidiuretic hormone secretion.

In cases where tumors are too small to be visualized by these noninvasive methods, angiography or selective venous sampling for hormone determination may provide anatomic localization. CT and magnetic resonance imaging (MRI) are the preferred means of assessing metastatic spread, since the liver and lymph nodes are the initial sites of tumor metastasis.

THERAPEUTIC CONSIDERATIONS Therapy of endocrine tumors has two goals: (1) to decrease or reverse the growth and spread of the tumor and (2) to relieve the symptoms of hormone overproduction. When the tumor is localized, both goals may be accomplished by surgical excision. However, most of these tumors are malignant and have spread by the time of diagnosis, and control of growth in such malignant tumors has proven difficult. Thus far, the greatest benefit has been seen with chemotherapeutic regimens that include streptozocin, alone or in combination with fluorouracil or doxorubicin. Interferon-alpha at high doses may also limit tumor growth. Control of hepatic metastases has been achieved with surgical resection of isolated lesions, hepatic artery embolization, or direct injection with cytotoxic agents (e.g., ethanol), although these approaches are palliative rather than curative.

Several approaches are used to control the effects of excess hormone production by these tumors. The most common is to block the function of the target tissue. For example, gastric acid hypersecretion induced by gastrin-producing tumors may be reversed by medications that inhibit acid secretion (e.g., H_2 receptor blockers or proton pump inhibitors) or by surgical resection of the stomach. Diazoxide is used to help reverse the effects of hyperinsulinemia, and hypomotility agents and inhibitors of intestinal chloride secretion may ameliorate the diarrhea caused by hypersecretion of vasoactive intestinal peptide (VIP), gastrin, somatostatin, neurotensin, or serotonin.

A second approach is to block release of the transmitter from the tumor cells. The success of this approach depends on the continued ability of the tumor cells to respond to such physiologic or pharmacologic stimuli. Initial trials used somatostatin, a peptide hormone that inhibits the release of numerous hormones and amine transmitters. While somatostatin controls the symptoms of many of these tumors, it has a short half-life and must be given intravenously. These limitations have been largely overcome by the use of octreotide, a longer-acting analogue of somatostatin with similar actions that can be administered subcutaneously. The chemical structures of somatostatin and octreotide are shown in Fig. 95-1 (see also Chap. 328). Octreotide frequently relieves the symptoms of several endocrine tumors that are inadequately controlled by tumor resection or ablation. In addition, tumor regression has oc-

curred in occasional patients, suggesting that the hormone agonist may have some growth-inhibiting effects. The major known side effects of octreotide are dose-dependent and are similar to symptoms of somatostatin excess, including steatorrhea, mild hyperglycemia, nausea, and abdominal pain. Patients on long-term therapy with this agent have an increased tendency to develop gallstones. The clinical disorders that respond to therapy with octreotide are summarized in Table 95-3.

CARCINOID TUMORS

Carcinoid tumors are the most protean and the most common gastrointestinal endocrine tumors, accounting for approximately 75 percent of such neoplasms. The incidence of carcinoid tumors in the United States is approximately 15 per 1 million population per year. They may present with gastrointestinal bleeding, abdominal pain, obstruction from tumor growth or tumor-induced mesenteric fibrosis, or symptoms arising from tumor-secreted hormones. The name *carcinoid* was applied to these tumors because slow growth and the homogeneous appearance of tumor cells led early investigators to underestimate their malignant potential. They pursue an indolent course, and the interval

FIGURE 95-1 Structures of somatostatin-14 and octreotide. The double circle denotes the substitution of D-tryptophan for the naturally occurring L-tryptophan. This substitution inhibits peptide degradation and prolongs serum half-life.

Table 95-3

Clinical Uses of Octreotide in Gastrointestinal Disease

Disease	Effect
Hormone-secreting tumors	
Carcinoid tumor	Inhibits cutaneous flushing, controls diarrhea, reverses hypotension, aids perioperative management, ?inhibits growth
VIPoma	Controls diarrhea
Insulinoma	Controls hypoglycemia acutely, aids perioperative management
Gastrinoma	Aids perioperative management, ?controls diarrhea
Glucagonoma	Controls necrolytic erythema
Dumping syndrome	Controls diarrhea, vasomotor symptoms
Diarrhea	Inhibits intestinal secretion, motility
Short-bowel syndrome	
Ileostomy	
Diabetic neuropathy	
AIDS	
Fistulas	Inhibits fluid and enzyme secretion, promotes healing
Pancreatic	
Enteric	
Crohn's disease	
Gastrointestinal bleeding	
Portal hypertensive gastropathy	Reduces portal pressure, splanchnic blood flow
Esophageal and gastric varices	Reduces portal pressure, splanchnic blood flow

between onset of symptoms and diagnosis averages 4.5 years. Carcinoid tumors arise from neuroendocrine cells throughout the body but are most prevalent in the gastrointestinal tract, pancreas, and pulmonary bronchi. Ninety percent of these tumors arise in the enterochromaffin, or Kulchitsky, cells within the gastrointestinal tract. The tumors can be found anywhere from the stomach to the rectum and are most common in the appendix, ileum, and rectum. In the small intestine, carcinoid tumors are one of the two most common malignancies, along with adenocarcinoma. Gastrointestinal carcinoids frequently cause abdominal pain, bleeding, or intestinal obstruction. Although they are rarely large, the tumors may become the leading point for intussusception. In addition, mesenteric and peritoneal spread stimulates a local fibrous reaction, causing intestinal kinking, obstruction, and vascular compromise. Rare sites of carcinoid tumors include the thymus, esophagus, biliary duct, Meckel's diverticulum, breast, and ovary. No risk factors have been clearly defined for these enterochromaffin cell tumors. Carcinoids of the bronchus, stomach, and duodenum may occur in association with MEN 1. Thymic carcinoids may be associated with hyperparathyroidism or Cushing's syndrome.

Gastric carcinoid tumors may arise from enterochromaffin cells or histamine-secreting enterochromaffin-*like* (ECL) cells. The incidence of ECL cell-derived tumors is increased in patients with chronic atrophic gastritis and achlorhydria associated with pernicious anemia or *Helicobacter pylori* infection. Gastrin is a growth factor for gastric ECL cells, and tumorigenesis appears to result from the *combination* of the chronic inflammation and profound hypergastrinemia associated with atrophic gastritis.

Appendiceal tumors make up nearly half of all carcinoid tumors and are incidental findings in 0.3 to 0.7 percent of routine appendectomy specimens. They are usually small, solitary, and benign. Local invasion is common, but metastatic spread is rare, and the presence of tumor does not appear to be associated with appreciable morbidity or mortality. Colorectal carcinoids have a similarly benign course and are usually asymptomatic. In contrast, small-bowel and bronchial carcinoids have a more malignant course. Local transmural invasion, early metastasis to lymph nodes and liver, and symptoms from hormone secretion are common. Other sites of metastatic spread include bone and, less commonly, heart, breast, and eye. The risk of metastatic

spread is dependent on tumor size. Metastases are found in fewer than 2 percent of tumors less than 1 cm in diameter but in nearly 100 percent of tumors greater than 2 cm. Additional primary tumor implants within the gastrointestinal tract are found in 40 percent of patients.

CARCINOID SYNDROME Enterochromaffin cells secrete a variety of hormones and are embryologically related to thyroid C cells, adrenal medullary cells, and melanocytes. Tumors of each of these cell types may produce syndromes of hormone excess. Hormone secretion by carcinoid cells can cause distinctive and debilitating effects (carcinoid syndrome) long before local growth or metastatic spread is otherwise apparent. Manifestations of the carcinoid syndrome include the "classic" triad of cutaneous flushing, diarrhea, and valvular heart disease and, less commonly, telangiectasias, wheezing, and paroxysmal *hypo*tension. Flushing, which is present in approximately 85 percent of patients with carcinoid syndrome, is also seen with many other conditions, including menopause, autonomic nervous system dysfunction, ethanol ingestion, disulfiram treatment, drug withdrawal, and a variety of hormone-secreting tumors, including pheochromocytoma, medullary thyroid carcinoma, VIPoma, and mastocytosis. It is estimated that approximately 5 percent of individuals presenting with the new onset of flushing will be found to have the carcinoid syndrome. Early in the course, symptoms are usually episodic and may be provoked by stress, catecholamines, and ingestion of food or alcohol. During acute paroxysms, systolic blood pressure typically falls 20 to 30 mmHg. Diarrhea may result from several mechanisms. The most common type is mixed secretory and hypermotility-induced, producing watery stools unresponsive to fasting. Other causes include partial mechanical obstruction from tumor or fibrosis and mesenteric vascular insufficiency from local fibrosis. Endocardial fibrosis can cause valvular heart disease, usually affecting the proximal side of the tricuspid and pulmonary valves and leading to tricuspid insufficiency, pulmonary stenosis, and secondary right-sided heart failure. Left-sided valvular disease may occur in association with bronchial carcinoids, presumably because venous effluent from these tumors passes directly into the pulmonary veins, evading inactivation of the hormone mediators in the lung.

Approximately 5 percent of all patients with carcinoid tumors experience one or more symptoms of the carcinoid syndrome. The likelihood that symptoms will develop depends strongly on the origin and behavior of the tumor. While 30 to 60 percent of small-bowel carcinoids are associated with systemic manifestations, only 3.5 percent of lung, 1 percent of appendix, and virtually no rectal carcinoids produce the syndrome. In patients with intestinal carcinoids, the humoral symptoms only develop in the setting of metastatic disease to the liver. Bronchial and other extraintestinal carcinoids, whose hormone products are not immediately cleared by the liver, may produce the carcinoid syndrome in the absence of metastasis.

Carcinoid tumors may be classified on the basis of embryonic origin (Table 95-4). Clinical features, secreted hormones, diagnostic evaluation, and prognosis vary according to whether a carcinoid arises in foregut, midgut, or hindgut structures. For example, carcinoid syndrome is less common in patients with foregut carcinoids than with midgut tumors, but the syndrome, when it occurs, is more likely to include wheezing. Patients with foregut carcinoid syndrome more often have dramatic cutaneous flushing involving the whole body than those with tumors of midgut or hindgut organs. The flush of bronchial carcinoids may be prolonged (lasting hours to days); may be associated with excessive lacrimation, salivation, and facial edema; and occasionally produces significant hypotension. The cutaneous manifestations of gastric enterochromaffin cell carcinoids, though lasting only minutes, are frequently well-circumscribed and associated with wheals, pruritus, and high levels of histamine secretion. In contrast, gastric ECL cell carcinoid tumors are rarely associated with carcinoid syndrome.

Midgut carcinoids commonly cause the carcinoid syndrome. Acute episodes of flushing tend to be less severe than those associated with foregut tumors, but facial telangiectasias may develop late in the course. Midgut tumors are more frequently associated with cardiac manifestations and peritoneal fibrosis. Hindgut tumors rarely cause the carcinoid syndrome. A rare variant syndrome associated with ovarian carcinoids causes severe peritoneal fibrosis.

Table 95-4

Characteristics of Carcinoid Tumors

Embryonic Origin	Site of Primary Tumor	Carcinoid Syndrome			
		Frequency, %	Characteristics		Monoamines
Foregut	Bronchus	3.5	Intense flush, lasting up to several hours; associated lacrimation, salivation, facial edema; wheezing; diarrhea; left- and right-sided cardiac lesions		5-HT, ± histamine
	Stomach	~5	Intense, patchy, whole-body flush, with defined borders, wheals, usually lasting several minutes; pruritus; wheezing; diarrhea		5-HTP, histamine, ± 5-HT
Midgut	Duodenum, jejunum	~40	Diarrhea		5-HT
	Pancreas, gallbladder	Rare	Occasional necrolytic erythema		5-HT, ± histamine
	Ileum	~40	Facial flush, usually lasting seconds to minutes; telangiectasias; cardiac lesions; peritoneal fibrosis; diarrhea		
	Appendix	~1			
Hindgut	Colon	Rare	Mild facial flush		5-HT
	Rectum	0	Diarrhea		

ABBREVIATIONS: 5-HT, 5-hydroxytryptamine (serotonin); 5-HTP, 5-hydroxytryptophan.

Serotonin (5-hydroxytryptamine, 5-HT) is the most common secretory product of carcinoid tumors. As shown in Fig. 95-2, carcinoid tumors synthesize serotonin by enzymatic modification of circulating tryptophan. Up to 50 percent of the dietary intake of tryptophan can be converted to serotonin by these cells, which may leave inadequate substrate for incorporation into proteins and conversion to niacin. As a result, patients with widely metastatic carcinoid tumors may suffer symptoms of protein malnutrition (see Chap. 74) or mild pellagra (see Chap. 79). Serotonin induces intestinal secretion, inhibits intestinal absorption, and stimulates intestinal motility. High serotonin levels are likely the cause of diarrhea in most cases of carcinoid syndrome. Serotonin also stimulates fibroblast growth and fibrogenesis and thus may mediate or accelerate the peritoneal and cardiac valvular fibrosis in this disease. Excess serotonin secretion alone does not account for cutaneous flushing. Multiple monoamine and peptide factors contribute to the vasomotor changes; the relative contributions of each mediator may vary from patient to patient.

Carcinoid tumors elaborate multiple monoamines and peptide hormones, including histamine, catecholamines, bradykinins, tachykinins, enkephalins and endorphins, vasopressin, gastrin, adrenocorticotrophin, and prostaglandins (Table 95-5). Many secrete somatostatin, neurotensin, substance P, neurokinin A, TRH-like peptide (EEP-NH$_2$) and motilin. The elevated circulating levels of these substances mediate many of the pathophysiologic changes of carcinoid syndrome, although the relative contributions of each remain to be identified.

DIAGNOSIS The diagnosis of carcinoid tumors is influenced by the presenting features of the tumor. Patients with nonfunctional tumors (i.e., without the carcinoid *syndrome*) usually present with symptoms due to the direct effects of the tumor in the gastrointestinal tract, including abdominal pain or tenderness, nausea, malaise, weight loss, intestinal or biliary obstruction, or gastrointestinal bleeding. Depending on the location of the tumor and on whether metastases are present, endoscopy, barium studies, or CT may allow anatomic localization. Radiographic studies should include small-bowel follow-through or direct instillation of radiographic contrast material into the small bowel (enteroclysis) to identify tumors in the jejunum and ileum. Despite the improved detection of tumors, however, their pathologic identity is usually not suspected before resection or liver biopsy.

Evaluation of patients with clinical features of carcinoid syndrome is based on the observation that serotonin is synthesized and secreted by the large majority of functional carcinoid tumors. As shown in Fig. 95-2, serotonin is metabolized in the blood to 5-hydroxyindoleacetic acid (5-HIAA), which is cleared by the kidneys. Plasma and platelet serotonin and urinary 5-HIAA levels are usually elevated in the setting of carcinoid syndrome. Measurement of urinary 5-HIAA excretion is the most useful diagnostic test, and approximately 75 percent of pa-

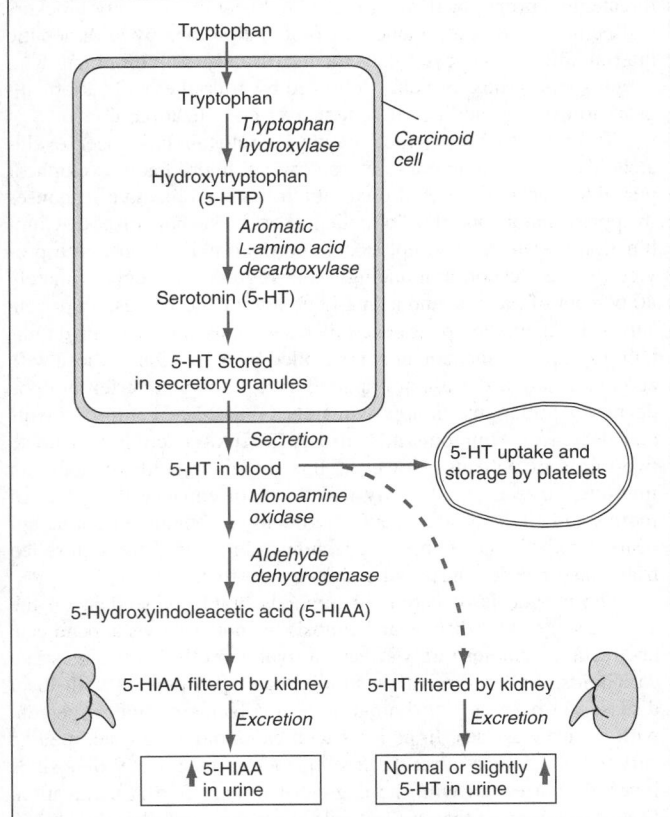

FIGURE 95-2 Metabolic pathway of serotonin in the carcinoid syndrome.

Table 95-5

Hormone Mediators of Carcinoid Syndrome

Clinical Feature	Frequency, %	Candidate Mediators
Diarrhea	78	5-HT, histamine, prostaglandins, VIP, glucagon, gastrin, calcitonin
Cutaneous flushing	94	5-HT, 5-HTP, kallikrein, NKA, histamine, SK, SP, prostaglandins
Telangiectasia	25	Unknown
Wheezing	18	5-HT, histamine
Abdominal pain	51	Tumor, hepatic enlargment, bowel ischemia (fibrosis)
Heart disease		5-HT
Right-sided	40	
Left-sided	13	
Pellagra dermatosis	7	Tryptophan depletion (5-HT synthesis)

ABBREVIATIONS: 5-HT, 5-hydroxytryptamine (serotonin): 5-HTP, 5-hydroxytryptophan; NKA, neurokinin A; SK, substance K; SP, substance P; VIP, vasoactive intestinal peptide.

SOURCE: After W Creutzfeldt and F Stockmann, Am J Med 82:4, 1987.

tients excrete more than 80 μmol/d (15 mg/d). The specificity of this test approaches 100 percent after exclusion of ingested substances known to elevate 5-HIAA levels; these include bananas, plantain, pineapple, kiwi fruit, walnuts, plums, pecans, avocados, guaifenesin, and acetaminophen. Conversely, aspirin and levodopa ingestion can cause a falsely depressed 5-HIAA level. In some patients with carcinoid syndrome and normal urinary 5-HIAA, documentation of elevated plasma or platelet serotonin concentrations may establish the diagnosis. However, many foregut carcinoid tumors lack aromatic L-amino acid decarboxylase and convert 5-hydroxytryptophan (5-HTP) to serotonin with low efficiency. Since 5-HTP is not metabolized to 5-HIAA, urinary studies may be misleading. These patients may have elevated urinary serotonin levels, since renal cells contain aromatic L-amino acid decarboxylase. Diagnosis in these cases may be confirmed by demonstrating elevated plasma 5-HTP, histamine, or peptide hormone levels, although it frequently rests on the anatomic detection of the tumor itself. Attempts to provoke cutaneous flushing are helpful for documenting flushing in cases when the clinical history is equivocal. Ethanol, pentagastrin, or *micro*gram quantities of epinephrine can be used for this purpose. CT, MRI, and selective angiography are the most sensitive tests for detecting metastatic disease in the liver. Since most patients with the humoral syndrome have metastases, liver biopsy is the most common access to histologic diagnosis. Additional information about bone metastases and cardiac sequelae may be obtained with bone scans and echocardiography, respectively. In patients in whom a tumor cannot be detected, scintigraphic imaging with radiolabeled octreotide is often helpful. Octreotide binds tightly to type 2 somatostatin receptors, which are expressed in large numbers by most carcinoid tumor cells. Octreotide scintigraphy identifies the sites of primary and metastatic tumor in approximately two-thirds of patients with carcinoid syndrome. The sensitivity of this method is improved with high doses (≥200 MBq) of radionuclide and single photon emission CT (SPECT) imaging. It is far more sensitive than scintigraphy with metaiodobenzyl guanidine (MIBG), which was previously used for this purpose.

℞ **TREATMENT**

Effective treatment of the carcinoid syndrome may require more than one approach. Therapy should be selected according to the severity of symptoms. Since nearly all patients with carcinoid syndrome have metastatic disease, resection is rarely curative. Mild diarrhea may be controlled with hypomotility agents such as loperamide or diphenoxylate/atropine. In patients who have undergone ileal resection, diarrhea can be exacerbated by bile salt malabsorption and frequently responds to cholestyramine. Flushing, if rare and mild, may not require therapy. Combination therapy with histamine H_1 and H_2 receptor antagonists (e.g., diphenhydramine and ranitidine) can inhibit the cutaneous flush associated with foregut carcinoids. Phenoxybenzamine may provide additional benefit by inhibiting the release of bradykinin. Methylxanthine bronchodilators and glucocorticoids are helpful in relieving the dyspnea and wheezing associated with bronchial carcinoids. Beta-adrenergic agonists should be avoided because they may provoke acute exacerbations. Serotonin antagonists, including cyproheptadine and methysergide, have been used to provide relief of diarrhea. Unfortunately, these agents have little effect on flushing and other vasomotor symptoms, and methysergide can induce fibrosis similar to that caused by the carcinoid itself.

Octreotide is a potent inhibitor of hormone secretion by carcinoid cells. At doses of 150 to 1500 μg/d, this agent provides effective control of diarrhea, flushing, and wheezing in more than 75 percent of cases. Octreotide is effective in the management of acute, life-threatening manifestations of the carcinoid syndrome, such as hypotension or resulting angina, as well as of the transient exacerbation of symptoms caused by hepatic artery embolization or the induction of general anesthesia. Octreotide must be administered in two or three subcutaneous injections each day. The development of long-

acting preparations of other somatostatin analogues, such as lanreotide, should provide even more convenient therapy. It is not yet known whether octreotide can prevent the observed cardiac (or mesenteric) fibrosis. Established valvular heart disease is not reversed by any form of medical therapy.

Surgery, hepatic artery embolization, and chemotherapy have been used to reduce the burden of tumor tissue. Surgery is the treatment of choice for small (<2 cm diameter) carcinoid tumors of the appendix or large bowel, as well as for the anatomic effects of these tumors (e.g., intestinal obstruction, ischemia, or bleeding). Curative resection also may be effective in patients with carcinoid syndrome from isolated bronchial or other extraintestinal carcinoids. Most patients with carcinoid syndrome, however, have gross metastatic disease. Hepatic resection generally provides only transient amelioration of symptoms and no improvement in survival. In isolated cases, however, long-term palliation has been achieved by resection of a *single* hepatic metastasis after removal of the primary tumor. Orthotopic liver transplantation for hepatic metastases has not provided long-term benefit. Several less invasive approaches have been tried to limit the hepatic tumor burden and control humoral symptoms, including local irradiation, selective hepatic artery infusion of chemotherapy, CT-guided instillation of ethanol into metastatic implants, CT-guided cryoablation, and hepatic arterial chemoembolization. Carcinoid tumors are generally radioresistant, although radiotherapy may provide transient relief of pain from bone metastases; they respond poorly to chemotherapy. Arterial occlusion by Gelfoam embolization provides rapid relief of symptoms for up to 1 year in approximately 90 percent of patients. Its success derives in part from the fact that the hepatic artery supplies less than half the blood supply of normal liver tissue but nearly all the blood supply of the tumor. Side effects of therapy include abdominal pain, fever, and occasional synthetic liver dysfunction. The effectiveness of therapy can be monitored by means of serum transaminase levels, which should rise substantially over the first 24 to 48 h after embolization. Patients undergoing embolization may experience acute exacerbation of carcinoid symptoms provoked by the sudden release of hormones from the tumor. Although such effects are rarely life-threatening, prophylactic treatment with histamine receptor blockers and octreotide is recommended. Combination therapy with hepatic arterial infusion of cytotoxic agents (usually 5-fluorouracil with streptozocin or doxorubicin), followed by arterial embolization, appears to offer no additional benefit over embolization alone.

Several systemic chemotherapeutic protocols have been evaluated. Various combinations of streptozocin, fluorouracil, cyclophosphamide, dacarbazine, and doxorubicin induce objective responses in approximately one-third of patients with metastatic disease. Combination therapy with streptozocin and doxorubicin appears to provide the best response, inducing tumor regression in approximately 40 percent of patients and a small but significant increase in patient survival. Chemotherapy is generally reserved for patients with debilitating symptoms inadequately controlled by octreotide or those with carcinoid cardiac disease or impaired liver function. Interferon-alpha decreases tumor size in approximately 10 to 20 percent of patients and decreases symptoms and urinary 5-HIAA excretion in up to two-thirds of patients. However, this immunomodulator does not improve survival significantly and does not enhance the effect of more standard chemotherapeutic regimens. Although octreotide appears to have induced objective responses in a few cases, controlled trials have not demonstrated a significant effect.

The prognosis of carcinoid tumor is highly dependent on the site and stage of the disease at diagnosis. As noted above, appendiceal and rectal carcinoids rarely affect survival. For other gastrointestinal carcinoids, 5-year survival is approximately 95 percent with local disease, 65 percent with lymph node involvement, and 20 percent with liver metastases. In patients with carcinoid syndrome, median survival is 2.5 years after the first episode of flushing. Prognosis is inversely correlated with the degree of urinary 5-HIAA elevation. Despite attempts at therapy, patients excreting >800 μmol/d (>150 mg/d) have a median survival of only 1 year.

The endocrine functions of the pancreas are mediated by the islets of Langerhans, which are distributed throughout the pancreatic parenchyma. Each mature islet is composed of four major classes of secretory cells: A cells, whose major secreted product is glucagon; B (or β) cells, which secrete insulin; D cells, which secrete somatostatin; and PP cells, which secrete pancreatic polypeptide. Each of these cells secretes additional regulatory peptides in lower concentrations. During development of the islets, precursors are transiently formed that secrete several additional regulatory peptides, including gastrin, VIP, adrenocorticotropin (ACTH), and others. Pancreatic islet cell tumors can arise from any of these cell populations. These tumors may therefore secrete one or more biologically active peptides, giving rise to a number of recognizable humoral syndromes (see Table 95-2).

GASTRINOMA (ZOLLINGER-ELLISON SYNDROME)

(See also Chap. 284) In 1955, Zollinger and Ellison reported the association of severe peptic ulcer disease and gastrin-secreting tumors of the pancreas. These gastrinomas generate high serum gastrin levels, leading to hypersecretion of gastric acid and consequent duodenal and jejunal ulcers. Gastrinomas are the most common of the hormone-secreting tumors of the pancreatic islets, constituting nearly one-tenth of gastroenteropancreatic endocrine tumors and occurring with a frequency of approximately 4 in 10 million in an unselected population in Ireland. Zollinger-Ellison syndrome may account for up to 0.1 percent of patients with duodenal ulcer disease in the United States. Ulcer disease develops in almost all patients with gastrinoma and is the presenting problem in approximately 70 percent. More than half of patients experience diarrhea (either watery stools or steatorrhea), and approximately 30 percent present with diarrhea alone. Radiologic and endoscopic examinations frequently reveal increased gastric fluid and thickened rugal folds. The age distribution of patients with gastrinoma is similar to that in ordinary acid peptic disease, with a broad peak in the fifth to eighth decades. Gastrinoma should be considered in all patients with recurrent or refractory ulcer disease, ulcers associated with gastric hypertrophy, ulcers in the distal duodenum or jejunum, ulcers in association with diarrhea, kidney stones, hypercalcemia, or pituitary disease, or a strong family history of duodenal ulcer disease or endocrine tumors.

Between one-fourth and one-half of gastrinomas occur in association with the MEN 1 syndrome (see Chap. 340). Hyperparathyroidism is the most common component of MEN 1 and occurs in about 80 percent of patients with this form of Zollinger-Ellison syndrome. All gastrinoma patients should be screened for possible MEN 1 by measurement of serum calcium, phosphorus, cortisol, and prolactin levels and imaging of the sella turcica. First-degree relatives of patients with MEN 1 should be similarly screened.

Approximately 80 percent of gastrin-secreting tumors arise in pancreatic islets, including nearly all those associated with MEN 1, and most are located in the pancreatic head. Another 10 to 15 percent arise from G cells in the duodenum, and the remainder are scattered in the distal small bowel, stomach, spleen, liver, lymph nodes, and ovary (mucinous cystadenoma). The tumors are usually small and are frequently multifocal, especially when associated with MEN 1. The biologic behavior may be variable. In most reported series, one-half to two-thirds of these tumors are malignant, with metastases to lymph nodes and liver and less frequently to bone. However, the prevalence of metastatic disease at the time of diagnosis appears to have decreased, perhaps owing to the more widespread consideration and earlier detection of these tumors. Such observations have important therapeutic implications, since isolated tumors are more likely to be cured by resection. Gastrinomas, like most other islet cell tumors, are generally slow-growing, but growth patterns vary widely, and metastases may be more aggressive than the primary tumor itself.

℞ TREATMENT

Treatment of Zollinger-Ellison syndrome is directed at the sequelae of excess gastrin secretion and at the tumor itself. The availability of potent inhibitors of gastric acid secretion, including H_2 receptor blockers and the H^+,K^+-ATPase inhibitors omeprazole and lansoprazole, has reduced the need for gastric surgery in these patients. The rare patient who fails to respond to medical therapy should be treated surgically. However, patients with coexistent hyperparathyroidism should undergo parathyroid resection before a decision is made about gastric surgery, since resolution of hypercalcemia may permit better medical control of gastric acid secretion.

Because of the effective control of hormone-mediated symptoms, morbidity and mortality from gastrinoma are increasingly related to the growth and spread of the tumor itself. Curative resection of the gastrinoma is possible in 15 to 20 percent of cases and is favored by an extrapancreatic location and by small tumor size. Gastrinomas in association with MEN 1 syndrome are not amenable to surgical cure, although these tumors generally have a benign natural history. A variety of imaging studies are used preoperatively to identify the primary tumor mass and exclude metastases. More than 90 percent of gastrinomas can be identified using a combination of CT, endoscopic ultrasonography, and octreotide scintigraphy. Each of these tests alone has a sensitivity of between 38 and 70 percent for detecting primary gastrinomas. (Transabdominal ultrasonography detects only 10 to 20 percent of these primary tumors, but it can identify approximately 50 percent of liver metastases.) In cases where these approaches fail to identify the tumor, angiography, selective venous hormone sampling, intraoperative palpation, and intraoperative ultrasonography are frequently effective. *Intraoperative* octreotide scintigraphy provides no additional diagnostic advantage.

Treatment of unresectable gastrinoma includes chemotherapy, hormonal therapy, and hepatic artery embolization. Chemotherapeutic regimens including streptozocin and fluorouracil, with or without doxorubicin, commonly induce partial responses. Interferon-alpha also may cause an objective response, but octreotide does not appear to be effective. Hepatic artery embolization may decrease hepatic tumor burden and ameliorate pain. Unfortunately, none of these approaches prolongs survival of patients with metastatic disease, which approximates 25 percent at 10 years.

INSULINOMA (β CELL TUMOR)

The hallmark of pancreatic β cell tumors is the development of symptomatic hypoglycemia from unregulated insulin hypersection (see also Chap. 335). Insulinomas are the second most common functioning islet cell tumors and have a reported prevalence of approximately 8 in 10 million in an unselected Irish population. They arise most frequently in the fifth to seventh decades, although cases have been reported at all ages. In infants and children, insulinoma must be distinguished from diffuse β cell adenomatosis and nesidioblastosis. Whipple's triad, the classic presentation of insulinoma, consists of fasting hypoglycemia, *symptoms* of hypoglycemia, and immediate relief after intravenous glucose administration. Weight gain may result from increased food ingested to combat symptoms of hypoglycemia. In the current era, the diagnosis of insulinoma is made by demonstrating fasting hypoglycemia in the presence of normal or elevated plasma insulin levels. Symptoms related to the hypoglycemia include headache, slurred speech, psychological alterations, visual disturbances, confusion, and, ultimately, coma and death. Hypoglycemia also induces the secondary release of catecholamines, leading to tremulousness, diaphoresis, pallor, palpitations, cardiac arrhythmias, and behavioral irritability. Because of the episodic release of insulin, symptoms early in the course may be intermittent or occur only after somewhat prolonged periods of fasting. However, symptoms do develop early, so that tumors are usually small and solitary at the time of diagnosis. Multiple primary tumors are found in approximately 10 percent of patients. An additional 10 percent of patients have malignant disease, with spread to the local lymph nodes and the liver. As with gastrinomas, insulinomas are frequently associated with MEN 1 (see Chaps. 335 and 340), and such tumors are more likely to be multifocal. Extrapancreatic insulin-secreting tumors are rare and usually arise in ectopic pancreatic tissue.

Diagnosis is made by demonstrating fasting hypoglycemia and an inadequate response of insulin to the hypoglycemia (see Chap. 335 for details). Patients are fasted under close supervision for up to 72 h, followed, if necessary, by an exercise tolerance test. Most patients with insulinoma develop hypoglycemia within 24 h, as evidenced by a serum glucose level of less than 2.8 mmol/L (50 mg/dL) in men or 2.5 mmol/L (45 mg/dL) in women. However, there is no absolute glucose level that defines hypoglycemia, so the diagnosis of insulinoma depends on the demonstration of inadequate insulin suppression in the face of falling glucose levels. Documentation of rising cortisol levels excludes hypoglycemia secondary to hypothalamic-pituitary-adrenal dysfunction. It is also necessary to exclude other causes of fasting hypoglycemia, including administration of exogenous insulin, sulfonylurea ingestion, severe liver failure, and tumors that secrete insulinlike growth factors (e.g., fibrosarcoma, mesothelioma, and hemangiopericytoma). Exogenous insulin administration can be excluded by measuring levels of the C peptide of proinsulin, which normally vary in parallel with the plasma insulin concentrations. Since insulin administration suppresses endogenous insulin secretion, detection of normal or elevated C-peptide levels is inconsistent with insulin abuse. In addition, because insulinoma cells often process proinsulin incompletely, the serum often has an increased ratio of proinsulin to insulin. A ratio greater than 20 percent in the appropriate clinical setting is suggestive of insulinoma. Serum levels of sulfonylureas should be elevated if hyperinsulinemic hypoglycemia is caused by these agents. Normal glucose/insulin ratios exclude liver failure and tumors that secrete insulin-like growth factors.

Rx TREATMENT

Once a diagnosis of insulinemia is established, acute treatment is supportive, with intravenous glucose infusion as required to maintain plasma levels within the normal range. Hyperglycemic agents, including diazoxide, beta-adrenergic receptor blockers, and phenytoin, can be used to support serum glucose levels, but their effects are variable and may last only a short time. Octreotide frequently inhibits insulin secretion by these tumors and may be an effective agent for acute management. Definitive therapy is accomplished by surgical resection. Because insulinomas are usually small (most are <2 cm in diameter), only half are detected by CT. Two-phase (arterial and parenchymal) contrast techniques improve the sensitivity of CT somewhat. In contrast, endoscopic ultrasonography detects 80 to 90 percent of tumors. Angiography with selective venous sampling for insulin levels is also about 80 percent sensitive, as is palpation during surgery. At surgery, all detectable tumors should be resected. The effectiveness of intervention is monitored by determination of intraoperative blood glucose levels. In cases where no tumors are detected by any of these methods, stepwise distal pancreatectomy is performed until frozen sections of resected specimens and/or blood glucose measurements indicate that all tumor has been removed. If no tumor is found, or if multiple tumors are present, pancreatectomy is limited to 70 to 80 percent to preserve digestive and endocrine pancreatic function.

Patients with metastatic disease and those whose insulinomas are not removed by partial pancreatectomy can frequently be managed with hyperglycemic agents such as diazoxide or octreotide. In one study, all seven patients with metastatic insulinoma showed a response to octreotide, although the degree of response varied. However, hypoglycemia may be worsened by octreotide administration, perhaps owing to inhibition of glucagon or growth hormone by this agent. Diazoxide, though frequently effective, can cause troubling side effects, including salt and fluid retention, hypertrichosis, and gastrointestinal upset. The combination of streptozocin and doxorubicin is the mainstay of chemotherapy for metastatic disease; it is superior to streptozocin-fluorouracil. These agents in-

duce objective remission in approximately half of patients and are associated with a modest but significant increase in survival. Patients with residual tumor should be followed carefully for changes in secretory profile which may affect therapy. Such changes may include development of hyperglycemia as a result of glucagon-secreting metastases.

VIPOMA [VERNER-MORRISON SYNDROME; WATERY DIARRHEA, HYPOKALEMIA, ACHLORHYDRIA (WDHA) SYNDROME] Verner and Morrison described a syndrome of watery diarrhea, hypokalemia, and renal failure in association with non-β-cell tumors of the pancreatic islets. The clinical features of this syndrome are caused by the high levels of VIP secreted by the tumors. VIPomas comprise approximately 2 percent of gastroenteropancreatic tumors and have a prevalence of approximately 1 in 10 million in the Irish population studied. The manifestations of VIPoma include secretory diarrhea, profound weakness, hypokalemia, and hypochlorhydria. Stool volume is greater than 3 L/d in most patients, and non-anion-gap acidosis usually occurs as a result of bicarbonate losses in the stool. Other electrolyte abnormalities include hypercalcemia (in approximately two-thirds of patients) and hypophosphatemia. Approximately half of patients develop hyperglycemia, which results from hypokalemia- and VIP-induced glycogenolysis in the liver, and a fifth of patients experience cutaneous flushing. Although most symptoms can be reproduced by infusion of exogenous VIP, these tumors also contain other peptide hormones, including the VIP-related peptide histidine-methionine (PHM), somatostatin, helodermin, and neurotensin, each of which may contribute to clinical features exhibited by individual patients. Diagnosis rests on the demonstration of high plasma VIP levels in the setting of a stool volume of at least 1 L/d. Lesser increases in VIP levels occur in patients with hepatic failure and intestinal ischemia.

VIPomas are most commonly pancreatic tumors. Unlike gastrinomas and insulinomas, however, VIPomas frequently grow to a large size before becoming clinically apparent. On average, the size of these tumors at the time of diagnosis is second only to that of nonfunctioning pancreatic islet cell tumors. Although they are slow-growing, these tumors are usually malignant. Approximately three-fifths are metastatic at the time of diagnosis. Most VIPomas are located in the body or tail of the pancreas. A few cases have been seen in association when MEN 1; however, there is no constant relation between the two syndromes. Between 10 and 15 percent of VIP-secreting tumors arise from neuroendocrine cells in the intestinal mucosa, and a few are ganglioneuroblastomas, mastocytomas, pheochromocytomas, or small cell carcinomas of the lung.

Rx TREATMENT

Treatment is surgical extirpation whenever possible. However, metastases may preclude this approach. Preoperative evaluation should include CT or MRI to localize the tumor and any metastases. In addition to supportive therapy with fluids and electrolytes, prednisone is frequently effective in reducing the volume of diarrhea, despite its inability to alter serum VIP levels. Octreotide inhibits the secretion of VIP and ameliorates symptoms in most patients, although most patients eventually become refractory to this agent. VIPomas often produce symptoms related to the large size of the tumor itself. Surgery may be indicated to relieve local effects or to remove a single large primary tumor. For patients with symptomatic metastatic disease, chemotherapy and hepatic artery embolization have the greatest benefit on tumor burden. Regimens combining streptozocin and doxorubicin or streptozocin-fluorouracil are the most effective chemotherapy, inducing objective partial remission in up to 90 percent of cases.

GLUCAGONOMA In 1966, McGovern described a rare syndrome of diabetes mellitus and necrolytic migratory erythema in association with a pancreatic islet cell tumor. The observation that these tumors secrete high levels of glucagon suggested a cause for the diabetes and the possibility that the peptide may have a role in the other clinical features. Although these tumors frequently synthesize and secrete additional peptides, including pancreatic polypeptide, somatostatin, insulin, and gastrin, the common link is hyperglucagonemia. Glucagonomas are characteristically single, large, and slow-growing. More than 75 percent have metastasized at the time of diagnosis, most commonly to the liver and bones. Glucagonoma has been reported in association with MEN 1 (see Chap. 340). A fasting plasma glucagon level of >1000 ng/L (>1000 pg/mL) establishes the diagnosis. More modest elevations of plasma glucagon levels may occur in diabetic ketoacidosis, renal failure, hepatic failure, sepsis, prolonged fasting, and gluten-sensitive enteropathy. Hypocholesterolemia and hypoaminoacidemia are common, with alanine, glycine, and serine levels usually less than 25 percent of normal. Glucagonoma may be distinguished from other hyperglucagonemic syndromes by the failure of glucose to suppress and the failure of arginine to increase serum glucagon concentrations.

The characteristic glucagonoma skin rash (necrolytic migratory erythema) is erythematous, raised, scaly, sometimes bullous, sometimes psoriatic, and ultimately crusted. It is located primarily on the face, abdomen, perineum, and distal extremities. After resolution, the regions of the acute eruption usually remain indurated and hyperpigmented. Patients also may experience glossitis, stomatitis, angular cheilitis, dystrophic nails, and hair thinning. The diabetes is usually mild or asymptomatic and may appear only as an abnormality on an oral glucose tolerance test. Ketoacidosis has not been reported. Weight loss, hypoaminoacidemia, anemia, and thromboembolic disease also occur in association with this syndrome. A causal association between hyperglucagonemia and skin disease has been difficult to prove, leading to speculation that the rash may result from nutritional deficiency. In some patients, the rash responds to oral zinc or to infusions of amino acids or essential fatty acids. Octreotide therapy also has yielded good results. However, dermatologic symptoms frequently recur after each of these therapies.

Because the primary tumor is usually large and found only in the pancreas, it is easily identified by CT, ultrasound, or angiography. Surgical therapy is curative in approximately 30 percent of patients. Resection is more frequently aimed at decreasing tumor burden. Despite occasional objective responses, attempts at chemotherapy with combinations of streptozocin, fluorouracil, doxorubicin, dacarbazine, octreotide, and interferon-alpha have little impact. As for other tumors described in this chapter, hepatic artery embolization, chemoembolization, cryotherapy, and direct instillation of ethanol can provide relief of symptoms. Fortunately, the slow-growing nature of the tumor allows for prolonged survival even in many cases of metastatic disease.

SOMATOSTATINOMA Somatostatin-secreting tumors are the most recent group to be identified with a defined clinical syndrome. The classic triad of somatostatinoma consists of diabetes mellitus, steatorrhea, and cholelithiasis. These symptoms derive from the widespread inhibitory actions of somatostatin, including inhibition of insulin release, pancreatic enzyme and bicarbonate secretion, and gallbladder motility, respectively. The diabetes is usually mild, and, in a few cases, *hypo*glycemia has been seen, perhaps from the concurrent secretion of other peptides. Individual somatostatinomas have been shown to secrete insulin, calcitonin, gastrin, VIP, ACTH, prostaglandins, substance P, motilin, and glucagon. Patients with somatostatinomas also may develop hypochlorhydria, weight loss, and paroxysmal hypertension.

Approximately 60 percent of reported somatostatinomas are located in the pancreas. The second most common site is in the small intestine, although intestinal tumors are associated with lower plasma somatostatin levels and are more commonly asymptomatic. Like glucagonomas and VIPomas, these tumors are usually single, large, and metastatic at the time of diagnosis. Somatostatinomas have not been reported in association with MEN 1. Curiously, the occasional coincidence of pheochromocytoma, café au lait spots, and neurofibromatosis suggests a possible association with MEN type 2b (see Chap. 340). Small cell lung carcinomas, medullary thyroid carcinomas, pheochromocytomas, and paragangliomas that secrete somatostatin also have been described.

MISCELLANEOUS FUNCTIONAL ISLET CELL TUMORS In addition to the diseases described above, islet cell tumors have been associated with several other syndromes of hormone excess, including acromegaly (growth hormone or growth hormone–releasing hormone), hypercalcemia (parathyroid hormone–related peptide), diarrhea and diabetes mellitus (neurotensin), and Cushing's syndrome (corticotropin-releasing factor or ACTH). Secretion by islet cell tumors of ACTH, alone or in combination with other peptides, appears to be a marker of more aggressive disease.

NONFUNCTIONING ISLET CELL TUMORS (See also Chap. 94) More than 15 percent of pancreatic islet cell tumors are not associated with any definable hormone-mediated syndrome. Nonetheless, many of these nonfunctioning islet cell tumors synthesize and secrete one or more regulatory peptides, including pancreatic polypeptide, substance P, and motilin. With increasing availability of radioimmunoassay and immunohistochemical reagents, protein products will probably be defined for more and more of these tumors. Nonetheless, most of these tumors behave in a similar fashion. They arise most commonly in the head or tail of the pancreas and are frequently large (5 to 10 cm in diameter) at the time of diagnosis. The most common clinical manifestations are abdominal pain, jaundice, a palpable mass, malaise, and bleeding esophageal or gastric varices (from splenic vein compression). Though slow-growing, at least half of these tumors present with metastases to the liver or lymph nodes. Surgical cure is achieved in approximately 20 percent. The remainder are poorly responsive to chemotherapy. Streptozocin with or without fluorouracil induces objective responses in approximately 60 percent of patients. Five-year survival for patients with these tumors is approximately 40 percent, with many long-term survivors despite known metastatic disease.

BIBLIOGRAPHY

CARCINOID TUMORS AND SYNDROME

ERICKSSON B, OBERG K: Peptide hormones as tumor markers in neuroendocrine gastrointestinal tumors. Acta Oncol 30:477, 1991

GODWIN JD: Carcinoid tumors: An analysis of 2837 cases. Cancer 36:560, 1975

JOENSUU H et al: Treatment of metastatic carcinoid tumor with recombinant interferon-alpha. Eur J Cancer 28A:1650, 1992

KVOLS LK et al: Treatment of the malignant carcinoid syndrome: Evaluation of a long-acting somatostatin analogue. N Engl J Med 315:663, 1986

MOERTEL CG et al: Carcinoid tumor of the appendix: Treatment and prognosis. N Engl J Med 317:1699, 1987

NORHEIM I et al: Malignant carcinoid tumors: An analysis of 103 patients with regard to tumor localization, hormone production, and survival. Ann Surg 206:115, 1987

PERRY RR, VINIK AI: Endocrine tumors of the gastrointestinal tract. Annu Rev Med 47:57, 1996

RUSNIEWSKI P et al: Treatment of the carcinoid syndrome with the long-acting somatostatin analogue lanreotide. Gut 39:279, 1996

SAINI A, WAXMAN J: Management of carcinoid syndrome. Postgrad Med 67:506, 1991

THORSON A et al: Malignant carcinoid of the small intestine with metastases to the liver, valvular disease of the right side of the heart, peripheral vasomotor symptoms, bronchoconstriction, and an unusual type of cyanosis: A clinical and pathologic syndrome. Am Heart J 47:795, 1954

ISLET CELL TUMORS

BIESMA B et al: Recombinant interferon alpha-2b in patients with metastatic apudomas: Effect on tumors and tumor markers. Br J Cancer 66:850, 1992

BLOOM SR, POLAK JM: Glucagonoma syndrome. Am J Med 82(Suppl 5B):25, 1987

BOSTWICK DG et al: Expression of opioid peptides in tumors. N Engl J Med 317:1439, 1987

GIBRIL F et al: Somatostatin receptor scintigraphy—its sensitivity compared with that of other imaging methods in detecting primary and metastatic gastrinomas. A prospective study. Ann Intern Med 125:26, 1996

GORDEN P et al: Somatostatin and somatostatin analogue (SMS 201-995) in treatment of hormone-secreting tumors of the pituitary and gastrointestinal tract and nonneoplastic diseases of the gut. Ann Intern Med 110:35, 1989

KLEIN S et al: In vivo assessment of the metabolic alterations in glucagonoma syndrome. Metabolism 41:1171, 1992

KREIS GJ: VIPoma syndrome. Am J Med 82(Suppl 5B):37, 1987

KVOLS LK et al: Treatment of metastatic islet cell carcinomas with a somatostatin analogue (SMS 201-995). Ann Intern Med 107:162, 1987

MOERTEL CG et al: Streptozocin-doxorubicin, streptozocin-fluorouracil or chlorozocin in the treatment of advanced islet cell carcinoma. N Engl J Med 326:519, 1992

OBERG K: Neuroendocrine gastrointestinal tumours. Ann Oncol 7:453, 1996

VINIK AI et al: Somatostatinomas, PPomas, neurotensinomas. Semin Oncol 14:263, 1987

WYNICK D et al: Symptomatic secondary hormone syndromes in patients with established malignant pancreatic endocrine tumors. N Engl J Med 319:605, 1988

96   *Howard I. Scher, Robert J. Motzer*

BLADDER AND RENAL CELL CANCER

BLADDER CANCER

Transitional epithelium lines the urinary tract starting at the renal pelvis and extending through the ureter, the urinary bladder, and the proximal two-thirds of the urethra. In the distal third of the urethra, a squamous epithelium is predominant. Carcinomas occur in all four sites, 90 percent developing in the bladder, 8 percent in the renal pelvis, and 2 percent in the ureter or urethra. Once diagnosed, these tumors tend to recur, and serial monitoring of the urothelial tract with cystoscopy and/or urinary cytology is essential. Bladder cancer is the fourth most common cancer in men and the ninth in women, with an estimated 52,900 new cases (38,300 in males and 14,600 in females) and 11,700 deaths (7800 males and 3900 females) predicted for 1996. The median age at diagnosis is 65 years.

EPIDEMIOLOGY The long latency period between exposure to putative carcinogens and the development of the clinical disease makes the establishment of causative links difficult. Nevertheless, estimates are that 25 percent of the cancers in men are related to occupational exposure, and 50 percent to cigarette smoking. Smoking duration is a key element in determining risk, which persists for up to 10 years after smoking cessation. The primary chemical compounds associated with increased risk are the polycyclic aromatic hydrocarbons such as 2-naphthylamine, 4-aminobiphenyl, and benzidine. They are detoxified by acetylation, and slow acetylators have a higher risk of bladder cancer. Individuals involved in the manufacture of aluminum and polychlorinated biphenyls and those who work as chimney sweeps and dry cleaners are also at increased risk. Dietary factors include a high consumption of fried meats and fats, while vitamin A supplements are protective. Chronic cyclophosphamide exposure increases the risk ninefold, while *Schistosoma haematobium* exposure is associated with an increased risk of squamous (70 percent) and transitional cell carcinomas (30 percent).

CLINICAL PRESENTATION, DIAGNOSIS, AND STAGING Hematuria is the first sign of bladder cancer in 80 to 90 percent of patients, followed by urinary frequency or irritative symptoms. Depending on the location of the tumor, ureteral obstruction may result in flank pain or discomfort. Less commonly, symptoms of metastatic disease occur. Screening of asymptomatic subjects for hematuria increases the likelihood that tumors will be diagnosed at an early stage but has not been shown to influence survival. The bladder is the most common source of gross hematuria (~40 percent), but benign cystitis (22 percent) is a more common cause than bladder cancer (15 percent) (see Chap. 48). Microscopic hematuria is more commonly of prostatic origin (25 percent); bladder cancer accounts for this sign in only 2 percent of cases. The evaluation of hematuria or of a suspected bladder tumor requires a urinary cytologic evaluation, visualization of the urothelial tract by sonography or an intravenous pyelogram, and cystoscopy. The endoscopic evaluation involves an examination under anesthesia to determine whether a palpable mass is present. A flexible endoscope is then inserted into the bladder, and the bladder is irrigated to evaluate for the presence of malignant cells. Visualized abnormal areas are biopsied, and an attempt is made to resect all visible tumors. Removal of all tumor is essential for both diagnostic and therapeutic purposes, and a portion of the muscle layer should be included to permit assessment of the depth of invasion of a tumor. As the endoscope is withdrawn, the urethra is inspected. Selective catheterization of the ureters with retrograde examination is used to evaluate for upper tract disease.

Computed tomography (CT) and magnetic resonance imaging (MRI) may assist in distinguishing tumors that extend to the perivesical fat (T3b) or to adjacent structures such as the prostate or vagina (T4) from those that do not (T3a) and in determining whether regional lymph nodes are involved (N +). Neither procedure accurately predicts the depth of invasion within the bladder wall. The presence of distant metastases is assessed by CT of the abdomen, chest x-rays, or radionuclide imaging of the skeleton. The need for these studies is based in part on the local extent of the lesion.

Staging follows the TNM (tumor, nodes, metastasis) staging system, which accounts for growth patterns observed clinically (Fig. 96-1). In general, tumors of stage T1 or below are managed by endoscopic means initially, while for those that invade muscle, surgical removal of the bladder is considered standard therapy.

PATHOLOGY In North America, 90 to 95 percent of bladder tumors are transitional; pure squamous tumors (with keratinization) make up 3 percent; adenocarcinomas, 2 percent; and small cell tumors (with paraneoplastic syndromes), <1 percent. Adenocarcinomas develop in the dome of the bladder in the urachal remnant or in the periurethral tissues. Some assume a signet cell histology. Lymphomas or melanomas are rare. Overall, 75 percent of tumors present as superficial lesions, 20 percent have muscle invasion, and in 5 percent there is metastatic disease. Among superficial lesions, the most frequent histologic subtype of transitional cell tumors is a low-grade papillary lesion that grows on a central stalk. These lesions are very friable, have a tendency to bleed, and have a high risk of recurrence. They rarely progress to the more lethal invasive variety. In contrast, carcinoma in situ (CIS) is a high-grade tumor and is believed to be the precursor of muscle-invasive disease. In other cases, the tumor invades directly and assumes a solid growth pattern.

Histologic grade provides prognostic information. Grade I lesions (highly differentiated tumors) rarely progress to a higher stage. In contrast, a Ta grade III tumor has a higher risk of progression to a more advanced stage. The risk of recurrence in the primary and distant sites correlates with lesion size, number of lesions, growth pattern, the presence of disease in the prostatic urethra or of carcinoma in situ in other sites, and the presence of hydronephrosis.

PATHOGENESIS Molecular genetic analyses of tumors of defined stage and grade have shown a number of *primary chromosomal aberrations* that are associated with tumor *development*, and *secondary abnormalities* that are related to *progression* to a more advanced stage. Evolving data suggest that superficial tumors that tend to recur but not invade and those that tend to invade and to metastasize result from distinct genetic defects (Table 96-1). Alterations on the long arm of chromosome 13, including those that affect the retinoblastoma gene locus on 13q14, occur more often in muscle-invasive than in non-muscle-invading tumors. Deletions of 17p (the *p53* locus), 18q (the *DCC* locus), and the *RB* gene are more frequent in invasive lesions, while 9q deletions appear to be an early event, given their high frequency in Ta and T1 recurring lesions. 3p and 5q deletions are more prevalent in invasive tumors but absent in superficial lesions. Patients with invasive disease whose tumors lack the *RB* gene have a poorer survival than those with *RB*-positive lesions. Similarly, *p53* overexpression is associated with a higher frequency of progression to a more advanced stage and a higher rate of death from bladder cancer for patients with Ta, T1, and CIS disease. In addition to the functional loss of tumor suppressor genes, bladder cancers often overexpress the epidermal growth factor receptor and the related receptor tyrosine kinase, HER-2/neu. Activating mutations of oncogenes (e.g., *ras*) are rare.

℞ TREATMENT

The choice of treatment is based on disease extent: superficial, invasive, or metastatic. Superficial tumors are treated by endoscopic resection with or without intravesical therapy. Once invasive disease is documented, the standard treatment is surgical removal of the bladder. Based on pathologic findings at surgery, systemic chemotherapy may or may not be advised. Combination chemotherapy is used to treat metastatic disease.

Superficial Disease Intravesical therapy is used to eliminate existing disease or more commonly as an adjuvant or as prophylaxis to prevent recurrence following endoscopic resection. Although transurethral resection is effective at completely eradicating disease in 80 percent of cases, 30 to 80 percent of patients develop recurrent disease, and grade and stage progression occurs in up to 30 percent. Indications for intravesical therapy vary, but treatment is generally advised for patients with four or more recurrences in a given year, involvement of more than 40 percent of the bladder surface by tumor, diffuse CIS, or T1 disease. Administration of the immune adjuvant bacillus Calmette-Guérin (BCG) is considered the standard therapy, but efficacy has also been observed for several chemotherapeutic agents including doxorubicin and mitomycin C. BCG reduces recurrence rates by 40 to 45 percent, compared to 8 to 18 percent for drug instillation. The most frequent symptoms of toxicity associated with intravesical therapy include bladder irritation, frequency, dysuria, and contact dermatitis (from mitomycin C). In rare cases, BCG treatment can result in a systemic infection that requires antituberculin therapy. Significant BCG toxicities occur in fewer than 6 percent of patients.

After an initial course of treatment, the patient is reevaluated at 3-month intervals to ensure that no recurrence has developed. Those with persistent or new tumors may be considered for more aggressive management including cystectomy. Recurrence may also occur in extravesical sites along the urothelial tract, including the distal ureter and/or urethra, supporting the concept of a "field change" in bladder carcinogenesis.

Muscle-Infiltrating Tumors Once a tumor involves muscle, the standard treatment is surgical removal of the entire organ by radical cystectomy. In 5 to 10 percent of cases, the tumor occurs in a location where only a partial cystectomy is required. Rarely, a transurethral resection alone is used. In males, radical cystectomy involves the removal of the bladder, prostate, seminal vesicles, proximal vas deferens, and proximal urethra, with a margin of adipose tissue and peritoneum. If the nervi errigentes, which are responsible for erectile capacity, are preserved, erectile function can be recovered. In females, the resection includes removal of the bladder, urethra, uterus, fallopian tubes, ovaries, anterior vaginal wall, and surrounding fascia. Grossly abnormal lymph nodes are sampled by frozen section. If spread is confirmed, the cystectomy is aborted unless a urinary diversion is required to relieve symptoms. This operation constitutes major surgery, and appropriate medical clearance is required.

Urinary flow is directed through a conduit diversion to the skin (Bricker procedure), or a low-pressure internal reservoir is created using a detubularized bowel segment and anastamosed to the skin

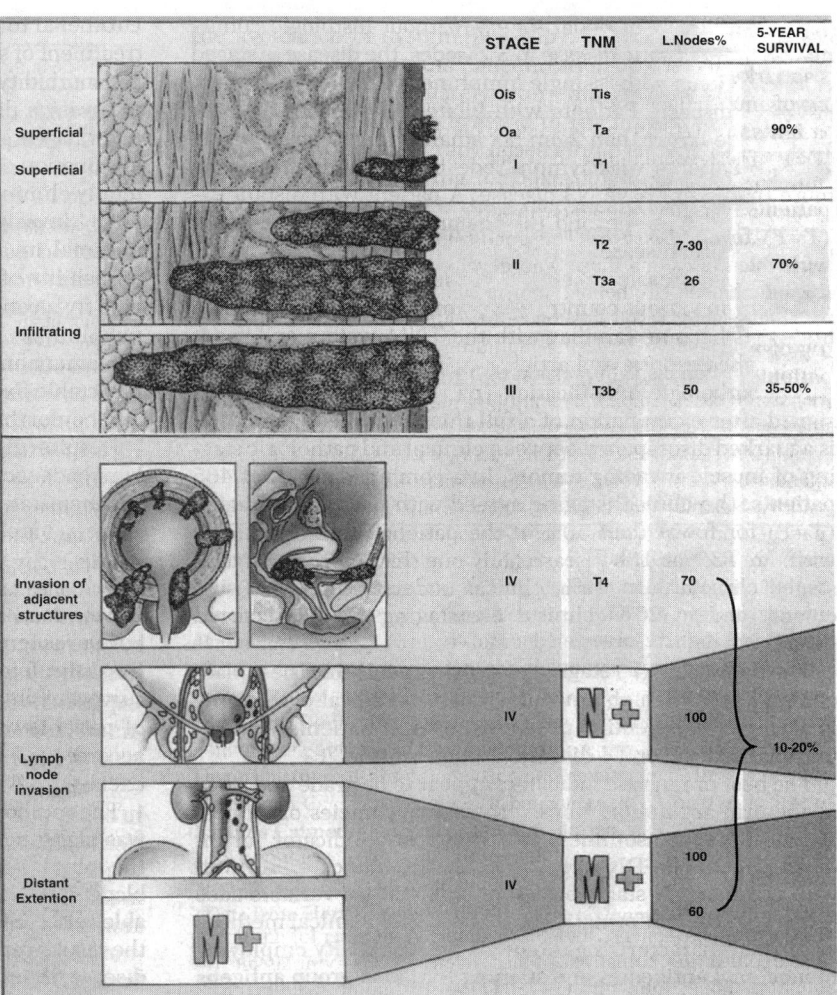

FIGURE 96-1 Clinical classification of the bladder. [Modified from WR Fair et al, Cancer of the bladder, in *Cancer: Principles and Practice of Oncology*, 4th ed, VT DeVita, Jr., et al (eds): Philadelphia, Lippincott, 1993].

(Koch pouch) or the urethra (Mainz or Indiana pouch). When an anastomosis to the urethra is created, the patient can void in a normal fashion. Reservoirs attached to the skin require intermittent catheterization. Contraindications to a continent reservoir include the presence of carcinoma in the prostatic urethra. An ileal conduit is the most widely used. A syndrome characterized by hypochloremic acidosis, hyperkalemia, hyponatremia, and uremia has been described when a segment of jejunum is used. Concurrent diseases in the bowel, such as ulcerative colitis or Crohn's disease, preclude the use of resected bowel.

The 5-year survival rate varies inversely with the depth of invasion and lymph node status. The 5-year survival rate is 70 percent for those with T2/3a (stage II) disese and 50 percent for those with T3b disese with no positive nodes, up to 35 percent for those with one node positive, and 10 percent for those with six or more positive

Table 96-1

Molecular Genetic Defects in Bladder Cancer

Chromosome Abnormality	Frequency, %	Phenotype
Loss of part or all of chromosome 9	55	Superficial recurrent
17p deletion ($\pm p53$ mutation)	40	Invasive
11p deletion	40	Invasive
13q deletion	20	Invasive

SOURCE: From Gordon-Cardo et al, with permission.

593

nodes. The influence of depth of invasion on survival after surgery is shown in Table 96-2. In some countries, external-beam radiation therapy is standard, but in the United States it is generalaly reserved for patients who are not suitable candidates for cystectomy. The 5-year survival after treatment with 5000 to 7000 cGy is 30 to 45 percent.

Metastatic Disease This cohort includes patients who present with metastases and those who develop metastases after definitive local treatment. Urothelial tumors are chemosensitive, and a number of single agents result in short-term regressions in 20 to 30 percent of cases (Table 96-3). Using multidrug combinations, in particular those based on cisplatin, responses have been observed in up to 70 percent of cases, and 20 percent of these responses are complete. On the basis of randomized trials, the M-VAC regimen [methotrexate, vinblastine, doxorubicin (Adriamycin), and cisplatin] is considered standard. Alternatively, a CMV regimen (cisplatin, methotrexate, and vinblastine) can be used. In general, a higher proportion of patients with only lymph node involvement than patients with metastases to visceral sites or to bone is rendered tumor-free. Patients with adverse features, such as a compromised performance status, visceral disease, or bone metastases, are rarely cured with chemotherapy alone. In these cases, median survival rarely exceeds 6 months, and the toxicities of treatment are significant. Long-term survival has been reported in 10 to 15 percent of patients with metastatic disease and in 20 to 25 percent of patients with unresectable nodal disease at presentation. Approximately 20 to 40 percent of patients develop neutropenic fever due to hematologic toxicity. Mucositis occurs in 10 to 20 percent, and a decrease in renal and auditory function as well as a peripheral neuropathy may be seen. Alopecia is universal; fatigue can be dose-limiting in some cases. For patients who relapse after first-line chemotherapy, activity has been seen with gallium nitrate, ifosfamide, gemcitabine, 5-fluorouracil-based combination regimens, and the taxanes. A number of groups are also exploring combinations of these agents (VIG—vinblastine, ifosfamide, and gallium nitrate—or ITP—ifosfamide, paclitaxel, and cisplatin) as initial treatment.

Chemotherapy for Invasive Disease Chemotherapy has also been integrated into the management of invasive bladder tumors either before (neoadjuvant) or after (adjuvant) definitive local therapy for patients with a high risk of metastases. It has also been used either alone or as part of combined-modality treatment with radiation therapy, with the aim of bladder preservation. Nonrandomized phase II trials have shown that the proportion of bladders rendered free of tumor varies inversely with T stage, with cumulative proportions in the range of 20 to 25 percent when the bladder is removed and examined pathologically. No survival benefit has been proved yet using a neoadjuvant approach.

An alternative approach preferred by many physicians is the removal of the bladder followed by a decision to use or omit chemotherapy based on the pathologic findings at surgery. Indications for chemotherapy include a finding of nodal disease, extravesical tumor extension, or vascular invasion in the resected specimen. Several trials, both nonrandomized and randomized, suggest a survival benefit using this approach. Most compare a policy of surgery followed by immediate chemotherapy (usually four cycles) with surgery followed by chemotherapy at the time of recurrence. None is definitive, however, because not enough patients have been enrolled and treated.

Table 96-2

Survival Relative to Pathologic Stage

5-Year Survival, %, for Stage:			
P2	**P3a**	**P3b**	**N+**
62–83	50–74	15–57	4–35

SOURCE: Modified from H Scher et al, *Principles and Practice of Oncology*, 5th ed, VT DeVita et al (eds). Philadelphia, Lippincott, 1997.

Table 96-3

Selected Single Agents with Activity in Urothelial Tract Malignancies

Agent	No. Responding/ No. Treated	Percent Responding	95% Confidence Interval, %
Cisplatin	200/706	28	26–32
Methrotrexate	8/236	45	37–50
Doxorubicin	47/274	17	13–22
Vinblastine	6/38	16	4–28
Ifosfamide	28/101	28	19–37
Gallium nitrate	9/29	29	13–45
Paclitaxel	11/26	42	23–61

Bladder Preservation Several groups are investigating bladder-sparing strategies. Most use a treatment policy that includes an aggressive transurethral resection followed by systemic chemotherapy either alone or in combination with external beam radiation therapy. The decision to leave the bladder in situ is based on the posttherapy assessment of response. A trial performed by Kaufman and colleagues involved giving two cycles of CMV and 4000 cGy of external beam radiation therapy with concurrent cisplatin. Patients with nonresponsive tumors were referred for cystectomy. After 4 years of follow-up, 45 percent of patients were alive with no evidence of disease. While these results, and those of others, show that bladder preservation is feasible in selected cases, any bladder left in situ must be monitored continuously for the development of new tumors. This approach should be undertaken with the caveat that survival equivalent to that achieved with the standard approach has not yet been proved. Quality of life is better with bladder preservation.

RENAL CELL CARCINOMA

Renal cell carcinoma accounts for 90 to 95 percent of malignant neoplasms arising from the kidney. Notable features include refractoriness to cytotoxic agents, infrequent but reproducible responses to biologic response modifiers such as interferon α and interleukin (IL) 2, and a variable clinical course for patients with metastatic disease, including anecdotal reports of spontaneous regression.

EPIDEMIOLOGY AND ETIOLOGY The incidence of renal cell carcinoma in the United States in 1996 was 30,600 cases (18,500 male; 12,100 female); the disease caused 12,000 deaths. The incidence peaks between the ages of 50 and 70, although this malignancy may be diagnosed at any age. Many environmental factors have been investigated as possible causal factors. The strongest associations are with cigarette smoking (accounting for as many as 20 to 30 percent of cases) and obesity. The risk of renal cell carcinoma is increased in patients who have acquired cystic disease of the kidney associated with end-stage renal disease.

Most cases are sporadic, although two familial forms have been reported: a rare form with autosomal dominant inheritance, and a form associated with von Hippel-Lindau syndrome. Nearly 35 percent of patients with von Hippel-Lindau disease develop renal cell cancers. An increased incidence has also been reported in patients with tuberous sclerosis and polycystic kidney disease.

Most of these cancers arise from the epithelical cells of the proximal tubules. A number of genetic alterations have been described, of which abnormalities on chromosome 3 are most frequent. A 3;8 translocation was first described in a pedigree of patients with the familial form of the disease, while deletions in 3p21-26 have been identified in familial as well as sporadic tumors. More recently, the gene for von Hippel-Lindau disease on chromosome 3p was cloned, and von Hippel-Lindau mutations can be identified in nearly 60 percent of sporadic, nonpapillary renal cell cancers and associated cell lines.

PATHOLOGY AND GENETICS In the past, renal cell cancers were grouped by cell type (clear, granular, oncocytic, and spindle) and growth pattern (acinar, sarcomatoid, and tubulopapillary). This

Table 96-4

CHAPTER 96
Bladder and Renal Cell Cancer

595

Signs and Symptoms in Patients with Renal Cell Cancer

Presenting Sign or Symptom	Incidence, %
Classic triad: hematuria, flank pain, flank mass	10–20
Hematuria	40
Flank pain	40
Palpable mass	25
Weight loss	33
Anemia	33
Fever	20
Hypertension	20
Abnormal liver function	15
Hypercalcemia	5
Erythrocytosis	3
Neuromyopathy	3
Amyloidosis	2
Increased erythrocyte sedimentation rate	55

schema has been abandoned because most tumors proved to contain mixtures of cell types and patterns. A current classification scheme based on the results of immunohistochemical and genetic studies consists of five variants: clear cell tumors, representing 75 percent of cases; chromophilic tumors (15 percent); chromophobic tumors (5 percent); oncocytic tumors (3 percent); and collecting duct or Bellini duct tumors (2 percent). Clear cell tumors are characterized by tumor cells with clear cytoplasm, which consistently show a 3p deletion. Chromophilic tumors, previously termed *tubulopapillary*, tend to be bilateral and multifocal. Trisomy 7 and/or trisomy 17 are the most frequent genetic abnormalities. Chromophobic tumors are characterized by multiple chromosomal losses but do not exhibit 3p deletions and have a more indolent clinical course. Similarly, oncocytomas have a characteristic morphology including a deeply eosinophilic cytoplasm, do not exhibit 3p deletions or trisomy 7 or 17, and rarely metastasize. In contrast, Bellini duct carcinomas are very rare and are believed to arise from the collecting ducts in the renal medulla. They tend to affect younger patients and have a very aggressive clinical course.

CLINICAL PRESENTATION

The presenting signs and symptoms include hematuria, abdominal pain, and a flank or abdominal mass. This classic triad occurs in 10 to 20 percent of patients. Other symptoms are fever, weight loss, anemia, and a varicocele; the tumor may also be found incidentally on a radiograph. A spectrum of paraneoplastic syndromes has been associated with these malignancies, including erythrocytosis, hypercalcemia, nonmetastatic hepatic dysfunction (Stauffers' syndrome), and acquired dysfibrinogenemia. Erythrocytosis is present at presentation in only about 3 percent of patients. More frequently, anemia, a sign of advanced disease, is reported (Table 96-4).

The standard evaluation of patients with suspected renal cell tumors includes an intravenous pyelogram (IVP), ultrasonography, CT of the abdomen and pelvis, a chest radiograph, urine analysis, and urine cytology (Fig. 96-2). CT of the chest is warranted if metastatic disease is suspected from the chest ra-

diograph, as it will detect significantly smaller lesions, and their presence may influence the approach to the primary tumor. MRI is useful in evaluating the status of the inferior vena cava in cases of suspected tumor involvement or invasion by thrombus, as well as for patients in whom iodinated contrast cannot be administered owing to either allergy or renal dysfunction. In clinical practice, any solid renal mass should be considered malignant until proven otherwise and requires a definitive diagnosis. If no metastases are demonstrated, surgery is indicated, even if there is invasion of the renal vein. The differential diagnosis of a renal mass includes cysts, benign neoplasms (adenoma, angiomyolipoma, oncocytoma), inflammatory lesions (pyelonephritis or abscesses), and other primary or metastatic malignant neoplasms. Other malignancies that may involve the kidney include transitional cell carcinoma of the renal pelvis, sarcoma, lymphoma, Wilms's tumor, and metastatic disease, especially from melanoma primaries. All of these are less common as kidney malignancies than is renal cell carcinoma.

STAGING AND PROGNOSIS The most widely used staging system in the United States is that developed by Robson. In this schema, stage I tumors are confined to the kidney; stage II tumors extend through the renal capsule but are confined by Gerota's fascia; stage III tumors involve the renal vein or vena cava (stage IIIA) or the hilar lymph nodes (stage IIIB); and stage IV disease includes tumors that are locally invasive to adjacent organs (excluding the adrenal gland) or distant metastases. Five-year survival varies by stage: 66 percent for stage I, 64 percent for stage II, 42 percent for stage

FIGURE 96-2 Standard evaluation of patients with suspected renal cell tumors.

III, and 11 percent for stage IV. The prognosis for stage IIIA lesions is similar to that for stage I or II disease, whereas the 5-year survival for stage IIIB lesions is only 20 percent, closer to that for stage IV tumors.

℞ **TREATMENT**

Localized Disease The standard management for stage I or II tumors and selected cases of stage III disease is radical nephrectomy. This procedure involves en bloc removal of Gerota's fascia and its contents, including the kidney, the ipsilateral adrenal gland, and adjacent hilar lymph nodes. The role of a regional lymphadenectomy is controversial. For patients with stage IIIA disease, the tumor should be resected from the renal vein or vena cava.

In selected patients who have only one kidney, and depending on the size and location of the lesion, a partial nephrectomy may be performed. Partial nephrectomy may also be performed in patients with bilateral tumors, accompanied by a radical nephrectomy on the opposite side. There is no proven role for adjuvant chemotherapy, immunotherapy, or radiation therapy following successful surgical removal of the tumor, even in cases with a poor prognosis.

Advanced Disease Metastatic renal cell carcinoma, for which there is no effective therapy, is associated with a dismal survival. A number of options have been explored, including hormonal therapy, chemotherapy (with cytotoxic agents), and immunotherapy. Responses to hormonal therapy (progestins) are rare (1 to 2 percent) and of short duration. No chemotherapy agent has been shown consistently to produce objective tumor regressions in >20 percent of patients. As a result, investigational agents in phase II trials are offered as first-line therapy.

Two biologic agents, interferon α and IL-2, have been studied extensively for the treatment of advanced disease. Both reproducibly produce a response in 10 to 20 percent of patients; in fewer than 5 percent of patients is the response durable. It was the observation of occasional durable complete remissions that resulted in approval by the Food and Drug Administration of IL-2 as a treatment for this disease. IL-2 is usually administered as a 24-h infusion of 18 MU/m^2 per day for 5 to 7 days. Toxicities from IL-2 include a capillary leakage syndrome, fever, chills, fatigue, and hypotension.

Surgery in the Setting of Metastases Nephrectomy may be indicated in highly selected cases for the alleviation of symptoms such as pain or recurrent urinary hemorrhage, particularly if the latter is severe or associated with obstruction. Some physicians advocate the performance of a nephrectomy in the presence of metastases in the hope either that a spontaneous regression will occur or that the sensitivity to a cytokine will be increased. In fact, the observed frequency of spontaneous regression, 0.8 percent, coupled with the morbidity and mortality of the procedure itself, does not justify the approach. Similarly, no data show a difference in response rates to a biologic agent depending on whether the primary is in place or has been removed. Removal of the primary as an adjunct to treatment with a biologic agent thus should not be considered standard practice.

In contrast, there are reports of long-term survival at rates of 15 to 50 percent for patients undergoing surgery who present with primary disease plus a solitary metastatic lesion or who relapse with a solitary lesion after nephrectomy and a long disease-free interval. Because renal cell tumors are radioresistant, surgical resection is also advised for palliation of solitary central nervous system metastases, repair of actual or impending pathologic fractures in weight-bearing bones, or relief of spinal cord compression. For the latter problem, resection should be considered before radiation.

Observation Alone Renal cell carcinoma is one of several malignancies in which spontaneous regressions have been reported anecdotally. A more frequent occurrence is prolonged periods of stable disease; up to 10 percent of patients with metastatic disease may show no progression for >12 months. Because responses to systemic therapy are uncommon and all systemic therapies are associated with treatment-related toxicity, an option for management in asymptomatic patients with metastases is close observation until disease progression or symptoms occur, at which time appropriate therapy is initiated.

CARCINOMA OF THE RENAL PELVIS AND URETER

About 500 cases of renal pelvis and ureter cancer occur each year, and over 90 percent are transitional cell carcinomas similar to bladder cancer in appearance. Smoking is a risk factor, as is chemical and hydrocarbon exposure. This tumor is also associated with chronic phenacetin abuse and with Balkan nephropathy, a chronic interstitial nephritis endemic in Bulgaria, Greece, Bosnia-Herzegovina, and Romania.

The most common symptom is painless gross hematuria, and the disease usually is detected on IVP during the workup for hematuria. Patterns of spread are like those in bladder cancer. For disease localized to the renal pelvis and ureter, nephroureterectomy (including excision of the distal ureter with a portion of the bladder) is associated with a 5-year survival rate of 80 to 90 percent for low-grade lesions. More invasive or histologically less well differentiated tumors are more likely to recur locally and metastasize. Metastatic disease is treated with M-VAC or CMV chemotherapy. The outcome is similar to that for metastatic transitional cell carcinoma of bladder origin.

BIBLIOGRAPHY

CORDON-CARDO C et al: Genetic alterations associated with bladder cancer, in *Important Advances in Oncology*, DeVita VT et al (eds). Philadelphia, Lippincott, 1994, pp 71–84

HERR HW et al: Intravesical Bacillus Calmette-Guerin therapy prevents tumor progression and death from superficial bladder cancer: Ten-year follow-up of a prospective randomized trial. J Clin Oncol 13:1404, 1995

MARTINS FE et al: Options in replacement cystoplasty following radical cystectomy: High hopes or successful reality. J Urol 153:1363, 1995

MINASIAN LM et al: Interferon alfa-2a in advanced renal cell carcinoma: Treatment results and survival in 159 patients with long-term follow-up. J Clin Oncol 11:1368, 1993

MOTZER RJ et al: Renal cell carcinoma. N Engl J Med 335:865, 1996

ROBSON CJ et al: The results of radical nephrectomy for renal cell carcinoma. J Urol 101:297, 1969

ROSENBERG SA et al: Treatment of 283 consecutive patients with metastatic melanoma or renal cell cancer using high dose bolus intravenous interleukin-2. JAMA 271:907, 1994

SCHER HI, NORTON L: Chemotherapy for urothelial tract malignancies: Breaking the deadlock. Semin Surg Oncol 8:316, 1992

SHUIN T et al: Frequent somatic mutations and loss of heterozygosity of the von Hippel-Lindau tumor suppressor gene in primary human renal cell carcinomas. Cancer Res 54:2852, 1994

STADLER W, VOGELZANG N (eds): Bladder cancer. Semin Oncol 23:533, 1996

VINEIS P et al: Molecular epidemiology of bladder cancer: Known chemical causes of bladder cancer: Occupation and smoking. Urol Oncol 1:137, 1995

97 *Arthur I. Sagalowsky, Jean D. Wilson*

HYPERPLASIA AND CARCINOMA OF THE PROSTATE

PROSTATIC HYPERPLASIA

Development of prostatic hyperplasia is an almost universal phenomenon in aging men. The prostate weighs only a few grams at birth; at puberty it undergoes androgen-mediated growth and reaches the adult size of about 20 g by age 20. It remains stable in size for about 25 years, and during the fifth decade a second growth spurt commences in the majority of men. Consequently, the disorder affects men over the age of 45 and increases in frequency with age so that by the eighth decade more than 90 percent of men have prostatic hyperplasia at autopsy. Because of the development of effective therapies the disorder is not a major cause of death, but it continues to be a leading cause of morbidity in elderly men. The prostate surrounds the urethra, and prostatic hyperplasia is the most common cause of obstruction to urinary outflow in men. The disorder occurs in all populations but may be less common in the Orient. The mean age for development of symptomatic disease is about 65 years for whites and about 60 years for blacks. It is not clear whether prostatic hyperplasia predisposes to the development of prostatic cancer.

PATHOGENESIS Unlike the pubertal growth spurt which involves the gland diffusely, prostatic hyperplasia begins in the periurethral region as a localized proliferation and progresses to compress the remaining normal gland. Histologically, the hyperplastic tissue is nodular and composed of varying amounts of glandular epithelium, stroma, and smooth muscle. The hyperplasia can compress and obstruct the urethra; the hyperplastic gland can also grow posteriorly to obstruct the rectum and cause constipation.

The pathogenesis is not well understood, but two necessary features for the process are aging and the presence of testes; whether the testes play a direct or permissive role is not known, but the active androgen that mediates prostatic growth at all ages is dihydrotestosterone, which is formed within the prostate from plasma testosterone (see Chap. 336). In the castrated dog, hormone replacement that increases dihydrotestosterone levels in the prostate causes prostatic enlargement comparable with that seen in spontaneous canine prostatic hyperplasia. Estradiol levels in men increase with age (absolutely or relative to testosterone levels), and in dogs estrogen acts synergistically with dihydrotestosterone to induce prostatic growth by enhancing the amount of androgen receptor protein in the tissue. Consequently, the role of aging in human prostatic hyperplasia might be due, at least in part, to the augmentation of dihydrotestosterone action by estrogen.

DIAGNOSIS Urethral obstruction results from the elongation, tortuosity, and compression of the posterior urethra, but there is no straightforward relationship between obstruction and prostate size or between symptoms and obstruction. Indeed, severe obstruction can occur when the hyperplasia has not yet caused an increase in the size of the normal gland, and some men with very large prostates are asymptomatic. Early symptoms can be minimal because compensatory hypertrophy of the detrusor musculature of the bladder can compensate for the resistance to urine flow. With increasing obstruction, diminution in the caliber and force of the urinary stream, hesitancy in initiating voiding, postvoiding dribbling, the sensation of incomplete emptying,

and on occasion urinary retention supervene. These *obstructive* symptoms must be distinguished from *irritative* symptoms such as dysuria, frequency, and urgency that also can result from inflammatory, infectious, or neoplastic causes. As the amount of residual urine increases, nocturia, overflow urinary incontinence, and a palpable bladder may be present. Eventually, the manifestations of chronic urinary retention and obstruction supervene, or acute urinary retention can be precipitated by infection, tranquilizing drugs, antihistamines, or alcohol. On occasion, profound obstruction can be compensated to the extent that symptoms are minimal or absent, and patients present with obstructive uropathy.

The natural history of this disorder is poorly understood, but it is clear that the majority of men with prostatic enlargement never develop significant obstruction and that in many men minor irritative and/or obstructive symptoms do not progress or progress very slowly. Consequently, it is not always clear when in the course to intervene, but increased size alone is not a valid reason to treat.

In the evaluation of the patient with prostatism a detailed *history* should focus on the urinary tract to identify other causes of voiding dysfunction. For quantification of symptoms the preferred questionnaire is the self-administered *AUA Symptom Index* in which the symptoms can be classified as mild, moderate, or severe on the basis of seven questions (Table 97-1). This index is useful in planning and in follow-up. On *digital rectal examination* (DRE), the prostate should be characterized with regard to size, consistency, and shape. Hyperplasia commonly produces a smooth, firm, elastic enlargement, but obstruction can occur in the absence of abnormalities on DRE. The measurement of prostate-specific antigen (PSA) is useful for excluding the diagnosis of advanced prostatic cancer, but the test does not discriminate between prostatic hyperplasia and early prostate cancer (see below). Several additional diagnostic tests are available, but it is not established whether any of them is of value in predicting the results of treatment. Such tests include *uroflowmetry*, which can identify those patients whose maximum flows are normal and who are unlikely to benefit from treatment; measurement of *postvoid residual urine volume*, which, although poorly reproducible in an individual patient, identifies those patients with a greater likelihood of failing a watchful-waiting strategy; *pressure-flow studies*, which are particularly helpful in patients at risk for primary bladder dysfunction; and *urethrocystoscopy*, which is of use in some patients before invasive treatment and

Table 97-1

AUA Symptom Index

Questions To Be Answered	Not at All	Less Than 1 Time in 5	Less Than Half the Time	About Half the Time	More Than Half the Time	Almost Always
			AUA Symptom Score (Circle 1 Number on Each Line)			
Over the past month, how often have you had a sensation of not emptying your bladder completely after you finished urinating?	0	1	2	3	4	5
Over the past month, how often have you had to urinate again less than 2 h after you finished urinating?	0	1	2	3	4	5
Over the past month, how often have you found you stopped and started again several times when you urinated?	0	1	2	3	4	5
Over the past month, how often have you found it difficult to postpone urination?	0	1	2	3	4	5
Over the past month, how often have you had a weak urinary stream?	0	1	2	3	4	5
Over the past month, how often have you had to push or strain to begin urination?	0	1	2	3	4	5
Over the past month, how many times did you most typically get up to urinate from the time you went to bed at night until the time you got up in the morning?	0 (None)	1 (1 time)	2 (2 times)	3 (3 times)	4 (4 times)	5 (5 times or more)

Sum of 7 circled numbers (AUA Symptom Score): _____

SOURCE: Barry, Fowler, O'Leary, et al. The American Urological Association symptom index for benign prostatic hyperplasia. J Urol 148:1549, 1992. Used with permission.

when there is some specific indication such as hematuria. Imaging of the upper urinary tract by ultrasonography or intravenous pyelography should be reserved for patients with indications such as hematuria, a history of stones, or prior urinary tract problems.

℞ TREATMENT

Asymptomatic patients with prostate enlargement generally do not require treatment. Those patients with specific complications of prostatic hyperplasia (inability to urinate, renal insufficiency, urinary tract infection, hematuria, or bladder stones) are clear candidates for prostate surgery. All other patients should, in consultation with their physician, decide on treatment based on the degree of incapacity and/or discomfort present and a consideration of the likely outcome of each potential treatment strategy. A variety of decision diagrams have been proposed for aiding physicians and patients in making decisions about the most appropriate management strategy, but ultimately the decision depends on the severity of symptoms and the patient's expectations and acceptance of the risks of treatment.

Watchful Waiting Watchful waiting is appropriate for most patients because the probability of disease progression or the development of complications is unknown. These patients should be monitored at least annually by reassessment of symptoms and clinical manifestations.

Medical Therapy Finasteride, a competitive inhibitor of the 5α-reductase enzyme, blocks the conversion of testosterone to dihydrotestosterone, the principal androgen in the prostate. In a dose of 5 mg/d by mouth the drug causes an average decrease in prostate size of around 24 percent, an increase in urine flow rates, and, in some, improvement in symptoms. Long-term efficacy has not been documented, but improvement is known to be sustained for as long as 3 years provided the therapy is continued. Patients who respond to this regimen may elect to continue indefinitely, and those whose symptoms are bothersome and do not improve or worsen are appropriate candidates for surgery. What is not clear is how to manage the half of patients whose symptoms do not change; indirect evidence suggests that the therapy halts the progression of the disease, but this is not proven. Alpha₁-adrenergic blockers such as terazosin relax smooth muscle of the bladder neck and cause an increase in peak urinary flow rate and a perceptible reduction in symptoms. However, there is no reason to expect that such agents will influence the progression of the disease.

Surgery Prostate surgery offers the best chance for improvement in symptoms but also has the highest rate of significant complications. Transurethral resection of the prostate is the most common surgical procedure. Transurethral incision of the prostate is of similar efficacy in men with relatively small prostates and can be performed in ambulatory settings. Open prostatectomy is usually reserved for men with massive prostates and may employ retropubic, suprapubic, or perineal approaches. Given proper patient selection, benefits are probably equivalent with each procedure, but complication rates differ. Open prostatectomy has a greater incisional morbidity and longer recovery time and a greater risk for impotence. Transurethral incision has the lowest morbidity and lowest rates of ejaculatory disturbances. Surgery is the appropriate initial therapy in many patients and appropriate as the second line of therapy for others who fail to respond to medical treatment or worsen with watchful waiting, but it should not be recommended on the grounds that surgical risk will increase with age. New technologies under evaluation include laser therapy, coils, stents, thermal therapy, and hyperthermia.

PROSTATIC CARCINOMA

Cancer of the prostate is the most common malignancy in men in the United States and the third most common cause of cancer death in men above age 55 (after carcinomas of the lung and colon). In the United States there are approximately 317,000 newly diagnosed cases

and more than 41,000 deaths from the disorder each year. Only about a third of cases identified at autopsy are manifest clinically. The disease is rare before age 50, and the incidence increases with age. The frequency varies in different parts of the world. The United States has 14 deaths per 100,000 men per year, compared with 22 for Sweden and 2 for Japan. However, Japanese immigrants to the United States develop prostatic cancer at a frequency similar to other men in this country, suggesting that environmental factors are the principal cause for population differences. The disease is more common among American blacks than whites; the reason for this difference is not known.

CLASSIFICATION Some carcinomas of the prostate are slow-growing and may persist for long periods without causing significant symptoms, whereas others behave aggressively. It is not known whether tumors can become more malignant with time. Insight into the natural history of a given tumor is provided by careful histopathologic grading, surgical evaluation of the pelvic lymph nodes, and measurement of the primary lesion, a size less than 1.5 mL in volume carrying a good prognosis.

Histologic Grading Over 95 percent of prostatic cancers are adenocarcinomas that arise in the prostatic acini. Adenocarcinoma may begin anywhere in the prostate but, in contrast to hyperplasia, has a predilection for the periphery. The tumors are frequently multifocal. Variability in cellular size, nuclear and nucleolar shape, glandular differentiation, and the content of acid phosphatase and mucin may occur within a single specimen, but the most poorly differentiated area of tumor (i.e., the area with the highest histologic grade) appears to determine its biologic behavior. In the Gleason grading scheme, the dominant and secondary glandular histologic patterns are independently assigned numbers from 1 to 5 (best to least differentiated), and these numbers are summed to give a total score of 2 to 10 for each tumor. Such grading is reproducible and correlates with the course of the disease and with patient survival.

The remaining prostatic cancers are divided among squamous cell and transitional cell carcinomas that arise in the prostatic ducts, carcinoma of the prostatic utricle (a müllerian duct remnant), carcinosarcomas that arise in the mesenchymal elements of the gland, and occasional metastatic tumors (usually carcinoma of the lung, melanoma, or lymphoma). These tumors will not be considered further.

DIAGNOSIS Symptoms and Signs Both early and advanced carcinoma of the prostate may be asymptomatic at the time of diagnosis, and in the past more than 80 percent of patients had locally advanced or metastatic disease at the time of diagnosis (see below). In symptomatic subjects, common presenting complaints (in descending order) include dysuria, difficulty in voiding, increased urinary frequency, complete urinary retention, back or hip pain, and hematuria. A high index of suspicion should be entertained in all men over age 40 with dysuria, frequency, or difficulty in voiding in the absence of mechanical urethral obstruction. Additional complications of advanced disease may include spinal cord compression from intradural metastases, deep venous thrombosis and pulmonary emboli, and myelophthisis.

Digital Rectal Examination Palpation of the prostate is an essential test for optimal detection of all stages of disease other than stage T1 (see "Staging and Assessment of Metastatic Disease"). Indeed, the importance of the DRE in the routine physical examination of men cannot be stressed too strongly. The posterior surfaces of the lateral lobes, where carcinoma begins most often, are easily palpable on DRE. Carcinoma characteristically is hard, nodular, and irregular, but induration also may be due to fibrous areas in benign prostatic hyperplasia, to focal infarcts, or to calculi as well as to tumor. The midline furrow between the lateral lobes may be obscured by either benign or malignant enlargement. Local extraprostatic extension of tumor into the seminal vesicles can often be detected by rectal examination. Scrotal and/or lower extremity lymphedema secondary to infiltration of pelvic lymph nodes indicates extensive disease.

Biochemical Markers The serum PSA level is the most sensitive test for early detection of prostatic cancer and is elevated in approximately 65 percent of cases. This antigen is an imperfect tumor marker because of insensitivity (approximate 35 percent false-negative rate) and lack of specificity (elevations can occur with benign prostatic hyperplasia, prostatitis, and prostatic infarction). Levels are higher in blacks and in men with prostatic hyperplasia. For these reasons, the value of routine screening is not established. However, the combined use of serum PSA measurements and DRE allows detection of more than 60 percent of cases of prostatic cancer while it is still localized. An approach to the use of DRE and PSA measurements for evaluating men at risk is shown in Fig. 97-1. If the DRE is abnormal or if the PSA level is >10 ng/mL, transrectal biopsy of the prostate under sonography should be performed; if the DRE is negative and the PSA level is <4 ng/mL, annual follow-up is appropriate. The issue of what to do if the DRE is negative and the PSA level is equivocal (4.1 to 10 ng/mL) is not clear; some surgeons biopsy all such patients, some biopsy only if the transrectal ultrasound is abnormal, and some utilize refinements of the PSA assay to determine the need for biopsy. Refinements in PSA testing that may improve the diagnostic accuracy and are under investigation include correlating absolute PSA levels with prostate volume (PSA density) or patient age (age-specific reference ranges); analysis of the rate of rise in PSA level with time (PSA velocity); and quantifying free and protein-bound forms of serum PSA. In patients with known prostatic cancer, PSA measurements are useful in staging (see below), in assessing response to therapy, and in detecting early relapse. Nevertheless, the correct management of patients with isolated PSA relapse is not clear.

Imaging With the use of transrectal prostatic sonography, carcinoma is revealed as hypoechoic densities within the peripheral zone. The procedure is a sensitive means of identifying prostate cancer but is not specific enough for use as a screening test. Ultrasonography is most useful for directing needle biopsy to assure uniform sampling of the prostate and for documenting the degree of extension of the tumor into the bladder and seminal vesicles. Magnetic resonance imaging (MRI) and to a lesser degree computed tomography (CT) of the prostate also may be helpful in defining the extent of tumor and locating nodes for aspiration needle biopsy. Transrectal prostatic sonography is recommended if either the DRE is positive or the PSA level is elevated. The findings on sonography, the amount of PSA elevation relative to prostate size, and the index of suspicion for carcinoma by history all affect the decision of whether or not to perform a biopsy. The combined use of these modalities allows early detection of large numbers of prostatic cancers and an increased proportion of localized and curable lesions. The biologic significance of individual lesions remains to be defined. Whether early diagnosis leads to improved survival and decreased morbidity from prostatic cancer requires further study.

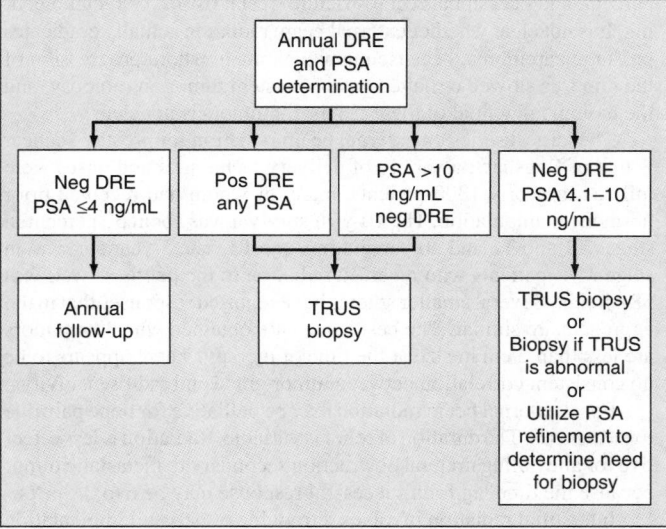

FIGURE 97-1 The use of the annual digital rectal examination (DRE) and measurement of prostate-specific antigen (PSA) as guides for deciding which men should have transrectal prostate biopsy under sonography (TRUS). There are at least three schools of thought about what to do if the DRE is negative and the PSA is equivocal (4.1 to 10 ng/mL).

Biopsy Biopsy of the prostate is essential for establishing the diagnosis and is indicated when an abnormality is detected by palpation or measurement of serum PSA level and/or by imaging or when lower urinary tract symptoms occur in men who have no known cause of obstruction. Core-needle biopsy may be performed transperineally or transrectally, with less risk of bacterial contamination with the former and more precise sampling with the latter. Transrectal prostatic biopsy with a rapid-fire spring-loaded needle under sonography provides the most accurate sampling of the index lesion and the remainder of the gland and is the preferred technique. Fine-needle aspiration cytology offers immediate diagnosis with minimal patient discomfort and morbidity. Open perineal biopsy is performed infrequently because it carries the risk of at least temporary impotence and is a more extensive surgical procedure. Transurethral biopsy is also used infrequently because most early lesions are in the peripheral regions of the gland.

Staging and Assessment of Metastatic Disease Adenocarcinoma of the prostate may spread by three routes: direct extension, the lymphatics, and the bloodstream. The prostatic capsule is a natural boundary against growth of tumor into adjacent structures, but direct extension occurs upward into the seminal vesicles and bladder floor. Lymphatic spread can best be assessed by surgical exploration; the frequency with which it occurs correlates with the size and histologic grade of the tumor and with the level of serum PSA. Only about one-tenth of tumors with a grade of less than 5 have lymph node involvement, while more than 70 percent of tumors with a Gleason grade of 9 or 10 have coexisting lymphatic invasion at the time of diagnosis. Lymphatic metastases are present in fewer than 10 percent of patients in whom the serum PSA level is <10 ng/mL. The route of lymphatic spread (in decreasing order) is to obturator, internal iliac, common iliac, presacral, and paraaortic nodes. Hematogenous metastases occur to bone (pelvis > lumbar vertebrae > thoracic vertebrae > ribs) more frequently than to viscera (lung > liver > adrenal gland). Diffuse pulmonary involvement is infrequent.

The TNM staging scheme involving assessment of primary *t*umor, *n*odes, and *m*etastases has replaced the Whitmore-Jewett system (Table 97-2). Stage T1 represents cancer not detectable by DRE and is subdivided into three groups. Stages T1a and T1b represent small but increasing amounts of well-differentiated tumor found in a surgical specimen removed at autopsy or during operation for prostatic hyperplasia, and stage T1c comprises the large number of nonpalpable tumors diagnosed by biopsy that was performed because of an elevated serum PSA level. Stage T2 disease is palpable but confined to the prostate. Stage T2a disease is a single nodule involving only one lobe and surrounded by tissue that is normal to palpation; stage T2b involves the majority of one lobe; and stage T2c involves both lobes of the gland. In stage T3 palpable tumor extends beyond the prostate, but there are no distant metastases. In all T stages, the presence of metastatic disease is designated M+. Stage M1-2 means that only pelvic nodes are involved with no other metastases, whereas the M2+ category means that metastatic disease is more widespread. Any of the primary stages (T1, T2, T3) may progress directly to stage M+. In the past, failure to include pelvic lymphadenectomy in the staging process resulted in marked underestimation of the frequency of lymph node metastases; for example, about one-fifth of tumors tentatively classified as T1b solely on the basis of prostate pathology were shown to be stage M+ disease when appropriate surgical staging was performed. The need for routine staging lymphadenectomy is being reassessed because large numbers of small-volume stage T1c tumors are being detected, and lymphatic metastases are rare in such patients with levels of serum PSA <10 ng/mL and with tumors of Gleason score <5. The frequency with which early hematogenous metastases are missed with the current staging procedures is uncertain. Utilizing a reverse transcriptase polymerase chain reaction to amplify PSA messenger RNA, it is now possible to detect small numbers of prostate cancer cells in the circulation, but the clinical significance of detecting such cells is not clear at present.

Table 97-2

Comparison of Clinical Stage by the TNM Classification System and
the Whitmore-Jewett Staging System

TNM Stage	Description	Whitmore-Jewett Stage	Description
T1a	Nonpalpable, with 5% or less of resected tissue with cancer	A1	Well differentiated tumor on few chips from 1 lobe
T1b	Nonpalpable, with >5% of resected tissue with cancer	A2	Involvement more diffuse
T1c	Nonpalpable, detected due to elevated serum PSA		
T2a	Palpable, half of one lobe or less	BIN	Palpable, < one lobe, surrounded by normal tissue
T2b	Palpable, > half of one lobe but not both lobes	B1	Palpable, < one lobes
T2c	Palpable, involves both lobes	B2	Palpable, one entire lobe or both lobes
T3a	Palpable, unilateral extracapsular extension	C1	Palpable, outside capsule, not into seminal vesicles
T3b	Palpable, bilateral extracapsular extension		
T3c	Tumor invades seminal vesicle(s)	C2	Palpable, seminal vesicle involved
MI	Distant metastases	D	Metastatic disease

SOURCE: Adapted from FF Schroder et al: TNM classification of prostate cancer. Prostate (Suppl) 4:129, 1992; and American Joint Committee on Cancer, 1992.

Bony metastases from prostatic carcinoma usually contain both osteoblastic and osteolytic components. The bony pelvis and lumbar vertebrae are involved most often, and metastases also occur in thoracic vertebrae, ribs, skull, and long bones. Skeletal survey has a low sensitivity of detection because a significant portion of bone must be involved to permit detection on a routine x-ray. Bone scans using radionuclides such as technetium 99 are more sensitive but not specific because positive scans may occur in any metabolically hyperactive bone; this includes sites of inflammation, healing fractures, osteoarthritis, and Paget's disease. Therefore, when a positive radionuclide scan is obtained during an initial survey for bone metastases, the presence of other lesions must be excluded by conventional radiography or biopsy of the affected site. Radionuclide bone scans are also useful for monitoring progression and response to therapy. Bone metastases are rare if the serum PSA level is <10 ng/mL. Consequently, bone scans are not necessary in initial staging or for the follow-up of every patient.

Surgical staging is still a common modality for assessing lymph node involvement and determining therapy. The procedure usually includes removal of the external iliac, internal iliac, and obturator lymph node chains and is either performed by open surgery or at laparoscopy. Pelvic lymphadenectomy may be performed by itself or in conjunction with prostatic surgery or implantation of radioactive beads. In patients at high risk for metastases and with a medical contraindication to lymphadenectomy, a pelvic CT scan or lymphangiogram can be obtained, followed when positive by confirmatory thin-needle biopsy of the affected lymph nodes.

℞ TREATMENT

Surgery Total prostatoseminovesiculectomy is the oldest treatment for carcinoma of the prostate. Radical perineal prostatectomy allows an easier vesicourethral anastomosis and less bleeding, while radical retropubic prostatectomy affords access to the pelvic lymph nodes. In experienced hands, both procedures have a low risk of major urinary incontinence. Formerly, both operations caused impotence in most patients, but improvements in surgical technique, particularly for the retropubic procedure, protect the neurovascular supply to the corpora cavernosa and preserve potency in most patients below age 60 without compromising the thoroughness of the operation.

Radical prostatectomy is not required for some stage T1a and T1c cancer, since the disease may be cured definitively by the simple prostatectomy at which the diagnosis is made. PSA determinations and sonographic biopsy of residual prostatic tissue aid in identifying those stage T1a and T1c patients with additional tumor who may require further therapy. True stage T1b disease in which pelvic nodes show no evidence of metastases may behave aggressively and be benefited by radical surgery, particularly when the neoplasm has a Gleason score ≥5. Indeed, 5- and 10-year survivals equivalent to those of age-matched controls have been reported following such treatment for stage T1b disease.

Radical prostatectomy has its clearest indication in stage T2 disease. Nearly all the apparent surgical cures in this stage are in men who have 1- to 2-cm nodules involving only one lobe of the prostate (i.e., stages T2a and T2b). Improvements in early diagnosis (see above) have increased the number of such patients diagnosed. In addition, subjects with stage T2c disease also may be candidates for radical prostatectomy.

The effectiveness of radical prostatectomy is less certain for locally advanced disease (stages T3 and M1). Clinical staging by DRE underestimates stage T2 and overestimates stage T3 disease in 40 to 50 percent of cases. Lymphadenectomy alone has no therapeutic benefit, but diminished surgical morbidity and renewed interest in early and total androgen ablation (see below) have spurred a reassessment of a role for radical prostatectomy in locally advanced disease. Morbidity rates from local pelvic symptoms, bladder outlet obstruction, hematuria, and ureteral obstruction may be decreased by radical prostatectomy in stage T3 and M1 disease, but controlled studies comparing morbidity rates after surgery with those following other therapies are lacking.

Radiation Radiation therapy was developed as a primary treatment in prostatic carcinoma because of a desire to avoid the impotence and occasional incontinence that may follow radical prostatectomy. The standard regimen is the administration of approximately 60 to 70 Gy (6000 to 7000 rad) to the prostate over 6 weeks by a variety of delivery patterns. Pelvic nodes may or may not be radiated. Acute proctitis and urethritis are common side effects but are usually controllable by local measures and adjustments in delivery pattern. Chronic complications after full courses of external beam radiation include impotence in 30 to 60 percent, chronic proctitis in 10 to 15 percent, and occasional rectal stricture, rectal fistula, or rectal bleeding. It is not clear whether external beam radiation actually eradicates prostatic carcinoma, because many patients in whom progression of the tumor is slowed or halted have persistent tumor on rebiopsy, and the biologic potential of these persistent tumors is not clear.

The largest series on external beam radiation for prostatic cancer is that of Bagshaw; a variety of delivery techniques and doses were utilized in nearly 1300 patients, many of whom had received prior hormone manipulation. The 10-year survival was about 50 percent in stages T1 and T2 and 30 percent in stage T3. The 5-year survival in stage M+ patients who received radiation to the pelvis as well was 58 percent. Several smaller studies have reported responses that in the aggregate are similar. The best results are obtained when the tumors are less than 2 cm in size at the time of therapy. There appears to be no consistent correlation between tumor grade and radiosensitivity.

Focal external beam radiation may be palliative for bone pain due to metastases. The duration of relief is variable. Radiation is less effective for alleviating ureteral obstruction secondary to metastatic tumor because the time lag for a successful response may be 6 to 8 weeks.

Interstitial radiation involves retropubic or perineal implantation of seeds of ^{125}I, ^{198}Au, ^{103}Pa, or ^{192}Ir. This treatment avoids major extirpative surgery and provides a concentrated delivery of radiation to the target tissue. Successful seed implantation requires a well-defined primary tumor with a diameter less than 5 cm, a tumor volume less than 30 to 40 mL, and uniform distribution of seeds throughout the prostate. In the initial reports, 5-year survival following staging pelvic lymphadenectomy and retropubic implantation of ^{125}I or ^{198}Au seeds was comparable with survival rates after other forms of treatment, but the incidence of tumor progression is higher. Potency is preserved in more than 90 percent, and early complications are fewer and less severe than after external beam radiation. Interstitial irradiation with seeds of palladium or iridium provides a higher radiation dose and a shorter half-life and may improve efficacy and decrease complications. Improvements in three-dimensional imaging of the prostate make it possible to distribute the seeds more evenly in the gland.

The efficacy and complication rates of several experimental therapies for the primary tumor, including hyperthermia, cryosurgery, and high-intensity focused ultrasound are under investigation.

In summary, except for impotence following external beam radiation, serious morbidity is infrequent following either form of radiation therapy. Practical considerations make ^{125}I or ^{198}Au seed implantation most suited to stage T2a disease. The long-term efficacy of either form of radiation as compared with radical prostatectomy for the treatment of localized carcinomas (stages T1 and T2) is not clear, but current data suggest that radiotherapy may be less curative than radical prostatectomy.

Androgen Deprivation   Because growth of the normal prostate is dependent on testicular androgens (see Chap. 336), it was logical to try androgen deprivation for treatment of advanced prostatic cancer. Androgen deprivation can be achieved in four ways: (1) surgical extirpation of the glands that synthesize androgens (castration and adrenalectomy); (2) inhibition of pituitary gonadotropin [and/or adrenocorticotropin (ACTH)] production [estrogen therapy, hypophysectomy, or treatment with luteinizing hormone–releasing hormone (LHRH) analogues such as leuprolide or buserelin]; (3) inhibition of androgen synthesis by the testes and adrenals (aminoglutethimide); and (4) inhibition of the binding of androgen to its receptor protein (cyproterone, flutamide, or bicalutamide).

Since testicular secretion accounts for more than 95 percent of testosterone production, bilateral orchiectomy results in a 90 percent decline of plasma levels. Estrogens such as diethylstilbestrol are potent inhibitors of the release from the pituitary gland of luteinizing hormone (LH), the gonadotropin that regulates testosterone production, and consequently, estrogen administration also causes a fall in plasma testosterone to castration levels. Maximum depression of plasma testosterone is achieved with 3 mg/d diethylstilbestrol. Other estrogens (conjugated estrogens, ethinyl estradiol, diethylstilbestrol diphosphate) are no more effective in the lowering of plasma testosterone level than is diethylstilbestrol.

Androgen deprivation by means of bilateral orchiectomy, diethylstilbestrol therapy, or combined orchiectomy plus diethylstilbestrol was a standard form of treatment for carcinoma of the prostate for many years, based largely on comparison of treatment groups with historical controls. Subsequently, in prospective control studies, the effectiveness of high-dose diethylstilbestrol or orchiectomy, alone or in combination, in enhancing survival in any stage of prostatic cancer was not clear-cut. Furthermore, death from cardiovascular disease was more frequent in patients treated with large doses of diethylstilbestrol. LHRH analogues have largely replaced estrogen therapy because of their safer cardiovascular profile. These analogues inhibit LH secretion and lower plasma testosterone levels.

Each of the above forms of androgen ablation still leaves a small amount of circulating adrenal androgen that may be detrimental in the control of advanced prostate cancer. Androgen depletion beyond that achieved by surgical castration, LHRH analogues, or estrogen administration can be accomplished by adrenalectomy or hypophysectomy. Adrenalectomy can be accomplished either by surgical ablation or by medical therapy with exogenous glucocorticoids, which inhibit ACTH secretion and the synthesis of adrenal androgen, or antiandrogens such as flutamide or nilutamide, which inhibit the binding of androgen to its cytoplasmic receptor protein. Extensive clinical trials in patients with metastatic disease comparing early androgen ablation alone with various forms of LHRH analogue

therapy versus androgen ablation with orchiectomy or LHRH analogues combined with antiandrogens have yielded inconsistent results. However, in most trials combination therapy resulted in a small but significant prolongation in both disease-free survival and overall survival; patients with the least amount of disease had the greatest degree of improvement with combination therapy. The modest improvement in outcomes in subsets of patients must be balanced against the added cost and the side effects of combination therapy. Although the appropriate time for initiating therapy remains controversial, the current trend is for early androgen ablation and, frequently, combination androgen ablation therapy in advanced prostatic cancer.

Even when there is no beneficial effect on survival, however, androgen deprivation decreases bone pain in two-thirds of symptomatic stage M+ patients and hence constitutes a major adjunctive therapy in the disease. Once the decision is made to institute such therapy, the choice must be made as to which form of androgen deprivation is appropriate. When acceptable to the patient, orchiectomy is safe and inexpensive and circumvents compliance problems. Diethylstilbestrol is also inexpensive and is usually safe in dosages of 3 mg/d or less in men who do not have preexisting cardiovascular disease. In men at risk for cardiovascular complications, LHRH analogues have similar response rates and fewer cardiovascular complications than diethylstilbestrol. The roles of intermittent androgen deprivation and of androgen blockers such as flutamide and bicalutamide in combination with each of the preceding means of establishing androgen deprivation are under study. In one study preoperative androgen deprivation in clinically localized prostate cancer resulted in a lower number of surgical specimens with positive margins. Whether such therapy improves rates of recurrence or survival is not clear.

As many as half of prostate cancers that have escaped from androgen ablation therapy have somatic mutations in the gene that encodes the androgen receptor in the prostate cancer cells. Many of these mutations cause amino acid substitutions in the hormone-binding domain of the protein that cause the loss of specificity for ligand, so that the receptor can respond to hormones such as progesterone that it would not ordinarily recognize or even to antiandrogens. The role of these mutations in the relentless progression of the disease is not established. Many prostate cancers express bcl 2 when they become androgen-independent.

Chemotherapy   Chemotherapy is reserved for hormone-unresponsive disease and is used for palliation. The age group at greatest risk for prostatic cancer has poor tolerance for chemotherapy. This feature, coupled with the variable course and long doubling time of the disease, makes it difficult to determine the effectiveness of such therapy. However, several comprehensive trials utilizing chemotherapy have been undertaken in stage M+ disease following relapse after hormonal treatment, a situation in which mean survival time is only 7 to 8 months. The agents studied most extensively are estramustine phosphate, prednimustine, and cisplatin; more limited trials have been conducted with 5-fluorouracil, melphalan, and hydroxyurea. Complete response is rare, and only one-tenth of stage M+ patients have an objective partial response. In other trials, combinations of chemotherapeutic agents have been tested in stage M+ disease, most commonly estramustine phosphate plus prednimustine and cisplatin; more limited trials have been conducted with 5-fluorouracil, melphalan, and hydroxyurea. Complete response is again rare, and only one-fourth of patients or fewer show any objective improvement. For progressive, symptomatic stage M+ prostatic cancer, endocrine ablation therapy should be undertaken first, but chemotherapeutic agents may provide some benefit when such patients relapse. Development of new forms of therapy for disease refractory to androgen deprivation is an urgent need in the management of prostatic carcinoma.

Palliation of Bone Metastases   Diffuse spread of metastases to bone limits the usefulness of external beam radiation therapy for relief of bone pain, which is a major cause of morbidity in the late phases of the disease when it is no longer responsive to androgen deprivation. Bone-seeking radiopharmaceuticals such as ^{89}Sr or diphosphonates unlabeled or labeled with samarium (^{153}Sm) can be of benefit in the control of pain even in the absence of objective response of the tumor.

BIBLIOGRAPHY

BENIGN PROSTATIC HYPERPLASIA

LEPOR H et al: The efficacy and safety of terazosin for the treatment of symptomatic BPH. Prostate 18:345, 1991

McCONNELL JD et al: *Clinical Practice Guideline Number 8: Benign Prostatic Hyperplasia: Diagnosis and Treatment*. US Dept of Health and Human Services AHCPR publication No. 94-0582. Rockville, MD, 1994

STONER E et al: Maintenance of clinical efficacy with finasteride therapy for 24 months in patients with benign prostatic hyperplasia. Arch Intern Med 154:83, 1994

WALSH PC: Benign prostatic hyperplasia, in *Campbell's Urology*, 6th ed, PC Walsh et al (eds). Philadelphia, Saunders, 1992, p 1007

WILSON JD: The pathogenesis of prostatic hyperplasia. Am J Med 68:745, 1980

CARCINOMA OF THE PROSTATE

ALBERTSON PC et al: Long-term survival among men with conservatively treated localized prostate cancer. JAMA 274:626, 1995

BAGSHAW MA: External radiation therapy of carcinoma of the prostate. Cancer 45:1912, 1980

BYAR DP, CORLE DK: VACURG randomized trial of radical prostatectomy for stages I and II prostate cancer. Urology 17(Suppl 4):7, 1981

CATALONA WJ: Screening for prostate cancer. JAMA 273:1174, 1995

————, BIGG SW: Nerve-sparing radical prostatectomy: Evaluation of results after 250 patients. J Urol 143:538, 1990

COONER WH et al: Prostate cancer detection in a clinical urological practice by ultrasonography, digital rectal examination and prostate specific antigen. J Urol 143:1146, 1990

CRAWFORD ED et al: A controlled trial of leuprolide with and without flutamide in prostatic carcinoma. N Engl J Med 321:419, 1989

EISENBERGER MA et al: A critical assessment of the role of chemotherapy for endocrine resistant prostatic carcinoma. AUA Update Series Lesson 28, vol 7, 1988

HENNRICKSSON P, JOHANSSON S-E: Prediction of cardiovascular complication in patients with prostatic cancer treated with estrogen. Am J Epidemiol 125:970, 1987

HERR HW: Iodine 125 implantation in the management of localized prostatic carcinoma. Urol Clin North Am 7:605, 1980

HUGOSSON J et al: Prostate cancer mortality in patients surviving more than 10 years after diagnosis. J Urol 154:2115, 1995

ISRAELI RS et al: Sensitive detection of prostatic hematogenous tumor cell dissemination using prostate specific antigen and prostate specific membrane-derived primers in the polymerase chain reaction. J Urol 153:573, 1995

JEWETT HJ: Radical perineal prostatectomy for palpable clinically localized, non-obstructive cancer: Experience at the Johns Hopkins Hospital, 1909–1963. J Urol 124:492, 1980

KATZ A et al: Enhanced reverse transcriptase-polymerase chain reaction for prostate specific antigen as an indicator of true pathologic stage in patients with prostate cancer. Cancer 75:1642, 1995

LAING AH et al: Strontium-89 chloride for pain palliation in prostatic skeletal malignancy. Br J Radiol 64:816, 1991

MORGAN TO et al: Age-specific reference ranges for serum prostate-specific antigen in black men. N Engl J Med 336:304, 1996

NATIONAL INSTITUTES OF HEALTH CONSENSUS DEVELOPMENT CONFERENCE: The management of clinically localized prostate cancer. J Urol 138:1369, 1987

OESTERLING JE et al: Free, complexed and total serum prostate specific antigen: The establishment of appropriate reference ranges for their concentrations and ratios. J Urol 154:1090, 1995

STAMEY TA, McNEAL JE: Adenocarcinoma of the prostate, in *Campbell's Urology*, 6th ed, PC Walsh et al (eds). Philadelphia, Saunders, 1992, p 1159

TAPLIN ME et al: Mutations of the androgen receptor gene in metastatic androgen-independent prostate cancer. N Engl J Med 332:1393, 1995

TYRRELL CJ et al: A multicenter randomized trial comparing the luteinizing hormone–releasing hormone analogue goserelin acetate alone and with flutamide in the treatment of advanced prostate cancer. J Urol 146:1321, 1991

98

Robert J. Motzer, George J. Bosl

TESTICULAR CANCER

TESTICULAR CANCER (GERM CELL TUMORS)

Primary germ cell tumors (GCTs) of the testis, arising by the malignant transformation of primordial germ cells, constitute 95 percent of all testicular neoplasms. Infrequently, GCTs arise from an extragonadal site, including the mediastinum, retroperitoneum and, very rarely, the pineal gland. This disease is notable for the young age of the afflicted patients, the totipotent capacity for differentiation of the tumor cells, and its curability; more than 90 percent of all newly diagnosed patients will be cured, and, since the advent of cisplatin-based chemotherapy, about 70 to 80 percent of patients with metastatic disease are cured.

INCIDENCE AND EPIDEMIOLOGY In 1996, approximately 7400 new cases of testicular GCT were diagnosed in the United States; the incidence of this malignancy has increased slowly over the past 40 years. The tumor occurs most frequently between the ages of 20 and 40. A testicular mass in a man aged 50 years or greater should be regarded as a lymphoma until proved otherwise. GCT is at least four to five times more common in white than in African-American males, and a higher incidence has been observed in Scandinavia and New Zealand than in the United States.

ETIOLOGY AND GENETICS Cryptorchidism is associated with a severalfold higher risk of GCT. Abdominal cryptorchid testes are at a higher risk than inguinal cryptorchid testes. Orchiopexy should be performed before puberty if possible. The protective effect of orchiopexy is difficult to quantify, but most studies suggest that early orchiopexy reduces the risk of GCT and improves the ability to save the testis. If an abdominal cryptorchid testis cannot be brought into the scrotum, it should be removed. Approximately 2 percent of men with GCTs of one testis will develop a primary tumor in the other testis. Testicular feminization syndromes increase the risk of testicular GCT, and Klinefelter's syndrome is associated with mediastinal GCT.

CLINICAL PRESENTATION A painless testicular mass is pathognomonic for a testicular malignancy. More commonly, patients present with testicular discomfort or swelling suggestive of epididymitis and/or orchitis. In this circumstance, a trial of antibiotics is reasonable. However, if symptoms persist or a residual abnormality remains, then testicular ultrasound examination is indicated. Back pain from retroperitoneal metastases is common and must be distinguished from musculoskeletal pain. Dyspnea from pulmonary metastases occurs infrequently. Patients with increased serum levels of human chorionic gonadotropin (hCG) may present with gynecomastia. A delay in diagnosis is associated with a more advanced stage and possibly worse survival.

Ultrasound examination of the testis is indicated whenever a testicular malignancy is considered and for persistent or painful testicular swelling. If this examination shows an intratesticular mass, a radical inguinal orchiectomy should be performed. Because the testis develops originally from the gonadal ridge in the peritoneal cavity, its blood supply and lymphatic drainage originate intraabdominally and descend with the testis into the scrotum. Cutting through the skin of the scrotum to remove the testis by a scrotal orchiectomy may breach anatomic barriers and permit tumor cells to spread by additional pathways; for this reason, the scrotal approach is discouraged. The staging evaluation for GCT includes a determination of serum levels of alpha fetoprotein (AFP) and hCG. Following orchiectomy, a chest radiograph and a computed tomography (CT) scan of the abdomen and pelvis should be performed. A chest CT scan is required if mediastinal or hilar disease is suspected. *Stage I disease* is defined as disease limited to the testis, epididymis, or spermatic cord. *Stage II disease* is defined as disease limited to retroperitoneal (regional) lymph nodes. *Stage III disease* is defined as disease outside the retroperitoneum, involving supradiaphragmatic nodal sites or viscera. The staging may be "clinical"—defined solely by physical examination, blood marker evaluation, and radiographs—or "pathologic"—defined by an operative procedure.

The regional draining lymph nodes for the testis are in the retroperitoneum, and the vascular supply originates from the great vessels (for the right testis) or the renal vessels (for the left testis). As a result, the lymph nodes that are involved first by a right testicular tumor are the interaortocaval lymph nodes just below the renal vessels. For a left testicular tumor, the first involved lymph nodes are lateral to the aorta (para-aortic) and below the left renal vessels. In both cases, further nodal spread is inferior and contralateral and, less commonly, above the renal hilum. Lymphatic involvement can extend cephalad to the retrocrural, posterior mediastinal, and supraclavicular lymph nodes. Treatment is determined by tumor histology (seminoma versus nonseminoma) and clinical stage (Table 98-1).

PATHOLOGY   GCTs are divided into nonseminoma and seminoma subtypes. Nonseminomatous GCTs are most frequent in the third decade of life and can display the full spectrum of embryonic and adult cellular differentiation. This entity comprises four histologies: embryonal carcinoma, teratoma, choriocarcinoma, and endodermal sinus (yolk sac) tumor. Choriocarcinoma, consisting of both cytotrophoblasts and syncytiophoblasts, represents malignant trophoblastic differentiation and is invariably associated with secretion of hCG. Endodermal sinus tumor is the malignant counterpart of the fetal yolk sac and is associated with secretion of AFP. Pure embryonal carcinoma may secrete AFP, or hCG, or both; this pattern is biochemical evidence of differentiation. Teratoma is composed of somatic cell types derived from two or more germ layers (ectoderm, mesoderm, or endoderm). Each of these histologies may be present alone or in combination with others. Nonseminomatous GCTs tend to metastasize early to sites such as the retroperitoneal lymph nodes and lung parenchyma. Approximately one-third of patients present with disease limited to the testis (stage I), one-third with retroperitoneal metastases (stage II), and one-third with more extensive supradiaphragmatic nodal or visceral metastases (stage III).

Seminoma represents about 50 percent of all GCTs, has a median age in the fourth decade, and generally follows a more indolent clinical course. Most patients (70 percent) present with stage I disease, about 20 percent with stage II disease, and 10 percent with stage III disease; lung or other visceral metastases are rare. Seminoma is radiosensitive, and radiotherapy is the treatment of choice in patients with stage I disease and stage II disease where the nodes are <5 cm in maximum diameter. When a tumor contains both seminoma and nonseminoma components, patient management is directed by the more aggressive nonseminoma component.

An isochromosome of the short arm of chromosome 12 [i(12p)] is a chromosomal marker specific for GCT. It has been found in all histologic types and has diagnostic and possibly prognostic significance. One clinical application of this marker is in the diagnosis of patients with midline tumors of uncertain histogenesis (see below).

TUMOR MARKERS   Careful monitoring of the serum tumor markers AFP and hCG is essential in the management of patients with GCT, as these markers are important for diagnosis, as prognostic indicators, in monitoring treatment response, and in the detection of early relapse. Approximately 70 percent of patients presenting with disseminated nonseminomatous GCT have increased serum concentra-

tions of AFP and/or hCG. While hCG concentrations may be increased in patients with either nonseminoma or seminoma histology, AFP is increased only in patients with nonseminoma histology. The finding of an increased AFP level in a patient whose tumor showed only seminoma indicates that an occult nonseminomatous component is present, and that the patient should be treated according to guidelines for a nonseminomatous GCT. The serum lactate dehydrogenase (LDH) level serves as an additional marker of all GCTs, but it is not as specific as either AFP or hCG. LDH levels will be increased in 50 to 60 percent of cases of metastatic nonseminoma and up to 80 percent of cases of advanced seminoma.

Determination of AFP, hCG, and LDH levels should be done before and after orchiectomy. Increased serum AFP and hCG concentrations decay according to first-order kinetics; the half-life is 24 to 36 h for hCG and 5 to 7 days for AFP. AFP and hCG should be assayed serially during and after treatment. Either reappearance of hCG and/or AFP or failure of these markers to decline according to the predicted half-life are indicators of persistent or recurrent tumor.

℞ **TREATMENT**

Stage 1 Nonseminoma   If, after an orchiectomy (for clinical stage I disease), radiographs and physical examination show no evidence of disease, and serum AFP and hCG concentrations either are normal or are declining to normal according to the known half-life, patients may be managed by either a nerve-sparing retroperitoneal lymph node dissection (RPLND) or surveillance. The retroperitoneal lymph nodes will be pathologically involved by GCT (pathologic stage II) in 20 to 50 percent of these patients. The decision between surveillance or RPLND is based on the pathology of the primary tumor. If the primary tumor shows no pathologic evidence for lymphatic or vascular invasion *and* is limited to the testis (T1), then either option is reasonable. If lymphatic or vascular invasion is present *or* the tumor extends into the tunica, spermatic cord, or scrotum (T2 through T4), then surveillance should not be offered. Either approach should cure more than 95 percent of patients.

A RPLND is the standard operation for removal of the regional lymph nodes of the testis (the retroperitoneal nodes). The operation removes the lymph nodes ipsilateral to the primary site and the nodal groups adjacent to the primary landing zone. The standard (modified bilateral) RPLND removes all node-bearing tissue down to the bifurcation of the great vessels, including the ipsilateral iliac nodes. The major long-term effect of this operation is retrograde ejaculation and infertility. A nerve-sparing RPLND, usually accomplished by identification and dissection of individual nerve fibers, avoids injury to the sympathetic nerves responsible for ejaculation. Normal ejaculation is preserved in approximately 90 percent of patients. Patients with pathologic stage I disease are observed, and only the 10 percent who relapse require additional therapy. If retroperitoneal nodes are found to be involved at RPLND, then a decision regarding adjuvant chemotherapy is made on the basis of the extent of retroperitoneal disease (see below).

Table 98-1

Germ Cell Tumor Staging System and Treatment

| Stage | Extent of Disease | Treatment | |
		Seminoma	Nonseminoma
I	Testis only, T1, no vascular/lymphatic invasion	Radiation therapy	RPLND or observation
	T2–4 or vascular/lymphatic invasion present	Radiation therapy	RPLND
IIA	Nodes <2 cm	Radiation therapy	RPLND
IIB	Nodes 2–5 cm	Radiation therapy	RPLND +/− adjuvant chemotherapy or chemotherapy followed by RPLND
IIC	Nodes >5 cm	Chemotherapy	Chemotherapy followed by RPLND
III	Distant metastases	Chemotherapy	Chemotherapy, often followed by surgery (biopsy or resection)

RPLND, retroperitoneal lymph node dissection

Surveillance is an option in the management of clinical stage I disease when no vascular/lymphatic invasion is found and the primary tumor is classified as T1. In this situation, only 20 to 30 percent of patients will have pathologic stage II disease, implying that most RPLNDs in this situation are not therapeutic. Although surveillance has not been compared to RPLND in a randomized trial, all large studies show that surveillance and RPLND lead to equivalent long-term survival. Patient compliance is essential if surveillance is to be successful. Patients must be carefully followed with periodic chest radiography, physical examination, CT scan of the abdomen, and serum tumor marker determinations. The median time to relapse is about seven months, and late relapses (later than 2 years) are rare. The 70 to 80 percent of patients who do not relapse require no intervention after orchiectomy; treatment is reserved for those who do relapse. When the primary tumor is classified as T2 through T4 *or* lymphatic/vascular invasion is identified, nerve-sparing RPLND is preferred. About 50 percent of these patients will have pathologic stage II disease and are destined to relapse.

Stage II Nonseminoma GCT Patients with limited, ipsilateral retroperitoneal adenopathy (nodes usually 3 cm in greatest diameter or smaller) generally undergo a modified bilateral RPLND as primary management. Nearly all patients with pathologic stage II disease whose disease is completely resected by RPLND are cured. The in-field recurrence rate after a properly performed RPLND is very low. Depending on the extent of disease, the postoperative management options include either surveillance or two cycles of adjuvant chemotherapy. Surveillance is the preferred approach for patients with resected "low-volume" metastases (all nodes with metastatic tumor are ≤2 cm in diameter, *and* fewer than six nodes are involved) because the probability of relapse is one-third or less. Because relapse occurs in 50 percent or more of patients with "high-volume" metastasis (fewer than six nodes involved, *or* any involved node >2 cm in largest diameter, *or* extranodal tumor extension), two cycles of adjuvant chemotherapy should be considered, as it results in cure in ≥98 percent of patients. Regimens consisting of etoposide (100 mg/m² daily on days 1 through 5) plus cisplatin (20 mg/m² daily on days 1 through 5) with or without bleomycin (30 units per day on days 2, 9, and 16) given at 3-week intervals are effective and well tolerated.

Stages I and II Seminoma Inguinal orchiectomy followed by retroperitoneal radiation therapy cures about 98 percent of patients with stage I seminoma. The dose of radiotherapy (2500 to 3000 cGy) is low and well tolerated, and the in-field recurrence rate is negligible. About 2 percent of patients will relapse with supradiaphragmatic or systemic disease. Surveillance has been proposed as an option, and studies have shown that there is an approximately 15 percent probability of relapse. The median time to relapse is 12 to 15 months, and late relapses during surveillance (>5 years) may be more frequent than with nonseminoma tumors. Chemotherapy is usually required to treat the relapse. Surveillance for clinical stage I seminoma is generally not recommended in the United States.

Nonbulky retroperitoneal disease (stage IIA and IIB) is also treated with radiotherapy alone. Prophylactic supradiaphragmatic radiotherapy is not indicated. Relapses in the anterior mediastinum are unusual, and the cumulative effect of infradiaphragmatic plus supradiaphragmatic radiotherapy causes extremely severe hematologic toxicity when chemotherapy is needed at relapse. The proportion of patients who achieve relapse-free survival with retroperitoneal masses <5 cm in diameter is about 90 percent. Because at least one-third of patients with bulkier disease relapse, initial chemotherapy is preferred for stage IIC disease.

Chemotherapy for Advanced GCT Regardless of histology, patients with stage IIC and stage III GCT are treated with chemotherapy. Combination chemotherapy programs developed in the 1970s and 1980s, based on bleomycin and cisplatin at doses of 100 to 120 mg/m² per cycle plus etoposide, showed that 70 and 80 percent, respectively, of such patients will be cured. Complete response (the complete disappearance of all clinical evidence of tumor on physical examination and radiography plus normal serum levels of AFP and hCG for 1 month or more) occurs after chemotherapy alone in about 60 percent of patients, and another 10 to 20 percent are rendered free of disease with surgical resection of all sites of residual disease. Randomized clinical trials have shown that lower doses of cisplatin result in inferior survival.

The toxicity of four cycles of the cisplatin/bleomycin/etoposide (BEP) regimen is substantial. Nausea, vomiting, and hair loss occur in most patients, although nausea and vomiting have been markedly ameliorated by modern antiemetic regimens. Myelosuppression is frequent, and symptomatic bleomycin pulmonary toxicity occurs in about 5 percent of patients. Treatment-induced mortality due to neutropenia with septicemia or bleomycin-induced pulmonary failure occurs in 1 to 3 percent of patients. Dose reductions for myelosuppression are rarely indicated. Long-term permanent toxicities include nephrotoxicity (reduced glomerular filtration and persistent magnesium wasting), ototoxicity, and peripheral neuropathy. When bleomycin is administered by weekly bolus injection, Raynaud's phenomenon appears in 5 to 10 percent of treated patients. Less often, other evidence of small blood vessel damage has been reported, including transient ischemic attacks and myocardial infarction.

Because not all patients are cured and significant treatment-related toxicities are known, it became necessary to stratify patients into "good-risk" and "poor-risk" groups. For good-risk patients, the goal is to achieve maximum efficacy with minimal toxicity. For poor-risk patients, the goal is to identify more effective therapy with tolerable toxicity. In general, good-risk patients have tumor of smaller extent with metastases limited to the retroperitoneum and lung and low serum levels of tumor markers. The presence of a primary mediastinal nonseminoma, high serum concentrations of hCG, and/or nonpulmonary visceral metastases indicate poor-risk disease (i.e., disease unlikely to be cured with standard therapy).

For patients with good-risk GCTs, four cycles of etoposide plus cisplatin (EP) or three cycles of BEP will result in a durable, complete response in about 90 percent of patients, with minimal acute and chronic toxicity. With these regimens, pulmonary toxicity is absent when bleomycin is not used and is rare when therapy is limited to 9 weeks; myelosuppression with neutropenic fever is less frequent; and treatment mortality is negligible. Randomized trials have shown that carboplatin, a less toxic analogue of cisplatin, is less effective than cisplatin. Bleomycin should not be deleted when treatment is limited to three cycles.

Only 35 to 50 percent of patients with poor-risk GCT are cured. No regimen has been found to be better than four cycles of BEP, a fact that emphasizes the need for more effective therapy. Randomized clinical trials have shown that the substitution of ifosfamide for etoposide and the use of higher doses of cisplatin (200 mg/m² per cycle) do not improve survival. Chemotherapy using a dose-intensive regimen of carboplatin, etoposide, and either cyclophosphamide or ifosfamide followed by hematopoietic stem cell rescue improves overall survival, and a randomized trial is in progress to test this hypothesis. If possible, patients with poor-risk GCT should be referred to centers and treated on clinical trials.

Postchemotherapy Surgery Resection of residual metastases after the completion of chemotherapy is an integral part of therapy. If the initial histology is nonseminoma and the marker values have normalized, all sites of residual disease should be resected. In general, residual retroperitoneal disease requires a modified bilateral RPLND, which is associated with retrograde ejaculation. Thoracotomy (unilateral or bilateral) and neck dissection are less frequently required to remove residual mediastinal, pulmonary parenchymal, or cervical nodal disease. Viable tumor (seminoma, embryonal carcinoma, yolk sac tumor or choriocarcinoma), mature teratoma, or necrotic debris and fibrosis will be present in about 15 percent, 40 percent, and 45 percent of resected specimens respectively. The frequency of teratoma or viable disease is highest in residual mediastinal tumors. If necrotic debris or mature teratoma is present, no further chemotherapy is necessary. If viable tumor is present but is completely excised, then two additional cycles of chemotherapy are needed.

If the initial histology is pure seminoma, mature teratoma is rarely present and the most frequent finding is necrotic debris. For residual retroperitoneal disease, a complete RPLND is technically difficult owing to extensive postchemotherapy fibrosis. Close observation is recommended when no radiographic abnormality exists or a residual mass smaller than 3 cm is present. Controversy exists over what to do when the residual mass exceeds 3 cm in diameter. About 25 percent of such masses will contain viable GCT. Some investigators prefer excision or biopsy, but radiotherapy or surveillance are alternatives.

Salvage Chemotherapy Of patients with advanced GCT, 20 to 30 percent fail to achieve a durable complete response to first-line chemotherapy. A combination of cisplatin, ifosfamide and, vinblastine (VeIP) will induce a durable complete response in 25 percent of patients as a second-line therapy. Patients are more likely to achieve a durable complete response to VeIP if they had a testicular primary tumor and have relapsed from a prior complete remission to first-line cisplatin-containing chemotherapy. In contrast, if the patient failed to achieve a complete response or has a primary mediastinal nonseminoma, then VeIP is rarely beneficial. Those patients are candidates for dose-intensive treatment.

Chemotherapy consisting of dose-intensive, high-dose carboplatin (≥ 1500 mg/m^2) plus etoposide (≥ 1200 mg/m^2), with or without cyclophosphamide or ifosfamide, with peripheral blood- or bone marrow–derived stem cell support will induce a complete response in 25 to 40 percent of patients who have failed ifosfamide-containing salvage chemotherapy. About one-half of the complete responses will be durable. High-dose therapy is the treatment of choice and standard of care for this patient population. Paclitaxel is active in previously treated patients. It is being studied as a new component in dose-intensive therapy.

EXTRAGONADAL GCT AND MIDLINE CARCINOMA OF UNCERTAIN HISTOGENESIS The prognosis and management of patients with extragonadal GCTs depends on the tumor histology and site of origin. All patients with a diagnosis of extragonadal GCT should have a testicular ultrasound examination. Nearly all patients with retroperitoneal or mediastinal seminoma achieve a durable complete response to BEP or EP. The clinical features of patients with primary retroperitoneal nonseminoma GCT are similar to those of patients with a primary of testis origin, and careful evaluation will find evidence of a primary testicular GCT in about two-thirds of cases. In contrast, a primary mediastinal nonseminomatous GCT is associated with a poor prognosis, with no more than one-third of patients being cured with standard therapy (four cycles of BEP). Patients with newly diagnosed mediastinal nonseminoma are considered to have poor-risk disease and should be considered for clinical trials testing regimens of possibly greater efficacy. In addition, mediastinal nonseminoma is associated with hematologic disorders, including acute myelogenous leukemia, myelodysplastic syndrome, and essential thrombocytosis unrelated to previous chemotherapy. An i(12p) isochromosome has been identified in both the primary GCT and leukemic cells, indicating a common clonal origin. These hematologic disorders are very refractory to treatment.

A group of patients with poorly differentiated tumors of unknown histogenesis has been reported. These tumors are most common in males, are midline in distribution, and are not associated with secretion of AFP or hCG; a minority of patients (10 to 20 percent) are cured by standard cisplatin-containing chemotherapy. Recently, conventional and molecular cytogenetic studies have shown that i(12p) is present in about 25 percent of such tumors, confirming their origin from primitive germ cells. This finding is also predictive of response to cisplatin-based chemotherapy and resulting long-term survival. Genetic analysis of these tumors has also identified other histologies, including neuroepithelial tumors and lymphoma, demonstrating the heterogeneity of this group of tumors.

FERTILITY Infertility is an important consequence of the treatment of GCTs. In addition, preexisting infertility or impaired fertility is often present. Azoospermia and/or oligospermia are present at diagnosis in at least 50 percent of patients with testicular GCTs. Ejaculatory dysfunction is associated with RPLND, and germ cell damage may result from cisplatin-containing chemotherapy. Nerve-sparing techniques to preserve the retroperitoneal sympathetic nerves have made retrograde ejaculation less likely in patient subgroups that are candidates for this operation. Spermatogenesis does recover in some patients after chemotherapy. However, because there is a significant risk of impaired reproductive capacity due either to a preexisting condition or to treatment, semen analysis and cryopreservation of sperm (in a "sperm bank") should be recommended to all patients before radiotherapy, chemotherapy, or RPLND.

BIBLIOGRAPHY

BAJORIN DF et al: Current perspectives on the role of adjunctive surgery in combined modality treatment for patients with germ cell tumors. Semin Oncol 19:148, 1992

——— et al: Randomized trial of etoposide and cisplatin versus etoposide and carboplatin in patients with good-risk germ cell tumors: A multiinstitutional study. J Clin Oncol 11:598, 1993

BOSL GJ et al: Clinical relevance of the i(12p) marker chromosome in germ cell tumors. J Natl Cancer Inst 86:349, 1994

——— et al: Cancer of the Testis, in *Cancer: Principles and Practice of Oncology*, 5th ed, VT DeVita, S Hellman, SA Rosenberg (eds). Lippincott, Philadelphia, 1997, pp 1397–1425

EINHORN LH et al: Evaluation of optimal duration of chemotherapy in favorable-prognosis disseminated germ cell tumors: A Southeastern Cancer Study Group protocol. J Clin Oncol 7:387, 1989

FELDMAN S et al: Low-risk metastatic gestational trophoblastic disease. Semin Oncol 22:166, 1995

MOTZER RJ, BOSL GJ: High-dose chemotherapy for resistant germ cell tumors: Recent advances and future directions. J Natl Cancer Inst 84:1703, 1992

99 *Robert C. Young*

GYNECOLOGIC MALIGNANCIES

OVARIAN CANCER

Incidence and Epidemiology Epithelial ovarian cancer is the leading cause of death from gynecologic cancer in the United States. In 1996 there were 26,700 new cases diagnosed and 14,800 deaths. The disease accounts for 5 percent of all cancer deaths in women in the United States; more women die of this disease than from cervical and endometrial cancer combined.

The age-specific incidence of the common epithelial type of ovarian cancer increases progressively and peaks in the eighth decade. It is uncommon before the age of 40. Epidemiologic studies suggest higher incidences in industrialized nations and an association with disordered ovarian function, including infertility, nulliparity, frequent miscarriages, and use of ovulation-inducing drugs such as clomiphene. Each pregnancy reduces the ovarian cancer risk by about 10 percent, and breast feeding and tubal ligation also appear to reduce the risk. Oral contraceptives reduce the risk of ovarian cancer in patients with a familial history of cancer and in the general population. Many of these risk reductions support the "incessant ovulation" hypothesis for ovarian cancer etiology, which implies that an aberrant repair process of the surface epithelium is central to ovarian cancer development. Estrogen replacement after menopause does not appear to increase the risk of ovarian cancer, although one study showed a modest increase in risk with more than 11 years of use.

Familial cases account for about 5 percent of all ovarian cancer, and a family history of ovarian cancer is a major risk factor. Compared to a life-time risk of 1.6 percent in the general population, women with one affected first-degree relative have a 5 percent risk. In families with two or more affected first-degree relatives, the risk may exceed 50 percent. Three types of autosomal dominant familial cancer are recognized: (1) site-specific in which only ovarian cancer is seen, (2) families with cancer of the ovary and breast, and (3) the Lynch type II cancer family syndrome with nonpolyposis colorectal cancer, endometrial cancer, and ovarian cancer.

Etiology and Genetics In women with hereditary breast-ovarian cancer, the susceptibility locus, BRCA-1, is located on chromosome 17q12-21. It is likely that BRCA-1 is a tumor suppressor gene and that its protein product acts as a negative regulator of tumor growth. A large number of mutations of BRCA-1 have now been described; most are frameshift or nonsense mutations, and 86 percent produce truncated protein products. The exact implications of the myriad of other mutations including many missense mutations are not known. Men in such families have an increased risk of prostate cancer.

Cytogenetic analysis of sporadic epithelial ovarian cancers generally reveals complex karyotypic rearrangements. Structural abnormalities frequently appear on chromosomes 1 and 11, and loss of heterozygosity (LOH) is common on 3q, 6q, 11q, 13q, and 17. Abnormalities of oncogenes are frequently found in ovarian cancer and include c-*myc*, H-*ras*, K-*ras*, and *neu*.

Ovarian tumors (usually not epithelial) are sometimes components of complex genetic syndromes. Peutz-Jeghers syndrome (mucocutaneous pigmentation and intestinal polyps) is associated with ovarian sex cord stromal tumors and Sertoli cell tumors in men. Patients with gonadal dysgenesis (46XY genotype or mosaic for Y-containing cell lines) develop gonadoblastomas, and women with nevoid basal cell carcinomas have an increased risk of ovarian fibromas.

Clinical Presentation and Differential Diagnosis Most patients with ovarian cancer are first diagnosed when the disease has already spread beyond the true pelvis. The occurrence of abdominal pain, bloating, and urinary symptoms usually indicates advanced disease. Localized ovarian cancer is generally asymptomatic. However, progressive enlargement of a localized ovarian tumor can produce urinary frequency or constipation, and rarely torsion of an ovarian mass causes acute abdominal pain or a surgical abdomen. In contrast to cervical or endometrial cancer, vaginal bleeding or discharge is rarely seen with early ovarian cancer. The diagnosis of early disease usually occurs with palpation of an asymptomatic adnexal mass during routine pelvic examination. However, most ovarian enlargements discovered this way are benign functional cysts that characteristically resolve over one to three menstrual cycles. Adnexal masses in premenarchal or postmenopausal women are more likely to be pathologic, and exploratory surgery is usually required. Other causes of adnexal masses include pedunculated uterine fibroids, endometriosis, benign ovarian neoplasms, and inflammatory lesions of the bowel.

Evaluation of patients with suspected ovarian cancer should include measurement of serum levels of the tumor marker CA-125. CA-125 determinants are glycoproteins with molecular masses from 220 to 1000 kDa, and a radioimmunoassay is used to determine circulating CA-125 antigen levels. Between 80 and 85 percent of patients with epithelial ovarian cancer have levels of CA-125 $\geq$35 U/mL. Other malignant tumors can also elevate CA-125 levels, including cancers of the endometrium, cervix, fallopian tubes, pancreas, breast, lung, and colon. Certain nonmalignant conditions that can elevate CA-125 levels include pregnancy, endometriosis, pelvic inflammatory disease, and uterine fibroids. One percent of normal females have serum CA-125 levels >35 U/mL. However, in postmenopausal women with an asymptomatic pelvic mass and CA-125 levels $\geq$65 U/mL, the test has a sensitivity of 97 percent and a specificity of 78 percent.

Screening In contrast to patients who present with advanced disease, patients with early ovarian cancers (stages I and II) are commonly curable with conventional therapy. For this reason, effective screening procedures would improve the cure rate in this disease. Although pelvic examination can occasionally detect early disease, it is a relatively insensitive screening procedure. Transvaginal sonography has replaced the slower and less sensitive abdominal sonography, but there are significant false-positive results, particularly in premenopausal women. In one study, 67 laparotomies were required to diagnose 1 primary ovarian cancer. Doppler flow imaging coupled with transvaginal ultrasound may improve accuracy and reduce the high rate of false positives.

CA-125 has been studied as a screening tool. Unfortunately, half of women with stages I and II ovarian cancer have CA-125 levels <65 U/mL. Other nonmalignant disorders can elevate the CA-125 level, and both false-negative and -positive results have been reported in most screening studies.

Attempts have been made to improve the sensitivity and specificity by combinations of procedures, commonly transvaginal ultrasound and CA-125 levels. In a screening study of 22,000 women, 42 had a positive screen and 11 had ovarian cancer (7 with advanced disease). In addition, eight women with a negative screen developed ovarian cancer. Thus, while screening can detect early ovarian cancer in asymptomatic women, the false-positive rate would lead to a large number of unnecessary (i.e., negative) laparotomies if each positive screen resulted in a surgical exploration. The National Institutes of Health Consensus Conference recommended against screening for ovarian cancer among the general population without known risk factors for the disease.

Pathology Common epithelial tumors comprise most (85 percent) of the ovarian neoplasms. These may be benign (50 percent), frankly malignant (33 percent), or tumors of low malignant potential (16 percent), or so-called tumors of borderline malignancy. Epithelial tumors of low malignant potential have the cytologic features of malignancy but do not invade the ovarian stroma. More than 75 percent present in early stage and generally occur in younger women. They have a natural history that is much better than their malignant counterpart.

There are five major subtypes of common epithelial tumors: serous (50 percent), mucinous (25 percent), endometroid (15 percent), clear cell (5 percent), and Brenner tumors (1 percent), the latter derived from the urothelial epithelium. Benign common epithelial tumors are almost always serous or mucinous and develop in women ages 20 to 60. They are frequently large (20 to 30 cm), bilateral, and typically cystic.

Malignant epithelial tumors are usually seen in women over 40. They present as solid masses, with areas of necrosis and hemorrhage. Masses larger than 10 to 15 cm have usually already spread into the intraabdominal space. Spread eventually results in intraabdominal carcinomatosis, which leads to bowel and renal obstruction and cachexia.

Although most ovarian tumors are epithelial, two other important ovarian tumor types exist—stromal and germ cell tumors. These tumors are distinct in their cell of origin but also have different clinical presentations and natural histories and are often managed differently (see below).

Metastasis to the ovary can occur from breast, colon, gastric, and pancreatic cancers, and the Krukenberg tumor was classically described as bilateral ovarian masses from metastatic mucin-secreting gastrointestinal cancers.

Staging and Prognostic Factors Although laparotomy is often the primary procedure used to establish the diagnosis, less invasive studies can often aid in defining the extent of spread. These include chest x-rays, abdominal computed tomography scans, and abdominal and pelvic sonography. If the woman has specific gastrointestinal symptoms, a barium enema or gastrointestinal series can be performed. Symptoms of bladder or renal dysfunction can be evaluated by cystoscopy or intravenous pyelography.

A careful staging laparotomy will establish the stage and extent of disease and allow for the cytoreduction of tumor masses in patients with advanced disease. Proper laparotomy requires a vertical incision of sufficient length to ensure adequate examination of the abdominal contents. The presence, amount, and cytology of any ascites fluid should be noted. The primary tumor should be evaluated for rupture, excrescences, or dense adherence. Careful visual and manual inspection of the diaphragm and peritoneal surfaces is required. In addition to total abdominal hysterectomy and bilateral salpingo-oophorectomy, a partial omentectomy should be performed and the paracolic gutters inspected. Pelvic lymph nodes as well as para-aortic nodes in the region of the renal hilus should be biopsied. Since this surgical procedure defines stage, establishes prognosis, and determines the necessity for subsequent therapy, it should be performed by a surgeon with special expertise in ovarian cancer staging. Studies have shown that patients operated upon by gynecologic oncologists were properly staged 97 percent of the time, compared to 52 and 35 percent of cases staged by obstetricians/gynecologists and general surgeons respectively. At the end of staging, 23 percent of women have stage I disease (cancer confined to the ovary or ovaries); 13 percent have stage II (disease confined to the true pelvis); 47 percent have stage III (disease spread into but confined to the abdomen); and 16 percent have stage IV disease (spread outside the pelvis and abdomen). The 5-year survival correlates with stage of disease: stage I—90 percent, stage II—70 percent, stage III—15 to 20 percent, and stage IV—1 to 5 percent (see Table 99-1).

Prognosis in ovarian cancer is dependent not only upon stage but on the extent of residual disease and histologic grade. Patients presenting with advanced disease but left without significant residual disease after surgery have a median survival of 39 months, compared to 17 months for those with suboptimal tumor resection.

Prognosis of epithelial tumors is also highly influenced by histologic grade but less so by histologic type. Some studies in early stage disease have suggested a better survival for mucinous adenocarcinoma than endometrial and serous types, and a worse prognosis for clear cell carcinomas. Although grading systems differ among pathologists, all grading systems show a better prognosis for well- or moderately differentiated tumors and a poorer prognosis for poorly differentiated histologies. Typical 5-year survivals for patients with all stages of disease are: well differentiated—88 percent, moderately differentiated—58 percent, poorly differentiated—27 percent.

The prognostic significance of pre- and postoperative CA-125 levels is uncertain. Serum levels generally reflect volume of disease, and high levels usually indicate unresectability and a poorer survival. Postoperative levels, if elevated, usually indicate residual disease. Nevertheless, on multivariate analysis, CA-125 is not an independent prognostic factor because of the association with volume of disease. The rate of decline of CA-125 levels during initial therapy or the absolute level after one to three cycles of chemotherapy correlates with prognosis but is not sufficiently accurate to guide individual treatment decisions. Even when the CA-125 level falls to normal after surgery or chemotherapy, "second-look" laparotomy identifies residual disease in 60 percent of women. Other more quantitative approaches to define prognosis include ploidy analysis and image cytometry (automated analysis of cell morphology), but, while promising, they remain investigational.

Genetic and biologic factors may influence prognosis. Increased tumor levels of p53 are associated with a worse prognosis in advanced disease. Epidermal growth factor receptors in ovarian cancer are associated with a high risk of progression, but the increased expression of HER-2/neu has given conflicting prognostic results, and expression of Mdr-1 has not been of prognostic value.

℞ TREATMENT

The selection of therapy for patients with epithelial ovarian cancer depends upon the stage, extent of residual tumor, and histologic grade. In general, patients are considered in three separate treatment groups: (1) those with early (stages I and II) ovarian cancer and microscopic or no residual disease; (2) patients with advanced (stage III) disease but minimal residual tumor (<1 cm) after initial surgery; and (3) patients with bulky residual tumor and advanced (stage III or IV) disease.

Patients with stage I disease, no residual tumor, and well or moderately differentiated tumors need no adjuvant therapy after definitive surgery and have a 5-year survival in excess of 95 percent. For all other patients with early disease and those stage I patients with poor prognosis histologic grade, adjuvant therapy is probably warranted, and total-abdominal irradiation, single-agent cisplatin, or drug combinations used in advanced disease are appropriate. Five-year survival for this group exceeds 80 percent.

For the patients with advanced (stage III) disease but with limited or no residual disease after definitive cytoreductive surgery (about 50 percent of all stage III patients), the primary therapy is combination chemotherapy. Approximately 70 percent of women respond to initial combination chemotherapy, and 40 to 50 percent have a complete regression of disease. Only about half of these patients are free of disease if surgically restaged. Although a variety of combinations are active, a randomized prospective trial of paclitaxel and cisplatin compared to cyclophosphamide and cisplatin in patients with more advanced disease demonstrated better results for the paclitaxel-cisplatin combination (response rate 77 versus 64 percent, complete remission rate 54 versus 33 percent, median survival 37.5 versus 24.4 months). This regimen of paclitaxel, 135 mg/m^2 body surface area over 24 h by infusion, followed by cisplatin, 75 mg/m^2, is now the standard therapy for advanced disease. Current trials are exploring the potential for reduction of cisplatin toxicity with substitution of carboplatin dosed to an AUC (area under the curve) of 7.5. The efficacy of this substitution and the appropriateness of alterations in the duration of paclitaxel infusion time have not been established through large randomized trials.

Patients with advanced disease (stages III and IV) and bulky residual tumor are generally treated with a paclitaxel-platinum combination regimen as well and, while the overall prognosis is poorer, 5-year survival may reach 10 to 15 percent. In some instances, cytoreductive surgery can be performed after initial response to chemotherapy, and a multicenter European trial demonstrated that this strategy led to a significant improvement in progression-free interval and survival.

Historically, patients who have had an excellent initial response to chemotherapy and have no clinical evidence of disease have had a second-look laparotomy. For patients with stage I ovarian cancer or for germ cell tumors, the operation rarely detects residual tumor and has been largely abandoned. For those with stages II and III epithelial tumors, the procedure can be appropriate in the context of a clinical trial or if unique therapy for minimal-residual disease is contemplated. However, there is no evidence that the second-look

Table 99-1

Staging and Survival in Gynecologic Malignancies

Stage	Ovarian	5-Year Survival, %	Endometrial	5-Year Survival, %	Cervix	5-Year Survival, %
0	—		—		Carcinoma in situ	100
I	Confined to ovary	90	Confined to corpus	89	Confined to uterus	85
II	Confined to pelvis	70	Involves corpus and cervix	80	Invades beyond uterus but not to pelvic wall	60
III	Intraabdominal spread	15–20	Extends outside the uterus but not outside the true pelvis	30	Extends to pelvic wall and/or lower third of vagina, or hydronephrosis	33
IV	Spread outside abdomen	1–5	Extends outside the true pelvis or involves the bladder or rectum	9	Invades mucosa of bladder or rectum or extends beyond the true pelvis	7

surgical procedure itself prolongs overall survival. The routine use of second-look laparotomy cannot be recommended. There is also no evidence that any form of maintenance therapy is beneficial in preventing recurrences in patients in complete remission.

Patients with advanced disease whose disease recurs after initial treatment are usually not curable but may benefit significantly from limited surgery to relieve intestinal obstruction, localized radiation therapy to relieve pressure or pain from mass lesions or metastasis, or palliative chemotherapy. The selection of chemotherapy for palliation depends upon the initial regimen used for treatment and evidence of drug resistance. Often patients who have a complete regression of disease that lasts 6 months or more respond to reinduction with the same agents. Patients relapsing within the first 6 months of initial therapy rarely do. Chemotherapeutic agents with ~20 percent activity in patients relapsing after initial combination chemotherapy include carboplatin, ifosfamide, hexamethylmelamine, and etoposide, and intraperitoneal chemotherapy may be used if a small residual volume (<1 cm^3) of tumor exists. Progestational agents and antiestrogens produce responses in 5 to 15 percent of patients and have minimal side effects. Experimental approaches with some promise include the agents gemcitabine and topotecan and high-dose chemotherapy with hematopoietic stem cell support.

OVARIAN GERM CELL TUMORS Fewer than 5 percent of all ovarian tumors are germ cell in origin. They include teratomas, dysgerminoma, endodermal sinus tumor, and embryonal carcinoma. Germ cell tumors of the ovary generally occur in younger women (75 percent of ovarian malignancies in women under 30), display an unusually aggressive natural history, were often fatal before the combination chemotherapy era, and now are commonly cured with less extensive nonsterilizing surgery and chemotherapy. There are now many reports of normal children born to women cured of these malignancies.

These neoplasms can be divided into three major groups: (1) benign tumors (usually dermoid cysts); (2) malignant tumors that arise from dermoid cysts; and (3) primitive malignant germ cell tumors including dysgerminoma, yolk sac tumors, immature teratomas, embryonal carcinomas, and choriocarcinoma.

Dermoid cysts are teratomatous cysts usually lined by epidermis and skin appendages. They often contain hair and calcified bone or teeth can sometimes be seen on conventional pelvic x-ray. They are almost always curable by surgical resection. Approximately 1 percent of these tumors have malignant elements, usually squamous cell carcinoma.

Malignant germ cell tumors are usually large (median—16 cm). Bilateral disease is rare except in dysgerminoma (10 to 15 percent bilaterality). Abdominal or pelvic pain in young women are the usual presenting symptoms. Serum human chorionic gonadoptropin (hCG) and alpha fetoprotein (αFP) levels are useful in the diagnosis and management of these patients. Before the advent of chemotherapy, extensive surgery was routine but has now been replaced by careful evaluation of extent of spread followed by resection of bulky disease and preservation of one ovary, uterus, and cervix if feasible. This allows many affected women to preserve fertility. After surgical staging 60 to 75 percent of women have stage I disease and 25 to 30 percent have stage III disease. Stages II and IV are infrequent.

Most of the malignant germ cell tumors are managed with chemotherapy after surgery. VAC (vincristine, actinomycin-D, cyclophosphamide) produces 70 to 90 percent cures in stage I disease but fewer than 50 percent for stage III disease. Regimens used in testicular cancer like PVB (cisplatin, vinblastine, bleomycin) and BEP (bleomycin 30 units IV weekly, etoposide 100 mg/m^2 days 1 to 5, and cisplatin 20 mg/m^2 days 1 to 5) with three or four courses given at 21-day intervals have produced excellent results. Postoperative chemotherapy with BEP in 93 patients (stages I to III) has achieved a 95 percent long-term survival (median follow-up >38 months). This regimen is the treatment of choice for all malignant germ cell tumors except grade I, stage I immature teratoma, where surgery alone is adequate, and per-

haps early stage dysgerminoma, where surgery and radiation therapy are used.

Dysgerminoma is the ovarian counterpart of testicular seminoma. The tumor has commonly been treated with radiation therapy and is very radiosensitive. Results in early disease are excellent (5-year disease-free survival—100 percent) but less so in stage III disease (5-year disease-free survival—61 percent). Unfortunately, the use of radiation therapy makes many patients infertile. BEP chemotherapy is equally or more effective and does not cause infertility. In incompletely resected patients with dysgerminoma, the 2-year disease-free survival was 95 percent and infertility was not observed. These data have led most physicians to replace postoperative radiation therapy with combination chemotherapy (BEP) in women with ovarian dysgerminoma.

OVARIAN STROMAL TUMORS Stromal tumors make up fewer than 10 percent of ovarian tumors. They are named for the stromal tissue involved: granulosa, theca, Sertoli, Leydig, and collagen-producing stromal cells. The granulosa and theca cell stromal cell tumors occur most frequently in the first three decades of life. Granulosa cell tumors frequently produce estrogen and cause menstrual abnormalities, bleeding, and precocious puberty. Endometrial carcinoma can be seen in 5 percent of these women, perhaps related to the persistent hyperestrogenism. Sertoli and Leydig cell tumors, when functional, produce androgens with resultant virilization or hirsutism. Seventy-five percent of these stromal cell tumors present in stage I and can be cured with total abdominal hysterectomy and bilateral salpingo-oophorectomy. Stromal tumors generally grow slowly, and recurrences can occur 5 to 10 years after initial surgery. Neither radiation therapy nor chemotherapy have been documented to be consistently effective, and surgical management remains the primary treatment.

CARCINOMA OF THE FALLOPIAN TUBE

The fallopian tube is the least common site of cancer in the female genital tract although its epithelial surface far exceeds that of the ovary, where epithelial cancer is 20 times more common. There are approximately 300 new cases yearly; 90 percent are papillary serous adenocarcinomas, with the remainder being mixed mesodermal, endometroid, and transitional cell tumors. The gross and microscopic characteristics and the spread of the tumor are similar to those of ovarian cancer but can be distinguished if the tumor arises from the endosalpinx, the tubal epithelium shows a transition between benign and malignant, and the ovaries and endometrium are normal or minimally involved. The differential diagnosis includes primary or metastatic ovarian cancer, chronic salpingitis, tuberculous salpingitis, salpingitis isthmica nodosa, and cautery artifact.

Unlike ovarian cancer, patients frequently present with early symptoms, usually postmenopausal vaginal bleeding, pain, and leukorrhea. Surgical staging is similar to that used for ovarian cancer, and prognosis is related to stage and extent of residual disease. Patients with stages I and II disease are generally treated with surgery alone or with surgery and pelvic radiation therapy, although there is no clear evidence for improved 5-year survival with irradiation (5-year survival stage I— 74 versus 75 percent, stage II—43 versus 48 percent). Patients with stages III and IV disease are treated with the same chemotherapy regimens used in advanced ovarian carcinoma, and 5-year survival is similar (stage III—20 percent, stage IV—5 percent).

UTERINE CANCER

Carcinoma of the endometrium is the most common female pelvic malignancy. Approximately 34,000 new cases are diagnosed yearly, although in most (75 percent) tumor is confined to the uterine corpus at diagnosis and therefore most can be cured. The 6000 deaths yearly make uterine cancer only the seventh leading cause of death from malignancy in females. It is primarily a disease of postmenopausal women, although 25 percent of cases occur in women below age 50 and 5 percent below age 40. The disease is common in Eastern Europe and the United States and uncommon in Asia.

Phenotypic characteristics and risk factors common in patients with endometrial cancer include obesity, altered menstruation, low fertility index, late menopause, anovulation, and postmenopausal bleeding. Many of these features suggest that exposure to unopposed estrogen from either endogenous or exogenous sources may play a central etiologic role. Women taking tamoxifen for breast cancer treatment or prevention are also at somewhat increased risk.

Endometrial carcinoma occurs most often in the sixth and seventh decades of life. Symptoms often include abnormal vaginal discharge (90 percent), abnormal bleeding (80 percent), which is usually postmenopausal, and leukorrhea (10 percent). Initial evaluation of patients suspected of endometrial cancer should include a history and physical and pelvic examination followed by an endometrial biopsy or a fractional dilation and curettage. Outpatient procedures such as endometrial biopsy or aspiration curettage can be used but are definitive only when positive.

Between 75 and 80 percent of all endometrial carcinomas are adenocarcinomas, and the prognosis depends upon stage, histologic grade, and extent of myometrial invasion. Grade I tumors are highly differentiated adenocarcinomas, grade II contain some solid areas, and grade III tumors are largely solid or undifferentiated. Adenocarcinoma with squamous differentiation is seen in 10 percent of patients; the most differentiated form is known as *adenoacanthoma*, and the poorly differentiated form is called *adenosquamous carcinoma*. Other less common pathologies include mucinous carcinoma (5 percent) and papillary serous carcinoma (<10 percent). This latter type has a natural history indistinguishable from ovarian carcinoma. Rarer histologies include secretory (2 percent), ciliated, clear cell, and undifferentiated carcinomas.

The staging of endometrial cancer requires surgery to establish the extent of disease and the depth of myometrial invasion. Peritoneal fluid should be sampled; the abdomen and pelvis explored; and pelvic and para-aortic lymphadenectomy performed depending upon the histology, grade, and depth of invasion in the uterine specimen on frozen section. After evaluation and staging, 74 percent of patients are stage I, 13 percent are stage II, 9 percent are stage III, and 3 percent are found to be stage IV. Five-year survival by stage is as follows: stage I—89 percent, stage II—80 percent, stage III—30 percent, and stage IV—9 percent (see Table 99-1).

Patients with uncomplicated endometrial carcinoma are effectively managed with total abdominal hysterectomy and bilateral salpingo-oophorectomy. Pre- or postoperative irradiation has been used, and although vaginal cuff recurrence is reduced, survival is not altered. In women with poor histologic grade, deep myometrial invasion, or extensive involvement of the lower uterine segment or cervix, intracavitary or external beam irradiation is warranted.

About 15 percent of women have endometrial carcinoma with extension to the cervix only (stage II), and management depends upon the extent of cervical invasion. Superficial cervical invasion can be managed like stage I disease, but extensive cervical invasion requires radical hysterectomy or preoperative radiotherapy followed by extrafascial hysterectomy. Once disease is outside the uterus but still confined to the true pelvis (stage III), management generally includes surgery and irradiation. Patients who have involvement only of the ovary or fallopian tubes generally do well with such therapy, and 5-year survivals of 80 percent have been reported. Other stage III patients with disease extending beyond the adnexa or those with serous carcinomas of the endometrium have a significantly poorer prognosis (5-year survival of 15 percent).

Patients with stage IV disease (outside the abdomen or invading the bladder or rectum) are generally treated symptomatically with irradiation, surgery, and/or progestational agents. Progestational agents are the most commonly used systemic treatment and produce responses in about 25 percent of patients. Well-differentiated tumors respond most frequently, and responses can be correlated with the level of progesterone-receptor expression in the tumor. The commonly used progestational agents hydroxyprogesterone (Dilalutin), megastrol (Megace), and deoxyprogesterone (Provera) all produce similar response rates, and the antiestrogen tamoxifen (Nolvadex) produces responses in 10 to 25 percent of patients in a salvage setting.

Chemotherapy is not very successful in advanced endometrial carcinoma. The most active single agents with consistent response rates of 20 percent or more include cisplatin, carboplatin, doxorubicin, epirubicin, and paclitaxel. Combinations of drugs with or without progestational agents have generally produced response rates similar to single agents.

CERVIX CANCER

Carcinoma of the cervix was once the most common cause of cancer death in women, but over the past 30 years, the mortality rate has decreased by 50 percent. Now, cervix cancer trails breast, lung, colorectal, endometrium, and ovarian cancers in incidence. In 1996, there were approximately 15,700 new cases of invasive cervix cancer, and more than 50,000 cases of carcinoma in situ. There were 4,900 deaths from the disease, and of those patients, approximately 85 percent had never had a Pap smear at any time in their lives. The disease remains the major gynecologic cancer in underdeveloped countries. It is more common in lower socioeconomic groups, women with early initial sexual activity, multiple sexual partners, and in smokers. Many of these factors suggest a venereal transmission. It appears that human papilloma virus (HPV) has an important etiologic role. Over 66 types of human papilloma viruses have been isolated, and many are associated with genital warts. Those types associated with cervical carcinoma are 16, 18, 31, 45, and 51 to 53. These, along with many other types, are also associated with cervical intraepithelial neoplasia (CIN). Of particular interest, the protein product of HPV-16, the E7 protein, binds and inactivates the tumor suppressor gene Rb, and the E6 protein of HPV-18 has sequence homology to the SV40 large T antigen and has the capacity to bind and inactivate the tumor suppressor gene p53. E6 and E7 are both necessary and sufficient to cause cell transformation in vitro. These binding and inactivation events may explain the carcinogenic effects of the viruses (see Chap. 190).

Uncomplicated HPV lower genital tract infection and condylomatous atypia of the cervix can progress to CIN. This lesion precedes invasive cervical carcinoma and is classified as low-grade squamous intraepithelial lesion (SIL), high-grade SIL, and carcinoma in situ. Carcinoma in situ demonstrates cytologic evidence of neoplasia without invasion through the basement membrane, can persist unchanged for 10 to 20 years, but eventually progresses to invasive carcinoma.

The Papanicolaou smear is 90 to 95 percent accurate in detecting early lesions such as CIN but is less sensitive in detecting cancer when frankly invasive cancer or fungating masses are present. Inflammation, necrosis, and hemorrhage may produce false-positive smears, and colposcopic-directed biopsy is required when any lesion is visible on the cervix, regardless of Pap smear findings. The American Cancer Society recommends that women after onset of sexual activity, or over age 20, have two consecutive yearly smears. If negative, smears should be repeated every 3 years. The American College of Obstetrics and Gynecology recommends yearly Pap smears with routine annual pelvic and breast examinations. Women with suspicious or abnormal Pap smears should have colposcopic-directed cervical biopsy. Colposcopy is a technique using a binocular microscope and 3% acetic acid applied to the cervix in which abnormal areas appear white and can be directly biopsied. This procedure has reduced the need for cone biopsy, which is still required when endocervical tumor is suspected, colposcopy is inadequate, the diagnosis of microinvasive carcinoma is made on biopsy, or when there is a discrepancy between the Pap smear and the colposcopic findings. Cone biopsy alone is therapeutic for CIN in many patients, although a less radical electrocautery excision may be sufficient.

Approximately 80 percent of invasive cervix carcinomas are squamous cell tumors; 10 to 15 percent are adenocarcinomas; 2 to 5 percent are adenosquamous with epithelial and glandular structures; and 1 to 2 percent are clear cell mesonephric tumors.

Patients with cervix cancer generally present with abnormal bleeding or postcoital spotting that may increase to intermenstrual or prominent menstrual bleeding. Yellowish vaginal discharge, lumbosacral back pain, and urinary symptoms can also be seen.

The staging of cervical carcinoma is clinical and generally completed with a pelvic examination under anesthesia with cystoscopy and proctoscopy. Chest x-rays, intravenous pyelograms, and computed tomography are generally required, and magnetic resonance imaging (MRI) may be used to assess extracervical extension. Stage 0 is carcinoma in situ; stage I is disease confined to the cervix; stage II disease invades beyond the cervix but not to the pelvic wall or lower third of the vagina; stage III disease extends to the pelvic wall or lower third of the vagina or causes hydronephrosis; stage IV is present when the tumor invades the mucosa of bladder or rectum or extends beyond the true pelvis. Five-year survivals are as follows: stage I—85 percent, stage II—60 percent, stage III—33 percent, and stage IV—7 percent (see Table 99-1).

Carcinoma in situ (stage 0) can generally be successfully managed by cone biopsy or by abdominal hysterectomy. For stage I disease, results appear equivalent for either radical hysterectomy or radiation therapy. Patients with stages II to IV disease are primarily managed with radical radiation therapy. Retroperitoneal lymphadenectomy is being investigated in clinical trials, but its benefit is unproven. Pelvic exenterations, although uncommon, are performed for centrally recurrent or persistent disease. Significant advances have been made in the reconstruction of the vagina, bladder, and rectum following this operation.

The majority of patients can be managed with either surgery, radiation therapy, or combinations of the two. Chemotherapy has been investigated in patients with unresectable advanced disease, recurrent disease, and as a radiation sensitizer. Active agents with ≥ 20 percent response rates include cisplatin, 5-fluorouracil (5-FU), hexamethylmelamine, and vincristine. Combination chemotherapy has been studied actively, but no combination has proved better than single agents. Intraarterial chemotherapy has been studied, either pre- or postoperatively, but is associated with substantial local toxicity and response rates of approximately 20 percent. Recent interest has centered on the use of chemotherapy as a radiosensitizer. Active agents include hydroxyurea, 5-FU, and cisplatin. Although definitive randomized trials have not been completed, concomitant chemoradiation is feasible, and response and survival rates appear to be better than in similar groups treated with radiation alone.

GESTATIONAL TROPHOBLASTIC NEOPLASIA

While gestational choriocarcinoma accounts for fewer than 1 percent of female gynecologic malignancies, it is important because it is cured with appropriate chemotherapy and represents one of the triumphs of modern cancer management. Before the use of chemotherapy, fewer than 10 percent of patients survived, but now with appropriate management, deaths from this disease have become rare in the United States. The spectrum of disease ranges from benign hydatidiform mole to trophoblastic malignancy (placental-site trophoblastic tumor and choriocarcinoma).

Epidemiology   In the United States, the incidence is about 1 per 1000 pregnancies; in Asia, 2 per 1000 pregnancies. Maternal age greater than 45 years is a risk factor for hydatidiform mole. A prior history of molar pregnancy is also a risk factor. Choriocarcinoma occurs approximately once in 25,000 pregnancies or once in 20,000 live births. Prior history of hydatidiform mole is a risk factor for choriocarcinoma. A woman with a molar pregnancy is 1000 times more likely to develop choriocarcinoma than a woman with a prior normal-term pregnancy.

Pathology and Etiology   The trophoblastic neoplasms have been divided by morphology into complete or partial hydatidiform mole, invasive mole, placental-site trophoblastomas, and choriocarcinomas. Hydatidiform moles contain clusters of villi with hydropic changes, hyperplasia of the trophoblast, and the absence of fetal vessels. Invasive moles differ only by invasion into the uterine myometrium. Placental-site trophoblastic tumors are predominately made up of cytotrophoblast

cells arising from the placental implantation site. Choriocarcinomas consist of anaplastic trophoblastic tissue with both cytotrophoblastic and syncytiotrophoblastic elements and no identifiable villi.

Complete moles result from uniparental disomy in which loss of the maternal genes (23 autosomes plus X) occurs by unknown mechanisms and is followed by duplication of the paternal haploid genome (23 autosomes plus X). Uncommonly (5 percent), moles result from dispermic fertilization of an empty egg, resulting in either 46XY or 46XX genotype. Partial moles result from dispermic fertilization of an egg with retention of the maternal haploid set of chromosomes, resulting in diandric triploidy (see Chap. 65).

Clinical Presentation   Molar pregnancies are generally associated with first-trimester bleeding, ectopic pregnancies, or threatened abortions. The uterus is inappropriately large for the length of gestation, and hCG levels are higher than expected. Fetal parts and heart sounds are not present. The diagnosis is generally made by the passage of grapelike clusters from the uterus, but ultrasound demonstration of the hydropic mole can be diagnostic. Patients suspected of a molar pregnancy require a chest film, careful pelvic examinations, and weekly serial monitoring of hCG levels.

℞ TREATMENT

Patients with hydatidiform moles require surgical evacuation coupled with postevacuation monitoring of hCG levels. In most women (80 percent), the hCG titer progressively declines within 8 to 10 days of evacuation (serum half-life is 24 to 36 h). Patients should be monitored on a monthly basis and should not become pregnant for at least a year. Patients found to have invasive mole at curettage are generally treated with hysterectomy and chemotherapy. Approximately half of patients with choriocarcinoma develop the malignancy after a molar pregnancy, and the other half develop the malignancy after abortion, ectopic pregnancy, or occasionally after a normal full-term pregnancy.

Chemotherapy is generally used for gestational trophoblastic neoplasia and is often used in hydatidiform mole if hCG levels rise or plateau or if metastases develop. Patients with invasive mole or choriocarcinoma require chemotherapy. Several regimens are effective, including methotrexate at 30 mg/m² intramuscularly on a weekly basis until hCG titers are normal. However, methotrexate (1 mg/kg) given every other day for 4 days followed by leukovorin (0.1 mg/kg) given intravenously 24 h after methotrexate is associated with a cure rate of ≥ 90 percent and low toxicity. Intermittent courses are generally continued until the hCG titer becomes undetectable for 3 consecutive weeks, and then patients are monitored monthly for a year.

Patients with high-risk tumors (high hCG levels, disease presenting ≥ 4 months after antecedent pregnancy, brain or liver metastasis, or failure of single-agent methotrexate) are initially treated with combination chemotherapy. MAC chemotherapy with methotrexate, actinomycin-D, and cyclophosphamide has been the most commonly used regimen, with cycles of therapy given every 3 weeks until complete remission. Other effective regimens include EMA-CO (a cyclic non-cross-resistant combination of etoposide, methotrexate, and dactinomycin alternating with cyclophosphamide and vincristine); cisplatin, bleomycin, and vinblastine; and cisplatin, etoposide, and bleomycin. EMA-CO is now the regimen of choice for patients with high-risk disease because of excellent survival rates (>80 percent) and less toxicity than MAC. Patients with brain or liver metastasis are usually treated with local irradiation to metastatic sites in conjunction with chemotherapy. Long-term studies of patients cured of trophoblastic disease have not demonstrated an increased risk of maternal complications or fetal abnormalities with subsequent pregnancies.

BIBLIOGRAPHY

Barakat RR et al: Corpus epithelial tumors, in *Principles and Practice of Gynecologic Oncology*, 2d ed, WJ Hoskins et al (eds). Philadelphia, Lippincott, 1996, pp 859–896

Bolis G et al: EMA/CO regimen in high-risk gestational trophoblastic tumor (GTT). Gynecol Oncol 31:439, 1988

Cressman WT, DiSaia PJ: Screening in ovarian cancer. Am J Obstet Gynecol 165:7, 1991

GOLDSTEIN DP: Gestational trophoblastic neoplasia in the 1990's. Yale J Biol Med 64:639, 1991

HACKER NF: Uterine cancer, in *Practical Gynecologic Oncology*, 2d ed, JS Berek, NF Hacker (eds). Baltimore, Williams & Wilkins, 1994, pp 285–326.

McGUIRE WP et al: Cyclophosphamide and cisplatin compared with paclitaxel and cisplatin in patients with stage III and stage IV ovarian cancer. N Engl J Med 334:1, 1996

OZOLS RF et al: Epithelial ovarian cancer, in *Principles and Practice of Gynecologic Oncology*, 2d ed, WJ Hoskins et al (eds). Philadelphia, Lippincott, 1996, pp 919–986.

SOPER VT: Identification and management of high-risk gestational trophoblastic disease. Semin Oncol 22:172, 1995

STEHMAN FB et al: Uterine cervix, in *Principles and Practice of Gynecologic Oncology*, 2d ed, WJ Hoskins et al (eds). Philadelphia, Lippincott, 1996, pp 785–857.

VANDERBURG ME et al: Intervention debulking surgery does improve survival in advanced epithelial ovarian cancer. N Engl J Med 332:629, 1995

WILLIAMS S et al: Adjuvant therapy of ovarian germ cell tumors with cisplatin, etoposide and bleomycin: A trial of the Gynecologic Oncology Group. J Clin Oncol 12:701, 1994

YOUNG RC et al: Adjuvant therapy in stage I and stage II epithelial ovarian cancer. Results of two prospective trials. N Engl J Med 327:1021, 1990

---

100   *Shreyaskumar R. Patel, Robert S. Benjamin*

SARCOMAS OF SOFT TISSUE AND BONE

Sarcomas are rare mesenchymal neoplasms that arise in bone and soft tissues. They constitute less than 1 percent of all malignancies. Most of these tumors are mesodermal in origin, although a few are derived from neuroectoderm, and they are biologically distinct from the more common epithelial malignancies. Sarcomas affect all age groups; 15 percent are found in children younger than age 15, and 40 percent occur after age 55. Sarcomas are one of the most common solid tumors of childhood and are the fifth most common cause of cancer deaths in children. Sarcomas may be divided into two groups, those derived from bone and those derived from soft tissues.

SOFT TISSUE SARCOMAS

Soft tissues include muscles, tendons, fat, fibrous tissue, synovial tissue, vessels, and nerves. Approximately 60 percent of soft-tissue sarcomas arise in the extremities, with the lower extremities involved three times as often as the upper extremities. Thirty percent arise in the trunk, the retroperitoneum accounting for 40 percent of all trunk lesions. The remaining 10 percent arise in the head and neck.

INCIDENCE Approximately 6400 new cases of soft tissue sarcomas occurred in the United States in 1996. The annual age-adjusted incidence is approximately 2 per 100,000 population, but the incidence varies with age and with the types of neoplasms included in the definition. Soft tissue sarcomas constitute 0.7 percent of all cancers in the general population and 6.5 percent of all malignancies in children.

EPIDEMIOLOGY Malignant transformation of a benign soft tissue tumor is extremely rare, with the exception that malignant peripheral nerve sheath tumors (neurofibrosarcoma, malignant schwannoma) can arise from neurofibromas in patients with neurofibromatosis. Several etiologic factors have been implicated in the pathogenesis of soft tissue sarcomas.

Environmental Factors Trauma or previous injury is rarely involved, but sarcomas can arise in scar tissue resulting from a prior operation, burn, fracture, or foreign body implantation. Chemical carcinogens such as polycyclic hydrocarbons, asbestos, and dioxin may be involved in the pathogenesis.

Iatrogenic Factors Sarcomas in bone or soft tissues occur in cancer patients who are treated with radiation and survive at least 5 years. The tumor nearly always arises in the irradiated field. The risk increases with time.

Viruses The association of Kaposi's sarcoma (KS) with human immunodeficiency virus (HIV) type 1 has led to studies of the role of viruses in the pathogenesis of KS. Herpesvirus-like DNA sequences have been documented in AIDS-associated KS, classic KS, and KS in HIV-negative homosexual men, leading to the hypothesis that this new herpes virus [human herpes virus (HHV8)] may be the common etiologic factor for all three variants of KS.

Immunologic Factors Congenital or acquired immunodeficiency, including therapeutic immunosuppression, is associated with or influences sarcoma development.

Genetic Factors Li-Fraumeni syndrome is a familial cancer syndrome in which affected individuals have germ-line abnormalities of the tumor suppressor gene *p53* and an increased incidence of soft tissue sarcomas and other malignancies, including breast cancer, osteosarcoma, brain tumors, leukemia, and adrenal carcinoma (Chap. 84). Neurofibromatosis 1 (NF-1, peripheral form, von Recklinghausen's disease) is characterized by multiple neurofibromas and café au lait spots. Neurofibromas occasionally undergo malignant degeneration to become malignant peripheral nerve sheath tumors. The gene for NF-1 is located in the pericentromeric region of chromosome 17 and encodes neurofibromin, a tumor suppressor protein with GTPase-activating activity that inhibits Ras function (Chap. 375). Germ-line mutation of the *Rb-1* locus (chromosome 13q14) in patients with inherited retinoblastoma is associated with the development of osteosarcoma in those who survive the retinoblastoma and of soft tissue sarcomas unrelated to radiation therapy. Other soft tissue tumors, including desmoid tumors, lipomas, leiomyomas, neuroblastomas, and paragangliomas, occasionally show a familial predisposition.

Insulin-like growth factor (IGF) type 2 is produced by some sarcomas and is thought to act both as an autocrine growth factor and as a motility factor that promotes metastatic spread. Antibodies to IGF-1 receptors block the stimulation of growth by IGF-2 in vitro but do not affect IGF-2–induced motility. If secreted in large amounts, IGF-2 may produce hypoglycemia (see Chaps. 102 and 335).

CLASSIFICATION Approximately 20 different types of sarcomas are recognized on the basis of the pattern of differentiation toward normal tissue. For example, rhabdomyosarcoma shows evidence of skeletal muscle fibers with cross-striations; leiomyosarcomas contain interlacing fascicles of spindle cells representing smooth muscle features; liposarcomas contain adipocytes; and angiosarcomas contain a rich network of blood vessels. When precise characterization of the type is not possible, the tumors are called *unclassified sarcomas*. All of the primary bone sarcomas also can arise from soft tissues (e.g., extraskeletal osteosarcoma, extraskeletal Ewing's sarcoma, and extraskeletal chondrosarcoma). The entity *malignant fibrous histiocytoma* includes a large number of tumors previously classified as fibrosarcomas or as pleomorphic variants of other sarcomas and is characterized by a mixture of spindle (fibrous) cells and round (histiocytic) cells arranged in a storiform pattern with frequent giant cells and areas of pleomorphism.

For purposes of treatment, most soft tissue sarcomas can be lumped together, with the choice of treatment depending mainly on the stage of disease. However, some aspects of the natural history require that specific histologic diagnoses be considered in planning treatment and follow-up. For example, the term *liposarcoma* indicates histogenesis from adipose tissue but gives no indication of biologic behavior. Pleomorphic liposarcomas and dedifferentiated liposarcomas behave like other high-grade sarcomas; in contrast, well-differentiated liposarcomas (better termed *atypical lipomatous tumors*) lack metastatic potential, and myxoid liposarcomas metastasize infrequently but, when they do, have a predilection for unusual metastatic sites containing fat, such as the retroperitoneum, mediastinum, and subcutaneous tissue. Rhabdomyosarcomas, Ewing's sarcoma, and other small cell sarcomas tend to be more aggressive, even when small, and are more responsive to chemotherapeutic agents than the more typical soft tissue sarcomas.

DIAGNOSIS The most common presentation is an asymptomatic mass. Mechanical symptoms referable to pressure, traction, or entrapment of nerves or muscles may be present, especially with large tumors. All new and persistent or growing masses should be biopsied, either by a cutting needle (core-needle biopsy) or preferably by a small incision, placed so that it can be encompassed in the subsequent excision without compromising a definitive resection. Sarcomas tend to metastasize through the blood rather than the lymphatic system. Consequently, the incidence of lymph node metastases is low (5 percent) for most of these tumors, although it is higher (17 percent) for certain tumors—e.g., synovial and epithelioid sarcomas, clear-cell sarcoma (melanoma of the soft parts), angiosarcoma, and rhabdomyosarcoma. The pulmonary parenchyma is the most common site of metastases in the vast majority of sarcomas. Exceptions are leiomyosarcomas arising in the gastrointestinal tract, which metastasize to the liver; myxoid liposarcomas, which seek fatty tissue: and clear-cell sarcomas, which may metastasize to bones. Central nervous system metastases are rare, except in the case of alveolar soft tissue sarcoma.

Radiographic Evaluation Imaging of the primary tumor is best accomplished by plain radiographs and magnetic resonance imaging (MRI) for tumors of the extremities or head and neck and by computed tomography (CT) for tumors of the chest, abdomen, or retroperitoneal cavity. A radiograph and CT scan of the chest are important for the detection of lung metastases. Other imaging studies may be indicated, depending on the symptoms, signs, or histology.

STAGING SYSTEMS The histologic grade and size of the primary tumor are the most important prognostic factors. Tumors are staged according to two systems, the American Joint Commission on Cancer (AJCC) staging system and the Musculoskeletal Tumor Society staging system.

AJCC Staging System The primary determinant of stage is *tumor histologic grade*. Grade 1 (well-differentiated) tumors are stage I; grade 2 (moderately well differentiated) tumors are stage II; and grade 3 (poorly differentiated) tumors are stage III. These stage designations are qualified further on the basis of tumor size as either A (tumor diameter <5 cm) or B (tumor diameter ≥5 cm). Tumors with lymph node metastases are stage IVA, and those with distant metastases are stage IVB.

Musculoskeletal Tumor Society Staging System This system is based on grade and compartmental localization. A Roman numeral reflects the tumor grade: stage I is low-grade, stage II is high-grade, and stage III includes tumors of any grade that have lymph node or distant metastases. In addition, the tumor is given a letter reflecting its compartmental localization. Tumors designated A are intracompartmental (i.e., confined to the same soft tissue compartment as the initial tumor), and tumors designated B are extracompartmental (i.e. extending into the adjacent soft tissue compartment or into bone). Thus, a stage IA tumor is a low-grade tumor confined to its compartment of origin, whereas a stage IB tumor is a low-grade tumor that extends outside its original compartment.

PROGNOSIS Prognosis is related to the stage, with 5-year survival rates averaging 75 percent for AJCC stage I, 55 percent for stage II, and 29 percent for stage III. The 5-year survival rate for stage IV disease is <20 percent, but a small number of patients in this category can be cured. Most patients with stage IV disease die within 6-12 months, but there is great variability in survival, and patients may live with slowly progressive disease for many years.

℞ TREATMENT

Surgery Soft tissue sarcomas tend to grow along fascial planes in the path of least resistance. As a result, the surrounding soft tissues are compressed to form a pseudocapsule that gives the sarcoma the appearance of a well-encapsulated lesion. This is invariably deceptive, because "shelling out" or marginal excision of such lesions results in a 50 to 90 percent probability of local recurrence. Radical excision with a negative margin, incorporating the biopsy site, is the standard surgical procedure for local disease. The adjuvant use of radiation therapy and/or chemotherapy improves the local control rate and per-

mits the use of limb-sparing surgery with a local control rate comparable to that achieved by radical excisions and amputations. The National Institutes of Health consensus conference in 1984 recommended limb-sparing surgery in conjunction with adjuvant irradiation and/or chemotherapy as effective therapy for local control except when negative margins are not obtainable, when the risks of radiation are prohibitive, or when neurovascular structures are involved so that resection will result in serious functional consequences to the limb. When appropriately performed, conservative limb-sparing procedures result in local failure rates of only 10 to 15 percent.

Radiation Therapy External beam radiation therapy is an adjuvant to limb-sparing surgery for improved local control. Preoperative administration of radiation therapy allows the use of smaller fields and smaller doses but results in a higher rate of wound complications. When radiation therapy is given postoperatively, the field of radiation must be larger, as the entire surgical bed must be encompassed, and the dose must be higher to compensate for hypoxia in the operated field. Brachytherapy or interstitial therapy, in which the radiation source is inserted into the tumor bed, is thought to be comparable in efficacy and also less time consuming and less expensive. Intraoperative irradiation has not been studied thoroughly.

Adjuvant Chemotherapy The role of adjuvant chemotherapy is controversial except for Ewing's sarcoma and rhabdomyosarcoma, where it is standard. Doxorubicin-based combination chemotherapy improves disease-free survival but has less effect on overall survival. Nevertheless, meta-analysis indicates that there is a significant decrease in the risk of disease recurrence (either local or distant) and death for patients with high-grade extremity saracomas who are treated with adjuvant chemotherapy. This approach is considered reasonable for high-risk primary tumors. An alternative approach is to treat such patients preoperatively with chemotherapy; the subset of patients who respond continue adjuvant therapy postoperatively, and the nonresponders can be spared the toxicity of systemic therapy to which they are unlikely to respond. Neither strategy has been proved superior.

Advanced Disease Metastatic soft tissue sarcomas are largely incurable, but up to 20 percent of patients who are rendered free of clinical evidence of disease become long-term survivors. The therapeutic intent, therefore, is to produce a complete remission with chemotherapy and/or surgery. Surgical resection of metastases, whenever possible, is an integral part of the management. Some patients benefit from repeated surgical excision of metastases. Despite their histologic heterogeneity, the sensitivity to chemotherapy of most soft tissue sarcomas is poor. The two most active chemotherapeutic agents are doxorubicin and ifosfamide, an analogue of cyclophosphamide. There is a steep dose-response relationship for these drugs in sarcomas. Dacarbazine (DTIC) has modest activity as a single agent but has better activity in combination with doxorubicin. Vincristine, etoposide, and dactinomycin are effective in Ewing's sarcoma and rhabdomyosarcoma, especially in children. Chondrosarcomas and leiomyosarcomas arising from the gastrointestinal tract are unresponsive to standard chemotherapeutic drugs.

Dose-intensive regimens (i.e., ones involving higher and more frequent doses) of doxorubicin and ifosfamide-based combinations, with growth factor support to ameliorate myelosuppression, may improve the rates of complete and partial response. Myeloablative doses of chemotherapy in combination with bone marrow transplantation have not been successful.

BONE SARCOMAS

INCIDENCE AND EPIDEMIOLOGY Bone sarcomas are rarer than soft tissue sarcomas; they accounted for only 0.2 percent of all new malignancies and approximately 2500 new cases in the United States in 1996. Several benign bone lesions have the potential for malignant transformation. Enchondromas and osteochondromas can transform into chondrosarcoma; and fibrous dysplasia, bone infarcts, and Paget's disease of bone can transform into either malignant fibrous histiocytoma or osteosarcoma.

CLASSIFICATION **Benign Tumors** The common benign bone tumors include enchondroma, osteochondroma, chondroblastoma, and chondromyxoid fibroma, all of cartilaginous origin; osteoid osteoma and osteoblastoma, of bone origin; fibroma and desmoplastic fibroma, of fibrous tissue origin; hemangioma, of vascular origin; and giant cell tumor, of unknown origin.

Malignant Tumors The most common malignant tumors of bone are plasma cell tumors (see Chap. 114). The four most common malignant tumors of nonhematopoietic origin are osteosarcoma, chondrosarcoma, Ewing's sarcoma, and malignant fibrous histiocytoma. Rare malignant tumors include chordoma (of notochordal origin), malignant giant cell tumor and adamantinoma (of unknown origin), and hemangioendothelioma (of vascular origin). Sarcomas of bone are staged according to the Musculoskeletal Tumor Society staging system outlined above.

OSTEOSARCOMA Osteosarcoma, accounting for almost 45 percent of all bone sarcomas, is a spindle cell neoplasm that produces osteoid (unmineralized bone) or bone. About 60 percent of all osteosarcomas occur in children and adolescents in the second decade of life, and about 10 percent occur in the third decade of life. Osteosarcomas in the fifth and sixth decades of life are frequently secondary to either radiation therapy or transformation in a preexisting benign condition, such as Paget's disease. Males are affected 1.5 to 2 times as often as females. Osteosarcoma has a predilection for metaphyses of long bones, and the most common sites of involvement are the distal femur, proximal tibia, and proximal humerus. The classification of osteosarcoma is complex, but 75 percent of osteosarcomas fall in the "conventional or classic" category, which include osteoblastic, chondroblastic, and fibroblastic osteosarcomas. The remaining 25 percent are classified as "variants" on the basis of (1) clinical characteristics, as in the case of osteosarcoma of the jaw, postradiation osteosarcoma, or Paget's osteosarcoma; (2) morphologic characteristics, as in the case of telangiectatic osteosarcoma, small cell osteosarcoma, or malignant fibrous histiocytoma; or (3) location, as in parosteal or periosteal osteosarcoma. Diagnosis usually requires a synthesis of clinical, radiologic, and pathologic features. Patients typically present with pain and swelling of the affected area. A plain radiograph reveals a destructive lesion with a moth-eaten appearance, a spiculated periosteal reaction (sunburst appearance), and a cuff of periosteal new bone formation at the margin of the soft tissue mass (Codman's triangle). A CT scan of the primary tumor is best for defining bone destruction and the pattern of calcification, whereas MRI is better for defining intramedullary and soft tissue extension. A chest radiograph and CT scan are used to detect lung metastases. Metastases to the bony skeleton should be imaged by a bone scan. Almost all osteosarcomas are hypervascular. Angiography is not helpful for diagnosis, but it is the most sensitive test for assessing the response to preoperative chemotherapy. Pathologic diagnosis is established either with a core-needle biopsy, where feasible, or with an open biopsy with an appropriately placed incision that does not compromise future limb-sparing resection. Most osteosarcomas are high-grade. The most important prognostic factor for long-term survival is response to chemotherapy. The 2-year survival of historical controls treated with surgery alone is <20 percent. The efficacy of adjuvant chemotherapy is better defined in osteosarcoma than in soft tissue sarcoma. Prospective, randomized trials have shown that adjuvant chemotherapy improves survival. The current state of the art, therefore, is preoperative chemotherapy followed by limb-sparing surgery (which can be accomplished in >80 percent of patients) followed by postoperative chemotherapy. The effective drugs are doxorubicin, ifosfamide, cisplatin, and high-dose methotrexate with leucovorin rescue. The various combinations of these agents that have been used have all been about equally successful. With the current management strategy, long-term survival rates in extremity osteosarcoma range from 60 to 70 percent. Osteosarcoma is radioresistant; radiation therapy has no role in the routine management. Malignant fibrous histiocytoma is considered a part of the spectrum of osteosarcoma and is managed similarly.

CHONDROSARCOMA Chondrosarcoma, which constitutes approximately 20 to 25 percent of all bone sarcomas, is a tumor of adulthood and old age with a peak incidence in the fourth to sixth decades of life. It has a predilection for the flat bones, especially the shoulder and pelvic girdles, but can also affect the diaphyseal portions of long bones. Chondrosarcomas can arise de novo or as a malignant transformation of an enchondroma or, rarely, of the cartilaginous cap of an osteochondroma. Chondrosarcomas have an indolent natural history and typically present as pain and swelling. Radiographically, the lesion may have a lobular appearance with mottled or punctate or annular calcification of the cartilaginous matrix. It is difficult to distinguish low-grade chondrosarcoma from benign lesions by x-ray or histologic examination. The diagnosis is therefore influenced by clinical history and physical examination. A new onset of pain, signs of inflammation, and progressive increase in the size of the mass suggest malignancy. The histologic classification is complex, but most tumors fall within the conventional or classic category. Like other bone sarcomas, high-grade chondrosarcomas spread to the lungs. Most chondrosarcomas are resistant to standard sarcoma chemotherapy, and surgical resection of primary or recurrent tumors, including pulmonary metastases, is the mainstay of therapy. There are two histologic variants for which this rule does not hold, however. Dedifferentiated chondrosarcoma is a low-grade tumor that dedifferentiates into a high-grade osteosarcoma or a malignant fibrous histiocytoma, a tumor that responds to chemotherapy. Mesenchymal chondrosarcoma, a rare variant composed of a small-cell element, also is responsive to systemic chemotherapy and is treated like Ewing's sarcoma.

EWING'S SARCOMA Ewing's sarcoma, which constitutes approximately 10 to 15 percent of all bone sarcomas, is common in adolescence and has a peak incidence in the second decade of life. It typically involves the diaphyseal region of long bones and also has an affinity for flat bones. The plain radiograph may show a characteristic "onion-peel" periosteal reaction with a generous soft tissue mass, which is better demonstrated by CT or MRI. This mass is composed of sheets of monotonous, small, round, blue cells and can be confused with lymphoma, embryonal rhabdomyosarcoma, and small cell carcinoma. The presence of p30/32, the product of the *mic-2* gene (which maps to the pseudoautosomal region of the X and Y chromosomes) is a cell-surface marker for Ewing's sarcoma [and other members of a family of tumors called *peripheral primitive neuroectodermal tumors* (PNETs)]. Most PNETs arise in soft tissues; they include peripheral neuroepithelioma, Askin's tumor (chest wall), and esthesioneuroblastoma. Glycogen-filled cytoplasm detected by immunohistochemical staining with periodic acid–Schiff is also characteristic of Ewing's sarcoma cells. The classic cytogenetic abnormality associated with this disease (and other PNETs) is a reciprocal translocation of the long arms of chromosomes 11 and 22, t(11;22), which creates a chimeric gene product of unknown function with components from the *fli-1* gene on chromosome 11 and *ews* on 22. This disease is very aggressive, and it is therefore considered a systemic disease. Common sites of metastases are lung, bones, and bone marrow. Systemic chemotherapy is the mainstay of therapy, often being used before surgery. Several chemotherapeutic drugs are active, including doxorubicin, cyclophosphamide or ifosfamide, etoposide, vincristine, and dactinomycin. Local treatment for the primary tumor includes surgical resection, usually with limb salvage or radiation therapy. Patients with lesions below the elbow and below the mid-calf have a 5-year survival of 80 percent with effective treatment. Ewing's sarcoma is a curable tumor, even in the presence of obvious metastatic disease, especially in children less than 11 years old. High-dose chemotherapy with hematopoietic support can cure a substantial fraction of patients with metastatic disease.

TUMORS METASTATIC TO BONE

Bone is a common site of metastasis for carcinomas of the prostate, breast, lung, kidney, bladder, and thyroid and for lymphomas and sarcomas. Prostate, breast and lung primaries account for 80 percent of all bone metastases. Metastatic tumors of bone are more common than primary bone tumors. Tumors usually spread to bone hematogenously, but local invasion from soft tissue masses also occurs. In descending order of frequency, the sites most often involved are the vertebrae, proximal femur, pelvis, ribs, sternum, proximal humerus, and skull. Bone metastases may be asymptomatic or may produce pain, swelling, symptoms of encroachment on a nerve root or the spinal cord, pathologic fracture, or myelophthisis (replacement of the marrow). Symptoms of hypercalcemia may be noted in cases of bony destruction.

Pain is the most frequent symptom. It usually develops gradually over weeks, is usually localized, and often is more severe at night. When patients with back pain develop neurologic signs or symptoms, emergency evaluation for spinal cord compression is indicated (see Chap. 104). Bone metastases exert a major adverse effect on quality of life in cancer patients.

Cancer in the bone may produce osteolysis, osteogenesis, or both. Osteolytic lesions result when the tumor produces substances that can directly elicit bone resorption (vitamin D–like steroids, prostaglandins, or parathyroid hormone–related peptide) or cytokines that can induce the formation of osteoclasts (interleukin 1 and tumor necrosis factor). Osteoblastic lesions result when the tumor produces cytokines that activate osteoblasts. In general, purely osteolytic lesions are best detected by plain radiography, but they may not be apparent until they are larger than 1 cm. These lesions are more commonly associated with hypercalcemia and with the excretion of hydroxyproline-containing peptides indicative of matrix destruction. When osteoblastic activity is prominent, the lesions may be readily detected using radionuclide bone scanning (which is sensitive to new bone formation), and the radiographic appearance may show increased bone density or sclerosis. Osteoblastic lesions are associated with higher serum levels of alkaline phosphatase, and, if extensive, may produce hypocalcemia. Although some tumors may produce mainly osteolytic lesions (e.g., kidney cancer) and others mainly osteoblastic lesions (e.g., prostate cancer), most metastatic lesions produce both types of lesion and may go through stages where one or the other predominates.

In older patients, particularly women, it may be necessary to distinguish metastatic disease of the spine from osteoporosis. In osteoporosis, the cortical bone may be preserved, whereas cortical bone destruction is usually noted with metastatic cancer.

Treatment of metastatic bone disease depends on the underlying malignancy and the symptoms. Some metastatic bone tumors are curable (lymphoma, Hodgkin's disease), and others are treated with palliative intent. Pain may be relieved by local radiation therapy. Hormonally responsive tumors are responsive to hormone inhibition (antiandrogens for prostate cancer, antiestrogens for breast cancer). Strontium 89 is a bone-seeking radionuclide that can exert antitumor effects and relieve symptoms. Bisphosphonates such as pamidronate may relieve pain and inhibit bone resorption. When the integrity of a weight-bearing bone is threatened by an expanding metastatic lesion that is refractory to radiation therapy, prophylactic internal fixation is indicated. Overall survival is related to the prognosis of the underlying tumor. Bone pain at the end of life is particularly common; an adequate pain relief regimen including sufficient amounts of narcotic analgesics is required.

→ *The management of hypercalcemia is discussed in Chap. 354.*

BIBLIOGRAPHY

BRENNAN MF, et al: The role of multi-modality therapy in soft tissue sarcoma. Ann Surg 214:328, 1991

———: Soft tissue sarcoma, in *Cancer: Principles and Practice of Oncology*, 5th ed, VT DeVita et al (eds). Philadelphia, Lippincott, 1997, pp 1738–1788

BURGERT EO et al: Multimodal therapy for the management of nonpelvic localized Ewing's sarcoma of bone: IESS II. J Clin Oncol 8:1514, 1990

CANGIR A et al: Ewing's sarcoma metastatic at diagnosis—Results and comparisons of two intergroup studies. Cancer 66:887, 1990

EVANS RG et al: Multimodal therapy for the management of localized Ewing's sarcoma of pelvic and sacral bones: A report from the second intergroup study. J Clin Oncol 9:1173, 1991

JABLONS D, et al: Metastasectomy for soft tissue sarcoma—further evidence for efficacy and prognostic indicators. J Thorac Cardiovasc Surg 97:695, 1989

LINDBERG RD, et al: Conservative surgery and post-operative radiotherapy in 300 adults with soft tissue sarcomas. Cancer 47:2391, 1981

LINK MP et al: The effect of adjuvant chemotherapy on relapse-free survival in patients with osteosarcoma of the extremity. N Engl J Med 314:1600, 1986

MALAWER MM et al: Sarcomas of bone, in *Cancer: Principles and Practice of Oncology*, 5th ed, VT DeVita et al (eds). Philadelphia, Lippincott, 1997, pp 1789–1852

PATEL SR, BENJAMIN RS: The role of chemotherapy in soft-tissue sarcomas. Cancer Control 1:599, 1994

———, ——— (eds): Sarcomas. Part I. Hematol Oncol Clin North Am 9:513, 1995

———, ——— (eds): Sarcomas. Part II. Hematol Oncol Clin North Am 9:707, 1995

NIH Consensus Development Panel on Limb Sparing Treatment of Adult Soft Tissue Sarcomas and Osteosarcomas. JAMA, 254:1791, 1985

ROTH JA: Resection of pulmonary metastases from osteogenic sarcoma. Cancer Bull 42:244, 1990

101 *Richard M. Stone*

METASTATIC CANCER OF UNKNOWN PRIMARY SITE

INCIDENCE AND EPIDEMIOLOGY The presenting findings in a patient with a newly discovered malignancy may not definitively reveal the site of origin of the neoplasm. Patients with cancer of unknown primary site (CUPS) present difficult diagnostic and therapeutic dilemmas. First, since the additional studies that could be ordered may be many, costly, and/or uncomfortable for the patient, the strategy used in searching for the primary must take into account what, if any, result the precise identification of the site of origin would have on the patient's treatment and length of survival. Second, while individuals with CUPS fare poorly overall (median survival is approximately 6 to 9 months), certain subgroups of patients are more likely to benefit from treatment and, in some cases, to enjoy long intervals without evidence of disease. The literature is a poor guide for the care of such patients, owing to the largely retrospective nature of the reports, the heterogeneity of the tumors, the selection bias in small, individual retrospective studies, and the variability in both the definition of the syndrome and the thoroughness of the evaluation performed to identify a primary site.

While there is no universally accepted definition of the CUPS syndrome, a truly occult neoplasm should fulfill all of the following criteria: (1) biopsy-proven malignancy, (2) unrevealing history, physical examination, chest film, abdominal and pelvic computed tomography (CT) scans, complete blood counts, chemistry survey, mammography (women), β human chorionic gonadotropin (βhCG) levels (men), alpha fetoprotein (AFP) levels (men), and prostate-specific antigen (PSA) levels (men), (3) histologic evaluation not consistent with a primary tumor at the biopsy site, and (4) failure of additional diagnostic studies (based only on findings from the laboratory and pathologic review) to identify the primary site. Such additional diagnostic tests could include, for example, colonoscopy in a patient whose rectal examination discloses guaiac-positive stool or a meticulous otolaryngologic examination in a patient who presents with squamous cell carcinoma in a cervical node. With increased understanding of the natural history of certain tumors and with the routine use of CT as well as detailed pathologic studies, there are many cases that fulfill the definition of CUPS but for which there is a reasonable suspicion that a given organ is the probable site of origin. Epidemiologic data suggest that the incidence of cancers for which the primary site is classified as unknown is decreasing. CUPS probably accounts for 2 to 3 percent of all cancer diagnoses currently, whereas it has been estimated that 10 to 15 percent of all cancers fell in this category in the last decade. Most patients with CUPS are over age 60.

BIOLOGIC CONSIDERATIONS The biologic behavior of CUPS is unique compared with that of other nonhematopoietic neoplasms. Such cancers as breast and prostate are relatively uncommon causes of CUPS. Breast primaries, for example, almost always are identified either before or simultaneously with their metastatic disease. Moreover, cancers presenting as CUPS often display unusual patterns of metastatic spread (e.g., pancreatic cancer presenting with bony metastases). The fact that more tumor bulk is present at distant sites than in the tissue of origin suggests that the genetic lesions underlying cases of CUPS produce a distinctly aggressive phenotype. Frequently, biopsy of an involved site will reveal a poorly differentiated histology, which is the morphologic correlate of this biologic behavior. The propensity of CUPS tumors to grow in distant locations also implies that the malignant cells can proliferate in the absence of the specific host factors (e.g., growth-promoting proteins, a vascular supply) that are important in the development of more typical cancers. Although physiologic and genetic data that might account for the distinctive natural history of CUPS neoplasms are scant, cell lines derived from such tumors may have abnormalities of chromosome 1, a finding generally associated with advanced malignancy.

CLINICAL PRESENTATION, DIAGNOSTIC EVALUATION, AND PATHOLOGY **History and Physical Examination** Patients present with a variety of symptoms and signs, including fatigue, weight loss, and other systemic symptoms, pain, abnormal bleeding, abdominal swelling, subcutaneous masses, and lymphadenopathy. Once it has been determined that metastatic cancer is present but that no primary site is obvious, the physician's approach must involve reasonable efforts to identify the primary site or to determine the histology or subcategory of the metastatic tumor to decide on the optimal therapy. Though usually unrevealing, a thorough history and physical examination should be carried out to elicit easily obtainable clues regarding the primary site. The patient should be questioned concerning epigastric pain, which, if present, would mandate careful exclusion of pancreatic carcinoma as well as other gastrointestinal malignancies. Symptoms referable to a given location (e.g., new cough, hematochezia, hemoptysis, change in bowel habits, unusual vaginal bleeding, nipple discharge) should prompt an aggressive specific diagnostic approach. Occupational exposure to asbestos, for example, would raise the suspicion of mesothelioma. The absence of prior smoking reduces the likelihood of lung cancer but does not exclude it. A history of fulguration of a skin lesion, colonic polypectomy, dilatation and curettage, or prostate biopsy should prompt a review of the original histology. Other than inferences drawn from the location of the involved area (see below), the physical examination will probably be unrevealing unless a thorough pelvic and rectal examination has not been performed previously.

Pathology Review The most important aspect of the workup of a patient with CUPS is the evaluation of the tissue obtained at biopsy. Vital clues pertaining to the primary site and the patient's management can be obtained by careful review of light-microscopic, immunohistochemical, ultrastructural, immunologic, karyotypic, and molecular biologic findings. First, if the original biopsy sample may be inadequate for either confirmation of malignancy or the performance of additional specialized studies, rebiopsy is mandatory. The clinician must have a close working relationship with a pathologist skilled in the evaluation of tumor specimens, especially when the organ of origin is uncertain. On either the initial or subsequent biopsy, plans may be made to process the tissue for (1) routine fixation for light-microscopic, histochemical, and immunohistochemical analysis, (2) freezing for DNA isolation or for additional immunologic evaluation (certain antibody-based detection methods, for example, cannot be applied to fixed, paraffin-embedded tissue), and (3) fixation, usually in glutaraldehyde, for ultrastructural analysis. Fresh tissue may be disaggregated into a single-cell suspension for short-term culture for purposes of cytogenetic analysis.

If routine histologic analysis fails to suggest the tissue of origin (e.g., gland formation in adenocarcinoma, psammoma bodies in ovarian or thyroid cancer, or spindle architecture in sarcomas), special histochemical studies may be helpful. For example, mucin positivity is helpful in recognizing a poorly differentiated adenocarcinoma. Light-microscopic review including histochemical analysis will show approximately 60 percent of CUPS tumors to be adenocarcinomas and 10 to 20 percent to be squamous cell carcinomas, usually of head and neck or lung origin. In the remaining poorly differentiated neoplasms, immunohistochemical, cytogenetic, and molecular biologic studies can be extremely useful in identifying sarcomas, germ cell carcinomas, lymphomas, neuroendocrine neoplasms (including melanoma), and other tumors whose diagnosis would suggest a more specific therapeutic approach.

Immunohistochemical Analysis Antibodies to specific cell components and the ability to detect binding by sensitive visualization methods such as peroxidase or streptavidin-biotin make it possible to characterize tumors that are not identified by standard techniques. Since in most situations no single antibody is specific enough to identify the primary site with certainty, a battery of such reagents must be employed. Table 101-1 provides a list of antigens that may be assessed by immunohistochemical analysis in undifferentiated or poorly differentiated specimens. It is particularly important to exclude the diagnosis of lymphoma by employing antibodies reactive to the leukocyte common antigen (LCA, CD45). The presence of LCA suggests that the patient has a lymphoid neoplasm and has the same chances of responding to therapy as if there were no diagnostic ambiguity. About half of patients with aggressive-histology lymphoma can be cured with combination chemotherapy (see Chap. 113). The immunohistochemical detection of specific types of filament proteins is helpful in the identification of carcinomas and sarcomas. The presence of keratin suggests carcinoma, since essentially all epithelial tumors contain this protein. However, certain sarcomas, mesotheliomas, and germ cell tumors are also keratin-positive, emphasizing the need for the judicious use of a battery of immunohistochemical markers. Sarcomas may react with antibodies to desmin. Prostate, breast, and thyroid carcinomas are suggested, respectively, by a reaction with antibodies to PSA or prostatic alkaline phosphatase, gross cystic fluid protein, or thyroglobulin. Immunohistochemistry may also identify sarcoma subgroups, including rhabdomyosarcoma (myoglobin) and angiosarcoma or Kaposi's sarcoma (factor VIII). The finding of AFP, βhCG, or placental alkaline phosphatase staining is very helpful in assigning a germ cell origin. The S-100 protein is present in virtually all primary and metastatic melanomas, including the amelanotic variety, the latter being difficult to classify by routine techniques. However, S-100 positivity is also found in many other tumors of neuroendocrine origin (e.g., small cell lung cancer, carcinoid, neuroepithelioma); a more specific marker for melanomas is the HMB45 (human melanoma black) antigen.

Other Diagnostic Approaches Ultrastructural analysis with electron microscopy can identify cell junctions (i.e., desmosomes, typical of epithelial cancers), neuroendocrine granules, melanosomes, and muscle filaments, which can be very helpful in identifying the tissue of origin. Cytogenetic analysis of solid tumors is a means of classifying neoplasms associated with specific chromosomal translocations or other genetic abnormalities and is used increasingly (Table 101-1). Cytogenetic abnormalities can also be determined by fluorescence in situ hybridization with chromosome-specific probes, a technique that does not require cells to divide, as is the case with traditional karyotype analysis. Fresh tissue may be required for detection of estrogen or progesterone receptors where breast cancer is a possibility or of antigens that are not fixation-resistant (such as those found on certain T cells). In addition to immunologic analysis, lymphomas can be diagnosed by using molecular approaches on DNA isolated from tumor tissue to detect lymphoid-specific gene rearrangements such as those of immunoglobulin, T-cell receptor, or *bcl*-2 genes. Since minimal amounts of template DNA are required for amplification by the polymerase chain reaction, paraffin-embedded tissue blocks may yield sufficient diagnostic material. As additional tumors are found to have specific acquired chromosomal rearrangements or mutations in genes controlling

Table 101-1

Possible Pathologic Evaluation of Biopsy Specimens from Patients with Metastatic Cancer of Unknown Primary Site

Evaluation/Findings	Suggested Primary Site or Neoplasm
HISTOLOGY (HEMATOXYLIN AND EOSIN STAINING)	
Psammoma bodies, papillary configuration	Ovary, thyroid
Signet ring cells	Stomach
IMMUNOHISTOLOGY	
Leukocyte common antigen (LCA, CD45)	Lymphoid neoplasm
Leu-M1	Hodgkin's disease
Epithelial membrane antigen	Carcinoma
Cytokeratin intermediate filaments	Carcinoma
CEA	Carcinoma
HMB45	Melanoma
Desmin	Sarcoma
Thyroglobulin	Thyroid carcinoma
Calcitonin	Medullary carcinoma of the thyroid
Myoglobin	Rhabdomyosarcoma
PSA/prostatic acid phosphatase	Prostate
AFP	Liver, stomach, germ cell
Placental alkaline phosphatase	Germ cell
B, T cell markers	Lymphoid neoplasm
S-100 protein	Neuroendocrine tumor, melanoma
Gross cystic fluid protein	Breast, sweat gland
Factor VIII	Kaposi's sarcoma, angiosarcoma
FLOW CYTOMETRY	
B, T cell markers	Lymphoid neoplasm
ULTRASTRUCTURE	
Actin-myosin filaments	Rhabdomyosarcoma
Secretory granules	Neuroendocrine tumors
Desmosomes	Carcinoma
Premelanosomes	Melanoma
CYTOGENETICS	
Isochromosome 12p; 12q($-$)	Germ cell
t(11;22)	Ewing's sarcoma, primitive neuroectodermal tumor
t(8;14)*	Lymphoid neoplasm
3p($-$)	Small cell lung carcinoma; renal cell carcinoma, mesothelioma
t(X;18)	Synovial sarcoma
t(12;16)	Myxoid liposarcoma
t(12;22)	Clear cell sarcoma (melanoma of soft parts)
t(2;13)	Alveolar rhabdomyosarcoma
1p($-$)	Neuroblastoma
RECEPTOR ANALYSIS	
Estrogen/progesterone receptor	Breast
MOLECULAR BIOLOGIC STUDIES	
Immunoglobulin, bcl-2, T-cell receptor gene rearrangement	Lymphoid neoplasm

* Or any other rearrangement involving an antigen-receptor gene

growth and differentiation, the detection of altered DNA and/or altered gene products will become increasingly useful in diagnosis.

Additional Studies If the pathology review fails to disclose a histology likely to be responsive to chemotherapy, it is unlikely that additional expensive diagnostic tests will benefit the patient, so they must be ordered only judiciously. In females with metastatic adenocarcinoma or poorly differentiated carcinoma, mammography should be performed, although the diagnostic yield will be quite low except in

patients with axillary metastases. The use of abdominal/pelvic CT scans leads to the identification of the primary site in as many as 35 percent of patients and will certainly reduce the number of cases of pancreatic cancer in which the primary site is obscure before death. Whether or not to measure routinely serum tumor markers such as AFP, βhCG, carcinoembryonic antigen (CEA), CA-125 (associated with ovarian cancer), and PSA is controversial. Many different adenocarcinomas elaborate CEA, CA-125, or both; these markers are useful for following the response to therapy rather than for identifying a primary site. Moreover, poorly differentiated colonic tumors frequently fail to produce CEA, and patients with benign prostate hypertrophy may have modestly elevated PSA levels, reducing the reliability of these markers in defining the primary site in a patient with metastatic cancer. Numerous studies have shown a lack of benefit of contrast studies (upper gastrointestinal series, barium enema or intravenous pyelogram) in patients with metastatic cancer of unknown primary who have no specific symptoms and no findings referable to the gastrointestinal or urinary tract. Moreover, autopsy series reveal that the most likely primary site of origin includes epithelial tissues such as lung, stomach, colon, and kidney, which give rise to tumors that respond poorly to chemotherapy, minimizing the therapeutic impact of such a diagnosis. Additional invasive diagnostic studies are indicated if the presentation strongly suggests a particular primary site. For example, radiographic evidence of lung or mediastinal involvement would mandate fiberoptic bronchoscopy to exclude lung cancer. In the relatively unusual case of metastatic squamous cell cancer presenting in an inguinal lymph node, anoscopy and colposcopy should be performed to detect carcinoma of the vulva, cervix, vagina, penis, or anus, all of which may be cured even with lymph node spread. A summary of a reasonable diagnostic approach is found in Table 101-2.

℞ **TREATMENT**

Prognostic Subgroups Regardless of patient age, the exclusion of treatable and potentially curable neoplasms is important. Patients with squamous cell carcinoma have a somewhat longer median survival (9 months) than do those with adenocarcinoma or unclassifiable neoplasms (4 to 6 months). If laboratory studies indicate a significant likelihood that the neoplasm is a lymphoma, germ cell tumor, sarcoma, neuroendocrine tumor, or breast or prostate cancer, then disease-appropriate therapy should be administered. Patients with lymphoma or a germ cell neoplasm may be cured with combination chemotherapy. In other malignancies, effective palliative chemotherapy (for sarcoma or a breast or neuroendocrine tumor) or hormonal therapy (for breast or prostate cancer) should be strongly considered. Although often requiring electron microscopy for diagnosis, neuroendocrine tumors (especially if anaplastic) are expected to respond to cisplatin-based chemotherapy.

Patients in whom the primary site can be identified fare somewhat better than those in whom it remains undefined. Generally favorable prognostic factors identified by multivariate analysis of large series of patients with CUPS include limited sites of involvement (especially if lymphadenopathy is present) and neuroendocrine histology. Patients often may be categorized as having one of several clinical features or syndromes suggesting a specific form of potentially beneficial therapy (Table 101-3).

Table 101-2

Suggested Clinical Evaluation of Patients with Metastatic Cancer of Unknown Primary Site

History: smoking history, asbestos exposure, abdominal pain
Physical examination: lymph nodes, thyroid, skin;
  Men: prostate
  Women: breasts, pelvic examination
Laboratory evaluation: stool evaluation for occult blood; urinalysis;
  complete blood count; liver function tests; measurement of serum levels of
  PSA, βhCG, AFP, CEA, and CA-125 (women); chest x-ray; abdominal
  and pelvic CT; mammography
Pathologic evaluation: see Table 101-1

Table 101-3

CHAPTER 101
Metastatic Cancer of Unknown Primary Site **617**

Presentations That Dictate Specific Therapies in Patients with CUPS

Clinicopathologic Features	Suspected Primary Site	Suggested Therapy
Squamous cell carcinoma, cervical node	Head and neck cancer	Radical neck dissection; radiotherapy ± chemotherapy
Carcinoma, axillary nodes (female)	Breast cancer	Breast radiotherapy or mastectomy, systemic adjuvant therapy
Peritoneal carcinomatosis (female)	Ovarian cancer	Debulking surgery, cisplatin-based chemotherapy
Poorly differentiated cancer, age <50, lung or retroperitoneal or mediastinal mass or lymph nodes, elevated serum βhCG or AFP levels	Germ cell tumor (extragonadal)	Cisplatin/VP-16-based chemotherapy
Bony metastases (male)	Prostate cancer	Androgen blockade (leuprolide plus flutamide)
Adenocarcinoma, liver metastases, elevated CEA level	Gastrointestinal malignancy	Colonoscopy with resection (if appropriate) of detected tumors; 5-fluorouracil/leucovorin

SYNDROME OF UNRECOGNIZED EXTRAGONADAL GERM CELL CANCER A subset of patients with poorly differentiated carcinoma of unknown primary site are extremely responsive to chemotherapy. These patients display one or more of the following features: age less than 50; tumor involving midline structures, lung parenchyma, or lymph nodes; an elevated serum AFP or βhCG level; evidence of rapid tumor growth; or tumor responsiveness to previously administered radiotherapy or chemotherapy. Cisplatin-based chemotherapy has led to long-term survival in a sizable fraction of patients with these features, especially those who have a favorable performance status at diagnosis, suggesting that their tumors behaved like germ cell neoplasms. If all patients with poorly differentiated carcinoma (including poorly differentiated adenocarcinoma) are treated with a chemotherapy regimen designed for those with germ cell cancer (e.g., cisplatin plus etoposide or vinblastine, often also with bleomycin) (see Chap. 98), about one-quarter will respond completely and one-third will experience a partial response. Patients whose disease does not respond to two cycles of therapy should not be committed to longer treatment. Approximately one in six patients is likely to survive more than 5 years without evidence of disease. Individuals with poorly differentiated carcinoma are more likely to respond to combination chemotherapy than those whose tumors display somewhat more mature features. Patients with poorly differentiated carcinoma or adenocarcinoma whose tumors have abnormalities of chromosome 12 similar to those described in patients with proven germ cell cancer are more likely to respond to platinum-based chemotherapy than are patients with a similar presentation whose tumors lack this cytogenetic abnormality.

PERITONEAL CARCINOMATOSIS IN WOMEN Women who present with increased abdominal girth and a pelvic mass or pain and who are found to have adenocarcinoma throughout the peritoneal cavity but without a clear site of origin also may benefit from platinum-based chemotherapy. This syndrome has been termed *primary peritoneal papillary serous carcinoma* or *multifocal extraovarian serous carcinoma*. While breast cancer or a gastrointestinal malignancy can produce these findings, peritoneal carcinomatosis is most commonly ascribed to ovarian cancer, even in patients with apparently normal ovaries at the time of laparotomy. Especially if psammoma bodies or a papillary configuration is noted in the pathology examination or if the CA-125 level is elevated, women with adenocarcinoma of the peritoneal cavity without a defined primary should receive maximum surgical cytoreduction followed by cisplatin-based ther-

apy. The stage-specific response to such therapy appears to be comparable to that for patients with proven ovarian cancer. Approximately 10 percent of patients who present in this fashion may remain free of disease 2 years after diagnosis.

CARCINOMA IN AN AXILLARY LYMPH NODE IN A FEMALE Women with an axillary mass proved to be adenocarcinoma or poorly differentiated carcinoma should receive treatment appropriate for stage II breast cancer whether or not a careful breast examination or mammography suggests the diagnosis of primary breast cancer and whether or not estrogen or progesterone receptors are detectable in the node. Even if no lesion is found in the breast, a breast recurrence will develop in one-half of these patients if no mastectomy is performed. Appropriate therapy generally includes either modified radical mastectomy or breast irradiation to reduce the risk of local recurrence. In addition, adjuvant systemic therapy (chemotherapy and/or tamoxifen, depending on menopausal status and whether or not estrogen receptor protein was found in the axillary tumor) to reduce the risk of developing evident metastatic breast cancer should be considered (see Chap. 91). Adjuvant systemic therapy may be administered before definitive local radiation treatment. Women with axillary metastases without an obvious breast primary appear to have the same likelihood of prolonged disease-free survival as patients with typical stage II breast cancer.

BONE METASTASES IN MALES Particularly if the lesions are osteoblastic, the serum PSA concentration should be measured, since the probability of prostate carcinoma is high in these patients. Empirical hormonal therapy (e.g., leuprolide and flutamide) should be strongly considered.

CERVICAL LYMPH NODE METASTASES Patients who present with a neck mass should be considered to have a primary tumor of the upper aerodigestive tract (usually termed *head and neck cancer*) until a different source is proven. Especially if the pathology analysis suggests a squamous histology and the node is located in a high or midcervical area, a careful ear, nose, and throat examination including direct laryngoscopy, nasopharyngoscopy, and random blind biopsies should be undertaken. A thyroid examination and scan also must be performed to rule out a primary thyroid tumor, especially if the histology is not definitely squamous. Particularly for patients in whom a primary site is discovered in the head or neck, definitive local therapy (external beam radiation or radical neck dissection) combined with platinum-based chemotherapy may lead to prolonged survival (see Chap. 89).

ADENOCARCINOMA AND LIVER METASTASES Although the entity of liver metastases proved to be adenocarcinoma is not as well characterized as the unrecognized germ cell cancer syndrome (nor as responsive to therapy), there is a significant likelihood of a primary stomach, biliary, or colorectal tumor. An elevated serum CEA level in this setting would be further evidence suggesting a gastrointestinal malignancy. It may be reasonable to perform a flexible sigmoidoscopy or colonoscopy to rule out a potentially obstructive colonic lesion. If a tumor is found, resection may be beneficial, depending on the tumor's size; even if none is found, treatment with a combination of 5-fluorouracil plus leucovorin is palliative for some patients with presumed metastatic gastrointestinal malignancy. Given both the severe and even life-threatening diarrhea that may be a consequence of this regimen and the relative resistance of gastrointestinal tumors to chemotherapy, patients should be made aware of the risks before embarking on such therapy.

Patients not falling into one of the preceding categories should be treated palliatively. In some patients, observation is appropriate. For example, individuals without evidence of additional metastatic disease who have undergone resection of a solitary pulmonary nodule containing malignant cells may actually have undergone definitive therapy for a small primary lung tumor. Radiation therapy is indicated in patients with local disease causing bony pain or neurologic compromise. The largest and most poorly responsive subgroup are those with moderate to well differentiated adenocarcinomas. Combination chemotherapy is frequently employed in such patients; however, response rates to "all-purpose" regimens [e.g., FAM (5-fluorouracil, doxorubicin, mitomycin C), FACP (5-fluorouracil, doxorubicin, cyclophosphamide, cisplatin)], or to ICE (ifosfamide, carboplatin, etoposide) are generally well under 50 percent, especially if patients with poorly differentiated adenocarcinoma, who have a higher response rate, are excluded; complete responses are rare. Regimens containing mitomycin C are associated with the risk of hemolytic uremic syndrome. In some series, patients with a good performance status whose disease is limited to soft tissue sites or extends only above the diaphragm have shown a better rate of response to therapy. While patients whose disease responds to treatment seem to have better survival than those whose disease does not respond, the difference may be related to inherent characteristics of the tumor rather than to a beneficial effect of chemotherapy.

Before combination chemotherapy is attempted in a patient with CUPS, the potential benefits must be weighed carefully against the certainty of toxicity. While some randomized studies have reported a benefit of one form of therapy over another, these reports are generally plagued by small numbers of patients and inadequate control of potential prognostic variables. Depending on motivation, eligibility, and availability, patients with CUPS may be candidates for evaluation of new (phase I) therapies.

BIBLIOGRAPHY

Abbruzzese JL et al: Analysis of a diagnostic strategy for patients with suspected tumors of unknown origin. J Clin Oncol 13:2094, 1995

——— et al: Unknown primary carcinoma: Natural history and prognostic factors in 657 consecutive patients. J Clin Oncol 12:1272, 1994

de Braud F, Al-Serraf M: Diagnosis and management of squamous cell carcinoma of unknown primary tumor site of the neck. Semin Oncol 20:273, 1993

Ellerbroek N et al: Treatment of patients with isolated axillary nodal metastases from an occult primary carcinoma consistent with breast origin. Cancer 66:1461, 1990

Fletcher JA et al: Diagnostic relevance of clonal cytogenetics in malignant soft tissue tumors. N Engl J Med 324:436, 1991

Hainsworth JD, Greco FA: Treatment of patients with cancer of an unknown primary site. N Engl J Med 329:257, 1993

Horning SJ et al: Lymphomas presenting as histologically unclassified neoplasms: Characteristics and response to treatment. J Clin Oncol 17:1281, 1989

Moertel CG et al: Treatment of neuroendocrine carcinomas with combined etoposide and cisplatin: Evidence of major therapeutic activity in the anaplastic variety of these neoplasms. Cancer 68:227, 1991

Motzer RJ et al: Molecular and cytogenetic studies in the diagnosis of patients with poorly differentiated carcinomas of unknown primary site. J Clin Oncol 13:274, 1995

Muggia FM, Baranda J: Management of peritoneal carcinomatosis of unknown primary tumor site. Semin Oncol 20:268, 1993

Sporn JR, Greenberg BR: Empirical chemotherapy for adenocarcinoma of unknown primary tumor site. Semin Oncol 20:261, 1993

102 *Bruce E. Johnson*

PARANEOPLASTIC SYNDROMES

ENDOCRINE SYNDROMES

There are three major classes of hormones: steroids, monoamines, and peptides/proteins. Production of steroid hormones by malignant tumors is rare; lymphomas may produce 1,25-dihydroxyvitamin D from circulating 1-hydroxyvitamin D, but most other steroid-producing tumors are benign tumors of the glands that normally secrete the steroid.

Monoamines such as norepinephrine and epinephrine are secreted by pheochromocytomas (see Chap. 333), but they are not secreted ectopically by malignant tumor cells.

Most hormonal syndromes in patients with cancer are related to the production of peptide or protein hormones. The most common of these endocrine syndromes are listed in Table 102-1, together with the protein hormones that mediate them and the tumors that most commonly produce the hormones. A peptide hormone generally is encoded by an mRNA that is translated into a larger prohormone molecule, which undergoes a number of posttranslational modifications, including cleavage, glycosylation, and/or other steps. For example, pro-opiomelanocortin can be cleaved to yield adrenocorticotropin (ACTH), lipotropin, endorphin, melanocyte-stimulating hormone, and/or enkephalin, with different cell types producing different products. In addition, some cells use alternatively spliced forms of the message to produce different proteins (e.g., calcitonin vs. calcitonin gene–related peptide).

Tumor cells of nonendocrine organs often lack certain components of the pathway that leads from prohormone to biologically active hormone to secreted product. As a result of defects in protein processing or post-translational changes, generally, tumor cells may produce proteins that are structurally related to but biologically less active than the normal hormones. Thus, cancer patients may have elevated levels of immunoreactive hormones in plasma in the absence of clinical syndromes of hormone excess.

The severity of paraneoplastic endocrine syndromes often parallels the clinical course of the cancer. However, with some benign or slowly growing tumors, the hormone syndrome can be the major cause of morbidity. Despite their production by tumor cells, hormones are not very good tumor markers. Human chorionic gonadotropin (hCG) is a reliable tumor marker in some forms of testicular cancer, but no other hormone is used to quantitate tumor mass.

Most endocrine cancer syndromes occur with tumors derived from neuroendocrine or neural crest tissue (small cell lung cancer, carcinoid tumors). The genetic mechanisms that account for the production of a hormone by a cell that does not usually produce it are not clear. Oncogenes may activate other cellular genes (including genes that encode hormones) that normally are silent. Alternatively, demethylation of normally methylated inactive genes may permit expression in rapidly dividing cells.

HYPERCALCEMIA OF MALIGNANCY   Hypercalcemia of malignancy, the most common paraneoplastic endocrine syndrome, is responsible for approximately 40 percent of all hypercalcemia (see Chap. 354). Hypercalcemia with cancer is classified as humoral hypercalcemia of malignancy (HHM), which is caused by circulating hormones, or local osteolytic hypercalcemia (LOH), which is caused by local paracrine factors secreted by cancers within bone. Parathyroid hormone–related peptide (PTHrP) causes nearly all cases of humoral hypercalcemia of malignancy, while the mediators of LOH in bone are heterogeneous.

Pathogenesis   Eighty percent of patients with hypercalcemia of malignancy have HHM. PTHrP is composed of 139 to 173 amino acids, and 8 of the first 13 amino acids at the amino-terminal end are identical to the amino-terminal portion of parathyroid hormone (PTH). PTHrP binds to PTH receptors in the bone and kidney and causes increased bone resorption, decreased bone formation, increased renal tubular reabsorption of calcium, increased phosphaturia, and increased urinary levels of cyclic adenosine monophosphate, leading to hypercalcemia. PTHrP is detected in the plasma in approximately 80 percent of cancer patients with hypercalcemia. Rare patients have been reported to have hypercalcemia caused by ectopically produced authentic PTH. HHM in lymphoma may be caused by the production of 1,25-dihydroxyvitamin D by the tumor.

Twenty percent of patients with hypercalcemia have LOH in which hypercalcemia is caused by the local production of hormones or cytokines by cancers that have spread to the bone or bone marrow; such factors increase bone resorption in the area around the cancer. The ectopically produced hormones that may play a role in LOH include transforming growth factors α and β, interleukin (IL) 1, IL-6, prostaglandins, and tumor necrosis factor.

Clinical Manifestations The initial symptoms and signs of hypercalcemia (calcium level $\geq$ 2.6 mmol/L)[1] include malaise, fatigue, confusion, anorexia, bone pain, polyuria, polydipsia, weakness, constipation, nausea, and vomiting. Neurologic symptoms and signs in profound hypercalcemia ($>$3.5 mmol/L) include confusion, lethargy, coma, and death. The cancers responsible for HHM in patients are non-small cell lung cancer and cancers of the breast, kidney, head and neck, and bladder. HHM is particularly common in patients with cancers of squamous cell histology. Hypercalcemia is uncommon at presentation ($<$1 percent of patients) with these tumors but becomes more common as the cancer progresses and is present in 10 to 20 percent of patients near the time of death. LOH is responsible for hypercalcemia in patients with breast cancer, myeloma, lymphoma, and leukemia. Among hypercalcemic patients with breast cancer, approximately half have HHM and half LOH.

Diagnosis The patient with cancer who develops hypercalcemia should be evaluated for other causes of hypercalcemia, including use of thiazide diuretics, vitamin D, or lithium, hyperthyroidism, and sarcoidosis. Elevation of serum PTH as measured by immunoassay suggests primary hyperparathyroidism, which may be responsible for as many as 10 percent of cases of hypercalcemia of cancer and which should be treated like other cases of hyperparathyroidism (see Chap. 356), if the underlying cancer is controlled. A normal PTH level and a low serum phosphorus level in the absence of bone metastases support the diagnosis of HHM, while a normal PTHrP level and normal phosphorus in a patient with bone metastases suggest LOH.

 TREATMENT

The median survival of patients with hypercalcemia of malignancy is only 1 to 3 months. Intervention to reverse hypercalcemia should be undertaken when the cancer is likely to be controlled with appropriate systemic or local treatment.

The treatment of HHM and LOH is similar (see Chap. 354). Patients with mild to moderate hypercalcemia (2.65 to 3.5 mmol/L) can be treated with 2 to 4 L of saline hydration per day and furosemide to prevent intravascular volume overload. The bisphosphonate pamidronate (60 to 90 mg intravenously) decreases osteoclastic bone resorption. Combined administration of diuretics and pamidronate reduces the serum calcium to normal values in 80 percent of patients within 7 days. Doses may be repeated as needed. In patients with LOH, glucocorticoids may inhibit the production of cytokines that promote bone resorption. Severe hypercalcemia [$>$3.50 mmol/L ($>$14 mg/dL)] with alteration of mental status can be treated with all of the above plus salmon calcitonin, 4 to 8 U/kg, administered intramuscularly or subcutaneously every 12 h. Calcitonin administration will decrease the serum calcium within 24 h, and its hypocalcemic effect can be prolonged in patients with LOH by adding glucocorticoids. If these agents are not effective in reducing the serum calcium, plicamycin and gallium nitrate may be added.

HYPONATREMIA OF MALIGNANCY Hyponatremia of malignancy (Na^+ level $<$ 130 mmol/L) is usually due to the inappropriate secretion of arginine vasopressin (AVP) and is termed the *syndrome of inappropriate antidiuretic hormone secretion* (SIADH). In rare cases, atrial natriuretic peptide produces hyponatremia.

Pathogenesis Small cell lung cancer is the malignancy chiefly responsible for producing ectopic AVP. AVP mRNA is expressed and translated, and the product is processed into the nonapeptide AVP, which is secreted into the circulation. The ectopically produced AVP binds to receptors in the kidney, causing retention of free water with resulting hypoosmolality in the plasma and hyperosmolality in urine (see Chap. 330).

About 15 percent of cancer patients with SIADH do not have evidence of ectopic production of AVP. In some of these patients, tumors secrete atrial natriuretic peptide. This hormone inhibits sodium reabsorption in the proximal tubule and inhibits release of renin and aldosterone. It is not yet clear how atrial natriuretic peptide leads to hyponatremia.

Clinical Manifestations SIADH is commonly recognized as asymptomatic hyponatremia on routine serum chemistry examination. It is present at the time of diagnosis in 15 percent of patients with small cell lung cancer, 3 percent of patients with head and neck cancer, and $<$1 percent of patients with non-small cell lung cancer. Hyponatremia may also occur with primary brain tumors, hematologic malignancies, melanoma, sarcoma, and gynecologic, gastrointestinal, breast, prostate, and bladder cancer. The symptoms of mild hyponatremia ($>$120 mmol/L) include difficulty focusing attention, fatigue, nausea, vomiting, anorexia, weakness, and headache. Profound hyponatremia ($<$120 mmol/L) can cause confusion, lethargy, coma, seizures, and death.

Diagnosis (See Chap. 330) SIADH is suspected in patients with hyponatremia (serum sodium $<$ 130 mmol/L) and a concentrated urine (osmolality $>$ 300 mmol/kg). Patients are euvolemic, are not using diuretics, and have normal thyroid and adrenal function. Polydipsia is excluded by the urine osmolality. Pseudohyponatremia can be present if serum glucose, triglyceride, or protein levels are high. Conditions other than cancer that can cause the SIADH include central nervous system disorders, pulmonary infections, positive-pressure breathing, pneumothorax, asthma, and a wide array of drugs, including chemotherapeutic agents (vincristine, vinblastine, cisplatin, cyclophosphamide, melphalan, levamisole), thiazide diuretics, carbamazepine, antidepressants, nicotine, and narcotics.

 TREATMENT

The treatment should be directed at the underlying cancer. Patients whose tumors have not been or cannot be controlled are candidates

Table 102-1

Common Paraneoplastic Endocrine Syndromes

Syndrome	Proteins	Tumors Typically Associated with Syndrome
Hypercalcemia of malignancy	Parathyroid hormone-related peptide (PTHrP)	Non-small cell lung cancer
		Breast cancer
	Parathyroid hormone (PTH)	Renal cell carcinoma
		Head and neck cancer
		Bladder cancer
		Myeloma
Syndrome of inappropriate vasopressin secretion (SIADH)	Arginine vasopressin (AVP)	Small cell lung cancer
	Atrial natriuretic peptide	Head and neck cancer
		Non-small cell lung cancer
Cushing's syndrome	Adrenocorticotropic hormone (ACTH)	Small cell lung cancer
		Carcinoid tumors
	Corticotropin-releasing hormone (CRH)	
Acromegaly	Growth hormone–releasing hormone (GHRH)	Carcinoid
		Small cell lung cancer
	Growth hormone (GH)	Pancreatic islet cell tumors
Gynecomastia	Human chorionic gonadotropin (hCG)	Testicular cancer
		Lung cancer
		Carcinoid tumors of the lung and gastrointestinal tract
Non-islet cell tumor hypoglycemia	Insulin-like growth factor-2 (IGF-2)	Sarcomas

[1] Calcium measurements given in millimoles per liter can be multiplied by 4 to convert to milligrams per deciliter or by 2 to convert to milliequivalents per liter.

for restriction of fluid intake to 500 mL/d. Such restriction corrects hyponatremia within 7 days in most patients, but it is difficult and uncomfortable for patients to maintain fluid restriction for extended periods. Oral demeclocycline (600 to 1200 mg/d) may be useful in blocking the effects of AVP but can cause renal insufficiency. Other agents that may be used for the treatment of hyponatremia include dilantin and lithium.

Rare patients develop profound hyponatremia and altered mental status. These patients should be treated with 0.9 percent saline hydration and furosemide diuresis. If that is not effective, 3 percent saline can be administered via a central line together with furosemide diuresis to prevent hypervolemia. Hypertonic saline is rarely required and must be given slowly; fluid balance and electrolytes should be monitored several times per day, and the increase in sodium should be limited to 0.5 mmol/L per hour to prevent pontine lysis (see Chap. 330).

ECTOPIC ACTH SYNDROME Ectopic production of ACTH by cancer cells is responsible for approximately 15 percent of all cases of Cushing's syndrome and for most cases of Cushing's syndrome that occur in cancer patients (see Chaps. 328 and 332). In rare patients, Cushing's syndrome is caused by ectopically produced corticotropin-releasing hormone (CRH), which in turn stimulates pituitary ACTH release.

Pathogenesis When pro-opiomelanocortin mRNA is expressed in cancer cells, the 241-amino-acid prohormone is translated and processed into a variety of molecules, including, in some cases, the 39-amino-acid hormone ACTH, which can be secreted into the circulation. The ectopically produced ACTH causes excessive secretion of glucocorticoids and mineralocorticoids by the adrenals.

Clinical Manifestations Women make up 50 percent of patients with ectopic ACTH syndrome and 90 percent of patients with pituitary Cushing's disease. Therefore, Cushing's syndrome in men is more likely to be caused by ectopic ACTH than by a pituitary tumor. Because of mineralocorticoid excess, patients with ectopic Cushing's syndrome usually have hypokalemic alkalosis at presentation, a rare finding in patients with Cushing's disease. Other common manifestations of ectopic ACTH syndrome include weakness, hypertension, and hyperglycemia. Ectopic ACTH syndrome in patients with slow-growing cancers (e.g., carcinoids) may develop typical features of central obesity, moon facies, hyperpigmentation, and hirsutism in addition to the metabolic abnormalities.

Ectopic ACTH syndrome is most commonly due to small cell lung cancer (50 percent of cases), bronchial carcinoid tumors (10 percent), thymic carcinoid tumors or thymomas (10 percent), pancreatic islet cell tumors (10 percent), pheochromocytoma or other neural crest tumors (5 percent), or medullary carcinoma of the thyroid (5 percent). About 2 percent of patients with small cell lung cancer and bronchial carcinoids have the ectopic ACTH syndrome at the time of diagnosis. Patients with small cell lung cancer and ectopic ACTH syndrome have shorter survival than patients without the syndrome and are more likely to develop opportunistic infections.

Diagnosis (See Chaps. 328 and 332) Ectopic ACTH syndrome is usually characterized by elevated levels of urinary free cortisol that do not decrease after administration of high doses of dexamethasone (8 mg/d). However, in one-third of patients with carcinoid tumors, urinary cortisol levels decrease by more than 50 percent after administration of high-dose dexamethasone. The plasma levels of ACTH are markedly elevated in more than half of patients. If these tests do not provide definitive evidence of ectopic ACTH syndrome, bilateral inferior petrosal vein sampling will show an elevated ACTH level in petrosal vein blood that does not increase after administration of CRH.

℞ TREATMENT
Treatment of the ectopic ACTH syndrome should be directed at the underlying cancer: chemotherapy for small cell lung cancer; surgical

resection or radiation therapy for carcinoids. Some patients with ectopic Cushing's syndrome have no evidence of tumor after extensive evaluation. These patients should be treated symptomatically and followed closely with periodic imaging studies, because they may have slow-growing tumors amenable to surgical resection.

Agents that inhibit steroidogenesis in the adrenal gland include ketoconazole (400 to 1200 mg/d), which reduces urinary cortisol excretion by more than half in two-thirds of patients, and metyrapone (1 to 4 g/d), which also reduces urinary cortisol excretion. Patients who are in good condition and whose manifestations are not controlled by drugs may be considered for adrenalectomy.

ECTOPIC ACROMEGALY Ectopic production of growth hormone-releasing hormone (GHRH) is the predominant cause of ectopic acromegaly (see Chap. 328).

Pathogenesis GHRH is processed into 40- and 44-amino-acid peptides and binds to receptors in the pituitary, causing them to increase production of growth hormone. Rare cases of ectopic acromegaly are due to ectopic production of growth hormone itself by tumors.

Clinical Manifestations The symptoms and signs of ectopic acromegaly develop over several years and include increasing glove and shoe size, facial disfigurement, arthralgias, amenorrhea-galactorrhea or impotence, hypertension, muscle weakness, and diabetes mellitus. Ectopic acromegaly has been reported in fewer than 100 patients and accounts for 1 percent or less of all cases of acromegaly. The cancers associated with ectopic acromegaly include carcinoid tumors of the bronchus, pancreatic islet cell tumors, and cancers of the lung, breast, colon, and adrenal glands.

Diagnosis If a clinical diagnosis of acromegaly is suspected in a patient with cancer, the serum levels of GHRH and insulin-like growth factor (IGF)-1 and the glucose-suppressed growth hormone (GH) serum level should be measured (see Chap. 328). Patients with elevated GHRH levels and acromegaly have ectopic acromegaly. Patients without evidence of cancer who have elevated GHRH levels should undergo imaging of the central nervous system, chest, and abdomen to look for an occult cancer. Patients with cancer, low GHRH levels, high GH levels, and elevated IGF-1 levels should undergo magnetic resonance imaging (MRI) of the pituitary and hypothalamus. If no pituitary tumor is detected, GH may be secreted directly by the known tumor. Not all GH-secreting tumors of the pituitary are demonstrable by imaging techniques, however.

℞ TREATMENT
The therapy of ectopic acromegaly should be directed at the underlying cancer and should consist of surgical resection or radiation therapy for patients with carcinoid and islet cell tumors. Agents for medical control of ectopic acromegaly include bromocriptine (20 to 60 mg/d) and octreotide (100 to 200 μg every 8 h), both of which can inhibit secretion of growth hormone by the pituitary. These agents produce symptomatic improvement in approximately half of patients.

GYNECOMASTIA Ectopic production of hCG or estrogens by tumors such as cancers of the lung and testis is responsible for approximately 3 percent of cases of gynecomastia detected in men (see Chap. 338). Ectopic production of hCG is the most common cause of paraneoplastic gynecomastia; the hCG acts by stimulating the Leydig cells of the testis to produce increased amounts of estrogen. Alternatively, on rare occasions, a tumor (such as a hepatoma or a germ cell tumor with choriocarcinoma elements) contains aromatase enzyme activity that converts circulating androgens to estrogen. Leydig cell or Sertoli cell tumors may also secrete estradiol. In all cases, the increased ratio of estrogen to testosterone leads to the proliferation of breast tissue and gynecomastia. Other tumors rarely associated with ectopic gynecomastia include carcinoid tumors of the bronchus, intestine, and small cell lung cancer.

The clinical manifestations of gynecomastia are described in Chap. 338. About 5 percent of men with testicular choriocarcinoma present with an enlarging breast mass. In the absence of an obvious cancer, men presenting with gynecomastia should have a careful examination of the testes and measurement of serum hCG. Patients with a testicular mass should undergo an inguinal orchiectomy for diagnosis and treatment. If no testicular mass is found by physical examination, the testes should be examined with ultrasound. Patients with an elevated hCG level and no testicular mass should undergo a workup for an extragonadal germ cell tumor.

 TREATMENT

The therapy of tumor-associated gynecomastia should be directed at the underlying cancer: Chemotherapy is used for testicular cancers, and surgical resection or radiation therapy for carcinoids and islet cell tumors. In patients with testicular cancer, gynecomastia completely resolves in three-fourths of cases.

NON-ISLET CELL TUMOR HYPOGLYCEMIA Hypoglycemia that is not caused by the ectopic production of insulin (as in patients with islet cell tumors of the pancreas) can occur with large, slow-growing sarcomas (see Chap. 335). Ectopic production of IGF-2 is responsible for hypoglycemia in most patients with non-islet cell tumors. The ectopically produced IGF-2 inhibits glycogenolysis and gluconeogenesis in the liver, suppresses lipolysis, and increases peripheral glucose utilization, thereby causing hypoglycemia. IGF-2 may also act as an autocrine growth factor for the tumor.

Patients with large sarcomas (1 to 10 kg) may develop hypoglycemia, particularly with fasting. Headache, fatigue, confusion, or seizures may occur. Patients with a large sarcoma and hypoglycemia are likely to have non-islet cell tumor hypoglycemia. Although IGF-2 protein or mRNA is detectable in tumor tissue, the diagnosis is usually made on clinical grounds, because the plasma levels of IGF-2 are typically not elevated. Levels of IGF binding proteins may be increased.

 TREATMENT

The therapy of non-islet cell hypoglycemia should be directed at the underlying cancer and should consist of surgical resection or radiation therapy. Patients whose tumor cannot be successfully resected or irradiated can be treated with frequent oral feedings or constant intravenous administration of glucose.

HEMATOLOGIC SYNDROMES

The elevation of granulocyte, platelet, and eosinophil counts in most patients with myeloproliferative disorders is caused by the proliferation of the myeloid elements due to the underlying disease rather than by a paraneoplastic syndrome. The paraneoplastic hematologic syndromes in patients with solid tumors are less well characterized than the endocrine syndromes, because the ectopic hormone(s) or cytokines responsible have not been identified in most of these tumors (Table 102-2). The severity of the paraneoplastic syndromes parallels the course of the cancer.

ERYTHROCYTOSIS Ectopic production of erythropoietin by cancer cells causes most paraneoplastic erythrocytosis. The ectopically produced erythropoietin stimulates the production of red blood cells in the bone marrow and raises the hematocrit. Other lymphokines and hormones produced by cancer cells may stimulate erythropoietin release but have not been proven to cause erythrocytosis.

Most patients with erythrocytosis have an elevated hematocrit (>52 percent in men and >48 percent in women) that is detected on a routine blood count. Approximately 3 percent of patients with renal cell cancers, 10 percent of patients with hepatocarcinomas, and 15 percent of patients with cerebellar hemangioblastomas have erythrocytosis. In most cases the erythrocytosis is asymptomatic.

Patients with erythrocytosis due to a renal cell cancer, hepatocarcinoma, or central nervous system cancer should have measurement of red cell mass. If the red cell mass is elevated, the serum erythropoietin level should be measured. Patients with an appropriate cancer, elevated erythropoietin levels, and no other explanation for erythrocytosis (e.g., a hemoglobinopathy that causes increased O_2 affinity, see Chap. 107) have the paraneoplastic syndrome.

Table 102-2

Paraneoplastic Hematologic Syndromes

Syndrome	Proteins	Cancers Typically Associated with Syndrome
Erythrocytosis	Erythropoietin	Renal cancers
		Hepatocarcinoma
		Cerebellar hemangioblastomas
Granulocytosis	G-CSF	Lung cancer
	GM-CSF	Gastrointestinal cancer
	IL-6	Ovarian cancer
		Genitourinary cancer
Thrombocytosis	IL-6	Lung cancer
		Gastrointestinal cancer
		Breast cancer
		Ovarian cancer
		Lymphoma
Eosinophilia	IL-5	Lymphoma
		Leukemia
		Lung cancer
Thrombophlebitis	Unknown	Lung cancer
		Pancreatic cancer
		Gastrointestinal cancer
		Breast cancer
		Genitourinary cancer
		Ovarian cancer
		Prostate cancer
		Lymphoma

 TREATMENT

Successful resection of the cancer usually causes the erythrocytosis to resolve. If the tumor neither can be resected nor treated effectively with radiation therapy or chemotherapy, phlebotomy may control any symptoms related to erythrocytosis.

GRANULOCYTOSIS Approximately 30 percent of patients with solid tumors have granulocytosis (granulocyte count > 8000/μL). In about half of patients with granulocytosis and cancer, the granulocytosis has an identifiable nonparaneoplastic etiology (infection, tumor necrosis, glucocorticoid administration, etc.). The other patients have proteins in urine and serum that stimulate the growth of bone marrow cells. A few tumors and tumor cell lines from patients with lung and bladder cancer have been documented to produce granulocyte colony stimulating factor (G-CSF), granulocyte-macrophage colony stimulating factor (GM-CSF), and/or IL-6. However, the etiology of granulocytosis has not been characterized in most patients.

Patients with granulocytosis are nearly all asymptomatic, and the differential white blood cell count does not have a shift to immature forms of neutrophils. Granulocytosis occurs in 40 percent of patients with lung and gastrointestinal cancers, 20 percent of patients with breast cancer, 30 percent of patients with brain tumors and ovarian cancers, and 10 percent of patients with renal cell carcinoma. Patients with advanced-stage disease are more likely to have granulocytosis than those with early-stage disease.

Paraneoplastic granulocytosis does not require treatment. The granulocytosis resolves when the underlying cancer is successfully treated.

THROMBOCYTOSIS Thirty-five percent of patients with thrombocytosis (platelet count > 400,000/μL) have an underlying diagnosis of cancer. IL-6, a candidate molecule for the etiology of paraneoplastic thrombocytosis, stimulates the production of platelets in vitro and in vivo. Some patients with cancer and thrombocytosis have elevated levels of IL-6 in plasma. Another candidate molecule is thrombopoietin, a peptide hormone that stimulates megakaryocyte proliferation and platelet production. The etiology of thrombocytosis has not been established in most cases.

Patients with thrombocytosis are nearly all asymptomatic. There is no clear link between thrombocytosis and thrombosis in patients with cancer. Thrombocytosis is present in 40 percent of patients with lung and gastrointestinal cancers, 20 percent of patients with breast and ovarian cancers, and 10 percent of patients with lymphoma and is most likely to be present in advanced-stage disease. Paraneoplastic thrombocytosis does not require treatment.

EOSINOPHILIA Eosinophilia is present in approximately 1 percent of patients with cancer. Tumors and tumor cell lines from patients with lymphomas or leukemia may produce IL-5, which stimulates eosinophil growth. Activation of IL-5 transcription in lymphomas and leukemias may involve translocation of the long arm of chromosome 5, to which the genes for IL-5 and other cytokines map.

Patients with eosinophilia are typically asymptomatic. Eosinophilia is present in 10 percent of patients with lymphoma, 3 percent of patients with lung cancer, and occasional patients with cervical, gastrointestinal, renal, and breast cancer. Patients with markedly elevated eosinophil counts ($>5000/\mu L$) can develop shortness of breath and wheezing. A chest radiograph may reveal diffuse pulmonary infiltrates from eosinophil infiltration and activation in the lungs.

℞ TREATMENT

Definitive treatment is directed at the underlying malignancy: Tumors should be resected or treated with radiation or chemotherapy. In most patients who develop shortness of breath related to eosinophilia, symptoms resolve with the use of oral or inhaled glucocorticoids.

THROMBOPHLEBITIS Approximately 15 percent of patients who develop deep venous thrombosis or pulmonary embolism have a diagnosis of cancer (see Chap. 118). The coexistence of peripheral venous thrombosis with visceral carcinoma, particularly pancreatic cancer, is called *Trousseau's syndrome.*

Pathogenesis Patients with cancer are predisposed to thromboembolism because they are often at bedrest or immobilized. In addition, clotting may be promoted by release of procoagulants or cytokines from tumor cells or associated inflammatory cells, or by platelet adhesion or aggregation. The specific molecules that mediate the increased risk of thromboembolism have not been identified.

Clinical Manifestations Patients with cancer who develop deep venous thrombosis usually develop swelling or pain in the leg, and physical examination reveals tenderness, warmth, and redness. Patients who present with pulmonary embolism develop dyspnea, chest pain, and syncope, and physical examination shows tachycardia, cyanosis, and hypotension. Approximately 5 percent of patients with no history of cancer who have a diagnosis of deep venous thrombosis or pulmonary embolism will have a diagnosis of cancer within 1 year. The most common cancers associated with thromboembolic episodes include lung, pancreatic, gastrointestinal, breast, ovarian, and genitourinary cancers, lymphomas, and brain tumors. Patients with cancer who undergo surgical procedures requiring general anesthesia have a 20 to 30 percent risk of deep venous thrombosis.

Diagnosis The diagnosis of deep venous thrombosis in patients with cancer is made by an evaluation with impedance plethysmography. If this evaluation suggests the presence of a clot in the vein, venography and/or Doppler ultrasound can confirm the diagnosis. Patients with symptoms and signs suggesting a pulmonary embolism should be evaluated with a chest radiograph, electrocardiogram, arterial blood gas analysis, and ventilation–perfusion scan. Patients with equivocal ventilation–perfusion findings should be considered for a pulmonary angiogram.

Patients without a diagnosis of cancer who present with an initial episode of thrombophlebitis or pulmonary embolus need no additional tests for cancer other than a careful history and physical exam. In light of the many possible primary sites, diagnostic testing in asymptomatic patients is wasteful. However, if the clot is refractory to standard treatment or is in an unusual site, or if the thrombophlebitis is migratory or recurrent, additional efforts to find an underlying cancer are indicated.

℞ TREATMENT

Patients with cancer and a diagnosis of deep venous thrombosis or pulmonary embolism should be treated initially with intravenous heparin. Patients with proximal deep venous thrombosis and a relative contraindication to heparin anticoagulation (brain metastases or pericardial effusion) should be considered for placement of a filter in the inferior vena cava (Greenfield filter) to prevent pulmonary embolism. Coumadin should be administered for 3 to 6 months. Patients with cancer who undergo a major surgical procedure should be considered for heparin prophylaxis or pneumatic boots. Breast cancer patients undergoing chemotherapy and patients with implanted catheters should be considered for prophylaxis (1 mg coumadin per day).

→ *Cutaneous paraneoplastic syndromes are discussed in Chap. 57. Neurologic paraneoplastic syndromes are discussed in Chap. 103. More extensive discussion of functional endocrine tumors is given in Chap. 95.*

BIBLIOGRAPHY

BARTTER F, SCHWARTZ W: The syndrome of inappropriate secretion of antidiuretic hormone. Am J Med 42:790, 1967

BECKER M, ARON DC: Ectopic ACTH syndrome and CRH-mediated Cushing's syndrome. Endocrinol Metab Clin North Am 23:585, 1994

BRAUNSTEIN GD: Gynecomastia. N Engl J Med 328:490, 1993

FAGLIA G et al: Ectopic acromegaly. Endocrinol Metab Clin North Am 21:575, 1992

GROSS AJ et al: Atrial natriuretic factor and arginine vasopressin production in tumor cell lines from patients with lung cancer and their relationship to serum sodium. Cancer Res 53:67, 1993

KAUSHANSKY K: Thrombopoietin: The primary regulator of platelet production. Blood 86:419, 1995

PRANDONI P et al: Deep-vein thrombosis and the incidence of subsequent symptomatic cancer. N Engl J Med 327:1128, 1992

RAUE F, PECHERSTORFER M: Drug therapy of hypercalcemia due to malignancy. Recent Results Cancer Res 137:138, 1994

SORENSEN JB et al: Syndrome of inappropriate secretion of antidiuretic hormone (SIADH) in malignant disease. J Intern Med 238:97, 1995

WINQUIST EW et al: Ketoconazole in the management of paraneoplastic Cushing's syndrome secondary to ectopic adrenocorticotropin production. J Clin Oncol 13:157, 1995

103   *Robert H. Brown*

PARANEOPLASTIC NEUROLOGIC SYNDROMES

Neoplasia can alter neurologic function in numerous ways, as outlined in Table 103-1. Several neurologic syndromes have been delineated that are a consequence of a remotely located neoplasm but do not arise from direct involvement of the nervous system by metastasis or from a known secondary complication of cancer or its therapy (e.g., malnutrition, opportunistic infection, drug-induced neuropathy). These paraneoplastic syndromes, outlined in Table 103-2, share several characteristics. They are clinically dramatic, arising subacutely in weeks or even days to produce neurologic symptoms that may be profoundly disabling. They may precede detection of the neoplasm by months or even years; their recognition should prompt a timely search for carcinoma. More than one syndrome may arise with a given neoplasm. In general, as outlined in Table 103-2, certain syndromes are associated with particular types of tumors. The diagnosis of a paraneoplastic neurologic disorder depends primarily on (1) the presence of a recognized clinical syndrome; (2) careful exclusion of other cancer-related

Table 103-1

CHAPTER 103
Paraneoplastic Neurologic Syndromes **623**

Effects of Malignancy on the Nervous System

Direct invasion
Metastatic invasion
  Parenchymatous
  Vascular (neoplastic angioendotheliosis)
  Meningeal (meningeal carcinomatosis)
Opportunistic infections
  Bacterial (e.g., listeriosis)
  Nonbacterial
    Typical and atypical viral (e.g., progressive multifocal
      leukoencephalopathy)
    Fungal (e.g., cryptococcosis)
Complications of antineoplastic therapy
  Complications of radiation therapy (e.g., radiation necrosis)
  Complications of chemotherapy (e.g., vincristine neuropathy)
Metabolic complications
  Nutritional deficiency
  Ectopic hormone production
Paraneoplastic syndromes

disorders, as in Table 103-1; and (3) in some instances, confirmatory laboratory studies, including measurement of serum or cerebrospinal fluid (CSF) antibodies with specific patterns of reactivity (Table 103-3) or electromyographic studies to detect findings typical of myasthenia gravis or myasthenic syndrome. CSF often shows protein elevation and a mild lymphocytic pleocytosis.

INCIDENCE Studies of the incidence of these syndromes are problematic because the syndromes are rare and because classifications vary among studies. In one series, these syndromes were detected in 7 percent of nearly 1500 patients with tumors, although recent studies suggest that the true incidence may be lower. Tumors that are most often associated with paraneoplastic neurologic syndromes are cancers of the lung (47 percent), stomach (12 percent), breast (12 percent), ovary (9 percent), and colon (6 percent). Paraneoplastic neurologic syndromes are encountered in one-sixth of all cases of ovarian tumors, one-seventh of lung tumor cases, and less frequently in cases of stomach, prostate, or breast cancer.

PATHOLOGIC CHANGES One group of paraneoplastic syndromes is characterized by *encephalomyelitis*, in which perivascular lymphocytosis, microglial proliferation, and loss of neurons occur. While these changes may be diffuse throughout the neuraxis, they often predominate in a specific anatomic location that dictates the resulting clinical abnormalities. Thus, as outlined below, the manifestations of limbic encephalitis may differ from those of brainstem encephalitis. Inflammatory destruction of the sensory neuronal cell bodies (*neuronopathy*) in the dorsal root ganglia results in wallerian degeneration of axons in peripheral nerves and corresponding ascending long tracts (posterior columns of the spinal cord).

In a second pathologic form of paraneoplastic disease, severe degeneration or loss of neurons occurs without inflammation. This is exemplified by the selective loss of Purkinje neurons in the cerebellum in subacute cortical cerebellar degeneration. This disorder may occur in isolation or concurrently with encephalomyelitis; thus, in cortical cerebellar degeneration there may be some accompanying cerebellar inflammation. In other paraneoplastic syndromes, the associated pathologic changes occur in the peripheral nervous system and consist of multifocal demyelination, myonecrosis, or ultrastructural changes in the neuromuscular junction.

PATHOGENESIS Several mechanisms have been invoked to explain these disorders, including release by the tumor of neurotoxic substances, viral or retroviral infections of tumor, and/or neural tissues, and an autoimmune response directed against common antigenic determinants expressed by the tumor and the affected neural cells. Some paraneoplastic disorders are characterized by serum and CSF antibodies with highly specific patterns of reactivity with neural tissue or muscle. These are exemplified by the Lambert-Eaton myasthenic syndrome and myasthenia gravis, in which circulating antibodies react with pre- and postsynaptic proteins, respectively. Both syndromes have been reproduced in animals by passive administration of fractionated immunoglobulins. In some cases of paraneoplastic cerebellar degeneration, serum and spinal fluid antibodies react specifically with cerebellar cytoplasmic antigens. In some instances, immunoglobulins from patients with different paraneoplastic neurologic syndromes may produce similar patterns of reactivity against neural tissue. Thus, antibodies recognizing neuronal nuclear antigens are common in patients with small cell carcinoma of the lung (SCLC), which may be associated with paraneoplastic encephalomyelitis or subacute sensory neuronopathy. In these cases, it appears that one or more pathogenic antibodies, possibly cross-reacting with antigens on the tumor, may provoke autoimmune neural injury in more than one region of the neuraxis. Detection of such antibodies may confirm that an evolving neurologic disorder is of paraneoplastic origin even though the antibodies are not diagnostic of a specific neurologic syndrome.

In general, treatment of the paraneoplastic disorders is difficult and is often unsuccessful. Resection of the underlying tumor is surprisingly ineffective, although there are isolated reports of symptomatic improvement following tumor removal. Immunosuppression is also of little benefit for most paraneoplastic disorders. Plasma exchange or immunosuppression may ameliorate some disorders such as Lambert-Eaton syndrome (see below). Otherwise, therapy is largely symptomatic.

The following is an outline of the salient features of the major paraneoplastic neurologic syndromes.

BRAIN, CEREBELLUM, AND SPINAL CORD **Visual Paraneoplastic Syndromes** Patients with carcinoma of the lung (and, rarely, of the breast, cervix, or endometrium) may develop progressive, painless loss of vision with photosensitivity due to loss of retinal photoreceptors. Lymphocytic inflammation of the retina accompanies loss of rods and cones. The electroretinogram is typically abnormal, and cells may be present in the spinal fluid. This cancer-associated retinopathy (CAR) is commonly associated with high titers of serum antibodies to one or more CAR antigens, including the 23-kDa photoreceptor protein recoverin, which is implicated in photoreceptor signal transduction.

Paraneoplastic Encephalomyelitis SCLC may precipitate an encephalomyelitis of variable distribution and, in consequence, variable but often overlapping clinical presentations. In addition, it is often accompanied by an inflammatory paraneoplastic sensory neuronopathy (see below). Serum and CSF from patients with paraneoplastic encephalomyelitis and neuropathy demonstrate antibodies to neuronal nuclear antigens. These antibodies recognize at least three closely homologous 35- to 40-kDa proteins (HuD, HuC, and Hel-N1) believed to be neuronal RNA-binding proteins required for normal neuronal differentiation.

Limbic Encephalitis In some cases, the encephalitis is most extensive in limbic structures such as the hippocampus and amygdala, producing affective changes in personality (anxiety and agitated depression), selective early memory loss suggestive of Korsakoff's psychosis, or confusion and hallucinations. In some cases, the initial presentation is an amnesic syndrome. The affective disorder often prompts psychiatric evaluation. Abnormalities of the electroencephalogram or overt seizures may be present early in the syndrome. While cognition may be spared initially, dementia is common as the disease progresses; symptoms referable to encephalitic involvement in other regions are often superimposed.

Brainstem Encephalitis Symptoms of brainstem encephalitis relate directly to the distribution of the inflammation. The predominant symptoms are due to medullary involvement producing nausea, vomiting, nystagmus, vertigo, and ataxia. A syndrome suggestive of progressive bulbar palsy with marked dysarthria and dysphagia is associated with pontine involvement. Mesencephalic inflammation and neuronal loss result in nuclear or internuclear eye movement abnormalities; diplopia and oscillopsia may be disabling. Rostral midbrain and nigral involvement may cause rigidity.

Cerebellar Encephalitis Inflammatory changes are rare in the cerebellar cortex but may be severe in deep cerebellar nuclei such as the dentate nucleus, causing myoclonus.

Table 103-2

Paraneoplastic Neurologic Syndromes

Site	Evolution	Clinical Features*	Cancer	Pathology
BRAIN AND CEREBELLUM				
Photoreceptor, retinal degeneration	Weeks to months	Painless visual loss progressing to blindness[1]	SCLC, rarely cervical cancer	Loss of rods and cones, infiltration of retina with mononuclear cells
Limbic encephalitis	Weeks to months	Agitated, confusional state, memory loss followed by dementia[2]	SCLC	Neuronal loss in medial temporal lobe and elsewhere in the limbic system, perivascular and meningeal lymphocytic infiltration
Brainstem encephalitis	Days to weeks	Nystagmus, diplopia, vertigo, ataxia, dysarthria, dysphagia[2]	SCLC	Neuronal loss in brainstem, inflammatory changes as above
Subacute cortical cerebellar degeneration	Weeks to months	Cerebellar ataxia, dysarthria[2,3]	SCLC, ovarian and breast cancer, Hodgkin's disease	Loss of Purkinje cells
Opsoclonus-myoclonus	Weeks	Dancing eyes and feet, cerebellar ataxia, and possibly encephalopathy in adults[2,4]	Neuroblastoma, bronchial carcinoma	In adults, degeneration of dentate nuclei
SPINAL CORD				
Necrotizing myelopathy	Hours, days, or weeks	Para- or quadriplegia with areflexia, sensory loss and bladder dysfunction	SCLC, lymphoma	Severe necrosis of gray and white matter
Subacute motor neuronopathy	Weeks or months	Flaccid weakness and muscle atrophy; legs affected more than arms	Non-Hodgkin's lymphoma	Inflammation of ventral horns, loss of anterior horn cells
PERIPHERAL NERVE				
Acute demyelinating polyneuropathy (Guillain Barré syndrome)	Hours to days	Ascending paralysis, areflexia, possibly ascending sensory loss, high spinal fluid protein level	Hodgkin's disease	Segmental demyelination, inflammation of peripheral nerves
Chronic demyelinating polyneuropathy	Weeks to months	Chronic progressive or relapsing weakness with sensory loss, high spinal fluid protein level	Rarely lung, breast, or gastric cancer; lymphoma, myeloma	As in acute demyelinating polyneuropathy
Neuropathy with paraproteinemia	Weeks to months	Chronic; may be predominantly sensory or motor[2,5]	Myeloma, osteosclerotic myeloma	As in chronic demyelinating polyneuropathy
Subacute sensory neuronopathy	Weeks to months	Severe sensory loss with areflexia and ataxia; paresthesias, pain[2]	SCLC and other lung tumors	Inflammation and neuronal degeneration in dorsal root ganglia; secondary axon loss
Sensorimotor neuropathy	Weeks to months	Distal motor and sensory loss[2]	SCLC and other tumors	Axonopathy, some segmental loss of myelin
NEUROMUSCULAR JUNCTION				
Lambert-Eaton myasthenic syndrome	Weeks to months	Proximal weakness, fatigability, dry mouth, possibly ptosis[6]	SCLC; cancers of the breast, prostate, stomach	Disruption of active zones on presynaptic terminals
Myasthenia gravis	Weeks to months	Weakness, fatigability, ptosis, diplopia[7]	Thymoma	Disruption of postsynaptic junctional membrane folds
MUSCLE				
Polymyositis	Months to years	Proximal weakness, myalgias, cardiomyopathy, high creatine phosphokinase level	Possible association with breast, ovary, lung tumors; lymphoma	Lymphocytic inflammation of muscle interstitium; myofiber necrosis, phagocytosis
Necrotizing myopathy	Days to weeks	Rapidly progressive proximal weakness, possibly dysphagia, dyspnea	Bronchial carcinoma, SCLC	Severe myonecrosis with minimal inflammation or phagocytosis

* Superscripts denote possible immunoglobulin reactivity as in Table 103-3.

Myelitis In paraneoplastic myelitis, the gray matter of the cord is diffusely infiltrated with leukocytes, leading to profound neuronal degeneration. The myelitis may be widespread through the cord or restricted to a few segmental levels. Anterior horn cell destruction typically produces muscle weakness and neurogenic atrophy, which is often asymmetric. There may be selective involvement of the neck and upper extremities or lower extremities alone. Corticospinal findings (hyperreflexia, weakness, Babinski signs) result from involvement

Table 103-3

CHAPTER 103
Paraneoplastic Neurologic Syndromes   **625**

Defined Antibodies Associated with Paraneoplastic Neurologic Syndromes*

Antibody†	Paraneoplastic Syndrome	Tumor	Antigen
[1]Anti-CAR	Retinopathy	SCLC	Recoverin, 25-kDa cone Ca^{2+} binding protein
[2]Anti-Hu	Encephalomyelitis, sensory neuronopathy	Mainly SCLC	35- to 40-kDa nuclear RNA-binding proteins
[3]Anti-Yo	Cerebellar degeneration	Gynecologic tumors, breast cancer	34- and 62-kDa leucine zipper proteins
[4]Anti-Ri	Opsoclonus-myoclonus	Breast cancer	55-kDa RNA-binding protein in motor system neurons
[5]Anti-MAG	Demyelinating neuropathy	Myeloma	Myelin-associated glycoprotein
[6]LEMS Ab	Lambert-Eaton myasthenic syndrome	SCLC	Voltage-sensitive calcium channel and associated proteins
[7]MG Ab	Myasthenia gravis	Thymoma	Acetylcholine receptor subunit

* Other patterns of reactivity have also been described for some of these antigens.
† Superscripts correspond to the antibody activities noted in Table 103-2.

of this tract in the cord or brainstem. The corticospinal tract dysfunction (and in some cases motor neuronopathy) should not be confused with motor neuron disease; typical amyotrophic lateral sclerosis does not appear to arise on a paraneoplastic basis. The presence of sensory signs with cancer denotes either dorsal root ganglioradiculitis or inflammation of the posterior horns.

Necrotizing Myelopathy   This is a rare complication of malignancy, presenting clinically as a subacute, transverse myelitis, often in a thoracic location. It can be distinguished from the less fulminant encephalomyelitis described above by the evolution of an intensely necrotic, central thoracic cord lesion which tails off rostrally and caudally over several segmental levels. In some instances, there are multiple necrotic foci within the cord. Clinical findings include leg (and possibly arm) plegia, sensory loss, and loss of sphincter control. The lesion frequently is asymmetrical initially, mimicking a Brown-Séquard syndrome. In severe cases, the protein concentration and cell count in the CSF are increased, and myelography demonstrates focal cord swelling. Although not all cases are associated with tumor, lung cancers, lymphoma, and leukemia are known to occur in such patients.

Opsoclonus-Myoclonus   A syndrome of opsoclonus, myoclonus, and ataxia ("dancing eyes–dancing feet") occurs in both children and adults. About one-half of affected children have differentiated neuroblastomas, usually in the thorax. In adults, the syndrome may be associated with solid tumors such as bronchial carcinoma. The onset is subacute, and in some instances the syndrome lasts for months and is followed by permanent encephalopathy or retardation. Pathologic findings in adults include prominent neuronal degeneration in the dentate nucleus of the cerebellum, suggesting a relationship to cortical cerebellar degeneration. Occasionally there is diffuse lymphocytic cuffing in the central nervous system and cerebrospinal fluid pleocytosis. In some individuals, this syndrome responds to glucocorticoids or treatment of the cancer. A subgroup of women developing opsoclonus with breast cancer have an antibody (anti-Ri) directed against a 55-kDa RNA-binding protein present in the nuclei of neurons and of the associated tumors.

Subacute Cortical Cerebellar Degeneration   Subacute cortical cerebellar degeneration (SCCD) is a subacutely progressive cerebellar disorder characterized by profound truncal and appendicular ataxia arising in association with gynecologic tumors (ovarian in 50 percent of cases; breast in 25 percent), SCLC, or Hodgkin's disease. Symptoms referable to the brainstem include vertigo, dysarthria, diplopia and nystagmus, and corticospinal signs. As a rule, any nonfamilial ataxia arising in a patient over the age of 45 should raise the suspicion of this entity. By contrast with paraneoplastic encephalomyelitis, described above, the predominant pathologic finding in SCCD is widespread loss of cerebellar Purkinje cell neurons with astrogliosis and secondary loss of Purkinje cell axons. Many cases are associated with dementia for which an anatomic basis has not been well established. The CSF commonly reveals a mild pleocytosis; cerebellar atrophy may be evident on magnetic resonance imaging or computed tomography scans.

Several types of anti-Purkinje cell antibodies have been detected in sera of patients with subacute cerebellar degeneration. Women with cancer of the breast or ovary and SCCD demonstrate antibodies (anti-Yo) recognizing a family of 34-kDa cytoplasmic leucine zipper proteins expressed in Purkinje cell neurons and in the gynecologic tumors. About a third of patients with Hodgkin's disease have anti-Purkinje cell antibodies that recognize an antigen distinct from that detected by anti-Yo antisera. A different cytoplasmic antigen is recognized by immunoglobulins from patients with SCCD and adenocarcinoma of the lung. In some patients with SCLC and SCCD, anti-Hu antibodies (see above) are present. Finally, a small subset of patients with SCCD and SCLC do not have anti-Hu or anti-Purkinje cell antibodies; in these patients, SCCD may coexist with Lambert-Eaton myasthenic syndrome (below).

PERIPHERAL NERVES   A number of clinical syndromes affecting the peripheral nerves occur in association with malignancy. Paraneoplastic *subacute sensory neuropathy*, arguably the most clinically distinctive of these syndromes, is a ganglioradiculitis which may arise with other manifestations of encephalomyelitis. Other paraneoplastic neuropathies are difficult to distinguish from noncarcinomatous neuropathies. However, their recognition is important, as they are relatively common and their manifestations often precede diagnosis of the underlying neoplasia. By electrodiagnostic criteria, neuropathy may be evident in as many as 50 percent of patients with lung cancer. In evaluating a possible paracarcinomatous neuropathy, it is particularly helpful to ascertain whether the neuropathy (1) affects motor fibers, sensory fibers, or both; (2) predominantly involves axons or myelin, or (3) occurs with an abnormal serum paraprotein.

Subacute Sensory Neuronopathy   This disorder primarily affects axons, with relative sparing of myelin. The typical pathology is a ganglioradiculitis, as noted earlier. Clinically, the onset is characterized by the subacute development of paresthesias and pain (sometimes severe) in the distal limbs and associated truncal sensory ataxia. The sensory ataxia may be profoundly disabling. Although often initially restricted only to arms and legs, the symptoms eventually affect all four extremities. In most cases, symptoms of the neuronopathy precede the diagnosis of the underlying malignancy by more than a year. The serum of some patients contains anti-Hu antibodies.

Acute Demyelinating Polyneuropathy   Acute inflammatory demyelinating polyneuropathy (Guillain-Barré syndrome), discussed in detail elsewhere (Chap. 381), is characterized by subacutely ascending paralysis, sensory loss which is often mild by comparison with the motor deficits, areflexia, and a characteristic elevation of spinal fluid protein concentration without pleocytosis. Histopathology reveals lymphocytic infiltration of nerves, segmental demyelination, and relative axonal sparing. This disorder is associated with Hodgkin's disease.

Chronic Demyelinating Polyneuropathy   Chronic demyelinating polyneuropathy includes a group of chronic progressive or relapsing, inflammatory demyelinating peripheral neuropathies that are distinguished from acute polyneuritis by their time course, more prominent involvement of sensory nerves, lack of involvement of autonomic nerves, and responsiveness to immunotherapy. As in acute demyelinating polyneuropathy, the demyelinating nature of these neuropathies is manifested physiologically by abnormalities such as slowed nerve conduction velocities or dispersion of compound muscle action potentials; the pathologic hallmark of both conditions is segmental loss of myelin with relative preservation of axons. In some cases, physiologic studies reveal only marginal slowing of conduction, while the biopsy clearly demonstrates selective myelin loss. Sural nerve biopsy may fail to reveal any alterations when the demyelination is proximal (and therefore detectable only with electrophysiologic methods). Elevation of the spinal fluid protein concentration helps confirm the diagnosis.

Chronic demyelinating polyneuropathy usually is not associated with neoplasia. Rarely, however, it occurs in association with solid tumors of the lung, breast, and stomach. It also occurs with Waldenstrom's macroglobulinemia, gamma heavy chain disease, and lymphoma. In many instances, the paraneoplastic form is characterized by the presence of a serum paraprotein, typically a monoclonal immunoglobulin ("M component"). As many as 10 to 15 percent of patients with monoclonal gammopathies of undetermined significance develop significant hematologic disease, including myeloma.

Two chronic demyelinating neuropathies are distinctive in this context. The first is associated with a monoclonal IgM that reacts with a myelin-associated glycoprotein (MAG) in peripheral nerve myelin. This pattern of reactivity occurs in about half of patients with an IgM gammopathy and neuropathy. This IgM anti-MAG neuropathy is more sensory than motor; it is only slowly progressive, as compared to the subacute sensory neuropathy (below). It remains to be established whether the anti-MAG antibody is a cause or consequence of the demyelination. The second distinctive subtype of chronic demyelinating polyneuropathy occurs with osteosclerotic myeloma and monoclonal IgG or IgA antibodies that do not react with MAG. This polyneuropathy is predominantly motor and often quite indolent, although it may eventually produce severe limb wasting. Sensory and autonomic findings are unusual. A related group of patients develop polyneuropathy, organomegaly, endocrinopathy, the M protein, and skin changes (POEMS syndrome); one-half have osteosclerotic myeloma and IgG or IgA M proteins with lambda light chains. Some patients with demyelinating neuropathies and IgM M proteins respond well to immunosuppressive therapy. Those with osteosclerotic myeloma may improve after treatment of the underlying plasmacytoma, particularly if it is solitary.

Sensorimotor Neuropathy This category of mixed sensory and motor axonopathy is perhaps the most common paraneoplastic neuropathy. Symptoms depend on the severity of the neuropathy and may include muscle wasting and weakness, distal limb paresthesias, and sometimes pain. Pathologically there is noninflammatory degeneration of axons and mild myelin loss, presumably secondary to the axonopathy. Paraneoplastic sensorimotor neuropathy has been reported with several types of tumors (SCLC, breast, stomach) and hematologic malignancies (Hodgkin's disease, lymphoma, multiple myeloma). In amyloidosis, itself often associated with myeloma, there may be an axonal neuropathy with intraneural deposition of amyloid fibrils derived from immunoglobulin light chains. Axonal neuropathy has been reported as a manifestation of occult insulinoma, possibly as a consequence of hypoglycemia. Infrequently, these neuropathies remit spontaneously; often they progress even with aggressive treatment of the underlying malignancy.

Subacute Motor Neuronopathy Another striking paracarcinomatous disorder of peripheral nerves is a subacutely progressive motor neuropathy that causes slowly evolving weakness of the legs heralding an otherwise occult lymphoma. Pathologic changes include loss of motorneurons in the anterolateral gray matter of the spinal cord, gliosis, loss of myelin in ventral roots, and some Schwann cell proliferation. Although there is no clearly effective treatment for this condition, many patients seem to improve following immunosuppressive therapy for the malignancy. In other patients, progression of the weakness may cease independently of the status of the lymphoma.

NEUROMUSCULAR JUNCTION Lambert-Eaton Myasthenic Syndrome (See also Chap. 382) Lambert-Eaton myasthenic syndrome (LEMS) occurs in association with either a malignancy or with other manifestations of autoimmune disease. It is characterized by weakness, myalgias, and fatigability, often most severe in the lower extremities and in the proximal muscles. Ptosis may be seen. Dysautonomic features are common and may include dryness of the mouth and eyes, impotence, diminished sweating, and orthostatic symptoms. The disorder afflicts men more often than women. The incidence of associated malignancy is 70 percent in men and 25 percent in women. In most cases the tumor is SCLC. The predominant clinical finding is a striking reduction in strength at rest with transient improvement in power on repetitive maximal exertion. Edrophonium chloride (Tensilon) has no effect or may marginally improve strength. Electromyography demonstrates motor unit potentials whose amplitude is low at rest but increases with exercise or tetanic stimulation; this contrasts with the electromyographic findings in myasthenia gravis. Electron microscopy of the presynaptic motor nerve terminals at the neuromuscular junction reveals a decrease in the number of active zones, which are believed to correspond to voltage-sensitive calcium channels. LEMS is believed to be an autoimmune disorder associated with diminished quantal release of acetylcholine. It is associated with other autoimmune disorders and appears to be HLA-linked (B8 and DRw3 antigens). In paraneoplastic LEMS, physiologic data incriminate antibodies directed against voltage-dependent calcium channels that are present both on tumor cells and on distal motor nerve terminals. Antibody activity has also been detected against the β subunits of these channels and against presynaptic proteins such as synaptotagmin. As noted, LEMS may arise concurrently with other paraneoplastic neurologic syndromes such as SCCD or sensory neuropathy. Treatment is directed toward the underlying neoplasm or autoimmune disease or toward augmenting acetylcholine release with drugs that prolong presynaptic depolarization and thereby enhance calcium influx. Guanidine hydrochloride and 3,4-diaminopyridine may be beneficial in either autoimmune or paraneoplastic LEMS; plasma exchange and immunosuppression may also be effective.

Myasthenia Gravis This disorder, discussed elsewhere in detail (Chap. 382), is characterized by exercise-induced muscle weakness caused by an antibody-mediated reduction in the numbers of acetylcholine receptors at the postsynaptic junction. About 15 percent of cases are associated with thymoma; other autoimmune disorders may coexist.

MUSCLE Polymyositis-Dermatomyositis This subject is discussed in Chap. 315. An increased incidence of malignancy exists in elderly patients with dermatomyositis.

Necrotizing Myopathy Carcinoma of the bronchus is associated rarely with a fatal, subacute, widespread, necrotizing myopathy that involves all muscles, including bulbar and diaphragmatic muscles. Intrafusal muscle fibers are also involved. Deep tendon reflexes are preserved. The muscle undergoes degeneration without phagocytosis or a significant inflammatory response. The cause of the necrotizing process is unknown.

OTHER Several other neurologic syndromes have been reported to be paraneoplastic but are less well characterized than the ones described above. *Stiff-man syndrome*—diffuse hypertonia with painful spasms due to loss of inhibitory spinal interneurons—may arise in association with carcinoma. In the nonneoplastic stiff-man syndrome, autoantibodies have been detected that react with glutamic acid decarboxylase (GAD). This enzyme is essential for the synthesis of gammaaminobutyric acid, a central nervous system inhibitory neurotransmitter. Similar autoantibodies are present in the serum of patients with insulin-dependent diabetes mellitus, although in stiff-man syndrome the antibodies are present in higher titer and react against different epitopes of GAD. Patients with stiff-man syndrome associated with breast cancer may also have antibodies against the synaptic vesicle–associated protein amphiphysin. Although paraneoplastic syndromes are rare with prostate cancer, a syndrome of *impaired horizontal gaze and orofacial spasm* has been associated with this tumor. Nonfamilial *subacute chorea* and *dystonia* occur with SCLC. *Optic neuritis* may develop as a paraneoplastic disorder, but it is difficult to exclude direct involvement of the optic nerve or chiasm by cancer cells or indirect effects of the underlying malignancy, as outlined in Table 103-1. Among the most striking autoimmune disorders of the nervous system is Rasmussen's encephalitis, a disorder characterized by slowly evolving focal encephalitis; some patients with this disorder have antibodies directed against a glutamate receptor subunit (GluR3). Cases of Rasmussen's disorder with neoplasia have not been reported, although focal, progressive limbic encephalitis (see above) is well documented to be a remote effect of cancer, and patients with paraneoplastic syndromes have been shown recently to possess antibodies against other glutamate receptor subunits (GluR1, GluR4, GluR5/6).

BIBLIOGRAPHY

BUCKANOVICH RJ et al: Nova, the paraneoplastic Ri antigen, is homologous to an RNA-binding protein and is specifically expressed in developing motor system. Neuron 11:657, 1993

DALMAU J, POSNER JB: Neurologic paraneoplastic antibodies (anti-Yo; anti-Hu; anti-Ri): The case for a nomenclature based on antibody and antigen specificity. Neurology 44:2241, 1994

DARNELL RB: Onconeural antigens and the paraneoplastic neurological disorders: At the intersection of cancer, immunity, and the brain. Proc Natl Acad Sci USA 93:4529, 1996

DECAMILLI P et al: The synaptic vesicle-associated protein amphiphysin is the 128-kD autoantigen of stiff-man syndrome with breast cancer. J Exp Med 178:2219, 1993

FURNEAUX HM et al: Characterization of a cDNA encoding a 34-kDa Purkinje neuron protein recognized by sera from patients with paraneoplastic cerebellar degeneration. Proc Natl Acad Sci USA 86:2873, 1989

GAHRING LC et al: Autoantibodies to neuronal glutamate receptors in patients with paraneoplastic neurodegenerative syndrome enhance receptor activation. Mol Med 1:245, 1995

HORMIGO A et al: Immunological and pathological study of anti-Ri-associated encephalopathy. Ann Neurol 36:896, 1994

KIM J et al: Higher autoantibody levels and recognition of a linear NH_2-terminal epitope in the autoantigen GAD_{65} distinguish stiff-man syndrome from insulin-dependent diabetes mellitus. J Exp Med 180:595, 1994

MARTIN-MOUTOT N et al: Synaptotagmin: A Lambert-Eaton myasthenic syndrome antigen that associates with presynaptic calcium channels. J Physiol 87:37, 1993

POLANS AS et al: Recoverin, a photoreceptor-specific calcium-binding protein, expressed by the tumor of a patient with cancer-associated retinopathy. Proc Natl Acad Sci USA 92:9176, 1995

POSNER JB, DALMAU J: Clinical enigmas of paraneoplastic neurologic disorders. Clin Neurol Neurosurg 97:61, 1995

104 *Rasim Gucalp, Janice Dutcher*

ONCOLOGIC EMERGENCIES

Emergencies in patients with cancer may be related directly to the underlying cancer or may result from its treatment. They can be classified into three groups: pressure or obstruction caused by a space-occupying lesion, metabolic or hormonal problems (paraneoplastic syndromes, see Chap. 102), and complications arising from the effects of treatment.

STRUCTURAL-OBSTRUCTIVE ONCOLOGIC EMERGENCIES

SUPERIOR VENA CAVA SYNDROME   Superior vena cava syndrome (SVCS) is the clinical manifestation of obstruction of the superior vena cava (SVC), with severe reduction in venous return from the head, neck, and upper extremities. Malignant tumors, such as lung cancer, lymphoma, and metastatic tumors, are responsible for more than 90 percent of all SVCS cases. Lung cancer, particularly of small-cell and squamous-cell histologies, accounts for approximately 85 percent of all cases of malignant origin. Metastatic cancers to the mediastinum, such as testicular and breast carcinomas, account for a small proportion of cases. Other causes include benign tumors, aortic aneurysm, thyroid enlargement, thrombosis, and fibrosing mediastinitis caused by prior irradiation or histoplasmosis.

Patients with SVCS usually present with complaints of neck and facial swelling (especially around the eyes), dyspnea, and cough. Other symptoms include hoarseness, tongue swelling, headaches, nasal con-

gestion, epistaxis, hemoptysis, dysphagia, pain, dizziness, syncope, and lethargy. Bending forward or lying down may aggravate the symptoms. The characteristic physical findings are dilated neck veins, an increased number of collateral veins covering the anterior chest wall, cyanosis, and edema of the face, arms, and chest. More severe cases include proptosis, glossal and laryngeal edema, and mental obtundation. The clinical picture is milder if the obstruction is located above the azygos vein.

Obstruction of recent onset is likeliest to be malignant in origin, whereas a longstanding obstruction is more likely to be of nonmalignant origin. The exception to this rule is SVC thrombosis due to a central venous line, in which the development of clinical symptoms and signs is rapid. The diagnosis of SVCS is essentially a clinical one. The most significant chest radiographic finding is widening of the superior mediastinum, most commonly on the right side. Pleural effusion occurs in only 25 percent of cases, often on the right side. However, a normal chest radiograph is still compatible with the diagnosis if other characteristic findings are present. Computed tomography (CT) provides the most reliable view of the mediastinal anatomy. The diagnosis of SVC syndrome requires diminished or absent opacification of central venous structures with prominent collateral venous circulation. Magnetic resonance imaging (MRI) has no advantages over CT. Invasive procedures, including bronchoscopy, percutaneous needle biopsy, mediastinoscopy, and even thoracotomy can be performed by a skilled clinician without any major risk of bleeding. For patients with a known malignancy, a detailed workup usually is not necessary, and appropriate treatment may be started after obtaining a CT scan of the thorax. For those with no history of malignancy, a detailed evaluation is absolutely necessary to rule out benign causes and also to determine a specific tumor histology to direct the appropriate therapy. This should be obtained before initiation of glucocorticoid or radiation therapy to obtain accurate diagnosis, since in rapidly responding tumors like lymphomas, delay in diagnostic procedures may result in inability to make an exact diagnosis.

 TREATMENT
The one potentially life-threatening complication of a superior mediastinal mass is tracheal obstruction. Upper airway obstruction demands emergent therapy. Diuretics with a low salt diet, head elevation, and oxygen may produce temporary symptomatic relief.

Radiation therapy is the primary treatment for SVC syndrome caused by non-small cell lung cancer and other metastatic solid tumors. Chemotherapy has been found to be an effective modality for the management of SVC syndrome with underlying malignancies such as small cell carcinoma of the lung or lymphoma. Because these tumors have a tendency to recur locally in areas of bulky disease, radiation therapy is recommended in addition. Surgery may provide immediate relief for patients in whom a benign process is causing obstruction of the SVC.

Clinical improvement occurs in most patients, although this improvement may be due to the development of adequate collateral circulation. The mortality associated with SVCS does not relate to caval obstruction, but rather to the underlying cause.

SVCS and Central Venous Catheters in Adults   The use of long-term central venous catheters has become common practice in patients with cancer. Major vessel thrombosis may occur. In these cases, catheter removal should be combined with anticoagulation to prevent embolization. SVCS in this setting, if detected early, can be treated successfully by fibrinolytic therapy without sacrificing the catheter. Monthly urokinase flushing may reduce the occlusive and infectious complications related to these catheters.

PERICARDIAL EFFUSION/TAMPONADE   Malignant pericardial disease is found at autopsy in 5 to 10 percent of patients with cancer, most frequently in patients with lung cancer, breast cancer, leukemias, and lymphomas. However, cardiac tamponade as the initial presentation of extrathoracic malignancy is rare. The origin is not malignancy in about 50 percent of cancer patients with symptomatic pericardial disease, but instead may be related to irradiation, drug-induced pericarditis, hypothyroidism, idiopathic pericarditis, infection, or autoimmune diseases. Two types of radiation pericarditis have been described: an acute inflammatory, effusive pericarditis occurring within months of irradiation, which usually resolves spontaneously, and a chronic effusive pericarditis that may appear up to 20 years after radiotherapy and is accompanied by a thickened pericardium.

Most patients with pericardial metastasis are asymptomatic. However, the common symptoms are dyspnea, cough, chest pain, orthopnea, and weakness. Pleural effusion, sinus tachycardia, jugular venous distension, hepatomegaly, peripheral edema, and cyanosis are the most frequent physical findings. Relatively specific diagnostic findings, such as paradoxical pulse, diminished heart sounds, pulsus alternans (pulse waves alternating in amplitude between those of greater and lesser volume with successive beats), and friction rub are less common than with nonmalignant pericardial involvement. Chest radiographs and electrocardiography reveal abnormalities in 90 percent of cases, but half of these abnormalities are nonspecific. Echocardiography is the most helpful diagnostic test. Pericardial fluid may be serous, serosanguineous, or hemorrhagic, and cytologic examination of pericardial fluid is diagnostic in most patients. False negative cytology may occur in patients with lymphoma and mesothelioma.

 TREATMENT

The treatment of malignant pericardial effusions includes pericardiocentesis with or without the introduction of sclerosing agents, the creation of a pericardial window, complete pericardial stripping, cardiac irradiation, or systemic chemotherapy. Acute pericardial tamponade with life-threatening hemodynamic instability requires immediate drainage of fluid. This can be quickly achieved by pericardiocentesis. Alternatively, subxyphoid pericardiotomy can be performed in 45 min under local anesthesia.

INTESTINAL OBSTRUCTION Intestinal obstruction and reobstruction is a common problem in patients with advanced cancer, particularly colorectal or ovarian carcinoma. However, other cancers, such as lung or breast cancer and melanoma, can metastasize within the abdomen, leading to intestinal obstruction. Intestinal pseudoobstruction is caused by infiltration of the mesentery or bowel muscle by tumor, involvement of the celiac plexus, or paraneoplastic neuropathy in patients with small cell lung cancer. Paraneoplastic neuropathy is associated with IgG antibodies reactive to neurons of the myenteric and submucosal plexuses of the jejunum and stomach. Ovarian cancer can lead either to authentic luminal obstruction or to pseudoobstruction that results when circumferential invasion of a bowel segment arrests the forward progression of peristaltic contractions.

The onset of obstruction is usually insidious. Pain is the most common symptom and is usually colicky in nature. Pain can also be due to abdominal distension, tumor masses, or hepatomegaly. Vomiting can be intermittent or continuous. Patients with complete obstruction usually have constipation. Physical examination may reveal abdominal distension with tympany, ascites, visible peristalsis, high-pitched bowel sounds, and tumor masses. Erect plain abdominal films may reveal multiple air-fluid levels and dilation of the small or large bowel. Acute cecal dilation to more than 12 to 14 cm is considered a surgical emergency because of the high likelihood of rupture. The overall prognosis for the cancer patient who develops intestinal obstruction is poor, with the median survival being about 3 to 4 months. About one-fourth to one-third of cases are found to have intestinal obstruction due to causes other than cancer. Adhesions from previous operations are a particularly common benign cause. Ileus induced by vincristine is another reversible cause of obstruction.

 TREATMENT

The management of intestinal obstruction in patients with advanced malignancy depends on the individual case. The extent of the underlying malignancy and the functional status of the major organs should be determined before decisions are made. The initial management should include surgical evaluation. Operation is not always successful and may lead to further complications with a substantial mortality rate (10 to 20 percent). Patients known to have advanced intraabdominal malignancy should receive a prolonged course of conservative management, including nasogastric decompression. Treatment with antiemetics, antispasmodics, and analgesics may allow patients to remain outside the hospital. The somatostatin analogue octreotide has been used successfully in the management of intestinal obstruction in cancer patients. The inhibitory effect of octreotide on gastrointestinal secretion reduces vomiting and pain.

URINARY OBSTRUCTION Urinary obstruction may occur in patients with prostatic or gynecologic malignancies, particularly cervical carcinoma, or metastatic disease from a variety of primary sites. Radiation therapy to pelvic tumors may cause fibrosis and subsequent ureteral obstruction. Bladder outlet obstruction is usually due to prostate and cervical cancers and may lead to bilateral hydronephrosis and subsequent renal failure.

Flank pain is the most common symptom. Persistent urinary tract infection, persistent proteinuria, or hematuria in patients with a cancer should alert the physician to the possibility of ureteral obstruction. Total anuria and/or anuria alternating with polyuria may occur. A slow, continuous rise in the serum creatinine value necessitates immediate evaluation in patients with cancer. Renal ultrasound examination is the safest and least expensive way to identify hydronephrosis. The function of an obstructed kidney can be evaluated by a nuclear scan. CT can be helpful in identifying a retroperitoneal mass or retroperitoneal adenopathy.

 TREATMENT

Bilateral ureteral or bladder outlet obstruction requires immediate attention. Obstruction associated with flank pain, sepsis, or fistula formation is an indication for palliative urinary diversion. There are many newer techniques by which internal ureteral stents can be placed under local anesthesia. Percutaneous nephrostomy offers an alternative approach for drainage. In the case of bladder outlet obstruction due to malignancy, a suprapubic cystostomy can be used for urinary drainage.

MALIGNANT BILIARY OBSTRUCTION This common clinical problem can be caused by a primary carcinoma arising in the pancreas, ampulla of Vater, bile duct, or liver or by metastatic disease to the periductal lymph nodes or liver parenchyma. The most common metastatic tumors causing biliary obstruction are gastric, colon, breast, and lung cancers. Jaundice, light-colored stools, dark urine, pruritus, and weight loss due to malabsorption are usual symptoms. Pain and secondary infection are uncommon in malignant biliary obstruction. Ultrasound, CT, or percutaneous transhepatic or endoscopic retrograde cholangiography will identify the site and nature of the biliary obstruction.

TREATMENT

Palliative intervention is indicated only in patients with disabling pruritus resistant to medical treatment, severe malabsorption, or infection. Therapeutic intervention by stenting under radiographic control, surgical bypass, or radiation therapy with or without chemotherapy may alleviate the obstruction. The choice of modality should be based on the site of obstruction (proximal versus distal), the type of tumor (sensitive to radiotherapy, chemotherapy, or neither), and the general condition of the patient. In the absence of pruritus, biliary obstruction may be a largely asymptomatic cause of death.

SPINAL CORD COMPRESSION Spinal cord compression occurs in 5 to 10 percent of patients with cancer. Epidural tumor is the first manifestation of malignancy in about 10 percent of patients. In most of these cases, the underlying cancer is identified during the initial evaluation; lung cancer is most commonly the primary malignancy.

Metastatic tumor involves the vertebral column more often than any other part of the bony skeleton. Lung, breast, and prostate cancer are the most frequent offenders. Multiple myeloma also has a high incidence of spine involvement. The thoracic spine is the most common site (70 percent), followed by the lumbosacral spine (20 percent) and the cervical spine (10 percent). Involvement of multiple sites is most frequent in patients with breast and prostatic carcinoma. By contrast, carcinoma of the lung almost invariably produces a single site of vertebral involvement. Cord injury develops when metastases to the vertebral body or pedicle enlarge and compress the underlying dura. Another cause of cord compression is direct extension of a paravertebral lesion through the intervertebral foramen. These cases usually involve a lymphoma, myeloma, or pediatric neoplasm. Parenchymal spinal cord metastasis due to hematogenous spread occurs in rare cases.

The most common initial symptom in patients with spinal cord compression is localized back pain and tenderness due to involvement of vertebrae by tumor. Pain is usually present for days or months before other neurologic findings appear. It is exacerbated by movement and by coughing or sneezing. It can be differentiated from the pain of disc disease by the fact that it worsens when the patient lies supine. Radicular pain is less common than localized back pain and usually develops later. Radicular pain in the cervical or lumbosacral areas may be unilateral or bilateral. Radicular pain from the thoracic roots is often bilateral and is described by patients as a feeling of tight, band-like constriction around the thorax and abdomen. Typical cervical radicular pain radiates down the arm; in the lumbar region, the radiation is down the legs. Loss of bowel or bladder control may be the presenting symptom.

On physical examination, pain induced by straight leg raising, neck flexion, or vertebral percussion may help to determine the level of cord compression. Patients develop numbness and paresthesias in the extremities or trunk. Loss of sensibility to pinprick is as common as loss of sensibility to vibration or position. The upper limit of the zone of sensory loss is often one or two vertebrae below the site of compression. Motor findings include weakness, spasticity, and abnormal muscle stretching. The presence of an extensor plantar reflex reflects significant compression. Deep tendon reflexes may be brisk. Motor and sensory loss usually precede sphincter disturbance. Patients with autonomic dysfunction may present with decreased anal tonus, decreased perineal sensibility, and a distended bladder. The absence of the anal wink reflex or the bulbocavernosus reflex confirms cord (conus or cauda equina) involvement. In doubtful cases, evaluation of post-voiding urinary residual volume can be helpful. A residual volume of more than 150 mL suggests bladder dysfunction. Autonomic dysfunction is an unfavorable prognostic factor. Patients with progressive neurologic symptoms should have frequent neurologic examinations and rapid therapeutic intervention.

Patients with known cancer who develop back pain should be evaluated for spinal cord compression as quickly as possible (Fig. 104-1). Treatment is more often successful in patients who are ambulatory and still have sphincter control at the time treatment is initiated. Patients should have a neurologic examination and plain films of the spine. Those whose physical examination suggests cord compression should receive dexamethasone (6 mg per os every 6 h), starting immediately. There is no specific upper limit to the dexamethasone dose. If neurologic function improves in response to 24 mg a day but examination still shows abnormalities, doubling the dose may lead to further improvement.

Erosion of the pedicles (the "winking owl" sign) is the earliest radiologic finding of vertebral tumor. Other radiographic changes include increased intrapedicular distance, vertebral destruction, lytic or sclerotic lesions, scalloped vertebral bodies, and vertebral body collapse. Vertebral collapse is not a reliable indicator of the presence of tumor; about 20 percent of cases of vertebral collapse, particularly those in older patients and postmenopausal women, are not due to

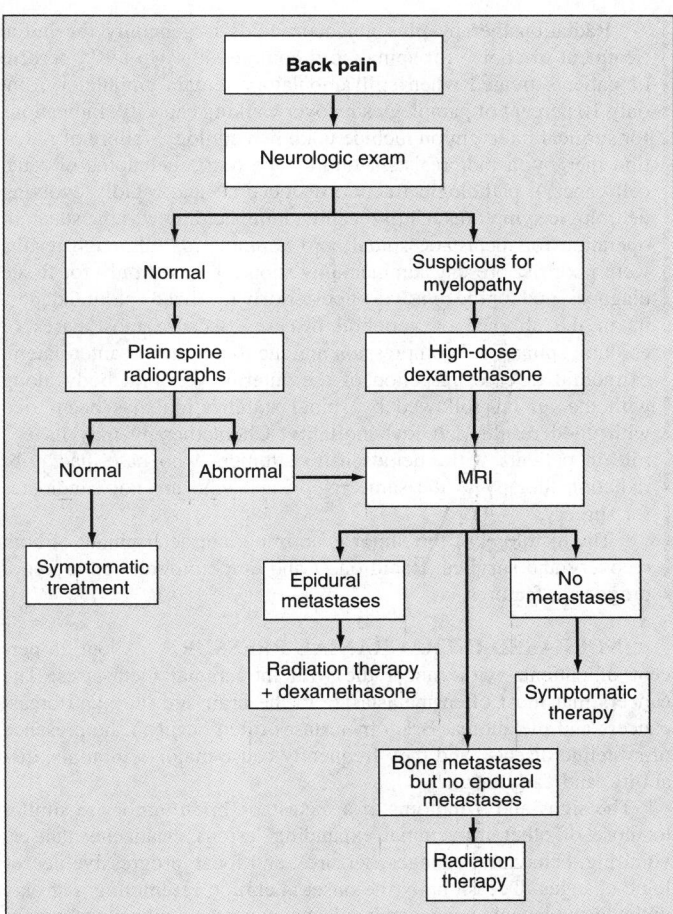

FIGURE 104-1 Management of cancer patients with back pain.

cancer. Also, a normal appearance on plain films of the spine does not exclude the diagnosis of cancer. The role of bone scans in the detection of cord compression is not clear. This method is sensitive, but it is less specific than spinal radiography.

The full-length image of the cord provided by MRI may be useful in the workup of patients with spinal cord compression. On T1-weighted images, there is good contrast between the cord, cerebrospinal fluid, and extradural lesions. Owing to their sensitivity in demonstrating the replacement of bone marrow by tumor, these MR images can show which parts of a vertebra are involved by tumor (the body, pedicle, lamina, spinous process, etc.). These images also visualize intraspinal extradural masses compressing the cord. T2-weighted images are most useful for the demonstration of intramedullary pathology. Gadolinium-enhanced MRI can help to characterize and delineate intramedullary disease. Comparative studies have shown that MRI is as good as or better than myelography plus postmyelogram CT in detecting metastatic epidural disease with cord compression. Myelography should be reserved for patients who have poor MR images or who cannot undergo MRI promptly. CT in conjunction with myelography clearly enhances the detection of small areas of spinal destruction.

In patients with spinal cord compression and an unknown primary tumor, a simple workup including chest radiography, mammography, measurement of prostate-specific antigen, and abdominal CT will usually reveal the underlying malignancy.

℞ TREATMENT

The treatment of patients with spinal cord compression is directed toward relief of pain and restoration of neurologic function (Fig. 104-1).

Radiation therapy plus glucocorticoids is generally the initial treatment of choice for spinal cord compression. Up to 75 percent of patients treated when still ambulatory remain ambulatory, but only 10 percent of paraplegics recover walking capacity. Indications for surgical intervention include unknown etiology, failure of radiation therapy, a radioresistant tumor type (e.g., melanoma or renal cell cancer), pathologic fracture dislocation, and rapidly evolving neurologic symptoms. Until recently, laminectomy was the standard operation for metastatic spinal cord compression, although results were poor. At present, laminectomy should be used only for tissue diagnosis and for the removal of posteriorly localized epidural deposits in the absence of vertebral disease. Because most cases of epidural spinal cord compression are due to anterior or anterolateral extradural disease, resection of the anterior vertebral body along with the tumor, followed by spinal stabilization, has been tried with good results and low mortality. Chemotherapy may have a role in patients with chemosensitive tumors who have had prior radiation therapy to the same region and who are not candidates for surgery.

The histology of the tumor is an important determinant of both recovery and survival. Rapid onset and quick progression are poor prognostic features.

INCREASED INTRACRANIAL PRESSURE About 25 percent of patients with cancer die with intracranial metastases. The cancers that most often metastasize to the brain are lung and breast cancers and melanoma. Brain metastases often occur in the presence of systemic disease, and they frequently cause major symptoms, disability, and early death.

The signs and symptoms of a metastatic brain tumor are similar to those of other intracranial expanding lesions: headache, nausea, vomiting, behavioral changes, seizures, and focal, progressive neurologic changes. Occasionally the onset is abrupt, resembling a stroke, with the sudden appearance of headache, nausea, vomiting, and neurologic deficits. This picture is usually due to hemorrhage into the metastasis. Of the metastatic tumors, melanoma, germ cell tumors, and renal cell cancers have a particularly high incidence of intracranial bleeding. The tumor mass and surrounding edema may cause obstruction of the circulation of cerebrospinal fluid, with resulting hydrocephalus. Patients with increased intracranial pressure may have papilledema with visual disturbances and neck stiffness. As the mass enlarges, brain tissue may be displaced through the fixed cranial openings, producing various herniation syndromes.

CT and MRI are equally effective in the diagnosis of brain metastases. CT with contrast should be used as a screening procedure. The CT scan shows brain metastases as multiple enhancing lesions of various sizes with surrounding areas of low-density edema. If there is a single lesion or if no metastases are visualized by contrast-enhanced CT, MRI of the brain should be performed. Gadolinium-enhanced MRI is more sensitive than CT at revealing small lesions, particularly in the brainstem or cerebellum.

℞ TREATMENT

If signs and symptoms of brain herniation (particularly headache, drowsiness, and papilledema) are present, the patient should be intubated and hyperventilated to maintain P_{CO_2} between 25 and 30 mmHg and should receive infusions of mannitol (1 to 1.5 g/kg) every 6 h. Dexamethasone is the best initial treatment for all symptomatic patients with brain metastases (see above). Patients with multiple lesions should receive whole-brain radiation therapy. Patients with a single brain metastasis and with controlled extracranial disease may be treated with surgical excision followed by whole-brain radiation therapy, especially if they are younger than 60 years. Radioresistant tumors should be resected if possible. Some patients with increased intracranial pressure associated with hydrocephalus may benefit from neurosurgical intervention.

SEIZURES Seizures occurring in a cancer patient can be caused by the tumor itself, by metabolic disturbances, by radiation injury, by cerebral infarctions, by chemotherapy-related encephalopathies, or by central nervous system infections. Metastatic disease to the central nervous system is the most common cause of seizures in cancer patients. The frequency with which seizures are a presenting symptom of intracranial metastasis ranges from 6 to 29 percent in published series. Approximately 10 percent of patients with intracranial metastasis eventually develop seizures. The presence of frontal lesions correlates with early seizures, and the presence of hemispheric symptomatology increases the risk for late seizures. Both early and late seizures are uncommon in patients with primarily posterior fossa lesions. Seizures are also common in patients with intracranial metastases from melanoma. Very rarely, cytotoxic drugs such as etoposide, busulfan, and chlorambucil cause seizures.

℞ TREATMENT

Patients in whom seizures due to intracranial metastases have been demonstrated should receive anticonvulsive treatment with diphenylhydantoin. Prophylactic anticonvulsant therapy is not recommended unless the patient is at a high risk for late seizures. In those cases, serum diphenylhydantoin levels should be monitored closely and the dosage adjusted accordingly.

INTRACEREBRAL LEUKOCYTOSTASIS Intracerebral leukocytostasis (Ball's disease) is a potentially fatal complication of acute leukemia (particularly myelogenous leukemia) that can occur when the peripheral blast cell count is greater than 100,000/μL. At such high blast cell counts, blood viscosity is increased and blood flow is slowed, and the primitive leukemic cells are capable of invading through endothelium and causing hemorrhage into the brain. Patients may experience stupor, dizziness, visual disturbances, ataxia, coma, or sudden death. Administration of 600cGy of whole-brain irradiation can protect against this complication and can be followed by rapid institution of antileukemic therapy. This complication is not a feature of the high white cell counts associated with chronic lymphocytic leukemia or chronic myelogenous leukemia.

HEMOPTYSIS While hemoptysis is usually caused by nonmalignant conditions, it may develop in older patients with lung cancer or lung metastases who have coagulation defects or thrombocytopenia. The volume of bleeding is often difficult to gauge. When respiratory difficulty occurs, hemoptysis should be treated emergently. Often patients can tell where the bleeding is occurring. They should be placed bleeding side down, given supplemental oxygen, and subjected to emergency bronchoscopy. If the site of the lesion is detected, either the patient undergoes a definitive surgical procedure or the lesion is treated with a neodymium:yttrium-aluminum-garnet (Nd:YAG) laser, endobronchial tamponade, or bronchial artery catheterization and embolization. The surgical option is preferred; the other procedures are less effective in the face of brisk bleeding, and complications are common with tamponade and embolization procedures. The thrombocytopenia and coagulation defects should be corrected, if possible.

AIRWAY OBSTRUCTION Generally, *airway obstruction* refers to a blockage at the level of the mainstem bronchi or above. It may result either from intraluminal tumor growth or from extrinsic compression of the airway. If the obstruction is proximal to the larynx, a tracheostomy may be life-saving. For more distal obstructions, surgery is preferred. However, radiation therapy (either external-beam irradiation or brachytherapy) given together with glucocorticoids may also open the airway. For intrinsic lesions, particularly incomplete centrally obstructing lesions, Nd:YAG laser treatment or photodynamic therapy (photosensitizers plus light) can be effective. Photodynamic therapy has the advantage of being suitable for use in patients who are not surgical candidates.

METABOLIC EMERGENCIES

HYPERCALCEMIA Hypercalcemia is the most common paraneoplastic syndrome (see Chaps. 102 and 353), occurring in about 10 percent of patients with advanced cancer. It is associated most often with cancers of the lung, breast, head and neck, and kidney and with multiple myeloma.

Increased release of calcium from bone is the main factor leading to hypercalcemia. Bone resorption is increased dramatically through stimulation of the proliferation and activity of osteoclasts, and bone formation is not stimulated in parallel. The kidney may play an important role through an increase in the reabsorption of calcium in the distal tubule. Parathormone-related protein (PTHrP) produced by tumors has a central role as a mediator of hypercalcemia in cancer. PTHrP shares 80 percent homology with the first 13 amino acids of parathormone (PTH), which are in the region responsible for binding to the PTH receptor. PTHrP acts via the PTH hormone receptors on osteoblasts and renal tubular cells to stimulate bone resorption and renal calcium conservation, leading to hypercalcemia. Elevated plasma PTHrP levels are also found in most hypercalcemic patients with bone metastases, in whom hypercalcemia has traditionally been explained by local osteolysis due to the production of osteolytic factors by tumors. Transforming growth factors, cytokines (interleukins 1 and 6), and other unknown factors could play a contributory role. True "ectopic" PTH production by malignant tumors is rare. In lymphoma, a vitamin D–related product of the tumor may also increase calcium absorption in the gut.

The clinical features of hypercalcemia in cancer patients are non-specific and include fatigue, anorexia, constipation, polydipsia, muscle weakness, nausea, and vomiting. They may easily be attributed to the malignancy itself or to its treatment. Laboratory assessment should include measurement of serum electrolytes, calcium, phosphate, and albumin. Hypoalbuminemia is common in malignancy and, if present, will affect the total serum concentration of calcium. If ionized calcium level cannot be obtained, then corrected serum calcium concentration should be calculated using the following formula:

$$\text{Corrected serum calcium} = \text{measured serum calcium} \\ + 0.8\,(4.0 - \text{measured serum albumin})$$

Most patients with hypercalcemia of malignancy have obvious evidence of malignancy, and their serum PTH levels are suppressed. Measurements of PTHrP and serum 1,25-dihydroxyvitamin D should be confined to research studies in patients with advanced cancer. The results of routine serum chemistry evaluations are not reliable alone for distinguishing between malignant and nonmalignant causes of hypercalcemia.

℞ TREATMENT

Not all patients with moderate to severe hypercalcemia (corrected calcium ≥12 mg/dL) should be treated. The decision of whether or not to treat will depend on the patient's quality of life, the current symptoms, and the prospect for further treatment. Treatment directed at hypercalcemia only extends life in patients for whom effective cancer treatment is available. Nonetheless, corrective therapy may be indicated on a palliative basis to improve symptoms and the quality of life. Treatment of symptomatic hypercalcemia begins with intravenous saline to restore the depleted intravascular volume, which may be 4 to 8 L below normal at presentation. However, rehydration usually has little effect on calcium levels, producing a median effective decrease of only 1 mg/dL. Antiresorptive agents are essential to decrease osteoclastic activity and control hypercalcemia. Bisphosphonates, which are potent inhibitors of bone resorption, have essentially replaced traditional agents such as calcitonin and mithramycin and have changed the therapeutic approach to this frequent complication of advancing cancer. Bisphosphonate therapy is easy to administer, is virtually free of side effects, and is rapidly effective in lowering serum calcium. Pamidronate is the most effective of the commercially available bisphosphonates. The recommended dose of pamidronate is 60 mg for moderate hypercalcemia (corrected calcium 12 to 13.5 mg/dL) and 90 mg for severe hypercalcemia (corrected calcium >13.5 mg/dL). The dose is given as a single infusion over 4 or 24 h.

Gallium nitrate inhibits osteoclast function, thus reducing serum calcium. Clinical use of this agent has been limited by the risk of nephrotoxicity and the inconvenient method of administration (200 mg/m² per day as a 5-day continuous intravenous infusion).

SYNDROME OF INAPPROPRIATE SECRETION OF ANTIDIURETIC HORMONE (SIADH)   SIADH is attributed to production of arginine vasopressin by the tumor cells and is characterized by hyponatremia, urine osmolarity inappropriately higher than plasma osmolarity, and high urinary sodium excretion in the absence of volume depletion. Renal, adrenal, and thyroid insufficiency must be excluded, because these disorders can also present with hyponatremia and impaired urinary dilution. Low serum levels of urea and uric acid are useful in distinguishing SIADH from conditions associated with renal hypoperfusion (see Chaps. 102 and 330).

A broad spectrum of malignant tumors have been reported to cause SIADH. Ectopic vasopressin secretion may occur in some 38 percent of small cell carcinomas of the lung; often there is cosecretion of adrenocorticotropic hormone. The presence of hyponatremia in patients with small cell lung cancer confers a poor prognosis. SIADH may also be caused by various other conditions, such as central nervous system and pulmonary disorders and some surgical procedures. A variety of drugs have also been shown to produce SIADH, including cytotoxic drugs such as vincristine, ifosfamide, cyclophosphamide, cisplatin, levamisole, and melphalan.

Most patients with SIADH are asymptomatic. The severity of symptoms and signs is related to the degree of hyponatremia and the rapidity with which it develops. Early changes include anorexia, depression, lethargy, irritability, confusion, muscle weakness, and marked personality changes. When the plasma sodium level falls below 110 mEq/L, extensor plantar responses, areflexia, and pseudobulbar palsy may be noted, and further reductions may cause coma, convulsions, and death.

℞ TREATMENT

The optimal therapy for SIADH is to treat the underlying malignancy. If that is not possible, other therapeutic approaches are available, such as water restriction or the administration of demeclocycline (900 to 1200 mg per os bid), urea, or lithium carbonate (300 mg per os tid). Demeclocycline is usually used first. It inhibits the effects of vasopressin on the distal renal tubule. Patients with seizure or coma from hyponatremia may require normal saline infusion plus furosemide to enhance free water clearance. The rate of sodium correction should be slow [0.5 to 1 (mEq/L)/h] to prevent rapid fluid shifts and central pontine myelinolysis. Serum calcium should be monitored closely to avoid hypocalcemia.

LACTIC ACIDOSIS   This is a rare and potentially fatal metabolic complication of cancer. Lactic acidosis associated with sepsis and circulatory failure is a common preterminal event in many malignancies. Lactic acidosis in the absence of hypoxemia may occur in patients with leukemia, lymphoma, or solid tumors. Extensive involvement of the liver by tumor is present in most cases. Alteration of liver function may be responsible for the lactate accumulation. Tachypnea, tachycardia, change of mental status, and hepatomegaly may be seen. The serum level of lactic acid may reach 10 to 20 mEq/L (90 to 180 mg/dL). Treatment is aimed at the underlying disease. The danger from lactic acidosis is from the acidosis, not the lactate. Sodium bicarbonate should be added if acidosis is very severe or if hydrogen ion production is very rapid and uncontrolled. The prognosis is poor.

HYPOGLYCEMIA   Persistent hypoglycemia occasionally is associated with tumors other than pancreatic islet cell tumors. Usually these tumors are large, and often they are of mesenchymal origin or are hepatomas or adrenocortical tumors. Mesenchymal tumors are usually located in the retroperitoneum or thorax. In these patients, obtundation, confusion, and behavioral aberrations occur in the postabsorptive period and may precede the diagnosis of the tumor. Hypoglycemia is due to unregulated overproduction of the insulin-like growth factors by a tumor or to the induction of autoantibodies to the insulin receptor. Treatment of the hypoglycemia has generally been symptomatic, relying on the administration of glucose.

ADRENAL INSUFFICIENCY In cancer patients, adrenal insufficiency may go unrecognized because the symptoms, such as nausea, vomiting, anorexia, and orthostatic hypotension, are nonspecific and may be mistakenly attributed to progressive cancer or to cancer therapy. In the cancer patient, primary adrenal insufficiency may develop owing to replacement of both glands by metastases (of lung, breast, colon, or kidney cancer) or infiltrating lymphoma, to removal of both glands, or to hemorrhagic necrosis in association with sepsis or anticoagulation. Impaired adrenal steroid synthesis occurs in patients being treated for cancer with mitotane, aminoglutethimide, ketoconazole, or the investigational agent suramin or undergoing rapid reduction in glucocorticoid therapy. Rarely, metastatic replacement will cause primary adrenal insufficiency as the first manifestation of an occult malignancy. Metastasis to the pituitary or hypothalamus is found at autopsy in up to 5 percent of patients with cancer, but associated secondary adrenal insufficiency is rare.

Acute adrenal insufficiency is potentially lethal. Treatment of suspected adrenal crisis is initiated after sampling serum cortisol and ACTH levels (see Chap. 332).

TREATMENT-RELATED EMERGENCIES

TUMOR LYSIS SYNDROME This is a well-recognized clinical entity that is characterized by various combinations of hyperuricemia, hyperkalemia, hyperphosphatemia, lactic acidosis, and hypocalcemia and is caused by the mass destruction of a large number of rapidly proliferating neoplastic cells. Frequently, acute renal failure develops as a result of tumor lysis syndrome.

Tumor lysis syndrome is most frequently associated with the treatment of Burkitt's lymphoma, acute lymphoblastic leukemia, and other high-grade lymphomas, but it also may be seen with chronic leukemias and, rarely, with solid tumors. This syndrome has been seen in patients with chronic lymphocytic leukemia after treatment with fludarabine. Tumor lysis syndrome usually occurs during or shortly (1 to 5 days) after chemotherapy. Rarely, spontaneous necrosis of malignancies causes tumor lysis syndrome.

Hyperuricemia may be present at the time of chemotherapy. Effective treatment accelerates the destruction of malignant cells and leads to increased serum uric acid levels from the turnover of nucleic acids. Owing to the acidic local environment, uric acid can precipitate in the tubules, medulla, and collecting ducts of the kidney, leading to renal failure. Lactic acidosis and dehydration may contribute to the precipitation of uric acid in the renal tubules. The finding of uric acid crystals in the urine is strong evidence for uric acid nephropathy. The ratio by weight of urinary uric acid to urinary creatinine is >1 in patients with acute hyperuricemic nephropathy and <1 in patients with renal failure due to other causes.

Hyperphosphatemia, which can be caused by the release of intracellular phosphate pools by tumor cell lysis, produces a reciprocal depression in serum calcium, which causes severe neuromuscular irritability and tetany. Deposition of calcium phosphate in the kidney and hyperphosphatemia may cause renal failure. Potassium is the principal intracellular cation, and massive destruction of malignant cells may lead to hyperkalemia. Hyperkalemia in patients with renal failure may rapidly become life-threatening. Hyperkalemia can cause ventricular arrhythmias and sudden death.

The likelihood that the tumor lysis syndrome will occur in patients with Burkitt's lymphoma is related to the tumor burden and renal function. Hyperuricemia and high serum levels of lactate dehydrogenase LDH (>1500 units per liter), both of which correlate with total tumor burden, also correlate with the risk of posttreatment tumor lysis

syndrome. In patients at risk for tumor lysis, pretreatment evaluations should include a complete blood count, serum chemistry evaluation, and urine analysis. High leukocyte and platelet counts may artificially elevate potassium levels ("pseudohyperkalemia") due to lysis of these cells after the blood is drawn. In these cases, plasma potassium instead of serum potassium should be followed. In pseudohyperkalemia, no electrocardiographic abnormalities will be present. In patients with abnormal baseline renal function, the kidneys and retroperitoneal area should be evaluated by sonography and/or CT. Urine output should be watched closely.

Recognition of risk and prevention are the most important steps in the management of this syndrome (Fig. 104-2). Despite aggressive pretherapy management, tumor lysis syndrome and/or oliguric or anuric renal failure may occur. Dialysis is often necessary and should be considered early in the course. Hemodialysis is preferred. The prognosis is excellent, and renal function recovers after the uric acid level is lowered by dialysis to less than 10 to 20 mg/dL.

HEMOLYTIC-UREMIC SYNDROME Hemolytic-uremic syndrome (HUS) and, less commonly, thrombotic thrombocytopenic purpura (TTP) occurring after treatment with antineoplastic drugs have been described. Mitomycin is by far the most common agent causing this peculiar syndrome. Other chemotherapeutic agents, particularly cisplatin and bleomycin, have also been reported to be associated with this syndrome. This syndrome occurs most often in patients with gastric, colorectal, and breast carcinoma. In one series, 35 percent of patients were without evident cancer at the time of the development of this syndrome. Secondary HUS/TTP has also been reported as a rare but sometimes fatal complication of bone marrow transplantation.

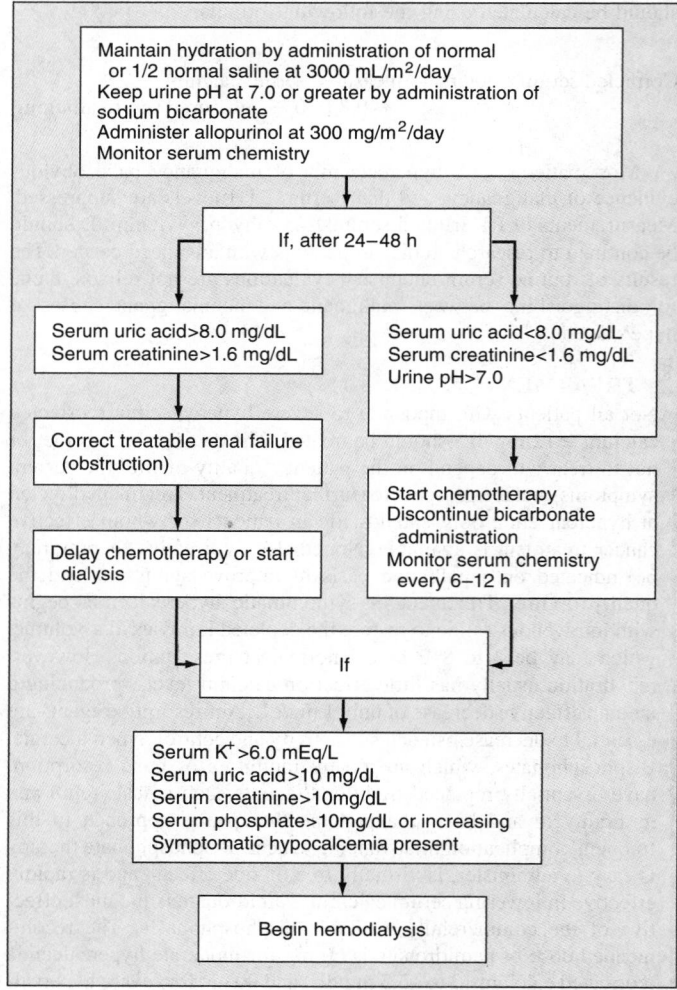

FIGURE 104-2 Management of patients at high risk for the tumor lysis syndrome.

HUS usually has its onset 4 to 8 weeks after the last dose of chemotherapy, but it is not rare to detect it several months later. HUS is characterized by microangiopathic hemolytic anemia, thrombocytopenia, and renal failure. Dyspnea, weakness, fatigue, oliguria, and purpura are also common initial symptoms and findings. Systemic hypertension and pulmonary edema commonly occur. Severe hypertension, pulmonary edema, and rapid worsening of hemolysis and renal function may occur after a blood transfusion. Cardiac findings include atrial arrhythmias, pericardial friction rub, and pericardial effusion. Raynaud's phenomenon has been reported as part of the syndrome in patients treated with bleomycin.

Laboratory findings include severe to moderate anemia associated with red cell fragmentation and numerous schistocytes on peripheral smear. Reticulocytosis, decreased plasma haptoglobin, and an elevated LDH level provide additional evidence of hemolysis. The serum bilirubin level is usually normal or slightly elevated. The Coombs test is negative. The white cell count is usually normal, and thrombocytopenia ($<100,000/\mu L$) is almost always present. Most patients have a normal coagulation profile, although some have mild elevations in thrombin time and in level of fibrin degradation products. The serum creatinine level is elevated at presentation and shows a pattern of subacute worsening within weeks of the initial azotemia. The urinalysis reveals hematuria, proteinuria, and granular or hyaline casts, and circulating immune complexes may be present.

The basic pathologic lesion appears to be deposition of fibrin in the walls of capillaries and arterioles, and these deposits are similar to those seen in HUS due to other causes. These microvascular abnormalities involve mainly the kidneys and rarely occur in other organs. The pathogenesis of chemotherapy-related HUS is unknown. Immune complexes have been proposed but not confirmed to be etiologic.

The case fatality rate is high, most patients dying within a few months. Plasmapheresis and plasma exchange may normalize the hematologic abnormalities, but renal failure is not reversed in most patients. Immunoperfusion over a staphylococcal protein A column is the most successful treatment. About half of the patients treated with immunoperfusion respond with resolution of thrombocytopenia, improvement in anemia, and stabilization of renal failure. Treatment is well tolerated. It is not clear how the treatment works.

NEUTROPENIA AND INFECTION These remain the most common serious complications of cancer therapy. → *They are covered in detail in Chap. 87.*

PULMONARY INFILTRATES Patients with cancer may present with dyspnea associated with diffuse interstitial infiltrates on chest radiographs. Such infiltrates may be due to progression of the underlying malignancy, to treatment-related toxicities, to infection, and/or to unrelated diseases. The cause may be multifactorial; however, most commonly they occur as a consequence of treatment. Infiltration of the lung by malignancy has been described in cases of leukemia, lymphoma, and breast and other solid cancers. Pulmonary lymphatics may be involved diffusely by neoplasm (pulmonary lymphangitic carcinomatosis), resulting in a diffuse increase in interstitial markings on chest radiographs. The patient is often mildly dyspneic at the onset, but pulmonary failure develops rapidly over a period of weeks. In some patients, dyspnea precedes changes on the chest radiographs and is accompanied by a nonproductive cough. This syndrome is characteristic of solid tumors. In leukemic patients, diffuse microscopic neoplastic peribronchial and peribronchiolar infiltration is frequent but may be asymptomatic. However, some patients present with diffuse interstitial infiltrates, an alveolar capillary block syndrome, and respiratory distress. In these situations, glucocorticoids can provide symptomatic relief, but specific chemotherapy should always be started promptly.

In addition, accumulation of leukemic blasts in the pulmonary capillary system may cause pulmonary distress and failure in patients with acute myelogenous leukemia. This complication is strongly related to high peripheral blast counts (more than $100,000/\mu L$) and a short tumor cell doubling time. Some patients with pulmonary leukostasis may have nodular and/or floccular, diffuse infiltrates on chest radiographs. In addition to dyspnea, patients may develop dizziness, confusion, tinnitus, ataxia, visual blurring, and retinal abnormalities due to leukostasis in cerebral vessels. Leukapheresis and/or chemotherapy should be started without delay. Pulmonary irradiation may reduce symptoms.

Several cytotoxic agents, such as bleomycin, methotrexate, busulfan, and the nitrosoureas, may cause pulmonary damage. The most frequent presentations are interstitial pneumonitis, alveolitis, and pulmonary fibrosis. Some cytotoxic agents, including methotrexate and procarbazine, may cause an acute hypersensitivity reaction. Cytosine arabinoside has been associated with noncardiogenic pulmonary edema. Administration of multiple cytotoxic drugs, as well as radiation therapy and preexisting lung disease, may potentiate the pulmonary toxicity. Supplemental oxygen may potentiate the effects of drugs and radiation injury. Patients should always be managed with the lowest $F_{I_{O_2}}$ that is sufficient to maintain hemoglobin saturation.

The onset of symptoms may be insidious, with symptoms including dyspnea, nonproductive cough, and tachycardia. Patients may have bibasilar crepitant rales, end-inspiratory crackles, fever, and cyanosis. The chest radiograph generally shows an interstitial and sometimes an intraalveolar pattern that is strongest at the lung bases and may be symmetric. A small effusion may occur. Hypoxemia with decreased carbon monoxide diffusing capacity is always present. Glucocorticoids may be helpful in patients in whom pulmonary toxicity is related to radiation therapy or to chemotherapy with mitomycin C, busulfan, methotrexate, or procarbazine. Treatment is otherwise supportive.

Radiation pneumonitis and/or fibrosis is a relatively frequent side effect of thoracic radiation therapy when the dosage exceeds 40 Gy and may be acute or chronic. It has its onset usually from 2 to 6 months after completion of radiation therapy. The clinical syndrome, which varies in severity, consists of dyspnea, cough with scanty sputum, low-grade fever, and an initial hazy infiltrate on chest radiographs. The infiltrate and tissue damage generally are confined to the radiation field. The patients subsequently may develop a patchy alveolar infiltrate and air bronchograms, which may progress to acute respiratory failure, sometimes fatal. A lung biopsy may be necessary to make the diagnosis. Asymptomatic infiltrates found incidentally after radiation therapy need not be treated. However, prednisone should be administered to patients with fever or other symptoms. The dosage should be tapered slowly after the resolution of radiation pneumonitis, as abrupt withdrawal of glucocorticoids may cause an exacerbation of pneumonia. Delayed radiation fibrosis may occur years after radiation therapy and is signaled by dyspnea on exertion. Often it is mild, but it can progress to chronic respiratory failure. Therapy is supportive.

Pneumonia is a common problem in patients undergoing treatment for cancer. Bacterial pneumonia typically causes a localized infiltrate on chest radiographs. Therapy is tailored to the causative organism. When diffuse interstitial infiltrates appear in a febrile patient, the differential diagnosis is extensive and includes pneumonia due to infection with *Pneumocystis carinii,* cytomegalovirus, or intracellular pathogens such as mycoplasma and *Legionella;* effects of drugs or radiation; tumor progression; nonspecific pneumonitis; and fungal disease. However, studies have shown that empirical intervention with trimethoprim-sulfamethoxazole plus erythromycin in nonneutropenic patients, with these antibiotics plus ceftazidime in neutropenic patients, covers nearly every treatable diagnosis (except tumor progression) and gives as good overall survival as a strategy based on early invasive intervention with bronchoalveolar lavage or open lung biopsy. If the patient does not improve in 4 days, open lung biopsy is the procedure of choice. Bronchoscopy with bronchoalveolar lavage may be used in patients who are poor candidates for surgery.

In patients with pulmonary infiltrates who are afebrile, heart failure and multiple pulmonary emboli form part of the differential diagnosis.

TYPHLITIS Typhlitis is the necrosis of the cecum and adjacent colon that may complicate the treatment of acute leukemia. The patient develops right lower quadrant abdominal pain, often with rebound tenderness and a tense, distended abdomen, in a setting of fever and neutropenia. Watery diarrhea and bacteremia are common, and bleeding may occur. Rapid institution of broad-spectrum antibiotic coverage and nasogastric suction may reverse the disease. Surgical intervention should be considered if there is no improvement by 24 h after the start of antibiotic treatment. If the localized abdominal findings become diffuse, the prognosis is poor.

HEMORRHAGIC CYSTITIS This condition can develop in patients receiving cyclophosphamide or ifosfamide. Both drugs are metabolized to acrolein, which is a strong chemical irritant that is excreted in the urine. Prolonged contact or high concentrations may lead to bladder irritation and hemorrhage. The best management is prevention. Maintaining a high rate of urine flow minimizes exposure. In addition, 2-mercaptoethanesulfonate (mesna) detoxifies the metabolites and can be coadministered with the instigating drugs. Mesna usually is given three times on the day of ifosfamide administration in doses that are each 20 percent of the total ifosfamide dose. If hemorrhagic cystitis develops, the maintenance of a high urine flow may be sufficient supportive care. If conservative management is not effective, irrigation of the bladder with an 0.37 to 0.74 percent formalin solution for 10 min stops the bleeding in most cases. *N*-acetylcysteine may also be an effective irrigant. In extreme cases, cystectomy may be necessary.

TREATMENT OF ACUTE PROMYELOCYTIC LEUKEMIA Therapy for this malignancy can produce two life-threatening syndromes. Chemotherapy acts by killing leukemic cells, and the dying cells release procoagulants from their cytoplasmic granules that can produce disseminated intravascular coagulation (see Chap 119). Heparin therapy may reverse this process. Cryoprecipitate and fresh-frozen plasma are used to replace depleted clotting factors. By contrast, treatment with all-*trans*-retinoic acid (ATRA, tretinoin) induces the leukemic cells to differentiate. This approach avoids bleeding complications but creates problems related to high white blood cell counts. The so-called ATRA syndrome includes fever, dyspnea, pleural and

pericardial effusion, and hypotension. Leukocytosis and the ATRA syndrome can be prevented by chemotherapy. The syndromes caused by treatment with either chemotherapy alone or ATRA alone each may cause death in about 15 to 20 percent of patients. The use of chemotherapy and tretinoin together may reduce the mortality by preventing both syndromes.

In summary, the diagnosis of cancer and its treatment carry risk of a multitude of medical problems. Knowledge of both the disease process and the potential hazards of the treatment is required to anticipate and treat these emergent complications.

BIBLIOGRAPHY

AHMANN FR: A reassessment of the clinical implications of the superior vena caval syndrome. J Clin Oncol 2:961, 1984

BOOGERD W et al: Diagnosis and treatment of spinal cord compression in malignant disease. Cancer Treat Rev 19:129, 1993

BROWNE MJ et al: A randomized trial of open lung biopsy versus empiric antimicrobial therapy in cancer patients with diffuse interstitial infiltrates. J Clin Oncol 8:222, 1990

GUCALP R et al: Treatment of cancer-associated hypercalcemia: Double blind comparison of rapid and slow intravenous infusion regimens of pamidronate and saline alone. Arch Intern Med 154:1935, 1994

IHDE JK et al: Adrenal insufficiency in the cancer patient: Implications for the surgeon. Br J Surg 77:1335, 1990

JONES DP et al: Tumor lysis syndrome: Pathogenesis and management. Pediatr Nephrol 9:206, 1995

LOKICH J et al: Biliary tract obstruction secondary to cancer: Management guidelines and selected literature review. J Clin Oncol 5:969, 1987

RIPAMONOTI C: Management of bowel obstruction in advanced cancer. Curr Opin Oncol 6:351, 1994

SNYDER HW et al: Treatment of cancer chemotherapy–associated thrombotic thrombocytopenic/hemolytic uremic syndrome by protein A immunoadsorption of plasma. Cancer 71:1882, 1993

SORENSON JB et al: Syndrome of inappropriate secretion of antidiuretic hormone (SIADH) in malignant disease. J Intern Med 238:97, 1995

VAITKUS PT et al: Treatment of malignant pericardial effusion. JAMA 272:59, 1994

SECTION 2
DISORDERS OF HEMATOPOIESIS

---

105 *Francis W. Ruscetti, Jonathan R. Keller, Dan L. Longo*

HEMATOPOIESIS

Hematopoiesis is the formation of blood cells. The cellular elements of the peripheral blood play a critical role in oxygen delivery to the tissues, hemostasis, and host defense. The turnover of differentiated hematopoietic cells in an adult weighing 70 kg (154 lbs) is over 0.5 trillion cells per day including 200 billion red blood cells (RBC) and 70 billion neutrophilic leukocytes. Under physiologic conditions, production and turnover are coordinated. The average RBC lives about 120 days; the average granulocyte lives 6 to 8 h; the average platelet survives 7 to 10 days. Lymphocytes may be very long-lived, indeed some may survive for many years. However, lymphopoiesis is marked by inefficiency. Many cells are generated but few (5 percent or so) survive to be selected from the marrow or the thymus into the periphery. Under conditions of stress, the production of one or more lineages must be increased to meet increased demand. Thus, the maintenance of normal numbers of peripheral blood components requires essentially continuous production of new cells. This continuous blood cell formation is supported by a small number of cells (0.01 percent) in the bone marrow termed hematopoietic stem cells (HSC), from which all the blood cells arise. When the marrow fails, clinical manifestations of the failure appear as a function of the turnover of the normal cellular endproduct. Thus, patients with marrow failure initially lose granulocytes, which may lead to susceptibility to infection, followed by bleeding related to decreased platelets. Generally pallor, weakness, and

dyspnea on exertion related to decreased RBC mass are the last to appear.

The anatomy and physiology of the hematopoietic organs regulating this remarkable process are complex. However, the understanding of blood cell formation, or hematopoiesis, has been enhanced by recent advances in cell culture techniques and applications of recombinant DNA technology.

HEMATOPOIETIC STEM CELLS HSC are capable of restoring normal hematopoiesis in irradiated animals (radioprotection); long-term multilineage reconstitution (LTRC), and formation of spleen colony forming units [day 12 colony forming units spleen (CFU-S)] that give rise to colonies containing granulocytic, monocytic, erythroid, megakaryocytic, and lymphoid lineages. These three assays have become endpoints for purifying stem cells. Stem cell purification techniques have exploited differences in physical properties (density centrifugation, countercurrent elutriation), cell surface antigen expression detected by monoclonal antibodies, and cell cycle status [Hoechst 33342, a DNA-binding dye, and Rhodamine 123 (Rh123), a mitochondrial-binding dye].

HETEROGENEITY OF STEM CELLS Using these purification methods, it has become clear that both LTRC and short-term repopulating cells (STRC) exist. STRC have radioprotective ability but not long-term persistence. Experiments using bone marrow cells (BMC) distinguishable by alloenzyme or retroviral integration showed that early after bone marrow transplant (BMT), numerous clones actively contributed to hematopoiesis only to be replaced by a few long-lived clones after 3 to 4 months. Using highly enriched Thy 1.1[lo], Sca-1 +, and lineage-specific marker-negative (lin −) BMC, it was shown that cells that stain brightly for Rh123 have STRC activity and lower proliferative potential, and cells that stain poorly for Rh123 are enriched for cells with LTRC and have higher growth potential. This suggests that repopulating cells are part of a continuum of HSC with different abilities to provide long- and short-term reconstitution. This is further supported by studies in which serially transplanted marrow was eventually depleted of LTRC, leaving only STRC. The loss of LTRC activity is likely a consequence of the pressure to produce differentiated progeny in a transplant setting, suggesting that rapidly dividing HSC have an advantage in competitive repopulation, but with reduced clonal longevity.

It is generally accepted that most stem cells are quiescent and only a few stem cells supply all the blood cells at a given time. Stem cell factor is a cytokine capable of promoting stem cell proliferation. Its receptor is c-kit (see Table 305-3). Separation of stem cells by elutriation was combined with separation into c-kit^{pos} and c-kit^{neg} fractions. While both cell types had LTRC, only the c-kit^{pos} cells proliferated in response to multiple cytokines in vitro, formed day 12 CFU-S in vivo, and could protect mice from radiation-induced death when transplanted in vivo. While c-kit^{neg} cells do not have primary day 12 CFU-S activity, transplantation of BMC from the primary recipient mice into secondary recipients gives rise to CFU-S. Thus, deeply quiescent c-kit^{neg} cells are pluripotent stem cells that can give rise to cells with CFU-S activity but require growth and differentiation in vivo, further subdividing the stem cell compartment (Fig. 105-1).

THE HEMATOPOIETIC MICROENVIRONMENT Bone marrow has an organized and structured architecture in which close relationships exist between a regulatory microenvironment and primitive hematopoietic cells. The more rapidly proliferating CFU-S are near the bone surface, while the more primitive, slowly cycling CFU-S are near the central axis. Thus, it is reasonable to conclude that specific positional effects exist and they are maintained and regulated by products of the microenvironment. Components of the microenvironment include adipocytes, fibroblastoid cells, and reticular-endothelioid cells as well as macrophages and T lymphocytes (Fig. 105-2). The role or even the presence of each cell type in the microenvironment in vivo is not clear.

The main evidence that stem cells bind to the stroma comes from in vitro long-term bone marrow cultures where data show that maturing precursors and terminally differentiated cells are present as nonadherent cells, while stem cells and primitive precursors bind tightly to the stroma. Similarly, aggregates of stroma and hematopoietic cells isolated from freshly explanted marrow are enriched in primitive hematopoietic cells. The differential expression of cell adhesion molecules plays a major role in cell-cell contact between hematopoietic cells and stroma. Antibodies to murine CD44 abrogate lympho- and myelopoiesis in long-term bone marrow cultures without any apparent effect on stroma formation. Similarly, antibodies to either vascular cell adhesion molecule 1 expressed on stromal cells or its ligand VLA-4 expressed on stem cells interfere with cell-cell interaction and cause the release of stem cells from stroma. Other adhesive interactions are mediated by cytokine receptors that specifically bind membrane-associated cytokines, such as stem cell factor, or extracellular matrix–bound ligands [proteoglycans can bind

granulocyte-macrophage (GM) colony stimulating factor (CSF); fibronectin can bind transforming growth factor β (TGFβ)]. Components of extracellular matrix include numerous types of collagen, laminin, fibronectin, hemonectin, and many proteoglycans. Extracellular matrix proteins can also serve as adhesion molecules. The multitude of these adhesive interactions suggests that they are physiologically important in the regulation of hematopoiesis. The processes by which stem cells remain quiescent, self-renew, or commit to lineage-specific differentiation are not well understood. It is likely that both intrinsic and extrinsic events contribute to these processes.

CYTOKINE REGULATION OF HEMATOPOIETIC PROGENITOR CELLS Progenitor cell production is regulated by combinations of cytokines. Dormant stem cells that have differentiated into a state capable of cycling can be purified by flow cytometry based on cell surface phenotype, blast morphology, and metabolic markers. While these cells show no proliferation to single cytokines, their maximal growth is promoted by combinations of factors that include, for example, one member of each of the following groups: (1) either stem cell factor or flt3 ligand; (2) interleukin (IL) 6, IL-11, IL-12, thrombopoietin (Tpo), or granulocyte (G) colony stimulating factor (G-CSF); and (3) IL-3, IL-4, or GM-CSF. These synergistic effects are direct (being observed in single cell assays). Synergy can be due to induction of cycling in resting cells and/or enhanced proliferative rate. The most primitive cells have the highest proliferative potential, eventually giving rise to multipotential colony forming cells; these give rise to mixed-lineage differentiated progeny but have little capacity for self-replicative divisions. Synergistic effects on progenitor cell colony formation were found to be consistently preceded by increased CSF receptor expression on enriched progenitor cells, which was not detectable on unfractionated marrow. The maximum upregulation of CSF receptor expression was observed by 24 h and occurred in a dose- and time-dependent manner.

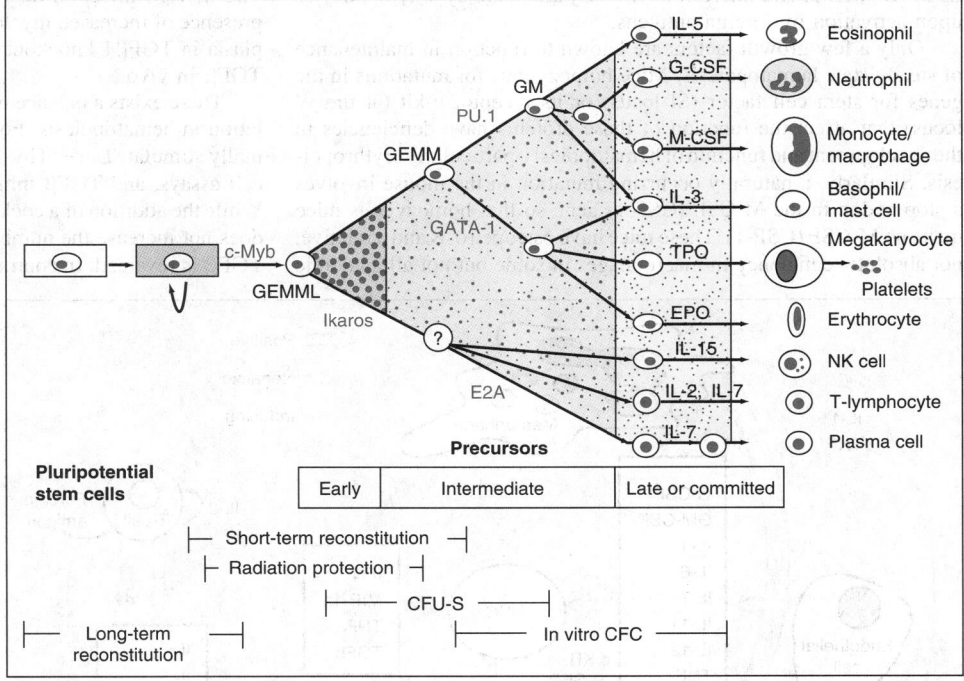

FIGURE 105-1 Cellular basis of hematopoiesis. Mature cells are derived from a common multipotent progenitor. Lineage development appears to occur as a consequence of the ordered expression of transcription factors (in blue). Thus, mice in which PU.1 expression has been blocked develop normal erythrocytes and megakaryocytes, but no other cell lineages. Once lineage commitment occurs, cytokines and colony-stimulating factors (in black) regulate development, again through the induction of transcription factors. Abbreviations: HSC, hematopoietic stem cell; GEMML, cell giving rise to granulocyte, erythroid, monocyte, megakaryocyte, and lymphoid cells; GEMM, cell giving rise to granulocytic, erythroid, monocyte, and megakaryocytic cells; GM, cell giving rise to granulocytic and monocyte cells.

MATURING CELLS—LATE-ACTING LINEAGE-SPECIFIC FACTORS The final proliferation cycles of the differentiated cells as they mature to become fully functional blood cells are stimulated by a number of factors that act in a lineage-specific manner (Fig. 105-1). For example, erythropoietin (Epo) and Tpo are the physiologic regulators for erythrocyte and megakaryocyte differentiation, respectively; however, both can also act on bipotent progenitors capable of differentiating into either lineage. IL-3, IL-5, and G-CSF drive basophilic, eosinophilic, and neutrophilic leukocyte maturation, respectively. IL-3 and G-CSF can also act on earlier cells. These mature cells exit the marrow environment via the central venous sinus and enter the peripheral circulation. The cells perform many functions (see Chap. 305). Also, many cell types are responsive to a variety of stress situations during which they perform their specialized functions.

PHYSIOLOGIC SOURCES OF HEMATOPOIETIC GROWTH FACTORS

Hematopoietic growth factors orchestrate the body's response to infection and other stresses (Fig. 105-2). In response to bacteria, several cytokines such as macrophage (M) colony stimulating factor (M-CSF or CSF-1), GM-CSF, and G-CSF are produced and secreted into the circulation. Furthermore, the inflammatory cytokines, IL-1, IL-6, and tumor necrosis factor α (TNFα) are released from a broad range of cells in the stroma (Fig. 105-2). Not only do they have direct effects on hematopoietic progenitors but they also initiate a cascade of cytokine production that stimulates the production of other cytokines. In addition, neuroendocrine hormones such as growth hormone and prolactin have growth-promoting activities on hematopoiesis that allow for improved myeloid recovery after BMT. The mechanism is partially direct and partially indirect through the stimulation of other growth factors like insulin-like growth factor-1. Another group of cytokines [IL-2, IL-3, IL-4, IL-5, and interferon (IFN) α] are made by T lymphocytes upon activation by foreign antigens.

Only a few growth factors are known to function in maintenance of steady state hematopoiesis. Mice homozygous for mutations in the genes for stem cell factor (Sl locus) or its receptor c-kit (at the W locus) that affect the function of these proteins have deficiencies in the development and function of hematopoiesis, particularly erythropoiesis. Similarly, a naturally occurring mutation in the mouse involves a stop codon in the M-CSF (CSF-1) gene so that homozygous mice make no M-CSF (CSF-1). These mice have osteopetrosis and a relative, not absolute, deficiency in macrophages in some but not all anatomic

sites. In addition, mice with either flt3 or IL-7 genes disrupted (so-called gene knockout mice) show deficiencies in development of lymphocyte lineages.

The steady-state regulation of erythropoietin is essential to the regulation of erythropoiesis. The primary site of Epo production after birth is the kidney, likely in peritubular interstitial cells located in the inner cortex and outer medulla. In response to sensing a lower oxygen pressure (hypoxia), Epo gene transcription increases, regulated by hypoxia responsive regions in 5' and 3' enhancers of the Epo gene. It is not known how cells detect changes in P_{O_2}. Evidence has been presented that a heme-carrying protein, cytochrome b_{559} in carotid bodies, might regulate superoxide ions that mediate sensing P_{O_2} changes. In hematopoietic tissues, elevated Epo results in increased erythroid cell production. This results in an increase in the oxygen-carrying capacity of the blood, thereby alleviating the hypoxic stimulus and providing a negative feedback loop shutting off Epo production. In patients with normal renal function, serum erythropoietin levels are inversely proportional to the hemoglobin concentration.

HEMATOPOIETIC CELL GROWTH INHIBITORS The growth and differentiation of hematopoietic cells have been shown to be negatively regulated both in vitro and in vivo by IFNα, -β and -γ, TNFα, macrophage inflammatory protein 1α, and several other chemokines as well as other agents such as prostaglandins, lactoferrin, and the heavy subunits of ferritin (H ferritin). It has been proposed that constitutive hematopoiesis is regulated, in part, by the balance of both positive and negative growth signals. The TGFβ family of proteins has potent hematopoietic regulatory properties, ranging from inhibitory effects on the growth of primitive stem cells to the differentiated functions of mature cells. TGFβ can have both inhibitory and stimulatory actions on these systems, depending on the differentiation state of the target cell and the other cytokines interacting with the cell. TGFβ has direct effects on cell surface expression of many cytokine receptors, suggesting that it is part of the mechanism of action of TGFβ. The major biologic effect of TGFβ on hematopoietic cell growth is the reversible inhibition of entry into the cell cycle. The in vivo injection of TGFβ mimics the in vitro effects, and the presence of increased myeloid cells and in some cases myeloid hyperplasia in TGFβ1 knockout mice supports the antiproliferative role of TGFβ in vivo.

There exists a balance between positive and negative growth regulation in hematopoiesis. For example, IL-3 and stem cell factor optimally stimulate Lin − Thy-1 + murine progenitor cell growth in single cell assays, and TGFβ inhibits more than 90 percent of this growth. While the addition of a cocktail of five additional stimulatory cytokines does not increase the number of responding progenitors, the effect of TGFβ is reversed. In contrast, TNFα and IFNγ cooperate with TGFβ to reverse the growth-promoting effects of these multiple growth factors. Thus, the overall biologic effect is determined by the contrasting effects and relative abundance of various cytokines.

GENERALITIES ABOUT CYTOKINE REGULATION Every cytokine (including hematopoietic growth factors and interleukins) has multiple biologic effects. Different cytokines may exert the same biologic effects, producing a system with redundancies. Cytokines are capable of both direct and indirect stimulatory (or inhibitory) effects. Cytokine action is often amplified by other factors. Cytokines that act on early lineage progenitors often act also on more mature lineage cells, though their effects may be different on cells at different stages of maturation. Cytokines work best in combinations. Cytokines and cytokine receptors each share certain structural features and signal

FIGURE 105-2 The cellular and humoral influences on hematopoietic stem/progenitor cells.

transduction pathways. In some instances cytokines share receptor components. Genetic alterations in cytokine or cytokine receptor genes can lead to dysregulation of hematopoiesis.

CHAPTER 105
Hematopoiesis

637

CLINICAL IMPLICATIONS OF STEM CELL BIOLOGY

CLONAL ORIGIN OF HEMATOPOIETIC MALIGNAN-CIES Hematologic malignancies arise as a clonal proliferation of one of the progenitor cells depicted in Fig. 105-1. The clinical manifestations of a particular malignancy depend on the stage of differentiation and lineage of the affected cell as well as on the specific nature of the initial mutation and of subsequent mutations that may appear during clonal evolution. In order for the abnormal clone of cells to attain sufficient tumor mass to produce clinical symptoms and signs, it must possess either a growth advantage or a block in apoptosis and/or differentiation over the normal cells. In lymphocyte proliferation, a block in fas-mediated apoptosis has been shown to be a causative mechanism.

Molecular techniques can be used to establish the clonal origin of known and suspected tumor cells. A monoclonal proliferation of cells can be distinguished from a polyclonal proliferation by morphologic examination of chromosomes, which may show clonal karyotypic abnormalities. Alternatively, analysis of DNA by Southern blot polymerase chain reaction can be used to identify (1) clonal immunoglobulin gene rearrangements in suspected B cell malignancies, (2) clonal T cell receptor gene rearrangements in T cells, and (3) diagnostic gene translocations such as the bcr-abl translocation seen in chronic myelogenous leukemia (Chap. 112). In females with the appropriate polymorphic loci on the X chromosome, clonality can be established by glucose-6-phosphate dehydrogenase isoenzyme patterns or analysis of DNA restriction fragments. This information is useful for several purposes: establishing a definitive diagnosis, providing insights into the cell of origin and steps in tumor progression, and providing a sensitive tool for assessing remission or relapse.

Clonal analysis of mature blood cells indicates that the many myeloproliferative and/or myelodysplastic disorders generally arise in the pluripotent stem cell.

BONE MARROW TRANSPLANTATION The ability of HSC to protect animals from death due to radiation-induced marrow failure has directly led to the use of high doses of both radiation and chemotherapy with BMT for the treatment of malignant disease (see Chap. 116). BMT has become the treatment of choice for several hematologic malignancies and is in use as a means of delivering dose-intensive therapy to patients with a variety of solid tumors, particularly those with poor prognosis.

In patients undergoing autologous BMT, the infused bone marrow may contain residual tumor cells. By using labeled cells, it has been demonstrated that these reinfused tumor cells are in some cases responsible for the subsequent disease relapse. The use of purified stem cell preparations in this setting of autologous BMT has the potential to reduce the rate of relapse secondary to the presence of tumor cells in the marrow.

In patients undergoing allogeneic BMT, the infusion of alloreactive donor cells is associated with two clinically important immunologic phenomena: (1) graft-versus-host disease (GVHD), caused by an immune response of donor T cells against host tissues (a major cause of both morbidity and mortality), and (2) the graft-versus-tumor (GVT) effect caused by the presence of either donor T cells or natural killer cells and responsible for the reduced risk of relapse of patients with leukemia and lymphoma.

Depleting the marrow of T cells to reduce the severity of GVHD in patients receiving an allograft has also increased the number of graft failures and reduced the GVT effects. Presumably the T cells play a role in producing important CSFs needed for marrow engraftment, or perhaps they inhibit the production of growth inhibitory cytokines that act to prevent engraftment. The use of positively selected purified stem cell populations devoid of alloreactive T cells may circumvent the development of GVHD. The addition back to the graft of T cell subsets that mediate the GVT effect (but not GVHD) could decrease the incidence of tumor recurrence and graft rejection. Addition of T cells cytotoxic to Epstein-Barr virus–infected cells to BMT has proven beneficial in reducing the development of Epstein-Barr virus–mediated lymphoma. The efficacy of this approach might be enhanced by vaccinating the marrow donor against the recipient's tumor in a specific fashion.

The treatment of patients with either chemotherapy or hematopoietic growth factors produces a dramatic mobilization of stem cell activity into the peripheral blood. Apheresis of peripheral blood mononuclear cells following growth factor mobilization yields cell preparations that provide engraftment as (or more) rapidly as (than) conventional BMT. The use of peripheral blood stem cells offers several potential advantages over bone marrow. Collection of these cells involves less invasive procedures than bone marrow harvest. Patients who are not candidates for a bone marrow harvest can now be transplanted with autologous peripheral blood–derived stem cells. In a variety of diseases, such as breast cancer and certain subtypes of lymphoma, significant contamination of the bone marrow by tumor cells may be avoided by using peripheral blood stem cells.

GENE THERAPY A variety of germ line mutations result in the development of a wide spectrum of hematologic diseases. A single nucleotide base substitution gives rise to hemoglobin S and produces sickle cell anemia (see Chap. 107). Similarly, the inheritance of impaired cellular and humoral immunity in many instances is attributable to mutations in a single gene, as in the case of adenosine deaminase deficiency.

Tissue-specific patterns of gene expression in these inherited hematologic diseases provide a clinical setting in which the transfer of genes into somatic cells could correct the underlying defect. The introduction of genes encoding enzymes critical for cellular immune function, such as adenosine deaminase, into HSCs should permit the development of functional T and B lymphocytes. However, at present several problems, including unsustained low levels of tissue-specific gene expression, prevent the broader application of this technology to inherited hematologic diseases.

THERAPEUTIC USE OF HEMATOPOIETIC GROWTH FACTORS—ERYTHROPOIETIN AND THROMBOPOIETIN Although it has been clearly shown that recombinant human Epo can increase the RBC mass in various patient groups as well as in normal individuals, the utility of recombinant human Epo depends on showing that it can be used to decrease the need for homologous RBC transfusions and/or to improve the quality of life. The two general areas in which recombinant Epo can be most effective are (1) in treatment of anemias due, at least in part, to an inadequate production of endogenous Epo (e.g., renal failure); and (2) stimulation of physiologic erythropoiesis to supranormal levels in the perioperative setting. In clinical trials in cancer patients, 32 to 85 percent of patients respond with a significant increase in hematocrit after 2 months of therapy. Epo is well tolerated, producing symptoms of hypertension or venous thrombosis only if given to patients with an elevated RBC mass. The starting dose is generally 50 units per kilogram of body weight subcutaneously three times weekly. Patients whose serum ferritin level is less than 400 µg/L (400 ng/mL) or whose serum Epo level is 100 units per liter or higher at the start of therapy are much less likely to respond. If the hemoglobin has not increased by at least 5 g/L (0.5 g/dL) after 2 weeks of therapy, the iron status should be checked. If the patient is not iron-deficient, Epo is unlikely to lead to improvement.

Tpo increased megakaryopoiesis and platelet production manyfold in both normal and myelosuppressed monkeys. Also red cell recovery was markedly enhanced in Tpo treated animals. Tpo is just entering clinical trials.

G-CSF AND GM-CSF The myeloid growth factors G-CSF and GM-CSF have been shown to stimulate neutrophil production in various clinical settings, but they are not universally effective. In cancer patients undergoing intensive cytotoxic chemotherapy, G-CSF stimulation of granulopoiesis translated into decreased incidence of neutro-

Table 105-1

Indications for the Clinical Use of G-CSF or GM-CSF

PREVENTIVE USES

With the first cycle of chemotherapy (so-called primary CSF administration)
    Not needed on a routine basis
    Use if the probability of febrile neutropenia is 40% or greater
    Use if patient has preexisting neutropenia or active infection
With subsequent cycles if febrile neutropenia has previously occurred (so-called secondary CSF administration)
    Not needed after short duration neutropenia without fever
    Use if patient had febrile neutropenia in previous cycle
    Use if prolonged neutropenia (even without fever) delays therapy

THERAPEUTIC USES

Afebrile neutropenic patients
    No evidence of benefit
Febrile neutropenic patients
    No evidence of benefit
    May feel compelled to use in the face of clinical deterioration from sepsis, pneumonia, or fungal infection, but benefit unclear
To augment dose-intensity of chemotherapy in patients with curable malignancies
    No evidence of benefit to date
In bone marrow or peripheral blood stem cell transplantation
    Use to mobilize stem cells from marrow
    Use to hasten myeloid recovery
In acute myeloid leukemia
    No evidence of benefit and may be harmful
In myelodysplastic syndromes
    Not routinely beneficial
    Use intermittently in subset with neutropenia and recurrent infection

WHAT DOSE AND SCHEDULE SHOULD BE USED?

G-CSF: 5 µg/kg per day subcutaneously
GM-CSF: 250 µg/m² per day subcutaneously

WHEN SHOULD CSF THERAPY START AND END?

    When indicated, start 24–72 h after chemotherapy
    Continue until absolute neutrophil count is 10,000/µL
    Do not use concomitantly with chemotherapy or radiation therapy

penia-associated fever and infection in patients with a high likelihood of developing granulocytopenia (Table 105-1). G-CSF has also been studied in patients with AIDS, congenital and cyclic neutropenia, myelodysplastic syndromes, and aplastic anemia; it increases the neutrophil count in many patients with these disorders. In neutropenic patients, G-CSF often increases the neutrophil count enough to decrease the frequency and severity of infection. G-CSF has been generally well tolerated, with no apparent dose-limiting toxicity. GM-CSF has been used in settings similar to those in which G-CSF was used. Although GM-CSF has proliferative effects on a broader range of hematopoietic progenitors in vitro, its primary clinical benefit in vivo has been on granulopoiesis. GM-CSF increases myeloid recovery following autologous BMT for lymphoid neoplasias and in patients who have undergone allogeneic or autologous BMT in whom engraftment has failed or is delayed. GM-CSF is more toxic than G-CSF, with bone pain, rash, fevers, fatigue, anorexia, phlebitis, thrombosis, and, at high doses, capillary leak syndrome with pleural and pericardial effusions and edema observed.

G-CSF-mobilized stem/progenitor cells collected by leukapheresis can be reinfused along with growth factors following intensive chemotherapy. In this setting, recovery of all blood lineages can be accelerated to 8 to 9 days rather than the 14 to 17 days seen with autologous marrow. These biologic effects will allow peripheral blood stem cell transplantation to be used more widely and safely.

IL-3, IL-6, IL-1 AND Pixy-321 IL-3 has been tested clinically in the hope that its effects on earlier progenitors might lead to beneficial effects on platelets as well as granulocytes. Clinical results have been disappointing. IL-3 has no significant effects on platelet recovery and

is not more effective than G-CSF in its effects on granulocytes, but it is toxic. IL-6 was also predicted to exert significant effects on platelets. However, its diverse biologic effects produce toxicity at doses that appear to have no effect on platelets.

IL-1 has been shown to have significant effects on both granulocyte and platelet recovery after cytotoxic chemotherapy. However, when it is given intravenously, it may produce hypotension and atrial arrhythmias at the biologically active doses. By contrast, subcutaneous administration preserves the beneficial effects on platelets and granulocytes and prevents the adverse side effects.

Pixy-321 is not a molecule found in nature. It is a chimeric fusion protein made in the laboratory and composed of active components of both IL-3 and GM-CSF. Although it appears to exert synergistic biologic effects on some cell types in vitro, clinical trials demonstrated only minor effects on granulocytes. In addition, its beneficial effects were restricted to the first cycle of administration because it elicits a potent neutralizing antibody response.

The future of hematopoietic growth factor therapy is difficult to predict. There is reason to hope that combinations of factors would be more effective than single agents. However, the tight physiologic regulation of hematopoiesis by both positive and negative growth regulators may make it difficult to achieve substantial beneficial effects. Hyperstimulation may simply lead to an amplification of inhibitory circuits. Some combination of stimulation plus inhibition of inhibitory pathways may be more successful. Even if such manipulations are successful, it is possible that the increase in proliferative demand on the stem cell population induced by repeated cycles of stem cell recruitment and chemotherapy could result in stem cell depletion and marrow aplasia or myelodysplasia.

BIBLIOGRAPHY

AMERICAN SOCIETY OF CLINICAL ONCOLOGY: Guidelines for the use of colony-stimulating factors. J Clin Oncol 12:2471, 1994

APPELBAUM FR: Allogeneic bone marrow transplantation and the use of hematopoietic growth factors. Stem Cells (Dayt) 13:344, 1995

BECKER AJ et al: Cytological demonstration of the clonal nature of spleen colonies derived from transplanted mouse marrow cells. Nature 197:452, 1963

CHEN S-J et al: Acute promyelocytic leukemia: From clinic to molecular biology. Stem Cells (Dayt)13:22, 1995

CROSS AR et al: Involvement of NAD(P)H oxidase as a P_{O_2} sensor protein in the rat carotid body. Biochem J 272:743, 1990

ESCHBACH JW et al: Treatment of the anemia of progressive renal failure with recombinant human erythropoietin. N Engl J Med 321:158, 1989

FARESE AM et al: Recombinant human megakaryocytic growth and differentiation factor stimulates thrombocytopoiesis in normal nonhuman primates. Blood 86:54, 1995

JACOBSEN SEW et al: Growth response of hematopoietic progenitors to cytokines is determined by the balance between the synergy of multiple stimulators and negative cooperation of multiple inhibitors. Exp Hematol 22:985, 1994

JONES RJ et al: Separation of pluripotent hematopoietic stem cells from spleen-colony forming cells. Nature 347:188, 1990

SPANGRUDE GJ et al: Purification and characterization of mouse hematopoietic stem cells. Science 241:58, 1988

106 *Robert S. Hillman*

IRON DEFICIENCY AND OTHER HYPOPROLIFERATIVE ANEMIAS

Normal erythropoiesis, including the expected proliferative response of the erythroid marrow to anemia, involves both the appropriate erythropoietin stimulation of a healthy erythroid marrow and an adequate supply of iron. A defect in one of these components results in a hypoproliferative or iron-deficiency anemia. This is a common and important mechanism of disease in clinical medicine. Hypoproliferative anemias are seen frequently in patients with renal insufficiency, marrow damage, iron deficiency, and acute and chronic inflammatory states. Furthermore, the pattern of the anemia can be of considerable value in diagnosis and management. Changes in red blood cell morphology and measurements of iron supply help in the differential diagnosis of the etiology of a hypoproliferative state. Effective management of patients with hypoproliferative anemias with hematinics and recombinant erythropoietin depends on a careful analysis of the defects involved.

CONTROL OF NORMAL ERYTHROPOIESIS

The pathophysiology of a hypoproliferative or iron-deficiency anemia is essentially a disruption of the control of normal erythropoiesis. The proliferative response of the erythron is a function of anemia severity and iron supply. Peritubular interstitial cells of the kidney produce erythropoietin in response to lower oxygen delivery. As the hemoglobin level falls below 100 g/L (10 g/dL), erythropoietin levels increase logarithmically, stimulating the erythroid marrow to proliferate and increase red blood cell production severalfold. The level of response can generally be predicted for the clinical situation. Blood-loss anemia in a patient with a healthy marrow and normal iron stores will usually generate a 2- to 3-fold increase in red cell production within 7 to 10 days. Higher levels of production are observed in patients with hemolytic anemias as the erythroid marrow expands within the marrow cavity. In fact, production levels in excess of five to six times normal can be observed in patients with congenital hemolytic anemias and inherited defects in hemoglobin synthesis.

Iron supply plays a key role in this production response. The bulk of the iron required for basal erythropoiesis is recycled from senescent red cells by the reticuloendothelial system (Fig. 106-1). This iron is transported through the plasma by transferrin, a plasma glycoprotein that binds two atoms of iron. The majority of iron-laden transferrin molecules are destined to bind to specific receptors on the surface of erythroid precursors and are subsequently internalized. The iron is then released, and the transferrin-receptor complex returns to the cell surface where transferrin molecules are released back to the circulation to complete the transport cycle. The erythroid precursor uses the delivered iron for the synthesis of hemoglobin, storing any excess as ferritin. A smaller amount of iron is taken up by other cells in the body, especially the liver parenchymal cells, for incorporation into heme enzymes and for ferritin storage.

FIGURE 106-1 Normal iron transport pathways. Iron recovered from senescent red cells and absorbed from food is bound to transferrin and transported to the erythroid marrow and other tissues. Iron-laden transferrin binds to transferrin receptors on the surface of erythroid precursors and is internalized. Once the iron is harvested for hemoglobin production, the transferrin–transferrin receptor complex returns to the cell surface, and the transferrin is released to complete the cycle. Males lose about 1 mg/d of iron and have iron stores in ferritin of about 1000 mg. Females may lose up to 2 mg/d of iron (particularly in menstruation) and have iron stores of 100 to 400 mg. (From Hillman and Ault, with permission.)

The amount of iron delivered to and accepted by the marrow is determined by several factors, including the level of iron stores, the amount of iron bound to transferrin, the blood flow to the marrow, the number of erythroid marrow precursors, and the expression of unoccupied transferrin receptor sites. The number of precursors and the expression of transferrin receptors on the cell surface are directly influenced by the level of erythropoietin stimulation. On the delivery side, the amount of iron available for transport is a function of available sources of iron supply, including the amount of reticuloendothelial iron stores, the level of food iron intake, and the rate of red blood cell turnover. To achieve a maximum proliferative response, iron supply and erythropoietin stimulation must be balanced. If iron delivery is suboptimal, the proliferative response of the marrow to erythropoietin is inhibited and normal hemoglobin synthesis is disrupted. The result is a hypoproliferative marrow response and, in situations of severe iron-supply deficiency, a microcytic, hypochromic anemia.

IRON-DEFICIENCY ANEMIA

While iron-deficiency anemia has traditionally been defined as a microcytic, hypochromic anemia secondary to a total-body iron deficit, a more sensitive definition of iron deficiency has to include the concepts of negative iron balance and iron-deficient erythropoiesis. By definition, iron-store depletion refers to an imbalance between normal physiologic demands such as body growth, menstrual blood loss, and pregnancy and the level of dietary iron intake. Iron-deficient erythropoiesis goes a step further and indicates a limitation in red blood cell production. Iron-deficiency anemia with microcytic, hypochromic red blood cell morphology indicates a prolonged period of negative iron balance and anemia severe enough to stimulate the production of poorly hemoglobinized cells. The incidence of each of these clinical states in any population depends on several variables, including the amount and character of dietary iron supply, the efficiency of iron absorption, and the incidence of disease states that result in iron loss.

NUTRITIONAL IRON BALANCE The amount of iron absorbed from the diet is a function of the kinds of foods eaten, the daily caloric intake, and the absorptive capacity of the small intestine. A key element is the heme iron content of the diet. Inorganic iron is toxic and not readily absorbed. Heme iron is much more available for absorption than inorganic forms of iron. Meat-eating individuals ingest more heme-containing myoglobin than do vegetarians. Populations existing on diets made up of primarily vegetables and grains are at a further disadvantage in maintaining iron homeostasis, because these foods contain certain compounds, such as phosphates and phytates, that inhibit iron absorption. In contrast, the ascorbic acid present in citrus fruits can promote iron absorption.

An adult male on a balanced diet containing both meat and vegetable products will ingest approximately 15 to 20 mg of iron each day, while the adult female will ingest 10 to 15 mg/d. In the male, only 1 to 2 mg needs to be absorbed to replace the iron lost from desquamation of skin and mucosal cells. The adult premenopausal female needs to absorb more from the diet to make up for menstrual blood loss. The same is true for the frequent blood donor. Infants, children, and adolescents may be unable to maintain normal iron balance because of the increased demands of body growth and much lower dietary intakes of iron. This is also true for the pregnant woman. During the last two trimesters of pregnancy, the daily iron requirement increases to 5 to 6 mg, a level that cannot be supported unless the diet is rich in heme iron or the woman receives an iron supplement. Some countries have taken to supplementing foods, such as bread, cereals, and bakery products, to help prevent negative iron balance in target populations. Multivitamins containing iron are recommended for patients at high risk, including adolescents, pregnant women, and regular blood donors.

Iron absorption by the proximal small intestine is a carefully regulated process that is tuned to the level of body iron stores and the demands of erythropoiesis. It becomes more efficient as body iron stores are depleted. Patients with certain types of anemias, especially those with high levels of ineffective erythropoiesis, have a tendency to absorb excess amounts of iron. In some cases, this can lead to iron overload and tissue iron damage. The normal individual, however, is capable of markedly reducing iron absorption in situations of excessive intake of either food or medicinal iron. This provides a considerable margin of safety when iron supplements are administered over a long period of time. Individuals at special risk of absorbing too much iron are those with idiopathic hemochromatosis, an inherited disorder where the normal regulation of iron absorption is defective (see Chap. 342).

Similar to the normal "range" of values for hemoglobin/hematocrit according to age and sex (Chap. 59), the distribution of body iron pools will depend on the patient's age, sex, and dietary content of iron (Table 106-1). The iron sequestered in red cells and in tissues as myoglobin or enzyme iron correlates with the patient's red blood cell mass and body size. The level of reticuloendothelial iron stores will reflect the balance between dietary intake and iron losses. An adult male will have from 600 to 1000 mg of reticuloendothelial iron stores, while women and adolescents generally have less than 300 mg of stores. Younger children, pregnant women, and women with very heavy menses will have little or no iron in their reticuloendothelial cells.

CLINICAL PRESENTATION There are situations where iron deficiency can be anticipated (Table 106-2). The delicate balance between iron intake and natural requirements means that any decreased intake or increased loss of iron may lead to deficiency. Significant chronic blood loss from any cause will deplete iron stores and exceed the capacity to absorb iron from the diet. Patients with severe malabsorption can also present with an iron-deficiency anemia regardless of the adequacy of their iron intake. The symptoms and signs of severe iron deficiency largely reflect the severity of the patient's anemia and include fatigue, pallor, and a decreased exercise capacity. When iron deficiency is severe and prolonged, the patient may complain of mouth soreness, difficulty swallowing, and a softening and curling of the nails called *spooning*. However, these findings are not very sensitive or specific; the diagnosis of an iron-deficiency state is basically a laboratory exercise.

LABORATORY IRON STUDIES The principal measurements of iron supply used in clinical diagnosis are the serum iron (SI), the transferrin iron-binding capacity (TIBC), and the serum ferritin level. Other useful studies include the inspection of the marrow aspirate or biopsy for reticuloendothelial iron stores and sideroblasts and red blood cell protoporphyrin and serum transferrin receptor levels. Measurements of plasma iron turnover and iron absorption are possible using tracer amounts of radioactive iron. From a research standpoint, such studies have been very important in defining the distribution of iron stores and the patterns of abnormal erythropoiesis. They do not play a significant role in clinical diagnosis.

Serum Iron Studies The SI is a measure of the amount of iron bound to transferrin, while the TIBC is a measure of the total binding capacity of transferrin. The normal SI falls between 9 and 27 μmol/L (50 and 150 μg/dL); the normal TIBC between 54 and 64 μmol/L (300 and 360 μg/dL). It is also routine to calculate the percent saturation of transferrin (SI ÷ TIBC = percent saturation). A normal

Table 106-1

Body Iron Distribution

	Iron Content, mg	
	Adult Male (80 kg)	**Adult Female (60 kg)**
Hemoglobin	2500	1700
Myoglobin/enzymes	500	300
Transferrin iron	3	3
Iron stores	600–1000	0–300

Table 106-2

Causes of Iron Depletion/Deficiency

Iron-Store Depletion	Iron-Deficient Erythropoiesis	Iron-Deficiency Anemia
Rapid growth	Blood loss	Blood loss
Infancy	Excessive menses or	GI hemorrhage
Adolescence	donation	Intravascular
Menstrual blood loss	Hemodialysis	hemolysis
Inadequate diet	GI hemorrhage	Surgical blood loss
Blood donation	Pregnancy	Hookworm
	Malabsorption	infestation
	Polycythemia vera treated	Severe malabsorption
	with phlebotomy	Gastrectomy
		Sprue
		Inflammatory bowel
		disease

NOTE: GI, gastrointestinal.

individual has a percent saturation of between 30 and 50 percent. Iron-deficiency states are associated with saturation levels below 20 percent, while clinically dangerous iron overload occurs if the saturation exceeds 50 to 60 percent (Fig. 106-2).

Serum Ferritin Level Iron is stored as ferritin or hemosiderin. The protein, apoferritin, binds to free ferrous ion and stores it as ferric ion. Iron plus apoferritin is ferritin. Apoferritin mRNA is present in the cell with a molecule of the protein bound to the message, which inhibits translation. Free iron leads to removal of the protein from the message, increased translation of apoferritin mRNA, and increased protein levels. When ferritin is taken up by cells in the reticuloendothelial system, it can be catabolized to hemosiderin. Iron in ferritin can be extracted for the synthesis of heme, whereas that in hemosiderin is less reliably available for metabolic needs. Ferritin found in the circulation is in equilibrium with tissue ferritins. The serum measurement correlates with the level of total-body iron stores. The normal value for a serum ferritin level will, therefore, vary according to the age and sex of the individual. The adult male has a serum ferritin level of 50 to 150 μg/L, while most adult women demonstrate levels between 15 and 50 μg/L. Once iron stores are depleted, the serum ferritin level declines to levels below 15 μg/L. This reduction correlates with a decrease in the intracellular synthesis of apoferritin protein because the free apoferritin binds again to its mRNA.

FIGURE 106-2 The patterns of serum iron (SI) and total iron-binding capacity [TIBC = unsaturated iron-binding capacity (UIBC) + SI] vary with different types of anemia. Normal individuals and patients with hemolytic anemias have SIs in the normal range of 50 to 150 μg/dL (9 to 27 μmol/L), and normal TIBCs. In contrast, iron-deficient patients have very low serum irons with TIBCs greater than 360 μg/dL (64 μmol/L). Inflammatory anemia patients have low SIs and low TIBCs. Finally, patients with ineffective erythropoiesis and iron overload have fully saturated iron-binding capacities. (From Hillman and Finch, with permission.)

Marrow Iron Stores Reticuloendothelial cell iron stores can be estimated from the Prussian blue stain of a marrow aspirate or a biopsy specimen. By convention, the stores are graded on a scale of 0 to 4+. While this is not quantitative, the visual grading of stores correlates fairly well with the ferritin and hemosiderin iron present in reticuloendothelial cells and available for erythropoiesis (Table 106-3). In situations of iron overload, the marrow iron stain is not as good as the serum ferritin level, which also reflects the level of iron sequestered in hepatocytes and other tissue cells. The marrow iron stain does provide information as to the delivery of iron to erythroid precursors. In a normal male, 50 to 60 percent of the more mature erythroid precursors will have a few visible ferritin iron granules in their cytoplasm. This represents excess iron not needed for hemoglobin formation. In disease states such as the sideroblastic anemias, the number and pattern of iron granules in marrow normoblasts is distinctly abnormal. In the case of ringed sideroblastic anemia, iron-encrusted mitochondria form a collar or ring of iron granules immediately around the nucleus (see Chap 110).

Red Cell Protoporphyrin Level Protoporphyrin is the molecule made in mitochondria to which iron is added to form heme (see Chap. 343). The level of red cell protoporphyrin is another sensitive indicator of iron-deficient erythropoiesis. Higher-than-normal levels indicate an inadequate iron supply to erythroid precursors to support the formation of heme. The assay can be performed on very small amounts of blood. Normal values fall below 0.53 μmol/L (30 μg/dL) of red blood cells, while iron-deficient individuals have values in excess of 1.77 μmol/L (100 μg/dL). Protoporphyrin levels also rise in children exposed to lead. This reflects the inhibition of heme synthetase, the enzyme required for the formation of heme (see Chap. 397).

Serum Transferrin Receptor Serum levels of serum transferrin receptor correlate with the level of erythroid precursor proliferation and the adequacy of iron supply to the marrow. Normal levels are 4 to 9 μg/L by immunoassay. Levels increase rapidly in patients with iron-deficient erythropoiesis and/or a proliferative marrow, including states of ineffective erythropoiesis. This test is not commonly employed.

STAGES OF IRON DEFICIENCY The several stages of iron deficiency, including iron-store depletion, iron-deficient erythropoiesis, and iron-deficiency anemia, can be distinguished using these measurements of iron supply (Fig. 106-3).

Iron-Store Depletion This is identified using the serum ferritin level and marrow iron stain. A ferritin level less than 20 μg/L and visible iron stores of only 0 to 1+ suggest usable iron stores of less than 100 to 300 mg. As long as some stores are still available, the SI, TIBC, and red cell protoporphyrin levels are within normal limits. Moreover, the patient is not anemic, and red blood cell morphology is normal.

Iron-Deficient Erythropoiesis This can be distinguished based on further changes in the serum ferritin level and marrow iron stain and abnormalities of the plasma iron, TIBC, and red cell protoporphyrin. By definition, marrow iron stores are no longer visible, and the serum ferritin level falls to levels below 15 μg/L. The SI also falls to levels below 11 μmol/L (60 μg/dL), while the TIBC increases, resulting in a percent saturation of less than 20 percent. The protoporphyrin level increases to greater than 1.77 μmol/L (100 μg/dL) of red blood cells. These abnormalities in iron supply are still not accompanied by a change in red blood cell morphology. There is, however,

Table 106-3

Iron Store Measurements

Iron Stores	Marrow Iron Stain, 0–4+	Serum Ferritin, μg/L
0	0	<15
1–300 mg	Trace to 1+	15–30
300–800 mg	2+	30–60
800–1000 mg	3+	60–150
1–2 g	4+	>150
Iron overload	—	>500–1000

	Normal	Iron-store depletion	Iron-deficient erythropoiesis	Iron-deficiency anemia
Iron stores				
Erythron iron				
Marrow iron stores	1–3+	0–1+	0	0
Serum ferritin (μg/L)	50–200	<20	<15	<15
TIBC (μg/dL)	300–360	>360	>380	>400
SI (μg/dL)	50–150	NL	<50	<30
Saturation (%)	30–50	NL	<30	<10
Marrow sideroblasts (%)	40–60	NL	<10	<10
RBC protoporphyrin (μg/dL)	30–50	NL	>100	>200
RBC morphology	NL	NL	NL	Microcytic/hypochromic

FIGURE 106-3 Laboratory studies in the evolution of iron deficiency. Measurements of marrow iron stores, serum ferritin, and TIBC are sensitive to early iron-store depletion. Iron-deficient erythropoiesis is recognized from additional abnormalities in the SI, percent saturation of transferrin, the pattern of marrow sideroblasts, and the red blood cell protoporphyrin level. Finally, patients with iron-deficiency anemia demonstrate all of these same abnormalities plus an anemia characterized by microcytic hypochromic morphology. (From Hillman and Finch, with permission.)

an impairment of the proliferative capacity of the marrow resulting in a mild normocytic, normochromic anemia, with hemoglobin levels of 100 to 120 g/L (10 to 12 g/dL).

Iron-Deficiency Anemia This is recognized from the combination of abnormal iron-supply studies and microcytic, hypochromic red blood cell morphology. The SI falls to very low levels [<4 μmol/L (<30 μg/dL)], while the TIBC increases, resulting in a percent saturation of less than 10 percent. The ferritin level is always less than 15 μg/L. Once the patient's hemoglobin level falls below 100 to 110 g/L (10 to 11 g/dL), poorly hemoglobinized cells begin to enter the circulation. When the anemia is only of moderate severity, the cells tend to be microcytic but not hypochromic. At lower hemoglobin levels, both microcytosis and hypochromia become more pronounced. Furthermore, red blood cell production becomes increasingly ineffective, resulting in greater degrees of aniso- and poikilocytosis. With very severe iron-deficiency anemia, cigar- or pencil-shaped red blood cells may be observed. As a rule, target cells are not seen with iron deficiency. When present, they suggest a globin chain production defect, one of the thalassemias. They may also be seen in the presence of liver disease.

Only a few diseases need to be considered in the differential diagnosis of an iron-deficiency anemia. Both α and β thalassemia are associated with microcytosis, hypochromia, and anemia of varying severity. The racial background and family history of the patient may be clues to the presence of thalassemia. However, this does not exclude the possibility of iron deficiency either alone or in combination with a globin production defect. Therefore, a full laboratory assessment is important (see Chap. 107). This should permit an accurate diagnosis of the cause of the microcytosis and hypochromia, whether a single or combined defect (Table 106-4). Morphologic clues that point to the diagnosis of thalassemia include the presence of target cells, a normal red cell distribution width indicating a uniform microcytosis, and microcytosis/hypochromia out of proportion to the severity of the anemia. In the latter case, thalassemia minor patients can demonstrate microcytosis (a mean corpuscular volume less than 75 to 80 fL) at hemoglobin levels above 130 to 140 g/L (13 to 14 g/dL). This is quite different from iron deficiency, where a moderate to severe anemia must be present before microcytosis appears. Any uncertainty about the diagnosis is usually resolved by measurements of iron supply and analysis of the hemoglobin pattern on electrophoresis. Unless iron deficiency is a complicating illness, patients with β thalassemia minor have normal to increased iron stores, SI, and TIBC and elevated hemoglobin A_2 levels. With iron deficiency, hemoglobin A_2 levels can be normal.

The more common diagnostic problem is the potential confusion between iron deficiency and an inflammatory block in iron delivery from the reticuloendothelial system to the erythroid progenitors (the anemia of chronic disease). Inflammatory cytokines, including tumor necrosis factor (TNF), interleukin (IL) 1, interferon (IFN) β, and IFNγ are capable of suppressing erythropoietin secretion, erythroid precursor proliferation, and the delivery of iron to the marrow. Both the SI and TIBC decline in patients with inflammatory anemias. The percent saturation of transferrin generally falls to levels between 10 and 20 percent. In patients who develop a moderately severe anemia, a hemoglobin level of 80 to 100 g/L (8 to 10 g/dL), this failure in iron delivery can produce a mild microcytic, hypochromic anemia, adding to the confusion about the diagnosis. A full study of the patient's iron supply should distinguish between the two conditions (Table 106-5). Inflammatory anemia patients typically show a low SI, low TIBC, a normal to high serum ferritin level, and, if a marrow aspiration is performed, normal to increased iron stores together with a hypoproliferative marrow morphology. The serum transferrin receptor assay can also distinguish between the two conditions. Transferrin receptor levels tend not to increase with inflammation as compared to a two- to four-fold increase seen with true iron deficiency.

Patients with a defect in mitochondrial function resulting in a sideroblastic anemia can also present with a microcytic, hypochromic anemia. Hereditary sideroblastic anemia is a rare condition that presents in childhood either as an X-linked or autosomally inherited condition. Red blood cell morphology is typically dimorphic, and measurements of iron supply make the distinction from iron deficiency quite easy (see Table 106-4). Patients who develop an acquired ringed sideroblastic anemia typically exhibit excessive iron accumulation, even to the point of tissue iron overload. Their red blood cell morphology can be quite variable, while marrow morphology demonstrates the pathognomonic finding of ringed sideroblasts. In children, lead poisoning can produce anemia with impaired hemoglobin formation and ringed sideroblasts. Lead poisoning makes the diagnosis of iron deficiency in children more difficult, because the inhibition of mitochondrial heme synthetase by lead results in very high red cell protoporphyrin levels. This must be kept in mind whenever the red cell protoporphyrin assay is used to screen for iron-deficient erythropoiesis.

℞ TREATMENT

The management of a patient with iron deficiency will be governed by the etiology of the deficiency state and the severity of the anemia (see Table 106-3). The ability of the patient to tolerate oral iron preparations will also be a factor. Higher dosages of oral iron result in significant gastrointestinal side effects. This can interfere with patient compliance and prevent a full and rapid recovery.

Situations of negative iron balance secondary to increased physiologic needs are readily corrected by dietary supplementation. Treatment of iron deficiency secondary to blood loss or malabsorption requires accurate diagnosis and effective control of the primary disease state. Continued blood loss can easily exceed the capacity of iron therapy to replenish iron supplies. In patients with gastrointestinal malabsorption, oral iron therapy will be ineffective. Response to iron therapy will also depend on the level of erythropoietin response and the health of the erythroid marrow. Patients with end-stage renal disease, a complicating inflammatory illness, or a damaged marrow will demonstrate a less than optimal response to treatment. In each of these situations, the clinician must decide between the judicious use of red blood cell transfusion and treatment with oral or parenteral iron therapy. Moreover, when the response to iron therapy is delayed or inadequate, a careful reevaluation of the patient is required to look for continued bleeding, the presence of an inflammatory disorder, or a defect in iron absorption.

Oral Iron Preparations Standard oral preparations of iron in tablet and elixir form are listed in Table 106-6. While the various preparations contain different amounts of ferrous iron, they are all readily absorbed and, therefore, quite effective in the treatment of iron-deficiency anemia. A number of other compoundings of iron are sold on the market. Some contain "absorption-enhancing" substances, such as amino acids and ascorbic acid. Others are advertised as delayed-release formulations aimed at prolonging iron absorption over several hours. All of these preparations tend to be more expensive. Moreover, attempts to enhance absorption can increase the incidence of gastrointestinal side effects.

To maximize the response to iron in an adult patient with a moderate to severe iron-deficiency anemia, a standard oral iron preparation such as ferrous sulfate should be given in tablet or elixir form, one tablet (325 mg) or 5 mL (300 mg) three to four times a day between meals. Patients who are achlorhydric or who have had gastric surgery should be treated with iron elixir, because the removal of the tablet coat depends on normal stomach acidity. A fourth dose of iron at bedtime will help maintain iron delivery to the marrow during late evening and night hours. Otherwise, the serum iron can decline to iron-deficient levels during the night, thereby dampening the marrow's proliferative response.

Three to four ferrous sulfate tablets should provide 200 to 250 mg of elemental iron per day, that is, 2 to 3 mg/kg in the average-sized adult. From this, the iron-deficient patient will absorb 40 to 60 mg of iron. This will support a red blood cell production level of up to three times normal in the patient with a normal erythroid marrow and a full erythropoietin response for the anemia. However, as the hemoglobin level rises, iron absorption declines and the rate of red blood cell production falls, regardless of the oral iron intake. Therefore, the dosage can be reduced as the hemoglobin rises to levels above 110 to 120 g/L (11 to 12 g/dL). This will help guarantee patient compliance for a therapy that must continue for several months. More than a quarter of individuals experience gastrointestinal distress, either abdominal pain, nausea, vomiting, constipation, or diarrhea, with the full treatment dose of three to four iron tablets per day. This will improve with smaller doses, although some patients have difficulty tolerating even one or two tablets a day. This can be a significant barrier in management, especially in reestablishing adequate iron stores. At least 6 months of iron supplementation is required in a normal adult to rebuild reticuloendothelial iron stores.

Usually the reticulocyte count increases 3 to 4 days after the initiation of therapy and reaches a peak at about 10 days. If a response does not occur, there are a number of possible explanations: patient noncompliance (common) or abnormal iron absorption (rare), persistent blood loss exceeding intake, and incorrect diagnosis or an additional diagnosis such as marrow damage or chronic inflammation. In any of the first three possibilities, it may be necessary (among other things) to increase iron delivery with a parenteral iron preparation.

Parenteral Iron Therapy Iron can be administered parenterally in patients who are unable to tolerate oral iron or who suffer from gastrointestinal malabsorption. Parenteral iron has also been used in the treatment of patients receiving recombinant erythropoietin to guarantee adequate iron delivery to support erythroid precursor proliferation. Iron for injection is formulated as ferric hydroxide–dextran compound and marketed as iron dextran injection, InFe D (Schein). Two preparations are available: one containing 0.5% phenol for intramuscular use and a second that is phenol-free for intramuscular or intravenous use. The phenol-containing compound should never be used for intravenous administration because it can produce phlebitis.

Small amounts of iron dextran can be administered by intramuscular injection, but care must be taken to prevent skin staining. The injection track should follow a Z pattern and no more than 2 mL (100 mg) of the iron dextran compound injected in each buttock site. For the treatment of an iron-deficiency anemia, the preferred method of administration is a bolus intravenous injection of the total dose required to correct the deficiency state. The amount of iron needed can be calculated as follows:

Body weight (kg) × 2.3 × (15 − patient's hemoglobin, g/dL) + 500 to 1000 mg (for stores) = Total dose (mg)

When administering intravenous iron dextran, care must be taken to anticipate and avoid an immediate anaphylactic-like reaction. If the patient gives a history of a past reaction to iron dextran, either an anaphylactic or a late serum sickness–like reaction with malaise, fever, arthralgias, skin rash, or lymphadenopathy, further exposure to iron dextran therapy should be avoided. When iron dextran is administered as a large intravenous bolus, it is best diluted in 100 to 250 mL of 0.9% sodium chloride solution and administered over 30 to 90 min. At the beginning of the infusion, a small test dose— less than 0.5 mL of the iron dextran solution—should be infused over 5 to 10 min while observing for any complaints of itching, shortness of breath, or chest or back pain. The blood pressure should be monitored during the test dose and throughout the period of administration. If the patient becomes hypotensive, the infusion should be stopped immediately. Dialysis patients on long-term erythropoietin therapy may require repeated injections of iron dextran to keep up with their iron needs. For this purpose, monthly intravenous injections of 100 to 200 mg of iron dextran will prevent iron deficiency and guarantee a steady supply of iron to the erythroid marrow.

OTHER HYPOPROLIFERATIVE ANEMIAS

Hypoproliferative anemias are common in patients with acute and chronic inflammatory disorders, end-stage renal disease, severe hypothyroidism, and other hormone deficiencies. In each case, the failure in the marrow proliferative response is primarily the result of a reduced erythropoietin response for the degree of anemia. With acute or chronic inflammatory disease, inhibition of iron delivery and erythroid precursor growth also contribute. However, the anemias of renal disease and chronic inflammation (the anemia of chronic disease) can usually be corrected with recombinant erythropoietin therapy if adequate iron stores are available. This reinforces the concept that the failure in erythropoietin stimulation is the most important factor.

INFLAMMATORY ANEMIAS The anemia associated with acute infections and chronic inflammatory diseases results from the release of inflammatory cytokines. TNF, IL-1, IFNβ, IFNγ, and neopterin all have suppressive effects on erythropoiesis. TNF and IFNβ are mediators in patients with bacterial infections and neoplasms, while IL-1 and IFNγ are involved in patients with chronic inflammatory states (the anemia of chronic disease). In both situations, these cytokines are capable of inhibiting the proliferative capacity of erythroid precursors, erythropoietin release by the kidney, and the delivery of iron from reticuloendothelial cells (Fig. 106-4). The impact is rapid and dramatic. With acute bacterial infections, a mild anemia [hemoglobin 100 to 120 g/L (10 to 12 g/dL)] can appear within 24 to 48 h. The initial drop

in hemoglobin is the result of a self-limited hemolytic event, where the oldest red blood cells in circulation are rapidly removed by the reticuloendothelial system. The persistence of the anemia over the next several days or weeks reflects the cytokine suppression of erythropoiesis.

With chronic inflammatory states, the nature of the primary disease will tend to determine the severity and pattern of the anemia. While a majority of patients demonstrate a normocytic, normochromic anemia, some will appear to have a more severe defect in iron supply and will develop a mild microcytosis and hypochromia. Patients with severe lupus erythematosus and rheumatoid arthritis can exhibit more severe hemolysis secondary to autoantibodies and a cytokine/T cell driven suppression of granulocytopoiesis (Felty syndrome).

Clinical and Laboratory Findings The inflammatory anemia associated with acute infection is generally of mild to moderate severity and, therefore, asymptomatic. However, this may not be true for older patients, in whom a modest anemia can provoke symptoms and signs of cardiovascular disease. It is usually first detected on the routine complete blood count as a normocytic, normochromic anemia [hemoglobin of 100 to 120 g/L (10 to 12 g/dL)], with a reticulocyte index of less than 2. The full erythropoietic profile that distinguishes this type of anemia from iron deficiency, renal disease, or a hypometabolic state is illustrated in Table 106-5. Iron-supply studies are the key to the diagnosis. They show an SI of less than 9 μmol/L (50 μg/dL) and a TIBC of less than 54 μmol/L (300 μg/dL), giving a percent saturation of 10 to 20%. This characteristic decline in both the SI and the TIBC is accompanied by an increase in the serum ferritin level. For adult males, the serum ferritin will increase to levels of between 150 and 350 μg/L, while females show a less impressive rise according to their basal serum ferritin level. This pattern is distinctly different from that seen with other hypoproliferative anemias. If a ferritin level is not available or there is confusion regarding the patient's iron status, a bone marrow examination can be used to document the presence of reticuloendothelial cell iron stores. A patient with an iron-deficiency anemia will have no visible stores, while inflammatory disease patients have normal to increased iron stores. Furthermore, with chronic inflammatory diseases, extra large hemosiderin granules form within the reticuloendothelial cells.

Direct measurements of inflammatory cytokines, serum erythropoietin, and levels of serum transferrin receptor, while feasible, are not

Table 106-4

Diagnosis of Microcytic Anemia

Tests	Iron Deficiency	Thalassemia	Sideroblastic Anemia
Smear	Micro/hypo	Micro/hypo with targeting	Variable
SI	Low	Normal to high	Normal to high
TIBC	High	Normal	Normal
Percent saturation	<10	30–80	30–80
Ferritin (μg/L)	<15	50–300	50–300
Hemoglobin pattern	Normal	Abnormal	Normal

Table 106-5

Diagnosis of Hypoproliferative Anemias

Tests	Iron Deficiency	Inflammation	Renal Disease	Hypometabolic States
Anemia	Mild to severe	Mild	Mild to severe	Mild
MCV (fL)	70–90	80–90	90	90
Morphology	Normo-microcytic	Normocytic	Normocytic	Normocytic
SI	<30	<50	Normal	Normal
TIBC	>360	<300	Normal	Normal
Saturation (%)	<10	10–20	Normal	Normal
Serum ferritin (μg/L)	<15	30–200	115–150	Normal
Iron stores	0	2–4 +	1–4 +	Normal

NOTE: MCV, mean corpuscular volume.

Table 106-6

Oral Iron Preparations

Generic Name	Tablet (Iron Content), mg	Elixir (Iron Content), mg in 5 mL
Ferrous sulfate	325 (65)	300 (60)
	195 (39)	90 (18)
Extended release	525 (105)	
Ferrous fumarate	325 (107)	
	195 (64)	100 (33)
Ferrous gluconate	325 (39)	300 (35)
Polysaccharide iron	150 (150)	100 (100)
	50 (50)	

necessary for the clinical diagnosis and differential diagnosis of an inflammatory anemia. One exception to this is the evaluation of anemia in patients with AIDS. With disease progression, AIDS patients develop a moderate to severe hypoproliferative anemia because of complicating infections and/or marrow damage secondary to involvement with human immunodeficiency virus or drug toxicity. Marrow damage may be suspected because of the appearance of a marked pancytopenia. However, a measurement of the serum erythropoietin level can help distinguish between marrow damage and an inflammatory anemia. The finding of a low serum erythropoietin level predicts a significant inflammatory component to the anemia. It is this type of patient who will respond to treatment with recombinant erythropoietin.

THE ANEMIA OF RENAL DISEASE Renal disease with progressive renal failure is almost always accompanied by a moderate to severe hypoproliferative anemia. In general, the severity of the anemia correlates with the severity of the renal failure. As the blood urea nitrogen (BUN) approaches 36 mmol/L (100 mg/dL) and creatinine is above 265 to 442 μmol/L (3 to 5 mg/dL), the hemoglobin will fall to levels below 70 g/L (7 g/dL). This reflects a combination of a significant reduction in circulating red blood cell life span secondary to the uremia and a failure of the erythropoietin response because of the kidney damage. There are certain situations of acute renal failure where the loss of renal function and the erythropoietin response do not correlate. For example, patients with hemolytic-uremic syndrome demonstrate a marked increase in red blood cell production in response to their hemolysis despite renal failure sufficient to require dialysis.

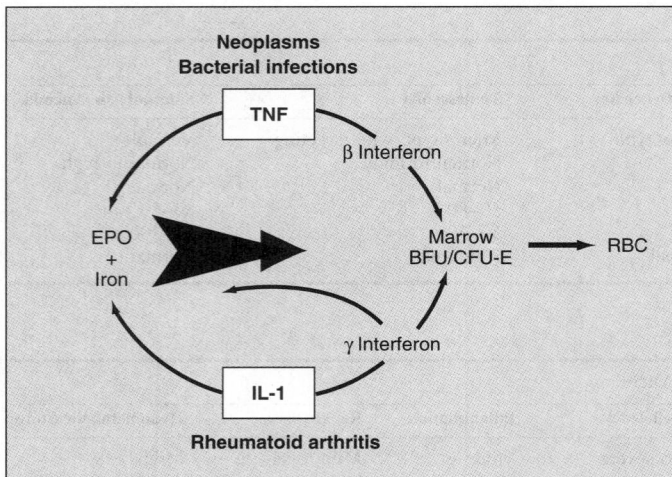

FIGURE 106-4 Suppression of erythropoiesis by inflammatory cytokines. Neoplasms and bacterial infections through the release of tumor necrosis factor (TNF) and interferon β suppress erythropoietin production, the release of iron from reticuloendothelial stores, and the proliferation of erythroid progenitors (BFU/CFU-E). The mediators in patients with vasculitis and rheumatoid arthritis include IL-1 and interferon γ. The blue arrows indicate sites of inflammatory cytokine inhibitory effects.

Polycystic renal disease is another situation where erythropoietin production can be preserved in the face of progressive renal failure. In contrast, patients with diabetes mellitus can demonstrate a more severe anemia than would be predicted from their BUN and creatinine, suggesting an early defect in erythropoietin production.

Clinical and Laboratory Findings Similar to other hypoproliferative anemias, the anemia of renal disease is typically a normocytic, normochromic anemia with a low reticulocyte production index. Moreover, there are no diagnostic clues provided by the red cell morphology. Exceptions to this rule include the appearance of burr cells (echinocytes) with liver disease and fragmented red cells in patients with vasculitic syndromes, especially hemolytic-uremic syndrome and thrombotic thrombocytopenic purpura (see Chap. 109).

Iron-supply studies provide the key to the diagnosis and successful management of the renal disease anemia patient. At presentation, the SI, TIBC, and serum ferritin levels should all be within the normal range, a pattern that is distinctly different from that seen with iron-deficiency or an inflammatory anemia (see Table 106-5). Subsequently, the pattern of iron studies will vary according to the clinical course. Patients maintained on chronic hemodialysis can become iron deficient secondary to procedural blood losses. Therefore, repeated iron studies are important in planning management, especially the use of recombinant erythropoietin to ameliorate the anemia. As with the other hypoproliferative states, a direct measurement of serum erythropoietin levels is not clinically useful. Measurable levels of serum erythropoietin are observed even in anephric patients. The underlying defect is not a total loss of erythropoietin production but a failure in the appropriate response for the degree of anemia.

HYPOMETABOLIC STATES A mild to moderate hypoproliferative anemia may be observed in patients who are hypometabolic secondary to protein starvation or hypothyroidism. The reduced erythropoietin response causing the anemia reflects a reduced oxygen requirement. It would appear that the sensor cells of the kidney are capable of assessing oxygen delivery according to their metabolic level.

Endocrine Deficiency States The measurable difference in hemoglobin levels between males and females is attributable to the effect of androgen and estrogen hormones on erythropoiesis. Testosterone and anabolic steroids enhance the erythropoietin stimulation of erythroid precursors, resulting in a mean hemoglobin level in adult males that is 10 to 30 g/L (1 to 3 g/dL) higher. Castration or estrogen administration will reduce the hemoglobin level in males by as much as 20 g/L (2 g/dL). Pituitary and thyroid function play an even more important role. Most patients who are clinically hypothyroid demonstrate a modest anemia, with a hemoglobin of 110 to 120 g/L (11 to 12 g/dL). Marked myxedema can be accompanied by a more severe anemia. In addition to the defect in erythropoietin stimulation, these patients can show abnormalities in iron and folic acid absorption as well as an overall reduction in dietary intake. This may result in a clinical presentation that is somewhat confusing, because one or another of the nutritional deficiencies may dominate. It is unlikely, however, that the anemia will resolve unless the hypometabolic state is corrected with appropriate thyroid replacement, reflecting the underlying impairment in erythropoietin response.

Addison's disease patients may present with a mild to moderate anemia, depending on the levels of impairment of thyroid function and androgen hormone production. When a patient presents in Addisonian crisis, shifts in plasma volume and total blood volume may obscure the anemia. In this situation, a rapid fall in the hemoglobin level will be observed as the patient receives cortisol and volume replacement. A mild hypoproliferative anemia has also been observed in patients with hyperparathyroidism. While the mechanism is not fully defined, it has been suggested that it is related either to an inhibition of erythroid progenitors or a defect in erythropoietin production secondary to renal calcification.

Protein Deprivation A very mild hypoproliferative anemia, with hemoglobin reduction of 10 to 30 g/L (1 to 3 g/dL), can result from protein deprivation. This has been suggested to play a role in elderly individuals on restricted diets. A more impressive reduction in red blood cell mass is observed with severe starvation. Marasmic individuals, who are both protein and calorie deprived, exhibit a reduced erythropoietin response that correlates with their reduced basal metabolism, although the severity of the red cell mass reduction may not be revealed until the patient is refed. With the recovery of albumin production and reconstitution of the plasma volume, the hemoglobin level will fall. The pattern of anemia in these patients is typically normocytic, normochromic with the low reticulocyte index of a hypoproliferative anemia. In situations of prolonged starvation, iron and vitamin deficiencies must also be considered. They may not be obvious from the pattern of anemia or the initial studies of iron supply. Therefore, the patient should be carefully monitored with repeated iron studies and measurements of folic acid and vitamin B_{12}.

Anemia in Liver Disease Patients with chronic liver disease from nearly any cause often develop a mild normocytic anemia. Patients with impaired lecithin cholesterol acyltransferase may accumulate excess cholesterol in the red blood cell membrane, leading to burr cells and stomatocytes. This may shorten red cell survival, but the marrow does not adequately compensate for the decreased life span of the cells. This form of anemia rarely requires treatment.

In alcoholic liver disease, this pathophysiology may be complicated by toxic effects of alcohol on bone marrow cells, nutritional folate deficiency, and iron deficiency related both to decreased dietary intake and increased blood loss.

℞ TREATMENT

The management of any hypoproliferative anemia must be tailored to the individual patient and the primary disease process. This makes accurate diagnosis very important. It also requires a careful evaluation of the mechanisms underlying the defect in erythropoiesis. A patient with an acute infection and a mild hypoproliferative anemia can be expected to recover spontaneously as the infection is treated. The same is true for a patient with chronic inflammatory anemia, unless the patient is elderly with cardiovascular disease. In this case, judicious transfusion therapy may be necessary to maintain the patient's exercise tolerance and well being. Patients with end-stage renal disease and severe anemia generally require therapy, either chronic transfusion or recombinant erythropoietin therapy. Selected AIDS patients can also benefit from treatment with erythropoietin. However, in both of these situations, careful monitoring of the patient's iron status is essential.

Transfusion Therapy Red blood cell transfusion should be reserved for those patients with anemia severe enough to result in cardiovascular compromise. Because younger individuals can easily tolerate hemoglobin levels as low as 70 to 80 g/L (7 to 8 g/dL), most acute and chronic inflammatory anemias in this age group should not be transfused. In elderly patients who experience worsening angina or congestive failure or who demonstrate a marked reduction in exercise tolerance, transfusion may be necessary to maintain a hemoglobin level above 110 to 120 g/L (11 to 12 g/dL). The amount of blood required will obviously depend on the severity of the initial anemia and the patient's red blood cell production level. A unit of packed red blood cells will increase the hemoglobin by approximately 10 g/L (1 g/dL). In general, a transfusion of 2 to 3 units of packed red cells will sustain the patient for several weeks to a month or longer as the patient adapts physiologically to lower hemoglobin levels. Repeat transfusions of red blood cells does run a small risk of transmission of infectious agents and alloimmunization (see Chap. 115). If a large number of red cell transfusions are given, the patient is at risk of iron overload.

Erythropoietin Therapy Recombinant erythropoietin therapy has proven to be very effective in the treatment of severe anemia in patients with end-stage renal disease. A majority of dialysis-dependent patients given a dose of erythropoietin of 50 to 150 U/kg three times a week by subcutaneous or intravenous injection will show a gradual increase in their hemoglobin to levels of 100 to 120 g/L (10 to 12 g/dL). The speed and level of response will depend on the individual patient and the level of iron supply. Hemodialysis patients are at risk for the development of iron deficiency secondary to procedural blood losses. They need to be monitored with iron

studies and continuously supplemented with either oral or parenteral iron to maximize iron delivery and guarantee a full production response. Once treatment has begun for patients with end-stage renal disease, they must be treated chronically with recombinant erythropoietin to sustain their hemoglobin in a range of 100 to 120 g/L (10 to 12 g/dL). The average maintenance dose is around 75 U/kg three times per week. However, individual patient requirements can be as little as 10 to more than 300 U/kg. Furthermore, any complicating inflammatory illness will interfere with the erythropoietin response. This needs to be recognized in the long-term care of a renal disease patient. While a higher dose of erythropoietin may overcome the impact of inflammatory cytokines on red blood cell production, it may make more sense to discontinue erythropoietin therapy during periods of acute inflammatory illness and maintain the patient's hemoglobin level with red blood cell transfusions. An increasing erythropoietin requirement or apparent refractoriness to treatment can also occur with aluminum toxicity or hyperparathyroidism. Here again, a return to transfusion therapy may be necessary.

See Chap. 53, Hematopoietic agents: Growth factors, minerals, and vitamins, in Goodman and Gilman's The Pharmacological Basis of Therapeutics, *9th ed, New York, McGraw Hill, 1996.*

BIBLIOGRAPHY

COOK JD, SKIKNE BS: Iron deficiency: Definition and diagnosis. J Intern Med 226:349, 1989
——— et al: Serum transferrin receptor. Annu Rev Med 44:63, 1993
FINCH CA, HUEBERS H: Perspectives in iron metabolism. N Engl J Med 306:1520, 1982
GUYATT GH et al: Laboratory diagnosis of iron-deficiency anemia. An overview. J Gen Intern Med 7:145, 1992
HILLMAN RS, AULT KA: *Hematology in Clinical Practice.* New York, McGraw-Hill, 1995
———, FINCH CA: *Red Cell Manual,* 7th ed. Philadelphia, Davis, 1996
MASSEY AC: Microcytic anemia. Differential diagnosis and management of iron deficiency anemia. Med Clin North Am 76:549, 1992
MEANS RT, KRANTZ SB: Progress in understanding the pathogenesis of the anemia of chronic disease. Blood 30:1639, 1992
NISSENSON AR et al: Recombinant human erythropoietin and renal anemia: Molecular biology, clinical efficacy, and nervous system effects. Ann Intern Med 114:402, 1991

107 *Ernest Beutler*

DISORDERS OF HEMOGLOBIN

In general, microcytic anemias result from abnormalities in hemoglobin production. The production of hemoglobin requires a supply of iron, synthesis of heme, and synthesis of globin. Problems with iron supply are discussed in Chap. 106, defects in heme synthesis are discussed in Chap. 343, and defects in globin synthesis will be discussed here. Lead interferes with heme synthesis (among other enzymatic processes), and lead intoxication is discussed in Chap. 397. When globin synthesis is defective, as in the thalassemias, the resulting red cells are microcytic. However, some abnormalities of hemoglobin do not produce microcytic anemia but lead to hemolysis, while others may not even cause anemia.

Hereditary disorders that result in a structurally abnormal hemoglobin (the hemoglobinopathies) or an insufficient quantity of hemoglobin (the thalassemias) are the most common genetic diseases of humans. Hemoglobin is not only essential for normal oxygen delivery by erythrocytes, but as the major component of these cells it also influences their shape, size, and deformability. Genetic and acquired alterations in hemoglobin structure can impair oxygen delivery and oxygen-carrying capacity, shorten cell life span, and impede passage through the microvasculature. Hemolytic anemia and localized tissue ischemia result. Because many changes in the hemoglobin molecule are compatible with life, and even with normal health, the physician encounters many disorders that are due to hereditary or acquired abnormalities of hemoglobin. Moreover, because of the ready availability of hemoglobin, it has been a favorite tool of the basic scientist, particularly in physiology, biochemistry, and genetics. Sickle cell disease was the first human disorder to be understood at the amino acid level, and the β-globin gene was the first human gene to be cloned.

STRUCTURE AND FUNCTION OF HEMOGLOBIN

Most of the hemoglobin in the red cells of adults exists as a tetramer of two α chains, each with 141 amino acids, and two β chains, each with 146 amino acids. Imbedded in each globin chain is one heme molecule; oxygen is carried by the iron of the heme. The iron must be in the ferrous state to bind oxygen. The α and β chains can undergo a change in conformation, both individually and in relation to one another, so that the molecule can exist in a series of forms with different oxygen affinities. The oxygen affinity of the oxygen-free molecule is low, and its affinity for additional oxygen molecules increases as oxygen begins to bind to heme. The result of this "cooperative interaction" is the well-known sigmoid oxygen association curve (Fig. 107-1). The position of this curve is affected by the pH (the Bohr effect); the CO_2 tension; the level of the metabolic intermediate 2,3-bisphosphoglycerate (2,3-BPG; formerly designated 2,3-DPG) and ATP; the temperature; and by mutations that may affect the globin chains.

The α- and β-globin chains are the products of a family of closely related genes. These genes exist as clusters of α-like genes on chromosome 16 and of β-like genes on chromosome 11 (Fig. 107-2). Normally, hemoglobins contain two α-like chains (α or ζ) and two β-like chains (β, δ, ε, or γ). During ontogeny, different globin genes are successively expressed so that the predominant hemoglobin changes during development. At birth, for example, very few β chains are expressed, and the predominant β-like chain is the γ chain, which complexes to α chains to form fetal hemoglobin ($\alpha_2\gamma_2$). As will be

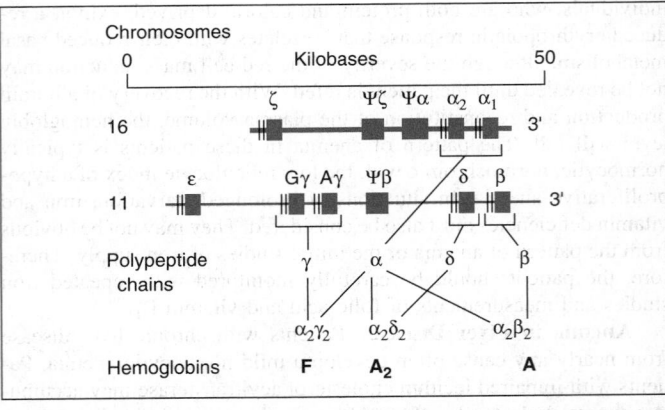

FIGURE 107-2 The globin genes. The α-like genes (α,ζ) are encoded on chromosome 16; the β-like genes (β,γ,δ,ε) are encoded on chromosome 11.

noted below, this normal pattern of activation of globin chains is altered in some disease states and may therefore be of diagnostic importance. Homotetramers of β-like chains can also exist: the γ-chain tetramer is designated *hemoglobin Barts*, and the β-chain tetramer *hemoglobin H*. Because these homotetramers are found in substantial quantities only in disorders in which insufficient α-like chains are produced (α thalassemias), their presence is of diagnostic importance.

REGULATION OF HEMOGLOBIN PRODUCTION

Despite their great importance in the understanding and treatment of the hemoglobinopathies, the mechanisms by which the appropriate globin genes are successively activated at the right moment in ontogenesis are not understood. A powerful upstream enhancer, designated the locus control region, apparently plays an important role and is required for the high level of globin synthesis needed during the development of red cells. When a globin gene is activated, its promoter binds factors necessary for transcription of DNA into the primary mRNA. Globin genes contain three exons and two introns. The introns are spliced from the primary messenger to provide the template for translation into the globin. Defects that prevent normal transcription of the gene, splicing of the messenger, or its translation into protein all have been identified as causes of thalassemias.

CLASSIFICATION, DEFINITIONS, AND NOMENCLATURE

A classification of hereditary or acquired disorders due to abnormal hemoglobins is presented in Table 107-1. Changes in the amino acid sequence of one of the globin chains give rise to what are usually designated *hemoglobinopathies*. Abnormalities in which there are no abnormal globin chains but rather a decrease in the quantity of normal globin chains produced are usually designated *thalassemias*. However, the thalassemic state is often also defined as a clinical syndrome, one that consists of a hereditary anemia characterized by small and poorly hemoglobinized (i.e., microcytic hypochromic) red cells. The distinction between hemoglobinopathies and thalassemias is not, in reality, an absolute one. Thalassemic clinical manifestations may also result from amino acid substi-

FIGURE 107-1 Hemoglobin-oxygen dissociation curve. The hemoglobin tetramer can bind up to four molecules of oxygen in the iron-containing sites of the heme molecules. As oxygen is bound, 2,3-BPG and CO_2 are expelled. Salt bridges are broken, and each of the globin molecules changes its conformation to facilitate oxygen binding. Oxygen release to the tissues is the reverse process, salt bridges being formed and 2,3-BPG and CO_2 bound. Deoxyhemoglobin does not bind oxygen efficiently until the cell returns to conditions of higher pH, the most important modulator of O_2 affinity (Bohr effect). When acid is produced in the tissues, the dissociation curve shifts to the right facilitating oxygen release and CO_2 binding. Alkalosis has the opposite effect, reducing oxygen delivery.

Table 107-1

CHAPTER 107
Disorders of Hemoglobin

647

A Classification of Disorders due to Hemoglobin Abnormalities

I. Hereditary
   A. Abnormal hemoglobins (hemoglobinopathies)
      1. Sickling and related disorders
      2. Unstable hemoglobins
      3. Hemoglobins with abnormal oxygen affinities
      4. Methemoglobins (hemoglobins M)
   B. Thalassemias
      1. α Thalassemias
      2. β Thalassemias, including hereditary persistence of fetal hemoglobin
   C. Methemoglobinemia due to NADH diaphorase (methemoglobin reductase) deficiency
II. Acquired
      1. Toxic sulfhemoglobinemia
      2. Toxic methemoglobinemia
      3. Toxic carboxyhemoglobinemia

tutions such as in the unstable hemoglobins; in read-through mutations such as hemoglobin Constant Spring (which produces a longer-than-normal globin chain because a stop codon is lost); and in the hemoglobins Lepore, in which a fusion gene composed of a portion of the δ- and a portion of the β-chain gene forms very little globin. In hemoglobin E disease, abnormal mRNA splicing occurs as a consequence of the very same mutation that produces an amino acid substitution.

Globin chains are represented by Greek letters, and mutations are shown as superscripts. The superscript A is used for normal hemoglobin, and for a common abnormal hemoglobin such as sickle hemoglobin (hemoglobin S), the designation β^S is commonly employed. More generally, however, the amino acid change is used, so that the mutation of hemoglobin S could also be designated $\beta^{6Glu \rightarrow Val}$. β Thalassemia mutations are usually categorized as β^0 thalassemia for those in which no β chains are made or β^+ when some β chains are produced. δβ Thalassemias are those in which the formation of δ chains as well as β chains is compromised, so that hemoglobin A_2 (i.e., $\alpha_2\delta_2$) levels are not increased in heterozygotes. In the α thalassemias the designation α^0 has been used for the deletion of both α loci, while a single deletion has been designated α^+. Alternatively, the double deletion is sometimes shown as $- -$ and a single deletion as $-\alpha$.

The inheritance of abnormal hemoglobins follows Mendelian genetics. Heterozygotes for abnormal hemoglobins or thalassemia have the *trait* corresponding to the homozygous disorder. Thus, a person with one normal β-globin gene and one sickle β-globin gene (genotype = β^A/β^S) has sickle trait, one who has the β^A/β^C genotype has hemoglobin C trait, and a heterozygote for β thalassemia has thalassemia trait. Those who are homozygous for abnormal hemoglobins have the *disease*. For example, one who has the β^C/β^C genotype has hemoglobin C disease. The thalassemias are divided clinically into thalassemia trait (thalassemia minor) and thalassemia major, based on disease severity. Patients with the trait are usually heterozygotes, while more severely affected patients are homozygotes or compound heterozygotes (that is, they have inherited different mutant alleles from each parent). Hereditary persistence of fetal hemoglobin may be considered as a subset of β thalassemia in which few β chains are synthesized, but the thalassemic features are mild or absent, and fetal hemoglobin represents much of the circulating hemoglobin.

Abnormal amounts of chemically altered hemoglobin molecules may appear in the circulating red cells after certain environmental stresses, resulting in syndromes known by the name of the abnormal pigment that accumulates. These include *methemoglobinemia* (oxidized hemoglobin with ferric rather than ferrous iron), *sulfhemoglobinemia* (sulfur is present in the porphyrin ring and alters its ability to bind oxygen), and *carboxyhemoglobinemia* (carbon monoxide bound to the heme iron). Methemoglobinemia may also occur as a hereditary disorder, either as a hemoglobinopathy in which oxidized hemoglobin resists reduction or as an enzyme defect (e.g., methemoglobin reductase or NADH diaphorase) in which the pathway for the reduction of hemoglobin is defective.

POPULATION GENETICS

The frequency of different hemoglobinopathies varies greatly among different populations. Common mutations, such as those of hemoglobin S, C, and E, and many of the mutations that cause thalassemia represent "balanced polymorphisms." Such mutations are concentrated in certain populations in which they have conferred a selective advantage upon the carrier. This advantage is generally resistance to infection with malaria, which counterbalances the deleterious effect of the homozygous state. In contrast, mutations that occur randomly are panethnic in their distribution and are each relatively rare.

Among African Americans, approximately 7.8 percent are carriers of the sickle mutation, i.e., they have sickle cell trait; 2.3 percent have hemoglobin C trait; and 0.8 percent have β-thalassemia trait. The predicted frequency of the homozygous state for sickle hemoglobin is approximately 1:650; for hemoglobin SC disease it is 1:1100, and for sickle-thalassemia it is 1:3200. In southeast Asia the incidence of hemoglobin E trait is as high as 30 percent in some areas, and that of β thalassemia is also very high in this region. β Thalassemias are very common in many parts of southern Europe. In Sardinia, for example, 12 percent of the population have thalassemia trait. Until the 1970s, 1 in every 250 newborns had thalassemia major, but, as indicated below, the birth incidence has been decreased considerably by organized genetic counseling.

There are many genetically neutral polymorphic sites throughout the genome, and when a new mutation occurs in an individual, it occurs in the context of other polymorphic sites in that region. Such an array of polymorphic sites has been termed a *haplotype*. Because rearrangements of nearby sites by crossing over during meiosis occur only very slowly, genes that have originated relatively recently in evolution (e.g., within 5000 years) are found in the context of the same haplotype in most or all of the descendants of the individual in whom the mutation first occurred. Haplotype identification may be important in several respects. It provides information regarding the number of times a mutation has arisen independently. The sickle mutation is found in five distinct haplotypes, four in Africa, designated Senegal, Benin, Central African Republic, and Cameroon, and one in India. This suggests that the sickle mutation arose independently at least five times. The severity of manifestations of the sickle gene is in part associated with the haplotype in which the mutation is found (see below). Because of the stable linkage between polymorphic sites and disease-producing mutations, haplotypes are also useful in prenatal diagnosis, even when the precise mutation itself is not, as may occur in the thalassemias; all affected children will have the same haplotype.

THE HEMOGLOBINOPATHIES

Mutations of the globin genes may produce abnormal protein molecules by a variety of mechanisms. The most common of these is a single base-pair change in the DNA code resulting in an amino acid substitution. Several hundred such mutations are now known. About half of the variants are clinically silent. Those that are not clinically silent generally either produce a change in oxygen affinity or a physically unstable hemoglobin molecule. The clinical manifestations observed are a function of which globin chain is affected and the consequence of the mutation on protein structure and function. Mutations of one of the α genes tend to have relatively mild clinical consequences because four copies of the α chain exist in the normal genome. β-Globin gene mutations tend to have more severe consequences because in the homozygous state all of the β chains will be abnormal. Mutations of embryonic ζ- and fetal γ-globin chains are of no clinical importance in adult medicine.

Mutations that decrease the stability of hemoglobin produce *Heinz body anemias*. The sickle cell mutation (see below) alters solubility of the deoxy form of hemoglobin and results in distortion of the

Table 107-2

Some Abnormal Hemoglobins

Designation	Mutation	Population	Main Clinical Effects
Sickle or S	$\beta^{6Glu\rightarrow Val}$	African	Anemia, ischemic infarcts
C	$\beta^{6Glu\rightarrow Lys}$	African	Mild anemia
E	$\beta^{26Glu\rightarrow Lys}$	Southeast Asian	Microcytic anemia, splenomegaly
Köln	$\beta^{98Val\rightarrow Met}$	Sporadic	Hemolytic anemia, Heinz bodies when splenectomized
Yakima	$\beta^{99Asp\rightarrow His}$	Sporadic	Polycythemia
Kansas	$\beta^{102Asn\rightarrow Lys}$	Sporadic	Mild anemia

erythrocytes when they are deoxygenated. Mutations that raise the oxygen affinity of hemoglobin result in hereditary polycythemia; those that lower oxygen affinity result in anemia. Hemoglobin mutants (hemoglobins M) that cannot be reduced by red cell enzymes result in methemoglobinemia.

SICKLE CELL DISORDERS **Definitions** *Sickle cell disorders* include all states in which a sickle gene has been inherited, but *sickle diseases* refer to states in which a morbid condition ensues, such as hemoglobin SC disease and hemoglobin S-β-thalassemia. The term *sickle cell anemia* is usually reserved for the homozygous state for hemoglobin S.

Pathophysiology Hemoglobin S is characterized by the substitution of a valine for glutamic acid as the sixth amino acid in the β-globin chain, resulting from a DNA substitution of thymine for adenine (Table 107-2). The diminished solubility of the deoxy form of this hemoglobin results in the formation of a gelatinous network of fibrous polymers, called *tactoids*, that stiffen and distort the cell, producing rigid, misshapen erythrocytes that traverse small blood vessels with great difficulty or not at all. After repeated episodes of sickling and unsickling, irreversible sickle cells may be formed. The removal of abnormal cells from the circulation at a rate that exceeds the capacity of the marrow to replace them results in a hemolytic anemia. The obstruction of small vessels by sickle cells results in repeated infarctions, leading to gradual involvement of all organ systems, most notably spleen, lungs, kidney, and brain. The obstruction of small blood vessels by sickle cells is not due entirely to their altered shape and rigidity. There are also membrane changes that may play an important role. Sickle cells adhere to endothelium.

The sickling of red cells containing sickle hemoglobin depends not only upon the degree of oxygenation of the hemoglobin in the cell but also upon the concentration of sickle hemoglobin in the cell, the pH, and the temperature. Moreover, the formation of the characteristic tubules that result when sickle hemoglobin molecules aggregate is not instantaneous; the time that has elapsed since conditions favoring sickling were achieved is of importance. Some hemoglobins interfere more with the sickling process than do others. Thus, fetal hemoglobin interferes with sickling more than does hemoglobin A. Hemoglobin C interacts so effectively with hemoglobin S that hemoglobin SC disease is clinically very similar and often indistinguishable from homozygous sickle cell disease.

Clinical Manifestations Patients with sickle cell disease manifest the signs and symptoms of chronic anemia with pallor of the mucous membranes, fatigue, and decreased exercise tolerance. Because most patients with sickle cell disease are of African origin, pallor is more readily appreciated on examining the mucus membranes than the skin, but the skin may have a grayish cast. Because of the chronic hemolysis, jaundice is commonly present and patients are prone to gallstone formation.

In addition to these general manifestations of anemia, symptoms and signs related more to the rheologic abnormalities than to the anemia are common. These include leg ulcers, priapism, repeated episodes of pulmonary infarction, and "acute chest syndrome" characterized by fever, chest pain, and pulmonary infiltrates. Damage to the pulmonary vasculature can produce pulmonary hypertension, heart failure, and death. Retinal vessel obstruction may result in hemorrhage, scarring, retinal detachment, and blindness. Renal papillary necrosis with hematuria occurs in sickle cell diseases and is one of the few clinical manifestations of the sickle cell trait. The hypertonic milieu in the renal medulla draws water out of the red blood cell and promotes sickling. Although the spleen may be enlarged in small children with sickle cell disease, repeated episodes of splenic infarction cause the spleen to be reduced to a small calcified remnant, a phenomenon that has been termed "autosplenectomy." As a result of the functional asplenic state, and for other poorly understood reasons, patients with sickle cell disease have an increased susceptibility to infection. Salmonella osteomyelitis is one such infection that is rarely seen in patients without sickling disorders. Stroke is a serious complication of sickle cell disease and may occur in very young children, leaving them permanently disabled. Progressive renal and pulmonary failure are of great importance in the fourth and fifth decades of life in patients with sickle diseases and are a common cause of death in these patients. Aseptic necrosis of the femoral head may occur, occasionally even in patients with sickle trait (see Table 107-3).

In addition to these chronic manifestations of sickle cell diseases, three types of acute episodes, termed *crises*, occur. By far the most common of these is the *infarctive or painful crisis*. This type of crisis is characterized by severe skeletal pain, which may persist for several days or even weeks. Fever is commonly present, but there is usually no change in the hemoglobin concentration of the blood. *Sequestration crises* are largely limited to infants and young children, although occasionally they may occur in the few adults who have splenomegaly. In this type of crisis, there is sudden massive pooling of red cells in

Table 107-3

Clinical Features of Sickle Hemoglobinopathies

Condition	Clinical Abnormalities	Hemoglobin Level, g/L (g/dL)	Mean Corpuscular Volume, fL	Hemoglobin Electrophoresis
Sickle cell trait	None; rare painless hematuria	Normal	Normal	Hb S/A:40/60
Sickle cell anemia	Vasoocclusive crises with infarction of spleen, brain, marrow, kidney, lung; aseptic necrosis of bone; gallstones; priapism; ankle ulcers	70–100 (7–10)	80–100	Hb S/A:100/0 Hb F:2–25%
S/β° thalassemia	Vasoocclusive crises; aseptic necrosis of bone	70–100 (7–10)	60–80	Hb S/A:100/0 Hb F:1–10%
S/β⁺ thalassemia	Rare crises and aseptic necrosis	100–140 (10–14)	70–80	Hb S/A:60/40
Hemoglobin SC	Rare crises and aseptic necrosis; painless hematuria	100–140 (10–14)	80–100	Hb S/A:50/0 Hb C:50%

the spleen with an acute fall in the hemoglobin concentration of the blood. It is not uncommon for such crises to have a fatal outcome. *Hemolytic crises* are uncommon and are characterized by a fall in the hemoglobin concentration of the blood with marked increase in jaundice. Crises may last a few hours or a few days.

Sickle trait, which occurs in nearly 8 percent of African Americans, is unaccompanied by anemia and is almost always clinically silent. Individuals with the trait have an impaired ability to concentrate urine and rarely may develop clinical signs under conditions of severe anoxia. For example, splenic infarction has occurred occasionally during unpressurized ascent to high altitudes.

Factors Influencing the Severity of Sickle Cell Disease Different genotypes can give rise to sickle cell disease. The classic form of the disease may be considered to be the homozygous state for hemoglobin S, i.e., SS disease or sickle cell anemia. However, the manifestations of SC disease, sickle cell β thalassemia, and hemoglobin SD disease are very similar. While, on the average, sickle cell anemia has the most severe clinical course and splenomegaly may be more likely to occur in hemoglobin SC disease and S thalassemia than in SS disease, there is a great deal of overlap between the severity and clinical manifestations of these disorders. The principal importance of the distinctions between different sickle disease genotypes is in their diagnosis and in genetic counseling.

A number of factors influence the course of sickle cell disease and may be important in precipitating crises. These include infection and fever, dehydration, and exposure to low oxygen tension. Even apart from these factors, the severity of the clinical manifestations of sickle cell disease varies greatly from patient to patient, not only in the degree to which they are affected but also with respect to which of the morbid manifestations predominate. Thus, some may suffer chiefly from anemia with few, if any, painful episodes, while others experience many painful crises but have hemoglobin levels that are nearly normal. In still other patients, strokes may be the predominant clinical events, and occasional patients have virtually no manifestations of the disease. The causes of this variability are unknown. Yet it is of great practical importance because of the high risk of some therapeutic measures that may be contemplated, particularly allogeneic bone marrow transplantation. There is a statistically significant association between the haplotype in which the sickle gene exists (Central African Republic is worst and Senegal is best) and the severity of disease. Concurrent α thalassemia seems to protect on the average against the clinical manifestations of sickle disease, and high levels of fetal hemoglobin are also protective. However, each of these predictors, individually or collectively, is weak, and good predictors of prognosis that can be applied to young children are badly needed.

Survival, though difficult to predict for an individual, correlates with the frequency of crises; the median age at death for those with more than three crises per year is 35 years, whereas those with fewer crises per year may live into their 50s.

Diagnosis The presence of sickle hemoglobin can be established by demonstrating that the red cells assume their characteristic morphologic form when the hemoglobin is deoxygenated, as by treatment with a reducing agent such as sodium metabisulfite. The classic sickling procedure does not distinguish between the different sickling disorders and is less well suited for large scale screening of blood samples than is electrophoretic separation of the hemoglobins. Electrophoresis of hemoglobins readily identifies the presence of the slow-moving hemoglobin S, but routine electrophoretic methods do not distinguish it from some other slow-moving hemoglobins such as hemoglobin D. Thus, the identity of the hemoglobin as hemoglobin S must be confirmed, usually by the use of a sickling or a solubility test. Quantitation of the different hemoglobins by electrophoresis also provides information regarding the genotype of the patient. If there is more hemoglobin A than hemoglobin S, then the patient has sickle cell trait. If hemoglobins S and A are present but hemoglobin S predominates, then the patient has sickle β⁺ thalassemia disease. When hemoglobin C is present with hemoglobin S, the patient has SC disease (Table 107-3).

Diagnosis of the genetic status of the unborn child is much more difficult than is postnatal diagnosis, both because of the difficulty and risk attendant upon obtaining fetal blood and because there is very meager expression of the β-globin locus during fetal life. DNA analysis is thus of principal value in prenatal diagnosis. DNA obtained either on chorionic villus biopsy or amniocentesis can be amplified by the polymerase chain reaction, and the sickle mutation readily ascertained.

℞ TREATMENT

Symptomatic Management The mainstays of management of patients with sickle disease are the avoidance of complications and their treatment when they do arise. Patients with sickle cell disease should be counseled to avoid high altitudes, to maintain an adequate fluid intake, and to treat infections promptly when they occur. They should be given folic acid—1 mg/day. *Haemophilus influenzae* type b vaccine and pneumococcal and meningococcal polysaccharide vaccines are recommended early (before spleen damage), and children with sickle cell disease should receive penicillin prophylaxis until the age of 6 years.

Leg ulcers may respond to prolonged bed rest and to surgical grafting. Priapism may be managed with pain medication and nifedipine. Priapism persisting for more than a day is usually managed surgically, and impotence is the common outcome in sexually mature males.

The management of painful crises is one of the most frequent and difficult challenges faced by the treating physician. Therapy consists of hydration, keeping the patient warm, and possibly the use of oxygen. Because of the renal papillary necrosis, patients have difficulty reabsorbing water from the urine and are particularly susceptible to dehydration. The use of analgesics in the treatment of painful crises represents a particularly difficult problem because of the propensity of patients with sickle cell disease, in common with patients with any type of chronic or recurrent pain, to become addicted to narcotics. Continuous infusions of morphine should be employed to keep the pain under control. Younger patients may require higher doses. Chronic transfusion therapy has been used to decrease the frequency of crises and may be useful in some severely affected patients. However, over the long term, this approach may lead to iron overload.

Patients with the acute chest syndrome require broad-spectrum antibiotics (ceftriaxone and erythromycin for *Mycoplasma*) in addition to hydration and O_2. In the face of respiratory insufficiency ($Pa_{O_2} < 60$ mmHg), exchange transfusion may be necessary.

A relatively high rate of fetal loss occurs during pregnancy. Maternal mortality was once about 33 percent but has declined to an average of 1.6 percent in areas where good prenatal care is available. The patient should be apprised of these risks. Chronic transfusion therapy has been attempted as a means of decreasing maternal and fetal mortality in sickle cell disease, but without success.

Specific Measures Many different antisickling agents have been tested therapeutically, but of these the only one that has proven to be clinically beneficial in controlled trials is hydroxyurea. This drug interferes with normal erythropoiesis in such a way as to increase the production of γ chains. The increased fetal hemoglobin levels interfere with the sickling process and decrease the incidence of crises. Its effects may be enhanced with the concomitant use of erythropoietin. Hydroxyurea administration should be limited to more severely affected patients with sickle cell disease.

Allogeneic bone marrow transplantation is the only currently available treatment that can cure sickle cell disease. Its use remains uncommon. Because the short- and intermediate-term mortality from bone marrow transplantation is 5 to 10 percent, the selection of patients to undergo this treatment is particularly difficult. Clearly, the risk is justified in patients who are destined to suffer the most severe manifestations of the disease, particularly strokes. Yet, as pointed out above, criteria for clearly identifying such patients do not yet exist.

Gene transfer therapy has the potential to provide marked improvement in or cure of patients with sickle cell disease while avoiding some of the risks of allogeneic transplantation. There was considerable optimism about this approach in the early 1980s. However, it is now apparent that for several reasons the difficulties in implementing gene therapy for sickle cell disease are much greater than those encountered in the treatment of enzyme defects such as adenosine deaminase deficiency, where gene transfer has been performed with some modest success. In sickle cell disease, the clinical manifestations are caused by the functioning of the abnormal gene, and merely placing a normal gene into the hematopoietic stem cell does not prevent the formation of sickle hemoglobin. Moreover, to be effective it is necessary for the transduced gene not only to function but to function at a very high level. The rate at which hemoglobin is normally synthesized is several orders of magnitude higher than that of most other proteins. Finally, it has been difficult to maintain continuing expression of genes transduced into primate hematopoietic stem cells. Prolonged activity would be essential for gene transfer therapy to be successful in sickle cell disease.

HEMOGLOBIN C DISORDERS   The most important clinical consequence of the hemoglobin C mutation is its interaction with the sickle mutation to cause hemoglobin SC disease, a form of sickle cell disease, as discussed above. Hemoglobin C trait is asymptomatic, and hemoglobin CC disease, the homozygous state, causes a mild anemia characterized by target-shaped, flattened, and sometimes folded erythrocytes. Characteristic intraerythrocytic crystals can sometimes be found, but the diagnosis of this disorder depends upon hemoglobin electrophoresis. A patient with manifestations of sickle cell disease who has splenomegaly and whose erythrocytes are target cells is likely to have SC disease.

HEMOGLOBIN E DISORDERS   The hemoglobin E mutation produces an amino acid substitution, 26Glu→Lys, through a G→A mutation in the 79th nucleotide of the coding sequence of the cDNA. It is unusual in that some of the mRNA bearing this mutation is spliced abnormally because of the substitution, and because the abnormally spliced message cannot be translated into globin, there is a marked β-globin deficiency. As a result, the hemoglobin E mutations cause a thalassemia-like state. Hemoglobin E trait is characterized by the presence of target cells, hypochromia, microcytosis, and mild anemia. The homozygous state for hemoglobin E is also clinically mild, with striking microcytosis usually without splenomegaly. The β thalassemia/hemoglobin E compound heterozygote has a somewhat more severe presentation than homozygous hemoglobin E disease; splenomegaly is usually present.

UNSTABLE HEMOGLOBINS   Some mutations cause the formation of unstable hemoglobin molecules that precipitate in vivo, causing hemolytic anemia. Most of these mutations affect the binding of heme by globin or the intermolecular contacts between the globin chain in the tetramer. A single copy of a gene for an unstable hemoglobin is sufficient to cause hemolytic disease, and thus these hemoglobinopathies are inherited as autosomal dominant disorders. Hemoglobins Geneva and Köln are examples. Hemolysis varies greatly in severity and may be accentuated by the ingestion of "oxidative" drugs, such as those that cause hemolysis in patients with glucose-6-phosphate dehydrogenase (G6PD) deficiency (see Chap. 109). Sulfonamides have been the chief offending agents. Heinz bodies, particles of denatured protein adhering to the cell membrane, are usually seen in patients who have been splenectomized.

Although unstable hemoglobins may be electrophoretically abnormal, they are best detected by the isopropanol stability test. In recent years a thalassemia-like state inherited as a dominant disorder and designated as a *hyperunstable hemoglobin syndrome* has been delineated. Here, the hemoglobin is so unstable that none of it can be detected

in red cells. Instead, the diagnosis must be established by showing a defect in the globin gene by DNA analysis. Even though only one of the copies of the β chain is abnormal, the very unstable hemoglobin apparently damages the erythrocytes sufficiently that severe hemolytic anemia occurs.

HEMOGLOBINS WITH ABNORMAL OXYGEN AFFINITY   The steady-state level of hemoglobin is presumably maintained by an as yet uncharacterized oxygen sensor. When an abnormal hemoglobin binds oxygen too tightly (i.e., has an increased oxygen affinity), the sensor causes more erythropoietin to be released. Consequently, the red cell mass increases. Patients with such mutations may become sufficiently polycythemic so as to require periodic phlebotomies. High-affinity hemoglobins are commonly also unstable, so that a compensated hemolytic state with a normal hemoglobin level results. Hemoglobins Zürich and Yakima are examples. Conversely, mutant hemoglobins with a decreased oxygen affinity cause a mild, usually asymptomatic anemia. Hemoglobin Kansas is an example.

These hemoglobinopathies are diagnosed by determining the oxygen dissociation of the hemoglobin freed of 2,3-BPG. This compound must be removed to distinguish high- and low-affinity hemoglobins from hereditary metabolic disorders of the red cell such as phosphofructokinase deficiency, which causes polycythemia by lowering the 2,3-BPG level, or pyruvate kinase deficiency, which increases the red cell 2,3-BPG level. Like the hemoglobinopathies caused by the unstable hemoglobins, the clinical syndromes caused by these mutant hemoglobins are inherited in an autosomal dominant fashion.

THE THALASSEMIAS

The thalassemias are divided into the α thalassemias, in which it is the production of α globin that is deficient, and the β thalassemias, in which β globin production is defective.

THE α THALASSEMIAS   Pathophysiology   α Thalassemias result in an excess production of β chains in adults and children and γ chains in newborns. The β chains that accumulate form tetramers—hemoglobin Barts (γ_4) in infants and hemoglobin H (β_4) in adults. These tetramers are abnormal hemoglobins with marked instability, a left-shifted oxygen dissociation curve with a lack of cooperativity, i.e., the normal sigmoid shape. The hematologic manifestations of the α thalassemias are a function principally of the extent to which these abnormal tetramers accumulate. This, in turn, depends upon how many of the four α loci have been deleted or inactivated by a mutation, as indicated below.

Clinical Manifestations (Table 107-4)   *Deletion or mutation of all four α loci*   Deletion of all of the α-globin genes is the most catastrophic form of α thalassemia. It is incompatible with extrauterine life, and the infants are either dead at birth with hydrops fetalis or die shortly after birth. They are severely edematous and have little circulating hemoglobin, which is almost entirely hemoglobin Barts.

Deletion or mutation of three of the four α loci   Hemoglobin H disease results from deletion of all but one of the α-globin genes. The disorder resembles an unstable hemoglobinopathy, because both hemoglobin Barts and hemoglobin H are, in fact, unstable hemoglobins. Patients have a microcytic hypochromic anemia with target cells and Heinz bodies on the blood smear. Onset may be apparent during childhood, but in milder cases it is often not until adult life. Hemolytic anemia with marked splenomegaly is the characteristic presentation. Reticulocytes are increased.

Deletion or mutation of two of the four α loci   Two α loci are sufficient for nearly normal erythropoiesis. This state has been called α-thalassemia trait and is characterized by mild anemia and moderate microcytosis and hypochromia. The hemoglobin concentration is usually within 10 or 20 g/L (1 or 2 g/dL) of normal, and the mean corpuscular volume (MCV) is in the 70 to 80 fL range. Because of the extraordinarily high prevalence (~30 percent) of deletion of one of the two α-globin loci on chromosomes of people of African origin, the inheritance of two such chromosomes is very common. This condition is very commonly mistaken for iron deficiency and treated inappropriately with iron.

Three α-globin loci are sufficient for essentially normal function. Anemia and hypochromia do not occur in these persons. They have been designated *silent carriers*.

Diagnosis   The diagnosis of the severe forms (three and four gene deletions) of α thalassemia is readily made by demonstrating the presence of the rapidly moving hemoglobin Barts in infants and hemoglobin H in adults. The erythrocytes show typical inclusions after incubation with an oxidant dye such as brilliant cresyl blue. Diagnosis of the milder forms is much more difficult, because the amounts of hemoglobins Barts and H are too small to detect reliably. Diagnosis is most reliably established by measuring the ratio of synthesis of α- to β-globin chain in isolated peripheral blood reticulocytes, a test that is, unfortunately, not widely available. Because most α thalassemias are due to deletions, Southern blotting of endonuclease-digested genomic DNA can be very useful but may be difficult to interpret in patients with the αα/− − genotype, in whom a normal pattern is seen.

℞ **TREATMENT**

There is currently no treatment for hydrops fetalis. However, the disease can be prevented by properly establishing the genotypes of parents. Only when two parents have a chromosome with the two-locus deletion, i.e., either αα/− − or α−/− −, is it possible to bear a child with no α-globin genes. The diagnosis can be established prenatally by examining DNA from a chorionic villus or from amniotic fluid cells.

Splenectomy is sometimes helpful in the treatment of patients with hemoglobin H disease, either when the anemia is quite severe or when massive splenomegaly is troublesome for the patient.

No treatment is required for deletions of only one or two α-globin loci.

THE β THALASSEMIAS   **Pathophysiology**   The excess α chains that are formed in β thalassemia do not self-associate to form tetramers but instead are bound to the red cell membrane, producing membrane damage. The severity of the β-thalassemic defect varies with different mutations. Some mutations (β°) prevent the formation of any β chains at all; others (β⁺) allow some β-chain formation to occur. Thus, depending on which two mutations are inherited, a broad range of compromise of β-chain formation can be encountered.

Hereditary persistence of fetal hemoglobin is a heterogeneous, clinically benign disorder characterized by elevated fetal hemoglobin levels. Both deletions and point mutations may cause this disorder, and exactly why some mutations produce this relatively innocuous disorder rather than thalassemia is not fully understood.

Clinical Manifestations   When both β-globin genes bear a thalassemic mutation, a severe anemia is generally present, associated, in the untreated patient, with bone changes due to expansion of the marrow space and often growth retardation. This increase in erythropoiesis produces a characteristic "chipmunk" facies. The skin may be a peculiar copper color from pallor, icterus, and melanin deposition. Hepatosplenomegaly may be massive. Many such patients with β thalassemia major (Cooley's anemia) are transfusion-dependent, and these patients, in particular, generally develop iron overload. In untreated patients this usually leads to death in the second decade.

β-Thalassemia trait β *thalassemia minor* presents as a modest anemia with striking microcytosis. The hemoglobin may be as much as 30 g/L (3 g/dL) below normal, and the MCV is often less than 70 fL. Patients with this trait sometimes complain of weakness and tiredness, which they are inclined to blame on their anemia, but it is by no means certain that such symptoms are more common in patients with β-thalassemia trait than in the general population.

Diagnosis   Most patients with β-thalassemia trait have twofold elevated levels of hemoglobin A₂ (α₂δ₂) (~5 percent of total). Exceptions are patients with concurrent iron deficiency and those with a less common form of thalassemia, δβ thalassemia, in which δ-chain as well as β-chain production is compromised. In about one-third of patients with β-thalassemia trait, hemoglobin F is elevated (1 to 3 percent), and in δβ thalassemia, hemoglobin F may account for 5 to 15 percent of the total hemoglobin. Measurement of globin chain synthetic ratios is a definitive method of diagnosis; however, it is difficult to perform and therefore not readily available. In β thalassemia major, greatly elevated levels of fetal hemoglobin, comprising nearly all of the pigment, are present.

℞ **TREATMENT**

Untreated severe β thalassemia is uniformly fatal in childhood. Life can be prolonged by periodic transfusions, and if the hemoglobin level of the blood is maintained adequately, the bone changes and growth impairment can be largely prevented. When the spleen is greatly enlarged splenectomy may produce a clinically significant decrease in the transfusion requirement. Iron overload then becomes a serious problem that can be ameliorated by treatment with regular intravenous or subcutaneous infusions of desferrioxamine at 50 mg per kilogram body weight. The drug may cause skin reactions at the injection site or neurologic side effects, particularly visual and auditory, but these effects are dose-related. Cure of the disease can be achieved with marrow transplantation. Although this carries some risk of death due to the procedure itself, and in some patients the thalassemic cells regrow, displacing the graft, marrow transplantation has an important place in the treatment of patients with this very serious disease (Fig. 107-3).

Heterozygotes for β-thalassemic mutations do not need to be treated, but in regions in which the incidence of these mutations is very high, as in Sardinia, screening for β thalassemia combined with skillful counseling has played an important role in greatly decreasing the incidence of the disease. Only a generation ago, the incidence of thalassemia was 1:250; now its occurrence is rare.

Table 107-4

The α Thalassemias

Condition	Hemoglobin A, %	Hemoglobin H (β⁴), %	Hemoglobin level, g/L (g/dL)	MCV, fL
Normal	97	0	150 (15)	90
Silent thalassemia: −α/αα	98–100	0	150 (15)	90
Thalassemia trait: −α/−α homozygous α-thal-2* or − −/αα heterozygous α-thal-1*	85–95	Rare red blood cell inclusions	120–130 (12–13)	70–80
Hemoglobin H disease: − −/−α heterozygous α-thal-1/α-thal-2	70–95	5–30	60–100 (6–10)	60–70
Hydrops fetalis: − −/− − homozygous α-thal-1	0	5–10†	Fatal in utero or at birth	

* When both α alleles on one chromosome are deleted, the locus is called α-thal-1; when only a single α allele on one chromosome is deleted, the locus is called α-thal-2.
† 90–95% of the hemoglobin is hemoglobin Barts (tetramers of γ chains).

FIGURE 107-3 The probability of survival for 271 thalassemic patients under 17 years of age. The patients received marrow transplantation from HLA-identical family members after conditioning with busulfan and cyclophosphamide. The degree of hepatomegaly and the presence of portal fibrosis was used to assign patients to risk classes. (*From G. Lucarelli and RA Clift, in SJ Forman et al (eds), Bone Marrow Transplantation, Boston, Blackwell Scientific, 1994, with permission.*)

COMPOUND HEMOGLOBINOPATHIES

HEMOGLOBIN E/THALASSEMIA Hemoglobin E (lysine for glutamic acid at position 26 of the β chain) results in a defect in mRNA processing and the production of an unstable hemoglobin. Both heterozygotes and homozygotes show microcytosis and hypochromia, but heterozygotes are not anemic. This form of hemoglobin is common in Cambodia and Thailand (30 to 40 percent). Patients who are compound heterozygotes for hemoglobin E and β thalassemia have the clinical features of β thalassemia major including severe hemolytic anemia and splenomegaly, require chronic transfusion, and suffer iron overload.

HEMOGLOBIN S/THALASSEMIA Compound heterozygotes of hemoglobin S and β thalassemia are most commonly seen in African and Mediterranean populations. They develop a clinical picture consistent with sickle cell anemia except that splenomegaly is usually present. Therapy consists of raising hemoglobin F levels with hydroxyurea.

HEMOGLOBIN C/THALASSEMIA Also noted in Mediterranean and African populations, hemoglobin C/β° thalassemia is associated with a moderately severe hemolytic anemia, splenomegaly, target cells, and a hypochromic microcytic peripheral blood smear. In blacks, hemoglobin C may occur with $β^+$ thalassemia, which produces a milder disease.

OTHER ACQUIRED AND INHERITED HEMOGLOBIN ABNORMALITIES

The most common cause of cyanosis is reduced arterial oxygen tension related to lung disease or right-to-left cardiac shunts. Hemoglobin can on rare occasions account for cyanosis either through mutations producing molecules with decreased oxygen affinity (e.g., hemoglobin Kansas-$β^{102Asn→Thr}$) or through the accumulation of methemoglobin or sulfhemoglobin.

METHEMOGLOBINEMIA AND SULFHEMOGLOBINE-MIA Accumulation of large amounts of the brown, reversibly oxidized methemoglobin in red cells can occur for three reasons: (1) a dominantly inherited abnormality in hemoglobin, one of the hemoglo-

bins M, in which the structural lesion prevents the reduction of methemoglobin to hemoglobin; (2) a recessively inherited deficiency in the enzyme methemoglobin reductase; and (3) exposure to hemoglobin-oxidizing chemicals or drugs such as nitrites, xylocaine, or benzene derivatives. Differentiation of these forms of methemoglobinemia from each other depends upon the clinical history; the pattern of transmission in the family; examination of the optical spectrum of the hemoglobin, which is abnormal in the hemoglobins M; and assay of the erythrocyte methemoglobin reductase.

The irreversible formation of another hemoglobin pigment with distinctively abnormal spectral properties, sulfhemoglobin, results from the administration of drugs, particularly sulfonamides. It produces marked cyanosis but disappears spontaneously as the cells containing the abnormal pigment are gradually removed from the circulation.

Methemoglobinemia induced by drugs or chemicals is spontaneously reversible when the agent is withdrawn. However, high levels of the pigment amounting to more than 30 to 40 percent of the total pigment can be life-threatening and are best treated by the infusion of methylene blue, 1 to 2 mg per kilogram body weight. This dye links the highly efficient NADP-linked methemoglobin-reducing system to methemoglobin and thus will result in rapid reduction of methemoglobin to hemoglobin in all but G6PD-deficient patients. Although methemoglobinemia due to methemoglobin reductase deficiency also responds to methylene blue treatment, this chronic disorder is best treated by the daily oral administration of 1 to 2 g ascorbic acid. Cyanosis due to hemoglobin M does not respond to treatment but is ordinarily a benign condition.

CARBOXYHEMOGLOBINEMIA Hemoglobin has an affinity for carbon monoxide (CO) that is about 200 times higher than its affinity for oxygen. The displacement of even one oxygen molecule by CO greatly increases the strength with which remaining oxygen molecules are bound. The left shift produced in the oxygen dissociation curve impairs delivery of oxygen to the tissues to an extent that is much greater than would otherwise occur from the decrease in the amount of oxygen carried by the blood. In contrast to methemoglobin, carboxyhemoglobin is cherry red in color and its presence may not be suspected by gross examination of the blood. Carbon monoxide poisoning may be caused by combustion of hydrocarbons such as by faulty heaters in poorly ventilated areas, in industrial accidents, and in fires. Smokers of cigarettes or cigar smokers who inhale the smoke may have carboxyhemoglobin levels as high as 20 percent. Displacement of more than 50 percent of the oxygen by CO can be fatal. Oxygen will gradually displace the CO from hemoglobin, so that in mildly affected patients administration of oxygen or no treatment at all may be sufficient. In severely compromised patients blood transfusions may be necessary.

BIBLIOGRAPHY

BEUTLER E: The sickle cell diseases and related disorders, in *Williams' Hematology*, 5th ed, E Beutler et al (eds). New York, McGraw-Hill, 1995, pp 616–654
————, SULLIVAN KM: Bone marrow transplantation for sickle cell disease, in *Bone Marrow Transplantation*, SJ Forman et al (eds). Boston, Blackwell Scientific, 1994, pp. 840–848
CAO A: 1993 William Allan Award address. Am J Hum Genet 54:397, 1994
CHARACHE S et al: Hydroxyurea: Effects on hemoglobin F production in patients with sickle cell anemia. Blood 79:2555, 1992
EHLERS KH et al: Prolonged survival in patients with beta-thalassemia major treated with deferoxamine. J Pediatr 118:540, 1991
EMBURY SH et al (eds): *Sickle Cell Disease: Basic Principles and Clinical Practice*. Hagerstown, MD, Lippincott-Raven, 1994
THEIN SL: Dominant beta thalassaemia: Molecular basis and pathophysiology. Br J Haematol 80:273, 1992
WALTERS MC et al: Bone marrow transplantation for sickle cell disease. N Engl J Med 335:369, 1996
WEATHERALL DJ: The thalassemias, in *Williams' Hematology*, 5th ed, E Beutler et al (eds). New York, McGraw-Hill, 1995, pp 581–615
WINTERBOURN CC: Oxidative denaturation in congenital hemolytic anemias: The unstable hemoglobins. Semin Hematol 27:41, 1990

MEGALOBLASTIC ANEMIAS

The megaloblastic anemias are disorders caused by impaired DNA synthesis. Cells primarily affected are those having relatively rapid turnover, especially hematopoietic precursors and gastrointestinal epithelial cells. Cell division is sluggish, but cytoplasmic development progresses normally, so megaloblastic cells tend to be large, with an increased ratio of RNA to DNA. Megaloblastic erythroid cells tend to be destroyed in the marrow. Thus, marrow cellularity is often increased but production of red blood cells (RBC) is decreased, an abnormality termed *ineffective erythropoiesis* (see Chap. 59).

Most megaloblastic anemias are due to a deficiency of cobalamin (vitamin B_{12}) and/or folic acid. The various clinical entities associated with megaloblastic anemia are listed in Table 108-1. This classification is easier to comprehend if the physiologic and biochemical principles discussed below are kept in mind.

PHYSIOLOGIC CONSIDERATIONS

FOLIC ACID   Folic acid is the common name for pteroylmonoglutamic acid. It is synthesized by many different plants and bacteria. Fruits and vegetables constitute the primary dietary source of the vitamin. Some forms of dietary folic acid are labile and may be destroyed by cooking. The minimum daily requirement is normally about $50\mu g$, but this may be increased severalfold during periods of enhanced metabolic demand such as pregnancy.

The assimilation of adequate amounts of folic acid is dependent on the nature of the diet and its means of preparation. Folates in various foodstuffs are largely conjugated to a chain of glutamic acid residues. This highly polar side chain impairs the intestinal absorption of the vitamin. However, conjugases (γ-glutamyl carboxypeptidases) in the lumen of the gut convert polyglutamates to mono- and diglutamates, which are readily absorbed in the proximal jejunum.

Plasma folate is primarily in the form of N^5-methyltetrahydrofolate, a monoglutamate. N^5-Methyltetrahydrofolate is transported into cells by a carrier that is specific for the tetrahydro forms of the vitamin. Once in the cell, the N^5-methyl group is removed in a cobalamin-requiring reaction (see below), and the folate is then reconverted to the polyglutamate form. The polyglutamate form may be useful for retention of folate by the cell.

A folate-binding protein occurs in plasma, milk, and other body fluids. The function of this folate binder and its membrane-bound precursor is unknown. Neither the binder nor its precursor is related to the tetrahydrofolate carrier.

Normal individuals have about 5 to 20 mg folic acid in various body stores, half in the liver. In light of the minimum daily requirement, it is not surprising that a deficiency will occur within months if dietary intake or intestinal absorption is curtailed.

COBALAMIN   This vitamin is a complex organometallic compound in which a cobalt atom is situated within a corrin ring, a structure similar to the porphyrin from which heme is formed. Unlike heme, however, cobalamin cannot be synthesized in the human body and must be supplied in the diet. The only dietary source of cobalamin is animal products: meat and dairy foods. The minimum daily requirement for cobalamin is about 2.5 μg.

During gastric digestion, cobalamin in food is released and forms a stable complex with gastric R binder, one of a closely related group of glycoproteins of unknown function that are found in secretions (e.g., saliva, milk, gastric juice, bile), phagocytes, and plasma. On entering the duodenum, the cobalamin–R binder complex is digested, releasing the cobalamin, which then binds to intrinsic factor (IF). This 50-kDa glycoprotein is produced by the parietal cells of the stomach. The secretion of intrinsic factor generally parallels that of hydrochloric acid. The cobalamin-IF complex is resistant to proteolytic digestion and travels to the distal ileum, where specific receptors on the mucosal brush border bind the cobalamin-IF complex, thereby enabling the

Table 108-1

Classification of the Megaloblastic Anemias

COBALAMIN DEFICIENCY

I. Inadequate intake: vegetarians (rare)
II. Malabsorption
  A. Inadequate production of intrinsic factor (IF)
    1. Pernicious anemia
    2. Gastrectomy
    3. Congenital absence or functional abnormality of IF (rare)
  B. Disorders of terminal ileum
    1. Tropical sprue
    2. Nontropical sprue
    3. Regional enteritis
    4. Intestinal resection
    5. Neoplasms and granulomatous disorders (rare)
    6. Selective cobalamin malabsorption (Imerslund's syndrome) (rare)
  C. Competition for cobalamin
    1. Fish tapeworm
    2. Bacteria: "blind loop" syndrome
  D. Drugs: *p*-aminosalicylic acid, colchicine, neomycin
III. Other
  A. Nitrous oxide
  B. Transcobalamin II deficiency (rare)

FOLIC ACID DEFICIENCY

I. Inadequate intake: unbalanced diet (common in alcoholics, teenagers, some infants)
II. Increased requirements
  A. Pregnancy
  B. Infancy
  C. Malignancy
  D. Increased hematopoiesis (chronic hemolytic anemias)
  E. Chronic exfoliative skin disorders
  F. Hemodialysis
III. Malabsorption
  A. Tropical sprue
  B. Nontropical sprue
  C. Drugs: Phenytoin, barbiturates, (?) ethanol
IV. Impaired metabolism
  A. Inhibitors of dihydrofolate reductase: methotrexate, pyrimethamine, triamterene, pentamidine, trimethoprim
  B. Alcohol
  C. Rare enzyme deficiencies: dihydrofolate reductase, others

OTHER CAUSES

I. Drugs that impair DNA metabolism
  A. Purine antagonists: 6-mercaptopurine, azathioprine, etc.
  B. Pyrimidine antagonists: 5-fluorouracil, cytosine arabinoside, etc.
  C. Others: procarbazine, hydroxyurea, acyclovir, zidovudine
II. Metabolic disorders (rare)
  A. Hereditary orotic aciduria
  B. Others
III. Megaloblastic anemia of unknown etiology
  A. Refractory megaloblastic anemia
  B. Di Guglielmo's syndrome*
  C. Congenital dyserythropoietic anemia

* A form of acute nonlymphocytic leukemia with atypical, dysplastic changes in erythroid series.

vitamin to be absorbed. Thus intrinsic factor, like transferrin for iron, serves as a cell-directed carrier protein. The receptor-bound cobalamin-IF complex is taken into the ileal mucosal cell, where the IF is destroyed and the cobalamin is transferred to another transport protein, transcobalamin (TC) II. The cobalamin–TC II complex is then secreted into the circulation, from which it is rapidly taken up by the liver, bone marrow, and other cells. The pathway of cobalamin absorption is shown in Fig. 108-1. Normally, about 2 mg cobalamin is stored in the liver, and another 2 mg is stored elsewhere in the body. In view of the minimum daily requirement, about 3 to 6 years would be required for a normal individual to become deficient in cobalamin if absorption were to cease abruptly.

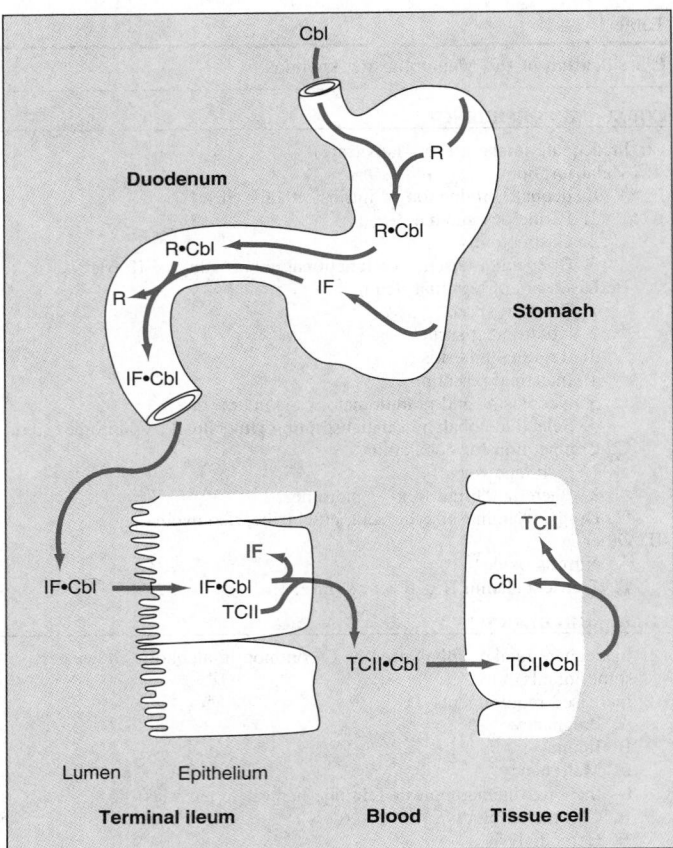

FIGURE 108-1 The assimilation of cobalamin. On entering the stomach, dietary cobalamin (Cbl) forms a complex with R binding protein. As this protein is digested, cobalamin is transferred to intrinsic factor (IF). This complex passes through the intestine until it reaches specific receptors on the mucosa of the distal ileum. The internalized Cbl is then transferred to transcobalamin II (TC II), which circulates in the plasma until it binds to receptors on cells throughout the body and is internalized.

Although TC II is the acceptor for newly absorbed cobalamin, most circulating cobalamin is bound to TC I, a glycoprotein closely related to gastric R binder. TC I appears to be derived in part from leukocytes. The paradox that most circulating cobalamin is bound to TC I rather than TC II, even though TC II initially carries all the cobalamin that is absorbed by the intestine, is explained by the fact that cobalamin bound to TC II is rapidly cleared from the blood ($t_{1/2}$ about 1 h), while clearance of cobalamin bound to TC I requires many days. The function of TC I is unknown.

BIOCHEMICAL CONSIDERATIONS

FOLATE   The prime function of this vitamin is to transfer 1-carbon moieties such as methyl and formyl groups to various organic compounds (see Fig. 108-2). The source of these 1-carbon moieties is usually serine, which reacts with tetrahydrofolate to produce glycine and $N^{5,10}$-methylenetetrahydrofolate. An alternative source is formiminoglutamic acid, an intermediate in histidine catabolism, which gives up its formimino group to tetrahydrofolate to yield N^5-formiminotetrahydrofolate and glutamic acid. These derivatives provide entry into an interconvertible donor pool consisting of tetrahydrofolate derivatives carrying various 1-carbon moieties. The constituents of this pool can donate their 1-carbon moieties to appropriate acceptor compounds to form metabolic intermediates, which are ultimately converted to building blocks used in the synthesis of biologic macromolecules. The most important building blocks are (1) purines, in which the C-2 and

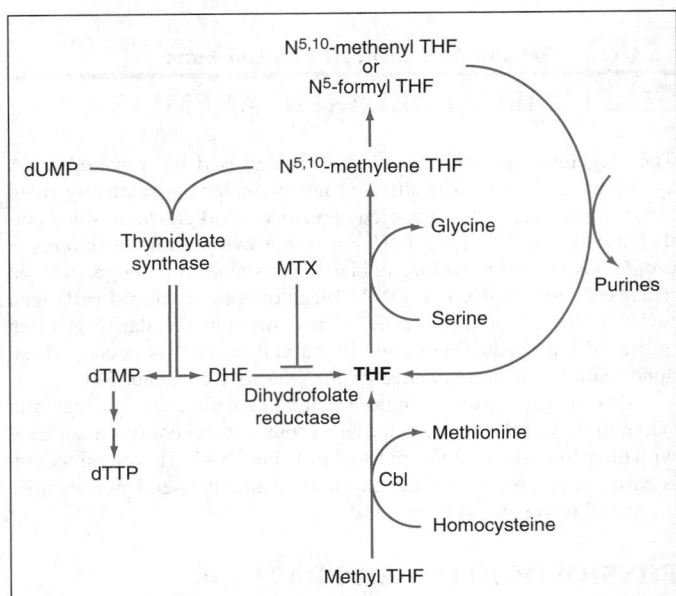

FIGURE 108-2   Folate metabolism. Folate is essential for the de novo synthesis of purines, deoxythymidylate monophosphate (dTMP) and methionine, serving as an intermediate carrier of 1-carbon fragments used in the biosynthesis of these compounds. Its active form is tetrahydrofolate (THF). THF acquires the 1-carbon fragment principally from serine, which is converted to glycine in the course of the reaction. For purine synthesis, the 1-carbon fragment is first oxidized to the level of formic acid, then transferred to substrate. For methionine synthesis, a cobalamin-requiring reaction, the 1-carbon fragment is first reduced to the level of a methyl group, then transferred to homocysteine. In these reactions the cofactor is released as THF, which can immediately participate in another 1-carbon transfer cycle. During the production of dTMP from dUMP, however, the 1-carbon fragment is reduced from formaldehyde to a methyl group in the course of the transfer reaction. The hydrogen atoms used for this reduction come from the cofactor, which is therefore released, not as THF, but as dihydrofolate (DHF). To participate further in the 1-carbon transfer cycle, the DHF has to be re-reduced to THF, a reaction catalyzed by dihydrofolate reductase.

The anemia of cobalamin deficiency is really due to tissue folate deficiency. This deficiency results from an impairment in the cobalamin-dependent transfer of the methyl group from N^5-methylTHF to homocysteine, leading to a delay in the attachment of a polyglutamate chain to the folate molecule (a process known as conjugation) and the leakage of the unconjugated folate out of the cell. Folate therefore corrects the anemia of cobalamin deficiency. The neurologic defects of cobalamin deficiency, however, are thought to result from inadequate methionine synthesis, leading to a deficiency of the methylating agent S-adenosylmethionine and an abnormality in the production of methylated phospholipids such as phosphatidylcholine. Folate does not correct the neurologic defects seen in cobalamin deficiency.

C-8 atoms are introduced in folate-dependent reactions, (2) deoxythymidylate monophosphate (dTMP), synthesized from $N^{5,10}$-methylenetetrahydrofolate and deoxyuridylate monophosphate (dUMP), and (3) methionine, formed by the transfer of a methyl group from N^5-methyltetrahydrofolate to homocysteine (two of these three reactions are shown in Fig. 108-2).

In all but one of the 1-carbon transfer reactions, tetrahydrofolate is produced. It can immediately accept a 1-carbon moiety and reenter the donor pool. The single exception is the thymidylate synthase reaction (dUMP → dTMP), in which dihydrofolate is the product (Fig. 108-2). This must be reduced to tetrahydrofolate by the enzyme dihydrofolate reductase before it can reenter the donor pool. A number of drugs are able to inhibit dihydrofolate reductase (Table 108-1), thereby diverting folate from the donor pool and producing what amounts to a state of folate deficiency in the face of normal tissue folate concentrations.

COBALAMIN   In humans there are two metabolically active forms of cobalamin, identified by the alkyl group attached to the sixth coordination position of the cobalt atom: methylcobalamin and adenosylcobalamin. The vitamin preparation that is used therapeutically is cyanocobalamin (also called vitamin B_{12}). Cyanocobalamin has no known physiologic role and must be converted to a biologically active form before it can be used by tissues.

Methylcobalamin is an essential cofactor in the conversion of homocysteine to methionine (Fig. 108-2). When this reaction is impaired, folate metabolism is deranged, and it is this derangement that is thought to underlie the defect in DNA synthesis and the megaloblastic maturation pattern in patients who are deficient in cobalamin. In cobalamin deficiency, the unconjugated N^5-methyltetrahydrofolate newly taken from the bloodstream cannot be converted to other forms of tetrahydrofolate by methyl transfer. This is the so-called folate trap hypothesis. Because N^5-methyltetrahydrofolate is a poor substrate for the conjugating enzyme, it largely remains in the unconjugated form and slowly leaks from the cell. Tissue folate deficiency therefore develops, and this results in megaloblastic hematopoiesis. This hypothesis explains why tissue folate stores in cobalamin deficiency are substantially reduced, with a disproportionate reduction in conjugated as compared with unconjugated folates, despite normal or supranormal serum folate levels. It also explains why large doses of folate can produce a partial hematologic remission in patients with cobalamin deficiency.

Plasma homocysteine levels are elevated in both folate and cobalamin deficiency, and high levels of plasma homocysteine appear to be a risk factor for thrombosis on both the venous and arterial side. It is not yet known, however, if hyperhomocysteinemia due to folate or cobalamin deficiency predisposes to thrombosis or alters its response to treatment.

Impairment in the conversion of homocysteine to methionine also may be partly responsible for the neurologic complications of cobalamin deficiency (see below). The methionine formed in this reaction is needed for the production of choline and choline-containing phospholipids. Nervous system damage is postulated to result at least in part from interference with these processes due to decreased methionine production in cobalamin deficiency.

Adenosylcobalamin is required for the conversion of methylmalonyl coenzyme A (CoA) to succinyl CoA. Lack of this cofactor leads to large increases in the tissue levels of methylmalonyl CoA and its precursor, propionyl CoA. As a consequence, nonphysiologic fatty acids containing an odd number of carbon atoms are synthesized and incorporated into neuronal lipids. This biochemical abnormality also may contribute to the neurologic complications of cobalamin deficiency (see below).

CLINICAL DISORDERS

CLASSIFICATION OF MEGALOBLASTIC ANEMIAS (See Table 108-1)
The cause of megaloblastic anemia varies in different parts of the world. In temperate zones, folate deficiency in alcoholics and pernicious anemia are the common types of megaloblastic anemias. In certain areas close to the equator, tropical sprue is endemic and an important cause of megaloblastic anemia, while in Scandinavia, it is occasionally secondary to infestations by the fish tapeworm, *Diphyllobothrium latum*.

The dietary intake of cobalamin is more than adequate for the body's requirements, except in true vegetarians (individuals who live on a purely vegetable diet) and their breast-fed infants. Thus deficiency of cobalamin is almost always due to malabsorption. As noted above, the absorption of cobalamin depends on a specific binding protein produced in the stomach and uptake by a specific receptor in the mucosa of the distal ileum. Accordingly, several steps in this process can go awry and lead to malabsorption. In contrast, the dietary intake of folic acid is marginal in many parts of the world. Furthermore, because the body's stores of folate are relatively low, folic acid deficiency can arise rather suddenly during periods of decreased dietary intake or increased metabolic demand. Finally, folic acid deficiency may be due to malabsorption. Often two or more of these factors coexist in a given patient.

Combined deficiencies of cobalamin and folic acid are not uncommon. Patients with tropical sprue are often deficient in both vitamins. The biochemical lesion that results in megaloblastic maturation of bone marrow cells also causes structural and functional abnormalities of the rapidly proliferating epithelial cells of the intestinal mucosa. Thus severe deficiency of one vitamin can lead to malabsorption of the other. Furthermore, as discussed above, a deficiency of cobalamin causes a secondary reduction in cellular folic acid.

Finally, megaloblastic anemias may occasionally be induced by factors unrelated to a vitamin deficiency. Most such cases are caused by one or more of the many drugs that interfere with DNA synthesis. Less commonly, megaloblastic maturation is encountered in certain acquired defects of hematopoietic stem cells. Rarest of all are specific congenital enzyme deficiencies.

COBALAMIN DEFICIENCY There are many conditions in which cobalamin deficiency may develop. Although each has its own characteristic manifestations, certain clinical features are common to all. These clinical features involve the blood, the gastrointestinal tract, and the nervous system.

The hematologic manifestations are almost entirely the result of anemia, although very rarely purpura may appear, due to thrombocytopenia. Symptoms of anemia may include weakness, light-headedness, vertigo, and tinnitus, as well as palpitations, angina, and the symptoms of congestive failure. On physical examination, the patient with florid cobalamin deficiency is pale, with slightly icteric skin and eyes. Elevated bilirubin levels are related to high RBC turnover in the marrow. The pulse is rapid, and the heart may be enlarged; auscultation will usually reveal a systolic flow murmur.

The gastrointestinal manifestations reflect the effect of cobalamin deficiency on the rapidly proliferating gastrointestinal epithelium. The patient sometimes complains of a sore tongue, which on inspection will be smooth and beefy red. Anorexia with moderate weight loss also may be evident, possibly accompanied by diarrhea and other gastrointestinal symptoms. These latter manifestations may be in part caused by megaloblastosis of the small-intestinal epithelium, which results in malabsorption.

The neurologic manifestations often fail to remit fully on treatment. They begin pathologically with demyelination, followed by axonal degeneration and eventual neuronal death; the final stage, of course, is irreversible. Sites of involvement include peripheral nerves; the spinal cord, where the posterior and lateral columns undergo demyelination; and the cerebrum itself. Signs and symptoms include numbness and paresthesias in the extremities (the earliest neurologic manifestations), weakness, and ataxia. There may be sphincter disturbances. Reflexes may be diminished or increased. The Romberg and Babinski signs may be positive, and position and vibration senses are usually diminished. Disturbances of mentation will vary from mild irritability and forgetfulness to severe dementia or frank psychosis. It should be emphasized that *neurologic disease may occur in a patient with a normal hematocrit* and normal RBC indexes.

In the classical patient, in whom hematologic problems predominate, the blood and bone marrow show characteristic megaloblastic changes (described under "Diagnosis" below). The anemia may be very severe—hematocrits of 15 to 20 are not infrequent—but is surprisingly well tolerated by the patient because it develops so slowly.

Pernicious Anemia The most common cause of cobalamin deficiency in temperate climates is pernicious anemia, in which intrinsic factor secretion ceases owing to atrophy of the gastric mucosa. It is most frequently seen in individuals of northern European descent and African-Americans and is much less common in southern Europeans and Asians. Men and women are equally affected. It is a disease of the elderly, the average patient presenting near age 60; it is rare under age 30, although typical pernicious anemia can be seen in children under age 10 (juvenile pernicious anemia). Inherited conditions in which a histologically normal stomach secretes either an abnormal intrinsic factor or none at all will induce cobalamin deficiency in infancy or early childhood.

There is considerable evidence for immunologic abnormalities in pernicious anemia. The incidence of pernicious anemia is substantially increased in patients with other diseases thought to be of immunologic origin, including Graves' disease, myxedema, thyroiditis, idiopathic adrenocortical insufficiency, vitiligo, and hypoparathyroidism. Patients with pernicious anemia also have abnormal circulating antibodies related to their disease: 90 percent have antiparietal cell antibody, while 60 percent have anti-intrinsic factor antibody. Antiparietal cell antibody is also found in 50 percent of patients with gastric atrophy without pernicious anemia, as well as in 10 to 15 percent of an unselected patient population, but anti-intrinsic factor antibody is usually absent from these patients. Relatives of patients with pernicious anemia have an increased incidence of the disease, and even clinically unaffected relatives may have anti-intrinsic factor antibody in their serum. Finally, treatment with glucocorticoids has been reported to reverse the disease both pathologically and clinically.

The destruction of parietal cells in pernicious anemia is thought to be mediated by complement-fixing antibodies against the parietal cell surface. The observation that pernicious anemia is unusually common in patients with agammaglobulinemia, however, suggests that the cellular immune system also may play a role in its pathogenesis. In contrast, *Helicobacter pylori* has little to do with parietal cell destruction in pernicious anemia.

Pathologically, the most characteristic finding in pernicious anemia is gastric atrophy affecting the acid- and pepsin-secreting portion of the stomach; the antrum is spared. Other pathologic changes are secondary to the deficiency of cobalamin; these include megaloblastoid alterations in the gastric and intestinal epithelium and the neurologic changes described above. The abnormalities in the gastric epithelium appear as cellular atypia in gastric cytology specimens, a finding that must be carefully distinguished from the cytologic abnormalities seen in gastric malignancy.

The *clinical manifestations* are primarily those of cobalamin deficiency, as described above. The disease is of insidious onset and progresses slowly. Laboratory examination will reveal hypergastrinemia and pentagastrin-fast achlorhydria as well as the hematologic and other laboratory abnormalities discussed under "Diagnosis."

Through appropriate replacement therapy, patients with pernicious anemia should experience complete and lifelong correction of all abnormalities that are due to cobalamin deficiency, except to the extent that irreversible changes in the nervous system may have occurred before treatment. These patients, however, are unusually subject to gastric polyps and have about twice the normal incidence of cancer of the stomach. Thus, patients should be followed with frequent stool guaiac examinations together with further diagnostic studies when indicated.

Postgastrectomy Following total gastrectomy or extensive damage to gastric mucosa as, for example, by ingestion of corrosive agents, megaloblastic anemia may develop because the source of intrinsic factor has been removed. In such patients, the absorption of orally administered cobalamin is impaired. Megaloblastic anemia also may follow partial gastrectomy, but the incidence is lower than after total gastrectomy, in which cobalamin malabsorption occurs in 100 percent of patients. The cause of cobalamin deficiency after partial gastrectomy may be intestinal overgrowth of bacteria, but it does not always respond to antibiotics.

Intestinal organisms Megaloblastic anemia may occur with intestinal stasis due to anatomic lesions (strictures, diverticula, anastomoses, "blind loops") or pseudoobstruction (diabetes mellitus, scleroderma, amyloid). This anemia is caused by colonization of the small intestine by large masses of bacteria that divert cobalamin from the host. Steatorrhea also may be seen under these circumstances, because bile salt metabolism is disturbed when the intestine is heavily colonized with bacteria. Hematologic responses have been observed after administration of oral antibiotics such as tetracycline and ampicillin.

Megaloblastic anemia is seen, in Scandinavia especially, in persons harboring the fish tapeworm, *D. latum*. The anemia has been attributed to competition by the worm for cobalamin. Destruction of the worm eliminates the problem.

Ileal Abnormalities Cobalamin deficiency is commonly found in tropical sprue, while it is an unusual complication of nontropical sprue (gluten-sensitive enteropathy; see Chap. 285). Virtually any disorder that compromises the absorptive capacity of the distal ileum can result in cobalamin deficiency. Specific entities include regional enteritis, Whipple's disease, and tuberculosis. Segmental involvement of the distal ileum by disease can cause megaloblastic anemia without any other manifestations of intestinal malabsorption such as steatorrhea. Cobalamin malabsorption is also seen after ileal resection. The Zollinger-Ellison syndrome (intense gastric hyperacidity due to a gastrin-secreting tumor) may cause cobalamin malabsorption by acidifying the small intestine. This will retard the transfer of the vitamin from R binder to intrinsic factor and will impair the binding of the cobalamin-IF complex to the ileal receptors. Chronic pancreatitis also may cause cobalamin malabsorption by impairing the transfer of the vitamin from R binder to intrinsic factor. This abnormality can be detected by tests of cobalamin absorption (see below, Schilling test), but it is invariably mild and never causes clinical cobalamin deficiency. Finally, there is a rare congenital disorder, Imerslund-Gräsbeck disease, in which a selective defect in cobalamin absorption is accompanied by proteinuria.

FOLIC ACID DEFICIENCY Patients with folic acid deficiency are more apt to be malnourished than those with cobalamin deficiency. Accordingly, they are likely to appear wasted. The gastrointestinal manifestations are similar to but may be more widespread and more severe than those of pernicious anemia. Diarrhea is often present, and cheilosis and glossitis are also encountered. However, in contrast to cobalamin deficiency, neurologic abnormalities do not occur.

The hematologic manifestations of folic acid deficiency are the same as those of cobalamin deficiency. Folic acid deficiency can generally be attributed to one or more of the following factors: inadequate intake, increased demand, and malabsorption.

Inadequate Intake Folic acid malnutrition is commonly encountered among a number of groups. Alcoholics frequently become folate deficient because their main source of caloric intake is alcoholic beverages. Distilled spirits are virtually devoid of folic acid, while beer and wine do not contain enough of the vitamin to satisfy the daily requirement. In addition, alcohol may interfere with folate metabolism. Narcotic addicts are also prone to become folate deficient because of malnutrition. Many indigent and elderly individuals who subsist primarily on canned foods or "tea and toast" and occasional teenagers whose diet consists of "junk food" develop folate deficiency.

Increased Demand Tissues with a relatively high rate of cell division such as the bone marrow or gut mucosa have a large requirement for folate. Therefore, patients with chronic hemolytic anemias or other causes of very active erythropoiesis may become deficient if their high folate requirement is not met by dietary intake. Likewise, a pregnant woman may become deficient in folic acid because of the high demand of the developing fetus. Deficiency in pregnancy can cause neural tube defects in newborns. Thus, pregnant women should receive oral folate supplementation. Folate deficiency also may occur during the growth spurts of infancy and adolescence. Patients on chronic hemodialysis may require supplementary folate to replace that lost in the dialysate.

Malabsorption Folic acid deficiency is a common accompaniment of tropical sprue. Both the gastrointestinal symptoms and malabsorption are improved by the administration of either folic acid or antibiotics by mouth. Patients with nontropical sprue (gluten-sensitive enteropathy) also may develop significant folic acid deficiency which parallels other parameters of malabsorption. Similarly, folate deficiency in alcoholics may be due in part to malabsorption. In addition, other primary small-bowel disorders are sometimes associated with vitamin deficiency. These entities are all discussed in Chap. 285.

DRUGS Next to deficiency of folate or cobalamin, the most common cause of megaloblastic anemia is drug ingestion. Drugs that cause megaloblastic anemia do so by interfering with DNA synthesis, either directly or by antagonizing the action of folate. They can be classified as follows:

1. *Direct inhibitors of DNA synthesis.* They include purine analogues (6-thioguanine, azathioprine, 6-mercaptopurine), pyrimidine analogues (5-fluorouracil, cytosine arabinoside), and other drugs that interfere with DNA synthesis by a variety of mechanisms (hydroxyurea, procarbazine). The antiviral agent zidovudine (AZT), used for treating the human immunodeficiency virus (HIV), often causes severe megaloblastic anemia.

2. *Folate antagonists.* The most toxic of these is methotrexate, an exceedingly powerful inhibitor of dihydrofolate reductase which is used in the treatment of certain malignancies. Much less toxic but still capable of inducing a megaloblastic anemia are several weak dihydrofolate reductase inhibitors that are used to treat a variety of nonmalignant conditions. These include pentamidine, trimethoprim, triamterene, and pyrimethamine.

The megaloblastic changes in methotrexate poisoning appear to result from a buildup of dUMP owing to impaired methylation to dTMP. The excess dUMP is partially phosphorylated to deoxyuridine triphosphate (dUTP), which accumulates in the cell and is incorporated into newly synthesized DNA. As a result, defective strands of DNA are produced in which T is partly replaced by U. U-rich DNA is also present in folate and cobalamin deficiency, suggesting a similar abnormality in DNA synthesis in the nutritional megaloblastic anemias.

3. *Nitrous oxide.* Nitrous oxide inhalation causes the destruction of endogenous cobalamin. As ordinarily used, this anesthetic does not destroy enough cobalamin to cause clinical manifestations. Repeated or protracted exposure, however, may lead to a megaloblastic anemia. Fatal megaloblastic anemia has been reported in patients with tetanus who were given nitrous oxide continuously for weeks.

4. *Others.* A number of drugs antagonize folate by mechanisms that are poorly understood but are thought to involve an effect on absorption of the vitamin by the intestine. In this category are the anticonvulsants phenytoin (Dilantin) and primidone (Mysoline) and phenobarbital (Luminal). Megaloblastic anemia induced by these agents is mild.

OTHER Hereditary Megaloblastic anemia may be seen in several hereditary disorders. It is a regular feature of orotic aciduria, a deficiency of orotidylic decarboxylase and phosphorylase, leading to a defect in pyrimidine metabolism and characterized by retarded growth and development as well as by the excretion of large amounts of orotic acid. Megaloblastic anemia has been reported in a single case of the Lesch-Nyhan syndrome, a condition resulting from a deficiency of hypoxanthine-guanine phosphoribosyltransferase whose clinical manifestations include gout, mental retardation, and self-mutilation. It also has been described in methylmalonic aciduria due to a combined defect in the biosynthesis of methyl and adenosyl cobalamins, although it is not seen in methylmalonic aciduria due to methylmalonyl CoA mutase deficiency. Congenital folate malabsorption causes megaloblastic anemia, accompanied by ataxia and mental retardation. Megaloblastic anemia has been reported to accompany the congenital deficiency of two other folate-metabolizing enzymes: dihydrofolate reductase and N^5-methyltetrahydrofolate:homocysteine methyltransferase. These deficiencies are less well documented than is congenital folate malabsorption. A thiamine-responsive megaloblastic anemia accompanied by nerve deafness and diabetes mellitus has been reported in several children. Megaloblastic changes as well as multinuclearity of red blood cell precursors are seen in the marrow of certain patients with congenital dyserythropoietic anemia, a group of inherited disorders characterized by mild to moderate anemia presenting at any age and pursuing a benign course.

Transcobalamin II deficiency, like the congenital abnormalities in cobalamin absorption described previously, causes pronounced deficiency in cobalamin in infancy or early childhood, with all the accompanying manifestations. Megaloblastic anemia is not seen in hereditary TC I deficiency.

Refractory Megaloblastic Anemia This is a form of myelodysplasia in which megaloblastic erythropoiesis may sometimes be seen. Megaloblastic changes are restricted to the RBC series; large granulocyte precursors and giant metamyelocytes are not seen (see below). As with other forms of myelodysplasia, refractory megaloblastic anemia is associated with an increased incidence of acute leukemia.

Megaloblastic changes are seen in erythremic myelosis and acute erythroleukemia (di Guglielmo), where RBC precursors are prominently involved. Here, the marrow is characterized by bizarre erythroid maturation, with multinuclearity and multipolar mitotic figures in the RBC precursors. Erythroleukemia is discussed further in Chap. 112.

MEGALOBLASTIC DISEASE WITHOUT ANEMIA Megaloblastic disease is easily overlooked in non-anemic patients. It can present in one of two ways.

Acute Megaloblastic Anemia Occasionally, a full-blown megaloblastic state can develop over the course of just a few days. This is usually seen following nitrous oxide anesthesia but may occur in any patient with a serious illness requiring intensive care, especially a patient receiving multiple transfusions, dialysis, or total parenteral nutrition. An acute megaloblastic state also can be precipitated by the administration of a weak antifolate (e.g., trimethoprim) to a patient with marginal tissue folate stores.

The condition resembles an immune cytopenia, with a rapidly developing thrombocytopenia and/or leukopenia in the absence of anemia. The blood smear may be completely normal, but the marrow is always floridly megaloblastic. Acute megaloblastic anemia responds rapidly to treatment with folate plus cobalamin in the usual therapeutic doses.

Cobalamin Deficiency without Anemia Cobalamin deficiency without hematologic abnormalities is surprisingly common, especially in the elderly. These patients may present with neuropsychiatric abnormalities, including peripheral neuropathies, gait disturbance, memory loss, and psychiatric symptoms, sometimes with abnormal evoked potentials. Serum cobalamin levels may be normal or low, but serum levels of methylmalonic acid are almost invariably increased due to a deficiency of cobalamin at the tissue level. The neuropsychiatric abnormalities tend to improve and serum methylmalonic acid levels generally return to normal after treatment with cobalamin.

DIAGNOSIS The finding of significant macrocytosis [mean corpuscular volume (MCV) > 100 fL] suggests the presence of a megaloblastic anemia. Other causes of macrocytosis include hemolysis, liver disease, alcoholism, hypothyroidism, and aplastic anemia. If the macrocytosis is marked (MCV > 110 fL), the patient is much more likely to have a megaloblastic anemia. Macrocytosis is less marked with concurrent iron deficiency or thalassemia. The reticulocyte count is low, and the leukocyte and platelet count also may be decreased, particularly in severely anemic patients. The blood smear **(see Plate IV-2)** demonstrates marked anisocytosis and poikilocytosis, together with macroovalocytes, which are large, oval, fully hemoglobinized erythrocytes typical of megaloblastic anemias. There is some basophilic stippling, and an occasional nucleated RBC may be seen. In the white blood cell series, the neutrophils show hypersegmentation of the nucleus. This is such a characteristic finding that a single cell with a nucleus of six lobes or more should raise the immediate suspicion of a megaloblastic anemia. A rare myelocyte also may be seen. Bizarre, misshapen platelets are also observed. The bone marrow examination is very helpful in the diagnosis of megaloblastic anemia. The marrow is hypercellular with a decreased myeloid/erythroid ratio and abundant stainable iron. RBC precursors are abnormally large and have nuclei that appear much less mature than would be expected from the development of the cytoplasm (nuclear-cytoplasmic asynchrony). The nuclear chromatin is more dispersed than it should be and consequently stains less intensely than normal. To the extent that it is aggregated, it condenses in a peculiar fenestrated pattern that is very characteristic of megaloblastic erythropoiesis. Abnormal mitoses may be seen. Granulocyte precursors are also affected, many being larger than normal, including giant bands and metamyelocytes. Megakaryocytes are decreased and show abnormal morphology.

Megaloblastic anemias are characterized by ineffective erythropoiesis (Chap. 59). In a severely megaloblastic patient, as many as 90 percent of the RBC precursors may be destroyed before they are released into the bloodstream, compared with 10 to 15 percent in the normal subject. Enhanced intramedullary destruction of erythroblasts results in an increase in unconjugated bilirubin and lactic acid dehydrogenase (isoenzyme 1) in plasma. Abnormalities in iron kinetics also attest to the presence of ineffective erythropoiesis, with increased iron turnover but low incorporation of labeled iron into circulating RBC.

In evaluating a patient with megaloblastic anemia, it is important to determine whether there is a specific vitamin deficiency by measuring serum cobalamin and folate levels. The normal range of cobalamin in serum is 200 to 900 pg/mL; values less than 100 pg/mL indicate clinically significant deficiency. The normal serum concentration of folic acid ranges from 6 to 20 ng/mL; values of 4 ng/mL or less are generally considered to be diagnostic of folate deficiency. Unlike serum cobalamin, serum folate levels may reflect recent alterations in dietary intake. Measurement of RBC folate level provides useful information because it is not subject to short-term fluctuations in folate intake and is, therefore, better than serum folate as an index of folate stores.

Once cobalamin deficiency has been established, its pathogenesis can be delineated by means of a Schilling test. A patient is given radioactive cobalamin by mouth, followed shortly thereafter by an intramuscular injection of unlabeled cobalamin. The proportion of the administered radioactivity excreted in the urine during the next 24 h provides an accurate measure of absorption of cobalamin, assuming that a complete urine sample has been collected. Because cobalamin deficiency is almost always due to malabsorption (see Table 108-1), this first stage of the Schilling test should be abnormal (i.e., small amounts of radioactivity in the urine). The patient is then given labeled cobalamin bound to intrinsic factor. Absorption of the vitamin will now approach normal if the patient has pernicious anemia or some other type of intrinsic factor deficiency. If cobalamin absorption is still decreased, the patient may have bacterial overgrowth (blind loop syndrome) or ileal disease (including an ileal absorptive defect secondary to the cobalamin deficiency itself). Cobalamin malabsorption due to bacterial overgrowth can frequently be corrected by the administration of antibiotics. The Schilling test can provide equally reliable information after the patient has had adequate therapy with parenteral cobalamin.

A normal Schilling test in a patient with documented cobalamin deficiency may indicate poor absorption of the vitamin when mixed with food. This can be established by repeating the Schilling test with radioactive cobalamin scrambled with an egg.

Serum methylmalonic acid and homocysteine are useful in the diagnosis of megaloblastic anemias. Levels of both are elevated in cobalamin deficiency, while elevated levels of homocysteine but not methylmalonic acid are seen in folate deficiency. These tests measure tissue vitamin stores and may demonstrate a deficiency even when the more traditional but less reliable folate and cobalamin levels are normal. Patients (particularly older patients) with normal serum cobalamin levels but elevated levels of serum methylmalonic acid may develop neuropsychiatric abnormalities. Treatment of patients with this "subtle" cobalamin deficiency may result in improvement.

℞ TREATMENT

Cobalamin Deficiency Apart from specific therapy related to the underlying disorder (e.g., antibiotics for intestinal overgrowth with bacteria), the mainstay of treatment for cobalamin deficiency is replacement therapy. Because the defect often is one of absorption, replacement should be administered parenterally, specifically in the form of intramuscular cyanocobalamin. (If intramuscular administration is contraindicated or refused, cobalamin deficiency can be managed by oral replacement therapy, but at doses of 300 to 1000 μg daily, it is an expensive mode of treatment that requires very close

medical supervision to avoid relapse.) Treatment should be started with 100 μg cobalamin per day for a week. The frequency of administration of the vitamin may then be decreased, the goal being to give a total of 2000 μg during the first 6 weeks. The patient may then be placed on 100 μg cyanocobalamin intramuscularly every month, a regimen that must be maintained for the rest of the patient's life. If necessary, larger doses may be given at less frequent intervals (e.g., 1 mg every 2 to 4 months), but the risk of relapse is substantially greater than if the vitamin is given monthly.

The response to treatment is gratifying. Shortly after treatment is begun, and several days before a hematologic response is evident in the peripheral blood, the patient will experience an increase in strength and an improved sense of well-being. Marrow morphology begins to revert toward normal within a few hours after treatment is initiated. Reticulocytosis begins 4 to 5 days after therapy is started and peaks at about day 7 (Fig. 108-3), with subsequent remission of the anemia over the next several weeks. If a reticulocytosis does not occur, or if it is less brisk than expected from the level of the hematocrit, a search should be made for other factors contributing to the anemia (e.g., infection, coexisting folate deficiency, or hypothyroidism). Hypokalemia and salt retention may occur early in the course of therapy. Thrombocytosis may also be seen.

In most cases, replacement therapy is all that is needed for the treatment of cobalamin deficiency. Occasionally, however, a patient with a severe anemia will have such a precarious cardiovascular status that emergency transfusion is necessary. This must be done with great care, because it is very easy to precipitate florid congestive failure in such patients by fluid overload. Blood must be administered slowly in the form of packed cells, with very close observation, giving as an initial dose no more than 100 mL. This small volume will frequently be enough to ameliorate the cardiovascular problems sufficiently that further therapy can be restricted to cobalamin replacement. If necessary, blood may be administered by exchanging patient blood (mostly plasma) for packed cells.

With lifelong treatment, patients should experience no further manifestations of cobalamin deficiency. As previously stated, neurologic symptoms may not be fully corrected even by optimal therapy. The potential for late development of gastric carcinoma in pernicious anemia necessitates careful follow-up of the patient.

Folate Deficiency As for cobalamin deficiency, folate deficiency is treated by replacement therapy. The usual dose of folate is 1 mg/d, by mouth, but higher doses (up to 5 mg/d) may be required for folate deficiency due to malabsorption. Parenteral folate is rarely necessary. The hematologic response is similar to that seen after replacement therapy for cobalamin deficiency—that is, a brisk reticulocytosis after about 4 days, followed by correction of the anemia over the next 1 to 2 months. The duration of therapy depends on the basis of the deficiency state. Patients with a continuously increased requirement (such as patients with hemolytic anemia) or those with malabsorption or chronic malnutrition should continue to receive oral

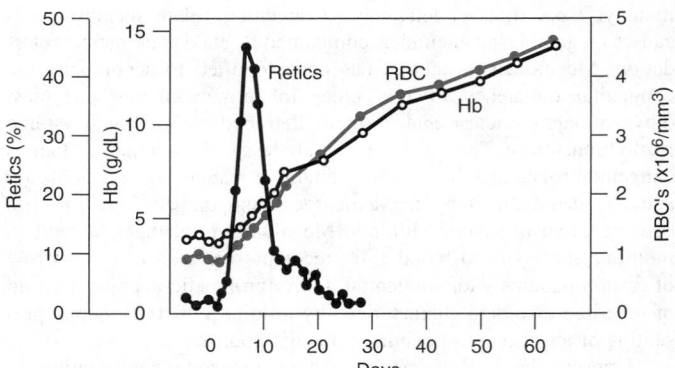

FIGURE 108-3 Hematologic response of a patient with pernicious anemia to an intramuscular injection of 100 μg cobalamin on day 0. (From A Erslev, TG Gabuzda, *Pathophysiology of Blood,* Philadelphia, Saunders, 1975, with permission.)

folic acid indefinitely. In addition, the patient should be encouraged to maintain an optimal diet containing adequate amounts of folate.

Folate, particularly in large doses, can correct the megaloblastic anemia of cobalamin deficiency without altering the neurologic abnormalities. The neurologic manifestations may even be aggravated by folate therapy. Cobalamin deficiency can thus be masked in patients who for one reason or another are taking large doses of folate. For this reason, a hematologic response to folate must never be used to rule out cobalamin deficiency in a given patient; cobalamin deficiency can be excluded only by appropriate laboratory evaluation.

Other Causes of Megaloblastic Anemia Megaloblastic anemia due to drugs can be treated, if necessary, by reducing the dose of the drug or eliminating it altogether. The effects of folate antagonists that inhibit dihydrofolate reductase can be counteracted by folinic acid [5-formyl tetrahydrofolate (THF)] in a dose of 100 to 200 mg/d (Fig. 108-2). It circumvents the block in folate metabolism imposed by dihydrofolate reductase inhibitors, replenishing the tissues with a form of folate that can directly enter the 1-carbon donor pool. Certain of the congenital megaloblastic anemia–producing enzyme deficiencies can be treated by appropriate specific therapeutic regimens. For the megaloblastic forms of sideroblastic anemia, pyridoxine in pharmacologic doses (as high as 300 mg/d) should be tried. Pyridoxalphosphate may also work presumably in part through promoting the conversion of THF to 5,10-methylene THF. A few patients will respond to one or the other vitamin B_6 congener. Simple supportive measures are all that appear to be in order for treatment of refractory megaloblastic anemia. Acute erythroleukemia (di Guglielmo's disease) is usually treated like other types of acute nonlymphocytic leukemia (see Chap. 112).

See Chap. 53, Hematopoietic agents: Growth factors, minerals, and vitamins, in Goodman & Gilman's The Pharmacological Basis of Therapeutics, 9th ed, New York, McGraw-Hill, 1996.

BIBLIOGRAPHY

ALLEN RH et al: Metabolic abnormalities in cobalamin [vitamin B_{12}] and folate deficiencies. FASEB J 7:1344, 1993

BABIOR BM: The megaloblastic anemias, in *Williams' Hematology*, 5th ed, E Beutler et al (eds). New York, McGraw-Hill, 1995, p 471

CARMEL R et al: The frequently low cobalamin levels in dementia usually signify treatable metabolic, neurologic and electrophysiologic abnormalities. Eur J Haematol 54:245, 1995

COOPER TR, ROSENBLATT DS: Inherited defects of vitamin B_{12} metabolism. Annu Rev Nutr 7:291, 1987

DICKINSON CJ: Does folic acid harm people with vitamin B_{12} deficiency? QJM 88:357, 1995

HSING AW et al: Pernicious anemia and subsequent cancer. Cancer 71:745, 1993

KAPADIA CR, DONALDSON RM: Disorders of cobalamin (vitamin B_{12}) absorption and transport. Annu Rev Med 36:93, 1985

LINDENBAUM J et al: Neuropsychiatric disorders caused by cobalamin deficiency in the absence of anemia or macrocytosis. N Engl J Med 318:1720, 1988

SAVAGE DG et al: Sensitivity of serum methylmalonic acid and total homocysteine determinations for diagnosing cobalamin and folate deficiencies. Am J Med 96:239, 1994

SCHILLING RF, WILLIAMS WJ: Vitamin B_{12} deficiency: Underdiagnosed, overtreated? Hosp Prac (Off Ed) 30:47, 1995

STABLER SP et al: Clinical spectrum and diagnosis of cobalamin deficiency. Blood 75:871, 1990

WATERS HM et al: High incidence of type II autoantibodies in pernicious anemia. J Clin Pathol 46:45, 1993

109   *Wendell Rosse, H. Franklin Bunn*

HEMOLYTIC ANEMIAS AND ACUTE BLOOD LOSS

Anemia may be caused by the loss of red cells either through hemorrhage or, less commonly, through premature destruction of the red cells (hemolysis) by a number of mechanisms. Hemolysis or blood loss will lead to an increase in red cell production, which is clinically manifested by an increase in the reticulocyte production index to greater than three times normal.

HEMOLYTIC ANEMIAS

Red blood cells (RBC) normally survive 90 to 120 days in the circulation. Red cell life span may be shortened in a number of disorders, often resulting in anemia if the bone marrow is not able to replenish adequately the prematurely destroyed red cells. The disorders associated with hemolytic anemias are generally identified by the abnormality that brings about the premature destruction of the red cells. In this chapter, we shall describe the general attributes of this important group of anemias, the diagnostic procedures useful in identifying the causes of the accelerated red cell breakdown, and the pathogenesis and management of specific hemolytic disorders.

In all patients with hemolytic anemia, a careful history and physical examination are important in the diagnosis. The patient may complain of fatigue and other symptoms of anemia (see Chap. 59). Less commonly, jaundice and even red-brown urine (hemoglobinuria) are reported. A complete drug and toxin exposure history and the family history are important in the diagnosis. The physical examination may show icterus and jaundice of skin and mucosae. The cardiac signs of anemia (flow murmurs, etc.) may be present. Splenomegaly is encountered in a variety of hemolytic anemias. As discussed in detail in this chapter, a wide array of other historical and physical findings is associated with specific hemolytic anemias.

Laboratory tests may be used initially to demonstrate the presence of hemolysis (Table 109-1) and then to demonstrate the cause of hemolysis. Elevation of the reticulocyte count in the anemic patient is the most useful indicator of hemolysis, reflecting erythroid hyperplasia of the bone marrow; biopsy of the bone marrow is often unnecessary. Reticulocytes are also elevated in patients with active blood loss, those with myelophthisis, and those who are recovering from suppression of erythropoiesis (see Chap. 59). The morphology of the red cells as seen on the peripheral blood film is often abnormal and may provide evidence both of hemolysis and of its cause; the characteristic abnormalities and their associated causes and syndromes are listed in Table 109-2. While the peripheral blood smear alone is rarely if ever truly pathognomonic, in many cases it is a low-cost, important clue to the presence of hemolysis and to diagnosis.

Red blood cells may be prematurely removed from the circulation by macrophages, particularly those of the spleen and liver (extravascular lysis), or less commonly by disruption of their membranes during their circulation (intravascular hemolysis). Both mechanisms result in increased heme catabolism and enhanced formation of the tetrapyrrole

Table 109-1

Laboratory Evaluation of Hemolysis

	Extravascular	Intravascular
HEMATOLOGIC		
Routine blood film	Polychromatophilia	Polychromatophilia
Reticulocyte count	↑	↑
Bone marrow examination	Erythroid hyperplasia	Erythroid hyperplasia
PLASMA OR SERUM		
Bilirubin	↑ Unconjugated	↑ Unconjugated
Haptoglobin	↓, Absent	Absent
Plasma hemoglobin	N – ↑	↑ ↑
Lactate dehydrogenase	↑ (Variable)	↑ ↑ (Variable)
URINE		
Bilirubin	0	0
Hemosiderin	0	+
Hemoglobin	0	+ in severe cases

Table 109-2

The Value of Red Blood Cell Morphology in Diagnosis of Hemolytic Anemia

Morphology	Cause	Syndromes
Spherocytes	Loss of membrane	Hereditary spherocytosis, autoimmune hemolytic anemia
Target cells	Increased ratio of RBC surface area to volume	Hemoglobin disorders: thalassemias, hemoglobin S, C, etc.; liver disease
Schistocytes	Traumatic disruption of membrane	Microangiopathic conditions, intravascular prostheses
Sickled cells	Polymerization of hemoglobin S	Sickle cell syndromes
Acanthocytes	?Abnormal membrane lipids	Severe liver disease (spur cell anemias)
Agglutinated cells	Presence of IgM antibody	Cold agglutinin disease
Heinz bodies	Precipitated hemoglobin	Unstable hemoglobin, oxidant stress

unconjugated bilirubin, which is normally metabolized by the liver by conjugation and subsequent excretion. The plasma level of unconjugated bilirubin may be high enough to produce readily apparent jaundice. The unconjugated (indirect) bilirubin level can be further elevated by a commonly encountered defect in transport of bilirubin (Gilbert's syndrome) (see Chap. 294). In patients with hemolysis, the level of unconjugated bilirubin never exceeds 70 to 85 μmol/L (4 to 5 mg/dL), unless liver function is impaired.

Other serum tests are also useful in the assessment of hemolysis. *Haptoglobin* is an alpha globulin that is present in high concentration (~1.0 g/L) in the plasma (and serum). It binds specifically and tightly to the protein (globin) in hemoglobin. The hemoglobin-haptoglobin complex is cleared within minutes by the mononuclear phagocyte system. Thus patients with significant hemolysis, either intravascular or extravascular, have low or absent levels of serum haptoglobin. Haptoglobin synthesis is decreased in patients with hepatocellular disease. Conversely, synthesis is enhanced in inflammatory states. These facts must be considered in the interpretation of serum haptoglobin. Intravascular hemolysis (which is relatively uncommon) results in the release of hemoglobin into the plasma. In these cases, plasma hemoglobin is increased in proportion to the degree of hemolysis but may be falsely elevated due to lysis of red cells in vitro. If the haptoglobin-binding capacity of the plasma is exceeded, free hemoglobin passes through renal glomeruli. This filtered hemoglobin is reabsorbed by the proximal tubule, where it is catabolized in situ, and the heme iron is incorporated into storage proteins (ferritin and hemosiderin). The presence of hemosiderin in the urine, detected by staining the sediment with Prussian blue, indicates that a significant amount of circulating free hemoglobin has been filtered by the kidneys. Hemosiderin appears 3 to 4 days after the onset of hemoglobinuria and may persist for weeks after its cessation. When the absorptive capacity of the tubular cells is exceeded, hemoglobinuria results. The presence of hemoglobinuria indicates severe intravascular hemolysis. Hemoglobinuria must be distinguished from hematuria (in which case red cells are seen in the examination of a fresh specimen of urine) and from myoglobin due to rhabdomyolysis; in all three cases, the urine will be positive with the benzidine reaction, commonly used in analysis of urine. The distinction between hemoglobinuria and myoglobinuria can best be made by specific tests that exploit immunologic differences or differences in solubility. After centrifugation of an anticoagulated specimen, the plasma of patients with hemoglobinuria has a reddish-brown color, whereas that of patients with myoglobinuria is normal in color. Because of its higher molecular weight, hemoglobin has

lower glomerular permeability than myoglobin and is less rapidly cleared by the kidneys.

CLASSIFICATION The hemolytic anemias can be conveniently grouped in three different ways, shown in Table 109-3. From an anatomic vantage point, the cause of accelerated red cell destruction can be regarded as either (1) a molecular defect (hemoglobinopathy or enzymopathy) inside the red cell, (2) an abnormality in membrane structure and function, or (3) an environmental factor such as mechanical trauma or an autoantibody. In *intracorpuscular types* of hemolysis, the patient's red cells have an abnormally short life span in a normal recipient (with a compatible blood type), while compatible normal red cells survive normally in the patient. The opposite is true in *extracorpuscular types* of hemolysis. Finally, as exemplified in the organization of the remainder of this chapter, hemolytic disorders can be conveniently classified as either inherited or acquired.

INHERITED HEMOLYTIC ANEMIAS The inherited hemolytic anemias are due to inborn defects in one of three main components of red cells: the membrane, the enzymes, or hemoglobin. With the advent of biochemical genetics, these defects are often known at the genomic level, but for the most part we still rely on the clinical and usual laboratory manifestations for their identification.

Red Cell Membrane Disorders These are usually readily detected by morphologic abnormalities of the red cells on examination of the blood film. There are three types of inherited abnormalities of the red cell membrane: hereditary spherocytosis, hereditary elliptocytosis (including hereditary pyropoikilocytosis), and hereditary stomatocytosis.

Hereditary spherocytosis This condition is characterized by spherical red cells due to a molecular defect in one of the proteins in the cytoskeleton of the red cell membrane, leading to a loss of membrane and hence decreased ratio of surface area to volume and consequently spherocytosis. This disorder usually has an autosomal dominant inheritance pattern and an incidence of approximately 1:1000 to 1:4500. In 20 percent of patients, the absence of hematologic abnormalities in family members suggests either autosomal recessive inheritance or, less commonly, a spontaneous mutation. The disorder is sometimes clinically apparent in early infancy but often escapes detection until adult life.

CLINICAL MANIFESTATIONS The major clinical features of hereditary spherocytosis are anemia, splenomegaly, and jaundice. The prominence of the last finding accounts for its prior designation as "congenital hemolytic jaundice" and is due to an increased concentration of unconjugated (indirect-reacting) bilirubin in plasma. Jaundice may be intermittent and tends to be less pronounced in early childhood. Because of the increased bile pigment production, gallstones of pigment type are common, even in childhood. Compensatory erythroid hyperplasia of the bone marrow occurs, with the extension of red marrow into the midshafts of long bones and occasionally with extramedullary erythropoiesis, at times leading to the formation of paravertebral masses visible on chest x-ray. Because the bone marrow's capacity to increase erythropoiesis by six- to eightfold exceeds the usual rate of hemolysis in this disease, anemia is usually mild or moderate and

Table 109-3

Classifications of Hemolytic Anemias

Intracorpuscular	1. Abnormalities of RBC interior
	  a. Enzyme defects
	  b. Hemoglobinopathies (Chap. 107)
	2. RBC membrane abnormalities
	  a. Hereditary spherocytosis etc.
	  b. Paroxysmal nocturnal hemoglobinuria
	  c. Spur cell anemia

Extracorpuscular	3. Extrinsic factors
	  a. Hypersplenism
	  b. Antibody: immune hemolysis
	  c. Microangiopathic hemolysis
	  d. Infections, toxins, etc.

Hereditary (items 1 and 2); Acquired (item 3)

FIGURE 109-1 Osmotic fragility of red blood cells in hereditary spherocytosis (HS). The cells of two patients are compared to normal red cells.

may even be absent in an otherwise healthy individual. Compensation may be temporarily interrupted by episodes of erythroid hypoplasia precipitated by infections, particularly parvovirus. Splenomegaly is a very common finding in hereditary spherocytosis. The hemolytic rate may increase transiently during systemic infections, which induce further splenic enlargement. Chronic leg ulcers, similar to those observed in sickle cell anemia, occur occasionally.

The characteristic erythrocyte abnormality is the spherocyte (**Plate IV-10**). The mean corpuscular volume (MCV) is usually normal or slightly decreased, and the mean corpuscular hemoglobin concentration (MCHC) is increased to 350 to 400 g/L. Spheroidicity may be quantitatively assessed by measurement of the osmotic fragility of the red cells upon exposure to hypoosmotic solutions causing a net influx of water (Fig. 109-1). Because spherocytes have a decreased surface area per unit volume, they are able to take in less water and hence lyse at a higher concentration of saline than normal cells. On microscopic examination, spherocytes are usually detected as small cells without central pallor. They will ordinarily not influence the osmotic fragility test unless they constitute more than 1 or 2 percent of the total cell population. An increase in the osmotic fragility of RBC following sterile incubation of whole blood for 24 h at 37°C is also characteristic of hereditary spherocytosis. The autohemolysis test which measures the amount of spontaneous hemolysis occurring after 48 h of sterile incubation is also useful. In hereditary spherocytosis, about 10 to 50

percent of the RBC are lysed (versus fewer than 4 percent of normal red blood cells). Autohemolysis of these RBC is largely prevented by the addition of glucose prior to incubation.

PATHOGENESIS The molecular abnormality in hereditary spherocytosis involves the proteins of the underlying cytoskeleton, primarily those responsible for tethering the lipid bilayer to the underlying cytoskeletal network. Nearly all patients have a significant deficiency of spectrin, which is sometimes secondary to an inherited molecular defect in that protein. About 50 percent of patients have a defect in ankyrin, the protein that forms a bridge between protein 3 and spectrin (Fig. 109-2). Those who have a recessive inheritance pattern for ankyrin deficiency have more severe anemia than those with the more common dominant form. About 25 percent of patients have a mutation of protein 3, resulting in a deficiency of that protein and mild anemia with dominant inheritance. Most of the remaining 25 percent have mutations of spectrin, leading to impaired synthesis or self-association; β-spectrin deficiency is generally mild, with dominant inheritance, while α-spectrin deficiency is severe, with a recessive inheritance pattern. Because the lipid bilayer is not well anchored when these proteins are defective, part of it is lost by vesiculation, resulting in a more spherical and less deformable cell. Because of their shape and rigidity, spherocytes cannot traverse the interstices of the spleen, especially those in the lining of the splenic venous sinuses, and they are exposed to an environment in which their increased metabolic rate cannot be sustained, causing a further loss of surface membrane. This "conditioning" produces a subpopulation of hyperspheroidal RBC in the peripheral blood.

DIAGNOSIS Hereditary spherocytosis must be distinguished primarily from the spherocytic hemolytic anemias associated with RBC antibodies. The family history of anemia and/or splenectomy is helpful, when present. The diagnosis of immune spherocytosis is usually readily established by a positive direct Coombs test (see below). Spherocytes are also seen in association with hemolysis induced by splenomegaly in patients with cirrhosis, in clostridial infections, and in certain snake envenomations (due to the action of phospholipases on the membrane). A few spherocytes are seen in the course of a wide variety of hemolytic disorders, particularly glucose-6-phosphate dehydrogenase (G6PD) deficiency.

FIGURE 109-2 Diagram of a cross section of the red blood cell membrane. Spectrin, actin, tropomyosin, and protein 4.1 form a meshwork that laminates the inner surface of the membrane. In contrast, other proteins such as the glycophorins (GP) and protein 3 (anion transport channel) traverse the lipid bilayer. Long polysaccharide chains are covalently attached to these proteins on the outer surface of the cell and also to glycolipid. Ankyrin and protein

4.2 form a bridge between spectrin and a fraction of the anion transport proteins. Protein 4.1 binds to GP. Phsopholipids in the lipd bilayer include phosphatidylcholine (PC) and sphingomyelin (SM), which are located primarily on the outer surface of the membrane, and phosphatidylserine (PS) and phosphatidylethanolamine (PE), which are located primarily on the inner surface of the membrane.

℞ TREATMENT

Splenectomy reliably corrects the anemia, although the RBC defect and its consequent morphology persist. The operative risk is low. RBC survival after splenectomy is normal or nearly so; if it is not, an accessory spleen or another diagnosis should be sought. Because of the potential for gallstones and for episodes of bone marrow hypoplasia or hemolytic crises, splenectomy should be performed in individuals in whom the disease causes symptoms; cholecystectomy should not be performed without splenectomy, as intrahepatic gallstones may result. Splenectomy in children should be postponed until age 4, if possible, in order to minimize the risk of severe infections with gram-positive encapsulated organisms. Polyvalent pneumococcal vaccine should be administered to all patients before they undergo splenectomy. In patients with hemolysis, folic acid (1 mg/d) should be administered prophylactically.

Hereditary elliptocytosis and hereditary pyropolkilocytosis Red blood cells of oval or elliptic shape are normally found in birds, reptiles, camels, and llamas; however, they occur in appreciable numbers in humans only in *hereditary elliptocytosis*, a disorder that is transmitted as an autosomal dominant trait and affects 1 per 4000 to 5000 of the population, a frequency similar to that of hereditary spherocytosis (rarely, patients with myelodysplastic disorders of the bone marrow may have acquired elliptocytosis). The elliptic shape is acquired as the cell deforms to traverse the microcirculation but does not spring back to its initial biconcave shape. In most affected individuals, this is due to a structural abnormality of erythrocyte spectrin that leads to impaired assembly of the cytoskeleton. In some families, affected individuals have a deficiency of erythrocyte membrane protein 4.1, which is important in stabilizing the interaction of spectrin and actin in the cytoskeleton (see Fig. 109-2); homozygotes with total absence of this protein have more marked hemolysis. In Southeast Asia there is a high incidence of hereditary ovalocytosis, in which a small internal deletion of protein 3 makes the membrane rigid and confers resistance against malaria.

The great majority of patients manifest only mild hemolysis, with hemoglobin levels above 120 g/L, reticulocytes less than 4 percent, depressed haptoglobin levels, and RBC survivals just under the normal range. In 10 to 15 percent of patients with more severe abnormalities, the rate of hemolysis is substantially increased, with median survival times of RBC as short as 5 days and reticulocytes ranging up to 20 percent. Hemoglobin levels rarely fall below 90 to 100 g/L. RBC destruction occurs predominantly in the spleen, which is enlarged in patients with overt hemolysis. Hemolysis is corrected by splenectomy.

In both the anemic and nonanemic varieties of this disorder, at least 25 percent and, more commonly, greater than 75 percent of RBC are elliptic, with an axial ratio (width/length) of less than 0.78. Patients with hemolysis frequently have microovalocytes, bizarre-shaped RBC, and red cell fragments, all of which increase in number following splenectomy. The degree of hemolysis does not correlate with the percentage of elliptocytes. Osmotic fragility is usually normal but may be increased in patients with overt hemolysis.

Hereditary pyropoikilocytosis is related to hereditary elliptocytosis, since both have been encountered in the same family. Hereditary pyropoikilocytosis is a rare disorder characterized by bizarre-shaped, microcytic red cells that undergo disruption at temperatures of 44 to 45°C (in contrast, normal red cells are stable up to 49°C). This results from a deficiency of spectrin and an abnormality of spectrin self-assembly. Hemolysis, which is usually severe, is recognized in childhood and is partially responsive to splenectomy.

Hereditary stomatocytosis Stomatocytes are RBC that are concave on one face and convex on the other. This results in a slitlike central zone of pallor on dried smears. The syndrome of hereditary hemolytic anemia and stomatocytic RBC is inherited in an autosomal dominant pattern. RBC have an increased permeability to sodium and potassium, which is compensated for by an increased active transport of these cations. In some patients, the RBC is swollen with an excess of ions and water and a decreased mean corpuscular hemoglobin concentration (overhydrated stomatocytes, "hydrocytosis"); many of these patients lack the red cell membrane protein 7.2 (stomatin). In other patients, the red cell is shrunken, with a decreased ion and water content and an increased mean corpuscular hemoglobin concentration (dehydrated stomatocytes, "desiccytosis" or "xerocytosis"). Those patients in whom the RBC are overhydrated have true stomatocytes on dried smears. Dehydrated stomatocytes assume the morphology of target cells on dried smears. In both instances, RBC are cup- or bowl-shaped when examined in wet preparation. Osmotic fragility is increased in overhydrated stomatocytes and decreased in underhydrated stomatocytes. Autohemolysis is increased and is corrected by glucose. Red cells lacking Rh proteins (Rh_{null} cells) are stomatocytic and have a shortened life span.

Most patients have splenomegaly and mild anemia. Splenectomy decreases but does not totally correct the hemolytic process; the indications for it are similar to those for hereditary spherocytosis.

Red Cell Enzyme Defects During its maturation, the RBC loses its nucleus, ribosomes, and mitochondria and thus its capability for protein synthesis and oxidative phosphorylation. The mature circulating RBC has a relatively simple pattern of intermediary metabolism (Fig. 109-3) in keeping with its modest metabolic obligations. ATP must be generated from the Embden-Meyerhof pathway to drive the cation pump which maintains the ionic milieu within the RBC. Smaller amounts of energy are needed for the preservation of hemoglobin iron in the ferrous (Fe^{2+}) state and perhaps for the renewal of the lipids in the RBC membrane. About 10 percent of the glucose consumed by the RBC is metabolized via the hexose-monophosphate shunt (Fig. 109-3). This pathway protects both hemoglobin and the membrane from exogenous oxidants, including certain drugs.

Studies of RBC enzyme defects have provided valuable information on the metabolic control of normal erythrocytes. In Fig. 109-3 is shown a large number of recognized specific enzyme deficiency states affecting the glycolytic pathway or the hexose-monophosphate shunt. Many of these enzyme abnormalities appear to be restricted to RBC. The long life span of the RBC and its inability to synthesize proteins pose a challenge to the stability of its enzymes. Therefore, a mutation resulting in decreased stability will be detected more readily in RBC compared with other tissues capable of renewing unstable enzymes.

Defects in the Embden-Meyerhof pathway Deficiencies of most of the enzymes of the Embden-Meyerhof (or glycolytic) pathway have been reported (Fig. 109-3). In general, all these enzymopathies have similar pathophysiologic and clinical features. Patients present with a congenital nonspherocytic hemolytic anemia of variable severity. The RBC are often relatively deficient in ATP, considering their young age. As a result, there is an increased leak of potassium ion from inside these cells. Abnormalities in RBC morphology (see below) indicate that the red cell membrane is secondarily affected by the enzyme defect. These RBC are apt to be rigid and thus more readily sequestered by the mononuclear phagocyte system.

Some of these glycolytic enzyme deficiencies such as pyruvate kinase (PK) deficiency and hexokinase deficiency are localized to the RBC, with no apparent metabolic abnormality in leukocytes or other cells that have been studied; in the case of PK deficiency, this is due to specific isozymes confined to the red cell. In other disorders, the enzyme deficiency is more widespread. Glucose phosphate isomerase deficiency and phosphoglycerate kinase deficiency also involve leukocytes, although affected individuals have no apparent abnormalities of white blood cell function. Individuals with deficiency of triose phosphate isomerase have decreased levels of enzyme in leukocytes, muscle cells, and cerebrospinal fluid. Furthermore, they have a progressive neurologic disorder. Some patients with phosphofructokinase deficiency have a myopathy.

Among the reported defects of glycolytic enzymes, about 95 percent are due to PK deficiency and about 4 percent are due to glucose phosphate isomerase deficiency. The remainder, shown in Fig. 109-3, are extremely rare. Most have been encountered in isolated families.

A number of different nucleotide substitutions and hence amino acid replacements result in PK deficiency. Some of these result in decreased reaction with substrate (phosphoenolpyruvate), an enhancing molecule (fructose 1,6 diphosphate), or ADP. Thus, there is considerable variability in the clinical manifestations and laboratory findings among individuals reported as having PK deficiency. Most of these patients are compound heterozygotes who have inherited a different defective enzyme from each parent. The clinical manifestations of the other less common glycolytic enzyme defects are also quite variable.

Most of the glycolytic enzyme defects are inherited in an autosomal recessive pattern. Thus, the parents of affected patients are heterozygotes. Heterozygotes generally possess half-normal levels of enzyme activity, which are more than adequate for normal metabolic function. Thus, these individuals are entirely asymptomatic. Since the gene frequency for this group of enzymopathies is low, it is not surprising that true homozygotes are often the offspring of a consanguineous mating. More often, affected individuals are compound heterozygotes. Phosphoglycerate kinase deficiency is inherited as a sex-linked disorder. Affected males have a severe hemolytic anemia, while female carriers may have a mild hemolytic process.

CLINICAL MANIFESTATIONS Patients with severe hemolysis usually present during early childhood with anemia, icterus, and splenomegaly. Other stigmata of chronic hemolysis are occasionally seen.

LABORATORY FINDINGS Patients have a normocytic (or slightly macrocytic), normochromic anemia with reticulocytosis. In those with PK deficiency, bizarre erythrocytes, including spiculated cells, are noted on the peripheral smear. Spherocytes are usually infrequent or absent. Hence the term *congenital nonspherocytic hemolytic anemia* has been applied to these disorders. Unlike hereditary spherocytosis, the osmotic fragility of freshly drawn blood is usually normal. Incubation brings out an osmotically fragile population of RBC, and this abnormality is not corrected by the addition of glucose.

The diagnosis of this group of anemias depends on specific enzymatic assays; care must be taken to provide an appropriate concentration of substrate so as to detect those variants with a low affinity for substrate or enhancing molecule. An abnormality in enzyme kinetics, differences in electrophoretic mobility, pH optimum, or heat stability may be found useful in documenting heterogeneity among enzyme variants.

℞ **TREATMENT**

Most patients do not require therapy. Those with severe hemolysis should be given a daily supplement of folic acid (1 mg/d). Blood transfusions may be necessary during a hypoplastic crisis. Women with PK deficiency may become very anemic during pregnancy, sometimes leading to the diagnosis for the first time.

Because of their enzymatic defect, the younger cells (reticulocytes) depend on mitochondrial respiration rather than glycolysis for maintenance of ATP. However, in the hypoxic environment of the spleen, aerobic metabolism is curtailed and the ATP-depleted cells are destroyed in situ. Reticulocytes are normally retained in the spleen for 24 to 48 h. Patients with PK deficiency may benefit from splenectomy as they may have a marked increase in circulating reticulocytes. Patients with deficiency of glucose phosphate isomerase also may improve after splenectomy. There is not sufficient information to indicate whether this operation would help individuals with other glycolytic enzymopathies.

Defects in the hexose-monophosphate shunt The normal RBC is well endowed to protect itself against oxidant stress. Upon exposure to a drug or toxin that results in the generation of oxygen radicals, the amount of glucose that is metabolized via the hexose-monophosphate shunt is normally increased severalfold. In this way reduced glutathione is regenerated, protecting the sulfhydryl groups of hemoglobin and the RBC membrane from oxidation. Individuals with an inherited defect in the hexose-monophosphate shunt are unable to maintain an adequate level of reduced glutathione in their RBC. As a result, hemoglobin sulfhydryl groups become oxidized, and the hemoglobin tends to precipitate within the RBC, forming Heinz bodies.

Among the congenital shunt defects, by far the most common is *G6PD deficiency*. It affects more than 200 million people throughout the world; like hemoglobin S, it probably partially protects the patient from malaria by providing a defective home for the merozoite. As with the glycolytic enzymopathies, there is considerable genetic heterogeneity among affected individuals, and over 400 variants of G6PD have been described. Abnormalities in primary DNA or protein sequence have been established in a number of the G6PD variants; in almost all cases, the alteration is one or more base substitutions, leading to an amino acid replacement and not a deletion in the protein. Evidence

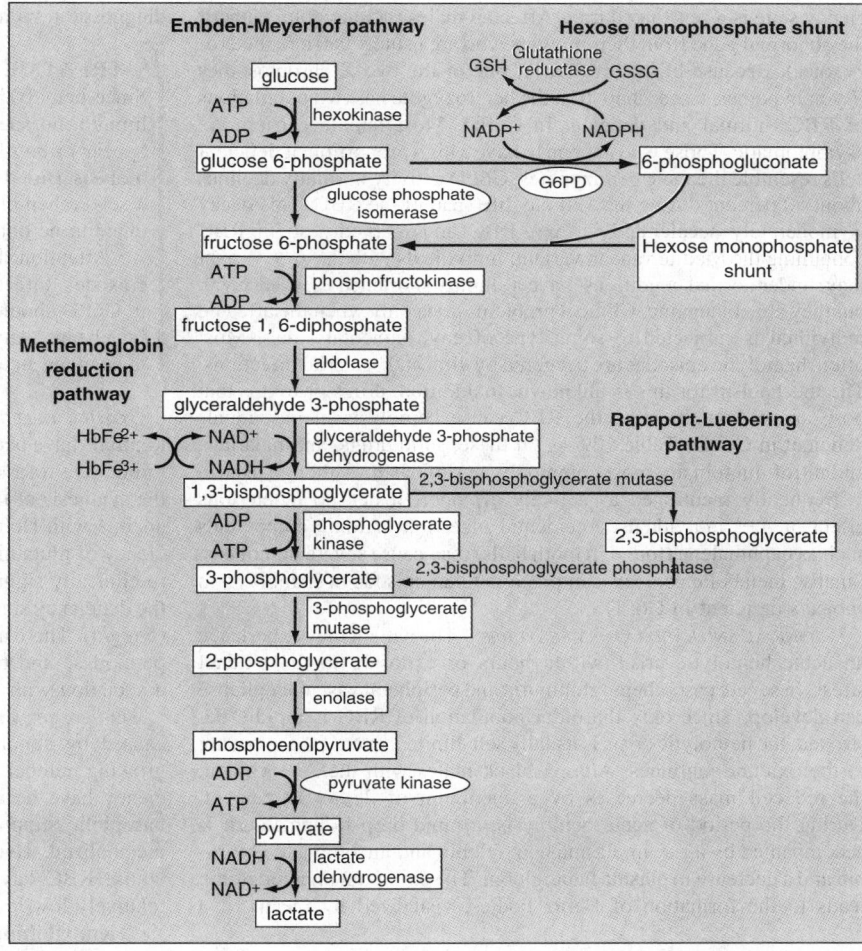

FIGURE 109-3 Red blood cell metabolic pathways. Four metabolic pathways maintain hemoglobin function and membrane integrity. The Embden-Meyerhof pathway (glycolysis) generates ATP for energy and membrane maintenance. The methemoglobin reduction pathway maintains hemoglobin in a reduced state. The hexose monophosphate shunt generates NADPH that is used to reduce glutathione, which protects the red cell against oxidant stress. The Rapaport-Luebering pathway controls the oxygen affinity of hemoglobin by regulating 2,3-bisphosphoglycerate levels. Enzyme deficiency states in order of prevalence: glucose-6-phosphate dehydrogenase (G6PD)>>>pyruvate kinase>glucose-6-phosphate isomerase>rare deficiencies of other enzymes in the pathway. The more common enzyme deficiencies are encircled.

of the abnormality in structure is seen in the differences in electrophoretic mobility, enzyme kinetics, pH optimum, and heat stability. These differences result in great variation of clinical severity, ranging from nonspherocytic hemolytic anemia without demonstrable oxidant stress (particularly shortly after birth), through hemolytic anemia only when stimulated by marked to mild oxidant stress, to no clinically detectable abnormality. The normal G6PD is designated as type B. About 20 percent of individuals of African descent have a G6PD (designated A+) that differs by a single amino acid and is electrophoretically distinguishable but functionally normal. Among the clinically significant G6PD variants, the most common, the so-called A− type, is due to two base substitutions and is encountered primarily in individuals with ancestral origins in central Africa. The A− G6PD has the same electrophoretic mobility as the A+ type, but it is unstable and has abnormal kinetic properties. This variant is found in about 11 percent of African-descended males in the United States. A second relatively common G6PD variant is encountered among peoples of the Mediterranean circumlittoral, particularly Sardinians and Sephardic Jews; this variant is more severe than the A− variant and may result in nonspherocytic hemolytic anemia. A third relatively common and slightly less severe variant occurs in southern Chinese populations.

The G6PD gene is located on the X chromosome. Thus the deficiency state is a sex-linked trait. Affected males (hemizygotes) inherit the abnormal gene from their mothers who are usually carriers (heterozygotes). Because of inactivation of one of the two X chromosomes (Lyon hypothesis: see Chap. 65), the heterozygote has two populations of RBC: normal and deficient in G6PD. Most female carriers are asymptomatic. Those who happen to have a high proportion of deficient cells resemble the male hemizygotes. G6PD activity normally declines about 50 percent during the 120-day life span of the RBC. This decay is moderately accelerated in A− RBC and markedly so in RBC containing the Mediterranean variant. Individuals with the A− variant may, under normal conditions, have a slightly shortened RBC survival, but they are not anemic. Clinical problems arise only when the affected individual is subjected to some type of environmental stress. Most often, hemolytic episodes are triggered by viral and bacterial infections. The mechanism for this is unknown. In addition, drugs or toxins that pose an oxidant threat to the RBC cause hemolysis in individuals deficient in G6PD (Table 109-4). Of these, sulfa drugs, antimalarials, and nitrofurantoin are most commonly incriminated. Although aspirin is frequently mentioned as a likely offender, it has no deleterious effect in A− individuals. Accidental ingestion of toxic compounds such as naphthalene (found in moth balls) may cause severe hemolysis. Finally, metabolic acidosis can precipitate an episode of hemolysis in subjects deficient in G6PD.

CLINICAL AND LABORATORY FEATURES   The patient may experience an acute hemolytic crisis within hours of exposure to the oxidant stress. In severe cases, hemoglobinuria and peripheral vascular collapse can develop. Since only the older population of RBC is rapidly destroyed, the hemolytic crisis is usually self-limited, even if the exposure to the oxidant continues. Among black males with the A− variant, the red cell mass decreases by a maximum of 25 to 30 percent. During the period of acute hemolysis, a rapid drop in hematocrit is accompanied by a rise in plasma hemoglobin and unconjugated bilirubin and a decrease in plasma haptoglobin. The oxidation of hemoglobin leads to the formation of Heinz bodies, visualized by means of a

Table 109-4

Drugs Causing Hemolysis in Subjects Deficient in G6PD

Antimalarials: Primaquine, pamaquine, dapsone
Sulfonamides: Sulfamethoxazole
Nitrofurantoin
Analgesics: Acetanilid
Miscellaneous: Vitamin K (water-soluble form), doxorubicin, methylene blue, nalidixic acid, furazolidone, niridazole, phenazopyridine

supravital stain such as crystal violet. However, Heinz bodies are usually not seen after the first day or so, since these inclusions are readily removed by the spleen. Their removal leads to the formation of "bite cells," red cells that have lost a peripheral portion of the cell. Multiple bites cause the formation of fragments. Small numbers of spherocytes also may be present. Individuals with the Mediterranean type G6PD have a more unstable enzyme and, therefore, a much lower overall enzyme activity than individuals with the A− variant. As a result, they have more severe clinical manifestations. Some have a chronic hemolytic anemia, even in the absence of any exposure to oxidants. A minority of patients are exquisitely sensitive to fava beans and will develop a fulminant hemolytic crisis following exposure. The oxidants in *Vicia fava* are two β-glycosides whose aglycones, when autooxidized, produce free radicals of oxygen. The incidence of favism is highly variable; this may be due to variations in concentration, in absorption, or in metabolism of the aglycones. Favism is not encountered in individuals with the A− variant.

The *diagnosis* of G6PD deficiency should be considered in any individual, particularly a male of African or Mediterranean descent, who experiences an acute hemolytic episode. The patient should be thoroughly questioned about possible exposure to oxidant agents. A number of screening tests are available to establish the diagnosis. However, since the deficiency occurs primarily in older RBC, a false-negative test may be seen during a hemolytic episode when there is a high proportion of young RBC. It may be necessary to repeat these diagnostic tests after the patient has recovered.

℞ TREATMENT

Since hemolysis in patients deficient in A− G6PD is usually self-limited, no specific treatment is necessary. Splenectomy does not appear to be of benefit to Mediterranean patients with chronic hemolysis. Blood transfusions are rarely indicated. If a patient develops a severe hemolytic episode with hemoglobinuria, maintaining adequate urine output is important.

Attention should be directed toward the *prevention* of hemolytic episodes. Infections ought to be treated promptly. Subjects deficient in G6PD should be warned about risks posed by oxidant drugs and fava beans. Any patient of African or Mediterranean ancestry about to be given an oxidant drug should be screened for G6PD deficiency.

OTHER DEFECTS OF THE HEXOSE-MONOPHOSPHATE SHUNT   A few kindreds have been found to have congenital deficiency in RBC glutathione due to a defect in either of the two enzymes responsible for the synthesis of this tripeptide. Affected individuals have a hemolytic anemia with Heinz bodies that is aggravated by oxidant drugs. Deficiency of glutathione reductase has been reported, but its relationship to clinically significant hemolysis is not well established. Sometimes the deficiency state can be corrected by the administration of riboflavin (5 mg/d). There are also isolated reports of deficiencies of glutathione peroxidase and 6-phosphogluconate dehydrogenase, but again, their association with hemolysis is uncertain.

Other enzyme defects   Hemolytic anemia may sometimes be caused by abnormalities in enzymes of nucleotide metabolism. A growing number of individuals with pyrimidine 5′-nucleotidase deficiency have been encountered. Their red cells have marked coarse basophilic stippling because the mRNA of the cell is not properly metabolized. Hemolytic anemia also has been noted in individuals whose RBC have supranormal levels of adenosine deaminase and relatively low levels of ATP.

Hemoglobinopathies   The sickling disorders constitute an important form of congenital hemolytic anemia. Less commonly, hemolysis may be due to the inheritance of an unstable hemoglobin variant. In β-thalassemia major or intermedia, anemia is due to a combination of ineffective erythropoiesis and hemolysis of circulating cells. → *For further discussion, see Chap. 107.*

ACQUIRED HEMOLYTIC ANEMIAS   In most patients with acquired hemolytic anemia, red cells are made normally but are prematurely destroyed because of damage acquired in the circulation. (The exceptions are rare disorders characterized by acquired dysplasia of the cells of the bone marrow and the production of structurally and functionally abnormal red cells.) The damage that occurs may be mediated by antibodies or toxins that mark the cell for premature death or may be due to vicissitudes encountered during the circulation, including an overactive mononuclear phagocyte system or traumatic lysis by natural or artificial impediments to smooth circulation. The acquired hemolytic anemias can be classified into five categories (see Table 109-5).

Hypersplenism The spleen is particularly efficient in trapping and destroying RBC that have minimal defects, often so mild as to be undetectable by in vitro techniques. This unique ability of the spleen to filter mildly damaged RBC results from its unusual vascular anatomy (see Chap. 61). Almost all the blood circulating through the spleen flows rapidly from arterioles in the white pulp to sinuses in the spleen's red pulp and then into the venous system. In contrast, a small portion of splenic blood flow (normally 1 to 2 percent) passes into the "marginal zone" of the lymphatic white pulp. Although the cells that occupy this zone are not phagocytic, they serve as a mechanical filter that hinders the progress of severely damaged blood cells. As RBC leave this zone and enter the red pulp, they flow into narrow cords, rich in macrophages, that end blindly but communicate with sinuses through small openings between the lining cells of the sinuses. These openings, averaging 3 μm in diameter, test the ability of RBC (4.5 μm in diameter) to undergo a deformation of shape. RBC that do not pass the stringent test imposed on them by the spleen filter are engulfed by phagocytic cells and destroyed (see Fig. 61-1).

The normal spleen retains reticulocytes for 1 to 2 days but otherwise poses no difficulties to normal RBC until they become senescent. However, the situation is different when splenomegaly exists. Splenomegaly is usually due to infiltrative diseases such as myeloproliferative disorders (Chap. 111), lymphomas (Chap. 113), and storage diseases such as Gaucher's disease (Chap. 346) as well as to systemic inflammatory diseases leading to splenic hypertrophy or diseases that cause congestive splenomegaly, particularly cirrhosis of the liver and thrombosis of the splenic, portal, or hepatic veins. Splenomegaly, therefore, may result in increased destruction of the cells of the blood, including the red cells. This is in part due to pooling of the blood in an environment relatively deprived of nutrients and full of phagocytic cells. Hemolysis is least predictable in infiltrative diseases of the spleen, where substantial splenomegaly may exist with no apparent hemolysis, whereas inflammatory and congestive splenomegaly is commonly associated with modest shortening of RBC survival, along with more marked granulocytopenia and thrombocytopenia (hypersplenism). Patients with cytopenia(s) sufficient to produce symptoms generally benefit from splenectomy.

Table 109-5

Causes of Acquired Hemolytic Anemia

I. Entrapment
II. Immune
   A. Warm-reactive (IgG) antibody
   B. Cold-reactive IgM antibody (cold agglutinin disease)
   C. Cold-reactive IgG antibody (paroxysmal cold hemoglobinuria)
   D. Drug-dependent antibody
     1. Autoimmune
     2. Haptene
III. Traumatic hemolytic anemia
   A. Impact hemolysis
   B. Macrovascular defects—prostheses
   C. Microvascular causes
     1. Thrombotic thrombocytopenic purpura/hemolytic-uremic syndrome
     2. Other causes of microvascular abnormalities
     3. Disseminated intravascular hemolysis
IV. Hemolytic anemia due to toxic effects on the membrane
   A. Spur cell hemolytic anemia
   B. External toxins
     1. Animal or spider bites
     2. Metals (e.g., copper)
     3. Organic compounds
V. Paroxysmal nocturnal hemoglobinuria

Immunologic Causes of Hemolysis Immune hemolysis in the adult is usually induced by IgG or IgM antibodies with specificity for antigens associated with the patient's red cells (often called "autoantibodies") (Table 109-6); rarely, transfused red cells may be hemolyzed by alloantibodies directed against foreign antigens on those cells (Chap. 115).

The Coombs antiglobulin test is the major tool for diagnosing autoimmune hemolysis. This test relies on the ability of antibodies specific for immunoglobulins (especially IgG) or complement components (especially C3) to agglutinate RBC when these human serum immunoproteins are present on the RBC surface. In the *direct Coombs test*, the ability of anti-IgG or anti-C3 antisera to agglutinate the patient's RBC is determined. The presence or absence of IgG and/or C3 may give important information about the origin of the immune hemolytic anemia (see Table 109-6). Rarely, neither IgG nor complement may be found on the red cells of the patient (Coombs-negative immune hemolytic anemia).

At times, it may be important to demonstrate antibody in the serum of the patient by reacting the serum with normal red cells bearing the antigen. IgM antibodies (usually cold-reacting) may be detected by agglutination of normal or fetal red cells. IgG antibodies may be detected by the *indirect Coombs test*, in which the serum of the patient is incubated with normal red cells and antibody is detected with anti-IgG, as in the direct Coombs test.

"Warm" antibodies Antibodies that react with protein antigens usually are IgG and react at body temperature; occasionally, they are IgA and rarely IgM. This acquired syndrome is frequently designated *autoimmune hemolytic (or immunohemolytic) anemia, warm antibody type.*

CLINICAL MANIFESTATIONS Immunohemolytic anemia of the warm antibody type is induced by IgG antibody and occurs at all ages but is more common in adults, particularly women. In approximately one-fourth of patients this disorder occurs as a complication of an underlying disease affecting the immune system, especially neoplasms of the immune system (chronic lymphocytic leukemia, non-Hodgkin's and Hodgkin's lymphoma); collagen vascular diseases, especially systemic lupus erythematosus (SLE); and congenital immunodeficiency diseases (Table 109-7). The presentation and course of IgG immunohemolytic anemia are quite variable. In its mildest form, the only manifestation is a positive direct Coombs test. In this instance, insufficient antibody is present on the RBC surface to permit the reticuloendothelial system to recognize the cell as abnormal.

Most symptomatic patients have a moderate to severe anemia [hemoglobin levels of 60 to 100 g/L and reticulocyte counts of 10 to 30 percent (200 to 600 × 10³/μL)], spherocytosis (**Plate IV-11**), and splenomegaly.

In its most severe form, immunohemolytic anemia presents with fulminant, overwhelming hemolysis associated with hemoglobinemia, hemoglobinuria, and shock; this syndrome may be rapidly fatal unless aggressively treated.

Table 109-6

Use of the Direct Coombs Test in Diagnosing the Cause of Autoimmune Hemolytic Anemia

Reaction with		
Anti-IgG	**Anti-C3**	**Causes**
Yes	No	Antibodies to Rh proteins, hemolysis caused by α-methyldopa or penicillin; not seen in SLE
Yes	Yes	Antibodies to glycoprotein antigens, SLE
No	Yes	Cold-reacting antibodies (agglutinins or Donath-Landsteiner antibody), most drug-related antibodies, IgM antibodies, IgG antibodies of low affinity, activation of complement by immune complexes

Table 109-7

Hemolysis due to Antibodies

WARM-ANTIBODY IMMUNOHEMOLYTIC ANEMIA

1. Idiopathic
2. Lymphomas: Chronic lymphocytic leukemia, non-Hodgkin's lymphomas, Hodgkin's disease (infrequent)
3. SLE and other collagen-vascular diseases
4. Drugs
   a. α-Methyldopa type (autoantibody to Rh antigens)
   b. Penicillin type (stable hapten)
   c. Quinidine type (unstable hapten)
5. Postviral infections
6. Other tumors (rare)

COLD-ANTIBODY IMMUNOHEMOLYTIC ANEMIA

1. Cold agglutinin disease
   a. Acute: *Mycoplasma* infection, infectious mononucleosis
   b. Chronic: Idiopathic, lymphoma
2. Paroxysmal cold hemoglobinuria

The direct Coombs test is positive in more than 98 percent of patients; usually IgG is detected with or without C3. Rarely, the cells may be agglutinated by the antibody, causing difficulty in analysis by flow cytometry.

Immune thrombocytopenia also may be present (*Evans's syndrome*), a disorder in which separate antibodies are directed against platelets and RBC. Occasionally, venous thrombosis occurs.

PATHOGENESIS IgG antibodies bring about the destruction of the cells by two mechanisms: (1) immune adherence of red cells to destructive cells of the immune system mediated by the antibody itself and by complement components that become fixed to the membrane (by far the more important mechanism of destruction), and (2) completion of the complement sequence, resulting in rupture of the membrane. In IgG-mediated immune adherence, the affixed antibody reacts with Fc receptors on macrophages; this binds the target to the destroyer and activates phagocytic processes that internalize the target, destroying it. If internalization is only partial, membrane is preferentially removed, resulting in the formation of spherocytes. These spherocytes are not able to pass through the fenestrations in the wall of the splenic sinus and thus accumulate in the spleen, where they are destroyed. Complement-mediated immune adherence involves the interaction of C3b and C4b with a series of receptors on the macrophage; this is much less likely to lead to destruction of the target by itself but markedly increases the immune adherence due to IgG. Immune adherence, particularly that due to the IgG antibody, is also enhanced by the transit of red cells into the cords and sinuses of the spleen, which brings cells into intimate contact with phagocytic cells. Significant lysis by the direct action of complement does not commonly occur.

℞ TREATMENT

In the initial evaluation of the patient, it is important to be sure that drugs that are known to cause immunohemolytic anemia are not involved (see below).

Patients having a mild degree of hemolysis usually do not require therapy. In those with clinically significant hemolysis, initial therapy consists of glucocorticoids (e.g., prednisone, 1.0 mg/kg per day). A rise in hemoglobin is frequently noted within 3 or 4 days and occurs in most patients within 1 to 2 weeks. Prednisone at this dosage is continued until the hemoglobin level has risen to normal values, and thereafter it is tapered rapidly to about 20 mg/d, then slowly over the course of several months. An algorithm for this tapering process is given in Fig. 109-4. For chronic therapy with prednisone, alternate-day administration is preferred. More than 75 percent of patients will achieve an initial significant and sustained reduction in hemolysis; however, in half these patients the disease will relapse,

FIGURE 109-4 Algorithm for the treatment of patients with IgG-mediated immune hemolytic anemia. The patient with minimal disease may be watched carefully. The patient with very severe disease may need all modalities of treatment applied at once. The more common patient with moderate disease may be treated with prednisone at a high dose; if no response is seen, then either splenectomy or chemotherapy is given. If a response is seen, the dose of prednisone is reduced over time. If relapse occurs during this process, splenectomy or chemotherapy may be needed.

either during the period of steroid tapering or following the cessation of steroid therapy. Steroids appear to have two modes of action: an immediate effect due to inhibition of the clearance of IgG-coated RBC by the mononuclear phagocyte system and a later effect due to steroid-induced inhibition of antibody synthesis. Splenectomy is the second line of therapy in immune hemolytic anemia due to IgG antibodies. It is recommended for patients who cannot tolerate or fail to respond to steroid therapy. Care must be taken that remnants of splenic tissue do not remain to cause trouble later.

Patients who have been refractory to steroid therapy and to splenectomy are treated with immunosuppressive drugs such as azathioprine and cyclophosphamide. A success rate of about 50 percent has been reported with each. Intravenous gamma globulin may be used when rapid cessation of hemolysis is required; however, it is not nearly as effective in this disorder as it is in immune thrombocytopenia.

Patients with severe anemia may require blood transfusions. Because the antibody in this disease is usually a "panagglutinin," reacting with nearly all normal donor cells, the usual compatibility tests (e.g., cross matching) are impossible. The goal in selecting blood for transfusion is to avoid administering red cells with antigens to which the patient may have *allo*antibodies. A common procedure is to adsorb the panagglutinin present in patient's serum using the patient's own red cells from which antibody has been previously eluted. Serum freed of autoantibody in this way can then be tested for the presence of alloantibody to specific donor blood groups. ABO-compatible red cells matched in this fashion are administered slowly, with attention paid to the possibility of an immediate-type hemolytic transfusion reaction.

PROGNOSIS In the majority of patients, this disease is controlled by steroid therapy alone, by splenectomy, or by a combination. In most of the remaining patients, a partial degree of control is achieved. Fatalities occur among three subsets of patients: (1) rare patients with overwhelming hemolysis in whom death is directly attributable to anemia; (2) those whose host defenses are impaired by glucocorticoids, splenectomy, and/or immunosuppressive agents; and (3) rarely, those with major thrombotic events coincident with active hemolysis.

In patients in whom immunohemolysis develops as a complication of an underlying disorder, the prognosis is often dominated by that of the primary disease.

Immunohemolytic anemia secondary to drugs Drugs that have been directly implicated in immunohemolytic anemia are of two kinds, as distinguished by their mechanisms of action: (1) drugs, such as α-methyldopa (an antihypertensive; Chap. 246), that induce a disorder identical almost in every respect to the warm-antibody immunohemolytic anemia described above, and (2) drugs that can become associated as haptenes with the RBC surface and induce the formation of an antibody directed against the RBC-drug complex. The association of drug and membrane protein may be relatively tight, as in the case of penicillin, or relatively loose, as in the case of quinidine and most other drugs.

A positive direct Coombs test is observed in up to 10 percent of patients receiving α-methyldopa therapy in doses of 2.0 g/d or higher. A small minority of these patients develop spherocytosis and hemolysis, which may be of severe degree. This "autoimmune" disorder is probably due to the fact that α-methyldopa alters the protein(s) of the Rh complex so that the protein becomes immunogenic; the resulting antibodies cross-react with the normal Rh protein. Thus the antibody does not react with the drug, and the indirect Coombs test is positive in almost all patients even when the drug is not added to the test. The red cells are coated with IgG but not C3. Hemolysis decreases over the course of several weeks after cessation of drug therapy, although the direct Coombs test may remain positive for more than 1 year.

In most other cases, when a drug induces an immune hemolytic reaction, the antibody is directed against the combination of the drug and the membrane glycoprotein to which it is attached. The hemolytic reaction in vivo is dependent on the presence of the drug and usually ceases shortly after the drug has been discontinued. Penicillin and its congeners may cause this type of reaction if the drug is given in very high doses (10 million units per day or more). In this case, the drug adheres relatively firmly to the protein of the red cell membrane. Complement is not usually fixed, and the hemolysis in vivo is usually not severe. Since the antibody is usually IgG, spherocytosis and splenic destruction may occur. Most other drugs (such as quinine, quinidine, sulfonamides, sulfonureas, phenacetin, stibophen, and dipyrone) do not adhere as tightly to their glycoproteins, and they and the antibodies that they have generated are removed during the washing steps of the direct and indirect Coombs reactions. Most of these antibodies are able to fix complement (especially those that are IgM), and these components remain on the red cell surface; thus the direct Coombs test is positive with anti-C3 but not anti-IgG. The antibody is detected in the *indirect* Coombs test only when the drug is added to the incubation mixture. Hemolysis may be quite severe, sometimes resulting in signs of intravascular hemolysis; resolution is usually prompt after the drug is discontinued.

Immune hemolysis due to cold-reactive antibodies Antibodies that react with polysaccharide antigens are usually IgM and react better at temperatures lower than 37°C, hence the name *cold-reactive antibodies*. Uncommonly, the antibody is IgG (the Donath-Landsteiner antibody of paroxysmal cold hemoglobinuria).

Cold agglutinins arise in two clinical settings: (1) monoclonal antibodies as the product of lymphocytic neoplasia or paraneoplasia and (2) polyclonal antibodies in response to infection. In many elderly patients, the "neoplasm" is benign monoclonal gammopathy, and, although chronic, it does not progress and the protein product remains its only manifestations. In a few patients, the lymphoma may be aggressive. Occasionally, cold agglutinins are found in patients with nonlymphocytic neoplasms.

Transient cold agglutinins occur commonly in two infections: *Mycoplasma pneumoniae* infection and infectious mononucleosis. In both, the titer of antibody is usually too low to cause clinical symptoms, but its presence is of diagnostic value; only occasionally is hemolysis present. Cold agglutinins are less frequently encountered in a number of other viral infections. Their manifestations are usually benign.

The specificity of the antibody may be of diagnostic value. Cold agglutinins reacting more strongly with adult cells than fetal (cord) cells are called *anti-I*; these antibodies are seen in benign lymphoproliferation (chronic cold agglutinin monoclonal gammopathy) and in *Mycoplasma* infections. Those reacting more strongly with cord cells

are called *anti-i*; these antibodies are seen in aggressive lymphomas and in infectious mononucleosis. Rarely, the antibody may react with other antigens that are equally expressed on adult and cord cells. The clinical manifestations elicited by the antibody upon exposure to cold are of two sorts: intravascular agglutination (acrocyanosis) and hemolysis. Acrocyanosis is the marked purpling of the extremities, ears, and nose when the blood becomes cold enough to agglutinate in the veins; it clears on warming and does not have the vasospastic characteristics of Raynaud's phenomenon (see Chap. 248). Patients may also have symptoms from the same cause when swallowing cold food or drinks.

The hemolysis is usually not severe and is manifest by a mild reticulocytosis, agglutination on the blood film, and agglutination during analysis of the blood by particle analysis (giving rise to a falsely high mean corpuscular volume). The degree of hemolysis depends on several variables.

1. *Antibody titer*. In general, the titer in symptomatic patients is above 1:2000 dilution of serum and may range to as high as 1:50,000. When collecting samples for testing the titer, great care must be taken that the serum is separated from the cells while maintaining the sample at 37°C so that the antibody will not adsorb onto the patient's own cells.
2. *Thermal amplitude of the antibody* (the highest temperature at which the antibody will react with the red cell). For most antibodies, this is 23 to 30°C. Those with a higher thermal amplitude (up to 37°C) will be more hemolytic, since it is more likely that these temperatures will be encountered during the circulation of the cells.
3. *Environmental temperature*. Since the reaction can only occur at temperatures below body temperature, frequency and degree of exposure to cold are major determinants of the rate of hemolysis.

The hemolysis that occurs is due primarily to the hemolytic action of complement, since there are no functional Fc receptors for the IgM antibody. Complement is readily fixed, since a single molecule of antibody is enough to effect binding of C1 and initiate the sequence of reactions. However, the normal human red cell is remarkably resistant to the hemolytic action of complement because of several defense mechanisms. Therefore, severe hemolysis with hemoglobinuria will occur only with massive activation of the antibody, such as by sudden chilling. The activation of complement is always marked by the accumulation of a degradation product of C3, C3dg, on the surface; this is what is detected with appropriate antisera in the direct Coombs test in all patients with significant cold agglutinin disease. The cutaneous manifestations of this disorder are best treated by maintaining the patient in a warm environment. This will also reduce hemolysis.

Splenectomy is usually not of value in this disorder. Glucocorticoids are of limited value, although patients with the panthermal variety of cold agglutinin disease may respond favorably to this therapy. Chlorambucil and cyclophosphamide are the most commonly employed agents in those patients with benign monoclonal gammopathy in whom therapy is indicated. Although some patients have experienced a dramatic improvement, the effectiveness of this therapy is usually marginal. Appropriate therapy of a malignant neoplasm responsible for the cold agglutinin will often reduce the titer of antibody and the severity of the hemolysis.

Chronic cold agglutinin disease tends to be unremitting. The overall prognosis is dominated by the underlying lymphoproliferative disease, if present. In those patients in whom cold agglutinin disease appears to arise spontaneously, malignant lymphoproliferative disease may become apparent after several years.

Paroxysmal cold hemoglobinuria (PCH) Now a rare disorder, PCH was more frequent at a time when tertiary syphilis was prevalent; now, most cases are either secondary to a viral infection or are autoimmune. It results from the formation of the Donath-Landsteiner antibody, an IgG antibody that is directed against the P antigen (see Chap.

115) and that can induce complement-mediated lysis. Attacks are precipitated by exposure to cold and are associated with hemoglobinemia and hemoglobinuria; chills and fever; back, leg, and abdominal pain; headache; and malaise. Recovery from the acute episode is prompt, and between episodes patients are usually asymptomatic. When this syndrome accompanies acute viral infections (e.g., measles and mumps in children), it is self-limited but may be severe. Although the direct Coombs test may show complement to be present (seldom IgG), this test may be completely negative. The diagnosis is made by demonstrating cold-reacting IgG antibodies either by lytic tests (when the titer is very high) or by special antiglobulin tests. When PCH is secondary to syphilis, it responds favorably to specific therapy for this disorder. Chronic autoimmune PCH may respond to prednisone or cytotoxic therapy (azathioprine or cyclophosphamide) but does not respond to splenectomy. Despite the severity of individual episodes, the natural history of this disease often extends over many years.

Hemolysis due to Trauma in the Circulation   Red cells may be fragmented by mechanical trauma as they circulate; this invariably leads to intravascular hemolysis and in most cases to red cell fragments called *schistocytes*. Schistocytes are identified by the sharp points that result from the faulty resealing of the fractured membrane (**Plate IV-7**). Such mechanical trauma leading to hemolysis occurs in three clinical settings: (1) when RBC flow through small vessels over the surface of bony prominences and are subject to external impact during various physical activities, (2) when they flow across a pressure gradient created by an abnormal heart valve or valve prosthesis and are disrupted by a shear stress (macrovascular), and (3) when the deposition of fibrin in the microvasculature exposes them to a physical impediment that fragments them (microvascular) (Table 109-8).

External impact   Hemoglobinemia and hemoglobinuria have been observed in a small proportion of individuals who have undergone a prolonged march or a prolonged jog, most typically on a hard surface and while wearing thin-soled shoes. The role of direct external trauma in this process has been demonstrated by the fact that hemolysis can be prevented by the insertion of a soft inner sole in the runner's shoes. Similar types of hemolysis have been described following karate and the playing of bongo drums. No abnormality of RBC morphology has been demonstrated, even during the acute episode, and no underlying RBC abnormality has been uncovered. Susceptible individuals will develop hemoglobinemia and hemoglobinuria when exposed to the conditions described above. As a result of muscle damage during some of these activities, myoglobinuria also may occur, but renal function is preserved. No specific therapy is required except to obtain better running shoes.

Macrovascular fragmentation hemolysis   Hemolysis associated with fragmented red blood cells (**Plate IV-7**) occurs in approximately 10 percent of patients with artificial aortic valve prostheses. This incidence is somewhat greater with valves having stellite rather than Silastic occluders, greater with small valves as compared with larger valves, and greater when valves are cloth-covered or when there is a paravalvular leak. Traumatic hemolysis is rare in recipients of porcine valves. Severe hemolysis may occur after repair of ostium primum or endocardial cushion defects with a prosthetic patch. Mitral valve prostheses also have been associated with hemolysis, but since the pressure gradient across these valves is lower than across aortic prostheses, the incidence is lower. A moderately shortened RBC survival with little or no anemia occurs in some patients with severe calcific aortic stenosis. Indeed, almost any intracardiac lesion that alters hemodynamics may lead to some shortening of RBC survival. In addition, traumatic hemolysis has been observed in patients who have undergone aortofemoral bypass.

CLINICAL MANIFESTATIONS   In severe cases, hemoglobin levels fall to 50 to 70 g/L with reticulocytosis, fragmented RBC in the peripheral blood, depressed haptoglobin, elevated serum lactate dehydrogenase (LDH), and hemoglobinemia and hemoglobinuria. Iron loss (as hemoglobin or hemosiderin) in the urine may lead to iron deficiency. The direct Coombs test may rarely become positive.

PATHOGENESIS   A number of factors combine to cause the fragmentation of RBC by prostheses: (1) the shear stress resulting from turbulent blood flow, particularly when blood is forced through a small aperture by high pressure (e.g., a paravalvular leak around an aortic valve); (2) direct mechanical trauma of RBC at the time of seating of the occluder of the prosthetic valve; and (3) the deposition of fibrin across disrupted attachment points.

℞ TREATMENT

Iron deficiency should be corrected by the administration of oral iron. The elevated hemoglobin that results may permit a decrease in the cardiac output and a slowing of the hemolytic rate. Limitation in physical activity also lessens the hemolytic rate. When these measures fail, any paravalvular leak must be repaired or the prosthetic valve replaced.

Microvascular causes of traumatic hemolysis   If fibrin is deposited in arteriolar sites, red cells may be trapped on the meshwork and fragmented by the force of the blood pressure. This may occur due to localized intravascular coagulation at sites of arteriolar wall injury, as in thrombotic thrombocytopenic purpura and the hemolytic-uremic syndrome, and in other disorders, such as malignant hypertension, eclampsia, rejection of a renal allograft, disseminated cancer, hemangiomas, or disseminated intravascular coagulation (DIC).

Abnormalities of the vessel wall   The degree of hemolysis induced by this family of disorders is usually quite mild, although the number of fragments in the peripheral blood may be striking. In some patients, thrombocytopenia may be severe. In each case, therapy is best directed at the primary disease. Thus reversal of renal graft rejection, treatment of malignant hypertension and eclampsia, control of cancer, etc., lead to a cessation of the hemolytic process. The relative importance of the primary vascular abnormality and of the deposition of fibrin in causing hemolysis is unclear.

Thrombotic thrombocytopenia purpura (TTP)   This disorder is characterized by arteriolar lesions in various organs that contain platelets and fibrin. This results in thrombocytopenia and hemolytic anemia due to fragmentation of the red cells. The tissue hypoxia resulting from the occlusion may cause organ dysfunction, most frequently manifest in the nervous system or the kidney. It affects individuals of all ages but primarily young adults, more often women.

CLINICAL MANIFESTATIONS   The classic pentad of TTP includes hemo-

Table 109-8

Disturbances of the Formed Elements of Blood Secondary to Intravascular Trauma

Etiology	Fragments	Hemolysis	Thrombocytopenia
Impact: march hemoglobinuria, etc.	0	+	0
Cardiac (turbulence):			
Aortic valve prosthesis	+ + + +	+ + + +	0
Mitral valve prosthesis	+ +	+ +	0
Calcific aortic stenoses	+	±	0
Vessel disease*	+ + +	+	+
Thrombotic thrombocytopenic purpura	+ + + +	+ + + +	+ + + +
Hemolytic-uremic syndrome	+ + + +	+ + + +	+ + + +
Adenocarcinoma	+ + + +	+ + + +	+ + + +
Disseminated intravascular coagulation	+ +	±	+ + + +

* Malignant hypertension, eclampsia, renal graft rejection, hemangiomas, immune disease (scleroderma).

lytic anemia with fragmentation of erythrocytes and signs of intravascular hemolysis, thrombocytopenia, diffuse and nonfocal neurologic findings, decreased renal function, and fever. These signs and symptoms occur variably, depending upon the number and sites of the arteriolar lesions. The anemia may be very mild to very severe, and the thrombocytopenia in general parallels it. The neurologic and renal symptoms are usually seen only when the platelet count is very significantly diminished (<20 to $30 \times 10^3/\mu L$). Fever is not reliably present. TTP may be very acute in onset, but its course spans days to weeks in most patients and occasionally continues for months. If the brain and kidneys are involved, their dysfunction is frequently the ultimate cause of death. Proteinuria and a moderate elevation of blood urea nitrogen may be found on initial presentation, and there can be a continued rise in blood urea nitrogen and a fall in urine output if the patient develops renal failure. Neurologic symptoms develop in more than 90 percent of patients whose disease terminates in death. Initially, there may be changes in mental status such as confusion, delirium, or altered states of consciousness. Focal findings include seizures, hemiparesis, aphasia, and visual field defects. These neurologic symptoms may fluctuate and terminate in coma. Involvement of myocardial blood vessels may be a cause of sudden death in some patients. The severity of the disorder can be estimated from the degree of anemia and thrombocytopenia as well as the serum LDH level, which is elevated as a result of the intravascular hemolysis. Tests of coagulation, such as the prothrombin time, partial thromboplastin time, fibrinogen concentration, and the level of fibrin split products are usually normal or only mildly abnormal. If the coagulation tests indicate a major consumption of procoagulants, the diagnosis of TTP is doubtful. A positive antinuclear antibody (ANA) determination is obtained in approximately 20 percent of patients.

PATHOGENESIS The cause of TTP is unknown, but the manifestations can be explained by *localized* platelet thrombi and fibrin deposition. Arterioles are filled with hyalin material, presumably fibrin and platelets, and similar material may be seen beneath the endothelium of otherwise uninvolved vessels. Immunofluorescence studies have shown the presence of immunoglobulin and complement in arterioles. Microaneurysms of arterioles are often present. An association with pregnancy, AIDS, SLE, scleroderma, and Sjögren's syndrome suggests an immunologic origin.

DIAGNOSIS The combination of hemolytic anemia with fragmented RBC, thrombocytopenia, normal coagulation tests, fever, neurologic disorders, and renal dysfunction is virtually pathognomonic of TTP. Although they are not usually required for diagnosis, biopsies of skin and muscle, gingiva, lymph node, or bone marrow may demonstrate the arteriolar abnormalities described above. TTP must be distinguished from idiopathic thrombocytopenic purpura or Evans's syndrome (the former plus immunohemolytic anemia) by the finding of fragmented but not spherocytic red blood cells in the peripheral blood and a negative direct Coombs test.

℞ TREATMENT

Until recently, this disease was almost universally fatal, but with the availability of plasmapheresis, more than 90 percent of patients can survive if therapy is promptly and aggressively instituted. Many patients require daily or even twice daily plasmapheresis with plasma replacement. If a response is obtained (as indicated by increasing platelet count and decreasing plasma LDH and fragmented red cells), plasmapheresis may be given progressively less frequently but often must be continued for several weeks to months. Most patients also receive high doses of glucocorticoids and may receive platelet-active agents (dipyridamole, sulfinpyrazone, dextran, aspirin), but the efficacy of these is not known. Immunosuppression with vincristine or cyclophosphamide as well as splenectomy has been used in patients who do not respond to plasmapheresis. Even deep coma is not a contraindication to therapy, since full neurologic recovery is the rule in patients responding to therapy. Relapses have been noted in approximately 10 percent of patients but are usually responsive to therapeutic intervention. Platelet transfusions should not be given because they can precipitate thrombotic events.

Hemolytic-uremic syndrome This disorder is similar to TTP and is characterized by the same arteriolar lesions, which may be confined to the kidney, and by similar laboratory findings. It is usually encountered in young children. Often the patient has a prodrome of a gastroenteritic bloody diarrhea caused by *Escherichia coli* 0157:H7, and the lesions are thought to be due to the elaboration of Shiga-like verotoxins that bind to the renal vascular endothelial cells and inhibit ribosomal activity. Several outbreaks of the disorder associated with undercooked meat have been reported. Very rarely, the disorder appears to be familial. Patients present with acute hemolytic anemia, thrombocytopenic purpura, and acute oliguric renal failure. Most patients have either hemoglobinuria or anuria. Unlike TTP, neurologic manifestations are uncommon. The peripheral blood findings and coagulation tests are usually indistinguishable from those of TTP.

Patients are treated with plasmapheresis, dialysis, and transfusions. The efficacy of glucocorticoids, dextran, and heparin is uncertain. The mortality in children ranges from 5 to 20 percent but is considerably higher in adults. A disorder resembling the hemolytic-uremic syndrome has been described in adults treated with the antineoplastic drug mitomycin C, usually in combination with other drugs. It may also occur in patients receiving high-dose chemotherapy with autologous stem cell transplantation.

Disseminated intravascular coagulation When the coagulation system is inappropriately activated in the plasma, the resulting accumulations of fibrin in small vessels may result in RBC fragmentation in the microvasculature (microangiopathic hemolytic anemia). This occurs in about one-fourth of patients with DIC (Chap. 118). The degree of hemolysis is much less in DIC than in either TTP or the hemolytic-uremic syndrome, and anemia with reticulocytosis and nucleated RBC is distinctly rare.

Environmental Alteration of the Red Cell Membrane by "Toxic" Effects Changes in the red cell membrane by external influences (chemical, bacterial, etc.) may result in hemolysis. A variety of infections may be associated with severe hemolysis. The microorganisms in bartonellosis (Chap. 165), malaria (Chap. 216), and babesiosis (Chap. 216) directly parasitize RBC. Other infectious organisms exert their damaging effects on RBC indirectly. The most striking is that resulting from septicemia with *Clostridium welchii* (Chap. 148). The phospholipase produced by this organism is capable of cleaving the phosphoryl bond of lecithin, thereby lysing human RBC. A mild, transient hemolysis frequently accompanies bacteremia with diverse organisms such as pneumococci, staphylococci, and *E. coli*.

Hemolysis may result from the direct action of snake and spider venoms on the RBC. Although cobra venom is directly lytic in vitro, the clinical disease induced by the bite of the cobra is one of moderate hemolysis associated with spherocytosis. Spider bites, particularly that of the brown recluse spider, are known to induce acute intravascular hemolysis associated with spherocytosis. The hemolytic disease continues for several days up to 1 week.

Copper has a direct hemolytic effect on RBC. Hemolysis has been observed following exposure of individuals to copper salts (such as during hemodialysis). In addition, the transient episodes of hemolysis observed in patients with Wilson's disease are probably due to copper toxicity.

The RBC membrane is unstable at temperatures above 49°C due to denaturation of the cytoskeletal protein spectrin. When studied in vitro, the RBC undergoes a process of budding, cleavage, and resealing above this temperature. The same process is observed in individuals who have suffered extensive burns. These patients have prominent spherocytosis as well as hemoglobinemia and sometimes hemoglobinuria.

Spur Cell Anemia Hemolytic anemia with bizarre-shaped RBC occurs in some patients with severe hepatocellular disease, usually advanced Laennec's cirrhosis.

It is observed in approximately 5 percent of patients with manifestations of severe cirrhosis and is a very poor prognostic sign. It has also been reported in neonatal hepatitis.

Clinical manifestations   Anemia is more severe than is observed in otherwise uncomplicated cirrhosis. Hematocrit levels range between 16 and 30 percent. Splenomegaly is always present and is greater than in patients who have cirrhosis but who do not have spur cell anemia. Jaundice may be severe because of the hemolysis and liver dysfunction, and hepatic encephalopathy is common. The characteristic RBC are irregularly shaped with multiple spicules, and a small number of bizarre-shaped fragments are commonly seen on peripheral blood smears (**Plate IV-8**). Reticulocytosis and other signs of hemolysis are present. The tests of liver function are similar to values obtained in most patients with severe cirrhosis.

RBC half-life is decreased to as short as 6 days (normal being 26 to 32 days), and red cell destruction is localized to the spleen. Normal transfused RBC acquire the defect and have a survival similar to that of the patient's own RBC.

Pathogenesis   The surface membrane of a spur cell contains 50 to 70 percent excess cholesterol, but its total phospholipid content is normal; this is distinct from the pattern seen in the more usual target RBC in liver disease, which possesses an excess of both cholesterol and phospholipid. This results from the presence in serum of an abnormal low-density lipoprotein with an increased mole ratio of free (unesterified) cholesterol to phospholipid. Cholesterol out of proportion to phospholipid decreases the fluidity of the spur cell membrane, and cell deformability is decreased.

These rigid, cholesterol-laden RBC cannot pass through the filtering system of the spleen, further impeded by congestive splenomegaly in cirrhosis.

Diagnosis   Spur cell anemia is characterized by evidence of hemolysis and the cells with the specific morphologic abnormality. Increasing anemia in a patient with chronic cirrhosis most commonly results from blood loss, folic acid deficiency, or iron deficiency.

RBC of similar morphologic appearance are seen in patients with abetalipoproteinemia. However, these individuals have a minimal amount of hemolysis.

Spur cells and acanthocytes must be distinguished from regularly scalloped, crenated red blood cells (echinocytes). These are a frequent artifact on blood smears, and they are present in some patients with uremia ("burr cells") (**Plate IV-9**). Small, dense crenated spheres (spheroechinocytes) are sometimes seen in congenital nonspherocytic hemolytic anemia due to enzyme deficiencies in the Embden-Meyerhof pathway (see above).

℞ **TREATMENT**
Since normal RBC acquire the spur abnormality when transfused into patients with this form of anemia, transfusion therapy is of limited benefit. Attempts to influence RBC cholesterol by the use of various lipid-lowering agents have been unsuccessful. Splenectomy has been reported to prevent both the conditioning of RBC in the spleen and their premature destruction. However, splenectomy carries a high risk in patients with severe liver disease complicated by portal hypertension and coagulation defects, and it must be reserved for selected patients in whom hemolysis is a major clinical problem and who appear to be relatively good surgical risks.

Prognosis   In most patients, spur cell anemia occurs during the late stages of cirrhosis, and more than 90 percent of patients succumb to their underlying liver disease within 1 year of the diagnosis of spur cell anemia.

Paroxysmal Nocturnal Hemoglobinuria (PNH)   This condition is distinctive among hemolytic disorders because it is an intracorpuscular defect acquired at the stem cell level.

Clinical manifestations   There are three common manifestations of PNH: hemolytic anemia, venous thrombosis, and deficient hematopoiesis. Anemia is of exceedingly variable degree, with hematocrit values of 20 percent and lower in occasional patients and normal values in others.

RBC are normochromic and normocytic unless iron deficiency has occurred owing to the chronic loss of iron in the urine.

Mild granulocytopenia and thrombocytopenia are commonly present and are manifestations of deficient hematopoiesis. Clinical hemoglobinuria is present only intermittently in most patients and never occurs in some, but hemosiderinuria is usually present in all patients. The lack of two proteins, decay-accelerating factor (DAF, CD55) and a membrane inhibitor of reactive lysis (MIRL, CD59) (see below) make the red cells more sensitive to the lytic effect of complement.

DAF normally disrupts the enzyme complexes from either the classical (antibody-driven) pathway or the alternative pathway that activate C3 and C5; CD59 inhibits the conversion of C9 by the membrane attack complex C5b-8 to a polymeric complex capable of penetrating the membrane.

The platelets also lack these proteins; however, the life span of the platelet is normal. On the other hand, the activation of complement indirectly stimulates platelet aggregation and hypercoagulability; this is probably responsible for the tendency to thrombosis seen in PNH.

Venous thrombosis is a common complication, affecting about 40 percent of patients at one time or another. It occurs primarily in intraabdominal veins (hepatic, portal, mesenteric, etc.) and results in the Budd-Chiari syndrome, congestive splenomegaly, and abdominal pain. It may occur in cerebral venous sinuses and is a common cause of death in patients with PNH. The deficit in hematopoiesis may not be clinically manifest by examination of the bone marrow cellularity but is evident in all patients when the growth of marrow progenitors is examined. About 15 to 30 percent of long-term survivors of aplastic anemia will have PNH cells manifest at some time or other; in some patients, the manifestations of PNH become dominant. Patients with PNH may have aplastic periods lasting from weeks to years. PNH may be seen in association with other stem cell disorders, including myelofibrosis, and (rarely) other myelodysplastic or myeloproliferative disorders.

Pathogenesis   PNH is an acquired clonal disease, probably arising from an inactivating somatic mutation in a single abnormal stem cell of a gene on the X-chromosome (*pig-A*) important for the biosynthesis of the glycosylphosphatidylinositol (GPI) anchor. This anchor is necessary for the attachment of a number of proteins to the external membrane surface, and its partial or complete absence results in the absence of those proteins; to date, about 20 proteins have been found to be missing on the blood cells of patients with PNH. The normal clone of stem cells and its descendants do not completely disappear, and the proportion of cells that are abnormal varies from patient to patient and from time to time in a single patient.

Diagnosis   PNH should be suspected in anyone with otherwise unexplained hemolytic anemia, especially with leukopenia and/or thrombocytopenia and with evidence of intravascular hemolysis (hemoglobinemia, hemoglobinuria, hemosiderinuria, elevated LDH of the erythrocyte type). Anyone recovering from aplastic anemia should be examined at intervals for the appearance of the diagnostic cells. The diagnosis is often delayed because (1) it is not considered, (2) hemoglobinuria is confused with hematuria, (3) elevation of the LDH is confused with that seen in liver disease, and (4) the tests commonly used (Ham's test and the sucrose lysis test) are not reliable.

Ham's test is performed by incubating the patient's RBC with normal serum acidified to a pH of 6.2. Complement is activated under these conditions, and the defective PNH cells are lysed but not normal cells (including the normal cells of the patient). The sensitivity of the test is increased by optimizing the Mg^{2+} concentration and by using sera of normal donors known to be potent in this test. The test may miss small populations of abnormal cells but is falsely positive only in a rare form of congenital dyserythropoietic anemia, which can be readily distinguished on clinical grounds. The sucrose lysis test, in which complement is activated by reduction of the ionic strength of the incubation medium, is more sensitive but less specific. The most sensitive and specific test is determination of the absence of the GPI-linked proteins on erythrocytes and granulocytes by flow cytometry (e.g., CD59, DAF).

TREATMENT

Transfusion therapy is useful in PNH not only for raising the hemoglobin level but also for suppressing the marrow production of RBC during episodes of sustained hemoglobinuria. Whole blood transfusions infrequently cause an exacerbation of the hemolytic process. This can be prevented by using washed RBC rather than whole blood. Therapy with androgens frequently results in a rise in hemoglobin level. Glucocorticoids also may be effective in reducing the rate of hemolysis but should be given in moderate doses (15 to 30 mg prednisone) *only on alternate days.*

Because of iron loss in the urine, iron deficiency is common. An exacerbation of hemolysis often follows the administration of iron because of the formation of a large number of young RBC, many of which are sensitive to complement. This may be minimized by giving prednisone (60 mg/d) or by suppressing the bone marrow with transfusions.

Acute thrombosis in PNH, particularly the Budd-Chiari syndrome and cerebral thrombosis, should be treated aggressively with thrombolytic agents. Heparin therapy should be instituted rapidly and maintained for several days before changing to coumadin therapy. Antithymoctye globulin is often of use in treating marrow hypoplasia, as it is in the related disease, aplastic anemia. A total dose of 150 mg/kg is given over 4 to 10 days; large doses of prednisone are usually needed to counteract the immune-complex disease that results from the administration of this foreign protein.

In patients, especially the younger ones, with either hypoplasia or thrombosis who have an appropriate sibling donor, marrow transplantation should be considered early in the course of the disease. The usual conditioning programs are sufficient to eradicate the aberrant clone.

ANEMIA OF ACUTE BLOOD LOSS

The normal capacity to compensate for acute blood loss involves cardiovascular mechanisms, an adjustment in the oxygen affinity of hemoglobin, and an increase in erythropoiesis in the marrow. The signs and symptoms of blood loss relate to the volume of the blood loss and the time frame over which the hemorrhage occurs (see Table 109-9). Blood losses of up to 20 percent of the blood volume are normally tolerated by redistribution of blood flow mediated by reflex venospasm, but the presence of fever or pain may interfere with this compensation. With larger blood losses, blood volume redistribution is not adequate to maintain normal blood pressure: initially, changes are only seen on standing, but with greater losses progressively greater problems are encountered maintaining blood pressure in sitting or supine positions. If the blood loss is more gradual, plasma volume may increase, but albumin production usually lags behind the fluid shifts. It may take 2 to 3 days for the liver to generate the albumin lost in a 1500-mL bleed.

The most rapid hematologic adjustment to acute blood loss is an increase in oxygen delivery to the tissues. This is first mediated by the Bohr effect, where the more acidic milieu of the hypoperfused tissues shifts the hemoglobin oxygen dissociation curve to the right. Over several hours the red cells increase their production of 2,3-bisphosphoglycerate, which also enhances the unloading of oxygen to tissues. These two mechanisms can nearly double the capacity of each red cell to deliver oxygen to the tissues.

The marrow response to hemorrhage is related to the generation of erythropoietin in the kidney in response to decreased oxygen tensions. A normal response depends upon the production of erythropoietin, the presence of normal erythroid progenitors in the marrow, and an adequate supply of iron. If these three elements are normal, reticulo-

Table 109-9

Signs and Symptoms of Blood Loss

Percent Blood Loss	Volume of Loss, mL*	Symptoms	Signs
<20	<1000	Restlessness	+/− Vasovagal reaction
20–30	1000–1500	Anxiety, DOE	Orthostatic hypotension, tachycardia on exertion
30–40	1500–2000	Syncope on sitting or standing	Orthostatic hypotension, tachycardia at rest
>40	>2000	Confusion, shortness of breath	Shock, poor perfusion

* Based on an estimated total blood volume of 5000 mL (70-kg adult).

cytes begin to increase in number in the first 2 days based upon early release of reticulocytes from the marrow. However, it takes 3 to 6 days for erythroid hyperplasia to appear and 7 to 10 days before the erythropoietic response is maximal, producing reticulocyte counts up to 20 to 30 percent, a reticulocyte index of 3 or greater, and a marked increase in the marrow erythoid/granulocytic ratio.

DIAGNOSIS Usually it is clear that a patient is bleeding; however, in some cases, large volumes of blood loss can occur internally from the gastrointestinal tract (esophageal varicies, cancer in the stomach or colon), a ruptured spleen, fractures and other trauma, or other lesions that can cause massive hemorrhage into the peritoneal cavity, pleural cavity, or the retroperitoneal space. Patients who have bled sufficiently to develop hypotension generally develop anemia, but this is only apparent after volume replacement. The granulocyte count may increase to 20,000 cells/µL or more and include immature cell types such as metamyelocytes and myelocytes. Epinephrine-induced demargination of peripheral granulocytes and release of cells from the marrow may account for this change. Nucleated RBC may appear in the circulation, and platelet counts may exceed 1×10^6/µL. The basis for the increased platelet count is unclear. Hemorrhage within an internal cavity is accompanied by a rise in unconjugated bilirubin and a fall in serum haptoglobin.

TREATMENT

Treatment of the underlying cause of the hemorrhage is of paramount importance. If the patient is severely anemic or sufficiently hypovolemic, packed red cells should be transfused. In less severe cases, if the patient has normal kidneys (and presumably a normal erythropoietin response to anemia), normal bone marrow function, and an adequate supply of iron, no specific therapy for the anemia is required.

BIBLIOGRAPHY

Amidon TM et al: Mitral and aortic paravalvular leaks with hemolytic anemia. Am Heart J 125:266, 1993

Becker PS, Lux SE: Disorders of the red cell membrane, in *Hematology of Infancy and Childhood,* DG Nathan, FA Oski (eds). Philadelphia, Saunders, 1992, pp 529–633

Beutler E: Study of glucose-6-phosphatedehydrogenase: History and molecular biology. Am J Hematol 42:53, 1993

Hirono A et al: Enzymatic diagnosis in non-spherocytic hemolytic anemia. Medicine 67:110, 1988

Miwa S, Fujii H: Molecular basis of erythroenzymopathies associated with hemolytic anemia: Tabulation of mutant enzymes. Am J Hematol 51:122, 1996

Palek J, Sahr SE: Mutations of the red blood cell membrane proteins: From clinical evaluation to detection of the underlying genetic defect. Blood 80:308, 1992

Robson WL et al: Hemolytic-uremic syndrome. Curr Probl Pediatr 23:16, 1993

Rose M et al: The changing course of thrombotic thrombocytopenic purpura and modern therapy. Blood Rev 7:94, 1993

Rosse WF: *Clinical Immunohematology.* Cambridge, Blackwell Scientific, 1990

———, Ware RE: The molecular basis of paroxysmal nocturnal hemoglobinuria. Blood 86:3277, 1995

Thompson CE et al: Thrombotic microangiopathies in the 1980s: Clinical features. Blood 80:1890, 1992

Table 110-2

110 | *Hugo Castro-Malaspina, Richard J. O'Reilly*

APLASTIC ANEMIA AND MYELODYSPLASTIC SYNDROMES

The anemias discussed in this chapter are usually normochromic and normocytic and associated with a low reticulocyte count. The hypoproliferative anemias associated with marrow damage include aplastic anemia, pure red cell aplasia, myelodysplastic syndromes, and myelophthisis (Fig. 59-4).

APLASTIC ANEMIA

Aplastic anemia is a disorder of hematopoiesis characterized by marked reduction or absence of erythroid, granulocytic, and megakaryocytic cells in the bone marrow with resultant pancytopenia. Hematopoiesis is markedly decreased, as shown by the marrow histology as well as the absent or reduced numbers of CD34 + cells and colony forming cells (see Plate IV-33). Hematopoietic stem cells in aplastic anemia are unable to proliferate and differentiate to give rise to mature blood cells and their precursors. The stem cell failure results in most cases from an acquired intrinsic stem cell defect and/or from an immune mechanism. Other potential mechanisms, such as growth factor deficiency and microenvironment defects, are rare and not well documented.

The overall incidence of aplastic anemia in Western countries has been estimated as 5 to 10 cases per million persons per year; about 1000 new cases are diagnosed every year in the United States. The disease can occur at any age, but is most common in young adults (15 to 30 years old) and elderly patients (>60 years old), with about the same incidence in males and females. The disease is more frequent in Asia than in North America and Europe, particularly in younger adults.

ETIOLOGY Most cases of aplastic anemia are acquired, but the disease may also occur as the result of inherited abnormalities, such as Fanconi's anemia. For acquired forms of aplastic anemia, a variety of causative factors, including certain drugs, viruses, organic compounds, and radiation, have been implicated (Table 110-1). However, for over half of patients, no cause can be determined (so-called idiopathic aplastic anemia). Even for patients in whom a well-defined association between exposure (e.g., to chloramphenicol) and subsequent development of aplastic anemia has been established, it remains unclear why only a small proportion of those exposed to a given agent develop the disease. Furthermore, the mechanisms by which certain agents or classes of agents (e.g., viruses, drugs) cause aplastic anemia are still poorly understood.

Table 110-1

Etiology of Aplastic Anemia

Acquired
  Drugs: antimetabolites, antimitotic agents, gold, chloramphenicol, phenyl-
    butazone, sulfonamides (see Table 110-2)
  Radiation
  Chemicals: benzene, solvents, insecticides
  Viruses: non-A, non-B, non-C hepatitis, human immunodeficiency virus,
    Epstein-Barr virus*
  Paroxysmal nocturnal hemoglobinuria
  Miscellaneous: pregnancy, connective tissue disorders, graft-versus-host
    disease
Hereditary
  Fanconi's anemia
  Dyskeratosis congenita
  Shwachman syndrome
Idiopathic: 50–65% of cases

* Parvovirus B19 may also produce transient aplastic crisis, but pure red cell aplasia is the more common manifestation.

Drugs Associated with Aplastic Anemia

Antineoplastic drugs
  Antimetabolites: fluorouracil, mercaptopurine, methotrexate
  Alkylating agents: busulfan, cyclophosphamide, nitrogen mustard,
    melphalan
  Cytotoxic antibiotics: daunorubicin, doxorubicin, mitoxantrone
Antimicrobial drugs
  Antibacterials: chloramphenicol, dapsone, β-lactam antibiotics
  Antifungals: amphotericin, flucytosine
  Antiprotozoals: quinacrine, chloroquine, pyrimethamine, mepacrine
Anti-inflammatory drugs: phenylbutazone, oxyphenbutazone, indomethacin,
  ibuprofen, naproxen, sulindac
Antiarthritic drugs: gold salts, colchicine
Anticonvulsant drugs: carbamazepine, phenytoin, ethosuximide, primidone
Analgesic drugs: phenacetin, salicylamide, aspirin
Antiarrhythmic drugs: quinidine, tocainamide
Antithyroid drugs: carbimazole, methimazole, methylthiouracil, potassium
  perchlorate, propylthiouracil, sodium thiocyanate
Sulfonamides and derivatives
  Antibacterials: sulfonamides
  Diuretics: acetazolamide, chlorothiazide, furosemide
  Hypoglycemics: chlorpropamide, tolbutamide
Antihypertensive drugs: captopril, methyldopa, enalapril
Antihistamine drugs: chlorpheniramine, pyrilamine, tripelennamine
Sedatives: chlordiazepoxide, chlorpromazine, lithium, meprobamate
Antiplatelet drugs: ticlopidine

Drugs Population-based case-control studies have shown an association between certain drugs and aplastic anemia. Drug-induced aplastic anemia may be dose-related or idiosyncratic. Table 110-2 shows some of the medications linked to aplastic anemia. The major classes of myelotoxic drugs are anticonvulsants, antibacterials, hypoglycemic and diuretic sulfonamides, antimetabolites, antimitotic agents, and synthetic antithyroid drugs. Certain classes of agents, such as antineoplastic drugs, antimetabolites, and sulfonamides, have a direct dose-dependent myelotoxic activity. However, for the other agents commonly associated with aplastic anemia, particularly chloramphenicol, phenylbutazone and oxyphenbutazone, indomethacin, and gold salts, aplasias are idiosyncratic and not dose related. The mechanisms contributing to aplasia are unclear. For instance, chloramphenicol produces a dose-related reversible suppression of erythropoiesis during treatment and an idiosyncratic, dose-independent global marrow suppression many weeks or months after cessation of therapy. Many other drugs have been linked to the development of aplastic anemia. For some of them, the incidence of aplastic anemia in exposed patients seems to be high enough to suggest an etiologic role, whereas with other drugs there is only a sporadic occurrence, and the causal relationship is difficult to establish.

Radiation Acute exposure causes a dose-related transient marrow suppression, which is reversible at low doses but is permanent and life-threatening at high doses. Chronic exposure to low-dose and localized radiation may cause late permanent marrow failure. For instance, patients irradiated for ankylosing spondylitis have a higher incidence of aplastic anemia. However, the incidence of aplastic anemia has been reported not to be increased in long-term survivors of the atomic bombings.

Benzene and Insecticides Benzene was the first organic solvent linked to aplastic anemia. There is a dose-effect relationship between exposure to benzene and the incidence of development of cytopenias. Chronic exposure has been associated with the development of aplastic anemia and leukemias. Benzene and related aryl hydrocarbons may generate catabolites that are directly toxic to stem cells. However, they may also induce formation of haptens that may stimulate immune responses. Benzene-induced aplasia in rabbits can be reversed following immunosuppression with antithymocyte globulin. DDT and lindane, well-recognized etiologic agents, are now outlawed as insecticides in the United States.

Viruses Viral illnesses are a precipitating event in some patients with aplastic anemia. The most common viral infection associated with aplastic anemia is viral hepatitis. Other viruses implicated in aplastic anemia include the Epstein-Barr virus, parvovirus B19, human immunodeficiency virus (HIV), and others. Approximately 1 to 5 percent of cases of aplastic anemia follow an overt hepatitis. Although hepatitis A, B, and C have been implicated in aplastic anemia in a small number of cases, most cases are not related to these viruses. Hepatitis G virus may be the major infection associated with marrow failure. Hepatitis preceding aplastic anemia is not usually severe, but posthepatitis aplastic anemia is commonly severe. While hepatitis viruses may induce lytic infection of primitive hematopoietic stem cells, the remissions of aplasia induced by immunosuppressive therapies in some cases of posthepatitis aplasia have suggested that immune responses induced by infection may also play a major role.

Parvovirus B19, the etiologic agent of erythema infectiosum (see Chap. 189), can cause transient erythroid aplasia in patients with underlying spherocytic anemias and hemoglobinopathies, and it can cause chronic marrow failure in immunodeficient patients. This virus infects and lyses hematopoietic stem cells. Persistent infection results from the inability to mount an adequate antibody response and is associated with pure red-cell aplasia. Epstein-Barr virus–induced infectious mononucleosis is rarely associated with aplastic anemia; blood counts usually recover spontaneously. Cytomegalovirus (CMV) has also been associated with marrow failure, particularly in marrow transplant recipients. Certain strains of CMV may infect the marrow stromal cells that support hematopoietic cell growth, thereby inducing secondary aplasia.

Pregnancy   Women may develop aplastic anemia during pregnancy. In a proportion of cases, aplasia has resolved with natural or premature termination of pregnancy, but it has sometimes recurred with a subsequent pregnancy. The pathogenesis and causal relationship between pregnancy and aplastic anemia is unknown.

Paroxysmal Nocturnal Hemoglobinuria   Paroxysmal nocturnal hemoglobinuria (PNH) is a clonal hemopathy caused by a defect in the *PIG-A* gene and is characterized by partial or complete inability to construct a glycosylphosphatidylinositol (GPI) anchor for the attachment of membrane proteins such as CD55, CD59, and others (see Chap. 109). Aplastic anemia can be the initial hematologic manifestation of this disease. PNH can also develop months to years after the diagnosis of aplastic anemia. The mechanisms whereby PNH induces aplastic anemia are unknown. The PNH clone may inhibit the growth of normal marrow progenitors. Alternatively, PNH clones may be less sensitive than normal counterparts to injury induced by viruses or toxins or the immune responses they elicit. A history of thrombosis and evidence of hemolysis in a patient with an aplastic anemia suggests the diagnosis of PNH. The diagnosis may be difficult to make, because the proportion of PNH cells in the blood may be too small to be detected by the Ham test (acidification of serum to pH 6.2 activates complement and lyses PNH cells). Flow cytometry using antibodies against cell-surface proteins, such as CD55 and CD59, which are lacking in this disease, are helpful in establishing this diagnosis. Aplastic patients with a positive Ham test may respond to anti-T-cell therapies such as cyclosporine and antithymocyte globulin.

Other Acquired Causes   Eosinophilic fasciitis, a rare connective tissue disease characterized by painful swelling and induration of the skin and subcutaneous tissue (see Chap. 383), has been associated with aplastic anemia. Myelosuppression is thought to be antibody-mediated. A similar mechanism has been implicated in systemic lupus erythematosus (SLE). However, patients with SLE and other autoimmune diseases are often treated with anti-inflammatory drugs and gold salts, which have been linked to aplastic anemia. Graft-versus-host disease may cause severe marrow suppression. Certain disorders of the immune system, including thymoma, X-linked lymphoproliferative disorder, and T-gamma lymphocyte proliferation have also been associated with marrow failure. Aplastic anemia also, in rare instances, precedes acute leukemia. The hypocellular variant of myelodysplastic syndrome (MDS) may present clinical and pathologic features difficult to distinguish from those of aplastic anemia.

Congenital Disorders   Fanconi's anemia (FA) is an autosomal recessive disorder characterized by a progressive pancytopenia, diverse congenital abnormalities, an increased predisposition to malignancy, and increased chromosomal fragility or cellular hypersensitivity to mutagenic chemicals. The features of FA include short stature, café-au-lait spots, kidney and urinary tract abnormalities, microphthalmia, mental retardation, and skeletal abnormalities, most often affecting the thumb and radius. Cells from FA patients are uniquely hypersensitive to the damaging effects of DNA-modifying agents such as diepoxybutane (DEB) and cyclophosphamide. Complementation analyses suggest that at least five different genetic defects may induce Fanconi's anemia. One genetic variant of this disease, type C, is due to a mutation of the *FACC* gene, which is involved in the cellular response to DNA damage.

Aplastic anemia also may occur as the result of other inherited disorders, such as Shwachman-Diamond syndrome and dyskeratosis congenita. Patients with Shwachman syndrome have pancreatic insufficiency, malabsorption, neutropenia, and an increased risk of aplastic anemia. Dyskeratosis congenita is a rare X-chromosome dermatologic syndrome characterized by reticular hyperpigmentation, mucous membrane leukoplakia, and dystrophic nails. About half of patients with this disease develop aplastic anemia.

PATHOGENESIS   The pathogenesis of this disease is complex and only partially understood. Acquired aplastic anemia results from two main pathogenic mechanisms: an acquired intrinsic stem cell defect and/or an immune suppressive mechanism. The fact that 40 to 50 percent of recipients of syngeneic transplants for aplastic anemia can achieve hematologic reconstitution without pretransplant immunosuppression suggests that a stem cell defect is responsible for the marrow failure in a significant proportion of patients. In the other 50 to 60 percent of recipients of syngeneic grafts, the donor marrow fails to engraft. However, use of immunosuppression before a second transplant can lead to prolonged hematologic recovery. Thus, in some cases, an immune mechanism contributes to the disease. The contribution of the immune system to the pathogenesis of aplastic anemia has been further supported by documentation of autologous recovery in patients receiving allogeneic bone marrow transplants after immunosuppressive conditioning and in patients with aplastic anemia who have achieved remission of disease following treatment with antithymocyte globulin and/or cyclosporine without transplantation. Activated cytotoxic T cells derived from the blood and the marrow of a significant proportion of patients with aplastic anemia overproduce cytokines such as interferon γ and tumor necrosis factor β (lymphotoxin) that suppress hematopoietic progenitors.

Approximately 25 percent of patients with aplastic anemia are cured by immunosuppressive therapy. However, 20 to 50 percent of patients with aplastic anemia who achieve a partial or, less commonly, a complete reconstitution of hematopoiesis following treatment with antithymocyte globulin develop myelodysplastic syndromes months to years after completion of immunosuppressive therapy. This high frequency has suggested the possibility that these patients develop aplastic anemia as a manifestation of an immune response directed against preexisting abnormal hematopoietic stem cells, or that these abnormal hematopoietic stem cells preferentially recover following immunosuppressive therapy. Whether stem cells in patients with aplastic anemia are normal or abnormal is under study.

CLINICAL MANIFESTATIONS   The onset of aplastic anemia is usually insidious. The most common presenting symptoms are those secondary to anemia and thrombocytopenia and include progressive weakness and fatigue and bleeding from the skin, nose, gums, vagina, or gastrointestinal tract. Although the patient may be severely neutropenic, infection is rarely the presenting symptom. The most frequent physical findings are cutaneous and conjunctival pallor and hemorrhages (petechiae, ecchymoses, and gum bleeding). If anemia is severe, tachycardia and murmurs associated with high-flow states may be present. Hepatosplenomegaly and lymphadenopathy are notably absent.

DIAGNOSIS   The diagnosis of aplastic anemia should be considered if a pancytopenic patient has a normochromic, normocytic (or slightly macrocytic) anemia, a low reticulocyte count (reticulocyte index < 2) indicative of a hypoproliferative mechanism, thrombocytopenia with normal-sized platelets, neutropenia, and the absence of abnormal cells in the leukocyte differential. Confirmation requires morphologic and cytogenetic evaluation of the bone marrow.

The bone marrow aspirate typically shows numerous spicules with empty fatty spaces and few hematopoietic cells. The hypocellularity is secondary to a marked decrease in megakaryocytes, granulocytes, and erythroid cells. Although sometimes the erythroid cells exhibit megaloblastic changes, the morphology of marrow elements is usually normal. The presence of overt dysplasia favors the diagnosis of hypocellular MDS. Lymphocytes, plasma cells, and mast cells are relatively increased and, in severe cases, constitute over 65 percent of the cells. Sometimes the cellularity appears normal because of isolated foci (hot spots) of hematopoiesis. The marrow biopsy allows a better assessment of the cellularity and permits evaluation for the presence of tumor cells, hairy cells, and fibrosis. Marrow cytogenetic studies distinguish aplastic anemia from MDS and Fanconi's anemia. The presence of clonal chromosomal abnormalities favors the diagnosis of MDS. However, a normal karyotype does not rule out this diagnosis. Assessment of clonality based on X chromosome inactivation in females suggests that stem cell abnormalities may be more frequent than originally suspected.

Serum levels of lactate dehydrogenase (LDH) and haptoglobin, Ham's test, and flow-cytometric analysis of peripheral blood cells using antibodies against the GPI-linked proteins are useful to establish or to rule out the diagnosis of PNH. In younger patients, the cytogenetics of marrow cells in the presence or absence of diepoxybutane may be diagnostic of FA, since patients with FA may not have a family history or other clinical findings of the disease.

CLASSIFICATION The International Aplastic Anemia Study Group distinguished severe and moderate forms of aplastic anemia. Aplasia is defined as *severe* when two or more of the following criteria are met: neutrophil count <500/μL, platelet count <20,000/μL, and reticulocyte count <20,000/μL. A new form with a worse prognosis characterized by a neutrophil count of <200/μL has been termed *super-severe* or *very severe*, aplastic anemia. This form has a lower response rate to and a poorer survival rate following immunosuppressive therapy.

DIFFERENTIAL DIAGNOSIS Patients with *hypocellular myelodysplastic syndrome* also have pancytopenia and a hypocellular bone marrow. However, the review of blood smears may show the presence of immature granulocytes or nucleated red cells. The few myeloid elements in the marrow have dysplastic changes, and the marrow karyotype may show a clonal abnormality. The differential diagnosis may be difficult when the dysplastic changes are subtle. *Hypocellular acute leukemia* can be misdiagnosed as aplastic anemia when the few mononuclear cells present in the bone marrow are not identified as blasts. Although *hairy cell leukemia* usually presents with splenomegaly and a hypercellular marrow, occasionally it presents without these features. The diagnosis is established by recognizing the few hairy cells by their typical morphology, as well as their cytochemical (tartrate-resistant acid phosphatase) and phenotypic (CD25+ monoclonal B cells) characteristics (see Chap. 113).

COURSE OF THE DISEASE AND PROGNOSIS The pancytopenia of aplastic anemia is progressive and life-threatening. With transfusion support alone, up to 80 percent of patients with severe aplastic anemia succumb to the disease within 18 to 24 months. Prognosis at diagnosis is closely correlated with the neutrophil count. The risk of infection, mainly bacterial and fungal, and associated mortality is high in patients with super-severe aplastic anemia. Before the advent of immunosuppressive therapy and allogeneic bone marrow transplantation, more than 25 percent of patients with severe aplastic anemia died within 4 months of diagnosis, and half died within one year. Treatment with androgens or glucocorticoids did not affect outcome.

Two therapeutic approaches, allogeneic bone marrow transplantation and immunosuppressive therapy, have radically improved the prognosis of patients with severe forms of aplastic anemia. Currently,

treatment with a human leukocyte antigen (HLA)-matched related marrow transplant is curative in 60 to 90 percent of patients. However, a proportion of long-term survivors suffer from chronic graft-versus-host disease. The success of bone marrow transplant correlates with age and degree of matching. The upper age limit for marrow transplantation continues to increase as better approaches are developed to prevent or treat transplant-related complications (see Chap. 116). Immunosuppressive therapy with antithymocyte or anti-thoracic duct lymphocyte globulin and/or cyclosporine can induce at least partial remission of disease in 60 to 80 percent of patients. However, about one-third of these responders relapse, and about 20 to 50 percent develop myelodysplastic syndromes. Patients who do not respond to immunosuppression can be maintained with supportive therapy, but their prognosis is poor. HLA-mismatched family member or unrelated donor marrow transplantation is an option for these patients.

℞ TREATMENT

Withdrawal of the etiologic agent is the most direct approach to the treatment of aplastic anemia. Discontinuation of a suspected drug, thymectomy in patients with thymoma, or delivery or therapeutic abortion in patients with pregnancy-associated aplastic anemia may result in recovery of blood counts. Unfortunately, these cases account for a very small proportion of patients.

Once the diagnosis of aplastic anemia is established, family HLA typing should be done as soon as possible, particularly in younger patients (<45 years), since these patients are most likely to benefit from bone marrow transplantation from a histocompatible sibling. Transfusions of blood products from family members should be avoided in transplant candidates to prevent sensitization to minor histocompatibility antigens, which increases the risk of graft rejection after transplantation. Whenever possible, only CMV-negative blood products should be given to CMV-seronegative potential transplant candidates to reduce the incidence of CMV infection in the post-transplant period. Immunosuppressive therapy is the treatment of choice for patients without a histocompatible sibling.

Supportive Therapy Blood and platelet transfusions should be used with caution because of short-term and long-term complications. The risk of bleeding should be carefully assessed, and platelet transfusions should be given only when the platelet count is less than 10,000/μL or if there is active bleeding with a higher platelet count. Pooled-donor platelets are usually used until sensitization occurs, as manifested by a failure of the transfusion to boost the platelet count. Ideally, single-donor platelets should be used from the beginning to minimize the risk of sensitization, but in practice, this alternative is difficult to carry out. Refractoriness to platelet transfusion is a major problem with long-term transfusion support. Refractory patients may need HLA-compatible platelet transfusions in case of severe hemorrhage.

Packed red cells also should be transfused when the hemoglobin concentration is <7 g/dL (70 g/L). Younger patients may tolerate lower values, whereas a higher threshold may be indicated in older patients. Packed red cells should be filtered to remove leukocytes and platelets to reduce sensitization. Chronic administration of red-cell transfusions results in secondary hemochromatosis, as each unit has approximately 200 to 250 mg of iron. Serum ferritin values should be monitored, and chelation therapy with deferoxamine should be given to reduce iron overload (see Chap. 342).

Patients with aplastic anemia who develop sepsis or other severe bacterial infections require intensive treatment with parenteral antibiotics. Leukocyte transfusions are likely only indicated in severely neutropenic (neutrophil count <200/μL) aplastic anemia patients with a documented fungal infection unresponsive to amphotericin, or bacterial infections with organisms that are resistant to most antibiotics. The modest benefits of such infusions should be weighed against the risks of sensitization and transmission of infectious agents, particularly CMV, which may compromise subsequent therapies (e.g., transplantation). Prophylactic use of antibiotics in afebrile neutropenic patients has no benefits and favors the emergence of resistant strains. *Staphylococcus epidermidis* is a common pathogen in patients with indwelling catheters. Neutropenic precautions should be used in patients who are hospitalized and have a neutrophil count of <500/μL. Menstruating females should be given suppressive doses of birth control pills to avoid severe blood losses.

Immunosuppressive Agents Several agents, including antithymocyte globulin (ATG) and cyclosporine (alone or in combination), glucocorticoids, and cyclophosphamide, have been used in aplastic anemia patients who do not qualify for transplantation because of their age or lack of a compatible donor. The licensed ATG preparations contain purified and concentrated gamma globulins, primarily monomeric IgG from hyperimmune serum of horses (also rabbits or goats) immunized with human thymocytes or thoracic duct lymphocytes. Several studies have recorded response rates to ATG treatment ranging from 50 to 70 percent. Of these responders, 20 to 30 percent achieve a complete and durable recovery of blood counts. The other 70 to 80 percent achieve a partial response and will be transfusion independent with platelet counts exceeding 20,000/μL and neutrophil counts exceeding 1000/μL.

The basis for the effects of ATG is unclear. Although ATG is an immunosuppressant, responses usually occur 8 to 12 weeks after its administration, long after the immunosuppressive effects of ATG have resolved. The response to ATG correlates with severity of the disease. Patients with the super-severe form have a lower response rate. Also, children have lower response rates than adults. The posttreatment survival is correlated with the severity of neutropenia and the level of response. Not surprisingly, complete responders have a better survival. Relapse occurs in approximately one-third of patients, particularly in those who achieve only a partial response. A second course of immunosuppressive therapy can induce a second response in a proportion of cases. The major long-term complication of therapy with ATG is the development of overt myelodysplastic syndrome or paroxysmal nocturnal hemoglobinuria in 30 to 60 percent of patients many months to years after therapy. These late complications are more frequent in patients who achieve a partial response. ATG is also associated with a higher incidence of secondary solid tumors, similar to that observed in aplastic anemia patients prepared for allogeneic bone marrow transplantation with regimens involving radiation therapy.

The experience with cyclosporine is less mature. Cyclosporine and ATG induce similar response rates. Combined therapy with ATG and cyclosporine induces higher and earlier response rates as compared to ATG alone, particularly in patients with the super-severe forms of aplasia. However, this combination has not significantly improved long-term survival. The impact of combined immunosuppressive therapy on the incidence of long-term complications is not known yet. Very-high-dose glucocorticoid treatment (prednisone at 10 to 20 mg/kg) can induce responses in a small proportion of patients with aplastic anemia, but glucocorticoids are no longer used as single agents because of their side effects and the better response rates achieved with other agents.

In one trial, therapy with cyclophosphamide alone was shown to induce complete responses in 7 of 10 patients with aplastic anemia. Strikingly, no MDS cases have been observed in long-term follow-up of this series, which contrasts with the 30 to 60 percent rates of MDS in patients treated with ATG. This treatment is not only immunosuppressive but also cytotoxic, and it may eliminate abnormal stem cell clones that give rise to MDS, thus favoring the expansion of suppressed normal stem cells.

Hematopoietic Growth Factors Recombinant hematopoietic growth factors have been explored as a first-line therapy for aplastic anemia and in the treatment of aplasia refractory to immunosuppressive therapy. Erythropoietin, granulocyte colony-stimulating factor (G-CSF), granulocyte-macrophage colony-stimulating factor (GM-CSF), interleukins (ILs) 1, 3, and 6, and stem cell factor can improve the blood counts, particularly the neutrophil counts, in only a small proportion of patients. Unfortunately, these increments are entirely dependent on the presence of residual normal hematopoietic progenitors. Patients with no neutrophils or very severe neutropenia (neutrophil count <200/μL) do not respond to growth factors. In patients who respond, blood counts drop to pretreatment values following discontinuation of the growth factor.

A common drawback to immunosuppressive treatments is that the response usually takes up to 12 weeks to appear, and, as a result, significant early mortality occurs, due in most cases to infections. The use of hematopoietic growth factors, particularly G-CSF, following intensive immunosuppression with ATG and cyclosporine, has resulted not only in a reduced frequency of infections because of rapid correction of neutropenia but also in a higher response rate. However, generalization of this approach awaits the results of randomized trials and long-term follow-up studies.

Data from randomized trials suggest that androgens are not beneficial in aplastic anemia; yet occasional patients who have failed other therapies respond to androgens.

Bone Marrow Transplantation Transplantation from an HLA-compatible sibling is a curative treatment for aplastic anemia. Unfortunately, this approach is only applicable to a minority of patients because the proportion of patients who have an HLA-matched sibling is about 25 to 30 percent. Current survival rates achievable with transplant (70 to 90 percent) reflect improvements in the management of transplant-related complications, particularly graft failure and graft-versus-host disease (GVHD). Early studies recorded a 20 to 30 percent incidence of graft failure in multiply transfused patients who were prepared for transplantation with cyclophosphamide alone. In contrast, the risk of graft failure in patients who had not been transfused was <5 percent. Subsequently, several approaches incorporating total-body or total-lymphoid irradiation in addition to cyclophosphamide administration were explored in an attempt to reduce the incidence of graft failure in sensitized patients. Although these treatments reduced the incidence of graft failure, long-term survival was not improved, because of the added transplant-related morbidity and mortality associated with these regimens. High-dose cyclophosphamide with ATG for pretransplant immunosuppression and cyclosporine prophylaxis for GVHD after transplantation has markedly reduced the incidence of graft failure and GVHD and has significantly improved the long-term survival (90 percent at 2 years after transplantation in one series).

What can be done for patients lacking sibling donors? Extended family searches, particularly in patients inheriting common HLA haplotypes, have led to the identification of donors who are HLA-matched or are mismatched in only a single HLA allele in a small proportion of cases (<5 percent). Transplants from such donors are associated with a higher incidence of acute and chronic GVHD. However, long-term survival is only slightly inferior to that achieved with matched related donor grafts. With the development of the National Marrow Donor Program and the European donor banks, over 2 million volunteer donors are now available for transplantation. Searches for donors in these pools has led to the identification of matched unrelated donors for up to 20 percent of patients. Matched unrelated donor transplants show a high incidence of acute and chronic GVHD. In addition, when the preparative regimen omitted total body irradiation, graft failure was common, and survival rates were only about 30 percent. Unrelated transplants should only be considered for patients who have failed immunosuppressive therapies and remain severely pancytopenic, particularly those who are affected with repeated infections and are refractory to platelet transfusions.

PURE RED CELL APLASIA

The selective absence of erythroid progenitors in an otherwise normal marrow is pure red cell aplasia (PRCA). Hereditary PRCA is the Diamond-Blackfan syndrome; anemia is detected within the first year of life, and other physical anomalies are present in about 30 percent of cases. The differential diagnosis includes in utero parvovirus infection and transient erythroblastopenia of childhood. PRCA in adults is usually an acquired disease. It may be idiopathic or associated with other medical problems such as thymoma, lymphoid malignancies, solid tumors, immunologic diseases like SLE and rheumatoid arthritis, or infections [especially viral; HIV, parvovirus, Epstein-Barr, hepatitis viruses, human T-lymphotropic virus type I (HTLV-I)]. Many of the drugs that may cause aplastic anemia (Table 110-2) may also cause PRCA, especially phenytoin, azathioprine, chloramphenicol, procainamide, and isoniazid. PRCA may complicate pregnancy. In some cases, immunoglobulin molecules directed at erythropoietin, at erythropoietin-responsive erythroid precursor cells, or at erythroblasts themselves may block the effects of erythropoietin or destroy erythroid cells. T-cell cytokines made by the tumor cells may block the response of erythroid precursors to erythropoietin in T-cell chronic lymphocytic leukemia and T-gamma lymphoproliferative disease. Parvovirus B19 may cause aplastic anemia acutely and transiently in people with underlying hemolytic anemia. The virus has a tropism for erythroid precursors and lyses them. In people who cannot mount an antibody response against the virus, the infection and destruction of erythroid progenitors persists, leading to PRCA. Parvoviral PRCA is usually detectable by the presence of giant pronormoblasts in the bone marrow, which are cells that are infected with parvovirus and are destined to die.

℞ **TREATMENT**

All medications should be stopped. A chest radiograph should be obtained to evaluate the presence of thymoma. Resection of thymoma usually reverses PRCA. Thymoma may be present in up to one-third of cases of PRCA. In the presence of evidence for persistent parvovirus infection (giant pronormoblasts, underlying immunosuppression), intravenous immunoglobulin is usually successful at treating the infection. PRCA that has been shown not to be due to thymoma, drugs, infection, or cancer is usually caused by an autoimmune mechanism and requires immunosuppressive therapy. Prednisone alone or with ATG, cyclosporine, azathioprine, or cyclophosphamide will successfully treat two-thirds of patients. Relapses may occur, but responses to a second or subsequent course of the same or alternative therapy are common. Progression to leukemia is rare (<5 percent).

MYELODYSPLASTIC SYNDROMES

Myelodysplastic syndromes, also referred to as preleukemic disorders, oligoblastic leukemia, or smoldering leukemia, are a group of acquired blood disorders that often progress to acute leukemia and are characterized by pancytopenias and low reticulocyte counts associated with a bone marrow that is typically normocellular or hypercellular with cells displaying overt morphologic abnormalities or dysplastic changes (alterations in size, shape, and organization of cells). Hematopoiesis in MDS is ineffective and, as a result, patients are pancytopenic in spite of having a cellular marrow.

In Western developed countries, MDSs are diagnosed in about 1 to 10 per 100,000 people every year; approximately 3000 new cases are expected each year in the United States. The rising incidence in recent years probably reflects increased awareness, better diagnostic criteria, and perhaps increased exposure to agents such as drugs or chemicals contributing to its etiology. Primary (or idiopathic) MDS may occur at any age, but is more common in elderly patients and is rare in children and young adults. The median age is usually between 70 and 80. Primary MDS is more common in males. The annual incidence is about 25 per 100,000 after age 70 years, comparable to that for chronic lymphocytic leukemia. The incidence of therapy-related (or secondary) MDS, particularly in younger patients, is increasing as more tumors are cured with radiation therapy and chemotherapy.

ETIOLOGY Although the causes of MDS are not well understood, certain factors are known to be contributory, including certain genetic and congenital anomalies, as well as exposure to radiation and to mutagenic chemicals.

Genetic and Congenital Factors Children with Down's syndrome have an increased risk of developing MDS and other forms of leukemia. Other genetic disorders prominently associated with MDS include Fanconi's anemia and von Recklinghausen's disease (neurofibromatosis).

Radiation Epidemiologic studies have linked MDS with exposure to high or repeated doses of ionizing radiation (x-rays and gamma rays). Atomic bomb survivors had 20- to 25-fold increase in the incidence of leukemia and MDS. Similarly, patients with cancers treated with high-dose radiation therapy, such as Hodgkin's disease and breast cancer, have a higher incidence of *therapy-related MDS*.

Chemicals and Drugs Individuals exposed over long periods to benzene have an increased higher incidence of MDS and other leukemias. Alkylating agents used in chemotherapy are known to induce therapy-related MDS.

Aplastic Anemia Of patients with aplastic anemia who are treated with immunosuppressive agents, 30 to 60 percent develop morphologic changes in the marrow cells and/or chromosome abnormalities consistent with the diagnosis of MDS, many years after the diagnosis of aplastic anemia. Similarly, a proportion of children with congenital neutropenia treated chronically with G-CSF develop this disorder.

PATHOGENESIS MDSs are clonal acquired disorders affecting the hematopoietic stem cells. Clonality has been demonstrated not only by the presence of clonal chromosome abnormalities but also through the study of glucose-6-phosphate dehydrogenase isoenzyme patterns and analysis of DNA polymorphism at X chromosome–linked loci. These studies have shown that MDS results from neoplastic transformation of the pluripotent stem cell with involvement of myeloid and, much less commonly, of lymphoid cell lineages.

The myeloid cells in MDS have not lost their ability to proliferate and differentiate, but they do undergo an abortive maturation resulting in an inadequate production of mature blood cells. As a result, most MDS patients have a cellular marrow but have low blood cell counts. Ineffective hematopoiesis is a hallmark of MDS. The ineffectiveness of the marrow cell production results from extensive intramedullary apoptotic cell death of myeloid precursors. The molecular basis of this phenomenon is not known.

CLINICAL MANIFESTATIONS MDSs are difficult to diagnose early in the course of the disease. The major difficulty in detecting MDS in its early stages is that patients are often asymptomatic. It is not uncommon for the disease to be discovered accidentally during a routine physical examination or a blood test. When symptoms do appear, they usually manifest in very subtle and varied forms of general malaise. Most common are complaints attributable to anemia, namely weakness, fatigue, palpitations, dizziness, headaches, and irritability. Thrombocytopenia may be manifested by excessive bleeding after a minor injury or surgical procedure, or by abnormal or unexplained skin bruises. Women may also present with heavy menstrual periods. Infections as a presenting symptom are less common and are usually associated with very severe neutropenia (neutrophil count <200/μL). A small proportion of patients present with a chronic or recurrent vasculitic skin rash.

The physical examination in patients with MDS is usually remarkable for anemia-related findings, such as pallor and tachycardia. Hepatosplenomegaly is rare and, if present, is usually moderate, except in patients with chronic myelomonocytic leukemia (CMML). Lymphadenopathy and purpura are uncommon.

DIAGNOSIS Since the symptoms outlined above are similar to those of other bone marrow failure syndromes, acute and chronic leukemia, and many other serious diseases, the diagnosis of MDS in patients with unexplained cytopenias requires careful morphologic evaluation of the blood and bone marrow cells.

Peripheral Blood The blood of a patient with MDS exhibits cytopenias involving one or multiple lineages. The reticulocyte count is low, indicating that the anemia is secondary to defective marrow production. Substantial anisocytosis with normocytic or mildly macrocytic indices is present. Some red blood cells may be macrocytic with a mean corpuscular volume of over 100 fL and exhibit abnormalities such as Howell-Jolly bodies, Abbott rings, and basophilic stippling. Nucleated red blood cells are not uncommon, and often they exhibit dysplastic changes. Mature neutrophils may have hypolobulated nuclei (pseudo Pelger-Huet anomaly) and very few or absent intracytoplasmic granules. In addition, immature granulocytes can be seen in the peripheral blood. A peculiar feature of MDS is an increase in the number of monocytes. Monocytosis is a distinctive feature of the CMML variant. Platelets in blood smears are often large and agranular. Rarely, micromegakaryocytes can be seen in peripheral blood.

Bone Marrow The confirmation of the diagnosis of MDS requires the morphologic examination of marrow elements. The bone marrow samples are analyzed for three important features: the cellularity, the number of blasts and ringed sideroblasts, and the presence of dysplastic changes. The marrow cellularity in MDS is typically normal or hypercellular. However, some cases present with a hypocellular marrow. The blast count and the number of ringed sideroblasts are important for defining the MDS subtype. The marrow cells of most patients with MDS exhibit dysplastic changes. Dyserythropoietic changes include nuclear abnormalities (multinuclearity, nuclear fragmentation, bizarre nuclear shape, abnormal mitosis, internuclear bridging, and abnormally dense chromatin), cytoplasmic abnormalities (Howell-Jolly bodies, defective hemoglobinization, and ringed sideroblasts), as well as nuclear-cytoplasmic asynchrony (dense chromatin nucleus with poorly hemoglobinized cytoplasm). The most common dysgranulopoietic changes are hypogranulation and hyposegmentation. The most frequent dysmegakaryopoietic changes are micromegakaryocytosis, megakaryocytes with multiple small nuclei, and hypolobulation. Sometimes dysplasia is subtle, requiring evaluation by an experienced hematologist.

Cytogenetic Studies Cytogenetic analysis of the marrow is an important diagnostic tool. Approximately half of patients with primary MDS and about 75 percent of patients with therapy-related MDS have chromosomal abnormalities. There is no single distinguishing chromosomal abnormality associated with MDS, but there are abnormalities that are more frequent, such as monosomy 7, 5q−, and trisomy 8. A variety of translocations are also common.

Molecular studies have also demonstrated an increased incidence of mutations involving the *ras, cFms* [monocyte colony-stimulating factor (M-CSF) receptor], *p53* and *RB* oncogenes in the hematopoietic cells of patients with MDS, and have identified some of the genes involved in specific chromosome deletions and translocations, such as loss of the interferon regulatory factor (IRF-1) gene in the 5q− abnormality, and the generation of a tel-PDGF-beta fusion gene in the t(5,12) translocation associated with CMML. The loss of a tumor suppressor gene such as *IRF-1* has been hypothesized to play a role in the pathogenesis of the disease.

CLASSIFICATION In 1976 and 1982, a group of hematologists from France, America, and Britain (FAB) published criteria providing a standardized and uniform basis for the diagnosis of MDS and a definition of subtypes. The FAB criteria are based on morphologic characteristics, including the blood and marrow blast count, the monocyte count, the presence of ringed sideroblasts, and the presence of Auer rods. There are five well-defined subtypes: *refractory anemia* (RA), *refractory anemia with ringed sideroblasts* (RARS), *refractory anemia with excess blasts* (RAEB), *refractory anemia with excess*

blasts in transformation (RAEB-t), and chronic myelomonocytic leukemia (CMML). The criteria used to distinguish the MDS subtypes are shown in Table 110-3.

In addition to these subtypes, there are less common variants of MDS, such as *hypocellular MDS* and *myelofibrotic MDS*, that are not included in this international classification. In contrast to most cases of MDS, the bone marrow of hypocellular MDS exhibits decreased cellularity, and the few remaining cells exhibit dysplasia. Myelofibrotic MDS is characterized by pancytopenia, minimal organomegaly, and a hypercellular bone marrow with fibrosis, trilineage dysplasia, and atypical megakaryocytic proliferation.

DIFFERENTIAL DIAGNOSIS Although the diagnosis of MDS is based on morphologic changes seen in the peripheral blood and bone marrow, none of these changes is specific for MDS. However, if these changes are associated with a clonal chromosomal abnormality, the diagnosis of MDS can be safely established. Cytopenias and dysplastic changes can also result from other etiologies, such as drugs, infections, toxic exposure, rheumatologic disorders, hypersplenism, vitamin deficiencies, tumors infiltrating the bone marrow, acute leukemia, and aplastic anemia.

Vitamin Deficiency Deficiencies of vitamins B_{12}, folic acid, and particularly vitamin B_6 can induce a hematologic picture similar to that of MDS. Therefore, serum levels of these vitamins should be measured, and attention should be paid to other symptoms that are associated with vitamin deficiency, e.g., neurologic symptoms in B_{12} deficiency.

Aplastic Anemia The blood and marrow picture of aplastic anemia and hypocellular MDS are very similar. Hypocellular MDS is sometimes difficult to distinguish from aplastic anemia, particularly when the dysplastic changes in the few remaining cells are subtle and there are no chromosomal abnormalities.

Paroxysmal Nocturnal Hemoglobinuria Although PNH more often presents with a picture of aplastic anemia, the blood and marrow picture is sometimes indistinguishable from that of MDS. Flow cytometry detects the absence of GPI-linked proteins.

Aleukemic Acute Leukemia Some patients with acute leukemia can present with pancytopenia without circulating blasts. The FAB has established that the diagnosis of acute leukemia should be made if the marrow blast count is >30 percent.

Acute and Chronic Myelofibrosis In acute myelofibrosis, the marrow is fibrotic, and the cells are mostly blasts, which in most instances are megakaryoblasts. In chronic myelofibrosis, organomegaly is prominent.

Other: Myelophthisic Anemia, Cirrhosis Metastasis of certain malignancies to the marrow may induce cytopenias with circulating immature marrow cells suggestive of MDS. The differential diagnosis of marrow metastasis from MDS requires a marrow biopsy study. Additional studies are usually necessary to exclude other pathologies.

COURSE OF THE DISEASE AND PROGNOSIS The course of MDS is closely related to two main factors: the severity of the cytopenia and the number of blasts. Patients with low-risk MDS (<5 percent blasts), which includes RA and RARS, usually have a long

Table 110-3

French-American-British (FAB) Classification of Myelodysplastic Syndromes

Fab Type	% of Cases	% Blasts Marrow	Blood	% Ringed Sideroblasts*	Monocytes	Dyspoiesis	Auer Rods
RA	28	<5	<1	<15	Rare	+	Absent
RARS	24	<5	<1	>15	Rare	+	Absent
RAEB	23	5–20	<5	<15	Rare	+ +	Absent
CMML	16	1–20	<5	<15	>1 × 10⁹/L	+ +	Absent
RAEB-t	9	20–30	>5	<15	Variable	+ +	+/−

* A ringed sideroblast is shown in **Plate IV-39**.

ABBREVIATIONS: RA, refractory anemia; RARS, refractory anemia with ringed sideroblasts; RAEB, refractory anemia with excess blasts; CMML, chronic myelomonocytic leukemia; RAEB-t, refractory anemia with excess blasts in transformation.

chronic phase with progressive worsening of the pancytopenia. Many patients succumb to complications associated with the pancytopenia or to the measures taken to treat them. For instance, patients who have received multiple red cell transfusions develop progressive hemochromatosis. Some of the low risk MDS patients eventually develop acute leukemia and die of its complications.

Patients with high-risk MDS usually have more severe cytopenias and a higher frequency of transformation to acute leukemia, which correlates with the number of blasts. However, many patients may die of complications associated with neutropenia, thrombocytopenia, and, less frequently, secondary hemochromatosis.

The prognosis for patients with MDS is shown in Table 110-4. Patients with RAEB and RAEB-t generally have a higher rate of progression to acute leukemia and a shorter survival. In contrast, patients with RA and RARS have a better prognosis. Patients with CMML have an intermediate prognosis. In addition to the FAB classification, the presence of chromosomal abnormalities has been shown the have a significant prognostic value. Patients with no chromosomal abnormalities have a lower chance of developing leukemia and a higher chance of longer survival. More refined prognostic scoring systems are based on the age, the number of blasts, the severity of pancytopenia, and the presence of chromosomal abnormalities.

℞ TREATMENT

Allogeneic bone marrow transplantation (BMT) is the only curative treatment for MDS. Unfortunately, this treatment is only applied to the minority of MDS patients who are under 55 years of age and have histocompatible donors. For all other patients, supportive therapy is the mainstay of the management. The results achieved with other approaches, such as chemotherapy, have not altered the natural history of the disease.

Supportive Therapy   Red cell and platelet transfusions and the use of antibiotics to treat infection constitute the most common therapies used in MDS patients. Although patients can receive many red cell and platelet transfusions, secondary hemochromatosis and alloimmunization limit repeated and prolonged use of these treatments. In heavily transfused patients, iron chelation with deferoxamine may prevent or delay the complications associated with hemochromatosis.

Hematopoietic Growth Factors   Hematopoietic growth factors can induce improvements in targeted cell counts in a relatively small proportion of patients. Those patients who do respond require continuous administration of growth factor to maintain the response. In some patients, progression to acute leukemia may be facilitated by chronic administration of cytokines. Erythropoietin and G-CSF are the most beneficial in MDS. Erythropoietin is effective in improving red cell production only in patients with low serum erythropoietin levels. G-CSF is beneficial in MDS patients who are neutropenic and have an infection. The increase in neutrophil counts in these cases can be lifesaving. The prophylactic use of G-CSF is not recommended unless the neutrophil count is <200/µL.

Vitamin Therapy, Steroid Hormones, and Immunosuppressive Agents   Certain vitamins, such as B_6, B_{12}, and folic acid, may be of help in some patients with MDS, since the increased but ineffective production of blood cells may deplete the body of these vitamins. Vitamin deficiency can worsen the pancytopenia. Glucocorticoids are of limited benefit in most patients with MDS, and their prolonged use can cause serious side effects. Androgens improve the blood counts of only a small proportion of patients with MDS. Administration of immunosuppressive agents, specifically antithymocyte globulin and/or cyclosporine, improves the blood counts of some patients with hypocellular MDS. These agents have not been systematically evaluated in patients with the other variants of MDS.

Differentiation Therapy   A prominent feature of MDS is the inability of the transformed marrow cells to fully differentiate to functional cells. Retinoic acids, vitamin D_3, and interferon α can induce the differentiation of immature malignant cell lines in vitro. Unfortunately, the use of these differentiation agents in the treatment of MDS has been disappointing. Most trials have demonstrated only a limited benefit in a very small proportion of patients.

Low-Dose Chemotherapy   Cytosine arabinoside, azacytidine, and topotecan, when given at low doses, can induce responses in some patients with MDS. These agents do not induce differentiation. They suppress the growth of the leukemic clone and allow the few remaining normal clones to repopulate the bone marrow and give rise to normal blood cells. Unfortunately, these responses are transient and are achieved in only a minority of patients.

Intensive (High-Dose) Chemotherapy   Chemotherapeutic agents given at high doses, as in the treatment of acute leukemia, can also induce remission in 40 to 60 percent of MDS patients. Such remissions are short-lived. Intensive chemotherapy often induces serious side effects, but it can be of some benefit in high-risk MDS patients who are candidates for BMT. Intensive chemotherapy is usually employed in patients with advanced forms of MDS, and it should not be used in older patients, since toxic side effects can be fatal in this age group.

Bone Marrow Transplantation   A bone marrow transplant from a histocompatible sibling can be curative in up to 60 percent of patients with MDS. The problems that have limited the success of BMT in MDS are mainly the transplant-related complications and recurrence of the disease in the post-transplant period. In MDS, GVHD is a common transplant-related complication, since the majority of MDS patients are older adults, in whom GVHD is more frequent. Post-transplant disease relapse is a major complication for those patients who have an excess of blasts at the time of transplantation. Of patients with RAEB and RAEB-t, 25 to 50 percent relapse within the first 2 years after the transplantation, versus <1 percent for patients with RA or RARS. Two approaches are being used to overcome this limitation. The first invokes intensive myeloablative treatments immediately before transplant in an attempt to eradicate the MDS. The higher intensity of these regimens is associated with a higher morbidity and mortality. Another approach invokes treatment of the patient with conventional induction chemotherapy to achieve remission or a phase of MDS without excess blasts and then perform BMT. Unfortunately, HLA-matched sibling donors are identified in no more than 25 to 30 percent of patients with MDS. Transplants from matched unrelated donors or partially mismatched related donors are associated with complications; particularly severe acute and chronic GVHD and infections have limited their success.

MYELOPHTHISIC ANEMIA

Replacement of the marrow with fibrosis (see **Plate IV-34**), often accompanied by a leukoerythroblastic response (neutrophilia, immature granulocytes, nucleated red cells, teardrop-shaped red cells) in the peripheral blood (see **Plate IV-12**), can occur as a primary hematologic disease called myeloid metaplasia or myelofibrosis (see Chap. 111) or as a secondary process called myelophthisis. The obliteration of the marrow space by fibrosis may be a reaction to invading tumor cells, infectious agents, particularly *Mycobacterium tuberculosis* or fungi, lipid storage diseases such as Gaucher's disease, or granulomas (e.g., sarcoidosis). In addition, in a rare congenital bone disease, osteopetrosis, the failure of osteoclasts to remodel bone can lead to

Table 110-4

Survival and Leukemic Transformation in Myelodysplastic Syndrome

Syndrome	Median Survival in Months (Range)	% Leukemic Transformation (Range)
RA	37 (19–64)	11 (0–20)
RARS	49 (21–76)	5 (0–15)
CMML	22 (8–60 +)	20 (3–55)
RAEB	9 (7–15)	23 (11–50)
RAEB-t	6 (5–12)	48 (11–75)

obliteration of the marrow space with bone and fibrous tissue. The tumors associated with marrow fibrosis are both hematopoietic (hairy cell leukemia, acute and chronic leukemia, lymphoma, Hodgkin's disease, myeloma) and epithelial (especially breast, lung, prostate, stomach) in origin. Many cytokines produced by tumor cells, during a chronic inflammatory response, or by cells resident in the bone marrow may stimulate fibroblast expansion including transforming growth factor β and platelet-derived growth factor. However, the cause of myelophthisis is usually not defined. Patients usually have normocytic, normochromic anemia with characteristic teardrop red cells suggesting membrane damage done by collagen fibers, low reticulocyte count, and circulating normoblasts. Platelet counts are reduced but granulocyte counts are normal or increased initially. The marrow fibrosis is often associated with extramedullary hematopoiesis (and sometimes hepatosplenomegaly) that maintains neutrophil production but fails to generate adequate red cells and platelets. Marrow may be difficult to aspirate ("dry tap"), but biopsy reveals fibrosis and usually the primary process—tumor or granuloma—is apparent. Therapy is aimed at the primary process. Some of the cancers that produce myelophthisis are more treatable than others. It is crucial to rule out tuberculosis and fungal infections that may be treatable.

BIBLIOGRAPHY

APLASTIC ANEMIA

BACIGALUPO A et al: Antithymocyte globulin, cyclosporine, and granulocyte colony-stimulating factor in patients with acquired severe aplastic anemia: A pilot study of the EBMT working party. Blood 85:1348, 1995

GLUCKMAN E et al: Marrow transplantation for severe aplastic anemia: Influence of conditioning and graft-versus-host disease prophylaxis regimens on outcome. Blood 79:269, 1992

MARSH JCW et al: Haemopoietic growth factors in aplastic anemia: A cautionary note. Lancet 344:172, 1994

STORB R et al: Cyclophosphamide combined with anti-thymocyte globulin in preparation for allogenic marrow transplants in patients with aplastic anemia. Blood 84:941, 1994

YOUNG N et al: The treatment of severe aplastic anemia. Blood 85:3367, 1995

MYELODYSPLASTIC SYNDROMES

ANDERSON JE et al: Allogeneic bone marrow transplantation for 93 patients with myelodysplastic syndromes. Blood 82:677, 1993

BENNETT JM et al: Proposals for the classification of the myelodysplastic syndromes. Br J Haematol 51:189, 1982

MOREL P et al: Cytogenetic analysis has strong independent prognostic value in the novo myelodysplastic syndromes and can be incorporated in a new scoring system: A report of 408 cases. Leukemia 7:1315, 1993

RAZA A et al: Apoptosis in bone marrow biopsy samples involving stromal and hematopoietic cells in 50 patients with myelodysplastic syndromes. Blood 86:268, 1995

SAN MIGUEL JF et al: Myelodysplastic syndromes. Crit Rev Oncol Hematol 23:57, 1996

SANZ GF et al: Two regression models and a scoring system for predicting survival and planning treatment in myelodysplastic syndromes: A multivariate analysis of prognostic factors in 370 patients. Blood 74:395, 1989

111   *Jerry L. Spivak*

POLYCYTHEMIA VERA AND OTHER MYELOPROLIFERATIVE DISEASES

Polycythemia vera, idiopathic myelofibrosis, essential thrombocytosis, and chronic myelogenous leukemia are commonly classified together under the rubric *the chronic myeloproliferative disorders*, because their pathophysiology involves the clonal expansion of a multipotent hematopoietic progenitor cell with the overproduction of one or more of the formed elements of the blood. These entities may transform into acute leukemia naturally or as a consequence of mutagenic treatment. However, while polycythemia vera, idiopathic myelofibrosis, essential thrombocytosis, and chronic myelogenous leukemia share similar phenotypic characteristics, chronic myelogenous leukemia is genotypically distinct from the other three disorders because it alone is associated with translocation of genetic material between the long arms of chromosomes 9 and 22, resulting in the production of the unique fusion protein, bcr-abl. Furthermore, in contrast to the other chronic myeloproliferative disorders, based on its natural history, chronic myelogenous leukemia is more appropriately considered as a form of leukemia. → *This is discussed in Chap. 112 with the leukemias.*

POLYCYTHEMIA VERA

Polycythemia vera is a clonal disorder involving a multipotent hematopoietic progenitor cell in which there is overproduction of phenotypically normal red cells, granulocytes, and platelets in the absence of a recognizable physiologic stimulus. Polycythemia vera is the most common of the chronic myeloproliferative disorders, with a frequency as high as 29 per 100,000. It spares no age group amongst adults. In several families, vertical transmission has been documented, establishing a genetic basis for the disorder. Although a slight overall male predominance has been observed, our experience suggests female predominance within the reproductive age range.

ETIOLOGY   The etiology of polycythemia vera is unknown. Although nonrandom chromosome abnormalities such as 20q-, trisomy 8 or 9 have been documented in a small percentage of untreated polycythemia vera patients, no consistent cytogenetic abnormality has been associated with the disorder and no specific genetic defect has yet been identified. In contrast to normal erythroid progenitor cells, polycythemia vera erythroid progenitor cells can grow in vitro in the absence of erythropoietin. However, this phenotypic abnormality is not specific for polycythemia vera and has been documented in essential thrombocytosis as well as in patients with erythrocytosis of undefined etiology in the presence of a normal or high serum erythropoietin level. Polycythemia vera erythroid progenitor cells are more resistant to apoptosis induced by erythropoietin deprivation, but the biochemical basis for this is unknown. Additionally, the transformed hematopoietic progenitor cells in polycythemia vera, as in other myeloproliferative disorders, exhibit clonal dominance and by an unknown mechanism suppress the proliferation of normal hematopoietic progenitor cells. As a consequence, eventually the circulating formed elements of the blood represent only progeny of the transformed clone.

CLINICAL FEATURES   Although massive splenomegaly may be the initial presenting sign in polycythemia vera, most often the disorder is first recognized by the discovery of a high hemoglobin or hematocrit, and with the exception of aquagenic pruritus, no symptoms distinguish polycythemia vera from other causes of erythrocytosis.

Uncontrolled erythrocytosis can, of course, lead to neurologic symptoms such as vertigo, tinnitus, headache, and visual disturbances. Systolic hypertension also accompanies an elevated red cell mass. In some patients venous or arterial thrombosis may be the presenting manifestation of polycythemia vera. Intraabdominal venous thrombosis is particularly common and may be catastrophic when there is sudden compromise of the hepatic vein. Indeed, polycythemia vera should be suspected in any patient who develops the Budd-Chiari syndrome. Digital ischemia may also occur. Easy bruising, epistaxis, or gastrointestinal hemorrhage may be observed, and given the overactive hematopoietic system, polycythemia vera patients are frequently hypermetabolic. Because isolated erythrocytosis is a common initial presentation for polycythemia vera but no clonal marker is available for the disease, the first task of the physician is to distinguish this autonomous clonal form of erythrocytosis from the many other types of erythrocytosis, most of which are correctable (Table 111-1). It is helpful in this regard to understand the physiology of erythropoietin, the primary regulator of erythropoiesis.

Table 111-1

Causes of Absolute Erythrocytosis

Hypoxia
  Carbon monoxide intoxication
  High altitude
  Pulmonary disease
  High-affinity hemoglobin
  Sleep-apnea syndrome
  Respiratory center dysfunction
  Supine hypoventilation
  Right-to-left cardiac shunts
Renal disease
  Renal cysts
  Hydronephrosis
  Renal artery stenosis
  Focal glomerulonephritis
  Renal transplantation
Tumors
  Hypernephroma
  Hepatoma
  Cerebellar hemangioblastoma
  Adrenal adenoma
  Pheochromocytoma
  Meningioma
  Uterine fibromyoma
Familial (with normal hemoglobin function)
Bartter's syndrome
Androgen therapy
Recombinant erythropoietin therapy
Polycythemia vera

Under normal circumstances, erythropoiesis is regulated by the glycoprotein hormone erythropoietin. Erythropoietin, which in adults is produced primarily in the kidneys and to a small extent in the liver, promotes the proliferation of erythroid progenitor cells, maintains their survival, and facilitates their differentiation. Because erythropoietin acts as a survival factor, it is constitutively produced and, like the red cell mass, its level in a given individual is constant as long as tissue oxygenation is adequate. The plasma erythropoietin level, like the red cell mass, does differ amongst individuals but in adults is not affected by either age or gender. Erythropoietin production is regulated at the level of gene transcription. Hypoxia is the only physiologic stimulus that increases the number of cells producing erythropoietin, and as a corollary, the production and metabolism of erythropoietin are independent of its plasma level. Thus, in the absence of renal or hepatic disease, plasma erythropoietin levels reflect erythropoietin production, and because there is only one form of erythropoietin in the circulation, the assay for plasma erythropoietin provides a measure of renal erythropoietin production and, therefore, a surrogate assay for tissue hypoxia. There is a caveat to this, however. Erythropoietin is a potent hormone, active at the picomolar level, and its production is tightly regulated. Thus, until the hemoglobin level falls below 105 g/L, the plasma erythropoietin level does not rise outside the normal range. This is not meant to imply that an increase in erythropoietin production does not occur as the hemoglobin level falls below normal, but because the normal range for plasma erythropoietin is wide (4 to 26 mU/mL), unless the patient's baseline level is known, any increase will not be recognized until the hemoglobin falls below 105 g/L. Thereafter, there is a log-linear inverse correlation between the levels of plasma erythropoietin and hemoglobin. With erythrocytosis, erythropoietin production is suppressed; this suppression reflects not only the increase in tissue oxygen transport associated with the increase in red cell number but also an additional negative-feedback mechanism that is independent of oxygen transport but is related to the erythrocytosis-induced increase in blood viscosity alone. The summation of both these mechanisms accounts for the paradoxical observation that many patients with hypoxic erythrocytosis due to cyanotic congenital heart disease or obstructive lung disease have a "normal" plasma erythropoietin

Table 111-2

Effect of Sampling Time on the Determination of the Red Cell Mass by Isotope Dilution

Time after Injection of ^{51}C-labeled Erythrocytes, min	Red Cell Mass, mL/kg
60	54
90	62
180	68
240	71

level. Of course, normal is relative in this circumstance because the normal range is so wide. Nevertheless, the plasma erythropoietin level is a useful diagnostic test in patients with isolated erythrocytosis, because an elevated level essentially excludes polycythemia vera as the cause for the erythrocytosis.

DIAGNOSIS When confronted with an elevated hemoglobin or hematocrit level, it is important to obtain previous values to determine the duration of this laboratory abnormality. Because the hemoglobin or hematocrit level is affected by the plasma volume, and there is not a linear correlation between hematocrit and red cell mass, a red cell mass determination must also be performed to distinguish absolute erythrocytosis from relative erythrocytosis due to a reduction in plasma volume alone (also known as *stress* or *spurious erythrocytosis* or *Gaisböck's syndrome*). The importance of red cell mass determination cannot be overemphasized because in polycythemia vera, in contrast to erythropoietin-driven erythrocytosis, the plasma volume is frequently elevated, not only masking the true extent of red cell mass expansion but often its presence. Indeed, a significant proportion of patients with polycythemia vera with a hematocrit within the normal range actually have an elevated red cell mass, and this is particularly true in patients with a substantial splenomegaly. Failure to recognize this phenomenon is undoubtedly the basis for many of the reported instances of hepatic or portal vein thrombosis in patients with a so-called undefined myeloproliferative disorder.

The only reliable method for determining the red cell mass is by isotope dilution using the patient's ^{51}C-tagged red cells; extrapolations made by determining directly only the plasma volume are unacceptable. Furthermore, to allow ample time for equilibration of the labeled red cells, measurements should be made over a period of no less than 90 min. Only in this manner can an adequate assessment of red cell mass be obtained (Table 111-2).

Once the presence of erythrocytosis has been established, its cause must be determined. An elevated plasma erythropoietin level suggests either an hypoxic cause for erythrocytosis or autonomous erythropoietin production, in which case assessment of pulmonary function and an abdominal computed tomography scan to evaluate renal and hepatic anatomy are appropriate. As mentioned above, a normal erythropoietin level does not exclude an hypoxic cause for erythrocytosis. In polycythemia vera, in contrast to hypoxic erythrocytosis, the arterial oxygen saturation is normal. However, a normal oxygen saturation does not exclude a high-affinity hemoglobin as a cause for erythrocytosis, and it is here that documentation of previous hemoglobin levels and a family study become important. Because there is no clonal marker for polycythemia vera, clinical guidelines have been proposed to define the disease. A modified version is provided in Table 111-3. However, it must be strongly emphasized that these are only guidelines; they do not establish clonality, and in some patients only with time will the

Table 111-3

Suggested Criteria for the Clinical Diagnosis of Polycythemia Vera*

Elevated red cell mass
Normal arterial oxygen saturation
Splenomegaly
In the absence of splenomegaly:
  Leukocytosis and thrombocytosis
Plasma erythropoietin level less than 4 mU/mL

---

* It must be emphasized that these criteria do not establish clonality.

underlying disorder become apparent. Diagnostic ambiguity, however, does not preclude the initiation of therapy as described below.

CHAPTER 111
Polycythemia Vera and Other Myeloproliferative Diseases
681

Other laboratory studies that may prove useful diagnostically include the red cell count, mean corpuscular volume, and red cell distribution width (RDW). Only three situations cause microcytic erythrocytosis: β-thalassemia trait, hypoxic erythrocytosis, and polycythemia vera. However, with β-thalassemia trait the RDW is normal, whereas with hypoxic erythrocytosis and polycythemia vera, the RDW is usually elevated. A properly made blood smear from a patient with erythrocytosis will be virtually unreadable due to the marked elevation in red cell count, but as mentioned above, there are no specific histologic abnormalities of the leukocytes or platelets in polycythemia vera. However, when these are also elevated the diagnosis is assured. In many patients, the leukocyte alkaline phosphatase is also increased, as is the uric acid. Elevated serum vitamin B_{12} or B_{12}-binding capacity may be present.

Although much has been written about bone marrow histology in polycythemia vera, a bone marrow aspirate and biopsy will provide no specific diagnostic information, and unless there is a need to establish the presence of myelofibrosis or exclude some other disorder, these procedures cannot be routinely recommended. The presence of a cytogenetic abnormality such as trisomy 8 or 9 or 20q- in the setting of an expansion of the red cell mass of course supports the existence of a clonal etiology for this expansion. However, as mentioned above, there is no specific cytogenetic abnormality associated with polycythemia vera, and the absence of a cytogenetic marker does not exclude the diagnosis.

COMPLICATIONS The major clinical complications of polycythemia vera relate directly to the increase in blood viscosity associated with elevation of the red cell mass and indirectly to the increased turnover of red cells, leukocytes, and platelets and the attendant increase in uric acid and histamine production. The latter appears to be responsible for the increase in peptic ulcer disease seen in patients with polycythemia vera and also for the pruritus associated with this disorder, although little formal proof for this has been obtained. A sudden massive increase in spleen size is another problem and can be associated with splenic infarction or progressive cachexia. Myelofibrosis and myeloid metaplasia can also develop with transfusion-dependent anemia, but the frequency with which these occur has never been established in a prospective study. Although acute nonlymphocytic leukemia is reported to have a higher incidence in polycythemia vera, the incidence of acute leukemia in untreated patients is low and there is no correlation between the development of leukemia and disease duration, suggesting that other factors such as the type of treatment employed may be more important in this regard than the disease itself.

Erythromelalgia is a curious syndrome of unknown etiology involving primarily the lower extremities and manifested usually by erythema, warmth, and pain of the affected appendage and occasionally digital infarction. It occurs with a variable frequency in patients with a myeloproliferative disorder and is usually responsive to salicylates. It is not unlikely that some of the central nervous system symptoms observed in patients with polycythemia vera represent a variant of erythromelalgia.

As mentioned earlier, if left uncontrolled, erythrocytosis can lead to intravascular thrombosis that frequently involves vital organs such as the liver, heart, brain, or lungs. Patients with massive splenomegaly are particularly prone to thrombotic events because the associated increase in plasma volume masks the true extent of the red cell mass elevation as measured by the hematocrit or hemoglobin level. A "normal" hematocrit or hemoglobin level in a polycythemia vera patient with massive splenomegaly should be considered as indicative of an elevated red cell mass until proven otherwise.

℞ **TREATMENT**
Polycythemia vera is generally an indolent disorder whose clinical course can run many decades, and its medical management should reflect the tempo of the disorder. Maintenance of the hemoglobin level at 140 g/L or less in men and 120 g/L or less in women is mandatory to avoid the thrombotic complications associated with an elevated red cell mass. It cannot be emphasized too strongly that thrombosis due to erythrocytosis is the most significant complication of this disorder. Statements to the effect that the erythrocytosis of polycythemia vera cannot be controlled by phlebotomy alone, or that phlebotomy-induced iron deficiency is detrimental metabolically as well as contributing to the hyperviscosity observed in this disorder, unfortunately reflect a total misunderstanding of the pathophysiology of polycythemia vera and its treatment. Phlebotomy serves initially to reduce hyperviscosity by bringing the red cell mass into the normal range. Periodic phlebotomies thereafter serve to maintain the red cell mass within the range of normal and to induce a state of iron deficiency, which prevents an accelerated reexpansion of the red cell mass. In most polycythemia vera patients, once an iron-deficient state is achieved, phlebotomy is usually required only at 3-month intervals. Although both phlebotomy and iron deficiency, in addition to the disease itself, tend to increase the platelet count, it cannot be emphasized enough that there is no correlation between thrombocytosis and thrombosis in polycythemia vera, in contrast to the strong correlation between erythrocytosis and thrombosis in this disease. Indeed, the use of salicylates as a tonic against thrombosis in polycythemia vera patients is potentially harmful, and salicylates should be employed only to treat erythromelalgia. There is also no routine indication for the use of oral anticoagulants, which may be difficult to employ owing to the artifactual imbalance between the test tube anticoagulant and plasma that occurs when blood from these patients is assayed for prothrombin or partial thromboplastin activity. Asymptomatic hyperuricemia requires no therapy, but allopurinol should be administered to avoid further elevation of the uric acid when chemotherapy is employed to reduce splenomegaly or leukocytosis-associated pruritus. Generalized pruritus intractable to antihistamines can be a major problem in polycythemia vera, and both hydroxyurea and psoralens with ultraviolet light in the A range (PUVA) therapy have been used effectively in this situation. Asymptomatic thrombocytosis requires no therapy. When it is necessary to lower the platelet count or reduce splenomegaly, hydroxyurea or recombinant interferon α have been useful, although each can be associated with significant side effects and neither is totally effective. Anagrelide, a quinazolin derivative and platelet antiaggregant that also lowers the platelet count, is currently under investigation for the treatment of thrombocytosis, but attention to the platelet count should not be allowed to divert attention from the important issues in polycythemia vera. A reduction in platelet number may be necessary in the treatment of erythromelalgia if salicylates are not effective, or if the thrombocytosis is associated with migraine-like symptoms, but any therapeutic decision in this regard should be made only after the red cell mass has been reduced to normal. Alkylating agents and ^{32}P are leukemogenic in polycythemia vera, and their use should be avoided. In some patients, massive splenomegaly unresponsive to reduction by hydroxyurea or interferon α therapy and associated with intractable weight loss will require splenectomy.

When approached from this perspective, patients with polycythemia vera can be expected to live long and useful lives, and reports of limited life expectancy due to thrombotic events appear to be primarily a consequence of inadequate control of the red cell mass, which in turn reflects a lack of understanding of the basic pathophysiology of this unique disorder. Furthermore, in those patients with isolated erythrocytosis for which the cause is not clear, potentially harmful treatment can be avoided because chemotherapy is never indicated to control the red cell mass unless venous access is impossible.

IDIOPATHIC MYELOFIBROSIS

Idiopathic myelofibrosis (other designations include *agnogenic myeloid metaplasia* or *myelofibrosis with myeloid metaplasia*) is a clonal disorder of a multipotent hematopoietic progenitor cell of unknown etiology characterized by marrow fibrosis, myeloid metaplasia with extramedullary hematopoiesis, and splenomegaly. Idiopathic myelofibrosis is uncommon, and in the absence of a specific clonal marker, establishing this diagnosis is difficult because myelofibrosis and myeloid metaplasia with splenomegaly are also features of both polycythemia vera and chronic myelogenous leukemia. Furthermore, myelofibrosis and splenomegaly occur in a variety of benign and malignant disorders (Table 111-4), many of which are amenable to specific therapies not effective in idiopathic myelofibrosis. In contrast to the other chronic myeloproliferative disorders and so-called acute or malignant myelofibrosis, which can occur at any age, idiopathic myelofibrosis primarily afflicts individuals in their sixth decade or later.

ETIOLOGY The etiology of idiopathic myelofibrosis is unknown. Although nonrandom chromosome abnormalities such as 20q-, 13q-, and trisomy 21 are not uncommon, no specific cytogenetic abnormality has been identified. There is also no correlation between the degree of myelofibrosis and the extent of extramedullary hematopoiesis. Analysis of collagen synthesis in this disorder has revealed overproduction of type III collagen, and this notion has been hypothetically linked to overproduction of platelet-derived growth factor or transforming growth factor β, but no biochemical substantiation for this notion has been forthcoming. Importantly, fibroblasts in idiopathic myelofibrosis are not part of the neoplastic clone, while the nature of collagen synthesis in other disorders complicated by myelofibrosis (Table 111-4) has not been evaluated to the same extent.

CLINICAL FEATURES There are no specific signs or symptoms associated with idiopathic myelofibrosis. Early in the course of the disease, most patients are asymptomatic and are usually detected by the discovery of splenic enlargement during a routine examination. Evaluation of a blood smear reveals the characteristic features of extramedullary hematopoiesis: teardrop-shaped red cells, nucleated red cells, myelocytes, and promyelocytes; myeloblasts may also be present but have no prognostic significance. Anemia, usually mild initially, is the rule, while the leukocyte and platelet counts are either normal or increased but either can be depressed. Mild hepatomegaly may accompany the splenomegaly, and both the LDH and serum alkaline phosphatase can be elevated. The leukocyte alkaline phosphatase can be low, normal, or elevated. Marrow may be unaspirable due to the myelofibrosis, and bone x-rays may reveal osteosclerosis. If it is exuberant, extramedullary hematopoiesis can cause ascites, pulmonary hypertension, intestinal or ureteral obstruction, intracranial hypertension, pericardial tamponade, spinal cord compression, or skin nodules. Splenic enlargement can be sufficiently rapid to cause splenic infarctions with fever and pleuritic chest pain. Hyperuricemia and secondary gout may ensue.

DIAGNOSIS While the clinical picture described above is characteristic of idiopathic myelofibrosis, it cannot be emphasized too strongly that all of the clinical features described can be observed in polycythemia vera or chronic myelogenous leukemia. Indeed, massive

Table 111-4

Causes of Myelofibrosis

Carcinoma metastatic to the marrow
Infection
Lymphoma
Hodgkin's disease
Acute leukemia (lymphocytic or myelocytic)
Hairy cell leukemia
Multiple myeloma
Chronic myelogenous leukemia
Polycythemia vera
Idiopathic myelofibrosis
Systemic mastocytosis
Thorium dioxide (Thorotrast) exposure
Systemic lupus erythematosus
Renal osteodystrophy

splenomegaly commonly masks erythrocytosis in polycythemia vera, and reports of intraabdominal thromboses in idiopathic myelofibrosis undoubtedly represent instances of unrecognized polycythemia vera. Furthermore, as mentioned above, many other disorders have features that overlap with idiopathic myelofibrosis but respond to distinctly different therapies. Therefore, the diagnosis of idiopathic myelofibrosis is one of exclusion, which requires that the disorders listed in Table 111-4 be ruled out.

The presence of teardrop-shaped red cells, nucleated red cells, myelocytes, and promyelocytes establishes the presence of extramedullary hematopoiesis; the presence of leukocytosis, thrombocytosis with large and bizarre platelets, as well as circulating myeloblasts suggests the presence of a myeloproliferative disorder as opposed to a secondary form of myelofibrosis (Table 111-4). Marrow is usually not aspirable due to increased marrow reticulin, but marrow biopsy will reveal a hypercellular marrow with trilineage hyperplasia and, in particular, increased megakaryocytes, but there are no characteristic morphologic abnormalities that distinguish idiopathic myelofibrosis from the other chronic myeloproliferative disorders. Splenomegaly due to extramedullary hematopoiesis may be sufficiently massive to cause portal hypertension and variceal formation. In some patients, as mentioned above, exuberant extramedullary hematopoiesis can dominate the clinical picture. An intriguing feature of idiopathic myelofibrosis is the occurrence of autoimmune abnormalities such as immune complexes, antinuclear antibodies, rheumatoid factor, or a positive Coombs' test. Whether these represent a host reaction to the disorder or are involved in its pathogenesis is unknown. Cytogenetic analysis, of either blood or marrow, if aspirable, is useful both to exclude chronic myelogenous leukemia and for prognostic purposes, because complex karyotype abnormalities portend a poor prognosis in idiopathic myelofibrosis.

COMPLICATIONS Idiopathic myelofibrosis is a chronic disorder but with a median survival of only 5 years, a duration much shorter than for polycythemia vera or essential thrombocytosis. The natural history of idiopathic myelofibrosis is one of inexorable marrow failure with transfusion-dependent anemia and increasing organomegaly. Patients with this disorder are prone to deep-seated tissue infections, particularly of the lungs. As with chronic myelogenous leukemia, idiopathic myelofibrosis can evolve from a chronic phase to an accelerated phase with constitutional symptoms and increasing marrow failure. In approximately 10 percent of patients, the disorder terminates in a rapidly progressive form of acute leukemia for which therapy is usually ineffective. Important prognostic factors with respect to disease acceleration include anemia, thrombocytopenia, age, the presence of complex cytogenetic abnormalities, and constitutional symptoms such as unexplained fever, night sweats, or weight loss. Any nonrandom cytogenetic abnormality is associated with a shortened life span, and the presence or development of multiple cytogenetic abnormalities is highly indicative of disease acceleration.

℞ TREATMENT

There is no specific therapy for idiopathic myelofibrosis. Anemia may be exacerbated by deficiency of folic acid or iron, and in rare instances, pyridoxine therapy has been effective. However, anemia is more often due to ineffective erythropoiesis not compensated for by the extramedullary hematopoiesis in the spleen and liver, and neither therapy with androgens nor recombinant erythropoietin has been consistently effective. A red cell splenic sequestration study can be useful in establishing the presence of hypersplenism, for which splenectomy is indicated. Splenectomy may also be necessary if splenomegaly impairs alimentation and should be performed before cachexia sets in. In this situation, splenectomy should not be avoided because of concern over rebound thrombocytosis, loss of hematopoietic capacity, or compensatory hepatomegaly. Such concerns have no clinical foundation. Allopurinol should be used to control significant hyperuricemia and hydroxyurea has proved useful in some patients for controlling organomegaly. The role of recombinant interferon α is still undefined, and its side effects are more pronounced in the older individuals who are affected with this disorder.

ESSENTIAL THROMBOCYTOSIS

Essential thrombocytosis (other designations include *essential thrombocythemia, idiopathic thrombocytosis, primary thrombocytosis, hemorrhagic thrombocythemia*) is a clonal disorder of unknown etiology involving a multipotent hematopoietic progenitor cell and is manifested clinically by the overproduction of platelets in the absence of a definable cause. Essential thrombocytosis is an uncommon disorder, but its frequency is unknown because there is no clinically applicable clonal marker with which to distinguish it from the more common nonclonal, reactive forms of thrombocytosis (Table 111-5). The epidemiology of essential thrombocytosis is also not well defined, not only because of the lack of a clonal marker but also because clinical recognition of thrombocytosis is unlikely in the largely asymptomatic persons affected by this disorder. As a consequence, essential thrombocytosis was formerly considered to be a disease of the elderly and to be responsible for significant morbidity due to hemorrhage or thrombosis. However, with the advent of electronic particle counters and the widespread application of platelet counting, it is now clear that not only can essential thrombocytosis occur at any age in adults but also in the absence of symptoms or disturbances of hemostasis. Furthermore, there is an unexplained female predominance, in contrast to the reactive forms of thrombocytosis where no gender bias exists. Because thrombocytosis is often a prominent feature of the other chronic myeloproliferative disorders, the treatment and prognosis of which differ from essential thrombocytosis, and because, as noted above, no clonal marker is available for the disorder, clinical criteria have been proposed to distinguish it from the other chronic myeloproliferative disorders (Table 111-6). It cannot be emphasized too strongly, however, that these criteria do not establish clonality; therefore, they are truly useful only in identifying disorders such as chronic myelogenous leukemia, polycythemia vera, or myelodysplasia, which can masquerade as essential thrombocytosis, as opposed to establishing the presence of essential thrombocytosis. Furthermore, it has not been sufficiently emphasized that, as with "primary" erythrocytosis, there may exist nonclonal, benign forms of thrombocytosis that have not been recognized simply because we currently lack the diagnostic tools to do so.

ETIOLOGY   Megakaryocytopoiesis and platelet production are still incompletely defined processes, but with the identification and molecular cloning of the genes for thrombopoietin and its receptor, the c-Mpl proto-oncogene, the physiology of thrombopoiesis should soon be clarified. As in the case of early erythroid and myeloid progenitor cells, early megakaryocytic progenitors require the presence of interleukin 3 and stem cell factor for optimal proliferation, and their subsequent development is enhanced by interleukins 6 and 11. However, megakaryocyte maturation and terminal differentiation still require the presence of thrombopoietin.

Table 111-5

Causes of Thrombocytosis

Iron-deficiency anemia
Hyposplenism
Postsplenectomy*
Malignancy
Collagen vascular disease
Inflammatory bowel disease
Infection
Hemolysis
Hemorrhage
Polycythemia vera
Idiopathic myelofibrosis
Essential thrombocytosis
Chronic myelogenous leukemia
Idiopathic sideroblastic anemia
Myelodysplasia (5q- syndrome)
Postsurgery
Rebound (cessation of ethanol intake, correction of vitamin B_{12}
   or folate deficiency)

* If the platelet count is greater than $2 \times 10^6/\mu L$, the etiology is most likely a myeloproliferative disorder.

Table 111-6

Suggested Criteria for the Clinical Diagnosis of Essential Thrombocytosis*

Platelet count $\geq$ 500,000/μL
Absence of a known cause of reactive thrombocytosis (see Table 111-5)
Absence of the Ph chromosome and the bcr-abl gene rearrangement
Normal red cell mass
Presence of marrow iron
Absence of myelofibrosis
Absence of myelodysplasia clinically and by cytogenetic analysis
Splenomegaly

* The concept that a platelet count greater than $1 \times 10^6/\mu L$ distinguishes essential thrombocytosis from other causes of thrombocytosis has no clinical validity.

Megakaryocytes are unique amongst hematopoietic progenitor cells because they undergo endomitotic as opposed to mitotic reduplication of their genome. In the absence of thrombopoietin, endomitotic megakaryocytic reduplication and, by extension, the cytoplasmic development necessary for platelet production are impaired. Like erythropoietin, thrombopoietin is produced in both the liver and the kidneys, and an inverse correlation between the platelet count and plasma thrombopoietic activity has been observed. However, whether thrombopoietin, like erythropoietin, behaves like a hormone and whether it acts as a mitogen, a survival factor, or both is unknown. In contrast to erythropoietin, but like its myeloid counterparts granulocyte and granulocyte-macrophage colony stimulating factors, thrombopoietin not only enhances the proliferation of its target cells but also activates their end-stage product, in this case the platelet. Whether thrombopoietin has a role in essential thrombocytosis or whether its production, like that of erythropoietin in polycythemia vera, is suppressed is also unknown.

The clonality of essential thrombocytosis has been established by the use of the isoenzymes of glucose-6-phosphate dehydrogenase in patients who are hemizygous for this gene, by the use of X-linked DNA polymorphisms, and by the identification of nonrandom, although variable cytogenetic abnormalities. Such studies together with in vivo clonal assays for hematopoietic progenitor cells have shown that the multipotent hematopoietic progenitor cell involved in this disorder can vary; in some patients lymphocytes contained the same clonal marker as the megakaryocytes, erythrocytes, and myeloid cells, whereas in others the lymphocytes were not involved. Similar observations have been made in polycythemia vera. Furthermore, a number of families have been described in which essential thrombocytosis was inherited, in one instance as an autosomal dominant trait. In one kindred, in addition to essential thrombocytosis, idiopathic myelofibrosis and polycythemia vera were also individually documented.

CLINICAL FEATURES   Clinically, essential thrombocytosis is most often identified incidentally when a platelet count is obtained during the course of a routine or diagnostic evaluation. Occasionally, review of previous platelet counts will reveal that an elevation was present but overlooked. There are no symptoms or signs specific for essential thrombocytosis, but these patients do have hemorrhagic and thrombotic tendencies expressed as easy bruising for the former or microvascular occlusions for the latter, which may be manifested by erythromelalgia, migraine, or transient ischemic attacks. Physical examination is generally unremarkable except for the presence of mild splenomegaly. Massive splenomegaly is more characteristic of the other myeloproliferative disorders, particularly polycythemia vera or idiopathic myelofibrosis.

Anemia is unusual, but a mild neutrophilic leukocytosis is not. The blood smear, however, is most remarkable for the number of platelets present, some of which may be very large. The leukocyte alkaline phosphatase score is either normal or elevated. The large mass of circulating platelets may prevent the accurate measurement of serum potassium due to the release of platelet potassium upon blood clotting. This hyperkalemia is a laboratory artifact and is not associated with any ECG abnormalities. Similarly, arterial oxygen measurements can be rendered inaccurate unless the blood is collected on ice. The prothrombin and partial thromboplastic times are normal, while abnormalities of platelet function such as a prolonged bleeding time and impaired platelet aggregation can be present. However, in spite of much study, there are neither characteristic nor consistent platelet function abnormalities associated with essential thrombocytosis, and there is no correlation between any platelet function test and the presence of clinically significant bleeding or thrombosis.

The elevated platelet count may hinder the collection of a marrow aspirate, but marrow biopsy usually reveals both megakaryocyte hyperplasia and hypertrophy, as well as an overall increase in marrow cellularity. An increase in marrow reticulin may be present, but if extensive, another diagnosis should be considered. The absence of stainable iron demands an explanation, because iron deficiency alone can cause thrombocytosis and absent marrow iron is a feature of polycythemia vera.

While nonrandom cytogenetic abnormalities have been identified in essential thrombocytosis, there is no consistently identifiable abnormality and, in particular, none involving chromosomes 3 and 1 where the genes for thrombopoietin and its receptor c-Mpl, respectively, are located.

DIAGNOSIS Given the important role for certain cytokines in megakaryocytopoiesis, it is not surprising that thrombocytosis is encountered in a variety of clinical disorders (Table 111-5) in which production of these cytokines is increased. Thus, the first obligation of the physician when confronted with a high platelet count is to determine if it is a consequence of another disorder. In this regard, a cytogenetic evaluation is mandatory to determine if the thrombocytosis is due to chronic myelogenous leukemia or a myelodysplastic disorder such as the 5q- syndrome. Because the bcr-abl translocation can be present in the absence of the Ph chromosome, it has been suggested that gene rearrangement studies should be performed in all patients with thrombocytosis in whom a cytogenetic study is normal. Anemia and ringed sideroblasts are not features of essential thrombocytosis, but they are features of idiopathic refractory sideroblastic anemia, in which thrombocytosis can also occur. The presence of massive splenomegaly should suggest the possibility of another myeloproliferative disorder, and in this setting a red cell mass determination is mandatory because substantial splenomegaly can mask the presence of erythrocytosis. In this regard, it should be noted that essential thrombocytosis can evolve into polycythemia vera and that often only the passage of time will resolve the true nature of the underlying myeloproliferative disorder.

COMPLICATIONS Perhaps no other situation in clinical medicine has caused otherwise astute physicians to intervene inappropriately more often than thrombocytosis, particularly if the platelet count is greater than 1×10^6 per microliter. It is commonly believed that a high platelet count must cause intravascular stasis and thrombosis; however, no controlled clinical study has ever established either association.

Indeed, quite to the contrary, very high platelet counts are associated primarily with hemorrhage, while platelet counts of less than a million are more often associated with thrombosis. In this regard, the role of platelet mass as opposed to platelet number has never been resolved. This is not meant to imply that an elevated platelet count cannot cause symptoms in a patient with essential thrombocytosis, but rather that the focus should be on the patient, not the platelet count. For example, some of the most dramatic neurologic problems in essential thrombocytosis are migraine-related but may respond only to lowering of the platelet count; other symptoms may be a manifestation of erythromelalgia and respond simply to platelet cyclooxygenase inhibitors such as aspirin, without resorting to a reduction in platelet number. Still others may represent an interaction between an atherosclerotic vascular system and a high platelet count, and others may have no

relationship to the platelet count whatsoever. A fundamental problem in this area is that the existing literature is largely uncritical and evolved in an era when not only was essential thrombocytosis often not distinguished from polycythemia vera but other causes for hypercoagulability, such as the lupus anticoagulant or factor V Leiden, were not yet appreciated.

℞ TREATMENT

An elevated platelet count per se in an asymptomatic patient requires no therapy, and before any therapy is initiated in a patient with thrombocytosis, the cause of symptoms must be clearly identified to be a consequence of the elevated platelet count. Although the literature is replete with extreme measures, such as plasmapheresis and cytotoxic therapy for reducing the platelet count in symptomatic patients with thrombocytosis, none of these measures has ever been documented to be more than anecdotally efficacious and none can be recommended. Furthermore, the development of acute leukemia in patients with essential thrombocytosis treated with ^{32}P or alkylating agents without any proof of benefit from such therapy should be a strong caution to their use. If platelet reduction is deemed necessary on the basis of neurologic symptoms refractory to salicylates, the physician currently has the choice of hydroxyurea, a mutagen, or recombinant interferon α, an immunosuppressive agent with substantial side effects. Anagrelide, a quinazolin derivative, can reduce the platelet count and is currently undergoing clinical trials, but it is neither uniformly effective nor without significant side effects. Bleeding associated with thrombocytosis usually responds to ε-aminocaproic acid, which can be given prophylactically before and after elective surgery. As more clinical experience is acquired, it appears that essential thrombocytosis is more benign than previously thought, and that evolution to acute leukemia is more likely to be a consequence of prior chemotherapy than of the disease itself. In managing patients with thrombocytosis, the physician's first obligation is to do no harm.

BIBLIOGRAPHY

ADAMSON JW et al: Polycythemia vera: Stem cell and probable clonal origin of the disease. N Engl J Med 295:913, 1976

BUSS DH et al: The incidence of thrombotic and hemorrhagic disorders in association with extreme thrombocytosis: An analysis of 129 cases. Am J Hematol 20:365, 1985

JACOBSON RJ et al: Agnogenic myeloid metaplasia: A clonal proliferation of hematopoietic stem cells with secondary myelofibrosis. Blood 51:189, 1978

MERTENS F et al: Karyotypic patterns in chronic myeloproliferative disorders: Report on 74 cases and review of the literature. Leukemia 5:214, 1990

SCHAFER AI: Bleeding and thrombosis in the myeloproliferative disorders. Blood 64:1, 1984

————: Essential thrombocythemia. Prog Hemost Thromb 10:69, 1991

VARKI A et al: The syndrome of idiopathic myelofibrosis: A clinicopathologic review with emphasis on the prognostic variables predicting survival. Medicine 62:353, 1983

112   *Meir Wetzler, Clara D. Bloomfield*

ACUTE AND CHRONIC MYELOID LEUKEMIA

The myeloid leukemias are a heterogeneous group of diseases characterized by infiltration of the blood, bone marrow, and other tissues by neoplastic cells of the hematopoietic system. In 1996, the estimated number of new myeloid leukemia cases in the United States was 12,800. These leukemias comprise a spectrum of malignancies that, untreated, range from among the most rapidly fatal to ones that are slowly growing. Based on their untreated course, the myeloid leukemias have traditionally been designated *acute* or *chronic*.

INCIDENCE The incidence of acute myeloid leukemia (AML) is approximately 2.3 per 100,000 people per year, and the age-adjusted incidence is higher in men than in women (2.9 versus 1.9). There has been no significant change in AML incidence over the past 20 years. The incidence of AML increases with age; under 65 years the incidence is 1.3, and above 65 the incidence is 12.2.

ETIOLOGY Heredity, radiation, chemical and other occupational exposures, and drugs have been implicated in the development of AML. There is no direct evidence of a viral etiology in AML.

Heredity Certain syndromes with somatic cell chromosome aneuploidy, e.g., Down (trisomy of chromosome 21), Klinefelter (XXY and variants), and Patau (trisomy of chromosome 13), are associated with an increased incidence of AML. Inherited diseases with excessive chromatin fragility, e.g., Fanconi anemia, Bloom syndrome, ataxia telangiectasia, and Kostmann syndrome, are also associated with an increased incidence of AML.

Radiation Survivors of the atomic bomb explosions in Japan during World War II had an increased incidence of myeloid leukemias that peaked 5 to 7 years following exposure. Therapeutic radiation alone seems to add little risk of acute leukemia but can increase the risk in people exposed to alkylating agents (see below).

Chemical and Other Exposures Benzene, used as a solvent in the chemical, plastic, rubber, and pharmaceutical industries, has been associated with an increased incidence of AML. Smoking and exposure to petroleum products, paint, embalming fluids, ethylene oxide, herbicides, pesticides, and electromagnetic fields have also been associated with an increased risk of AML.

Drugs Antineoplastic drugs are the leading cause of drug-related (or treatment-associated) AML. Alkylating agent–associated leukemias occur on average 48 to 72 months after exposure and demonstrate aberrations in chromosomes 5 and 7. Topoisomerase II inhibitor–associated leukemias occur 1 to 3 years after exposure and usually have aberrations involving chromosome band 11q23. Similarly, chloramphenicol, phenylbutazone, and less commonly chloroquine and methoxypsoralen have been reported to result in bone marrow failure that may evolve into AML.

CLASSIFICATION The categorization of acute leukemia into biologically distinct groups is based on morphology, cytochemistry, and immunophenotype as well as cytogenetic and molecular techniques.

Morphologic and Cytochemical Classification The diagnosis of AML is established by the presence of at least 30 percent myeloblasts in blood and/or bone marrow. Myeloblasts have nuclear chromatin that is uniformly fine or lacelike in appearance and large nucleoli (two to five per cell). If specific cytoplasmic granules, Auer rods, or the nuclear folding and clefting characteristic of monocytoid cells are not present, the morphologic features observed under light microscopy may not be sufficient to clarify the diagnosis.

AML is classified based on morphology and cytochemistry according to the French, American, and British (FAB) schema, which includes eight major subtypes, M0 to M7 (Table 112-1). In AML of the M1 variety, a positive myeloperoxidase reaction (i.e., presence of myeloperoxidase in 3 percent or more of the blast cells) may be the only distinguishing characteristic separating it from L2 acute lymphoblastic

Table 112-1

The French-American-British (FAB) Classification of AML

FAB subtype	% of Cases	Morphology	Cytochemistry[a] Peroxidase/ Sudan Black	Nonspecific Esterase[b]	Flow Cytometry[c]	Cytogenetic Association[d]
M0: Minimally differentiated leukemia	2–3	Immature morphology	−	−	CD13 or 33	
M1: Myeloblastic leukemia without maturation	20	Few blasts with azurophilic granules, Auer rods, or both	3% or more	−	CD13, 33, 34, HLA-DR+	
M2: Myeloblastic leukemia with maturation	25–30	Azurophilic granules, Auer rods are often present Variant: M2Baso: blasts with basophil granules	+	−	CD13, 15, 33, 34, HLA-DR+	t(8;21) (q22;q22)[e]
M3: Hypergranular promyelocytic leukemia	8–15	Hypergranular promyelocytes with multiple Auer rods Variant: hypogranular	+	−	CD13, 15, 33, HLA-DR−	t(15;17) (q22;q11-12)
M4: Myelomonocytic leukemia	20–25	Granulocytic and monocytic blasts Variant: M4Eo: increase in abnormal marrow eosinophils	+/−	+	CD11b, 13, 14[f], 15, 33, HLA-DR+	M4Eo: inv(16) (p13q22)
M5: Monocytic leukemia	20–25	M5a undifferentiated M5b differentiated	−	+	CD11b, 13, 14[f], 15, 33, HLA-DR+	11q23 translocations
M6: Erythroleukemia (Di Guglielmo's disease)	5	Erythroblasts >50% of nucleated cells, myeloblasts >30% of nonerythroid cells	+/−	−	CD33, HLA-DR+	
M7: Megakaryoblastic leukemia	1–2	Megakaryoblasts >30% of all nucleated cells	−	−	CD33, 41	

[a] Periodic acid Schiff staining is characteristic of the neoplastic erythroid precursors of M6.
[b] With fluoride inhibition.
[c] The antigens listed are the most commonly expressed in the given FAB subtype.
[d] A subset of M2 and M5 demonstrate the listed cytogenetic abnormality.
[e] CD19 positivity is characteristically associated with t(8;21).
[f] CD14, if present denotes monocytic lineage.

SOURCE: JM Bennett et al, Ann Intern Med 103:620, 1985; BD Cheson et al, J Clin Oncol 8:813, 1990.

leukemia (ALL). The M2 and M3 types are most strongly peroxidase positive, while M4 exhibits less intense activity, and the peroxidase reaction occurs to a limited extent or not at all in M5 and M7 subtypes. Other cytochemical stains useful in diagnosis are shown in Table 112-1.

Immunophenotypic Classification The phenotype of human myeloid leukemia cells can be studied by multiparameter flow cytometry following labeling with monoclonal antibodies to cell-surface antigens. Results are useful both for diagnosis and prognosis. For example, M0, which is characterized by immature morphology and no lineage-specific cytochemical reactions, is diagnosed by flow cytometric demonstration of the myeloid-specific antigens cluster designation (CD) 13 or 33. Similarly, M7 can often be diagnosed only by expression of the platelet-specific antigen CD41 or by electron-microscopic demonstration of myeloperoxidase. An example of the use of immunophenotyping for prognosis is the poor outcome shown in patients whose leukemic cells coexpress CD13, CD14, and CD34. In addition, the use of multiparameter flow cytometry to detect residual disease following therapy in AML is under investigation by several groups.

Chromosomal Classification Chromosomal analysis of the leukemic cell currently provides the most important pretreatment prognostic information in AML. Only two cytogenetic abnormalities have been invariably associated with a specific FAB group: t(15;17)(q22;q11-12) with M3 and inv(16)(p13q22) with M4Eo. However, many chromosomal abnormalities have been associated primarily with one FAB group, including t(8;21)(q22;q22) with M2, and t(9;11)(p22;q23), and other translocations involving 11q23, with M5. Many of the recurring chromosomal abnormalities in AML have been associated with specific clinical characteristics. More commonly associated with younger age are t(8;21) and t(15;17), and with older age, del(5q) and del(7q). Lymphadenopathy is associated with inv(16); chloromas with t(8;21); disseminated intravascular coagulation (DIC) with t(15;17); central nervous system involvement with inv(16); and diabetes insipidus, fever, and infection, all with monosomy 7. The reasons for most associations of chromosomal abnormalities with specific clinical features are unknown.

Molecular Classification The many recurring cytogenetic abnormalities led to molecular studies, which have revealed several genes that may play a causative role in leukemogenesis. The 15;17 translocation, characteristic of M3 leukemia, encodes a chimeric protein, Pml/Rarα, which is formed by the fusion of the retinoic acid receptor α (RARα) gene from chromosome 17 and the promyelocytic leukemia (PML) gene from chromosome 15. The RARα gene encodes a member of the steroid/thyroid hormone receptor family of transcription factors. After binding retinoic acid, Rarα can bind to specific DNA sequences in the promoters of a variety of genes. The 15;17 translocation juxtaposes PML with RARα in a head-to-tail configuration that is under the transcriptional control of PML. There are three different breakpoints within the PML gene leading to various fusion proteins, which may correlate with remission duration. The molecular data are intriguing given the excellent clinical response of M3 patients with t(15;17) to tretinoin (all-*trans*-retinoic acid or ATRA). In a rare form of M3 which has a related translocation, t(11;17)(q23;q21), the RARα gene is juxtaposed to the promyelocytic leukemia zinc finger gene from chromosome 11, resulting in a chimeric gene that renders the cells unresponsive to ATRA.

The inv(16), characteristic of M4Eo, results in a fusion of the core-binding factor β (CBFB) gene on the q arm and the myosin heavy chain (MYH11) gene on the p arm. The CBFB gene encodes a subunit of the transcription factor complex core-binding factor, also known as polyomavirus enhancer binding protein 2 gene. This gene is involved in the determination of differentiation-dependent and cell type–specific expression of the polyomavirus enhancer. Interestingly, Cbf proteins are composed of an α subunit, the Aml1 protein, and a β subunit, the Pebp2 protein. The 8;21 translocation involves the core-binding factor α (CBFA) gene on chromosome 21, more commonly

designated as the AML1 gene, which encodes a transcription factor that regulates myeloid cell differentiation. Unraveling the interactions between CBFA and CBFB may explain the differences and the similarities between inv(16)- and t(8;21)-associated leukemia.

Most translocations that involve 11q23 rearrange the ALL1 gene (also known as myeloid-lymphoid or mixed-lineage leukemia gene). The ALL1 gene has two regions that encompass multiple zinc fingers, and has at least two additional potential DNA-binding motifs. Abnormalities in the ALL1 gene are relatively common in patients with AML who do not have 11q23 rearrangements cytogenetically.

These various molecular aberrations are increasingly being used for diagnosis and detection of residual disease following treatment. At this point, the molecular information is useful for therapy only for M3 leukemia. However, antisense techniques to block translation of the specific transcripts are being developed for gene-directed therapy.

CLINICAL PRESENTATION **Symptoms** Patients with AML most often present with nonspecific symptoms that begin gradually or abruptly and are the consequence of anemia, leukocytosis, leukopenia or leukocyte dysfunction, or thrombocytopenia. Nearly half have had symptoms for 3 months or more before the leukemia is diagnosed.

Half mention fatigue as the first symptom, but most complain of fatigue or weakness at the time of diagnosis. Other nonspecific complaints, such as anorexia and weight loss, are common. Fever, with or without an identifiable infection, is the initial symptom in approximately 10 percent of patients. Similarly, signs of abnormal hemostasis (bleeding, easy bruising) are noted first in 5 percent of all cases. On occasion, bone pain, lymphadenopathy, nonspecific cough, headache, or diaphoresis are the presenting symptoms.

Rarely patients may present with symptoms from a mass lesion located in the soft tissues, breast, uterus, ovary, cranial or spinal dura, gastrointestinal tract, lung, mediastinum, prostate, bone, or other organs. The mass lesion represents a tumor of leukemic cells and is called a *granulocytic sarcoma*, or *chloroma*. Typical AML may occur simultaneously, later, or not at all in these patients. This rare presentation is more common in patients with t(8;21) translocations.

Physical Findings Fever, splenomegaly, hepatomegaly, lymphadenopathy, sternal tenderness, and evidence of infection and hemorrhagic tendencies are often found at diagnosis. Significant gastrointestinal bleeding, intrapulmonary hemorrhage, or intracranial hemorrhage occur most often in M3 leukemia. Bleeding associated with coagulopathies may also occur in M5 leukemia and with extreme degrees of leukocytosis or thrombocytopenia in other FAB subtypes. Retinal hemorrhages are detected in 15 percent of patients. Infiltration of the gingivae, skin, soft tissues, or the meninges with leukemic blasts at diagnosis is characteristic of the monocytic subtypes (M4 and M5).

Hematologic Findings Anemia is usually present at diagnosis and can be severe. The degree varies considerably irrespective of other hematologic findings, splenomegaly, or the duration of symptoms. The anemia is usually normochromic normocytic. Decreased erythropoiesis often results in a reduced reticulocyte count, and erythrocyte survival is decreased by accelerated destruction. Active blood loss also contributes to the anemia.

The median presenting leukocyte count is about 15,000/μL. Twenty-five to 40 percent of patients will have counts less than 5000/μL, and 20 percent will have counts greater than 100,000/μL. Fewer than 5 percent will have no detectable leukemic cells in the blood. There can be poor neutrophil function, demonstrated functionally by impaired phagocytosis and migration and morphologically by abnormal lobulation and deficient granulation.

Platelet counts under 100,000/μL are found at diagnosis in about 75 percent of patients, and about 25 percent of patients will have counts less than 25,000/μL. Both morphologic and functional platelet abnormalities can be observed. These include, for example, large and bizarre shapes with abnormal granulation and inability of platelets to aggregate or adhere normally to one another.

Pretreatment Evaluation Once the diagnosis of AML is suspected, a rapid evaluation and initiation of appropriate therapy should follow (Table 112-2). In addition to clarifying the subtype of leukemia,

Table 112-2

CHAPTER 112
Acute and Chronic Myeloid Leukemia

687

Diagnostic Evaluation of Patients with AML

History and physical examination
Hemoglobin level, leukocyte count (differential), platelet count
Bone marrow aspirate and biopsy
   Morphology
   Cytochemistry
   Cell membrane immunophenotyping
   Cytogenetics
   Molecular studies
   Cryopreservation of viable cells
Blood chemistries
   Hepatic enzymes, creatinine, serum electrolytes, lactic dehydrogenase,
     uric acid, calcium, phosphorus, lysozyme
Coagulation profile
   Prothrombin time, partial thromboplastin time, thrombin time, fibrinogen,
     fibrin split products
Chest roentgenogram
Electrocardiogram and evaluation of left ventricular ejection fraction
Blood type and HLA determination (also evaluate family members as poten-
   tial blood component and allogeneic bone marrow donors)
Lumbar puncture (in symptomatic patients only)

initial studies should evaluate the overall functional integrity of the major organ systems, including the cardiovascular, pulmonary, hepatic, and renal systems. Factors that have prognostic significance, either for achieving complete remission (CR) or for predicting the duration of CR, should also be assessed before initiating treatment. Leukemic cells should be obtained from all patients and cryopreserved for future use as new tests become available. All patients should be evaluated for overt or inapparent infection.

The majority of patients are anemic and thrombocytopenic at presentation. Immediately after results of the initial studies are known, prompt replacement of the appropriate blood components, if necessary, should begin. Because qualitative platelet dysfunction or the presence of an infection may increase the likelihood of bleeding, evidence of hemorrhage justifies the immediate use of platelet transfusion, even if the platelet count is only moderately decreased.

Liver function tests will be abnormal in approximately 20 percent of patients at diagnosis. Because some chemotherapeutic agents are detoxified and excreted by the liver, drug dosages in patients with hepatic dysfunction may require modification. Some drugs, such as purine analogues and anthracyclines, can also be hepatotoxic and aggravate underlying liver disease.

Approximately 50 percent of patients will have a mild to moderate elevation of serum uric acid at presentation. Only 10 percent have marked elevations, but renal precipitation of uric acid and the nephropathy that may result are serious potential complications. The initiation of chemotherapy may aggravate hyperuricemia, and patients are usually immediately started on allopurinol and bicarbonate at diagnosis. Finally, lysozyme, a marker for monocytic differentiation, when present in high concentrations may be etiologic in renal tubular dysfunction, which could intensify other renal problems that often arise during the initial phases of the therapy.

PROGNOSTIC FACTORS The single most important factor related to an improved survival is attainment of CR. CR is defined following examination of both blood and bone marrow and should last ≥4 weeks. For a patient to be considered to have achieved CR, the blood neutrophil count must be ≥1500/μL and the platelet count ≥100,000/μL. Neither hemoglobin concentration nor hematocrit are considered in determining CR. Circulating blasts should not be present. While a rare blast may be detected in the blood during marrow regeneration, they should disappear on successive studies. Bone marrow cellularity should be >20 percent with trilineage maturation. The bone marrow should contain <5 percent blasts, and Auer rods should not be detected. Extramedullary leukemia should not be present. For patients in CR, reverse transcriptase polymerase chain reaction (RT-PCR) to detect AML-associated molecular abnormalities, and fluorescence in situ hybridization (FISH) to detect AML-associated cytogenetic aberrations are currently employed to detect residual disease. Although

further study is needed, such detection of minimal residual disease may become a reliable discriminator between patients in CR who do or do not require additional and/or alternative therapies.

Many factors have been identified that influence the likelihood of entering CR. More recently, factors specifically related to the length of CR and curability have been determined. It is important to remember that prognostic factors are highly dependent on the treatment used. Age at diagnosis remains among the most important pretreatment risk factors, with advanced age (>60 years) being associated with a poorer prognosis primarily because of its influence on the patient's ability to survive induction therapy and thus achieve a CR. Chronic and intercurrent diseases impair tolerance to rigorous therapy; acute medical problems at diagnosis negatively influence the likelihood of survival. Performance status, independent of age, also influences ability to survive induction therapy and thus respond to treatment. Age may also influence outcome because AML in older patients may differ biologically. The leukemic cells in elderly patients more commonly express CD34 and the mdr1 efflux pump that conveys resistance to natural product-derived agents such as the anthracyclines (see below). Data also suggest that with each successive decade of age, a greater proportion of patients will have more resistant disease.

Chromosome findings at diagnosis are another important independent prognostic factor. Patients with t(8;21) and inv(16) have extremely good prognoses, while those with no cytogenetic abnormality or with t(15;17) have moderately favorable outcomes with high-dose cytarabine. Patients with del(5q), -7, and abnormalities involving 12p have a very poor prognosis. Patients with certain abnormalities, such as inv(3), do not achieve CR with standard induction chemotherapy.

A prolonged symptomatic interval preceding diagnosis is another pretreatment clinical feature that remains strongly associated with a lower CR rate and shorter survival. The duration of symptoms before diagnosis and the documented presence of an antecedent hematologic disorder before the emergence of leukemia are related factors. The CR rate has been lower in patients who have had anemia, leukopenia, and/or thrombocytopenia for more than 1 month before the diagnosis of acute leukemia when compared to those without such a history. In fact, responsiveness to chemotherapy appears to decline steadily as the duration of the antecedent disorder(s) increases. In addition, secondary AML developing following treatment with cytotoxic agents and/or irradiation for other malignancies has proved extremely difficult to treat successfully.

A number of prognostic factors have been reported in some series but not in others. An inverse relationship between the duration of CR and the presenting leukocyte count or absolute circulating myeloblast count has been reported. Among patients with hyperleukocytosis (>100,000/μL), those who are older or have pulmonary leukostasis, hepatomegaly, hyperbilirubinemia or hypofibrinogenemia, have been reported to be at a greater risk for early death during induction.

Although the FAB classification has not usually been found to be an independent prognostic factor, other characteristics of the leukemic cell have been reported, in some studies, to have prognostic significance. These include Auer rods, ultrastructural features, in vitro and in vivo growth characteristics and chemotherapeutic sensitivity, and immunophenotype. Recently, the importance of the multidrug resistance gene 1 has been suggested in several studies. This gene encodes a protein that actively pumps out a variety of lipophilic compounds (e.g., anthracyclines) from the cell. Patients whose leukemic cells express multidrug resistance gene 1 have had lower CR rates and decreased CR duration.

In addition to pretreatment variables, several treatment factors have been reported to correlate with prognosis in AML, in particular with CR duration. One is the rapidity with which the blast cells disappear from the blood following the institution of therapy. In addition, patients who achieve CR following one induction cycle have longer CR than those requiring multiple cycles. Patients whose marrow at the time of CR has fewer than 1 percent blasts also fare better.

℞ **TREATMENT**

Treatment of the newly diagnosed patient with AML is usually divided into two phases, induction and postremission management (Fig. 112-1). The initial goal in treatment is to eradicate the leukemia quickly and induce CR. Once CR is obtained, further strategies must be applied to prolong survival and establish cure.

Induction Chemotherapy The most commonly used CR induction regimens (for patients with all FAB subtypes except M3) consist of combination chemotherapy with cytarabine (cytosine arabinoside) and an anthracycline. Cytarabine is a cell cycle S-phase-specific antimetabolite that becomes phosphorylated to an active triphosphate form that interferes with DNA synthesis. Anthracyclines are DNA intercalaters. Their primary mode of action is considered to be interaction with topoisomerase II, leading to breakage of DNA. Cytarabine is usually administered as a continuous intravenous infusion at 100 to 200 mg/m² per day for 7 days. Anthracycline therapy generally consists of daunorubicin, 45 mg/m² intravenously on days 1, 2, and 3 of cytarabine given as above (*the 7 and 3 regimen*). Treatment with idarubicin, a new anthracycline, at 12 or 13 mg/m² per day for 3 days in conjunction with cytarabine by 7-day continuous infusion is at least as effective and may be superior to daunorubicin, according to several randomized trials.

Following induction chemotherapy, the bone marrow is examined when the blood counts reach normal levels or plateau to determine CR or residual leukemia. CR is usually achieved within 4 weeks of initiation of chemotherapy. If there is unequivocal persistent or recurrent leukemia in the bone marrow on day 14 or subsequently,

the patient has traditionally been retreated with cytarabine and an anthracycline in doses similar to those given initially but for 5 and 2 days, respectively. Our recommendation, however, is to change therapy in this setting. We prefer to give high-dose cytarabine (3 g/m² over 1 h every 12 h for a total of 12 doses, with a reduction to 1.5 g/m² for patients over 50 years of age) and an anthracycline (e.g., idarubicin 12 mg/m² daily for 3 days) as a second course of induction therapy for patients with clear-cut persistent or recurrent leukemia in a cellular marrow after one cycle of standard dose cytarabine and daunorubicin therapy. We also recommend consideration of bone marrow transplantation (BMT) early in the management of these patients.

With the 7 and 3 cytarabine/daunorubicin regimen outlined above, CR is achieved in 65 to 75 percent of adults with de novo AML. Two-thirds achieve CR after a single course of therapy, and one-third require two courses. Approximately 50 percent of patients who do not achieve a CR have a leukemia that is resistant to the therapy administered, and 50 percent do not achieve CR because of fatal complications of bone marrow aplasia or impaired recovery of normal stem cells.

High-dose cytarabine–based regimens have been used as initial remission-induction therapy in several single-arm clinical trials with very high CR rates reported following a single cycle of therapy. When given in high doses, more cytarabine may enter the cells, saturate the cytarabine-inactivating enzymes, and increase the intracellular levels of 1-β-D-arabinofuranylcytosine-triphosphate, the active metabolite incorporated into the DNA. Thus higher doses of cytarabine may increase the inhibition of DNA synthesis and thereby overcome resistance to standard-dose cytarabine. In two randomized studies, one by the Southwest Oncology Group (SWOG) and one by the Australian Leukemia Study Group (ALSG), high-dose cytarabine with an anthracycline produced CR rates similar to those seen with standard 7 and 3 regimens. However, the ALSG demonstrated that the CR duration was much longer following high-dose cytarabine as compared to standard-dose cytarabine. Another approach to using high-dose cytarabine would be as induction therapy in patients whose leukemic cells contain the inv(16), t(8;21), or RAS (named after the rat sarcoma virus) mutations, because these groups appear particularly likely to benefit from it.

The hematologic toxicity of high-dose cytarabine–based induction regimens has typically been greater than that associated with 7 and 3 regimens. A current trial at Roswell Park Cancer Institute suggests that administration of recombinant human granulocyte colony stimulating factor (G-CSF) beginning 12 h following completion of chemotherapy accelerates count recovery following high-dose cytarabine and anthracycline chemotherapy, such that hematologic toxicity does not exceed and is often less than that associated with 7 and 3 regimens without growth factor. When high-dose cytarabine regimens are used for patients over 50 years old, the cytarabine dose must be reduced (maximum dose 1.5 to 2 g/m²) because of the higher risk of cerebellar toxicity in older patients. All patients treated with high-dose cytarabine must be closely monitored for cerebellar toxicity. Full cerebellar testing should be performed before each dose, and further high-dose cytarabine should be withheld if evidence of cerebellar toxicity develops. For treatment-associated AML, the high-dose cytarabine and anthracycline combination has yielded better results than 7 and 3 in some, but not all, studies.

Because of the synergy between cytarabine and etoposide, etoposide was added to the 7 and 3 induction regimen in a randomized trial by the ALSG. Etoposide interacts with topoisomerase II, an enzyme that binds to DNA, producing temporary double strand breaks to control the degree of supercoiling. Etoposide stabilizes the DNA/topoisomerase II complex leading to permanent double strand DNA breaks. The results showed improved CR duration but no change in overall survival.

Supportive Care Measures geared to supporting patients through several weeks of granulocytopenia and thrombocytopenia are critical to the success of AML therapy. Patients with AML should be treated in centers expert in providing supportive measures for their management.

FIGURE 112-1 Flow chart for the therapy of newly diagnosed AML. For all forms of AML except M3, standard therapy includes a 7-day continuous infusion of cytarabine (100–200 mg/m² per day) and a 3-day course of daunorubicin (45 mg/m² per day) or idarubicin (12–13 mg/m² per day). Patients who achieve complete remission undergo some form of maintenance therapy with either high-dose cytarabine or high-dose combination chemotherapy with allogeneic marrow transplantation. Patients with AML M3 usually receive tretinoin together with combination chemotherapy for remission induction.

Recombinant hematopoietic growth factors have been incorporated into clinical trials in AML. These trials have been designed either to lower the infection rate after chemotherapy, to sensitize (prime) the leukemic blasts to chemotherapy, or to achieve both goals. Both G-CSF and granulocyte-macrophage colony stimulating factor (GM-CSF) have reduced the median time to neutrophil recovery by an average of 5 to 7 days. This accelerated rate of neutrophil recovery, however, has not always translated into significant reductions in infection rates. A randomized study from 22 centers in Europe demonstrated a higher CR rate, especially in patients with unfavorable cytogenetics, with G-CSF, as compared to placebo, used following completion of induction chemotherapy. A placebo-controlled, randomized study from the Eastern Cooperative Oncology Group has demonstrated longer median survival in patients treated with GM-CSF following induction therapy. The positive effects on CR rate and survival reported could reflect either reduced fatal infection rates or changes in leukemic cell proliferation. Effects on disease-free survival are not significant. The priming hypothesis is based on in vitro data showing enhanced sensitivity to cell cycle–specific chemotherapeutic agents by increasing the number of cells in S-phase. The use of growth factors for a short time (1 to 2 days) before and/or during chemotherapy has not supported this hypothesis. We favor the use of growth factors following chemotherapy for AML only in the setting of clinical trials, so that long-term follow-up data can be obtained to monitor for late adverse effects.

Megakaryocyte growth and development factor, thrombopoietin, may have a beneficial effect on treatment outcome by shortening the duration of thrombocytopenia. Clinical trials are ongoing.

Multilumen right atrial catheters should be inserted through a subcutaneous tunnel as soon as patients with newly diagnosed AML have been stabilized. They should be used thereafter for administration of intravenous medications and transfusions, as well as for blood drawing. The separation between the vascular access site and the exit site and the presence of a Dacron cuff in the subcutaneous channel reduce the risk of infectious complications. With meticulous attention to sterile technique in catheter placement and maintenance, catheters may often be left in place for months.

Adequate and prompt blood bank support is critical to therapy of AML. Platelet transfusions should be given as needed to maintain a platelet count above 20,000/μL. We believe that the platelet count should be kept at higher levels in febrile patients and during episodes of active bleeding or DIC. Measures that may be used in patients with poor posttransfusion platelet count increments include administration of platelets from human leukocyte antigen (HLA)-matched donors and intravenous immunoglobulin therapy. Red blood cell transfusions should be administered to keep the hemoglobin above 85 g/L (8.5 g/dL). Blood products leukodepleted by filtration should be used to avert or delay alloimmunization as well as febrile reactions. Blood products should also be irradiated to prevent graft-versus-host disease (GVHD). Cytomegalovirus (CMV)-negative blood products should be used for CMV-seronegative patients who are potential candidates for allogeneic BMT. Leukodepleted products are also effective for these patients if CMV-negative products are not available.

Infectious complications remain the major cause of morbidity and of death during induction and postremission chemotherapy for AML. Prophylactic administration of antibacterial antibiotics in the absence of fever is controversial. Oral nystatin or clotrimazole are recommended to prevent localized candidiasis. For patients who are herpes simplex virus–positive, acyclovir prophylaxis is effective in preventing reactivation of latent herpes infections.

Fever develops in the vast majority of AML patients, but infections are documented in only half of febrile patients. Early initiation of empiric broad-spectrum antibacterial and antifungal antibiotics has significantly reduced the number of patients dying of infectious complications (see Chap. 87). A combination of antibiotics adequate to treat both gram-negative and -positive organisms should be instituted at the onset of fever in a granulocytopenic patient, following clinical evaluation and procurement of cultures and roentgenograms aimed at documenting the source of fever. Specific antibiotic regimens should be based on antibiotic sensitivity data obtained from the institution at which the patient is being treated. We prefer to use imipenem-cilastatin with vancomycin as first-line therapy. Other acceptable regimens include an antipseudomonal semisynthetic penicillin (e.g., piperacillin) combined with an aminoglycoside, a third-generation cephalosporin with antipseudomonal activity (i.e., ceftazidine) or double β-lactam combinations (ceftazidine and piperacillin), with or without vancomycin. Aminoglycosides should be avoided if possible in patients with renal insufficiency. For patients with known immediate type hypersensitivity reactions to penicillin, aztreonam may be substituted for β-lactams. Aztreonam should be combined with an aminoglycoside rather than used alone. Empiric amphotericin B therapy should be initiated in neutropenic patients who remain febrile without a known source for 7 days or who develop new fever while on broad-spectrum antibacterial antibiotics. Antibacterial and antifungal antibiotics should be continued until patients are no longer neutropenic, regardless of whether a specific source has been found for the fever.

Treatment of M3 Leukemia Daily oral ATRA during induction has been shown to improve outcome in patients with t(15;17). The cells in this subtype are induced to differentiate, and complications of cytotoxic therapy (e.g., DIC) are usually averted. However, retinoic acid syndrome may develop within the first 3 weeks of therapy. The syndrome includes fever, chest pain, dyspnea, pulmonary infiltrates, and progressive hypoxemia. Unless reversed, it can rapidly be fatal. It must be aggressively managed with early initiation of glucocorticoid therapy, oxygen, and supportive care measures. Patients with elevated leukocyte counts are at particular risk for this syndrome, but it may also develop in the setting of low white blood cell counts. Some investigators advocate the addition of chemotherapy if the leukocyte count rises above 10,000/μL. It is important that patients induced into CR with ATRA receive consolidation chemotherapy, as essentially all patients treated with ATRA alone relapse.

In M3 leukemia patients treated with 7 and 3, a second course of chemotherapy should be withheld despite persistence of leukemic promyelocytes in the bone marrow on days 14 to 28, as CR frequently follows one course of standard 7 and 3 therapy in this subtype of AML, despite persistence of leukemic cells in the bone marrow during the initial weeks of therapy.

The importance of ATRA for M3 leukemia was demonstrated in a National Cancer Institute–sponsored intergroup study, where patients were randomized to receive either ATRA or standard 7 and 3 for induction. This was followed by one cycle of standard 7 and 3 therapy and one cycle of high-dose cytarabine and daunorubicin for all patients and a second randomization for the maintenance phase between ATRA or observation. Although the follow-up is relatively short, almost all patients who received chemotherapy alone followed by observation have relapsed. Patients receiving ATRA mostly remain in CR. This study demonstrates the importance of ATRA therapy in patients with t(15;17), although the best time for administering it is still not clear.

The clinical relevance of RT-PCR in detecting residual disease in M3 leukemia has been shown by several groups. With current assays, the complete and sustained disappearance of the PML-RARα transcript by RT-PCR is associated with a high probability of maintaining disease-free survival. Persistence of the RT-PCR product predicts for relapse, suggesting that the disease was not eradicated, and further therapy is indicated.

Postremission Therapy Induction of a durable first CR is critical to long-term disease-free survival in AML. Once relapse has occurred, AML is generally curable only by BMT.

Postremission therapy is designed to eradicate any residual leukemic cells. Therefore it should prevent relapse and prolong survival.

Approaches to postremission therapy in AML include intensive chemotherapy and allogeneic or autologous BMT. Initial postinduction chemotherapy studies demonstrated a dose-response effect for cytarabine, and randomized studies have substantiated the superiority of high-dose over standard-dose cytarabine. The Cancer and Leukemia Group B, for example, compared the duration of CR in patients randomized to four cycles of either high (3 g/m² every 12 h on days 1, 3, and 5), intermediate (400 mg/m² for 5 days by continuous infusion), or standard (100 mg/m² per day for 5 days by continuous infusion) doses of cytarabine postremission. A dose-response effect for cytarabine in patients with AML who were 60 years of age or younger was demonstrated. High-dose cytarabine significantly prolonged CR and increased the fraction cured in patients with favorable [t(8;21) and inv(16)] and normal cytogenetics but had no significant effect on patients with other abnormal karyotypes.

Allogeneic BMT in first CR, in patients under age 65 years without major organ dysfunction (e.g., renal, pulmonary, cardiac, or hepatic damage) who have an HLA-compatible related bone marrow donor or in those under age 55 years with an HLA-compatible unrelated donor, results in cure in 40 to 60 percent of patients. However, toxicity is relatively high with treatment-related complications, including venoocclusive disease, GVHD, and infections. To test whether allogeneic BMT is superior to postremission intensive chemotherapy in first CR, several groups have prospectively studied AML patients at diagnosis for an HLA-compatible sibling and genetically randomized them between the two treatment options. Patients with an HLA-compatible sibling have been offered an allogeneic BMT as early as possible after CR achievement, and patients without an HLA-compatible sibling have received high-dose intensive chemotherapy. Attempts have been made to minimize biases related to patient selection, transplantation center referral, and time delay between CR achievement and BMT. Although there is a tendency toward a lower risk of relapse in the BMT arm of these studies, no significant differences have generally been detected in overall survival rate between the treatment approaches. This may be because (1) some patients with a compatible donor do not undergo BMT, (2) there is a higher incidence of treatment-related complications after BMT, and (3) the availability of better salvage therapy for patients who relapse after intensive chemotherapy (i.e., allogeneic BMT) as compared to patients who relapse after BMT. The use of predictive models based on prognostic factors may help to select patients for whom BMT is recommended in first CR.

Autologous BMT for postinduction therapy uses the same high-dose chemotherapy as in allogeneic BMT, except that the patients subsequently receive their own cells, collected while in remission and temporarily stored. In a study from the European Organization for Research and Treatment of Cancer and the Gruppo Italiano Malattie Ematologiche Maligne dell'Adulto, in which patients without an HLA-identical related donor were randomly assigned to undergo autologous BMT with unpurged marrow or a second course of high-dose cytarabine and daunorubicin, the projected rate of disease-free survival at 4 years was 48 percent and 30 percent, respectively. The overall survival, using an intent-to-treat analysis, was not different between the two groups. Stratifying patients according to risk groups and the development of more sensitive methods to detect minimal residual disease might help to discern a population more likely to benefit from autologous BMT.

For autologous BMT, ex vivo purged marrow has been used in an attempt to avoid reinfusing residual viable leukemic cells. However, this method results in a significantly higher risk, for a prolonged time, of infection and bleeding. In some patients, blood stem cells that do not appear to contain the malignant clone, even when sensitive molecular techniques such as RT-PCR are used, can be harvested early in the recovery period following dose-intensive chemotherapy and can be used to restore normal hematopoiesis after myeloablative

therapy. Because stem cells collected from the blood during the recovery phase after chemotherapy (mobilization) appear to be enriched for normal CD34+ cells, they also may be better starting material than bone marrow for subsequent selection of CD34+ subsets or other ex vivo manipulation designed to eliminate leukemic cells that may remain after mobilization. Studies in first CR of this and other approaches to decrease the incidence of relapse, such as the ex vivo use of monoclonal antibodies (against the leukemic cells) with or without chemotherapy to purge the chemotherapy-mobilized stem cells, are ongoing.

A major focus of current research is detection of residual leukemic cells in the bone marrow of CR patients using techniques such as RT-PCR, FISH, and multiparameter flow cytometry. The availability of sensitive and specific methods for detection of occult residual leukemia cells during CR would allow optimization of postinduction management for individual patients. The use of immune modulation postremission is another experimental approach. It is based on the following observations: (1) natural killer cells are defective in patients with leukemia, (2) allogeneic transplant recipients who develop significant GVHD have a decreased risk of leukemic relapse compared with patients in whom GVHD does not develop, and (3) infusions of donor leukocytes alone (without prior conditioning or GVHD prophylaxis) for relapse after allogeneic BMT induces CR. These have led to speculation that an adoptive immune response, termed *graft-versus-leukemia* (GVL), mediated by cytotoxic T cells, and possibly natural or lymphokine-activated killer cells, may be the reason for the enhanced antileukemia effect seen in unmanipulated allografts as compared to T cell–depleted allografts. Thus stimulation of a GVL or immunologic effect in patients with AML in remission may lead to a decreased relapse rate. The hypothesis from these observations is that the immune system is an important element in the cure of AML. Several approaches are under investigation that attempt to stimulate the immune system postremission. One such approach is the use of low-dose (1.2 × 10⁶ units/m²) interleukin (IL) 2,[1] administered subcutaneously for 10 days, to induce natural killer cell expansion, followed by continuous infusion IL-2 (3 × 10⁶ units/m²) to induce natural killer cell cytotoxicity.

Another postremission approach being used by several groups has emerged from the findings on the role of the multidrug resistance gene in AML. Modulators (e.g., cyclosporine) that can block drug efflux are being administered along with postremission chemotherapy.

Relapse   Once relapse occurs following the standard induction and postremission chemotherapy approach described above and outlined in Fig. 112-1, patients are rarely cured with further standard-dose chemotherapy. Patients eligible for allogeneic or autologous BMT should be expeditiously transplanted at the first sign of relapse. Long-term disease-free survival is approximately the same (30 percent) using allogeneic BMT in first relapse or in second remission. The most important factors predicting response at relapse are the length of the previous CR, whether initial CR was achieved with one or two courses of chemotherapy, and the type of postremission therapy. Because of the poor outcome of patients in early (<6 months) first relapse, it is justified (for patients without HLA-compatible donors) to explore innovative approaches, such as new drugs. Patients with longer (>12 months) first CR generally relapse with drug-sensitive disease and may achieve a second remission with the original induction regimen. However, for these patients too, long-term disease-free survival requires treatment with additional agents, not previously received, or BMT. Salvage regimens used for relapsed disease, as well as for initially refractory disease, include high-dose cytarabine with an anthracycline or mitoxantrone (for patients who have not received high-dose cytarabine in induction or postremission) and high-dose etoposide in conjunction with high-dose cyclophosphamide.

---

[1] This drug has not been approved for this purpose by the Food and Drug Administration at the time of publication.

INCIDENCE The incidence of chronic myeloid leukemia (CML) is approximately 1.3 per 100,000 people per year, and the age-adjusted incidence is higher in men than in women (1.7 versus 1.0). There was a slight decrease in the incidence of CML between 1973 and 1991 (1.5 versus 1.3). The incidence of CML increases slowly with age until the middle forties, when the incidence starts to rise rapidly.

DEFINITION The diagnosis of CML is established by identifying cytogenetically or molecularly a clonal expansion of a hematopoietic stem cell possessing a reciprocal translocation between chromosomes 9 and 22. This translocation results in the head-to-tail fusion of the breakpoint cluster region (BCR) gene on chromosome 22 at band q11 with the ABL (named after the abelson murine leukemia virus) gene located on chromosome 9 at band q34. The disease is characterized by the inevitable transition from a chronic phase to an accelerated phase and on to blast crisis.

ETIOLOGY No clear correlation with exposure to cytotoxic drugs, such as alkylating agents, has been found, and there is no direct evidence of a viral etiology. Cigarette smoking has been shown to accelerate the progression to blast crisis and therefore has an adverse effect on survival in CML. The effect of radiation was demonstrated in the study of the atomic bomb survivors, where it has been estimated that the development of a CML cell mass of $10,000/\mu L$ takes 6.3 years. The Chernobyl nuclear facility accident and the availability of more sensitive techniques to detect the product of the t(9;22) may teach us more about initiation events in the pathogenesis of CML.

PATHOPHYSIOLOGY The product of the fusion gene resulting from the t(9;22) is believed to play a central role in the initial development of CML. This chimeric gene is transcribed into a hybrid BCR-ABL mRNA in which exon 1 of ABL is replaced by variable numbers of 5′ BCR exons. Bcr-Abl fusion proteins, $p210^{BCR-ABL}$, are produced that contain NH_2-terminal domains of Bcr and the COOH-terminal domains of Abl. The oncogenic potential of the Bcr-Abl fusion proteins has been validated by their ability to transform hematopoietic progenitor cells in vitro. Furthermore, there is a model where reconstituting lethally irradiated mice with bone marrow cells infected with retrovirus carrying the gene encoding the $p210^{BCR-ABL}$ leads to the development of a myeloproliferative syndrome resembling CML in 50 percent of the experimental animals. Another approach that supports a role for Bcr-Abl in the growth of t(9;22)-positive leukemic cells involves the use of specific antisense oligomers to the BCR-ABL junctions. After exposure to BCR-ABL antisense, suppression of leukemia colony formation was detected, whereas granulocyte-macrophage colony formation from normal marrow progenitors was unaffected. Taken together, these data provide cogent evidence for BCR-ABL gene participation in leukemogenesis.

The mechanism(s) by which $p210^{BCR-ABL}$ promotes the transition from the benign state to the fully malignant one is still unclear. However, attachment of the BCR sequences to ABL results in three critical functional changes: (1) the Abl protein becomes constitutively active as a tyrosine kinase enzyme, (2) the DNA protein–binding activity of Abl is attenuated, and (3) the binding of Abl to cytoskeletal actin microfilaments is enhanced.

Disease Progression The events associated with transition to the acute phase are poorly understood. Chromosomal instability of the malignant clone, resulting, for example, in the acquisition of an additional t(9;22), trisomy 8, or 17p-, is a fundamental characteristic of CML. It is generally believed that acquisition of resultant genetic and/or molecular abnormalities are critical to the phenotypic transformation. Several groups have reported that the site of the breakpoint within the BCR gene predicts the time to development of blast crisis, but these results have been refuted by others. Heterogeneous structural alterations of the p53 gene, as well as structural alterations and lack of protein production of the retinoblastoma gene, have been associated with disease progression in a subset of patients. Similarly, several reports have demonstrated rare cases with alterations in the RAS gene. Sporadic reports also exist indicating the presence of an altered MYC (named after the myelocytomatosis virus) gene or the appearance of

$p190^{BCR-ABL}$, the protein commonly found in adult ALL and occasionally in AML, during the clinical evolution of small numbers of patients with CML. Progressive de novo DNA methylation at the BCR-ABL locus has also been shown to herald blastic transformation. Finally, IL-1β may be involved in the progression of CML to the blastic phase. In summary, multiple pathways to disease transformation exist, although the exact timing and the relevance of each of these remains unclear.

CLINICAL PRESENTATION **Symptoms** The clinical onset of the chronic phase is generally insidious. Accordingly, some patients are diagnosed while still asymptomatic, during health screening tests; other patients present with fatigue, malaise, and weight loss or have symptoms resulting from splenic enlargement, such as early satiety and left upper quadrant pain or mass. Less common are features related to granulocyte or platelet dysfunction, such as infections, thrombosis, or bleeding. Occasionally, patients present with leukostatic manifestations due to severe leukocytosis or thrombosis such as vasoocclusive disease, cerebrovascular accidents, myocardial infarction, venous thrombosis, priapism, visual disturbances, and pulmonary insufficiency.

Progression of CML is associated with worsening symptoms. Unexplained fever, significant weight loss, increasing dose requirement of the drugs controlling the disease, bone and joint pain, bleeding, thrombosis, and infections suggest transformation into accelerated or blastic phases. Presentation with accelerated disease or with de novo blastic phase CML represents fewer than 10 to 15 percent of newly diagnosed cases.

Physical Findings In most patients the abnormal finding on physical examination at diagnosis is minimal to moderate splenomegaly; mild hepatomegaly is found occasionally. Persistent splenomegaly despite continued therapy is a sign of disease acceleration. Lymphadenopathy and extramedullary leukemic deposition (chloromas) are unusual except late in the course of the disease, and when present, the prognosis is poor.

Hematologic Findings Elevated white blood cell counts, with various degrees of immaturity of the granulocytic series, are observed at diagnosis. Usually there are fewer than 5 percent circulating blasts and fewer than 10 percent blasts and promyelocytes. Cycling of the counts may be observed when following patients without treatment. Platelet counts are almost always elevated at diagnosis, and a mild degree of normochromic normocytic anemia is present. Leukocyte alkaline phosphatase is characteristically low in CML cells. Serum levels of vitamin B_{12} and vitamin B_{12}–binding proteins are generally elevated. Phagocytic functions are usually normal at diagnosis and remain normal during the chronic phase. Increased histamine production secondary to basophilia occurs in later stages, causing diarrhea and flushing.

At diagnosis, increased bone marrow cellularity, primarily of the myeloid and megakaryocytic lineages, with a greatly altered myeloid to erythroid ratio, is found in almost all CML patients. The marrow blast percentage is generally normal or slightly elevated. Marrow or blood basophilia, eosinophilia, and monocytosis may be observed. While collagen fibrosis in the marrow is unusual at presentation, significant degrees of reticulin stain–measured fibrosis are noted in about half of the patients.

Disease acceleration is defined by the development of increasing degrees of anemia unaccounted for by bleeding or chemotherapy, cytogenetic clonal evolution, blood or marrow blasts ≥15 percent but <30 percent, blood or marrow blasts and promyelocytes ≥30 percent, blood or marrow basophils ≥20 percent, or platelet count <100,000/ μL. *Blast crisis* is defined as acute leukemia, with blood or marrow blasts ≥30 percent. Hyposegmented neutrophils may appear (Pelger-Huët anomaly). Blast cells can be classified as myeloid, lymphoid, erythroid, or undifferentiated, based on morphologic, cytochemical, and immunologic features. About half of the cases are acute myeloid leukemia, one-third are acute lymphoid leukemia, 10 percent are acute erythroleukemia, and the rest are undifferentiated.

Chromosomal Findings The cytogenetic hallmark of CML, found in 90 to 95 percent of the cases, is the t(9;22)(q34;q11). Originally, this was recognized by the presence of a shortened chromosome 22 (22q-), designated as the *Philadelphia chromosome*, that arises from the reciprocal 9;22 translocation. Some patients may have complex translocations (designated as *variant translocations*) involving three, four, or five chromosomes (usually including chromosomes 9 and 22). However, the molecular consequences of these chromosomal changes appear similar to those resulting from the typical t(9;22).

PROGNOSTIC FACTORS The clinical outcome of patients with CML is variable. Death is expected in 10 percent of patients within 2 years and in somewhat fewer than 20 percent yearly thereafter. The median survival is about 4 years. Therefore, several prognostic models that identify different risk groups in CML have been developed. The most commonly used staging systems have been derived from multivariate analyses of prognostic factors. The Sokal index identified percentage of circulating blasts, spleen size, platelet count, cytogenetic clonal evolution, and age as the most important prognostic indicators. Two models, that of Tura and the combined model of Kantarjian, divide patients according to the number of negative prognostic factors. Age ≥60, spleen ≥10 cm below the costal margin, blasts ≥3 percent in blood or ≥5 percent in marrow, basophils ≥7 percent in blood or ≥3 percent in marrow, platelets ≥700,000/mL, or any of the characteristics of accelerated disease are associated with a very poor short-term prognosis and a threefold higher hazard rate, or risk of death per unit of time, in the first year.

℞ TREATMENT

The goal of therapy in CML is to achieve prolonged, durable, nonneoplastic nonclonal hematopoiesis, which entails the eradication of any residual cells containing the BCR-ABL transcript. Hence the goal is complete molecular remission and cure (Table 112-3). A proposed treatment plan for the newly diagnosed CML patient is presented in Fig. 112-2.

Allogeneic BMT Allogeneic BMT is the only curative therapy for CML and, when feasible, is the treatment of choice. However, it is complicated by a high early mortality rate owing to the transplant procedure. When the outcome of all patients undergoing allogeneic BMT reported to the International Bone Marrow Transplant Registry was compared to the outcome of all patients treated with hydroxyurea or interferon (IFN) α by the German CML Study Group, the survival for the former group was statistically better, but only starting 5 years from the time of transplant. When only low-risk patients (by Sokal's criteria) were evaluated, the benefit in survival for allogeneic BMT was seen after 6 years. Outcome of BMT depends on multiple factors

Table 112-3

Response Criteria in CML

Hematologic	
Complete response*	White blood cell count <10,000/μL, normal morphology
	Normal hemoglobin and platelet counts
Incomplete response	White blood cell count ≥10,000/μL
Cytogenetic	Percentage of bone marrow metaphases with t(9;22)
Complete response	0
Partial response	≤35
Minor response	36–85†
No response	85–100
Molecular	Presence of BCR-ABL transcript by RT-PCR
Complete response	None
Incomplete response	Any

* Complete hematologic response requires the disappearance of splenomegaly.

† Up to 15% normal metaphases are occasionally seen at diagnosis (when 30 metaphases are analyzed).

NOTE: RT-PCR, reverse transcriptase polymerase chain reaction.

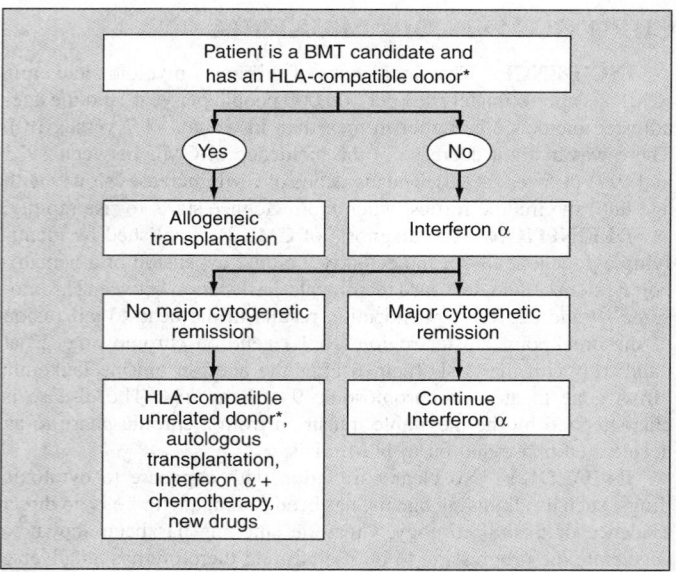

FIGURE 112-2 Flow chart for the therapy of newly diagnosed CML. Patients with an HLA-compatible donor often receive high-dose therapy plus an allogeneic marrow transplant as initial therapy. The asterisk denotes that some centers employ allogeneic marrow transplant only if interferon-α fails to induce a response. Most data suggest that treatment outcome is superior if marrow transplantation is performed earlier rather than later in the course of disease.

including: (1) the patient (i.e., age and phase of disease); (2) the type of donor [i.e., syngeneic (monozygotic twins) or HLA-compatible allogeneic, related or unrelated]; (3) the preparative regimen; (4) GVHD; and (5) posttransplantation treatment.

THE PATIENT As experience has been gained, and safety and efficacy established, it has become clear that patients should be relatively young (<65 years) and have a healthy and histocompatible donor. Furthermore, survival following BMT in the accelerated and blastic phases of the disease is significantly worse and is associated with a very high rate of relapse. The Seattle data demonstrate that transplantation early in the chronic phase (1 to 2 years from diagnosis) is superior to later transplant. It has been shown that the overall survival, disease-free survival, incidence and severity of acute and chronic GVHD, and relapse rates are not influenced by prior IFNα treatment.

THE DONOR Transplantation from a family donor, who is either fully matched or mismatched at only one HLA locus, should be considered standard therapy for any CML patient who is a candidate for an HLA-related sibling transplant. Syngeneic transplantation in chronic phase CML patients has been reported from the Seattle group to result in 7-year disease-free survival in 55 percent, with a 30 percent relapse rate. With HLA-identical sibling transplantation in the chronic phase, many groups have reported 5-year disease-free survival in 40 to 70 percent of patients, with a 25 percent relapse rate. Transplantation from an HLA-matched unrelated donor has been reported by the Seattle group to result in a 74 percent probability of surviving 3 years for patients who are in chronic phase, less than 1 year from diagnosis, and younger than 50 years old. A 2-year actuarial incidence of disease-free (based on hematologic analyses) survival of 45 percent (±21 percent) for unrelated transplants, matched or mismatched at only one locus, transplanted less than 1 year from diagnosis was reported by the National Marrow Donor Program. Patients in the age group of 40 to 50 fared poorly (15 of 55 survived). The probability of 2-year disease-free (based on cytogenetic analyses) survival in a report on unrelated transplants from the Medical College of Wisconsin, using a standardized conditioning regimen and T cell depletion, was 52 percent for patients transplanted in chronic phase (regardless of the time from diagnosis). Unrelated transplants have higher rates of graft failure and acute and chronic GVHD and prolonged convalescence following treatment, compared to related allogeneic transplants. Peripheral blood is now being studied as a source of allogeneic hematopoietic progenitor cells; it may offer rapid engraftment and less risk for the donor.

PREPARATIVE REGIMENS These have been studied by several groups. A randomized study from the Seattle group compared cyclophosphamide and total-body irradiation with busulphan and cyclophosphamide. They found no significant differences in the 3-year probabilities of survival, relapse, event-free survival, speed of engraftment, or incidence of venoocclusive disease of the liver. Significantly more patients in the total-body irradiation arm experienced major creatinine elevations, acute GVHD, longer periods of fever, positive blood cultures, hospital admissions, and longer inpatient hospital stays. These data suggest that the combination of busulphan and cyclophosphamide is the preferred regimen. Other preparative regimens are being tested with the primary goal of reducing the relapse rate.

THE DEVELOPMENT AND TYPE OF GVHD Development of grade I GVHD, as compared to no GVHD, has been shown by The European Group for Blood and Marrow Transplantation to decrease the incidence of relapse. A lower relapse rate was observed also in patients with grade II GVHD but was accompanied by a substantially higher transplant-related mortality. The decreased relapse rate may be caused by a GVL effect. Depletion of T lymphocytes from donor marrow can prevent GVHD but results in an increased risk of relapse, which exceeds the relapse rate following syngeneic BMT. Thus, T lymphocytes from the donor marrow mediate a significant antileukemic, or GVL, effect, and even syngeneic marrow may exhibit limited GVL activity in CML.

POSTTRANSPLANTATION TREATMENT Further support for the existence of an immunologically mediated GVL effect comes from the observation that donor leukocyte infusions (without prior conditioning or GVHD prophylaxis) can induce hematologic and cytogenetic remissions in CML patients who have relapsed after allogeneic BMT.

The activity of IFNα in patients with early chronic-phase CML was the basis for the use of IFNα after BMT, either to induce cytogenetic remissions in relapsed patients or to prevent relapse after BMT for high-risk patients. The main concern about IFNα use after allogeneic BMT has been the development or worsening of GVHD, because IFNα is known to act as an immunomodulator. However, in published reports comprising 52 allogeneic recipients who were free of GVHD and were either at high risk for relapse or had already relapsed, only 6 subsequently developed GVHD after IFNα therapy was initiated. IFNα has also been combined with mononuclear cells obtained from donor blood to induce cytogenetic remissions in relapsed patients. Cytogenetic remissions have been achieved, but the exact role of IFNα as opposed to the mononuclear cells is unclear. IL-2, with or without IFNα, is also being evaluated for its ability to restore complete cytogenetic remission in patients relapsing following BMT.

IFNα has also been used following BMT to prevent relapse in patients with advanced disease at time of transplant (patients at high risk for relapse). Maintenance of cytogenetic CR as long as 2 years posttransplantation in patients with blast crisis or second chronic phase has been reported in small numbers of patients. Similarly, IL-2 (2.5×10^6 to 6×10^6 units/m² per day) has been given following T cell–depleted allogeneic BMT in an effort to induce GVL without GVHD, and thus prevent relapse. Preliminary data suggest that, compared with historical controls, patients treated with IL-2 have a lower risk of disease relapse. A randomized trial is warranted.

Interferons When allogeneic BMT is not feasible, IFNα therapy is the treatment of choice. The interferons are a complex group of naturally occurring proteins produced by eukaryotic cells in response to viruses, antigens, and mitogens. Three distinct groups of IFN species have been identified: IFNα, -β, and -γ. Although a variety of interferons have become available for clinical investigation, the most data have been generated using IFNα preparations.

Interferons have potent, pleiotropic biological effects, spanning a spectrum of antiviral, microbicidal, immunomodulatory, and anti-

proliferative properties. While interferons have been shown to downregulate the expression of several oncogenes and cytokines, they also upregulate the expression of interferon regulatory factor-1 (a transcriptional activator with antioncogenic activity), adhesion molecules, and the histocompatibility genes. Interferons have also been shown to inhibit angiogenesis and to induce a cellular immune response. Although bench research has revealed a diverse array of possibilities for interferons, a clear knowledge of their mode(s) of action is still lacking.

The initial studies of IFNα in the treatment of CML were single-agent, single-arm trials that attempted to determine an effective dose, the patient population that would benefit from the treatment, and toxicity. An association between IFNα dose and the quality of response became clear from these studies. The effective dose was found to be 5 million units subcutaneously daily. Treatment with IFNα was found to be effective only when initiated within the first year of diagnosis. Experience with IFNα suggests that segregation of patients into IFNα-sensitive and -resistant subgroups correlates strongly with time from diagnosis and prognosis at diagnosis.

Patients develop both acute and chronic side effects from IFNα therapy. Acute side effects (flulike symptoms) appear early in the course of the treatment. Most flulike symptoms respond to acetaminophen, and tachyphylaxis develops within 1 to 2 weeks. Chronic reactions, such as fatigue and lethargy, weight loss, myalgias, and arthralgias, occur in approximately half of the patients and may require dose reduction. Patients also report cough, postnasal drip, and dryness of the skin. Infrequently, immune-mediated thrombocytopenia and anemia develop. In addition, long-term therapy has been associated with late autoimmune side effects, such as hypothyroidism and occasionally generalized autoimmune phenomena.

The most important persistent side effects in CML patients treated with IFNα are neurologic. All IFNα-treated patients are subject to some neurologic toxicity, the most common symptom being lethargy. Up to 20 percent of patients have neurologic side effects that are associated with compromised quality of life and reduction in their ability to carry out their regular activity, such as full-time work. In addition, at the required doses, impotence in men is not infrequent. In an effort to modify the side effects, the role of antidepressant agents such as amitriptyline hydrochloride is currently being tested. Furthermore, because IFNα has been shown to have opioid-like effects, and the opioid antagonist naloxone modifies IFNα-induced changes both in vitro and in vivo, a trial with naltrexone (an opioid antagonist) has been initiated at the M.D. Anderson Cancer Center.

Hematologic remissions are generally achieved within 1 to 2 months of starting IFNα. However, some patients show a cyclic response pattern with progressively lower peak and nadir counts over a period of months. The increase in counts during the cycling that occurs in the first few months of therapy should not be confused with resistance. Cytogenetic responses generally start at 3 to 12 months, and complete cytogenetic responses may require 6 months to 4 years of therapy. However, most complete cytogenetic responses are achieved within 12 to 18 months, and in single-agent, single-arm studies they have been seen in up to 26 percent of patients.

Randomized trials of IFNα versus chemotherapy have found that both treatment modalities are effective in achieving hematologic remissions. The incidence of IFNα-induced hematologic and cytogenetic responses have been considerably lower in the randomized trials than in the single-arm studies. These results are probably explained by lower IFNα doses, patient population heterogeneity (some studies have included high-risk patients, as defined by Sokal's criteria), multicenter participation without a unified policy on dose modification, and premature discontinuation of treatment.

Three randomized studies (those of the Italian Cooperative Study Group, the United Kingdom Medical Research Council, and the Kouseisho Leukemia Study Group) have demonstrated an association between IFNα therapy and improved survival. Interestingly, in the first two of these studies, a survival advantage for achieving a cytogenetic response in the IFNα-treated groups was seen, but this advantage was unrelated to the degree of that response. A fourth trial, by the German CML Study Group, did not show an increase in survival for IFNα-treated patients. These results probably differ from those of the previous studies because of the inclusion of patients with more advanced CML.

Chemotherapy   Initial management of patients with chemotherapy is currently reserved for rapid lowering of white blood cell counts, reduction of symptoms, and reversal of symptomatic splenomegaly. Hydroxyurea, a ribonucleotide reductase inhibitor, induces rapid disease control. The initial dose is 1 to 4 g/d, and the dose should be reduced by half with each 50 percent reduction of the leukocyte count. Unfortunately, cytogenetic remissions with hydroxyurea are uncommon. Busulphan, an alkylating agent that acts on early progenitor cells, has a more prolonged effect. However, we do not recommend its use because of its serious side effects. These include unexpected, and occasionally fatal, myelosuppression in 5 to 10 percent of patients; pulmonary, endocardial, and marrow fibrosis; and an Addison-like wasting syndrome.

Intensive combination chemotherapy has also been used in chronic phase CML, with 30 to 50 percent of patients achieving complete cytogenetic responses. However these cytogenetic remissions have been short lived. Consequently, intensive combination chemotherapy regimens are being used today only to mobilize normal progenitors in the blood in order to collect circulating stem cells for autologous transplantation. Another role for chemotherapy (e.g., homoharringtonine or low-dose cytarabine) is in combination with IFNα. An M.D. Anderson Cancer Center trial has shown an improved survival for CML patients who were more than 1 year from diagnosis and who were treated with low-dose cytarabine and IFNα, as compared to a historical control population treated with IFNα alone.

Autologous BMT   Autologous hematopoietic stem cell transplantation could potentially cure CML if a means to select the residual normal progenitors, which are known to coexist with their malignant counterparts, could be developed. As a source of autologous hematopoietic stem cells for transplantation, blood offers certain advantages over marrow (e.g., faster engraftment and no general anesthesia). Normal hematopoietic stem cells appear with increased frequency in the blood of patients with CML during the recovery phase after chemotherapy and G-CSF.

A retrospective analysis of over 200 autologous progenitor cell transplants performed for CML at eight centers worldwide suggests that autologous transplantation prolongs survival in chronic- or accelerated-phase patients when compared retrospectively with conventional therapy. Disease phase at transplant included 93 patients in chronic phase, 25 in accelerated phase, and 114 in blast crisis or second chronic phase. Patients received autologous bone marrow and/or blood hematopoietic stem cells. In 42 cases the hematopoietic progenitors were subjected to ex vivo manipulation, either by long-term bone marrow culture, by incubation with recombinant IFNγ, or by chemotherapy. In 49 cases the hematopoietic progenitors were harvested during the recovery phase following various chemotherapy regimens. Following autologous stem cell transplantation, 29 of 93 (31 percent) patients in first chronic phase achieved complete cytogenetic remissions. The median duration of cytogenetic remission was 14 months, with a range of 2 to 68 months. Approaches to treat minimal residual disease following autologous transplantation, such as immune modulation, are currently being investigated.

Leukapheresis and Splenectomy   Intensive leukapheresis may control the blood counts in chronic phase CML; however, it is expensive and cumbersome. It is useful in emergencies where leukostasis-related complications such as pulmonary failure or cerebrovascular accidents are likely. It may also have a role in pregnant women in whom it is important to avoid potentially teratogenic drugs.

Splenectomy was used in CML in the past because of the suggestion that evolution to the acute phase might occur in the spleen. However, this does not appear to be the case, and splenectomy is now reserved for symptomatic relief of painful splenomegaly unresponsive to chemotherapy or for significant anemia or thrombocytopenia associated with hypersplenism. Splenic radiation is used on rare occasions to reduce the size of the spleen.

Minimal Residual Disease   The correlation between residual cells with the t(9;22) and disease recurrence is not completely understood. Initial studies using RT-PCR to predict disease recurrence following IFNα therapy found residual disease in all samples tested from patients with complete cytogenetic remissions. Later studies demonstrated the elimination of the BCR-ABL mRNA transcript after more prolonged IFNα treatment in some cases. It is now possible to quantify transcripts, and longer follow-up may indicate whether quantitation of the BCR-ABL transcript is useful for predicting cytogenetic and clinical relapse.

The nature of the complete molecular remission after IFNα therapy was studied at the M.D. Anderson Cancer Center. Blood, bone marrow, and individually plucked soft agar colonies were simultaneously analyzed for the presence of the BCR-ABL transcript in patients with complete cytogenetic and molecular responses. The RT-PCR-amplified BCR-ABL transcripts were detected only in myeloid or erythroid colonies. These observations demonstrate that residual disease resides in myeloid or erythroid colony forming cells; whether they have the potential to repopulate the bone marrow and thus induce a relapse is unknown. It is possible that IFNα induces tumor dormancy in CML.

Following allogeneic BMT, RT-PCR analysis may be positive for residual disease during the first 6 months in patients who subsequently achieve a long-lasting remission. However, late persistence of RT-PCR positivity appears to indicate a reduced probability of cure. RT-PCR positivity at any single time point is not predictive of imminent relapse. Patients are often divided according to RT-PCR results following allogeneic BMT into one of three groups: (1) persistently positive, (2) intermittently negative, and (3) persistently negative. These three groups have a low, intermediate, and high probability of maintaining remission and disease free-survival, respectively. This suggests that patients who are persistently RT-PCR positive more than 6 months following allogeneic BMT need additional therapeutic interventions. Further, in patients who do not have any evidence for GVHD and are intermittently RT-PCR negative, GVL may be induced by alloreactive donor cells (without the side effects of GVHD) to suppress the proliferation of the leukemic cells.

Future Directions   The use of BCR-ABL antisense oligonucleotides to purge residual leukemic cells from autologous hematopoietic progenitors before reinfusion, as well as approaches to induce GVL in the setting of minimal residual disease without inducing GVHD, are underway.

Treatment of Blast Crisis   The treatment for all forms of blast crisis is generally ineffective. Treatment is tailored to the phenotype of the blast cell. Myeloid crises are treated as for AML, but remissions occur in only a minority of cases and are generally short lived. Patients may present without having had a chronic phase. AML with a t(9;22) is probably blast crisis of CML and carries a poor prognosis. Erythroid blast crisis is treated like AML and also has a poor outcome.

Lymphoid blast crisis is treated like ALL (Chap. 113) with vincristine (1.4 mg/m^2 weekly) plus prednisone (60 mg/m^2 PO qd) induction therapy. About one-third of patients will reenter chronic phase after 2 to 3 weeks of treatment, but the remissions last only a median of about 4 months. Even marrow transplantation is poorly effective during blast crises. Novel treatment approaches are needed.

BIBLIOGRAPHY

APPELBAUM FR et al: Bone marrow transplantation for chronic myelogenous leukemia. Semin Oncol 22:405, 1995

BLOOMFIELD CD, HERZIG GP (eds): Advances in the management of acute leukemia. Hematol Oncol Clin North Am 7:1, 1993

DEGOS L et al: All-trans-retinoic acid as a differentiation agent in the treatment of acute promyelocytic leukemia. Blood 85:2643, 1995

KHOURI I et al: Chronic myeloid leukemia, in *Clinical Oncology*, MD Abeloff et al (eds). New York, Churchill Livingstone, 1995, pp 2035–2051

STONE RM, MAYER RJ: Acute myeloid leukemia in adults, in *Clinical Oncology*, MD Abeloff et al (eds). New York, Churchill Livingstone, 1995, pp 1959–1976

WETZLER M et al: Interferon-α therapy for chronic myelogenous leukemia. Am J Med 99:402, 1995

113

Arnold S. Freedman, Lee M. Nadler

MALIGNANCIES OF LYMPHOID CELLS

DEFINITION Lymphoid leukemias and malignant lymphomas are malignant counterparts of normal lymphoid cells at distinct stages of differentiation. The precursor B and T cell lymphoblastic leukemias correspond to normal pre-B and pre-T cells, respectively. Consequently, these malignant cells originate in the bone marrow, where their normal cellular counterparts reside. In contrast, malignant lymphomas are neoplastic transformations of cells that reside predominantly in lymphoid tissues. Although both leukemias and lymphomas involve reticuloendothelial organs, they are biologically and clinically distinct (Table 113-1).

CELLULAR AND DEVELOPMENTAL ASPECTS OF MALIGNANCIES OF LYMPHOCYTES Lymphoid leukemias, non-Hodgkin's lymphomas, and Hodgkin's disease are classified morphologically (as shown in Tables 113-2, 113-3, and 113-4). Multiple classification schemes have been employed over the past 30 years. The most widely used have been the FAB (French-American-British) classification for acute leukemias, the "Working Formulation" or the Kiel classification for lymphomas, and the Rye classification for Hodgkin's disease.

A classification known as the Revised European-American Classification of Lymphoid Neoplasms (R.E.A.L.) has been created that encompasses all of the lymphoid malignancies. The R.E.A.L. classification has included clinical and pathologic entities that were not included in the other schemes and utilizes detailed immunologic studies and cytogenetics to further characterize various diseases. Since it is hypothesized that acute and chronic lymphoid leukemias and non-Hodgkin's lymphomas represent neoplastic counterparts of normal populations of cells that reside in lymphoid tissues and the bone marrow, it is within the context of normal B and T cell [and natural killer (NK) cell] differentiation (see Chap. 305) that the R.E.A.L. classification has subgrouped the various pathologic entities. In this chapter the R.E.A.L. classification will be presented within a clinical context. General aspects of lymphocytic leukemias and lymphomas will be presented, followed by specific discussions of chronic leukemias/lymphomas, non-Hodgkin's lymphoma with detailed discussion of the indolent and aggressive forms, acute lymphoblastic leukemias/lymphomas, and Hodgkin's disease.

Leukemias and Lymphomas of B Cell Origin Some 80 percent of lymphoblastic leukemias and 90 percent of non-Hodgkin's lymphomas are of B cell derivation, based upon the expression of B lineage–restricted antigens and clonal rearrangements of immunoglobulin heavy and light chain genes. These tumors correspond to major and minor subpopulations of pre-B and mature B cells (Fig. 113-1). Within the context of lineage derivation of these diseases, it

is important that they be viewed within a clinically meaningful perspective. For this reason, the lymphoid leukemias and non-Hodgkin's lymphomas will be discussed as being clinically indolent or aggressive in behavior.

Indolent B cell malignancies Chronic lymphocytic leukemia (CLL) is the most common type of indolent leukemia. The malignant cells correspond to a minor subpopulation of B cells that express cell surface immunoglobulins IgM/D and the T cell–associated antigen CD5. Small lymphocytic lymphoma, like B cell CLL, appears to correspond to a unique subpopulation of B cells that express pan-B cell antigens, surface IgM/D, CD23, and CD5. In contrast to CLL, small lymphocytic lymphomas express the adhesion molecule CD11a/CD18, which may account for the differences in anatomic sites of involvement of the two diseases. Hairy cell leukemia is a rare disorder with characteristics of activated B cells, with expression of interleukin (IL) 2 receptors (CD25) and specific adhesion molecules involved in localizing cells to the spleen and marrow. Prolymphocytic leukemias have morphologic and phenotypic characteristics of transformed B cells and have stronger expression of sIg than do CLL cells. The majority of indolent lymphomas are the follicular lymphomas. Follicular lymphomas include the grade I (small cleaved cell), grade II (mixed small cleaved and large cell), and grade III (large cell) subtypes. Follicular large cell lymphoma has a more rapid natural history and is grouped with the aggressive B cell lymphomas. Follicular lymphomas are thought to correspond to germinal center B cells, which express pan-B cell antigens, surface immunoglobulin (IgM, 60 percent; IgG, 40 percent), and CD10. Consistent with their ability to disseminate widely, these tumors express the molecules that are involved in lymphocyte homing and recirculation—CD44 and L-selectin.

Lymphoplasmacytoid lymphoma/Waldenström's macroglobulinemia is an indolent lymphoma in which cells have characteristics of B cells that are differentiating toward plasma cells. The marginal zone lymphomas, which are hypothesized to be lymphomas of the memory B cell compartment, lack surface IgD and can occur in the following locations: lymph nodes, where they are known as monocytoid B-cell lymphoma; extranodal tissues, where they are referred to as lymphomas of mucosal-associated lymphoid tissues (MALT); and the spleen (splenic lymphoma with or without villous lymphocytes).

Aggressive B cell malignancies Diffuse large cell lymphoma is the most common histologic type of aggressive lymphoma. These tumors express pan-B cell antigens and several B cell activation antigens and resemble transformed activated B cells. Within this category there are patients who present with predominantly mediastinal tumors, which are thought to arise from thymic B cells. From a clinical point of view the follicular large cell (grade III) lymphomas are considered aggressive diseases. Like grade I follicular lymphoma, follicular large cells express pan-B cell antigens, variable surface Ig, and CD10,

Table 113-1

Lymphoid Leukemias and Lymphomas

	Lymphoblastic Leukemia	Non-Hodgkin's	Hodgkin's
Cellular derivation	80% B	90% B	Unresolved
	20% T	10% T	
Sites of disease			
Localized	Uncommon	Uncommon	Common
Nodal spread	Common	Discontiguous	Contiguous
Extranodal	Common	Common	Uncommon
Mediastinal	Common (T cell)	Uncommon	Common
Abdominal	Uncommon	Common	Uncommon
Bone marrow	Always	Common	Uncommon
B symptoms	Common	Uncommon	Common
Chromosomal abnormalities	Common (translocations, deletions)	Common (translocations, deletions)	Common (aneuploidy)
Curability	40–60%	30–40%	75–85%

whereas B cell diffuse large cell lymphomas are generally CD5− and CD10−. Mantle cell lymphomas, which include many cases of "diffuse small cleaved cell lymphoma," express surface IgM/D and CD5, characteristics of normal B cells that reside in the mantle zone of lymphoid follicles. Burkitt's lymphomas are related to normal germinal center B cells and follicular lymphomas in that they express pan-B cell antigens, B cell activation antigens, and CD10. The endemic (African) Burkitt's lymphoma cells, which have the Epstein-Barr virus (EBV) genome present in the tumor cells, express the EBV receptor CD21, whereas the nonendemic (American) variant cells do not. The aggressive Burkitt-like lymphomas are similar to Burkitt's lymphoma

Table 113-2

Histologic Classification of Lymphoid Leukemias and Non-Hodgkin's Lymphoma

R.E.A.L. Classification	Working Formulation	Kiel Classification	Rappaport Terminology	Cellular Lineage, %	Chromosomal Abnormalities
INDOLENT					
B cell CLL, small lymphocytic, prolymphocytic leukemia	A: Small lymphocytic	Lymphocytic (CLL), prolymphocytic leukemia	Diffuse well-differentiated lymphocytic (DWDL)	B	Trisomy 12; t(11;14), t(14;19), t(9;14)
T cell CLL, prolymphocytic leukemia	A: Small lymphocytic E: Diffuse small cleaved cell	Lymphocytic (CLL), prolymphocytic leukemia	DWDL, diffuse poorly differentiated lymphocytic (DPDL)	T	
Large granular lymphocyte leukemia	A: Small lymphocytic E: Diffuse small cleaved cell	Lymphocytic (CLL), prolymphocytic leukemia	DWDL, DPDL	T	
Hairy cell leukemia		Hairy cell leukemia		B	
Follicular center (grade I)	B: Follicular, predominantly small cleaved cell	Centroblastic/ centrocytic	Nodular poorly differentiated lymphocytic (NPDL)	B	t(14;18); del(6)
Follicular center (grade II)	C: Follicular mixed, small cleaved and large cell	Centroblastic/ centrocytic	Nodular mixed lymphocytic histiocytic (NM)	B	t(14;18); del(2) Trisomy 8
Marginal zone B cell (nodal/extranodal-MALT)		Monocytoid/ immunocytoma (nodal/extranodal)		B	
Mycosis fungoides		Small cell cerebriform (mycosis fungoides)		T	
AGGRESSIVE					
Follicular center (grade III)	D: Follicular, predominantly large cell	Centroblastic (follicular)	Nodular histiocytic (NH)	B	t(14;18); Trisomy 7
Mantle cell	E: Diffuse small cleaved cell	Centrocytic	DPDL	B	t(11;14)
Diffuse large B cell	F: Diffuse mixed, small and large cell G: Diffuse large cell H: Large cell immunoblastic	Centroblastic	Diffuse mixed lymphocytic-histiocytic (DM); diffuse histiocytic (DH)	B	t(14;18)/IgH-bcl 2 t(3;22)/bcl 6 t(3;14) t(2;3); Trisomy 4, 7, 21; del(6), (8), (13)
Primary mediastinal (thymic) B cell	G: Diffuse large cell	Large cell, sclerosing B cell lymphoma of mediastinum	DH	B	
Peripheral T cell	F: Diffuse mixed, small and large cell G: Diffuse large cell H: Large cell immunoblastic	Lymphoepithelioid, pleiomorphic (small, medium, or large cell)	DM, DH	T	t(14;14)(q11;q32)/ TCR-tcl 1 inv (14)(q11;q32) t(8;14)(q24;q11) t(10;14)(q24;q11)
Angioimmunoblastic T cell		Angioimmunoblastic		T	
Adult T cell lymphoma/leukemia		Pleiomorphic (small, medium, or large cell HTLV+)		T	
Angiocentric			DH	T	
Intestinal T cell		Pleiomorphic (small, medium, or large cell)		T	
Anaplastic large cell	H: Large cell immunoblastic	Large cell anaplastic (Ki-1+)		T (70) Null (30)	t(2;5)
Precursor T/B cell lymphoblastic lymphoma	I: Lymphoblastic	T lymphoblastic, lymphoblastic	Diffuse lymphoblastic (LL)	T (90) B (10)	
Precursor T/B cell lymphoblastic leukemia				B (80) T (20)	pre-B: t(9;22), t(4;11), t(1;19) T cell: 14q11 or 7q34 B cell: t(8;14), t(2;8), t(8;22)
Burkitt's	J: Small noncleaved cell; Burkitt's	Burkitt's	Diffuse undifferentiated (DUL)	B (95) T (5)	t(8;14), t(2;8), t(8;22)

Table 113-3

Classification of Acute Lymphoblastic Leukemia (ALL)

Immunologic Subtype	% of Cases	FAB Subtype	Cytogenetic Abnormalities
Pre-B ALL	75	L1, L2	t(9;22), t(4;11), t(1;19)
T cell ALL	20	L1, L2	14q11 or 7q34
B cell ALL	5	L3	t(8;14), t(8;22), t(2;8)

NOTE: FAB, French-American-British classification.

Table 113-4

Rye Classification of Hodgkin's Disease

Histologic Subgroup	Incidence, %	Pathology	
		Reed-Sternberg Cell	Other
Lymphocyte-predominant	2–10	Rare	Predominance of normal-appearing lymphocytes
Nodular sclerosis	40–80	Frequent "lacunar variants"	Lymphoid nodules, collagen bands
Mixed cellularity	20–40	Numerous	Pleiomorphic infiltrate
Lymphocyte-depleted	2–15	Numerous, often bizarre	Lymphocytes, pleiomorphic fibrosis

(BL) except they lack surface Ig and probably correspond to an activated peripheral B cell. The vast majority of acute lymphoblastic leukemias (ALL) in the R.E.A.L. classification are pre-B lymphoblastic leukemias, which express characteristics of pre-B cells. Pre-B cell (L1, L2) ALL express CD19 and in most cases CD10 (Fig. 113-1; Table 113-3). Approximately 50 percent of pre-B ALL also express CD20. The B cell (L3) surface Ig+ ALL are morphologically and phenotypically identical to Burkitt's lymphoma cells. Approximately 20 to 30 percent of adult ALL express myeloid antigens (CD13 and or CD33), which are associated with a worse prognosis in some studies.

Malignant Leukemias and Lymphomas of T Cell Origin The most widely expressed T cell antigens that define lineage are CD2 and CD7. As depicted in Fig. 113-2, T cell malignancies reflect distinct stages of T cell ontogeny.

Indolent T cell malignancies The indolent-behaving T cell lymphoproliferative disorders include T cell CLL, T cell prolymphocytic leukemia (PLL) and the large granular lymphocytic (LGL) leukemias (T and NK types), and the cutaneous T cell lymphomas. Fewer than 5 percent of CLL and about 20 percent of PLL are of T cell origin. Most cases of T-CLL and T-PLL have mature T helper cell phenotypes (CD2+, CD3+, CD4+, CD5+, CD7+, CD11a+), with occasional cases having cells coexpressing CD4 and CD8. LGL leukemias are clonal expansions of either CD3+/CD8+ cytotoxic T cells or CD3− NK, cells which express other characteristic antigens of NK cells, including CD16 (Fcγ receptor) and CD56. The cutaneous T cell lymphomas express a mature activated T helper cell phenotype: CD2, CD3, CD4, CD5, CD7, CD25 (IL-2 receptor), and CD71 (transferrin receptor).

Aggressive T cell malignancies Nearly all T cell lymphomas are considered aggressive diseases. Peripheral T cell lymphomas have been previously classified within the Working Formulation as diffuse small cleaved cell, diffuse mixed small and large cell, and diffuse large cell.

The tumor cells variably express the mature T cell antigens CD2, CD3, CD5, CD6, and CD7. Most express CD4, with a small fraction expressing CD8. Within this category are other specific histologic subtypes with unique clinical presentations, including the following: angioimmunoblastic T cell lymphoma and angiocentric lymphoma (nasal T cell/NK type and pulmonary angiocentric lymphoma-lymphomatoid granulomatosis), which are EBV-related diseases; intestinal T cell lymphoma (± gluten enteropathy-associated); hepatosplenic γδ T cell lymphoma; and subcutaneous panniculitis-like T cell lymphoma. The adult T cell lymphomas associated with human T cell leukemia/lymphoma virus (HTLV) I are similar to the cutaneous T cell lymphomas in that they express CD2, CD3, CD4, CD5, CD7, and CD25. The anaplastic large cell lymphomas characteristically involve the sinusoids of lymph nodes. These tumors express the CD30 (Ki-1) antigen and generally express the phenotype of mature activated T cells (HLA-DR, CD25), although a minor subset have no clear T or B cell lineage by immunophenotyping. Lymphoblastic lymphomas correspond to stage II thymocytes, and the majority express CD1, CD2, CD4, CD7, and CD8. Rarely, lymphoblastic lymphomas will have an immature B cell phenotype. Approximately 20 percent of adult lymphoblastic leukemias are of T cell lineage. Precursor T cell leukemias, although heterogeneous, have immunophenotypic characteristics of early thymocytes, expressing CD2 along with CD5 and CD7, with expression of cytoplasmic CD3, which is associated with the T cell antigen receptor complex. In contrast to T cell lymphoblastic lymphoma, T cell ALL are often CD4− and CD8−.

LYMPHOCYTIC LEUKEMIAS AND NON-HODGKIN'S LYMPHOMA— GENERAL ASPECTS

EPIDEMIOLOGY AND ETIOLOGY The majority of patients with ALL are children and young adults. The incidence in adults is about 1/100,000 persons per year. ALL is more common in males than females and in whites more than in blacks. In contrast to ALL, CLL is the most common adult leukemia in western countries. The

FIGURE 113-1 Correlation of B cell differentiation and B cell malignancies.

T CELL DIFFERENTIATION

THYMUS

T CELL MALIGNANCIES

Stage I
Prothymocyte
CD: 2, 7, 38, 71
— Majority of T cell ALL

Stage II
Thymocyte
CD: 1, 2, 4, 7, 8, 38
— Minority of T-ALL
Majority of T-LL

Stage III
Thymocyte
CD: 2, 3, 4/8, 5, 6, 7; TCR
— Minority of T-LL
Rare T-ALL

PERIPHERAL BLOOD

Mature T Helper Cell
CD: 2, 3, 4, 5, 6, 7; TCR
— Majority of T-CLL, CTCL, Sezary Cell, NHL

Mature T Cytotoxic/
Suppressor Cell
CD: 2, 3, 4, 5, 6, 7; TCR
— Minority of T-CLL, NHL

FIGURE 113-2 Correlation of T cell differentiation and T cell malignancies.

incidence of CLL is over 10/100,000 for persons over 70 but less than 1/100,000 for those under 50. CLL is also more common in males and in whites.

About 45,000 new cases of non-Hodgkin's lymphoma occur each year in the United States, and this number is increasing. Although the total number of patients is relatively small compared to some of the more common solid tumors, non-Hodgkin's lymphoma ranks as the sixth most common cause of cancer-related death in the United States. For males, non-Hodgkin's lymphoma ranks as the fourth leading cause of cancer mortality for individuals under the age of 15. In the decades between 15 and 34, it ranks second for males and fifth for females as the leading cause of death from cancer. Even for males between the ages of 35 and 54, it still ranks as the third leading cause of cancer-related mortality. There is little difference in 5-year survival rates for non-Hodgkin's lymphoma between whites and blacks. Non-Hodgkin's lymphomas rank fourth in the total number of person-years of life lost each year from cancer, demonstrating the profound personal and economic impact of this disease. This is true even if one subtracts the exponential increase resulting from cases of AIDS-related lymphomas.

There is evidence that infectious agents are involved in the pathogenesis of some non-Hodgkin's lymphomas, but no direct evidence exists in pre-B or T cell ALL or CLL. EBV has a strong association with development of Burkitt's lymphoma and leukemia (L3 ALL); some lymphomas associated with immunodeficiency, including human immunodeficiency virus (HIV) 1–related lymphoma; and angiocentric lymphomas (see Chap. 186). HTLV-I is the causative agent of the adult T cell leukemia/lymphoma endemic to the Caribbean and southern Japan (see Chap. 192). Gastric MALT lymphoma occurs as a consequence of *Helicobacter pylori* infection (see Chap. 156).

A number of primary diseases have an increased incidence of subsequently developing ALL, non-Hodgkin's lymphoma, and, to a lesser extent, Hodgkin's disease (Table 113-5). Individuals with Down's and Wiskott-Aldrich syndrome are at increased risk of developing ALL. There is also an increased incidence of ALL and CLL among family members who have these diseases. Diseases of inherited and acquired immunodeficiency as well as autoimmune diseases are associated with an increased incidence of lymphoma (Table 113-5).

Non-Hodgkin's lymphomas occur in the context of drug-induced immunosuppression and acquired or congenital immunodeficiency. Non-Hodgkin's lymphomas develop in up to 30 percent of HIV-1 infected individuals and between 40 and 50 percent are EBV-associated. EBV is also present in virtually all the primary central nervous system (CNS) lymphomas seen in HIV-1 patients. The association between immunosuppression and induction of non-Hodgkin's lymphomas appears to be compelling; if the immunosuppression can be reversed (e.g., by discontinuing immunosuppressive agents following organ transplantation), a percentage of these lymphomas regress spontaneously. The incidence of lymphoma in iatrogenic immune suppression, HIV-1 infection, and autoimmune disease argues strongly for the contribution of immune dysregulation to the development of lymphoma. It is controversial as to whether certain chemical exposures including dioxin, phenoxyherbicides, pesticides, and hair dyes are involved in the pathogenesis of non-Hodgkin's lymphoma. Other potential environmental associations include exposure to arsenic, phenoxyacetic acids, chlorophenols, organic solvents, halomethane, lead, vinyl chloride, or asbestos. Occupational exposures associated with an increased risk include farming, welding, and work in the lumber industry. There is an increased incidence of ALL and non-Hodgkin's lymphoma in survivors of nuclear explosions or reactor accidents and of other radiation exposures. Moreover, non-Hodgkin's lymphoma has been observed as a late complication of prior chemotherapy and/or radiation therapy. Specifically, patients with Hodgkin's disease treated with radiation therapy and chemotherapy exhibit an increased risk of developing secondary large cell lymphomas. Lymphoma-like syndromes have also been found in patients treated with phenytoin. Although in most cases this disease regresses when the drug is stopped, a significant number of patients still develop malignant lymphomas.

MOLECULAR GENETICS Although limited progress has been made in identifying agents that might be involved in inducing ALL and non-Hodgkin's lymphomas, exciting advances have been made in identifying those genes that appear to be involved in the pathogenesis of these diseases. Cytogenetic abnormalities have been

Table 113-5

Diseases or Exposures Associated with Increased Risk of Development of Malignant Lymphoma

Inherited immunodeficiency disease
   Klinefelter's syndrome
   Chédiak-Higashi syndrome
   Ataxia telangiectasia syndrome
   Wiscott-Aldrich syndrome
   Common variable immunodeficiency disease
Acquired immunodeficiency diseases
   Iatrogenic immunosuppression
   HIV-1 infection
   Acquired hypogammaglobulinemia
Autoimmune disease
   Sjögren's syndrome
   Celiac sprue
   Rheumatoid arthritis and systemic lupus erythematosus
Chemical or drug exposures
   Phenytoin
   Dioxin, phenoxyherbicides
   Radiation
   Prior chemotherapy and radiation therapy
Infectious agent association (other than HIV)
   Epstein-Barr virus
   Human T cell leukemia/lymphoma virus-I
   Helicobacter pylori

well documented in a number of non-Hodgkin's lymphomas and ALL (Tables 113-2, 113-3). DNA sequence analysis of several of these chromosomal translocations has demonstrated that genes that normally regulate heavy and light chain immunoglobulin synthesis have been juxtaposed to genes that regulate normal cellular activation and proliferation. It is postulated that these transforming genes, or *oncogenes*, have come under the control of those regulatory elements that normally control B cell proliferation and differentiation. The best-studied example is the t(8;14) or variant t(2;8) or t(8;22) translocations of Burkitt's lymphoma present in over 90 percent of Burkitt's lymphomas and a subgroup of pre-B cell ALL. In this disease, the c-*myc* oncogene on chromosome 8 is joined to either the immunoglobulin heavy chain locus on chromosome 14, the κ light chain locus on chromosome 2, or the λ light chain locus on chromosome 22, leading to activation and overexpression of the c-*myc* gene product. Another example is the t(14;18) translocation, which is seen in approximately 85 percent of patients with follicular lymphomas and 25 percent of patients with diffuse lymphomas. In t(14;18), the gene *bcl*-2 (chromosome 18) is juxtaposed to the immunoglobulin heavy chain locus (chromosome 14). The *bcl*-2 gene product prevents programmed cell death, or *apoptosis*. By blocking apoptosis, the overexpression of the *bcl*-2 protein can lead to prolonged cell survival, and additional genetic changes are more likely to occur. Moreover, transgenic mice which overexpress the *bcl*-2 gene in their B cells develop a unique benign polyclonal lymphoproliferative syndrome. It is hypothesized that this alteration in *bcl*-2 expression is involved in the pathogenesis of the follicular lymphomas. Two other genes on chromosomes 11 and 3, when joined to immunoglobulin gene loci on chromosome 14, are associated with certain non-Hodgkin's lymphomas. On chromosome 11q13 a number of breakpoints have been identified, and one of the sequences has been identified as the *bcl*-1 gene. This translocation, seen in mantle cell lymphoma, leads to dysregulated expression of the gene that encodes for cyclin D1, which is involved in cell cycle regulation. More recently, a candidate oncogene, termed *bcl*-6, has been identified at the 3q27 breakpoint in a subset of diffuse large B cell non-Hodgkin's lymphomas. The protein encoded by this gene is homologous to zinc finger transcription factors and may be involved in activating certain growth-promoting genes. The t(2;5) in anaplastic large cell lymphoma produces a fusion protein consisting of the nucleophosmin (NPM) nucleolar phosphoprotein gene on chromosome 5q35 fused to a protein tyrosine kinase gene, ALK (for anaplastic large cell lymphoma kinase) on chromosome 2p23.

The t(9;22) BCR-ABL rearrangement leading to the formation of the abnormal tyrosine kinase (p190 or p210 BCR-ABL) is seen in about 30 percent of adult pre-B cell ALL. Chromosomal translocations involving 11q23 (MLL, HRX, ALL-1 gene) are seen in about 5 percent of adult pre-B ALL. These translocations lead to the development of abnormal DNA binding proteins, consequently to abnormal gene transcription. Translocations involving 11q23 are also involved in predominantly acute myeloid leukemias following epipodophyllotoxin exposures. Other translocations include t(1;19) in a subset of pre-B ALL and translocations involving the T cell antigen receptor genes (14q11, 7q34) in about half of the cases of T cell ALL. Analogous to those involving immunoglobulin genes, these T cell antigen receptor translocations lead to abnormal expression of certain transcription factors.

CHRONIC LEUKEMIAS/LYMPHOMAS

CLINICAL FEATURES AND NATURAL HISTORY Chronic Lymphocytic Leukemia/Small Lymphocytic Lymphoma The most common chronic leukemia/lymphoma is B cell CLL, which presents with asymptomatic lymphocytosis in patients with a median age of 60. A reactive lymphocytosis, which is usually of normal T cells, is the major diagnosis that must be excluded. Approximately 40 percent of patients with B cell CLL have only lymphocytosis, with no anemia, thrombocytopenia, lymphadenopathy, or organomegaly. Constitutional symptoms are uncommon unless there is intercurrent infection, very extensive bulky disease, or histologic transformation

to a more aggressive lymphoma, usually diffuse large B cell lymphoma (Richter's syndrome). In Richter's syndrome, which occurs in ~5% of cases, patients also have rapidly growing nodal and extranodal masses. With more extensive marrow compromise and/or splenic involvement, patients with B cell CLL can develop cytopenias or immunosuppression, which can lead to symptoms. The white cell count usually ranges between 10 and 200 × 10⁹/L with 70 to 95 percent small lymphocytes. The minimum lymphocytosis to make the diagnosis of CLL is 5 × 10⁹/L. The absolute neutrophil count is usually normal, and red cell and platelet counts mildly decreased. The marrow is universally involved, and the extent of involvement influences survival, with a nodular infiltration being more favorable than diffuse involvement. Most patients have depressed serum immunoglobulin levels, which worsen with disease progression. Autoimmune phenomena can occur in up to 20 percent of patients, most commonly hemolytic anemia and less frequently thrombocytopenia or pure red cell aplasia. In B cell CLL the clinical staging of patients is of prognostic importance (Table 113-6). Other prognostic factors that predict for a shorter survival include a lymphocyte doubling time of <12 months, initial absolute lymphocyte count >50,000/μL, and an abnormal karyotype, most commonly trisomy 12.

Small lymphocytic lymphoma is the lymphomatous presentation of CLL and therefore occurs in middle-aged and older patients. Patients usually present with asymptomatic generalized lymphadenopathy. Unlike in CLL, the peripheral blood may appear normal or reveal only a mild lymphocytosis (60 percent will have absolute lymphocytosis of >4000/μL at diagnosis). In contrast, the bone marrow is involved in 75 to 95 percent of patients. A serum paraprotein is found in about 20 percent of patients, and hypogammaglobulinemia is also common. These patients can often be observed without treatment for 3 to 4 years; median survival is 8 to 10 years.

Other Chronic Leukemias There are other chronic leukemias that can present with lymphocytosis, including T cell CLL, PLL, LGL leukemia, hairy cell leukemia, splenic lymphoma with villous lymphocytes, and non-Hodgkin's lymphoma in leukemic phase. These "other" chronic leukemias are rare disorders. Patients with T cell CLL often present with prominent splenomegaly and extensive skin lesions and can have a rapidly progressive course. PLL can be of T or B cell lineage, with malignant cells that are larger than those in CLL and with prominent nucleoli. In contrast to CLL, patients with PLL present with higher levels of lymphocytosis, splenomegaly with minimal adenopathy, and a poor response to treatment. The LGL leukemias consist of two distinct clinical and pathologic entities. Patients with T cell LGL have a median age of 55 and present with recurrent bacterial infections due to severe neutropenia. Patients will have marrow involvement and splenomegaly. About one-third of patients will have rheumatoid arthritis resembling patients with Felty's syndrome. Most patients have a more indolent disease, with 60 percent alive more than 2 years from diagnosis. In contrast, patients with NK cell LGL leukemia have a median age of 39 and often present with fever in

Table 113-6

Staging of B Cell CLL and Relation to Survival

Stage	Clinical Features	Median Survival, years
RAI		
0	Lymphocytosis	12
I	Lymphocytosis + adenopathy	9
II	Lymphocytosis + splenomegaly	7
III	Anemia	1–2
IV	Thrombocytopenia	1–2
BINET		
A	No anemia/thrombocytopenia, <3 involved sites	>10
B	No anemia/thrombocytopenia, >3 involved sites	5
C	Anemia and/or thrombocytopenia	2

the absence of infection and no signs or symptoms of rheumatoid arthritis. These patients have significant hepatosplenomegaly as well as marrow involvement. Neutropenia is less severe than in T cell LGL leukemia, but anemia and thrombocytopenia are more pronounced. NK cell LGL leukemia is a very aggressive disease with a poor response to therapy.

Hairy cell leukemia is a rare disease occurring predominantly in males over age 40; it presents with cytopenias, splenomegaly, and large malignant B cells with characteristic morphologic and immunologic features. The presentation of patients can range from asymptomatic lymphocytosis to profound granulocytopenia, and some patients have vasculitis-like syndromes. The bone marrow biopsy is usually hyperplastic, with fibrosis common. An indolent course is commonly seen, with a median survival of over 4 years. The indications for treatment include pancytopenia, recurrent infections (including bacterial and opportunistic pathogens), and symptomatic splenomegaly.

℞ TREATMENT

The approach to patients with B cell CLL is very similar to that for patients with indolent non-Hodgkin's lymphoma, such as follicular lymphoma (see below). Since most patients are asymptomatic at presentation, with a disease that can have a very long natural history without treatment, initial observation is generally recommended. Randomized trials in very early stage patients (Binet A, Rai 0, I, II) involving no therapy versus initial treatment with an alkylating agent (chlorambucil) with prednisone suggested no benefit for early treatment. The indications for treating patients include symptomatic lymphadenopathy or organ involvement, cytopenia due to progressive disease or autoimmune phenomena, or systemic symptoms. The choices for initial therapy are many but generally involve alkylating agents given daily or in pulse fashion, with or without prednisone. Randomized trials suggest that chlorambucil is equivalent to combination therapy with cyclophosphamide, vincristine, and prednisone (CVP) in terms of complete response (CR) rate (25 percent), response duration (2 years), and median survival (4 years). Although controversial, some trials have demonstrated that in Binet stage B patients, more aggressive combination chemotherapy with cyclophosphamide, doxorubicin, vincristine, and prednisone (CHOP) was superior to CVP.

The nucleoside analogues fludarabine, pentostatin, and cladribine are very active in CLL. In previously treated patients, the response rate to fludarabine is around 50 percent [15 percent CR, including "nodular CRs" in the marrow; 40 percent partial response (PR)]. In previously untreated patients, the CR rates are over 30 percent, with 45 percent PRs. When one takes into account "nodular CRs" with residual "normal" nodules in the marrow, the CR rates are even higher. This has led to a randomized trial comparing fludarabine to alkylating agent–based treatment. Early analysis shows superiority for fludarabine in previously treated patients, but results are presently not clear for previously untreated patients. The toxicities of fludarabine and other purine analogues can be profound, with marked immunosuppression, depression of CD4+ T cells, opportunistic infections, and myelosuppression. Although not as extensively studied, results with cladribine are similar to fludarabine, while responses to pentostatin appear inferior to fludarabine. It is unlikely that patients who are resistant to fludarabine will respond to cladribine.

Intravenous immunoglobulin has been given to patients who are hypogammaglobulinemic. In these studies there is a significant decrease in serious infections; however, the treatment is costly. High-dose therapy and bone marrow transplantation (BMT) are being investigated in CLL using both purged autologous as well as allogeneic marrow. Early results are encouraging, but the follow-up is relatively short. There are several scenarios in which splenectomy is indicated in patients with CLL, including marked cytopenias often with symptomatic splenomegaly. Patients can have dramatic improvement in anemia and thrombocytopenia that can last for years

(median survival of responders >3 years). Splenectomy has also been used in the 25 percent of patients with autoimmune hemolytic anemia or thrombocytopenia that has not responded to glucocorticoids or intravenous immunoglobulin. Palliative radiation therapy to the spleen can be of limited benefit to some patients, as can radiation of bulky nodal masses.

The treatment of the other chronic leukemias with the exception of hairy cell leukemia has been largely unsuccessful. PLL and the NK and T cell LGL leukemias are generally resistant to combination chemotherapy. The standard treatment for cytopenias due to hairy cell leukemia used to be splenectomy, with a median duration of response of 8 months. The treatment of hairy cell leukemia has been revolutionized by the purine analogues, specifically cladribine. Cladribine induces a high CR rate (>80 percent) often with one course of treatment, with long clinical remissions, many in excess of 3 years. Cladribine is very active in patients previously treated with pentostatin or interferon α. It remains unknown if these patients will be cured, since minimal residual disease can be detected in patients in long clinical remissions.

NON-HODGKIN'S LYMPHOMA— GENERAL CONSIDERATIONS

CLINICAL PRESENTATION AND DIFFERENTIAL DIAGNOSIS More than two-thirds of patients with non-Hodgkin's lymphoma present with persistent, painless peripheral lymphadenopathy (see Chap. 61). At the time of presentation, the differential diagnosis of generalized lymphadenopathy necessitates the exclusion of infectious etiologies including bacteria, viruses (e.g., infectious mononucleosis, cytomegalovirus, and HIV), and parasites (toxoplasmosis). It is generally agreed that a firm lymph node larger than 1 cm that is not associated with a documentable infection and that persists longer than 4 weeks should be considered for biopsy. However, lymph nodes in several histopathologic subtypes of non-Hodgkin's lymphomas frequently wax and wane. Therefore, incomplete regression does not exclude a diagnosis of non-Hodgkin's lymphoma. In teenagers and young adults, infectious mononucleosis and Hodgkin's disease should be placed high in the differential diagnosis. A number of clinical features are suggestive of the diagnosis of non-Hodgkin's lymphoma. Involvement of Waldeyer's ring, epitrochlear, and mesenteric nodes are more frequently observed in patients with non-Hodgkin's lymphoma than with Hodgkin's disease. Unlike patients with Hodgkin's disease who present with weight loss, fever, or night sweats, fewer than 20 percent of patients with non-Hodgkin's lymphoma present with systemic complaints. Systemic symptoms are more common in patients with diffuse aggressive histologies, especially in those with hepatic and extranodal involvement. Less frequent presenting symptoms include fatigue, malaise, and pruritus, occurring in fewer than 10 percent of patients.

Non-Hodgkin's lymphomas also present with thoracic, abdominal, and/or extranodal symptoms. Although much less common than with Hodgkin's disease, approximately 20 percent of patients with non-Hodgkin's lymphoma present with mediastinal adenopathy. These patients most frequently present with persistent cough or chest discomfort or without clinical symptoms but having an abnormal chest x-ray. Occasionally, a superior vena caval syndrome is noted at presentation. Differential diagnosis of mediastinal presentation includes infections (e.g., histoplasmosis, tuberculosis, infectious mononucleosis), sarcoidosis, Hodgkin's disease, and other neoplasms. Involvement of retroperitoneal, mesenteric, and pelvic nodes is common in most histologic subtypes of non-Hodgkin's lymphoma. Unless massive or leading to obstruction, nodal enlargement in these sites usually does not produce symptoms. In contrast, patients who come to medical attention because of an abdominal mass, massive splenomegaly, or primary gastrointestinal lymphoma present with complaints similar to those caused by other abdominal space-occupying lesions. These complaints include chronic pain, abdominal fullness, early satiety, symptoms associated with visceral obstruction, or even acute perforation and gastrointestinal hemorrhage. Symptoms due to extralymphatic disease are common in some subtypes of aggressive non-Hodgkin's lymphoma but are uncommon in indolent lymphomas. Rarely, patients present with symptoms of unexplained anemia. Those with aggressive non-Hodgkin's lymphomas can present with primary cutaneous lesions, testicular masses, acute spinal cord compression, solitary bone lesions, and, rarely, lymphomatous meningitis. Primary non-Hodgkin's lymphoma of the CNS constitutes only 1 percent of all non-Hodgkin's lymphomas. However, with increasing incidence of HIV-1 infection, as well as increasing use of high-dose immunosuppressive therapy, primary CNS lymphoma has become as common as glioblastoma multiforme.

When non-Hodgkin's lymphoma is present in an extranodal site, the differential diagnosis is more difficult. Patients with non-Hodgkin's lymphoma uncommonly present with bronchovascular-lymphangitic, nodular, or alveolar patterns of involvement in the lung. In contrast, hepatic infiltration is common, although frequently not clinically evident. Between 25 and 50 percent of patients with non-Hodgkin's lymphoma present with hepatic infiltration, although relatively few present with large hepatic masses. Nearly 75 percent of patients with advanced-stage indolent lymphomas have microscopic hepatic infiltration at presentation. In contrast, primary hepatic lymphoma is extremely rare and is nearly always an aggressive histology tumor. Another extranodal presentation occurring in fewer than 5 percent of patients is primary lymphoma of bone. This is virtually always diffuse large B cell lymphoma, which presents as a painful bony site. Most frequently, lytic lesions are observed on bone x-ray. The most common sites of primary lymphoma of bone include femur, pelvis, and vertebrae. Approximately 5 percent of non-Hodgkin's lymphomas occur as primary gastrointestinal lymphoma. These patients present with hemorrhage, pain, or obstruction since the stomach is most frequently infiltrated, followed by small intestine and colon, respectively. Most gastrointestinal lymphomas have diffuse aggressive histologies, with a subset being low-grade non-Hodgkin's lymphoma (MALT lymphoma). An uncommon presentation of non-Hodgkin's lymphoma is renal infiltration, and even less common is localized presentation in the prostate, testis, or ovary. Localized skin infiltration by lymphoma is another uncommon site of presentation, usually of aggressive histology lymphoma. CNS presentation is relatively uncommon, although primary spinal cord and brain lymphomas are the most frequent areas of involvement. Primary CNS symptoms include headache, lethargy, focal neurologic symptoms, seizures, or paralysis. Rare sites of primary lymphoma include the orbit, heart, breast, salivary glands, thyroid, and adrenal gland.

STAGING AND DISEASE DETECTION The Ann Arbor staging system developed for Hodgkin's disease has also been used in staging non-Hodgkin's lymphomas. This staging system focuses on the number of tumor sites (nodal and extranodal), location, and the presence or absence of systemic symptoms. Table 113-7 summarizes this staging system. In stages I and II, sites of disease are on the same side of the diaphragm. Stage III disease involves both sides of the diaphragm, whereas stage IV is defined as extranodal lymphomatous involvement, most frequently of the bone marrow and liver. Systemic symptoms (fever, weight loss of >10 percent of body weight, and night sweats; i.e., B symptoms) are less common in non-Hodgkin's lymphomas (about 20 percent of cases) than in Hodgkin's disease. This staging scheme was specifically developed for Hodgkin's

disease, which disseminates by contiguous lymphatic extension and to a much lesser extent hematogenously. Since non-Hodgkin's lymphomas most frequently disseminate hematogenously, this staging system has proven to be less useful in this type of lymphoma.

The concept of staging has a small impact on treatment strategy in patients with non-Hodgkin's lymphomas. Only 10 percent of patients with follicular lymphoma have localized disease and are candidates for local radiation therapy. For the diffuse aggressive lymphomas, even patients with localized disease now receive systemic treatment. Therefore, staging is undertaken in non-Hodgkin's lymphomas to identify those small numbers of patients who can be treated with local therapy and to identify prognostic subgroups within histologic subtypes.

Staging Procedures after Biopsy Diagnosis Staging must be undertaken in the context of histology. A suggested staging workup for patients with non-Hodgkin's lymphoma is summarized in Table 113-8. After the initial excisional biopsy and documentation of the pathologic and immunologic subtype of disease, blood tests should be obtained, including complete blood count, routine chemistries, liver function tests including lactic dehydrogenase (LDH), serum protein electrophoresis to document the presence of circulating monoclonal paraprotein, and serum β_2-microglobulin, which has been shown to predict prognosis in both indolent and aggressive lymphomas. Waldeyer's ring involvement is often associated with intestinal involvement, and gastrointestinal contrast studies or endoscopy are indicated if the patient appears to have localized disease. Chest radiography is used to exclude mediastinal and hilar adenopathy, pleural effusions, and pulmonary parenchymal infiltration. Computed tomography (CT)

Table 113-7

Ann Arbor Staging System

Stage I	Involvement in single lymph node region or single extralymphatic site
Stage II	Involvement of two or more lymph node regions on the same side of diaphragm
	Localized contiguous involvement of only one extralymphatic site and lymph node region (stage IIE)
Stage III	Involvement of lymph node regions on both sides of diaphragm; may include spleen
Stage IV	Disseminated involvement of one or more extralymphatic organs with or without lymph node involvement

Table 113-8

Staging Evaluation for Non-Hodgkin's Lymphoma

Essential
1. Pathologic documentation by hematopathologist
2. Physical examination
3. Documentation of B symptoms
4. Laboratory evaluation
   a. Complete blood counts
   b. Liver function tests including LDH
   c. Renal function tests
   d. Uric acid
   e. Calcium
   f. Serum protein electrophoresis
   g. Serum β_2-microglobulin
5. Chest radiograph
6. CT scan of abdomen and pelvis
7. Bone marrow biopsy

Essential Under Certain Circumstances
1. Chest CT scan
2. Head CT scan
3. Lumbar puncture
4. Barium studies of gastrointestinal tract
5. Endoscopic examination
6. Cytologic examination of effusion
7. Gallium scan (planar or SPECT)

Useful But Not Essential Tests
1. Cell surface marker phenotypic analysis
2. Cytogenetic analysis
3. Gene rearrangement analysis
4. Polymerase chain reaction analysis of minimal residual disease
5. Flow cytometry for DNA analysis
6. Liver scan
7. Liver biopsy
8. Bone scan
9. Thallium scan
10. Lymphangiography
11. Ultrasonography
12. Magnetic resonance imaging
13. Echocardiogram
14. Laparotomy

scan of the chest is used to assess the extent of disease more precisely and is strongly recommended for patients with abnormal chest radiographs. It is not indicated if the chest x-ray is normal. However, abdominal/pelvic CT scan is essential for accurate staging to assess lymphadenopathy in retroperitoneal, mesenteric, and retrocrural areas. Lymphangiography is less useful than in Hodgkin's disease, since common sites of disease in non-Hodgkin's lymphoma include nodes in the mesentery, hilum of liver, spleen, or kidneys as well as nodes in the deep bony pelvis, none of which are detected by this procedure. The major advantage of lymphangiography over abdominal/pelvic CT is its ability to detect infiltrated but normal-sized retroperitoneal nodes and the ability to monitor the progress of treatment cheaply with a plain abdominal film. The primary indication for lymphangiography in non-Hodgkin's lymphoma is for patients with localized inguinal disease who may be candidates for local radiotherapy, where CT scanning for intraabdominal disease may be falsely negative. Bilateral percutaneous bone marrow biopsies must be performed, since the likelihood of lymphomatous involvement of the marrow is relatively high, especially in low-grade lymphoma, where marrow involvement occurs in up to 70 percent of cases. With any indication of hepatic abnormalities on blood tests or on liver scan, a percutaneous liver biopsy may be indicated in patients who would otherwise have stage I disease. In patients with aggressive lymphomas with marrow, bone, testicular, or paranasal sinus involvement, or if clinically indicated, examination of the cerebrospinal fluid by lumbar puncture should be performed.

More invasive tests are reserved for the uncommon presentation with stage I or II non-Hodgkin's lymphoma. While staging laparotomy may be performed in Hodgkin's disease, this is not so in the non-Hodgkin's lymphomas. In the aggressive non-Hodgkin's lymphomas, all stages can be considered to reflect disseminated disease and are therefore usually treated with chemotherapy. In contrast, only stages I and II indolent-histology lymphoma will be considered as localized and treated with radiation alone. Therefore, for most patients with non-Hodgkin's lymphoma it is less critical to ascertain the precise pathologic stage of disease. Moreover, it is common for these patients to exhibit disseminated disease after routine staging tests (e.g., bone marrow or liver biopsy). For example, within follicular lymphoma (grades I and II), following clinical staging and bone marrow biopsy, more than 85 percent of these patients will have stage III or stage IV disease. Thus, surgical staging should never be considered a routine procedure in patients with non-Hodgkin's lymphoma.

A number of other tests are becoming more important both in staging and in advancing our knowledge of the biology of non-Hodgkin's lymphoma. Gallium radionuclide scans appear to have clinical utility. Gallium scans are positive in virtually all intermediate- and high-grade lymphomas and in about 50 percent of low-grade lymphomas. Gallium scans, with high doses of isotope which permit delayed imaging, combined with single photon emission computed tomography (SPECT) are very sensitive in detecting tumor infiltration. These tests are also very useful in monitoring response to therapy. Magnetic resonance imaging appears to be most valuable for detecting occult marrow involvement and for evaluation of the brain and spinal cord. Thallium scanning may be a useful diagnostic modality to assess tumor infiltration by low-grade follicular lymphomas. There is little, if any, thallium uptake by high- or intermediate-grade lymphomas. Immunologic and molecular biologic studies are proving increasingly useful in confirming diagnosis. For example, in cases with difficult histopathologic patterns, cell-surface markers can distinguish between non-Hodgkin's lymphoma and carcinoma (leukocyte common antigen, CD45, is specific for lymphoid cells). Similarly, monoclonal antibodies directed against lineage-restricted antigens and detection of rearrangement of immunoglobulin or T cell receptor genes are useful in identifying lymphoid tumors. The delineation of the cell-surface phenotype is becoming important because an increasing number of treatment approaches employ monoclonal antibodies for purging of autologous stem cells for support of high-dose therapy and as part of investigational antibody-based treatments. Definition of a specific chromosomal abnormality in some studies appears to be of prognostic significance in certain histologic subtypes.

Sensitive Techniques to Detect Minimal Residual Disease The development of molecular techniques to define immunoglobulin and T cell receptor gene rearrangements has resulted in very sensitive tools with which to assess tumor cell infiltration more accurately. The most common and accessible tissues to be tested include peripheral blood and bone marrow. Whereas conventional histologic analysis of the bone marrow can detect 1 lymphoma cell infiltrating 20 normal cells, immunologic flow cytometric and Southern blot analysis each improve this level of detection to 1 lymphoma cell in approximately 100 normal cells. Similarly, flow cytometry has been used to detect "clonal excess" in the blood of patients with B cell non-Hodgkin's lymphoma. More recently, molecular biologic techniques have demonstrated that minimal disease detection can be markedly improved. For those non-Hodgkin's lymphomas with a known chromosomal translocation, it is now possible to identify a unique chromosomal "breakpoint." This has been most elegantly accomplished for the t(14;18) translocation present in the majority of follicular lymphomas and in about 25 percent of diffuse lymphomas. Based on DNA sequence, it is possible to amplify this unique stretch of DNA using specific oligonucleotide primers and the polymerase chain reaction (PCR). For those cases where a classic translocation is not known, PCR analysis of the IgH chain CDRIII region may be used. With this approach, 1 tumor cell in 10^5 to 10^6 normal cells can be detected. Thus, while other tests may be negative, PCR may demonstrate that the blood or bone marrow is contaminated by lymphoma cells. These techniques are presently being compared to more conventional staging methods. Considering their sensitivity, they may be useful in assessing complete remission more accurately and, more importantly, in determining whether treatment should be prolonged, truncated, or intensified. On the other hand, the presence of cells bearing the t(14;18) may not imply impending disease relapse or progression. Some normal people without a history of lymphoma have cells bearing t(14;18), and even patients with lymphoma in remission for many years may have such cells. Additional data are needed to assess the meaning of PCR-detected clonal cells.

PATHOLOGIC CLASSIFICATION The histologic classification of the non-Hodgkin's lymphomas is based on assessment of the overall pattern of lymph node architecture as well as on the cytologic classification of the neoplastic cell. It is clear that immunophenotype, genetic analysis, and cytogenetic analysis can, in many cases, refine the diagnosis. As the diagnostic techniques are improved, an increasing number of discrete clinicopathologic entities have been defined. Many of the entities are very rare. Thus, it has become necessary to group certain lymphomas together based on their likely natural history. Over time, it is anticipated that specialized treatment approaches will be developed for each disease entity. Table 113-2 compares the R.E.A.L., Working Formulation, modified Kiel, and the Rappaport classifications. In current clinical practice these classification schemes are frequently used interchangeably. However, disease entities are not necessarily easily translated from one to the other. For example, mantle cell lymphoma may be classified in five different Working Formulation categories. The crucial attributes of a pathologic diagnosis are accuracy and reproducibility, for it has been found that the histologic diagnosis provides critical predictors of clinical pattern of disease, response to treatment, and prognosis.

INDOLENT LYMPHOMAS Clinical Features and Natural History *Follicular center lymphoma* Follicular lymphomas account for approximately 50 percent of the non-Hodgkin's lymphomas; the grade I (small cleaved cell) type is the most common. Patients usually present with painless peripheral adenopathy in cervical, axillary, inguinal, and femoral regions. Patients frequently note that lymph node enlargement has been present for long periods of time, often years, and the nodes have "waxed and waned." Less typically, there is enlargement of Waldeyer's ring and epitrochlear nodes. Some patients present with asymptomatic large abdominal and retroperitoneal masses, with or without evidence of gastrointestinal and/or renal obstruction. Although patients may present with one or more sites of nodal disease, noninvasive workup usually demonstrates widely disseminated disease with involvement of spleen and bone marrow in over 80 percent of patients. Bone marrow involvement in follicular lymphoma reveals a unique pattern of paratrabecular infiltration. Peripheral blood involvement is seen in about 20 percent of patients, and CNS disease is rare, although epidural disease can be seen. In contrast to aggressive lymphomas, about 20 percent of patients present with extramedullary extranodal disease, and fewer than 10 percent present with B symptoms. The course of this disease is quite variable. The conventional approach for most patients is that they can be observed with waxing and waning disease for an average of 3 years without the need for therapy. In patients with stage I or limited stage II disease, local radiation therapy may provide long-term remissions or possible cure. Some patients demonstrate more disseminated and rapid growth and require treatment because massive nodal or organ enlargement leads to pain, lymphatic obstruction, organ obstruction, or, more rarely, neurologic symptoms. At the time of increasing generalized disease or rapid growth at a single site, involved nodes should be considered for rebiopsy. A significant number of rapidly progressing patients will demonstrate a "conversion" or "transformation" to a more aggressive histologic pattern, often diffuse large cell. This conversion is associated with acquisition of additional genetic abnormalities and occurs in about 7 percent of patients per year. Nearly all patients with follicular lymphoma who die of lymphoma have undergone histologic progression. Histologic conversion is associated with infiltration of extranodal sites, the development of systemic symptoms, and a poor prognosis since the tumor is much less responsive to treatment. Historically, both disease-free and overall survivals of patients with follicular lymphoma have not improved despite many different therapeutic approaches. Although 40 to 80 percent of patients achieve complete remissions (noninvasively staged) with conventional single-agent or aggressive combination chemotherapy, the median duration of remission is between 2 and 3 years. Following relapse, patients can be observed or retreated; however, the median survival after first relapse is 5 years. Patients with follicular non-Hodgkin's lymphoma survive long periods of time, with median overall survivals for patients with stages III and IV disease approaching 7 to 9 years. The grade II (mixed small and large cell) type can have a slightly different clinical presentation. Bone marrow infiltration at diagnosis is less frequent than in grade I (small cell) type, but large abdominal masses are more commonly seen. Since these patients generally progress faster if not treated and some studies suggest that a subset of these patients may be cured with conventional therapy, these patients are generally not observed but are treated soon after diagnosis with combination chemotherapy.

Marginal zone lymphomas These lymphomas present in nodal or extranodal sites and are then referred to as monocytoid B cell lymphomas or MALT lymphomas, respectively. A third related disease, splenic lymphoma (± circulating villous lymphocytes), presents as splenomegaly. Many patients with marginal zone lymphomas present with stage I or II disease. There is no age predilection for the extranodal tumors, which can involve the gastrointestinal tract, respiratory tract, lacrimal and salivary glands, thyroid, breast, or lung but usually not peripheral blood and marrow. Patients can present with peptic ulcer disease, abdominal pain, and sicca syndrome (Sjögren's syndrome). The clinical behavior of this disease is similar to that of the indolent follicular lymphomas.

Mycosis fungoides The cutaneous T cell lymphomas are diseases of middle-aged adults, with a slight male predominance. Major variants include mycosis fungoides and the Sézary syndrome, characterized by peripheral blood involvement. These diseases present with cutaneous manifestations and lymphadenopathy and follow an indolent course. Later, patients will develop hepatic, splenic, gastrointestinal tract, pulmonary, and renal involvement. Infiltration of the bone marrow and circulating leukemia cells (Sézary cells), usually in the presence of generalized erythroderma, are also frequent late manifestations. The median survival from diagnosis is about 10 years, with infection being the most common cause of death.

 TREATMENT

The majority of patients with indolent non-Hodgkin's lymphomas present with advanced disease, with fewer than 10 percent having pathologic stage I/II. Early-stage patients treated with radiotherapy have 5-year relapse-free survival of 60 to 80 percent, with overall 5-year survivals approaching 100 percent. In early-stage disease, chemotherapy alone has rarely been used due to the radioresponsiveness of these tumors, and there is no significant advantage of combined modality over local radiotherapy.

The long natural history of indolent non-Hodgkin's lymphomas and the lack of symptoms in the majority of patients at diagnosis have led to close observation as the initial approach to some of these patients. The advantages of this approach include a prolonged period free of treatment during which tumor cells will not be selected for drug resistance by continuous exposure to drugs. Moreover, spontaneous remissions of longer than 1 year have been reported to occur in 23 percent of patients. When treatment is started, these diseases are very sensitive to both single-agent and combination chemotherapy. The complete response rates of previously untreated patients to single alkylating agents such as cyclophosphamide or chlorambucil range between 30 and 60 percent, with a median duration of remission of about 2 years. More aggressive chemotherapy regimens have produced more rapid and higher percentages of complete remissions but unfortunately have not clearly changed the overall survival of patients with these diseases. Attempts to treat patients for prolonged periods of time with single-agent therapy or the addition of long-term "maintenance" treatment also have not improved survival. Following relapse, most patients can be successfully retreated; however, the ability to achieve third and subsequent remissions becomes more difficult, and the duration of those remissions is usually shorter. The implications on prognosis of conversion from indolent to aggressive histology continues to be controversial. Although most patients do poorly when treated with combination chemotherapy, the subset of patients with sensitive disease who achieve a CR may experience prolonged remission and survival. In addition to its curative potential in stage I patients, radiotherapy is frequently used in conjunction with systemic therapy to treat sites of bulk disease and to palliate sites of symptomatic disease. However, it remains controversial whether the addition of radiotherapy increases the overall disease-free survival. A subset of patients with follicular center lymphoma, grade II (mixed small cleaved and large cell lymphoma), are reported to experience long-term remissions and possible cure following treatment with combination chemotherapy; however, this remains controversial. The combinations used are either cyclophosphamide, Oncovin (vincristine), prednisone, and procarbazine (C-MOPP) or CHOP.

The subtype of indolent lymphoma that is associated with MALT, known as *extranodal marginal zone lymphoma*, is often treated surgically with or without local radiotherapy. Since these diseases tend to remain localized for long periods of time before systemic spread, surgery remains a highly effective approach. For patients with advanced disease, the use of chemotherapy with alkylating agents for MALT lymphomas has received limited attention but appears to be effective at inducing remissions. Primary gastric MALT lymphomas associated with *H. pylori* gastritis respond to omeprazole and amoxycillin, suggesting that eradication of infection induces regression of lymphoma. Unfortunately, for most sites of disease, the stimulating antigen, if any, has not been defined.

Local and systemic therapy are used in the treatment of mycosis fungoides. Patients with disease limited to the skin may be cured with electron beam radiation therapy. Topical treatment of skin lesions with chemotherapeutic agents such as nitrogen mustard can induce remissions in up to 90 percent of patients with disseminated disease. Systemic therapy with either drugs alone or combined modality therapy can induce high response rates (up to 80 percent), but few long-term remissions are seen in advanced-stage patients. Oral psoralens combined with ultraviolet light often induce PR. Interferon α is one effective second-line palliative therapy. Monoclonal antibodies (unconjugated and conjugated to toxins or radioisotopes), extracorporeal phototherapy, and the adenosine deaminase inhibitor pentostatin remain investigational. Fludarabine and cladribine may also be active.

Several new agents have been examined in advanced-stage follicular lymphomas. Interferon α is an active agent. Several prospective randomized trials have examined the role of interferon when added to combination chemotherapy in patients with advanced-stage disease and have found a significant prolongation of remission duration. However, a prolongation of survival was seen in only one trial. The purine analogues cladribine and fludarabine induced responses in 40 to 50 percent of previously treated patients. A humanized anti-CD20 antibody appears to induce PR in 50 percent and CR in 5 to 10 percent of patients, with little or no toxicity.

If these diseases are to be cured, either more aggressive high-dose chemotherapy regimens must be evaluated or new therapeutic modalities must be employed. Patients with advanced-stage follicular lymphomas are being treated earlier in the course of their disease with aggressive chemotherapy combined with total nodal irradiation or high-dose chemoradiotherapy and autologous stem cell transplantation. These studies suggest that high CR rates in the range of 80 percent or greater are possible. However, the impact of these studies on long-term disease-free survival and overall survival remain uncertain due to limited follow-up.

AGGRESSIVE LYMPHOMAS Clinical Features and Natural History *Follicular center lymphoma (large cell)* Although the follicular architecture of these tumors is preserved, this disease behaves much more like diffuse large B cell lymphoma. In contrast to other follicular lymphomas, this histologic variant has less frequent infiltration of the marrow and liver and presents with large masses and, frequently, extranodal disease. A finite cure rate has been reported in selected series. Follicular large cell lymphomas often evolve into diffuse large B cell lymphoma.

Mantle cell lymphoma This entity has also been called *diffuse intermediate lymphocytic lymphoma* and *centrocytic lymphoma*. However, it does not develop from centrocytes and no "intermediate" stage of differentiation has been defined. Typical sites of involvement include lymph nodes, spleen, liver, gastrointestinal tract, and bone marrow. Peripheral blood involvement has been reported in approximately 25 percent of patients at presentation, and systemic B symptoms are observed in approximately one-third of patients. Mantle cell lymphoma can involve any region of the gastrointestinal tract, occasionally presenting as multiple intestinal polyposis. Lymphomas with a mantle zone pattern, pseudoproliferation centers, and low growth fraction (Ki-67 expression) are reported to have a better prognosis, whereas those with a more diffuse form and higher proliferation index are thought to have a poorer prognosis. However, median survival is about 3 years.

Diffuse large B cell lymphoma Patients, who are generally middle-aged or older, present with either nodal enlargement (especially in the neck or abdomen) or extranodal disease (in the gastrointestinal tract, testes, bone, thyroid, salivary glands, skin, or brain). During the course of the disease, the liver, kidneys, and lung may be involved. Diffuse large B cell lymphoma is highly invasive, with local compression of vessels or airways, involvement of peripheral nerves, and destruction of bone. Although bone marrow involvement is found in only 10 to 20 percent of patients initially, its detection is important because of its strong correlation with later spread to the CNS. Later in the disease, some patients demonstrate both extensive bone marrow infiltration and peripheral blood involvement. A subset of patients present with predominantly mediastinal disease, known as *primary mediastinal (thymic) B cell lymphoma*. Mediastinal B cell lymphoma affects young females predominantly and is locally aggressive.

Aggressive T cell lymphomas These diseases are rare and consist of a number of distinct pathologic and clinical entities. *Peripheral T cell lymphomas*, so called because of their shared immunophenotype with peripheral blood T cells, clinically resemble diffuse large B cell lymphomas. *Angioimmunoblastic T cell lymphoma* is a disease of older adults, presenting with the acute onset of generalized lymphadenopathy, rash, hepatosplenomegaly, and B symptoms. Immunologic abnormalities are common and include plasmacytosis, polyclonal hypergammaglobulinemia, and a positive Coombs' test. This disease is progressive and frequently fatal, with median survival of 30 months. Angiocentric lymphomas clinically present as two entities: (1) *nasal T cell lymphoma*, probably associated with EBV and previously known as lethal midline granuloma; and (2) *pulmonary angiocentric lymphoma*, previously in the spectrum of lymphomatoid granulomatosis. The nasal lymphomas tend to be locally aggressive and recur locally after therapy. Patients with gluten-sensitive enteropathy are at risk of developing *intestinal T cell lymphomas*. They involve the ileum predominantly. These diseases present with abdominal pain, obstruction, and perforation, and surgical debulking is often indicated in their management. The *anaplastic large cell lymphomas* are either of T cell or null cell lineage. These diseases present with extranodal disease, often skin, and at nodal sites as well. Clinically these patients present with symptoms similar to those with aggressive diffuse large B cell lymphoma.

AIDS-related lymphomas Although not a separate pathologic entity, non-Hodgkin's lymphoma occurs in 10 to 30 percent of patients with AIDS. Virtually all cases are diffuse large B cell or Burkitt's type. In these cases extranodal involvement is common, with CNS, bone marrow, liver, and gastrointestinal tract the most frequent sites. Most patients present with widespread disease, rapid nodal enlargement, and B symptoms. A subset present with an effusion, without a mass. Primary CNS lymphoma—a disease with a short survival—is common in advanced AIDS patients. When treated with the most aggressive combinations of chemotherapy, results have been poor, largely due to the high death rate from intercurrent infections associated with severe immunodeficiency.

℞ TREATMENT

To decide the appropriate treatment regimen, the clinician must know the histology and extent of disease. Most patients with aggressive-histology lymphoma should be treated initially with curative intent. Choice of therapy may be influenced by age and the presence of comorbid diseases (cardiac, renal, pulmonary, hepatic), which might significantly affect end-organ toxicity.

The treatment of diffuse large B cell lymphoma is one of the major success stories of modern chemotherapy. The first successful regimen for this disease was C-MOPP, which induced complete remissions in approximately 45 percent of patients and with long-term disease-free survival for about one-third of patients. The CHOP regimen achieves complete remissions in about 50 percent of patients, with long-term disease-free survival of 35 percent. Success with this and subsequent regimens requires attention to administering full doses and adhering to schedules as strictly as possible. Over the past 15 years, attempts have been made to improve the percentage of complete remissions and overall cure rate. Additional agents have been added to those in CHOP including bleomycin, methotrexate, procarbazine, nitrogen mustard, cytosine arabinoside, and etoposide (e.g., M-BACOD, m-BACOD, ProMACE-MOPP, COP-BLAM, MACOP-B, ProMACE/CytaBOM). With these approaches, the complete remission rate now approaches 80 percent for the most aggressive regimens. However, toxicities have also increased (e.g., infections as well as cardiac and pulmonary complications). Within individual institutional studies, the results with some of these third-generation regimens has been far superior to CHOP, with approximately 70 percent of patients appearing to be cured. However, a multi-institutional randomized trial comparing CHOP to m-BACOD, ProMACE/CytaBOM, or MACOP-B found no difference in the overall survival, response rate, or time to treatment failure between the four treatment arms. Confidence in this trial is undermined by the 30 percent lower than expected CR rates obtained with MACOP-B and ProMACE-CytaBOM. Prolonged "maintenance" therapy has not improved overall survival. A significant proportion of patients with diffuse aggressive lymphoma are over age 60, and the outcome for patients over age 60 is worse than for younger patients. The reasons for these differences may be related to less intensive treatment delivered as well as to the presence of comorbid diseases. In some studies, increased deaths unrelated to lymphoma or its treatment have been reported, whereas in others, an increased treatment-related mortality has been reported. Attempts to modify regimens and improve supportive care may improve the treatment of aggressive lymphomas in elderly patients. Selected patients with localized aggressive diffuse large B cell lymphomas have been treated in the past with local radiation therapy, with 50 to 60 percent attaining long-term disease-free survival; however, the use of four cycles of chemotherapy with local radiation results in cure of 85 to 90 percent of such patients. Local radiation therapy may also improve the effect of chemotherapy on the aggressive nasal T cell lymphomas, which have a high propensity to recur locally. However, for the vast majority of patients with aggressive lymphoma, radiation therapy is of no proven benefit.

AIDS-related lymphomas are among the most aggressive of the non-Hodgkin's lymphomas. Initial studies with aggressive regimens yielded dismal results, with only one-third of patients achieving complete remission, and a high frequency of CNS relapse and fatal opportunistic infection. Subsequent studies using modified doses of chemotherapy and CNS prophylaxis have given CR rates of 50 percent, with a median survival of 15 months for those patients in complete remission. Since neutropenia was a major problem even in modified-dose therapy, the addition of the hematopoietic growth factors has permitted tolerable escalation of chemotherapy doses. Response rates appear to be related to clinical factors, including history of AIDS, CD4 T cell counts, and performance status. For patients who do not respond or who relapse, the results of salvage treatment are very poor, with short survival.

Prognostic Factors CLINICAL PROGNOSTIC FACTORS Without question, the response to treatment is one of the most important prognostic indicators, particularly in patients with aggressive non-Hodgkin's lymphoma. Patients with aggressive non-Hodgkin's lymphoma who do not respond to first-line therapy generally have very short survival. In contrast, patients with diffuse large B cell lymphoma who rapidly attain a clinical complete remission have a 70 to 80 percent likelihood of having long-term disease-free survival.

Analysis of a large group (2031) of patients with aggressive non-Hodgkin's lymphomas, largely diffuse large B cell lymphomas, has led to the establishment of a prognostic factor model that appears to apply to both indolent and aggressive lymphomas. A large number of factors were examined for all patients studied: age (≤60 vs. >60), serum LDH (normal vs. >1 × normal), performance status (0 or 1 vs. 2 to 4), stage (I or II vs. III or IV), and extranodal involvement (≤1 site vs. >1 site) were independently prognostic for overall survival. For the patients age 60 or less, only stage, LDH, and performance status were of prognostic significance. For relapse-free survival, age, stage, and performance status were significant parameters for predicting outcome. These data permitted the identification of four risk groups based on the number of risk factors: low risk with no or one factor; low-intermediate with two factors; high-intermediate with three factors; and high with four or five factors (Table 113-9).

LABORATORY PROGNOSTIC FACTORS Markers of proliferating cells such as expression of specific proteins (Ki-67, PCNA) and thymidine uptake have been associated with decreased survival. Similarly, it remains unclear whether the expression of certain cell surface markers such as adhesion molecules or T or B cell antigens is associated with clinical presentation or outcome. High serum levels of β_2-microglobulin are associated with poor prognosis.

A number of chromosomal abnormalities have been reported to influence prognosis: absence of normal metaphase cells, complexity of the karyotype, the presence of specific chromosomal abnormalities such as t(8;14), abnormality of the short arm of chromosome 1,

Table 113-9

The International Index and Prognosis in Diffuse Aggressive Non-Hodgkin's Lymphoma

Risk Group (Patients of All Ages)	Risk Factors*	Distribution of Cases, %	Complete Response Rate, %	5-Year Survival Rate, %
Low	0, 1	35	87	73
Low-intermediate	2	27	67	51
High-intermediate	3	22	55	43
High	4, 5	16	44	26

* Age (≤60 vs. >60); serum LDH (normal vs. >1 × normal); performance status (0 or 1 vs. 2–4); stage (I or II vs. III or IV); and extranodal involvement (≤1 site vs. >1 site)
SOURCE: Adapted from Shipp.

trisomy 7, trisomy 18, deletions of chromosome 6, and the presence of abnormalities of chromosome 17. Rearrangement of the *bcl*-6 gene, present in approximately one-third of diffuse large B cell lymphomas, may be a favorable independent prognostic variable.

SIGNIFICANCE OF MINIMAL RESIDUAL DISEASE Following aggressive therapy of patients with follicular lymphoma using high-dose ablative therapy and autologous BMT, those patients who consistently lack a *bcl*-2 translocation in the bone marrow and the peripheral blood have a significantly better disease-free survival than patients with PCR-detectable disease. The presence of abnormal cells after therapy of aggressive lymphoma may also predict relapse. The meaning of a "molecular" complete response as compared to the usual clinical criteria for complete response is being assessed. Currently, molecular assessment of remission is a research tool.

Salvage Chemotherapy The prognosis for patients with intermediate- and high-grade non-Hodgkin's lymphoma who fail to achieve a complete remission or who relapse following aggressive therapy is very poor. Salvage chemotherapy employing drugs such as cytosine arabinoside, cisplatin, etoposide, ifosfamide, given as single agents or in combination, have been used to induce remissions. Depending upon the histology and regimen, approximately 20 to 30 percent of patients attain a complete remission after conventional dose salvage therapy, with partial remissions in another 30 percent. Unfortunately, these remissions tend to be short-lived (approximately 2 to 6 months), with fewer than 3 percent of patients in remission beyond 2 years.

Stem Cell Transplantation (BMT) Patients with disease resistant to conventional or salvage therapeutic regimens can still be induced into a complete remission with very high doses of chemotherapy or the combination of high-dose chemotherapy and radiotherapy. A steep dose-response curve persists in non-Hodgkin's lymphomas, even after relapse. This treatment approach is complicated by very significant and prolonged myelosuppression. Bone marrow as a source of hematopoietic stem cells can be infused from an identical twin (syngeneic), an HLA-matched relative (allogeneic), or from the patient (autologous). Alternatively, hematopoietic stem cells can be isolated from peripheral blood. The vast majority of transplants for patients with lymphoma have employed autologous stem cells. Stem cell transplantation has become widespread in the treatment of patients with refractory or relapsed non-Hodgkin's lymphoma. Patients whose disease has never responded to primary therapy are presently not salvaged by this approach. Following relapse from remission, fewer than 15 percent of patients whose disease is resistant to all forms of salvage therapy have long-term disease-free survival. In contrast, approximately 40 percent of those patients whose disease is still responsive to therapy have long-term disease-free survival with high-dose therapy and BMT. High-dose therapy and autologous BMT are superior to conventional-dose salvage therapy with DHAP (cisplatin, cytarabine, dexamethasone) in relapsed patients with diffuse large B cell lymphoma. While the majority of patients undergoing BMT have intermediate- and high-grade non-Hodgkin's lymphoma, studies in those with low-grade lymphomas suggest that a subset of patients experience long-term disease-free survival. Early studies with BMT reported treatment-related deaths in the range of 20 to 30 percent; however, as patients with no associated comorbid disease are treated, this mortality has significantly decreased to less than 5 percent. The use of recombinant hematopoietic growth factors to hasten myeloid cell recovery has also significantly reduced morbidity and length of hospitalization following high-dose therapy and stem cell transplantation.

Lower treatment-related mortality has led some groups to use high-dose therapy as consolidation therapy in patients with poor prognosis non-Hodgkin's lymphomas in first remission. Patients who are at high risk for relapse following conventional therapy have a significantly better disease-free survival with consolidation autologous BMT than with conventional treatment alone. Although this modality is capable of curing some patients with relapsed non-Hodgkin's lymphomas, many issues still remain, including optimal therapeutic regimen, timing of transplantation, source of hematopoietic stem cells, the need to purge autologous marrow, and methods to minimize morbidity and mortality.

New Therapeutic Approaches Although great strides have been made in the treatment of non-Hodgkin's lymphoma with conventional, salvage, and high-dose ablative therapy, many patients are not cured. However, unlike most other cancers, many patients can achieve a complete remission. This suggests that the major obstacle to cure is subpopulations of resistant neoplastic cells. There are a number of newer approaches to the treatment of non-Hodgkin's lymphomas that may overcome resistance. There are a growing number of cytokines that may be either cytostatic or cytotoxic to neoplastic cells. Monoclonal antibodies (unconjugated, conjugated to toxins, or conjugated to a radionuclide) are being used to treat patients with non-Hodgkin's lymphomas. Anti-B cell (anti-CD20) monoclonal antibodies conjugated to ^{131}I have shown promising results with limited follow-up. Endogenously or exogenously activated lymphocytes or NK cells can be used to attack lymphoma cells specifically. Infusion of cytokines (such as IL-12) that augment antitumor immunity are in clinical trials and may well have a role in the minimal disease state. Vaccination studies are underway using the tumor Ig idiotype to induce specific immunity against residual tumor cells. Another approach is to modify the tumor cells to make them more immunogenic and more susceptible to endogenous effector mechanisms.

ACUTE LEUKEMIA/LYMPHOMA

CLINICAL FEATURES AND NATURAL HISTORY **Lymphoblastic Leukemia** Patients with lymphoblastic leukemia present with signs and symptoms of marrow failure. These include pallor and fatigue, bleeding and bruising, and fever and infection—due to anemia, thrombocytopenia, and neutropenia, respectively. The risk of bleeding increases with platelet counts less than $20 \times 10^5/\mu L$ and often involves skin and mucosal sites. With platelet transfusions, hemorrhage is no longer a major cause of death, although alloimmunization can limit optimal platelet support of patients, particularly when patients have been heavily transfused. The increased risk of infection occurs with absolute neutrophil counts less than $500/\mu L$ and is the leading cause of death. Febrile patients should be promptly treated with broad-spectrum antibiotics, and these should be continued until neutropenia is resolved. Infections commonly involve mucosal sites such as the pharynx and perianal area as well as the lungs and skin (particularly intravenous line sites). The most common bacterial organisms are *Staphylococcus* spp. and gram-negative organisms. Patients in relapse or under treatment, particularly when on broad-spectrum antibiotics, are susceptible to opportunistic organisms such as anaerobic bacteria, yeast (*Candida* spp.), fungi (*Aspergillus*, *Mucor*, *Pneumocystis*), and viruses (such as herpesviruses).

Patients with ALL can present with infiltration of spleen, lymph nodes, liver, skin, or CNS (particularly as a site of relapse). Patients with leukemic meningitis generally present with headache, nausea, and cranial nerve palsies. Involvement of the testis as an extramedullary site of relapse is not uncommon. A mediastinal mass is a frequent presentation of T cell lymphoblastic leukemia/lymphoma (see below). Bone pain, particularly sternal tenderness, is seen in many patients with lymphoblastic leukemia.

Several metabolic abnormalities are seen in patients with ALL. Uric acid nephropathy is caused by the rapid turnover of acute leukemia cells. This is aggravated by dehydration, acidosis, and therapy leading to tumor cell lysis. The use of hydration, alkalinization of the urine, and allopurinol can prevent urate nephropathy. Both hypokalemia and hyperkalemia can occur in patients with ALL. The cause of the hypokalemia is unknown in ALL but is caused by an unknown renal tubular defect. Hyperkalemia is seen along with hypocalcemia and hyperphosphatemia as part of the tumor lysis syndrome following initiation of therapy (see Chap. 104). This syndrome is most commonly seen in L3 ALL/Burkitt's lymphoma and is aggravated by renal failure.

In order to make a diagnosis of acute leukemia, the marrow must be involved, with >30 percent lymphoblasts, although a similar number of blasts in the peripheral blood also makes the diagnosis. There is some relationship between immunophenotype with subtype of ALL and clinical findings. Patients with pre-B ALL (French-American-British L1, L2), the "classic" childhood ALL, often have splenomegaly and rarely have white blood counts over $25,000/\mu L$. T cell ALL (L1, L2) has a male predominance and CNS and mediastinal disease. B cell ALL (L3) often has extramedullary presentation with metabolic abnormalities. The distribution of subtypes of ALL differs between adults and children. In contrast to childhood ALL, where L1 morphology is most common, L2 is the most common subtype in adults. T cell phenotype is also more common in adults (20 percent of cases) than in children. Finally, t(9;22) is seen in about 20 percent of adults but is rare in childhood ALL.

Precursor T Cell/B Cell Lymphoblastic Lymphoma Although lymphoblastic lymphomas represent a major subgroup of childhood non-Hodgkin's lymphomas, they are much less common in adults (fewer than 5 percent of adult non-Hodgkin's lymphomas). Such patients are usually males in their twenties and thirties who present with lymphadenopathy in cervical, supraclavicular, and axillary regions (50 percent) or with a mediastinal mass (50 to 70 percent). In most patients the mediastinal mass is anterior, >10 cm, is symptomatic often with superior vena cava syndrome, and is associated with pleural effusions. Less commonly, patients present with extranodal disease (e.g., skin, testicular, or bony involvement). More than 90 percent of patients present with stage III or stage IV disease, and half have B symptoms. Although the bone marrow can be normal at presentation, approximately 60 percent of patients develop bone marrow infiltration and a subsequent leukemic phase indistinguishable from T cell ALL. Before current aggressive acute leukemia–like therapy, this disease was rapidly fatal.

Burkitt's Lymphoma Burkitt's lymphoma is a childhood tumor that has two major clinical presentations. The endemic (African) form generally presents as a jaw or abdominal tumor that spreads to extranodal sites, especially to the bone marrow and meninges. The nonendemic (American) form has an abdominal presentation with massive disease; ascites; and skin, bone, and peripheral node involvement. Like the African form, it also spreads to the bone marrow and CNS (although less than in the African form). Before aggressive therapeutic programs, all children died rapidly. These tumors are now treated with very aggressive chemotherapeutic programs with more gratifying results. Burkitt's lymphoma is uncommon in adults but is occasionally seen in patients up to age 35. In contrast, the high-grade Burkitt-like lymphomas are heterogeneous and aggressive and frequently present like diffuse large B cell lymphoma in extranodal sites. Burkitt-like lymphoma behaves more like diffuse large cell lymphoma.

Adult T Cell Leukemia/Lymphoma This entity has been observed in southwestern Japan, the Caribbean, and in blacks in the southeastern United States and is associated with the HTLV-I retrovirus. Adult T cell leukemia/lymphoma (ATLL) presents with generalized lymphadenopathy, hepatosplenomegaly, cutaneous infiltration, hypercalcemia, lytic bone lesions, elevated LDH, and a leukemia characterized by pleomorphic CD4+ T cells. The skin lesions can vary from papules to plaques to tumors to ulcerations. Marrow involvement is not marked, and anemia and thrombocytopenia are not common. This disease has a fulminant course, and its natural history has been minimally altered by aggressive combination chemotherapy. Although 50 to 70 percent of patients will achieve a complete remission, the median duration of remission is about 12 months. The incidence of infection, often opportunistic, is very high in patients with ATLL because of an underlying immunodeficiency in these HTLV-I-infected patients. A chronic form has also been described with skin lesions, mild lymphocytosis without significant numbers of circulating blasts, and absence of hepatosplenomegaly or lymphadenopathy. These patients can survive for years before converting to the more aggressive form of the disease.

℞ TREATMENT

Although the clinical distinction between lymphoblastic leukemia and lymphoma is based upon the percentage of marrow involvement, both diseases require similar aggressive therapy with induction, consolidation, CNS prophylaxis, and maintenance therapy. With this approach, 40 percent or more of patients are cured. Optimum induction therapy for adults with ALL must include an anthracycline in addition to vincristine and prednisone (±L-asparaginase). This improves the CR rate from 50 percent to as high as 85 percent in some series. The use of more intensive induction regimens has added no significant benefit to date. Once CR is achieved, postremission therapy (which in some studies is very intensive) is critical to improving the duration of CR in patients with ALL. CNS prophylaxis is more optimally given early rather than late during postremission therapy. Cranial radiation with intrathecal methotrexate or intrathecal and high-dose systemic methotrexate are effective methods of prophylaxis. Maintenance therapy lasting about 2 years, similar to that given to children, generally includes methotrexate, 6-mercaptopurine, vincristine, and prednisone. However, the optimal duration and intensity of maintenence therapy in adults are unclear.

Precursor T cell or B cell lymphoblastic lymphoma in adults has been treated with some success, although inferior to that seen in children. When treated with regimens initially developed for childhood ALL with intrathecal therapy, about 40 percent of adults are reported to survive at 5 years. CNS prophylaxis is critical in treating these diseases since the CNS is a sanctuary site for recurrence. Similarly, Burkitt's lymphoma in adults has been treated with regimens designed for the pediatric populations, which involve the use of high doses of cyclophosphamide, cytosine arabinoside, and CNS prophylaxis with methotrexate. The cure rate is about 60 percent in experienced centers.

Prognostic Factors   As is the case in non-Hodgkin's lymphoma, age remains an independent prognostic variable in ALL, with older adults (>35) having a worse prognosis. Other adverse factors include delay in achieving CR; B cell phenotype (L3 or Burkitt's morphology); high white cell count at presentation (>50,000/μL); and presence of certain cytogenetic abnormalities, specifically t(9;22), t(8;14), t(1;19), and t(4;11). T cell phenotype was previously thought to be a poor prognostic factor, although with more intensive induction regimens the prognosis for patients with T cell ALL is no worse than for B cell ALL. With the identification of these prognostic factors, distinct treatment approaches have evolved for patients with poor-prognosis subtypes of ALL. The major focus has been on myeloablative therapy for patients with suitable marrow donors.

Treatment of Recurrent ALL and the Role of BMT   Despite postremission therapy and CNS prophylaxis, remission duration in adults with ALL is shorter than in children. The prognosis of patients who fail to achieve remission or who relapse on therapy is very poor. Although second remissions can be obtained, they are usually of very short duration. Patients who relapse after maintenance have

a greater likelihood of attaining a second CR, but virtually all relapse. Patients who have isolated extramedullary relapses, such as in the CNS or testis, are treated with radiation, and intrathecal therapy, or radiation, respectively, but they should also receive reinduction to prevent systemic relapse. In general, due to the poor prognosis of patients with relapsed adult ALL, consideration should be made for BMT. For selected patients in second remission, the long-term leukemia-free survival following BMT from a matched sibling donor is 20 to 30 percent.

The role of allogeneic BMT in adults with ALL in first remission is unclear. It appears from retrospective and prospective studies that the 3-year disease-free survivals are similar after chemotherapy and allogeneic BMT—around 45 percent. However, patient selection, high transplant-related mortality, and late relapses after chemotherapy alone have contributed to the failure to define the need for transplantation. Patients with unfavorable cytogenetics, L3 morphology, and very high presenting white cell counts should be considered for allogeneic transplantation in first remission. For example, patients with t(9;22) ALL (a disease that has evolved from Ph' CML), who have a dismal prognosis with chemotherapy alone, have a disease-free survival of 38 percent with BMT. Similar results are reported with patients with t(4;11) ALL. For patients without suitable allogeneic or matched unrelated donors, high-dose therapy with either purged or unpurged autologous marrow has been performed. In highly selected patients, the long-term leukemia-free survival with autologous BMT in second remission is approximately 30 percent. Although the treatment-related mortality in these studies is significantly lower than in allogeneic transplants, a high relapse rate remains in patients undergoing autologous transplantation, related in part to the absence of a graft-vs.-tumor effect.

HODGKIN'S DISEASE

CELLULAR ORIGIN OF THE REED-STERNBERG CELL OF HODGKIN'S DISEASE   Reed-Sternberg (RS) cells, in the appropriate cytoarchitectural milieu, are required for the diagnosis of Hodgkin's disease. In Hodgkin's disease tissues, the majority of cells are small lymphocytes with a mature T cell phenotype (CD2, CD3, CD4 > CD8, CD5) together with a variable number of B cells. RS cells and their variants may be immunologically distinguished from the neoplastic cells of most non-Hodgkin's lymphomas by their lack of a characteristic pattern of expression of T and B cell–associated antigens. The exception is lymphocyte-predominant Hodgkin's disease; the malignant cells in this subset express B cell markers. RS cells of lymphocyte-predominant Hodgkin's disease also express the leukocyte common antigen (CD45RB), whereas RS cells in other subtypes of Hodgkin's disease are CD45RB negative.

Two antigens expressed on the RS cell have proven to be diagnostically useful. The first is CD15 (identified by monoclonal antibody Leu M1), which is the Lewis X blood group antigen and functions as an adhesion receptor. CD15 is expressed on RS cells in all subtypes of Hodgkin's disease except for the lymphocyte-predominant variant. The second antigen is the CD30 antigen (Ki-1), which is present on virtually all RS cells. The CD30 antigen also is expressed on some activated B cells, activated T cells, dendritic cells, EBV-transformed cell lines, and tumor cells isolated from some patients with anaplastic large cell lymphomas.

Molecular studies of RS-enriched populations and in situ hybridization studies have provided conflicting results about the origin of these cells. RS cells may have monoclonal or polyclonal immunoglobulin gene rearrangements. In some cases, T cell receptor β-chain rearrangements have been demonstrated. Sensitive in situ hybridization studies have identified a clonal form of the EBV genome in RS cells in about 30 percent of cases examined. This supports a role for EBV in some cases of Hodgkin's disease, usually the mixed cellularity subtype. RS cells are certainly of hematopoietic lineage, but specific lineage assignment is difficult. Hodgkin's disease is a heterogeneous disease, derived from subpopulations of activated lymphohematopoietic cells. The distinct biologic and clinical behaviors (Table 113-1) of Hodgkin's and non-Hodgkin's lymphomas may be a reflection of their divergent cellular origins.

EPIDEMIOLOGY AND ETIOLOGY Approximately 7500 new cases of Hodgkin's disease are diagnosed annually in the United States. In non-Hodgkin's lymphomas, there is a linear increase in incidence with age. In contrast, in Hodgkin's disease the age-specific incidence curve is characteristically bimodal, with an initial peak in young adults (15 to 35 years) and a second peak after age 50. However, in Japan, there is an absence of the early peak, and in some third world countries, there is a shift of the first peak into childhood as well as a shift of histology from nodular sclerosis to mixed cellularity and lymphocyte predominant. Hodgkin's disease is more prevalent in males, and when the age-specific incidence curve is compared to the sex distribution of the patients, the increased male prevalence is most prominent in young adults. A disproportionate number of patients in the first modal peak exhibit nodular sclerosis histology. In childhood Hodgkin's disease, this male predominance is even more striking, with over 80 percent of patients being male. This has led some investigators to hypothesize a sex-linked genetic or hormonally related increase in susceptibility.

Hodgkin's disease is 99-fold more common in an identical twin of an affected case than in the general population, fueling suspicion of a genetic contribution.

Although controversial, clustering of patients with Hodgkin's disease has been reported. Increased risk has been associated with decreased number of siblings, single family dwellings, decreased number of playmates, early birth order, a sibling with Hodgkin's disease, tonsillectomy, and certain HLA antigens. These findings have been used to suggest that Hodgkin's disease is caused by a virus possessing low oncogenic potential that increases with age from the time of infection. However, exhaustive search has yielded nothing. There is strong evidence for a role of EBV in the pathogenesis of a subset of cases. The EBV genome is present and is monoclonal in some cases, dependent upon histologic subtype: 60 percent of mixed cellularity, 30 percent of nodular sclerosis and lymphocyte-depleted subtypes. As in non-Hodgkin's lymphomas, there is an increased risk of Hodgkin's disease in patients with immunodeficiencies and autoimmune diseases (Table 113-5). In contrast to non-Hodgkin's lymphoma, where chromosomal deletions and translocations are common, cytogenetic studies have uncommonly found clonal hyperdiploid abnormalities in the neoplastic Hodgkin's disease CD30 + cells, though aneuploidy is common.

CLINICAL FEATURES AND DIFFERENTIAL DIAGNOSIS Hodgkin's disease usually presents as a localized disease and subsequently spreads to contiguous lymphoid structures; ultimately, it disseminates to nonlymphoid tissues, with a potentially fatal outcome. Hodgkin's disease commonly presents with a newly detected mass or group of lymph nodes that are firm, freely moveable, and usually nontender. Approximately half of patients present with adenopathy in the neck or supraclavicular area, and over 70 percent of patients present with superficial lymph node enlargement. Because these are frequently not painful, detection by the patient may be delayed until the lymph nodes are quite large. Approximately 60 percent of patients present with mediastinal adenopathy. This is sometimes first detected on a routine chest x-ray. Nodes involved by Hodgkin's disease tend to be centripetal or axial, in contrast to non-Hodgkin's lymphomas, which have a tendency to be centrifugal and involve epitrochlear, Waldeyer's Ring, and abdominal nodes. In 2 to 5 percent of patients, lymph nodes or other tissues involved with Hodgkin's disease can become painful after the ingestion of alcoholic beverages. The growth of lymph nodes may be quite variable; some lesions can remain stable for long periods of time, while spontaneous and temporary regression of some nodes may also occur.

The majority of patients presenting with Hodgkin's disease have few or no symptoms related to their disease. However, 25 to 30 percent

of patients have some constitutional symptoms; the most common is low-grade fever, which can be associated with recurrent night sweats. For some patients, night sweats may be the sole complaint. A small number of patients may have high fluctuating fevers accompanied by drenching night sweats. These fevers can persist for several weeks followed by afebrile intervals (Pel-Epstein fevers). Fevers and night sweats are more commonly seen in older patients and in those with more advanced stage disease. Some patients with extensive abdominal but limited peripheral adenopathy are first evaluated for fever and night sweats. They undergo a workup for fever of unknown origin and usually are found to have mixed cellularity or lymphocyte-depleted Hodgkin's disease. Another important presenting symptom is unexplained weight loss of greater than 10 percent over 6 months or less. Other frequent symptoms include fatigue, malaise, and weakness. Pruritus occurs in approximately 10 percent of patients at initial diagnosis; it is usually generalized, may be associated with a skin rash, and rarely may be the only disease manifestation. It is not a B symptom. Mediastinal, pulmonary, pleural, or pericardial involvement may be associated with cough, chest pain, shortness of breath, or hypertrophic osteoarthropathy; bone involvement may be associated with bone pain. Occasionally a patient will present with obstruction of the superior vena cava as the first symptom. Sudden spinal cord compression can be a presenting complaint but is usually a complication of advanced progressive disease. Headache or visual disturbances may be seen in the very rare patient with intracranial Hodgkin's disease, and abdominal involvement may result in abdominal pain, bowel disturbances, and even ascites.

The differential diagnosis is similar to that described for non-Hodgkin's lymphoma. In patients with cervical adenopathy, infections including bacterial or viral pharyngitis, infectious mononucleosis, and toxoplasmosis must be excluded. Other malignancies such as non-Hodgkin's lymphomas, nasopharyngeal cancers, and thyroid cancers can also present with localized cervical adenopathy. Axillary adenopathy must be differentiated from non-Hodgkin's lymphoma and breast cancer. Mediastinal adenopathy must be distinguished from infections, sarcoid, and other tumors. In older patients, the differential diagnosis includes tumors of the lung and mediastinum, specifically small cell and non-small cell carcinomas. Reactive mediastinitis and hilar adenopathy from histoplasmosis can be confused with lymphoma since it occurs in otherwise asymptomatic people. Primary abdominal disease with hepatomegaly, splenomegaly, and massive adenopathy is uncommon, and other neoplastic diseases, especially non-Hodgkin's lymphoma, must be excluded under these circumstances.

DIAGNOSIS AND PATHOLOGIC CLASSIFICATION The diagnosis of Hodgkin's disease requires a biopsy that contains sufficient tissue to permit an accurate microscopic diagnosis. Biopsy specimens are usually from lymph nodes but may occasionally be from other tissues. Needle aspirations or needle biopsies are not adequate for the primary histologic diagnosis of Hodgkin's disease or any other lymphoma.

The criteria for the diagnosis and classification of Hodgkin's disease have remained unchanged since 1966 when the Rye classification was adopted (Table 113-4). Central to the diagnosis is the presence of the RS cell, a large cell with a bilobed or multilobulated nucleus with prominent inclusion-like nucleoli. **(See Plate IV-25.)** There are several morphologic variants of RS cells, and it is the frequency of these variants as well as the cellular and stromal background of the node that help to establish the histologic subtypes of Hodgkin's disease. RS cells may occasionally be found in other conditions such as infectious mononucleosis and non-Hodgkin's lymphomas. Thus, an accurate diagnosis of Hodgkin's disease depends on additional cellular and architectural features of the tissue.

Hodgkin's disease is subdivided into four types: (1) lymphocyte predominant, (2) nodular sclerosis, (3) mixed cellularity, and (4) lymphocyte depleted. The R.E.A.L. classification includes these four major subtypes. Treatment and prognosis in Hodgkin's disease is dependent on the stage of disease, whereas in non-Hodgkin's lymphoma, treatment is largely based on histologic subtype.

STAGING AND OTHER LABORATORY ABNORMALITIES Ann Arbor Classification Following biopsy and histopathologic classification of Hodgkin's disease, one must define the extent of the disease (i.e., staging), which is essential for the selection of optimal therapy. In the Ann Arbor staging classification (Table 113-7), the patient receives both a clinical and a pathologic stage. The clinical stage is defined by the extent of disease based on physical examination and other noninvasive studies. The pathologic stage is defined by data obtained from invasive tests including biopsy specimens obtained from different sites, usually during a staging laparotomy. The presence of localized extralymphatic disease is designated by the suffix *E*. Such extralymphatic involvement may include solitary involvement of lung or bone. Multifocal involvement in these organs usually is defined as disseminated disease. Bone involvement must be separated from bone marrow involvement, since bone marrow and liver involvement are always defined as stage IV disseminated disease.

The presence of systemic symptoms (fever, night sweats, weight loss) is designated by the suffix *B* and their absence by the suffix *A*. The presence of both fevers and weight loss results in a less favorable prognosis, while night sweats are currently thought to be of no independent prognostic importance. Patients with early-stage disease, such as pathologic stage IA or IIA, are treated effectively with radiotherapy alone; patients with more disseminated disease, such as pathologic stage III, IVA, or IVB, are most effectively treated with combination chemotherapy alone. Patients of any stage with a very large mediastinal mass are usually treated with combined modality therapy.

Staging Procedures After Biopsy Diagnosis The diagnostic studies recommended for complete staging are outlined in Table 113-10. Detailed physical examination with attention to documentation of all sites of nodal involvement and splenomegaly is essential. The chest radiograph is usually sufficient to exclude mediastinal, hilar, pleural, and parenchymal involvement. However, in patients with demonstrable thoracic disease, chest CT more accurately defines the extent of disease. CT of the abdomen and pelvis may assess certain groups of nodes but is not sensitive for detecting splenic and hepatic disease or node involvement that does not produce enlargement. CT scanning can detect the exact location and extent of all enlarged nodes including iliac, mesenteric, and retrocrural nodal areas. A lymphangiogram evaluates the paraaortic and common internal and external iliac nodes and is essential if radiation therapy alone is a treatment option.

Radiation therapy is a local treatment. Disease not within a treatment portal is not eradicated. For this reason, a number of more invasive diagnostic tests are required if patients are clinically stage I, II, or IIIA and radiation therapy is a treatment option. Lymphangiograms are more sensitive than abdominal/pelvic CT scans. Moreover, lymphangiograms are useful before staging laparotomy to direct the surgeon to the nodes to be biopsied. However, the accuracy of this procedure is highly dependent on the experience of the radiologist. If a staging laparotomy is considered, patients should undergo bilateral bone marrow biopsies to exclude stage IV disease. The frequency of a positive bone marrow biopsy in clinical stage IA or IIA disease is low, but if present, makes laparotomy unnecessary. Staging laparotomy includes biopsy of selected lymph nodes in the retroperitoneum, splenectomy, and several needle and wedge biopsies of the liver. Traditionally, all patients without obvious stage IV disease underwent laparotomy, and nearly one-third had their initial clinical stage changed as a result of the procedure. For example, one-third of patients with normal-sized spleens had demonstrable tumor infiltration at laparotomy, whereas 35 percent of patients with clinical splenomegaly had no histologic evidence of disease. Liver involvement is more common in patients with positive lymphangiograms and enlarged spleens. Laparotomy should be utilized in patients whose clinical stages make them candidates for treatment with radiation therapy alone and in whom evidence of unsuspected abdominal disease will significantly change treatment. Approximately one-third of patients with clinical stage I or II (with or without B symptoms) will have occult upper abdominal or spleen disease not dectected by noninvasive studies. A staging laparotomy should not be performed in patients who are to receive chemotherapy based upon the presence of bulky chest disease, more than four nodal sites, bulky abdominal involvement, or clinical stage III or stage IV disease. A staging laparotomy with splenectomy should be performed by a surgeon who is skilled in this procedure after careful review of clinical, laboratory, pathologic, and radiologic studies. Finally, a number of ancillary studies may be very useful in selected patients and are listed in Table 113-10. Gallium scintigraphy is most useful in following response to treatment and to detect early recurrences; it is not useful at the time of initial staging.

Laboratory Abnormalities Routine blood counts, liver function tests, and renal function tests are all necessary parts of the medical workup but do not provide information about the extent of Hodgkin's disease or of specific organ involvement. A moderate, normochromic, normocytic anemia associated with low serum iron and low iron-binding capacity, but with normal or increased iron stores in the bone marrow, may be present in patients with Hodgkin's disease as well as in other neoplastic and chronic diseases. This reflects a cytokine-mediated inhibition of iron reutilization. A moderate to marked leukemoid reaction is common, particularly in symptomatic patients and usually disappears with treatment. Mild peripheral absolute eosinophilia is not uncommon, especially in patients with pruritus. Absolute monocytosis is also observed. Absolute lymphocytopenia (<1000 cells/μL) usually occurs in patients with more advanced disease. Many tests have been evaluated as indicators of disease activity. To date, the erythrocyte sedimentation rate still is the best monitor, but it suffers from its lack of specificity and can return to normal when residual disease is still demonstrable. Other abnormal tests include increased serum levels of copper, calcium, lactic acid, alkaline phosphatase, lysozyme, globulins, C-reactive protein, and other acute-phase reactants. Soluble CD30, soluble CD25, and soluble CD4 have been suggested as tumor markers.

Immunologic Abnormalities Hodgkin's disease is associated with a well-described but poorly understood immunologic defect. Untreated patients, including those with limited disease, have defective cellular immunity characterized by anergy to routine skin tests. They also have a reversal of the CD4:CD8 ratio, suggesting that this anergy may be due to increased numbers of suppressor T cells as well as decreased numbers of CD4+ cells. T cells from patients with Hodgkin's disease have defects in signal transduction, including decreased T cell receptor ζ chain and decreased tyrosine kinase activation. In

---

Table 113-10

Staging Evaluation for Hodgkin's Disease

Essential
1. Pathologic documentation by hematopathologist
2. Physical examination
3. Documentation of B symptoms
4. Laboratory evaluation
   a. Complete blood counts
   b. Liver function tests
   c. Renal function tests
   d. Uric acid
   e. Erythrocyte sedimentation rate
5. Chest radiograph
6. CT scan of chest, abdomen, and pelvis
7. Bone marrow biopsy

Essential Under Certain Circumstances
1. Liver biopsy
2. Bipedal lymphangiogram
3. Gallium scan
4. Staging laparatomy
5. Bone scan
6. Bone radiographs

Useful But Not Essential Tests
1. Cell-surface marker phenotypic analysis
2. Gene rearrangement analysis
3. Ultrasonography
4. Magnetic resonance imaging
5. Delayed-hypersensitivity skin tests

several studies, decreased immune reactivity correlates with both advanced stages of disease and the presence of systemic symptoms. However, anergy to recall and neoantigens appears to have no prognostic significance. Following successful therapy, anergy to recall antigens reverses but is still present in some patients to neoantigens. In addition to anergy, other tests of T cell function, including responses to mitogens and suppressor cell function, suggest a defect in immune function before and following treatment. Humoral immunity with antibody production to soluble antigens is normal in untreated patients. Thus, patients who undergo staging laparotomy and splenectomy will develop humoral immunity to pneumococcal antigens if immunized with the pneumococcal vaccine before splenectomy, but not after. The clinical impact of these immune defects is limited. Except for a higher than normal incidence of herpes zoster and development of warts, these patients are not plagued by opportunistic infections.

NATURAL HISTORY ACCORDING TO HISTOLOGIC SUBTYPE Patients with lymphocyte-predominant Hodgkin's disease are usually asymptomatic at presentation and tend to have localized disease. These patients are usually young, rarely have systemic symptoms or mediastinal mass, and are predominantly males. Nodular sclerosis Hodgkin's disease is found most frequently in adolescents and young adults who usually have localized disease; a preponderance are young women who present with a large mediastinal mass. Lymphocyte-depleted Hodgkin's disease is usually disseminated at the time of diagnosis and occurs in older patients who frequently have systemic symptoms. The mixed cellularity type occurs in all age groups and stages and is only slightly more common in males. There is a tendency toward an older age peak (30 to 40 years) than with nodular sclerosis, and approximately half of these patients have advanced disease. Patients with lymphocyte-predominant and nodular sclerosis Hodgkin's disease, if untreated, have a more indolent disease associated with a longer survival and are more likely to be cured with radiotherapy.

℞ TREATMENT

With appropriate treatment, about 85 percent of patients with Hodgkin's disease are curable. Radiotherapy may cure over 80 percent of patients with localized Hodgkin's disease, and chemotherapy over 70 percent of those with disseminated disease. Nearly half of those not cured by primary treatment are cured with salvage therapy. The choice of treatment is dependent on stage of disease. As with all neoplasms, the therapy of Hodgkin's disease is constantly being reevaluated to improve disease-free survival and decrease toxicity.

Treatment of Early-Stage Disease The mainstay of therapy for early-stage (I and II) Hodgkin's disease has been radiation therapy. With the knowledge that Hodgkin's disease spreads by lymphatic contiguity, three radiation fields were devised to cover likely sites of disease—the mantle field, paraaortic field, and the pelvic field. The mantle field includes the submandibular, cervical, supraclavicular, infraclavicular, axillary, mediastinal, and hilar lymph nodes. The paraaortic field covers the transverse processes of the abdominal vertebral bodies and the spleen, if it has not been removed. Pelvic irradiation includes the common iliac, hypogastric, external iliac, and inguinal nodes. When there is gross pelvic nodal involvement, the femoral nodes are also treated. Sometimes the pelvic and paraaortic fields are treated as one unit, which is commonly called the "inverted-Y" field. The use of pelvic irradiation has been recently reduced since stages I and II supradiaphragmatic Hodgkin's disease can be treated without pelvic irradiation. Patients now receive mantle and paraaortic irradiation and only rarely total nodal irradiation (i.e., all three fields). Patients receive doses of 3000 to 3600 cGy with an additional "cone down" dose for a total of 4000 cGy to areas of bulk disease.

Patients with localized nodal Hodgkin's disease (pathologic stages IA and IIA) treated with mantle or paraaortic radiation therapy have nearly an 80 percent long-term disease-free survival beyond 10 years, with less than a 10 percent mortality from Hodgkin's

disease. Randomized trials comparing radiation therapy to combination chemotherapy plus radiation show a relapse-free survival advantage for combined-modality treatment but no survival advantage. Although the disease-free survival is somewhat higher, salvage therapy after relapse from radiation is very efficacious and overall survival is not improved. Patients with stages IB and IIB have a slightly reduced disease-free survival (70 percent); however, most patients who relapse can be successfully treated with combination chemotherapy.

The very high rate of radiation therapy–related fatal complications, including second malignancies (0.5 to 1 percent risk per year up to at least 30 years after treatment) and a greater than threefold increased risk of fatal myocardial infarction (see below), has led to consideration of using primary combination chemotherapy in patients with early-stage Hodgkin's disease after clinical staging. The success of this approach is at least equal to using radiation therapy and spares the patient the unpleasant consequences of splenectomy for staging (i.e., infectious risk) and radiation therapy.

Treatment of Advanced-Stage Disease Chemotherapy with the combination of mechlorethamine (nitrogen mustard), vincristine (Oncovin), procarbazine, and prednisone (MOPP) produces CR in 85 to 90 percent of patients; about two-thirds of the CR are durable. MOPP therapy has been associated with significant toxicity. Nearly all patients experience some degree of nausea and vomiting and bone marrow suppression. About 2 percent of patients treated with MOPP develop myelodysplasia and/or acute leukemia 4 to 6 years after treatment. However, those who survive 10 years or more without developing leukemia are unlikely to do so. Infertility is another important toxicity.

Other multiple-drug regimens have been developed for the treatment of advanced Hodgkin's disease. However, none of the "MOPP-derived combinations" have been superior to the original MOPP administered at optimal dose and schedule. Substitution of chlorambucil for mechlorethamine and vinblastine for vincristine (ChlVPP) yields a regimen that is associated with less gastrointestinal and neurotoxicity with similar efficacy. Several regimens have been developed to treat MOPP-resistant patients. The best known of these is Adryamicin (doxorubicin), bleomycin, vinblastine, and dacarbazine (ABVD). ABVD has some efficacy in MOPP treatment failures and is comparable to MOPP in activity in previously untreated patients. Several randomized trials have attempted to determine optimum initial therapy, comparing MOPP, ABVD, and combinations of MOPP/ABVD. MOPP alternating with ABVD appears to be superior to a modified version of MOPP, achieving a higher CR rate (89 percent vs. 74 percent) as well as improved disease-free survival (68 percent vs. 46 percent) and overall survival (69 percent vs. 58 percent). However, alternating MOPP/ABVD gave similar results to ABVD alone. Studies that have compared a combination including all the MOPP/ABVD drugs into each cycle (hybrid) rather than alternating each monthly regimen have found no difference in response rate or duration or survival. ABVD has the advantage of sparing fertility but the disadvantage of a 3 percent risk of fatal pulmonary toxicity. The seven- (MOPP/ABV) or eight-drug (MOPP/ABVD) regimens produce no risk of acute leukemia or fatal pulmonary fibrosis but induce infertility in half the men and in 25 percent of the women. Thus, the choice of therapy involves trade-offs of toxicity risk. If fertility is the overriding issue, ABVD is the treatment of choice. If minimizing the risk of fatal toxicity is overriding, MOPP/ABV hybrid or MOPP/ABVD is the treatment of choice.

Prognostic Factors Prognostic factors have been identified that alter therapy for early-stage patients. Early-stage patients with large mediastinal involvement appear to have a higher risk of relapse after radiation therapy alone (disease-free survival of 40 to 55 percent) compared to patients with minimal or no mediastinal disease; they should be managed with chemotherapy followed by involved-field or mantle irradiation. Patients over age 40 also have a decreased survival. Finally, patients with pathologic stage IB or IIB and who have fevers and weight loss (but not night sweats) and are treated with radiation alone have a decreased disease-free and overall survival. They might best be treated with combination chemotherapy. Prognostic variables have been identified for patients who are clinical stages I and II. The factors that adversely affect outcome include male sex, multiple sites, high erythrocyte sedimentation rate, bulky mediastinal disease, mixed cellularity and lymphocyte-depleted histologies, and treatment with involved-field radiation. In advanced-stage patients who would be treated with combination chemotherapy, several clinical and laboratory parameters are independently significant for an unfavorable survival. These include stage IV disease, B symptoms, inguinal node involvement, large mediastinal mass, male gender, bulky disease, anemia, leukocytosis, lymphocytosis, and anemia. Even placing all of these factors together, the group with the worst prognosis has a 5-year survival of 54 percent. Thus, there is no single group of patients who are obvious candidates for primary high-dose therapy with hematopoietic support. Using these parameters, clinical investigations are focused on minimizing or intensifying therapy in appropriate patients.

Salvage Therapy   After proper restaging, further radiotherapy can be delivered (if technically feasible) to a subset of patients with early-stage disease who have relapsed outside of a radiation field or following combination chemotherapy. In patients not achieving a complete remission or relapsing after MOPP, second-line non-cross-resistant regimens are available. If patients relapse more than 12 months after the completion of primary chemotherapy, they can be retreated with the original treatment regimen; if they relapse in less than 12 months, they should be treated with an alternative salvage regimen, such as ABVD for MOPP, MOPP for ABVD, and mini BEAM (carmustine, etoposide, cytarabine, and melphalan) for MOPP/ABVD or MOPP/ABV. Conventional-dose salvage regimens will produce complete response in 30 to 40 percent of patients and long-term survival in 10 to 25 percent. Poor prognostic variables for salvage include stage IV disease at diagnosis, B symptoms at relapse, poor performance status, or remission lasting <12 months. Various salvage regimens containing combinations of cisplatin, etoposide, and ifosfamide have been used for patients who have failed two regimens such as MOPP and ABVD, with good responses that unfortunately are not durable. As is the case with non-Hodgkin's lymphoma, autologous or allogeneic BMT or peripheral blood stem transplantation is an effective salvage treatment for many relapsed patients. Hodgkin's disease patients whose disease remains sensitive to chemotherapeutic agents are more likely to experience long-term disease-free survival in the range of 50 percent, while resistant patients have disease-free survivals of 15 to 25 percent. In contrast to non-Hodgkin's lymphoma, total body irradiation has limited value, and virtually all ablative regimens include high-dose chemotherapy. The acute lethal pulmonary and hepatic toxicity from these high-dose regimens, however, can be as high as 25 percent in patients previously treated with radiation therapy, although with better patient selection and supportive care, mortality is now less than 5 percent. Any patient with a short initial remission should have high-dose therapy as a component of their salvage treatment.

Complications of Treatment   Radiation therapy can lead to acute and late complications. Acute side effects of mantle irradiation include transient xerostomia, pharyngitis, fatigue, and weight loss. Within several months of mantle irradiation, approximately 15 percent of patients develop paresthesia in the lower extremities upon flexion of the neck or thighs (Lhermitte's syndrome). This syndrome usually resolves spontaneously; there is no correlation between this syndrome and irreversible spinal injury. Other long-term side effects include radiation pneumonitis (severe in fewer than 5 percent of patients) and symptomatic pulmonary fibrosis (<1 percent). Late complications of mantle radiation include cardiac damage such as pericardial effusion and myocardial damage. Cardiac irradiation accelerates coronary artery disease and induces a greater than threefold risk of fatal myocardial infarctions. Anthracycline cardiomyopathy can occur but usually not with the doses administered with the ABVD or MOPP/ABVD regimens. It remains unclear whether long-term cardiac toxicity will occur in patients treated with combined-modality therapy that includes doxorubicin. Hypothyroidism may

occur in up to 30 percent of patients following mantle irradiation. Paraaortic irradiation is rarely associated with significant side effects. Pelvic irradiation acutely induces transient diarrhea and bladder irritation associated with frequency. Chronic effects include potential long-term bone marrow suppression and sterility; therefore, pelvic irradiation is infrequently employed. Gonadal dysfunction is also a significant problem in patients treated with MOPP or other regimens containing alkylating agents. Infertility is about one-half as frequent in patients who received MOPP/ABVD and is rare in patients treated with ABVD alone. Increasing numbers of secondary tumors are being observed in patients treated for Hodgkin's disease. In 15-year survivors with Hodgkin's disease treated with radiation therapy, a cumulative risk of development of second tumors 2.8 fold higher than expected has been observed. MOPP chemotherapy has not been associated with the development of second solid tumors. The most common cancers involve breast, thyroid, lung (in smokers), stomach, and skin as well as sarcomas and primary bone tumors. Secondary acute nonlymphocytic leukemia (usually seen between 5 and 10 years later) occurs in about 2 percent of MOPP-treated patients and in 8 percent of patients treated with MOPP plus radiation therapy. These leukemias usually have an antecedent myelodysplastic syndrome characterized by chromosomal deletions involving 5q and 7q. Leukemias associated with epipodophyllotoxins are seen rarely, but with a shorter latent period. High-grade non-Hodgkin's lymphomas are also seen with increased frequency, independent of the type of therapy. This complication may be related to the underlying immune defect in Hodgkin's disease patients.

Therapeutic Recommendation by Stage   STAGES IA AND IIA, NONBULKY DISEASE   Following staging laparotomy in patients with supradiaphragmatic disease, mantle or mantle and paraaortic irradiation is the treatment of choice. In patients with subdiaphragmatic lymphoma, radiotherapy is delivered to an inverted-Y field including the splenic pedicle in stage I disease and through total nodal irradiation in stage II disease. Some studies suggest that treatment with involved-field radiotherapy combined with chemotherapy produces comparable results, but most do not consider this the best treatment choice. For patients with subdiaphragmatic stage II disease of paraaortic nodes, chemotherapy is recommended. Chemotherapy alone is an appropriate treatment for patients who are clinically staged.

STAGES IB AND IIB, NONBULKY DISEASE   The therapy is the same as for stages IA and IIA Hodgkin's disease; however, the relapse rate is higher (20 percent). Relapse can usually be salvaged with chemotherapy. Subtotal or combination chemotherapy with involved-field irradiation remains an alternative treatment for these patients. Chemotherapy alone is an appropriate treatment for patients who are clinically staged.

STAGE II, BULKY DISEASE   Stage II disease with bulky mediastinal/hilar adenopathy should be managed with combined-modality therapy. This should include six cycles of combination chemotherapy and radiotherapy (usually a mantle field) to sites of bulk disease.

STAGES IIIA, IIIB, AND IV   Combination chemotherapy is recommended, consisting of two cycles beyond achieving complete remission. For most patients, six cycles of therapy are adequate; 15 percent of patients may require eight cycles. Although only 10 to 15 percent of patients fail to achieve a CR with combination chemotherapy, about half of the partial responders may be converted to CR with the addition of involved-field radiation therapy.

BIBLIOGRAPHY

BHATIA S et al: Breast cancer and other second neoplasms after childhood Hodgkin's disease. N Engl J Med 334:745, 1996

BIERMAN P et al: Autologous transplantation for Hodgkin's disease. Blood 83:1161, 1994

CANELLOS GP et al: Chemotherapy of advanced Hodgkin's disease with MOPP, ABVD, or MOPP alternating with ABVD. N Engl J Med 327:1478, 1992

COPELAN EA, MCGUIRE EA: The biology and treatment of acute lymphoblastic leukemia in adults. Blood 85:1151, 1995

FREEDMAN AS, NADLER LM: Immunologic markers in non-Hodgkin's lympho-
    mas. Hematol Oncol Clin North Am 5:871, 1991

HARRIS N et al: A revised European-American classification of lymphoid neo-
    plasms: A proposal from the International Lymphoma Study Group. Blood
    84:1361, 1994

KAPLAN HS: *Hodgkin's Disease*, 2d ed. Cambridge, MA, Harvard University
    Press, 1980

LEVINE AM: Acquired immunodeficiency syndrome–related lymphomas.
    Blood 80:8, 1992

LONGO DL: What's the deal with follicular lymphomas? J Clin Oncol
    11:202, 1993

O'BRIEN S et al: Advances in the biology and treatment of B-cell chronic
    lymphocytic leukemia. Blood 85:307, 1995

SHIPP MA: Prognostic factors in aggressive non-Hodgkin's lymphoma: Who
    has "high risk" disease? Blood 83:1165, 1994

URBA WJ, LONGO DL: Hodgkin's disease. N Engl J Med 326:678, 1992

114   *Dan L. Longo*

PLASMA CELL DISORDERS

GENERAL PRINCIPLES   The *plasma cell disorders* are
monoclonal neoplasms related to each other by virtue of their development from common progenitors in the B lymphocyte lineage. Multiple
myeloma, Waldenström's macroglobulinemia, primary amyloidosis
(see Chap. 309), and the heavy chain diseases comprise this group
and may be designated by a variety of synonyms such as *monoclonal
gammopathies*, *paraproteinemias*, *plasma cell dyscrasias*, and *dysproteinemias*. Normal development of B lymphocytes is discussed in
Chap. 305. Mature B lymphocytes destined to produce IgG bear surface
immunoglobulin molecules of both M and G heavy chain isotypes
with both isotypes having identical idiotypes (variable regions). Under
normal circumstances, maturation to antibody-secreting plasma cells
is stimulated by exposure to the antigen for which the surface immunoglobulin is specific; however, in the plasma cell disorders the control
over this process is lost. The clinical manifestations of all the plasma
cell disorders relate to the expansion of the neoplastic cells, to the
secretion of cell products (immunoglobulin molecules or subunits,
lymphokines), and to some extent to the host's response to the tumor.

There are three categories of structural variation among immunoglobulin molecules that form antigenic determinants, and these are
used to classify immunoglobulins (Chap. 305). *Isotypes* are those
determinants that distinguish among the main classes of antibodies of
a given species and are the same in all normal individuals of that
species. Therefore, isotypic determinants are, by definition, recognized
by antibodies from a distinct species (heterologous sera) but not by
antibodies from the same species (homologous sera). There are five
heavy chain isotypes (M, G, A, D, E) and two light chain isotypes
(kappa, lambda). *Allotypes* are distinct determinants that reflect regular
small differences between individuals of the same species in the amino
acid sequences of otherwise similar immunoglobulins. These differences are determined by allelic genes, and by definition, they are
detected by antibodies made in the same species. *Idiotypes* are the third
category of antigenic determinants. They are unique to the molecules
produced by a given clone of antibody-producing cells. Idiotypes
are formed by the unique structure of the antigen-binding portion of
the molecule.

Antibody molecules (see Fig. 305-8) are composed of two heavy
chains (mol wt ~50,000) and two light chains (mol wt ~25,000).
Each chain has a constant portion (limited amino acid sequence variability) and a variable region (extensive sequence variability). The
light and heavy chains are linked by disulfide bonds and are aligned
so that their variable regions are adjacent to one another. This variable
region forms the antigen recognition site of the antibody molecule;
its unique structural features form a particular set of determinants, or
idiotypes, that are reliable markers for a particular clone of cells
because each antibody is formed and secreted by a single clone.
Each chain is specified by distinct genes, synthesized separately, and
assembled into an intact antibody molecule after translation (see Fig.
114-1). Because of the mechanics of the gene rearrangements necessary
to specify the immunoglobulin variable regions (VDJ joining for the
heavy chain, VJ joining for the light chain; see Fig. 114-1), a particular
clone rearranges only one of the two chromosomes to produce an
immunoglobulin molecule of only one light chain isotype and only
one allotype (allelic exclusion). After exposure to antigen, the variable
region may become associated with a new heavy chain isotype (class
switch). Each clone of cells performs these sequential gene arrangements in a unique way. This results in each clone producing a unique
immunoglobulin molecule. In most cells, light chains are synthesized
in slight excess, are secreted as free light chains by plasma cells, and
are cleared by the kidney, but less than 10 mg of such light chains is
excreted per day.

FIGURE 114-1   Immunoglobulin heavy chains are encoded by four distinct
genetic elements, variable (Igh-V), diversity (Igh-D), joining (Igh-J), and constant (Igh-C) genes. The variable region of the immunoglobulin heavy chain
is encoded by the V, D, and J genes. The same variable region may be associated
with any of the 10 heavy chain constant region genes. In the germline genome
(all cells except B cells) the V, D, and J genes are widely separated and exist
in numerous forms. Once a cell becomes committed to B cell differentiation,
a single V gene and a single D gene translocate to a single J gene, and the
intervening genetic material is excised (VDJ joining). The newly formed VDJ
gene is transcribed into a single message along with either an M or D isotype
C gene. Upon exposure to antigen, another rearrangement may occur so that
the VDJ gene may be associated with a G, A, or E isotype C gene. In light
chain genes there appear to be no D genes, and thus light chain variable regions
are formed by VJ joining.

Electrophoretic analysis of components of the serum proteins permits determination of the amount of immunoglobulin in the serum (Fig. 114-2). The variety of immunoglobulins move heterogeneously in an electric field and form a broad peak in the gamma region. The gamma globulin region of the electrophoretic pattern is usually increased in the sera of patients and animals with plasma cell tumors. There is a sharp spike in this region called an *M component* (M for monoclonal). Less commonly, the M component may appear in the beta$_2$ or alpha$_2$ globulin region. The antibody must be present at a concentration of at least 5 g/L (0.5 g/dL) to be detectable by this method. This corresponds to approximately 10^9 cells producing the antibody. Confirmation that such an M component is truly monoclonal relies on the use of immunoelectrophoresis that shows a single light and heavy chain type. Hence immunoelectrophoresis and electrophoresis provide qualitative and quantitative assessment of the M component, respectively. Once the presence of an M component has been confirmed, electrophoresis provides the more practical information for managing patients with monoclonal gammopathies. In a given patient, the amount of M component in the serum is a reliable measure of the tumor burden. This makes the M component an excellent tumor marker, yet it is not specific enough to be used to screen asymptomatic patients. In addition to the plasma cell disorders, M components may be detected in other lymphoid neoplasms such as chronic lymphocytic leukemia and lymphomas of B or T cell origin; nonlymphoid neoplasms such as chronic myelogenous leukemia, breast and colon cancer; a variety of nonneoplastic conditions such as cirrhosis, sarcoidosis, parasitic diseases, Gaucher's disease, and pyoderma gangrenosum; and a number of autoimmune conditions, including rheumatoid arthritis, myasthenia gravis, and cold agglutinin disease. A very rare skin disease known as lichen myxedematosus or papular mucinosis is associated with a monoclonal gammopathy. Highly cationic IgGλ is deposited in the dermis of patients with this disease. It is unclear whether this organ specificity reflects the specificity of the antibody for some antigenic component of the dermis.

The nature of the M component is variable in plasma cell disorders. It may be an intact antibody molecule of any heavy chain subclass, or it may be an altered antibody or fragment. Isolated light or heavy chains may be produced. In some plasma cell tumors such as extramedullary or solitary bone plasmacytomas, less than a third of patients will have an M component. In about 20 percent of myelomas, only light chains are produced and in most cases are secreted in the urine

as Bence Jones proteins. The frequency of myelomas of a particular heavy chain class is roughly proportional to the serum concentration, and therefore IgG myelomas are more common than IgA and IgD myelomas.

MULTIPLE MYELOMA **Definition** Multiple myeloma represents a malignant proliferation of plasma cells derived from a single clone. The terms *multiple myeloma* and *myeloma* may be used interchangeably. The tumor, its products, and the host response to it result in a number of organ dysfunctions and symptoms of bone pain or fracture, renal failure, susceptibility to infection, anemia, hypercalcemia, and occasionally clotting abnormalities, neurologic symptoms, and vascular manifestations of hyperviscosity.

Etiology The cause of myeloma is not known. Myeloma occurred with increased frequency in those exposed to the radiation of nuclear warheads in World War II after a 20-year latency. In contrast to most other B cell tumors, consistent chromosomal alterations have not been found in patients with myeloma, though cytogenetic abnormalities are noted in a substantial fraction of cases. Overexpression of *myc* or *ras* genes has been noted in some cases. Mutations in p53 and Rb-1 have also been described, but no common molecular pathogenesis has yet emerged. The murine plasmacytoma models suggest that the induction of plasmacytomas (e.g., with mineral oil injection) may require exposure to foreign antigens as well as a cellular event. Thus chronic antigenic stimulation may play a role in the transformation of a particular B cell clone. This is supported by evidence that M proteins from different persons sometimes share idiotypes. There is also some evidence for a genetic predisposition to myeloma in humans. Myeloma has been seen more commonly than expected among farmers, wood workers, leather workers, and those exposed to petroleum products. The neoplastic event in myeloma may involve cells earlier in B cell differentiation than the plasma cell. Circulating B cells bearing surface immunoglobulin that share the idiotype of the M component are present in myeloma patients. It is possible that the malignant clone escapes normal control mechanisms at a pre-plasma cell stage of differentiation and the chronic exposure to a particular antigenic stimulus drives the cell to terminal differentiation. Interleukin (IL) 6 may play a role in driving myeloma cell proliferation; a large fraction of myeloma cells exposed to IL-6 in vitro respond by proliferating. It remains difficult to distinguish benign from malignant plasma cells on the basis of morphologic criteria in all but a few cases. **(See Plate IV-27)**

Incidence and Prevalence About 14,400 cases of myeloma were diagnosed in 1996, and 10,400 people died from the disease. Myeloma increases in incidence with age. The median age at diagnosis is 68 years. It is rare under age 40. The yearly incidence is around 4 per 100,000 and remarkably similar in countries throughout the world. Males are slightly more commonly affected than females, and blacks have nearly twice the incidence of whites. In the age group over 25 the incidence is 30 per 100,000. Myeloma accounts for about 1 percent of all malignancies in whites and 2 percent in blacks; 13 percent of all hematologic cancers in whites and 33 percent in blacks.

Pathogenesis and Clinical Manifestations (Table 114-1) Bone pain is the most common symptom in myeloma, affecting nearly 70 percent of patients. The pain usually involves the back and ribs, and unlike the pain of metastatic carcinoma, which often is worse at night, the pain of myeloma is precipitated by movement. Persistent localized pain in a patient with myeloma usually signifies a pathologic fracture. The bone lesions of myeloma are caused by the proliferation of the tumor cells and the activation of osteoclasts that destroy the bone. The osteoclasts respond to osteoclast activating factors (OAF) made by the myeloma cells [OAF activity can be mediated by several cytokines, including IL-1, lymphotoxin, and tumor necrosis factor (TNF)]. However, production of these factors stops following administration of glucocorticoids or interferon (IFN)-γ. The bone lesions are lytic in nature and are rarely associated with osteoblastic new bone formation; therefore, radioisotopic bone scanning is less useful in diagnosis than

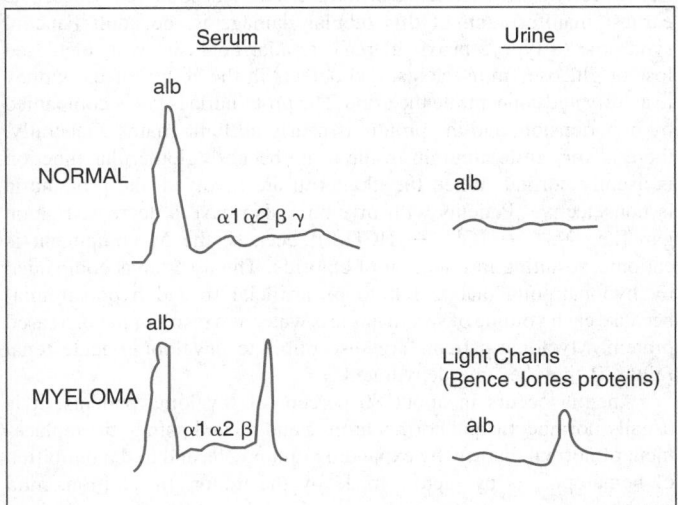

FIGURE 114-2 Representative electrophoretic patterns of serum and urine. The upper panel illustrates the normal pattern of serum and urine protein on electrophoresis. Since there are many different immunoglobulins in the serum, their differing mobilities in an electric field produce a broad peak. The lower panel illustrates the patterns of serum and urine proteins in a patient with myeloma. The predominance of a product of a single cell is reflected by a "church spire" sharp peak. The presence of free light chains in the urine is reflected in a peak as well.

Table 114-1

Pathogenesis and Clinical Manifestations of Multiple Myeloma

Clinical Finding	Underlying Cause	Pathogenic Mechanism
Hypercalcemia, pathologic fractures, cord compression, lytic bone lesions, osteoporosis, bone pain	Skeletal destruction	Tumor expansion; production of osteoclast activating factors (OAF) by tumor cells
Renal failure	Light chain proteinuria, hypercalcemia, urate nephropathy, amyloid glomerulopathy (rare) Pyelonephritis	Toxic effects of tumor products, light chains, OAF, DNA breakdown products Hypogammaglobulinemia
Anemia	Myelophthisis, decreased production, increased destruction	Tumor expansion; production of inhibitory factors and autoantibodies by tumor cells
Infection	Hypogammaglobulinemia, decreased neutrophil migration	Decreased production due to tumor-induced suppression; increased IgG catabolism
Neurologic symptoms	Hyperviscosity, cryoglobulins, amyloid deposits Hypercalcemia, cord compression	Products of tumor; properties of M component; light chains OAF
Bleeding	Interference with clotting factors, amyloid damage of endothelium, platelet dysfunction	Products of tumor; antibodies to clotting factors; light chains; antibody coating of platelets
Mass lesions		Tumor expansion

FIGURE 114-3 Bony lesions in multiple myeloma. The skull demonstrates the typical "punched out" lesions characteristic of multiple myeloma. The lesion represents a purely osteolytic lesion with little or no osteoblastic activity. *(Courtesy of Dr. Geraldine Schechter.)*

plain radiography. The bony lysis results in substantial mobilization of calcium from bone, and serious acute and chronic complications of hypercalcemia may dominate the clinical picture (see below). Localized bone lesions may expand to the point that mass lesions may be palpated, especially on the skull (Fig. 114-3), clavicles, and sternum, and the collapse of vertebrae may lead to symptoms of spinal cord compression.

The next most common clinical problem in patients with myeloma is susceptibility to bacterial infections. The most common infections are pneumonias and pyelonephritis, and the most frequent pathogens are *Streptococcus pneumoniae*, *Staphylococcus aureus*, and *Klebsiella pneumoniae* in the lungs and *Escherichia coli* and other gram-negative organisms in the urinary tract. In about 25 percent of patients, recurrent infections are the presenting features, and over 75 percent of patients will have a serious infection at some time in their course. The susceptibility to infection has several contributing causes. First, patients with myeloma have diffuse hypogammaglobulinemia if the M component is excluded. The hypogammaglobulinemia is related to both decreased production and increased destruction of normal antibodies. Moreover, some patients generate a population of circulating regulatory cells in response to their myeloma that can suppress normal antibody synthesis. In the case of IgG myeloma, normal IgG antibodies are broken down more rapidly than normal because the catabolic rate for IgG antibodies varies directly with the serum concentration. The large M component results in fractional catabolic rates of 8 to 16 percent instead of the normal 2 percent. These patients have very poor antibody responses, especially to polysaccharide antigens such as those on bacterial cell walls. Such responses are normally T cell–independent. Most measures of T cell function in myeloma are normal, but a subset of CD4+ cells may be decreased. Granulocyte lysozyme content is low, and granulocyte migration is not as rapid as normal in patients with my-

eloma, probably the result of a product of the tumor. There are also a variety of abnormalities in complement functions in myeloma patients. All these factors contribute to the immune deficiency of these patients.

Renal failure occurs in nearly 25 percent of myeloma patients, and some renal pathology is noted in over half. There are many contributing factors. Hypercalcemia is the most common cause of renal failure. Glomerular deposits of amyloid, hyperuricemia, recurrent infections, and occasional infiltration of the kidney by myeloma cells all may contribute to renal dysfunction. However, tubular damage associated with the excretion of light chains is almost always present. Normally, light chains are filtered, reabsorbed in the tubules, and catabolized. With the increase in amount of light chains presented to the tubule, the tubular cells become overloaded with these proteins, and tubular damage results either directly from light chain toxic effects or indirectly from the release of intracellular lysosomal enzymes. The earliest manifestation of this tubular damage is the adult Fanconi syndrome (a type 2 proximal renal tubular acidosis) with increased loss of glucose, amino acids, and defects in the ability of the kidney to acidify and concentrate the urine. The proteinuria is not accompanied by hypertension, and the protein is nearly all light chains. Generally, there is very little albumin in the urine because glomerular function is usually normal. When the glomeruli are involved, the proteinuria is nonselective. Patients with myeloma also have a decreased anion gap [i.e., $Na^+ - (Cl^- + HCO_3^-)$] because the M component is cationic, resulting in retention of chloride. This is often accompanied by hyponatremia that is felt to be artificial (pseudohyponatremia) because each volume of serum has less water as a result of the increased protein. Myeloma patients are susceptible to developing acute renal failure if they become dehydrated.

Anemia occurs in about 80 percent of myeloma patients. It is usually normocytic and normochromic and related both to the replacement of normal marrow by expanding tumor cells and to the inhibition of hematopoiesis by factors made by the tumor. In addition, mild hemolysis may contribute to the anemia. A larger than expected fraction of patients may have megaloblastic anemia due to either folate or vitamin B_{12} deficiency. Granulocytopenia and thrombocytopenia are very rare. Clotting abnormalities may be seen due to the failure of antibody-coated platelets to function properly or to the interaction of the M component with clotting factors I, II, V, VII, or VIII. Raynaud's phenomenon and impaired circulation may result if the M component forms cryoglobulins, and hyperviscosity syndromes may develop depending on the physical properties of the M component (most common with IgM, IgG3, and IgA paraproteins). Hyperviscosity is defined on the basis of the relative viscosity of serum as compared with water. Normal relative serum viscosity is 1.8 (i.e., serum is normally almost twice as viscous as water). Symptoms of hyperviscosity occur at a level of 5 to 6, a level usually reached at paraprotein concentrations of around 40 g/L (4 g/dL) for IgM, 50 g/L (5 g/dL) for IgG3, and 70 g/L (7 g/dL) for IgA.

Although neurologic symptoms occur in a minority of patients, they may have many causes. Hypercalcemia may produce lethargy, weakness, depression, and confusion. Hyperviscosity may lead to headache, fatigue, visual disturbances, and retinopathy. Bony damage and collapse may lead to cord compression, radicular pain, and loss of bowel and bladder control. Infiltration of peripheral nerves by amyloid can be a cause of carpal tunnel syndrome and other sensorimotor mono- and polyneuropathies.

Many of the clinical features of myeloma, e.g., cord compression, pathologic fractures, hyperviscosity, sepsis, and hypercalcemia, can present as medical emergencies. Despite the widespread distribution of plasma cells in the body, tumor expansion is dominantly within bone and bone marrow and, for reasons unknown, rarely causes enlargement of spleen, lymph nodes, or gut-associated lymphatic tissue.

Diagnosis and Staging The classic triad of myeloma is marrow plasmacytosis (>10 percent), lytic bone lesions, and a serum and/or urine M component. The diagnosis may be made in the absence of bone lesions if the plasmacytosis is associated with a progressive increase in the M component over time or if extramedullary mass lesions develop. There are two important variants of myeloma, solitary bone plasmacytoma and extramedullary plasmacytoma. These lesions are associated with an M component in fewer than 30 percent of the cases, they may affect younger individuals, and both are associated with median survivals of 10 or more years. Solitary bone plasmacytoma is a single lytic bone lesion without marrow plasmacytosis. Extramedullary plasmacytomas usually involve the submucosal lymphoid tissue of the nasopharynx or paranasal sinuses without marrow plasmacytosis. Both tumors are highly responsive to local radiation therapy. If an M component is present, it should disappear after treatment. Solitary bone plasmacytomas may recur in other bony sites or evolve into myeloma. Extramedullary plasmacytomas rarely recur or progress.

The most difficult differential diagnosis in patients with myeloma involves their separation from individuals with benign monoclonal gammopathies or monoclonal gammopathies of uncertain significance (MGUS). MGUS are vastly more common than myeloma, occurring in 1 percent of the population over age 50 and in up to 10 percent over age 75. Patients with MGUS usually have <10 percent bone marrow plasma cells; <30 g/L (3 g/dL) of M components; no urinary Bence Jones protein; and no anemia, renal failure, lytic bone lesions, or hypercalcemia. When bone marrow cells are exposed to radioactive thymidine in order to quantitate dividing cells, patients with MGUS always have a labeling index <1 percent and patients with myeloma always have a labeling index >1 percent. Other discriminators include plasma cell acid phosphatase and β-glucuronidase, both of which are low in MGUS patients, and the salmon calcitonin stimulation test, which is positive only in patients with active ongoing bone destruction. With long-term follow-up, about 25 percent of patients with MGUS go on to develop myeloma. Typically, patients with MGUS require no therapy. Their survival is about 2 years shorter than age-matched controls without MGUS.

The clinical evaluation of patients with myeloma includes a careful physical examination searching for tender bones and masses. It is paradoxical that only a small minority of patients have an enlargement of the spleen and lymph nodes, the physiologic sites of antibody production. Chest and bone radiographs may reveal lytic lesions or diffuse osteopenia. A complete blood count with differential may reveal anemia. Erythrocyte sedimentation rate is elevated. Very rare patients (~2 percent) may have plasma cell leukemia with more than 2000 plasma cells per microliter. This may be seen in disproportionate frequency in IgD (~12 percent) and IgE (~25 percent) myelomas. Serum calcium, urea nitrogen, creatinine, and uric acid levels may be elevated. Protein electrophoresis and measurement of serum immuno-

globulins are useful for detecting and characterizing M spikes, supplemented by immunoelectrophoresis, which is especially sensitive for identifying low concentrations of M components not detectable by protein electrophoresis. A 24-h urine specimen is necessary to quantitate protein excretion, and a concentrated aliquot is used for electrophoresis and immunologic typing of any M component. Serum alkaline phosphatase is usually normal even with extensive bone involvement because of the absence of osteoblastic activity. It is also important to quantitate serum β$_2$-microglobulin (see below). Serum-soluble IL-6 receptor levels and C-reactive protein may reflect physiologic IL-6 levels in the patient.

The serum M component will be IgG in 53 percent of patients, IgA in 25 percent, and IgD in 1 percent, and 20 percent of patients will have only light chains in serum and urine. Dipsticks for detecting proteinuria are not reliable at identifying light chains, and the heat test for detecting Bence Jones protein is falsely negative in about 50 percent of patients with light chain myeloma. Fewer than 1 percent of patients have no identifiable M component, and these patients usually have light chain myelomas in which renal catabolism has made the light chains undetectable in the urine. IgD myeloma may also present as light chain myeloma. About two-thirds of patients with serum M components also have urinary light chains. The light chain isotype may have an impact on survival. Patients secreting lambda light chains have a significantly shorter overall survival than those secreting kappa light chains. It is not clear whether this is due to some genetically important determinant of cell proliferation or because lambda light chains are more likely to cause renal damage and form amyloid than are kappa light chains. The heavy chain isotype may have an impact on patient management as well. About half of patients with IgM paraproteins develop hyperviscosity compared with only 2 to 4 percent of patients with IgA and IgG M components. Among IgG myelomas, it is the IgG3 subclass that has the highest tendency to form both concentration- and temperature-dependent aggregates, leading to hyperviscosity and cold agglutination at lower serum concentrations.

The staging system for patients with myeloma is a functional system for predicting survival and is based on a variety of clinical and laboratory tests, unlike the anatomic staging systems for solid tumors. Details of the staging system are given in Table 114-2. Based on the hemoglobin, calcium, M component, and degree of skeletal involvement, the total-body tumor burden is estimated to be low (stage I, <0.6 × 10^{12} cells per square meter), intermediate (stage II, 0.6 to 1.2 × 10^{12} cells per square meter), or high (stage III, >1.2 × 10^{12} cells per square meter), and the stages are further subdivided on the basis of renal function [A if serum creatinine < 177 μmol/L (<2 mg/dL), B if > 177 (>2)]. Patients in stage IA have a median survival of more than 5 years and those in stage IIIB about 15 months. β$_2$-Microglobulin is a protein of 11,000 mol wt with homologies with the constant region of immunoglobulins that is the light chain of the class I major histocompatibility antigens (HLA-A, -B, -C) on the surface of every cell. Serum β$_2$-microglobulin is the single most powerful predictor of survival and can substitute for staging. Patients with β$_2$-microglobulin levels less than 0.004 g/L have a median survival of 43 months and those with levels higher than 0.004 g/L only 12 months. It is also felt that once the diagnosis of myeloma is firm, histologic features of atypia may also exert an influence on prognosis. IL-6 may be an autocrine and/or paracrine growth factor for myeloma cells; elevated levels are associated with more aggressive disease. High labeling index and high levels of lactate dehydrogenase and thymidine kinase are also associated with poor prognosis.

℞ TREATMENT

About 10 percent of patients with myeloma will have an indolent course demonstrating only very slow progression of disease over many years. Such patients only require antitumor therapy when the serum myeloma protein level rises above 50 g/L (5 g/dL) or

Table 114-2

Myeloma Staging System

Stage	Criteria	Estimated Tumor Burden, $\times 10^{12}$ cells/m^2

I	All the following:
	1. Hemoglobin >100 g/L (>10 g/dL)
	2. Serum calcium <3 mmol/L (<12 mg/dL)
	3. Normal bone x-ray or solitary lesion
	4. Low M-component production
	   a. IgG level <50 g/L (<5 g/dL)
	   b. IgA level <30 g/L (<3 g/dL)
	   c. Urine light chain <4 g/24 h
		<0.6 (low)

II	Fitting neither I nor III	0.6–1.20 (intermediate)

III	One or more of the following:
	1. Hemoglobin <85 g/L (<8.5 g/dL)
	2. Serum calcium >3 mmol/L (>12 mg/dL)
	3. Advanced lytic bone lesions
	4. High M-component production
	   a. IgG level >70 g/L (>7 g/dL)
	   b. IgA level >50 g/L (>5 g/dL)
	   c. Urine light chains >12 g/24 h
		>1.20 (high)

SUBCLASSIFICATION BASED ON SERUM CREATININE LEVELS

Level	Stage	Median Survival, Months
A < 177 µmol/L (<2 mg/dL)	IA	61
B > 177 µmol/L (>2 mg/dL)	IIA,B	55
	IIIA	30
	IIIB	15

STAGING BASED ON SERUM β$_2$-MICROGLOBULIN LEVELS

Level	Stage	Median Survival, Months
<0.004 g/L (<4 µg/mL)	I	43
>0.004 g/L (>4 µg/mL)	II	12

progressive bone lesions develop. Patients with solitary bone plasmacytomas and extramedullary plasmacytomas may be expected to enjoy prolonged disease-free survival after local radiation therapy to a dose of around 40 Gy. There is a low incidence of occult marrow involvement in patients with solitary bone plasmacytoma. Such patients are usually detected because their serum M component falls slowly or disappears initially only to return after a few months. These patients respond well to systemic chemotherapy.

The vast majority of patients with myeloma require therapeutic intervention. In general, such therapy is of two sorts: systemic chemotherapy to control the progression of myeloma, and symptomatic supportive care to prevent serious morbidity from the complications of the disease. All patients with stage II or III disease and stage I patients exhibiting Bence Jones proteinuria, progressive lytic bone lesions, vertebral compression fractures, recurrent infections, or rising serum M component should be treated with systemic combination chemotherapy. Therapy can prolong and improve the quality of life for myeloma patients.

The standard treatment has consisted of intermittent pulses of an alkylating agent [L-phenylalanine mustard (L-PAM, melphalan), cyclophosphamide, or chlorambucil] and prednisone administered for 4 to 7 days every 4 to 6 weeks. The alkylating agents appear to be roughly equally active, but resistance to one agent is often accompanied by resistance to the others. The usual doses are as follows: melphalan, 8 mg/m^2 of body surface area per day; cyclophosphamide, 200 mg/m^2 per day; chlorambucil, 8 mg/m^2 per day; prednisone, 25 to 60 mg/m^2 per day. Melphalan is used most commonly, but because of their near equivalence in antitumor efficacy,

we favor cyclophosphamide as the alkylating agent because it is less toxic to the marrow stem cell compartment and results in a lower incidence of acute myelodysplastic syndromes than do the other alkylating agents. Doses may need adjustment based on marrow tolerance. However, there are few constraints on the dose of the steroid pulse, and it appears that more is better. Patients responding to therapy generally have a prompt and gratifying reduction in bone pain, hypercalcemia, and anemia and often have fewer infections. The serum M component lags substantially behind the symptomatic improvement, often taking 4 to 6 weeks to fall. This fall depends on the rate of tumor kill and the fractional catabolic rate of immunoglobulin, which in turn depends on the serum concentration (for IgG). Light chain excretion, with a functional half-life of approximately 6 h, may fall within the first week of treatment. However, since urine light chain levels may relate to renal tubular function, they are not a reliable measure of tumor cell kill. Calculations of tumor cell kill are made by extrapolation of the serum M component level and rely heavily on the assumption that every tumor cell produces immunoglobulin at a constant rate. About 60 percent of patients will achieve at least a 75 percent reduction in serum M component level and tumor cell mass in response to an alkylating agent and prednisone. Although this is a tumor reduction of less than one log, clinical responses may last many months. The important feature of the level of the M protein is not how far or how fast it falls, but the rate of its increase after therapy. Efforts to improve the fraction of patients responding and the degree of response have involved adding other active chemotherapeutic agents to the treatment program. Patients with more advanced disease may benefit most from such an approach. High-dose therapy with hematopoietic support is also being tested in younger patients. Sequential treatment with combination chemotherapy regimens followed by two successive high-dose melphalan treatments, each supported with peripheral blood stem cell transplants, have achieved complete responses in 50 percent of patients treated within a year of diagnosis. Complete responses are rare (<10 percent) with standard therapy. Long-term follow-up is not yet available. Allogeneic transplants may also produce high response rates, but treatment-related mortality may be as high as 40 percent.

The ideal duration of therapy has not been determined. Most physicians treat every 4 to 6 weeks for 1 or 2 years. Cessation of therapy is followed by relapse, usually within a year. Retreatment may be associated with a second response in up to 80 percent of patients. Maintenance therapy (e.g., with IFNα) may prolong the duration of response, but this therapy is toxic and has generally not prolonged survival. The regrowth rate of the tumor during relapse accelerates with each relapse. This observation suggests that kinetic resistance to therapy (i.e., increase in cycling cells) is perhaps more important than drug resistance controlled by mdr-1 expression. Patients often respond to treatment, but the length of the response progressively shortens. Patients primarily resistant to initial therapy have a median survival of less than a year. High-dose pulsed steroids used alone (200 mg prednisone every other day or 1 g/m^2 per day methylprednisolone for 5 days) or VAD combination chemotherapy (vincristine, 0.4 mg/d in a 4-day continuous infusion; doxorubicin, 9 mg/m^2 per day in a 4-day continuous infusion; dexamethasone, 40 mg/d for 4 days per week for 3 weeks) may offer useful palliation in patients resistant to primary therapy.

About 15 percent of patients die within the first 3 months after diagnosis, and subsequently, the death rate is about 15 percent per year. The disease usually follows a chronic course for 2 to 5 years before developing an acute terminal phase, usually marked by the development of pancytopenia with a cellular marrow that is refractory to treatment. Widespread organ infiltration by myeloma cells occurs, and survival is less than 6 months. About 46 percent of patients die in the chronic phase of disease from progressive myeloma (16 percent) and renal failure (10 percent), sepsis (14 percent), or both (6 percent). Death in the acute terminal phase (26 percent) is chiefly from progressive myeloma (13 percent) and sepsis (9 percent). Five percent of patients die of acute leukemia, myeloblastic or monocytic, and although it has been debated that this is related to the primary disease, it appears more likely to be the result of chronic therapy with alkylating agents. Nearly 23 percent of patients die of myocardial infarction, chronic lung disease, diabetes, or stroke, all intercurrent illnesses related more to the age of the patient group than to the tumor.

Supportive care directed at the anticipated complications of the disease may be as important as primary antitumor therapy. The hypercalcemia generally responds well to glucocorticoid therapy, hydration, and natriuresis. Calcitonin may add to the inhibitory effects of steroids on bone resorption. Bisphosphonates (e.g., pamidronate 90 mg once a month) reduce osteoclastic bone resorption and preserve performance status and quality of life. Treatments aimed at strengthening the skeleton, such as fluorides, calcium, and vitamin D, with or without androgens, have been suggested but are not of proven efficacy. Iatrogenic worsening of renal function may be prevented by the use of allopurinol during chemotherapy to avoid urate nephropathy and by maintaining a high fluid intake to prevent dehydration and to help excrete light chains and calcium. In the event of acute renal failure, plasmapheresis is approximately 10 times more effective at clearing light chains than peritoneal dialysis, and acutely reducing the protein load may result in functional improvement. Urinary tract infections should be watched for and treated early. Chronic dialysis probably should not be initiated in patients who have failed to respond to antitumor therapy. Plasmapheresis may be the treatment of choice for hyperviscosity syndromes. Although the pneumococcus is a dreaded pathogen in myeloma patients, pneumococcal polysaccharide vaccines may not elicit an antibody response. The advent of intravenous gamma globulin preparations raises some hope that prophylactic administration may prevent some serious infections, but this has not been tested. Chronic oral antibiotic prophylaxis is probably not warranted. Patients developing neurologic symptoms in the lower extremities, severe localized back pain, or problems with bowel and bladder control may need emergency myelography and radiation therapy for palliation. Most bone lesions respond to analgesics and chemotherapy, but certain painful lesions may respond most promptly to localized radiation. The chronic anemia may respond to hematinics (iron, folate, cobalamin), and some have responded to androgens. The pathogenesis of the anemia should be established and specific therapy instituted, where possible.

WALDENSTRÖM'S MACROGLOBULINEMIA In 1948, Waldenström described a malignancy of lymphoplasmacytoid cells that secreted IgM. In contrast to myeloma, the disease was associated with lymphadenopathy and hepatosplenomegaly, but the major clinical manifestation was the hyperviscosity syndrome. The disease resembles the related diseases chronic lymphocytic leukemia, myeloma, and lymphocytic lymphoma. Waldenström's macroglobulinemia and IgM myeloma both follow a similar clinical course. The diagnosis of IgM myeloma is usually reserved for patients with lytic bone lesions and is important only because of the hazard of pathologic fractures.

The cause of macroglobulinemia is unknown. The disease is similar to myeloma in being slightly more common in men and occurring with increased incidence with age (median 64 years). There have been reports that the IgM in some patients with macroglobulinemia may have specificity for myelin-associated glycoprotein (MAG), a protein that has been associated with demyelinating disease of the peripheral nervous system and may be lost earlier and to a greater extent than the better known myelin basic protein in patients with multiple sclerosis. Sometimes patients with macroglobulinemia develop a peripheral neuropathy before the appearance of the neoplasm. There is speculation that the whole process begins with a viral infection that may elicit an antibody response that cross-reacts with a normal tissue component.

Like myeloma, the disease involves the bone marrow, but unlike myeloma, it does not cause bone lesions or hypercalcemia. Like myeloma, a serum M component is present in the serum in excess of 30 g/L (3 g/dL), but unlike myeloma, the size of the IgM paraprotein results in little renal excretion and only around 20 percent of patients excrete light chains. Therefore, renal disease is not common. The light chain isotype is kappa in 80 percent of the cases. Patients present with weakness, fatigue, and recurrent infections, similar to myeloma patients, but epistaxis, visual disturbances, and neurologic symptoms such as peripheral neuropathy, dizziness, headache, and transient paresis are much more common in macroglobulinemia. Physical examination reveals adenopathy and hepatosplenomegaly, and ophthalmoscopic examination may reveal vascular segmentation and dilatation of the retinal veins characteristic of hyperviscosity states. Patients may have a normocytic, normochromic anemia, but rouleaux formation and a positive Coombs' test are much more common than in myeloma. Malignant lymphocytes are usually present in the peripheral blood. About 10 percent of macroglobulins are cryoglobulins. These are pure M components and are not the mixed cryoglobulins seen in rheumatoid arthritis and other autoimmune diseases. Mixed cryoglobulins are composed of IgM or IgA complexed with IgG, for which they are specific. In both cases, Raynaud's phenomenon and serious vascular symptoms precipitated by the cold may occur, but mixed cryoglobulins are not commonly associated with malignancy. Patients suspected of having a cryoglobulin based on history and physical examination should have their blood drawn into a warm syringe and delivered to the laboratory in a container of warm water to avoid errors in quantitating the cryoglobulin.

℞ TREATMENT

Control of serious hyperviscosity symptoms such as an altered state of consciousness or paresis can be achieved acutely by plasmapheresis because 80 percent of the IgM paraprotein is intravascular. Fludarabine (25 mg/m^2 per day for 5 days every 4 weeks) or cladribine (0.1 mg/kg per day for 7 days every 4 weeks) are highly effective single agents. About 80 percent of patients respond to chemotherapy, and their median survival is over 3 years. The absence of other serious organ toxicities results in a longer life span of patients with macroglobulinemia compared with those with myeloma.

POEMS SYNDROME The features of this syndrome are *p*olyneuropathy, *o*rganomegaly, *e*ndocrinopathy, *m*ultiple myeloma, and *s*kin changes (POEMS). Patients usually have a severe, progressive sensorimotor polyneuropathy associated with sclerotic bone lesions from myeloma. Polyneuropathy occurs in about 1.4 percent of myelomas, but the POEMS syndrome is only a rare subset of that group. Unlike typical myeloma, hepatomegaly and lymphadenopathy occur in about two-thirds of patients and splenomegaly is seen in one-third. The lymphadenopathy frequently resembles Castleman's disease histologically, a condition that has been linked to IL-6 overproduction. The endocrine manifestations include amenorrhea in women and impotence and gynecomastia in men. Hyperprolactinemia due to loss of normal inhibitory control by the hypothalamus may be associated with other central nervous system manifestations such as papilledema and elevated cerebrospinal fluid pressure and protein. Type 2 diabetes mellitus occurs in about one-third of patients. Hypothyroidism and adrenal insufficiency are occasionally noted. Skin changes are diverse: hyperpigmentation, hypertrichosis, skin thickening, and digital clubbing. Other manifestations include peripheral edema, ascites, pleural effusions, fever, and thrombocytosis.

The pathogenesis of the disease is unclear, but high circulating levels of the proinflammatory cytokines IL-1β, IL-6, and TNFα have been documented and levels of the inhibitory cytokine transforming growth factor β (TGFβ) are lower than expected. Treatment of the myeloma may result in an improvement in the other disease manifestations.

HEAVY CHAIN DISEASES The heavy chain diseases are rare lymphoplasmacytic malignancies. Their clinical manifestations vary with the heavy chain isotype. Patients secrete a defective heavy chain that usually has an intact Fc fragment and a deletion in the Fd region. Gamma, alpha, and mu heavy chain diseases have been described, but no reports of delta or epsilon heavy chain diseases have appeared. Molecular biologic analysis of these tumors has revealed structural genetic defects that may account for the aberrant chain secreted.

Gamma Heavy Chain Disease (Franklin's Disease) This disease affects people of widely different age groups and countries of origin. It is characterized by lymphadenopathy, fever, anemia, malaise, hepatosplenomegaly, and weakness. Its most distinctive symptom is palatal edema, resulting from node involvement of Waldeyer's ring, and this may progress to produce respiratory compromise. The diagnosis depends on the demonstration of an anomalous serum M component [often <20 g/L (<2 g/dL)] that reacts with anti-IgG but not anti-light chain reagents. *The M component is typically present in both serum and urine.* Most of the paraproteins have been of the gamma₁ subclass, but other subclasses have been seen. The patients may have thrombocytopenia, eosinophilia, and nondiagnostic bone marrow. Patients usually have a rapid downhill course and die of infection; however, some patients have survived 5 years with chemotherapy.

Alpha Heavy Chain Disease (Seligmann's Disease) This is the most common of the heavy chain diseases. It is closely related to a malignancy known as *Mediterranean lymphoma*, a disease that affects young people in parts of the world such as the Mediterranean, Asia, and South America in which intestinal parasites are common. The disease is characterized by an infiltration of the lamina propria of the small intestine with lymphoplasmacytoid cells that secrete truncated alpha chains. Demonstrating alpha heavy chains is difficult because the alpha chains tend to polymerize and appear as a smear instead of a sharp peak on electrophoretic profiles. Despite the polymerization, hyperviscosity is not a common problem in alpha heavy chain disease. Without J chain–facilitated dimerization, viscosity does not increase dramatically. Light chains are absent from serum and urine. The patients present with chronic diarrhea, weight loss, and malabsorption and have extensive mesenteric and paraaortic adenopathy. Respiratory tract involvement occurs rarely. Patients may vary widely in their clinical course. Some may develop diffuse aggressive histologies of malignant lymphoma. Chemotherapy may produce long-term remissions. Rare patients appear to have responded to antibiotic therapy, raising the question of the etiologic role of antigenic stimulation perhaps by some chronic intestinal infection. Chemotherapy plus antibiotics may be more effective than chemotherapy alone.

Mu Heavy Chain Disease The secretion of isolated mu heavy chains into the serum appears to occur in a very rare subset of patients with chronic lymphocytic leukemia. The only features that may distinguish patients with mu heavy chain disease are the presence of vacuoles in the malignant lymphocytes and the excretion of kappa light chains in the urine. The diagnosis requires ultracentrifugation or gel filtration to confirm the nonreactivity of the paraprotein with the light chain reagents because some intact macroglobulins fail to interact with these serums. The tumor cells seem to have a defect in the assembly of light and heavy chains because they appear to contain both in their cytoplasm. There is no evidence that such patients should be treated differently from other patients with chronic lymphocytic leukemia (see Chap. 113).

BIBLIOGRAPHY

ALEXANIAN R, DIMOPOULOS M: The treatment of multiple myeloma. N Engl J Med 330:484, 1994

ATTAL M et al: A prospective, randomized trial of autologous bone marrow transplantation and chemotherapy in multiple myeloma. N Engl J Med 335:91, 1996

BERENSON JR et al: Efficacy of pamidronate in reducing skeletal events in patients with advanced multiple myeloma. N Engl J Med 334:488, 1996

DIMOPOULOS MA, ALEXANIAN R: Waldenström's macroglobulinemia. Blood 83:1452, 1994

GHERARDI RK et al: Overproduction of proinflammatory cytokines imbalanced by their antagonists in POEMS syndrome. Blood 87:1458, 1996

GREGORY WM et al: Combination chemotherapy versus melphalan and prednisone in the treatment of multiple myeloma: An overview of published trials. J Clin Oncol 10:334, 1992

GRIEPP PR: Prognosis in myeloma. Mayo Clin Proc 69:895, 1994

HOLLAND J et al: Plasmacytoma. Treatment results and conversion to myeloma. Cancer 69:1513, 1992

KYLE RA: "Benign" monoclonal gammopathy—after 20–35 years of follow-up. Mayo Clin Proc 68:26, 1993

——— (ed): Myeloma and related disorders, in *Neoplastic Diseases of the Blood*. New York, Churchill Livingstone, 1996, pp 411–705

LUST JA: Role of cytokines in the pathogenesis of monoclonal gammopathies. Mayo Clin Proc 69:691, 1994

NORDIC MYELOMA STUDY GROUP: Interferon-α2b added to melphalan-prednisone for initial and maintenance therapy in multiple myeloma. A randomized, controlled trial. Ann Intern Med 124:212, 1996

VESOLE DH et al: High-dose therapy for refractory multiple myeloma: Improved prognosis with better supportive care and double transplants. Blood 85:950, 1994

115   *Jeffery S. Dzieczkowski, Kenneth C. Anderson*

TRANSFUSION BIOLOGY AND THERAPY

BLOOD GROUP ANTIGENS AND ANTIBODIES

The study of red blood cell (RBC) antigens and antibodies reactive with them forms the foundation of transfusion medicine. Serologic studies initially characterized these antigens, but now the molecular composition and structure of many are known. These antigens are assigned to blood group systems based upon the structure and the similarity of the determinant epitopes. The composition of antigens may be carbohydrate or protein. Other cellular blood elements and plasma proteins are also antigenic and can result in *alloimmunization*, the production of antibodies directed against the blood group antigens of another individual. These antibodies are called *alloantibodies*.

Antibodies directed against RBC antigens may result from "natural" exposure, particularly to carbohydrates that mimic some blood group antigens. Those antibodies that occur via natural stimuli are usually produced by a T cell–independent response (thus, generating no memory) and are IgM isotype. *Autoantibodies* (antibodies against autologous blood group antigens) arise spontaneously or as the result of infectious sequelae (e.g., from *Mycoplasma pneumoniae*) and are also often IgM. These antibodies are often clinically insignificant due to their low affinity for antigen at body temperature. However, IgM antibodies can activate the complement cascade and result in hemolysis. Antibodies that result from allogeneic exposure, such as transfusion or pregnancy, are usually IgG. IgG antibodies commonly bind to antigen at warmer temperatures and may hemolyze RBCs. Unlike IgM antibodies, IgG antibodies can cross the placenta and bind fetal erythrocytes bearing the corresponding antigen, resulting in hemolytic disease of the newborn, or *hydrops fetalis*.

Alloimmunization to leukocytes, platelets, and plasma proteins may also result in transfusion complications such as fevers and urticaria but generally does not cause hemolysis. Assay for these other alloantibodies is not routinely performed; however, they may be detected using special assays.

ABO ANTIGENS AND ANTIBODIES The first blood group antigen system, recognized in 1900, was ABO, the most important in transfusion medicine. The major blood groups of this system are A, B, AB, and O. The latter includes red cells that lack A or B antigens. These antigens are carbohydrates attached to a precursor backbone, may be found on the cellular membrane either as glycosphingolipids or glycoproteins, and are secreted into plasma and body fluids as glycoproteins. H substance is the immediate precursor upon which the A and B antigens are added. This H substance is formed by the addition of fucose to the glycolipid or glycoprotein backbone. The subsequent addition of *N*-acetylgalactosamine creates the A antigen, while the addition of galactose produces the B antigen.

The genes that determine the A and B phenotypes are found on chromosome 9p and are expressed in a Mendelian codominant manner. The gene products are glycosyl transferases, which confer the enzymatic capability of attaching the specific antigenic carbohydrate. Individuals who lack the "A" and "B" transferases are phenotypically type

"O," while those who inherit both transferases are type "AB." Rare individuals lack the H gene, which codes for fucose transferase, and cannot form H substance. These individuals are homozygous for the silent h allele (hh) and have Bombay phenotype (O_h).

The ABO blood group system is important because essentially all individuals produce antibodies to the ABH carbohydrate antigen that they lack. The naturally occurring anti-A and anti-B antibodies are termed *isoagglutinins*. Thus, type A individuals produce anti-B, while type B individuals make anti-A. Neither isoagglutinin is found in type AB individuals, while type O individuals produce both anti-A and anti-B. Thus, persons with type AB are "universal recipients" because they do not have antibodies against any ABO phenotype, while persons with type O blood can donate to essentially all recipients because their cells are not recognized by any ABO isoagglutinins. The rare individuals with Bombay phenotype produce antibodies to H substance (which is present on all red cells except those of hh phenotype) as well as to both A and B antigens and are therefore compatible only with other hh donors.

In most people, A and B antigens are secreted by the cells and are present in the circulation. Nonsecretors are susceptible to a variety of infections (e.g., *Candida albicans*, *Neisseria meningitidis*, *Streptococcus pneumoniae*, *Haemophilus influenzae*). Many organisms may bind to polysaccharides on cells; soluble blood group antigens may block this binding.

Rh SYSTEM The Rh system is the second most important blood group system in pretransfusion testing. The Rh antigens are found on a 30- to 32-kDa RBC membrane protein, which has no defined function. Although more than 40 different antigens in the Rh system have been described, five determinants account for the vast majority of phenotypes. The presence of the D antigen confers Rh "positivity," while people who lack the D antigen are Rh negative. Two allelic antigen pairs, E/e and C/c, are also found on the Rh protein. The three Rh genes, E/e, D, and C/c, are arranged in tandem on chromosome 1 and inherited as a haplotype, i.e., cDE or Cde. Two haplotypes can result in the phenotypic expression of two to five Rh antigens.

The D antigen is a potent alloantigen. About 15 percent of people lack this antigen. Exposure of these Rh-negative people to even small amounts of Rh-positive cells, by either transfusion or pregnancy, can result in the production of anti-D alloantibody.

OTHER BLOOD GROUP SYSTEMS AND ALLOANTIBODIES There are more than 100 recognized blood group systems, composed of more than 500 antigens. The presence or absence of certain antigens has been associated with various diseases and anomalies; antigens also act as receptors for infectious agents. Alloantibodies of importance in routine clinical practice, and their respective antigens, are listed in Table 115-1.

Antibodies to *Lewis system* carbohydrate antigens are the most common cause of incompatibility during pretransfusion screening. The Lewis gene product is a fucosyl transferase and maps to chromosome 19. The antigen is not an integral membrane structure but is adsorbed to the RBC membrane from the plasma. Antibodies to Lewis antigens are usually IgM and cannot cross the placenta. Lewis antigens may be adsorbed onto tumor cells and may be targets of therapy.

I system antigens are also oligosaccharides related to H, A, B, and Le. I and i are not allelic pairs but are carbohydrate antigens that differ only in the extent of branching. The i antigen is an unbranched chain that is converted by the I gene product, a glycosyltransferase, into a branched chain. The branching process affects all the ABH antigens, which become progressively more branched in the first 2 years of life. Some patients with cold agglutinin disease or lymphomas can produce anti-I autoantibodies that cause RBC destruction. Occasional patients with mononucleosis or *Mycoplasma* pneumonia may develop cold agglutinins of either anti-I or anti-i specificity. Most adults lack i expression; thus, finding a donor for patients with anti-i is not difficult. Even though most adults express I antigen, binding is generally low at body temperature. Thus, administration of warm blood prevents isoagglutination.

The *P system* is another group of carbohydrate antigens controlled by specific glycosyltransferases. Its clinical significance is in rare cases of syphilis and viral infection that lead to paroxysmal cold hemoglobinuria. In these cases, an unusual autoantibody to P is produced that binds to RBCs in the cold and fixes complement upon warming. Antibodies with these biphasic properties are called *Donath-Landsteiner antibodies*. The P antigen is also expressed on urothelial cells and may be a receptor for *Escherichia coli* binding.

The *MNSsU system* is regulated by genes on chromosome 4. M and N are determinants on glycophorin A, an RBC membrane protein, and S and s are determinants on glycophorin B. Anti-S and anti-s IgG antibodies may develop after pregnancy or transfusion and lead to hemolysis. Anti-U antibodies are rare but create a situation in which virtually every donor is incompatible because nearly all persons express U.

The *Kell* protein is very large (720 amino acids) and its secondary structure contains many different antigens. The immunogenicity of Kell is third behind the ABO and Rh systems. The absence of the Kell precursor protein (controlled by a gene on X) is associated with acanthocytosis, shortened RBC survival, and a progressive form of muscular dystrophy that includes cardiac defects. This rare condition is called the *McLeod phenotype*. The K_x gene is linked to the 91-kDa component of the NADPH-oxidase on the X chromosome, deletion or mutation of which accounts for about 60 percent of cases of chronic granulomatous disease.

The *Duffy* antigens are codominant alleles, Fy^a and Fy^b, that also serve as receptors for *Plasmodium vivax*. More than 70 percent of persons in malaria-endemic areas lack these antigens, probably as a result of selective influences of the infection on the population.

The *Kidd* antigens, Jk^a and Jk^b, may elicit antibodies transiently. A delayed hemolytic transfusion reaction that occurs with blood tested as compatible is often related to delayed appearance of anti-Jk^a.

PRETRANSFUSION TESTING

Pretransfusion testing of a potential recipient consists of the "type and screen." The "forward type" determines the ABO and Rh phenotype of the recipient by using reagent antisera directed against the A, B, and D antigens. The "reverse type" detects isoagglutinins in the patient's serum and should correlate with the ABO phenotype, or forward type.

The alloantibody screen identifies antibodies directed against other RBC antigens. The detection and characterization of alloantibodies before transfusion is important to ensure the selection of antigen-negative red cell components. The alloantibody screen is performed by mixing patient serum with type O RBC that contain the major antigens of most blood group systems and whose extended phenotype is known. The specificity of the alloantibody is identified by correlating the presence or absence of antigen with the results of the agglutination.

Cross matching is ordered when there is a high probability that the patient will require a packed RBC transfusion. Blood selected for cross matching must be ABO compatible and lack antigens for which

Table 115-1

RBC Blood Group Systems and Alloantigens

Blood Group System	Antigen	Alloantibody	Clinical Significance
Rh (D, C/c, E/e)	RBC protein	IgG	HTR, HDN
Lewis (Le^a, Le^b)	Oligosaccharide	IgM/IgG	Rare HTR
Kell (K/k)	RBC protein	IgG	HTR, HDN
Duffy (Fy^a/Fy^b)	RBC protein	IgG	HTR, HDN
Kidd (Jk^a/Jk^b)	RBC protein	IgG	HTR (often delayed), HDN (mild)
I/i	Carbohydrate	IgM	None
MNSsU	RBC protein	IgM/IgG	Anti-M rare HDN, anti-S, -s, and -U HDN, HTR

NOTE: RBC, red blood cell; HDN, hemolytic disease of the newborn; HTR, hemolytic transfusion reaction.

the patient has clinically significant alloantibodies. Nonreactive cross matching confirms the absence of any major incompatibility and reserves that unit for the patient.

In the case of Rh-negative patients, every attempt must be made to provide Rh-negative blood components to prevent alloimmunization to the D antigen. In an emergency, Rh-positive blood can be safely transfused to a Rh-negative patient who lacks anti-D; however, the recipient is then at risk for becoming alloimmunized and producing anti-D. Rh-negative women with child-bearing potential who are inadvertently transfused with products containing Rh-positive RBCs should receive passive immunization with anti-D (RhoGam or WinRho) to reduce or prevent sensitization.

BLOOD COMPONENTS

Blood products intended for transfusion are routinely collected as whole blood (450 mL) in various anticoagulants. Most donated blood is processed into components: packed red blood cells (PRBC), platelets, and fresh frozen plasma (FFP) or cryoprecipitate (Table 115-2). Whole blood is first separated into PRBC and platelet-rich plasma by slow centrifugation. The platelet-rich plasma is then centrifuged at high speed to yield one unit of random donor (RD) platelets and one unit of FFP. Cryoprecipitate is produced from FFP by slowly thawing to precipitate the plasma proteins, which are then separated by centrifugation.

Apheresis technology, in addition to its therapeutic applications, is used for the collection of multiple units of platelets from a single donor. These single-donor apheresis platelets (SDAP) contain the equivalent of at least six units of RD units and often have fewer contaminating leukocytes than pooled RD platelets.

Plasma may also be collected by apheresis. Plasma derivatives such as albumin, intravenous immunoglobulin, antithrombin 3, and coagulation factor concentrates are prepared from very large plasma pools (~20,000 donors per pool) but are unlikely to transmit infections because of the use of various methods of postcollection sterilization.

WHOLE BLOOD Whole blood provides both oxygen-carrying capacity and volume expansion. It is the ideal component for patients who have sustained acute hemorrhage of 25 percent or greater total blood volume loss. Whole blood is stored at 4°C to maintain erythrocyte viability, but platelet dysfunction and degradation of some coagulation factors occurs. In addition, 2,3-BPG levels fall over time, leading to an increase in the oxygen affinity of the hemoglobin and a decreased capacity to deliver oxygen to the tissues, a problem with all red cell storage. Whole blood is not readily available because of the need to process blood into components that can be used for different recipients.

PACKED RED BLOOD CELLS This product increases oxygen-carrying capacity in the anemic patient. Adequate oxygenation can be maintained with a hemoglobin content of 70 g/L in the well-perfused patient (normovolemic, able to increase cardiac output); however, comorbid factors often necessitate transfusion at a higher threshold. The decision to transfuse should be guided by the clinical situation and not by an arbitrary laboratory value.

PRBC may be modified to prevent or reduce the incidence of certain adverse reactions. Contaminating donor leukocytes are responsible for inducing fevers in the recipient and causing alloimmunization to HLA antigens. Contaminating leukocytes can be removed by several methods, with varying degrees of success. These methods include filtration and centrifugation. Although bedside filtration is the most popular method of leukocyte depletion and removes 99.9 percent of donor leukocytes, recent studies suggest it may not be effective in avoiding reactions or alloimmunization. Due to the difficulty of quality control of bedside filtration and the evolving role of cytokines that accumulate during storage of cellular blood components in mediating transfusion reactions, leukoreduction is more commonly being done in the blood bank before storage of cellular components.

Donor plasma may cause transfusion complications such as allergic reactions. Plasma can be removed from cellular blood components by washing.

PLATELETS Thrombocytopenia is a risk factor for hemorrhage, and platelet transfusion has been shown to reduce the incidence of bleeding. While the threshold for prophylactic platelet transfusion remains controversial, 10,000 to 20,000/μL has been widely used. Recently, 5000/μL has been suggested as sufficient to prevent spontaneous hemorrhage. However, 50,000/μL platelets is the usual minimum target level for hemostasis during invasive procedures.

Platelets are given either as pools prepared from five to eight RD or as SDAP from a single donor. In an unsensitized patient without increased platelet consumption [splenomegaly, fever, disseminated intravascular coagulation (DIC)], six to eight units of RD platelets are pooled and transfused, and each unit is anticipated to increase the platelet count 5000 to 10,000/μL. Patients who have received multiple transfusions are exposed to many HLA- and platelet-specific antigens, which may result in alloimmunization. These sensitized patients often have little or no increase in their posttransfusion platelet counts and are thus considered to be refractory. Patients who are anticipated to require multiple transfusions are best served by receiving SDAP and leukocyte-reduced components to lower the risk of alloimmunization.

Refractoriness to platelet transfusion may be evaluated using the corrected count increment (CCI):

$$\text{CCI} = \frac{\text{posttransfusion count} - \text{pretransfusion count}}{\text{number of platelets transfused} \times 10^{11}} \times \text{BSA}$$

where BSA is body surface area measured in square metres. The posttransfusion count performed 1 h after the transfusion is acceptable if the CCI is 10×10^9/mL, and after 18 to 24 h an increment of 7.5×10^9/mL is expected. Patients who have suboptimal responses are likely to have received multiple transfusions and have antibodies directed against class I HLA antigens. Refractoriness can be investigated by detecting anti-HLA antibodies in the recipient's serum. Patients who are sensitized will often react with 100 percent of the lymphocytes used for the HLA-antibody screen, and HLA-matched SDAP should be considered for those patients who require transfusion. Although ABO-identical HLA-matched SDAP provide the best chance for increasing the platelet count, locating these products is difficult. Additional clinical causes for a low platelet CCI should be considered, such as fever, bleeding, splenomegaly, DIC, or medications in the recipient.

FRESH FROZEN PLASMA FFP contains stable coagulation factors and plasma proteins: fibrinogen, antithrom-

Table 115-2

Characteristics of Selected Blood Components

Component	Volume, mL	Content	Clinical Response
PRBC	180–200	RBCs with variable leukocyte content and small amount of plasma	Increase hemoglobin 10 g/L and hematocrit 3%
Platelets	50–70	5.5×10^{10}/RD unit	Increase platelet count 5000–10,000/μL
	200–400	$\geq 3.0 \times 10^{11}$/SDAP product	CCI $\geq 10 \times 10^9$/L within 1 h and $\geq 7.5 \times 10^9$/L within 24 h posttransfusion
FFP	200–250	Plasma proteins—coagulation factors, proteins C and S, antithrombin	Increases coagulation factors about 2%
Cryoprecipitate	10–15	Cold-insoluble plasma proteins, fibrinogen, factor VIII, vWF	Topical fibrin glue, also 80 IU factor VIII

NOTE: PRBC, packed red blood cells; RBC, red blood cell; CCI, corrected count increment; FFP, fresh frozen plasma; vWF, von Willebrand factor.

bin, albumin, as well as proteins C and S. Indications for FFP transfusion include correction of coagulopathies, including the rapid reversal of coumadin; supplying deficient plasma proteins; and treatment of thrombotic thrombocytopenic purpura. Although FFP is an excellent volume expander, it should not be routinely used in this role. FFP is an acellular component and therefore does not transmit intracellular infections, i.e., cytomegalovirus (CMV). Patients who are IgA-deficient and require plasma support should receive FFP collected from IgA-deficient donors because the risk of anaphylaxis is increased with normal donors (see below).

CRYOPRECIPITATE Cryoprecipitate is a source of fibrinogen, factor VIII, and von Willebrand factor (vWF). It is ideal for supplying fibrinogen to the volume-sensitive patient. Cryoprecipitate is also used as a source of fibrinogen to create fibrin glue, a topical hemostatic sealant used in the surgical setting. When factor VIII concentrates are not available, cyroprecipitate is an option since each unit contains approximately 80 units of factor VIII. vWF may also be supplied to patients with dysfunctional vWF multimers (type II von Willebrand disease) and those who lack the capacity to generate vWF altogether (type III).

PLASMA DERIVATIVES Plasma from thousands of donors may be pooled to derive specific protein concentrates. These products include albumin, intravenous immunoglobulin, antithrombin, and coagulation factor concentrates. In addition, donors who have high titer antibodies to specific agents or antigens provide hyperimmune globulins, such as anti-D (RhoGam, WinRho), and antisera to hepatitis B virus (HBV), varicella-zoster virus, CMV, and a number of other infectious agents.

ADVERSE REACTIONS TO BLOOD TRANSFUSION

Adverse reactions to transfused blood components occur despite multiple tests, inspections, and checks. Fortunately, the most common reactions are not life-threatening, although serious reactions can present with mild symptoms and signs. Some reactions can be reduced or prevented by modified (filtered, washed, or irradiated) blood components. When an adverse reaction is suspected, the transfusion should be stopped and reported to the blood bank for investigation.

Transfusion reactions may result from immune and nonimmune mechanisms. Immune-mediated reactions are often due to preformed donor or recipient antibody; however, cellular elements may also cause adverse effects. Nonimmune causes of reactions are due to the chemical and physical properties of the stored blood component and its additives.

Infectious complications of transfusion have become less frequent, although fear of these complications remains the primary concern of both patients and clinicians. The incidence of transfusion-related infections has been reduced substantially due to improved donor screening and testing of collected blood. Infections, like any adverse transfusion reaction, must be brought to the attention of the blood bank for appropriate "look-back" studies (Table 115-3).

IMMUNE-MEDIATED REACTIONS Acute Hemolytic Transfusion Reactions Immune-mediated hemolysis occurs when the recipient has preformed antibodies that bind and lyse donor erythrocytes. The ABO isoagglutinins are responsible for the majority of these reactions, although alloantibodies directed against other red blood cell antigens, i.e., Rh, Kell, and Duffy, may result in intravascular hemolysis.

Acute hemolytic reactions may present with hypotension, tachypnea, tachycardia, fever, chills, hemoglobinemia, hemoglobinuria, chest and/or flank pain, and discomfort at the catheter or infusion site. Monitoring the patient's vital signs before and during the transfusion is important to identify these reactions promptly. When acute hemolysis is suspected, the transfusion must be immediately stopped, intravenous access maintained, and the reaction reported to the blood bank. A correctly labeled posttransfusion blood sample and any untransfused blood should be sent to the blood transfusion service for investigation. The laboratory evaluation for hemolysis includes the measurement of haptoglobin, lactate dehydrogenase (LDH), and indirect bilirubin levels in the recipient's serum.

Table 115-3

Risks of Transfusion Complications

	Frequency, Episodes : Unit
Reactions	
Febrile (FNHTR)	1–4:100
Allergic	1–4:100
Delayed hemolytic	1:1,500
Acute hemolytic	1:12,000
Fatal hemolytic	1:100,000
Anaphylactic	1:150,000
Infections*	
Hepatitis C	1:103,000
Hepatitis B	1:200,000
HIV-1	1:490,000
HIV-2	None reported
HTLV-I (II)	1:641,000
Malaria	1:4,000,000
Other complications	
RBC allosensitization	1:100
HLA allosensitization	1:10
Graft-versus-host disease	Rare
Hypervolemia	NQ†
Iron overload	NQ
Hypothermia	NQ

* Infectious agents rarely associated with transfusion or theoretically possible, unknown risk include parvovirus B-19, *Babesia microti* (babesiosis), *Borrelia burgdorferi* (Lyme disease), *Trypanosma cruzi* (Chagas' disease), and *Treponema pallidum*.
† NQ, not quantified.
NOTE: FNHTR, febrile nonhemolytic transfusion reaction; HIV, human immunodeficiency virus; HTLV, human T lymphotropic virus; RBC, red blood cell.

The immune complexes that result in RBC lysis can cause renal compromise and failure. Diuresis should be induced, using furosemide or mannitol with intravenous fluids, to prevent or minimize this complication. Tissue factor released from the lysed erythrocytes may initiate DIC. Coagulation studies including prothrombin time (PT), activated partial thromboplastin time (aPTT), fibrinogen, and platelet count should be monitored in patients with hemolytic reactions.

Errors at the patient's bedside, such as mislabeling the sample or transfusing an incorrect patient, are responsible for the majority of these reactions. The blood bank investigation of these reactions includes examination of the pre- and posttransfusion samples for hemolysis, repeat typing of the patient samples; direct antiglobulin test (DAT), sometimes called the direct Coombs test, of the posttransfusion sample; repeating the cross matching of the blood component; and checking all clerical records for errors. DAT detects the presence of antibody or complement bound to RBCs in vivo. In addition to confirming whether an immune hemolytic reaction has taken place, detecting or preventing the reciprocal error, i.e., patient A received blood intended for patient B and vice versa, is important.

Delayed Hemolytic and Serologic Transfusion Reactions Delayed hemolytic transfusion reactions (DHTR) are not completely preventable. A good transfusion history by the clinician can lower the risk. If the patient has had past transfusion or cross matching difficulties, the blood bank may be able to trace the problem. These reactions occur in patients previously sensitized to RBC alloantigens who have a negative alloantibody screen due to low antibody levels. When the patient is transfused with antigen-positive blood, an anamnestic response results in the early production of alloantibody that binds donor RBCs. The alloantibody is detectable 1 to 2 weeks following the transfusion, and the posttransfusion DAT may become positive due to circulating donor RBCs coated with antibody or complement. The transfused, alloantibody-coated erythrocytes are removed by the reticuloendothelial system, resulting in their extravascular clearance. Most commonly these reactions are detected in the blood bank when a subsequent patient sample, often there for additional cross matching, reveals a positive alloantibody screen or a new alloantibody in a recently transfused recipient.

No specific therapy is usually required, although additional RBC transfusions may be necessary to treat the falling hematocrit. Delayed serologic transfusion reactions (DSTR) are similar to DHTR, as the DAT is positive and alloantibody is detected; however, there is no evidence of RBC clearance.

Febrile Nonhemolytic Transfusion Reaction The most frequent reaction associated with the transfusion of cellular blood components is a febrile nonhemolytic transfusion reaction (FNHTR). These reactions are characterized by chills and rigors and a 1°C or greater rise in temperature. Since FNHTR is primarily a diagnosis of exclusion, it is important to rule out other causes of fever in the transfused patient. Classically, antibodies directed against donor leukocyte and HLA antigens have been proposed to mediate these reactions, and multiply transfused patients and multiparous women therefore are felt to be at increased risk. Although it is sometimes possible to demonstrate the offending antibodies in the recipient's serum, this is not necessary because of the mild nature of most FNHTR. The use of leukocyte-reduced blood products may prevent or delay sensitization to leukocyte antigens and thereby reduce the incidence of these febrile episodes. Of note, cytokines that accumulate within stored cellular blood components may mediate FNHTR, suggesting the utility of leukoreduction before storage to prevent these reactions. The incidence and severity of these reactions can be decreased by premedicating the patient with acetaminophen or other antipyretic agents, but this should be reserved only for patients with recurrent reactions.

Allergic Reactions Urticarial reactions, characterized by a pruritic rash, edema, headache, and dizziness, are related to plasma proteins found in transfused components. Mild reactions may be treated symptomatically by temporarily stopping the transfusion and administering antihistamines (diphenhydramine, 50 mg by mouth or intramuscularly). The transfusion may be completed after the signs and/or symptoms resolve. Patients with a history of allergic transfusion reaction should be premedicated with an antihistamine. Cellular components can be washed to remove residual plasma for the extremely sensitized patient.

Anaphylactic Reaction This severe reaction presents after transfusion of only a few milliliters of the blood component. Symptoms and signs include difficulty breathing, coughing, nausea and vomiting, hypotension, bronchospasm, respiratory arrest, shock, and loss of consciousness. Treatment includes stopping the transfusion, maintaining vascular access, and administering epinephrine (0.5 to 1.0 mL of 1:1000 dilution SQ). Glucocorticoids may be required in severe cases.

Patients who are IgA-deficient may be sensitized to this Ig class and are at risk for anaphylactic reactions associated with plasma transfusion. Individuals with severe IgA deficiency should therefore receive only IgA-deficient plasma and washed cellular blood components. Patients who have anaphylactic or repeated allergic reactions to blood components should be tested for IgA deficiency.

Graft-Versus-Host Disease Graft-versus-host disease (GVHD) is a frequent complication of allogeneic bone marrow transplantation, in which setting viable lymphocytes derived from donor marrow cannot be eliminated by an immunodeficient host. Transfusion-related GVHD is mediated by donor T lymphocytes that recognize host HLA antigens as foreign and mount an immune response, which is manifested clinically by the development of fever, a characteristic cutaneous eruption, diarrhea, and liver function abnormalities. GVHD can also occur when blood components that contain viable T lymphocytes are transfused to immunodeficient recipients or to immunocompetent recipients who share HLA antigens with the donor. In addition to the aforementioned clinical features, transfusion-associated (TA-GVHD) GVHD is further characterized by marrow aplasia and pancytopenia. In contrast to GVHD that develops in the setting of allogeneic marrow transplantation, TA-GVHD is notoriously resistant to treatment with immunosuppressive therapies, including glucocorticoids, cyclosporine, antithymocyte globulin, and ablative therapy followed by allogeneic bone marrow transplantation. Clinical manifestations appear at 8 to 10 days,

and death occurs at 3 to 4 weeks posttransfusion. The resistance to treatment and fatal outcome highlight the need for identification of patient groups at risk for TA-GVHD and use of methods for its prevention.

TA-GVHD can be prevented by irradiation of cellular components (minimum of 2500 cGy) before transfusion to patients at risk. At present, patients at risk for TA-GVHD include fetuses receiving intrauterine transfusions, selected immunocompetent (e.g., lymphoma patients) or immunocompromised recipients, recipients of donor units known to be from a blood relative, and recipients who have undergone marrow transplantation. Directed donations by family members should be discouraged (they are not less likely to transmit infection); lacking other options, the blood products from family members should always be irradiated.

Transfusion-Related Acute Lung Injury This uncommon reaction results from the transfusion of donor plasma that contains high titer anti-HLA antibodies that bind the corresponding antigens on recipient leukocytes. The leukocytes are thought to aggregate in the pulmonary vasculature and release mediators that increase capillary permeability. The recipient develops symptoms of respiratory compromise and signs of noncardiogenic pulmonary edema, including bilateral interstitial infiltrates on chest x-ray. Treatment is supportive, and patients usually recover without sequelae. Testing the donor's plasma for anti-HLA antibodies can support this diagnosis. The implicated donors are frequently multiparous women, and transfusion of their plasma component should be avoided.

Posttransfusion Purpura This reaction presents as thrombocytopenia 7 to 10 days after platelet transfusion and occurs predominantly in women. Platelet-specific antibodies are found in the recipient's serum, and the most frequently recognized antigen is HPA-1a found on the platelet glycoprotein IIIa receptor. The delayed thrombocytopenia is due to the production of antibodies that react to both donor and recipient platelets. Additional platelet transfusions can worsen the thrombocytopenia and should be avoided. Treatment with intravenous immunoglobulin may neutralize the offending antibodies, or plasmapheresis can be used to remove the antibodies should therapy be required.

Alloimmunization Cellular blood elements and plasma proteins bear a number of antigens to which the recipient may become alloimmunized. Alloantibodies to RBC antigens are detected during pretransfusion testing, and their presence may delay finding antigen-negative crossmatch-compatible products for transfusion. Women of child-bearing age who are sensitized to certain RBC antigens (i.e., D, c, E, Kell, or Duffy) are at risk for bearing a fetus with hemolytic disease of the newborn. Matching for D antigen is the only pretransfusion selection test to prevent RBC alloimmunization.

Alloimmunization to antigens on leukocytes and platelets can result in refractoriness to platelet transfusions. Once alloimmunization has developed, identifying and supplying HLA-compatible platelets from donors who share similar antigens with the recipient may be time-consuming and often futile. Hence, prudent transfusion practice is directed at preventing sensitization through the use of leukocyte-reduced cellular components, as well as limiting antigenic exposure by the judicious use of transfusions and transfusion of SDAP.

NONIMMUNOLOGIC REACTIONS **Fluid Overload** Blood components are excellent volume expanders, and transfusion may quickly lead to volume overload. Monitoring the rate and volume of the transfusion, along with the use of a diuretic, can minimize this problem.

Hypothermia Blood components stored either refrigerated (4°C) or frozen (−18°C or below) can result in hypothermia when rapidly infused. Particular attention is required when transfusing via a central venous catheter, because cardiac dysrhythmias can result from exposing the sinoatrial node to cold fluid. Use of an in-line warmer will prevent this complication.

Electrolyte Toxicity RBC leakage during storage increases the plasma concentration of potassium in the unit. Neonates and patients in renal failure are at risk for hyperkalemia. Measuring the recipient's serum potassium level or noting electrocardiographic changes characteristic of hyperkalemia is diagnostic. Preventive measures, such as using fresh or washed RBCs, are warranted for neonatal transfusions because this complication can be fatal.

Citrate, commonly used to anticoagulate blood components, chelates calcium and thereby inhibits the coagulation cascade. Hypocalcemia, manifested by circumoral numbness and/or tingling sensation of the fingers and toes, may result from multiple rapid transfusions. Because citrate is quickly metabolized to bicarbonate, calcium supplementation is seldom required in this setting. If calcium or any other intravenous infusion is necessary, it must be given through a separate intravenous line or site.

Iron Overload Each unit of RBCs contains 200 to 250 mg of iron. The transfused iron is added to the normal body store of 1 to 3 g, because excretion mechanisms are inadequate for the iron excess. Symptoms and signs of iron overload affecting endocrine, hepatic, and cardiac function are common after 100 units of RBCs have been transfused (total body iron load of 20 g). Preventing this complication by using alternative therapies (i.e., erythropoietin) and judicious transfusion is preferable and cost effective. Deferoxamine and other chelating agents are available, but the response is often suboptimal.

INFECTIOUS COMPLICATIONS **Viral Infections** *Hepatitis C virus* (HCV) The major etiologic agent of what was previously termed non-A non-B hepatitis remains the most common cause of transfusion-associated viral hepatitis. Testing donated blood for the presence of antibodies to HCV, using the first-generation assay, reduced the incidence of posttransfusion HCV infection to 3 in 10,000 transfusion episodes. Since the implementation of an improved screening assay for HCV antibodies, this risk has been lowered further (1 in 103,000). Infection with HCV may be asymptomatic or lead to chronic active hepatitis, cirrhosis, and liver failure.

Hepatitis B virus Increased and improved donor selection and screening, along with increased vaccination of the donor and recipient population, has markedly reduced the incidence of this transfusion-associated infection. Vaccination of individuals who require long-term transfusion therapy can prevent this complication.

Human immunodeficiency virus (HIV) type 1 Intensive donor screening and testing has dramatically reduced the risk of HIV-1 infection via blood transfusion. The risk of HIV-1 infection per transfusion episode is 1 in 490,000. The use of donor testing for HIV-1 p24 antigen may further reduce this risk. HIV-2 may also be transmitted via blood; accordingly, in 1992 a specific assay to detect antibodies to HIV-2 was added to the serologic tests performed on donated blood. There have been no reported cases of HIV-2 infection related to transfusion in the United States, and to date only two donors have tested positive for HIV-2 antibodies.

Cytomegalovirus This ubiquitous virus infects 50 percent or more of the general population and is transmitted by the infected "passenger" white blood cells found in transfused PRBC or platelet components. Donated blood is not routinely tested for serologic evidence of donor exposure. Classically, blood components harvested from CMV-seronegative donors have been utilized to avoid transfusion-related infection, but more recently, cellular components that are leukoctye-reduced have been shown to have a decreased risk of transmitting CMV, regardless of the serologic status of the donor. Groups at risk for CMV infectious complications include immunosuppressed patients, CMV-seronegative transplant recipients, and neonates; these patients should receive seronegative or leukoreduced components.

Human T lymphotropic virus (HTLV) type I This virus is associated with adult T cell leukemia/lymphoma and tropical spastic paraparesis in a small percentage of infected persons (see Chap. 192). The reported risk of HTLV-I infection via transfusion is 1 in 641,000 transfusion episodes. HTLV-II may also be transmitted by blood products, although to date it is unclear what diseases may be associated with the virus.

Parvovirus B-19 Blood components and products derived from pooled plasma can transmit this virus, the etiologic agent of erythema infectiosum, or fifth disease, in children. Parvovirus B-19 shows tropism for erythroid precursors and inhibits both erythrocyte production

and maturation. Pure red cell aplasia, presenting either as acute aplastic crisis or chronic anemia with shortened RBC survival, may occur in individuals with an underlying hematologic disease, such as sickle cell disease or thalassemia. The fetus of a seronegative woman is at risk for developing hydrops if infected with this virus.

Bacterial Contamination Blood components may be contaminated with bacteria (1) at the time of donation due to inadequate skin cleansing before venipuncture, (2) during component processing, or (3) from the bacteremic donor. Because most bacteria do not grow well at cold temperatures, packed RBCs and frozen plasma are not common sources of bacterial contamination. However, some gram-negative bacteria, notably *Yersinia* and *Pseudomonas* species, can grow at 1 to 6°C. Platelet concentrates, which are stored at room temperature, are more likely to be contaminated with skin contaminants such as gram-positive organisms, including coagulase-negative staphylococci.

Recipients of transfusions contaminated with bacteria may develop fever and chills, which can progress to septic shock and DIC. These reactions may occur abruptly, within minutes of initiating the transfusion, or after several hours. Characteristically the onset of symptoms and signs is sudden and fulminant, which will aid in differentiating bacterial contamination from a FNHTR. The reactions, particularly those related to gram-negative contaminants, are the result of infused endotoxins formed within the contaminated stored component.

When contaminated transfusions are suspected (i.e., when there is sudden development of shock), the transfusion must be stopped immediately. Therapy is directed at supporting the recipient's blood pressure, cardiac output, oxygenation, and renal function. The laboratory investigation should include cultures of any untransfused component, along with the routine blood bank clerical checks and serologic studies. Broad-spectrum antibiotic coverage should be started immediately and may be adjusted after the culture and sensitivity reports are available.

Parasites Various parasites including those causing malaria, babesiosis, and Chagas' disease have been or potentially can be transmitted by blood transfusion. Geographical migration and travel of donors can shift the incidence of these rare infections. Because these infections can prove fatal, they should be considered in the transfused patient in the appropriate clinical setting.

ALTERNATIVES TO TRANSFUSION

There is much interest in finding alternatives to allogeneic blood transfusions and thereby avoiding homologous donor exposures with attendant immunologic and infectious risks. When transfusion support is required, autologous blood is the best available option. However, the benefit-to-cost ratio of autologous transfusion has been challenged. No transfusion is a zero-risk event, and even with autologous transfusions clerical errors and bacterial contamination remain potential complications. Additional methods of autologous transfusion in the surgical patient include preoperative hemodilution, recovery of shed blood from sterile surgical sites, and postoperative drainage collection. Directed or designated donation, from friends and family of the potential recipient, has not proven to reduce the risk of transfusion-related infection below that of volunteer donor component transfusions. Such directed donations may in fact place the recipient at higher risk for complications, such as GVHD and alloimmunization.

Oxygen-carrying blood substitutes, such as perfluorocarbons and aggregated hemoglobin solution, are presently in various stages of clinical trials. Granulocyte- and granulocyte-macrophage colony stimulating factor (G- or GM-CSF) are clinically useful to hasten leukocyte recovery in patients with leukopenia related to high-dose chemotherapy. Erythropoietin stimulates erythrocyte production in patients with anemia of chronic renal failure and other conditions, thus avoiding or reducing the need for transfusion. This hormone can also stimulate erythropoiesis in the autologous donor to enable additional donation.

Thrombopoietin, the hormonal stimulus for megakaryocyte proliferation and maturation, is anticipated to play a similar role in stimulating thrombopoiesis in thrombocytopenic patients, thereby avoiding homologous platelet transfusion.

Finally, synthetic products, such as DDAVP (a vasopressin analogue) and recombinant factor VIII, provide therapeutic options that also avoid homologous donor exposure for patients with coagulopathies.

BIBLIOGRAPHY

AGRE P, CARTRON JP: Molecular biology of the Rh antigens. Blood 78:551, 1991

ANDERSON KC, NESS PM (eds): *Scientific Basis of Transfusion Medicine, Implications for Clinical Practice.* Philadelphia, Saunders, 1994

DZIECZKOWSKI JS et al: Characterization of reactions after exclusive transfusion of white cell–reduced cellular blood components. Transfusion 35:20, 1995

ETCHSON J et al: The cost effectiveness of preoperative autologous blood donations. N Engl J Med 332:719, 1995

KAUSHANSKY K: Thrombopoietin: The primary regulator of platelet production. Blood 86:419, 1995

PISCIOTTO PT et al: Prophylactic versus therapeutic platelet transfusion practices in hematology and/or oncology patients. Transfusion 35:498, 1995

SCHREIBER GB et al: The risk of transfusion-transmitted viral infections. N Engl J Med 334:1685, 1996

SHULMAN IA: Parasitic infections and their impact on blood donor selection and testing. Arch Pathol Lab Med 118:366, 1994

WALKER RR et al: *The Technical Manual,* 11th ed. Arlington, VA, American Association of Blood Banks, 1993

YAMAMOTO F et al: Molecular genetic basis of the histo-blood group ABO system. Nature 345:229, 1990

116   *James O. Armitage*

BONE MARROW TRANSPLANTATION

Hematopoietic stem cell transplantation is usually carried out for one of two reasons: (1) to replace an abnormal but not malignant marrow that has been purposefully destroyed with either radiation or chemotherapy, or (2) to allow for the administration of higher than usual doses of myelotoxic chemotherapy and/or radiation therapy to treat a malignancy. The types of bone marrow abnormalities treated with this procedure include both congenital and acquired diseases; the malignancies treated with hematopoietic support include acute leukemias and lymphomas, as well as solid tumors that appear to have a dose-response curve to chemotherapy (Table 116-1). The source of hematopoietic stem cells may be the bone marrow, peripheral blood, cord blood, or fetal liver of another individual, generally one who is immunologically matched at the major histocompatibility complex (see Chap. 306). Cord blood is usually available in too small a volume to reconstitute an adult; thus, cord blood transplants are performed nearly exclusively in children. Fetal liver between 10 and 14 weeks of gestation is a rich source of hematopoietic stem cells, but such transplants are rare because of the scarcity of material. When another individual is the stem cell donor, the transplantation is termed *allogeneic.* Autologous bone marrow and peripheral blood may also be stored before marrow ablation for reinfusion after myeloablative therapy. Such transplants are termed *autologous.* In the special case where the donor is an identical twin, i.e., genetically identical to the recipient, the transplantation is termed *syngeneic.* In all these types of transplants, hematopoietic stem cells are infused into a peripheral vein of the recipient and the stem cells home to the marrow to reestablish hematopoiesis.

The beginning of modern bone marrow transplantation can be traced to animal experiments in which mice were saved from a lethal dose of whole-body irradiation by shielding of the spleen. It was subsequently shown that intravenous infusion of bone marrow could also rescue such lethally irradiated animals. Allogeneic bone marrow transplantation was first performed successfully in the late 1960s and was gradually accepted as a legitimate therapy in the 1970s. Autologous bone marrow transplantation was first successfully employed to cure patients with lymphoma in the late 1970s, and its use became widespread in the 1980s. The annual number of autologous transplants now surpasses that of allogeneic transplants.

ALLOGENEIC AND SYNGENEIC BONE MARROW TRANSPLANTATION

Allogeneic bone marrow transplantation is usually restricted to persons less than 60 years of age. The results tend to be poorer in older patients because of increased complications associated with graft-versus-host disease (GVHD) in this population. However, the patient's general health is also very important, and many transplantation groups make decisions about intervening on the basis of the patient's physiologic rather than chronologic age.

For patients without a twin, an HLA-matched sibling donor is the best choice for an allogeneic bone marrow transplantation. The genes for the HLA antigens are found on chromosome 6. One would expect that the HLA type would follow the rules of mendelian genetics, namely, that any two siblings would have one chance in four of sharing the same HLA type. Except for an approximate 1 percent chance of crossover (a switch in genetic material between chromosomes during meiosis), this is in fact the case, forming the basis for HLA family

Table 116-1

Diseases Treated with Hematopoietic Stem Cell Transplantation

	Allogeneic	Autologous
MALIGNANCIES		
Acute leukemia (lymphoblastic or myelogenous)	+	+
Chronic myelogenous leukemia	+	+
Myelodysplastic syndrome	+	–
Lymphoma	+	+
Hodgkin's disease	+	+
Multiple myeloma	+	+
Chronic lymphocytic leukemia	+	+
Myelofibrosis	+	–
Breast cancer	–	+
Testicular cancer	–	+
Ovarian cancer	–	+
Neuroblastoma	+	+
Peripheral neuroepithelial tumors	–	+
Wilms's tumor	–	+
Ewing's sarcoma	–	+
NONMALIGNANT CONDITIONS		
Aplastic anemia	+	–
Pure red cell aplasia	+	–
Paroxysmal nocturnal hemoglobinuria	+	–
Fanconi's anemia	+	–
Sickle cell anemia	+	–
Thalassemia	+	–
Severe combined immunodeficiency	+	–
Leukocyte adhesion defects	+	–
Glanzmann's thrombasthenia	+	–
Gaucher's disease	+	–
Chronic granulomatous disease	+	–
Chédiak-Higashi syndrome	+	–
Hurler's syndrome	+	–
Hunter's syndrome	+	–
Metachromatic leukodystrophy	+	–
Adrenoleukodystrophy	+	–
Lesch-Nyhan syndrome	+	–
Type IIa glycogen storage disease	+	–
Osteopetrosis	+	–
Radiation accidents	+	–
Others	+	–

typing. Because of the relatively small size of American families, only about 30 percent of Americans have an HLA-identical sibling. The formula for calculating the chance that a particular person has an HLA-matched sibling is $1 - (0.75)^n$, where n denotes the number of potential sibling donors.

For patients who may benefit from an allogeneic bone marrow transplant but lack an HLA-matched sibling donor, there are two possible solutions. One is to identify an unrelated but closely HLA-matched person willing to donate marrow or peripheral blood, and the other is to use marrow from a related donor who is less than perfectly matched. The extremely large number of possible HLA phenotypes (the number of theoretical possibilities is larger than the total world population) makes the search for an unrelated donor a difficult undertaking. Fortunately, in patients with a similar genetic background, certain HLA phenotypes occur more frequently than might be expected based upon random population genetics.

For example, for a person of European ancestry, it has been estimated that a registry of 200,000 potential donors also of European ancestry would provide a 40 to 50 percent chance of containing an HLA-matched donor. The National Marrow Donor Program has been developed to facilitate the search for unrelated donors in the United States. Because of the imprecision of traditional serologic studies, HLA typing at the molecular level has been widely adopted as a technique for identifying HLA-matched unrelated donors.

Bone marrow transplantation using unrelated donors has become a widely applied therapy. While the results remain somewhat inferior to those seen when using an HLA-matched sibling donor, treatment outcomes with this approach have been improving as the techniques to manage GVHD and graft rejection have been refined (see below).

An alternative approach is to identify a related individual who shares most, but not all, of the patient's HLA antigens. Successful allogeneic transplantation can be performed using marrow from such donors, but the risk of graft rejection and GVHD increases with the level of mismatch. Long-term survival for recipients of marrow with one antigen mismatched is about the same as that for recipients of HLA-identical marrow. There is a somewhat higher rate of death from GVHD, but there is a somewhat lower rate of death from tumor relapse because the mismatched marrow exerts a greater graft-versus-tumor effect. However, with more than one gene mismatched, more serious complications are encountered; results deteriorate substantially with two or three antigen mismatched marrow.

Once a donor has been identified, the actual transplantation procedure begins. It consists of three phases: preparation for transplant, transplant, and management after transplant.

PREPARATION FOR TRANSPLANT High doses of chemotherapy with or without radiation therapy are delivered to the recipient with two main goals: destruction of the residual malignant or dysfunctional cells and destruction of the immune system of sufficient degree to avoid rejection of the allograft by residual, immunoglogically active cells in the host. In some cases, this therapy also serves to create space in the marrow for the new cells to engraft, but this is debated.

The choice of drugs for the preparative regimen is somewhat limited because higher doses of myelotoxic drugs often cause other serious organ toxicities. For example, doses of doxorubicin cannot be significantly increased because of cardiac toxicity. Most preparative regimens include alkylating agents such as cyclophosphamide, ifosfamide, busulfan, or melphalan; topoisomerase II inhibitors such as etoposide; antimetabolites such as cytarabine; and nitrosoureas such as carmustine. Even high doses of combinations of these agents may not be myeloablative. When allogeneic transplants are performed using T cell–depleted donor marrow to lower the risk of GVHD (Table 116-2), engraftment is not as efficient. Many such patients develop so-called mixed chimerism in which cells of both donor and host origin are present, indicating survival of host hematopoietic cells. No single preparative regimen has been proven superior to others.

THE TRANSPLANTATION PROCEDURE Collection of bone marrow from a donor is referred to as *harvesting*. Marrow is usually harvested by repeated aspiration from the posterior iliac crest until an adequate number of cells has been removed. If a sufficient

Table 116-2

Prevention of Acute Graft-versus-Host Disease

Histocompatibility matching of donor and recipient
Sterile environment
In vivo prophylaxis
    Cyclosporine ± methotrexate ± prednisone
    Antithymocyte globulin
    FK-506
In vitro marrow T cell depletion
    Antibodies ± complement
    Immunotoxins
    E-rosette depletion
    Lectin treatment
    Immunoadsorbent column separation
    Elutriation

number of cells cannot be obtained from the posterior iliac crest, marrow can also be harvested from the anterior iliac crest and sternum. If peripheral blood stem cells are being harvested, the donor may receive a colony stimulating factor (CSF) to augment the number of circulating stem cells and then will undergo repetitive apheresis procedures lasting several hours on consecutive days. The risk to the donor is very slight and predominantly associated with the risk of the anesthesia used. The procedure is usually accomplished on an outpatient basis, and donors usually return promptly to their usual activities, requiring only oral analgesia.

The smallest number of nucleated marrow cells required for long-term hematopoietic repopulation in humans is not precisely known. Operationally, the number of marrow cells harvested is usually 1 to 3×10^8 per kilogram of recipient body weight. 10^8 marrow cells usually contain 1 to 3×10^6 CD34 + stem cells. When peripheral blood cells are used, 5 to 8×10^8 cells/kg are infused, which corresponds to 1 to 3×10^6 CD34 + cells/kg. For a number of conditions, it appears that the more marrow cells given, the better the outcome. In nonmalignant hematologic disorders, a larger number of donor cells may be compensating for the use of a somewhat less intensive preparative regimen. A larger number of donor cells is also required when the donor marrow is depleted of T cells or when the donor and host are HLA-mismatched.

Marrow is sometimes treated in vitro to remove unwanted cells before being administered to the patient. When the donor and patient have a major ABO red cell incompatibility, it is necessary to remove the mature erythrocytes from the graft to avoid a hemolytic transfusion reaction. Alternatively, one may avoid a hemolytic transfusion reaction by performing a plasma exchange and removing anti-A or anti-B antibodies from the recipient's circulation. While this may seem more drastic than depleting red cells from the donor marrow, all manipulations of the marrow result in a loss of stem cells. In settings where the number of marrow cells is low and may be limiting, the plasma exchange approach is sometimes taken. The removal of T cells from an allograft can reduce the incidence and severity of GVHD, but this has never been shown to translate into better long-term survival, probably because T cell depletion also increases the risk of graft rejection and tumor relapse.

MANAGEMENT AFTER TRANSPLANT All patients undergoing bone marrow transplantation require intense supportive care between the time that the hematopoietic progenitor cells are infused and when they are able to produce adequate numbers of granulocytes, platelets, and erythrocytes. Early after the transplant, therapy is focused on prophylaxis against infection, bleeding, and GVHD. Acute GVHD prophylaxis measures are shown in Table 116-2. Beyond careful HLA matching, some combination of methotrexate, cyclosporine, and prednisone appears to be the most effective prophylactic drug regimen. In addition, supportive care usually includes blood components as needed to keep the platelet count above 20,000/μL and the hemoglobin above 80 g/L (8 g/dL), protective isolation, and broad-spectrum antibiotics (see Table 116-3). Blood components should be irradiated to avoid inducing GVHD mediated by lymphocytes from an HLA-incompatible donor. The average time to recovery of granulocyte counts greater than 500/μL is 10 to 20 days. Platelets are usually the slowest to recover. Platelet recovery is measured as time to independence from platelet transfusions, but a normal platelet count may not be achieved until day 100 or later. In some centers, patients routinely receive parenteral hyperalimentation and almost all patients receive CSFs. Despite intensive efforts to prevent complications, patients undergoing transplantation may develop serious medical problems (see Table 116-4 and Fig. 116-1).

Acute Graft-versus-Host Disease Even when the donor and host are completely matched at the HLA loci, there are usually differences between the donor and the host at minor histocompatibility loci. The infusion of functional lymphocytes from the donor into the host, whose cells express antigens perceived as foreign by the donor lymphocytes, results in the stimulation of an immune response in which donor CD4 + and CD8 + T cells and natural killer cells participate. The activated T cells and natural killer cells produce cytokines such as interferon γ and tumor necrosis factor α that are thought to mediate the tissue destruction associated with acute GVHD. The disease is manifested by a skin rash, liver function test abnormalities, and diarrhea. Histologically, the skin disease is a lichenoid reaction, the liver shows bile duct inflammation, and the gastrointestinal tract shows inflammation of crypts and mucosal inflammation and sloughing. The onset of the disease is usually within the first 2 months post transplant. The severity of the disease is graded based upon the organ dysfunction. It is not clear why some organs are spared damage in this systemic immune response. In addition to the damage to the affected end organs, florid acute GVHD is associated with immunosuppression and susceptibility to infection.

This complication is more frequent and more rapid in onset when the donor and host are mismatched at two or more HLA loci. With appropriate prophylaxis, GVHD of grades II to IV occurs in fewer than 40 percent of patients. The frequency is increased when marrow from an alloimmunized female (e.g., a woman who has given birth) is given to a male recipient. In addition, those receiving transplants from donors with cytotoxic T cell precursors that respond to recipient type cells are at greater risk. When acute GVHD develops, it is usually treated with high doses of methylprednisolone. Antibodies to T cells may be a useful second-line treatment. Experimental agents aimed at counteracting the cytokine effects (such as pentoxyfylline and thalidomide) have not yet been proven useful.

Paradoxically, despite our efforts to prevent acute GVHD, it appears that some low-grade disease may actually be beneficial through the mediation of a graft-versus-tumor effect. Reduction in the incidence and grade of GVHD is associated with higher rates of tumor relapse.

Chronic GVHD Although chronic GVHD may occasionally develop in the absence of acute GVHD, it is clear that the diseases are

Table 116-3

Antimicrobial Prophylaxis in Allogeneic Marrow Transplantation

Pathogen	Prophylaxis	Timing
Bacteria	Variable	By onset of neutropenia until engraftment
Fungi	Fluconazole, 100 mg PO qd	Day −7 to engraftment
Pneumocystis carinii	Bactrim-DS, 2 PO twice weekly	Engraftment to day 180*
Viruses		
Herpes simplex	Acyclovir, 250 mg/m² IV q 8 h	Day −1 to engraftment
Cytomegalovirus†	Ganciclovir, 5 mg/kg twice weekly	Engraftment to day 100

* Or until immunosuppressive therapy is stopped.
† In seropositive patients or recipients of seropositive marrow; it is best to use seronegative blood products in seronegative patients or to filter white cells from seropositive donors.

Table 116-4

Complications of Allogeneic Bone Marrow Transplantation

EARLY COMPLICATIONS

Regimen-related toxicity	Venoocclusive disease of the liver
Cystitis	Idiopathic pneumonia syndrome
Mucositis	Graft failure
Pulmonary complications	Infection
Renal toxicity	Immunodeficiency
Neurologic toxicity	Acute graft-vs.-host disease
	Bleeding

LATE COMPLICATIONS

Regimen-related toxicity	Immunodeficiency
Cataracts	Infection
Neurologic toxicity	Chronic graft-vs.-host disease
Gonadal toxicity	Relapse of primary tumor
Endocrine toxicity	Second malignancy
Abnormal growth and development	

largely related. Chronic GVHD usually develops more than 3 months after transplant. It is characterized by skin rash, sclerodermatitis, alopecia, hepatic dysfunction, oral lichenoid lesions, and a sicca complex (dry eyes and mouth) and may involve obliterative bronchiolitis and gastrointestinal motility disorders. The disease is mediated by donor T cells, most of which are recognizing minor histocompatibility complex differences in the host. In addition, there may be autoreactive donor T cells that recognize a self-antigen shared by the donor and host, especially when there is tissue damage. The activated T cells produce a variety of cytokines, including interleukin (IL) 4, which has been suggested as a primary mediator of the disease. Apparently newly developed T cells in the adoptive host do not undergo normal negative selection to delete autoreactive cells and induce self-tolerance. Patients who had grade II or greater acute GVHD and those who are older are at increased risk. For the majority of patients, the disease is self-limited. Treatment is with immunosuppressive agents. By 3 years after transplant, very few patients have persistent chronic GVHD and can be tapered off their chronic immunosupression. The basis for this late development of self-tolerance is not understood. The greatest threat to life from chronic GVHD is opportunistic infection related both to the underlying autoimmune disease and its treatment. Patients produce few antibodies to carbohydrates and are susceptible to bacterial infections. Prophylactic cotrimoxazole and intravenous immunoglobulin may reduce serious infectious sequelae. Thrombocytopenia and hyperbilirubinemia are adverse prognostic factors.

Infections Infections that complicate allogeneic bone marrow transplantation are discussed in Chap. 136.

Delayed Immune Recovery After bone marrow transplantation, donor stem cells attempt to recapitulate the ontogeny of the immune

FIGURE 116-1 Timing of major complications of bone marrow transplantation.

system. However, in adults, thymic involution often leads to inadequate generation of new T cells. The T cell function of the transplant recipient is dependent upon peripheral expansion of the relatively few T cells transferred with the marrow graft. T cell recovery after transplantation may take 18 months or more. The initial T cells detected in the peripheral blood are not fully functional, often failing to produce IL-2 upon stimulation. With time, normal T cell responses may develop; however, the use of live viral vaccines is to be avoided.

Regimen-Related Toxicities The toxicities associated with chemotherapy and radiation therapy are discussed in Chap. 86.

Graft Rejection Rejection of a bone marrow graft in most cases represents destruction of the graft by functional host lymphocytes that survived the preparative regimen. This complication is most frequent in patients with aplastic anemia who do not receive total-body radiation therapy. Predisposing factors include previous blood transfusions (which sensitize the host), less intensive preparative regimens (which fail to kill host lymphocytes), and the removal of T cells from the allograft (donor T cells produce CSFs and may interfere with host cell rejection). Graft rejection is less likely to occur when patients undergo transplantation before any blood products are transfused, but this is often not practical. Infusion of buffy coat preparations from the donor in the days following the transplant reduces the frequency of graft rejection but increases the frequency of severe acute GVHD. The primary approach to the prevention of graft rejection is the use of more immunosuppressive preparative regimens. CSFs are not useful in preventing graft rejection.

Tumor Recurrence In general, tumor recurrence is an authentic recurrence of malignant cells of host origin. Although several approaches to this problem may be taken, the infusion of large numbers of donor T cells, obtained by leukapheresis or aspiration of buffy coat of donor blood, often induces complete remission in relapsed leukemia, particularly chronic granulocytic leukemia. Such donor T cells may also worsen GVHD. Experimental efforts to further improve the efficacy of donor T cells include the administration of IL-2 after transplant and immunizing the donor against the tumor before the transplant.

Pulmonary Complications After transplantation, between 5 percent and 10 percent of patients develop a nonbacterial, nonfungal interstitial pneumonitis characterized by fever, interstitial infiltrates, hypoxia, and the adult respiratory distress syndrome. Cytomegalovirus (CMV) is the most common pathogen, and the pneumonitis occurs more commonly in the setting of GVHD in the second month or later after transplantation. In CMV-seropositive patients, the prophylactic use of ganciclovir can reduce the risk of developing CMV pneumonia. In CMV-seronegative patients, scrupulous use of blood products only from CMV-seronegative donors will minimize the risk. If only CMV-seropositive donor blood is available, leukocyte filters to remove donor leukocytes will usually prevent transmission. Some cases may be caused by the human herpesvirus 6. When this syndrome occurs early (within the first 2 weeks) and an infectious etiology is not defined, the idiopathic pneumonia syndrome may be related to the use of pulmonary toxins in the preparative regimen. It has a mortality rate of 50 percent or greater. Pathologically, the lesion is diffuse alveolar hemorrhage. Frequently beneficial results may be obtained with high-dose glucocorticoids.

Venoocclusive Disease of the Liver Up to 50 percent of patients undergoing transplantation may develop two of the three primary symptoms of hepatic venoocclusive disease (jaundice, tender hepatomegaly, and ascites or unexplained weight gain) within the first few weeks following transplant. The disease is caused by damage to the hepatocytes, endothelial cells, and sinusoids surrounding the central vein of the liver mediated by radiation or chemotherapy. About 70 percent of patients recover, but the disease can be fatal, especially in patients who develop the hemolytic-uremic syndrome. Thrombolytic therapy with tissue plasminogen activator appears to reduce the fatality rate of established disease. Criteria for intervening are not yet clear.

Psychosocial Complications The great majority of patients who survive bone marrow transplantation, who do not develop significant chronic GVHD and do not experience disease recurrence return to full activity and resume a normal life. Full recovery may take more

than 1 year. The most common persisting abnormalities are infertility and sexual dysfunction.

AUTOLOGOUS BONE MARROW TRANSPLANTATION

Autologous bone marrow transplantation involves the use of the patient's own hematopoietic progenitor cells to reestablish hematopoietic cell function after the administration of high-dose chemotherapy and/or radiation therapy. The reinfused hematopoetic progenitors may come from the patient's bone marrow or peripheral blood. When the latter source is used, the procedure is called peripheral blood stem cell transplantation. Generally, before peripheral stem cell harvest, the stem cell content of the blood is augmented by treating the patient with chemotherapy and CSFs, especially granulocyte CSF, a manipulation that results in marrow stem cells being released into the peripheral blood.

Autologous bone marrow transplantation differs from allogeneic transplantation in several ways. Although many of the complications are similar to those encountered in allogeneic transplants, usually the incidence is lower and there are no complications related to GVHD. The early clinical problems arise mainly from regimen-related toxicity. Interstitial pneumonitis may occur in 10 to 15 percent of patients but is more likely to be idiopathic than CMV-related. In addition, hematopoietic reconstitution is often more rapid than in allogeneic transplants (granulocyte recovery in 8 to 14 days, platelet recovery in 14 to 21 days). CSFs are essentially always used in autologous transplants. Because of this more favorable toxicity profile, autologous transplantation may be employed safely in older patients.

Increasingly, autologous stem cell transplantation is being performed on an outpatient basis. Patients are treated with prophylactic antibiotics and see the physician in clinic daily. The development of neutropenic fever or overt infection is the stimulus to admission.

A concern related specifically to autologous transplantation is the possible presence of contaminating tumor cells in the graft. A number of approaches have been employed to rid the graft of tumor cells, including purging tumor cells with antibody plus complement, an immunotoxin, and incubating the marrow with chemotherapeutic agents. In addition, positive selection methods have been employed to enrich for CD34+ stem cells. It has also been observed that the act of freezing the marrow and thawing it for delivery to the patient may preferentially kill tumor cells. Despite all this concern, there is little evidence that purging techniques influence disease-free survival. When relapses occur, they are generally at previous sites of disease rather than widely disseminated, as might be expected by hematogenous distribution. Nevertheless, three pieces of data support the concern that the graft may be a source of tumor. Retrospective analysis has suggested that purging leads to a reduced rate of relapse in patients with acute myeloid leukemia or malignant lymphoma. When tumor cells can be cultured from histologically negative marrow in patients with lymphoma, leukemia, or breast cancer, those patients have a higher rate of relapse than those with negative cultures. Finally, early attempts to introduce genetic markers into stem cells (contaminated with tumor cells) in vitro and trace their fate in vivo have suggested that some patients relapse with cells from the graft. However, purging techniques are not generally employed.

DISEASES TREATED BY BONE MARROW TRANSPLANTATION

Interpretation of the results of trials of bone marrow transplantation is always complicated by the problem of patient selection. The efficacy of transplantation can be underestimated if only patients with the worst prognosis are studied and overestimated if only those with the best prognosis are studied. Randomized trials, which might help resolve problems in interpretation, have been very difficult to conduct. Even with imperfect data, however, it is necessary to make the best possible recommendations to patients.

NONMALIGNANT DISEASES **Aplastic Anemia, Thalassemia, and Sickle Cell Anemia** Allogeneic bone marrow transplantation leads to disease-free survival in up to 85 to 90 percent of patients with severe aplastic anemia. As compared with immunosuppression induced by antithymocyte globulin with or without cyclosporine, allogeneic transplantation is more likely to produce a complete hematologic remission. However, many centers recommend a trial of immunosuppressive therapy before proceeding to bone marrow transplantation in older patients (i.e., 40 to 55 years of age) and in patients with only moderately severe disease. Allogeneic bone marrow transplantation is effective in the treatment of all forms of aplastic anemia, including that following paroxysmal nocturnal hemoglobinuria. However, Fanconi's anemia poses special problems, and patients with this disorder require modified preparative regimens because of an increase in the toxic effects of treatment to liver and lungs.

The effectiveness of allogeneic bone marrow transplantation in patients with thalassemia was demonstrated more than a decade ago. Busulfan and cyclophosphamide are most often used as a preparative regimen, rather than total-body radiotherapy and cyclophosphamide, in an attempt to avoid long-term complications. Treatment-related deaths are unusual when transplantation is performed before severe complications related to iron overload develop. Disease-free survival is approximately 75 percent. Adverse prognostic factors include hepatomegaly and portal fibrosis—complications presumably related to previous transfusions.

Sickle cell anemia is another serious hematologic disorder that is potentially curable with allogeneic bone marrow transplantation. Available reports suggest that allogeneic transplantation can establish normal hematopoiesis and alleviate the symptoms of the disorder; it is especially useful in patients with frequent crises who do not respond to hydroxyurea.

Immunodeficiency Disorders Allogeneic bone marrow transplantation was first successfully utilized in treating children with life-threatening immunodeficiency disorders. The procedure can replace defective stem cells with normal cells in patients with severe combined immunodeficiency, Wiskott-Aldrich syndrome, and Chédiak-Higashi syndrome. When an HLA-identical sibling is available as a donor for a child recognized to have any of these lethal disorders, allogeneic bone marrow transplantation is the treatment of choice. Unfortunately, such donors are often not available, but transplants are often attempted with less than perfectly matched family donors.

Other Genetic Disorders In principle, allogeneic bone marrow transplantation should be a successful therapy for any genetic disorder involving the immunologic or hematopoietic system. Examples of its application include the reversal of infantile malignant osteopetrosis, Gaucher's disease, infantile metachromatic leukodystrophy, and X-linked adrenoleukodystrophy. One lesson learned from the experience with these disorders is that damage to the extramedullary organs, once inflicted, sometimes cannot be reversed by replacing hematopoietic stem cells, and transplantation may therefore have to be performed very early in the course of the disease.

MALIGNANT DISEASES Well over 90 percent of all bone marrow transplants are performed for the treatment of malignant disease. Table 116-1 identifies those disorders in which bone marrow transplantation has been shown to be curative or to prolong survival.

Leukemia Acute myeloid leukemia was one of the first disorders to be shown to be curable with allogeneic bone marrow transplantation. In patients with end-stage, refractory leukemia, cure rates of approximately 10 percent are possible. When patients are treated in second or subsequent remission, 20 to 40 percent cure rates are achievable, and patients transplanted in their first complete remission can be cured 40 to 70 percent of the time. However, because some patients can be cured with standard chemotherapy regimens alone, the relative advantages of transplanting all patients who have matched donors and

are in first complete remission versus only transplanting those patients who eventually relapse are still debated. Autologous bone marrow transplantation has also been used in patients with acute myeloid leukemia but has been associated with a higher relapse rate and, in most series, a lower cure rate.

Myelodysplastic syndrome frequently develops into acute myeloid leukemia. This disorder is more common in elderly patients but is occasionally seen in younger adults. When an HLA-identical sibling donor is available, allogeneic bone marrow transplantation offers a potentially curative therapy.

Acute lymphoblastic leukemia can also be cured with allogeneic bone marrow transplantation. Results of standard intensive chemotherapy in children with this disorder are sufficiently good so that bone marrow transplantation should be reserved only for those with very high risk cytogenetic abnormalities—for example, Philadelphia chromosome–positive acute lymphoblastic leukemia. However, children who have early relapse after a standard chemotherapy regimen should undergo allogeneic bone marrow transplantation if they have a donor. Adults with acute lymphoblastic leukemia have poorer results with standard chemotherapy than do children. However, use of bone marrow transplantation in first complete remission has not been shown to improve treatment outcome. Autologous transplantation has been performed in acute lymphoblastic leukemia, but, as in acute myeloid leukemia, the relapse rate is higher than with allogeneic transplantation, although long-term disease-free survival can be achieved in some patients.

Chronic myelogenous leukemia is the most common indication for allogeneic bone marrow transplantation. In a patient of appropriate age who has an HLA-matched sibling donor, allogeneic bone marrow transplantation should be performed within the first year of diagnosis. If an HLA-matched sibling donor is not available, transplants using unrelated donors are frequently used, but with somewhat poorer results. Autologous transplantation has also been used in patients unable to undergo allogeneic bone marrow transplantation with some positive results.

Chronic lymphocytic leukemia rarely occurs in young patients who might be candidates for bone marrow transplantation. However, allogeneic bone marrow transplantation has been demonstrated to produce complete remissions in some patients. It will take many years to determine whether bone marrow transplantation can be curative in this type of leukemia because of the indolent natural history of the disorder.

Lymphoma and Myeloma The most common diseases treated by autologous transplantation are non-Hodgkin's lymphoma and Hodgkin's disease. Long-term disease-free survival and cure can be achieved in patients with aggressive non-Hodgkin's lymphoma and Hodgkin's disease. The chances for cure are related to the timing of the transplantation. Patients with end-stage, refractory disease are cured infrequently, while patients with chemotherapy-sensitive disease at relapse are cured 30 to 50 percent of the time. Autologous transplantation has been shown in a randomized trial to be superior to chemotherapy at standard doses for patients with relapsed aggressive non-Hodgkin's lymphoma (Fig. 116-2). Currently, studies are under way testing the utility of bone marrow transplantation as part of the primary therapy of these disorders. At the present time, transplantation is the treatment of choice for patients with aggressive non-Hodgkin's lymphoma and Hodgkin's disease who relapse after an effective chemotherapy regimen.

The use of bone marrow transplantation to treat patients with low-grade non-Hodgkin's lymphoma is a more recent development. Studies using either purged bone marrow or peripheral blood progenitor cells in patients with first relapse of low-grade follicular lymphoma has demonstrated a 40 to 50 percent disease-free survival 5 years after treatment. Because late relapses tend to occur in these disorders, a very long follow-up will be necessary to determine whether transplantation is curative.

Allogeneic bone marrow transplantation is also performed for patients with non-Hodgkin's lymphoma and Hodgkin's disease. In general, allogeneic bone marrow transplants have been selected in younger patients and those in whom blood and marrow involvement by the lymphoma make collection of uncontaminated hematopoietic progenitors difficult or impossible. Also, certain patients who have

FIGURE 116-2 The curves depict the treatment outcome for patients with chemotherapy sensitive, relapsed aggressive non-Hodgkin's lymphoma randomly assigned to continue standard dose therapy or undergo autologous bone marrow transplantation. *A*. Event-free survival, $p = .001$. *B*. Overall survival, $p = .038$.

developed myelodysplasia from their initial therapy for their lymphoma are also candidates for allogeneic bone marrow transplantation.

Both allogeneic and autologous bone marrow transplantation have been performed for the treatment of multiple myeloma. Few patients with multiple myeloma are young enough to be good candidates for allogeneic bone marrow transplantation. However, for those few patients, long-term disease-free survival might be possible. Autologous bone marrow transplantation incorporated into the primary treatment of patients with multiple myeloma has been tested in a randomized trial. This study showed prolonged survival for the patients undergoing autologous transplantation as compared to further standard therapy.

Solid Tumors   Breast cancer has become the individual disease most frequently treated by autologous transplantation in the United States. The use of this treatment has been controversial. At the present time, autologous bone marrow transplantation as adjuvant treatment for patients with high-risk breast cancer is undergoing randomized clinical trials measured against standard-dose therapy. One randomized trial has been completed comparing autologous bone marrow transplantation with standard-dose chemotherapy in patients with metastatic breast cancer. Although it was unclear if patients in either group were cured, the median survival was approximately doubled with autologous bone marrow transplantation.

Neuroblastoma in children has often been treated with allogeneic and autologous bone marrow transplantation. Disease-free survival rates as high as 40 percent at 2 years for patients with stage IV disease have been reported. However, the occurrence of late relapses and improved results of chemotherapy not requiring bone marrow transplantation have raised questions about the role of transplantation in the treatment of this disorder.

Autologous bone marrow transplantation has been used in patients with testicular cancer who were not able to be cured with platinum-based chemotherapy regimens. Approximately 10 to 20 percent of such patients with advanced, refractory disease can be cured when transplanted. This is similar to the outcome reported for patients with lymphoma.

Autologous bone marrow transplantation has been used to treat patients with malignant melanoma, soft tissue sarcoma, ovarian or

uterine cancer, brain tumors, small cell lung cancer, and colon cancer. For the treatment of malignant melanoma, colon cancer, and small cell lung cancer, the results of transplantation have been discouraging. For gynecologic cancers, soft tissue sarcoma, and brain tumors, however, transplantation has had more positive results, stimulating further trials.

PATIENT FOLLOW-UP AFTER BONE MARROW TRANSPLANTATION

While only a few physicians actually perform bone marrow transplantation, many physicians are involved in the care of these patients after a successful transplant. Usually the referring physician expects to accept a major part of the patient's care by 3 months after a patient has undergone bone marrow transplantation. By this time most patients will have recovered normal hematopoietic function, although a few patients will demonstrate chronic marrow injury—usually with low platelet counts. A significant proportion of patients undergoing allogeneic bone marrow transplantation will still be receiving therapy for chronic GVHD.

The most important long-term complications that need to be monitored are infection and the development of relapse of the underlying disorder. In patients treated for malignant disease, recurrence of the malignancy is the major cause of death after autologous bone marrow transplantation and an important cause of death after allogeneic bone marrow transplantation. Late infections, particularly herpes zoster, are not infrequent. Patients with chronic GVHD sometimes have functional asplenia and are at risk for overwhelming infection by encapsulated bacteria. Patients who receive radiotherapy as part of their primary treatment or as part of the transplant regimen are at risk for the development of hypothyroidism. This diagnosis can be difficult and requires an alert physician. Patients who have total-body radiotherapy as part of their preparative regimen need to be monitored for cataracts. Most patients who undergo bone marrow transplantation will be infertile. However, this is not always the case, and patients sometimes recover fertility following transplantation. Fertility is most likely to return in patients who did not have extensive alkylating agent therapy before coming to transplantation, those who did not receive total-body radiotherapy as part of their preparative regimen, and those who came to transplantation at a younger age. Women seem more likely to recover fertility than men. It is important to make patients aware of this possibility.

Patients exposed to alkylating agents, etoposide, and radiotherapy are at increased risk to develop second malignancies. Acute leukemia seems to be a risk for patients who undergo autologous transplantation for Hodgkin's disease or non-Hodgkin's lymphoma—particularly if they receive total body radiotherapy as part of their preparative regimen. All patients who have been irradiated as part of their primary treatment or as part of the bone marrow transplant preparative regimen are at risk for the development of late solid tumors. This increased risk should lead to early institution of appropriate screening maneuvers, such as regular mammography in young women who received radiotherapy to the mediastinum that included the breast. It is useful to know that Pap smears done early after bone marrow transplantation will often be abnormal because of dysplastic cells induced by the high-dose chemotherapy/radiotherapy. This should not be overinterpreted.

CONCLUSIONS

Allogeneic bone marrow transplantation is likely to remain an important treatment of leukemia, aplastic anemia, and certain genetic disorders for many years to come. Autologous bone marrow transplantation as a treatment for malignant disease might be avoided in some patients as effective new chemotherapeutic agents are developed and/

or new generations of hematopoietic growth factors become available. The most important improvement today in the use of autologous bone marrow transplantation could come from identifying those patients at high risk for treatment failure with standard therapies and the early institution of this treatment. If genetic manipulation of hematopoietic progenitor cells becomes practical, autologous bone marrow transplantation might become a common treatment for a variety of nonmalignant disorders.

BIBLIOGRAPHY

CHAO NJ et al: Cycolosporine, methotrexate and prednisone compared with cyclosporine and prednisone for prophylaxis of acute graft-vs-host disease. N Engl J Med 329:1225, 1993

CLIFT RA et al: Allogeneic marrow transplantation during untreated first relapse of acute myeloid leukemia. J Clin Oncol 10:1723, 1992

DAVIES SM et al: Unrelated donor bone marrow transplantation: Influence of HLA A and B incompatibility on outcome. Blood 86:1636, 1995

GLUCKMAN E et al: Bone marrow transplantation for severe aplastic anemia: Influence of conditioning and graft-versus-host disease prophylaxis regimens on outcome. Blood 79:269, 1992

KENNEDY MJ: High-dose chemotherapy of breast cancer: Is the question answered? J Clin Oncol 13:2477, 1995

KOLB HJ et al: Graft-versus-leukemia effect of donor lymphocyte transfusions in marrow grafted patients. Blood 86:2041, 1995

LINCH DC et al: Dose intensification with autologous bone marrow transplantation in relapsed and resistant Hodgkin's disease: Results of a BNLI randomized trial. Lancet 341:1051, 1993

LUCARELLI G et al: Bone-marrow transplantation in patients with thalassemia. N Engl J Med 322:417, 1990

PHILIP T et al: Autologous bone marrow transplantation as compared with salvage chemotherapy in relapses of chemotherapy-sensitive non-Hodgkin's lymphoma. N Engl J Med 333:1540, 1995

THOMAS ED et al: Marrow transplantation for the treatment of chronic myelogenous leukemia. Ann Intern Med 104:155, 1986

VOSE J et al: Long-term sequelae of autologous bone marrow of peripheral stem cell transplantation for lymphoid malignancies. Cancer 69:784, 1992

ZHANG M et al: Long-term follow-up of adults with acute lymphoblastic leukemia in first remission treated with chemotherapy or bone marrow transplantation. Ann Intern Med 123:428, 1995

SECTION 3
DISORDERS OF HEMOSTASIS

117

Robert I. Handin

DISORDERS OF THE PLATELET AND VESSEL WALL

Patients with platelet or vessel wall disorders usually bleed into superficial sites such as the skin, mucous membranes, or genitourinary or gastrointestinal tract. Bleeding begins immediately after trauma and either responds to simple measures such as pressure and packing or requires systemic therapy with glucocorticoids, plasma fractions, or platelet concentrates. The most common platelet/vessel wall disorders are (1) various forms of thrombocytopenia, (2) von Willebrand's disease (vWD), and (3) drug-induced platelet dysfunction. This chapter reviews the diagnosis and treatment of quantitative and qualitative platelet disorders as well as vessel wall defects that cause bleeding. The physiology of normal hemostasis and the cardinal manifestations of bleeding arising from hemostatic disorders have been reviewed in Chap. 60.

PLATELET DISORDERS

Platelets arise from the fragmentation of megakaryocytes, which are very large, polyploid bone marrow cells produced by the process of endomitosis. They undergo from three to five cycles of chromosomal duplication without cytoplasmic division. After leaving the marrow space, approximately one-third of the platelets are sequestered in the spleen, while the other two-thirds circulate for 7 to 10 days. Normally, only a small fraction of the platelet mass is consumed in the process of hemostasis, so most platelets circulate until they become senescent and are removed by phagocytic cells. The normal blood platelet count is maintained between 150,000 and 450,000 per microliter. A decrease in platelet mass stimulates an increase in the number, size, and ploidy of megakaryocytes, releasing additional platelets into the circulation. This process is regulated by thrombopoietin (TPO) binding to its megakaryocyte receptor, a proto-oncogene called c-mpl. TPO, also called the c-mpl ligand, is secreted continuously at a low level and binds tightly to circulating platelets. A reduction in platelet mass increases the level of free TPO and thereby stimulates megakaryocyte and platelet production. Recombinant TPO is being tested in clinical trials as a means to prevent or reduce thrombocytopenia in patients receiving cytotoxic chemotherapy.

The platelet count varies during the menstrual cycle, rising following ovulation and falling at the onset of menses. It is also influenced by the patient's nutritional state and can be decreased in severe iron, folic acid, or vitamin B_{12} deficiency. Platelets are *acute-phase reactants*, and patients with systemic inflammation, tumors, bleeding, and mild iron deficiency may have an increased platelet count, a benign condition called *secondary* or *reactive thrombocytosis*. The cytokines interleukin (IL)-3, IL-6, and IL-11 may stimulate platelet production in acute inflammation. In contrast, the increase in platelet count that is characteristic of the myeloproliferative disorders such as polycythemia vera, chronic myelogenous leukemia, myeloid metaplasia, and essential thrombocytosis can cause either severe bleeding or thrombosis. In these patients, unregulated platelet production is secondary to a clonal stem cell abnormality affecting all the bone marrow progenitors.

THROMBOCYTOPENIA   Thrombocytopenia is caused by one of three mechanisms—decreased bone marrow production, increased splenic sequestration, or accelerated destruction of platelets. In order to determine the etiology of thrombocytopenia, each patient should have a careful examination of the peripheral blood film, an assessment of marrow morphology by examination of an aspirate or biopsy, and an estimate of splenic size by bedside palpation supplemented, if necessary, by ultrasonography or computed tomographic (CT) scan. Occasional patients have "pseudothrombocytopenia," a benign condition in which platelets agglutinate or adhere to leukocytes when blood is collected with EDTA as anticoagulant. This is a laboratory artifact, and the actual platelet count in vivo is normal. A scheme for classifying patients with thrombocytopenia based on these clinical observations and laboratory tests is outlined in Fig. 117-1.

Impaired Production   Disorders that injure stem cells or prevent their proliferation in marrow frequently cause thrombocytopenia. They usually affect multiple hematopoietic cell lines so that thrombocytopenia is accompanied by varying degrees of anemia and leukopenia. Diagnosis of a platelet production defect is readily established by examination of a bone marrow aspirate or biopsy, which should show a reduced number of megakaryocytes. The most common causes of decreased platelet production are marrow aplasia, fibrosis, or infiltration with malignant cells, all of which produce highly characteristic marrow abnormalities. Occasionally, thrombocytopenia is the presenting laboratory abnormality in these disorders. Cytotoxic drugs, which are frequently used in cancer chemotherapy, impair megakaryocyte proliferation and maturation and frequently cause thrombocytopenia. There are also rare marrow disorders such as congenital amegakaryocytic hypoplasia and *t*hrombocytopenia with *a*bsent *r*adii (TAR syndrome), which selectively decrease megakaryocyte production.

Splenic Sequestration Since one-third of the platelet mass is normally sequestered in the spleen, splenectomy will increase the platelet count by 30 percent. Postsplenectomy thrombocytosis is a benign self-limited condition that does not require specific therapy. In contrast, when the spleen enlarges, the fraction of sequestered platelets increases, lowering the platelet count. The most common causes of splenomegaly are portal hypertension secondary to liver disease and splenic infiltration with tumor cells in myeloproliferative or lymphoproliferative disorders or with macrophages in storage disorders such as Gaucher's disease. Isolated splenomegaly is rare, and in most patients, splenomegaly is accompanied by other

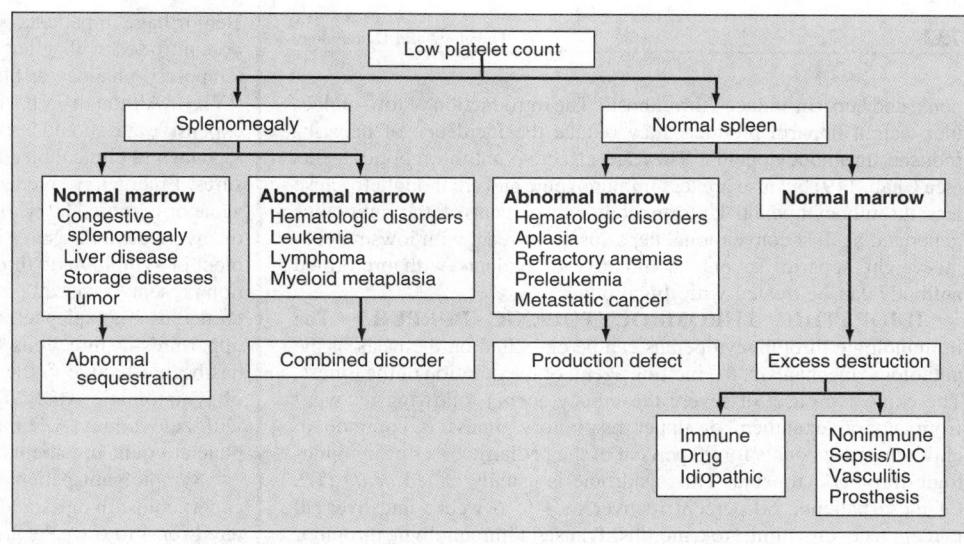

FIGURE 117-1 Clinical evaluation of patients with thrombocytopenia. *[Modified from RI Handin, in W Beck (ed), Hematology, 4th ed, Cambridge, MA, MIT Press, 1985.]*

clinical manifestations of an underlying disease. Many patients with leukemia, lymphoma, or a myeloproliferative syndrome have both marrow infiltration and splenomegaly and develop thrombocytopenia from a combination of impaired marrow production and splenic sequestration of platelets.

Accelerated Destruction Abnormal vessels, fibrin thrombi, and intravascular prostheses can all shorten platelet survival and cause *nonimmunologic thrombocytopenia*. For example, thrombocytopenia is common in patients with vasculitis, the hemolytic uremic syndrome (HUS), thrombotic thrombocytopenic purpura (TTP), as one manifestation of disseminated intravascular coagulation (DIC), and in patients with prosthetic cardiac valves. In addition, platelets coated with antibody, immune complexes, or complement are rapidly cleared by mononuclear phagocytes in the spleen or other tissues inducing *immunologic thrombocytopenia*. The most common causes of immunologic thrombocytopenia are viral or bacterial infections, drugs, and a chronic autoimmune disorder referred to as *idiopathic thrombocytopenic purpura* (ITP). Patients with immunologic thrombocytopenia do not usually have splenomegaly and have an active bone marrow with an increased number of megakaryocytes.

DRUG-INDUCED THROMBOCYTOPENIA Many common drugs can cause thrombocytopenia (Table 117-1). As previously mentioned, many chemotherapeutic agents are cytotoxic and depress megakaryocyte production. Ingestion of large quantities of alcohol has a similar marrow-depressing effect leading to transient thrombocytopenia. The syndrome is particularly common in binge drinkers. Thiazide diuretics, which are used commonly to treat hypertension or congestive heart failure, impair megakaryocyte production and can produce mild thrombocytopenia (50,000 to 100,000/µL), which may persist for several months after the drug is discontinued.

Most drugs induce thrombocytopenia by eliciting an immune response in which the platelet is an innocent bystander. The platelet is damaged by complement activation following the formation of drug-antibody complexes. Current laboratory tests can identify the causative agent in 10 percent of patients with clinical evidence of drug-induced thrombocytopenia. The best proof of a drug-induced etiology is a prompt rise in the platelet count when the suspected drug is discontinued. Patients with drug-induced platelet destruction also may have a secondary increase in megakaryocyte number without other marrow abnormalities.

Although most patients recover within 7 to 10 days and do not require therapy, occasional patients with platelet counts below 10,000 to 20,000/µL have severe hemorrhage and may require temporary support with glucocorticoids, plasmapheresis, or platelet transfusions while waiting for the platelet count to rise. A patient who has recovered from drug-induced immunologic thrombocytopenia should be in-

structed to avoid the offending drug in the future, since only minute amounts of drug are needed to set up subsequent immune reactions. Certain drugs such as phenytoin and gold salts may induce prolonged thrombocytopenia, since the drugs are cleared from body storage depots quite slowly. Heparin deserves special mention because it is a common cause of thrombocytopenia in hospitalized patients. It is estimated that 10 to 15 percent of patients receiving therapeutic doses of heparin develop thrombocytopenia and, occasionally, may have severe bleeding or intravascular platelet aggregation and paradoxical thrombosis. Heparin-induced thrombosis, sometimes called the "white clot syndrome," can be fatal unless recognized promptly. Most cases of heparin thrombocytopenia are due to drug-antibody binding to platelets, although some may be secondary to direct platelet agglutination by heparin. The offending antigen is a complex formed between heparin and the platelet-derived heparin neutralizing protein, platelet factor four. Prompt cessation of heparin will reverse both thrombocyto-

Table 117-1

Drugs Implicated in Thrombocytopenia

SUPPRESSION OF PLATELET PRODUCTION

Myelosuppressive drugs
  Severe: cytosine arabinoside, daunorubicin
  Moderate: cyclophosphamide, busulfan, methotrexate, 6-mercaptopurine
  Mild: vinca alkaloids
Thiazide diuretics
Ethanol
Estrogens

IMMUNOLOGIC PLATELET DESTRUCTION

Clinical suspicion plus convincing experimental evidence
  Antibiotics: sulfathiazole, novobiocin, *p*-aminosalicylate
  Cinchona alkaloids: quinidine, quinine
  Foods: beans
  Sedatives, hypnotics, anticonvulsants: apronalide, carbamazepine
  Arsenical drugs used to treat syphilis
  Digitoxin
  Methyldopa
  Stibophen
Clinical suspicion (major drugs implicated)
  Aspirin
  Chlorpropamide
  Chloroquine
  Chlorothiazide and hydrochlorothiazide
  Gold salts
  Insecticides
  Sulfadiazine, sulfisoxazole, sulfamerazine, sulfamethazine, sulfamethoxypyridazine, sulfamethoxazole, sulfatolamide

penia and heparin-induced thrombosis. The introduction of low-molecular-weight heparin products may reduce the incidence of heparin-induced thrombocytopenia. They are effective antithrombotic agents (see Chap. 119) but also are less immunogenic and are thought to cause less thrombocytopenia. Unfortunately, 80 percent of the antibodies generated against conventional heparins cross-react with low-molecular-weight heparin, so only a minority of patients with preformed antibody can be treated with this product.

IDIOPATHIC THROMBOCYTOPENIC PURPURA The immunologic thrombocytopenias can be classified on the basis of the pathologic mechanism, the inciting agent, or the duration of the illness. The explosive onset of severe thrombocytopenia following recovery from a viral exanthem or upper respiratory illness is common in children and accounts for 90 percent of the pediatric cases of immunologic thrombocytopenia. This syndrome is usually called *acute ITP*. Of these patients, 60 percent recover in 4 to 6 weeks and over 90 percent recover within 3 to 6 months. Transient immunologic thrombocytopenia also complicates some cases of infectious mononucleosis, acute toxoplasmosis, or cytomegalovirus infection and can be part of the prodromal phase of viral hepatitis and infection with the human immunodeficiency virus (HIV). Acute ITP is rare in adults and accounts for fewer than 10 percent of postpubertal patients with immune thrombocytopenia. Acute ITP is caused by immune complexes containing viral antigens that bind to platelet Fc receptors or by antibodies produced against viral antigens that cross-react with the platelet. In addition to the viral disorders described above, the differential diagnosis should include atypical presentations of aplastic anemia, acute leukemias, or metastatic tumor. A bone marrow examination is essential to exclude these disorders, which can occasionally mimic acute ITP.

Most adults present with a more indolent form of thrombocytopenia that may persist for many years and is referred to as *chronic ITP*. Women aged 20 to 40 are afflicted most commonly and outnumber men by a ratio of 3:1. They may present with an abrupt fall in platelet count and bleeding similar to patients with acute ITP. More often they have a prior history of easy bruising or menometrorrhagia. These patients have an autoimmune disorder with antibodies directed against target antigens on the glycoprotein IIb-IIIa or glycoprotein Ib-IX complex (see Fig. 60-2). Although most antibodies function as opsonins and accelerate platelet clearance by phagocytic cells, occasional antibodies bind to epitopes on critical regions of these glycoproteins and impair platelet function. A number of tests have been introduced to measure platelet-associated IgG. Although the tests are quite sensitive, their specificity is a problem. First, there is a high "background" level of IgG on normal platelets. Second, an elevation in plasma immunoglobulin levels or in circulating immune complexes will nonspecifically increase platelet-associated IgG.

Since a low platelet count may be the initial manifestation of systemic lupus erythematosus (SLE) or the first sign of a primary hematologic disorder, all patients with chronic ITP should have a bone marrow examination and an antinuclear antibody determination. In addition, patients with hepatic or splenic enlargement, lymphadenopathy, or atypical lymphocytes should have serologic studies for hepatitis, cytomegalovirus, Epstein-Barr virus, toxoplasma, and HIV. HIV infection has rapidly become a common cause of immunologic thrombocytopenia and should be considered in the differential diagnosis of thrombocytopenia, especially in high-risk groups—homosexuals, hemophiliacs, intravenous drug abusers, and heterosexual individuals with multiple partners. Thrombocytopenia can be the initial symptom of HIV infection or a complication of fully developed clinical AIDS.

℞ **TREATMENT**

Treatment of patients with ITP must take into account the age of the patient, the severity of the illness, and the anticipated natural history. Although adults have a higher incidence of intracranial bleeding than children, specific therapy may not be necessary unless the platelet count is under 20,000/μL or there is extensive bleeding.

Hemorrhage in patients with either acute or chronic ITP usually can be controlled with glucocorticoids but, in rare cases, may require temporary phagocytic blockade with intravenous immunoglobulin (IVIG). Although IVIG is an effective form of therapy, it is quite expensive and should be reserved for patients with severe thrombocytopenia and clinical bleeding who have not responded to other measures. Emergency splenectomy is usually reserved for patients with acute or chronic ITP who are desperately ill and have not responded to any medical measures designed to improve hemostasis. The treatment of symptomatic thrombocytopenia in patients with HIV infection presents a special problem because the administration of glucocorticoids or splenectomy may increase susceptibility to the opportunistic infections that threaten these patients. Splenectomy has been effective in the course of HIV infection prior to the onset of symptomatic AIDS. There is increasing evidence that treatment with zidovudine (AZT) and other antiviral agents can improve the platelet count in patients with HIV-induced thrombocytopenia.

Symptomatic patients with chronic ITP are usually placed on glucocorticoids. In one standard regimen, 60 mg prednisone is administered for 4 to 6 weeks and then decreased slowly over another few weeks. Approximately 50 percent of patients with chronic ITP will normalize their platelet count on high doses of prednisone. However, the majority will have a fall in platelet count following steroid withdrawal. Patients with chronic ITP who fail to maintain a normal platelet count after a course of steroids are eligible for elective splenectomy. These steroid-responsive but steroid-dependent patients are very likely to respond to splenectomy, and 70 percent will have a normal platelet count within 1 week after surgery. Some patients who do not respond to glucocorticoids may still respond to splenectomy. Occasionally, patients may fail to respond to splenectomy because of the failure to remove an accessory spleen. In other patients, a small inactive accessory spleen may grow or new splenic foci may develop from splenic cells shed at the time of surgery and cause the late onset of thrombocytopenia. In either case, the presence of splenic tissue can be diagnosed by examination of the blood smear for Howell-Jolly bodies that appear in the red cells of asplenic individuals. Persistent splenic tissue can be confirmed by a radionuclide scan.

Patients who are still thrombocytopenic after steroid therapy or splenectomy or who relapse months to years after initial therapy have received a variety of immunosuppressive drugs including azathioprine, cyclophosphamide, vincristine, and vinblastine. Danazol has also been used with some success. Although each of these drugs may be beneficial, it is important to use some restraint because they have serious side effects. IVIG has become a popular therapy, although it is only transiently effective and quite expensive. It should be used to temporarily raise the platelet count and to support patients before surgery or labor and delivery. Anti-RhD therapy appears to be equally effective and is now available commercially as WinPro. If a patient is not bleeding and maintains a platelet count over 20,000/μL, consideration should be given to withholding therapy, since there are many patients with severe chronic thrombocytopenia who have lived with their disease for two or three decades.

FUNCTIONAL PLATELET DISORDERS As described in Chap. 60, normal hemostasis requires three critical platelet reactions—adhesion, aggregation, and granule release. Clinical bleeding can result from a failure of any of these important functions. Table 117-2 provides an outline of the major functional platelet disorders discussed below. Table 117-3 discusses the methods to assess platelet function.

Von Willebrand's Disease vWD is the most common inherited bleeding disorder, occurring in as many as 1 in 800 to 1000 individuals. The von Willebrand factor (vWF) is a heterogeneous multimeric plasma glycoprotein with two major functions. It facilitates platelet adhesion under conditions of high shear stress by linking platelet membrane receptors to vascular subendothelium; it also serves as the plasma carrier for factor VIII, the antihemophilic factor, a critical blood coagulation protein. Discrete domains in each vWF subunit mediate each of these important functions. The normal plasma vWF level is 10 mg/L. The vWF activity is distributed among a series of

Table 117-2

CHAPTER 117
Disorders of the Platelet and Vessel Wall   **733**

Classification of Functional Platelet Disorders

I. Disorders of adhesion
    A. Inherited
        1. Bernard-Soulier syndrome
        2. von Willebrand's disease (vWD)
    B. Acquired
        1. Uremia
        2. Acquired vWD
II. Disorders of aggregation
    A. Inherited
        1. Glanzmann's thrombasthenia
        2. Afibrinogenemia
    B. Acquired
        1. Fibrin degradation product inhibition
        2. Dysproteinemias
        3. Drug ingestion—e.g., ticlopidine, anti-IIb/IIIa antibodies
           (RheoPro)
III. Disorders of granule release
    A. Inherited
        1. Oculocutaneous albinism (Hermansky-Pudlak syndrome)
        2. Chédiak-Higashi syndrome
        3. Isolated dense (δ) granule deficiency
        4. Gray-platelet syndrome—combined α and δ granule deficiency
    B. Acquired
        1. Cardiopulmonary bypass
        2. Myeloproliferative disorders
        3. Drugs—aspirin and other nonsteroidal anti-inflammatory agents

plasma multimers with estimated molecular weights ranging from 400,000 to over 20 million. A single large vWF precursor subunit is synthesized in endothelial cells and megakaryocytes, where it is cleaved and assembled into the disulfide-linked multimers present in plasma, platelets, and vascular subendothelium. A modest reduction in plasma vWF concentration or a selective loss in the high-molecular-weight multimers decreases platelet adhesion and causes clinical bleeding.

Although vWD is heterogeneous, there are certain clinical features that are common to all the syndromes. With one exception (type III disease), all forms are inherited as autosomal dominant traits, and affected patients are heterozygous with one normal and one abnormal vWF allele. In mild cases, bleeding occurs only after surgery or trauma. More severely affected patients have spontaneous epistaxis or oral mucosal, gastrointestinal, or genitourinary bleeding. The laboratory findings are variable. The most diagnostic pattern is the combination of (1) a prolonged bleeding time, (2) a reduction in plasma vWF concentration, (3) a parallel reduction in biologic activity as measured with the ristocetin cofactor assay, and (4) reduced factor VIII activity.

Table 117-3

Evaluation of Platelet Function

Bleeding time
  Modified Ivy method
  Skin incision—time to stop bleeding
  Global screen of platelet role in hemostasis
von Willebrand factor assays
  vWF Ag—immunoassay of total vWF protein
  vWF R:Cof—bioassay of vWF that measures ability of patient plasma to
    support agglutination of normal platelets in the presence of ristocetin
  Factor VIII—coagulation assay of factor VIII bound and carried by
    plasma vWF
Platelet aggregometry
  Measures platelet aggregation in response to a panel of agonists, usually
    ADP, collagen, arachidonic acid, and epinephrine
Membrane glycoproteins
  Presence of glycoproteins Ib-IX and IIb-IIIa can be measured using
    monoclonal antibodies and flow cytometry
Platelet granule content
  Dense granules—electron microscopy or uptake and retention of
    radiolabeled serotonin
  Alpha granules—electron microscopy and/or immunoassays for platelet-
    associated proteins—vWF, fibrinogen, platelet factor four

NOTE: vWF, von Willebrand factor; ADP, adenosine diphosphate; Ag, antigen; R:Cof, ristocetin cofactor.

FIGURE 117-2 Pattern of inheritance and laboratory findings in von Willebrand's disease. The assays of platelet function include a coagulation assay of factor VIII bound and carried by von Willebrand factor (vWF), abbreviated as VIII; immunoassay of total vWF protein, abbreviated vWF:Ag; bioassay of the ability of patient plasma to support ristocetin-induced agglutination of normal platelets, abbreviated vWF:RCoF; and ristocetin-induced aggregation of patient platelets abbreviated RIPA. The multimer pattern illustrates the protein bonds present when plasma is electrophoresed in a polyacrylamide gel. The II-1 and II-2 columns refer to the phenotypes of the second generation offspring.

The variability in laboratory tests is related to both the heterogeneous nature of the defects in vWD and the fact that plasma levels are influenced by ABO blood group type, central nervous system disorders, systemic inflammation, and pregnancy. Since vWD is an autosomal dominant disorder, some vWF is produced by the remaining normal allele. Thus patients with mild defects may have laboratory values that fluctuate over time and may occasionally be within the normal range.

There are three major types of vWD. Their mode of inheritance and laboratory findings are summarized in Fig. 117-2. Patients with *type I disease*, the most common abnormality, have a mild to moderate decrease in plasma vWF. In the milder cases, although hemostasis is clearly impaired, the vWF level is just below the lower limit of normal (50 percent activity, or 5 mg/L). In type I disease, there is a parallel decrease in vWF antigen, factor VIII activity, and ristocetin cofactor activity, with a normal spectrum of multimers detected by sodium dodecyl sulfate (SDS)–agarose gel electrophoresis. Cultured endothelial cells derived from the umbilical cords of patients with vWD synthesize and secrete reduced quantities of vWF multimer and have a two- to fourfold reduction in vWF mRNA.

The variant forms of vWD (*type II disease*), which are much less common, are characterized by normal or near-normal levels of a dysfunctional protein. Patients with the *type IIa variant* of vWD have a deficiency in the high- and medium-molecular-weight forms of vWF multimer detected by SDS-agarose electrophoresis. This is due either to an inability to secrete the high-molecular-weight vWF multimers or to proteolysis of the multimers soon after they leave the endothelial cell and enter the circulation. Mutations in a localized region of the vWF A-2 domain have been identified in families with type IIa vWD (see Fig. 117-3). The quantity of vWF antigen and the amount of associated factor VIII are usually normal. In the *type IIb variant*, there is also a loss in high-molecular-weight multimers. However, in type IIb disease, it is due to the inappropriate binding of vWF to platelets. This forms intravascular platelet aggregates that are rapidly cleared from the circulation, causing mild, cyclic thrombocytopenia. Mutations in a disulfide-bonded loop in the A-1 domain that binds to glycoprotein Ib-IX have been identified as the cause of the type IIb defect (Fig. 117-3). A few patients have been described with a platelet membrane disorder that mimics type IIb vWD—*platelet-type vWD*. It is due to mutations in the portion of glycoprotein Ib-IX that interacts with vWF. Levels of total vWF antigen and factor VIII are normal.

Approximately 1 in 1 million individuals have a very severe form of vWD that is phenotypically recessive (*type III disease*). Type III patients are usually the offspring of two parents with mild type I disease. However, in many cases, the parents are very mildly affected or are asymptomatic. Type III patients may inherit a different abnormality from each parent (a doubly heterozygous or compound heterozygous state) or be homozygous for a single defect. Type III patients have severe mucosal bleeding, no detectable vWF antigen or activity, and may have sufficiently low factor VIII that they have occasional hemarthroses like mild hemophiliacs. Several type III families have been described who have major deletions in the vWF gene. In addition, families with nonsense mutations and the combination of a deleted and nonsense mutant allele have been described.

℞ TREATMENT

Appropriate therapy of vWD depends on the symptoms and the underlying type of disease. There are two therapeutic options. One involves the use of cryoprecipitate, a plasma fraction enriched in vWF, or factor VIII concentrates, which retain high-molecular-weight vWF multimers (Humate-P, Koate HS). The factor VIII concentrates are highly purified and heat-treated to destroy HIV and are appropriate treatments for all the inherited forms of vWD. During surgery or after major trauma, patients should receive cryoprecipitate or factor VIII concentrate twice daily. This regimen should be continued for 48 to 72 h to ensure optimal hemostasis. Minor bleeding episodes such as prolonged epistaxis or severe menorrhagia may respond to a single infusion. Recurrent menorrhagia, a major problem for women with severe vWD, can be treated effectively with oral contraceptive agents that suppress menses.

A second therapeutic option, which avoids the use of plasma, is the use of 1-desamino-8-D-arginine vasopressin (DDAVP) or desmopressin, a vasopressin analogue that has minimal blood pressure–elevating and fluid-retaining properties and raises the plasma vWF level in both normal individuals and patients with mild vWD. Patients with type I disease are the best candidates for DDAVP therapy. However, they must be tested for an adequate response before anticipated surgery, and vWF levels must be monitored closely during therapy, since the patient may develop tachyphylaxis when therapy is continued for more than 48 h. DDAVP should not be given to patients with variant forms of vWD without prior testing, since it may not improve multimer pattern or hemostasis in type IIa patients and it may actually worsen the defect by depleting high-molecular-weight multimers, inducing intravascular platelet aggregation, and lowering the platelet count in type IIb patients. It is also ineffective therapy for patients with the severe (type III) form of vWD.

Acquired vWD   Although most cases of vWD are inherited, there are also acquired forms of vWD caused by antibodies that inhibit vWF function or by lymphoid or other tumors that selectively adsorb vWF multimers onto their surfaces. Anti-vWF antibodies have developed in patients with severe vWD following multiple transfusions, as well as in patients with autoimmune and lymphoproliferative disorders. Adsorption of vWF to tumor surfaces has been documented in patients with Waldenström's macroglobulinemia and Wilms' tumor and inferred in other patients with lymphoma. Treatment of acquired vWD should focus on controlling the underlying disease, since plasma derivatives and DDAVP are often not effective and the disorder can be fatal.

Platelet Membrane Defects   Receptors that modulate platelet adhesion and aggregation are located on the two major platelet surface glycoproteins. As previously discussed (see Chap. 60), vWF facilitates platelet adhesion by binding to glycoprotein Ib-IX, while fibrinogen links platelets into aggregates via sites on the glycoprotein IIb-IIIa complex. There are two rare but well-defined platelet defects characterized by a loss of or a defect in these glycoprotein receptors. Patients with the *Bernard-Soulier syndrome* have markedly reduced platelet adhesion and cannot bind vWF to their platelets owing to deficiency or dysfunction of the glycoprotein Ib-IX complex. They also have reduced levels of several other membrane proteins, mild thrombocytopenia, and extremely large, lymphocytoid platelets. Platelets from patients with *Glanzmann's disease* or *thrombasthenia* are deficient in or have a defect in the glycoprotein IIb-IIIa complex. Their platelets do not bind fibrinogen and cannot form aggregates, although the platelets undergo shape change and secretion and are of normal size.

Both these disorders are inherited as autosomal recessive traits and are characterized by markedly impaired hemostasis and recurrent episodes of severe mucosal hemorrhage. In keeping with the selective nature of the defects, Bernard-Soulier platelets react normally to all stimuli except ristocetin. In contrast, thrombasthenic platelets adhere normally and will agglutinate with ristocetin but will not aggregate with any of the agonists that require fibrinogen binding, such as adenosine diphosphate (ADP), thrombin, or epinephrine.

The only effective therapy for hemorrhagic episodes in these two disorders is transfusion with normal platelets. This is usually effective, although alloimmunization will eventually limit the life span of infused platelets. In addition, a few patients have developed inhibitor antibodies with specificity for the missing protein. These antibodies bind to the protein that is expressed on the transfused normal platelets and impair their function.

Platelet Release Defects   The most common mild bleeding disorders arise from the ingestion of aspirin and

FIGURE 117-3   Location of mutations in types IIa and IIb von Willebrand's disease. Mutations in the region of the protein between amino acids 742 and 875 have been identified in patients with type IIa disease. These result in a deficiency in high- and medium-molecular-weight multimers either due to failure to secrete high-molecular-weight forms of vWF or to their proteolytic degradation in the circulation. In type IIb disease, there is also a decrease in high-molecular-weight vWF, but the defect is due to the failure of vWF with mutations in the A-1 domain of the protein (amino acids 509–695) to bind properly to platelet glycoprotein Ib-IX.

other nonsteroidal anti-inflammatory drugs (NSAIDs) that inhibit platelet production of thromboxane A_2, an important mediator of platelet secretion and aggregation (see Figs. 60-3 and 60-4). These drugs are inhibitors of the enzyme cyclooxygenase, which converts arachidonic acid to a labile endoperoxide intermediate that is critical for thromboxane formation. Aspirin is the most potent agent, since it irreversibly acetylates the platelet enzyme so that a single dose impairs hemostasis for 5 to 7 days. The other agents are competitive and reversible inhibitors with more transient effects. Blocking thromboxane A_2 synthesis partially inhibits platelet release and aggregation with weak agonists such as ADP and epinephrine and produces a mild hemostatic defect. The administration of high doses of certain antibiotics, particularly penicillin, can coat the platelet surface, block platelet release, and impair hemostasis.

Patients generally have minimal symptoms such as easy bruising, and bleeding is usually confined to the skin. Occasional patients will have prolonged oozing after surgery, particularly with procedures involving mucous membranes such as periodontal, oral, or reconstructive plastic surgery. Not surprisingly, the antiplatelet effect of drugs such as aspirin is more dramatic when they are administered to patients with underlying defects like vWD or hemophilia. Patients with drug-induced cyclooxygenase deficiency often but not always have a mildly prolonged bleeding time, and their platelets fail to aggregate when incubated with arachidonic acid, epinephrine, or low doses of ADP. Since the bleeding time is not entirely reliable, if patients have taken aspirin, they should be treated as if they have a mild hemostatic defect for the next 5 to 7 days. Platelet responses to collagen and thrombin are impaired at low doses but normal at higher doses. Symptomatic patients should be encouraged to use drugs such as acetaminophen that do not impair platelet function. Although most cases of cyclooxygenase deficiency are drug-induced, occasional patients have inherited disorders in platelet cyclooxygenase activity that impair thromboxane production or receptor level defects that prevent platelets from responding to thromboxane A_2.

Although a number of metabolic disorders can perturb hemostasis, uremic platelet dysfunction is clinically the most important. The mechanism by which uremia impairs platelet function is not well understood, and retention of phenolic and guanidinosuccinic acids, excess prostacyclin production, or impaired vWF-platelet interactions have all been implicated. There is a good correlation between the degree of uremia and bleeding symptoms and the degree of anemia and bleeding. Bleeding can usually be reversed by dialysis and often improves after red cell transfusion or treatment with erythropoietin. In addition, the administration of cryoprecipitate or DDAVP, which raise plasma vWF levels, can also improve hemostasis. Conjugated estrogens improve hemostasis and can be used as long-term therapy.

Storage Pool Defects Platelet granules have considerable amounts of adenine nucleotides, calcium, and adhesive glycoproteins such as thrombospondin, fibronectin, and vWF, all of which promote platelet adhesion and aggregation. Thus, it is not surprising that patients with defective platelet granules have a mild bleeding disorder. Platelet storage pool defects may be inherited as an isolated disorder or be part of systemic granule packaging defects such as oculocutaneous albinism or the Hermansky-Pudlak or Chédiak-Higashi syndromes. Clinically, these patients cannot be distinguished from those with other functional platelet disorders, since they all have easy bruising, mucosal bleeding, and a prolonged bleeding time. They can be differentiated from patients with the cyclooxygenase defects because their platelets will usually aggregate in response to arachidonic acid. In addition, their platelets have decreased levels of specific granule constituents such as ADP and serotonin and abnormalities in granule morphology that are best visualized by electron microscopy.

Occasionally, patients with acute or chronic leukemia or one of the myeloproliferative disorders develop an acquired storage pool disorder due to dysplastic megakaryocyte development. In addition, patients with liver disease and some patients with SLE or other immune-complex–mediated disorders may have circulating platelets that have degranulated prematurely. Platelet degranulation and a transient storage pool disorder also have been described following pro-

longed cardiopulmonary bypass. Fortunately, most patients with storage pool defects have only mildly impaired hemostasis. They can be treated with platelet transfusions. Occasional patients have responded to DDAVP.

VESSEL WALL DISORDERS

Bleeding from vascular disorders (nonthrombocytopenic purpura) is usually mild and confined to the skin and mucous membranes. The pathogenesis of bleeding is poorly defined in many of the syndromes, and classical tests of hemostasis, including the bleeding time and tests of platelet function, are usually normal. Vascular purpura arises from damage to capillary endothelium, abnormalities in the vascular subendothelial matrix or extravascular connective tissues that support blood vessels, or from the formation of abnormal blood vessels. There are also several idiopathic disorders that involve the vessel wall and can cause more severe bleeding and organ dysfunction.

THROMBOTIC THROMBOCYTOPENIC PURPURA TTP is a fulminant, often lethal disorder that may be initiated by endothelial injury and subsequent release of vWF and other procoagulant materials from the endothelial cell. Causes include pregnancy, metastatic cancer, mitomycin C, and high-dose chemotherapy. Characteristic findings include the microvascular deposition of hyaline thrombi that stain for fibrin, thrombocytopenia, microangiopathic hemolytic anemia, fever, renal failure, fluctuating levels of consciousness, and evanescent focal neurologic deficits. The presence of hyaline thrombi in arterioles, capillaries, and venules without any inflammatory changes in the vessel wall is diagnostic. Gingival biopsies are positive in 30 to 40 percent of patients, and marrow biopsies are occasionally helpful. The presence of a severe Coombs-negative hemolytic anemia with schistocytes or fragmented red blood cells in the peripheral blood smear, coupled with thrombocytopenia, and minimal activation of the coagulation system help to confirm the clinical suspicion of TTP. This disorder should be distinguished from vasculitis and SLE, which can predispose patients to TTP. Levels of platelet-associated IgG and complement are usually normal in TTP.

The treatment of acute TTP has changed radically in the past few years. Steroids and heparin or emergency splenectomy have been abandoned, and the enthusiasm for antiplatelet therapy has diminished. Increasingly, treatment has focused on the use of exchange transfusion or intensive plasmapheresis coupled with infusion of fresh frozen plasma. With this therapeutic approach, the overall mortality has been markedly reduced, and the majority of patients with TTP are recovering from this formerly fatal disorder. Most patients surviving the acute illness recover completely with no residual renal or neurologic disease. Occasional patients with a chronic, relapsing form of TTP require maintenance plasmapheresis and plasma infusion, and a few patients are only controlled with glucocorticoids.

HEMOLYTIC-UREMIC SYNDROME HUS is a disease of infancy and early childhood that closely resembles TTP. Patients present with fever, thrombocytopenia, microangiopathic hemolytic anemia, hypertension, and varying degrees of acute renal failure. In many cases, onset is preceded by a minor febrile or viral illness, and an infectious or immune-complex–mediated cause has been proposed. As in TTP, there is no evidence of disseminated intravascular coagulation. In contrast to TTP, the disorder remains localized to the kidney, where hyaline thrombi are seen in the afferent arterioles and glomerular capillaries. Such thrombi are not present in other vessels, and neurologic symptoms, other than those associated with uremia, are uncommon. There is no effective therapy; however, with dialysis for acute renal failure, the initial mortality is only 5 percent. Between 10 and 50 percent of patients are left with some chronic renal impairment.

HENOCH-SCHÖNLEIN PURPURA Henoch-Schönlein or anaphylactoid purpura is a distinct, self-limited type of vasculitis that occurs in children and young adults. Patients have an acute inflammatory reaction in capillaries, mesangial tissues, and small arterioles that leads to increased vascular permeability, exudation, and hemorrhage. Vessel lesions contain IgA and complement components. The syndrome may be preceded by an upper respiratory infection or streptococcal pharyngitis or be associated with food or drug allergies. Patients develop a purpuric or urticarial rash on the extensor surfaces of the arms and legs and on the buttocks; they also have polyarthralgias or arthritis, colicky abdominal pain, and hematuria from focal glomerulonephritis. Despite the hemorrhagic features, all coagulation tests are normal. A small number of patients may develop fatal acute renal failure, and 5 to 10 percent develop chronic nephritis. Glucocorticoids provide symptomatic relief of the joint and abdominal pains but do not alter the course of the illness.

METABOLIC AND INFLAMMATORY DISORDERS A number of acute febrile illnesses cause capillary fragility and skin bleeding. Immune complexes containing viral antigens or the viruses themselves may damage endothelial cells. In addition, certain pathogens such as the rickettsiae that cause Rocky Mountain spotted fever replicate in endothelial cells and damage them. Thrombocytopenia is also a frequent finding in acute infectious disorders and may contribute to skin bleeding. In addition, whenever the platelet count falls below 10,000 per microliter, gaps that develop between endothelial cells allow the diapedesis of red cells into the dermis, leading to the formation of petechiae. Drugs such as the sulfonamides, penicillin, and allopurinol may cause vascular inflammation resulting in maculopapular or urticarial rashes. Some of these mechanisms are additive, and drug reactions in thrombocytopenic individuals cause an intensely hemorrhagic rash.

Occasionally, patients with diffuse polyclonal hyperglobulinemia will develop purpuric lesions on the lower limbs—a benign condition referred to as *hyperglobulinemic purpura*. Vascular purpura may occur in patients with various monoclonal plasma protein abnormalities, including Waldenström's macroglobulinemia, multiple myeloma, and cryoglobulinemia. These proteins markedly increase serum viscosity and may impair blood flow through capillaries. Thus retinal hemorrhage, central nervous system dysfunction, and skin necrosis have all been described in these syndromes due to the marked elevation in viscosity. In addition, the globulins may impair platelet aggregation and adhesion and interfere with fibrin polymerization. Patients with mixed cryoglobulinemia develop a more extensive maculopapular lesion due to immune-complex–mediated damage to the vessel wall. The mixed cryoglobulinemia (usually IgG and anti-IgG) may be associated with arthralgias, diffuse weakness, and unexplained nephritis. Plasmapheresis will temporarily lower the level of globulins, remove immune complexes, and improve symptoms in these patients. However, long-term management must include control of the underlying disease that produces the abnormal globulins or immune complexes.

Patients with *scurvy* (vitamin C deficiency) develop painful episodes of perifollicular skin bleeding as well as bleeding into muscles and, occasionally, into the gastrointestinal and genitourinary tracts. The diagnosis is confirmed by the presence of hyperkeratosis of skin, gum swelling, and low levels of the vitamin in leukocytes. Vitamin C–deficient patients have markedly defective collagen synthesis, since ascorbic acid is needed to synthesize hydroxyproline, an essential constituent of collagen. Patients with *Cushing's syndrome*, which is characterized by excess production of glucocorticoids, or patients on large doses of glucocorticoids develop generalized protein wasting and may show skin bleeding or easy bruising due to atrophy of the supporting connective tissue around blood vessels. Aging causes a similar atrophy of perivascular connective tissue on the extensor surfaces of the hands and arms, leading to "senile purpura." These individuals develop dark purple, irregularly shaped hemorrhagic areas due to abnormal skin mobility that tears small blood vessels.

Patients with inherited disorders of the connective tissue matrix such as *Marfan's syndrome*, *Ehlers-Danlos syndrome*, and *pseudoxanthoma elasticum* also have easy bruising. In addition to having fragile skin vessels and easy bruising, patients with Ehlers-Danlos syndrome

may develop aneurysms in intraabdominal vessels and apoplectic rupture and hemorrhage due to defects in the vascular collagen network. Primary vascular abnormalities also can lead to bleeding. Patients with *Osler-Weber-Rendu disease* (hereditary hemorrhagic telangiectasia), an inherited autosomal dominant disorder, have frequent episodes of nasal and gastrointestinal bleeding from abnormal telangiectatic capillaries; patients with *angiodysplasia* of the colon have increased incidence of gastrointestinal bleeding. In the *Kasabach-Merritt syndrome*, patients may have very extensive and progressively enlarging vascular malformations that may involve large portions of their extremities. Bleeding is secondary to disseminated intravascular coagulation triggered by stagnant blood flow through the tortuous abnormal vessels.

BIBLIOGRAPHY

EWENSTEIN BM, HANDIN RI: von Willebrand's disease, in *Blood: Principles and Practice of Hematology*, RI Handin et al (eds). Philadelphia, Lippincott, 1994, pp 1069–1094

WARKENTON TE, KELTON J: The platelet life cycle: Quantitative disorders in blood, in *Blood: Principles and Practice of Hematology*, RI Handin et al (eds). Philadelphia, Lippincott, 1994 pp 973–1049

118 | *Robert I. Handin*

DISORDERS OF COAGULATION AND THROMBOSIS

Patients with congenital plasma coagulation defects characteristically bleed into muscles, joints, and body cavities hours or days after an injury. Most of the *inherited* plasma coagulation disorders are due to defects in single coagulation proteins, with the two X-linked disorders, factors VIII and IX deficiency, accounting for the majority of the congenital coagulation disorders. These patients merit special attention because they may have severe bleeding and chronic disability and require specialized medical therapy. With rare exceptions, the known disorders prolong either the prothrombin time (PT), partial thromboplastin time (PTT), or both of these important laboratory screening tests. If they are abnormal, quantitative assays of specific coagulation proteins are then carried out using the PT or PTT tests with plasma from congenitally deficient individuals as substrate. The corrective effect of varying concentrations of patient plasma is measured and expressed as a percentage of a normal pooled plasma standard. The interval range for most coagulation factors is from 50 to 150 percent of this average value, and the minimal level of most individual factors needed for adequate hemostasis is 25 percent.

Acquired coagulation disorders are both more frequent and more complex, arising from deficiencies of multiple coagulation proteins and simultaneously affecting both primary and secondary hemostasis. The most common acquired hemorrhagic disorders are (1) disseminated intravascular coagulation (DIC), (2) the hemorrhagic diathesis of liver disease, and (3) vitamin K deficiency and complications of anticoagulant therapy.

Although congenital and acquired bleeding disorders are relatively rare, venous and arterial thrombosis and embolism are common medical disorders that have been recognized for over 100 years. Although risk factors such as atherosclerotic vascular disease, congestive heart failure, malignancy, and immobility predispose patients to thrombosis, specific coagulation defects have not yet been identified in most patients with thromboembolism. Several inherited coagulation abnormalities have now been described that induce a hypercoagulable or prethrombotic state and predispose patients to thrombosis. These disorders merit special attention because they affect young people, cause recurrent episodes of thromboembolism, and may involve multiple members of a single family. An understanding of the biochemical basis of thromboembolism is also important because anticoagulant and antithrombotic regimens are based on the premise that modifying critical coagulation reactions will reduce the incidence of thrombosis. This chapter will review the diagnosis, natural history, and therapy of congenital and acquired plasma coagulation disorders, as well as the inherited prethrombotic disorders. → *The physiology of normal hemostasis and the cardinal manifestations of the hemorrhagic and thrombotic disorders are described in Chap. 60.*

FACTOR VIII DEFICIENCY—HEMOPHILIA A   Pathogenesis and Clinical Manifestations   The antihemophilic factor (AHF), or factor VIII coagulant protein, is a large (265-kDa), single-chain protein that regulates the activation of factor X by proteases generated in the intrinsic coagulation pathway (see Figs. 60-5 and 60-6). It is synthesized in liver parenchymal cells and circulates complexed to the von Willebrand factor (vWF) protein. Previous efforts to purify and characterize the factor VIII molecule were limited by its low concentration (10 μg/L) and susceptibility to proteolysis. However, the cloning and sequencing of complementary DNA (cDNA) encoding the factor VIII molecule and the mapping of the factor VIII gene on the X chromosome have provided a detailed picture of its structure and have led to improved methods for carrier detection and prenatal diagnosis of hemophilia A.

One in 10,000 males is born with deficiency or dysfunction of the factor VIII molecule. The resulting disorder, hemophilia A, is characterized by bleeding into soft tissues, muscles, and weight-bearing joints. Although normal hemostasis requires at least 25 percent factor VIII activity, symptomatic patients usually have factor VIII levels below 5 percent, with a close correlation between the clinical severity of hemophilia and plasma AHF level. Patients with <1 percent factor VIII activity have *severe* disease; they bleed frequently even without discernible trauma. Patients with levels between 1 and 5 percent have *moderate* disease with less frequent bleeding episodes. Those with levels over 5 percent have *mild* disease with infrequent bleeding that is usually secondary to trauma. Occasional patients with factor VIII levels as high as 25 percent are discovered when they bleed after major trauma or surgery. The majority of patients with hemophilia A have factor VIII levels below 5 percent.

Hemophilic bleeding occurs hours or days after injury, can involve any organ, and, if untreated, may continue for days or weeks. This can result in large collections of partially clotted blood putting pressure on adjacent normal tissues and can cause necrosis of muscle (compartment syndromes), venous congestion (pseudophlebitis), or ischemic damage to nerves. For example, hemophiliacs often develop femoral neuropathy due to pressure from an unsuspected retroperitoneal hematoma. They also can develop large calcified masses of blood and inflammatory tissue that are mistaken for soft tissue sarcomas (pseudotumor syndrome).

Patients with severe hemophilia are usually diagnosed shortly after birth because of an extensive cephalhematoma or profuse bleeding at circumcision. However, young children with moderate disease may not bleed until they begin to walk or crawl, and individuals with mild hemophilia may not be diagnosed until they are adolescents or young adults. Typically, a hemophiliac patient presents with pain followed by swelling in a weight-bearing joint, such as the hip, knee, or ankle. The presence of blood in the joint (hemarthrosis) causes synovial inflammation, and repetitive bleeding erodes articular cartilage and causes osteoarthritis, articular fibrosis, joint ankylosis, and eventually muscle atrophy. Although bleeding may occur into any joint, after a joint has been damaged, it may become a site for subsequent bleeding episodes.

Hematuria, in the absence of any genitourinary pathology, is also common. It is usually self-limited and may not require specific therapy. The most feared complications of hemophilia are oropharyngeal and central nervous system bleeding. Patients with oropharyngeal bleeding may require emergency intubation to maintain an adequate airway. Central nervous system bleeding can occur without antecedent trauma or without evidence of a specific lesion.

Patients suspected of having hemophilia should have screening tests of hemostasis, including a platelet count, bleeding time, PT, and PTT. Typically, the patient will have a prolonged PTT with all other tests normal. Because of the clinical similarity of factor VIII deficiency and factor IX deficiency, any male with an appropriate bleeding history and a prolonged PTT should have specific assays for factor VIII and factor IX.

 TREATMENT

There are several tenets regarding the treatment of bleeding in hemophiliac patients: (1) Symptoms often precede objective evidence of bleeding. (2) Signs of bleeding may not appear until several days after well-documented trauma. Physicians caring for these patients have learned to rely on their patients to inform them of early symptoms, usually pain, and to begin treatment at that time. Early treatment is more effective, less costly, and can be lifesaving. (3) It is critical to avoid the use of aspirin or aspirin-containing drugs, which impair platelet function and may cause severe hemorrhage.

Plasma products enriched in factor VIII have revolutionized the care of hemophilia patients, reduced the degree of orthopedic deformity, and permitted virtually any form of elective and emergency surgery. The widespread use of factor VIII concentrates also has produced serious complications, including viral hepatitis, chronic liver disease, and AIDS. *Cryoprecipitate*, which contains about half the factor VIII activity of fresh frozen plasma in one-tenth the original volume, is simple to prepare and is produced in hospital or regional blood banks. It must be stored frozen and is thawed and pooled before administration. Partially purified *factor VIII concentrate*, which is prepared from multiple donors and supplied as a lyophilized powder, can be refrigerated and reconstituted just before use.

Three developments have increased the safety of factor VIII therapy and have changed medical practice. First, heating of lyophilized factor VIII concentrates under carefully controlled conditions can inactivate human immunodeficiency virus (HIV) without destroying factor VIII coagulant activity. Second, highly purified factor VIII can be produced by adsorbing and eluting factor VIII from monoclonal antibody columns. Third, recombinant factor VIII is now available. Patients with hemophilia should receive either monoclonal purified or recombinant factor VIII to minimize viral infections and exposure to irrelevant proteins.

It has been determined empirically that each unit of factor VIII infused, defined as the amount present in 1 mL normal plasma, will raise the plasma level of the recipient by 2 percent per kilogram of body weight. Factor VIII has a half-life of 8 to 12 h, making it necessary to infuse it continuously or at least twice daily to sustain a chosen factor VIII level. In patients with mild hemophilia, an alternative to the use of plasma products is desmopressin (DDAVP), which transiently increases the factor VIII level. Desmopressin, in general, will increase the factor level two- to threefold. Although generally safe, it occasionally causes hyponatremia or may precipitate thrombosis in elderly patients.

An uncomplicated episode of soft tissue bleeding or an early hemarthrosis can be treated with one infusion of sufficient factor VIII concentrate to raise the factor VIII level to 15 or 20 percent. A more extensive hemarthrosis or retroperitoneal bleeding requires twice-daily or continuous infusions in order to keep the factor VIII level between 25 and 50 percent for at least 72 h. Life-threatening bleeding into the central nervous system or major surgery may require therapy for 2 weeks with levels kept at a minimum of 50 percent of normal. In addition to the prompt infusion of factor VIII–enriched plasma products, patients need skilled orthopedic care with immobilization of inflamed joints to promote healing and to prevent contractures and physical therapy to strengthen muscles and maintain joint mobility. Before surgery, every patient should be screened for the presence of an inhibitor to factor VIII.

Patients with hemophilia who do not have an inhibitor should receive factor VIII infusions just before surgery and will require daily monitoring so that the factor VIII level is maintained above 50 percent for 10 to 14 days after surgery. When patients undergo joint replacement or other major orthopedic surgery, therapy should be continued for 3 weeks. This permits adequate wound healing and the institution of necessary joint mobilization and physical therapy.

Hemophiliacs also require treatment before dental procedures. Filling of a carious tooth can be managed by a single infusion of cryoprecipitate or factor VIII concentrate coupled with the administration of 4 to 6 g of ϵ-aminocaproic acid (EACA) four times daily for 72 to 96 h after the dental procedure. EACA is a potent antifibrinolytic agent that will inhibit plasminogen activators present in oral secretions and stabilize clot formation in oral tissue. Alternatives include tranexamic acid, a longer-acting antifibrinolytic. EACA is also effective when used as a mouthwash. For major oral and periodontal surgery and extractions of permanent teeth, patients should probably be hospitalized briefly and also treated with factor VIII concentrates. Therapy should begin just before surgery and be continued for a minimum of 48 to 72 h.

Many centers have organized home care programs so that patients can administer their own factor VIII infusions with the onset of symptoms. Occasional patients with very frequent bleeding receive regularly scheduled infusions. However, the expense and inconvenience usually limit the use of "prophylactic" infusions. Concern regarding transmission of AIDS has complicated therapy of hemophilia, and some patients are reluctant to treat themselves, despite the fact that current blood products carry a very low or no risk of transmitting HIV.

Complications Most hemophiliac patients have had multiple episodes of hepatitis, and a majority have elevated hepatocellular enzyme levels and abnormalities on liver biopsy. Between 10 and 20 percent of patients also have hepatosplenomegaly, and a small number develop chronic active or persistent hepatitis or cirrhosis. A few patients with hemophilia and end-stage liver disease have received liver transplants with cure of both diseases. Along with homosexuals and intravenous drug abusers, hemophiliacs are at high risk for AIDS because they frequently receive blood products. Hemophiliacs also can present with the full range of AIDS-related syndromes, including diffuse lymphadenopathy and immune thrombocytopenia. Although as many as 80 percent of multiply transfused hemophiliacs are HIV-positive and some have clinical AIDS, the advances in factor VIII concentrate technology discussed previously should prevent future HIV infection.

Despite frequent bleeding, severe iron-deficiency anemia is uncommon because most of the bleeding is internal and iron is effectively recycled. Mild iron deficiency from chronic epistaxis or gastrointestinal bleeding has been noted in some patients. In addition, after receiving large doses of the partially purified factor VIII concentrates, some patients have developed a mild Coombs-positive hemolytic anemia due to small amounts of anti-A and anti-B antibody that are present in commercial concentrates.

Following multiple transfusions, between 10 and 20 percent of patients with severe hemophilia develop inhibitors to factor VIII. Inhibitors are, generally, IgG antibodies that rapidly neutralize factor VIII activity. There are two types of inhibitors which have different biologic characteristics and lead to different clinical presentations. Patients with type I inhibitors have a typical anamnestic response and raise their antibody titer following exposure to factor VIII. Patients with a type II inhibitor have a low antibody titer that cannot be stimulated by factor VIII infusion. Patients with the type I inhibitor should not receive factor VIII. Control of bleeding may require the infusion of either porcine factor VIII concentrates, which may not cross-react with inhibitors, or prothrombin complex concentrates, which contain trace quantities of activated coagulation factors and can bypass the block in coagulation produced by the inhibitor. Patients with low-titer type II antibodies may respond to higher than normal doses of factor VIII.

Genetic Counseling and Carrier Detection Carrier detection formerly required biologic and immunologic assays that compared the ratio of factor VIII to vWF protein and were predictive in only 70 to 80 percent of cases. It is now possible to trace the defective allele in some families by examining the inheritance of restriction fragment length polymorphisms (RFLP) linked to the factor VIII gene. In addition, in families in which a specific mutation has been defined in the factor VIII gene, it can be readily detected by gene amplification and allele-specific oligonucleotide hybridization. For example, 45 percent of patients with severe hemophilia A have a chromosomal inversion arising from recombination between homologous sequences in intron 22 and an upstream gene. The inversion is readily detected by polymerase chain reaction (PCR) or Southern blotting. Previously, prenatal diagnosis required sampling fetal blood for coagulant activity. Now, in families with an identifiable RFLP linked to the gene or a known mutation, precise diagnosis is possible early in pregnancy from either chorionic villus biopsy or amniocentesis. The amount of material required for diagnosis has decreased, and the rapidity of diagnosis has increased with the introduction of PCR to amplify desired segments of genes.

Female carriers of hemophilia, who are heterozygotes, usually produce sufficient factor VIII from the factor VIII allele on their normal X chromosome for normal hemostasis. However, occasional hemophilia carriers will have factor VIII levels far below 50 percent due to random inactivation of normal X chromosomes in tissue producing factor VIII. These symptomatic carriers may bleed with major surgery or bleed occasionally with menses. Rarely, true female hemophiliacs arise from consanguinity within families with hemophilia or from concomitant Turner's syndrome or XO mosaicism in a carrier female.

FACTOR IX DEFICIENCY—HEMOPHILIA B Factor IX is a single-chain, 55-kDa proenzyme that is converted to an active protease (IXa) by factor XIa or by the tissue factor–VIIa complex. Factor IXa then activates factor X in conjunction with activated factor VIII. Factor IX is one of a group of six proteins synthesized in the liver that require vitamin K for biologic activity. As previously discussed (see Chap. 60), vitamin K is a cofactor for a unique posttranslational modification that inserts a second carboxyl group onto certain glutamic acid residues on factor IX. This modification permits calcium binding and adsorption onto phospholipid surfaces. Factor IX cDNA has been cloned and the gene locus mapped to the X chromosome. Many patients with deletions and mutations in the IX gene have now been described.

Factor IX deficiency or dysfunction (hemophilia B, Christmas disease) occurs in 1 in 100,000 male births. Accurate laboratory diagnosis is critical, since it is indistinguishable clinically from factor VIII deficiency (hemophilia A) but requires treatment with a different plasma fraction. Either fresh frozen plasma or a plasma fraction enriched in the prothrombin complex proteins is used. Monoclonally purified or recombinant factor IX preparations are undergoing clinical trials. In addition to the expected complications of hepatitis, chronic liver disease, and AIDS, the therapy of factor IX deficiency has a special hazard. Trace quantities of activated coagulation factors in prothrombin complex concentrates may activate the coagulation system and cause thrombosis and embolism. This is particularly common in immobilized surgical patients and patients with liver disease. As a result, some centers have returned to fresh frozen plasma for factor IX–deficient surgical patients, while others have recommended the addition of small doses of heparin to the concentrate to activate antithrombin III during the infusion and reduce hypercoagulability. The recombinant or monoclonally purified products are unlikely to be thrombogenic.

FACTOR XI DEFICIENCY Factor XI is a 160-kDa dimeric protein that is activated via the intrinsic coagulation pathway. It is converted to an active protease (XIa) by factor XIIa, in conjunction with high-molecular-weight kininogen and kallikrein (see Figs. 60-5 and 60-6). Factor XI deficiency is inherited as an autosomal recessive trait and is especially common in Ashkenazi Jews. In contrast to factors VIII and IX deficiency, the correlation between factor level and propensity to bleed is not as precise, there is less spontaneous bleeding, and hemarthroses are rare. Many patients with factor XI deficiency present with posttraumatic bleeding or with bleeding in the perioperative period, and occasional factor XI–deficient women have menorrhagia. Daily infusions of fresh frozen plasma are sufficient, since the half-life of factor XI is approximately 24 h. The majority of defective factor XI alleles were accounted for by a limited number of mutations in one large study.

OTHER FACTOR DEFICIENCIES Deficiencies in factors V, VII, X, and prothrombin (factor II) are all exceedingly rare autosomal recessive disorders. Although spontaneous or posttraumatic musculo-skeletal bleeding or menorrhagia can occur with these deficiencies, hemarthroses are uncommon. Fresh frozen plasma is the appropriate therapy, although prothrombin concentrates may be employed for patients with severe prothrombin or factors VII and X deficiency as long as the risks of hepatitis and thrombosis are recognized.

Defects in the contact activation pathway involving Hageman factor (factor XII), high-molecular-weight kininogen, and prekallikrein cause laboratory abnormalities but no clinical bleeding. Despite dramatic prolongation of the PTT, which is often greater than 100 s, deficient individuals have normal hemostasis and can undergo major surgery without plasma replacement therapy. It is important to recognize and diagnose these disorders because the patients should neither be treated inappropriately with plasma nor denied indicated surgery on the basis of these laboratory abnormalities. As discussed in Chap. 60, direct activation of factor IX by the tissue factor–VIIa complex may bypass this defective step in coagulation (Fig. 60-7).

AFIBRINOGENEMIA AND DYSFIBRINOGENEMIA Fibrinogen is a 340-kDa dimeric molecule made up of two sets of three covalently linked polypeptide chains. Thrombin sequentially cleaves fibrinopeptides A and B from the Aα and Bβ chains of fibrinogen to produce fibrin monomer, which then polymerizes to form a fibrin clot. Although fibrinogen is needed for platelet aggregation and fibrin formation, severe fibrinogen deficiency, paradoxically, does not usually cause serious bleeding except after surgery. Patients with afibrinogenemia, who have no detectable fibrinogen in plasma or platelets, may have infrequent, mild bleeding episodes. Preliminary genetic analyses do not show any gross deletion or structural changes in the genes encoding the α, β, and γ chains of fibrinogen despite the total absence of plasma fibrinogen.

Fibrinogen is an abundant plasma protein (2.5 g/L) that has been very well characterized. Mutations have been identified that alter the release of fibrinopeptides from the Aα and Bβ chains of fibrinogen, the rate of polymerization of fibrin monomers, and the sites for fibrin cross-linking. These dysfibrinogenemias are almost always inherited as autosomal dominant traits, so patients have approximately equal concentrations of normal and mutant fibrinogen in their plasma. Patients with dysfibrinogenemia have a slightly prolonged PT and PTT, a prolonged thrombin time, and a disparity between the quantity of fibrinogen measured with functional and immunologic assays. Despite these abnormalities, most patients have no symptoms, while other patients have moderate bleeding. A few dysfibrinogenemias induce a hypercoagulable state and increase the risk of thrombosis, and others have been associated with an increased incidence of abortion (see Chap. 119). Some patients with liver disease, AIDS, and lymphoproliferative disorders developed an acquired form of dysfibrinogenemia.

FACTOR XIII DEFICIENCY AND DEFECTIVE FIBRIN CROSS-LINKING Factor XIII is a transglutaminase that stabilizes fibrin clots by forming ϵ-amino–γ-glutamyl cross-links between adjacent α and γ chains of fibrin. Factor XIII deficiency is an extremely rare inherited syndrome with only a few hundred documented cases. Patients usually bleed in the neonatal period from their umbilical stump or circumcision. In addition to hemorrhage, these patients may have poor wound healing, a high incidence of infertility among males and abortion among affected females, and a high incidence of intracerebral hemorrhage. These observations suggest that the enzyme may be important in other physiologic and pathologic processes beyond hemostasis, including placental implantation, spermatogenesis, and wound healing. Several drugs, including isoniazid, may bind to cross-linking sites on fibrinogen and mimic factor XIII deficiency by blocking enzyme activity. Normal hemostasis requires only 1 percent of normal enzyme activity, which can be achieved with a single infusion of fresh frozen plasma or a purified factor XIII-rich product

derived from human placenta called Fibrogammin. Factor XIII has a 14 day half-life.

VITAMIN K DEFICIENCY Vitamin K is a fat-soluble vitamin that plays a critical role in hemostasis. Dietary vitamin K is absorbed in the small intestine and stored in the liver. The vitamin is also synthesized by endogenous bacterial flora resident in the small intestine and colon; however, there is controversy regarding the quantity of endogenous vitamin K that is absorbed from the large intestine. Following absorption and transport, vitamin K is converted to an active epoxide in liver microsomes and serves as a cofactor in the enzymatic carboxylation of glutamic acid residues on prothrombin complex proteins (Fig. 118-1).

There are three major causes of vitamin K deficiency—inadequate dietary intake, intestinal malabsorption, and loss of storage sites due to hepatocellular disease. Neonatal vitamin K deficiency, which causes hemorrhagic disease of the newborn, has disappeared from western countries with the routine administration of vitamin K to all newborn infants. Although there is, theoretically, a 30-day store of vitamin K in the normal liver, acutely ill patients can become deficient within 7 to 10 days. Acute vitamin K deficiency is particularly common in patients recovering from biliary tract surgery who have no dietary intake of vitamin K, have T-tube drainage of bile, and are on broad-spectrum antibiotics. Vitamin K deficiency is also seen in chronic liver disease, particularly primary biliary cirrhosis, and in some malabsorption states (see Chaps. 285 and 298). The cephalosporin antibiotics induce vitamin K deficiency in a manner analogous to the coumarin anticoagulants—they inhibit the reduction and recycling of vitamin K.

With the onset of vitamin K deficiency, plasma levels of all the prothrombin complex proteins (factors II, VII, IX, X; protein C and protein S) decrease. Factor VII and protein C, which have the shortest half-lives, decrease first. Because of the rapid fall in factor VII, patients with mild vitamin K deficiency may have a prolonged PT and a normal PTT. Later, as the levels of the other factors fall, the PTT also will become prolonged. Parenteral administration of 10 mg vitamin K rapidly restores vitamin K levels in the liver and permits normal production of prothrombin complex proteins within 8 to 10 h. Severe hemorrhage can be treated with fresh frozen plasma, which immediately corrects the hemostatic defect. If the cause of vitamin K deficiency cannot be eliminated, patients may need monthly injections. Purified prothrombin complex concentrates should be avoided because they contain trace quantities of activated forms of the prothrombin complex proteins and can cause thrombosis in patients with liver disease. They also will expose patients to an increased risk of hepatitis.

DISSEMINATED INTRAVASCULAR COAGULATION DIC can be either an explosive and life-threatening bleeding disorder or a relatively mild or subclinical disorder. Although there is a long list of diseases complicated by DIC, it is most frequently associated with obstetrical catastrophes, metastatic malignancy, massive trauma,

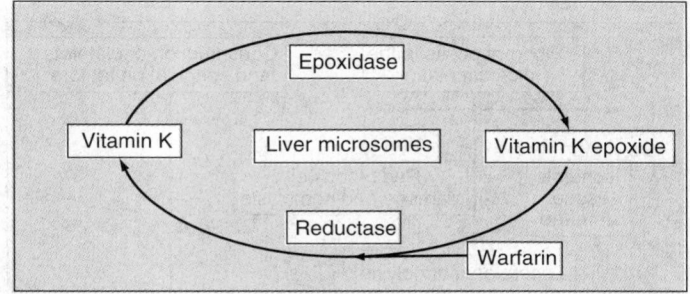

FIGURE 118-1 The mechanism of action of vitamin K, a cofactor in the formation of di-γ-carboxyglutamic acid residues on coagulation proteins, is depicted. Vitamin K is converted to an epoxide in liver microsomes. The epoxide is the active form and is reduced back to vitamin K by a liver membrane reductase. Warfarin blocks the action of the reductase and competitively inhibits the effects of vitamin K.

Table 118-1

Etiologic Factors and Disorders Causing Disseminated Intravascular Coagulation

Liberation of tissue factors	Obstetrical syndromes—abruptio placentae, amniotic fluid embolism, retained dead fetus, second trimester abortion
	Hemolysis
	Neoplasms, particularly mucinous adenocarcinomas, acute promyelocytic leukemia
	Intravascular hemolysis
	Fat embolism
	Tissue damage—burns, frostbite, head injury, gunshot wounds
Endothelial damage	Aortic aneurysm
	Hemolytic uremic syndrome
	Acute glomerulonephritis
	Rocky Mountain spotted fever
Vascular malformation and decreased blood flow	Kasabach-Merritt syndrome
Infections	Bacterial: staphylococci, streptococci, pneumococci, meningococci, gram-negative bacilli
	Viral: arboviruses, varicella, variola, rubella
	Parasitic: malaria, kala-azar
	Rickettsial: Rocky Mountain spotted fever
	Mycotic: acute histoplasmosis

SOURCE: Modified from RI Handin, RD Rosenberg, in *Hematology*, 4th ed, WS Beck (ed), Cambridge, MA, MIT Press, 1985.

and bacterial sepsis (Table 118-1). In each case, a tentative triggering mechanism has been identified. For example, tumors and traumatized or necrotic tissue release tissue factor into the circulation, while endotoxin from gram-negative bacteria activates several steps in the coagulation cascade. In addition to a direct effect on the activation of Hageman factor (factor XII), endotoxin induces the expression of tissue factor on the surface of monocytes and endothelial cells. These activated cell surfaces then accelerate coagulation reactions. These potent thrombogenic stimuli cause the deposition of small thrombi and emboli throughout the microvasculature. This early thrombotic phase of DIC is then followed by a phase of procoagulant consumption and secondary fibrinolysis. Continued fibrin formation and fibrinolysis lead to hemorrhage from the depletion of coagulation proteins and platelets and the antihemostatic effects of fibrin degradation products (Fig. 118-2).

The clinical presentation varies with the stage and severity of the syndrome. Most patients have extensive skin and mucous membrane bleeding and hemorrhage from multiple sites—usually surgical incisions or venipuncture or catheter sites. Less often, patients present with peripheral acrocyanosis, thrombosis, and pregangrenous changes in digits, genitalia, and nose—areas where blood flow is markedly

FIGURE 118-2 The pathophysiology of disseminated intravascular coagulation (DIC). Shown are the interactions between coagulation and fibrinolytic pathways that result in bleeding in patients with DIC.

reduced by vasospasm or microthrombi. Some patients, particularly those with chronic DIC secondary to malignancy, have laboratory abnormalities without any evidence of thrombosis or hemorrhage.

The laboratory manifestations include thrombocytopenia and the presence of schistocytes or fragmented red blood cells that arise from cell trapping and damage within fibrin thrombi; prolonged PT and PTT and thrombin time and a reduced fibrinogen level from depletion of coagulation proteins; and elevated fibrin degradation products (FDP) from intense secondary fibrinolysis. The D dimer immunoassay, which specifically measures cross-linked fibrin derivatives, is a more specific FDP assay. The cardinal manifestation of DIC which correlates most closely with bleeding is the plasma fibrinogen level; low fibrinogen levels are associated with more bleeding.

℞ TREATMENT

DIC, although sometimes indolent, can cause life-threatening hemorrhage and may require emergency treatment. This should include (1) an attempt to correct any reversible cause of DIC; (2) measures to control the major symptom, either bleeding or thrombosis; and (3) a prophylactic regimen to prevent recurrence in cases of chronic DIC. Treatment will vary with the clinical presentation. In patients with an obstetric complication such as abruptio placentae or acute bacterial sepsis, the underlying disorder is easy to correct, and prompt delivery of the fetus and placenta or treatment with appropriate antibiotics will reverse the DIC syndrome. In patients with metastatic tumor causing DIC, control of the primary disease may not be possible, and long-term prophylaxis may be necessary.

Patients with bleeding as a major symptom should receive fresh frozen plasma to replace depleted clotting factors and platelet concentrates to correct thrombocytopenia. Those with acrocyanosis and incipient gangrene or other thrombotic problems need immediate anticoagulation with intravenous heparin. The use of heparin in the treatment of bleeding is still controversial. Although it is a logical way to reduce thrombin generation and prevent further consumption of clotting proteins, it should be reserved for patients with thrombosis or those who continue to bleed despite vigorous treatment with plasma and platelets.

Patients who initially have mild DIC and may not be symptomatic may begin to bleed following surgery or chemotherapy. For example, mild DIC, without clinical bleeding, has been documented during saline- or prostaglandin-induced midtrimester abortions. Prophylactic treatment of patients with heparin may prevent progression of a mild DIC syndrome and has been used in the treatment of patients with acute promyelocytic leukemia and in some patients with a retained dead fetus who require surgical extraction. However, most patients with low-grade DIC can be managed simply with plasma and platelet replacement and do not require heparin. Chronic DIC does not respond to oral warfarin anticoagulants, but it can be controlled with long-term heparin infusion. Occasional patients with indolent tumors and severe DIC have been maintained on heparin administered by intermittent subcutaneous injection or continuous infusion with portable pumps.

Despite our detailed understanding of the pathophysiology of DIC and a vigorous approach to therapy, there is little evidence that its treatment will change the natural history of the underlying disorder. Therapy will only stabilize the patient, prevent exsanguination or massive thrombosis, and permit institution of definitive therapy.

COAGULATION DISORDERS IN LIVER DISEASE Since the liver plays a central role in the synthesis and metabolism of coagulation proteins, liver dysfunction is frequently accompanied by a hemostatic defect. The major causes of hemorrhage in patients with liver disease are outlined in Table 118-2. It is important to recognize that bleeding is usually due to an anatomic lesion, which can then be exacerbated by a hemostatic defect. Most patients bleed from complications of portal hypertension such as esophageal varices or from gastritis and peptic ulceration of the gastrointestinal tract. Portal hypertension also causes splenomegaly, with splenic sequestration of plate-

Table 118-2

CHAPTER 118
Disorders of Coagulation and Thrombosis   **741**

Causes of Bleeding in Liver Disease

ANATOMIC FACTORS

Portal hypertension
   Varices
   Splenomegaly and secondary thrombocytopenia
Peptic ulceration
Gastritis

HEPATIC FUNCTION ABNORMALITIES

Decreased synthesis of procoagulant proteins: fibrinogen, prothrombin,
  factors V, VII, IX, X, XI
Decreased synthesis of coagulation inhibitors: protein C, protein S,
  antithrombin III
Impaired absorption and metabolism of vitamin K
Failure to clear activated coagulation proteins leading to:
  Disseminated intravascular coagulation
  Systemic fibrinolysis

COMPLICATIONS OF THERAPY

Dilution of platelets and coagulation proteins from massive transfusions
Infusion of activated coagulation proteins in prothrombin complex
  concentrates
Bleeding from heparin; thrombosis from ε-aminocaproic acid (EACA)

---

lets and thrombocytopenia, which contributes to the hemostatic defect (see Chap. 298).

Patients with hepatocellular liver disease cannot store vitamin K optimally and may have some degree of vitamin K deficiency. Cholestasis, which is a frequent feature of liver disease, impairs vitamin K absorption and further decreases liver vitamin K stores. Abnormalities in the gamma carboxylation of prothrombin complex proteins independent of vitamin K and the production of abnormal proteins also have been described. Patients also may have decreased production of other coagulation proteins, including fibrinogen and factor V. The liver also produces inhibitors of coagulation such as antithrombin III and proteins C and S and is the clearance site for activated coagulation factors and fibrinolytic enzymes. Thus patients with liver disease are also "hypercoagulable" and predisposed to developing DIC or systemic fibrinolysis. For these reasons, coagulation defects in advanced liver failure are often difficult to distinguish from those of DIC.

Each patient with hemorrhage and liver disease should have a PT, PTT, platelet count, and fibrinogen determination, although it is not always possible to determine the major hemostatic abnormality from a single set of laboratory values. It is helpful to have previous laboratory data available for patients with chronic liver disease who develop an acute complication. There is a good correlation between the degree of prolongation of the PT and the risk of bleeding. Most patients present with moderate prolongation of the PT and PTT, mild thrombocytopenia, and a normal fibrinogen level. However, they also may present with a more complex defect combining defective synthesis, abnormal clearance, and active consumption of coagulation proteins. Since vitamin K deficiency is so common, it is advisable to administer a single parenteral dose of vitamin K after initial laboratory studies have been obtained, even though this may only partially correct the laboratory abnormalities. The presence of severe thrombocytopenia or a low fibrinogen level suggests the additional complication of DIC and may require further studies and therapy.

The safest replacement therapy for a patient with liver disease is fresh frozen plasma, since it supplies all known coagulation factors. However, even this form of therapy has drawbacks, since large quantities of plasma may precipitate hepatic encephalopathy and cause fluid and sodium overload. Prothrombin complex concentrates should be avoided because they only replace the vitamin K–dependent factors, may be contaminated with hepatitis and AIDS virus, and contain trace quantities of activated coagulation proteins. Similarly, fibrinogen concentrates (or cryoprecipitate) which are rich in factor VIII and fibrinogen should not be used without additional fresh frozen plasma. Anticoagulation with heparin has been advocated to control DIC, but this is particu-

larly hazardous and not recommended in cirrhosis because heparin is metabolized erratically and may thus lead to severe bleeding.

FIBRINOLYTIC DEFECTS Bleeding also can occur from defects in the fibrinolytic system. Patients with alpha$_2$ plasmin inhibitor deficiency or plasminogen activator inhibitor (PAI)1 have rapid fibrinolysis following fibrin deposition after trauma or surgery and so may experience recurrent hemorrhage. Similarly, patients with cirrhosis have an impaired clearance of tissue plasminogen activator (tPA) and systemic fibrinolysis that may contribute to their hemorrhagic defect. Rarely, patients with tumors such as metastatic prostatic carcinoma may develop diffuse bleeding from primary fibrinolysis rather than DIC. Clues to the diagnosis include a disproportionately low fibrinogen level with a relatively normal PT and PTT and the presence of a normal or nearly normal platelet count. Although there are some exceptions, patients with primary fibrinolysis should have an elevated titer of FDP but a normal D dimer level. However, it is sometimes difficult or impossible to differentiate primary fibrinolysis from the secondary fibrinolysis accompanying DIC. Patients with clearly established primary fibrinolysis should not receive heparin; they do require plasma therapy and, occasionally, fibrinolytic inhibitors such as EACA. However, EACA should not be given to patients suspected of having DIC unless they are also receiving heparin, since EACA can cause massive, often fatal, thrombosis in a patient with DIC.

CIRCULATING ANTICOAGULANTS Circulating anticoagulants, or inhibitors, are usually IgG antibodies that interfere with coagulation reactions. Specific inhibitors inactivate individual coagulation proteins and may cause severe hemorrhage. As previously discussed, they arise in 15 to 20 percent of patients with factor VIII or factor IX deficiency who have received plasma infusions. *Specific* inhibitors also occur in previously normal individuals. Although the most common target protein is factor VIII, inhibitors have been described with specificity for each of the coagulation proteins. In addition to hemophiliacs, anti-factor VIII antibodies are seen in postpartum females, in patients on various drugs, as part of the spectrum of autoantibodies in systemic lupus erythematosus (SLE) patients, and in normal elderly individuals. Circulating anticoagulants also have been reported in patients with AIDS.

Nonspecific (lupus-like) inhibitors prolong coagulation tests by binding to phospholipids. They are assayed by their anticoagulant effect [lupus anticoagulant (LA) activity] or their ability to bind to the complex phospholipid cardiolipin [anticardiolipin antibody (ACLA) activity]. While they are most often encountered in patients with SLE, these nonspecific inhibitors have also been noted in patients with many other disorders and also in otherwise normal individuals.

The critical laboratory feature, which identifies the presence of either type of inhibitor, is the failure of normal plasma to correct a prolonged PT, PTT, or both. Plasma from patients with a specific inhibitor will progressively inactivate a coagulation protein and thus prolong whichever of these screening tests requires the participation of that clotting factor. This effect persists after dilution. Nonspecific inhibitors immediately prolong the PT and PTT and, at low dilution, block multiple coagulation reactions. However, these effects can be overcome by altering the quantity or type of phospholipid or by diluting the plasma.

Hemorrhage in patients with specific inhibitors may require treatment with massive plasma or concentrate infusion, the use of activated prothrombin complex concentrates to bypass the antibodies against factors VIII or IX, and plasmapheresis or exchange transfusion to lower antibody titer. Chronic immunosuppressive regimens have been sometimes employed and have been particularly useful in otherwise normal individuals with an acquired factor VIII antibody. Many patients lose their antibody and recover within 6 to 12 months, although the acute mortality rate from uncontrollable bleeding may approach 10 percent.

Patients with LA activity have normal hemostasis and will not bleed unless they have concomitant thrombocytopenia or prothrombin deficiency. Both thrombocytopenia and hypoprothrombinemia are secondary to autoantibodies that bind either to platelets or the prothrombin molecule. While these antibodies have no effect on function, they accelerate clearance of the coated platelets or the antibody-prothrombin complexes.

There is increasing evidence that the presence of LA activity may predispose patients to thromboembolism and may cause midtrimester abortions. However, it is difficult to make firm predictions about the risk of thrombosis and the appropriate therapy for individual patients. First, tests for either LA or ACLA activity are not well standardized, and results vary among patients and can vary with serial measurements. The best predictor is a consistent prolongation of more than one coagulation test coupled with a high titer of ACLA activity. Second, the risk of thrombosis is increased in patients who have SLE compared with those with idiopathic LA or ACLA activity. There is little evidence that prophylactic therapy is beneficial or that treatments aimed at reducing the titer of antibody are superior to conventional antithrombotic therapy.

Although therapy should be individualized, the following general guidelines may be helpful. They are based on personal experience and review of a rapidly expanding and changing literature. Patients with SLE and either LA or ACLA activity who have had a thrombotic episode are at high risk for a recurrence and should receive long-term anticoagulant therapy. Women who have had more than one midtrimester abortion, especially those with SLE, should have a trial of anticoagulant therapy. Patients with a single thrombotic episode and no other risk factor except LA or ACLA activity may be treated, but the evidence for efficacy in this setting is minimal. Asymptomatic patients with laboratory abnormalities only should not be treated. Glucocorticoids should only be administered in conjunction with antithrombotic agents and are not of proven efficacy.

INHERITED PRETHROMBOTIC DISORDERS As previously discussed (see Chap. 60), coagulation is carefully regulated by a series of inhibitors that limit thrombin generation and fibrin formation and by the fibrinolytic system which effectively removes fibrin thrombi (see Figs. 60-5 and 60-6). Inherited defects in the natural coagulation inhibitors (i.e., antithrombin, protein C, and protein S), abnormalities in the fibrinolytic system, and certain dysfibrinogenemias predispose patients to thrombosis (see Table 60-5). A single point mutation in the factor V gene (factor V Leiden), which converts arginine 506 to glutamine and makes the molecule resistant to degradation by activated protein C, may account for 25 percent of inherited prethrombotic states. Antithrombin, protein C, and protein S defects are all autosomal dominant traits, so heterozygous individuals, who have a 50 percent reduction in protein concentration or a mixture of mutant and normal molecules, will have an increased risk of thrombosis. The effect of inheriting one or two factor V Leiden alleles is discussed in detail below. The patients all have similar clinical presentations with a strong family history of thrombosis, episodes of recurrent venous thromboembolism, and symptoms by their early twenties. Any patient with this distinctive history should be tested for the molecule abnormalities described below.

ANTITHROMBIN DEFICIENCY Antithrombin complexes with activated coagulation proteins and blocks their biologic activity (see Fig. 60-5). The rate of this reaction is enhanced by heparin-like molecules within the vessel wall or on endothelial cells. Plasma antithrombin III content varies from 5 to 15 mg/L (50 to 150 percent), with values only slightly below normal increasing the risk of thrombosis. For optimal screening, it is important to assess both the antithrombin III concentration by immunoassay and the plasma antithrombin and heparin cofactor activity with functional assays. The most common defect is mild (heterozygous) antithrombin deficiency, which occurs in 1 in 2000 individuals. In addition, dysfunctional antithrombin molecules, with mutations affecting either the serine protease–binding site or the heparin-binding site, or activation of inhibitor by heparin have been described.

Patients with antithrombin deficiency who develop acute thrombosis or embolism can be treated with intravenous heparin, since there is usually sufficient normal antithrombin to act as a heparin cofactor. Following their first episode of thromboembolism, patients should be placed on oral anticoagulants for life to prevent recurrent thrombosis. Family studies should be conducted when an antithrombin-deficient individual is discovered, since up to half the members of a kindred may be affected. Asymptomatic individuals with antithrombin deficiency should receive prophylactic anticoagulation with heparin or plasma infusions to raise their antithrombin level before medical or surgical procedures that may increase their risk of thrombosis. Chronic oral anticoagulation is not recommended until individuals at risk have a clinical thrombotic episode.

DEFICIENCIES OF PROTEINS C AND S Protein C is a vitamin K–dependent hepatic protein that binds to the endothelial cell surface protein thrombomodulin and is converted to an active protease by thrombin (see Fig. 60-5). Activated protein C, in conjunction with protein S, proteolyzes factors Va and VIIIa, which shuts off fibrin formation. Activated protein C also may stimulate fibrinolysis and accelerate clot lysis. Deficiencies of proteins C and S are usually autosomal dominant disorders, and deficiencies in the two proteins cause an identical syndrome of recurrent venous thrombosis and pulmonary embolism. Dysfunctional molecules also have been definitely identified in some patients with thrombosis. In addition, rare patients with homozygous protein C deficiency have fulminant neonatal intravascular coagulation and require prompt diagnosis and treatment.

The correlation between protein C and S levels and the risk of thrombosis is not as precise as for antithrombin III deficiency. In fact, as large surveys have been completed, asymptomatic individuals with protein C "deficiency" have been discovered. Protein C levels in these individuals overlap those with recurrent thromboembolism. In addition, in some well-studied protein C–deficient kindreds, asymptomatic individuals may have protein C levels as low as or lower than relatives with recurrent thrombosis. These observations raise the possibility that an as yet undiscovered comorbid condition is present in symptomatic patients. Finally, since a fraction of the available protein S is bound to C4b-binding protein and is unavailable for coagulation reactions, it may be important to measure both free and total protein S or to have a concomitant measurement of C4b-binding protein for maximum accuracy.

Heterozygous patients with protein C or S deficiencies who develop acute thrombosis should be heparinized and then placed on oral anticoagulants. There are, however, two potential problems with the use of coumarin anticoagulants in these patients. First, these vitamin K antagonists (see Fig. 118-1 and Fig. 60-5), which lower the level of the procoagulant factors II, VII, IX, and X, also may reduce the concentration of proteins C and S sufficiently to nullify the desired antithrombotic effect. In addition, there are patients with coumarin-induced skin necrosis who are protein C–deficient, suggesting that this defect may predispose patients to a rare but serious complication of oral anticoagulants. Patients with homozygous protein C deficiency require periodic plasma infusions rather than oral anticoagulants to prevent recurrent intravascular coagulation and thrombosis.

RESISTANCE TO ACTIVATED PROTEIN C AND THE FACTOR V LEIDEN MUTATION Several years ago there was an intriguing clinical observation that some patients with familial or recurrent venous thromboembolism did not prolong their PTT when activated protein C was added to their plasma. It has subsequently been shown that these patients all have an identical mutation in which arginine 506 in factor V is converted to glutamine. This amino acid substitution abolishes a protein C cleavage site in factor V and, thus, prolongs the thrombogenic effect of factor V activation. Approximately 3 percent of the population worldwide is heterozygous for this mutation, and presence of this mutation may account for 25 percent of patients with recurrent deep venous thrombosis or pulmonary embolism.

There is a clear relationship between inheritance of this defect and other thrombogenic stimuli. For example, heterozygosity at this allele increases an individual's lifetime risk of venous thromboembolism sevenfold. The risk also rises steadily with age. A homozygote has a 20-fold increased risk of thrombosis. In addition, heterozygosity coupled with ingestion of oral contraceptives or pregnancy increases the risk at least 15-fold. Coinheritance of factor V Leiden and another low-penetrance defect such as protein C or S deficiency are also additive. Many previous studies of risk factors predisposing patients to venous thromboembolism are being reevaluated to take into account this common mutation.

Approach to the Patient

With Venous Thromboembolism The following approach is suggested for the evaluation of patients who present with deep venous thrombosis or pulmonary embolism. Patients who develop venous thromboembolism without a clear predisposing factor, have a strong family history, present under the age of 30, or have more than one episode should definitely have studies sent for antithrombin III, proteins C and S, and factor V Leiden. Patients who present with deep venous thrombosis or pulmonary embolism during pregnancy or while using oral contraceptives have a 30 percent chance of having factor V Leiden and probably also deserve screening upon presentation.

Recommendations regarding treatment of patients with the inherited prethrombotic disorders are more controversial. All patients should receive standard initial therapy with heparin, either conventional or low dose (see Chap. 119), followed by 3 months of an oral anticoagulant such as warfarin. This regimen should allow for maximal healing and reendothelialization of the thrombosed vessels and minimize recurrence in the damaged vascular beds. There is not yet general agreement about which patients should go on to receive long-term (perhaps lifelong) anticoagulation, a judgment that depends on a careful balancing of the risk/benefit ratio.

The following approach is recommended based on current information about the natural history of these disorders. Patients with antithrombin III deficiency who become symptomatic have a high likelihood of recurrent events and should be placed on lifelong anticoagulation. Patients with protein C or S deficiency or heterozygous factor V Leiden patients have a lower likelihood of recurrent disease and do not need long-term anticoagulation until their second or subsequent episode of thromboembolism. Homozygous factor V Leiden patients should be placed on long-term anticoagulation after their initial episode, and all patients should receive replacement therapy or receive heparin prophylaxis during surgery or after trauma; women with these defects should avoid the use of oral contraceptives. The asymptomatic relatives of patients who are shown to have these disorders should receive appropriate prophylaxis but not start anticoagulation until they are symptomatic. In the absence of a congenital defect predisposing a patient to thrombosis, recurring or migratory thrombophlebitis may indicate an underlying malignancy.

DYSFIBRINOGENEMIAS AND FIBRINOLYTIC DEFECTS
Several families have now been described with recurrent venous thrombosis and embolism due to defects in fibrinogen or plasminogen or with decreased synthesis or release of tPA. While the majority of dysfibrinogenemias cause bleeding, several variants are characterized by excessively rapid release of fibrinopeptides and recurrent thromboembolism. Patients with this disorder as well as those with an abnormal plasminogen that resists activation by streptokinase and urokinase have been treated successfully with heparin and oral anticoagulants. Defects in tPA content or release have not been completely characterized. One group of patients with recurrent venous thrombosis and embolism failed to increase venous blood fibrinolytic activity when challenged with local ischemia or physical exercise. The other group had impaired fibrinolytic activity in extracts prepared from biopsied veins. The cloning of cDNA for tPA coupled with the availability of immunoassays for tPA should facilitate more detailed studies of this class of defects. There is also evidence that young

patients with acute myocardial infarction may have impaired fibrinolysis due to increased plasma levels of PAI, a serine protease inhibitor that binds to tPA and is derived from endothelial cells.

In addition to the inherited disorders that predispose patients to thromboembolism, many common illnesses are associated with an increased risk of thrombosis (see Table 60-5). These patients are said to have a "hypercoagulable" or "prethrombotic" state. This increased risk is seen in patients with chronic congestive heart failure and metastatic malignancy and in patients undergoing major surgery. In these patients, the generation of tissue factor activity in damaged or ischemic tissue or metastatic tumor, coupled with venous stasis and endothelial injury, induces the formation of venous and, more rarely, arterial thrombi. There are also several hematologic disorders including paroxysmal nocturnal hemoglobinuria, essential thrombocythemia, and polycythemia vera in which poorly defined abnormalities in circulating leukocytes and platelets or changes in blood flow and viscosity predispose patients to venous and arterial thrombosis. Diseases that affect the endothelial cell, such as Behçet's syndrome, Kawasaki's disease, and homocystinuria, or the administration of drugs such as the oral contraceptives, which lower antithrombin III levels, or L-asparaginase, which inhibits production of multiple coagulation factors, also may predispose patients to thrombosis. Infusion of granulocyte-macrophage colony stimulating factor (GM-CSF) has been associated with thrombosis as well.

There is increasing interest in the relationship between plasma homocysteine levels and the risk of both venous and arterial thromboembolism. It is well recognized that individuals with the congenital homocystinuria syndrome have, in addition to their Marfanoid habitus, an increased incidence of strokes and coronary artery disease. These patients have well-recognized enzyme defects (see Chap. 349), excrete homocysteine in their urine, and have very high plasma levels of the amino acid. There are also patients with early-onset cerebral vascular events who have mild homocystinuria that can be brought out by a methionine loading test. Epidemiologic studies show a relationship between homocysteine levels that are nearer to the normal range and coronary arterial disease. Although this correlation is not yet definitive, the relationship remains intriguing and of potential clinical relevance.

BIBLIOGRAPHY

ANTONARAKIS SE: The molecular genetics of hemophilia A and B in man. Factor III and factor IX deficiency. Adv Hum Genet 17:17, 1988

DESTEFANO V et al: Inherited thrombophilia: Pathogenesis, clinical syndromes and management. Blood 87:3531, 1996

FEINSTEIN DI: Lupus anticoagulant, anticardiolipin antibodies, fetal loss and systemic lupus erythematosus. Blood 80:859, 1992

GIDDINGS JC, PEAKE IR: Laboratory support in the diagnosis of coagulation disorders. Clin Haematol 14:571, 1985

GINSBURG KJ et al: Anticardiolipin antibodies and the risk for ischemic stroke and venous thrombosis. Ann Intern Med 117:997, 1992

KANE WH, DAVIE EW: Blood coagulation factors V and VIII: Structural and functional similarities and their relationship to hemorrhagic and thrombotic disorders. Blood 71:539, 1988

KASPER CK, DIETRICH SL: Comprehensive management of haemophilia. Clin Haematol 14:489, 1985

LAKICH D et al: Inversions disrupting the factor VIII gene are a common cause of servere hemophilia A. Nat Genet 5:226, 1993

LAWN R: The molecular genetics of hemophilia. Sci Am 254:48, 1986

LUSHER JM et al: Recombinant factor VIII for the treatment of untreated patients with hemophilia A: Safety, efficacy and development of inhibitors. N Engl J Med 328:453, 1993

MAMMEN E: Congenital coagulation disorders. Semin Thromb Hemost 9:1, 1983

PIERCE GF et al: The use of purified clotting factor concentrates in hemophilia. Influence of viral safety, cost and supply on therapy. JAMA 261:3434, 1989

WHITE GC, SHOEMAKER CB: Factor VIII gene and hemophilia A. Blood 73:1, 1989

119 *Robert I. Handin*

ANTICOAGULANT, FIBRINOLYTIC, AND ANTIPLATELET THERAPY

ANTICOAGULANT AND FIBRINOLYTIC THERAPY

Anticoagulation with heparin, followed by treatment with oral vitamin K antagonists, is the standard treatment for acute venous thrombosis and pulmonary embolism. In addition, chronic oral anticoagulation is used to prevent cerebral arterial embolism from cardiac sources such as ventricular mural thrombi, atrial thrombi, or from an atherosclerotic, partially stenosed carotid or vertebral artery. Anticoagulants are also used, less successfully, to treat peripheral or mesenteric arterial thrombosis. These agents retard fibrin deposition on established thrombi and prevent the formation of new thrombi. The induction of a fibrinolytic state by the infusion of plasminogen activators such as recombinant tissue plasminogen activator (rtPA), streptokinase (SK), or urokinase (UK) has become an accepted mode of therapy for some thromboembolic disorders. Fibrinolytic therapy has been proposed for patients with massive pulmonary embolism and systemic hypotension and to restore the patency of acutely occluded peripheral and coronary arteries. Prompt fibrinolytic therapy can reduce both myocardial damage and mortality following acute coronary occlusion (see Chap. 243). Fibrinolytic therapy may also be effective in acute thrombotic strokes and in venoocclusive disease of the liver.

ACUTE ANTICOAGULATION WITH HEPARIN Heparin is a naturally occurring mucopolysaccharide polymer with tetrasaccharide sequences that bind to and activate antithrombin III. It is an extremely potent anticoagulant that can dramatically reduce thrombin generation and fibrin formation in patients with acute venous and arterial thrombosis or embolism (Table 119-1). Heparin is administered to patients with acute thrombosis or embolism by continuous intravenous infusion at a rate sufficient to raise the activated partial thromboplastin time (APTT) to 1.5 to 2 times the patient's preheparin APTT. This requires infusion of approximately 1000 U.S.P. units per hour and is continued while patients are begun on oral anticoagulants and achieve appropriate prolongation of the prothrombin time. The usual duration of combined heparin-warfarin therapy is 5 to 7 days. Heparin is then discontinued, and the patient is maintained on warfarin. Alternatives to a continuous infusion include the administration of 5000 U.S.P. units of heparin four times a day either subcutaneously or intravenously. Commercial heparin preparations are heterogeneous, with only 20 percent of the product biologically active. In addition, active heparin fractions may vary considerably in molecular weight.

Table 119-1

Anticoagulant Therapy with Heparin

Clinical Indication	Dose, U.S.P. Units	Route
Prophylaxis in general surgery	5000 q 12 h	SC
Prophylaxis in medical patients with congestive heart failure, cardiomyopathy, or myocardial infarction	10,000 q 12 h	SC
Venous thromboembolism (acute)	5000 (bolus), then 1000 qh	IV
Venous thromboembolism (prophylaxis in pregnancy, warfarin failures, or chronic disseminated intravascular coagulation)	1000 qh	SC pump

ABBREVIATION: SC, subcutaneous

Biologically active, low-molecular-weight heparin preparations, while more expensive than unfractionated heparin, have several advantages: (1) they can be administered subcutaneously once or twice daily, (2) their pharmacokinetics are so predictable that APTT monitoring is not necessary, and (3) they are less immunogenic and less likely to cause thrombocytopenia. Many patients with deep venous thrombosis, a frequent cause for hospitalization, can be given low-molecular-weight heparin as outpatients. Given their other advantages and equivalent efficacy, low-molecule-weight heparin preparations may replace unfractionated heparin.

Long-term heparin administration via portable external or implantable pumps is occasionally needed for patients with recurrent thromboembolism that is refractory to oral anticoagulants, for pregnant women with thromboembolism, and for patients with chronic disseminated intravascular coagulation (DIC). Lower doses of heparin (5000 U.S.P. units every 12 h) have also been used to prevent deep venous thrombosis in high-risk surgical and medical patients. Patients with congestive heart failure, myocardial infarction, or cardiomyopathy may require 10,000 U.S.P. units every 12 h for similar protection.

The major complication of heparin therapy is bleeding—especially from surgical sites and into the retroperitoneum. Aspirin or aspirin-containing drugs impair platelet function. Thus, intramuscular injections in patients on both heparin and an antiplatelet drug may cause significant bleeding. Heparin's anticoagulant effect can be rapidly reversed by the administration of protamine sulfate. However, this is usually not necessary, since reduction or omission of a heparin dose usually improves hemostasis and stops bleeding. Thrombocytopenia occurs in about 10 percent of heparin recipients and is usually mild, with the platelet count falling to 50,000 to 100,000/μL. Thrombocytopenia is more common in patients receiving heparin derived from beef lung as opposed to porcine intestinal mucosa. Thus, porcine heparin is the preferred agent. As previously discussed, low-molecular-weight heparin is less likely to cause thrombocytopenia. Unfortunately, the majority of the antibodies arising from exposure to unfractionated heparin cross-react, so low-molecular-weight heparin cannot usually be used to treat patients with established thrombocytopenia. Occasionally, thrombocytopenia can be severe and may be accompanied by intravascular platelet agglutination and arterial thrombosis. Recognition of the rare complication of thrombocytopenia and paradoxical thrombosis is critical, since discontinuing heparin can promptly reverse the syndrome and may be lifesaving. Heparin administration for longer than 5 months also carries a risk of osteoporosis, perhaps through its activation of osteoclasts.

CHRONIC ORAL ANTICOAGULATION The coumarin anticoagulants, which include warfarin and dicumarol (dicoumarol), prevent the reduction of vitamin K epoxides in liver microsomes and induce a state analogous to vitamin K deficiency (see Fig. 118-1). They slow thrombin generation and clot formation by impairing the biologic activity of the prothrombin complex proteins and are used to prevent the recurrence of venous thrombosis and pulmonary embolism. Although regimens employing loading doses of drug have been advocated, the simplest way to induce anticoagulation is to administer a single dose of a coumarin compound and monitor the prothrombin time (PT) until the desired prolongation is achieved. For example, treatment can be initiated with 5 to 10 mg/d of warfarin or equivalent, with the goal of prolonging the PT to 1.5 to 2 times the control value. Although the PT may reach this value after a few days of therapy, effective anticoagulation, with stable reduction of all the prothrombin complex proteins, requires at least 1 week of warfarin administration. Most patients require a daily maintenance dose of 2.5 to 7.5 mg of warfarin to remain anticoagulated. As discussed above, patients should remain on heparin until the appropriate dose of a coumarin anticoagulant, such as warfarin, is established.

There is increasing concern that a more precise method is needed to assess the intensity of anticoagulation with warfarin. Commercial thromboplastins have different potencies and markedly affect the resulting PT. The International Normalized Ratio (INR) method has been adopted by most hospital laboratories and clinicians. In this reporting method, the ratio of the patient's PT is compared to the

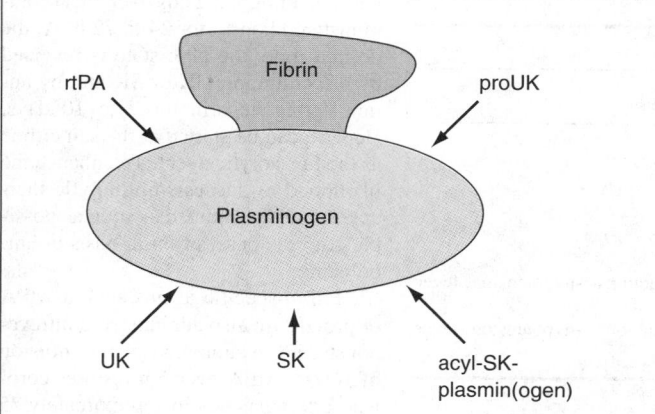

FIGURE 119-1 The mechanism of action of various plasminogen activators used for thrombolytic therapy. Recombinant tissue plasminogen activator (rtPA) and pro-urokinase (proUK) preferentially activate plasminogen bound to fibrin and are called "fibrin-specific" activators. Urokinase (UK), streptokinase (SK), and acylated streptokinase-plasminogen conjugates activate both free and fibrin-bound plasminogen.

mean PT for a group of normal individuals. The ratio is adjusted for the sensitivity of the laboratory's thromboplastin determined by the International Sensitivity Index (ISI). Thus, INR = $(PT_{patient}/PT_{normal})^{ISI}$. Use of the INR permits physicians to obtain the appropriate level of anticoagulation independent of laboratory reagents and to follow published recommendations for intensity of anticoagulation. The intensity of anticoagulation may be varied somewhat depending on the clinical indication. For example, the goal for anticoagulation in patients with venous thrombosis is to achieve an INR of 2 to 3. Patients with paroxysmal atrial fibrillation or a porcine bioprosthetic valve, who are taking a warfarin anticoagulant as a prophylactic measure, may be protected with an INR of 1.5 to 2. In contrast, patients with lupus-like anticoagulants and thromboembolism or those patients with mechanical cardiac valves require more intense anticoagulation. Satisfactory control requires an INR of 3 to 4. Patients with chronic indwelling venous catheters may be maintained on 1 mg/d of warfarin to prevent clot formation at the catheter tip; such a dose has no effect on the PT.

Although warfarin anticoagulants reduce the recurrence of deep venous thrombosis and pulmonary or cerebral embolism, they may also cause bleeding. Any patient who takes oral anticoagulants requires frequent monitoring of the PT. Despite the most careful management, fluctuations in PT can occur. Various drugs that alter liver microsomal metabolism of coumarins or compete for albumin-binding sites can increase or decrease the potency of these drugs (Table 119-2).

There is a direct relation between the duration of anticoagulation and the risk of recurrent thrombosis. Although recommendations vary somewhat, most patients with a single uncomplicated thromboembolic event have maximal benefit after 3 to 6 months of anticoagulation. About 10 percent of patients on an oral anticoagulant for 1 year have a serious complication requiring medical supervision, and 0.5 to 1 percent have a fatal hemorrhagic event despite careful medical management. The anticoagulant effects of coumarins can be reversed by infusion of fresh frozen plasma or by the administration of vitamin K. In many cases, reduction or omission of several doses improves hemostasis and stops hemorrhage. Despite the risk of bleeding, patients with prosthetic heart valves, severe mitral stenosis, cardiomyopathy, chronic congestive heart failure, recurrent or persistent atrial fibrillation, or an inherited "prethrombotic" disorder may require lifelong anticoagulation.

One devastating complication of oral anticoagulation is hemorrhagic skin necrosis. Some patients with this complication are deficient in protein C, a natural anticoagulant protein whose activity is reduced by vitamin K antagonists. Patients with suspected protein C deficiency should not begin oral anticoagulant therapy unless they simultaneously

Table 119-2

Effect of Drugs and Metabolic Changes on Oral Anticoagulant Potency

I. Factors leading to enhanced potency and increased prothrombin time
  A. Reduced coumarin clearance
    1. Disulfiram
    2. Metronidazole
    3. Trimethoprim-sulfamethoxazole
  B. Reduced albumin binding
    Phenylbutazone
  C. Additive hemostatic effect of certain drugs or disorders
    1. Aspirin
    2. Heparin
    3. Liver disease
    4. Thrombocytopenia
    5. Vitamin K deficiency
  D. Increased turnover of vitamin K
    1. Clofibrate
    2. Hypermetabolism (e.g., hyperthyroidism)
II. Factors leading to diminished potency and decreased prothrombin time
  A. Accelerated coumarin clearance—induction of hepatic metabolizing enzymes
    1. Barbiturates
    2. Rifampin
  B. Reduced absorption
    Cholestyramine
  C. Impaired metabolism
    Genetic coumarin resistance

receive heparin or plasma infusions to restore protein C levels to normal. Patients with an inherited trait that causes coumarin resistance may require extremely high doses to get an anticoagulant effect. Psychologically disturbed patients may surreptitiously ingest coumarin and present with unexplained bleeding and a prolonged PT. Plasma coumarin levels can be measured to confirm such ingestion.

FIBRINOLYTIC THERAPY Fibrinolysis, an important part of the normal hemostatic process, is initiated by the release of either tissue plasminogen activator (tPA) or pro-urokinase (proUK) from endothelial cells. These agents preferentially activate plasminogen, which is adsorbed onto fibrin clots. This serves to direct and localize the lytic process to sites that contain fibrin thrombi. Although fibrinolysis begins immediately after vascular injury, clot lysis and vessel recanalization may not be complete for 7 to 10 days. As previously discussed (see Chap. 60), the fibrinolytic pathway is important in normal hemostasis, as defects can predispose patients to either hemorrhage or recurrent thrombosis (see Chap. 118). Activators of the fibrinolytic system are frequently used to accelerate clot lysis in patients with thromboembolism (see Fig. 119-1, Table 119-3).

The pharmacologic agents being used to accelerate clot lysis are either derived from natural products or are chemically modified derivatives. They differ with respect to fibrin specificity and some types of complications (see Table 119-3). For example, many individuals have antistreptococcal antibodies that react with streptokinase and reduce its potency and cause febrile reactions. All fibrinolytic agents cause hemorrhage. tPA, proUK, and several other agents are relatively "fibrin-specific" and preferentially activate plasminogen in the presence of fibrin. Although this makes it theoretically possible to achieve selective clot lysis, in practice there is little difference in either the efficacy or toxicity of the "specific" and "nonspecific" fibrinolytic agents. There is, however, a substantial difference in cost, with equivalent doses of rtPA costing ten times that of SK.

It is important to remember that there is always some systemic fibrinolysis after the infusion of clinically effective doses of fibrin-specific agents. In fact, the fibrinogen level falls approximately 25 percent after infusion of lytic doses of rtPA. In addition, both the fibrin-specific and -nonspecific agents can cause hemorrhage as they cannot differentiate between vital hemostatic plugs and pathologic thrombi. To minimize the risk of bleeding, systemic lytic therapy is

Table 119-3

Fibrinolytic Activators

Product	Source	Molecular Weight	Fibrin	Complications
Recombinant tissue plasminogen activator (rtPA)	Recombinant	70,000	+	Bleeding
Pro-urokinase (proUK)	Melanoma cell cultures	55,000	+	Bleeding
Urokinase (UK)	Renal tubular cell cultures	33,000	+	Bleeding
Streptokinase (SK)	β-Hemolytic streptococci	47,000	−	Immune reactions—hypotension, fever Bleeding
Acyl-SK-plasmin(ogen)	Chemical synthesis	139,000	+/−	Immune reactions—hypotension, fever Bleeding

not recommended for patients with recent surgery or a history of neurologic lesions, gastrointestinal bleeding, or hypertension.

The current indications for fibrinolytic therapy are listed in Table 119-4. Fibrinolytic agents have been given to patients with pulmonary embolism for over 30 years. Such therapy is currently recommended for patients with massive pulmonary embolism that is complicated by hypotension, hypoxemia, and right heart strain. It is also used for selected patients with peripheral arterial embolism or occlusion and for patients with extensive iliofemoral thrombophlebitis. While lytic therapy may hasten the resolution of venous thrombi, the long-term benefit still remains unproven, and there is no firm evidence that lytic therapy reduces postphlebitic complications. In contrast, fibrinolytic therapy may be of distinct benefit in patients with axillary vein thrombosis, a condition that does not usually respond to conventional anticoagulation. Fibrinolytic agents are also used to restore the patency of occluded venous catheters and dialysis shunts. For this indication the agents are instilled locally. The extensive literature on the use of fibrinolytic agents to treat patients with coronary artery disease and myocardial infarction is reviewed in Chap. 243. When given within a few hours of infarction, fibrinolytic therapy reduces mortality and myocardial damage.

Although the doses and mode of administration may differ slightly, the general principles and complications are the same for all the fibrinolytic agents. SK and UK are the oldest and most extensively studied fibrinolytic agents. SK is a bacterial enzyme, and UK is a product of renal tubular epithelial cells. SK is an indirect plasminogen activator that interacts with circulating plasminogen to form an equimolar complex with proteolytic activity. The SK-plasminogen complex then activates additional plasminogen molecules that initiate fibrinolysis. In contrast, UK has intrinsic proteolytic activity and can activate plasminogen directly.

In the case of SK, a loading dose of 250,000 units is usually given irrespective of body weight. Since patients may have antistreptococcal antibodies, the loading dose may need to be repeated. In addition, patients may develop acute allergic symptoms including urticaria and, occasionally, serum sickness reactions. With UK, a loading dose of 4400 units per kilogram body weight is administered over 10 to 30 min. Both regimens induce an intense lytic state as evidenced by a drop in fibrinogen, prolongation of the thrombin time, and a prolongation of the euglobulin lysis time—an in vitro measure of fibrinolytic activity. After the initial loading dose, 100,000 units of SK or 4400 units of

Table 119-4

Indications for Fibrinolytic Therapy

Acute coronary occlusion/infarction
Acute peripheral arterial occlusion
Massive pulmonary embolism
Axillary vein thrombosis
Massive iliofemoral vein thrombosis
Occluded arteriovenous shunt
Arterial or venous cannulae
Venoocclusive disease of the liver

UK per kilogram body weight are administered hourly for 24 to 72 h. At the desired time, the lytic state is reversed by discontinuing UK or SK and by administering heparin for 7 to 10 days. Heparin can be started at the same time as the fibrinolytic agent. To enhance the likelihood of success, fibrinolytic therapy should be initiated as soon as possible after the onset of thrombosis or embolism.

Fibrin-specific agents such as rtPA or proUK are also administered intravenously. For example, systemic infusion of 100 mg rtPA over 6 h restores coronary artery patency in approximately 75 percent of patients. Patients are then maintained on heparin for several days. ProUK given in a similar manner has almost identical effects.

ANTIPLATELET DRUG THERAPY

Antiplatelet drugs have a role to play in the management of patients with arterial vascular disease and thromboembolism (see Table 119-5). Aspirin is the most widely studied of these drugs because of its unique pharmacology. A single dose of aspirin irreversibly acetylates and inactivates the enzyme cyclooxygenase and thereby inhibits platelet production of thromboxane A_2. Although aspirin may also inactivate cyclooxygenase in some tissues, including endothelial cells, such cells recover rapidly by synthesizing new enzyme. Platelets, which are anucleate, cannot synthesize new enzyme and remain inactive for the rest of their life span. As little as one 160-mg tablet of aspirin daily or a 325-mg tablet every other day inhibits platelet thromboxane production and aggregation.

Patients with coronary artery disease who have unstable angina are at high risk for myocardial infarction (Chap. 243). In two large clinical trials, the prompt administration of aspirin dramatically reduced progression to myocardial infarction in this group, although aspirin had no effect on the frequency, intensity, or duration of chronic angina. Aspirin also reduces the incidence of second infarction by 25 percent when administered to men who have had a myocardial infarct. In a large study of male physicians, daily aspirin therapy also reduced the incidence of first infarcts and is now widely used for prevention of myocardial infarction. The preliminary results of large-scale clinical and epidemiologic studies carried out in women suggest that the same beneficial effects of aspirin may be expected. The combination of aspirin and dipyridamole, when begun before surgery, may also increase the patency of coronary bypass grafts, and the same combination reduces the incidence of cerebral emboli in patients on warfarin who have prosthetic intracardiac valves. Although dipyridamole has been a popular antithrombotic agent, it has little efficacy when given alone. There is abundant evidence that aspirin is probably the only active agent in the combination aspirin-dipyridamole trials. Thus, dipyridamole can be eliminated in favor of aspirin alone.

Table 119-5

Indications for Antiplatelet Drug Therapy

A. Cerebrovascular disease
  1. Transient ischemic attacks
  2. Secondary prevention of cerebrovascular accidents
B. Cardiovascular disease
  1. Unstable angina pectoris
  2. Primary prevention of myocardial infarction
  3. Secondary prevention of myocardial infarction
  4. Following coronary bypass grafting
  5. Following insertion of a prosthetic valve
C. Renal disease
  1. To maintain the patency of arteriovenous cannulas
  2. ? To slow the progression of glomerular disease

Aspirin also reduces the frequency of transient ischemic attacks in patients with occlusive cerebrovascular disease. It has largely supplanted anticoagulation with the coumarin compounds in patients with transient ischemia. Aspirin also reduces the incidence of a second stroke by 25 percent when administered to men following the first cerebrovascular accident. Aspirin is also effective in maintaining the patency of arteriovenous cannulas inserted into patients with renal failure who require hemodialysis. Aspirin plus dipyridamole may also slow the progression of some forms of glomerulonephritis, although these drugs are not widely used in the treatment of renal disease. However, aspirin appears not to be effective in maintaining the patency of vessels following percutaneous angioplasty.

Although aspirin is clearly the most efficacious antiplatelet agent in clinical use today, there are a large number of new drugs being tested that may soon supplement aspirin therapy. Ticlopidine, which is a potent inhibitor of platelet function, has shown efficacy in several clinical trials. It is being used as an alternative to aspirin in patients with cerebrovascular disease and is superior to aspirin or warfarin-type anticoagulants in maintaining coronary stent patency. Monoclonal antibodies and both recombinant and chemically synthesized peptides that block either platelet adhesion or aggregation are being tested in clinical trials. A monoclonal antibody that blocks fibrinogen binding to platelet GpIIb/IIIa and thereby inhibits platelet aggregation (RheoPro) has been thoroughly tested and is now licensed for use in patients with coronary artery disease who undergo angioplasty. RheoPro is also being evaluated in other settings, e.g., as an adjunct to fibrinolytic therapy in patients with an acute myocardial infarction. There are also several orally active GpIIb/IIIa inhibitors in clinical trials that could be used chronically in patients with various coronary artery syndromes.

See Chap. 54, Anticoagulant, thrombolytic and antiplatelet drugs, *in* Goodman & Gilman's The Pharmacological Basis of Therapeutics *9th ed, New York, McGraw-Hill, 1966, pp 1341–1359.*

BIBLIOGRAPHY

AMERICAN COLLEGE OF CHEST PHYSICIANS: Fourth Consensus Conference on Antithrombotic Therapy. Chest 108(Suppl): 2255, 1995

COLLER BS: Platelets and thrombolytic therapy. N Engl J Med 322:33, 1990

LEVINE MN, HIRSH J: Hemorrhagic complications of anticoagulation therapy. Semin Thromb Hemost 12L:39, 1986

SAOUR JN et al: Trial of different intensities of anticoagulation in patients with prosthetic heart valves. N Engl J Med 322:428, 1990

SCHWARTZ L, SEIDELIN PH: Antithrombotic and thrombolytic therapy in patients undergoing coronary artery intervention: A review. Prog Cardiovasc Dis 38:67, 1995

120   *Lawrence C. Madoff, Dennis L. Kasper*

INTRODUCTION TO INFECTIOUS DISEASES: HOST-PARASITE INTERACTION

Despite decades of dramatic progress in their treatment and prevention, infectious diseases remain a major cause of death and debility and are responsible for worsening the living conditions of many millions of people around the world. Infections frequently challenge the physician's diagnostic skill and must be considered in the differential diagnoses of syndromes affecting a multitude of organ systems.

With the advent of antimicrobial agents, some medical leaders believed that infectious diseases would soon be eliminated and become of historic interest only. Indeed, the hundreds of chemotherapeutic agents developed since World War II, most of which are potent and safe, include drugs effective not only against bacteria but also against viruses, fungi, and parasites. Nevertheless, we now realize that, as we developed antimicrobial agents, microbes developed the ability to elude our best weapons and to counterattack with new survival strategies. Antibiotic resistance occurs at an alarming rate among all classes of mammalian pathogens. Diseases once thought to have been nearly eradicated from the developed world—tuberculosis, cholera, and rheumatic fever, for example—have rebounded with renewed ferocity. Newly discovered and emerging infectious agents appear to have been brought into contact with humans by changes in the environment and movements of populations. Many of these agents have been discovered only in recent decades. Ebola virus, hantavirus, the agent of human granulocytic ehrlichiosis, and retroviruses such as human immunodeficiency virus (HIV) humble us despite our deepening understanding of pathogenesis at the most basic molecular level. Even in developed countries, infectious diseases have made a resurgence. Between 1980 and 1992, age-adjusted mortality from infectious diseases in the United States increased by 39 percent. The role of infectious agents in the etiology of diseases once believed to be noninfectious is being increasingly recognized. For example, it is now widely accepted that *Helicobacter pylori* is the causative agent of peptic ulcer disease and perhaps of gastric malignancy. Human papillomavirus is likely to be the most important cause of invasive cervical cancer. A new human herpesvirus (HHV-8) is believed to be the cause of most cases of Kaposi's sarcoma. Epstein-Barr virus is a likely cause of certain lymphomas and may play a role in the genesis of Hodgkin's disease. The possibility certainly exists that other diseases of unknown cause, such as rheumatoid arthritis, sarcoidosis, or inflammatory bowel disease, have infectious etiologies.

Medical advances over infectious diseases have been hindered by changes in the patient population. Immunocompromised hosts now constitute a significant proportion of the seriously infected population. Physicians immunosuppress their patients to prevent the rejection of transplants and to treat neoplastic and inflammatory diseases. Some infections, most notably that caused by HIV, immunocompromise the host in and of themselves. Lesser degrees of immunosuppression are associated with other infections, such as influenza and syphilis. Infectious agents that coexist peacefully with immunocompetent hosts wreak havoc in those who lack a complete immune system. AIDS has brought to prominence once-obscure organisms such as *Pneumocystis carinii, Cryptosporidium parvum,* and *Mycobacterium avium.*

For any infectious process to occur, the parasite and the host must first encounter each other. Factors such as geography, environment, and behavior thus influence the likelihood of infection. Though the initial encounter between a susceptible host and a virulent organism frequently results in disease, some organisms can be harbored in the host for years before disease becomes clinically evident. For a complete view, individual patients must be considered in the context of the population. Infectious diseases often do not occur in isolation; rather, they spread through a group exposed from a point source (e.g., a contaminated water supply) or from individual to individual (e.g., via respiratory droplets). Thus, the clinician must be alert to infections prevalent in the community as a whole. A detailed history, including information on travel, behavioral factors, exposures to animals or potentially contaminated environments, and living and occupational conditions, must be elicited. For example, the likelihood of infection by *Plasmodium falciparum* can be significantly affected by altitude, climate, terrain, season, and even time of day. Antibiotic-resistant strains are localized to specific geographic regions, and a seemingly minor alteration in a travel itinerary can dramatically influence the likelihood of acquiring chloroquine-resistant malaria. If such important details in the history are overlooked, inappropriate treatment may result in the death of the patient. Likewise, the chance of acquiring a sexually transmitted disease can be greatly affected by relatively minor variation in sexual practices, such as the method used for birth control. Knowledge of the relationship between specific risk factors and disease allows the physician to influence a patient's health even before the development of infection by modification of these risk factors and—when a vaccine is available—by immunization.

Many specific host factors influence the likelihood of acquiring an infectious disease. Age, immunization history, prior illnesses, level of nutrition, pregnancy, coexisting illness, and perhaps emotional state all have some impact on the risk of infection after exposure to a potential pathogen. The importance of individual host defense mechanisms, either specific or nonspecific, becomes apparent in their absence, and our understanding of these immune mechanisms is enhanced by studies of clinical syndromes developing in immunodeficient patients (Table 120-1). For example, the frequent occurrence of meningococcal disease in people with deficiencies in specific complement proteins of the "membrane attack complex" underscores the importance of an intact complement system in the prevention of meningococcal infection.

Medical care itself increases the patient's risk of acquiring an infection in several ways: (1) through contact with pathogens during hospitalization; (2) through breaching of the skin (with intravenous devices or surgical incisions) or mucosal surfaces (with endotracheal tubes or bladder catheters); (3) through introduction of foreign bodies; (4) through alteration of the natural flora with antibiotics; and (5) through treatment with immunosuppressive drugs.

Infection involves complicated interactions of parasite and host and inevitably affects both. In most cases, a pathogenic process consisting of several steps is required for the development of infections. Since the competent host has a complex series of barricades in place to prevent infection, the successful parasite must utilize specific strategies at each of these steps. The specific strategies used by bacteria (see Chap. 139), viruses (see Chap. 182), and parasites have some remarkable conceptual similarities, but the strategic details are unique not only for each class of organism but also for individual species within a class.

Table 120-1

Infections Associated with Common Defects in Inflammatory or Immunologic Response

Host Defect	Disease or Therapy Associated with Defect	Common Etiologic Agent of Infection
NONSPECIFIC IMMUNITY		
Impaired cough	Rib fracture, neuromuscular dysfunction	Bacteria causing pneumonia, aerobic and anaerobic oral flora
Loss of gastric acidity	Achlorhydria, histamine blockade	*Salmonella* spp., enteric pathogens
Loss of cutaneous integrity	Penetrating trauma, athlete's foot	*Staphylococcus* spp., *Streptococcus* spp.
	Burn	*Pseudomonas aeruginosa*
	Intravenous catheter	*Staphylococcus* spp., *Streptococcus* spp., gram-negative rods, coagulase-negative staphylococci
Implantable device	Heart valve	*Streptococcus* spp., coagulase-negative staphylococci, *Staphylococcus aureus*
	Artificial joint	*Staphylococcus* spp., *Streptococcus* spp., gram-negative rods
Loss of normal bacterial flora	Antibiotic use	*Clostridium difficile*, *Candida* spp.
Impaired clearance		
Poor drainage	Urinary tract infection	*Escherichia coli*
Abnormal secretions	Cystic fibrosis	Chronic pulmonary infection with *P. aeruginosa*
INFLAMMATORY RESPONSE		
Neutropenia	Hematologic malignancy, cytotoxic chemotherapy, aplastic anemia, HIV infection	Gram-negative enteric bacilli, *Pseudomonas* spp., *Staphylococcus* spp., *Candida* spp.
Chemotaxis	Chédiak-Higashi syndrome, Job's syndrome, protein-calorie malnutrition	*S. aureus*, *Streptococcus pyogenes*, *Haemophilus influenzae*, gram-negative bacilli
Phagocytosis (cellular)	Systemic lupus erythematosus, chronic myelogenous leukemia, megaloblastic anemia	*Streptococcus pneumoniae*, *H. influenzae*
Splenectomy	—	*H. influenzae*, *S. pneumoniae*, other streptococci, *Capnocytophaga* spp., *Babesia microti*, *Salmonella* spp.
Microbicidal defect	Chronic granulomatous disease	Catalase-positive bacteria and fungi: staphylococci, *E. coli*, *Klebsiella* spp., *P. aeruginosa*, *Aspergillus* spp., *Nocardia* spp.
	Chédiak-Higashi syndrome	*S. aureus*, *S. pyogenes*
	Interferon γ-receptor defect	*Mycobacterium* spp., *Salmonella* spp.
COMPLEMENT SYSTEM		
C3	Congenital liver disease, systemic lupus erythematosus, nephrotic syndrome	*S. aureus*, *S. pneumoniae*, *Pseudomonas* spp., *Proteus* spp.
C5	Congenital	*Neisseria* spp., gram-negative rods
C6, C7, C8	Congenital, systemic lupus erythematosus	*Neisseria meningitidis*, *Neisseria gonorrhoeae*
Alternative pathway	Sickle cell disease	*S. pneumoniae*, *Salmonella* spp.
IMMUNE RESPONSE		
T lymphocyte deficiency/ dysfunction	Thymic aplasia, thymic hypoplasia, Hodgkin's disease, sarcoidosis, lepromatous leprosy	*Listeria monocytogenes*, *Mycobacterium* spp., *Candida* spp., *Aspergillus* spp., *Cryptococcus neoformans*, herpes simplex virus, varicella-zoster virus
	AIDS	*Pneumocystis carinii*, cytomegalovirus, herpes simplex virus, *Mycobacterium avium-intracellulare*, *C. neoformans*, *Candida* spp.
	Mucocutaneous candidiasis	*Candida* spp.
	Purine nucleoside phosphorylase deficiency	Fungi, viruses
B cell deficiency/dysfunction	Bruton's X-linked agammaglobulinemia	*S. pneumoniae*, other streptococci
	Agammaglobulinemia, chronic lymphocytic leukemia, multiple myeloma, dysglobulinemia	*H. influenzae*, *N. meningitidis*, *S. aureus*, *Klebsiella pneumoniae*, *E. coli*, *Giardia lamblia*, *P. carinii*, enteroviruses
	Selective IgM deficiency	*S. pneumoniae*, *H. influenzae*, *E. coli*
	Selective IgA deficiency	*G. lamblia*, hepatitis virus, *S. pneumoniae*, *H. influenzae*
Mixed T and B cell deficiency/ dysfunction	Common variable hypogammaglobulinemia	*P. carinii*, cytomegalovirus, *S. pneumoniae*, *H. influenzae*, various other bacteria
	Ataxia-telangiectasia	*S. pneumoniae*, *H. influenzae*, *S. aureus*, rubella virus, *G. lamblia*
	Severe combined immunodeficiency	*S. aureus*, *S. pneumoniae*, *H. influenzae*, *Candida albicans*, *P. carinii*, varicella-zoster virus, rubella virus, cytomegalovirus
	Wiskott-Aldrich syndrome	Agents of infections associated with T and B cell abnormalities

SOURCE: Adapted from H Masur and A Fauci, in *Harrison's Principles of Internal Medicine*, 13th ed, KJ Isselbacher et al (eds), New York, McGraw-Hill, 1994.

SURFACE CONTACT Most often, the first contact between host and parasite is at a mucosal or cutaneous surface. In order to prevent the initiation of the infectious process during such contact, the host has developed highly effective defense mechanisms operating at the body's interface with the outside world. Many of these initial mechanisms of host defense are not specifically directed at individual species of organisms. Mechanical barriers, for example, including the tough cornified epithelium of the skin and the flow of secretions from glands, tend to prevent infection by any potential pathogen. Chemical barriers, such as the acidic environment of the stomach and urinary bladder, represent hostile environments for most microorganisms. The

CHAPTER 120
Introduction to Infectious Diseases: Host-Parasite Interaction **751**

normal microflora, composed of nonpathogenic organisms that inhabit mucosal surfaces, makes colonization by pathogens more difficult by competing for environmental resources. Behavioral and neurologic mechanisms, such as gagging and coughing, help prevent infection of the lower respiratory tract.

We recognize the importance of these mechanisms by the diseases that arise when they are impaired (Table 120-1). Patients with a suppressed cough (e.g., due to pain associated with a fractured rib) are very susceptible to pneumonia. Achlorhydric individuals are particularly likely to develop salmonellosis after the ingestion of contaminated food or drink because a lower inoculum is required for organisms to reach the intestine. The abnormal bronchial secretions in patients with cystic fibrosis usually permit chronic pulmonary infection with *Pseudomonas aeruginosa*. A break in the skin resulting from an animal or insect bite, a burn, a scratch, trauma, or surgery allows the entry of pathogenic or opportunistic agents. The eradication of the normal bowel flora by antibiotics may render organisms such as *Clostridium difficile* pathogenic.

The host has also evolved an organism-specific immune system that functions at mucosal surfaces. Specialized macrophages and lymphocytes, which play a role in the specific defense system, reside in the epithelium of the gut, in the nasal and vaginal mucosae, and at other sites that interface with the environment. This mucosa-associated lymphoid tissue appears to play a role in trapping antigens and allowing them to be presented to lymphocytes at the mucosal surface. In certain areas, these tissues become anatomically distinct; examples include the oropharyngeal tonsil and—in the gastrointestinal tract—Peyer's patches and the appendix. Central to this defense system is the elaboration of surface immunoglobulins, particularly secretory IgA, which prevents adherence and penetration of organisms.

Pathogens have evolved an array of methods for breaching this well-developed boundary between the host and the outside world. In order to invade, most pathogens must first attach. Many microorganisms have developed a highly specialized apparatus for binding to the surface of the host. For example, pili of uropathogenic *Escherichia coli* recognize certain host glycoproteins that serve as sites for bacterial attachment to epithelial cells. The binding of Epstein-Barr virus to a specific complement receptor (CR2) on B lymphocytes allows the subsequent internalization of the virus. HIV binds to the CD4 complex present in certain human T lymphocytes. Many bacterial pathogens produce enzymes or surface components that bind to or inactivate secretory IgA. Other organism factors impair ciliary motility, thus hindering clearance.

Some potentially pathogenic organisms are capable of living symbiotically with the host, colonizing but not infecting for extended periods. It is important for the astute clinician to distinguish colonization from infection. *E. coli* is normally present in large numbers in the colon, where it contributes to the synthesis of vitamin K and induces natural immunity to other bacteria. It is only when *E. coli* penetrates the mucosal barriers and enters normally sterile sites that it becomes an opportunistic pathogen. The penetration of *E. coli* into the peritoneum through a mechanical breach in the bowel wall, its entry into the urinary bladder, and its invasion of the bloodstream are events associated with infection and disease. Some virulent pathogens, such as group A streptococci and *Neisseria meningitidis*, are able to colonize most individuals for prolonged intervals without untoward effects. In these cases, the individuals involved may already have developed specific immunity following colonization with antigenically similar nonpathogenic organisms, or invasion may be prevented by nonspecific host defenses while specific immunity is being stimulated. Certain viruses (e.g., herpesviruses) inhabit tissue for the life of the host, causing little harm as long as the host's immune system is intact but inducing severe symptomatic disease if the immune status is altered.

INVASION Microorganisms attached to a mucosal surface use specific mechanisms to invade deeper host structures. Meningococci and gonococci penetrate and traverse mucosal epithelial cells by transcytotic mechanisms. *Haemophilus influenzae* enters the vascular system by squeezing through the junction between epithelial cells. Salmo-

nellae induce their own phagocytosis by the host's gastrointestinal macrophages (i.e., in Peyer's patches); these bacteria then resist killing by the phagolysosome of the unactivated macrophage and subsequently proliferate, spilling into the bloodstream. Schistosomal cercariae penetrate the epidermis of the host in contaminated fresh water and are able to uncoat, mature, and enter the circulation. Other pathogens, including bacteria (e.g., *Rickettsia rickettsii* and *Yersinia pestis*), viruses (e.g., dengue and eastern equine encephalitis virus), and parasites (e.g., *Plasmodium* and *Trypanosoma*), may enlist the aid of an insect vector to breach the protective skin and enter the circulation.

Infection has a substantial impact on the microorganism as well as the host. It is increasingly recognized that the invading microbe senses and adapts to changes in its environment through complex regulatory mechanisms, "turning on" the virulence factors necessary for invasion and survival in the host. For example, *Yersinia* spp., *Shigella* spp., and *Bordetella pertussis* all express virulence factors in response to exposure to the 37°C temperature likely to be encountered at the time of infection. Other virulence determinants—the Shiga-like toxin of enterohemorrhagic *E. coli*, for example—are expressed in response to low levels of free iron that exist in the host, where iron is tightly bound by transferrin and other proteins. Many such bacterial virulence factors are controlled by two-component regulatory systems: one protein component senses environmental changes and then signals (often by phosphorylation) a second protein that coordinately regulates the expression of a group of genes whose products facilitate survival in the host milieu.

TROPISM In order to infect a host successfully, many pathogens occupy highly specific niches within the host and thus are tropic to a particular body site or cell type. This tropism has many implications for the life cycle of the pathogen, for the immune system of the host, and for the disease process. Malaria sporozoites, for example, are rapidly cleared from the blood into hepatocytes, where they undergo maturation and release into the circulation; trophozoites, in turn, can infect only the erythrocyte. The bacterial pathogen *H. pylori* produces the enzyme urease, which, by cleaving urea to form ammonium ion, may allow the organism to inhabit a neutral microenvironment within the highly acidic gastric mucosa. Many viruses are tropic for specific tissues; for example, the hepatitis viruses are tropic for hepatocytes, HIV is tropic for CD4-bearing T lymphocytes, herpesviruses are tropic for neural tissues, and rhinoviruses are tropic for the nasal epithelium.

The central nervous system (CNS) is uniquely protected from perturbations in the environment by a blood-brain barrier—a system of tight junctions in capillaries of the CNS that resists the entry of inflammatory cells, pathogens, and even macromolecules into the subarachnoid space. Certain pathogens have devised highly specialized, and as yet poorly understood, mechanisms for breaching this barricade. One strategy employed by organisms such as rabies virus and herpes simplex virus in humans and by reovirus in experimental animals is to travel within peripheral nerves into the CNS. Other organisms, such as certain highly encapsulated bacteria and fungi, enter from the bloodstream and possess surface components that allow them to traverse the capillary tight junctions. The degree of specialization required for this mechanism is demonstrated by the predilection of certain serotypes of organisms within a species to cause meningitis. Type III strains account for the vast majority of cases of neonatal meningitis caused by group B *Streptococcus*, even though other serotypes cause much of the invasive disease outside the CNS. This disparity appears to be due solely to the arrangement of the component sugars of the capsular polysaccharide: other serotypes of group B *Streptococcus* rarely cause neonatal meningitis even though their capsules possess the same four component sugars in different structural arrangements.

MICROBIAL VIRULENCE STRATEGIES Microbes have developed a variety of strategies for escaping host immunity. Many bacteria are encapsulated with polysaccharides that allow them to evade complement deposition in the absence of specific antibodies. These organisms proliferate freely until the host is able to generate capsule-specific antibodies. Several species of gram-positive bacteria possess surface proteins that bind immunoglobulins, thereby perhaps interfering with immune recognition. Other organisms even employ the host's immune response as a survival strategy. *Schistosoma mansoni* recognizes the host cytokine tumor necrosis factor (TNF) and responds to it by depositing eggs. Some pathogenic organisms elaborate toxins and enzymes that facilitate invasion of the host and are often responsible for the disease state. Pathogenic strains of *Vibrio cholerae* (Chap. 161) elaborate a potent and well-characterized toxin that enters the host's enterocytes via a specific receptor (the monosialyl GM$_1$ ganglioside) and then enzymatically activates the host cell's adenylate cyclase system. This event in turn leads to the copious electrolyte and fluid secretion by the enterocyte and the voluminous watery diarrhea that are characteristic of cholera. *Staphylococcus aureus* expresses a large number of extracellular proteins that contribute to the variety of disease states associated with this bacterium (Chap. 142). Enterotoxins cause staphylococcal food poisoning, even though viable organisms may never enter the host. Toxic shock syndrome toxin 1 (TSST-1) is responsible for the many systemic effects of toxic shock syndrome, even though the organism is confined to a mucosal surface or a wound. Toxin-mediated damage to mucosal surfaces sometimes permits proliferation of a pathogen at a mucosal site, whether or not the organism invades. Pertussis toxin impairs the ability of ciliated epithelium to clear the pathogen from the host's bronchial tree. Enteropathogenic *E. coli* and *V. cholerae* are examples of toxin-producing bacteria that normally do not invade. In contrast, other toxins are clearly capable of promoting invasion and spread. The extracellular enzymes of *Streptococcus pyogenes*, such as hyaluronidase, facilitate movement through tissue planes, and streptolysins O and S disrupt leukocyte membranes and thus impair the host's defense.

Integral components of pathogens are often responsible for much of the disease process that results from infection. Lipopolysaccharides of gram-negative bacteria act as a potent endotoxin (*endo-* in this case indicating that the lipopolysaccharides are part of the bacterial membrane, not a secreted product) that is the proximate cause of the sepsis syndrome. The cell walls of gram-positive bacteria appear to elicit a similar host inflammatory response. The anaerobic pathogen *Bacteroides fragilis* possesses a capsular polysaccharide that promotes abscess formation by the host.

IMMUNE RESPONSE   Once in the bloodstream or a normally sterile body site, the microorganism faces the host's tightly integrated cellular and humoral immune systems. Cellular immunity (Chap. 305), comprising T lymphocytes, macrophages, and natural killer cells, primarily recognizes and combats pathogens that proliferate intracellularly. Cellular immune mechanisms are important in immunity to all classes of infectious agents, including most viruses and many bacteria (e.g., *Mycoplasma*, *Chlamydia*, *Listeria*, *Salmonella*, *Mycobacterium*), parasites (e.g., *Trypanosoma*, *Toxoplasma*, *Leishmania*), and fungi (e.g., *Histoplasma*, *Cryptococcus*, and *Coccidioides*). Usually, T lymphocytes are activated by macrophages and B lymphocytes, which present foreign antigens along with the host's own major histocompatibility complex antigen. Activated T cells may then act in several ways to fight infection. Cytotoxic T cells may directly attack and lyse host cells that express foreign antigens. Helper T cells stimulate the proliferation of B cells and the production of immunoglobulins. T cells elaborate cytokines (e.g., interferon), which directly inhibit the growth of pathogens or stimulate killing by host macrophages and cytotoxic cells. Cytokines also augment the host's immunity by stimulating the inflammatory response (fever, the production of acute-phase serum components, and the proliferation of leukocytes). Cytokine stimulation does not always result in a favorable response in the host; septic shock (see Chap. 124) and toxic shock syndrome (see Chaps. 142 and 143) are among the conditions that are mediated by these inflammatory substances.

The reticuloendothelial system comprises monocyte-derived phagocytic cells that are located in the liver (Kupffer cells), lung (alveolar macrophages), spleen, kidney (mesangial cells), brain (microglia), and lymph nodes and that clear circulating microorganisms. Although these tissue macrophages and polymorphonuclear leukocytes (PMNs) are capable of killing microorganisms without help, they function much more efficiently when pathogens are first *opsonized* (from the Greek for "to prepare for eating") by components of the complement system such as C3b and/or by antibodies.

Extracellular pathogens, including most encapsulated bacteria, are attacked by the humoral immune system, which includes antibodies, the complement cascade, and phagocytic cells. Antibodies are complex glycoproteins (also called immunoglobulins) that are produced by mature B lymphocytes, circulate in body fluids, and are secreted on mucosal surfaces. Antibodies specifically recognize and bind to foreign antigens. One of the most impressive features of the immune system is the ability to generate an incredible diversity of antibodies capable of recognizing virtually every foreign antigen yet not reacting with self. In addition to being exquisitely specific for antigens, antibodies come in different structural and functional classes: IgG predominates in the circulation and persists for many years after exposure; IgM is the earliest specific antibody to appear in response to infection; secretory IgA is important in immunity at mucosal surfaces, while monomeric IgA appears in the serum; and IgE is important in allergic and parasitic diseases. Antibodies may act by directly impeding the function of an invading organism, by neutralizing secreted toxins and enzymes, or by facilitating the removal of the antigen (invading organism) by phagocytic cells. Immunoglobulins participate in cell-mediated immunity by promoting the antibody-dependent cellular cytotoxicity functions of certain T lymphocytes. Antibodies also promote the deposition of complement components on the surface of the invader.

The complement system (see Chap. 305) consists of a group of serum proteins that function as a cooperative, self-regulating cascade of enzymes that adhere to—and in some cases disrupt—the surface of invading organisms. Some of these surface-adherent proteins (e.g., C3b) can then act as opsonins for destruction of microbes by phagocytes. The later, "terminal" components (C7, C8, and C9) can directly kill some bacterial invaders (notably, many of the neisseriae) by forming a "membrane attack complex" and disrupting the integrity of the bacterial membrane, thus causing bacteriolysis. Other complement components, such as C5a, act as chemoattractants for PMNs. Complement activation and deposition occur by either or both of two pathways: the classic pathway is activated primarily by immune complexes (i.e., antibody bound to antigen), and the alternative pathway is activated by microbial components, frequently in the absence of antibody. PMNs have receptors for both antibody and C3b, and antibody and complement function together to aid in the clearance of infectious agents.

PMNs, short-lived white blood cells that engulf and kill invading microbes, are first attracted to inflammatory sites by chemoattractants such as C5a, which is a product of complement activation at the site of infection. PMNs localize to the site of infection by adhering to cellular adhesion molecules expressed by endothelial cells. Endothelial cells express these receptors, called *selectins* (CD-62, ELAM-1), in response to inflammatory cytokines such as TNFα and interleukin 1. The binding of these selectin molecules to specific receptors on PMNs results in the adherence of the PMN to the endothelium. Cytokine-mediated upregulation and expression of intercellular adhesion molecule 1 (ICAM 1) on endothelial cells then take place, and this latter receptor binds to β$_2$ integrins on the PMN, thereby facilitating diapedesis into the extravascular compartment. Once the PMNs are in the extravascular compartment, various molecules such as arachidonic acids further enhance the inflammatory process.

Approach to the Patient

The clinical manifestations of infectious diseases at presentation are myriad, varying from fulminant life-threatening processes to brief and self-limited conditions to indolent chronic maladies. The clinician must use all the skills of medicine to diagnose the infection and prescribe appropriate treatment. First, a careful history is essential and must include details on underlying chronic diseases; medications; occupation; travel; and risk factors for exposure to certain types of pathogens, such as those associated with sexual contacts, family illnesses, illicit drug use, particular animals, blood transfusions, ingestion of contaminated liquids or foods, or bites of insect vectors. Since infectious diseases may involve many organ systems, a careful review of systems may elicit important clues as to the disease process. The physical examination must be thorough, and attention must be paid to seemingly minor details: a soft heart murmur that might indicate bacterial endocarditis; an evanescent skin rash that suggests rheumatic fever; or a retinal lesion that suggests disseminated candidiasis or cytomegalovirus (CMV) infection.

LABORATORY INVESTIGATIONS Laboratory studies must be carefully considered and directed toward establishing an etiologic diagnosis in the shortest possible time, at the lowest possible cost, and with the least possible discomfort to the patient. Cultures must be performed in a manner that minimizes the likelihood of contamination with normal flora while maximizing the yield. A sputum sample is far more likely to be valuable when elicited with careful coaching by the clinician than when collected in a container simply left at the bedside with cursory instruction. Gram's stains of specimens should be interpreted carefully, and the quality of the specimen assessed. The findings on Gram's staining should correspond to the results of culture; a discrepancy may suggest diagnostic possibilities such as infection due to fastidious or anaerobic bacteria.

The microbiology laboratory must be an ally in the diagnostic endeavor (see Chap. 121). Astute laboratory personnel will suggest optimal culture and transport conditions or alternative tests to facilitate diagnosis. If informed about specific potential pathogens, an alert laboratory staff will allow sufficient time for these organisms to become evident in culture, even when present in small numbers or when slow-growing. The parasitology technician who is attuned to the specific diagnostic considerations relevant to a particular case may be able to detect the rare, otherwise-elusive egg or cyst in a stool specimen. In cases where a diagnosis appears difficult, serum should be stored during the early acute phase of the illness so that a diagnostic rise in titer of antibody to a specific pathogen can be detected later. Bacterial and fungal antigens can sometimes be detected in body fluids, even when cultures are negative or are rendered sterile by antibiotic therapy. Techniques such as the polymerase chain reaction allow the amplification of specific DNA sequences so that minute quantities of foreign nucleic acids can be recognized in host specimens.

℞ TREATMENT

Optimal therapy for infectious diseases requires a broad knowledge of medicine and careful clinical judgment. Life-threatening infections such as bacterial meningitis or sepsis, viral encephalitis, or falciparum malaria must be treated immediately, often before a specific causative organism is identified. Antimicrobial agents must be chosen empirically and must be active against the range of potential infectious agents consistent with the clinical scenario. In contrast, good clinical judgment sometimes dictates withholding of antimicrobials in a self-limited process or until a specific diagnosis is made. The dictum *primum non nocere* should be adhered to, and it should be remembered that all antimicrobials carry a risk (and a cost) to the patient. Direct toxicity may be encountered—e.g., ototoxicity due to aminoglycosides, bone marrow toxicity due to zidovudine, and hepatotoxicity due to antituberculous agents such as isoniazid and rifampin. Allergic reactions are common and can be serious. Since superinfection sometimes follows the eradication of the normal flora and colonization by a resistant organism, one invariable principle is that infectious disease therapy should be directed toward as narrow a spectrum of infectious agents as possible. Treatment specific for the pathogen should result in as little perturbation as possible of the host's microflora. With few exceptions, abscesses require surgical or percutaneous drainage for cure. Foreign bodies, including medical devices, must generally be removed in order to eliminate an infection of the device or of the adjacent tissue. Other infections, such as necrotizing fasciitis, peritonitis due to a perforated organ, gas gangrene, and chronic osteomyelitis, require surgery as the primary means of cure; in these conditions, antibiotics play only an adjunctive role.

Recently, the role of immunomodulators in the management of infectious diseases has received increasing attention. Glucocorticoids have been shown to be of benefit in the treatment of *H. influenzae* meningitis in children and in therapy for *P. carinii* pneumonia in patients with AIDS. The use of these agents in other infectious processes remains less clear and in some cases (in cerebral malaria and septic shock, for example) is detrimental. Other agents that modulate the immune response include prostaglandin inhibitors, specific lymphokines, and TNF inhibitors. Specific antibody therapy has been shown to play a role in the treatment and prevention of many diseases. Specific immunoglobulins have long been known to prevent the development of symptomatic rabies and tetanus. More recently, CMV immune globulin has been recognized as important not only in preventing the transmission of the virus during organ transplantation but also in treating CMV pneumonia in bone marrow transplant recipients. There is a strong need for well-designed clinical trials to evaluate each new interventional modality.

PERSPECTIVE The genetic simplicity of many infectious agents allows them to undergo rapid evolution and to develop selective advantages that result in constant variation in the clinical manifestations of infection. Moreover, changes in the environment and the host can predispose new populations to a particular infection. An epidemic of lethal respiratory failure—later identified as hantavirus pulmonary syndrome—on a Navajo reservation in the southwestern United States in 1993 caused nationwide alarm exemplifying the fear that new plagues induce in the human psyche. The potential for infectious agents to emerge in novel and unexpected ways requires that physicians and public health officials be knowledgeable, vigilant, and open-minded in their approach to the consideration of unexplained illness. The emergence of antimicrobial-resistant pathogens (e.g., enterococci that are resistant to all known antimicrobial agents and cause infections that are essentially untreatable) has led some to conclude that we are entering the "postantibiotic era." Others have held to the perception that infectious diseases no longer represent as serious a concern to world health as they once did. The progress that science, medicine, and society as a whole have made in combating these maladies is impressive, and it is ironic that, as we stand on the threshold of an understanding of the most basic biology of the microbe, infectious diseases are posing renewed problems. We are threatened by the appearance of new diseases such as AIDS, hepatitis C, and Ebola virus infection and by the reemergence of old foes like tuberculosis, cholera, plague, and *S. pyogenes* infection. True students of infectious diseases were perhaps less surprised than anyone else by these developments. Those who know pathogens are aware of their incredible adaptability and diversity. As ingenious and successful as therapeutic approaches may be, our ability to develop methods to counter infectious agents so far has not matched the myriad strategies employed by the sea of microbes that surrounds us. Their sheer numbers and the rate at which they can evolve are daunting. Moreover, environmental changes, rapid global travel, population movements, and medicine itself—through its use of antibiotics and immunosuppressive agents—all increase the impact of infectious diseases. Although new vaccines, new antibiotics, improved global communication, and new modalities for treating and preventing infection will be developed, pathogenic microbes will continue to develop new strategies of their own, presenting us with an unending and dynamic challenge.

BIBLIOGRAPHY

BERKELMAN RL, HUGHES JM: The conquest of infectious diseases: Who are we kidding? Ann Intern Med 119:426, 1993
BUCKLEY RH: Immunodeficiency diseases. JAMA 268:2797, 1992
FIELDS BN: Pathogenesis of viral infections, in *Virology*, BN Fields (ed). New York, Raven, 1996, pp 191–239

MAHMOUD A: Parasitic protozoa and helminths. Science 246:1015, 1989

NEWPORT MJ et al: A mutation in the interferon-γ-receptor gene and susceptibility to mycobacterial infection. N Engl J Med 335:1941, 1996

NICAS TI, EISENSTEIN BI: Introduction to bacterial diseases, in *Principles and Practice of Infectious Diseases*, 4th ed, GL Mandell et al (eds). New York, Wiley, 1995, pp 1484–1489

PINNER RW et al: Trends in infectious diseases mortality in the United States. JAMA 275:189, 1996

QUAGLIARELLO V, SCHELD MW: Bacterial meningitis: Pathogenesis, pathophysiology, and progress. N Engl J Med 327:864, 1992

Report of the Task Force on Microbiology and Infectious Diseases. NIH Publication No. 92-3320. Bethesda, MD: National Institute of Allergy and Infectious Diseases, April 1992

121 *Andrew B. Onderdonk*

LABORATORY DIAGNOSIS OF INFECTIOUS DISEASES

The laboratory diagnosis of infection requires the demonstration, either direct or indirect, of viral, bacterial, mycotic, or parasitic agents in tissues, fluids, or excreta of the host. Clinical microbiology laboratories are responsible for processing these specimens and also for determining the antibiotic susceptibility of bacterial pathogens. Traditionally, detection of pathogenic agents largely relies on either the microscopic visualization of pathogens in clinical material or the growth of microorganisms in the laboratory. Identification is generally based on phenotypic characteristics, such as fermentation profiles for bacteria, cytopathic effects in tissue culture for viral agents, and microscopic morphology for fungi and parasites. These techniques are reliable but are often time-consuming.

DETECTION METHODS Reappraisal of the methods employed in the clinical microbiology laboratory has led to the development of strategies for detecting pathogenic agents through nonvisual biologic signal detection systems. Much of this methodology is based on computerization of detection systems with relatively inexpensive but sophisticated computers. In this chapter, both the methods currently available and those under development will be discussed. → *Chapter 213 discusses the detection of parasitic agents.*

Biologic Signals A *biologic signal* is a material that can be reproducibly differentiated from other substances present in the same physical environment. Key issues in the use of biologic (and electronic) signals are distinguishing the signal from background "noise" and translating it into meaningful information. Examples of biologic signals applicable to clinical microbiology include structural components of bacteria, fungi, and viruses; specific antigens; metabolic end products; unique DNA or RNA base sequences; enzymes; toxins or other proteins; and surface polysaccharides.

Detection Systems A detector is used to sense (or detect) a signal and to discriminate between the signal and background noise. Detection systems range from the trained eyes of a technologist assessing morphologic variations to sensitive electronic instruments, such as gas-liquid chromatographs coupled to computer systems for signal analysis. The sensitivity with which signals can be detected varies widely. It is essential to use a detection system that discerns small amounts of signal even when biologic background noise is present—i.e., a system that is both sensitive and specific. Some common detection systems used in microbiology are immunofluorescence, the detection of substrate utilization or end-product formation as color changes, the detection of enzyme activity as a change in light absorbance, chemiluminescence for DNA/RNA probes, flame ionization detection of short- or long-chain fatty acids, and the detection of turbidity changes, cytopathic effects in cell lines, and agglutination of particles.

Amplification Amplification of weak signals enhances the sensitivity with which the signals can be detected. The most common

microbiologic amplification technique is growth of a single bacterium into a discrete colony on an agar plate or into a suspension containing many identical organisms. The advantage of growth as an amplification method is that it requires nothing but an appropriate medium; the disadvantage is the amount of time required for amplification. More rapid, specific amplification of biologic signals can be achieved with techniques such as polymerase (ligase) chain reactions (for DNA/RNA), enzyme immunoassays (EIAs, for antigens and antibodies), electronic amplification (for gas-liquid chromatography assays), antibody capture methods for concentration and/or separation, and selective filtration or centrifugation.

Although a variety of methods are available for the amplification and detection of biologic signals on a research basis, thorough testing is required before they are validated as diagnostic assays.

DIRECT DETECTION **Microscopy** The field of microbiology has been defined largely by the development and use of the microscope. The examination of specimens by microscopic methods often provides useful diagnostic information rapidly. Staining techniques permit organisms to be seen more clearly.

The simplest method for microscopic evaluation is the wet mount, which is used, for example, to examine cerebrospinal fluid (CSF) for the presence of *Cryptococcus neoformans*, with India ink as a background against which to visualize large-capsuled yeast cells. Wet mounts with dark-field illumination are also used to detect spirochetes from genital lesions. Skin scrapings and hair samples can be examined with use of either 10% KOH wet-mount preparations or the calcofluor white method and ultraviolet (UV) illumination to detect fungal elements as fluorescing structures. Staining of wet mounts—for example, with lactophenol cotton blue stain for fungal elements—is often used for morphologic identification. These techniques enhance signal detection and decrease the background by making it easier to identify specific fungal structures.

Staining *Gram's stain* Without staining, bacteria are difficult to see at the magnifications (400 to 1000×) usually used for their detection. Although simple one-step stains can be used, differential stains are more common. Gram's stain differentiates between those organisms with thick peptidoglycan cell walls (gram-positive) and those whose outer membranes can be dissolved with alcohol or acetone (gram-negative).

Gram's stain is particularly useful for examining sputum for the presence of polymorphonuclear leukocytes (PMNs) and bacteria. Sputum specimens with 25 or more PMNs and fewer than 10 epithelial cells per low-power field often provide clinically useful information. However, the presence in "sputum" samples of more than 10 epithelial cells per low-power field and of multiple bacterial types suggests contamination with oral microflora. Despite the difficulty of discriminating between normal microflora and pathogens, Gram's stain may prove useful for specimens from areas with a large resident microflora if a useful biologic marker (signal) is available. Gram's staining of vaginal swab specimens is useful for detecting epithelial cells covered with gram-positive bacteria, which are regarded as a sign of bacterial vaginosis. Similarly, examination of stained stool specimens for the presence of leukocytes is useful as a screening procedure before testing for *Clostridium difficile* toxin or other enteric pathogens.

The examination of CSF and joint, pleural, or peritoneal fluid with Gram's stain is useful for determining whether bacteria and/or PMNs are present. The sensitivity is such that >10⁴ bacteria per milliliter should be detected. Centrifugation is often performed before staining to concentrate specimens suspected of containing low numbers of organisms. The pellet is then examined after staining. This simple method is particularly useful for examination of CSF for bacteria and white blood cells or of sputum for acid-fast bacilli.

Acid-fast stain The acid-fast stain identifies organisms capable of retaining carbol fuchsin dye after acid/organic solvent disruption (e.g., *Mycobacterium* species). Modifications of this procedure also allow the differentiation of *Actinomyces* from *Nocardia* or other weakly acid-fast organisms. The acid-fast stain is employed for sputum, gastric aspirates, other fluids, or tissue samples when acid-fast bacilli (AFB; e.g., *Mycobacterium* species) are suspected. The identification of the pink/red AFB against the blue background of the counterstain requires a trained eye, since few AFB may be detected in an entire smear, even when the specimen has been concentrated by centrifugation. An alternative method is the auramine-rhodamine combination fluorescent dye technique.

Fluorochrome stains Fluorochrome stains, such as acridine orange, are used to identify white blood cells, yeasts, and bacteria in body fluids. Other specialized stains, such as Dappe's stain, may be used in the detection of *Mycoplasma* in cell cultures designated for this purpose. Capsular, flagellar, and spore stains are also used for identification or demonstration of characteristic structures.

Immunofluorescent stains The direct immunofluorescent antibody (DFA) technique uses antibody that is coupled to a fluorescing compound, such as fluorescein, and directed at a specific antigenic target to visualize organisms or subcellular structures. When samples are examined under appropriate conditions, the fluorescing compound absorbs the UV light and reemits light at a higher (visible) wavelength that can be detected by the human eye. In the indirect immunofluorescent antibody (IFA) technique, an unlabeled (target) antibody binds a specific antigen. The specimen is then stained with labeled polyclonal antibody directed at the target antibody. Because each unlabeled target antibody attached to the appropriate antigen has multiple sites for attachment of the second antibody, the visual signal can be intensified (i.e., amplified). This form of staining is called *indirect* because a two-antibody system is used to generate the signal for detection of the antigen. Both direct and indirect fluorescence methods can be used to detect viruses such as cytomegalovirus and herpes simplex virus within cultured cells as well as many difficult-to-grow bacterial agents (e.g., *Legionella pneumophila*) directly in clinical specimens.

Macroscopic Antigen Detection Latex agglutination assays and EIAs are rapid and inexpensive methods for identifying organisms or extracellular toxins and viral agents by means of protein and polysaccharide antigens. Such assays may be performed directly on clinical samples or after growth of organisms on agar plates or in viral cell cultures. The biologic signal in each case is the antigen to be detected. Monoclonal or polyclonal antibodies are used.

Techniques such as direct agglutination of bacterial cells with specific antibody are simple but relatively insensitive, while latex agglutination procedures and EIAs are more sensitive. Some cell-associated antigens, such as capsular polysaccharides, lipopolysaccharides, and other surface-expressed antigens, can be detected by agglutination of a suspension of bacterial cells when antibody is added, a method useful for typing of the somatic antigens of *Shigella* and *Salmonella*. In systems such as EIAs, which employ monoclonal antibodies coupled to an enzyme, an antigen-antibody reaction results in the conversion of a colorless substrate to a colored product. Because the coupling of an enzyme to the monoclonal antibody can amplify a weak biologic signal, the sensitivity of such assays is often high. In each instance, the basis for antigen detection is antigen-antibody binding, with the detection system changed to accommodate the biologic signal. Most such assays provide information as to whether antigen is present but do not quantify the antigen. EIAs have also proved to be useful for detecting the presence of bacterial toxins. For instance, this technique is commonly employed for detecting *C. difficile* toxin in stool, as the presence of the organism alone is not diagnostic for toxin-mediated disease.

DETECTION OF PATHOGENIC AGENTS BY CULTURE

Specimen Collection and Transport To culture bacterial, mycotic, or viral pathogens, an appropriate sample must be placed into the proper medium for growth (amplification). The success or failure of efforts to identify a specific microbial pathogen often depends on the collection and transport process. Appendix B lists procedures for collection and transport of common specimens. Because there are many pathogen-specific paradigms for these procedures, it is important to seek advice from the microbiology laboratory when in doubt about a particular situation.

Isolation of Bacterial Pathogens The isolation of the suspect pathogen(s) from clinical material relies on the use of artificial media designed to support the growth of bacteria in vitro. Such media are composed of agar, which is not metabolized by bacteria, and nutrients to support the growth of the microbial species of interest, often in combination with substances to inhibit the growth of other bacteria. Broth for growth (amplification) of organisms is employed for specimens with low numbers of bacteria, such as peritoneal dialysis fluid, CSF, or samples in which anaerobes may be present. Two basic strategies are used to isolate pathogenic bacteria. The first is to employ enriched media for the growth of any bacteria that may be present in a sample such as blood or CSF. Since bacteria are not present in such fluids under normal conditions, the finding of organisms is usually significant. Broths that allow the growth of small numbers of organisms may be subcultured to solid media when growth is detected. The second strategy is to isolate (amplify) specific bacterial species from stool, genital tract secretions, or sputum—sites that contain large numbers of bacteria under normal conditions. For this purpose, antimicrobial agents or other inhibitory substances are incorporated into the agar medium to inhibit growth of all but the bacteria of interest. After incubation, organisms that grow on such media are further characterized to determine whether they are pathogens. Selection for organisms that may be pathogens from the normal microflora shortens the time required to make the diagnosis.

Isolation of Viral Agents (See Chap. 182) Pathogenic viral agents often are cultured when the presence of serum antibody is not a criterion of active infection or when an increase in serum antibody may not be detected during infection. The biologic signal, virus, is thus amplified to a level at which detection is possible. Although a number of techniques are available, the essential elements include a monolayer of cultured mammalian cells sensitive to infection with the suspected viral pathogen. These cells serve as the amplification system by allowing the proliferation of viral particles. Virus may be detected by direct observation of the cultured cells for cytopathic effects or by immunofluorescent detection of viral antigens following incubation. Culture methods are particularly useful for detection of rapidly propagated agents, such as cytomegalovirus or herpes simplex virus.

IDENTIFICATION METHODS Once bacteria are isolated, traditional methods of phenotypic characterization are often used for the identification of specific isolates. Phenotypic characteristics include the traits of the organism that are readily detectable after growth on agar media (colony size, color, hemolytic reactions, odor), use by the organism of specific substrates and carbon sources (such as carbohydrates), formation of specific end products during growth, and microscopic appearance. Broth tubes containing specific substrates are commonly employed for such characterization procedures.

Classic Phenotyping Automated systems allow identification of bacterial pathogens on the basis of phenotypic characteristics in a matter of hours. Most such systems are based on biotyping techniques, in which isolates are grown in multiple substrates and the pattern of reactions is compared with known patterns for various bacterial species. This procedure is relatively fast, and commercially available systems include a coding system to simplify recording of results, probability calculations for the most likely candidate pathogens, and miniaturized fermentation methods. If the biotyping approach is automated and the reading process is coupled to computer-based data analysis, rapidly growing organisms, such as the Enterobacteriaceae, can be identified within hours of detection on agar plates.

Several systems use preformed enzymes for speedier identification (within 2 to 3 h). Such systems do not rely on bacterial growth per se to determine whether a substrate has been used or not. They employ a heavy inoculum in which enzymes are present in sufficient quantity to convert substrate to product rapidly. In addition, some systems use fluorogenic substrate/end-product detection methods to increase sensitivity (through signal amplification).

Gas-Liquid Chromatography Gas-liquid chromatography is used for the detection of metabolic end products of bacterial fermentations. A common application of this technique is identification of the short-chain fatty acids produced by obligate anaerobes during the fermentation of glucose. Because the types of volatile acids and their relative concentrations differ among the various genera and species that make up this group of organisms, such information serves as a metabolic "fingerprint" for a particular isolate.

Gas-liquid chromatography can be coupled to a sophisticated signal-analysis computer software system for identification and quantitation of long-chain fatty acids (LCFAs) in the outer membranes and cell walls of bacteria and fungi. For any given species, the types and relative concentrations of LCFAs are different enough to allow identification of even closely related species. An organism may be identified definitively within a few hours after the start of growth on appropriate media. LCFA analysis is one of the most advanced procedures currently available for phenotypic characterization.

Nucleic Acid Probes In recent years, techniques for the detection of specific DNA and RNA base sequences in clinical specimens have become powerful tools for the diagnosis of bacterial, viral, parasitic, and fungal infections. The basic strategy is to detect a relatively short sequence of bases specific for a particular pathogen on single-stranded DNA or RNA by hybridization of a complementary sequence of bases (probe) coupled to a "reporter" molecule that serves as the signal for detection. Detection of an organism by nucleic acid probes does not depend on its viability. Thus, this approach offers a decided advantage over culture methods for difficult-to-grow organisms. Current technology encompasses a wide array of methods for amplification and signal detection, some of which have been approved by the Food and Drug Administration for clinical diagnosis.

Use of nucleic acid probes generally involves lysis of intact cells and denaturation of the DNA or RNA to render it single-stranded. The probe may be hybridized to the target sequence in a solution or on a solid support, depending on the system employed. In situ hybridization of a probe to a target is also possible and allows the use of probes with agents that are present in tissue specimens. Once the probe has been hybridized to the target (biologic signal), a variety of strategies may be employed to amplify and/or detect the target-probe complex (Fig. 121-1).

Probes for direct detection of pathogens in clinical specimens Nucleic acid probes for the direct detection in clinical specimens of various bacterial pathogens (including *L. pneumophila*, *Chlamydia trachomatis*, *Neisseria gonorrhoeae*, group A *Streptococcus*, and *Gardnerella vaginalis*) are available commercially. In addition, probes for the direct detection of human papillomavirus, *Candida* spp., and *Trichomonas vaginalis* have been approved for use. An assortment of probes for confirming the identity of cultured pathogens, such as *Mycobacterium* and *Salmonella* spp., are also available. Probes for the direct detection of bacterial pathogens are often directed at highly conserved 16S ribosomal RNA sequences, because there are many more copies of the ribosomal RNA sequence than there are of any single genomic DNA sequence in a bacterial cell. The sensitivity and specificity of probe assays for direct detection are comparable to those of more traditional assays, including EIA and culture methods. Many laboratories have developed their own probes for the detection of microbial and viral pathogens; however, unless a method-validation protocol for diagnostic use has been performed, the use of such probes is restricted to research by federal law.

Nucleic acid probe amplification strategies In theory, a single target nucleic acid sequence can be amplified to detectable levels. There are several strategies for target and/or probe amplification, including the polymerase chain reaction (PCR), the ligase chain reaction, strand displacement amplification, and self-sustaining sequence replication. In each case, a target sequence or hybridized probe is amplified exponentially to obtain a signal that can be detected, usually by the attachment of chemiluminescent reporter groups. The PCR strategy requires repeated heating of the DNA or RNA to separate the two complementary strands of the double helix, hybridization of the primer sequence to the appropriate target sequence, target amplification using the PCR for complementary strand extension, and signal detection via a labeled probe. The sensitivity of such assays is far greater than that of traditional assay methods such as cul-

FIGURE 121-1 Strategies for amplification and/or detection of a target-probe complex. DNA or RNA extracted from microorganisms is heated to create single-stranded (ss) DNA/RNA containing appropriate target sequences. These target sequences may be hybridized directly (direct detection) with probes attached to reporter molecules; they may be amplified by repetitive cycles of complementary strand extension (polymerase chain reaction) before attachment of a reporter probe; or the original target-probe signal may be amplified via hybridization with an additional probe containing multiple copies of a secondary reporter target sequence (branched-chain DNA, or bDNA).

ture. However, the care with which the assays are performed is important, because cross-contamination of clinical material with DNA or RNA from other sources (even at low levels) can cause false-positive results. At present, amplification assays for the detection of *Mycobacterium tuberculosis* and *C. trachomatis* are available. As is the case for direct detection probes, many laboratories have used commercially available heat-stable *taq* polymerase, probe sequences, and reagents to develop "in-house" assays for diagnostic use. Issues related to quality control, interpretation of results, sample processing, and regulatory requirements have slowed the commercial development of diagnostic assay kits.

In other systems, probes attached to complementary target sequences are amplified by the attachment of a second probe and an amplification multimer to the original probe. One such system, termed *branched-chain DNA* (bDNA)-*based amplification*, attaches bDNA to a site different from the target-binding sequence of the original probe. Enzyme-labeled oligonucleotides can then bind to multiple repeating sequences on the bDNA. The amplified bDNA signal is detected by chemiluminescence. The advantage of this system over PCR is that only a single step is required to hybridize the target-binding probe to the target sequence.

Application of nucleic acid probe technology Nucleic acid probe technology is currently being applied to the identification of difficult-to-grow bacterial pathogens such as *Mycobacterium* spp. Further applications of these techniques in the clinical microbiology laboratory will likely include the replacement of culture methods for the identification of many pathogens in clinical material, the detection of antibiotic resistance markers, and the detection of a variety of difficult-to-cultivate or noncultivable pathogens, such as *Ehrlichia*, *Rickettsia*, *Babesia*, *Borrelia*, and *Rochalimaea*. Probe technology also has the potential to detect viral pathogens faster than is possible with current culture techniques. However, if clinical microbiology laboratories are to take full advantage of probe technology, the cost of reagents and automation of the assays must be competitive with the cost and automation of existing methodology. At present, the detection of agents such as *C. trachomatis* or *N. gonorrhoeae* by probe technology is more expensive for most laboratories than detection by traditional culture or EIA methods. Moreover, because automated processing equipment has not yet been designed for clinical use, PCR methods are both more labor-intensive and more expensive than other detection systems. In the absence of clear documentation of clinical utility, many laboratories continue to wait for approval of commercially available DNA probe assays rather than validating in-house assays.

SUSCEPTIBILITY TESTING One of the principal responsibilities of the clinical laboratory is to determine which antimicrobial agents are inhibitory for a specific bacterial isolate. Two approaches are useful for this purpose. The first is to use a qualitative assessment of susceptibility, categorizing responses as susceptible, resistant, or intermediate. This qualitative approach can involve either the placement of paper disks containing antibiotics on an agar surface inoculated with the bacterial strain to be tested (Kirby-Bauer or disk/agar-diffusion method) or the use of broth tubes containing a set concentration of antibiotic (breakpoint method). These methods have been carefully calibrated against quantitative methods and clinical experience with each antibiotic.

The second approach is to inoculate the test strain of bacteria into a series of broth tubes (or agar plates) with increasing concentrations of antibiotic. The lowest concentration of antibiotic that inhibits microbial growth in this test system is known as the *minimum inhibitory concentration* (MIC). If tubes in which no growth occurs are subcultured, the minimum concentration of antibiotic required to kill the starting inoculum can also be determined. This measurement is called the *minimum bactericidal concentration* (MBC). Quantitative susceptibility testing using the *microbroth dilution technique*, a miniaturized version of the macrobroth dilution technique using microwell plates, lends itself to automation and is used commonly in larger clinical laboratories.

A novel version of the disk/agar-diffusion method employs a quantitative diffusion gradient, or epsilometer (E-test), and uses an absorbent strip with a known gradient of antibiotic concentrations along its

length. When the strip is placed on the surface of an agar plate seeded with a bacterial strain to be tested, antibiotic diffuses into the medium, and bacterial growth is inhibited. The MIC is estimated by determining the lowest concentration on the gradient strip that inhibits microbial growth.

AUTOMATION OF MICROBIAL DETECTION IN BLOOD The detection of microbial growth in blood is difficult because the numbers of organisms present in the sample are often low and because the integrity of the organisms and their ability to replicate may be damaged by humoral defense mechanisms or antimicrobial agents. Over the years, systems that rely on the detection of CO_2 produced by the organisms in blood culture bottles have allowed the automation of the detection procedure. The most common system involves inserting a sampling device into each bottle at periodic intervals and drawing off the head-space gas of the bottle. An infrared monitor is used to determine the CO_2 level. The system interprets levels exceeding a set concentration as indicative of microbial growth. Such methods are no more sensitive than the human eye in detecting a positive culture, but because the bottles in an automated system are generally monitored more frequently, a positive culture is often detected more rapidly than by manual techniques, and important information, including the results of Gram's stain and preliminary susceptibility assays, can be obtained sooner.

One technique for automated blood-culture monitoring uses reflectance optics consisting of a photodiode and a light-emitting diode to monitor the amount of CO_2 produced in each blood-culture bottle every 10 min through a self-contained sensor that is part of each bottle. Each reflectance measurement is then stored in computer memory. When an appropriate change in reflectance occurs, the system alerts the clinical laboratory to the presence of a positive culture via audible and visible alarms. The continuous scanning of bottles used in this system shortens detection times and permits early reporting of positive cultures. In addition, the noninvasive monitoring procedure decreases the likelihood of laboratory contamination.

Automated systems also have been applied to the detection of microbial growth from specimens other than blood, such as peritoneal and other normally sterile fluids. *Mycobacterium* spp. can be detected in certain automated systems if appropriate media are used for culture.

DETECTION OF PATHOGENIC AGENTS BY SEROLOGIC METHODS Measurement of serum antibody provides an indirect marker for past or current infection with a specific viral agent or with other pathogens, including *Brucella*, *Legionella*, *Rickettsia*, and *Chlamydia*. The biologic signal is usually either IgM or IgG antibody directed at surface-expressed antigen(s). The detection systems include those used for bacterial antigens (agglutination reactions, immunofluorescence, and EIA) and unique systems such as hemolysis inhibition and complement fixation. Serologic methods generally fall into two categories: those that determine protective antibody levels and those that measure changing antibody titers to detect current infection. Determination of an antibody response as a measure of current immunity is important for viral agents such as rubella virus or varicella-zoster virus; assays for this purpose normally use one or two dilutions of serum for a qualitative determination of protective antibody levels. Quantitative serologic assays to detect increases in antibody titers most often employ paired serum samples obtained 10 to 14 days apart (i.e., acute- and convalescent-phase samples). Since the incubation period before symptoms are noted may be long enough for an antibody response to occur, the demonstration of acute-phase antibody alone is often not enough to establish the diagnosis of active infection as opposed to past exposure. In such circumstances, the finding of IgM may be useful as a measure of an early, acute-phase antibody response. A fourfold increase in total antibody titer or in EIA activity between the acute- and convalescent-phase samples is also regarded as evidence for active infection.

For certain viral agents, such as Epstein-Barr virus, the antibodies produced may be directed at different antigens during different phases of the infection. For this reason, most laboratories test for antibody directed at both viral capsid antigens and antigens associated with recently infected host cells to determine the stage of infection.

BIBLIOGRAPHY

COLLINS ML et al: Preparation and characterization of RNA standards for use in quantitative branched DNA hybridization assays. Anal Biochem 226:120, 1995

HALONNEN P et al: Detection of enteroviruses and rhinoviruses in clinical specimens by PCR and liquid-phase hybridization. J Clin Microbiol 33:648, 1995

HERMANN JE: Immunoassays for the diagnosis of infectious diseases, in *Manual of Clinical Microbiology*, 6th ed, P Murray et al (eds). Washington, American Society for Microbiology, 1995

MILLER JM et al: Specimen collection, transport and storage, in *Manual of Clinical Microbiology*, 6th ed, B Murray et al (eds). Washington, American Society for Microbiology, 1995

PFYFFER GE et al: Diagnostic performance of amplified *Mycobacterium tuberculosis* direct test with cerebrospinal fluid, other nonrespiratory and respiratory specimens. J Clin Microbiol 34:834, 1996

PODZORSKI RP et al: Molecular detection and identification of microorganisms, in *Manual of Clinical Microbiology*, 6th ed, P Murray et al (eds). Washington, Americal Society for Microbiology, 1995

SCHOCHETMAN G et al: Polymerase chain reaction. J Infect Dis 158:1154, 1988

WILSON ML: General principles of specimen collection and transport. Clin Infect Dis 22:766, 1996

---

122 | Gerald T. Keusch, Kenneth J. Bart

IMMUNIZATION PRINCIPLES AND VACCINE USE

Most humans live their lives ignoring the certainty of their own mortality. Perhaps this fact explains why the adage "an ounce of prevention is worth a pound of cure" has so little effect on their everyday behavior. Even when it comes to acting to protect their young, parents are capable of ignoring the potential for mortality among their children (in the developed world) and of accepting the certainty of childhood deaths (in the developing world). In both settings, parents all too often fail to seek out and demand the best preventive measures available. Unless mandated by the law in the former setting or provided by benevolent organizations or governments in the latter, universal immunization has invariably remained an unattained goal. Compulsion and benevolence, it seems, are two essential components of immunization.

However, the integration of immunization practices (a major component of primary disease prevention) into routine health care services has provided caregivers with control over a substantial proportion of the disease and mortality that plagued the United States during the first half of the twentieth century (Table 122-1). For society today, immunization represents one of the most cost-effective means of preventing infectious disease. For every dollar spent, diphtheria/tetanus/pertussis (DTP) vaccine saves $29, measles/mumps/rubella (MMR) vaccine saves $21, trivalent oral poliovirus vaccine (OPV) saves $6, varicella vaccine saves $5, and *Haemophilus influenzae* type b (Hib) vaccine saves $2. At present, more than 50 biologic products are licensed in the United States, and 6 vaccines (12 antigens) are used for routine immunization in the young, including diphtheria/tetanus/acellular pertussis vaccine (DTaP), OPV, MMR, Hib vaccine, hepatitis B virus (HBV) vaccine, and varicella vaccine. Five vaccines are designed for routine use in adults, including tetanus/diphtheria (Td) toxoids, adsorbed, for adult use; HBV vaccine; influenza virus vaccine; polyvalent pneumococcal polysaccharide vaccine; and varicella vaccine. Some preparations are designated as special-use vaccines (e.g., hepatitis A vaccine for travelers). Unfortunately, vaccines for eukaryotic pathogens (protozoa and helminths), which affect a large proportion of the world's population, have been difficult to develop and remain only a hope for the future.

Table 122-1

Changes in the Incidence of Vaccine-Preventable Diseases in the United States

Disease	Peak Incidence Year	Peak Incidence No. of Cases	No. of Cases in 1995[a]	Decrease from Maximum as of 1995, %
Diphtheria	1921	206,939	0	100.00
Measles	1941	894,134	288	99.97
Mumps	1968	152,209	840	99.45
Pertussis	1934	265,269	4315	98.37
Poliomyelitis (paralytic)	1952	21,269	0[b]	100.00
Rubella	1969	57,686	146	99.75
Congenital rubella syndrome	1965	20,000[c]	7	99.97
Tetanus[d]	1923	1560	43	97.24
Haemophilus influenzae type b[e]	—	20,000[f]	270	98.65

[a] Provisional.
[b] Projected to be 5 to 10 vaccine-associated cases.
[c] Estimated.
[d] All ages.
[e] Invasive disease, children <5 years old.
[f] Not notifiable before 1991; estimated prevaccine-era annual incidence, all ages.

SOURCE: Centers for Disease Control and Prevention.

IMPACT OF IMMUNIZATION The epidemiologically appropriate use of vaccines has resulted in the global eradication of smallpox; the elimination of poliomyelitis in the Americas; the virtual elimination of congenital rubella syndrome, tetanus, and diphtheria in the United States; and a dramatic reduction in pertussis, rubella, measles, and mumps in the United States. Figure 122-1 shows the effect of vaccines on the incidence of Hib meningitis. The Hib conjugate vaccines in particular have exerted a remarkable influence on invasive *Haemophilus* infections, presumably because they reduce nasopharyngeal carriage of Hib and induce protection before the period of greatest vulnerability in infancy.

DEFINITIONS *Vaccination* and *immunization* are often used as interchangeable terms. However, the former denotes only the administration of a vaccine or toxoid, whereas the latter describes the process of inducing or providing immunity by any means, whether active or

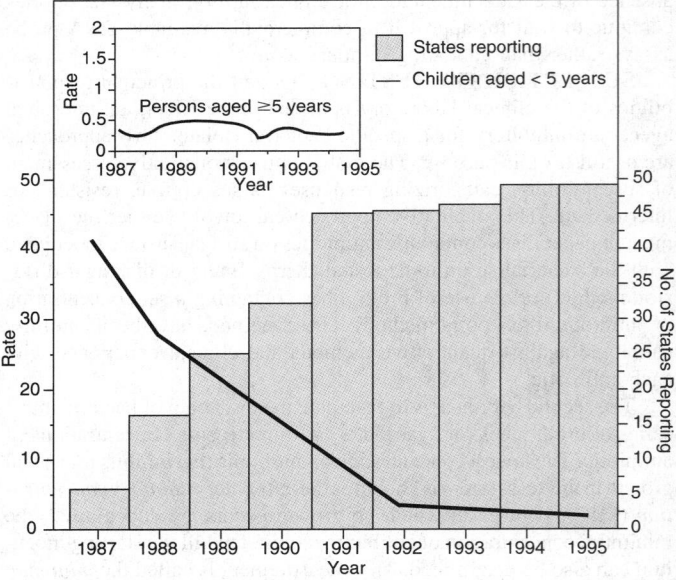

FIGURE 122-1 Incidence rate of invasive *Haemophilus influenzae* disease per 100,000 children <5 years of age and number of states reporting to the CDC *H. influenzae* surveillance system. The insert shows the incidence rate among persons ≥5 years of age. Because of the low number of states reporting surveillance data during 1987–1990, rates for those years were race-adjusted on the basis of the 1990 U.S. population. *(From the Centers for Disease Control and Prevention.)*

immunization refers to the induction of immune defenses by the administration of antigens in appropriate forms, whereas *passive immunization* involves the provision of temporary protection by the administration of exogenously produced immune substances. Immunizing agents thus include vaccines, toxoids, and antibody-containing immunoglobulin preparations from human or animal donors (Table 122-2).

PRINCIPLES OF IMMUNIZATION Artificial induction of immunity closely follows two well-tested principles of nature. The first, active immunization, can be traced at least as far back as Thucydides, who noted that people surviving epidemics of plague in Athens were spared during later outbreaks of the same disease. The second, passive immunization, is a natural process as well and is exemplified by the transplacental transmission of maternal antibodies to the fetus to provide protection against several diseases during the first months of life. Use of the two measures together may produce a complementary effect (as with HBV vaccine plus hepatitis B immune globulin) or may actually interfere with the development of immunity (as when measles vaccine is administered within 6 weeks of immunoglobulin). Depending on whether there are multiple species or serotypes of an organism and—if so—whether there are common, cross-reactive, protective antigens, a specific vaccine may induce protection against all representative forms of an infectious agent or against the immunizing strain only. One of the intrinsic virtues of whole-organism vaccines is that they potentially contain all protective antigens of the organism. However, this virtue is counterbalanced by an inherent problem with such vaccines: the possibility of adverse responses to reactive but nonprotective antigens present in the mix. Because the immune response to specific antigens is controlled genetically, all individuals cannot be expected to respond identically to the same vaccine.

APPROACHES TO ACTIVE IMMUNIZATION The two principal approaches to active immunization are (1) the use of live, generally attenuated, infectious agents (e.g., measles virus) and (2) the use of inactivated agents, detoxified extracts or toxins from these agents, or specific antigens obtained by genetic recombination (e.g., HBV). For many diseases (e.g., poliomyelitis, influenza), both approaches have been employed. Live attenuated vaccines are believed to induce an immunologic response more nearly like that resulting from natural infection than the response induced by killed vaccines. Currently available inactivated or killed vaccines consist of inactivated whole organisms (e.g., plague vaccine); detoxified protein exotoxins (e.g., tetanus toxoid); recombinant protein antigens (e.g., HBV vaccine); or carbohydrate antigens, either present as soluble purified capsular material (e.g., *Streptococcus pneumoniae* polysaccharides) or conjugated to a protein carrier (e.g., Hib polysaccharide conjugated to diphtheria or tetanus toxoids).

APPROACHES TO PASSIVE IMMUNIZATION Passive immunization is generally used to provide temporary immunity in an unimmunized subject exposed to an infectious disease when active immunization either is unavailable (e.g., for cytomegalovirus infection) or has not been implemented before exposure (e.g., for rabies). Passive immunization is used in the treatment of certain disorders associated with toxins (e.g., diphtheria), in certain bites (those of snakes and spiders), and as a specific or nonspecific immunosuppressant [Rho(D) immune globulin and antilymphocyte globulin, respectively].

Three types of preparations are used in passive immunization: (1) standard human immune serum globulin for general use (e.g., gamma globulin), administered intramuscularly or intravenously; (2) special immune serum globulins with a known content of antibody for specific agents (e.g., HBV or varicella-zoster immune globulin); and (3) animal sera and antitoxins.

ROUTE OF ADMINISTRATION The route of administration in part determines the rapidity and nature of the immune responses to vaccines. Vaccines can be administered orally, intranasally, intradermally, subcutaneously, or intramuscularly. Parenterally administered vaccine may not induce mucosal secretory IgA, and mucosal immunization may not induce good systemic responses. Vaccines must be administered by the licensed route to ensure immunogenicity and safety. For example, administration of HBV vaccine into the gluteal rather than the deltoid muscle often fails to induce an adequate immune response, while subcutaneous rather than intramuscular administration of DTP increases the risk of reactions.

AGE The age of the individual influences the response to vaccines. Therefore, recommended schedules for immunization are based on age-dependent responses determined empirically from clinical trials. The presence of high levels of maternal antibody and/or the immaturity of the immune system in the early months of life impairs the initial immune response to some antigens (e.g., measles vaccine but not HBV vaccine). In the elderly, vaccine responses may be diminished because of natural waning of the immune system. Hence, larger amounts of an antigen may be required to produce the desired response (e.g., in vaccination against influenza).

ADJUVANT POTENTIATION The immune response to some antigens is potentiated by the addition of adjuvants such as aluminum salts or, in the case of polysaccharides (e.g., the polyribose phosphate oligosaccharide of Hib), by conjugation to a peptide. Adjuvants, nonspecific boosters of immune responses, are used with inactivated products such as diphtheria and tetanus toxoids, acellular pertussis (aP) vaccine, and HBV vaccine. The mechanism for adjuvant enhancement of antigenicity is not well defined but relates in part to the rendering of soluble antigens into a particulate form, the mobilization of phagocytes to the site of antigen deposition, and the slowing down of the release of antigens, which prolongs stimulation of the immune response.

THE IMMUNE RESPONSE Although many constituents of infectious microorganisms and their products, such as exotoxins, are or can be made to be antigenic, only a limited number stimulate a protective immune response. The immune system is complex, and antigen composition and presentation are critical for stimulation of the desired immune responses.

The Primary Response In the primary response to a vaccine antigen, an apparent latent period of several days precedes the detection of humoral and cell-mediated immunity, although the immune response is turned on by contact with the antigen and the immune system. Circulating antibodies do not appear for 7 to 10 days. The immunoglobulin class of the response also changes over time. Early-appearing IgM antibodies generally exhibit only low affinity for the antigen, whereas later-appearing IgG antibodies display high affinity. For "thymus-dependent" antigens, T helper lymphocytes control the switch from IgM to IgG. Some individuals do not respond, even when presented repeatedly with a vaccine antigen, perhaps because they lack the major histocompatibility complex determinants required to recognize the antigen. This situation is known as *primary vaccine failure*.

The Secondary Response Heightened humoral or cell-mediated responses are elicited by a second exposure to the same antigen. These secondary responses occur rapidly, usually within 4 or 5 days, and

Table 122-2

Definitions of Immunizing Agents

Term	Definition
Vaccine	A suspension of attenuated live or killed microorganisms or antigenic portions of these agents presented to a potential host to induce immunity and prevent disease
Toxoid	A modified bacterial toxin that has been made nontoxic but retains the capacity to stimulate the formation of antitoxin
Immune globulin	An antibody-containing solution derived from human blood by cold ethanol fractionation of large pools of plasma and used primarily for maintenance of the immunity of immunodeficient persons or for passive immunization; intramuscular and intravenous preparations available
Antitoxin	An antibody derived from the serum of animals after stimulation with specific antigens and used to provide passive immunity

result in increased titers of IgG antibody. The secondary response depends on immunologic memory after the first exposure and is characterized by a marked proliferation of antibody-producing B lymphocytes and/or effector T cells. Polysaccharide vaccines, such as that for *S. pneumoniae*, evoke immune responses that are independent of T cells and are not enhanced by repeated administration. Linking of polysaccharides to proteins converts the former to T cell–dependent antigens that induce immunologic memory and secondary responses to revaccination. Although levels of vaccine-induced antibodies may decline over time (*secondary vaccine failure*), revaccination or exposure to the organism may elicit a rapid protective secondary response consisting of IgG antibodies with little or no detectable IgM. This *anamnestic response* indicates that immunity has persisted. The lack of measurable antibody does not necessarily mean that the individual is unprotected. Furthermore, the mere presence of detectable antibodies after the administration of some vaccines and toxoids does not ensure clinical protection. A minimal circulating level of antibody is known to be required for protection from some diseases (e.g., 0.01 IU/mL for tetanus antitoxin).

Hypersensitivity Reactions Independent of antibody production, the stimulation of the immune system by vaccination may elicit unanticipated responses, especially hypersensitivity reactions. In the past, killed measles vaccine induced incomplete humoral immunity and cell-mediated hypersensitivity, resulting in the development of a syndrome of atypical measles in some children after subsequent exposure; thus this type of vaccine is no longer in use.

Mucosal Immunity Some pathogens are confined to and replicate only at mucosal surfaces (e.g., *Vibrio cholerae*), while others are able to penetrate the mucosa and replicate (e.g., poliovirus, rubella virus, and influenza virus). At the mucosal site, these organisms induce secretory IgA. The induction of secretory IgA by vaccines may be an efficient way to block the essential first steps in pathogenesis, whether the organism is restricted to mucosal surfaces or systemically invades the host across mucosal surfaces.

Measurement of the Immune Response Immune responses to vaccines are often gauged by the concentration of specific antibody in serum. While seroconversion serves as a dependable indicator of an immune response, it measures only one immunologic parameter and does not necessarily indicate protection. The development of circulating antibodies after immunization often correlates directly with clinical protection (e.g., against measles or rubella). Some responses may not in themselves confer immunity but may be sufficiently associated with protection that they remain useful proxy measures of protective immunity (e.g., vibriocidal serum antibodies in cholera).

HERD IMMUNITY It is not necessary to immunize every person in order to stop transmission of an infectious agent through a population. For those organisms dependent on person-to-person transmission, there may be a definable prevalence of immunity in the population above which it becomes difficult for the organism to circulate and reach new susceptibles. This prevalence is called *herd immunity*. When herd immunity is operative, the goals of immunization are converted from the immunization of every person in the community to the immunization of a specified minimum percentage of persons at risk. Herd immunity may be lost when immunity wanes (as in diphtheria in the new independent states of the former Soviet Union) or when a sufficient percentage of individuals refuse to be immunized. The latter situation developed with regard to pertussis in the United Kingdom and Japan in the 1970s because concern about infrequent—albeit severe—vaccine reactions came to exceed the fear of the disease itself. In both situations, loss of herd immunity has led to renewed increases in the circulation of the organism and susceptibility to infection, with subsequent large outbreaks.

TARGET POPULATIONS AND TIMING OF IMMUNIZATION For common and highly communicable childhood diseases like measles, the target population is the universe of susceptible individuals, and the time to immunize is as early in life as is feasible.

Epidemiologic differences in measles in different settings, however, dictate different strategies of immunization. In the industrialized world, immunization with live-virus vaccine at 12 to 15 months of age has been the norm because the vaccine protects more than 95 percent of those immunized at this age and there is little measles morbidity/mortality among very young infants. In contrast, in the developing world, measles accounts for a significant proportion of deaths of young infants. Thus it is desirable to immunize children during the first few months of life in order to narrow the window of vulnerability between the rapid decline of maternal antibody after 4 to 6 months and the development of vaccine-induced active immunity.

Hib causes meningitis, epiglottitis, and pneumonia in early childhood. As in measles, the majority of cases of severe Hib disease occur in this age group, with rates rising sharply after the disappearance of maternally derived antibody. However, the first Hib vaccines were subject to primary failure when administered during infancy; this failure was due mainly to an age-related inability to respond to polysaccharide antigens. To overcome this problem, the protective polysaccharide was coupled to protein and was thereby converted to a T cell–dependent antigen to which young infants could respond.

In contrast to measles and Hib infection, rubella is primarily a threat to the fetus; young infants and children are not at risk of serious illness. Given the risk to the fetus, immunization of all women of reproductive age before pregnancy would be an ideal strategy. However, it is difficult to systematically vaccinate adolescent and young-adult females. Thus, to assure the protection of as many women as possible, the rubella component is included in a combination vaccine with mumps and measles (MMR) that is administered during infancy.

Some vaccines are now used primarily for adults. For example, influenza virus and polyvalent pneumococcal polysaccharide vaccines are used to prevent pneumonia deaths in the elderly. Unfortunately, these vaccines are underutilized, in part because physicians and otherwise healthy individuals in the target group ignore the indications and in part because there is still a tendency to think about disease prevention with vaccines as a strategy for children. Pneumococcal polysaccharide vaccine is also recommended for children over 2 years of age who are at risk of severe or even life-threatening pneumococcal infection, such as those with sickle cell disease, asplenia (whether functional or anatomic), renal failure with nephrotic syndrome, cerebrospinal fluid leak, and human immunodeficiency virus (HIV) infection or other immunosuppressive disease states.

THE DEVELOPMENT OF VACCINES

BIOLOGIC IMPEDIMENTS There are often major technical problems to overcome in vaccine development. Influenza virus, characterized biologically by its antigenic drift, periodically emerges in a new antigenic version capable of causing a global pandemic for which a new vaccine must be rapidly devised, produced, and distributed. In contrast to the circulation of one major antigenic type of influenza A virus at any one time is the circulation of many prevalent pneumococcal polysaccharide serotypes at all times. However, because immunity to the pneumococcus is serotype specific, an individual is susceptible to all serotypes against which he or she lacks antibody. Serotype-specific protection made it more difficult to develop an effective pneumococcal vaccine than it was to develop a vaccine against *H. influenzae*, of which one capsular serotype (type b) is associated with a significant portion of cases of severe disease. To overcome this problem, pneumococcal vaccine currently includes 23 polysaccharides that represent approximately 80 percent of the virulent serotypes commonly encountered in the United States. Unfortunately, some serotypes are poorly immunogenic, and immunized individuals remain susceptible to the serotypes not included in the vaccine.

STRATEGY FOR VACCINE DEVELOPMENT Vaccine development depends on the systematic application of a four-phase strategy: (1) studies in animals to identify protective antigen, (2) determination of how to present this antigen effectively to the immune system, (3) assessment of the safety and immunogenicity of the preparation in small and then in large human populations at various ages, and (4) evaluation of safety and efficacy in the target population. Each of these steps is simple in concept but difficult in execution, not least because of the clinical trials necessary to assess safety and efficacy; failure at any level stops the process. Thus, in 1995, more than 190 candidate vaccines were under investigation, but just 5 new products were licensed in the United States. Progress in immunology has taught us much about the organization and function of the immune system (see Chap. 305); it has also taught us that the immune system is complicated and that details of antigen composition and presentation are critical for stimulating desired immune responses.

In the development of vaccines, initial studies are typically carried out in animal models, if available, to demonstrate the production of immune responses, an ability to protect the host, and relative safety. Ultimately, vaccines for humans must be tested in humans. When initial in vitro and animal data look promising, graded doses of vaccine are given to small numbers of humans to assess immune responses, optimal dosage, and safety. Human clinical trials of vaccine efficacy are then performed with a larger group, often consisting of informed volunteers who are challenged with a virulent strain. After clinical trials in the community, typically involving 1000 to 10,000 vaccinees, licensure may be sought. Because of their limited size, however, these trials cannot be expected to detect rare adverse effects. Thus, licensing does not guarantee that a new vaccine is completely safe, and post-licensing monitoring is needed to ensure effectiveness and to document the occurrence of adverse events of low frequency.

The development of vaccines goes beyond technology and proof of principle to issues such as development costs, manufacturers' liability and indemnity, perceived public health needs, and the likelihood that a product will be used or sold. Given the complex science required, the costs of vaccine development are high and success is uncertain, adding risk to the development decision. It is unfortunate that the one sure implication of uncertainty in vaccine development is increased cost. In addition, a rational assignment of costs for development between the public and private sectors in the United States has never been achieved.

VACCINE FORMULATIONS Studies of clinical immunology have shown that living and dead antigens do not necessarily induce the same immune responses and that the requirements for the development of protective immunity differ with the organism. These insights, together with the refinement of epidemiologic concepts surrounding immunization, have changed the strategy of vaccine development. The goal is not only to select the correct antigens but also to ensure that the vaccines will result in the type of immune response needed for protection, whether the T cell–mediated activation of macrophages or the generation of cytotoxic T cells, B cell–mediated secretory IgA, or a particular IgG subtype response to a specific polysaccharide epitope.

Live vaccines consist of selected or genetically altered organisms that are avirulent or dramatically attenuated yet remain immunogenic. These agents are expected to cause a subclinical illness that mimics natural infection except for the lack of clinically significant disease. They offer the advantage of replication in vivo, which increases the antigenic load presented to the host's immune system; they are believed to confer lifelong protection with one dose; they present a diversity of antigens, thus overcoming immunogenetic restrictions in some hosts; they may reach the local sites most relevant to the induction of protective immunity; and they may produce important protective antigens in vivo that are not efficiently expressed in vitro.

In contrast, with nonviable vaccines, what is presented to the host in terms of antigen load and specific antigenic determinants defines the ultimate response. Nonviable preparations may fail to elicit mucosal IgA-mediated immunity, as they lack a delivery system that will transport them to local antigen-processing cells as effectively as living organisms are conveyed. Moreover, except for pure polysaccharide antigens, these preparations must almost always be given in multiple doses to induce effective responses. However, killed vaccines can be extremely effective. For example, the nonviable hepatitis A vaccine formulation appears to be close to 100 percent effective in inducing protective immunity.

In spite of their advantages, live vaccines are not always to be preferred. For example, live OPV is contraindicated for use in children with immune-deficiency diseases and in their adult contacts. In addition, even though killed poliovirus vaccine does not completely immunize the gut and can neither reduce the circulation of wild-type poliovirus nor immunize contacts of vaccine recipients, this vaccine is preferred for the immunization of adults when urgency of protection is not an issue because of the greater risk of vaccine-associated polio posed by live OPV. In some countries (e.g., Denmark and Israel), a combination schedule of killed and live poliovirus vaccine has been recommended.

To create a deliverable vaccine, constituents other than the antigens are required (Table 122-3). These constituents can affect the immunogenicity, efficacy, and safety of a vaccine and can render one formulation superior to another.

PRODUCTION OF VACCINES As products to be given to healthy individuals to prevent disease, vaccines not only must be efficacious but also must lack the capacity to cause harm. In the United States, quality assurance is the responsibility of vaccine manufacturers. Standards of manufacture of biologics [known as good manufacturing practices (GMPs)] are regulated and supervised by the Food and Drug Administration (FDA). Proof of the safety, efficacy, sterility, and purity of products is required before licensure, and sterility and purity are continually monitored for all lots of vaccine after licensure. Post-marketing studies of safety (phase IV studies) are part of routine regulatory control. On rare occasions, either GMP or quality assurance is inadequate; for example, the release of incompletely killed Salk polio vaccine in 1955 caused an outbreak of poliomyelitis in nearly 200 vaccine recipients and their contacts. Unregulated and uncontrolled manufacture of vaccines in developing countries has sometimes led to the release and use of inactive products that fail to provide the expected protective immunity.

Another problem in the production of vaccines has unexpectedly cropped up in the past decade. For various reasons, including the high costs of vaccine development and the prospect of much higher profitability from investments in other products, the number of vaccine manufacturers in the United States has declined and the cost of some basic childhood vaccines has increased. Concern therefore exists about the future availability of these essential biologics for national use. Furthermore, pricing decisions made within the private-sector pharmaceutical industry can have a major impact on vaccine use. This situation has stimulated an initiative toward increased public involvement in the supplying of vaccine to individuals for whom price is an issue (as in the Vaccines for Children Program discussed below) as well as in oversight of the vaccine supply and of price negotiations with the industry.

ADMINISTRATION OF VACCINES Health care workers administering vaccines must take the precautions necessary to minimize the risk of spreading disease. They should be immunized against hepatitis B, measles, rubella, influenza, and varicella, and they should wash their hands before seeing each new patient. The syringes and

Table 122-3

Constituents of Vaccines

Constituent(s)	Examples/Purpose
Preservatives, stabilizers, antibiotics	These components are used to prevent the vaccine's deterioration before use, to inhibit or prevent bacterial growth, or to stabilize the antigen. Any of these additives may elicit allergic reactions.
Adjuvants	An aluminum salt is used in some vaccines (e.g., toxoids, hepatitis B vaccine) to enhance the immune response.
Suspending fluid	The suspending fluid can be sterile water, saline, buffer, or more complex fluids derived from the growth medium or biologic system in which the agent is produced (e.g., egg antigens, cell culture ingredients, serum proteins).

needles they use for injection must be sterile and preferably disposable to minimize the risk of contamination. Different vaccines should not be mixed in the same syringe unless such a practice is specifically endorsed by licensure. Disposable needles and syringes should be discarded in labeled, puncture-proof containers to prevent inadvertent needlestick injury or reuse.

The recent addition of new, individually injectable vaccines to the immunization schedule has heightened parental concerns about the administration of up to four injections at a single clinic visit. The development and use of combinations of vaccines are intended to mitigate these concerns. Even when multiple injections are required, providers must make every effort to administer all indicated vaccines at each visit.

Wherever effective primary health care systems ensure access to medical services for the majority and the population is educated about the need for and efficacy of vaccines, coverage rates for basic immunization are usually high, regardless of the route of vaccine administration or the number of doses necessary. However, without systematic attention to the completion of multiple-dose vaccine schedules, coverage rates for second, third, and booster doses may drop off significantly.

USE OF VACCINES

Until recently, recommendations for vaccine use in the United States were developed by several different groups. In order to establish a single childhood immunization schedule, the American Academy of Pediatrics (AAP) and the Advisory Committee on Immunization Practices (ACIP) have unified their vaccine recommendations, and this unified version has been approved by the American Academy of Family Practice (AAFP). These recommendations are the result of a collaborative process among the recommending groups, the pharmaceutical industry, and the FDA.

Vaccines recommended in 1996 for routine administration to infants, children, and adults are shown in Table 122-4; vaccines recommended for special use are shown in Table 122-5; and schedules for immunization of children and adults are shown in Fig. 122-2 and Table 122-6, respectively. The recommendations on route, site, and dosages for vaccination are derived from theoretical considerations, experimental trials, and clinical experience; deviation from these recommendations can result in inadequate protection. The administration of doses at intervals longer than those recommended does not diminish the ultimate protective response but merely delays it. It is not necessary to restart an interrupted series from the beginning or to add an extra dose. In contrast, giving vaccines at shorter-than-recommended intervals may result in poor responses.

RECORDING AND REPORTING REQUIREMENTS Certain aspects of vaccine use are regulated by the National Childhood Vaccine Injury Act (NCVIA) of 1986 (modified in 1995). The act requires that all mandated childhood vaccinations be recorded by health care providers in the child's permanent medical record, including date of administration, manufacturer and lot number, and name of the provider administering the vaccine. State-based immunization information systems and registries are being developed to help public and private providers manage their immunization activities and particularly to address the problem of assessing immunization coverage when an individual's records are divided among multiple medical facilities.

Parents should maintain an up-to-date immunization record on their children. The NCVIA requires that the potential for reactions to vaccines and the benefits of vaccination to the child be explained to parents. Educational materials providing the required information are available from the AAP or the Centers for Disease Control and Prevention (CDC).

VACCINES FOR ROUTINE USE Infants and Children Recommended routine-use vaccines and schedules for their administration to infants and children are shown in Table 122-4 and Fig. 122-2, respectively. It is current practice for all children in the United States to receive DTaP, poliovirus, MMR, Hib, HBV, and varicella vaccines

Table 122-4

Routinely Recommended Vaccines for Infants, Children, and Adults

Vaccine	Year Licensed	Type of Immunizing Agent	Protective Antibody	Route of Administration	Efficacy, %	Adverse Events
DT	1949	Toxoid	Diphtheria and tetanus neutralizing antitoxins, ≥0.1 IU/mL each	IM	D: 95	Local reactions
Td	1955				T: 95	Hypersensitivity to tetanus toxoid
aP	1993	Inactivated bacterial antigen	Not known	IM	80–90	Reduced local reactions compared with whole-cell vaccines; no serious reactions reported
	1996	Acellular (DTaP)				
Hib	1987	Bacterial polysaccharide-protein conjugate	Antibody to capsular polysaccharide, 0.15 μg/mL	IM	90	Few local, no serious reactions
HBV	1981	Inactivated serum-derived viral antigen	Antibody to surface antigen, 10 mIU/mL	IM	80–95	Few (? Guillain-Barré syndrome)
	1987	Recombinant antigen				
Influenza	1945	Inactivated virus or viral components	Neutralizing antibody	IM	40–60	? Guillain-Barré syndrome with swine influenza vaccine
MMR	1971	Live viruses	Neutralizing measles antibody, ≥200 mIU/mL; not known for mumps or rubella	SC	M: 95	Acute encephalopathy (measles)
					Mu: 90	Rare parotitis or orchitis (mumps)
					R: 95	Arthralgia and rare arthropathy (rubella)
Pneumococcus	1983	Bacterial polysaccharide of 23 types	Antibody to capsular polysaccharide	IM or SC	60–80	Local reactions; rare anaphylaxis
Poliomyelitis	1963	OPV, live virus of 3 serotypes	Neutralizing antibody at any detectable titer	Oral	95*	Rare vaccine-associated polio
	1967	IPV-e, inactivated virus of 3 serotypes		SC	95	No significant reactions

* In developing countries, OPV efficacy is only 70 to 90 percent, presumably because of interfering enteroviruses in the intestinal tract.

NOTE: DT, diphtheria and tetanus toxoids, adsorbed; Td, tetanus and diphtheria toxoids, adsorbed, for adult use; aP, acellular pertussis; Hib, *Haemophilus influenzae* type b; HBV, hepatitis B virus; MMR, measles-mumps-rubella; OPV, trivalent oral poliovirus vaccine; IPV-e, inactivated poliovirus vaccine, enhanced; IM, intramuscular; SC, subcutaneous.

SOURCE: Recommendations of the Advisory Committee on Immunization Practices, the American Academy of Pediatrics, and the American College of Physicians.

unless there are specific contraindications. A four-dose schedule of DTaP and *either* a four-dose poliovirus vaccine schedule consisting of two doses of inactivated poliovirus vaccine, enhanced (IPV-e), followed by two doses of OPV *or* a four-dose schedule of either OPV or IPV-e, including a booster dose at 4 to 6 years of age, constitute the full series. The combined IPV-e/OPV schedule is intended to reduce the incidence of vaccine-associated poliomyelitis. DTaP (Connaught, Tripedia) was first licensed in 1996 for primary immunization of infants. DTaP is now the preferred vaccine, although DTP may still be used. A booster dose is recommended at 4 to 6 years of age. Adult-formulation Td boosters are recommended every 10 years thereafter. One dose of MMR vaccine along with varicella vaccine is recommended at 15 months. MMR is given again at school entry or in middle school. DTaP, MMR, varicella, poliovirus, and Hib vaccines may be given simultaneously at 15 months of age without increasing rates of adverse reactions or impairing the immune response. Unvaccinated children who lack a reliable history of chickenpox should receive varicella vaccine before the teenage years.

Adults (See Table 122-6)   All adults should be immune to diphtheria and tetanus. If not previously immunized, adults require a primary immunizing course of three doses of Td, with the second dose

4 to 8 weeks after the first, the third dose at 12 months, and boosters every 10 years thereafter. Many individuals remain immune to tetanus into adulthood because they have received tetanus toxoid rather than Td after injuries, but they are commonly at risk of diphtheria because of the decline in titer of diphtheria antitoxin and the lack of boosting against diphtheria. Routine immunization against polio is not recommended for adults unless they are at particular risk of exposure (e.g., through travel to endemic regions, as discussed below) or are the parents or guardians of a child with an immunodeficiency disorder. Adults should be protected from measles, mumps, and rubella; they should be vaccinated unless they are known to have received vaccine on or after their first birthday or to have had physician-diagnosed disease. Rubella vaccine should be given to all women of childbearing age unless they have documentary proof of immunization after their first birthday or laboratory evidence of immunity. An unsupported history of rubella disease is unreliable and should not be accepted. Adults without a clear history of chickenpox should receive varicella vaccine.

Table 122-5

Special-Use Vaccines

Vaccine	Year Licensed in United States	Type of Immunizing Agent	Route of Administration	Indications	Efficacy	Adverse Events
Anthrax	1970	Inactivated avirulent bacteria	SC (6 doses primary; annual booster)	For high risk of exposure (i.e., persons in contact with or involved in manufacture of animal hides, furs, bone meal, wool, goat hair)	90% antibody response but efficacy uncertain	No serious adverse effects known
Tuberculosis (BCG)	1950	Living bacteria (attenuated *Mycobacterium bovis*)	ID	PPD-negative individuals in prolonged contact with active TB patient	Controversial; reduces disseminated disease in children (0–80% protection against pulmonary TB; 75–86% protection against miliary and meningitic TB)	Regional adenitis, disseminated BCG infection, osteitis
Hepatitis A	1995	Killed virus antigen	IM	Travelers or persons living in high-risk areas	94%	Local reactions
Cholera	1914	Inactivated bacteria	SC or IM	Not recommended for public health use	50% (short-lived)	Frequent fever, local pain, swelling
Meningococcus A, C, Y, W135	1981	Bacterial polysaccharide of 4 serotypes	SC	Military personnel; principally travelers to epidemic areas	90% for 2- to 3-year-olds	Rare
Plague	1911	Inactivated bacteria	IM	Laboratory workers; foresters in endemic areas; travelers	90% antibody response but efficacy uncertain	10% local reactions; rare sterile abscesses and hypersensitivity
Rabies (human diploid)	1980	Inactivated virus	IM or ID	Travelers; laboratory workers; veterinarians	Virtually 100%	25% local reactions; 6% arthropathy, arthritis, angioedema
Yellow fever	1953	Live virus	SC	Laboratory workers; travelers	High	Encephalitis; encephalopathy
Japanese encephalitis	1993	Inactivated virus	SC	Travelers	80–90%	Anaphylactic/severe delayed allergic reactions common; recipient should be observed for 10 days
Typhoid						
Phenol and heat-killed	1952	Killed whole bacteria	IM	Not routinely recommended in U.S.; used for travelers, contacts of carriers	50–70% (short-lived)	Frequent fever, local swelling, pain
Ty21a	1992	Live mutant bacteria	Oral	Travelers, contacts of carriers	50–70%	None
Vi	1995	Vi capsular polysaccharide	IM	Travelers	70–75%	Local reactions

NOTE: SC, subcutaneous; BCG, bacille Calmette-Guérin; ID, intradermal; PPD, purified protein derivative; TB, tuberculosis; IM, intramuscular.
SOURCE: Recommendations of the Advisory Committee on Immunization Practices, the American Academy of Pediatrics, and the American College of Physicians.

Age ▶ Vaccine[1] ▼	Birth	1 mo	2 mos	4 mos	6 mos	12 mos	15 mos	18 mos	4-6 yrs	11-12 yrs	14-16 yrs
Hepatitis B[2,3]	Hep B-1									Hep B[3]	
		Hep B-2		Hep B-3							
Diphtheria, tetanus, pertussis[4]			DTaP or DTP	DTaP or DTP	DTaP or DTP		DTaP or DTP[4]		DTaP or DTP	Td	
H. influenzae type b[5]			Hib	Hib	Hib[5]	Hib[5]					
Polio[6]			Polio[6]	Polio	Polio[6]				Polio		
Measles, mumps, rubella[7]						MMR			MMR[7] or MMR[7]		
Varicella[8]						Var			Var[8]		

FIGURE 122-2 Recommended childhood immunization schedule in the United States for January through December 1997. Vaccines are listed under the routinely recommended ages. Shaded bars indicate a range of acceptable ages for vaccination; clear bars indicate timing of catch-up vaccination: at 11 or 12 years of age, hepatitis B vaccine should be administered to children not previously vaccinated, and varicella vaccine should be administered to children not previously vaccinated who lack a reliable history of chickenpox. Vaccine abbreviations: Hep B, hepatitis B; DTaP, diphtheria/tetanus/acellular pertussis; DTP, diphtheria/tetanus/pertussis; Hib, *Haemophilus influenzae* type b; Td, tetanus/diphtheria toxoids, adsorbed; MMR, measles/mumps/rubella; Var, varicella-zoster. **Key to footnotes:** [1] *This schedule indicates the recommended age* for routine administration of currently licensed childhood vaccines. Some combination vaccines are available and may be used whenever administration of all components of the vaccine is indicated. Providers should consult the manufacturers' package insert for detailed recommendations. [2] *The hepatitis B surface antigen (HBsAg) status of pregnant women,* if not known, should be determined as soon as possible during pregnancy. Infants born to HBsAg-negative mothers should receive 2.5 μg of Recombivax HB (Merck, Sharpe and Dohme) or 10 μg of Engerix-B (Smith-Kline Beecham) at birth or within the first 2 months of life. The second dose should be administered ≥1 month after the first dose. In this setting a *combination Hep B/Hib vaccine (Comvax, Merck) released in January 1997 may be used* and may be given along with other recommended pediatric vaccines. *Infants born to HBsAg-positive mothers* should receive immunoprophylaxis with 0.5 mL of hepatitis B immune globulin along with 5 μg of Recombivax or 10 μg of Engerix-B within 12 h of birth. The second dose of vaccine is recommended at 1 to 2 months of age and the third dose at 6 months of age. *Infants born to mothers whose HBsAg status remains unknown at delivery* should receive either 5 μg of Recombivax or 10 μg of Engerix-B within 12 h of birth. The second dose of vaccine is recommended at 1 month of age and the third dose at 6 months of age. Blood should be drawn at the time of delivery to determine the mother's HBsAg status; if it is positive, the infant should receive hepatitis B immune globulin as soon as possible and no later than 1 week of age. The size and timing of subsequent vaccine doses are based on the mother's HBsAg status. [3] *Adolescents who have not previously received three doses of Hep B vaccine* should have the series initiated or completed at 11 or 12 years of age. The second dose should be administered at least 1 month after the first dose, and the third dose should be administered at least 4 months after the first dose and 2 months after the second dose. [4] *DTaP is the preferred vaccine for all doses,* including completion of the series in children who have received ≥1 dose of whole-cell DTP. Whole-cell DTP is an acceptable alternative to DTaP. The fourth dose of DTaP may be administered at 12 months, provided that 6 months have elapsed since the third dose, and if the child is unlikely to return at 15 to 18 months of age. A booster dose of DTaP (or DTP) is given at 4 to 6 years. Td is recommended at 11 or 12 years of age if at least 5 years have elapsed since the last dose of DTaP, DTP, or DT. [5] *Three Hib conjugate vaccines* are licensed for infant use. If PRP-OMP (PedVaxHIB [Merck]) is administered at 2 and 4 months of age, no dose is required at 6 months. After completion of the primary series, any Hib conjugate vaccine may be used as a booster. [6] *Two poliovirus vaccines are currently licensed in the United States:* enhanced inactivated poliovirus vaccine (IPV-e) and oral poliovirus vaccine (OPV). Three schedules are acceptable, and parents and providers may choose among them: (1) IPV-e at 2 and 4 months; OPV at 12 to 18 months and 4 to 6 years; (2) IPV-e for all four doses; (3) OPV for all four doses. IPV is the only poliovirus vaccine recommended for persons with a congenital or acquired immunodeficiency disease or an altered immune status resulting from disease or immunosuppressive therapy and for their household contacts. [7] *The second dose of MMR vaccine* is routinely recommended at 4 to 6 years of age or at 11 or 12 years of age but may be administered at any visit, provided that at least 1 month has elapsed since receipt of the first dose. [8] *Varicella-zoster virus vaccine* can be administered to susceptible children at any time after 12 months of age. Unvaccinated children who lack a reliable history of chickenpox should be vaccinated at 11 to 12 years of age. *(From the Advisory Committee on Immunization Practices, the American Academy of Pediatrics, and the American Academy of Family Practice in conjunction with the Food and Drug Administration and the pharmaceutical industry.)*

Current recommendations also include influenza vaccine for routine annual administration to adults ≥65 years of age and to individuals with chronic illness at any age. Polyvalent pneumococcal polysaccharide vaccine is similarly recommended for the elderly or chronically ill. HBV vaccine is recommended for individuals at high risk of exposure, including health care workers exposed to potentially infected blood or blood products, homosexuals, injection drug users, individuals living and working in institutions for the mentally retarded, and household contacts of known carriers of hepatitis B surface antigen.

Adverse Events Modern vaccines, while safe and effective, are associated with adverse effects that range from infrequent and very mild to rare and life-threatening. The decision to use a vaccine involves an assessment of the risks of disease, the benefits of vaccination, and the risks associated with vaccination. Because these factors may change over time, continued assessment is essential. Table 122-7 lists valid and invalid contraindications to immunization and describes appropriate precautions in the use of specific vaccines.

Vaccine components, including protective antigens, animal proteins introduced during vaccine production, and antibiotics or other preservatives or stabilizers, can cause allergic reactions in some recipients. These reactions may be local or systemic and may include urticaria and serious anaphylaxis. The most common extraneous allergen is egg protein introduced when vaccines such as those for measles, mumps, influenza, and yellow fever are prepared in embryonated eggs. Local or systemic reactions can result from too-frequent administration of vaccines such as Td, diphtheria/ tetanus (DT), or rabies; these reactions are probably due to antigen-antibody complexes. In addition, live-virus vaccines can interfere with tuberculin test responses. When a tuberculin skin test is indicated, it should be done either on the day of immunization or 6 weeks later.

All detected adverse events temporally related to vaccination are expected to be reported to both the local health department and the vaccine manufacturer. The NCVIA requires health care providers to report certain suspected adverse events following the receipt of a mandated vaccine to the FDA's Vaccine Adverse Events Reporting System (Table 122-8). Although a temporal relationship does not establish cause and effect, this surveillance system remains the only mechanism for collecting the data needed to form conclusions and make decisions.

USE OF VACCINES IN SPECIAL CIRCUMSTANCES **Pregnancy** Because of theoretical risk to the fetus and real risk of litigation to the practitioner, routine immunization of pregnant women is best avoided. However, wherever hygienic conditions during delivery cannot be guaranteed, it is essential to ensure that pregnant women are immune to tetanus: the transfer of maternal antitoxin is an important means of preventing neonatal tetanus, and pregnant women can safely receive tetanus as well as diphtheria toxoids. Although live-virus vaccines in general should be withheld during pregnancy, polio and yellow fever vaccines are exceptions and may be administered if the risk of exposure to disease is great. If indicated, some inactivated-virus vaccines (e.g., HBV, influenza, and pneumococcal vaccines) are safe for pregnant women. Known pregnancy is considered a contraindication to the receipt of rubella, measles, mumps, and varicella vaccines. Although of theoreti-

Table 122-6

CHAPTER 122
Immunization Principles and Vaccine Use

765

Adult Immunization Schedule

Vaccine	Timing of Immunization
Hepatitis A*	Two doses are recommended for individuals requiring long-term protection, with the second dose 6–12 months after the first.
Hepatitis B*	Three doses are given, with the second dose 1 month after the first and the third dose 5 months after the second.
Measles/mumps/ rubella	One dose is given to adults born in 1957 or later **and not previously immunized.** A second dose may be required in some work or school settings.
Tetanus/diphtheria toxoids, adsorbed	A three-dose schedule applies for individuals who **have not received an initial immunization series in childhood.** The second dose is given 1 month after the first and the third dose 6 months after the second. Boosters are then given every 10 years.
Varicella	Two doses are given to individuals ≥13 years of age who have not had chickenpox. The second dose is given 1–2 months after the first.
Influenza	Vaccine is administered yearly to individuals ≥65 years of age; to younger people with chronic medical problems, such as heart disease and diabetes; and to those who work or live with high-risk persons.
Streptococcus pneumoniae	Vaccine is usually given once to individuals ≥65 years of age. A repeat dose may be given 5 years later for those at highest risk. Immunization is also recommended for younger people with chronic medical problems, such as heart disease, diabetes, renal failure, and sickle cell anemia, and for those who work or live with high-risk persons.

* For individuals at risk.
SOURCE: National Coalition for Adult Immunization.

cal concern, no cases of congenital rubella syndrome or abnormalities attributable to rubella vaccine virus have been observed in infants born to susceptible mothers who received rubella vaccine during pregnancy. A registry for susceptible women who have inadvertently received varicella vaccine during pregnancy has been established for the purpose of data collection.

Breast Feeding Neither killed nor live vaccine affects the safety of breast feeding for either mother or infant. Breast-fed infants can be immunized on a normal schedule. Breast feeding does not adversely affect the immune response and is not a contraindication for any vaccine. Although live vaccine viruses multiply within the mother's body, most are not excreted in breast milk. Mothers may therefore receive OPV or yellow fever vaccine without interrupting breast feeding. Rubella vaccine virus may be transmitted in breast milk; however, the virus usually does not infect the infant, and if it does the infection is well tolerated.

Occupational Exposure Immunization recommendations for most occupational groups remain to be developed. Specific practices are now mandated by the Occupational Safety and Health Administration for the immunization of health care workers against hepatitis B in the United States. Those at particular risk of exposure to hepatitis B, such as surgeons and health care workers dealing with blood products, must be immunized. Many medical institutions now give HBV vaccine to all health care workers and to all medical, dental, and nursing students. Rubella is transmitted to and from health care workers in medical facilities, particularly in pediatric practice. Health care workers who might transmit rubella to pregnant patients should be immune to rubella; it is prudent to screen these employees for antibodies to rubella virus and to immunize susceptible individuals. Persons providing health care are also at greater risk from measles and varicella than the general public, and those who are likely to come into contact with measles- and varicella-infected patients should be immune. Persons employed in caring for patients with chronic diseases can transmit influenza; such workers should be vaccinated annually. Unfortunately, these recommendations often are not fully implemented, even in academic institutions.

HIV Infection and Other Immunocompromised States Limited studies in HIV-infected individuals have found no increase in the risk of adverse events from live or inactivated vaccines. However, immune responses may not be as vigorous in immunocompromised individuals as in subjects with a normal immune system. Persons known to be infected with HIV should be immunized with recommended vaccines—except for poliovirus vaccine—in the same manner as individuals with a normal immune system and as early in the course of their disease as possible, before immune function becomes significantly impaired. Live attenuated MMR vaccine can be administered to this group, but OPV cannot (Table 122-9). IPV-e should be used when vaccination against polio is indicated because the risk of vaccine-associated poliomyelitis is too great with OPV. Household contacts of immunocompromised individuals should be immune to polio; when vaccinated, they should receive IPV-e and not OPV. In practice, it is not necessary to test for HIV before making decisions about the immunization of asymptomatic individuals from known HIV risk groups.

Live attenuated vaccines are normally contraindicated in immunocompromised patients, including those with congenital immunodeficiency syndromes and those receiving immunosuppressive therapy. Passive immunization with immunoglobulin preparations or antitoxins can be considered in individual cases, either as postexposure prophylaxis or as part of the treatment of established infection.

Postexposure Immunization For certain infections, active or passive immunization soon after exposure prevents or attenuates disease expression. The immune globulins and antitoxins currently available in the United States are listed in Table 122-10, and the recommended postexposure immunization regimens are compiled in Table 122-11. Measles immune globulins given within 6 days of exposure may prevent or modify infection, and measles vaccine given within the first few days after exposure may prevent symptomatic infection. Although clinical manifestations of rubella in pregnant women are minimized by postexposure passive immunization, this approach may not prevent maternal viremia, fetal infection, and congenital rubella syndrome. Therefore, the administration of immune globulin is recommended only for women developing rubella during pregnancy who will not consider abortion under any circumstances. Tetanus immune globulin can be used in patients with tetanus. Survivors with no history of tetanus immunization should receive a primary series of toxoid injections since disease does not result in the development of protective levels of antitoxin. Administration of rabies immune globulin plus rabies vaccine in the immediate postexposure period is highly effective in preventing disease. Similarly, for persons who have not been actively immunized, the use of immune globulin within 2 weeks of exposure to hepatitis A is likely to prevent clinical illness. Good data indicate the efficacy of human hepatitis B immune globulin in preventing disease after exposure. While no high-titer preparation is available for postexposure protection against non-A, non-B hepatitis, standard human immune serum globulin is efficacious.

Simultaneous Administration of Multiple Vaccines The simultaneous administration of the most widely used live and inactivated vaccines has not resulted in impaired antibody responses or in increased rates of adverse reactions. Simultaneous administration of vaccines is advantageous in that it increases the probability that a child will ultimately be fully immunized; it is also useful in any age group when the potential exists for exposure to multiple infectious diseases during travel to endemic countries. Inactivated vaccines can often be given together in a single injection or at separate sites at the same time. Administration of the combined MMR vaccine yields results comparable to those obtained with the administration of the individual vaccines at different sites; combined administration has greatly facilitated effective immunization for the three infections with little increase in cost. Although recent administration of OPV is not a contraindication to the use of MMR, other live-virus vaccines not given together on the same day should generally be administered at least 30 days apart.

Neither the response to OPV nor that to yellow fever vaccine is altered by the administration of immune globulins. In contrast, since high doses of immune globulin may inhibit the efficacy of measles and rubella vaccines, an interval of at least 3 months is recommended between the administration of immune globulin and that of MMR or its components. Postpartum vaccination of rubella-susceptible women should not be delayed because of the administration of anti-Rho(D) immune globulin or any other blood product during the last trimester or at delivery. Should administration of an immune globulin preparation become necessary after vaccination, it should be postponed, if possible, for at least 14 days to allow time for vaccine-virus replication and

development of immunity. In general, there is little interaction of immune globulin with inactivated vaccines, and postexposure passive prophylaxis can be given together with HBV vaccine or tetanus toxoid, resulting in both immediate and long-lasting protection.

Travel The International Sanitary Regulations allow countries to impose requirements for yellow fever and killed cholera vaccines as a condition for admission, even though the latter is not an effective public health tool. Travelers should know whether these vaccines are required for entry into the countries on their itinerary to avoid being turned back or immunized on the spot. Infants, children, and adults should have all routine immunizations updated before traveling, with

Table 122-7

Immunization Contraindications and Precautions

Vaccine	Contraindication or Precaution[a]	
	Valid	Invalid
General[b]	Anaphylactic reaction to vaccine (contraindication to further doses of that vaccine)	Mild to moderate local reaction (soreness, redness, swelling) following dose of injectable antigen
	Anaphylactic reaction to vaccine constituent (contraindication to use of vaccines containing that substance)	Mild acute illness, with or without low-grade fever
	Moderate or severe illnesses, with or without fever	Current antimicrobial therapy
		Convalescent phase of illness
		Prematurity (same dosage and indications as for normal, full-term infants)
		Recent exposure to an infectious disease
		History of penicillin or other nonspecific allergies or family history of such allergies
DTaP/DTP	Encephalopathy within 72 h after dose	Temperature of <40.5°C (105°F) after dose
	Fever of ≥40.5°C (105°F) within 48 h after dose (P)	Family history of convulsions[c]
	Collapse or shocklike state (hypotonic-hyporesponsive episode) within 48 h after dose (P)	Family history of an adverse event following vaccination
	Seizures within 3 days after dose (P)	Family history of sudden infant death syndrome
	Persistent, inconsolable crying lasting ≥3 h within 48 h after dose (P)	
OPV[d]	Infection with HIV or a household contact infected with HIV	Breast feeding
	Known immunodeficiency (hematologic and solid tumors, congenital immunodeficiency, and long-term immunosuppressive therapy)	Current antimicrobial therapy
		Diarrhea
	Immunodeficient household contact	
	Pregnancy[e] (P)	
IPV/IPV-e	Anaphylactic reactions to neomycin or streptomycin	—
	Pregnancy[e]	
MMR	Anaphylactic reactions to eggs or to neomycin[f]	Tuberculosis or positive PPD test
	Pregnancy	Simultaneous TB skin testing[g]
	Known immunodeficiency (hematologic and solid tumors, congenital immunodeficiency syndrome, and long-term immunosuppressive therapy)	Breast feeding
		Pregnancy of mother of recipient
		Immunodeficient family member or household contact
	Recent IG administration (P)	Infection with HIV
		Nonanaphylactic reactions to eggs or neomycin
Hib	None identified	History of Hib disease
HBV	None identified	Pregnancy
Influenza	First trimester of pregnancy (vaccination avoided on theoretical grounds)	—
	Anaphylactic reactions to eggs	
Pneumococcus	Has not been evaluated in pregnancy	—
Varicella	Primary acquired immunodeficiency	Contact dermatitis in response to neomycin
	History of anaphylactic reaction to neomycin	
	Pregnancy	

[a] Precautions are followed by "(P)." The events or conditions listed as precautions, although not contraindications, should be carefully reviewed. The benefits and risks of administering a specific vaccine to an individual under the circumstances should be considered. If the risks are believed to outweigh the benefits, the vaccine should be withheld; if the benefits are believed to outweigh the risks (for example, during an outbreak or foreign travel), the vaccine should be administered. Whether and when to administer DTaP to children with proven or suspected underlying neurologic disorders should be decided on an individual basis.
[b] For DTP/DTaP, OPV, IPV/IPV-e, MMR, Hib, HBV, influenza, pneumococcus, and varicella.
[c] If a child has a precaution to the receipt of a subsequent dose of whole-cell DTP, the child should not routinely receive DTaP. If a child has a contraindication to the receipt of a subsequent dose of whole-cell DTP, the child should not receive DTaP. Acetaminophen given before DTaP and thereafter every 4 h for 24 h should be considered for children with a personal or family (sibling or parent) history of convulsions.
[d] No data exist to substantiate the theoretical risk of a suboptimal immune response when OPV and MMR are given within 30 days of each other.
[e] It is prudent on theoretical grounds to avoid vaccinating pregnant women. However, if immediate protection against poliomyelitis is needed, OPV is preferred, although IPV may be considered if vaccination can be completed before the anticipated imminent exposure.
[f] Persons with a history of anaphylactic reactions following egg ingestion should be vaccinated only with caution. Protocols have been developed for vaccinating such persons and should be consulted (J Pediatr 102:196, 1983; J Pediatr 113:504, 1988).
[g] Measles vaccination may temporarily suppress tuberculin reactivity. If skin testing cannot be done on the day of MMR vaccination, the test should be postponed for 4 to 6 weeks.
NOTE: IPV, inactivated polio vaccine; PPD, purified protein derivative; TB, tuberculosis; IG, immunoglobulin.
SOURCES: Standards for Pediatric Immunization Practices, Centers for Disease Control and Prevention; ACIP: Morb Mort Week Rep 38:73, 1989; ACIP: Morb Mort Week Rep 42:1, 1993. This information is based on the recommendations of the Advisory Committee on Immunization Practices (ACIP) and those of the Committee on Infectious Diseases (Red Book Committee) of the American Academy of Pediatrics (AAP). Sometimes these recommendations vary from those contained in the manufacturers' package inserts. For more detailed information, providers should consult the published recommendations of the ACIP and the AAP as well as the manufacturers' package inserts.

Table 122-8

CHAPTER 122
Immunization Principles and Vaccine Use **767**

Reportable Events Following Vaccination, as Required by the National Childhood Vaccine Injury Act of 1986 (Modified in 1995)*

Vaccine/Toxoid	Event	Interval from Vaccination
DTaP; P; DTP-Hib; DT; Td or TT	Anaphylaxis	4 h
	Encephalopathy (or encephalitis)	72 h
MMR, MR, or M	Anaphylaxis	4 h
	Encephalopathy (or encephalitis)	5–15 days
	Residual seizure disorder	5–15 days
Rubella-containing vaccines (MMR, MR, R)	Chronic arthritis	42 days
	Anaphylaxis	4 h
	Encephalopathy (or encephalitis)	5–15 days
	Residual seizure disorder	5–15 days
OPV	Paralytic poliomyelitis	
	In an immunocompetent recipient	30 days
	In an immunocompromised recipient	6 months
	In a vaccine-associated community case	No limits
Inactivated polio vaccine	Anaphylaxis	4 h

* Compensation (under the NCVIA) is effective for claims filed on or after March 10, 1995. Any acute complications or sequelae of an illness, disability, injury, or condition that arose within the prescribed period (including deaths) are also covered.

NOTE: P, pertussis; TT, tetanus toxoid; MR, measles/rubella; M, measles; R, rubella.

particular attention to polio, measles, and DTP/DTaP or Td vaccines. The use of hepatitis A vaccine or pooled human gamma globulin may be advisable for travelers to some locales. Special-use vaccines (Table 122-5), including rabies, meningococcal A and C polysaccharide, typhoid (oral live or Vi polysaccharide), Japanese encephalitis, and plague vaccines, should be considered for those individuals who expect to go beyond the usual tourist routes or to spend extended periods in rural areas in disease-endemic regions. Most U.S. cities have at least one travel clinic that maintains up-to-date epidemiologic information and can provide the appropriate vaccines. Military personnel, some laboratory personnel, and some individuals subject to occupational hazards (e.g., veterinarians) may receive special-use vaccines when indicated.

DELIVERY OF VACCINES Over the past 20 years, considerable progress has been made to ensure that every child in the United States is fully immunized by the time of school entry. All 50 states now require immunization for school entry, and most have laws addressing attendance at preschools and day-care centers. Survey data (collected before the widespread use of Hib conjugate vaccine and HBV vaccine) indicated that up to 98 percent of all children were immunized against five vaccine-preventable diseases by the time they entered school. The impact of immunization and of other improvements in the health care provided to the American population on the incidence of vaccine-preventable illness is shown in Table 122-1 and Fig. 122-1.

By the mid-1980s, however, it was recognized that large numbers of preschool children were not fully immunized by 15 months of age. Only 37 to 56 percent of preschoolers in the United States had been completely immunized,[1] and this rate was as low as 10 percent in some communities. The failure to vaccinate preschool children was largely responsible for the resurgence of measles between 1989 and 1991, with 55,467 cases, more than 11,200 admissions to the hospital, more than 44,100 days of hospitalization, and more than 130 measles-related deaths. The number of cases of congenital rubella syndrome increased from 6 in 1988 to 47 in 1991. Outbreaks of pertussis and mumps were on the rise for the same reason: low immunization rates among preschool children.

ACCESS TO IMMUNIZATION Four major barriers to infant and childhood immunization have been identified within the health care system: (1) low public awareness and lack of public demand for immunization, (2) inadequate access to immunization services, (3) missed opportunities to administer vaccines, and (4) inadequate resources for public health and preventive programs. These problems are sources of public concern, and their solution is a priority for national health policy in the United States. In response, the Children's Immunization Initiative was begun in 1990. At the national level, this program includes outreach and educational campaigns to promote parental awareness of the value of vaccination and to encourage health care providers to use every opportunity to vaccinate the children in their care. At the state and local levels, community and business groups, religious and service groups, schools, and the media have joined together in community-based networks. A National Immunization Week each April has been established to focus attention on the vaccination needs of infants and children. To improve the quality and quantity of vaccination services, expanded immunization-clinic hours and computerization of immunization records are being implemented as well.

One of the national health objectives for the millennium established under the Healthy People 2000 plan—a set of national health promotion and disease prevention objectives for the year 2000—is to achieve full coverage with the recommended vaccines for 90 percent of children under 2 years of age. By 1995, the National Immunization Survey showed vaccination coverage estimates to be at an all-time high (Table 122-12), while vaccine-preventable childhood diseases were at an all-time low (Table 122-13). Despite this success, about 25 percent of toddlers in the United States (or almost 1.4 million children from 19 to 35 months of age) still lacked one or more doses of the 4 DTP/3 polio/1 MMR series.

[1] By the second birthday, a fully immunized child will have received four doses of DTP/DTaP, three or four doses of a poliovirus vaccine (IPV-e and/ or OPV), one dose of MMR, three doses of HBV vaccine, one dose of varicella vaccine, and three or four doses of a suitable Hib conjugate vaccine.

Table 122-9

Recommendations for Routine Immunization of HIV-Infected Persons in the United States

Vaccine	HIV Clinical Status		Comments
	Asymptomatic	Symptomatic	
DTaP/Td	Yes	Yes	No change in usual immunization schedule
OPV	No	No	Increased risk of vaccine virus proliferation and paralytic polio; IPV-e used for household contacts of HIV-infected persons
IPV-e	Yes	Yes	Antibody response potentially impaired in symptomatic patients
MMR	Yes	Yes	No change in usual immunization schedule; with high risk of exposure to measles, first dose given at 6–11 months of age, second dose at >12 months of age; with documented infection, measles immune globulin potentially administered (see Table 122-11)
Hib conjugate	Yes	Yes	No change in usual immunization schedule
HBV	Yes	Yes	Antibody response potentially impaired; higher-dose vaccine available, but no data address optimal dose; possibly wise to check antibody titer after immunization and give additional doses if titer is inadequate
Pneumococcus	Yes	Yes	Should be given to all ≥2 years old
Influenza	Yes	Yes	Antibody response potentially impaired in symptomatic patients
Varicella	No	No	Vaccine use in asymptomatic HIV persons not studied

SOURCE: Centers for Disease Control and Prevention.

There has been only modest progress towards the goals for adult immunization in the United States promulgated under Healthy People 2000. Adult-immunization goals are important: as many as 60,000 adults die each year of vaccine-preventable diseases for which effective vaccines are not being optimally used. As few as 41 percent of persons ≥65 years of age receive influenza vaccine each year, and fewer than 30 percent of this group have ever received pneumococcal vaccine (Table 122-14). Health care providers more often miss vaccination opportunities with adults than with infants and children. Sixty to 90 percent of adults hospitalized for or dying of influenza-associated respiratory disease have received medical care during the previous year and could have been immunized at that time. Medicare reimbursement for excess hospitalization during influenza epidemics ranges from $750 million to $1 billion. Additional efforts are required to ensure that adults receive pneumococcal, Td, and HBV vaccines as well.

Financing Immunization Many private health insurance policies do not provide adequate coverage for immunization, and physicians and other health care providers pass these costs directly on to patients. In 1994, as a part of the Children's Immunization Initiative, the Vaccines for Children Program was implemented to remove critical barriers to protection against nine vaccine-preventable diseases. The program is designed to reach more children with free vaccine at public clinics and at the offices of their primary care providers. Moreover, states can buy vaccines at reduced prices from the Federal government. Thus, cost is no longer a barrier for the poorest children, and free

Table 122-10

Immune Globulins and Antitoxins* Available in the United States and Indications for Their Use, 1996

Immunobiologic Preparation	Indication(s)
Botulinum antitoxin (equine)	Treatment of botulism
Cytomegalovirus immune globulin, intravenous	Prophylaxis for liver, kidney, and possibly bone marrow transplant recipients
Diphtheria antitoxin (equine)	Treatment of respiratory diphtheria
Immune globulin	Hepatitis A pre- and postexposure prophylaxis; measles postexposure prophylaxis
Intravenous immune globulin	Replacement therapy for antibody deficiency disorders; immune thrombocytopenic purpura; hypogammaglobulinemia in chronic lymphocytic leukemia; Kawasaki disease
Hepatitis B immune globulin	Hepatitis B postexposure prophylaxis
Rabies immune globulin†	Rabies postexposure management of persons not previously immunized
Tetanus immune globulin	Tetanus treatment; postexposure prophylaxis for persons not adequately immunized with tetanus toxoid
Vaccinia immune globulin	Treatment of eczema vaccinatum, vaccinia necrosum, and ocular vaccinia
Varicella-zoster immune globulin	Postexposure prophylaxis of susceptible immunocompromised persons, certain susceptible pregnant women, and perinatally exposed newborns

* Immune globulins and antitoxins are administered intramuscularly unless indicated otherwise.
† Rabies immune globulin is administered around the wound in addition to being injected intramuscularly.

Table 122-11

Recommended Postexposure Immunization with Immunoglobulin Preparations in the United States

Disease	Indicated	Comments
Measles	Yes	Standard human immune globulin is recommended for exposed infants and adults with normal immunocompetence (but with a contraindication to measles vaccine) and for immunocompromised patients exposed to measles (regardless of immunization status). Patients should be immunized 3–6 months after immunoglobulin administration. Recommended dose: 0.25–0.5 mL/kg (40–80 mg of IgG/kg) IM; 80 mg of IgG/kg for immunocompromised contact; maximum, 15 mL.
Rubella	No	Efficacy is unreliable; therefore, standard human immune globulin is recommended for administration only to antibody-negative pregnant women in the first trimester who have a documented rubella exposure and who will not consider terminating the pregnancy. Recommended dose: 0.55 mL/kg (90 mg of IgG/kg) IM.
Tetanus	Yes	Human tetanus immune globulin (TIG) has replaced equine tetanus antitoxin because of the risk of serum sickness with equine serum. Recommended dose for postexposure prophylaxis: 250–500 units of TIG (10–20 mg of IgG/kg) IM. Recommended dose for treatment of tetanus: 500–3000 units of TIG IM.
Rabies	Yes	Human rabies immune globulin (RIG) is preferred over equine rabies antiserum because of the risk of serum sickness. RIG or antiserum is recommended for nonimmunized individuals with animal bites in which rabies cannot be ruled out and with other exposures to known rabid animals. Recommended dose of RIG: 20 IU/kg (22 mg of IgG/kg). Recommended dose of antiserum: 40 IU/kg. Rabies vaccine is given as well at 0, 3, 7, 14, and 28 days.
Hepatitis A	Yes	Standard immune serum globulin is given in a single dose of 0.02–0.04 mL/kg or (for continuous exposure) in a dose of up to 0.06 mL/kg every 5 months. Postexposure treatment with hepatitis A immune globulin has not been studied.
Hepatitis B	Yes	Standard immune serum globulin is not reliably effective. Special human hepatitis B immune globulin is useful and is recommended for neonates born to an infected mother and after mucous-membrane or parenteral contact with infected persons or infected blood or serum. Recommended dose for neonates: 0.5 mL IM within 12 h of birth. Recommended dose for percutaneous or mucosal exposure: 0.06 mL/kg (10 mg of IgG/kg) IM.
Non-A, non-B hepatitis	Yes	Standard immune serum globulin may be valuable. Recommended dose: 0.12 mL/kg (10 mg of IgG/kg) IM, up to 10 mL.

SOURCES: Advisory Committee on Immunization Practices (ACIP), Morb Mort Week Rep 42(RR-4):1, 1993; ACIP, 1991b; ACIP, Morb Mort Week Rep 40(RR-3):1, 1991; ACIP, 1991c; ACIP, Morb Mort Week Rep 39(RR-15):1, 1990.

vaccines are available from the provider of choice.

In contrast, gaps for immunization of adults exist under Medicare. Medicare coverage includes the cost of influenza and pneumococcal vaccines and their administration to all enrolled individuals; it also includes HBV vaccine for those at high risk of exposure (i.e., renal dialysis patients). However, reimbursement is not adequate to encourage vaccine use among providers, and the program does not cover other vaccines, such as Td.

STANDARDS FOR IMMUNIZATION PRACTICES National standards of immunization for adult and pediatric practice have been established to define common policies and practices for public health clinics and in physicians' private offices (Table 122-15). These guidelines highlight the need to distinguish between valid contraindications and conditions that are often considered but are not in fact contraindications (Table 122-7). Among the valid contraindications applicable to all vaccines are a history of anaphylaxis or other serious allergic reactions to a vaccine or vaccine component and the presence of a moderate or severe illness, with or without fever. Infants who develop encephalopathy within 72 h of a dose of DTP or DTaP should not receive further doses; those who develop a "precaution" (Table 122-7) should not normally receive further doses. Because of theoretical risks to the fetus, pregnant women should not receive MMR or varicella vaccine. Diarrhea, minor respiratory ill-

Table 122-12

CHAPTER 122
Immunization Principles and Vaccine Use 769

Vaccination Levels Among Children Aged 19 to 35 Months, by Vaccine—National Immunization Survey, United States, April 1994 through March 1995

Vaccine/Dose	1996 Goal, %	Year 2000 Objective, %	Coverage in April 1994–March 1995 (95% confidence interval)
DTP/DT			
≥3 doses	90	90	94 (±0.6%)
≥4 doses	—	90	77 (±1.0%)
Poliovirus, ≥3 doses	90	90	84 (±0.9%)
Hib, ≥3 doses	90	90	90 (±0.7%)
MMR, ≥1 dose	90	90	89 (±0.8%)
HBV, ≥3 doses	70	90	42 (±1.2%)
19–24 months			58 (±1.4%)
25–30 months			41 (±1.4%)
31–35 months			24 (±1.3%)
Combined series			
4 DTP/3 polio/1 MMR	—	90	75 (±1.0%)
4 DTP/3 polio/1 MMR/3 Hib	—	90	72 (±1.1%)

SOURCE: Centers for Disease Control and Prevention.

ness with or without fever, mild to moderate local reactions to a previous dose of vaccine, the concurrent or recent use of antimicrobial agents, mild to moderate malnutrition, or the convalescent phase of an acute illness are not valid contraindications to routine immunization. Failure to vaccinate children because of these conditions is increasingly being viewed as a missed opportunity for immunization.

THE ROLE OF INDUSTRY Except in the states of Michigan and Massachusetts, which manufacture certain vaccines and immune globulin preparations, the American public is entirely dependent upon the willingness of the commercial sector to make and market vaccines. This willingness has declined over the past two decades, and many manufacturers no longer produce vaccines. There are currently just one or two U.S.-based commercial sources for most childhood vaccines.

THE NATIONAL VACCINE INJURY COMPENSATION PROGRAM The use of mandated vaccines benefits society as a whole by reducing morbidity and the cost of care for preventable diseases and by reducing childhood mortality. Thus, in the United States, society has assumed the obligation to care for those injured by the administration of mandated vaccines. The NCVIA of 1986 (modified in 1995) is the instrument in use to ensure fairness to injured persons as well as protection for Federal, state, and local immunization programs; private immunization providers; and vaccine manufacturers. The act was designed to implement two vital public policies: (1) to provide prompt and fair compensation to the families of children who have died or have been injured as a result of routine mandated immunization; and (2) to reduce the adverse impact of the tort system

Table 122-13

Vaccine-Preventable Disease Targets

Disease	1987 Baseline	1995	2000 Target
Diphtheria among people aged 25 and younger	1	0	0
Tetanus among people aged 25 and younger	3	5	0
Polio (wild-type virus)	0	0	0
Measles	3058	288	0
Rubella	225	146	0
Congenital rubella syndrome	6	7	0
Mumps	4866	840	<500
Pertussis	3450	4315	<1000
Haemophilus influenzae type b	20,000*	1164	0

* Not notifiable before 1991; estimated prevaccine-era annual incidence.

SOURCE: *Healthy People 2000: National Health Promotion and Disease Prevention Objectives,* Washington, DC, Department of Health and Human Services, 1990.

on vaccine supply, cost, and innovation/development. The success of immunization programs in the United States depends upon the continued viability of the National Vaccine Injury Compensation Program.

CONTROL OF VACCINE-PREVENTABLE DISEASE

A continuing task of public health practice is to maintain individual and herd immunity. The job is not over once a population is fully vaccinated; rather, it is imperative to immunize each subsequent generation as long as the threat of the disease persists. Ongoing surveillance and prompt reporting of disease to local or state health departments are essential to this goal, ensuring a continuing awareness of the possibility of vaccine-preventable illness. Nearly all vaccine-preventable diseases are now notifiable, and individual case data are routinely forwarded to the CDC. These data are used to detect outbreaks or other unusual events that require investigation and to evaluate prevention and control policies, practices, and strategies.

As a direct consequence of successes in immunization, vaccine-preventable diseases have become less visible; ironically, this situation may foster complacency among parents and health care providers about routine immunization of children. Even among the affluent and educated, immunization levels may be low, reflecting a misunderstanding of the continuing threat of disease with which parents and health care providers have limited experience or perhaps an unjustifiably greater fear of adverse reactions to vaccination than of the potential for illness and death due to vaccine-preventable diseases. Health care workers play an essential role in influencing the attitudes of patients regarding appropriate immunization; therefore, it is essential that these professionals continually update their own knowledge about vaccines and about the epidemiology of vaccine-preventable illnesses.

RESEARCH ON VACCINES AND IMMUNIZATION

To accomplish the preventive goals of Healthy People 2000, current immunization recommendations in the United States call for every child to receive 10 different vaccines (many at the same time and most requiring more than one dose) between birth and entry into kindergarten. This agenda requires at least five visits to a health care provider by age 2, with an additional visit before entry into school. This is a formidable task, particularly for persons with limited access to health care, and compliance can be expected to become more difficult as new vaccines are licensed.

THE CHILDREN'S VACCINE INITIATIVE The potential to eradicate selected diseases and to build sustainable immunization programs that reach every child is not being fulfilled with existing vaccines and delivery technology. New vaccines or new formulations that will not only improve protective responses but also simplify the

Table 122-14

Estimates of Vaccine Coverage or Immunity Among Adults

Vaccine	Percent
Influenza (age 65+)	41*
Pneumococcus (age 65+)	28†
Hepatitis B (age 65+)	1–60‡
Tetanus	16–59§
Diphtheria	34–51§
Measles	85–95§
Rubella	80–90‡
Mumps	91‡
Varicella	93

* Year 2000 target is 60%. ‡ Varies by risk group.
† Year 2000 target is 60%. § Varies by study.

SOURCE: Centers for Disease Control and Prevention.

Table 122-15

Standards for Immunization Practices

Standard Number	Standard

PEDIATRIC PRACTICE

1. Immunization services are readily available.
2. There are no barriers to or unnecessary prerequisites for the receipt of vaccines.
3. Immunization services are available free or for a minimal fee.
4. Providers use all clinical encounters to screen and, when indicated, immunize children.
5. Providers educate parents and guardians about immunization in general terms.
6. Providers question parents or guardians about contraindications and, before immunizing a child, inform them in specific terms about the risks and benefits of the immunizations their child is to receive.
7. Providers follow only true contraindications.
8. Providers administer simultaneously all vaccine doses for which a child is eligible at the time of each visit.
9. Providers use accurate and complete recording procedures.
10. Providers coschedule immunization appointments in conjunction with appointments for other child health services.
11. Providers report adverse events following immunization promptly, accurately, and completely.
12. Providers operate a tracking system.
13. Providers adhere to appropriate procedures for vaccine management.
14. Providers conduct semiannual audits to assess immunization coverage levels and to review immunization records for the patient populations they serve.
15. Providers maintain up-to-date, easily retrievable medical protocols at all locations where vaccines are administered.
16. Providers operate with patient-oriented and community-based approaches.
17. Vaccines are administered by properly trained individuals.
18. Providers receive ongoing education and training on current immunization recommendations.

ADULT PRACTICE

1. Appropriate vaccine use is promoted through information campaigns for health care practitioners and trainees, employers, and the public about the benefits of immunizations.
2. Providers are completely immunized to protect themselves and prevent transmission to patients.
3. Providers routinely determine the immunization status of their adult patients, offer vaccines to those for whom they are indicated, and maintain complete immunization records.
4. Providers identify high-risk patients in need of influenza vaccine and develop a system to recall them for annual immunization.
5. Providers and institutions identify high-risk adult patients in hospitals and other treatment centers and ensure that appropriate vaccination is considered either before discharge or as part of discharge planning.
6. Licensing/accreditation agencies support the development by health care institutions of comprehensive immunization programs for staff, trainees, volunteer workers, inpatients, and outpatients.
7. States establish preenrollment immunization requirements for colleges and other institutions of higher education.
8. Institutions that train health care professionals, deliver health care, or provide laboratory or other medical support services require appropriate immunizations for persons at risk of contracting or transmitting vaccine-preventable illnesses.
9. Health care benefit programs, third-party payers, and government health care programs provide coverage for adult immunization services.
10. A standard personal and institutional immunization record is adopted as a means of verifying the immunization status of patients and staff.

SOURCE: For pediatric standards: Ad Hoc Working Group for the Development of Standards for Pediatric Immunization Practices. JAMA 269:1817, 1993; for adult standards: The National Coalition for Adult Immunization.

immunization schedule are needed. The Children's Vaccine Initiative is an international effort to attain these ends. The ideal is to develop vaccines that can be administered orally early in life, that provide lifelong protection against multiple infections, that can be given as one or only a few doses, and that are less reactive and more heat stable than current vaccines. To attain these ambitious goals may take years or decades, but progress is already being made in the development of new combinations of current vaccines to facilitate complete immunization. Strategies for research directed toward improved vaccine delivery are listed in Table 122-16. The results will be applicable to immunization programs in both developed and developing countries.

REEMERGENCE OF CONTROLLED DISEASE AND EMERGENCE OF NEW DISEASE The emergence of new pathogens is fostered by the genetic potential of microbes to evolve as well as by rapid changes in human demographics and behavior and in a global ecology that creates new or more favorable hosts. Proof of the need for continuing vaccine research is found in the emergence of new infectious diseases such as HIV infection, Lyme borreliosis, hantavirus pulmonary syndrome, and hepatitis C; the appearance of a new epidemic cholera strain (serotype O139 Bengal) that exhibits no cross-immunity with the traditional O1 serotype; and the increase in global incidence and in drug resistance of familiar diseases that were once considered under control, such as tuberculosis and malaria. In addition, some common illnesses without a previously known etiology, such as peptic ulcer disease and cervical and nasopharyngeal cancer, have now been epidemiologically linked to specific infectious agents and have thus become potentially vaccine-preventable conditions.

DEVELOPMENT OF NEW VACCINES For many serious or even life-threatening infectious diseases, no effective vaccines are available. Although many new vaccines are undergoing human trials (Table 122-17), the task of developing vaccines is proving very complex. Priorities for the United States currently include research on the following vaccines: HIV, pneumococcus (conjugate), group B *Streptococcus*, respiratory syncytial virus, rotavirus, *Mycobacterium tuberculosis*, herpes simplex virus, influenza A and B viruses, and hepatitis C virus. Also of high priority are vaccines for two virus-associated tumors: cervical cancer (human papillomavirus) and nasopharyngeal cancer (Epstein-Barr virus).

INTERNATIONAL CONSIDERATIONS

Since the establishment of the World Health Organization's Expanded Programme on Immunization in 1981, levels of coverage for the recommended basic children's vaccines (bacille Calmette-Guérin, polio, DTP, measles, and hepatitis B) have risen from 5 percent to approximately 80 percent worldwide. Each year, at least 2.7 million deaths from measles, neonatal tetanus, and pertussis and 200,000 cases of paralysis due to polio are prevented by immunization. Despite the successes of this program, many vaccine-preventable diseases remain prevalent in the developing world. Measles, for example, continues to kill an estimated 1.5 million children each year, and cases of diphtheria, whooping cough, polio, and neonatal tetanus still occur at unacceptably high rates. It is estimated that between 20 and 35 percent of all deaths of children under the age of 5 years are still associated with vaccine-preventable diseases.

In addition to the antigens included in the Expanded Programme for routine use in the developing world, others (Hib, Japanese B encephalitis, yellow fever, group A meningococcus, mumps, and rubella) are used regionally, depending on disease epidemiology and resources. Polio has been targeted for eradication by the year 2000; this disease has already been eliminated in the Americas and is close to elimination in the Western Pacific.

Because infectious diseases know no geographic or political boundaries, uncontrolled disease anywhere in the world poses a threat to the United States. Vaccines offer the opportunity to control and even eradicate some diseases, and eradication means that vaccines are no longer needed. The experience with smallpox has shown that the eradication of disease is a remarkably good economic investment.

Table 122-16

Examples of Scientific Research Directed Toward Improved Vaccine Delivery

Delivery System Change Desired	Scientific Input	Products in Process
Decrease number of visits required for full immunization	Development of new combination vaccines	MMRV; DTaP-Hib
	Research on recombinant live multiantigen vaccines	Canarypox-measles, Canarypox-RSV, vaccinia-rabies, vaccinia-influenza, *Salmonella*-BCG
Decrease number of doses	Development of time-release products	Microencapsulated forms of tetanus toxoid, hepatitis B, pertussis, influenza
Decrease number of injections	Research on oral vaccines	Pertussis
	Research on mucosal immunity	Cholera
	Research on antigen presentation	Influenza
Immunize as early in life as possible	Research on maternal immunization	Hib, meningococcus, pneumococcus
	Research on neonatal immunity	Group B *Streptococcus*, measles
Decrease rates of adverse events	Research on mechanisms of adverse events	Pertussis, OPV
Increase protection	Research on more immunogenic antigens	Group B *Streptococcus*
	Development of conjugate vaccines	Meningococcus, pneumococcus
	Research on adjuvants	Typhoid, influenza
Increase thermal stability	Research on stabilizers	Chemical stabilizers, freeze drying
Immunize by the oral route	Development of oral delivery systems	Iscoms, liposomes, polylactic and polyglycolic acid polymers, etc.

NOTE: MMRV, measles/mumps/rubella/varicella; RSV, respiratory syncytial virus; BCG, bacille Calmette-Guérin.

Table 122-17

Vaccines Undergoing Human Trials

Bacterial	Viral
Vibrio cholerae	Respiratory syncytial
Mycobacterium leprae	Dengue
Salmonella typhi	Rotavirus
Salmonella paratyphi	Japanese B encephalitis
Neisseria meningitidis	Influenza A and B
Streptococcus pneumoniae	Parainfluenza
Group B *Streptococcus*	Measles
Shigella spp.	Cytomegalovirus
Enterotoxigenic *Escherichia coli*	Rabies
Enterohemorrhagic *E. coli*	Junin
Borrelia burgdorferi	Chikungunya
Fungal	Rift Valley fever
Cryptococcus neoformans	Herpes simplex
Parasitic	Yellow fever
Plasmodium spp.	

The entire sum that the United States spent for the global smallpox eradication campaign has been recouped, in 1968 dollars, every 2.5 months since 1971. The global eradication of polio will save the United States over $300 million a year in vaccine and associated delivery costs and will save over $1.5 billion a year worldwide.

SOURCES OF INFORMATION ON IMMUNIZATION

- Official vaccine package circulars
- Report of the Committee on Infectious Diseases of the American Academy of Pediatrics ("Red Book")
- Recommendations of the Advisory Committee on Immunization Practices (ACIP), Centers for Disease Control and Prevention
- Guide for Adult Immunization, American College of Physicians
- Health Information for International Travel (published yearly) and Advisory Memoranda on Travel (published periodically), Centers for Disease Control and Prevention
- Control of Communicable Diseases in Man, American Public Health Association
- Technical Bulletin of the College of Obstetrics and Gynecology

BIBLIOGRAPHY

ADVISORY COMMITTEE ON IMMUNIZATION PRACTICES: General recommendations on immunization: Recommendations of the Immunization Practices Advisory Committee (ACIP). Morb Mort Week Rep 38:205, 1989

————: Diphtheria, tetanus, and pertussis: Recommendations for vaccine use and other preventive measures. Immunization Practices Advisory Committee (ACIP). Morb Mort Week Rep 40:1, 1991a

————: Update on adult immunization. Recommendations of the Immunization Practices Advisory Committee (ACIP). Morb Mort Week Rep 40(RR-12):1, 1991b

————: Hepatitis B virus: A comprehensive strategy for elimination of transmission in the United States through universal childhood vaccination. Recommendations of the Immunization Practices Advisory Committee (ACIP). Morb Mort Week Rep 40(RR-13):1, 1991c

————: Pertussis vaccination: Acellular pertussis vaccine for the fourth and fifth doses of the DTP series: Update to the supplementary ACIP statement: Recommendations of the Advisory Committee on Immunization Practices. Morb Mort Week Rep 41(RR-15):1, 1992

————: Recommendations for use of *Haemophilus* b conjugate vaccines and a combined diphtheria, tetanus, pertussis, and *Haemophilus* b vaccine. Morb Mort Week Rep 42(RR-13):1, 1993

————: General recommendations on immunization: Recommendation of the Advisory Committee on Immunization Practices (ACIP). Morb Mort Week Rep 1995;44(RR-5):1, 1995

————: Recommended childhood immunization schedule—United States, January 1995. Morb Mort Week Rep 43:959, 1995

————: National, state and urban area vaccination coverage levels among children 19–35 months—United States, April 1994–March 1995. Morb Mort Week Rep 45:145, 1996

AMERICAN ACADEMY OF PEDIATRICS: *Report of the Committee on Infectious Diseases ("Red Book")*, 22d ed, G Peter et al (eds). Elk Grove Village, IL, 1994

AMERICAN COLLEGE OF PHYSICIANS: *Guide for Adult Immunization*, 2d ed. Philadelphia, American College of Physicians, 1994

AMERICAN PUBLIC HEALTH ASSOCIATION: *Control of Communicable Diseases in Man*, 16th ed, AS Benenson (ed). Washington, DC, American Public Health Association, 1995

BRICKMAN HF et al: The timing of tuberculin tests in relation to immunization with live viral vaccines. Pediatrics 55:392, 1975

CHANDER J, SUBRAHMANYAN S: Mass polio vaccination. Eradication by 2000 is a realistic goal. BMJ 312:1178, 1996

DE QUADROS CA et al: Measles elimination in the Americas. Evolving strategies. JAMA 275:224, 1996

KING GE, HADLER SC: Simultaneous administration of childhood vaccines: An important public health policy that is safe and efficacious. Pediatr Infect Dis J 13:394, 1994

NINANE J et al: Disseminated BCG in HIV infection. Arch Dis Child 63:1268, 1988

SIBER GR et al: Interference of immune globulin with measles and rubella immunization. J Pediatr 122:204, 1993

SOMANI J, LARSON RA: Reimmunization after allogeneic bone marrow transplantation. Am J Med 98:389, 1995

VETTER RT, JOHNSON GM: Vaccination update. Hib, hepatitis, polio, varicella, influenza, pneumococcal and meningococcal disease. Postgrad Med 98:141, 1995

WATSON BM et al: Safety and immunogenicity of a combined live attenuated measles, mumps, rubella, and varicella vaccine (MMR$_{II}$V) in healthy children. J Infect Dis 173:731, 1996

WHITE CJ: Clinical trials of varicella vaccine in healthy children. Infect Dis Clin North Am 10:595, 1996

123 J.S. Keystone, P.E. Kozarsky

HEALTH RISKS TO TRAVELERS

In 1991, the World Health Organization estimated that more than 30 million persons traveled from industrialized countries to the developing world. Studies show that between 50 and 75 percent of short-term travelers to the tropics or subtropics report some health impairment. Most of these health problems are minor, with only 5 percent requiring medical attention and fewer than 1 percent requiring hospitalization.

Although infectious agents contribute substantially to morbidity in travelers, these pathogens account for only about 1 percent of deaths among this population. Cardiovascular disease and injuries are the most frequent causes of death among travelers from the United States, accounting for 49 and 22 percent of deaths, respectively. Age-specific rates of mortality due to cardiovascular disease are similar to those among nontravelers. In contrast, rates of death due to injury—the majority from motor vehicle, drowning, or aircraft accidents—are several times higher among travelers. Figure 123-1 summarizes the monthly incidence of health problems during travel in developing countries.

TRAVELER'S DIARRHEA Diarrhea is the leading cause of illness in travelers (see Chap. 128) and is usually a short-lived, self-limited condition; however, 40 percent of affected individuals need to alter their scheduled activities, and another 20 percent are confined to bed. The most important determinant of risk is the destination of the traveler. Incidence rates per 2-week stay have been reported to be as low as 8 percent in industrialized countries and as high as 55 percent in parts of Africa, Central and South America, and Southeast Asia. Infants and young adults are at particularly high risk. The incidence of diarrhea is proportional to the number of dietary indiscretions. Studies of U.S. students in Mexico showed that eating meals in restaurants and cafeterias or consuming food from street vendors was associated with increased risk.

The most frequently identified pathogen causing traveler's diarrhea is toxigenic *Escherichia coli*, although in some parts of the world (notably North Africa and Southeast Asia), *Campylobacter* infections appear to predominate. Other common causative organisms include *Salmonella*, *Shigella*, rotavirus, and the Norwalk agent. Except for

giardiasis, parasitic infections are uncommon causes of traveler's diarrhea. A growing problem for travelers is the development of antibiotic resistance in many bacterial pathogens; examples include strains of *Campylobacter* resistant to quinolones and strains of *E. coli*, *Shigella*, and *Salmonella* resistant to trimethoprim-sulfamethoxazole.

Although extremely common, acute traveler's diarrhea is usually self-limited or amenable to antibiotic therapy. Travelers who have chronic bowel problems after their return home are more likely to seek medical attention from a specialist, because the etiology of this problem is less well defined. Infectious agents appear to be responsible for only a small proportion of cases with chronic bowel symptoms; of the pathogens detected in these instances, *Giardia intestinalis* (also called *Giardia lamblia*; see Chap. 220) is by far the most common, whereas *Cyclospora cayetanensis*, *Cryptosporidium* species, and *Entamoeba histolytica* are rare. By far the most frequent causes of chronic diarrhea after travel are postinfectious sequelae, such as lactose intolerance or an irritable bowel syndrome. When no infectious etiology can be identified, a trial of metronidazole therapy for presumed giardiasis, a strict lactose-free diet for 1 week, or a several-week trial of high-dose hydrophilic mucilloid relieves the symptoms of many patients.

MALARIA It is estimated that more than 30,000 American and European travelers develop malaria each year (see Chap. 216). The risk of malaria is highest in sub-Saharan Africa and Oceania (1:50 to 1:1000) and during the past decade has increased more than fivefold for travelers to Kenya. The risk is intermediate (1:1000 to 1:12,000) for travelers to Haiti and the Indian subcontinent and is low (less than 1:50,000) for travelers to Asia and to Central and South America. Of the 1000 cases of malaria reported annually in the United States, 90 percent of those due to *Plasmodium falciparum* occur in travelers returning or immigrating from Africa and Oceania. With the worldwide increase in chloroquine- and multidrug-resistant falciparum malaria, decisions about chemoprophylaxis have become more difficult. In addition, the spread of malaria due to primaquine- and chloroquine-resistant strains of *Plasmodium vivax* has added to the complexity of treatment. The case-fatality rate of falciparum malaria in the United States is 4 percent; however, in only one-third of patients who die is the diagnosis of malaria considered before death. Compliance with antimalarial chemoprophylaxis regimens and use of personal protection measures to prevent mosquito bites are keys to the prevention of malaria. Several recent studies indicate that fewer than 50 percent of travelers adhere to basic recommendations for malaria prevention.

VACCINE-PREVENTABLE DISEASES *Immunizations of Worldwide Importance* *Diphtheria, tetanus, and polio* Diphtheria continues to be a problem worldwide, with recent large outbreaks in the new independent states formerly encompassed by the Soviet Union (see Chap. 144). Serosurveys now show that tetanus antitoxin is lacking in many North Americans, especially those over the age of 50 (see Chap. 146). Although the risk of polio to the international traveler is extremely low, studies in the United States have found varying levels of immunity in the general population, and recent data indicate that 12 percent of adult American travelers are unprotected against at least one serogroup (see Chap. 195). Foreign travel is an ideal opportunity to have these immunizations updated (see Chap. 122).

Measles Measles (rubeola) continues to be a major cause of morbidity and mortality in the developing world (see Chap. 196). Several outbreaks of measles in the United States have been linked to imported cases. The group at highest risk consists of persons born after 1956 and vaccinated before 1980, in many of whom primary vaccination failed. Travelers in this group should be reimmunized.

Influenza Influenza occurs year-round in the tropics and during the summer months in the Southern Hemisphere (i.e., the winter months in the Northern Hemisphere). Vaccination should be considered for all travelers to these regions, particularly those who are elderly or chronically ill (see Chap. 193).

Special Immunizations for Travelers *Hepatitis A and B* Hepatitis A (see Chap. 295) is the most frequent vaccine-preventable infection of travelers; the incidence of symptomatic infection during a 1-month stay in a developing country ranges from 3 to 6 cases per 1000. The risk is six times greater for those who stray from the usual

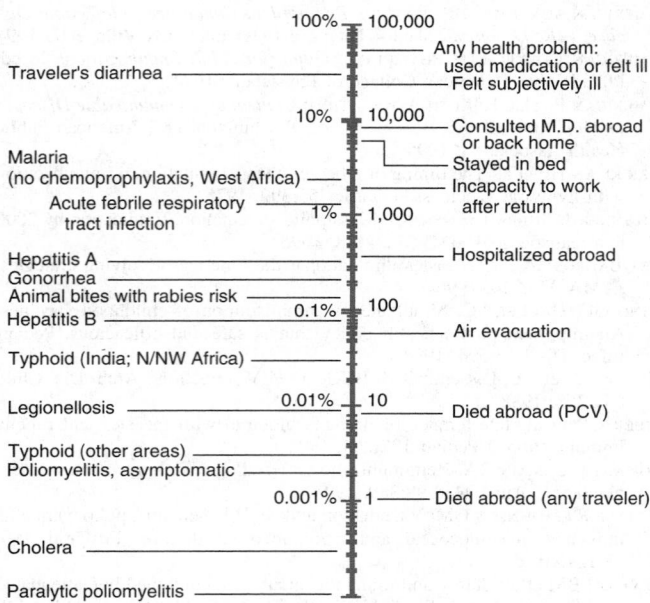

FIGURE 123-1 Incidence rate, per month, of health problems during a stay in developing countries. PCV, Peace Corps volunteer. (*From Steffen and Lobel*, with permission from Chapman and Hall, New York.)

tourist routes. The monthly incidence of hepatitis B infection, both symptomatic and asymptomatic, is 80 to 240 cases per 100,000. For reasons that are not entirely clear, long-stay overseas workers are at considerable risk for hepatitis B infection.

Typhoid and cholera The attack rate for typhoid fever is 1 case per 30,000 per month of travel to the developing world (see Chap. 158). However, the rates in India, Senegal, and North Africa are 10-fold higher, and, within these areas, rates are especially high among travelers to more remote destinations and among persons who are returning to their homeland to visit and stay with relatives or friends. These same groups, because they are more likely than other travelers to commit dietary indiscretions, are at higher risk for cholera as well. Overall, the risk of cholera to travelers is extremely low: approximately 1 case per 500,000 journeys to endemic areas (see Chap. 161). Cholera vaccine is not indicated for most travelers.

Miscellaneous infections The incidence of yellow fever among travelers is extremely low, probably because the vaccine is highly efficacious and is required by health authorities for entry into most countries of sub-Saharan Africa and South America in which this infection exists (see Chap. 200). Many cases of rabies have been reported in travelers, but there are no data on the risk of infection. Domestic animals are the major transmitters of rabies in developing countries (see Chap. 199). Countries where canine rabies is highly endemic include Mexico, the Philippines, Sri Lanka, India, Thailand, and Vietnam. Almost half of the cases of rabies reported in the United States in recent years have been acquired outside of the country. The risk of Japanese encephalitis, an infection transmitted by mosquitoes in rural Asia and Southeast Asia, is approximately 1:5000 per month of stay in an endemic area (see Chap. 200). Most symptomatic infections in U.S. residents have been in military personnel or their families. Although the risk of meningococcal disease in travelers has not been quantified, it appears to be highest among travelers who live with the indigenous population in overcrowded conditions (see Chap. 149).

PREGNANCY AND TRAVEL A woman's medical history and itinerary, the quality of medical care at her destinations, and her degree of flexibility determine whether travel is wise during pregnancy. According to the American College of Obstetrics and Gynecology, the safest part of pregnancy in which to travel is the second trimester (between 18 and 24 weeks), when there is the least danger of spontaneous abortion or premature labor. Some obstetricians prefer that women stay within a few hundred miles of home after the 28th week of pregnancy in case problems arise; in general, however, healthy women may be advised that it is acceptable to travel.

Despite this general recommendation, there are some relative contraindications to international travel during pregnancy, including certain obstetrical risk factors: a history of miscarriage, premature labor, incompetent cervix, or toxemia. General medical problems such as diabetes, heart failure, severe anemia, or a history of thromboembolic disease should also prompt the pregnant woman to postpone her travels. Finally, regions in which the pregnant woman and her fetus may be at excessive risk (e.g., those at high altitudes and those where live-virus vaccines are required or where multidrug-resistant malaria is endemic) are not ideal destinations during any trimester.

Malaria Malaria during pregnancy carries a significant risk of morbidity and death. Levels of parasitemia are highest and failure to clear the parasites after chloroquine treatment are most frequent among primigravidae. Severe disease, with complications such as cerebral malaria, massive hemolysis, and renal failure, is especially likely in pregnancy. Fetal sequelae include spontaneous abortion, stillbirth, preterm delivery, and congenital infection.

Traveler's Diarrhea Because dehydration due to traveler's diarrhea can lead to inadequate placental blood flow, pregnant travelers must be extremely cautious regarding their food and beverage intake. The exclusive consumption of bottled (carbonated) or boiled drinks without ice, the eating of well-cooked meats and pasteurized dairy products, and the avoidance of pre-prepared salad items should help protect against traveler's diarrhea due to the usual causes as well as against infections such as toxoplasmosis and listeriosis, which can have serious sequelae in pregnancy.

The mainstay of therapy for traveler's diarrhea is rehydration. Kaolin-pectin combinations and loperamide may be used if necessary, but many of the usual antibiotics (e.g., quinolones) are contraindicated during pregnancy. Ampicillin alone or with clavulanic acid may be used, but many strains of *E. coli* and other organisms implicated in traveler's diarrhea are resistant. An oral third-generation cephalosporin may be the best option.

Because of the major problems encountered when infants are given local foods and beverages, women are strongly encouraged to breast-feed when traveling with a neonate. A nursing mother with traveler's diarrhea should not stop breast-feeding but should increase her fluid intake.

Air Travel and High-Altitude Destinations Commercial air travel is not a risk to the healthy pregnant woman or to the fetus. Fetal oxygenation is not adversely affected by the decreased cabin pressures because of the fetal hemoglobin dissociation curve; the higher radiation levels reported at altitudes of more than 35,000 feet should pose no problem to the healthy traveler. Since each airline has a policy regarding pregnancy and flying, it is best to check with the specific carrier when booking reservations. Domestic air travel is usually permitted until the 36th week, whereas international air travel is generally curtailed after the 32d week.

There are no known risks for pregnant women who travel to high-altitude destinations and stay for short periods. However, there are likewise no data on the safety of pregnant women at altitudes of greater than 15,000 feet. Because of the harsh conditions usually associated with such trips, they are generally contraindicated for other reasons.

THE HIV-INFECTED TRAVELER The traveler infected with human immunodeficiency virus (HIV) is at special risk of serious infections due to a number of pathogens that may be more prevalent at travel destinations than at home. However, the degree of risk depends primarily on the state of the immune system at the time of travel. For persons whose CD4+ cell counts are normal or above 500/μL, no data suggest a greater risk during travel than for persons without HIV infection. Individuals with AIDS (CD4+ counts of <200/μL) and others who are symptomatic need special counseling and should visit their primary care physician before traveling, especially to the developing world.

Several countries now deny routine entry to HIV-positive individuals, even though no data show that these restrictions decrease rates of transmission of the virus. In general, HIV testing is required of those individuals who wish to stay abroad longer than 3 months or who intend to work or study abroad. Some countries will accept an HIV serologic test done within 6 months of departure, whereas others will not accept a blood test done at any time in the traveler's home country. In addition, border officials often have the authority to make inquiries of individuals entering a country and to check the medications they are carrying. If a drug such as zidovudine is identified, the person may be barred from entering the country. Information on testing requirements for specific countries is available from consular offices but is subject to frequent change.

Health insurance policies should be checked to make sure they are valid for care in other countries. The HIV-positive traveler should strongly consider obtaining trip cancellation insurance and evacuation insurance in case of illness. It is ideal to have the name of a physician at the travel destination who is familiar with the treatment of patients with AIDS, as the clinical findings associated with infection may be atypical in a patient with AIDS, and several infections may exist simultaneously. The traveler should be encouraged to visit the physician promptly if problems arise.

Immunizations All of the HIV-infected traveler's routine immunizations should be up to date (see Chap. 122). The response to immunization may be impaired at CD4+ cell counts of <200/μL (and in some cases at even higher counts). However, when the risk of illness is high or the sequelae of illness are serious, immunization is recommended. In certain circumstances, it may be prudent to check the adequacy of the serum antibody response before departure (e.g., yellow fever neutralization if exposure is unavoidable).

Because of the increased risk of infections due to *Streptococcus pneumoniae* and other bacterial pathogens that cause pneumonia following influenza, pneumococcal polysaccharide and influenza vaccines should be administered. The estimated rates of response to influenza vaccine are more than 80 percent among persons with asymptomatic HIV infection and less than 50 percent among those with AIDS.

In general, live attenuated vaccines are contraindicated for persons with immune dysfunction. Live oral polio vaccine should not be given to HIV-infected patients or to members of their households. Instead, inactivated polio vaccine (eIPV) should be used; most HIV-infected individuals without AIDS will develop protective antibody levels in response to this vaccine.

Because measles (rubeola) can be a severe and lethal infection in HIV-positive patients, the measles vaccine (or the combination measles-mumps-rubella vaccine) should be given to these individuals. Although this is a live vaccine, there have been no reports of serious complications in this population. Between 18 and 58 percent of symptomatic HIV-infected vaccinees develop adequate antibody titers, and between 50 and 100 percent of those who are infected but asymptomatic seroconvert.

The decision of whether or not to administer any of the special vaccines to an HIV-infected traveler should be based on the individual's risk. Inactivated vaccines can be administered without concern for safety but with concern about adequate protection. For example, data suggest that HIV-infected persons do not have as strong an antibody response to the meningococcal meningitis vaccine as do uninfected persons. Moreover, few data are available on the efficacy of many of the other vaccines (e.g., those for hepatitis A, typhoid, and cholera).

It is recommended that live yellow-fever vaccine not be given to HIV-infected travelers. Nevertheless, when inadvertently administered to HIV-positive military personnel, this vaccine elicited no adverse reactions. Therefore, if the traveler's CD4+ count is >200/μL and travel in an endemic area is absolutely necessary, the vaccine can probably be administered safely. HIV-infected persons whose CD4+ count is <200/μL should be discouraged from traveling to these regions. If the traveler is passing through or traveling to an area where the vaccine is required but the disease risk is low, a physician's waiver should be issued. Bacille Calmette-Guérin vaccine should not be given because of reports of disseminated infection in HIV-infected persons.

A transient (days to weeks) burst of viremia has been demonstrated in HIV-infected individuals following immunization with vaccines for such diseases as influenza, pneumococcal infection, and tetanus (see Chap. 308). However, at this point, there is no evidence that this transient increase in viremia is detrimental over time. Furthermore, it is likely that immune activation associated with infection with the live organisms in question would result in increases in viremia of greater magnitude and duration than those associated with vaccination. Therefore, the vaccination recommendations discussed above need not be modified at this time.

Gastrointestinal Illness Decreased levels of gastric acid, abnormal gastrointestinal mucosal immunity, and other complications of HIV infection, as well as medications taken by HIV-infected patients, make traveler's diarrhea especially problematic in these individuals. Traveler's diarrhea is likely to occur more frequently, be more severe, and be more difficult to treat in association with HIV infection. *Salmonella*, *Shigella*, and *Campylobacter* infections also are more protracted and more often accompanied by bacteremia in HIV-infected persons. *Cryptosporidium* (see Chap. 220), a common cause of diarrhea in tropical countries, produces severe chronic diarrhea and cholecystitis with increased mortality among patients with AIDS. *Isospora belli* also causes infections at high rates among AIDS patients in the developing world. This infection is associated with malabsorption, weight loss,

and relapses after treatment. Persistent diarrhea due to microsporidiosis has also been reported.

Because of these potential problems, the HIV-infected traveler needs to be careful to consume only appropriately prepared foods and beverages. In addition, this group of individuals may benefit from prophylaxis for traveler's diarrhea, using bismuth subsalicylate or a daily antibiotic (ideally a quinolone derivative) for short-term travel to the developing world. If the traveler is already taking a sulfonamide preparation for prophylaxis of *Pneumocystis* pneumonia, a regimen of self-treatment with a quinolone would be appropriate.

Other Travel-Related Infections Data are lacking on the severity of vector-borne diseases in HIV-infected individuals. Malaria is more severe in asplenic and certain immunocompromised hosts, although increased severity has not been demonstrated in AIDS. *Babesia* infection is known to cause serious illness and to recur in HIV-infected patients; this tick-transmitted illness occurs in parts of the United States but is not known to be a widespread problem.

Visceral leishmaniasis (see Chap. 217) has been reported in numerous HIV-infected travelers. Because the usual signs—splenomegaly and hyperglobulinemia—are nonspecific and may even be lacking, the diagnosis is difficult to make. In addition, serological results are often negative. This infection is hard to treat, and its associated mortality is high. Even short-term travelers to southern Europe have developed the illness; thus, the avoidance of sandfly bites is critical.

Certain respiratory illnesses, such as histoplasmosis and coccidioidomycosis, cause greater morbidity and mortality among patients with AIDS than in the general population. Though tuberculosis is common among HIV-infected persons (especially in developing countries), the acquisition of this infection by the short-term traveler is not a major concern. The possibility of acquiring *Legionella* infections from spas should be considered, although no data confirm an increase in the severity of such infections in AIDS.

Finally, the HIV-infected traveler should always be cautioned about safe sexual practices, which may help prevent both the transmission of HIV to others and the acquisition by the traveler of other sexually transmitted diseases that may be drug resistant or may result in serious sequelae (e.g., syphilis).

Medications Adverse events due to medications and drug interactions are common and raise complex issues for HIV-infected persons. In addition, rates of cutaneous reaction are unusually high among patients with AIDS. Physicians advising these travelers need to consider the problems that may arise from the use of agents such as antimalarial drugs, medications for altitude acclimatization, or antidiarrheal compounds; one example is increased cutaneous sensitivity to sulfonamides. Since zidovudine (AZT) is metabolized by hepatic glucuronidation, inhibitors of this process may elevate serum levels of the drug. Though quinine does not affect levels of zidovudine, there are no relevant data on chloroquine, primaquine, or mefloquine. Furthermore, it is not known whether the antagonistic effect of zidovudine on pyrimethamine has clinical relevance in the treatment or prevention of plasmodial infections.

CHRONIC ILLNESS, DISABILITY, AND TRAVEL

Chronic health problems should not prevent travel, but special attention can make it safer and more comfortable.

Heart Disease Cardiovascular events are the main cause of deaths among travelers and of in-flight emergencies on commercial aircraft. Persons with underlying heart disease should review their itineraries with a physician prior to departure; travel in harsh environments or to remote destinations is not wise. Extra supplies of all medications should be kept in carry-on luggage, along with a recent copy of an electrocardiogram and the name and telephone number of the traveler's physician at home. Pacemakers are not affected by airport security devices, but electronic telephone checks of pacemaker function cannot be transmitted by international satellites. The traveler may benefit from supplemental oxygen, which should be ordered by a physician (since oxygen delivery systems are not standardized) 48 to 72 h before flight time. Personal oxygen tanks are not permitted on aircraft. Travelers should request aisle seating and should walk, perform stretching and flexing exercises, and remain hydrated during the flight to prevent venous thrombosis and pulmonary embolism.

Chronic Lung Disease Chronic obstructive pulmonary disease (COPD) is one of the most common diagnoses in patients who require emergency-room evaluation for symptoms occurring during airline flights. Patients with COPD experience dyspnea, edema, wheezing, cyanosis, and chest pain. The best predictor of the development of these symptoms is the sea level Pa_{O_2}. A Pa_{O_2} of at least 72 mmHg corresponds to an in-flight arterial Pa_{O_2} of 55 mmHg when the cabin is pressurized to 8000 ft. Therefore, if the traveler's baseline Pa_{O_2} is <72 mmHg, the provision of supplemental oxygen during the flight should be considered. Pulmonary function is also maximized by continuing bronchodilator treatment and the use of steroids as prescribed. Contraindications to flight include active bronchospasm, lower respiratory infection, phlebitis, pulmonary hypertension, and recent thoracic surgery (within the preceding 3 weeks) or pneumothorax. Consideration should be given to decreasing the amount of outdoor activity at the destination if there is excessive air pollution.

Diabetes Mellitus Alterations in glucose control and changes in insulin requirements are common problems when diabetics travel. Changes in time zone, in the amount and timing of food intake, and in physical activity demand more vigilant assessment of metabolic control. The diabetic traveler should pack medication (including a bottle of regular insulin for emergencies), insulin syringes and needles, equipment and supplies for glucose monitoring, and snacks in carry-on luggage. Insulin is stable for about 3 months at room temperature but should be kept as cool as possible. The name and telephone number of the home physician and a card and necklace listing the medical problems and the type and dose of insulin used should accompany the traveler. When six or more time zones are crossed, insulin requirements may be temporarily altered, depending on food intake and physical activity. In traveling eastward (e.g., from the United States to Europe), the morning insulin dose on arrival may need to be decreased. The blood glucose can then be checked during the day to determine whether additional insulin is required. For flights westward, with lengthening of the day, an additional dose of regular insulin may be required. Comfortable footwear is essential for the diabetic traveler.

Other Special Groups Other groups for whom special travel measures are now being encouraged include patients undergoing dialysis, those with transplants, and those with other disabilities. Up to 13 percent of travelers have some disability, but few advocacy groups and tour companies dedicate themselves to this growing population. The key to safe travel in each case is adequate research ahead of time. Patients undergoing chronic ambulatory peritoneal dialysis may ship their dialysis solutions to their destinations before traveling. They should carry essential medical records as well as antibiotics for self-treatment of presumed peritonitis. Hemodialysis patients need to reserve appointments at dialysis centers prior to their departure from home. Travel by transplant recipients to distant destinations should ideally be scheduled at least 1 year after surgery, as most rejection episodes occur early. Medication interactions are a source of serious concern for these travelers, and appropriate medical information should be carried, along with the home physician's name and telephone number. Some travelers taking steroids carry stress doses in case they become ill. Immunization of these immunocompromised travelers may result in less than adequate protection against certain diseases. Thus, the traveler and physician must carefully consider which destinations are appropriate.

PROBLEMS AFTER RETURN The most frequent medical problems encountered by travelers after their return home are diarrhea, fever, respiratory illnesses, and skin diseases. Frequently ignored problems are fatigue and emotional stress, especially in long-stay travelers. The approach to diagnosis requires some knowledge of geographic medicine, in particular the epidemiology and clinical presentation of infectious disorders. A geographic history should focus on the traveler's exact itinerary, including dates of arrival and departure, exposure history (food indiscretions, drinking-water sources, freshwater contact, sexual activity, animal contact, insect bites), location and style of travel (urban vs. rural, first-class hotel

accommodation vs. camping), immunization history, and use of antimalarial chemosuppression.

Fever Because death from *P. falciparum* malaria can occur after an illness of only several days, fever in a traveler who has returned from a malarious area should be considered a medical emergency. Although "fever from the tropics" does not always have a tropical cause, malaria should be the first diagnosis considered. The risk of *P. falciparum* malaria is highest among travelers returning from Africa or Oceania and among those who become symptomatic within the first 2 months after return. Other important causes of fever after travel include viral hepatitis (hepatitis A and E), typhoid fever, bacterial enteritis, arbovirus infections (e.g., dengue fever), rickettsial infections (including tick and scrub typhus or Q fever) and—in rare instances—leptospirosis, acute HIV infection, and amebic liver abscess. In at least 25 percent of cases, no etiology can be found, and the illness resolves spontaneously. Clinicians should keep in mind that no present-day antimalarial agent guarantees protection from malaria and that some immunizations—notably, those against typhoid and cholera—are only partially protective.

Skin Diseases Pyodermas, sunburn, insect bites, skin ulcers, and cutaneous larva migrans are the most frequent skin conditions encountered in travelers after their return home. In those with persistent skin ulcers, the diagnoses of cutaneous leishmaniasis, mycobacterial infection, or fungal infection should be considered. Careful, complete inspection of the skin is important in detecting the rickettsial eschar in a febrile patient or the central breathing hole in a "boil" due to myiasis.

Emerging Infectious Diseases In recent years, travel and commerce have fostered the worldwide spread of HIV infection, led to the reemergence of cholera as a global health threat, and created considerable fear about the possible spread of Ebola virus infection and plague. For travelers, there are more realistic concerns. One of the largest outbreaks of dengue fever ever documented is now raging in Latin America; schistosomiasis is being described in previously unaffected lakes in Africa; and antibiotic-resistant strains of sexually transmitted and enteric pathogens are emerging at an alarming rate in the developing world. As Nobel Laureate Dr. Joshua Lederberg pointed out, "The microbe that felled one child in a distant continent yesterday can reach yours today and seed a global pandemic tomorrow." The vigilant clinician understands that the importance of a thorough travel history cannot be overemphasized.

BIBLIOGRAPHY

Barry M, Bia F: Pregnancy and travel. JAMA 261:728, 1989

Bia FS, Barry M: Special health considerations for travelers. Med Clin North Am 76:1295, 1992

Caumes E et al: Dermatoses associated with travel to tropical countries: A prospective study of the diagnosis and management of 269 patients presenting to a tropical disease unit. Clin Infect Dis 20:542, 1995

DuPont HL, Capsuto EG: Persistent diarrhea in travelers. Clin Infect Dis 22:124, 1996

Kelsall BL, Guerrant RL: Evaluation of diarrhea in the returning traveler. Infect Dis Clin North Am 6:413, 1992

Laguna F et al: Gastrointestinal leishmaniasis in human immunodeficiency virus–infected patients: Report of five cases and review. Clin Infect Dis 19:48, 1994

Phillips–Howard PA, Wood D: The safety of antimalarial drugs in pregnancy. Drug Safety 14:131, 1996

Rhoads JL et al: Safety and immunogenicity of multiple conventional immunizations administered during early HIV infection. J Acquir Immune Defic Syndr 4:724, 1991

Schwartz JS et al: Air travel and hypoxemia with chronic obstructive lung disease. Ann Intern Med 100:473, 1984

Steffen R, Lobel HO: Epidemiologic basis for the practice of travel medicine. J Wilderness Med 5:56, 1994

Strickland GT: Fever in the returned traveler. Med Clin North Am 76:1375, 1992

Svenson JE et al: Imported malaria. Clinical presentation and examination of symptomatic travelers. Arch Intern Med 155:861, 1995

Wilson ME et al: Infections in HIV-infected travelers: Risks and prevention. Ann Intern Med 114:582, 1991

124   *Robert S. Munford*

SEPSIS AND SEPTIC SHOCK

DEFINITIONS   (See Table 124-1) The host's reaction to invading microbes involves a rapidly amplifying polyphony of signals and responses that may spread beyond the invaded tissue. Fever or hypothermia, tachypnea, and tachycardia often herald the onset of *sepsis*, the systemic inflammatory response to microbial invasion. When counterregulatory control mechanisms are overwhelmed, often as the microbe moves from a local site to invade the bloodstream, homeostasis may fail, and dysfunction of major organs may supervene (*severe sepsis*). Further failure of counterregulatory control leads to *septic shock*, which is characterized by hypotension as well as organ dysfunction. As sepsis progresses to septic shock, the risk of dying increases substantially. Early sepsis is usually reversible, whereas patients with septic shock often succumb despite aggressive therapy.

The *systemic inflammatory response syndrome* (SIRS), as defined recently by critical-care specialists, may have an infectious or a noninfectious etiology. If infection is suspected or proven, a patient with SIRS is said to have sepsis.

ETIOLOGY   Sepsis can be a response to any class of microorganism. Microbial invasion of the bloodstream is not essential for the development of sepsis; local or systemic spread of microbial signal molecules or toxins can also elicit the response. Blood cultures yield bacteria or fungi in approximately 20 to 40 percent of cases of severe sepsis and 40 to 70 percent of cases of septic shock. Individual gram-

Table 124-1

Definitions Often Used to Describe the Condition of Septic Patients

Bacteremia (fungemia)	Presence of viable bacteria (fungi) in the blood, as evidenced by positive blood cultures
Septicemia	Systemic illness caused by the spread of microbes or their toxins via the bloodstream
Systemic inflammatory response syndrome (SIRS)*	At least 2 of the following 4 conditions: (1) oral temperature of >38°C or <36°C; (2) respiratory rate of >20 breaths/min or Pa_{CO_2} of <32 torr; (3) heart rate of >90 beats/min; (4) leukocyte count of >12,000/μL or <4,000/μL or >10% bands
Sepsis*	SIRS that has a proven or suspected microbial etiology
Severe sepsis* (similar to "sepsis syndrome")	Sepsis with one or more signs of organ dysfunction, hypoperfusion, or hypotension, such as metabolic acidosis, acute alteration in mental status, oliguria, or adult respiratory distress syndrome
Hypotension*	Systolic blood pressure <90 mmHg—or 40 mmHg less than patient's baseline blood pressure—in the absence of other reasons for hypotension
Septic shock*	Sepsis with hypotension that is unresponsive to fluid resuscitation plus organ dysfunction or perfusion abnormalities as listed above for severe sepsis
Refractory septic shock	Septic shock that lasts for >1 h and does not respond to fluid and pressor administration
Multiple-organ dysfunction syndrome (MODS)*	Dysfunction of more than one organ, requiring intervention to maintain homeostasis

* Term preferred by the American College of Chest Physicians/Society of Critical Care Medicine Consensus Conference, 1992.

negative or gram-positive bacteria account for approximately 75 to 85 percent of these isolates; the remainder are fungi or a mixture of microorganisms. In patients whose blood cultures are negative, the etiologic agent is often established by culture or microscopic examination of infected material from a local site. In some case series, a majority of patients with a clinical picture of severe sepsis or septic shock have had negative microbiological results.

EPIDEMIOLOGY   Sepsis is now a contributing factor in more than 100,000 deaths per year in the United States. The annual incidence is probably between 300,000 and 500,000 cases. Approximately two-thirds of cases occur in patients hospitalized for other illnesses. Factors that predispose to gram-negative bacillary bacteremia include diabetes mellitus, lymphoproliferative diseases, cirrhosis of the liver, burns, invasive procedures or devices, and treatment with drugs that cause neutropenia. Major risk factors for gram-positive bacteremia include vascular catheterization, the presence of indwelling mechanical devices, burns, and intravenous drug use. Fungemia occurs most often in immunosuppressed patients with neutropenia, often after broad-spectrum antimicrobial therapy. The increasing incidence of sepsis in the United States is attributable to the aging of the population, the increasing longevity of patients with chronic diseases, and the relatively high frequency of this condition among patients with AIDS. The widespread use of antimicrobial agents, glucocorticoids, indwelling catheters, mechanical devices, and mechanical ventilation also plays a role.

PATHOPHYSIOLOGY   The septic response is usually triggered when microorganisms spread from the gastrointestinal tract or skin into contiguous tissues. Localized tissue infection may then lead to bacteremia or fungemia. Alternatively, microorganisms may be introduced directly into the bloodstream (for example, via intravenous catheters). In a minority of cases, no primary site of infection is apparent. In general, the septic response occurs when an invading microbe has circumvented the host's innate and acquired immune defenses. Host factors that allow microbial growth (such as deficiencies of antibody, complement factors, or cell-mediated immunity) are therefore critical.

Microbial Signals   Animals recognize certain microbial molecules as signals that microorganisms have invaded. Lipopolysaccharide (LPS, also called endotoxin) is the most potent and best-studied gram-negative bacterial signal molecule. A plasma protein (LPS-binding protein, or LBP) transfers LPS to CD14 on the surfaces of monocytes, macrophages, and neutrophils. This interaction rapidly triggers the production and release of mediators, such as tumor necrosis factor (TNF) α (see below), that amplify the LPS signal and transmit it to other cells and tissues. Soluble CD14 may also bind LPS in plasma and transfer it to vascular endothelial cells, which lack cell-surface CD14. The peptidoglycan and lipoteichoic acids of gram-positive bacteria, certain polysaccharides, extracellular enzymes, and toxins elicit responses in animals that are similar to those induced by LPS. The molecular basis for the stimulatory potency of these molecules is poorly understood, although some of them may also bind cell-surface or soluble CD14 before activating cells. CD14 may therefore be a receptor that facilitates responses to many microbial signals. Other innate immune mechanisms that recognize microbial molecules include complement (principally the alternative pathway; see Chap. 305), mannose-binding protein, and C-reactive protein.

Host Responses   The septic response involves complex interactions among microbial signal molecules, leukocytes, humoral mediators, and the vascular endothelium.

Cytokines   Inflammatory cytokines amplify and diversify the response. These proteins can exert endocrine, paracrine, and autocrine effects (Chap. 305). TNFα stimulates leukocytes and vascular endothelial cells to release other cytokines (as well as additional TNFα), to express cell-surface adhesion molecules, and to increase arachidonic acid turnover. Blood levels of TNFα are high in most patients with severe sepsis. Moreover, intravenous infusion of TNFα can elicit many of the characteristic abnormalities of sepsis, including fever, tachycardia, tachypnea, leukocytosis, myalgias, and somnolence. In animals, large doses of TNFα induce shock, disseminated intravascular coagulation (DIC), and death. Specific TNFα antagonists can abrogate the septic response and prevent the deaths of experimental animals challenged with endotoxin.

Although TNFα is a central mediator, it is only one of many cytokines that contribute to the septic process. Interleukin (IL)-1β, for example, which exhibits many of the same activities as TNFα, seems to play an increasingly significant role as the septic process intensifies. TNFα, IL-1β, interferon γ, IL-8, and other cytokines probably interact synergistically with one another and with additional mediators. Moreover, some mediators (such as IL-1β and TNFα) may enhance their own rates of synthesis by positive feedback. As sepsis progresses, the mixture of cytokines and other mediators becomes very complex: elevated blood levels of more than 30 pro- and anti-inflammatory molecules have been found in patients with septic shock. In animal models, the septic response can be interrupted by early interventions that neutralize one or another of its many components; this observation testifies to the importance of mediator interactions in the overall outcome. Unfortunately, it has been much more difficult to rescue animals from severe sepsis and septic shock.

Phospholipid-derived mediators Arachidonic acid, released from membrane phospholipids by phospholipase A₂, is converted by the cyclooxygenase pathway into prostaglandins and thromboxanes. Prostaglandin E₂ and prostacyclin cause peripheral vasodilation, whereas thromboxane is a vasoconstrictor and promotes platelet aggregation. Leukotrienes are also potent mediators of ischemia and shock; the fact that the reaction to endotoxin challenge is normal in mice that lack the 5-lipoxygenase gene, however, casts doubt on the role of leukotrienes in the septic response.

Another important phospholipid-derived mediator is platelet-activating factor (PAF, or 1-*O*-alkyl-2-acetyl-*sn*-glycerol-3-phosphocholine). PAF potently stimulates neutrophil aggregation and degranulation, promotes platelet aggregation, and may contribute to tissue injury.

Coagulation factors Intravascular fibrin deposition, thrombosis, and DIC are important features of the septic response. TNFα promotes intravascular coagulation initially by inducing blood monocytes to express tissue factor (see Chap. 60). When tissue factor is expressed on monocytes, it binds to factor VIIa to form an active complex that can convert factors X and IX to enzymatically active forms. The result is activation of both extrinsic and intrinsic clotting pathways, culminating in the generation of fibrin. Clotting is also favored by impaired function of the protein C–protein S inhibitory pathway, while fibrinolysis is prevented by increased plasma levels of plasminogen activator inhibitor 1. Thus, there may be a striking propensity for intravascular fibrin deposition, thrombosis, and bleeding. Contact-system activation occurs during sepsis but contributes more to the development of hypotension than to DIC.

Complement C5a and other products of complement activation may promote neutrophil reactions such as chemotaxis, aggregation, degranulation, and oxygen-radical production. When administered to animals, C5a induces hypotension, pulmonary vasoconstriction, neutropenia, and vascular leakiness due in part to endothelial damage.

Activation of the vascular endothelium Many tissues may be damaged by sepsis. The probable underlying mechanism is widespread vascular endothelial injury, with fluid extravasation and microthrombosis that decrease oxygen and substrate utilization by the affected tissues. Leukocyte-derived mediators and platelet-leukocyte-fibrin thrombi contribute to this injury, but the vascular endothelium itself seems to play an active role. Stimuli such as TNFα induce vascular endothelial cells to produce and release cytokines, procoagulant molecules, PAF, endothelium-derived relaxing factor (nitric oxide), and other mediators. In addition, regulated cell-adhesion molecules promote the adherence of leukocytes to endothelial cells. While these responses may attract phagocytes to infected sites and activate their antimicrobial arsenals, endothelial cell activation can also promote increased vascular permeability, microvascular thrombosis, DIC, and hypotension. Moreover, vascular integrity may be damaged by neutro-

phil enzymes (such as elastase) and toxic oxygen metabolites so that local hemorrhage ensues. Blocking the adhesion of leukocytes to endothelial cell surfaces, as with monoclonal antibodies to intercellular adhesion molecule 1, can prevent tissue necrosis in response to endotoxin administration in animals.

Septic shock Much evidence now implicates nitric oxide, produced by inducible nitric oxide synthase (*iNOS*), as a mediator of septic shock in experimental animals and probably in humans. Mice that lack the *iNOS* gene may not be resistant to endotoxic shock, however. Other prominent hypotensive molecules are β-endorphin, bradykinin, PAF, and prostacyclin. Agents that inhibit the synthesis or action of each of these mediators can prevent or reverse endotoxic shock in animals.

Control mechanisms Elaborate host mechanisms regulate both microbial signals and the inflammatory response. While plasma LBP promotes the inflammatory response by facilitating the interaction of LPS with monocyte cell-surface CD14, LBP and soluble CD14 can also prevent LPS signaling by transferring LPS molecules into plasma lipoprotein particles. The relative plasma concentrations of LPS, LBP, CD14, and lipoprotein therefore may determine LPS signal intensity. The mechanisms that control the inflammatory response are complex, overlapping, and poorly understood. Glucocorticoids inhibit cytokine synthesis by monocytes in vitro and, when administered with or shortly after an inflammatory stimulus, may protect animals from septic shock. The increase in blood cortisol levels early in the septic response presumably plays a similar inhibitory role. Certain cytokine antagonists also may contribute. Blood levels of IL-1 receptor antagonist often greatly exceed those of circulating IL-1β, and this excess may result in inhibition of the binding of IL-1β to its receptors. Transforming growth factor β (TGFβ) and IL-10 also can inhibit LPS-induced responses of human monocytes in vitro and prevent endotoxic death in animals. Blood and tissue levels of prostaglandin E₂, TGFβ, α-melanocyte-stimulating hormone, cortisol, IL-1 receptor antagonist, soluble TNF receptors, and IL-10 increase during the septic response, and these molecules probably act in concert to diminish its intensity. Indeed, blood leukocytes from patients with severe sepsis may be hyporesponsive to agonists such as LPS. The fact that plasma concentrations of many of these anti-inflammatory molecules may be very high in the patient with septic shock, however, indicates that they are unable to control the inflammatory response when it is most severe.

CLINICAL MANIFESTATIONS The systemic inflammatory response often intensifies over time from mild (sepsis) to extremely severe (septic shock). The rate at which the response increases may differ from patient to patient, and there are striking individual variations in its manifestations. For example, some septic patients have a normal temperature or are hypothermic; the absence of fever is most common among neonates, elderly patients, and persons with uremia or alcoholism.

Hyperventilation is often an early sign. Disorientation, confusion, and other manifestations of encephalopathy may also develop early in the septic response, particularly in the elderly and in individuals with preexisting neurologic impairment. Focal neurologic signs are uncommon, although preexisting focal deficits may become more prominent.

Hypotension and DIC predispose to acrocyanosis and ischemic necrosis of peripheral tissues, most commonly the digits. Cellulitis, pustules, bullae, or hemorrhagic lesions may develop when hematogenous bacteria or fungi seed the skin or underlying soft tissue. Bacterial toxins may also be distributed hematogenously, eliciting diffuse cutaneous reactions. On occasion, skin lesions may be suggestive of specific pathogens. When sepsis is accompanied by cutaneous petechiae or purpura, infection with *Neisseria meningitidis* (or, less commonly, *Haemophilus influenzae*) should be suspected; in a patient who has been bitten by a tick while in an endemic area, petechial lesions also suggest Rocky Mountain spotted fever. A cutaneous lesion seen almost exclusively in neutropenic patients is ecthyma gangrenosum, usually caused by *Pseudomonas aeruginosa* or *Aeromonas hydrophila*. It is a bullous lesion, surrounded by edema, that undergoes central hemorrhage and necrosis. Histopathologic examination shows bacteria in and around the wall of a small vessel, with little or no neutrophilic response. Hemorrhagic or bullous lesions in a septic patient who has recently eaten raw oysters suggest *Vibrio vulnificus* bacteremia, while such lesions in a patient who has recently suffered a dog bite may indicate bloodstream infection due to *Capnocytophaga canimorsus* or *Capnocytophaga cynodegmi*. Generalized erythroderma in a septic patient suggests the toxic shock syndrome due to *Staphylococcus aureus* or *Streptococcus pyogenes*.

Gastrointestinal manifestations such as nausea, vomiting, diarrhea, and ileus may be indicative of acute gastroenteritis. Stress ulceration can lead to upper gastrointestinal bleeding. Cholestatic jaundice, with elevated levels of serum bilirubin (mostly conjugated) and alkaline phosphatase, may precede other signs of sepsis. Hepatocellular or canalicular dysfunction appears to underlie most cases, and the results of hepatic function tests return to normal with resolution of the infection. Prolonged or severe hypotension may induce acute hepatic injury or ischemic bowel necrosis.

Blood lactate levels rise early, in part because of increased glycolysis with impaired clearance of the resulting lactate and pyruvate by the liver and kidneys. As hypoperfusion develops, tissue hypoxia generates more lactic acid, contributing to metabolic acidosis. The blood glucose concentration often increases, particularly in diabetics, although impaired gluconeogenesis and excessive insulin release on occasion produce hypoglycemia. The cytokine-driven acute-phase response inhibits the synthesis of albumin and transthyretin while enhancing the production of C-reactive protein, LBP, fibrinogen, and complement components. Protein catabolism is often markedly accelerated.

MAJOR COMPLICATIONS Cardiopulmonary Complications Ventilation-perfusion mismatching produces a fall in arterial P_{O_2} early in the course. Increasing alveolar capillary permeability results in an increased pulmonary water content, which decreases pulmonary compliance and interferes with oxygen exchange. Progressive diffuse pulmonary infiltrates, decreasing compliance, and arterial hypoxemia (whose frequent refractoriness to supplemental oxygen therapy indicates right-to-left shunting) signal the development of the adult respiratory distress syndrome (ARDS, or "shock lung"). ARDS develops in 20 to 50 percent of patients with sepsis, and sepsis is the leading cause of this syndrome. The failure of the respiratory muscles can exacerbate hypoxemia and hypercapnia. An elevated pulmonary capillary wedge pressure (>18 mmHG) suggests fluid volume overload or cardiac failure rather than ARDS. Pneumonia caused by viruses or *Pneumocystis carinii* infection may be clinically indistinguishable from ARDS.

Septic shock usually results from a severe decrease in systemic vascular resistance, a generalized maldistribution of blood flow, and functional hypovolemia that is due, at least in part, to diffuse capillary leakage of intravascular constituents. Other factors that may decrease effective intravascular volume include dehydration from antecedent disease or insensible fluid losses, vomiting or diarrhea, and polyuria. Cardiac output is initially normal or elevated. Indeed, normal or increased cardiac output and decreased systemic vascular resistance distinguish septic shock from cardiogenic, extracardiac obstructive, and hypovolemic shock; other processes that can produce this combination include anaphylaxis, beriberi, cirrhosis of the liver, and overdoses of nitroprusside or narcotics.

Depression of myocardial function, manifested as increased end-diastolic and systolic ventricular volumes with a decreased ejection fraction, develops within 24 h in most patients with advanced sepsis. Cardiac output is maintained despite the low ejection fraction because ventricular dilation permits a normal stroke volume. In survivors, myocardial function returns to normal over several days. While myocardial dysfunction may contribute to hypotension, refractory hypotension is usually due to a low systemic vascular resistance, and death results from refractory shock or the failure of multiple organs rather than from cardiac dysfunction per se.

Renal Complications Oliguria, azotemia, proteinuria, and nonspecific urinary casts are frequently found. Many patients are inappropriately polyuric; hyperglycemia may exacerbate this tendency. Most renal failure is due to acute tubular necrosis induced by hypotension or capillary injury, although some patients also have glomerulonephritis, renal cortical necrosis, or interstitial nephritis. Drug-induced renal damage may complicate therapy, particularly when hypotensive patients are given aminoglycoside antibiotics.

Coagulation Although thrombocytopenia occurs in 10 to 30 percent of patients, the underlying mechanism(s) are not understood. Platelet counts are usually very low (i.e., below 50,000/μL) in patients with DIC; these low counts typically reflect diffuse endothelial injury (see Chap. 315).

Neurologic Complications When the septic illness lasts for weeks to months, "critical-illness" polyneuropathy may prevent weaning from ventilatory support and produce distal motor weakness. Electrophysiologic studies are diagnostic. Guillain-Barré syndrome, metabolic disturbances, and toxin activity must be ruled out.

LABORATORY FINDINGS In early sepsis, abnormalities may include leukocytosis with a left shift, thrombocytopenia, hyperbilirubinemia, and proteinuria. Leukopenia may develop. The neutrophils may contain toxic granulations, Döhle bodies, or cytoplasmic vacuoles. As the septic response becomes more severe, thrombocytopenia worsens (often with prolongation of the thrombin time, a decrease in fibrinogen, and the presence of D-dimers, suggesting DIC), azotemia and hyperbilirubinemia become more prominent, and levels of aminotransferases rise. Active hemolysis suggests clostridial bacteremia, malaria, a drug reaction, or DIC; in the case of DIC, microangiopathic changes may be seen on a blood smear.

During early sepsis, hyperventilation induces respiratory alkalosis. With respiratory-muscle fatigue and the accumulation of lactate, metabolic acidosis (with an increased anion gap) typically supervenes. Evaluation of arterial blood gases reveals hypoxemia, which is initially correctable with supplemental oxygen but whose later refractoriness to 100% oxygen inhalation indicates right-to-left shunting. The chest radiograph may be normal or may show evidence of underlying pneumonia, volume overload, or diffuse infiltrates of ARDS. The electrocardiogram may show only sinus tachycardia or nonspecific ST-T wave abnormalities.

Most diabetics with sepsis develop hyperglycemia. Severe infection may precipitate diabetic ketoacidosis, which may exacerbate hypotension (see Chap. 334). Hypoglycemia occurs rarely. The serum albumin level, initially within the normal range, declines as sepsis continues. Serum lipid concentrations are often elevated. Hypocalcemia is rare.

DIAGNOSIS There is no specific test. Diagnostically sensitive findings in a patient with suspected or proven infection include fever or hypothermia, tachypnea, tachycardia, and leukocytosis or leukopenia (see Table 124-1); acutely altered mental status, thrombocytopenia, or hypotension also suggest the diagnosis. The septic response can be quite variable, however. In one study, 36 percent of patients with sepsis had a normal temperature, 40 percent had a normal respiratory rate, 10 percent had a normal pulse rate, and 33 percent had normal white blood cell counts. Moreover, the systemic responses of uninfected patients with other conditions may be similar to those characteristic of sepsis. Noninfectious etiologies of SIRS (see Table 124-1) include pancreatitis, burns, trauma, adrenal insufficiency, pulmonary embolism, dissecting or ruptured aortic aneurysm, myocardial infarction, occult hemorrhage, cardiac tamponade, post-cardiopulmonary bypass syndrome, anaphylaxis, and drug overdose.

Definitive etiologic diagnosis requires the isolation of the microorganism from the blood or a local site of infection. At least two blood samples (10 mL each) should be obtained (from different venipuncture sites) for culture. Because gram-negative bacteremia is typically low-grade (fewer than 10 organisms per milliliter of blood), multiple blood cultures or prolonged incubation of cultures may be necessary;

S. aureus grows more readily and is detectable in blood cultures within 48 h in most instances. In many cases, blood cultures are negative; this result can reflect prior antibiotic administration, the presence of slow-growing or fastidious organisms, or the absence of microbial invasion of the bloodstream. In these cases, Gram's staining and culture of material from the primary site of infection or from infected cutaneous lesions may help establish the microbial etiology. The skin and mucosae should be examined carefully and repeatedly for lesions that might yield diagnostic information. With overwhelming bacteremia (e.g., pneumococcal sepsis in splenectomized individuals or fulminant meningococcemia), microorganisms are sometimes visible on buffy-coat smears of peripheral blood.

Detection of endotoxin in blood by the limulus lysate test may portend a poor outcome, but this assay is not useful for diagnosing gram-negative bacterial infections, including gram-negative bacteremia. Although blood levels of IL-6 also may correlate with prognosis, cytokine assays are poorly standardized and currently have limited clinical value.

℞ TREATMENT

Sepsis can kill quickly. Successful management requires urgent measures to treat local infection, to provide hemodynamic and respiratory support, and to eliminate the offending microorganism. The outcome is also influenced by the patient's underlying disease, which should be managed aggressively.

Antimicrobial agents Antimicrobial chemotherapy should be initiated as soon as samples of blood and other relevant sites have been cultured. The choice of initial therapy is based on knowledge of the likely pathogens at specific sites of local infection. Available information about patterns of antimicrobial susceptibility among bacterial isolates from the community, the hospital, and the patient also should be taken into account. It is important, pending culture results, to initiate empirical antimicrobial therapy that is effective against both gram-positive and gram-negative bacteria (see Table 124-2). Maximal recommended doses of antimicrobial drugs should be given intravenously, with adjustment for impaired renal function when necessary. When culture results become available, the regimen can often be simplified, as a single antimicrobial agent is frequently adequate for the treatment of a known pathogen. Most patients require antimicrobial therapy for at least 1 week; the duration of treatment is typically influenced by factors such as the site of tissue infection, the adequacy of surgical drainage, the patient's underlying disease (see Chap. 136), and the antimicrobial susceptibility of the bacterial isolate(s).

Removal of the source of infection Removal or drainage of a focal source of infection is essential. Sites of occult infection should be sought carefully. Indwelling intravenous catheters should be removed, the tip rolled over a blood agar plate for quantitative culture, and a new catheter inserted at a different site. Foley and drainage catheters should be replaced. The possibility of paranasal sinusitis (often caused by hospital-acquired gram-negative bacteria) should be considered if the patient has undergone nasal intubation. In the neutropenic patient, cutaneous sites of tenderness and erythema, particularly in the perianal region, must be carefully sought. In patients with sacral or ischial decubitus ulcers, it is important to exclude pelvic or other soft-tissue pus collections (by computed tomography or magnetic resonance imaging, if necessary). In patients with severe sepsis arising from the urinary tract, sonography or computed tomography should be used to rule out ureteral obstruction, perinephric abscess, and renal abscess. These studies are not so urgent in patients with less severe urosepsis, provided that a clinical response is evident within 48 to 72 h.

Hemodynamic, respiratory, and metabolic support (See also Chap. 38) Here the primary goal is to restore adequate oxygen and substrate delivery to the tissues. Adequate organ perfusion is essential. Effective intravascular volume depletion is common in septic patients, and the initial management of hypotension should include the administration of intravenous fluids—typically 1 to 2 L of normal saline over 1 to 2 h. The pulmonary capillary wedge

Table 124-2

Initial Antimicrobial Therapy for Severe Sepsis with No Obvious Source in Adults with Normal Renal Function

Type of Patient	Antimicrobial Regimens*
Immunocompetent adult	The many acceptable regimens include (1) ticarcillin-clavulanate *or* piperacillin-tazobactam (6.2 and 7.5 g q6h, respectively) *plus* gentamicin or tobramycin (1.5 mg/kg q8h); (2) ampicillin (30 mg/kg q4h) *plus* gentamicin (1.5 mg/kg q8h) *plus* clindamycin (900 mg q8h); and (3) imipenem-cilastatin (0.5 g q6h). If the patient is allergic to β-lactam agents, ciprofloxacin (400 mg q12h) *or* aztreonam (2 g q8h) should be substituted for ampicillin in regimen 2.
Neutropenic patient (<500 neutrophils/μL)	Regimens include (1) ticarcillin, mezlocillin, or piperacillin (3 g q4h) *or* ceftazidime (2 g q8h) *plus* tobramycin (1.5 mg/kg q8h) and (2) imipenem-cilastatin (0.5 g q6h) *or* ceftazidime. If the patient is allergic to β-lactam agents, aztreonam or ciprofloxacin should be used with tobramycin. If the patient has an infected vascular catheter or if the involvement of staphylococci is suspected, vancomycin (15 mg/kg q12h) should be added.
Splenectomized patient	Cefotaxime (2 g q4h) *or* ceftriaxone (2 g q12h) should be used. If the local prevalence of cephalosporin-resistant pneumococci is high, add vancomycin. If the patient is allergic to β-lactam drugs, vancomycin (15 mg/kg q12h) *plus* ciprofloxacin (400 mg q12h) *or* aztreonam (2 g q8h) should be used.
Intravenous drug user	Nafcillin *or* oxacillin (2 g q4h) *plus* gentamicin (1.5 mg/kg q8h) should be used. If the local prevalence of methicillin-resistant *Staphylococcus aureus* is high or if the patient is allergic to β-lactam drugs, vancomycin (15 mg/kg q12h) with gentamicin should be used.
AIDS patient	Ticarcillin-clavulanate (3 g q4h) *plus* tobramycin (1.5 mg/kg q8h) should be used. If the patient is allergic to β-lactam drugs, ciprofloxacin (400 mg q12h) *plus* vancomycin (15 mg/kg q12h) *plus* tobramycin should be used.

* All administered intravenously.

pressure or the central venous pressure must be monitored in patients with refractory shock or underlying cardiac or renal disease. To avoid pulmonary edema, the pulmonary capillary wedge pressure should be maintained at 14 to 18 mmHg or the central venous pressure at 10 to 12 cmH$_2$O. The urine output should be kept above 30 mL/h by continuing fluid administration; a diuretic such as furosemide may be used if needed. In about one-third of patients, hypotension and organ hypoperfusion respond to fluid resuscitation; a reasonable goal is to maintain a mean arterial blood pressure of >60 mmHg (systolic pressure, >90 mmHg) and a cardiac index of ≥4 (L/min)/m². If these guidelines cannot be met by volume infusion, inotropic and vasopressor therapy is indicated (see Chap. 38).

Adrenal insufficiency should be considered in septic patients with refractory hypotension, fulminant *N. meningitidis* bacteremia, prior glucocorticoid use, disseminated tuberculosis, or AIDS. The cosyntropin (α^{1-24}-ACTH) stimulation test (see Chap. 332) may suggest absolute or partial adrenal insufficiency. Supplemental hydrocortisone (50 mg intravenously every 6 h) may be given while the results of the cosyntropin test are awaited.

Ventilator therapy is indicated for progressive hypoxemia, hypercapnia, neurologic deterioration, or respiratory muscle failure.

Intubation is often undertaken to ensure adequate oxygenation, divert blood from the muscles of respiration, and reduce the cardiac afterload. Blood or erythrocyte transfusion is indicated if oxygen delivery is compromised by a low hemoglobin concentration (<8 to 10 g/dL).

Bicarbonate is sometimes administered for severe metabolic acidosis (arterial pH < 7.2). DIC, if complicated by major bleeding, should be treated with transfusion of fresh frozen plasma and platelets. Successful treatment of the underlying infection is essential for the reversal of both acidosis and DIC. In patients with prolonged sepsis, nutritional supplementation may reduce the impact of protein hypercatabolism.

These are consensus recommendations; none of these generally accepted components of resuscitative care has been validated in randomized clinical trials.

Other measures Despite aggressive management, many patients with severe sepsis or septic shock die. Two kinds of agents that may help prevent these deaths are being investigated: (1) drugs that neutralize bacterial endotoxin and that thereby may benefit the fraction (approximately half) of septic patients who have gram-negative bacterial infections and (2) drugs that interfere with one or more mediators of the inflammatory response and may benefit all patients with sepsis.

ANTIENDOTOXIN AGENTS Lipid A, the toxic moiety of endotoxin, is conserved in the LPS of gram-negative bacteria. Despite much effort to develop drugs that bind lipid A and neutralize endotoxin in vivo, the potential of endotoxin as a target for therapeutic intervention remains controversial. In placebo-controlled clinical trials, two monoclonal antibodies to endotoxin failed to prevent the death of patients with severe gram-negative bacterial sepsis. In retrospective studies, these antibodies did not bind to LPS with high affinity, and one was reported to be a polyreactive autoantibody. Antibodies with improved binding properties are being evaluated. A theoretically more promising agent is bactericidal permeability-increasing protein, a human neutrophil protein that neutralizes the toxicity of lipid A and may be bactericidal to many gram-negative microorganisms. Other investigational drugs include nontoxic lipid A analogs that reduce host responses to endotoxins, a polymyxin B–dextran conjugate that binds endotoxins, and lipoproteins (such as high-density lipoprotein) that bind and neutralize endotoxin in the circulation.

ANTIMEDIATOR AGENTS Other adjunctive therapies are intended to control the inflammatory response, regardless of the microbial stimulus. Unfortunately, numerous agents that interfere directly or indirectly with the actions of inflammatory mediators have not prevented the death of patients with severe sepsis or septic shock. Anticytokine drugs tested in unsuccessful clinical trials include methylprednisolone, recombinant IL-1 receptor antagonist, genetically engineered soluble receptors for TNFα, and monoclonal antibodies to TNFα. Because TNFα and IL-1β doubtless play key roles in antimicrobial host defense, antagonizing these cytokines could be detrimental in some cases. In fact, recent studies suggest that many anti-inflammatory molecules may already be present at high concentrations in the plasma of patients with septic shock. Identifying beneficial regimens of treatment with drugs that neutralize TNFα and IL-1β may therefore be very difficult. Other compounds tested in recent clinical trials include PAF antagonists, bradykinin antagonists, and ibuprofen. Additional investigational agents include pentoxifylline, α-melanocyte-stimulating hormone, ketoconazole, inhibitors of *iNOS*, and recombinant anticoagulant proteins.

All of the recent clinical trials have enrolled patients with severe sepsis or septic shock. Neither the ability of adjunctive agents to *prevent* severe sepsis or septic shock in high-risk patients nor the value of combination therapy with two or more adjunctive drugs has been tested.

PROGNOSIS Approximately 25 to 35 percent of patients with severe sepsis and 40 to 55 percent of patients with septic shock die within 30 days. Others die within the ensuing 5 months. Late deaths often result from poorly controlled infection, complications of intensive care, failure of multiple organs, or underlying disease.

Several prognostic stratification systems that factor in the patient's age, underlying condition, and various physiologic variables yield estimates of the risk of dying of severe sepsis. Of the individual covariates, underlying disease most strongly influences the risk of dying. Septic shock is also a strong predictor of short- and long-term mortality. Case-fatality rates are similar for culture-positive and culture-negative severe sepsis and septic shock.

PREVENTION Prevention offers the best opportunity to reduce morbidity and mortality from sepsis. Most episodes of severe sepsis and septic shock are nosocomial. These cases might be prevented by reducing the number of invasive procedures undertaken, by limiting the use (and duration) of indwelling vascular and bladder catheters, by reducing the incidence and duration of profound neutropenia (<500 neutrophils/μL), and by more aggressively treating localized nosocomial infections. Increasing evidence supports the administration of enteral feeding supplements to traumatized patients at risk for infection. Indiscriminate use of antimicrobial agents and glucocorticoids should be avoided, and optimal infection-control measures (see Chap. 138) should be used. In addition, prompt and aggressive management of patients with early sepsis is imperative. Research is needed to identify patients at high risk for severe sepsis and to develop adjunctive agents that can damp the septic response before organ dysfunction or hypotension develops.

BIBLIOGRAPHY

AMERICAN COLLEGE OF CHEST PHYSICIANS/SOCIETY OF CRITICAL CARE MEDICINE CONSENSUS CONFERENCE COMMITTEE: Definitions for sepsis and organ failure and guidelines for the use of innovative therapies in sepsis. Crit Care Med 20:864, 1992

ASTIZ ME et al: Intravascular volume and fluid therapy for severe sepsis. New Horizons 1:127, 1993

BERNARD GR: Sepsis trials. Intersection of investigation, regulation, funding, and practice. Am J Respir Crit Care Med 152:4, 1995

BOLTON CF et al: The neurological complications of sepsis. Ann Neurol 33:94, 1993

EIDELMAN LA et al: The spectrum of septic encephalopathy. Definitions, etiologies, and mortalities. JAMA 275:470, 1996

HARRIS RL et al: Manifestations of sepsis. Arch Intern Med 147:1895, 1987

LEVI M et al: Pathogenesis of disseminated intravascular coagulation in sepsis. JAMA 270:975, 1993

LYNN WA, COHEN J: Adjunctive therapy for septic shock: A review of experimental approaches. Clin Infect Dis 20:143, 1995

MARTIN MA et al: Gram-negative sepsis and the adult respiratory distress syndrome. Clin Infect Dis 14:1213, 1992

PERL TM et al: Long-term survival and function after suspected gram-negative sepsis. JAMA 274:338, 1995

PINNER RW et al: Trends in infectious disease mortality in the U.S. JAMA 275:189, 1996

RANGEL-FRAUSTO MS et al: The natural history of the systemic inflammatory response syndrome (SIRS). A prospective study. JAMA 273:117, 1995

125   *Jeffrey A. Gelfand, Charles A. Dinarello*

FEVER OF UNKNOWN ORIGIN*

DEFINITION AND CLASSIFICATION

Fever of unknown origin (FUO) was defined by Petersdorf and Beeson in 1961 as (1) temperatures higher than 38.3°C (101°F) on several occasions, (2) a duration of fever of more than 3 weeks, and (3) failure to reach a diagnosis despite 1 week of inpatient investigation. While this classification has stood for more than 30 years, Durack and Street have proposed a new system for classification of FUO: (1) classic FUO, (2) nosocomial FUO, (3) neutropenic FUO, and (4) FUO associated with human immunodeficiency virus (HIV) infection (Table 125-1).

* Sheldon M. Wolff, M.D., now deceased, was an author in the previous edition of this revised chapter, and it is to his memory that the chapter is dedicated.

Table 125-1

Categories of FUO*

	Category of FUO			
Feature	Nosocomial	Neutropenic	HIV-Associated	Classic
Patient's situation	Hospitalized, acute care, no infection when admitted	Neutrophil count either less than 500/μL or expected to reach that level in 1–2 days	Confirmed HIV-positive	All others with fevers for ≥3 weeks
Duration of illness while under investigation	3 days†	3 days†	3 days† (or 4 weeks as outpatient)	3 days† or three outpatient visits
Examples of cause	Septic thrombophlebitis, sinusitis, *Clostridium difficile* colitis, drug fever	Perianal infection, aspergillosis, candidemia	MAI‡ infection, tuberculosis, non-Hodgkin's lymphoma, drug fever	Infections, malignancy, inflammatory diseases, drug fever

* All require temperatures of ≥38.3°C (101°F) on several occasions.
† Includes at least 2 days' incubation of microbiology cultures.
‡ *M. avium/M. intracellulare.*
SOURCE: Modified from Durack and Street.

CLASSIC FUO This category corresponds closely to the earlier definition of FUO, differing only with regard to the prior requirement for 1 week's study in the hospital; the new definition is broader, stipulating three outpatient visits or 3 days in the hospital without elucidation of a cause or 1 week of "intelligent and invasive" ambulatory investigation. In our opinion, a 2-week period of fever is sufficient grounds for entertaining the diagnosis of FUO when other criteria have been met.

NOSOCOMIAL FUO In nosocomial FUO, a temperature of ≥38.3°C (101°F) develops on several occasions in a hospitalized patient who is receiving acute care and in whom infection was not manifest or incubating on admission. Three days of investigation, including at least 2 days' incubation of cultures, is the minimum requirement for this diagnosis. In hospitalized patients, occult nosocomial infections, infected intravascular lines, recurrent pulmonary embolism, transfusion-related viral infection, and drug-related fever are possible diagnoses. In this setting, the approach is to focus on sites where occult infections might be sequestered (such as the sinuses of intubated patients and prosthetic devices) or on nosocomial complications such as acalculous cholecystitis, *Clostridium difficile* toxin in the stool (in cases including diarrhea), and drug reactions. Blood cultures are mandatory. Appropriate diagnostic maneuvers include ultrasonography and computed tomography (CT) of the abdomen, indium 111–labeled white blood cell or immunoglobulin scans, sinus x-rays, and discontinuation of treatment with suspect drugs.

NEUTROPENIC FUO This condition is defined as a temperature of ≥38.3°C (101°F) on several occasions in a patient whose neutrophil count is <500/μL or is expected to fall to that level in 1 to 2 days. The diagnosis of neutropenic FUO is invoked if a specific cause is not identified after 3 days of investigation, including at least 2 days' incubation of cultures. Neutropenic patients are susceptible to focal bacterial and fungal infections, to bacteremic infections, to infections involving catheters (including septic thrombophlebitis), and to perianal infections. *Candida* and *Aspergillus* infections are common.

Infections due to herpes simplex virus or cytomegalovirus (CMV) are sometimes causes of FUO in this group. While the duration of illness is far shorter in these patients, the consequences of untreated infection may be catastrophic.

HIV-ASSOCIATED FUO This disorder is defined by a temperature of ≥38.3°C (101°F) on several occasions over a period of more than 4 weeks for outpatients or more than 3 days for hospitalized patients with HIV infection. This diagnosis is invoked if appropriate investigation over 3 days, including 2 days' incubation of cultures, reveals no source. In this group of patients, HIV infection alone may be a cause of fever. Infection due to *Mycobacterium avium* or *Mycobacterium intracellulare* (together known as MAI), toxoplasmosis, CMV infection, tuberculosis, *Pneumocystis carinii* infection, salmonellosis, cryptococcosis, histoplasmosis, non-Hodgkin's lymphoma, and (of particular importance) drug fever are all possible causes of FUO.

Adoption of these categories of FUO on a wide scale in the literature would allow a more rational compilation of data regarding these disparate groups. In the remainder of this chapter, the discussion will focus on classic FUO unless otherwise specified.

CAUSES OF CLASSIC FUO

Table 125-2 summarizes the findings of a number of large studies of FUO carried out since the advent of the antibiotic era. Coincident with the widespread use of antibiotics, increasingly useful diagnostic technologies—both noninvasive and invasive—have been developed. Newer studies reflect not only changing patterns of disease but also the impact of diagnostic techniques that make it possible to eliminate many patients with specific illness from the FUO category. The ubiquitous use of microbiologic cultures and the widespread use of potent broad-spectrum antibiotics may have decreased the number of infections causing FUO. The wide availability of ultrasonography, CT, and magnetic resonance imaging (MRI) has enhanced the detection of occult neoplasms and lymphomas in patients previously thought to

Table 125-2

Classic FUO in Adults

Authors	Years of Study	No. of Cases	Infections (%)	Neoplasms (%)	Collagen Vascular Diseases (%)	Causes (%)	
						Miscellaneous Causes	Undiagnosed Causes
Petersdorf and Beeson	1952–57	100	36	19	13	25	7
Jacoby and Swartz	1957–71	128	40	20	15	17	8
Howard et al.	1969–76	100	37	31	19	8	5
Larson and Featherstone	1970–80	105	30	31	16	10	12
Knockaert and Vanneste	1980–89	199	22.5	7	21.5*	26.5*	2.5*

* Authors' raw data retabulated to conform to prior diagnostic categories.

have FUO. Likewise, the widespread availability of highly specific and sensitive immunologic testing has reduced the number of undetected cases of systemic lupus erythematosus (SLE) and other autoimmune diseases.

Several generalizations can be made. Infections, especially extrapulmonary tuberculosis, remain the leading cause of FUO. Prolonged mononucleosis syndromes caused by Epstein-Barr virus, CMV, or HIV are conditions whose consideration as a cause of FUO is sometimes confounded by delayed antibody responses. Intraabdominal abscesses (sometimes poorly localized) and renal, retroperitoneal, and paraspinal abscesses continue to be difficult to diagnose. Renal malacoplakia, with submucosal plaques or nodules involving the urinary tract, may cause FUO and is often fatal if untreated. It is associated with coliform infection, is seen most often in patients with defects of intracellular bacterial killing, and is treated with fluoroquinolones or trimethoprim-sulfamethoxazole. Occasionally, other organs may be involved. Osteomyelitis, especially where prosthetic devices have been implanted, and infective endocarditis must be considered. Although true culture-negative infective endocarditis is rare, one may be misled by slow-growing organisms of the HACEK group (*Haemophilus aphrophilus, Actinobacillus actinomycetemcomitans, Cardiobacterium hominis, Eikenella corrodens,* and *Kingella kingae*; see Chap. 152), *Bartonella* species (previously *Rochalimaea*), *Legionella* species, *Coxiella burnetii, Chlamydia psittaci,* and fungi. Prostatitis, dental abscesses, sinusitis, and cholangitis continue to be sources of occult fever.

Fungal disease, most notably histoplasmosis involving the reticuloendothelial system, may cause FUO. FUO with headache should prompt examination of spinal fluid for *Cryptococcus neoformans.* Malaria (which may result from transfusion, the failure to take a prescribed prophylactic agent, or infection with a drug-resistant strain) continues to be a cause, particularly of nonsynchronized FUO.

In most early series, neoplasms were the next most common cause of FUO after infections (Table 125-3). In a series of 199 patients studied between 1980 and 1989, a decrease in the percentage of FUO cases due to malignancy was attributed to the improvement in diagnostic technologies. This observation does not diminish the importance of considering neoplasia in the initial diagnostic evaluation of a patient with fever. A large number of patients in this series had diseases such as temporal arteritis, adult Still's disease, drug-related fever, and factitious fever. In most series, approximately 10 percent of cases of FUO remained undiagnosed. The general term "collagen vascular diseases" is used somewhat loosely to apply not only to SLE and temporal arteritis but also to systemic rheumatologic or vasculitic diseases such as polymyalgia rheumatica and adult Still's disease.

In the elderly, multisystem disease is the most frequent cause of FUO, giant-cell arteritis being the leading etiologic entity in this category. Tuberculosis is the most common infection causing FUO in the elderly, and colon cancer is an important cause of FUO with malignancy.

Many diseases have been grouped in the various studies as "miscellaneous." At the top of this list are the granulomatous diseases, including sarcoidosis, Crohn's disease, and granulomatous hepatitis. Additional diagnoses include drug fever, erythema multiforme, pulmonary embolism, factitious fever, familial Mediterranean fever, Behçet's syndrome, Fabry's disease, and Whipple's disease (now attributed to the bacillus *Tropheryma whippelii*).

Table 125-3

Malignancies That Commonly Cause FUO

Hodgkin's disease
Non-Hodgkin's lymphoma
Leukemia (including preleukemic and aleukemic phases)
Renal cell carcinoma
Hepatoma

Table 125-4

Causes of FUO Lasting More than 6 Months

Cause	Percentage of Cases
None identified	19
Miscellaneous causes	13
Factitious causes	9
Granulomatous hepatitis	8
Neoplasm	7
Still's disease	6
Infection	6
Collagen vascular disease	4
Familial Mediterranean fever	3
No fever*	27

* No actual fever observed during 2 to 3 weeks of inpatient observation. Includes patients with exaggerated circadian rhythm.

SOURCE: From a study of 347 patients referred to the National Institutes of Health from 1961 to 1977 with a presumptive diagnosis of FUO of >6 months' duration (Aduan et al).

A drug-related etiology must be considered in any case of prolonged fever. Any febrile pattern may be elicited by a drug, and both relative bradycardia and hypotension are uncommon. Eosinophilia and/or rash is found in only one-fifth of patients with drug fever. Fever usually begins 1 to 3 weeks after the start of therapy and remits 2 to 3 days after therapy is stopped. Virtually all classes of drugs cause fever, but antimicrobials (especially β-lactam antibiotics), cardiovascular drugs (e.g., quinidine), antineoplastic drugs, and drugs acting on the central nervous system (e.g., phenytoin) are particularly common causes.

It is axiomatic that, as the duration of fever increases, the likelihood of an infectious cause decreases (Table 125-4). In a series of 347 patients referred to the National Institutes of Health from 1961 to 1977, only 6 percent had an infection. A significant number (9 percent) had *factitious fevers*—i.e., fevers due either to false elevations of temperature or to self-induced disease. A substantial number of these factitious cases were in young women in the health professions. It is worth noting that 8 percent of the patients with prolonged fevers (some of whom had completely normal liver function studies) had granulomatous hepatitis, and 6 percent had adult Still's disease. After prolonged investigation, 19 percent of cases still had no specific diagnosis. A total of 27 percent of patients either had no actual fever during the weeks of inpatient observation or had an exaggerated circadian temperature rhythm without chills, elevated pulse, or other abnormalities. The conditions that may be considered in a differential diagnosis of classic FUO in adults are listed in Table 125-5. While this list applies strictly to the United States, the frequency of global travel underscores the need for a detailed travel history.

SPECIALIZED DIAGNOSTIC STUDIES IN CLASSIC FUO

Certain specific diagnostic maneuvers become critical in dealing with prolonged fevers. If factitious fever is suspected, numbered thermometers should be used, temperature-taking should be supervised, and simultaneous urine and body temperatures should be measured. Any tissue removed during prior relevant surgery should be reexamined; slides should be requested and, if need be, paraffin blocks of fixed pathologic material should be reexamined and additional special studies performed. Relevant x-rays should be reexamined; reviewing of prior radiologic reports may be insufficient. Serum should be set aside in the laboratory as soon as possible and retained for future examination for rising antibody titers. *Febrile agglutinins* is a vague term that in most laboratories refers to serologic studies for salmonellosis, brucellosis, and rickettsial diseases. These studies are seldom useful, having low sensitivity and variable specificity. Rising titers of antibody to *Brucella* are usually diagnostic, but false-positive results may be obtained in typhoid fever, tularemia, and yersinial infections. Infection with *Brucella canis* may be missed with standard antibody tests for

Brucella. Salmonella infection elevates antibody titers to the H and O antigens. High titers of antibody to the H antigen persist for years and may reflect previous infection or immunization. The measurement of specific antirickettsial titers should be requested for the diagnosis of Rocky Mountain spotted fever and Q fever. Multiple blood samples—no fewer than three, rarely more than six—should be cultured in the laboratory for at least 2 weeks to ensure that any HACEK-group organisms that may be present have ample time to grow (see Chap. 152). Lysis-centrifugation blood culture techniques should be employed in cases where prior antimicrobial therapy or fungal or atypical mycobacterial infection is suspected. Blood culture media should be supplemented with L-cysteine or pyridoxal to assist in the isolation of nutritionally variant streptococci. It should be noted that sequential cultures positive for multiple organisms may reflect self-injection of contaminated substances. Urine cultures, including cultures for mycobacteria, fungi, and CMV, are indicated. Liver biopsy, even when the results of liver function studies are normal, should be considered and pursued if the diagnosis remains elusive. Specimens should be cultured for mycobacteria and fungi. Likewise, bone marrow

Table 125-5

Causes of FUO in Adults in the United States

Infections
  Localized pyogenic infections
    Appendicitis
    Cat-scratch disease
    Cholangitis
    Cholecystitis
    Dental abscess
    Diverticulitis/abscess
    Lesser sac abscess
    Liver abscess
    Mesenteric lymphadenitis
    Osteomyelitis
    Pancreatic abscess
    Pelvic inflammatory disease
    Perinephric/intrarenal abscess
    Prostatic abscess
    Renal malacoplakia
    Sinusitis
    Subphrenic abscess
    Suppurative thrombophlebitis
    Tuboovarian abscess
  Intravascular infections
    Bacterial aortitis
    Bacterial endocarditis
    Vascular catheter infection
  Systemic bacterial infections
    Bartonellosis
    Brucellosis
    Campylobacter infection
    Cat-scratch disease/bacillary angiomatosis
      (*B. henselae*)
    Gonococcemia
    Legionnaires' disease
    Leptospirosis
    Listeriosis
    Lyme disease
    Melioidosis
    Meningococcemia
    Rat-bite fever
    Relapsing fever
    Salmonellosis
    Syphilis
    Tularemia
    Typhoid fever
    Vibriosis
    Yersinia infection
  Mycobacterial infections
    M. avium/M. intracellulare infections
    Other atypical mycobacterial infections
    Tuberculosis
  Fungal infections
    Aspergillosis
    Blastomycosis
    Candidiasis
    Coccidioidomycosis
    Cryptococcosis
    Histoplasmosis
    Mucormycosis
    Paracoccidioidomycosis
    Sporotrichosis

  Other bacterial infections
    Actinomycosis
    Nocardiosis
    Whipple's disease
  Rickettsial infections
    Ehrlichiosis
    Murine typhus
    Q fever
    Rickettsialpox
    Rocky Mountain spotted fever
  Mycoplasmal infections
  Chlamydial infections
    Lymphogranuloma venereum
    Psittacosis
    TWAR (*C. pneumoniae*) infection
  Viral infections
    Colorado tick fever
    Coxsackievirus group B infection
    Cytomegalovirus infection
    Dengue
    Epstein-Barr virus infection
    Hepatitis A, B, C, D, and E
    Human immunodeficiency virus infection
    Lymphocytic choriomeningitis
    Parvovirus B19 infection
  Parasitic infections
    Amebiasis
    Babesiasis
    Chagas' disease
    Leishmaniasis
    Malaria
    P. carinii infection
    Strongyloidiasis
    Toxocariasis
    Toxoplasmosis
    Trichinosis
  Presumed infections, agent undetermined
    Kawasaki's disease (mucocutaneous lymph
      node syndrome)
    Kikuchi's disease (necrotizing
      lymphadenitis)

Neoplasms
  Malignant
    Colon cancer
    Hepatoma
    Hodgkin's lymphoma
    Immunoblastic lymphadenopathy
    Leukemia
    Lymphomatoid granulomatosis
    Malignant histiocytosis
    Nephroma
    Non-Hodgkin's lymphoma
    Pancreatic cancer
    Sarcoma
  Benign
    Atrial myxoma
    Renal angiomyolipoma

Collagen vascular/hypersensitivity diseases
  Adult Still's disease
  Behçet's disease
  Erythema multiforme
  Erythema nodosum
  Giant-cell arteritis/polymyalgia rheumatica
  Hypersensitivity pneumonitis (e.g., "metal
    fume fever," "farmer's lung," "air-
    conditioner lung")
  Hypersensitivity vasculitis
  Mixed connective-tissue disease
  Polyarteritis nodosa
  Relapsing polychondritis
  Rheumatic fever
  Rheumatoid arthritis
  Systemic lupus erythematosus
  Takayasu's aortitis
  Weber-Christian disease
  Wegener's granulomatosis
Granulomatous diseases
  Crohn's disease
  Idiopathic granulomatous hepatitis
  Midline granuloma
  Sarcoidosis
Miscellaneous conditions
  Aortic dissection
  Drug fever
  Gout
  Hematomas
  Hemolytic diseases/hemoglobinopathies
  Laennec's cirrhosis
  Postmyocardial infarction syndrome
  Recurrent pulmonary emboli
  Subacute thyroiditis (de Quervain's)
  Tissue infarction/necrosis
Inherited and metabolic diseases
  Adrenal insufficiency
  Cyclic neutropenia
  Deafness, urticaria, and amyloidosis
  Fabry's disease
  Familial Mediterranean fever
  Hyperimmunoglobulinemia D and periodic
    fever
  Type V hypertriglyceridemia
Thermoregulatory disorders
  Central
    Brain tumor
    Cerebrovascular accident
    Encephalitis
    Hypothalamic dysfunction
  Peripheral
    Hyperthyroidism
    Pheochromocytoma
Factitious fevers
"Afebrile" FUO (<38.3°C)
Habitual hyperthermia (exaggerated circadian rhythm)

SOURCE: Modified from RK Root, RG Petersdorf, in *Harrison's Principles of Internal Medicine,* 12th ed, JD Wilson et al (eds). New York, McGraw-Hill, 1991.

biopsy (not simple aspiration) should be used to obtain specimens for histology and culture. The blood smear should be examined for *Plasmodium, Babesia, Trypanosoma, Leishmania,* and *Borrelia.*

In an FUO workup, the erythrocyte sedimentation rate (ESR) should be determined. Striking elevation of the ESR and anemia of chronic disease are frequently seen in association with giant-cell arteritis or polymyalgia rheumatica, common causes of FUO in patients over 50 years of age. Still's disease is also suggested by elevations of ESR, leukocytosis, and anemia and is often accompanied by arthralgias, polyserositis (pleuritis, pericarditis), lymphadenopathy, splenomegaly, and rash. Antinuclear antibody should be measured to rule out other collagen vascular diseases. Another cause of an extremely high ESR may be a "false-positive" value attributable to a cold agglutinin with a broad thermal amplitude. The ESR test is nonspecific, yielding values that depend on certain serum proteins (most notably fibrinogen) known to interfere with the zeta-potential that keeps erythrocytes from clumping. When fibrinogen levels go up, the zeta-potential is inhibited, erythrocytes clump, and the ESR is high. A cold agglutinin, by binding to erythrocytes, can produce a "false-positive" agglutinin that mimics an acute-phase response; cold agglutinins may be seen in *Mycoplasma* and Epstein-Barr virus infections and in lymphomas.

With rare exceptions, the intermediate-strength purified protein derivative (PPD) skin test should be used to screen for tuberculosis in patients with classic FUO. Concurrent control tests, such as the CMI test (Connaught Labs, Swiftwater, PA), which is especially effective, should be employed. It should be kept in mind that a negative PPD skin test plus negative results of the control tests may be seen with miliary tuberculosis, sarcoidosis, Hodgkin's disease, malnutrition, or AIDS. Noninvasive procedures should include an upper gastrointestinal contrast study with small-bowel follow-through and barium enema to include the terminal ileum and cecum. Chest x-rays should be repeated if new symptoms arise. In some cases, pulmonary function studies may be necessary. A diminished carbon monoxide diffusing capacity (DL_{CO}) may indicate a restrictive lung disease such as sarcoidosis, even with a normal chest x-ray. In such cases, transbronchial biopsy may prove diagnostic. Flexible colonoscopy may be advisable, since colon carcinoma is a cause of FUO and easily escapes detection by ultrasound and CT.

CT of the chest and abdomen should be performed. If a spinal or paraspinal lesion is suspected, however, MRI is preferred. MRI may be superior to CT in demonstrating intraabdominal abscesses and aortic dissection, but the relative utility of MRI and CT in the diagnosis of FUO is unknown. At present, it would appear that abdominal CT should be used unless MRI is specifically indicated. Ultrasonography of the abdomen is useful for the investigation of the hepatobiliary tract, kidneys, spleen, and pelvis. Echocardiography may be helpful in an evaluation for bacterial endocarditis, pericarditis, nonbacterial thrombotic endocarditis, and atrial myxomas. Transesophageal echocardiography is especially sensitive for these lesions.

Radionuclide scanning procedures using technetium (Tc)-99m sulfur colloid, gallium (Ga) citrate, or indium (In) 111–labeled leukocytes or immunoglobulin may be useful in identifying and/or localizing inflammatory processes. In a recent study, Ga scintigraphy yielded useful diagnostic information in almost one-third of cases, and it was suggested that this procedure might actually be used before other imaging techniques if no specific organ is suspected of being abnormal. Tc bone scan should be undertaken to look for osteomyelitis or bony metastases; Ga scan may be used to identify sarcoidosis or *P. carinii* in lungs or Crohn's disease in the abdomen. ^{111}In-labeled white blood cell scan may be used to locate abscesses; ^{111}In-labeled immunoglobulin scan also shows promise in this regard. With both Ga and In white blood cell scans, false-positive and false-negative findings are common.

Biopsy of the liver and bone marrow should be considered routine in the workup of FUO if the studies mentioned above are unrevealing or if fever is prolonged. It goes without saying that areas of suspected abnormality should be sampled for pathologic examination whenever

practical. When possible, a section of the tissue block should be retained for further sections or stains. Polymerase chain reaction technology makes it possible to identify and speciate mycobacterial DNA in paraffin-embedded, fixed tissues. Thus, in some cases, it is possible to make a retrospective diagnosis based on studies of long-fixed pathologic tissues. In a patient over age 50 (or occasionally in a younger patient) with the appropriate symptoms and laboratory findings, "blind biopsy" of one or both temporal arteries may yield a diagnosis of arteritis. If noted, tenderness or decreased pulsation should guide the selection of a site for biopsy. Lymph node biopsy may be helpful if nodes are enlarged, but inguinal nodes are often palpable and are seldom diagnostically useful.

Exploratory laparotomy has been performed when all other diagnostic procedures fail but has largely been replaced by modern imaging and guided-biopsy techniques.

℞ TREATMENT

Patients with neutropenic FUO may be treated by a variety of empirical protocols. The regimen usually combines an aminoglycoside with an antipseudomonal β-lactam antibiotic or consists of imipenem or ceftazidime alone. Vancomycin should be added to the regimen if intravenous catheter–associated infection is suspected. If vancomycin is administered and fever continues, the addition of amphotericin B should be considered.

Empirical therapy for nosocomial FUO must be guided by the clinical situation. While empirical antibiotic therapy may be indicated, it should be remembered that complications of drug therapy (including *C. difficile*–associated colitis and drug-related fever), rather than infection, may be the cause of the fever.

The treatment of HIV-associated FUO depends on many factors and is discussed in Chap. 308. MAI, CMV, drugs administered to the patient, and HIV itself are probably the most common causes of FUO in this group once *P. carinii* infection, cryptococcosis, toxoplasmosis, tuberculosis, and bacterial sinusitis have been ruled out. Discontinuing or changing drugs is often necessary, and empirical therapy for these infections may be indicated.

The emphasis in patients with classic FUO is on continued observation and examination, with the avoidance of "shotgun" empirical therapy. Empirical treatment for endocarditis, for example, should be avoided unless there are specific reasons beyond fever to invoke this diagnosis. Every patient with FUO should undergo an exhaustive examination for tuberculosis. If the PPD skin test is positive or if granulomatous hepatitis or other granulomatous disease is present with anergy (and sarcoid seems unlikely), then a therapeutic trial with isoniazid and rifampin (and possibly a third drug) should be undertaken, with treatment usually continued for up to 6 weeks. A failure of the fever to respond over this period suggests an alternative diagnosis.

Q fever may cause noncaseating granulomatous hepatitis. Doxycycline is the drug of choice for a therapeutic trial if this etiology is suspected.

The response of rheumatic fever and Still's disease to aspirin and nonsteroidal anti-inflammatory agents (NSAIDs) may be dramatic. The effects of glucocorticoids on temporal arteritis, polymyalgia rheumatica, and granulomatous hepatitis are equally dramatic. Colchicine is highly effective in preventing attacks of familial Mediterranean fever but is of little use once an attack is well under way. The ability of glucocorticoids and NSAIDs to mask fever while permitting the spread of infection dictates that their use be avoided unless infection has been largely ruled out and unless inflammatory disease is both probable and debilitating or threatening.

When no underlying source of FUO is identified after prolonged observation (>6 months), the prognosis is generally good, however vexing the fever may be to the patient. Under such circumstances, debilitating symptoms are treated with NSAIDs, and glucocorticoids are the last resort. The initiation of empirical therapy does not mark the end of the diagnostic workup; rather, it commits the physician to continued thoughtful reexamination and evaluation. Patience, compassion, equanimity, and intellectual flexibility are indispensable attributes for the clinician in dealing successfully with FUO.

BIBLIOGRAPHY

ADUAN R et al: Prolonged fever of unknown origin. Clin Res 26:558A, 1978
—— et al: Factitious fever and self-induced infection. Ann Intern Med 90:230, 1979

CUNHA BA: Fever of unknown origin. Infect Dis Clin North Am 10:111, 1996

DATA FL, THORNE DA: Gastrointestinal tract radionuclide activity on In-111 labeled leukocyte imaging: Clinical significance in patients with fever of unknown origin. Radiology 160:635, 1986

DEKLEIJN EM et al: Utility of scintigraphic methods in patients with fever of unknown origin. Arch Intern Med 155:1989, 1995

DINARELLO CA, WOLFF SM: Fever of unknown origin, in *Principles and Practice of Infectious Diseases,* 3d ed, GL Mandell et al (eds). New York, Wiley, 1990, pp 468–479

DURACK DT, STREET AC: Fever of unknown origin—reexamined and redefined, in *Current Clinical Topics in Infectious Diseases,* JS Remington, MN Swartz (eds). Cambridge, MA, Blackwell, 1991

GRANOWITZ EV et al: Interleukin-1 receptor antagonist production during experimental endotoxaemia. Lancet 338:1423, 1991

HOLTZ T et al: Liver biopsy in fever of unknown origin. J Clin Gastroenterol 17:29, 1993

HOWARD P JR et al: Fever of unknown origin: A prospective study of 100 patients. Tex Med 73:56, 1977

HUGGINS JW et al: Prospective, double-blind, concurrent placebo-controlled clinical trial of intravenous ribavirin therapy of hemorrhagic fever with renal syndrome. J Infect Dis 164:1119, 1991

HUGHES WT et al: Guidelines for the use of antimicrobial agents in neutropenic patients with unexplained fever. J Infect Dis 161:381, 1990

ISAAC B et al (eds): *Unexplained Fever.* Boca Raton, CRC Press, 1991

JACOBY GA, SWARTZ MN: Fever of undetermined origin. N Engl J Med 289:1407, 1973

KNOCKAERT DC, VANNESTE LJ: Fever of unknown origin in the 1980s. Arch Intern Med 152:51, 1992
—— et al: Fever of unknown origin in elderly patients. J Am Geriatr Soc 41:1187, 1993
—— et al: Clinical value of gallium-67 scintigraphy in evaluation of fever of unknown origin. Clin Infect Dis 18:601, 1994

LARSON EB, FEATHERSTONE HJ: Fever of undetermined origin: Diagnosis and follow-up of 105 cases, 1970–80. Medicine 61:269, 1982

MEYERS SP, WIENER SN: Diagnosis of hematogenous pyogenic vertebral osteomyelitis by magnetic resonance imaging. Arch Intern Med 151:683, 1991

MITCHELL MA et al: Bilateral renal parenchymal malacoplakia presenting as fever of unknown origin: Case report and review. Clin Infect Dis 18:704, 1994

ORR PH et al: Febrile urinary infection in the institutionalized elderly. Am J Med 100:71, 1996

PETERSDORF RC: Fever of unknown origin. An old friend revisited [editorial]. Arch Intern Med 152:21, 1992
—— RG, BEESON PB: Fever of unexplained origin. Medicine 40:1, 1961

ROSENBERG MR, GREEN M: Neuroleptic malignant syndrome. Arch Intern Med 149:1927, 1989

ROWLAND MD, DEL BENE VE: Use of body computed tomography to evaluate fever of unknown origin. J Infect Dis 156:408, 1987

RUBIN RH et al: ¹¹¹In-labeled nonspecific immunoglobulin scanning in the detection of focal infection. N Engl J Med 321:935, 1989

SABBOOR SA et al: Detection of mycobacterial DNA in sarcoidosis and tuberculosis with polymerase chain reaction. Lancet 339:1012, 1992

SCHMIDT KG et al: Indium-111 granulocyte scintigraphy in the evaluation of patients with fever of undetermined origin. Scand J Infect Dis 19:339, 1987

SIMON HB, WOLFF SM: Granulomatous hepatitis and prolonged fever of unknown origin: A study of 13 patients. Medicine 52:1, 1973

SMITH JW: Southwestern internal medicine conference: Fever of undetermined origin: Not what it used to be. Am J Med Sci 292:56, 1986

SPACH DH et al: *Bartonella (Rochalimaea) quintana* bacteremia in inner-city patients with chronic alcoholism. N Engl J Med 332:424, 1995

STEINMETZ HT et al: Increase in interleukin-6 serum level preceding fever in granulocytopenia and correlation with death from sepsis. J Infect Dis 171:225, 1995

WEINSTEIN L: Clinically benign fever of unknown origin: A personal retrospective. Rev Infect Dis 7:692, 1985

WILSON ME: *A World Guide to Infections: Diseases, Distribution, Diagnosis.* New York, Oxford University Press, 1991

WOLFF SM et al: A syndrome of periodic hypothalamic discharge. Am J Med 36:956, 1964
—— et al: Unusual etiologies of fever and their evaluation. Annu Rev Med 26:277, 1975

ZANGWILL KM et al: Cat scratch disease in Connecticut—epidemiology, risk factors, and evaluation of a new diagnostic test. N Engl J Med 329:8, 1993

126 *Donald Kaye*

INFECTIVE ENDOCARDITIS

Infective endocarditis is a disease that produces vegetations on the endocardium. It is virtually always fatal if untreated. A heart valve is usually involved, but the infection may develop on a septal defect or on the mural endocardium. Infection of an arteriovenous shunt or coarctation of the aorta is more properly called *endarteritis* but produces a similar clinical syndrome. The discussion of endocarditis in this chapter also applies to endarteritis.

CLASSIFICATION

Endocarditis can be classified in three categories: native valve endocarditis, endocarditis in intravenous drug abusers, and prosthetic valve endocarditis. These categories have different infecting microorganisms and run different courses. Endocarditis also can be classified as acute or subacute. Acute endocarditis most frequently is caused by *Staphylococcus aureus*, occurs on a normal heart valve, is rapidly destructive, produces metastatic foci, and, if untreated, is fatal in less than 6 weeks. Subacute endocarditis usually is caused by viridans streptococci, occurs on damaged valves, does not produce metastatic foci, and, if untreated, takes more than 6 weeks—perhaps as long as a year—to be fatal. Correlations between organism and course are not perfect; viridans streptococci can be associated with an acute course and *S. aureus* with a subacute course. The most important basis for classification is the infecting organism (e.g., *S. aureus* endocarditis), because the organism has implications for therapy as well as course.

NATIVE VALVE ENDOCARDITIS Etiology Although almost any bacteria can produce endocarditis, streptococci, enterococci, and staphylococci account for the vast majority of cases.

Streptococci Streptococci cause about 55 percent of cases of native valve endocarditis in patients who do not abuse intravenous drugs. Viridans streptococci [most commonly *Streptococcus sanguis*, *Streptococcus mutans*, *Streptococcus mitis* (formerly *S. mitior*), or *Streptococcus milleri*] account for about 75 percent of these cases; *Streptococcus bovis* and other streptococci cause 20 and 5 percent, respectively. Viridans streptococci are normal inhabitants of the oropharynx and generally are highly susceptible to penicillin. Two group D streptococci, *S. bovis* and *Streptococcus equinus*, are also highly susceptible to penicillin G. *S. bovis* endocarditis occurs in elderly individuals; 80 percent of cases are in persons over 60 years of age. More than a third of these individuals have a malignant or premalignant gastrointestinal lesion, most often colonic cancer or a villous adenoma or polyp of the colon.

Group A beta-hemolytic streptococci attack normal or damaged heart valves and may cause their rapid destruction. Group B streptococci, which have been reported more frequently as a cause of endocarditis in recent years, also attack normal valves and result in large, friable vegetations and large emboli. Other streptococci are much more likely to infect damaged valves and rarely cause rapid valve destruction. *S. milleri* can cause metastatic abscesses, which are uncommon with other streptococci.

Enterococci Enterococci cause about 6 percent of cases of native valve endocarditis. Enterococci are alpha-, beta-, or gamma-hemolytic and are normal inhabitants of the gastrointestinal tract, the anterior urethra, and occasionally the mouth. All enterococci are in Lancefield's group D and can be distinguished from streptococci by biochemical tests. They are relatively resistant to penicillin G; an aminoglycoside must be added to achieve a bactericidal effect. Enterococcal endocarditis is more common among males, who develop infection at an average age of 60 years. Many patients have a recent history of genitourinary tract manipulation, trauma, or disease (e.g., cystoscopy, urethral catheterization, prostatectomy, abortion, pregnancy, or cesarean section).

Staphylococci Staphylococci cause about 30 percent of cases of native valve endocarditis (with *S. aureus* 5 to 10 times more frequent than *Staphylococcus epidermidis*). *S. aureus* attacks normal or damaged heart valves, often causing rapid destruction. The course is often fulminant, with death from bacteremia within days or from heart failure within weeks. Abscesses are common at multiple sites (e.g., kidneys, lungs, and brain). *S. epidermidis* usually infects prosthetic valves.

HACEK organisms The HACEK group of bacteria (*Haemophilus, Actinobacillus, Cardiobacterium, Eikenella,* and *Kingella*) are part of the oropharyngeal flora. They produce endocarditis with a subacute presentation and large vegetations. HACEK organisms are difficult to isolate from blood (see Chap. 152).

Other bacteria Almost all species of bacteria are occasional causes of acute or subacute endocarditis, including *Streptococcus pneumoniae, Neisseria gonorrhoeae,* enteric gram-negative bacilli, *Pseudomonas, Salmonella, Streptobacillus, Serratia marcescens, Bacteroides, Brucella, Mycobacterium, Neisseria meningitidis, Listeria, Legionella,* and *Corynebacterium.*

Fungi Fungi rarely cause native valve endocarditis in persons who do not abuse intravenous drugs. However, *Candida* and *Aspergillus* endocarditis can occur in patients with intravascular catheters who frequently have received glucocorticoids, broad-spectrum antimicrobial drugs, or cytotoxic agents. The course is usually subacute. Large friable vegetations are common and give rise to large emboli, often to the lower extremities. The prognosis is grave, partly because of the relatively poor activity of available antifungal agents.

Other microorganisms Spirochetes (e.g., *Spirillum minus*), cell wall–deficient bacteria, rickettsiae (*Coxiella burnetii*), and chlamydiae (*Chlamydia psittaci, Chlamydia pneumoniae,* and *Chlamydia trachomatis*) are rare causes of endocarditis.

Epidemiology Of patients with native valve endocarditis, more are male than female, and most are over age 50. Endocarditis is uncommon in children.

Between 60 and 80 percent of patients have an identifiable predisposing cardiac lesion. *Rheumatic valvular disease* accounts for about 25 percent of cases. The mitral valve is most commonly involved and the aortic valve next most commonly. The tricuspid valve is involved in rare cases.

Congenital heart disease other than mitral valve prolapse is the underlying lesion in about 10 to 20 percent of patients with endocarditis. Predisposing lesions include patent ductus arteriosus, ventricular septal defect, tetralogy of Fallot, coarctation of the aorta, pulmonary stenosis, and bicuspid aortic valve but not uncomplicated atrial septal defect. *Mitral valve prolapse* is the underlying lesion in about 10 to 33 percent of cases.

Degenerative heart disease predisposes to endocarditis. *Calcific aortic stenosis* (from degenerative disease or bicuspid valve) is an important lesion in the elderly. Other predisposing but unusual lesions are *asymmetric septal hypertrophy, Marfan's syndrome,* and *syphilitic aortic valve. Arterioarterial* or *arteriovenous fistulas* are also reported as underlying lesions. In 20 to 40 percent of patients with infective endocarditis, *no underlying heart disease* can be recognized.

ENDOCARDITIS IN INTRAVENOUS DRUG ABUSERS Drug abusers with endocarditis are frequently young males. The skin is most often the source of microorganisms responsible for endocarditis in these cases; contamination of drugs is less common. *S. aureus* causes more than 50 percent of cases, streptococci and enterococci about 20 percent, and fungi (mainly *Candida*) and gram-negative bacilli (usually *Pseudomonas* species) about 6 percent each. Infection with multiple organisms is common. The onset is usually acute. Only about 20 percent of addicts experiencing their first episode of endocarditis have previously damaged heart valves. The tricuspid valve is infected in about 50 percent of cases, the aortic valve in 25 percent, the mitral valve in about 20 percent, and multiple valves in the rest. More than 75 percent of patients with *S. aureus* infection and a much lower percentage of those infected with other organisms have tricuspid valve endocarditis. Pulmonary emboli or pneumonia consequent to septic pulmonary emboli is common in tricuspid valve endocarditis, and murmurs are frequently absent.

PROSTHETIC VALVE ENDOCARDITIS Any intravascular prosthesis predisposes to endocarditis and makes cure difficult. Infections of prosthetic valves now account for 10 to 20 percent of cases of endocarditis. Intravascular sutures, pacemaker wires, and Teflon-Silastic tubes also can be foci of infection. Most patients with prosthetic valve endocarditis are males over age 60. Endocarditis occurs in 1 to 2 percent of these patients during the first year after surgery and in about 0.5 percent per year thereafter. Aortic valve prostheses are much more likely to be involved than mitral valve prostheses. The infection is usually on the suture line.

Early-onset endocarditis (onset of symptoms within 60 days of surgery) is usually a consequence of valve contamination during the procedure or of perioperative bacteremia. *Late-onset endocarditis* (onset of symptoms after 60 days) may have the same pathogenesis as early endocarditis (especially during the first year) but with a long incubation period; it also may result from transient bacteremia.

About half of all episodes of early-onset endocarditis and one-third of all episodes of late-onset endocarditis are caused by staphylococci, and *S. epidermidis* is more frequently involved than *S. aureus.* Gram-negative bacilli cause up to 15 percent, and fungi (most commonly *Candida*) up to 10 percent, of early-onset cases; they are less common in late-onset endocarditis. A prosthetic valve may malfunction because of large vegetations (often fungal). Streptococci are the most frequent single cause of late-onset endocarditis (about 40 percent of cases) but are uncommon in early-onset endocarditis.

Early-onset prosthetic valve endocarditis is often associated with valvular dysfunction or dehiscence and a fulminant course. Although late-onset endocarditis may be similarly fulminant, the course is commonly indistinguishable from that of endocarditis in patients without prosthetic valves, especially when the infecting organism is a streptococcus.

PATHOGENESIS AND PATHOLOGY

The characteristic lesions of infective endocarditis are vegetations on valves or elsewhere on the endocardium. The disease usually is secondary to the colonization by microorganisms of sterile vegetations composed of platelets and fibrin. Sterile vegetations, which represent *nonbacterial thrombotic endocarditis,* form over areas of trauma to the endothelium (from intracardiac foreign bodies, for example), in areas of turbulence (as on deformed valves), over scars, or in the setting of wasting disease, particularly malignancy (marantic endocarditis).

Infection of a sterile vegetation is most likely when bacteremia involves bacteria that adhere well to platelets, fibrin, and fibronectin. The vegetation of infective endocarditis then results from deposition of platelets and fibrin over the bacteria, which forms a "protected site" into which phagocytic cells penetrate poorly.

Endocarditis tends to occur in high-pressure areas (i.e., on the left side of the heart) and downstream from sites where blood flows at high velocity through a narrow orifice from a high- to a low-pressure chamber (e.g., distal to the constriction in coarctation of the aorta). Endocarditis is unusual in sites with a small pressure gradient, as in atrial septal defects. The disease occurs more frequently in patients with valvular incompetence than in those with pure stenosis, and the lesion characteristically is located on the atrial side of a regurgitant mitral valve and on the ventricular surface of a regurgitant aortic valve. A high-velocity stream of blood can produce satellite infected lesions at distant points of impact.

Microorganisms that possess little pathogenicity in other situations (e.g., viridans streptococci) usually implant only on deformed heart valves exhibiting nonbacterial thrombotic endocarditis, but more virulent microorganisms (e.g., *S. aureus* and *S. pneumoniae*) can infect apparently normal valves.

Transient bacteremia is common in various infections and during traumatic procedures involving epithelial surfaces that are colonized by a bacterial flora (oropharynx, genitourinary and gastrointestinal tracts, and skin). For example, after trauma to tissues of the mouth, viridans streptococci are the most common bacteria isolated from blood, either alone or—more often—mixed with other bacteria. The frequency and magnitude of bacteremia are related to the severity of periodontal disease and the severity of trauma. The portal of entry for the infecting organism in the initiating episode of bacteremia is usually not apparent in viridans streptococcal endocarditis. Dental procedures, the most common cause of apparent portals of entry, precede viridans streptococcal endocarditis in only 15 to 20 percent of cases.

Bacteremia also is common with prostatic surgery, cystoscopy, urethral dilation or catheterization, and procedures involving the female reproductive tract. The infecting organisms are usually enterococci and gram-negative bacilli. About 50 percent of patients with enterococcal endocarditis have recently undergone surgery or instrumentation of the genitourinary or gastrointestinal tract. About 35 percent of patients with staphylococcal endocarditis have had a preceding staphylococcal infection at a remote site.

The clinical features of endocarditis result from the vegetations and from an immune reaction to the infection. Extensive vegetations, especially in fungal endocarditis, may occlude the valve orifice. Rapid valve destruction with consequent regurgitation may occur, especially with *S. aureus*. Healing may cause scar formation, with subsequent valvular stenosis or regurgitation. Infection may extend into the myocardium, producing burrowing abscesses. Conduction abnormalities, fistulas (between chambers of the heart and the pericardium or major vessels), or rupture of the chordae, of a papillary muscle, or of the ventricular septum may result.

Pieces of vegetation may break off and cause embolisms in the heart, brain, kidney, spleen, liver, extremities, and lung (in right-sided endocarditis). Infarcts and occasionally abscesses result. Septic embolization to the vasa vasorum or direct bacterial invasion of the arterial wall may lead to the formation of mycotic aneurysms, which may rupture. Mycotic aneurysms most often develop in the cerebral arteries, aorta, sinuses of Valsalva, ligated ductus arteriosus, and superior mesenteric, splenic, coronary, and pulmonary arteries.

Patients with endocarditis usually have high titers of antibody to the infecting microorganism. This factor contributes to formation of circulating immune complexes that may result in glomerulonephritis (focal, membranoproliferative, or diffuse), arthritis, or various mucocutaneous manifestations of vasculitis.

Myocarditis may be due to small coronary-artery emboli, myocardial abscesses, or immune-complex vasculitis.

CLINICAL MANIFESTATIONS

Symptoms of endocarditis generally start within 2 weeks of the precipitating event. The frequencies of occurrence of some prominent clinical manifestations are shown in Table 126-1. With organisms of low pathogenicity (e.g., viridans streptococci), the *onset* is usually gradual, with mild fever and malaise. With organisms of high pathogenicity (e.g., *S. aureus*), the onset is often acute, with high fever. *Fever* is present in almost all patients with endocarditis (except occasionally in the elderly or in patients with renal failure, congestive heart failure, or severe debility). The fever is usually low-grade (less than 39.4°C) except in acute disease. Arthralgias and myalgias, especially low-back pain, are common, and arthritis develops occasionally.

Cardiac murmurs are almost always present except in patients with early acute endocarditis and in intravenous drug abusers with tricuspid valve infection. True changes in murmurs or the appearance of a new murmur is uncommon except in acute endocarditis, where a new murmur (particularly aortic regurgitation) is frequent. Changes in intensities of murmurs are often due to changes in heart rate and/or cardiac output (e.g., from anemia) and not necessarily to progressive valvular damage.

Splenomegaly and *petechiae* tend to occur in disease of long duration. Petechiae are most frequently found on the conjunctivae, palate, buccal mucosa, and upper extremities. *Splinter hemorrhages* are subungual, linear, dark-red streaks that may appear in endocarditis but also commonly result from trauma. *Roth's spots* are oval, retinal hem-

Table 126-1

Frequencies of Occurrence of Prominent Clinical and Laboratory Manifestations in Endocarditis

Manifestation	Percentage of Cases
CLINICAL MANIFESTATIONS	
Fever	>95
Arthralgias and/or myalgias	25–45
Murmur	>85
Splenomegaly	25–60
Petechiae	20–40
Splinter hemorrhages	10–30
Roth's spots	<5
Osler's nodes	10–25
Janeway lesions	<5
Clubbing	10–20
Clinically apparent emboli	25–45
Neurologic manifestations	20–40
LABORATORY MANIFESTATIONS	
Anemia	70–90
Leukocytosis	20–30
Proteinuria	50–65
Microscopic hematuria	30–50
Elevated serum creatinine level	10–20
Elevated erythrocyte sedimentation rate	>90
Rheumatoid factor	50
Circulating immune complexes	65–100
Decreased serum complement level	5–40

orrhages with a clear, pale center; they may also occur in connective tissue disease and severe anemia. Likewise, *Osler's nodes* (small, tender nodules, usually on the finger or toe pads, which persist for hours to days) may also develop in other diseases. *Janeway lesions* are small hemorrhages with a slightly nodular character on the palms and soles and are most commonly seen in acute endocarditis. *Clubbing* of the fingers is reported in some patients with long-standing disease. *Embolic episodes* may occur during or after therapy. Emboli to large arteries (e.g., femoral arteries) are often the result of fungal endocarditis, with its large, friable vegetations. Pulmonary emboli are common in drug abusers with right-sided endocarditis and may be seen in patients with left-sided endocarditis who have left-to-right cardiac shunts.

Mycotic aneurysms occur in about 10 percent of patients. Symptoms are usually lacking but may be those of an expanding mass. The aneurysms can rupture during or even years after therapy. *Neurologic manifestations* are more common with left-sided endocarditis than with right-sided disease and with *S. aureus* infection than with viridans streptococcal infection. Clinically apparent cerebral emboli occur in about 20 percent of patients; encephalopathy (from microemboli with or without microabscess formation) in 10 percent; leakage from a mycotic aneurysm in fewer than 5 percent; and meningitis or a macroscopic brain abscess in fewer than 5 percent. Major cerebral emboli as well as mycotic aneurysms usually involve the middle cerebral artery system. Most patients with brain abscess or purulent meningitis have *S. aureus* endocarditis.

Heart failure may occur during the course of endocarditis or long after its cure. Contributing factors are valve destruction, myocarditis, coronary artery emboli with infarction, and myocardial abscesses. *Myocardial abscess* is most common in acute endocarditis (particularly that caused by *S. aureus*) or with a prosthesis. Conduction defects may result from ventricular septal invasion secondary to extension from a valve (most frequently the aortic valve). A valve-ring abscess—or, less commonly, a myocardial abscess—may extend into the epicardium and cause pericarditis. Echocardiography may be helpful in the diagnosis of myocardial abscess, and surgery is often indicated, especially with a prosthesis. *Renal disease* exists in most patients with endocarditis and is due to renal emboli or immune-complex glomerulonephritis. Renal insufficiency may result.

LABORATORY FEATURES

The frequencies of occurrence of some laboratory manifestations are shown in Table 126-1. Normocytic normochromic anemia is usual in infective endocarditis. The white blood cell and differential counts are often normal. However, in acute disease, leukocytosis without anemia may be present. Proteinuria and/or microscopic hematuria is found in most patients, and the serum creatinine level may be elevated. The erythrocyte sedimentation rate is almost always elevated except in cases with heart failure.

About 50 percent of patients with endocarditis of at least 6 weeks' duration have a positive serum test for rheumatoid factor, and most have circulating immune complexes, which tend to disappear with cure. The serum complement level may be decreased, especially with diffuse glomerulonephritis. Bacteria can be seen inside leukocytes in buffy-coat preparations of blood in about 50 percent of cases of endocarditis.

The critical diagnostic finding in endocarditis is bacteremia or fungemia. Blood cultures are positive in more than 95 percent of patients. The bacteremia is continuous; if any cultures are positive, all are likely to be positive. There is no advantage to obtaining samples for cultures at any particular time or body temperature. Arterial blood or bone marrow offers no advantage over antecubital vein blood.

In suspected subacute disease and in the absence of previous therapy, three sets of blood samples for culturing should be obtained over 3 to 6 h and therapy initiated. With previous therapy, it is justifiable to delay treatment until an attempt has been made to obtain positive blood cultures. In general, in acute disease, therapy should not be delayed for more than 2 to 3 h while cultures are obtained. Only one culture should be performed for each venipuncture; anaerobic as well as aerobic techniques should be used. Samples should be collected at least 30 to 60 min apart to demonstrate continuous bacteremia. The rate of positive cultures is increased by observation of the cultures over 3 weeks, with periodic sampling for Gram's stain and subculture even in the absence of turbidity.

Blood cultures may be negative in infections with fastidious organisms, such as *Haemophilus parainfluenzae*. Fifty percent of patients with *Candida* endocarditis and almost all with *Aspergillus, Histoplasma,* or *C. burnetii* endocarditis have negative blood cultures. With fungi, large peripheral emboli are common, necessitating embolectomy. Histologic examination and culture of the embolus may be diagnostic. Serologic tests for *C. burnetii* and *C. psittaci* are positive in endocarditis caused by these organisms.

Echocardiography has added a great deal to the ability to confirm or reject a diagnosis of infective endocarditis. All patients in whom infective endocarditis is suspected should at least undergo baseline transthoracic echocardiography (TTE) to determine the size and location of the vegetation, to obtain a picture that can be used for comparative purposes should cardiac complications arise, and to define underlying cardiac abnormalities. Transesophageal echocardiography (TEE) can detect vegetations as small as 1 to 1.5 mm, whereas the smallest size detectable by TTE is 2 to 3 mm. It follows that TEE is much more sensitive than TTE in detecting vegetations (90 percent vs. about 65 percent). This difference is even greater for the detection of prosthetic valve vegetations (about 75 percent vs. about 25 percent) and myocardial abscesses (85 percent vs. 25 percent). TEE should be performed for any patient with suspected infective endocarditis who has a prosthetic valve, for any patient with suspected myocardial or valve-ring abscess, and for any patient in whom TTE is technically unsatisfactory. In addition, any candidate for cardiac surgery should undergo TEE to delineate the cardiac architecture. Finally, a negative result of TEE

Clinical Diagnosis of Infective Endocarditis

I. *Definite infective endocarditis:* Two major criteria *or* one major and three minor criteria *or* five minor criteria
  A. Major criteria
    1. Isolation of viridans streptococci, *S. bovis,* HACEK-group organisms, or (in the absence of a primary focus) community-acquired *S. aureus* or *Enterococcus* from two separate blood cultures *or* isolation of a microorganism consistent with endocarditis in (1) blood cultures ≥12 h apart or (2) all of three or most of four or more blood cultures, with first and last at least 1 h apart
    2. Evidence of endocardial involvement on echocardiography: oscillating intracardiac mass or abscess or new partial dehiscence of prosthetic valve *or* new valvular regurgitation
  B. Minor criteria
    1. Predisposing lesion or intravenous drug use
    2. Fever of ≥38.0°C
    3. Major arterial emboli, septic pulmonary infarcts, mycotic aneurysm, intracranial hemorrhage, conjunctival hemorrhages, Janeway lesions
    4. Glomerulonephritis, Osler's nodes, Roth's spots, rheumatoid factor
    5. Positive blood cultures not meeting the major criterion (excluding single cultures positive for organisms that do not typically cause endocarditis) or serologic evidence of active infection with an organism that causes endocarditis
    6. Echocardiogram consistent with endocarditis but not meeting the major criterion
II. *Possible infective endocarditis:* Findings that fall short of "definite" but do not fall into the "rejected" category
III. *Rejected:* Alternative diagnosis or resolution of syndrome or no evidence of infective endocarditis at surgery or autopsy with ≤4 days of antibiotic therapy

SOURCE: After Durack et al.

is strong evidence against infective endocarditis in patients with an equivocal syndrome.

Serial phonocardiography and cineradiography may be useful in evaluating infection on prosthetic valves. Disappearance of an opening click or sound produced by a closing valve suggests the presence of a vegetation. With dehiscence, cineradiography of the valve will show abnormal motion.

DIAGNOSIS

Recently introduced clinical criteria for the definitive diagnosis of infective endocarditis are shown in Table 126-2. These criteria depend heavily on blood culture and cardiac echocardiography.

Endocarditis should be suspected in patients who have a heart murmur and unexplained fever lasting for at least 1 week and in febrile intravenous drug abusers, even in the absence of a murmur.

Atrial myxoma, nonbacterial thrombotic endocarditis, acute rheumatic fever, lupus erythematosus, and sickle cell disease can duplicate the syndrome of infective endocarditis. Any patient with an existing heart murmur can develop fever related to another occult illness or to drugs. Therefore, in the absence of positive blood cultures and/or echocardiographic evidence, a search must be made for other causes of fever.

Following cardiac surgery, fever may be related to infection at other sites, to the postcardiotomy syndrome, or to a "postpump syndrome."

 TREATMENT

Principles of Therapy Cure of endocarditis requires eradication of all microorganisms from the vegetation. Therefore, microbicidal drug regimens must be used in high enough concentrations and for a long enough duration to sterilize the vegetation. Regimens including penicillins, cephalosporins, and vancomycin give far better results than are obtained when these agents cannot be used because of resistant organisms or drug reactions.

The minimal inhibitory concentration (MIC) and minimal bactericidal concentration (MBC) should be determined. In monitoring the therapeutic efficacy of a drug regimen, it may be useful to measure the bactericidal activity of the patient's serum against his or her isolate. A bactericidal titer of ≥1:8 in serum drawn 30 min after drug infusion probably indicates adequate therapy. While this determination is not necessary in most cases, it may be useful when infection is caused by organisms other than gram-positive cocci, when treatment has failed, or when the regimens being used do not include penicillins, cephalosporins, or vancomycin. Except in unusual circumstances, antibiotic administration should be parenteral to guarantee adequate absorption of drugs. The infecting microorganism should be saved for future testing (e.g., assessment of serum antibacterial activity, evaluation of different antibiotics, or comparison with a strain isolated during relapse).

Specific Antimicrobial Regimens THERAPY BEFORE CULTURE RESULTS ARE KNOWN The treatment of subacute infective endocarditis on a native valve while culture results are awaited should cover enterococci, which are more resistant to antibiotics than streptococci.

With an acute course, therapy should be directed against *S. aureus*. In intravenous drug abusers, initial therapy should be directed against *S. aureus*, and gentamicin (in a dose of 1.7 mg/kg every 8 h) should be included for the coverage of gram-negative bacilli. In many cities, most *S. aureus* isolates from drug abusers are methicillin-resistant, and vancomycin must be used. With prosthetic valves, vancomycin plus gentamicin should be used because of the high incidence of methicillin-resistant *S. epidermidis* and the need to cover enterococci.

Once the organism is isolated, the regimen should be altered appropriately. If cultures remain sterile and culture-negative endocarditis is likely, treatment is continued provided that the response is adequate.

STREPTOCOCCI WITH PENICILLIN G MICs OF ≤0.1 μg/mL Most streptococci are inhibited by concentrations of penicillin G of 0.1 μg/mL. Suggested regimens are listed in Table 126-3. Penicillin G or ceftriaxone alone for 4 weeks (regimens A and C in Table 126-3) gives cure rates of 98 percent. Addition of gentamicin to penicillin (regimen B) results in a more rapid bactericidal effect and gives equivalent cure rates in 2 weeks. Regimen B should be standard for uncomplicated infection treated in the hospital, but regimen A or C is preferred in patients likely to have side effects with aminoglycosides (i.e., those with renal insufficiency or eighth-nerve disease and those older than 65 years). Regimen B should not be used in patients with complications (e.g., metastatic abscesses). Regimen C is preferred for home treatment and can also be used in patients with a history of a delayed rash in response to penicillin. Regimen D should be used in patients with a history of anaphylaxis to penicillin.

STREPTOCOCCI WITH PENICILLIN G MICs OF >0.1 μg/mL BUT < 0.5 μg/mL Endocarditis caused by streptococci with MICs of penicillin G of >0.1 but <0.5 μg/mL is managed with regimen E.

ENTEROCOCCI OR STREPTOCOCCI WITH PENICILLIN G MICs OF ≥0.5 μg/mL OR NUTRITIONALLY VARIANT VIRIDANS STREPTOCOCCI Penicillin, ampicillin, and vancomycin are not bactericidal for most enterococci. However, the addition of an aminoglycoside results in a synergistic bactericidal effect. Enterococcal endocarditis requires penicillin, ampicillin, or vancomycin plus an aminoglycoside for cure in most cases (regimens F and G, with G used for patients hypersensitive to penicillin G). An alternative to regimen G consists of skin testing with major and minor determinants of penicillin, with subsequent attempts at desensitization to penicillin. This process involves a scratch test through a drop of penicillin G (100 units per

Table 126-3

Therapy for Infective Endocarditis

STREPTOCOCCI WITH PENICILLIN G MICs OF ≤0.1 μg/mL

Regimen A	Penicillin G, 12–18 million units per day IV in divided doses q4h × 4 weeks
Regimen B	Penicillin as in regimen A plus gentamicin, 1 mg/kg IV q8h, both × 2 weeks
Regimen C	Ceftriaxone, 2 g IV or IM once daily × 4 weeks
Regimen D	Vancomycin, 15 mg/kg IV q12h × 4 weeks

STREPTOCOCCI WITH PENICILLIN G MICs OF >0.1 BUT <0.5 μg/mL

Regimen E	Penicillin G, 18 million units per day IV in divided doses q4h × 4 weeks, plus gentamicin, 1 mg/kg IV q8h for the first 2 weeks; or regimen D if patient is allergic to penicillin

ENTEROCOCCI OR STREPTOCOCCI WITH PENICILLIN G MICs OF ≥0.5 μg/mL OR NUTRITIONALLY VARIANT VIRIDANS STREPTOCOCCI

Regimen F	Penicillin G, 18–30 million units per day IV, or ampicillin, 12 g/d IV, in divided doses q4h, plus gentamicin, 1 mg/kg IV q8h, both × 4–6 weeks
Regimen G	Vancomycin, 15 mg/kg IV q12h, plus gentamicin as in regimen F, both × 4–6 weeks

METHICILLIN-SUSCEPTIBLE STAPHYLOCOCCI ON A NATIVE VALVE

Regimen H	Nafcillin or oxacillin, 2 g IV q4h × 4–6 weeks, with or without gentamicin, 1 mg/kg IV q8h × the first 3–5 d
Regimen I	Cefazolin*, 2 g IV q8h × 4–6 weeks, with or without gentamicin as in regimen H
Regimen J	Vancomycin, 15 mg/kg IV q12h × 4–6 weeks, with or without gentamicin as in regimen H

METHICILLIN-RESISTANT STAPHYLOCOCCI OR *CORYNEBACTERIUM* SPP. ON A NATIVE VALVE

Regimen K	Vancomycin as in regimen J, with or without gentamicin as in regimen H, for staphylococci; continue gentamicin × 4–6 weeks for *Corynebacterium* spp.

THE ABOVE ORGANISMS ON A PROSTHETIC VALVE

Streptococci or enterococci: Regimen F or G. Streptococci: Penicillin or vancomycin × 6 weeks, with gentamicin × the first 2 weeks or longer. Enterococci: Penicillin or vancomycin plus an aminoglycoside × 6–8 weeks
Methicillin-susceptible staphylococci: Regimen H, I, or J × 6–8 weeks, with gentamicin × the first 2 weeks and rifampin (300 mg orally q8h) for the entire course
Methicillin-resistant staphylococci: Regimen J × 6–8 weeks, with gentamicin × the first 2 weeks and rifampin (300 mg orally q8h) for the entire course

HACEK BACTERIA

Regimen L	Use regimen C

* Another first-generation cephalosporin may be used instead of cefazolin.

NOTE: Serum concentrations of gentamicin should be about 3 μg/mL 1 h after a 20- to 30-min IV infusion or IM injection. Streptomycin may be substituted for gentamicin in regimens B, E, F, and G at 7.5 mg/kg IM every 12 h; serum concentrations should be about 20 μg/mL 1 h after injection. The maximal dose of vancomycin is 1 g every 12 h; serum concentrations of vancomycin 1 h after completion of the infusion should be 30–45 μg/mL.

milliliter), followed in 30 min by intradermal inoculation of graded amounts of penicillin, beginning at 0.01 unit in 0.1 mL of saline solution and continuing in tenfold increments every 30 min; with increasing amounts, administration is changed to the subcutaneous, the intramuscular, and finally the intravenous route. An oral desensitization regimen is also available, as described by Wendel et al. Epinephrine and diphenhydramine should be on hand for emergency use during the procedure in case of anaphylaxis, and, if possible, the procedure should be carried out in an intensive care unit. If a reaction occurs, alternative therapy should be initiated.

Therapy is usually given for 4 weeks but is prolonged to 6 weeks when symptoms have been present for longer than 3 months or the course is complicated. Cephalosporins cannot be used in enterococcal endocarditis because these organisms are highly resistant.

Penicillin and aminoglycosides exert a synergistic bactericidal effect against enterococci only when growth is inhibited by gentamicin at 500 μg/mL or streptomycin at 2000 μg/mL. Synergism is most likely with gentamicin. However, enterococci resistant to gentamicin at 500 μg/mL are now common. Some of these gentamicin-resistant strains are inhibited by streptomycin at 2000 μg/mL, but most are resistant to all aminoglycosides. With aminoglycoside-resistant strains, it is best to exclude aminoglycosides from the regimen and treat for 6 to 8 weeks. However, relapses may occur. Isolates of enterococci that are highly resistant to penicillin (owing to either production of penicillinase or other mechanisms) or to vancomycin have been observed with increasing frequency. A high percentage of strains of *Enterococcus faecium* and occasional strains of *Enterococcus faecalis* are highly resistant to penicillin and/or vancomycin. *E. faecium* accounts for about 15 percent of all enterococcal isolates from cases of endocarditis and *E. faecalis* for close to 85 percent. In vitro susceptibility testing of enterococci is required in the selection of appropriate therapy.

Endocarditis caused by streptococci with MICs of penicillin G of ≥0.5 μg/mL or by nutritionally variant viridans streptococci is managed in the same way as enterococcal endocarditis.

STAPHYLOCOCCI Methicillin-susceptible *S. aureus* and *S. epidermidis* are treated with regimen H or I. Methicillin-resistant staphylococci are resistant to all penicillins and cephalosporins. In these instances and in those involving patients who cannot tolerate penicillins or cephalosporins, vancomycin must be used as in regimens J and K. Some experts advocate addition of gentamicin for the first 3 to 5 days because of an increase in the rate of bactericidal activity. However, clinical evidence of improved outcome is lacking, and routine use of this drug is not recommended. Four weeks' therapy is standard, but with metastatic or intracardiac abscess (or other complications), therapy should be extended to 6 weeks or even longer.

Evidence is mounting that vancomycin is inferior to β-lactam antibiotics in the treatment of staphylococcal endocarditis. Possible explanations include vancomycin's unpredictable pharmacokinetics, slower bactericidal activity, and poorer penetration into vegetations.

In intravenous drug users with *S. aureus* endocarditis localized to the tricuspid valve, excellent cure rates have been achieved with 2 weeks of treatment with nafcillin (but not vancomycin) plus an aminoglycoside.

STREPTOCOCCI, ENTEROCOCCI, AND STAPHYLOCOCCI IN PROSTHETIC VALVE ENDOCARDITIS Prolonged therapy (Table 126-3) and combinations with an aminoglycoside for streptococci or enterococci and with an aminoglycoside plus rifampin for staphylococci are recommended for prosthetic valve infection.

OTHER ORGANISMS Endocarditis due to HACEK organisms should be treated with regimen L and that due to *Corynebacterium* spp. with regimen K. In endocarditis caused by other organisms, bactericidal antibiotics—preferably a penicillin, a cephalosporin, or vancomycin with or without an aminoglycoside—should be given and therapy continued for 4 to 6 weeks. With gram-negative bacilli,

the penicillin or cephalosporin that displays the greatest potency against the infecting bacteria in vitro should be administered in large doses intravenously along with an aminoglycoside to which the bacterium is susceptible—e.g., ampicillin (2 g every 4 h), piperacillin (3 g every 4 h), cefotaxime (2 g every 4 to 6 h), or ceftazidime (2 g every 8 h) plus gentamicin (1.7 mg/kg every 8 h). A quinolone such as ciprofloxacin alone, which is bactericidal for gram-negative bacilli, also may be useful.

Therapy for fungal endocarditis with amphotericin B or an imidazole, such as fluconazole, usually has been unsuccessful. Such therapy plus cardiac surgery has generally been required for cure.

When the infecting organisms are resistant to penicillins, cephalosporins, quinolones, and vancomycin, therapy will probably be unsuccessful. Under these circumstances, treatment should consist of the bactericidal drug grouping with the best activity in vitro. If the response is poor or relapse occurs, antimicrobial therapy plus valve replacement will probably be necessary.

Home Therapy Home Therapy is cost-effective and has been used successfully with stable individuals who are not intravenous drug users and are highly motivated, able to administer the therapy, and living with someone else. Regimen C or D has been used most frequently for streptococcal endocarditis and regimen J for staphylococcal endocarditis.

Surgery in the Management of Endocarditis When curative microbicidal therapy is not available (as in most cases of fungal endocarditis), when positive blood cultures persist during therapy, or when relapse occurs after appropriate therapy, replacement of the valve should be considered. Ideally, surgery should be performed only after several days of the best available antimicrobial therapy. With organisms that tend to produce metastatic foci, therapy should then be continued long enough to eradicate these foci. Persistence of infection with the same organism following valve replacement has been uncommon. Immediate replacement (even after only hours of therapy) is essential in patients developing heart failure secondary to severe valvular regurgitation. Surgery is necessary to drain myocardial or valve-ring abscesses. Surgery should be considered when there are recurrent emboli despite adequate antimicrobial therapy. However, the frequency of emboli decreases dramatically with the initiation and continuation of antimicrobial therapy. Surgery also should be considered in patients with aortic valve endocarditis who develop first- and second-degree atrioventricular block. In some centers, the presence of a large vegetation on echocardiography has been considered an indication for surgery, but this point is controversial.

Replacement of a prosthesis is often necessary for infections with organisms other than streptococci. Some indications are valvular dysfunction or dehiscence and myocardial invasion. The latter is common with prosthetic valves and is suggested by continued fever after 10 days of therapy, a new regurgitant murmur, and/or atrioventricular conduction disturbance.

COURSE

Defervescence usually follows 3 to 7 days of antimicrobial therapy. Blood cultures should be obtained periodically during treatment; they generally become negative after several days of therapy. Both defervescence and the eradication of bacteremia have been slower when *S. aureus* endocarditis is treated with regimens containing vancomycin. Lack of response of fever and bacteremia may be associated with myocardial or metastatic abscess formation (especially associated with *S. aureus*).

The most common cause of persistent or recurrent fever during therapy is a drug reaction; less commonly, emboli are responsible. If a rash develops, therapy can be continued, and antihistamines or even glucocorticoids can be given to suppress the reaction. If the rash is severe, therapy should be altered.

Weight gain and a rise in hemoglobin may not be seen until weeks after therapy has been completed. Petechiae, Osler's nodes, and emboli may occur during and for weeks after successful antimicrobial therapy.

Mycotic aneurysms may regress during drug therapy or may rupture weeks to years later. Heart failure may occur during or after therapy and is the principal cause of death.

Anticoagulants should not be used in an attempt to prevent embolization from vegetations. Rather, they should be used only with a pressing indication (such as the presence of certain prosthetic valves) because of an increased risk of hemorrhage (especially intracranial). Warfarin is preferable to heparin. Blood cultures performed 2 and 4 weeks after discontinuation of therapy detect the vast majority of relapses. However, relapses are almost always clinically apparent.

PROGNOSIS

Factors that predispose to a poor prognosis are (1) nonstreptococcal disease, (2) development of heart failure, (3) aortic valve involvement, (4) infection on a prosthetic valve, (5) older age, and (6) valve-ring or myocardial abscess. The cure rate in streptococcal endocarditis is about 90 percent. Failures of therapy are due not to uncontrolled infection but to death from heart failure, embolus, rupture of a mycotic aneurysm, or renal failure. The mortality rate in nonaddicts with *S. aureus* endocarditis is at least 40 percent, and most deaths are due to overwhelming infection or heart failure. In drug addicts with *S. aureus* infection on the tricuspid valve, cure rates are over 90 percent. Results are poor in endocarditis caused by fungi and gram-negative bacilli resistant to penicillins and cephalosporins. Large vegetations (detected by echocardiography) may indicate a poorer prognosis than small or no vegetations. About 10 percent of patients will have additional episodes of endocarditis months or years later. The prognosis in early prosthetic valve endocarditis is much worse than that in late disease, with mortality rates of 40 to 80 percent versus 20 to 40 percent.

ANTIMICROBIAL PROPHYLAXIS OF ENDOCARDITIS

Although the risk of endocarditis is small and there is no proof of the efficacy of preventive therapy, prophylaxis is recommended for patients with predisposing cardiac lesions who are undergoing procedures known to cause bacteremia. The conditions in which prophylaxis is recommended are valvular or congenital heart disease (except uncomplicated atrial septal defect), intracardiac prostheses, asymmetric septal hypertrophy, and previous endocarditis. Mitral valve prolapse is associated with a low to moderate increase in the risk of endocarditis. However, this condition is so common that it is neither risk- nor cost-effective to give prophylaxis to all patients with prolapse for all procedures. It is, however, reasonable to use prophylaxis in individuals with mitral valve prolapse who have mitral regurgitation and who presumably are at greatest risk. Patients who have thickened, redundant mitral valve leaflets on echocardiography also appear to be at high risk.

Oral hygiene must be as good as possible in patients with cardiac lesions that predispose to endocarditis, especially those who are to have prosthetic cardiac valves implanted. For dental and other procedures in the mouth, nose, or throat that are likely to cause bleeding or significant trauma, prophylaxis is aimed at viridans streptococci. The regimen recommended by the American Heart Association is amoxicillin, 3 g orally 1 h before the procedure and 1.5 g 6 h after the initial dose. With penicillin allergy, the recommendation is 800 mg of oral erythromycin ethylsuccinate or 1.0 g of erythromycin stearate 2 h before the procedure or 300 mg of oral clindamycin 1 h before the procedure, in each case followed by half the dose 6 h after the initial dose. In high-risk patients (e.g., those with prosthetic valves), an alternative but optional and more stringent regimen is ampicillin (2 g intramuscularly or intravenously) plus gentamicin (1.5 mg/kg intramuscularly or intravenously)—both 30 min before the procedure—followed by amoxicillin (1.5 g orally) 6 h later or, with penicillin allergy, vancomycin (1 g intravenously) over 1 h starting 1 h before the procedure.

For genitourinary and gastrointestinal tract procedures likely to cause significant trauma (e.g., cystoscopy, prostatic surgery, and colonic or gallbladder surgery), prophylaxis is directed against enterococci. The recommended regimen is ampicillin plus gentamicin followed by amoxicillin, as delineated above. With penicillin allergy, the vancomycin regimen described above is given, but gentamicin at 1.5 mg/kg, given intravenously or intramuscularly, is added 1 h before the procedure. For low-risk patients, amoxicillin (3 g orally) may be used 1 h before the procedure, with 1.5 g administered 6 h later. Fiberoptic endoscopy, even with biopsy, carries such a low risk of endocarditis that prophylaxis is difficult to justify. Prophylaxis should be used only in high-risk patients, if at all.

Prophylaxis for cardiac surgery involving the placement of intracardiac prostheses, patches, or sutures is directed against staphylococci and has usually consisted of 2 g of cefazolin intravenously plus gentamicin at 1.5 mg/kg intravenously starting immediately preoperatively, with repeated doses 8 and 16 h later. However, since hospital strains of *S. epidermidis* and *S. aureus* may be methicillin-resistant, substitution of vancomycin for cefazolin (15 mg/kg intravenously over 1 h, starting 1 h before the procedure; 10 mg/kg after completion of bypass; and then 7.5 mg/kg every 6 h for 3 doses) is reasonable. Vancomycin also can be used when patients are hypersensitive to penicillins and cephalosporins.

Patients with coronary artery bypass grafts or transvenous pacemakers in place do not require prophylaxis for endocarditis, nor do patients undergoing cardiac catheterization.

BIBLIOGRAPHY

BAYER AS: Infective endocarditis. Clin Infect Dis 17:313, 1993

DAJANI AS et al: Prevention of bacterial endocarditis: Recommendations by the American Heart Association. JAMA 264:2919, 1990

DANIEL WG et al: Comparison of transthoracic and transesophageal echocardiography for detection of abnormalities of prosthetic and bioprosthetic valves in the mitral and aortic positions. Am J Cardiol 71:210, 1993

DINUBILE MJ: Short-course antibiotic therapy for right-sided endocarditis caused by *Staphylococcus aureus* in injection drug users. Ann Intern Med 121:873, 1994

DURACK D: Prophylaxis of infective endocarditis, in *Principles and Practice of Infectious Diseases*, 4th ed, GL Mandell et al (eds). New York, Churchill Livingstone, 1995

—— et al: New criteria for diagnosis of infective endocarditis: Utilization of specific echocardiographic findings. Am J Med 96:200, 1994

FRANCIOLI PB: Ceftriaxone and outpatient treatment of infective endocarditis. Infect Dis Clin North Am 7:97, 1993

HEINLE S et al: Value of transthoracic echocardiography in predicting embolic events in active infective endocarditis. Am J Cardiol 74:799, 1994

KAYE D (ed): *Infective Endocarditis*, 2d ed. New York, Raven Press, 1992

——: Treatment of infective endocarditis. Ann Intern Med 124:606, 1996

MULLANY CJ et al: Early and late survival after surgical treatment of culture-positive active endocarditis. Mayo Clin Proc 70:517, 1995

SCHELD M, SANDE M: Endocarditis and intravascular infections, in *Principles and Practice of Infectious Diseases*, 4th ed, GL Mandell et al (eds). New York, Churchill Livingstone, 1995

STECKELBERG JM et al: Emboli in infective endocarditis. The prognostic value of echocardiography. Ann Intern Med 114:635, 1991

STEWART WJ, SHAN K: The diagnosis of prosthetic valve endocarditis by echocardiography. Semin Thorac Cardiovasc Surg 7:7, 1995

THRELKELD M, COBBS G: Infectious disorders of prosthetic valves and intravascular devices, in *Principles and Practice of Infectious Diseases*, 4th ed, GL Mandell et al (eds). New York, Churchill Livingstone, 1995

TUNKEL AR, KAYE D: Neurologic complications of infective endocarditis. Neurol Clin 11:419, 1993

WENDEL GD JR et al: Penicillin allergy and desensitization in serious infections during pregnancy. N Engl J Med 312:1229, 1985

WILSON WR et al: Antibiotic treatment of adults with infective endocarditis due to viridans streptococci, enterococci, staphylococci, and HACEK microorganisms. JAMA 274:1706, 1995

YU VL et al: Prosthetic valve endocarditis: Superiority of surgical valve replacement versus medical therapy only. Ann Thorac Surg 58:1073, 1994

127 | Dori F. Zaleznik, Dennis L. Kasper

INTRAABDOMINAL INFECTIONS AND ABSCESSES

Intraperitoneal infections generally arise because a normal anatomic barrier is disrupted. This disruption may occur when the appendix, a diverticulum, or an ulcer ruptures; when the bowel wall is weakened by ischemia, tumor, or inflammation (e.g., in inflammatory bowel disease); or with adjacent inflammatory processes, such as pancreatitis or pelvic inflammatory disease, in which enzymes (in the former case) or organisms (in the latter) may leak into the peritoneal cavity. Whatever the inciting event, once inflammation develops and organisms usually contained within the bowel or another organ enter the normally sterile peritoneal space, a predictable series of events takes place. Intraabdominal infections occur in two stages: peritonitis and—if it goes untreated—abscess formation. The types of microorganisms predominating in each stage of infection are responsible for the pathogenesis of disease.

PERITONITIS

The peritoneal cavity is large but is divided into compartments. The upper and lower peritoneal cavities are divided by the transverse mesocolon; the greater omentum extends from the transverse mesocolon and from the lower pole of the stomach to line the lower peritoneal cavity. The pancreas, duodenum, and ascending and descending colon are located in the anterior retroperitoneal space; the kidneys, ureters, and adrenals are found in the posterior retroperitoneal space. The other organs, including liver, stomach, gallbladder, spleen, jejunum, ileum, transverse and sigmoid colon, cecum, and appendix, are found within the peritoneal cavity itself. Normally the cavity is lined with a serous membrane that can serve as a conduit for fluids—a property utilized in peritoneal dialysis. A small amount of fluid, sufficient to allow movement of organs, is normally present in the peritoneal space. This fluid is serous, with a protein content (consisting mainly of albumin) of <30 g/L and fewer than 300 white blood cells (WBCs, generally mononuclear cells) per microliter. In the presence of infection, some of these compartments collect fluid or pus more often than others. These compartments include the pelvis (the lowest portion), the subphrenic spaces on the right and left sides, and Morrison's pouch, which is a posterosuperior extension of the subhepatic spaces and is the lowest part of the paravertebral groove when a patient is recumbent. The falciform ligament separating the right and left subphrenic spaces appears to act as a barrier to the spread of infection; consequently, it is unusual to find bilateral subphrenic collections.

SPONTANEOUS BACTERIAL PERITONITIS Peritonitis is either primary (without an apparent source of contamination) or secondary. The types of organisms found and the clinical presentation of these two processes are different. In adults, primary or spontaneous bacterial peritonitis (SBP) occurs most commonly in conjunction with cirrhosis of the liver (frequently the result of alcoholism). It virtually always develops in patients with ascites. Nevertheless, it is not a common event, occurring in no more than 10 percent of cirrhotic patients. The cause of SBP has not been established definitively but is believed to involve hematogenous spread of organisms in a patient in whom a diseased liver and altered portal circulation result in a defect in the usual filtration function. Organisms are able to multiply in ascites, a good medium for growth. The proteins of the complement cascade have been found in peritoneal fluid, with lower levels in cirrhotic patients than in patients with ascites of other etiologies. The opsonic and phagocytic properties of neutrophils are decreased in patients with advanced liver disease.

The presentation of SBP differs from that of secondary peritonitis. The most common manifestation is fever, which is reported in as many as 80 percent of patients. Ascites is found but virtually always predates infection. Abdominal pain, an acute onset of symptoms, and peritoneal irritation detected during physical examination can be helpful diagnostically, but the absence of any of these findings does not exclude this often-subtle diagnosis. It is vital to sample the peritoneal fluid of any cirrhotic patient with ascites and fever. The finding of more than 300 polymorphonuclear leukocytes (PMNs) per microliter is diagnostic for SBP, according to Conn. The microbiology of SBP also is distinctive. While enteric gram-negative bacilli such as *Escherichia coli* are the organisms most commonly encountered, gram-positive organisms such as streptococci, enterococci, or even pneumococci are sometimes found. The characteristic microbiologic features of SBP are that generally only a single organism is recovered and anaerobes are found infrequently. This microbiologic picture contrasts with that of secondary peritonitis, in which a mixed flora including anaerobes is the rule. In fact, if SBP is suspected and multiple organisms including anaerobes are recovered from the peritoneal fluid, the diagnosis must be reconsidered and a source of secondary peritonitis sought.

The diagnosis of SBP is not easy. The level of suspicion needs to be high. It may be difficult to recover organisms from cultures of peritoneal fluid, presumably because the burden of organisms is low. The yield can be improved if 10 mL of peritoneal fluid is placed directly into a blood culture bottle. Bacteremia may accompany SBP; therefore, blood should be cultured simultaneously. No specific radiographic studies are helpful in the diagnosis of SBP. A plain film of the abdomen would be expected to show ascites. Chest and abdominal radiography should be performed in patients with abdominal pain to exclude free air, which signals a perforation.

Treatment for SBP is directed at the isolate from blood or peritoneal fluid. Gram's staining of peritoneal fluid often gives negative results in primary peritonitis; therefore, until culture results become available, empirical therapy should cover gram-negative aerobic bacilli and gram-positive cocci. Ampicillin plus gentamicin is a reasonable initial regimen. Third-generation cephalosporins, carbapenems, or broad-spectrum penicillin/β-lactamase inhibitor combinations also are options. Empirical coverage for anaerobes is not necessary. After the infecting organism is identified, therapy should be narrowed to treat that specific pathogen.

SECONDARY PERITONITIS Secondary peritonitis develops when bacteria contaminate the peritoneum as a result of spillage from an intraabdominal viscus. The organisms found almost always constitute a mixed flora in which facultative gram-negative bacilli and anaerobes predominate, especially when the contaminating source is colonic. Early in the course of infection, when the host response is directed toward containment of the infection, exudate containing fibrin and PMNs is found. Early death in this setting is attributable to gram-negative bacillary sepsis and to potent endotoxins circulating in the bloodstream (see Chap. 124). Gram-negative bacilli, particularly *E. coli*, are common bloodstream isolates, but *Bacteroides fragilis* bacteremia occurs as well. The severity of abdominal pain and the clinical course depend on the inciting process. The species of organisms isolated from the peritoneum also vary with the source of the initial process and the normal flora present at that site. Peritonitis can result primarily from chemical irritation or bacterial contamination. For example, as long as the patient is not achlorhydric, a ruptured gastric ulcer will release low-pH gastric contents that will serve as a chemical irritant. The normal flora of the stomach comprises the same organisms found in the oropharynx (see Chap. 169) but in lower numbers. The surfaces of teeth contain approximately 10^7 aerobic and 10^7 anaerobic organisms per milliliter of saliva; the normally acidic stomach contains an equal ratio of aerobic and anaerobic species, but in concentrations more in the range of 10^5 per milliliter. After meals, when gastric acidity is highest, this number may fall to 10^3. Thus, the bacterial burden in a ruptured gastric ulcer—or even a duodenal ulcer—is negligible compared with that in a ruptured appendix. The normal flora of the colon below the ligament of Treitz contains about 10^{11} anaerobic organisms per gram of feces but only 10^8 aerobes per gram; therefore, anaerobic species account for 99 percent of the bacteria.

Leakage of colonic contents (pH 7 to 8) does not cause significant chemical peritonitis, but infection is intense because of the heavy bacterial load.

Depending on the inciting event, local symptoms may initially be found in secondary peritonitis—for example, epigastric pain from a ruptured gastric ulcer. In appendicitis (see Chap. 290), the initial presenting symptoms often are vague, with periumbilical discomfort and nausea followed in a number of hours by pain more localized to the right lower quadrant. Unusual locations of the appendix (including a retrocecal position) can complicate this presentation further. Once infection has spread to the peritoneal cavity, however, pain increases, particularly with infection involving the parietal peritoneum, which is innervated extensively. Patients usually lie motionless, often with knees drawn up to avoid stretching the nerve fibers of the peritoneal cavity. Coughing and sneezing, which increase pressure within the peritoneal cavity, are associated with sharp pain. There may or may not be pain localized to the infected or diseased organ from which secondary peritonitis has arisen. Patients with secondary peritonitis generally have abnormal findings on abdominal examination, with marked voluntary and involuntary guarding of the anterior abdominal musculature. Later findings include tenderness, especially rebound tenderness. In addition, there may be localized findings in the area of the inciting event. In general, patients are febrile, with marked leukocytosis and a left shift of the WBCs to earlier granulocyte forms.

While recovery of organisms from peritoneal fluid is easier in secondary than in primary peritonitis, a tap of the abdomen is rarely the procedure of choice in secondary peritonitis. An exception is in cases involving trauma, where the possibility of a hemoperitoneum may need to be excluded early. Treatment for secondary peritonitis includes early administration of antibiotics aimed particularly at aerobic gram-negative bacilli and anaerobes (see below) as well as etiologic studies. Secondary peritonitis usually requires both surgical intervention to address the inciting process and antibiotic administration to treat early bacteremia, to decrease the incidence of abscess formation and wound infection, and to prevent more distant spread of infection. In SBP in adults, surgery is rarely indicated. In secondary peritonitis, surgery may be life-saving.

PERITONITIS IN PATIENTS UNDERGOING CAPD   A third type of peritonitis arises in patients who are undergoing continuous ambulatory peritoneal dialysis (CAPD). Unlike primary and secondary peritonitis, which are caused by endogenous bacteria, peritonitis in CAPD patients usually involves skin organisms. The pathogenesis of infection is similar to that of intravascular-device infection, in which skin organisms migrate along the catheter, which both serves as an entry point and exerts the effects of a foreign body. Exit-site or tunnel infection may or may not accompany CAPD peritonitis. Like primary peritonitis, CAPD peritonitis is usually caused by a single organism. Peritonitis is, in fact, the most common reason for discontinuation of CAPD. Improvements in equipment design, especially that of the Y-set connector, have resulted in a decrease from one case of peritonitis per 9 months of CAPD to one case per 15 months.

The clinical presentation of CAPD peritonitis resembles that of secondary peritonitis in that diffuse pain and peritoneal signs are common. The dialysate is usually cloudy and contains more than 100 WBCs per microliter, more than 50 percent of which are neutrophils. The most common etiologic organism is coagulase-negative *Staphylococcus*, which accounts for approximately 30 percent of cases. *Staphylococcus aureus* causes about 10 percent of cases and is more commonly identified among patients who are nasal carriers of the organism. Gram-negative bacilli and fungi such as *Candida* species are also found. The finding of more than one organism in dialysate culture should prompt a search for a cause of secondary peritonitis. As with primary peritonitis, culture of dialysate fluid in blood culture bottles improves the yield.

Empirical treatment is directed at coagulase-negative *Staphylococcus*, *S. aureus*, and gram-negative bacilli; intraperitoneal vancomycin plus gentamicin is a commonly used regimen. Vancomycin, when administered at a dose of 2 g and allowed to remain in the peritoneal cavity for 6 h, produces a reasonable level for 7 days. A loading dose

of 70 to 140 mg of gentamicin is followed by maintenance therapy with 20 mg/L for a single daily exchange or with 4 to 8 mg/L per exchange for multiple daily exchanges. The clinical response is rapid; if the patient has not responded after 48 h of treatment, catheter removal should be considered.

INTRAPERITONEAL ABSCESSES

Abscess formation is common in untreated peritonitis if overt gram-negative sepsis either does not develop or develops but is not fatal. In experimental models of abscess formation, mixed aerobic and anaerobic organisms have been implanted intraperitoneally. Without therapy directed at anaerobes, animals develop intraabdominal abscesses. As in humans, these experimental abscesses may stud the peritoneal cavity, lie within the omentum or mesentery, or even develop on the surface of or within viscera such as the liver.

PATHOGENESIS AND IMMUNITY   There is often disagreement about whether an abscess represents a disease state or a host response. In a sense, it represents both: While an abscess is an infection in which viable infecting organisms and PMNs are contained in a fibrous capsule, it is also a process by which the host confines microbes to a limited space, thereby preventing further spread of infection. Experimental work has helped to define both the host cells and the bacterial virulence factors responsible—most notably, in the case of *B. fragilis*. This organism, although accounting for only 0.5 percent of the normal colonic flora, is the anaerobe most frequently isolated from intraabdominal infections and is the most common anaerobic bloodstream isolate. On clinical grounds, therefore, *B. fragilis* appears to be uniquely virulent. Moreover, *B. fragilis* causes abscesses in animal models of intraabdominal infection, whereas most other *Bacteroides* species must act synergistically with a facultative organism to induce abscess formation.

Of the several virulence factors identified in *B. fragilis*, one is critical—the capsular polysaccharide complex (CPC) found on the bacterial surface. The CPC comprises two distinct surface polysaccharides, PS A and PS B. Structural analysis of each polysaccharide in the CPC has shown an unusual motif of oppositely charged sugars. Polysaccharides having these zwitterionic characteristics evoke a host response in the peritoneal cavity that localizes bacteria into abscesses. Although abscesses characteristically contain PMNs, the process of abscess induction depends on the stimulation of T lymphocytes by these unique polysaccharides. Animals depleted of CD4+/CD8+ T cells cannot form abscesses. The other host factors that have been found to participate in abscess formation include the alternative pathway of complement and fibrinogen.

While antibodies to the CPC are not critical in immunity to abscesses, they enhance bloodstream clearance of *B. fragilis*. When administered subcutaneously, *B. fragilis* PS A has immunomodulatory characteristics and stimulates T cells to inhibit the host response of abscess formation to intraperitoneal challenge with *B. fragilis*. Treatment of experimental animals with PS A can actually prevent the formation of abscesses, even in the face of provocation by the complete contents of the cecum, with its hundreds of bacterial species.

CLINICAL PRESENTATION   Most intraperitoneal abscesses result from SBP due to fecal spillage from a colonic source, such as an inflamed appendix. Of all intraabdominal abscesses, 74 percent are intraperitoneal or retroperitoneal and are not associated with a specific organ. Abscesses also can arise from a number of other processes. They usually form within weeks of the development of peritonitis and may be found in a variety of locations, from omentum to mesentery, pelvis to psoas muscles, and subphrenic space to a visceral organ such as the liver, where they may develop either on the surface of the organ or within it. Infections of the female genital tract and pancreatitis are among the more common causative events. When abscesses occur in the female genital tract—either as a primary infection (e.g., tubo-ovarian abscess) or as an infection extending into the pelvic cavity or peritoneum—*B. fragilis* figures prominently among the organisms isolated. *B. fragilis* is not found in large numbers in the normal vaginal flora. It is encountered less commonly in pelvic inflammatory disease and endometritis, for example, without an associated abscess. In pancreatitis with leakage of damaging pancreatic enzymes, inflammation is prominent. Therefore, clinical findings such as fever, leukocytosis, and even abdominal pain do not distinguish pancreatitis itself from complications such as pancreatic pseudocyst, pancreatic abscess, or intraabdominal collections of pus. Some authors have advocated early needle aspiration of pancreatic collections under computed tomographic (CT) guidance as a means of distinguishing pseudocysts from abscesses, but this procedure is somewhat hazardous, and the recovery of organisms is not of clear significance.

The psoas muscle of the anterior back is another location in which abscesses are encountered. These abscesses may arise from a presumed hematogenous source, by contiguous spread from an intraabdominal or pelvic process, or by contiguous spread from nearby bony structures such as vertebral bodies. Associated osteomyelitis due to spread from bone to muscle or from muscle to bone is common in psoas abscesses. When Pott's disease was common, *Mycobacterium tuberculosis* was a frequent cause of psoas abscess. Currently in the United States, the usual isolates from psoas abscesses are either *S. aureus* or a mixture of enteric organisms including aerobic gram-negative bacilli. *S. aureus* is most likely to be isolated when a psoas abscess arises from hematogenous spread or a contiguous focus of osteomyelitis; a mixed enteric flora is most likely when the abscess has an intraabdominal or pelvic source.

DIAGNOSIS A variety of scanning procedures have considerably facilitated the diagnosis of intraabdominal abscesses. Abdominal CT scans probably have the highest yield, although ultrasonography is particularly useful for the right upper quadrant, kidneys, and pelvis. Both indium-labeled WBCs and gallium tend to localize in abscesses and may be useful in finding a collection. Since gallium is taken up in the bowel, indium-labeled WBCs may have a slightly greater yield for abscesses near the bowel. Neither indium-labeled WBC nor gallium scans serve as a basis for a definitive diagnosis, however; both need to be followed by other, more specific studies, such as CT, if an area of possible abnormality is identified. Abscesses contiguous with or contained within outpouchings of bowel are particularly difficult to diagnose with scanning procedures. Occasionally, a barium enema may detect a diverticular abscess not diagnosed by other procedures, although barium should not be injected if a free perforation is suspected. If one study is negative, a second study sometimes reveals a collection. On occasion, exploratory laparotomy still must be undertaken if an abscess is strongly suspected on clinical grounds, although this procedure has been less commonly used since the advent of CT.

℞ TREATMENT
The treatment of intraabdominal infections involves the determination of the initial focus of infection, the administration of broad-spectrum antibiotics targeted at organisms involved in the associated infection, and the performance of a drainage procedure if one or more definitive abscesses have formed already. It cannot be overemphasized that antimicrobial therapy, in general, is adjunctive to drainage and/or surgical correction of an underlying lesion or process in intraabdominal abscesses. Unlike the intraabdominal abscesses precipitated by most infections, for which drainage of some kind generally is required, abscesses associated with diverticulitis usually wall off locally after rupture of a diverticulum, so that surgical intervention is not routinely required.

A number of antimicrobial agents exhibit excellent activity against aerobic gram-negative bacilli. Since mortality in intraabdominal sepsis is linked to gram-negative bacteremia, empirical therapy for intraabdominal infection always needs to include adequate coverage of gram-negative aerobic and facultative organisms. Aminoglycosides and second- and third-generation cephalosporins are the agents most widely tested and used in intraabdominal processes. Newer antibiotics, such as aztreonam, imipenem, ticarcillin/clavulanic acid, piperacillin/tazobactam, and quinolones (e.g., ciprofloxacin), cover these organisms as well, although at a higher cost. Second-generation cephalosporins, such as cefoxitin or cefotetan, are not as uniformly active as the other agents against all of the aerobic gram-negative species. Aztreonam, ciprofloxacin, aminoglycosides, and most of the third-generation cephalosporins are not active against anaerobes; for the treatment of intraabdominal infections, these drugs need to be used in combination with another antibiotic. Since a number of antibiotics highly effective against anaerobes are available, third-generation cephalosporins generally should not be considered for use against the anaerobic bacteria involved in intraabdominal sepsis.

The most active and cost-effective antibiotic for anaerobic coverage currently is metronidazole (see Chap. 169). Only rare isolates of *B. fragilis* have been reported to be resistant to this drug. In a recent study from 10 geographic locations in the United States over a 5-year period, rates of resistance and susceptibility among *B. fragilis* isolates were analyzed for a number of antibiotics. The three that were most consistently active in vitro were metronidazole, imipenem, and piperacillin/tazobactam, with resistance rates of 0, 0.1, and 0.2 percent, respectively. In contrast, cefoxitin resistance was found in 6 percent of the 2800 isolates tested, and clindamycin resistance in 14 percent. Of the cephamycins, cefoxitin was more active than cefotetan or cefmetazole, with resistance observed in 27 and 20 percent of isolates, respectively. *Bacteroides* species other than *B. fragilis* often are highly resistant to the latter two drugs. Despite increasing reports of in vitro resistance of *B. fragilis* to a number of agents, clinical failures are still limited to case reports; therefore, the clinical significance of antimicrobial resistance in anaerobes is uncertain. One report describes a bloodstream isolate of *B. fragilis* with resistance to metronidazole and with reduced susceptibility to imipenem and amoxicillin/clavulanic acid that became resistant to both of the latter two drugs after treatment of the patient with imipenem. Among newer agents, imipenem, ticarcillin/clavulanic acid, piperacillin/tazobactam, meropenem, and ampicillin/sulbactam are highly active against anaerobes. Chloramphenicol, which exhibits strong activity against *B. fragilis* in vitro, nevertheless should probably not be considered a first-line drug for use against anaerobes, since failures of treatment have been documented in both experimental and clinical intraabdominal infections. Neither metronidazole nor clindamycin covers aerobic gram-negative bacilli; thus, these drugs must be combined with other agents for use in this setting.

VISCERAL ABSCESSES **Liver Abscesses** The liver is the organ most subject to the development of abscesses. Altemeier and associates studied 540 intraabdominal abscesses over a 12-year period. Of these abscesses 26 percent were visceral. Liver abscesses made up 13 percent of the total number of abscesses, or 48 percent of all visceral abscesses. Liver abscesses may be solitary or multiple; they may arise from hematogenous spread of bacteria or from local spread from contiguous sites of infection within the peritoneal cavity. In the past, appendicitis with rupture and subsequent spread of infection was the most common route for the development of a liver abscess. Currently, associated disease of the biliary tract is most often the etiology. Suppurative pylephlebitis, arising usually from infection in the pelvis but sometimes from infection elsewhere in the peritoneal cavity, is another common source for bacterial seeding of the liver.

Fever is the most common presenting sign of liver abscess. Some patients, particularly those with active associated disease of the biliary tract, have symptoms and signs localized to the right upper quadrant, including pain, guarding, punch tenderness, and even rebound tenderness. Nonspecific symptoms, such as chills, anorexia, weight loss, nausea, and vomiting, also may develop. Only 50 percent of patients with liver abscesses, however, have hepatomegaly, right-upper-quadrant tenderness, or jaundice; thus, half of patients have no symptoms or signs that would direct attention to the liver. Fever of unknown origin (FUO) may be the only presenting manifestation of liver abscess, especially in the elderly. Diagnostic studies of the abdomen, especially the right upper quadrant, should be a part of any FUO workup. The single most reliable laboratory finding is an elevated serum concentration of alkaline phosphatase, which is documented in 90 percent of patients with liver abscesses. Other tests of liver function may yield normal results, but 50 percent of patients have elevated serum levels of bilirubin, and 48 percent have elevated concentrations of aspartate aminotransferase. Other associated laboratory findings include leukocytosis in 77 percent of patients, anemia (usually normochromic, normocytic) in 50 percent, and hypoalbuminemia in 33 percent. Concomitant bacteremia is found in one-third of patients. A liver abscess is sometimes suggested by chest radiography, especially if a new elevation of the right hemidiaphragm is seen; other suggestive findings include a right basilar infiltrate and a right pleural effusion.

Imaging studies are the most reliable methods for diagnosing liver abscesses. These studies include ultrasonography, CT scan, indium-labeled WBC or gallium scans, and even magnetic resonance imaging. In an occasional case, more than one such study may be required. Organisms recovered from liver abscesses vary with the etiology. In liver infection arising from the biliary tree, enteric gram-negative aerobic bacilli and enterococci are common isolates. Unless previous surgery has been performed, anaerobes are not generally involved in liver abscesses arising from biliary infections. In contrast, in liver abscesses arising from pelvic and other intraperitoneal sources, a mixed flora including aerobic and anaerobic species (especially *B. fragilis*) is common. With hematogenous spread of infection, usually only a single organism is encountered; this species may be *S. aureus* or a streptococcal species such as *Streptococcus milleri*.

Liver abscesses also may be caused by *Candida* species; such abscesses usually follow fungemia in patients receiving chemotherapy for cancer and often present as a return of neutrophils after a period of neutropenia. Treatment of candidal liver abscesses usually entails lengthy administration of amphotericin B, although recent reports have described successful maintenance therapy with fluconazole after an initial course of amphotericin (see Chap. 207).

Amebic liver abscesses are not an uncommon problem (see Chap. 215). Amebic serologic testing gives positive results in more than 95 percent of cases; thus, a negative result helps to exclude this diagnosis.

While drainage—either percutaneous (with a pigtail catheter kept in place) or surgical—remains the mainstay of therapy for intraabdominal abscesses (including liver abscesses), there is growing interest in medical management alone for pyogenic liver abscesses. The drugs used in empirical broad-spectrum antibiotic therapy include the same ones used in intraabdominal sepsis. Usually, a diagnostic aspirate of abscess contents should be obtained before the initiation of empirical therapy, and antibiotic choices adjusted when the results of Gram's staining and culture become available. Cases treated without definitive drainage generally require longer courses of antibiotic therapy. When percutaneous drainage was compared with open surgical drainage, the average length of hospital stay for the former was almost twice that for the latter, although both the time required for fever to resolve and mortality were the same for the two procedures. Mortality was appreciable despite treatment, averaging 15 percent. Several factors may predict the failure of percutaneous drainage and therefore may favor primary surgical intervention. These factors include the presence of multiple, sizable abscesses; viscous abscess contents that tend to plug the catheter; associated disease (e.g., disease of the biliary tract) that requires surgery; or the lack of a clinical response to percutaneous drainage in 4 to 7 days.

Splenic Abscesses   Splenic abscesses are much less common than liver abscesses. In fact, no splenic abscesses were observed in Altemeier's series of 540 intraabdominal abscesses. The incidence of splenic abscesses has ranged from 0.14 to 0.7 percent in various autopsy series. The clinical setting and the organisms isolated usually differ from those for liver abscesses. The degree of clinical suspicion for splenic abscess needs to be high, as this condition frequently is fatal if left untreated. Even in the most recently published series, diagnosis was made only at autopsy in 37 percent of cases. While splenic abscesses may arise occasionally from contiguous spread of infection or from direct trauma to the spleen, hematogenous spread of infection is the usual mode of development. Bacterial endocarditis is the most common associated infection. Splenic abscesses can develop in patients who have received extensive immunosuppressive therapy (particularly those with malignancy involving the spleen) and in patients with hemoglobinopathies or other hematologic disorders (especially sickle cell anemia).

While approximately 50 percent of patients with splenic abscesses have abdominal pain, the pain is localized to the left upper quadrant in only half of these cases. Splenomegaly is found in approximately 50 percent of patients. Fever and leukocytosis generally are present; the development of fever preceded diagnosis by an average of 20 days in one series. Left-sided chest findings may include abnormalities to auscultation, and chest radiographic findings may include an infiltrate or a left-sided pleural effusion. When splenic abscesses are being considered in a differential diagnosis, CT scan of the abdomen has been the most sensitive diagnostic tool. Ultrasonography can yield the diagnosis, but cases have been missed with this modality. Liver-spleen scan or gallium scan also may be useful. Streptococcal species are the most common bacterial isolates from splenic abscesses, and *S. aureus* is the next most common; presumably these prevalences reflect the bacterial cause of the associated endocarditis. An increase in the frequency of isolation of gram-negative aerobic organisms from splenic abscesses has been reported; these organisms often derive from a urinary tract focus, with associated bacteremia, or from another intraabdominal source. *Salmonella* species are seen fairly commonly, especially in patients with sickle cell hemoglobinopathy. Anaerobic species accounted for only 5 percent of isolates in the largest collected series, but the reporting of a number of "sterile abscesses" may indicate that optimal techniques for the isolation of anaerobes were not employed. Because of the high mortality figures reported for splenic abscesses, the treatment of choice is splenectomy with adjunctive antibiotics. However, percutaneous drainage has been successful. The most important factor in successful treatment of splenic abscesses is early consideration of the diagnosis.

Perinephric and Renal Abscesses   Perinephric and renal abscesses are not common: The former accounted for only about 0.02 percent of hospital admissions and the latter for about 0.2 percent in Altemeier's series of 540 intraabdominal abscesses. While liver abscesses generally arise from contiguous foci of infection or track from other intraabdominal sources and splenic abscesses usually arise from hematogenous spread (e.g., spread from bacterial endocarditis), perinephric and renal abscesses have a different pathogenesis. Before antibiotics became available, most renal and perinephric abscesses were hematogenous in origin, with *S. aureus* most commonly recovered. Now, in contrast, more than 75 percent of perinephric and renal abscesses arise from an initial urinary tract infection. Infection ascends from the bladder to the kidney, with pyelonephritis occurring first. Bacteria may directly invade the renal parenchyma from medulla to cortex. Local vascular channels within the kidney may also facilitate the transport of organisms. Areas of abscess developing within the parenchyma may rupture into the perinephric space. The kidneys and adrenal glands are surrounded by a layer of perirenal fat that, in turn, is surrounded by Gerota's fascia, which extends superiorly to the diaphragm and inferiorly to the pelvic fat. When abscesses extend into the perinephric space, tracking may occur through Gerota's fascia into the psoas or transversalis muscles, into the anterior peritoneal cavity, superiorly to the subdiaphragmatic space, or inferiorly to the pelvis. Of the several risk factors that have been associated with the development of perinephric abscesses, the most important is the presence of concomitant nephrolithiasis producing local obstruction to urinary flow. Of patients with perinephric abscess, 20 to 60 percent have renal stones. In addition, other structural abnormalities of the urinary tract, a history of urologic surgery, trauma, and diabetes mellitus all have been identified as risk factors.

The organisms most frequently encountered in perinephric and renal abscesses are *E. coli*, *Proteus* species, and *Klebsiella* species. *E. coli*, the aerobic species most commonly found in colonic flora, seems to have unique virulence properties in the urinary tract, including factors promoting adherence to uroepithelial cells. The urease of *Proteus* species splits urea, thereby creating a more alkaline and hospitable environment for bacterial proliferation. *Proteus* species frequently are found in association with large struvite stones caused by the precipitation of magnesium ammonium sulfate in an alkaline environment. These stones serve as a nidus for recurrent urinary tract infection. While a single bacterial species usually is recovered from a perinephric or renal abscess, multiple species also may be found. If a urine culture is not contaminated with periurethral flora and is found to contain more than one organism, a perinephric abscess or renal abscess should be considered in the differential diagnosis. Urine cultures also may be polymicrobial in cases of bladder diverticulum.

Candida species should be considered in the etiology of renal abscesses. This fungus may spread to the kidney via the hematogenous route or by ascension from the bladder. The hallmark of the latter route of infection is ureteral obstruction with large fungal balls.

The presentation of perinephric and renal abscesses is quite non-specific. Flank pain and abdominal pain are common. At least 50 percent of patients are febrile. Pain may be referred to the groin or leg, particularly with extension of infection. The diagnosis of perinephric abscess, like that of splenic abscess, is frequently delayed, and mortality in some series is appreciable, although lower than in the past. Perinephric or renal abscess should be most seriously considered when a patient presents with symptoms and signs of pyelonephritis and remains febrile after 4 or 5 days, by which time the fever should have resolved. Moreover, when a urine culture yields a polymicrobial flora, when a patient is known to have renal stone disease, or when fever and pyuria coexist with a sterile urine culture, the diagnosis of perinephric or renal abscess should be entertained.

Renal ultrasonography and abdominal CT scan are the most useful diagnostic modalities. If a renal abscess or perinephric abscess is diagnosed, nephrolithiasis should be excluded, especially when a high urinary pH suggests the presence of a urea-splitting organism. Treatment for perinephric or renal abscesses, like that for other intraabdominal abscesses, includes drainage of pus and antibiotic therapy directed at the organism(s) recovered. For perinephric abscesses, percutaneous drainage usually is successful.

BIBLIOGRAPHY

ALDRIDGE KE et al: A five-year multicenter study of the susceptibility of the *Bacteroides fragilis* group isolates to cephalosporins, cephamycins, penicillins, clindamycin, and metronidazole in the United States. Diagn Microbiol Infect Dis 18:235, 1994

ALTEMEIER WA et al: Intra-abdominal abscesses. Am J Surg 125:70, 1973

CHUN CH et al: Splenic abscess. Medicine 59:50, 1980

FINEGOLD SM: Anaerobic bacteria: General concepts, in *Mandell, Douglas and Bennett's Principles and Practice of Infectious Diseases*, 4th ed, GL Mandell et al (eds). New York, Churchill Livingstone, 1995

HUTCHISON FN, KAYSEN GA: Perinephric abscess: The missed diagnosis. Med Clin North Am 72:993, 1988

LEVISON ME, BUSH LM: Peritonitis and other intra-abdominal infections, in *Mandell, Douglas and Bennett's Principles and Practice of Infectious Diseases*, 4th ed, GL Mandell et al (eds). New York, Churchill Livingstone, 1995

MAHER JA et al: Successful medical treatment of pyogenic liver abscess. Gastroenterology 77:681, 1979

McDOWELL RK, DAWSON SL: Evaluation of the abdomen in sepsis of unknown origin. Radiol Clin North Am 34:177, 1996

SHULER FW et al: Nonoperative management for intra-abdominal abscesses. Am Surg 62:218, 1996

SOLOMKIN JS et al: Results of a randomized trial comparing sequential intravenous/oral treatment with ciprofloxacin plus metronidazole to imipenem/cilastatin for intra-abdominal infections. Ann Surg 223:303, 1996

TURNER et al: Simultaneous resistance to metronidazole, co-amoxiclav, and imipenem in clinical isolates of *Bacteroides fragilis*. Lancet 345:1275, 1995

TZIANABOS AO et al: Structural features of polysaccharides that induce intraabdominal abscesses. Science 262:416, 1993

——— et al: Polysaccharide-mediated protection against abscess formation in experimental intra-abdominal sepsis. J Clin Invest 96:2727, 1995

128 *Joan R. Butterton, Stephen B. Calderwood*

ACUTE INFECTIOUS DIARRHEAL DISEASES AND BACTERIAL FOOD POISONING

Ranging from mild annoyances during vacations to devastating dehydrating illnesses that can kill within hours, acute gastrointestinal illnesses rank second only to acute upper respiratory illnesses as the most common diseases worldwide. In children less than 5 years old, attack rates range from 2 to 3 illnesses per child per year in developed countries to as high as 10 to 18 illnesses per child per year in developing countries. In Asia, Africa, and Latin America, acute diarrheal illnesses are not only a leading cause of morbidity in children—with an estimated 1 billion cases per year—but also the major cause of mortality, being responsible for 4 to 6 million deaths per year, or a sobering total of 12,600 deaths per day. In some areas, more than 50 percent of deaths of children are directly attributable to acute diarrheal illnesses. In addition, by contributing to malnutrition and thereby reducing resistance to other infectious agents, gastrointestinal illnesses may be indirect factors in a far greater burden of disease.

The wide range of clinical manifestations of acute gastrointestinal illnesses is matched by the wide variety of infectious agents involved, including viruses, bacteria, and parasitic pathogens (Table 128-1). This chapter will discuss factors that enable gastrointestinal pathogens to cause disease, will review host defense mechanisms, and will delineate an approach to the evaluation and treatment of patients presenting with acute diarrhea. Individual organisms causing acute gastrointestinal illnesses are discussed in detail in subsequent chapters.

PATHOGENIC MECHANISMS Enteric pathogens have developed a variety of tactics to overcome host defenses. Understanding the virulence factors employed by these organisms is important in the diagnosis and treatment of clinical disease.

Inoculum Size The number of microorganisms that must be ingested to cause disease varies considerably from species to species. In the case of *Salmonella* or *Vibrio cholerae*, for example, 10^5 to 10^8 organisms must be ingested orally to cause disease, whereas for *Shigella*, *Giardia lamblia*, or *Entamoeba*, as few as 10 to 100 bacteria or cysts can produce infection. The ability of organisms to overcome host defenses has important implications for transmission; *Shigella*, *Entamoeba*, and *Giardia* can spread by person-to-person contact, whereas bacteria such as *Salmonella* may have to grow in food for several hours before reaching an effective infectious dose.

Adherence Many organisms must adhere to the gastrointestinal mucosa as an initial step in the pathogenic process; thus, organisms that can compete with the normal bowel flora and colonize the mucosa have an important advantage in causing disease. Specific cell-surface proteins involved in attachment of bacteria to intestinal cells are important virulence determinants. *V. cholerae*, for example, adheres to the brush border of small-intestinal enterocytes via specific surface adhesins, including the toxin-coregulated pilus and other accessory colonization factors. Enterotoxigenic *Escherichia coli* produces an adherence protein called *colonization factor antigen* that is necessary for colonization of the upper small intestine by the organism prior to the production of enterotoxin. Enteropathogenic and enterohemorrhagic strains of *E. coli* produce virulence determinants that allow these organisms to attach to and efface the brush border of the intestinal epithelium.

Toxin Production The production of one or more exotoxins is important in the pathogenesis of numerous enteric organisms. Such toxins include *enterotoxins*, which cause watery diarrhea by acting directly on secretory mechanisms in the intestinal mucosa; *cytotoxins*, which cause destruction of mucosal cells and associated inflammatory diarrhea; and *neurotoxins*, which act directly on the central or peripheral nervous system. Some exotoxins act by more than one mechanism; *Shigella dysenteriae* type 1, for example, produces an exotoxin that has both enterotoxic and cytotoxic activities.

The prototypical enterotoxin is cholera toxin, a heterodimeric protein composed of one A and five B subunits. The A subunit contains the enzymatic activity of the toxin, while the B subunit pentamer binds holotoxin to the enterocyte surface receptor, the ganglioside G_{M1}. After the binding of holotoxin, a fragment of the A subunit is translocated across the eukaryotic cell membrane into the cytoplasm, where it catalyzes the ADP-ribosylation of a GTP-binding protein and causes persistent activation of adenylate cyclase. The end result is an increase of cyclic AMP in the intestinal mucosa, which increases Cl^- secretion and decreases Na^+ absorption, leading to loss of fluid and the production of diarrhea.

Enterotoxigenic strains of *E. coli* may produce a protein called *heat-labile enterotoxin* (LT) that is similar to cholera toxin and causes secretory diarrhea by the same mechanism. Alternatively, enterotoxigenic strains of *E. coli* may produce *heat-stable enterotoxin* (ST), one form of which causes diarrhea by activation of guanylate cyclase and elevation of intracellular cyclic GMP. Some enterotoxigenic strains produce both LT and ST.

Bacterial cytotoxins, in contrast, destroy intestinal mucosal cells and produce the syndrome of dysentery, with bloody stools containing inflammatory cells. Enteric pathogens that produce such cytotoxins include *S. dysenteriae*, *Vibrio parahaemolyticus*, and *Clostridium difficile*. Enterohemorrhagic strains of *E. coli*, most commonly serotype O157:H7 in the United States, also produce potent cytotoxins that are highly related to Shiga toxin from *S. dysenteriae* and have been termed *Shiga-like toxins*. Such strains of *E. coli* have been associated with outbreaks of hemorrhagic colitis and hemolytic-uremic syndrome.

Neurotoxins usually are produced by the responsible organism outside the host and therefore cause symptoms soon after ingestion. Included are the staphylococcal and *Bacillus cereus* toxins, which act on the central nervous system to produce vomiting.

Invasion   Dysentery may result not only from the production of cytotoxins but also from bacterial invasion and destruction of intestinal mucosal cells. Infections due to *Shigella* and enteroinvasive *E. coli*, for example, are characterized by the organisms' invasion of mucosal epithelial cells, intraepithelial multiplication, and subsequent spread to adjacent cells. *Salmonella*, on the other hand, causes inflammatory diarrhea by invasion of the bowel mucosa but generally is not associated with the destruction of enterocytes or the full clinical syndrome of dysentery. *Salmonella typhi* and *Yersinia enterocolitica* can penetrate intact intestinal mucosa, multiply intracellularly in Peyer's patches and intestinal lymph nodes, and then disseminate through the bloodstream to cause enteric fever, a syndrome characterized by fever, headache, relative bradycardia, abdominal pain, splenomegaly, and leukopenia.

HOST DEFENSES   Given the enormous number of microorganisms ingested with every meal, it is evident that the normal host must possess effective defense mechanisms to combat a constant influx of potential enteric pathogens. Studies of infections in patients with alterations in these defenses have led to a greater understanding of the variety of ways in which the normal host can protect itself against disease.

Normal Flora   The large numbers of bacteria that normally inhabit the intestine act as an important host defense by preventing colonization by potential enteric pathogens. Persons with fewer intestinal bacteria, such as infants who have not yet developed normal enteric colonization or patients receiving antibiotics, are at significantly greater risk of developing infections with enteric pathogens. The composition of the intestinal flora is as important as the number of organisms present. More than 99 percent of the normal colonic flora is made up of anaerobic bacteria, and the acidic pH and volatile fatty acids produced by these organisms appear to be critical elements in the resistance to colonization conferred by the normal enteric flora.

Gastric Acid   The acidic pH of the stomach is an important barrier to enteric pathogens, and an increased frequency of infections

Table 128-1

Gastrointestinal Pathogens Causing Acute Diarrhea

Mechanism	Location	Illness	Stool Findings	Examples of Pathogens Involved
Noninflammatory (enterotoxin)	Proximal small bowel	Watery diarrhea	No fecal leukocytes	*Vibrio cholerae* Enterotoxigenic *Escherichia coli* (LT and/or ST) *Clostridium perfringens* *Bacillus cereus* *Staphylococcus aureus* *Aeromonas hydrophila* *Plesiomonas shigelloides* Rotavirus Norwalk-like viruses Enteric adenoviruses *Giardia lamblia* *Cryptosporidium*
Inflammatory (invasion or cytotoxin)	Colon or distal small bowel	Dysentery or inflammatory diarrhea	Fecal polymorphonuclear leukocytes	*Shigella* spp. *Salmonella* spp. *Campylobacter jejuni* Enterohemorrhagic *E. coli* Enteroinvasive *E. coli* *Yersinia enterocolitica* *Vibrio parahaemolyticus* *Clostridium difficile* ?*Aeromonas hydrophila* ?*Plesiomonas shigelloides* *Entamoeba histolytica*
Penetrating	Distal small bowel	Enteric fever	Fecal mononuclear leukocytes	*Salmonella typhi* *Yersinia enterocolitica*

SOURCE: After Guerrant.

due to *Salmonella*, *Shigella*, *G. lamblia*, and a variety of helminths has been reported among patients who have undergone gastric surgery or are achlorhydric for some other reason. Neutralization of gastric acid with antacids or with H_2 blockers—common among hospitalized patients—similarly increases the risk of enteric colonization. Some microorganisms, however, can survive the extreme acidity of the gastric environment; rotavirus, for example, is highly stable to acidity.

Intestinal Motility Normal peristalsis is the major mechanism for clearance of bacteria from the proximal small intestine, although gastric acidity and secreted immunoglobulins also play a role in limiting the number of organisms present. When intestinal motility is impaired—for example, by treatment with opiates or other antimotility drugs, anatomic abnormalities (diverticula, fistulas, or afferent-loop stasis following surgery), or hypomotility states (as in diabetes mellitus or scleroderma)—the frequency of bacterial overgrowth and infection of the small bowel with enteric pathogens is much increased. Some patients in whom *Shigella* infection is treated with diphenoxylate hydrochloride with atropine (Lomotil) experience prolonged fever and shedding of organisms, while patients treated with opiates for mild *Salmonella* gastroenteritis have a higher frequency of bacteremia than those not treated with opiates.

Immunity Both cellular immune responses and antibody production play important roles in protecting susceptible hosts from enteric infections. The wide spectrum of viral, bacterial, parasitic, and fungal gastrointestinal infections in patients with AIDS highlights the significance of cell-mediated immunity in protecting the normal host from these pathogens. Humoral immunity is also important and consists of systemic IgG and IgM as well as secretory IgA. Growing evidence supports the concept of a mucosal immune system for secretory IgA in which binding of bacterial antigens to the luminal surface of M cells in the distal small bowel and subsequent presentation of the antigens to subepithelial lymphoid tissue lead to the proliferation of sensitized lymphocytes. These lymphocytes circulate and populate all of the mucosal tissues of the body as IgA-secreting plasma cells.

Approach to the Patient

The approach to the patient with possible infectious diarrhea or bacterial food poisoning is shown in Fig. 128-1.

History The answers to questions with high discriminating value can quickly narrow the range of potential causes of diarrhea and help determine whether treatment is needed. Important elements of the narrative history are detailed in Fig. 128-1.

Physical Examination The examination of patients for signs of dehydration provides essential information about the severity of the diarrheal illness and the need for rapid therapy. Mild dehydration is indicated by thirst, dry mouth, decreased axillary sweat, decreased urine output, and slight weight loss. Signs of moderate dehydration include an orthostatic fall in blood pressure, skin tenting, and sunken eyes (or, in infants, a sunken fontanelle). Signs of severe dehydration range from hypotension and tachycardia to confusion and frank shock.

Diagnostic Approach After the severity of illness is assessed, the most important distinction that the clinician must make is between *inflammatory* and *noninflammatory* disease. Using the history and epidemiologic features of the case as guides in making this distinction, the clinician can rapidly evaluate the need for further efforts to define a specific etiology and for therapeutic intervention. Examination of a stool sample is an important supplement to the narrative history. Grossly bloody or mucoid stool suggests an inflammatory process, but all stools should be examined for fecal leukocytes; the latter task is accomplished by the preparation of a thin smear of the stool on a glass slide, the addition of a drop of methylene blue, and examination of the wet mount. Causes of acute infectious diarrhea, categorized as inflammatory and noninflammatory, are listed in Table 128-1.

EPIDEMIOLOGY **Travel History** Of the 12 to 20 million people who travel from temperate industrialized countries to tropical regions of Asia, Africa, and Central and South America each year, 20 to 50 percent will experience a sudden onset of abdominal cramps, anorexia, and watery diarrhea; thus *traveler's diarrhea* is the most common travel-related illness (see Chap. 123). The time of onset is usually 3 days to 2 weeks after the traveler's arrival in a tropical area; most cases begin within the first 3 to 5 days. The illness is generally self-limited, lasting 1 to 5 days. The high rate of diarrhea among travelers to underdeveloped areas is related to the ingestion of contaminated food or water.

The organisms that cause traveler's diarrhea vary considerably with location. In all areas, enterotoxigenic *E. coli* is the most common isolate from persons with the classic secretory traveler's diarrhea syndrome; the proportion of cases accounted for by this organism ranges from a high of approximately 50 percent in Latin America to a low of 15 percent in Asia. *Shigella*, *Salmonella*, and *Campylobacter* spp. are classically considered to cause more invasive dysenteric disease than enterotoxigenic *E. coli*, but clinical differentiation of infections attributable to these organisms can be difficult. *Shigella*, *Salmonella*, and *Campylobacter* are isolated in 1 to 15 percent of cases, with different organisms being more common in different locations. *Vibrio* species are most common in Asia, although *V. cholerae* disease reached epidemic proportions in parts of Central and South America in 1991 and has become a significant concern to travelers to these regions. Less common bacteria are *Aeromonas hydrophila* and *Plesiomonas shigelloides*, which have been isolated from travelers to Thailand. Parasitic causes of traveler's diarrhea include *Entamoeba histolytica*, which is responsible for up to 5 percent of cases in Mexico and Thailand, and *G. lamblia*, which has been associated with contaminated freshwater supplies in many areas of the world. *Giardia* is found in association with zoonotic reservoirs in the northern United States and poses a risk to hikers and campers who drink from freshwater streams. A striking association of *Giardia* with contaminated water supplies has likewise been noted in St. Petersburg in the former Soviet Union. *Cryptosporidium* has been recognized as a problem in travelers to the Commonwealth of Independent States, Mexico, and Africa and has caused large-scale urban outbreaks of infection in the United States. Viruses such as rotavirus and Norwalk-like viruses have been isolated from up to 12 percent of visitors to Latin America, Asia, and Africa.

Location Day-care centers are sites of particularly high attack rates of enteric infections. Rotavirus is most common among children less than 2 years old, with attack rates of 75 to 100 percent among those exposed. *G. lamblia* is more common among older children, with somewhat lower attack rates. Other common organisms, often spread by fecal-oral contact, are *Shigella*, *Campylobacter jejuni*, and *Cryptosporidium*. A characteristic feature of infection in day-care centers is the high rate of secondary cases among family members.

Similarly, hospitals are sites for concentrations of enteric infections. In medical intensive-care units and pediatric wards, diarrhea is among the most common nosocomial infections. *C. difficile* and *Salmonella* species are predominant causes of nosocomial diarrhea in the United States; viral pathogens, especially rotavirus, can spread rapidly in pediatric wards. Enteropathogenic *E. coli* has been associated with outbreaks of diarrhea in newborn nurseries. One-third of elderly patients in chronic-care institutions develop a significant diarrheal illness each year. Surveillance stool cultures suggest that 25 percent of the residents of these institutions harbor cytotoxin-producing *C. difficile*, which causes more than half of all cases of diarrhea in this population. Antimicrobial therapy can predispose to pseudomembranous colitis by altering the normal colonic flora and allowing the multiplication of *C. difficile*.

Age Most of the morbidity and mortality from enteric pathogens involves children less than 5 years of age. Breast-fed infants are protected from contaminated food and water and derive some protection from maternal antibodies, but their risk of infection rises dramatically when they begin to eat solid foods. Infants and younger children are more likely than adults to develop rotaviral disease, while older children and adults are more commonly infected with Norwalk-like viruses. Other organisms with higher attack rates among children than among adults include enterotoxigenic and enteropathogenic *E. coli*,

C. jejuni, and *G. lamblia*. In children, the incidence of *Salmonella* infections is highest among infants under 1 year of age, while the attack rate for *Shigella* infections is greatest among children aged 6 months to 4 years.

Bacterial Food Poisoning   If the history and the stool examination indicate a noninflammatory etiology of diarrhea and there is evidence of a common-source outbreak, questions concerning the ingestion of specific foods and the time of onset of the diarrhea after a meal can provide clues to the bacterial cause of the illness. Potential causes of bacterial food poisoning are shown in Table 128-2.

Bacterial disease caused by an enterotoxin elaborated outside the host, such as that due to *Staphylococcus aureus* or *B. cereus*, has the shortest incubation period (1 to 6 h) and generally lasts less than 12 h. Most cases of staphylococcal food poisoning are caused by contamination from infected human carriers. Staphylococci can multiply at a wide range of temperatures; thus, if food is left to cool slowly and remains at room temperature after cooking, the organisms will have the opportunity to form enterotoxin. Outbreaks following picnics where potato salad, mayonnaise, and cream pastries have been served offer classic examples of staphylococcal food poisoning. Diarrhea, nausea, vomiting, and abdominal cramping are common, while fever is less so.

B. cereus can produce either a syndrome with a short incubation period—the *emetic* form, mediated by a staphylococcal type of enterotoxin—or one with a longer incubation period (8 to 16 h)—the *diarrheal* form, caused by an *E. coli* LT type of enterotoxin, in which diarrhea and abdominal cramps are characteristic but vomiting is uncommon. The emetic form of *B. cereus* food poisoning is associated with contaminated fried rice; the organism is common in uncooked rice, and its heat-resistant spores survive boiling. If cooked rice is not refrigerated, the spores can germinate and produce toxin. Frying before serving may not destroy the preformed, heat-stable toxin.

Food poisoning due to *Clostridium perfringens* also has a slightly longer incubation period (8 to 14 h) and results from the survival of heat-resistant spores in inadequately cooked meat, poultry, or legumes. After ingestion, toxin is produced in the intestinal tract, causing moderately severe abdominal cramps and diarrhea; vomiting is rare, as is fever. The illness is self-limited, rarely lasting for more than 24 h.

Not all food poisoning has a bacterial cause. Diagnostic confusion can result from diarrhea caused by nonbacterial agents of short-incubation food poisoning, including capsaicin, which is found in hot peppers, and a variety of toxins found in fish and shellfish (Table 128-3).

LABORATORY EVALUATION   Many cases of noninflammatory diarrhea are self-limited or can be treated empirically, and in these instances the clinician may not need to determine a specific etiology. Potentially pathogenic *E. coli* cannot be distinguished from normal fecal flora by routine culture. Special tests to detect LT and

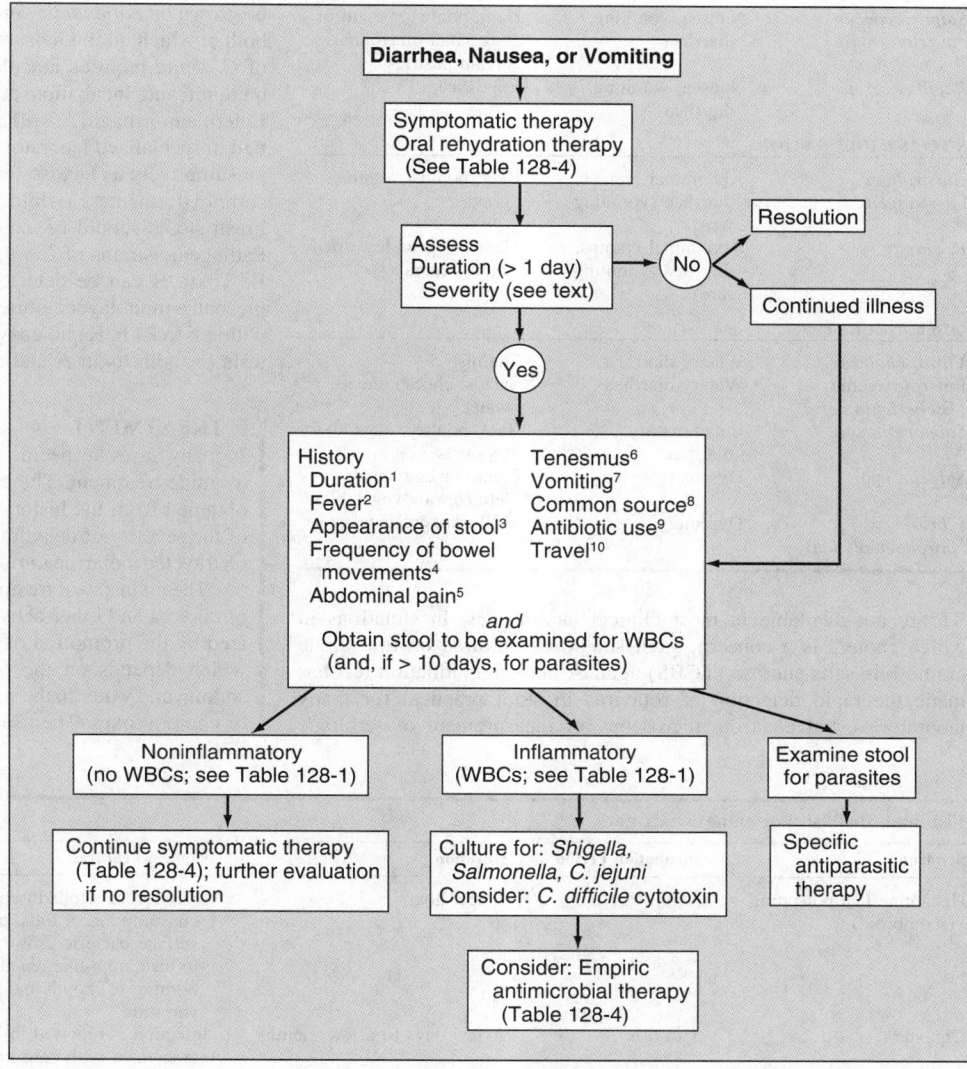

FIGURE 128-1   Clinical algorithm for the approach to patients with possible infectious diarrhea or food poisoning. Key to superscripts: 1. Diarrhea lasting more than 2 weeks generally is defined as chronic; in such cases, many of the causes of acute diarrhea are much less likely, and a new spectrum of causes needs to be considered. 2. Fever often implies invasive disease, although fever and diarrhea also may result from infection outside the gastrointestinal tract, as in malaria. 3. Stools that contain blood or mucus indicate ulceration of the large bowel. Bloody stools without fecal leukocytes should alert the laboratory to the possibility of infection with Shiga-like toxin–producing enterohemorrhagic *Escherichia coli*. Bulky white stools suggest a small intestinal process that is causing malabsorption. Profuse "rice-water" stools suggest cholera or a similar toxigenic process. 4. The number of stools over a given period can be the first warning of impending dehydration. 5. Abdominal pain may be most severe in inflammatory processes like those due to *Shigella, Campylobacter,* and necrotizing toxins. Painful abdominal muscle cramps, caused by electrolyte loss, can develop in severe cases of cholera. Bloating is common in giardiasis. An appendicitis-like syndrome should prompt a culture for *Yersinia enterocolitica* with cold enrichment. 6. Tenesmus (cramps in the rectum felt after a bowel movement) may be a feature of cases with inflammation of the rectum, as in shigellosis. 7. Vomiting implies an acute infection (e.g., a toxin-mediated illness or food poisoning) but can also be prominent in a variety of systemic illnesses (e.g., malaria) and in intestinal obstruction. 8. Asking patients whether anyone else they know is sick is a more efficient means of identifying a common source than is constructing a list of recently eaten foods. If a common source seems likely, specific foods can be investigated. See text for a discussion of bacterial food poisoning. 9. Stop antibiotic treatment if possible and consider culture for cytotoxigenic *Clostridium difficile*. Antibiotic use may increase the risk of other infections, such as salmonellosis. 10. See text for a discussion of traveler's diarrhea. (*After Guerrant and Guerrant and Bobak.*)

Table 128-2

Bacterial Food Poisoning

Organisms	Symptoms	Common Food Sources
1 TO 6 h INCUBATION		
Staphylococcus aureus	Nausea, vomiting, diarrhea	Ham, poultry, potato or egg salad, mayonnaise, cream pastries
Bacillus cereus	Nausea, vomiting, diarrhea	Fried rice
8 TO 16 h INCUBATION		
Clostridium perfringens	Abdominal cramps, diarrhea (vomiting rare)	Beef, poultry, legumes, gravies
B. cereus	Abdominal cramps, diarrhea (vomiting rare)	Meats, vegetables, dried beans, cereals
>16 h INCUBATION		
Vibrio cholerae	Watery diarrhea	Shellfish
Enterotoxigenic *Escherichia coli*	Watery diarrhea	Salads, cheese, meats, water
Salmonella spp.	Inflammatory diarrhea	Beef, poultry, eggs, dairy products
Shigella spp.	Dysentery	Potato or egg salad, lettuce, raw vegetables
Vibrio parahaemolyticus	Dysentery	Mollusks, crustaceans

ST are not available in most clinical laboratories. In situations in which cholera is a concern, stool should be cultured on thiosulfate citrate bile salts sucrose (TCBS) agar. A latex agglutination test has made the rapid detection of rotavirus in stool practical for many laboratories, but electron microscopy or measurement of serologic

response with a radioimmunoassay is still necessary for the identification of Norwalk-like viruses. At least three stool specimens should be examined for *Giardia* cysts or stained for *Cryptosporidium* if the level of clinical suspicion regarding the involvement of these organisms is high.

All patients with fever and evidence of inflammatory disease should have stool cultured for *Salmonella*, *Shigella*, and *Campylobacter*. *Salmonella* and *Shigella* can be selected on MacConkey's agar as non-lactose-fermenting (colorless) colonies or can be grown on *Salmonella-Shigella* agar or in selenite enrichment broth, both of which inhibit most organisms except these pathogens. Isolation of *C. jejuni* requires inoculation of fresh stool onto selective growth medium and incubation at 42°C in a microaerophilic atmosphere. Enterohemorrhagic *E. coli* strains of serotype O157:H7 can be identified in specialized laboratories by serotyping but also can be identified presumptively as lactose-fermenting, indole-positive colonies of non-sorbitol fermenters (white colonies) on sorbitol MacConkey plates. Fresh stools should be examined for amebic cysts and trophozoites. Pathogenic strains of *C. difficile* generally produce two toxins, A and B. Toxin B can be detected with a cytotoxin assay; if the toxin is present, a monolayer culture of fibroblasts will show cytopathic effects within 6 to 24 h. Rapid enzyme immunoassays and latex agglutination tests for both toxin A and toxin B have recently been developed.

TREATMENT

In many cases, a specific diagnosis is not necessary or not available to guide treatment. The clinician can proceed with the information obtained from the history, by stool examination, and by evaluation of the severity of dehydration. Empirical regimens for the treatment of traveler's diarrhea are listed in Table 128-4.

The mainstay of treatment is adequate rehydration. The treatment of cholera and other dehydrating diarrheal diseases was revolutionized by the promotion of oral rehydration solutions, the efficacy of which depends on the fact that glucose-facilitated absorption of sodium and water in the small intestine remains intact in the presence of cholera toxin. The use of oral rehydration solutions has reduced

Table 128-3

Fish and Shellfish Poisoning Syndromes

Syndrome	Incubation Period	Duration	Clinical Features
Histamine fish poisoning (scombroid)	5 min to 1 h	A few hours	Infection develops in coastal states and Hawaii and is associated with consumption of tuna, mackerel, and dolphin. Toxin is formed when surface bacteria grow on flesh, releasing free histidine, which leads to histamine-like reactions, with flushing, headache, dizziness, burning of mouth and throat, palpitations, nausea, diarrhea, and vomiting.
Ciguatera	1 to 6 h	A few days to a few months	Infection is reported in Hawaii, Florida, and the Caribbean and is associated with consumption of carnivorous reef fish such as barracuda and grouper. Toxin is produced by dinoflagellates and acquired by fish through the food chain. Vomiting, watery diarrhea, and cramps develop. Other symptoms include numbness and tingling of the lips and extremities, a reversal of hot and cold sensation, tooth pain, blurred vision, tremor, ataxia, hypotension, and bradycardia.
Paralytic shellfish poisoning	5 min to 4 h	A few hours to a few days	Infection is acquired in temperate coastal areas. Toxin is produced by dinoflagellates and concentrated in bivalve mollusks, often in association with "red tides." Symptoms include paresthesias of the mouth and extremities, headache, ataxia, vertigo, cranial-nerve dysfunction, and muscle paralysis. The case-fatality rate due to respiratory failure is 8 to 9 percent.
Neurotoxic shellfish poisoning	5 min to 4 h	A few hours to a few days	Infection is found in coastal Florida. Toxin is produced by dinoflagellates and concentrated in mollusks. Illness is milder than in paralytic shellfish poisoning, with paresthesias, ataxia, vomiting, and diarrhea but no paralysis.
Tetrodotoxin poisoning	10 min to 3 h	A few days	Infection is acquired in Japan and is caused by a neurotoxin concentrated in the skin and viscera of puffer fish (*Fugu*). Symptoms include lethargy, paresthesias, hyperemesis, salivation, weakness, ataxia, and dysphagia; severe cases may include ascending paralysis, respiratory failure, hypotension, and bradycardia. Mortality is 59 percent.

SOURCE: After Tauxe and Hughes.

Table 128-4

Treatment of Traveler's Diarrhea on the Basis of Clinical Features

Clinical Syndrome	Suggested Therapy
Watery diarrhea (no blood in stool or fever), 1–2 unformed stools per day without distressing enteric symptoms	Oral fluids (Pedialyte, Lytren, or flavored mineral wateR) and saltine crackers
Watery diarrhea (no blood in stool or fever), 1–2 unformed stools per day with distressing enteric symptoms	Bismuth subsalicylate (for adults): 30 mL or 2 tablets (262 mg/tablet) every 30 min for 8 doses; or loperamide*: 4 mg initially followed by 2 mg after passage of each unformed stool, not to exceed 8 tablets (16 mg) per day (prescription dose) or 4 caplets (8 mg) per day (over-the-counter dose); drugs can be taken for 2 days
Watery diarrhea (no blood in stool, distressing abdominal pain, or fever), >2 unformed stools per day	Antibacterial drug† plus (for adults) loperamide* (see dose above)
Dysentery (passage of bloody stools) or fever (>37.8°C)	Antibacterial drug†
Vomiting, minimal dirrhea	Bismuth subsalicylate (for adults; see dose above)
Diarrhea in infants (<2 y old)	Fluids and electrolytes (Pedialyte, Lytren); continue feeding, especially with breast milk; seek medical attention for moderate dehydration, fever lasting >24 h, bloody stools, or diarrhea lasting more than several days
Diarrhea in pregnant women	Fluids and electrolytes; can consider attapulgite, 3 g initially, with dose repeated after passage of each unformed stool or every 2 h (whichever is earlier), for a total dosage of 9 g/d
Diarrhea despite trimethoprim-sulfamethoxazole prophylaxis	Fluoroquinolone—with loperamide (see dose above) if no fever or blood in stool, alone in cases of fever/dysentery
Diarrhea despite fluoroquinolone prophylaxis	Bismuth subsalicylate (see dose above) for mild to moderate disease; consult physician for moderate to severe disease or if disease persists

* Loperamide should not be used by patients with fever or dysentery; its use may prolong diarrhea in patients with infection due to *Shigella* or other invasive organisms.
† The recommended antibacterial drugs are as follows:

Travel to Mexican interior, summer   *Adults:* Trimethoprim-sulfamethoxazole (TMP-SMZ), 160 mg/800 mg bid for 3 days
    Children: TMP-SMZ, 4/20 mg/kg/d, given bid for 3 days
Travel to other areas in other seasons   *Adults:* Norfloxacin, 400 mg bid; ciprofloxacin, 500 mg bid; ofloxacin, 300 mg bid; or fleroxacin, 400 mg/d, for 3 days
    Children: TMP-SMZ (above dose) plus erythromycin at dose based on weight (<11 kg, 250 mg/d; 11–18 kg, 375 mg/d; 18.5–25 kg, 500 mg/d; 25.5–36 kg, 750 mg/d; and >36 kg, 1000 mg/d) in four divided doses for 5 days; alternative single agent: furazolidone, 7.5 mg/kg/d in four divided doses for 5 days

All patients should take oral fluids (Pedialyte, Lytren, or flavored mineral water) plus saltine crackers. If moderate to severe diarrhea develops, if fever persists, or if bloody stools or dehydration develops, the patient should seek medical attention.

SOURCE:After Dupont.

mortality due to cholera from greater than 50 percent (in untreated cases) to less than 1 percent. The World Health Organization recommends a solution containing 3.5 g of sodium chloride, 2.5 g of sodium bicarbonate, 1.5 g of potassium chloride, and 20 g of glucose (or 40 g of sucrose) per liter of water. Patients who are severely dehydrated or in whom vomiting precludes the use of oral therapy should receive intravenous solutions such as Ringer's lactate.

Although most secretory forms of traveler's diarrhea—usually due to enterotoxigenic *E. coli*—can be treated effectively with rehydration, bismuth subsalicylate, or antiperistaltic agents, antimicrobial agents can shorten the duration of illness from 3 to 4 days to 24 to 36 h.

PROPHYLAXIS Improvements in hygiene to limit fecal-oral spread of enteric pathogens will be necessary if the prevalence of diarrheal diseases is to be significantly reduced in developing countries. Travelers can reduce their risk of diarrhea by eating only hot, freshly cooked food; by avoiding raw vegetables, salads, and unpeeled fruit; and by drinking only boiled or treated water and avoiding ice.

Bismuth subsalicylate is an inexpensive agent for the prophylaxis of traveler's diarrhea; it is taken at a dosage of 2 tablets (525 mg) four times a day. Treatment appears to be effective and safe for up to 3 weeks. Prophylactic antimicrobial agents, although effective, are not generally recommended for the prevention of traveler's diarrhea. The risk of side effects and the possibility of developing an infection with a drug-resistant organism or with more harmful, invasive bacteria make it more reasonable to institute a short course of treatment once symptoms have developed.

The possibility of exerting a major impact on the worldwide morbidity and mortality associated with diarrheal diseases has led to intense efforts to develop effective vaccines against the common bacterial and viral enteric pathogens. Recent research has shown promising advances in the development of vaccines against rotavirus, *Shigella*, *V. cholerae*, *S. typhi*, and enterotoxigenic *E. coli*.

BIBLIOGRAPHY

Advice for travelers. Med Lett Drugs Ther 38:17, 1996

ALTEKRUSE SF, SWERDLOW DL: The changing epidemiology of foodborne diseases. Am J Med Sci 311:23, 1996

DUPONT HL: Travelers' diarrhea, in *Infections of the Gastrointestinal Tract*, MJ Blaser et al (eds). New York, Raven Press, 1995, chap 22

———, ERICSSON CD: Prevention and treatment of traveler's diarrhea. N Engl J Med 328:1821, 1993

EASTAUGH J, SHEPHERD S: Infectious and toxic syndromes from fish and shellfish consumption. Arch Intern Med 149:1735, 1989

GUERRANT RL: Principles and syndromes of enteric infection, in *Mandell, Douglas and Bennett's Principles and Practice of Infectious Diseases*, 4th ed, GL Mandell et al (eds). New York, Churchill Livingstone, 1995, chap 75

———, BOBAK DA: Bacterial and protozoal gastroenteritis. N Engl J Med 325:327, 1991

TAUXE RV, HUGHES JM: Food-borne disease, in *Mandell, Douglas and Bennett's Principles and Practice of Infectious Diseases*, 4th ed, GL Mandell et al (eds). New York, Churchill Livingstone, 1995, chap 81

129

King K. Holmes, H. Hunter Handsfield

SEXUALLY TRANSMITTED DISEASES: OVERVIEW AND CLINICAL APPROACH

In all societies, sexually transmitted diseases (STDs) are among the most common of all infections. Moreover, STDs figure prominently among the world's major emerging/reemerging infections. Many new sexually transmitted pathogens have been recognized and characterized since 1980, including human immunodeficiency virus (HIV) types 1 and 2, human T cell lymphotropic virus (HTLV) types I and II, many genotypes of human papillomavirus (HPV), *Mycoplasma genitalium*, two species of *Mobiluncus*, and the Kaposi's sarcoma–associated herpesvirus. Certain well-known STD pathogens, including *Neisseria gonorrhoeae* and *Haemophilus ducreyi*, often lead the way in acquiring resistance to new antimicrobials. In developing countries, such factors as the population explosion (especially in the adolescent and young-adult age groups), rural-to-urban migration, wars, and poverty create steady pressure that favors the emergence of new STDs. In addition, in the developing countries, HIV infection and three bacterial STDs—gonorrhea, chlamydial infection, and syphilis—rank among the top 10 to 20 diseases causing the loss of years of healthy, productive life. Among the viral STDs, infection with HIV has become the leading cause of death in persons 25 to 44 years of age in the United States and in developing countries. Two of the most common sexually transmitted viruses—HPV and hepatitis B virus (HBV)—are important causes of cervical, vaginal, vulvar, and penile carcinomas and of hepatocellular carcinoma, respectively. In industrialized nations, sexually transmitted herpes simplex virus (HSV) infections are the most common cause of genital ulceration that may facilitate HIV transmission, and perinatally transmitted HSV frequently causes serious morbidity among infants. There is also growing evidence of the sexual transmission of HTLV-I in many developing countries of Latin America, Africa, and the Caribbean. Although the bacterial STDs remain extremely common in developing countries, their incidence is now rapidly declining in most industrialized countries. However, rates of gonorrhea, chancroid, and syphilis remain higher in the United States than in any other industrialized country except for Russia and several other eastern European nations that are now experiencing major epidemics of STDs. The Centers for Disease Control and Prevention (CDC) in Atlanta estimates that at least 12 million U.S. residents acquire an STD each year, and some authorities estimate that at least half of all Americans acquire a sexually transmitted infection by age 35. The total annual costs attributable to STDs other than HIV infection for the United States in 1994 have been estimated at $10 billion. In industrialized countries, certain incurable viral STDs [e.g., HPV infection, genital herpes, and cytomegalovirus (CMV) infection] remain very common in all segments of the adult population. The marked enhancement of the efficiency of transmission of HIV by both the genital ulcerative and the genital mucosal STDs adds to the urgency of STD prevention and control.

CLASSIFICATION AND GENERAL APPROACH

STDs can be classified on the basis of either cause or clinical manifestations. Table 129-1 summarizes the etiologic classification of STDs. Several of the pathogens listed are also transmitted nonsexually, but in each instance sexual transmission is clinically and epidemiologically important.

No single STD can be regarded as an isolated problem because multiple infections are common and because the presence of one STD denotes high-risk sexual behavior that is often associated with other, more serious infections. Most STDs are rarely if ever transmitted by fomites, food, flies, or casual contact. *At least one sexual partner is always infected*; the apparent exceptions usually can be attributed to prolonged subclinical infection in one or both partners. Therefore, risk assessment (including elicitation of a sexual history) and management of sexual partners are of paramount importance.

Persons with overt genital discharge, lesions, or pain usually cease sexual activity and seek medical care. Accordingly, those who transmit infection usually are asymptomatic or have mild symptoms and do not seek medical attention spontaneously. Physicians must examine and treat or refer such partners. In the United States, local health departments will usually help to identify and treat or counsel contacts of patients with syphilis, gonorrhea, and (in some jurisdictions) chlamydial or HIV infection; for most STDs, however, this responsibility is shared by the patient and the clinician.

In general, persons with a new-onset STD have a *source contact* from whom it was acquired; in addition, they may have a *secondary contact* (also known as a *spread contact* or *exposed contact*). The identification and treatment of both types of contacts are important but generally for different reasons. Treatment of the source contact (often a casual contact who, by definition, is transmitting infection) benefits the community by preventing further transmission. Treatment of the recently exposed secondary contact (more often a spouse or another steady sexual partner) prevents both the development of serious complications, such as pelvic inflammatory disease (PID), in the partner and reinfection of the index patient.

The increasing importance of the viral STDs, most of which are incurable and lifelong, underscores the central role of preventing infection. Whereas early detection and curative treatment can help curtail the spread of the bacterial STDs, control of the viral STDs depends entirely on the avoidance of unprotected exposure to infected persons; the sole exception is vaccination against HBV infection.

STDs disproportionately affect women and newborn children. Many STDs (e.g., genital herpes, gonorrhea, and HIV infection) are transmitted more efficiently from men to women than from women to men. Once infection occurs, many STDs produce complications more often in women than in men, for several reasons. For anatomic or physiologic reasons, for example, women appear to be intrinsically more susceptible to genital cancers complicating HPV infection, to upper genital tract infections, and to puerperal complications. Furthermore, early in the course, women are more likely than men to have subclinical infections or minor, nonspecific symptoms—a situation that can result in delayed diagnosis. The lesser specificity of clinical findings and the lesser sensitivity of several microbiologic tests in women than in men make the diagnosis of STDs more difficult in women. Thus prevention of STDs is a women's health issue. CDC epidemiologists identified 150,737 deaths attributable to STDs in

Table 129-1

Sexually Transmitted Pathogens

Bacteria	Viruses	Other*
TRANSMITTED IN ADULTS PREDOMINANTLY BY SEXUAL INTERCOURSE		
Neisseria gonorrhoeae	Human immunodeficiency virus (types 1 and 2)	*Trichomonas vaginalis*
Chlamydia trachomatis		*Phthirus pubis*
Treponema pallidum	Human T cell lymphotropic virus type I	
Haemophilus ducreyi	Herpes simplex virus type 2	
Calymmatobacterium granulomatis	Human papillomavirus (multiple genotypes)	
Ureaplasma urealyticum	Hepatitis B virus†	
	Cytomegalovirus	
	Molluscum contagiosum virus	
SEXUAL TRANSMISSION REPEATEDLY DESCRIBED BUT NOT WELL DEFINED OR NOT THE PREDOMINANT MODE		
Mycoplasma hominis	Human T cell lymphotropic virus type II	*Candida albicans*
Mycoplasma genitalium	(?) Hepatitis C, D viruses	*Sarcoptes scabiei*
Gardnerella vaginalis and other vaginal bacteria	Herpes simplex virus type 1	
	(?) Epstein-Barr virus	
Group B *Streptococcus*	Kaposi's sarcoma–associated herpesvirus	
TRANSMITTED BY SEXUAL CONTACT INVOLVING ORAL-FECAL EXPOSURE; OF DECLINING IMPORTANCE IN HOMOSEXUAL MEN		
Shigella spp.	Hepatitis A virus	*Giardia lamblia*
Campylobacter spp.		*Entamoeba histolytica*

* Includes protozoa, ectoparasites, and fungi.
† Among U.S. patients for whom a risk factor can be ascertained, most hepatitis B virus infections are sexually transmitted.

U.S. women from 1973 to 1992; 29 percent of these deaths were attributable to HIV, 59 percent to cervical cancer, 11 percent to hepatitis, and the remainder to other STDs. STDs are propagated most efficiently in populations with frequent changes of sexual partners and with poor access to or low motivation in obtaining early treatment. In most of the United States, these groups consist predominantly of young unmarried individuals of low socioeconomic status. These individuals often reside within circumscribed, deteriorating, crowded urban neighborhoods, although rates of STDs are also high in some rural areas (in the southeastern United States, for example). The treatable bacterial STDs, such as syphilis, gonorrhea, and chancroid, are increasingly concentrated in "core populations" and increasingly affect prostitutes and their sexual partners as well as persons involved in the use of illicit drugs, particularly crack cocaine in the United States. Members of these core populations have been difficult to reach for the purposes of education and contact tracing and may continue to be sexually active despite STD symptoms. Other STDs are more evenly distributed in society. For example, in the absence of diagnostic testing and partner treatment, chlamydial infections can persist for many months (often asymptomatically) and can be propagated widely in populations that do not share all of the characteristics of core groups associated with gonorrhea, syphilis, chancroid, or HIV infection. Similarly, genital HPV infection is incurable and therefore persists and spreads efficiently in relatively low-risk populations.

Various STDs differ in the extent to which their spread and persistence in the population depend on high rates of sexual partner change. In general, the initial rate of spread of any STD pathogen within a population depends on the product of three factors: rate of exposure, efficiency of transmission per exposure, and duration of infectivity of those infected. For any given sexually transmitted infection, Anderson and May express this idea as $R_0 = c \times \beta \times D$, where R_0 represents the "reproductive rate" of a pathogen (i.e., the average number of new secondary cases arising from an infected person); c reflects the average rate and variance in the rate of partner change in the population and patterns of partner mixing; β represents the average efficiency of transmission per exposure of a susceptible person to an infected person; and D is the mean duration of infectivity for infected persons. For diseases with a high efficiency of transmission and/or a long duration of infectiousness, rates of partner change need not be very high to sustain an epidemic. For STDs with a low efficiency of transmission (e.g., HIV infection) or a short duration of infectiousness (e.g., chancroid), high rates of partner change may be necessary to sustain an epidemic. Efforts to prevent and control STDs involve attempts to decrease the duration of infectiousness (through early diagnosis and treatment), to decrease the efficiency of transmission (e.g., through promotion of condom use), and to decrease the rate of partner change (e.g., through provision of information, health education, and counseling and efforts to change the norms of sexual behavior).

MANAGEMENT OF COMMON STD SYNDROMES

Table 129-2 lists some of the most common clinical STD syndromes and their associated complications. Strategies for the management of some of the common STD syndromes are outlined below. Infections with human retroviruses are discussed in Chaps. 192 and 308.

An overall approach to the management of a patient with an STD begins with risk assessment (of sexual orientation, number of recent and current sexual partners, sexual practices, recent STD history of the partner, STD history of the patient, and sociodemographic and other markers for high risk) and clinical assessment (elicitation of information on specific current symptoms and signs of STDs). Confirmatory diagnostic tests or screening tests (e.g., culture, antigen detection tests, genetic probe or amplification tests, serologic tests) may then be ordered. In developing countries and in office practices in most industrialized countries, initial treatment is usually syndrome-based and is selected to cover the most likely causes. For certain syndromes in industrialized countries, rapid tests may be used to narrow the spectrum of this initial therapy (e.g., wet mount of vaginal

Table 129-2

Common STD Syndromes and Sexually Transmitted (ST) Etiologic Agents

Syndrome	Primary ST Agents
AIDS	HIV types 1 and 2
Urethritis: males	*Neisseria gonorrhoeae, Chlamydia trachomatis, Ureaplasma urealyticum, Trichomonas vaginalis*, HSV
Epididymitis	*C. trachomatis, N. gonorrhoeae*
Lower genital tract infections: females	
Cystitis/urethritis	*C. trachomatis, N. gonorrhoeae*, HSV
Mucopurulent cervicitis	*C. trachomatis, N. gonorrhoeae*
Vulvovaginitis	*Candida albicans, T. vaginalis*
Bacterial vaginosis (BV)	BV-associated bacteria (see text)
Acute pelvic inflammatory disease	*N. gonorrhoeae, C. trachomatis,* BV-associated bacteria
Infertility	*N. gonorrhoeae, C. trachomatis,* BV-associated bacteria
Ulcerative lesions of the genitalia	HSV-1, HSV-2, *Treponema pallidum, Haemophilus ducreyi, C. trachomatis* (LGV strains), *Calymmatobacterium granulomatis*
Intestinal infections	
Proctitis	*C. trachomatis, N. gonorrhoeae*, HSV, *T. pallidum*
Proctocolitis or enterocolitis	*Campylobacter* spp., *Shigella* spp., *Entamoeba histolytica*, other enteric pathogens
Enteritis	*Giardia lamblia, Cryptosporidium,* Microsporidia
Acute arthritis with urogenital infection or viremia	*N. gonorrhoeae* (e.g., DGI), *C. trachomatis* (e.g., Reiter's syndrome), HBV
Genital and anal warts	HPV (genital types)
Mononucleosis syndrome	CMV, HIV, EBV
Viral hepatitis	HBV, *T. pallidum*, CMV, EBV
Neoplasias	
Squamous cell dysplasias and cancers of the cervix, anus, vulva, vagina, or penis	HPV (especially types 16, 18, 31, 45)
Kaposi's sarcoma (KS), body-cavity lymphomas	KS-associated herpesvirus
T cell leukemia	HTLV-I
Hepatocellular carcinoma	HBV
Tropical spastic paraparesis	HTLV-I
Scabies	*Sarcoptes scabiei*
Pubic lice	*Phthirus pubis*

NOTE: HIV, human immunodeficiency virus; HSV, herpes simplex virus; LGV, lymphogranuloma venereum; DGI, disseminated gonococcal infection; HPV, human papillomavirus; CMV, cytomegalovirus; EBV, Epstein-Barr virus; HBV, hepatitis B virus; HTLV, human T cell lymphotropic virus.

fluid for women with vaginal discharge, Gram's stain of urethral discharge for men with such a discharge). After the institution of syndrome-based treatment or (when rapid tests have been diagnostic) of specific treatment, it is essential to complete the first phase of STD management with proper measures for prevention and control (see below). The following approach to the management of common STD syndromes is geared toward clinicians in industrialized countries, where rapid tests and confirmatory tests are widely available but less widely used than they should be.

URETHRITIS IN MEN Urethritis is the most commonly recognized STD syndrome in men. During the past decade, the incidence of gonococcal urethritis has fallen precipitously in nearly all industrialized countries, while that of nongonococcal urethritis (NGU) remains high—a pattern suggesting that measures for control of NGU have so far been relatively ineffective. Gonorrhea and NGU occur with similar frequencies among men seen in STD clinics in the United

States, whereas NGU is much more common than gonorrhea among men seen by physicians in most other clinical settings.

About 30 to 40 percent of NGU cases are caused by *Chlamydia trachomatis*, although the proportion of cases due to this organism may have declined in populations where chlamydial control programs have been implemented. HSV and *Trichomonas vaginalis* each cause a small proportion of NGU cases in the United States, but most cases cannot be attributed to any of these three pathogens. *Ureaplasma urealyticum* has been implicated in case-control studies as a probable cause of many *Chlamydia*-negative cases, and *M. genitalium* was found by polymerase chain reaction (PCR) tests of urethral specimens to be associated with NGU in two recent case-control studies. A few cases are caused by coliform bacteria in men who are the insertive partners in unprotected anal intercourse. The initial diagnosis of urethritis in men usually does not include specific tests for pathogens aside from *N. gonorrhoeae* and *C. trachomatis*. The following steps should be taken in evaluating sexually active men with symptoms of urethral discharge and/or dysuria.

1. *Establish the presence of urethritis.* The first step is examination for purulent or mucopurulent urethral discharge. Sometimes the urethra must be milked after the patient has not voided for several hours, preferably overnight. Whether or not an abnormal discharge is evident, inflammation should be evaluated by examination of a Gram-stained smear after passage of a small swab 2 to 3 cm into the urethra; the presence of 5 or more neutrophils per 1000× field in areas containing cells suggests urethritis. Alternatively, the centrifuged sediment of the first 20 to 30 mL of voided urine can be examined for inflammatory cells, either by microscopy or by the leukocyte esterase test. Patients with symptoms who lack objective evidence of urethritis may have functional rather than organic problems and generally do not benefit from repeated courses of antibiotics.

2. *Evaluate for complications or alternative diagnoses.* Epididymitis and systemic complications, such as disseminated gonococcal infection and Reiter's syndrome, should be excluded by a brief history and examination. Bacterial prostatitis and cystitis should be excluded by appropriate testing of men with dysuria who lack evidence of urethritis and of sexually inactive men with urethritis. Digital examination of the prostate gland is seldom informative in the evaluation of sexually active young men with urethritis.

3. *Evaluate for gonococcal and chlamydial infection.* Gonorrhea is diagnosed by the demonstration of typical gram-negative diplococci within neutrophils, and a preliminary diagnosis of NGU is warranted if gram-negative diplococci are not found. However, as the incidence of gonorrhea declines and the infection becomes uncommon in many clinical settings, fewer clinicians and laboratories may have sufficient expertise to rely solely on stained smears for diagnosis or exclusion of gonococcal infection. Therefore, culture or genomic detection tests for *N. gonorrhoeae* and culture, antigen, or genomic detection tests for *C. trachomatis* should be routinely used in most clinical settings. Genetic amplification using ligase chain reaction or PCR appears to be sensitive and highly specific for either organism; such tests are likely to become widely used for screening and perhaps in diagnostic testing for chlamydial infection and gonorrhea. Diagnostic testing for *C. trachomatis* is recommended, even if empirical treatment for chlamydial infection is planned, because the results predict the patient's prognosis and guide the counseling given to the patient and the management of the patient's sexual partner(s).

4. *Treat the urethritis.* In practice, if gonorrhea is excluded by Gram's stain, urethritis is treated with a regimen effective for NGU—e.g., doxycycline (100 mg orally twice daily for 7 days) or azithromycin (1.0 g orally in a single dose). If gonococci are demonstrated by Gram's stain or if no diagnostic tests are performed, treatment should also include one of the single-dose regimens for gonorrhea

(see Chap. 150) plus azithromycin or a 7-day course of doxycycline for possible chlamydial infection. Sexual partners should be tested for gonorrhea and chlamydial infection and should receive the regimen given to the male index case.

EPIDIDYMITIS Acute epididymitis is almost always unilateral and must be differentiated from testicular torsion, tumor, and trauma. Torsion, a surgical emergency, usually occurs in the second or third decade of life and is suggested by a sudden onset of pain, elevation of the testicle within the scrotal sac, rotation of the epididymis from a posterior to an anterior position, and absence of blood flow on Doppler examination or ^{99m}Tc scan. Testicular tumor is suggested by the persistence of symptoms after a course of therapy. In sexually active men under age 35, acute epididymitis is caused most frequently by *C. trachomatis* and less commonly by *N. gonorrhoeae* and is usually associated with overt or subclinical urethritis. Acute epididymitis in older men or following urinary tract instrumentation is usually caused by gram-negative bacilli or other urinary pathogens. Similarly, epididymitis in men who have been the insertive partners in rectal intercourse is often caused by Enterobacteriaceae. Urethritis is usually absent in these cases, but bacteriuria is detected.

Antimicrobial agents are the mainstays of therapy; an optimal agent for syndrome-based treatment of epididymitis is ofloxacin (300 mg orally, twice daily for 10 days), which is effective against both *N. gonorrhoeae* and *C. trachomatis* as well as against Enterobacteriaceae. Alternatively, ceftriaxone (250 mg intramuscularly) followed by doxycycline (100 mg orally, twice daily for 10 days) is effective for epididymitis caused by *N. gonorrhoeae* or *C. trachomatis*.

LOWER GENITOURINARY TRACT INFECTION IN WOMEN Infections of the female lower urinary tract, cervix, vulva, and vagina produce various combinations of dysuria, vulvar irritation, dyspareunia, and increased or altered vaginal discharge. Two steps are required in the evaluation of symptoms of the lower genitourinary tract in women: (1) differentiation among cystitis, urethritis, vulvovaginitis, and cervicitis and (2) exclusion of associated upper tract disease (e.g., pyelonephritis, salpingitis).

Urethritis and the Urethral Syndrome *C. trachomatis, N. gonorrhoeae,* and occasionally HSV cause symptomatic urethritis—known as the *urethral syndrome*—characterized by "internal" dysuria (usually without urinary urgency or frequency) and pyuria, with *Escherichia coli* or other uropathogens not present at counts of ≥10^2 per milliliter of urine. In contrast, the dysuria associated with vulvar herpes or vulvovaginal candidiasis (and perhaps with trichomoniasis) is often described as "external," being caused by painful contact of urine with the inflamed labia or introitus.

Among women with acute dysuria and frequency, costovertebral pain and tenderness or fever suggest acute pyelonephritis. The management of bacterial urinary tract infection (UTI) is discussed in Chap. 131. Signs of vulvovaginitis, coupled with symptoms of external dysuria, suggest vulvar or vaginal infection. Among women without signs of vulvovaginitis, bacterial UTI must be differentiated from the urethral syndrome by assessment of risks, evaluation of the pattern of symptoms and signs, and specific microbiologic testing. An STD etiology is suggested by young age, more than one current sexual partner or a new partner within the past month, or coexisting mucopurulent cervicitis (see below). Bacterial cystitis is suggested by acute onset, association with urinary urgency or frequency, hematuria, or suprapubic bladder tenderness. The finding of a single conventional urinary pathogen, such as *E. coli* or *Staphylococcus saprophyticus*, in a concentration of ≥10^2/mL in a properly collected specimen of midstream urine from a symptomatic woman with pyuria indicates probable bacterial UTI, whereas pyuria with <10^2 conventional uropathogens per milliliter of urine ("sterile" pyuria) suggests acute urethral syndrome due to *C. trachomatis* or *N. gonorrhoeae*. Gonorrhea and chlamydial infection should be evaluated by cervical culture or other specific tests. Among women with "sterile" pyuria caused by chlamydial infection, treatment with doxycycline (100 mg twice daily for 7 days) alleviates dysuria.

Vulvovaginal Infections Vulvovaginal symptoms rank among the most common reasons for visits to physicians by young women.

Further, certain vulvovaginal infections may have serious sequelae, and trichomoniasis and vulvovaginal candidiasis may increase the rate of sexual transmission of HIV. Vaginal trichomoniasis and bacterial vaginosis early in pregnancy are independent predictors of premature onset of labor. Bacterial vaginosis also appears to be a risk factor for anaerobic bacterial infection of the upper genital tract. Vaginitis may be an early and prominent feature of toxic shock syndrome, and recurrent or chronic vulvovaginal candidiasis develops with increased frequency among women with systemic illnesses, such as diabetes mellitus or HIV infection with impaired immunity (although only a very small proportion of women with recurrent vulvovaginal candidiasis in the United States actually have a serious predisposing illness). Vaginal discharge may be the presenting manifestation of genital herpes and occasionally reflects mucopurulent cervicitis or PID caused by gonorrhea or chlamydial infection.

Thus vulvovaginal symptoms or signs warrant careful evaluation and appropriate therapy that is specific for the anatomic site and type of infection. A careful pelvic examination should usually precede more invasive or expensive tests in the evaluation of women with vulvovaginal, pelvic, or abdominal symptoms.

Bacterial vaginosis is the most common cause of vulvovaginal symptoms in most clinical settings; it is closely followed in frequency by vulvovaginal candidiasis. Trichomoniasis is much less common in most settings in developed countries. Vaginal infection may be characterized by one or more of the following: increased volume of discharge; abnormal yellow color of discharge caused by increased concentration of polymorphonuclear leukocytes; vulvar pruritus, irritation, or burning, often with external dysuria; vulvar dyspareunia; and vaginal malodor. An important component of the clinical evaluation of vaginal discharge is ascertaining by speculum examination whether this discharge emanates from the vagina or the cervix and whether it is objectively abnormal. The diagnosis and treatment of the three common types of vaginal infection are summarized in Table 129-3. A DNA probe test for the detection of *T. vaginalis*, *Candida albicans*, and the increased vaginal concentrations of *Gardnerella vaginalis* found in bacterial vaginosis is now commercially available but has not been extensively evaluated. The general approach to the management of these conditions is outlined below.

Vaginal trichomoniasis (See also Chap. 220)   *T. vaginalis* is sexually transmitted. Although many infected women and most infected men are asymptomatic, treatment of asymptomatic as well as symptomatic cases reduces rates of transmission and prevents later development of symptoms.

Table 129-3

Diagnostic Features and Management of Vaginal Infection

Feature	Normal Vaginal Examination	Vulvovaginal Candidiasis	Trichomonal Vaginitis	Bacterial Vaginosis
Etiology	Uninfected; lactobacilli predominant	*Candida albicans*	*Trichomonas vaginalis*	Associated with *Gardnerella vaginalis*, various anaerobic bacteria, and mycoplasmas
Typical symptoms	None	Vulvar itching and/or irritation	Profuse purulent discharge; vulvar itching	Malodorous, slightly increased discharge
Discharge				
Amount	Variable; usually scant	Scant	Profuse	Moderate
Color*	Clear or white	White	Yellow	White or gray
Consistency	Nonhomogeneous, floccular	Clumped; adherent plaques	Homogeneous	Homogeneous, low viscosity; uniformly coats vaginal walls
Inflammation of vulvar or vaginal epithelium	None	Erythema of vaginal epithelium, introitus; vulvar dermatitis common	Erythema of vaginal and vulvar epithelium; colpitis macularis	None
pH of vaginal fluid†	Usually ≤4.5	Usually ≤4.5	Usually ≥5.0	Usually >4.5
Amine ("fishy") odor with 10% KOH	None	None	May be present	Present
Microscopy‡	Normal epithelial cells; lactobacilli predominant	Leukocytes, epithelial cells; mycelia or pseudomycelia in up to 80% of *C. albicans* culture-positive persons with typical symptoms	Leukocytes; motile trichomonads seen in 80% to 90% of symptomatic patients, less often in the absence of symptoms	Clue cells; few leukocytes; lactobacilli outnumbered by profuse mixed flora, nearly always including *G. vaginalis* plus anaerobic species on Gram's stain
Usual treatment	None	Miconazole or clotrimazole intravaginally, 100 mg nightly for 3 to 7 nights. Fluconazole, 150 mg orally (single dose)	Metronidazole, 2 g orally (single dose). Metronidazole, 500 mg orally, twice daily for 7 days	Metronidazole, 500 mg orally, twice daily for 7 days. Clindamycin, 2% vaginal cream, each night for 7 days. Metronidazole, 0.75% vaginal gel, twice daily for 5 days. Metronidazole, 2 g orally (single dose)§
Usual management of sexual partner	None	None; topical treatment if candidal dermatitis of penis is detected	Examination for STD; treatment with metronidazole, 2 g orally (single dose)	Examination for STD; no treatment if normal

* Color of discharge is best determined by examination against the white background of a swab.
† pH determination is not useful if blood is present.
‡ To detect fungal elements, vaginal fluid is digested with 10% KOH prior to microscopic examination; to examine for other features, fluid is mixed (1:1) with physiologic saline. Gram's stain is also excellent for detecting yeasts and pseudomycelia and for distinguishing normal flora from the mixed flora seen in bacterial vaginosis, but it is less sensitive than the saline preparation for detection of *T. vaginalis*.
§ Single-dose regimen is less effective than 7-day metronidazole regimen.

Symptomatic trichomoniasis characteristically produces a profuse, yellow, purulent, homogeneous vaginal discharge and vulvar irritation. The vaginal and vulvar epithelium may be visibly inflamed, and colposcopy reveals petechial lesions on the cervix ("strawberry cervix") in about 50 percent of cases. The pH of vaginal fluid is usually 5.0 or greater. In women with typical symptoms and signs of trichomoniasis, microscopic examination of vaginal discharge mixed with saline usually reveals motile trichomonads and polymorphonuclear leukocytes. In such cases, wet-mount examination is at least 80 percent as sensitive as culture. However, in women without symptoms or signs, culture is often required for detection of the organism. In men, the diagnosis of *T. vaginalis* infection requires culture of early-morning first-voided urine sediment or of a urethral swab specimen obtained before voiding. Methods of identifying *T. vaginalis* by immunofluorescence or by use of oligonucleotide probes are under investigation and may prove diagnostically helpful for cases in both men and women.

Only nitroimidazoles consistently cure trichomoniasis. A single 2.0-g oral dose of metronidazole is the treatment of choice and is as effective as more prolonged regimens. Other nitroimidazoles such as tinidazole and ornidazole have longer half-lives than metronidazole but do not clearly give better results in trichomoniasis. Routine treatment of sexual partners reduces both the risk of reinfection and the reservoir of infection. Vaginal treatment with 0.75% metronidazole gel, although effective for bacterial vaginosis (see below), is not highly effective for vaginal trichomoniasis. Metronidazole is not recommended during the first trimester of pregnancy but is considered safe thereafter. Alcohol must be avoided for 24 h after its use because of occasional disulfiram-like effects. When practical, the partners of patients with trichomoniasis (or with any sexually transmitted infection, for that matter) should be seen in person, examined, and counseled, but it is common practice to dispense metronidazole to the male partner via the infected female patient.

Bacterial vaginosis Vaginal discharge not associated with *T. vaginalis*, yeast, or cervical infection is usually due to bacterial vaginosis. This syndrome (formerly termed *nonspecific vaginitis, anaerobic vaginitis,* or *Gardnerella-associated vaginal discharge*) is characterized by vaginal malodor and a slightly to moderately increased white discharge that is homogeneous, is low in viscosity, and smoothly coats the vaginal mucosa. The syndrome is associated with STD risk factors, such as multiple sexual partners and recent intercourse with a new partner, but no single sexually transmitted pathogen has been clearly implicated as the cause, and antibiotic treatment of male partners so far has not reduced the rate of recurrence among affected women. Formerly considered a benign condition, bacterial vaginosis has been implicated as a risk factor for acute salpingitis, premature labor, and related neonatal and perinatal complications.

The prevalence and concentrations of *G. vaginalis, Mycoplasma hominis,* and several anaerobic bacteria [e.g., *Mobiluncus* spp., *Prevotella* spp. (formerly *Bacteroides* spp.), and some *Peptostreptococcus* spp.] are markedly greater in vaginal fluid of women with bacterial vaginosis than in that of women without this syndrome. However, none of these organisms is found only among women with bacterial vaginosis, and *G. vaginalis* has been isolated in low concentrations from the vagina of up to 50 percent of healthy women. Hydrogen peroxide–producing *Lactobacillus* spp., which constitute most of the normal vaginal flora, are usually absent from the vagina in bacterial vaginosis. This situation may permit overgrowth of the vagina by anaerobic bacteria, *M. hominis,* and *G. vaginalis.* Vaginal douching, use of intravaginal nonoxynol-9 spermicide, and new sexual partners are associated with loss of vaginal colonization by hydrogen peroxide–producing lactobacilli.

Bacterial vaginosis is conventionally diagnosed by demonstration of any three of the following four abnormalities:

1. *Objective signs of increased white homogeneous vaginal discharge and exclusion of candidal and trichomonal vaginitis and*

mucopurulent cervicitis. This process must include the collection of endocervical specimens to be tested for *C. trachomatis* and *N. gonorrhoeae.*

2. *Liberation of a distinct fishy odor immediately after mixing of vaginal secretions with a 10% solution of KOH.* This odor is attributable to volatile amines (e.g., trimethylamine, putrescine, and cadaverine) resulting from anaerobic bacterial metabolism in the vaginal fluid.

3. *A vaginal discharge pH of >4.5.* The elevated pH may be partly due to the presence of amines as well as to the decreased production of lactate. (Testing of cervical secretions, which typically have a pH of about 7.0, should be avoided.)

4. *Microscopic demonstration of "clue cells."* Clue cells are vaginal epithelial cells coated with coccobacillary organisms. On a wet mount prepared by mixing of vaginal secretions with normal saline in a ratio of approximately 1:1, clue cells have a granular appearance and indistinct borders (Fig. 129-1). Alternatively, the laboratory diagnosis of bacterial vaginosis can be based upon the detection of clue cells in a Gram-stained smear of vaginal discharge. The normally predominant lactobacilli (large, gram-positive rods) are mostly or completely replaced by a profusion of bacterial morphotypes consistent with *G. vaginalis* and anaerobic organisms. The demonstration of many clue cells by wet-mount microscopy and the documentation of a characteristically altered vaginal flora by Gram's stain are the most sensitive, specific, and objective criteria for the diagnosis of bacterial vaginosis in women with symptoms and/or signs of this condition.

Attempts to isolate *G. vaginalis,* genital mycoplasmas, or anaerobic bacteria are of little use in the diagnosis of bacterial vaginosis because these organisms are components of the vaginal flora in many women without the syndrome.

FIGURE 129-1 *A.* Vaginal epithelial "clue cells." Note granular appearance due to adherent *G. vaginalis* and indistinct cell margins (400×). *B.* Normal vaginal epithelial cells. The cell margins are distinct and lack granularity.

The standard regimen for the treatment of bacterial vaginosis has been metronidazole (500 mg orally, twice daily for 7 days). Clindamycin (300 mg orally, twice daily for 7 days) is also effective but not preferred. Intravaginal treatment with 2% clindamycin cream [one applicator full (5 g containing 100 mg of clindamycin phosphate) each night for 7 nights] or 0.75% metronidazole gel [one applicator full (5 g containing 37.5 mg of metronidazole) twice daily for 5 days] is also effective and does not elicit systemic adverse reactions. A single 2-g oral dose of metronidazole can also be used but produces short-term recurrence rates somewhat higher than those obtained with the 7-day metronidazole regimen. Long-term recurrence (i.e., after several months) is distressingly common, and its frequency is not reduced by treatment of male partners with metronidazole. Nonetheless, a new sexual partner has been implicated as a risk factor for recurrence.

No controlled data support the use of vaginal or oral preparations of *Lactobacillus* spp. in the treatment or prevention of recurrence of bacterial vaginosis. However, few if any of the available commercial preparations of lactobacilli contain hydrogen peroxide–producing vaginal strains that adhere to vaginal epithelium. Since adherence may be required for successful colonization, studies with such isolates will be of interest.

Vulvovaginal candidiasis The predominant symptom in vulvovaginal candidiasis is vulvar pruritus or irritation. There is usually no distinct odor, and symptoms of vaginal discharge are not characteristic. Signs of vulvar erythema, edema, and fissures are common. The vaginal discharge typically is white and scant and sometimes takes the form of white thrushlike plaques or cottage cheese–like curds adhering loosely to the vaginal mucosa. *C. albicans* accounts for at least 80 percent of yeasts isolated from the vagina, while *Torulopsis glabrata* and less commonly encountered *Candida* spp. are found in the remainder. Most cases of vulvovaginal candidiasis probably arise from endogenous strains of *C. albicans* that have colonized the vagina or the intestinal tract. Some men whose partners have vulvovaginal candidiasis develop symptomatic candidal dermatitis of the penis.

The diagnosis of vulvovaginal candidiasis involves the demonstration of fungi by microscopic examination of vaginal fluid in saline or 10% KOH or by Gram's stain. Demonstration of pseudohyphae or hyphae strengthens the diagnosis of vaginitis due to *C. albicans*. Polymorphonuclear leukocytes usually are present. Microscopic examination is less sensitive than culture but correlates better with symptoms. Culture does identify *C. albicans* in some women with symptoms and signs of vulvovaginal candidiasis in conjunction with negative results upon microscopic examination but also commonly detects coincidental colonization in women without such symptoms or signs. The pH of vaginal secretions is usually ≤4.5, and no amine odor is produced when vaginal secretions are mixed with 10% KOH. The superficial vulvar erosions or fissures of vulvovaginal candidiasis must be differentiated from the manifestations of genital herpes and other causes of genital ulcer.

In most circumstances, therapy for candidal vaginal infection is indicated only if the patient is symptomatic or has signs of vulvovaginitis. The usual treatment is intravaginal administration of any of several imidazole antibiotics (e.g., miconazole or clotrimazole) for 3 to 7 days. Over-the-counter marketing of such preparations has reduced the cost of care and made treatment more convenient for many women with recurrent yeast vulvovaginitis. However, the symptoms of this condition are nonspecific, and self-treatment of presumed vulvovaginal candidiasis may delay detection and treatment of more serious infections. Therefore, self-treatment should be strictly limited to women with classic symptoms of vulvar pruritus in whom previous episodes of yeast vulvovaginitis have been documented by an experienced clinician. Single-dose oral treatment with fluconazole (150 mg) is also effective and is preferred by many patients. Prolonged or periodic oral therapy with fluconazole or ketoconazole may be indicated for especially severe or frequently recurrent cases or for those that do not respond to intravaginal or single-dose oral therapy. Such patients probably should be evaluated for diabetes or HIV infection, although such systemic illnesses are uncommon explanations for recurrent vulvovaginal candidiasis. Treatment of sexual partners is not routinely indicated.

Mucopurulent Cervicitis *Mucopurulent cervicitis* refers to inflammation of the columnar epithelium and subepithelium of the endocervix and of any contiguous columnar epithelium that lies exposed in an ectopic position on the exocervix. Mucopurulent cervicitis in women is the "silent partner" of urethritis in men, being equally common and caused by the same agents but more difficult to recognize. It is the most common major STD syndrome in women, can be a harbinger or sign of PID, and—in pregnant women—can lead to obstetric complications. Mucopurulent cervicitis is caused most commonly by *C. trachomatis* and sometimes by *N. gonorrhoeae*; the relative proportions of cases due to these two organisms depend on their prevalence in the community. In the United States, however, at least half of all cases are associated with neither of these organisms and currently remain idiopathic. The syndrome usually can be differentiated clinically from cervicitis caused by HSV, which produces ulcerative lesions on the stratified squamous epithelium of the exocervix as well as on the columnar epithelium.

The diagnosis is based on the detection of yellow mucopurulent discharge from the cervical os or of increased numbers of polymorphonuclear leukocytes in Gram-stained or Papanicolaou smears of endocervical mucus. Edematous cervical ectopy (see below) and endocervical bleeding induced by gentle swabbing are also common signs of mucopurulent cervicitis due to *C. trachomatis*. The color of cervical mucus on a white swab removed from the endocervix should be noted; a yellow color indicates the presence of polymorphonuclear leukocytes. The mucus should be rolled *thinly* on a slide for Gram's staining. The presence of 20 to 30 or more polymorphonuclear cells per 1000× microscopic field within strands of cervical mucus not contaminated by vaginal squamous epithelial cells or vaginal bacteria suggests cervicitis. When carefully collected endocervical specimens are examined by experienced personnel, Gram's staining of endocervical mucus is also an insensitive but fairly specific test for gonorrhea; intracellular gram-negative diplococci indicate gonococcal infection. Culture or other specific and sensitive tests for *N. gonorrhoeae* and *C. trachomatis* are also indicated.

Treatment usually should be administered when the clinical diagnosis is made—i.e., before the etiology is known. In settings where both gonorrhea and chlamydial infection are common, therapy should include a single-dose regimen effective for gonorrhea, such as cefixime (400 mg orally), followed by doxycycline (100 mg orally, twice daily for 1 week) or by azithromycin (1.0 g orally in a single dose). In settings where gonorrhea is much less common than chlamydial infection, initial therapy for mucopurulent cervicitis may cover chlamydial infection only (e.g., a regimen of azithromycin or doxycycline). The sexual partner(s) of a woman with mucopurulent cervicitis should be examined and given a regimen similar to that chosen for the woman unless results of tests for gonorrhea or chlamydial infection in either partner warrant a change in therapy.

Cervical Ectopy Cervicitis must be differentiated from *cervical ectopy*, which is often mislabeled "cervical erosion." Ectopy represents the presence of the one-cell-thick columnar epithelium extending from the endocervix out onto the visible ectocervix. In ectopy, the cervical os may contain clear or slightly cloudy mucus but usually does not contain yellow mucopus. Colposcopy shows that the epithelium is intact and not ulcerated. Ectopy is normally found during early adolescence and gradually recedes as squamous metaplasia replaces the ectopic columnar epithelium. Oral contraceptive use favors the persistence or reappearance of ectopy. Cauterization for the elimination of ectopy is not warranted. Ectopy may make the cervix more susceptible to infection with *N. gonorrhoeae* or *C. trachomatis* by exposing a larger area of susceptible columnar epithelium. Moreover, ectopy appears to enhance susceptibility to HIV infection. If mucopurulent cervicitis supervenes, the area of ectopy becomes edematous and fragile. Edema may result in eversion of the os, with enlargement of the apparent area of ectopy.

PELVIC INFLAMMATORY DISEASE The term *PID* refers to various combinations of endometritis, salpingitis, and pelvic peritonitis resulting from ascending genital infection, which usually arises from gonococcal or chlamydial mucopurulent cervicitis and/or from bacterial vaginosis. PID predominantly affects sexually active adolescents and young women, in whom at least 90 percent of cases are sexually acquired. Although sometimes clinically severe, with overt pelvic peritonitis or tuboovarian abscess (especially, it now appears, among women with HIV infection), most cases of acute PID are relatively mild or even subclinical. However, even subclinical PID can result in significant tubal damage, as evidenced by the frequent lack of history of clinically diagnosed PID in *Chlamydia*-seropositive women with tubal infertility or ectopic pregnancy. Accordingly, the clinician must not be slow to consider PID in the differential diagnosis of mild or even trivial abdominal pain in young women. This approach represents a shift in thinking from the days when PID was considered likely only in women with severe adnexal tenderness plus an elevation in temperature, white blood cell count, or erythrocyte sedimentation rate.

The proportion of cases of PID caused by *N. gonorrhoeae* recently has declined in most industrialized countries, a trend reflecting the declining incidence of gonococcal infections in general. *C. trachomatis* remains a common cause of PID in many settings. However, in geographic areas and health maintenance organizations that have implemented widespread screening of sexually active young women for chlamydial infection, the incidence of chlamydial PID has declined. Numerous other pathogens contribute to PID, including *M. hominis* and various anaerobic members of the vaginal flora found in bacterial vaginosis. PID occurs with increased frequency for a short period after insertion of an intrauterine contraceptive device, and endometritis can result from induced abortion or from childbirth (especially after cesarean section). Vaginal douching has been found to be an important risk factor for ascending pelvic infection, perhaps because the practice depletes hydrogen peroxide–producing *Lactobacillus* spp. Clinicians should not prescribe douching (which has not been demonstrated to be effective for treatment or prevention of any condition) and should strongly discourage douching for genital hygiene. PID is discussed in detail in Chap. 130.

ULCERATIVE LESIONS OF THE GENITALIA The etiology of genital ulcer disease has not been systematically studied in industrialized countries for more than 20 years except in recent outbreaks involving syphilis and chancroid in New Orleans, Louisiana, and Jackson, Mississippi. Table 129-4 approximates the differential diagnosis in patients attending STD clinics and, by extension, in young, sexually active persons in other clinical settings.

The incidence and etiology of ulcerative lesions of the genitalia vary greatly in different areas of the world. In Asia and Africa, genital

Table 129-4

Etiologies of Genital Ulcer Disease in Industrialized and Tropical Developing Countries

	Percent of Cases	
Diagnosis	Industrialized Countries	Tropical Developing Countries
Genital herpes	50–70	10–30*
Syphilis	10–20	10–30
Chancroid	0–10†	50–60
Lymphogranuloma venereum	<1	0–5
Donovanosis	<1	<1‡
Other/unknown	5–20	5–30

* The proportion of genital ulcers caused by HSV appears to be increasing as the prevalence of HIV infection increases in developing countries.
† The proportion is highly variable, depending on time, place, and population group. Chancroid may account for more than 25% of cases in STD clinic populations in selected U.S. cities during chancroid outbreaks.
‡ Donovanosis accounts for higher proportions of cases in some geographic areas (e.g., southern Africa, western Australia, Papua New Guinea, and the Indian subcontinent) than in others.

ulcers are seen as frequently as gonorrhea in some STD clinics; chancroid is the most common cause. Genital herpes was considered relatively uncommon until serologic studies and PCR testing of genital ulcers showed it to be common, especially among persons infected with HIV. In industrialized western countries, genital ulcers are considerably less common than urethritis, mucopurulent cervicitis, and vaginitis; genital herpes is the most common cause, and chancroid is relatively uncommon. Syphilis is the second most common form of genital ulcer in most areas of the world, and the possibility of syphilis must always be excluded. Lymphogranuloma venereum (LGV) and donovanosis (granuloma inguinale) are very rare in North America and Europe, although an unusual outbreak of LGV occurred in the Bahamas during the 1980s in association with crack cocaine use and epidemic HIV infection. Other causes of genital ulcer include candidiasis and traumatized genital warts, both of which usually are readily recognized. Trauma per se is an uncommon cause of genital ulcer unless there is a clear history of definite injury accompanied by bleeding. The differential diagnosis of genital ulceration is broad, and other conditions are more common in older patients, those at low risk for STDs, and those who present with lesions due to genital involvement of more widespread dermatoses, such as genital mucosal ulceration in Stevens-Johnson syndrome.

Chancroid, syphilis, genital herpes, and probably all causes of genital ulcer enhance the efficiency of sexual transmission and acquisition of HIV. Moreover, genital ulcers, especially those of chancroid and syphilis, are most common in sexually active inner-city populations with low socioeconomic status and high rates of prostitution and illicit drug use—independent risk factors for HIV infection. In the late 1980s in the United States, chancroid and syphilis spread at epidemic rates in such populations, although these rates declined rapidly from 1990 through 1995.

In industrialized countries, the differential diagnosis of genital ulceration in young, sexually active patients usually includes genital herpes, syphilis, and chancroid; together, these infections probably account for more than 90 percent of cases in which discrete genital ulcers are present in patients without generalized dermatoses. The clinical findings are occasionally definitive (e.g., the presence of herpetic vesicles), and clinical findings plus epidemiologic considerations can usually guide initial therapy pending the results of further studies. Nevertheless, most genital ulcerations cannot be diagnosed confidently on clinical grounds. It is axiomatic to exclude syphilis in all cases. Although syphilis serology should be routine, about one-quarter of patients with primary syphilis have not yet seroconverted when they first present for medical attention. All lesions except those highly characteristic of infection with HSV should therefore be subjected to dark-field examination or a direct immunofluorescence test for *Treponema pallidum*. Selective enrichment media are available for isolation of *H. ducreyi*. Use of simultaneous multiple PCR tests (e.g., for HSV, *T. pallidum*, and *H. ducreyi*) has proven valuable in recent studies of genital ulcer, identifying an etiologic agent in up to 95 percent of cases. Such tests are not yet commercially available.

The following general guidelines are recommended for management of ulcerative genital lesions.

Lesions Typical of Genital Herpes A clinical diagnosis of genital herpes is warranted if typical vesicles or pustules are evident or if there is a cluster of painful ulcers that was preceded by vesiculopustular lesions. These clinical presentations are sufficiently typical that confirmation of the diagnosis by isolation of HSV or immunochemical detection of the virus is optional. A serologic test for syphilis should be performed not only for diagnostic purposes but also because screening is indicated in all patients with a newly diagnosed STD.

All Other Acute Genital Ulcers The appearance of genital herpetic lesions is highly variable, and—except in the relatively clearcut cases described above—a specific test for HSV is required to establish a diagnosis. "Nonspecific" or clinically trivial ulcers may be more common manifestations of genital herpes than classic vesiculopustular lesions. Isolation of HSV by culture, immunochemical identification of antigens, or detection of genetic material should be attempted. Culture or direct immunofluorescence tests allow typing of

HSV if it is detected, while enzyme-linked immunosorbent assays currently do not. Type-specific serologic tests are available for research and are now being developed to aid in the identification of HSV-2-seronegative persons who might benefit from future vaccines. However, commercially available serologic tests do not distinguish between antibodies to the two types of HSV and are of little use (see Chap. 184). Cytologic methods (Tzanck preparation with Wright-Giemsa or Papanicolaou staining) for the detection of HSV-infected multinucleated cells are insensitive except in the presence of intact vesicles and are seldom useful in diagnosing genital ulcer disease.

An attempt should be made to isolate *H. ducreyi* if the genital ulcer is painful and is not typical of herpes, especially when inguinal lymphadenopathy with fluctuance or overlying erythema is noted; if chancroid is prevalent in the community; if the patient is at high risk for chancroid (e.g., through the use of injection drugs or crack cocaine or through prostitution); or if the patient has recently had a sexual exposure in a chancroid-endemic area (e.g., a developing country or certain North American cities). Enlarged, fluctuant lymph nodes should be aspirated for culture and Gram's staining to detect *H. ducreyi* and pyogenic bacteria. A diagnosis of syphilis should be excluded by dark-field examination and serologic testing, and the latter should be repeated 1 to 2 weeks later if the results are initially negative and if another diagnosis cannot be established.

Lesions Typical of Syphilis If lesions are at all suggestive of syphilis (e.g., painless, nontender, indurated); if there is firm, nontender inguinal adenopathy; or if there are epidemiologic reasons to suspect syphilis (e.g., recent exposure), dark-field examination and a rapid serologic test for syphilis should be performed. If the results are negative and the patient is reliable in terms of follow-up and sexual abstinence, two more dark-field examinations should be conducted on successive days before treatment is attempted, and the serologic test should be repeated 1, 2, and 6 weeks later. Direct immunofluorescence staining of *T. pallidum* is quite reliable and should be used if dark-field examination by experienced examiners is impossible.

Chronic Genital Ulceration When genital ulcers persist beyond the usual course of herpes (2 to 3 weeks) or chancroid or syphilis (up to 6 weeks) and do not resolve with syndrome-based antimicrobial therapy, then—in addition to the usual tests for herpes, syphilis, and chancroid—biopsy is indicated to exclude donovanosis, carcinoma, and other nonvenereal dermatoses. A test for HIV infection should be done, since chronic, persistent genital herpes is common in HIV infection with immunosuppression.

Treatment of Genital Ulcers Ideally, treatment for genital ulceration should be withheld until the diagnosis is secure. However, immediate syndrome-based treatment for acute genital ulcerations (after collection of all necessary diagnostic specimens) is sometimes necessary—e.g., when it is believed that a patient may not return for follow-up or may continue to be sexually active. Initial treatment in such cases should generally include 2.4 million units of benzathine penicillin G for possible primary syphilis. Immediate empirical therapy for chancroid also is indicated if the patient has been exposed in an area where chancroid is endemic and especially if regional lymph node suppuration is evident or appears imminent. Prompt systemic therapy with acyclovir is indicated for patients with initial episodes of genital or anorectal herpes (see Chap. 184). Finally, empirical antimicrobial therapy may be indicated if ulcers persist and the diagnosis remains unclear after 1 to 2 weeks of observation and repeated attempts to diagnose herpes, syphilis, and chancroid.

Candidate vaccines against HSV-2 are undergoing clinical trials; one candidate subunit vaccine recently appeared to be ineffective in preventing HSV-2 infection. If any vaccine proves effective in preventing genital herpes, potential target populations for HSV-2 immunization include the uninfected partners of persons with genital herpes and perhaps all young persons before the onset of sexual activity. Candidate vaccines are also being investigated for their efficacy in moderating the course of recurrent genital herpes.

PROCTITIS, PROCTOCOLITIS, ENTEROCOLITIS, AND ENTERITIS Sexually acquired proctitis, or inflammation limited to the rectal mucosa, results from direct rectal inoculation of typical STD pathogens. In contrast, inflammation extending from the rectum to the colon (proctocolitis), involving both the small and the large bowel (enterocolitis), or involving the small bowel alone (enteritis) can result from ingestion of typical intestinal pathogens through oral-fecal exposure during sexual contact. Anorectal pain and mucopurulent, bloody rectal discharge suggest proctitis or proctocolitis. Proctitis is commonly associated with tenesmus (causing frequent attempts to defecate, but not true diarrhea) and constipation, whereas proctocolitis and enterocolitis are more often associated with true diarrhea. In all three conditions, anoscopy usually shows mucosal exudate and easily induced mucosal bleeding (i.e., a positive "wipe test"), sometimes with petechiae or mucosal ulcers. Exudate should be sampled for microbiologic studies and Gram's staining. Sigmoidoscopy or colonoscopy shows inflammation limited to the rectum (in proctitis) or disease extending at least into the sigmoid colon (in proctocolitis).

Most cases of sexually transmitted intestinal infection in the past have involved homosexual men. During the AIDS era, however, there has been an extraordinary shift in the clinical and etiologic spectrum of intestinal infections among homosexual men. The number of AIDS-related opportunistic intestinal infections has risen rapidly; most such infections are associated with chronic rather than acute intestinal symptoms. At the same time, the number of cases of the usually more acute sexually transmitted intestinal infections described below has fallen rapidly as high-risk sexual behaviors have become less common in this group.

Most infectious proctitis is due to the acquisition of *N. gonorrhoeae*, HSV, or *C. trachomatis* during receptive anorectal intercourse. Primary and secondary syphilis also can produce anal or anorectal lesions, with or without symptoms. Proctitis due to *N. gonorrhoeae* or to common strains of *C. trachomatis* typically involves the most distal rectal mucosa and the anal crypts and is clinically mild, without systemic manifestations. In contrast, primary proctitis due to HSV and proctocolitis due to the strains of *C. trachomatis* that cause LGV usually produce severe anorectal pain and often cause fever. Perianal ulcers and inguinal lymphadenopathy, most commonly due to HSV, also can occur in LGV or syphilis. Sacral nerve root radiculopathies, usually presenting as urinary retention, laxity of the anal sphincter, or constipation, are common in primary herpetic proctitis. In LGV, biopsy typically shows crypt abscesses, granulomas, and giant cells—findings resembling those in Crohn's disease. Syphilis also can produce rectal granulomas, usually in association with infiltration by plasma cells or other mononuclear cells.

Diarrhea and abdominal bloating or cramping pain without anorectal symptoms and with normal findings on anoscopy and sigmoidoscopy occurs with inflammation of the small intestine (enteritis) or with proximal colitis. In homosexual men without HIV infection, enteritis is often attributable to *Giardia lamblia*. Sexually acquired proctocolitis is most often due to *Campylobacter* spp., *Shigella* spp., or *Entamoeba histolytica*.

ACUTE ARTHRITIS The gonococcal arthritis-dermatitis syndrome and Reiter's syndrome are among the most common forms of acute arthritis in sexually active young adults. These two syndromes must be differentiated from each other, from other forms of infective arthritis, from various diseases associated with immune-complex deposition, from crystal-induced arthritis, from acute rheumatoid arthritis, and from other, less common rheumatic disorders, such as systemic lupus erythematosus. Meningococcemia, infection with *Yersinia*, sarcoidosis, and syphilis are other occasional causes of acute arthritis in young adults.

Demonstration of *N. gonorrhoeae* by culture or by a specific immunochemical method in synovial fluid, blood, skin lesions, or cerebrospinal fluid is diagnostic of disseminated gonococcal infection (DGI). Even when such tests fail to detect the organism, gonococcal arthritis is highly probable if *N. gonorrhoeae* is recovered from a mucosal site of infection or from the patient's sexual partner in the presence of typical pustular or hemorrhagic skin lesions distributed primarily on the extremities. Suspected and confirmed cases of DGI should be treated promptly with an antibiotic effective against antibiotic-sensitive and antibiotic-resistant gonococci, such as ceftriaxone (see Chap. 150).

Reiter's syndrome occurs in a sporadic (apparently sexually transmitted) form that usually follows chlamydial infection and in a postdysenteric form that usually follows infection with *Yersinia*, *Campylobacter*, or *Shigella* spp. Discrete epidemics of the latter form are sometimes documented (see Chap. 317).

HUMAN PAPILLOMAVIRUS INFECTION AND GENITAL WARTS Genital warts and infection with HPV were long considered inconvenient but benign conditions. Most genital warts are caused by HPV types 6 and 11, which are rarely if ever associated with invasive cancers. However, evolving evidence implicates some strains of HPV—e.g., types 16, 18, 31, 33, 35, 39, 45, 52, 55, 56, and 58—in the development of moderate to severe squamous dysplasia and of overt cancer of the cervix, anus, vulva, vagina, and penis. Accordingly, HPV infection is now recognized as one of the most important STDs. The number of visits to clinicians because of genital warts has been estimated at more than 1.2 million each year in the United States. However, most HPV infections are subclinical, and increasingly sensitive tools for the detection of HPV (e.g., PCR) show that most sexually active young men and women seen at STD clinics have genital HPV infection, usually without visible clinical abnormalities. A recent study of university women followed from their initial sexual intercourse through their first two or three sexual partners suggested that about half became infected with HPV, many with oncogenic HPV types. Genital HPV infection was five times as common as all other sexually transmitted infections combined in this population.

Treatment of symptomatic external genital warts usually consists of provider-administered cryotherapy or podophyllin resin (10 to 25 percent resin in tincture of benzoin) or of patient-administered podophyllotoxin (podophylox), which is available as a 0.5 percent solution or gel. In special circumstances, surgery is used (e.g., scissor excision, electrodesiccation, laser vaporization). However, surgery does not cure subclinical infection of adjacent tissues. Thus the primary goal of treatment of genital warts is cosmetic, and therapy should be conservative. Although genital warts are no more predictive than other STDs of severe cervical dysplasia (since the types of HPV that commonly cause genital warts are not the types that cause severe dysplasia or invasive cancer), women with any STD should undergo routine cervical cytologic screening. These conditions are addressed further in Chap. 190.

HEPATITIS B VIRUS INFECTION Sexually transmitted HBV infection (Chap. 295) was an extremely common problem among homosexual and bisexual men until the mid-1980s, and sexual contact among men continues to account for 5 to 10 percent of adult HBV infections in the United States. About 25 percent of cases of hepatitis B in U.S. adults currently are attributed to heterosexual transmission and 30 percent to sharing of injection equipment by illicit drug users. The route of acquisition is unknown in 35 to 40 percent of cases, but the age distribution and other behavioral characteristics are consistent with sexual acquisition. Hepatitis B is the only STD for which an effective vaccine is available, and current recommendations in the United States include not only universal vaccination of infants but also targeted vaccination of adolescents in high-risk communities, people with multiple sexual partners or other STDs, sexual partners of individuals with acute hepatitis B, and seronegative sexual partners of chronic carriers of the hepatitis B surface antigen.

CYTOMEGALOVIRUS CMV is carried in blood and shed in semen and cervical secretions; it can be transmitted through sexual and perinatal exposure. Sexual contact is the most important mode of transmission of CMV between adults in many settings in industrialized countries. Among initially seronegative women attending STD clinics, the annual incidence of seroconversion is 8 to 30 percent. CMV (Chap. 187) is among the most common causes of congenital neurodevelop-

mental abnormalities and of life-threatening morbidity in patients with advanced cellular immunodeficiency due to HIV, malignancy, or chemotherapy. Until an effective vaccine is developed, the prevention of sexually transmitted CMV infection will be problematic.

HUMAN T-CELL LYMPHOTROPIC VIRUS HTLV-I is transmitted perinatally, especially through breast feeding, and parenterally, especially through blood transfusions; it is also endemic as a sexually transmitted virus in parts of the Caribbean, Latin America, Asia, and Africa. HTLV-I (Chap. 192) is associated with T cell leukemia and tropical spastic paresis (HTLV-I–associated myelopathy), although only the latter has been seen after adult acquisition. HTLV-II is found in up to 15 to 20 percent of injection drug users in the United States, in whom it appears to be parenterally transmitted, and is also found in some Native American tribes. The clinical consequences of infection with HTLV-II have yet to be defined. Small case-control studies have implicated other sexually transmitted infections as possible risk factors for sexual acquisition of HTLV-I and HTLV-II.

KAPOSI'S SARCOMA–ASSOCIATED HERPESVIRUS (See Chap. 187) Early in the AIDS era, epidemiologic studies suggested that Kaposi's sarcoma in HIV-infected persons was due to a separate sexually transmissible agent. More recently, DNA sequences consistent with a previously unrecognized gamma herpes-group virus were identified in Kaposi's sarcoma lesions of homosexually active men with AIDS. This Kaposi's sarcoma–associated herpesvirus has since been associated with body-cavity lymphomas and Castleman's disease in preliminary studies. Rapid progress in cultivation and characterization of this virus and future development of specific serologic tests will eventually elucidate the epidemiologic features of the agent and will help to define whether and how it is involved in the pathogenesis of Kaposi's sarcoma and other conditions.

PREVENTION AND CONTROL OF STDs

Although rates of all curable STDs have been falling in the United States during the 1990s, all other industrialized countries of comparable economic development have made greater progress. For example, Sweden has virtually eliminated the transmission of gonorrhea, syphilis, and chancroid and has achieved very low rates of HIV transmission. Elimination of syphilis as an endemic disease might also be a plausible intermediate-term objective in the United States, but much stronger efforts toward prevention and control of all STDs are necessary.

Prevention and control of STDs rest on the reduction of the average risk of sexual exposure through (1) reduction of the average rate of partner change in all population groups; (2) reduction of the efficiency of transmission by promoting safer sexual practices, use of condoms during casual or commercial sex, hepatitis B immunization, and many other approaches; and (3) shortening of the duration of infectivity of STDs through early detection and curative or suppressive treatment.

Many barriers stand in the way of each of these three approaches. For example, sex education of children and young adults is hindered by the taboo surrounding the discussion of sexuality in the United States. Opposition to use of schools and the media as vehicles for sex education contrasts with frequent use of the media for the promulgation of explicit sexual messages in programs and advertising.

Clinicians have traditionally focused on early detection and treatment of curable STDs to reduce the duration of infectivity. They generally have relatively little training or experience in or time for counseling on risk reduction, treatment of sexual contacts, or condom promotion. Certain constraints imposed on time and finances by managed-care practice patterns may further curtail prevention efforts. Even the efforts of clinicians simply to detect and treat STDs are severely limited at several steps, as outlined in Fig. 129-2. As implied by this figure, improved detection and treatment of STDs depend in part on societal efforts to teach young people how to recognize symptoms of STDs; to motivate those with symptoms to seek care promptly; and to make such care accessible, affordable, and acceptable, especially to the young indigent patients most likely to acquire an STD. Clinicians must develop and maintain their skills in recognition of symptoms and signs of STDs and in treatment. The primary care clinician is

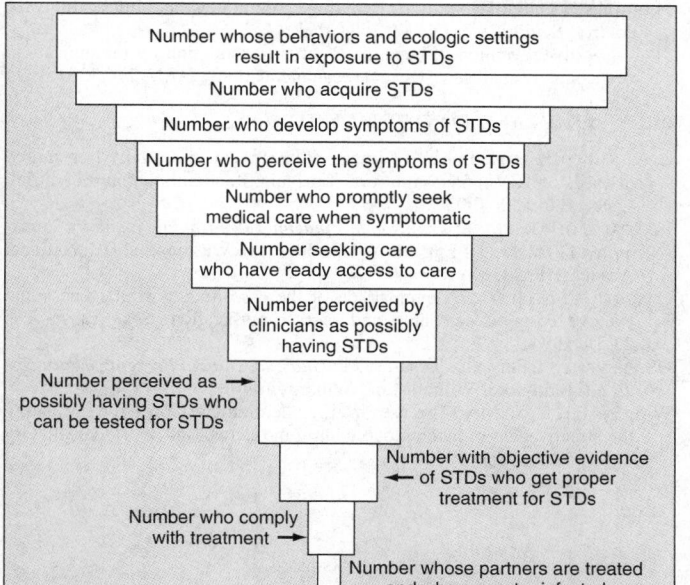

FIGURE 129-2 Schematic representation of the levels of potential breakdown in the steps required for preventing and controlling STDs. Each level represents an important point for public health or clinical intervention. *(Adapted from Waller and Piot and from "Resource allocation model for public health planning—a case study of tuberculosis control," a supplement to volume 84 of the Bulletin of the World Health Organization, 1973.)*

also responsible for "the 4 Cs" of STD case management: ensuring *c*ompliance with therapy, arranging treatment of *c*ontacts, promoting the use of *c*ondoms, and *c*ounseling on risk reduction. Further, given that many infected individuals develop no symptoms or fail to recognize and report symptoms, clinicians should routinely perform an STD risk assessment for teenagers and young adults and should use the information obtained to selectively screen for STDs, to interpret symptoms and signs, and to identify individuals in need of counseling.

Screening tests for gonorrhea, chlamydial infection, and HIV as well as cervical cytology should be used in populations at risk in the United States according to the U.S. Preventive Services Task Force Guidelines. With few exceptions, sexually active females from 14 to 20 years of age should be tested for *C. trachomatis* whenever they present for health care (at least once a year), regardless of whether their sexual behavior appears to place them at risk; older women should be tested if they have more than one sexual partner, if they have begun a new sexual relationship since the previous test, or if they have another STD diagnosed. In other countries and in a few locations in the United States, widespread selective screening of young women for cervical *C. trachomatis* infection has been associated with a 50 to 60 percent drop in the prevalence of chlamydial infection; as noted above, such screening protects the individual woman from PID. Sexually active young men also can be screened for urethral *C. trachomatis* infection. Although definitive selective screening criteria have not yet been published, sensitive urine-based genetic amplification tests permit expansion of screening to men and teenage boys and to women in settings where a pelvic examination is not planned or is impractical.

Although gonorrhea is substantially less common than chlamydial infection, some persons should still be screened routinely, including women and teenage girls attending STD clinics and sexually active teens and women from impoverished environments, settings of substance abuse, or areas of high gonorrhea prevalence. Routine screening of asymptomatic men for urethral gonorrhea usually is unproductive in the primary care setting. However, if genetic amplification tests for *N. gonorrhoeae* become available at sufficiently low cost, combination with *C. trachomatis* testing in a single assay may facilitate the prevention and control of both infections in the populations at highest risk.

All patients with STDs or at high risk for STDs and all pregnant women should be routinely encouraged to undergo serologic testing for syphilis and HIV infection, with appropriate counseling before and after testing. In the primary care setting, such counseling is usually straightforward and can present opportunities for further risk-reduction counseling. Serologic tests for syphilis and HIV infection currently are not advocated for routine premarital use. Preimmunization serologic testing for antibody to HBV is indicated for unvaccinated persons who are known to be at high risk, such as homosexually active men and injection drug users. In most young persons, however, it is more cost-effective to vaccinate against HBV without serologic screening.

In summary, clinicians and public health agencies share responsibility for the prevention and control of STDs, including HIV infection, and it is likely in the managed-care era that the role of primary care clinicians will become increasingly important in prevention as well as in diagnosis and treatment.

BIBLIOGRAPHY

GENERAL

ANDERSON RM, MAY R: *Infectious Diseases of Humans: Dynamics and Control.* New York, Oxford Univ Press, 1991
BOEKELOO BO et al: Frequency and thoroughness of STD/HIV risk assessment by physicians in a high-risk metropolitan area. Am J Public Health 81:1645, 1991
BRANDT AM: *No Magic Bullet: A Social History of Venereal Disease in the United States Since 1890,* 2d ed. New York, Oxford Univ Press, 1989
CENTERS FOR DISEASE CONTROL AND PREVENTION: 1993 sexually transmitted disease treatment guidelines. Morb Mort Week Rep 42(RR-14):1, 1993
———: Update: Barrier protections against HIV infection and other sexually transmitted diseases. Morb Mort Week Rep 42:589, 1993
———: *Sexually Transmitted Disease Surveillance, 1994.* Atlanta, U.S. Public Health Service, 1995
Drugs for sexually transmitted diseases. Med Lett Drugs Ther 37:117, 1995
EBRAHIM SH et al: Mortality related to sexually transmitted diseases in women, US, 1973–1992. Am J Public Health, 1997
HANDSFIELD HH: *Color Atlas and Synopsis of Sexually Transmitted Diseases.* New York, McGraw-Hill, 1992
HOLMES KK: Human ecology and behavior and sexually transmitted bacterial infections. Proc Natl Acad Sci USA 91:2448, 1994
——— et al (eds): *Sexually Transmitted Diseases,* 3d ed. New York, McGraw-Hill, 1997
LAUMANN EO et al: *The Social Organization of Sexuality: Sexual Practices in the United States.* Chicago, Univ of Chicago Press, 1994
LEE HH et al: Diagnosis of *Chlamydia trachomatis* genitourinary infection in women by ligase chain reaction assay of urine. Lancet 345:213, 1995
MORSE SA et al: *Atlas of Sexually Transmitted Diseases,* 2d ed. Baltimore, Mosby-Wolfe, 1996
ORIEL JD: *The Scars of Venus: A History of Venereology.* London, Springer-Verlag, 1994
ROSS PE, LANDIS SE: Development and evaluation of a sexual history-taking curriculum for first- and second-year family practice residents. Fam Med 26:293, 1994
SMITH KR et al: Evaluation of ligase chain reaction for use with urine for identification of *Neisseria gonorrhoeae* in females attending a sexually transmitted disease clinic. J Clin Microbiol 33:455, 1995
WASSERHEIT JN: Effect of changes in human ecology and behavior on patterns of sexually transmitted diseases, including human immunodeficiency virus infection. Proc Natl Acad Sci USA 91:2430, 1994

URETHRITIS IN MALES

BOWIE WR et al: Etiology of nongonococcal urethritis. Evidence for *Chlamydia trachomatis* and *Ureaplasma urealyticum.* J Clin Invest 59:735, 1977
KRIEGER JN et al: Clinical manifestations of trichomoniasis in men. Ann Intern Med 118:844, 1993
MARTIN DH, BOWIE WR: Urethritis in males, in *Sexually Transmitted Diseases,* 3d ed, KK Holmes et al (eds). New York, McGraw-Hill, 1997, Chap 60
——— et al: A controlled trial of a single dose of azithromycin for the treatment of chlamydial urethritis and cervicitis. N Engl J Med 327:921, 1992
SHAFER MA et al: Urinary leukocyte esterase screening test for asymptomatic chlamydial and gonococcal infection in males. JAMA 262:2562, 1989
STAMM WE et al: Azithromycin for empirical treatment of the nongonococcal urethritis syndrome in men: A randomized double-blind study. JAMA 274:545, 1995

TAYLOR-ROBINSON D: The history and role of *Mycoplasma genitalium* in sexually transmitted diseases. The Harrison Lecture, Genitourin Med 71:1, 1995

EPIDIDYMITIS

BERGER RE: Epididymitis, in *Sexually Transmitted Diseases*, 3d ed, KK Holmes et al (eds). New York, McGraw-Hill, 1997, Chap 61

URETHRAL SYNDROME

STAMM WE, HOOTON TM: Management of urinary tract infections in adults. N Engl J Med 329:1328, 1993

VAGINAL INFECTIONS

ESCHENBACH DA et al: Diagnosis and clinical manifestations of bacterial vaginosis. Am J Obstet Gynecol 158:819, 1988

HAUTH JC et al: Reduced incidence of preterm delivery with metronidazole and erythromycin in women with bacterial vaginosis. N Engl J Med 333:1732, 1995

HAWES SE et al: Hydrogen peroxide–producing lactobacilli and acquisition of vaginal infections. J Infect Dis 174:1058, 1996

HILLIER SL et al: The relationship of hydrogen peroxide–producing lactobacilli to bacterial vaginosis and genital microflora in pregnant women. Obstet Gynecol 79:369, 1992

——— et al: Association between bacterial vaginosis and preterm delivery of a low-birth-weight infant. N Engl J Med 333:1737, 1995

WØLNER-HANSSEN P et al: Clinical manifestations of vaginal trichomoniasis. JAMA 261:571, 1989

MUCOPURULENT CERVICITIS

BRUNHAM RC et al: Mucopurulent cervicitis—the ignored counterpart in women of urethritis in men. N Engl J Med 311:1, 1984

GENITAL ULCERS

COREY L: The current trends in genital herpes: Progress in prevention. Sex Transm Dis 21(Suppl 2):S38, 1994

KOUTSKY LA et al: Underdiagnosis of genital herpes by current clinical and viral isolation procedures. N Engl J Med 326:1533, 1992

ORLE KA et al: Simultaneous PCR detection of *Haemophilus ducreyi, Treponema pallidum*, and herpes simplex virus types 1 and 2 from genital ulcers. J Clin Microbiol 34:49, 1996

WALD A et al: Virologic characteristics of subclinical and symptomatic genital herpes infections. N Engl J Med 333:770, 1995

PROCTITIS, PROCTOCOLITIS, ENTEROCOLITIS, AND ENTERITIS

QUINN TC et al: The polymicrobial etiology of intestinal infections in homosexual men. N Engl J Med 309:576, 1983

ARTHRITIS

RICE P, HANDSFIELD HH: Arthropathies, in *Sexually Transmitted Diseases*, 3d ed, KK Holmes et al (eds). New York, McGraw-Hill, 1997, Chap 68

PELVIC INFLAMMATORY DISEASE

HILLIER SL et al: Role of bacterial vaginosis–associated microorganisms in endometritis. Am J Obstet Gynecol 175:435, 1996

SCHOLES D et al: Prevention of pelvic inflammatory disease by screening for cervical chlamydial infection. N Engl J Med 334:1362, 1996

SOPER DE: Diagnosis and laparoscopic grading of acute salpingitis. Am J Obstet Gynecol 164:1370, 1991

HPV/WARTS

BAKEN LA et al: Genital human papillomavirus infection among male and female sex partners: Prevalence and type-specific concordance. J Infect Dis 171:429, 1995

KOUTSKY LA et al: A cohort study of the risk of cervical intraepithelial neoplasia grade 2 or 3 in relation to papillomavirus infection. N Engl J Med 327:1272, 1992

HBV, CMV, HTLV-I, AND HTLV-II

COLLIER AC et al: Cytomegalovirus infection in women attending a sexually transmitted disease clinic. J Infect Dis 162:46, 1990

GOTUZZO E et al: HTLV-I infection among female sex workers in Peru. J Infect Dis 169:754, 1994

MARGOLIS HS et al: Hepatitis B: Evolving epidemiology and implications for control. Semin Liver Dis 11(2):84, 1991

——— et al: Prevention of hepatitis B virus transmission by immunization. An economic analysis of current recommendations. JAMA 274:1201, 1995

PREVENTION AND CONTROL OF STDs

GROSSKURTH H et al: Impact of improved treatment of sexually transmitted diseases on HIV infection in rural Tanzania: Randomised controlled trial. Lancet 346:530, 1995

INSTITUTE OF MEDICINE: *The Hidden Epidemic: Confronting Sexually Transmitted Diseases*, TR Eng and WT Butler (eds). Washington, DC, National Academy Press, 1997

OXMAN GL, DOYLE L: A comparison of the case finding effectiveness and average costs of screening and partner notification. Sex Transm Dis 23:51, 1996

US PREVENTIVE SERVICES TASK FORCE: *Guide to Clinical Preventive Services*, 2d ed. Baltimore, Williams and Wilkins, 1996

WALLER HT, PIOT MA: The use of an epidemiologic model for estimating the effectiveness of tuberculosis control measures. Bull World Health Org 41:75, 1969; 43:1, 1970

130 PELVIC INFLAMMATORY DISEASE

King K. Holmes

DEFINITION   The term *pelvic inflammatory disease* (PID) usually refers to ascending infection of the endometrium and/or fallopian tubes. Intrauterine infection can be primary (spontaneously occurring and usually sexually transmitted) or secondary to invasive intrauterine surgical procedures (e.g., dilatation and curettage, termination of pregnancy, insertion of an intrauterine device, or hysterosalpingography) or to parturition. Endometritis or endomyometritis is particularly common following delivery by cesarean section.

PID is uncommon during pregnancy itself. The uterotubal junction is closed as early as the seventh week of pregnancy, and the chorioamnion becomes approximated to the endocervical os, sealing off the intrauterine cavity, at the twelfth to fifteenth week of gestation. As a consequence, ascending intrauterine infection prior to the twelfth week of gestation may be associated (as either cause or effect) with endometritis and spontaneous abortion, while ascending infection after the twelfth week may be associated with chorioamnionitis. In rare instances, infection extends secondarily to the pelvic organs from adjacent foci of inflammation (e.g., sites of appendicitis, regional ileitis, or diverticulitis), as a result of hematogenous dissemination (e.g., of tuberculosis), or as a rare complication of certain tropical diseases (e.g., schistosomiasis).

Spontaneously occurring PID can be of the chronic or the acute type. Chronic PID due to *Mycobacterium tuberculosis* has become uncommon in industrialized countries. However, subacute or chronic PID caused by chronic infection with *Chlamydia trachomatis* is thought to be common.

The term *PID* is most often used today to refer to cases of acute, spontaneously occurring infection ascending from the cervix or vagina. The clinical diagnosis of PID is imprecise. Use of endometrial biopsy together with laparoscopy provides evidence of a continuum progressing from cervicitis alone to endometritis, to salpingitis, to pelvic peritonitis, and finally to generalized peritonitis, perihepatitis, or pelvic abscess. In this chapter, *PID* is used to refer to the clinical syndrome that includes each of these conditions, and the term *salpingitis* is restricted to cases of visually or histopathologically confirmed inflammation of the fallopian tubes. The distinction between endometritis and salpingitis and the distribution of cases of each infection may be important, because long-term sequelae are common after salpingitis. These sequelae include infertility due to bilateral tubal occlusion, peritubal adhesions, ectopic pregnancy due to tubal damage without occlusion, chronic pelvic pain, and recurrent PID.

ETIOLOGY The etiology of PID has seemed to vary greatly in several studies for reasons related to the selection of patients, the prevalence of sexually transmitted disease (STD) pathogens at the time and place of the study, and methodology. As is summarized in Table 130-1, the agents most often implicated in acute PID include those that are primary causes of cervicitis (*Neisseria gonorrhoeae* and *C. trachomatis*) and those that can be regarded as normal components of the vaginal flora.

During the 1980s, *N. gonorrhoeae* and/or *C. trachomatis* were found in 65 percent of women with a clinical diagnosis of PID at San Francisco General Hospital and in 85 percent of patients with proven salpingitis and endometritis in Seattle; in both studies, gonorrhea was nearly twice as common as chlamydial infection and dual infection was common. However, in Scandinavian countries, where gonococcal infection is under much better control, endocervical gonococcal infection has been found in a declining proportion of women with PID during the past decade, while chlamydial infection remains more common in this group. In general, PID is most often associated with gonorrhea where there is a high incidence of gonorrhea—e.g., in developing countries and in indigent, inner-city populations in developed countries. In several studies of women with PID, up to two-thirds of women with endocervical cultures positive for *N. gonorrhoeae* have also had endometrial, peritoneal, or tubal cultures positive for this organism. Similarly, studies of women with proven PID have shown that *C. trachomatis* can be demonstrated by culture or immunofluorescent staining in the endometrium or tubes of the majority of those who have endocervical chlamydial infection.

Anaerobic and facultative anaerobic organisms (especially *Prevotella* species, peptostreptococci, *Escherichia coli*, and group B streptococci) and genital mycoplasmas have been isolated from specimens obtained at laparoscopy from the peritoneal fluid or fallopian tubes in a varying proportion—typically one-fourth to one-third—of women with PID studied in the United States. These vaginal organisms can be found in association with chlamydial or gonococcal infection as well as in the absence of such infection. The importance of vaginal organisms in salpingitis has probably been overestimated in studies based on culture of specimens obtained by culdocentesis or endometrial aspiration, procedures in which contamination of the aspirated specimen by vaginal flora is possible. However, specimens obtained by laparoscopy from some patients with PID also have contained anaerobic and facultative species. It is extremely difficult to determine the exact microbial etiology of an individual case of PID because of the frequency of mixed infection, the difficulty in sampling the fallopian tube itself, and the complexity of the microbiologic techniques required to detect the various fastidious pathogens involved.

In general, first episodes of acute PID are particularly likely to be caused by *N. gonorrhoeae* and/or *C. trachomatis*. These sexually transmitted pathogens are implicated somewhat less often in recurrent bouts of acute PID, in episodes occurring in women with intrauterine devices (IUD), and in episodes precipitated by invasive intrauterine diagnostic or therapeutic procedures, which are often associated with ascending infection caused by certain components of the endogenous vaginal flora.

EPIDEMIOLOGY It has been estimated that about 850,000 cases of PID occurred in the United States each year during the mid-1970s. PID is not a reportable disease in the United States; surveillance of physicians in private practice and of hospital discharges suggests that the incidence of PID increased from the mid-1960s through the mid-1970s and may then have decreased. Hospitalization for acute PID declined steadily from 1982 through 1993, but visits to physicians' offices remained constant during that period.

Acute PID is almost exclusively a disease of sexually active women. Important risk factors include a history of salpingitis, a recent history of vaginal douching, and the use of an IUD, particularly the Dalkon shield. In most studies, the relative risk of PID among IUD users is higher in nulliparous than in parous women and is greatest during the first few months after IUD insertion. The increased risk of PID among IUD users is evident mainly among those with multiple sex partners. In contrast, women using oral contraceptives appear to be at decreased risk of PID. Barrier methods of contraception also make PID less likely by reducing the risk of chlamydial and gonococcal infection. Tubal sterilization reduces (but does not completely eliminate) the risk of salpingitis by preventing intraluminal spread of infection into the tubes.

PATHOGENESIS Factors cited as possibly contributing to intracanalicular upward spread of gonococci and chlamydiae from the endocervix to the endometrium and endosalpinx include estrogen-dominated (thin) cervical mucus, attachment to sperm that migrate upward into the tubes, use of an IUD, vaginal douching, and menstruation. The onset of symptoms of *N. gonorrhoeae*–associated and *C. trachomatis*–associated PID often occurs during or soon after the menstrual period. In fallopian tube organ cultures in vitro, gonococci attach to the surface of the secretory columnar cells (but not the ciliated cells) of the endosalpinx. Gonococcal pili and perhaps other surface proteins are important in this attachment. Gonococci then are taken into the secretory cells by endocytosis. They pass through the cells—and perhaps between cells—and are extruded through the base of the cell into the submucosal connective tissue. Ciliary motion ceases, and then ciliated cells, although not directly invaded by gonococci, are sloughed from the mucosa—a factor that may render the tubes more susceptible to superinfection by other organisms. It is uncertain whether this loss of ciliated cells is irreversible in vivo. Gonococcal endotoxin and peptidoglycan as well as certain cytokines appear to be responsible for these cytotoxic effects. Gonococci associated with PID are significantly less susceptible to penicillin and less likely to belong to the Arg-Hyx-Ura auxotype than are strains causing uncomplicated gonorrhea.

C. trachomatis also infects the columnar cells of the fallopian tube but produces little damage in tubal organ cultures, perhaps because the host response is more important than directly toxic effects of bacterial products in the pathogenesis of chlamydial salpingitis. In chlamydial mucopurulent cervicitis (MPC), cervical biopsies show inclusions containing chlamydiae within columnar cells; columnar epithelial infiltration by neutrophils; submucosal and stromal infiltration by plasma cells, lymphocytes, histiocytes, and neutrophils; and lymphoid aggregates containing transformed lymphocytes. Routine endometrial biopsies from consecutive women with chlamydial MPC show endometritis in approximately one-half of cases. Although endometritis detected in this way is sometimes associated with uterine tenderness, abnormal menstrual bleeding, and leukocytosis, symptoms of abdominal pain and fever as well as signs of adnexal tenderness are usually lacking; this point underscores the subclinical nature or minimal clinical manifestations of many cases of upper genital tract chlamydial infection. It is not known what proportion of women with endometritis also have salpingitis, since laparoscopy has not been performed in the absence of more suggestive symptoms and signs of salpingitis. However, among women with chlamydial MPC who do have such symptoms and signs, the great majority of those who undergo endometrial biopsy and laparoscopy have both endometritis and salpingitis. Chlamydial inclusions are demonstrable by direct immunofluorescence in columnar epithelial cells of the endometrium and endosalpinx. The endometrial biopsies usually show neutrophils infiltrating

Table 130-1

Cervical and Vaginal Organisms Most Often Implicated in Acute PID

Cervical Pathogens	Vaginal Flora Components
Neisseria gonorrhoeae	Anaerobic bacteria
Chlamydia trachomatis	*Prevotella*, *Peptostreptococcus*, *Mobiluncus*, and *Actinomyces* species
	Facultative bacteria
	Enterobacteriaceae, *Haemophilus influenzae*, *Gardnerella vaginalis*, group B *Streptococcus*
	Mycoplasmas
	Mycoplasma hominis, *Ureaplasma urealyticum*

the epithelium and plasma cells infiltrating the stroma, findings also seen in gonococcal endometritis but not in the uninfected endometrium. Other inflammatory changes analogous to those seen in the cervix are also found in the endometrium with chlamydial infection. Experimental inoculation of the fallopian tubes of lower primates produces mild acute salpingitis and ciliary sloughing that is transient and reversible. However, if experimental tubal inoculation is preceded by repeated inoculation of the fallopian tubes or cervix, a more intense salpingitis results and progresses to peritubular scarring. The implication is that in the female genital tract, as in the eye, repeated exposure to *C. trachomatis* leads to the greatest degree of tissue inflammation and damage.

The pathogenesis of PID attributable to mycoplasmas or other vaginal anaerobic or facultative organisms is less well studied. It is possible that other vaginal organisms implicated in PID often cause tubal infection in women whose tubes have already been damaged by a primary sexually transmitted pathogen (i.e., *N. gonorrhoeae* or *C. trachomatis*). The vaginal organisms implicated in PID are found in the vagina most often and in greatest concentration in bacterial vaginosis, and there is epidemiologic evidence that bacterial vaginosis itself is a predisposing factor for PID (just as poor oral hygiene is a risk factor for aspiration pneumonia).

Certain other iatrogenic factors, such as dilatation and curettage or cesarean section, are known to increase the risk of PID in women with endocervical gonococcal or chlamydial infection. Recent evidence indicates that among women undergoing cesarean section, the presence of bacterial vaginosis increases the risk of postpartum endometritis.

CLINICAL MANIFESTATIONS   Tuberculous Salpingitis
Unlike nontuberculous salpingitis, genital tuberculosis often occurs in older women, about half of whom are postmenopausal. In a large review in Sweden, 38 percent of women with tuberculous salpingitis had had tuberculosis diagnosed previously. The most common presenting symptoms were abnormal vaginal bleeding, pain (including dysmenorrhea), and infertility. Most of these women had normal findings on bimanual pelvic examination, though about one-quarter had adnexal masses. The most common basis for diagnosis was endometrial biopsy showing tuberculous granulomas, often in association with a positive culture.

Nontuberculous Salpingitis   The evolution of symptoms of nontuberculous salpingitis classically proceeds from a mucopurulent vaginal discharge caused by cervicitis to midline abdominal pain and abnormal vaginal bleeding caused by endometritis and then to bilateral lower abdominal and pelvic pain caused by salpingitis, with nausea and vomiting and increased abdominal tenderness caused by peritonitis. Some patients have diffuse abdominal pain caused by generalized peritonitis or pleuritic right upper quadrant pain caused by perihepatitis. The pattern in which symptoms evolve varies from patient to patient and is also related to the etiology of the PID.

The onset of IUD-associated PID is typically gradual and may be preceded by the malodorous vaginal discharge characteristic of bacterial vaginosis. The onset of gonococcal PID has been more acute than that of chlamydial PID in some but not all studies, and PID of either etiology usually presents during the first half of the menstrual cycle.

The abdominal pain in nontuberculous salpingitis is usually described as dull or aching. In some cases, pain is lacking or is atypical, and active inflammatory changes are found in the course of an unrelated evaluation or procedure, such as a tubal ligation or a laparoscopic evaluation for infertility. Abnormal uterine bleeding precedes or coincides with the onset of pain in about 40 percent of women with PID, symptoms of urethritis (dysuria) occur in 20 percent, and symptoms of proctitis (anorectal pain, tenesmus, and rectal discharge or bleeding) occasionally are seen in women with gonococcal or chlamydial infection.

Speculum examination shows evidence of MPC in the majority of women with gonococcal or chlamydial PID. Cervical motion tenderness is produced by stretching of the adnexal attachments on the side toward which the cervix is pushed. Bimanual examination reveals uterine fundal tenderness due to endometritis and abnormal adnexal

tenderness due to salpingitis that is usually, but not necessarily, bilateral. Adnexal swelling is palpable in about one-half of women with acute salpingitis, but evaluation of the adnexae in a patient with marked tenderness—even by an experienced examiner—is not reliable. The initial temperature is >38°C in only about one-third of patients with acute salpingitis; thus fever is not required for the diagnosis.

Laboratory findings include elevation of the erythrocyte sedimentation rate (ESR) in 75 percent of patients with acute salpingitis and elevation of the peripheral white blood cell count in up to 60 percent. Microscopic examination of a saline wet-mount preparation of vaginal fluid has revealed either more than one polymorphonuclear leukocyte per vaginal epithelial cell or findings consistent with bacterial vaginosis in nearly all patients with laparoscopically confirmed salpingitis in Swedish studies. However, exceptions have not been uncommon in U.S. studies.

Certain clinical manifestations of acute PID have been correlated with etiologic findings. For example, the onset of salpingitis is related to menses in women with gonococcal or chlamydial infection. Women with *N. gonorrhoeae*– or *C. trachomatis*–associated salpingitis are significantly younger than women with salpingitis of other etiologies. In a Swedish study, women with *Chlamydia*-associated salpingitis had more indolent disease, with mild symptoms of significantly longer duration and less fever, than women with gonorrhea-associated salpingitis. It is suspected that, for all recognized cases of symptomatic acute chlamydial salpingitis, there is a comparable number of unrecognized cases of indolent or mildly symptomatic chlamydial salpingitis. Furthermore, it is thought that subclinical chronic or recurrent chlamydial salpingitis may be a major cause of female infertility.

IUD-associated PID has been much less common since withdrawal of the Dalkon shield from the market. This infection tends to be indolent and is associated less often with fever, but more often with adnexal masses, than is PID not associated with IUD use.

Perihepatitis and Periappendicitis   Symptoms of perihepatitis, including pleuritic upper abdominal pain and tenderness (usually localized to the right upper quadrant), develop in 3 to 10 percent of women with acute PID. The onset of symptoms of perihepatitis takes place during or after the onset of symptoms of PID and may overshadow lower abdominal symptoms, thereby leading to a mistaken diagnosis of cholecystitis. In perhaps 5 percent of cases of acute salpingitis, early laparoscopy reveals inflammation ranging from edema and erythema of the liver capsule to exudate with fibrinous adhesions between the visceral and parietal peritoneum. When treatment is delayed and laparoscopy is performed late, dense "violin-string" adhesions are seen over the liver; chronic exertional or positional right upper quadrant pain ensues when traction is placed on the adhesions. Although perihepatitis, also known as the *Fitz-Hugh–Curtis syndrome*, was for many years attributed to gonococcal PID, most cases are now associated with chlamydial salpingitis. In patients with chlamydial salpingitis, serum titers of microimmunofluorescent antibody to *C. trachomatis* are typically much higher when perihepatitis is present than when it is absent, and it has been suggested that repeated chlamydial infections are responsible for perihepatitis.

Physical findings include right upper quadrant tenderness and usually include adnexal tenderness and cervicitis, even in patients whose symptoms are not suggestive of salpingitis. Liver function tests are nearly always normal, since inflammation is largely limited to the liver capsule and usually spares the parenchyma. Oral cholecystography may show nonfunction of the gallbladder, but ultrasonography of the right upper quadrant is normal. The presence of MPC and pelvic tenderness in a young woman with subacute pleuritic right upper quadrant pain and normal ultrasonography of the gallbladder points to a diagnosis of perihepatitis.

Periappendicitis (appendiceal serositis without involvement of the intestinal mucosa) has been found in approximately 5 percent of patients undergoing appendectomy for suspected appendicitis and can occur as a complication of gonococcal or chlamydial salpingitis.

Influence of Human Immunodeficiency Virus Infection   Several studies have yielded inconsistent results with regard to the influence of infection with human immunodeficiency virus (HIV) on certain clinical manifestations of PID, such as fever, clinical severity, and etiology. However, HIV-infected women with PID do appear to be more likely than women without HIV infection to present with tubo-ovarian abscess, to require hospitalization, and to require surgery for PID.

DIAGNOSIS Early diagnosis and initiation of therapy are essential to minimize tubal scarring. Recent reanalysis of Weström's cohort of Swedish women with proven salpingitis showed that those who delayed seeking care were three times more likely than those who sought care promptly to experience subsequent infertility or ectopic pregnancy. Appropriate treatment must not be withheld from patients who have an equivocal diagnosis. Since delay in therapy may lead to progression of tubal scarring, it is better to err on the side of overdiagnosis and overtreatment. On the other hand, it is essential to differentiate between salpingitis and other pelvic pathology, particularly surgical emergencies such as appendicitis and ectopic pregnancy.

No clinical finding or laboratory test short of laparoscopy definitively identifies salpingitis, and routine laparoscopy to confirm suspected salpingitis is generally impractical. Most patients with acute PID have lower abdominal pain of less than 3 weeks' duration, pelvic tenderness on bimanual pelvic examination, and evidence of lower genital tract infection (e.g., white blood cells outnumbering all other cells in the vaginal fluid). Approximately 60 percent of such patients have salpingitis at laparoscopy. Among the patients with these findings, a rectal temperature above 38°C, a palpable adnexal mass, and elevation of the ESR over 15 mm/h also raise the probability of salpingitis, which has been found at laparoscopy in 68 percent of patients with one of these additional findings, 90 percent of patients with two or fewer, and 96 percent of patients with three or fewer. However, only 17 percent of all patients with laparoscopy-confirmed salpingitis have had all three additional findings.

MPC is probably responsible for the presence of neutrophils in vaginal fluid in PID. In a woman with pelvic pain and tenderness, demonstration of an increased number of neutrophils ($\geqslant$30 per 1000 $\times$ microscopic field in strands of cervical mucus) increases the predictive value of a clinical diagnosis of acute PID.

Several clinical features other than the presence of cervicitis also favor the diagnosis of acute PID. These include onset with menses, history of recent menstrual bleeding, presence of an IUD, history of salpingitis, and sexual exposure to a male with urethritis. Detection of polymorphonuclear leukocytes in fluid aspirated by culdocentesis supports a diagnosis of suspected salpingitis. Urethritis or proctitis may occur in chlamydial or gonococcal infection but also may represent a urinary tract source or an intestinal source, respectively, for the patient's symptoms. Appendicitis or another disorder of the gut is favored by the early onset of anorexia, nausea, or vomiting; the onset of pain later than day 14 of the menstrual cycle; or unilateral pain limited to the right or left lower quadrant. A missed menstrual period dictates an evaluation for ectopic pregnancy. The more sensitive assays for human beta-chorionic gonadotropin are usually positive. Ultrasonography is sometimes useful for the identification of tuboovarian or pelvic abscess, and intravaginal ultrasound assessment of the tubes has recently been reported to show increased tubal diameter, intratubal fluid, or tubal wall thickening in some cases of salpingitis.

Laparoscopy is the most specific method for diagnosis of acute salpingitis. Although laparoscopic findings may be normal if inflammation is limited to the endosalpinx or the endometrium, patients with suspected PID who have a normal laparoscopy have a better prognosis (with no sequelae at all or fewer sequelae) than patients who have abnormal laparoscopic findings. The primary and uncontested value of laparoscopy in women with lower abdominal pain is for the exclusion of other surgical problems. Table 130-2 clearly shows that the most common and serious problems that may be confused with salpingitis are usually unilateral. Unilateral pain or pelvic mass, though not incompatible with PID, is a strong indication for laparoscopy unless the clinical picture warrants laparotomy instead. Atypical clinical findings, such as the absence of lower genital tract infection, a missed menstrual period, or failure to respond to appropriate therapy, are other frequent indications for laparoscopy.

Table 130-2

Laparoscopic Findings in Patients with False-Positive or False-Negative Clinical Diagnoses of Acute PID

False-Positive Clinical Diagnosis		False-Negative Clinical Diagnosis, Unexpected PID at Laparoscopy	
Laparoscopic Diagnosis	Percent	Clinical Diagnosis	Percent
Acute appendicitis	24	Ovarian tumor	20
Endometriosis	16	Acute appendicitis	18
Corpus luteum bleeding	12	Ectopic pregnancy	16
Ectopic pregnancy	11	Chronic salpingitis	6
Pelvic adhesions only	7	Acute peritonitis	6
Benign ovarian tumor	7	Endometriosis	5
Chronic salpingitis	6	Uterine myoma	5
Miscellaneous	15	Atypical pelvic pain	6
		Miscellaneous	6

Laparoscopic criteria used for the diagnosis of salpingitis include (1) erythema of the fallopian tube, (2) edema of the fallopian tube, and (3) seropurulent exudate or fresh, easily lysed adhesions at the fimbriated end or on the serosal surface of a fallopian tube.

Endometrial biopsy is relatively sensitive and specific for the diagnosis of endometritis when the endometrial changes described above are found, and the presence of endometritis correlates well with the presence of salpingitis. Endometritis is found in at least three-fourths of women with laparoscopically confirmed salpingitis and is not found in women without PID.

The etiologic diagnosis of PID can be further studied by culture or other testing of specimens obtained by endocervical swab, endometrial aspiration, or culdocentesis or by laparoscopy or laparotomy. Endocervical swab specimens should be examined by Gram's staining for neutrophils and gram-negative diplococci and by culture or DNA amplification test for *N. gonorrhoeae*. Compared with culture, the sensitivity of Gram's staining is about 60 percent, and the specificity is more than 95 percent. The endocervical swab specimen also should be tested for *C. trachomatis* by culture, antigen detection, or assays for chlamydial DNA or RNA. Although detection of either *N. gonorrhoeae* or *C. trachomatis* in the endocervix does not prove that either agent is also present in the upper genital tract, this finding strongly supports the diagnosis of PID. The clinical diagnosis of PID made by expert gynecologists is confirmed by laparoscopy or endometrial biopsy in only about 60 percent of all consecutive patients but in about 90 percent of those who also have cultures positive for *N. gonorrhoeae* or *C. trachomatis*. There is no evidence that the isolation of anaerobes or facultative aerobes from the cervix or vagina correlates with the presence of these organisms in the upper genital tract in acute PID, but this point has not been well studied. The value of culture of culdocentesis and endometrial aspirate specimens is disputed because of the risk of contamination of the specimen with components of the vaginal flora. When laparoscopy is performed, material can be obtained directly from the cul-de-sac or the fimbriated opening of the tube or by tubal aspiration if pyosalpinx is present. Such specimens should be cultured for anaerobic and facultative pathogens as well as for *N. gonorrhoeae* and *C. trachomatis*.

TREATMENT

Hospitalization should be considered in all cases of PID and is strongly recommended when (1) the diagnosis is uncertain and surgical emergencies such as appendicitis and ectopic pregnancy cannot be excluded, (2) pelvic abscess is suspected, (3) severe illness or nausea and vomiting preclude outpatient management, (4) the patient is pregnant, (5) the patient is an adolescent (since the compliance of adolescents is less predictable than that of adults), (6) the patient has HIV infection, (7) the patient is assessed as unable to follow or tolerate an outpatient regimen, (8) the patient has failed to respond to outpatient therapy, or (9) clinical follow-up after 48 to 72 h of antibiotic treatment cannot be arranged. Treatment should cover *N. gonorrhoeae*, *C. trachomatis*, gram-negative facultative bacteria (especially *E. coli*), vaginal anaerobes, and group B streptococci. No single agent is active against the entire spectrum of pathogens (Table 130-3). Several antimicrobial combinations do provide a broad spectrum of activity against the major pathogens in vitro, but many have not been adequately evaluated for clinical efficacy in PID.

Examples of Combination Regimens with Broad Activity Against Major Pathogens in PID Clinicians have had extensive experience with the following two inpatient regimens, which have given nearly identical results in a multicenter randomized trial:

1. Doxycycline [100 mg twice a day, given intravenously (IV) or orally] plus cefoxitin (2.0 g IV every 6 h) or cefotetan (2.0 g IV every 12 h). Administration of these drugs by the IV route should be continued for at least 48 h after the patient's condition improves, then followed with doxycycline (100 mg by mouth, twice a day) to complete 14 days of therapy. This regimen provides excellent coverage for *N. gonorrhoeae*, including penicillinase-producing strains, and for *C. trachomatis*.
2. Clindamycin (900 mg IV every 8 h) plus gentamicin (2.0 mg/kg IV followed by 1.5 mg/kg IV every 8 h) in patients with normal renal function. Treatment with these drugs should be continued for at least 48 h after the patient's condition improves, then followed with doxycycline (100 mg orally twice a day) or with clindamycin (450 mg orally four times a day) to complete 14 days of therapy. This regimen is active against anaerobes and facultative gram-negative rods as well as against *C. trachomatis* and *N. gonorrhoeae*. In cases with tuboovarian abscess, many experts use clindamycin rather than doxycycline for continued therapy in order to provide better coverage for anaerobic infection.

Patients who are not hospitalized also should receive a combined regimen with broad activity, such as ceftriaxone [250 mg intramuscularly (IM)] followed by doxycycline (100 mg by mouth, twice a day for 14 days). Cefoxitin (2.0 g IM) given concurrently with probenecid (1.0 g orally) or another parenteral third-generation cephalosporin (e.g., ceftizoxime or cefotaxime) can be used in place of ceftriaxone. An alternative outpatient regimen that provides good coverage of the major pathogens is ofloxacin (400 mg twice daily) plus either metronidazole (500 mg twice daily) or clindamycin (450 mg four times daily) for 14 days.

Management of Sexual Partners Sexual partners of patients with acute PID—particularly those who have been partners within the 1 to 2 months before the onset of symptoms of PID—should be examined for STDs and promptly treated with a regimen effective against uncomplicated gonococcal and chlamydial infection. Treatment of PID should be considered inadequate until sexual partners have been properly evaluated and treated.

Follow-Up Hospitalized patients should show substantial clinical improvement within 3 to 5 days. Women treated as outpatients should be clinically reevaluated within 72 h. A follow-up telephone survey of women seen in an emergency room and given a prescription for 10 days of oral doxycycline for PID found that 28 percent never filled the prescription and 41 percent stopped taking medication early (after an average of 4.1 days), often because of persistent symptoms, lack of symptoms, or side effects. Women not responding favorably to ambulatory therapy should be hospitalized. After completion of treatment, tests for persistent or recurrent infection with *N. gonorrhoeae* or *C. trachomatis* should be performed if symptoms persist or recur or if the patient has not complied with therapy or has been reexposed to an untreated sex partner.

Removal of an IUD Although a beneficial impact of IUD removal on the response of acute salpingitis to antimicrobial therapy and on the risk of recurrent salpingitis has not been proven, removal of the IUD 2 or 3 days after antimicrobial therapy has been initiated seems reasonable. When an IUD is removed, contraceptive counseling is essential.

Surgery Surgery is necessary for the treatment of salpingitis only in the face of life-threatening infection (such as rupture or threatened rupture of a tuboovarian abscess) or for drainage of an abscess. Ultrasonography is useful for diagnosing and monitoring pelvic abscesses. When surgery is performed, conservative procedures are usually sufficient. Pelvic abscesses often can be drained by posterior colpotomy, and peritoneal lavage can be used if there is generalized peritonitis.

PROGNOSIS Among 900 women who underwent long-term follow-up for a mean period of 8 years after successful treatment of an acute episode of PID with various regimens in Sweden, late sequelae included infertility due to bilateral tubal occlusion, ectopic pregnancy due to tubal scarring without occlusion, chronic pelvic pain, and recurrent salpingitis. Chronic pain lasting longer than 6 months was seen in 18 percent of patients and infertility due to tubal occlusion in 17 percent; 4 percent of the pregnancies that did occur were ectopic, representing approximately a sixfold increase over the expected rate of ectopic pregnancies. The rate of infertility after salpingitis was found to be related to the age of the patient, the duration of symptoms when treatment was started, the severity of salpingitis (as determined by laparoscopy) at the time of diagnosis, and the number of episodes of salpingitis. The postsalpingitis risk of infertility due to tubal occlusion among sexually active women not using contraceptives was 14 percent at 15 to 24 years of age and 26 percent at 25 to 34 years of age; the risk for women of all ages combined was 11 percent after one episode of salpingitis, 23 percent after two episodes, and 54 percent after three or more episodes. The risk of infertility after gonococcal salpingitis was comparable to the risk after chlamydial salpingitis in one small prospective study. A study of outcomes of PID at the University of Washington found a sevenfold increase in the risk of ectopic pregnancy and an eightfold increase in the rate of hysterectomy after PID.

In several countries, a striking relationship has also been found between

Table 130-3

Relative Activities of the Antimicrobial Agents Most Commonly Used to Treat PID

Agent	N. gonorrhoeae	C. trachomatis	Vaginal Anaerobes GPC†	Vaginal Anaerobes GNR‡	PID-Associated Facultative GNR	M. hominis
Ampicillin/amoxicillin	2+	2+	4+	2+	2+	0
Doxycycline	2+	4+	2+	1+	1+	2+
Cefoxitin, cefotetan	3+	0	4+	3+	3+	0
Ceftriaxone§	4+	0	3+	2+	4+	0
Gentamicin/tobramycin	2+	0	1+	0	4+	2+?
Ofloxacin	4+	3+	1+	1+	4+	1+
Azithromycin	2+	4+	2+	?+	2+	?
Clindamycin	1+	3+	4+	4+	0	3+
Metronidazole	0	0	4+	4+	0	0

* No single antimicrobial agent offers optimal activity against all of these pathogens, but certain combinations (e.g., cefoxitin plus doxycycline, gentamicin plus clindamycin, and ofloxacin plus metronidazole) have complementary activity. Relative activity is indicated on a scale of 0 to 4+.
† GPC, gram-positive cocci (peptostreptococci).
‡ GNR, gram-negative rods (anaerobic GNR include *Prevotella*; facultative GNR include Enterobacteriaceae and *Haemophilus influenzae*).

infertility due to tubal occlusion and the prevalence and titer of antibody to *C. trachomatis*. Recurrent salpingitis has been seen in approximately 15 to 25 percent of women treated for salpingitis in various studies.

PREVENTION Prevention of PID depends first on the effective control of gonococcal and chlamydial infection in the general population. Effective methods include the promotion of changes in sexual behavior and the use of barrier contraceptives in the context of ready access to modern methods of diagnosis and effective treatment of sex partners to control further spread. The decline in popularity of the IUD, particularly among nulliparous women, has undoubtedly helped to reduce the incidence of PID. It is also possible, but not proven, that the use of oral contraceptives and the avoidance of vaginal douching may reduce the risk of PID.

A 1996 report presented the results of a randomized controlled trial designed to determine whether selective screening for chlamydial infection reduced the risk of subsequent PID. Women at high risk for chlamydial infection were identified by means of a questionnaire mailed to all women 18 to 34 years of age who were enrolled in the Group Health Cooperative of Puget Sound in Washington. Women randomized to undergo chlamydial screening had a 56 percent lower rate of PID over the following year than did women receiving the usual care without screening. This report strongly supports risk-based screening for *Chlamydia* among young women receiving health care in managed-care organizations or other settings.

The complications of salpingitis can be minimized by early diagnosis and prompt treatment. It seems logical, but is unproven, that broad-spectrum therapy effective against all of the common causes of PID offers the best outcome. Although few methodologically sound clinical trials (especially with prolonged follow-up) have been conducted, one meta-analysis by Dodson showed a benefit of providing good coverage against anaerobes. Similarly, hospitalization to ensure rest and adequate compliance may improve the rather dismal long-term prognosis for tubal function. One placebo-controlled study showed that concurrent anti-inflammatory therapy with prednisolone hastened the reduction of acute inflammatory changes but did not improve the end results, as measured by fertility, hysterosalpingographic findings, or chronic pain. The potential value of anti-inflammatory therapy remains to be evaluated adequately.

BIBLIOGRAPHY

CATES WJ et al: Worldwide patterns of infertility: Is Africa different? Lancet 2:596, 1985

CENTERS FOR DISEASE CONTROL AND PREVENTION: Policy guidelines for the prevention and management of pelvic inflammatory disease. Morb Mort Week Rep 40(RR-5):1, 1992

————: 1993 Sexually transmitted disease treatment guidelines. Morb Mort Week Rep 42(RR-14):T-102, 1993

DODSON MG: Antibiotic regimens for treating acute pelvic inflammatory disease. An evaluation. J Reprod Med 39:285, 1994

ESCHENBACH DA et al: Polymicrobial etiology of acute pelvic inflammatory disease. N Engl J Med 293:166, 1975

FALK V et al: Genital tuberculosis in women. Am J Obstet Gynecol 138:974, 1980

FERRIS DG et al: Women's use of over-the-counter antifungal medications for gynecologic symptoms. J Fam Pract 42:595, 1996

GERMAINE A et al: *Reproductive Tract Infections: Global Impact and Priorities for Women's Reproductive Health*. New York, Plenum, 1992

HASSELQUIST MB, HILLIER S: Susceptibility of upper-genital tract isolates from women with pelvic inflammatory disease to ampicillin, cefpodoxime, metronidazole, and doxycycline. Sex Transm Dis 18:146, 1991

HEMSELL DL et al: Comparison of three regimens recommended by the Centers for Disease Control and Prevention for the treatment of women hospitalized with acute pelvic inflammatory disease. Clin Infect Dis 19:729, 1994

HILLIER SL et al: Role of bacterial vaginosis–associated microorganisms in endometritis. Am J Obstet Gynecol 175:435, 1996

HILLIS SD et al: Delayed care of pelvic inflammatory disease as a risk factor for impaired fertility. Am J Obstet Gynecol 168:1503, 1993

KAMENGA MC et al: The impact of human immunodeficiency virus infection on pelvic inflammatory disease: A case-control study in Abidjan, Ivory Coast. Am J Obstet Gynecol 172:919, 1995

KIMANI J et al: Risk factors for *Chlamydia trachomatis* pelvic inflammatory disease among sex workers in Nairobi, Kenya. J Infect Dis 173:1437, 1996

KIVIAT N et al: Endometrial histopathology in patients with culture-proven upper genital tract infection and laparoscopically diagnosed acute salpingitis. Am J Surg Pathol 14:167, 1990

LANDERS DV et al: Combination antimicrobial therapy in the treatment of acute pelvic inflammatory disease. Am J Obstet Gynecol 164:849, 1991

PEIPERT JF et al: Laboratory evaluation of acute upper genital tract infection. Obstet Gynecol 87(pt 1):730, 1996

PLUMMER FA et al: Postpartum upper genital tract infections in Nairobi, Kenya: Epidemiology, etiology, and risk factors. J Infect Dis 156:92, 1987

REED SD et al: Antibiotic treatment of tuboovarian abscess: Comparison of broad-spectrum beta-lactam agents versus clindamycin-containing regimens. Am J Obstet Gynecol 164:1556, 1991

SCHOLES D et al: Prevention of pelvic inflammatory disease by screening for cervical chlamydial infection. N Engl J Med 334:1362, 1996

ST JOHN RK, BROWN ST (eds): International symposium on pelvic inflammatory disease. Am J Obstet Gynecol 138:845, 1980

SVENSSON L et al: Infertility after acute salpingitis—with special reference to *Chlamydia trachomatis*–associated infections. Fertil Steril 40:322, 1983

WALKER CK et al: Pelvic inflammatory disease: Meta-analysis of antimicrobial regimen efficacy. J Infect Dis 168:969, 1993

WASHINGTON AE, KATZ P: Cost of and payment source for pelvic inflammatory disease: Trends and projections, 1983 through 2000. JAMA 266:2565, 1991

WASSERHEIT JN et al: Microbial causes of proven pelvic inflammatory disease and efficacy of clindamycin with tobramycin. Ann Intern Med 104:187, 1986

WØLNER-HANSSEN P: Silent pelvic inflammatory disease: Is it overstated? Obstet Gynecol 86:321, 1995

131 *Walter E. Stamm*

URINARY TRACT INFECTIONS AND PYELONEPHRITIS

DEFINITIONS Acute infections of the urinary tract can be subdivided into two general anatomic categories: lower tract infection (urethritis, cystitis, and prostatitis) and upper tract infection (acute pyelonephritis and intrarenal and perinephric abscesses). Infections at these various sites may occur together or independently and may either be asymptomatic or present as one of the clinical syndromes outlined below. Infections of the urethra and bladder are often considered superficial (or mucosal) infections, while prostatitis, pyelonephritis, and renal suppuration signify tissue invasion.

From a microbiologic perspective, urinary tract infection exists when pathogenic microorganisms are detected in the urine, urethra, bladder, kidney, or prostate. In most instances, growth of more than 10^5 organisms per milliliter from a properly collected midstream "clean-catch" urine sample indicates infection. However, significant bacteriuria is lacking in some cases of true urinary infection. Especially in symptomatic patients, a smaller number of bacteria (10^2 to 10^4 per milliliter of midstream urine) may signify infection. In urine specimens obtained by suprapubic aspiration or "in-and-out" catheterization and in samples from a patient with an indwelling catheter, colony counts of 10^2 to 10^4 per milliliter generally indicate infection. Conversely, colony counts in excess of 10^5 per milliliter of midstream urine are occasionally due to specimen contamination. That is especially likely to be the explanation when multiple species are found.

Infections that recur after antibiotic therapy can be due to the persistence of the originally infecting strain (as judged by species, antibiogram, serotype, and molecular type) or to reinfection with a new strain. "Same-strain" recurrent infections that become evident within 2 weeks of cessation of therapy can be the result of unresolved renal or prostatic infection (termed *relapse*) or of persistent vaginal or intestinal colonization leading to rapid reinfection of the bladder.

Symptoms of dysuria, urgency, and frequency that are unaccompanied by significant bacteriuria have been termed the *acute urethral syndrome*. Although widely used, this term lacks anatomic precision

818

PART SEVEN
Infectious Diseases

because many cases so designated are actually bladder infections. Moreover, since the causative agent can usually be identified in these patients, the term *syndrome*—implying unknown causation—is inappropriate.

Chronic pyelonephritis refers to chronic interstitial nephritis believed to result from bacterial infection of the kidney (see Chap. 276). Many noninfectious diseases also cause an interstitial nephritis that is indistinguishable pathologically from chronic pyelonephritis.

ACUTE INFECTIONS OF THE URINARY TRACT: URETHRITIS, CYSTITIS, AND PYELONEPHRITIS

EPIDEMIOLOGY Epidemiologically, urinary tract infections should be subdivided into catheter-associated (or nosocomial) infections and non-catheter-associated (or community-acquired) infections. Infections in either category may be symptomatic or asymptomatic. Acute infections are very common in noncatheterized patients (more so among women than among men) and account for more than 6 million office visits annually in the United States. These infections occur in 1 to 3 percent of schoolgirls and then increase markedly in incidence with the onset of sexual activity in adolescence. The vast majority of acute symptomatic infections involve young women. Acute symptomatic urinary infections are unusual in men under the age of 50. The development of asymptomatic bacteriuria parallels that of symptomatic infection and is rare among men under 50 but common among women between 20 and 50. Asymptomatic bacteriuria is quite common among elderly men and women, with rates as high as 40 to 50 percent in some studies.

ETIOLOGY Many different microorganisms can infect the urinary tract, but by far the most common agents are the gram-negative bacilli. *Escherichia coli* causes approximately 80 percent of acute infections in patients without catheters, urologic abnormalities, or calculi. Other gram-negative rods, especially *Proteus* and *Klebsiella* and occasionally *Enterobacter*, account for a smaller proportion of uncomplicated infections. These organisms, plus *Serratia* and *Pseudomonas*, assume increasing importance in recurrent infections and in infections associated with urologic manipulation, calculi, or obstruction. They play a major role in nosocomial, catheter-associated infections (see below). *Proteus* species, by virtue of urease production, and *Klebsiella* species, through the production of extracellular slime and polysaccharides, predispose to stone formation and are isolated more frequently from patients with calculi.

Gram-positive cocci play a lesser role in urinary tract infections. However, *Staphylococcus saprophyticus*, a novobiocin-resistant, coagulase-negative staphylococcus, accounts for 10 to 15 percent of acute symptomatic urinary tract infections in young females. Enterococci occasionally cause acute uncomplicated cystitis in women. More commonly, enterococci and *Staphylococcus aureus* cause infections in patients with renal stones or previous instrumentation. Isolation of *S. aureus* from the urine should arouse suspicion of bacteremic infection of the kidney.

About one-third of women with dysuria and frequency have either an insignificant number of bacteria in midstream urine cultures or completely sterile cultures and have been previously defined as having the urethral syndrome. About three-quarters of these women have pyuria, while one-quarter have no pyuria and little objective evidence of infection. In the women with pyuria, two groups of pathogens account for most infections. Low quantities (10^2 to 10^4 bacteria per milliliter) of typical bacterial uropathogens such as *E. coli*, *S. saprophyticus*, *Klebsiella*, or *Proteus* are found in midstream urine specimens from most of these women. These bacteria are probably the causative agents in these infections because they can usually be isolated from a suprapubic aspirate, are associated with pyuria, and respond to appropriate antimicrobial therapy. In other women with acute urinary symptoms, pyuria, and urine that is sterile (even when obtained by

suprapubic aspiration), sexually transmitted urethritis-producing agents such as *Chlamydia trachomatis*, *Neisseria gonorrhoeae*, and herpes simplex virus are etiologically important. These agents are found most frequently in young, sexually active women with new sexual partners.

The causative role of nonbacterial pathogens in urinary tract infections remains poorly defined. *Ureaplasma urealyticum* has frequently been isolated from the urethra and urine of patients with acute dysuria and frequency but is also found in specimens from many patients without urinary symptoms. Ureaplasmas probably account for some cases of urethritis and cystitis. *U. urealyticum* and *Mycoplasma hominis* have been isolated from prostatic and renal tissues of patients with acute prostatitis and pyelonephritis and are probably responsible for some of these infections as well. Adenoviruses cause acute hemorrhagic cystitis in children and in some young adults, often in epidemics. Although many other viruses can be isolated from urine (cytomegalovirus, for example), they are thought not to cause urinary infection. Colonization of the urine of catheterized patients or diabetics by *Candida* and other fungal species is common and sometimes progresses to symptomatic invasive infection (see Chap. 207). → *Mycobacterial infection of the genitourinary tract is discussed in Chap. 171.*

PATHOGENESIS AND SOURCES OF INFECTION The urinary tract should be viewed as a single anatomic unit that is united by a continuous column of urine extending from the urethra to the kidney. In the vast majority of urinary tract infections, bacteria gain access to the bladder via the urethra. Ascent of bacteria from the bladder may follow and is probably the pathway for most renal parenchymal infections.

The vaginal introitus and distal urethra are normally colonized by diphtheroids, streptococcal species, lactobacilli, and staphylococcal species but not by the enteric gram-negative bacilli that commonly cause urinary tract infections. In females prone to the development of cystitis, however, enteric gram-negative organisms residing in the bowel colonize the introitus, the periurethral skin, and the distal urethra before and during episodes of bacteriuria. The factors that predispose to periurethral colonization with gram-negative bacilli remain poorly understood but probably include alteration of the normal perineal flora by antibiotics, other genital infections, or contraceptives, especially diaphragms and spermicide. Small numbers of periurethral bacteria probably gain entry to the bladder frequently, a process that is facilitated in some cases by urethral massage during intercourse. Whether bladder infection ensues depends on interacting effects of the pathogenicity of the strain, the inoculum size, and the local and systemic mechanisms of host defense.

Under normal circumstances, bacteria placed in the bladder are rapidly cleared, partly through the flushing and dilutional effects of voiding but also as a result of the antibacterial properties of urine and the bladder mucosa. Owing mostly to a high urea concentration and high osmolarity, the bladder urine of many normal persons inhibits or kills bacteria. Prostatic secretions possess antibacterial properties as well. Polymorphonuclear leukocytes in the bladder wall also appear to play a role in clearing bacteriuria. The role of locally produced antibody remains unclear.

Hematogenous pyelonephritis occurs most often in debilitated patients who either are chronically ill or are receiving immunosuppressive therapy. Metastatic staphylococcal or candidal infections of the kidney may follow bacteremia or fungemia, spreading from distant foci of infection in the bone, skin, endothelium, or elsewhere.

CONDITIONS AFFECTING PATHOGENESIS Gender and Sexual Activity The female urethra appears to be particularly prone to colonization with colonic gram-negative bacilli because of its proximity to the anus, its short length (about 4 cm), and its termination beneath the labia. Sexual intercourse causes the introduction of bacteria into the bladder and is temporally associated with the onset of cystitis; it thus appears to be important in the pathogenesis of urinary infections in younger women. (Voiding after intercourse has been shown to reduce the risk of cystitis, probably because it promotes the clearance of bacteria introduced during intercourse.) In addition, use of a diaphragm and/or a spermicide dramatically alters the normal introital bacterial flora and has been associated with marked increases in vaginal colonization with *E. coli* and in the risk of urinary infection. In males, prostatitis and urethral obstruction due to prostatic hypertrophy are important factors predisposing to bacteriuria. Homosexuality also is associated with an increased risk of cystitis, which probably is related to rectal intercourse. Men infected with human immunodeficiency virus (HIV) who have CD4 + T cell counts of <200/μL have recently been shown to be at increased risk of both bacteriuria and symptomatic urinary tract infection. Finally, lack of circumcision has been identified as a risk factor for urinary tract infection in both neonates and young men.

Pregnancy Urinary infections are detected in 2 to 8 percent of pregnant women, the exact figure depending on socioeconomic status. Symptomatic upper tract infections, in particular, are unusually common during pregnancy; fully 20 to 30 percent of pregnant women with asymptomatic bacteriuria subsequently develop pyelonephritis. This predisposition to upper tract infection during pregnancy results from decreased ureteral tone, decreased ureteral peristalsis, and temporary incompetence of the vesicoureteral valves. Bladder catheterization during or after delivery causes additional infections. Cystitis and pyelonephritis are no more common among women with toxemia of pregnancy than among other pregnant women. Increased prevalences of premature delivery and newborn mortality may result from urinary infections during pregnancy, particularly those involving the upper urinary tract.

Obstruction Any impediment to the free flow of urine—tumor, stricture, stone, or prostatic hypertrophy—results in hydronephrosis and a greatly increased frequency of urinary tract infection. Infection superimposed on urinary tract obstruction may lead to rapid destruction of renal tissue. It is of utmost importance, therefore, when infection is present, to repair obstructive lesions. On the other hand, when an obstruction is minor and is not progressive or associated with infection, great caution should be exercised in attempting surgical correction. The introduction of infection in such cases may be more damaging than an uncorrected minor obstruction that does not significantly impair renal function.

Neurogenic Bladder Dysfunction Interference with the nerve supply to the bladder, as in spinal cord injury, tabes dorsalis, multiple sclerosis, diabetes, and other diseases, may be associated with urinary tract infection. The infection may be initiated by the use of catheters for bladder drainage and is favored by the prolonged stasis of urine in the bladder. An additional factor often operative in these cases is bone demineralization due to immobilization, which causes hypercalciuria, calculus formation, and obstructive uropathy.

Vesicoureteral Reflux Defined as reflux of urine from the bladder cavity up into the ureters and sometimes into the renal pelvis, vesicoureteral reflux occurs during voiding or with elevation of pressure in the bladder. In practice, this condition is demonstrated by the finding of retrograde movement of radiopaque or radioactive material during a voiding cystourethrogram. An anatomically impaired vesicoureteral junction facilitates reflux of bacteria and thus upper tract infection. However, since a fluid connection between the bladder and the kidney always exists, even in the normal urinary system, some retrograde movement of bacteria probably takes place during infection but is not detected by radiologic techniques.

Vesicoureteral reflux is common among children with anatomic abnormalities of the urinary tract as well as among children with anatomically normal but infected urinary tracts. In the latter group, reflux disappears with advancing age and probably is attributable to factors other than urinary infection. Long-term follow-up of children with urinary tract infection who have reflux has established that renal damage correlates with marked reflux, not with infection.

The routine search for reflux would be aided by the development of noninvasive tests applicable to young children, in whom the need for an effective technique is greatest. In the meantime, it appears reasonable to search for reflux in anyone with unexplained failure of renal growth or with renal scarring, because urinary tract infection per se is an insufficient explanation for these abnormalities. On the other hand, it is doubtful that all children who have recurrent urinary tract infections but whose urinary tract appears normal on pyelography

should be subjected to voiding cystoureterography merely for the detection of the rare patient with marked reflux not revealed by the intravenous pyelogram.

Bacterial Virulence Factors Bacterial virulence factors markedly influence the likelihood that a given strain, once introduced into the bladder, will cause urinary tract infection. Not all strains of *E. coli*, for example, are equally able to infect the intact urinary tract. Most strains that cause symptomatic urinary tract infections in noncatheterized patients belong to a small number of specific O, K, and H serogroups, produce hemolysin, and share certain other "uropathogenic" properties. Adherence of bacteria to uroepithelial cells is a critical first step in the initiation of infection. For both *E. coli* and *Proteus*, fimbriae (hairlike proteinaceous surface appendages) mediate the attachment of bacteria to specific receptors on epithelial cells. Nearly all strains of *E. coli* that cause pyelonephritis in patients with anatomically normal urinary tracts possess a particular pilus (the P pilus or gal-gal pilus) that mediates attachment to the digalactoside portion of glycosphingolipids present on uroepithelium. In addition, strains that cause pyelonephritis usually produce hemolysin, have aerobactin (a siderophore for scavenging iron), and are resistant to the bactericidal action of human serum. Since most strains that produce acute pyelonephritis in the intact host possess all or nearly all of these virulence factors, the concept has arisen that only a few uropathogenic clones cause most such cases of infection. In contrast, infections in patients with structural or functional abnormalities of the urinary tract are generally caused by bacterial strains that lack these uropathogenic properties; the implication is that these properties are not needed for infection of the compromised urinary tract.

Genetic Factors Increasing evidence suggests that host genetic factors influence susceptibility to urinary infection. The number and type of receptors on uroepithelial cells to which bacteria may attach are at least in part genetically determined. Many of these structures are components of blood group antigens and are present on both erythrocytes and uroepithelial cells. For example, P fimbriae mediate attachment of *E. coli* to P-positive erythrocytes and are found on nearly all strains causing acute uncomplicated pyelonephritis. Conversely, P blood group–negative individuals, who lack these receptors, have a decreased likelihood of pyelonephritis. It has also been demonstrated that nonsecretors of blood group antigens are at increased risk of recurrent urinary infection; this predisposition may relate to a different profile of genetically determined glycolipids on uroepithelial cells.

LOCALIZATION OF INFECTION Infections involving the upper urinary tract usually cause a significant rise in serum antibodies to the O antigen of the infecting strain. They also produce a temporary defect in renal concentrating ability in many patients and may be associated with the formation of leukocyte casts. Lower tract infections rarely result in increased antibody titers, concentrating defects, or white cell casts. Unfortunately, these methods of distinguishing renal parenchymal infection from cystitis are neither reliable nor convenient enough for routine clinical use. More sensitive tests for distinguishing pyelonephritis from cystitis (bilateral ureteral catheterization and the bladder washout technique originated by Fairley) are inherently invasive and are too complex for routine clinical practice. A simpler, noninvasive test by which to distinguish upper from lower tract infections on the basis of antibody coating of bacteria in the urine is not sufficiently sensitive or specific to be of value in the routine clinical management of patients. An elevated level of C-reactive protein often accompanies acute pyelonephritis and is rare in cystitis, but this acute-phase reactant is nonspecific since it is also detectable in infections other than pyelonephritis.

CLINICAL PRESENTATION Clinical signs and symptoms cannot be relied on as an accurate basis for the diagnosis or localization of urinary tract infection. Many patients with significant bacteriuria (including some with upper tract infection) have no symptoms at all. Of those with significant bacteriuria and symptoms of cystitis, about two-thirds have lower tract infection and about one-third have clinically silent upper tract infection that becomes evident only on the performance of localization studies. Clinical symptoms and signs of pyelonephritis, though usually suggestive, do not always indicate upper tract infection. Finally, among women presenting with acute dysuria and frequency, only 60 to 70 percent have significant bacteriuria, but most of those without significant bacteriuria also have infections of the kidneys, bladder, or urethra.

Enumeration of the number and type of bacteria in the urine is an extremely important diagnostic procedure. In symptomatic infections of the urinary tract, uropathogenic bacteria are usually demonstrable in the urine in large numbers. As a rule, quantitative estimation of the number of bacteria in voided urine specimens makes it possible to distinguish contamination from true bacteriuria, and a bacterial colony count of $\geq 10^5$/mL has been the criterion traditionally used for this purpose. However, in symptomatic women with pyuria, colony counts of 10^2 to 10^4 *E. coli*, *Klebsiella*, *Proteus*, or *S. saprophyticus* per milliliter of midstream urine usually indicate infection, not contamination, and should not be disregarded. In asymptomatic patients, two consecutive urine specimens should be examined bacteriologically before therapy is instituted, and 10^5 or more bacteria of a single species per milliliter should be demonstrable in both specimens. Since the large number of bacteria in the bladder urine is due in part to bacterial multiplication during residence in the bladder cavity, samples of urine from the ureters or renal pelvis may contain fewer than 10^5 bacteria per milliliter and yet indicate infection. Similarly, the presence of bacteriuria of any degree in suprapubic aspirates or of 10^2 or more bacteria per milliliter of urine obtained by catheterization usually indicates infection. In some circumstances (antibiotic treatment, high urea concentration, high osmolarity, low pH), urine inhibits bacterial multiplication, resulting in relatively low bacterial colony counts despite infection. For this reason, antiseptic solutions should not be used in washing the periurethral area before collection of the urine specimen. Water diuresis or recent voiding also reduces bacterial counts in urine.

Rapid methods of detection of bacteriuria have been developed as alternatives to standard culture methods. These methods detect bacterial growth by photometry, bioluminescence, or other means and provide results rapidly, usually in 1 to 2 h. Compared with urine cultures, these techniques generally exhibit a sensitivity of 95 to 98 percent and a negative predictive value of >99 percent when bacteriuria is defined as 10^5 colony forming units per milliliter. However, the sensitivity of these tests falls to 60 to 80 percent when 10^2 to 10^4 colony forming units per milliliter is the standard of comparison.

Microscopy of urine from symptomatic patients can be of great diagnostic value. Microscopic bacteriuria, which is best assessed with Gram-stained uncentrifuged urine, is found in more than 90 percent of specimens from patients whose infections are associated with colony counts of at least 10^5/mL, and this finding is very specific. However, bacteria cannot usually be detected microscopically in infections with lower colony counts (10^2 to 10^4/mL). The detection of bacteria by urinary microscopy constitutes firm evidence of infection, but the absence of microscopically detectable bacteria does not exclude the diagnosis. When carefully sought by means of chamber-count microscopy, pyuria is a highly sensitive indicator of urinary tract infection in symptomatic patients. Pyuria is demonstrated in nearly all acute bacterial urinary tract infections, and its absence calls the diagnosis into question. The leukocyte esterase "dipstick" method is less sensitive than microscopy in identifying pyuria but is a useful alternative where microscopy is not feasible. Pyuria in the absence of bacteriuria (sterile pyuria) may indicate infection with unusual bacterial agents such as *C. trachomatis*, *U. urealyticum*, and *Mycobacterium tuberculosis* or with fungi. Alternatively, sterile pyuria may be demonstrated in noninfectious urologic conditions such as calculi, anatomic abnormality, nephrocalcinosis, vesicoureteral reflux, interstitial nephritis, or polycystic disease.

Cystitis Patients with dysuria, frequency, urgency, and suprapubic pain usually have cystitis. The urine often becomes grossly cloudy and malodorous, and it is bloody in about 30 percent of cases. White cells and bacteria can be detected by examination of unspun urine in most cases. However, some women with cystitis have only 10^2 to 10^4 bacteria per milliliter of urine, and in these instances bacteria cannot be seen in a Gram-stained preparation of unspun urine. Physical examination generally reveals only tenderness of the urethra or the suprapubic area. If a genital lesion or a vaginal discharge is evident, especially in conjunction with fewer than 10^5 bacteria per milliliter on urine culture, then pathogens that may cause urethritis, vaginitis, or cervicitis, such as *C. trachomatis*, *N. gonorrhoeae*, *Trichomonas*, *Candida*, and herpes simplex virus, should be considered. Prominent systemic manifestations such as a temperature of >38.3°C (>101°F), nausea, and vomiting usually indicate concomitant renal infection, as does costovertebral angle tenderness. However, the absence of these findings does not ensure that infection is limited to the bladder and urethra.

Acute Pyelonephritis Symptoms of acute pyelonephritis generally develop rapidly over a few hours or a day and include a temperature of ≥ 39.4°C (≥ 103°F), shaking chills, nausea, vomiting, and diarrhea. Symptoms of cystitis may or may not develop. Besides fever, tachycardia, and generalized muscle tenderness, physical examination reveals marked tenderness on deep pressure in one or both costovertebral angles or on deep abdominal palpation. In some patients, signs and symptoms of gram-negative sepsis predominate. Most patients have significant leukocytosis, pyuria with leukocyte casts in the urine, and bacteria detectable in Gram-stained unspun urine. Hematuria may be demonstrated during the acute phase of the disease; if it persists after acute manifestations of infection have subsided, a stone, a tumor, or tuberculosis should be considered.

Except in individuals with papillary necrosis or urinary obstruction, the manifestations of acute pyelonephritis usually respond to therapy within 48 to 72 h. However, despite the absence of symptoms, bacteriuria or pyuria may persist. In severe pyelonephritis, fever subsides more slowly and may not disappear for several days, even after appropriate antibiotic treatment has been instituted.

Urethritis Approximately 30 percent of women with acute dysuria, frequency, and pyuria have midstream urine cultures that show either no growth or insignificant bacterial growth. Clinically, these women cannot readily be distinguished from those with cystitis. In this situation, a distinction should be made between women infected with sexually transmitted pathogens, such as *C. trachomatis*, *N. gonorrhoeae*, or herpes simplex virus, and those with low-count *E. coli* or staphylococcal infection of the urethra and bladder. Chlamydial or gonococcal infection should be suspected in women with a gradual onset of illness, no hematuria, no suprapubic pain, and more than 7 days of symptoms. The additional history of a recent sex-partner change, especially if the patient's partner has recently had chlamydial or gonococcal urethritis, should heighten the suspicion of a sexually transmitted infection, as should the finding of mucopurulent cervicitis. Gross hematuria, suprapubic pain, an abrupt onset of illness, a duration of illness of less than 3 days, and a history of previous urinary tract infections favor the diagnosis of *E. coli* urinary tract infection.

Catheter-Associated Urinary Tract Infections Bacteriuria develops in at least 10 to 15 percent of hospitalized patients with indwelling urethral catheters. The risk of infection is about 3 to 5 percent per day of catheterization. *Proteus*, *Pseudomonas*, *Klebsiella*, and *Serratia*, in addition to *E. coli*, usually cause these infections. Many infecting strains display markedly greater antimicrobial resistance than organisms that cause community-acquired urinary infections. Factors associated with an increased risk of infection include female sex, prolonged catheterization, severe underlying illness, disconnection of the catheter and drainage tube, other types of faulty catheter care, and lack of systemic antimicrobial therapy.

Infection occurs when bacteria reach the bladder by one of two routes: by migrating through the column of urine in the catheter lumen (intraluminal route) or by moving up the mucous sheath outside the catheter (periurethral route). Hospital-acquired pathogens reach the patient's catheter or urine-collecting system on the hands of hospital personnel, in contaminated solutions or irrigants, and via contaminated instruments or disinfectants. Bacteria usually enter the catheter system at the catheter–collecting tube junction or at the drainage bag portal. The organisms then ascend intraluminally into the bladder within 24 to 72 h. Alternatively, the patient's own bowel flora may colonize the perineal skin and periurethral area and reach the bladder via the external surface of the catheter. This route is particularly common in women. Recent studies have demonstrated the importance of the attachment and growth of bacteria on the inner surface of the catheter in the pathogenesis of catheter-associated urinary tract infection. Such bacteria growing in biofilms on the inner surface of the catheter eventually produce encrustations consisting of bacteria, bacterial glycocalyces, host urinary proteins, and urinary salts. These encrustations provide a refuge for bacteria and may protect them from antimicrobials and phagocytes.

Clinically, most catheter-associated infections cause minimal symptoms and no fever and often resolve after withdrawal of the catheter. The frequency of upper tract infection associated with catheter-induced bacteriuria is unknown. Gram-negative bacteremia, which follows catheter-associated bacteriuria in 1 to 2 percent of cases, is the most significant recognized complication of catheter-induced urinary infections. The catheterized urinary tract has repeatedly been demonstrated to be the most common source of gram-negative bacteremia in hospitalized patients, generally accounting for about 30 percent of cases.

Catheter-associated urinary tract infections can sometimes be prevented in patients catheterized for less than 2 weeks by use of a sterile closed collecting system, by attention to aseptic technique during insertion and care of the catheter, and by measures to minimize cross-infection. Other preventive approaches, including short courses of systemic antimicrobial therapy, topical application of periurethral antimicrobial ointments, use of preconnected catheter–drainage tube units, and addition of antimicrobials to the drainage bag, have all been protective in one or more controlled trials but are not recommended for general use. Despite precautions, the majority of patients catheterized for longer than 2 weeks eventually develop bacteriuria. The need for treatment as well as the optimal type and duration of treatment for such patients with asymptomatic bacteriuria have not been established. Removal of the catheter in conjunction with a short course of antibiotics to which the organism is susceptible probably constitutes the best course of action and nearly always eradicates bacteriuria. Treatment of asymptomatic catheter-associated bacteriuria may be of greatest benefit to elderly women, who most often develop symptoms if left untreated. If the catheter cannot be removed, antibiotic therapy usually proves to be unsuccessful and may in fact result in infection with a more resistant strain. In this situation, the bacteriuria should be ignored unless the patient develops symptoms or is at high risk of developing bacteremia. In these cases, use of systemic antibiotics or urinary bladder antiseptics may reduce the degree of bacteriuria and the likelihood of bacteremia. Because of spinal cord injury, incontinence, or other factors, some patients in hospitals or nursing homes require long-term or semipermanent bladder catheterization. Measures intended to prevent infection have been largely unsuccessful, and essentially all such chronically catheterized patients develop bacteriuria. If feasible, intermittent catheterization by a nurse or by the patient appears to reduce the incidence of bacteriuria and associated complications in such patients. Treatment should be provided when symptomatic infections arise, but treatment of asymptomatic bacteriuria in such patients has no apparent benefit.

DIAGNOSTIC TESTING Although many authorities have recommended that urine culture and antimicrobial susceptibility testing be performed for any patient with a suspected urinary tract infection, it may be more practical and cost-effective to manage women who have symptoms characteristic of acute uncomplicated cystitis without an initial urine culture. Two approaches to presumptive therapy have generally been used. In the first, treatment is initiated solely on the basis of a typical history and/or typical findings on physical examination. In the second, women with symptoms and signs of acute cystitis and without complicating factors are managed with urinary microscopy (or, alternatively, with a leukocyte esterase test). A positive result for pyuria and/or bacteriuria provides enough evidence of infection to indicate that urine culture and susceptibility testing can be omitted

and the patient treated empirically. Urine should be cultured, however, when a woman's symptoms and urine-examination findings leave the diagnosis of cystitis in question. Pretherapy cultures and susceptibility testing also are essential in the management of all patients with suspected upper tract infections and of those with complicating factors, as in these situations any of a variety of pathogens may be involved and antibiotic therapy is best tailored to the individual organism.

℞ **TREATMENT**

The following principles underlie the treatment of urinary tract infections:

1. In most circumstances, a quantitative urine culture, a Gram stain, or an alternative rapid diagnostic test should be performed to confirm infection before treatment is begun. When culture results become available, antimicrobial sensitivity testing should be used to direct therapy.
2. Factors predisposing to infection, such as obstruction and calculi, should be identified and corrected if possible.
3. Relief of clinical symptoms does not always indicate bacteriologic cure.
4. Each course of treatment should be classified after its completion as a failure (symptoms and/or bacteriuria not eradicated during therapy or in the immediate posttreatment culture) or a cure (resolution of symptoms and elimination of bacteriuria). Recurrent infections should be classified as same-strain or different-strain and as early (occurring within 2 weeks of the end of therapy) or late.
5. In general, uncomplicated infections confined to the lower urinary tract respond to short courses of therapy, while upper tract infections require longer treatment. After therapy, early recurrences due to the same strain may result from an unresolved upper tract focus of infection but often (especially after short-course therapy for cystitis) result from persistent vaginal colonization rather than from recurrent bladder infection. Recurrences more than 2 weeks after the cessation of therapy nearly always represent reinfection with a new strain.
6. Community-acquired infections, especially initial infections, are usually due to antibiotic-sensitive strains.
7. In patients with repeated infections, instrumentation, or recent hospitalization, the presence of antibiotic-resistant strains should be suspected.

The anatomic location of a urinary tract infection greatly influences the success or failure of a therapeutic regimen. Bladder bacteriuria (cystitis) can usually be eliminated with nearly any antimicrobial to which the infecting strain is sensitive; in the past, it was demonstrated that as little as a single dose of 500 mg of intramuscular kanamycin eliminated bladder bacteriuria in most cases. With upper tract infections, however, single-dose therapy fails in the majority of cases, and even a 7-day course is unsuccessful in many instances. Longer periods of treatment (2 to 6 weeks) aimed at eradicating a persistent focus of infection may be necessary in some cases.

In *acute uncomplicated cystitis*, more than 80 percent of infections are due to *E. coli*, and, although resistance patterns vary geographically, most strains are sensitive to many antibiotics. Single doses of trimethoprim-sulfamethoxazole (four single-strength tablets), trimethoprim alone (400 mg), sulfa alone (2.0 g), and most fluoroquinolones (norfloxacin, ciprofloxacin, ofloxacin) have been used successfully to treat acute uncomplicated episodes of cystitis. A single 3-g dose of amoxicillin appears to result in lower cure rates than these other agents, especially when infection is due to amoxicillin-resistant strains. In most areas, about one-third of *E. coli* strains causing acute cystitis are amoxicillin-resistant.

The advantages of single-dose therapy include less expense, ensured compliance, fewer side effects, and perhaps less intense pressure favoring the selection of resistant organisms in the intestinal, vaginal, or perineal flora. However, several studies have suggested that more recurrences develop shortly after single-dose therapy than after 3 to 7 days of treatment and that single-dose therapy does not eradicate vaginal colonization with *E. coli*. Nevertheless, single-dose therapy does appear to be safe and efficacious for women presenting with acute uncomplicated cystitis. Single-dose therapy should be used only for reliable patients whose posttreatment follow-up can be ensured and for patients who have had symptoms for less than 7 days. A 3-day course of therapy with trimethoprim-sulfamethoxazole, trimethoprim, norfloxacin, ciprofloxacin, or ofloxacin appears to preserve the low rate of side effects of single-dose therapy while improving efficacy. Neither single-dose nor 3-day therapy should be used for women with symptoms or signs of pyelonephritis, urologic abnormalities or stones, or previous infections due to antibiotic-resistant organisms. Males with urinary tract infection often have urologic abnormalities or prostatic involvement and hence are not candidates for single-dose or 3-day therapy. They should generally receive a 7- to 14-day course.

The choice of treatment for women with acute urethritis depends on the etiologic agent involved. In chlamydial infection, doxycycline (100 mg orally bid for 7 days) should be used. Women with acute dysuria and frequency, negative urine cultures, and no pyuria usually do not respond to antimicrobial agents.

In women, *acute uncomplicated pyelonephritis* without accompanying clinical evidence of calculi or urologic disease is due to *E. coli* in most cases. Although the optimal route and duration of therapy have not been established, a 14-day course of trimethoprim-sulfamethoxazole, a fluoroquinolone, an aminoglycoside, or a third-generation cephalosporin is usually adequate. Ampicillin or amoxicillin should not be used as initial therapy because 20 to 30 percent of strains of *E. coli* are now resistant to these drugs in vitro. In some areas, more than 20 percent of *E. coli* strains causing acute pyelonephritis are resistant to trimethoprim-sulfamethoxazole; alternative therapies should be used in such areas. For at least the first few days of treatment, antibiotics should probably be given intravenously to most patients, but patients with mild symptoms can be treated with 2 weeks of an oral antibiotic (usually trimethoprim-sulfamethoxazole, ciprofloxacin, or ofloxacin). Patients who fail to respond to treatment within 72 h or who relapse after therapy should be evaluated for unrecognized suppurative foci, calculi, or urologic disease. If the results are negative, re-treatment for 2 to 6 weeks to eliminate a presumed upper tract focus causing recurrent bacteriuria should be given.

Complicated urinary tract infections (those arising in a setting of catheterization, instrumentation, urologic anatomic or functional abnormalities, stones, obstruction, immunosuppression, renal disease, or diabetes) are typically due to hospital-acquired bacteria, including *E. coli*, *Klebsiella*, *Proteus*, *Serratia*, *Pseudomonas*, enterococci, and staphylococci. Many of the infecting strains are antibiotic-resistant. Empirical antibiotic therapy ideally provides broad-spectrum coverage against these pathogens. In patients with minimal symptoms, oral therapy with a fluoroquinolone, such as ciprofloxacin or ofloxacin, can be administered until culture results and antibiotic sensitivities are known. In patients with more severe illness, including acute pyelonephritis or suspected urosepsis, hospitalization and parenteral therapy should be undertaken. Commonly used empirical regimens include imipenem alone, a penicillin or cephalosporin plus an aminoglycoside, and (when the involvement of enterococci is unlikely) ceftriaxone or ceftazidime. When information on the antimicrobial sensitivity pattern of the infecting strain becomes available, a more specific antimicrobial regimen can be selected. Therapy should generally be administered for 7 to 21 days, with the exact duration depending on the severity of the infection and the susceptibility of the infecting strain. Follow-up cultures 2 to 4 weeks after cessation of therapy should be performed to demonstrate cure.

In *pregnancy*, acute cystitis can be managed with 3 to 7 days of treatment with amoxicillin, nitrofurantoin, or a cephalosporin. All pregnant women should be screened for asymptomatic bacteriuria during the first trimester and, if bacteriuric, should be treated with one of the regimens just outlined. After treatment, a culture should be performed to ensure cure, and cultures should be repeated monthly thereafter until delivery. Acute pyelonephritis in pregnancy should be managed with hospitalization and parenteral antibiotic therapy, generally with a cephalosporin or an extended-spectrum penicillin. Continuous low-dose prophylaxis with nitrofurantoin should be given to women who have recurrent infections during pregnancy.

Asymptomatic bacteriuria should be documented by at least two positive cultures before treatment is given. Seven days of therapy with an oral agent to which the organism is sensitive should be given initially. If bacteriuria persists, it can be monitored without further treatment in most patients. High-risk patients with neutropenia, renal transplants, or other complicating conditions may require longer treatment.

UROLOGIC EVALUATION Very few women with recurrent urinary tract infections have correctable lesions discovered at cystoscopy or upon intravenous pyelography, and these procedures should not be undertaken routinely in such cases. Urologic evaluation should be performed in selected instances—namely, in women with relapsing infection, a history of childhood infections, stones or painless hematuria, or recurrent pyelonephritis. Most males with urinary infection should be considered to have complicated infection and thus should be evaluated urologically. Possible exceptions include young men who have cystitis associated with sexual activity, who are uncircumcised, or who have AIDS. Men or women presenting with acute infection and signs or symptoms suggestive of an obstruction or stones should undergo urologic evaluation, generally by means of ultrasound.

PROGNOSIS In patients with uncomplicated cystitis or pyelonephritis, treatment ordinarily results in complete resolution of symptoms. Lower tract infections in women are of concern mainly because they cause discomfort, morbidity, loss of time from work, and substantial health-care costs. Cystitis also may result in upper tract infection or in bacteremia (especially during instrumentation), but little evidence suggests that renal impairment follows. When repeated episodes of cystitis occur, they are nearly always reinfections, not relapses.

Acute uncomplicated pyelonephritis in adults rarely progresses to renal functional impairment and chronic renal disease. Repeated upper tract infections often represent relapse rather than reinfection, and a vigorous search for renal calculi or an underlying urologic abnormality should be undertaken. If neither is found, 6 weeks of chemotherapy may be useful in eradicating an unresolved focus of infection.

Repeated symptomatic urinary tract infections in children and in adults with obstructive uropathy, neurogenic bladder, structural renal disease, or diabetes progress to chronic renal disease with unusual frequency. Asymptomatic bacteriuria in these groups as well as in adults without urologic disease or obstruction predisposes to increased numbers of episodes of symptomatic infection but does not result in renal impairment in most instances.

PREVENTION Patients with frequent symptomatic infections may benefit from long-term administration of low-dose antibiotics directed at preventing recurrences. Daily or thrice-weekly administration of a single dose of trimethoprim/sulfamethoxazole (80/400 mg), trimethoprim alone (100 mg), or nitrofurantoin (50 mg) has been particularly effective. Prophylaxis should be initiated only after bacteriuria has been eradicated with a full-dose treatment regimen. Women who have more than two infections every 6 months are candidates for such prophylaxis. The same regimens can be used after sexual intercourse to prevent episodes of symptomatic infection in women in whom these episodes are temporally related to intercourse. Other patients for whom prophylaxis appears to have some merit include men with chronic prostatitis; patients undergoing prostatectomy, both during the operation and in the postoperative period; and pregnant women with asymptomatic bacteriuria. All pregnant women should be screened for bacteriuria in the first trimester and should be treated if bacteriuria is demonstrated.

PAPILLARY NECROSIS

When infection of the renal pyramids develops in association with vascular diseases of the kidney or with urinary tract obstruction, renal papillary necrosis is likely to result. Patients with diabetes, sickle cell disease, chronic alcoholism, and vascular disease seem peculiarly susceptible to this complication. Hematuria, pain in the flank or abdomen, and chills and fever are the most common presenting symptoms. Acute renal failure with oliguria or anuria sometimes develops. Rarely, sloughing of a pyramid may take place without symptoms in a patient with chronic urinary infection, and the diagnosis is made when the necrotic tissue is passed in the urine or identified as a "ring shadow" on pyelography. If renal function deteriorates suddenly in a diabetic individual or a patient with chronic obstruction, the diagnosis of renal papillary necrosis should be entertained, even in the absence of fever or pain. Renal papillary necrosis is often bilateral; when it is unilateral, however, nephrectomy may be a life-saving approach to the management of overwhelming infection.

RENAL AND PERINEPHRIC ABSCESS

See Chap. 127

PROSTATITIS

The term *prostatitis* has been used for various inflammatory conditions affecting the prostate, including acute and chronic infections with specific bacteria and, more commonly, instances in which signs and symptoms of prostatic inflammation are present but no specific organisms can be detected. Patients with acute bacterial prostatitis can usually be identified on the basis of typical symptoms and signs, pyuria, and bacteriuria. To classify a patient with suspected chronic prostatitis correctly, first-void and midstream urine specimens, a prostatic expressate, and a postmassage urine specimen should be quantitatively cultured and evaluated for numbers of leukocytes. On the basis of the results of these studies, patients can be classified as having chronic bacterial prostatitis, chronic nonbacterial prostatitis, or prostatodynia. Patients with suspected chronic prostatitis usually have low back pain, perineal or testicular discomfort, mild dysuria, and lower urinary obstructive symptoms. Microscopic pyuria may be the only objective manifestation of prostatic disease.

ACUTE BACTERIAL PROSTATITIS   When it occurs spontaneously, this disease generally affects young men; however, it may also be associated with an indwelling urethral catheter. It is characterized by fever, chills, dysuria, and a tense or boggy, extremely tender prostate. Although prostatic massage usually produces purulent secretions with a large number of bacteria on culture, bacteremia may result from manipulation of the inflamed gland. For this reason and because the etiologic agent can usually be identified by Gram's staining and culture of urine, vigorous prostatic massage should be avoided. In non-catheter-associated cases, the infection is generally due to common gram-negative urinary tract pathogens (*E. coli* or *Klebsiella*). Initially, intravenous trimethoprim-sulfamethoxazole, a cephalosporin, a fluoroquinolone, or an aminoglycoside can be administered if gram-negative rods are visible in urine, and a cephalosporin or nafcillin can be given if gram-positive cocci are detected. Although many of these drugs do not readily diffuse into the noninflamed prostate gland, the response to antibiotics in acute bacterial prostatitis is usually prompt, perhaps because drugs penetrate more readily into the acutely inflamed prostate. In catheter-associated cases, the spectrum of etiologic agents is broader, including hospital-acquired gram-negative rods and enterococci. The urinary Gram stain may be particularly helpful in such cases. Imipenem, an aminoglycoside, a fluoroquinolone, or a third-generation cephalosporin should be used for initial therapy until the organism has been isolated and its susceptibilities have been determined. The long-term prognosis is good, although in some instances acute infection may result in abscess formation, epididymoorchitis, seminal vesiculitis, septicemia, and residual chronic bacterial prostatitis. Since the advent of antibiotics, the frequency of acute bacterial prostatitis has diminished markedly. In many instances, infections diagnosed as acute prostatitis are probably cases of posterior urethritis.

CHRONIC BACTERIAL PROSTATITIS   This entity is now infrequent but should be considered in men with a history of recurrent bacteriuria. Symptoms are usually lacking, and the prostate usually feels normal on palpation. Obstructive symptoms or perineal pain develops in some patients. Intermittently, infection spreads to the bladder, producing frequency, urgency, and dysuria. A pattern of relapsing infection in a middle-aged man strongly suggests chronic bacterial prostatitis. Classically, the diagnosis is established by culture of *E. coli*, *Klebsiella*, *Proteus*, or other uropathogenic bacteria from the expressed prostatic secretion or postmassage urine in higher quantities than are found in first-void or midstream urine. Antibiotics promptly relieve the symptoms associated with acute exacerbations but have been less effective in eradicating the focus of chronic infection in the prostate. The relative ineffectiveness of antimicrobials for long-term cure results in part from the poor penetration of the prostate by most of these drugs; the low pH that prevails in this organ precludes the passage of most agents. Fluoroquinolones, including ciprofloxacin and ofloxacin, have been more successful than other antimicrobials, but they must be given for at least 12 weeks to be effective. Patients with frequent episodes of acute cystitis can be managed with prolonged courses of antimicrobials (usually a sulfonamide, trimethoprim, or nitrofurantoin), with a view toward suppressing symptoms and keeping the bladder urine sterile. Total prostatectomy obviously results in the cure of chronic prostatitis but is associated with considerable morbidity. Transurethral prostatectomy is safer but cures only one-third of patients.

NONBACTERIAL PROSTATITIS   Patients who present with symptoms and signs of prostatitis, increased leukocytes in expressed prostatic secretion and postmassage urine, no bacterial growth in cultures, and no history of recurrent episodes of bacterial prostatitis are classified as having nonbacterial prostatitis. Prostatic inflammation can be considered present when the expressed prostatic secretion and postmassage urine contain at least 10-fold more leukocytes than the first-void and midstream urine specimens or when the expressed prostatic secretion contains ≥1000 leukocytes per microliter.

The presumably infectious etiology of this condition remains unidentified. Evidence for a causative role of both *U. urealyticum* and *C. trachomatis* has been presented but is not conclusive. Since most cases of nonbacterial prostatitis occur in young, sexually active men and since many cases follow an episode of nonspecific urethritis, the causative agent may well be sexually transmitted. The effectiveness of antimicrobial agents in this condition remains uncertain. Some patients benefit from a 4- to 6-week course of treatment with erythromycin, doxycycline, trimethoprim-sulfamethoxazole, or a fluoroquinolone, but controlled trials are lacking.

PROSTATODYNIA   Patients who have symptoms and signs of prostatitis but no evidence of prostatic inflammation (normal leukocyte counts) and negative urine cultures are classified as having prostatodynia. Despite their symptoms, these patients most likely do not have prostatic infection and should not be given antimicrobial agents.

BIBLIOGRAPHY

AGACE W et al: Host resistance to urinary tract infection, in *Molecular Pathogenesis and Clinical Management,* HLT Mobley, JW Warren (eds). Washington, DC, ASM Press, 1996, pp 221–245

BAILEY RR: Management of lower urinary tract infections. Drugs 45(Suppl 3):139, 1993

BERGERON MG: Treatment of pyelonephritis in adults. Med Clin North Am 79:619, 1995

EISENSTADT J, WASHINGTON JA: Diagnostic microbiology for bacteria and yeasts causing urinary tract infections, in *Molecular Pathogenesis and Clinical Management,* HLT Mobley, JW Warren (eds). Washington, DC, ASM Press, 1996, pp 29–67

GRATACOS E et al: Screening and treatment of asymptomatic bacteriuria in pregnancy prevent pyelonephritis. J Infect Dis 169:1390, 1994

HOOTON TM et al: A prospective study of risk factors for symptomatic urinary tract infection in young women. N Engl J Med 335:468, 1996

JOHNSON JR: Virulence factors in *E. coli* urinary tract infections. Clin Microbiol Rev 4:80, 1991

————: Treatment and prevention of urinary tract infections, in *Molecular Pathogenesis and Clinical Management*, HLT Mobley, JW Warren (eds). Washington, DC, ASM Press, 1996, pp 95–118

KUNIN CM: Urinary tract infection in females. Clin Infect Dis 18:1, 1994

LIPSKY BA: Urinary tract infections in men. Ann Intern Med 110:138, 1989

SCHAEFFER AJ: Urinary tract infection in men—state of the art. Infection (Suppl 1):S19, 1994

STAMM WE, HOOTON TM: Management of urinary tract infections in adults. N Engl J Med 329:1328, 1993

————: Catheter-associated urinary tract infections: Epidemiology, pathogenesis, prevention. Am J Med 91(Suppl 3B):655, 1991

132 *James H. Maguire*

OSTEOMYELITIS

Osteomyelitis, an infection of bone, is caused most commonly by pyogenic bacteria and mycobacteria. Classification of cases on the basis of the causative agent and the route, duration, and anatomic location of infection provides a useful framework for evaluating the patient and planning treatment.

PATHOGENESIS AND PATHOLOGY Microorganisms enter bone by the hematogenous route, by direct introduction from a contiguous focus of infection, or by a penetrating wound. Trauma, ischemia, and foreign bodies enhance the susceptibility of bone to microbial invasion by exposing sites to which bacteria can bind. Phagocytes attempt to contain the infections and, in the process, release enzymes that lyse bone. Pus spreads into vascular channels, raising intraosseous pressure and impairing the flow of blood; as the untreated infection becomes chronic, ischemic necrosis of bone results in the separation of large devascularized fragments (*sequestra*). When pus breaks through the cortex, subperiosteal or soft tissue abscesses form, and the elevated periosteum deposits new bone (the *involucrum*) around the sequestrum. Bacteria escape host defenses by adhering tightly to damaged bone and by coating themselves and underlying surfaces with a protective polysaccharide-rich biofilm.

Microorganisms, infiltrates of neutrophils, and congested or thrombosed blood vessels are the principal histologic findings of acute osteomyelitis. The distinguishing feature of chronic osteomyelitis is necrotic bone, which is characterized by the absence of living osteocytes. Mononuclear cells predominate in chronic infections, and granulation and fibrous tissues replace bone that has been resorbed by osteoclasts. In the chronic stage, organisms may be too few to be seen.

HEMATOGENOUS OSTEOMYELITIS Hematogenous infection accounts for approximately 20 percent of cases of osteomyelitis and primarily affects children, in whom the long bones are infected, and older adults and intravenous drug users, in whom the spine is the usual site of infection.

Acute Hematogenous Osteomyelitis Infection usually involves a single bone, most commonly the tibia, femur, or humerus. Bacteria settle in the well-perfused metaphysis, where functioning phagocytes are scarce, a network of venous sinusoids slows the flow of blood, and fenestrations in capillaries allow organisms to escape into the extravascular space. Because vascular anatomy changes with age, hematogenous infection of long bones is uncommon during adulthood and, when it occurs, usually involves the diaphysis.

In children, the source of bacteremia is often inapparent, although there may have been recent blunt trauma to the extremity leading to a small intraosseous hematoma or vascular obstruction. On presentation, the child usually appears acutely ill, with high fever, chills, localized pain and tenderness, and leukocytosis. Cutaneous erythema and swelling indicate extension of pus through the cortex. During infancy and after puberty, infection may spread through the epiphysis into the joint space. In children of other ages (i.e., between infancy and puberty), extension of infection through the cortex results in involvement of joints if the metaphysis is intracapsular. Thus, septic arthritis of the elbow, shoulder, and hip may complicate osteomyelitis of the proximal radius, humerus, and femur, respectively.

Plain radiographs initially show soft tissue swelling, but the first change in bone—a periosteal reaction—is not evident until at least 10 days after the onset of infection. Lytic changes can be detected after 2 to 6 weeks, when 50 to 75 percent of bone density has been lost. Rarely, a well-circumscribed lytic lesion, or *Brodie's abscess*, is seen in a child who has been in pain for several months but has had no fever.

Chronic Hematogenous Osteomyelitis With prompt treatment, fewer than 5 percent of cases of acute hematogenous osteomyelitis progress to chronic osteomyelitis. On average, 10 days are required for the formation of necrotic bone, but plain radiographs are unable to detect sequestra or sclerotic new bone for many weeks.

A protracted clinical course, long periods of quiescence, and recurrent exacerbations are characteristic of chronic osteomyelitis. Sinus tracts between bone and skin may drain purulent material and occasionally pieces of necrotic bone. An increase in drainage, pain, or the erythrocyte sedimentation rate (ESR) signals an exacerbation. Fever is unusual except when obstruction of a sinus tract leads to soft tissue infection. Rare late complications include pathologic fractures, squamous cell carcinoma of the sinus tract, and amyloidosis.

Vertebral Osteomyelitis Organisms reach the well-perfused vertebral body of adults via spinal arteries and quickly spread from the end plate into the disk space and then to the adjacent vertebral body. The infection may originate in the urinary tract and reach the spine via the prostatic venous (Baston's) plexus; such cases develop particularly often among elderly men. Other sources of bacteremia include endocarditis, soft tissue infection, and a contaminated intravenous line; these sources usually are obvious. Diabetes mellitus, hemodialysis, and intravenous drug use carry an increased risk of spinal infection. Penetrating injuries and surgical procedures to the spine may cause nonhematogenous vertebral osteomyelitis or infection localized to the disk.

Most patients with vertebral osteomyelitis report neck or back pain; 15 percent describe atypical pain in the chest, the abdomen, or an extremity that is due to irritation of nerve roots. Symptoms are localized to the lumbar spine more often than to the thoracic spine (more than 50 percent vs. 35 percent of cases) or the cervical spine in pyogenic infections, but the thoracic spine is involved most commonly in tuberculous spondylitis (Pott's disease). Percussion over the involved vertebra elicits tenderness, and physical examination may reveal spasm of the paraspinal muscles and a limitation of motion. More than 50 percent of patients experience a subacute illness in which a vague, dull pain gradually intensifies over the course of 2 to 3 months; fever is low grade or absent, and the white blood cell count is normal. An acute presentation with high fever and toxicity is less common and suggests ongoing bacteremia.

Usually, by the time the patient seeks medical attention, the ESR is elevated, and plain radiographs show irregular erosions in the end plates of adjacent vertebral bodies and narrowing of the intervening disk space. This radiographic pattern is virtually diagnostic of bacterial infection because tumors and other diseases of the spine rarely cross the disk space. Computed tomography (CT) or magnetic resonance imaging (MRI) may demonstrate epidural, paraspinal, retropharyngeal, mediastinal, retroperitoneal, or psoas abscesses that originate in the spine. An epidural abscess may evolve suddenly or over the course of several weeks; irreversible paralysis may be the consequence of failure to recognize the classic clinical presentation of a spinal epidural abscess, consisting of spinal pain progressing to radicular pain and weakness.

Microbiology More than 95 percent of cases of hematogenous osteomyelitis are caused by a single organism. *Staphylococcus aureus* accounts for 50 percent of isolates. Other common pathogens include group B streptococci and *Escherichia coli* during the newborn period and group A streptococci and *Haemophilus influenzae* in early childhood. Vertebral osteomyelitis is due to *E. coli* and other enteric bacilli in approximately 25 percent of cases. *S. aureus, Pseudomonas aeruginosa,* and *Serratia* infections are associated with intravenous drug use in some parts of the United States and may involve the sacroiliac, sternoclavicular, or pubic joints as well as the spine. *Salmonella* spp. and *S. aureus* are the major causes of long-bone osteomyelitis complicating sickle cell anemia and other hemoglobinopathies. Tuberculosis and brucellosis affect the spine more often than other bones. Other common sites of tuberculous osteomyelitis include the small bones of the hands and feet, the metaphyses of long bones, the ribs, and the sternum.

Unusual causes of hematogenous osteomyelitis include disseminated histoplasmosis, coccidioidomycosis, and blastomycosis in endemic areas. Immunocompromised persons on rare occasions develop osteomyelitis due to atypical mycobacteria or to species of *Candida, Cryptococcus, Aspergillus,* or *Pneumocystis.* Syphilis, yaws, varicella, and vaccinia may involve bone. The etiology of chronic relapsing multifocal osteomyelitis, an inflammatory condition of children that is characterized by recurrent episodes of painful lytic lesions in multiple bones, has not yet been identified.

OSTEOMYELITIS SECONDARY TO A CONTIGUOUS FOCUS OF INFECTION   Clinical Features   This broad category of osteomyelitis includes infections introduced by penetrating injuries and surgical procedures and by direct extension of infection from adjacent soft tissues. It accounts for the greatest number of cases of osteomyelitis and occurs most commonly in adults.

Frequently, the diagnosis is not made until the infection has already become chronic. The pain, fever, and inflammatory signs due to acute osteomyelitis may be attributed to the original injury or soft tissue infection. An indolent infection may become apparent only weeks or months later, when a sinus tract develops, a surgical wound breaks down, or a fracture fails to heal. It may be impossible to distinguish radiographic abnormalities due to osteomyelitis from those due to the precipitating condition.

A special type of contiguous-focus osteomyelitis occurs in the setting of peripheral vascular disease and nearly always involves the small bones of the feet of adult diabetic patients. Diabetic neuropathy exposes the foot to frequent trauma and pressure sores, and the patient may be unaware of infection as it spreads into bone. Poor tissue perfusion impairs normal inflammatory responses and wound healing and creates a milieu that is conducive to anaerobic infections. It is often during the evaluation of a nonhealing ulcer, a swollen toe, or acute cellulitis that a radiograph provides the first evidence of osteomyelitis. If bone is palpable during examination of the base of an ulcer with a blunt surgical probe, osteomyelitis is likely.

Microbiology   *S. aureus* is a pathogen in more than half of cases of contiguous-focus osteomyelitis. However, in contrast to hematogenous osteomyelitis, these infections often are polymicrobial and are more likely to involve gram-negative and anaerobic bacteria. Hence a mixture of staphylococci, streptococci, enteric organisms, and anaerobic bacteria may be isolated from a diabetic foot infection or pelvic osteomyelitis underlying a decubitus ulcer. Aerobic and anaerobic bacteria cause osteomyelitis following surgery or soft tissue infection of the oropharynx, paranasal sinuses, gastrointestinal tract, or female genital tract. *S. aureus* is the principal cause of postoperative infections; coagulase-negative staphylococci are common pathogens after implantation of orthopedic appliances; and these organisms as well as gram-negative enteric bacilli, atypical mycobacteria, and *Mycoplasma* may cause sternal osteomyelitis after cardiac surgery. Infection with *P. aeruginosa* is frequently associated with puncture wounds of the foot or with thermal burns, and *Pasteurella multocida* infection commonly follows cat bites (see Chap. 135).

DIAGNOSIS   Early diagnosis of acute osteomyelitis is critical because prompt antibiotic therapy may prevent the necrosis of bone. The evaluation usually begins with plain radiographs because of their ready availability, although they frequently show no abnormalities during early infection. The ESR and C-reactive protein levels are

elevated in most cases of active osteomyelitis, including those in which constitutional symptoms and leukocytosis are lacking. These findings are not specific to osteomyelitis, however, and the ESR is occasionally normal in early infections. In 95 percent of cases, the technetium radionuclide scan using ^{99m}Tc diphosphonate is positive within 24 h of the onset of symptoms. Falsely negative scans usually indicate obstruction of blood flow to the bone. Because the uptake of technetium reflects osteoblastic activity and skeletal vascularity, the bone scan cannot differentiate osteomyelitis from fractures, tumors, infarction, or neuropathic osteopathy. ^{67}Ga citrate– and ^{111}In-labeled leukocyte or immunoglobulin scans, which have greater specificity for inflammation, may help distinguish infectious from noninfectious processes and indicate inflammatory changes within bones that for other reasons are already abnormal on radiography and technetium scanning. Ultrasound can be used to diagnose osteomyelitis by the detection of subperiosteal fluid collections, soft tissue abscesses adjacent to bone, and periosteal thickening and elevation.

MRI is as sensitive as the bone scan for the diagnosis of acute osteomyelitis because it is able to detect changes in the water content of marrow. MRI yields better anatomic resolution of epidural abscesses and other soft tissue processes than CT and is currently the imaging technique of choice for vertebral osteomyelitis (see Fig. 132-1).

The role of diagnostic imaging in chronic osteomyelitis is to determine the presence of active infection and delineate the extent of debridement necessary to remove necrotic bone and abnormal soft tissues. Although plain films accurately reflect chronic changes, the CT scan is more sensitive for the detection of sequestra, sinus tracts, and soft tissue abscesses. Both CT and ultrasound are useful for

FIGURE 132-1   Osteomyelitis of the lumbar spine demonstrated on a sagittal T1-weighted magnetic resonance image after the administration of intravenous gadolinium. At L2–L3 there is involvement of the adjacent vertebral bodies and intervening disk. An epidural abscess compresses the thecal sac (open arrow), and the inflammatory process extends into the anterior prevertebral space (closed arrows).

guiding percutaneous aspiration of subperiosteal and soft tissue fluid collections. Sequential technetium and gallium or indium scans may help determine whether infection is active and may distinguish infection from noninflammatory bone changes; these methods do not, however, provide good anatomic detail. MRI provides detailed information about the activity and the anatomic extent of infection but does not always distinguish osteomyelitis from healing fractures and tumors. MRI is particularly useful in distinguishing cellulitis from osteomyelitis in the diabetic foot; however, no imaging modality consistently distinguishes infection from neuropathic osteopathy.

Appropriate samples for microbiologic studies should be obtained in all cases of suspected osteomyelitis before the initiation of antimicrobial therapy. Blood cultures are indicated in acute cases and are positive in more than one-third of cases of hematogenous osteomyelitis in children and in 25 percent of cases of vertebral osteomyelitis in adults. If the clinical picture demands immediate antibiotic therapy or if blood cultures are negative, samples from needle aspiration of pus in bone or soft tissues or from a bone biopsy should be obtained for culture.

The results of culture of specimens obtained by swabbing of a sinus tract or the base of an ulcer correlate poorly with the organisms infecting the bone. For this reason, in cases of chronic osteomyelitis and contiguous-focus osteomyelitis, samples for aerobic and anaerobic culture should be obtained from several sites by percutaneous needle aspiration, percutaneous biopsy, or intraoperative biopsy at the time of debridement. Isolates of coagulase-negative staphylococci and other organisms of low virulence should not automatically be disregarded as contaminants, especially in the presence of prosthetic materials. Special culture media may be necessary for the isolation of mycobacteria, fungi, and other, less common pathogens. In some cases, histopathologic examination of biopsy specimens may be the only way to make a diagnosis.

℞ TREATMENT

Antibiotic Therapy Antibiotics are administered only after appropriate specimens have been obtained for culture. The antibiotics selected should be bactericidal and, at least initially, should be given intravenously. When necessary, empirical therapy is guided by findings on Gram's staining of a specimen from the bone or abscess or is chosen to cover the most likely pathogens. Empirical therapy in most cases should include high doses of an agent active against *S. aureus* (such as oxacillin, nafcillin, a cephalosporin, or vancomycin) and, if gram-negative organisms are likely to be involved, a third-generation cephalosporin, an aminoglycoside, or a fluoroquinolone.

Specific intravenous therapy is based on the in vitro susceptibility of the organism(s) isolated from bone or blood. Penicillin G (3 to 4 million units every 4 h) is the drug of choice for the treatment of infections due to penicillin-sensitive staphylococci and streptococci; nafcillin or oxacillin (2 g every 4 h) is preferred for penicillin-resistant, methicillin-sensitive staphylococci. Cefazolin (1 to 2 g every 8 h) or vancomycin [15 mg/kg (up to 1 g) every 12 h] is an alternative for persons allergic to penicillins. Infections due to methicillin-resistant staphylococci are treated with vancomycin. Regimens for infections due to susceptible gram-negative rods include ampicillin (2 g every 4 h), cefazolin, a second-generation cephalosporin such as cefuroxime (1.5 g every 8 h), or a fluoroquinolone such as ciprofloxacin (400 mg every 12 h). Initial therapy for osteomyelitis due to *P. aeruginosa* or *Enterobacter* spp. should not consist of a β-lactam antibiotic alone because of the potential for these organisms to develop resistance during therapy. Appropriate intravenous therapies for *P. aeruginosa* infections include tobramycin (1.7 mg/kg every 8 h, or 5 to 7 mg/kg every 24 h) and a broad-spectrum β-lactam compound such as ticarcillin (3 g every 4 h), ceftazidime (1 to 2 g every 8 h), or aztreonam (1 to 2 g every 8 h); a fluoroquinolone may be substituted for one of the latter. *Enterobacter* infections can be treated with a fluoroquinolone alone or with combinations of a broad-spectrum β-lactam antibiotic and

gentamicin in the same doses as tobramycin. Serum levels of aminoglycosides should be monitored closely to avoid toxicity.

The duration of therapy is typically 4 to 6 weeks; at-home intravenous administration of antibiotics or oral therapy is appropriate for motivated and medically stable patients. Antibiotics that require infrequent dosing, such as ceftriaxone and vancomycin, facilitate home therapy. Children with acute hematogenous osteomyelitis routinely receive oral antibiotics after 5 to 10 days of parenteral therapy if signs of active infection have resolved; such treatment has been as successful as standard parenteral therapy. The doses of oral penicillins or cephalosporins required for the treatment of osteomyelitis are several times higher than the doses of these drugs given for common infections. Adults may not tolerate these high doses as well as children, and, except in the case of the fluoroquinolones, few data support the use of oral antibiotics by adults. Oral administration of an agent such as ciprofloxacin (750 mg every 12 h) or ofloxacin (400 mg every 12 h) has been as successful as intravenous administration of β-lactam antibiotics. Caution should be exercised in the use of fluoroquinolones as the sole agents for treatment of infection due to *S. aureus* or *P. aeruginosa* because resistance may develop during therapy. Oral administration of clindamycin (300 to 450 mg every 6 h) or metronidazole (500 mg every 8 h) results in high drug levels in serum and can take the place of intravenous regimens for the treatment of *Bacteroides* infections. Oral clindamycin has produced good results in therapy for osteomyelitis due to *S. aureus*, especially in children.

Serum minimal bactericidal concentrations (MBCs) against isolates of the responsible pathogen can be measured to document compliance and adequate serum levels in patients who receive an oral antibiotic. Otherwise, few data support the routine use of the MBC to monitor therapy for osteomyelitis.

Acute Osteomyelitis Early treatment of acute hematogenous osteomyelitis of childhood with 4 to 6 weeks of an appropriate antibiotic is usually successful; treatment for less than 3 weeks has resulted in a 10-fold greater rate of failure. Surgical intervention in childhood cases is indicated for intraosseous or subperiosteal abscesses, concomitant septic arthritis, and failure of the acute signs of infection to improve in 24 to 48 h. Acute hematogenous osteomyelitis of bones other than the spine in adults often requires surgical debridement.

Vertebral Osteomyelitis A 4- to 6-week course of treatment with an appropriate antibiotic is usually sufficient to cure vertebral osteomyelitis. Failure of the ESR to drop to no more than two-thirds of pretreatment levels is an indication for longer treatment. Surgery is seldom necessary, even in cases of many months' duration, except in instances of spinal instability, new or progressive neurologic deficits, large soft tissue abscesses that cannot be drained percutaneously, or a failure of medical treatment. Patients should maintain bed rest until back pain has declined to the point at which ambulation is possible. Body casts are no longer used. Spontaneous fusion of involved vertebrae occurs in the majority of cases after successful treatment.

Contiguous-Focus Osteomyelitis Even when diagnosed early, contiguous-focus osteomyelitis usually requires surgery in addition to 4 to 6 weeks of appropriate antibiotic therapy because of underlying soft tissue infection or damage to bone from an injury or surgery.

Chronic Osteomyelitis The risks and benefits of aggressive therapy for chronic osteomyelitis should be weighed before any attempt is made to eradicate the infection. Some patients with extensive disease prefer to live with their infections rather than undergo multiple surgical procedures, take prolonged courses of antimicrobial therapy, and face the risk of loss of an extremity. Such persons often benefit from intermittent courses of oral antibiotics to suppress acute exacerbations.

Once the decision has been made to treat chronic osteomyelitis aggressively, the patient's nutritional and metabolic status should be optimized to expedite healing of soft tissues and bone. Antibiotic administration should be started several days before surgery to reduce inflammation if the etiology of the infection is known preoperatively.

If not, antibiotic therapy should be withheld until surgical debridement. An empirical antibiotic regimen is started intraoperatively after culture specimens are obtained. A 4- to 6-week course of appropriate antibiotic therapy is given postoperatively on the basis of the susceptibility pattern of organisms isolated from the bone. The benefit of prolonged oral antibiotic therapy after 4 to 6 weeks of parenteral therapy remains unproven. There is insufficient information to recommend the routine use of hyperbaric oxygen to enhance the killing of microorganisms by phagocytes or of instillation pumps and antibiotic-impregnated methacrylate beads to deliver high levels of antibiotics to the bone.

The success of therapy for chronic osteomyelitis rests largely on the complete surgical removal of necrotic bone and abnormal soft tissues. Modern imaging techniques allow accurate preoperative delineation of tissues to be debrided, but it remains difficult for the surgeon to determine intraoperatively whether all necrotic and infected tissue has been removed. In the past, the inability to repair large defects in bone and soft tissue limited the extent of debridement. Muscle flaps and skin grafts are now used routinely to cover large soft tissue defects and fill dead space, and bone grafts and vascularized bone transfer may restore a seriously compromised bone to a functional state.

In infections of recent fractures, internal fixators are often left in place, and the infection is controlled by limited debridement and suppressive antibiotic therapy. Definitive surgical/antimicrobial therapy is delayed until after bony union of the fracture is achieved. If there is nonunion of the fracture or loosening of the fixator, the appliance should be removed, the bone debrided, and an external fixator or a new internal fixator applied.

Osteomyelitis of the small bones of the feet in persons with vascular disease also requires surgical treatment. The effectiveness of the surgery is limited by the blood supply to the site and the body's ability to heal the wound. Revascularization of the extremity is indicated if the vascular disease involves large arteries. In cases of decreased perfusion due to small-vessel disease, foot-sparing surgery may fail, and the best option is suppressive therapy or amputation. The duration of antibiotic therapy depends on the surgical procedure performed. When the infected bone is removed entirely but residual infection of soft tissues remains, antibiotic therapy should be given for 2 weeks; if amputation eliminates infected bone and soft tissue, standard surgical prophylaxis is given; otherwise, postoperative antibiotics must be given for 4 to 6 weeks.

BIBLIOGRAPHY

BRYSON YJ et al: High dose oral dicloxacillin treatment of acute staphylococcal osteomyelitis in children. J Pediatr 94:673, 1979

CAPUTO GM et al: Assessment and management of foot disease in patients with diabetes. N Engl J Med 331:854, 1994

CUNNINGHAM R et al: Clinical and molecular aspects of the pathogenesis of *Staphylococcus aureus* bone and joint infections. J Med Microbiol 44:157, 1996

DAROUICHE RO et al: Osteomyelitis associated with pressure sores. Arch Intern Med 154:753, 1994

ECKARDT JJ et al: An aggressive surgical approach to the management of chronic osteomyelitis. Clin Orthop 298:229, 1994

ESOLEN LM et al: *Pneumocystis carinii* osteomyelitis in a patient with common variable immunodeficiency. N Engl J Med 326:999, 1992

HENRY SL, GALLOWAY KP: Local antibacterial therapy for the management of orthopaedic infections. Pharmacokinetic considerations. Clin Pharmacokinet 29:36, 1995

HOPKINS KL et al: Gadolinium-DPTA-enhanced magnetic resonance imaging of musculoskeletal infectious processes. Skeletal Radiol 24:325, 1995

JAUREGUI LE: *Diagnosis and Management of Bone Infections.* New York, Marcel Dekker, 1995

LEW DP, WALDVOGEL FA: Quinolones and osteomyelitis: State-of-the-art. Drugs 49(Suppl 2):100, 1995

MAUCERI AA: Treatment of bone and joint infections utilizing a third-generation cephalosporin with an outpatient drug delivery device. HIAT Study Group. Am J Med 97(2a):14, 1995

MAY JW JR et al: Treatment of chronic traumatic bone wounds. Microvascular free tissue transfer: A 13-year experience in 96 patients. Ann Surg 214:241, 1991

MEIER JL, BEEKMANN SE: Mycobacterial and fungal infections of bones and joints. Curr Opin Rheumatol 7:329, 1995

NORDEN C et al: *Infections in Bones and Joints.* Boston, Blackwell Scientific, 1994

OSTERMANN PA et al: Local antibiotic therapy for severe open fractures. J Bone Joint Surg [Br] 77:93, 1995

SAPICO FL et al: Bone and joint infections in patients with infective endocarditis: Review of a 4-year experience. Clin Infect Dis 22:783, 1996

TORDA AJ et al: Pyogenic vertebral osteomyelitis: Analysis of 20 cases and review. Clin Infect Dis 20:320, 1995

WALDVOGEL FA et al: Osteomyelitis: A review of clinical features, therapeutic considerations, and unusual aspects. N Engl J Med 282:198, 1970

————, VASEY H: Osteomyelitis: The past decade. N Engl J Med 303:360, 1980

133 *Dennis L. Stevens*

INFECTIONS OF THE SKIN, MUSCLE, AND SOFT TISSUES

ANATOMIC RELATIONSHIPS: CLUES TO THE DIAGNOSIS OF SOFT TISSUE INFECTIONS Protection against infection of the epidermis is dependent on the mechanical barrier afforded by the stratum corneum, since the epidermis itself is devoid of blood vessels (Fig. 133-1). Disruption of this layer by burns, bites, abrasions, or foreign bodies allows penetration of bacteria to the deeper structures. Similarly, the hair follicle can serve as a portal either for components of the normal flora (e.g., *Staphylococcus*) or for extrinsic bacteria (e.g., *Pseudomonas* in hot-tub folliculitis). Intracellular infection of the squamous epithelium with vesicle formation may arise from cutaneous inoculation [as in infection with herpes simplex virus (HSV) type 1], from the dermal capillary plexus (as in varicella and infections due to other viruses associated with viremia), or from cutaneous nerve roots (as in herpes zoster). Bacteria infecting the epidermis, such as *Streptococcus pyogenes*, may be translocated laterally to deeper structures via lymphatics, an event that results in the rapid superficial spread of erysipelas. Later, engorgement or obstruction of lymphatics causes flaccid edema of the epidermis, another characteristic of erysipelas.

The rich plexus of capillaries beneath the dermal papillae provides nutrition to the stratum germinativum, and physiologic responses of this plexus produce important clinical signs and symptoms. For exam-

FIGURE 133-1 Structural components of the skin and soft tissue are identified at the left. Superficial infections are depicted along the top of the figure, and infections of the deeper structures of the soft tissue at the right. The rich capillary network beneath the dermal papillae plays a key role in the localization of infection and in the development of the acute inflammatory reaction.

ple, infective vasculitis of the plexus results in petechiae, Osler's nodes, Janeway lesions, and palpable purpura, which are important clues to the existence of endocarditis (Chap. 126). In addition, metastatic infection within this plexus can result in cutaneous manifestations of disseminated fungal infection (Chap. 207), gonococcal infection (Chap. 150), *Salmonella* infection (Chap. 158), *Pseudomonas* infection (i.e., ecthyma gangrenosum) (Chap. 157), meningococcemia (Chap. 149), and staphylococcal infection (Chap. 142). The plexus also provides access for bacteria to the circulation, thereby facilitating local spread or bacteremia. The postcapillary venules of this plexus are a major site of polymorphonuclear leukocyte sequestration, diapedesis, and chemotaxis to the site of cutaneous infection.

Exaggeration of these physiologic mechanisms by excessive levels of cytokines or bacterial toxins causes leukostasis, venous occlusion, and pitting edema. Edema with purple bullae and ecchymosis suggests loss of vascular integrity and necessitates exploration of the deeper structures for evidence of necrotizing fasciitis or myonecrosis. To make an early diagnosis, one must exercise a high level of suspicion in instances of unexplained fever and of pain and tenderness in the soft tissue, even in the absence of acute cutaneous inflammation.

INFECTIONS ASSOCIATED WITH VESICLES (Table 133-1)

Vesicle formation due to infection is caused by viral proliferation within the epidermis. In varicella and variola, viremia precedes the onset of a diffuse centrifugal rash that progresses from macules to vesicles, then to pustules, and finally to scabs over the course of 1 to 2 weeks. Vesicles of varicella have a "dewdrop" appearance and develop in crops randomly about the trunk, extremities, and face over 3 to 4 days. Herpes zoster occurs in a single dermatome; the appearance of vesicles is preceded by pain for several days. Zoster may occur in persons of any age but is most common among immunosuppressed individuals and elderly patients, whereas most cases of varicella occur in young children. Vesicles due to HSV are found on or around the lips (HSV-1) or genitals (HSV-2) but may appear on the head and neck of young wrestlers (herpes gladiatorum) or on the digits of health care workers (herpetic whitlow). Coxsackievirus A16 characteristically causes vesicles on the hands, feet, and mouth of children. Orf is caused by a DNA virus related to smallpox virus and infects the fingers of individuals who work around goats and sheep. Molluscum contagiosum virus induces flaccid vesicles on the skin of healthy and immunocompromised individuals.

INFECTIONS ASSOCIATED WITH BULLAE (Table 133-1)

Staphylococcal scalded-skin syndrome (SSSS) in neonates is caused by a toxin (exfoliatin) from phage group II *Staphylococcus aureus*. SSSS must be distinguished from toxic epidermal necrolysis (TEN), which occurs primarily in adults, is drug-induced, and has a higher mortality. Punch biopsy with frozen section is useful in making this distinction since the cleavage plane is the stratum corneum in SSSS (Fig. 133-1) and the stratum germinativum in TEN. Necrotizing fasciitis and gas gangrene also induce bulla formation (see "Necrotizing Fasciitis" below). Halophilic vibrio infection (see Chap. 161) can be as aggressive and fulminant as necrotizing fasciitis; a helpful clue in its diagnosis is a history of exposure to waters of the Gulf of Mexico or the Atlantic seaboard or (in a patient with cirrhosis) the ingestion of raw seafood. This organism is highly susceptible to tetracycline.

INFECTIONS ASSOCIATED WITH CRUSTED LESIONS (Table 133-1)

Impetigo contagiosa is caused by *S. pyogenes*, and bullous impetigo is due to *S. aureus*. Both skin lesions may have an early bullous stage but then appear as thick crusts with a golden-brown color. Streptococcal lesions are most common among children 2 to 5 years of age, and epidemics may occur in settings of poor hygiene, particularly among children of lower socioeconomic status in tropical climates. It is important to recognize impetigo contagiosa because of its relationship to poststreptococcal glomerulonephritis. Superficial dermatophyte infection (ringworm) can occur on any skin surface, and skin scrapings with KOH staining are diagnostic. Primary infections with dimorphic fungi such as *Blastomyces* (Chap. 205) and

Table 133-1

Skin and Soft Tissue Infections

Lesion, Clinical Syndrome	Infectious Agent	Chapter
Vesicles		
Smallpox	Variola virus	188
Chickenpox	Varicella-zoster virus	185
Shingles (herpes zoster)	Varicella-zoster virus	185
Cold sores, herpetic whitlow, herpes gladiatorum	Herpes simplex virus	184
Hand-foot-and-mouth disease	Coxsackievirus A16	195
Orf	Parapoxvirus	188
Molluscum contagiosum	Pox-like virus	188
Bullae		
Staphylococcal scalded-skin syndrome	*Staphylococcus aureus*	142
Necrotizing fasciitis	*Streptococcus pyogenes, Clostridium* spp., mixed aerobes and anaerobes	169
Gas gangrene	*Clostridium* spp.	148
Halophilic vibrio	*Vibrio vulnificus*	161
Crusted lesions		
Bullous impetigo	*S. aureus*	142
Impetigo contagiosa	*S. pyogenes*	143
Ringworm	Superficial dermatophyte fungi	210
Sporotrichosis	*Sporothrix schenckii*	210
Histoplasmosis	*Histoplasma capsulatum*	203
Coccidioidomycosis	*Coccidioides immitis*	204
Blastomycosis	*Blastomyces dermatitidis*	205
Cutaneous leishmaniasis	*Leishmania* spp.	216
Cutaneous tuberculosis	*Mycobacterium tuberculosis*	171
Nocardiosis	*Nocardia asteroides*	167
Folliculitis		
Furunculosis	*S. aureus*	142
Hot-tub folliculitis	*Pseudomonas aeruginosa*	157
Swimmer's itch	*Schistosoma* spp.	224
Acne vulgaris	*Propionibacterium acnes*	55
Ulcers with or without eschars		
Anthrax	*Bacillus anthracis*	144
Ulceroglandular tularemia	*Francisella tularensis*	163
Bubonic plague	*Yersinia pestis*	164
Buruli ulcer	*Mycobacterium ulcerans*	173
Leprosy	*Mycobacterium leprae*	172
Cutaneous tuberculosis	*M. tuberculosis*	171
Erysipelas	*S. pyogenes*	143
Necrotizing fasciitis		
Streptococcal gangrene	*S. pyogenes*	143
Fournier's gangrene	Mixed aerobic and anaerobic bacteria	169
Myositis and myonecrosis		
Pyomyositis	*S. aureus*	142
Streptococcal necrotizing myositis	*S. pyogenes*	143
Gas gangrene	*Clostridium* spp.	148
Nonclostridial (crepitant) myositis	Mixed aerobic and anaerobic bacteria	169
Synergistic nonclostridial anaerobic myonecrosis	Mixed aerobic and anaerobic bacteria	169

Sporothrix schenckii (Chap. 210) can initially present as crusted skin lesions resembling ringworm. Disseminated infection with *Coccidioides immitis* (Chap. 204) also can involve the skin, and biopsy and culture should be performed on crusted lesions in patients from endemic areas. Crusted nodular lesions caused by *Mycobacterium chelonae* have recently been described in patients positive for human immunodeficiency virus. Treatment with clarithromycin looks promising.

FOLLICULITIS (Table 133-1)

Hair follicles serve as a portal of entry for a number of bacteria, though *S. aureus* is the most common cause of localized folliculitis. Sebaceous glands empty into hair follicles and ducts and if blocked form sebaceous cysts, which may resemble staphylococcal abscesses or may become secondarily infected. Infection of sweat glands (hidradenitis suppurativa) can also mimic infection of hair follicles, particularly in the axillae. Chronic folliculitis is uncommon except in acne vulgaris, where constituents of the normal flora (e.g., *Propionibacterium acnes*) may play a role.

Diffuse folliculitis occurs in two settings. "Hot-tub folliculitis" is caused by *Pseudomonas aeruginosa* in waters that are insufficiently chlorinated and maintained at temperatures between 37 and 40°C. Infection is usually self-limited, though bacteremia and shock have been reported. Swimmer's itch occurs when a skin surface is exposed to water infested with freshwater avian schistosomes. Warm water temperatures and alkaline pH are suitable for molluscs that serve as intermediate hosts between bird and human. Free-swimming schistosomal cercariae (see Chap. 224) readily penetrate human hair follicles or pores but quickly die and elicit a brisk allergic reaction causing intense itching and erythema.

ULCERS WITH OR WITHOUT ESCHARS (Table 133-1) Cutaneous anthrax begins as a pruritic papule, which develops within days into an ulcer with surrounding vesicles and edema and then into an enlarging ulcer with black eschar. Cutaneous diphtheria may cause chronic nonhealing ulcers with an overlying dirty-gray membrane, though lesions may also mimic psoriasis, eczema, or impetigo. Ulceroglandular tularemia may have associated ulcerated skin lesions with painful regional adenopathy. Although buboes are the major cutaneous manifestation of plague (see Chap. 164), in 25 percent of cases ulcers with eschars, papules, or pustules are also present.

Mycobacterium ulcerans typically causes chronic skin ulcers on the extremities of individuals living in the tropics. *Mycobacterium leprae* may be associated with cutaneous ulcerations in patients with lepromatous leprosy related to Lucio's phenomenon or during reversal reactions. *Mycobacterium tuberculosis* may also cause ulcerations, papules, or erythematous macular lesions of the skin in both normal and immunocompromised patients.

Decubitus ulcers are due to tissue hypoxia secondary to pressure-induced vascular insufficiency and may become secondarily infected with components of the skin and gastrointestinal flora, including anaerobes. Ulcerative lesions on the anterior shins may be due to pyoderma gangrenosum, which must be distinguished from similar lesions of infectious etiology by histologic evaluation of biopsy sites.

ERYSIPELAS (Table 133-1) Erysipelas is due to *S. pyogenes* (see Chap. 143) and is characterized by an abrupt onset of fiery-red swelling of the face or extremities. The distinctive features of erysipelas are well-defined indurated margins, particularly along the nasolabial fold; rapid progression; and intense pain. Flaccid bullae may develop during the second or third day of illness, but extension to deeper soft tissues is rare. Treatment with penicillin is effective; swelling may progress despite appropriate treatment, though fever, pain, and the intense red color diminish. Desquamation of the involved skin occurs 5 to 10 days into the illness. Infants and elderly adults are most commonly afflicted, and the severity of systemic toxicity varies.

CELLULITIS Cellulitis is an acute inflammatory condition of the skin that is characterized by localized pain, erythema, swelling, and heat. Cellulitis may be caused by indigenous flora colonizing the skin and appendages (e.g., *S. aureus* and *S. pyogenes*) or by a wide variety of exogenous bacteria. Because the exogenous bacteria involved in cellulitis occupy unique niches in nature, a thorough history provides important clues to etiology (see Table 133-1 and text below).

Bacteria may gain access to the epidermis through cracks in the skin, abrasions, cuts, burns, insect bites, surgical incisions, and intravenous catheters. Cellulitis caused by *S. aureus* spreads from a central localized infection, such as an abscess, folliculitis, or an infected foreign body (e.g., a splinter, a prosthetic device, or an intravenous catheter). In contrast, cellulitis due to *S. pyogenes* is a more rapidly spreading, diffuse process frequently associated with lymphangitis and fever. Recurrent streptococcal cellulitis of the lower extremities may be caused by organisms of group A, C, or G in association with chronic venous stasis or with saphenous venectomy for coronary artery bypass surgery. Streptococci also cause recurrent cellulitis among patients with chronic lymphedema resulting from elephantiasis, lymph node dissection, or Milroy's disease. Recurrent staphylococcal cutaneous infections are more common among individuals who have eosinophilia and elevated serum levels of IgE (Job's syndrome) and among nasal

carriers of staphylococci. Cellulitis caused by *Streptococcus agalactiae* (group B streptococci) occurs primarily in patients with diabetes mellitus or peripheral vascular disease. *Haemophilus influenzae* typically causes periorbital cellulitis in children in association with sinusitis, otitis media, or epiglottitis. It is unclear whether this form of cellulitis will (like meningitis) become less common as a result of the impressive efficacy of the *H. influenzae* type b vaccine.

Many other bacteria also cause cellulitis. Fortunately, these organisms occur in such characteristic settings that a good history provides useful clues to the diagnosis. Cellulitis associated with cat bites and, to a lesser degree, with dog bites is commonly caused by *Pasteurella multocida*, though in the latter case *Staphylococcus intermedius* and *Capnocytophaga canimorsus* (DF-2) must also be considered. Sites of cellulitis and abscesses associated with dog bites and human bites also contain a variety of anaerobic organisms. *Pasteurella* is notoriously resistant to dicloxacillin and nafcillin but is sensitive to all other β-lactam antimicrobials as well as to quinolones, tetracycline, and erythromycin. Ampicillin/clavulanate, ampicillin/sulbactam, and cefoxitin are good choices for the treatment of animal or human bite infections. *Aeromonas hydrophila* causes aggressive cellulitis in tissues surrounding lacerations sustained in fresh water (lakes, rivers, and streams). This organism remains sensitive to aminoglycosides, fluoroquinolones, chloramphenicol, trimethoprim-sulfamethoxazole, and third-generation cephalosporins; it is resistant to ampicillin, however.

P. aeruginosa causes three types of soft tissue infection: ecthyma gangrenosum in neutropenic patients, hot-tub folliculitis, and cellulitis following penetrating injury. Most commonly, *P. aeruginosa* is introduced into the deep tissues when a person steps on a nail; this scenario is referred to as the "sweaty tennis shoe syndrome." Treatment includes surgical inspection and drainage, particularly if the injury also involves bone or joint capsule. Choices for empirical treatment while antimicrobial susceptibility data are awaited include an aminoglycoside, a third-generation cephalosporin (ceftazidime, cefoperazone, or cefotaxime), a semisynthetic penicillin (ticarcillin, mezlocillin, or piperacillin), or a fluoroquinolone (though drugs of the last class are not indicated for the treatment of children less than 13 years old).

Gram-negative bacillary cellulitis, including that due to *P. aeruginosa*, is most common among hospitalized, immunocompromised hosts. Cultures and sensitivity tests are critically important in this setting because of multidrug resistance (see Chap. 157).

The gram-positive aerobic rod *Erysipelothrix rhusiopathiae*, which causes cellulitis in bone renderers and fishmongers, remains susceptible to penicillin, erythromycin, clindamycin, tetracycline, and cephalosporins but is resistant to sulfonamides and chloramphenicol. Fish food containing the water flea *Daphnia* is sometimes contaminated with *Mycobacterium marinum*, which can cause cellulitis or granulomas on skin surfaces exposed to the water in aquariums or injured in swimming pools. Rifampin plus ethambutol has been an effective combination in some cases, though no comprehensive studies have been undertaken. In addition, some strains of *M. marinum* are susceptible to tetracycline or to trimethoprim-sulfamethoxazole.

The etiology of cellulitis can be suggested by epidemiologic data (see above). When there is drainage, an open wound, or an obvious portal of entry, Gram's stain and culture provide a definitive diagnosis. In the absence of these findings, the bacterial etiology of cellulitis is difficult to establish. Even with needle aspiration of the leading edge or a punch biopsy of the cellulitis tissue itself, cultures are positive in only 20 percent of cases. This observation suggests that relatively low numbers of bacteria may cause cellulitis and that the expanding area of erythema within the skin may be a direct effect of extracellular toxins or of the soluble mediators of inflammation elicited by the host.

NECROTIZING FASCIITIS (Table 133-1) Necrotizing fasciitis, formerly called streptococcal gangrene, may be associated with group A *Streptococcus* or mixed aerobic-anaerobic bacteria or may occur as part of gas gangrene caused by *Clostridium perfringens*. Early diagnosis may be difficult when pain or unexplained fever is the only presenting manifestation. Swelling then develops and is followed by brawny edema and tenderness. With progression, dark red induration of the epidermis appears along with bullae filled with blue or purple fluid. Later the skin becomes friable and takes on a bluish, maroon, or black color. By this stage, thrombosis of blood vessels in the dermal papillae is extensive (see Fig. 133-1). Extension of infection to the level of the deep fascia causes it to take on a brownish-gray appearance. Rapid spread occurs along fascial planes, through venous channels and lymphatics. Patients in the later stages are toxic and frequently manifest shock and multiorgan failure.

Necrotizing fasciitis caused by mixed aerobic-anaerobic bacteria begins with a breach in the integrity of a mucous membrane barrier, such as the mucosa of the gastrointestinal or genitourinary tract. The portal can be a malignancy, diverticulum, hemorrhoid, anal fissure, or urethral tear. Other predisposing factors include peripheral vascular disease, diabetes mellitus, surgery, and penetrating injury to the abdomen. Leakage into the perineal area results in a syndrome called *Fournier's gangrene*, characterized by massive swelling of the scrotum and penis with extension into the perineum or the abdominal wall and legs.

Necrotizing fasciitis caused by *S. pyogenes* has increased in frequency and severity since 1985. It frequently begins deep at the site of a nonpenetrating minor trauma such as a bruise or a muscle strain. Seeding of the site via transient bacteremia is likely, though most patients deny antecedent streptococcal infection. Alternatively, *S. pyogenes* may reach the deep fascia from a site of cutaneous infection or penetrating trauma. Toxicity is severe, and renal impairment may precede the development of shock. In 20 to 40 percent of cases, myositis occurs concomitantly, and, as in gas gangrene (see below), serum creatinine phosphokinase values may be markedly elevated. Necrotizing fasciitis due to mixed aerobic-anaerobic bacteria may be associated with gas in the deep tissue, but gas is not usually present when the cause is *S. pyogenes*. Prompt surgical exploration down to the deep fascia and muscle is essential. Necrotic tissue must be surgically removed, and Gram's staining and culture of excised tissue are useful in establishing whether group A streptococci, mixed aerobic-anaerobic bacteria, or *Clostridium* spp. are present (see "Treatment" below).

MYOSITIS (Table 133-1)   Muscle involvement can occur with virus infection [influenza, dengue, coxsackievirus B (pleurodynia)]; or parasitic invasion [*Trichinella spiralis* (trichinosis), *Taenia solium* (cysticercosis), *Toxoplasma gondii* (toxoplasmosis)]. Although myalgia can occur in most of these infections, severe muscle pain is the hallmark of pleurodynia, trichinosis, and bacterial infection. Acute rhabdomyolysis predictably occurs with clostridial and streptococcal myositis but may also be associated with influenza virus, echovirus, coxsackievirus, Epstein-Barr virus, and *Legionella* infection.

Pyomyositis is usually due to *S. aureus*, is common in tropical areas, and generally has no known portal of entry. Infection remains localized, and, unless organisms produce toxic shock syndrome toxin 1 or certain enterotoxins, shock does not develop. In contrast, *S. pyogenes* may induce primary myositis referred to as *streptococcal necrotizing myositis*, which is associated with severe systemic toxicity. Myonecrosis occurs concomitantly with necrotizing fasciitis in about 50 percent of cases. Both are part of the streptococcal toxic shock syndrome.

Gas gangrene usually follows severe penetrating injuries that result in interruption of the blood supply and introduction of soil into wounds. Such cases of traumatic gangrene are usually caused by *C. perfringens*, *Clostridium septicum*, or *Clostridium histolyticum*. Rarely, latent or recurrent gangrene can occur years after penetrating trauma, most likely owing to dormant spores that reside at the site of previous injury. Spontaneous nontraumatic gangrene among patients with neutropenia, gastrointestinal malignancy, diverticulosis, or recent radiation therapy to the abdomen is caused by *C. septicum*. The tolerance of this anaerobe to oxygen probably explains why it can initiate infection spontaneously in normal tissue anywhere in the body.

Synergistic nonclostridial anaerobic myonecrosis, also known as necrotizing cutaneous myositis and synergistic necrotizing cellulitis, is a variant of necrotizing fasciitis caused by mixed aerobic and anaerobic bacteria with the exclusion of clostridial organisms (see "Necrotizing Fasciitis" above).

℞ TREATMENT

Early and aggressive surgical exploration is essential in patients with suspected necrotizing fasciitis, myositis, or gangrene in order to (1) visualize the deep structures, (2) remove necrotic tissue, (3) reduce compartment pressure, and (4) obtain suitable material for Gram's staining and for aerobic and anaerobic cultures. Appropriate empirical antibiotic treatment for mixed aerobic-anaerobic infections could consist of ampicillin/sulbactam, cefoxitin, or the following combination: (1) clindamycin (600 to 800 mg intravenously every 8 h) or metronidazole (750 mg every 6 h) plus (2) ampicillin or ampicillin/sulbactam (2 to 3 g intravenously every 6 h) plus (3) gentamicin (1.0 to 1.5 mg/kg every 8 h). Group A streptococcal and clostridial infection of the fascia and/or muscle carries a mortality rate of 20 to 50 percent with penicillin treatment. In experimental models of streptococcal and clostridial necrotizing fasciitis/myositis, clindamycin has exhibited markedly superior efficacy, but no comparative trials have been performed in humans. Hyperbaric oxygen treatment may also be useful in gas gangrene due to clostridial species. Antibiotic treatment should be continued until all signs of systemic toxicity have resolved, all devitalized tissue has been removed, and granulation tissue has developed (Chaps. 143, 148, and 169).

In summary, infections of the skin and soft tissues are diverse in presentation and severity and offer a great challenge to the clinician. This chapter provides an approach to diagnosis and understanding of the pathophysiologic mechanisms involved in these infections. More in-depth information is found in chapters on specific infections.

BIBLIOGRAPHY

BISNO AI, STEVENS DL: Streptococcal infections in skin and soft tissues. N Engl J Med 334:240, 1996

FRANCIS JS, NEFF J: Viral infections of the skin and soft tissues, in *Atlas of Infectious Diseases*, DL Stevens (ed). Philadelphia, Churchill Livingstone, 1994

GOLDSTEIN EJC: Bite wounds and infection. Clin Infect Dis 14:633, 1992

HOOK EW et al: Microbiologic evaluation of cutaneous cellulitis in adults. Arch Intern Med 146:295, 1986

SIMMONS RL, AHRENHOLZ DH: Infections of the skin and soft tissue, in *Surgical Infectious Diseases*, 2d ed, RJ Howard, RL Simmons (eds). Norwalk, CT, Appleton & Lange, 1988, p 377

STEVENS DL et al: Effect of antibiotics on toxin production and viability of *Clostridium perfringens*. Antimicrob Agents Chemother 31:213, 1987

——— et al: Spontaneous, nontraumatic gangrene due to *Clostridium septicum*. Rev Infect Dis 12:286, 1990

———: Invasive group A streptococcus infections. Clin Infect Dis 14:2, 1992

——— et al: Evaluation of hyperbaric oxygen therapy for treatment of experimental *Clostridium perfringens* infection. Clin Infect Dis 17:231, 1993

——— et al: Penicillin binding protein expression at different growth stages determines penicillin efficacy in vitro and in vivo: An explanation for the inoculum effect. J Infect Dis 167:1401, 1993

———: Necrotizing infections of the skin and soft tissues, in *Atlas of Infectious Diseases*, DL Stevens (ed). Philadelphia, Churchill Livingstone, 1994

———: Streptococcal toxic shock syndrome: Spectrum of disease, pathogenesis and new concepts in treatment. Emerging Infect Dis 1:69, 1995

WALLACE RJ et al: Clinical trial of clarithromycin for cutaneous (disseminated) infection due to *Mycobacterium chelonae*. Ann Intern Med 119:482, 1993

INFECTIONS (EXCLUDING AIDS) IN INJECTION DRUG USERS

The injection of illicit drugs is a widespread practice whose prevalence has increased dramatically since the 1950s in association with successive epidemics of heroin and cocaine use. Injection drug users are a hidden population, engaging in an illegal activity of which society disapproves. It is impossible to determine their precise number or, consequently, the true incidence of infectious complications in this population.

A markedly higher age-specific mortality rate among injection drug users than in the general population was documented even before the epidemic of infection with human immunodeficiency virus (HIV) and AIDS (see Chap. 308). For example, in New York City between 1965 and 1972, the death rate among relatively young (20- to 54-year-old) adult heroin addicts not involved in drug-treatment programs was estimated to be five times greater than that among age-matched, non-heroin-addicted adults (28.2 per 1000 versus 5.6 per 1000). A substantial portion of this excess mortality was the result of infectious complications of injection drug use. Data from the New York City Medical Examiner during the 1960s indicated that 27 percent of narcotic-related deaths were associated with infections. During this period, a wide array of infectious complications of injection drug use were described. More recently, as a consequence of the HIV epidemic, overall mortality and cause-specific mortality secondary to both AIDS and bacterial infections have dramatically increased in this population. Mortality rates of 3.41 per 100 person-years from AIDS and 1.08 per 100 person-years from bacterial infection preceding AIDS have been reported in HIV-infected injection drug users.

Most infectious complications in injection drug users reflect the events surrounding drug injection and associated life-style issues rather than the direct effects of the illicit drugs themselves. Drugs are purchased in powdered form and often contain adulterants such as quinine, talc, and dextrose. The drugs are dissolved in water (obtained from any available source) or occasionally in saliva in bottle caps or "cookers," filtered through cotton wool or gauze, aspirated into tuberculin or diabetic syringes, and injected intravenously or subcutaneously. Skin preparation is usually minimal and may consist of rubbing saliva on the injection site. A small amount of blood may remain in the needle and syringe after use and may merely be diluted by rinsing in tap water or bleach. Needles and syringes are often shared among injection drug users, either by a few friends or relatives or by larger numbers of users sequentially and anonymously in "shooting galleries." These clandestine locations, where injection drug users gather to rent injection equipment and administer drugs, are ideal sites for the transmission of bloodborne infectious agents.

In this setting, the characteristics of injection drug users that increase the risk of infection are (1) increased rates of skin, mucous membrane, and nasopharyngeal carriage of pathogenic organisms, particularly staphylococci; (2) unsterile injection technique resulting in the introduction of components of the dermal or nasopharyngeal flora into soft tissues or the bloodstream; (3) contamination of injection equipment or drugs with viral, bacterial, and parasitic microorganisms, which may be present in residual blood in shared injection equipment or in contaminated water used to dissolve drugs before injection or to rinse equipment afterward; (4) humoral, cell-mediated, and phagocytic defects induced by HIV infection and/or drug use (even before the HIV/AIDS epidemic, injection drug users were known to have abnormal immunologic parameters, including high levels of globulins, false-positive serologic reactions to multiple antigens, and abnormalities in phagocytosis, and these defects have been markedly exacerbated by HIV-induced B- and T-cell dysfunction); (5) poor dental hygiene and drug-induced impairment of gag and cough reflexes; (6) alteration of the normal microbial flora owing to intermittent antibiotic use; (7) low socioeconomic status, with increased prevalence of exposure to certain pathogens (notably *Mycobacterium tuberculosis*); (8) behaviors associated with injection drug use, such as cigarette smoking, alcohol use, or exchange of sex for drugs or money; and (9) decreased access to and/or lack of appropriate use of preventive and primary health care services, resulting in low levels of immunization and prophylaxis and delay in the diagnosis and treatment of minor infectious complications.

SPECIFIC INFECTIONS AMONG INJECTION DRUG USERS

SKIN AND SOFT TISSUE INFECTIONS (See also Chap. 133) Infections of the skin and soft tissues are the most common bacterial infectious complication of injection drug use and, before the AIDS epidemic, were the most common cause of hospital admissions of injection drug users. The clinical spectrum of infection is broad, ranging from simple cellulitis and abscess to life-threatening necrotizing fasciitis and septic thrombophlebitis. The high frequency of skin and soft tissue infections is attributable to several factors: the practice of injecting drugs subcutaneously ("skin popping"), the extravasation of drugs into soft tissue during intravenous injection, the presence in injected material of adulterants that may cause tissue necrosis, and the increased skin carriage of pathogenic organisms.

Most skin and soft tissue infections occur on the upper and lower extremities, but occasionally atypical sites (e.g., the abdomen or back, groin, scrotum, and neck) may be involved as a result of injection into the jugular or femoral veins. Cellulitis may extend from a fresh injection site or may result from superinfection of an open wound sustained earlier. The clinical appearance is often atypical because of chronic damage to the skin and to venous and lymphatic systems in both the upper and the lower extremities, with resultant underlying lymphedema, hyperpigmentation, scarring, and regional lymphadenopathy. Nevertheless, careful examination often reveals characteristic redness, warmth, and tenderness, with tender inguinal or axillary lymph nodes. Fever is variable and bacteremia infrequent.

Uncomplicated cellulitis is most often due to group A streptococci, other streptococci, or *Staphylococcus aureus*. Unless an associated open draining wound is present or bacteremia develops, the precise microbial etiology is difficult to determine. For localized abscesses presenting either as draining lesions or as fluctuant subcutaneous masses, Gram's staining and culture of pus or aspirated material are required. Although these abscesses are usually staphylococcal in etiology, they are sometimes due to a complex mixture of anaerobic and aerobic bacteria. A foul odor and characteristic findings on Gram's staining of pus suggest a polymicrobial etiology.

Treatment of skin infections consists of hospitalization in most cases, incision and drainage in instances of abscess formation, and administration of intravenous antistaphylococcal β-lactam antibiotics such as oxacillin or nafcillin. Cefazolin (4 to 6 g/d) may be an alternative choice. In areas where methicillin-resistant *S. aureus* is highly prevalent, vancomycin should be used empirically, pending the results of susceptibility tests. The total duration of therapy should be 10 to 14 days; for the latter part of this course, oral agents may or may not be used, depending on the individual's clinical response. For injection drug users who have an established relationship with a health care provider, mild infections may be treated with oral agents on an outpatient basis; therapy should be followed by frequent visits at which the response is assessed.

Indolent skin ulcers are common. These lesions are shallow and indurated and may become superinfected. Their etiology is unclear, but they are likely the result of foreign-body inflammatory changes, necrosis, and low-grade infection. They usually respond to local wound care and oral or topical antibiotic treatment. Occasionally, these ulcers are extensive enough to require skin grafting. When the lesions heal, they leave depressed, hyperpigmented scars.

Necrotizing fasciitis and myositis and septic thrombophlebitis are life-threatening local complications of injection drug use. Although infrequent, they should always be considered when skin or soft tissue infection develops in injection drug users. The presence of fasciitis and myositis is associated with exquisite pain and tenderness at the injection site and with toxicity and hemodynamic instability out of proportion to the local lesion. Crepitus may be noted, and soft tissue radiographs may reveal gas in tissues. Immediate surgical exploration, with extensive drainage and debridement of infected and nonviable tissue, is required. These infections often have a polymicrobial etiology that includes *S. aureus*, aerobic and anaerobic streptococci, enteric gram-negative bacilli, and other anaerobes. Parenteral antibiotic therapy aimed at gram-positive and gram-negative organisms, with anaerobic coverage, is essential. Several regimens—including vancomycin or nafcillin plus metronidazole or clindamycin plus an aminoglycoside, a third-generation cephalosporin, or a broad-spectrum penicillin—are indicated.

Septic thrombophlebitis of extremity, jugular, or femoral veins often appears as septic pulmonary emboli. Bacteremia is invariably found, and pus may be expressed from injection sites of infected vessels. Parenteral antibiotic therapy as well as ligation and excision of infected thrombosed veins (if technically feasible) are advocated. The value of heparin remains unproved, and its use is generally not recommended.

Other, infrequent complications of injection drug use under unsterile circumstances include wound botulism, tetanus, malaria, and disseminated candidiasis. The first two have been sporadically reported, usually in long-term users and often in "skin poppers," whereas outbreaks of malaria have resulted from the sharing of needles contaminated with infected blood. Botulism should be considered in patients with unusual, progressive cranial nerve palsies; wounds should be cultured for *Clostridium botulinum*. Tetanus should be suspected in drug users with seizures, muscle rigidity, and autonomic hyperactivity.

ENDOCARDITIS (See Chap. 126) The potential for life-threatening complications and the usual need for prolonged intravenous antibiotic therapy in the hospital make bacterial endocarditis a disease of great consequence in injection drug users. In several studies of consecutive hospital admissions of injection drug users before the AIDS epidemic, endocarditis accounted for 5 to 16 percent of admissions and for 2 to 8 percent of all deaths.

Microbiology The predominant organism causing endocarditis in injection drug users is *S. aureus*. In various published series, this organism has caused from 60 to more than 90 percent of cases. In many geographic locations, a substantial and increasing proportion of *S. aureus* isolates are resistant to methicillin. Although the organism was originally believed to be a contaminant of drugs and injection paraphernalia, it is now clear that *S. aureus* is part of the patient's own flora, carried in the nares and oropharynx and on the skin and subsequently introduced into the bloodstream by unsterile injection.

Right-sided endocarditis is caused by *S. aureus* in more than 80 percent of cases in injection drug users, whereas the organisms isolated in aortic or mitral valve endocarditis are more similar to those found in other patients. Streptococci and enterococci, including alpha-hemolytic viridans streptococci and *Enterococcus faecalis*, are the second most common organisms but account for only 5 to 10 percent of cases of endocarditis in various series. Geographic and temporal clustering of more unusual infecting organisms has occasionally been reported. These organisms include *Pseudomonas aeruginosa*, *Pseudomonas cepacia*, *Serratia marcescens*, enterococci, and, recently, methicillin-resistant *S. aureus*. Infrequent cases of endocarditis due to *Candida* spp., *Bacillus* spp., diphtheroids, and fastidious gram-negative or anaerobic components of the oral flora have been described as well. Polymicrobial endocarditis due to both gram-positive and gram-negative organisms has been documented.

Pathogenesis and Clinical Presentation Longer duration and higher frequency of drug injection are associated with increased risk of endocarditis. The site most frequently involved is the tricuspid valve, possibly because of its proximity to the injection site. Injection of particulate matter, including talc and cotton, may cause pitting and disruption of the smooth endothelial lining—changes that may facilitate the attachment of pathogenic organisms. Left-sided endocarditis may occur with or without right-sided involvement and usually develops in the setting of underlying valvular heart disease.

The various characteristic clinical presentations depend on the site of valvular involvement. In tricuspid valve endocarditis, the predominant picture is one of an abrupt illness with persistent high fever, pulmonary involvement, and an absence of systemic embolic or microvascular phenomena. Approximately 50 percent of patients present with cough and pleuritic chest pain, and some exhibit hemoptysis—all the result of multiple septic pulmonary emboli and infarctions. The characteristic murmur of tricuspid regurgitation may be heard in 50 percent of patients. This is a medium-pitched, midsystolic murmur at the lower left sternal border that increases in intensity with inspiration. Characteristically, chest radiography shows multiple patchy or nodular infiltrates that progress to cavitation during therapy and eventually resolve.

Endocarditis involving the mitral and aortic valves also has an acute onset, with high fever, toxicity, and signs and symptoms resulting from multiple systemic emboli (including arterial emboli and septic infarcts of the skin, liver, spleen, kidneys, and central nervous system). Toxic encephalopathy, focal neurologic abnormalities (the result of mycotic aneurysm or brain abscess), and bacterial meningitis may ensue. Petechiae and splenomegaly occur in approximately 50 percent of patients, and aortic and mitral regurgitant murmurs are reported in almost all cases.

Diagnosis The diagnosis of endocarditis in injection drug users can be problematic, even in the emergency room setting, where most febrile drug users are evaluated and this diagnosis is often suspected. Right-sided endocarditis may be particularly difficult to diagnose because systemic emboli and a regurgitant murmur are usually absent. The diagnosis rests on a composite of clinical, microbiologic, radiologic, and imaging data.

The clinical criteria used include sustained bacteremia involving an organism likely to cause endocarditis and the presence of compatible pulmonary, systemic, or cardiac findings. The diagnostic accuracy of emergency room evaluation in predicting endocarditis in febrile injection drug users is quite low. Of 87 consecutive febrile injection drug users in one study, 13 percent ultimately met the case definition for definite or probable endocarditis. Only 4 of the 12 injection drug users suspected of having endocarditis in the emergency room proved to have this diagnosis, while 8 of 30 admitted with other diagnoses ultimately proved to have endocarditis. Bacterial pneumonia and minor illnesses were more frequent than endocarditis. The authors concluded that the accuracy of emergency room diagnosis is insufficient to distinguish between endocarditis and other conditions and that febrile injection drug users seen in emergency rooms should therefore be admitted for observation and/or therapy.

Injection drug users may self-medicate with oral antibiotics. This behavior, which is not always disclosed when the patient's medical history is taken, may be critically important in the evaluation of patients with suspected endocarditis because blood cultures may be falsely negative. The use of nonprescribed antibiotics before admission to the hospital is an important factor predicting endocarditis due to methicillin-resistant *S. aureus* among drug injectors.

All febrile injection drug users should have a careful history taken, with an emphasis on the frequency and type of drug injection and on antibiotic use. The physical examination should focus attention on the presence of septic emboli in the skin and on mucosal surfaces and the existence of regurgitant murmurs. Chest radiography should be used to detect the characteristic septic emboli or focal infections that may result in bacteremia. Ideally, three sets of blood samples—collected over several hours, as clinical exigency permits—should be cultured. Cardiac imaging studies are a valuable adjunct to diagnosis, although they cannot usually be undertaken at the time of initial presentation and are of variable sensitivity and specificity; false-negative results are frequent in right-sided involvement, and false-positive results also have been documented. Echocardiography may be invaluable in following patients with potentially unstable lesions (i.e., valvular incompetence or intramyocardial abscess).

℞ TREATMENT

After blood has been obtained for cultures, empirical antibiotic therapy should be instituted if patients are acutely ill, if left-sided endocarditis is strongly suspected, and/or if septic pulmonary emboli are seen on radiographs. However, it is not necessary to institute therapy for endocarditis in all injection drug users with fever. In fact, it is often reasonable to withhold antibiotics and to observe the patient carefully until the results of blood cultures are known. Some patients will be found to have a minor transient illness or a pyrogenic or hypersensitivity reaction to injected drugs and will defervesce within 24 h. In others, an alternative diagnosis will become apparent.

Appropriate empirical antibiotic therapy should be given parenterally and should always include an antistaphylococcal agent. Depending on local susceptibility patterns and the severity of the patient's illness, the agent selected is usually either a β-lactam antibiotic, such as oxacillin or nafcillin, or—if infection with methicillin-resistant *S. aureus* is suspected—vancomycin. If local patterns warrant, gram-negative coverage with an added aminoglycoside may be appropriate. For endocarditis due to methicillin-susceptible staphylococci, conventional therapy consists of 4 weeks of oxacillin or nafcillin at a dose of 1.5 to 2 g every 4 hours. In severe endocarditis, some clinicians add an aminoglycoside, usually gentamicin (1.5 mg/kg every 8 h) for the first 2 weeks of therapy; this addition may result in more rapid resolution of bacteremia, although an improved outcome has never been shown. In cases of allergy to penicillin or infection with methicillin-resistant *S. aureus*, vancomycin (1 g every 12 h) is given. Therapy targeting other organisms should be selected on the basis of antimicrobial susceptibility patterns. Treatment is usually given for 4 weeks. Successful treatment of uncomplicated right-sided endocarditis with a 2-week course of a β-lactam antibiotic plus an aminoglycoside has been reported. Given the difficulty of obtaining long-term secure intravenous access, this alternative regimen may prove valuable in selected cases. Most experts advocate parenteral therapy for the duration of the course, although this decision often necessitates the placement of an indwelling central line.

The prognosis of right-sided staphylococcal endocarditis in this population is excellent, with only rare deaths and an infrequent lack of response to medical therapy. Endocarditis caused by other organisms and left-sided involvement carry a more serious prognosis, with higher complication and fatality rates. The role of surgery remains controversial in this as in other populations with endocarditis (see Chap. 126). The criteria for surgical intervention should be the same as in other populations: intractable heart failure, undrained myocardial abscess, and failure of medical therapy, particularly in candidal or fungal endocarditis. The surgical approach varies with the cardiac valve(s) involved. Valve excision alone appears to be sufficient for severe tricuspid endocarditis. In mitral and aortic valve endocarditis, valve replacement is required and usually can be accomplished safely. Concerns about subsequent reinfection in the setting of continued injection drug use engender heated debates and require joint decisions by medical and surgical personnel and the patient.

PNEUMONIA (See also Chap. 255)   Community-acquired bacterial pneumonia, most often caused by *Streptococcus pneumoniae* and *Haemophilus influenzae*, was commonly described among drug injectors in the 1960s and 1970s. These infections were thought to be more frequent among drug users than among the general population. The putative risk factors in drug users included pulmonary aspiration resulting from intermittent overdose, deleterious effects of opiates on lung defenses and cough reflex, hypoventilation due to respiratory depression, and smoking.

These factors have all been outweighed by HIV infection, which has dramatically increased the risk of bacterial pneumonia in drug injectors. Beginning in the mid-1980s, epidemiologic surveillance data from New York City showed rising mortality from bacterial pneumonia and other bacterial infections among drug injectors—a phenomenon linked to HIV infection. In some cases, HIV-infected drug users died

from pyogenic bacterial infections even before the diagnosis of AIDS. Prospective studies demonstrated that even when they were not actively injecting drugs, HIV-infected drug users had a four- to fivefold greater risk of bacterial pneumonia and sepsis (up to 10 cases per 100 person-years) than their HIV-seronegative counterparts. Among febrile drug users presenting to an emergency room, pneumonia was the single largest diagnostic category, accounting for 38 percent of admissions.

The 1993 Revised AIDS Case Definition of the Centers for Disease Control and Prevention includes recurrent bacterial pneumonia in persons with HIV infection as an AIDS-defining condition. The organisms involved in HIV-related pneumonia among drug injectors are predominantly those reported in the earlier literature on community-acquired pneumonia in this group—*S. pneumoniae* and *H. influenzae*.

The clinical presentation of bacterial pneumonia and the strategies for its diagnosis and therapy are similar in injection drug users and in other populations, despite a wider array of differential diagnostic possibilities in the former group. The typical presentation includes fever, productive cough, pleuritic chest pain, and findings of consolidation and segmental or lobar infiltrates on chest radiography. Specific etiologic diagnosis requires cultures of sputum and/or blood. For uncomplicated community-acquired bacterial pneumonia, therapy aimed at *S. pneumoniae* and/or *H. influenzae*, given for 10 days to 2 weeks, is recommended. Many clinicians begin therapy with cefuroxime (1.5 g every 8 h). Therapeutic modifications are based on Gram's stain and culture results and on the clinical presentation and course. For uncomplicated pneumococcal pneumonia caused by a susceptible organism, penicillin G in a dose of 2 to 3 million units daily remains the drug of choice.

Among the infectious entities to be considered in the differential diagnosis of pulmonary infiltrates in this population of patients are septic pulmonary emboli, tuberculosis, and *Pneumocystis carinii* pneumonia (in patients infected with HIV). Noninfectious pulmonary complications of injection drug use also should be considered. Heroin-induced pulmonary edema, the most common of these complications, occurs most often in drug-use neophytes but also develops in experienced users exposed to particularly potent opiates and in persons who have resumed drug injection after a period of abstinence; this complication rapidly causes death by asphyxiation unless treated promptly with a narcotic antagonist (e.g., naloxone) and respiratory support.

The virtual universality of heavy cigarette smoking among drug injectors may not only predispose them to the usual sequelae of this behavior but also complicate the differential diagnosis of pulmonary symptoms (e.g., cough, shortness of breath, sputum production).

TUBERCULOSIS (See also Chap. 171)   The other important pulmonary infection described in drug injectors is tuberculosis. Infections due to *M. tuberculosis* were well documented in drug users before the AIDS epidemic, accounting for greater morbidity and mortality in this population than in the non-drug-using population. Although some authors attributed this greater impact to poverty, poor housing, and the social and demographic factors associated with both drug use and tuberculosis, others found an elevated risk of tuberculosis among drug users even after attempting to control for these other factors. AIDS has now overwhelmed all other potential risk factors and has resulted in a new epidemic of resurgent tuberculosis among HIV-infected drug users and their contacts (see Chaps. 171 and 308). Among persons with HIV infection, tuberculosis has disproportionately affected injection drug users. This observation may reflect higher levels of latent infection with *M. tuberculosis* in drug-using populations and associated environmental factors. In parts of the urban northeastern United States, where 20 percent of drug injectors have evidence of latent *M. tuberculosis* infection and 50 percent are infected with HIV, the overlap of these two endemic infections has resulted in an unprecedented increase in the incidence of tuberculosis since 1985. Both high rates of reactivation of latent infection (8 percent per 100 person-years) and increased transmission to susceptibles in community and hospital settings are responsible. Aggressive chemoprophylaxis with isoniazid, active case finding, and therapy are all essential.

Pulmonary tuberculosis should always be suspected and included in the differential diagnosis of pneumonia in injection drug users. Particularly among those with HIV infection, extrapulmonary tuberculosis has increased greatly in frequency. The unusually high incidence of both single-drug-resistant and multidrug-resistant (MDR) tuberculosis among injection drug users further complicates diagnosis and treatment in this population. MDR tuberculosis should be suspected in individuals with a history of treatment for tuberculosis, recent hospitalization or incarceration, or contact with a known case. The therapy administered to injection drug users is similar to that given to other populations. For nonresistant tuberculosis, a 2-month course of treatment with four drugs—isoniazid (5 mg/kg daily; maximum, 300 mg/d), rifampin (10 mg/kg daily; maximum, 600 mg/d), ethambutol (15 mg/kg daily; maximum, 1200 mg/d), and pyrazinamide (25 mg/kg daily; maximum, 2 g/d)—is followed by a 4-month course of isoniazid and rifampin alone. In patients with HIV infection, the duration of treatment is usually extended to 9 to 12 months. The treatment of MDR tuberculosis requires multiple additional drugs, usually including a quinolone and ethionamide. Special efforts must be made to ensure long-term adherence to the regimen, including direct observation of compliance with therapy.

SKELETAL INFECTIONS (See Chap. 132) Skeletal infections in injection drug users result both from hematogenous dissemination and, less commonly, from contiguous spread from chronically infected skin and soft tissue sites to underlying bone. In one series, skeletal infections represented 9 percent of admissions of injection drug users to a large urban hospital. Septic arthritis of large synovial joints may be seen during the course of staphylococcal endocarditis or of bacteremia arising from other infected sites and may appear as a complication of disseminated gonococcal disease. The joints most frequently involved are the knees, hips, shoulders, and elbows, but there is a predilection for the involvement of unusual joints as well—e.g., the vertebral column; the symphysis pubis; and the sternoclavicular, sternochondral, and sacroiliac joints. These infections are usually unilateral and subacute, with an indolent, progressive course characterized by pain, limitation of motion, and absence of fever. The diagnosis may be easily overlooked. Point tenderness over the affected joint is usually elicited. Sternoarticular infections are often associated with soft tissue swelling of the chest wall and bacteremia. Vertebral osteomyelitis may be associated with paraspinal soft tissue masses and (in cases of posterior extension) with the formation of spinal epidural abscesses. Radiologic and imaging studies may suggest the diagnosis by findings that are most characteristic of vertebral osteomyelitis, where the disk space is lost, contiguous bone erosion and new bone formation are evident, and several vertebrae are involved. Infection of the sacroiliac joints and symphysis pubis results in joint-space separation and erosion of the articular surfaces.

S. aureus is the pathogen most commonly isolated from sites of skeletal infection, but gram-negative organisms—notably *P. aeruginosa*, *S. marcescens*, and fungi—also have been well documented. *M. tuberculosis* should be included in the differential diagnosis, particularly in cases of vertebral osteomyelitis. Because etiologic agents and their antimicrobial susceptibilities vary, efforts should be made to obtain a specific microbiologic diagnosis. This process may involve diagnostic aspiration or closed or open biopsy, with fluid or material sent for staining and culture for bacterial, mycobacterial, and fungal pathogens.

Treatment consists of a combination of drainage of the synovial joints and the contiguous soft tissue collections and prolonged administration of appropriate high-dose antimicrobial therapy. For *S. aureus*, oxacillin—or, in cases of intolerance or resistance, vancomycin—is given for 4 to 6 weeks. *Pseudomonas* infections require an active third-generation cephalosporin and an aminoglycoside.

CENTRAL NERVOUS SYSTEM COMPLICATIONS The nervous system—in particular, the central nervous system—is an important site for adverse sequelae of drug injection. Drug injectors are at increased risk for certain noninfectious complications, including intracerebral hemorrhage and other stroke syndromes (especially with cocaine and amphetamine use), particulate emboli to the brain and spinal cord, vasculitis, and the consequences of head trauma. Among the infectious complications, the most common is systemic embolization to the brain as a result of bacterial endocarditis or bacteremia, which frequently involves multiple small septic emboli from either aortic or mitral valve vegetations. Patients may present with focal neurologic deficits, seizures, altered mental status, and/or meningismus. *S. aureus* and other bacteria that cause endocarditis in drug injectors are most commonly involved in these manifestations. Cerebral mycotic aneurysms and spinal and epidural abscesses also have been described as complications of endocarditis in this population. Less commonly, drug users have been reported to be at risk for focal brain abscesses that are unrelated to endocarditis and are caused by organisms such as *Aspergillus*, *Mucor*, other fungi, and *Nocardia*. There is also evidence that tuberculous meningitis and focal tuberculomas of the brain may be more common among drug users than among other patients with tuberculosis, with or without HIV infection. Finally, ocular infections, including episcleritis, chorioretinitis, and endophthalmitis, have been well described in drug injectors, involving such organisms as *Bacillus cereus*, *Aspergillus*, and *Candida albicans*.

HEPATITIS (See also Chaps. 295 and 297) Injection drug users have long been known to be at high risk for hepatitis, primarily through parenteral transmission. The acquisition of hepatitis B is a relatively early event for most drug injectors, occurring within the first several years of illicit drug use. Since the 1970s, seroprevalence studies in a wide range of drug-using populations have indicated that 75 to 90 percent of long-term drug injectors have serologic evidence of past exposure to hepatitis B. Approximately 5 to 10 percent of these individuals will remain chronic carriers of hepatitis B surface antigen; the remainder will develop immunity to hepatitis, producing antibody to hepatitis B core antigen and/or to hepatitis B surface antigen.

Another infectious agent commonly found in drug injectors is hepatitis D virus, previously referred to as the *delta agent*. This defective hepatotropic RNA virus depends on coexisting infection with hepatitis B virus for expression and replication. Antibody to hepatitis D virus has been found in 10 to 15 percent of patients with antibody to hepatitis B surface or core antigen and in as many as 50 to 70 percent of patients with chronic carriage of hepatitis B surface antigen. Fulminant hepatitis B may show a characteristic biphasic pattern in the setting of hepatitis D coinfection. Moreover, hepatitis D has been associated among drug users with chronic active hepatitis and persistent abnormalities of liver function.

The third significant bloodborne agent of hepatitis in injection drug users is hepatitis C virus. In seroprevalence studies in the United States and Europe, antibody to hepatitis C virus has been detected at levels of 70 percent or higher among drug injectors—a rate reflecting a level of infection comparable to that for hepatitis B. Like hepatitis B, hepatitis C appears to be acquired relatively soon after the start of illicit drug injection. Hepatitis C has been associated with chronic active hepatitis, persistent abnormalities of liver function, and cirrhosis. Interferon α may be of benefit in patients with progressive hepatitis B or hepatitis C. Treatment with interferon α has not yet been widely administered to drug users, however, and its requisite duration is unknown.

Although not considered to be a bloodborne infection, hepatitis A has been associated with injection drug use. Several surveillance-based investigations have indicated that injection drug users may have up to a 50-fold higher risk of acquiring hepatitis A than non-injection drug users. In addition, recent outbreaks of hepatitis A have been linked to groups of injection drug users in both the United States and Europe. Investigation of these outbreaks has suggested that fecal-oral contamination, close personal contact, and poor hygiene were more likely than viral contamination of drugs or injection equipment to be responsible for spread of the disease.

These observations suggest that in long-term drug injectors with known past exposure to hepatitis B and/or hepatitis C, hepatitis A (and—for chronic carriers of hepatitis B—hepatitis D) should be strongly considered in the differential diagnosis of new-onset acute hepatitis syndromes. The acquisition of bloodborne hepatitis soon after the start of illicit injection drug use suggests the importance of developing public health strategies that will reach adolescent and young-adult drug users with information about preventive interventions (such as hepatitis B vaccine) and risk-reducing behaviors.

While most hepatitis infections in drug users do not progress to chronic forms of clinically significant hepatitis or cirrhosis, at least 40 percent of most series of entrants into drug-treatment programs exhibit abnormalities of liver function. In addition to infectious causes, the toxic effects of adulterants used in the production of illicit drugs and the hepatotoxic effects of alcohol are responsible in part for these abnormalities. Hepatic cirrhosis in drug users is most often associated with coexisting alcohol abuse.

HTLV-I/II Injection drug users are at relatively high risk not only for infection with HIV but also for that with human T-cell lymphotropic virus (HTLV) types I and II (see Chap. 192). In the United States, injection drug use has been the most important behavioral factor associated with the presence of antibody to HTLV-I/II in blood donors screened for retroviral infection. Seroprevalence studies in the United States have documented HTLV-I/II infection in more than 10 percent of certain populations of drug users. HTLV infection has often been associated with black race, older age, and a history of heroin injection. Rates of infection have shown wide geographic variation. More than three-fourths of the HTLV infections in drug injectors are due to HTLV-II; this observation may account for the relatively low rate of clinical disease reported to date in patients with such infections. Two studies have suggested, however, that coinfection with HTLV-I/II and HIV may be associated with more rapid progression of HIV infection and earlier mortality.

HARM REDUCTION FOR INJECTION DRUG USERS

The myriad infectious consequences of injection drug use mandate the development of preventive harm-reduction strategies based on the principle that, since many drug users will continue to inject drugs, they should do so in a way that minimizes harm to themselves and others. Prevention of the infectious complications of injection and education about more hygienic injection practices are primary goals. Legalization of the purchase and possession of needles and syringes and institution of needle- and syringe-exchange programs are the most obvious examples of the harm-reduction approach. In addition to the distribution or exchange of injection equipment, needle-exchange programs typically include AIDS education, condom distribution, and enrollment in a variety of medical and social services.

Provision of primary medical care services linked to drug-abuse treatment is a way to promote preventive regimens to enhance harm reduction. In this and all other clinical settings, injection drug users should be routinely screened for hepatitis B, latent *M. tuberculosis* infection, and syphilis and other sexually transmitted diseases. They should be offered pneumococcal, influenza, tetanus, and hepatitis B immunization and (when appropriate) prophylaxis for tuberculosis and complications of HIV disease.

Clearly, the ultimate goal of harm-reduction strategies should be the reduction or prevention of illicit drug use itself, with the elimination of its root causes. Nonetheless, a high priority must also be assigned to the development of strategies that will minimize the serious medical consequences of drug abuse.

BIBLIOGRAPHY

ALCABES P, FRIEDLAND G: Injection drug use and human immunodeficiency virus infection. Clin Infect Dis 20:1467, 1995

ALLAND D et al: Transmission of tuberculosis in New York City: An analysis by DNA fingerprinting and conventional epidemiologic methods. N Engl J Med 330:1710, 1994

CENTERS FOR DISEASE CONTROL AND PREVENTION: Initial therapy for tuberculosis in the era of multi-drug resistance. Morb Mort Week Rep 42(RR-7):1, 1993

————: National action plan to combat multi-drug-resistant tuberculosis; meeting the challenge of multi-drug-resistant tuberculosis; management of persons exposed to multi-drug-resistant tuberculosis. Morb Mort Week Rep 41(RR-11):1, 1992

CHAMBERS HF et al: *Staphylococcus aureus* endocarditis: Clinical manifestations in addicts and non-addicts. Medicine 62:170, 1983

———— et al: Right-sided *Staphylococcus aureus* endocarditis in intravenous drug users: Two-week combination therapy. Ann Intern Med 109:619, 1988

CHANDRASEKAR PH, NARULA AP: Bone and joint infections in intravenous drug abusers. Rev Infect Dis 8:904, 1986

CHERUBIN CE, SAPIRA JD: The medical complications of drug addiction and the medical assessment of the intravenous drug user: 25 years later. Ann Intern Med 119:1017, 1993

FELTON CP: Pulmonary infections in the addict, in *Medical Aspects of Drug Abuse*, RW Richter (ed). Hagerstown, MD, Harper & Row, 1975

FRIEDEN TR et al: The emergence of drug-resistant tuberculosis in New York City. N Engl J Med 328:521, 1993

HAVERKOS HW, LANGE WR: Serious infections other than human immunodeficiency virus among intravenous drug users. J Infect Dis 161:894, 1990

HIRSCHTICK RE et al: Bacterial pneumonia in persons infected with the human immunodeficiency virus. N Engl J Med 333:845, 1995

ISEMAN MD et al: Directly observed treatment of tuberculosis. N Engl J Med 328:576, 1993

KHABBAZ RA et al: Seroprevalence of HTLV-I and HTLV-II among intravenous drug persons in clinics for sexually transmitted diseases. N Engl J Med 326:375, 1992

LETTAU LA et al: Outbreak of severe hepatitis due to delta and hepatitis B viruses in parenteral drug abusers and their contacts. N Engl J Med 317:1256, 1987

LEVINE DP, SOBEL JD (eds): *Infections in Intravenous Drug Abusers.* New York, Oxford University Press, 1991

LURIE P et al: *The Public Health Impact of Needle-Exchange Programs in the United States and Abroad.* San Francisco, University of California, 1993

MARANTZ PR et al: Inability to predict diagnosis in febrile intravenous drug abusers. Ann Intern Med 106:823, 1978

SANDE MA et al: Endocarditis in intravenous drug users, in *Infective Endocarditis,* 2d ed, D Kaye (ed). New York, Raven Press, 1992, pp 345–359

SELWYN PA et al: Clinical manifestations and predictors of disease progression in drug users with human immunodeficiency virus infection. N Engl J Med 327:1697, 1992

STONEBURNER RL et al: A larger spectrum of severe HIV-1 related disease in intravenous drug users in New York City. Science 242:916, 1988

135

Lawrence C. Madoff

INFECTIONS FROM BITES, SCRATCHES, AND BURNS

The skin is an essential component of the nonspecific immune system, protecting the host from potential pathogens in the environment. Breaches in this protective barrier thus represent a form of immunocompromise that predisposes the patient to infection. Bites and scratches from animals and humans allow the inoculation of microorganisms past the skin's protective barrier into deeper, susceptible host tissues. Thermal burns may cause massive destruction of the integument as well as derangements in humoral and cellular immunity, enabling environmental opportunists and components of the host's own skin flora to cause infection.

ANIMAL BITES AND SCRATCHES Each year in the United States, between 1 and 2 million animal-bite wounds are sustained; the vast majority are inflicted by pet dogs and cats, which number more than 100 million. Other bite wounds are a consequence of encounters with animals in the wild or in occupational settings. While many of these wounds require minimal or no therapy, a significant number result in infection, which may be life-threatening. The microbiology of bite-wound infections in general reflects the oropharyngeal flora of the biting animal, although organisms from the soil, the skin of the animal and victim, and the animal's feces may also be involved.

Dog Bites Dogs are responsible for approximately 80 percent of bite wounds, an estimated 15 to 20 percent of which become infected. Most dog bites are provoked and inflicted by the victim's pet or by a dog known to the victim. These bites frequently occur during efforts to break up a dogfight. Victims tend to be male, and bites most often involve a lower extremity. Infection typically manifests 8 to 24 h after the bite as pain at the site of injury with cellulitis accompanied by purulent, sometimes foul-smelling discharge. Septic arthritis and osteomyelitis may develop if the canine tooth penetrates synovium or bone. Systemic manifestations such as fever, lymphadenopathy, and lymphangitis also may occur. The microbiology of dog-bite wound infections is usually mixed and includes alpha-hemolytic streptococci, *Staphylococcus* species, *Pasteurella multocida*, *Eikenella corrodens*, and *Capnocytophaga canimorsus* (formerly designated DF-2). Many wounds also include anaerobic bacteria such as *Actinomyces*, *Fusobacterium*, *Prevotella*, and *Porphyromonas* species.

While most infections resulting from dog-bite injuries are localized to the area of injury, many of the microorganisms involved are capable of causing systemic infection, including bacteremia, meningitis, brain abscess, endocarditis, and chorioamnionitis. These infections are particularly likely in hosts with edema or compromised lymphatic drainage in the involved extremity (e.g., after radical or modified radical mastectomy) and in patients who are immunocompromised by medication or disease (e.g., glucocorticoid use, systemic lupus erythematosus, acute leukemia, or hepatic cirrhosis). In addition, dog bites and scratches may result in systemic illnesses such as rabies (Chap. 199) and tetanus (Chap. 146).

Infection with *C. canimorsus* following dog-bite wounds may result in fulminant sepsis, disseminated intravascular coagulation, and renal failure, particularly in hosts who have impaired hepatic function, who have undergone splenectomy, or who are immunosuppressed. This organism is a thin gram-negative rod that is difficult to culture on most solid media but grows in a variety of liquid media. The bacteria are occasionally seen within polymorphonuclear leukocytes on Wright-stained smears of peripheral blood from septic patients.

Cat Bites Although less common than dog bites, more than half of all cat bites and scratches result in infection. Because the narrow, sharp feline incisors penetrate deeply into tissue, cat bites are more likely than dog bites to cause septic arthritis and osteomyelitis; the development of these conditions is particularly likely when punctures are located over or near a joint, especially in the hand. Women sustain cat bites more frequently than do men. These bites most often involve the hands and arms. Both bites and scratches from cats are prone to infection from organisms in the cat's oropharynx. *P. multocida*, a normal component of the feline oral flora, is a small gram-negative coccobacillus implicated in the majority of cat-bite wound infections. Like that of dog-bite wound infections, however, the microflora of cat-bite wound infections is usually mixed. Other microorganisms causing infection after cat bites are similar to those causing dog-bite wound infections.

The same risk factors for systemic infection following dog-bite wounds apply to cat-bite wounds. *Pasteurella* infections tend to advance rapidly, often within hours, causing severe inflammation accompanied by purulent drainage; *Pasteurella* may also be spread by respiratory droplets from animals, resulting in pneumonia or bacteremia. Like dog-bite wounds, cat-bite wounds may result in the transmission of rabies or in the development of tetanus. Infection with *Bartonella henselae* causes cat-scratch disease (Chap. 165) and is an important late consequence of cat bites and scratches. Tularemia (Chap. 163) has also been reported to follow cat bites.

Other Animal Bites Infections have been attributed to bites from many animal species, often as a consequence of occupational exposure (farmers, laboratory workers, veterinarians) or recreational exposure (hunters and trappers, wilderness campers, owners of exotic pets). Generally, the microflora of bite wounds reflects the oral flora of the biting animal. Most members of the cat family, including feral cats, harbor *P. multocida*. Bite wounds from aquatic animals such as alligators or piranhas may contain *Aeromonas hydrophila*. Venomous snakebites (Chap. 392) result in severe inflammatory responses and tissue necrosis, which renders these injuries prone to infection. The snake's oral flora includes many species of aerobes and anaerobes, such as *Pseudomonas aeruginosa*, *Proteus* species, *Staphylococcus epidermidis*, *Bacteroides fragilis*, and *Clostridium* species. Bites from nonhuman primates are highly susceptible to infection with pathogens similar to those isolated from human bites (which are discussed later in this chapter). Bites from Old World monkeys (*Macaca*) may also result in the transmission of B virus (*Herpesvirus simiae*, cercopithecine herpesvirus), a cause of serious infection of the human central nervous system. Bites of seals, walruses, and polar bears may cause a chronic suppurative infection known as seal finger, which is probably due to one or more species of *Mycoplasma* colonizing these animals.

Rat-bite fever Small rodents, including rats, mice, and gerbils, as well as animals that prey on rodents may transmit *Streptobacillus moniliformis* (a microaerophilic, pleomorphic gram-negative rod) or *Spirillum minor* (a spirochete), which cause a clinical illness known as rat-bite fever. The vast majority of cases in the United States are streptobacillary, whereas *Spirillum* infection occurs mainly in Asia.

In the United States, the risk of rodent bite mainly affects laboratory workers or inhabitants of rodent-infested dwellings (particularly children). Rat-bite fever is distinguished from acute bite-wound infection by its typical manifestation after the initial wound has healed. Streptobacillary disease follows an incubation period of 3 to 10 days. Fever, chills, myalgias, headache, and severe migratory arthralgias are usually followed by a maculopapular rash, which characteristically involves the palms and soles and may become confluent or purpuric. Complications include endocarditis, myocarditis, meningitis, pneumonia, and abscesses in many organs. *Haverhill fever* is an *S. moniliformis* infection acquired from contaminated milk or drinking water and has similar manifestations. Streptobacillary rat-bite fever was frequently fatal in the preantibiotic era. The differential diagnosis includes Rocky Mountain spotted fever, Lyme disease, leptospirosis, and secondary syphilis. The diagnosis is made by direct observation of the causative organisms in tissue or blood, by culture on enriched media, or by serologic testing with specific agglutinins.

Spirillum infection (referred to in Japan as *sodoku*) causes pain and purple swelling at the site of the initial bite, with associated lymphangitis and regional lymphadenopathy, after an incubation period of 1 to 4 weeks. The systemic illness includes fever, chills, and headache. The original lesion may eventually progress to an eschar. The infection is diagnosed by direct visualization of the spirochetes in blood or tissue or by animal inoculation.

Erysipeloid This distinctive skin infection is caused by direct cutaneous inoculation with *Erysipelothrix rhusiopathiae*. Because this organism is most often associated with fish and domestic swine, erysipeloid most commonly results from an occupational injury related to fishing ("fish-handler's disease") or slaughterhouse work; it may also follow contact with other animals or contact with fish or meat in a household setting. After an incubation period of several days, pain (often severe), edema, and a well-demarcated, purplish-red lesion develop. Systemic manifestations are unusual, but bacteremia and endocarditis have occasionally been reported. Definitive diagnosis requires isolation of the bacteria from a biopsy specimen, a tissue aspirate, or blood.

Human bite infections Human bites may be self-inflicted, may be sustained by medical personnel caring for patients, or may take place during fights or domestic abuse or during sexual activity. Human bites more frequently become infected than do bites inflicted by other animals. These infections reflect the diverse oral microflora of humans, which includes multiple species of aerobic and anaerobic bacteria. Common aerobic isolates include viridans streptococci, *Staphylococcus aureus*, *E. corrodens* (which is particularly common in clenched-fist injury; see below), and *Haemophilus influenzae*. Anaerobic species, including *Fusobacterium nucleatum* and *Prevotella*, *Porphyromonas*, *Peptococcus*, and *Peptostreptococcus* species, are isolated from 50 percent of human-bite wound infections; many of these isolates produce β-lactamases. The oral flora of hospitalized and debilitated patients often includes Enterobacteriaceae in addition to the usual organisms. Human immunodeficiency virus and hepatitis B virus have both been reported to be transmitted by human bite, but these instances appear to be quite rare.

Human bites are categorized as *occlusional* injuries, which are inflicted by actual biting, and *clenched-fist* injuries, which are sustained when the fist of one individual strikes the teeth of another, causing traumatic laceration of the hand. For several reasons, clenched-fist injuries result in particularly serious infections. The deep spaces of the hand, including the bone, joint, and tendons, are frequently inoculated with organisms in the course of such injuries. The clenched position of the fist during injury, followed by extension of the hand, may further promote the introduction of bacteria as contaminated tendons retract beneath the skin's surface. Moreover, medical attention often is sought only after frank infection develops.

TREATMENT

Initial Assessment A careful history should be elicited, including the type of biting animal, the type of attack (provoked or unprovoked), and the amount of time elapsed since injury. Local and regional authorities should be contacted to determine whether an individual species could be rabid and/or to locate and observe the biting animal when rabies prophylaxis may be indicated. Suspicious human-bite wounds should provoke careful questioning regarding domestic or child abuse. Details on antibiotic allergies, immunosuppression, splenectomy, liver disease, mastectomy, and immunization history should be obtained. The wound should be inspected carefully for evidence of infection, including redness, exudate, and foul odor. The type of wound (puncture, laceration, or scratch), the depth of penetration, and the possible involvement of joints, tendons, nerves, and bone should be assessed. It is often useful to include a diagram or photograph of the wound in the medical record. In addition, a general physical examination should be conducted and should include an assessment of vital signs as well as an evaluation for evidence of lymphangitis, lymphadenopathy, dermatologic lesions, and functional limitations. Injuries to the hand warrant consultation with a hand surgeon for the assessment of tendon, nerve, and muscular damage. Radiographs should be obtained when the bone may have been penetrated or a tooth fragment may be present. Culture and Gram's staining of all infected wounds are essential; anaerobic cultures should be undertaken if abscesses, devitalized tissue, or foul-smelling exudate is present. A small-tipped swab may be used to culture deep punctures or small lacerations. It is also reasonable to culture samples from uninfected wounds due to bites inflicted by animals other than dogs and cats, since the microorganisms causing disease are less predictable in these cases. A white blood cell count should be determined and blood cultured if systemic infection is suspected.

Wound Management Wound closure is controversial in bite injuries. Many authorities prefer not to attempt primary closure of wounds that are or may become infected, preferring to irrigate these wounds copiously, debride devitalized tissue, remove foreign bodies, and approximate the wound edges. Delayed primary closure may be undertaken after the risk of infection is over. Small uninfected wounds may be allowed to close by secondary intention. Puncture wounds due to cat bites should be left unsutured because of the high rate at which they become infected. Facial wounds are usually sutured after thorough cleaning and irrigation because of the importance of a good cosmetic result in this area and because anatomic factors such as an excellent blood supply and the absence of dependent edema lessen the risk of infection.

Antibiotic Therapy Antibiotics should be administered in all established bite-wound infections and should be chosen in light of the most likely potential pathogens, as indicated by the biting species and by Gram's stain and culture results (Table 135-1). For dog and cat bites, antibiotics should be effective against *S. aureus*, *P. multocida*, *C. canimorsus*, streptococci, and oral anaerobes. For human bites, agents with activity against *S. aureus*, *H. influenzae*, and β-lactamase-positive oral anaerobes should be used. The combination of an extended-spectrum penicillin with a β-lactamase inhibitor (amoxicillin/clavulanic acid, ticarcillin/clavulanic acid, ampicillin/sulbactam) appears to offer the most reliable coverage for these pathogens. Second-generation cephalosporins (cefuroxime, cefoxitin) also offer substantial coverage. The choice of antibiotics in penicillin-allergic patients (particularly those in whom immediate-type hypersensitivity makes the use of cephalosporins hazardous) is more difficult and is based primarily on in vitro sensitivity since data on clinical efficacy are inadequate. The combination of an antibiotic active against gram-positive cocci and anaerobes (such as clindamycin) with trimethoprim-sulfamethoxazole or a fluoroquinolone, which has activity against many of the other potential pathogens, would appear reasonable.

Antibiotics are normally given for 10 to 14 days, but the response to therapy must be carefully monitored. Failure to respond should prompt a consideration of diagnostic alternatives and surgical evaluation for possible drainage or debridement. Complications such as osteomyelitis or septic arthritis mandate a longer duration of therapy.

Management of *C. canimorsus* sepsis requires a 2-week course of intravenous penicillin G (2 million units intravenously every 4 h) and supportive measures. Alternative agents for the treatment of *C. canimorsus* infection include cephalosporins and fluoroquinolones. Serious infection with *P. multocida* (e.g., pneumonia, sepsis, or meningitis) should also be treated with intravenous penicillin G. Alternative agents include second- or third-generation cephalosporins or ciprofloxacin.

Bites by venomous snakes may not require antibiotic treatment, but it is often difficult to distinguish signs of infection from tissue damage caused by the envenomation. Thus many authorities continue to recommend treatment directed against the snake's oral flora—i.e., the administration of broadly active agents such as ceftriaxone (1 to 2 g intravenously every 12 to 24 h) or ampicillin/sulbactam (1.5 to 3.0 g intravenously every 6 h).

Seal finger appears to respond to doxycycline (100 mg twice daily). *E. rhusiopathiae* is sensitive to most β-lactam antibiotics, including penicillin, as well as to ciprofloxacin. Its resistance to vancomycin, which is unusual among gram-positive bacteria, is of potential clinical significance since this agent is sometimes used in empirical therapy for skin infection.

The use of antibiotics in patients presenting early after bite injury (within 8 h) is controversial. Although symptomatic infection will not yet be manifest in many of these wounds at this point, many early wounds will harbor pathogens, and many will become infected. Studies of the use of prophylactic antibiotics in wound infections are limited and have often included small numbers of cases in which various types of wounds have been managed according to various protocols. A recent meta-analysis of eight randomized trials of prophylactic antibiotics in patients with dog-bite wounds demonstrated a reduction of the rate of infection by approximately 50 percent with prophylaxis. However, in the absence of sound clinical trials, many clinicians base the decision to treat bite wounds presumptively with empirical antibiotics on the species of the biting animal; the location, severity, and extent of the bite wound; and the existence of comorbid conditions in the host (Table 135-1). All human- and monkey-bite wounds should be treated presumptively because of the high rate of infection. Most cat-bite wounds, particularly those involving the hand, should be treated. Other factors favoring treatment for bite wounds include severe injury, as in crush wounds; potential bone or joint involvement; involvement of the hands or genital region; host immunocompromise, including that due to liver disease or splenectomy; and prior mastectomy on the side of an involved upper extremity. When prophylactic antibiotics are administered, they are usually given for 3 to 5 days.

Rabies prophylaxis, consisting of both passive administration of rabies immune globulin and active immunization with the human diploid vaccine, should be given in consultation with local and regional public health authorities for many wild-animal (and some domestic-animal) bites and scratches as well as for certain nonbite exposures (see Chap. 199). Rabies is endemic in a variety of animals, including dogs and cats in many areas of the world. Many local

Table 135-1

Management of Wound Infections Following Animal Bites

Biting Species	Commonly Isolated Pathogens	Preferred Antibiotic(s)*	Alternative Agent for Penicillin-Allergic Patient	Recommendation for Prophylaxis in Patients with Recent Uninfected Wounds	Other Considerations
Dog	*Staphylococcus aureus, Pasteurella multocida,* anaerobes, *Capnocytophaga canimorsus*	Amoxicillin/clavulanic acid (250–500 mg PO tid); or ampicillin/ sulbactam (1.5–3.0 g IV q6h)	Clindamycin (150–300 mg PO qid) plus either TMP-SMZ (1 double-strength tablet bid) or ciprofloxacin (500 mg PO bid)	Sometimes†	Consider rabies prophylaxis.
Cat	*P. multocida, S. aureus,* anaerobes	Amoxicillin/clavulanic acid or ampicillin/ sulbactam, as for dog bite	Clindamycin plus either TMP-SMZ or a fluoroquinolone	Usually	Consider rabies prophylaxis; carefully evaluate for joint/bone penetration.
Human; occlusional bite	Viridans streptococci, *S. aureus, Haemophilus influenzae,* anaerobes	Amoxicillin/clavulanic acid or ampicillin/ sulbactam, as for dog bite	Erythromycin, fluoroquinolone	Always	—
Human; clenched-fist injury	As for occlusional bite plus *Eikenella corrodens*	Ampicillin/sulbactam as for dog bite or imipenem	Cefoxitin‡ (1.5 g IV q6h)	Always	Examine for tendon/nerve/ joint involvement.
Monkey	As for human bite	As for human bite	As for human bite	Always	For macaque monkeys, consider B virus prophylaxis with acyclovir.
Snake	*Pseudomonas aeruginosa, Proteus* species, *Bacteroides fragilis, Clostridium* species	Ampicillin/sulbactam as for dog bite	Clindamycin plus either TMP-SMZ or a fluoroquinolone	Sometimes, especially for venomous snakebite	Use antivenin for venomous snakebite.
Rodent	*Streptobacillus moniliformis, Leptospira* species, *P. multocida*	Penicillin VK (500 mg PO bid)	Doxycycline (100 mg PO qd)	Sometimes†	—

* Antibiotic choices should be based on culture data, when available. These suggestions for empirical therapy need to be tailored to individual circumstances and local conditions. Intravenous regimens should be used for hospitalized patients. When the patient is to be discharged after initial management, a single intravenous dose of antibiotic may be given and followed by oral therapy. TMP-SMZ, trimethoprim-sulfamethoxazole.

† Prophylactic antibiotics are suggested for severe or extensive wounds, facial wounds, or crush injuries; when bone or joint may be involved; or when comorbidity exists (see text).

‡ Cefoxitin may be hazardous to patients with immediate-type hypersensitivity to penicillin.

health authorities require the reporting of all animal bites. A tetanus booster immunization should be given if the patient has undergone primary immunization but has not received a booster dose in the past 5 years. Patients who have not previously undergone primary immunization should be immunized and should also receive tetanus immune globulin. Elevation of the site of injury is an important adjunct to antimicrobial therapy. Immobilization of the infected area, especially the hand, is also beneficial.

INFECTIONS CAUSED BY *AEROMONAS* AND *PLESIO-MONAS* Two species of gram-negative bacilli, members of the family Pseudomonadaceae, are found in fresh and brackish coastal waters and are occasional causes of human disease. *Aeromonas* species may be inoculated into wounds exposed to salt water or freshwater or into injuries caused by fish or shellfish implicated in skin and soft tissue infection. Bacteremic illness may occur in immunocompromised patients and in those with hepatobiliary disease. *Aeromonas* has also been associated with diarrhea, particularly among travelers. *Plesiomonas shigelloides* has also been implicated in diarrhea, usually that developing in association with exposure to contaminated food or water. This organism can cause bacteremia and meningitis; most cases involve immunocompromised patients. Both *Aeromonas* and *Plesiomonas* exhibit variable antibiotic sensitivities but are most often susceptible to chloramphenicol, trimethoprim-sulfamethoxazole, quinolones, imipenem, and third-generation cephalosporins.

BURNS **Epidemiology** More than 2 million burn injuries are brought to medical attention in the United States each year. While many burn injuries are minor and require little or no intervention, approximately 70,000 persons are hospitalized for these injuries, and 20,000 of this number are burned severely enough to require admission to a specialized burn unit. Scalds, structural fires, and flammable liquids and gases are the major causes of burns, but electrical, chemical, and smoking-related sources are also important. Burns predispose to infection by damaging the protective barrier function of the skin, thus facilitating the entry of pathogenic microorganisms, and by inducing systemic immunosuppression. It is therefore not surprising that infectious complications are the major cause of morbidity and mortality in serious burn injury and that as many as 10,000 patients in the United States die of burn-related infections each year.

Pathophysiology Loss of the cutaneous barrier facilitates entry of the patient's own flora and of organisms from the hospital environment into the burn wound. The wound often contains devitalized or frankly necrotic tissue that quickly becomes contaminated with bacteria. Invasive infection—localized and/or systemic—occurs when bacteria penetrate viable tissue, usually below the eschar. Streptococci and staphylococci were the predominant causes of burn-wound infection in the preantibiotic era and remain important pathogens at present. With the advent of antimicrobial agents, *P. aeruginosa* became a major problem in burn-wound management. As antibiotics more effective against *Pseudomonas* have become available, fungal infections (particularly those due to *Candida albicans, Aspergillus* species, and the agents of mucormycosis) have emerged as increasingly important pathogens in burn-wound patients. Herpes simplex virus infection has also been found in burn wounds, especially on the face.

The frequency of infection parallels the extent and severity of burn injury. Severe burns cause defects in both cellular and humoral immunity that have a major impact on infection. For example, decreases in the number and activity of circulating helper T cells, increases in suppressor T cells, and diminution in levels of immunoglobulin follow major burns. Neutrophil function has also been shown to be impaired after burns. The increased levels of multiple cytokines detected in burn patients are compatible with the widely held belief that the inflammatory response becomes dysregulated in these individuals. Increased permeability of the gut wall to bacteria and their components, such as endotoxin, also contributes to immune dysregulation and sepsis. Thus, the burn patient is predisposed to infection at remote sites (see below) as well as at the sites of burn injury.

Clinical Manifestations Since clinical indications of wound infection are difficult to interpret, wounds must be monitored carefully for changes that may reflect infection. A margin of erythema frequently surrounds the sites of burns and by itself is not usually indicative of infection. Signs of infection include the conversion of a partial-thickness to a full-thickness burn, color changes (e.g., the appearance of a dark brown or black discoloration of the wound), the new appearance of erythema or violaceous edema in normal tissue at the wound margins, the sudden separation of the eschar from subcutaneous tissues, and the degeneration of the wound with the appearance of a new eschar. The appearance of a green discoloration of the wound or subcutaneous fat or the development of ecthyma gangrenosum at a remote site points to a diagnosis of invasive *P. aeruginosa* infection. Changes in body temperature, hypotension, tachycardia, altered mentation, neutropenia or neutrophilia, thrombocytopenia, and renal failure may result from invasive burn wounds and sepsis. However, because profound alterations in homeostasis occur as a consequence of burns per se and because inflammation without infection is a normal component of these injuries, the assessment of these changes is complicated. Alterations in body temperature, for example, are attributable to thermoregulatory dysfunction; tachycardia and hyperventilation accompany the metabolic changes induced by extensive burn injury and are not necessarily indicative of bacterial sepsis.

Given the difficulty of evaluating burn wounds solely on the basis of clinical observation and laboratory data, wound biopsies are necessary for definitive diagnosis of infection. The timing of these biopsies can be guided by clinical changes, but in some centers burn wounds are routinely biopsied at 48-h intervals. The biopsy specimen is examined for histologic evidence of bacterial invasion, and quantitative microbiologic cultures are performed. The presence of $>10^5$ viable bacteria per gram of tissue is highly suggestive of invasive infection and of a dramatically increased risk of sepsis. Histopathologic evidence of invasion of viable tissue by microorganisms is a more definitive indicator of infection. A blood culture positive for the same organism seen in high quantities in biopsied tissue is a reliable indicator of burn sepsis. Surface cultures may provide some indication of the microorganisms present in the hospital environment but are not indicative of the etiology of infection.

In addition to infection of the burn wound itself, a number of other infections due to the immunosuppression caused by extensive burns and the manipulations necessary for clinical care put burn patients at risk. Pneumonia, now the most common infectious complication among hospitalized burn patients, most often is nosocomially acquired via the respiratory route; septic pulmonary emboli may also occur. Suppurative thrombophlebitis may complicate the vascular catheterization necessary for fluid and nutritional support in burns. Endocarditis, urinary tract infection, bacterial chondritis (particularly in patients with burned ears), and intraabdominal infection also complicate serious burn injury.

TREATMENT

The ultimate goal of burn-wound management is closure and healing of the wound. Early surgical excision of burned tissue, with extensive debridement of necrotic tissue and grafting of skin or skin substitutes, greatly decreases the mortality associated with severe burns. In addition, the three widely used topical antimicrobial agents—silver sulfadiazene cream, mafenide acetate cream, and silver nitrate—dramatically decrease the bacterial burden of burn wounds and re-

duce the incidence of burn-wound infection; they are routinely applied to partial- and full-thickness burns. All three agents are broadly active against many bacteria and against some fungi and are useful before bacterial colonization is established. Silver sulfadiazene is often used initially, but its value can be limited by bacterial resistance. Mafenide acetate has broader activity; the cream penetrates eschars and thus can prevent or treat infection beneath the eschars. The foremost disadvantages of this agent are that it can inhibit carbonic anhydrase, resulting in metabolic acidosis, and that it elicits hypersensitivity reactions in up to 7 percent of patients. This agent is most often used when gram-negative bacteria invade the burn wound and when treatment with silver sulfadiazene fails.

When invasive wound infection is diagnosed, topical therapy should be changed to mafenide acetate. Subeschar clysis (the direct instillation of an antibiotic, often piperacillin, under the eschar into wound tissues) is a useful adjunct to surgical and systemic antimicrobial therapy. Systemic treatment with antibiotics active against the pathogens present in the wound should be instituted. In the absence of culture data, treatment with an antibiotic active against gram-positive pathogens, such as oxacillin (2 g intravenously every 4 h), and with antibiotics active against *P. aeruginosa*, such as mezlocillin (3 g intravenously every 4 h) and gentamicin (5 mg/kg intravenously per day), should be started. In the penicillin-allergic patient, vancomycin (1 g intravenously every 12 h) may be substituted for oxacillin (and is efficacious when methicillin-resistant *S. aureus* is present), and ciprofloxacin (400 mg intravenously every 12 h) may be substituted for mezlocillin. It has frequently been noted that patients with burn wounds have alterations in metabolism and renal clearance mechanisms that mandate the monitoring of serum antibiotic levels; the levels achieved with standard doses are often subtherapeutic.

In general, prophylactic systemic antibiotics have no role in the management of burn wounds (except for minor burns in outpatients) and can in fact lead to colonization with resistant microorganisms. An exception involves cases requiring burn-wound manipulation. Since procedures such as debridement, excision, or grafting frequently result in bacteremia, prophylactic systemic antibiotics are administered at the time of burn-wound manipulation; the particular agents used should be chosen on the basis of data obtained by wound culture or data on the hospital's resident flora. All burn-injury patients should undergo tetanus booster immunization if they have completed primary immunization but have not received a booster dose in the past 5 years. Patients without prior immunization should receive tetanus immune globulin and undergo primary immunization. Infection control measures play a major role in preventing burn-wound infection and limiting the spread of antibiotic-resistant nosocomial pathogens.

BIBLIOGRAPHY

CUMMINGS P: Antibiotics to prevent infection in patients with dog bite wounds: A meta-analysis of randomized trials. Ann Emerg Med 23:535, 1994

FALLOUJI MA: Traumatic love bites. Br J Surg 77:100, 1990

GOLDSTEIN EJ: Bite wounds and infection. Clin Infect Dis 14:633, 1992

HOLMES GP et al: Guidelines for the prevention and treatment of B-virus infections in exposed persons. The B Virus Working Group. Clin Infect Dis 20:421, 1995

KULLBERG BJ et al: Purpura fulminans and symmetrical peripheral gangrene caused by *Capnocytophaga canimorsus* (formerly DF-2) septicemia—a complication of dog bite. Medicine (Baltimore) 70:287, 1991

MCMANUS WF et al: Subeschar antibiotic infusion in the treatment of burn wound infection. J Trauma 20:1021, 1980

PRUITT BJ et al: The changing epidemiology of infection in burn patients. World J Surg 16:57, 1992

WEBER DJ et al: Infections resulting from animal bites. Infect Dis Clin North Am 5:663, 1991

YOUN YK et al: The role of mediators in the response to thermal injury. World J Surg 16:30, 1992

YURT R: Burns, in *Mandell, Douglas and Bennett's Principles and Practice of Infectious Diseases*, 4th ed, G. Mandell et al (eds). New York, Churchill Livingstone, 1995, pp 2761–2765

136 *Robert Finberg, Joyce Fingeroth*

INFECTIONS IN TRANSPLANT RECIPIENTS

The evaluation of infections in transplant recipients involves consideration of both the donor and the recipient of the transplanted organ. Infections following transplantation are complicated by the use of drugs that are necessary to enhance the likelihood of survival of the transplanted organ but that also cause the host to be immunocompromised. Thus what might have been a latent or asymptomatic infection in an immunocompetent donor becomes a life-threatening problem for the immunocompromised recipient.

A variety of organisms have been transmitted by organ transplantation (Table 136-1). Careful attention to the sterility of the medium used to handle the organ combined with meticulous culturing to detect contamination may reduce rates of transmission of infectious material. From 2 percent to more than 20 percent of donor kidneys are estimated to be contaminated with bacteria—in most cases, the organisms that colonize the skin or grow in the tissue culture medium used to bathe the donor kidney while it awaits transplantation. The reported rate of bacterial contamination of transplanted bone marrow is as high as 17 percent but is most commonly around 1 percent. It is not surprising that the use of enrichment columns and monoclonal-antibody depletion procedures results in a higher incidence of contamination. Approximately 2 percent of cryopreserved marrow and peripheral blood stem cells transfused as part of treatment for cancer are contaminated. In one series of patients receiving contaminated products, 14 percent had fever or positive blood cultures, but none died. Results of cultures performed at the time of cryopreservation and at the time of thawing were helpful in guiding therapy for the recipient.

In many organ transplantation centers, transmission of diseases that may be latent or clinically inapparent in the donor has resulted in the development of specific protocols for the screening of transplanted organs. In addition to ordering serologic studies focusing on viruses such as herpes simplex virus (HSV), varicella-zoster virus (VZV), cytomegalovirus (CMV), Epstein-Barr virus (EBV), hepatitis B and C viruses, and human immunodeficiency virus (HIV) and on parasites such as *Toxoplasma gondii*, clinicians caring for organ donors should also consider assessing stool (for parasites) and testing for tuberculosis. In this chapter, we will consider aspects unique to various transplant settings.

INFECTIONS IN BONE MARROW TRANSPLANT RECIPIENTS

Bone marrow transplantation for either immune deficiency or cancer results in a transient state of complete immune incompetence. Immediately after transplantation, both phagocytes and immune cells (T cells and B cells) are absent, and the host is extremely susceptible to infection. The reconstitution that follows transplantation has been likened to maturation of the immune system in neonates. The analogy does not entirely predict infections seen in bone marrow transplant (BMT) recipients, however, because the new marrow is usually expressed in an old host who has several latent infections already.

TIMING OF INFECTIONS In the first month after bone marrow transplantation, infectious complications are similar to those in granulocytopenic patients receiving chemotherapy for acute myelocytic or acute lymphocytic leukemia (see Chap. 87 and Fig. 136-1). Because of the anticipated 2- to 4-week duration of neutropenia in this population, many centers give prophylactic antibiotics to patients with the initiation of chemotherapy. Prophylactic trimethoprim-sulfamethoxazole or ciprofloxacin decreases the incidence of gram-negative bacteremia among these patients.

In the second month after transplantation, a major concern (particularly in allogeneic BMT recipients) is CMV disease (see Chap. 187), which rarely has its onset earlier than 14 days after transplantation and may become evident up to 4 months after the procedure. In cases in which the donor marrow is depleted of T cells [to prevent graft-versus-host disease (GVHD) or to eliminate a T cell tumor], the disease may be manifested earlier. Patients who are treated with ganciclovir (either prophylactically or because of positive antigen tests or cultures) may develop CMV infection even later than 4 months after transplantation; treatment appears to delay the development of the normal immune response to CMV infection. Although CMV infection may present as isolated fever or gastrointestinal disease, the cause of death from CMV infection in this setting is pneumonia.

The diagnosis of pneumonia in BMT recipients poses some special problems (see Table 87-5). Because they have undergone treatment with multiple chemotherapeutic agents as well as irradiation, their differential diagnosis should include CMV pneumonitis, diffuse alveolar hemorrhage, pneumonia of viral or fungal etiology, and parasitic infection. Since fungal disease and viruses such as adenovirus are also causes of pneumonia in this setting, it is important to diagnose CMV specifically (see below).

The late posttransplantation period (6 months after bone marrow reconstitution) is marked by episodes of bacteremia due to encapsulated organisms and reactivation of VZV. Because of the high risk of *Pneumocystis carinii* pneumonia (especially among patients being treated for hematologic malignancies), most patients should be maintained on prophylactic doses of trimethoprim-sulfamethoxazole. Such prophylaxis may also protect patients seropositive for *T. gondii*, which may cause pneumonia in the early weeks after transplantation or central nervous system (CNS) lesions later on. The advantages of maintaining patients on daily trimethoprim-sulfamethoxazole for 1 year after transplantation include protection against late bacterial infections with pneumococci and *Haemophilus influenzae*, which are a consequence of the inability of the immature bone marrow to respond to polysaccharide antigens (Fig. 136-1).

VIRAL INFECTIONS FOLLOWING BONE MARROW TRANSPLANTATION BMT recipients are susceptible to infection with a variety of viruses, including reactivation syndromes caused by most human herpesviruses (Table 136-2) and infections caused by viruses that circulate in the community.

Herpes Simplex Virus Within the first 6 weeks after transplantation, most patients who are seropositive for HSV type 1 excrete the virus in the oropharynx. The ability to isolate HSV declines with time. Because of the association between cultivability of virus and severity of mucositis, many clinicians administer prophylactic acyclovir to seropositive BMT recipients in order to reduce mucositis and prevent HSV pneumonia (a rare condition reported almost exclusively in BMT recipients). Both esophagitis (usually due to HSV-1) and anogenital disease (induced by HSV-2) may be prevented by acyclovir prophylaxis. → *For further discussion, see Chap. 184.*

Table 136-1

Organisms Transmitted by Organ Transplantation

Viruses	Parasites
Cytomegalovirus	*Plasmodium falciparum*
Epstein-Barr virus	*Toxoplasma gondii*
Herpes simplex virus	*Strongyloides stercoralis*
Hepatitis B and C viruses	*Trypanosoma cruzi*
Human immunodeficiency virus	
Fungi	
Candida albicans	
Histoplasma capsulatum	
Cryptococcus	

Bacteria	
Staphylococci and strep-tococci	
Pseudomonas species	Haemophilus influenzae
Enterobacte-riaceae	Streptococcus pneumoniae

Parasites

Toxoplasma gondii

Fungi

Pneumocystis carinii

Candida species

Aspergillus species

Viruses

Herpes simplex virus

Cytomegalovirus

Varicella-zoster virus

0 10 20 30 40 50 60 70 80 90 100	Beyond 120
Early	Middle	Late

Days after transplantation

FIGURE 136-1 Infections after bone marrow transplantation.

Cytomegalovirus The onset of CMV infection usually comes between 30 and 90 days after transplantation, when the granulocyte count is adequate but immunologic reconstitution has not occurred. CMV infection may cause interstitial pneumonia, bone marrow suppression, or graft failure. With the standard use of CMV-negative or filtered blood products, primary CMV infection should be a risk in allogeneic transplantation only when the donor is CMV-seropositive and the recipient is CMV-seronegative. Reactivation disease or superinfection with another strain from the donor is also common in CMV-positive recipients, and most seropositive patients who undergo bone marrow transplantation excrete CMV, with or without clinical findings.

Table 136-2

Herpes-Group Virus Syndromes in Transplant Recipients

Virus	Reactivation Disease
Herpes simplex virus type 1	Oral lesions, sometimes with spread (pneumonia described in bone marrow transplant recipients)
Herpes simplex virus type 2	Severe and/or persistent anogenital lesions
Varicella-zoster virus	Zoster (with possible dissemination)
Cytomegalovirus	Associated with graft rejection, fever, esophagitis, colitis, pneumonitis, hepatitis, neuropathy, glomerulopathy, and bone marrow failure
Epstein-Barr virus	Runaway infectious mononucleosis and B cell lymphoproliferative disease
Human herpesvirus 6	Fever, rash,* pneumonitis, bone marrow suppression
Human herpesvirus 7	Undefined
Kaposi's sarcoma–associated virus (human herpesvirus 8)	Kaposi's sarcoma

* A characteristic rash (seen in primary infection) has not been well defined.

Serious CMV disease is much more common among allogeneic BMT recipients and is often associated with GVHD. In addition to pneumonia and graft failure (or marrow suppression), manifestations of CMV disease in BMT recipients include fever with or without arthralgias, myalgias, hepatitis, and esophagitis. CMV ulcerations occur in both the lower and the upper gastrointestinal tract, and it is often difficult to distinguish diarrhea due to GVHD from that due to CMV infection. The finding of CMV in the liver of a patient with GVHD does not necessarily mean that CMV is responsible for hepatic enzyme abnormalities.

Because of the high fatality rate associated with CMV pneumonia in bone marrow transplantation and the difficulty of early diagnosis of CMV infection, prophylactic ganciclovir is given in some centers during the period of maximal vulnerability (from engraftment to day 120 after transplantation). The foremost problem with the administration of this drug relates to its adverse effects, which include dose-related neutrophil and platelet suppression. Because the frequency of CMV pneumonia is lower among autologous BMT recipients (2 to 7 percent) than among allogeneic BMT recipients (10 to 40 percent), prophylaxis in the former group will not become the rule until a less toxic antiviral agent becomes available. A common practice at many centers treating allogeneic BMT patients is to culture blood and urine (and bronchial secretions in some cases) and to give ganciclovir as prophylaxis for CMV pneumonia to those patients who have cultures positive for CMV. The use of the leukocyte antigen test for CMV disease (fluorescent staining of leukocytes for CMV antigens) permits earlier diagnosis but leads to the treatment of more patients, which is associated with an increase in very late disease (>120 days after transplantation). Treatment of CMV pneumonia in BMT recipients requires both intravenous immunoglobulin and ganciclovir, although ganciclovir alone is effective prophylactically. Transfusion of CMV-specific T cells from the donor decreased viral replication in one small series of patients. This result suggests that, in the future, immunotherapy may play a role in the treatment of this disease. → *For further discussion, see Chap. 187.*

Varicella-Zoster Virus Reactivation of herpes zoster may occur as early as 1 month but more commonly occurs several months after transplantation (see Plate ID-38). Reactivation rates are approximately 40 percent for allogeneic BMT recipients and 25 percent for autologous BMT recipients. Localized zoster can spread in an immunosuppressed patient. Fortunately, disseminated disease can usually be controlled with high doses of acyclovir. Because of the high incidence of dissemination of herpes zoster among patients with skin lesions, acyclovir is given prophylactically in some centers to prevent severe disease. Low doses of acyclovir (400 mg orally, three times daily) appear to be effective in preventing reactivation of VZV. However, acyclovir also inhibits the development of VZV-specific immunity. Thus, its administration for only 6 months after transplantation does not prevent zoster from occurring when treatment is stopped. Some data suggest that administration of low doses of acyclovir for an entire year after transplantation is effective and may eliminate most cases of posttransplantation zoster. → *For further discussion, see Chap. 185.*

Epstein-Barr Virus Primary EBV infection can be fatal to transplant recipients; EBV reactivation can cause B cell lymphoproliferative disease (EBV lymphoproliferative syndrome), which may also be fatal to patients taking immunosuppressive drugs. The localization of EBV to B cells leads to several interesting phenomena in marrow transplants. The marrow ablation that occurs as part of the bone marrow transplantation procedure may eliminate latent EBV from the host. The disease can then be reacquired after transplantation when a susceptible pool of B cells is regenerated.

The EBV lymphoproliferative syndrome can develop in the recipient's B cells (if any should survive marrow ablation) but is more likely to be a consequence of reactivation in donor cells. Reactivation of EBV is more likely during immunosuppression (e.g., it is associated with GVHD and the use of antibodies to T cells). Although less likely in autologous transplantation, reactivation can occur in T cell–depleted autologous BMT recipients (e.g., patients being treated for a T cell lymphoma with marrow depletion using antibodies to T cells). The EBV lymphoproliferative syndrome, which usually becomes apparent 1 to 3 months after engraftment, can cause high fevers and cervical adenopathy resembling the symptoms of infectious mononucleosis but more commonly resembles disseminated lymphoma. The incidence of 0.6 percent among allogeneic BMT recipients contrasts with figures of approximately 5 percent for renal transplant recipients and up to 20 percent for cardiac transplant patients. In all cases, EBV lymphoproliferative syndrome is more likely to occur with continued immunosuppression (especially that caused by the use of antibodies to T cells and cyclosporine). EBV-specific T cells generated from the donor have been used to treat EBV lymphoproliferative syndrome in the recipient. → *For further discussion, see Chap. 186.*

Other (Nonherpes) Viruses Both respiratory syncytial virus (RSV) and parainfluenza virus type 3 can cause severe or even fatal pneumonia in BMT recipients. Infections with both of these agents sometimes occur as disastrous nosocomial epidemics. Therapy with ribavirin reportedly lessens the severity of disease. Influenza is also seen in BMT recipients and generally mirrors the presence of infection in the community. In addition, adenovirus can be isolated from BMT recipients at rates varying from 5 to 18 percent. Although hemorrhagic cystitis, pneumonia, and fatal disseminated infection have been reported, adenovirus infection, which (like CMV infection) usually occurs in the first or second month after transplantation, is often asymptomatic. Infections with parvovirus B19 (presenting as anemia) and enteroviruses (sometimes fatal) can occur, rotaviruses are a common cause of gastroenteritis, and BK and JC viruses (polyomavirus hominis 1 and 2, respectively) are sometimes found in urine.

INFECTIONS IN SOLID ORGAN TRANSPLANT RECIPIENTS

Morbidity and mortality among solid organ transplant recipients have been reduced by the use of more effective antibiotics. The most important cause of early death among kidney transplant recipients, for example, was infection with organisms not susceptible to conventional antibiotic therapy. These infections developed in patients requiring prolonged courses of glucocorticoids and other immunosuppressive drugs.

The organisms that cause infections in recipients of solid organ transplants are different from those that infect BMT recipients because solid organ recipients do not go through a period of neutropenia. On the other hand, since organ transplant patients are immunosuppressed for more prolonged periods (usually permanently), they are susceptible to the same organisms as cancer patients with impaired T cell

immunity (see Chap. 87, Table 87-1). In addition, since the transplantation procedure involves surgery, the recipients are subject to wound infections.

During the early period (less than 1 month after transplantation), infections are most often caused by extracellular bacteria (staphylococci, streptococci, *Escherichia coli*, other gram-negative organisms), which frequently originate in surgical wound or anastomotic sites. Thus these infections are largely determined by the type of transplant.

In subsequent weeks, the consequences of the administration of agents that suppress cell-mediated immunity and of the acquisition (from the transplanted organ) or reactivation of parasites and viruses become apparent. CMV infection is often a problem at this time and may present as severe systemic disease or as an infection of the transplanted organ. CMV is associated not only with generalized immunosuppression but also (in some series) with organ-specific, rejection-related syndromes: glomerulopathy in kidney transplant recipients, bronchiolitis obliterans in lung transplant recipients, premature atherosclerosis in heart transplant recipients, and the vanishing bile duct syndrome in liver transplant recipients. Whether these syndromes are actually caused by CMV, which itself is an opportunistic invader, or are merely associated with it has not been established. It is clear that the presence of CMV infection and/or disease is associated with a poor outcome after transplantation. For this reason, considerable attention has been focused on the diagnosis, treatment, and prophylaxis of CMV infection in organ transplant recipients.

Beyond 6 months after transplantation, infections characteristic of patients with defects in cell-mediated immunity—e.g., infections with *Listeria monocytogenes*, *Nocardia*, various fungi, and other intracellular parasites—may be a problem. Elimination of these late infections will not be possible until specific tolerance to the transplanted organ can be achieved without the administration of drugs that lead to generalized immunosuppression. Meanwhile, vigilance, prophylaxis (when indicated), and rapid diagnosis and treatment of infections can be lifesaving in solid organ transplant recipients, who, unlike most BMT recipients, continue to be immunosuppressed.

Solid organ transplant recipients are susceptible to EBV lymphoproliferative disease from as early as 2 months to many years after transplantation. The prevalence of this complication is increased by potent immunosuppressive drugs; the condition may be reversed (in some cases) by decreasing the degree of immunosuppression. Among organ transplant patients, those with lung and heart transplants are most likely to develop EBV-induced B cell proliferation, particularly in the lungs. Whether the tendency of EBV lymphoproliferation to take place in the transplanted organ relates to local factors (e.g., lack of access of host T cells to the transplanted organ because of disturbed lymphatics) or to the differences in major histocompatibility loci between the host T cells and the organ (which may lead to lack of cell migration or lack of effective T cell/macrophage cooperation) has not been established.

KIDNEY TRANSPLANTATION

(Table 136-3) **Early Infections** Infections developing soon after kidney transplantation are often caused by bacteria associated with skin or wound infections. Some data indicate a role for perioperative antibiotic prophylaxis, and many centers give cephalosporins or a penicillin with an aminoglycoside to decrease the risk of postoperative complications. Urinary tract infections manifesting immediately after transplantation are usually related to anatomic alterations resulting from surgery. Such early infections may require prolonged treatment (e.g., 6 weeks of antibiotic administration for pyelonephritis). Urinary tract infections that occur more than 6 months after transplantation do not seem to be associated with the high rate of

Table 136-3

Infections After Kidney Transplantation

Site	Infections in Indicated Period after Transplantation		
	Early, <1 Month	Middle, 1–6 Months	Late, >6 Months
Urinary tract	Bacteria (*Escherichia coli*, *Klebsiella*, Enterobacteriaceae, *Pseudomonas*, *Enterococcus*), associated with bacteremia and pyelonephritis, *Candida*	CMV (fever alone is common)	Bacteria; late UTIs usually not associated with bacteremia
Lungs	Bacteria (including *Legionella* in endemic settings)	CMV diffuse interstitial pneumonitis, *Pneumocystis carinii*, *Aspergillus*, *Legionella*	*Nocardia*, *Aspergillus*, *Mucor*
Central nervous system	—	*Listeria monocytogenes*, bacteremia and meningitis, CMV encephalitis, toxoplasmosis	CMV retinitis, listerial meningitis, cryptococcal meningitis, *Aspergillus*, *Nocardia*

NOTE: CMV, cytomegalovirus; UTIs, urinary tract infections.

pyelonephritis or relapse seen with infections that occur in the first 3 months and therefore may be treated for shorter periods.

Prophylaxis with trimethoprim-sulfamethoxazole [1 double-strength tablet (160 mg of trimethoprim and 800 mg of sulfamethoxazole) per day] for the first 4 months after transplantation decreases the incidence of early and middle-period infections (see below, Table 136-4).

Middle-Period Infections Because of continuing immunosuppression, kidney transplant recipients are predisposed to lung infections characteristic of those in patients with T cell deficiencies (i.e., infections with *Listeria*, *Mycobacterium*, *Nocardia*, fungi, viruses, and parasites). The high mortality associated with *Legionella pneumophila* infection (Chap. 153) led to the closing of renal transplant units in hospitals with endemic *Legionella*. Fifty percent of all renal transplant recipients presenting with fever 1 to 4 months after transplantation have evidence of CMV disease; CMV itself accounts for the fever in more than two-thirds of cases and thus is the predominant pathogen during this period. CMV infection (Chap. 187) may also present as arthralgias or myalgias. This infection can result in primary disease (in the case of a seronegative recipient who receives a kidney from a seropositive donor) or can present as either reactivation disease or superinfection during this interval. Patients may have atypical lymphocytosis. Unlike immunocompetent patients, however, they often do not have lymphadenopathy or splenomegaly. Therefore, clinical suspicion (and laboratory confirmation) are necessary for diagnosis. The clinical syndrome may be accompanied by bone marrow suppression (particularly leukopenia). CMV also causes glomerulopathy and is associated with an increased incidence of other opportunistic infections (e.g., fungal infections). Because of the frequency and severity of CMV disease, a considerable effort has been made to prevent and treat it in renal transplant recipients. Administration of an immune globulin preparation enriched with antibodies to CMV (CMV-Ig) decreases the incidence in the group at highest risk for severe infections (seronegative recipients of seropositive kidneys). Ganciclovir is useful for the treatment of serious CMV disease.

Infection with the other herpes-group viruses may become evident within 6 months after transplantation or later. Early after transplantation, HSV may cause either oral or anogenital lesions that are usually responsive to acyclovir. Large ulcerating lesions in the anogenital area may lead to bladder and rectal dysfunction as well as predisposing to bacterial infection. VZV may cause fatal disseminated infection in nonimmune kidney transplant recipients, but in immune patients reactivation zoster usually does not disseminate outside the dermatome; thus disseminated VZV infection is a less fearsome complication in kidney transplantation than in bone marrow transplantation.

EBV reactivation disease is more serious; it often presents as a polyclonal proliferation of B cells that invade the CNS, nasopharynx, liver, small bowel, heart, and transplanted kidney. The disease is diagnosed by the finding of a proliferation of EBV-positive B cells. The incidence of the syndrome is higher among patients given high doses of cyclosporine. Fortunately, the B cells usually regress, with or without antiviral therapy (acyclovir), when immunocompetence is restored. Human herpesvirus 6 infection and reactivation also follow renal transplantation.

The papovaviruses BK (polyomavirus hominis 1) and JC (polyomavirus hominis 2) have been cultured from the urine of kidney transplant recipients (as they have from that of BMT recipients). The excretion of BK virus is associated with ureteral strictures and that of JC virus with progressive multifocal leukoencephalopathy. Adenoviruses may persist with continued immunosuppression in these patients.

Kidney transplant recipients are also subject to infections with other intracellular organisms. These patients are likely to have pulmonary infections with *Nocardia*, *Aspergillus*, and *Mucor* as well as infections with other pathogens in which the T cell/macrophage axis plays an important role. In patients without intravenous catheters, *L. monocytogenes* is the most common cause of bacteremia 1 month or more after transplantation. Kidney transplant recipients may have *Salmonella* bacteremia, which can lead to endovascular infections and require prolonged therapy. Pulmonary infections with *P. carinii* are common unless the patient is maintained on trimethoprim-sulfamethoxazole prophylaxis. The addition of cyclosporine to azathioprine and prednisone is probably associated with an increased risk of *P. carinii* pneumonia. *Nocardia* infection (Chap. 167) may present in the skin, bones, lungs, or CNS (where it usually takes the form of single or multiple brain abscesses). *Nocardia* infection generally occurs 1 month or more after transplantation and may follow immunosuppressive treatment for an episode of rejection. Pulmonary findings are nonspecific: localized disease with or without cavities is most common, but the disease may disseminate. The diagnosis is made by culture of the organism from sputum or from the involved nodule. Most of these infections are now cured with prolonged sulfonamide therapy. Prophylaxis with trimethoprim-sulfamethoxazole also appears to be efficacious in the prevention of disease. The occurrence of *Nocardia* infections more than 2 years after transplantation suggests that a long-term prophylaxis regimen is justified.

Toxoplasmosis develops in seropositive patients, usually in the first few months after kidney transplantation. In endemic areas, histoplasmosis, coccidioidomycosis, and blastomycosis may cause pulmonary infiltrates or disseminated disease.

Late Infections Late infections (more than 6 months after transplantation) include CMV retinitis and a variety of CNS complications. Patients (particularly those whose degree of immunosuppression has been increased) are at risk for subacute meningitis due to *Cryptococcus*. Cryptococcal disease may present in an insidious manner (sometimes as a skin infection before the development of clear CNS findings). *Listeria* meningitis may have an acute presentation and requires prompt therapy to avoid a fatal outcome.

Patients who continue to take glucocorticoids are predisposed to infection. "Transplant elbow" is a recurrent bacterial infection in and around the elbow that is thought to result from a combination of poor tensile strength of the skin of steroid-treated patients and steroid-induced proximal myopathy that requires patients to push themselves up with their elbows to get out of chairs. Bouts of cellulitis (usually caused by *Staphylococcus aureus*) recur until patients are provided with elbow protection.

Table 136-4

Prophylaxis of Infections in Transplant Recipients

Risk Factor	Infection or Organism	Prophylactic Antibiotics	Examinations
Travel or residence in area with known risk of fungal infection	Coccidioidomycosis, histoplasmosis, blastomycosis	Imidazoles or amphotericin B	Chest radiography
Latent viruses	HSV, VZV, EBV, CMV	Acyclovir after BMT for HSV and VZV; ganciclovir in some settings	Serologic testing for HSV, VZV, CMV, EBV
Latent fungi/parasites	*Pneumocystis carinii*, *Toxoplasma gondii*	Trimethoprim-sulfamethoxazole or dapsone plus pyrimethamine	Serologic testing for *Toxoplasma*
History of exposure to tuberculosis	*Mycobacterium tuberculosis*	Isoniazid in cases with recent conversion of chest x-ray to positive and no previous treatment	PPD skin testing and chest radiography

NOTE: HSV, herpes simplex virus; VZV, varicella-zoster virus; EBV, Epstein-Barr virus; CMV, cytomegalovirus; BMT, bone marrow transplantation; PPD, purified protein derivative.

Kidney transplant recipients are susceptible to other fungal infections—with *Aspergillus* and *Rhizopus*, for example, which may present as superficial lesions before dissemination. Mycobacterial infection (particularly that with *Mycobacterium marinum*) can be diagnosed by skin examination. Infection with *Prototheca wickerhamii* (an achlorophyllic alga) has been diagnosed by skin biopsy. Warts caused by human papillomaviruses are a late consequence of persistent immunosuppression; local therapy is usually satisfactory.

HEART TRANSPLANTATION **Early Infections** Mediastinitis is an early complication of heart transplantation. An indolent course is common, with fever or a mildly elevated white blood cell count preceding the development of site tenderness or drainage. Clinical suspicion based on evidence of sternal instability and failure to heal may lead to the diagnosis. Although common residents of the skin, such as *S. aureus* and *Staphylococcus epidermidis*, are often involved, mediastinitis in these patients can also be due to *Mycoplasma hominis* (Chap. 180). Since this organism requires an anaerobic environment for growth and may be difficult to see on conventional medium, the laboratory should be alerted that *M. hominis* infection is suspected. *M. hominis* mediastinitis has been cured with a combination of surgical debridement (sometimes requiring muscle-flap placement) plus clindamycin and tetracycline. Other organisms, including *Pseudomonas aeruginosa* and *Candida*, can cause mediastinitis. The organisms may be cultured from accompanying pericardial fluid.

Middle-Period Infections *T. gondii* (Chap. 219) may be transmitted to a seronegative recipient in the heart of a seropositive donor. Thus serologic screening for *T. gondii* infection is important in the months after transplantation. The incidence of disease is so high in this setting that some centers have advocated prophylaxis with pyrimethamine. CMV and HIV have also been transmitted by heart transplantation. CNS infections can be caused by *Toxoplasma*, *Nocardia*, and *Aspergillus*. *L. monocytogenes* meningitis should be considered in heart transplant recipients with fever and headache.

CMV infection is associated with poor outcomes after heart transplantation. The virus is usually cultivable 1 to 2 months after transplantation, causes manifestations (usually fever and atypical lymphocytosis, often associated with leukopenia and thrombocytopenia) at 2 to 3 months, and produces severe disease (e.g., pneumonia) at 3 to 4 months. Seropositive recipients usually develop cultivable virus faster than patients whose primary CMV infection is a consequence of transplantation. Between 40 and 70 percent of patients develop symptomatic CMV disease: (1) CMV pneumonia, the most likely form of CMV disease to be fatal; (2) CMV esophagitis and gastritis, sometimes accompanied by abdominal pain with or without ulcerations and bleeding; and (3) the CMV syndrome consisting of CMV in the blood, fever, leukopenia, thrombocytopenia, and hepatic enzyme abnormalities. Ganciclovir is efficacious in the treatment of CMV infection; prophylaxis with ganciclovir may reduce the incidence of CMV-related disease.

Late Infections EBV infection usually presents as a lymphoma-like proliferation of B cells late after heart transplantation, particularly with increased immunosuppression. A subset of heart-lung transplant recipients may develop early (within 2 months) fulminant EBV lymphoproliferative disease, often in the transplanted lung. Prophylaxis for *P. carinii* infection is required for these patients (see below).

LUNG TRANSPLANTATION **Early Infections** It is not surprising that lung transplants are predisposed to the development of pneumonia. The combination of ischemia and the resulting mucosal damage together with accompanying denervation and lack of lymph drainage probably contributes to the high rate of pneumonia (66 percent in one series). The prophylactic use of high doses of broad-spectrum antibiotics for the first 3 or 4 days after surgery decreases the incidence of pneumonia. Gram-negative pathogens (Enterobacteriaceae and *Pseudomonas* species) are troublesome in the first 2 weeks after surgery (the period of maximal vulnerability). Pneumonia can also be caused by *Candida* (possibly as a result of colonization of the donor lung), *Aspergillus*, and *Cryptococcus*.

Mediastinitis may occur at an even higher rate among lung transplant recipients than among heart transplant recipients. *Staphylococcus*, *M. hominis*, and *Candida albicans* are common causes of mediastinitis that develops within 2 weeks of surgery. Mediastinitis due to CMV (which may be transmitted as a consequence of transplantation) usually presents between 2 weeks and 3 months after surgery, with primary disease occurring later than reactivation disease. The incidence of CMV infection, either reactivated or primary, is between 75 and 100 percent if either the donor or the recipient is seropositive for CMV. CMV-induced disease appears to be most severe in recipients of lung and heart-lung transplants. Whether this severity relates to the mismatch in lung antigen-presenting and host immune cells or is attributable to other (nonimmune) factors is not known. More than half of lung transplant recipients with symptomatic CMV disease have pneumonia, and difficulty in distinguishing the radiographic picture of CMV infection from organ rejection further complicates therapy. CMV can also cause bronchiolitis obliterans in lung transplants. The development of pneumonitis related to HSV has led to the prophylactic use of acyclovir. Such prophylaxis may also decrease rates of CMV disease and isolation. Ganciclovir is routinely used in therapy for CMV disease in lung transplant recipients.

Late Infections The incidence of *P. carinii* infection (which may present with a paucity of findings) is high among lung and heart-lung transplant recipients. Some form of prophylaxis for *P. carinii* pneumonia is indicated in all organ transplant situations (Table 136-4). Trimethoprim-sulfamethoxazole prophylaxis for 12 months after transplantation may be sufficient to prevent *P. carinii* disease in patients whose degree of immunosuppression is not increased.

As in other transplant recipients, infection with EBV may cause either a mononucleosis-like syndrome or lymphoproliferative disease in recipients of lung transplants. The tendency of the B cell blasts to present in the lung appears to be greater after lung transplantation than after the transplantation of other organs. Allograft disease may be of donor origin. Reduction of the cyclosporine dosage causes remission in some cases, but lymph node compression can be fatal. Prophylactic use of acyclovir or ganciclovir may prevent the spread of EBV to naive recipients and decrease the rate of development of runaway mononucleosis as well as other manifestations of lymphoproliferative disease.

LIVER TRANSPLANTATION **Early Infections** As in other types of transplantation, early bacterial infections are a major problem after liver transplantation. Many centers administer systemic broad-spectrum antibiotics for the first 5 days after surgery, even in the absence of documented infection. However, despite prophylaxis, infectious complications are common and are correlated with the duration of the surgical procedure and the type of biliary drainage. An operation lasting longer than 12 h is associated with an increased likelihood of infection. Patients who have a choledochojejunostomy with drainage of the biliary duct to a Roux-en-Y jejunal bowel loop have more fungal infections than those whose bile is drained via a choledochocholedochostomy (with anastomosis of the donor common bile duct to the recipient common bile duct).

Peritonitis and intraabdominal abscesses are common complications of liver transplantation. Bacterial peritonitis may result from biliary leaks and primary or secondary infection after leakage of bile. Peritonitis in liver transplant recipients is often polymicrobial, commonly involving enterococci, aerobic gram-negative bacteria, staphylococci, anaerobes, or *Candida*. Only one-third of patients with intraabdominal abscesses have bacteremia. Abscesses within the first month after surgery may occur not only over the liver but also in the spleen, pericolic area, and pelvis. Treatment includes antibiotic administration and drainage as necessary.

Like other transplant recipients, liver transplant patients have a high incidence of fungal infections, and the occurrence of fungal infection (often candidiasis) correlates with the preoperative use of glucocorticoids, a long duration of treatment with antibacterial agents, and posttransplantation use of immunosuppressive agents.

Middle-Period Infections The development of postsurgical biliary stricture predisposes patients to cholangitis. These patients may lack the characteristic signs and symptoms of cholangitis: fever, abdominal pain, and jaundice. Alternatively, these findings may be present but may suggest graft rejection. The diagnosis of cholangitis in liver transplant recipients therefore requires documentation of bacteremia or demonstration of aggregated neutrophils in bile duct biopsy specimens. Unfortunately, invasive studies of the biliary tract (either T-tube cholangiography or endoscopic retrograde cholangiopancreatography) may lead to cholangitis. For this reason, many clinicians recommend prophylaxis with antibiotics covering gram-negative organisms and anaerobes when these procedures are performed in liver transplant recipients.

Viral Infections Viral hepatitis is a common complication of liver transplantation (see Chap. 295). As in other transplant settings, reactivation disease with herpes-group viruses is common (Table 136-2). HSV, human herpesvirus 6, and CMV can be transmitted in donor organs. Although CMV hepatitis occurs in about 4 percent of liver transplant recipients, it is usually not so severe as to require retransplantation. CMV disease develops in the majority of seronegative recipients of organs from CMV-positive donors, but fatality rates are lower in liver transplant recipients than in lung or heart-lung transplant recipients. Disease due to CMV is associated with the vanishing bile duct syndrome after liver transplantation. Patients respond to treatment with ganciclovir; prophylaxis with CMV-Ig and acyclovir may modify disease. EBV lymphoproliferative disease after liver transplantation shows a propensity for involvement of the liver, and such disease may be of donor origin.

PANCREAS TRANSPLANTATION Transplantation of the pancreas is complicated by early abdominal infection in approximately 20 percent of cases. To prevent contamination of the allograft with enteric bacteria and yeasts, some surgeons, instead of draining the pancreas through the bowel, drain secretions into the urinary tract or bladder. A cuff of duodenum is often used in the anastomosis between the pancreatic graft and the bladder. In addition to bicarbonate loss, this technique causes a high rate of urinary tract infection (30 to 40 percent) that may be related to the retention of the duodenum. An alternative method—the transplantation of islet cells only—may eliminate the problems characteristically posed by wound and urinary tract sepsis in pancreas transplant recipients.

Issues related to the development of CMV infection, EBV lymphoproliferative disease, and infection with opportunistic pathogens in patients receiving a pancreas are similar to those discussed for other solid organ transplant recipients.

VACCINATION OF TRANSPLANT RECIPIENTS

In addition to receiving antibiotic prophylaxis, transplant recipients should be vaccinated against likely pathogens (Table 136-5). In the case of BMT recipients, optimal responses cannot be achieved until after reconstitution; despite previous immunization of both donor and recipient, recipients of allogeneic BMTs must be reimmunized if they are to be protected against pathogens. The situation is complex in the case of autologous transplantation. T and B cells in the peripheral blood may reconstitute the response if they are transferred in adequate numbers. However, cancer patients (particularly those with Hodgkin's disease, in whom vaccination has been extensively studied) who are undergoing chemotherapy do not respond normally to immunization, and titers of antibodies to infectious agents fall more rapidly than in healthy individuals. Therefore, even immunosuppressed patients who have not had marrow transplants may need booster vaccine injections. If memory cells are specifically eliminated as part of a marrow "cleanup" procedure, it will be necessary to reimmunize the recipient with a new primary series. Optimal times for immunizations of different transplant populations are being evaluated.

In the absence of compelling data as to optimal timing, it is reasonable to administer the pneumococcal and *H. influenzae* conjugate vaccines to both autologous and allogeneic BMT recipients 12 months after transplantation and again 12 months later (since the response to the initial vaccine dose is weak in the early posttransplantation period). These two vaccines are particularly important for patients who have undergone splenectomy. In addition, *Neisseria meningitidis* polysaccharide vaccine, diphtheria vaccine, tetanus vaccine, and inactivated polio vaccine can all be given at these same intervals (12 and 24 months after transplantation). Some authorities recommend instead a new primary series for tetanus-diphtheria and inactivated polio vaccine (vaccination 12, 14, and 16 months after transplantation). Because of the risk of spread, household contacts of BMT recipients (or of patients immunosuppressed as a result of chemotherapy) should also receive inactivated polio vaccine. Live virus measles/mumps/rubella vaccine (MMR) can be given to autologous BMT recipients 24 months after transplantation and to most allogeneic BMT recipients at the same point if they are not receiving maintenance therapy with immunosuppressive drugs and do not have ongoing GVHD. The risk of spread from a household contact is lower for MMR than for polio vaccine. In patients who have active GVHD and/or are taking high maintenance doses of glucocorticoids, it may be prudent to avoid all live virus vaccines.

In the case of solid organ transplant recipients, administration of all the usual vaccines and of the indicated booster doses should be completed before immunosuppression, if possible, to maximize responses. For patients taking immunosuppressive agents, the administration of pneumococcal vaccine should be repeated every 6 years. No data are available for meningococcal polysaccharide vaccine, but it is probably reasonable to administer it along with the pneumococcal vaccine. *H. influenzae* conjugate vaccine is safe and should be efficacious in this population; therefore, its administration before transplantation is recommended. Booster doses of this vaccine are not recommended for adults. Solid organ transplant recipients who continue to receive immunosuppressive drugs (glucocorticoids, cyclosporine) should not receive live virus vaccines. Thus a person in this group exposed to measles should be given immune globulin. Similarly, an immunocompromised patient who is seronegative for varicella and who comes into contact with a person who has chickenpox should be given varicella-zoster immune globulin as soon as possible (certainly within 96 h).

Table 136-5

Vaccination for Bone Marrow or Solid Organ Transplant Recipients

Vaccine	Use with Indicated Type of Transplantation	
	Bone Marrow	**Solid Organ**
Streptococcus pneumoniae, Haemophilus influenzae, Neisseria meningitidis infections	Immunize after transplantation (optimal timing not established); preimmunize*	Immunize before transplantation and every 6 years for Pneumovax (others not established)
Seasonal influenza	Vaccinate in the fall	Vaccinate before transplantation if possible
Poliomyelitis	Administer inactivated vaccine	Administer inactivated vaccine; live vaccine may be given before immunosuppression
Measles/mumps/rubella	Immunize 24 months after transplantation if graft-versus-host disease does not develop	Immunize before transplantation
Tetanus, diphtheria	Reimmunize after transplantation	Immunize before transplantation; give boosters at 10 years or as required; a new primary series is not required

* Studies indicate that it is possible to "immunize the graft" before transplantation.

Immunocompromised patients who travel benefit from some but not all vaccines. In general, they should receive any killed or inactivated vaccine preparation appropriate to the area they are visiting; this recommendation includes the vaccines for Japanese encephalitis, hepatitis A and B, poliomyelitis, meningococcal infection, and typhoid. The live typhoid vaccines are not recommended for use in most immunocompromised patients, but inactivated typhoid or the purified polysaccharide vaccine can be used. Live yellow fever vaccine should not be administered. Phenol-inactivated cholera vaccine is probably of little use in this setting. On the other hand, immunization with the purified protein hepatitis B vaccine is reasonable if patients are likely to be exposed. Inactivated hepatitis A vaccine should be used in the appropriate setting (see Chap. 122). If hepatitis A vaccine is not administered, travelers should consider receiving passive protection with immune globulin (the dose depending on the duration of travel in the high-risk area). Patients who will remain for longer than 6 months in areas where hepatitis B is common (Africa, Southeast Asia, the Middle East, eastern Europe, parts of South America, and the Caribbean) should receive hepatitis B vaccine.

BIBLIOGRAPHY

BRAYMAN KL: Analysis of infectious complications occurring after solid-organ transplantation. Arch Surg 127:38, 1992

FOX BC et al: A prospective, randomized, double-blind study of trimethoprim-sulfamethoxazole for prophylaxis of infection in renal transplantation: Clinical efficacy, absorption of trimethoprim-sulfamethoxazole, effects on the microflora, and the cost-benefit of prophylaxis. Am J Med 89:255, 1990

GOTTESDIENER KM: Transplanted infections: Donor-to-host transmission with the allograft. Ann Intern Med 110:1001, 1989

HOYLE C et al: Life-threatening infections occurring more than 3 months after BMT. Bone Marrow Transplant 14:247, 1994

KEATING MR et al: Strategies for prevention of infection after cardiac transplantation. May Clin Proc 67:676, 1992

LJUNGMAN P et al: Immunisations after bone marrow transplantation: Results of a European survey and recommendations from the Infectious Diseases Working Party of the European Group for Blood and Marrow Transplantation. Bone Marrow Transplant 15:455, 1995

MARTINEZ-MARCOS F et al: Prospective study of renal transplant infections in 50 consecutive patients. Eur J Clin Microbiol Infect Dis 13:1023, 1994

MOLRINE DC et al: Donor immunization with Haemophilus influenzae type b (HIB) conjugate vaccine in allogeneic bone marrow transplantation. Blood 87:3012, 1996

ROONEY CM et al: Use of gene-modified virus-specific T lymphocytes to control Epstein-Barr virus–related lymphoproliferation. Lancet 345:9, 1995

WEBB IJ et al: Sources and sequelae of bacterial contamination of hematopoietic stem cell products: Implications for safety and hematotherapy and graft engineering. Transfusion 36:782, 1996

137 Dori F. Zaleznik

HOSPITAL-ACQUIRED AND INTRAVASCULAR DEVICE–RELATED INFECTIONS

Nosocomial infections are defined as infections acquired during or as a result of hospitalization. Generally, a patient who has been in the hospital for less than 48 h and develops an infection is considered to have been incubating the infection before hospital admission. Most infections that become manifest after 48 h are considered to be nosocomial. A patient may develop a nosocomial infection after being discharged from the hospital if the organism apparently was acquired in the hospital. Surgical wound infection developing in the weeks after hospital discharge is an example of such nosocomial infection.

INCIDENCE AND COSTS Nosocomial infections contribute significantly to morbidity and mortality as well as to excess costs for hospitalized patients. It is estimated that 5 percent of patients admitted to an acute care hospital in the United States acquire a new infection, with more than 2 million nosocomial infections per year and an annual cost in excess of $2 billion. Some authorities estimate that the odds of death are doubled for patients who develop a nosocomial infection, although clearly such factors as underlying disease and severity of illness also play an important role in outcome.

Although immunosuppressed hosts are especially vulnerable to infections acquired in a hospital, common nosocomial infections occur even in immunocompetent hosts. The National Nosocomial Infections Surveillance (NNIS) Registry has been monitoring nosocomial infection rates since 1970. Its most recent report covers the period from January 1993 to April 1995 and includes both teaching and nonteaching hospitals and both small and large facilities. While the most common nosocomial infections have remained the same, the frequency distribution has altered in recent years. Urinary tract infection remains the most common type but now accounts for only 28 percent of hospital-acquired infections (as opposed to 40 percent in the past). Surgical wound infection and pneumonia—at 19 and 17 percent, respectively—are the next most common nosocomial infections. The frequency of primary bloodstream infection, often associated with intravascular devices, has risen from 7 to 16 percent.

The potential impact of nosocomial infections is considerable when assessed in terms of incidence, morbidity, mortality, and financial burden. Analyses of these factors examine nosocomial infections as both medical and economic issues. The clinical problem facing the physician is the development of a new fever in a patient in the hospital. In the evaluation of such a patient, information about the most common categories of infection may not be sufficient. Rather, the clinician must also use clinical clues from the patient's presentation and hospitalization to diagnose a nosocomial infection.

The evaluation of a hospitalized patient with new fever should include a careful history. Particular attention should be paid to symptoms of headache, cough, abdominal pain, diarrhea, flank pain, dysuria, urinary frequency, and leg pain. Other features related to the patient's hospitalization also are important, such as the presence and type of intravenous devices, the past or current use of a urinary catheter, the surgical procedure conducted (if any), and the new medications administered, including those for surgical prophylaxis. The physical examination should be directed at possible sources of infection and should focus particularly on the skin (with a search for rash or embolic lesions); the lungs; the abdomen (especially the right upper quadrant); the costovertebral angles; surgical wounds; the calves; and current and old intravenous access sites (for signs of phlebitis). The laboratory evaluation of all hospitalized patients with new fever should include a complete blood count with differential, a chest radiograph, and blood and urine cultures. Other diagnostic tests to consider include liver function tests; plain-film or other studies of the abdomen; routine aerobic cultures of sputum, stool, or other relevant body fluids; and (in cases of diarrhea) testing of stool for Clostridium difficile toxin.

CATEGORIES OF INFECTION **Pneumonia** Certainly the astute clinician will question the patient thoroughly and perform a rapid comprehensive physical examination. One way to continue the approach to the development of fever in a hospitalized patient is to consider potential infections that may be life-threatening, such as pneumonia. Most at risk for developing nosocomial pneumonia are patients in an intensive care unit (ICU), especially those who are intubated; patients with an altered level of consciousness, especially those with nasogastric tubes; elderly patients; patients with chronic lung disease; postoperative patients; and any of the above patients taking H_2 blockers or antacids. Nosocomial pneumonia in the NNIS Registry is diagnosed 4 to 7 times per 1000 hospitalizations. Among patients on ventilators, the occurrence of pneumonia is estimated at 15 cases per 1000 ventilator days in medical and surgical ICUs. Mortality figures for nosocomial pneumonia are as high as 50 percent.

Oropharyngeal and gastric colonization plays a critical role in the pathogenesis of pneumonia in hospitalized patients. The oropharynx can become colonized by many species of aerobic gram-negative organisms within 48 h of the patient's hospitalization; aspiration occurs commonly during sleep and is increased by such factors as a nasogastric tube, altered consciousness, decreased gag reflex, or delayed gastric emptying. As for gastric colonization, bacterial counts in the stomach rise in the presence of medications that raise gastric pH, such as H_2 blockers and antacids, as well as in malnourished, achlorhydric, and some elderly patients. The prevalence of pneumonia is reportedly two to three times higher among intubated patients receiving H_2 blockers or antacids for stress-ulcer prophylaxis than among intubated patients receiving sucralfate, a medication that heals ulcers without altering gastric pH. Gastric colonization is believed to influence the development of pneumonia by retrograde colonization of the oropharynx. Ventilated patients are also at risk of developing pneumonia by exposure to bacteria leaking around the cuff of the endotracheal tube or to bacteria from nebulizers, condensate within ventilator circuits, or humidifiers.

Outside the ICU, pneumonia should be suspected when a patient develops a new cough, fever, leukocytosis, sputum production, and a new infiltrate on chest x-ray. Diagnosis can be complicated in patients with congestive heart failure who have concomitant chest x-ray abnormalities or in patients with chronic sputum production. Some organisms, such as *Legionella* spp., may not be associated with peripheral leukocytosis.

In ICU patients, especially those who are intubated, the signs of pneumonia are relatively subtle, and thus the diagnosis often is relatively complex. In particular, the chest x-ray films are difficult to interpret, because fluid overload, congestive heart failure, and adult respiratory distress syndrome (ARDS) are all common findings in intubated patients. Polymorphonuclear leukocytes (PMNs) often are present on Gram-stained preparations of the purulent secretions commonly obtained from these patients. An important clue to pneumonia is a change in the output or character of these secretions. If their volume or thickness increases or their color changes, a sputum Gram's stain should be performed and pneumonia seriously considered in the differential diagnosis. Serial Gram's stains are useful, as the number of PMNs may increase substantially and the type(s) of organisms may shift with the development of pneumonia. For example, the baseline sputum sample from an intubated patient may contain about 25 PMNs per high-power field and have mixed gram-positive and gram-negative organisms of several morphologic types in moderate numbers. On the day of a new fever, the same patient may have copious amounts of more tenacious sputum with more PMNs and a predominance of enteric-appearing gram-negative rods. Even without distinct changes in the chest x-ray, this patient would be considered to have developed pneumonia. Another subtle sign of pneumonia in the intubated patient is a requirement for change in ventilator settings in the absence of fluid overload, a mechanical alteration (e.g., a shift in endotracheal tube placement), or a pneumothorax.

The major organisms of concern in nosocomial pneumonia are gram-negative aerobic bacteria. *Pseudomonas aeruginosa, Staphylococcus aureus,* and *Klebsiella pneumoniae* are frequent pathogens in nosocomial pneumonia. While surveys of organisms are useful, it is essential to know which pathogens are common in a given institution, as hospitals and especially ICUs differ in their resident flora. In some institutions, methicillin-resistant *S. aureus, Stenotrophomonas* (formerly *Xanthomonas) maltophilia, Flavobacterium* spp., and even *Legionella* spp. may be of particular concern. Viruses such as respiratory syncytial virus and adenovirus are receiving increased attention as etiologic agents of nosocomial pneumonia in both adults and children. In the past, viruses have been underrepresented in statistics on the agents of nosocomial pneumonia because the diagnosis of viral infection is more difficult and because many microbiology laboratories do not have the capability to isolate viruses.

Antibiotic resistance is another important issue to address in the management of a hospitalized patient. In addition to knowing the sensitivity patterns of the hospital flora, one must consider whether a patient has received continuous or multiple courses of antibiotic therapy. To reduce the likelihood of altering the sensitivity patterns of the patient's flora, antibiotic courses for pneumonia should be kept as short as possible, with coverage as narrow as is possible for the organism(s) involved.

Bacteremia Another potentially life-threatening nosocomial infection to consider in the evaluation of the patient with a new fever is bacteremia, which usually is related to the presence of an intravascular device (see also Chap. 138). While many common nosocomial infections such as pneumonia or urinary tract infection can be accompanied by bacteremia, primary bacteremia is defined by isolation of a recognized pathogen from the blood without an infection at another site. One carefully controlled study reported bloodstream infection in 2.7 percent of admissions to a surgical ICU, with 50 percent mortality and a prolongation of hospitalization by 24 days in survivors.

One difficulty in assessing the significance of bacteremia is to distinguish true pathogens from contaminating skin flora. This distinction is especially important in establishing an infection of an indwelling intravascular catheter because organisms that inhabit the skin, such as coagulase-negative staphylococci, also frequently cause infection. The most common point of entry for infection related to intravascular devices is the insertion site, with spread of the infection along the outside of the device initially. Other means of entry for infecting organisms include introduction via contaminated infusates or tubing, ports, or leaking connections and hematogenous seeding of a catheter during bacteremia. While gram-negative aerobic bacilli are probably the most feared nosocomial bloodstream pathogens, the NNIS data for 1980 through 1989 showed that the isolation of these organisms had not increased in frequency over the decade. The frequency of bloodstream isolation increased the most for coagulase-negative staphylococci, with the next highest increase for *Candida* spp. Other leading causes of line-related bacteremia were *S. aureus* and enterococci. Recent studies have confirmed these findings.

Establishing an infection of an intravascular device or primary bacteremia as the cause of fever in a hospitalized patient is a diagnosis of exclusion. If a patient has a fever and signs of cutaneous involvement (erythema, induration, tenderness, or purulent drainage) at the insertion site of a catheter, full cultures should be performed, the vascular-access line removed, and the catheter tip sent for quantitative culture. Studies have correlated the growth of 15 colonies or more from a catheter tip with infection of the line. More commonly, the exit site does not show signs of infection, and there is considerable debate about the necessity of removing a line from a febrile patient at that point. Unless another site of infection is obvious, it is generally advisable to remove the line when a patient develops a new fever. While central-line changes over a guidewire have been shown to be safe, it is not clear that maintaining the same insertion site is wise in cases of possible line infection. In general, when a line is removed because of possible infection, the site should be changed. If vascular access is a problem and one wishes to continue intravascular therapy despite the intravascular-device infection, it is probably not necessary to change the line over a guidewire. The traditional teaching is that an infected intravenous device should be removed. In current practice, however, especially with surgically implanted intravenous catheters, a decision may be made to attempt treatment with antibiotics while leaving the catheter in place. This practice is often successful when the infecting organism is a coagulase-negative *Staphylococcus* but is less often effective with other organisms, particularly *Candida* spp.

Another controversial management issue is whether to draw blood for culture through a line. While some studies report a correlation in the 90 percent range between culture results for blood drawn through vascular-access lines and those for peripheral blood, the former cultures can be either false-positive or false-negative. If the line culture is positive and no peripheral blood has been drawn, it is impossible to determine whether the patient has true bacteremia or the culture merely reflects bacteria associated with the line. Conversely, if multiple peripheral blood cultures are positive, it is reasonable to assume that the line is at least infected secondarily. Whether bacteremia is high- or low-grade and whether it is sustained or transient may influence the duration of antibiotic therapy and cannot be determined from cultures of specimens obtained through a line.

Surgical Wound Infection   Evaluation of fever in the postoperative patient must include careful evaluation of the surgical wound. Although surgical wound infection reportedly accounts for 19 percent of nosocomial infections, the true incidence of postoperative wound infection is difficult to assess, particularly at a time when many patients are hospitalized for relatively short periods. In a number of studies, careful follow-up for the development of wound infections after discharge—especially observation of the wound by a trained observer, such as a nurse—has shown the actual rates of wound infections in all categories of surgery to be greater than the reported rates. Surgical procedures have long been classified as clean, clean-contaminated, contaminated, and dirty-infected. A more sophisticated risk index is based on the American Society of Anesthesiologists preoperative assessment score, the surgery classification (as either contaminated or dirty-infected), and the duration of surgery. With this index, rates of surgical wound infection have varied from 1.5 to 13 per 100 operations.

Other risk factors for the development of postoperative wound infection include the presence of a drain; a long preoperative length of stay, with the rates doubling for each week of preoperative hospitalization; preoperative shaving of the field, especially if performed 24 h or more beforehand; a long duration of surgery; the presence of an untreated remote infection; and the surgeon. Perioperative antibiotic prophylaxis has been shown to decrease rates of wound infection in a number of careful studies, including those of clean surgical procedures. Antibiotic coverage after the surgical wound is closed has not been shown to provide additional benefit.

A surgical wound should be examined for erythema extending more than 2 cm beyond the margin of the wound, localized tenderness and induration, fluctuance, drainage of purulent material, and dehiscence of sutures. Mechanical factors, as well as infection, can cause wound dehiscence. Sternal wounds following cardiac surgery are of special concern because the consequences of infection can be severe. The surface of the wound may not present an obvious cause for concern, but, in some patients, ongoing fevers and especially the development of rocking or instability of the sternum may be sufficient cause for surgical exploration of the wound. Mediastinitis or sternal osteomyelitis is a severe complication of cardiac surgery. Wounds associated with the placement of prosthetic devices such as mechanical joints also are of special concern. Infection of these wounds can lead to infection of the prosthesis, and clearance of prosthetic joint infections generally requires surgical removal of the device.

Urinary Tract Infection   Urinary tract infection (UTI), the most common type of nosocomial infection, generally is the easiest to treat and has the least severe sequelae. Four principal risk factors have been associated repeatedly with the development of UTI in hospitalized patients: female sex, prolonged urinary catheterization, lack of systemic antibiotic therapy, and breach of appropriate catheter care. The administration of systemic antibiotics to patients with urinary catheters in place for 1 to 5 days has been associated with a decrease in rates of bacteriuria. For patients with catheters in place for 6 or more days, however, this benefit is not observed.

The pathogenesis of catheter-associated UTI appears to differ in men and women. In women, the typical mechanism involves periurethral colonization with fecal flora and tracking of organisms up the catheter to the bladder and thus resembles the pathogenesis of UTI in noncatheterized female patients, in whom bacteria track up the short female urethra. In contrast, periurethral colonization often cannot be demonstrated in men; most infections seem to arise from intraluminal spread of organisms to the bladder. Some organisms, such as *Proteus* and *Pseudomonas* spp., appear to facilitate the growth along the inside of the urinary catheter of a biofilm that encrusts and obstructs the flow of urine.

UTI is certainly an extremely common nosocomial infection; however, it is important to define this type of infection precisely. Especially in the evaluation of a febrile hospitalized patient, it is crucial to think carefully about all possible sources of infection and not to assume that UTI is the probable cause. In patients who have had urinary catheters in place for a number of days, fever, dysuria, frequency, leukocytosis, and especially flank pain or costovertebral angle tenderness are highly suggestive of bladder infection or pyelonephritis. In patients with fever but no other symptoms or signs referable to the urinary tract, one should look for ancillary findings suggestive of urinary tract involvement, such as white blood cells without epithelial cells in the urine sediment or leukocyte esterase or nitrite on urinalysis. A urine culture positive for a single organism should not be accepted as definitive evidence of UTI in an asymptomatic patient. While one might treat the febrile patient who has a positive urine culture with antibiotics, it is prudent to repeat the culture before the institution of therapy. Inability to recover any organism or the same organism on repeat culture, particularly if the patient does not respond to antibiotics, should raise questions about the validity of the diagnosis of UTI. In addition, isolation of two or more bacteria from a single specimen is most likely due to contamination unless there is reason to suspect a bladder diverticulum or a perinephric abscess.

Other Infectious Sources of Fever   Several other types of infection may cause fever in the hospitalized patient and should be considered in the differential diagnosis of new fever. In patients who have received antibiotics (even a single dose as surgical prophylaxis), antibiotic-associated diarrhea may develop. This condition is usually caused by the spore-forming organism *C. difficile*, which produces toxins that cause diarrhea. Some patients may appear quite toxic with this infection, with high fevers, leukocytosis, and profuse diarrhea. The organism is quite hardy and is difficult to eradicate from the hospital environment. The hands of hospital personnel have been implicated as a mode of transmission of this organism, as have electronic rectal thermometers (despite the use of individual covering sheaths for each patient). The colon may become colonized with *C. difficile* while the patient is in the hospital, but—particularly if the patient is still taking antibiotics when sent home—diarrhea may not develop until after discharge.

Other infections to consider in the hospitalized patient include decubitus ulcers, particularly in patients in chronic-care wards or confined to bed rest for prolonged periods, and sinusitis, especially in intubated patients.

NONINFECTIOUS SOURCES OF FEVER   A consideration of several common noninfectious causes of fever in hospitalized patients is part of a thorough evaluation of new fever. Drug treatment is the foremost noninfectious cause of fever. Drug fever may occur with or without an accompanying rash or eosinophilia and can be caused by a new medication or by medications the patient has been receiving for some time. Particular agents associated with drug fever include phenytoin, H_2 blockers, procainamide, and antibiotics, most notably sulfonamides. Even drug-associated fevers can be quite high in some patients and may take up to 5 days to resolve after discontinuation of treatment with the offending agent. Other noninfectious causes of fever include phlebitis, often at the site of an old intravenous line and sometimes followed by suppurative thrombophlebitis with clots or septic emboli, and pulmonary emboli, especially in patients undergoing prolonged bed rest; prophylactic heparin or mechanical boots often are used to reduce the risk of pulmonary embolism in the latter patients.

CONCLUSION   The range of possibilities for the etiology of a new fever in a hospitalized patient is quite broad. An attention to detail, a careful history and physical examination, and a knowledge of the infections and organisms likely to cause nosocomial problems usually lead to an accurate diagnosis.

BIBLIOGRAPHY

BRONSEMA DA et al: Secular trends in rates and etiology of nosocomial urinary tract infections at a university hospital. J Urol 150:414, 1993

CRAVEN DE, STEGER KA: Epidemiology of nosocomial pneumonia: New perspectives on an old disease. Chest 108:1S, 1995

CULVER DH et al: Surgical wound infection rates by wound class, operative procedure, and patient risk index. Am J Med 91(S3B):152S, 1991

FAGON J-Y et al: Mortality attributable to nosocomial infections in the ICU. Infect Control Hosp Epidemiol 15:428, 1994

GEORGE DL: Nosocomial pneumonia, in *Hospital Epidemiology and Infection Control*, CG Mayhall (ed). Baltimore, Williams & Wilkins, 1996, p 175

JARVIS WR: Epidemiology of nosocomial fungal infections, with emphasis on *Candida* species. Clin Infect Dis 20:1526, 1995

National Nosocomial Infections Surveillance (NNIS) Semiannual Report, May 1995. Am J Infect Control 23:377, 1995

PITTET D et al: Nosocomial bloodstream infection in critically ill patients. JAMA 271:1598, 1994

---

138   *Robert A. Weinstein*

INFECTION CONTROL IN THE HOSPITAL

The costs of nosocomial (hospital-acquired) infections are great, whether measured in dollars or in morbidity and mortality (see Chap. 137). Although infection-control and hospital epidemiology activities have been the subjects of increasing scientific study over the past 25 years, efforts to lower infection risks have been continually challenged by the growing numbers of immunocompromised patients, of antibiotic-resistant bacteria, of fungal and viral superinfections, and of invasive devices and procedures. Three international decennial conferences on infection control, organized by the Centers for Disease Control and Prevention (CDC), have clearly documented these formidable trends. This chapter reviews the basic surveillance and prevention activities that have been developed to deal with these problems and that form the foundation for current hospital epidemiology programs.

ORGANIZATION AND RESPONSIBILITIES OF INFECTION-CONTROL PROGRAMS The standards of the Joint Commission on Accreditation of Healthcare Organizations require all accredited hospitals to have an active program for surveillance, prevention, and control of nosocomial infections; a multidisciplinary infection-control committee usually oversees the program. The agents of the committee are the chairperson, who is preferably an infectious disease physician, and the infection-control practitioners, who are usually trained in nursing or medical technology and in epidemiology and public health. Education of physicians in infection control and hospital epidemiology is offered in some infectious disease fellowship programs and is available in courses provided by professional societies, primarily the Society for Healthcare Epidemiology of America.

In the 1970s, the CDC's extensive Study on the Efficacy of Nosocomial Infection Control found that nosocomial infection rates fell by 32 percent in hospitals that established programs with organized surveillance and control activities; a trained, effectual infection-control physician; and one infection-control practitioner per 250 beds. In contrast, rates in hospitals without effective programs increased by 18 percent. Since that study, however, the responsibilities and roles of hospital epidemiology programs have expanded in several directions. Diagnosis-related reimbursement has led hospital administrators to place increased emphasis on cost containment and on documentation of the cost-effectiveness of infection control. The quality-improvement movements and the Joint Commission's Agenda for Change have redirected infection-control attention, in part, beyond the mere writing of policies and procedures to improvement of the actual processes and optimization of outcomes. In a few hospitals, epidemiology programs have even taken on additional pharmacoepidemiologic and antibiotic-use review responsibilities. Finally, all programs must now respond to increasing governmental regulation of hospital waste and to Occupational Safety and Health Administration (OSHA)–mandated standards for protecting health care workers from occupational exposure to bloodborne pathogens and tuberculosis.

SURVEILLANCE Traditionally, infection-control practitioners survey inpatients for nosocomial infections (defined as those neither present nor incubating at the time of admission). Surveillance involves a review of microbiology laboratory results, "shoe-leather" epidemiology on the nursing wards, application of standardized definitions of infection, ongoing dialogue with hospital workers, and com-

mon sense. Some innovative infection-control programs have taken advantage of the increased use of computerized pharmacy, microbiology, and other databases in hospitals to create algorithm-driven surveillance activities.

Because total hospital surveillance leaves little time for data analysis and education, most hospitals now aim surveillance at infections that are associated with a high level of morbidity [e.g., intensive care unit (ICU)–related infections and nosocomial pneumonia], are costly (e.g., cardiac surgery wound infections) or difficult to treat (e.g., infections due to antibiotic-resistant bacteria), pose recurring epidemic problems (e.g., *Clostridium difficile*–related diarrhea), and are potentially preventable (e.g., vascular access–related infections). Quality-assurance activities in infection control have led to increased surveillance of the compliance of personnel with policies (e.g., monitoring of the actual adherence to isolation precautions).

The results of surveillance are expressed as rates; for example, 5 to 10 percent of patients develop nosocomial infections. Although such overall statistics are often requested of hospitals by administrators or surveyors, they have little value unless qualified by site of infection, by patient population, and by exposure to risk factors. Meaningful denominators for infection rates include the number of patients exposed to a specific risk (e.g., rates of pneumonia among patients using mechanical ventilators) and the number of intervention days (e.g., rates of pneumonia per 1000 patient-days on a ventilator).

Temporal trends in rates should be reviewed, and rates ideally should be compared with regional and national norms. However, even comparison rates generated by the CDC's ongoing National Nosocomial Infection Surveillance System, which collects data from more than 200 hospitals that use standardized definitions of nosocomial infections, have not been validated independently and represent a nonrandom sample of hospitals. Interhospital comparisons are easily confounded by the wide range in risk factors and in severity of underlying illnesses; unless rates are adjusted for these factors, comparisons may be misleading. Unfortunately, systems for making such adjustments either are rudimentary or have not been well validated.

The ongoing analysis of an individual hospital's infection rates helps to determine whether control efforts are succeeding and where increased education and control measures should be focused. Knowledge of infection rates is also useful in discussions with the hospital administration regarding areas to which additional resources should be directed.

PREVENTION AND CONTROL MEASURES **Epidemiologic Basis and General Measures** Nosocomial infections follow basic epidemiologic patterns that can help to direct prevention and control measures. Nosocomial pathogens have reservoirs, follow predictable routes of transmission, and require susceptible hosts. Reservoirs and sources exist in the inanimate environment (e.g., tap water contaminated with *Legionella*) and in the animate environment (e.g., infected or colonized health care workers, patients, and hospital visitors). The mode of transmission most often is either cross-infection (e.g., indirect spread of pathogens from one patient to another on the inadequately washed hands of hospital personnel) or autoinoculation (e.g., aspiration of oropharyngeal flora into the lung along an endotracheal tube). Occasionally, pathogens (e.g., group A streptococci and many respiratory viruses) are spread indirectly from person to person via infectious droplets released by coughing or sneezing. Much less common—but often devastating in terms of epidemic risk—is true airborne spread of droplet nuclei (as in nosocomial chickenpox) or common-source spread by contaminated materials (e.g., iodophors contaminated with *Pseudomonas*). Factors that increase host susceptibility include underlying conditions (discussed elsewhere in this text) and the many medical-surgical interventions and procedures that bypass or compromise normal host defenses.

The hospital's infection-control committee, through its infection-control program, must determine the general and specific measures used to control infections and must review and recommend specific antiseptics and disinfectants for hospital use. Given the prominence of cross-infection, hand washing is the single most important preventive measure in hospitals. Many studies have examined the antimicrobial activity of a wide variety of antiseptic-containing hand-washing agents. The use of such agents is important before invasive procedures and possibly in ICU settings. Given the poor general compliance with hand-washing recommendations, the importance of using any hand cleanser between patient contacts cannot be overemphasized (Table 138-1).

The fact that 25 to 50 percent of nosocomial infections are due to the combined effect of the patient's own flora and invasive devices highlights the importance of improvements in the use and design of such devices. Intensive educational programs can be associated with at least a temporary reduction in infection rates through improved asepsis in handling and earlier removal of invasive devices, but the maintenance of such gains is often difficult. It is encouraging that epidemiologic studies have been used increasingly to assess the value of newer devices and site-specific control measures (discussed below) and to debunk some traditional yet ineffective and costly measures, such as routine culturing of the environment and personnel for "pathogens."

Urinary Tract Infections Approaches to the prevention of urinary tract infections (UTIs) have included the use of topical meatal antimicrobials, drainage bag disinfectants, antimicrobial-coated catheters, and sealed catheter–drainage tube junctions to eliminate inadvertent breaks in the system. Because of conflicting study results, none of these measures is considered routine. Systemic antimicrobials given for other purposes decrease the risk of UTI during the first 4 days of catheterization, after which resistant bacteria or yeasts emerge as pathogens. Selective decontamination of the gut also is associated with a reduced risk. Again, however, neither approach is routine. Moreover, irrigation of catheters, with or without antimicrobials, may actually increase the risk of infection.

Pneumonia Control measures for pneumonia are aimed at the remediation of risk factors in general patient care (e.g., minimizing aspiration-prone supine positioning and possibly avoiding prophylactic gastric alkalization because of the increased risk of colonization with gram-negative rods when the gastric pH is >4) and at meticulous aseptic care of respirator equipment (e.g., disinfecting or sterilizing all in-line reusable components such as nebulizers, replacing tubing circuits at intervals of more than 48 h—rather than more frequently—to lessen the number of breaks in the system, and teaching aseptic technique for suctioning). More controversial is the infection-control benefit of sucralfate, which provides stress-ulcer prophylaxis without

altering gastric pH, and of selective decontamination of the oropharynx and gut with nonabsorbable antimicrobials. Each approach merits further investigation.

Surgical Wound Infections The most important control measures for surgical wound infections include the use of antimicrobial prophylaxis at the start of high-risk procedures, attention to technical surgical issues and operating-room asepsis (e.g., not shaving the operative site until surgery and avoiding open or prophylactic drains), and preoperative therapy for any active infection. Reporting of surveillance results to surgeons has been associated with reductions in infection rates. This association, in conjunction with the increasingly extensive review of infection rates by regulatory agencies and third-party payers, emphasizes the importance of stratifying rates by patient-related risk factors and of developing meaningful systems for interhospital comparisons and for wound surveillance after the patient's discharge from the hospital or clinic (when more than 50 percent of infections first become apparent).

Infections Related to Vascular Access and Monitoring (See also Chap. 137) Control measures for infections associated with vascular access and monitoring include the moving of peripheral or arterial catheters to a new site at specified intervals (e.g., every 72 h for peripheral intravenous catheters), which may be facilitated by use of an intravenous team; the application of disposable transducers and aseptic technique for the accessing of transducers or other vascular ports; and the removal of "idle" catheters. Unresolved issues include the best frequency for the rotation of central venous catheter sites (guidewire-assisted catheter changes at the same site do not lessen infection risk); the best antiseptics for site preparation and for catheter dressing; the appropriate role for mupirocin ointment, a topical antibiotic with excellent antistaphylococcal activity, in site care; the relative degrees of risk posed by percutaneous central catheters and by newer designs—tunneled, totally implanted, or peripherally inserted central catheters (PICC lines); and the role of other costly catheter innovations, such as the impregnation of the catheter with antimicrobials or the attachment of subcutaneous cuffs that contain bactericidal silver. In several studies, the use of semitransparent polyurethane dressings has increased infection rates, although these dressings can offer nursing benefits (ease of bathing and site inspection and protection of the site from secretions).

Isolation Techniques Written policies for the isolation of infectious patients are a standard component of infection-control programs. The CDC is in the process of revising its isolation guidelines; their current system recommends that hospitals use either category-specific isolation (based on suspected infection) or disease-specific isolation (based on likely mode of transmission). The category-specific system includes *strict isolation* (e.g., for chickenpox), *contact isolation* (e.g., for staphylococcal wound infections), *respiratory isolation* (e.g., for untreated bacterial meningitis), and *acid-fast bacillus isolation* (for *Mycobacterium tuberculosis* infection, which has specific ventilation requirements, as described below), as well as *enteric precautions* (e.g., for *C. difficile*–associated bacterial diarrhea) and *drainage/secretion precautions* (e.g., for minor wound infections). Some hospitals also use blood and body-fluid precautions, although universal precautions have largely supplanted these measures. For each of the six category-specific modes, a door sign lists the necessary protective measures (e.g., gown, gloves, and mask for strict isolation). In the disease-specific system, the caregiver checks off the appropriate measures on a generic isolation sign on the basis of an understanding of the patient's infection and its specific mode(s) of transmission. The pending revision of the CDC's recommendations will offer greater guidance in the isolation of patients on the basis of presenting syndromes (before the recovery of specific infectious agents); will emphasize more standard, routine use of barrier precautions; and will simplify the categories of isolation.

In body-substance isolation, the preceding systems are abandoned in favor of instructing personnel to wear gloves for contact with any body substance or mucous membrane. Other barriers, such as gowns, are required if soiling or splashing is anticipated. For patients with airborne pathogens such as *M. tuberculosis*, additional isolation precautions are required (see below).

Table 138-1

Examples of Ways in Which Physicians Can Contribute to Infection-Control Efforts

- Act as role models for other personnel by paying careful attention to hand-washing recommendations and barrier precautions during contact with patients and by observing posted isolation precautions.
- Give corrective feedback to caregivers who do not adhere to hand-washing recommendations or isolation precautions.
- Place invasive devices based on clinical need (not just on convenience).
- Remove invasive devices promptly when they are no longer needed clinically.
- Limit surgical antimicrobial prophylaxis to the perioperative period.
- Exercise care in initial empirical antibiotic selection (avoid "shotgun" approaches).
- Narrow the spectrum of antibiotic therapy once a pathogen is recovered.
- Discontinue antibiotic therapy in a timely fashion.
- Become familiar with the hospital's bloodborne pathogen and tuberculosis control plans.
- Order appropriate isolation precautions promptly for infected patients.
- During patient rounds, alert nursing staff to lapses in asepsis (e.g., soiled dressings at sites of intravascular catheters) and to infection-predisposing situations (e.g., aspiration-prone positioning of patients).
- Notify infection-control practitioners of potential infection-control problems (e.g., surgical wound infections that manifest after a patient's discharge).

In addition to these three alternative systems, all hospitals are required by OSHA to provide annual in-service training in, and to monitor compliance with, universal precautions to protect health care workers from bloodborne pathogens, including human immunodeficiency virus (HIV) and hepatitis B and C viruses. In essence, these precautions require gloves, gown, mask, and/or eye protection, varying with the likelihood of contact or splashing with blood or *any* other potentially contaminated body fluid. Some hospitals use additional guidelines for infected mothers and their newborns and antibiotic-resistance precautions for patients colonized or infected with problematic strains.

EPIDEMIC PROBLEMS Outbreaks are always big news but probably account for fewer than 5 percent of nosocomial infections. The investigation and control of epidemics in hospitals require that infection-control personnel develop a case definition, confirm that an outbreak really exists (since many apparent epidemics are actually pseudo-outbreaks due to surveillance or laboratory artifacts), review aseptic practices and disinfectant use, determine the extent of the outbreak, perform an epidemiologic investigation to determine modes of transmission, work closely with microbiology personnel to culture for common sources or personnel carriers as appropriate and to type epidemiologically important isolates, and heighten surveillance to judge the effect of control measures. Control measures generally include the early reinforcement of routine aseptic practices during a search for compliance problems that may have fostered the outbreak, the ensuring of the appropriate isolation of cases (and the institution of cohort isolation and nursing if needed), and the implementation of further controls on the basis of the findings of the investigation. Examples of some potential epidemic problems follow.

Chickenpox When health care workers are exposed to chickenpox in the community or through patients with initially unrecognized infections, or when these employees work during the 24 h before developing chickenpox, infection-control practitioners institute a varicella exposure investigation and control plan. In this plan, the names of exposed workers and patients are obtained; medical histories are reviewed, and (if necessary) serologic tests for immunity are conducted; physicians are notified of susceptible exposed patients; prophylactic varicella-zoster immune globulin and/or early acyclovir treatment (where appropriate) is administered; and susceptible exposed employees are furloughed during the at-risk period for disease. The recently approved varicella vaccine should markedly decrease risk for susceptible employees.

Tuberculosis The resurgence of pulmonary tuberculosis in the United States since 1987 and a series of nosocomial outbreaks of infection with multidrug-resistant strains—primarily involving patients with AIDS and their caregivers—have led to a reevaluation of tuberculosis control. Important control measures include prompt recognition, isolation, and treatment of cases; recognition of atypical presentations (e.g., lower-lobe infiltrates without cavitation); use of negative pressure, 100 percent exhaust, private isolation rooms with closed doors, and six air changes per hour; use of face masks (approved by the National Institute for Occupational Safety and Health) by caregivers entering isolation rooms; possible use of HEPA (high-efficiency particulate air) filter units and/or ultraviolet lights for disinfecting air when other engineering controls are not feasible or reliable; and follow-up skin-testing of susceptible personnel who have been exposed to infectious patients before isolation.

Group A Streptococci The potential for a group A streptococcal outbreak should be considered when even a single nosocomial case occurs. Most outbreaks involve surgical wounds and are due to the presence of an asymptomatic carrier in the operating room. Investigation can be confounded by carriage at extrapharyngeal sites such as the rectum and vagina. Health care workers in whom carriage has been linked to nosocomial transmission of group A streptococci are removed from the patient-care setting and are not permitted to return until carriage has been eliminated by antimicrobial therapy.

Aspergillus *Aspergillus* spores are common in the environment, particularly on dusty surfaces. When hospital ceiling tiles are removed to provide access for electrical wiring or plumbing or when dusty areas are disturbed during hospital renovation, the spores become airborne. Inhalation of spores by immunosuppressed (particularly neutropenic) patients creates a risk of pulmonary and/or paranasal sinus infection and disseminated aspergillosis. Routine surveillance among neutropenic patients for infections with filamentous fungi, such as *Aspergillus* and *Fusarium*, helps hospitals to determine whether they have unduly large environmental loads of these organisms. To lower the risk, hospitals should inspect and clean air-handling equipment on a routine schedule, review all planned hospital renovations with infection-control personnel and subsequently construct appropriate barriers, remove immunosuppressed patients from renovation sites, and consider the use of HEPA filters for air supplied to rooms housing immunosuppressed patients.

Legionella Sporadic and epidemic cases of nosocomial *Legionella* pneumonia are most often due to the contamination of potable water or air-handling systems and predominantly affect immunosuppressed patients, particularly those receiving glucocorticoid medication. The risk varies greatly among geographic regions and within a given region, depending on the extent of hospital hot-water contamination, on the presence or absence of high-risk patient populations, and on specific hospital practices (e.g., inappropriate use of nonsterile water in respiratory therapy equipment). Laboratory-based surveillance for nosocomial *Legionella* should be performed, and a diagnosis of legionellosis should probably be considered more often than it is. If cases are detected, environmental samples (e.g., hot-water tank sediment, faucets, and showerheads) should be cultured. If cultures yield *Legionella* and if typing of clinical and environmental isolates reveals a correlation, eradication measures should be pursued (see Chap. 153). An alternative approach is to periodically culture water tanks and water on wards housing high-risk patients. If *Legionella* is found, a concerted effort should be made to culture samples from all patients with nosocomial pneumonia for *Legionella*.

Antibiotic-Resistant Bacteria Outbreaks of antibiotic resistance begin with Darwinian selection of bacterial chromosomal mutations, spread of plasmid- and/or transposon-borne resistance among bacterial species, and/or (re)admission to the hospital of patients chronically infected with resistant bacteria. After the introduction of resistant strains, dissemination occurs by cross-infection on unwashed hands of caregivers or, occasionally, via personnel carriage and/or environmental contamination. Outbreak control depends on close laboratory surveillance, with early detection of problems; on the reinforcement of routine asepsis (e.g., hand washing); on the implementation of barrier precautions for all colonized and/or infected patients; on the use of patient-surveillance cultures to more fully ascertain the extent of patient colonization; and on the timely initiation of an epidemiologic investigation when rates increase. Colonized personnel who are implicated in nosocomial transmission and patients who pose a threat may be decontaminated; for example, colonization with methicillin-resistant *Staphylococcus aureus* may be controlled with oral antibiotics, including trimethoprim-sulfamethoxazole and rifampin, and with topical agents, including hexachlorophene or chlorhexidine and mupirocin. In a few ICUs, selective decontamination has been used successfully as a temporary emergency control measure for outbreaks of infection due to gram-negative bacilli.

The most recent bacterial-resistance problem to plague hospitals is the emergence of vancomycin-resistant enterococci (VRE). Initially an ICU problem, VRE have now spread onto general wards in many hospitals. VRE are particularly problematic because of a substantial "iceberg" effect (i.e., the fact that, for each individual with a clinical infection, many other patients are colonized); the occurrence of both gastrointestinal and skin colonization (reflecting fecal contamination on the skin of ill, hospitalized patients); and the propensity for these organisms to contaminate the patient's environment, which may increase the risk of cross-infection. Control of VRE requires strict attention to hand washing by personnel, concerted use of barrier precautions for patients known to be colonized or infected, and emphasis on thorough cleaning of the rooms of these patients.

Because the excessive use of broad-spectrum antibiotics underlies many resistance problems, antibiotic-control policies (Table 138-2) must be considered a cornerstone of resistance-control efforts. Although the efficacy of antibiotic-control measures in reducing rates of antimicrobial resistance has not been proved in prospective controlled trials, it seems worthwhile to restrict the use of particular agents to narrowly defined indications or to cycle the use of antibiotic classes to limit the selective pressure on the nosocomial flora. Timely examples include the replacement of oral vancomycin with metronidazole for the treatment of *C. difficile* diarrhea, the elimination of oral vancomycin from prophylactic regimens administered to neutropenic patients, and the limitation of the empirical use of parenteral vancomycin for the treatment of fever in neutropenic patients.

EMPLOYEE HEALTH SERVICE ISSUES An institution's employee health service (EHS) is a critical component of its infection-control efforts. New employees should be processed through the EHS, where a contagious-disease history can be taken; evidence of immunity to a variety of diseases, such as hepatitis B, chickenpox, measles, and rubella, can be sought; immunizations for hepatitis B, measles, rubella, and varicella can be given as needed, and a reminder about the need for yearly influenza immunization can be imparted; a baseline PPD (purified protein derivative of tuberculin) skin test can be performed; and education about personal responsibility for infection control can be initiated. Evaluations of employees should be codified to meet the requirements of accrediting and regulatory agencies; for example, the CDC recommends at least annual PPD skin testing of susceptible caregivers, and OSHA requires that employees who may be exposed to blood or blood-containing fluids either receive hepatitis B vaccine at no cost or sign a specific refusal form.

The EHS must have protocols for dealing with employees who have been exposed to contagious diseases. A new problem is the counseling, treatment, and monitoring of personnel after percutaneous or mucosal exposure to the blood of patients infected with HIV or hepatitis C virus. The available data indicate that postexposure HIV prophylaxis with zidovudine is beneficial. Protocols are also needed for dealing with caregivers who have common contagious diseases, such as chickenpox, group A streptococcal infections, respiratory infections, and infectious

Table 138-2

Elements of an Antibiotic-Control Program

- Review antimicrobial agents and select a basic formulary.
- Establish prophylactic, empirical, and therapeutic guidelines.
- Restrict the use of agents that have special limited indications, cause excessive toxicity, or are costly.
- Release restricted agents for use in predetermined circumstances or after prospective approval.
- Ensure that the antibiotics on the formulary are the same as those being used for susceptibility testing by the microbiology laboratory.
- Monitor patterns of antibiotic susceptibility and trends in antibiotic use, providing regular feedback to the medical staff.
- Audit the use of specific antibiotics.
- Conduct ongoing educational programs.
- Regulate in-hospital promotional efforts of pharmaceutical companies.

SOURCE: After JP Flaherty, RA Weinstein, Infect Control Hosp Epidemiol 17:236, 1996.

diarrhea, and for those who have less common but high-visibility public health problems, such as chronic hepatitis B or C or HIV infection, for which exposure-control guidelines have been published by the CDC and by the Society for Healthcare Epidemiology of America.

BIBLIOGRAPHY

BENNETT JV, BRACHMAN PS (eds): *Hospital Infections*, 4th ed. Boston, Little, Brown, 1996

CENTERS FOR DISEASE CONTROL: Report of the National Nosocomial Infections Surveillance (NNIS) System: Nosocomial infection rates for interhospital comparison: Limitations and possible solutions. Infect Control Hosp Epidemiol 12:609, 1991

CENTERS FOR DISEASE CONTROL AND PREVENTION: Draft guideline for isolation precautions in hospitals. Part I. Evolution of isolation precautions. Part II. Recommendations for isolation precautions in hospitals. Fed Regist 59:55552, 1994

GOLDMANN DA et al: Strategies to prevent and control the emergence and spread of antimicrobial-resistant microorganisms in hospitals—A challenge to hospital leadership. JAMA 275:234, 1996

MARTONE WJ, GARNER JS (eds): Proceedings of the Third Decennial International Conference on Nosocomial Infections. Am J Med 91(Suppl 3B):1S, 1991

MAYHALL CG (ed): *Hospital Epidemiology and Infection Control.* Baltimore, Williams & Wilkins, 1995

SECTION 4

BACTERIAL DISEASES: GENERAL CONSIDERATIONS

---

139   *Gerald B. Pier*

MOLECULAR MECHANISMS OF BACTERIAL PATHOGENESIS

The past decade has seen an explosion of information about the bacterial and host molecules that contribute to the processes of infection and disease. These processes are thought by many to occur in three stages: (1) bacterial entry and colonization of the host; (2) bacterial invasion and growth in host tissues, along with elaboration of toxic substances; and (3) the host response. These three stages reflect the more traditional concepts of *infection* (presence of bacteria in a host) and *disease* (reaction to the infection)—terms that are often used interchangeably. Bacterial pathogenesis is the measure of an organism's capacity to cause disease and is a function of the myriad pathogenic or virulence factors elaborated by bacteria. These virulence factors may be classified in two groups: those that promote bacterial colonization and infection (usually surface molecules) and those that cause disease (often, but not exclusively, secreted toxins or toxic

metabolites). In addition, the host's inflammatory response to infection can contribute greatly to the observed disease and its attendant clinical signs and symptoms. Knowledge of the molecular architecture of the bacterial surface (Fig. 139-1), its interaction with the host, and the host response is critical to an understanding of the basic processes of infection and disease.

CELL WALL STRUCTURE OF GRAM-POSITIVE AND GRAM-NEGATIVE BACTERIA

GRAM-POSITIVE BACTERIA Gram-positive bacteria have a typical lipid bilayer cytoplasmic membrane surrounded by a rigid cell wall, which gives the organisms their characteristic shape, differentiates them from eukaryotic cells, and allows them to survive in osmotically unfavorable environments. The cell wall is composed mainly of peptidoglycan, a polymer of N-acetylglucosamine and its lactyl ether, N-acetylmuramic acid, with peptide side chains covalently bound to the lactyl group. The peptide chains consist of alternating D and L amino acids and are usually linked to each other by a pentaglycine bridge that binds a terminal D-alanine on one peptide substituent to the penultimate L-lysine on a neighboring peptide. Variations in this basic structure have been described for a number of bacterial genera.

In addition, the cell walls of gram-positive bacteria contain teichoic acids, phosphate-linked polymers of ribitol or glycerol that can have additional compounds linked to available side groups. Lipid tails anchor these acids to the cytoplasmic membrane, giving rise to lipoteichoic acids. Various substituents on teichoic acids are often responsible for the biologic and immunologic properties associated with disease due to pathogenic gram-positive bacteria.

Most pathogenic gram-positive bacteria have additional extracellular structures. These include surface polysaccharides (such as the group antigens of streptococci), capsular polysaccharides, and surface proteins and polypeptide capsules, which are needed for survival in blood and are useful for epidemiologic classification.

GRAM-NEGATIVE BACTERIA   In addition to having a cytoplasmic membrane and a peptidoglycan layer similar to but thinner than the one found in gram-positive organisms, gram-negative bacteria are characterized by an outer membrane that is covalently linked to the tetrapeptides of the peptidoglycan layer by a lipoprotein; this protein also contains a special lipid substituent on the terminal cysteine that embeds the lipoprotein in the outer membrane. The external surface of the outer membrane contains the lipopolysaccharide (LPS) constituent, and embedded in this membrane are special proteins that have important functions, including maintaining the outer membrane's integrity, acting as a selective barrier for diffusion of molecules into the cell, serving as receptors for bacteriophages, and binding siderophores that scavenge iron for transport into the bacterial cell.

Lipopolysaccharide   The LPS comprises lipid A and a polysaccharide. Lipid A is made up of a relatively conserved di-*N*-acetylglucosamine backbone that is linked β1→6 and has phosphate groups on the reducing 1 and nonreducing 4' carbons. Hydroxyl and amino groups on various carbons are esterified with fatty acids of varying length. Lipid A likely possesses most of the important biologic properties associated with LPS or endotoxin. Attached to carbon 6' is the inner polysaccharide core, which is usually, but not always, composed of a di- or trisaccharide of 2-keto-3-deoxyoctonate (KDO). Additional sugar substituents are linked to the inner core, forming a complete core that is somewhat conserved among related gram-negative pathogens. Attached to the complete core of LPS-smooth strains are the O-polysaccharide side chains, which, when present, confer serologic variability on different strains within a species and protect the cell from host proteins such as lytic complement components. O polysaccharides can be composed of a variety of monosaccharides, ranging from the common pentoses and hexoses to more complex and often unique sugars. These sugars can be substituted by a variety of components, such as formyl, acetyl, and hydroxybutyryl side chains; amino acids or peptides; and phosphate groups. This high level of chemical variability is thought to be central to bacterial pathogenesis, in that it allows various strains of pathogenic organisms to avoid host defenses.

Pili   Pili or fimbriae extend through the outer membrane into the external environment. They are seen in electron micrographs as hair-

FIGURE 139-1   Schematic representations of bacterial surface structures. *A*. Cytoplasmic membrane and cell wall typical of gram-positive bacteria. *B*. Outer structure of a gram-negative organism (OM = outer membrane). *C*. Detailed structure of peptidoglycan showing backbone of *N*-acetylmuramic acid (MurNac) and *N*-acetylglucosamine (GlcNac); tetrapeptide bridges composed of L-alanine (L-ala), D-glutamate (D-glu-N), L-lysine (L-lys), and D-alanine (D-ala); and pentaglycine [Gly(5)] cross-bridges. *D*. Teichoic acid backbone. *E*. Detailed structure of lipopolysaccharide typical of *Salmonella* spp., including the lipid A sugars glucosamine (GlcN) and 4-amino arabinose (AraN) and the core sugars 2-keto-3-deoxyoctonate (KDO), heptose (Hep), glucose (Glc), galactose (Gal), and *N*-acetylglucosamine (GlcNAc). Hexagons depicting the O-specific chain represent variable monosaccharide residues that comprise this structure. (*Drawing courtesy of T. J. DiCesare.*)

like projections, which may be confined to one end of the organism (polar pili) or distributed more evenly over the surface, with up to several hundred per cell. An individual cell may make multiple pili with different functions. Most pili consist of a major pilin protein subunit with a molecular weight of 17,000 to 30,000 that polymerizes to form the pilus. Some pili, such as the gal-gal–binding pili of *Escherichia coli*, have additional proteins located at their tips that are functionally critical. The major function attributed to pili to date is mediation of the binding of bacteria to host tissues.

Flagella Flagella are long appendages attached to either one or both ends of the bacterial cell (polar flagella) or distributed over the entire cell surface (peritrichous flagella). Flagella, like pili, are composed of a polymerized or aggregated basic protein. In flagella, the protein subunits form a tight helical structure and show serologic variability among different species. Spirochetes such as *Treponema pallidum* and *Borrelia burgdorferi* have axial filaments similar to flagella running down the long axis of the center of the cell and swim by rotation around these filaments. Some bacteria can glide over a surface in the absence of obvious motility structures.

INITIAL STAGE OF BACTERIAL INFECTION: COLONIZATION OF HOST SURFACES

Most bacterial pathogens initially enter the host through a mucosal surface of the respiratory, ocular, gastrointestinal, or genitourinary tract. The skin can be an important site of bacterial colonization (particularly for staphylococci), and direct inoculation of pathogens into the host is always a risk factor for subsequent disease. Successful colonization usually requires bacterial adherence to the mucosal surface. The ability to adhere is most often attributed to the pili, capsular polysaccharides, and lipoteichoic acids exposed on the cell surface, although any surface structure is capable of mediating adherence to host tissues. Host targets for bacterial adherence are either the epithelial cells lining mucosal tracts or the mucous layer itself. In the latter case, the bacteria must circumvent the host's normal ability to clear mucus-embedded cells. Such circumvention is thought to occur in states like ciliary dyskinesia in the respiratory tract or chronic *Pseudomonas aeruginosa* colonization of the respiratory tract of individuals with cystic fibrosis.

It now appears that an individual bacterial cell expresses multiple, often serologically variable adhesins and that the cell uses different adhesins during different stages of colonization. For example, most strains of *E. coli* express type 1 pili, whose binding to host tissues is inhibited by D-mannose. These pili appear to help these organisms bind to mucus. Strains of *E. coli* causing pyelonephritis express a different adhesin, the Pap or P pilus, that mediates binding to digalactose residues on globosides of the human P blood groups. Adherence here is due to minor components of the pilus proteins that are found only on the tip. In a recent study, a mutant strain of *E. coli* that (owing to a single base-pair mutation in the gene *papG*) lacked the pilus tip protein mediating bacterial binding to renal tissues failed to cause pyelonephritis in cynomolgus monkeys but did cause bladder infections. *E. coli* cells causing diarrheal disease express receptors for enterocytes on the small bowel, along with other receptors termed *colonization factors*. These receptors include the S and G fimbriae and a family of adhesins that bind to the complement regulatory factor designated *decay-accelerating factor*, a protein that also expresses the human Dr blood-group antigen.

A common type of pilus found in *Neisseria* spp., *Moraxella* spp., *Vibrio cholerae*, and *P. aeruginosa* appears to be involved in adherence of these organisms to target surfaces. These pili tend to have a relatively conserved amino-terminal region and a more variable carboxy-terminal region. For some species, such as *Neisseria gonorrhoeae* and *Neisseria meningitidis*, the pili are critical for attachment to mucosal epithelial cells; recent work shows that the principal pilus subunit of *Neisseria* also contains a minor component, the PilC protein, that is crucial for bacterial binding to host tissue. For other species, such as *P. aeruginosa*, the pili mediate only some of the epithelial cell adherence. *V. cholerae* cells appear to use two different types of pili for intestinal colonization. While interference with this stage of colonization would appear to be an effective antibacterial strategy, attempts to develop pilus-based vaccines for human diseases have not been highly successful to date. Although there are claims that pilus vaccines prevent diarrhea due to *E. coli* in pigs, calves, and lambs, this ability has not been validated in a clinical trial, and a trial of a gonococcal pilus vaccine in humans failed to demonstrate efficacy. The serologic variability among pili is one barrier to this approach.

Other bacterial structures involved in adherence to host tissues include specific proteins found among staphylococci that bind to human proteins such as fibrin, fibronectin, laminin, and collagen and that have been called MSCRAMMs (microbial surface components recognizing adhesive matrix molecules). These bacterial structures probably promote the normal colonization of the nares and skin. Fibronectin appears to be a commonly used receptor for various pathogens; a particular sequence—Arg-Gly-Asp, or RGD—is critical to binding. Surface lipoteichoic acids promote adherence of streptococci to mucosal surfaces. The mucoid exopolysaccharide or alginate capsule of *P. aeruginosa* promotes binding of mucoid strains to respiratory mucins. Coagulase-negative staphylococci have emerged as important pathogens through their ability to colonize prosthetic devices and catheters commonly used in medical care; the surface capsular polysaccharide of these organisms promotes binding to the prosthetic material.

TISSUE INVASION AND TISSUE TROPISM

TISSUE INVASION Bacteria may invade deeper layers of mucosal tissue via intracellular uptake by epithelial cells or via traversal of epithelial cell junctions. Among virulent *Shigella* strains and invasive *E. coli*, outer-membrane proteins are critical to epithelial cell invasion and bacterial multiplication. Staphylococci and streptococci elaborate a variety of extracellular enzymes, such as hyaluronidase, lipases, nucleases, and hemolysins, that are probably important in breaking down cellular and matrix structures and allowing the bacteria access to deeper tissues and blood. Organisms that colonize the gastrointestinal tract can often translocate through the mucosa into the blood and, under circumstances in which host defenses are inadequate, cause bacteremia. *Yersinia enterocolitica* can invade the mucosa through the activity of the invasin protein. Some bacteria (e.g., *Brucella*) can be carried from a mucosal site to a distant site by phagocytic cells (e.g., polymorphonuclear leukocytes, or PMNs) that ingest but fail to kill the organisms. However, it has been shown that shedding of viable epithelial cells with bound and ingested bacteria can protect tissues such as the bladder from bacterial infection.

A number of major pathogens cause disease without further invasion of host tissues; these include *Bordetella pertussis*, *V. cholerae*, *Clostridium tetani*, *Clostridium botulinum*, *Corynebacterium diphtheriae*, *Mycobacterium tuberculosis*, and *Mycobacterium leprae*. Other pathogens can cause both local disease (such as pharyngitis and epiglottitis, skin ulcerations, or diarrhea) and disease due to tissue invasion. Some pathogens require a breach in host tissues to cause deeper infections; an example of this situation is peritonitis due to *Bacteroides fragilis* or other intestinal organisms after bursting of the appendix or intestinal trauma. In such cases, bacterial factors are not critical for invasion.

TISSUE TROPISM The propensity of certain bacteria to cause disease by infecting specific tissues has been known since the early days of bacteriology, yet the molecular basis for this propensity is much less well understood than is viral tissue tropism. By analogy, receptor-ligand interactions may be expected to underlie bacterial tissue tropism, and some good evidence from studies of gastrointestinal infection supports this possibility. However, there is no well-accepted explanation of why *N. gonorrhoeae* colonizes and infects the human genital tract, while the closely related species *N. meningitidis* principally colonizes the human oropharynx. *N. gonorrhoeae* can use the enzyme sialyltransferase from host tissues to add *N*-acetylneuraminic acid (sialic acid) to its LPS O side chain, and this alteration appears to make the organism resistant to host defenses. Whether this enzyme is present in a special form or amount in the genital tract of humans is not known. Bacteria with sialic acid sugars in their capsules, such as *N. meningitidis*, *E. coli* K1, and group B streptococci, have a propensity to cause meningitis, but this generalization has many exceptions. For example, all six recognized serotypes of group B streptococci contain sialic acid in their capsules, but only one of these serotypes (type III) is responsible for most cases of meningitis due to infection by these organisms. In addition, both *Haemophilus influenzae* and pneumococci can readily cause meningitis, and these organisms do not have sialic acid in their capsules.

COMPONENTS OF THE DISEASE PROCESS

Disease is a complex phenomenon resulting from bacterial colonization, invasion, and toxin elaboration and the host's response to these events. Toxin elaboration is one of the best-characterized molecular mechanisms of bacterial pathogenesis, while host factors such as interleukin (IL) 1 and IL-6, tumor necrosis factor (TNF) α, kinins, inflammatory proteins and products of complement activation, and mediators derived from arachidonic acid metabolites (leukotrienes) and cellular degranulation (histamines) readily contribute to the severity of disease.

TOXINS Among the first diseases caused by bacterial infection to be understood were those due to toxin-elaborating organisms. Diphtheria, botulism, and tetanus toxins are responsible for the disease associated with local infections due to *C. diphtheriae*, *C. botulinum*, and *C. tetani*, respectively. Enterotoxins produced by *E. coli*, *Salmonella*, *Shigella*, *Staphylococcus*, and *V. cholerae* contribute to diarrheal disease caused by these organisms. Staphylococci, streptococci, *P. aeruginosa*, and *Bordetella* elaborate a variety of toxins that cause or contribute to disease, including toxic shock syndrome toxin 1 (TSST-1), erythrogenic toxin, exotoxin A, and pertussis toxin. A number of toxins (e.g., cholera toxin, diphtheria toxin, pertussis toxin, *E. coli* heat-labile toxin, and *P. aeruginosa* exotoxin) have adenosine diphosphate (ADP)–ribosyltransferase activity, wherein the toxins enzymatically catalyze the transfer of the ADP-ribosyl portion of nicotinamide adenine diphosphate to target proteins and inactivate them. The staphylococcal enterotoxins, TSST-1, and streptococcal pyogenic exotoxins are known as "superantigens," stimulating certain T cells to proliferate without processing of the protein toxin by antigen-presenting cells. Part of this process involves stimulation of the antigen-presenting cells to produce IL-1 and TNFα, which have been implicated in many of the clinical features of diseases such as staphylococcal toxic shock syndrome, scarlet fever, and the increasingly recognized streptococcal toxic shock syndrome.

ENDOTOXIN The lipid A portion of gram-negative LPS has potent biologic activities that are thought to cause many of the clinical features seen in gram-negative bacterial sepsis. These include fever, muscle proteolysis, uncontrolled intravascular coagulation, and shock. This effect appears to be mediated by production from mononuclear cells of IL-1, TNFα, and perhaps IL-6. These molecules exhibit potent hyperthermic activity via effects in the hypothalamus, increase vascular permeability, alter the activity of endothelial cells, and induce these cells to show procoagulant activity. Unfortunately, to date, most therapeutic strategies aimed at neutralizing the effects of endotoxin—including the use of antibodies to lipid A and to TNF and the administration of the IL-1 receptor antagonist, which blocks the binding of IL-1 to its cellular receptor—have not proved clinically useful.

BACTERIAL INVASION Some diseases are likely caused primarily by the presence of bacteria in tissue sites that are normally sterile. Invasion of the bloodstream by gram-negative rods gives rise to sepsis and bacteremia without obvious exotoxin involvement, although endotoxin is very important in this situation. Pneumococcal pneumonia is mostly attributed to the growth of *Streptococcus pneumoniae* in the lung and the attendant host inflammatory response. Disease following bacteremia and invasion of the meninges by meningitis-producing bacteria such as *N. meningitidis*, *H. influenzae*, *E. coli* K1, and group B streptococci appears to be due solely to the ability of these organisms

to get into these tissues and multiply. Most of the tissue destruction here results from bacterial growth and host inflammation.

If organisms are to effectively invade host tissues (particularly the blood), they must avoid the major host defenses of complement and phagocytic cells. This avoidance is most often accomplished through the presence of cell-surface polysaccharides—either capsular polysaccharides or long O-side-chain antigens characteristic of the smooth LPS of gram-negative bacteria. These polysaccharides appear to function by preventing activation and/or deposition of complement opsonins or by limiting access of phagocytic cells with receptors for complement opsonins to these molecules when they are deposited on the bacterial surface below the capsular layer. Another potential mechanism of microbial virulence is the ability of some organisms to present the capsule as an apparent self-antigen via molecular mimicry. For example, the polysialic acid capsule of group B *N. meningitidis* is chemically identical to an oligosaccharide found on human brain cells. The M proteins of group A streptococci appear to convey resistance to phagocytic activity in blood. Some bacteria, such as *Brucella*, *Yersinia*, *Listeria*, *Francisella*, and *Mycobacterium*, resist destruction inside phagocytic cells. Even when an obvious bacteremic phase is lacking (as, for example, in shigellosis), production of a smooth LPS is critical for bacterial pathogenesis and disease.

Immunochemical studies of capsular polysaccharides have led to an appreciation of the tremendous chemical diversity that can result from the linking of a few monosaccharides. For example, three different hexoses can link up in more than 300 different and potentially serologically distinct ways, while three different amino acids have only six possible peptide combinations. This immunochemical diversity may be the reason why many pathogenic bacteria use capsular polysaccharides to avoid host defenses. Capsular polysaccharides have been employed as effective vaccines against meningococcal meningitis as well as pneumococcal and *H. influenzae* infections and are currently under development as vaccines against infections due to group B streptococci, *P. aeruginosa*, *Klebsiella*, *Staphylococcus aureus*, and *Staphylococcus epidermidis*. In fact, capsular polysaccharides can function as a vaccine against any organism expressing a nontoxic, immunogenic capsular polysaccharide. In addition, most encapsulated pathogens become virtually avirulent when capsule production is interrupted via genetic manipulation; this observation emphasizes the importance of this structure in bacterial pathogenesis. Some encapsulated bacteria may alter their expression of capsular antigens during pathogenesis, producing a capsule when avoiding host defenses (such as during bloodstream dissemination) but not when adhering to and invading an epithelial cell during mucosal colonization.

HOST RESPONSE The inflammatory response of the host is critical for interruption and resolution of the infectious process but also is often responsible for the signs and symptoms of disease. Bacterial infection promotes a complex series of host responses involving the complement, kinin, and coagulation pathways. Most likely, the initial recognition of a foreign pathogen involves the activation of complement, and the generation of molecules such as C3a and C5a initiates inflammation. Consequently, changes take place in endothelial membranes; receptors for inflammatory cells are produced on the luminal side of the blood vessel, causing these cells to adhere to the endothelium and migrate through the vessel wall to the site of infection. The subsequent production of factors such as IL-1, IL-6, and TNF leads to fever, muscle proteolysis, and other effects noted above. An inability to kill or contain the microbe usually results in further damage due to the progression of inflammation and infection. For example, in many chronic infections, degranulation of host inflammatory cells can lead to release of host proteases, elastases, histamines, and other toxic substances that can degrade host tissues. Chronic inflammation in any tissue will eventually lead to the destruction of that tissue and to clinical disease associated with loss of organ function, such as sterility from pelvic inflammatory disease caused by chronic infection with *N. gonorrhoeae*.

The nature of the host response is often a critical factor in the type of pathology associated with a particular infection. Most bacterial pathogens provoke either local or systemic inflammation or the formation of a granuloma or an abscess. Local inflammation, as noted above, produces local tissue damage, while systemic inflammation, such as that seen during sepsis, can result in the signs and symptoms of septic shock. The latter can occur with either gram-negative or gram-positive infections, and its severity is associated with the degree of production of host effectors such as IL-1 and TNFα. Disease due to intracellular parasitism arising from infection with bacteria that cause tuberculosis, leprosy, or brucellosis results from the formation of granulomas, wherein the host attempts to wall off the parasite inside a fibrotic lesion surrounded by fused epithelial cells that make up so-called multinucleated giant cells. Levels of the cytokine IL-1α produced by macrophages can markedly affect the fate of intracellular microbes. A number of pathogens, particularly anaerobic bacteria, staphylococci, and streptococci, provoke the formation of an abscess. It has been shown that bacterial polysaccharides that contain both a positive and a negative charge (i.e., a free amino acid and a free carboxylate group) can induce abscesses following inoculation into the peritoneum of experimental animals. *B. fragilis*, a frequent cause of peritoneal abscesses, actually produces two surface polysaccharides capable of inducing these abscesses. IL-8 plays a role in recruiting and activating PMNs during abscess formation. The outcome of a bacterial infection will depend on the balance between an effective host response that eliminates a pathogen and an excessive inflammatory response that is associated with an inability to eliminate a pathogen and with the resultant tissue damage that leads to disease.

BIBLIOGRAPHY

BITTERSUERMANN D: Influence of bacterial polysialic capsules on host defense: Masquerade and mimicry, in *Polysialic Acid*, J Roth et al (eds). Basel, Birkhauser-Verlag, 1993, p 11

BOSLEGO JW et al: Efficacy trial of a parenteral gonococcal pilus vaccine in men. Vaccine 9:154, 1991

DAVIS BD: Bacterial architecture, in *Microbiology*, 4th ed, BD Davis et al (eds). Philadelphia, Lippincott, 1990, p 21

GLAUSER MP et al: Pathogenesis and potential strategies for prevention and treatment of septic shock: An update. Clin Infect Dis 18(Suppl 2):S205, 1994

MEKALANOS JJ: Environmental signals controlling expression of virulence determinants in bacteria. J Bacteriol 174:1, 1992

MELULENI GJ et al: Mucoid *Pseudomonas aeruginosa* growing in a biofilm in vitro are killed by opsonic antibodies to the mucoid exopolysaccharide capsule but not by antibodies produced during chronic lung infection in cystic fibrosis patients. J Immunol 155:2029, 1995

PATTI JM et al: MSCRAMM-mediated adherence of microorganisms to host tissues. Annu Rev Microbiol 48:585, 1994

ROBERTS JA et al: The Gal(alpha 1-4)Gal-specific tip adhesin of *Escherichia coli* P-fimbriae is needed for pyelonephritis to occur in the normal urinary tract. Proc Natl Acad Sci USA 91:11889, 1994

RUDEL T et al: Neisseria PilC protein identified as type-4 pilus tip-located adhesin. Nature 373:357, 1995

SCHAFER R et al: Superantigens and their role in infectious disease. Adv Pediatr Infect Dis 10:369, 1995

SCHLIEVERT PM et al: Severe invasive group A streptococcal disease: Clinical description and mechanisms of pathogenesis. J Lab Clin Med 127:13, 1996

SOUTHWICK FS, PURICH DL: Intracellular pathogenesis of listeriosis. N Engl J Med 334:770, 1996

STEVENS DL: Streptococcal toxic-shock syndrome. Emerging Infect Dis 1:69, 1995

TZIANABOS AO et al; Structural features of polysaccharides that induce intraabdominal abscesses. Science 262:416, 1993

Gordon L. Archer, Ronald E. Polk

TREATMENT AND PROPHYLAXIS OF BACTERIAL INFECTIONS

The development of drugs able to prevent and cure bacterial infections is one of the twentieth century's major contributions to human longevity and quality of life. Antibacterial agents are among the most commonly prescribed drugs of any kind worldwide. Used appropriately, these drugs are lifesaving. However, their indiscriminate use drives up the cost of health care, leads to a plethora of side effects and drug interactions, and fosters the emergence of bacterial resistance, rendering previously valuable drugs useless. The rational use of antibacterial agents is dependent on an understanding of their mechanisms of action, pharmacokinetics, toxicities, and interactions; bacterial strategies for resistance; and bacterial susceptibility in vitro. In addition, patient-associated parameters, such as the site of infection and the immune and the excretory status of the host, are critically important to appropriate therapeutic decisions.

This chapter provides specific data required for making an informed choice of antibacterial agent. Throughout the chapter the term *antibacterial agent* is used to refer to all natural, synthetic, and semi-synthetic compounds that kill bacteria or inhibit their growth. The term *antibiotic* is reserved for those compounds produced by living organisms.

MECHANISMS OF ACTION

Antibacterial agents, like all antimicrobial drugs, are directed against unique targets not present in mammalian cells. The goal is to limit toxicity to the host and maximize chemotherapeutic activity affecting invading microbes only. The mechanisms of action of the antibacterial agents to be discussed in this section are summarized in Table 140-1.

INHIBITION OF CELL-WALL SYNTHESIS One major difference between bacterial and mammalian cells is the presence in bacteria of a rigid wall external to the cell membrane. The wall protects bacterial cells from osmotic rupture, which would result from the fact that the cell is usually markedly hyperosmolar (by up to 20 atm) to the host environment. The structure conferring cell-wall rigidity and resistance to osmotic lysis in both gram-positive and gram-negative bacteria is peptidoglycan, a large, covalently linked sacculus that surrounds the bacterium. In gram-positive bacteria, peptidoglycan is the only layered structure external to the cell membrane and is thick (20 to 80 nm); in gram-negative bacteria, there is an outer membrane external to a very thin (1-nm) peptidoglycan layer.

Chemotherapeutic agents directed at any stage of the synthesis, export, assembly, or cross-linking of peptidoglycan lead to inhibition of bacterial cell growth and, in most cases, to cell death. Peptidoglycan is composed of (1) a backbone of two alternating sugars, *N*-acetylglucosamine and *N*-acetylmuramic acid; (2) a chain of four amino acids that extends down from the backbone (stem peptides); and (3) a peptide bridge that cross-links the peptide chains. Peptidoglycan is formed by the addition of subunits (a sugar with its five attached amino acids) that are assembled in the cytoplasm and transported through the cytoplasmic membrane to the cell surface. Subsequent cross-linking is driven by cleavage of the terminal stem-peptide amino acid. Antibacterial agents act to inhibit cell-wall synthesis in several ways, as described below.

Bacitracin, a cyclic peptide antibiotic, inhibits the conversion to its active form of the lipid carrier that moves the water-soluble cytoplasmic peptidoglycan subunits through the cell membrane to the cell exterior. Cell-wall subunits accumulate in the cytoplasm and cannot be added to the growing peptidoglycan chain.

Glycopeptides (vancomycin and teicoplanin) are high-molecular-weight antibiotics that bind to the terminal D-alanine–D-alanine component of the stem peptide while the subunits are external to the cell membrane but still linked to the lipid carrier. This binding sterically inhibits the addition of subunits to the peptidoglycan backbone.

β-*Lactam antibiotics* (penicillins, cephalosporins, carbapenems, and monobactams; see Table 140-2), characterized by a four-membered β-lactam ring, prevent the cross-linking reaction called *transpeptidation*. The energy for attaching a peptide cross-bridge from the stem peptide of one peptidoglycan subunit to another is derived from the cleavage of a terminal D-alanine residue from the subunit stem peptide. The cross-bridge amino acid is then attached to the penultimate D-alanine by transpeptidase enzymes. The β-lactam ring of the antibiotic forms an irreversible covalent acyl bond with the transpeptidase enzyme (probably because of the antibiotic's steric similarity to the enzyme's D-alanine–D-alanine target), preventing the cross-linking reaction. Transpeptidases and similar enzymes involved in cross-linking are called *penicillin-binding proteins (PBPs)* because they all have active sites that bind β-lactam antibiotics.

Virtually all the antibiotics that inhibit bacterial cell-wall synthesis are bactericidal. That is, they eventually result in the cell's death due to osmotic lysis. However, much of the loss of cell-wall integrity following treatment with cell wall–active agents is due to the bacteria's own cell-wall remodeling enzymes (autolysins) that cleave peptidoglycan bonds in the normal course of cell growth. In the presence of antibacterial agents that inhibit cell-wall growth, autolysis proceeds without normal cell-wall repair; weakness and eventual cellular lysis occur.

INHIBITION OF PROTEIN SYNTHESIS Most of the antibacterial agents that inhibit protein synthesis interact with the bacterial ribosome. The difference between the composition of bacterial and mammalian ribosomes gives these compounds their selectivity.

Aminoglycosides (gentamicin, kanamycin, tobramycin, streptomycin, netilmicin, neomycin, and amikacin) are a group of structurally related compounds containing three linked hexose sugars. They exert a bactericidal effect by binding irreversibly to the 30S subunit of the bacterial ribosome and blocking initiation of protein synthesis. The reason for the lethal effect of aminoglycosides (as opposed to the largely bacteriostatic effect of other protein synthesis–inhibiting antibacterial drugs, including the macrolides, the lincosamides, chloramphenicol, and tetracycline) is not completely understood. Uptake of aminoglycosides and their penetration through the cell membrane constitute an aerobic, energy-dependent process. Thus, aminoglycoside activity is markedly reduced in an anaerobic environment. *Spectinomycin*, an aminocyclitol antibiotic, also acts on the 30S ribosomal subunit but has a different mechanism of action from the aminoglycosides and is bacteriostatic rather than bactericidal.

Macrolides (erythromycin, clarithromycin, and azithromycin) are antibiotics that consist of a large lactone ring to which sugars are attached. They bind specifically to the 50S portion of the bacterial ribosome. After attachment of mRNA to the initiation site of the 30S ribosomal subunit (the process blocked by aminoglycosides), the 50S subunit becomes bound to the 30S component to form the 70S ribosomal complex, and protein chain elongation proceeds. Binding of macrolides to the 50S ribosomal subunit inhibits protein chain elongation.

Table 140-1

Mechanisms of Action of and Resistance to Major Classes of Antibacterial Agents

Antibacterial Agent*	Major Cellular Target	Mechanism of Action	Major Mechanisms of Resistance
β-Lactams (penicillins and cephalosporins)	Cell wall	Inhibit cell-wall cross-linking	1. Drug inactivation (β-lactamase) 2. Insensitivity of target (altered penicillin-binding proteins) 3. Decreased permeability (altered gram-negative outer-membrane porins)
Vancomycin	Cell wall	Interferes with the addition of new cell-wall subunits (muramyl pentapeptides)	Alteration of target (substitution of terminal amino acid of peptidoglycan subunit)
Bacitracin	Cell wall	Prevents addition of cell-wall subunits by inhibiting recycling of membrane lipid carrier	Not defined
Macrolides (erythromycin)	Protein synthesis	Bind to 50S ribosomal subunit	1. Alteration of target (ribosomal methylation) 2. Drug interaction 3. Decreased intracellular drug accumulation (active efflux)
Lincosamides (clindamycin)	Protein synthesis	Bind to 50S ribosomal subunit	Alteration of target (ribosomal methylation)
Chloramphenicol	Protein synthesis	Binds to 50S ribosomal subunit	Drug inactivation (chloramphenicol acetyltransferase)
Tetracyclines	Protein synthesis	Bind to 30S ribosomal subunit	1. Decreased intracellular drug accumulation (active efflux) 2. Insensitivity of target
Aminoglycosides (gentamicin)	Protein synthesis	Bind to 30S ribosomal subunit	Drug inactivation (aminoglycoside-modifying enzyme)
Mupirocin	Protein synthesis	Inhibits isoleucine tRNA synthetase	Insensitivity of target (mutation of target gene or acquisition of gene for new, insensitive enzyme)
Sulfonamides and trimethoprim	Cell metabolism	Competitively inhibit enzymes involved in two steps of folic acid biosynthesis	Production of insensitive targets (dihydropteroic acid [sulfonamides] and dihydrofolic acid [trimethoprim]) that bypass metabolic block
Rifampin	DNA synthesis	Inhibits DNA-dependent RNA polymerase	Insensitivity of target (mutation of polymerase gene)
Metronidazole	DNA synthesis	Intracellularly generates short-lived reactive intermediates by electron transfer system	Not defined
Quinolones (ciprofloxacin)	DNA synthesis	Inhibit DNA gyrase (A subunit)	1. Insensitivity of target (mutation of gyrase genes) 2. Decreased intracellular drug accumulation (active efflux)
Novobiocin	DNA synthesis	Inhibits DNA gyrase (B subunit)	Not defined
Polymyxins (polymyxin B)	Cell membrane	Disrupt membrane permeability by charge alteration	Not defined
Gramicidin	Cell membrane	Forms pores	Not defined

* Compounds in parentheses are major representatives for the class.

Lincosamides (clindamycin and lincomycin), although structurally unrelated to macrolides, bind to a site on the 50S ribosome nearly identical to the binding site for macrolides. Although the mechanism and site of action of macrolides and lincosamides are similar, the number and types of bacteria against which these two groups of agents are active differ.

Chloramphenicol, a small antibiotic with a single aromatic ring and short side chain, binds reversibly to the 50S portion of the bacterial ribosome at a site close to but not identical with the binding sites of the macrolides and lincosamides. The ribosomal binding of chloramphenicol inhibits peptide bond formation.

Tetracyclines (tetracycline, doxycycline, and minocycline) consist of four aromatic rings with various substituent groups. They interact reversibly with the bacterial 30S ribosomal subunit, blocking the binding of aminoacyl tRNA to the mRNA-ribosome complex. This mechanism is markedly different from that of the aminoglycosides, which also bind to the 30S subunit. The specificity of tetracyclines for bacteria depends both on their selectivity for bacterial ribosomes and on their requirement for active, energy-dependent transport into the bacterial cell by a system not found in mammalian cell membranes.

Mupirocin (pseudomonic acid) is produced by the bacterium *Pseudomonas fluorescens*. Its mechanism of action is unique in that it inhibits the enzyme isoleucine tRNA synthetase by competing with bacterial isoleucine for its binding site on the enzyme. Inhibition of this enzyme depletes cellular stores of isoleucine-charged tRNA and therefore leads to a cessation of protein synthesis. The antibiotic is selective for bacteria because mammalian isoleucine tRNA synthetase lacks affinity for the compound.

INHIBITION OF BACTERIAL METABOLISM The *antimetabolites* are all synthetic compounds that interfere with bacterial synthesis of folic acid. Products of the folic acid synthesis pathway function as coenzymes for the one-carbon transfer reactions that are essential for the synthesis of thymidine, all purines, and several amino acids. Inhibition of folate synthesis leads to cessation of cell growth and, in some cases, to bacterial cell death. The principal antibacterial antimetabolites are sulfonamides (sulfisoxazole, sulfadiazine, and sulfamethoxazole) and trimethoprim.

Sulfonamides are structural analogues of *p*-aminobenzoic acid (PABA), one of the three structural components of folic acid (the other two being pteridine and glutamate). The first step in the synthesis of folic acid is the addition of PABA to pteridine by the enzyme dihydropteroic acid synthetase. Sulfonamides compete with PABA as substrates for the enzyme. The selective effect of sulfonamides is due to the fact that bacteria synthesize folic acid, while mammalian cells cannot synthesize the cofactor and must have exogenous supplies. However, the activity of sulfonamides can be greatly reduced in the presence of excess PABA or by the exogenous addition of end products of one-carbon transfer reactions (e.g., thymidine and purines). High concentrations of the latter substances may be present in some infections as a result of tissue and white cell breakdown, compromising sulfonamide activity.

Trimethoprim is a diaminopyrimidine, a structural analogue of the pteridine moiety of folic acid. It is a competitive inhibitor of dihydrofolate reductase, the enzyme responsible for reduction of dihydrofolic acid to tetrahydrofolic acid, the essential final component in the folic acid synthesis pathway that is necessary for all one-carbon transfer reactions. Like the sulfonamides, trimethoprim is bactericidal in the absence of thymine but is only bacteriostatic when this pyrimidine is present in high concentration. The selective antibacterial activity of trimethoprim is based on the extreme sensitivity of bacterial dihydrofolate reductase to inhibition by this drug in comparison with the mammalian enzyme. The bacterial enzyme is approximately 50,000 times more sensitive to such inhibition.

INHIBITION OF NUCLEIC ACID SYNTHESIS OR ACTIVITY Numerous antibacterial compounds have disparate effects on nucleic acids. The *quinolones*, including nalidixic acid and its fluorinated derivatives (norfloxacin, ciprofloxacin, ofloxacin, and lomefloxacin), are synthetic compounds that inhibit the activity of one of the subunits (the A subunit) of the bacterial enzyme DNA gyrase. DNA gyrase is responsible for negative supercoiling of DNA, an essential conformation for DNA replication in the intact cell. Inhibition of the activity of DNA gyrase is lethal to bacterial cells. The antibiotic *novobiocin* also interferes with the activity of DNA gyrase, but it interferes with the B subunit.

Rifampin, used primarily as an antituberculous agent, is an antibiotic that is also active against a variety of bacteria other than *Mycobacterium tuberculosis*. Rifampin binds tightly to bacterial DNA-dependent RNA polymerase, thus inhibiting transcription of DNA into RNA. Mammalian-cell RNA polymerase is not sensitive to the compound.

Nitrofurantoin, a synthetic compound, causes DNA damage. The nitrofurans, compounds containing a single five-membered ring, are reduced by a bacterial enzyme to highly reactive, short-lived intermediates that are thought to cause DNA strand breakage, either directly or indirectly.

Metronidazole, a synthetic compound, is an imidazole that has activity against a wide range of anaerobic bacteria and protozoa. This activity is totally dependent on the organism's system for anaerobic energy production. In the presence of the anaerobic electron-transport system, the nitro group of metronidazole is reduced to a series of transiently produced, reactive intermediates that are thought to cause DNA damage. Although the unique redox system of anaerobes accounts for the selective antibacterial activity of metronidazole, this

Table 140-2

Classification of β-Lactam Antibiotics

Class	Route of Administration	
	Parenteral	Oral
Penicillins		
β-Lactamase–susceptible		
Narrow-spectrum	Penicillin G	Penicillin V
Enteric-active	Ampicillin	Amoxicillin, ampicillin
Enteric-active and antipseudomonal	Carbenicillin, ticarcillin, mezlocillin, azlocillin, piperacillin	Indanyl carbenicillin
β-Lactamase–resistant		
Antistaphylococcal	Methicillin, oxacillin, nafcillin	Cloxacillin, dicloxacillin
Combined with β-lactamase inhibitors	Ticarcillin plus clavulanic acid, ampicillin plus sulbactam, piperacillin plus tazobactam	Amoxicillin plus clavulanic acid
Cephalosporins		
First-generation	Cefazolin, cephalothin, cephapirin	Cephalexin, cephradine, cefadroxil
Second-generation		
Haemophilus-active	Cefamandole, cefuroxime, cefonicid, ceforanide	Cefaclor, cefuroxime axetil, cefixime,* cefprozil, cefpodoxime,* loracarbef
Bacteroides-active	Cefoxitin, cefotetan, cefmetazole	None
Third-generation		
Extended-spectrum	Ceftriaxone, cefotaxime, ceftizoxime	None
Extended-spectrum and antipseudomonal	Ceftazidime, cefoperazone	None
Carbapenems	Imipenem-cilastatin	None
Monobactams	Aztreonam	None

* Some sources classify cefixime and cefpodoxime as third-generation oral agents because of a marginally broader spectrum.

compound is also a mutagen and a radiosensitizer of hypoxic mammalian cells.

ALTERATION OF CELL-MEMBRANE PERMEABILITY

The *polymyxins* (polymyxin B and colistin, or polymyxin E) are cyclic, basic polypeptides. They behave as cationic, surface-active compounds that disrupt the permeability of both the outer and the cytoplasmic membranes of gram-negative bacteria.

Gramicidin A is a polypeptide of 15 amino acids that acts as an ionophore, forming pores or channels in lipid bilayers.

MECHANISMS OF RESISTANCE

Some bacteria are *intrinsically resistant* to certain classes of antibacterial agents (e.g., obligate anaerobic bacteria to aminoglycosides and gram-negative bacteria to vancomycin). Clearly these agents can never be used alone in the treatment of infections caused by resistant bacteria. In addition, bacteria that are ordinarily susceptible to antibacterial agents can acquire resistance. *Acquired resistance* is one of the major limitations to effective antibacterial chemotherapy. Resistance can develop by mutation of resident genes or by acquisition of new genes. New genes mediating resistance are usually spread from cell to cell by way of mobile genetic elements such as plasmids, transposons, and bacteriophages. The resistant bacterial populations flourish in areas of high antimicrobial use, where they enjoy a selective advantage over susceptible populations.

The major mechanisms used by bacteria to resist the action of antimicrobial agents are inactivation of the compound, alteration or overproduction of the antibacterial target, decreased permeability of the cell envelope to the agent, and active elimination of the compound from the interior of the cell. Specific mechanisms of bacterial resistance to the major antibacterial agents are outlined below and are summarized in Table 140-1.

β-LACTAMS Bacteria develop resistance to β-lactam antibiotics by a variety of mechanisms. Most common is the destruction of the drug by β-lactamases. These enzymes have a higher affinity for the antibiotic than the antibiotic has for its target. Binding results in hydrolysis of the β-lactam ring. Genes encoding β-lactamases have been found in both chromosomal and extrachromosomal locations and in both gram-positive and gram-negative bacteria; these genes are often on mobile genetic elements. One strategy that has been devised for circumventing resistance mediated by β-lactamases is to combine the susceptible β-lactam with an inhibitor that avidly binds the inactivating enzyme, preventing its attack on the antibiotic. Unfortunately, the inhibitors (e.g., clavulanic acid and sulbactam) do not bind all classes of β-lactamase and thus cannot be depended on to prevent the inactivation of β-lactam antibiotics by all β-lactamases. No β-lactam antibiotic or inhibitor has been produced that can resist all of the many β-lactamases that have been identified.

A second mechanism of bacterial resistance to β-lactam antibiotics is an alteration in PBP targets so that the PBPs have a markedly reduced affinity for the drug. While this alteration may occur by mutation of existing genes, the acquisition of new PBP genes (as in staphylococcal resistance to methicillin) or of new pieces of PBP genes (as in pneumococcal, gonococcal, and meningococcal resistance to penicillin) is more important.

A final resistance mechanism is the alteration by gram-negative bacteria of their outer membrane so that it is no longer permeable to the antibiotic. Mutations of genes encoding the outer-membrane proteins called *porins* mediate this alteration in permeability. The resistance of Enterobacteriaceae to some cephalosporins and that of *Pseudomonas* spp. to ureidopenicillins are the best examples of this mechanism. Two or more resistance mechanisms commonly coexist in the same bacterial cell.

VANCOMYCIN Clinically important resistance to vancomycin was first described among enterococci in France in 1988. Vancomycin-resistant enterococci have subsequently become disseminated worldwide. The genes encoding resistance are carried on plasmids that can transfer themselves from cell to cell. Resistance is mediated by enzymes that substitute a different molecule for the terminal amino acid on the peptidoglycan stem peptide so that there is no longer an appropriate target for vancomycin binding. This alteration does not appear to affect cell-wall integrity, however. Acquired vancomycin resistance is so far confined to enterococci. Most clinically important staphylococci (i.e., *S. aureus* and *S. epidermidis*) remain susceptible.

AMINOGLYCOSIDES The most common resistance mechanism is inactivation of the antibiotic. Aminoglycoside-modifying enzymes, usually encoded on plasmids, transfer phosphate, adenyl, or acetyl residues from intracellular molecules to hydroxyl or amino side groups on the antibiotic. The modified antibiotic is less active because of decreased transport across the cytoplasmic membrane and diminished binding to its ribosomal target. Modifying enzymes that can inactivate any of the available aminoglycosides have been found in both gram-positive and gram-negative bacteria.

A second resistance mechanism that is uncommon but has been identified in clinical isolates of *Pseudomonas aeruginosa* is decreased antibiotic uptake, presumably due to alterations in the outer membrane.

MACROLIDES AND LINCOSAMIDES Resistance in gram-positive bacteria, the usual target organisms for macrolides and lincosamides, is due to the production of an enzyme—most commonly plasmid-encoded—that methylates ribosomal RNA, interfering with binding of the antibiotics to their target. Methylation mediates resistance to erythromycin, newer macrolides, and clindamycin.

CHLORAMPHENICOL Most bacteria resistant to this antibiotic produce a plasmid-encoded enzyme, chloramphenicol acetyltransferase, that inactivates the compound by acetylation.

TETRACYCLINES The most common mechanism of resistance in gram-negative bacteria is a plasmid-encoded active-efflux pump that is inserted into the cytoplasmic membrane and extrudes antibiotic from the cell. Resistance in gram-positive bacteria is due either to active efflux or to ribosomal alterations that diminish binding of the antibiotic to its target. Genes involved in ribosomal protection are found on mobile genetic elements.

MUPIROCIN Although this topical compound was only recently introduced into clinical use, resistance is already becoming widespread in some areas. The mechanisms appear to be mutation of the target isoleucine tRNA synthetase so that it is no longer inhibited by the antibiotic and plasmid-encoded production of a form of the target enzyme that binds mupirocin poorly.

TRIMETHOPRIM AND SULFONAMIDES The most prevalent resistance mechanism in both gram-positive and gram-negative bacteria is the acquisition of plasmid-encoded genes that produce a new, drug-insensitive target. Bacteria produce an insensitive dihydrofolate reductase for trimethoprim and an altered dihydropteroate synthetase for sulfonamides.

QUINOLONES Resistance to the newer fluoroquinolones emerged rapidly among *Staphylococcus* and *Pseudomonas* species after the introduction of these agents. The most common mechanism is the development of one or more mutations in target DNA gyrases so that the antibacterial agent no longer interferes with the activity of the enzyme. Some gram-negative bacteria also acquire mutations in their outer-membrane porins so that cells are no longer permeable to the drugs; some gram-positive bacteria develop a mutation that allows them to actively pump the antibacterial agents from the cell.

RIFAMPIN Bacteria rapidly become resistant to rifampin by developing mutations in RNA polymerase that render the enzyme unable to bind the antibiotic. The rapid selection of resistant mutants is the major limitation to the use of this antibiotic against otherwise susceptible staphylococci and requires that it be used in combination with another antistaphylococcal agent.

MULTIPLE ANTIBIOTIC RESISTANCE The acquisition by one bacterium of resistance to multiple antibacterial agents is becoming increasingly common. The two major mechanisms are the acquisition of multiple unrelated resistance genes and the development of mutations in a single gene or gene complex that mediate resistance to a series of unrelated compounds. The construction of multiresistant strains by acquisition of multiple genes occurs by sequential steps of gene transfer and environmental selection in areas of high antimicrobial use. In contrast, mutations in a single gene can conceivably be selected in a single step. Bacteria that are multiresistant by virtue of the acquisition of new genes include hospital-associated gram-negative bacteria, enterococci, and staphylococci and community-acquired strains of salmonellae, gonococci, and pneumococci. Most of the latter bacterial isolates originated in other countries but have become established in some areas of the United States. Mutations that confer resistance to multiple unrelated antimicrobial agents occur in the outer-membrane proteins (porins) of gram-negative bacteria. These mutations affect the permeability of these bacteria to β-lactams, quinolones, tetracycline, chloramphenicol, and trimethoprim. Multiresistant bacterial isolates pose increasing problems in U.S. hospitals; strains resistant to all available antibacterial chemotherapy have already been identified.

PHARMACOKINETICS

The *pharmacokinetic profile* of an antibacterial agent refers to concentrations in serum and tissue versus time after administration and reflects the processes of absorption, distribution, metabolism, and excretion. Important characteristics include peak and trough serum concentrations and mathematically derived parameters such as half-life, clearance, and distribution volume. Pharmacokinetic information is useful for estimating the appropriate antibacterial dose and frequency of administration, for adjusting dosages in patients with impaired excretory capacity, and for comparing one drug with another.

ABSORPTION Data on absorption can refer to oral, intramuscular, or intravenous administration.

Oral Administration Most patients with infection are treated with oral antibacterial agents in the outpatient setting. Advantages of oral therapy over parenteral therapy include lower cost, generally fewer adverse effects (including complications of indwelling lines), and greater acceptance by patients. The percentage of an orally administered antibacterial agent that is absorbed (i.e., the agent's *bioavailability*) ranges from as little as 10 to 20 percent (erythromycin and penicillin G) to nearly 100 percent (clindamycin, metronidazole, doxycycline, and trimethoprim-sulfamethoxazole). These differences in bioavailability are not clinically important as long as concentrations at the site of infection are sufficient to inhibit or kill the pathogen. However, therapeutic efficacy may be compromised when absorption is reduced as a result of physiologic or pathologic conditions (such as the presence of food for some drugs or the shunting of blood away from the gastrointestinal tract in patients with hypotension), drug interactions (such as that of quinolones and metal cations), or noncompliance. The oral route is usually used for patients with relatively mild infections in whom absorption is not thought to be compromised by the preceding conditions.

Intramuscular Administration Although the intramuscular route of administration usually results in 100 percent bioavailability, it is not as widely used in the United States as the oral and intravenous routes, in part because of the pain often associated with intramuscular injections and the relative ease of intravenous access in the hospitalized patient. Intramuscular injection may be suitable for specific indications requiring an "immediate" and reliable effect (e.g., with long-acting forms of penicillin, including benzathine and procaine, and with single doses of ceftriaxone for uncomplicated gonococcal infection).

Intravenous Administration The intravenous route is appropriate when oral antibacterial agents are not effective against a particular pathogen, when bioavailability is uncertain, or when larger doses are required than are feasible with the oral route. After intravenous administration, bioavailability is 100 percent, and serum concentrations peak at the end of the infusion. For many patients requiring long-term therapy, outpatient intravenous administration with the use of convenient portable pumps may be cost-effective and safe when oral therapy is not feasible. Alternatively, some newer oral antibacterial drugs are sufficiently active against some organisms to rival parenteral therapy; their use may allow the patient to return home earlier or to avoid hospitalization entirely.

DISTRIBUTION After absorption, the serum concentrations of most antibacterial agents must exceed the minimum concentration required to inhibit bacterial growth (MIC; see Chap. 121) to be effective. Since most infections are extravascular, an antibiotic also must *distribute* to the site of infection. Concentrations of most antibacterials in interstitial fluid are similar to free drug concentrations in serum. However, when the infection is located in a "protected" site where penetration is poor, such as cerebrospinal fluid (CSF), the eye, the prostate, or infected cardiac vegetations, high parenteral doses or local administration for prolonged periods may be required for cure. In addition, even though an antibacterial agent may penetrate to the site of infection, its activity may be antagonized by local factors, such as an unfavorable pH or inactivation by cellular degradation products. For example, since the activity of aminoglycosides is reduced at acidic pH, the acidic environment in many infected tissues may be partly responsible for the relatively poor efficacy of aminoglycoside monotherapy. In addition, the abscess milieu reduces the activity of many antibacterial compounds, so that surgical drainage is required for cure.

Most bacteria that cause human infections are located extracellularly. Intracellular pathogens such as *Legionella*, *Chlamydia*, *Brucella*, and *Salmonella* may persist or cause relapse if the antibacterial agent does not enter the cell. In general, β-lactams, vancomycin, and aminoglycosides penetrate cells poorly, whereas macrolides, tetracyclines, metronidazole, chloramphenicol, rifampin, trimethoprim-sulfamethoxazole, and quinolones penetrate cells well.

METABOLISM AND ELIMINATION Like other drugs, antibacterial agents are disposed of by hepatic elimination (metabolism or biliary elimination), by renal excretion in unchanged or metabolized form, or by a combination of the two processes. For most antibacterial drugs, metabolism leads to loss of in vitro activity, although some agents, such as cefotaxime, rifampin, and clarithromycin, have bioactive metabolites that may contribute to their overall efficacy.

The most practical consequence of the mode of excretion of an antibacterial agent is the need to adjust the dosage when elimination capability is impaired. Direct, nonidiosyncratic toxicity from antibacterial drugs most often results from failure to reduce the dosage appropriately in a patient with impaired elimination. For agents that are primarily cleared intact by glomerular filtration, drug clearance is linearly correlated with creatinine clearance. Commonly used antibacterial drugs that require dosage adjustment in patients with renal impairment are listed in Table 140-3. Unfortunately, for drugs whose elimination is primarily hepatic, no simple marker (such as serum creatinine) is useful for dosage adjustment in subjects with liver disease. Even in patients with severe hepatic disease, residual metabolic capability is usually sufficient for the avoidance of accumulation and toxic effects. However, for drugs that undergo hepatic metabolism and have a narrow therapeutic index (such as chloramphenicol), alternative therapy may be warranted in patients with liver disease, since the technology for the monitoring of serum levels is not widely available.

PRINCIPLES OF ANTIBACTERIAL CHEMOTHERAPY

The choice of an antibacterial compound for a particular patient and a specific infection involves more than just a knowledge of the agent's mechanism of action and pharmacokinetic profile. The basic tenets of chemotherapy, to be elaborated below, include the following: First, whenever possible, material containing the infecting organism(s) should be obtained so that presumptive identification can be made by microscopic examination of stained specimens and the organism can be grown for definitive identification and susceptibility testing. Second, once the organism is identified and its susceptibility to antibacterial agents is determined, the regimen with the narrowest effective spectrum should be chosen. Third, the choice of antibacterial agent is guided by the pharmacokinetic and adverse-reaction profile of active compounds, the site of infection, the immune status of the host, and evidence of efficacy from well-performed clinical trials. Finally, if all other factors are equal, the antibacterial regimen that is the least expensive should be chosen.

SUSCEPTIBILITY OF BACTERIA TO ANTIBACTERIAL DRUGS IN VITRO

The determination of the susceptibility of the patient's infecting organism to a panel of appropriate antibacterial agents is an essential first step in devising a chemotherapeutic regimen. The details of susceptibility testing are discussed elsewhere (Chap. 121). Such testing is designed to estimate the susceptibility of a bacterial isolate to an antibacterial drug under standardized conditions that favor rapidly growing aerobic or facultative organisms and to assess bacteriostasis only. Specialized testing is required for the assessment of bactericidal antimicrobial activity; for the detection of resistance among such fastidious organisms as obligate anaerobes, *Haemophilus* spp., and pneumococci; and for the determination of resistance phenotypes with variable expression, such as resistance to methicillin or oxacillin among staphylococci.

RELATIONSHIP OF PHARMACOKINETICS AND IN VITRO SUSCEPTIBILITY TO CLINICAL RESPONSE

The relationship between the report of susceptibility in vitro and the clinical pharmacokinetics of the antibacterial agent helps predict clinical response. Bacteria are usually considered to be *susceptible* to a drug if the achievable peak serum concentration exceeds the MIC by at least fourfold. The *breakpoint* is the concentration of the antibiotic that separates susceptible from resistant bacteria. When a majority of the isolates of a given bacterial species are inhibited at concentrations below the breakpoint, the species is within the spectrum of the drug (see "Choice of Antibacterial Therapy" below). Antibacterial agents are frequently administered every three to four half-lives, since serum concentrations will by then be below the breakpoint and may be below the MIC for the organism. These relationships are illustrated in Fig. 140-1. *Pharmacodynamics* refers to the quantitative relationship among drug concentrations in serum and tissues, in vitro susceptibility, and microbial response at the site of infection. Pharmacodynamic parameters that appear to correlate with reduction in the number of bacteria at the site of infection include the ratio of the area under the serum concentration curve to the MIC (especially for aminoglycosides and quinolones), the length of time that concentrations exceed the MIC (especially for β-lactams), and the postantibiotic effect (PAE, or length of time that bacterial growth is inhibited after concentrations fall below the MIC). For some drugs with a PAE, such as the aminoglycosides, it may not be necessary to maintain serum concentrations above the MIC for the entire dose interval. Newer dosage regimens, such as the administration of the entire daily dosage of an aminoglycoside in a single dose, are designed to take advantage of this property. Many microbiology laboratories report quantitative susceptibilities (MICs); Table 140-3 lists peak serum concentrations and breakpoints for some common antibacterial agents.

STATUS OF THE HOST

Various host factors must be considered when devising antibacterial chemotherapy. The host's antibacterial *immune function* is of importance, particularly as it relates to opsonophagocytic function. Since the major host defense against acute, overwhelming bacterial infection is the polymorphonuclear leukocyte, patients with neutropenia must be treated aggressively and empirically with bactericidal drugs for suspected infection (see Chap. 87). Like-

Table 140-3

Pharmacokinetics of Selected Antibacterial Agents

Drug	Dose, Route	Peak Serum Concentration, μg/mL	Breakpoint,* μg/mL	Half-life, h	Dose Alteration in Renal Disease
Penicillin G	2×10^6 units, IV	60	0.1†	0.5	Yes
Ampicillin	1000 mg, IV	40	8‡	1	Yes
Dicloxacillin	500 mg, PO	15	2	1	No
Nafcillin	1000 mg, IV	40	2	1	No
Ticarcillin	3000 mg, IV	160	16‡	1	Yes
Cefazolin	1000 mg, IV	188	8	2	Yes
Cefaclor	500 mg, PO	15	8	1	Yes
Cephalexin	500 mg, PO	15	8	1	Yes
Cefoxitin	1000 mg, IV	110	8	1	Yes
Cefuroxime	1000 mg, IV	100	8	1.5	Yes
Ceftriaxone	1000 mg, IV	150	8	8	Slight
Ceftazidime	2000 mg, IV	170	8	2	Yes
Aztreonam	2000 mg, IV	200	8	2	Yes
Imipenem	500 mg, IV	43	4	1	Yes
Gentamicin	1.5 mg/kg, IV	8	4	2	Yes
Amikacin	7.5 mg/kg, IV	35	16	2	Yes
Doxycycline	100 mg, PO	2.5	4	18	Yes
Tetracycline	500 mg, PO	4	4	8	§
Erythromycin	500 mg, PO	1	0.5	0.5–2.0	No
Clindamycin	600 mg, IV	10	0.5	2.4	No
Metronidazole	500 mg, PO	10	NA¶	6	No
Vancomycin	1000 mg, IV	30	4	6	Yes
Trimethoprim-sulfamethoxazole	160/800 mg, PO	2/40	2/38	11/9	Yes
Ciprofloxacin	500 mg, PO	3	1	4	Yes
Ofloxacin	400 mg, PO	6	2	6	Yes

* For fully susceptible organisms.
† For most gram-positive organisms.
‡ For Enterobacteriaceae.

§f Contraindicated in renal impairment.
¶ NA = not applicable.

wise, patients who have deficient humoral immunity (e.g., those with chronic lymphocytic leukemia and multiple myeloma) and individuals with surgical or functional asplenia (e.g., those with sickle cell disease) should be treated empirically for infections with encapsulated organisms, especially the pneumococcus.

Pregnancy increases the risk of toxicity of certain antibacterial drugs for the mother (e.g., the hepatic toxicity of tetracycline), affects drug disposition and pharmacokinetics, and—because of the risk of fetal toxicity—severely limits the choice of agents for treating infections. Certain antibacterials are contraindicated in pregnancy either because their safety has not been established or because they are known to be toxic. These agents include all fluoroquinolones, clarithromycin, erythromycin estolate (but not erythromycin base), and tetracyclines. Data on the safety of many other antibacterial drugs are limited, but these drugs may be used cautiously when there is no suitable alternative and the perceived benefit outweighs the risk. These agents include the

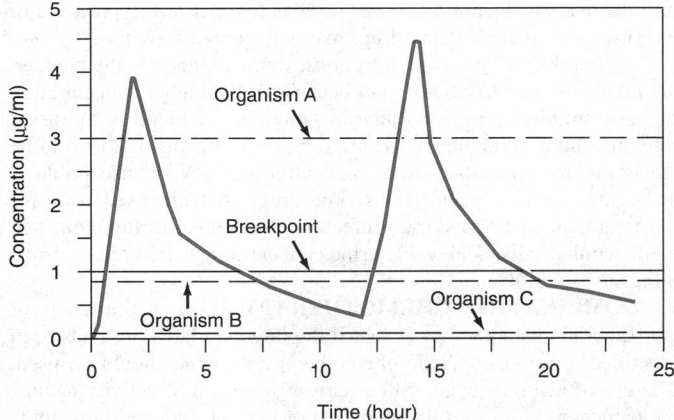

FIGURE 140-1 Relationship between pharmacokinetics of an antibiotic and susceptibility. Organism A is resistant, organism B is moderately susceptible, and organism C is very susceptible.

aminoglycosides, azithromycin, clindamycin, imipenem, metronidazole, trimethoprim, and vancomycin. The following drugs are contraindicated in the third trimester but can be used cautiously in the first two trimesters: chloramphenicol, nitrofurantoin, and the sulfonamides.

In patients with *concomitant viral infections*, the incidence of adverse reactions to antibacterial drugs may be unusually high. For example, persons with infectious mononucleosis and those infected with human immunodeficiency virus (HIV) may react more often to ampicillin and folic acid synthesis inhibitors, respectively.

In addition, the patient's age, sex, racial heritage, and excretory status all determine the incidence and type of side effects that can be expected with certain antibacterial agents.

SITE OF INFECTION   The location of the infected site may play a major role in the choice and dose of antimicrobial drug. Patients with suspected *meningitis* should receive drugs that can cross the blood-CSF barrier; in addition, because of the relative paucity of phagocytes and opsonins at the site of infection, the agents should be bactericidal. Chloramphenicol, one of the standard drugs used in the treatment of meningitis, is bactericidal for common organisms causing meningitis (i.e., meningococci, pneumococci, and *Haemophilus influenzae*, but *not* enteric gram-negative bacilli), is highly lipid-soluble, and enters the CSF well. However, β-lactams, the mainstay of therapy for most of these infections, do not normally reach high levels in CSF. Their efficacy is based on the increased permeability of the blood-brain and blood-CSF barriers to hydrophilic molecules during inflammation and the extreme susceptibility of most infectious organisms to even small amounts of β-lactam drug.

The vegetation that is the major site of infection in *bacterial endocarditis* is also a focus that is protected from normal host-defense mechanisms. Antibacterial therapy needs to be bactericidal, with the selected agent administered parenterally over a long period and at a dose that produces serum levels at least eight times higher than the minimum bactericidal concentration (MBC) for the infecting organism. Likewise, *osteomyelitis* involves a site that is somewhat resistant to opsonophagocytic removal of infecting bacteria; furthermore, avascular bone (sequestrum) represents a foreign body that thwarts normal host-defense mechanisms. *Chronic prostatitis* is exceedingly difficult to cure because most antibiotics do not penetrate the nonfenestrated capillaries serving the prostate, especially when acute inflammation is absent. Drugs that are "ion trapped" after entering prostatic tissue, such as trimethoprim and fluoroquinolones, may be uniquely effective because of this mechanism. *Intraocular infections*, especially endophthalmitis, are difficult to treat because drug penetration into the vitreous from blood is hindered by retinal capillaries lacking fenestration. Inflammation does little to disrupt this barrier. Thus, direct injection into the vitreous is necessary in many cases. Antibiotic penetration into *abscesses* is usually poor. Even when an antibiotic does penetrate into the abscess, local conditions, such as low pH or the presence of enzymes that hydrolyze the drug, may antagonize activity.

In contrast, *urinary tract infections*, when confined to the bladder, are relatively easy to cure, in part because of the higher concentration of most antibiotics in urine than in blood. Since blood is the usual reference fluid in defining susceptibility, even organisms found to be "resistant" to achievable serum concentrations may be susceptible to achievable urine concentrations. For drugs that are used only for the treatment of urinary tract infections, such as nitrofurantoin and methenamine salts, achievable urine concentrations are used to determine susceptibility.

COMBINATION CHEMOTHERAPY   One of the tenets of antibacterial chemotherapy is that if the infecting bacterium has been identified, the most specific chemotherapy possible should be used. The use of a single agent with a narrow spectrum of activity against the pathogen diminishes the alteration of normal flora and thus limits the overgrowth of resistant nosocomial organisms (e.g., *Candida albicans*, enterococci, *Clostridium difficile*, or methicillin-resistant staphylococci), avoids the potential toxicity of multiple-drug regimens, and

reduces cost. However, certain circumstances call for the use of more than one antibacterial agent. These are summarized below.

1. *Prevention of the emergence of resistant mutants.* Spontaneous mutations occur at a detectable frequency in certain genes encoding the target proteins for some antibacterial agents. The use of these agents can eliminate the susceptible population, select out resistant mutants at the site of infection, and result in the failure of chemotherapy. Resistant mutants are usually selected when the MIC of the antibacterial agent for the infecting bacterium is close to achievable levels in serum or tissues and/or when the site of infection limits the access or activity of the agent. The most common examples are rifampin for staphylococci, imipenem for *Pseudomonas*, and ciprofloxacin for staphylococci and *Pseudomonas*. Small-colony variants of staphylococci resistant to aminoglycosides also emerge during monotherapy with these antibiotics. A second antibacterial agent with a mechanism of action different from that of the first is added to prevent the emergence of these resistant mutants (e.g., imipenem plus an aminoglycoside for systemic *Pseudomonas* infections). However, since resistant mutants have emerged following combination chemotherapy, this approach is not uniformly successful.

2. *Synergistic or additive activity.* Against some bacteria, two antibacterial agents are clearly more active than one; whether or not this is the case is usually judged on the basis of testing in vitro. *Synergistic* or *additive activity* is defined as a lowering of the MIC or MBC of *each* of two drugs tested in combination against a specific bacterium. Thus *each* agent is more active when combined with a second drug than it would be alone. The best examples of a synergistic or additive effect, confirmed both in vitro and by animal studies, are the enhanced bactericidal activities of certain β-lactam–aminoglycoside combinations against enterococci, viridans streptococci, and *P. aeruginosa*. The synergistic or additive activity of these combinations also has been demonstrated for selected isolates of enteric gram-negative bacteria and staphylococci. The combination of trimethoprim and sulfamethoxazole also has synergistic or additive activity against many enteric gram-negative bacteria. Most other antimicrobial combinations show indifferent activity (i.e., the combination is *no better* than the more active of the two agents alone), and some combinations (e.g., penicillin plus tetracycline against pneumococci) may be antagonistic (i.e., the combination is *worse* than either drug alone).

3. *Therapy directed against multiple potential pathogens.* For certain infections, either a mixture of pathogens is suspected or the patient is desperately ill with an as-yet-unidentified infection. In these situations, the most important of the likely infecting bacteria need to be covered by therapy until culture and susceptibility results become available. Examples of the former infections are intraabdominal or brain abscesses and infections of limbs in diabetic patients with microvascular disease. The latter situations include fevers in neutropenic patients, acute pneumonia from aspiration of oral flora by hospitalized patients, and septic shock or sepsis syndrome. However, in circumstances where empirical therapy with more than one agent is begun, monotherapy should always be given subsequently if a single infecting bacterium that can be treated effectively with one agent is identified.

CHOICE OF ANTIBACTERIAL THERAPY

The antibacterial spectrum of specific agents and the infections for which they represent the treatment of choice are detailed below. No attempt has been made to include all the potential situations in which antibacterial agents may be used. A more detailed discussion of specific bacteria and infections that they cause can be found elsewhere in this volume.

β-LACTAMS (Table 140-2)   All *penicillins* (except for the semisynthetic, penicillinase-resistant antistaphylococcal agents) are hydrolyzed by β-lactamases and are ineffective against isolates that produce these enzymes. Penicillin G has a spectrum that includes spirochetes (*Treponema pallidum*, *Borrelia*, and *Leptospira*), streptococci (groups A and B, viridans, and *Streptococcus pneumoniae*), enterococci, most *Neisseria* species, a few staphylococci, many fastidious oral bacteria [*Bacteroides* (*Porphyromonas* and *Prevotella*), streptococci, *Actinomyces*, and *Fusobacterium*], *Clostridium* species (except *C. difficile*), *Pasteurella multocida*, *Erysipelothrix rhusiopathiae*, and *Streptobacillus moniliformis*. However, resistance is widespread among staphylococci; is increasing rapidly among gonococci, enterococci, and pneumococci; and is emerging among meningococci and oral anaerobes such as *Porphyromonas* and *Prevotella*. Penicillin G is the drug of choice for syphilis, yaws, leptospirosis, group A and B streptococcal infections, actinomycosis, oral and periodontal infections, meningococcal meningitis and meningococcemia, viridans streptococcal endocarditis, clostridial myonecrosis, tetanus, anthrax, rat-bite fever, *P. multocida* infections, and erysipeloid (*E. rhusiopathiae*).

Ampicillin extends the spectrum of penicillin G to some gram-negative rods. It is active against some isolates of *Escherichia coli*, *Proteus mirabilis*, *Salmonella*, *Shigella*, and *H. influenzae* and is one of the drugs of choice for susceptible organisms causing urinary tract infections, salmonellosis, *H. influenzae* meningitis and epiglottitis, and *Listeria monocytogenes* meningitis. High rates of resistance have lessened its value as empirical therapy in some situations. For example, more than 80 percent of isolates of *E. coli* and *P. mirabilis* are resistant in some hospitals, as are 10 to 30 percent of isolates of *H. influenzae*; moreover, in some outbreaks of infection due to salmonellae, all isolates are ampicillin-resistant.

The *penicillinase-resistant penicillins* are used solely for the treatment of staphylococcal infections and are the drugs of choice for systemic or deep staphylococcal infections caused by susceptible organisms. Unfortunately, on average, approximately 20 percent of *S. aureus* isolates and more than 60 percent of coagulase-negative staphylococcal isolates acquired in U.S. hospitals are resistant to these agents (i.e., methicillin-resistant). The spectrum of these agents also includes most of the same gram-positive bacteria that are susceptible to penicillin G.

The spectrum of the *antipseudomonal penicillins* includes the bacteria covered by ampicillin as well as some additional nonpseudomonal enteric gram-negative bacilli. For example, piperacillin is active against many indole-positive *Proteus*, *Enterobacter*, *Klebsiella*, *Providencia*, and *Serratia* species. However, the susceptibility of these penicillins to β-lactamase markedly limits their utility as empirical therapy when infections caused by gram-negative enteric organisms are suspected. The major use of these compounds is in the treatment of proven or suspected infections with *P. aeruginosa* and *Acinetobacter*, for which they are among the drugs of choice. Their relative antipseudomonal activities can be ranked as follows: piperacillin > mezlocillin/ticarcillin > carbenicillin.

The addition of β-*lactamase inhibitors* (clavulanic acid, sulbactam, or tazobactam) to ampicillin, amoxicillin, ticarcillin, or piperacillin extends the spectrum of these agents to include many organisms that are resistant by virtue of β-lactamase production. These organisms include *E. coli*, *Klebsiella*, all *Proteus* species, *H. influenzae*, *Moraxella* (formerly *Branhamella*) *catarrhalis*, *Providencia*, and *Bacteroides fragilis*. Such combinations are also active against staphylococci that produce β-lactamase but are not methicillin-resistant. However, the efficacy of these combinations in serious staphylococcal infections has not been adequately proven. Furthermore, *Enterobacter*, *Pseudomonas*, *Acinetobacter*, and various enteric gram-negative isolates either produce β-lactamases not inhibited by these compounds or develop resistance attributable to non-β-lactamase-mediated mechanisms.

The *first-generation cephalosporins* have a spectrum that includes penicillinase-producing, methicillin-susceptible staphylococci and streptococci. While these drugs may be used when infections with gram-positive bacteria are suspected, they are *not* the drugs of choice for such infections. They have excellent activity against many isolates of *E. coli*, *Klebsiella pneumoniae*, and *P. mirabilis* and are among the drugs of choice in presumptive therapy for non-hospital-acquired urinary tract infections. They have no activity against *B. fragilis*, enterococci, methicillin-resistant staphylococci, *Pseudomonas*, *Aci-*

netobacter, *Enterobacter*, indole-positive *Proteus*, and *Serratia* and poor activity against *H. influenzae*.

The *parenteral second-generation cephalosporins* extend the gram-negative spectrum of first-generation compounds. The various second-generation agents have differing activities. Cefuroxime and cefamandole retain activity against gram-positive cocci and are also active against *H. influenzae*, *Neisseria*, some *Enterobacter* isolates, and indole-positive *Proteus* but exhibit poor activity against *B. fragilis*. Cefoxitin and cefotetan have reasonably good activity against *B. fragilis*, but cefotetan is less effective against some other *Bacteroides* species (see Chaps. 127 and 169). Both of the latter drugs display poor activity against gram-positive cocci and *Enterobacter*. No second-generation cephalosporin is active against *Pseudomonas* or *Acinetobacter*.

Oral second-generation cephalosporins have fair activity against gram-positive cocci and *H. influenzae* and are widely used in outpatient therapy for otitis media, sinusitis, and lower respiratory tract infections, although cheaper agents that are equally effective are preferable. Cefixime, cefuroxime axetil, and cefpodoxime are among the drugs of choice for single-dose treatment of gonococcal urethritis.

Third-generation cephalosporins all have a broad spectrum of activity against enteric gram-negative rods and are especially useful for treating hospital-acquired infections caused by multiresistant organisms. In addition, ceftazidime has excellent antipseudomonal activity. Cefoperazone has modest antipseudomonal activity, and the other third-generation cephalosporins have poor antipseudomonal activity. Since resistance to third-generation cephalosporins is increasing among all nosocomial gram-negative rods, the use of these agents should be guided by susceptibility testing. The gram-positive spectrum of the third-generation cephalosporins is variable, the relative rank being cefotaxime/ceftizoxime/ceftriaxone > cefoperazone > ceftazidime. Because of its excellent gram-negative spectrum, its activity against *Haemophilus*, *S. pneumoniae*, and penicillin-resistant *Neisseria*, its long serum half-life, and its high serum and CSF levels, ceftriaxone has become one of the drugs of choice for empirical therapy for bacterial meningitis (except that caused by *Listeria*), all gonococcal infections, salmonellosis, and typhoid fever. It is also a drug of choice for nonpseudomonal hospital-acquired pneumonia. Third-generation cephalosporins have poor activity against *B. fragilis* and no activity against methicillin-resistant staphylococci, *Enterococcus*, *Acinetobacter*, or *Xanthomonas*.

The only *carbapenem* currently available in the United States is imipenem. This drug is marketed in combination with the renal dipeptidase inhibitor cilastatin, which enables imipenem to escape renal inactivation and thus to reach higher urinary levels. Imipenem has excellent activity in vitro against virtually all bacterial pathogens except *Xanthomonas*, methicillin-resistant staphylococci, and *Enterococcus faecium*. Limitations to its use are its relatively low blood levels, short serum half-life, central nervous system side effects, and high cost. Resistance to imipenem is a problem only among nosocomial isolates of *P. aeruginosa*, approximately 20 percent of which are resistant. Imipenem is *not* the drug of choice for any bacterial infection, but, because of its broad spectrum, it can be used as empirical therapy for serious nosocomial infections thought to be caused by multiple bacterial species or multiresistant organisms. This antibiotic often is held in reserve as therapy for nosocomial infections due to gram-negative pathogens resistant to third-generation cephalosporins.

The only *monobactam* currently available is aztreonam. This antibiotic has a spectrum limited to facultative gram-negative enteric bacilli. It has no activity against any gram-positive or anaerobic bacterium. Its gram-negative spectrum is similar to that of ceftazidime, with equally good activity against *Pseudomonas*. Its primary advantages are its theoretical ability to preserve the normal gram-positive and anaerobic flora and the lack of cross-reactive immediate hypersensitivity in patients who have had this type of reaction to other β-lactam antibiotics.

VANCOMYCIN The spectrum of vancomycin is limited to gram-positive cocci, especially enterococci, streptococci, and staphylococci. Vancomycin serves as second-line therapy for most gram-positive bacterial infections but is the drug of choice for infections caused by methicillin-resistant staphylococci or *Corynebacterium jeikeium* and for serious infections in penicillin-allergic patients. Given orally (a route by which it is not absorbed), vancomycin can be used to treat antibiotic-associated pseudomembranous colitis caused by *C. difficile* in patients who have failed to respond to metronidazole, the drug of choice. Resistance to vancomycin is increasing rapidly among isolates of *E. faecium* in large hospitals, particularly in areas of high-level vancomycin use. Because of the growing threat of vancomycin-resistant enterococci and the potential for staphylococci to acquire resistance genes, a national advisory committee has established guidelines for appropriate and limited use of this antibiotic.

AMINOGLYCOSIDES The aminoglycosides are rapidly bactericidal in vitro at low concentrations, with activity limited to facultative gram-negative bacteria and staphylococci. They have no activity against anaerobic bacteria and are not effective in environments that are acidic or have a low oxygen tension. However, their spectrum includes virtually all gram-negative bacteria that are not strict anaerobes, and they are among the drugs of choice for any suspected gram-negative bacteremic infection, particularly in neutropenic patients. Aminoglycosides are synergistically bactericidal in combination with a penicillin for the treatment of staphylococcal, enterococcal, or viridans streptococcal endocarditis and are usually combined with a β-lactam antibiotic for the treatment of gram-negative bacteremia. Aminoglycosides are also among the drugs of choice for severe infections of the upper urinary tract. The major limitations to use of aminoglycosides are their renal and otic toxicity, their diminished activity at certain sites of infection (e.g., abscesses and the central nervous system), the resistance of target bacteria, and the need to monitor serum levels. Among the available agents, gentamicin is generally preferred because of its low cost; however, tobramycin has slightly greater activity against *P. aeruginosa*, and amikacin retains activity against many tobramycin- and gentamicin-resistant gram-negative bacteria because it is inactivated by fewer aminoglycoside-modifying enzymes. Streptomycin is still one of the drugs of choice in initial therapy for tularemia, plague, glanders, and brucellosis and is a second-line agent for the treatment of tuberculosis.

MACROLIDES Erythromycin has broad-spectrum activity against gram-positive bacteria, with additional activity against *Legionella*, *Mycoplasma*, *Campylobacter*, and some *Chlamydia* isolates. It is the drug of choice for infections due to *Legionella*, *Campylobacter*, and *Mycoplasma* and is among the drugs of choice for pneumococcal pneumonia and pharyngitis and for skin and soft-tissue infections due to group A streptococci in penicillin-allergic patients. However, resistance to erythromycin among group A streptococci and pneumococci is increasing in some countries. Erythromycin also appears to be one of the drugs of choice for infections caused in immunocompromised patients by the newly identified agent of bacillary angiomatosis (*Bartonella henselae*). The newer macrolides clarithromycin and azithromycin have an antibacterial spectrum similar to that of erythromycin in vitro. However, azithromycin has greater activity against *Chlamydia*. Clarithromycin, in combination with a proton pump inhibitor, has been designated a drug of choice for the treatment of gastric infections due to *Helicobacter pylori* (gastritis, gastric and duodenal ulcers). Both are active against nontuberculous mycobacteria, and both appear to have fewer gastrointestinal side effects than does erythromycin.

LINCOSAMIDES The only lincosamide used in the United States is clindamycin. It shares the gram-positive coccal spectrum of erythromycin but is more active, in some cases showing bactericidal activity, against susceptible staphylococci. However, resistance among staphylococci and many streptococci, mediated by the same genes responsible for macrolide resistance, limits clindamycin's usefulness against gram-positive cocci. In general, all gram-positive cocci resistant to erythromycin should be considered resistant to clindamycin regardless of the results of in vitro susceptibility testing. Clindamycin is one of the drugs of choice for anaerobic infections because of its broad spectrum of activity against both gram-positive and gram-negative strict anaerobes. In contrast, clindamycin, like erythromycin, has no clinically significant activity against facultative gram-negative enteric bacilli. Appropriate use is limited only by resistance or the development of pseudomembranous colitis, the major serious side effect of this drug.

CHLORAMPHENICOL Chloramphenicol has a broad spectrum of activity against gram-positive and gram-negative bacteria, although plasmid-mediated resistance has diminished its effective spectrum. This antibiotic is rarely used in adult infections because of the rare idiosyncratic side effect of irreversible bone-marrow aplasia and the availability of other agents with similar activity. It remains one of the drugs of choice for the treatment of typhoid fever and plague and is still useful for the treatment of brucellosis and both pneumococcal and meningococcal meningitis in penicillin-allergic patients.

TETRACYCLINES Tetracyclines have a broad spectrum of bacteriostatic activity against gram-positive and gram-negative bacteria and are widely used in a variety of non-hospital-acquired infections. These agents are among the drugs of choice for chronic bronchitis, granuloma inguinale, brucellosis (with streptomycin), tularemia, glanders, melioidosis, spirochetal infections caused by *Borrelia* (Lyme disease and relapsing fever; doxycycline), infections caused by *Vibrio vulnificus*, some *Aeromonas* infections, infections caused by *Xanthomonas* (minocycline), plague, and ehrlichiosis (doxycycline). The tetracyclines are also used in penicillin-allergic patients for the treatment of leptospirosis, syphilis, actinomycosis, and skin and soft-tissue infections caused by gram-positive cocci. They are among the drugs of choice for infections due to chlamydiae (doxycycline), rickettsiae, and ehrlichiae and for granulomatous skin infection due to *Mycobacterium marinum* (minocycline).

SULFONAMIDES AND TRIMETHOPRIM The folic acid synthesis inhibitors have a broad spectrum of bacteriostatic activity individually; in combination, they can be bactericidal against facultative gram-negative bacteria and staphylococci. The fixed combination of sulfamethoxazole and trimethoprim, the major folic acid synthesis inhibitors used in therapy for bacterial infections, has only modest activity against some streptococci and no activity against strict anaerobes. The individual sulfonamides are rarely used in the treatment of bacterial infections but are among the drugs of choice for the treatment of nocardial infections, leprosy (dapsone, a sulfone), and toxoplasmosis (sulfadiazine). Trimethoprim-sulfamethoxazole is the drug of choice for the treatment of uncomplicated urinary tract infections (except for those caused by enterococci) and is widely used in the treatment of otitis media. It can be used in therapy for upper respiratory tract infections in which *H. influenzae* and *M. catarrhalis* are suspected, gonococcal and meningococcal infections, chancroid, and infections thought to be caused by *Aeromonas*, *Xanthomonas*, *Pseudomonas cepacia*, *Acinetobacter*, and *Yersinia enterocolitica*. For nosocomial infections due to *Xanthomonas*, trimethoprim-sulfamethoxazole is the drug of choice.

FLUOROQUINOLONES The fluoroquinolones have excellent activity against most facultative gram-negative rods, fair activity against staphylococci, variable to poor activity against streptococci, and no activity against obligate anaerobes. They are the oral agents with greatest activity against *P. aeruginosa*; ciprofloxacin is the most active against this species. The oral absorption of all the quinolones is good to excellent; ciprofloxacin and ofloxacin are also administered as intravenous formulations. Treatment with norfloxacin can be used for urinary tract infections and has been recommended for infectious diarrhea. However, quinolones other than norfloxacin should be used for systemic gram-negative infections. The quinolones are among the drugs of choice for complicated urinary tract infections, bacterial gastroenteritis, and enteric fever and may be useful in therapy for chronic infections caused by gram-negative organisms, such as osteomyelitis and chronic otitis externa in adults. The use of quinolones is limited by the development of resistance among staphylococci and *P. aeruginosa* and by interactions with other drugs.

RIFAMPIN Rifampin has been used in combinations for the treatment of serious infections due to methicillin-resistant staphylococci (e.g., coagulase-negative staphylococcal foreign-body infections). Because the spontaneous selection of rifampin-resistant mutants occurs rapidly, rifampin should never be used alone in the treatment of staphylococcal infections. Rifampin is also used for chemoprophylaxis in persons at risk of meningococcal meningitis and for the treatment of *Legionella* pneumonia.

METRONIDAZOLE Metronidazole has a spectrum limited to anaerobic bacteria. It is one of the drugs of choice for the treatment of any abscess in which the involvement of obligate anaerobes is suspected (e.g., lung, brain, or intraabdominal abscesses) because of its spectrum and its ability to penetrate into the area of infection. Other antibacterial agents should be used in combination with metronidazole if additional facultative and aerobic pathogens are thought to be involved. Metronidazole is the drug of choice for the treatment of bacterial vaginosis and antibiotic-associated pseudomembranous colitis.

URINARY TRACT ANTISEPTICS Urinary tract antiseptics are active only in the lower urinary tract and cannot be used for the treatment of upper urinary tract or systemic infections. Their activity is limited to susceptible gram-negative enteric bacteria. The available agents in this category include nitrofurantoin and methenamine salts.

TOPICAL ANTIBACTERIAL AGENTS Mupirocin is available only as a topical preparation for use against staphylococci and streptococci. Its major applications are for impetigo and eradication of the staphylococcal carrier state. It is the drug of choice for the elimination of nasal carriage of both methicillin-susceptible and methicillin-resistant staphylococci. Unfortunately, the emergence of resistance is limiting its usefulness in some hospitals.

Although their efficacy has never been well documented, topical preparations that include sulfonamides, polymyxin B, neomycin, bacitracin, gramicidin, and novobiocin in a variety of combinations are widely used as eye drops, irrigation solutions, and ointments for superficial skin infections.

ADVERSE REACTIONS

Adverse drug reactions are frequently classified by mechanism as either dose-related ("toxic") effects or unpredictable reactions. Unpredictable reactions are further categorized as either idiosyncratic or allergic. Dose-related reactions include aminoglycoside-induced nephrotoxicity, penicillin-induced seizures, and vancomycin-induced anaphylactoid reactions. Many of these reactions can be avoided by reducing dosage, limiting the duration of therapy, or reducing the frequency or rate of administration. Adverse reactions to antibacterial agents are a common cause of morbidity, requiring alteration in therapy and additional expense, and they occasionally result in death. The elderly, often those with the more severe infections, may be especially prone to certain adverse reactions. These reactions to antibacterial agents are summarized below.

β-LACTAMS The therapeutic index for β-lactam antibiotics is broad, and dose-related adverse reactions are uncommon and largely preventable. The greatest concern is allergic reactions. All types can occur, including anaphylaxis (type 1, hypersensitivity reactions), nephritis and Coombs-positive hemolytic anemia (type 2, cytotoxic reactions), drug fever and serum sickness (type 3, immune-complex formation), contact dermatitis (type 4, cell-mediated effects), and maculopapular eruption (type 5, idiopathic reactions). Approximately 1 to 4 percent of treatment courses result in an allergic reaction, and approximately 0.004 to 0.015 percent of treatment courses result in anaphylaxis. Fewer than half the patients who claim an allergy to penicillin react to skin testing with the major and minor determinants (penicilloyl-polylysine and benzylpenicillin degradation products, respectively); those with negative skin tests only rarely react adversely to subsequent therapeutic doses. Generally, a suitable alternative to β-lactams is available for patients who have a severe allergy, and penicillin desensitization can be carefully undertaken if there is no suitable alternative. A small proportion (fewer than 2 percent) of persons who are allergic to penicillin react similarly when a cephalosporin is administered; thus, cephalosporins are contraindicated in patients with a history of an immediate reaction to penicillin, although

they are often used in patients with a history of mild reactions. The same precaution applies to imipenem, but aztreonam is antigenically distinct and can be administered safely to the penicillin-allergic patient.

Other reactions thought to have an allergic basis include nephritis (associated with methicillin), hepatitis (related to oxacillin), leukopenia (following high doses of most β-lactams administered for prolonged periods), and severe skin rashes (toxic epidermal necrolysis and Stevens-Johnson syndrome). These reactions are not IgE-mediated, and skin testing is not predictive of their occurrence. For unclear reasons, most patients who have infectious mononucleosis develop a rash when given ampicillin.

Miscellaneous reactions to β-lactams include gastrointestinal side effects ranging in severity from mild diarrhea (5 to 10 percent) to pseudomembranous colitis (<1 percent). Drugs excreted to a large extent through the bile, such as ampicillin, ceftriaxone, and cefoperazone, may be especially prone to cause diarrhea. The addition of clavulanic acid to amoxicillin further increases the frequency of diarrhea. Ceftriaxone, because of extremely high concentrations in bile, can cause "sludging" in the gallbladder and occasionally produces symptoms compatible with acute cholecystitis.

In high doses—and most often in patients with renal impairment who receive an excessive dose—penicillins (especially ticarcillin and penicillin G) can cause bleeding from impaired platelet aggregation. Bleeding also is associated occasionally with the use of cephalosporins containing a methylthiotetrazole group at the 3' position (most commonly, cefamandole and cefoperazone); this reaction may result from impairment of prothrombin formation. These same cephalosporins can cause a disulfiram-like reaction if ethanol is ingested concurrently. Carbenicillin and ticarcillin are disodium salts and in high doses can cause hypokalemia and fluid overload.

Seizures are occasionally observed with β-lactams, especially penicillin G and imipenem. This reaction is most common when excessive doses relative to renal function are administered or in patients with a history of seizures.

VANCOMYCIN When vancomycin was first used clinically in 1956, local intolerance at the infusion site was common, as were systemic reactions, including ototoxicity and nephrotoxicity. Current formulations are of higher purity and, when proper dosage guidelines are followed, are very safe, although phlebitis can still be troublesome. The most common adverse reaction is called *red man syndrome* and is characterized by pruritus, flushing, and erythema of the head and upper torso. This anaphylactoid reaction usually follows the first dose, is dependent on dose and infusion time, and results from vancomycin-induced release of histamine. The reaction is usually mild in adult patients who receive 1 g over 60 min and diminishes with repeated doses. If vancomycin is mistakenly given as a bolus, severe hypotension may result. In unusually sensitive patients, extending the infusion time or administering H₁ receptor antagonists is usually effective in preventing this reaction or reducing its severity. Patients with this reaction must not be mislabeled as having an allergy to vancomycin, since vancomycin may be the only effective treatment for certain infections, such as those due to methicillin-resistant staphylococci.

Nephrotoxicity from vancomycin is mild and occurs in fewer than 5 percent of patients. Although some data suggest that aminoglycosides and vancomycin are synergistically nephrotoxic, this point is difficult to prove, and the simultaneous use of these agents should not be avoided if clinically indicated, as in the treatment of enterococcal endocarditis in penicillin-allergic patients.

Ototoxicity from vancomycin is rare as long as doses are appropriately reduced in patients with renal insufficiency. Other uncommon adverse reactions include leukopenia, skin rashes, and true allergy.

AMINOGLYCOSIDES Aminoglycoside antibiotics have a narrow therapeutic index. The two most common adverse reactions are nephrotoxicity and ototoxicity. Rarely, respiratory depression is observed. Nephrotoxicity results from accumulation of the aminoglycoside in the peritubular space, with damage to the proximal tubule and a corresponding reduction in the glomerular filtration rate. The incidence of nephrotoxicity, defined as a greater than 0.5 percent increase over baseline in the serum creatinine level, is approximately 5 to 10 percent among adult patients who receive a therapeutic course for 10 to 14 days. However, many cofactors also influence the frequency of toxicity, such as extremes of age (toxicity is uncommon among children, more common among the elderly), concomitant drug therapy, and hydration status. Nephrotoxicity is manifested clinically by a gradual rise in serum creatinine levels after a few days of therapy and is reversible if the dosage is reduced or treatment is discontinued. Serum creatinine levels should be monitored every 3 to 5 days or more often if changes are seen. There is not an important difference among the most useful agents (gentamicin, tobramycin, and amikacin) in terms of the frequency of nephrotoxicity; streptomycin is a rare cause of nephrotoxicity.

Ototoxicity from aminoglycoside therapy presents as either auditory or vestibular damage. Since the aminoglycosides can destroy hair cells in the inner ear, ototoxicity may be permanent. The risk of ototoxicity increases with prolonged therapy, higher serum concentrations (especially in patients with renal impairment), hypovolemia, and concurrent treatment with other ototoxins, especially ethacrynic acid. Clinically apparent ototoxicity, manifested by diminished acuity or vestibular imbalance, is uncommon (probably occurring in fewer than 1 percent of cases) when serum concentrations are monitored and the duration of therapy is kept to a minimum. With more sensitive monitoring (e.g., audiograms), asymptomatic high-tone hearing loss is more commonly noted. There are no clinically important differences among the aminoglycosides in the overall frequency of ototoxicity.

Neuromuscular depression from aminoglycosides is caused by reduced acetylcholine activity at postsynaptic membranes and can result in rare but severe respiratory depression. Risk factors include hypocalcemia, peritoneal administration, use of neuromuscular blockers, and preexisting respiratory depression. This complication can be largely avoided if the aminoglycoside is administered intravenously over 30 min or by intramuscular injection; if respiratory depression occurs, it is reversed by the administration of calcium.

Fear of toxicity should not prevent the use of aminoglycosides for a legitimate indication, since toxicity is usually mild and reversible. Serum concentrations are monitored both to minimize the risk of toxicity and to ensure that sufficient drug is administered to treat targeted infections.

MACROLIDES Serious adverse reactions to the macrolide antibiotics are very rare. Gastrointestinal effects, such as burning, nausea, and vomiting, are the most common adverse reactions to the macrolides; depending on dosage, these reactions may occur in up to 50 percent of patients, occasionally requiring early discontinuation of therapy. The mechanism is thought to be the binding of erythromycin to motilin receptors, with a consequent increase in gastrointestinal motility. Gastrointestinal side effects appear equally common for all the oral formulations and also occur with intravenous administration. Clarithromycin and azithromycin are better tolerated than erythromycin, although gastrointestinal distress is still their most common adverse effect.

Less common reactions include hepatotoxicity and ototoxicity. Hepatotoxicity is a rare, nonfatal complication that is usually associated with erythromycin estolate and presents as an allergic cholestatic jaundice. Ototoxicity is rare after oral administration but may occur in a dose-dependent pattern in up to 20 percent of adults who receive intravenous erythromycin (4 g/d) and have audiograms performed. Ototoxicity is usually reversible and mild. Allergic cutaneous reactions are observed in rare cases.

LINCOSAMIDES The most common adverse effect of clindamycin is gastrointestinal distress. Diarrhea has been reported in up to 20 percent of patients, and pseudomembranous colitis in 0.01 to 10 percent. The mechanism of pseudomembranous colitis is production of a toxin by *C. difficile* (see Chap. 148). *C. difficile* colonizes the gastrointestinal tract and may produce a toxin when the normal flora

is suppressed by clindamycin. This toxin causes mucosal damage that results in cramps, pain, and diarrhea that may be bloody. Pseudomembranous colitis may follow both intravenous and oral administration and may not become manifest until after completion of therapy. Oral metronidazole or oral vancomycin is effective in treating symptomatic patients with toxin-positive stools, but some spores may survive, and relapse is frequent. Although diarrhea and pseudomembranous colitis can be caused by most antibacterial agents, the incidence in relation to the amount used appears to be highest for clindamycin. Allergic reactions (such as rashes and fever), hepatotoxicity, and neutropenia are observed only rarely.

CHLORAMPHENICOL Chloramphenicol causes two types of bone marrow suppression; a dose-related, reversible suppression of all elements, which occurs commonly during therapy at the maximal recommended doses (4 g/d in adults), and an idiosyncratic, irreversible aplastic anemia, which occurs in approximately 1 in every 25,000 to 40,000 exposures. The irreversible form has been reported to follow all types of chloramphenicol treatment, including ocular administration, and often develops months after therapy is discontinued.

In premature neonates and infants, chloramphenicol can cause a dose-related "gray syndrome" that is characterized by cyanosis, hypotension, and death and that results from an inability of the newborn to metabolize the drug. These potentially serious toxicities and the availability of newer drugs have substantially reduced the indications for chloramphenicol.

TETRACYCLINES Gastrointestinal effects are the most common adverse reactions to the tetracyclines. These problems may be related to a direct irritant effect, since tetracyclines also can cause esophageal ulceration when they dissolve before reaching the stomach. Concurrent food intake may improve tolerance, but absorption of tetracycline HCl is impaired when it is taken with food.

Hepatotoxicity has been reported after administration of more than 2 g of tetracycline intravenously and at lower doses during pregnancy. There are currently no indications for intravenous tetracycline treatment in pregnancy. All tetracyclines can cause phototoxic skin reactions; these reactions are most common with doxycycline. Other dermal reactions, including rash, are uncommon. Tetracyclines are contraindicated in children less than 8 years of age because of mottling of the permanent teeth; doxycycline may be less likely than the other tetracyclines to cause this problem. Worsening of renal function in patients with preexisting renal dysfunction has been reported with use of tetracycline, although some of the increased azotemia may be due to amino acid catabolism. Doxycycline and perhaps minocycline appear to be free from these renal side effects. Alternative effective agents are nearly always available for use in patients with renal dysfunction. Minocycline can cause vertigo in up to 70 percent of women receiving therapeutic doses and in a lower percentage of men.

SULFONAMIDES AND TRIMETHOPRIM The sulfonamides are generally safe, but the list of possible adverse reactions is very long. These compounds occasionally cause a number of allergic reactions, from relatively minor skin rashes (including maculopapular rashes and urticarial reactions typically appearing after a week of therapy) to severe or even life-threatening reactions such as erythema multiforme, Stevens-Johnson syndrome, and toxic epidermal necrolysis. The severe hypersensitivity reactions have occurred most commonly after treatment with the long-acting sulfonamides, such as sulfamethoxypyridazine, which are no longer used. Pyrimethamine plus sulfadoxine (Fansidar), used for malaria prophylaxis, may cause severe allergic reactions, including hepatic and hematologic toxicities, in addition to dermatologic toxicity. Photosensitivity reactions are also relatively common with sulfonamides.

Many patients infected with HIV who receive trimethoprim-sulfamethoxazole have adverse dermatologic reactions. These reactions are usually not life-threatening and appear to regress in many cases despite continuation of therapy. In high doses, trimethoprim interferes with the renal secretion of potassium. Hyperkalemia is relatively common among HIV-positive patients and is most often found after 7 days of trimethoprim-sulfamethoxazole therapy for pneumonia caused by *Pneumocystis carinii*.

Sulfonamides and trimethoprim also may cause severe hematologic complications, including agranulocytosis, hemolytic and megaloblastic anemia, and thrombocytopenia. These dose-related side effects may be greater in patients with renal insufficiency. Hemolytic anemia is most common in patients with glucose-6-phosphate dehydrogenase deficiency who take long-acting compounds; trimethoprim-sulfamethoxazole rarely causes hemolysis in such subjects. Granulocytopenia from trimethoprim-sulfamethoxazole is especially common in HIV-infected patients, occurring in 10 to 50 percent of subjects.

Renal insufficiency, caused by crystals of the relatively insoluble acetyl metabolite, is observed primarily with the long-acting sulfonamides. Many cases of crystalluria in HIV-infected patients taking sulfadiazine for toxoplasmosis have been reported. A high level of fluid intake may prevent this complication.

It is recommended that sulfonamides not be administered to the newborn because of concerns that bilirubin may be displaced from protein-binding sites, with subsequent jaundice and kernicterus.

In addition to the preceding problems, sulfonamides may occasionally cause drug fever with serum sickness, hepatic toxicity (including necrosis), and systemic lupus erythematosus.

FLUOROQUINOLONES Fluoroquinolones are relatively safe; adverse reactions rarely require discontinuation of therapy. The most common reactions include gastrointestinal distress, such as nausea or diarrhea (<5 percent), and central nervous system effects, including insomnia and dizziness (<5 percent). Phototoxicity can be severe, especially with lomefloxacin. Rarely, hepatic and renal dysfunction and anaphylactoid and allergic reactions are observed. The use of these drugs is contraindicated in children less than 18 years of age because of evidence in animals of cartilage damage in developing joints. In carefully selected situations in which the perceived benefits outweigh the risks, such as in adolescent patients with cystic fibrosis who have pulmonary exacerbations, fluoroquinolones may be useful for short-term therapy. They are contraindicated in pregnancy because of concern for the developing fetus.

RIFAMPIN Rifampin is generally well tolerated but has several important side effects. Some patients have transient rises in hepatic aminotransferases, but these levels usually return to normal without discontinuation of the drug. Although hepatitis from rifampin itself develops only rarely, the drug is thought by some investigators to potentiate the hepatic toxicity of concomitantly administered isoniazid. Intermittent administration of rifampin, usually less than three times per week, has been associated with symptoms that seem to have an immunologic basis. These include flulike symptoms and (rarely) hemolysis, thrombocytopenia, shock, and renal failure. Minor gastrointestinal side effects, skin rashes, and interstitial nephritis also have been reported. Patients should be warned that rifampin and its metabolites cause secretions such as urine, tears, sweat, and saliva to turn orange and that contact lenses may be stained.

METRONIDAZOLE Serious adverse reactions to metronidazole are uncommon. Gastrointestinal side effects such as nausea are most frequent but rarely necessitate discontinuation of therapy. Pseudomembranous colitis in association with metronidazole has been reported but is very rare. A metallic taste is relatively common, and stomatitis and glossitis are occasionally reported. Disulfiram-like reactions can occur if ethanol is ingested concurrently. Peripheral neuropathy develops in some patients, and seizures and encephalopathy have been reported after high doses and in patients with hepatic failure.

Concerns about mutagenicity and carcinogenicity from metronidazole have led to recommendations that it not be used in pregnancy (especially during the first trimester) when alternative agents are available. Although retrospective studies have found no association between metronidazole and carcinogenesis, long-term administration of high doses should be avoided when therapeutic alternatives exist.

DRUG INTERACTIONS

Historically, clinically important interactions involving antibacterial drugs were generally of little concern, since β-lactams were the most widely used agents and rarely interacted with other drugs in a manner that affected the patient adversely. However, fluoroquinolones, macrolides, and rifampin are now more widely used, and interactions are of increasing concern. Table 140-4 lists the most common and best-documented interactions of antibacterial agents with other drugs and characterizes the clinical relevance of these interactions. Coadministration of drugs paired in Table 140-4 does not necessarily have clinically important adverse consequences. The result depends on the timing of administration, the dose and duration of therapy, the baseline serum concentration of the non-antibacterial drug administered, the patient's susceptibility to the pharmacologic effect of the non-antibacterial drug, and other, less well described cofactors. Recognition of the potential for an interaction before the administration of an antibacterial agent is crucial to the rational use of these drugs, since adverse consequences often can be prevented if the interaction is anticipated. Table 140-4 is intended only to heighten awareness of the potential for an interaction. Additional sources should be consulted to identify appropriate options.

MACROLIDES Erythromycin can inhibit the hepatic metabolism of many concurrently administered drugs, such as theophylline, carbamazepine, terfenadine, warfarin, and ergot alkaloids—an effect leading to increased serum concentrations and toxicity. The magnitude of the theophylline interaction is highly variable and is proportional to the dose and duration of erythromycin treatment. In contrast, cyclosporine levels predictably increase when erythromycin is admin-

Table 140-4

Interactions of Antibacterial Agents with Other Drugs

Antibacterial Agent (A), Drug (B)	Effect	Clinical Relevance*
Erythromycin		
Theophylline	Increased levels of B	1
Carbamazepine	Increased levels of B	1
Digoxin	Increased levels of B	3
Triazolam	Increased levels of B	2
Ergotamine	Increased levels of B	1
Warfarin	Increased levels of B	2
Cyclosporine	Increased levels of B	1
Terfenadine/astemizole	Increased levels of B	1
Valproate	Increased levels of B	2
Fluoroquinolones		
Theophylline	Increased levels of B†	2
Divalent/trivalent cations (Al, Fe, Mg, etc.)	Decreased levels of A	1
Tetracyclines		
Divalent/trivalent cations	Decreased levels of A	1
Digoxin	Increased levels of B	3
Sulfonamides		
Oral hypoglycemic agents	Increased levels of B	2
Phenytoin	Increased levels of B	2
Warfarin	Increased levels of B	2
Metronidazole		
Ethanol	Disulfiram-like reaction	2
Warfarin	Increased levels of B	2
Rifampin		
Warfarin	Decreased levels of B	1
Oral contraceptives	Decreased levels of B	1
Cyclosporine	Decreased levels of B	1
Oral hypoglycemic agents	Decreased levels of B	1
Glucocorticoids	Decreased levels of B	1
Methadone	Decreased levels of B	1
Digoxin/digitoxin	Decreased levels of B	1
Quinidine	Decreased levels of B	1
Azole antifungal agents	Decreased levels of B	2
Phenytoin	Decreased levels of B	2
Zidovudine	Decreased levels of B	1
Diltiazem	Decreased levels of B	1
Verapamil	Decreased levels of B	1

* 1 = a well-documented interaction with clinically important consequences; 2 = an interaction of uncertain frequency but possible clinical importance; 3 = an unusual interaction of possible clinical importance in some patients.
† Enoxacin > ciprofloxacin > norfloxacin/ofloxacin > lomefloxacin.

istered, since erythromycin inhibits the specific enzyme responsible for cyclosporine metabolism. Decreased metabolism of terfenadine and probably of astemizole has been reported to cause severe cardiac dysfunction. Clarithromycin appears to be similar to erythromycin in its inhibitory potential, although azithromycin may have little effect on the metabolism of other drugs. In approximately 10 percent of patients receiving digoxin, concentrations increase when erythromycin is also given; the mechanism is increased absorption of digoxin because of the killing of digoxin-metabolizing bacteria by erythromycin.

TETRACYCLINES The most important interaction involving tetracyclines is the reduction in absorption when these drugs are coadministered with di- and trivalent cations, such as antacids, iron compounds, or dairy products. A similar interaction is seen with quinolones (see below). Food also adversely affects absorption of most tetracyclines. Inducers of hepatic isoenzymes, such as phenytoin and barbiturates, increase the clearance of doxycycline; although the clinical significance of this effect is unknown, use of an alternative antibiotic may be appropriate.

SULFONAMIDES Sulfonamides may increase the hypoprothrombinemic effect of warfarin by inhibition of metabolism of the more potent isomer of this agent and possibly by protein-binding displacement. Sulfonamides also may potentiate the effects of oral hypoglycemic agents and phenytoin through reduction in metabolism or displacement from serum protein.

FLUOROQUINOLONES There are two clinically important drug interactions involving fluoroquinolones. First, like tetracyclines, all fluoroquinolones are chelated by divalent and trivalent cations, which prevent most of the dose from being absorbed. Second, certain fluoroquinolones (enoxacin, ciprofloxacin, and to a lesser extent norfloxacin and ofloxacin, but not lomefloxacin) can inhibit hepatic en-

zymes that metabolize theophylline, with resultant theophylline toxicity. The same mechanism accounts for increases in serum caffeine concentrations, but the clinical significance of this interaction is unknown. Scattered reports indicate that quinolones also can potentiate the nephrotoxicity of cyclosporine, exaggerate the effects of warfarin, and increase neurotoxicity when coadministered with nonsteroidal anti-inflammatory agents. However, these interactions have not been confirmed by controlled trials.

RIFAMPIN Rifampin is an excellent inducer of many cytochrome P450 enzymes and increases the hepatic clearance of a number of drugs, including the following (with the indicated predictable outcomes): oral contraceptives (pregnancy), warfarin (decreased prothrombin times), cyclosporine and prednisone (organ rejection or exacerbations of any underlying inflammatory condition), and verapamil and diltiazem (increased dosage requirements).

METRONIDAZOLE Metronidazole can cause a disulfiramlike syndrome when alcohol is ingested; thus, patients taking metronidazole should be instructed to avoid alcohol. Inhibition of the metabolism of warfarin by metronidazole leads to significant rises in prothrombin times.

PROPHYLAXIS OF BACTERIAL INFECTIONS

Antibacterial agents are occasionally indicated for use in patients who have no evidence of infection but who have been or are expected to be exposed to bacterial pathogens under circumstances that constitute a major risk of infection. The basic tenets of antimicrobial prophylaxis are as follows: First, the risk or potential severity of infection should be greater than the risk of side effects from the antibacterial agent. Second, the antibacterial agent should be given for the shortest period necessary to prevent target infections. Third, the antibacterial agent should be given before the expected period of risk (e.g., surgical prophylaxis) or as soon as possible after contact with an infected individual (e.g., prophylaxis for meningococcal meningitis).

Table 140-5 lists the major indications for antibacterial prophylaxis in adults. (The use of antibacterial agents in children to prevent rheumatic fever and otitis media under certain circumstances is also common practice.) The table includes only those indications that are widely accepted, supported by well-designed studies, or recommended by expert panels. Prophylaxis is also used but is less widely accepted for recurrent cellulitis in conjunction with lymphedema, recurrent pneumococcal meningitis in conjunction with deficiencies in humoral immunity or CSF leaks, traveler's diarrhea, gram-negative sepsis in conjunction with neutropenia, and spontaneous bacterial peritonitis in conjunction with ascites.

The major use of antibacterial prophylaxis in the United States is for infections following surgical procedures. Antibacterial agents are administered just before the surgical procedure—and, for long operations, during the procedure as well—to ensure high levels in serum and tissues during surgery. The objective is to eradicate bacteria originating from the air of the operating suite, the skin of the surgical team, or the patient's own flora that may contaminate the wound. In all but colorectal surgical procedures, prophylaxis is predominantly directed against staphylococci. Prophylaxis is in-

Table 140-5

Prophylaxis of Bacterial Infections in Adults

Condition	Antibacterial Agent	Timing or Duration of Prophylaxis
Nonsurgical		
Cardiac lesions susceptible to bacterial endocarditis	Amoxicillin*	Before and after procedures causing bacteremia
Recurrent *S. aureus* infections	Mupirocin	5 days (intranasal)
Contact with patient with meningococcal meningitis	Rifampin Ciprofloxacin or ofloxacin	2 days Single dose
Bite wounds†	Penicillin V or amoxicillin–clavulanic acid	3–5 days
Recurrent cystitis	Trimethoprim-sulfamethoxazole	3 times per week for up to 1 year or after sexual intercourse
Surgical		
Clean (cardiac, vascular, neurologic, or orthopedic surgery)	Cefazolin (vancomycin)‡	Before and during procedure
Ocular	Topical combinations and subconjunctival cefazolin	During and at end of procedure
Clean-contaminated (head and neck, high-risk gastroduodenal or biliary tract surgery; cesarean section; hysterectomy)	Cefazolin (or clindamycin for head and neck)	Before and during procedure
Clean-contaminated (colorectal surgery or appendectomy)	Cefoxitin or cefotetan (add oral neomycin + erythromycin for colorectal)	Before and during procedure
Dirty† (ruptured viscus)	Cefoxitin or cefotetan ± gentamicin (clindamycin + gentamicin) or another appropriate regimen directed at anaerobes and gram-negative aerobes	Before and for 3–5 days after procedure
Dirty† (traumatic wound)	Cefazolin	Before and for 3–5 days after trauma

* Gentamicin should be added to the amoxicillin regimen for high-risk gastrointestinal and genitourinary procedures.
† In these cases, use of antibacterial agents actually constitutes treatment of infection rather than prophylaxis.
‡ Vancomycin is recommended only in institutions that have a high incidence of infection with methicillin-resistant staphylococci.

tended to prevent wound infection or infection of implanted devices, not all infections that may occur during the postoperative period (e.g., urinary tract infections or pneumonia). Prolonged prophylaxis merely alters the normal flora and favors infections with organisms resistant to the antibacterial agents used.

ANTIBACTERIAL COSTS AND INAPPROPRIATE USE

Use of antibacterial agents in hospitals in the United States accounts for 20 to 50 percent of all drug costs and represents the largest expenditure for any pharmacologic class. In the outpatient setting, the costs of antibacterial drugs are second only to those of cardiovascular agents. A survey of office-based physicians found that between 1980 and 1992 there was a marked increase in the use of expensive broad-spectrum antimicrobials. It is not unusual for the purchase cost (in 1995 dollars) of a newer parenteral antibiotic to be $1000 to $2000 for a 10- to 14-day course of treatment. Therapy with a new oral antibiotic can easily cost $50 to $60. Administration costs, monitoring costs, and pharmacy charges must be added to these figures. While some newer antibacterial agents undeniably represent important advances in therapy, many newer drugs offer no advantage over older, less expensive agents.

Clinicians are understandably confused by the bewildering array of available drugs. Numerous surveys have reported that approximately 50 percent of antibiotic use is in some way "inappropriate." Aside from the monetary cost of unnecessary antibiotics, there are the costs of excess morbidity from adverse effects and drug interactions and the eventual costs of treating more resistant organisms. The following suggestions are intended to provide guidance through the antibiotic maze.

First, objective evidence regarding the merits of newer drugs is available through publications such as *The Medical Letter*, including the annual update of *Drugs of Choice*. Second, clinicians should become comfortable using a few drugs recommended by independent experts and should resist the temptation to use a new drug unless the merits are clear. A new antibacterial agent with a "broader spectrum and greater potency" or a "longer half-life and higher tissue levels" does not necessarily mean greater clinical efficacy. Third, the clinician must become familiar with local bacterial susceptibility profiles. It may not be necessary to use a new drug with "improved activity against *P. aeruginosa*" if that pathogen is rarely encountered or if it retains full susceptibility to older drugs. Finally, with regard to inpatient use of antibacterial drugs, appropriate empirical treatment with one or more broad-spectrum agents may often be simplified, with use of a narrower-spectrum agent or even an oral drug, once the results of cultures and susceptibility tests become available. While there is an understandable temptation not to alter effective therapy, switching to a more specific agent, once the patient has improved clinically, does not compromise eventual outcome. If these guidelines are followed, the care of patients will not be undermined, many unnecessary complications and expenses will be avoided, and the useful life of valuable drugs will be extended.

BIBLIOGRAPHY

Anné S, Reisman RE: Risk of administering cephalosporin antibiotics to patients with histories of penicillin allergy. Ann Allergy Asthma Immunol 74:167, 1995

Antimicrobial prophylaxis in surgery. Med Lett Drugs Ther 37:79, 1995

Gillum JG et al: Pharmacokinetic drug interactions with antimicrobial agents. Clin Pharmacokinet 25:450, 1993

Hooper DC, Wolfson JS: Fluoroquinolone antimicrobial agents. N Engl J Med 324:384, 1991

Hospital Infection Control Practices Advisory Committee: Recommendations for preventing the spread of vancomycin resistance. Infect Control Hosp Epidemiol 16:105, 1995

McCaig LF, Hughes JM: Trends in antimicrobial drug prescribing among office-based physicians in the United States. JAMA 273:214, 1995

Neu HC: The crisis in antibiotic resistance. Science 257:1064, 1992

Nicolau DP et al: Antibiotic kinetics and dynamics for the clinician. Med Clin North Am 79:477, 1995

The choice of antibacterial drugs. Med Lett Drugs Ther 38:25, 1996

SECTION 5

DISEASES CAUSED BY GRAM-POSITIVE BACTERIA

---

141   *Daniel M. Musher*

PNEUMOCOCCAL INFECTIONS

HISTORY AND DEFINITION *Streptococcus pneumoniae* (the pneumococcus) was recognized as a major cause of pneumonia in the 1880s and has been a central focus of study leading to a modern understanding of humoral immunity. Before the start of the twentieth century, immunization with killed pneumococci was shown to protect rabbits against subsequent challenge with viable pneumococci. Serum from immunized rabbits or from humans who had recovered from pneumococcal pneumonia conferred protection. Early in the twentieth century, field trials of vaccination of South African miners with killed pneumococci demonstrated protection. Shortly thereafter, evidence implicated the capsule as the basis for resistance to phagocytosis; in the 1920s, antibody specific for capsular polysaccharide was determined to facilitate the ingestion and killing of *S. pneumoniae*. In 1936, pneumococcal capsular polysaccharide vaccine was used to abort an epidemic of pneumococcal pneumonia. In the 1940s, experiments involving capsular transformation among pneumococci first identified DNA as the material that carries genetic information.

The name *Diplococcus pneumoniae* was assigned to the organism in 1926 on the basis of its appearance in Gram-stained sputum. In 1974, the organism was renamed *Streptococcus pneumoniae* because of its growth in chains in liquid medium. Around 1900, pneumococcal serotypes were recognized after it was observed that the injection of killed organisms into a rabbit stimulated the production of serum antibody that agglutinated and caused increased capsular density of the immunizing strain as well as of some but not all other pneumococcal isolates. Ninety serotypes are now known to exist, each possessing a unique polysaccharide capsule.

MICROBIOLOGY Pneumococci are identified in the clinical laboratory as gram-positive cocci that grow in chains and are catalase-negative. They produce alpha hemolysin, a toxin that breaks down hemoglobin into a greenish degeneration product and causes alpha hemolysis on blood agar. More than 98 percent of pneumococcal isolates are susceptible to ethylhydrocupreine (optochin), and virtually all pneumococcal colonies are dissolved by bile salts.

Peptidoglycan and teichoic acid are the principal constituents of the pneumococcal cell wall. The cell wall's integrity depends on the presence of numerous peptide side chains cross-linked by the activity of enzymes such as trans- and carboxypeptidases. β-Lactam antibiotics inactivate these enzymes by covalent binding at their active site. Unique to *S. pneumoniae* and uniformly present in all strains is C-substance, a polysaccharide that is a teichoic acid containing a phosphorylcholine residue. An antigenically variable protein, PspA, is partially exposed on the cell surface. Nearly every clinical isolate of *S. pneumoniae* has a polysaccharide capsule. There are two systems for numbering the 90 known distinct capsules of *S. pneumoniae*. In the American system, serotypes are numbered in the order in which they were identified. The strains that most frequently cause human disease were generally the earliest to be identified and thus tend to have lower numbers. The more widely accepted Danish system places serotypes into groups based on antigenic similarities; for example, Danish group 19 includes types 19F, 19A, 19B, and 19C, which in the American system would be types 19, 57, 58, and 59, respectively. Serotyping was clinically relevant in the 1930s, when type-specific antisera were administered as therapy, and (although genetic typing is more specific) it has again become important for epidemiologic studies of the spread of antibiotic-resistant isolates in communities and among countries.

EPIDEMIOLOGY *S. pneumoniae* colonizes the nasopharynx and can be isolated from 5 to 10 percent of healthy adults and from 20 to 40 percent of healthy children. Once the organisms have colonized an adult, they are likely to persist for 2 to 6 months. Pneumococci spread from one individual to another as a result of extensive close contact; transmission may be enhanced by poor ventilation. Day-care centers have been a site of spread of penicillin-resistant strains, especially those of serotypes 6B, 14, 19F, and 23F. Epidemics among adults are associated with crowded living conditions—e.g., in military barracks, prisons, and shelters for the homeless. The risk of pneumococcal pneumonia is not increased by contact in schools or workplaces (including hospitals).

The incidence of pneumococcal bacteremia is relatively high among infants up to 2 years of age and low among teenagers and young adults; rates increase steadily beginning at around age 55. A recent surveillance study in South Carolina showed the incidences of pneumococcal bacteremia among infants, young adults, and persons ≥70 years of age to be 160, 5, and 70 cases per 100,000 population, respectively. Most cases of pneumococcal bacteremia in adults are due to pneumonia, and there are three to four cases of nonbacteremic pneumonia for every bacteremic case. Thus, it is estimated that there are 20 cases of pneumonia annually per 100,000 young adults and 280 cases annually per 100,000 persons over the age of 70. The incidence of pneumococcal bacteremia among adults exhibits a distinct midwinter peak and a striking dip in summer. In children, the incidence of otitis media increases in midwinter, but bacteremia is relatively constant throughout the year except for a marked dip in midsummer.

PATHOGENETIC MECHANISMS *S. pneumoniae* attaches to human nasopharyngeal cells through the specific interaction of bacterial surface adhesins with epithelial cell receptors that contain the disaccharide GlcNAcβ1–4Gal. Once the nasopharynx has been colonized, infection results if the organisms are carried into anatomically contiguous areas such as the eustachian tubes or the nasal sinuses and if their clearance is hindered by mucosal edema (for example, due to allergy or viral infection). Similarly, pneumonia ensues if organisms are inhaled or aspirated into the bronchioles or alveoli and then are not cleared—in many cases, because viral infection or cigarette smoke or other toxic substances have damaged ciliary action and other mechanisms of clearance. A mechanism by which pneumococci may bind to pneumocytes after viral infection has been suggested. Pneumocytes activated by cytokines have been shown to express the receptor for platelet-activating factor. This receptor binds the phosphorylcholine residue on pneumococcal C-substance, facilitating the adherence of pneumococci, which is coupled to invasion. Studies suggest that pneumococci may invade tissues by penetrating mucosal layers; the clinical significance of this finding remains to be determined.

Once pneumococci reach an area where they do not naturally belong, they activate complement by classic and alternative pathways and stimulate cytokine production, which leads to the attraction of polymorphonuclear neutrophils (PMNs). The polysaccharide capsule, however, renders the organisms resistant to phagocytosis. In the absence of anticapsular antibody, alveolar macrophages have a limited capacity to ingest and kill pneumococci; a large bacterial inoculum and/or the compromise of phagocytic function allows the initiation of lung infection. Infection of the meninges, joint spaces, bones, and peritoneal cavity results from the spread of pneumococci through the bloodstream, usually but not always from a recognized focus of infection in the respiratory tract.

The capacity to cause disease reflects the ability of pneumococci to escape ingestion and killing by host phagocytic cells, on the one hand, and to stimulate an inflammatory response, on the other. Some pneumococcal constituents may directly damage mammalian tissues. Encapsulated pneumococci are poorly ingested and killed in vivo in the immunologically naive host or in vitro by mammalian phagocytic cells in the absence of anticapsular antibody and complement. Unencapsulated pneumococci virtually never cause invasive disease (although they can cause conjunctivitis), and mutants lacking a capsule are essentially avirulent in experimental animals. Symptoms of disease are largely attributable to the generation of an inflammatory response that may cause pain by increasing pressure (as in otitis media) or may interfere with vital bodily functions, such as oxygenation of blood (as in pneumonia) or cerebral function (as in meningitis). Cell-wall constituents of *S. pneumoniae*, probably including both teichoic acid and peptidoglycan, activate complement by the alternative pathway; the reaction between cell-wall structures and antibody also activates the classic complement pathway. The result is the release of C5a, a potent attractant for PMNs, into the surrounding medium. Inflammation is also facilitated by the ability of peptidoglycan to stimulate cytokine production, which activates endothelial cells to express selectin and integrin receptors for inflammatory cells. Inflammation in the central nervous system (CNS) during meningitis is a major contributor to neuronal cell injury. Pneumolysin, a thiol-activated toxin, exerts a variety of effects on ciliary cells and PMNs and also activates the classic complement pathway by direct binding of C1q. Injection of pneumolysin into the lungs of experimental animals produces the histologic features of pneumonia; in mice, immunization with this substance or challenge with genetically engineered mutants that do not produce pneumolysin is associated with a significant reduction in virulence. Autolysin may contribute to the pathogenesis of pneumococcal disease by lysing the bacteria, thereby releasing bacterial constituents and heightening the reaction with human tissues. The release of excitatory amino acids in neuronal tissue may contribute to damage caused by meningitis.

HOST DEFENSE MECHANISMS Mechanisms of host defense may be immunologically nonspecific or specific. Nonspecific mechanisms include laminar airflow across mucous layers that filter inspired air, the glottal reflex, laryngeal closure, the cough reflex, the clearance of organisms from the lower airways by ciliated cells, and the ingestion by pulmonary macrophages and PMNs of small bacterial inocula that manage to reach alveolar spaces. Respiratory virus infection, chronic pulmonary disease, or heart failure compromises these mechanisms, predisposing to the development of pneumococcal pneumonia. Antibody to PspA and other pneumococcal constituents such as pneumolysin may be prevalent in the population and may contribute to nonspecific immunity to infection.

Anticapsular antibody provides serotype-specific protection against pneumococcal infection. However, most healthy adults lack IgG antibody to most pneumococcal capsular polysaccharides. Antibody appears after colonization, infection, or vaccination. In the first few weeks after colonization, nonspecific mechanisms probably protect the host from infection. Thereafter, newly developed anticapsular antibody provides a high degree of specific protection. In contrast to this normal situation, adults who are at risk of aspirating pharyngeal contents and/or who have diminished mechanisms of lower airway clearance are at risk of developing pneumonia before antibody is produced, and children whose nasal mucosal membranes become acutely congested around the time of colonization are at risk of developing otitis media. Persons with a diminished capacity to form antibody remain susceptible for as long as they are colonized.

The risk of serious pneumococcal infection is greatly increased in persons with conditions that compromise IgG synthesis and/or phagocytic function of PMNs and macrophages (Table 141-1). The susceptibility of elderly individuals to pneumococcal pneumonia may reflect senescence of the immune system, especially that due to diminished production of immunoglobulin, but debilitation, malnutrition, and comorbid diseases undoubtedly contribute to this susceptibility as well. Prior hospitalization either predisposes to or serves as a strong

Table 141-1

CHAPTER 141
Pneumococcal Infections

871

Common Conditions Predisposing to Pneumococcal Infection

Defective antibody formation
    Common variable hypogammaglobulinemia
    Selective IgG-subclass deficiency
    Multiple myeloma
    Chronic lymphocytic leukemia
    Lymphoma
Defective complement function
Defective clearance of pneumococcal bacteremia*
    Congenital asplenia, hyposplenia
    Splenectomy
    Sickle cell disease
Multifactorial conditions
    Infancy and aging
    Chronic disease, hospitalization
    Glucocorticoid treatment
    Malnutrition
    Infection with human immunodeficiency virus
    Alcoholism
    Cirrhosis of the liver
    Renal insufficiency
    Diabetes mellitus
    Fatigue, stress, and/or exposure to cold
Increased risk of exposure
    Day-care centers
    Military training camps
    Prisons
    Shelters for the homeless
Respiratory infection, inflammation†
    Influenza, other viral respiratory infections
    Air pollution
    Allergies
    Cigarette smoking
    Chronic obstructive pulmonary disease
    Other causes of chronic pulmonary inflammation or obstruction
Anatomic disruption of meninges (dural tear)‡

* The absence of a spleen predisposes to more fulminant infection (see text).
† Predisposes specifically to infections of the upper or lower respiratory tract.
‡ Predisposes to recurrent bacterial meningitis.

marker for pneumococcal infection. Once a pneumococcal infection has been initiated, the absence of a spleen predisposes to fulminant disease. The liver is able to remove opsonized (antibody-coated) pneumococci from the circulation; in the absence of antibody, however, only the slow passage of blood through the splenic sinuses and prolonged contact with reticuloendothelial cells in the cords of Billroth allow time for bacterial clearance. Patients without spleens may die of pneumococcal pneumonia and sepsis at such an early stage of the illness that pulmonary consolidation is not evident on x-ray but rather is found only at autopsy.

SPECIFIC INFECTIONS CAUSED BY *S. PNEUMONIAE*

S. pneumoniae causes infections of the middle ear, sinuses, trachea, bronchi, and lungs (Table 141-2) by spreading directly from the nasopharyngeal site of colonization. Infections of the CNS, heart valves, bones, joints, and peritoneal cavity usually arise by hematogenous spread; in rare cases peritoneal infection develops via ascent through the fallopian tubes. The CNS may also be infected by contiguous spread of organisms, as in patients who have a tear in the dura. Primary bacteremia—i.e., the presence of pneumococci in the blood with no

Table 141-2

Most Common Infections Caused by *Streptococcus pneumoniae*

Acute sinusitis	Osteomyelitis
Pneumonia	Septic arthritis
Acute purulent	Peritonitis
tracheobronchitis	Endocarditis
Otitis media	Pericarditis
Empyema	Endometritis
Meningitis	Cellulitis
Primary bacteremia	Brain abscess

NOTE: The order of the list very roughly approximates the order of frequency among adults, from most to least common.

apparent source—occurs commonly in children under 2 years of age and infrequently in adults; if no therapy is given, a source may become apparent. Pleural infection results either from direct extension of pneumonia to the visceral pleura or from hematogenous spread of bacteria from a pulmonary or extrapulmonary focus; the route cannot be determined in any individual case.

Otitis Media and Sinusitis When fluid from the middle ear is cultured during acute otitis media or fluid from a paranasal sinus is cultured during acute sinusitis, *S. pneumoniae* is the most common isolate or is second only to nontypable *Haemophilus influenzae*. Whether in adults or in children, pneumococci are identified in about 40 to 50 percent of cases of otitis in which an etiologic agent is isolated. Prior infection by a respiratory virus or allergy is thought to contribute significantly to these pneumococcal infections by causing congestion of the openings to the eustachian tubes or the paranasal sinuses. Prospective studies of young children have shown that colonization precedes infection in most cases. For reasons that are unclear, serotypes 6, 14, 19F, and 23F predominate both as colonizing and as infecting organisms of children; therefore, these serotypes are currently being studied most intensively for use in vaccines to be administered to young children.

Meningitis Except during outbreaks of meningococcal infection, *S. pneumoniae* is the most common etiologic agent of bacterial meningitis in adults. Because of the remarkable success of *H. influenzae* type b vaccine, *S. pneumoniae* now predominates among cases in infants and toddlers as well (but not among those in newborns). Meningitis develops either by the direct extension of infection from the sinuses or the middle ear or as a result of bacteremia with seeding of the choroid plexus. Favoring the former possibility are the association between acute otitis media and meningitis as well as the well-documented role of *S. pneumoniae* as the most common cause of recurrent bacterial meningitis associated with head trauma, cerebrospinal fluid (CSF) leak, and/or dural tear. Favoring the latter are the association between pneumococcal bacteremia from any source and meningitis as well as an autopsy study of temporal bone from children who died of bacterial meningitis, which yielded no evidence of extension from the middle ear. In the meninges and subarachnoid space, pneumococcal cell-wall antigens like peptidoglycan stimulate an intense inflammatory response mediated by the release of C5a, tumor necrosis factor, interleukins, and other proinflammatory cytokines. This inflammatory response and the local effect of pneumococci result in raised intracranial pressure, brain edema, and decreased blood flow leading to meningismus, drowsiness, or coma. Focal neurologic signs may result from suppurative vasculitis with venous or arterial thrombosis, from cranial neuropathy due to entrapment or infarction, from local cerebritis, from subdural effusion, or from brain herniation (see Chap. 377).

No distinctive clinical or laboratory feature differentiates meningitis due to *S. pneumoniae* from that due to other bacteria. Patients note the sudden onset of fever, headache, and stiffness or pain in the neck. Without treatment, there is a progression, over 24 to 48 h, to confusion and then obtundation. On physical examination, the patient looks acutely ill and has a rigid neck. In these cases lumbar puncture should not be delayed for computed tomography (CT) of the head unless papilledema or focal neurologic signs are evident. Typical CSF findings consist of pleocytosis (500 to 10,000 cells/μL) with a predominance of PMNs, an elevated protein level (100 to 500 mg/dL), and a decrease in glucose content. If antibiotics have not been given, large numbers of pneumococci can be seen in a Gram-stained specimen of CSF in nearly all cases. If an effective antibiotic has already been administered, the number of bacteria may be greatly decreased; in this situation, immunologic methods for the detection of pneumococcal capsule in the CSF may identify an etiologic agent in up to two-thirds of cases. However, these methods have fallen out of favor. Cultures will eventually turn positive in the great majority of cases, and most physicians prefer to continue empirical broad-spectrum antibiotic therapy until the etiologic agent has been definitively identified.

Pneumonia The distinctive symptoms and signs of pneumococcal pneumonia are (1) cough and sputum production, which reflect the proliferation of bacteria and the resulting inflammatory response in the alveoli; (2) fever; and (3) radiographic detection of an infiltrate.

Predisposing conditions Pneumococcal pneumonia is most common at the extremes of age. Despite the undisputed role of *S. pneumoniae* as a major pathogenic bacterium for humans, the great majority of adults with pneumococcal pneumonia have underlying diseases that predispose to infection. Otherwise healthy military recruits involved in outbreaks of infection may be an exception to this rule; however, many of those affected have an antecedent viral-type illness that may reduce normal host resistance. In addition to prior viral respiratory illness, the most common predisposing conditions are alcoholism, malnutrition, chronic pulmonary disease of any kind, infection with human immunodeficiency virus (HIV), diabetes mellitus, cirrhosis of the liver, renal insufficiency, and congestive heart failure. HIV infection is such an important predisposing factor that some authorities recommend that any young adult with pneumococcal pneumonia be tested for antibody to HIV.

Presenting symptoms Patients often present with a preexisting respiratory condition that has distinctly deteriorated. If a viral upper respiratory illness is the predisposing factor, the patient may have felt unwell for several days, with coryza or a nonproductive cough and low-grade fever; at the time of onset of pneumonia, the temperature rises to 38.9 to 39.4°C (102 to 103°F), and sputum production becomes prominent. In a patient who has chronic bronchitis, the sputum may increase in volume, become yellow or green and thicker than usual, and be associated with a fever that becomes progressively higher over 48 to 72 h. In a small proportion of cases, the onset of disease follows a hyperacute pattern in which the patient—often a healthy young individual—suddenly has a single episode of shaking chills followed by sustained fever and a cough productive of blood-tinged sputum. This clinical picture is unfortunately called "classic," a vague term that is best avoided because many physicians believe that it means "most common," which is clearly not the case. In elderly subjects, the onset of disease may be especially insidious and may not suggest pneumonia at all. Persons in their 80s may have minimal cough, no sputum production, and even no fever, instead appearing tired or confused or simply becoming hypothermic and going into shock. For the reasons noted above, the most abrupt progression of pneumococcal disease is that in patients who have previously undergone splenectomy; these individuals may go from apparent good health to death in as little as 24 h. In pneumonia, pleuritic chest pain may result from extension of the inflammatory process to the visceral pleura; persistence of this pain, especially after the first day or two of treatment, raises concern about empyema (see "Complications," below). Nausea and vomiting or diarrhea, sometimes quite prominent, occur in up to 20 percent of cases. Clearly, the range of symptoms is sufficiently broad that there is no characteristic presentation to distinguish pneumococcal from other types of bacterial pneumonia (and from some types of nonbacterial pneumonia).

Physical findings Patients with pneumococcal pneumonia usually appear ill and have a grayish, anxious appearance that differs from that of persons with viral or mycoplasmal pneumonia. Typically, the temperature is 38.9 to 39.4°C (102 to 103°F), the pulse 90 to 110 beats per minute, and the respiratory rate >20 breaths per minute. Elderly patients may have only a slight temperature elevation or be afebrile. A lack of fever in young or middle-aged adults is associated with increased morbidity and mortality, as is hypothermia. Herpes labialis appears in a small percentage of cases. Pain may cause diminished respiratory excursion (splinting) on the affected side. Dullness to percussion is noted in about half of cases, and vocal fremitus is increased. Breath sounds may be bronchial or tubular, and crackles are heard regularly on careful auscultation. Flatness to percussion at the lung base and inability to detect the expected degree of diaphragmatic motion suggest the presence of pleural fluid, which raises the possibility of empyema; the failure to assess fremitus, to distinguish dullness

from flatness by percussion, or to examine for diaphragmatic excursion may leave the physician at the mercy of often ambiguous radiologic interpretations. The finding of a heart murmur raises concern about endocarditis, a rare but serious complication. Confusion may result from hypoxia or the generalized response to pneumonia; obtundation or neck stiffness should lead to an immediate consideration of meningitis.

Radiographic findings In most cases of pneumococcal pneumonia, the chest x-ray reveals an area of infiltration involving less than a full segment. Whereas true consolidation with an air bronchogram is common among relatively healthy young adults, pneumonia superimposed on severe chronic lung disease causes a more moth-eaten, less homogeneous appearance. Segmental or lobar consolidation is apparent in fewer than half of cases, although most bacteremic patients exhibit such a radiologic pattern. Multilobar involvement is not uncommon. In rare instances, pneumococcal pneumonia leads to a lung abscess. Although some pleural fluid may actually be present in half of cases, no more than 20 percent of patients have a sufficient volume of fluid to allow aspiration, and in only a minority of these patients is empyema documented.

General laboratory findings The peripheral-blood white blood cell (WBC) count is >12,000/μL in the great majority of patients with pneumococcal pneumonia. However, the count is <6000/μL in 5 to 10 percent of persons hospitalized for pneumococcal pneumonia. Such a low count is often but not always associated with bone marrow suppression due to alcohol ingestion; this finding connotes a high risk of death. The serum bilirubin level may be increased to 4 mg/dL (68 μmol/L); hypoxia, inflammatory changes in the liver, and breakdown of red blood cells in the lung are all thought to contribute to this increase. Levels of lactate dehydrogenase may be elevated. A variety of other abnormalities may be present, reflecting the contributory role of underlying diseases. → *Abnormalities of pleural fluid in empyema are reviewed in Chap. 255.*

Diagnostic microbiology An etiologic role for the pneumococcus in pneumonia is strongly suggested by the demonstration of large numbers of PMNs and slightly elongated gram-positive cocci in pairs and chains in the sputum (Fig. 141-1). Examined areas of the slide must be free of epithelial cells, because organisms found in these locations may represent contamination by the oral bacterial flora. Capsules may be seen surrounding the bacterial forms. In this setting, the diagnosis can be confirmed by the identification of *S. pneumoniae* in sputum culture. However, culture is less sensitive than Gram's staining for identifying pneumococci. Since most pneumococci do not produce distinctively mucoid colonies, their identification in the laboratory depends on the ability to select putative pneumococcal colonies for further study from among alpha-hemolytic streptococci of the mouth. In short, laboratory diagnosis by sputum culture relies on the quality of the specimen provided, the care with which the relevant purulent component is separated for culture, and the assiduity with which alpha-hemolytic colonies are studied. These factors need

FIGURE 141-1 The microbiologist can easily identify *Streptococcus pneumoniae* as the etiologic agent of pneumonia when microscopic examination of a Gram-stained sputum specimen reveals this kind of picture.

to be considered when sputum cultures from patients who appear to have pneumococcal pneumonia are said to yield only "normal mouth flora" and when the medical literature describes what appear to be poor results of sputum culture. Because of the central role of Gram's stain in diagnosis, physicians should review the slides with the microbiologist. Blood cultures yield *S. pneumoniae* in about 20 percent of cases of pneumococcal pneumonia. Modern, automated systems often yield positive blood cultures within 12 h after the sample is obtained.

Complications Empyema is the most common complication of pneumococcal pneumonia, occurring in about 2 percent of cases. As noted above, some fluid appears in the pleural space in a substantial proportion of cases of pneumococcal pneumonia, but this parapneumonic effusion usually reflects an inflammatory response to infection that has been contained within the lung, and its presence is self-limited. When bacteria reach the pleural space—either hematogenously or as a result of contiguous spread, possibly across lymphatics of the visceral pleura—empyema results. The finding of frank pus, a positive result on Gram's staining, or the presence of fluid with a pH of ≤7.1 indicates the need for aggressive and complete drainage, preferably by prompt insertion of a chest tube, with verification by CT that fluid has been removed. If there is no response, thoracotomy is indicated. Persistence of fever (even if low-grade) and leukocytosis after 4 or 5 days of appropriate antibiotic treatment for pneumococcal pneumonia suggests empyema; in this setting, the diagnosis is exceedingly likely if the x-ray shows the persistence of pleural fluid; at this stage, thoracotomy is often needed for cure. Aggressive drainage is likely to reduce morbidity and mortality from empyema.

Other Syndromes The appearance of pneumococcal infection at other, usually sterile body sites indicates hematogenous spread, either during frank pneumonia or, in a smaller proportion of cases, from an inapparent focus of infection. A case of pneumococcal endocarditis is seen every few years at large tertiary-care hospitals. Purulent pericarditis due to this organism, occurring as a separate entity or together with endocarditis, is even rarer. Most cases of spontaneous bacterial peritonitis in children and some cases in adults are caused by *S. pneumoniae*. Peritonitis in women may be related to the use of an intrauterine contraceptive device, and pneumococcal infections of the female reproductive organs continue to be described. Septic arthritis can arise spontaneously in a natural or prosthetic joint or as a complication of rheumatoid arthritis. Osteomyelitis in adults tends to involve vertebral bones. Epidural and brain abscesses are rarely described. Cellulitis can develop and does so most often in persons who have connective tissue diseases or HIV infection. The appearance of any of these unusual pneumococcal infections in a young adult may suggest that tests for HIV infection should be undertaken.

℞ TREATMENT

Antibiotic Susceptibility β-Lactam antibiotics, the cornerstone of therapy for serious pneumococcal infection, act by binding covalently to and thereby blocking the action of the cell-membrane enzymes (endo-, trans-, and carboxypeptidases) that are responsible for cell-wall synthesis. These enzymes were identified by their reaction with radiolabeled penicillin and thus are called penicillin-binding proteins. In the 1960s, virtually all clinical isolates of *S. pneumoniae* were susceptible to penicillin (i.e., were inhibited in vitro by concentrations of <0.06 µg/mL). During the past 15 years in Europe and the past 5 years or so in the United States, a steadily increasing number of pneumococcal isolates have shown some degree of resistance to penicillin, often together with resistance to other antibiotics (Table 141-3). Resistance results from spontaneous mutation or acquisition of new genetic material leading to the alteration of penicillin-binding proteins in a manner that necessitates a higher concentration of penicillin for their saturation. The genetic information acquired also conveys resistance to other antibiotics. Mutation and selection of strains in communities in the United States—especially in areas of high antibiotic use, such as day-care centers—and spread of identifiable strains from other countries where antibiotics are available without prescription have both contributed to the prevalence of resistance.

For most of the antibiotic era, pneumococcal susceptibility was not studied in vitro because of the organism's high degree of susceptibility to virtually all antibiotics. Clearly, the situation has changed, and it seems reasonable to expect routine study of pneumococcal isolates, as of other organisms, for antibiotic susceptibility. In 1995, about 15 to 20 percent of strains isolated in the United States showed intermediate resistance to penicillin [minimum inhibitory concentration (MIC), 0.1 to 1.0 µg/mL], and 2 to 5 percent exhibited high-level resistance (MIC ≥2 µg/mL). A varying proportion of intermediately resistant isolates are also resistant to erythromycin and the newer macrolides, tetracyclines, trimethoprim-sulfamethoxazole, and clindamycin (Table 141-3), as are a greater proportion of highly resistant strains; certain of the latter isolates are also resistant to second-generation and some third-generation cephalosporins. So far, the majority of strains have retained susceptibility to cefotaxime, ceftriaxone, and imipenem. Given the relatively poor activity of ciprofloxacin against *S. pneumoniae*, most experts do not consider ciprofloxacin or ofloxacin reliable for the treatment of pneumococcal infection. Better alternative agents are almost always available, even for use against resistant strains. Some of the newer quinolones appear to be more effective in vitro against penicillin-resistant pneumococcal strains. Nearly all pneumococcal isolates remain susceptible to vancomycin, although the acquisition of resistance to this antibiotic is feared because of the increasing prevalence of vancomycin resistance among enterococci and among other gram-positive bacteria that may eventually transfer genetic material to pneumococci. The reader must be warned that this situation is fluid and that susceptibility patterns may vary greatly between and even within individual communities.

General Therapy Despite increased emphasis on outpatient therapy in the past decade, the author prefers to hospitalize all patients with pneumococcal pneumonia when it is feasible to do so. Patients who are elderly, have undergone splenectomy, appear sick, have oxygen desaturation, are confused, or have underlying lung disease, heart failure, cirrhosis, or renal insufficiency should certainly be hospitalized. Direct admission to an intensive care unit should be considered for all persons thought to have pneumococcal pneumonia who have hypotension, substantial oxygen desaturation or an increase in P_{CO_2} relative to their own baseline, radiographic involvement of more than one lobe, or a low peripheral WBC count (<6000/µL), even though it has been difficult to prove that such care enhances outcome.

Specific Antibiotic Therapy PNEUMONIA Pneumonia caused by penicillin-susceptible or intermediately penicillin-resistant pneu-

Table 141-3

Penicillin Susceptibility Status of Pneumococci Resistant to Other Antimicrobial Agents

Status of Strain	Percentage of Isolates Resistant to Indicated Agent											
	Amox	Amox/ Clav	Tet	Em	TMP-SMZ	Cfur	Ctax or Ctri	Cm	Newer Mac	Quin	Imi	Vm
Pen-S	0	0	20	2	10	0	0	0	0	?0	0	0
Pen-I	?	?	40	10	25	0	0	<10	10	?0	0	0
Pen-R	100	100	50	50	50	25	10	50	50	?0	10	0

Abbreviations: Pen-S, sensitivity to penicillin; Pen-I, intermediate resistance to penicillin; Pen-R, resistance to penicillin; Amox, amoxicillin; Clav, clavulanate; Tet, tetracycline; Em, erythromycin; TMP-SMZ, trimethoprim-sulfamethoxazole; Cfur, cefuroxime; Ctax, cefotaxime; Ctri, ceftriaxone; Cm, clindamycin; Mac, macrolides; Quin, quinolones; Imi, imipenem; Vm, vancomycin.

NOTE: These percentages reflect a composite of the data available in October 1995; actual results vary with the time and locale studied. A question mark indicates that the clinical significance of in vitro susceptibility results is uncertain, as discussed in the text.

mococcal isolates appears to be readily treatable with penicillin. The dosages that follow are acceptable for use against intermediately resistant strains and are somewhat excessive for susceptible isolates; it is a problem that pneumococcal susceptibility-test results do not become available until 24 to 72 h after treatment has begun (see below). Most patients hospitalized for pneumococcal pneumonia are treated with intravenous medications; 1 million units of penicillin every 4 h is excellent for this purpose. A first-generation cephalosporin given intravenously (for example, 1 g of cefazolin every 8 h) or procaine penicillin G given intramuscularly (2.4 million units to start, followed by 1.2 million units every 12 h) should be adequate. Amoxicillin has a substantially broader spectrum than is necessary for the treatment of pneumococcal infection. Nevertheless, its reliable and complete absorption after oral administration, substantially longer half-life, and antibacterial effect exceeding that of penicillin make this drug a good choice for the oral treatment of pneumococcal pneumonia in a dosage of 500 mg to start and then 250 mg every 8 h. Clindamycin is also highly effective against susceptible and intermediately resistant strains. Many isolates are resistant to tetracycline, and increasing numbers are resistant to erythromycin, newer macrolides, and trimethoprim-sulfamethoxazole; thus, the emphasis on "empirical" treatment of pneumonia is likely to become increasingly problematic. For highly penicillin-resistant isolates, intravenous treatment with cefotaxime (1 g every 6 h), ceftriaxone (1 g every 12 h), or imipenem (500 mg every 6 h) will be effective in about 90 percent of cases, and the course of therapy can be concluded with oral cefpodoxime. Vancomycin must be administered when the isolate is resistant to these drugs. Newer quinolones, streptogramins, oxazolidinones, and advanced tetracyclines are currently being studied in vivo, having shown in vitro activity against antibiotic-resistant *S. pneumoniae*.

Because the degree of susceptibility of a pneumococcal strain is not known when therapy is begun, it seems reasonable to treat a patient who has any of the markers that specifically suggest life-threatening pneumococcal pneumonia with cefotaxime or ceftriaxone. If resistance to ceftriaxone becomes prevalent, it may be necessary to administer vancomycin as well. Since bacteremic pneumococcal pneumonia is a life-threatening disease, this initial approach might be considered in all patients hospitalized for presumed pneumococcal pneumonia. Subsequent therapy should be based on the results of susceptibility testing. Patients with severe allergic reactions to β-lactam antibiotics should receive an advanced macrolide, clindamycin, or vancomycin until the results of susceptibility testing become available. The lack of a prompt response to therapy should raise the possibility of resistance, even if the laboratory has reported susceptibility, and treatment with vancomycin should be begun. In such instances, susceptibility testing should be repeated, and evidence of loculated infections (such as empyema) and/or other causes of fever should be sought.

The optimal duration of treatment for pneumococcal pneumonia is still uncertain. Pneumococci disappear from sputum within several hours of the first dose of penicillin, and a single dose of procaine penicillin, which produces an effective antimicrobial level persisting for 24 h, has been said to be curative in otherwise healthy young adults. Most older physicians treated pneumococcal pneumonia for 5 to 7 days. Although the failure of such therapy has not been reported, younger physicians seem to be treating this infection for 10 to 14 days. Prolongation of therapy is a two-edged sword, especially in debilitated patients, because the risk of complications increases with each day of antibiotic treatment, particularly in the hospital. Three to five days of close observation with parenteral therapy and a final few days of oral treatment—in all, not exceeding 5 days after the patient has become afebrile [temperature <37.2°C (<99°F)]—may be the best approach.

OTITIS MEDIA Treatment of acute otitis media may be more difficult than that of pneumonia. In the absence of diagnostic tympanocentesis, the etiologic diagnosis is nearly always presumptive

rather than proven. Many authorities continue to recommend amoxicillin. However, because penetration into a closed space is required for therapeutic efficacy, infection caused by intermediately resistant strains may not respond to penicillin or amoxicillin, and cefuroxime or cefpodoxime may be preferable. Once therapy has been initiated, patients must be monitored closely to be certain that they are responding. Although pneumococcal DNA has been detected by molecular analysis in middle-ear fluid, chronic serous otitis ("glue ear") is probably not due to active infection and does not require antibiotic therapy.

MENINGITIS Meningitis is the most life-threatening of pneumococcal infections. The author recommends that pneumococcal meningitis be treated initially with cefotaxime (2 g every 6 h) or ceftriaxone (1 g every 12 h) plus vancomycin (500 mg every 6 h or 1 g every 12 h) unless resistance to third-generation cephalosporins has not been reported in the community. Two drugs are given because the cephalosporin is likely to be effective against most isolates and readily penetrates the blood-brain barrier, whereas vancomycin is uniformly effective but has a somewhat unpredictable capacity to enter the CSF. Once an isolate is shown to be penicillin-susceptible, treatment can be continued with 24 million units of penicillin every 24 h, given every 4 h in divided doses or continuously. If the isolate exhibits intermediate resistance to penicillin but is susceptible to cefotaxime or ceftriaxone, the administration of vancomycin may be discontinued. Rifampin inhibits the bactericidal activity of β-lactam antibiotics and probably should not be added to the regimen. The total duration of therapy for pneumococcal meningitis is 10 to 14 days. Despite the central pathogenic role of inflammation in meningitis, the use of glucocorticoids or other anti-inflammatory agents is controversial, even in children, in whom most of the relevant studies have been done. Data simply do not exist on which to base an informed decision regarding the administration of glucocorticoids or cyclooxygenase inhibitors to adults with pneumococcal meningitis (see Chap. 377).

ENDOCARDITIS Pneumococcal endocarditis is associated with rapid destruction of heart valves. Vancomycin should be given pending assays for the minimal bactericidal concentrations of β-lactam antibiotics. There is no clear evidence that the addition of another antibiotic to the regimen is beneficial; aminoglycosides are somewhat synergistic and rifampin or quinolones are antagonistic with β-lactams. Endocarditis and meningitis should be treated initially in an intensive care unit, with the participation of appropriate consultants. Patients with meningitis should probably be seen by a neurologist as well as by a specialist in infectious diseases; those with endocarditis should be observed by an infectious disease consultant and a cardiologist, with a cardiovascular surgeon notified.

Other Therapeutic Modalities A variety of agents that block the action of tumor necrosis factor α, interleukin 1, or platelet-activating factor have conferred no benefit in and may have had a detrimental effect on pneumococcal sepsis. Similar results have been obtained with glucocorticoids.

PREVENTION Pneumococcal vaccine contains 25 μg of capsular polysaccharide from the 23 most prevalent serotypes; vaccination stimulates antibody to most serotypes in most recipients. In adults under 55 years old, protection rates are at least 85 percent, even 5 years or longer after vaccination. The level and duration of protection decrease with advancing age, such that persons in their eighties have 50 percent protection for 3 years and very little or no protection thereafter. In subgroups of the population who are most at risk (e.g., debilitated elderly persons and individuals with severe chronic lung disease), vaccine has not been shown conclusively to be effective. Persons who most need the vaccine because of compromised immunity are not likely to respond to immunization with significant increases in antibody level. Nevertheless, the poor average rate of response should not deter the physician from administering vaccine to a person at increased risk of pneumococcal infection. In light of the data demonstrating the safety, low cost, and efficacy of vaccine and the emergence of antibiotic-resistant strains, the failure to vaccinate elderly persons and individuals who have conditions predisposing to pneumococcal disease can be viewed as a missed opportunity in public health policy.

The Immunization Practices Advisory Committee of the Centers for Disease Control and Prevention recommends that pneumococcal vaccine be administered to adults who are generally regarded as immunocompetent but who are unusually likely to develop pneumococcal infection and/or a serious complication of such infection; this category includes (but is not limited to) persons with chronic pulmonary disease, advanced cardiovascular disease, diabetes mellitus, alcoholism, cirrhosis, chronic renal insufficiency, or CSF leak as well as all persons older than 65 years. A second category includes (but is not limited to) persons in whom immunosuppression is associated with an increased risk of pneumococcal disease or its complications, such as those with splenic dysfunction or asplenia, multiple myeloma, lymphoma, Hodgkin's disease, HIV infection, or organ transplantation.

There are, at the time of this writing, no official recommendations regarding revaccination. Nevertheless, in light of available data on the decline of antibody levels, the author believes that persons in these categories, especially those who have undergone splenectomy, should be revaccinated every 5 to 7 years.

With the increasing prevalence of penicillin-resistant pneumococci, the conditions under which the vaccine is administered may be liberalized. For example, pneumococcal vaccine could be given routinely to members of ethnic or racial groups that appear to have a particularly high incidence of pneumococcal infection (e.g., certain Native American populations) or to persons living in crowded settings, such as military camps or prisons. Adults over the age of 60 could be vaccinated and then revaccinated every 7 to 10 years or (after the age of 75) every 3 to 5 years. If penicillin-resistant pneumococci continue to increase in prevalence, routine immunization of children over the age of 2 should also be considered. Pneumococcal vaccine is not useful in children younger than 2 years because they do not respond well to polysaccharide antigens. Protein conjugate vaccines, currently under investigation, may eventually provide protection for infants and children.

BIBLIOGRAPHY

AFESSA B et al: Pneumococcal bacteremia in adults: A 14-year experience in an inner-city university hospital. Clin Infect Dis 21:345, 1995

AVERY OT et al: Studies on the chemical nature of the substance inducing transformation of pneumococcal types: Induction of transformation by a desoxyribonucleic acid fraction isolated from pneumococcus type III. J Exp Med 79:137, 1944

BOULNOIS GJ: Pneumococcal proteins and the pathogenesis of disease caused by Streptococcus pneumoniae. J Gen Microbiol 138:249, 1992

BREIMAN RF et al: Pneumococcal bacteremia in Charleston County, South Carolina: A decade later. Arch Intern Med 150:1401, 1990

—— et al: Emergence of drug-resistant pneumococcal infections in the United States. JAMA 271:1831, 1994

BURMAN LA et al: Invasive pneumococcal infections: Incidence, predisposing factors, and prognosis. Rev Infect Dis 7:133, 1985

DiNUBILE MJ et al: Pneumococcal soft-tissue infections: Possible association with connective tissue diseases. J Infect Dis 63:897, 1991

FEDSON DS, MUSHER DM: Pneumococcal vaccine, in Vaccines, 2d ed, SA Plotkin, EA Mortimer Jr (eds). Philadelphia, Saunders, 1994, p 517

FRANKLIN C et al: Reduced mortality of pneumococcal bacteremia after early intensive care. J Intensive Care Med 6:302, 1991

FRIEDLAND IR, McCRACKEN GH JR: Management of infections caused by antibiotic-resistant Streptococcus pneumoniae. N Engl J Med 331:377, 1994

GRAY BM, DILLON HC JR: Epidemiological studies of Streptococcus pneumoniae in infants: Antibody to types 3, 6, 14, and 23 in the first two years of life. J Infect Dis 158:948, 1988

HEFFRON R: Pneumonia: With special reference to pneumococcus lobar pneumonia. A Commonwealth Fund Book, © 1939. Reprinted by Harvard University Press, Cambridge, MA, 1979

JANOFF EN et al: Streptococcus pneumoniae colonization, bacteremia, and immune response among persons with human immunodeficiency virus infection. J Infect Dis 167:49, 1993

KIM PE et al: Invasive pneumococcal disease and the association with season, atmospheric temperature and isolation of respiratory viruses. Clin Infect Dis 20:100, 1996

MARKIEWICZ A, TOMASZ A: Variation in penicillin-binding protein patterns of penicillin-resistant clinical isolates of pneumococci. J Clin Microbiol 27:405, 1989

MURPHY TF, SETHI S: Bacterial infection in chronic obstructive pulmonary disease. Am Rev Respir Dis 146:1067, 1992

MUSHER DM: Streptococcus pneumoniae, in Mandell, Douglas and Bennett's Principles and Practice of Infectious Diseases, 4th ed, GL Mandell et al (eds). New York, Churchill Livingstone, 1994, p 1811

—— et al: Antibody to capsular polysaccharides of Streptococcus pneumoniae in adults: Prevalence, persistence, relation to carriage, and resistance to infection. Clin Infect Dis 17:66, 1993

ORT S et al: Pneumococcal pneumonia in hospitalized patients. JAMA 249:214, 1983

ORTQVIST A: Prognosis in community-acquired pneumonia requiring treatment in hospital. Importance of predisposing and complicating factors, and of diagnostic procedures. Scand J Infect Dis (Suppl) 65:1, 1990

POWDERLY WG et al: Pneumococcal endocarditis: Report of a series and review of the literature. Rev Infect Dis 8:786, 1986

RODRIGUEZ MC et al: Unusual manifestations of pneumococcal infection in HIV-infected individuals: The past revisited. Clin Infect Dis 14:192, 1992

SHAPIRO ED et al: The protective efficacy of polyvalent pneumococcal polysaccharide vaccine. N Engl J Med 325:1453, 1991

SIMBERKOFF MS et al: Efficacy of pneumococcal vaccine in high risk patients: Results of a Veterans Administration cooperative study. N Engl J Med 315:1318, 1986

SPANGLER SK et al: Activities of RPR 106972 (a new oral streptogramin), cefditoren (a new oral cephalosporin), two new oxazolidinones (U-100592 and U-100766), and other oral and parenteral agents against 203 penicillin-susceptible and -resistant pneumococci. Antimicrob Agents Chemother 40:481, 1996

TUOMANEN EI et al: Pathogenesis of pneumococcal infection. N Engl J Med 332:1280, 1995

VERSALOVIC J et al: Penicillin-resistant Streptococcus pneumoniae strains recovered in Houston: Identification and molecular characterization of multiple clones. J Infect Dis 167:850, 1993

VIÐARSSON G et al: Opsonization and antibodies to capsular and cell wall polysaccharides of Streptococcus pneumoniae. J Infect Dis 170:592, 1994

142   Robert L. Deresiewicz, Jeffrey Parsonnet

STAPHYLOCOCCAL INFECTIONS

The staphylococci are hardy and ubiquitous colonizers of human skin and mucous membranes and were among the first human pathogens identified. They cause a variety of syndromes, including superficial and deep pyogenic infections, systemic intoxications, and urinary tract infections. Staphylococci are the leading cause of bacteremia, surgical wound infections, and infections of bioprosthetic materials in the United States; in addition, they are the second leading cause of nosocomial infections overall. Organisms of this genus are also a significant cause of bacterial food poisoning.

Staphylococcus aureus is the most important human pathogen in the genus. It remains a major public health concern due to its tenacity, potential destructiveness, and increasing resistance to antimicrobial agents. Although less virulent, the coagulase-negative staphylococci (CNS), especially *Staphylococcus epidermidis*, adhere avidly to prosthetic materials and are increasingly important nosocomial pathogens, especially of compromised hosts. Another CNS species, *Staphylococcus saprophyticus*, is a common cause of urinary tract infections.

TAXONOMY AND MICROBIOLOGY   Members of the genus *Staphylococcus* are nonmotile, nonsporulating gram-positive cocci, 0.5 to 1.5 μm in diameter, that occur singly and in pairs, short chains, and the irregular three-dimensional clusters from which their name is derived (Greek *staphulé*, "grape-like"). Staphylococci can grow over a wide range of environmental conditions, but they grow best at temperatures between 30°C and 37°C and at a pH around neutrality. They are resistant to desiccation and to chemical disinfectants, and they tolerate NaCl concentrations up to 12%. With rare exceptions, the staphylococci are facultatively anaerobic and catalase-positive. The more virulent staphylococci can clot plasma (coagulase-positive), while the less virulent cannot (coagulase-negative). Of the five recognized coagulase-positive staphylococcal species, the only important human pathogen is *S. aureus*, whose colonies are larger than those of *S. epidermidis*, are often pigmented (golden yellow), and are usually β-hemolytic on sheep blood agar. Twenty-seven species of CNS are recognized. Of these, *S. epidermidis* is by far the most common nonurinary human isolate. Strains of *S. epidermidis* are typically white and nonhemolytic and may be tenaciously adherent as a result of their production of polysaccharide adhesin. *S. epidermidis* is followed in frequency by *Staphylococcus haemolyticus* and *Staphylococcus warneri*. *S. saprophyticus* is the most common staphylococcal urinary isolate.

STAPHYLOCOCCUS AUREUS

EPIDEMIOLOGY Humans constitute the major reservoir of *S. aureus* in nature; the cross-sectional carriage rate in adults is 15 to 40 percent. The mucous membranes of the anterior nasopharynx are the principal site of carriage; other sites include the axillae, the vagina, and the perineum and occasionally the gastrointestinal tract. Among postmenarcheal U.S. women, the rate of vaginal colonization by *S. aureus* ranges from 5 to 15 percent but rises to 30 percent during menses—a change that is relevant to the pathogenesis of the toxic shock syndrome (TSS). Colonization by *S. aureus* may be intermittent or persistent and is probably influenced by both microbial and host factors as well as by the nature of the competing nonstaphylococcal flora. Carriage is more common among persons with frequent staphylococcal exposure and those with habitual or chronic disruption of cutaneous epithelial integrity. Thus, health care workers, dialysis patients, diabetic patients, injection drug users, and persons with chronic dermatologic conditions are often colonized. Colonization of mucocutaneous sites is an important risk factor for staphylococcal infection; for example, wound infection following cardiothoracic surgery is more frequent among patients who harbor *S. aureus* in the nares preoperatively than among those who do not.

In reference laboratories, a number of techniques are available to assess strain relatedness in potential epidemic situations. These include phage typing, determination of plasmid profile or antibiotic resistance pattern, DNA fingerprinting, ribotyping, and polymerase chain reaction–based genetic polymorphism analysis. At present, no one technique is clearly superior to the others.

PATHOGENESIS AND HOST DEFENSE *S. aureus* causes two types of syndrome: *intoxications* and *infections*. The clinical manifestations of intoxications are attributable solely to the action of one or a few secreted products of the microorganism (toxins), and these clinical features can be reproduced by administration of the toxin(s) in the absence of the microorganism. The toxin can be produced either in vivo (as in TSS or staphylococcal scalded skin syndrome) or in a suitable vector that subsequently delivers it to the host (as in staphylococcal food poisoning). Infections, on the other hand, involve bacterial proliferation, invasion or destruction of host tissues, and—in most cases—local and systemic responses by the host to these events. Although the ability of a microorganism to infect is predicated on its capacity to produce certain products that enable it to survive and prosper in the host (*virulence factors*), no single product is responsible for all manifestations of the infection. *S. aureus* is a particularly well-armed bacterium and produces an array of putative virulence factors.

Steps in Pathogenesis The pathogenesis of staphylococcal intoxications is straightforward and involves four steps: colonization by a toxigenic strain of the bacterium, toxin production, toxin absorption, and intoxication. The pathogenesis of staphylococcal infections is more complex and the steps less discrete. They include colonization, invasion of the bacterium across epithelial barriers, adherence to materials in the extracellular matrix, evasion or neutralization of host defenses, and destruction of host tissues. For both intoxications and infections, the entire process is carefully orchestrated by the bacterium in response to specific environmental conditions.

Physical preservation of cellular integrity Staphylococci are robust and adaptable organisms that can survive under relatively harsh environmental conditions. A rigid cell wall confers shape and strength to the organisms. The major component of the cell wall, *peptidoglycan*, is responsible for its physical properties. Disruption of peptidoglycan cross-linking by cell wall–active antibiotics (β-lactams or glycopeptides) renders the staphylococci susceptible to lysis mediated by endogenous peptidoglycan hydrolases (*autolysins*). Other important components of the staphylococcal cell wall include ribitol teichoic acid and protein A.

The osmotolerance exhibited by *S. aureus* enables the organism to grow without microbial competition in foods of low water activity and so sets the stage for contamination of food by staphylococcal enterotoxins. If ingested, these toxins can cause staphylococcal food poisoning.

Colonization Staphylococcal adherence to the nasal mucosa is mediated by cell wall and cell membrane teichoic acid. Whether teichoic acid also mediates adherence to other mucosal surfaces (e.g., the vaginal mucosa) is unknown. After colonization, the production of certain staphylococcal toxins [toxic shock syndrome toxin 1 (TSST-1), exfoliative toxins, or enterotoxins] can ensue if the appropriate environmental signals are present. Other circumstances (e.g., toxin absorption, a nonimmune host) can lead to systemic intoxication. Alternatively, colonization may persist for a while before the organism is cleared. If in the meantime the organism gains access to deeper tissues, the process of infection may begin.

Invasion and adherence to the extracellular matrix Staphylococci generally cannot invade through intact epithelial surfaces, which represent the primary line of antistaphylococcal defense. Invasion is facilitated by a mechanical break in the epithelium or by plugging of a gland or hair follicle. Once the epithelial barrier is breached, *S. aureus* can adhere to any of several molecules present either on cell surfaces or in the extracellular matrix. These molecules include fibrinogen, fibronectin, laminin, thrombospondin, collagen, elastin, vitronectin, and bone sialoprotein.

Destruction of host cells and alteration of the host microenvironment A number of products of *S. aureus* alter the host environment in a way that benefits the bacterium. *Coagulase* is a secreted enzyme that binds prothrombin and thereby causes the conversion of fibrinogen to fibrin; it may aid in the establishment of an environment within host tissues that is protected from cells of the immune system or from antibiotics. *S. aureus* also produces a number of *lipases*, which may enhance the organism's survival in sebaceous areas of the human body. *Hyaluronidase* hydrolyzes hyaluronic acid, a mucopolysaccharide present in extracellular ground substance; its action may ease the spread of the organism through the extracellular matrix. *Fatty acid–modifying enzyme* inactivates mammalian staphylocidal lipids, which accumulate during development of the staphylococcal abscess and which are thought to be a component of the body's nonspecific antistaphylococcal defense. *Staphylokinase*, *thermonuclease*, and *serine protease* are other extracellular enzymatic products that may play roles in pathogenesis.

S. aureus also produces a number of membrane-active toxins that probably contribute to pathogenesis by damaging host cells. These toxins include α-, β-, and δ-hemolysins and the synergohymenotropic toxins (γ-hemolysin and Panton-Valentine leukocidin). α-*Hemolysin* (α-toxin) is the prototypic pore-forming toxin; it inserts into the cell membrane, creating ion-conductive channels that destroy membrane integrity. The toxin is dermonecrotic on subcutaneous injection. It is responsible for the β-hemolytic phenotype exhibited by many *S. aureus* strains when they are grown on sheep erythrocytes. β-*Hemolysin* is a sphyngomyelinase that exhibits species-specific hemolytic activity dependent on the sphyngomyelin content of the target cell membrane. Little is known about δ-*hemolysin*, although it appears to exert a detergent-like effect on cell membranes. The *synergohymenotropic toxins* are a newly described family of bicomponent toxins. Their name derives from the fact that their two components, which are secreted separately, are tropic for cell membranes and are synergistically active against them. Like α-toxin, the synergohymenotropic toxins are pore-forming toxins. *Panton-Valentine leukocidin* is most active against polymorphonuclear cells, monocytes, and macrophages. It is dermonecrotic to rabbit skin, and strains producing it are strongly associated with human furunculosis. γ-*Hemolysin* is active against a wide range of mammalian erythrocytes.

Evasion of host defense Once staphylococci have breached mucosal or epithelial barriers, the host's immune response is directed at containing and eliminating them, principally by polymorphonuclear recruitment and phagocytic killing. The bacteria fight back by cloaking antigenic determinants on their surface, by interfering with the function of opsonins, by directly killing the phagocytes, and by developing strategies to survive within them. The pyogenic abscess, the histologic hallmark of staphylococcal infection, represents the battlefield for this encounter and in some sense benefits both the microorganism and the host—the microorganism by providing an environment in which leukocyte function is impaired and into which antibiotics penetrate poorly, and the host by containing the spread of the bacteria.

Certain staphylococcal components and products are direct chemoattractants for polymorphonuclear leukocytes; others provoke the release of chemoattractant cytokines that recruit phagocytic cells to the infected area. Histologic sections of early lesions typically reveal a central focus of organisms surrounded by a zone of necrotic debris, which in turn is surrounded by a zone of viable inflammatory cells. The toxic action of staphylococcal leukocidin may in part explain the zone of necrosis. After several days, fibroblasts populate the margin of the abscess and there elaborate collagen, which creates a true capsule around the abscess.

Staphylococcal cell wall peptidoglycan activates complement, which is an important opsonin in persons lacking antibody to staphylococcal surface components. Peptidoglycan also acts as a general stimulator of inflammatory cytokine release but is much weaker in this regard than gram-negative lipopolysaccharide.

Opsonic antibodies specific for peptidoglycan or capsule also mediate phagocytosis. There is considerable interstrain variation in susceptibility to opsonization, and acquired protective immunity to staphylococcal infection is generally thought not to develop. At least two staphylococcal products mitigate against opsonization. *Polysaccharide capsule* is produced by about 80 percent of clinical isolates and lies external to the cell wall; it physically interferes with opsonization by complement. *Protein A*, an important cell surface component, binds the Fc portion of IgG subclasses 1, 2, and 4 and thereby interferes with antibody-mediated opsonization. Acquired antibody-mediated immunity to systemic staphylococcal intoxications (as opposed to infections) does occur.

Opsonized organisms are efficiently ingested by polymorphonuclear leukocytes and macrophages. Most are then killed rapidly by the oxidative burst within the phagosome. Staphylococcal catalase, which converts hydrogen peroxide to oxygen and water, detoxifies oxygen radicals and potentiates intracellular bacterial survival. Staphylococci are also taken up by nondedicated phagocytes, such as endothelial cells and osteoblasts, and may survive within them. Yet another staphylococcal strategy for intracellular survival is the genesis of so-called small-colony variants. These slow-growing cells exhibit alterations in electron transport and generally produce reduced amounts of virulence determinants such as α-toxin. They are relatively resistant to antibiotics and appear capable of persisting intracellularly for extended periods. Their existence may in part explain the startling capacity of certain *S. aureus* infections (e.g., chronic osteomyelitis) to recrudesce after years of dormancy.

Hosts at particular risk for staphylococcal infection include those with frequent or chronic disruptions in epithelial integrity, such as injection drug users or persons with chronic onychomycoses of the fingers or toes; those with disordered leukocyte chemotaxis, such as patients with the Chédiak-Higashi or Wiskott-Aldrich syndrome; those whose phagocytes are defective in oxidative killing, as in chronic granulomatous disease; and those with indwelling foreign bodies, which provide a matrix for staphylococcal adherence and biofilm formation. Patients with disorders of immunoglobulin or complement

are also at increased risk for *S. aureus* infection, as are patients infected with human immunodeficiency virus.

Superantigens The superantigens are V_β-restricted T cell mitogens: they bind directly and without prior processing to major histocompatibility class II molecules on the surface of antigen-presenting cells, thereby stimulating T cells on the basis of the sequence of the variable region of the β chain of the T cell receptor rather than on the basis of the epitope specified by this receptor. Accordingly, a superantigen may be able to stimulate up to about 10 percent of the T cells in a given individual—a percentage much higher than the approximately 1 in 10^6 cells stimulated by conventional antigens. This massive T cell stimulation provokes an exuberant and dysregulated immune response characterized by the release of the cytokines interleukins 1 and 2, tumor necrosis factor, and interferon γ. *S. aureus* produces a number of superantigens, including the staphylococcal enterotoxins (SEs), TSST-1, and possibly the exfoliative toxins (ETs). Eight SEs are currently known (enterotoxins A, B, C_{1-3}, D, E, and H) and are the causative agents of staphylococcal food poisoning. The mechanism by which the SEs cause vomiting is uncertain but may involve direct neural stimulation of the autonomic nervous system rather than a local effect on the gastrointestinal mucosa. The superantigenic properties of TSST-1 are thought to explain its ability to cause TSS, although the exact mechanism by which it crafts the various clinical manifestations of TSS is uncertain. There is conflicting evidence as to whether the ETs, which cause scalded skin syndrome, are superantigens; structural data suggest that they may instead be related to the serine proteases.

Genetic Regulation of Virulence Genes The production of virulence factors by bacteria is typically tightly and coordinately regulated by genetic apparatuses that sense and respond to environmental cues. Such coordinate regulation enables an organism to rapidly tailor its repertoire of proteins to suit its changing needs, either as it passes between microenvironments or as the environment evolves around it. Many of the staphylococcal exoproteins are typical virulence factors in this regard. For example, α-, β-, and δ-hemolysins, TSST-1, staphylococcal enterotoxin B, serine protease, and thermonuclease are all produced during the late logarithmic phase of growth in batch culture, at a time when nutrients become scarce and cell density reaches saturation. Their production is coordinately regulated and occurs reciprocally to that of the cell wall–associated staphylococcal proteins protein A and coagulase. Several genetic regulatory loci modulate these events, as do specific environmental conditions that presumably operate through those genetic loci. Foreign materials that increase the risk of TSS and conditions in food that predispose to staphylococcal food poisoning probably do so by presenting microenvironments that stimulate production of the relevant toxins. Similar events are undoubtedly operative within the environment of host tissues during infection, even in the absence of a foreign body.

At least three separate genetic loci regulate exoprotein production in *S. aureus*: *agr* (accessory gene regulator), *xpr* (extracellular protein regulator), and *sar* (staphylococcal accessory regulator). All three loci affect gene expression primarily at the level of transcription, and all three activate the expression of secreted proteins and diminish the expression of cell wall–associated proteins during the late logarithmic phase of bacterial growth. Recent data suggest that *agr* may function primarily as a "quorum sensor," an apparatus that informs the bacterium of the density of staphylococci in its environment. Exoprotein regulation in *S. aureus* apparently results from a complex interplay of environmental factors and gene products.

STAPHYLOCOCCAL INTOXICATIONS Toxic Shock Syndrome TSS is an acute, life-threatening intoxication characterized by fever, hypotension, rash, multiorgan dysfunction, and desquamation during the early convalescent period (Fig. 142-1). The disease was first characterized in 1978 but gained notoriety in 1980 upon the recognition of a large outbreak in menstruating women. It is a relatively uncommon illness, with a reported incidence (among menstruating

FIGURE 142-1 Cutaneous manifestations of toxic shock syndrome. The patient was a 7-year-old child with osteomyelitis and nonmenstrual TSS. *Top:* Diffuse erythroderma. The rubor was intense on the chest wall of this patient and is accurately represented in this black-and-white photograph. Circumoral pallor is evident. *Bottom:* Desquamation of the fingers during convalescence. *(From Deresiewicz, with permission.)*

women) of 1 case per 100,000; it is likely, however, that the disease is substantially underreported. About half of all cases occur in settings other than menstruation and are distributed among individuals of both sexes and all ages. Menstrual and nonmenstrual cases are clinically indistinguishable. Among cases reported to the Centers for Disease Control and Prevention between 1985 and 1994, the minimum case-fatality rate was 2.5 percent for menstrual cases and 6.4 percent for nonmenstrual cases.

TSS is caused by any of several related toxic exoproteins produced by *S. aureus*. TSST-1 is the toxin most frequently implicated and staphylococcal enterotoxin B the second most frequent. For illness to develop, an individual must be colonized or infected with a toxigenic strain of *S. aureus* and must lack a protective level of antibody to the toxin made by that strain. That TSS is primarily a disease of the young reflects the fact that more than 90 percent of individuals have antibodies to TSS toxins by adulthood.

Menstruation remains the most common setting for TSS, but the disease can also complicate the use of barrier contraceptives, the puerperium, septic abortion, and nonobstetric gynecologic surgery. Moreover, nonmenstrual TSS can complicate skin lesions of many types, including chemical or thermal burns, insect bites, varicella lesions, and surgical wounds. Postoperative disease can develop from

hours to weeks after a surgical procedure. Overt infection with *S. aureus* is not required for the development of TSS; mere colonization with a toxigenic strain may suffice. Accordingly, the primary site of toxin production in TSS may appear entirely benign. TSS has also been associated with musculoskeletal infections and respiratory infections caused by *S. aureus* and occasionally with staphylococcal bacteremia.

TSS remains a clinically defined syndrome (Table 142-1); patients meeting the case definition are severely ill. The illness begins precipitously, with high fever and a complex of symptoms that may include nausea, vomiting, abdominal pain, diarrhea, muscular pain, sore throat, and headache. Dizziness is a common manifestation of orthostatic or frank hypotension. The characteristic macular erythroderma develops over the first 2 days of illness. It is usually generalized but is sometimes locally confined; it can be evanescent or persistent. The patient's mental status is often abnormal to a degree that is out of proportion to the degree of hypotension. Conjunctival suffusion, pharyngeal injection, and peripheral edema are evident in many cases; a so-called strawberry tongue develops in up to half of patients. In menstrual disease, the vaginal mucosa may be erythematous and a purulent vaginal discharge may be present, but these findings are not universal. Common laboratory abnormalities include azotemia, hypoalbuminemia, hypocalcemia, hypophosphatemia, creatine phosphokinase elevation, leukocytosis or leukopenia with a left shift, thrombocytopenia, and pyuria.

The early signs and symptoms of TSS resolve within the first few days of illness, after which complications of organ hypoperfusion, such as renal and myocardial dysfunction, massive edema, and adult respiratory distress syndrome, dominate the picture. After about a week of illness, desquamation begins with superficial flaking of the skin of the torso, face, and extremities, which is followed by full-thickness desquamation of the palms, soles, and digits. Common late sequelae include peripheral gangrene, reversible nail and hair loss, muscle weakness, and neuropsychiatric dysfunction.

The differential diagnosis of TSS is that of a severe febrile exanthem with hypotension. In the setting of menstruation accompanied by purulent vaginal discharge, the diagnosis may be obvious. The challenge is to recognize the less obvious cases, in which the exanthem may be fleeting, multiorgan dysfunction may be subtle, or (in nonmenstrual cases) a primary site of infection may be inapparent. Other

Table 142-1

Staphylococcal Toxic Shock Syndrome: Case Definition

1. Fever: temperature of ≥38.9°C (102°F)
2. Rash: diffuse macular erythroderma ("sunburn" rash)
3. Hypotension: systolic blood pressure of ≤90 mmHg (adults) or <5th percentile for age (children under 16 years of age); or orthostatic hypotension (orthostatic drop in diastolic blood pressure by ≥15 mmHg, orthostatic dizziness, or orthostatic syncope)
4. Involvement of at least three of the following organ systems
   a. Gastrointestinal: vomiting or diarrhea at onset of illness
   b. Muscular: severe myalgias or serum creatine phosphokinase level at least twice the upper limit of normal
   c. Mucous membranes: vaginal, oropharyngeal, or conjunctival hyperemia
   d. Renal: blood urea nitrogen or creatinine level at least twice the upper limit of normal; or pyuria (≥5 leukocytes per high-power field) in the absence of urinary tract infection
   e. Hepatic: total serum bilirubin or aminotransferase (alanine or aspartate) level at least twice the upper limit of normal
   f. Hematologic: thrombocytopenia (platelet count, ≤100,000/μL)
   g. Central nervous: disorientation or alteration in consciousness but no focal neurologic signs at a time when fever and hypotension are absent
5. Desquamation: 1 to 2 weeks after the onset of illness (typically palms and soles)
6. Evidence against an alternative diagnosis: negative results of cultures of blood, throat, or CSF (if performed);* no rise in titers of antibody to the agents of Rocky Mountain spotted fever, leptospirosis, and rubeola (if obtained)

*Blood culture may be positive for *S. aureus*.
SOURCE: AL Reingold et al, Ann Intern Med 96(part 2):875, 1982.

diagnoses to consider include streptococcal TSS (toxic shock-like syndrome), staphylococcal scalded skin syndrome, Kawasaki syndrome, Rocky Mountain spotted fever, leptospirosis, meningococcemia, gram-negative sepsis, exanthematous viral syndromes, and severe drug reactions. Staphylococcal TSS and streptococcal TSS (see Chap. 143) can be clinically indistinguishable.

Treatment of TSS involves decontamination of the site of toxin production, aggressive fluid resuscitation, and administration of antistaphylococcal drugs. Recent surgical wounds should be explored and irrigated, even when signs of inflammation are lacking. Pressors should be used for sustained hypotension that is unresponsive to fluids. Electrolyte abnormalities, particularly hypocalcemia and hypomagnesemia, must be corrected. Semisynthetic penicillins (nafcillin, oxacillin) have been widely used in TSS; however, a growing body of clinical and laboratory evidence indicates that a protein synthesis inhibitor, such as clindamycin, might be superior. The authors recommend therapy with clindamycin (900 mg intravenously every 8 h), either alone or in combination with a β-lactam antibiotic or vancomycin. For a seriously ill patient in whom the diagnosis is uncertain, broad-spectrum antibiotics are appropriate until the diagnosis is confirmed. A 14-day course of therapy—some of which may be administered perorally—is reasonable. Patients whose illness is severe enough to warrant vasopressors, who require mechanical ventilation, who have worsening renal function, or who have an undrainable focus of infection should be treated with intravenous immunoglobulin, which contains high levels of neutralizing antibody to TSS toxins. A single infusion of 400 mg/kg generates a protective level of antibody to TSST-1 that persists for weeks. Steroids should not be administered routinely.

Because vaginal staphylococcal carriage can be sustained or recurrent and because in more than half of all cases TSS does not elicit immunity, recurrent menstrual TSS is a concern; recurrent nonmenstrual TSS has also been reported. The risk of recurrent illness can be assessed by tests for seroconversion to TSST-1. Women who do not seroconvert after acute illness (or who are not tested for antibody) should refrain indefinitely from using tampons or barrier contraceptives.

Staphylococcal Scalded Skin Syndrome This syndrome encompasses a range of cutaneous diseases of varying severity caused by ET-producing strains of *S. aureus*. The most severe form of staphylococcal scalded skin syndrome is termed *Ritter's disease* in newborns and *toxic epidermal necrolysis* (TEN) in older individuals. Milder and more common forms include *pemphigus neonatorum* and (in children and adults) *bullous impetigo* (see "Skin and Soft Tissue Infections" below). A portion of cases of so-called *staphylococcal scarlet fever* are also due to intoxication with ETs, although others are probably mild cases of TSS.

Persons over the age of 5 years rarely develop staphylococcal TEN; those who do almost invariably have underlying disease (renal insufficiency, systemic immunosuppression). The rarity of the syndrome in adults has been ascribed to acquired immunity to the inciting toxins, to enhanced renal clearance of the toxins, and perhaps to diminished sensitivity to the action of the toxins. Most adults have antibodies to the ETs as they do to other staphylococcal exotoxins. The syndrome has followed infections in a variety of sites, the most common being purulent rhinitis. Staphylococcal bacteremia is detected in only about 3 percent of children with this syndrome but in up to half of adults.

Staphylococcal TEN or Ritter's disease often begins with a nonspecific prodrome. The acute phase starts with the onset of an erythematous rash. The erythema begins in the periorbital and perioral areas and spreads to the trunk and centrifugally to the limbs. Pastia's lines may be apparent. The skin has a sandpaper texture and is often tender to the touch. Periorbital edema is common. In infants and children, fever and irritability or lethargy are common, but systemic toxicity is not. Within hours or days, wrinkling and sloughing of the epidermis begins; sloughing can be provoked by gentle stroking of the skin (Nikolsky's sign), even in areas that appear uninvolved. The denuded areas are red and glistening but not purulent, and staphylococci are not present. Exfoliation may continue in large sheets or in ragged snippets of tissue. Large, flaccid bullae may develop. As in thermal

burns, significant fluid and electrolyte loss can occur at this stage, as can secondary infection. Within about 48 h, the exfoliated areas dry and secondary desquamation begins. The entire illness resolves within about 10 days. Mortality (from hypovolemia or sepsis) is about 3 percent among children but approaches 50 percent among adults. Treatment includes the administration of antistaphylococcal agents, fluid and electrolyte management, and local care to the denuded skin.

Staphylococcal Food Poisoning Between 2 and 6 h after ingestion of contaminated food, staphylococcal food poisoning begins abruptly with nausea, vomiting, crampy abdominal pain, and diarrhea. The diarrhea is usually noninflammatory and is of lower volume than that in cholera or toxigenic *Escherichia coli* infection. Fever and rash are absent, and the patient is neurologically normal. The majority of cases are self-limited and resolve between 8 and 24 h after onset. In severe cases, hypovolemia and hypotension can develop. Although most cases probably do not come to medical attention or are not diagnosed, staphylococcal intoxication is the second or third leading cause of diagnosed food poisoning in the United States.

Food poisoning is caused by the ingestion of any of the SEs, which are produced by *S. aureus* in contaminated food before it is eaten. The presence of SEs in the food vector before its consumption accounts for the short incubation period of this illness. The SEs are heat stable, thus tolerating cooking conditions that kill the organisms that produced them. The disease has a high attack rate and is somewhat more common during the summer than at other times of the year. Processed meats and custard-filled baked goods are common food vectors, perhaps because staphylococci can tolerate conditions of high protein, salt, or sugar and so grow without competition in these environments. The most important epidemiologic risk factor in outbreaks of this disease is the ingestion of food that has been left at room temperature for prolonged periods, thereby allowing toxin production to occur before consumption. Contaminated preparation equipment and poor personal hygiene of food handlers are frequently implicated as well.

When a common-source food-borne outbreak of staphylococcal food poisoning is suspected, health authorities should be promptly consulted so that they can determine the etiology, isolate the source, and correct the conditions that led to the outbreak. A variety of immunologic techniques are available for the detection of SEs in foodstuffs.

STAPHYLOCOCCAL INFECTIONS *S. aureus* causes invasive disease by breaching host defense barriers, often after disruption or dysfunction of such barriers. The most common portals of entry leading to staphylococcal invasion are the skin and associated structures. A nidus for staphylococcal colonization and subsequent invasion is provided by chronic skin conditions, such as eczema and psoriasis; acute breaks in the skin, such as puncture wounds, abrasions, and lacerations; and abnormalities of skin appendages, such as hair follicles and nails. Colonization of the nasopharynx predisposes to respiratory tract infection after aspiration, obstruction (e.g., of a bronchus by carcinoma or of sinus ostia by trauma, edema, or polyps), or impaired ciliary function (e.g., in chronic bronchitis or acute viral infection). Intubation of the trachea provides a conduit by which upper respiratory flora, including pathogens such as *S. aureus*, can reach the lower respiratory tract. Less common portals of entry for *S. aureus* are the urinary and gastrointestinal tracts.

Skin and Soft Tissue Infections *S. aureus* is the most common etiologic agent of skin and soft tissue infections. Such infections are usually caused by endogenous flora—i.e., strains of *S. aureus* that are harbored in the nares or other sites of colonization. Infection may represent a primary pathologic process, with direct invasion of skin and adjacent tissues, or a secondary process complicating preexisting lesions.

Staphylococcal infections originating in hair follicles range in severity from trivial to life-threatening. *Folliculitis* is an infection of follicular ostia; the appearance is that of domed, yellow pustules with a narrow red margin. Infection is often self-limited, although healing may be hastened by topical antiseptics and more severe cases may benefit from topical or systemic antibiotics. A *furuncle* (often called a *boil*) is a deep-seated necrotic infection of a hair follicle, most often located on the buttocks, face, or neck. Furuncles are painful and tender, and their appearance is often accompanied by fever and constitutional symptoms. Surgical drainage and systemic antibiotic treatment are often required to hasten recovery and limit scar formation. Furunculosis may recur if there is continued colonization with a pathogenic strain of *S. aureus*. Deep infection of a group of contiguous follicles is called a *carbuncle*. This type of painful necrotic lesion, which is often accompanied by high fever and malaise, occurs most commonly on the back of the neck, shoulders, hips, and thighs, typically in middle-aged or elderly men. There is intense inflammation of surrounding and underlying connective tissue, and illness may be complicated by bacteremia. Surgical drainage and systemic antibiotic administration are indicated. *S. aureus* is also the most common cause of acute *paronychia*, infection of the lateral nail folds.

S. aureus causes *bullous impetigo*, a superficial cutaneous disorder occurring predominantly in children. An epidermal split caused by ET results in the formation of 1- to 2-cm bullae containing neutrophils and organisms. *Nonbullous impetigo* is most frequently caused by β-hemolytic streptococci, but *S. aureus* can secondarily infect impetiginous lesions. Treatment of impetigo with a topical antibiotic, such as mupirocin, may suffice for mild and localized infection, whereas systemic therapy is indicated for widespread or severe disease or for infection accompanied by lymphadenopathy.

Cellulitis, a spreading infection of subcutaneous tissue, is occasionally caused by *S. aureus*, but β-hemolytic streptococci are much more common agents of this disease (see Chap. 143). Secondary infection of surgical and traumatic wounds is more likely to be staphylococcal in etiology than is cellulitis arising from minor or inapparent breaks in the skin, and empiric treatment directed against both *S. aureus* and streptococci is reasonable in these settings. *Erysipelas*, the hallmark of which is a well-demarcated raised border, is a more superficial infection of the dermis and subcutaneous tissue; it is usually caused by group A streptococci and only rarely, if ever, by *S. aureus*.

Respiratory Tract Infections *S. aureus* can gain access to the lung parenchyma by two routes: aspiration of upper respiratory flora and hematogenous spread. Staphylococcal pneumonia is a relatively uncommon but severe infection, characterized clinically by chest pain, systemic toxicity, and dyspnea and pathologically by intense neutrophilic infiltration, necrosis, and abscess formation. Only rarely does *S. aureus* cause pneumonia without predisposing epidemiologic or host factors that favor colonization of the respiratory tract and/or that impair defense mechanisms. Residence in a chronic care facility, recent use of antibiotics, and hospitalization favor colonization—and hence respiratory tract infection—with *S. aureus*. Staphylococcal pneumonia most commonly follows tracheal intubation of a hospitalized patient or viral infection of the respiratory tract. Influenza virus is known both to increase respiratory colonization by *S. aureus* and to impair ciliary function (and therefore clearance of staphylococci). In a classic scenario, a patient (often elderly and/or institutionalized) develops a flulike respiratory illness and then, after several days, deteriorates rapidly, with high fever, dyspnea, productive cough, and obtundation. The diagnosis is readily established by Gram's staining of expectorated sputum, which reveals abundant clusters of gram-positive cocci.

Hematogenous seeding of the lungs with *S. aureus* follows embolization from an intravascular nidus of infection. Common settings for septic pulmonary embolization are right-sided endocarditis (especially common among injection drug users) and septic thrombophlebitis, which is most often a complication of an indwelling venous catheter. Pneumonia is heralded by the acute onset of pleuritic chest pain and dyspnea; although diagnostic sputum may be lacking, a chest radiograph typically shows multiple nodular infiltrates and thus provides an important clue to both the diagnosis and the pathogenesis of disease. *Empyema* is a common sequela of staphylococcal pneumonia and increases the already-considerable morbidity associated with this infection.

Although not typically considered in the differential diagnosis of sore throat, *S. aureus* is occasionally isolated as the dominant organism from patients (especially children) with exudative *pharyngitis*. The illness may be accompanied by a scarlatiniform rash and may result in severe toxicity (like that seen in TSS). Staphylococcal *tracheitis* may be diagnosed in patients who have systemic toxicity and positive respiratory cultures but who lack pulmonary infiltrates. *S. aureus* is a prominent cause of *chronic sinusitis*, typically following the selection pressure of antimicrobial regimens that lack activity against this organism. Finally, *S. aureus* is a major etiologic agent of *sphenoid sinusitis*.

Infections of the Central Nervous System *S. aureus* gains access to structures of the central nervous system by hematogenous spread or by direct extension from contiguous structures. This organism is a prominent cause of *brain abscess*, especially as a result of embolization during mitral or aortic valve endocarditis. Such abscesses are often multiple, small, and scattered diffusely throughout the brain. Brain abscess can also develop by direct extension from frontoethmoid or sphenoid sinuses or from infected soft tissue after surgery or penetrating trauma. Patients with staphylococcal brain abscesses are more likely to have fever, meningismus, and other signs of infection than are patients with anaerobic bacterial or mixed-etiology brain abscesses. Purulent *meningitis* may accompany staphylococcal brain abscess or may develop during bacteremia in the absence of demonstrable abscesses.

S. aureus is the organism most likely to cause a variety of other space-occupying, suppurative intracranial infections. *Subdural empyema* usually develops by direct extension of osteomyelitis of the skull, after surgery or trauma, or in the setting of sinusitis. This condition may be accompanied by meningitis, epidural abscess, or intracranial phlebitis. The cardinal features of subdural empyema are fever, headache, vomiting, and signs of meningeal irritation. As the infection progresses, cerebral edema, often with infarction, may ensue and may be accompanied by alteration in mental status, seizures, and focal neurologic signs, which sometimes progress rapidly. The diagnosis should be suspected in any patient with meningeal signs and focal neurologic findings. Magnetic resonance imaging (MRI) is the diagnostic procedure of choice; lumbar puncture is contraindicated because of the danger of brainstem herniation. Early surgical drainage and treatment with an antibiotic that penetrates well into the central nervous system may be curative, although neurologic sequelae are not uncommon.

S. aureus is the most common cause of *spinal epidural abscess*, which develops most often in association with vertebral osteomyelitis or diskitis. The diagnosis is suggested by fever, back pain, radicular pain, lower-extremity weakness, bowel or bladder dysfunction, and leukocytosis, but the presentation is often subtle. Patients may report only difficulty in walking or weakness, and objective findings may initially be lacking. The principal danger is the potential for necrosis of the spinal cord by compression and/or venous involvement. Early recognition of this condition is critical if long-term sequelae, such as paraplegia, are to be averted. An MR scan of the spine establishes whether or not an epidural collection is present; if it is, needle aspiration or open drainage confirms the infectious etiology. Prompt surgical decompression by laminectomy is often required for preservation of neurologic function, although a trial of antibiotic therapy alone may be considered if no focal neurologic deficits are detected. The pathogenesis of *intracerebral epidural abscess* is similar to that of subdural empyema, with staphylococcal infection usually following sinusitis, craniotomy, or trauma. Clinical manifestations reflect the anatomy of the underlying osteomyelitis plus the mass effect of the abscess, cerebral edema, and (often) secondary involvement of the subdural space. Emergent surgical drainage is usually required for cure.

Finally, *S. aureus* is the most common cause of *septic intracranial thrombophlebitis*, typically following sinusitis, mastoiditis, or soft tissue infection of the face. Clinical manifestations reflect the underlying condition and the anatomic structures in contiguity with the infected vein or sinus. Focal neurologic deficits, particularly of cranial nerve function, are characteristic of cavernous sinus thrombosis. Sagittal sinus thrombosis may be manifested by leg and arm weakness and by altered mental status; infections of the lateral and petrosal sinuses also produce characteristic clinical syndromes. Intracranial phlebitis may accompany epidural abscess, subdural empyema, and meningitis and is sometimes clinically indistinguishable from other types of intracranial infection. MRI is the diagnostic procedure of choice.

Urinary Tract Infections *S. aureus* is an uncommon cause of urinary tract infection. Ascending infection almost exclusively follows instrumentation of the bladder (e.g., cystoscopy or placement of an indwelling catheter). Under other circumstances, the presence of *S. aureus* in the urine, even in low numbers, suggests staphylococcal bacteremia and hematogenous seeding of the kidneys, with or without abscess formation; staphylococcal endocarditis should be considered in this setting.

Endovascular Infections *S. aureus* is the most common cause of acute bacterial *endocarditis* of both native and prosthetic valves. Staphylococcal endocarditis presents as an acute febrile illness, rarely of more than a few weeks' duration; complications such as meningitis, brain or visceral abscess, peripheral vascular embolization, valvular incompetence with heart failure, myocardial abscess, and purulent pericarditis have often developed by the time a patient seeks medical attention. The valves most commonly involved are the mitral and/or the aortic except among injection-drug users, in whom infection of the tricuspid valve is most common. The diagnosis is suggested by a heart murmur and the presence of conjunctival hemorrhages, subungual petechiae, or purpuric lesions on the distal extremities; it is readily confirmed by multiple positive blood cultures and echocardiography showing valvular vegetations. Echocardiography also helps establish which valve(s) are infected, the degree of valvular dysfunction or destruction, the quality of left ventricular function, and the presence or absence of annular or myocardial abscess.

Staphylococcal endocarditis carries a high mortality rate (on the order of 40 to 60 percent) and mandates prompt initiation of antimicrobial therapy. In addition to blood cultures and echocardiography, evaluation may include computed tomography (CT) of the head and lumbar puncture if brain abscess or meningitis is suspected; a radionucleotide study if osteomyelitis is suspected; and abdominal CT if visceral abscesses are suggested by abdominal pain or persistent fever or bacteremia. Indications for valve replacement are the same as those in endocarditis caused by other organisms: persistent bacteremia (beyond 5 to 7 days of therapy), valvular dysfunction resulting in heart failure, perivalvular or myocardial abscess, or recurrent embolization. Early consultation with a cardiothoracic surgeon is advisable because of the high percentage of patients with *S. aureus* endocarditis (around half) who develop one of these complications and therefore require valve replacement, often urgently. Once there is an indication for removal of an infected valve, nothing is gained and much can be lost by delaying surgery.

Right-sided endocarditis, which most often develops in association with injection drug use or venous catheterization, is frequently complicated by septic pulmonary emboli but otherwise carries a lower rate of serious complications than left-sided disease. Surgery is rarely required for right-sided disease. A relatively short course of parenteral therapy (2 weeks) may be curative, and the prognosis is relatively good. In contrast, *S. aureus* infection of a prosthetic valve (as an early or a late complication of valve replacement) almost always requires surgery for one of the above indications.

The propensity of *S. aureus* to adhere to and infect damaged tissues makes it the foremost cause of endovascular infections other than endocarditis. Vascular infection may be a consequence of hematogenous seeding of damaged vessels, especially large arteries with atheromatous plaques, resulting in the development of a mycotic aneurysm. It may also develop by spread from a contiguous focus of infection (e.g., after vascular surgery), often resulting in an infected pseudoaneurism, or by contamination of an intravascular device, resulting in septic phlebitis. Staphylococcal infection of an atherosclerotic artery (most commonly the abdominal aorta or iliac arteries), which may be aneurysmal to begin with, is a potentially catastrophic event. Such infections are associated with high-grade bacteremia, may result in rupture and massive hemorrhage, and are almost never curable without surgical

resection and bypass of the infected vessel. Septic phlebitis is also associated with high-grade bacteremia and systemic toxicity but is less likely than arteritis to result in rupture. Persistent bacteremia suggests the need for surgical removal of infected thrombus or vein, but the technical difficulty of such surgery may warrant an attempt at cure with antibiotics and anticoagulants alone.

A classic clinical scenario is that of a patient presenting with *S. aureus* bacteremia but without a demonstrable primary site of infection. Even in the absence of a changing murmur, peripheral embolic lesions, or a diagnostic echocardiogram, the possibility of endocarditis must be considered carefully in this situation. It is often hard to differentiate between endocarditis and bacteremia arising from another primary site; in addition, *S. aureus* may secondarily seed endovascular sites, such as heart valves or atheromatous plaques. Several criteria increase the probability that a patient has endocarditis as opposed to simple bacteremia: community (vs. nosocomial) acquisition of infection, absence of a primary site of infection, and evidence of metastatic infection. The evaluation of a bacteremic patient should be tailored to the individual but may include (in addition to an echocardiogram) an abdominal CT scan and a bone scan or gallium scan to detect an occult visceral abscess or osteomyelitis. Persistent bacteremia in conjunction with negative results in these studies may warrant a transesophageal echocardiogram, which is more sensitive than a transthoracic echo in detecting valvular vegetations.

Complications of *S. aureus* bacteremia include abscesses of abdominal viscera, brain abscess, meningitis, septic arthritis, osteomyelitis, endocarditis (if not already present), and mycotic aneurysm. High-grade or persistent bacteremia mandates a thorough evaluation for these complications, even if a primary site of infection has been identified.

Musculoskeletal Infections *S. aureus* is the most common cause of *acute osteomyelitis* in adults and one of the leading causes in children. Acute osteomyelitis develops as a result of either hematogenous seeding of bone (especially damaged bone) or direct extension from a contiguous focus of infection. The most common sites of hematogenous staphylococcal osteomyelitis in adults are the vertebral bodies; in children, the highly vascular metaphyses of long bones are most often affected. Acute osteomyelitis in adults usually presents as constitutional symptoms and pain over the affected area, often developing over several weeks or months; the diagnosis may be subtle, however, in the absence of localizing symptoms. Leukocytosis and an elevated erythrocyte sedimentation rate are laboratory clues to the diagnosis. Bacteremia may or may not be demonstrable. Four to six weeks of parenteral antibiotic therapy is usually curative.

S. aureus is also a prominent cause of *chronic osteomyelitis*, which develops at sites of previous surgery, trauma, or devascularization. In light of the hectic pace of many infections caused by *S. aureus*, chronic staphylococcal osteomyelitis can be impressively indolent; the infection may be asymptomatic for years or even decades, only to reawaken spontaneously and cause pain, sinus tract formation, and purulent drainage. A plain film of the affected area usually reveals bony destruction. The staphylococcal etiology of infection is best established by biopsy and culture of bone, as cultures of superficial or sinus tract drainage may yield misleading results. Cure requires surgical debridement of necrotic bone followed by a prolonged course of antibiotics.

A special form of osteomyelitis is that associated with prosthetic joints or with internal or external fixation devices. Pain, fever, swelling, and decreased range of motion are cardinal features of an infected prosthesis. A plain film may suggest loosening of the prosthesis, often as radiolucency at the interface between bone and cement. *S. aureus* osteomyelitis associated with a prosthesis can rarely be cured by antibiotics alone. Clinical sepsis, persistent bacteremia, or clinical or radiologic evidence of loosening is an absolute indication for removal of the prosthesis. *S. aureus* infection of fixation devices requires their removal, although this procedure is frequently delayed long enough to allow healing of the underlying fracture. Late relapses after apparent medical cure are not uncommon. A strategy of microbial suppression with oral antibiotics after a course of high-dose parenteral therapy is occasionally employed when removal of hardware is deemed too aggressive a measure for a particular patient.

S. aureus is a major cause of *septic arthritis* in adults. Predisposing factors include injection drug use, rheumatoid arthritis, use of systemic or intraarticular steroids, penetrating trauma, and joints previously damaged by trauma or disease. Knees, hips, and sacroiliac joints are most frequently infected. In addition to parenteral antibiotics, cure requires either repeated joint aspirations—the end points being sterilization of the joint space, a decrease in the number of leukocytes in the joint aspirate, and no reaccumulation of fluid—or open or arthroscopic debridement and drainage. Failure to adequately drain joints infected with *S. aureus* poses a risk of permanent loss of function. *S. aureus* is also the most common cause of *septic bursitis*.

S. aureus infection of muscle (*pyomyositis*) is relatively uncommon in temperate climates. *Psoas abscess* is the main exception. The psoas muscle is seeded either hematogenously or by direct extension from the site of vertebral osteomyelitis; the results are pain upon extension of the hip and fever. Although formerly an occasional cause of fever of unknown origin, psoas abscess is now relatively easy to diagnose by abdominal CT or MRI. Psoas abscesses are occasionally amenable to drainage via a percutaneous catheter; if not, then surgical drainage is indicated. For reasons that are not well understood, most other cases of staphylococcal pyomyositis occur in the tropics (tropical pyomyositis); in the United States, pyomyositis is seen most often in patients with underlying conditions such as diabetes mellitus, alcoholism, immunosuppressive therapy, or hematologic malignancy.

DIAGNOSIS The diagnosis of *S. aureus* infection is generally straightforward and is based on the isolation of the organism either from purulent material or from a normally sterile body fluid. Rarely if ever should *S. aureus* growing from even a single blood culture be considered a contaminant. Clinical samples require no special transport media to preserve the viability of the organisms. Gram's staining of purulent material from a staphylococcal abscess invariably reveals abundant neutrophils and intra- and extracellular cocci, which may be found singly or in pairs, short chains, tetrads, or clusters. *S. aureus* grows readily on standard laboratory media such as blood and chocolate agar. Colonies that are catalase positive and coagulase or thermonuclease positive may be identified presumptively as *S. aureus*. Many commercial kits are now available for the identification of gram-positive cocci and are generally reliable for the identification of *S. aureus*.

The diagnosis of staphylococcal intoxications may be more difficult and may in fact rely entirely on clinical data (e.g., the diagnosis of TSS). The contribution of the laboratory may be confirmatory—for example, the demonstration of seroconversion to TSST-1 following a compatible illness, the demonstration of toxin production in vitro by a strain isolated from a patient, or the detection of SE in a food sample.

℞ **TREATMENT**

The essential elements of therapy for staphylococcal infections are drainage of purulent collections of pus, debridement of necrotic tissue, removal of foreign bodies, and administration of antimicrobial agents. The importance of adequate drainage cannot be overemphasized; all but the smallest of staphylococcal abscesses require drainage for cure. In skin and soft tissue infections, surgical drainage is occasionally all that is required for cure. It is almost impossible to eradicate *S. aureus* infection in the presence of a foreign body, such as a piece of orthopedic hardware, an intravascular catheter or other device, or a pacemaker. Only under extraordinary circumstances should an attempt be made to cure such infections without removal or debridement of foreign material.

Antimicrobial Resistance The relentless spread of antibiotic resistance among strains of *S. aureus* is one of the great challenges facing clinicians today. Within 4 years of the introduction of penicil-

lin G into clinical practice in 1941, β-lactamase-mediated resistance to penicillin was reported. As additional antibiotics (chloramphenicol, tetracyclines, macrolides, aminoglycosides) became available in the 1950s, resistance rapidly emerged to them as well. Penicillin resistance in *S. aureus* is due to the production of β-lactamase, a serine peptidase that enzymatically degrades penicillin's β-lactam ring, thereby inactivating the drug. β-Lactamase is related to the penicillin-binding proteins (PBPs), a group of transpeptidases that catalyze the terminal steps in peptidoglycan assembly. Methicillin-sensitive *S. aureus* (MSSA) produces four PBPs, all of which are inhibited by β-lactam antibiotics and three of which are essential for bacterial multiplication. Unlike β-lactamases from gram-negative organisms, some of which are more active against cephalosporins than against penicillins, the staphylococcal β-lactamases are principally penicillinases. Their transcription is induced by the presence of β-lactam molecules in the medium. Today, all but a very small percentage of *S. aureus* strains produce β-lactamase.

Methicillin, the first β-lactamase-stable semisynthetic penicillin, was introduced in 1960; the very next year, a methicillin-resistant strain of *S. aureus* (MRSA) was isolated. In recent years, the percentage of staphylococcal isolates from U.S. hospitals that are methicillin resistant has risen substantially, a trend that has been driven by indiscriminate antibiotic use. In some tertiary care institutions, more than 40 percent of *S. aureus* isolates are now resistant to methicillin, although rates of 5 to 10 percent are more typical. Community-acquired MRSA carriage remains rare except in certain high-risk groups, such as injection drug users.

Methicillin resistance is most accurately determined by the standard agar screen for MRSA. Classic methicillin resistance is encoded by the methicillin resistance determinant (*mec*), a 30- to 50-kb transposon-like segment of DNA that is present in MRSA strains and absent in MSSA strains. The *mecA* gene, which resides on *mec*, encodes a variant PBP called *PBP2'* or *PBP2a*. PBP2' has reduced affinity for β-lactam antibiotics and is able to substitute for the essential PBPs if they have been inactivated by β-lactams. MRSA strains are resistant to the action of all β-lactam antibiotics, including penicillins, cephalosporins, and carbapenems. These strains tend to be resistant to most other antibiotics as well, most often because they carry large conjugative plasmids bearing multiple resistance determinants. They remain uniformly sensitive to vancomycin, although the days of glycopeptide resistance may soon be upon us: transfer of such resistance from *Enterococcus faecalis* to *S. aureus* has been demonstrated in the laboratory.

An additional mechanism is responsible for a borderline methicillin-resistant phenotype (the so-called borderline-resistant, or BORSA, phenotype): hyperproduction of β-lactamase. These strains lack the *mecA* gene and are killed by oxacillin at the level used in the standard agar screen for methicillin resistance. BORSA infections can probably be treated successfully with high doses of semisynthetic penicillins.

Selection of Antibiotics Although most pathogenic strains of *S. aureus* are resistant to penicillin, the development of penicillins and cephalosporins that are resistant to β-lactamase has enabled these classes of antibiotics to remain useful for treatment of *S. aureus* infections. Nafcillin and oxacillin, both of which are β-lactamase-resistant penicillins, are the drugs of choice for parenteral treatment of serious staphylococcal infections. Penicillin remains the drug of choice for infections caused by susceptible organisms. Drug combinations consisting of a penicillin plus a β-lactamase inhibitor are also effective but are best reserved for treatment of mixed infections. Penicillin-allergic patients can usually be given a cephalosporin, although caution should be exercised if the adverse reaction to penicillin was anaphylaxis. Of the cephalosporins, the first-generation agents (e.g., cefazolin) are preferred for reasons related to cost, potency, and breadth of spectrum. The best alternative for parenteral administration is vancomycin. Dicloxacillin and cephalexin are recommended for oral treatment of minor infections or for continuation therapy. Several other agents are also available for use against susceptible strains.

In most clinical settings, no significant benefit is attained by treating *S. aureus* infections with more than one drug to which the organism is known to be susceptible. Synergy has been demonstrated in vitro for aminoglycoside/β-lactam combinations, which hasten sterilization of the blood in endocarditis. Accordingly, therapy for *S. aureus* bacteremia is often initiated with such a combination for a brief period (e.g., 5 to 7 days)—a strategy to which the authors are sympathetic. Thereafter, the toxicity of an aminoglycoside cannot be justified on the basis of available data. Use of rifampin in conjunction with a β-lactam antibiotic (or vancomycin) occasionally results in sterilization of sites of otherwise refractory infections, particularly those involving foreign bodies or avascular tissue; the results can be dramatic. Nevertheless, routine use of rifampin for serious *S. aureus* infections is not recommended because of potential added toxicity and theoretical antimicrobial antagonism. Rifampin should be reserved for refractory, usually inoperable infections and should never be administered as monotherapy, which rapidly leads to resistance.

Route and Duration of Therapy Because of poor bioavailability or tolerability of most oral antistaphylococcal agents, parenteral therapy should be used for infections that require high concentrations of antibiotic, such as endovascular infections, infections of poorly vascularized tissue, and infections of the central nervous system. Given the propensity of *S. aureus* to adhere to endovascular and devitalized or damaged tissues, high doses of antibiotics (e.g., 12 g of nafcillin per day) should be used for bacteremic infections. When high serum levels of antibiotic are required to produce adequate tissue levels (e.g., in endocarditis or osteomyelitis), the parenteral route should be used for the duration of therapy. Oral agents may suffice for the treatment of nonbacteremic infections in which high serum levels of antibiotic are not requisite (e.g., skin, soft tissue, and upper respiratory tract infections).

With the notable exceptions of bacteremia and osteomyelitis, the duration of therapy for *S. aureus* infections can be tailored to the severity of illness, the immunologic status of the host, and the response to treatment. Because antibiotics penetrate bone poorly, treatment of acute osteomyelitis in adults requires 4 to 6 weeks of parenteral therapy, with the actual duration depending on the vascular supply at the site of infection and the response to treatment. Chronic osteomyelitis is occasionally treated with 6 to 8 weeks of parenterally administered antibiotics followed by several months of oral therapy, especially if the adequacy of debridement is uncertain.

Acute endocarditis and other endovascular infections caused by *S. aureus* should be treated with parenteral antibiotics for 4 weeks (6 weeks in the case of prosthetic valves). Simple bacteremia, as might occur with a removable or drainable focus of infection, requires a shorter duration of therapy, but a 2-week course of *parenteral* therapy is recommended *for all patients* with *S. aureus* bacteremia, even under these circumstances. The cost and effort implicit in this recommendation are apparent, but shorter courses of therapy are associated with an unacceptable rate of secondary complications. One of the more challenging aspects of treating staphylococcal bacteremia is deciding whether to administer parenteral therapy for 2 or 4 weeks. A conservative approach (one that is supported by numerous studies) dictates that *4 weeks* should be standard unless specific criteria are met (Table 142-2).

PREVENTION AND CONTROL Nosocomial staphylococcal outbreaks and the spread of resistant strains of *S. aureus* are serious global problems. Within an institution, the most important vector of transmission of *S. aureus* is the hands of health care workers. Patients with exposed wounds or with nasal colonization are important reservoirs of the organisms. Transmission of *S. aureus*—and hence the incidence of staphylococcal infection within an institution—can be reduced most effectively by meticulous hand washing before and after contact with patients.

More stringent infection-control measures must be taken to prevent the nosocomial spread of MRSA. Such measures include assigning patients colonized or infected with MRSA to private rooms, wearing gloves for contact with contaminated wounds and mucous membranes

Table 142-2

Criteria for the Selection of Short-Course (2-Week) Parenteral Antibiotic Therapy for Patients with *S. aureus* Bacteremia

Subjects with *S. aureus* bacteremia who meet *all* criteria may be treated with parenteral antibiotics for 2 rather than 4 weeks.
1. No serious underlying condition, such as hematologic malignancy, poorly controlled diabetes, cirrhosis, severe malnutrition, rheumatoid arthritis, or AIDS
2. No hemodynamically significant valvular dysfunction
3. No "seedable sites," such as prosthetic heart valve, aortic aneurysm, necrotic bone, transvenous pacemaker, or prosthetic joint
4. A primary focus of infection that is readily apparent and amenable to removal (e.g., intravenous catheter) or surgical drainage
5. A short interval between the presumed onset of bacteremia and initiation of therapy (e.g., removal of catheter and start of antibiotics)
6. A staphylococcal isolate that proves to be susceptible to antibiotic(s) chosen initially
7. A prompt response to removal of the catheter and initiation of antibiotic treatment: defervescence within 72 h, negative blood cultures after catheter removal
8. No suppurative phlebitis at the catheter entry site
9. No evidence of metastatic foci of infection during the first 2 weeks of therapy

as well as a gown if contamination of clothing is likely, and hand washing with an antiseptic after patient contact. Patients who are colonized but not infected with MRSA should not be treated with vancomycin merely for the sake of eliminating carriage of this organism. *S. aureus* is the most common cause of postoperative wound infection. The incidence of staphylococcal infection in this situation can be reduced by perioperative administration of any of a number of antibiotics with favorable pharmacokinetic properties, including cefazolin, cefuroxime, and vancomycin.

Staphylococcal skin and soft tissue infections may recur once a person has been colonized with a virulent strain. In this context, therapy directed at the elimination of staphylococcal colonization may be warranted, especially for patients at particular risk for complications of infection. Use of an oral β-lactam antibiotic alone is ineffective, but combination therapy for 10 days with dicloxacillin or cephalexin (500 mg four times a day) plus rifampin (300 mg twice a day) plus mupirocin (2% ointment applied topically to both nares) is usually effective at clearing the carrier state.

COAGULASE-NEGATIVE STAPHYLOCOCCI

CNS are a major cause of nosocomial infection and are the organisms most frequently isolated from the blood of hospitalized patients. The frequency with which they cause opportunistic infection in immunocompromised hosts attests more to the increased vulnerability of such hosts in modern medical practice than to the intrinsic virulence of the organisms. Despite the weak pathogenicity of these bacteria, the global impact of CNS infection is considerable, including increased length and cost of hospital stay; increased use of antibiotics in general; and increased use of vancomycin in particular, which has contributed to the recent emergence of vancomycin-resistant enterococci.

Although the variety of clinical syndromes caused by CNS is impressive, several characteristics apply to most such infections (with notable exceptions). First, they tend to be *indolent*. There is often a long latent period between the time of contamination (e.g., of a medical device) and the onset of clinical illness; bacteremia in neutropenic patients can be an exception to this rule. Second, most CNS infections are nosocomial in origin; important exceptions are native valve endocarditis and *S. saprophyticus* infections of the urinary tract. Third, most clinically significant infections are caused by strains of CNS that are resistant to multiple antibiotics, including penicillins and cephalosporins. Finally, most CNS infections are associated with a medical device of some kind, and removal of such devices is usually required for cure.

EPIDEMIOLOGY AND PATHOGENESIS CNS, particularly *S. epidermidis*, are invariable and prominent constituents of the normal human skin flora. Infection most often results from direct inoculation of a foreign body at the time it is inserted, although hematogenous seeding can also occur. Patients and hospital personnel are the principal reservoirs for strains in the nosocomial environment.

CNS are the quintessential pathogens of medical devices. The array of virulence factors produced by CNS is meager compared with that of the virulence factors produced by *S. aureus*, but among these few factors are substances that promote bacterial adherence to and persistence on foreign bodies. A variety of surface antigens that promote colonization of medical devices by CNS (particularly *S. epidermidis*) have been identified; the best-studied of these is polysaccharide adhesin, which promotes the initial interaction of the bacteria and a foreign body. *S. epidermidis* also produces an exopolysaccharide known as *slime*, which is important in the persistence of infection; slime thwarts host defenses by coating foreign materials and impairing phagocytic killing. CNS appear not to make important exoproteins or toxins; rather, they cause disease by tenaciously persisting on foreign materials, resulting in a local and occasionally a systemic inflammatory response.

The most important risk factor for infection with CNS is the presence of a foreign body, especially an indwelling catheter. The likelihood of catheter-related infection depends upon a number of variables, including the experience and skill of the person who inserts the catheter, the length of time that a catheter is left in place, the adequacy of host immunity (especially granulocyte number and function), and the quality of postinsertion care of the catheter site. A second major risk factor for infection is deficient phagocyte function—especially neutropenia, which is most often an iatrogenic complication of chemotherapy for cancer but may also reflect an underlying disease process (such as leukemia). CNS only rarely cause infections in immunologically normal hosts and typically do so only under extenuating circumstances—e.g., subacute endocarditis involving an abnormal native valve or sternal osteomyelitis following cardiac surgery.

CLINICAL SYNDROMES Because CNS can adhere to a variety of materials, virtually all *foreign bodies* are susceptible to colonization by these organisms. CNS are the most common pathogens complicating the use of intravenous catheters, hemodialysis shunts and grafts, cerebrospinal fluid (CSF) shunts, peritoneal dialysis catheters, pacemaker wires and electrodes, prosthetic joints, vascular grafts, and prosthetic valves. CNS infection of intravenous catheters may or may not be accompanied by signs of inflammation at the site of catheter insertion, and the degree of systemic toxicity (including fever) ranges from minimal to considerable. The diagnosis can be established by the performance of multiple cultures of blood drawn from the catheter and by venipuncture. Infection of CSF shunts is usually evident within several weeks of implantation. Signs of meningitis are sometimes readily apparent but more often are subtle or absent. Malfunction of the shunt may be the only manifestation of shunt infection. CNS infection of a prosthetic joint often does not become evident until long after implantation, although the inciting contamination usually occurs at the time of implantation. Infection of vascular grafts may result in the development of an aneurysm or a pseudoaneurysm, with catastrophic consequences.

CNS are a prominent cause of *bacteremia* in immunosuppressed patients. While such infections in immunocompetent hosts are relatively benign, patients with neutropenia may have high-grade bacteremia that results in significant systemic toxicity and even death. A serious consequence of bacteremia is the seeding of a secondary foreign body, such as a prosthetic heart valve or joint or a pacemaker.

CNS are the organisms most commonly responsible for *prosthetic valve endocarditis*, causing the majority of infections that develop within several months of implantation as well as a substantial percentage of late infections. CNS are a less frequent but important cause of *native valve endocarditis*, accounting for fewer than 5 percent of such infections and usually affecting abnormal valves. The syndrome generally consists of subacute endocarditis (thus contrasting with the syndrome produced by *S. aureus*), with an illness that is clinically indistinguishable from that caused by viridans streptococci. Infection of prosthetic valves is often complicated by valvular dysfunction secondary either to dehiscence of the sewing ring or obstruction of the valve's orifice by bulky vegetations.

S. saprophyticus is a prime cause of *urinary tract infection*, especially among sexually active young women, in whom it is second only to *E. coli* in frequency. *S. saprophyticus* produces a syndrome indistinguishable from that caused by other etiologic agents, with pyuria and symptoms of dysuria, frequency, and abdominal pain. Infection with *S. saprophyticus* is readily amenable to therapy with most agents commonly used to treat urinary tract infections. CNS can also cause urinary tract infection in hospitalized patients who have undergone invasive procedures; such infections are especially likely to be asymptomatic and may be difficult to treat because of antimicrobial resistance.

DIAGNOSIS Although CNS are the most common cause of nosocomial bacteremia, they are also the most common contaminant of blood cultures; differentiation between infection and contamination often poses a challenge with major therapeutic implications. Positive blood cultures are more likely to be "true positives" when there is a clinical illness suggestive of infection, when there is an indwelling catheter or some other risk factor for CNS infection, and when cultures of blood drawn from multiple sites are positive for phenotypically similar organisms with the same antimicrobial susceptibility patterns. Except in the setting of neutropenia, physicians often have the luxury of awaiting the results of repeat cultures when the significance of CNS growing from a blood culture is questionable.

℞ **TREATMENT**

Removal of the foreign body (especially when it is an intravenous catheter) often constitutes adequate therapy for CNS infection related to that device. Most infections of a foreign body require the removal of the device—whether a prosthetic valve, prosthetic joint, CSF shunt, vascular graft, pacemaker and associated hardware, or hemodialysis shunt. Cures of all such infections with antibiotics alone have been reported, however, and a patient's poor medical condition or the hazards of surgery occasionally warrant an attempt at medical cure without extirpation of the device (see below). Infections of peritoneal dialysis catheters can be cured with antibiotics alone often enough that an attempt should be made to do so. CNS infections of central venous catheters are also amenable to medical therapy, although relapses are common. Persistent bacteremia during therapy is an absolute indication for removal of a catheter, and bacteremia after a catheter's removal suggests seeding of a secondary site.

It is difficult to make generalizations about the optimal duration of therapy for CNS infections. In general, the duration of treatment is the same as for infection syndromes caused by other bacteria. For example, native valve endocarditis should be treated for 4 weeks, prosthetic valve endocarditis for 6. Transient bacteremia in an immunocompetent host may require no antimicrobial therapy after removal of an offending catheter. The efficacy of therapy can occasionally be enhanced by the delivery of antibiotics directly to the site of infection—e.g., by intraventricular administration of vancomycin and gentamicin for central nervous system infections or by intraperitoneal administration of these drugs for infections of peritoneal dialysis catheters.

Despite the low degree of pathogenicity of CNS, treatment of serious infections due to these organisms is usually problematic because of the high percentage of strains that are resistant to commonly used antibiotics, including most oral agents. Most strains of CNS isolated from patients in U.S. hospitals are resistant not only to penicillin but also to the penicillinase-resistant penicillins and cephalosporins. Nosocomial isolates are usually resistant to other classes of antibiotics as well. Vancomycin, to which CNS remain uniformly susceptible, is of necessity the drug of choice for *empiric* therapy for serious CNS infections. Strains proven to be susceptible to nafcillin (oxacillin) or penicillin should be treated with one of these agents or with a first-generation cephalosporin.

Synergistic combinations of antibiotics are often useful in the treatment of CNS infections. Rifampin plays a unique role in this endeavor by virtue of its potency against most staphylococci, its excellent penetration into tissues (including those that are poorly vascularized), and the high levels it reaches within human cells. Unfortunately, rifampin must be used in combination with other antibiotics because of the frequent and rapid emergence of microbial resistance to the drug when it is used alone. If an effort must be made to eradicate infection of a medical device without its removal, the concomitant use of a β-lactam antibiotic to which the organism is susceptible plus rifampin (300 mg twice daily by mouth) plus an aminoglycoside (usually gentamicin) affords the best chance for success. Vancomycin can be substituted for the β-lactam agent if so dictated by an organism's susceptibility pattern or by a patient's drug allergy.

BIBLIOGRAPHY

BAILEY CJ et al: The epidermolytic (exfoliative) toxins of *Staphylococcus aureus.* Med Microbiol Immunol 184:53, 1995

DERESIEWICZ RL: Staphylococcal toxic shock syndrome, in *Superantigens: Molecular Biology, Immunology, and Relevance to Human Disease,* DYM Leung et al (eds). New York, Marcel Dekker, 1997, pp 435–479

GUANGYONG J et al: Cell density control of staphylococcal virulence mediated by an octapeptide pheromone. Proc Natl Acad Sci USA 92:12055, 1995

JERNIGAN JA, FARR BM: Short-course therapy of catheter-related *Staphylococcus aureus* bacteremia: A meta-analysis. Ann Intern Med 119:304, 1993

MARRACK P, KAPPLER J: The staphylococcal enterotoxins and their relatives. Science 248:705, 1990

MULLIGAN ME et al: Methicillin-resistant *Staphylococcus aureus*: A consensus review of the microbiology, pathogenesis, and epidemiology with implications for prevention and management. Am J Med 94:313, 1993

MUSHER DM et al: The current spectrum of *Staphylococcus aureus* infection in a tertiary care hospital. Medicine 73:186, 1994

NEU HC: The crisis of antibiotic resistance. Science 257:1064, 1992

PRASAD GS et al: Structure of toxic shock syndrome toxin 1. Biochemistry 32:13761, 1993

RUPP ME, ARCHER GL: Coagulase-negative staphylococci: Pathogens associated with medical progress. Clin Infect Dis 19:231, 1994

SHEAGREN JN: *Staphylococcus aureus*: The persistent pathogen. N Engl J Med 310:1368, 1437, 1984

143   *Michael R. Wessels*

STREPTOCOCCAL AND ENTEROCOCCAL INFECTIONS

Many varieties of streptococci are found as part of the normal human flora colonizing the respiratory, gastrointestinal, and genitourinary tracts. Several species are important causes of human disease. Group A *Streptococcus*, or *Streptococcus pyogenes*, is the organism responsible for streptococcal pharyngitis, one of the most common bacterial infections of school-age children, and for the postinfectious syndromes of acute rheumatic fever and poststreptococcal glomerulonephritis. Group B *Streptococcus*, or *Streptococcus agalactiae*, is the leading cause of bacterial sepsis and meningitis in newborn infants and a major cause of endometritis and fever in parturient women. Enterococci are significant causes of urinary tract infection, intraabdominal infection, and endocarditis. Viridans streptococci are the most common cause of bacterial endocarditis.

Streptococci are gram-positive bacteria of spherical to ovoid shape that characteristically form chains when grown in liquid media. Most streptococci that cause human infections are facultative anaerobes, although some are strict anaerobes. Streptococci are relatively fastidious organisms, requiring enriched media for growth in the laboratory. No single scheme for classification of streptococci is entirely satisfactory. Consequently, clinicians and clinical microbiologists often identify streptococci by any of several classification systems, including

hemolytic pattern, Lancefield group, species name, and common or trivial name. Many of the streptococci associated with human infection produce a zone of complete hemolysis around the bacterial colony when cultured on blood agar, a pattern known as beta hemolysis. The beta-hemolytic streptococci can be classified by the Lancefield system, a serologic grouping based on the reaction of specific antisera with cell-wall carbohydrate antigens of the bacteria. With rare exceptions, organisms belonging to Lancefield groups A, B, C, and G are all beta-hemolytic streptococci, and each is associated with characteristic patterns of human infection. Other streptococci produce a zone of partial, or alpha, hemolysis, often imparting a greenish appearance to the agar. These alpha-hemolytic streptococci are identified more specifically by biochemical testing and include *Streptococcus pneumoniae*, an important cause of pneumonia, meningitis, and other infections (discussed in Chap. 141), and several species of streptococci referred to collectively as the viridans streptococci, which are part of the normal oral flora and are prominent as agents of subacute bacterial endocarditis. Finally, some streptococci are nonhemolytic, a pattern sometimes called gamma hemolysis. The classification of the major groups of streptococci responsible for human infections is outlined in Table 143-1. Among the organisms classified serologically as group D streptococci, the enterococci are now considered to constitute a separate genus on the basis of DNA homology studies. Thus, species previously designated as *Streptococcus faecalis* and *Streptococcus faecium* have been renamed *Enterococcus faecalis* and *Enterococcus faecium*, respectively.

GROUP A STREPTOCOCCI

Lancefield group A consists of a single species, *S. pyogenes*. As its species name implies, this organism is associated with a variety of suppurative infections. In addition, group A streptococci have the

Table 143-1

Classification of Streptococci Responsible for Human Infections

Lancefield Group	Representative Species	Hemolytic Pattern	Typical Infections
A	*S. pyogenes*	Beta	Pharyngitis, impetigo, cellulitis, scarlet fever
B	*S. agalactiae*	Beta	Neonatal sepsis and meningitis, puerperal infection, urinary tract infection, diabetic ulcer infection, endocarditis
C	*S. equi*	Beta	Cellulitis, bacteremia, endocarditis
D	Enterococci: *E. faecalis* *E. faecium*	Usually nonhemolytic	Urinary tract infection, wound infection, endocarditis
	Nonenterococci: *S. bovis*	Usually nonhemolytic	Bacteremia, endocarditis
G	*S. canis*	Beta	Cellulitis, bacteremia, endocarditis
Variable or nongroupable	Viridans streptococci: *S. mutans* *S. sanguis*	Alpha	Endocarditis, dental abscess, brain abscess
	Intermedius or *milleri* group: *S. intermedius*	Variable	Brain abscess, visceral abscess
	Anaerobic streptococci: *Peptostreptococcus magnus*	Usually nonhemolytic	Sinusitis, pneumonia, empyema, brain abscess, liver abscess

capacity to trigger the postinfectious syndromes of acute rheumatic fever and poststreptococcal glomerulonephritis, which are uniquely associated with these organisms. → *Acute rheumatic fever and glomerulonephritis are discussed in Chap. 236 and Chap. 274, respectively.*

PATHOGENESIS Group A streptococci elaborate a number of cell-surface components and extracellular products important both in the pathogenesis of infection and in the immune response of the human host. The cell wall contains a carbohydrate antigen that may be released by treatment with acid. The reaction of such acid extracts with group A–specific antiserum is the basis for the definitive identification of a streptococcal strain as *S. pyogenes*. The major surface protein of group A streptococci is M protein, which occurs in more than 80 antigenically distinct types and is the basis for the serotyping of strains with specific antisera. The M protein molecules are fibrillar structures anchored in the cell wall of the organism and extending as hairlike projections away from the cell surface. The amino acid sequence of the distal or amino-terminal portion of the M protein molecule is quite variable, accounting for the antigenic variation of the different M types, while more proximal regions of the protein are relatively conserved. The presence of M protein correlates with the capacity of a strain to resist phagocytic killing in fresh human blood; this phenomenon appears to be due, at least in part, to the binding of plasma fibrinogen to M protein molecules on the streptococcal surface, which interferes with complement activation and deposition of opsonic complement fragments on the bacterial cell. This resistance to phagocytosis may be overcome by M protein–specific antibodies, and thus individuals with antibodies to a given M type acquired as a result of prior infection are protected against subsequent infection with organisms of the same M type but not against that with different M types. Group A streptococci also elaborate (to varying degrees) a polysaccharide capsule composed of hyaluronic acid. The production of large amounts of hyaluronic acid capsule by certain strains results in a characteristic mucoid appearance of the bacterial colonies. The capsular polysaccharide also plays an important role in protecting the organisms from ingestion and killing by phagocytes. In contrast to M protein, the hyaluronic acid capsule is a weak immunogen, presumably because of the apparent structural identity between streptococcal hyaluronic acid and the hyaluronic acid of mammalian connective tissues. Antibodies to hyaluronate have not been shown to be important in protective immunity.

Group A streptococci produce a large number of extracellular products that may be important in local and systemic toxicity and in the spread of infection through tissues. These products include streptolysins S and O, toxins that damage cell membranes and account for the hemolysis produced by the organisms; streptokinase; DNases; protease; and pyrogenic exotoxins A, B, and C. The pyrogenic exotoxins, previously known as erythrogenic toxins, cause the rash of scarlet fever. Relatively recently, pyrogenic exotoxin-producing strains of group A *Streptococcus* have been linked to unusually severe invasive infections, including necrotizing fasciitis and a systemic syndrome termed the *streptococcal toxic shock-like syndrome*. Several extracellular products stimulate specific antibody responses useful in the serodiagnosis of recent streptococcal infection. Tests for these antibodies are used primarily for the detection of preceding streptococcal infection in cases of suspected acute rheumatic fever or poststreptococcal glomerulonephritis.

PHARYNGITIS Although seen in patients of all ages, group A streptococcal pharyngitis is one of the most common bacterial infections of childhood, accounting for 20 to 40 percent of all cases of exudative pharyngitis in children. It is rare among those under the age of 3, who may manifest streptococcal infection with a syndrome of fever, malaise, and lymphadenopathy without exudative pharyngitis. Infection is acquired through contact with another individual carrying the organism. Respiratory droplets are the usual mechanism of spread, although other routes, including food-borne outbreaks, have been well described.

The incubation period of streptococcal pharyngitis is 1 to 4 days. Symptoms include sore throat, fever and chills, malaise, and sometimes abdominal complaints and vomiting, particularly in children. Both symptoms and signs are quite variable, ranging from mild throat discomfort with minimal physical findings to high fever and severe sore throat associated with intense erythema and swelling of the pharyngeal mucosa and the presence of purulent exudate over the posterior pharyngeal wall and tonsillar pillars. Enlarged, tender anterior cervical lymph nodes commonly accompany exudative pharyngitis.

The differential diagnosis of streptococcal pharyngitis encompasses the many other bacterial and viral causes of pharyngitis. Other infections that frequently produce exudative pharyngitis include infectious mononucleosis and adenovirus infection. Now rare in the United States, the pseudomembrane of diphtheria may give a similar appearance. *Corynebacterium (Arcanobacterium) haemolyticum* may cause pharyngitis, often in association with a scarlet fever-like rash. Other causes of pharyngitis, usually without a purulent exudate, include infections with coxsackievirus, influenza virus, mycoplasmas, or *Neisseria gonorrhoeae* and acute infection with human immunodeficiency virus. Because of the range of clinical presentations of streptococcal pharyngitis and the large number of other agents that can produce the same clinical picture, the diagnosis of streptococcal pharyngitis on clinical grounds alone is not reliable.

The throat culture remains the gold standard for diagnosis. Culture of a throat specimen that is properly collected (i.e., by vigorous rubbing of a sterile swab over both tonsillar pillars) and properly processed is the most sensitive and specific means available by which to make a definitive diagnosis. Rapid diagnostic kits using latex agglutination or enzyme immunoassay of swab specimens are now widely available and can serve as a useful adjunct to the throat culture. While precise figures on sensitivity and specificity vary among studies, the rapid diagnostic kits generally are highly (more than 95 percent) specific. Thus a positive result can be relied on for definitive diagnosis and eliminates the need for a throat culture. However, because the rapid diagnostic tests are less sensitive than throat culture (with a relative sensitivity ranging from 55 to 90 percent in comparative studies), a negative result should be confirmed with a throat culture.

In the usual course of uncomplicated streptococcal pharyngitis, symptoms resolve after 3 to 5 days. The course is shortened little by treatment, which is given primarily to prevent suppurative complications and rheumatic fever. Prevention of rheumatic fever depends on eradication of the organism from the pharynx, not simply on resolution of symptoms, and requires penicillin treatment—either a single intramuscular dose of benzathine penicillin G or a 10-day course of oral penicillin (Table 143-2). Erythromycin may be substituted for penicillin in the treatment of individuals allergic to penicillin. Follow-up culture after treatment is no longer routinely recommended but may

Table 143-2

Treatment of Group A Streptococcal Infections

Infection	Treatment*
Pharyngitis	Benzathine penicillin G, 1.2 million units IM; or penicillin V, 250 mg PO qid × 10 days (Children <27 kg: Benzathine penicillin G, 600,000 units IM; or penicillin V, 125 mg PO qid × 10 days)
Impetigo	Same as pharyngitis
Erysipelas/cellulitis	Severe: Penicillin G, 1–2 million units IV q4h Mild to moderate: Procaine penicillin, 1.2 million units IM bid
Necrotizing fasciitis/ myositis	Surgical debridement plus penicillin G, 2–4 million units IV q4h
Pneumonia/empyema	Penicillin G, 2–4 million units IV q4h plus drainage of empyema

* Penicillin allergy: Erythromycin (10 mg/kg PO qid up to a maximum of 250 mg per dose) may be substituted for oral penicillin. Alternative agents for parenteral therapy include first-generation cephalosporins—if the penicillin allergy does not manifest as immediate hypersensitivity (anaphylaxis or urticaria) or as another potentially life-threatening reaction (e.g., severe rash and fever)—and vancomycin.

be warranted in selected cases, such as those involving patients or families with frequent streptococcal infections or those occurring in situations in which the risk of rheumatic fever is thought to be high (for example, when cases of rheumatic fever have recently been reported in the community).

Suppurative complications of streptococcal pharyngitis have become uncommon with the widespread use of antibiotics for most cases of symptomatic streptococcal infection. These complications result from the spread of infection from the pharyngeal mucosa to deeper tissues, either by direct extension or by the hematogenous or lymphatic route, and may include cervical lymphadenitis, peritonsillar or retropharyngeal abscess, sinusitis, otitis media, meningitis, bacteremia, endocarditis, and pneumonia. Local complications, such as abscess formation in the peritonsillar or parapharyngeal space, should be considered in a patient with unusually severe or prolonged symptoms or localized pain associated with high fever and a toxic appearance.

ASYMPTOMATIC CARRIER STATE Surveillance cultures have shown that up to 20 percent of individuals in certain populations may have asymptomatic pharyngeal colonization with group A streptococci. There are no definitive guidelines for management of these asymptomatic carriers or of asymptomatic individuals who still have a positive throat culture after a full course of treatment for symptomatic pharyngitis. A reasonable course of action is to give a single 10-day course of penicillin for symptomatic pharyngitis and, if positive cultures persist, not to re-treat unless symptoms recur. Studies of the natural history of streptococcal carriage and infection have shown that the risk both of developing rheumatic fever and of transmitting infection to others is substantially lower among asymptomatic carriers than among individuals with symptomatic pharyngitis. Therefore, aggressive attempts to eradicate carriage probably are not justified under most circumstances. An exception to this general statement is the situation in which an asymptomatic carrier is a potential source of infection to others. Outbreaks of food-borne infection and nosocomial puerperal infection have been traced to asymptomatic carriers who may harbor the organisms in the throat, on the skin, or in the vagina or anus. In cases in which a carrier is transmitting infection, attempts to eradicate carriage are warranted, although data are limited on the best regimen to use to clear the organism after penicillin alone has failed. The combination of penicillin and rifampin has been used to eliminate pharyngeal carriage, and the addition of oral vancomycin has led to success in eradicating rectal colonization; however, experience is not extensive with any regimen for this indication.

SCARLET FEVER Scarlet fever consists of streptococcal infection, usually pharyngitis, accompanied by a characteristic rash. The rash arises from the effects of one of three toxins, which are currently designated streptococcal pyrogenic exotoxins A, B, and C and previously were known as erythrogenic or scarlet fever toxins. In the past, scarlet fever was thought to reflect infection of an individual lacking toxin-specific immunity with a toxin-producing strain of group A *Streptococcus*. Susceptibility to scarlet fever was correlated with results of the Dick test. A small amount of erythrogenic toxin injected intradermally produced local erythema in susceptible individuals but elicited no reaction in those with specific immunity. Subsequent studies have suggested that development of the scarlet fever rash may reflect a hypersensitivity reaction requiring prior exposure to the toxin. For reasons that are not clear, scarlet fever has become less common in recent years, although strains of group A streptococci that produce pyrogenic exotoxins continue to be prevalent in the population.

The symptoms of scarlet fever are the same as those of pharyngitis alone. The rash typically begins on the first or second day of illness over the upper trunk, spreading to involve the extremities but sparing the palms and soles. The rash is made up of minute papules, giving a characteristic "sandpaper" texture to the skin. Associated findings include circumoral pallor, "strawberry tongue" (enlarged papillae on a coated tongue, which later may become denuded), and accentuation of the rash in the skin folds (Pastia's lines). Subsidence of the rash after 6 to 9 days is followed after several days by desquamation of the palms and soles. The differential diagnosis of scarlet fever includes other causes of fever and generalized rash, such as measles and other viral exanthems, Kawasaki disease, toxic shock syndrome, and systemic allergic reactions (e.g., drug eruptions).

SKIN AND SOFT TISSUE INFECTIONS Group A streptococci—and occasionally other streptococcal species—cause a variety of infections involving the skin, subcutaneous tissues, muscles, and fascia. While several clinical syndromes, recognized according to the tissues involved, offer a useful means for classification of skin and soft tissue infections, not all cases fit exactly into a single category. The classic syndromes should be considered as general guides to predicting the level of tissue involvement in a particular patient, the probable clinical course, and the likelihood that surgical intervention or aggressive life-support measures will be required.

Impetigo (Pyoderma) Impetigo is a superficial infection of the skin caused primarily by group A streptococci and occasionally by other streptococci or by *Staphylococcus aureus*. This condition is seen most often in young children, tends to occur during the warmer months, and is more common in semitropical or tropical climates than in cooler regions. The infection occurs especially often among children living under conditions of poor hygiene. Prospective studies have shown that colonization of unbroken skin with group A streptococci precedes the development of clinical infection. Minor trauma, such as a scratch or an insect bite, may then serve to inoculate organisms into the skin. Impetigo is best prevented, therefore, by attention to adequate hygiene. The usual sites of involvement are the face (particularly around the nose and mouth) and the legs, although lesions may occur at other locations. Individual lesions begin as red papules, which evolve quickly into vesicular and then pustular lesions that break down and coalesce to form characteristic honeycomb-like crusts. Lesions generally are not painful, and patients do not appear ill. Fever is not a feature of impetigo and, if present, suggests either infection extending to deeper tissues or another diagnosis.

The classic presentation of impetigo usually poses little diagnostic difficulty. Cultures of impetiginous lesions often yield *S. aureus* as well as group A streptococci, but longitudinal studies have shown that, in almost all cases, streptococci can be isolated initially, with staphylococci appearing later, presumably as secondary colonizing flora. Previously, the nearly universal effectiveness of penicillin in these infections, despite the resistance of most staphylococcal strains, supported the primary role of streptococci. More recent studies, however, have reported treatment failures with penicillin and have suggested that *S. aureus* has become a significant cause of impetigo. *Bullous impetigo* is a distinctive form of *S. aureus* infection characterized by the presence of more extensive, bullous lesions that break down and leave thin paperlike crusts instead of the thick amber crusts of streptococcal impetigo. Other skin lesions that may be confused with impetigo include herpetic lesions—either those of orolabial herpes simplex or those of chickenpox or zoster. Herpetic lesions can generally be distinguished by their appearance as more discrete, grouped vesicles and by a positive Tzanck test (see Chap. 184). In diagnostically difficult cases, cultures of vesicle fluid should yield group A streptococci in impetigo and the responsible virus in herpes virus infection.

Agents active against *S. aureus* and streptococci (such as dicloxacillin, cephalexin, or topical mupirocin ointment) provide the most reliable treatment for impetigo, although penicillin or erythromycin is cheaper and equally effective in cases due to group A streptococci. Rheumatic fever is not a sequel to streptococcal skin infections (as opposed to pharyngitis), although poststreptococcal glomerulonephritis may follow either skin or throat infection. The reason for this difference is not known. One hypothesis is that the immune response necessary for the development of rheumatic fever occurs only after infection of the pharyngeal mucosa. In addition, the strains of group A streptococci that cause pharyngitis generally have a different type of M protein than those associated with skin infections; thus, the strains that cause pharyngitis may have rheumatogenic potential, while the skin-infecting strains may not.

Cellulitis Inoculation of organisms into the skin may lead to infection involving the skin and subcutaneous tissues, or cellulitis. The portal of entry may be a traumatic or surgical wound, an insect bite, or any other break in the skin's integrity. Often, no entry site is apparent.

One form of streptococcal cellulitis, known as *erysipelas*, is characterized by a bright red appearance of the involved skin, which forms a plateau sharply demarcated from the surrounding normal skin. The lesion is warm to the touch, may be tender, and appears shiny and swollen. The skin often has a *peau d'orange* texture, which is thought to reflect involvement of superficial lymphatics; superficial blebs or bullae may form, usually 2 or 3 days after onset. The lesion typically develops over a few hours and is associated with fever and chills. Erysipelas tends to occur in certain characteristic locations: the malar area of the face (often with extension over the bridge of the nose to the contralateral malar region) and the lower extremities. After one episode, recurrence at the same site—sometimes years later—is not uncommon.

Classic cases of erysipelas, with the typical features described above, are almost always due to group A streptococci. Often, however, the appearance of streptococcal cellulitis is not sufficiently distinctive to permit a specific diagnosis on clinical grounds. The area of involvement may not be one of the typical sites for erysipelas; the lesion may be less intensely red than usual and may fade into surrounding skin; and/or the patient may appear only mildly ill. In such cases, it is prudent to broaden the spectrum of empirical antimicrobial therapy to include other pathogens, particularly *S. aureus*, that can produce cellulitis with the same appearance.

Streptococcal cellulitis tends to develop at anatomic sites in which normal lymphatic drainage has been disrupted, such as sites of prior episodes of cellulitis, the arm ipsilateral to a mastectomy and axillary lymph-node dissection, a lower extremity previously involved in deep venous thrombosis or chronic lymphedema, and the leg from which a saphenous vein has been harvested for coronary artery bypass grafting. The organism may enter via a breach in the dermal barrier at a location some distance from the eventual site of clinical cellulitis. For example, some patients with recurrent episodes of leg cellulitis following saphenous vein removal have stopped having recurrent episodes only after treatment of tinea pedis on the foot of the affected extremity, fissures in the skin presumably having served as a portal of entry for streptococci, which then produced infection more proximally in the leg at the site of previous injury. Streptococcal cellulitis may also involve recent surgical wounds. Group A streptococci are among the few bacterial pathogens that typically produce signs of wound infection and surrounding cellulitis within the first 24 h after surgery. These wound infections are usually associated with a thin exudate and may spread rapidly, either as cellulitis in the skin and subcutaneous tissue or as a deeper tissue infection (see below). Streptococcal wound infection or localized cellulitis may also be associated with *lymphangitis*, manifested by red streaks extending proximally along superficial lymphatics from the site of infection.

Deep Soft Tissue Infections *Necrotizing fasciitis*, also referred to as *hemolytic streptococcal gangrene*, is an infection involving the superficial and/or deep fascia investing the muscles of an extremity or the trunk. The source of the infection is either the skin, with organisms introduced into the tissue as a result of trauma (which may be trivial), or the bowel flora, with organisms released during abdominal surgery or from an occult enteric source, such as a diverticular or appendiceal abscess. The site of inoculation in both forms of necrotizing fasciitis may be inapparent and often is some distance from the site of clinical involvement; for example, the introduction of organisms via minor trauma to the hand may be associated with clinical infection of the tissues overlying the shoulder or chest. In cases associated with the bowel flora, the infection is usually polymicrobial, involving a mixture of anaerobic bacteria (such as *Bacteroides fragilis* or anaerobic streptococci) and facultative organisms (usually gram-negative bacilli). Cases unrelated to contamination from bowel organisms are most commonly caused by group A streptococci, either alone or in combination with other organisms (most often *S. aureus*). Overall, group A streptococci are implicated in about 60 percent of cases of necrotizing fasciitis.

The onset of symptoms is usually quite acute and is marked by severe pain at the site of involvement, malaise, fever, chills, and a toxic appearance. The physical findings, particularly early in the illness, may not be striking, with only minimal erythema of the overlying skin. Pain and tenderness are usually severe; in contrast, in more superficial cellulitis, the appearance of the skin is more abnormal, but pain and tenderness are only mild or moderate. As the infection progresses (often in a matter of several hours), the severity and extent of symptoms worsen, and skin changes become more evident, with the appearance of dusky or mottled erythema and edema. The marked tenderness of the involved area may evolve into anesthesia as the spreading inflammatory process produces infarction of cutaneous nerves. Once the diagnosis is suspected, early surgical exploration is both diagnostically and therapeutically indicated. Surgery reveals necrosis and inflammatory fluid tracking along the fascial planes above and between muscle groups, without involvement of the muscles themselves. The process usually is found to extend beyond the area of clinical involvement, and extensive debridement is required. Drainage and debridement are central to the management of necrotizing fasciitis; antibiotic treatment is a useful adjunct (Table 143-2), but surgery is life-saving.

Although this syndrome is due more commonly to *S. aureus* infection, group A streptococci occasionally produce abscesses in skeletal muscles (*streptococcal myositis*), with little or no involvement of the surrounding fascia or overlying skin. The presentation is usually subacute, but a fulminant form has been described in association with severe systemic toxicity, bacteremia, and a high mortality rate. The fulminant form may reflect the same basic disease process as that seen in necrotizing fasciitis, but with the necrotizing inflammatory process extending into the muscles themselves rather than remaining limited to the fascial layers. Treatment for streptococcal myositis consists of surgical drainage—usually by an open procedure that permits evaluation of the extent of the infection and ensures adequate debridement of involved tissues—and high-dose penicillin (Table 143-2).

PNEUMONIA AND EMPYEMA Group A streptococci are an occasional cause of pneumonia, generally in previously healthy individuals. The onset of symptoms may be abrupt or gradual. Pleuritic chest pain, fever, chills, and dyspnea are the characteristic symptoms. Cough is usually present but may not be prominent. Approximately one-half of patients with group A streptococcal pneumonia have an accompanying pleural effusion. In contrast to the sterile parapneumonic effusions typically seen with pneumococcal pneumonia, the effusions that complicate streptococcal pneumonia are almost always infected. The empyema fluid is usually visible by chest radiography on initial presentation and may increase rapidly in volume. These pleural collections should be drained early, as they tend to become loculated quickly, resulting in a chronic fibrotic reaction that may necessitate thoracotomy for removal.

BACTEREMIA, PUERPERAL SEPSIS, AND STREPTOCOCCAL TOXIC SHOCK-LIKE SYNDROME Group A streptococcal bacteremia is usually associated with an identifiable local infection. Bacteremia occurs rarely with otherwise uncomplicated pharyngitis, occasionally with cellulitis or pneumonia, and relatively frequently with necrotizing fasciitis. Bacteremia without an identified source raises the possibility of endocarditis, an occult abscess, or osteomyelitis. A variety of focal infections may arise secondarily from streptococcal bacteremia, including endocarditis, meningitis, septic arthritis, osteomyelitis, peritonitis, and visceral abscesses.

Group A streptococci are occasionally implicated in infectious complications of childbirth, usually endometritis and associated bacteremia. In the preantibiotic era, puerperal sepsis was commonly caused by group A streptococci, but currently it is more often caused by group B streptococci. Several nosocomial outbreaks of puerperal infection due to group A streptococci have been traced to an asymptomatic carrier, usually an individual present at the time of delivery of the infant. The site of carriage may be the skin, throat, anus, or vagina.

Beginning in the late 1980s, several reports described patients who had group A streptococcal infections associated with shock and multisystem organ failure. This syndrome has been called the *streptococcal toxic shock-like syndrome* because it shares certain features with staphylococcal toxic shock syndrome. In 1993, a case definition for streptococcal toxic shock syndrome was formulated by a working group of clinicians, microbiologists, and epidemiologists in conjunction with the Centers for Disease Control and Prevention (Table 143-3). The general features of the illness include fever, hypotension, renal impairment, and respiratory distress syndrome. Various types of rash have been described, but rash usually does not develop. Laboratory abnormalities include a marked shift to the left in the white blood cell differential, with many immature granulocytes; hypocalcemia; hypoalbuminemia; and thrombocytopenia, which usually becomes more pronounced on the second or third day of illness. In contrast to those with staphylococcal toxic shock, most patients with the streptococcal syndrome are bacteremic. The most common associated infection is a soft tissue infection—necrotizing fasciitis, myositis, or cellulitis—although a variety of other local infections have been described in association with the syndrome, including pneumonia, peritonitis, osteomyelitis, and myometritis. Streptococcal toxic shock syndrome is associated with a mortality rate of 30 percent, with most deaths secondary to shock and respiratory failure. Because of its rapidly progressive and lethal course, early recognition of the syndrome is essential. Patients should be given aggressive supportive care in the form of fluid resuscitation, pressors, and mechanical ventilation in addition to antimicrobial therapy and, in cases associated with necrotizing fasciitis, surgical debridement. Exactly why certain patients develop this fulminant syndrome is not known; however, early studies of the streptococcal strains isolated from these patients demonstrated a strong association with the production of pyrogenic exotoxin A. In more recent case series, particularly from Europe, the syndrome has also been associated with strains producing either exotoxin B or exotoxin C.

Table 143-3

Proposed Case Definition for the Streptococcal Toxic Shock Syndrome*

I. Isolation of group A streptococci (*Streptococcus pyogenes*)
   A. From a normally sterile site (e.g., blood, cerebrospinal fluid, pleural or peritoneal fluid, tissue biopsy, surgical wound)
   B. From a nonsterile site (e.g., throat, sputum, vagina, superficial skin lesion)

II. Clinical signs of severity
   A. Hypotension: Systolic blood pressure of ≤90 mmHg in adults or in the 5th percentile for age in children

and

   B. Two or more of the following signs:
      1. Renal impairment: Serum creatinine level of ≥177 μmol/L (≥2 mg/dL) for adults or at least twice the upper limit of normal for age; in patients with preexisting renal disease, an elevation over the baseline level by a factor of 2 or more
      2. Coagulopathy: Platelet count of $\leq 100 \times 10^9$ per liter (100,000/μL) or disseminated intravascular coagulation defined by prolonged clotting times, low fibrinogen level, and the presence of fibrin degradation products
      3. Liver involvement: Alanine aminotransferase (SGOT), aspartate aminotransferase (SGPT), or total bilirubin level at least twice the upper limit of normal for age; in patients with preexisting liver disease, an elevation over the baseline level by a factor of 2 or more
      4. Adult respiratory distress syndrome, defined by acute onset of diffuse pulmonary infiltrates and hypoxemia in the absence of cardiac failure; or evidence of diffuse capillary leakage manifested by acute onset of generalized edema; or pleural or peritoneal effusions with hypoalbuminemia
      5. Generalized erythematous macular rash that may desquamate
      6. Soft-tissue necrosis, including necrotizing fasciitis or myositis, or gangrene

---

* An illness fulfilling criteria IA, IIA, and IIB is defined as a *definite* case. An illness fulfilling criteria IB, IIA, and IIB is defined as a *probable* case if no other etiology is identified.

SOURCE: Working Group on Severe Streptococcal Infections, 1993.

In light of the possible role of these or other streptococcal toxins in streptococcal toxic shock syndrome, treatment of the affected patients with clindamycin has been advocated by some authorities, who argue that, through its direct action on protein synthesis, clindamycin is more effective in rapidly terminating toxin production than penicillin—a cell-wall agent. Support for this view comes from studies of an experimental model of streptococcal myositis, in which mice treated with clindamycin had a higher rate of survival than those given penicillin. Comparable data on the treatment of human infections are not available.

Intravenous immunoglobulin has been suggested as adjunctive therapy for streptococcal toxic shock; pooled immunoglobulin preparations are likely to contain antibodies capable of neutralizing the effects of streptococcal toxins. Anecdotal reports have suggested favorable clinical responses to intravenous immunoglobulin, but no controlled trials of this modality of therapy have yet been reported.

STREPTOCOCCI OF GROUPS C AND G

Group C and group G streptococci are beta-hemolytic bacteria that occasionally cause human infections similar to those caused by group A streptococci, including pharyngitis, pneumonia, cellulitis and soft-tissue infection, bacteremia, septic arthritis, and endocarditis. Group C or G streptococcal bacteremia occurs most often in patients who are elderly or chronically ill and, in the absence of an obvious local infection, is likely to reflect endocarditis. Septic arthritis due to these organisms, sometimes involving multiple joints, may complicate endocarditis or may develop in the absence of endocarditis. The response to treatment is slow, and patients with joint infections often require repeated aspiration or open drainage and debridement for cure. Penicillin is the drug of choice for therapy of infections due to group C or G streptococci. Because of the poor clinical response of some patients treated with penicillin alone, the addition of gentamicin (1 mg/kg every 8 h for patients with normal renal function) is recommended for the treatment of endocarditis or septic arthritis.

GROUP B STREPTOCOCCI

Identified first as a cause of mastitis in cows, streptococci belonging to Lancefield group B have since been recognized as a major cause of sepsis and meningitis in human neonates. Group B streptococci also are a frequent cause of peripartum fever in women and an occasional cause of serious infection in nonpregnant adults. Lancefield group B consists of a single species, *S. agalactiae*. This organism is definitively identified by means of serologic studies with antiserum specific for the group B cell wall–associated carbohydrate antigen. A streptococcal isolate can be classified presumptively as belonging to group B on the basis of biochemical tests, including hydrolysis of sodium hippurate (in which 99 percent of isolates are positive), hydrolysis of bile esculin agar (in which 99 to 100 percent are negative), bacitracin susceptibility (in which 92 percent are resistant), and production of CAMP factor (in which 98 to 100 percent are positive). CAMP factor is a phospholipase produced by group B streptococci that results in synergistic hemolysis with beta lysin produced by certain strains of *S. aureus*. Its presence can be demonstrated by cross-streaking of the test isolate and an appropriate staphylococcal strain on a blood agar plate. Group B streptococci causing human infections are encapsulated by one of nine antigenically distinct polysaccharides. The capsular polysaccharide has been shown experimentally to be important in the virulence of the organism. Antibodies to the capsular polysaccharide afford protection against group B streptococci of the same (but not of a different) capsular type.

INFECTION IN NEONATES Two general types of group B streptococcal infection in infants are defined by the age of the patient at presentation. Early-onset infections occur within the first week of life, with a median age of 20 h at the onset of illness. Approximately half of these infants have signs of group B streptococcal disease at birth. The infection is acquired during or shortly before birth from organisms colonizing the maternal genital tract. Surveillance studies have shown that 5 to 40 percent of women are vaginal or rectal carriers of group B streptococci. Approximately 50 percent of infants delivered vaginally by carrier mothers become colonized, although only 1 to 2 percent of those colonized develop clinically evident infection. Prematurity and maternal risk factors (prolonged labor, obstetric complications, and maternal fever) are often involved. The presentation of early-onset infection is the same as that of other forms of neonatal sepsis. Typical findings include respiratory distress, lethargy, and hypotension. Essentially all infants with early-onset disease are bacteremic, one-third to one-half have pneumonia and/or respiratory distress syndrome, and one-third have meningitis.

Late-onset infections occur in infants between 1 week and 3 months of age, with a mean age at onset of 3 to 4 weeks. The infecting organism may be acquired during birth (as in early-onset cases) or during later contact with a colonized mother, nursery personnel, or another source. Meningitis is the most common manifestation of late-onset infection and in most cases is associated with a strain of capsular type III. Infants present with fever, lethargy or irritability, poor feeding, and seizures. Poor prognostic signs include presentation with hypotension, coma, status epilepticus, or neutropenia. Up to 50 percent of survivors have some degree of long-term neurologic impairment, ranging from mild language delay or hearing loss to profound mental retardation, blindness, and uncontrolled seizures. A variety of other types of late-onset infection occur, including bacteremia without an identified source, osteomyelitis, septic arthritis, and facial cellulitis associated with submandibular or preauricular adenitis.

Penicillin is the treatment of choice for all group B streptococcal infections. Empirical broad-spectrum therapy for suspected neonatal bacterial sepsis, consisting of ampicillin and gentamicin, is generally administered until culture results become available. If cultures yield group B streptococci, many pediatricians continue to administer gentamicin, along with ampicillin or penicillin, for a few days until clinical improvement becomes evident. This practice is based on in vitro studies showing synergistic killing of group B streptococci by gentamicin and either of the latter two agents in combination. For infants with group B streptococcal meningitis, combined therapy for the first few days certainly is recommended, although rigorous clinical data to support this view are lacking. Therapy with penicillin alone should be continued for 10 days for bacteremia and local infections and for a minimum of 14 days for meningitis because of the risk of relapse in patients treated with shorter courses.

The incidence of group B streptococcal infection is unusually high among infants of women with risk factors: preterm delivery, early rupture of membranes (>24 h before delivery), prolonged labor, fever, or chorioamnionitis. Because the usual source of the organisms infecting a neonate is the mother's birth canal, efforts have been made to prevent group B streptococcal infections by the identification of high-risk carrier mothers and the administration of various forms of antibiotic or immunoprophylaxis. Prophylactic administration of ampicillin or penicillin to such patients during delivery has been shown to reduce the risk of infection in the newborn. This approach has been hampered by the logistical difficulties of identifying colonized women before delivery, since the results of vaginal cultures early in pregnancy are poor predictors of carrier status at the time of delivery. The Centers for Disease Control and Prevention have suggested the following approach to the prevention of neonatal group B streptococcal infection: Women should be screened for anogenital colonization at 35 to 37 weeks of pregnancy by means of a swab culture of the lower vagina and anorectum, and intrapartum chemoprophylaxis should be offered to all carriers and *recommended* to those carriers with any of the risk factors noted above, those anticipating multiple births, and those who have previously given birth to an infant with group B streptococcal infection. The recommended regimen is 5 million units of penicillin

G followed by 2.5 million units every 4 h until delivery. Clindamycin or erythromycin may be substituted in women allergic to penicillin.

There is controversy about whether to recommend chemoprophylaxis to carriers without risk factors: Although 25 percent of neonatal infections occur in infants born to women without risk factors, the risk of infection in such neonates is much lower than that in infants delivered to women with risk factors. Treatment of all carriers will result in the exposure of 15 to 25 percent of pregnant women and newborns to antibiotics, with the attendant risks of allergic reactions and selection for resistant organisms. A group B streptococcal vaccine—still in the developmental stages—ultimately may offer a better method of prevention. Because transplacental passage of maternal antibodies produces protective antibody levels in the newborn, efforts are under way to develop a vaccine against group B streptococci that can be given to women of childbearing age before or during pregnancy.

INFECTION IN ADULTS The majority of group B streptococcal infections in adults are related to pregnancy and parturition. Peripartum fever, the most common manifestation, is sometimes accompanied by symptoms and signs of endometritis or chorioamnionitis (abdominal distention and uterine or adnexal tenderness). Blood cultures often are positive, as are cultures of vaginal swabs. Bacteremia is usually transitory but occasionally results in meningitis or endocarditis. Infections in adults that are not associated with the peripartum period generally involve individuals who are elderly or have some underlying chronic illness, such as diabetes mellitus or a malignancy. Infections that develop with some frequency in adults include cellulitis and soft-tissue infection (including infected diabetic skin ulcers), urinary tract infection, pneumonia, endocarditis, and septic arthritis. Less commonly reported infections include meningitis, osteomyelitis, and intra-abdominal or pelvic abscesses.

Group B streptococci are less sensitive to penicillin than group A organisms, requiring drug concentrations 10 to 100 times higher for inhibition of growth in vitro. Therefore, somewhat higher doses of penicillin are needed for the treatment of group B infections. Adults with serious localized infections (pneumonia, pyelonephritis, abscess) should receive doses in the range of 12 million units of penicillin G daily, while patients with endocarditis or meningitis should receive 18 to 24 million units per day in divided doses. Vancomycin is an acceptable alternative for patients allergic to penicillin.

ENTEROCOCCI AND GROUP D STREPTOCOCCI

Lancefield group D includes the enterococci, organisms now classified in a separate genus from other streptococci, and nonenterococcal group D streptococci. Enterococci are distinguished from nonenterococcal group D streptococci by their ability to grow in the presence of 6.5 percent sodium chloride and by the results of other biochemical tests. The enterococcal species that are significant pathogens for humans are *E. faecalis* and *E. faecium*. These organisms tend to produce infection in patients who are elderly or debilitated or in whom mucosal or epithelial barriers have been disrupted or the balance of the normal flora altered by antibiotic treatment. Urinary tract infections due to enterococci are quite common, particularly among patients who have received antibiotic treatment or undergone instrumentation of the urinary tract. Enterococci account for 10 to 20 percent of cases of bacterial endocarditis on both native and prosthetic valves. The presentation of enterococcal endocarditis is usually subacute but may also be acute, with rapidly progressive valve destruction. Enterococci frequently are cultured from bile and are involved in infectious complications of biliary surgery and in liver abscesses. Moreover, enterococci often are isolated from polymicrobial infections arising from the bowel flora (e.g., intraabdominal abscesses), from abdominal surgical wounds, and from diabetic foot ulcers. While such mixed infections frequently are cured by antimicrobials not active against enterococci, specific therapy directed against enterococci is warranted when these organisms are the predominant species or are isolated from blood cultures.

Unlike other streptococci, enterococci are not reliably killed by penicillin or ampicillin alone at concentrations achieved clinically in the blood or tissues. Because in vitro testing has shown evidence of synergistic killing of most enterococcal strains by the combination of penicillin or ampicillin with an aminoglycoside, combined therapy is recommended for serious enterococcal infections. Ampicillin reaches sufficiently high urinary concentrations to constitute adequate single-drug therapy for uncomplicated urinary tract infections. For other types of enterococcal infection, however, the addition of gentamicin at moderate doses (e.g., 1 mg/kg every 8 h for patients with normal renal function) is recommended. Vancomycin, in combination with gentamicin, may be substituted for penicillin in the treatment of allergic patients. Enterococci are resistant to all cephalosporins; therefore, this class of antibiotics should not be used for the treatment of enterococcal infections.

The antimicrobial susceptibility of enterococcal isolates from patients with serious infections should be evaluated routinely and therapy adjusted according to the results (Table 143-4). Most enterococci are resistant to streptomycin, and this drug should not be used for the treatment of enterococcal infection unless in vitro testing of the strain indicates susceptibility. Though less widespread than streptomycin resistance, high-level resistance to gentamicin [minimum inhibitory concentration (MIC), greater than 2000 μg/mL] has become common. Gentamicin-resistant enterococci should be tested for susceptibility to other aminoglycosides; occasional gentamicin-resistant enterococci are sensitive to streptomycin. If the isolate is resistant to all aminoglycosides, treatment with penicillin or ampicillin alone may be successful. The prolonged administration (i.e., for at least 6 weeks) of high-dose ampicillin (e.g., 12 g/day) is recommended for endocarditis due to these highly resistant enterococci.

Enterococci may be resistant to penicillins by two distinct mechanisms. The first is the production of β-lactamase (mediating resistance to penicillin and ampicillin), which has been reported for E. faecalis isolates from several locations in the United States and other countries. Because the amount of β-lactamase produced by enterococci may be insufficient for detection by routine antibiotic susceptibility testing, isolates from serious infections should be screened specifically for β-lactamase production with use of a chromogenic cephalosporin or by another method. For the treatment of infections caused by β-lactamase–producing strains, vancomycin, ampicillin/sulbactam, amoxicillin/clavulanate, or imipenem may be used in combination with gentamicin.

The second mechanism of penicillin resistance is not mediated by β-lactamase and may be due to altered penicillin-binding proteins. This intrinsic penicillin resistance is common among isolates of E. faecium, which routinely are more resistant to β-lactam antibiotics than are isolates of E. faecalis. Moderately resistant enterococci (MICs of penicillin and ampicillin, 16 to 64 μg/mL) may be susceptible to high-dose penicillin or ampicillin in combination with gentamicin, but strains with MICs of ≥200 μg/mL must be considered resistant to clinically achievable levels of β-lactam antibiotics, including imipenem. Vancomycin plus gentamicin is the recommended regimen for infections due to enterococci with high-level intrinsic resistance to β-lactams.

Vancomycin-resistant enterococci, first reported from clinical sources in the late 1980s, have become relatively common in many hospitals. Three major vancomycin resistance phenotypes have been described: VanA, VanB, and VanC. The VanA phenotype is associated with high-level resistance to vancomycin and to teicoplanin, a related glycopeptide antibiotic not currently available in the United States. VanB and VanC strains are resistant to vancomycin but susceptible to teicoplanin, although teicoplanin resistance may develop during treatment in VanB strains. For enterococci resistant to both vancomycin and β-lactams, there are no established therapies. Regimens that have been tried with some success in individual cases or experimentally include ciprofloxacin plus rifampin plus gentamicin; ampicillin plus vancomycin (particularly if in vitro testing shows synergistic bacteriostatic activity); and chloramphenicol or tetracycline (if the strain is susceptible in vitro).

The main nonenterococcal group D streptococcal species that causes human infections is Streptococcus bovis. S. bovis endocarditis is often associated with neoplasms of the gastrointestinal tract—most frequently a colon carcinoma or polyp. When occult gastrointestinal lesions are carefully sought, abnormalities are found in at least 60 percent of patients with S. bovis endocarditis. In contrast to the enterococci, nonenterococcal group D streptococci like S. bovis are reliably killed by penicillin as a single agent, and penicillin is the treatment of choice for S. bovis infections.

VIRIDANS AND OTHER STREPTOCOCCI

Consisting of multiple species of alpha-hemolytic streptococci, the viridans streptococci are a heterogeneous group of organisms that are important as agents of bacterial endocarditis. Several species of viridans streptococci, including Streptococcus salivarius, Streptococcus mutans, Streptococcus sanguis, and Streptococcus mitis, are part of the normal flora of the mouth, where they live in close association with the teeth and gingiva. Some species contribute to the development of dental caries. The transient viridans streptococcal bacteremia induced by eating, tooth-brushing, flossing, and other sources of minor trauma, together with adherence to biologic surfaces, is thought to account for the tendency of these organisms to cause endocarditis. Viridans streptococci are also isolated, often as part of a mixed flora, from sites of sinusitis, brain abscess, and liver abscess.

Viridans streptococcal bacteremia occurs relatively frequently in neutropenic patients, particularly after bone marrow transplantation or high-dose chemotherapy for cancer. Some of these patients develop a sepsis syndrome with high fever and shock. Risk factors for viridans streptococcal bacteremia include antibiotic prophylaxis with trimethoprim-sulfamethoxazole or a fluoroquinolone, mucositis, treatment with antacids or histamine antagonists, and profound neutropenia. Because many of the viridans streptococci isolated from the blood in the setting of neutropenia are resistant to penicillin, neutropenic patients with bacteremia should be treated presumptively with vancomycin until the results of susceptibility testing become available.

The organisms referred to as the Streptococcus intermedius or Streptococcus milleri group (Streptococcus intermedius, Streptococcus anginosus, and Streptococcus constellatus) often are considered to be viridans streptococci, although they differ somewhat from other viridans streptococci in both their hemolytic pattern (they are often beta-hemolytic) and the disease syndromes they cause. These organisms commonly produce suppurative infections, particularly abscesses of brain and abdominal viscera.

As noted above, isolates from neutropenic patients with bacteremia frequently are resistant to penicillin; viridans streptococci isolated in other clinical settings usually are sensitive to penicillin. Occasional isolates cultured from the blood of patients with endocarditis fail to grow when subcultured on solid media. These *nutritionally variant*

Table 143-4

Treatment Options for Antibiotic-Resistant Enterococcal Infections

Resistance Pattern	Recommended Therapy
β-Lactamase production	Gentamicin plus ampicillin/sulbactam, amoxicillin/clavulanate, imipenem, or vancomycin
β-Lactam resistance, but no β-lactamase production	Gentamicin plus vancomycin
High-level gentamicin resistance	Streptomycin-sensitive isolate: Streptomycin plus ampicillin or vancomycin Streptomycin-resistant isolate: No proven therapy (continuous-infusion ampicillin, prolonged treatment)
Vancomycin resistance	Ampicillin plus gentamicin
Vancomycin and β-lactam resistance	Unknown; teicoplanin active against strains with low-level vancomycin resistance (VanB or VanC phenotype, but not VanA)

streptococci require supplemental thiol compounds or active forms of vitamin B$_6$ (pyridoxal or pyridoxamine) for growth in the laboratory. Because treatment failure and relapse appear to be more common for cases of endocarditis due to nutritionally variant streptococci than for those due to nutritionally standard viridans streptococci, the addition of gentamicin (1 mg/kg every 8 h for patients with normal renal function) to the penicillin regimen is recommended for therapy of endocarditis due to these organisms.

Streptococcus suis is an important pathogen in swine and has been reported to cause meningitis in humans, usually in individuals with occupational exposure to pigs. Strains of *S. suis* associated with human infections have generally reacted with Lancefield group R typing serum and sometimes with group D typing serum as well. Isolates may be alpha- or beta-hemolytic and have been shown to be sensitive to penicillin.

Anaerobic streptococci, or peptostreptococci, are part of the normal flora of the oral cavity, bowel, and vagina. They are involved, usually along with other organisms, in brain abscess, sinusitis, dental abscess, and other odontogenic infections (Ludwig's angina, abscesses of the retropharyngeal or lateral pharyngeal space); in aspiration pneumonia, lung abscess, and empyema; and in intraabdominal and pelvic abscesses. Anaerobic and microaerophilic streptococci, together with facultative bacteria, may also play a role in invasive soft-tissue infections—generally those related to trauma or surgical wounds. Management of these infections involves debridement of infected tissues and treatment with high-dose penicillin (12 to 18 million units per day for serious infections).

BIBLIOGRAPHY

BASILIFRE JL et al: Streptococcal pneumonia. Am J Med 44:580, 1968

BISNO AL: Group A streptococcal infections and acute rheumatic fever. N Engl J Med 325:783, 1991

————, STEVENS DL: Streptococcal infections of skin and soft tissues. N Engl J Med 334:240, 1996

CENTERS FOR DISEASE CONTROL AND PREVENTION: Prevention of perinatal group B streptococcal disease: A public health perspective. Morb Mort Week Rep 45(RR-7):1, 1996

EDWARDS MS, BAKER CJ: *Streptococcus agalactiae* (group B *Streptococcus*), in *Principles and Practice of Infectious Diseases*, 4th ed, GL Mandell et al (eds). New York, Churchill Livingstone, 1995, p 1835

ELIOPOULOS GM: Increasing problems in the therapy of enterococcal infections. Eur J Clin Microbiol Infect Dis 12:409, 1993

ELTING LS et al: Septicemia and shock syndrome due to viridans streptococci: A case-control study of predisposing factors. Clin Infect Dis 14:1201, 1992

KLEIN RS et al: Association of *Streptococcus bovis* with carcinoma of the colon. N Engl J Med 297:800, 1977

LANCEFIELD RC: A serological differentiation of human and other groups of hemolytic streptococci. J Exp Med 57:571, 1933

MOELLERING RC JR: Emergence of *Enterococcus* as a significant pathogen. Clin Infect Dis 14:1173, 1992

STEVENS DL et al: Severe group A streptococcal infections associated with a toxic shock-like syndrome and scarlet fever toxin A. N Engl J Med 321:1, 1989

VARTIAN C et al: Infections due to Lancefield group G streptococci. Medicine 6:75, 1985

VIGLIONESE A et al: Recurrent group A streptococcal carriage in a health care worker associated with widely separated nosocomial outbreaks. Am J Med 91(Suppl 3B):329S, 1991

WANNAMAKER LW: Differences between streptococcal infections of the throat and of the skin. N Engl J Med 282:23, 78, 1970

WELLS VD et al: Infections due to beta-lactamase-producing, high-level gentamicin-resistant *Enterococcus faecalis*. Ann Intern Med 116:285, 1992

WORKING GROUP ON SEVERE STREPTOCOCCAL INFECTIONS: Defining the group A streptococcal toxic shock syndrome. JAMA 269:390, 1993

YODER EL et al: Spontaneous gangrenous myositis induced by *Streptococcus pyogenes*: Case report and review of the literature. Rev Infect Dis 9:382, 1987

DIPHTHERIA, OTHER CORYNEBACTERIAL INFECTIONS, AND ANTHRAX

DIPHTHERIA

DEFINITION Diphtheria is a localized infection of mucous membranes or skin caused by *Corynebacterium diphtheriae*. A characteristic pseudomembrane may be present at the site of infection. Some strains of *C. diphtheriae* produce diphtheria toxin, a protein that can cause myocarditis, polyneuritis, and other systemic toxic effects. Respiratory diphtheria is usually caused by toxinogenic (tox$^+$) *C. diphtheriae*, but cutaneous diphtheria is frequently caused by nontoxinogenic (tox$^-$) strains.

ETIOLOGIC AGENT *C. diphtheriae* is an aerobic, nonmotile, nonsporulating, irregularly staining, gram-positive rod. The bacteria are 2 to 6 μm long, 0.5 to 1 μm wide, club-shaped, and often arranged in clusters (*Chinese letters*) or parallel arrays (*palisades*). *C. diphtheriae* forms gray to black colonies on selective media containing tellurite. Three biotypes, designated *gravis*, *mitis*, and *intermedius*, are distinguished on the basis of colonial morphology and laboratory tests. Both tox$^+$ and tox$^-$ strains cause infections, and tox$^+$ strains of all three biotypes can cause severe disease.

The gene for diphtheria toxin is present in specific corynephages. Nontoxinogenic *C. diphtheriae* acquires the ability to produce diphtheria toxin by infection with tox$^+$ phages, a process termed *phage conversion*. Growth of *C. diphtheriae* under low-iron conditions mimicking the environment of host tissues induces the synthesis of diphtheria toxin and the expression of a siderophore-dependent, high-affinity iron uptake system.

IMMUNOLOGY Treatment of diphtheria toxin with formaldehyde converts it to a nontoxic product called *diphtheria toxoid*. Immunization with toxoid elicits antibody (*antitoxin*) that neutralizes the toxin and prevents diphtheria. No specific amount of antitoxin provides absolute protection against diphtheria, but the attack rate and the mortality rate for diphtheria are much lower in individuals with >0.01 unit of antitoxin per milliliter. This antitoxin level is often used, therefore, as an index of immunity in epidemiologic studies. Antitoxin neither prevents colonization by *C. diphtheriae* nor eradicates the carrier state. If most individuals in a population have antitoxic immunity, however, the carriage of tox$^+$ strains of *C. diphtheriae* decreases to a low level. Thus, herd immunity reduces the risk that nonimmune individuals in the population will be exposed to tox$^+$ *C. diphtheriae*. Nonimmune individuals may contract diphtheria if they travel to regions where the disease is present or if tox$^+$ strains of *C. diphtheriae* are introduced into their community.

EPIDEMIOLOGY AND IMMUNITY Humans are the reservoir for *C. diphtheriae*. The organism is transmitted primarily by close contact of diphtheria patients or carriers with susceptible individuals, but the risk of transmission from patients appears to be substantially greater than that of transmission from asymptomatic carriers. Transmission involving fomites and indirect routes is less common, although *C. diphtheriae* can survive for weeks to months in the environment. The incubation period for respiratory diphtheria is typically 2 to 5 days and rarely up to 8 days. Cutaneous diphtheria is usually a secondary infection whose signs develop an average of 7 days (range, 1 to >21 days) after the appearance of primary skin lesions.

In populations in temperate climates, diphtheria primarily involves the respiratory tract; occurs throughout the year, with a peak incidence in colder months; and is usually caused by tox$^+$ strains. Before the introduction of active immunization, diphtheria was generally a disease of children; it affected up to 10 percent of individuals in this group and sometimes occurred in devastating epidemics. Most infants were immune because of transplacental transfer of maternal IgG antitoxin, but children became susceptible by 6 to 12 months of age. Approximately 75 percent of individuals became immune by age 10 as a result of clinical or subclinical infection with *C. diphtheriae*. Mortality rates of 30 to 40 percent were common in untreated disease and sometimes exceeded 50 percent in epidemics. Treatment with antitoxin reduced the case-fatality rate to 5 to 10 percent.

Routine immunization of children in the United States resulted in a progressively decreasing incidence of diphtheria (from more than 206,000 cases in 1921 to few or no cases per year recently) that was accompanied by a shift of cases to older age groups; however, the case-fatality rate remained at 5 to 10 percent. High rates of immunization (96 percent) are now achieved by the time of school entry, but rates for younger children are substantially lower. Among adults over 20 years of age, 20 to 60 percent are susceptible to diphtheria. Large local outbreaks of diphtheria occurred in San Antonio, TX, in 1969 to 1970 (201 cases) and in Seattle, WA, in 1972 to 1982 (1100 cases). Alcoholism, low socioeconomic status, crowded living conditions, and Native American ethnic background were significant risk factors in these and other recent outbreaks. A report from England in 1992 described pharyngeal infections with tox$^-$ *C. diphtheriae* developing predominantly among homosexual men; they often caused symptomatic pharyngitis and sometimes resulted in a tonsillar exudate.

A massive and expanding epidemic of diphtheria has been under way since 1990 in 14 of the 15 new independent states of the former Soviet Union, with 47,802 cases and 1746 deaths reported for 1994. Approximately 70 percent of cases have occurred in persons ≥15 years of age. Case-fatality rates have varied from 2.8 percent in the Russian Federation to 23 percent in Lithuania and Turkmenistan. Twenty imported cases related to this epidemic have already been reported in European countries, and two cases have been acquired by U.S. citizens in Russia and Ukraine.

In the tropics, cutaneous diphtheria is more common than respiratory diphtheria, occurs throughout the year, and often develops as a secondary infection complicating other dermatoses. Isolates of *C. diphtheriae* from skin lesions are more often tox$^-$ than tox$^+$. A study in Rangoon, Burma, demonstrated *C. diphtheriae* (18.5 percent tox$^+$ strains) in more than 60 percent of bacterially infected skin lesions in patients under 12 years of age. Eighty percent of isolates were from impetiginous scabies, and most other isolates were from impetiginous eczema or impetigo. Cutaneous diphtheria has also been recognized increasingly in temperate climates during the past two decades; it accounted for 86 percent of the 1100 cases in the Seattle outbreak of 1972 to 1982.

PATHOLOGY AND PATHOGENESIS *C. diphtheriae* infects mucous membranes, most commonly in the respiratory tract, and also invades open skin lesions resulting from insect bites or trauma. In infections caused by tox$^+$ *C. diphtheriae*, initial edema and hyperemia are often followed by epithelial necrosis and acute inflammation. Coagulation of the dense fibrinopurulent exudate produces a pseudomembrane, and the inflammatory reaction accompanied by vascular congestion extends into the underlying tissues. The pseudomembrane contains large numbers of *C. diphtheriae*, but the bacterium is rarely isolated from the blood or internal organs.

Diphtheria toxin acts both locally and systemically. Very small amounts cause dermonecrosis, and toxin presumably contributes to pseudomembrane formation. The lethal dose of diphtheria toxin for nonimmune humans and highly susceptible animals is about 0.1 μg/kg of body weight. Absorbed toxin can cause myocarditis, neuritis, and focal necrosis in various organs, including the kidneys, liver, and adrenal glands. Early changes in diphtheritic myocarditis include cloudy swelling of muscle fibers and interstitial edema. These changes are followed within weeks by hyaline and granular degeneration of muscle fibers (sometimes with fatty degeneration of the myocardium) progressing to myolysis and finally to the replacement of lost muscle by fibrosis. Thus, diphtheria can cause permanent cardiac damage. In diphtheritic polyneuritis, pathologic changes include patchy breakdown of myelin sheaths in peripheral and autonomic nerves, but recovery of nerve damage is the rule if the patient survives.

Diphtheria toxin is produced by *C. diphtheriae* as an extracellular polypeptide. It is cleaved by proteases to form nicked toxin consisting of fragments A and B. Fragment B binds to a plasma-membrane receptor (a precursor of a heparin-binding growth factor resembling epidermal growth factor) on cells from humans or susceptible animals, and the bound toxin is internalized by receptor-mediated endocytosis. Fragment A is translocated across the endosomal membrane and released into the cytoplasm, where it catalyzes the transfer of the adenosine diphosphate ribose moiety from nicotinamide adenine dinucleotide (NAD) to a modified histidine residue (diphthamide) on elongation factor 2 (EF-2), thereby inactivating EF-2 and inhibiting protein synthesis. One molecule of fragment A in the cytoplasm can kill a cell. Other metabolic alterations in intoxicated cells are secondary to inhibition of protein synthesis.

CLINICAL MANIFESTATIONS Patients with *C. diphtheriae* in the respiratory tract are classified as diphtheria cases if they have symptoms consistent with local infection and as diphtheria carriers if they are asymptomatic. Signs and symptoms vary with the site and severity of the local infection, the patient's age, and the patient's status with regard to preexisting nasopharyngeal disease and concomitant systemic disease. The onset is often gradual, but most patients seek medical care within a few days of becoming ill. Sore throat is the most common symptom, but children are less likely than adults to complain of sore throat and are more likely to have nausea and vomiting. Fever of 37.8 to 38.9°C (100 to 102°F) and dysphagia are documented in about half of patients; cough, hoarseness, chills, and rhinorrhea are less common. Systemic manifestations are due primarily to the effects of diphtheria toxin. Patients without toxicity exhibit discomfort and malaise associated with local infection, whereas severely toxic patients may develop listlessness, pallor, and tachycardia that can progress rapidly to vascular collapse.

Primary infection in the respiratory tract is most often tonsillopharyngeal (one-half to two-thirds of cases) but also may be (in decreasing order of frequency) laryngeal, nasal, and tracheobronchial. Multiple sites are frequently involved, and secondary spread of pharyngeal infection upward to the nasal mucosa or downward to the larynx and tracheobronchial tree is much more common than primary infection at those sites. Systemic toxicity is usually less severe in nasal diphtheria than in tonsillopharyngeal diphtheria and is most severe when pseudomembrane extends from the tonsils and pharynx into contiguous regions. A small percentage of patients present with malignant, or "bull-neck," diphtheria, with abrupt onset, extensive pseudomembrane formation, foul breath, massive swelling of the tonsils and uvula, thick speech, cervical lymphadenopathy, striking edematous swelling of the submandibular region and anterior neck, and severe toxicity.

In tonsillopharyngeal diphtheria, only erythema may be noted initially, but isolated spots of gray or white exudate are common. These spots often extend and coalesce within a day to form a confluent, sharply demarcated pseudomembrane that becomes progressively thicker, more tightly adherent to the underlying tissue, and darker gray. Unlike the exudate in streptococcal pharyngitis, the diphtheritic pseudomembrane often extends beyond the margin of the tonsils onto the tonsillar pillars, palate, or uvula. Dislodgement of the membrane is likely to cause bleeding. Estimates of the proportion of patients with pharyngeal diphtheria who develop typical pseudomembranes vary widely, from as few as one-third to almost all. Patients with nasal diphtheria often present with serosanguineous nasal discharge, which may be unilateral or bilateral and may cause irritation of the nares or the lip. Laryngeal diphtheria often presents as hoarseness and cough. Demonstration of laryngeal pseudomembrane by laryngoscopy is helpful for distinguishing diphtheria from other infectious forms of laryngitis. Primary or secondary diphtheritic infection occasionally involves other mucous membranes, including the conjunctiva and the membranes of the genitourinary and gastrointestinal tracts.

Cutaneous diphtheria usually presents as an infection by *C. diphtheriae* of preexisting dermatoses involving, in decreasing order of frequency, the lower extremities, upper extremities, head, or trunk. The clinical features are similar to those of other secondary cutaneous bacterial infections. In the tropics, the presentation of cutaneous diphtheria occasionally includes morphologically distinct "punched-out" ulcers that are covered by necrotic slough or membrane and have well-demarcated edges.

C. diphtheriae is an occasional cause of invasive infections, including endocarditis and septic arthritis. Risk factors for such infections include preexisting cardiac abnormalities, abuse of intravenous drugs, and alcoholic cirrhosis.

COMPLICATIONS Obstruction of the respiratory tract, presenting as tachypnea, dyspnea, stridor, cyanosis, and use of accessory muscles of respiration, can be caused by extensive pseudomembrane formation and swelling during the first few days of the disease or by sloughed pseudomembrane that becomes lodged in the airways at a later stage in the disease. The risk of respiratory obstruction is greater when infection involves the larynx or the tracheobronchial tree and is higher in children because of the small size of the airways.

Myocarditis and polyneuritis are the most prominent toxic manifestations of diphtheria. The risk of developing these manifestations is proportional to the severity of local disease, and the two can occur together in the same patient. Myocarditis may present during the acute phase of illness, develop as local disease is resolving, or begin insidiously after several weeks. One-half to two-thirds of patients with typical diphtheria have subtle evidence of cardiac dysfunction, including electrocardiographic abnormalities, but clinically apparent myocarditis develops in 10 to 25 percent of patients and is usually more severe when the onset is early. Electrocardiographic abnormalities include ST-T-wave changes, varying degrees of heart block, and arrhythmias, including atrial fibrillation, ventricular premature beats, ventricular tachycardia, and ventricular fibrillation. Clinical signs include diminished heart sounds, gallop rhythm, systolic murmurs, and (less commonly) acute or insidiously progressive congestive heart failure. Serum levels of aspartate aminotransferase reflect the intensity of myocardial damage and can be used to monitor its course.

Polyneuritis is uncommon in mild diphtheria but occurs in approximately 10 percent of cases of average severity and in up to 75 percent of severe cases. Bulbar dysfunction typically develops during the first 2 weeks. Palatal and pharyngeal paralysis usually develop first. Swallowing is difficult, the voice sounds nasal, and ingested fluids may be regurgitated through the nose. With unilateral pharyngeal infection, ipsilateral palatal paralysis is more common than contralateral or bilateral paralysis. Additional bulbar signs may develop over several weeks, with oculomotor and ciliary paralysis occurring more often than facial or laryngeal paralysis. Peripheral polyneuritis typically begins from 1 to 3 months after the onset of diphtheria with proximal weakness of the extremities that spreads distally. The severity of this condition varies from mild weakness of the pelvic muscles with unsteady gait to total paralysis, including failure of respiration. Paresthesias may develop and most often have a glove-and-stocking distribution. Approximately half of patients with diphtheritic neuropathy have evidence of cardiac vagal denervation, and fewer have abnormal baroreceptor function. Polyneuritis usually resolves completely, with the time needed for improvement approximately equal to that elapsing from exposure to the development of symptoms. Since severe muscular weakness may develop 1 to 2 weeks before maximal abnormalities in peripheral-nerve conduction velocity are demonstrated, there may be a striking dissociation between clinical and electrophysiologic findings. Cerebrospinal fluid (CSF) most often contains moderately increased levels of albumin, occasionally with pleocytosis, but the abnormalities in CSF do not determine prognosis.

Pneumonia occurs in more than half of fatal cases of diphtheria. Less common complications include renal failure, encephalitis, cerebral infarction, pulmonary embolism, and bacteremia or endocarditis due to invasive infection by *C. diphtheriae*. Serum sickness may result from antitoxin therapy.

COURSE AND PROGNOSIS Most cases of diphtheria develop in nonimmunized patients. The attack rate, severity of disease, and risk of complications are much lower in immunized patients. The

pseudomembrane may continue to increase in size during the first day after administration of antitoxin. During the next several days to a week, it becomes softer, less adherent, and nonconfluent and eventually disappears. In the preantibiotic era, *C. diphtheriae* persisted in the throat for about 2 weeks in one-half of patients and for 1 month or more in about one-fifth. Mortality increases with the severity of local disease, the extent of pseudomembrane formation, and the interval between onset of local disease and administration of antitoxin. The death rate is highest during the first week of illness; among patients with bull-neck diphtheria; among patients with myocarditis who develop ventricular tachycardia, atrial fibrillation, or complete heart block; among patients with laryngeal or tracheobronchial involvement; among infants and patients over 60 years of age; and among alcoholics. Both mortality and the risk of myocarditis or peripheral neuropathy are significantly lower in cutaneous diphtheria than in respiratory diphtheria.

DIAGNOSIS A characteristic pseudomembrane on the mucosa of the oropharynx, palate, nasopharynx, nose, or larynx suggests diphtheria but is not uniformly present. Diphtheritic pseudomembrane must be distinguished from other pharyngeal exudates, including those of group A beta-hemolytic streptococcal infections, infectious mononucleosis, viral pharyngitides, fusospirochetal infection, and candidiasis. A diagnosis of diphtheria should be considered in patients with sore throat, cervical adenopathy or swelling, and low-grade fever, especially when these manifestations are accompanied by systemic toxicity, hoarseness, stridor, palatal paralysis, or serosanguineous nasal discharge with or without demonstrable pseudomembrane. Treatment with diphtheria antitoxin should be begun as soon as the clinical diagnosis of diphtheria is made.

The definitive diagnosis of diphtheria depends on the isolation of *C. diphtheriae* from local lesions. The laboratory should be notified that diphtheria is suspected to ensure the use of selective tellurite medium appropriate for the isolation of *C. diphtheriae*. All isolates of *C. diphtheriae* should be subjected to toxicity testing. Primary isolates can be screened rapidly for toxinogenicity by the polymerase chain reaction, although occasional strains of *C. diphtheriae* that carry an inactive toxin gene give false-positive results. The biochemical tests needed to differentiate *C. diphtheriae* from corynebacteria of the normal flora (diphtheroids) require several days. Group A beta-hemolytic streptococci and *Staphylococcus aureus* are also isolated frequently from patients with diphtheria.

Cutaneous diphtheria may present as a characteristic punched-out ulcer with a membrane, but it is more often indistinguishable from other inflammatory dermatoses. Its diagnosis depends on a high degree of suspicion and on culture of cutaneous lesions on laboratory media appropriate for the isolation of *C. diphtheriae*. Throat samples from all patients with cutaneous diphtheria should be cultured for *C. diphtheriae*.

℞ TREATMENT
The decision to administer diphtheria antitoxin must be based on the clinical diagnosis of diphtheria without definitive laboratory confirmation, since each day of delay in treatment is associated with increased mortality. Because diphtheria antitoxin is produced in horses, it is necessary to inquire about possible allergy to horse serum and to perform a conjunctival or intracutaneous test with diluted antitoxin for immediate hypersensitivity. Epinephrine must be available for immediate administration to patients with severe allergic reactions. Patients with immediate hypersensitivity should be desensitized before a full therapeutic dose of antitoxin is given. The dose of diphtheria antitoxin currently recommended by the Committee on Infectious Diseases of the American Academy of Pediatrics is based on the site of the primary infection and the duration and severity of disease: 20,000 to 40,000 units for disease that has been present for 48 h or less and involves the pharynx or larynx; 40,000 to 60,000 units for nasopharyngeal infections; and 80,000 to 100,000 units for disease that is extensive, has been present for 3 days or longer, or is accompanied by diffuse swelling of the neck. Antitoxin is administered intravenously by infusion in saline over 60 min to neutralize unbound toxin rapidly. The approximately 10 percent risk of serum sickness is acceptable because of the estab-

lished therapeutic value of antitoxin in decreasing mortality from respiratory diphtheria.

CHAPTER 144
Diphtheria, Other Corynebacterial Infections, and Anthrax

895

During the early phase of the Seattle epidemic, all patients with cutaneous diphtheria received 20,000 units of antitoxin. Later, when most isolates were tox⁻, antitoxin was withheld initially and administered only to patients from whom tox⁺ strains were isolated. The potential systemic complications of cutaneous diphtheria must be weighed against the potential adverse effects of antitoxin treatment; authorities are not unanimous in recommending antitoxin therapy for cutaneous diphtheria.

Antibiotics have little demonstrated effect on the healing of local infection in diphtheria patients treated with antitoxin. The primary goal of antibiotic therapy for patients or carriers is therefore to eradicate *C. diphtheriae* and prevent its transmission from the patient to susceptible contacts. Erythromycin, penicillin G, rifampin, or clindamycin is recommended by most authorities. The commonly recommended regimen for the treatment of adults with respiratory diphtheria is erythromycin (500 mg four times daily, given parenterally or orally) or intramuscular procaine penicillin G (600,000 units at 12-h intervals) for 14 days. Patients with cutaneous diphtheria and carriers can be treated orally with erythromycin (500 mg four times daily) or rifampin (600 mg once daily) for 7 days. If compliance is in question, a single dose of benzathine penicillin G (1.2 to 2.4 million units intramuscularly) can be substituted. Eradication of *C. diphtheriae* should be documented by negative cultures of samples taken on two or three successive days, beginning at least 24 h after the completion of antibiotic therapy. Some authorities also recommend a repeat throat culture 2 weeks later. The small percentage of patients who continue to be infected with *C. diphtheriae* after treatment should receive an additional 10-day course of oral erythromycin or rifampin. Plasmid-mediated erythromycin resistance of the MLS type emerged transiently in *C. diphtheriae* during the Seattle epidemic, but its frequency declined dramatically after the routine use of erythromycin was discontinued.

Patients with respiratory or cutaneous diphtheria caused by tox⁺ strains or by strains of unknown toxinogenicity should be hospitalized, kept in bed initially, handled with isolation procedures appropriate for the site of infection, and given supportive care as needed. Respiratory and cardiac function must be monitored closely. Early intubation or tracheostomy is recommended when the larynx is involved or signs of impending airway obstruction are detected. Tracheobronchial membrane can sometimes be removed mechanically via the endotracheal tube or tracheostomy. Primary or secondary pneumonia should be diagnosed and treated promptly. Sedative or hypnotic drugs that may mask respiratory symptoms are contraindicated. Close electrocardiographic monitoring, treatment of arrhythmias, and electrical pacing for heart block are essential. Congestive heart failure should be treated as described in Chap. 233. Glucocorticoids do not reduce the risk of diphtheritic myocarditis or polyneuritis. Oral therapy with DL-carnitine (100 mg/kg per day, given in twice-daily doses for 4 days) may have a beneficial effect in diphtheritic myocarditis, but such therapy should be considered experimental until additional data become available. Ulcerative or ecthymatous cutaneous lesions should be treated with Burow's solution applied on wet compresses after debridement of necrotic areas, and treatment for associated conditions such as pediculosis, scabies, or underlying dermatoses should be instituted.

PREVENTION Vaccines available in the United States for immunization against diphtheria include diphtheria and tetanus toxoids and pertussis vaccine adsorbed (DTP), diphtheria and tetanus toxoids and acellular pertussis vaccine adsorbed (DTaP), diphtheria and tetanus toxoids adsorbed (DT; for pediatric use), and tetanus and diphtheria toxoids adsorbed (Td; for adult use). The adsorbent is alum, which functions as an adjuvant and enhances the immunogenicity of the vaccines. Td contains less diphtheria toxoid than DTP, DTaP, or DT and causes fewer adverse reactions in adults.

The recommended schedule for primary immunization against diphtheria for children from 2 months of age up to the seventh birthday consists of five doses of vaccine administered intramuscularly: three doses of DTP at 2-month intervals beginning at age 2 months, a fourth dose 6 to 12 months after the third dose, and a fifth dose at the age of 4 to 6 years—before entry into kindergarten or elementary school. DTaP can be substituted for DTP for doses 4 and 5 in children aged 15 months or older. Some preparations of DTP and *Haemophilus influenzae* type b conjugate vaccine are approved for administration as a single injection to children scheduled to receive the two vaccines separately. DT is substituted for DTP if pertussis vaccine is contraindicated. The fifth (preschool) dose of DTP, DTaP, or DT is omitted if the fourth dose is administered after the fourth birthday.

If immunization is delayed until after the seventh birthday, the recommended primary series consists of two doses of Td given 1 to 2 months apart and followed by a third dose 6 to 12 months after the second dose. If primary immunization is interrupted, the series should simply be completed; there is no need to start a new series. Adults with an uncertain history of immunization against diphtheria should receive a primary series.

Periodic booster doses of diphtheria toxoid are required to maintain immunity. The Task Force on Adult Immunization currently supports two regimens. Either doses of Td should be given at 10-year intervals after the completion of primary immunization and throughout adult life, or a single dose of Td should be given at age 50 to individuals who have completed a full primary series and have received a teenage/young adult booster dose. Among patients who require tetanus toxoid for wound management, use of DTP, DTaP, DT, or Td as appropriate, given the individual's age and specific contraindications, is recommended for the maintenance of immunity to diphtheria as well as tetanus. All patients should undergo active immunization after treatment for diphtheria, since infection does not necessarily confer immunity.

Close contacts of patients with diphtheria should be cultured for *C. diphtheriae*, kept under surveillance for 1 week, and treated with appropriate antibiotics if cultures are positive. Previously immunized close contacts should receive an appropriate booster injection including diphtheria toxoid if their last booster dose was given more than 5 years previously. If their immunization status is uncertain, close contacts should receive an antibiotic regimen appropriate for carriers and a primary immunization series appropriate for their age.

OTHER CORYNEBACTERIAL INFECTIONS

DEFINITION Medically important *coryneform bacteria* (formerly called *diphtheroids*) include members of the normal flora that cause opportunistic infections, human pathogens of relatively low virulence, and animal pathogens that cause occasional zoonotic infections. Reported infections caused by coryneform bacteria have increased substantially in number over the past two decades. Isolates of *Corynebacterium jeikeium* and group D-2 coryneform bacteria are often resistant to multiple antibiotics.

ETIOLOGIC AGENTS AND LABORATORY DIAGNOSIS Because coryneform bacteria are potential pathogens, it is important not to dismiss them as constituents of the normal flora or as contaminants when they are found in clinical specimens. Laboratory differentiation of coryneform bacteria is important when they are isolated repeatedly, when they are recovered in pure culture or in large numbers, or when they form pigmented or hemolytic colonies.

The coryneform bacteria are a large, taxonomically heterogeneous, poorly classified group of gram-positive, pleomorphic, irregularly staining bacilli or coccobacilli that superficially resemble *C. diphtheriae*. The scheme recommended by the Centers for Disease Control and Prevention (CDC) for the classification of coryneform bacteria assigns them to several genera, including *Actinomyces*, *Arcanobacterium*, *Corynebacterium*, *Oerskovia*, and *Rhodococcus*, as well as to several groups that have not yet been categorized at the genus and species level.

ECOLOGY AND EPIDEMIOLOGY Humans are the probable natural reservoir for *Corynebacterium xerosis*, *Corynebacterium* *pseudodiphtheriticum* (formerly *Corynebacterium hofmannii*), *Corynebacterium striatum*, *Corynebacterium minutissimum*, *Corynebacterium jeikeium* (fomerly CDC group JK), *Arcanobacterium haemolyticum* (formerly *Corynebacterium haemolyticum*), and members of CDC coryneform groups A-4, D-2, G, I, 1, and 2. Animals are the probable natural reservoir for *Actinomyces pyogenes* (formerly *Corynebacterium pyogenes*; cows, sheep, pigs), *Corynebacterium ulcerans* (cows, horses), and *Corynebacterium pseudotuberculosis* (sheep, goats, horses). The natural habitat for *Rhodococcus equi* (formerly *Corynebacterium equi*) is soil. The ecologic niches for most other coryneform bacteria of medical importance are not well defined.

The coryneform bacteria found most frequently as components of the normal flora include *C. pseudodiphtheriticum* (pharynx, skin), *C. xerosis* (conjunctival sac, nasopharynx, skin), and *C. striatum* (anterior nares, skin). Coryneform bacteria that frequently colonize the skin of hospitalized patients include *C. jeikeium* (axilla, groin, perineum) and CDC group D-2. *C. jeikeium* most frequently colonizes patients with malignancies or severe immunodeficiency; it is also isolated from environmental sources (surfaces, air) in hospitals and from the hands of ward staff. *C. ulcerans* infections are acquired by consumption of raw milk. *C. pseudotuberculosis* infections are acquired by contact with animals or animal products or by consumption of raw milk.

PATHOGENESIS AND CLINICAL MANIFESTATIONS

C. jeikeium was recognized in 1976 as a cause of infections in immunocompromised hosts. It also causes infections in immunocompetent hosts, but severe infections continue to be most frequent in patients with hematologic malignancies and neutropenia. Colonization of the skin precedes clinical infection. Additional risk factors for nosocomial *C. jeikeium* sepsis include prolonged hospitalization, breaks in the integument, chronic intravascular catheterization, and prior treatment with broad-spectrum antibiotics. Other presentations of *C. jeikeium* infection include endocarditis, device-related infections, pulmonary infiltrates, cutaneous septic emboli, soft tissue infections, and rashes. Endocarditis due to *C. jeikeium* occurs primarily in patients with prosthetic heart valves. *C. jeikeium* is a rare cause of central nervous system infections in patients with ventricular shunts.

Group D-2 coryneform bacteria were identified in 1985 as a significant cause of nosocomial urinary tract infections, including acute and chronic cystitis and pyelonephritis. These organisms closely resemble *C. jeikeium* but differ from the latter in that they produce urease and fail to convert glucose to acidic metabolites. Hydrolysis of urea by urease causes alkalinization of the urine and formation of ammonium magnesium phosphate (struvite) stones. Group D-2 bacteria cause alkaline-encrusted cystitis in patients with preexisting bladder lesions, which serve as foci for precipitation of struvite crystals. Risk factors associated with symptomatic urinary tract infections include preexisting immunosuppression, recent urologic procedures (including renal transplantation), underlying disorders of the genitourinary tract, and a history of urinary tract infections.

A. haemolyticum causes pharyngitis, with 90 percent of cases occurring in patients between 10 and 30 years old. In this age group, *A. haemolyticum* pharyngitis is 5 to 13 percent as frequent as *Streptococcus pyogenes* pharyngitis. An erythematous rash is present in 30 to 67 percent of cases. The rash is usually scarlatiniform and most pronounced on the extremities, but it sometimes resembles urticaria or erythema multiforme. Because rash is more frequent in *A. haemolyticum* infections than in *S. pyogenes* infections, older children and adults presenting with the scarlet fever syndrome are as likely to have *A. haemolyticum* as *S. pyogenes* infection. Infection due to *A. haemolyticum* can also present as extensive pharyngeal exudate and can mimic diphtheria. *A. haemolyticum* occasionally causes peritonsillar abscess, sepsis, endocarditis, or meningitis.

C. minutissimum is frequently isolated from the lesions of erythrasma, a common superficial skin infection characterized by the presence in intertriginous areas of reddish-brown, scaly, pruritic, macular patches that exhibit coral-red fluorescence under a Wood's light.

The etiology of erythrasma has not been definitively established; infection of the skin by *C. minutissimum* has been shown to follow the onset of maceration and scaling. Deep infections caused by *C. minutissimum* are rare and include abscesses, bacteremia, and endocarditis.

Among coryneform bacteria that cause disease in animals and occasionally in humans, *R. equi* is emerging as a potentially important, intracellular, opportunistic pathogen in immunocompromised patients. Most reported cases are pulmonary infections that resemble tuberculosis in patients with severely defective cell-mediated immunity. Several cases of *R. equi* infection have recently been documented in patients with AIDS. *A. pyogenes* causes bovine mastitis, a disease transmitted by flies. Yearly epidemics of leg ulcers infected with *A. pyogenes* occurred among schoolchildren in Thailand between 1979 and 1984 and were postulated to have resulted from introduction of the organism into traumatic skin lesions by flies. Reported *A. pyogenes* infections among adults in Denmark have included abscesses, cystitis, intraabdominal infections, and mastoiditis with bacteremia. *C. ulcerans* infections in humans usually present as pharyngitis and can mimic respiratory diphtheria, whereas infections caused by *C. pseudotuberculosis* typically present as suppurative granulomatous lymphadenitis. Some strains of *C. ulcerans* and *C. pseudotuberculosis* can produce diphtheria toxin. Human infections caused by tox$^+$ strains of *C. ulcerans*—but not by tox$^+$ strains of *C. pseudotuberculosis*—have been reported.

C. pseudodiphtheriticum, a commensal of low virulence, is an uncommon cause of pneumonia in men with AIDS and of endocarditis, necrotizing tracheitis, tracheobronchitis, and urinary tract infection in patients without known immune deficiencies. Likewise, *C. xerosis* and *C. striatum* only occasionally cause human infections.

DIAGNOSIS The clinical features of *C. jeikeium* infections are not pathognomonic. The diagnosis of these infections is based on a high index of suspicion, identification of the organism by culture from appropriate clinical specimens, and exclusion of other likely causes of infection.

Group D-2 coryneform bacteria often are not detected by routine urine cultures; rather, it is necessary to incubate the cultures for 24 to 48 h on blood agar or on special media. Cultivation should be prolonged in selected cases—i.e., those involving patients (especially elderly men with preexisting genitourinary abnormalities) who have alkaline urine, ammonium magnesium phosphate stones, gram-positive bacilli in the urine, or negative standard urine cultures despite clinical evidence of bacteriuria. Other microbes that can cause urinary tract infections with alkaline urine include *Proteus*, *Ureaplasma*, and some staphylococci and streptococci. Alkaline-encrusted cystitis is an anatomic diagnosis made by cystoscopy.

The differential diagnosis of *A. haemolyticum* pharyngitis with rash includes scarlet fever; rubella; staphylococcal and streptococcal toxic shock syndromes; infections caused by Epstein-Barr virus, cytomegalovirus, and enteroviruses (especially coxsackieviruses); disseminated gonococcal infection; secondary syphilis; and drug allergy. Routine diagnostic methods for throat cultures are not ideal for the detection of *A. haemolyticum*, nor is this organism detected by the rapid tests for *S. pyogenes* that are sometimes substituted for throat cultures. Pharyngitis caused by *A. haemolyticum* in adolescents and adults is likely to be underdiagnosed until improved tests for the organism are used by diagnostic laboratories.

Erythrasma is diagnosed clinically. Because of uncertainty about the etiologic role of *C. minutissimum*, culture of erythrasma lesions is not currently recommended. Pharyngitis caused by tox$^+$ strains of *C. ulcerans* may be clinically indistinguishable from diphtheria. The presentations of infections caused by other coryneform bacteria are not usually diagnostic; cultures are required for identification of the causal organisms.

℞ TREATMENT

Strains of *C. jeikeium* are typically resistant to most antibiotics except vancomycin, which is the drug of choice for the treatment of infections caused by this organism. Some recent isolates of *C. jeikeium* are susceptible or only moderately resistant to β-lactam antibiotics; infections due to fully susceptible strains can be treated with β-lactam antibiotics alone, and those due to moderately resistant strains can be treated with β-lactam antibiotics plus an aminoglycoside. Quinolones, especially ciprofloxacin, have excellent in vitro activity against *C. jeikeium*. For device-related *C. jeikeium* infections, removal of the infected device is usually required in addition to appropriate antibiotic therapy.

Group D-2 coryneform bacteria are often resistant to the antibiotics used commonly for the treatment of urinary tract infections. Early isolates were uniformly susceptible to vancomycin and quinolones, but recent isolates have exhibited increasing resistance to norfloxacin and ciprofloxacin. Isolates are often susceptible to erythromycin, rifampin, novobiocin, and tetracyclines. Treatment of urinary tract infections due to group D-2 strains is often difficult; several courses of antibiotic therapy may be necessary for bacteriologic cure. Patients with alkaline-encrusted cystitis require resection of the encrusted lesions in addition to antibiotic therapy.

Controlled trials of treatment for infections caused by *A. haemolyticum* have not been performed. In vitro tests have demonstrated susceptibility to erythromycin but tolerance or relative resistance to penicillin. Limited data suggest that the clinical course of *A. haemolyticum* pharyngitis may be shortened by treatment with erythromycin.

Infections with *C. ulcerans* that present like diphtheria or that are known to be caused by tox⁺ strains of *C. ulcerans* should be treated like diphtheria. Oral erythromycin is usually effective for the treatment of erythrasma. Initial treatment of infections caused by other coryneform bacteria should be based on the identity of the organism and on published data regarding antibiotic susceptibility. Therapy should be modified, when necessary, in light of the results of antibiotic susceptibility tests. All isolates of *Corynebacterium* and of coryneform bacteria reported to date have been susceptible to vancomycin.

ANTHRAX

DEFINITION Anthrax is an acute bacterial infection caused by *Bacillus anthracis*. It occurs most frequently in herbivorous animals. Humans become infected when spores of *B. anthracis* are introduced into the body by contact with infected animals or contaminated animal products, insect bites, inhalation, or ingestion. In humans, the most common form is cutaneous anthrax, which is characterized by the development of a localized skin lesion with a central eschar surrounded by marked nonpitting edema. Inhalation anthrax (woolsorters' disease) typically involves hemorrhagic mediastinitis, rapidly progressive systemic infection, and a very high mortality rate. Gastrointestinal anthrax is rare and is associated with a high mortality rate.

ETIOLOGIC AGENT *B. anthracis* is a large (1 to 1.5 μm by 4 to 10 μm), nonmotile, encapsulated, chain-forming, aerobic, gram-positive rod that forms oval spores. Oxygen is required for sporulation but not for germination of spores, and sporulation does not take place in living animals. The rectangular shape of the individual bacteria gives chains of *B. anthracis* a boxcar-like appearance. On blood agar, virulent *B. anthracis* usually forms nonhemolytic or weakly hemolytic, grayish-white, rough colonies; however, if the medium contains bicarbonate and incubation takes place in the presence of excess CO_2, the colonies are smooth and mucoid. Virulent strains of *B. anthracis* are pathogenic for animals, including mice and guinea pigs. Known virulence factors include three proteins collectively called *anthrax toxin* (see below) and an antiphagocytic capsular polypeptide composed of D-glutamic acid residues linked by peptide bonds involving the gamma carboxyl group. The genes that determine the production of anthrax toxin and that of capsular polypeptide are located on separate plasmids of *B. anthracis*. Determination of susceptibility to bacillus phage gamma and demonstration of species-specific antigens are helpful in laboratory identification of *B. anthracis*. Spores of *B. anthracis* can survive for years in dry earth but are destroyed by boiling for about 10 min, by treatment with oxidizing agents such as potassium permanganate or hydrogen peroxide, or by dilute formaldehyde. Most strains of *B. anthracis* are susceptible to penicillin.

EPIDEMIOLOGY The distribution of anthrax is worldwide. All animals are susceptible to varying degrees, but the disease is most prevalent among domestic herbivores (including cattle, sheep, horses, and goats) and wild herbivores.

Grazing animals become infected when they are foraging for food in areas contaminated with spores of *B. anthracis* under appropriate climatic conditions. Anthrax in herbivores tends to be severe, with a high mortality rate. Terminally ill animals have overwhelming bacteremic infections and often bleed from the nose, mouth, and bowel, thereby contaminating soil or watering places with vegetative *B. anthracis* that can subsequently sporulate and persist in the environment. The carcasses of infected animals provide additional potential foci of contamination. Epidemics among animals may spread from an initial focus to contiguous geographic areas in a pattern consistent with the movement of infected animals. Biting flies have also been implicated as vectors for the spread of anthrax, and vultures that feed on infected carcasses occasionally spread spores from a contaminated area to noncontiguous areas, probably by the contamination of surface water pools.

The natural resistance of humans to anthrax is greater than that of herbivorous animals. It is difficult to determine the annual worldwide incidence of human anthrax, because many cases do not receive medical attention and are not reported; estimates of 20,000 to 100,000 cases per year have been made. Human cases are classified as agricultural or industrial on the basis of the epidemiologic setting in which they occur. Agricultural cases result most often from contact with animals that have anthrax (for example, during skinning, butchering, or dissecting), from bites of contaminated or infected flies, and (in rare instances) from consumption of contaminated meat. Industrial cases are associated with exposure to contaminated hides, goat's hair, wool, or bones. Anthrax in animals has been a long-standing problem in Iran, Turkey, Pakistan, and Sudan, and the probability is high that animal products (especially goat's hair) originating from these areas will be contaminated with anthrax spores.

Only three cases of cutaneous anthrax were reported to the CDC in the United States from 1984 through 1993, and gastrointestinal anthrax has never been documented in this country. Large epidemics of anthrax occurred in the former Soviet Union at Sverdlovsk in 1979 and in Zimbabwe between 1978 and the early 1980s. Initially, the cases in Sverdlovsk were reported to be cutaneous and gastrointestinal anthrax and were attributed to exposure to meat from infected animals. Intense international interest was stimulated by the suspicion that the release of *B. anthracis* from a nearby military facility was responsible for the outbreak. Recent analyses of epidemiologic data from the Sverdlovsk outbreak and autopsy findings on most of the fatal cases determined that the disease was, in fact, inhalation anthrax. The outbreak in Zimbabwe involved more than 9700 cases of agricultural anthrax in humans. This massive outbreak occurred during wartime and was associated with disruption of the veterinary and medical infrastructure and the cessation of veterinary anthrax vaccination programs (see below).

PATHOGENESIS *B. anthracis* is an extracellular pathogen that can evade phagocytosis, invade the bloodstream, multiply rapidly to a high population density in vivo, and kill quickly. Capsular polypeptide and anthrax toxin are the principal virulence factors of *B. anthracis*. The capsule of *B. anthracis* consists of poly-D-glutamic acid and confers resistance to phagocytosis. Anthrax toxin consists of three proteins called *protective antigen* (PA), *edema factor* (EF), and *lethal factor* (LF). The toxin was discovered in studies demonstrating that the transfer of sterile blood from guinea pigs dying of anthrax to uninfected guinea pigs killed the recipients.

PA binds to plasma membranes of target cells and is cleaved by a cellular protease into two fragments. The larger fragment remains on the cell surface, displays a single binding site for a domain that is present in both EF and LF, and serves as a specific receptor that mediates endocytic entry of EF or LF into the target cells. The activity of EF, a calmodulin-dependent adenylate cyclase, is expressed within human or animal cells that provide both the calmodulin activator and the ATP substrate for EF. The biologic effects of EF, which include formation of edema in anthrax lesions and the inhibition of polymorphonuclear leukocyte functions, are mediated by the cyclic AMP that is formed intracellularly by the enzymatic action of EF. PA-mediated entry of LF into susceptible cells leads to cell death by an unknown mechanism.

Cutaneous anthrax is initiated when spores of *B. anthracis* are introduced into the skin through cuts or abrasions or by biting flies. The spores germinate within hours, and the vegetative cells multiply and produce anthrax toxin. Histologically, the lesion in cutaneous anthrax is characterized by necrosis, vascular congestion, hemorrhage, and gelatinous edema. The number of leukocytes is disproportionately small in comparison with the amount of tissue damage. The clinical description of this lesion as a "malignant pustule" is not in concordance with the pathologic findings.

In inhalation anthrax, *B. anthracis* spores in airborne particles <5 μm in diameter are deposited directly into the alveoli or alveolar ducts. The spores are phagocytized by alveolar macrophages, and some are carried to and germinate in mediastinal nodes. Hemorrhagic necrosis of the nodes, in association with hemorrhagic mediastinitis and overwhelming *B. anthracis* bacteremia, may develop rapidly. Secondary pneumonia sometimes occurs.

Gastrointestinal anthrax usually results from ingestion of inadequately cooked meat from animals with anthrax. Primary infection can be initiated in the intestine by organisms that survive passage through the stomach, but an oropharyngeal form of the disease also has been described. Lesions in the throat or intestine are usually accompanied by hemorrhagic lymphadenitis.

B. anthracis bacteremia can develop in any form of anthrax and occurs in almost all fatal cases. Autopsies reveal large numbers of bacteria in blood vessels, lymph nodes, and many organs.

CLINICAL MANIFESTATIONS Approximately 95 percent of human cases of anthrax are the cutaneous form and about 5 percent the inhalation form. Gastrointestinal anthrax is rare. Anthrax meningitis occurs in a small percentage of all cases and is a frequent complication of overwhelming *B. anthracis* bacteremia.

Cutaneous Anthrax The cutaneous lesion in anthrax is most often found on exposed areas of skin. In Zimbabwe, lesions in children under 5 years old were significantly more likely to be on the head, neck, or face and less likely to be on the upper limbs than lesions in adults. This distribution correlates with the fact that children have less contact with carcasses of infected animals and are more likely to acquire infection through fly bites.

Within days after inoculation of *B. anthracis* spores into the skin, a small red macule appears. During the next week, the lesion typically progresses through papular and vesicular or pustular stages to the formation of an ulcer with a blackened necrotic eschar surrounded by a highly characteristic, expanding zone of brawny edema. The early lesion may be pruritic, and the fully developed lesion is painless. Small satellite vesicles may surround the original lesion, and painful nonspecific regional lymphadenitis is common. Most patients are afebrile, with mild or no constitutional symptoms; in severe cases, however, edema may be extensive and associated with shock. Spontaneous healing occurs in 80 to 90 percent of untreated cases, but edema may persist for weeks. In the 10 to 20 percent of untreated patients who have progressive infection, bacteremia develops and is often associated with high fever and rapid death. The differential diagnosis includes staphylococcal skin infections, tularemia, plague, and orf. Cutaneous anthrax should be considered when patients have painless ulcers associated with vesicles and edema and have had contact with animals or animal products.

Inhalation Anthrax The frequent similarity of the presenting symptoms of inhalation anthrax (woolsorters' disease) to those of severe viral respiratory diseases makes early diagnosis difficult. After

1 to 3 days, an acute phase supervenes, with increasing fever, dyspnea, stridor, hypoxia, and hypotension usually leading to death within 24 h. Occasionally, patients present with fulminant disease. A characteristic radiologic finding associated with hemorrhagic mediastinitis is symmetric mediastinal widening.

Gastrointestinal Anthrax Symptoms of gastrointestinal anthrax are variable and include fever, nausea and vomiting, abdominal pain, bloody diarrhea, and sometimes rapidly developing ascites. Diarrhea is occasionally massive in volume, causing hemoconcentration and severe contraction of intravascular volume. The major features of oropharyngeal anthrax are fever, sore throat, dysphagia, painful regional lymphadenopathy, and toxemia; respiratory distress may be evident. The primary lesion is most often on the tonsils.

LABORATORY DIAGNOSIS *B. anthracis* is present in large numbers in cutaneous lesions of anthrax and can be demonstrated by Gram's staining, direct fluorescent antibody staining, or culture unless the patient has been treated with antibiotics. A small proportion of patients with anthrax have bacteremia, but the disease may progress to death before blood cultures become positive. Patients with anthrax meningitis have bloody spinal fluid containing large numbers of *B. anthracis* organisms demonstrable by staining or culture. The virulence of suspected isolates of *B. anthracis* can be demonstrated by inoculation of guinea pigs; death occurs within 24 h with positive cultures of heart blood. Patients with mild disease usually have normal leukocyte counts, but patients with disseminated disease typically have polymorphonuclear leukocytosis. Tests for antibody to *B. anthracis* are useful in confirming the diagnosis of anthrax. A sensitive and specific polymerase chain reaction method developed for the detection of spores of *B. anthracis* may be useful for rapid testing of potentially contaminated animal or agricultural products.

℞ **TREATMENT**

Viable *B. anthracis* organisms disappear from the lesions of cutaneous anthrax within 5 h of the initiation of treatment with parenteral penicillin G. The recommended therapeutic regimen for adults is 2 million units of penicillin G at intervals of 6 h until edema subsides, with the subsequent administration of oral penicillin to complete a 7- to 10-day course. For penicillin-sensitive adults, treatment with ciprofloxacin, erythromycin, tetracycline, or chloramphenicol can be substituted. Antibiotics decrease local edema and systemic toxicity in cutaneous anthrax but do not prevent eschar formation. Cutaneous lesions should be cleaned and covered, and used dressings should be decontaminated. For inhalation anthrax, high-dose penicillin therapy (2 million units at 2-h intervals) is recommended; for gastrointestinal anthrax or anthrax meningitis, the recommended regimen is the same. A rational case can be made for passive immunization with anthrax antitoxin in addition to antibiotic therapy in severely ill patients with anthrax, but no appropriate antitoxin is commercially available.

PREVENTION Inhalation anthrax was essentially eliminated in England before 1940 through the development of methods to decontaminate wool and goat's hair and the improvement of working conditions for handlers of animal products.

Nonliving vaccines consisting of alum-precipitated or aluminum hydroxide–adsorbed extracellular components of unencapsulated *B. anthracis* are used in the United Kingdom and the United States for the immunization of agricultural workers, veterinary personnel, and others at risk of exposure to anthrax. The major active component of these vaccines is PA. Live attenuated vaccines containing spores of *B. anthracis* are used in both developed and developing countries to immunize domestic herbivores; these preparations are also used to immunize humans in Russia but not in the United States. The probable basis for attenuation of the original Pasteur spore vaccine is partial loss of the plasmid that encodes anthrax toxin during prolonged incubation of *B. anthracis* cultures at 42°C. The basis for attenuation of the current Sterne spore vaccine is loss of the plasmid that encodes capsular polypeptide.

Improved anthrax vaccines for humans are needed, because the current vaccines are impure and chemically complex, elicit only slow-onset protective immunity, provide incomplete protection, and cause significant adverse reactions. In addition to agricultural and industrial anthrax, the possible use of *B. anthracis* as an agent of biological warfare is a stimulus for the development of an improved vaccine. Current strategies for vaccine development include purification of candidate protective antigens, expression of protective antigens in recombinant microbial vaccines, and construction of improved live attenuated strains of *B. anthracis*.

Carcasses of animals that succumb to anthrax should be buried intact or cremated. Necropsy or butchering of infected animals should be avoided, because sporulation of *B. anthracis* occurs only in the presence of oxygen.

PROGNOSIS The mortality rate for cutaneous anthrax is 10 to 20 percent in the absence of treatment but is very low with appropriate antibiotic therapy. In contrast, the mortality rate for inhalation anthrax approaches 100 percent, and therapy is usually unsuccessful. The mortality rate for treated gastrointestinal anthrax is approximately 50 percent. Anthrax meningitis is usually fatal.

BIBLIOGRAPHY

ACP TASK FORCE ON ADULT IMMUNIZATION AND INFECTIOUS DISEASES SOCIETY OF AMERICA: *Guide for Adult Immunization*, 3d ed. Philadelphia, American College of Physicians, 1994, p 19

AKSARAY N et al: Cutaneous anthrax. Trop Geogr Med 42:168, 1990

CENTERS FOR DISEASE CONTROL AND PREVENTION: Diphtheria epidemic—new independent states of the former Soviet Union, 1990–1994. Morb Mort Week Rep 44(10):177, 1995

———: Diphtheria acquired by U.S. citizens in the Russian Federation and Ukraine—1994. Morb Mort Week Rep 44(12):237, 1995

COHEN Y et al: *Corynebacterium pseudodiphtheriticum* pulmonary infection in AIDS patients. Lancet 340:114, 1992

COMMITTEE ON INFECTIOUS DISEASES: Diphtheria, in *Report of the Committee on Infectious Diseases*, 23d ed. Elk Grove Village, IL, American Academy of Pediatrics, 1994, p 177

COYLE MB, LIPSKY BA: Coryneform bacteria in infectious diseases: Clinical and laboratory aspects. Clin Microbiol Rev 3:227, 1990

CREANGE A et al: Diphtheritic neuropathy. Muscle Nerve 18:1460, 1995

DAMADE R et al: Septic arthritis due to *Corynebacterium diphtheriae*. Clin Infect Dis 16:446, 1993

FARIZO KM et al: Fatal respiratory disease due to *Corynebacterium diphtheriae*: Case report and review of guidelines for management, investigation, and control. Clin Infect Dis 16:59, 1993

GEORGE S et al: An outbreak of anthrax meningoencephalitis. Trans R Soc Trop Med Hyg 88:206, 1994

HARDY IRB et al: Current situation and control strategies for resurgence of diphtheria in newly independent states of the former Soviet Union. Lancet 347:1739, 1996

HEDLUND KW: Anthrax toxin: History and recent advances and perspectives. J Toxicol Toxin Rev 11:41, 1992

HÖFLER W: Cutaneous diphtheria. Int J Dermatol 30:845, 1991

KAIN KC et al: *Arcanobacterium haemolyticum* infection: Confused with scarlet fever and diphtheria. J Emerg Med 9:33, 1991

LAFORCE FM: Anthrax. Clin Infect Dis 19:1009, 1994

MESELSON M et al: The Sverdlovsk anthrax outbreak of 1979. Science 266:1202, 1994

POPOVIC T et al: Molecular epidemiology of diphtheria in Russia, 1985–1994. J Infect Dis 174:1064, 1996

RAKHMANOVA AG et al: Diphtheria outbreak in St. Petersburg: Clinical characteristics of 1,860 adult patients. Scand J Infect Dis 28:37, 1996

ROZDZINSKI E et al: *Corynebacterium jeikeium* bacteremia at a tertiary care center. Infection 19:201, 1991

SORIANO F et al: Urinary tract infection caused by *Corynebacterium* group D2: Report of 82 cases and review. Rev Infect Dis 12:1019, 1990

TILEY SM et al: Infective endocarditis due to nontoxigenic *Corynebacterium diphtheriae*: Report of seven cases and review. Clin Infect Dis 16:271, 1993

TURNBULL PCB: Anthrax vaccines: Past, present and future. Vaccine 9:533, 1991

WILSON APR et al: Unusual non-toxigenic *Corynebacterium diphtheriae* in homosexual men. Lancet 339:998, 1992

145   *Anne Schuchat, Claire V. Broome*

INFECTIONS CAUSED BY *LISTERIA MONOCYTOGENES*

Listeria monocytogenes is a gram-positive rod that can be isolated from soil, vegetation, and many animal reservoirs. Human disease due to *L. monocytogenes* generally occurs in the setting of pregnancy or immunosuppression caused by illness or medication. Increasing evidence suggests that a substantial portion of cases of human listeriosis are attributable to the food-borne transmission of *L. monocytogenes*. Unlike most food-borne pathogens, which cause primarily gastrointestinal illness, *L. monocytogenes* causes invasive syndromes, such as meningitis, sepsis, chorioamnionitis, and stillbirth.

ETIOLOGY Listeriae are aerobic or facultatively anaerobic nonsporulating bacilli that grow at 1 to 45°C and typically have tumbling motility when cultured at 20 to 25°C. Characteristics that help distinguish *L. monocytogenes* from other *Listeria* species include the formation of a narrow zone of beta hemolysis on sheep blood agar and the production of acid from glucose, maltose, L-rhamnose, and α-methyl-D-mannoside but not from D-xylose. Determination of the serotype of *L. monocytogenes* is based on somatic (O) and flagellar (H) antigens. Most cases of human disease are caused by serotypes 1/2a, 1/2b, and 4b. Molecular subtyping techniques, including multilocus enzyme electrophoresis, phage typing, and DNA fingerprinting methods, have made it easier to discriminate among strains of *Listeria* and thus to link environmental or food isolates with clinical infections.

PATHOGENESIS *L. monocytogenes* is an intracellular pathogen, a characteristic consistent with its predilection for causing illness in persons with deficient cell-mediated immunity. The organism can be found as part of the gastrointestinal flora in healthy individuals. Lack of gastric acidity and abnormal gastrointestinal functioning may increase the risk of invasive disease following exposure to the organism in the gastrointestinal tract. Invasion, intracellular multiplication, and cell-to-cell spread of the organism appear to be mediated through proteins such as internalin, the hemolysin listeriolysin O, and phospholipase C. The increased risk of *L. monocytogenes* infection in pregnant women may be due to both systemic and local immunologic changes associated with pregnancy. For example, local immunosuppression at the maternal-fetal interface of the placenta may facilitate intrauterine infection following transient maternal bacteremia.

EPIDEMIOLOGY Long recognized as a veterinary pathogen, *L. monocytogenes* causes basilar meningitis ("circling disease") and stillbirth in sheep and cattle. The occurrence of listeriosis among humans has received increasing attention as the role of contaminated foods in the pathogenesis of epidemic listeriosis has been recognized and reports of disease associated with the expanding immunosuppressed population have accumulated.

Invasive listeriosis—confirmed by culture of blood or cerebrospinal fluid—occurs in approximately 4.4 individuals per million population annually in the United States, for an estimated 1092 cases per year. Perinatal listeriosis complicates 9 births per 100,000. A 40 percent decline in incidence since the period from 1986 through 1990 may be attributable to aggressive food regulation and industrial clean-up efforts. Multistate surveillance for sporadic listeriosis suggests that 23 percent of infections are fatal or result in stillbirth, although higher case-fatality rates have been reported during listeriosis epidemics and were described in early series. Most cases of disease due to *L. monocytogenes* are sporadic; however, investigation of several outbreaks of listeriosis during the 1980s and 1990s demonstrated common-source food-borne transmission as a cause of human illness and showed that the incubation period for disease following consumption of contaminated food can be 2 to 6 weeks. The largest North American outbreak, which took place in Los Angeles in 1985, involved more than 100 cases and 48 deaths or stillbirths. A nationwide outbreak in France in

1992 involved 279 cases and 63 deaths. Foods implicated in outbreaks of listeriosis include contaminated coleslaw, pasteurized milk, soft cheeses, pâté, and ready-to-eat pork products, while epidemiologic studies have implicated undercooked chicken, uncooked hot dogs, soft cheeses, and food from store delicatessen counters in sporadic disease. Listerial contamination of foods is relatively common. Among foods contaminated with the organism, those that are purchased ready to eat, are contaminated with serotype 4b, and are contaminated at a relatively high level may be the most likely to cause illness. The long incubation period associated with listeriosis contributes to the difficulty of implicating specific foods as the cause of either common-source outbreaks or sporadic cases.

Although food-borne transmission appears to be the foremost cause of epidemic and sporadic disease, several clusters of late-onset neonatal infection suggest nosocomial transmission of *L. monocytogenes*. Contaminated multiuse materials and equipment have been suggested as causes of some nosocomial clusters. Listeriosis has been reported in veterinarians and other persons in close contact with infected animals.

CLINICAL PRESENTATION *Pregnancy-associated listeriosis* may occur during any stage of pregnancy, although most infections are detected during the third trimester, possibly because of failure to obtain specimens for bacterial culture earlier during gestation in instances of abortion and stillbirth. One-half to two-thirds of pregnant women with perinatal listeriosis experience a mild illness that is characterized by fever, myalgias, malaise, and backache, which sometimes are accompanied by diarrhea, abdominal pain, nausea, and/or vomiting during the bacteremic phase. Blood cultures should be used for diagnosis, since isolation of the organism from rectal or vaginal culture is not diagnostic. Transplacental spread of the organism results in intrauterine infection, which can lead to chorioamnionitis, premature labor, intrauterine fetal demise, or early-onset disease of the newborn. Women with listeriosis diagnosed during pregnancy have a favorable clinical outcome after antibiotic therapy or delivery. Although often included in the differential diagnosis of recurrent spontaneous abortion, infection with *L. monocytogenes* appears to cause fewer than 2 percent of stillbirths.

Neonatal listeriosis can be classified under the same categories used for group B streptococcal infection, with early-onset disease evident during the first week of life and late-onset disease developing thereafter. Infants may be symptomatic at birth; most infants with early-onset disease are symptomatic by the second day of life. Aspiration of infected amniotic fluid contributes to the pathogenesis. Early-onset disease may include sepsis, respiratory distress, skin lesions, and the syndrome called *granulomatosis infantisepticum*, which is characterized by disseminated abscesses involving the liver, spleen, adrenal glands, lungs, and other sites. Infants with late-onset neonatal disease are more likely than those with early-onset disease to develop meningitis. While early-onset disease is often associated with obstetrical complications such as premature delivery and chorioamnionitis, late-onset disease typically affects infants born at term by uncomplicated deliveries. Infants may acquire *L. monocytogenes* during passage through the birth canal; except in several clusters of late-onset neonatal infections linked to nosocomial transmission, the pathogenesis of late-onset disease is not well understood.

Listeriosis not associated with pregnancy usually affects persons with immunosuppressive conditions, although invasive disease can also affect immunocompetent adults, particularly elderly persons. The most common underlying conditions in nonpregnant adults with listeriosis are chronic glucocorticoid therapy, solid or hematologic malignancies, diabetes mellitus, renal disease, liver disease, and AIDS. Although the prevalence of listeriosis among persons infected with human immunodeficiency virus (HIV) is much higher than that in the general population, listeriosis is a relatively uncommon opportunistic infection in AIDS.

Sepsis Recent studies of clinical series have shown that bacteremic infection without an evident focus is the most common clinical manifestation of listeriosis among immunocompromised hosts, while infection of the central nervous system (CNS) ranks second in frequency. Listerial sepsis cannot be distinguished clinically from bacteremia involving other organisms. Patients are usually febrile, often appear extremely ill, and may have prodromal symptoms including myalgia, nausea, vomiting, and diarrhea. Immunocompromised patients with listeriosis are less likely than other adults to present with CNS infection. Immunocompromised patients may be especially likely to have blood cultured during febrile episodes, whereas in other adults transient bacteremia due to *L. monocytogenes* may go unrecognized.

CNS Infection The most common presentation of CNS infection due to *L. monocytogenes* is meningitis. Meningitis due to *L. monocytogenes* is not distinguishable clinically from other types of bacterial meningitis; presenting symptoms include fever, headache, and an altered level of consciousness. Examination of cerebrospinal fluid (CSF) usually reveals pleocytosis, increased protein concentrations, and normal glucose levels, although other patterns are sometimes found. As in other forms of bacterial meningitis, Gram's stain may not be revealing. The diagnosis is made when *L. monocytogenes* is identified on culture. Despite its name, *L. monocytogenes* is rarely associated with monocytosis of either CSF or blood. Other syndromes seen in CNS infection include meningoencephalitis; cerebritis; and brainstem, spinal cord, or intracranial abscesses. The unusual syndrome of rhombencephalitis includes asymmetrical cranial nerve palsies, altered consciousness, cerebellar signs, and motor or sensory loss. Symptoms of other nonmeningitic CNS infections include fever, ataxia, seizures, personality changes, and coma. Nuchal rigidity is rare in nonmeningitic infections. CSF cultures may be sterile; blood cultures are usually diagnostic.

Endocarditis Like most forms of bacterial endocarditis, endocarditis due to *L. monocytogenes* typically occurs in patients with prosthetic or previously damaged valves. The organism has a predilection for the left side of the heart. Endocarditis due to *L. monocytogenes* is often associated with systemic embolization.

Focal Infections Other focal infections that can follow unrecognized bacteremia include endophthalmitis, peritonitis, osteomyelitis, visceral abscess, pleuropulmonary infection, and cholecystitis. Cutaneous lesions may develop without systemic involvement and have been reported in veterinarians and poultry workers.

Recurrences Recurrent infection with *L. monocytogenes* has been reported but is rare. Many recurrences are due to the subtype responsible for the initial infection, which suggests that recurrence results either from insufficient treatment of a focus of primary infection or from repeated exposure to a persistently contaminated source.

Gastrointestinal Illness Recent investigations of common-source outbreaks of acute gastroenteritis suggest that *L. monocytogenes* can cause an acute diarrheal syndrome in persons without immunocompromising conditions. The importance of *L. monocytogenes* in sporadic diarrheal illness is unclear. Although the organism is not identified by the culture methods routinely used for stool specimens, studies using selective enrichment media for evaluation of consecutive specimens from patients hospitalized with acute diarrhea have suggested that *L. monocytogenes* is not a major cause of sporadic diarrhea.

DIAGNOSIS Invasive listeriosis is diagnosed when the organism is cultured from a site that is usually sterile, such as blood, CSF, or amniotic fluid. The organism will grow readily within 36 h on routine culture media, but morphologic similarities between *Listeria* and both diphtheroids and streptococci make it necessary to use biochemical tests to identify the species. Serologic assays with whole-cell antigens have not been useful for the diagnosis of listeriosis, both because exposure to the organism (and thus the presence of antibody) may be common and because infected individuals may not produce antibody after infection. Assays for antibody to listeriolysin O have been applied in epidemiologic investigations and, retrospectively, in the diagnosis of culture-negative CNS infection. Culture of the organism from nonsterile sites such as the vagina and rectum is not useful for clinical diagnosis, as the organism may be carried at these sites by approximately 5 percent of healthy individuals.

Differential diagnosis of prematurity, spontaneous abortion, or stillbirth includes infectious diseases such as group B streptococcal infection, congenital syphilis, and toxoplasmosis; pathogens such as group B streptococci and *Escherichia coli* are more common than *L. monocytogenes* as causes of meningitis and sepsis in the newborn period. Because *L. monocytogenes* is not sensitive to cephalosporins, these agents should not be used for single-agent empirical treatment of neonatal sepsis and meningitis. Listerial infection should always be considered in the differential diagnosis of meningitis in immunosuppressed persons, particularly transplant recipients and others receiving glucocorticoid treatment, patients with hematologic malignancy, and HIV-infected patients. Among healthy adults, meningitis is much more likely to be caused by *Neisseria meningitidis*, *Streptococcus pneumoniae*, or viral pathogens than by *L. monocytogenes*.

℞ TREATMENT

The treatment of choice for listeriosis is intravenous administration of either ampicillin or penicillin, often in combination with an aminoglycoside for synergy. Trimethoprim-sulfamethoxazole is bactericidal against *L. monocytogenes* and has been used successfully in the treatment of patients with penicillin allergy. *L. monocytogenes* is susceptible in vitro to penicillin G, ampicillin, erythromycin, trimethoprim-sulfamethoxazole, chloramphenicol, rifampin, tetracyclines, aminoglycosides, and imipenem. However, chloramphenicol and rifampin may antagonize the bactericidal effect of penicillins. Cephalosporins are not recommended.

Dosages and durations of therapy have not been subjected to controlled trials. For nonpregnant adults with listeriosis, the therapy of choice is either ampicillin (12 g intravenously per day in six divided doses) or penicillin G (15 to 20 million units intravenously per day in six divided doses); for immunosuppressed patients with meningitis, some experts add gentamicin (1.3 mg/kg intravenously every 8 h) for synergy. Penicillin-allergic patients may be treated with trimethoprim-sulfamethoxazole (15/75 mg/kg intravenously per day in three equal portions every 8 h). Meningitis in an immunocompetent patient may require 2 to 3 weeks of antibiotic therapy after defervescence. Meningitis, bacteremia, endocarditis, and nonmeningitic listeriosis in immunosuppressed patients should be treated longer, probably for 4 to 6 weeks. Neonatal listeriosis can be treated with a 2-week course of ampicillin. Infants weighing less than 2000 g should receive 100 mg/kg per day in two equal doses during the first week of life and 150 mg/kg per day during the second week. Infants weighing 2000 g or more should receive 150 mg/kg per day in three equal doses during the first week of life and 200 mg/kg per day during the second week. The addition of an aminoglycoside should be considered for neonatal infection (gentamicin, 5 mg/kg per day in two divided doses during the first week of life; 7.5 mg/kg per day in three equal doses during the second week). For listeriosis in pregnant women, a 2-week course of ampicillin (4 to 6 g per day in four equal doses) is recommended. During the last month of pregnancy, infected women with serious penicillin allergies may be treated with erythromycin.

PROGNOSIS Treatment of maternal bacteremia during pregnancy can prevent neonatal infection. Antibiotic therapy for the newborn can limit sequelae, although the widely disseminated disease characteristic of granulomatosis infantisepticum is frequently fatal regardless of treatment. Early-onset disease carries a higher mortality risk than late-onset infection, and immunocompromised hosts have a worse prognosis than do otherwise healthy adults with listeriosis.

PREVENTION *L. monocytogenes* is frequently isolated from food; the Food and Drug Administration, the U.S. Department of Agriculture, and manufacturers are pursuing further measures to reduce *L. monocytogenes* contamination of foods that have been subjected to listericidal processing. Prevention of listeriosis requires dietary counseling of persons at increased risk of disease (Table 145-1). There is no role for the administration of prophylaxis to contacts of patients with listeriosis. Clinicians are encouraged to report cases of listeriosis to local or state health departments and thus to facilitate early recognition of outbreaks and prevention of subsequent cases.

Table 145-1

Dietary Recommendations for the Prevention of Food-Borne Listeriosis

Recommendations to all individuals:
1. Thoroughly cook raw food from animal sources, such as beef, pork, and poultry.
2. Wash raw vegetables thoroughly before eating them.
3. Keep uncooked meats separate from vegetables and from cooked and ready-to-eat foods.
4. Avoid raw (unpasteurized) milk or foods made from raw milk.
5. Wash hands, knives, and cutting boards after handling uncooked foods.

Additional recommendations to high-risk individuals*:
• Avoid soft cheeses such as Mexican-style, feta, Brie, Camembert, and blue-veined cheese. There is no need to avoid hard cheeses, cream cheese, cottage cheese, or yogurt.
• Leftover foods or ready-to-eat foods, such as hot dogs, should be reheated until steaming hot before being eaten.
• Although the risk of listeriosis associated with foods from delicatessen counters is relatively low and poorly characterized, pregnant women and immunosuppressed persons may choose to avoid these foods or to thoroughly reheat cold cuts before eating them.

* Persons immunocompromised by illness or medications; pregnant women.

BIBLIOGRAPHY

BERCHE P et al: Detection of anti-listeriolysin O for serodiagnosis of human listeriosis. Lancet 335:624, 1990

CHERUBIN CE et al: Epidemiologic spectrum and current treatment of listeriosis. Rev Infect Dis 13:1108, 1991

NIEMAN RE, LORBER B: Listeriosis in adults: A changing pattern. Report of eight cases and review of the literature, 1968–1978. Rev Infect Dis 2:207, 1980

PINNER RW et al: Role of foods in sporadic listeriosis: II. Microbiologic and epidemiologic investigation. JAMA 267:2046, 1992

PORTNOY DA et al: Molecular determinants of *Listeria monocytogenes* pathogenesis. Infect Immun 60:1263, 1992

RIEDO FX et al: A point-source foodborne listeriosis outbreak: Documented incubation period and possible mild illness. J Infect Dis 170:693, 1994

SCHLECH WF et al: Epidemic listeriosis—evidence for transmission by food. N Engl J Med 308:203, 1983

SCHUCHAT A et al: Role of foods in sporadic listeriosis: I. Case-control study of dietary risk factors. JAMA 267:2041, 1992

——— et al: Epidemiology of human listeriosis. Clin Microbiol Rev 4:169, 1991

SEELIGER HPR: *Listeriosis*. Basel, Karger, 1961

SKOGBERG K et al: Clinical presentation and outcome of listeriosis in patients with and without immunosuppressive therapy. Clin Infect Dis 14:815, 1992

SOUTHWICK FS, PURICH DL: Intracellular pathogenesis of listeriosis. N Engl J Med 334:770, 1996

SWAMINATHAN B et al: *Listeria*, in *Manual of Clinical Microbiology*, PR Murray et al (eds). Washington, DC, ASM Press, 1995, p 341

TAPPERO JW et al: Reduction in the incidence of human listeriosis in the United States—effectiveness of prevention efforts? JAMA 273:1118, 1995

146 *Elias Abrutyn*

TETANUS

DEFINITION Tetanus is a neurologic disorder, characterized by increased muscle tone and spasms, that is caused by tetanospasmin, a powerful protein toxin elaborated by *Clostridium tetani*. Tetanus occurs in several clinical forms, including generalized, neonatal, and localized disease.

ETIOLOGIC AGENT *C. tetani* is an anaerobic, motile grampositive rod that forms an oval, colorless, terminal spore and thus assumes a shape resembling a tennis racket or drumstick. The organism is found worldwide in soil, in the inanimate environment, in animal feces, and occasionally in human feces. Spores may survive for years in some environments and are resistant to various disinfectants and to boiling for 20 min. Vegetative cells, however, are easily inactivated and are susceptible to several antibiotics (metronidazole, penicillin, and others).

Tetanospasmin is formed in vegetative cells under plasmid control. It is a single-polypeptide chain. With autolysis, the single-chain toxin is released and cleaved to form a heterodimer consisting of a heavy chain (100 kDa), which mediates binding to nerve-cell receptors and entry into these cells, and a light chain (50 kDa), which acts to block neurotransmitter release. The amino acid structures of the two most powerful toxins known, botulinum toxin and tetanus toxin, are partially homologous.

EPIDEMIOLOGY Tetanus occurs sporadically and almost always affects nonimmunized persons, partially immunized persons, or fully immunized individuals who fail to maintain adequate immunity with booster doses of vaccine. Although tetanus is entirely preventable by immunization, the burden of disease is large worldwide. The disease is common in areas where soil is cultivated, in rural areas, in warm climates, during summer months, and among males. In countries without a comprehensive immunization program, tetanus occurs predominantly in neonates and other young children; an estimated 515,000 neonates died of tetanus worldwide in 1993. In the United States and other nations with successful immunization programs, neonatal tetanus is rare and the disease affects other age groups and groups inadequately covered by immunization (such as nonwhites). The elderly in particular are prominently involved. Only 27 percent of persons aged 70 years or older have a protective level of antibody to *C. tetani*, whereas 88 percent of children 6 to 11 years of age are protected. Overall, fewer than 60 cases of tetanus were reported to the Centers for Disease Control and Prevention each year during the period 1991 through 1994; 95 percent of all cases involved persons 20 years of age or older, and 53 percent involved persons 70 years of age or older. The burden of illness, however, is greater than the statistics indicate because reporting is incomplete.

In the United States, most cases of tetanus follow an acute injury, such as a puncture wound, laceration, or abrasion. Tetanus is often acquired indoors or during farming, gardening, and other outdoor activities. The injury may be major but often is trivial, so that medical attention is not sought; in some instances no injury can be identified. The disease may complicate chronic conditions such as skin ulcers, abscesses, and gangrene. Tetanus is also associated with burns, frostbite, middle-ear infection, surgery, abortion, childbirth, and drug abuse, notably "skin popping." In some patients no portal of entry for the organism can be identified.

PATHOGENESIS Contamination of wounds with spores of *C. tetani* is probably frequent. Germination and toxin production, however, take place only in wounds with low oxidation-reduction potential, such as those with devitalized tissue, foreign bodies, or active infection. *C. tetani* does not itself evoke inflammation, and the portal of entry retains a benign appearance unless infection with other organisms is present.

Toxin released in the wound binds to peripheral motor neuron terminals, enters the axon, and is transported to the nerve-cell body in the brainstem and spinal cord by retrograde intraneuronal transport. The toxin then migrates across the synapse to presynaptic terminals, where it blocks release of the inhibitory neurotransmitters glycine and gamma-aminobutyric acid (GABA). The blocking of neurotransmitter release by tetanospasmin, a zinc metalloprotease, involves the cleavage of protein(s) critical to proper function of the synaptic vesicle release apparatus. With diminished inhibition, the resting firing rate of the alpha motor neuron increases, producing rigidity. With lessened activity of reflexes, which limits polysynaptic spread of impulses (a glycinergic activity), agonists and antagonists may be recruited rather than inhibited, with the consequent production of spasms. Loss of inhibition also may affect preganglionic sympathetic neurons in the lateral gray matter of the spinal cord and produce sympathetic hyperactivity and high circulating catecholamine levels. Tetanospasmin, like botulinum toxin, may block neurotransmitter release at the neuromuscular junction and produce weakness or paralysis; recovery requires sprouting of new nerve terminals.

In local tetanus, only the nerves supplying the affected muscles are involved. Generalized tetanus occurs when toxin released in the wound enters the lymphatics and bloodstream and is spread widely to distant nerve terminals; the blood-brain barrier blocks direct entry into the central nervous system. If it is assumed that intraneuronal transport times are equal for all nerves, short nerves are affected before long nerves: this fact explains the sequential involvement of nerves of the head, trunk, and extremities in generalized tetanus.

CLINICAL MANIFESTATIONS Generalized tetanus, the most common form of the disease, is characterized by increased muscle tone and generalized spasms. The median time of onset after injury is 7 days; 15 percent of cases occur within 3 days and 10 percent after 14 days.

Typically, the patient first notices increased tone in the masseter muscles (trismus, or lockjaw). Dysphagia or stiffness or pain in the neck, shoulder, and back muscles appears concurrently or soon thereafter. The subsequent involvement of other muscles produces a rigid abdomen and stiff proximal limb muscles; the hands and feet are relatively spared. Sustained contraction of the facial muscles results in a grimace or sneer (risus sardonicus), and contraction of the back muscles produces an arched back (opisthotonos). Some patients develop paroxysmal, violent, painful, generalized muscle spasms that may cause cyanosis and threaten ventilation. These spasms occur repetitively and may be spontaneous or provoked by even the slightest stimulation. A constant threat during generalized spasms is reduced ventilation or apnea or laryngospasm. The severity of illness may be mild (muscle rigidity and few or no spasms), moderate (trismus, dysphagia, rigidity, and spasms), or severe (frequent explosive paroxysms). The patient may be febrile, although many have no fever; mentation is unimpaired. Deep tendon reflexes may be increased. Dysphagia or ileus may preclude oral feeding.

Autonomic dysfunction commonly complicates severe cases and is characterized by labile or sustained hypertension, tachycardia, arrhythmia, hyperpyrexia, profuse sweating, peripheral vasoconstriction, and increased plasma and urinary catecholamine levels. Periods of bradycardia and hypotension also may be documented. Sudden cardiac arrest sometimes occurs, but its basis is unknown. Other complications include pneumonia, fractures, muscle rupture, deep vein thrombophlebitis, pulmonary emboli, decubitus ulcer, and rhabdomyolysis.

Neonatal tetanus usually occurs as the generalized form and is usually fatal if left untreated. It develops in children born to inadequately immunized mothers, frequently after unsterile treatment of the umbilical cord stump. Its onset generally comes during the first 2 weeks of life. Poor feeding, rigidity, and spasms are typical features of neonatal tetanus.

Local tetanus is an uncommon form in which manifestations are restricted to muscles near the wound. The prognosis is excellent.

Cephalic tetanus, a rare form of local tetanus, follows head injury or ear infection. Trismus and dysfunction of one or more cranial nerves, often the seventh nerve, are found. The incubation period is a few days and the mortality is high.

DIAGNOSIS The diagnosis of tetanus is based entirely on clinical findings. Tetanus is unlikely if a reliable history indicates the completion of a primary vaccination series and the receipt of appropriate booster doses. Wounds should be cultured in suspected cases. However, *C. tetani* can be isolated from wounds of patients without tetanus and frequently cannot be recovered from wounds of those with tetanus. The leukocyte count may be elevated. Cerebrospinal fluid examination yields normal results. Electromyograms may show continuous discharge of motor units and shortening or absence of the silent interval normally seen after an action potential. Nonspecific changes may be evident on the electrocardiogram. Muscle enzyme levels may be raised. Serum antitoxin levels of 0.01 unit/mL or higher are considered protective and make tetanus unlikely, although cases developing despite protective antitoxin levels have been reported.

The differential diagnosis includes local conditions also producing trismus, such as alveolar abscess, strychnine poisoning, dystonic drug reactions (e.g., to phenothiazines and metoclopramide), and hypocalcemic tetany. Other conditions sometimes confused with tetanus include meningitis/encephalitis, rabies, and an acute intraabdominal process (because of the rigid abdomen). Markedly increased tone in central muscles (face, neck, chest, back, and abdomen) with superimposed generalized spasms and relative sparing of the hands and feet strongly suggests tetanus.

℞ TREATMENT

General Measures The goals of therapy are to eliminate the source of toxin, neutralize unbound toxin, prevent muscle spasms, and provide support—especially respiratory support—until recovery. Patients should be admitted to a quiet room in an intensive care unit, where observation and cardiopulmonary monitoring can be maintained continuously but stimulation can be minimized. Protection of the airway is vital. Wounds should be explored, carefully cleansed, and thoroughly debrided.

Antibiotic Therapy Although of unproven value, antibiotic therapy is administered to eradicate vegetative cells—the source of toxin. The use of penicillin (10 to 12 million units intravenously, given daily for 10 days) has been recommended, but metronidazole (500 mg every 6 h or 1 g every 12 h) is preferred by some experts on the basis of this drug's excellent antimicrobial activity, a survival rate higher than that obtained with penicillin in one nonrandomized trial, and the absence of the GABA antagonistic activity seen with penicillin. Clindamycin and erythromycin are also alternatives for the treatment of penicillin-allergic patients. Additional specific antimicrobial therapy should be given for active infection with other organisms.

Antitoxin Given to neutralize circulating toxin and unbound toxin in the wound, antitoxin effectively lowers mortality; toxin already bound to neural tissue is unaffected. Human tetanus immune globulin (TIG) is the preparation of choice and should be given promptly. The dose is 3000 to 6000 units intramuscularly, usually in divided doses because the volume is large. The optimal dose is not known, however, and results from one study indicated that a 500-unit dose was as effective as higher doses. Pooled intravenous immunoglobulin may be an alternative to TIG. It may be best to administer antitoxin before manipulating the wound; the value of injecting a dose proximal to the wound or infiltrating the wound is unclear. Additional doses are unnecessary because the half-life of antitoxin is long. Antibody does not penetrate the blood-brain barrier. Intrathecal administration should be considered experimental. Equine tetanus antitoxin (TAT) is also available. It is cheaper than human antitoxin, but its half-life is shorter and its administration commonly elicits hypersensitivity and serum sickness. Doses of up to 100,000 units are given, part intramuscularly and part intravenously, but 10,000 units may suffice.

Control of Muscle Spasms Many agents, alone and in combination, have been used to treat the muscle spasms, which are painful and can threaten ventilation by causing laryngospasm or sustained contraction of ventilatory muscles. The ideal therapeutic regimen would abolish spasmodic activity without causing oversedation and hypoventilation. Diazepam, a benzodiazepine and GABA agonist, is in wide use. The dose is titrated, and large doses (250 mg/d or more) may be required. Lorazepam, with a longer duration of action, and midazolam, whose short half-life necessitates administration by continuous intravenous infusion, are other options. Barbiturates and chlorpromazine are considered second-line agents. Mechanical ventilation and therapeutic paralysis with a nondepolarizing neuromuscular blocking agent may be required for the treatment of spasms unresponsive to medication or spasms that threaten ventilation. However, prolonged paralysis after the discontinuation of therapy with such agents has been described, and both the need for continued paralysis and the occurrence of complications should be assessed daily. Alternative agents include propofol, which is expensive, and dantrolene and baclofen, which are being investigated in the hope of shortening the period of therapeutic paralysis.

Respiratory Care Intubation or tracheostomy, with or without mechanical ventilation, may be required for hypoventilation due to oversedation or laryngospasm or for the avoidance of aspiration by patients with trismus, disordered swallowing, or dysphagia. The need for these procedures should be anticipated, and they should be undertaken electively and early.

Autonomic Dysfunction The optimal therapy for sympathetic overactivity has not been defined. Agents that have been considered include labetalol (an alpha- and beta-adrenergic blocking agent that is recommended by some experts but that reportedly has caused sudden death), esmolol administered by continuous infusion (a beta blocker whose short half-life may be advantageous in the event of severe hypertension from unopposed alpha-adrenergic activity), clonidine (a central-acting antiadrenergic drug), and morphine sulfate. Parenteral magnesium sulfate and continuous spinal or epidural anesthesia have been used but may be more difficult to administer and monitor. The relative efficacy of these modalities has yet to be determined. Hypotension or bradycardia may require volume expansion, use of vasopressors or chronotropic agents, or pacemaker insertion.

Vaccine Patients recovering from tetanus should be actively immunized (see below) because immunity is not induced by the small amount of toxin that produces disease.

Additional Measures Additional therapeutic measures include hydration to control insensible and other fluid losses, which may be significant; the meeting of the patient's increased nutritional requirements by enteral or parenteral means; physiotherapy to prevent contractures; and administration of heparin or another anticoagulant to prevent pulmonary emboli. Bowel, bladder, and renal function must be monitored. Gastrointestinal bleeding and decubitus ulcers must be prevented, and intercurrent infection should be treated.

PREVENTION **Active Immunization** All partially immunized and unimmunized adults should receive vaccine, as should those recovering from tetanus. The primary series for adults consists of three doses: the first and second doses are given 4 to 8 weeks apart, and the third dose is given 6 to 12 months after the second. A booster dose is required every 10 years and may be given at mid-decade ages—35, 45, and so on. Combined tetanus and diphtheria toxoid (Td) adsorbed (for adult use), rather than single-antigen tetanus toxoid, is preferred for persons over 7 years of age.

Wound Management Proper wound management requires consideration of the need for (1) passive immunization with TIG and (2) active immunization with vaccine, preferably Td in persons over age 7. For clean minor wounds, Td is administered to persons who have (1) unknown tetanus immunization histories; (2) received fewer than three doses of adsorbed tetanus toxoid; (3) received three or more doses of adsorbed vaccine, with the last dose given more than 10 years previously; and (4) received three doses of *fluid* (nonadsorbed) vaccine. The recommendations for contaminated or severe wounds are identical, except that vaccine should be given to those who have received three or more doses of adsorbed tetanus toxoid if more than 5 years have elapsed since the last dose. Passive immunization with TIG is not recommended for clean minor wounds but is given for all other wounds if the patient's vaccination history indicates unknown or partial immunization. The dose of TIG for passive immunization of persons with wounds of average severity is 250 units intramuscularly, which produces a protective antibody level in the serum for at least 4 to 6 weeks; the appropriate dose of TAT is 3000 to 6000 units. Vaccine and tetanus antitoxin should be administered at separate sites in separate syringes.

Neonatal Tetanus Measures aimed at preventing neonatal tetanus include maternal vaccination, even during pregnancy; efforts to increase the proportion of births that take place in the hospital; and the provision of training for nonmedical birth attendants.

PROGNOSIS The application of methods to support respiration has markedly improved the prognosis in tetanus; mortality rates as low as 10 percent have been reported from units accustomed to handling such cases. In the United States, 11 deaths from tetanus were reported in 1990, 11 in 1991, and 9 in 1992. The outcome is poor in neonates and the elderly and in patients with a short incubation period, a short interval from the onset of symptoms to admission, or a short period from onset of symptoms to the first spasm (period of onset).

The course of tetanus extends over 4 to 6 weeks, and patients may require ventilatory support for 3 weeks during this period. Increased tone and minor spasms can last for months, but recovery is usually complete.

BIBLIOGRAPHY

ABRUTYN E, BERLIN JA: Intrathecal therapy of tetanus: A meta-analysis. JAMA 266:2262, 1991

AHMADSYAH I, SALIM A: Treatment of tetanus: An open study to compare the efficacy of procaine penicillin and metronidazole. BMJ 291:648, 1985

BAGETTA G, NISTICO B: Tetanus toxin as a neurobiological tool to study mechanisms of neuronal cell death in the mammalian brain. Pharmacol Ther 62:29, 1994

BLECK TP: *Clostridium tetani*, in *Principles and Practice of Infectious Diseases*, vol 2, 4th ed, GL Mandell et al (eds). New York, Churchill Livingstone, 1995

CENTERS FOR DISEASE CONTROL: Diphtheria, tetanus, and pertussis: Recommendations for vaccine use and other preventive measures. Recommendations of the Immunization Practices Advisory Committee. Morb Mort Week Rep 40(RR-10):1, 1991

CRONE NE, REDER AT: Severe tetanus in immunized patients with high antitetanus titers. Neurology 42:761, 1992

GERGEN PJ et al: A population-based serologic survey of immunity to tetanus in the United States. N Engl J Med 332:761, 1995

LEE DC, LEDERMAN HM: Anti-tetanus toxoid antibodies in intravenous gamma globulin: An alternative to tetanus immune globulin. J Infect Dis 166:642, 1992

SANFORD JP: Tetanus—forgotten but not gone. N Engl J Med 332:812, 1995

SCHIAVO G et al: Intracellular targets and metalloprotease activity of tetanus and botulinum neurotoxins. Curr Top Microbiol Immunol 195:257, 1995

WASSILAK SGF et al: Tetanus toxoid, in *Vaccines,* 2d ed, SA Plotkin and EA Mortimer Jr (eds). Philadelphia, Saunders, 1994

WESLEY AG, PATHER M: Tetanus in children: An 11-year review. Ann Trop Paediatr 7:32, 1987

YEN JM et al: Role of quinine in the high mortality of intramuscular injection tetanus. Lancet 344:786, 1994

147 | *Elias Abrutyn*

BOTULISM

DEFINITION Botulism is a paralytic disease that begins with cranial nerve involvement and progresses caudally to involve the extremities. It is caused by potent protein neurotoxins elaborated by *Clostridium botulinum*. Cases may be classified as (1) *food-borne botulism*, from ingestion of preformed toxin in food contaminated with *C. botulinum*; (2) *wound botulism*, from toxin produced in wounds contaminated with the organism; (3) *infant botulism*, from ingestion of spores and production of toxin in the intestine of infants; or (4) *undetermined classification*, a group that includes some cases in older children and adults in which disease is produced by a mechanism similar to that described for infant botulism.

ETIOLOGIC AGENT *C. botulinum*, a heterogeneous group of anaerobic gram-positive organisms that form subterminal spores, is found in soil and marine environments throughout the world and elaborates the most potent bacterial toxin known. Organisms of types A through G have been distinguished by the antigenic specificities of their toxins; a classification system based on physiologic characteristics has also been described. Rare strains of other clostridial species—*C. butyricum* and *C. baratii*—also have been found to produce toxin. *C. botulinum* strains with proteolytic activity can digest food and produce

a spoiled appearance; nonproteolytic types leave the appearance of food unchanged.

Of the eight distinct toxin types described (A, B, C_1, C_2, D, E, F, and G), all except for C_2 are neurotoxins; C_2 is a cytotoxin of unknown clinical significance. Botulinum neurotoxin, whether ingested or produced in the intestine or a wound, enters the vascular system and is transported to peripheral cholinergic nerve terminals, including neuromuscular junctions, postganglionic parasympathetic nerve endings, and peripheral ganglia. The central nervous system is not involved. Active neurotoxin (150 kDa) is composed of a heavy chain (100 kDa) and a light chain (50 kDa). The steps involved in neurotoxin activity include (1) specific binding to presynaptic nerve cells at the myoneural junction, (2) internalization of the toxin inside the nerve cell in vesicles of unknown nature, (3) translocation of the toxin into the cytosol, and (4) proteolysis by toxin (a zinc endopeptidase) of components of the neuroexocytosis apparatus that curtails the release of the neurotransmitter acetylcholine. Cure follows sprouting of new nerve terminals.

Toxin can be inactivated during home cooking by exposure to a temperature of 100°C for 10 min. In the gastrointestinal tract, toxin is complexed with nontoxin proteins and resists degradation. Spores are highly heat-resistant, and their inactivation requires exposure to a temperature of 120°C (e.g., in steam sterilizers or pressure cookers).

Toxin types A, B, E, and (in rare instances) F cause human disease; type G (now called *C. argentinense*) has been associated with sudden death, but not with neuroparalytic illness, in a few patients in Switzerland; and types C and D cause animal disease.

EPIDEMIOLOGY Human botulism occurs worldwide. In the United States, the geographic distribution of cases by toxin type parallels the distribution of organism types found in the environment. Type A predominates west of the Rocky Mountains; type B is generally distributed but is more common in the East; and type E is found in the Pacific Northwest, Alaska, and the Great Lakes area. In the United States, food-borne botulism has been associated primarily with home-canned food, particularly vegetables, fruit, and condiments, and less commonly with meat and fish. Type E outbreaks are frequently associated with fish products. Commercial products occasionally cause outbreaks, but some of these outbreaks have resulted from improper handling after purchase. Outbreaks in restaurants, schools, and private homes have been traced to uncommon sources (commercial potpies, beef stew, turkey loaf, sauteed onions, baked potatoes, and chopped garlic in oil). Food-borne botulism can occur when (1) a food to be preserved is contaminated with spores, (2) preservation does not inactivate the spores but kills other putrefactive bacteria that might inhibit the growth of *C. botulinum* and provides anaerobic conditions at a pH and temperature that allow germination and toxin production, and (3) food is not heated to a temperature that destroys toxin before being eaten.

CLINICAL MANIFESTATIONS **Food-Borne Botulism** Following ingestion of food containing toxin, illness varies from a mild condition for which no medical advice is sought to very severe disease that can result in death within 24 h. The incubation period is usually 18 to 36 h but, depending on toxin dose, can extend from a few hours to several days. Symmetric descending paralysis is characteristic and can lead to respiratory failure and death. Cranial nerve involvement, which almost always marks the onset of symptoms, usually produces diplopia, dysarthria, and/or dysphagia; weakness progresses, often rapidly, from the head to involve the neck, arms, thorax, and legs; the weakness is occasionally asymmetric. Nausea, vomiting, and abdominal pain may precede or follow the onset of paralysis. Dizziness, blurred vision, dry mouth, and very dry, occasionally sore throat are common. Patients are generally alert and oriented, but they may be drowsy, agitated, and anxious. Typically, they have no fever. Ptosis is frequent; the pupillary reflexes may be depressed, and fixed or dilated pupils are noted in half of patients. The gag reflex may be suppressed, and deep tendon reflexes may be normal or decreased. Paralytic ileus, severe constipation, and urinary retention are common.

Wound Botulism When wounds are contaminated with *C. botulinum* spores, the spores may germinate into vegetative organisms that produce toxin. This rare condition resembles food-borne illness except that the incubation period is longer, averaging about 10 days, and gastrointestinal symptoms are lacking. Wound botulism has been documented after traumatic injury involving contamination with soil, in chronic drug abusers, and after cesarean delivery. The illness has occurred even after antibiotics have been given to prevent wound infection. When present, fever is probably attributable to concurrent infection with other bacteria. The wound may appear benign.

Infant Botulism In infant botulism, the most common form of the disease, toxin is produced in and absorbed from the intestine after the germination of ingested spores. The severity ranges from mild illness with failure to thrive to fulminant severe paralysis with respiratory failure and may be one cause of sudden infant death. The identification of contaminated honey as one source of spores has led to the recommendation that honey not be fed to children less than 12 months of age. Most cases cannot be attributed to a particular food source. The factors permitting intestinal colonization with *C. botulinum* are not fully defined, but cases usually involve infants under 6 months of age; susceptibility may decrease as the normal intestinal flora develops.

Undetermined Classification This group of cases includes those in which a specific food cannot be implicated. In some cases, the disease resembles infant botulism in that toxin is produced in the intestine of persons colonized with the organism. Toxin and organisms may be found in the stool over prolonged periods, and spores—but not toxin—may be found in the suspect food. Gastrointestinal disease or surgery may predispose to illness. Descriptive names for this illness include *adult enteric infectious botulism*, *adult infectious botulism of unknown source*, and *adult infant botulism*.

DIAGNOSIS A diagnosis of botulism must be considered in afebrile, mentally intact patients who have symmetric descending paralysis without sensory findings. The diagnosis must be suspected on clinical grounds in the context of an appropriate history. Conditions often confused with botulism include myasthenia gravis, which may be ruled out by electromyography and antibody studies, and Guillain-Barré syndrome, which is characterized by ascending paralysis, sensory abnormalities, and elevation of the protein concentration in cerebrospinal fluid. The Fisher variant of Guillain-Barré—a descending paralysis—can indeed be difficult to differentiate from botulism. Other conditions that may resemble botulism include Lambert-Eaton syndrome, poliomyelitis, tick paralysis, diphtheria, and intoxications from mushrooms, medications, or chemicals. Hypermagnesemia should be considered.

The demonstration of toxin in serum by bioassay in mice is definitive, but this test may be negative, particularly in wound and infant botulism. It is performed only by specific laboratories, which can be identified through regional public health authorities. The demonstration of the organism or its toxin in vomitus, gastric fluid, or stool is strongly suggestive of the diagnosis, because intestinal carriage is rare. Isolation of the organism from food without toxin is insufficient grounds for the diagnosis. Wound cultures yielding the organism are suggestive of botulism. The edrophonium chloride (Tensilon) test for myasthenia gravis may be falsely positive in botulism but is usually less dramatically positive than in the former condition. Nerve conduction velocity is normal, but action potentials on routine electromyography are decreased with a supramaximal stimulus, and facilitation is evident after repetitive stimulation at high frequency. Single-fiber electromyography may be helpful. The white blood cell count and sedimentation rate are normal.

℞ TREATMENT

Patients should be hospitalized and monitored closely, both clinically and by spirometry, pulse oximetry, and measurement of arterial blood gases for incipient respiratory failure. Intubation and mechanical ventilation should be strongly considered when the vital capacity is less than 30 percent of predicted, especially when paralysis is progressing rapidly and hypoxemia with absolute or relative hypercarbia is documented (see Chap. 266). Serial measurements of the maximal static inspiratory pressure may be useful in predicting respiratory failure.

In food-borne illness, trivalent (types A, B, and E) equine antitoxin should be administered as soon as possible after specimens are obtained for laboratory analysis. The initiation of treatment should not await laboratory confirmation, which may take days. After testing for hypersensitivity to horse serum, two vials of antitoxin are given, one intravenously and one intramuscularly; repeated doses probably are not necessary but may be given 2 to 4 h later. Anaphylaxis and serum sickness are risks inherent in use of the equine product, and desensitization of allergic patients may be required. If there is no ileus, cathartics and enemas may be given to purge the gut of toxin; emetics or gastric lavage can also be used if the time since ingestion is brief (only a few hours). Use of antibiotics to eliminate an intestinal source for possible continued toxin production and of guanidine hydrochloride and other drugs to reverse paralysis is of unproven value. In the United States, antitoxin as well as help in clinical management and laboratory confirmation are available at *any* time from state health departments or the Centers for Disease Control and Prevention.

Treatment of infant botulism requires supportive care. Neither equine antitoxin nor antibiotics have been shown to be beneficial, and the value of human botulism immune globulin, an experimental preparation, is still being evaluated. In wound botulism, equine antitoxin is administered. The wound should be thoroughly explored and debrided, and an antibiotic such as penicillin should be given to eradicate *C. botulinum* from the site, even though the benefit of this therapy is unproven. Results of wound cultures should guide the use of other antibiotics.

PROGNOSIS Type A disease is generally more severe than type B, and mortality from botulism is higher among patients above age 60 than among younger patients. With improved respiratory and intensive care, the case-fatality rate in food-borne illness has been reduced to about 7.5 percent and is low in infant botulism as well. Artificial respiratory support may be required for months in severe cases. Some patients experience residual weakness and autonomic dysfunction for as long as a year after disease onset.

BOTULINUM TOXIN THERAPY Botulinum toxin is being used as therapy for strabismus, blepharospasm, and other dystonias and appears safe and effective.

BIBLIOGRAPHY

CARDOSO F, JANKOVIC J: Clinical use of botulinum neurotoxins. Curr Top Microbiol Immunol 195:123, 1995

DAVIS LE: Botulinum toxin: From poison to medicine. West J Med 158:25, 1993

FERRARI ND III, WEISSE ME: Botulism. Adv Pediatr Infect Dis 10:81, 1995

HATHEWAY CL: Botulism: The present status of disease. Curr Top Microbiol Immunol 195:55, 1995

JAHN R, NIEMANN H: Molecular mechanisms of clostridial neurotoxins. Ann NY Acad Sci 733:245, 1994

McCROSKEY LM, HATHEWAY CL: The large intestine as the site of *Clostridium botulinum* colonization in human infant botulism. J Clin Microbiol 26:1052, 1988

MECHEM CC, WALTZER FG: Wound botulism. Vet Hum Toxicol 36:233, 1994

OGUMA K et al: Structure and function of *Clostridium botulinum* toxins. Microbiol Immunol 39:161, 1995

ROBLOT P et al: Retrospective study of 108 cases of botulism in Poitiers, France. J Med Microbiol 40:379, 1994

SCHIAVO G et al: Intracellular targets and metalloprotease activity of tetanus and botulism neurotoxins. Curr Top Microbiol Immunol 195:257, 1995

SCHWARZ PJ, ARNON SS: Botulism immune globulin for infant botulism arrives—one year and a Gulf War later. West J Med 156:197, 1991

SMITH LDS, SUGIYAMA H: *Botulism: The Organism, Its Toxins, the Disease,* 2d ed. Springfield, IL, Charles C Thomas, 1988

WEBER JT et al: Wound botulism in a patient with a tooth abscess: Case report and review. Clin Infect Dis 16:635, 1993

Wound botulism—California, 1995. Morb Mortal Wkly Rep 44:889, 1995

148 *Dennis L. Kasper, Dori F. Zaleznik*

GAS GANGRENE, ANTIBIOTIC-ASSOCIATED COLITIS, AND OTHER CLOSTRIDIAL INFECTIONS

DEFINITION Bacteria of the genus *Clostridium* are gram-positive, spore-forming, obligate anaerobes that are ubiquitous in nature. There are more than 60 recognized species of clostridia, many of which are generally considered saprophytic. Some of these species are pathogenic for humans and animals, particularly under conditions of lowered oxidation-reduction potential. Infections associated with these organisms range from localized wound contamination to overwhelming systemic disease. The four major disease categories for which clostridia are responsible are intestinal disorders, deep tissue suppurative infections, skin and soft tissue infections, and bacteremia (see Table 148-1). Toxins play a major role in some of these syndromes.

ETIOLOGY In humans, clostridia normally reside in the gastrointestinal tract and in the female genital tract, although they occasionally are isolated from the skin or the mouth. Of the known species of the genus *Clostridium*, at least 30 have been isolated from human infections. Like several other pathogenic anaerobic bacterial species, clostridia are quite aerotolerant, but they do not grow on artificial media in the presence of oxygen. Clostridia characteristically produce abundant gas in artificial media and form subterminal endospores. *Clostridium perfringens*, one of the most important species, is encapsulated and nonmotile and rarely sporulates in artificial media; the spores usually can be destroyed by boiling. *Clostridium tetani* and *Clostridium botulinum* are discussed in detail in Chaps. 146 and 147, respectively.

Clostridia are present in the normal colonic flora at concentrations of 10^9 to 10^{10} per gram. Of the 30 or more species that normally colonize humans, *Clostridium ramosum* is the most common and is followed in frequency by *C. perfringens*. These organisms are universally present in soil at concentrations of up to 10^4 per gram. Clostridia are gram-positive organisms; however, in clinical specimens or stationary-phase cultures, many species may appear to be gram-negative. Therefore, the results of Gram's staining of cultures or clinical material should be interpreted with great care.

C. perfringens is the most common of the clostridial species isolated from tissue infections and bacteremias; next in frequency are *Clostridium novyi* and *Clostridium septicum*. In the category of enteric infections, *Clostridium difficile* is an important cause of antibiotic-associated colitis, and *C. perfringens* is associated with food poisoning and enteritis necroticans.

PATHOGENESIS Despite the isolation of clostridial species from many serious traumatic wounds, the prevalence of severe infections due to these organisms is low. Two factors that appear to be essential to the development of severe disease are tissue necrosis and a low oxidation-reduction potential. *C. perfringens* requires about 14 amino acids and at least six additional growth factors for optimal growth. These nutrients are not found in appreciable concentrations in normal body fluids but are present in necrotic tissue. When *C. perfringens* grows in necrotic tissue, a zone of tissue damage due to the toxins elaborated by the organism allows for progressive growth. In contrast, when only a few bacteria leak into the bloodstream from a small defect in the intestinal wall, the organisms do not have the opportunity to multiply rapidly because blood as a medium for growth is relatively deficient in certain amino acids and growth factors. Therefore, in a patient without tissue necrosis, bacteremia is usually benign.

C. perfringens possesses at least 17 possible virulence factors, including 12 active tissue toxins and enterotoxins. This species has been divided into five types (A through E) on the basis of four major toxins: alpha, beta, epsilon, and iota. The alpha toxin is a phospholipase C (lecithinase) that splits lecithin into phosphorylcholine and diglyceride. This alpha toxin has been associated with gas gangrene and is known to be hemolytic, to destroy platelets and polymorphonuclear leukocytes, and to cause widespread capillary damage. When injected intravenously, it causes massive intravascular hemolysis and damages liver mitochondria. Alpha toxin may be important in the initiation of muscle infections that may progress to gas gangrene. Experimentally, the higher the concentration of alpha toxin present in the culture fluid, the smaller the dose of *C. perfringens* required to produce infection. The protective effect of antiserum is directly proportional to its content of alpha antitoxin. Beta, epsilon, and iota toxins are also known to increase capillary permeability.

C. difficile produces two major toxins, designated A and B. In experimental models of intestinal inflammation, toxin A mediates alteration in fluid secretion, enhances inflammation, and induces postcapillary venules to leak albumin. Toxin B appears to be more active than toxin A in causing damage to and exfoliation of superficial epithelial cells. Toxin B inhibits ADP ribosylation of Rho proteins. Both toxins cause disruption and condensation of F actin, which result in electrophysiologic alterations of colonic tissue. Diarrheal disease due to *C. difficile* is toxin mediated. Earlier teaching about the pathogenesis of this disease centered on the overgrowth of *C. difficile* when antibiotics suppress the normal bowel flora. Actually, the mechanism is probably more complex, since many of the antibiotics that cause this disease are active against *C. difficile* as well as other members of the bowel flora and since many patients who become colonized with *C. difficile* do not develop diarrhea. Critical features in the pathogenesis of this disease include mechanisms of toxin production and the interaction of *C. difficile* with other components of the bowel flora. Some antibiotics may actually trigger toxin production by the organism. In turn, other constituents of the bowel flora may suppress or inhibit toxin production. *Clostridium sordellii*, for example, neutralizes cytotoxin B in vitro. In addition, when antibiotics eliminate more sensitive members of the bowel flora, more resistant organisms may produce enzymes such as β-lactamases that can inactivate antibiotics and thereby facilitate the growth of *C. difficile*.

CLINICAL MANIFESTATIONS Intestinal Disorders *Food poisoning* *C. perfringens* is the second or third most common cause of food poisoning in the United States (see Chap. 128). Outbreaks generally have resulted from problems in the cooling and storage of food cooked in bulk. The food sources primarily involved are meat, meat products, and poultry. Generally, the implicated meats have been cooked, allowed to cool, and then recooked the following day, often in a stew or hash. Strains of *C. perfringens* that contaminate meat manage to survive initial cooking. During reheating, the organisms sporulate and germinate. The disease is associated with an attack rate that is often as high as 70 percent. Symptoms of food poisoning from type A strains develop 8 to 24 h after ingestion of foods heavily contaminated with the organism. The primary symptoms include epigastric pain, nausea, and watery diarrhea usually lasting 12 to 24 h. Fever and vomiting are uncommon. Diarrhea appears to be caused by a heat-labile protein enterotoxin. The enterotoxin inhibits glucose

Table 148-1

Classification of Diseases Caused by Clostridia

1. Intestinal syndromes
   a. Food poisoning
   b. Enteritis necroticans
   c. Antibiotic-associated colitis
2. Suppurative deep tissue infections
   a. Mixed bacterial infections
   b. Monobacterial infections
3. Skin and soft tissue infections
   a. Simple contamination
   b. Local infection without systemic signs
   c. Spreading cellulitis and fasciitis
   d. Myonecrosis (gas gangrene)
4. Bacteremia
   a. Transient bacteremia
   b. Sepsis

transport, damages the intestinal epithelium, and causes protein loss into the intestinal lumen.

C. perfringens has also been implicated in a more severe form of diarrhea than that of classic food poisoning. This more severe disease tends to occur in the elderly and has been associated with antibiotic use in hospitalized populations. In this form of disease, diarrhea is generally more profuse, of longer duration, and accompanied by abdominal pain. Blood and mucus have been detected in the feces of the affected patients. In one hospital-based study of a cluster of cases, widespread environmental contamination with *C. perfringens* spores was documented.

Enteritis necroticans Necrotizing enteritis (enteritis necroticans, or *pigbel*) is caused by beta toxin produced by type C strains of *C. perfringens* following ingestion of a high-protein meal in conjunction with trypsin inhibitors (e.g., in sweet potatoes) by a susceptible host who has limited intestinal proteolytic activity. This disease has been reported among children and adults in New Guinea. A similar disease, *darmbrand*, was epidemic in Germany after World War II. Clinical features of pigbel include acute abdominal pain, bloody diarrhea, vomiting, shock, and peritonitis; 40 percent of patients die. Pathologic studies reveal an acute ulcerative process of the bowel restricted to the small intestine. The mucosa is lifted off the submucosa, with the formation of large denuded areas. Pseudomembranes composed of sloughed epithelium are common, and gas may dissect into the submucosa. The source of the organisms may be the patient's own intestinal flora; cultures of ingested pork have failed to yield the organism. Antibodies to the beta toxin of *C. perfringens* have been of considerable benefit in changing the course of established disease. In a large-scale trial, children immunized with *C. perfringens* beta toxoid were protected.

Antibiotic-associated colitis Currently, strains of *C. difficile* that produce toxins detectable in the stool are the only identified cause of colitis induced by antibiotic use. The diagnosis of this type of colitis requires that there be no other identifiable cause of diarrhea and that the onset of symptoms occur either during antimicrobial administration or within 4 weeks after treatment with the implicated agent has been discontinued. Essentially any antibiotic can cause this syndrome; even metronidazole and vancomycin, which are used to treat the disease, have been implicated as etiologic agents in some cases. On a per-use basis, clindamycin, which was the first antibiotic described to cause this entity, is the most commonly implicated antibiotic. However, since other antibiotics are prescribed more often than clindamycin in the United States, cephalosporins are currently the antibiotics that most commonly cause *C. difficile* enterocolitis, and penicillins rank next in frequency.

Antimicrobial-associated diarrhea can be divided into four categories based on the appearance of the colon: (1) normal colonic mucosa; (2) mild erythema with some edema; (3) granular, friable, or hemorrhagic mucosa; and (4) pseudomembrane formation. Most patients with antibiotic-associated diarrhea have a normal, minimally erythematous colonic mucosa with some edema. Occasionally, colitis is more severe and is characterized by a granular, friable, or hemorrhagic mucosa. Examination of stool from the affected patients may reveal large numbers of red blood cells and some leukocytes. Biopsy shows subepithelial edema with round cell infiltration of the lamina propria and focal extravasation of erythrocytes. *C. difficile* cytotoxin B has been found in 15 to 75 percent of stools from patients in the first three categories, which suggests that other factors are involved in the pathogenesis of antibiotic-associated diarrhea.

The most characteristic form of antibiotic-associated colitis caused by *C. difficile* is pseudomembranous colitis (PMC). More than 95 percent of patients with documented PMC have positive stool toxin assays. Close inspection of pseudomembranes reveals exudative, punctate, raised plaques with skip areas or edematous hyperemic mucosa. These plaques can enlarge and coalesce over large segments of intestine in the later stages of disease. The clinical spectrum of antibiotic-associated PMC is diverse. Diarrhea is the key feature and is usually watery, voluminous, and without gross blood or mucus. Most patients have abdominal cramps and tenderness, fever, and leukocytosis. However, the symptoms vary considerably. At one end of the spectrum

are many patients with annoying diarrhea but no systemic signs or symptoms, while at the other end are those with severe systemic toxicity, fever (temperatures of 40 to 40.6°C, or 104 to 105°F), and peripheral white blood cell counts of up to 50,000/μL with a marked left shift. Fecal examination frequently reveals leukocytes. Without specific therapy, the course is highly variable. Some patients, particularly those with clinically mild disease, experience prompt resolution of symptoms with discontinuation of drug treatment, while others have protracted diarrhea with large stool volumes for up to 8 weeks, with resultant hypoalbuminemia and electrolyte imbalance. Severely ill patients with toxic megacolon and colonic perforation have been reported. Among patients who are severely ill mortality rates may be as high as 30 percent, while in most of those with minimal symptoms disease may resolve with the discontinuation of antibiotic treatment alone. In the majority of patients, symptoms begin 4 to 10 days after antibiotic therapy is initiated. However, about 25 percent of patients do not develop symptoms until use of the implicated antimicrobial has been discontinued, in some instances as long as 4 weeks afterward. Some cases have been reported within hours after initiation of antibiotic therapy or after a single dose of antibiotic administered for surgical prophylaxis.

Suppurative Deep Tissue Infections Clostridia are recovered frequently from various suppurative conditions in conjunction with other anaerobic and aerobic bacteria but also can be the only organisms isolated. These suppurative conditions, which exist with severe local inflammation but usually without the characteristic systemic signs induced by clostridial toxins, include intraabdominal sepsis, empyema, pelvic abscess, subcutaneous abscess, frostbite with gas gangrene, infection of a stump in an amputee, brain abscess, prostatic abscess, perianal abscess, conjunctivitis, infection of a renal cell carcinoma, and infection of an aortic graft.

Clostridia are isolated from approximately two-thirds of patients with intraabdominal infections resulting from intestinal perforation. *C. ramosum*, *C. perfringens*, and *Clostridium bifermentans* are the most commonly isolated species. The presence of clostridial species does not affect the clinical presentation or outcome of these infections (see Chap. 169).

An association has been made between malignancy and the isolation of *C. septicum* in the absence of grossly contaminated deep traumatic wounds. A major site for such a malignancy is the gastrointestinal tract, particularly the colon. An association with leukemia or with other solid tumors also has been noted. Some of these patients present with *C. septicum* bacteremia; these cases have a fulminant clinical course (discussed below). Others develop localized suppurative infection in the abdomen or the abdominal wall without bacteremia. Presumably, this infection arises from a silent perforation that leads to intraabdominal abscess formation.

Clostridia have been isolated from suppurative infections of the female genital tract, particularly tuboovarian and pelvic abscesses. The major species involved has been *C. perfringens*. Most of these are mild suppurative infections without evidence of uterine gangrene. *C. perfringens* has been isolated from as many as 20 percent of diseased gallbladders at surgery. One clinical syndrome, emphysematous cholecystitis, is caused by clostridial species at least 50 percent of the time. In this syndrome, gas forms in the biliary radicles and the wall of the gallbladder. It is seen most often in diabetic patients. Although the mortality rate in this entity is higher than in more common forms of cholecystitis, there is no evidence of myonecrosis.

Clostridia are among the many organisms found in empyema fluid or isolated by transtracheal aspiration from patients with lung abscesses. There is no unique clinical clue to the presence of clostridia (as opposed to other organisms) in these infections. *C. perfringens* has been reported as a cause of empyema arising from aspiration pneumonia, pulmonary emboli, and infarction. However, the majority of cases of clostridial empyema are secondary to trauma.

Skin and Soft Tissue Infections Various categories of traumatic wound infections due to clostridia have been described: simple contamination, anaerobic cellulitis, fasciitis with or without systemic manifestations, and anaerobic myonecrosis.

Simple contamination Clostridia are cultured most often from wounds in the absence of clinical signs of sepsis. As many as 30 percent of battle wounds are contaminated by clostridia without signs of suppuration, and 16 percent of penetrating abdominal wounds yield clostridia on culture despite treatment with cephalothin and kanamycin. In cases of trauma, clostridia are isolated with equal frequency from suppurative and well-healing wounds. Thus the diagnosis of clostridial infection should be based on clinical rather than bacteriologic criteria.

Localized infection of the skin and soft tissue without systemic signs This condition, originally referred to as *anaerobic cellulitis*, is a localized infection involving the skin and soft tissue and is due to clostridia alone or with other bacteria. There are no systemic signs of toxicity, although the infection may invade locally, producing necrosis. These infections tend to be relatively indolent, spreading slowly to contiguous areas. Localized infections are relatively free of pain and edema. Perhaps because of the lack of edema, gas that is limited to the wound and the immediately surrounding tissue may be more evident than in gas gangrene. In these localized infections, gas is never found intramuscularly. Cellulitis, perirectal abscesses, and diabetic food ulcers are typical infections from which clostridial species can be isolated. If inadequately treated, these localized infections advance by extension through subcutaneous tissue and fascial planes into muscle and may produce severe systemic disease with signs of toxemia.

A localized form of suppurative myositis has been described in heroin addicts. These patients develop local pain and tenderness in discrete areas (particularly the thigh and forearm), with the subsequent appearance of fluctuance and crepitance that require surgical drainage. The unusual aspect of these infections is that they remain localized without systemic signs of toxicity. Moreover, the affected local areas are not necessarily sites of trauma or heroin injection. Pathologic examination reveals subcutaneous abscesses, purulent myositis, and fasciitis from which clostridia are recovered in pure culture; on occasion, mixed infections involving aerobes and anaerobes are found.

Spreading cellulitis and fasciitis with systemic toxicity This condition involves diffuse spreading cellulitis and fasciitis, without myonecrosis and with only mild inflammation in muscle. Patients present with the abrupt onset of a syndrome that progresses rapidly (within hours) through the fascial planes. In cases with suppuration and gas in soft tissues as well as overwhelming toxemia, the infection is rapidly fatal. On physical examination there is subcutaneous crepitance but little localized pain. Surgery is of no proven value because there are no discretely involved tissues amenable to resection, as may be the case in myonecrosis. However, in rapidly advancing fasciitis, incision of the affected area is still the cornerstone of therapy. The initial local lesion may be quite innocuous and arises from an area involved by tumor or other infection and not by injury. The systemic toxic effects include hemolysis and injury of capillary membranes. Usually, this infection is uniformly fatal within 48 h, despite intensive therapy involving antitoxin and exchange transfusion. This syndrome is seen most commonly in patients with carcinoma, especially of the sigmoid or the cecum. Presumably, the tumor invades the fascia, and colonic contents leak into the abdominal wall. Patients present with extreme toxicity and occasionally with total-body crepitance. The syndrome differs from necrotizing fasciitis caused by other organisms in three respects: (1) rapid mortality, (2) rapid tissue invasion, and (3) the systemic effects of the toxin, typified by massive hemolysis.

Clostridial myonecrosis (gas gangrene) Clostridial myonecrosis occurs when bacteria invade healthy muscle from adjacent traumatized muscle or soft tissue. The infection originates in a wound contaminated with clostridia. Although more than 30 percent of deep wounds are infected with clostridia, the incidence of clostridial myonecrosis is quite low. These infections occur in both military and civilian settings. An essential factor in the genesis of gas gangrene appears to be trauma, particularly involving deep muscle laceration. The entity of clostridial

myonecrosis is relatively uncommon after simple, through-and-through bullet wounds without shattering of bone and is relatively common following shrapnel fragmentation wounds, particularly when deep muscle is involved. In civilian cases, gas gangrene can follow trauma, surgery, or intramuscular injection. The trauma need not be severe; however, the wound must be deep, necrotic, and without communication to the surface.

The incubation period of gas gangrene is usually short: almost always less than 3 days and frequently less than 24 h. Eighty percent of cases are caused by *C. perfringens*, while *C. novyi*, *C. septicum*, and *Clostridium histolyticum* cause most of the other cases. Typically, gas gangrene begins with the sudden onset of pain in the region of the wound, which helps to differentiate it from spreading cellulitis. Once established, the pain increases steadily in severity but remains localized to the infected area and spreads only if the infection spreads. Soon after pain develops, local swelling and edema—accompanied by a thin, often hemorrhagic exudate—appear. Patients frequently develop marked tachycardia, but elevation in temperature may be only minimal. Gas usually is not obvious at this early stage and may be completely absent. Frothiness of the wound exudate may be noted. The skin is tense, white, often marbled with blue, and cooler than normal. The symptoms progress rapidly; swelling, edema, and toxemia increase, and a profuse serous discharge, which may have a peculiar sweetish smell, appears. Gram's staining of the wound exudate shows many gram-positive rods with relatively few inflammatory cells.

At surgery, muscle may appear pale because of the intensity of edema, but it does not contract when probed with a scalpel. When dissected, the muscle is beefy red and nonviable and can progress to become black, friable, and gangrenous. It is important to establish a diagnosis early, preferably by frozen-section biopsy of muscle.

Despite hypotension, renal failure, and (often) body crepitance, patients with myonecrosis frequently have a heightened awareness of their surroundings until just before death, when they lapse into toxic delirium and coma. In untreated cases, as the local wounds progress, the skin becomes bronzed; bullae appear, become filled with dark red fluid, and are accompanied by dark patches of cutaneous gangrene. Gas appears in later phases but may not be as obvious as in anaerobic cellulitis. Jaundice is rare in wound gas gangrene (in contrast to uterine infections) and, when it does appear, is almost invariably associated with hemoglobinuria, hemoglobinemia, and septicemia. Cases of clostridial myonecrosis without a history of trauma have been reported. These patients have bullous lesions and crepitance of the skin; they present with a rapidly worsening course that includes myonecrosis, especially of the extremities.

Bacteremia and Clostridial Sepsis The relatively common entity of transient clostridial bacteremia can arise in any hospitalized patient but is most common with a predisposing focus in the gastrointestinal tract, biliary tract, or uterus. Fever frequently resolves within 24 to 48 h without therapy. Despite the finding of clostridial bacteremia following septic abortions and the frequent isolation of clostridia from the lochia, most of the patients involved do not have evidence of sepsis. In one series of 60 patients with clostridial bacteremia, half had an infected site that could be associated with the bacteremia, while the other half had a totally unrelated illness, such as tuberculous pneumonia, meningitis, or benign gastroenteritis. By the time blood culture reports are returned, patients frequently are completely well and sometimes have been discharged. Therefore, when a blood culture is positive for clostridia, the patient must be assessed clinically rather than simply treated on the basis of the culture result.

Clostridial sepsis is an uncommon but almost invariably fatal illness following clostridial infection—primarily that of the uterus, colon, or biliary tract. This entity must be differentiated from transient clostridial bacteremia, which is much more common. *C. perfringens* causes the majority of cases of sepsis as well as the majority of cases of transient bacteremia. *C. septicum*, *C. sordellii*, and *C. novyi* account for most of the remainder of cases. Clostridia account for 1 to 2.5 percent of all positive blood cultures in major hospital centers.

The majority of cases of clostridial sepsis originate from the female genital tract and follow septic abortion. Introduction of a foreign body is a common antecedent event. In the uterus, residual necrotic fetal and placental tissues and traumatized endometrium may allow the growth of clostridia. Only a small fraction of cases of septic abortion (1 percent) are followed by serious sepsis. In these patients, sepsis, fever, and chills begin from 1 to 3 days after the attempted abortion. The initial signs are malaise, headache, severe myalgias, abdominal pain, nausea, vomiting, and occasionally diarrhea. Frequently, a bloody or brown vaginal discharge is noted. Patients may rapidly develop oliguria, hypotension, jaundice, and hemoglobinuria. The hemolysis, which is secondary to *C. perfringens* alpha toxin, causes a characteristic bronzing of the skin. As in myonecrosis, the mental status of severely ill patients is characterized by increased alertness and apprehension. Local examination of the pelvis reveals foul cervical discharge, occasionally with gas. Frequently, laceration marks around the cervix or perforation of the cervical segment are evident. If the infection involves the myometrium or has spread to the adnexa, extreme tenderness, guarding, and an adnexal mass may be found.

Laboratory studies in patients with sepsis reveal an elevated white blood cell count and may show pink, hemoglobin-tinged plasma. Anemia is proportional to the degree of hemolysis, and the hematocrit may be extremely low. Platelet counts may be reduced, and there is often evidence of disseminated intravascular coagulation. Oliguria or anuria, increasingly refractory hypotension, and hemorrhage and bruising may develop.

Clostridia may enter the bloodstream from the gastrointestinal or biliary tract. This occurrence is associated with ulcerative lesions or obstruction of the small or large intestine, necrotic or infiltrating malignancy, bowel surgery, or various abdominal catastrophes. The patient may present with an acute febrile illness, with chills and fever but no other signs of localized infection. Intravascular hemolysis occurs in as many as half of such cases. Biliary or gastrointestinal symptoms, if present, may be the only clue to the etiology. Positive blood cultures provide the definitive clue to the diagnosis.

Patients with malignant disease also can develop rapidly fatal clostridial sepsis, particularly from a gastrointestinal focus. The most common species in this setting is *C. septicum*. Characteristic signs and symptoms include fever, tachycardia, hypotension, abdominal pain or tenderness, nausea, vomiting, and (preterminally) coma. The tachycardia may be out of proportion to the fever. Only about 20 to 30 percent of patients develop hemolysis. A striking feature of this syndrome is the rapidity of death, which frequently occurs in less than 12 h.

DIAGNOSIS The diagnosis of clostridial disease, in association with positive cultures, must be based primarily on clinical findings. Because of the presence of clostridia in many wounds, their mere isolation from any site, including the blood, does not necessarily indicate severe disease. Smears of wound exudates, uterine scrapings, or cervical discharge may show abundant large gram-positive rods as well as other organisms. Cultures should be placed in selective media and incubated anaerobically for identification of clostridia. The diagnosis of clostridial myonecrosis can be established by frozen-section biopsy of muscle.

The urine of patients with severe clostridial sepsis may contain protein and casts, and some patients may develop severe uremia. Profound alterations of circulating erythrocytes are seen in severely toxemic patients. Patients have hemolytic anemia, which develops extremely rapidly, along with hemoglobinemia, hemoglobinuria, and elevated levels of serum bilirubin. Spherocytosis, increased osmotic and mechanical red blood cell fragility, erythrophagocytosis, and methemoglobinemia have been described. Disseminated intravascular coagulation may develop in patients with severe infection. In patients with severe sepsis, Wright's or Gram's staining of a smear of peripheral blood or buffy coat may demonstrate clostridia.

X-ray examination sometimes provides an important clue to the diagnosis by revealing gas in muscles, subcutaneous tissue, or the uterus. However, the finding of gas is not pathognomonic for clostridial infection. Other anaerobic bacteria, frequently mixed with aerobic organisms, may produce gas.

The diagnosis of *C. difficile*–associated colitis is made by the identification of *C. difficile* toxin in stool. Diagnostic evaluation of patients with PMC should include examination of the stool for *C. difficile* cytotoxin. Although several assays are available, the tissue culture assay is the most practical and sensitive. The assay is performed by incubation of stool filtrates with tissue culture cells and monitoring for a cytopathic effect that can be neutralized by antitoxin to either *C. sordellii* (which is cross-reactive with *C. difficile* but does not cause PMC) or *C. difficile*. Identical cytopathic and actinomorphic changes in fibroblasts are induced by toxins A and B; however, the standard assay is about 1000-fold more sensitive for toxin B. Most strains produce both toxins when grown under similar conditions. Endoscopy, although useful in establishing the presence of PMC, does not establish the etiology and should be reserved for cases with more serious disease manifestations, in which it can be used to exclude alternative diagnoses. Isolation of *C. difficile* from stool cultures is difficult. Moreover, *C. difficile* may be part of the "normal" flora of asymptomatic patients, particularly infants.

℞ **TREATMENT**

Traditionally, the treatment of choice for severe clostridial infection has been penicillin G (20 million units a day in adults). Recently, penicillin G treatment of gas gangrene has become more controversial because of increasing resistance to this drug and data obtained from animal models of infection. In a mouse model of gas gangrene, Stevens et al. demonstrated that antibiotics that inhibit protein synthesis may be preferable to cell wall–active drugs. Clindamycin treatment enhanced survival more than therapy with penicillin. The combination of clindamycin and penicillin was superior to penicillin alone. For severe clostridial sepsis, clindamycin may be used at a dose of 600 mg every 6 h in combination with high-dose penicillin. Although no clinical trials validate this choice, it is gaining acceptance in the infectious disease community.

In cases of penicillin sensitivity or allergy, other antibiotics should be considered, but all should be tested for in vitro activity because of the occasional isolation of resistant strains. Clostridia are frequently, but not universally, susceptible in vitro to cefoxitin, carbenicillin, chloramphenicol, clindamycin, metronidazole, doxycycline, imipenem, minocycline, tetracycline, third-generation cephalosporins, and vancomycin. For severe clostridial infections, sensitivity testing should be done before an antimicrobial with unpredictable activity is used. Simple contamination of a wound with clostridia should not be treated with antibiotics. Localized skin and soft tissue infection can be managed by debridement rather than with systemic antibiotics. Drugs are required when the process extends into adjacent tissue or when fever and systemic signs of sepsis are present. Surgery is a mainstay of therapy for clostridial myonecrosis or gas gangrene. Amputation may be required for rapidly spreading infection involving a limb. Hysterectomy is required for uterine myonecrosis. Abdominal wall myonecrosis usually continues despite initial aggressive surgery and antibiotic therapy and requires repeated surgical debridement of all involved muscle.

Suppurative infections should be treated with antibiotics. Frequently, broad-spectrum antibiotics must be used because of the mixed flora involved in these infections. Aminoglycosides can be used for the aerobic gram-negative bacteria involved in mixed infections.

The use of a polyvalent gas gangrene antitoxin is still recommended by some authorities. At present, no such antitoxin is produced in the United States, and most centers have discontinued its use in the management of patients with suspected gas gangrene or clostridial postabortion sepsis because of questionable efficacy and the substantial risk of hypersensitivity to horse serum, from which the antitoxin is derived.

The use of hyperbaric oxygen in the treatment of gas gangrene is also controversial. Studies in humans are not well designed to answer questions on efficacy, but several knowledgeable authors believe that hyperbaric oxygen therapy has contributed to dramatic clinical improvement. Such therapy may, however, be associated with untoward effects due to oxygen toxicity and high atmospheric pressure. Some centers without hyperbaric chambers have reported acceptable mortality rates; thus expert surgical and medical management and control of complications are probably the most important factors in the treatment of gas gangrene.

The treatment of *C. difficile*–associated colitis requires discontinuation of therapy with the offending antimicrobial agent. In some patients, symptoms will resolve over a period of 2 weeks if the infection is left untreated. However, specific therapy shortens the duration of symptoms.

The most widely used agent in the treatment of antibiotic-associated diarrhea ascribed to *C. difficile* is oral vancomycin. Most strains of *C. difficile* are susceptible to achievable concentrations of this agent. Vancomycin is poorly absorbed after oral administration and reaches high levels in the stool. The usual initial schedule is 125 mg orally four times a day for 7 to 10 days, but in cases of extremely severe disease the dose may be increased to 500 mg orally four times a day. A randomized trial comparing vancomycin with metronidazole demonstrated equal efficacy and relapse rates of 8 to 9 percent for the two regimens. The dose of metronidazole used was 250 mg four times a day, although 500 mg three times a day should be equally effective. Both because metronidazole is considerably less costly than vancomycin and because oral vancomycin has been implicated in the emergence of vancomycin-resistant enterococci, treatment should begin with metronidazole. If diarrhea persists, therapy should be changed to vancomycin. In patients with refractory symptoms and fever unresponsive to either regimen, the combination of rifampin with vancomycin has sometimes been beneficial. Since resistance to rifampin can develop, this agent should not be used alone.

A number of patients who respond to initial therapy present with a relapse of symptoms and a repeat positive toxin assay. Relapses following therapy are much more frequent than failures to respond to initial therapy. Most relapses occur 3 to 10 days after discontinuation of treatment. Most relapsing patients respond to a second course of antibiotics, but some go on to suffer multiple relapses. A number of options are available in this situation. Some patients have been shown to acquire a different strain of *C. difficile* despite the appearance of relapsing disease. These patients respond to a second course of the same agent used to treat the first episode. Alternatively, patients who receive vancomycin and who then have a relapse can be treated with metronidazole, and vice versa. Some authors report success with tapering regimens of vancomycin given daily or every other day for 1 to 2 months to avoid relapse. The resin cholestyramine binds the cytotoxin of *C. difficile* and has been used with some success to treat severe cases. Since cholestyramine also binds vancomycin, the two agents should not be used in combination. Repopulation of the normal colonic flora has also been tried in relapsing disease. Ingestion of capsules of the yeast *Saccharomyces boulardii* showed some promise in one trial. It appears that all of these regimens are effective in some cases but that no regimen is universally efficacious in relapsing disease.

BIBLIOGRAPHY

BARTLETT JG: *Clostridium difficile:* History of its role as an enteric pathogen and the current state of knowledge about the organism. Clin Infect Dis 18:S265, 1994

————: Antibiotic-associated diarrhea. Clin Infect Dis 15:573, 1992

————: Gas gangrene (other clostridium-associated diseases), in *Principles and Practice of Infectious Diseases,* 3d ed, GL Mandell et al (eds). New York, Churchill Livingstone, 1990

———— et al: Antibiotic-associated pseudomembranous colitis due to toxin-producing clostridia. N Engl J Med 298:531, 1978

BORRIELLO SP: Clostridial disease of the gut. Clin Infect Dis 20:S242, 1995

FINEGOLD SM: *Anaerobic Bacteria in Human Disease.* New York, Academic, 1977

————: Anaerobic infections and *Clostridium difficile* colitis emerging during antibacterial therapy. Scand J Infect Dis (Suppl) 49:160, 1986

GORBACH SL, THADEPALLI H: Isolation of *Clostridium* in human infections: Evaluation of 114 cases. J Infect Dis 131:S81, 1975

JENDRZEJEWSKI JW et al: Nontraumatic clostridial myonecrosis. Am J Med 65:542, 1978

JOHNSON S et al: Enteritis necroticans among Khmer children at an evacuation site in Thailand. Lancet 2:496, 1987

JUST I et al: Glucosylation of Rho proteins by *Clostridium difficile* toxin B. Nature 375:500, 1995

KORANSKY JR et al: *Clostridium septicum* bacteremia. Am J Med 66:63, 1979

KUROSE I et al: *Clostridium difficile* toxin A–induced microvascular dysfunction: Role of histamine. J Clin Invest 94:1919, 1994

PRITCHARD JA, WHALLEY PJ: Abortion complicated by *Clostridium perfringens* infection. Am J Gynecol 111:484, 1971

RIEGLER M et al: *Clostridium difficile* toxin B is more potent than toxin A in damaging human colonic epithelium in vitro. J Clin Invest 95:2004, 1995

SMITH LDS: Virulence factors of *Clostridium perfringens.* Rev Infect Dis 1:254, 1979

STEVENS DL et al: Comparison of clindamycin, rifampin, tetracycline, metronidazole, and penicillin for efficacy in prevention of experimental gas gangrene due to *Clostridium perfringens.* J Infect Dis 155:220, 1987

————: Effect of antibiotics on toxin production and viability of *Clostridium perfringens.* Antimicrob Agents Chemother 31:213, 1987

————: Comparison of single and combination antimicrobial agents for prevention of experimental gas gangrene caused by *Clostridium perfringens.* Antimicrob Agents Chemother 31:312, 1987

TEASLEY DG et al: Prospective, randomized trial of metronidazole versus vancomycin for *Clostridium difficile*–associated diarrhea and colitis. Lancet 2:1043, 1983

TIBBLES PM, EDELSBERG JS: Medical progress: Hyperbaric-oxygen therapy. N Engl J Med 334:1642, 1996

SECTION 6

DISEASES CAUSED BY GRAM-NEGATIVE BACTERIA

149 *Claus O. Solberg*

MENINGOCOCCAL INFECTIONS

DEFINITION *Neisseria meningitidis* can cause a variety of infections; bacteremia and meningitis are by far the most common. Meningococcal disease remains a worldwide problem and occurs sporadically, as localized outbreaks, or as widespread epidemics. The clinical manifestations are varied and range from transient bacteremia to fulminant disease culminating in death within hours of the onset of symptoms. Few, if any, infectious diseases rival severe meningococcemia in fulminance.

ETIOLOGIC AGENT *N. meningitidis* is a gram-negative diplococcus whose adjacent sides are flattened to produce its characteristic biscuit shape. The microorganism grows best on enriched media such as Mueller-Hinton or chocolate agar and at 37°C in an atmosphere of 5 to 10% CO_2. Because meningococci are highly susceptible to drying or chilling, cultures should be promptly inoculated and incubated. *Neisseria* spp. are differentiated by their ability to use sugars as sources of energy. Typically, meningococci use glucose and maltose and not sucrose or lactose.

In contrast to other neisseriae, meningococci are surrounded by a polysaccharide capsule. On the basis of antigenic differences among their capsular polysaccharides, the microorganisms are divided into at least 13 serogroups. Although encapsulated meningococci from all serogroups frequently colonize the nasopharynx and have the potential to cause systemic disease, more than 99 percent of meningococcal infections are caused by strains of serogroups A, B, C, 29E, W-135, and Y. The serogroups are further divided into serotypes, subtypes, and immunotypes according to differences in outer-membrane proteins and lipopolysaccharides (LPSs). In addition to being classified serologically, the meningococci are divided into clonal types based on characterization of the bacterial genome. These classification systems have been of great value for epidemiologic surveillance.

EPIDEMIOLOGY Meningococci are confined entirely to humans; the natural habitat of these bacteria is the nasopharynx. The organisms are presumably transmitted from person to person through the inhalation of droplets of infected nasopharyngeal secretions and by direct or indirect oral contact. In nonepidemic periods, the overall rate of nasopharyngeal carriage is about 10 percent but may approach 60 to 80 percent in closed populations, such as those at military recruit camps or schools. Rates of carriage are also high among family members and other close contacts of patients with meningococcal disease. Carriage usually persists for a few months; chronic carriage is not uncommon. Nasopharyngeal acquisition is followed by a rise in titers of specific serum antibodies to the colonizing strain, and colonization only rarely proceeds to disease. Observations during epidemics suggest that invasive meningococcal disease is most likely to occur within a few days of acquisition of a new strain, i.e., before the development of specific serum antibodies.

In temperate climates, the annual incidence of meningococcal infection is generally 1 to 2 cases per 100,000 population; the attack rate is highest in the first quarter of the year. Most infections occur among children 6 months to 3 years of age. The annual attack rate in this group is usually 10 to 15 cases per 100,000 population, with the peak incidence at 6 to 12 months of age. A second group at risk is the adolescent population between 14 and 20 years of age. As in infectious mononucleosis, the girls in this risk group who develop meningococcal infection are on average 2 years younger than the boys. In epidemics, the age distribution of the patients is shifted to older individuals, and more cases develop among individuals 3 to 20 years of age. When sporadic cases occur in families, the attack rate among household contacts may increase dramatically to 1 in 1000.

Major outbreaks of meningococcal disease are regularly reported from Africa, China, and South America. These epidemics may involve thousands of individuals and cause many deaths. Serogroup A meningococci are the primary cause of the epidemics. In the "meningitis belt" of sub-Saharan Africa, the incidence of meningococcal disease rises sharply towards the end of the dry and dusty season and falls with the onset of rains. It has been postulated that the presence of dust interferes with local IgA secretion in the nasopharynx, reducing host defenses against meningococci.

Serogroup A strains caused most outbreaks of meningococcal disease in Europe and the United States in the first half of the twentieth century. Since World War II, meningococci of serogroups B and C have become predominant. Currently, group B strains account for 50 percent of sporadic cases. Serogroup C strains have caused more infections in older age groups, and serogroup B strains have been especially common in very young children. Outbreaks occur more frequently among the poorest segments of the population, where overcrowding and poor sanitation are common.

PATHOGENESIS Meningococcal infection begins in the nasopharynx. Shortly after adherence to the nasopharyngeal mucosa, encapsulated meningococci are transported through nonciliated epithelial cells in large, membrane-bound phagocytic vacuoles. Within 24 h the microorganisms are observed in the submucosa in close proximity to local immune cells and blood vessels. In most instances, this nasopharyngeal infection is subclinical, but mild symptoms occasionally develop. After mucosal penetration and presumably a phase of adaptation, the bacteria may gain access to the circulation. In the vascular compartment, the invading meningococci either may be killed by the combined actions of serum bactericidal antibodies, complement, and phagocytic cells or may multiply, initiating the bacteremic stage. The symptoms and signs of systemic disease appear concurrently with meningococ-

cemia and usually precede symptoms of meningitis by 24 to 48 h. Meningococci are capable of replicating at an astonishing rate; within hours, a patient may deteriorate from good health to irreversible shock, marked hemorrhagic diathesis, and death.

Role of LPS Endotoxin (LPS) of the meningococcal outer membrane seems to play a central role in the development of severe disease. LPS is released into the circulation during multiplication and autolysis of meningococci, and a fair correlation has been established between LPS levels in plasma and disease severity: patients with minor symptoms have low or undetectable levels of LPS, while patients with fulminant meningococcemia have among the highest LPS levels detected in human plasma. In fulminant disease, major cascade systems associated with inflammation (including the coagulation, complement, fibrinolysis, and kallikrein-kinin systems) as well as the production of cytokines [tumor necrosis factor α (TNFα), interleukin (IL) 1, IL-6, IL-8, and IL-10] and nitric oxide are all triggered and upregulated simultaneously by native LPS. This dose-dependent inflammatory response results in marked vasodilation, reduced cardiac performance, platelet aggregation, disseminated intravascular coagulation (DIC), and capillary leak. The end results of these complicated processes are septic shock, adult respiratory distress syndrome, and multiple-organ failure (Chap. 124).

Although systemic meningococcal infection is primarily a bacteremic disease, *N. meningitidis* exhibits marked tropism for the meninges and skin and to a lesser degree for synovia, serosal surfaces, and adrenal glands. The most common clinical presentation is a composite of bacteremia and meningitis. Infection of the central nervous system may begin in the vicinity of the ependyma that lines the cerebral ventricles, subsequently spreading to the subarachnoid space. Meningococci appear to adhere readily to the cerebrovascular endothelium and (by yet poorly defined mechanisms) to penetrate the vessel walls. Later, the permeability of the blood-brain barrier may be further increased by locally produced inflammatory mediators such as TNFα, IL-1, and IL-6 induced by increasing levels of LPS in the cerebrospinal fluid (CSF). In patients with meningococcal meningitis, LPS levels in CSF are 100 to 1000 times higher than those in simultaneously collected plasma. This compartmentalized bacterial growth is also reflected in the higher CSF levels of bioactive TNFα, IL-1, IL-6, and IL-10 in patients with meningitis than in patients with septic shock or mild bacteremia.

Host Immunity The development of invasive disease is most dependent on host factors. Invasive meningococcal disease occurs almost exclusively in individuals who lack protective bactericidal antibodies to the infecting strain. Infants are protected from meningococcal disease for the first few months of life by passively transferred maternal antibodies and by a very low rate of meningococcal acquisition. As maternal antibodies are lost, susceptibility rises, peaking at 6 to 12 months; it then falls progressively as antibodies are acquired through colonization with closely related but nonpathogenic bacteria such as *N. lactamica*, avirulent *N. meningitidis*, or other bacteria expressing surface antigens in common with virulent meningococcal strains. *N. lactamica* colonizes the nasopharynx earlier during life than *N. meningitidis*, and colonized infants develop antibodies that prompt complement-mediated lysis and opsonophagocytosis of a broad spectrum of potentially pathogenic meningococci.

As children grow older, colonization with *N. meningitidis* gradually replaces that with *N. lactamica*, whose carriage is rare among teenagers. Colonization with *N. meningitidis* induces antibodies to the infecting strain and to other strains; thus naturally acquired immunity is reinforced and broadened. Many enteric bacteria have capsules or other antigens that are chemically similar to those of meningococci. Colonization with these unrelated yet immunologically similar bacteria may be important in the development of natural immunity to meningococci.

Immunologic Deficiencies The complement system plays a critical role in host defenses against invasive meningococcal disease, and activated complement brings about bacterial cell death by direct lysis or opsonophagocytosis. Occasional individuals who experience recurrent attacks of meningococcal disease have a high prevalence of a familial deficiency in a terminal complement component. This deficiency results in an inability to assemble the membrane attack complex (C5 to C9). The population prevalence of terminal complement-component deficiency is very low (about 0.03 percent), but approximately 50 percent of affected individuals experience an attack of meningococcal disease at some time. In these individuals the infection is usually mild and the mortality low. This milder illness may be due to intact opsonophagocytic mechanisms that do not require the terminal cascade and to diminished release of LPS from invading bacteria as a consequence of the host's inability to directly lyse bacteria in the serum. Patients with complement deficiency tend to be infected with strains of the less common W-135, X, Y, Z, and 29E serogroups. Several systemic diseases (e.g., systemic lupus erythematosus and membranoproliferative glomerulonephritis) can lead to secondary complement-component deficiencies and sporadic meningococcal disease.

Individuals with properdin deficiency, a sex-linked inherited disorder, have an intact classic complement pathway but impaired alternative pathway activation. More than half of the males in this group develop meningococcal disease, the course of which is frequently fulminant, with a case-fatality rate approaching 75 percent. Vaccination of properdin-deficient individuals is likely to reduce the risk of meningococcal disease as the generation of complement-fixing antibodies leads to the activation of complement via the classic pathway and to the consequent lysis and opsonophagocytosis of bacteria. Individuals with hypogammaglobulinemia, primary isolated IgM deficiency, and functional asplenia are also at increased risk of sporadic meningococcal disease, although pneumococcal infection is a more common complication in this group.

Other Risk Factors   An association between respiratory virus infections and meningococcal infection has been postulated. While infection with influenza A virus seems to predispose to meningococcal disease, this association appears to be less likely for other viral infections.

Reasons for epidemics of meningococcal disease are poorly understood. Overcrowding is clearly a prominent risk factor. Moreover, it has been suggested that epidemic meningococcal strains are clonal and that important surface structures vary cyclically, providing a new bacterial surface that allows evasion of host defense systems.

CLINICAL MANIFESTATIONS   *N. meningitidis* typically causes an acute infective illness, and more than 90 percent of the patients who become ill have meningococcemia and/or meningitis. A sequential development of clinical manifestations can be discerned, the usual sequence consisting of initial infection of the upper respiratory tract followed by meningococcemia, meningitis, and less common focal manifestations.

Upper Respiratory Tract Infection   The portal of entry of meningococci is the nasopharynx. Most patients are asymptomatic or report fever alone before the onset of systemic manifestations. Some patients with invasive meningococcal disease describe mild prodromal symptoms of sore throat, rhinorrhea, cough, headache, and conjunctivitis in the week before hospital admission. Whether these manifestations are due to infection with the meningococcus or with other microorganisms that may facilitate meningococcal invasion is not known.

Meningococcemia   Between 30 and 40 percent of patients with meningococcal disease have meningococcemia without clinical signs of meningitis. The clinical manifestations vary from minor symptoms of transient bacteremia to fulminating disease of a few hours' duration. The onset is usually sudden, with fever, chills, nausea, vomiting, rash, myalgia, and arthralgia. Fever, usually between 39 and 41°C, is almost universal, although occasional patients with fulminant disease may be afebrile or even hypothermic. Most patients suffer from nausea and vomiting and are distressed. One-third of patients have myalgias and/or arthralgias. The most striking feature is rash, which develops in

three-fourths of patients and may be maculopapular, petechial, or ecchymotic. The maculopapular rash appears soon after the onset of disease; the lesions are pink, 2 to 10 mm in diameter, and sparsely distributed on the trunk and extremities. Often petechiae appear in the center of the macules. The rash may progress within hours to become hemorrhagic as the general condition of the patient deteriorates. The petechial lesions are 1 to 2 mm in diameter and are distributed mainly on the trunk and lower extremities but also on the face, palate, and conjunctivae. In relatively severe cases, petechiae may become confluent and develop into hemorrhagic bullae, with extensive ulcerations. Widespread petechial eruption, hypotension, reduced peripheral circulation, and lack of meningism are all indicators of poor prognosis. Ecchymoses and fulminant purpuric rash are common among patients with fulminant meningococcemia.

Fulminant meningococcemia, previously called Waterhouse-Friderichsen syndrome, differs from the milder form in its rapid progression and overwhelming character. It occurs in 10 to 20 percent of patients with meningococcal disease and is characterized by the development of shock, DIC, and multiple-organ failure. The onset is abrupt; purpuric lesions, hypotension, and peripheral vasoconstriction with cold cyanotic extremities frequently develop within hours. The state of consciousness is variable, but many patients remain alert despite hypotension. The purpuric lesions enlarge rapidly and involve skin, mucous membranes, and internal organs such as skeletal muscle, adrenal glands, and occasionally the pituitary gland. Myocardial depression contributing to shock is evidenced by impaired myocardial contractility, lowered cardiac index, increased wedge pressure, and elevated serum levels of creatinine phosphokinase. Metabolic acidosis, serum electrolyte derangement, oliguria, leukopenia, and low levels of coagulation factors are common. Despite advanced intensive care management, 50 to 60 percent of patients die, usually from cardiac and/or respiratory failure. Patients who recover may have severe skin lesions necessitating plastic surgery or loss of parts of limbs due to gangrene.

Chronic meningococcemia makes up only 1 to 2 percent of all cases of meningococcal disease. This syndrome of recurrent fever, maculopapular rash, and arthralgia may last for weeks to months. The rash may also be petechial. During afebrile periods, patients appear remarkably well. Failure to diagnose and treat chronic meningococcemia may result in the development of systemic disease.

Meningitis   Meningitis is frequently associated with meningococcemia; in patients with systemic disease, the onset of meningitis may be inapparent. However, most patients with meningitis soon develop symptoms of meningeal inflammation, including severe headache, confusion, lethargy, and vomiting. Signs of meningeal irritation are present in most but not all cases. The symptoms and signs associated with meningococcal meningitis cannot be differentiated from those associated with meningitis due to other organisms (see Chap. 377). Infants present particularly often with nonspecific symptoms and without localizing signs, although they may have a tense, bulging fontanelle. Meningitis may also occur without specific signs in elderly patients or in those with fulminant meningococcemia. As the infection advances, lethargy may progress to coma, and seizures, cranial nerve palsies, and hemiparesis or other focal neurologic signs may appear.

Less Common Manifestations   A number of less common manifestations of meningococcal infections have been reported. These include arthritis, pneumonia, sinusitis, otitis media, conjunctivitis, endophthalmitis, endocarditis, pericarditis, urethritis, and endometritis. Arthritis occurs in 5 to 10 percent of patients and may develop at any stage of the acute illness. Large joints are most commonly affected, particularly the knee. Meningococci are infrequently isolated from the synovial fluid, and the majority of cases, especially when arthritis develops after the initiation of therapy, are immunologically mediated. Sequelae are rare. Primary meningococcal pneumonia is well recognized, particularly in association with serogroup Y strains. The clinical syndrome is similar to that of other bacterial pneumonias. Since the introduction of antibiotics, endocarditis and pericarditis have become very unusual features of acute meningococcal disease.

Complications The complications of meningococcal infections include intercurrent infections and damage to the central nervous system. Most pyogenic complications have become uncommon. However, superinfection of the respiratory tract with microorganisms other than meningococci may develop, particularly during assisted ventilation of seriously ill patients. Neurologic complications may result from direct infection of brain parenchyma (cerebritis or brain abscess), injury to cranial nerves as they pass through the inflamed meninges, venous or arterial infarction (seizures, focal deficits), cerebral edema (raised intracranial pressure), interruption of CSF pathways (hydrocephalus), or effusions into the subdural space producing mass effects. Nonetheless, permanent neurologic sequelae are infrequent, occurring in fewer than 5 percent of survivors of acute meningococcal meningitis. As in other severe infections, herpes labialis is prevalent in the acute stage of meningococcal disease.

LABORATORY FINDINGS Meningococci usually can be isolated from blood and CSF of patients with meningococcal disease and occasionally are found in petechial aspirate and synovial, pleural, or pericardial fluid. The growth of meningococci in blood culture bottles can be inhibited by sodium polyanetholesulfonate, a frequent additive to media. Gram-negative diplococci may be demonstrated in CSF, petechiae, or buffy coat smears from at least half of patients. Group-specific capsular polysaccharides can be detected in CSF, synovial fluid, serum, or urine by counterimmunoelectrophoresis or latex agglutination assays. However, these tests give false-negative results in 50 percent of culture-proven cases. The combined use of cultures, gram-stained smears, and immunoassays will provide a diagnosis in more than 95 percent of cases. The immunoassays may be particularly useful in situations where cultures are of limited value because of prior antibiotic administration. The polymerase chain reaction (PCR) may also be a valuable tool in these situations. CSF examinations indicate that the specificity and sensitivity of PCR for the diagnosis of meningococcal meningitis are at least 90 percent. A specific antibody response during convalescence may also be diagnostic.

Other laboratory data offer limited support in the diagnosis of meningococcal disease. Elevated counts of polymorphonuclear leukocytes with a left shift are common, but normal counts are not unusual. Patients with fulminant meningococcemia usually have neutropenia and markedly reduced platelet counts; prothrombin and partial thromboplastin times are prolonged, plasma fibrinogen levels are diminished, and fibrinogen degradation product titers are elevated as a result of DIC (see Chap. 124). Decreased P_{CO_2} and metabolic acidosis secondary to tissue hypoperfusion are frequent. CSF findings in meningitis include increased pressure, increased protein content, low glucose concentrations, and (in most cases) 100 to 20,000 polymorphonuclear leukocytes per microliter (see Chap. 377).

DIAGNOSIS Meningococcal infections in their early stages may resemble any acute systemic infection, including influenza or another common viral infection, and the distinction between the latter infections and early meningococcemia may be most difficult. In contrast to the prevalence of neurologic symptoms in meningococcal meningitis, the lack of such symptoms in meningococcemia may prevent early recognition of this severe form of meningococcal disease. However, early in meningococcal disease there is often a generalized, mottled erythema or a light pink maculopapular rash resembling the rose spots of typhoid fever. By careful examination of the patient, the physician can detect these lesions and establish a presumptive diagnosis. As the disease progresses, a petechial or purpuric rash usually develops, and the diagnosis becomes more obvious. The rash seen in some common viral exanthems, *Mycoplasma* infection, Rocky Mountain spotted fever, endemic typhus, and vascular purpura may be confused with that of meningococcemia. In the absence of rash or other manifestations of bacteremia, meningococcal meningitis is indistinguishable from meningitis caused by other pathogens (see Chap. 377). The ultimate diagnosis of meningococcal disease depends on the recovery of *N. meningitidis* or the detection of its antigens in various body fluids or petechial aspirates. Isolation of meningococci from the nasopharynx only confirms the carrier state and cannot be used alone to establish the diagnosis of systemic infection.

TREATMENT

Despite the availability of potent antibiotics and advances in intensive care management, overall mortality from meningococcal disease is about 10 percent, rising to as high as 50 to 60 percent among patients with meningococcemia and shock. To improve the prognosis, early diagnosis and treatment are of utmost importance, particularly in patients with meningococcemia. Any febrile patient with a petechial rash should be considered to have meningococcal infection. Blood for cultures should be taken immediately and treatment begun without awaiting confirmation. If the patient is not initially seen in the hospital, intravenous penicillin G (60,000 to 100,000 units per kilogram) should be given and the patient immediately admitted. In the outpatient setting, if vascular access is problematic, antibiotics can be given intramuscularly (at several injection sites in light of the large volume). If the patient is first seen in the hospital, intravenous access should be established immediately, blood obtained for cultures, and antibiotics administered as soon as possible. Initiation of therapy in patients with signs of circulatory insufficiency or rapid deterioration in cerebral condition should not await lumbar puncture.

Antibiotics Penicillin G remains the drug of choice for meningococcal disease. Prior to the identification of the etiologic agent, the choice of antibiotics depends upon the age of the patient, the status of the patient's underlying host-defense system, and the prevalence of antimicrobial resistance in the community. *Streptococcus pneumoniae* as well as *Haemophilus influenzae* and other gram-negative bacteria may cause a clinical picture similar to that of meningococcal infection. The third-generation cephalosporins cefotaxime and ceftriaxone are recommended as empiric therapy. Although mortality and long-term morbidity among patients given cephalosporins for the treatment of meningococcal disease are similar to those among patients treated with penicillin, the cephalosporins are preferred because of their high level of activity against other common meningeal pathogens, including most penicillin-resistant pneumococci; their excellent penetration into the CSF; their lack of toxicity; and the convenience of using a single agent that can be administered three times daily (cefotaxime) or once or twice daily (ceftriaxone).

As part of their empiric regimen, patients undergoing immunosuppressive therapy, newborns, and the elderly should receive high-dose penicillin to cover *Listeria monocytogenes*. The cephalosporins are also highly active against *N. meningitidis* strains with reduced sensitivity to penicillin. Such strains have been reported from several countries and have been described especially often in reports from South Africa and Spain. The usual daily dosage of cefotaxime is 150 to 200 mg/kg intravenously up to a maximum daily dosage of 12 g; that of ceftriaxone is 75 to 100 mg/kg intravenously up to a maximum daily dosage of 5 g. Once meningococci have been isolated and shown to be sensitive to penicillin G, the therapeutic regimen can be changed to penicillin G. Chloramphenicol is as effective as penicillin G for the treatment of meningococcal disease and can be used in patients allergic to penicillins or cephalosporins. The usual daily dosage of penicillin G is 200,000 to 300,000 units per kilogram intravenously in divided doses every 6 h up to a maximum daily dosage of 24 million units; that of chloramphenicol is 75 to 100 mg/kg intravenously in divided doses every 6 h up to a maximum daily dosage of 4 g. A 7-day course of high-dose parenteral therapy is adequate for both meningococcal meningitis and meningococcemia. The dose should not be tapered over the course of therapy.

Supportive Care The course of meningococcal disease is highly unpredictable. All patients with invasive meningococcal infection, whatever their clinical condition on admission, should be considered to have potentially life-threatening infection and should be carefully observed during the first 48 h in the hospital, with monitoring of arterial blood pressure, pulse, perfusion, urine output, and core and peripheral temperature. Many patients who do not appear acutely ill on admission may deteriorate suddenly in the following hours, with the development of severe shock and profound DIC. Patients with a rapidly progressive purpuric rash, a low peripheral white cell count, and no evidence of meningeal involvement are likely to deteriorate very soon after admission.

The most important manifestation requiring urgent intervention is severe meningococcemia with shock. Patients with this form of meningococcal disease have a severe capillary leak syndrome and myocardial dysfunction. Strategies to reverse circulatory failure include optimizing preload, decreasing afterload, and improving myocardial contractility. Intravenous fluid administration together with ionotropic support with dobutamine (1 to 10 μg/kg per minute) or dopamine (2 to 10 μg/kg per minute) should be started immediately and tailored to the needs of each patient on the basis of clinical assessment and of monitoring of systemic arterial pressure and central venous or pulmonary wedge pressure (see Chap. 38). Vasodilators should be administered with extreme caution to patients with severe shock. In marked tissue edema in adults, the administration of as much as 8 to 10 L of intravenous fluid may be necessary during the first 24 h. Because the risk of pulmonary edema is considerable, patients in severe shock should be electively ventilated, even if they are ventilating adequately. Several controlled studies of patients with septic shock have demonstrated no beneficial effect of high-dose glucocorticoid treatment. Although these studies have included only small numbers of patients with meningococcemia, a beneficial effect of glucocorticoids in fulminant meningococcemia seems unlikely.

Some patients present in profound respiratory failure, even if they have not received intravenous fluid. Such patients should be ventilated immediately to prevent acute respiratory collapse. Adult respiratory distress syndrome is heralded by an increase in oxygen requirement and a reduction of pulmonary compliance and tends to follow initial resuscitation and correction of hypovolemia. Management in this situation depends on measures to improve myocardial function, assisted ventilation, and removal of extravascular fluid (if necessary, by dialysis).

Patients with severe meningococcemia usually have a complex derangement of serum electrolytes, acid-base balance, and metabolism. Metabolic acidosis is a result of poor tissue perfusion in shock. Serum electrolytes and acid-base balance should be measured frequently and abnormalities corrected immediately. Correction is often hampered by oliguria or anuria, and dialysis is often required. Because dialysis is a highly effective means of reducing extravascular fluid accumulation and correcting electrolytic and metabolic derangements, it should be instituted early in patients with severe meningococcemia. Continuous plasma filtration or dialysis may also be necessary in proximal tubular necrosis due to meningococcal disease.

Virtually all patients with severe meningococcemia have marked DIC. Routine heparinization for patients with DIC has failed to improve prognosis and is not recommended. However, in patients with impending peripheral gangrene and severe coagulopathy, the administration of low-dose heparin (10 units/kg per hour) together with fresh frozen plasma may be tried. The administration of large quantities of fresh frozen plasma may also restore depleted levels of antithrombin III, protein C, and protein S.

Brain damage in bacterial meningitis may result in part from cytokines produced in the inflammatory response to bacterial products, and the reduction of brain injury by anti-inflammatory agents has been demonstrated in animals. In studies of children with *H. influenzae* meningitis, dexamethasone has significantly reduced the severity of neurologic sequelae, particularly deafness. Firm conclusions on the efficacy of dexamethasone in reducing neurologic sequelae in meningococcal meningitis cannot be derived from these studies, and the use of this agent in meningococcal meningitis remains controversial (see Chap. 377).

Symptom-based treatment of raised intracranial pressure is best administered in an intensive care setting. Elevation of the head to 30°, modest hyperventilation, and fluid restriction may be useful. Infusion of mannitol (0.25 to 1 g/kg) results in a rapid shift of fluid from the extravascular to the intravascular space and may be associated with a prompt reduction of intracranial pressure. In patients whose condition is unstable, insertion of an intracranial pressure monitor may aid in the management of this complication of meningitis. Airway obstruction, cardiac insufficiency, and convulsions may lead to hypoxia, impaired brain perfusion, and enhanced cerebral edema. Measures to optimize respiration and cardiac output and to control convulsions also are important in reducing intracranial pressure.

A number of experimental forms of therapy, including the use of monoclonal antibodies to endotoxin, TNFα, IL-1, and leukocyte adhesion molecules, have shown promise in animal models of meningitis or septic shock. The results of clinical trials have been less promising, but several trials are still in progress.

PROGNOSIS Meningococcal disease was usually fatal before the antibiotic era. After the introduction of antibiotics, overall mortality declined to 10 to 15 percent and has remained at about 10 percent despite early appropriate chemotherapy and advances in intensive care management. The mortality rate is less than 5 percent among patients with meningococcal meningitis but can be as high as 50 to 60 percent among patients with fulminant meningococcemia, primarily because these patients are often in severe shock when admitted to the hospital. Most deaths from fulminant meningococcemia occur within 24 to 48 h of admission. Permanent sequelae of meningococcal meningitis, including deafness, cranial nerve paralysis, and mental deficiency, are uncommon.

PREVENTION Attack rates are approximately 100-fold higher among household contacts of patients with meningococcal disease than in the general population. The risk is highest in the first week after the index case has presented with infection. Chemoprophylaxis helps avert secondary cases of infection and should be administered to intimate contacts in the household, day-care center, and nursery school and also to anyone who has had oral contact with the index case (kissing, mouth-to-mouth resuscitation). The recommended regimen for prophylaxis consists of rifampin at a dosage of 10 mg/kg (up to 600 mg) every 12 h for 2 days for adults and children over 1 year of age and 5 mg/kg every 12 h for 2 days for children less than 1 year old. Ciprofloxacin or ofloxacin (a single oral dose of 500 or 400 mg, respectively) is a suitable alternative for adults but is not recommended for children or pregnant women. A single 250-mg intramuscular dose of ceftriaxone is recommended for pregnant contacts; for children less than 12 years of age, 125 mg of ceftriaxone can be given.

Vaccines are available against four serogroups of meningococci: A, C, W-135, and Y. No effective serogroup B vaccine is presently available. The efficacy rate of a single dose of serogroup A or serogroup C vaccine is at least 90 percent in adults and children over 2 years of age, and routine immunization of recruits has eliminated nearly all disease among military personnel. To prevent late secondary cases, close contacts of patients with sporadic disease caused by strains of serogroup A or C should receive a single dose of polysaccharide vaccine. Travelers to areas where disease is epidemic as well as individuals with splenic dysfunction or deficiencies in complement or properdin should be immunized. Conjugate serogroup A and serogroup C vaccines have been developed and are now undergoing clinical trials. If these vaccines provide young infants with long-lasting protection, they may be used in outbreak management as well as in routine infant-immunization programs. Serogroup B vaccines are also being developed.

BIBLIOGRAPHY

BRANDTZAEG P: Pathogenesis of meningococcal infections, in *Meningococcal Disease*, K Cartwright (ed). Chichester, John Wiley, 1995, pp 71–114

CARTWRIGHT K: Meningococcal carriage and disease, in *Meningococcal Disease*, K Cartwright (ed). Chichester, John Wiley, 1995, pp 115–146

DENSEN P et al: Familial properdin deficiency and fatal meningococcemia: Correction of the bactericidal defect by vaccination. N Engl J Med 316:922, 1987

FRASCH CE: Meningococcal vaccines: Past, present and future, in *Meningococcal Disease*, K Cartwright (ed). Chichester, John Wiley, 1995, pp 245–283

GRIFFISS JM: Mechanisms of host immunity, in *Meningococcal Disease*, K Cartwright (ed). Chichester, John Wiley, 1995, pp 35–70

GUTTORMSEN H-K et al: Cross-reacting serum opsonins in patients with meningococcal disease. Infect Immun 60:2777, 1992

HALSTENSEN A et al: Case fatality of meningococcal disease in western Norway. Scand J Infect Dis 19:35, 1987

LYNN WA, COHEN J: Adjunctive therapy of septic shock: A review of experimental approaches. Clin Infect Dis 20:143, 1995

NAESS A et al: Sequelae one year after meningococcal disease. Acta Neurol Scand 89:139, 1994

PARILLO JE: Pathogenetic mechanisms of septic shock. N Engl J Med 328:1471, 1993

ROSS SC et al: Killing of *Neisseria meningitidis* by human neutrophils: Implications for normal and complement-deficient individuals. J Infect Dis 155:1266, 1987

SCHILDKAMP RL et al: Clinical manifestations and course of meningococcal disease in 562 patients. Scand J Infect Dis 28:47, 1996

---

150 *King K. Holmes, Stephen A. Morse*

GONOCOCCAL INFECTIONS

DEFINITION Gonorrhea, an infection of columnar and transitional epithelium caused by *Neisseria gonorrhoeae*, is the most common reportable communicable disease in the United States. Anatomic sites that can be infected directly by the gonococcus include the urethra, rectum, conjunctiva, pharynx, and endocervix. Local complications include endometritis, salpingitis, peritonitis, perihepatitis, and bartholinitis in the female and periurethral abscess and epididymitis in the male. Systemic manifestations of gonoccemia include arthritis, dermatitis, endocarditis, and meningitis as well as myopericarditis and hepatitis.

ETIOLOGIC AGENT *N. gonorrhoeae* is a gram-negative coccus usually found in pairs with flattened adjacent sides. It forms oxidase-positive colonies and is differentiated from other *Neisseria* species by its ability to utilize glucose but not maltose, sucrose, or lactose; by nucleic acid probes; and by specific immunologic reactions.

Organisms present in colonies examined within 20 h of inoculation from clinical specimens are covered by fimbriae (*pili*). Pili mediate attachment to various epithelial cells and interfere with neutrophil phagocytosis. Each pilus is composed of repeating peptide (*pilin*) subunits, which have a molecular weight of about 20,000. The pilin subunits consist of conserved and variable regions. Pili undergo both antigenic and phase variation. Chromosomal rearrangements, leading to expression of any one of a large number of incomplete (silent) pilin genes, lead to *antigenic variation* in pili. If the rearrangement involves a defective pilin gene, piliated gonococci (pil⁺) produce nonpiliated variants (pil⁻), a process known as *phase variation*. Piliated organisms cause infection and urethritis after inoculation into the urethras of male volunteers, whereas nonpiliated organisms do not. Binding to epithelial cells requires the presence of another phase-variable protein, PilC, which is located at the tip of the pili. Antigenic variation of pilin subunits may allow gonococci to attach to different types of epithelial surfaces and to evade the

host's antibody response to pilin. Phase variation from pil⁺ to pil⁻ may permit gonococcal detachment and facilitate spread. The synthesis of pilin is essential for competence in transformation of *N. gonorrhoeae*. Genetic transformation presumably is responsible for recombination between chromosomal genes of different gonococcal lineages.

The trilaminar outer-membrane of the gonococcus contains several classes of proteins, including proteins I, II, and III, and lipopolysaccharide (LPS) (Fig. 150-1). Like pili, protein II [now referred to as *opacity-associated outer-membrane proteins* (OPAs)] is thought to function as a ligand, mediating the attachment of gonococci to various types of human cells. An individual gonococcus can possess about a dozen OPA genes and can express zero to three or more OPAs at a time. Gonococci possessing certain OPAs adhere to and are phagocytosed by human neutrophils in the absence of serum. Certain OPAs may be responsible for the clumping of gonococci that is so evident on Gram-stained smears of urethral exudate.

Opaque colonies contain organisms that express OPAs and predominate in isolates from the male urethra and in cervical isolates obtained from women in midcycle. Transparent colonies often lack OPAs and predominate in cervical isolates obtained from women during menses and in isolates from blood, synovial fluid, or fallopian tubes.

From a quantitative point of view, protein I is the major outer-membrane protein; it exhibits intrastrain differences in molecular mass, with variation between 34.6 and 37.7 kDa. Protein I molecules associate in a trimeric structure, forming anion-selective transmembrane channels (*porins*) that permit the exchange of hydrophilic molecules through the outer membrane. Protein I also interacts with other outer-membrane components, such as protein III and LPS, to form complex outer-membrane structures. Protein I molecules have been shown to move rapidly from gonococcal outer membranes to the more fluid cytoplasmic membrane of human cells, where they form pores. This process may initiate endocytosis of the gonococcus, the first step in gonococcal invasion of the epithelium.

The LPS of the gonococcus contains lipid A and an oligosaccharide. Features that distinguish gonococcal LPS from enteric LPS are the highly branched oligosaccharide structure and the absence of repeating O-antigen subunits; thus gonococcal LPS is often referred to as *lipooligosaccharide* (LOS). Gonococcal LOS exhibits antigenic variation, which may be a mechanism for evading host defenses. The type of LOS produced can be altered by a mechanism that is not well understood but is thought to have to do with transcriptional regulation

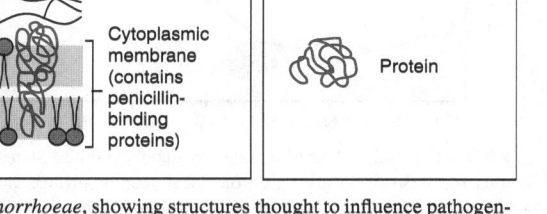

FIGURE 150-1 Diagram of the envelope of *N. gonorrhoeae*, showing structures thought to influence pathogenesis, antimicrobial susceptibility, and antigenicity.

of glycosyltransferases involved in LOS biosynthesis. Host-derived cytidine monophospho-*N*-acetylneuraminic acid can be used by gonococci to sialylate the oligosaccharide component of a LOS. This sialylation results in the conversion of a serum-sensitive organism into one that is serum-resistant and markedly reduces nonopsonic interactions of OPA-expressing gonococci with human neutrophils. The fact that gonococci observed in urethral exudate are sialylated indicates that sialylation occurs in vivo. Recent structural and immunochemical analyses of gonococcal LOS have revealed that the antigenicity and immunogenicity of the LOS is complex, in part because of the structural similarity of the oligosaccharide to host glycosphingolipids. No capsular polysaccharide has been isolated, but high-molecular-weight surface polyphosphates that may have functions similar to those of capsular polysaccharides in other organisms have been demonstrated.

For the past decade, gonococcal strains have been typed for epidemiologic studies on the basis of nutritional requirements (*auxotyping*) or antigenic differences of protein I (*serotyping*). Unlike pili and protein II, the protein I expressed by any single strain of gonococcus is antigenically stable, although there is considerable antigenic heterogeneity of protein I between strains. There are two structurally related forms of protein I, known as IA and IB; individual strains contain either but not both. Protein IA and IB genes are alleles of the same gene. Monoclonal antibodies to different epitopes of protein IA and protein IB can be used to classify gonococci into a large number of serovariants, known as serovars IA1 to IA24 and IB1 to IB32. In most populations, only a limited number of auxotype/serovar classes account for the majority of isolates. New techniques based on DNA polymorphism [e.g., restriction fragment length polymorphism (RFLP)] or OPA typing permit enhanced discrimination.

EPIDEMIOLOGY The only natural hosts for *N. gonorrhoeae* are humans. In the United States, the annual age-specific incidence rates tripled from 1963 to 1975, when more than 1 million cases were reported and an equal number probably went unreported. During this period of epidemic gonorrhea, the incidence increased fastest among young white females. As shown in Fig. 150-2, the reported incidence of gonorrhea has decreased from a peak of 473 cases per 100,000 in 1975 to about 150 per 100,000 in 1995—approximately the same incidence as when the epidemic began 30 years ago. Nonetheless, this incidence is unsurpassed by that of any other industrialized country. For example, it is 50 times higher than the incidence of 3 per 100,000 in 1995 in Sweden, which has essentially eliminated endemic transmission of gonorrhea.

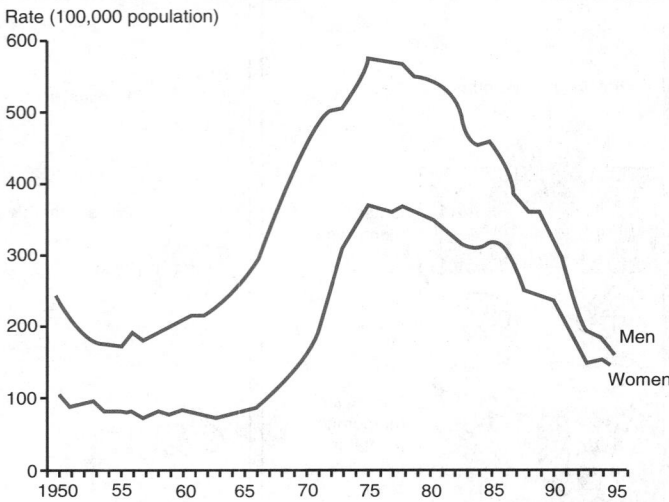

FIGURE 150-2 Gonorrhea rates by gender: United States, 1950–1995. Figures for 1950–1955 are based on fiscal-year reporting; those for 1956–1995 are based on calendar-year reporting. (*Unpublished data courtesy of Russell Roegner, Centers for Disease Control and Prevention, Atlanta.*)

Gonorrhea incidence and prevalence rates are known to be related to age, sex, sexual preference, race, socioeconomic status, marital status, residential setting (urban, suburban, rural), and level of education—risk factors that influence sexual behavior, illness-related behavior, and accessibility of health care. Among sexually active individuals, the rates are highest in teenagers, in nonwhites, in the poor and poorly educated, in residents of large cities, and in unmarried persons—particularly those who live alone. Many such individuals make up a core group of "efficient transmitters" who play a disproportionate role in the spread of gonorrhea. The incidence of gonorrhea has continued to fall among white and Hispanic men and women since 1985 and has declined among black men and women since 1990. Beginning in the mid-1980s and continuing through the mid-1990s, gonorrhea, like syphilis and chancroid, has been associated with the "crack" cocaine epidemic and with the exchange of sex by women for illegal drugs such as cocaine. The incidence of gonorrhea is higher among men than among women, while the prevalence is higher among women. Routine testing by endocervical culture or newer methods is still advocated for gonorrhea case detection in asymptomatic young women who are considered to be at high risk because of their sexual behavior or the demographic factors cited above. Outreach to such women in selected settings, such as teen clinics, juvenile detention centers, jails, and drug treatment centers, remains most productive and often involves combined testing for gonorrhea and chlamydial infection. However, as the incidence and prevalence of gonorrhea continue to fall, greater reliance should be placed on partner notification (contact tracing) than on routine endocervical tests, which are expensive and often do not focus on the individuals most likely to transmit the infection. The single most important axiom about the epidemiology of this disease is that *gonorrhea is usually spread by carriers who have developed no symptoms or have ignored symptoms*. Symptomatic patients, male or female, have usually been recently infected by such carriers, who must in turn be traced and treated to prevent further transmission. *Men and women with symptomatic gonorrhea should always be interviewed to identify their recent sexual contacts, who should be examined and treated if infected.*

There are interesting regional differences in the antibiotic resistance of *N. gonorrhoeae*. In 1976, penicillinase-producing strains of *N. gonorrhoeae* (PPNG) that were completely resistant to penicillin and ampicillin appeared almost simultaneously in West Africa and Asia. PPNG first became established and then spread in areas of the world where prostitution is exceptionally common and where access to subcurative antimicrobial therapy is unrestricted. PPNG now account for 50 percent or more of all gonococci in many areas of Africa, Asia, and Latin America and have become well established in many regions of the United States and Europe. Plasmid-borne penicillin resistance results from the presence of a TEM-1-type β-lactamase gene on one of five small R factors that make up a very closely related family of plasmids. Plasmid-borne tetracycline resistance results from the introduction of the streptococcal resistance determinant *tetM* into *N. gonorrhoeae*, where it resides on a plasmid derived in part from a gonococcal conjugative plasmid. This plasmid is self-transmissible and retains the capacity to mobilize some of the β-lactamase plasmids. Strains of *N. gonorrhoeae* with tetracycline resistance plasmids (TRNG) are clinically resistant to tetracycline, minocycline, and doxycycline. Strains possessing both penicillin and tetracycline resistance plasmids are now widespread; one or both of these two types of plasmid were present in about 14 percent of gonococcal isolates in the United States by 1994 (Fig. 150-3). Of equal importance has been the spread of gonococci with chromosomally mediated resistance to penicillin and tetracycline, referred to as chromosomally mediated resistant *N. gonorrhoeae* (CMRNG). Overall, one-third of U.S. gonococcal strains are resistant to penicillin and/or tetracycline. Recently, strains with high-level fluoroquinolone resistance have been reported from Australia, Hong Kong, the Philippines, the United Kingdom, and the United States. Resistance to fluoroquinolones is not yet widespread in the United States. Auxotyping, monoclonal antibody serotyping, and RFLP analysis have shown that in a midsized metropolitan city, as many as 60 to 100 different gonococcal strains are circulating, and

FIGURE 150-3 Antimicrobial resistance in *N. gonorrhoeae*. PPNG, penicillinase-producing *N. gonorrhoeae* (plasmid-mediated); TRNG, tetracycline-resistant *N. gonorrhoeae* [minimal inhibitory concentration (MIC), ≥ 16 μg/mL; presumably plasmid-mediated]; PP/TR, penicillinase-producing and tetracycline-resistant *N. gonorrhoeae*; CMR-PEN, chromosomal resistance to penicillin (MIC, ≥ 2 μg/mL); CMR-TET, chromosomal resistance to tetracycline (MIC, 2.0–8.0 μg/mL); CMR-PEN/TET, chromosomal resistance to penicillin and tetracycline; CIP-DS, decreased susceptibility to ciprofloxacin (MIC, ≥ 0.125–0.5 μg/mL; two isolates with MICs of 4.0 and 8.0 μg/mL, respectively). [*U.S. CDC Gonococcal Isolate Surveillance Project 1994 (5000 isolates). Courtesy of Kimberly Fox and W. L. Whittington.*]

new strains are being continuously introduced. Against this background, local outbreaks of infection due to PPNG, TRNG, CMRNG, or strains with high-level fluoroquinolone resistance belonging to a single auxotype-serovar class have been identified. Public health efforts have at times been successfully focused on the control of such strains.

Recent epidemiologic studies have shown interesting relationships between gonorrhea and human immunodeficiency virus (HIV) infection. Gonorrhea in female prostitutes has been associated with increased susceptibility to HIV infection; gonococcal urethritis has been related to increased shedding of cell-free HIV in the seminal plasma and of cell-associated HIV in the urethral exudate of HIV-seropositive men; in both instances, shedding is eliminated or decreased by treatment and cure of the urethritis. HIV infection in prostitutes has been associated with both increased risk of gonococcal reinfection and increased risk of clinical signs of salpingitis when gonococcal infection occurs.

IMMUNOLOGY AND PATHOGENESIS Epidemiologic data suggest that only about one-third of men become infected after a single exposure to *N. gonorrhoeae*; under experimental conditions an inoculum of about 10^3 organisms appears necessary to establish urethral infection in 50 percent of male volunteers. Various gonococcal virulence factors influence the size of the inoculum required. Factors that may confer resistance to infection remain undefined. However, components of the urethral or vaginal flora, such as *Candida albicans*, *Staphylococcus epidermidis*, and certain types of lactobacilli, can inhibit *N. gonorrhoeae* in vitro and may provide some natural resistance in vivo.

In humans, most extracellular iron is bound by the major iron-binding proteins transferrin and lactoferrin. The resulting concentration of free iron (10^{-18} M) is far too low to support gonococcal growth. Under these iron-limiting conditions, gonococci produce iron-repressible proteins that help remove iron from transferrin and lactoferrin. Gonococci bind only human transferrin and lactoferrin. This specificity may explain why gonococci in nature infect only humans. *N. gonorrhoeae* presumably competes with the lactoferrin present at mucosal surfaces for the iron required for growth of the organism. Gonococcal strains requiring arginine, hypoxanthine, and uracil for growth (AHU auxotype) are generally unable to remove iron from lactoferrin;

this inability may in part explain the tendency of such strains to cause asymptomatic mucosal infections.

Gonococci infect mucus-secreting epithelial surfaces, and mucus may be a physical barrier or a competitive inhibitor. Pili and protein II partially mediate the attachment of gonococci to mucosal cells. Local antibody to pili or protein II can partially block attachment. Pili also impede phagocytosis of gonococci by neutrophils, and antibody to pili (as well as antibody to protein II) is opsonic. An enzyme produced by the pathogenic neisseriae—IgA1 protease, which inactivates sIgA1—may interfere with IgA-mediated antiadherence activity, resulting in increased attachment.

After attachment to columnar or transitional epithelium, gonococci penetrate through or between cells to reach the subepithelial connective tissue. Transfer of gonococcal protein I into the host cell may initiate endocytosis into the epithelial cell. Gonococcal LOS produces mucosal damage in fallopian tube organ cultures. Recent evidence suggests that gonococcal LOS stimulates the production of tumor necrosis factor in fallopian tube organ cultures; inhibition of tumor necrosis factor with specific antiserum prevents tissue damage. Peptidoglycan fragments also damage the fallopian tube mucosa and may contribute to the intense inflammatory reactions characteristic of gonococcal disease. Gonococci produce several proteases, peptidases, and phospholipases that may play a role in pathogenesis. In subepithelial tissue as well as in blood, gonococci presumably interact with serum antibody, including natural IgM antibody to LOS antigens. These immune complexes activate complement, with generation of the chemotactic factor C5a and formation of the bactericidal C5b-C9 attack complex. Insertion of the attack complex into the outer membrane of serum-sensitive gonococci results in gonococcal cell lysis, making antibody to LOS (like antibody to protein I) bactericidal. Certain gonococci that tend to be associated with gonococcal bacteremia resist killing by normal human serum. The attack complex formed when serum interacts with such gonococci has an abnormal configuration, and its insertion into the outer membrane of the organism does not result in the usual rapid cell lysis. Furthermore, some human sera contain complement-fixing IgG antibody to epitopes on protein III, which blocks bactericidal antibodies to other gonococcal antigens. Protein III has extensive homology to the enterobacterial OmpA protein and the meningococcal class 4 protein. Since Enterobacteriaceae and *Neisseria meningitidis* are common commensal microorganisms, it is possible that the protein III–blocking antibodies result from prior exposure to cross-reacting proteins from other microbial species.

Oxygen-independent antimicrobial mechanisms contribute significantly to intraleukocytic killing of gonococci following their phagocytosis by neutrophils. Despite effective intraleukocytic killing of gonococci in vitro, a small but reproducible number of organisms survive. Whether gonococci survive within neutrophils in vivo remains a subject of controversy.

Spread of gonococci from the cervix to the endometrium and salpinges may be enhanced in women using an intrauterine device. Menstruation further increases the risk of intraluminal ascent from the cervix and also predisposes to gonococcal bacteremia.

CLINICAL MANIFESTATIONS The clinical spectrum of gonococcal infection depends on the site of inoculation, the duration of infection, the virulence of the infecting strain, and whether or not the organism spreads locally or systemically. The influence of inoculum size, variations in host susceptibility, and coinfection with *Chlamydia trachomatis* or other genital pathogens on clinical manifestations has not been well defined.

Gonorrhea in the Male The usual incubation period of gonococcal urethritis ("clap") in the male is 2 to 5 days, although the interval can be longer and some men never develop symptoms. In one study, one auxotype—the AHU auxotype—was associated with 96 percent of asymptomatic infections and with only 40 percent of symptomatic infections. Symptoms of urethritis include a purulent urethral discharge, which develops in 90 to 95 percent of men with urethral gonococcal infection and is usually associated with dysuria, and meatal erythema. Most symptomatic men seek treatment and are removed from the infectious pool. The remaining men—who never develop symptoms or who ignore their symptoms—accumulate in number over time and constitute about two-thirds of all infected men at any point in time. Together with those who have just become infected, have begun to shed organisms, but have not yet developed symptoms, they serve as the source of spread of infection to women. Before antibiotic treatment became available, symptoms of urethritis persisted for an average of 8 weeks, and unilateral epididymitis occurred in 5 to 10 percent of untreated men. Epididymitis is now an uncommon complication (see below), and gonococcal prostatitis occurs rarely if at all. Other local complications of gonococcal urethritis that are now unusual include inguinal lymphadenitis, edema of the penis due to dorsal lymphangitis or thrombophlebitis, submucous inflammatory "soft" infiltration of the urethral wall, periurethral abscess or fistula, unilateral inflammation or abscess of Cowper's gland (which lies between the thumb and forefinger when the forefinger is in the anal canal and the thumb is positioned anteriorly on the perineum), and (in rare cases) seminal vesiculitis. Urethral stricture presumably results from poorly managed urethritis due to gonococci, chlamydiae, or less common causes.

Among homosexual men, the frequency of gonococcal infection fell by 90 percent or more throughout the United States during the early AIDS era of the 1980s, but a disturbing resurgence of gonorrhea in young homosexual men has been seen in several cities during the 1990s. Gonococcal isolates from homosexual men tend to be more resistant to antimicrobials than are isolates from heterosexuals. The reason may be that certain highly susceptible strains are rapidly killed by bile salts and fatty acids in feces and thus are rarely found in homosexual men, while gonococci with a mutation resulting in multidrug resistance (*mtr*) are more resistant to bile salts and fatty acids and thus are found with increased frequency in homosexual men. The *mtr* mutation involves a DNA-binding protein and results in the derepression of genes encoding an efflux mechanism of resistance. Rectal infection may be asymptomatic from the outset or may produce anorectal pain, pruritus, tenesmus, and a bloody, mucopurulent rectal discharge. Proctoscopy and appropriate laboratory studies are essential to exclude several other conditions that cause similar symptoms (see Chap. 129). These symptoms may subside without treatment, leaving a chronic asymptomatic carrier state. Pharyngeal gonococcal infection occurs in approximately 20 percent of homosexual men or heterosexual women exposed via fellatio and in a smaller proportion of heterosexual men exposed via cunnilingus. Pharyngeal infection may produce exudative tonsillitis but frequently is asymptomatic; asymptomatic pharyngeal gonococcal infection usually clears spontaneously over several weeks, even without therapy.

Gonorrhea in the Female Gonococcal infection in the female involves the endocervix, urethra, rectum, and pharynx, in decreasing order of frequency. Endocervical inflammation produces mucopurulent (yellow) endocervical discharge, which may result in a yellow vaginal discharge, and causes easily induced cervical bleeding. Upward extension of infection from the endocervix to the fallopian tubes occurs in at least 15 percent of women with gonorrhea. This extension tends to come soon after the acquisition of infection or during menstruation and results in *acute endometritis*—with abnormal menstrual bleeding, midline low-abdominal pain and tenderness, and dyspareunia—followed by *acute salpingitis*, the major complication of gonorrhea. Salpingitis can be subclinical but typically produces symptoms of bilateral lower-quadrant pain and tenderness and signs of cervical motion and abnormal adnexal mass. Endometritis and salpingitis may cause fever, leukocytosis, and abnormalities in serum acute-phase reactants (e.g., elevation of the erythrocyte sedimentation rate or of levels of C-reactive protein). Coexisting *C. trachomatis* infection may increase the rate of pelvic inflammatory disease (PID). Extension of infection to the pelvis may produce symptoms and signs of pelvic peritonitis accompanied by nausea and vomiting and may lead to pelvic abscess.

Early antibiotic treatment (before the development of adnexal masses) restores normal tubal function and fertility in nearly all cases of gonococcal salpingitis. However, if adnexal swelling is prominent before treatment is begun, bilateral tubal damage occurs in 15 to 25 percent of cases.

Spread of gonococci or chlamydiae into the upper abdomen may cause *perihepatitis* (Fitz-Hugh–Curtis syndrome), manifested by right upper quadrant or bilateral upper-abdominal pain and tenderness and occasionally by a hepatic friction rub.

Acute gonorrhea in the female often causes dysuria due to urethritis as well as anorectal discomfort due to proctitis; the mucopurulent cervical discharge due to endocervicitis may cause perceptible yellow vaginal discharge. Whereas dysuria in a young man arouses the suspicion of gonococcal urethritis, the same symptom in a young woman is often automatically attributed to "cystitis." Actually, some of those without bacteriuria have gonococcal or chlamydial infection of the urethra. Young women with dysuria should undergo a thorough pelvic examination. Compression of the urethra through the anterior vaginal wall against the symphysis pubis may express urethral exudate that can be examined by Gram's staining and culture. Symptomatic young women with "sterile pyuria" (i.e., ≥ 10 neutrophils per $100\times$ microscopic field in the centrifuged sediment of clean-catch midstream urine or a positive urine leukocyte esterase test, with no uropathogens isolated from the urine) should be evaluated for gonococcal and chlamydial infection. Acute symptoms of gonococcal urethritis in the female may subside spontaneously or after subcurative therapy with sulfonamides or urinary antiseptics. The proportion of women with gonorrhea who never develop symptoms is undefined but may be one-half or more.

Acute inflammation of Bartholin's gland is usually unilateral and frequently is due to gonococcal infection. The acutely infected duct is surrounded by a red halo and exudes pus at the posterior third of the labium majus. Occlusion of the duct results in formation of a Bartholin abscess. Chronic Bartholin cysts are rarely caused by active gonococcal infection.

There is evidence that peripartum endocervical gonococcal infection is associated with premature rupture of membranes, preterm delivery, and postpartum endometritis. In a recent randomized trial comparing a single dose of ceftriaxone with a single dose of placebo given at 28 to 34 weeks of gestation to women in Nairobi, the ceftriaxone regimen resulted in a significant increase in birth weight and a significant reduction in rates of postpartum endometritis and postpartum gonorrhea.

Gonorrhea in the Child During childbirth, the gonococcus may infect the conjunctiva, pharynx, respiratory tract, or anal canal of the newborn. The risk of infection increases with prolonged rupture of membranes. Prevention of gonococcal ophthalmia by prophylactic use of 1% silver nitrate eyedrops or ophthalmic preparations containing erythromycin or tetracycline is a cost-effective measure in most areas of the world, including the United States. However, it is not certain whether ophthalmic tetracycline prophylaxis is effective in preventing neonatal conjunctivitis caused by TRNG. Since neonates and young infants lack bactericidal IgM antibody to *N. gonorrhoeae*, they may be at increased risk for gonococcal bacteremia. During the first year of life, infection of the infant usually results from accidental contamination of the eye or vagina by organisms from an adult under very poor hygienic conditions. In the United States, many cases of gonorrhea in children between 1 year of age and puberty involve vulvovaginitis in females who have been molested, and medicolegal considerations necessitate a complete bacteriologic diagnosis and a child welfare consultation. Auxotyping and serotyping of isolates from the sexual assault victim and the accused assailant have been used as evidence in court.

Disseminated Gonococcal Infection The incidence of disseminated gonococcal infection (DGI) varies with time and place in relation to the local incidence of infection with strains of gonococci that have a propensity to produce bacteremia and to produce few or no symptoms or signs of inflammation at the local mucosal site of infection. Approximately two-thirds of patients with DGI are women, and symptoms of bacteremia often begin during menses.

Patients typically present either with manifestations of gonococcemia or with purulent arthritis affecting one or two joints. The onset of gonococcemia is characterized by fever, polyarthralgias, and the appearance (usually on the distal extremities) of 3 to 20 papular, petechial, pustular, hemorrhagic, or necrotic skin lesions. Initial joint manifestations are characteristically limited to tenosynovitis involving several joints asymmetrically. The wrists, fingers, knees, and ankles are most often involved. Circulating immune complexes have been demonstrated at this stage of infection, but serum complement levels are normal (except in individuals with complement deficiency), and the role of immune complexes, if any, is uncertain. Without treatment, the duration of gonococcemia is variable; the systemic manifestations of bacteremia can subside spontaneously within a week. Alternatively, septic arthritis can ensue, often without prior symptoms of fever, polyarthralgias, or skin lesions. Pain and swelling then increase in one or (very occasionally) more joints, with accumulation of purulent synovial fluid leading to progressive destruction of the joint if treatment is delayed.

IgM antibody to gonococcal LOS, present in normal human serum, is bactericidal for most strains of gonococci in the presence of complement. Gonococci isolated from patients with DGI exhibit stable resistance to normal human serum. Isolates from patients with tenosynovitis and skin lesions are even more serum-resistant than are isolates from patients with purulent arthritis; this difference suggests that the two DGI syndromes may be determined by characteristics of the causative organism. Gonococci associated with DGI usually contain outer-membrane protein IA and are highly susceptible to penicillin unless they produce β-lactamase. They often belong to the AHU auxotype. The decline in the incidence of such strains in the United States during the past two decades has been associated with a sharp decline in the incidence of DGI as well. Patients deficient in complement components C5, C6, C7, and C8 are uniquely susceptible to gonococcemia and meningococcemia because they cannot mount a serum bactericidal response to gonococci or meningococci. Although only perhaps 5 percent of patients with a first episode of gonococcemia or meningococcemia are complement-deficient, the proportion is higher among those with recurrent gonococcemia or meningococcemia. Strains isolated from complement-deficient patients may not be resistant to normal human serum.

The probability of positive blood cultures decreases after 48 h of illness, and the probability of recovery of gonococci from synovial fluid increases with the duration of illness. Gonococci are infrequently recovered from early effusions containing fewer than 20,000 leukocytes/μL but are usually recovered from effusions containing more than 80,000 leukocytes/μL. The organisms are seldom recovered simultaneously from blood and synovial fluid of the same patient.

Other common manifestations of DGI include mild myopericarditis and "toxic" hepatitis. Endocarditis and meningitis are infrequent but severe complications. Endocarditis is suggested by pathologic or changing heart murmurs, major embolic phenomena, severe myocarditis, deterioration of renal function, or an unusually large number of skin lesions.

DIFFERENTIAL DIAGNOSIS Gonococcal infection produces several common clinical syndromes that have multiple possible etiologies or that mimic other conditions. In particular, the epidemiologic and clinical features of C. trachomatis infections closely resemble those of gonococcal infections. The differential diagnosis of urethritis, epididymitis, and proctitis in men; cervicitis in women; vaginitis in prepubertal girls; and acute arthritis in young adults is discussed in Chap. 129. The differential diagnosis of PID is discussed in Chap. 130.

LABORATORY DIAGNOSIS The presence of intracellular gram-negative diplococci within leukocytes on Gram-stained smears of urethral or endocervical exudate warrants a presumptive diagnosis of gonorrhea. The diagnosis is equivocal if only extracellular or atypical gram-negative diplococci are seen and is ruled out if no gram-negative diplococci are seen. When experienced microbiologists employ these criteria, the sensitivity and specificity of Gram's staining of the urethral exudate approach 100 percent. The specificity of Gram's staining of purulent cervical exudate also is high, but the sensitivity is only about 50 percent. A presumptive diagnosis of gonorrhea cannot be made on the basis of gram-negative diplococci in smears from the pharynx, where other Neisseria species are components of the normal flora.

The "gold standard" for diagnosis of gonorrhea is the isolation of the organism by culture, which allows testing of isolates for antimicrobial resistance. Selective media (i.e., regular or modified Thayer-Martin medium), which contain antibiotics that selectively inhibit most other organisms, are most useful for recovering the gonococcus from the urethra, endocervix, pharynx, and rectum. After inoculation, the medium should be placed in a chamber with 70 percent humidity and an atmosphere containing 3 to 10% CO_2 to permit growth of the gonococcus. Inoculated media should be incubated at 35 to 37°C for 24 to 48 h, and putative gonococcal colonies should be confirmed by oxidase reaction; Gram's staining; and sugar utilization tests, rapid enzyme tests, nucleic acid probes, or agglutination reactions with antibodies specific for N. gonorrhoeae. The last four tests are especially important for isolates from the pharynx and rectum; for isolates obtained from populations with a low prevalence of gonorrhea, such as prenatal patients; and for isolates from victims of rape or sexual child abuse.

For diagnosis in men with incubating or chronic asymptomatic urethral infection without exudate or as a test of cure following treatment, a very thin urogenital swab should be inserted 2 cm into the anterior urethra and used to inoculate Thayer-Martin or another selective medium. Samples from the pharynx and rectum of homosexual men with suspected gonorrhea should be obtained for culture.

The endocervical culture is positive on a single examination in approximately 80 to 90 percent of women with gonorrhea. This diagnostic yield can be increased by the performance of a second endocervical culture and cultures of the rectum, urethra, and pharynx.

Another diagnostic approach has been the detection of gonococcal antigen in urethral or cervical secretions by enzyme-linked immunosorbent assay. In men with urethritis, Gram's staining is just as accurate, quicker, and cheaper; in women, the positive predictive value of antigen detection tests has been poor in populations with a low prevalence of gonorrhea. A nucleic acid probe test appears to be quite sensitive and specific in the detection of urethral and endocervical infections in populations with a relatively high prevalence of gonorrhea. Experience with pharyngeal and rectal specimens suggests that the probe test may be less sensitive than culture. The results of the probe test should be considered presumptive, particularly in low-prevalence populations. Promising DNA amplification tests, which make use of polymerase chain reaction or ligase chain reaction technology, have been developed for the diagnosis of gonococcal and chlamydial infections. The eventual utility of these tests may be greater for the diagnosis of chlamydial infection than for the diagnosis of gonorrhea, but the possibility of a single technology that could be used to detect either infection is attractive.

Standard blood-culture broth medium should be used for the culture of blood and is also recommended for the culture of synovial fluid. The broth should be vented and incubated under increased CO_2 tension. Synovial fluid also can be plated onto chocolate agar rather than a selective medium because it is not likely to be contaminated with commensal bacteria. In pus from skin lesions, N. gonorrhoeae is often demonstrable by immunofluorescent staining, but this test is seldom performed.

Techniques designed to detect gonococcal infection by testing of a single serum sample for antibody to N. gonorrhoeae have been limited by an inability to differentiate antibody due to past gonorrhea from antibody due to current infection and by false-positive results caused by cross-reactive antibody to N. meningitidis. For these reasons, serologic tests for gonorrhea have had a very low predictive value and are not used in clinical practice.

A false-positive diagnosis of gonorrhea can have medicolegal and psychosocial implications for both the physician and the patient.

 TREATMENT

Although long-acting forms of penicillin (such as benzathine penicillin G) are effective in therapy for syphilis, they have *no place* in the treatment of gonorrhea. Penicillin V and the isoxazolyl penicillins are not recommended for the treatment of gonococcal infection.

Similarly, first-generation cephalosporins are not used for gonorrhea. In 1993, the Centers for Disease Control and Prevention (CDC) published new guidelines for the treatment of gonorrhea. These 1993 guidelines are based on several observations: the importance of single-dose efficacy; the substantial proportion (over 30 percent in the United States and over 50 percent in many developing countries) of infections due to gonococci that are resistant to the penicillins (including ampicillin and amoxicillin) and/or the tetracyclines; the high frequency of coexisting chlamydial infections in persons with gonorrhea; and the severity of complications of gonococcal and chlamydial infections. The guidelines do not represent a comprehensive list of all possible treatment regimens.

As is shown in Table 150-1, for uncomplicated urethral, endocervical, rectal, or pharyngeal gonococcal infections in adults, the 1993 CDC guidelines recommend a regimen combining a single dose of any of the four most effective drugs for gonorrhea (ceftriaxone, cefixime, ciprofloxacin, or ofloxacin) with a 7-day course of doxycycline (for potential coinfection with chlamydiae). A single 1-g oral dose of azithromycin is a highly effective and convenient—but more expensive—alternative to doxycycline for chlamydial infections; potential drug interactions and adverse reactions resulting from the use of azithromycin in combination with gonorrhea therapy have not yet been well studied. These combination regimens can be expected to provide adequate therapy for gonorrhea at any site and will eliminate coexisting infections due to *C. trachomatis*. Although gonococci with high-level resistance to the fluoroquinolones remain uncommon in the United States as of 1997, an increasing incidence of such strains in the future could limit the usefulness of ciprofloxacin or ofloxacin, which can no longer be considered highly reliable for

gonorrhea in parts of Southeast Asia (e.g., the Philippines, Malaysia, Hong Kong, and Cambodia). A 2-g dose of azithromycin appears to be effective so far for gonorrhea but causes unacceptable gastrointestinal side effects.

Pregnant women who cannot tolerate a cephalosporin can receive a single dose of spectinomycin (2 g intramuscularly) for gonorrhea. Pregnant women should not receive doxycycline for chlamydial coverage but can instead take erythromycin base or stearate (500 mg by mouth four times daily for 7 days) or equivalent doses of erythromycin ethylsuccinate. If these doses of erythromycin are not well tolerated, 250 mg four times daily can be given for 14 days. Amoxicillin (500 mg orally three times daily for 7 to 10 days) can also be used for coexisting chlamydial infection in pregnancy.

All patients with gonorrhea should have a serologic test for syphilis at the time of diagnosis and should be offered confidential testing for HIV infection. Patients who have incubating seronegative syphilis without clinical signs of syphilis are likely to be cured of syphilis by the recommended ceftriaxone/doxycycline regimen. The quinolones are not effective for the treatment of syphilis, and the efficacy of cefixime for incubating syphilis has not been established, but the administration of doxycycline for 1 week to cure coexisting chlamydial infection also undoubtedly cures many cases of incubating syphilis. Nonetheless, patients with gonorrhea who also have syphilis or who are established contacts of someone with syphilis should be given additional treatment appropriate to the stage of syphilis (see Chap. 174).

Follow-Up and Treatment Failure Failure of combined therapy with ceftriaxone or cefixime and doxycycline is exceedingly rare. In the United States, the same is still true for therapy with ciprofloxacin or ofloxacin plus doxycycline. Therefore, at present, a follow-up culture is not essential after treatment with any of the recommended regimens for uncomplicated gonococcal infection. Patients should be advised to return for reexamination if any symptoms persist or recur after completion of treatment. Persistent or recurrent symptoms or signs after treatment for gonorrhea should be evaluated by culture for *N. gonorrhoeae* and by a specific test for chlamydial infection. Any posttreatment gonococcal isolate should be tested for antibiotic susceptibility. Recurrent gonococcal infections after treatment with the recommended schedule are almost always due to reinfection and indicate a need for improved referral of patients' sexual partners and education of patients themselves.

Postgonococcal urethritis (PGU) usually becomes apparent about 2 to 3 weeks after treatment of gonorrhea with a penicillin or a cephalosporin. PGU often is caused by *C. trachomatis*, which sometimes is acquired at the same time as *N. gonorrhoeae* but does not produce clinical symptoms until later because of a longer incubation period. When PGU occurs, it can be managed, like nongonococcal urethritis, with doxycycline (100 mg orally twice daily) or tetracycline (0.5 g four times a day) for 7 days. Similarly, mucopurulent cervicitis in women often persists or appears after treatment of gonorrhea with a single dose of a cephalosporin, a fluoroquinolone, or spectinomycin. This condition is frequently caused by *C. trachomatis* and can be treated like PGU. Men and women exposed to gonorrhea should be examined, have specimens obtained for culture, and be treated according to one of the recommended schedules.

Gonococcal arthritis can be treated satisfactorily with several regimens. Gonococci recovered from patients with gonococcal arthritis are generally less resistant to penicillin or tetracycline than isolates from patients with uncomplicated gonorrhea. However, several cases of DGI caused by PPNG have been reported. Because of the threat of endocarditis, meningitis, and joint sepsis, patients with DGI should be hospitalized and treated with ceftriaxone intravenously (1 g once a day) or with an alternative listed in Table 150-1. Patients without endocarditis or meningitis whose compliance is reliable can be discharged 24 to 48 h after symptoms resolve and can then complete a 7- to 10-day course of therapy with oral cefixime (400 mg twice a day) or ciprofloxacin (500 mg twice a day). A patient's failure to improve despite the administration of appropriate antimicrobial regimens strongly suggests a diagnosis other than DGI.

Table 150-1

Recommended Treatment for Gonococcal Infection: 1993 Guidelines of the Centers for Disease Control and Prevention

Diagnosis	Treatment of Choice
Uncomplicated infection of urethra, cervix, rectum, or pharynx	Ceftriaxone, 125-mg single IM dose *or* Cefixime, 400-mg single PO dose *or* Ciprofloxacin, 500-mg single PO dose *or* Ofloxacin, 400-mg single PO dose *plus* A regimen effective against possible coinfection with chlamydiae, such as: Doxycycline, 100 mg PO bid for 7 days *or* Azithromycin, 1-g single PO dose
Treatment failure	True treatment failure with ceftriaxone or cefixime is rare so far. Evaluate for reinfection or alternative diagnosis. In cases of ciprofloxacin or ofloxacin failure, also evaluate for gonococcal resistance to quinolones.
Alternative regimens	Spectinomycin, 2-mg single IM dose Ceftizoxime, 500-mg single IM dose Cefotaxime, 500-mg single IM dose
Disseminated gonococcal infection, initial therapy*	Ceftriaxone, 1 g IV or IM q 24 h *or* Cefotaxime or ceftizoxime, 1 g IV q 8 h *or†* Spectinomycin, 2 g IM q 12 h
Pelvic inflammatory disease	See Chap. 130.
Epididymitis	See Chap. 129.
Pediatric gonococcal infection	See text.

* Hospitalization is recommended to exclude endocarditis, meningitis, and other diagnoses. See text for information on duration of inpatient and subsequent outpatient therapy.
† Spectinomycin is given if the patient is allergic to β-lactam agents.

Repeated joint aspiration or closed irrigation of the joint with sterile saline may be required to reduce inflammation in patients with high synovial-fluid leukocyte counts. Open drainage is seldom if ever required for gonococcal arthritis except in infants with hip infection. Temporary immobilization of the joint may reduce discomfort and may facilitate walking by patients with persistent effusions of the knee or ankle. Antibiotics should not be injected directly into the joint. Once the diagnosis of gonococcal arthritis is proven, occasional patients benefit from treatment with anti-inflammatory agents along with antimicrobial drugs. However, if the diagnosis is suspected but not proven, the early use of anti-inflammatory drugs will make it impossible to monitor the response to antimicrobial therapy, which is usually rapid and often of diagnostic importance in gonococcal arthritis.

Meningitis and endocarditis caused by the gonococcus require high-dose intravenous therapy with an agent effective against the strain causing the disease. Ceftriaxone (1 to 2 g intravenously every 12 h) is given for 10 to 14 days for meningitis and for at least 1 month for endocarditis. Patients with gonococcal endocarditis or meningitis—and perhaps all patients with DGI—should be evaluated for complement deficiency.

Gonococcal conjunctivitis in adults or in children weighing more than 20 kg should be managed by prompt irrigation of the conjunctiva with saline and administration of a single 1-g intramuscular dose of ceftriaxone, which was found to be effective in all of 12 adults with gonococcal conjunctivitis in a recent North American study. All patients must undergo careful ophthalmologic evaluation, including slit-lamp examination.

Treatment of Pediatric Gonococcal Infection The infant born to a mother with gonorrhea is at high risk of infection and requires prophylaxis with a single dose of ceftriaxone (25 to 50 mg/kg intravenously or intramuscularly, not to exceed 125 mg). Ceftriaxone should be given with caution to hyperbilirubinemic infants, especially premature babies. Topical prophylaxis for neonatal ophthalmia does not provide adequate protection against infections at other sites. Infants with gonococcal infection at any site (e.g., the eye) should be hospitalized and evaluated for signs of DGI (e.g., sepsis, arthritis, meningitis). Those with DGI should be treated for 7 days with ceftriaxone (25 to 50 mg/kg in a single daily intravenous or intramuscular dose); a treatment duration of 10 to 14 days is recommended if meningitis is documented. Alternatively, cefotaxime can be administered intravenously or intramuscularly in a dose of 25 mg/kg twice daily. Limited data suggest that uncomplicated gonococcal ophthalmia in the infant can be cured with a single injection of ceftriaxone (25 to 50 mg/kg, with a maximum dose of 125 mg). Irrigation of the eyes with saline or buffered ophthalmic solutions should be performed immediately and then repeated as often as necessary to eliminate discharge. Topical antibiotic preparations alone are neither sufficient nor required when appropriate systemic antibiotic therapy is given. Both parents of a newborn with gonococcal ophthalmia should be evaluated and treated for gonorrhea. The parents and infant also should be tested for chlamydial infection.

Children who weigh 45 kg or more should be treated with adult regimens. Children who weigh less than 45 kg should be treated as follows: For uncomplicated vulvovaginitis, cervicitis, urethritis, proctitis, and pharyngitis, the recommended regimen is a single intramuscular dose of ceftriaxone (125 mg), and the alternative regimen is a single intramuscular dose of spectinomycin (40 mg/kg, with a maximum dose of 2 g). In addition, children 8 years of age or older can be given doxycycline (100 mg twice a day for 7 days). Children with suspected gonorrhea should be evaluated by standard culture systems for isolation and identification of *N. gonorrhoeae* and should be tested for coexisting syphilis and chlamydial infection. Sexual abuse is the most common cause of gonococcal infection in prepubescent children after the age of 1 year; anorectal and pharyngeal sites are most often infected and are frequently asymptomatic.

Topical and/or systemic estrogen therapy is of no benefit in gonococcal vulvovaginitis. All children should have follow-up cultures, and the source of infection should be identified, examined, and treated. The possibility of sexual abuse should be carefully considered and evaluated. For the treatment of complicated disease, the alternative regimens recommended for adults may be used in appropriate pediatric dosages.

Treatment of Gonorrhea in Developing Countries The proportion of gonococcal infections caused by PPNG, TRNG, CMRNG, or strains resistant to ciprofloxacin is highest in developing countries, which can least afford ceftriaxone, cefixime, spectinomycin, or other new antimicrobials effective against these strains and where the newer cephalosporins are not widely available in any case. Inexpensive alternatives to penicillin G and tetracycline, the traditional mainstays of gonorrhea therapy, have been disappointing. For example, a sulfonamide-trimethoprim combination that initially cured more than 95 percent of cases of gonorrhea in African countries was found to be effective in fewer than 75 percent of cases within 2 years after it became a popular regimen in Kenya. Norfloxacin, ciprofloxacin, and ofloxacin are increasingly prescribed or dispensed without prescription for urethritis and other conditions in developing countries. Ciprofloxacin has been on the UNICEF essential-drug list and is widely available. However, none of these drugs is effective as a single-dose regimen for chlamydial urethritis. Furthermore, the emergence of high-level fluoroquinolone resistance in Asia means that one of the few relatively inexpensive, widely available, oral antimicrobials is no longer reliable for the treatment of gonorrhea in Asia. Another approach has been the administration of 4.8 million units of procaine penicillin G intramuscularly plus 1.0 g of probenecid orally together with 125 mg of clavulanic acid (in the form of one capsule of amoxicillin/clavulanate) to inhibit gonococcal β-lactamase. This inexpensive regimen was effective in small-scale trials in Kenya, even against PPNG infections, but would not be highly effective again CMRNG. Gentamicin, in a single 280-mg intramuscular dose, also has been used in this setting. Use of newer cephalosporins in lower-than-recommended doses to reduce cost should be discouraged. There is a growing need for less expensive regimens and for ongoing surveillance of in vitro sensitivity of *N. gonorrhoeae*.

PREVENTION AND CONTROL Gonorrhea probably provides the most striking illustration of the failure of a specific treatment alone to eradicate a communicable disease. No vaccine is available. A field trial of a purified gonococcal pilus vaccine in U.S. soldiers in Korea showed that the vaccine was not effective. Use of a condom can prevent transmission. The extensive use of condoms for contraception may be responsible for the low rates of gonorrhea in some countries (e.g., Japan). Spermicidal preparations used with a diaphragm or cervical sponges impregnated with nonoxynol-9 offer some protection against gonorrhea and chlamydial infection. Prophylactic antibiotics (e.g., 200 mg of minocycline or doxycycline taken soon after sexual exposure) have reduced the risk of infection but are not recommended for general use or for use by individuals with known exposure to gonorrhea, who should receive one of the regimens recommended for established gonorrhea.

To contain the increasing spread of antimicrobial-resistant gonococci, several measures are important: (1) routine use of highly effective antibiotics, such as ceftriaxone, to prevent gonorrhea treatment failures; (2) rapid identification and treatment of sexual partners of patients with gonorrhea, particularly partners of those with recurrent infection and those known to be infected with resistant strains; (3) in patients in whom treatment appears to have failed, routine diagnosis by cultures and testing of isolates for antimicrobial resistance or β-lactamase production; and (4) much greater emphasis on prevention by methods other than diagnosis and treatment—for example, by public health education and individual patient counseling to promote fewer sexual partners and condom use during casual and commercial sexual encounters.

BIBLIOGRAPHY

BRITIGAN BE, SPARLING PF: Gonococcal infection: A model of molecular pathogenesis. N Engl J Med 312:1683, 1985

CENTERS FOR DISEASE CONTROL AND PREVENTION: 1993 Sexually transmitted diseases treatment guidelines. Morb Mort Week Rep 42(RR-14):1, 1993

———: Fluoroquinolone resistance in Neisseria gonorrhoeae—Colorado and Washington, 1995. Morb Mort Week Rep 44:761, 1995

COHEN MS, SPARLING PF: Mucosal infection with Neisseria gonorrhoeae. Bacterial adaptation and mucosal defenses. J Clin Invest 89:1699, 1992

——— et al: Human experimentation with Neisseria gonorrhoeae: Rationale, methods, and implications for the biology of infection and vaccine development. J Infect Dis 169:532, 1994

HANDSFIELD HH et al: A comparison of single-dose cefixime with ceftriaxone as treatment for uncomplicated gonorrhea. N Engl J Med 325:1337, 1991

——— et al: Multicenter trial of single-dose azithromycin vs. ceftriaxone in the treatment of uncomplicated gonorrhea. Sex Transm Dis 21:107, 1994

HOLMES KK et al: Impact of a gonorrhea control program, including selective mass treatment, in female sex workers. J Infect Dis 174(Suppl 2):S230, 1996

KNAPP JS et al: Serologic classification of Neisseria gonorrhoeae using monoclonal antibodies directed against outer membrane protein I. J Infect Dis 150:44, 1985

MANALASTOS R et al: Fluoroquinolone resistance in Neisseria gonorrhoeae in the Republic of the Philippines. Antimicrob Agents Chemother 1997, in press

MORAN JS, LEVINE WC: Drugs of choice for the treatment of uncomplicated gonococcal infection. Clin Infect Dis 20(Suppl 1):S47, 1995

MORSE SA et al: High-level tetracycline resistance in Neisseria gonorrhoeae is result of acquisition of streptococcal tetM determinant. Antimicrob Agents Chemother 30:664, 1986

——— et al (eds): Perspectives on pathogenic Neisseria spp. Clin Microbiol Rev 2(Suppl 1S), 1989

MOSS G et al: Human immunodeficiency virus DNA in urethral secretions in men: Association with gonococcal urethritis and CD4 cell depletion. J Infect Dis 172:1469, 1995

O'ROURKE M et al: Opa-typing: A high-resolution tool for studying the epidemiology of gonorrhea. Mol Microbiol 17:865, 1995

PETERSEN BH et al: Neisseria meningitidis and Neisseria gonorrhoeae bacteremia associated with C6, C7, or C8 deficiency. Ann Intern Med 90:917, 1979

RICE PA et al: Immunoglobulin G antibodies directed against protein III block killing of serum-resistant Neisseria gonorrhoeae by immune serum. J Exp Med 164:1735, 1986

——— et al: Sociodemographic distribution of gonorrhea incidence: Implications for prevention and behavioral research. Am J Public Health 81:1252, 1991

SMITH KR et al: Evaluation of ligase chain reaction for use with urine for identification of Neisseria gonorrhoeae in females attending a sexually transmitted disease clinic. J Clin Microbiol 33:455, 1995

TEMMERMAN M et al: Mass antimicrobial treatment in pregnancy. A randomized placebo-controlled trial in a population with high rates of sexually transmitted diseases. J Reprod Med 40:176, 1995

VAN PUTTEN JPM: Iron acquisition and the pathogenesis of meningococcal and gonococcal disease. Med Microbiol Immunol 179:289, 1990

YORKE JA et al: Dynamics and control of the transmission of gonorrhea. Sex Transm Dis 5:51, 1978

151   Daniel M. Musher

MORAXELLA (BRANHAMELLA) CATARRHALIS, OTHER MORAXELLA SPECIES, AND KINGELLA

MORAXELLA (BRANHAMELLA) CATARRHALIS

The gram-negative coccus now known as *Moraxella catarrhalis* has undergone three changes of name in as many decades. Originally called *Micrococcus catarrhalis*, it was renamed *Neisseria catarrhalis* in the 1960s because of its morphologic similarity to *Neisseria* species. Then, in 1970, it was elevated to the status of a distinct genus, *Branhamella*, on the basis of DNA homology. In 1979 this organism was placed into the genus *Moraxella*, of which *Branhamella* may be a subgenus. Some authorities continue to call it *Moraxella (Branhamella) catarrhalis*. A component of the normal bacterial flora of the upper airways, *M. catarrhalis* has been increasingly recognized as a cause of otitis media, sinusitis, and bronchopulmonary infection.

BACTERIOLOGY AND IMMUNITY   On Gram's staining, *M. catarrhalis* appears as gram-negative cocci, often occurring in pairs and retaining the side-by-side kidney-bean configuration of *Neisseria*. These cocci tend to retain crystal violet during the decolorizing step and may be confused with *Staphylococcus aureus*. Colonies grow well on blood or chocolate agar and are readily distinguishable from *Neisseria* species by biochemical tests.

M. catarrhalis shows a surprising degree of homogeneity of outer-membrane proteins. Antibody to certain of these proteins is generally present in serum of children over the age of 4 years; however, colonizing isolates or those that cause disease may survive in serum despite this naturally present antibody and complement. Bactericidal antibody emerges following natural infection and may be directed against one or more conserved outer-membrane proteins, a property of potential value in vaccine development. An 81-kDa outer-membrane protein is associated with virulence in mice; antibody to this protein is protective.

EPIDEMIOLOGY   With the use of selective media, *M. catarrhalis* can be isolated from the upper respiratory tract or saliva of 50 percent of healthy schoolchildren and up to 7 percent of healthy adults. The rate of nasopharyngeal colonization is higher among children who have otitis media. Investigators in both the Northern and Southern Hemispheres have reported a striking seasonal variation in the isolation of this organism from clinical specimens, with a peak in late winter/early spring and a nadir in late summer/early fall. Direct contact has not been shown to contribute to community-acquired infection, but nosocomial spread of infection has been documented occasionally.

OTITIS MEDIA, SINUSITIS   *M. catarrhalis* has repeatedly been shown to be the third most common bacterial isolate from middle-ear fluid of children who have otitis media, being surpassed only by *Streptococcus pneumoniae* and nontypable *Haemophilus influenzae*. Recent studies have shown this organism to be a prominent isolate from sinus cavities in acute and chronic sinusitis.

PURULENT TRACHEOBRONCHITIS, PNEUMONIA   *M. catarrhalis* causes acute exacerbations of chronic bronchitis (increased production and/or purulence of sputum), purulent tracheobronchitis (the latter also involving fever and leukocytosis), and pneumonia. The great majority of infected persons are older than 50 years and have a long history of cigarette smoking and underlying chronic obstructive pulmonary disease (COPD); lung cancer is often present as well. In one recent study, 76 percent of affected persons had COPD (often severe), and one-third of those with COPD had lung cancer; most patients also had clinical evidence of malnutrition. In one extensive series of cases, *M. catarrhalis* pneumonia did not occur in otherwise healthy hosts.

Symptoms of patients with *M. catarrhalis* pneumonia have been regarded as modest in severity, perhaps more because of a diminished febrile response (due to the advanced age and underlying diseases of the affected individuals) than because of any lack of pathogenic capacity of this organism. Both cough and the amount and purulence of the sputum are usually increased above baseline. Chills are reported in one-quarter of patients, pleuritic pain in one-third, and malaise in 40 percent. Most patients have peak temperatures of <101°F (38.3°C), and peripheral white blood cell counts are <10,000/μL in nearly one-quarter of cases. Microscopic examination of a good sputum specimen following Gram's staining regularly reveals profuse organisms (approximately 2×10^8 colony forming units per milliliter). The radiologic appearance is variable; in one study, 43 percent of subjects had segmental or lobar infiltrates, and the remainder had a mixed pattern of subsegmental, segmental, interstitial, and diffuse involvement. These clinical, laboratory, and radiographic findings do not differ from those of pneumococcal pneumonia in an older patient population. However, a far lesser degree of bloodstream invasion occurs in *M. catarrhalis* infection; in one series, none of 25 patients with *M. catarrhalis* pneumonia had bacteremia. Nevertheless, pneumonia due to *M. catarrhalis* is a marker for severe underlying disease, in that nearly one-half of patients die within 3 months of onset.

OTHER SYNDROMES Local extension causing empyema is very uncommon, and, as might be inferred from the low rate of bacteremia, metastatic complications of *M. catarrhalis* pneumonia, such as septic arthritis, are exceedingly rare. As of 1990, 27 cases of bacteremic infection due to *M. catarrhalis* had been reported, mainly in children less than 10 years old or adults more than 60 years old; most of these patients were immunocompromised. The syndromes reported have included bacteremia with no apparent focus, endocarditis, and meningitis. A petechial or purpuric rash, reminiscent of that observed in meningococcal sepsis and associated with disseminated intravascular coagulation, has been described in a few cases, nearly all in children.

℞ TREATMENT

Treatment of presumed *M. catarrhalis* infection with a penicillin/clavulanic acid combination seems highly appropriate. Penicillin resistance first appeared in *Branhamella* isolates in the mid-1970s and is now found in 85 percent of clinical isolates. Resistance is mediated by two closely related β-lactamases, BRO-1 and BRO-2 (acronyms derived from *Branhamella* and *Moraxella*), which are present in 90 and 10 percent, respectively, of resistant isolates. These enzymes are active against penicillin, ampicillin, and amoxicillin but less so against cephalosporins, especially third-generation cephalosporins, and they bind avidly to clavulanic acid and sulbactam.

Cephalosporins, especially those of the second and third generations, are effective alternatives. A 5-day course of therapy has been shown to cure respiratory infection, although a slightly longer course may be required in sinusitis. Isolates in the United States are nearly uniformly susceptible to tetracycline, erythromycin, trimethoprim-sulfamethoxazole, quinolones, and chloramphenicol, although tetracycline resistance, perhaps due to TetB determinants, is increasing in Europe and Asia and has been documented in two isolates in the United States.

During the period between the identification of gram-negative cocci in a Gram-stained specimen and the final identification of the organisms by culture, the severity of the condition and the potential presence of other infecting organisms should dictate antibiotic selection. For example, an exacerbation of bronchitis caused by *M. catarrhalis* might be treated with tetracycline or trimethoprim-sulfamethoxazole; however, in a patient with pneumonia, the possibility that pneumococci resistant to these agents also might be present dictates the choice of ampicillin/sulbactam or a third-generation cephalosporin, at least until results of culture are available.

OTHER *MORAXELLA* SPECIES AND *KINGELLA KINGAE*

Other *Moraxella* species cause a wide range of infections, including bronchitis, pneumonia, empyema, endocarditis, meningitis, conjunctivitis, urinary tract infection, septic arthritis, and wound infection. In a report of all *Moraxella* isolates submitted to the Centers for Disease Control and Prevention (CDC) between 1953 and 1980, certain clinical associations were apparent (Table 151-1). *M. osloensis* and *M. nonliquefaciens* were the most common species, having been cultured from a wide range of normally sterile body sites, including blood, cerebrospinal fluid, and joints. *M. osloensis* was the *Moraxella* species most commonly isolated from blood; *M. nonliquefaciens* tended to be isolated from the ears, nose, or throat (47 percent) or the sputum (8 percent). *M. canis* (formerly *Moraxella* M-5) had a striking association with infected wounds from dog bites (72 percent of all isolates), whereas *M. lacunata* was associated with conjunctivitis and keratitis (70 percent of isolates). *M. urethralis* was isolated most often from urine and the genital tract and probably represents the *Moraxella* species implicated previously in urethritis. More than one-half of isolates of *M. phenylpyruvica* and *M. atlantae* were obtained from normally sterile sites. The clinical features of infections due to *Moraxella* species other than *M. catarrhalis* and the nature of the hosts in which they occur have not been fully characterized.

Table 151-1

Moraxella Species and *Kingella kingae*

Species	Number of Isolates	Common Sites/Clinical Association	Number (Percent) for Each Site
*M. osloensis**	199	Blood	44 (22)
		CSF	18 (9)
		Urine	17 (9)
		Respiratory tract	24 (12)
M. nonliquefaciens	356	Blood	27 (8)
		CSF	6 (2)
		Respiratory tract	196 (55)
M. canis	74	Dog-bite wound	53 (72)
M-6	47	Blood, bone	15 (32)
M. lacunata	33	Conjunctivitis, keratitis	23 (70)
M. urethralis	28	Urine	16 (57)
		Genital tract	3 (11)
M. phenylpyruvica	73	Blood	19 (26)
		CSF	8 (11)
		Urine	12 (16)
M. atlantae	44	Blood	20 (45)
		CSF	5 (11)
Kingella kingae	79	Blood	38 (48)
		Joint	10 (13)
		Bone	11 (14)

* Some of these isolates would now be distinguished as a new species, *M. lincolnii*.
SOURCE: Adapted from a summary of CDC experience (Graham et al).

Kingella kingae was originally designated *Moraxella* new species 1 (M-1) and was subsequently named in honor of Dr. Elizabeth King of the CDC, who first described it. A fastidious organism, *K. kingae* has been found to cause endocarditis, arthritis, and osteomyelitis (see Table 151-1); isolated instances of other infections have been recorded. Most bone and joint infections occur in young children. One-half of all cases of septic arthritis in one recently reported series of children younger than 24 months were due to *K. kingae*. The fact that this organism is not implicated more frequently as a cause of pneumonia may indicate a true tissue tropism for heart valve, bones, and joints, or it may reflect the difficulty of separating *Kingella* from the normal respiratory flora on sputum culture.

Most moraxellae and kingellae remain susceptible to penicillins, cephalosporins, tetracyclines, and chloramphenicol, but some strains of *Moraxella* produce BRO β-lactamases, and clinical specimens must be tested for lactamase production and antibiotic susceptibility. Initial therapy with a penicillin or cephalosporin is reasonable pending susceptibility testing.

BIBLIOGRAPHY

CATLIN BW: *Branhamella catarrhalis:* An organism gaining respect as a pathogen. Clin Microbiol Rev 3:293, 1990

DEGROOT R et al: Bone and joint infections caused by *Kingella kingae:* Six cases and review of the literature. Rev Infect Dis 10:998, 1988

GRAHAM D et al: Infections caused by *Moraxella, Moraxella urethralis, Moraxella*-like groups M-5 and M-6, and *Kingella kingae* in the United States, 1953–1980. Rev Infect Dis 12:423, 1990

HAGER H et al: *Branhamella catarrhalis* respiratory infections. Rev Infect Dis 9:1140, 1987

HELMINEN ME et al: A large, antigenically conserved protein on the surface of *Moraxella catarrhalis* is a target for protective antibodies. J Infect Dis 170:867, 1994

IOANNIDIS JPA et al: Spectrum and significance of bacteremia due to *Moraxella catarrhalis*. Clin Infect Dis 21:390, 1995

KIBSEY PC et al: Disk diffusion versus broth microdilution susceptibility testing of *Haemophilus* species and *Moraxella catarrhalis* using seven oral antimicrobial agents: Application of updated susceptibility guidelines of the National Committee for Clinical Laboratory Standards. J Clin Microbiol 32:2786, 1994

MORRISON VA, WAGNER KF: Clinical manifestations of *Kingella kingae* infections: Case report and review. Rev Infect Dis 11:776, 1989

VERGHESE A, BERK SL: *Moraxella (Branhamella) catarrhalis*. Infect Dis Clin North Am 5:523, 1991

WALLACE RJ JR et al: Antibiotic susceptibilities and drug resistance in *Moraxella (Branhamella) catarrhalis*. Am J Med 88(Suppl 5A):46S, 1990

WRIGHT PW et al: A descriptive study of 42 cases of *Branhamella catarrhalis* pneumonia. Am J Med 88(Suppl 5A):2S, 1990

YAGUPSKY P et al: Epidemiology, etiology, and clinical features of septic arthritis in patients younger than 24 months. Arch Pediatr Adolesc Med 149:537, 1994

152   *Timothy F. Murphy, Dennis L. Kasper*

INFECTIONS DUE TO *HAEMOPHILUS INFLUENZAE*, OTHER *HAEMOPHILUS* SPECIES, THE HACEK GROUP, AND OTHER GRAM-NEGATIVE BACILLI

HAEMOPHILUS INFLUENZAE

MICROBIOLOGY   *Haemophilus influenzae* was first recognized in 1892 by Pfeiffer, who erroneously concluded that the bacterium was the cause of influenza. The bacterium is a small (~1- by 0.3-μm) gram-negative organism of variable shape; hence, it is often described as a pleomorphic coccobacillus. In clinical specimens such as cerebrospinal fluid (CSF) and sputum, it frequently stains only faintly with phenosafranin and therefore can easily be overlooked.

H. influenzae grows both aerobically and anaerobically. Its aerobic growth requires two factors: hemin (X factor) and nicotinamide adenine dinucleotide (V factor). These requirements are used in the clinical laboratory to identify the bacterium. Six major serotypes of *H. influenzae* have been identified; designated *a* through *f*, they are based on antigenically distinct polysaccharide capsules. In addition, some strains lack a polysaccharide capsule and are referred to as *nontypable* strains. Type b and nontypable strains are the most relevant strains clinically, although encapsulated strains other than type b can cause disease. *H. influenzae* is the first free-living organism whose entire genome has been sequenced.

The antigenically distinct type b capsule is a linear polymer composed of ribosyl-ribitol phosphate. Strains of *H. influenzae* type b (Hib) cause disease primarily in infants and children under the age of 6 years. Nontypable strains are primarily mucosal pathogens, although the incidence of invasive disease caused by these strains is increasing.

EPIDEMIOLOGY AND TRANSMISSION   *H. influenzae* is an exclusively human pathogen. Nontypable strains colonize the upper respiratory tract of up to three-fourths of healthy adults. Colonization with nontypable *H. influenzae* is a dynamic process; new strains are acquired and other strains are replaced periodically.

Hib strains colonize the nasopharynx of children at a rate of 3 to 5 percent; before the introduction of type b vaccine, higher rates were seen in day-care centers. The rate of nasopharyngeal colonization by Hib strains is decreasing with the widespread use of conjugate vaccines to prevent invasive infections caused by Hib. The organism is spread by airborne droplets or by direct contact with secretions or fomites.

Certain population groups have a higher incidence of invasive Hib disease than the general population. The incidence of meningitis due to Hib has been three to four times higher among black children than among white children in several studies. In some Native American groups, the incidence of invasive Hib disease is 10 times higher than that in the general population. Although this increased incidence has not yet been accounted for, several factors may be relevant, including age at exposure to the bacterium, socioeconomic conditions, and genetic differences in the ability to mount an immune response.

PATHOGENESIS   Hib strains cause systemic disease by invasion and hematogenous spread to distant sites such as the meninges, bones, and joints. The type b polysaccharide capsule is an important virulence factor affecting the bacterium's ability to avoid opsonization and cause systemic disease.

Nontypable strains cause disease by local invasion of mucosal surfaces. Otitis media results when bacteria reach the middle ear by way of the eustachian tube. Lower respiratory infection develops in adults with chronic bronchitis when nontypable strains gain access to and colonize the lower respiratory tract. The incidence of invasive disease caused by nontypable strains is low but increasing.

IMMUNE RESPONSE   Antibody to capsule is important in protection from infection by Hib strains. The level of (maternally acquired) serum antibody to the capsular polysaccharide, which is a polymer of polyribitol ribose phosphate and thus is sometimes designated PRP, declines from birth to 6 months of age and, in the absence of vaccination, remains low until around 2 or 3 years of age. The age at the antibody nadir correlates with that of the peak incidence of type b disease. Antibody to PRP then appears partly as a result of exposure to Hib or cross-reacting antigens. Systemic Hib disease is unusual after the age of 6 years because of the presence of protective antibody. Vaccines in which PRP is conjugated to protein carrier molecules have been developed and are now used widely. These vaccines generate an antibody response to PRP in infants and are effective in preventing invasive infections in infants and children.

Since nontypable strains lack a capsule, the immune response to infection is directed at noncapsular antigens. These noncapsular antigens of *H. influenzae* have generated considerable interest as targets of the human immune response and as potential vaccine components.

CLINICAL MANIFESTATIONS   *H. influenzae* **Type b**   The most serious manifestation of infection with Hib is meningitis. The age of peak incidence varies somewhat among populations, depending in part on the use of vaccine, but this infection primarily affects infants under 2 years of age. The clinical manifestations of meningitis caused by Hib are similar to those of meningitis caused by other bacterial pathogens. Fever and altered central nervous system function are the most common features at presentation. Nuchal rigidity may or may not be evident. Subdural effusion, the most common complication, is suspected when, despite 2 or 3 days of appropriate antibiotic therapy, the infant has seizures, hemiparesis, or continued obtundation. The overall mortality from meningitis caused by Hib is approximately 5 percent, and the rate of morbidity is high. Six percent of survivors have permanent sensorineural hearing loss, and about one-fourth have a significant handicap of some type. If more subtle handicaps are sought, up to half of survivors are found to have some neurologic sequelae, such as partial hearing loss and delay in language development.

Epiglottitis is a life-threatening infection involving cellulitis of the epiglottis and supraglottic tissues. It can lead to acute upper airway obstruction. Its unique epidemiologic features are its occurrence in an older age group (2 to 7 years old) than other Hib infections and its absence among Navajo Indians and Alaskan Eskimos. Sore throat and fever rapidly progress to dysphagia, drooling, and airway obstruction.

Cellulitis due to Hib occurs in young children. The most common location is on the head or neck, and the involved area sometimes takes on a characteristic bluish-red color. Most patients have bacteremia, and 10 percent have an additional focus of infection.

Hib causes pneumonia in infants. The infection is clinically indistinguishable from other types of bacterial pneumonia (e.g., pneumococcal pneumonia) except that it is more likely to involve the pleura.

Several less common invasive conditions can be important clinical manifestations of Hib infection in children. These include osteomyelitis, septic arthritis, pericarditis, orbital cellulitis, endophthalmitis, urinary tract infection, abscesses, and bacteremia without an identifiable focus. As has already been mentioned, infections due to Hib are unusual among patients older than 6 years.

Nontypable *H. influenzae*   Nontypable *H. influenzae* is the second most common cause (after *Streptococcus pneumoniae*) of community-acquired bacterial pneumonia in adults. Nontypable *H. influenzae* pneumonia is especially common among patients with chronic obstructive pulmonary disease (COPD) or AIDS. The clinical features of pneumonia due to *H. influenzae* are similar to those of other types of bacterial pneumonia (including pneumococcal pneumonia). Patients present with fever, cough, and purulent sputum, usually of several days' duration. Chest radiography reveals alveolar infiltrates in a patchy or lobar distribution. Gram-stained sputum contains a predominance of small, pleomorphic, coccobacillary gram-negative bacteria.

Exacerbations of COPD caused by nontypable *H. influenzae* are characterized by increased cough, sputum production, and shortness of breath. Fever is low-grade, and no infiltrates are evident on chest x-ray.

Nontypable *H. influenzae* is one of the three most common causes of childhood otitis media (the other two being *S. pneumoniae* and *Moraxella catarrhalis*). Infants are febrile and irritable, while older children report ear pain. Symptoms of viral upper respiratory infection often precede otitis media. The diagnosis is made by pneumatic otoscopy. An etiologic diagnosis, although not routinely sought, can be established by tympanocentesis and culture of middle-ear fluid. Nontypable *H. influenzae* also causes puerperal sepsis and is an important cause of neonatal bacteremia. Nontypable strains tend to be of biotype IV and cause invasive disease after colonizing the female genital tract.

Nontypable *H. influenzae* causes sinusitis in adults and children. In addition, the bacterium is a less common cause of various invasive infections that are reported primarily as small series descriptions and case reports. These infections include empyema, adult epiglottitis, pericarditis, cellulitis, septic arthritis, osteomyelitis, endocarditis, cholecystitis, intraabdominal infections, urinary tract infections, mastoiditis, aortic graft infection, and bacteremia without a detectable focus. Before the early 1980s, nontypable strains were frequently misidentified as Hib because of their autoagglutination when serotypes were determined in agglutination assays.

DIAGNOSIS   The most reliable method for establishing a diagnosis of Hib infection is recovery of the organism in culture. The CSF of a patient in whom meningitis is suspected should be subjected to Gram's staining and culture. The presence of gram-negative coccobacilli in Gram-stained CSF is strong evidence for Hib meningitis. Recovery of the organism from CSF confirms the diagnosis. Cultures of other normally sterile body fluids, such as blood, joint fluid, pleural fluid, pericardial fluid, and subdural effusion, are confirmatory in other infections.

Detection of PRP is an important adjunct to culture in rapid diagnosis. Immunoelectrophoresis, latex agglutination, coagglutination, and enzyme-linked immunosorbent assay are effective in detecting PRP. These assays are particularly helpful when patients have received prior antimicrobial therapy and thus are especially likely to have negative cultures.

Since nontypable *H. influenzae* is primarily a mucosal pathogen, it is a component of a mixed flora; this situation makes etiologic diagnosis challenging. Nontypable *H. influenzae* infection is strongly suggested by the predominance of gram-negative coccobacilli among abundant polymorphonuclear leukocytes in a Gram-stained sputum specimen from a patient in whom pneumonia or tracheobronchitis is suspected. A sputum culture is helpful when interpreted along with the results of Gram's staining. Although bacteremia is detectable in a small proportion of patients with pneumonia due to nontypable *H. influenzae*, most such patients have negative blood cultures.

A diagnosis of otitis media is based on the detection by pneumatic otoscopy of fluid in the middle ear. An etiologic diagnosis requires tympanocentesis but is not routinely sought. An invasive procedure is also required to determine the etiology of sinusitis; thus, treatment is often empirical once the diagnosis is suspected in light of clinical symptoms and sinus radiographs.

℞ TREATMENT

Initial therapy for meningitis due to Hib should consist of a cephalosporin such as ceftriaxone or cefotaxime. An alternative regimen for initial therapy is ampicillin plus chloramphenicol. Therapy should continue for a total of 1 to 2 weeks.

Administration of glucocorticoids to patients infected with *H. influenzae* reduces the incidence of neurologic sequelae. The presumed mechanism is reduction of the inflammation induced by bacterial cell-wall mediators of inflammation when cells are killed by antimicrobial agents. Dexamethasone (0.6 mg/kg per day intravenously in four divided doses for 4 days) is recommended for the treatment of Hib meningitis in children over 2 months of age.

Invasive infections other than meningitis are treated with the same antimicrobial agents. Epiglottitis constitutes a medical emergency, and maintenance of an airway is critical. The duration of therapy is determined by the clinical response. A course of 1 to 2 weeks is usually appropriate.

Many infections caused by nontypable strains of *H. influenzae*, such as otitis media, sinusitis, and exacerbations of COPD, can be treated with oral antimicrobial agents. Approximately 25 percent of nontypable strains produce β-lactamase and are resistant to ampicillin. Infections caused by ampicillin-resistant strains can be treated with a variety of agents, including trimethoprim-sulfamethoxazole, erythromycin/sulfisoxazole, amoxicillin/clavulanic acid, various extended-spectrum cephalosporins, fluoroquinolones, and clarithromycin.

PREVENTION   Vaccination   The development of conjugate vaccines that prevent invasive infections by Hib in infants and children has been a dramatic success. Four such vaccines are licensed in the United States. In addition to eliciting protective antibody, these vaccines prevent disease by reducing pharyngeal colonization with Hib.

All children should be immunized with an Hib conjugate vaccine, receiving the first dose at approximately 2 months of age, the rest of the primary series between 2 and 6 months of age, and a booster dose at 12 to 15 months of age. Specific recommendations vary for the different conjugate vaccines. The reader is referred to the recommendations of the American Academy of Pediatrics.

Currently no vaccines are available for the prevention of disease caused by nontypable *H. influenzae*.

Chemoprophylaxis   The risk of secondary disease is greater than normal among household contacts of patients with Hib disease. The attack rate is as high as 4 percent among susceptible infants. Therefore, all members (children and adults) of households where there are contacts less than 4 years old should receive prophylaxis with oral rifampin. (This rule does not apply when all household contacts under the age of 4 years have been completely immunized with conjugate vaccine.) Children under 12 years old should receive rifampin at a dose of 20 mg/kg once daily for 4 days, and adults should receive 600 mg daily for 4 days. The index case should receive rifampin before or at the time of discharge from the hospital because antimicrobial agents used for the treatment of meningitis do not reliably eradicate Hib from the nasopharynx.

The data on secondary cases among contacts outside the household (e.g., in day-care settings) are conflicting. The administration of rifampin prophylaxis to contacts in day-care centers should be considered, but each decision should be individualized and in part based on the contacts' immunization history, the size of the center, the extent of contact, and whether the exposure is to a single case or to multiple cases.

HAEMOPHILUS INFLUENZAE BIOGROUP AEGYPTIUS

H. influenzae biogroup aegyptius was formerly called *Haemophilus aegyptius* because of phenotypic characteristics distinct from those of *H. influenzae*. However, more recent studies involving DNA hybridization and DNA transformation have demonstrated that *H. aegyptius* and *H. influenzae* are members of the same species.

H. influenzae biogroup aegyptius has long been associated with conjunctivitis. Moreover, this strain is now known to be the cause of Brazilian purpuric fever (BPF), which was first recognized in 1984 in the rural Brazilian town of Promissao. The sharing of many phenotypic and genotypic characteristics by the various strains of *H. influen-*

zae biogroup aegyptius that cause BPF indicates that these strains represent a clone of *H. influenzae*. The age of peak incidence of BPF is 1 to 4 years, with a range of 3 months to 8 years. The illness can occur sporadically or in outbreaks. Typically, after an episode of purulent conjunctivitis, high fever occurs in association with vomiting and abdominal pain. Within 12 to 48 h after onset, the patient develops petechiae, purpura, and peripheral necrosis and experiences vascular collapse. The characteristic laboratory features are thrombocytopenia, prolonged prothrombin time, uniformly unrevealing CSF findings, and blood cultures positive for *H. influenzae* biogroup aegyptius. Initial reports cited high mortality (~70 percent), but subsequent studies have indicated that milder forms of the illness exist. Most patients have resolved or resolving purulent conjunctivitis, and culture of the conjunctiva is positive in approximately one-third of cases. BPF has been seen in several towns in Brazil and on two occasions in Australia.

HAEMOPHILUS DUCREYI

Haemophilus ducreyi is the etiologic agent of chancroid, a sexually transmitted disease characterized by genital ulceration and inguinal adenitis. *H. ducreyi* poses a significant health problem in developing countries. Although this infection is less common in the United States, its incidence has increased dramatically in the past several years. In addition to being a cause of morbidity in itself, chancroid is associated with infection with human immunodeficiency virus (HIV) because of the role of genital ulceration in the transmission of HIV.

MICROBIOLOGY *H. ducreyi* is a highly fastidious coccobacillary gram-negative bacterium whose growth requires X factor (hemin). Although, in light of this requirement, the bacterium has been classified in the genus *Haemophilus*, DNA homology and chemotaxonomic studies have established substantial differences between *H. ducreyi* and other *Haemophilus* species. Taxonomic reclassification of the organism is likely in the future but awaits further study.

EPIDEMIOLOGY AND PREVALENCE Chancroid is a common cause of genital ulcers in developing countries. Several large outbreaks of chancroid have occurred in the United States since 1981. Recurring epidemiologic themes have been apparent in these outbreaks: (1) transmission has been predominantly heterosexual, (2) males have outnumbered females by ratios of 3:1 to 25:1, and (3) prostitutes have been important in transmission of the infection. The incidence of chancroid in the United States will undoubtedly increase in the coming years, and the genital ulcers associated with this infection will continue to play a role in the transmission of HIV.

CLINICAL MANIFESTATIONS Infection is acquired as the result of a break in the epithelium during sexual contact with an infected individual. After an incubation period of 4 to 7 days, the initial lesion—a papule with surrounding erythema—appears. In 2 to 3 days, the papule evolves into a pustule, which spontaneously ruptures and forms a sharply circumscribed ulcer that is generally not indurated. The ulcers are painful and bleed easily; little or no inflammation of the surrounding skin is evident. Approximately half of patients develop enlarged, tender inguinal lymph nodes, which frequently become fluctuant and spontaneously rupture.

The presentation of chancroid does not usually include all of the typical clinical features and is sometimes atypical. Multiple ulcers can coalesce to form giant ulcers. Ulcers can appear and then resolve, with inguinal adenitis and suppuration following 1 to 3 weeks later; this clinical picture can be confused with that of lymphogranuloma venereum. Multiple small ulcers can resemble folliculitis. Other differential diagnostic considerations include the various infections causing genital ulceration, such as primary syphilis, condyloma latum of secondary syphilis, genital herpes, and donovanosis. In rare cases chancroid lesions become secondarily infected with bacteria; the result is extensive inflammation.

DIAGNOSIS Clinical diagnosis of chancroid is often inaccurate, and laboratory confirmation should be attempted in suspected cases. Gram's staining of a swab of the lesion may reveal a predominance of characteristic gram-negative coccobacilli, but the presence of other bacteria often makes it difficult to interpret this result. An accurate diagnosis of chancroid relies on cultures of *H. ducreyi* from the lesion. Since the organism can be difficult to grow, the use of selective and supplemented media is necessary.

 TREATMENT
Clinical isolates of *H. ducreyi* often exhibit plasmid-mediated resistance to ampicillin, chloramphenicol, tetracyclines, and sulfonamides. Nevertheless, chancroid can be treated effectively with several regimens, including (1) ceftriaxone, 250 mg intramuscularly as a single dose; (2) erythromycin, 500 mg orally four times daily for 7 days; (3) trimethoprim-sulfamethoxazole, one double-strength tablet twice daily for 7 days (in regions where resistant strains are not prevalent); and (4) ciprofloxacin, 500 mg orally twice daily for 3 days. Isolates from patients who do not respond promptly to treatment should be tested for antimicrobial susceptibility.

OTHER HAEMOPHILUS SPECIES

Haemophilus species are often recovered as components of the flora of the normal human upper respiratory tract. However, these bacteria are infrequent causes of infection because of their low pathogenic potential. *Haemophilus* species have fastidious growth requirements and are generally rather slow-growing. The species implicated in human infections include *Haemophilus parainfluenzae*, *Haemophilus aphrophilus*, and *Haemophilus paraphrophilus* (see "HACEK Group Organisms" below); *Haemophilus parahaemolyticus*; *Haemophilus haemolyticus*; and *Haemophilus segnis*. *Haemophilus* species are differentiated from one another by several characteristics, primarily their requirements for X and V factors. Species designated *para-* require V factor but not X factor for growth, whereas the others require either X and V or X only.

A variety of infections involving almost all organ systems can be caused by *Haemophilus* species. Most of these unusual manifestations have been reported as single cases and small series.

The antimicrobial susceptibility characteristics of other *Haemophilus* species are similar to those of *H. influenzae*. Some strains produce β-lactamase and are thereby resistant to ampicillin. Other strains are sensitive to ampicillin, and this agent has been used successfully to treat many infections. Alternative agents with good activity against most *Haemophilus* species include trimethoprim-sulfamethoxazole, third-generation cephalosporins, tetracycline, chloramphenicol, and aminoglycosides. Endocarditis caused by ampicillin-sensitive strains should be treated with ampicillin plus an aminoglycoside.

HACEK GROUP ORGANISMS

HACEK organisms are a group of fastidious, slow-growing, gram-negative organisms whose growth requires an atmosphere of carbon dioxide. Species belonging to this group include several *Haemophilus* species (the most important of which are *H. aphrophilus*, *H. parainfluenzae*, and *H. paraphrophilus*), *Actinobacillus actinomycetemcomitans*, *Cardiobacterium hominis*, *Eikenella corrodens*, and *Kingella kingae*. These organisms frequently require prolonged incubation for isolation from blood cultures (at least 7 days). Cultures of blood from patients with suspected endocarditis due to HACEK organisms may require up to 30 days to become positive. These organisms are found less commonly in clinical specimens than *H. influenzae*, perhaps because they are less virulent. HACEK bacteria normally reside in the oral cavity and have been associated with local infections in the mouth. They are also known to cause severe systemic infections—most often bacterial endocarditis.

Of the HACEK group, the *Haemophilus* species, *A. actinomycetemcomitans*, and *C. hominis* are most frequently associated with endocarditis, which can develop on either native or prosthetic valves. In large series of cases of infective endocarditis, about 1 percent of cases are attributable to HACEK organisms, with the *Haemophilus* species most commonly isolated. The clinical course of HACEK endocarditis tends to be subacute; however, embolization is common. The overall prevalence of major emboli associated with endocarditis due to these organisms is 28 percent; rates have been as high as 60 percent in some series.

Thirty-three percent of patients with HACEK native-valve endocarditis due to *Haemophilus* species have a history of cardiac valvular disease, 60 percent have been ill for less than 2 months before presentation, and 50 percent are anemic at presentation. Nineteen percent of patients develop congestive heart failure. Mortality rates as high as 30 percent (with most deaths attributed to cerebral embolism) have been reported. Despite these grim statistics for endocarditis on native valves, the cure rate for HACEK prosthetic-valve endocarditis appears to be high. Frequently (in more than 80 percent of cases), cure is achieved with antibiotic treatment alone and without surgical intervention. The better success in prosthetic-valve than in native-valve endocarditis is most likely due to earlier detection of infection.

Therapy for HACEK endocarditis due to *Haemophilus* species should be based on antibiotic sensitivity testing. Empirical combination therapy with ampicillin and gentamicin, which tend to be synergistic against some isolates, is a reasonable initial approach. Ceftriaxone (2 g/d) has also been used successfully.

A. actinomycetemcomitans, another slow-growing inhabitant of the oral cavity, can be isolated from soft tissue infections and abscesses in association with *Actinomyces israelii*. About 30 percent of actinomycotic lesions also yield *A. actinomycetemcomitans* on culture. *A. actinomycetemcomitans* has been associated with severe destructive periodontal disease, characterized by loss of alveolar bone of the molars and incisors, in both children and adults. This organism has also been associated with endocarditis, especially in patients with severe periodontal disease and underlying cardiac valvular damage; high rates of embolic phenomena are associated with endocarditis. *A. actinomycetemcomitans* has been isolated from patients with brain abscesses, meningitis, parotitis, osteomyelitis, urinary tract infection, pneumonia, and empyema, among other infections. Most isolates are susceptible to third-generation cephalosporins, semisynthetic penicillins like mezlocillin, trimethoprim-sulfamethoxazole, quinolones, and azithromycin. However, because of variability among strains, susceptibility testing should be undertaken. Endocarditis should be treated for 4 weeks, whereas prosthetic-valve infections or infections in patients with complications such as embolization justify 6 weeks of therapy.

C. hominis primarily causes endocarditis in patients with underlying valvular heart disease or with prosthetic valves. Many patients have signs and symptoms of long-standing infection before diagnosis. As in endocarditis due to other HACEK organisms, embolization, mycotic aneurysms, and congestive heart failure are frequent. Antibiotic sensitivity testing of *C. hominis* is difficult. Most cases of infection due to *C. hominis* are treated with penicillin, either alone or in combination with an aminoglycoside. The value of the aminoglycoside in this situation has not been established.

E. corrodens, a fastidious facultative gram-negative organism, is part of the endogenous flora of the mouth and nasopharynx. It is most frequently recovered from sites of infection in conjunction with other bacterial species. Clinical sources of *E. corrodens* include sites of human bite wounds (clenched-fist injuries), endocarditis, soft tissue infections of the head and neck, soft tissue infections in drug abusers, osteomyelitis, respiratory infections, chorioamnionitis, gynecologic infections associated with intrauterine devices, meningitis and brain abscesses, and visceral abscesses. *E. corrodens*–associated infections can be treated with ampicillin or with second- or third-generation cephalosporins. The organism is susceptible to the fluoroquinolones in vitro but is resistant to metronidazole and clindamycin. → *Kingella kingae* is discussed in Chap. 151.

OTHER GRAM-NEGATIVE BACILLI

ALCALIGENES XYLOSOXIDANS   This gram-negative bacillus is probably part of the endogenous intestinal flora and has been isolated from water sources. Immunocompromised hosts appear to be

at increased risk for infection with this organism. Nosocomial sources to which outbreaks of infection with *A. xylosoxidans* have been attributed include contaminated intravenous fluids, pressure transducers, and disinfectants. Clinical illness has been associated with isolates from many sites, including blood, urine, respiratory secretions, peritoneal and pleural fluids, and endocarditic prosthetic valves. In vitro susceptibility testing of all clinically relevant isolates is essential to the selection of appropriate therapy.

AGROBACTERIUM TUMEFACIENS   This organism has been associated with intravascular catheter–related infections in immunocompromised hosts, especially individuals infected with HIV. Clinically important infections associated with *A. tumefaciens* include prosthetic-joint and prosthetic-valve infections, bacteremia, peritonitis, and urinary tract infections. Antibiotic sensitivity testing is essential in the choice of therapy.

***CAPNOCYTOPHAGA* SPECIES**   This genus of fusiform, long, thin gram-negative rods is facultatively anaerobic and requires an atmosphere enriched in carbon dioxide for optimal growth. *Capnocytophaga ochracea*, *Capnocytophaga gingivalis*, and *Capnocytophaga sputigena* are normal inhabitants of the human oral cavity and have been isolated from the female genital tract. Their isolation has also been reported from blood, CSF, and respiratory fluids (including pleural collections). These organisms have been associated with sepsis in immunocompromised hosts; particularly at risk are patients with acute myelogenous leukemia or acute lymphocytic leukemia. In the immunocompetent host, these three species probably play a role in localized juvenile periodontitis; however, they have been isolated from many other sites as well, usually as part of a polymicrobial infection. In vitro sensitivity testing of these organisms is difficult because they are slow-growing and fastidious. Although penicillin has been considered first-line therapy, an increasing number of isolates reportedly produce β-lactamase. Clindamycin or drug combinations including a penicillin derivative plus a β-lactamase inhibitor—such as ampicillin/sulbactam or amoxicillin/clavulanate—are currently recommended for empiric therapy.

Capnocytophaga canimorsus and *Capnocytophaga cynodegmi* are endogenous to the canine mouth. Patients infected with these species frequently have a history of dog bites or of exposure to dogs without scratches or bites. Asplenia, glucocorticoid therapy, and alcohol abuse are predisposing conditions and are associated with relatively fulminant infections. The interval from dog bite to presentation averages 5 days but ranges from 1 day to 1 month. *C. canimorsus* causes a wide range of infections, including severe sepsis with shock and disseminated intravascular coagulation, meningitis, endocarditis, cellulitis, and septic arthritis. In the asplenic individual who has recently sustained a dog bite, infection with this organism must be considered early because of a potentially rapid progression to death. Penicillin is the drug of choice for infections with *C. canimorsus*. This agent should also be given prophylactically to asplenic patients sustaining dog-bite injuries. Patients with suspected *C. canimorsus* infection should be treated empirically, because identification of this organism and determination of its antibiotic sensitivity can take many days. Other drugs to which *C. canimorsus* is reportedly susceptible include clindamycin, imipenem, quinolones, and third-generation cephalosporins.

CHROMOBACTERIUM VIOLACEUM   This organism is rarely a human pathogen but reportedly has been responsible for life-threatening infections with severe sepsis and metastatic abscesses. A slender, slightly curved, gram-negative rod that is facultatively anaerobic, *C. violaceum* inhabits tropical water and soil and causes infection after contamination of skin wounds. Patients with defective neutrophil function (e.g., those with chronic granulomatous disease) are infected by this organism with unusual frequency. The mortality rate in the United States from infection with *C. violaceum* has been reported at >60 percent. The organism is generally susceptible to ciprofloxacin, trimethoprim-sulfamethoxazole, gentamicin, and chloramphenicol.

FLAVOBACTERIUM MENINGOSEPTICUM   The most important of the *Flavobacterium* species isolated from humans, *F. menin-*

gosepticum is associated with nosocomial infections transmitted by fluids such as disinfectants and arterial catheter flush solutions. This organism has also been associated with neonatal sepsis and meningitis. Adults have sometimes developed infection after receiving aerosolized antibiotics or while immunocompromised. *F. meningosepticum* has been reported to cause meningitis, endocarditis, bacteremia, and respiratory infections. Antibiotic treatment should be based on susceptibility results because of the high likelihood that *F. meningosepticum* will produce β-lactamase.

PLESIOMONAS SHIGELLOIDES This freshwater organism is a cause of acute diarrhea (see Chap. 128) and occasionally of serious extraintestinal disease. *P. shigelloides* is transmitted to humans via contaminated water or food. This motile, facultatively anaerobic gram-negative rod most often produces mild diarrhea with mucoid, bloody feces containing leukocytes. Severe extraintestinal infections have been reported most commonly in immunocompromised hosts and include bacteremia, cellulitis, neonatal sepsis and meningitis, and septic arthritis. There is great variability among strains in terms of antibiotic sensitivity patterns, and isolates must be tested before appropriate therapy can be selected.

MISCELLANEOUS ORGANISMS Many other gram-negative rods have been reported to cause occasional infections in hosts who are immunologically unprepared to deal with relatively avirulent organisms or who are unfortunate enough to encounter an exceptionally large inoculum. Such organisms include *Weeksella* species; various CDC groups, such as EF-4, Ve-2 (*Flavimonas* species), IVc-2, NO-1, WO-1, and Gilardi Group WO-1; *Sphingobacterium* species; *Protomonas* species; *Ochrobactrum anthropi*; *Oligella urethralis*; and *Achromobacter* species. The reader is advised to consult subspecialty texts and references for further guidance on these organisms.

BIBLIOGRAPHY

BARBOUR ML et al: The impact of conjugate vaccine on carriage of *Haemophilus influenzae* type b. J Infect Dis 171:93, 1995

BILGRAMI S et al: *Capnocytophaga* bacteremia in a patient with Hodgkin's disease following bone marrow transplantation: Case report and review. Clin Infect Dis 14:1045, 1992

BRUCKNER DA, COLONNA P: Nomenclature for aerobic and facultative bacteria. Clin Infect Dis 16:598, 1993

CAMPBELL JR, EDWARDS MS: *Capnocytophaga* species infections in children. Pediatr Infect Dis J 10:944, 1991

CIESLAK TJ, RASZKA WV: Catheter-associated sepsis due to *Alcaligenes xylosoxidans* in a child with AIDS. Clin Infect Dis 16:592, 1993

CLARK RB et al: Fatal *Plesiomonas shigelloides* septicaemia in a splenectomized patient. J Infect 23:89, 1991

COLDING H et al: Ribotyping for differentiating *Flavobacterium meningosepticum* isolates from clinical and environmental sources. J Clin Microbiol 32:501, 1994

COMMITTEE ON INFECTIOUS DISEASES: *Haemophilus influenzae* infections, in *1994 Red Book, Report of the Committee on Infectious Diseases,* G Peter et al (eds). Elk Grove Village, IL, American Academy of Pediatrics, 1994

DECRE D et al: A beta-lactamase-overproducing strain of *Alcaligenes denitrificans* subsp. *xylosoxidans* isolated from a case of meningitis. J Antimicrob Chemother 30:769, 1992

FARLEY MM et al: Invasive *Haemophilus influenzae* disease in adults. Ann Intern Med 116:806, 1992

FLEISCHMANN RD et al: Whole-genome random sequencing and assembly of *Haemophilus influenzae* Rd. Science 269:496, 1995

FLOOD JM et al: Multistrain outbreak of chancroid in San Francisco, 1989–91. J Infect Dis 167:1106, 1993

FUJII T et al: Purification and properties of inducible penicillin beta-lactamase isolated from *Alcaligenes faecalis*. Antimicrob Agents Chemother 27:608, 1985

HARABUCHI Y et al: Nasopharyngeal colonization with nontypeable *Haemophilus influenzae* and recurrent otitis media. J Infect Dis 170:862, 1994

HOLMBERG SD et al: *Plesiomonas* enteric infections in the United States. Ann Intern Med 105:690, 1986

HULSE M et al: *Agrobacterium* infection in humans: Experience at one hospital and review. Clin Infect Dis 16:112, 1993

JANDA JM, ABBOTT SL: Expression of hemolytic activity by *Plesiomonas shigelloides*. J Clin Microbiol 31:1206, 1993

KULLBERG JB et al: Purpura fulminans and symmetrical peripheral gangrene caused by *Capnocytophaga canimorsus* (formerly DF-2) septicemia—a complication of dog bite. Medicine 70:287, 1991

KURIKKA S et al: Comparison of five different vaccination schedules with *Haemophilus influenzae* type b–tetanus toxoid conjugated vaccine. J Pediatr 128:524, 1996

MURPHY TF, SETHI S: Bacterial infection in chronic obstructive pulmonary disease. Am Rev Respir Dis 146:1067, 1992

——— et al: Declining incidence of *Haemophilus influenzae* type b disease since introduction of vaccination. JAMA 269:246, 1993

PATRICK WD et al: Infective endocarditis due to *Eikenella corrodens:* Case report and review of the literature. Can J Infect Dis 1:139, 1990

PICKETT MJ et al: Miscellaneous gram-negative bacteria, in *Manual of Clinical Microbiology,* 5th ed, A Balows et al (eds). Washington, DC, American Society for Microbiology, 1991, pp 410–428

POKRYUKA M et al: A *Flavobacterium meningosepticum* outbreak among intensive care patients. Am J Infect Control 21:139, 1993

POLLNER JH et al: Severe soft-tissue infection caused by *Eikenella corrodens*. Clin Infect Dis 15:740, 1992

RAMIREZ FC et al: *Agrobacterium tumefaciens* peritonitis mimicking tuberculosis. Clin Infect Dis 15:938, 1992

ROBISON WJ, VITELLI AS: Infectious endocarditis caused by *Cardiobacterium hominis*. South Med J 78:1020, 1985

ROSCOE DL et al: Antimicrobial susceptibilities and β-lactamase characterization of *Capnocytophaga* species. Antimicrob Agents Chemother 36:2197, 1992

SCHEIFELE DW: Recent trends in pediatric *Haemophilus influenzae* type b infections in Canada. Immunization Monitoring Program, Active (IMPACT) of the Canadian Paediatric Society and the Laboratory Centre for Disease Control. Can Med Assoc J 154:1041, 1996

SORENSON RU et al: *Chromobacterium violaceum* adenitis acquired in the northern United States as a complication of chronic granulomatous disease. Pediatr Infect Dis 4:701, 1985

STEINHART R et al: Invasive *Haemophilus influenzae* infections in men with HIV infection. JAMA 268:3350, 1992

TAVERAS JM III et al: Apparent culture-negative endocarditis of the prosthetic valve caused by *Cardiobacterium hominis*. South Med J 86:1439, 1993

TI T-Y et al: Nonfatal and fatal infections caused by *Chromobacterium violaceum*. Clin Infect Dis 17:505, 1993

VADHEIM CM et al: Eradication of *Haemophilus influenzae* type b disease in southern California. Arch Pediatr Adolesc Med 148:51, 1994

WALSH RD et al: *Achromobacter xylosoxidans* osteomyelitis. Clin Infect Dis 16:176, 1993

WILSON ME: Prosthetic valve endocarditis and paravalvular abscess caused by *Actinobacillus actinomycetemcomitans*. Rev Infect Dis 11:665, 1989

153

Lutfiye Mulazimoglu, Victor L. Yu

LEGIONELLA INFECTION

DEFINITION *Legionellosis* refers to the two clinical syndromes caused by bacteria of the genus *Legionella*. *Pontiac fever* is an acute, febrile, self-limited illness that has been serologically linked to *Legionella* species, whereas *Legionnaires' disease* is the designation for pneumonia caused by these species.

HISTORY Legionnaires' disease was first recognized in 1976, when an outbreak of pneumonia took place at a hotel in Philadelphia during the American Legion Convention. Investigators from the Centers for Disease Control and Prevention (CDC) identified the causative aerobic gram-negative bacterium in lung specimens obtained from the victims at autopsy and named this organism *Legionella pneumophila*. Retrospective studies of stored serum samples revealed that an epidemic of Legionnaires' disease had occurred in 1957 in Austin, Minnesota. In this epidemic (the earliest documented so far), 78 persons were hospitalized with acute respiratory infection. Antibody determinations showed seroconversion to *L. pneumophila* in most cases.

MICROBIOLOGY At present, the family Legionellaceae comprises 41 species with 63 serogroups. The species *L. pneumophila* causes 80 to 90 percent of human infections and includes at least 14 serogroups; serogroups 1, 4, and 6 are most commonly implicated in human infections. To date, 17 species other than *L. pneumophila* have been associated with human infections, among which *L. micdadei* (Pittsburgh pneumonia agent), *L. bozemanii*, *L. dumoffii*, and *L. longbeachae* are the most common.

Members of the Legionellaceae are aerobic, thin, gram-negative bacilli that do not grow on routine microbiologic media. Buffered charcoal yeast extract (BCYE) agar is the medium used to grow *Legionella*. This highly enhanced medium contains the amino acid L-cysteine, which is an absolute growth requirement for *Legionella*. Growth of the organism on BCYE medium is usually visible in 3 to 5 days at 35 to 37°C. *L. micdadei* and *L. maceachernii* produce blue colonies on BCYE medium containing bromocresol purple and bromothymol blue dyes, while the other species produce green colonies.

Antimicrobial agents, including polymyxin B, cefamandole, and vancomycin, are used in *Legionella*-selective media to suppress competing components of the microflora. Although *L. pneumophila* is relatively tolerant to these antibiotics, the drugs may inhibit the growth of other legionellae; for example, cefamandole-containing media suppress the growth of *L. micdadei*.

Traditional biochemical tests are not particularly helpful in distinguishing one *Legionella* species from another. Fatty-acid profile determination by gas-liquid chromatography and ubiquinone analysis allow identification to the genus level. The direct fluorescent antibody (DFA) test can definitively identify a number of individual species. In *L. pneumophila*, lipopolysaccharide is a prominent constituent of the outer membrane, and the serogroup-specific antigen and antibodies detected by immunofluorescence are directed primarily at the lipopolysaccharide. Both polyclonal and monoclonal DFA reagents are commercially available. The monoclonal antibody reagent (Genetic Systems, Seattle, WA) is less cross-reactive but is specific for *L. pneumophila*. Genetic analysis has been considered the definitive arbiter for the identification of individual species, with the degree of DNA sequence homology the most common criterion employed. A nucleic-acid hybridization probe reactive to *Legionella* ribosomal RNA, used with a single reagent, can identify a member of the genus within hours.

ECOLOGY AND TRANSMISSION The natural habitats for *L. pneumophila* are aquatic bodies, including lakes and streams; *L. longbeachae* has been isolated from soil. Legionellae can survive under a wide range of environmental conditions; for example, the organisms can live for years in refrigerated water samples. Natural bodies of water contain only small numbers of legionellae. However, once the organisms enter human-constructed aquatic reservoirs (such as cooling towers or water-distribution systems), they can grow and proliferate. Factors known to enhance colonization by and amplification of legionellae include warm temperatures (25 to 42°C), stagnation, and scale and sediment. The presence of symbiotic microorganisms, including algae, amebas, ciliated protozoa, and other water-dwelling bacteria, likewise promotes growth of *L. pneumophila*.

Hot-water tanks colonized with *L. pneumophila* are significantly more likely than uncolonized tanks to be cooler (<60°C), to have a vertical configuration, to be older, and to have higher concentrations of calcium and magnesium. Vertical tanks, especially those that are electric coil-heated rather than gas-heated, have a pronounced temperature stratification and thick sediment accumulation at the bottom. Studies have shown that neither a high degree of outward cleanliness nor routine application of maintenance measures decreases the frequency or intensity of *Legionella* colonization. Thus, engineering guidelines and building codes, although often advocated as preventive measures, have relatively little impact on *Legionella* colonization.

The source of *Legionella* is water, but the mode of transmission from the environmental reservoir to the patient remains controversial. Early investigations that implicated cooling towers antedated the discovery that the organism could also exist in potable water distribution systems. It is now known that, in many outbreaks, cases of Legionnaires' disease continued to occur despite disinfection of cooling towers and the potable water supply was the actual source. Koch's postulates have been fulfilled in epidemiologic studies using molecular fingerprinting methods to link potable water sources (unlike cooling

towers) to *Legionella* infection in humans. Community-acquired Legionnaires' disease has been linked to colonization of residential and industrial water supplies.

The modes of transmission of *Legionella* to humans are probably multiple: evidence exists for transmission due to aerosolization, aspiration, and direct instillation into the lung during respiratory tract manipulations. Aspiration may be the predominant mode of transmission, but it is unclear whether *Legionella* enters the lung via oropharyngeal colonization or directly via the drinking of contaminated water. Nasogastric tubes have been linked to nosocomial Legionnaires' disease in several reports; microaspiration of contaminated water was the hypothesized mode of transmission. Surgery with general anesthesia is a known risk factor that is consistent with aspiration. Especially compelling is the reported 30 percent incidence of postoperative *Legionella* pneumonia among patients undergoing head and neck surgery in a hospital with a contaminated water supply; aspiration is a recognized sequela in such cases. Studies of patients with hospital-acquired Legionnaires' disease showed that these individuals underwent endotracheal intubation significantly more often and for a significantly longer duration than patients with nosocomial pneumonia of other etiologies.

Aerosolization of legionellae by devices filled with tap water, including nebulizers and humidifiers, has caused cases of Legionnaires' disease. An ultrasonic mist machine in the produce section of a grocery store was implicated in a community outbreak. Pontiac fever has been linked to *Legionella*-containing aerosols from water-using machinery, a cooling tower, air-conditioners, and whirlpools.

EPIDEMIOLOGY The incidence of Legionnaires' disease depends on the degree of contamination of the aquatic reservoir, the susceptibility and immune status of the persons exposed to the water from that reservoir, the intensity of exposure, and the availability of specialized laboratory tests on which the correct diagnosis can be based.

Numerous prospective studies have found *Legionella* to rank among the top three microbial causes of community-acquired pneumonia (*Streptococcus pneumoniae* and *Haemophilus influenzae* usually ranking first and second), accounting for 3 to 15 percent of cases. On the basis of a multihospital study of community-acquired pneumonia in Ohio, the CDC has estimated that only 3 percent of sporadic cases of Legionnaires' disease are correctly diagnosed. Legionellae are responsible for 10 to 50 percent of nosocomial pneumonias when a hospital's water system is colonized with the organisms. One situation in which the diagnosis of Legionnaires' disease should be considered is that in which the presenting patient has been hospitalized within 10 days before the onset of symptoms. In one study, a number of patients had been discharged from the hospital and readmitted with Legionnaires' disease; molecular fingerprinting showed that the isolates obtained from patients and the isolate from the hospital's water supply were similar.

The most common risk factors for Legionnaires' disease are cigarette smoking, chronic lung disease, advanced age, and immunosuppression. The disease most often develops in elderly men; this predilection is probably related to cigarette smoking. Surgery is a prominent predisposing factor in nosocomial infection, with transplant recipients at highest risk. Nosocomial cases are now being recognized among neonates and among children with immunosuppression or underlying pulmonary disease.

Pontiac fever occurs in epidemics. The high attack rate (above 90 percent) reflects airborne transmission.

PATHOGENESIS Legionellae enter the lungs via aspiration or direct inhalation. The organisms possess pili that may mediate adherence to respiratory tract epithelial cells. Thus, conditions that impair mucociliary clearance, including cigarette smoking, lung disease, or alcoholism, predispose to Legionnaires' disease.

Cell-mediated immunity is the primary mechanism of host defense against *Legionella*, as it is against other intracellular pathogens, including *Mycobacterium tuberculosis*, *Listeria*, and *Toxoplasma*. Alveolar macrophages readily phagocytose legionellae. However, the organisms are not killed and proliferate intracellularly until the cells rupture; the bacteria are then phagocytosed again by newly recruited phagocytes, and the cycle begins anew. Legionnaires' disease is more common and the disease manifestations are more severe in patients with depressed cell-mediated immunity, including transplant recipients, patients infected with human immunodeficiency virus, and patients receiving glucocorticoids. The disease also occurs with unusual frequency among patients with hairy cell leukemia (which is characterized by monocyte deficiency and dysfunction) but not among patients with other types of leukemia.

The role of neutrophils in immunity appears to be minimal: neutropenic patients are not predisposed to Legionnaires' disease. Although *L. pneumophila* is susceptible to oxygen-dependent microbiologic systems in vitro, it resists killing by neutrophils.

The humoral immune system is active against *Legionella*. Type-specific IgM and IgG antibodies are measurable within weeks of infection. In vitro, antibodies promote killing of legionellae by phagocytes (neutrophils, monocytes, and alveolar macrophages). However, antibodies neither enhance lysis by complement nor inhibit intracellular multiplication within phagocytes. Immunized animals develop a specific antibody response, with subsequent resistance to *Legionella* challenge.

Some *L. pneumophila* strains are clearly more virulent than others, although the precise factors mediating virulence remain uncertain. For example, although multiple strains may colonize water-distribution systems, only a few cause disease in patients exposed to that water. At least one surface epitope of *L. pneumophila* serogroup 1 is associated with virulence. *L. pneumophila* serogroup 6 is more commonly involved in nosocomial Legionnaires' disease and is more likely to be associated with a poor outcome.

PATHOLOGY The consistent pathologic features of Legionnaires' disease are confined to the lungs. Findings in infected lung tissue range from multifocal pneumonia with patchy lobular inflammation to extensive multilobar consolidation. Visible abscesses with central necrosis were seen in 20 percent of autopsied cases in one study. On histologic examination, fibrinopurulent pneumonia with intensive alveolitis and bronchiolitis is evident. Lesions of longer standing can have a nodular appearance with a central area of necrosis surrounded by macrophages and other cells. The alveoli are filled with fibrin, neutrophils, and alveolar macrophages.

Usual tissue stains, including Gram's, hematoxylin and eosin, Brown-Brenn, and methenamine silver, do not reveal the organism. Giminez stain can be used for imprints on fresh or fixed tissue. Dieterle's silver stain or modified Giminez stain, although nonspecific and relatively insensitive, can be used for paraffin-fixed specimens. The DFA stain is not only specific but also the most sensitive option for visualization of the organism in tissues. Polyvalent DFA stains but not monoclonal DFA stain can be used for formalinized specimens. Because the DFA stains are species and serogroup specific, false-negative results can be obtained if the incorrect reagent is used. Thus culture is the preferred method for diagnosis based on clinical specimens.

CLINICAL AND LABORATORY FEATURES **Pontiac Fever** Pontiac fever is an acute, self-limiting, flulike illness with a 24- to 48-h incubation period. Pneumonia does not develop in Pontiac fever. Malaise, fatigue, and myalgias are the most frequent symptoms, occurring in 97 percent of cases. Fever (usually with chills) develops in 80 to 90 percent of cases and headache in 80 percent. Other symptoms (seen in fewer than 50 percent of cases) include arthralgias, nausea, cough, abdominal pain, and diarrhea. Modest leukocytosis with a neutrophilic predominance is sometimes detected. Complete recovery takes place within only a few days without antibiotic therapy; a few patients may experience lassitude for many weeks thereafter. The diagnosis is established by antibody seroconversion.

Table 153-1

Clinical Clues Suggestive of Legionnaires' Disease

Diarrhea
High fever (>40°C)
Numerous neutrophils but no organisms revealed by Gram's staining of respiratory secretions
Hyponatremia (serum sodium level of <131 meq/L)
Failure to respond to β-lactam drugs (penicillins or cephalosporins) and aminoglycoside antibiotics
Occurrence of illness in an environment in which the potable water supply is known to be contaminated with *Legionella*
Onset of symptoms within 10 days after discharge from the hospital

Legionnaires' Disease (Pneumonia) Clinical findings that raise the possibility of Legionnaires' disease are summarized in Table 153-1. Although these manifestations may provide clues to the diagnosis, prospective comparative studies have shown that they are generally nonspecific and do not serve to distinguish Legionnaires' disease from pneumonia of other etiologies. Legionnaires' disease is often included in the differential diagnosis of "atypical pneumonia," along with infection due to *Chlamydia pneumoniae*, *Chlamydia psittaci*, *Mycoplasma pneumoniae*, *Coxiella burnetii*, and some viruses. The clinical similarities among these types of pneumonia include a relatively nonproductive cough and a low incidence of grossly purulent sputum. However, the clinical manifestations of Legionnaires' disease are usually more severe than those of most "atypical" pneumonias, and the course and prognosis of *Legionella* pneumonia more resemble those of bacteremic pneumococcal pneumonia than those of pneumonia due to other "atypical" pathogens. Patients with community-acquired Legionnaires' disease are significantly more likely than patients with pneumonia of other etiologies to be admitted to an intensive care unit upon presentation.

The incubation period for Legionnaires' disease is 2 to 10 days. The symptoms and signs may range from a mild cough and a slight fever to stupor with widespread pulmonary infiltrates and multisystem failure. Nonspecific symptoms—malaise, fatigue, anorexia, and headache—are seen early in the illness. Myalgias and arthralgias are uncommon but are unusually marked in a few patients. Upper respiratory symptoms, including coryza, are rare.

The mild cough of Legionnaires' disease is only slightly productive. Sometimes the sputum is streaked with blood. Chest pain—either pleuritic or nonpleuritic—can be a prominent feature and, when coupled with hemoptysis, can lead to an incorrect diagnosis of pulmonary embolism. Shortness of breath is reported by one-third to one-half of patients.

Gastrointestinal difficulties are often pronounced; abdominal pain, nausea, and vomiting affect 10 to 20 percent of patients. Diarrhea (watery rather than bloody) is reported in 25 to 50 percent of cases. The most common neurologic abnormalities are confusion or changes in mental status; however, the multitudinous neurologic symptoms reported range from headache and lethargy to encephalopathy.

Patients with Legionnaires' disease virtually always have fever. Temperatures in excess of 40.5°C were recorded in 20 percent of the cases in one series. Relative bradycardia has been overemphasized as a useful diagnostic finding; it occurs infrequently, primarily affecting older patients with severe pneumonia. Chest examination reveals rales early in the course and evidence of consolidations as the disease progresses. Abdominal examination may reveal generalized or local tenderness.

Diarrhea and hyponatremia occur significantly more often in Legionnaires' disease than in other forms of pneumonia. Hyponatremia is most common in severe cases. The mechanism of hyponatremia does not appear to be related to inappropriate secretion of antidiuretic hormone but instead to salt and water loss. Besides hyponatremia, other laboratory abnormalities include abnormal liver function tests, hypophosphatemia, hematuria, hematologic abnormalities, and thrombocytopenia; although common, these abnormalities are not found significantly more frequently in Legionnaires' disease than in pneumonias of other etiologies.

Extrapulmonary Legionellosis Since the portal of entry for legionellae is the lung in virtually all cases, extrapulmonary manifestations usually result from bloodborne dissemination from the lung. In a prospective survey of patients with Legionnaires' disease diagnosed by isolation of the organism from sputum, legionellae were isolated from the blood by a special culture method in 38 percent of cases.

Legionella has been identified in the spleen, liver, or kidneys in 50 percent of autopsied cases of Legionnaires' disease. The organism has also been isolated from intrathoracic and inguinal lymph nodes—a finding suggesting dissemination by lymphatic pathways. Extrapulmonary involvement, including sinusitis, peritonitis, pyelonephritis, cellulitis, and pancreatitis, has been documented predominantly in immunosuppressed patients.

The most common extrapulmonary site of legionellosis is the heart; numerous reports have described myocarditis, pericarditis, postcardiotomy syndrome, and prosthetic-valve endocarditis. Most cases have been hospital-acquired. Since many of the patients involved have not had overt pneumonia, the lung may not have been the portal of entry. Rather, in these cardiac infections, the organisms may have gained entry via a postoperative sternal wound exposed to contaminated tap water or via a mediastinal-tube insertion site.

Various other sources of or factors promoting *Legionella* infection at various extrapulmonary sites have been postulated, including the presence of foreign bodies, such as sutures and draining tubes (wound infection following cardiothoracic surgery); immersion in a Hubbard tank (superinfection of a hip wound); bloodborne dissemination from a pulmonary infection site (perirectal abscess); and ingestion of contaminated water (peritonitis).

Chest Radiographic Abnormalities Virtually all patients with Legionnaires' disease have abnormal chest radiographs showing pulmonary infiltrates at the time of clinical presentation. In a few cases of nosocomial disease, fever and respiratory tract symptoms have preceded the appearance of the infiltrate on chest radiography. Findings on chest radiography are nonspecific and do not serve to distinguish Legionnaires' disease from pneumonias of other etiologies. Pleural effusion is evident in one-third of cases, and the diagnosis is often based on culture and antigen testing (by the method designed for use with urine) of pleural fluid obtained by thoracentesis.

In immunosuppressed patients, especially those receiving glucocorticoids, distinctive rounded nodular opacities may be seen; these lesions may expand and cavitate (Fig. 153-1). Likewise, pulmonary abscesses can occur in immunosuppressed hosts. The progression of infiltrates on chest radiography despite appropriate antibiotic therapy is common, and radiographic improvement lags behind clinical improvement by several days. Complete clearing of infiltrates requires 1 to 4 months.

DIAGNOSIS The diagnosis of Legionnaires' disease requires special microbiologic tests (Table 153-2). The sensitivity of bronchoscopy specimens is approximately the same as that of sputum samples; if sputum is not available, bronchoscopy specimens may yield the

Table 153-2

Utility of Special Laboratory Tests for the Diagnosis of Legionnaires' Disease

Test	Sensitivity, %	Specificity, %
Culture		
Sputum*	80	100
Transtracheal aspirate	90	100
DFA staining of sputum	50–70	96–99
Urinary antigen testing†	70	100
Antibody serology‡	40–60	96–99

* Use of multiple selective media with dyes.
† Serogroup 1 only.
‡ IgG and IgM testing of both acute- and convalescent-phase sera. A single titer of ≥1:128 is considered presumptive, while a single titer of ≥1:256 or fourfold seroconversion is considered definitive.

organism. Bronchoalveolar lavage fluid gives higher yields than bronchial wash specimens. Thoracentesis should be performed if pleural effusion is found, and the fluid should be evaluated by DFA staining, culture, and the antigen test designed for use with urine.

Staining Gram's staining of material from normally sterile sites, such as pleural fluid or lung tissue, occasionally suggests the diagnosis; efforts to detect legionellae in sputum by Gram's staining typically reveal numerous leukocytes, but no organisms. When they are visualized, the organisms appear as small, pleomorphic, faint, gram-negative bacilli. *L. micdadei* organisms can be detected as weakly or partially acid-fast bacilli in clinical specimens. Modified acid-fast staining substitutes 1% sulfuric acid for the traditional 3% hydrochloric acid; the less aggressive decolorizer increases the yield of *L. micdadei*. *Legionella*-infected patients have often been treated empirically with antituberculosis medications because of false-positive acid-fast smears.

Culture The definitive method for diagnosis of *Legionella* infection is isolation of the organism from respiratory secretions or other specimens. As has been mentioned, BCYE agar supplemented with antibiotics and dyes is the most sensitive medium, and colonies grow slowly, requiring 3 to 5 days to become grossly visible. When culture plates are overgrown with other microflora, pretreatment of the specimen with acid or heat can markedly improve the yield. *L. pneumophila* is often isolated from sputum that is not grossly or microscopically purulent; sputum containing more than 25 epithelial cells per high-power field (a finding that classically suggests contamination) may still yield *L. pneumophila*.

DFA The DFA test is rapid and highly specific but is less sensitive than culture because large numbers of organisms are required for microscopic visualization. This test is more likely to be positive in advanced than in early disease.

FIGURE 153-1 Chest radiographic findings in a 52-year-old man who presented with pneumonia subsequently diagnosed as Legionnaires' disease. The patient was a cigarette smoker with chronic obstructive pulmonary disease and alcoholic cardiomyopathy; he had received glucocorticoids. *L. pneumophila* was identified by DFA staining and culture of sputum. *Left:* Baseline chest radiograph showing long-standing cardiomegaly. *Center:* Admission chest radiograph showing new rounded opacities. *Right:* Chest radiograph taken 3 days after admission, during treatment with erythromycin. *(Courtesy of Dr. Feng-Yee Chang.)*

Antibody Detection   Antibody testing of both acute- and convalescent-phase sera may be necessary. A fourfold rise in titer is diagnostic; 4 to 12 weeks are often required for the detection of an antibody response, and some patients never seroconvert. A single titer of 1:128 in a patient with pneumonia constitutes presumptive (but not definitive) evidence for Legionnaires' disease. Serology is of use primarily in epidemiologic studies. The specificity of serology for the non–*L. pneumophila* species is uncertain; there is cross-reactivity with *L. pneumophila* and some gram-negative bacilli.

Urinary Antigen   The assay for *Legionella* soluble antigen in urine (Binax, South Portland, ME) is rapid, relative inexpensive, easy to perform, second only to culture in terms of sensitivity, and highly specific (Table 153-2). Its use in every clinical laboratory is recommended. The test is available only for *L. pneumophila* serogroup 1, which, as has been mentioned, causes about 80 percent of *Legionella* infections. Antigen in urine is detectable 3 days after the onset of clinical disease, even if specific therapy has been started; furthermore, urinary antigen persists for several weeks.

Molecular Methods   Polymerase chain reaction (PCR) with DNA probes may prove more sensitive and specific than other methods. PCR has proved useful in the identification of legionellae from environmental water specimens. Evaluation of the sensitivity of this technique for the testing of clinical specimens is under way.

℞ TREATMENT

Regimens of value in the treatment of *Legionella* infections are listed in Table 153-3. Prospective, controlled evaluations of therapy for Legionnaires' disease have not been conducted. In the 1976 American Legion outbreak, cases treated with erythromycin and tetracycline appeared to have a better outcome than those treated with other agents. These two antibiotics also exhibit intracellular activity against legionellae and, unlike other antimicrobials, are effective in animal models.

The preference for erythromycin in the treatment of *Legionella* infections has evolved over time, although use of the intravenous dosage recommended specifically for Legionnaires' disease (4 g/d) has unmasked adverse effects that have led to management problems. These problems include the necessity for a large fluid volume, which is challenging because so many patients with Legionnaires' disease have underlying cardiac disease and prolongation of the QT interval. Symptomatic ototoxicity was confirmed by audiography in 21 percent of patients receiving the 4-g dose as empirical therapy for community-acquired pneumonia; ototoxicity was reversible when the administration of erythromycin was discontinued. Gastrointestinal side effects are especially troublesome, given the promi-

nent gastrointestinal symptoms in some cases of Legionnaires' disease.

Compared with erythromycin, the new macrolides (azithromycin, clarithromycin, roxithromycin, josamycin) display superior in vitro activity against legionellae and greater intracellular and lung tissue penetration. Clinical experience is most extensive with azithromycin, but anecdotal reports have indicated that all of the newer macrolides are effective in the treatment of Legionnaires' disease. Given that adverse effects are notably less pronounced with the newer macrolides than with erythromycin and that the improved pharmacokinetics of the newer agents allows once- or twice-daily administration, it is anticipated that—once intravenous formulations become available—these drugs will supplant erythromycin as the antibiotics of choice for Legionnaires' disease.

Moreover, the newer macrolides (especially azithromycin) may be preferred for the treatment of immunocompetent patients with community-acquired pneumonia in whom Gram's staining of sputum shows many neutrophils but a paucity or absence of organisms. Such a result is compatible not only with infection due to *Legionella* but also with that due to *M. pneumoniae* or *C. pneumoniae*, which can also be treated with these new macrolides. Finally, the newer macrolides are active against *S. pneumoniae*, *H. influenzae*, *Moraxella catarrhalis*, and *Staphylococcus aureus*—common pathogens in community-acquired pneumonia. (Clarithromycin is the least active of these drugs against *H. influenzae*.)

The quinolones (ciprofloxacin, ofloxacin, pefloxacin) are highly active against *Legionella* in vitro, in dilution susceptibility tests and intracellular models, and in animal models. Furthermore, in open noncomparative studies of pneumonia, numerous cases of Legionnaires' disease have been successfully treated with quinolones. Ciprofloxacin is the preferred antibiotic for *Legionella*-infected transplant recipients because both macrolides and rifampin interact pharmacologically with transplant-immunosuppressive medications, including cyclosporine and tacrolimus.

For severely ill patients with Legionnaires' disease, the combination of rifampin plus a macrolide or a quinolone is recommended as initial treatment. Alternative agents include tetracycline and its analogues (doxycycline, minocycline) and trimethoprim-sulfamethoxazole. Anecdotal reports have described success with imipenem and clindamycin, but these agents probably should not be used until more experience in the treatment of humans has accumulated.

The clinical response to intravenous treatment usually occurs within 3 to 5 days, after which the switch to oral therapy can be made. The recommended total duration of therapy is 10 to 14 days; a longer course (3 weeks) may be appropriate for immunosuppressed patients with advanced disease. With appropriate and timely antibiotic therapy, mortality is low among immunocompetent patients (although in nosocomial infection the figure has sometimes approached 40 to 50 percent).

Pontiac fever requires only symptom-based treatment, not antimicrobial therapy.

PREVENTION   Disinfection of the water supply is the ultimate preventive measure. Although many disinfection modalities have been tried, only two methods have proved reliable and cost-effective. The superheat and flush method requires heating of the water so that the distal-outlet temperature is 70 to 80°C and flushing of the distal outlets with hot water for at least 30 min. This method is ideal for emergency situations. A commercial copper and silver ionization method has proved effective in numerous hospitals. Hyperchlorination is no longer recommended because of its expense, carcinogenicity, corrosive effects on piping, and unreliable efficacy.

Table 153-3

Antibiotic Therapy for *Legionella* Infection

Antimicrobial Agent	Dose, mg*	Route	Frequency
Azithromycin	500†	PO, IV‡	q 24 h
Clarithromycin	500	PO, IV‡	q 12 h
Roxithromycin	300‡	PO	q 12 h
Erythromycin	1000 (1 g)	IV	q 6 h
	500	PO	q 6 h
Ciprofloxacin	400	IV	q 8 h
	750	PO	q 12 h
Ofloxacin	400	PO, IV	q 12 h
Doxycycline	100†	PO, IV	q 12 h
Minocycline	100†	PO, IV	q 12 h
Tetracycline	500	PO, IV	q 6 h
Trimethoprim- sulfamethoxazole	160/800	IV	q 8 h
	160/800	PO	q 12 h
Rifampin	600	PO, IV	q 12 h

* Except as indicated.
† Doubling first dose should be considered.
‡ Investigational in the United States.

BIBLIOGRAPHY

BARBAREE JM et al: *Legionella: Current status and emerging perspectives.* Washington, DC, American Society for Microbiology, 1993

CARRATALA J et al: Risk factors for nosocomial *Legionella pneumophila* pneumonia. Am J Respir Crit Care Med 149:625, 1994

EDELSTEIN PH: Antimicrobial chemotherapy for Legionnaires' disease: A review. Clin Infect Dis 21:5265, 1995

FALCO V et al: *L. pneumophila*—a cause of severe community acquired pneumonias. Chest 100:1007, 1991

FANG GD: Disease due to *Legionella* (other than *Legionella pneumophila*): Historical, microbiological, clinical and epidemiologic review. Medicine 68:116, 1989

——— et al: New and emerging etiologies for community-acquired pneumonia with implications for therapy: A prospective multicenter study of 359 cases. Medicine 69:37, 1990

HEATH CH et al: Delay in appropriate therapy of *Legionella* pneumonia associated with increasing mortality. Eur J Clin Microbiol Infect Dis 15:286, 1996

LOWRY PW, TOMPKINS LS: Nosocomial legionellosis: A review of pulmonary and extrapulmonary syndromes. Am J Infect Control 21:21, 1993

ROIG J et al: Legionnaires' disease. Chest 105:1827, 1994

STRAUSS WL et al: Risk factors for domestic acquisition of Legionnaires' disease. Arch Intern Med 156:1685, 1996

YU VL: Could aspiration be the major mode of transmission for *Legionella*? Am J Med 95:13, 1993

154

George R. Siber, Matthew H. Samore

PERTUSSIS

DEFINITION   Pertussis, or whooping cough, is an acute infection of the respiratory tract caused by *Bordetella pertussis*. The name *pertussis*, coined by Sydenham in 1679, means "violent cough" and describes the most characteristic feature of this disease. The Chinese call this illness "the cough of 100 days" because of the chronic nature of the cough. A dramatic inspiratory whoop following a paroxysmal cough is a hallmark of severe pertussis in children but is frequently lacking, particularly in infants and adults. Thus the term *whooping cough* may mislead clinicians by implying that whoops are an essential feature of the disease.

The clinical features that should suggest pertussis are a chronic cough lasting 2 weeks or longer and coughing spells that are typically sudden in onset and paroxysmal in nature. The episodes may, in severe cases, be followed by a whoop or by vomiting. Fever is absent or low except in cases of superinfection. An absolute lymphocytosis may provide an additional clue to the diagnosis, particularly in unimmunized children.

MICROBIOLOGY   *B. pertussis* was first isolated by Bordet and Gengou in 1900 from the medium that bears their names. Humans are the only known host of *B. pertussis*. Other species in the genus *Bordetella* include *B. parapertussis*, which is associated with a milder respiratory illness in humans, and *B. bronchiseptica*, an animal pathogen that on rare occasions causes respiratory or opportunistic infections in humans.

B. pertussis is a small, nonmotile, gram-negative coccobacillus that is slow growing and fastidious in its growth requirements. After 3 to 16 days of growth at 36°C on special medium such as Bordet-Gengou agar, glistening pinpoint colonies with surrounding zones of hemolysis appear. Preliminary identification is accomplished by direct fluorescent antibody staining or by agglutination with antiserum to *B. pertussis*. This species is distinguished from *B. bronchiseptica* and *B. parapertussis* by further tests, such as motility and nitrate reduction. *B. pertussis*, *B. parapertussis*, and *B. bronchiseptica* show extensive DNA homology and share many enzymes not related to virulence as well as some virulence factors. However, only *B. pertussis* expresses pertussis toxin.

Like many other bacterial pathogens, *B. pertussis* possesses a precise mechanism for coordinated regulation of its virulence factors. Antigenic modulation involves reversible downregulation of virulence factors (i.e., pertussis toxin, filamentous hemagglutinin, pertactin, fimbriae, adenyl cyclase, dermonecrotic toxin) and upregulation of other proteins in response to a variety of environmental stimuli. Phase variation, which abolishes the expression of virulence factors, involves mutations of a regulatory locus at a frequency of 10^{-3} to 10^{-6} organisms. Both antigenic modulation and phase variation occur in vitro

and in vivo, but their role in the ecology of *B. pertussis* is unknown. It has been suggested that phase variation or antigenic modulation may facilitate expulsion of the organism from the respiratory tract by lowering its adherence, may enable it to survive hostile environmental conditions during transmission, or may allow it to survive intracellularly in a quiescent state, protected from attack by immune mechanisms directed toward its virulence factors.

PATHOGENESIS   *B. pertussis* initiates colonization of the respiratory tract by adhering to ciliated epithelial cells; grows to high numbers, causing local mucosal damage; and induces the paroxysmal cough that enhances its expulsion and transmission to contacts. A number of virulence factors responsible for this cycle of events have been described. Fimbriae, hairlike appendages on the surface of the organism, may play a role in the initial stages of adherence to ciliated cells. The fimbriae induce serotype-specific agglutinating antibodies (agglutinins) and are therefore called *agglutinogens*. Filamentous hemagglutinin (a large, 220-kDa, rodlike surface protein) and pertactin (a 69-kDa protein residing in the outer membrane) enable the organism to adhere closely to ciliated and other mammalian cells. Both of these adherence factors have arginine-glycine-aspartic acid repeat sequences (RGD) typical of eukaryotic adhesins that stick to the integrin family of mammalian cell-surface proteins.

A variety of toxins then impair local defenses (tracheal cytotoxin by inducing ciliostasis and adenyl cyclase by inhibiting phagocytes) and cause local tissue damage (tracheal cytotoxin and dermonecrotic toxin), thereby enhancing the supply of nutrients and perhaps facilitating systemic absorption of pertussis toxin. Pertussis toxin conforms to the general A/B model of enzymatic bacterial exotoxins. It contains an enzymatic moiety, the A subunit, which consists of a single peptide (S1), and a binding moiety, the B oligomer, which consists of four peptides (S2, S3, S4, and S5) in a molar ratio of 1:1:2:1. The B oligomer adheres to mammalian cells and delivers the A subunit to its targets; it exerts some biologic functions directly (e.g., mitogenesis of T cells) and may contribute to adherence of the whole organism to mammalian cells. The A subunit transfers ADP-ribose from NAD to certain members of a family of guanine nucleotide–binding regulatory membrane proteins (G proteins) in target cells. By this mechanism, pertussis toxin produces a variety of biologic effects, including lymphocytosis (lymphocytosis-promoting factor); the sensitization of mice to histamine and serotonin (histamine-sensitizing factor); the enhancement of insulin secretion in response to regulatory signals, such as beta-adrenergic stimulation (islet-activating protein); and the enhancement of certain immune functions, such as the production of IgG and IgE antibodies.

The mechanisms whereby *B. pertussis* produces the paroxysmal cough typical of pertussis have not been elucidated. The best evidence that pertussis toxin plays a critical role in producing the pertussis syndrome was provided by studies in which infants immunized only with pertussis toxoid had an 80 to 90 percent lower rate of severe pertussis than did controls.

EPIDEMIOLOGY   Pertussis is a highly communicable disease, with attack rates of 90 to 100 percent among nonimmune household contacts. Transmission of the organism is mediated by exposure to respiratory droplets expelled in large numbers by symptomatic individuals.

Before the introduction of pertussis vaccine in the late 1940s, 115,000 to 270,000 cases of pertussis were reported annually in the United States (average incidence, 150 cases/100,000 population per year). Epidemics of pertussis recurred at intervals of 3 to 4 years without significant seasonality. During the years 1940 to 1948, pertussis caused more deaths among infants than did diphtheria, polio, measles, meningitis, and scarlet fever combined.

The incidence of pertussis declined 100- to 150-fold after the adoption of universal whole-cell pertussis vaccination, and mortality rates decreased even more dramatically, primarily as a result of improvements in health care. Discontinuation or reduction of pertussis vaccination was associated with a rapid resurgence of pertussis in Great Britain, Sweden, and Japan. In the United States, the incidence of pertussis fell to a nadir in the mid-1970s, with 1010 cases reported in 1976, and subsequently increased, with peaks in 1983, 1986, 1990, and 1993. In 1992 to 1994, a total of 15,286 cases of pertussis were reported to the Centers for Disease Control and Prevention (CDC). Infants <1 year of age accounted for 41 percent of these reported pertussis cases and for 78 percent of pertussis deaths. The case-fatality rate was 0.2 percent overall but was 0.6 percent among infants <6 months of age. Of children between 7 months and 4 years of age who developed pertussis, approximately half had not received the appropriate number of doses of vaccine for their age group.

Persons aged 20 years or older accounted for 11 percent of pertussis cases reported during 1992 to 1994. However, epidemiologic studies suggest that the actual incidence of pertussis in this age group is much higher than is indicated by estimates based on passive reporting to the CDC. Serologic studies show that 12 to 30 percent of episodes of persistent paroxysmal cough (i.e., episodes lasting longer than 2 weeks) in healthy adults are due to pertussis. In a recent seroprevalence study, the incidence of pertussis among U.S. adults was estimated to be 176 cases/100,000 person-years—a figure 500- to 1000-fold higher than that based on reported cases.

The high degree of transmissibility of *B. pertussis* in susceptible adolescent and adult populations is demonstrated by the large outbreaks of pertussis that have occurred in schools, nursing homes, hospitals, and residential facilities. Furthermore, careful studies of household contacts of pertussis cases show that 40 to 80 percent of family members have serologic evidence of infection and that only one-third to one-half of these infections are clinically symptomatic. It is now widely recognized that symptomatic undiagnosed pertussis in adults is an important source of transmission to infants and children and a mechanism for perpetuation of the disease in the population.

Studies of pertussis outbreaks suggest that protective immunity induced by whole-cell vaccine wanes rapidly. Child contacts appear to resist transient colonization and seroconversion for 2 years after their last vaccination, transiently develop asymptomatic or minimally symptomatic colonization and seroconvert at 3 to 5 years, and develop prolonged cough—frequently along with other symptoms of pertussis—at 6 to 12 years. The whole-cell vaccine does not offer protection beyond 12 years after immunization. Although it was once thought that natural pertussis offered lifelong protection, recent studies show that adults who have had pertussis again become susceptible to the disease after 20 years. Indeed, the rate of adult pertussis in Germany, where most adults are immune as a result of natural infection, resembles that in the United States (133 cases/100,000 population per year).

CLINICAL MANIFESTATIONS   Pertussis is typically a prolonged illness, with an average duration of 6 to 8 weeks. The incubation period ranges from 5 to 14 days but is usually 7 to 10 days. The symptoms of pertussis generally evolve through three stages: the catarrhal, the paroxysmal, and the convalescent. The *catarrhal stage* lasts 1 and 2 weeks and is characterized by nonspecific symptoms of coryza, mild cough, lacrimation, malaise, and low-grade fever. The *paroxysmal stage*, which usually lasts 2 to 4 weeks, is characterized by paroxysmal cough, defined as sudden, forceful, repetitive coughing. The number of coughs per spasm is variable, ranging from 10 to 30; the paroxysms of pertussis characteristically occur during a single exhalation, a feature useful in distinguishing this illness from the repetitive cough caused by other pathogens, in which there are inspirations between coughs. In severe cases, the physical effort associated with each spasm may be extreme, with neck-vein distention, bulging of the eyes, and cyanosis. The distinctive whoop is heard in half of pediatric cases and is due to sudden inspiration against a closed glottis at the end of the paroxysm. Often resulting in the expectoration of viscous respiratory secretions, the paroxysm may be triggered by external stimuli, such as loud noises or physical contact. Typically, 10 to 25 paroxysms occur per 24-h period, with disruption of nocturnal

sleep. Posttussive vomiting is common and should be considered suggestive of pertussis. Fever is generally absent during the paroxysmal stage except in cases of bacterial superinfection. Most complications of pertussis develop during the paroxysmal stage. The *convalescent stage* is defined by the gradual waning in intensity of the cough. Complete resolution of the cough may require several months. Superimposed viral or bacterial respiratory infections may lead to severe clinical exacerbations, with the recurrence of paroxysmal coughing.

An absolute lymphocytosis is a characteristic but not universal laboratory finding in children with pertussis. Typically, the total white blood cell count ranges from 10,000 to 30,000 cells/μL, with 50 to 75 percent lymphocytes. Lymphocytosis is much less common among teenagers and adults, presumably because of antitoxin immunity.

The most common presentation of pertussis in adolescents and adults is cough, with or without paroxysms, persisting for 2 weeks or more (Table 154-1). Whooping is less common than it is among children, and lymphocytosis is rare. Useful clinical clues include shortness of breath during coughing spells, nocturnal cough, a tingling sensation in the back of the throat, posttussive vomiting, and a history of exposure to other patients with prolonged coughing illness.

B. pertussis has been isolated from human immunodeficiency virus–infected patients with chronic respiratory symptoms and may persist in these patients for many months. It is not known whether the incidence of pertussis is unusually high in this group.

COMPLICATIONS   Minor complications of pertussis secondary to increased intrathoracic pressure include subconjunctival hemorrhage and upper torso petechiae. Episodes of cyanosis and apnea are common among infants and small children (prevalence, 20 to 50 percent). Malnutrition and weight loss may result from inadequate caloric intake. The major respiratory complication of pertussis is pneumonia, usually due to superinfection by encapsulated bacterial pathogens such as *Streptococcus pneumoniae* and *Haemophilus influenzae*. Pneumonia is more common among infants (incidence, 21 percent) than among children between 1 and 2 years of age (12 percent) or among adults (3 percent). Nonimmune infants may develop severe primary pneumonia due to *B. pertussis*. Neurologic complications, which are infrequent, include encephalopathy (0.7 percent) and seizures (2 percent). The potential mechanisms of pertussis-associated encephalopathy, though unknown, are postulated to include hypoxia and/or hypoglycemia due to pertussis toxin, hemorrhages secondary to increased venous pressure, direct neurotoxic effects, and coinfection by neurotoxic viruses.

DIAGNOSIS   Laboratory confirmation should be attempted in all cases of suspected pertussis. The standard diagnostic test is the isolation of *B. pertussis* from nasopharyngeal swab culture. A calcium alginate swab is inserted into the nares and maintained in contact with the nasopharynx for 10 s to permit moistening. The swab should be placed immediately into transport medium (such as Regan-Lowe charcoal medium) or plated directly onto fresh Bordet-Gengou agar or another suitable agar. A nasopharyngeal aspirate collected with a syringe attached to a fine plastic catheter is a suitable alternative specimen. Growth typically requires 3 to 5 days of incubation at

Table 154-1

Clinical Features of Pertussis in Adolescents and Adults

Feature	Percentage of Patients
Cough	100
Prolonged (>14–21 days)	60–90
Paroxysmal	60–90
Worse at night	50–80
Whooping	5–20
Posttussive vomiting	15–60
Cold symptoms	60–75
Lymphocytosis	<5
Laboratory evidence of *B. pertussis*	
Culture	50–80 early, <5 late
Polymerase chain reaction	50–80 early, <5 late
Serology	20–50 early, 50–80 late

36°C. Suspicious colonies may be presumptively identified by direct fluorescent antibody staining or agglutination. Nasopharyngeal cultures are positive in 70 to 80 percent of children and in 30 to 60 percent of adults when specimens are obtained within 2 weeks of the onset of symptoms (during the catarrhal or early paroxysmal stage). The diagnostic yield declines rapidly thereafter. By 4 weeks, cultures are rarely positive. Detection of *B. pertussis* DNA in nasopharyngeal specimens by the polymerase chain reaction (PCR) may increase the diagnostic yield over that obtained by culture, particularly when the patient has received antibiotics. Again, however, the rate of positive results in PCR declines rapidly with the increasing duration of symptoms.

Thus, serologic assays are the only method currently available for the diagnosis of pertussis in patients with cough persisting for longer than 2 to 3 weeks. Enzyme-linked immunosorbent assays (ELISAs) for IgG or IgA antibodies to pertussis toxin and filamentous hemagglutinin are most frequently used. Seroconversion (a two- to fourfold rise in titer) is useful in previously nonimmune individuals, but previously immune individuals typically have already mounted an anamnestic response by the time the diagnosis is considered. Therefore, a single high titer (≥2 standard deviations above the mean for appropriately matched controls) is the most useful diagnostic test in such patients and has a sensitivity of 50 to 80 percent. Unfortunately, adequately standardized serologic assays for pertussis are not yet available in most areas of the United States.

DIFFERENTIAL DIAGNOSIS The classical presentation of pertussis—the constellation of prolonged paroxysmal cough accompanied by whoops and lymphocytosis—is highly specific. *B. parapertussis* typically causes a milder respiratory illness and is not associated with lymphocytosis. Although the organisms are distinct species, *B. parapertussis* and *B. pertussis* are occasionally associated epidemiologically. They have been isolated from the same patients simultaneously or sequentially. Although viruses such as respiratory syncytial virus and adenovirus have been isolated from patients with clinical pertussis (with or without the isolation of *B. pertussis*), it is unlikely that these viruses alone can cause the full pertussis syndrome with whooping and lymphocytosis.

The infectious and noninfectious differential diagnosis of prolonged cough without whooping and lymphocytosis, a typical presentation of pertussis in adolescents and adults, is much broader. Influenza virus, adenovirus, *Mycoplasma pneumoniae*, *Chlamydia pneumoniae*, and pyogenic bacteria such as *S. pneumoniae* are common causes of acute respiratory infection. In general, the diagnosis of pertussis should be considered when an individual has an unexplained cough lasting for more than 2 weeks, has severe paroxysmal coughing of any duration, or has cough or upper respiratory symptoms of any duration after contact with a patient with pertussis.

℞ **TREATMENT**

Antibiotics The major aim of antibiotic therapy for pertussis is to eradicate *B. pertussis* from the respiratory tract. Erythromycin (preferably in the estolate form), at a dose of 50 mg/kg per day (maximum, 2 g/d) in two to four divided doses, reliably eradicates the organism from the nasopharynx within 5 days. Treatment should be continued for a full 14 days to prevent bacteriologic relapse. Therapy with erythromycin ameliorates clinical illness when begun during the catarrhal phase and may also reduce the severity of the disease when begun within 2 weeks of the onset of paroxysmal cough.

Other macrolide antibiotics, such as azithromycin and clarithromycin, have exhibited excellent in vitro activity against *B. pertussis*, but clinical data on their effectiveness are currently lacking. Another alternative of unproven efficacy for patients unable to tolerate erythromycin is trimethoprim-sulfamethoxazole (8/40 mg/kg per day in two divided doses). Resistance to erythromycin has been described in only a single instance; in this case a *B. pertussis* strain recovered from an infant who deteriorated clinically during erythromycin treatment proved to be fully resistant to the drug.

Supportive Care Infants have the highest rates of complications and death due to pertussis. Accordingly, most infants and those older patients with severe pertussis should be hospitalized. Supportive care includes monitoring for apnea and cyanosis, gentle nasotracheal suctioning, oxygen supplementation, hydration, and nutritional support. Glucocorticoids and the beta-adrenergic stimulant albuterol (salbutamol) have been advocated but have not been proved to be effective. Cough suppressants are ineffective.

Isolation of Hospitalized Patients Persons caring for hospitalized patients with pertussis should use precautions appropriate for infectious agents transmitted by large respiratory droplets. Wearing of a surgical-type mask within 3 ft of the infected patient is considered to provide adequate protection. Isolation should be continued for 5 days after initiation of erythromycin treatment or for 3 weeks if the patient is unable to tolerate antimicrobial therapy.

PREVENTION **Management of Contacts** All household and other close contacts, irrespective of age or immunization status, should receive chemoprophylaxis with erythromycin (preferably the estolate) at 40 to 50 mg/kg per day in four divided doses (maximum, 2 g/d) for 14 days. Erythromycin is effective in limiting secondary transmission if administered within 2 weeks of the onset of symptoms in the index case. For children younger than 7 years, pertussis immunization should be initiated or continued according to the recommended schedule.

Vaccines Diphtheria-tetanus-pertussis (DTP) vaccine, which is currently used for primary immunization of infants, consists of killed whole-cell *B. pertussis* organisms combined with diphtheria and tetanus toxoids adsorbed to aluminum phosphate adjuvant. The standard schedule involves three primary doses at 2-month intervals (with the first dose given at 6 to 8 weeks of age) and booster doses given at 15 to 18 months and 4 to 6 years of age. Vaccination above the age of 6 years is not recommended but has been used in special circumstances for the control of nosocomial outbreaks.

The best whole-cell vaccines are 80 to 95 percent efficacious in protecting individuals from pertussis for 2 to 3 years. Thereafter, protective immunity wanes, with attack rates reaching 90 percent among household contacts exposed more than 12 years after immunization. Some whole-cell vaccines are less efficacious, perhaps because of their low content of protective antigens. Widespread administration of whole-cell vaccines to children reduces the incidence of clinical pertussis in the population by >90 percent.

Injection of DTP vaccine containing the whole-cell pertussis component is associated with high rates of local reactions and fever (30 to 50 percent). In rare instances, reactions are more severe; these reactions include a temperature of >40.5°C, persistent crying, unusual high-pitched crying, seizures, hypotonic hyporesponsive episodes, and anaphylaxis. The occurrence of the more severe of these adverse events constitutes a contraindication to further use of DTP vaccine. The physician should refer to package inserts for details.

The risk of acute encephalopathy appears to be unusually high during the 7 days after DTP immunization (1 in 140,000 doses; excess risk, 0 to 10.5 per 1 million doses). Children with DTP-related acute encephalopathy are at excess risk of subsequent chronic neurologic disease and death; their risk is similar to that of children with DTP-unrelated acute encephalopathy. It remains uncertain whether DTP causes encephalopathy or triggers the disease in children with underlying brain or metabolic abnormalities.

In recently completed trials, a variety of acellular pertussis vaccines have exhibited a degree of efficacy similar to that of whole-cell vaccines in infants, with significantly fewer side effects. Pertussis vaccines containing only pertussis toxoid appear to be about as efficacious as multicomponent vaccines in preventing severe pertussis (i.e., >3 weeks of paroxysmal cough). However, the inclusion of the adherence factors pertactin, fimbriae, and filamentous hemagglutinin appears to contribute additional protection against milder illness, particularly in the setting of household exposure or epidemic disease.

Two acellular pertussis (aP) vaccines formulated with diphtheria and tetanus toxoids (DTaP) are licensed in the United States for use as booster doses at 15 to 18 months and 4 to 6 years of age in children previously immunized with three primary doses of whole-cell DTP vaccine. A variety of DTaP vaccines are expected to be licensed for the primary immunization of infants.

Neither DTaP vaccine nor whole-cell DTP vaccine is currently approved for use in adults. Whole-cell vaccine has been used rarely in the control of hospital outbreaks of pertussis but is associated with high rates of adverse reactions in adults. Both DTaP and aP vaccines are associated with much lower rates of adverse reactions and induce strong antibody responses in adults.

The Future of Immunoprophylaxis   Key issues that will need to be evaluated include (1) whether the various acellular vaccines differ in terms of the rates at which they elicit severe adverse reactions; (2) whether these vaccines differ detectably in efficacy or effectiveness in the United States, where pertussis is endemic rather than epidemic; (3) whether aP vaccine, perhaps formulated with adult doses of tetanus and diphtheria toxoids (TdaP), should be introduced into the routine immunization schedules for adolescents and adults to reduce the high rates of disease in these age groups and to reduce transmission of infection to young infants; and (4) whether immunization of mothers reduces the frequency or severity of pertussis in young infants.

B. pertussis is known to be a pathogen only in humans and is believed to be spread primarily by symptomatic individuals. Thus routine immunization of the entire population with aP vaccine has the potential to eradicate this pathogen.

BIBLIOGRAPHY

Aoyama T et al: Pertussis in adults. Am J Dis Child 146:163, 1992

Cattaneo LA et al: The seroepidemiology of *Bordetella pertussis* infections: A study of persons ages 1–65 years. J Infect Dis 173:1256, 1996

Centers for Disease Control and Prevention: Pertussis—United States, January 1992–1995. Morb Mort Week Rep 44:28, 1995

Deen JL et al: Household contact study of *Bordetella pertussis* infections. Clin Infect Dis 21:1211, 1995

Deville JG et al: Frequency of unrecognized *Bordetella pertussis* infections in adults. Clin Infect Dis 21:639, 1995

Greco D et al: A controlled trial of two acellular vaccines and one whole-cell vaccine against pertussis. N Engl J Med 334:341, 1996

Gustafsson L et al: A controlled trial of a two-component acellular, a five-component acellular, and a whole-cell pertussis vaccine. N Engl J Med 334:349, 1996

He Q et al: Outcomes of *Bordetella pertussis* infection in different age groups of an immunized population. J Infect Dis 170:873, 1994

Marchant CD et al: Pertussis in Massachusetts, 1981–1991: Incidence, serologic diagnosis, and vaccine effectiveness. J Infect Dis 169:1297, 1994

Mink CAM et al: A search for *Bordetella pertussis* infection in university students. Clin Infect Dis 14:464, 1992

Nennig ME et al: Prevalence and incidence of adult pertussis in an urban population. JAMA 275:1672, 1996

Olson LC: Pertussis. Medicine 54:427, 1975

Pittman M: The concept of pertussis as a toxin-mediated disease. Pediatr Infect Dis J 3:467, 1984

Schmitt-Grohe S et al: Pertussis in German adults. Clin Infect Dis 21:860, 1995

Shefer A et al: Use and safety of acellular pertussis vaccine among adult hospital staff during an outbreak of pertussis. J Infect Dis 171:1053, 1995

Trollfors B et al: A placebo-controlled trial of a pertussis-toxoid vaccine. N Engl J Med 333:1045, 1995

Weber DJ, Rutala WA: Management of healthcare workers exposed to pertussis. Top Occup Med 15:411, 1994

Wirsing von König CH et al: Pertussis in adults: Frequency of transmission after household exposure. Lancet 346:1326, 1995

Wright SW et al: Pertussis infection in adults with persistent cough. JAMA 273:1044, 1995

155

Barry I. Eisenstein, Vish Watkins

DISEASES CAUSED BY GRAM-NEGATIVE ENTERIC BACILLI

The gram-negative enteric bacilli are a diverse group of bacteria that reside in the human colon. They also colonize a number of other habitats with which many hospitalized patients come into contact. Because of their ubiquity, they often cause opportunistic infections such as pneumonia in debilitated patients. As a group, the enteric bacteria account for about one-third of all septicemia isolates, two-thirds of bacterial gastroenteritis isolates, and three-quarters of urinary tract infection isolates. One of these organisms, *Escherichia coli*, is the most frequent cause of urinary tract infection and one of the most important causes of bacterial diarrhea.

GENERAL PROPERTIES

CLASSIFICATION AND PHYSIOLOGY   On a genetic basis, the gram-negative enteric bacilli belong to the family Enterobacteriaceae, which includes other pathogens (*Shigella, Edwardsiella, Salmonella, Citrobacter, Yersinia*) discussed elsewhere in this volume. Members of this family lack the ability to form spores, can grow both aerobically and anaerobically (i.e., are facultative anaerobes), can ferment glucose to acid, are oxidase negative, and have variable motility (depending on the presence or absence of flagella).

STRUCTURE   Like all typical bacteria, Enterobacteriaceae have a peptidoglycan-containing cell wall, a single circular chromosome consisting of double-stranded DNA that is located throughout the cytoplasm, and prokaryote-type ribosomes. What distinguishes gram-negative bacteria from other bacteria is the unique multilayered nature of the cell envelope, which, in addition to the inner (or cytoplasmic) membrane and the surrounding polymeric peptidoglycan, also has a complex outer membrane. The medically important elements of the outer layer include lipopolysaccharide (LPS, or endotoxin), which is toxic to humans, and porins, multimeric proteins that form channels for the passage of antimicrobial agents and nutrients. The LPS of all gram-negative bacteria has a core that contains the moiety lipid A, which triggers endotoxic septic shock (see Chap. 124). Most pathogenic strains (at least those of *E. coli*) also have repeating polysaccharide side chains (O antigens) attached to the core LPS (see Chap. 139).

Three classes of surface antigens have been used in serologic tests for the clonal identification of *E. coli* and *Salmonella* strains: (1) the O (somatic) antigens of LPS, (2) the H (flagellar) antigens, and (3) the K (capsular) antigens. Clonal identification is of taxonomic and epidemiologic importance. In *E. coli*, a number of the O, H, and K serogroupings act as markers for clones capable of causing particular infectious diseases; these clones possess other virulence factors required for pathogenesis of those diseases. The O serogroups may be markers for a specific clustering of virulence properties. Thus, some O serogroups possess adhesive factors and toxins needed to cause urinary tract infections, while other O serogroups have adhesins and toxins needed to produce gastroenteritis. The O157:H7 serogroup is associated with hemorrhagic colitis and the hemolytic-uremic syndrome. The K, or capsular, antigen of the K1 type is an epidemiologic marker (and virulence factor) for neonatal meningitis, bacteremia, and urinary tract infection. Today, genetics-based tests are supplanting analysis of surface antigens as the preferred method of differentiating bacterial clones.

THE HOST-PARASITE INTERACTION   Many enteric bacteria colonize the gastrointestinal tract without causing symptoms. Significant disease requires an exceptionally virulent organism, a defect in host defenses, or a combination of the two. Thus, a virulent bacterium like *Shigella dysenteriae* can produce dysentery even in normal hosts. A commensal strain of *E. coli* can produce peritonitis in a healthy individual with a ruptured appendix (a breach in physical defenses) or bacteremia in a person who is granulocytopenic from treatment with an antineoplastic drug (a defect in host immunity).

Regardless of the initial state of the host defenses, disease due to enteric bacterial infection consists of several sequential stages, beginning with entry into and colonization of the gastrointestinal tract, nasopharynx, oropharynx, or urinary tract. Those bacteria that are successful at colonizing the gastrointestinal tract, whether they are pathogenic or commensal, must survive the harsh environmental excesses of high acidity in the stomach and then the alkalinity and high concentrations of detergent (bile salts) and digestive enzymes in the small intestine, not to mention the immune system's IgA and phagocytic and lymphocytic cells. The compact texture of the cell wall of gram-negative bacteria enables them to cope with these challenges. To avoid being dislodged by the passing intestinal contents, these bacteria attach to specific receptors on the epithelial cell or in the cell-associated mucus by hairlike, proteinaceous organelles known as fimbriae or pili, which cover the entire surface of each bacterium. Strains of *E. coli* that cause gastroenteritis have fimbriae that bind specifically to receptors in the gastrointestinal tract. Other strains of *E. coli* that are associated with urinary tract infections contain P fimbriae (so called because of affinity for the P blood-group antigen found on uroepithelial cells) that bind specifically to receptors in the urinary tract. P fimbriae are also called PAP, for *p*yelonephritis-*a*ssociated *p*ili.

The normal host defenses limit most bacterial interactions to benign commensalism. To produce disease in healthy hosts, these organisms need special attributes, known as virulence factors. For localized diseases (e.g., diarrhea, dysentery), the bacteria use secretory and cytologic toxins and, occasionally, cellular invasive factors. For survival in the bloodstream, the organisms have capsules (e.g., K1) that enable them to resist opsonization. In addition, the polysaccharide chains of O antigens, along with particular outer-membrane proteins, enable the bacteria to resist the bactericidal activity of serum by preventing the cylindrical membrane-attack complex of the terminal components of complement from inserting efficiently into the bacterial membrane and thus causing bacterial lysis.

In contrast to infections in normal hosts, those in debilitated individuals are often caused by relatively avirulent organisms. Such organisms are robust enough to survive in various hospital environments, including water supplies and the hands of caregivers, and are sufficiently drug resistant to be part of the flora of an antibiotic-treated host. A debilitated host recovering from surgery or trauma can become ill merely from the inadvertent relocation of a commensal strain to a site either normally sterile or normally not colonized with enteric bacteria. For example, aspiration of gram-negative bacteria colonizing the upper airways can lead to pneumonia, and contamination of surgical wounds or previously sterile intravascular or urinary catheters can cause wound infection, bacteremia, and urinary tract infection, respectively. These "opportunistic" infections can be severe if the debilitated host cannot mount a normal immune response. Moreover, the bacteria in the antimicrobial-laden hospital environment are preselected for drug resistance and may be particularly difficult to treat.

Whether the pathogen is a virulent invader or an opportunistic commensal, the host response, together with appropriate antimicrobial therapy, mediates recovery. Paradoxically, the normal immune response can also potentiate the disease by mediating inflammatory responses beyond those needed for bacterial containment. Complement activation, the liberation of cytokines (e.g., tumor necrosis factor and the numerous interleukins), leukocyte mobilization and degranulation, and platelet and coagulation-pathway activation can mediate the lethal manifestations of endotoxemia, including excessive fluid extravasation and circulatory collapse, renal tubular necrosis, adult respiratory distress syndrome, and (when the organism has entered the cerebrospinal fluid) meningitis. Recent efforts to treat severe gram-negative infection have been directed not only at eliminating the invading microbe but also at attenuating the immune response.

DRUG RESISTANCE AND VIRULENCE FACTORS   The success of therapy for bacterial infection depends on the use of antimicrobial agents to which the infecting microbe is susceptible. Unfortunately, bacteria have an evolutionary ability to avoid the effects of these drugs (see Chap. 140) by mechanisms that include alteration of the antibacterial target site, decreased permeability to influx of drug,

active export of drug to the outside, and enzymatic destruction of drug. Mutation of preexisting DNA can result in drug resistance, particularly through target-site alteration but also through alteration of the amount or affinity of drug-destroying enzymes. Most drug resistance results from the acquisition of new genes, usually in the form of transposons. Transposons are usually found on R-plasmids, which are self-replicating, nonchromosomal units of DNA that can be transferred by conjugation from one bacterial cell to another (even to a cell of a different species).

The genetic organization of these genes promotes their spread throughout the Enterobacteriaceae. Since R-plasmids move across bacterial populations readily, the presence of several antimicrobials in the environment selects those bacteria that contain multiple drug-resistance elements. With time and the continued use of different drugs in hospitals and in agriculture, R-plasmids have become larger; each now consists of many different transposons strung together like pearls on a necklace. The genes encoding many virulence factors, including colonization factors, enterotoxins, and hemolysin, are found on plasmids (occasionally on R-plasmids), and this situation promotes their spread.

ESCHERICHIA COLI INFECTIONS

ETIOLOGY, EPIDEMIOLOGY, AND MANIFESTATIONS
Enteric Infections   *E. coli* is a major cause of bacterial gastroenteritis in U.S. residents traveling abroad. This organism comes in many pathogenic varieties, each with a different mechanism of disease production. The most important are enterotoxigenic *E. coli* (ETEC), an important cause of traveler's diarrhea; enteropathogenic or enteroadherent *E. coli* (EPEC), an important cause of childhood diarrhea; enteroinvasive *E. coli* (EIEC), which causes a dysentery-like disease; and enterohemorrhagic *E. coli* (EHEC), which causes hemorrhagic colitis and has been associated with the hemolytic-uremic syndrome (HUS) in children.

Traveler's diarrhea occurs in individuals from industrialized countries who visit tropical or subtropical regions that lack advanced hygienic conditions. The organism, commonly ETEC, is acquired through the fecal-oral route, usually through consumption of unbottled water or uncooked vegetables. The inoculum of organisms must be high enough to resist destruction by acid in the stomach. (Individuals with achlorhydria are especially susceptible.) The major manifestations are a consequence of the copious outpouring of fluid from the gastrointestinal tract due to the action of one of two types of enterotoxin on the gastrointestinal mucosa. The heat-labile toxin activates intracellular adenylate cyclase, with a subsequent increase in intracellular levels of cyclic adenosine monophosphate. The heat-stable toxin activates guanylate cyclase, with the subsequent elevation of intracellular levels of cyclic guanosine monophosphate. The elevated cyclic monophosphate levels stimulate chloride secretion and inhibit sodium chloride absorption—effects that result in net intestinal secretion. Within 1 or 2 days of exposure in most cases, the patient develops abdominal cramps and frequent explosive bowel movements; these symptoms last 3 to 4 days. Traveler's diarrhea is treated with oral trimethoprim-sulfamethoxazole or a fluoroquinolone. For social convenience or for medical reasons (e.g., for diabetics prone to dehydration with serious consequences or for persons with underlying inflammatory bowel disease), chemoprophylaxis with bismuth subsalicylate, trimethoprim-sulfamethoxazole, or fluoroquinolones may be reasonable.

EPEC strains cause childhood diarrhea, especially in underdeveloped countries and in nursery outbreaks. These bacteria bind to the membranous cells of Peyer's patches and disrupt the overlying mucous gel of the host cell. In contrast to ETEC and EPEC, EIEC strains (rare in the United States) invade the host cell and provoke a significant inflammatory response. The manifestations are those of bacterial dysentery, with fever and bloody diarrheal stool containing polymorphonuclear leukocytes. Treatment consists of fluid replacement. Because these organisms are often resistant to antibiotics, the role of specific treatment is limited. Antibiotics usually are not needed. In severe cases, trimethoprim-sulfamethoxazole, fluoroquinolones, and sometimes intravenous third-generation cephalosporins may be indicated.

Every year, EHEC strains, typically of serotype O157:H7, cause about 20,000 cases of colitis (often hemorrhagic) in the United States. Young children and the elderly can develop HUS characterized by microangiopathic hemolytic anemia, thrombocytopenia, and acute renal failure; central nervous system manifestations, including seizures, hemiparesis, and coma, may develop. Hemorrhage and edema in the lamina propria, accompanied by focal necrosis, hemorrhage, and inflammation of the superficial mucosa, are found in the colon. Injury to the glomerular capillary endothelial cell and microvascular angiopathy elsewhere, especially in the central nervous system, are the predominant pathologic features of HUS. Shiga-like cytotoxins produced by the organisms are thought to participate in the pathogenesis of this disease by their lethality to human colonic cells and their ability to damage endothelial cells. The diagnosis is confirmed by culture from stool of *E. coli* strains that, unlike most commensal strains, fail to ferment sorbitol. These strains also agglutinate with antiserum to O157. Treatment consists of supportive measures. Patients are monitored for signs of HUS for 1 week after the onset of diarrhea. In young children and the elderly, blood counts, peripheral-blood smears, serum creatinine levels, and the urinary sediment are monitored. Antimotility agents should be avoided, as they exacerbate illness and facilitate the development of HUS. Patients with renal failure may need dialysis.

Urinary Tract Infection (See Chap. 131) Unlike the gastrointestinal tract, the urinary tract is normally sterile. Most uncomplicated infections are due to *E. coli*. The typical acute infection occurs in a sexually active female following bacterial colonization of the periurethral region and ascension up the urethra; disease includes asymptomatic bacteriuria, urethritis, cystitis, pyelitis, and pyelonephritis. Complications, including obstruction of the urinary tract, the presence of foreign bodies or anatomic defects, prior surgery, pregnancy, or stones, increase a patient's chance of infection with other Enterobacteriaceae and strains of *Pseudomonas* and of chronic or relapsing infection, loss of renal tissue, and bacteremia.

Intraabdominal Infections (See Chap. 127) *E. coli* represents a small part of the normal bowel flora—more than 99 percent of the bacteria in this population are strict anaerobes—yet it is a significant pathogen in infections resulting from spillage of normal bowel contents into previously sterile environments. Studies of experimental infections in animals suggest that the aerobic bowel flora (including *E. coli*) is responsible for the often lethal early septicemia associated with bowel spillage, whereas anaerobic species cause late-onset abscesses (with aerobic bacteria acting as potentiators). Thus, in cases of peritonitis resulting from a perforated viscus, *E. coli* is usually cultured from the local site and, in severe cases, from the blood. It can also be associated with intraabdominal abscesses in any location as well as with cholecystitis and ascending cholangitis. Intraabdominal infections can be particularly severe in patients with ischemia of the bowel or other organs—e.g., many patients with diabetes and atherosclerotic vascular disease. Such individuals are at unusually high risk of developing acute emphysematous cholecystitis, which is characterized by gangrene and perforation, and septic thrombophlebitis of the portal vein (pyelophlebitis), which leads to liver abscesses. *E. coli* is a prominent pathogen in each of these processes.

Bacteremia Because of its association with septic shock (Chap. 124), bloodstream invasion by *E. coli* is the most serious event associated with this pathogen and the one most likely to lead to multiorgan failure and death. In these cases, the sequential biologic responses of the host to the invading pathogen or to its circulating constituents (e.g., LPS) result in the clinical progression of disease from a systemic inflammatory response syndrome (SIRS) through syndromes of sepsis and severe sepsis to septic shock. *SIRS* is defined as the combination of any two of the following: fever or hypothermia; tachycardia (>90 beats per minute); tachypnea (>20 breaths per minute); and leukocyto-

sis, leukopenia, or >10 percent immature leukocytes in a differential white blood cell count. *Septic shock* is sepsis-induced hypotension that persists in spite of fluid resuscitation and involves hypoperfusion abnormalities, including lactic acidosis, oliguria, and an acute change in mental status, accompanied by organ dysfunction. In a significant proportion of patients, combinations of uremia, hepatic failure, respiratory failure (adult respiratory distress syndrome), and stupor and coma develop. Antecedent diseases include urinary tract infection, biliary or intraperitoneal sepsis, and nosocomial infections such as pneumonia and intravascular catheter–related infections. Patients in whom bacteremia persists despite adequate therapy often have an undrained abscess, most typically intraabdominal. Some patients, especially those with poor filtering capacity in the liver (i.e., those with cirrhosis or portosystemic shunts), diminished reticuloendothelial function, or diminished numbers of circulating phagocytic cells, have no obvious portal of bacterial entry. In most of these cases, the gastrointestinal tract is the source.

Other Manifestations As a consequence of bacteremia or contiguous spread, *E. coli* can be found in abscesses anywhere in the body. Individuals with vascular disease (which is especially common in conjunction with diabetes mellitus) are prone to infections of the distal extremities and surgical wounds, whereas those with diminished numbers of circulating phagocytes are prone to perianal abscesses. Many of these subcutaneous infections are polymicrobial, involving anaerobic as well as aerobic organisms. *E. coli* may cause septic arthritis, perinephric abscess, endophthalmitis, suppurative thyroiditis, brain abscess, endocarditis, osteomyelitis, sinusitis, pneumonia, and other infections. Neonates, particularly premature infants, are especially susceptible to bacteremia and meningitis with K1 encapsulated *E. coli*.

DIAGNOSIS The diagnosis of *E. coli* infection depends on the combination of suspicious clinical findings (e.g., signs and symptoms of urinary tract infection) and isolation of *E. coli* by the clinical microbiology laboratory. Infection with *E. coli* can be a monomicrobial condition developing either at a previously sterile site (e.g., urinary tract infection, meningitis) or in a nonsterile setting (e.g., gastroenteritis); alternatively, it can be part of a polymicrobial process (e.g., a ruptured appendix, or an infected foot in a diabetic). These distinctions are important in the interpretation of laboratory results. Because *E. coli* is present normally in stool, the diagnosis of *E. coli* gastroenteritis is problematic, but it can be made with techniques that exploit unique properties of specific strains that cause these infections (e.g., sorbitol negativity in EHEC). Whether the recovery of *E. coli* from tracheal aspirates in intubated patients indicates colonization or infection (i.e., tracheitis from local inflammation induced by the endotracheal tube or bacterial pneumonia) must be decided in the context of the patient's clinical state. In contrast, any growth of *E. coli* in a normally sterile locale—the bloodstream, cerebrospinal fluid, biliary tract, pleural fluid, or peritoneal cavity—should be assumed to be diagnostic of *E. coli* infection at that site.

Gram's staining can rapidly identify gram-negative bacilli at the site of infection. Unfortunately, this technique cannot differentiate *E. coli* from other gram-negative bacteria that cause similar infectious diseases. Newer techniques, particularly those incorporating amplification of nucleic acid, show promise in identifying virulence genes associated with specific microbes or drug-resistance genes. Although the culture method is slow, isolation of the microbe can be followed by antimicrobial susceptibility testing, which is particularly important with the emergence of drug-resistant pathogens.

R̆ **TREATMENT**

As for any infectious disease, the mainstay of treatment for *E. coli* infections is twofold: antimicrobial therapy and elimination of pus, necrotic tissue, and foreign bodies. General principles of treatment will be discussed here. For treatment of specific infections and for information about specific antibiotics, the reader is referred to the chapters on particular infectious syndromes and to the chapter on antimicrobial chemotherapy (Chap. 140).

Several classes of antibiotics and various antibiotics within those classes have recently become available for the treatment of infections caused by members of the Enterobacteriaceae, including *E. coli*

(Table 155-1). The antibiotic selected, its dose, and the duration of treatment depend on (1) the site of infection, (2) the presence or absence of complicating illnesses, (3) the susceptibility or resistance of the isolated strain, (4) the severity of illness, (5) a history—or lack thereof—of allergy to a potentially useful antibiotic, (6) the cost of the regimen, and (7) other factors (such as whether or not the patient is pregnant and how old the patient is). Urinary tract infections serve as an example to show how these factors influence therapy. Uncomplicated cystitis in a healthy woman is treated for 3 days with oral trimethoprim-sulfamethoxazole. A patient allergic to sulfonamides may be treated with a fluoroquinolone for 3 days. A diabetic or pregnant patient with this infection requires 7 days of treatment. For the pregnant patient, the choice of agents is limited to amoxicillin, macrocrystalline nitrofurantoin, or cefpodoxime proxetil. The patient with mild uncomplicated pyelonephritis can be treated with oral trimethoprim-sulfamethoxazole or a fluoroquinolone for 10 to 14 days. The pregnant patient with pyelonephritis and any patient with severe pyelonephritis should be given intravenous antibiotics in the hospital; the choices are ceftriaxone, ciprofloxacin, gentamicin with or without ampicillin, aztreonam, imipenem/cilastatin, or an extended-spectrum penicillin. After acute symptoms resolve, an oral antibiotic should replace the intravenous antibiotic for a total duration of 14 to 21 days. Again, the choice is dictated by the factors mentioned above—e.g., avoidance of aminoglycosides if the patient has diabetes mellitus; avoidance of imipenem if the patient has renal failure; and, if the patient is pregnant, avoidance of fluoroquinolones and caution with gentamicin (which may cause eighth-cranial-nerve toxicity in the fetus).

KLEBSIELLA, ENTEROBACTER, AND SERRATIA INFECTIONS

Klebsiella, Enterobacter, and *Serratia* belong to the tribe Klebsielleae. These genera are typically differentiated only by certain amino acid decarboxylase tests and the facts that strains of *Klebsiella* are usually nonmotile and form large mucoid colonies when grown on solid media. Like *E. coli,* all of these organisms colonize the human gastrointestinal tract, yet they rarely cause disease in the normal host; rather, they are a major cause of nosocomial and opportunistic infection. In many hospitals, strains of *Klebsiella* are among the most antimicrobial-resistant microbes isolated; they readily acquire R-plasmids carrying aminoglycoside-inactivating enzymes, a wide variety of β-lactamases, and other drug-resistance genes.

Klebsiella pneumoniae (Friedlander's bacillus) is a well-recognized cause of community-acquired lobar pneumonia found typically in alcoholic men over 40 years of age with such underlying conditions as diabetes mellitus and chronic obstructive pulmonary disease. Pneumonia due to *K. pneumoniae* mimics pneumococcal pneumonia except for the greater tendency of *Klebsiella* pneumonia to progress to lung abscess and empyema. Occasionally, this necrotic process causes the radiographic features of bulging fissures and loss of lung volume, which are sometimes seen in severe bacterial pneumonia of any etiology. Gram's staining of the sputum can help in the diagnosis; it shows a predominance of short, plump, gram-negative bacilli, often surrounded by a capsule that appears as a clear space.

In the hospital, *K. pneumoniae* and its tribal relatives are major causes of infections of the urinary tract, lower respiratory tract, biliary tract, and surgical wounds. Many of these infections are associated with bacteremia and life-threatening septic shock. *K. pneumoniae* infections are usually treated with a cephalosporin. In severe infections, some specialists add an aminoglycoside for synergy, usually for a short duration (e.g., 3 or 4 days). The antibiotic selected, its dosage, and the duration of therapy depend on the factors discussed above in the section on treatment of *E. coli* infections. Treatment of infections due to resistant organisms depends on the results of susceptibility tests. Less common conditions caused by strains closely related to *K. pneumoniae* include rhinoscleroma, a chronic granulomatous disease that involves the mucosa of the upper respiratory system, occasionally leads to bony invasion and airway obstruction, and is associated with *Klebsiella rhinoscleromatis;* and ozena, a chronic severe rhinitis involving turbinate atrophy and progressive anosmia that is associated with *Klebsiella ozaenae.* DNA-relatedness studies have shown that these strains, which are indole negative, actually belong to the species *K. pneumoniae* and that indole-positive strains of *K. pneumoniae* belong to a new species, *Klebsiella oxytoca.*

The genus *Enterobacter* consists of *Enterobacter aerogenes, Enterobacter cloacae, Enterobacter agglomerans* (formerly called *Erwinia*), and several other species. *E. cloacae* accounts for most hospital-acquired infections with this genus. Like *Enterobacter, Serratia* is

Table 155-1

Antibiotics Used in the Treatment of Infections with Enterobacteriaceae

Antibiotic Class	Representative Antibiotics	Properties to Consider
Early penicillins	Ampicillin (parenteral), amoxicillin (oral)	Resistance (30%) among bacteria causing urinary infections in the U.S.; inexpensive; bactericidal
Extended-spectrum penicillins	Ticarcillin, piperacillin	Useful in some infections with resistant *Enterobacter* spp. when combined with an aminoglycoside; useful in some polymicrobial infections (e.g., diabetic foot infections) when combined with a β-lactamase inhibitor
First-generation cephalosporins	Cephalothin, cefazolin	Inexpensive; bactericidal; useful in many infections with *Escherichia coli* and in some infections with *Klebsiella* spp. and *Proteus mirabilis*
Third-generation cephalosporins	Ceftriaxone, cefotaxime, ceftizoxime, cefpodoxime (oral)	Broad-spectrum; bactericidal; intravenous forms excellent for treating meningitis; resistance in many *Enterobacter* spp.; oral agents useful in uncomplicated urinary infections caused by susceptible bacteria (most *E. coli, Klebsiella pneumoniae*)
Carbacephems	Loracarbef (oral)	Similar to oral third-generation cephalosporins, with activity against common urinary tract pathogens but not *Enterobacter* spp.
Carbapenems	Imipenem/cilastatin	Broad-spectrum; may cause seizures in patients with renal failure or central nervous system lesions; useful in infections with resistant *Enterobacter* spp.
Sulfonamides	Trimethoprim-sulfamethoxazole	Inexpensive; useful in urinary infections; intravenous form useful in serious infections (meningitis) caused by *Enterobacter* spp.
Monobactams	Aztreonam	Useful in patients allergic to penicillin; may be used in pregnant patients
Quinolones	Ciprofloxacin, ofloxacin, norfloxacin, lomefloxacin, enoxacin	Useful in traveler's diarrhea, urinary infections, osteomyelitis, and infections with resistant *Enterobacter* spp.; should not be used by pregnant patients
Aminoglycosides	Gentamicin, tobramycin, amikacin	Once-daily dosing may reduce toxicity; should not be used by patients with renal dysfunction and diabetes mellitus unless absolutely necessary; prolonged therapy to be avoided; useful in infections with resistant *Enterobacter* spp.

an opportunist that has been recognized as a human pathogen only since the 1960s. *Serratia marcescens* and *Serratia liquefaciens* have been predominantly associated with human disease. The epidemiology of *S. marcescens* differs from that of other Enterobacteriaceae in that *S. marcescens* appears less likely to colonize the gastrointestinal tract but more likely to colonize the respiratory and urinary tracts of hospitalized adults.

Numerous strains of *Enterobacter*, *Serratia*, and *Klebsiella* have become resistant to many of the β-lactam antibiotics by three different mechanisms. The use of newer cephalosporins has led to a higher frequency of *Enterobacter* strains that are resistant to β-lactam antibiotics, a higher frequency of infections caused by these strains, and a higher rate of mortality from infections caused by the resistant strains than by the sensitive strains. The basis of this resistance is an enzyme that inactivates all clinically available cephalosporins. Unless there is prior exposure to cephalosporins, the gene encoding this cephalosporinase lies dormant in the bacterial chromosome; the fact that the enzyme is not expressed gives the erroneous impression on susceptibility testing that the organism is sensitive to the newer cephalosporins. This *inducible* gene is also present in *Citrobacter freundii*, *Serratia* spp., and indole-positive *Proteus*. Mutations in this gene have enabled many *Enterobacter* strains to produce large amounts of the cephalosporinase constitutively (i.e., continuously, without the need for induction). A second form of resistance is the production of plasmid-encoded enzymes, the extended-spectrum β-lactamases, which cause resistance to all available β-lactam antibiotics except the carbapenems. A third form of resistance has recently been identified in which some strains, by exposure to the carbapenems, acquire mutant porins that no longer allow these antibiotics to enter the bacterial cells. Thus, the carbapenems can no longer reach their normal target sites and kill the bacteria. Table 155-1 provides suggestions for treating *Enterobacter* infections.

PROTEUS, MORGANELLA, AND *PROVIDENCIA* INFECTIONS

Proteeae are actively motile bacteria that do not ferment lactose. DNA studies show this tribe to consist of at least three genera—*Proteus*, *Morganella*, and *Providencia*—and seven species: *Proteus vulgaris*, *Proteus mirabilis*, *Proteus myxofaciens*, *Morganella morganii* (previously *Proteus morganii*), *Providencia alcalifaciens*, *Providencia stuartii*, and *Providencia rettgeri* (previously *Proteus rettgeri*). Virtually all strains of *P. mirabilis*, which causes most *Proteus* infections, are indole negative, whereas virtually all other strains in the tribe are indole positive. *Proteus* strains are unique in their ability to swarm on moist agar media, which is due to the presence of hundreds of flagella per cell. These organisms are part of the normal fecal flora and are found in soil, water, and sewage. Except for urinary tract infections, *Proteus* rarely causes primary disease in otherwise healthy individuals. *Proteus* is an important cause of chronic urinary tract infection, in part because it possesses the enzyme urease, which splits urea into ammonium hydroxide and raises urinary pH to levels that promote the formation of struvite stones. These stones act as foreign bodies that obstruct urinary flow, serve as a nidus for persistent infection, and exacerbate destruction of the renal parenchyma. *Proteus* species are common opportunistic invaders in debilitated individuals undergoing broad-spectrum antimicrobial therapy. Like other gram-negative bacteria, they can contaminate burns, decubitus ulcers, and surgical wounds. Similarly, they have been associated with destructive chronic infections of the middle ear and mastoid, occasionally leading to deafness or malignant extension to the central nervous system with lateral sinus thrombosis, meningitis, brain abscess, and death. Following trauma to the eye, these organisms can cause corneal ulcers, leading to panophthalmitis. Like other gram-negative bacteria, *Proteus* can cause bacteremia and septic shock. The urinary tract serves as the portal of entry in most cases; next in frequency are the biliary tree, the gastrointestinal tract, and other foci. A surgical procedure often

precedes bloodstream invasion. Like *Proteus*, *P. rettgeri* and *P. stuartii* are important nosocomial urinary tract pathogens. The latter organisms are often resistant to many antibiotics.

Treatment of these infections is similar to that of infections due to other gram-negative bacteria, with two differences. Most strains of *P. mirabilis* are sensitive to most β-lactam antibiotics and aminoglycosides and are less difficult to treat. Nevertheless, the association of struvite stones with urinary tract infections due to these urea-splitting organisms poses compensatory challenges. Because contaminated stones provide a nidus of bacterial persistence, surgical intervention is often required for the eradication of infection. Untreated obstruction leads to rapid renal destruction and sepsis.

ACINETOBACTER INFECTIONS

Acinetobacter organisms are saprophytes ubiquitous in water and soil that, along with the genera *Moraxella*, *Neisseria*, and *Kingella*, make up the family Neisseriaceae. The two well-characterized variants are *Acinetobacter calcoaceticus* var. *lwoffii*, formerly called *Mima polymorpha*, and *Acinetobacter calcoaceticus* var. *anitratus*, formerly called *Herellea vaginicola*. Like other family members, these organisms have the appearance of gram-negative diplococci when grown on agar but differ from the latter by their typically negative oxidase reaction, their simple growth requirements, and their bacillary appearance when grown in broth. Unlike Enterobacteriaceae, they give a negative nitrate reaction.

The infections caused by *Acinetobacter* are similar to those caused by the Enterobacteriaceae, particularly nosocomial and community-acquired infections of the urinary tract, meninges, and lower respiratory tract and bacteremia. *Acinetobacter* strains also cause both subacute and acute bacterial endocarditis. With their low innate virulence but high prevalence on the skin of normal individuals, these bacteria are opportunistic and tend to invade the bloodstream of patients with intravenous catheters, surgical wounds, or burns. Occasionally, a bacteremic episode may be fulminant and suggestive of meningococcemia, with high fever, shock, and petechiae. Many cases of bacteremia are polymicrobial.

Given the ubiquity of *Acinetobacter*, disease due to this organism must be distinguished from mere colonization. True infection may be difficult to treat because it occurs in debilitated patients and because these bacteria have grown increasingly resistant to standard antimicrobials. While the results of sensitivity testing are awaited, treatment with an extended-spectrum β-lactam plus an aminoglycoside should be provided in conjunction with the removal of foreign bodies and the debridement of necrotic tissue.

BIBLIOGRAPHY

ENTEROBACTERIACEAE: GENERAL

BONE RC: The pathogenesis of sepsis. Ann Intern Med 115:457, 1991

MURRAY BE: New aspects of antimicrobial resistance and the resulting therapeutic dilemmas. J Infect Dis 163:1184, 1991

NICOLLE LE et al: Infections and antibiotic resistance in nursing homes. Clin Microbiol Rev 9:1, 1996

RANGEL-FRAUSTO MS et al: The natural history of the systemic inflammatory response syndrome (SIRS). JAMA 273:117, 1995

SANDERS CS, SANDERS WE: Resistance in gram-negative bacteria: Global trends and clinical impact. Clin Infect Dis 15:824, 1992

SCHABERG DR et al: Major trends in the microbial etiology of nosocomial infection. Am J Med 91(Suppl 3B):72S, 1991

ESCHERICHIA COLI INFECTIONS

GRANSDEN WR et al: Bacteremia due to *Escherichia coli*: A study of 861 episodes. Rev Infect Dis 12:1008, 1990

RUBINOFF MJ, FIELD M: Infectious diarrhea. Annu Rev Med 42:403, 1991

KLEBSIELLA-ENTEROBACTER-SERRATIA INFECTIONS

BODEY GP et al: Bacteremia caused by *Enterobacter*: 15 years of experience in a cancer hospital. Rev Infect Dis 13:550, 1991

CARPENTER JL: *Klebsiella* pulmonary infections: Occurrence at one medical center and review. Rev Infect Dis 12:672, 1990

CHOW JW et al: *Enterobacter* bacteremia: Clinical features and emergence of antibiotic resistance during therapy. Ann Intern Med 115:585, 1991

JOHNSON MP, RAMPHAL R: β-Lactam-resistant *Enterobacter* bacteremia in febrile neutropenic patients receiving monotherapy. J Infect Dis 162:981, 1990

SCHWIMMBECK PL, OLDSTONE MB: Molecular mimicry between human leukocyte antigen B27 and *Klebsiella*. Consequences for spondyloarthropathies. Am J Med 85:51, 1988

WOLFF MA et al: Antibiotic therapy for enterobacter meningitis: A retrospective review of 13 episodes and review of the literature. Clin Infect Dis 16:772, 1993

PROTEUS INFECTIONS

RAIMONDI A et al: Imipenem- and meropenem-resistant mutants of *Enterobacter cloacae* and *Proteus rettgeri* lack porins. Antimicrob Agents Chemother 35:1174, 1991

ACINETOBACTER INFECTIONS

BERGOGNE-BÉRÉZIN E, TOWNER KJ: *Acinetobacter* spp. as nosocomial pathogens: Microbiological, clinical, and epidemiological features. Clin Microbiol Rev 9:148, 1996

156   *John C. Atherton, Martin J. Blaser*

HELICOBACTER INFECTIONS

DEFINITION Most human *Helicobacter* infections are caused by *Helicobacter pylori* and a few by *Helicobacter heilmanii* (formerly *Gastrospirillum hominis*) and other *Helicobacter* species (for example, *Gastrospirillum suis*). The current level of interest in *H. pylori* infection is high because of its etiologic importance in peptic ulcer disease and in gastric malignancy.

ETIOLOGIC AGENTS Helicobacters are gram-negative, spiral, flagellate bacilli. Many species exist, most of which colonize specific animal hosts. *H. pylori* naturally infects humans and monkeys and has recently been described in domestic cats. It is noninvasive, living in the mucus that overlies gastric-type mucosae; a small proportion of the bacterial cells are adherent to the mucosa. Its spiral shape and flagellae render *H. pylori* motile in the mucous environment, and its efficient urease protects it against acid by catalyzing urea hydrolysis to produce ammonia. Urease plays a role in colonization and may be important in the maintenance of infection, although the deep gastric mucus is far less acidic than the gastric lumen. In vitro, *H. pylori* is microaerophilic and requires complex growth media; its major metabolic pathways are still poorly understood. It grows slowly, and old cultures contain slowly metabolizing coccoid forms that may or may not be important in the natural history of the infection. *H. heilmanii* is a longer, more tightly coiled spiral and also produces urease. It cannot be cultured in vitro by current techniques. Unlike *H. pylori* and most other helicobacters, *H. heilmanii* readily colonizes a range of animal species.

EPIDEMIOLOGY The prevalence of *H. pylori* infection is about 30 percent in the United States and other developed countries as opposed to 80 percent in most developing countries. In the United States, prevalence varies with age: the figure is around 50 percent among 60-year-old persons and 25 percent among those 30 years old. Most studies show that spontaneous acquisition or loss of infection in adulthood is uncommon; thus most infections are thought to be acquired in childhood. The age association is largely but not exclusively due to a cohort effect. In other words, persons who are now 60 years old more commonly acquired the infection as children than did those who are now 30 years old. Other than age, the main risk factor for infection is low income. Humans are the major—if not the only—reservoir of *H. pylori,* but the exact route and source of infection are unknown. The fact that members of a family often carry the same strain of *H. pylori* implies that they acquire the infection from one another or from a common source; children may be the usual source of infection. Given that the bacteria can be cultured from feces, fecal-oral spread is likely, but oral-oral spread also is possible, and the relative contribution of each route to overall transmission is not known. *H. pylori* DNA has been identified in water sources, and cats may harbor the infection; however, whether either water sources or cats are important reservoirs of infection is unknown.

The prevalence of *H. heilmanii* infection is less than 1 percent. This *Helicobacter* species colonizes a number of animals, including domestic pets, and infection in humans is thought to be a zoonosis. Concurrent infection of the same human host with *H. pylori* and *H. heilmanii* has been described.

CLINICAL MANIFESTATIONS Although *H. pylori* infection is usually asymptomatic, essentially all *H. pylori*–infected persons have gastric inflammation (Fig. 156-1). *H. pylori* infection is the foremost cause of peptic ulcer disease, which occurs at some point in the lifetime of about 15 percent of infected persons in developed countries. The main lines of evidence for a causal role of *H. pylori* are (1) that the presence of infection is a risk factor for the development of ulcers, (2) that ulcers do not develop in the absence of infection (except in cases with other known etiologic factors, such as treatment with nonsteroidal anti-inflammatory drugs), (3) that cure of the infection results in a dramatic drop in the rate of ulcer relapse (from about 80 percent to 15 percent in the first year, with even lower rates thereafter), and (4) that experimental infection of gerbils and mice causes gastroduodenal injury.

Prospective case-control studies have shown that *H. pylori* also is a risk factor for adenocarcinomas of the stomach other than those arising in the gastric cardia. The relative risk of these adenocarcinomas associated with *H. pylori* infection is about ninefold after adjustment for the inaccuracy of serologic testing in the elderly. The attributable risk of noncardia gastric adenocarcinoma to *H. pylori* has been estimated to be 75 percent in the United States and 85 percent in some developing countries. Infection due to *H. pylori* appears to be a major risk factor for primary gastric non-Hodgkin's lymphoma. It is strongly associated with low-grade B cell mucosa-associated lymphoid tissue (MALT) lymphoma, which is antigen driven and regresses in about half of cases when *H. pylori* infection is eradicated with antimicrobial agents. *H. pylori* infection may also increase the risk of aggressive diffuse large cell lymphoma of the stomach; patients with this tumor are 7.4 times more likely than controls to have been infected.

Whether *H. pylori* infection causes symptoms in the absence of ulcers or malignancy is unknown. The prevalence of *H. pylori* is

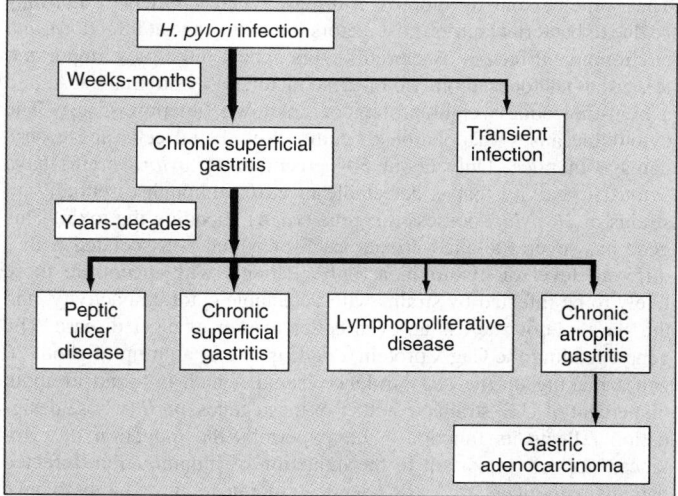

FIGURE 156-1 Natural history of infection with *Helicobacter pylori*. Some infected persons develop transient infection after exposure to *H. pylori*, while others develop chronic superficial gastritis within months after acquisition of the organism. In the absence of antimicrobial treatment, this process persists in most hosts for life. A minority of hosts develop clinically relevant conditions such as peptic ulceration, lymphoproliferative disease, or severe chronic atrophic gastritis leading to adenocarcinoma of the distal stomach. (*After Blaser and Parsonnet, with permission.*)

approximately 20 percent higher among patients with so-called non-ulcer dyspepsia than among matched controls; some but not all trials of *H. pylori* eradication in nonulcer dyspepsia have documented the alleviation of symptoms in some proportion of patients. Thus, some patients with nonulcer dyspepsia may benefit from treatment targeting *H. pylori*, but at present there is no prospective method for identifying this group. Peptic ulcers and nonulcer dyspepsia have been described in association with *H. heilmanii* infection, but it is unclear whether this association is causal.

PATHOLOGY AND PATHOGENESIS Infection with *H. pylori* induces chronic superficial gastritis, which includes both mononuclear and polymorphonuclear cell infiltration of the mucosa and injury to epithelial cells. (The term *gastritis* should be used specifically to describe histologic features; it has also been used to describe endoscopic appearances and even symptoms, neither of which have been linked to microscopic findings or to *H. pylori* infection.) The immune response to *H. pylori* infection includes both the production of antibody (local and systemic) and a cell-mediated response but is ineffective in clearing the infection. *H. pylori* and associated inflammation are most evident in the stomach but are also found elsewhere in areas of gastric metaplasia and heterotopia (e.g., the duodenal bulb). In the United States, the most common pattern of gastric inflammation is antral-predominant, and this is the pattern most closely linked with duodenal ulceration. In developing countries, the predominant form is pangastritis, which is epidemiologically linked with gastric ulceration and gastric carcinoma. Longitudinal analyses of gastric biopsy specimens taken from the same patient on occasions many years apart show that inflammation may progress to atrophy, intestinal metaplasia, and dysplasia and then, by implication, to carcinoma. Patients with atrophic gastritis are at risk of developing vitamin B$_{12}$ deficiency with the associated hematologic and neurologic sequelae. The individual's age at acquisition of the infection may influence the pattern of infection in the stomach and the pattern of disease. Thus, infection during early childhood may lead to gastric ulcers and gastric carcinoma, whereas infection later in childhood may lead to antral-predominant gastritis and duodenal ulceration.

Like *H. pylori*, *H. heilmanii* is associated with chronic gastritis. However, infection due to *H. heilmanii* is patchier and may clear spontaneously.

Most *H. pylori*–infected persons do not develop clinical sequelae. That some persons develop overt disease whereas others do not may be due to bacterial factors, host factors (including age at infection), and environmental factors. Bacterial factors appear to be most important. Research has focused on two of these factors: a cytotoxin, VacA, and a high-molecular-weight protein of unknown function, CagA. The cytotoxin causes vacuolation of cultured epithelial cells and gastric damage in mice. Only about 50 percent of *H. pylori* strains have cytotoxin activity that is detectable in vitro, although essentially all strains of *H. pylori* possess the gene (*vacA*) encoding the toxin. This gene has several allelic variants, each of which is associated with a different level of cytotoxin activity. Patients with ulcers are more likely to be infected by strains with detectable cytotoxin activity, and the sla allele of *vacA* is an even better marker of ulcer disease. The gene encoding the CagA protein, *cagA*, is one of a group of about 20 genes making up the *cag* virulence island, which is found in about 60 percent of U.S. strains. Another of these genes, *picB* (whose designation reflects its function—i.e., it *p*ermits the *i*nduction of *c*ytokines), appears important in the induction of inflammation. Infected patients with ulcers or gastric adenocarcinoma are more likely to have CagA-positive strains than persons without these conditions.

One puzzling question regarding *H. pylori* has been how a gastric infection causes duodenal ulceration. Colonization of areas of gastric heterotopia or metaplasia in the duodenum appears important, as does an *H. pylori*–induced increase in acid secretion. The latter phenomenon is due both to hypergastrinemia and to increased responsivity of the parietal cell mass to gastrin. The number of antral G cells (which produce gastrin) is unchanged, but the number of D cells (which

produce somatostatin) is decreased. Somatostatin has a negative feedback on gastrin release and on stimulated acid production, and the reduction of this negative feedback may account for the observed changes. Whether the resulting hyperacidity causes duodenal ulceration per se or induces gastric metaplasia in the duodenum—which subsequently becomes infected and inflamed, then ulcerates—is still unclear. After the eradication of *H. pylori* in patients with duodenal ulcer disease, the level of acid secretion falls.

DIAGNOSIS Tests for *H. pylori* infection can be divided into two groups: invasive tests, which require upper gastrointestinal endoscopy and are based on the analysis of gastric biopsy specimens, and noninvasive tests (Table 156-1). At present, invasive tests are preferred in the initial management of dyspeptic patients because the decision about whether to treat the infection depends on ulcer disease status. The most convenient endoscopy-based test is the biopsy urease test. In this procedure, two antral biopsy specimens are put into a gel containing urea and an indicator. The presence of *H. pylori* urease elicits a color change, which often takes place within minutes but can require up to 24 h; a complicating issue is that at 24 h the result of the test is sometimes falsely positive. Histologic examination of biopsy specimens is accurate. Special stains (e.g., a modified Giemsa or silver stain) permit optimal visualization of *H. pylori*. Histologic study also yields additional information, including the degree and pattern of inflammation, atrophy, metaplasia, and dysplasia. However, these details are rarely of clinical use. Microbiologic culture is most specific, although failure of this test is common except in expert hands. The identity of *H. pylori* can be confirmed by its typical appearance on Gram's staining and its positive reactions in oxidase, catalase, and urease tests. Once bacteria have been cultured, antibiotic sensitivities can be determined, but this information is not used routinely at present in the selection of treatment regimens. Biopsy specimens containing *H. heilmanii* are only weakly positive in the urease test. The diagnosis of *H. heilmanii* infection is based on the characteristic histologic appearance of the organism since it cannot be cultivated in vitro.

The simplest tests for *H. pylori* infection are serologic, involving the assessment of specific IgG levels in serum. Both standard and rapid office tests are available. When these tests are properly done, their diagnostic accuracy parallels that of invasive tests, although not all tests are equally accurate. A drop in antibody titer between matched serum samples taken before and 6 months after treatment (no sooner because of a lag in antibody decline) accurately indicates that *H. pylori* infection has been eradicated. The other major noninvasive tests are the ^{13}C and ^{14}C urea breath tests. In these simple tests, the patient drinks a labeled urea solution and then blows into a tube. The urea is labeled with either the nonradioactive isotope ^{13}C or a minute dose of the radioactive isotope ^{14}C (which exposes the patient to less radiation than a standard chest x-ray). If *H. pylori* urease is present, the

Table 156-1

Tests Commonly Used in the Diagnosis of *Helicobacter pylori* Infection

Test	Advantages	Disadvantages
INVASIVE (ENDOSCOPY- AND BIOPSY-BASED)		
Biopsy urease	Quick, simple	Rapid test not fully sensitive, 24-h test not fully specific
Histology	Widely available; may give additional histologic information	Sensitivity dependent on experience
Culture	Permits determination of antibiotic susceptibilities	Sensitivity dependent on experience
NONINVASIVE		
Serology	Cheap and convenient	Cannot be used for early follow-up
Urea breath	Safer and cheaper than endoscopy	Low-dose irradiation required for ^{14}C test

urea is hydrolyzed and labeled carbon dioxide is detected in breath samples. Both urea breath tests and serology may be more accurate than biopsy-based tests, as they are not subject to the sampling error involved in the collection of biopsy specimens. Unlike serologic tests, urea breath tests can be used to assess the outcome of treatment 1 month after its completion and thus may replace endoscopy for this purpose. Neither urea breath tests nor endoscopy-based tests can be used to assess treatment outcome earlier since, even when treatment is unsuccessful, the load of organisms may be too small to render the test positive.

℞ TREATMENT

At present, the only clear indications for treatment are *H. pylori*–related duodenal and gastric ulceration and the rare low-grade B cell MALT lymphoma. *H. pylori* infection should be treated in patients with ulcer disease, whether or not the ulcers are currently active, to reduce the likelihood of relapse. In the future, the indications for therapy may be broader, but at present treatment is not recommended for nonulcer dyspepsia. Neither is routine prophylaxis against ulcers or gastric adenocarcinoma recommended, although it may be reasonable to treat the infection in persons with a strong family history of gastric cancer. Reasons for avoiding treatment for "soft" indications include the expense, the induction of morbidity in otherwise healthy people, and the risk of widespread antibiotic resistance.

Treatment of *H. pylori* infection is becoming increasingly simple and effective, although multidrug regimens are required. *H. pylori* is susceptible to many antibiotics in vitro, but these drugs often fail in vivo, perhaps because they are not delivered to the site of infection in effective concentrations and in a fully active form. Initial failure of monotherapy has led to the use of multidrug regimens (still not approved by the Food and Drug Administration), the most widely tested of which is "standard triple therapy" with bismuth subsalicylate, tetracycline, and metronidazole, which is given for 2 weeks and eradicates *H. pylori* in about 90 percent of cases (Table 156-2). However, good compliance is crucial to the success of this complex regimen and is difficult to ensure. Thus, there is much interest in simpler 1-week triple-therapy regimens involving agents that inhibit gastric acidity (Table 156-2). These regimens have yielded promising early results, and the newly approved ranitidine bismuth citrate may be a reasonable substitute for proton pump inhibitors. Problems remain, for example, with regimens containing metronidazole or clarithromycin: resistance to these agents often arises in *H. pylori* after treatment failure, and the previous use of metronidazole for the treatment of an intercurrent infection, even many years earlier, commonly leads to metronidazole resistance. Paradoxically, metronidazole-containing regimens are still effective against around 60 percent of resistant infections. Resistance to amoxicillin, tetracycline, bismuth compounds, and proton pump inhibitors has not been described for *H. pylori*.

Successful treatment of *H. heilmanii* infections with bismuth compounds alone has been reported. However, it is unclear whether this treatment has been truly successful or whether the good outcome has merely reflected the natural history of the infection.

Because of the uncertainties surrounding the efficacy of treatment for *H. pylori* infection, it is reasonable to retest for the infection; to this end, the urea breath test or endoscopy should be undertaken no sooner than 1 month after treatment. The knowledge gained will elucidate prognosis and facilitate management. Once treatment regimens with confirmed efficacy are available, such a strategy may be unnecessary except when there is good reason to suspect that treatment has failed. Matched pretreatment and late posttreatment serology may then become the norm.

PREVENTION   *H. pylori* infection is a major public health problem in developing countries, and gastric adenocarcinoma is the second leading cause of cancer death worldwide. The most immediate solution is vaccination, and experimental immunization of animals has given promising results. In the United States and other developed countries, the incidences of *H. pylori* infection and its clinical sequelae are dropping, possibly because of improvements in living standards. Thus the prevention of infection in these countries may be necessary for populations at high risk of gastric cancer. In the United States, these groups include African, Asian, Hispanic, and Native Americans.

BIBLIOGRAPHY

ATHERTON JC, SPILLER RC: The urea breath test for *Helicobacter pylori*. Gut 35:723, 1994

BLASER MJ, PARSONNET J: Parasitism by the "slow" bacterium *Helicobacter pylori* leads to altered gastric homeostasis and neoplasia. J Clin Invest 94:4, 1994

———: The bacteria behind ulcers. Sci Am 274:104, 1996

DOOLEY CP et al: Prevalence of *Helicobacter pylori* infection and histologic gastritis in asymptomatic persons. N Engl J Med 321:1562, 1989

HANSSON L-E et al: The risk of stomach cancer in patients with gastric or duodenal ulcer disease. N Engl J Med 335:242, 1996

KUIPERS E et al: Atrophic gastritis and *Helicobacter pylori* infection in patients with reflux esophagitis treated with omeprazole or fundoplication. N Engl J Med 334:1018, 1996

MARSHALL BJ, WARREN JR: Unidentified curved bacilli in the stomach of patients with gastritis and peptic ulceration. Lancet 1:1311, 1984

NIH CONSENSUS DEVELOPMENT PANEL: *Helicobacter pylori* and peptic ulcer disease. JAMA 272:65, 1994

NOMURA A et al: *Helicobacter pylori* infection and gastric carcinoma in a population of Japanese-Americans in Hawaii. N Engl J Med 325:1132, 1991

PARSONNET J et al: *Helicobacter pylori* infection and gastric lymphoma. N Engl J Med 330:1267, 1994

——— et al: Modelling cost-effectiveness of *Helicobacter pylori* screening to prevent gastric cancer: A mandate for clinical trials. Lancet 348:150, 1996

WOTHERSPOON AC et al: *Helicobacter pylori*–associated gastritis and primary B cell gastric lymphoma. Lancet 338:1175, 1991

Table 156-2

Recommended Regimens for the Eradication of *Helicobacter pylori* Infection

Drug 1	Drug 2	Drug 3	Duration
STANDARD TRIPLE-THERAPY REGIMEN			
Bismuth subsalicylate (2 tabs qid)	Tetracycline HCl (500 mg qid*)	Metronidazole (250 mg tid)	2 weeks
TRIPLE-THERAPY REGIMENS WITH ACID REDUCTION			
Omeprazole (20 mg bid)	Clarithromycin (250 mg bid)	Metronidazole (500 mg bid)	1 week
Omeprazole (20 mg bid)	Clarithromycin (500 mg bid)	Amoxicillin (1 g bid)	1 week

* Amoxicillin (500 mg qid) may be substituted for tetracycline, although meta-analysis suggests that this substitution results in a small drop in efficacy.

NOTE: These regimens have not yet been approved for this indication by the Food and Drug Administration.

---

157   *Matthew Pollack*

INFECTIONS DUE TO *PSEUDOMONAS* SPECIES AND RELATED ORGANISMS

Pseudomonas species and phylogenetically related bacteria are ubiquitous, free-living, opportunistic gram-negative pathogens. *Pseudomonas aeruginosa*, the most common human pathogen in this group, is the primary subject of this chapter. Also discussed are *Burkholderia cepacia* (formerly *Pseudomonas cepacia*), primarily an opportunistic pathogen; *Stenotrophomonas maltophilia* (formerly *Xanthomonas maltophilia*), which primarily infects hospitalized patients; *Burkholderia pseudomallei* (formerly *Pseudomonas pseudomallei*), an organism that inhabits soil and water (primarily in the tropics) and that causes melioidosis—a systemic disease with acute or chronic manifestations—in nonimmunocompromised patients; and *Burkholderia mallei* (formerly *Pseudomonas mallei*), a pathogen of animal origin that occasionally produces glanders in humans.

INFECTIONS DUE TO *P. AERUGINOSA*

P. aeruginosa is a small, aerobic gram-negative rod belonging to the family Pseudomonadaceae. It is motile by virtue of its single polar flagellum. More than half of all clinical isolates produce the blue-green pigment pyocyanin; this pigment is helpful in the identification of the organism and accounts for the species name *aeruginosa*, which refers to the distinctive color of copper oxide. *P. aeruginosa* is readily identified in the clinical laboratory. It is a straight or slightly curved, nonsporulating, motile gram-negative rod that grows aerobically on most common media.

EPIDEMIOLOGY   *P. aeruginosa* is widespread in nature, inhabiting soil, water, plants, and animals (including humans). It has a predilection for moist environments. This organism occasionally colonizes the skin, external ear, upper respiratory tract, or large bowel of healthy humans. Rates of carriage are relatively low, however, except among patients who have serious underlying disease, whose host defenses have been naturally or iatrogenically compromised, who have previously received antibiotic therapy, and/or who have been exposed to the hospital environment. Under these circumstances, colonization with *P. aeruginosa* frequently precedes infection, and factors that predispose to the former also increase the likelihood of the latter.

Most *P. aeruginosa* infections are hospital acquired. Many potential reservoirs of infection have been identified, including respiratory equipment, cleaning solutions, disinfectants, sinks, vegetables, flowers, endoscopes, and physiotherapy pools. Most reservoirs are associated with moisture. It is assumed that the organism is transmitted to patients via the hands of hospital personnel or via fomites.

While some infecting strains of *P. aeruginosa* appear to be endemic within the hospital environment, others are traced to a common source associated with a specific outbreak or epidemic. Epidemiologic investigation is facilitated by serotyping (immunotyping) of strains on the basis of differences in lipopolysaccharide structure and by the use of DNA or RNA probes.

PATHOGENESIS   That the pathogenesis of infections due to *P. aeruginosa* is complex is evidenced by the clinical diversity of the diseases related to this organism and by the multiplicity of virulence factors it produces. *P. aeruginosa* rarely causes disease in the healthy host. It may undergo a "malignant" transformation, however, when normal cutaneous or mucosal barriers have been breached or bypassed (e.g., as a result of burn injury, penetrating trauma, surgery, endotracheal intubation, urinary bladder catheterization, or intravenous drug abuse); when immunologic defense mechanisms have been compromised (e.g., by chemotherapy-induced neutropenia, hypogammaglobulinemia, extremes of age, diabetes mellitus, cystic fibrosis, cancer, or AIDS); when the protective function of the normal bacterial flora has been disrupted by broad-spectrum antibiotic therapy; and/or when the patient has been exposed to reservoirs associated with a hospital environment. The ubiquity of the organism, its flexible nutritional and metabolic requirements, its environmental resiliency, and its relative resistance to antibiotics help account for the frequency and success with which it acts as an opportunistic pathogen.

Infections caused by *P. aeruginosa* usually begin with bacterial attachment and superficial colonization of cutaneous or mucosal surfaces and progress to localized bacterial invasion and damage to underlying tissues. This process may continue with bloodstream invasion, dissemination, systemic inflammatory-response syndrome (SIRS), multiple-organ dysfunction, and ultimately death. Alternatively, the infection may remain anatomically localized or may spread by direct extension to contiguous structures. The organism and its products may cause tissue injury at primary and secondary sites of infection, while the release of systemically acting toxins or inflammatory mediators

of the infected host may contribute directly or indirectly to the sepsis syndrome.

The initial attachment of *P. aeruginosa* to the respiratory epithelium and other epithelial surfaces appears to be mediated by bacterial organelles called *pili* or *fimbriae* and by the mucoid exopolysaccharide *alginate*, which is produced by mucoid strains. Receptors for these adhesins are found, for example, on tracheal epithelial cells and tracheobronchial mucin and are composed, at least in part, of *N*-acetylneuraminic acid (sialic acid) and *N*-acetylglucosamine, respectively.

Surface moieties of *P. aeruginosa*, including exopolysaccharide and lipopolysaccharide, may protect the organism from direct antibody- and complement-mediated bactericidal mechanisms and from opsonophagocytosis. Meanwhile, the organism produces a number of extracellular enzymes, including alkaline protease, elastase, phospholipase, cytotoxin, and exoenzymes (or exotoxins) A and S. The breakdown of host tissues by these extracellular bacterial products creates conditions conducive to enhanced bacterial proliferation, invasion, and tissue injury.

The preceding process is particularly likely to culminate in bloodstream invasion and dissemination in the face of immune compromise such as that resulting from profound neutropenia. The sepsis syndrome, or SIRS, due to *P. aeruginosa* shares many of the features of gram-negative sepsis caused by other bacteria, and the lipopolysaccharide or endotoxin produced by this organism, like that produced by other bacterial species, is thought to play a pivotal role in the pathogenesis of this syndrome.

In addition to lipopolysaccharide, which is a structural component of the bacterial outer membrane, the extracellular enzyme exotoxin A—a diphtheria-like toxin—is produced by most clinical isolates of *P. aeruginosa*. Exotoxin A inhibits mammalian protein synthesis by transferring the adenosine diphosphate (ADP) ribose moiety of the nicotinamide adenine dinucleotide into covalent linkage with elongation factor 2, an enzyme that catalyzes the elongation step in polypeptide assembly but is inactivated by exotoxin-mediated ADP ribosylation. Exotoxin A appears to cause both local and systemic disease. It is cytotoxic in vitro and necrotizing in vivo and produces fatal shock in experimental animals, including nonhuman primates. Toxigenic clinical isolates are more virulent than nontoxigenic strains. Moreover, the rate of survival is higher among patients with *P. aeruginosa* bacteremia in the presence than in the absence of adequate preexisting levels of exotoxin A–specific serum antibodies.

CLINICAL MANIFESTATIONS AND DIAGNOSIS   Respiratory Tract Infections   Lower respiratory tract infections due to *P. aeruginosa* occur mainly in immunocompromised patients. *Primary or nonbacteremic pneumonia* results from aspiration of upper respiratory tract secretions; often develops in patients with chronic lung disease, congestive heart failure, or AIDS; and is most common in an intensive care setting in association with mechanical ventilator use. *Bacteremic pneumonia*, in contrast, complicates hematopoietic malignancies, especially after chemotherapy that induces severe neutropenia. Chronic infection of the lower respiratory tract with *P. aeruginosa* is prevalent among patients with cystic fibrosis. It occurs typically in older children or young adults and is caused almost exclusively by mucoid strains.

Primary or nonbacteremic pneumonia caused by *P. aeruginosa* may present as an acute, life-threatening infection characterized by fever, chills, severe dyspnea, cyanosis, productive cough, apprehension, confusion, and other signs of severe systemic toxicity. Chest roentgenograms typically show bilateral bronchopneumonia with nodular infiltrates and small areas of radiolucency; pleural effusions are common; empyema is relatively uncommon; and lobar consolidation is occasionally seen. Pathologic lesions include alveolar necrosis, focal hemorrhages, and microabscesses. Cavitary lesions are particularly common in AIDS patients with *P. aeruginosa* pneumonia.

Bacteremic pneumonia due to *P. aeruginosa*, typically associated with neutropenia, begins as a respiratory infection, but subsequent bloodstream invasion and resulting metastatic spread produce characteristic lesions in the lung and other viscera. Alveolar hemorrhage and necrosis are common. The signs and symptoms of this fulminant disease include those described for nonbacteremic pneumonia caused by this organism as well as those associated with gram-negative sepsis.

Chest roentgenograms characteristically demonstrate a rapid progression from pulmonary vascular congestion to interstitial edema, then to pulmonary edema, and finally to diffuse necrotizing bronchopneumonia with cavity formation. The patient typically dies 3 or 4 days after initial presentation.

Mucoid strains of *P. aeruginosa* infect the lower respiratory tract of patients with cystic fibrosis, contributing to the acute exacerbations and chronic progression that characterize pulmonary disease in these individuals. Colonization with *P. aeruginosa* correlates with bronchial airway disease in cystic fibrosis patients. It is unclear whether mucus plugging precedes infection or vice versa. The uncertainty notwithstanding, airway obstruction appears to begin with bronchiolitis, which causes mucus plugging and predisposes to *P. aeruginosa* infection. The latter produces more mucus plugging, chronic suppuration, bronchiectasis, atelectasis, and ultimately fibrosis. This process progresses to pulmonary insufficiency, hypoxemia, and alterations in cardiopulmonary dynamics resulting in pulmonary hypertension and cor pulmonale.

Clinical manifestations of lower respiratory tract infections due to *P. aeruginosa* in cystic fibrosis vary with the severity and duration of underlying lung disease and with the frequency and intensity of acute episodes. Early in the disease, patients may experience recurrent upper respiratory symptoms followed by a lingering cough. Episodes of pneumonia develop later, with persistent cough between acute episodes. Eventually, patients exhibit a chronic productive cough, diminished appetite, weight loss, growth retardation, and decreased activity. Other symptoms may include wheezing, tachypnea, and irritability. Acute exacerbations are typically accompanied by low-grade fever and heightened respiratory symptoms. Physical signs include evidence of malnutrition, an increase in anteroposterior diameter, intercostal retractions, cyanosis, inspiratory and expiratory wheezing, rhonchi, moist rales, abdominal distention, and clubbing of the fingers and toes. Laboratory abnormalities include leukocytosis with a left shift and hypoxemia with or without hypercarbia. Tests of pulmonary function demonstrate obstructive and restrictive defects. Chest roentgenograms reveal overaeration, patchy atelectasis, peribronchial fibrosis, and patchy infiltrates associated with pneumonia. In more advanced disease, there may be evidence of severe overaeration, depressed diaphragm, increased anteroposterior diameter, extensive peribronchial infiltration, generalized bronchiectasis, and cyst formation.

Bacteremia *P. aeruginosa* causes one of the most common and life-threatening gram-negative bloodstream infections in immunocompromised patients. *P. aeruginosa* bacteremia is usually associated with nosocomial infections and is frequently iatrogenic. It is either primary (with no identifiable source) or secondary to a discrete extravascular focus. *P. aeruginosa* bacteremia is associated with underlying conditions such as hematologic malignancies, neutropenia, immunoglobulin deficiencies, severe burns, dermatitis, diabetes mellitus, AIDS, and prematurity. Predisposing iatrogenic factors include cancer chemotherapy resulting in neutropenia or mucosal ulceration, genitourinary instrumentation or catheterization, placement of intravascular hardware, recent surgery, steroid therapy, and antibiotic administration.

The clinical features of *P. aeruginosa* bacteremia are similar to those of other forms of bacteremia. Common primary sites of infection include the urinary tract, gastrointestinal tract, lungs, intravascular foci, skin, and soft tissues. Fever, tachypnea, tachycardia, and prostration are common. Disorientation, confusion, or obtundation may be evident. Hypotension can progress to refractory shock. Renal failure, adult respiratory distress syndrome, or disseminated intravascular coagulation sometimes occurs as a complication. Jaundice is seen more commonly in *P. aeruginosa* bacteremia than in other forms of gram-negative sepsis.

Pathognomonic skin lesions termed *ecthyma gangrenosum* develop in a relatively small minority of patients with *P. aeruginosa* bacteremia. The lesions begin as small hemorrhagic vesicles surrounded by a rim of erythema and undergo central necrosis with subsequent ulceration. They occur singly or in small numbers on the perineum, buttocks, and extremities; in the axillae; or elsewhere. Ecthyma-like lesions are occasionally noted on the mucous membranes of the mouth or gingiva. Histologic study shows that these lesions contain numerous bacteria invading blood vessels but few inflammatory cells. Bacteria are readily visible on Gram's staining and may be cultured from aspirated material.

Endocarditis *P. aeruginosa* infects native heart valves in intravenous drug users as well as prosthetic heart valves. The source of *P. aeruginosa* strains infecting drug users appears to be standing water contaminating drug paraphernalia. Moreover, foreign materials that are mixed with heroin may cause injury to valve leaflets or mural endocardium, with consequent fibrosis. These factors, combined with the apparent high affinity of the organism for human endocardium, may explain the association between *P. aeruginosa* endocarditis and intravenous drug use. The particularly frequent exposure of the tricuspid valve to both trauma and bacteria apparently accounts for the high incidence of tricuspid involvement in association with intravenous drug use.

The pulmonic, mitral, or aortic valve or the mural endocardium of either atrium also may be affected in *P. aeruginosa* endocarditis. Multiple-valve infections are common. Tricupsid or right-sided involvement is often associated with septic pulmonary emboli. Right-sided *P. aeruginosa* endocarditis usually presents subacutely, while the appearance of left-sided disease is likely to be more acute or even fulminant. Fever is a virtually invariable feature, and murmurs are usually detectable at initial presentation or shortly thereafter. Septic pulmonary emboli associated with right-sided disease result in cough, pleuritic chest pain, sputum production, pulmonary infiltration (with or without abscess formation), and pleural effusion. Left-sided infections may present as intractable heart failure or large systemic emboli. Mycotic aneurysms, cerebritis, or brain abscess may occur; septic infarcts are occasionally found in the spleen; but skin and soft tissue manifestations, including Janeway lesions, Osler's nodes, and ecthyma gangrenosum, are relatively uncommon.

The diagnosis of *P. aeruginosa* endocarditis is based on a positive blood culture in the absence of an extracardiac source; an indication of valvular dysfunction or vegetation on an echocardiogram; evidence of septic pulmonary lesions on a chest roentgenogram (in right-sided disease); and the actual demonstration of infected heart valves at the time of surgery.

Central Nervous System Infections *P. aeruginosa* infections of the central nervous system include meningitis and brain abscess. These infections follow extension from a contiguous parameningeal structure such as the ear, mastoid, or paranasal sinus; direct inoculation into the subarachnoid space or brain through head trauma, surgery, or diagnostic procedures; or bacteremic spread from a distant site such as the urinary tract, lung, or heart valve. Like *P. aeruginosa* infections at other anatomic sites, central nervous system infections are documented almost exclusively in patients with compromised local or systemic immune-defense mechanisms. Predisposing factors include recent neurosurgical procedures, penetrating head trauma, lumbar puncture or spinal anesthesia, cancer of the head and neck, parameningeal infection, and *P. aeruginosa* infections at distant sites in association with bloodstream invasion.

The clinical signs of *P. aeruginosa* meningitis, like those of other forms of acute bacterial meningitis, include fever, headache, stiff neck, confusion, and obtundation. The onset of illness may be acute or even fulminant, particularly in bacteremic patients, with a precipitous downhill course, shock, coma, and early death. In nonbacteremic patients, *P. aeruginosa* meningitis or brain abscess may present more insidiously, with a paucity of systemic symptoms. This presentation is especially common in infections resulting from recent neurosurgery, cancer of the head and neck, or direct extension from a parameningeal focus of chronic infection. Occasionally, *P. aeruginosa* meningitis runs a subacute or relapsing course that is thought to be related to the intermittent release of bacteria from a loculated site of infection. Chronic or recurrent meningitis may result from altered cranial anatomy associated with central nervous system tumors, traumatic injury, neurosurgical procedures, indwelling hardware, or cerebrospinal fluid leaks.

Ear Infections *P. aeruginosa* is often found in the external auditory canal, particularly under moist conditions and in the presence of inflammation or maceration (as in "swimmer's ear"). Moreover, this organism is the predominant pathogen associated with external otitis, a usually benign inflammatory process affecting the external auditory canal. This self-limited condition provides a local environment conducive to the growth of *P. aeruginosa*, which, in turn, appears to contribute to the inflammatory process. The ear is painful or merely itchy, there is a purulent discharge, and pain is elicited by pulling on the pinna. The external canal appears edematous and is filled with detritus that often prevents visualization of the tympanic membrane.

P. aeruginosa occasionally penetrates the epithelium overlying the floor of the external auditory canal at the junction between bone and cartilage and invades underlying soft tissue. The ensuing invasive process, which involves soft tissue, cartilage, and cortical bone, is typically slow but destructive. Termed *malignant external otitis*, this condition occurs predominantly in elderly diabetic patients but is reported occasionally in infants with other underlying diseases and rarely in elderly nondiabetic patients. Virtually all cases of malignant external otitis are caused by *P. aeruginosa*. From the external ear, the infection advances to the retromandibular area or parotid space and enters the mastoid air cells and temporal bone. Advancing osteomyelitis at the base of the skull often involves the seventh, ninth, tenth, and eleventh cranial nerves. The cavernous sinus can become involved, as can the contralateral petrous apex. The middle ear is commonly spared; meningitis and brain abscess are relatively rare complications.

Otalgia and otorrhea are common presenting symptoms of malignant external otitis. Facial-nerve paralysis tends to occur early, while other cranial-nerve palsies appear later. There may be a loss of hearing, the pinna of the ear is typically tender, and trismus indicates temporomandibular involvement. Constitutional symptoms such as fever and weight loss are relatively uncommon. Physical examination almost always reveals abnormalities of the external auditory canal, including swelling, erythema, purulent discharge, debris, and granulation tissue in the canal wall. The tympanic membrane is often hidden from view and is sometimes perforated. Inflammation may involve the pinna as well as the periauricular, retromandibular, and mastoid areas. Bilateral disease is unusual but does occur.

Peripheral leukocytosis is relatively infrequent in malignant external otitis, while the erythrocyte sedimentation rate usually is markedly elevated. Cerebrospinal fluid occasionally exhibits pleocytosis and an elevation in the protein level. Computed tomography (CT) or polytomography of the mastoid or temporal bone typically reveals bony erosions and new bone formation, while the floor of the skull may have soft tissue densities associated with areas of cellulitis. Magnetic resonance imaging (MRI) may delineate soft tissue involvement with greater sensitivity and accuracy than CT. In addition, technetium 99m bone scans and gallium 67 scans frequently give positive results. Cultures of samples from the external auditory canal and of surgical specimens are almost always positive for *P. aeruginosa*.

P. aeruginosa is commonly implicated in chronic suppurative otitis media in children and adults. It either is the sole bacterial isolate or is among the organisms isolated from the middle or external ear in a majority of cases, and it is thought to play a central pathogenic role.

Eye Infections (See also Chap. 28)   *P. aeruginosa* causes bacterial keratitis or corneal ulcer and endophthalmitis in the human eye. Keratitis due to *P. aeruginosa* may result from even minor corneal injury, which interrupts the integrity of the superficial epithelial surface and permits bacterial access to the underlying stroma. Corneal ulcer may complicate contact lens use, particularly when extended-wear soft contact lenses are involved. Contact lens solutions or the lenses themselves may be the source of the organism, which is probably inoculated into the eye at sites of minor lens-induced corneal damage. Patients who have sustained serious burns, have undergone ocular irradiation or tracheostomy, have been exposed to the intensive care environment, and/or are in a coma are also susceptible to *P. aeruginosa*–associated corneal ulcers. *P. aeruginosa* keratitis usually starts

as a small central ulcer; spreads concentrically to involve a large portion of the cornea, sclera, and underlying stroma; and in some cases progresses to posterior corneal perforation.

The clinical manifestations of *P. aeruginosa* keratitis include a rapidly expanding, necrotic stromal infiltrate in the bed of an epithelial injury; surrounding epithelial edema; an anterior chamber reaction; and mucopurulent discharge adherent to the ulcer's surface. Corneal ulcer due to *P. aeruginosa* may advance rapidly to involve the entire cornea in 2 days or less or may evolve subacutely over several days. Systemic symptoms are uncommon. Complications include corneal perforation, anterior chamber involvement, and endophthalmitis.

P. aeruginosa endophthalmitis may complicate penetrating injuries of the eye, intraocular surgery, hematogenous spread from other sites of *Pseudomonas* infection, or posterior perforation of corneal ulcers. It is typically a rapidly progressive, sight-threatening condition that demands immediate therapeutic intervention. Clinical manifestations may include eye pain, conjunctival hyperemia, chemosis, lid edema, decreased visual acuity, hypopyon, severe anterior uveitis, and signs of possible vitreous involvement. Panophthalmitis may result from this intraocular infection.

Bone and Joint Infections   Vertebral osteomyelitis due to *P. aeruginosa* is associated with complicated urinary tract infection, genitourinary instrumentation or surgery, and intravenous drug abuse. Vertebral infections associated with a urinary tract source most often develop in the elderly and usually affect the lumbosacral spine. Drug use–related infections typically occur in younger patients and may affect the cervical or lumbosacral spine. *P. aeruginosa* vertebral osteomyelitis is usually an indolent disease. Accordingly, symptoms may develop weeks or even months before diagnosis. Back or neck pain is generally reported, while fever and systemic symptoms are relatively uncommon. Local tenderness and decreased range of motion of the affected spine are typical. Neurologic deficits are documented in a minority of patients. Leukocytosis may be noted, the erythrocyte sedimentation rate is almost always markedly elevated, and blood cultures are sometimes positive. Roentgenograms reveal loss of bone density, narrowed intervertebral space, destruction of vertebral end plates, lytic lesions of vertebral bodies, sclerosis, and possible osteophyte formation. CT or MRI may be the most sensitive means of defining lesions. Technetium bone scans and gallium scans usually yield positive results, while myelograms are revealing only if granulation tissue impinges on the epidural space. An etiologic diagnosis requires the culture of material obtained by needle aspiration or biopsy of the affected spine under fluoroscopic guidance; open biopsy is occasionally needed.

Sternoclavicular pyarthrosis caused by *P. aeruginosa* is another complication of intravenous drug abuse; in some cases it is associated with *P. aeruginosa* endocarditis, but more often it is not. Joint involvement is usually monoarticular, with the sternoclavicular joint more often affected than sternochondral joints. Localized pain in the anterior chest wall is the usual presenting complaint, movement of the homolateral shoulder may be restricted by discomfort, associated fever is common, and symptoms typically last for months (although some cases do have more acute presentations). Physical examination reveals tenderness, erythema, and swelling over the affected joint. Leukocytosis is common, and the erythrocyte sedimentation rate is almost invariably elevated. Roentgenograms show soft tissue edema, bone demineralization, lytic lesions, and periosteal elevation of the clavicular head, rib, or sternum. Material obtained by arthrocentesis or synovial biopsy yields *P. aeruginosa* in culture.

P. aeruginosa infections of the symphysis pubis are associated with pelvic surgery and intravenous drug use. The symphysis pubis, like other fibrocartilaginous joints, exhibits a peculiar susceptibility to bloodborne infection with *P. aeruginosa*. Affected patients report pain in the groin, hip, thigh, and/or lower abdomen that is made worse by walking. Fever is variable, and the duration of symptoms before diagnosis ranges from days to months. As in other bone and joint infections caused by *P. aeruginosa*, leukocytosis is variable, while the erythrocyte sedimentation rate is markedly elevated. Roentgenograms show irregularities of the pubic margins, separation of the symphysis pubis, and osteomyelitic abnormalities of the pubic rami that may be extensive. Bone scans are usually positive. Needle aspiration or biopsy

CHAPTER 157
Infections due to *Pseudomonas* Species and Related Organisms   **947**

extensive. Bone scans are usually positive. Needle aspiration or biopsy is necessary to obtain material for culture. A positive culture is particularly important for the discrimination of *P. aeruginosa* infections and other pyogenic infections from osteitis pubis, which is thought to be a noninfectious condition complicating pelvic surgery, childbirth, or trauma.

P. aeruginosa osteochondritis of the foot follows puncture wounds of the foot, primarily in children. The organism infects the small joints and bones of the foot, including the proximal phalanges, metatarsals, metatarsophalangeal joints, tarsal bones, and calcaneus. *P. aeruginosa* shows a particular predilection for cartilage. Systemic symptoms are usually lacking. On average, symptoms last for several weeks. There may be plantar cellulitis over the involved area or tenderness upon deep palpation. Results of roentgenograms and bone scans are generally positive. Aspiration of the affected joint usually yields purulent material in which *P. aeruginosa* can be demonstrated by Gram's staining and by culture.

P. aeruginosa is one of the most common causative agents in a variety of other, less specific syndromes involving nonhematogenous infections of bones and joints and collectively referred to as *chronic contiguous osteomyelitis*. These infections may result, for example, from compound fractures, contamination associated with open reduction and fixation of closed fractures, sternotomy performed in conjunction with cardiac surgery, contiguous spread from infected ischemic ulcers related to peripheral vascular disease or diabetes mellitus, and cellulitis in general. The chronicity, indolence, and heterogeneity of these infections explain their varied clinical manifestations and the frequent need for complicated long-term management.

Gastrointestinal Infections   *P. aeruginosa* infections involving virtually every portion of the human gastrointestinal tract—from oropharynx to rectum—have been documented. *P. aeruginosa*–associated gastrointestinal disease is most common among infants and among adults with hematologic malignancies and neutropenia. Moreover, asymptomatic large-bowel colonization resulting from prolonged exposure to the hospital environment and the selective pressure of antibiotics may be a silent source of organisms that subsequently invade the bloodstream during severe chemotherapy-induced neutropenia or other forms of immunosuppression.

P. aeruginosa causes necrotizing enterocolitis in infants and a similar disease in neutropenic patients with cancer. The most common sites of involvement are the distal ileum, cecum, and colon. The pathologic lesions are hemorrhagic and necrotic ulcers that begin in the bowel mucosa and extend into the submucosa. Vascular invasion by bacteria may be documented in the submucosa in association with bacteremia, local spread to the muscularis and serosa, and subsequent perforation leading to peritonitis. Necrotic ulcers are also documented occasionally in the oropharynx, esophagus, stomach, or proximal small bowel. Typhlitis, a disease developing most frequently in patients with leukemia, involves localized lesions of the cecum that are associated with necrosis and gangrene and that sometimes result in perforation, bacterial peritonitis, and early death; *P. aeruginosa* is the agent most commonly identified in this condition. This organism is also among the pathogens most frequently isolated from rectal abscesses in neutropenic patients with cancer. These lesions, which may be associated with few signs and symptoms, must be carefully sought in susceptible patients because they may give rise to life-threatening sepsis if not surgically drained.

P. aeruginosa has been implicated in epidemics of moderate to severe diarrhea in children, in a form of enteric fever sometimes referred to as *Shanghai fever*, and in a cholera-like illness attributed to a putative but still-unidentified *Pseudomonas* enterotoxin.

Urinary Tract Infections   *P. aeruginosa* is one of the most common causes of complicated and nosocomial infections of the urinary tract. These infections may result from urinary tract catheterization, instrumentation, surgery, or obstruction; they may arise from persistent foci (e.g., the prostate or stones) and may be chronic or recurrent. The urinary tract may be a target for bloodborne infection in patients with *P. aeruginosa* bacteremia but more often is the source of bacteremia. Chronic *P. aeruginosa* infections of the urinary tract are relatively common among patients with indwelling Foley catheters, altered urinary tract anatomy secondary to diversionary procedures, and paraplegia.

The clinical features of urinary tract infections due to *P. aeruginosa* are usually indistinguishable from those of other bacterial infections. However, *P. aeruginosa* infections exhibit a propensity for persistence, chronicity, resistance to antibiotic therapy, and recurrence. More unusual forms of urinary tract involvement peculiar to *P. aeruginosa* include ulcerative lesions of the renal pelvis, ureters, and bladder that cause sloughing of vesical membrane in the urine and bacterial invasion of renal blood vessels that produces ecthyma-like lesions in association with *Pseudomonas* sepsis.

Skin and Soft Tissue Infections   As indicated above, *P. aeruginosa* bacteremia may be associated with ecthyma gangrenosum. These disseminated skin lesions, which frequently begin as small vesicles, are characterized by hemorrhage, necrosis, surrounding erythema, and histologic evidence of blood vessel invasion by bacteria. *P. aeruginosa* can almost always be cultured from the lesions. Less common skin manifestations of *P. aeruginosa* sepsis include vesicular or pustular lesions, bullae, subcutaneous nodules, deep abscesses, and cellulitis. Metastatic lesions of the skin or mucous membranes complicate *Pseudomonas* sepsis and occasionally produce massive necrosis or gangrene of the extremities, perineum, face, or oropharynx.

Primary *P. aeruginosa* pyoderma occurs when the skin breaks down secondary to trauma, burn injury, dermatitis, or ulcers related to peripheral vascular disease or pressure sores. Moist conditions, such as those in the perineum or diaper area of infants, contribute to the development of *P. aeruginosa* pyoderma. Neutropenia also may predispose to this condition. The clinical appearance of primary *P. aeruginosa* pyoderma, which frequently includes hemorrhage and necrosis, resembles that of metastatic *P. aeruginosa* skin lesions. Histologic studies document vascular invasion by bacteria in both diseases. A rare distinguishing feature of *P. aeruginosa* pyoderma is its association with a blue-green exudate and a characteristic fruity odor.

P. aeruginosa wound sepsis complicating extensive third-degree burn injuries results from colonization of the burn site or burn eschar, invasion of the subeschar space and underlying dermis, vascular invasion, and systemic spread. The development and progression of *P. aeruginosa* burn wound sepsis are facilitated by the injury-associated breakdown of normal skin, antibiotic selection, and burn-related immune defects. Local manifestations include black, dark brown, or violaceous discoloration of the burn eschar; degeneration of underlying granulation tissue, hemorrhage, and premature eschar separation; edema, hemorrhage, and necrosis of skin adjacent to the burn site; erythematous nodular lesions in unburned skin; and formation of brown or black neoeschars. Systemic manifestations include fever or hypothermia, confusion or obtundation, oliguria, hypotension, ileus, and sometimes respiratory failure or pneumonia. The diagnosis of *P. aeruginosa* burn sepsis is based on these local and systemic clinical manifestations and on a burn wound biopsy that reveals both $>10^5$ colony-forming units of *P. aeruginosa* per gram of tissue and histologic evidence of bacterial invasion of unburned tissue, vasculitis, or intense inflammation at the burn margin.

P. aeruginosa causes diffuse pruritic maculopapular and vesiculopustular rashes associated with exposure to contaminated hot tubs, spas, whirlpools, and swimming pools. Most cases of *P. aeruginosa* dermatitis have occurred as part of a common-source outbreak. At least two nosocomial common-source outbreaks—one related to a physiotherapy pool—have been reported. Skin rashes may be limited to areas covered by swimsuits or may be more diffuse, sparing only the head and neck. Associated symptoms may include dizziness, headache, earache, sore eyes, sore nose, sore throat, swollen breasts, or abdominal cramps. Low-grade fever is uncommon. The illness is usually self-limited, and the rash resolves without specific therapy after cessation of exposure. One nosocomial outbreak involving immunocompromised patients, however, resulted in *P. aeruginosa* folliculitis evolving into full-blown ecthyma gangrenosum.

℞ TREATMENT

Most types of *P. aeruginosa* disease are treated with one or more antibiotics to which the infecting organism is sensitive. Exceptions are external otitis (nonmalignant) and dermatitis associated with exposure to contaminated water. Both of these infections are self-limited and usually require no specific antimicrobial therapy.

In general, the choice of antibiotics with antipseudomonal activity includes the aminoglycosides (e.g., gentamicin, tobramycin, netilmicin, amikacin), selected third-generation cephalosporins (e.g., ceftazidime, cefoperazone), selected extended-spectrum penicillins (e.g., ticarcillin, ticarcillin/clavulanate, piperacillin, piperacillin/tazobactam, mezlocillin, azlocillin), carbapenems (e.g., imipenem, meropenem), monobactams (e.g., aztreonam), and fluoroquinolones (e.g., ciprofloxacin, ofloxacin, enoxacin, lomefloxacin, norfloxacin). (For information on dosages and schedules, see Chap. 140.) All these agents except enoxacin, lomefloxacin, and norfloxacin are available in parenteral form; ciprofloxacin and ofloxacin are available in both oral and intravenous forms. It is noteworthy that because of sometimes variable antimicrobial activity against *P. aeruginosa* or distinctive pharmacokinetic properties, different members of a particular antibiotic class are not always interchangeable in the treatment of all *P. aeruginosa* infections. Ciprofloxacin, for example, demonstrates somewhat higher in vitro activity against many clinical isolates of *P. aeruginosa* than do other fluoroquinolones. Conversely, certain multiresistant strains of *P. aeruginosa* exhibit cross-resistance to antibiotics of different classes. Thus, local patterns of antimicrobial susceptibility should influence the initial choice of antibiotic agents, while the susceptibility profile of the isolate from a particular case should dictate definitive antibiotic therapy.

In most severe or life-threatening infections due to *P. aeruginosa*, two antibiotics to which the infecting strain is (or is likely to be) sensitive should be administered together. The combination of an aminoglycoside and a β-lactam antibiotic is usually appropriate. The goals of combined therapy are to achieve additive or synergistic killing, to exploit the pharmacologic strengths and offset the pharmacologic limitations of each agent, and to prevent the emergence of antibiotic resistance. Particularly in acute or fulminant infections, antibiotics should be employed at the maximal doses consistent with safety. Likewise, when sites of infection are relatively inaccessible (e.g., the central nervous system or the heart), maximal or even supramaximal antibiotic doses may be required for the attainment of therapeutic concentrations in infected tissues. In relatively indolent, self-limited, and often chronic infections due to *P. aeruginosa* (e.g., certain cases of chronic contiguous osteomyelitis or malignant external otitis), a single antimicrobial agent may be employed; an oral fluoroquinolone such as ciprofloxacin or ofloxacin may be appropriate under these circumstances, although such oral therapy must often be protracted if infection is to be eradicated. In addition, certain urinary tract infections due to *P. aeruginosa*, which are limited to the lower urinary tract, may be amenable to short-term treatment with a single antibiotic active against *P. aeruginosa*.

The appropriate duration of antibiotic therapy for disease caused by *P. aeruginosa* depends on the type, location, and severity of infection. Precise, prospectively defined treatment guidelines are sometimes problematic; it may be more appropriate to tailor the duration of therapy to the specific circumstances of a case, including the initial response to treatment. In general, chronic infections associated with extensive tissue injury, disruption of normal anatomy, foreign or prosthetic material, or suboptimal antibiotic accessibility require therapy for weeks or even months rather than days. More acute infections may be treated aggressively but for shorter periods.

P. aeruginosa infections of the lower respiratory tract in patients with cystic fibrosis pose a special challenge because these infections represent long-standing, chronic conditions complicated by acute exacerbations and a downhill course. Antibiotic therapy for acute exacerbations clearly results in clinical improvement. A more aggressive approach featuring periodic expectant courses of antimicrobial therapy may limit disease progression. Frequent pulmonary toileting is important in the management of this disease, while periodic bronchial lavage has been employed to good effect to relieve symptoms associated with mucus plugging. Aerosolized antibiotics also have been used successfully in some instances. Finally, lung transplantation has been employed with good results in selected cystic fibrosis patients with severe progressive lower respiratory tract infections due to *P. aeruginosa*.

Optimal management of infections due to *P. aeruginosa* often requires surgical intervention as well as antimicrobial therapy. The presence of necrotic tissue or of prosthetic or foreign material necessitates surgical debridement (e.g., in malignant external otitis and in some cases of chronic osteomyelitis or osteochondritis); loculated pus demands drainage (e.g., in sternoclavicular pyarthrosis, brain abscess, and endophthalmitis); left-sided endocarditis is an indication for early valve replacement; perforated bowel requires laparotomy and bowel resection (e.g., in necrotizing enterocolitis); and urinary tract obstruction may necessitate appropriate surgery.

PROGNOSIS All infections caused by *P. aeruginosa* are treatable and—with the possible exception of lung infections in patients with cystic fibrosis—are potentially curable. The heterogeneity of these infections, however, accounts for substantial differences in short- and long-term prognosis. At one end of the spectrum are acute fulminant infections such as bacteremic pneumonia, septicemia, burn wound sepsis, and meningitis, which are associated with extremely high mortality despite appropriate therapy. At the other end of the spectrum are more chronic, indolent infections, including certain cases of chronic contiguous osteomyelitis, malignant external otitis, and lower respiratory tract infections in patients with cystic fibrosis. Although the latter infections may not be imminently life-threatening, they are often difficult to eradicate and (as in the case of cystic fibrosis lung disease) may end fatally in the longer term.

INFECTIONS CAUSED BY OTHER *PSEUDOMONAS* SPECIES OR RELATED BACTERIA

Burkholderia cepacia (formerly *P. cepacia*), like *P. aeruginosa*, is primarily an opportunistic pathogen that is implicated in both endemic infections and occasional nosocomial outbreaks. Hospital epidemics are most frequently associated with a liquid reservoir or a moist environmental surface. Under these circumstances, the organism may colonize various body sites, with the subsequent development of invasive disease. The distinction between colonization and true infection is often difficult and may hinge on the presence of clinical signs of infection as well as a positive culture. *B. cepacia* has been reported to cause pneumonia, urinary tract infections, meningitis, peritonitis, surgical and burn wound infections, bacteremia, and endocarditis related to injection drug use. In addition, *B. cepacia* has been implicated, either alone or together with *P. aeruginosa*, in chronic infections of the lower respiratory tract in patients with cystic fibrosis. In some of these patients, the appearance of *B. cepacia* has been associated with fulminant necrotizing pneumonia, bacteremia, and a rapid downhill course.

The treatment of *B. cepacia* infections is complicated by the resistance of the organism to aminoglycosides and to many β-lactam agents. Although trimethoprim-sulfamethoxazole and chloramphenicol have been used successfully in the treatment of *B. cepacia* infections, resistance to these two antimicrobial agents has been reported. Third-generation cephalosporins and fluoroquinolones have variable activity against *B. cepacia*. However, ciprofloxacin and ampicillin/sulbactam may be considered as alternative agents for use against sensitive strains. While in vitro synergy has been demonstrated for certain antibiotic combinations, such as ciprofloxacin, imipenem, and rifampin, the clinical efficacy of such combinations has not been fully documented.

Stenotrophomonas maltophilia (formerly *X. maltophilia*) is a ubiquitous, free-living opportunistic pathogen that colonizes and occasionally infects hospitalized patients, particularly in an intensive care setting. This organism has been associated with pneumonia, urinary tract infection, wound infection, peritonitis, cholangitis, meningitis, bacteremia, and endocarditis. *S. maltophilia*, like *Pseudomonas* species, has been implicated in pseudoinfections, particularly pseudobacteremia related to contaminated blood-drawing materials. It is thus essential to consider clinical signs and symptoms in distinguishing exogenous contamination or simple colonization from genuine infection. Urinary tract infection is usually associated with a chronic indwelling urinary catheter or with urinary tract instrumentation; line-related sepsis complicates intravenous therapy; peritonitis has occurred in patients undergoing chronic ambulatory peritoneal dialysis; native valve endocarditis has been described in intravenous drug users; and prosthetic valve endocarditis also has been reported. Acute *S. maltophilia* pneumonia, an often devastating disease associated with bacteremia, is being seen with increasing frequency in debilitated patients on intensive care units.

Antibiotic resistance in *S. maltophilia*, based on both low outer-membrane permeability and inducible β-lactamases, is at least partly responsible for the emergence of this organism as a nosocomial pathogen under the selective pressure of antibiotic treatment. Trimethoprim-sulfamethoxazole is often useful for the treatment of infections due to drug-resistant strains. Alternative agents include ticarcillin/clavulanate, ciprofloxacin, and minocycline or doxycycline. The third-generation cephalosporins cefoperazone and ceftazidime may be active against *S. maltophilia* in some instances, but in vitro susceptibilities should be tested in each case. The aminoglycosides and imipenem are usually inactive.

Pseudomonas fluorescens occasionally causes human disease; it is implicated particularly often in infections related to the administration of contaminated (stored) blood products and in pseudoinfections. Additional bacterial species that are associated only rarely with human infections include *Pseudomonas putida*, *Pseudomonas stutzeri*, *Pseudomonas pseudoalcaligenes*, and (all formerly *Pseudomonas* species) *Burkholderia pickettii*, *Comamonas acidovorans*, *Comamonas testosteroni*, *Brevundimonas diminuta*, and *Brevundimonas vesicularis*.

MELIOIDOSIS Infections caused by *B. pseudomallei* constitute a broad spectrum of acute and chronic, local and systemic, clinical and subclinical disease processes collectively called *melioidosis*. *B. pseudomallei* and the infections it causes are found mainly in the tropics and are endemic in Southeast Asia and surrounding areas. *B. pseudomallei* is a free-living, small, motile, aerobic gram-negative rod previously classified in the rRNA homology group II of *Pseudomonas* and related species. The organism is a saprophyte that is normally found in soil, ponds, and rice paddies and on produce from endemic areas. It is occasionally a pathogen for animals. Humans contract the disease through soil contamination of abrasions, ingestion, nasal instillation, or inhalation. Person-to-person transmission is apparently rare.

Acute infections most often involve the lungs, although lesions sometimes develop in other organs. Pulmonary lesions tend to be more extensive and dissemination to other organs tends to be more widespread in subacute melioidosis. Acute abscesses exhibit necrosis, polymorphonuclear leukocyte infiltration, and surrounding hemorrhage; multinucleated histiocytes are observed in areas of necrosis. Subacute lesions, in contrast, are characterized by caseation necrosis, with mononuclear and plasma cell infiltration.

Melioidosis presents in different forms. High rates of seropositivity in endemic areas such as Vietnam, Thailand, and Malaysia suggest that many infections are clinically inapparent. The occasional diagnosis based solely on abnormal routine chest roentgenograms represents asymptomatic pulmonary infection. Acute, localized, suppurative skin infections associated with nodular lymphangitis and regional lymphadenitis result from direct inoculation at sites of minor skin trauma. Acute pulmonary infections may originate in the respiratory tract or result from hematogenous spread, their severity varying from mild bronchitis to extensive necrotizing pneumonia. Onset may be sudden or gradual. Fever, productive cough, and marked tachypnea are frequent. Chest roentgenograms typically reveal upper lobe consolidation or thin-walled cavities. Progressive upper lobe disease mimics tuberculosis.

Acute suppurative infections or pulmonary disease may give rise to hematogenous dissemination and the acute septicemic form of melioidosis. This progression is more likely in chronically debilitated patients, such as those with diabetes mellitus or alcoholism. Patients with pulmonary infections in particular may present with severe tachypnea, confusion, headache, pharyngitis, diarrhea, and pustular lesions of the head, trunk, and extremities. The skin may be flushed or cyanotic; signs of meningitis or arthritis may be apparent; the liver and spleen may be enlarged; and muscle tenderness may be striking. Chest roentgenograms show diffuse nodular densities that may expand, coalesce, and finally cavitate. The acute septicemic form of melioidosis usually follows a rapid downhill course, ending in early death unless arrested by early and aggressive therapy.

Chronic suppurative melioidosis is characterized by acute or chronic abscesses of the skin and various organs. Recrudescent disease arising from inactive sites of infection and perhaps triggered by intercurrent illness or other events may present in any acute or chronic form.

The diagnosis of melioidosis should be entertained when a febrile patient who has been in an endemic area presents with an acute lower respiratory tract illness associated with tachypnea, exhibits unusual skin or subcutaneous lesions, or has a chest roentgenogram suggesting tuberculosis in the absence of sputum-associated tubercle bacilli. An etiologic diagnosis may be made by microscopic demonstration of small, irregularly staining, gram-negative rods in exudate material; by characteristic bipolar ("safety-pin") staining of organisms with methylene blue; and by a culture positive for *B. pseudomallei* and/or a fourfold or greater rise in the titer of serum antibody to the organism.

℞ TREATMENT

The mainstay of treatment for melioidosis is antibiotic administration combined with appropriate surgical drainage of abscesses and aggressive support for patients with septicemic forms of the disease. The guidelines for antibiotic therapy are somewhat imprecise. Subclinical infection or mere seropositivity does not usually require specific therapy. Ceftazidime appears to be the agent of choice for clinical disease, while trimethoprim-sulfamethoxazole, cefotaxime, imipenem, and amoxicillin/clavulanate are possible alternatives. Therapy with a combination such as ceftazidime plus trimethoprim-sulfamethoxazole is indicated in severe forms of melioidosis. However, the resistance of many strains of *B. pseudomallei* to trimethoprim-sulfamethoxazole, particularly in Southeast Asia, necessitates other antibiotic choices. Acute septicemic infections probably should be treated with combinations of multiple agents administered parenterally. Patients with acute pulmonary infections should receive antibiotics for 60 to 150 days, while chronic disease associated with persistently positive sputum cultures may require longer treatment. Extrapulmonary suppurative disease is appropriately treated for 6 months to 1 year. When initial therapy for acute infections involves a third-generation cephalosporin such as ceftazidime, a switch can often be made after 30 days to an oral agent such as trimethoprim-sulfamethoxazole or amoxicillin/clavulanate.

Most cases of melioidosis are curable if appropriately treated. However, septicemic infections are still associated with very high mortality despite optimal therapy, while all forms of melioidosis are subject to possible early or very late recrudescence.

GLANDERS Glanders is primarily a systemic equine disease that is caused by *B. mallei* and is associated with pulmonary involvement, subcutaneous ulcerative lesions, and lymphangitis. Once widespread, glanders still occurs in Africa, Asia, and South America but not in the United States or western Europe. The infection may be communicated to humans during close contact with horses, mules, or donkeys, probably by cutaneous inoculation or nasal exposure to contaminated discharges. Glanders assumes the following forms in humans: acute localized suppurative infection, acute pulmonary infection, acute septicemic infection, and chronic suppurative infection. Inoculation of *B. mallei* into the skin usually produces a nodule with an area of lymphangitis. Fever, malaise, and prostration are common. Mucous membrane infection results in the production of a mucopurulent discharge from the eye, nose, or lips, with the subsequent development of granulomatous ulcers. Pulmonary infection secondary to inhalation of the organism is accompanied by typical local and systemic signs and symptoms of pneumonia. Lymphadenopathy and splenomegaly may be documented. Chest roentgenograms reveal circumscribed densities suggesting early lung abscesses; bronchopneumonia or lobar consolidation also may be evident. Chronic suppurative infection presents as multiple subcutaneous and intramuscular abscesses, particularly often involving the extremities; visceral lesions are documented in some patients. The acute septicemic form of glanders may be associated with a diffuse papular or pustular eruption, severe systemic symptoms, and early death.

The diagnosis of glanders may be suggested by the clinical setting (including a history of close contact with equines) and confirmed by culture of the causative agent from clinical material and by demonstration of *B. mallei*–specific seroconversion.

℞ TREATMENT

Optimal antimicrobial therapy for glanders has not been adequately defined. Sulfadiazine has proven effective historically both in animals and in humans. It has been suggested, however, that rational therapy consists of the same antibiotics recommended for the treatment of melioidosis, with the specific agent chosen on the basis of in vitro susceptibility testing. Antibiotics are administered for at least 30 days in uncomplicated infections and longer in complicated cases. Abscesses may require surgical drainage, and appropriate supportive measures are necessary in acute septicemic forms of the disease.

BIBLIOGRAPHY

P. AERUGINOSA INFECTIONS

BALTCH AL, SMITH RP (eds): *Pseudomonas aeruginosa Infections and Treatment.* New York, Marcel Dekker, 1994

BARKER LF: The clinical symptoms, bacteriologic findings and postmortem appearances in cases of infection of human beings with the *Bacillus pyocyaneus.* JAMA 29:213, 1897

BODEY GP et al: *Pseudomonas* bacteremia: Retrospective analysis of 410 episodes. Arch Intern Med 145:1621, 1985

FICK RB (ed): *Pseudomonas aeruginosa: The Opportunist, Pathogenesis and Disease.* Boca Raton, CRC, 1992

KORVICK JA, YU VL: Antimicrobial agent therapy for *Pseudomonas aeruginosa.* Antimicrob Agents Chemother 35:2167, 1991

MORRISON AF, WENZEL RP: Epidemiology of infections due to *Pseudomonas aeruginosa.* Rev Infect Dis 6(Suppl):S267, 1984

POLLACK M: The virulence of *Pseudomonas aeruginosa.* Rev Infect Dis 6(Suppl):S617, 1984

————: *Pseudomonas aeruginosa,* in *Principles and Practice of Infectious Diseases,* 4th ed, GL Mandell et al (eds). New York, Churchill Livingstone, 1995, pp 1980–2003

INFECTIONS DUE TO RELATED ORGANISMS

ELTING LS, BODEY GP: Septicemia due to *Xanthomonas* species and non-*aeruginosa Pseudomonas*species: Increasing incidence of catheter-related infections. Medicine 69:296, 1990

GOLDMANN DA, KLINGER JD: *Pseudomonas cepacia:* Biology, mechanisms of virulence, epidemiology. J Pediatr 108:806, 1986

MURRAY AR et al: Blood transfusion–associated *Pseudomonas fluorescens* septicemia: Is this an increasing problem? J Hosp Infect 9:243, 1987

POLLACK M: *Pseudomonas,* in *Infectious Diseases,* SL Gorbach et al (eds). Philadelphia, Saunders, 1992, pp 1502–1513

TOMASHEFSKI JF et al: *Pseudomonas cepacia*–associated pneumonia in cystic fibrosis. Arch Pathol Lab Med 112:166, 1988

MELIOIDOSIS

LEELARASAMEE A, BOVORNKITTI S: Melioidosis: Review and update. Rev Infect Dis 11:413, 1989

SANFORD JP: *Pseudomonas* species (including melioidosis and glanders), in *Principles and Practice of Infectious Diseases,* 4th ed, GL Mandell et al (eds). New York, Churchill Livingstone, 1995, pp 2003–2009

158 Gerald T. Keusch

SALMONELLOSIS

The prototypic *Salmonella, S. choleraesuis,* mistakenly described by Theobald Smith in 1894 as the cause of the viral disease hog cholera, was named in honor of Smith's supervisor, Dr. Daniel Salmon. The genus is both vast and diverse. Of its more than 2300 distinguishable organisms, some can cause infections in humans, including typhoid fever (also known as enteric fever); focal systemic infections; septicemia; and (most commonly) diarrhea, varying from acute watery diarrhea to bloody diarrhea or dysentery. Salmonellae are ecologically entrepreneurial and exist in a multiplicity of habitats; this characteristic adaptability, which accounts for the ubiquity of the organisms in nature and for the many ways in which they encounter potential new human hosts, is related to their genetic plasticity.

ETIOLOGY Salmonellae are gram-negative bacillary members of the family Enterobacteriaceae that are almost always motile by means of multiple peritrichous flagella and with two exceptions are nonencapsulated. (*S. typhi* and *S. paratyphi* C express the Vi capsular polysaccharide.) The salmonellae are facultatively anaerobic and typically do not ferment lactose; these properties form the basis for their identification during initial screening in the microbiology laboratory. Taxonomy, typically the staid and stable domain of a few cognoscenti, has been in a state of flux for *Salmonella* in recent years, as the number of recognized species classified within the genus has varied from one to a few thousand. The current classification, based on DNA relatedness, recognizes only two species, *S. enterica* and *S. bongori,* the latter of which is not a human pathogen (Table 158-1). The choice of the designation *S. enterica* reflects a desire to avoid confusion with the prototypic organism described by Smith, *S. choleraesuis,* and the fact that none of the named isolates has previously been called *enterica. S. enterica* encompasses six subspecies, each of which includes multiple members (serovars). Most human pathogenic salmonellae fall within subspecies *enterica.*

The huge number of salmonellae distinguishable by serologic methods reflects the ability of the organisms to create mosaic flagellin genes through multiple recombinational events and horizontal transfer, point mutations, and gene duplications and alterations in length, all of which together may constitute an adaptive response to host immune defense systems. Since subspecies members are distinguished by serologic markers on polysaccharide somatic O antigens and protein flagellar H antigens, individual salmonellae are properly considered *serovars.* Thus, *S. typhi* should be called *S. enterica* subspecies *enterica* serovar typhi, while *S. typhimurium* would properly be designated *S. enterica* subspecies *enterica* serovar typhimurium. Because the majority of serovars have been named after the place in which they were first detected (for example, Heidelberg or Newport), *Salmonella* nomenclature seems more geographic than microbiologic. Nevertheless,

Table 158-1

Taxonomy of the Genus *Salmonella,* with Serogroups and Representative Serovars

Species	Subspecies		Serogroup	Common Serovars
S. enterica	(I)	*enterica*	A	paratyphi A
			B	typhimurium, agona, derby, heidelberg, paratyphi B
			C	choleraesuis, infantis, virchow
			D	dublin, enteritidis, typhi
			E	anatum
	(II)	*salamae*		
	(IIIa)	*arizonae*		
	(IIIb)	*diarizonae*		
	(IV)	*houtenae*		
	(VI)	*indica*		
*S. bongori**	—			

* Formerly subspecies V of *S. enterica.*

clinicians continue to use convenient abbreviated names such as *S. heidelberg* or *S. newport* to refer to these organisms. Therefore, this chapter also makes use of this shorthand system.

Another commonly used historic classification system for salmonellae groups isolates on the basis of the major representatives of the 60 phase-1 somatic antigens they express. These *serogroups* are designated by letters (A, B, C, etc.). Most human pathogenic salmonellae are members of groups A through D (Table 158-1); indeed, the serogroup designation is typically the first piece of specific data about an isolate to emerge from the clinical microbiology laboratory. Because just a few serovars cause most cases of human disease (see below), serogrouping offers a useful initial clue to the exact identity of the organism involved and also provides clinically useful diagnostic, prognostic, and therapeutic information.

Some salmonellae are highly adapted to human or other animal hosts. Animal-adapted strains generally do not cause human disease, while human-adapted strains often cause typhoid fever. The rest of the salmonellae are non-host-adapted organisms that may infect both humans and other animals. These organisms are the most common causes of *Salmonella* diarrhea.

TYPHOID FEVER

Typhoid fever is a distinctive acute systemic febrile infection of the mononuclear phagocytes and deserves separate consideration. Since it may be caused by several serovars (*S. typhi*, *S. paratyphi* A, *S. paratyphi* B, and occasionally *S. typhimurium*), many clinicians prefer the term *enteric fever*. However, because typhoid is fundamentally not an enteric disease, this term is also inappropriate. On balance, *typhoid fever* is still the best term, for it is understood by nearly all clinicians to describe a particular syndrome that is, in fact, due primarily to *S. typhi*.

EPIDEMIOLOGY Because the cause of clinical typhoid fever is almost always a human-adapted *Salmonella*, most cases can be traced to a human carrier. The proximate cause is most often water but may also be food contaminated by a human carrier. Chronic carriers are generally over 50 years old, are more commonly women than men, and often have gallstones. *S. typhi* resides in the bile (even inside stones), intermittently reaches the lumen of the bowel, and is excreted in the stool, thereby contaminating water or food.

With improvements in environmental sanitation in the United States, the incidence of *S. typhi* infection has dropped to a low level. From 1930 to 1950, the typhoid incidence—initially around 22 per 100,000—diminished by 90 percent (Fig. 158-1). From 1985 to 1994, an average of only 508 cases per year were identified in the United States, accounting for just over 1 percent of all *Salmonella* isolates.

FIGURE 158-1 Incidence of typhoid fever and nontyphoidal salmonellosis in the United States, 1930–1994. *(Courtesy of Robert V. Tauxe, M.D., Centers for Disease Control and Prevention, Atlanta.)*

Even this small number greatly exceeds the figures for the isolation of paratyphoid organisms in the United States, of which two-thirds are *S. paratyphi* B. The majority of *S. typhi* infections take the form of active disease or convalescent carriage rather than chronic asymptomatic carriage. This pattern is consistent with the decline of domestically acquired infections in the United States. Most active cases are now acquired during travel abroad and involve children, adolescents, and young adults, whereas chronic carriers are most often in the seventh decade of life. In New York City, the proportion of typhoid cases that were related to travel increased from two-thirds to four-fifths from 1980 to 1990, and most of these cases followed travel to southern and Southeast Asia. Mexico remains the leading source of typhoid among residents of the United States, especially those in border states and traveling students; because there are so many travelers to Mexico, this problem is seen frequently even though the rate of acquisition of typhoid in Mexico is relatively low. Known global hotspots for typhoid fever include Peru, Alexandria (Egypt), Jakarta (Indonesia), India, Pakistan, and Nepal. In Santiago, Chile, the previously high endemic rate of typhoid has recently been reduced markedly by improvements in water quality and in the sanitation infrastructure.

Typhoid contracted in the United States is usually due either to contact with carriers or to large (common-source) or small (family-related) food-borne outbreaks, which are often associated with food handlers or domestic workers who are immigrants from endemic countries. Also at continuing risk of typhoid are bacteriology laboratory workers. The number of patients in the United States is clearly underestimated, and an unknown proportion of cases escape detection because appropriate cultures are not done or antibiotic treatment is administered before samples for culture can be obtained.

In *S. typhi*–endemic regions, the rate of clinical typhoid among persons positive for human immunodeficiency virus (HIV) is approximately 25-fold higher than that among HIV-negative individuals in the 15- to 35-year-old age group and is as much as 60-fold higher than that in the general population. Asymptomatic HIV-positive patients have a typical clinical presentation and response to therapy; AIDS patients can present with fulminant diarrhea and/or colitis and are far more likely to relapse. While this enhanced sensitivity has little practical significance for AIDS patients in countries with a low typhoid incidence, it may become a problem for those who travel to highly endemic countries.

PATHOGENESIS Infection is initiated by oral ingestion of organisms, which must pass the gastric acid barrier to establish infection. While experiments with volunteers have suggested that 10^5 organisms are required for the initiation of infection, buffering of acid by food lowers the necessary inoculum in natural exposures, and the actual infectious dose is probably considerably less than 10^5. Analysis of multiple studies of experimental *S. typhi* infection in healthy young adults, which generally have used a single laboratory strain (Quailes), has suggested no significant association between dose and severity of illness, although both a direct relation between dose and attack rate and an indirect relation between dose and incubation period exist (Table 158-2). Severity is determined by both host and microbial properties (as discussed below).

Salmonella exhibits a genetic adaptive acid-tolerance response: exposure to acid leads to synthesis of at least 40 proteins, some of which may play a role in pathogenesis. Bacteria successfully evading

Table 158-2

Response of Volunteers to Experimental Infection with *S. typhi*

Inoculum	Attack Rate		Mean Incubation Period, days
10^3	0/13	(0)	—
10^5	77/200	(38.5)	9.3
10^7	13/27	(48.1)	7.4
10^8–10^9	24/25	(96.0)	4.7

"acid death" in the stomach pass on to the distal ileum and colon, where they penetrate the mucosal barrier. Most new information about *Salmonella* pathogenesis has been derived from a combination of studies in cell culture and experimental infection with *S. typhimurium* in mice (which results in a typhoid-like illness in this species). It is curious that the infection of mice with *S. typhi* produces no clinical illness. The mechanism of penetration of mammalian cells by *S. typhi* appears to be similar to that for nontyphoidal salmonellae and is discussed below in relation to the latter organisms.

Initial bacterial invasion results in transient asymptomatic bacteremia, as organisms are rapidly ingested by mononuclear phagocytes within which they survive and multiply. This process is favored by a lack of bactericidal antibodies in the susceptible host; in contrast, opsonized salmonellae are taken up by neutrophils and killed. Opsonophagocytosis is limited by the capsular Vi polysaccharide of *S. typhi* (also expressed by *S. paratyphi* C and *Citrobacter freundii*), which enhances resistance to complement activation and bacterial lysis by the alternative pathway as well as to peroxide-mediated killing. Another apparent microbial determinant of the host-pathogen interaction is flagellar type. Flagellar type H1-j bacteria, which have been associated with infection only in Indonesia, affect older individuals and cause milder illness than flagellar type H1-d bacteria. The fate of organisms within macrophages depends both on microbial factors that promote resistance to killing and on specific host T lymphocyte–activated, cell-mediated immune mechanisms that are under the genetic control of the *ity* locus in mice. This locus, which was identified in studies of the resistance of inbred mouse strains to infection with *S. typhimurium*, turned out to be of more general relevance and identical to the *lsh* and *bcg* loci mediating resistance to other intracellular pathogens such as *Leishmania* species and *Mycobacterium bovis* strain BCG. The human variant of the *ity/lsh/bcg* locus, *Nramp* (natural resistance-associated macrophage protein), is present on chromosome 2q35. *Nramp*, which is actually a family of at least three genes linked to the genes for the interleukin (IL) 1 receptor and the IL-8 receptor gene cluster, encodes a macrophage-specific membrane transport protein needed for the early killing of intracellular pathogens by a mechanism that remains uncertain but is distinct from those of activated macrophages.

When intracellular multiplication has proceeded enough to permit the initiation of persistent bacteremia, the clinical phase of typhoid fever begins with invasion of the gallbladder and Peyer's patches of the intestine. The sustained bacteremia is responsible for the persistent fever of clinical typhoid, while inflammatory responses to tissue invasion determine the pattern of clinical expression (cholecystitis, intestinal hemorrhage, or perforation). With invasion of the gallbladder and Peyer's patches, bacteria regain entry to the bowel lumen and may be recovered in stool cultures beginning in the second week of clinical disease. Seeding of the kidney leads to positive urine cultures, albeit in a much lower percentage of patients than have positive blood cultures. The lipopolysaccharide (endotoxin) of *S. typhi* may contribute to fever, leukopenia, and other systemic symptoms, but the occurrence of such symptoms in individuals rendered tolerant to endotoxin supports a role for other factors, such as cytokines released from infected mononuclear phagocytes, that can mediate inflammation (see Chap. 17).

CLINICAL MANIFESTATIONS The incubation period of typhoid fever is variable and depends on both the inoculum size and the state of the host's defenses. A range of 3 to 60 days has been reported. The disease classically presents with a steplike daily increase in temperature (up to 40 to 41°C) associated with headache, malaise, and chills. The hallmark of typhoid fever is prolonged, persistent fever (4 to 8 weeks in untreated patients). The illness may be mild and brief; however, in some cases, acute, severe infection with disseminated intravascular coagulation and central nervous system involvement rapidly results in death. In other instances, necrotizing cholecystitis or intestinal bleeding and perforation can occur in the third or fourth week of illness, when the patient is otherwise improving. In most cases, the onset of these complications is dramatic and clinically

obvious. Intestinal perforation appears to be less common among children under 5 years of age.

Early intestinal manifestations include constipation (especially in adults) or mild diarrhea (in children) associated with abdominal tenderness. Mild hepatosplenomegaly is detectable in the majority of patients. Bradycardia relative to the height of the fever may be a clinical clue to typhoid but is present in only a minority of patients. Epistaxis may be noted in the early stages of illness. "Rose spots," appearing as small, pale red, blanching, slightly raised macules, are occasionally seen on the chest and abdomen during the first week. They can evolve into nonblanching small hemorrhages that are difficult to see in dark-skinned patients. The major characteristics of untreated typhoid are persistent high fever, severe anorexia, weight loss, and changes in sensorium, but a variety of other complications also may develop, including hepatitis, meningitis, nephritis, myocarditis, bronchitis, pneumonia, arthritis, osteomyelitis, parotitis, and orchitis. Except for that of relapse, the frequency of all these complications, including hemorrhage and perforation, is reduced by prompt use of appropriate antibiotics. Typhoid, long considered to be uncommon and typically mild in young children, may in reality be frequent and severe in this group. Neonatal typhoid, which can be acquired vertically from infected mothers or from exogenous sources, is often a severe, life-threatening septicemic illness with a high case-fatality rate.

Multidrug-resistant *S. typhi* is becoming more prevalent in many endemic countries. Patients infected with resistant strains present with more severe illness, look "toxic," and have a higher incidence of disseminated intravascular coagulation and hepatomegaly and a three-fold higher mortality rate that is thought to be related to the longer duration of disease and to prior ineffective oral antibiotic therapy.

Around 3 to 5 percent of patients become long-term asymptomatic carriers, some for life unless treated. Many carriers give no history of typhoid fever and probably have had an undiagnosed mild infection.

LABORATORY FINDINGS AND DIAGNOSIS In around 25 percent of patients, leukopenia and neutropenia are evident. In most patients, the white blood cell count is normal, albeit low in relation to the degree of fever; this pattern may be a clue to the diagnosis. Severe leukopenia (<2000 cells/µL) is found in rare instances. In the event of intestinal perforation or pyogenic complications, secondary leukocytosis develops. The anemia of blood loss may be superimposed on the anemia of chronic infection.

Whereas definitive diagnosis still depends on isolation of the organism, the overall yield of culture is disappointingly low. The yield is affected by several variables: when the cultures are performed, what is cultured, and whether the patient has taken antibiotics. The rate of recovery of organisms from blood is highest in the first week of illness, approaching 90 percent among untreated patients; the figure falls to less than 50 percent by the third week. Yields can approach 100 percent when blood and bone marrow both are cultured; bone marrow cultures are frequently positive even when the patient is taking antibiotics. Buffy-coat culture can shorten the time required for a positive result, but this technique is rarely used. Stool cultures are often negative in the first week, when it is most urgent to make the diagnosis; they become positive in 75 percent of cases during the third week, when the organism reinvades the bile and Peyer's patches. The recovery rate diminishes to 10 percent by the eighth week, and one-third to one-half of the patients with positive stool cultures at this point will continue to have positive cultures for at least 1 year. Sampling of the upper-small-bowel secretions by means of the string test increases the yield over that of stool culture at this stage of illness.

Other diagnostic tests are available. The simplest is the measurement of agglutinating antibodies to O or H antigens (the Widal test). In the absence of recent immunization, a high titer of antibody to O antigen (>1:160) is consistent with acute typhoid, and higher titers (>1:640) are even more suggestive of this condition. However, other serogroup D salmonellae, along with some organisms in groups A and B, share the antigen used in the Widal test, which therefore is not specific. Antibodies to H antigens may be found in even higher titer but, because of their broad cross-reactivity, are difficult to interpret. A fourfold rise in antibody titer between paired serum samples is strong evidence for infection; however, such a rise is of little use in the management of the acutely ill patient, and the antibody response may be blunted by early, effective antibiotic therapy. Recently developed latex agglutination or coagglutination tests for antibody to the Vi antigen appear to be much more specific and sensitive than classic Widal tests. Sensitivities are 95 percent or higher, with very low rates of false negativity; however, these new tests either are not commercially available or are not in common use. In some studies in developing countries with high incidences of typhoid fever, coagglutination is much more reliable than culture because so many patients have already taken antibiotics before being seen by a physician. Promising new enzyme immunoassays that detect *S. typhi* outer-membrane proteins are being evaluated. A sensitive and specific multiplex polymerase chain reaction for Vi antigen promises to be highly sensitive and specific, but its value has not been proved in clinical studies, nor is it available yet.

DIFFERENTIAL DIAGNOSIS When all the classic clinical manifestations are present, including rose spots, prolonged fever, relative bradycardia, and leukopenia, the diagnosis of typhoid will be strongly suggested. However, most cases do not fit this "typical" profile. Differential diagnosis includes infections associated with prolonged fever, such as the rickettsioses, brucellosis, tularemia, leptospirosis, miliary tuberculosis, viral hepatitis, infectious mononucleosis, cytomegalovirus infections, and malaria, as well as noninfectious causes of fever, such as lymphoma (see Chap. 17). In the United States, typhoid should be considered in any patient with prolonged, unexplained fever, especially after recent travel to places with endemic typhoid fever.

℞ TREATMENT

Since its introduction, chloramphenicol has been the antimicrobial "gold standard" for treatment. No drug has been better in promoting a favorable clinical response, which usually becomes apparent within 24 to 48 h of the start of treatment in the appropriate dosages (3 to 4 g/d in adults or 50 to 75 mg/kg of body weight per day in young children). The drug is given orally for 2 weeks; the dose may be reduced to 2 g/d or 30 mg/kg per day when the patient becomes afebrile—usually by day 5 of treatment. However, because of the specter of aplastic anemia associated with chloramphenicol, the drug is little used in the United States. Other effective oral regimens include amoxicillin (4 to 6 g/d in four divided doses in adults or 100 mg/kg per day in children), trimethoprim-sulfamethoxazole (640 and 3200 mg, respectively, in two divided doses daily in adults or 185 mg of the trimethoprim component per square meter of body surface area per day in children), or—for patients over 17 years of age—a 4-fluoroquinolone such as ciprofloxacin or ofloxacin.

A variety of intravenous drugs are also effective. Both chloramphenicol and trimethoprim-sulfamethoxazole can be given intravenously to patients who cannot take oral medications. Other effective parenteral antimicrobials include high-dose ampicillin, cefotaxime, cefoperazone, and the 4-fluoroquinolones. However, none has been as rapidly acting or as effective as ceftriaxone, which rivals or betters chloramphenicol in rapidity of defervescence. Initial recommendations for a 7-day course of ceftriaxone have been pared down (to 3 days of 2 to 4 g once daily in adults or 5 days of 50 to 80 mg/kg once daily in children) without apparent loss of efficacy. In addition, compared with that for other drugs, the relapse rate for ceftriaxone appears lower.

The prevalence of resistance to multiple first-line oral drugs has been rising among strains of *S. typhi* in developing countries, especially in the Indian subcontinent and Southeast Asia, due to the acquisition of plasmids encoding inactivating β-lactamases and chloramphenicol acetyl transferases. Where multidrug resistance is a problem, ceftriaxone or a 4-fluoroquinolone should be administered initially to adults over 17 years of age, and ceftriaxone is the best choice for children because of concerns about quinolone-induced arthropathy and cartilage damage in this age group. Recent safety studies employed magnetic resonance imaging in the evaluation of children 8 months to 13 years of age who had received ciprofloxacin

at a daily dosage of 15 to 25 mg/kg for 9 to 16 days; these studies found no bone or cartilage damage, and follow-up measurements 2 years later detected no abnormality in height. Short-course (3-day) quinolone therapy has been shown to be effective against multidrug-resistant typhoid in children, and its use further reduces the likelihood of drug toxicity. Alternative oral agents that reportedly are effective for this indication include furazolidone (7.5 mg/kg per day) and cefixime (5 mg/kg every 12 h). The high cost of ceftriaxone is somewhat offset by the efficacy of a short course and the economy of once-daily dosing.

Studies in Indonesia of patients with severe typhoid who presented with central nervous system manifestations and/or evidence of disseminated intravascular coagulation suggested that intravenous dexamethasone (3 mg/kg as a loading dose over 30 min, followed by 1 mg/kg every 6 h for 24 to 48 h), used along with parenteral antimicrobials, reduces mortality. Salicylates should be avoided to diminish the danger of intestinal hemorrhage. Prompt surgical management of bleeding and bowel perforation reduces mortality, since a fatal outcome is associated primarily with peritonitis. Bowel perforations should be closed in two layers for best results. The antibiotics selected should cover not only *S. typhi* but also the facultative and anaerobic bowel flora. Selective angiography, radioisotopic scanning methods, and sometimes endoscopy (see Chap. 282) to localize the bleeding site can facilitate operative repair. In developing countries, however, patients often present late after perforation, are poor surgical candidates, and may be severely malnourished, and only limited surgical and postoperative care may be available. Supportive medical care and antibiotics alone have been recommended in this setting, although limited surgery to close the perforation site without bowel resection is increasingly favored. With double-layer closure of the lesion, aggressive fluid replacement, and administration of an inexpensive broad-spectrum antibiotic regimen including chloramphenicol, gentamicin, and metronidazole, mortality rates have been reduced from 25 to 30 percent to well under 10 percent.

The early use of effective antimicrobials is associated with a relatively high rate of relapse; relapse rates of 20 percent can be expected, whereas the figure is only 5 to 10 percent in untreated patients. Presumably, prompt therapy inhibits the development of an adequate immune response. Relapses are usually milder than the initial attack and respond to the same antimicrobial used initially.

Eradication of the chronic carrier state, especially in the presence of gallstones, is notoriously difficult. Traditional regimens have used ampicillin or amoxicillin (100 mg/kg per day) plus probenecid (30 mg/kg per day) or trimethoprim-sulfamethoxazole (160/800 mg twice daily) plus rifampin (600 mg once daily) for at least 6 weeks. Recent studies suggest that a 4-week course of a 4-fluoroquinolone is at least as good and probably much better because the organism is exquisitely sensitive in vitro and the drugs reach the gut lumen, liver, gallbladder, and bile in active form. The new quinolones provide the best chance of eradicating *S. typhi* in the presence of gallstones; for reasons of simplicity and safety, they should be the first-choice agents for the treatment of patients without stones as well. The optimal dose and duration of quinolone treatment have yet to be defined. These drugs are the best choice for chronic suppression of typhoid relapse in AIDS patients.

PREVENTION AND CONTROL Worldwide experience has shown that improvement of environmental sanitation, including sewage disposal and water supplies, will sharply reduce the incidence of typhoid fever. Where this approach is not yet possible and for travelers, immunization has been used. Traditional heat-killed, phenol-extracted whole typhoid vaccine is no longer recommended because of its limited efficacy and duration of protection and the high frequency of local reactions and fever. One option for children over 6 years of age and adults consists of three doses of a first-generation live oral vaccine (Ty21a), which is invasive but metabolically defective and dies after a few cycles of replication. This vaccine is safe, provides as much protection as the killed vaccine, and continues to be protective for at least several years. One dose of purified Vi polysaccharide vaccine has proved as effective and long-lasting as multiple doses of Ty21a and may be used in children over 2 years of age and in at-risk HIV-infected patients. New genetically engineered live typhoid vaccine strains are being developed, not only for immunization against typhoid but also for use as live vectors into which extraneous genes can be cloned for oral delivery of protective antigens from unrelated species. In addition, Vi-protein conjugates are being evaluated as immunogens suitable for infants, especially in endemic regions where infantile typhoid is prevalent and remains a dangerous disease.

Typhoid is a reportable disease in the United States. Patients should be monitored for prolonged carriage and treated if necessary. Precautions in food handling by carriers and in disposal of their stools are obviously important (see Chap. 138).

PROGNOSIS Appropriate therapy for typhoid fever, especially if patients present for medical care in the early stage of disease, is highly successful. The mortality rate should be under 1 percent, and few complications other than relapse should occur.

NONTYPHOIDAL SALMONELLOSIS

An infection caused by any *Salmonella* organism other than *S. typhi* is termed *nontyphoidal salmonellosis*. Such an infection can present as acute diarrhea, a septicemic syndrome, focal abscesses, meningitis, osteomyelitis, endocarditis, or mycotic aneurysm or can be asymptomatic.

EPIDEMIOLOGY The species *S. enterica* includes a diverse group of host-adapted and non-host-adapted serovars. Two human-adapted serovars, *S. paratyphi* A and *S. schottmuelleri* (more often called *S. paratyphi* B), mimic *S. typhi* and cause a mild form of typhoid fever. Of the more than 2300 known serovars, just 10 account for two-thirds of all human-disease isolates in the United States, and four serovars (*S. typhimurium, S. enteritidis, S. heidelberg,* and *S. newport*) cause about three-fifths of all disease cases (Table 158-3). Periodic increases in the recovery of certain serovars represent either the introduction of a new transmission source or the occurrence of a large outbreak. A fivefold increase in the recovery of *S. enteritidis* isolates between 1976 and 1986 was due to ingestion of contaminated intact grade-A eggs, primarily in the northeastern United States. The number of infections from this source continued to increase, and by 1992 *S. enteritidis* overtook *S. typhimurium* as the most frequently isolated *Salmonella* serovar in the United States and in all countries of Europe. These changes suggested a new global pandemic related primarily to infected poultry eggs.

Surveillance data in the United States indicate that not only the number but also the incidence of nontyphoidal *Salmonella* isolates is increasing (Fig. 158-1). The incidence of disease is five times higher among young children than among older subjects and increases again in adults over 70 years of age. Between 1970 and 1986, the median age of infected individuals rose from 6 years to 20 years and has since remained the same. The greatest increase has been in the 20- to 39-year-old population; this observation suggests that foods consumed by young adults are important vehicles or that persons in this age group are traveling more to endemic areas. For example, the emergence of serious systemic infections in southern California due to *S. dublin* carrying a high-virulence plasmid has been associated with the ingestion of unpasteurized dairy products or nontraditional nutritional treatments containing raw calf-liver extracts contaminated with this serotype. A reasonable estimate of the total incidence of symptomatic nontyphoidal *Salmonella* infection in the United States is around 2 million cases per year. The degree of morbidity represented by this figure implies a significant economic impact in terms of lost productivity and medical costs and, by extension, a serious and underestimated cause of mortality.

Because nontyphoidal salmonellae are so often non-host-adapted, many kinds of domestic animals can harbor the organisms and serve as a source for human infection. From 50 to 75 percent of broiler and layer chicken flocks in Canada are infected with a wide variety of *Salmonella* serovars, many of which are virulent for humans. At laying, intact eggs of naturally infected layer flocks may be positive for low numbers of organisms belonging to serovars virulent for humans; however, growth to large numbers quickly takes place if the eggs are not kept at 4°C. At such levels of contamination, viable organisms will survive cooking by any method. If an egg rests for a short time on infected hen feces or even on the dry bedding of an infected hen, *Salmonella* can penetrate the surface of the shell through microscopic pores normally present in the shell. Because the epidemic due to *S. enteritidis* is so extensive and thus so unlike salmonellosis associated with cracked eggs, and because it has involved free-range as well as commercial henhouse eggs, a transovarian route is most likely and poses a problem for infection control. The conditions in which raising, shipping, slaughtering, and marketing take place contribute to the spread of *Salmonella* in the food supply. Introduction of the organism into processed foods, including commercial milk-chocolate products, can result in widespread dissemination, and contamination of such common foods as eggs or milk leads to large-scale outbreaks, including nosocomial epidemics. Dried or frozen foods preserve viable salmonellae. For these reasons, salmonellosis is more a disease of the industrialized world than of the developing world. Additional sources of human infection are animals sold as pets, including baby chicks, ducks, and turtles, and medical products of animal origin, such as carmine dye (from insects), pancreatin, bile salts, or tissue extracts from thyroids, adrenals, stomachs, or rattlesnakes.

A potentially serious problem is the selection of antibiotic-resistant salmonellae by unregulated drug use in animal husbandry. Persistent and severe salmonellosis also has been recognized as a problem among patients with AIDS (see Chap. 308).

PATHOGENESIS As with *S. typhi*, the events following ingestion of other salmonellae are determined by environmental factors (dose), microbial factors (the ability to invade epithelial cells, to multiply within mononuclear phagocytes, and to resist intestinal peptide antibiotic defensins), and host resistance factors (the effects of gastric acid, the rapid mobilization of phagocytic cells, and the activation and expansion of clones of T cells involved in protection, such as V gamma 9–bearing γ/δ T cells). As few as 10^3 virulent organisms may cause disease, especially in persons who have achlorhydria or who have recently received antimicrobial therapy. Systemic invasion is more likely in patients with "reticuloendothelial blockade" due to hemolysis (e.g., in malaria, barto-

Table 158-3

The Ten Most Common *S. enterica* Isolates in the United States in 1994

Rank	Serovar	Serogroup	No. of Isolations	Percentage (Cumulative Percentage) of All *Salmonella* Isolations
1	enteritidis	D	10,009	26.1 (26.1)
2	typhimurium	B	8479	22.1 (48.2)
3	heidelberg	B	1855	4.8 (53.0)
4	newport	C_2	1698	4.4 (57.4)
5	hadar	C_2	1033	2.7 (60.1)
6	agona	B	766	2.0 (62.1)
7	montevideo	C_1	639	1.7 (63.8)
8	oranienburg	C_1	616	1.6 (65.4)
9	muenchen	C_2	562	1.5 (66.9)
10	thompson	C_1	560	1.5 (68.4)

SOURCE: Centers for Disease Control and Prevention, Annual Surveillance Report, 1994.

nellosis, leptospirosis, or sickle cell anemia) or intracellular infections (e.g., histoplasmosis) and may be facilitated by the expression of bacterial plasminogen receptors, the conversion of bound plasminogen to enzymatically active plasmin, and subsequent degradation of the extracellular matrix. Documented bacteremia varies in incidence from 5 to 45 percent but is assumed to occur early in the course of many, and possibly all, *Salmonella* infections. Bacteremia is quickly cleared by patients infected with most *S. enteritidis* serovars. *S. dublin*, *S. infantis*, *S. virchow*, *S. panama*, and *S. newport* may be especially invasive; virulence is associated with an 80-kb plasmid in *S. dublin*. *S. typhimurium* isolates from the bloodstream are significantly more likely to hybridize with a probe from the highly conserved *Eco*RI fragment of the *S. dublin* plasmid than are fecal isolates (rate of hybridization, 76 vs. 42 percent). Bacteremia may lead to focal tissue infections. *S. choleraesuis*, a highly invasive serotype, usually causes a septicemia syndrome and is commonly isolated from blood but not from stool. Microbial factors that determine the invasiveness of salmonellae include motility and the presence of chromosomal and plasmid genes needed for invasion and replication within mononuclear phagocytes. Many of these genes are turned on by contact of the organism with host cells and are regulated by a two-component sensing/signaling system, *Pho*P/*Pho*Q.

Invasion occurs across the small-intestinal mucosa. In *Shigella* infection, the organism multiplies within epithelial cells; in contrast, in *Salmonella* infection, epithelial cells represent a barrier to be crossed by the organism, not an ecologic niche for its survival. Invading salmonellae induce a dramatic ruffling of the plasma membrane of the mammalian cell that is regulated by *Pho*P/*Pho*Q and reflects cytoskeletal rearrangements leading to uptake of the organism within phagosome-like vesicles, its transit across the cell, and its release into the lamina propria. A multigene chromosomal locus, *inv*, encodes the invasive phenotype and shares homology with genes of other invasive bacteria. *Pho*P/*Pho*Q also regulates the resistance of salmonellae to host intestinal antibacterial defensins. Invasion activates cell signaling pathways, including mitogen-activated protein kinase; phospholipase A_2; release of arachidonic acid; production of prostaglandins and leukotrienes (especially leukotriene D_4); and a sharp increase in intracellular calcium level. Many of these changes are known to alter electrolyte transport and may cause diarrhea. Invasion and inflammation are necessary but not sufficient to cause *Salmonella* diarrhea in experimental animal models, and transepithelial signals that recruit neutrophils are also involved via induced local chemokine (IL-8) production. Some salmonellae appear to produce a molecule similar to cholera toxin that increases electrolyte and fluid secretion. However, the importance of this molecule in causing diarrhea remains uncertain.

CLINICAL MANIFESTATIONS **Gastroenteritis** The incubation period of *Salmonella* gastroenteritis is generally short (24 to 48 h). Sporadic illness is likely to go undiagnosed because specimens are not taken for culture. Large outbreaks, often considered "food poisoning" and characterized by self-limited fever and diarrhea, are more likely to be investigated and diagnosed. Diarrhea may be associated with nausea, vomiting, and abdominal cramps and occasionally is bloody or even dysenteric when the colon becomes involved. Direct microscopic examination of stool shows many leukocytes, which offer a clue to the invasive nature of the infection. The illness is generally mild and resolves without specific therapy, but it may cause severe dehydration or disseminate and lead to death in debilitated elderly patients or neonates. Blood cultures obtained initially often become positive as the patient's condition is improving. Treatment may be discontinued after identification of the organism unless there is an underlying immunosuppressive disease (e.g., sickle cell disease, AIDS, or a malignancy such as a lymphoma) or the patient is receiving glucocorticoid or immunosuppressive drug therapy. In these conditions, an appropriate antibiotic should be administered for 7 to 10 days. Carriage of salmonellae in the stool continues for several weeks after the resolution of symptomatic disease but rarely persists for longer than 2 months.

Localization of Systemic Infections Bloodborne salmonellae can invade any tissue or organ. The most common isolates are *S.* *typhimurium*, *S. enteritidis*, *S. virchow*, *S. dublin*, and *S. choleraesuis*. Localized infections usually follow intestinal infection, although there may be no prior diarrhea. Endocarditis is rare but, when it occurs, may include destructive cardiac lesions such as valve perforations or ring or septal abscesses. Therapy may require both the administration of appropriate antimicrobials and surgery (see Chap. 126).

Arterial infection generally occurs in persons with preexisting arteriosclerotic infrarenal aortic aneurysms and is especially likely in men over the age of 50 years. *S. choleraesuis* accounts for about 20 percent of arterial infections but is isolated from fewer than 1 percent of patients with *Salmonella* diarrhea; this distribution reflects the capacity of this organism to cause systemic invasive disease. *S. typhimurium* accounts for approximately 25 percent of isolates in arterial infections—a finding consistent with its high prevalence in gastrointestinal salmonellosis. In addition to treatment with antimicrobials, eradication usually requires prompt excision and drainage with bypass through uninvolved tissue. The disease should be suspected when elderly men develop prolonged fever accompanied by back, abdomen, or chest pain following gastroenteritis; when bacteremia occurs or recurs after therapy for the initial illness; or when bacteremia develops in patients with vertebral osteomyelitis or prosthetic valves.

Cholecystitis, other *hepatobiliary infection*, and *splenic abscess* are the most common intraabdominal localized infections due to *Salmonella*. In addition to *S. typhimurium* and *S. enteritidis*, *S. typhi* is an important cause.

Urinary tract infections due to *Salmonella* sometimes develop. These illnesses are especially likely in patients who have urolithiasis, structural abnormalities, or immunosuppressive diseases or who are receiving immunosuppressive therapy. *Salmonella* urinary tract infections can coexist with renal tuberculosis or with *Schistosoma haematobium* infection.

Pneumonia or *empyema* caused by *Salmonella* is rare. These conditions usually involve patients with preexisting abnormalities of the lungs or pleura or with conditions that predispose to infection, including malignancy, diabetes, glucocorticoid use, sickle cell disease, or alcohol abuse.

Meningitis caused by *Salmonella* is also rare and is most prevalent among infants and young children. Gram's stains of cerebrospinal fluid are usually positive. Mortality rates of 40 and 60 percent are reported for children and adults, respectively. In survivors, residua include seizures, hydrocephalus, subdural empyemas, and permanent disabilities such as retardation, paresis, athetosis, and visual disturbances.

Septic arthritis due to *Salmonella* is associated with positive joint-fluid cultures and should not be confused with reactive arthritis (a culture-negative inflammatory joint disease following invasive diarrheas, especially in HLA-B27–positive patients). Common underlying conditions include glucocorticoid or immunosuppressive drug therapy, sickle cell disease, prosthetic joints, or aseptic necrosis. Drainage may be needed in addition to appropriate antibiotic therapy.

Salmonella osteomyelitis is predictably associated with sickle cell disease. It generally affects the long bones and occurs primarily in young patients. Blood cultures are often positive; the most common isolate is *S. typhimurium*.

Bacteremia Sepsis, with prolonged fever and positive blood cultures but generally without prior diarrhea, occurs most commonly with *S. choleraesuis* or *S. dublin* infection. While this presentation is "typhoidal," typical manifestations of typhoid (rose spots, relative bradycardia, leukopenia) are lacking, and the illness is more acute in onset than typhoid. *S. choleraesuis* or *S. dublin* sepsis is a severe disease that is associated with high mortality.

Intermittent symptomatic *Salmonella* bacteremia is seen in patients with hepatosplenic or urinary schistosomiasis. Clinically severe *Salmonella* sepsis due to *S. typhimurium* also occurs in AIDS patients (see Chap. 308), is often recurrent, and is an AIDS-defining event. The infection may be refractory to treatment or recurrent despite appropriate therapy. The incidence of salmonellosis among AIDS patients in the United States is estimated at 46 to 384 per 100,000, which is 100- to 1000-fold greater than the incidence in the general population (0.3 per 100,000).

DIAGNOSIS Specific diagnosis depends on the isolation of salmonellae from stool, blood, or tissue fluids. All clinical laboratories should be able to make the initial isolation and identify common serovars. Uncommon serovars usually must be sent to reference laboratories for identification.

℞ TREATMENT

Choice of antibiotic is complicated by the increasing prevalence of antimicrobial resistance (including multiple-drug resistance) among nontyphoidal salmonellae as well as in *S. typhi*. The use of antibiotics in commercial animal rearing, the prevalence of *Salmonella* in the global food chain, and the growing international commerce in meat, poultry, and processed food products are contributing to the wider distribution of resistant clones.

In the face of these complications, treatment for focal systemic infections requires the selection of the most appropriate antibiotic and, at times, drainage or resection of infected tissue. Bactericidal antibiotics, administered by the parenteral route, are usually chosen. The regimen may include ampicillin (6 to 12 g/d for adults or 100 mg/kg for young children, in divided doses) or appropriate doses of third-generation cephalosporins such as ceftriaxone. Unless resistance is prevalent, chloramphenicol (2 to 4 g/d for adults or 50 mg/kg for children, in divided doses) remains a good choice in developing countries because it can be given orally and is inexpensive. The new quinolones are highly effective, in part because they act on the intracellular compartment and thus affect bacteria within host mononuclear cells; while concerns remain about their safety in infants and children, increasing evidence suggests that the risk of cartilage damage is small.

The proper treatment of *Salmonella* gastroenteritis is not clear; the traditional dogma has been that antibiotics do not shorten the illness but do increase the duration of convalescent carriage. For this reason, it has generally been recommended that antimicrobial agents not be used in this illness. Initial highly favorable results with the new quinolones are now balanced by a number of contradictory studies. The best recommendation at present is that antimicrobial therapy be reserved for patients with severe disease and for patients at high risk of invasive disease.

Positive blood cultures in the setting of otherwise uncomplicated gastroenteritis do not warrant antibiotic therapy. When an infant under 3 months of age has diarrhea and signs of systemic invasion, a workup to localize the septic process should be initiated and presumptive treatment with a third-generation cephalosporin administered until culture results are available. Fever is often absent in very young infants and is not a reliable indicator of systemic infection. Asymptomatic patients with salmonellae other than *S. typhi* in the stool should *not* receive antimicrobial treatment, since active disease may be provoked and the carriage state is generally self-limiting. A quinolone would be a good choice for the treatment of long-term carriers.

PREVENTION AND CONTROL It is not possible to eradicate nontyphoidal salmonellosis because the organisms are so widespread in nature. Reduced animal-feed use of antimicrobials employed for the treatment of human infection and improved animal-rearing and animal-marketing practices would be useful. Vigilance in food preparation and in quality testing of the known and commonly contaminated foods should help as well. It is recommended that eggs not be eaten raw or partially cooked, especially by persons at high risk of infection; however, even fully cooked eggs can harbor viable *Salmonella*. If universal body-substance precautions are not routinely utilized, hospital staff caring for patients with salmonellosis should observe "enteric precautions," wearing gowns and gloves when handling stool and urine and carefully washing their hands after patient contact (see Chap. 138).

During outbreaks, food handlers may be responsible for transmission. Much effort is given to the identification (by stool culture) of asymptomatic food handlers who are carriers during food-borne outbreaks; these individuals are usually kept away from work until they become culture-negative. (The predictive value of three consecutive stool cultures negative for *Salmonella* is 95 percent.) However, it is more important that standards are maintained to ensure the environmental and personal hygiene of food handlers and thus to prevent the problem in the first place, since carriage may be intermittent and is often not uniform within a single stool sample and since foods contaminated with the organism require improper handling to permit the growth of a sufficient inoculum to cause disease. It may be justifiable to restrict carriers from the workplace only in the course of a hospital outbreak or when workers refuse to improve their personal hygiene.

The development of effective vaccines for nontyphoidal salmonellosis may be difficult because of the great number of serovars involved in infection. Some progress has been made with galactose epimerase and aroA vaccine mutants of *S. typhimurium* for use in animals, and these vaccines may ultimately be tested in humans. It would be most useful to have vaccines for *S. choleraesuis*, *S. typhimurium*, and *S. enteritidis*. *S. dublin* and *S. virchow*, while quite virulent, are still uncommon causes of human disease.

BIBLIOGRAPHY

ACHARYA G et al: Treatment of typhoid fever: Randomized trial of a three-day course of ceftriaxone versus a fourteen-day course of chloramphenicol. Am J Trop Med Hyg 52:162, 1995

CELLIER M et al: Human natural resistance–associated macrophage protein: cDNA cloning, chromosomal mapping, genomic organization, and tissue-specific expression. J Exp Med 180:1741, 1994

DUPONT HL: Quinolones in *Salmonella typhi* infection. Drugs 45(Suppl 3):119, 1993

GLYNN JR et al: Infecting dose and severity of typhoid: Analysis of volunteer data and examination of the influence of the definition of illness used. Epidemiol Infect 115:23, 1995

GRUNEWALD R et al: Relationship between human immunodeficiency virus infection and salmonellosis in 20- to 59-year-old residents of New York City. Clin Infect Dis 18:358, 1994

GUINEY DG et al: Plasmid-mediated virulence genes in non-typhoid *Salmonella* serovars. FEMS Microbiol Lett 124:1, 1994

HENNESSY TW et al: A national outbreak of *Salmonella enteritidis* infections from ice cream. N Engl J Med 334:1281, 1996

IVANOFF B et al: Vaccination against typhoid fever: Present status. Bull World Health Organ 72:957, 1994

LAHTEENMAKI K et al: Bacterial plasminogen receptors: In vitro evidence for a role in degradation of the mammalian extracellular matrix. Infect Immun 63:3659, 1995

LEE LA et al: Increase in antimicrobial-resistant *Salmonella* infections in the United States, 1989–1990. J Infect Dis 170:128, 1994

MCCORMICK BA et al: Transepithelial signaling to neutrophils by salmonellae: A novel virulence mechanism for gastroenteritis. Infect Immun 63:2302, 1995

MILLS SD, FINLAY BB: Comparison of *Salmonella typhi* and *Salmonella typhimurium* invasion, intracellular growth and localization in cultured human epithelial cells. Microb Pathog 17:409, 1994

PAVIA AT et al: Epidemiologic evidence that prior antimicrobial exposure decreases resistance to infection by antimicrobial-sensitive *Salmonella*. J Infect Dis 161:255, 1990

PRADHAN KM et al: Safety of ciprofloxacin therapy in children: Magnetic resonance images, body fluid levels of fluoride and linear growth. Acta Paediatr 84:555, 1995

RIESENBERG-WILMES MR et al: Role of the acid tolerance response in virulence of *Salmonella typhimurium*. Infect Immun 64:1085, 1996

SCHAAD UB: Use of the quinolones in paediatrics. Drugs 45(Suppl 3):37, 1993

TRAN TH et al: Short-course ofloxacin for treatment of multidrug-resistant typhoid. Clin Infect Dis 20:917, 1995

TUMBARELLO M et al: The impact of bacteraemia on HIV infection. Nine years experience in a large Italian university hospital. J Infect 31:123, 1996

WILCOX MH, SPENCER RC: Quinolones and *Salmonella* gastroenteritis. J Antimicrob Chemother 30:221, 1992

WORKMAN MR et al: *Salmonella* bacteraemia in sickle cell disease at King's College Hospital: 1976–1991. J Hosp Infect 27:195, 1994

159 *Gerald T. Keusch*

SHIGELLOSIS

DEFINITION *Shigellosis* is an acute infectious inflammatory colitis due to one of the members of the genus *Shigella*. Although the disease is often referred to as "bacillary dysentery," many patients have only mild watery diarrhea and never develop dysenteric symptoms. Less severe illness predominates in industrialized countries such as the United States, whereas more severe, often fatal dysentery occurs in patients in developing countries.

ETIOLOGIC AGENT Shigellae are slender, gram-negative, nonmotile bacilli and are members of the family Enterobacteriaceae and the tribe Escherichieae. They are so closely related to *Escherichia coli* that the two genera cannot be distinguished by DNA hybridization methods. In fact, *Shigella* can be thought of as a differentiated pathogenic *E. coli*. The four *Shigella* species (*S. dysenteriae*, *S. flexneri*, *S. boydii*, and *S. sonnei*) are defined on the basis of surface somatic O antigens and carbohydrate fermentation patterns. Most are lactose-negative (*S. sonnei* is a late lactose fermenter) and produce acid but not gas from glucose, resulting in a typical acid butt and alkaline slant in triple sugar iron agar without H_2S production. The genus is characterized by its ability to invade intestinal epithelial cells and to cause infection and illness in humans, even when the inoculum is small (a few hundred to a few thousand organisms).

EPIDEMIOLOGY Worldwide, it is estimated that at least 140 million cases of shigellosis and almost 600,000 deaths due to shigellosis occur annually among children under the age of 5 years, primarily in developing countries. The organism is found everywhere in the world but is most common where poor environmental sanitation and crowding facilitate transmission from person to person. A major outbreak took place in the makeshift camps for refugees fleeing the Rwandan civil war in 1994, with thousands of cases and high mortality.

Data collected by the Centers for Disease Control and Prevention in the United States from 1967 through 1988 suggest an average annual incidence of 6 *Shigella* infections per 100,000 population, with periodic hyperendemic increases (primarily due to large outbreaks of *S. sonnei* infection) raising the rate to between 9 and 10 per 100,000. On the basis of these data, the annual number of episodes of shigellosis in the United States is estimated at 25,000 to 30,000. Incidence rates approximate 27 per 100,000 among children 1 to 4 years of age but are only 2.6 per 100,000 among persons 20 years of age or older. Cases are detected most commonly in counties with a relatively high proportion of low-income minority-group residents, including African Americans, Hispanics, and Native Americans; rates are especially high in poor urban communities, in day-care centers, and among retarded children in custodial care.

A comparison with rates among rural Guatemalan Indian children during the same period puts this disease burden into perspective. A prospective surveillance study among 321 such children revealed an annual incidence of nearly 10,000 per 100,000.

Since the description of the genus *Shigella*, major global shifts in the prevalence of its four species have been noted. Until World War I, *S. dysenteriae* type 1 was the predominant isolate, frequently causing devastating epidemics with high mortality until it was replaced by *S. flexneri*. Since World War II, however, *S. flexneri* has been steadily replaced by *S. sonnei* in the industrialized countries. The reasons for these shifts are not clear. *S. boydii*, the fourth species, has remained largely confined to the Indian subcontinent.

Shigella is highly host-adapted and is a natural pathogen only of humans and a few other primates. Transmission from person to person takes place by the fecal-oral route, generally via direct contact but sometimes through contaminated vectors such as food, water, flies, and fomites. The organism can even be transmitted during participation in recreational water sports in fecally contaminated pools or lakes and can spread rapidly among confined populations in close contact—for example, in day-care centers, in institutions for the mentally retarded, on cruise ships, or among military personnel. *Shigella* is one of several pathogens associated with *gay bowel syndrome*. These cases are commonly transmitted by anal-oral sexual practices and are almost always due to *S. flexneri*; homosexual young men may be a major reservoir for these organisms in the United States (see Chap. 308).

Shigellosis is associated with a high rate of secondary household transmission. As many as 40 percent of children and 20 percent of adults who are household contacts of a case (generally a preschool child) will develop *Shigella* infection; the infection is often symptomatic in children but asymptomatic in adults, who seem to have an acquired immunity. In contrast, epidemic disease affects all ages, with clusters of severe and fatal cases in the very young and the very old. Since 1969, epidemic *S. dysenteriae* type 1 has reappeared in Latin America, in the Indian subcontinent and elsewhere in Asia, and in central and southern Africa and has been associated with relatively high mortality rates due to antimicrobial resistance and inadequate diagnosis and case management. Prolonged asymptomatic carriage is uncommon; unless there is underlying malnutrition, the organisms are generally cleared in a few weeks.

PATHOGENESIS AND PATHOLOGY Shigellae are orally ingested and, because they survive low pH more easily than other enteric pathogens (a genetically regulated property), seem to have little difficulty in passing the gastric acid barrier. An essential step in pathogenesis is invasion of colonic epithelial cells and cell-to-cell spread of infection. This step involves initial attachment of the organism to colonic cells, entry by an endocytic mechanism in which organisms are initially encased in and then escape from plasma membrane–enclosed vesicles, and a jet propulsion–like movement to the epithelial cell surface that is powered by bacterium-induced actin polymerization at the trailing end of the organism. This sequence of events not only provides the organism with a means to evade host defenses but also allows its effective local spread. Although invasion is initially innocuous, subsequent intracellular multiplication causes cell damage and death, ultimately resulting in characteristic mucosal ulcerations.

These events are extremely complicated and require the functions of multiple genes and regulatory elements encoded on both the chromosome and a large 120- to 140-MDa plasmid present in all virulent shigellae as well as on enteroinvasive *E. coli* (EIEC), which cause a *Shigella*-like disease. The number of structural and regulatory genes known to be involved in pathogenesis continues to increase as the process continues to be dissected. Some of these gene products induce the phagocytosis-like uptake of the organism by causing rearrangements of the host cell's cytoskeleton. Once a single *Shigella* organism has invaded a single host cell, the entire process of bacterial escape from the phagocytic vesicle into the host cell's cytoplasm, multiplication, and cell-to-cell spread can take place without exposure of the bacterium to the extracellular milieu and to the host's defenses.

It was originally thought that shigellae invade the host across the intestinal epithelial cells; however, recent studies using cell culture or a rabbit-ileum in vivo model suggest that the initial invasion may occur via the antigen-sampling M cell. The resulting limited penetration by organisms initiates an inflammatory response and alters the functional integrity of tight junctions between epithelial cells. These changes allow more organisms to breach the mucosal barrier at intercellular junctions. Subsequent neutrophil infiltration of the lamina propria appears to be essential to the development of illness and is associated with dramatically increased invasion. If neutrophil migration is directly inhibited by the treatment of animals with antibody to CD18, the escalating invasion by microorganisms does not take place.

Escape from the phagocytic vesicle is necessary for the virulence of shigellae and permits multiplication of the organisms in the cytoplasm. The multiplying organisms spread within the cytoplasm to the plasma membrane of the host cell and then from cell to cell. This spread is achieved by the polymerization of actin at the back end of the dividing bacteria (defined relative to the subsequent direction of motion). Binding and cross-linking by the host protein plastin result in a sphincter-like contraction that provides a forward propulsive force. This so-called actin motor is energized by ATP generated by a microbial-encoded ATPase called *IcsA*, which is, at the same time, phosphorylated and regulated by cyclic nucleotide-dependent protein kinases of the host. Phosphorylation may serve as a molecular host-defense mechanism to modulate virulence, limiting microbial spread.

Another important host protein involved in pathogenesis of shigellosis is the cadherin L-CAM, which is essential in the cell-to-cell spread of infection. Mutations in L-CAM alter the long finger-like protrusions induced by shigellae when they reach the plasma membrane and impair their subsequent fusion with the plasma membrane of the adjacent cell, thus inhibiting the transfer of the bacterium from one cell to another. Ultimately, the invaded host cell dies, possibly as a result of apoptosis induced by or during the process of microbial invasion.

Another property of apparent importance in virulence for *S. dysenteriae* type 1 is the ability to produce Shiga toxin, which is encoded by the iron-regulated chromosomal gene *stx*. Shiga toxin is composed of two distinct peptide subunits, each with highly conserved active regions. The first, located on the larger A subunit, is an *N*-glycosidase that hydrolyzes adenine from specific sites of ribosomal RNA of the mammalian 60S ribosomal subunit, irreversibly inhibiting protein synthesis. The second common region is a binding site on the B subunit that recognizes glycolipids of target cell membranes that terminate in a galactose $\alpha 1 \rightarrow 4$-galactose disaccharide. The glycolipid Gb3, containing a gal-gal-glu trisaccharide, is a specific receptor present on toxin-sensitive rabbit intestinal villus cells but not crypt cells, and toxin action is specific for the former.

Wild-type toxigenic *S. dysenteriae* causes more severe illness in primates than does an isogenic toxin-negative mutant. The toxin of this organism, the prototype of a family of related toxin proteins produced by enterohemorrhagic *E. coli* (EHEC), appears to play a role in the pathogenesis of microangiopathic complications, hemolytic-uremic syndrome (HUS), and thrombotic thrombocytopenic purpura: only toxin-producing shigellae and *E. coli* are associated with these systemic illnesses. Two new *Shigella* enterotoxins, ShET-1 and -2, have been described; the former is restricted almost exclusively to *S. flexneri* 2a, whereas the latter is distributed more widely (e.g., on the physiologically similar EIEC). The two enterotoxins are encoded by chromosomal and plasmid genes, respectively. Both toxins alter electrolyte transport by segments of gut in vitro and cause net fluid secretion in vivo in ligated rabbit ileal loops. Moreover, both toxins induce antibody in infected humans. However, their role (if any) in the pathogenesis of the watery diarrhea phase of shigellosis remains uncertain.

In shigellosis, the epithelial surface of the human colon shows extensive ulcerations, with an exudate consisting of desquamated colonic cells, polymorphonuclear leukocytes, and erythrocytes; the ulcerations may resemble a pseudomembrane in severely affected areas. Marked mucus depletion and increased mitotic activity are evident in the crypt regions and presumably reflect a response to the loss of surface colonic cells. The lamina propria is edematous and hemorrhagic and is infiltrated by neutrophils and plasma cells. There is also swelling of capillary and venular endothelial cells, with margination of neutrophils. At the ultrastructural level, bacteria can be seen within vesicles as well as free in the cytoplasm. Histologic examination of colon from dysenteric humans shows an alteration of mucosal endothelial cells similar to that induced by endotoxin (lipopolysaccharide, or LPS). Shiga toxin (protein) targets endothelial cells as well, especially when toxin receptor expression is upregulated by exposure to LPS or proinflammatory cytokines. Levels of circulating LPS are high in *S. dysenteriae* type 1 infection and somewhat lower in *S. flexneri* infection, even without bacteremia. The frequency of endotoxemia in shigellosis suggests a broader role for LPS in the pathogenesis of the disease. One likely mechanism is related to the ability of LPS to induce cytokine gene transcription and the strong association of cyto-

kine secretion and inflammation. However, bacterial invasion of the mucosa itself activates the transcription factor NF-kappa B, which is involved in regulation of cytokine synthesis. Cytokine-producing cells are present in the mucosa of patients infected with *S. dysenteriae* or *S. flexneri* and in their stools as well. In fact, the number of cells producing interleukin 1, interleukin 6, interferon α, and tumor growth factor β is directly related to the severity of the inflammation. Inflammatory changes in *Shigella* infection thus appear to be components of the pathogenesis of dysentery as much as they are a consequence of the bacterial invasive process.

Epidemiologic evidence indicates that immunity develops and is serotype specific. The precise nature of this immunity is not known. Common surface outer-membrane proteins involved in invasion elicit serum antibodies; however, these are cross-reactive among *Shigella* species and serotypes and do not seem to be protective. The serotype-specific determinants are likely to be somatic antigens, as serum antibody to LPS predicts resistance to infection, and there is evidence of IgA-mediated mucosal responses to LPS during convalescence from shigellosis.

CLINICAL MANIFESTATIONS The spectrum of clinical shigellosis was shown in a study in which volunteers ingested 10,000 organisms of *S. flexneri* type 2a. While approximately one-quarter of the volunteers never became ill, over the first 24 to 48 h approximately 25 percent developed transient fever, another 25 percent had fever and self-limited watery diarrhea, and the remaining 25 percent had fever and watery diarrhea that progressed to bloody diarrhea and dysentery. In young children in particular, the temperature can rise rapidly to 40° to 41°C, and fever sometimes results in generalized seizures. These seizures rarely recur or result in serious sequelae. Dysentery is characterized by frequent passage (usually 10 to 30 times per day) of small-volume stools consisting of blood, mucus, and pus; this diarrhea is accompanied by abdominal cramps and tenesmus—the painful straining with stooling that may lead to rectal prolapse, especially in young children. Severe dysentery is most likely in infection due to *S. dysenteriae* type 1 or *S. flexneri* and least likely in *S. sonnei* infection. Patients with mild disease generally recover without specific therapy in a few days to a week. Severe shigellosis can progress to toxic dilatation and colonic perforation, which may be fatal.

Endoscopy shows the mucosa to be hemorrhagic, with mucous discharge and focal ulcerations and sometimes with overlying exudate. The majority of lesions are in the distal colon and progressively diminish in the more proximal segments of large bowel. Mild dehydration is common among patients with watery diarrhea; severe dehydration is very rare. With extensive colonic involvement, protein-losing enteropathy can occur and can have important adverse nutritional consequences, especially for already poorly nourished children.

A variety of *extraintestinal complications* of shigellosis have been described. The majority arise in patients in developing countries and are related both to the prevalence of infections due to *S. dysenteriae* type 1 and *S. flexneri* and to the poor nutritional state of the host. For example, bacteremia, thought to be relatively infrequent in the United States, develops in up to 8 percent of patients hospitalized for shigellosis in Dacca, Bangladesh. The causative *Shigella* species is isolated from half the patients; other Enterobacteriaceae are found in the remainder. Bacteremia is associated with higher-than-usual mortality and is more common among infants under 1 year of age and among persons with protein-energy malnutrition. Persistent and clinically severe *Shigella* bacteremia has been encountered in the United States in patients with AIDS (see Chap. 308).

HUS may occur with *S. dysenteriae* type 1 infection. In the United States, the more likely cause of HUS is one of the hemorrhagic colitis-causing strains of *E. coli* (such as *E. coli* O157:H7) that produce high levels of Shiga-family toxins. HUS usually develops toward the end of the first week of shigellosis, when dysentery is already resolving. Oliguria and a marked drop in hematocrit (by as much as 10 percent within 24 h) are the first signs and may progress to anuria with renal failure and to severe anemia with congestive heart failure, respectively. Even with advanced therapy, 5 to 10 percent of patients with HUS die of the acute illness. In addition, renal damage progresses slowly over several decades in survivors, an estimated 50 percent of whom develop significant renal failure and most of whom require long-term dialysis or renal transplantation. Leukemoid reactions, with leukocyte counts of more than 50,000/μL, may occur along with HUS; thrombocytopenia (with 30,000 to 100,000 platelets/μL) is common. Profound hyponatremia and severe hypoglycemia may be documented. Central nervous system abnormalities include encephalopathic symptoms, seizures, altered consciousness, and bizarre posturing.

Less common extraintestinal manifestations include seizures in some patients and reactive arthritis in others; both of these manifestations are usually due to infection with *S. flexneri* strains. In patients expressing histocompatibility antigen HLA-B27, the full triad of Reiter's syndrome sometimes develops (see Chap. 317). Pneumonia, meningitis, vaginitis (in prepubertal girls), keratoconjunctivitis, and "rose spot" rashes are rare events.

DIAGNOSIS AND LABORATORY FINDINGS Shigellosis is the principal bacterial cause of dysentery and should be considered whenever a patient presents with bloody diarrhea. However, in the United States, because *S. sonnei* is the most common species, most patients present with fever and nonbloody watery diarrhea indistinguishable from signs caused by other bacterial or viral agents of mild to moderate diarrhea, while many patients with bloody diarrhea have EHEC as the cause. The specific diagnosis is based on culture of *Shigella* from the stool; however, diagnosis by the polymerase chain reaction is possible, and a commercial enzyme immunoassay to detect Shiga-family toxins in stool can identify most patients infected with *S. dysenteriae* type 1 or EHEC within 3 h. The yield of *Shigella* is increased if the organism is sought by stool culture when the patient has fecal leukocytes or bloody diarrhea. The organism is very labile and must be transferred quickly to plates or holding media (such as buffered glycerol saline) if it is to survive. Stool samples are preferable to swabs; when the latter are used, a rectal sample should be obtained. More than one selective medium should be used for culture—i.e., MacConkey and one other, such as Hektoen enteric or xylose-lysine-deoxycholate.

Serologic tests can be performed, since antibodies to somatic antigens develop early in the acute phase of disease. However, the resources for such tests are not generally available, and serologic assessments usually are used only for epidemiologic studies.

The differential diagnosis includes inflammatory colitis due to other microbial agents: EHEC, EIEC, *Campylobacter jejuni*, *Salmonella enteritidis*, *Yersinia enterocolitica*, *Clostridium difficile*, and the protozoan *Entamoeba histolytica*. Ulcerative colitis and Crohn's colitis are among the conditions with "noninfectious" causes that should be considered (see Chap. 286). All these infections except that due to *E. histolytica* are associated with the presence of large numbers of fecal leukocytes. Amebiasis can be diagnosed by the detection of erythrophagocytic trophozoites in the stool (see Chap. 215).

Other laboratory studies are nonspecific and may disclose neutrophilic leukocytosis, anemia due to blood loss with hemorrhagic diarrhea, prerenal azotemia, or (if watery diarrhea has been pronounced) hyperchloremic acidosis. Laboratory findings in shigellosis complicated by HUS are discussed above.

℞ TREATMENT
The mild to moderate dehydration in shigellosis is readily corrected with oral rehydration solutions (see Chap. 161). The role of antibiotic therapy is variable and depends on the organism and the severity of disease. Since *S. sonnei* infection is usually self-limited, culture results generally do not become available until the patient is better and there is little clinical need for further therapy. The use of antibiotics in severe cases with bloody diarrhea or dysentery reduces the duration of illness and can shorten the carriage state. Resistance to sulfonamides, streptomycin, chloramphenicol, and tetracyclines is almost universal, and many shigellae are now resistant to ampicillin and trimethoprim-sulfamethoxazole as well. Knowledge of the pattern of resistance in a given population, which can change with time, is useful. In the United States, multiresistant strains are most likely to be acquired during travel abroad, and either ampicillin (50 to 100 mg/kg per day in children or 2 g/d in adults, in divided doses) or trimethoprim-sulfamethoxazole (8/40 mg/kg per day in children or 2 regular-strength tablets twice a day in adults, given for 5 days) is generally recommended. Short courses of treatment (1 or 3 days) or even single doses of drugs like tetracycline and ciprofloxacin have been employed with success and may soon become the standard. Amoxicillin should *not* be substituted for ampicillin because it is not effective against shigellosis. In developing countries, where resistance to both of these drugs is commonplace, the drug of choice for the treatment of multiresistant *S. dysenteriae* type 1 infections has been nalidixic acid (55 mg/kg per day for 5 days); however, resistance to the latter agent is increasing in prevalence. The 4-fluoroquinolones (e.g., ciprofloxacin) are highly effective against all strains (see Chap. 140) but are currently too costly in the Third World and are not yet approved for use in children under 17 in the United States; these drugs have caused cartilage damage in young rodents during toxicity tests, although there is no evidence for a similar effect of therapeutic doses in humans. Alternative drugs shown to be effective include oral pivamdinocillin (amdinocillin, pivoxil, pivmecillinam; still not available in the United States) and intravenous ceftriaxone (50 mg/kg per day for 5 days). In small-scale clinical trials, cephalexin has had no effect in limiting symptoms; single doses of ceftriaxone may be effective, but more information is needed. No antibiotic treatment is recommended for the convalescent carrier state, which usually lasts no more than several weeks. Patients with AIDS may develop chronic carriage of *Shigella* and may be subject to relapsing infection with bacteremia (see Chap. 308). This cycle may be interrupted by prolonged (several weeks') treatment with a quinolone.

The role of antimotility agents such as atropine sulfate and diphenoxylate (Lomotil) and loperamide (Imodium) in the early phases of shigellosis is controversial. Loperamide, in particular, may reduce diarrhea and in one study was highly effective in combination with antimicrobials. However, these antimotility drugs are suspected of enhancing the severity of disease by delaying excretion of organisms and thus facilitating further invasion of the mucosa. Therefore, they are contraindicated for the treatment of infants and young children. In adults, these agents are contraindicated for use in the dysenteric phase of disease.

Treatment of complications of shigellosis often differs in developed and developing countries. For example, antibiotic-unresponsive toxic megacolon, with or without perforation, is often managed by colectomy in the United States. Surgery is less often employed in developing countries because of a lack of availability or difficulties in ileostomy management. HUS often requires dialysis. In developing countries, dialysis may be needed relatively infrequently because azotemia is slow to develop and the risk of significant hyperkalemia is often diminished by a preexisting deficiency in total-body potassium, with malnutrition and wasting of lean body mass. The management of hyponatremia, usually caused by inappropriate secretion of antidiuretic hormone (vasopressin), is governed by the severity of the condition and the symptomatic state of the patient, as outlined in Chap. 49. Infusion of glucose can reverse clinical manifestations caused by hypoglycemia, and responses can be monitored by fingerstick blood glucose tests if no biochemistry laboratory is available. Optimal nutritional management is needed to correct deficiencies due to underlying malnutrition as well as the superimposed catabolic stress and protein-losing enteropathy of shigellosis. Nutritional support should begin during the acute illness and may be required for months thereafter (see Chap. 78).

PREVENTION Direct-contact transmission of shigellosis can be prevented by appropriate environmental and personal hygiene. Hand washing with soap and water, decontamination of water supplies, use of sanitary latrines or toilets, and precautions in the preparation and storage of food can all reduce the primary and secondary transmission of *Shigella* infection. In highly endemic developing countries, infants are protected during the period of exclusive breast feeding, which should be encouraged. Any measures that reduce the burden of malnutrition will also reduce the burden of shigellosis in the population. Stool precautions should be instituted for hospitalized infected patients to ensure safe disposal of infected excreta and linens, and hospital personnel must wash their hands and medical instruments (such as stethoscopes) after each contact with an infected patient. Cohorting of asymptomatic infected children, use of antibiotics to reduce infectiousness, and scrupulous attention to hygiene are usually successful in nosocomial outbreaks. Children in day care must be kept at home while clinically ill and ideally should have a negative stool culture before returning to the day-care facility. Likewise, food handlers who develop shigellosis should be culture-negative before returning to work. Antibiotic treatment is not indicated for the asymptomatic carrier state. No effective vaccine is available.

BIBLIOGRAPHY

ACHESON DWK et al: The family of Shiga and Shiga-like toxins, in *Sourcebook of Bacterial Protein Toxins*, JE Alouf, JH Freer (eds). London, Academic Press, 1991, pp 415–433

BENNISH ML, SALAM MA: Rethinking options for the treatment of shigellosis. J Antimicrob Chemother 30:243, 1992

BRIAN MJ et al: Evaluation of the molecular epidemiology of an outbreak of multiply resistant *Shigella sonnei* in a day-care center by using pulsed-field gel electrophoresis and plasmid DNA analysis. J Clin Microbiol 31:2152, 1993

COLES FB et al: Shigellosis outbreaks at summer camps for the mentally retarded in New York State. Am J Epidemiol 130:966, 1989

CRUZ JR et al: Infection, diarrhea and dysentery caused by *Shigella* species and *Campylobacter jejuni* among Guatemalan rural children. Pediatr Infect Dis J 13:216, 1994

FASANO A et al: Shigella enterotoxin 1: An enterotoxin of *Shigella flexneri* 2a active in rabbit small intestine in vivo and in vitro. J Clin Invest 95:2853, 1995

GOLDBERG MB, SANSONETTI PJ: *Shigella* subversion of the cellular cytoskeleton: A strategy for epithelial colonization. Infect Immun 61:4941, 1993

GOMA EPIDEMIOLOGY GROUP: Public health impact of Rwandan refugee crisis: What happened in Goma, Zaire, in July 1994? Lancet 345:339, 1995

HOFFMAN RE, SHILLAM PJ: The use of hygiene, cohorting, and antimicrobial therapy to control an outbreak of shigellosis. Am J Dis Child 144:219, 1990

KRISTJANSSON M et al: Polymicrobial and recurrent bacteremia with *Shigella* in a patient with AIDS. Scand J Infect Dis 26:411, 1994

LEE LA et al: Hyperendemic shigellosis in the United States: A review of surveillance data for 1967–1988. J Infect Dis 164:894, 1991

LEVINE OS, LEVINE MM: Houseflies (*Musca domestica*) as mechanical vectors of shigellosis. Rev Infect Dis 13:688, 1991

LINDBERG AA, PAL T: Strategies for development of potential candidate *Shigella* vaccines. Vaccine 11:168, 1993

MATHAN MM, MATHAN VI: Morphology of rectal mucosa of patients with shigellosis. Rev Infect Dis 13(Suppl 4):S314, 1991

PERDOMO OJ et al: Acute inflammation causes epithelial invasion and mucosal destruction in experimental shigellosis. J Exp Med 180:1307, 1994

RAQUIB R et al: Persistence of local cytokine production in shigellosis in acute and convalescent stages. Infect Immun 63:289, 1995

SANSONETTI PJ et al: Role of interleukin-1 in the pathogenesis of experimental shigellosis. J Clin Invest 96:884, 1995

SCHAAD UB et al: Use of fluoroquinolones in pediatrics: Consensus report of an International Society of Chemotherapy commission. Pediatr Infect Dis J 14:1, 1995

TAUXE RV et al: The persistence of *Shigella flexneri* in the United States: The increased role of the adult male. Am J Public Health 78:1432, 1988

ZYCHLINSKY A et al: Molecular and cellular mechanisms of tissue invasion by *Shigella flexneri*. Ann NY Acad Sci 730:197, 1994

160 *Martin J. Blaser*

INFECTIONS DUE TO *CAMPYLOBACTER* AND RELATED SPECIES

DEFINITION Bacteria of the genus *Campylobacter* and of the related genera *Arcobacter* and *Helicobacter* cause a variety of pyogenic infections. Although acute diarrheal illnesses are most common, these organisms may cause infections in virtually all parts of the body, especially in compromised hosts, and these infections may have late nonsuppurative sequelae. The designation *Campylobacter* comes from the Greek for "curved rod" and refers to the organism's vibrio-like morphology.

ETIOLOGY Campylobacters are motile, non-spore-forming, curved gram-negative rods. Originally known as *Vibrio fetus*, these bacilli were reclassified as a new genus in 1973 after it was recognized that they were quite dissimilar from other vibrios. Since then, more than 15 species have been identified. These species are currently divided into three genera: *Campylobacter*, *Arcobacter*, and *Helicobacter*. Not all of the species are pathogens of humans. The human pathogens can be divided into two major groups: those that primarily cause diarrheal disease and those that cause extraintestinal infection. The principal diarrheal pathogen is *Campylobacter jejuni*, which accounts for 80 to 90 percent of all cases of recognized illness due to campylobacters. Other organisms that cause diarrheal disease include *Campylobacter coli*, *Campylobacter upsaliensis*, *Campylobacter lari*, and *Campylobacter fetus*. The major species causing extraintestinal illnesses is *C. fetus*; however, any of the diarrheal agents may cause systemic or localized infection as well. Neither aerobes nor strict anaerobes, these microaerophilic organisms are adapted for survival in the gastrointestinal mucous layer. This chapter will focus on *C. jejuni* and *C. fetus* as the major pathogens and prototypes for their groups; the key features of infection are listed by species (excluding *C. jejuni*, described in detail in the text below) in Table 160-1.

EPIDEMIOLOGY Campylobacters are found in the gastrointestinal tract of many animals used for food (including poultry, cattle, sheep, and swine) and of many household pets (including birds, dogs, and cats). These microorganisms usually do not cause illness in their animal hosts. In most cases, campylobacters are transmitted to humans in raw or undercooked food products or through direct contact with infected animals. In the United States and other developed countries, ingestion of contaminated poultry that has not been sufficiently cooked is the most common means of acquiring infection (50 to 70 percent of cases). Other modes of transmission include ingestion of raw (unpasteurized) milk or untreated water, contact with infected household pets, travel to developing countries (campylobacters being among the causes of traveler's diarrhea), and (occasionally) contact with an index case who is incontinent of stool.

Campylobacter infections are not rare. Several studies indicate that, in the United States, diarrheal disease due to campylobacters is more common than that due to *Salmonella* and *Shigella* combined. Infections occur throughout the year, but their incidence peaks during summer and early autumn. Persons of all ages are affected; however, attack rates for *C. jejuni* are highest among young children and young adults, while those for *C. fetus* are highest at the extremes of age. Systemic infections due to *C. fetus* (and to other *Campylobacter* and related species) are most common in compromised hosts. Persons at increased risk include those with AIDS, hypogammaglobulinemia, neoplasia, liver disease, diabetes mellitus, and generalized atherosclerosis as well as pregnant women. However, apparently healthy nonpregnant persons occasionally develop transient *Campylobacter* bacteremia.

In developing countries, *C. jejuni* infections are hyperendemic, with the highest rates among children <2 years old. Infection rates fall with age, as does the illness-to-infection ratio; these observations suggest that frequent exposure to *C. jejuni* leads to the acquisition of immunity.

Many *C. jejuni* infections are subclinical, especially in partially immune hosts. Most illnesses occur within 2 to 4 days (range, 1 to 7 days) of exposure to the organism in food or water. The sites of tissue injury include the jejunum, ileum, and colon. Biopsies show an acute nonspecific inflammatory reaction, with neutrophils, monocytes, and eosinophils in the lamina propria, as well as damage to the epithelium, including loss of mucus, glandular degeneration, and crypt abscesses. Biopsy findings may be consistent with Crohn's disease or ulcerative colitis, but these "idiopathic" chronic inflammatory diseases should not be diagnosed unless infectious colitis, *specifically including* that due to infection with *Campylobacter*, has been ruled out.

The high frequency of *C. jejuni* infections and their severity and recurrence among hypogammaglobulinemic patients suggest that antibodies are important in protective immunity. The pathogenesis of infection is uncertain. Both the motility of the strain and its capacity to adhere to host tissues appear to favor disease, but classic enterotoxins and cytotoxins (although described) do not appear to play any substantial role in tissue injury or disease production. In contrast, the organisms have been visualized in the epithelium, albeit in low numbers. The documentation of a significant tissue response and occasionally of *C. jejuni* bacteremia further suggests that tissue invasion is clinically significant.

The pathogenesis of *C. fetus* infections is better defined. Virtually all clinical isolates of *C. fetus* possess a proteinaceous capsule-like structure (an S layer) that renders the organism resistant to complement-mediated killing and opsonization. As a result, *C. fetus* can cause bacteremia and can seed sites beyond the intestinal tract. The ability of the organism to switch the S-layer proteins expressed, a phenomenon that results in antigenic variability, may contribute to the chronicity and high rate of recurrence of these infections in compromised hosts.

CLINICAL MANIFESTATIONS OF *C. JEJUNI* AND *C. FETUS* INFECTIONS The clinical features of infections due to all of the *Campylobacter* and related species causing enteric disease appear to be highly similar. There is often a prodrome, with fever, headache, myalgia, and/or malaise, 12 to 48 h before the onset of diarrheal symptoms. The most common symptoms of the intestinal phase are diarrhea, abdominal pain, and fever. The degree of diarrhea varies from several loose stools to grossly bloody stools; most patients presenting for medical attention have 10 or more bowel movements

on the worst day of illness. Abdominal pain usually consists of cramping and may be the most prominent symptom. Pain usually is generalized but may become localized; *C. jejuni* infection may cause pseudo-appendicitis. Fever may be the only initial manifestation of *C. jejuni* infection, a situation mimicking the early stages of typhoid fever. Febrile young children may develop convulsions. *Campylobacter* enteritis generally is self-limited; however, symptoms persist for longer than 1 week in 10 to 20 percent of patients seeking medical attention, and relapses occur in 5 to 10 percent of untreated patients.

C. fetus may cause a diarrheal illness similar to that due to *C. jejuni*, especially in normal hosts, or may cause either intermittent diarrhea or nonspecific abdominal pain without localizing signs. Sequelae are uncommon, and outcome is benign. *C. fetus* also may cause a prolonged relapsing systemic illness (with fever, chills, and myalgias) that has no obvious primary source; this manifestation is especially common in compromised hosts. Secondary seeding of an organ (e.g., meninges, brain, bone, urinary tract, or soft tissue) complicates the course, which may be fulminant. *C. fetus* infections have a tropism for vascular sites: endocarditis, mycotic aneurysm, and septic thrombophlebitis all may occur. Infection during pregnancy often leads to fetal death. *Helicobacter cinaedi* causes recurrent cellulitis with fever and bacteremia in immunocompromised hosts.

COMPLICATIONS Except in the case of infection with *C. fetus* or *H. cinaedi*, bacteremia is uncommon, developing most often in immunocompromised hosts and at the extremes of age. Three patterns of extraintestinal infection have been noted: (1) transient bacteremia in a normal host with enteritis (benign course, no specific treatment needed); (2) sustained bacteremia or focal infection in a normal host (bacteremia originating from enteritis, with patients responding well to antimicrobial therapy); and (3) sustained bacteremia or focal infection in a compromised host. Enteritis may not be demonstrated. Antimicrobial therapy, possibly prolonged, is necessary for suppression or cure of the infection.

Campylobacter infections in patients with AIDS or hypogammaglobulinemia may be severe, persistent, and extraintestinal; relapse after cessation of therapy is common. Hypogammaglobulinemic patients also may develop osteomyelitis and an erysipelas-like rash.

Table 160-1

Clinical Features Associated with Infection due to "Atypical" *Campylobacter* and Related Species Implicated as Causes of Human Illness

Species	Common Clinical Features	Less Common Clinical Features	Additional Information
Campylobacter coli	Fever, diarrhea, abdominal pain	Bacteremia	Clinically indistinguishable from *C. jejuni*
Campylobacter fetus	Bacteremia, sepsis, meningitis, vascular infections	Diarrhea, relapsing fevers	Not usually isolated from media containing cephalothin
Campylobacter upsaliensis	Watery diarrhea, low-grade fever, abdominal pain	Bacteremia, abscesses	Difficult to isolate because of cephalothin susceptibility
Campylobacter lari	Abdominal pain, diarrhea	Colitis, appendicitis	Seagulls frequently colonized; organism often transmitted to humans via contaminated water
Campylobacter hyointestinalis	Watery or bloody diarrhea, vomiting, abdominal pain	Bacteremia	Causes proliferative enteritis in swine
Helicobacter fennelliae	Chronic mild diarrhea, abdominal cramps, proctitis	Bacteremia*	Best treated with fluoroquinolones
Helicobacter cinaedi	Chronic mild diarrhea, abdominal cramps, proctitis	Bacteremia*	Best treated with fluoroquinolones; identified in healthy hamsters
Campylobacter jejuni subspecies *doylei*	Diarrhea	Chronic gastritis, bacteremia†	Uncertain role as human pathogen
Arcobacter cryaerophila	Diarrhea	Bacteremia	Cultured under aerobic conditions
Arcobacter butzleri	Fever, diarrhea, abdominal pain, nausea	Bacteremia, appendicitis	Cultured under aerobic conditions; enzootic in nonhuman primates
Campylobacter sputorum	Pulmonary, perianal, groin, and axillary abscesses	None described	Three clinically relevant biovars: *C. sputorum* subspecies *sputorum*, *C. sputorum* subspecies *bubulus*, and *Campylobacter mucosalis*

* In children and HIV-infected persons.
† In children.

SOURCE: Allos and Blaser.

Local suppurative complications of infection include cholecystitis, pancreatitis, and cystitis; distant complications include meningitis, endocarditis, arthritis, peritonitis, cellulitis, and septic abortion. All are rare. Hepatitis, interstitial nephritis, and the hemolytic-uremic syndrome occasionally complicate acute infection. Reactive arthritis and other rheumatologic complaints may develop several weeks after infection, especially in persons with the HLA-B27 phenotype. Guillain-Barré syndrome follows *Campylobacter* infections uncommonly (i.e., in 1 of every 1000 to 2000 cases). However, because of their high incidence, it is now estimated that *Campylobacter* infections may trigger 20 to 40 percent of all cases of Guillain-Barré syndrome.

LABORATORY FINDINGS In patients with *Campylobacter* enteritis, peripheral leukocyte counts reflect the severity of the inflammatory process. However, stools from nearly all patients presenting for medical attention in the United States contain leukocytes or erythrocytes. Fecal smears should be treated with Gram's or Wright's stain and examined in all suspected cases. When the diagnosis of *Campylobacter* enteritis is suspected on the basis of findings of inflammatory diarrhea (fever, fecal leukocytes), clinicians can ask the laboratory to attempt the visualization of organisms with characteristic vibrioid morphology by direct microscopic examination of stools with Gram's staining or to use phase-contrast or dark-field microscopy to identify the organisms' characteristic "darting" motility. Confirmation of the diagnosis of *Campylobacter* infection is based on identification of an isolate from cultures of stool, blood, or another site. *Campylobacter*-specific media should be used to culture stools from all patients with inflammatory or bloody diarrhea. Since all *Campylobacter* species are fastidious, they will not be isolated unless selective media or other selective techniques are used. Not all media are equally useful for isolation of the broad array of campylobacters; therefore, failure to isolate campylobacters from stool does not entirely rule out their presence. The detection of the organisms in stool almost always implies infection; there is a brief period of postconvalescent fecal carriage and no commensalism. In contrast, *Campylobacter sputorum* and related organisms found in the oral cavity are commensals without known pathogenic significance.

DIFFERENTIAL DIAGNOSIS The symptoms of *Campylobacter* enteritis are not sufficiently unusual to distinguish this illness from that due to *Salmonella*, *Shigella*, or *Yersinia*, among other pathogens. The combination of fever and fecal leukocytes or erythrocytes is indicative of inflammatory diarrhea, and definitive diagnosis is based on culture. Similarly, extraintestinal *Campylobacter* illness is diagnosed by culture. Infection due to *Campylobacter* should be suspected in the setting of septic abortion and that due to *C. fetus* specifically in the setting of septic thrombophlebitis. It is important to reiterate that the presentation of *Campylobacter* enteritis may mimic that of ulcerative colitis or Crohn's disease, that *Campylobacter* enteritis is much more common than either of the latter (especially among young adults), and that biopsy may not distinguish among these entities. Thus a diagnosis of inflammatory bowel disease should not be made until *Campylobacter* infection has been ruled out, especially in persons with a history of foreign travel, significant animal contact, immunodeficiency, or practices incurring a high risk of transmission.

℞ TREATMENT

Fluid and electrolyte replacement is central to the treatment of diarrheal illnesses (see Chap. 128). Even among patients presenting for medical attention with *Campylobacter* enteritis, fewer than half will clearly benefit from specific antimicrobial therapy. Indications for such therapy include high fever, bloody diarrhea, severe diarrhea, persistence for more than 1 week, and worsening of symptoms. A 5- to 7-day course of erythromycin (250 mg orally four times daily or—for children—30 to 50 mg/kg per day, in divided doses) is the regimen of choice. Although no relevant clinical trials have been conducted, the in vitro susceptibility of *Campylobacter* species to macrolides such as clarithromycin and azithromycin suggests that

these organisms also would be useful therapeutic agents. An alternative regimen for adults is ciprofloxacin (500 mg orally twice daily) for 5 to 7 days, but resistance to this agent is increasing. Other alternatives include tetracycline, norfloxacin, and furazolidone. Use of antimotility agents, which may prolong the duration of symptoms and has been associated with deaths, is not recommended.

For systemic infections, treatment with gentamicin, imipenem, or chloramphenicol should be started empirically, but susceptibility testing should then be performed. Ciprofloxacin and amoxicillin/clavulanate are alternative agents. For immunocompromised patients with systemic infections due to *C. fetus*, prolonged therapy is usually necessary.

PROGNOSIS Nearly all patients recover fully from *Campylobacter* enteritis, either spontaneously or after antimicrobial therapy. Volume depletion likely contributes to the few deaths that are reported. As stated above, occasional patients develop reactive arthritis or Guillain-Barré syndrome. Systemic infection with *C. fetus* is much more often fatal than that due to related species; this higher mortality reflects in part the population affected. Prognosis is dependent on the rapidity with which appropriate therapy is begun. Otherwise healthy hosts usually survive *C. fetus* infections without sequelae. Compromised hosts often have recurrent infections.

BIBLIOGRAPHY

ALLOS BM, BLASER MJ: *Campylobacter jejuni* and the expanding spectrum of related infections. Clin Infect Dis 20:1092, 1995

BLASER MJ et al: *Campylobacter* enteritis in the United States: A multicenter study. Ann Intern Med 98:360, 1983

NACHAMKIN I et al (eds): *Campylobacter jejuni: Current Strategy and Future Trends.* Washington, American Society for Microbiology, 1992, pp 1–300

<table>
<tr><td>161</td></tr>
</table>

Gerald T. Keusch, Robert L. Deresiewicz

CHOLERA AND OTHER VIBRIOSES

Members of the genus *Vibrio* cause a number of important infectious syndromes. Classic among them is cholera, a devastating diarrheal disease caused by *Vibrio cholerae* group O1 that has been responsible for seven global pandemics and much suffering over the past two centuries. Epidemic cholera remains a major public health concern and is dealt with at length in this chapter. Recently, other vibrioses have been described, including syndromes of diarrhea, soft tissue infection, or primary sepsis caused by additional named species in the genus *Vibrio*. These, too, are considered below.

All members of the genus are actively motile, facultatively anaerobic, curved gram-negative rods with one or more polar flagella. Except for *V. cholerae* and *Vibrio mimicus*, all require salt for growth ("halophilic vibrios"). In nature, vibrios most commonly reside in tidal rivers and bays under conditions of moderate salinity. They proliferate in the summer months when water temperatures exceed about 20°C. As might be expected, the illnesses they cause also increase in frequency during the warm months.

CHOLERA

DEFINITION Cholera is an acute diarrheal disease that can, in a matter of hours, result in profound, rapidly progressive dehydration and death. Accordingly, cholera gravis (the severe form of cholera) is a much-feared disease, particularly in its epidemic presentation. Fortunately, prompt, aggressive fluid repletion and supportive care can obviate the high mortality that it has historically wrought. While the term *cholera* occasionally has been applied to any severely dehydrating secretory diarrheal illness, whether infectious in etiology or not, it generally refers to disease caused by *V. cholerae* serogroup O1. Epidemic and endemic O1 cholera has raged in Africa since the early 1970s and appeared in Latin America for the first time in this century in 1991. In 1992, a new epidemic serotype emerged on the Indian subcontinent and has since killed thousands of people.

ETIOLOGY AND EPIDEMIOLOGY The species *V. cholerae* comprises a host of organisms classified on the basis of the carbohydrate determinants of their somatic O antigens. Some 140 serogroups have been recognized. They are divided into those that agglutinate in antisera to the O1 group antigen (*V. cholerae* O1) and those that do not (non-O1 *V. cholerae*). Although some strains of non-O1 *V. cholerae* occasionally cause sporadic outbreaks of diarrhea, serogroup O1 was, until recently, the exclusive cause of epidemic cholera. That paradigm changed in late 1992 with the identification of serogroup O139 Bengal as the cause of a large epidemic of cholera in southern India and Bangladesh along the Bay of Bengal. *V. cholerae* O139 Bengal is discussed in greater detail below.

V. cholerae O1 exists in two biotypes, *classic* and *El Tor*, that are distinguished on the basis of a number of characteristics, including phage susceptibility and hemolysin production. Each biotype is further subdivided into two serotypes, termed *Inaba* and *Ogawa*. Serotyping is a useful tool in field epidemiologic studies. Newer molecular epidemiologic techniques, such as ribotyping and other gene-based methods, now make it possible to trace the source and origin of cholera strains from around the world.

The natural habitat of *V. cholerae* is coastal salt water and brackish estuaries, where the organism lives in close relation to plankton and where it may survive in a viable but noncultivable form. Humans become infected incidentally but, once infected, can act as vehicles for spread. Ingestion of water contaminated by human feces is the most common means of acquisition of *V. cholerae*. Consumption of contaminated food in the home, in restaurants, or from street vendors can also contribute to spread. There is no known animal reservoir. While the infectious dose is relatively high, it is markedly reduced in hypochlorhydric persons, in those using antacids, and when gastric acidity is buffered by a meal. Cholera is predominantly a pediatric disease in endemic areas, but it affects adults and children equally when newly introduced into a population. In endemic areas, the disease is more common in the summer and fall months. While this seasonality has not been explained fully, it may be due to environmental conditions that affect the multiplication of vibrios or to seasonal alterations in human behavior that affect contact with water. Asymptomatic infections are frequent and more common with the El Tor than the classic biotype. In endemic areas, children under 2 years of age are less likely to develop severe cholera than are older children, perhaps because of passive immunity acquired from breast milk. For unexplained reasons, susceptibility to cholera is significantly influenced by ABO blood group status; those with type O blood are at greatest risk, while those with type AB are at least risk.

Cholera is native to the Ganges delta in the Indian subcontinent. Since 1817, seven global pandemics have occurred. The current (seventh) pandemic, the first due to the El Tor biotype, began in Indonesia in 1961 and spread throughout Asia, with *V. cholerae* El Tor displacing the endemic classic strain in many areas. It briefly invaded Europe, but effective public health measures and the high level of sanitation combined to limit its impact. In the early 1970s, El Tor cholera struck in Africa, causing major epidemics before becoming a persistent endemic problem. Its recent history in Africa has been punctuated by severe outbreaks, often fed by the chaos of war and genocide. Such was the case in the camps for Rwandan refugees set up in 1994 around Goma, Zaire. Tens of thousands of cases occurred and mortality was high. In 1995, the occurrence of hundreds of cases in Romania and the Black Sea states of the former Soviet Union demonstrated the epidemic potential of this organism whenever public health measures break down.

Since 1973, sporadic endemic infections due to vibrios related to the seventh-pandemic strain have been recognized along the U.S. Gulf Coast of Louisiana and Texas. These infections are typically associated with the consumption of contaminated, locally harvested shellfish. Occasionally, cases in U.S. locations remote from the Gulf Coast have been linked to shipped-in Gulf Coast seafood.

Although the event was long expected, it was not until 1991 that the current cholera pandemic reached Latin America. Beginning along the Peruvian coast in January 1991, the disease was carried by fishermen to Ecuador and Colombia. It then spread in an explosive epidemic to virtually all of South and Central America and to Mexico (Fig. 161-1). About 400,000 cases were reported in the first year of the outbreak, and more than 1 million had been reported by the end of 1994. While the cumulative mortality rate has been under 1 percent, the mortality rate approached 30 percent in the communities first affected, where a lack of familiarity with the disease led initially to the deployment of wholly ineffective treatment. Intensive education of health care providers and of the community at large has enhanced awareness of the disease and its appropriate management and has greatly diminished mortality. As it did in Africa two decades earlier, the epidemic El Tor strain proved capable of establishing itself in inland waters rather than in its classic niche of coastal salt waters; the organism has already become endemic in many of the Latin American countries into which it was recently introduced.

Cases linked to the Latin American epidemic have occurred in the United States. For example, 11 people in New York and New Jersey were infected in two separate outbreaks in 1991 after eating boiled crabmeat illegally transported by travelers from Ecuador. Although secondary spread of this strain has not taken place in the United States, these events underscore the need for vigilance among health care professionals, even in locations remote from an epidemic.

In October 1992, a large-scale outbreak of clinical cholera occurred in the port city of Madras and surrounding towns in southern India. The etiologic agent proved to be a novel strain of *V. cholerae* belonging neither to the O1 serogroup that typically causes epidemic cholera nor to any of the 137 other serogroups known at the time. This strain spread rapidly up and down the coast of the Bay of Bengal, reaching Bangladesh in December 1992. There alone, it caused more than 100,000 cases of cholera in the first 3 months of 1993. It subsequently

FIGURE 161-1 Spread of *Vibrio cholerae* O1 in the Americas, 1991–1994. (Courtesy of Dr. Robert V. Tauxe, Centers for Disease Control and Prevention, Atlanta.)

spread across the Indian subcontinent and to neighboring countries, affecting Pakistan, Nepal, western China, Thailand, and Malaysia by the end of 1994 (Fig. 161-2). The organism has since been designated *V. cholerae* O139 Bengal, in recognition of its novel somatic O antigen and its geographic origin.

The clinical manifestations and epidemiologic features of the disease caused by strain O139 Bengal are indistinguishable from those of O1 cholera. Immunity to the latter, however, is not protective against the former. Thus, although O139 Bengal cholera has been restricted almost exclusively to O1-endemic areas, it has affected patients of all ages, with most cases in adults. Moreover, populations into which strain O139 Bengal has been introduced have responded as virgin populations with respect to severe, lethal cholera. Because naturally acquired immunity to *V. cholerae* O1 does not cross-protect against the O139 Bengal strain, vaccines being developed against the former are unlikely to be effective against the latter.

Like the O1 epidemics in cholera-naive areas before it, the O139 epidemic was initially devastating. Some authorities believed that the emergence of *V. cholerae* O139 signaled the beginning of the eighth global cholera pandemic. Indeed, just as O1 El Tor replaced the classic biotype that preceded it, O139 Bengal in 1993 rapidly replaced O1 El Tor as the most common environmental isolate and the predominant cause of clinical cholera in the areas in which it had appeared (Fig. 161-3). Surprisingly and unexpectedly, however, by the beginning of 1994, O1 El Tor had resumed its dominance in Bangladesh, relegating O139 Bengal cholera to the status of a background endemic infection. This trend continued in 1995. That notwithstanding, the potential for global spread of O139 Bengal was underscored by an intercontinental food-borne outbreak that occurred in early 1994 among passengers on a cruise ship in Southeast Asia. Six of the 630 travelers (five from the United States and one from Great Britain) became ill, their symptoms beginning only after they returned home. They likely acquired the organism during a stopover in Thailand. A specific rice dish eaten during a specific meal at a specific restaurant was the probable source.

PATHOGENESIS In the final analysis, cholera is a toxin-mediated disease. Its characteristic watery diarrhea is due to the action of

FIGURE 161-3 Isolations of *Vibrio cholerae* O1 and *V. cholerae* O139 in Bangladesh, 1993–1994, by month. (Courtesy of Dr. John Albert and Dr. A S G Faruque, International Centre for Diarrhoeal Disease Research, Bangladesh.)

cholera toxin (CTX), a potent protein enterotoxin elaborated by the organism in the small intestine. However, for *V. cholerae* to colonize the small intestine and produce CTX, it must first recognize, contend with, and traverse several hostile environments. The first of these is the acidic milieu of the stomach. *V. cholerae* lacks genetically controlled mechanisms of acid resistance (such as those that exist in *Shigella*). Rather, it relies on a large inoculum size to allow some organisms to elude the bactericidal effects of gastric acidity.

If successful, it must next traverse the mucous layer of the upper small bowel. Several properties of the organism enhance its ability to accomplish this feat, including its motility, its chemotaxis, and its production of hemagglutinin/protease. This last substance, originally named cholera lectin, is closely related to the *Pseudomonas aeruginosa* elastase and is both an agglutinin and a zinc-dependent protease. It is able to cleave mucin and fibronectin as well as the A subunit of CTX. Hemagglutinin/protease may also serve to detach vibrios bound to the small-bowel surface, thus facilitating their spread within the intestine and excretion in the stool.

Having successfully negotiated the barriers of gastric acidity and small-intestinal mucus, the vibrios must finally adhere to the bowel wall. Their attachment is mediated by the toxin-coregulated pilus (TCP), so named because its synthesis is regulated in parallel with that of CTX.

CTX, TCP, and several other virulence factors, including an accessory colonization factor and various hemagglutinins, are coordinately regulated by the *toxR* gene product. ToxR protein is a "master switch" that modulates the expression of virulence genes in response to signals that it senses in the environment, the most important of which, at least in vitro, are changes in osmolarity and pH and the presence of certain free amino acids. Coordinate regulation presumably enables the organism to tailor its repertoire of proteins to suit its needs as it passes from one microenvironment to another. Regulation of the *toxR* type has become a paradigm for similar systems that have been discovered in a wide range of pathogenic bacteria.

FIGURE 161-2 Spread of *Vibrio cholerae* O139 in the Indian subcontinent and elsewhere in Asia, 1992–1994. (Courtesy of Dr. Robert V. Tauxe, Centers for Disease Control and Prevention, Atlanta.)

Once established, the organism produces CTX, which consists of a monomeric enzymatic moiety (the A subunit) and a pentameric binding moiety (the B subunit). The B pentamer binds to G_{M1} ganglioside, a glycolipid receptor on the surface of jejunal epithelial cells, and this binding makes possible the delivery of the A subunit to its cytosolic target. The activated A subunit (A_1) irreversibly transfers ADP-ribose from nicotinamide adenine dinucleotide to its specific target protein, the GTP-binding regulatory component of adenylate cyclase in intestinal epithelial cells. When ADP-ribosylated, this G protein up-regulates the cyclase catalytic subunit; the result is the intracellular accumulation of high levels of cyclic AMP. In turn, cyclic AMP inhibits the absorptive sodium transport system in villus cells and activates the excretory chloride transport system in crypt cells, and these events lead to the accumulation of sodium chloride in the intestinal lumen. Since water moves passively to maintain osmolality, isotonic fluid accumulates in the lumen. When the volume of that fluid exceeds the capacity of the rest of the gut to resorb it, watery diarrhea results. Unless the wasted fluid and electrolytes are adequately replaced, shock (due to profound dehydration) and acidosis (due to loss of bicarbonate) follow.

Although perturbation of the adenylate cyclase pathway is the primary mechanism by which CTX causes excess fluid secretion, it is not the only one. Increasing evidence indicates that CTX also enhances intestinal secretion via prostaglandins and/or neural histamine receptors. It is possible that the redundancy of secretory mechanisms activated by CTX accounts for the profound diarrhea and dehydration characteristic of severe cholera.

The genes encoding CTX (*ctxAB*) have for some time been known to reside on the so-called CTX *genetic element*, a 7- to 9.7-kb segment of DNA occupying a particular position on the chromosomes of toxigenic strains and absent in nontoxigenic strains. The element carries at least four open reading frames in addition to *ctxAB*: *cep* (encoding core-encoded pilin), *orfU* (encoding a product for which no function has been assigned), *ace* (encoding accessory cholera enterotoxin), and *zot* (encoding zonula occludens toxin). On the basis of the element's structural organization and its failure readily to self-transmit in vitro, it had been assumed to represent a transposon. Recent work has demonstrated conclusively that the element is not a transposon but a lysogenic filamentous bacteriophage (CTXΦ). Cep, the *orfU* gene product, Ace, and Zot, which were originally thought to be accessory virulence factors, may actually function in phage morphogenesis.

The surface receptor for CTXΦ on *V. cholerae* is TCP. Accordingly, the phage is transferred far more efficiently under conditions of high rather than low TCP expression. Moreover, enhanced transmission of CTXΦ has been detected in vivo in a murine intestinal colonization model. This finding provides strong genetic evidence for expression of TCP in vivo and demonstrates the critical role of environmental signaling in shaping the behaviors of these microorganisms. The discovery of CTXΦ establishes that horizontal transfer of virulence genes takes place in *V. cholerae* and may be one mechanism by which novel virulent serogroups emerge. Whether transfer to attenuated vaccine strains of *V. cholerae* can also occur remains to be determined. The attenuated strain currently in use, which is discussed in more detail below, has been carefully studied in field trials and appears to have an excellent safety profile.

Molecular analysis of *V. cholerae* O139 Bengal has suggested the basis of its origin and the reasons it was able to cause an explosive epidemic of cholera. Both phenotypically and genotypically, strain O139 Bengal is closely related to the O1 El Tor strains of the seventh pandemic, and it seems to have arisen from them by horizontal gene transfer. It shares the virulence attributes and general pathogenic mechanisms of O1 vibrios, including possession of the same CTX genetic element, the same TCP, and the *toxR* regulon. In all ways but two, strain O139 Bengal is virtually identical to the seventh-pandemic strain of *V. cholerae* O1 El Tor. Those differences are its production of the novel O139 lipopolysaccharide (LPS) and of an immunologically related O-antigen polysaccharide capsule. Both are putative virulence factors, independently enhancing colonization in a murine infection model. The ability to produce the O139 LPS is due to a replacement of the DNA in the central region of the O1 antigen biosynthetic complex with an 11-kb segment containing the genes encoding O139

LPS. At least one of those genes is involved in the production of both the O139 LPS and the capsule. Encapsulation is not a feature of O1 strains and may explain the resistance of O139 strains to human serum in vitro as well as the occasional development of O139 bacteremia.

CLINICAL MANIFESTATIONS   After a 24- to 48-h incubation period, cholera begins with the sudden onset of painless watery diarrhea that may quickly become voluminous and often is followed shortly by vomiting. In severe cases, stool volume can exceed 250 mL/kg in the first 24 h. If fluids and electrolytes are not replaced, hypovolemic shock and death ensue. Fever is usually absent. Muscle cramps due to electrolyte disturbances are common. The stool has a characteristic appearance: a nonbilious, gray, slightly cloudy fluid with flecks of mucus, no blood, and a somewhat sweet, inoffensive odor. It has been called "rice-water" stool because of its resemblance to the water in which rice has been washed. Clinical symptoms parallel volume contraction: At losses of 3 to 5 percent of normal body weight, thirst develops; at 5 to 8 percent, postural hypotension, weakness, tachycardia, and decreased skin turgor; and above 10 percent, oliguria, weak or absent pulses, sunken eyes (and, in infants, sunken fontanelles), wrinkled ("washerwoman") skin, somnolence, and coma. Complications derive exclusively from the effects of volume and electrolyte depletion and include renal failure due to acute tubular necrosis. Thus, if the patient is adequately treated with fluid and salt, complications are averted and the process is self-limited, resolving in a few days.

Laboratory data usually reveal an elevated hematocrit (due to hemoconcentration) in nonanemic patients; mild neutrophilic leukocytosis; elevated levels of blood urea nitrogen and creatinine consistent with prerenal azotemia; normal sodium, potassium, and chloride levels; a markedly reduced bicarbonate level (<15 mmol/L); and an elevated anion gap (due to increases in serum lactate, protein, and phosphate). Arterial pH is usually low (about 7.2).

DIAGNOSIS   The clinical suspicion of cholera can be confirmed by the identification of *V. cholerae* in stool; however, the organism must be specifically sought. In experienced hands, it can be detected directly by dark-field microscopy on a wet mount of fresh stool, and its serotype can be discerned by immobilization with Inaba- or Ogawa-specific antiserum. Laboratory isolation of the organism requires the use of a selective medium. The best of these is thiosulfate–citrate–bile salts–sucrose (TCBS) agar, on which the organism grows as a flat yellow colony. If a delay in sample processing is expected, Carey-Blair transport medium and/or alkaline-peptone water-enrichment medium should be inoculated as well. In endemic areas there is little need for biochemical confirmation and characterization, although these tasks may be worthwhile in places where *V. cholerae* is an uncommon isolate. Standard microbiologic biochemical testing for Enterobacteriaceae will suffice for identification of *V. cholerae*. All vibrios are oxidase-positive. *V. cholerae* can be distinguished from the otherwise similar *V. mimicus* by its ability to ferment sucrose.

The yield of stool cultures for the diagnosis of *V. cholerae* infection declines late in the course of the illness or when effective antibacterial therapy is initiated. Although not generally evaluable in clinical laboratories, serum vibriocidal antibody titers can be used to confirm the diagnosis in non-cholera-endemic regions of the world. Monoclonal antibody–based diagnostic kits and methods based on the polymerase chain reaction and on DNA probes have been developed for *V. cholerae* O1 and O139 but are unlikely to become available in U.S. clinical laboratories.

℞ **TREATMENT**

Cholera is simple to treat; only the rapid and adequate replacement of fluids, electrolytes, and base is required. The mortality rate for appropriately treated disease is usually less than 1 percent. However, analysis of a large outbreak of cholera among airline travelers from an endemic country to the United States revealed frequent misdiagnoses by U.S. health professionals and poor appreciation on their part of the principles of management. Compounding these problems was the general unavailability of appropriate oral fluids. Even intravenous fluid therapy typically was not optimal.

It has been proved conclusively that fluid may be given orally. This approach takes advantage of the hexose-Na^+ cotransport mechanism to move Na^+ across the gut mucosa together with an actively transported molecule such as glucose. Since Na^+ losses in the stool are high, a fluid containing Na^+ at 90 mmol/L has been recommended by the World Health Organization (WHO) (Table 161-1). This amount of Na^+ is higher than that needed to treat diarrhea due to most other causes. The solution is safe, even for infants, if its intake is alternated with the consumption of sodium-free fluids such as breast milk or water. For the sake of simplicity, WHO advises routine use of this single solution for diarrheal disease rather than attempts to choose among multiple formulations according to etiology.

Cereal-based formulations are receiving increased attention as alternative oral rehydration solutions. Because of their lower osmolarity, they may reduce stool output. A mixture with a lower sugar and salt content has also been evaluated in cholera patients, with favorable results. However, concerns have been raised over the safety of its use—in particular, whether it could cause significant hyponatremia in patients with moderate or severe diarrhea. Because commercial oral rehydration solutions also contain concentrations of glucose and sodium lower than those of the WHO formulation, they should not yet be used routinely to treat cholera.

For initial management of severely dehydrated patients, intravenous fluid replacement is preferable, if available. Because profound acidosis (pH < 7.2) is common in this group, Ringer's lactate is the best choice among commercial products (Table 161-2). It must be used with additional potassium supplements, preferably given by mouth. The total fluid deficit in severely dehydrated patients (10 percent or more of body weight) can be replaced safely within the first 4 h of therapy, half within the first hour. Thereafter, oral therapy usually can be initiated, with the goal of maintaining fluid intake equal to fluid output. However, patients with continued large-volume diarrhea may require prolonged intravenous treatment to keep up with gastrointestinal fluid losses. Severe hypokalemia can develop but will respond to potassium given either intravenously or orally. In the absence of adequate staff to monitor the patient's progress, the oral route of rehydration and potassium replacement is safer than the intravenous route and is physiologically regulated by thirst and urine output.

Although not necessary for cure, the use of an antibiotic to which the organism is susceptible will diminish the duration and volume of fluid loss and will hasten clearance of the organism from the stool. Single-dose tetracycline (2 g) or doxycycline (300 mg) is effective in adults but is not recommended for children under 8 years of age because of possible deposition in bone and developing teeth. Emerging drug resistance is an ever-present concern. For adults with cholera in areas where tetracycline resistance is prevalent,

ciprofloxacin—either in a single dose (30 mg/kg, not to exceed a total dose of 1 g) or in a short course (15 mg/kg bid for 3 days, not to exceed a total daily dose of 1 g)—or erythromycin (a total of 40 mg/kg daily in three divided doses for 3 days) is a clinically effective substitute. Both drugs are highly effective in reducing total stool output, and each is significantly better than trimethoprim-sulfamethoxazole. Because of the high cost of quinolones, WHO recommends erythromycin as the first alternative to tetracycline. For children, furazolidone has been the recommended agent and trimethoprim-sulfamethoxazole the second choice. It is of note that *V. cholerae* O139 is resistant to both of these drugs but is susceptible to quinolones, erythromycin, tetracycline, and ampicillin (among others). Because of cost and/or toxicity issues related to the other drugs, erythromycin is a good choice for pediatric cholera, especially where O139 Bengal is present. The efficacy of single-dose erythromycin therapy for cholera has not been demonstrated.

CONTROL In outbreaks, efforts should first be made to identify case contacts and to treat incubating carriers. Next, epidemiologic studies should be undertaken to establish the modes of transmission to define the best strategy to interrupt them. Both the establishment of rehydration centers and instruction in rehydration techniques are essential to the reduction of mortality.

PREVENTION Provision of safe water and facilities for sanitary disposal of feces, improved nutrition, and attention to food preparation and storage in the household could significantly reduce the incidence of cholera. Much effort has been devoted to the development of a cholera vaccine over the past two decades, with a particular focus on the use of live oral vaccine strains. Traditional killed cholera vaccine given intramuscularly provides little protection to nonimmune subjects and predictably causes adverse effects, including pain at the injection site, malaise, and fever. The vaccine's limited efficacy is at least partially due to its failure to induce a local immune response at the intestinal mucosal surface.

Two types of oral cholera vaccines are under development. The first is the killed whole-cell vaccine, which has been prepared both with and without the inclusion of the nontoxic B subunit of CTX (WC/BS and WC vaccine, respectively). The second is the live attenuated vaccine. In trials in Bangladesh, both of the killed vaccines were compared with placebo and conferred about 50 percent protection over a 3-year evaluation period. The protective efficacy of WC/BS was superior to that of WC during the initial 8 months of follow-up (69 versus 41 percent) but equivalent or inferior thereafter. Immunity was relatively sustained in persons vaccinated at an age of >5 years but not well sustained in younger vaccinees.

Live attenuated vaccine strains are being developed in several laboratories, with the use of various starting strains and attenuation strategies. A strain can be attenuated by the isolation or creation of mutants lacking certain virulence factors. Three criteria must be met in live vaccine design: The vaccine strain must induce protective immunity, it must be safe to administer, and it must be minimally reactogenic. *Safety* refers to the vaccine strain's potential to regain virulence, either spontaneously or via horizontal gene transfer from environmental strains. *Reactogenicity* refers to its potential to cause symptoms such as fever or diarrhea in vaccinees.

Table 161-2

Electrolyte Composition of Cholera Stool and of Intravenous Rehydration Solution

Substance	Concentration, mmol/L			
	Na^+	K^+	Cl^-	Base
Stool				
Adult	135	15	90	30
Child	100	25	90	30
Ringer's lactate	130	4*	109	28

* Potassium supplements, preferably administered by mouth, are required to replace the usual potassium losses from stool.

Table 161-1

Composition of World Health Organization Oral Rehydration Solution (ORS)*,†

Constituent	Concentration, mmol/L
Na^+	90
K^+	20
Cl^-	80
Citrate‡	10
Glucose	110

* Contains (per package, to be added to 1 L of drinking water): NaCl, 3.5 g; $Na_3C_6H_5O_7 \cdot 2H_2O$, 2.9 g; KCl, 1.5 g; and glucose, 20 g.
† If prepackaged ORS is unavailable, a simple homemade alternative can be prepared by combining 5 g NaCl (about 1 level teaspoon) with either 50 g precooked rice cereal or 40 g sucrose in 1 L of drinking water. In that case, potassium must be supplied separately (e.g., in orange juice or coconut water).
‡ 10 mmol citrate per liter, which supplies 30 mmol HCO_3/L.

Strain CVD 103-HgR, an oral live cholera vaccine licensed in Europe, was created from a classic strain of *V. cholerae* by the deletion of the CTX A subunit gene and the insertion in the hemolysin gene of a mercury resistance marker. Although poorly excreted in the stool of human vaccinees, CVD 103-HgR produces a significant increase in the titer of vibriocidal antibody in about 75 percent of recipients, including children between the ages of 2 and 4 years, when given in single dose. This vaccine is more effective against classic than against El Tor cholera. It is marketed in Europe by the Swiss Serum and Vaccine Institute but is unavailable in the United States. This vaccine has an acceptable safety record. Nevertheless, the recent discoveries of CTXΦ and of its capacity for horizontal transfer in vivo mandate reconsideration of vaccine strategies that utilize live cholera strains attenuated only by deletion of toxin genes. Such strains are presumably still capable of infection by wild-type CTXΦ and therefore have at least the theoretical potential for reversion to virulence.

Other vaccine candidate strains have been prepared from El Tor and from O139 vibrios. These strains have been attenuated by the removal of the entire CTX genetic element and its flanking site-specific RS1 insertion sequences, as well as attRS1, the chromosomal target for insertion of the CTX operon. The *recA* gene, which mediates homologous recombination, has also been deleted. These modifications make it virtually impossible for the organisms to regain virulence. To enhance the protective immune response elicited by these strains, the gene encoding the CTX B subunit has been restored to their chromosomes under the control of a strong promoter. In some formulations, spontaneously arising motility-deficient strains have been used to further reduce the potential for reactogenicity. These vaccines are all still years away from licensing. At present, because of the minimal efficacy of existing parenteral vaccines, cholera immunization is recommended for U.S. travelers only if it is mandated by the countries they plan to visit.

OTHER *VIBRIO* SPECIES

In recent years, the taxonomic, epidemiologic, pathophysiologic, and clinical features of the non-O1 vibrios have become increasingly well understood. Ten human pathogens are currently recognized in the genus *Vibrio*. Included are species associated primarily with gastrointestinal illness (*V. parahaemolyticus*, non-O1 *V. cholerae*, *V. mimicus*, *V. fluvialis*, *V. hollisae*, and *V. furnissii*) and species associated primarily with soft tissue infections (*V. vulnificus*, *V. alginolyticus*, and *V. damsela*). In addition, *V. vulnificus* has emerged as a cause of primary sepsis in certain compromised hosts. Vibrios are abundant in coastal waters the world over and tend to concentrate in the tissues of filter-feeding mollusks. Under optimal conditions, some can double in number in as little as 9 min. Consequently, seawater and raw or undercooked shellfish are important sources of human infection (Table 161-3). Vibrios grow best at temperatures between about 28°C and 44°C but not at all below 4°C or above 60°C. Most can be cultured on blood or MacConkey agar, each of which contains enough salt to support the growth of the halophilic organisms (≥0.5 percent). As with *V. cholerae*, TCBS is the best selective medium. The species can be differentiated in the laboratory by standard biochemical tests. The most important members of the group are *V. parahaemolyticus*, a major cause of gastroenteritis in the Far East, and *V. vulnificus*, a notable cause of sepsis in certain immunosuppressed patients in the United States. These and selected other species are considered below in greater detail.

SPECIES ASSOCIATED PRIMARILY WITH GASTROINTESTINAL ILLNESS *V. parahaemolyticus*
First implicated as a cause of enteritis by Japanese workers in 1953, *V. parahaemolyticus* is now recognized as an important intestinal pathogen in

many parts of the world. In one study from Japan, 24 percent of reported cases of food poisoning were attributed to this organism, presumably owing to the widespread consumption of raw seafood there. In the United States, *V. parahaemolyticus* has been responsible for several well-documented common-source outbreaks of diarrhea, typically linked to ingestion of undercooked or improperly handled seafood or of other foods that have been contaminated by seawater. Most reports have come from the Atlantic Coast, the Gulf of Mexico, and Hawaii. The organism is ubiquitous in marine environments and is able to grow in saline concentrations up to about 8 to 10 percent. The ability to cause hemolysis on Wagatsuma agar (the so-called Kanagawa phenomenon) is closely linked to enteropathogenicity. In one study, 96.5 percent of isolates from patients with diarrhea were hemolytic versus only about 1 percent of isolates from seawater. Hemolysis is attributed to a 42-kDa heat-stable protein, the exact pathophysiologic role of which is uncertain. The mechanism by which *V. parahaemolyticus* causes diarrhea is not clear.

V. parahaemolyticus has been associated with two distinct gastrointestinal presentations. The more common is a syndrome of watery diarrhea, accompanied in most cases by abdominal cramps, nausea, and vomiting and in about one-quarter of cases by fever and chills. The incubation period ranges from 4 h to 4 days, and the symptomatic period lasts for a median of 3 days. The vast majority of North American cases have been of this type. The less common syndrome is one of dysentery, described in India and Bangladesh and characterized by severe abdominal cramps, nausea, vomiting, and bloody or mucoid stools. Most cases of either type are self-limited and require neither antimicrobial treatment nor hospitalization. The occasional severe case should be treated with fluid replacement and antibiotics, as described above for cholera. Death is very rare. There are no reliable differential diagnostic features. *V. parahaemolyticus* should be considered as a possible cause in all cases of diarrhea that can be epidemiologically linked to seafood consumption or to the sea itself.

In addition to gastrointestinal disease, *V. parahaemolyticus* is a rare cause of extraintestinal infections, including wound infections, otitis, and—very rarely—sepsis.

Non-O1 *V. cholerae* The heterogeneous non-O1 *V. cholerae* organisms are biochemically indistinguishable from *V. cholerae* O1 on routine testing but fail to agglutinate in O1 antiserum. While technically a non-O1 vibrio, *V. cholerae* O139 Bengal is not grouped with these pathogens because of its epidemic potential, as detailed above. Non-O1 *V. cholerae* strains have been responsible for several well-described food-borne outbreaks of gastroenteritis as well as for sporadic cases of otitis media, wound infection, and bacteremia. About half of all U.S. isolates are obtained from stool specimens. Like other vibrios, non-O1 *V. cholerae* organisms are widely distributed in marine environments; unlike most other vibrios, however, they require only trace amounts of NaCl to survive (i.e., they are nonhalophilic). Recognized U.S. cases invariably have been associated either with the consumption of raw oysters or with recent travel, typically to Mexico. The clinical spectrum of diarrheal disease caused by non-O1 *V. cholerae* is

Table 161-3

Features of Selected Noncholera Vibrioses

Organism	Vehicle or Activity	Host at Risk	Syndrome
V. parahaemolyticus	Shellfish, seawater	Normal	Gastroenteritis
	Seawater	Normal	Wound infection
Non-O1 *V. cholerae*	Shellfish, travel	Normal	Gastroenteritis
	Seawater	Normal	Wound infection, otitis media
V. vulnificus	Shellfish	Immunosuppressed*	Sepsis, secondary cellulitis
	Seawater	Normal	Wound infection, cellulitis
V. alginolyticus	Seawater	Normal	Wound infection, cellulitis, otitis
	Seawater	Burned, other immunosuppressed	Sepsis

* Especially with liver disease or hemochromatosis.

broad and likely reflects the heterogeneous virulence attributes of the group. Occasional isolates make a protein enterotoxin very similar to CTX. Others produce cytotoxins, hemolysins, or invasins.

Gastroenteritis due to non-O1 *V. cholerae* typically has an incubation period of less than 2 days. Stools may be copious and watery, and their passage may leave the patient severely dehydrated, as in cholera; alternatively, the stools may be partly formed, less voluminous, and bloody or mucoid. Abdominal cramps, nausea, vomiting, and fever are often reported. In one series, 11 percent of patients were hospitalized; in another, the figure was 50 percent. The duration of illness ranges from about 2 to 7 days. As in cholera, patients with significant dehydration should be treated with oral or intravenous fluids. The role of antibiotics is uncertain.

Wound infection and otitis media each account for about 10 percent of non-O1 *V. cholerae* isolates. Bacteremia accounts for another 20 percent. Patients with extraintestinal infection often have a history of occupational or recreational exposure to seawater. Bacteremia is more likely to develop in the presence of liver disease. Extraintestinal infections should be treated with antibiotics. There is a paucity of information to guide the choice of a specific agent and schedule. Most strains are sensitive in vitro to tetracycline, chloramphenicol, and other agents.

SPECIES ASSOCIATED PRIMARILY WITH SOFT TISSUE INFECTION OR BACTEREMIA *V. vulnificus* Though it represents only a small minority of the *Vibrio* species found in nature (4 percent of Atlantic Coast isolates in one study), *V. vulnificus* is perhaps the most important cause of severe *Vibrio* infections in the United States (0.8 cases per 100,000 population in one study from Louisiana). Formerly included in the species *V. parahaemolyticus*, *V. vulnificus* was distinguished in the 1970s by its ability to ferment lactose and to cause distinct clinical syndromes. Like most vibrios, it proliferates in the warm summer months. It requires a saline environment for growth but prefers concentrations lower than those preferred by *V. parahaemolyticus* and *V. alginolyticus* (range, up to about 8 percent; optimal, about 1 percent). Infections in humans typically occur in coastal states between May and October and most often involve men over age 40. *V. vulnificus* has been linked unequivocally to two distinct syndromes: primary sepsis, typically in patients with antecedent liver disease, and primary wound infections, usually in people without underlying disease. Some authors have suggested that this organism causes gastroenteritis, but the evidence for this association is tenuous.

V. vulnificus is remarkably invasive in animal models. It is endowed with a number of virulence attributes, including an antiphagocytic capsule, serum resistance, a cytotoxin/hemolysin (the organism is Kanagawa-positive), collagenase, elastolytic protease, phospholipase, and siderophores. Its virulence, as measured by the 50 percent lethal dose in mice, is markedly enhanced under conditions of iron overload, a fact consonant with its propensity to infect patients with hemochromatosis.

Primary sepsis occurs most commonly in patients with cirrhosis or hemochromatosis but also has developed in patients with hematopoietic disorders or chronic renal insufficiency, in persons using immunosuppressive medications or alcohol, and (rarely) in individuals without apparent underlying disease. Most of those affected have ingested raw oysters within 2 days of onset (median incubation period, 16 h). The process begins precipitously with malaise, chills, fever (mean temperature, 39.8°C), and prostration. Hypotension develops in one-third of cases, often by the time of admission. Cutaneous manifestations, which develop in three-quarters of cases (usually by 36 h after onset), typically involve the extremities—lower more often than upper. A common sequence is the evolution of erythematous patches followed by ecchymoses, vesicles, and bullae. (Indeed, the presence of sepsis and bullous skin lesions suggests the diagnosis in an appropriate setting.) Necrosis and sloughing may occur. Laboratory study reveals leukopenia more often than leukocytosis, thrombocytopenia, and (occasionally) elevated levels of fibrin split products. *V. vulnificus* can be cultured from blood or cutaneous lesions.

Mortality approaches 50 percent, with most deaths due to uncontrolled sepsis. Accordingly, prompt treatment is critical and should include empirical antibiotic administration, aggressive debridement, and general supportive care. *V. vulnificus* is sensitive to a number of antimicrobials in vitro, including tetracycline, gentamicin, and third-generation cephalosporins. No compelling clinical data from studies of humans support the preferential use of any one of these agents. Tetracycline is demonstrably superior in a murine model and on that basis is considered the drug of choice (0.5 to 1 g intravenously every 12 h), either alone or in combination with gentamicin. The duration of therapy is guided by the clinical response.

Wound infections with *V. vulnificus* can develop in patients with or without underlying disease and invariably follow contact of seawater with either a prior or a fresh wound. The incubation period is brief (4 h to 4 days; mean, 12 h). The disease begins with swelling, erythema, and—in many cases—intense pain around the wound. Rapidly spreading cellulitis follows, with vesicular, bullous, or necrotic lesions developing in some instances. Metastatic events do not generally occur. Fever (median temperature, 38.9°C) and leukocytosis are demonstrable in most cases. The organism can be cultured from skin lesions and occasionally from blood. Prompt antibiotic therapy and debridement are usually curative.

V. alginolyticus This species was first recognized as a human pathogen in 1973 and is now known to cause occasional wound, ear, and eye infections. It is the most salt-tolerant of the vibrios, able to grow in concentrations exceeding 10 percent. Most clinical isolates come from superinfected wounds, which presumably became contaminated at the beach. Infection varies in severity but is generally not serious and responds well to antibiotic therapy and drainage. A few reports have described otitis externa, otitis media, or conjunctivitis. Therapy with tetracycline is usually curative. *V. alginolyticus* is a rare cause of bacteremia in immunocompromised hosts.

BIBLIOGRAPHY

ALI A et al: *Vibrio vulnificus* sepsis in solid organ transplantation: A medical nemesis. J Heart Lung Transplant 14:598, 1995

BEGUE RE et al: Community-based assessment of safety and immunogenicity of the whole cell plus recombinant B subunit (WC/rBS) oral cholera vaccine in Peru. Vaccine 13:691, 1995

BESSER RE et al: Diagnosis and treatment of cholera in the United States. Are we prepared? JAMA 272:1203, 1994

BHAN MK et al: Clinical trials of improved oral rehydration salt formulations: A review. Bull WHO 72:945, 1994

COLWELL RR, HUQ A: Environmental reservoir of *Vibrio cholerae*, the causative agent of cholera. Ann NY Acad Sci 740:44, 1994

COSTER TS et al: Safety immunogenicity, and efficacy of live attenuated *Vibrio cholerae* O139 vaccine prototype. Lancet 345:949, 1995

HOGE CW et al: Epidemiological study of *Vibrio cholerae* O1 and O139 in Thailand: At the advancing edge of the eighth pandemic. Am J Epidemiol 143:263, 1996

KAPER JB et al: Cholera. Clin Microbiol Rev 8:48, 1995

KHAN WA et al: Comparative trial of five antimicrobial compounds in the treatment of cholera in adults. Trans R Soc Trop Med Hyg 89:103, 1995

LACEY SW: Cholera: Calamitous past, ominous future. Clin Infect Dis 20:1409, 1995

LEVINE WC, GRIFFIN PM: Vibrio infections on the Gulf Coast: Result of first year of regional surveillance. J Infect Dis 167:479, 1993

MEKALANOS JJ, SADOFF JC: Cholera vaccines: Fighting an ancient scourge. Science 265:1387, 1994

MORRIS JG JR: Non-O1 *V. cholerae*: A look at the epidemiology of an occasional pathogen. Epidemiol Rev 12:179, 1990

TAYLOR DN et al: Cholera among Americans living in Peru. Clin Infect Dis 22:1108, 1996

WALDOR MK et al: Emergence of a new cholera pandemic: Molecular analysis of virulence determinants in *Vibrio cholerae* O139 and development of a live vaccine prototype. J Infect Dis 170:278, 1994

———— et al: The *Vibrio cholerae* O139 serogroup antigen includes an O-antigen capsule and lipopolysaccharide virulence determinants. Proc Natl Acad Sci USA 91:11388, 1994

————, MEKALANOS JJ: Lysogenic conversion by a filamentous phage encoding cholera toxin. Science 272:1910, 1996

WEBER JT et al: Cholera in the United States, 1965–1991. Risks at home and abroad. Arch Intern Med 154:551, 1994

BRUCELLOSIS

DEFINITION   Brucellosis is a zoonosis transmitted to humans from infected animals. Its clinical features are not disease specific. Brucellosis and its etiologic agents are named after David Bruce, a Scottish physician who discovered the latter in 1887 while stationed in Malta. *Brucellosis* has many synonyms derived from the geographical regions in which the disease occurs (e.g., Mediterranean fever, Malta fever, Gibraltar fever, Cyprus fever); from the remittent character of its fever (e.g., undulant fever); or from its resemblance to malaria and typhoid (e.g., typhomalarial fever, intermittent typhoid).

ETIOLOGIC AGENTS   Human brucellosis can be caused by any of four species: *Brucella melitensis* (the most common cause worldwide) is acquired primarily from goats, sheep, and camels; *Brucella abortus* from cattle; *Brucella suis* from hogs; and *Brucella canis* from dogs. These small aerobic gram-negative bacilli are unencapsulated, nonmotile, non-spore-forming, facultative intracellular parasites. Brucellae are killed by boiling or pasteurization of milk and milk products. They survive for up to 8 weeks in unpasteurized, white, soft cheese made from goat's milk and are not killed by freezing. The organisms remain viable for up to 40 days in dried soil contaminated with infected-animal urine, stool, vaginal discharge, and products of conception and for longer periods in damp soil.

EPIDEMIOLOGY   The global incidence of human brucellosis is not known because of the variable quality of disease reporting and notification systems in many countries. Worldwide, the only countries believed to be free of brucellosis are Norway, Sweden, Finland, Denmark, Iceland, Switzerland, the Czech and Slovak republics, Romania, the United Kingdom (including the Channel Islands), the Netherlands, Japan, Luxembourg, Cyprus, and Bulgaria; the U.S. Virgin Islands are also free of the disease. Reports indicate that, even in developed nations, the true incidence of brucellosis may be up to 26 times higher than official figures suggest. In the United States, about 200 new cases are reported every year; however, it is estimated that only 4 to 10 percent of cases are recognized and reported. Consumption of imported cheese, travel abroad, and occupation-related exposures are the most frequently identified sources of infection. In communities where brucellosis occurs in children, the disease may be endemic and family members of infected persons are at risk. Even in countries where animal brucellosis is controlled, the disease occasionally develops among farmers, meat-processing workers, veterinarians, and laboratory workers.

Brucella is transmitted most commonly through the ingestion of untreated milk or milk products, raw meat, or bone marrow. However, the organism can be contracted via inhalation during contact with animals, especially by children and by slaughterhouse, farm, and laboratory workers. Other routes of infection for at-risk workers include skin abrasion, autoinoculation, and conjunctival splashing. The organism has been transmitted from person to person through the placenta, during breast feeding, and (in rare instances) during sexual activity.

IMMUNITY AND PATHOGENESIS   Immunity to *Brucella* is determined by phagocytosis mediated by specific antibodies and by cell-mediated mechanisms. *Brucella* organisms are phagocytosed by polymorphonuclear leukocytes and by activated macrophages. *Brucella* antigens are capable of inducing the production of specific antibodies. Serum IgM antibodies appear early after infection and are followed later by IgG and IgA. Inflammatory responses or granulomas may develop, and caseation, necrosis, and abscess formation have been described. Endogenous interleukin (IL)-12 has a strong inducing effect on interferon γ–producing T cells (see Chap. 305), which also play a key role in the host's defense against *Brucella* infection; in contrast, IL-10 downregulates protective immunity to *Brucella*. Intracellular multiplication of the organism takes place in lymph nodes and reticuloendothelial tissues. Other organs may also be affected through hematogenous spread.

CLINICAL FEATURES   The protean manifestations of brucellosis may mimic the features of other febrile illnesses. The incubation period lasts for about 1 to 3 weeks but may be as long as several months. The onset of symptoms may be either abrupt (over 1 to 2 days) or gradual (over 1 week or more). The most common symptoms are fever, chills, diaphoresis, headaches, myalgia, fatigue, anorexia, joint and low-back pain, weight loss, constipation, sore throat, and dry cough. Physical examination often reveals no abnormalities, and patients can look deceptively well. Some patients, in contrast, are acutely ill, with pallor, lymphadenopathy, hepatosplenomegaly, arthritis, spinal tenderness, epididymoorchitis, skin rash, meningitis, cardiac murmurs, or pneumonia. The fever of brucellosis has no distinctive pattern but may exhibit diurnal variation, with normal temperatures in the morning and high temperatures in the afternoon and evening. Table 162-1 lists the frequencies of key historical features, symptoms, and signs among 500 patients with brucellosis due to *B. melitensis*.

Bones and Joints   Although monarticular septic arthritis occurs, 30 to 40 percent of patients have reactive asymmetric polyarthritis involving the knees, hips, shoulders, and sacroiliac and sternoclavicular joints. The total white cell count in synovial fluid ranges from 4000 to 40,000/μL, with 60 percent polymorphonuclear leukocytes. The synovial fluid glucose concentration may be reduced and the protein concentration elevated; cultures of synovial fluid are positive in about 50 percent of cases.

Brucella osteomyelitis commonly affects the lumbar vertebrae, starting at the superior end plate (an area with a rich blood supply) and occasionally progressing to involve the entire vertebra, disk space, and adjacent vertebrae. Extraspinal *Brucella* osteomyelitis is rare. In *Brucella* septic arthritis and osteomyelitis, the peripheral white cell

Table 162-1

Relevant Historical Features and Symptoms and Signs in 500 Patients with Brucellosis due to *Brucella melitensis*

Feature	No. (%) of Patients
HISTORY	
Animal contact	368 (74)
Raw milk/cheese ingestion	350 (70)
Raw liver ingestion	147 (29)
Family history of brucellosis	188 (38)
SYMPTOM/SIGN	
Fever	464 (93)
Chills	410 (82)
Sweats	437 (87)
Aches	457 (91)
Lack of energy	473 (95)
Joint and back pain	431 (86)
Arthritis	202 (40)
Spinal tenderness	241 (48)
Headache	403 (81)
Loss of appetite	388 (78)
Weight loss	326 (65)
Constipation	234 (47)
Abdominal pain	225 (45)
Diarrhea	34 (7)
Cough	122 (24)
Testicular pain/epididymoorchitis	62 (21*)
Rash	72 (14)
Sleep disturbances	185 (37)
Ill appearance	127 (25)
Pallor	110 (22)
Lymphadenopathy	160 (32)
Splenomegaly	125 (25)
Hepatomegaly	97 (19)
Jaundice	6 (1)
Central nervous system abnormalities	20 (4)
Cardiac murmur	17 (3)
Pneumonia	7 (1)

* Among 290 males.

count is normal, while the erythrocyte sedimentation rate may be either normal or elevated.

Heart Cardiovascular complications of brucellosis include endocarditis, myocarditis, pericarditis, aortic root abscess, mycotic aneurysms, thrombophlebitis with pulmonary aneurysm, and pulmonary embolism. *Brucella* endocarditis may develop on valves previously damaged by rheumatic fever or congenital malformation but also occurs on previously normal valves. The clinical features are indistinguishable from those of endocarditis caused by other organisms (see Chap. 126). In the past, endocarditis was the leading cause of death in brucellosis. In recent years, the outcome of *Brucella* endocarditis has been more favorable because of advances in early diagnosis, antibiotic treatment, and cardiac surgery. Physicians of patients with culture-negative endocarditis who, because of environmental exposure, may be at risk for *Brucella* infection should notify the bacteriology laboratory performing the blood culture so that extended incubation, specific media, and biohazard precautions can be employed.

Respiratory Tract *Brucella* can produce respiratory symptoms. A flulike illness with sore throat, tonsillitis, and dry cough is common and usually mild. Hilar and paratracheal lymphadenopathy, pneumonia, solitary or multiple pulmonary nodules, lung abscesses, and empyema have been reported.

Gastrointestinal Tract Gastrointestinal manifestations of *Brucella* infection are generally mild and may include nausea, vomiting, constipation, acute abdominal pain, and/or diarrhea. Pathologic examination of the liver may reveal any of several changes, including noncaseating granuloma, suppurative abscesses, or mononuclear cell infiltration. Hepatic and splenic enlargement may be documented in 15 to 20 percent of cases, and abscesses may develop in the liver and spleen. Mild jaundice may be evident, with elevated levels of bilirubin and hepatic enzymes.

Genitourinary Tract Various genitourinary infections have been attributed to *Brucella*, including unilateral or bilateral epididymoorchitis, which is a self-limiting manifestation. Prostatitis, seminal vesiculitis, dysmenorrhea, tuboovarian abscess, salpingitis, cervicitis, and acute pyelonephritis have also been documented. *Brucella* has been cultured from the urine in up to 50 percent of cases of genitourinary tract infection.

Central Nervous System Neurobrucellosis is uncommon but serious and includes meningoencephalitis, multiple cerebral or cerebellar abscesses, ruptured mycotic aneurysms, myelitis, Guillain-Barré syndrome, cranial nerve lesions, hemiplegia, sciatica, myositis, and rhabdomyolysis. Papillitis, papilledema, retrobulbar neuritis, optic atrophy, and ophthalmoplegia due to lesions in cranial nerves III, IV, and VI may occur in *Brucella* meningoencephalitis. Cerebrospinal fluid (CSF) pressure is usually elevated; the fluid may appear clear, turbid, or hemorrhagic; the protein concentration and cell count (predominantly lymphocytes) are elevated; and the glucose concentration may be either reduced or normal. In *Brucella* meningitis, the organism may be cultured from the CSF.

Other Manifestations Splashing of the eyes with virulent brucellae or with organisms in veterinary vaccines may result in keratitis, corneal ulcers, uveitis, retinal detachment, and endophthalmitis.

Skin manifestations of brucellosis are uncommon. They include maculopapular eruptions, purpura and petechiae, chronic ulcerations, multiple cutaneous and subcutaneous abscesses, discharging sinuses, superficial thrombophlebitis, erythema nodosum, and pemphigus.

Brucellosis during human pregnancy can cause fetal death. *Brucella* has been isolated from the human placenta and fetus.

Endocrinologic findings in brucellosis include thyroiditis, adrenal insufficiency, and the syndrome of inappropriate secretion of antidiuretic hormone.

DIAGNOSIS The combination of potential exposure, consistent clinical features, and raised levels of *Brucella* agglutinin (with or without positive cultures of blood or tissues) confirms the diagnosis

of brucellosis. Serum antibodies to *Brucella* can be detected by several methods, including standard tube agglutinins (STA), the 2-mercaptoethanol agglutination test, Coombs' test, and an enzyme-linked immunosorbent assay. *B. abortus* antigens, which are commonly used for serologic tests, cross-react with *B. melitensis* and *B. suis* but not with *B. canis*. Specific antigen is required for the diagnosis of *B. canis* infection; although the materials required for testing are not commercially available, *B. canis* antibody titers can be determined in the United States at the Centers for Disease Control and Prevention in Atlanta. A false-negative result in the STA may be obtained because of the presence of IgA and IgG blocking antibodies. This so-called prozone phenomenon can be avoided by testing of sera at both low and high dilutions. In endemic areas a *Brucella* antibody titer of 1:320 or 1:640 is significant, while in nonendemic areas an antibody titer of 1:160 is considered significant. Detection of elevated levels of antibody to *Brucella* in the absence of symptoms during the screening of potential blood donors is common in endemic areas. To establish a diagnosis in these regions, clinical and serologic evaluation should be repeated after 2 to 4 weeks and a further rise in titer sought. A high titer of specific IgM suggests recent exposure, while a high titer of specific IgG suggests active disease. Lower titers of IgG may indicate past exposure or treated infection. Several studies have demonstrated that the polymerase chain reaction is specific and highly sensitive for the detection of *Brucella*.

Cooperation and consultation with a microbiologist are important when brucellosis is suspected. It may be necessary to hold culture bottles for up to 6 weeks. Subcultures should be prepared on duplicate blood agar plates (with and without an atmosphere of 10% CO_2) and special media. Cultures of blood or bone marrow are positive in 50 to 70 percent of cases. The peripheral white cell count is usually normal but may be low, with relative lymphocytosis. Thrombocytopenia and disseminated intravascular coagulation may be documented. Levels of hepatic enzymes and serum bilirubin may be raised.

Radiologic investigations aimed at detecting skeletal involvement include plain radiography, bone scintigraphy, computed tomography (CT), and magnetic resonance imaging (MRI). Bone scintigraphy is more sensitive than conventional radiography in detecting areas of spinal and extraspinal involvement, particularly in the early stage of infection. CT is useful for further evaluation of spinal lesions and of the extension of infection into the spinal canal. MRI is the modality of choice for the assessment of *Brucella* spondylitis and is more sensitive than scintigraphy or CT for demonstration of the extent of disease.

Plain lateral radiography of the spine may reveal bone sclerosis, with destruction and erosion of the superior end plate anteriorly. As the disease progresses, healing with osteophyte formation and reduction of disk space may take place. In *Brucella* septic monarthritis, plain radiography may show effusion and soft tissue swelling without bone or joint destruction. Scintigraphy may document increased uptake in sacroiliac joints or lumbar vertebrae even when plain radiography gives normal results. MRI shows diffuse, high signal intensity of the affected vertebrae and may reveal narrowing of the spinal canal as well as loss of definition of the posterior aspect of the vertebrae.

℞ TREATMENT

Single-agent therapy for brucellosis has now been abandoned because of the high incidence of failure and relapse and the potential development of resistance. Relatively short courses (less than 8 weeks) of treatment with antibiotic combinations have similarly been associated with high rates of relapse. The combination of doxycycline and an aminoglycoside (streptomycin, gentamicin, or netilmicin) for 4 weeks followed by the combination of doxycycline and rifampin for 4 to 8 weeks is the most effective regimen. Doxycycline (which is preferred over tetracycline) is given orally in a dose of 100 mg twice daily. Netilmicin (which is preferred to streptomycin) is given (intramuscularly to outpatients, intravenously to inpatients) in a dose of 2 mg/kg every 12 h; trough levels in plasma should be monitored regularly and maintained at ≤2 µg/mL. Streptomycin is given intramuscularly in a dose of 1 g once daily to patients under 45 years of age and in a dose of 0.5 to 0.75 g/d to older patients. Gentamicin is given intramuscularly or as a slow intravenous infusion (3 to 5 mg/kg per day in divided doses every 8 h). Tetracycline is given orally in a dose of 250 mg every 6 h and rifampin as a single daily dose of 600 to 900 mg. An alternative regimen consists of the doxycycline/rifampin combination given for 8 to 12 weeks. The doxycycline/netilmicin (or doxycycline/ streptomycin) combination is more effective than the doxycycline/ rifampin combination in that rifampin reduces levels of doxycycline in plasma.

When used alone, fluoroquinolones—antibiotics with good intracellular penetration and efficacy against *Brucella* in vitro—have been associated with the development of quinolone resistance and with high rates of failure and relapse. At present, clinical data are inadequate for the formulation of recommendations regarding the combination of fluoroquinolones with doxycycline, rifampin, or streptomycin.

Third-generation cephalosporins (e.g., ceftriaxone), although active in vitro against *Brucella* when used alone, have also been associated with a high incidence of clinical failure and relapse. These agents may be useful in combination with other drugs for the treatment of *Brucella* meningitis.

In pregnancy, trimethoprim-sulfamethoxazole (TMP-SMZ) can be given in combination with rifampin for 8 to 12 weeks. Children below the age of 7 years can also be treated with rifampin and TMP-SMZ for 8 to 12 weeks, while older children should receive the same antibiotics as adults in the following doses: doxycycline, 100 mg/d orally; an aminoglycoside; and rifampin, 15 mg/kg per day orally or by slow intravenous infusion. TMP-SMZ is given orally every 12 h in a dose that depends on the patient's age (birth to 6 months, 120 mg; 6 months to 6 years, 240 mg).

In cases of neurobrucellosis, aortic root abscess, and endocarditis, rifampin should be added to the doxycycline/aminoglycoside combination. Cardiac surgery may be needed along with antibiotic therapy in the acute stage, particularly in cases of *Brucella* endocarditis and aortic root abscess. In instances of renal failure, doxycycline can be used safely. In contrast, the use of aminoglycosides requires facilities for the monitoring of plasma levels; if such facilities are not available, then the doxycycline/rifampin combination should be administered for 8 to 12 weeks.

Within 4 to 14 days after the initiation of therapy, patients become afebrile and constitutional symptoms disappear. The enlarged liver and spleen return to their normal size within 2 to 4 weeks. An acute, intense flare-up of symptoms may follow the start of treatment, especially that with tetracyclines. This reaction is transient and does not necessitate the discontinuation of therapy. In endemic areas the coexistence of brucellosis and tuberculous spondylitis may result in a failure to respond to appropriate treatment. Treated patients whose infections are apparently cured should be followed up clinically and serologically, with repeat blood cultures, every 3 to 6 months for 2 years.

PREVENTION Efforts at prevention should be aimed at the source of infection. Immunization of animals and boiling or pasteurization of milk and milk products are important. Workers in the meat and dairy industries in the former Soviet Union, China, and France have been vaccinated; the vaccine (two injections given 2 weeks apart, each containing 1 mg of an insoluble fraction of phenol-extracted bacteria) has markedly reduced the rate of infection. However, immunity is short-lived, and vaccination should be repeated every 2 years. This vaccine is not used in the United States.

PROGNOSIS Deaths attributable to brucellosis should be avoidable. Even before the discovery of antibiotics, mortality was less than 2 percent and endocarditis was most frequently the cause of death. Morbidity due to brucellosis remains significant; its severity depends on the infecting *Brucella* species and is greatest with *B. melitensis*. Spinal damage, paraplegia, and other neurologic deficits may occur. Nerve deafness due to meningitis or secondary to treatment with streptomycin has been documented.

BIBLIOGRAPHY

AL-KASAB S et al: Management of *Brucella* endocarditis with aortic root abscess. Chest 98:1532, 1990

AL MAJED SA et al: Use of antibiotics in the treatment of human brucellosis. Curr Ther Res Clin Exp 57:175, 1996

ARIZA J et al: Treatment of human brucellosis with doxycycline plus rifampin or doxycycline plus streptomycin: A randomized double-blind study. Ann Intern Med 117:25, 1992

CENTERS FOR DISEASE CONTROL AND PREVENTION: Brucellosis outbreak at a pork processing plant—North Carolina, 1992. JAMA 271:1734, 1994

CHEVALIER P et al: Fatal *Brucella* pancarditis. Presse Med 25:628, 1996

CHOMEL BB et al: Changing trends in the epidemiology of human brucellosis in California from 1973 to 1992: A shift toward foodborne transmission. J Infect Dis 170:1216, 1994

COMENERO JD et al: Possible implications of doxycycline-rifampin interaction for treatment of brucellosis. Antimicrob Agents Chemother 38:2798, 1994

GARCIA-RODRIGUEZ JA et al: Susceptibilities of *Brucella melitensis* to clinafloxacin and four other new fluoroquinolones. Antimicrob Agents Chemother 39:1194, 1995

HADJICHRISTODOVLOV C et al: Tolerance of the human brucellosis vaccine and the intradermal reaction test for brucellosis. Eur J Clin Microbiol Infect Dis 13:129, 1994

MADKOUR MM: *Brucellosis*. London, Butterworths, 1989

——— et al: Osteoarticular brucellosis; results of bone scintigraphy in 140 patients. Am J Roentgenol 150:1101, 1988

——— et al: Occupational related infectious arthritis, in *Baillier's Clinical Rheumatology: Occupational Rheumatic Diseases*, GP Balint (ed). London, Saunders, 1989, pp 157–192

ROMERO C et al: Specific detection of *Brucella* DNA by PCR. J Clin Microbiol 33:615, 1995

ZHAN Y, CHEERS C: Endogenous interleukin-12 is involved in resistance to *Brucella abortus* infection. Infect Immun 63:1387, 1995

163   *Richard F. Jacobs*

TULAREMIA

DEFINITION Tularemia is a zoonosis caused by *Francisella tularensis*, so named in 1974 in recognition of the contributions of Edward Francis. Humans of any age, sex, or race are universally susceptible to this systemic infection. Tularemia is primarily a disease of wild animals and persists in contaminated environments, ectoparasites, and animal carriers. Human infection is incidental and usually results from interaction with biting or blood-sucking insects, wild or domestic animals, or the environment. Tularemia is common in Arkansas, Oklahoma, and Missouri, where more than 50 percent of the cases in the United States occur. An increasing number of cases of tularemia have been reported from the Scandinavian countries, eastern Europe, and Siberia. The illness is characterized by various clinical syndromes, the most common of which consists of an ulcerative lesion at the site of inoculation, with regional lymphadenopathy and lymphadenitis. Systemic manifestations, including pneumonia, typhoidal tularemia, and fever without localizing findings, pose a greater diagnostic challenge.

ETIOLOGY AND EPIDEMIOLOGY *F. tularensis* is the etiologic agent of tularemia, which, with rare exceptions, is the only disease produced by this genus. The organism is a small, gram-negative, pleomorphic, nonmotile, non-spore-forming bacillus measuring 0.2×0.2 to 0.7 μm. Bipolar staining results in a coccoid appearance. The organism is a thinly encapsulated, nonpiliated strict aerobe that invades host cells.

In nature, *F. tularensis* is a hardy organism that persists for weeks or months in mud, water, and decaying animal carcasses. Dozens of biting and blood-sucking insects, especially ticks and tabanid flies, serve as vectors. Ticks and wild rabbits are the source for most of the human cases in the endemic areas of the southeastern United States and the Rocky Mountain states. In Utah, Nevada, and California, tabanid flies are the most common vectors. Animal reservoirs include wild rabbits, squirrels, birds, sheep, beavers, muskrats, and domestic dogs and cats.

The two main biovars of *F. tularensis*—*tularensis* (type A) and *palearctica* (type B)—are both found in the United States. Type A produces more serious disease in humans; without treatment, the associated fatality rate is approximately 5 percent. Type B produces a milder, often subclinical infection that is usually contracted from water or marine mammals.

Ticks pass the organism to their offspring via a transovarian route. The organism is found in tick feces but not in large quantities in tick salivary glands. In the United States, the disease can be carried by *Dermacentor andersoni* (Rocky Mountain wood tick), *Dermacentor variabilis* (American dog tick), *Dermacentor occidentalis* (Pacific coast dog tick), and *Amblyomma americanum* (Lone Star tick). *F. tularensis* is transmitted frequently during blood meals taken by embedded ticks following hours of attachment. It is the taking of a blood meal through a fecally contaminated field that transmits the organism. Tularemia is more common among men. Person-to-person transmission is rare or nonexistent. Transmission of the organism by ticks and tabanid flies takes place mainly in the spring and summer. However, continued transmission in the winter months by trapped or hunted animals has been documented. The organism is extremely infectious. Biosafety level 2 is recommended for clinical laboratory work with material whose contamination is suspected, and biosafety level 3 is required for culture of the organism in large quantities.

PATHOGENESIS AND PATHOLOGY The most common portal of entry for human infection is through skin or mucous membranes, either directly—through the bite of a tick, other arthropods, or other animals—or via inapparent abrasions. Inhalation or ingestion of *F. tularensis* can also result in infection. Although more than 10^8 organisms are usually required to produce infection via the oral route (oropharyngeal or gastrointestinal tularemia), fewer than 50 organisms will result in infection when injected into the skin (ulceroglandular/glandular tularemia) or inhaled (pneumonia). After inoculation into the skin, the organism multiplies locally; within 2 to 5 days (range, 1 to 10 days), it produces an erythematous, tender, or pruritic papule. The papule rapidly enlarges and forms an ulcer with a black base (chancriform lesion). The bacteria spread to regional lymph nodes, producing lymphadenopathy (buboes), and, with bacteremia, may spread to distant organs.

Tularemia is characterized by mononuclear cell infiltration with pyogranulomatous pathology. The histopathologic findings can be quite similar to those in tuberculosis, although tularemia develops more rapidly. As a facultatively intracellular bacterium, *F. tularensis* is capable of parasitizing both phagocytic and nonphagocytic host cells and of surviving intracellularly for prolonged periods. In the acute phase of infection, the primary organs affected (skin, lymph nodes, liver, and spleen) include areas of focal necrosis, initially surrounded by polymorphonuclear leukocytes. Subsequently, granulomas form, with epithelioid cells, lymphocytes, and multinucleated giant cells surrounded by areas of necrosis. These areas may resemble caseation necrosis but later coalesce to form abscesses.

Conjunctival inoculation can result in infection of the eye, with regional lymph node enlargement (preauricular lymphadenopathy, Parinaud's complex). Aerosolization and inhalation or hematogenous spread of organisms can result in pneumonia. In the lung, an inflammatory reaction—with foci of alveolar necrosis and cell infiltration (initially polymorphonuclear and later mononuclear) with granulomas—develops. Chest roentgenograms usually reveal bilateral patchy infiltrates rather than large areas of consolidation. Pleural effusions are common and may contain blood. Lymphadenopathy occurs in regions draining infected organs. Therefore, in pulmonary infection, mediastinal adenopathy may be evident, while patients with oropharyngeal tularemia develop cervical lymphadenopathy. In gastrointestinal or typhoidal tularemia, mesenteric lymphadenopathy may follow the in-

gestion of large numbers of organisms. The term *typhoidal tularemia* may be used to describe severe bacteremic disease, irrespective of the mode of transmission or portal of entry. Meningitis has been reported as a primary or secondary manifestation of bacteremia. Patients may also present with fever and no localizing signs.

IMMUNOLOGY Infection with *F. tularensis* stimulates the host to produce antibodies. However, this antibody response probably plays only a minor role in the containment of infection. In contrast, cell-mediated immunity, which develops over 2 to 4 weeks, plays a major role in containment and eradication of the infection. Macrophages, once activated, are capable of killing *F. tularensis*.

Immunospecific protection against tularemia can be afforded either by natural infection or by vaccination with live attenuated strains of *F. tularensis*. Killed vaccines, on the other hand, induce no protection against virulent *F. tularensis*. After natural infection or vaccination, serum antibodies to surface-exposed carbohydrate antigens predominate, whereas T cell determinants are located on membrane proteins beneath the bacterial capsule. T cell responses are thought to be due to priming by the organism. The anamnestic T cell response to *F. tularensis* seems to involve a multitude of microbial proteins, each with a distinct set of T cell determinants. A predominant role for CD4+ T cells is supported by the results of experiments in mice, which indicated that resistance to infection was restricted at the level of the MHC class II determinants. Humans primed to *F. tularensis* (like those primed to *Mycobacterium tuberculosis*) show a T_H1-like response. T cell proliferation is associated with the production of interleukin (IL) 2 and interferon γ but with little or no production of IL-4.

Recent investigations of neutrophils in cases of tularemia have suggested that polymorphonuclear neutrophils (PMNs) are needed for defense against primary infection. PMNs may restrict the growth of *F. tularensis* before the organism becomes intracellular.

CLINICAL MANIFESTATIONS Tularemia often starts with a sudden onset of fever, chills, headache, and generalized myalgias and arthralgias (Table 163-1). This onset takes place when the organism penetrates the skin, is ingested, or is inhaled. An incubation period of 2 to 10 days is followed by the formation of an ulcer at the site of penetration, with local inflammation. The ulcer may persist for several months as organisms are transported via the lymphatics to the regional lymph nodes. These nodes enlarge and may become necrotic and suppurating. If the organism enters the bloodstream, widespread dissemination as well as signs and symptoms of endotoxemia may result.

In the United States, most patients with tularemia (75 to 85 percent) acquire the infection by inoculation of the skin. In adults, the most common localized form is inguinal/femoral lymphadenopathy; in children, it is cervical lymphadenopathy. About 20 percent of patients develop a generalized maculopapular rash, which occasionally becomes pustular. Erythema nodosum occurs infrequently. The clinical manifestations of tularemia have been divided into various syndromes, which are listed in Table 163-2.

Ulceroglandular/Glandular Tularemia These two forms of tularemia account for approximately 75 to 85 percent of cases. The predominant form in children involves cervical or posterior auricular lymphadenopathy and is usually related to tick bites on the head and neck area. In adults, the most common form is inguinal/femoral

Table 163-1

Clinical Presentation of Tularemia

Sign or Symptom	Rate of Occurrence, %	
	Children	Adults
Lymphadenopathy	96	65
Fever ($\geq$38.3°C)	87	21
Ulcer/eschar/papule	45	51
Myalgias/arthralgias	39	2
Headache	9	5
Cough	9	5
Pharyngitis	43	—
Diarrhea	43	—

SOURCE: Adapted from Jacobs et al.

Table 163-2

CHAPTER 163
Tularemia

973

Clinical Syndromes of Tularemia

Syndrome	Rate of Occurrence, %	
	Children	Adults
Ulceroglandular	45	51
Glandular	25	12
Pulmonary (pneumonia)	14	18
Oropharyngeal	4	—
Oculoglandular	2	—
Typhoidal	2	12
Unclassified	6	11

SOURCE: Adapted from Jacobs et al.

lymphadenopathy resulting from insect and tick exposures on the lower limbs. In cases related to wild game, the usual portal of entry for *F. tularensis* is either an injury sustained while skinning or cleaning an animal carcass or a bite (usually on the hand). Epitrochlear lymphadenopathy/lymphadenitis is common in patients with bite-related injuries.

In ulceroglandular tularemia, the ulcer is erythematous, indurated, and nonhealing, with a punched-out appearance that lasts from 1 to 3 weeks. The papule may begin as an erythematous lesion that is tender or pruritic; it evolves over several days into an ulcer with sharply demarcated edges and a yellow exudate. The ulcer gradually develops a black base, and simultaneously the regional lymph nodes become tender and severely enlarged. The affected lymph nodes may become fluctuant and drain spontaneously, but usually the condition resolves with effective treatment. Late suppuration of lymph nodes has been described in up to 25 percent of patients with ulceroglandular/glandular tularemia. Examination of material taken from these late fluctuant nodes after successful antimicrobial treatment has revealed sterile necrotic tissue. In 5 to 10 percent of patients, the skin lesion may be inapparent, with lymphadenopathy plus systemic signs and symptoms the only physical findings. This clinical syndrome is designated *glandular tularemia*. Conversely, a tick or deerfly bite on the trunk may result in an ulcer without evident lymphadenopathy.

Oculoglandular Tularemia In about 1 percent of patients, the portal of entry for *F. tularensis* is the conjunctiva. Usually, the organism reaches the conjunctiva through contact with contaminated fingers. The inflamed conjunctiva is painful, with numerous yellowish nodules and pinpoint ulcers. Purulent conjunctivitis with regional lymphadenopathy (preauricular, submandibular, or cervical) is evident. Because of debilitating pain, the patient may seek medical attention before regional lymphadenopathy develops. Painful preauricular lymphadenopathy is unique to tularemia and distinguishes it from cat-scratch disease, tuberculosis, sporotrichosis, and syphilis. Corneal perforation may occur.

Oropharyngeal and Gastrointestinal Tularemia Rarely, tularemia follows the ingestion of contaminated undercooked meat, the oral inoculation of *F. tularensis* from the hands in association with the skinning and cleaning of animal carcasses, or the consumption of contaminated food or water. Oral inoculation may result in acute, exudative, or membranous pharyngitis associated with cervical lymphadenopathy or in ulcerative intestinal lesions associated with mesenteric lymphadenopathy, diarrhea, abdominal pain, nausea, vomiting, and gastrointestinal bleeding. Infected tonsils become enlarged and develop a yellowish-white pseudomembrane, which can be confused with that of diphtheria. The clinical severity of gastrointestinal tularemia varies from mild, unexplained, persistent diarrhea with no other symptoms to a rapidly fulminant, fatal disease. In fatal cases, the extensive intestinal ulceration found at autopsy suggests an enormous inoculum.

Pulmonary Tularemia Tularemia pneumonia presents as variable parenchymal infiltrates that are unresponsive to treatment with β-lactam antibiotics. Tularemia must be considered in the differential diagnosis of atypical pneumonia in a patient with a history of travel to an endemic area. The disease can result from either inhalation of an infectious aerosol or spread to the lungs and pleura after bloodstream

dissemination. Inhalation-related pneumonia has been described in laboratory workers after exposure to contaminated materials and is associated with a relatively high mortality rate. Exposure to *F. tularensis* in aerosols from live domestic animals or dead wildlife (including birds) has been reported to cause pneumonia. Hematogenous dissemination to the lungs occurs in 10 to 15 percent of cases of ulceroglandular tularemia and in about half of cases of typhoidal tularemia. Previously, tularemia pneumonia was thought to be a disease of older patients, but as many as 10 to 15 percent of children with clinical manifestations of tularemia have parenchymal infiltrates detected by chest roentgenography. Patients with pneumonia usually have a nonproductive cough and may have dyspnea or pleuritic chest pain. Roentgenograms of the chest usually reveal bilateral patchy infiltrates (described as ovoid or lobar densities), lobar parenchymal infiltrates, and cavitary lesions. Pleural effusions may have a predominance of mononuclear leukocytes or PMNs and sometimes red blood cells. Empyema may develop. Patients with tularemia pneumonia can have blood cultures positive for *F. tularensis*.

Typhoidal Tularemia Once thought to represent up to 10 percent of all cases of tularemia, the typhoidal presentation is now considered to be rare in the United States. In this presentation, fever develops without apparent skin lesions or lymphadenopathy. In the absence of a history of possible contact with a vector, diagnosis can be extremely difficult. Blood cultures may be positive and patients may present with classic sepsis or septic shock in this acute systemic form of the infection. Typhoidal tularemia is usually associated with a huge inoculum or with a preexisting compromising condition. High continuous fevers, signs of endotoxemia, and severe headache are common findings. The patient may be delirious and may develop prostration and shock. If presumptive antibiotic therapy in culture-negative cases does not include an aminoglycoside, the mortality rate can approach 30 percent.

Other Manifestations *F. tularensis* infection has been associated with meningitis, pericarditis, hepatitis, peritonitis, endocarditis, osteomyelitis, and sepsis and septic shock with rhabdomyolysis and acute renal failure. In the rare cases of tularemia meningitis, a predominantly lymphocytic response can be demonstrated in cerebrospinal fluid.

DIFFERENTIAL DIAGNOSIS When patients in endemic areas present with fever, chronic ulcerative skin lesions, and large tender lymph nodes, a diagnosis of tularemia should be made presumptively, and confirmatory diagnostic testing and appropriate therapy should be undertaken. When the possibility of tularemia is considered in a patient with this presentation in a nonendemic area, an attempt should be made to determine whether the individual has come into contact with a potential animal vector. The level of suspicion of tularemia should be especially high in hunters, trappers, game wardens, veterinarians, laboratory workers, and individuals with a history of exposure to an insect or other animal vector. However, up to 40 percent of patients with tularemia have no known history of epidemiologic contact with an arthropod or other animal vector.

The characteristic presentation of ulceroglandular tularemia does not pose a diagnostic problem, but a less classic progression of regional lymphadenopathy or glandular tularemia must be differentiated from other diseases. The skin lesion may resemble those seen in sporotrichosis; skin infection with *Staphylococcus aureus*, *Streptococcus pyogenes*, or *Mycobacterium marinum*; syphilis; anthrax; rat-bite fever (due to *Spirillum minus*); or rickettsiosis (scrub typhus). In the latter infections, regional lymphadenopathy is usually not as impressive as in tularemia. The lymphadenopathy of tularemia (especially glandular tularemia) must be differentiated from that of plague, lymphogranuloma venereum, and cat-scratch disease. In children, the differentiation from cat-scratch disease is made more difficult by the chronic papulovesicular lesion associated with *Bartonella henselae* infection (see Chap. 165).

Oropharyngeal tularemia can resemble and must be differentiated from pharyngitis due to group A beta-hemolytic streptococci, *Arcano-*

bacterium haemolyticum, or *Corynebacterium diphtheriae* as well as from infectious mononucleosis. Tularemia pneumonia may resemble any of the atypical pneumonias, including those due to various viruses, *Mycoplasma pneumoniae, Chlamydia pneumoniae, Chlamydia psittaci, Legionella pneumophila, Coxiella burnetii,* and (occasionally) *Histoplasma capsulatum.* Typhoidal tularemia may resemble typhoid fever, other *Salmonella* bacteremias, rickettsial infections (Rocky Mountain spotted fever, ehrlichiosis), brucellosis, infectious mononucleosis, acquired toxoplasmosis, miliary tuberculosis, sarcoidosis, and hematologic or reticuloendothelial malignancies.

LABORATORY DIAGNOSIS   Direct microscopic examination of polychromatically stained tissue smears or clinical specimens reveals *F. tularensis* organisms, singly and in groups, both intra- and extracellularly. Gram's staining of clinical or biopsy material is of little value, as the small, weakly staining organisms cannot be readily distinguished from the background. An indirect fluorescent antibody test with commercially available antisera can be useful, although false-positive results due to *Legionella* species have been reported.

The diagnosis of tularemia is most frequently confirmed by serologic testing. In the standard tube agglutination test, a single titer of ≥1:160 is interpreted as a presumptive positive result. A fourfold increase in titer between paired serum samples collected 2 to 3 weeks apart is considered diagnostic. False-negative serologic responses are obtained early in infection; up to 30 percent of patients infected for 3 weeks have sera that test negative. Late in infection, titers into the thousands are common, and titers of 1:20 to 1:80 may persist for years. A microagglutination test that may be as much as 100-fold more sensitive than the standard tube agglutination test has been described and is currently being used in many clinical microbiology laboratories. Enzyme-linked immunosorbent assays have proven useful for the detection of both antibodies and antigens. Analysis of urine for *F. tularensis* antigen has yielded promising results in clinical trials, but facilities for this type of analysis are not widely available. A skin test for delayed hypersensitivity to *F. tularensis* turns positive during the first week of illness and remains positive for years. The skin-test antigen, which is not commercially available, can boost titers of agglutinating antibody.

Culture and isolation of *F. tularensis* are difficult. In one study the organism was isolated in only 10 percent of more than 1000 human cases, 84 percent of which were confirmed by serology. The medium of choice is cysteine-glucose-blood agar. *F. tularensis* can be isolated directly from infected ulcer scrapings, lymph-node biopsy specimens, gastric washings, sputum, and blood cultures. Colonies are blue-gray, round, smooth, and slightly mucoid. On media containing blood, a small zone of alpha hemolysis usually surrounds the colony. Slide agglutination tests or direct fluorescent antibody tests with commercially available antisera can be applied directly to culture suspensions for identification.

The polymerase chain reaction has been used to detect *F. tularensis* DNA, primarily in blood. However, this test has not been shown to be more sensitive than direct culture and at present remains a research tool.

℞ TREATMENT

F. tularensis cannot be subjected to standardized antimicrobial susceptibility testing because the organism will not grow on the media used. A wide variety of antibiotics, including all β-lactam antibiotics and the newer cephalosporins, are ineffective for the treatment of this infection. Recent studies indicated that third-generation cephalosporins were active against *F. tularensis* in vitro, but clinical case reports suggested a nearly universal failure rate of ceftriaxone in pediatric patients with tularemia. Although in vitro data indicate that imipenem may be active, therapy with imipenem, sulfanilamides, and macrolides is not presently recommended because of the lack of clinical data. Fluoroquinolones have shown promise in terms of their relatively low toxicity and their potential for oral administration. Chloramphenicol

and tetracycline have been used successfully for treatment of the acute stages of tularemia but have been associated with higher relapse rates (up to 20 percent) than conventionally used agents.

Streptomycin, given intramuscularly at a dose of 7.5 to 10 mg/kg every 12 h, is considered the drug of choice for adults. In severe cases, 15 mg/kg every 12 h may be used for the first 48 to 72 h. Streptomycin is also considered the drug of choice for children; the appropriate dose is 30 to 40 mg/kg daily in two divided doses administered intramuscularly. In children, after a clinical response is demonstrated at 3 to 5 days, the dose can be reduced to 10 to 15 mg/kg daily in two divided doses. Therapy is typically continued for 7 to 10 days; however, in mild to moderate cases of tularemia in which the patient becomes afebrile within the first 48 to 72 h of streptomycin treatment, a 5- to 7-day course has been successful.

Gentamicin, at a dose of 1.7 mg/kg given intravenously or intramuscularly every 8 h, is also effective. The published experience in adults consists of two reports describing, respectively, nine and eight patients who were treated effectively with gentamicin. The eight patients in one of the reports all had fever before treatment, and all eight became afebrile within 24 to 72 h. In a recent pediatric study, other symptoms, such as tender lymphadenitis and pharyngitis, also responded within 24 to 72 h of the start of gentamicin therapy.

Virtually all strains of *F. tularensis* are susceptible to streptomycin and gentamicin. In successfully treated patients, defervescence usually occurs within 2 days, but skin lesions and lymph nodes may take 1 to 2 weeks to heal. When therapy is not initiated within the first several days of illness, defervescence may be delayed. Relapses are uncommon with streptomycin or gentamicin therapy. Late lymphnode suppuration, however, occurs in approximately 40 percent of children, regardless of the treatment received. These nodes have typically been found to contain sterile necrotic tissue without evidence of active infection. Patients with fluctuant nodes should receive several days of antibiotic therapy before drainage to minimize the risk to hospital personnel. Unlike streptomycin and gentamicin, tobramycin is ineffective in the treatment of tularemia and should not be used.

PROGNOSIS   If tularemia goes untreated, symptoms usually last 1 to 4 weeks but may continue for months. The mortality rate from severe untreated infection (including all cases of untreated tularemia pneumonia and typhoidal tularemia) can be as high as 30 percent. However, the overall mortality rate for untreated tularemia is less than 8 percent. Mortality is less than 1 percent with appropriate treatment. Poor outcomes are often associated with long delays in diagnosis and treatment. Lifelong immunity usually follows tularemia.

PREVENTION   The prevention of tularemia is based on avoidance of exposure to biting and blood-sucking insects, especially ticks and deerflies. An intradermal vaccine made from live attenuated *F. tularensis* is available from the Centers for Disease Control and Prevention. This vaccine is effective in reducing the frequency and severity of infection. Vaccination of high-risk individuals working with large quantities of cultured organisms is recommended. Others who come into contact with the organisms, such as veterinarians, hunters, or game wardens, should consider vaccination, particularly if they live in endemic areas. The avoidance of skinning wild animals, especially rabbits, and the wearing of gloves while handling animal carcasses decrease the risk of transmission. Use of insect repellents and preparations that prevent tick attachment as well as prompt removal of ticks can be helpful. Prophylaxis of tularemia has not proved effective in patients with embedded ticks or insect bites. However, in patients who are known to have been exposed to large quantities of organisms (e.g., in the laboratory) and who have incubating infection with *F. tularensis*, early treatment can prevent the development of significant clinical disease.

BIBLIOGRAPHY

BAKER CN et al: Antimicrobial susceptibility testing of *Francisella tularensis* with a modified Mueller-Hinton broth. J Clin Microbiol 22:212, 1985

BERNARD K et al: Early recognition of atypical *Francisella tularensis* strains lacking a cysteine requirement. J Clin Microbiol 32:551, 1994

CROSS JT, JACOBS RF: Tularemia: Treatment failures with outpatient use of ceftriaxone. Clin Infect Dis 17:976, 1993

ENDERLIN G et al: Streptomycin and alternative agents for the treatment of tularemia: Review of the literature. Clin Infect Dis 19:42, 1994

JACOBS RF, NARAIN JP: Tularemia in children. Pediatr Infect Dis J 2:487, 1983

———— et al: Tularemia in adults and children: A changing presentation. Pediatrics 76:818, 1985

LONG GW et al: Detection of *Francisella tularensis* in blood by polymerase chain reaction. J Clin Microbiol 31:152, 1993

MASON WL et al: Treatment of tularemia, including pulmonary tularemia, with gentamicin. Am Rev Respir Dis 121:39, 1980

PENN RL, KINASEWITZ GT: Factors associated with a poor outcome in tularemia. Arch Intern Med 147:265, 1987

RUBIN SA: Radiographic spectrum of pleuropulmonary tularemia. Am J Roentgenol 131:277, 1978

SCHMID GP et al: Granulomatous pleuritis caused by *Francisella tularensis*: Possible confusion with tuberculous pleuritis. Am Rev Respir Dis 128:314, 1983

SJOSTEDT A et al: Neutrophils are critical for host defense against primary infection with the facultative intracellular bacterium *Francisella tularensis* in mice and participate in defense against reinfection. Infect Immun 62:2779, 1994

TARNVIK A: Nature of protective immunity to *Francisella tularensis*. Rev Infect Dis 11:440, 1989

———— et al: *Francisella tularensis*—a model for studies of the immune response to intracellular bacteria in man. Immunology 76:349, 1992

TAYLOR JP et al: Epidemiologic characteristics of human tularemia in the southwest-central states, 1981–1987. Am J Epidemiol 133:1032, 1991

| 164 | *Grant L. Campbell, David T. Dennis* |

PLAGUE AND OTHER *YERSINIA* INFECTIONS

PLAGUE

DEFINITION Plague is an acute, febrile, zoonotic disease caused by infection with *Yersinia pestis*. Although human cases are infrequent and are curable with antibiotics, plague is one of the most virulent and potentially lethal infectious diseases known. The plague bacterium occurs in widely scattered foci in Asia, Africa, and the Americas, where its usual hosts are wild and peridomestic rodents. It is transmitted to humans typically by flea bite and less commonly by direct contact with infected animal tissues or by airborne droplet. The principal clinical forms of plague are bubonic, septicemic, and pneumonic. Most cases are sporadic, occurring singly or in small clusters, although the potential for epidemic spread still exists in some countries.

ETIOLOGIC AGENT *Y. pestis* is a gram-negative coccobacillus in the family Enterobacteriaceae. It is microaerophilic, nonmotile, nonsporulating, oxidase and urease negative, and biochemically unreactive. The organism is nonfastidious and infective for laboratory rodents. It grows well, if slowly, on routinely used microbiologic media (e.g., sheep blood agar, brain-heart infusion broth, and Mac-Conkey agar). *Y. pestis* can multiply within a wide range of temperatures ($-2°C$ to $45°C$) and pH values (5.0 to 9.6), but optimal growth occurs at $28°C$ and at pH ~7.4. When incubated on agar plates, colonies are pinpoint in size at 24 h and 1 to 2 mm in diameter at 48 h. Colonies are gray-white with irregular surfaces that are often described as having a "hammered-metal" appearance when viewed microscopically. In broth culture, *Y. pestis* grows without turbidity in clumps clinging to the sides of tubes. When stained with a polychromatic stain (e.g., Wayson or Giemsa), *Y. pestis* isolated from clinical specimens exhibits a characteristic bipolar appearance, often resembling closed safety pins. The bacterium is nonencapsulated but when grown at $\geq30°C$ produces an immunogenic cell-surface envelope glycoprotein, fraction 1 (F1).

HISTORIC BACKGROUND Plague's deadly epidemic potential is notorious and well documented. The Justinian pandemic (542 to 767 A.D.) spread from central Africa to the Mediterranean littoral and thence to Asia Minor, causing an estimated 40 million deaths. The second pandemic began in central Asia, was carried to Sicily by ship from Constantinople in 1347, and swept through Europe and the British Isles in successive waves over the next four centuries. At its height, it killed as many as a quarter of the affected population and became known as the Black Death. In the third (modern) pandemic, plague appeared in Yunnan, China, in the latter half of the nineteenth century; established itself in Hong Kong in 1894; and spread by ship to Bombay in 1896 and subsequently to major port cities throughout the world, including San Francisco and several other West Coast and Gulf Coast ports in the United States. The plague bacillus was first cultured by Alexandre Yersin in Hong Kong in 1894. In 1898, Paul-Louis Simond, a French scientist sent to investigate epidemic bubonic plague in Bombay, identified the bacillus in the tissues of dead rats and proposed transmission by rat fleas. Waldemar Haffkine, also in Bombay at that time, developed a crude vaccine.

By 1910, plague had circled the globe and established itself in rodent populations on all inhabited continents other than Australia. After 1920, however, the spread of plague was largely halted by international regulations that mandated control of rats in harbors and inspection and rat-proofing of ships. Before the third pandemic subsided, it resulted in an estimated 26 million plague cases and more than 12 million deaths, the vast majority in India. By 1950, plague outbreaks around the world had become isolated, sporadic, and manageable with modern techniques of surveillance, flea and rat control, and antimicrobial treatment of patients. From 1969 through 1993, a median of 1356 human plague cases were reported annually to the World Health Organization, with around 10 to 15 countries reporting cases each year. Plague has practically disappeared from cities and now occurs mostly in rural and semirural areas, where it is maintained in wild rodents. In the United States, the last outbreak of urban plague occurred in Los Angeles in 1924 and 1925, and human cases since then have resulted from zoonotic exposures in rural areas of western states.

Plague, because of its pandemic history, remains one of three quarantinable diseases subject to international health regulations (the other two being cholera and yellow fever). The alarm that plague is still able to evoke was highlighted by the public panic over and exaggerated international response to reports of outbreaks of bubonic and pneumonic plague in India in 1994.

EPIDEMIOLOGY *Y. pestis* is maintained in enzootic cycles involving relatively resistant wild rodents and their fleas in mostly remote, lightly populated areas of Asia, Africa, and the Americas and in limited rural foci in extreme southeastern Europe near the Caspian Sea. Humans and other nonrodent mammals are incidental hosts. Enzootic transmission places humans at low risk, and cases are typically infrequent and sporadic. Epizootic transmission involving susceptible rodents and efficient flea vectors (both are amplifying hosts) results in local or even widespread depopulation of susceptible rodents and poses a more serious threat to humans than does enzootic transmission. In the United States, the principal epizootic hosts are various ground squirrels, prairie dogs, and chipmunks; a variety of burrowing rodents act as epizootic hosts in rural areas elsewhere in the world. *Y. pestis* occasionally spills over from wild rodents to commensal rat species that inhabit cultivated fields and adjacent homes, villages, and towns. The organism can then be transported from towns to cities by these relatively cosmopolitan rats and their fleas. Urban plague is reported from a few countries in southern Asia, such as Vietnam and Myanmar, and occurs only sporadically elsewhere.

Plague in populated areas is most likely to develop when sanitation is poor and rats are numerous—especially the common black or roof rat (*Rattus rattus*) and the larger brown sewer or Norway rat (*R. norvegicus*). A high mortality rate from plague in these susceptible rat populations forces their fleas to seek alternative hosts, including humans. The virtually ubiquitous oriental rat flea *Xenopsylla cheopis* and (in southern Africa and Brazil) the related species *X. brasiliensis* are efficient vectors of the plague bacillus among rats and are also efficient vectors to humans. *Y. pestis* can multiply to enormous numbers in the foregut (proventriculus) of these fleas, resulting in a bolus of organisms and clotted blood that blocks the passage of subsequent blood meals. Regurgitation by a "blocked" flea while it feeds facilitates transmission of the plague bacillus to the new host.

Except for large outbreaks of pneumonic plague in Manchuria in the early part of the twentieth century, person-to-person respiratory transmission of plague during and since the third pandemic has occurred only sporadically and has been limited to clusters of close contacts of pneumonic plague patients, such as household members and caregivers. The 1994 outbreak of pneumonic plague in the city of Surat, India, although reported to be extensive, most likely involved fewer than 100 cases and 50 deaths.

International health regulations require immediate reporting of plague cases. From 1979 through 1993, 16,312 human plague cases and 1668 deaths (mortality, 10 percent) were reported by 20 countries to the World Health Organization. In the same 15-year period, the United States reported 227 plague cases (mean, 15 cases per year) and 32 deaths (mortality, 14 percent). Cases reported by the United States are confirmed by the plague laboratory at the Centers for Disease Control and Prevention (CDC). Enzootic and epizootic plague occurs in 17 contiguous western states, extending from the Great Plains states and eastern Texas to the Pacific Coast; around 80 percent of human cases in this country occur in New Mexico, Arizona, and Colorado and around 10 percent in California. Although plague in the United States is a rural disease, more than 50 percent of cases are thought to be caused by peridomestic exposures, especially in the southwestern states, where homes are often situated in natural surroundings that provide a favorable habitat for plague-susceptible animals (such as rock squirrels and wood rats) and their fleas. In the Sierra Nevadas of California and Nevada, epizootic plague in chipmunks and ground squirrels poses a risk to visitors in public parks. Hikers, campers, and hunters in natural areas throughout the western states are at a small but finite risk of exposure to plague, especially in the summer months.

Plague can be transmitted during the skinning and handling of carcasses of wild animals such as rabbits and hares, prairie dogs, wildcats, and coyotes. Such direct inoculation of mammal-adapted organisms is associated with primary septicemia and high mortality. Oropharyngeal plague can result from the ingestion of undercooked contaminated meat and perhaps from the manual transfer of infected fluids to the mouth during the handling of infected animal tissues.

Carnivores, including dogs and cats, can become infected with *Y. pestis* by eating infected rodents and perhaps by being bitten by fleas from infected rodents. Although clinical plague commonly develops in infected cats, it rarely does so in infected dogs, which thus do not directly expose humans to infection. However, both dogs and cats may transport infected fleas from rodent-infested areas to the home environment.

From 1950 through 1994, 373 plague cases were reported in the United States. Of the 364 evaluable cases, 313 cases (86 percent) presented as primary lymphadenitic (bubonic) plague, almost all of them thought to be associated with flea bites; 44 cases (12 percent) presented as primary septicemic plague, many of them following direct animal exposures; and 7 cases (2 percent) presented as primary pneumonic plague, 6 resulting from the inhalation of respiratory droplets released by infected cats. The last case of human-to-human plague transmission in the United States occurred in the Los Angeles outbreak of 1924/1925.

PATHOGENESIS AND PATHOLOGY *Y. pestis* is among the most invasive bacteria known. The mechanisms by which the organism causes disease are incompletely understood, but both chromosome- and plasmid-encoded gene products are probably involved. Three plasmids encode for a variety of known or presumed virulence factors, including the F1 envelope antigen, which confers bacterial resistance to phagocytosis by polymorphonuclear leukocytes (PMNs) in vitro; a murine exotoxin; the V antigen, which is essential for virulence, may immunocompromise the host by suppressing the synthesis of interferon γ and tumor necrosis factor α, and stimulates

protective immunity in laboratory animals; pesticin, a bactericidal protein of unknown function and importance; a protease that can activate plasminogen and degrade serum complement and that is thought to play a role in the dissemination of *Y. pestis* from peripheral sites of infection; a coagulase; and a fibrinolysin. A lipopolysaccharide endotoxin, believed to be chromosomally encoded, is probably important in the pathogenesis of septicemic plague and disseminated intravascular coagulation (DIC).

Y. pestis organisms inoculated through the skin or mucous membranes usually invade cutaneous lymphatic vessels and reach regional lymph nodes, although direct bloodstream inoculation may take place. Mononuclear phagocytes, which can phagocytize *Y. pestis* organisms without destroying them, may play a role in dissemination of the infection to distant sites. Plague can involve almost any organ, and untreated plague generally results in widespread and massive tissue destruction. In the early stages, infected lymph nodes (buboes, Fig. 164-1) are characterized by edema and congestion without inflammatory infiltrates or apparent vascular injury. Fully developed buboes contain huge numbers of infectious plague organisms and show distorted or obliterated lymph node architecture with vascular destruction and hemorrhage, serosanguineous effusion, necrosis, and a mild neutrophilic infiltration. At this stage, the effusion often involves perinodal tissues. If several adjacent lymph nodes are involved, a boggy edematous mass can result.

Primary septicemic plague results from the direct inoculation of infected fluids or tissues or from an infective flea bite in the apparent absence of a bubo; secondary septicemic plague occurs when lymphatic and other host defenses are breached and the plague bacillus multiplies within the bloodstream. In either primary or secondary septicemic plague, renal glomeruli often contain fibrin thrombi. Diffuse interstitial myocarditis with cardiac dilatation may develop. Multifocal necrosis of the liver is common, as is diffuse hemorrhagic splenic necrosis. If DIC ensues, vascular necrosis may lead to widespread cutaneous, mucosal, and serosal ecchymoses and petechiae.

Pneumonic plague arises from primary exposure to infective respiratory droplets from a person or cat with respiratory plague or secondary to hematogenous spread in a patient with bubonic or septicemic plague. Pneumonic plague can also result from accidental inhalation of *Y. pestis* in the laboratory. Primary plague pneumonia generally begins as a lobular process and then extends by confluence, becoming lobar and then multilobar (Fig. 164-2). Plague organisms typically are most numerous in the alveoli. Secondary plague pneumonia begins more diffusely, with organisms usually most numerous in the interstitium. In untreated cases of both primary and secondary plague pneumo-

FIGURE 164-1 Left inguinal and femoral buboes, with surrounding edema and overlying desquamation.

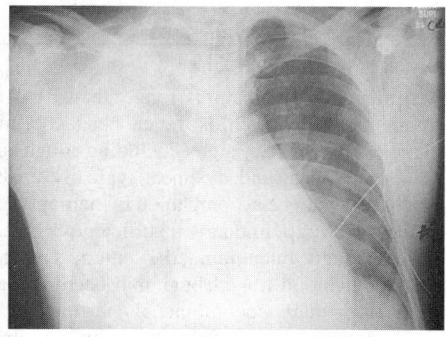

FIGURE 164-2 Sequential chest radiographs of a patient with fatal primary plague pneumonia. *Left:* Upright posteroanterior film taken at admission to hospital emergency department on third day of illness, showing segmental consolidation of right upper lobe. *Center:* Portable anteroposterior film taken 8 h after admission, showing extension of pneumonia to right middle and right lower lobes. *Right:* Portable anteroposterior film taken 13 h after admission (when patient had clinical ARDS), showing diffuse infiltration throughout right lung and patchy infiltration of left lower lung. A cavity later developed at the site of initial right upper lobe consolidation.

nia, diffuse hemorrhage, necrosis, and scant neutrophilic infiltration develop.

MANIFESTATIONS Plague is characterized by a rapid onset of fever and other systemic manifestations of gram-negative bacterial infection. If it is not quickly and correctly treated, plague can follow a toxic course, resulting in shock, multiple-organ failure, and death. In humans, the three principal forms of plague are bubonic, septicemic, and pneumonic. Bubonic plague, the most common form, is almost always caused by the bite of an infected flea but occasionally results from direct inoculation of infectious tissues or fluids. Septicemic and pneumonic plague can be either primary or secondary to metastatic spread. Unusual secondary forms include plague meningitis, endophthalmitis, and lymphadenitis at multiple sites. Primary plague pharyngitis has been documented by culture of organisms from throat swabs, but its clinical and epidemiologic features have not been completely described.

Bubonic plague usually has an incubation period of 2 to 6 days, occasionally longer. Typically, the patient experiences chills; fever, with temperatures that rise within hours to 38°C or higher; myalgias; arthralgias; headache; and a feeling of weakness. Soon—usually within 24 h—the patient notices tenderness and pain in one or more regional lymph nodes proximal to the site of inoculation of the plague bacillus (Fig. 164-1). Because fleas often bite the legs, femoral and inguinal nodes are most commonly involved; axillary and cervical nodes are next most commonly affected. The enlarging bubo becomes progressively painful and tender, sometimes exquisitely so. The patient usually guards against palpation and limits movement, pressure, and stretch around the bubo. The surrounding tissue often becomes edematous, sometimes markedly so, and the overlying skin may be erythematous, warm, and tense. Inspection of the skin surrounding or distal to the bubo sometimes reveals the site of a flea bite marked by a small papule, pustule, scab, or ulcer. Large eschars develop rarely (Fig. 164-3). A list of lymphadenitic conditions that could be confused with a plague bubo would include *Staphylococcus aureus* and group A beta-hemolytic streptococcal infections, cat-scratch disease, and tularemia. The bubo of plague is distinguishable from lymphadenitis of most other causes, however, by its rapid onset, its extreme tenderness, the accompanying signs of toxemia, and the absence of cellulitis or obvious ascending lymphangitis.

Treated in the uncomplicated state with an appropriate antibiotic, bubonic plague usually responds quickly, with defervescence and alleviation of other systemic manifestations over 2 to 5 days. Buboes often remain enlarged and tender for a week or more after the initiation of treatment and can become fluctuant. Without effective antimicrobial treatment, patients with typical bubonic plague manifest an increasingly toxic state of fever, tachycardia, lethargy leading to prostration, agitation and confusion, and (occasionally) convulsions and delirium. Secondary plague sepsis may result in an alarmingly rapid and refractory cascade of DIC, bleeding, shock, and organ failure. Mild forms of bubonic plague, called *pestis minor*, have been described in South America and elsewhere; in these cases, the patients are ambulatory, are only mildly febrile, and have subacute buboes.

Septicemic plague is a progressive, overwhelming bacterial infection. Primary septicemia develops in the absence of apparent regional lymphadenitis, and the diagnosis of plague often is not suspected until preliminary blood culture results are reported to be positive by the laboratory. *Y. pestis*, however, can also be cultured from the blood of most bubonic plague patients, and bacteremia should be distinguished from septicemia, in which the patient is desperately ill and requires aggressive care. Patients with septicemic plague often present with gastrointestinal symptoms of nausea, vomiting, diarrhea, and abdominal pain, which may further confound the correct diagnosis. If not treated early with appropriate antibiotics, septicemic plague can be fulminant and fatal. In the United States in 1950 through 1994, 64 cases of septicemic plague and 18 deaths were reported, for a case-fatality rate of 28 percent. Petechiae, ecchymoses, bleeding from puncture wounds and orifices, and gangrene of acral parts are manifestations of DIC; refractory hypotension, renal shutdown, obtundation, and other signs of shock are preterminal events. Adult respiratory distress syndrome (ARDS), which can occur at any stage of septicemic plague, is sometimes confused with other conditions such as Hantavirus pulmonary syndrome.

Of all forms of the disease, pneumonic plague develops most rapidly and is most frequently fatal. The incubation period for primary

FIGURE 164-3 Large abdominal ulceration with eschar at presumed site of inoculation of *Y. pestis* by flea bite, accompanied by right inguinal bubo and erythema of overlying skin.

pneumonic plague is rarely longer than 1 to 4 days. The onset is most often sudden, with chills, fever, headache, myalgias, weakness, and dizziness. Pulmonary signs, including cough, sputum production, chest pain, tachypnea, and dyspnea, typically arise on the second day of illness and may be accompanied by hemoptysis, increasing respiratory distress, cardiopulmonary insufficiency, and circulatory collapse. In primary plague pneumonia, the sputum is most often watery or mucoid, frothy, and blood-tinged, but it may become frankly bloody. Pulmonary signs in primary pneumonic plague may indicate involvement of a single lobe in the early stage, with rapidly developing segmental consolidation before bronchopneumonic spread to other lobes of the same and opposite lungs. Liquefaction necrosis and cavitation may occur early in areas of consolidation and may or may not leave significant residual scarring.

Secondary plague pneumonia manifests first as diffuse interstitial pneumonitis in which sputum production is scant; since the sputum is more likely to be inspissated and tenacious in character than the sputum found in primary pneumonia, it may be less infectious. In the United States in 1950 through 1994, 39 cases of secondary pneumonic plague and 7 cases of primary pneumonic plague were reported, with no known transmission to contacts and an overall case-fatality rate of 41 percent. Observers in the early twentieth century remarked on the relative lack of auscultatory findings, the usual presence of toxemia, and the frequency of sudden death in patients with pneumonic plague as compared to patients with other bacterial pneumonias.

Meningitis is an unusual manifestation of plague. In the United States, there were 12 meningitis cases among the 373 plague cases reported in 1950 through 1994. All cases of meningitis were complications of bubonic plague, and all patients survived. Although meningitis may be a part of the initial presentation of plague, its onset is often delayed and is a manifestation of insufficient treatment. Recent cases in the United States have occurred during the first and second weeks of antibiotic treatment for bubonic plague. Chronic relapsing meningeal plague over periods of weeks or even months was described in the preantibiotic era. The affected patients typically presented with fever, headache, meningismus, and pleocytosis.

Plague pharyngitis presents as fever, sore throat, cervical lymphadenitis, and headache and is often indistinguishable clinically from pharyngitis of other infectious etiologies. Caregivers working in plague-endemic areas must be alert to the possibility of plague to avoid misdiagnosis leading to delayed and/or inappropriate treatment.

LABORATORY FINDINGS AND DIAGNOSIS Since plague is a rare disease in the United States, a high index of clinical suspicion as well as the elicitation of a thorough clinical and epidemiologic history and a careful physical examination are required for timely diagnosis and prompt institution of specific therapy. When the diagnosis of plague is delayed or missed altogether, a high case-fatality rate results; infected travelers who seek medical care after they have left endemic areas (peripatetic plague cases) are at especially high risk. Plague should always be considered when a previously healthy person presents with septic shock in the southwestern United States. When the diagnosis of plague is being considered, close communication between clinicians and the diagnostic laboratory and between the diagnostic laboratory and a qualified reference laboratory is essential. Tests for plague are highly reliable when conducted by laboratory personnel experienced with *Y. pestis*, but such expertise is usually limited to selected reference laboratories, including state health department laboratories in some plague-endemic states and the CDC plague laboratory.

When plague is suspected, specimens should be collected promptly for laboratory studies, chest roentgenograms should be obtained, and specific antimicrobial therapy should be initiated pending confirmation. Appropriate diagnostic specimens for smear and culture include citrated or heparinized whole blood from all patients with suspected plague, bubo aspirates from those with suspected buboes, sputum samples or tracheal aspirates from those with suspected pneumonic

plague, and cerebrospinal fluid (CSF) from those with suspected plague meningitis. Since early buboes are often exquisitely tender and are seldom fluctuant or necrotic, these lesions usually require aspiration under local anesthesia and after surface decontamination with an injection of 1 to 2 mL of normal saline (sterile but nonbacteriostatic) through a 20- to 22-gauge needle. A variety of appropriate culture media (including brain-heart infusion broth, sheep blood agar, and MacConkey agar) should be inoculated with a portion of each specimen. Moreover, for each specimen, at least one smear should be examined immediately with Wayson or Giemsa stain and at least one with Gram's stain; a smear should also be submitted for direct fluorescent antibody testing. An acute-phase serum specimen should be tested for antibody to *Y. pestis*; whenever possible, a convalescent-phase serum specimen collected 3 to 4 weeks later should also be tested. When a patient dies and plague is suspected, appropriate autopsy tissues for culture and fluorescent antibody testing include buboes, all solid organs (especially liver, spleen, and lung), and bone marrow. If culture of such specimens is to be attempted, they should be sent to the laboratory either fresh or frozen on dry ice, not in preservatives or fixatives. If necessary, Cary-Blair or a similar medium can be used to transport *Y. pestis*–infected tissues.

Laboratory confirmation of plague depends on the isolation of *Y. pestis* from cultures of body fluids or tissues. Cultures of three blood samples taken over a 45-minute period before treatment will usually result in isolation of the bacterium. *Y. pestis* strains are readily distinguished from those of the closely related species *Yersinia pseudotuberculosis* by differences in biochemical profile, temperature-dependent susceptibility to lysis by a *Y. pestis*–specific bacteriophage, and motility. Automated bacteriologic test systems can be used to assist in the identification of isolates as *Y. pestis*, but such strains can be misidentified (e.g., as *Y. pseudotuberculosis*) or overlooked if these systems are improperly programmed.

In the absence of isolation of *Y. pestis*, plague cases can be confirmed by the demonstration of seroconversion (a fourfold or greater titer rise) to *Y. pestis* F1 antigen by passive hemagglutination testing of acute- and convalescent-phase serum specimens or by detection of an antibody titer of >128 in a single serum sample from a patient with a plague-compatible illness who has not received plague vaccine. The specificity of a positive passive-hemagglutination test requires confirmation with the F1 antigen hemagglutination-inhibition test. A few plague patients seroconvert to F1 antigen as early as 5 days after the onset of illness. Most seroconvert between 1 and 2 weeks after onset; a few seroconvert 3 weeks or more after onset; and a few (fewer than 5 percent) fail to seroconvert at all. Early, specific antibiotic treatment may delay seroconversion by several weeks. After seroconversion, positive serologic titers diminish gradually over months to years. Enzyme-linked immunosorbent assays (ELISAs) for IgM and IgG antibodies to *Y. pestis* have only recently been developed.

Detection of F1 antigen in tissues or fluids by direct fluorescent antibody testing is presumptive evidence of plague, as is an F1 antibody titer of >10 in a single serum sample from a patient with a plague-compatible illness who has not received plague vaccine. Visualization of characteristic bipolar bacilli in a Giemsa- or Wayson-stained smear constitutes supportive evidence of plague. Tularemia, especially the glandular, typhoidal, and pneumonic forms, can sometimes be confused clinically and epidemiologically with plague, but the results of microbiologic and serologic tests should readily distinguish these two diseases.

Patients with plague typically have white blood cell (WBC) counts of 15,000 to 25,000/μL, with a predominance of PMNs and a left shift. Leukemoid reactions with WBC counts as high as 100,000/μL can occur. Modest thrombocytopenia is usually documented, and fibrin-fibrinogen split products are often detected even in patients without frank DIC. Serum levels of aminotransferases and bilirubin may be elevated. Chest roentgenograms of patients with pneumonic plague usually show patchy bronchopneumonic infiltrates as well as lobar or segmental consolidation with or without confluence (Fig. 164-2); they occasionally show cavitation. Stained sputum samples usually contain PMNs and characteristic bipolar-staining bacilli. In

FIGURE 164-4 Peripheral blood smear from a patient with fatal plague septicemia and shock, showing characteristic bipolar-staining *Y. pestis* bacilli (Wright's stain, oil immersion).

Y. pestis septicemia, visualization of the characteristic bacilli in a routine blood smear or a buffy-coat smear is an uncommon but grave prognostic sign (Fig. 164-4). In patients with plague meningitis, pleocytosis with a predominance of PMNs is the rule, and the characteristic bacilli are usually visible in stained CSF smears.

℞ TREATMENT

Left untreated, plague is fatal in more than 50 percent of cases of bubonic disease and in nearly all cases of septicemic, pneumonic, and meningeal disease. The overall mortality rate for plague cases in the United States in the past 25 years has been ~15 percent; deaths are almost always due to delays in seeking treatment, misdiagnosis, delays in the institution of treatment, or incorrect treatment. Rapid diagnosis and appropriate antimicrobial therapy are essential.

Guidelines for the treatment of plague are given in Table 164-1. Streptomycin is the drug of choice. Alternative antibiotics include the tetracyclines and chloramphenicol; these agents are usually given orally with initial loading doses but may be given intravenously to critically ill patients and to patients unable to tolerate oral medication. Gentamicin is increasingly used for the treatment of plague in the United States because of its ready availability; it is probably as effective as streptomycin, although results of controlled studies have not yet been published. Penicillins, cephalosporins, and macrolides are suboptimal and should not be used. Doxycycline may be as effective as other tetracyclines or even more so, but comparative evaluations have not been made. Trimethoprim-sulfamethoxazole

has been used successfully to treat bubonic plague but is not considered a first-line choice. Chloramphenicol is indicated for the treatment of plague meningitis, pleuritis, endophthalmitis, and myocarditis because of its superior tissue penetration; it is used alone or in combination with streptomycin. In general, antimicrobial treatment should be continued for 10 days or for at least 3 days after the patient has become afebrile and has made a clinical recovery. Patients initially given intravenous antibiotics may be switched to oral regimens upon clinical improvement. Such improvement is usually evident 2 or 3 days after the start of treatment, even though fever may continue for several more days; as noted earlier, buboes can persist for days or even weeks.

Consequences of delayed treatment of plague include DIC, ARDS, and other complications of gram-negative sepsis. Patients with these disorders require intensive monitoring and close physiologic support, as outlined elsewhere (see Chaps. 118 and 265). Buboes may require surgical drainage. Abscessed nodes can cause recurrent fever in patients who have apparently recovered; this relation may be occult if intrathoracic or intraabdominal nodes are involved. Viable *Y. pestis* organisms have been isolated from affected nodes 1 to 2 weeks after clinical recovery from acute disease. Antibiotic-resistant strains of *Y. pestis* have rarely been identified, and the plague bacillus is considered to be genetically stable.

PREVENTION AND CONTROL Persons at greatest risk for plague in the United States are those who live, work, and participate in outdoor recreational activities in areas of those western states in which plague is enzootic. Surveillance, education, and environmental management are the cornerstones of prevention and control. A network of biologists and public health specialists coordinates these activities through local and state health departments and the CDC. Personal protective measures include the avoidance of areas with known epizootic plague (which may be posted) and of sick or dead animals; the use of repellents, insecticides, and protective clothing when at risk of exposure to rodents' fleas; and the wearing of gloves when handling animal carcasses. Short-term antibiotic prophylaxis (Table 164-2) is recommended for persons known to have had face-to-face or other direct contact with a patient with suspected or confirmed pneumonic plague; it may also be advisable occasionally for persons who are unable to avoid an area where a plague outbreak is in progress or who are caring for patients with plague. To decrease the risk of pneumonic transmission, all patients in whom plague is suspected should be placed in respiratory isolation (to prevent droplet spread) until pneumonia has been ruled out or until 48 h of specific antimicrobial therapy has been administered, after which only standard precautions are generally necessary.

Rodent food (garbage, pet food) and habitats (brush piles, junk heaps, woodpiles) should be eliminated in domestic, peridomestic,

Table 164-1

Guidelines for the Treatment of Plague

Drug	Daily Dosage	Interval, h	Route(s) of Administration
Streptomycin			
Adults	2 g	12	IM
Children	30 mg/kg	12	IM
Gentamicin			
Adults	4.5 mg/kg	8	IM or IV
Children	6.0–7.5 mg/kg	8	IM or IV
Infants/neonates	7.5 mg/kg	8	IM or IV
Tetracycline			
Adults	2 g	6	PO or IV
Children ≥9 y	25–50 mg/kg	6	PO or IV
Doxycycline			
Adults	200 mg	12 or 24	PO or IV
Children ≥9 y	4 mg/kg	12 or 24	PO or IV
Oxytetracycline			
Adults	250–300 mg	8, 12, or 24	PO or IM
Children ≥9 y	15–25 mg/kg	8, 12, or 24	PO or IM
Chloramphenicol			
Adults	75–100 mg/kg	6	PO or IV
Children ≥1 y	75–100 mg/kg	6	PO or IV

* Maximum, 250 mg/d.

SOURCE: Adapted with permission from DT Dennis, in *Conn's Current Therapy 1996*, RE Rakel (ed). Philadelphia, Saunders, 1996.

Table 164-2

Guidelines for Plague Prophylaxis

Drug	Daily Dosage	Interval, h	Route of Administration
Tetracycline			
Adults	1–2 g	6 or 12	PO
Children ≥9 y	25–50 mg/kg	6 or 12	PO
Doxycycline			
Adults	100–200 mg	12 or 24	PO
Children ≥9 y	2–4 mg/kg	12 or 24	PO
Trimethoprim-sulfamethoxazole			
Adults	1.6–3.2 g*	12	PO
Children ≥2 mo	40 mg/kg*	12	PO

* Sulfamethoxazole component.

SOURCE: Adapted with permission from DT Dennis, in *Conn's Current Therapy 1996*, RE Rakel (ed). Philadelphia, Saunders, 1996.

and working environments; buildings and food stores should be rodent-proofed. The control of fleas with insecticides is a key public health measure in situations where epizootic plague activity places humans at high risk; this effort includes dusting and spraying of rodent burrows, rodent runs, and other sites where rodents and their fleas are found. In plague-endemic areas of the western United States, persons should keep their dogs and cats free of fleas and restrained. The decision to control plague by killing rodents should be left to public health authorities, and such a program should be carried out only in conjunction with effective flea control. Killing of rodents has no lasting benefit without environmental sanitation.

A killed, whole-cell plague vaccine is available in the United States. The efficacy of this vaccine in humans has not been evaluated in controlled studies, although reviews of vaccine use during the Vietnam War provide indirect evidence that it is at least partially protective against plague transmitted by fleas. The vaccine does not appear to offer protection against primary pneumonic plague. As recommended by the manufacturer, primary immunization consists of a series of three injections followed by booster doses as warranted (at intervals of 6 months or more). The degree and duration of the immune response vary, and persons at continuing risk may need to have their antibody levels monitored. Adverse reactions are usually mild after injection of the first dose but may increase with repeated doses. Vaccination is recommended for laboratory personnel who routinely work with *Y. pestis* and should also be considered for persons whose vocation brings them into regular contact with wild rodents and their fleas in areas experiencing enzootic or epizootic plague. Military personnel in some situations are vaccinated, but vaccination is not routinely indicated for civilians living in areas with enzootic plague (such as the western United States), for medical personnel, for travelers to countries that have reported plague cases, or for the control of plague epidemics.

OTHER *YERSINIA* INFECTIONS

DEFINITION Yersiniosis is an uncommon bacterial zoonosis caused by infection with either of the two enteropathogenic *Yersinia* species: *Yersinia enterocolitica* or *Yersinia pseudotuberculosis*. Reservoir hosts of these bacteria include swine and other wild and domestic animals. These yersiniae are transmitted to humans predominantly via the oral route. Both sporadic cases and common-source outbreaks occur. The most frequent acute clinical manifestations are (1) enteritis or enterocolitis with self-limited diarrhea (especially with *Y. enterocolitica*), and (2) mesenteric adenitis and terminal ileitis (especially with *Y. pseudotuberculosis*), which can be difficult to distinguish from acute appendicitis. Septicemia and metastatic focal infections are less common. Some cases of yersiniosis are complicated by nonsuppurative, extraintestinal, inflammatory sequelae (e.g., reactive arthritis and erythema nodosum).

ETIOLOGIC AGENTS *Y. enterocolitica* and *Y. pseudotuberculosis* are pleomorphic gram-negative bacilli in the family Enterobacteriaceae. They are aerobic or facultatively anaerobic, motile at 25°C, nonmotile at 37°C, oxidase negative, urease positive, able to ferment glucose, unable to ferment lactose, and usually able to reduce nitrates. They grow well, if slowly, on nonselective media (e.g., blood agar) and on most of the routine media used to select for enteric bacteria (e.g., MacConkey agar). They can multiply within a wide temperature range (-1°C to 45°C). The most clinically and epidemiologically useful methods for identifying pathogenic *Y. enterocolitica* isolates are biotyping based on biochemical profiles and serotyping according to somatic O and H antigens. Six biotypes and more than 60 serotypes of *Y. enterocolitica* are recognized. A separate serotyping system for *Y. pseudotuberculosis* (also based on somatic antigens) has distinguished six major serotypes (I through VI) and their subtypes.

EPIDEMIOLOGY *Y. enterocolitica* is distributed worldwide and has been isolated from soil, fresh water, contaminated foodstuffs (e.g., meat, milk, and vegetables), and a wide variety of wild and domestic animals, including mammals, birds, amphibians, fish, and shellfish. Many serotypes isolated from environmental sources, however, evidently are not human pathogens. Most human infections have been caused by *Y. enterocolitica* serotypes O:3, O:5, O:8, and O:9, which are primarily associated with wild and domestic mammals. The incidence of these infections and their sequelae is highest in Scandinavia and some other northern European countries, but this observation may be in part an artifact of underrecognition in other countries. Because many individuals with enteric *Y. enterocolitica* infection are asymptomatic or minimally symptomatic and do not seek medical attention, reliable population-based estimates of incidence are unavailable. However, in many clinical microbiology laboratories in recent decades, *Y. enterocolitica* has been the fourth most common bacterial pathogen isolated from patients' fecal specimens, trailing *Salmonella* (the most frequently isolated), *Campylobacter*, and *Shigella* species. In one multistate pediatric study in the United States, *Y. enterocolitica* strains were isolated from 1 percent of submitted fecal specimens and accounted for 16 percent of all bacterial pathogens isolated from fecal samples. This yield was comparable to that of *Shigella* or *Campylobacter* and about 40 percent as great as that of *Salmonella*.

All age groups are susceptible to *Y. enterocolitica* infections, but the majority of cases of enterocolitis are in children aged 1 to 4. Moreover, these infections show a modest predilection for males. Mesenteric adenitis and terminal ileitis are most common among older children and young adults. Risk factors for *Y. enterocolitica* septicemia and metastatic focal infections include chronic liver disease, malignancy, diabetes mellitus, immunosuppressive therapy, alcoholism, malnutrition, advanced age, iron overload (see below), and hemolytic anemias (including the thalassemias). The nonsuppurative sequelae of yersiniosis are most common among adults. HLA-B27 is expressed in 70 to 80 percent of patients who develop reactive arthritis associated with yersiniosis. HLA-B27 is not a risk factor for *Yersinia*-induced erythema nodosum; females with this condition outnumber males by 2 to 1. In Europe, *Y. enterocolitica* infections are more common in the cooler months than in warmer weather. In North America, no consistent seasonal pattern has been documented.

For several decades, serotypes O:3 and O:9 have predominated among *Y. enterocolitica* isolates from patients in Europe. Serotype O:3 has also predominated in Canada and Japan. In the United States, serotype O:3 emerged in the 1980s to surpass serotype O:8 in frequency of isolation from patients. The incidence of *Yersinia*-induced nonsuppurative sequelae reportedly is 10 to 30 percent in Scandinavia and much lower in most other countries, including the United States. No convincing explanation for this observation has been confirmed, but reasonable possibilities include population genetic factors and geographic strain variation.

Common-source outbreaks of *Y. enterocolitica* enteritis have been traced to such vehicles as raw milk, contaminated pasteurized milk, and foods prepared with contaminated fresh water. In Belgium, the ingestion of ground raw pork (a regional custom) is a significant risk factor for sporadic infection with *Y. enterocolitica* serotypes O:3 and O:9. These serotypes commonly colonize the oral cavity and intestines of European swine, and *Y. enterocolitica* infection is an occupational risk of swine butchers in Europe. In the United States, sporadic cases and one outbreak of *Y. enterocolitica* O:3 infection have been associated with the preparation or ingestion of raw pork intestines (chitterlings). In some cases of yersiniosis, circumstantial evidence suggests transmission via contact with dogs and cats or their feces. Several nosocomial outbreaks of *Y. enterocolitica* infection have been described; fecal-oral transmission from person to person was suspected. Fecal-oral transmission among family members may also explain occasional secondary cases in households. In a prospective study of 50 children with *Y. enterocolitica* enteritis, fecal excretion of the organism persisted for an average of 27 days (range, 4 to 79 days) after the cessation of symptoms. A chronic carrier state, however, has not been demonstrated. *Y. enterocolitica* is a rare but often lethal cause of transfusion-associated septicemia. The explanation is that blood donors occasionally have transient, occult *Y. enterocolitica* bacteremia and that this organism can slowly multiply to high concentrations in blood refrigerated for at least 10 to 20 days.

The ecology of *Y. pseudotuberculosis* seems to parallel that of *Y. enterocolitica* closely. *Y. pseudotuberculosis* is also widespread in wild and domestic animals and is isolated from many environmental sources. Human infections with *Y. pseudotuberculosis*, however, appear to be rare. In North America and Europe, most such infections have been with serotype I, but outbreaks involving other serotypes have occurred in Japan and Scandinavia. Swine appear to be an important reservoir for pathogenic strains of *Y. pseudotuberculosis*.

PATHOGENESIS AND PATHOLOGY Except in rare instances of transmission via contaminated blood products or direct cutaneous inoculation, the enteropathogenic yersiniae are thought to enter the host via the oral route. The 50 percent infectious dose in humans is uncertain but may be $\geq 10^9$. The incubation period averages 5 days (range, 1 to 11 days). Studies of animals have shown that the organisms initially invade the ileal epithelium, then are translocated via M cells into the lamina propria, and finally enter Peyer's patches, where they are able to replicate. They subsequently drain into the mesenteric lymph nodes, which undergo hyperplasia and from which the bacteria can be distributed systemically. The mesenteric lymph nodes can become intensely swollen and matted and are occasionally detected on physical examination as a tender right lower quadrant mass. Intestinal inflammation (most commonly of the distal ileum and less commonly of the ascending colon) develops and may be accompanied by mucosal ulcerations and by the shedding of PMNs and red blood cells into the intestinal lumen. In relatively severe cases, thrombosis of mesenteric blood vessels, intestinal hemorrhage, and necrosis can occur. In patients with enteropathogenic yersinial infections who undergo exploratory laparotomy, the appendix usually is histologically normal or shows only lymphoid hyperplasia, but frank suppuration is sometimes evident.

A plasmid of ~70 kb is essential for virulence of the enteropathogenic yersiniae because it encodes at least six *Yersinia* outer-membrane proteins, some of which confer to bacterial strains such properties as cytotoxicity; resistance to phagocytosis by PMNs; and the ability to suppress the host's expression of tumor necrosis factor α, to interfere with platelet aggregation and host complement activation, and to dephosphorylate host proteins. A chromosomal gene (*inv*) encodes for the surface protein invasin, which is necessary for yersinial invasion of nonphagocytic host cells (e.g., epithelial cells) in vitro and which facilitates the translocation of bacteria across the intestinal epithelium. Both *Y. enterocolitica* and *Y. pseudotuberculosis* can express at least one protein superantigen that selectively stimulates the proliferation of T cells. Many strains of *Y. enterocolitica* produce a heat-stable enterotoxin that is similar to *Escherichia coli* enterotoxin. The cell walls of *Y. enterocolitica* and *Y. pseudotuberculosis* contain a lipopolysaccharide (endotoxin). The roles of superantigens, enterotoxin, and endotoxin in the pathogenesis of yersiniosis are unclear. Some *Yersinia* strains are unable to synthesize bacterial iron chelators called *siderophores*. However, they can exploit host-chelated iron stores and the drug deferoxamine (a siderophore produced by *Streptomyces pilosus*). Therefore, iron overload (e.g., caused by hemodialysis or multiple transfusions) and deferoxamine therapy appear to be independent risk factors for *Y. enterocolitica* bacteremia (especially that involving serotypes O:3 and O:9) and to a lesser degree for *Y. pseudotuberculosis* bacteremia.

Immunogenetic factors are clearly involved in the pathogenesis of reactive arthritis following infection with the enteropathogenic yersiniae. As noted above, most patients with *Yersinia*-induced reactive arthritis express HLA-B27. In addition, *Y. pseudotuberculosis* shares at least one cross-reactive epitope with HLA-B27. In patients with reactive arthritis following *Y. enterocolitica* infection, yersinial antigens are commonly detectable in synovial fluid cells in the apparent absence of whole organisms. Thus, it is unknown whether the arthritis results from occult bacterial persistence through self-tolerance of HLA-B27 with a failure of cross-reactive immune responses to yersiniae, from an immune response to common antigenic determinants shared by the bacteria and host HLA-B27 (i.e., molecular mimicry), or from other mechanisms. Local T cell immune responses appear to be particularly important in the pathogenesis of reactive arthritis. The pathogenesis of *Yersinia*-induced erythema nodosum is obscure.

In some assays, patients with Graves' disease have an increased prevalence of serum antibodies to *Y. enterocolitica*, and the immunoglobulins of patients recovering from *Y. enterocolitica* infections react with the human thyroid-stimulating hormone receptor. However, a link between *Y. enterocolitica* infection and the subsequent development of autoimmune thyroiditis has not been convincingly demonstrated.

MANIFESTATIONS The principal clinical manifestations of *Y. enterocolitica* infection are enteritis, enterocolitis, mesenteric adenitis, and terminal ileitis. Less common manifestations include exudative pharyngitis, septicemia, metastatic focal infections, reactive polyarthritis, and erythema nodosum. When age groups are combined, the most common presentation of *Y. enterocolitica* infection is acute diarrhea from enteritis or enterocolitis. Low-grade fever and cramping abdominal pain occur in most cases, nausea and vomiting in 15 to 40 percent, hematochezia in up to 30 percent, and a generalized maculopapular skin rash in a few cases. Diarrhea persists for an average of 2 weeks (range, 1 day to many months), during which the frequency of bowel movements diminishes. Uncommonly, enteritis or enterocolitis can be complicated by severe abdominal pain and high fever. Rare (and sometimes fatal) complications include diffuse inflammation, ulceration, hemorrhage, and necrosis of the small bowel and colon; intestinal perforation; peritonitis; ascending cholangitis; mesenteric vein thrombosis; diverticulitis; toxic megacolon; and ileocecal intussusception.

The syndrome of mesenteric adenitis and terminal ileitis without diarrhea is easily confused with appendicitis. Low-grade fever and right lower quadrant pain, tenderness, guarding, and rebound tenderness are common. During six recognized common-source outbreaks in the United States, 10 percent of 444 patients with symptomatic undiagnosed *Y. enterocolitica* infections underwent laparotomy for suspected appendicitis; surgical incisions became infected with *Y. enterocolitica* in a few of these cases.

Acute pharyngitis and pharyngotonsillitis, with or without cervical adenitis or intestinal illness, are less common but potentially lethal manifestations of *Y. enterocolitica* infection, particularly in adults. *Y. enterocolitica* septicemia generally presents as a severe illness with fever and leukocytosis, often with abdominal pain and jaundice and without localized signs of infection. Metastatic focal *Y. enterocolitica* infections can occur with or without clinically apparent bacteremia and can affect almost any organ system. Examples include abscess formation (e.g., in liver, spleen, kidney, lung, skeletal muscle, lymph node, or cutaneous tissue), osteomyelitis, meningitis, peritonitis, urinary tract infection, pneumonia, empyema, endocarditis, pericarditis, mycotic aneurysm, septic arthritis, suppurative conjunctivitis, panophthalmitis, Parinaud's oculoglandular syndrome, and cutaneous pustules or bullae.

In Scandinavia, the incidence of reactive arthritis following *Y. enterocolitica* infection among adults is estimated to be at least 10 percent. About 80 percent of these patients have preceding symptoms such as fever, diarrhea, or abdominal pain. Typically, these symptoms precede the arthritis by 1 week and are of short duration. The most commonly affected joints are the knees and ankles, but other joints can be involved. Typically, multiple (two to eight) joints become involved sequentially and asymmetrically over a period of a few days to 2 weeks, after which no additional joints are affected. Monoarticular arthritis occurs less commonly. In two-thirds of cases, the acute arthritis remits spontaneously within 1 to 3 months. Chronic joint disease is documented in a minority of cases. A few HLA-B27-positive patients with *Y. enterocolitica*–induced arthritis have subsequent ankylosing spondylitis, but this development is best explained by the fact that HLA-B27 is a major risk factor for each of these diseases. Mild, self-limited myocarditis accompanies about 10 percent of cases of *Yersinia*-induced arthritis and can occur independently. Typical manifestations include cardiac murmurs and transient electrocardiographic abnormalities, including prolongation of the PR interval and nonspecific ST-segment and T-wave changes. The syndrome of *Yersinia*-induced arthritis and carditis can be confused with acute rheumatic fever. In Scandinavia, erythema nodosum occurs in 15 to 20 percent of patients with yersiniosis, usually within a few days to 3 weeks after the onset of intestinal illness. Lesions typically are located on the lower extremities and resolve within 1 month. Less commonly reported nonsuppurative sequelae of *Y. enterocolitica* infections include reactive uveitis, iritis, conjunctivitis, urethritis, and glomerulonephritis. The complete triad of Reiter's syndrome (arthritis, conjunctivitis, and urethritis) is seen in 5 to 10 percent of patients with *Yersinia*-induced arthritis.

The most common clinical presentation of *Y. pseudotuberculosis* infection is fever and abdominal pain caused by mesenteric adenitis; diarrheal illness is less common than in *Y. enterocolitica* infection. Systemic manifestations, including septicemia, focal infections, reactive arthritis, and erythema nodosum, generally are similar to those associated with *Y. enterocolitica* infection. In addition, *Y. pseudotuberculosis* has been associated with a scarlet fever–like syndrome, acute interstitial nephritis, and hemolytic-uremic syndrome.

LABORATORY FINDINGS AND DIAGNOSIS Results of routine laboratory tests in most patients with yersiniosis are nonspecific. Leukocyte counts are usually normal or slightly elevated, often with a modest left shift. Standard microbiologic methods are sufficient to isolate *Y. enterocolitica* and *Y. pseudotuberculosis* from otherwise-sterile sites, such as blood, CSF, lymph node tissue, and peritoneal fluid, and from abscesses. Isolation of these organisms from feces is impeded by their slow growth and the overgrowth of normal fecal flora on culture media routinely used to select for enteric bacteria. When routine enteric media are used, the yield of yersinial isolates from feces is increased by incubation at 22 to 25°C for 48 h. The yield from feces and other grossly contaminated specimens can be further increased by the use of *Yersinia*-selective cefsulodin-Irgasan-novobiocin (CIN) agar and by cold enrichment (i.e., inoculation of feces into buffered saline and incubation at 4°C for 2 to 4 weeks, with periodic plating onto enteric media). Because bacteriologic procedures designed to isolate yersiniae from feces are not considered cost-effective, many laboratories undertake them by special request only.

The results of serologic tests can be used to support a diagnosis of yersiniosis. Agglutination tests or ELISAs are used most commonly. The existence of multiple serotypes makes routine serologic tests laborious; thus these tests are generally conducted only in research laboratories or large commercial laboratories. Since these tests are experimental and are neither standardized nor well validated, and since some strains of *Yersinia* cross-react with other bacteria (e.g., *Brucella*, *Salmonella*, and *Vibrio*) and with serum from some patients with thyroiditis, results should be interpreted with caution. In typical uncomplicated cases of yersiniosis, agglutinin titers begin to rise within the first week of illness, peak in the second week, and then gradually diminish and return to normal within 3 to 6 months, although agglutinating antibody may remain detectable for several years in some cases. Because an initial serum specimen is often collected a week or more after the onset of illness, when agglutinin titers are already high, it is usually impossible to document a fourfold or greater rise in titer between paired specimens (although a fourfold or greater fall in titer may be found).

In patients with *Yersinia*-induced reactive arthritis, synovial fluid is sterile and the leukocyte count ranges from a few hundred to 60,000/µL, with a majority of PMNs. The erythrocyte sedimentation rate is often >100 mm/h. Rheumatoid factor and antinuclear antibodies are usually absent. The diagnosis of *Yersinia*-induced reactive arthritis or other nonsuppurative inflammatory sequelae can be difficult, especially when triggering infections are asymptomatic or clinically mild or occur several weeks before the diagnosis is attempted. Because the isolation of a pathogenic *Yersinia* strain from feces is the most specific diagnostic test in such cases, it should be attempted. Since culture is of limited sensitivity in this clinical setting, a high index of suspicion and positive results of serologic tests for *Y. enterocolitica* or *Y. pseudotuberculosis* usually are required for diagnosis.

℞ **TREATMENT**
The effectiveness of antimicrobial agents in the treatment of yersinial enteritis, enterocolitis, mesenteric adenitis, or terminal ileitis has not been established. These conditions are usually self-limited, and their treatment is symptom-based and supportive. In uncomplicated cases, diarrhea should be treated with fluid and electrolyte replacement, with the route of delivery dependent on clinical severity. Enteric precautions are advisable for patients hospitalized with yersinial diarrhea. In general, antimicrobial treatment should be reserved for patients with septicemia, metastatic focal infections, or immunosuppression and enterocolitis. Controlled clinical comparisons of antimicrobial agents in the treatment of severe cases of yersiniosis have not yet been conducted. In such cases, drug selection should ultimately be guided by clinical response and bacterial sensitivity patterns. Clinical isolates of *Y. enterocolitica* and *Y. pseudotuberculosis* are usually susceptible in vitro to aminoglycosides, third-generation cephalosporins, chloramphenicol, quinolones, tetracyclines, and trimethoprim-sulfamethoxazole. In laboratory animals infected with enteropathogenic yersiniae, the fluoroquinolones have exerted the strongest bactericidal effects in vivo; clinical experience with these drugs against these pathogens in humans is promising but limited. Because they produce β-lactamases, isolates typically are resistant to penicillin, ampicillin, carbenicillin, and first-generation and most second-generation cephalosporins. Optimal dosages and durations of therapy have not been established. Mortality from *Y. enterocolitica* septicemia has been estimated at 25 to 50 percent despite treatment. However, in a recent retrospective, population-based study of 53 cases in France, mortality was 7.5 percent. Focal extraintestinal infections may require at least 3 weeks of therapy. No role for antimicrobial agents in the management of the nonsuppurative inflammatory manifestations of yersiniosis has been established. Patients with reactive arthritis may benefit from treatment with nonsteroidal anti-inflammatory drugs, intraarticular steroid injections, and physical therapy.

PREVENTION AND CONTROL The importance of safe food-handling and food-preparation practices in the prevention of yersiniosis cannot be overemphasized. Caution is particularly warranted in the case of pork and other animal products. The consumption of raw or undercooked meats, especially pork, should be avoided. Increased efforts to prevent the spread of enteric pathogens in household, pet-care, day-care, and hospital settings and in the food industry would be likely to decrease the incidence of yersiniosis. Current regulations of the Food and Drug Administration require visual inspection of packed red cell units before transfusion, with the discarding of units in which bacterial contamination is suspected on the basis of darkening (reflecting decreased oxygen saturation and hemolysis). Since the risk is minimal, more specific measures to further decrease the likelihood of transfusion of *Y. enterocolitica*–contaminated blood products (e.g., limiting the period for which red cells can be stored before transfusion) are not considered cost-effective.

Yersiniosis is not routinely reportable to public health authorities in most jurisdictions. However, clinicians who suspect a common-source outbreak (e.g., because they have documented a familial case cluster or have diagnosed the disease in several apparently unrelated patients over a short period) or some other public health threat (e.g., because they have found occult *Y. enterocolitica* bacteremia in a recent blood donor) should consult promptly with local public health officials.

BIBLIOGRAPHY

PLAGUE

BARNES AM: Surveillance and control of bubonic plague in the United States, in *Animal Disease in Relation to Animal Conservation*, MA Edwards, U McDonnell (eds). New York, Academic Press, 1982, p 237

BRUBAKER RR: Factors promoting acute and chronic diseases caused by yersiniae. Clin Microbiol Rev 4:309, 1991

Butler T: *Yersinia* infections: Centennial of the discovery of the plague bacillus. Clin Infect Dis 19:655, 1994

Campbell GL, Hughes JM: Plague in India: A new warning from an old nemesis; editorial. Ann Intern Med 122:151, 1995

Centers for Disease Control and Prevention: Prevention of plague: Recommendations of the Advisory Committee on Immunization Practices (ACIP). Morb Mort Week Rep 45(RR-14):1, 1996

Craven RB et al: Reported cases of human plague infections in the United States, 1970–1991. J Med Entomol 30:758, 1993

Leary SE et al: Active immunization with recombinant V antigen from *Yersinia pestis* protects mice against plague. Infect Immun 63:2854, 1995

Nakajima R et al: Suppression of cytokines in mice by protein A-V antigen fusion peptide and restoration of synthesis by active immunization. Infect Immun 63:3021, 1995

Politzer R: *Plague.* WHO monograph series 22:1. Geneva, World Health Organization, 1954

Russell P et al: Doxycycline or ciprofloxacin prophylaxis and therapy against experimental *Yersinia pestis* infection in mice. J Antimicrob Chemother 37:769, 1996

OTHER YERSINIA INFECTIONS

Beuscher HU et al: Bacterial evasion of host immune defense: *Yersinia enterocolitica* encodes a suppressor for tumor necrosis factor alpha expression. Infect Immun 63:1270, 1995

Bottone EJ: *Yersinia enterocolitica.* A panoramic view of a charismatic microorganism. CRC Crit Rev Microbiol 5:211, 1977

——— (ed): *Yersinia enterocolitica.* Boca Raton, FL, CRC Press, 1981

Brubaker RR: Factors promoting acute and chronic diseases caused by yersiniae. Clin Microbiol Rev 4:309, 1991

Cover TL, Aber RC: *Yersinia enterocolitica.* N Engl J Med 321:16, 1989

Gayraud M et al: Antibiotic treatment of *Yersinia enterocolitica* septicemia: A retrospective review of 43 cases. Clin Infect Dis 17:405, 1993

Hermann E et al: HLA-B27-restricted CD8 T cells derived from synovial fluids of patients with reactive arthritis and ankylosing spondylitis. Lancet 342:646, 1993

Kihlstrom E et al: Intestinal symptoms and serological response in patients with complicated and uncomplicated *Yersinia enterocolitica* infections. Scand J Infect Dis 24:57, 1992

Lee LA et al: *Yersinia enterocolitica* O:3: An emerging cause of pediatric gastroenteritis in the United States. J Infect Dis 163:660, 1991

Leino R et al: Yersiniosis as a gastrointestinal disease. Scand J Infect Dis 19:63, 1987

Ostroff SM et al: Clinical features of sporadic *Yersinia enterocolitica* infections in Norway. J Infect Dis 166:812, 1992

Pepe JC, Miller VL: *Yersinia enterocolitica* invasin: A primary role in the initiation of infection. Proc Natl Acad Sci USA 90:6473, 1993

Preston MA et al: Antimicrobial susceptibility of pathogenic *Yersinia enterocolitica* isolated in Canada from 1972 to 1990. Antimicrob Agents Chemother 38:2121, 1994

Resetkova E et al: Seroreactivity to bacterial antigens is not a unique phenomenon in patients with autoimmune thyroid diseases in Canada. Thyroid 4:269, 1994

Tauxe RV et al: *Yersinia enterocolitica* infections and pork: The missing link. Lancet 1:1129, 1987

Zhang Y et al: Antibiotic prophylaxis and treatment of reactive arthritis. Lessons from an animal model. Arthritis Rheum 39:1238, 1996

165 *Lucy Stuart Tompkins*

BARTONELLA INFECTIONS, INCLUDING CAT-SCRATCH DISEASE

Bartonella species, including *B. bacilliformis, B. henselae,* and *B. quintana,* are tiny gram-negative bacilli that can invade mammalian cells, including endothelial cells and erythrocytes. Previously classified as *Rochalimaea* species within the rickettsia group, *Bartonella* species have now been removed from the order Rickettsiales on the grounds that they are not obligate intracellular parasites. These agents cause a wide spectrum of clinical illnesses, including trench fever, cat-scratch disease (CSD), bacillary angiomatosis, endocarditis, Oroya fever, and verruga peruana. The pathologic manifestations of *Bartonella* disease vary with the immune status of the host.

OROYA FEVER AND VERRUGA PERUANA

DEFINITION Oroya fever and verruga peruana are caused by *B. bacilliformis.* Oroya fever is characterized by fever, profound anemia, and—unless antibiotic treatment is given—high mortality. The lesions referred to as verruga peruana may develop during the convalescent phase of Oroya fever or during chronic infection with *B. bacilliformis.* In 1885 Daniel Carrión, a Peruvian medical student, inoculated himself with blood from a patient with verruga peruana and subsequently died of Oroya fever, thus proving that both diseases are caused by a single agent.

EPIDEMIOLOGY Infection with *B. bacilliformis* follows the bite of the sandfly vector *Phlebotomus,* an insect found in the river valleys of the Andes Mountains at altitudes of 600 to 2500 m. Oroya fever develops in nonimmune individuals who are not residents of the endemic region, whereas verruga peruana occurs in persons who apparently have been exposed in the past, including those who have recently had Oroya fever. The disease has rarely been described in the United States.

PATHOLOGY During initial infection in the nonimmune host, *B. bacilliformis* cells adhere to erythrocytes and produce indentations in the cell membrane; the bacteria subsequently enter the erythrocytes and cause persistent deformation of the cytoskeleton. The parasitized erythrocytes are ultimately phagocytosed and destroyed. Although the life span of infected erythrocytes is markedly shortened, not all of this change can be attributed to the mechanical fragility induced by the internalization of bacteria. Decreased bone marrow erythropoiesis also contributes to anemia.

CLINICAL MANIFESTATIONS The onset of symptoms in Oroya fever may be either insidious or abrupt, after an incubation period of approximately 3 weeks. The subacute presentation may include low-grade fever, malaise, headache, and anorexia. Sudden-onset disease commences with high fever, chills, diaphoresis, headaches, and changes in mental status. These manifestations are followed by the sudden development of profound anemia, which is due to a marked decrease in erythrocyte numbers and is associated with macrocytic changes, poikilocytosis, Howell-Jolly bodies, nucleated erythrocytes, and immature myeloid cells. The leukocyte differential usually shifts to the left, although the total leukocyte count may be normal. The erythrocyte count may fall to extremely low levels. In eosin/thiazine-stained peripheral-blood smears, numerous microorganisms can be seen adhering to most erythrocytes.

During the acute phase, muscle and joint pain and headache may be severe; central nervous system changes include insomnia, delirium, and decreased level of consciousness. Thrombocytopenic purpura may develop. If the patient survives, a convalescent phase ensues, characterized by the sudden disappearance of bacteria from blood smears, declining fever, and an increase in the erythrocyte count. While much of the mortality associated with Oroya fever is due to profound anemia and toxicity, secondary bacterial infections (including salmonellosis and other enteric infections, malaria, and tuberculosis) are often an important contributing factor.

After convalescence from acute Oroya fever, verrugas may develop. These red or purple cutaneous lesions may be either tiny and sessile or large, pedunculated, and nodular. They bear a marked resemblance to the lesions of bacillary angiomatosis and to Kaposi's sarcoma.

DIAGNOSIS During acute infection, bacteria can be cultured from the blood on agar containing rabbit blood, with incubation at 28°C. The hallmark of verruga peruana is the formation of new blood vessels (angiogenesis) at the sites of bacterial replication.

℞ **TREATMENT**

Oroya fever responds to a variety of antimicrobial agents, including chloramphenicol, tetracyclines, penicillin, and streptomycin. Chloramphenicol is used most often because of its efficacy against most

Salmonella infections (as salmonellosis may develop intercurrently). Verruga peruana may respond similarly; however, failure to respond to therapy and relapse are common and require the reinstitution of prolonged therapy.

BACILLARY ANGIOMATOSIS

DEFINITION AND ETIOLOGY Bacillary angiomatosis was initially described as a condition occurring primarily in patients with AIDS and characterized by vascular cutaneous lesions resembling Kaposi's sarcoma. The disease can disseminate to involve virtually any organ system. Immunocompromised individuals, especially those infected with human immunodeficiency virus (HIV), are at particularly high risk for bacillary angiomatosis, although in rare instances the patient is not obviously immunosuppressed. Both *B. henselae* and *B. quintana* (the infectious agent initially associated with trench fever) produce bacillary angiomatosis in persons with immunodeficiency.

EPIDEMIOLOGY Acquisition of *B. henselae* has been significantly associated with exposure to young cats infested with fleas (*Ctenocephalides felis*). Since a high percentage of cats are seropositive, it has been suggested that patients with HIV infection avoid exposure to these animals. The recent finding that a large proportion of cats with fleas have persistent asymptomatic *B. henselae* bacteremia suggests that the domestic cat is the animal reservoir of this microorganism. The flea may serve as a transmitting vector in the cross-infection of cats, but its role in human infection is not clear. Tick-associated cases of *B. henselae* bacteremia have been reported in healthy immunocompetent individuals.

Person-to-person transmission of *B. quintana* by the human body louse (*Pediculus humanis corporis*) was documented during World War I under conditions of poor personal hygiene and sanitation. Recent cases of infection have most often involved homeless people; the implication is that ectoparasites, including mites and lice, may transmit infection from person to person. However, this point has not been proven, and the reservoir of *B. quintana* has not been identified.

MICROBIOLOGY *B. henselae* can be demonstrated in tissue by Warthin-Starry staining. Clumps and clusters of pleomorphic bacilli appear as purple deposits in tissue stained with hematoxylin and eosin. Although the bacteria may be difficult to cultivate in the laboratory, they can eventually be isolated from cultures of blood and of material from other sites. Colonies develop after prolonged incubation (1 to 4 weeks) on blood-containing media; bacterial cells are gram-negative.

Classification of *B. henselae* was first accomplished when molecular techniques were used to analyze bacterial ribosomal genes extracted from tissue samples. Definitive identification of *Bartonella* species is based on sequence analysis of 16S ribosomal DNA.

PATHOGENESIS AND PATHOLOGY Bacillary angiomatosis is characterized by a lobular proliferation of new blood vessels (angiogenesis) and a neutrophilic inflammatory response to myriad bacilli located within collagen-rich microscopic and macroscopic nodules. The endothelial cells lining the vascular spaces have a typical epithelioid appearance, and the lesions may resemble Kaposi's sarcoma histopathologically, although the characteristic spindle cell of the latter disease is usually absent. The bacterial and eukaryotic host factors that elicit the pathologic response are unknown.

CLINICAL MANIFESTATIONS The skin lesions of bacillary angiomatosis (also called *epithelioid angiomatosis*) are vascular nodules, papules, or tumors that range from tiny lesions resembling cherry angiomas or pyogenic granulomas to large, pedunculated, exophytic masses (Fig. 165-1). Characteristically, the lesions are red or purple, resembling Kaposi's sarcoma; they may be surrounded by an epithelial collarette, may be located anywhere on the skin, and may involve mucous membranes. The overlying epidermis may be focally ulcerated, and the underlying bone may be invaded and destroyed.

Dissemination of *B. henselae* infection occurs primarily in patients with cellular immune defects. Clinical manifestations accompanying

FIGURE 165-1 Characteristic skin lesion of bacillary angiomatosis in an HIV-positive young woman. This large, pedunculated tumor exhibits the typical angiomatous appearance. The patient was treated with oral erythromycin, with nearly complete resolution of the lesion; however, upon discontinuation of antibiotic therapy after a 4-week course, the lesion recurred.

dissemination are often nonspecific and include persistent fever, abdominal pain, weight loss, and malaise. Although the liver, spleen, bone marrow, and lymph nodes are primarily affected, HIV-infected patients may also develop central nervous system abnormalities (including psychiatric disorders and brain lesions), which are responsive to antibiotic therapy. Skin lesions usually are not evident in disseminated infection. Involvement of the liver or spleen may produce bacillary peliosis hepatis. Patients with the latter condition may report localized pain on palpation of the abdomen. Nodular lesions of variable size can be demonstrated by computed tomography or magnetic resonance imaging, with or without contrast agents.

DIAGNOSIS The diagnosis of bacillary angiomatosis is based primarily on the typical histopathologic findings of angiomas in association with clumps of tiny bacilli revealed by Warthin-Starry silver stain. Infection due to *B. henselae* can also be established by culture or by identification of specific DNA sequences. *B. henselae* is most easily isolated from blood through a lysis-centrifugation system. Colonies may be detected on blood-containing agar (rabbit blood is preferred) incubated with 5 to 10% CO_2 at 37°C for 2 to 4 weeks. *B. quintana* may be isolated from BACTEC (Becton Dickinson, Sparks, MD) aerobic bottles containing resin. Isolation from skin lesions and other tissues is more difficult but should be attempted when feasible. Initial reports suggested that cocultivation with endothelial cell monolayers was necessary; however, isolation by direct plating onto freshly prepared agar media has also been successful. Bacilli picked from new colonies but not subcultured may not stain, even with acridine orange; they stain weakly with safranin. Identification of *B. henselae* and *B. quintana* is based primarily on cellular fatty-acid analysis and on polymerase chain reaction (PCR)-based restriction fragment length polymorphism analysis. Definitive identification of *Bartonella* species depends on DNA sequence analysis of 16S ribosomal RNA genes. The diagnosis of CSD (see next section) can be made by specific serologic testing that detects *B. henselae*-specific antibodies, but the sensitivity and specificity of this method in patients with cutaneous and disseminated bacillary angiomatosis have not been determined.

DIFFERENTIAL DIAGNOSIS The differential diagnosis of cutaneous bacillary angiomatosis includes Kaposi's sarcoma, angiomas, and pyogenic granulomas. These conditions can be distinguished by histopathologic examination of biopsied material.

Cutaneous bacillary angiomatosis caused by *B. henselae* or *B. quintana* resembles verruga peruana, which is not seen outside of South America. In patients with AIDS, Kaposi's sarcoma lesions and bacillary angiomatosis may coexist.

 TREATMENT

Cutaneous lesions have been treated with a wide variety of antimicrobial drugs, including macrolides, tetracyclines, and antituberculous agents; *B. henselae* is susceptible to most antibiotics in vitro. Erythromycin (2 g/d), given orally for 3 weeks, is usually effective; however, relapse may require prolonged therapy with antibiotics that reach an intracellular compartment, such as erythromycin (2 g/d), ciprofloxacin (1 to 1.5 g/d), or doxycycline (200 mg/d). Patients with peliosis hepatis should be treated with intravenous antibiotics, and those with disseminated disease or bacteremia should be treated with a prolonged course (3 weeks to 2 months) of systemic antibiotics, such as macrolides (erythromycin, 2 g/d) or quinolones (ciprofloxacin, 800 mg/d). Cutaneous lesions may or may not regress spontaneously, perhaps depending on the status of the host's immunity. The safety of ciprofloxacin in pregnant or lactating women has not been established. Moreover, no antimicrobial has been studied prospectively, and information on efficacy comes from only a few case reports.

CAT-SCRATCH DISEASE

DEFINITION AND ETIOLOGY Typical CSD is manifested by painful regional lymphadenopathy persisting for several weeks or months after a cat scratch. Occasionally, infection may disseminate and produce more generalized lymphadenopathy and systemic manifestations, which may be confused with the manifestations of lymphoma. *B. henselae* is the causative agent of CSD. There is no evidence that *B. quintana* or *Afipia felis* (originally proposed as the agent of CSD) can cause this disease, nor are those two species carried by cats.

EPIDEMIOLOGY Approximately 60 percent of cases of CSD in the United States occur in children. Exposure to bacteremic young cats that either are flea-infested or have been in contact with another cat carrying fleas poses a significant risk of infection. Most infections are caused by a scratch and only rare cases by a bite or by licking. Most cases occur in the warmer months, when fleas are active. Regions of the United States where fleas are endemic have higher rates of infection. The flea may serve to transmit infection between cats; it is not known whether humans can be infected through the bite of an infected flea.

CLINICAL MANIFESTATIONS A localized papule, progressing to a pustule that often crusts over, develops 3 to 5 days after a cat scratch. Tender regional lymphadenopathy develops within 1 to 2 weeks after inoculation; by this time, the papule may have healed spontaneously. Scratches are most often sustained on the hands or face, producing epitrochlear, axillary, pectoral, and cervical lymph node involvement. The involved nodes occasionally become suppurative; bacterial superinfection with staphylococci or other cutaneous pathogens may develop. Although most patients do not have fever, systemic symptoms are frequent and include malaise, anorexia, and weight loss. Without treatment, lymphadenopathy persists for weeks or even months and may be confused with lymphatic malignancy. Other manifestations in apparently immunocompetent patients include encephalitis, seizures and coma (especially in children), meningitis, transverse myelitis, granulomatous hepatitis and splenitis, osteomyelitis, and disseminated infection. Conjunctival inoculation may cause Parinaud's oculoglandular syndrome, with conjunctivitis and preauricular lymphadenopathy.

PATHOLOGY The histopathologic hallmark of CSD is granulomatous inflammation with stellate necrosis but no evidence of angiogenesis. Thus, infection by *B. henselae* can produce two entirely different pathologic reactions, depending on the immune status of the host: CSD or bacillary angiomatosis.

DIAGNOSIS CSD should be suspected if the patient has a history of exposure to cats and develops lymphadenopathy and a skin lesion. The diagnosis can be confirmed by pathologic examination of the involved nodes. Tiny bacilli in clusters can sometimes be seen in biopsy samples stained with Warthin-Starry silver. The CSD skin test, in which lymph node material obtained from patients with CSD serves as an antigen, is no longer used for diagnosis because of concerns about the transmission of viral agents. A specific serologic test has been developed recently and may produce a positive result in 70 to 90 percent of patients with intact immunity. The identification of *B. henselae* 16S ribosomal RNA genes in biopsy material by PCR amplification with specific oligonucleotide primers can also be diag-

nostically useful; however, these methods are not yet commercially available. Cultures of lymph nodes, cerebrospinal fluid, or other tissues are rarely positive.

TREATMENT

Although CSD is generally self-limited, tender regional lymphadenopathy and systemic symptoms may be debilitating. Patients with encephalitis or other serious manifestations should be treated with antibiotics, even though the efficacy of such therapy is unclear. No comparative trials of antibiotic treatment have been performed, and no anecdotal reports of treatment failures have appeared. Several reports suggest that aminoglycoside treatment (e.g., intravenous gentamicin at standard doses calculated to result in therapeutic levels) is effective in patients with encephalitis and other systemic infections. The oral agents that appear to be useful are those that also are most effective for the treatment of bacillary angiomatosis; they include ciprofloxacin, doxycycline, and possibly erythromycin (at the dosages recommended for bacillary angiomatosis). Many patients with established CSD have no apparent response to antibiotics; the necessary duration of therapy is variable.

TRENCH FEVER

Trench fever was first described as a debilitating febrile illness associated with prolonged *B. quintana* bacteremia in soldiers fighting in Europe during World War I. Although not usually fatal, the illness accounted for substantial morbidity. In recent years, trench fever has reemerged in the United States and has been caused by either *B. henselae*—the agent of CSD and bacillary angiomatosis—or *B. quintana.*

EPIDEMIOLOGY Although trench fever was thought to have disappeared from the United States, recent cases have been diagnosed in homeless persons (*B. quintana*) and in persons bitten by ticks (*B. henselae*). During World War I, trench fever was transmitted from person to person by the human body louse. Transmission by ectoparasites is suspected in the recent cases of *B. quintana* infection but has not been firmly documented. Patients with trench fever have apparently normal immune defenses.

CLINICAL MANIFESTATIONS Trench fever is characterized by the sudden onset of headache, aseptic meningitis, persistent fever (which can be high-grade and is commonly paroxysmal), malaise, weight loss, and other nonspecific symptoms. Severe musculoskeletal pain is more common among immunocompetent than among immunocompromised patients. Bacteremia can persist for days or weeks, and relapses have followed short courses of antibiotic therapy. Localized findings are uncommon.

DIAGNOSIS Trench fever is diagnosed by the finding of sustained bacteremia. *B. henselae* and *B. quintana* grow slowly. Colonies develop on rabbit blood agar after 1 to 4 weeks of incubation under conditions of increased CO_2. Serologic tests for this disease have not yet been standardized.

TREATMENT

A prolonged course (4 weeks) of antimicrobial therapy may be required. Agents that can cross the mammalian cell membrane are most effective, including erythromycin (2 g/d) or azithromycin (500 mg/d). Data on the efficacy of these agents come from a limited number of case reports.

OTHER *BARTONELLA* INFECTIONS

The application of molecular methods to the detection of microorganisms that are difficult to cultivate in the laboratory has revealed new *Bartonella* species and has established *Bartonella* species as a cause of endocarditis cases previously classified as being of unknown etiology. One new species, *Bartonella elizabethae*, has been identified as an agent of endocarditis, and cases of endocarditis associated with *B. quintana* and *B. henselae* have been reported recently. Therefore, the possibility of *Bartonella* infection should be considered and appropriate laboratory methods employed in an effort to isolate and identify *Bartonella* species in cases of "culture-negative" endocarditis or bacteremia.

BIBLIOGRAPHY

ARIAS-STELLA J et al: Histology, immunohistochemistry, and ultrastructure of the verruga in Carrion's disease. Am J Surg Pathol 10:595, 1986

BOGUE CW et al: Antibiotic therapy for cat-scratch disease? JAMA 262:813, 1989

CARITHERS HA: Cat scratch disease: An overview based on a study of 1,200 patients. Am J Dis Child 139:1124, 1985

COCKERELL DJ, LeBOIT PE: Bacillary angiomatosis: A newly characterized, pseudoneoplastic, infectious, cutaneous vascular disorder. J Am Acad Dermatol 22:501, 1990

DOLAN MJ et al: Syndrome of *Rochalimaea henselae* adenitis suggesting cat scratch disease. Ann Intern Med 118:331, 1993

HOLLEY HP Jr: Successful treatment of cat-scratch disease with ciprofloxacin. JAMA 265:1563, 1991

KOEHLER JE et al: Isolation of *Rochalimaea* species from cutaneous and osseous lesions of bacillary angiomatosis. N Engl J Med 23:1625, 1992

————, TAPPERO JW: AIDS commentary: Bacillary angiomatosis and bacillary peliosis in patients infected with human immunodeficiency virus. Clin Infect Dis 17:612, 1993

———— et al: *Rochalimaea henselae* infection: A new zoonosis with the domestic cat as reservoir. JAMA 271:531, 1994

LUCEY D et al: Relapsing illness due to *Rochalimaea henselae* in immunocompetent hosts: Implication for therapy and new epidemiological associations. Clin Infect Dis 14:683, 1992

PERKOCHA LA et al: Clinical and pathological features of bacillary peliosis hepatis in association with human immunodeficiency virus infection. N Engl J Med 323:148, 1990

REGNERY RL et al: Characterization of a novel *Rochalimaea* species, *R. henselae*, sp.nov., isolated from blood of a febrile, human immunodeficiency virus–positive patient. J Clin Microbiol 30:265, 1992

RELMAN DA et al: The agent of bacillary angiomatosis: An approach to the identification of uncultured pathogens. N Engl J Med 323:1573, 1990

RICKETTS WE: Clinical manifestations of Carrion's disease. Arch Intern Med 84:751, 1949

SHINALL EA: Cat-scratch disease: A review of the literature. Pediatr Dermatol 7:11, 1990

SLATER LN et al: A newly recognized fastidious gram-negative pathogen as a cause of fever and bacteremia. N Engl J Med 323:1587, 1990

SPACH DH et al: *Bartonella (Rochalimaea) quintana* bacteremia in inner-city patients with chronic alcoholism. N Engl J Med 332:425, 1995

STRONG RO (ed): *Trench Fever: Report of Commission, Medical Research Committee, American Red Cross.* Oxford, Oxford University Press, 1918, p 40

TAPPERO JW et al: The epidemiology of bacillary angiomatosis and bacillary peliosis. JAMA 269:770, 1993

ZANGWILL KM et al: Cat scratch disease in Connecticut: Epidemiology, risk factors, and evaluation of a new diagnostic test. N Engl J Med 329:8, 1993

166 | *King K. Holmes*

DONOVANOSIS (GRANULOMA INGUINALE)

DEFINITION Donovanosis (granuloma inguinale) is a mildly contagious, chronic, indolent, progressive, autoinoculable, ulcerative disease involving the skin and lymphatics of the genital or perianal areas. The disease appears to be sexually transmitted and is associated with the presence in affected tissues of an intracellular microorganism, identified morphologically as the Donovan body.

ETIOLOGY Donovanosis was described by McLeod in India in 1882. In 1905 Donovan described the intracellular bodies that are thought to cause the disease. During the 1940s, encapsulated bacteria resembling Donovan bodies were recovered from pseudobuboes of granuloma inguinale by inoculation of chick embryo yolk sacs or yolk-agar medium. These bacteria, which are known as *Calymmatobacterium granulomatis*, measure 1.5 by 0.7 μm. Since such isolates are no longer available and *C. granulomatis* has not been reproducibly cultivable, the organism has not been characterized. However, investigators in South Africa have recently reported cultivation and propagation of a *C. granulomatis*–like organism in mononuclear cells, and other researchers have used polymerase chain reaction amplification of the *phoE* or ribosomal genes of material obtained directly from donovanosis ulcers in attempts to identify the causative organism. Definitive characterization of *C. granulomatis* awaits further research. Electron-microscopic studies of Donovan bodies show their morphologic resemblance to gram-negative bacteria.

EPIDEMIOLOGY Donovanosis is endemic in the tropics, particularly in Papua New Guinea, southern India, southern Africa, and parts of Australia, Brazil, and the Caribbean. In the United States, the disease is rare. In reported cases, the sex ratio of males to females is nearly 10:1. The disease is uncommon in Caucasians. The frequency of donovanosis in sexual partners of chronically infected patients is highly variable, ranging from 1 percent to over 50 percent. Evidence for sexual transmission includes the age-specific incidence, which corresponds to that of other sexually transmitted diseases; the frequent concomitant presence of syphilis; the predilection for genital involvement in heterosexuals and for anorectal infection in homosexually active men; and the fact that outbreaks of clusters of cases of donovanosis have been traced to sexual exposure to a single-source contact. A significant association of human immunodeficiency virus (HIV) infection with donovanosis has been found among men in Durban, South Africa.

CLINICAL MANIFESTATIONS The incubation period for donovanosis ranges from 8 days to 12 weeks, but most lesions appear within 30 days after sexual exposure. The disease begins as a papule that ulcerates and develops into a painless elevated zone of clean, beefy-red, friable granulation tissue. The edges are irregular and spread by continuity or by autoinoculation of approximated skin surfaces. Secondary anaerobic infection may produce pain and a foul-smelling exudate. Less common complications of the disease include deep ulcerations, chronic cicatricial lesions, phimosis, lymphedema, and exuberant epithelial proliferation that grossly resembles carcinoma. In men, the lesions are usually located on the glans, prepuce, or shaft of the penis or in the perianal area, while infection of the labia is most common in women. Lesions in women often arise at the fourchette and progress anteriorly in a V pattern along the vulva. Extragenital lesions may develop, involving the face, neck, mouth, and/or other sites. The chronicity of the disease is of diagnostic importance, since several months often elapse before patients seek treatment. Extension to the inguinal region by autoinoculation, by continuity, or via the lymphatics results in a diffuse intradermal and subcutaneous swelling or suppuration known as a *pseudobubo* because involvement of the underlying lymph nodes is minimal. Locally destructive lesions and secondary infection may cause severe morbidity or death. Fatal disseminated disease involving the bones, joints, or liver has been reported. Rates of disseminated infection are apparently elevated during pregnancy. The relationship of donovanosis to subsequent carcinoma of the genitalia is uncertain.

DIAGNOSIS Early donovanosis may be mistaken for the primary chancre or condyloma latum of syphilis. Epithelial proliferation resembling carcinoma in the genital or perianal region in a young individual should always raise the suspicion of donovanosis if unnecessary destructive surgery is to be avoided. Chronic ulcerative or cicatricial changes may resemble those of lymphogranuloma venereum.

Amebiasis can produce penile lesions resembling the lesions of donovanosis. In the United States, *Haemophilus ducreyi* frequently has been isolated from lesions resembling those of donovanosis; these *H. ducreyi*–associated lesions have been termed *pseudo–granuloma inguinale chancroid*. Histologic studies in donovanosis reveal marked acanthosis and pseudoepitheliomatous hyperplasia. The dermis contains an inflammatory infiltrate consisting mainly of plasma cells and histiocytes. Because Donovan bodies are seldom detectable in sections stained with hematoxylin and eosin, these changes may lead to an erroneous diagnosis of carcinoma and to unnecessary and destructive surgery. Although silver impregnation techniques are useful for the demonstration of Donovan bodies in sections, the diagnosis is best made by examination of impression smears prepared from specimens obtained by punch biopsy of granulation tissue from the periphery of a lesion; the deep portion of the specimen is removed and crushed between two slides, which are air-dried, fixed in methanol, and stained with Wright-Giemsa. In these stained smears, Donovan bodies appear as rounded coccobacilli of 1 by 2 μm lying within cystic spaces in the cytoplasm of large mononuclear cells. The capsule stains as a dense acidophilic zone surrounding the bacterium, which resembles a closed safety pin because of bipolar condensation of chromatin. The pathognomonic mononuclear cell is 25 to 90 μm in diameter and has many cystic areas containing Donovan bodies. Donovan bodies also have been identified within histiocytes in cervical Papanicolaou smears.

Perianal donovanosis may resemble condylomata lata of secondary syphilis. Other venereal diseases, particularly syphilis, frequently co-exist with donovanosis. Repeated negative dark-field examinations of lesions and negative serologic tests exclude syphilis but should not be rigidly required while treatment is withheld from potentially non-compliant patients. In countries where donovanosis is endemic, the persistence of suspected condylomata lata after appropriate penicillin therapy for syphilis is highly suggestive of donovanosis.

℞ TREATMENT
The antimicrobials currently effective in the treatment of dono-vanosis in various parts of the world include trimethoprim-sulfameth-oxazole, tetracycline, erythromycin, newer quinolones, gentamicin, and chloramphenicol or the related drug thiamphenicol (not available in the United States). Recent studies have found azithromycin or ceftriaxone to be effective. Streptomycin, once commonly used for this condition, is not widely used today. Ampicillin is not recom-mended for the treatment of donovanosis. Unfortunately, no compar-ative trials have been conducted with the currently used antimicrobi-als, and in vitro susceptibility testing is not possible. The minimum duration of treatment is not well established; it is customary, though perhaps not essential, to continue therapy until lesions have com-pletely healed over. Thus treatment for large lesions is generally more prolonged than that for small lesions, whose healing is usually apparent within 3 weeks. As the lesions heal, they become pale and flatter and peripheral reepithelialization begins. Lack of an objective clinical response within 7 days should lead to reassessment of the diagnosis and therapy. Donovan bodies disappear from lesions within a few days after the initiation of therapy. Typical dosages of the commonly used drugs include 500 mg four times daily for tetracy-cline or erythromycin and 160/800 mg twice daily for trimethoprim-sulfamethoxazole.

BIBLIOGRAPHY

Bassa AG et al: Granuloma inguinale (donovanosis) in women. An analysis of 61 cases from Durban, South Africa. Sex Transm Dis 20:164, 1993

Bowden FJ et al: Pilot study of azithromycin in the treatment of genital donovanosis. Genitourin Med 72:17, 1996

Kuberski T: Granuloma inguinale (donovanosis). Sex Transm Dis 7:29, 1980

Mein J et al: Donovanosis: Sequelae of severe disease and successful azithro-mycin treatment. Int J STD AIDS 7:448, 1996

Merianos A et al: Ceftriaxone in the treatment of chronic donovanosis in central Australia. Genitourin Med 70:84, 1994

O'Farrell N: Clinico-epidemiological study of donovanosis in Durban, South Africa. Genitourin Med 69:108, 1993

——— et al: A rapid stain for the diagnosis of granuloma inguinale. Genitourin Med 66:200, 1990

——— et al: HIV-1 infection among heterosexual attendees of a sexually transmitted disease clinic in Durban. S Afr Med J 80:17, 1991

Ramanan C et al: Treatment of donovanosis with norfloxacin. Int J Dermatol 29:298, 1990

Richens J: The diagnosis and treatment of donovanosis (granuloma inguinale). Genitourin Med 67:441, 1991

Rosen T et al: Granuloma inguinale. J Am Acad Dermatol 11:433, 1984

SECTION 7
MISCELLANEOUS BACTERIAL INFECTIONS

---

167   *Gregory A. Filice*
NOCARDIOSIS

DEFINITION The term *nocardiosis* refers to invasive disease associated with *Nocardia* species, aerobic actinomycetes that cause several characteristic syndromes. Pneumonia and disseminated dis-ease, both thought to follow inhalation of fragmented bacterial mycelia, are most common. Three syndromes follow transcutaneous inocula-tion: cellulitis, a lymphocutaneous syndrome, and actinomycetoma. Keratitis follows inoculation into the eye at the time of corneal trauma.

ETIOLOGIC AGENTS Nocardiae are common bacterial in-habitants of soil, where they contribute to the decay of organic matter. Seven *Nocardia* species have been associated with human disease: *N. asteroides*, *N. brasiliensis*, *N. otitidiscaviarum* (formerly *N. caviae*), *N. farcinica*, *N. nova*, *N. transvalensis*, and *N. pseudobrasiliensis*.

EPIDEMIOLOGY Nocardiosis occurs throughout the world. Approximately 1000 cases are diagnosed annually in the United States, 85 percent of them pulmonary and/or systemic. The disease is more common among adults than among children and among males than among females. Outbreaks are rare, and person-to-person spread has not been well documented.

The risk of pulmonary or disseminated disease is greater than usual among people with deficient cell-mediated immunity, especially deficiency associated with lymphoma, transplantation, or AIDS. No-cardiosis has also been associated with pulmonary alveolar proteinosis, tuberculosis, and chronic granulomatous disease.

Nocardia is one of the several actinomycete genera associated with antinomycetoma, which occurs mainly in tropical and subtropical regions, especially those of Mexico, Central and South America, Africa, and India. The most important risk factor for actinomycetoma is frequent contact with soil or vegetable matter.

PATHOLOGY AND PATHOGENESIS The characteristic histologic feature of pulmonary or systemic nocardial infection is an abscess extensively infiltrated with neutrophils. Granulation tissue usually surrounds the lesions, but extensive fibrosis or encapsulation is uncommon. Actinomycetoma is characterized by suppurative in-flammation with sinus tract formation. The lesions of actinomycetoma and their drainage contain granules composed of dense masses of bacterial filaments.

Nocardiae have evolved a number of properties that enable them to survive within phagocytes, including neutralization of oxidants, prevention of phagosome-lysosome fusion, and prevention of phago-some acidification. Neutrophils phagocytose the organisms and limit their growth but do not kill them efficiently. Cell-mediated immunity is important for definitive control and elimination of the organisms.

CLINICAL MANIFESTATIONS **Pulmonary Disease** No-cardial pneumonia is typically subacute; persons generally seek med-ical care several days or weeks after the development of symptoms.

The onset may be more acute in immunosuppressed patients. Cough is prominent and productive of small amounts of thick, purulent sputum that is not malodorous. Fever, anorexia, weight loss, and malaise are common; dyspnea, pleuritic pain, and hemoptysis are less common. Tracheitis and bronchitis are uncommon. Obstructive bronchial masses have been reported. Remissions and exacerbations over periods of several weeks are frequent.

Roentgenologic patterns are variable. Infiltrates vary in size and are usually of moderate or greater density. Nodules and cavitation are common. Empyema is evident in one-third of cases.

Pulmonary nocardiosis may spread directly from the lungs to involve adjacent tissues. Pericarditis, mediastinitis, and the superior vena cava syndrome have all been reported. Spread through the chest wall is rare.

Nocardia species are sometimes isolated from respiratory secretions of patients without apparent nocardial disease. Most of these patients have chronic pulmonary disease with abnormal airways or parenchyma.

Extrapulmonary Dissemination In half of all cases of pulmonary nocardiosis, disease appears outside the lungs. One-fifth of patients with disseminated disease present only with extrapulmonary disease, which has probably spread hematogenously from an inapparent or healed pulmonary focus. The most common sites are the brain, skin and supporting structures, kidneys, bone, and muscle, but dissemination to nearly every organ has been reported. Peritonitis and endocarditis have been described. The typical manifestation of extrapulmonary dissemination is a subacute or chronic abscess. A minority of abscesses outside the lungs or central nervous system (CNS) form fistulas and discharge small amounts of pus. All *Nocardia* species are associated with disseminated disease, but most invasive strains previously classified as *N. brasiliensis* have been grouped in the new species *N. pseudobrasiliensis*.

The CNS is the most common location for disseminated disease. Usually there are one or more supratentorial brain abscesses, often multiloculated. Brain abscesses tend to burrow into the ventricles or out into the subarachnoid space. The symptoms and signs are somewhat more indolent than those of brain abscess due to other bacteria. Meningitis without apparent brain abscess is rare. The organism is not easily recovered from cerebrospinal fluid.

Disease Following Transcutaneous Inoculation As has already been mentioned, infection following transcutaneous inoculation usually takes one of three forms: cellulitis, lymphocutaneous syndrome, or actinomycetoma. Cellulitis generally begins 1 to 3 weeks after a recognized breach of the skin. Often the wound has been contaminated with soil. Subacute cellulitis, with pain, swelling, erythema, and warmth, develops over days or weeks. The lesions are usually firm and nonfluctuant. The process may progress to involve underlying muscles, tendons, bones, and joints. Dissemination is rare. *N. asteroides* is common in colder climates, while *N. brasiliensis* predominates in warmer climates.

In the lymphocutaneous syndrome, there is typically a pyodermatous lesion at the site of inoculation, with central ulceration and purulent or honey-colored drainage. Subcutaneous nodules often appear along lymphatics that drain the primary lesion. The lymphangitic form closely resembles lymphocutaneous sporotrichosis (see Chap. 210). Most cases of the lymphocutaneous syndrome are associated with *N. brasiliensis*.

Actinomycetoma usually begins with a nodular swelling, sometimes in conjunction with local trauma. Lesions typically develop on the feet or the hands but may involve the posterior part of the neck, the upper back, the head, and other sites. The nodule eventually breaks down and a fistula appears. This fistula is soon accompanied by others. The fistulas tend to come and go, with new ones forming as old ones disappear. The discharge is serous or purulent, may be bloody, and often contains 0.1- to 2-mm white granules consisting of masses of mycelia. The lesions spread slowly along fascial planes to involve adjacent areas of skin, subcutaneous tissue, and bone. Over a period

of months to years, there may be extensive deformation of the affected part. Lesions involving soft tissues are only mildly painful, whereas those affecting bones or joints are more so. Systemic symptoms are minimal or lacking altogether. Infection rarely disseminates from actinomycetoma, and lesions on the hands and feet usually cause only local disability. Lesions on the head, neck, and trunk can invade locally to involve deep organs and result in severe disability or death.

Keratitis *Nocardia* species (most often *N. asteroides*) are uncommon causes of subacute keratitis. The infection usually follows eye trauma. Nocardial infection of lacrimal glands has been reported. Disease involving deeper eye structures is usually a manifestation of dissemination.

DIAGNOSIS The first step in the diagnosis of nocardiosis is the examination of sputum or pus for crooked, branching, beaded, gram-positive filaments 1 μm in width and up to 50 μm long. Most nocardiae are acid-fast in direct smears if a weak acid is used for decolorization (e.g., in the modified Kinyoun, Ziehl-Neelsen, and Fite-Faraco methods). The organisms often take up silver stains. Nocardiae grow relatively slowly; colonies may take up to 2 weeks to appear and may not develop their characteristic appearance for up to 4 weeks. Their pattern of growth is quite different from those of more common pathogens; thus, the laboratory should always be alerted when nocardial infection is suspected so that the likelihood of its recovery is maximized. In difficult cases, paraffin baiting can be employed, as nocardiae are among the few aerobic microorganisms that can use paraffin as a carbon source.

Smears are often negative. In such cases, invasive procedures are necessary for diagnosis. Transtracheal aspiration should be avoided, as it frequently leads to nocardial cellulitis in tissues around the puncture wound.

Growth of nocardiae from sputum may represent colonization and not disease. Findings that make disease more likely are the detection of nocardiae on Gram-stained preparations and the isolation of the organisms from multiple cultures. A positive culture of sputum from an immunosuppressed patient usually reflects disease.

A careful history should be obtained and a thorough physical examination performed to evaluate the possibility of dissemination in patients with nocardial pneumonia. Suggestive symptoms or signs should be pursued with further diagnostic tests. Computed tomography or magnetic resonance imaging of the head, with and without contrast material, should be undertaken if there are signs or symptoms suggesting brain involvement.

Biphasic culture bottles incubated aerobically for up to 30 days often yield nocardiae, but routine blood cultures are usually negative. If clinically indicated, specimens of cerebrospinal fluid or urine should be concentrated and then cultured. In cases of actinomycetoma, an effort should be made to find granules in the discharge. Suspect particles should be washed in saline, examined microscopically, and cultured.

Several presumptive diagnostic tests have been studied, including tests for antibodies and nocardial metabolites in serum or cerebrospinal fluid. None of these tests is ready for clinical use at this time.

℞ TREATMENT

Sulfonamides are the drugs of choice for nocardiosis. Initially, 6 to 8 g of sulfadiazine or sulfisoxazole per day in four divided doses should be used. After the disease is under control, 4 g per day can be used to complete the course of therapy. (For durations, see below.) In difficult cases, sulfonamide levels in serum should be measured and dosages adjusted to keep serum concentrations between 100 and 150 μg/mL. The combination of sulfamethoxazole and trimethoprim is equivalent or possibly slightly more effective but poses a modestly greater risk of hematologic toxicity. Initially, 10 to 20 mg of trimethoprim per kilogram and 50 to 100 mg of sulfamethoxazole per kilogram should be given each day in two divided doses. Later, the daily dose can be dropped to as little as 5 mg of trimethoprim and 25 mg of sulfamethoxazole per kilogram. Sulfonamides given for prophylaxis of other infectious diseases appear to reduce the risk of nocardiosis.

Antimicrobial susceptibility testing has not been developed to the point where its clinical relevance is certain, and initial choices of antimicrobials should be based on published clinical experience. However, isolates should be sent to a reference laboratory for definitive identification and susceptibility testing with methods developed specifically for *Nocardia*. The results may help guide therapy if initial choices do not work or if toxicity develops. Nocardiae are generally susceptible to sulfonamides, minocycline, amikacin, cefotaxime, ceftizoxime, ceftriaxone, and imipenem and resistant to ampicillin and erythromycin. *N. farcinica* strains differ in that most are resistant to cephalosporins and one-fifth are resistant to imipenem. Strains of *N. pseudobrasiliensis* often show resistance to minocycline or amoxicillin/clavulanic acid and exhibit susceptibility to ciprofloxacin or clarithromycin.

Minocycline is the best-established alternative oral drug for use against all species and should be given in doses of 100 to 200 mg twice a day. Other tetracyclines are usually ineffective. Infections due to *N. nova* can be treated with erythromycin (500 to 750 mg four times a day) and/or ampicillin (1 g four times a day), but other *Nocardia* species are usually resistant to both of these drugs. Amoxicillin combined with clavulanate (500 and 125 mg, respectively, given three times a day) can be used except against *N. nova*, in which clavulanate induces β-lactamase production. Ofloxacin (400 mg twice a day) and clarithromycin (500 mg twice a day) have each been used successfully in a few cases.

Amikacin, the best-established drug for parenteral use, is given in doses of 5 to 7.5 mg/kg every 12 h. Serum levels should be monitored if therapy is prolonged, if renal function is diminished, or if the patient is elderly. Newer β-lactam antibiotics, including cefotaxime, ceftizoxime, ceftriaxone, and imipenem, are usually effective except against *N. farcinica*.

The administration of immunosuppressive agents should be continued if necessary for the treatment of underlying disease or the prevention of organ-transplant rejection. In many cases, two or more antimicrobials have been used to treat nocardiosis, often in combinations including a sulfonamide or minocycline. Whether therapy with two or more agents is better than therapy with a single agent is not known, however, and therapy with multiple drugs increases the risk of toxicity.

A brain abscess should be aspirated, drained, or excised if the diagnosis is unclear, if the abscess is large and accessible, or if it fails to respond to chemotherapy. Small abscesses and those in inaccessible or critical locations should be treated medically. In cases managed medically, clinical improvement should be noticeable within 1 to 2 weeks. Anatomic resolution often lags behind clinical improvement and should be monitored with repeated imaging.

Antimicrobial therapy usually suffices for nocardial actinomycetoma. In cases of deep or extensive disease, drainage or excision of heavily involved tissue may facilitate healing, but structure and function should be preserved whenever possible.

Because nocardial infections tend to relapse, long courses of antimicrobial therapy are necessary. Nocardiosis is particularly tenacious and likely to relapse in people with chronic granulomatous disease. When the patient is immunocompetent, the treatment of pulmonary or systemic nocardiosis outside the CNS should be continued for 6 to 12 months. Ordinarily, treatment of CNS nocardiosis should be continued for 1 year. If all apparent sites of CNS disease have been excised, it may be possible to reduce the duration of therapy to 6 months. When the patient is immunosuppressed, the treatment of pulmonary or systemic nocardiosis should be continued for 1 year. In some patients with AIDS, it has been necessary to continue therapy indefinitely. If nocardial disease is unusually extensive or if the response to therapy is slow, these recommendations should be exceeded.

Patients with cellulitis or the lymphocutaneous syndrome should be treated for 2 months if the infection is limited to soft tissues and for 4 months if bone is involved. Unusually extensive cases or cases in immunosuppressed people should be treated longer. Therapy for actinomycetoma should be continued for 6 to 12 months after clinical cure. Keratitis should be treated with oral and topical sulfonamides until the infection appears to be cured and then with oral sulfonamides alone for an additional 2 to 4 months.

PROGNOSIS The mortality for pulmonary or disseminated nocardiosis outside the CNS should be less than 5 percent. CNS disease poses a greater risk of death. Patients should be followed carefully for at least 6 months after therapy has ended. Any child with nocardiosis and no known cause of immunosuppression should undergo tests to determine the adequacy of the phagocytic respiratory burst.

BIBLIOGRAPHY

ARDUINO RC et al: Nocardiosis in renal transplant recipients undergoing immunosuppression with cyclosporine. Clin Infect Dis 16:505, 1993

BERKEY P, BODEY GP: Nocardial infection in patients with neoplastic disease. Rev Infect Dis 11:407, 1989

FILICE GA, SIMPSON GS: Management of *Nocardia* infections, in *Current Clinical Topics in Infectious Diseases*, JS Remington, MN Swartz (eds). New York, McGraw-Hill, 1984, vol 5, pp 49–64

KING CT et al: Recurrent nocardiosis in a renal transplant recipient. South Med J 86:225, 1993

LEBLANG SD et al: CNS *Nocardia* in AIDS patients: CT and MRI with pathologic correlation. J Comput Assist Tomogr 19:15, 1995

MCNEIL MM et al: Infections due to *Nocardia transvalensis*: Clinical spectrum and antimicrobial therapy. Clin Infect Dis 15:453, 1992

PALMER DL et al: Diagnostic and therapeutic considerations in *Nocardia asteroides* infection. Medicine 53:391, 1974

PETERSON EA et al: Minocycline treatment of pulmonary nocardiosis. JAMA 250:930, 1983

RUIMY R et al: *Nocardia pseudobrasiliensis* sp. nov., a new species of *Nocardia* which groups bacterial strains previously identified as *Nocardia brasiliensis* and associated with invasive diseases. Int J Syst Bacteriol 46:259, 1996

SATTERWHITE TK, WALLACE RJ JR: Primary cutaneous nocardiosis. JAMA 242:333, 1979

TIGHT RR, BARTLETT MS: Actinomycetoma in the United States. Rev Infect Dis 3:1139, 1981

UTTAMCHANDANI RB et al: Nocardiosis in 30 patients with advanced human immunodeficiency virus infection: Clinical features and outcome. Clin Infect Dis 18:348, 1994

WALLACE RJ JR et al: Antimicrobial susceptibility patterns of *Nocardia asteroides*. Antimicrob Agents Chemother 32:1776, 1988

———— et al: Cefotaxime-resistant *Nocardia asteroides* strains are isolates of the controversial species *Nocardia farcinica*. J Clin Microbiol 28:2726, 1990

———— et al: Clinical and laboratory features of *Nocardia nova*. J Clin Microbiol 29:2407, 1991

———— et al: New *Nocardia* taxon among isolates of *Nocardia brasiliensis* associated with invasive disease. J Clin Microbiol 33:1528, 1995

168 *Thomas A. Russo*

ACTINOMYCOSIS

Actinomycosis is an indolent, slowly progressive bacterial infection caused by a variety of gram-positive, non-spore-forming anaerobic or microaerophilic rods, most of which are of the genus *Actinomyces*. Actinomycosis was common in the preantibiotic era but is less frequent now, and consequently so is its timely recognition. The clinical presentations of this disease, which can affect nearly every organ and body site, are myriad, but most characteristic are the formation of "sulfur granules" and the violation of normal tissue plane barriers as infection spreads and creates draining sinuses. Actinomycosis has been called "the most misdiagnosed disease," and it has been said that "no disease is so often missed by experienced clinicians." An awareness of the full spectrum of the disease is needed to expedite its diagnosis and treatment and to minimize the unnecessary morbidity and mortality that are reported all too often.

ETIOLOGIC AGENTS Actinomycosis is most commonly caused by *Actinomyces israelii*. *Actinomyces naeslundii*, *Actinomyces odontolyticus*, *Actinomyces viscosus*, *Actinomyces meyeri*, *Actinomyces gerencseriae*, and *Propionibacterium propionicum* (formerly *Arachnia propionica*) are established but less common causes of disease.

Most if not all actinomycotic infections are polymicrobial. *Actinobacillus actinomycetemcomitans*, *Eikenella corrodens*, Enterobacteriaceae, and species of *Fusobacterium*, *Bacteroides*, *Capnocytophaga*, *Staphylococcus*, and *Streptococcus* are commonly isolated with actinomycetes in various combinations, depending on the site of infection. The contribution of these other species to pathogenesis in actinomycosis is uncertain.

EPIDEMIOLOGY   The agents of actinomycosis are members of the normal oral flora and are often cultured from the bronchi, the gastrointestinal tract, and the female genital tract. Infection occurs throughout life, with a peak incidence in the middle decades. Males have a threefold higher incidence of infection, possibly because of poorer dental hygiene and/or more frequent trauma. Likely contributing factors to the decrease in the incidence of actinomycosis since the start of the antibiotic era include improved dental hygiene and the initiation of antimicrobial treatment early on—before the full development of the disease. Individuals who do not have access to health care may well be at higher risk.

PATHOGENESIS AND PATHOLOGY   A vital step in the development of actinomycosis is disruption of the mucosal barrier, which allows the actinomycetes to invade beyond their endogenous habitat in the mouth, lower gastrointestinal tract, and female genitourinary tract. Local infection, subsequent extension, and (in rare instances) distant hematogenous seeding may ensue. Initial acute inflammation is followed by the characteristic chronic, indolent phase. Lesions usually appear as single or multiple indurations. Cental fluctuance, with pus containing neutrophils and sulfur granules, may develop. Granules are gritty in vivo conglomerations of organisms that are virtually diagnostic of actinomycosis (Fig. 168-1). The fibrous walls of the mass are typically described as woody and, in the absence of suppuration, are sometimes confused with neoplasms. Once established, actinomycosis spreads contiguously in a slow, progressive manner. Tissue planes are ignored; with time, sinus tracts that can spontaneously close and reopen will form and extend to skin, adjacent organs, or bone.

FIGURE 168-1 Actinomycotic sulfur granule surrounded by inflammatory cells. The delicate branched filaments of *Actinomyces* are surrounded by the proteinaceous eosinophilic coating of the granule (Slendore-Hoeppli phenomenon).

An association of pelvic actinomycosis with use of an intrauterine contraceptive device (IUD) suggests that this foreign body contributes to pathogenesis. In addition, an increasing number of reports have described an association of actinomycosis with infection due to human immunodeficiency virus (HIV). Ulcerative mucosal infections (caused, for example, by herpes simplex virus or cytomegalovirus) and abnormalities in host defenses may facilitate the development of actinomycosis in the latter setting.

CLINICAL MANIFESTATIONS Oral-Cervicofacial Disease   Actinomycosis occurs most frequently at an oral, cervical, or facial site, usually as a soft tissue swelling, abscess, or mass lesion that is often mistaken for a neoplasm. The angle of the jaw is generally involved, but a diagnosis of actinomycosis should be considered with any mass lesion or relapsing infection in the head and neck. Otitis, sinusitis, and canaliculitis can also develop. Pain, fever, and leukocytosis are variably reported. Contiguous extension to the cranium, cervical spine, or thorax is a potential sequela.

Thoracic Disease   Thoracic actinomycosis usually follows an indolent, progressive course, with involvement of the pulmonary parenchyma and/or the pleural space. Chest pain, fever, and weight loss are common. A cough, when present, is variably productive. The usual radiographic appearance is either a mass lesion or pneumonitis. Cavitary disease or hilar adenopathy may develop. More than 50 percent of cases include pleural thickening, effusion, or empyema. Rarely, pulmonary nodules or endobronchial lesions occur. Pulmonary lesions suggestive of actinomycosis may cross fissures or pleura; may involve the mediastinum, contiguous bone, or chest wall; or may be associated with a sinus tract. In the absence of these findings, thoracic actinomycosis is usually mistaken for a neoplasm or for pneumonitis due to more usual causes (see Chap. 255).

Mediastinal infection is uncommon, usually arising from thoracic extension but rarely resulting from perforation of the esophagus, from trauma, or from head-and-neck or abdominal disease. The structures in the mediastinum and the heart can be involved in various combinations; consequently, the possible presentations are diverse. Isolated disease of the breast has been described.

Abdominal Disease   Abdominal actinomycosis poses a great diagnostic challenge. Months or years usually pass from the inciting event (e.g., appendicitis, diverticulitis, peptic ulcer disease, foreign-body perforation, or bowel surgery) to the clinical recognition of disease. Because of the flow of peritoneal fluid and/or the direct extension of primary disease, virtually any abdominal organ, region, or space can be involved. The disease usually presents as an abscess or a mass lesion that is often fixed to underlying tissue and mistaken for a tumor. Infiltrative disease with irregular contrast enhancement may be seen on computed tomography. Sinus tracts to the abdominal wall or perianal region may develop. Recurrent disease or a wound or fistula that fails to heal (in the absence of inflammatory bowel disease) suggests actinomycosis.

Hepatic infection usually presents as single or multiple abscesses or masses. Isolated disease presumably develops via hematogenous seeding from cryptic foci. The imaging and percutaneous techniques that now are available have resulted in improved diagnosis and treatment.

All levels of the urogenital tract can be infected. Renal disease usually presents as pyelonephritis and/or renal and perinephric abscess. Bladder involvement, usually due to extension of pelvic disease, may result in ureteral obstruction or fistulas to bowel, skin, or uterus.

Pelvic Disease   Actinomycotic involvement of the pelvis occurs most commonly in association with an IUD. Although the risk has not yet been quantified, it appears to be small. The disease rarely develops unless the IUD has been in place for at least 2 years, but it can present months after the removal of the device. Symptoms are typically indolent, with fever, weight loss, abdominal pain, and abnormal vaginal bleeding or discharge being the most common. The earliest stage of disease—often endometritis—commonly progresses to limited pelvic masses or a tubo-ovarian abscess. Unfortunately, because diagnosis is often delayed, a "frozen pelvis" mimicking malignancy or endometriosis can develop by the time of recognition.

An unresolved issue is whether the isolation of *Actinomyces*-like organisms (ALOs) from cultures of screening cervical or endometrial specimens or the detection of ALOs by immunofluorescence is correlated with IUD-associated disease. Until more quantitative data become available, detection of ALOs or immunofluorescence-positive organisms in conjunction with symptoms that cannot be accounted for appears to warrant removal of the IUD and initiation of a 14-day course of empirical treatment for possible early pelvic actinomycosis. If such organisms are detected in the absence of symptoms, education of the patient and close follow-up are warranted, but removal of the IUD is not required.

Central Nervous System Disease Actinomycosis of the central nervous system is rare. Single or multiple brain abscesses are most common, usually appearing on computed tomography as a ring-enhancing lesion with a thick wall that may be irregular or nodular.

Musculoskeletal Infection Actinomycotic infection of the bone is usually due to adjacent soft-tissue infection but may be associated with trauma (e.g., fracture of the mandible) or hematogenous spread. Because of slow disease progression, new-bone formation and bone destruction are seen concomitantly. Infection of an extremity is uncommon and is usually a result of trauma. Skin, subcutaneous tissue, muscle, and bone (with periostitis or acute or chronic osteomyelitis) are involved alone or in various combinations.

Disseminated Disease Hematogenous dissemination of disease from any location rarely results in multiple-organ involvement. The lungs and the liver are most commonly affected, with the presentation of multiple nodules mimicking disseminated malignancy. The clinical presentation may be surprisingly indolent given the extent of disease.

DIAGNOSIS Actinomycotic sulfur granules consist of aggregated microorganisms; are usually yellow; can be oval, round, or U-shaped; and, if sought, can be identified macroscopically and/or microscopically in drainage from sinus tracts or other purulent material. Their detection makes the diagnosis of actinomycosis likely. Botryomycosis, mycetoma, and pseudoactinomycotic radiate granules need to be excluded. The isolation of an agent of actinomycosis from granules or from a sterile site confirms the diagnosis. Microbiologic identification is possible in only a minority of cases, often being precluded by prior antimicrobial therapy. Therefore, for optimal yield, the avoidance of even a single dose of antibiotics is mandatory. The microbiology laboratory should be alerted so that cultures are processed appropriately. Primary isolation usually requires 5 to 7 days but may take as long as 2 to 4 weeks. Immunofluorescence testing for *A. israelii*, *A. naeslundii*, and *P. propionicum* (available through the Centers for Disease Control and Prevention in Atlanta) has become a useful diagnostic alternative. Because these organisms are components of the normal oral and genital-tract flora, their identification in sputum, bronchial washings, and cervicovaginal secretions is of little significance in the absence of sulfur granules. *Actinomyces* can be detected in urine by means of appropriate staining and culture.

℞ **TREATMENT**

Actinomycosis must be treated with high doses of antimicrobials for a prolonged period. Although therapy needs to be individualized, the intravenous administration of 18 to 24 million units of penicillin for 2 to 6 weeks, followed by oral therapy with penicillin or amoxicillin for 6 to 12 months, is a reasonable guideline for serious infections. Less extensive disease, particularly that involving the oral-cervicofacial region, may require less intensive therapy. If therapy is extended beyond the point of resolution of measurable disease, the risk of relapse—one of the clinical hallmarks of this infection—will be minimized. For the treatment of penicillin-allergic patients, tetracycline has been used most extensively; erythromycin, minocycline, and clindamycin are other suitable alternatives. First-generation cephalosporins may be an option, depending on the nature of the penicillin allergy and the degree of infection. Of the newer antimicrobial agents, imipenem and ceftriaxone have been described as successful in anecdotal reports. Metronidazole and the aminoglycosides are unreliable. Although the role of "companion" microbes in actinomycosis is unclear, many of these isolates are pathogens in their

own right; therefore, an initial therapeutic regimen that covers these organisms is reasonable.

Combined medical-surgical therapy is still advocated by some authorities. Since antimicrobial therapy alone can cure extensive disease, it is unclear how often surgical intervention is actually necessary. Moreover, percutaneous drainage has become an additional option. If the patient's condition is stable and the response to therapy can be monitored, an attempt to cure the infection with medical therapy alone seems justified. However, when the patient is critically ill or disease is documented at a critical site (e.g., central nervous system), a combined approach seems prudent.

BIBLIOGRAPHY

BENNHOFF D: Actinomycosis: Diagnostic and therapeutic considerations and a review of 32 cases. Laryngoscope 94:1198, 1984

CINTRON JR et al: Abdominal actinomycosis. Dis Colon Rectum 39:105, 1996

FIORINO AS: Intrauterine contraceptive device–associated actinomycotic abscess and *Actinomyces* detection on cervical smear. Obstet Gynecol 87:142, 1996

GOODMAN HM, CENTENO BA: Case records of the Massachusetts General Hospital, Case 10-1992. N Engl J Med 326:692, 1992

RUSSO TA: Actinomycosis, in *Principles and Practice of Infectious Diseases*, 4th ed, GL Mandell et al (eds). New York, Churchill Livingstone, 1995, p 2280

169 *Dennis L. Kasper*

INFECTIONS DUE TO MIXED ANAEROBIC ORGANISMS

DEFINITIONS *Anaerobic* bacteria are organisms that require reduced oxygen tension for growth, failing to grow on the surface of solid media in 10% CO_2 in air. *Microaerophilic* bacteria can grow in 10% CO_2 in air or under anaerobic or aerobic conditions; however, these organisms grow best in the presence of only a small amount of atmospheric oxygen. *Facultative* bacteria can grow in the presence or absence of air. This chapter describes infections caused by nonsporulating anaerobic bacteria. In general, anaerobes associated with human infections are relatively aerotolerant. They can survive for as long as 72 h in the presence of oxygen, although generally they will not multiply in this environment. A far smaller number of pathogenic anaerobic bacteria (which are also part of the normal flora) die after brief contact with oxygen, even in low concentrations.

The nonsporulating anaerobic bacteria exist as components of the normal flora on the mucosal surfaces of humans and animals. The major reservoirs of these bacteria are the mouth, gastrointestinal tract, skin, and female genital tract. Among the constituents of the oral flora, anaerobes are the predominant commensal organisms, ranging in concentration from 10^9/mL in saliva to 10^{12}/mL in gingival scrapings. In the oral cavity, the ratio of anaerobic to aerobic bacteria ranges from 1:1 on the surface of a tooth to 1000:1 in the gingival crevice. Anaerobic bacteria are not found in appreciable numbers in the normal intestine until the distal ileum. In the colon, the proportion of anaerobes increases significantly, as does the overall bacterial count. For example, in the colon there are 10^{11} to 10^{12} organisms per gram of stool, with a ratio of anaerobes to aerobes of approximately 1000:1. In the female genital tract, there are approximately 10^9 organisms per milliliter of secretions, with a ratio of anaerobes to aerobes of approximately 10:1.

Hundreds of species of anaerobic bacteria have been identified as part of the normal flora of humans. Identification of as many as 500 different anaerobic species in fecal specimens reflects the diversity of the anaerobic flora. Despite the complex array of bacteria in the normal flora, relatively few species are isolated commonly from human infection.

Anaerobic infections occur when the harmonious relationship between the host and the bacteria is disrupted. Any site in the body is susceptible to infection with these indigenous organisms when a mucosal barrier or the skin is compromised by surgery, trauma, tumor, or ischemia or necrosis, which reduce local tissue redox potentials. Because the sites that are colonized by anaerobic bacteria contain many species of bacteria, disruption of anatomic barriers allows penetration of many organisms, resulting in mixed infections involving multiple species of anaerobes combined with facultative or microaerophilic organisms. Such mixed infections are seen in the head and neck (chronic sinusitis, chronic otitis media, Ludwig's angina, and periodontal abscesses). Brain abscesses and subdural empyema are the most frequent anaerobic infections of the central nervous system. Anaerobes are responsible for pleuropulmonary diseases such as aspiration pneumonia, necrotizing pneumonia, lung abscess, and empyema. These organisms also play an important role in various intraabdominal infections, such as peritonitis and intraabdominal and liver abscesses (see Chap. 127). They are isolated frequently in female genital tract infections, such as salpingitis, pelvic peritonitis, tuboovarian abscess, vulvovaginal abscess, septic abortion, and endometritis (see Chaps. 129 and 130). Anaerobic bacteria also are frequently found in infections of the skin, soft tissues, and bones and in bacteremia.

ETIOLOGY   The major anaerobic gram-positive cocci that produce disease are *Peptostreptococcus* species. The major species involved in infections are *P. magnus*, *P. asaccharolyticus*, *P. anaerobius*, and *P. prevotii*. Clostridia are gram-positive rods that are isolated from wounds, abscesses, sites of abdominal infection, and blood; they are discussed in Chap. 148. The principal anaerobic gram-negative bacilli are the members of the *Bacteroides* "family," which includes the *Bacteroides fragilis* group, fusobacteria, *Prevotella*, and *Porphyromonas*.

The *B. fragilis* group contains the anaerobic pathogens most frequently isolated from clinical infections. Members of this group are part of the normal bowel flora; they include several distinct species, such as *B. fragilis*, *B. thetaiotaomicron*, *B. distasonis*, *B. vulgatus*, *B. uniformis*, and *B. ovatus*. Of this group, *B. fragilis* is the most important clinical isolate. However, *B. fragilis* is isolated from the normal fecal flora at a lower frequency than other *Bacteroides* species.

A second major group of phenotypically similar organisms is part of the indigenous oral flora. These are primarily pigment-producing bacteria that were previously classified under the species *Bacteroides melaninogenicus*, now known as *Prevotella melaninogenica*. The nomenclature of this group has changed so that several distinct species are recognized, including *Porphyromonas gingivalis*, *Porphyromonas asaccharolytica*, and *P. melaninogenica*. The asaccharolytic pigmented *Porphyromonas* species seldom cause systemic infections in humans.

In female genital tract infections, *Prevotella bivia* and *Prevotella disiens* are the most frequent isolates, although *B. fragilis* is not uncommon. Fusobacteria are also isolated from clinical infections, including necrotizing pneumonia and abscesses. *Bilophila wadsworthia* is an anaerobic, gram-negative organism that is frequently resistant to several antimicrobials, including imipenem, cefoxitin, and other beta-lactam agents. This organism has been reported to cause serious infections, including bacteremia, necrotizing fasciitis, and abscesses.

Infections caused by anaerobic bacteria most frequently are due to more than one organism. These infections may be due to one or several anaerobic species or to a combination of anaerobic organisms and aerobic bacteria acting synergistically.

Approach to the Patient

The physician must consider several points when approaching the patient with presumptive infection due to anaerobic bacteria. (1) Most of these organisms are harmless commensals; very few cause disease. (2) For these organisms to cause infection, they must spread beyond the normal mucosal barriers. (3) Conditions favoring the propagation of these bacteria, particularly a lowered oxidation-reduction potential, are necessary. These conditions exist at sites of trauma, tissue destruction, compromised vascular supply, and complication of preexisting infection that produces necrosis. (4) There is a complex array of infecting flora. For example, as many as 12 different types of organisms can be isolated from a suppurative site. (5) Anaerobic organisms tend to be found in abscess cavities or in necrotic tissue. The failure of an abscess to yield organisms on routine culture is a clue that the abscess is likely to contain anaerobic bacteria. Often smears of this "sterile pus" are found to be teeming with bacteria when Gram's stain is applied. Malodorous pus suggests anaerobic infection. Although some facultative organisms, such as *Staphylococcus aureus*, also are capable of causing abscesses, abscesses in organs or deeper body tissues should call to mind anaerobic infection. (6) Treatment need not be directed at all the organisms in the infectious site. However, some species (the best example being the *B. fragilis* group) require specific therapy. Many of these synergistic infections can be cured with antibiotics directed at some but not all of the organisms involved. Antibiotic therapy, combined with debridement and drainage, disrupts the interdependent relationship among the bacteria, and some species that are resistant to the antibiotic do not survive without the coinfecting organisms. (7) Manifestations of disseminated intravascular coagulation are unusual in patients with anaerobic infection.

EPIDEMIOLOGY   Difficulties in the performance of appropriate cultures, contamination of cultures by aerobic bacteria or components of the normal flora, and the lack of readily available, reliable culture techniques have made it impossible to obtain accurate incidence or prevalence data. However, these infections are encountered frequently in hospitals with active surgical, trauma, and obstetric and gynecologic services. In some centers, anaerobic bacteria, particularly *B. fragilis*, account for approximately 8 to 10 percent of positive blood cultures.

PATHOGENESIS   Anaerobic bacterial infections usually occur when an anatomic barrier becomes disrupted and constituents of the local flora enter a site that was previously sterile. The bacteria isolated from infected sites have survived changes in oxidation-reduction potential and exposure to host defenses. Because of the specific growth requirements of anaerobic organisms and their presence as commensals on mucosal surfaces, conditions must arise that allow these organisms to penetrate mucosal barriers and enter tissue with a lowered oxidation-reduction potential. Therefore, tissue ischemia, trauma, surgery, perforated viscus, shock, and aspiration provide environments conducive to the proliferation of anaerobes. Some highly fastidious anaerobes lack the enzyme superoxide dismutase, which in other organisms reduces toxic superoxide radicals and thereby lessens the potentially lethal effects of superoxide. In the case of a perforated viscus, hundreds of species of anaerobic bacteria are spilled into the peritoneal cavity, but many of these organisms are unable to survive because the highly vascularized tissue provides an adequate oxygen supply. The entry of oxygen into the environment results in the selection of aerotolerant organisms.

The ability of an organism to adhere to host tissues is important to the establishment of infection. Some oral species adhere to crevicular epithelium in the oral cavity. *P. melaninogenica* actually attaches to other microorganisms; *P. gingivalis* is a common isolate in periodontal disease. These organisms have fimbriae that facilitate attachment. Some unencapsulated *Bacteroides* strains appear to be piliated, a characteristic that may account for their ability to adhere.

The most extensively studied virulence factor of the nonsporulating anaerobes is the polysaccharide capsule of *B. fragilis*. This polysaccharide possesses distinct biologic properties, such as the ability (owing to a unique motif of charged sugars) to promote abscess formation in a rodent model of intraabdominal sepsis. Abscess induction is a T cell–dependent phenomenon. Immunization with the capsule confers protection against abscess induction following challenge with *B. fragilis* or other intestinal microorganisms capable of inducing abscesses. This protection is mediated by a T cell circuit that blocks the tissue response of abscess formation. Although some clinicians have viewed abscess formation as a protective host response that localizes and contains infecting bacteria, abscess formation in patients with sepsis often results in severe and chronic illness that requires surgical drainage in combination with antimicrobial therapy.

Anaerobic bacteria produce a number of exoproteins that are capable of enhancing the organisms' virulence. These enzymes include a heparinase elaborated by *B. fragilis* that may contribute to intravascular clotting and necessitate increased doses of heparin for patients receiving heparin therapy. Collagenase, produced by *P. gingivalis*, may enhance tissue destruction. Alteration of the secretory cytoskeleton of intestinal epithelial cells by an enterotoxin from *B. fragilis* has been described. Both *B. fragilis* and *P. melaninogenica* possess lipopolysaccharides (endotoxins) that lack the biologic potency characteristic of endotoxins associated with aerobic gram-negative bacteria. The biologic inactivity of the endotoxin may account for the lower frequency of disseminated intravascular coagulation and purpura in *Bacteroides* bacteremia than in facultative and aerobic gram-negative bacillary bacteremia.

CLINICAL MANIFESTATIONS Anaerobic Infections of the Mouth, Head, and Neck

(See Chap. 30) Infections of the mouth can arise from either the supragingival or the subgingival dental plaque. Supragingival plaque formation begins with the adherence of gram-positive bacteria to the tooth surface. This form of plaque is influenced by salivary and dietary components, oral hygiene, and local host factors. Once the supragingival plaque is established, the acquisition of pathogenic bacteria and an increase in the amount of plaque are responsible for the ultimate development of gingivitis. Early bacteriologic changes in the supragingival plaque initiate an inflammatory response in the gingiva, including edema, swelling, and increase in gingival fluid, and cause the development of caries and endodontic (pulp) infections. In addition, these changes contribute to the subsequent pathogenic alteration in the subgingival plaque that arises from poor or inadequate oral hygiene.

Subgingival plaque is associated with periodontal disease and disseminated infection arising from the oral cavity. Bacteria that colonize the subgingival area are primarily anaerobic. The black-pigmented gram-negative anaerobic bacilli, principally *P. gingivalis* and *P. melaninogenica*, are the most important. Infections in this area are frequently mixed and involve both anaerobic and aerobic bacteria. After establishment of local infection either in root canals or in the periodontal area, infection may extend into the mandible, causing osteomyelitis; to the maxillary sinuses; or to local tissues in the submandibular or submental spaces, depending on which teeth are involved. Periodontitis also may result in spreading infection that can involve adjacent bone or soft tissues.

Gingivitis Gingivitis may become a necrotizing infection (trench mouth, Vincent's stomatitis). The onset of disease is usually sudden and is associated with tender bleeding gums, foul breath, and a bad taste. The gingival mucosa, especially the papillae between the teeth, becomes ulcerated and may be covered by a gray exudate, which is removable with gentle pressure. Patients may become systemically ill, developing fever, cervical lymphadenopathy, and leukocytosis. Occasionally, ulcerative gingivitis can spread to the buccal mucosa, the teeth, and the mandible or maxilla, resulting in widespread destruction of bone and soft tissue. This infection is termed *acute necrotizing ulcerative mucositis* (cancrum oris, noma). It destroys tissue rapidly, causing the teeth to fall out and large areas of bone—or even the whole mandible—to be sloughed. A strong putrid odor is frequently detected, although the lesions are not painful. The gangrenous lesions eventually heal, leaving large disfiguring defects. This infection is seen most commonly following a debilitating illness or in severely malnourished children. It has been known to complicate leukemia or to develop in individuals with a genetic deficiency of catalase.

Acute necrotizing infections of the pharynx These infections usually occur in association with ulcerative gingivitis. Symptoms include an extremely sore throat, foul breath, and a bad taste accompanied by fever and a sensation of choking. Examination of the pharynx demonstrates that the tonsillar pillars are swollen, red, ulcerated, and covered with a grayish membrane that peels easily. Lymphadenopathy and leukocytosis are common. The disease may last for only a few days or, if not treated, may persist for weeks. Lesions begin unilaterally but may spread to the other side of the pharynx or the larynx. Aspiration of the infected material by the patient can result in lung abscesses. Soft tissue infection of the oral-facial area may or may not be odontogenic. *Ludwig's angina*, a periodontal infection usually arising from the tissues surrounding the third molar, may produce submandibular cellulitis that results in marked local swelling of tissues, with pain, trismus, and superior and posterior displacement of the tongue. Submandibular swelling of the neck can impair swallowing and cause respiratory obstruction. In some cases, tracheotomy may be life-saving.

Fascial infections These infections arise from the spread of organisms originating in the upper airways to potential spaces formed by the fascial planes of the head and neck. Perimandibular space infection most commonly involves the submandibular, peritonsillar, and parapharyngeal spaces. Peritonsillar abscesses occur in association with pharyngitis. Complicated dental infections spread to the submandibular and buccal spaces. Entry of organisms by either portal can result in parapharyngeal space infections. Although there are few well-documented reports on the microbiology of these syndromes, anaerobes from the oral flora have been implicated in many cases. *S. aureus* and *Streptococcus pyogenes* infections may arise from boils or impetigo, whereas anaerobes are associated with space infections either occurring spontaneously or arising from diseases of the mucous membranes or from dental manipulations.

Sinusitis and otitis The role of anaerobic bacteria in acute sinusitis may be underestimated because of improper collection of specimens. In a study of chronic sinusitis, anaerobic bacteria were found in 52 percent of specimens collected during external frontoethmoidotomy or radical antrotomy. Anaerobic bacteria are much more easily implicated in chronic suppurative otitis media than in acute otitis media. Purulent exudate from chronically draining ears has been found to contain anaerobes, particularly *Bacteroides* species, in up to 50 percent of cases. *B. fragilis* has been isolated from up to 28 percent of patients with chronic otitis media.

Complications of anaerobic head and neck infections Contiguous craniad spread of these infections may result in osteomyelitis of the skull or mandible or in intracranial infections such as brain abscess and subdural empyema. Caudad spread can produce mediastinitis or pleuropulmonary infection. Hematogenous complications also may result from anaerobic infections of the head and neck. Bacteremia, which occasionally is polymicrobial, can lead to endocarditis or other distant infections. When infections spread to produce suppurative thrombophlebitis of the internal jugular vein, a destructive syndrome—with prolonged fever, bacteremia, septic emboli to both the lung and the brain, and multiple metastatic foci of suppurative infection—may develop. This syndrome has been reported with fusobacterial septicemia following exudative pharyngitis but is uncommon in this era of antimicrobial agents.

Central Nervous System Infections Brain abscesses are frequently associated with anaerobic bacteria (see Chap. 377). If optimal bacteriologic techniques are employed, as many as 85 percent of brain abscesses yield anaerobic bacteria—most often anaerobic gram-positive cocci, which are followed in frequency by fusobacteria and *Bacteroides* species. Facultative or microaerophilic streptococci and coliforms often are part of a mixed infecting flora in brain abscesses.

Pleuropulmonary Infections Anaerobic pleuropulmonary infections result from the aspiration of oropharyngeal contents, often in the context of an altered state of consciousness or an absent gag reflex. Four clinical syndromes are associated with anaerobic pleuropulmonary infection produced by aspiration: simple aspiration pneumonia, necrotizing pneumonia, lung abscess, and empyema.

Aspiration pneumonitis Aspiration pneumonitis must be distinguished from two other clinical syndromes associated with aspiration that are not of bacterial etiology. One syndrome results from aspiration of solids, usually food. Obstruction of major airways typically results in atelectasis and moderate nonspecific inflammation. Therapy consists of removal of the foreign body.

The second aspiration syndrome is more easily confused with bacterial aspiration. This is the so-called Mendelson's syndrome, resulting from regurgitation of stomach contents and aspiration of chemical material, usually gastric juices. Pulmonary inflammation—including the destruction of the alveolar lining, with transudation of fluid into the alveolar space—occurs with remarkable rapidity. Typically this syndrome develops within hours, often following anesthesia when the gag reflex is depressed. The patient becomes tachypneic, hypoxic, and febrile. The leukocyte count may rise, and the chest x-ray may evolve suddenly from normal to a complete "whiteout" bilaterally within 8 to 24 h. Sputum production is minimal. The pulmonary signs and symptoms can resolve quickly with symptom-based therapy or can culminate in respiratory failure with the subsequent development of bacterial superinfection over a period of days. Antibiotic therapy is not indicated unless bacterial infection supervenes. The signs of bacterial infection include sputum production, persistent fever, leukocytosis, and clinical evidence of sepsis.

In contrast to these syndromes, bacterial aspiration pneumonia develops more slowly. It is seen in patients who are hospitalized and have a depressed gag reflex, impaired swallowing, or a tracheal or nasogastric tube; elderly patients; or those with transient impaired consciousness in the wake of seizures, cerebrovascular accidents, or alcoholic blackouts. Patients who enter the hospital with this syndrome typically have been ill for several days and generally complain of low-grade fever, malaise, and sputum production. Usually the history reveals a predisposition for aspiration, such as alcohol overdose or residence in a nursing home. Sputum characteristically is not malodorous unless the process has been going on for at least a week. A mixed bacterial flora with many polymorphonuclear leukocytes is evident on Gram's staining; cultures are reliable only if contamination with the normal oral flora is avoided—that is, by transtracheal aspiration. In general, this procedure is not indicated in the evaluation of these patients. The most commonly encountered anaerobes in these infections are pigmented and nonpigmented *Prevotella* spp., *Fusobacterium nucleatum*, *Peptostreptococcus* spp., and *Bacteroides* spp. Chest x-rays show consolidation in dependent pulmonary segments: in the basilar segments of the lower lobes if the patient has aspirated while upright or sitting and in either the posterior segment of the upper lobe (usually on the right side) or the superior segment of the lower lobe if the patient has aspirated while supine. The organisms isolated reflect the pharyngeal flora; *P. melaninogenica*, *Fusobacterium* species, and anaerobic cocci are the most frequent isolates. The patient who aspirates in the hospital also may have a mixed infection involving enteric gram-negative rods.

Necrotizing pneumonitis This form of anaerobic pneumonitis is characterized by numerous small abscesses that spread to involve several pulmonary segments. The process can be indolent or fulminating. This syndrome is less common than either aspiration pneumonia or lung abscess and includes features of both types of infection.

Anaerobic lung abscesses These abscesses result from subacute anaerobic pulmonary infection. The clinical syndrome typically involves a history of constitutional symptoms, including malaise, weight loss, fever, chills, and foul-smelling sputum, perhaps over a period of weeks (see Chap. 255). Patients who develop lung abscesses characteristically have dental infection and periodontitis, but lung abscesses in edentulous patients have been reported. Abscess cavities may be single or multiple and generally occur in dependent pulmonary segments. Anaerobic abscesses must be distinguished from those associated with tuberculosis, neoplasia, and other conditions. Oral anaerobes predominate, although *B. fragilis* is isolated in up to 10 percent of cases. *S. aureus* may be found as well.

For many years penicillin was considered the gold standard of therapy for lung abscesses. Recent clinical trials have shown that clindamycin therapy results in a better clinical outcome than penicillin,

presumably because clindamycin has a better spectrum of activity against oral anaerobes. Thus, a combination of penicillin and metronidazole or another antibiotic combination that treats both oral anaerobes and aerobes is likely to be as effective as clindamycin. Bronchoscopy is indicated only to rule out the presence of airway obstruction, but it should be delayed until the antimicrobial has begun to affect the disease process so that it does not spread the infection. Bronchoscopy has no role in enhancing drainage. Surgery is almost never indicated because of the danger of spilling the abscess contents into the lungs.

Empyema Empyema is a manifestation of long-standing anaerobic pulmonary infection. The clinical presentation, which includes the presence of foul-smelling sputum, resembles that of other anaerobic pulmonary infections. Patients may complain of pleuritic chest pain and marked chest-wall tenderness.

Empyema may be masked by overlying pneumonitis and should be considered especially in cases of persistent fever in a patient receiving antibiotic therapy. Diligent physical examination and the use of ultrasound to localize a loculated empyema are important diagnostic tools. The collection of a foul-smelling exudate by thoracentesis is typical. Cultures of infected pleural fluid yield an average of 3.5 anaerobes and 0.6 facultative or aerobic bacterial species. Drainage is required. Defervescence, a return to a feeling of well-being, and resolution of the process may require several months.

Extension from a subdiaphragmatic infection also may result in anaerobic empyema. Septic pulmonary emboli may originate from intraabdominal or female genital tract infections and can produce anaerobic pneumonia.

Intraabdominal Infections (See Chap. 127) Enterotoxigenic *B. fragilis* has been associated with watery diarrhea in a small number of young children and adults. In case-control studies of children with undiagnosed diarrheal disease, enterotoxigenic *B. fragilis* was isolated from as many as 20 percent of the children with diarrhea but from fewer than 5 percent of the control children. The role of this enterotoxin and of enterotoxigenic *B. fragilis* in diarrheal disease remains unclear.

Pelvic Infections The vagina of a healthy woman is one of the major reservoirs of anaerobic and aerobic bacteria. In the normal flora of the female genital tract, anaerobes outnumber aerobes by a ratio of approximately 10:1 and include anaerobic gram-positive cocci and *Bacteroides* species. Anaerobes are isolated from most patients with infections of the genital tract not caused by a sexually transmitted pathogen. The major anaerobic pathogens are *B. fragilis*, *P. bivia*, *P. disiens*, *P. melaninogenica*, anaerobic cocci, and clostridial species. Anaerobes frequently are encountered in tuboovarian abscess, septic abortion, pelvic abscess, endometritis, and postoperative wound infection, particularly following hysterectomy. Although these infections are frequently mixed, involving both anaerobes and coliforms, pure anaerobic infections without coliform or other facultative bacterial species occur more often in pelvic than in intraabdominal sites and are characterized by drainage of foul-smelling pus or blood from the uterus, generalized uterine or local pelvic tenderness, and continued fever and chills. Suppurative thrombophlebitis of the pelvic veins may complicate the infections and lead to repeated episodes of septic pulmonary emboli. Anaerobic bacteria have been thought to be contributing factors in the etiology of bacterial vaginosis. This syndrome is characterized by a profuse malodorous discharge and an increase in the number of bacteria in the vagina, including *Gardnerella vaginalis*, *Prevotella* spp., *Mobiluncus* spp., peptostreptococci, and genital mycoplasmas. Anaerobic bacteria are thought to play a role in the etiology of pelvic inflammatory disease (see Chap. 130), and several investigations have shown an association between bacterial vaginosis and the development of pelvic inflammatory disease.

Skin and Soft Tissue Infections Injury to skin, bone, or soft tissue by trauma, ischemia, or surgery creates a suitable environment for anaerobic infections. These infections are most frequently found in sites prone to contamination with feces or with upper airway secretions—for example, wounds associated with intestinal surgery, decubitus ulcers, or human bites. Anaerobic bacteria can be isolated in cases of crepitant cellulitis, synergistic cellulitis, or gangrene and necrotizing fasciitis. Moreover, these organisms have been isolated from cutaneous abscesses, rectal abscesses, and axillary sweat gland infections (hydradenitis suppurativa). Anaerobes frequently have been cultured from foot ulcers in diabetic patients.

These soft tissue or skin infections are usually polymicrobial. A mean of 4.8 bacterial species are isolated, with a roughly 3:2 ratio of anaerobes to aerobes. The most frequently isolated organisms include *Bacteroides* species, anaerobic streptococci, enterococci, clostridial species, and *Proteus* species. The presence of anaerobes in these types of infections is associated with a higher frequency of fever, foul-smelling lesions, or visible foot ulcer.

Anaerobic bacterial *synergistic gangrene* (Meleney's gangrene) is characterized by exquisite pain, redness, and swelling followed by induration. Erythema surrounds a central zone of necrosis. A granulating ulcer, which may heal, forms at the original center as necrosis and erythema extend outward. Symptoms are limited to pain; fever is not typical. These infections usually involve a combination of anaerobic cocci and *S. aureus;* the usual site of infection is an abdominal surgical wound or the area surrounding an ulcer on an extremity. Treatment includes surgical removal of necrotic tissue and antimicrobial therapy.

Necrotizing fasciitis This rapidly spreading destructive disease of the fascia is usually attributed to group A streptococci but can also be caused by anaerobic bacteria, including *Peptostreptococcus* and *Bacteroides* species. Similarly, myonecrosis can be associated with mixed anaerobic infection. Fournier's gangrene consists of cellulitis involving the scrotum, perineum, and anterior abdominal wall, with mixed anaerobic organisms spreading along deep external fascial planes and causing extensive loss of skin.

Bone and Joint Infections Although *actinomycosis* (see Chap. 168) accounts on a worldwide basis for most anaerobic infections in bone, organisms including anaerobic or microaerophilic cocci, *Bacteroides* species, *Fusobacterium* species, and *Clostridium* species can also be found. These infections frequently arise adjacent to soft tissue infections. Hematogenous seeding of bone is uncommon. Oral *Bacteroides* species are seen in infections involving the maxilla and mandible, whereas *Clostridium* species have been reported as anaerobic pathogens in cases of osteomyelitis of the long bones following fracture or trauma. Fusobacteria have been isolated in pure culture from sites of osteomyelitis adjacent to the perinasal sinuses. Anaerobic and microaerophilic cocci have been reported as significant pathogens in infections involving the skull or mastoid.

In cases of anaerobic septic arthritis, the most common isolates are *Fusobacterium* species. Most of the patients involved have uncontrolled peritonsillar infections progressing to septic cervical venous thrombophlebitis and resulting in hematogenous dissemination with a predilection for the joints. Antibiotic treatment of peritonsillar abscess has decreased the prevalence of dissemination to the joints; thus, since the beginning of the antibiotic era, the isolation of *Fusobacterium* species from joints has been less common. Unlike anaerobic osteomyelitis, anaerobic pyoarthritis in most cases is not polymicrobial and may be acquired hematogenously. Anaerobes are important pathogens in infections involving prosthetic joints; in these infections, the causative organisms (such as anaerobic gram-positive cocci and *Propionibacterium acnes*) are part of the normal skin flora.

In patients with osteomyelitis (see Chap. 132), the most reliable source of culture is a bone biopsy sample free of normal uninfected skin and subcutaneous tissue. If a mixed flora is isolated from a bone biopsy specimen, all isolates should be covered by the regimen selected for treatment. When an anaerobic isolate is recognized as a major or sole pathogen infecting a joint, the duration of treatment should be similar to that used for arthritis caused by aerobic bacteria. Therapy includes the management of underlying disease states, appropriate antimicrobial therapy, temporary joint immobilization, percutaneous drainage of effusions, and usually the removal of infected prostheses or internal fixation devices. Surgical drainage and debridement procedures such as sequestrectomy are essential for the removal of necrotic tissue that would sustain anaerobic infections.

Bacteremia Transient bacteremia is a well-known event in healthy people whose anatomic mucosal barriers have been injured (e.g., during dental extractions or dental scaling). These bacteremic episodes, which are often due to anaerobes, have no pathologic consequences. However, anaerobic bacteria are found in cultures of blood from clinically ill patients when proper culture techniques are used. *B. fragilis* is the single most common anaerobic isolate. In recent years, the rate of isolation of anaerobic bacteria from blood cultures has been decreasing. Studies from the 1970s and early 1980s found that 10 to 15 percent of positive blood cultures yielded anaerobes. More recently, similar surveys have found lower rates. The cause of this change is unknown but may be related to the administration of antibiotic prophylaxis before intestinal surgery, the earlier recognition of localized infections, and the empirical use of broad-spectrum antibiotics for presumed infection.

Once the organism has been identified, both the portal of bloodstream entry and the underlying problem that probably led to seeding of the bloodstream can often be deduced from an understanding of the organism's normal place of residence. For example, mixed anaerobic bacteremia including *B. fragilis* usually implies colonic pathology with mucosal disruption from neoplasia, diverticulitis, or some other inflammatory lesion. The initial manifestations are determined by the portal of entry and reflect the localized condition. When bloodstream invasion occurs, patients can become extremely ill, with rigors and hectic fevers ranging up to 40.6°C (105°F). The clinical picture may be quite similar to that seen in sepsis involving aerobic gram-negative bacilli. Although other complications of anaerobic bacteremia, such as septic thrombophlebitis and septic shock, have been reported, the incidence of these complications in association with anaerobic bacteremia is low. Anaerobic bacteremia is potentially fatal and requires rapid diagnosis and appropriate therapy. Mortality appears to increase with the age of the patient (with reported rates of more than 66 percent among patients over 60 years old), with the isolation of multiple species from the bloodstream, and with the failure to surgically remove a focus of infection.

Endocarditis (See Chap. 126) Endocarditis due to anaerobes is uncommon. However, anaerobic streptococci, which are often classified incorrectly, are responsible for this disease more frequently than is generally appreciated. Gram-negative anaerobes are unusual causes of endocarditis.

DIAGNOSIS Because of the time and difficulty involved in the isolation of anaerobic bacteria, diagnosis of these infections must frequently be based on presumptive evidence. Certain sites (such as avascular necrotic tissues) with lowered oxidation-reduction potential favor the diagnosis of an anaerobic infection. When infections occur in proximity to mucosal surfaces normally harboring an anaerobic flora, such as the gastrointestinal tract, female genital tract, or oropharynx, anaerobes should be considered as potential etiologic agents. A foul odor is often indicative of anaerobes, which produce certain organic acids as they proliferate in necrotic tissue. Although the presence of these odors is nearly pathognomonic for anaerobic infection, the absence of odor does not exclude these organisms as etiologic agents. Because anaerobes often coexist with other bacteria to cause mixed or synergistic infection, Gram's staining of exudate frequently reveals numerous pleomorphic cocci and bacilli suggestive of anaerobes. Sometimes these organisms will have morphologic characteristics associated with specific species.

The presence of gas in tissues is highly suggestive, but not diagnostic, of anaerobic infection. When cultures of obviously infected sites yield no growth, streptococci only, or a single aerobic species such as *Escherichia coli*, and Gram's staining reveals a mixed flora, the implication is that the anaerobic microorganisms failed to grow because of inadequate transport and/or culture techniques. Failure of a patient to respond to antibiotics that are not active against anaerobes—for example, aminoglycosides and in some circumstances penicillin, cephalosporins, or tetracyclines— suggests the possibility of anaerobic infection.

There are three critical steps in the diagnosis of anaerobic infection: (1) proper specimen collection; (2) rapid transport of the specimens to the microbiology laboratory, preferably in anaerobic transport media; and (3) proper handling of the specimens by the laboratory.

Specimens must be collected by meticulous sampling of infected sites and avoidance of contamination with the normal flora. When contamination of a specimen with the normal flora is likely, the specimen is unacceptable for processing by the bacteriology laboratory. Examples of specimens unacceptable for anaerobic culture include (1) sputum collected by expectoration or nasal tracheal suction, (2) bronchoscopy specimens, (3) samples collected directly through the vaginal vault, (4) urine collected by voiding, and (5) feces. Specimens that can be cultured for anaerobes include blood, pleural fluid, transtracheal aspirates, pus obtained by direct aspiration from an abscess cavity, fluid obtained by culdocentesis, suprapubic bladder aspirates, cerebrospinal fluid, and lung puncture specimens.

Because even brief exposure to oxygen may kill some anaerobic organisms and result in a failure to isolate them in the laboratory, air must be expelled from the syringe used to aspirate the abscess cavity, and the needle must be capped with a sterile rubber stopper. Proper precautions should be used in the handling of contaminated needles. Specimens can be injected into transport bottles containing a reduced medium or taken immediately in syringes to the laboratory for direct culture on anaerobic media. In general, swabs should not be used. If a swab must be used, it should be placed in a reduced semisolid carrying medium before transport to the laboratory. Delays in transport may lead to a failure to isolate anaerobes due to exposure to oxygen or overgrowth of facultative organisms, which may eliminate or obscure the anaerobes that are present. All clinical specimens from suspected anaerobic infections should be Gram-stained and examined for organisms with characteristic morphology. It is not unusual for organisms to be observed on Gram's staining but not isolated in culture. If purulent materials are found to be sterile or organisms are seen on Gram's staining but do not grow in the culture, the involvement of anaerobes should be suspected.

℞ TREATMENT

Successful therapy for anaerobic infections involves a combination of appropriate antibiotics, surgical resection, debridement of devitalized tissues, and drainage. Perforations must be closed promptly, closed spaces drained, tissue compartments decompressed, and an adequate blood supply established. Abscess cavities should be drained as soon as fluctuation or localization occurs. While surgery was formerly required to establish drainage, with the advent of computed tomography, magnetic resonance imaging, and ultrasound, diagnostic radiologists now are able to drain a number of abscess sites percutaneously.

Patients with infections due to anaerobic bacteria require treatment with appropriate antibiotics. Antibiotic susceptibility testing of anaerobic bacteria has been difficult and controversial. Owing to the slow growth rate of many anaerobes, the lack of standardized methodology, the lack of clinically related standards for resistance, and the generally good results obtained with empirical therapy, susceptibility testing has been recommended only for the study of resistance patterns in regional centers or local hospitals, for the prediction of the efficacy of new antibiotics, and for the management of selected patients. The selection of initial antibiotic therapy should be based on knowledge of the pathogens likely to be present in a specific clinical condition in combination with the Gram's stain findings, which should suggest the likelihood of certain species of organisms. In many infections, anaerobes tend to be mixed with coliforms and other facultative organisms. The best therapeutic regimens, therefore, are usually those with activity against both aerobic and anaerobic bacteria. The choice of empirical antibiotics for the anaerobes can nearly always be made reliably, since patterns of antimicrobial susceptibility are usually predictable (see Chap. 140 and Table 169-1).

Anaerobic gram-negative rods that are frequently resistant to penicillin are listed in Table 169-2. Organisms belonging to the *B. fragilis* group are essentially all resistant to penicillin. This clinically significant resistance mandates that anaerobic infections arising be-

Table 169-1

Antimicrobial Therapy for Infections Involving Commonly Encountered Anaerobic Gram-Negative Rods

Group 1 (<1% Resistance)	Group 2 (<15% Resistance)	Group 3 (Variable Resistance)	Group 4 (Resistance)
Metronidazole*	Clindamycin	Penicillin	Aminoglycosides
Ampicillin/sulbactam	Cefoxitin	Cephalosporins	Quinolones
Ticarcillin/clavulanic acid	High-dose	Tetracycline	Monobactams
Piperacillin/tazobactam	antipseudo-	Vancomycin	
Imipenem	monal peni-	Erythromycin	
Meropenem	cillins		
Chloramphenicol†			

* Usually needs to be given in combination with aerobic bacterial coverage. For infections originating below the diaphragm, aerobic gram-negative coverage is essential. For infections from an oral source, aerobic gram-positive coverage is added. Metronidazole also is not active against *Actinomyces* or *Propionibacterium* and is unreliable against peptostreptococci.
† Chloramphenicol is probably not as effective as other group 1 antimicrobials in treating anaerobic infections.

low the diaphragm be treated with specific therapy directed at *B. fragilis* (see Table 169-1). Recently, β-lactamase production has been reported in strains that are usually isolated from infections originating above the diaphragm. Forty to sixty percent of the clinical isolates classified as *Prevotella* or *Porphyromonas*, non–*B. fragilis* species of *Bacteroides*, or *Fusobacterium* species have been reported as producing β-lactamase. The clinical implications of this resistance have not been completely clarified. However, clindamycin does appear to be superior to penicillin for the treatment of lung abscesses. Although most oral anaerobic infections and cases of anaerobic pneumonia still respond to penicillin therapy, some infections due to oral organisms fail to respond, and in these cases the use of a drug that is effective against penicillin-resistant anaerobes is recommended (see Table 169-1). Life-threatening infections involving the anaerobic flora of the mouth, such as space infections of the head and neck, should be treated empirically as if penicillin-resistant anaerobes are involved. Less serious infections involving the oral microflora can be treated with penicillin alone; metronidazole can be added (or clindamycin can be substituted) if the patient responds poorly to therapy. If metronidazole is used in the treatment of mixed anaerobic and aerobic infections, it is imperative that other appropriate antibiotics be used in conjunction. Metronidazole is inactive against aerobic bacteria, *Actinomyces*, and *Propionibacterium*. The sensitivity of peptostreptococci to metronidazole is unpredictable. Therapy for intraabdominal sepsis (see Chap. 127) must include drugs active against the aerobic flora of the bowel. Combinations of antibiotics used in the treatment of mixed infections of oral origin must include antibiotics active against the aerobic flora of the mouth.

Table 169-2

Frequency of Penicillin Resistance among Commonly Encountered Anaerobic Gram-Negative Rods

Organism	Frequency of Penicillin Resistance*
Bacteroides fragilis	High
Bacteroides thetaiotaomicron	High
Bacteroides ovatus	High
Bacteroides distasonis	High
Bacteroides vulgatus	High
Bacteroides gracilis	High
Bilophila wadsworthia	High
Fusobacterium nucleatum	Low
Fusobacterium necrophorum	Low
Fusobacterium mortiferum	Low
Fusobacterium varium	Low
Prevotella species	Moderate
Porphyromonas species	Low

* High: >90 percent of strains; moderate: 5 to 90 percent of strains; low: <5 percent of strains.

Infections arising from a colonic source are likely to involve *B. fragilis*. Many therapeutic failures have been noted in patients with documented *B. fragilis* infection who are treated with penicillin or first-generation cephalosporins. In intraabdominal sepsis, the use of antibiotics effective against penicillin-resistant anaerobes has clearly reduced the incidence of postoperative infection and serious infectious complications. The number of antimicrobial agents effective against *B. fragilis* has expanded, and there are currently several useful choices (see Table 169-1). In general, cure rates of greater than 80 percent can be achieved in patients with *B. fragilis* infection by means of appropriate antimicrobial therapy and drainage.

Recommendations for the treatment of anaerobic infections with antibiotics are usually based on known resistance patterns in certain species and the likelihood of encountering a given species in the case at hand. Antibiotics active against the *B. fragilis* group, penicillin-resistant *Prevotella* and *Porphyromonas*, non–*B. fragilis* species of *Bacteroides*, and *Fusobacterium* species can be grouped into four categories on the basis of their predicted activity against anaerobes (see Table 169-1).

Resistance of *B. fragilis* to metronidazole has been reported rarely. This well-tolerated drug reaches significant levels in serum and also can be found at high levels in abscess cavities. It should be considered first-line therapy against *B. fragilis* infection. If a patient fails to respond to one of the group 1 or 2 drugs (Table 169-1), consideration should be given to alternative therapy and to determination of the resistance patterns among *B. fragilis* group isolates. Although in vitro resistance to chloramphenicol has not been reported, this drug may not be as effective as other group 1 drugs. Ampicillin/sulbactam, ticarcillin/clavulanic acid, piperacillin/tazobactam, imipenem, and meropenem have been effective in the treatment of *B. fragilis* infection. Ciprofloxacin and other currently available quinolones should not be used as primary agents against *B. fragilis*. Penicillin remains the drug of choice for use against peptostreptococci.

Specific regimens must be tailored to the initial infecting site in clinical situations. In the treatment of intraabdominal sepsis, a group 1 drug must be included for broad-spectrum coverage (see Chap. 127). If the involvement of gram-positive bacteria is suspected, an appropriate penicillin should be added. Chloramphenicol has been used successfully in patients with anaerobic central nervous system infections at a dose of 30 to 60 mg/kg per day, depending on the severity of illness. However, penicillin G and metronidazole also cross the blood-brain barrier and are bactericidal for many anaerobic organisms (see Chap. 377).

Nearly all the drugs mentioned have toxic side effects, which are described in detail in Chap. 140.

Anaerobic infections that have failed to respond to treatment or that have relapsed should be reassessed. Consideration should be given to additional surgical drainage or debridement. Superinfections with resistant gram-negative facultative or aerobic bacteria should be ruled out. The possibility of drug resistance also must be entertained; repeated cultures should yield the pathogenic organism.

Other supportive measures in the management of anaerobic infections include careful attention to fluid and electrolyte balance (since extensive local edema may lead to hypoalbuminemia); hemo-dynamic support for septic shock; immobilization of infected extremities; maintenance of adequate nutrition during chronic infections by parenteral hyperalimentation; relief of pain; and anticoagulation with heparin for thrombophlebitis. Hyperbaric oxygen therapy is advocated by some experts but is of no proven value.

BIBLIOGRAPHY

APPELBAUM PC et al: β-Lactamase production and susceptibilities to amoxicillin, amoxicillin-clavulanate, ticarcillin, ticarcillin-clavulanate, cefoxitin, imipenem, and metronidazole of 320 non–*Bacteroides fragilis Bacteroides* isolates and 129 fusobacteria from 28 U.S. centers. Antimicrob Agents Chemother 34:1546, 1990

BARTLETT JG: Infections caused by anaerobic bacteria, in *Infectious Diseases*, SL Gorbach et al (eds). Philadelphia, Saunders, 1992

———, FINEGOLD SM: Anaerobic infections of the lung and pleural space. Am Rev Respir Dis 110:56, 1974

CRABB JH et al: T-cell regulation of *Bacteroides fragilis*–induced intraabdominal abscesses. Rev Infect Dis 12:S178, 1990

DORSHER CW et al: Anaerobic bacteremia: Decreasing rate over a 15-year period. Rev Infect Dis 13:633, 1991

FINEGOLD SM: Anaerobic bacteria: General concepts, in *Principles and Practice of Infectious Diseases*, 4th ed, GL Mandell et al (eds). New York, Churchill Livingstone, 1995

———: Overview of clinically important anaerobes. Clin Infect Dis 20:S205, 1995

———, GEORGE WL: *Anaerobic Infections in Humans*. San Diego, Academic, 1989

GIBBS RS: Microbiology of the female genital tract. Am J Obstet Gynecol 156:491, 1987

HORN J et al: Role of anaerobic bacteria in perimandibular space infections. Ann Otol Rhinol Laryngol (Suppl) 154:34, 1991

LEVIN S, GOODMAN LJ: Selected overview of nongynecologic surgical intraabdominal infections: Prophylaxis and therapy. Am J Med 79:146, 1985

MATHISEN GE et al: Brain abscess and cerebritis. Rev Infect Dis 6:S101, 1984

NAKATA MN, LEWIS RP: Anaerobic bacteria in bone and joint infections. Rev Infect Dis 6:S165, 1984

NEWMAN MG: Anaerobic oral and dental infections. Rev Infect Dis 6:S107, 1984

NICHOLS RL: Surgical infections: Prevention and treatment—1965 to 1995. Am J Surg 172:68, 1996

ONDERDONK AB et al: Animal model system for studying virulence of and host response to *Bacteroides fragilis*. Rev Infect Dis 12:S169, 1990

PANTOSTI A et al: Immunochemical characterization of two surface polysaccharides of *Bacteroides fragilis*. Infect Immun 59(5):1690, 1991

SEARS CL et al: Enterotoxigenic *Bacteroides fragilis*. Clin Infect Dis 20:S142, 1995

SUMMANEN PH et al: *Bilophila wadsworthia* isolates from clinical specimens. Clin Infect Dis 20:S210, 1995

SWEET RL: Role of bacterial vaginosis in pelvic inflammatory disease. Clin Infect Dis 20:S271, 1995

THORNSBERRY C: Antimicrobial susceptibility testing of anaerobic bacteria: Review and update on the role of the National Committee for Clinical Laboratory Standards. Rev Infect Dis 12:S218, 1990

TZIANABOS AO et al: Structural features of polysaccharides that induce intraabdominal abscesses. Science 262:416, 1993

ZALEZNIK DF: Role of bacterial virulence factors in pathogenesis of anaerobic infections, in *Anaerobic Infections in Humans*, S Finegold (ed). Orlando, Academic, 1989

SECTION 8
MYCOBACTERIAL DISEASES

170

Paul W. Wright, Richard J. Wallace, Jr.

ANTIMYCOBACTERIAL AGENTS

The physician is greatly challenged to provide optimal therapy for mycobacterial illnesses because of the advent of AIDS, the increase in both drug-susceptible and multidrug-resistant tuberculosis, and the plethora of new antibiotics with antimycobacterial potential. This chapter reviews the agents used for the treatment of tuberculosis, leprosy (Hansen's disease), and diseases caused by pathogenic nontuberculous mycobacteria including *Mycobacterium avium-intracellulare* (MAI), *Mycobacterium kansasii*, the rapidly growing mycobacteria, and *Mycobacterium marinum*. The use of antimycobacterial agents in patients with renal or hepatic disease and in pregnant women is summarized in Table 170-1. The effects of major antimycobacterial agents on the levels, activity, and toxicity of other commonly used drugs are summarized in Table 170-2.

Table 170-1

Use of Antimycobacterial Agents in Patients with Renal or Hepatic Disease and in Pregnant Women

| | | Use in Indicated Circumstances | | |
| | | Renal Disease: Creatinine Clearance Rate | | |
Agent	Severe Hepatic Disease	>30 mL/min	≤30 mL/min	Pregnancy*
Azithromycin	No change	No change	?Decrease dose	No evidence of risk (B)
Clarithromycin	No change	No change	Decrease dose	Risk cannot be ruled out (C)
Ethambutol	No change	No change	Decrease dose	Risk cannot be ruled out (?C)
Isoniazid	Avoid use or decrease dose	No change	Decrease dose	Risk cannot be ruled out (?C)
Pyrazinamide	Avoid use or decrease dose	No change	Decrease dose†	Risk cannot be ruled out (C)
Rifabutin	No change	No change	No change	No evidence of risk (B)
Rifampin	Avoid use or decrease dose	No change	No change	Risk cannot be ruled out (C)
Streptomycin	No change	Decrease dose	Decrease dose and frequency	Definite evidence of risk (D)

* Based on Food and Drug Administration pregnancy categories of A–D, X.
† Prudent but not absolutely necessary.

TUBERCULOSIS

Drugs used to treat tuberculosis are classified as first-line and second-line agents. *First-line essential* antituberculous agents are the most effective and are a necessary component of any short-course therapeutic regimen. The two drugs in this category are isoniazid and rifampin. *First-line supplemental* agents either can shorten chemotherapy (e.g., pyrazinamide) or are highly effective and infrequently toxic (ethambutol and streptomycin). *Second-line* antituberculous drugs are clinically much less effective than first-line agents and much more frequently elicit severe reactions. These drugs are rarely used in therapy and then only by caregivers experienced with their use. They include para-aminosalicylic acid (PAS), ethionamide, cycloserine, kanamycin, amikacin, capreomycin, viomycin, and thiacetazone. *Newer* antitubercular drugs, which have not yet been placed in the above categories, include rifabutin and the quinolones, especially ciprofloxacin, ofloxacin, and sparfloxacin.

FIRST-LINE ESSENTIAL DRUGS Isoniazid Perhaps the best antituberculous drug available, isoniazid should be included in all tuberculosis treatment regimens unless the organism is resistant. It is inexpensive, readily synthesized, available worldwide, very selective for mycobacteria, and well tolerated, with only 5 percent of patients exhibiting adverse effects.

Mechanism of action Isoniazid is the hydrazide of isonicotinic acid, a small water-soluble molecule that easily penetrates the cell. Its mechanism of action involves inhibition of mycolic acid cell-wall synthesis via oxygen-dependent pathways such as the catalase-peroxidase reaction. Isoniazid is bacteriostatic against resting bacilli and bactericidal against rapidly multiplying organisms, both extracellularly and intracellularly. The minimal inhibitory concentrations (MICs) of isoniazid for wild-type (untreated) strains of *Mycobacterium tuberculosis* are <0.1 μg/mL, while those for *M. kansasii* usually are 0.5 to 2.0 μg/mL. The MICs of this drug for other mycobacteria are much higher.

Pharmacology Both oral and intramuscular preparations of isoniazid are readily absorbed. A 300-mg oral dose generally produces peak serum levels of 3 to 5 μg/mL. Isoniazid diffuses well throughout the body and reaches therapeutic concentrations in serum, cerebrospinal fluid (CSF), and infected tissue, including caseous granulomas. Isoniazid is metabolized in the liver via acetylation and hydrolysis; its metabolites are excreted into the urine. The rate of acetylation is genetically controlled. The usual daily dose for the treatment of tuberculosis is 5 mg/kg for adults and 10 to 20 mg/kg for children, with a maximal daily dose of 300 mg for both groups. For intermittent therapy (usually directly observed), a maximal dose of 900 mg twice or three times weekly is used. Even in moderate or severe renal failure, the adult dose rarely needs to be reduced below 200 mg/d.

Adverse effects (Table 170-3) The two most important adverse effects of isoniazid therapy are hepatotoxicity and peripheral neuropathy. Other adverse reactions are either rare or less significant and include rash (2 percent), fever (1.2 percent), anemia, acne, arthritic symptoms, a systemic lupus erythematosus–like syndrome, optic atrophy, seizures, and psychiatric symptoms. Isoniazid-associated hepatitis is idiosyncratic and increases in incidence with age. It occurs in 0.3 percent of treated persons under 35 years of age, 1.2 percent of those under 49 years of age, and 2.3 percent of those over 50 years of age. The risk of isoniazid-associated hepatitis is increased by daily alcohol consumption,

Table 170-2

Effect of Major Antimycobacterial Agents on Levels/Activity/Toxicity of Other Commonly Used Drugs

Rifampin	Isoniazid	Clarithromycin	Rifabutin*	Agents with No/Minimal Drug Effects
Analgesics (↓)	Alcohol (↑ risk of hepatitis)	Astemizole (↑)	(↓ In same drugs as rifampin but to a lesser degree)	Amikacin
Anticonvulsants (↓)		Carbamazepine (↑)		Azithromycin
Barbiturates (↓)	Carbamazepine (↑)	Digoxin (↑)		Capreomycin
β blockers (↓)		Rifabutin (↑)		Ethambutol
Chloramphenicol (↓)	Diphenylhydantoin (↑)	Ritonavir (↑)		Streptomycin
Clarithromycin (↓)		Terfenadine (↑)		Pyrazinamide
Clofibrate (↓)	Enflurane (↑ risk of renal failure)	Zidovudine (↓)		
Cyclosporine (↓)	Warfarin (↑)			
Dapsone (↓)				
Diazepam (↓)				
Digoxin (↓)				
Disopyramide (↓)				
Glucocorticoids (↓)				
Halothane (↓)				
Indinavir (↓)				
Ketoconazole (↓)				
Mexiletine (↓)				
Narcotics (↓)				
Oral contraceptives (↓)				
Oral hypoglycemic agents (↓)				
Probenecid (↓)				
Progestins (↓)				
Quinidine (↓)				
Ritonavir (↓)				
Saquinavir (↓)				
Theophylline (↓)				
Verapamil (↓)				
Warfarin (↓)				
Zidovudine (↓)				

* Rifabutin induces the cytochrome P450 system but to a lesser degree than rifampin. All drugs whose half-life is decreased by rifampin induction of hepatic microsomal enzymes may be subject to the same effect when coadministered with rifabutin; however, this point has not yet been studied.

concomitant rifampin administration, and slow acetylation of isoniazid. Mortality from isoniazid-induced hepatitis has been reported to be 6 to 12 percent, but the real risk is certainly much lower: the reported rates were documented in high-risk patients who continued to take the drug despite progressive symptoms of hepatitis and without monitoring of liver enzyme levels. Liver enzymes are monitored in most settings among high-risk patients, and administration of the drug is discontinued at the onset of hepatitis. The American Thoracic Society recommends that serum concentrations of aspartate or alanine aminotransferase (AST or ALT) be determined at baseline in patients over 35 years of age who are receiving isoniazid for chemoprophylaxis, with monthly determinations thereafter. The benefit of such routine monitoring remains controversial, however. Measurement of the ALT or AST level is certainly mandatory whenever a patient notices the onset of symptoms suggestive of isoniazid-associated hepatitis (e.g., fever, anorexia, nausea, vomiting, and/or a flulike syndrome including fever and myalgias), and treatment should immediately be discontinued until the relationship between therapy and symptoms is ascertained. The American Thoracic Society also recommends that, even in the absence of these symptoms, discontinuation of isoniazid be strongly considered whenever an AST or ALT level exceeds 150 to 200 IU (three to five times the upper limit of normal) in a high-risk patient. When these guidelines are followed, death from isoniazid-associated hepatitis has occurred at a rate of only 14 per 100,000 treated patients. Twelve percent of patients who have initially normal liver function and take isoniazid may experience transient elevations of AST. If AST elevation persists, if AST is elevated to more than five times the normal level, or if symptoms of hepatitis develop, therapy must be discontinued. Several recent studies have demonstrated that many patients with isoniazid intolerance can be desensitized.

Peripheral neuritis associated with isoniazid develops at a dose-dependent rate of 2 to 20 percent and probably relates to interference with pyridoxine metabolism. This rate can be reduced to 0.2 percent with the prophylactic administration of 10 to 50 mg of pyridoxine (vitamin B_6) daily.

Resistance Isoniazid-resistant mutants of *M. tuberculosis* occur spontaneously at a rate of 1 in 10^5 to 10^6 organisms. The molecular sites of isoniazid resistance have recently been detailed. Almost all isoniazid-resistant strains have amino acid changes in the catalase-peroxidase gene (*katG*) or a two-gene locus known as *inhA*. Missense mutations or deletion of *katG* are also associated with reduced catalase and peroxidase activity. Primary isoniazid resistance is detected in 7 percent of untreated patients in native U.S. populations, but the percentage is much higher in many immigrant populations.

Rifampin Rifampin, a semisynthetic derivative of *Streptomyces mediterranei*, is the second most important antituberculous agent, exhibiting efficacy against *M. tuberculosis* comparable to that of isoniazid. It is also active against a wide spectrum of other organisms, including some gram-positive and gram-negative bacteria, *Legionella* species, *M. kansasii*, *M. marinum*, and some strains of MAI.

Pharmacology Rifampin is a fat-soluble complex macrocyclic antibiotic that is absorbed readily either orally or intravenously. Serum levels of 10 to 20 μg/mL follow a standard oral dose of 600 mg. Rifampin distributes well throughout most body tissues, including inflamed meninges. The fact that rifampin turns body fluids (urine, saliva, sputum, tears) to a red-orange color makes it simple and inexpensive to check on a patient's compliance with therapy. Rifampin is excreted primarily through the bile and the entero-hepatic circulation, while 30 to 40 percent of a dose is excreted via the kidneys. The drug is administered either twice weekly or daily at a dose of 600 mg for adults (10 mg/kg) and 10 to 20 mg/kg for children.

Mechanism of action Rifampin has both intracellular and extracellular bactericidal activity. It blocks RNA synthesis by specifically binding and inhibiting DNA-dependent RNA polymerase. Susceptible strains of *M. tuberculosis* as well as *M. kansasii* and *M. marinum* are inhibited by ≤1 μg/mL.

Adverse effects (Table 170-3) Rifampin is generally well tolerated; the most common adverse event is gastrointestinal upset. Patients with chronic liver disease, especially those with alcoholism and those who are elderly, appear to be at unusually high risk for the most serious adverse reaction: hepatitis. Concomitant administration of rifampin increases the risk of isoniazid-associated hepatitis. Other adverse effects of rifampin include rash (0.8 percent), hemolytic anemia (<1 percent), thrombocytopenia, and immunosuppression of unknown clinical importance. Rifampin is a potent inducer of the hepatic microsomal enzymes and thereby decreases the half-life of a number of drugs, including digoxin, warfarin, prednisone, cyclosporine, methadone, oral contraceptives, clarithromycin, zidovudine, and quinidine (Table 170-2).

Resistance Resistance to rifampin results from spontaneous point mutations that alter the β subunit of the RNA polymerase (*rpoB*) gene. Recent studies have shown that 96 percent of rifampin-resistant strains have a missense mutation within a 91-bp central core region of the gene. Rifampin-resistant strains of *Mycobacterium leprae* have similar mutations that alter a single serine residue (Ser-425) in the same core region of the *rpoB* gene.

Rifabutin Rifabutin, a semisynthetic rifamycin spiropiperidyl derivative, shares many characteristics with rifampin, including activity against *M. tuberculosis*. Rifabutin is active against some strains of rifampin-resistant *M. tuberculosis* and is more active than rifampin against MAI and other nontuberculous mycobacteria. To date, rifabutin has been most useful in the prophylaxis of disseminated MAI infection and in the treatment of drug-resistant tuberculosis. Because it seems

Table 170-3

Monitoring Side Effects of Common Antituberculous Drugs

Drug	Side Effect	Management
Isoniazid	Hepatitis	Monitor AST/limit alcohol consumption/monitor for hepatitis symptoms/educate patient/stop drug at first symptoms of hepatitis (nausea, vomiting, anorexia, flulike syndrome)
	Peripheral neuritis	Administer vitamin B_6
	Optic neuritis	Administer vitamin B_6
	Seizures	Administer vitamin B_6
Rifampin	Rash	Observe patient
	Liver dysfunction	Monitor AST/limit alcohol consumption/monitor for hepatitis symptoms
	Flulike syndrome	Administer at least twice weekly/limit dose to 10 mg/kg (adults)
	Red-orange urine	Reassure patient
	Drug interactions	Consider monitoring drug levels when possible, especially with contraceptives, anticoagulants, and digoxin/avoid use with protease inhibitors
Pyrazinamide	Hepatitis	Monitor AST/limit dosage to 15–30 mg/kg/d
	Hyperuricemia	Monitor uric acid level only in cases of gout or renal failure
Ethambutol	Optic neuritis	Use lower dose (15 mg/kg/d) when possible/monitor visual acuity (eye chart) and red-green color vision (Ishihara Color Book) monthly and with any visual complaint/educate patient/stop drug at first change in vision
Streptomycin, amikacin, capreomycin	Ototoxicity, renal toxicity	Limit dose and duration of therapy as much as possible/avoid daily therapy in patients >50 years old/monitor BUN and serum creatinine levels and possibly conduct audiometry before and as needed during therapy/question patient regularly about tinnitus, dizziness, vertigo, and decreased hearing/measure serum drug levels if possible/educate patient/stop drug at first development of adverse effect

NOTE: AST, aspartate aminotransferase; BUN, blood urea nitrogen.

to show more antituberculous activity than rifampin in vitro and in animals, its possible advantages over rifampin are being evaluated. In a multinational trial with either rifampin (600 mg/d) or rifabutin (150 mg/d) in combination with isoniazid plus 2 months of pyrazinamide and ethambutol, rifampin and rifabutin were equally effective and well tolerated in the treatment of newly diagnosed pulmonary tuberculosis. Rifabutin may be preferable to rifampin in the treatment of individuals positive for human immunodeficiency virus (HIV) who are also taking a protease inhibitor.

Pharmacology The pharmacology of rifabutin is dramatically different from that of rifampin. Rifabutin is readily absorbed after a single oral dose of 300 mg and reaches peak serum levels (0.35 μg/mL) in 2 to 4 h. This lipophilic drug distributes best to tissue: tissue levels are 5 to 10 times higher than plasma levels. CSF concentrations are 30 to 70 percent of plasma levels in HIV-infected patients who have meningitis. The drug's slow clearance via hepatic metabolism and renal excretion results in a mean serum half-life of 45 h, which is much longer than the 3- to 5-h half-life of rifampin. Clarithromycin (but not azithromycin) and fluconazole appear to block the hepatic metabolism of rifabutin, with consequent increases in serum levels. When rifabutin is administered orally with food, its rate of absorption is slowed, but the extent of absorption is unchanged. Adjustment of dosage is usually unnecessary in elderly patients and in patients with reduced hepatic or renal function.

Mechanism of action In *Escherichia coli* and *Bacillus subtilis*, rifabutin inhibits DNA-dependent RNA polymerase in the same manner as rifampin. Its mode of action against mycobacteria is believed to be the same.

Adverse effects Most adverse effects of rifabutin are dose related and occur most frequently in patients receiving >300 mg/d. Discontinuation of therapy because of adverse reactions is reported in 16 percent of patients receiving rifabutin as opposed to 8 percent of those receiving a placebo. The most common symptoms are gastrointestinal; other reactions include rash, fever, headache, asthenia, chest pain, myalgia, and insomnia. Like those taking rifampin, most patients taking rifabutin have discolored (orange to tan) urine and other body fluids. Less common adverse reactions include a flulike syndrome, hepatitis, *Clostridium difficile*–associated diarrhea, and skin discoloration. After a rifabutin dose of 450 or 600 mg in combination with clarithromycin, anterior uveitis is reported in up to 40 percent of patients; also reported are hyperpigmentation and a polymyalgia/arthralgia syndrome, both of which are reversible when treatment is discontinued. Laboratory abnormalities include neutropenia, leukopenia, thrombocytopenia, and increased levels of liver enzymes.

Rifabutin induces the hepatic cytochrome P450 enzymes but does so much less strongly than rifampin. Drugs whose metabolism is enhanced by rifabutin include anticoagulants, quinidine, oral contraceptives, sulfonylureas, analgesics, dapsone, narcotics, glucocorticoids, clarithromycin, zidovudine, and cardiac glycosides.

Resistance Resistance to rifabutin occurs by the same mechanism as that to rifampin—i.e., spontaneous point mutations involving the *rpoB* gene. However, of the 14 mutant *rpoB* alleles that confer resistance to rifampin, only nine confer high-level resistance to rifabutin, while the remaining five result in only small changes in rifabutin MICs (all remain at ≤0.5 μg/mL). The MIC of rifabutin for susceptible strains of *M. tuberculosis* is low (<0.06 μg/mL), and the drug is considered clinically active against partially resistant strains that are inhibited by plasma levels of ≤0.5 μg/mL. Thus rifabutin inhibits about one-quarter of rifampin-resistant strains of *M. tuberculosis*.

FIRST-LINE SUPPLEMENTAL DRUGS **Pyrazinamide** A derivative of nicotinic acid, pyrazinamide is an important bactericidal drug used in short-course therapy for tuberculosis.

Pharmacology Pyrazinamide is well absorbed after oral administration, with a plasma concentration of 45 μg/mL in 2 h and excellent distribution throughout the body. The drug is hydrolyzed in the liver into several metabolites, one of which, pyrazinoic acid, is considered

the active form. Pyrazinoic acid is then hydroxylated to 5-hydroxypyrazinoic acid, which is subsequently excreted by renal glomerular filtration.

Mechanism of action Pyrazinamide is similar to isoniazid in its narrow spectrum of antibacterial activity, which essentially includes only *M. tuberculosis*. At plasma levels of 12.5 μg/mL, the drug is bactericidal to slowly metabolizing organisms located within the acidic environment of the phagocyte or caseous granuloma (being active only at a pH of <6.0). The mode of action of pyrazinamide and the mechanism of resistance to pyrazinamide are unknown.

Adverse effects (Table 170-3) At the high dosages used in the past, hepatotoxicity was a prominent complication of pyrazinamide therapy. However, at the currently recommended daily dosage of 15 to 30 mg/kg, with a maximum of 2 g (which can be given in one dose), the frequency of hepatotoxicity is not higher than that for concomitant isoniazid and rifampin therapy. Hyperuricemia is a common adverse effect of pyrazinamide therapy that is probably reduced by concurrent rifampin therapy. Clinical gout is seen only rarely in patients receiving pyrazinamide. Polyarthralgias are encountered fairly commonly but are not related to hyperuricemia.

Ethambutol A derivative of ethylenediamine, ethambutol is a water-soluble compound that is active only against mycobacteria. Susceptible species include *M. tuberculosis*, *M. marinum*, *M. kansasii*, and MAI. Among first-line drugs, it is the least potent against *M. tuberculosis*. It is used most often with rifampin in the treatment of tuberculosis in patients who are unable to tolerate isoniazid or who are thought or known to be infected with isoniazid-resistant organisms.

Mechanism of action Ethambutol is bacteriostatic against rapidly growing mycobacteria. Neither the mechanism of action nor the mechanism of resistance has been elucidated for this drug.

Pharmacology After oral administration, 75 to 80 percent of a dose of ethambutol is absorbed from the gastrointestinal tract. Serum levels peak at 2 to 4 μg/mL 2 to 4 h after a dose of 15 mg/kg. The drug's distribution throughout the body is adequate except in the CSF, where it reaches only low levels. However, ethambutol can reach CSF levels up to 50 percent as high as peak plasma levels when administered at a dose of 25 mg/kg to a patient with inflamed meninges. Almost all of the dose is excreted by the kidneys within 24 h of ingestion, either unchanged or as metabolites. The usual daily adult dosage of ethambutol is 25 mg/kg (which may be given in one dose) for the first 2 months, with a subsequent reduction to 15 mg/kg. In cases where retreatment is necessary, the higher dose may be given for the duration. For intermittent therapy, the dosage is 50 mg/kg twice weekly or 30 mg/kg three times weekly. The dosage must be lowered for patients with renal insufficiency (a creatinine clearance rate of <25 mL/min) to prevent drug accumulation and toxicity.

Adverse effects (Table 170-3) Ethambutol is usually well tolerated. Retrobulbar optic neuritis is the most serious adverse effect; axial or central neuritis—the only form reported in patients taking daily doses of <30 mg/kg—involves the papillomacular bundle of fibers and results in reduced visual acuity, central scotoma, and loss of the ability to see green. Symptoms of ocular toxicity typically develop several months after the initiation of therapy, but rapid-onset optic neuritis has been reported. The risk of optic neuritis depends on the dose and duration of therapy: this reaction develops in 5 percent of patients receiving a daily dose of 25 mg/kg but in fewer than 1 percent of patients given a daily dose of 15 mg/kg. Patients should be tested monthly (and whenever there is a subjective visual change) for visual acuity and red-green color discrimination. Optic neuritis with associated visual loss is usually reversible, but recovery may take 6 months or longer.

Other adverse effects of ethambutol are infrequent. Hyperuricemia occurs but is usually asymptomatic. The drug is not recommended for young children, in whom visual complications are difficult to monitor.

Streptomycin An aminoglycoside isolated from *Streptomyces griseus*, streptomycin is available for intramuscular and intravenous administration only. In the United States, it is the least used first-line supplemental drug for tuberculosis because of its toxicity, the difficulty in obtaining adequate CSF levels, and the inconvenience of its parenteral administration. In developing countries, however, streptomycin is frequently used because of its low cost. The drug is active against untreated strains of *M. tuberculosis*, *M. kansasii*, and *M. marinum* and against some strains of MAI at readily achievable serum levels.

Pharmacology Serum levels of streptomycin peak at 25 to 40 μg/mL after a 1.0-g dose. Streptomycin is bactericidal for rapidly dividing extracellular mycobacteria but is ineffective in the acidic environment within the macrophage. It diffuses poorly into the meninges and reaches CSF levels in patients with meningitis that are only 20 percent of serum levels.

The usual adult dose of streptomycin is 0.5 to 1.0 g (10 to 15 mg/ kg) daily or five times per week; the pediatric dose is 20 to 40 mg/kg per day, with a maximum of 1 g/d. Because streptomycin is eliminated almost exclusively by the kidneys, the dosage must be lowered and the frequency of administration reduced (to only two or three times per week) in most patients over 50 years of age and in any patient with renal impairment.

Mechanism of action Streptomycin inhibits protein synthesis by disruption of ribosomal function.

Adverse effects (Table 170-3) Adverse reactions to streptomycin therapy occur in 10 to 20 percent of patients. Ototoxicity and renal toxicity are the most common and the most serious. Renal toxicity, usually manifested as nonoliguric renal failure, is less common with streptomycin than with other commonly used aminoglycosides, such as gentamicin. Ototoxicity involves both hearing loss and vestibular dysfunction. The latter is more common and includes loss of balance, vertigo, and tinnitus. Patients receiving streptomycin must be monitored carefully for these adverse effects. Less serious effects include perioral paresthesias, eosinophilia, rash, and drug fever.

Resistance Spontaneous resistance to streptomycin occurs in 1 in 10^5 to 10^7 organisms. In two-thirds of streptomycin-resistant strains of *M. tuberculosis*, mutations have been identified in one of two targets: a 16*S* rRNA gene (*rrs*) and the gene encoding ribosomal protein S12 (*rpsL*). Both targets are believed to be involved in streptomycin ribosomal binding. No mutational change has been identified in the other one-third of resistant isolates. Strains of *M. tuberculosis* that are resistant to streptomycin are not cross-resistant to capreomycin or amikacin.

SECOND-LINE DRUGS Second-line antituberculous agents are used either for drug-resistant tuberculosis or when first-line supplemental drugs are not available. The more important second-line drugs are discussed below in the general (descending) order of usefulness.

Quinolones A surprisingly large number of fluorinated quinolones are being developed and studied as inhibitors of mycobacteria. Their mode of action presumably is the prevention of DNA synthesis through the inhibition of DNA gyrase. Ofloxacin and ciprofloxacin, the best-studied quinolones, are active against many mycobacteria, including *M. tuberculosis*, *M. marinum*, *M. kansasii*, and *Mycobacterium fortuitum*. These two drugs are well absorbed orally, reach high serum levels, and distribute well to body tissues and fluids. While not approved for antituberculous therapy in the United States, ofloxacin—used in combination with isoniazid and rifampin for the treatment of pulmonary tuberculosis—was shown to be as active and safe as ethambutol in initial trials. Adverse effects are relatively uncommon, occurring in 0.5 to 10 percent of cases, and consist mostly of benign reactions such as gastrointestinal intolerance, rashes, dizziness, and headache. However, more serious adverse effects are now being reported and include confusion, seizures, interstitial nephritis, skin vasculitis, and acute renal failure.

Mycobacterial resistance to the fluoroquinolones develops rapidly. Its molecular basis is complex; only some strains exhibit missense mutations in the A subunit (*gyrA* gene) of DNA gyrase. Fluoroquinolone-resistant tuberculosis is a source of growing concern: 22 such cases were reported recently from New York City. Antituberculous therapy with quinolones should be reserved for patients with multidrug resistance or those who are intolerant to first-line drugs.

Capreomycin Capreomycin, a complex cyclic polypeptide antibiotic derived from *Streptomyces capreolus*, is similar to streptomycin in terms of dosing, mechanism of action, pharmacology, and toxicity. It is administered only by the intramuscular route in doses of 10 to 15 mg/kg daily or five times per week (maximum daily dose, 1 g), with peak blood levels of 20 to 40 μg/mL. After 2 to 4 months, the dosage should be reduced to 1 g two or three times a week. Cross-resistance to kanamycin and amikacin—but not to streptomycin—is common. After streptomycin, capreomycin is the injectable drug of choice for tuberculosis.

Amikacin and Kanamycin These well-known aminoglycosides are bactericidal to extracellular organisms. Kanamycin is rarely used because of its toxicity. Amikacin is active against *M. tuberculosis* and several of the nontuberculous species, including the rapidly growing mycobacteria, *Mycobacterium scrofulaceum*, *M. leprae*, and MAI. The usual adult dosage is 10 to 15 mg/kg intramuscularly or intravenously three to five times a week.

Para-Aminosalicylic Acid PAS, a calcium or sodium salt that inhibits the growth of *M. tuberculosis* by impairing folate synthesis, is rarely indicated for the treatment of tuberculosis because of its low level of antituberculous activity and its high gastrointestinal toxicity (manifesting as nausea, vomiting, and diarrhea). A recently approved PAS formulation, enteric-coated PAS granules (4 g every 8 h), may be better tolerated and results in higher therapeutic blood levels. PAS is well absorbed after oral administration but reaches only low concentrations in the CSF. The drug has a short half-life (1 h), and 80 percent of the dose is excreted in the urine.

Thiacetazone Also called amithiozone, thiacetazone is not available in the United States but—because it is inexpensive and readily available—is widely used in the developing world as a single-tablet combination with isoniazid to treat tuberculosis. The usual daily dosage is 150 mg. Thiacetazone is structurally related to isoniazid but is bacteriostatic and more toxic. The World Health Organization advises against the use of thiacetazone by HIV-infected patients because of an unacceptably high rate of severe adverse (gastrointestinal) and fatal (skin) reactions.

Viomycin A complex basic polypeptide antibiotic, viomycin has properties similar to those of capreomycin, amikacin, and kanamycin and must be administered by intramuscular injection. Ninety percent of strains of multidrug-resistant *M. tuberculosis* are inhibited by viomycin levels of 1 to 10 μg/mL. Toxic effects are more common and severe than with other polypeptide antibiotics. This drug is not available in the United States.

Ethionamide Like isoniazid and pyrazinamide, ethionamide is a derivative of isonicotinic acid. This agent is bacteriostatic against metabolizing *M. tuberculosis* and some nontuberculous mycobacteria. It is most useful in therapy for multidrug-resistant tuberculosis. However, its use is severely limited by its toxicity and frequent side effects, which include intense gastrointestinal intolerance (anorexia, vomiting, and dysgeusia), serious neurologic reactions, reversible hepatitis (5 percent of cases), hypersensitivity reactions, and hypothyroidism. Ethionamide is well absorbed orally and is widely distributed throughout the body at sites including the CSF.

Cycloserine Cycloserine (D-4-amino-3-isoxazolidinone) is produced by *Streptomyces orchidaceus* and is active against a broad spectrum of bacteria, including *M. tuberculosis*. Cycloserine is well absorbed after oral administration and is widely distributed throughout the body fluids, including the CSF. Serious side effects limit the use of this drug and include psychosis (with suicide in some cases), seizures, peripheral neuropathy, headaches, somnolence, and allergic reactions. Cycloserine should not be given to patients with epilepsy, active alcohol abuse, severe renal insufficiency, or a history of depression or psychosis.

Miscellaneous Drugs A number of other drugs are being evaluated for their antituberculous activity. This group includes amoxicillin/ clavulanic acid, clofazimine, clarithromycin, and new rifamycins such as rifapentine and KRM-1648 (a newly synthesized benzoxazinorifamycin).

LEPROSY (HANSEN'S DISEASE)

Therapy for leprosy remains difficult, especially in developing countries, because of the long duration of therapy required, the high cost and low availability of most drugs, the frequency of adverse reactions to drugs, the acquisition of drug resistance, the difficulty of determining a disease end point or cure, and (given that *M. leprae* still cannot be grown in vitro) the difficulty of conducting susceptibility testing. While many drugs are active against *M. leprae*, efficacy in the treatment of leprosy has been established only for dapsone, rifampin, clofazimine, and ethionamide.

Dapsone Dapsone (4,4′-diaminodiphenylsulfone) inhibits bacterial folic acid synthesis. It is considered the drug of choice in most cases of Hansen's disease because of its ready availability, low cost, and low toxicity and the susceptibility of untreated strains of *M. leprae* to very low concentrations.

Pharmacology Dapsone is well absorbed orally and distributes well throughout the body. The usual daily dosage is 100 mg for adults and 0.9 to 1.4 mg/kg for children. Plasma concentrations peak within 1 to 3 h. The median half-life of elimination is 22 h. Dapsone is cleared by acetylation in the liver, with genetic variation similar to that documented for the acetylation of isoniazid. The drug is 70 percent bound to plasma protein. Usual daily doses produce serum concentrations of 10 to 15 μg/mL, which far exceed the MIC for *M. leprae* (0.01 to 0.001 μg/mL).

Adverse effects Hemolysis and methemoglobinemia are common untoward reactions to dapsone. Patients should be screened for glucose-6-phosphate dehydrogenase deficiency to prevent drug-induced hemolysis. However, most patients tolerate dapsone therapy well with adequate clinical and laboratory supervision. Other side effects include gastrointestinal intolerance, headache, pruritus, peripheral neuropathies, nephrotic syndrome, fever, and rash. In lepromatous and borderline lepromatous leprosy, erythema nodosum leprosum (ENL) may occur. This reaction may be difficult to distinguish from reactions of leprosy, including drug reactions and the infectious mononucleosis–like dapsone syndrome.

Rifampin The use of rifampin, the second most useful drug in leprosy therapy, is limited by its cost. This drug is markedly bactericidal against *M. leprae* and rapidly reduces the number of viable bacilli in the patient's tissues. It must be combined with other antileprosy drugs to prevent the development of resistance. For reasons of cost, the drug is given at a dose of 600 mg once a month (supervised) outside the United States, but it is given daily in the United States.

Clofazimine A phenazine iminoquinone dye, clofazimine is weakly bactericidal against *M. leprae*. It is useful in treating dapsone-resistant leprosy and may lessen the severity of ENL. Clofazimine's mode of action is not well understood, but the drug may inhibit DNA binding. It is absorbed orally and is distributed to the fatty tissues and the reticuloendothelial system. Its serum half-life is about 60 to 70 days; only a small proportion of the dose is excreted daily into the urine or bile. Bactericidal activity is very slow and is evident for about 50 days after administration. The usual adult dosage is 50 to 100 mg daily, 100 mg three times a week, or 300 mg/d for treatment of ENL. Untoward effects include skin discoloration and, less commonly, gastrointestinal intolerance. Recently, clofazimine was reported to be responsible for a case of cardiotoxicity induced via ventricular arrhythmia. Even though clofazimine-resistant disease has been reported only rarely when this agent is used alone, it should be used with other effective antibiotics. Clofazimine is active in vitro against some of the nontuberculous mycobacterial species, including MAI, *M. kansasii*, *Mycobacterium simiae*, and *Mycobacterium abscessus*.

Ethionamide While ethionamide (250 mg/d) has not been approved by the Food and Drug Administration for the treatment of leprosy, it is sometimes used in the United States in combination with rifampin (600 mg/d) to treat dapsone-resistant leprosy in patients who cannot accept the skin-depigmentation effect of clofazimine. Because resistance to ethionamide develops quickly when the drug is used alone, it must be used with other effective agents. Patients should be monitored closely for hepatotoxicity when taking ethionamide (especially in combination with rifampin), and treatment should be discontinued if the patient's ALT levels exceed 2.5 times the normal value.

Prothionamide, a congener of ethionamide that is not available in the United States, has pharmacologic properties similar to those of ethionamide and is widely used throughout the world.

Other Agents A number of other drugs exhibit significant activity against *M. leprae*, but clinical experience with these agents is lacking. Thalidomide may be useful in suppressing ENL but acts as a tranquilizer and also is extremely teratogenic; it is available as an investigational drug in the United States (Gillis W. Long Hansen's Disease Center, Carville, LA). The newer macrolide antibiotics (particularly clarithromycin), minocycline (a long-acting tetracycline), and a number of the fluoroquinolones (including ofloxacin, sparfloxacin, and pefloxacin) have shown promising bactericidal activity against *M. leprae* in studies of mice and in early clinical trials. All of these newer leprosy drugs have low toxicity profiles, modes of action different from those of the established agents, and powerful bactericidal activity against *M. leprae*. However, their levels of bactericidal activity are still lower than that of rifampin.

NONTUBERCULOUS MYCOBACTERIA

Although less pathogenic than *M. tuberculosis*, the nontuberculous mycobacteria can cause pulmonary, skin, bone and joint, lymph node, and soft tissue infection as well as disseminated disease in immunocompromised hosts, including patients with AIDS. MAI and *M. kansasii* are the two most common causes of nontuberculous mycobacterial pulmonary infection. Up to 40 percent of AIDS patients develop disseminated disease with MAI.

Clarithromycin Clarithromycin (6-*O*-methylerythromycin) is a new macrolide that is similar to erythromycin in its mechanism of action. However, unlike erythromycin, it is well absorbed with or without meals and elicits little gastrointestinal intolerance at low doses. Clarithromycin distributes well into body tissues and fluids and is highly concentrated in macrophages. The drug is metabolized in the liver, and approximately 30 percent of a given dose is excreted in the urine. The dosage should be reduced if the creatinine clearance rate is ≤30 mL/min. Like erythromycin, clarithromycin binds with plasma proteins (65 to 70 percent) and can raise the levels of drugs such as theophylline and carbamazepine. As noted earlier, serum levels of clarithromycin are reduced by the concomitant administration of rifampin and to a lesser degree by that of rifabutin; clarithromycin treatment increases serum levels of rifabutin and some antihistamines (e.g., terfenadine), thus increasing their toxicity. Clarithromycin and (probably) azithromycin are the most active agents for the treatment of MAI infections; one of these drugs is considered an essential component of any regimens used for this purpose. However, because of mutational drug resistance, clarithromycin should be given in combination with other agents, such as ethambutol and rifampin or rifabutin. The drug is also highly active against almost all other nontuberculous mycobacteria, including *M. marinum*, *M. kansasii*, *M. haemophilum*, *M. genavense*, *M. xenopi*, *M. abscessus*, *M. chelonae*, and most isolates of *M. fortuitum*. Standard antimycobacterial doses have been 500 mg twice daily; doses of 1000 mg twice daily have been associated with increased mortality in patients with AIDS and disseminated MAI disease. The more common side effects of high doses include nausea, vomiting, a bitter taste, and (occasionally) abnormal liver-function tests. Most side effects can be minimized by reducing the dose, usually by 50 percent. Clarithromycin is teratogenic in laboratory animals and is in category C for use in pregnancy (Table 170-1). Mutational resistance occurs in one in 10^8 to 10^9 organisms and develops rapidly with monotherapy, especially that for disseminated MAI disease. Resistance results from point mutations involving A2058 or A2059 in the 23*S* ribosomal binding site.

Azithromycin Azithromycin is a macrolide that belongs to the family of azalides. It reaches much lower serum levels than clarithromycin (usually ≤0.5 μg/mL) but attains high tissue and macrophage concentrations and has a longer half-life that suggests the feasibility of intermittent therapy. Azithromycin appears to be as active as clarithromycin against MAI. It is involved in few drug interactions since it does not affect the cytochrome P450 system. No alteration in dose is required in renal failure. The usual dose is 250 to 500 mg/d. The most common side effects are gastrointestinal symptoms and reversible hearing loss. Resistance to azithromycin develops by the same mechanism as that to clarithromycin, with cross-resistance between the two macrolides.

THERAPY FOR SPECIFIC NONTUBERCULOUS MYCOBACTERIA

MAI First-line antituberculous drugs are much less active against MAI than against *M. tuberculosis*. Therapy for MAI is controversial because of the lack of controlled clinical trials. In 1990 the American Thoracic Society recommended the following four-drug regimen for MAI lung disease in HIV-negative patients: 18 to 24 months of isoniazid (300 mg), rifampin (600 mg), and ethambutol (25 mg/kg, then 15 mg/kg beginning in the third month), with intermittent streptomycin. However, two subsequent events—the demonstration of the dramatic activity of clarithromycin against both pulmonary and disseminated MAI infection and the introduction of rifabutin—have altered the therapeutic approach to MAI infection. Clarithromycin (500 mg twice daily) now replaces isoniazid, and rifabutin (300 mg/d) is often used in place of rifampin. Therapy for pulmonary disease is generally continued until cultures have been negative for 12 months.

For disseminated disease in AIDS, one of the newer macrolides (clarithromycin or azithromycin) plus ethambutol (15 mg/kg) are considered essential components of any treatment regimen, with rifabutin (300 mg) a commonly used third drug in patients not taking a protease inhibitor for their HIV infection. Other alternative drugs include ciprofloxacin, streptomycin, and amikacin. Clofazimine appears to increase mortality and should be avoided. For the prophylaxis of disseminated MAI disease, rifabutin (300 mg/d), clarithromycin (500 mg twice daily), and azithromycin (1200 mg once weekly) have all been demonstrated to be effective in controlled or comparative clinical trials.

Mycobacterium kansasii *M. kansasii* is usually sensitive to most antituberculous drugs except for pyrazinamide. Current recommendations for the treatment of *M. kansasii* pulmonary disease are 18 to 24 months of daily isoniazid (300 mg), rifampin (600 mg), and ethambutol (15 mg/kg). The potential advantages of the highly active rifabutin and the newer macrolides have not been studied.

Rapidly Growing Mycobacteria *M. fortuitum*, *M. abscessus*, and *M. chelonae* account for more than 80 percent of cases of clinical disease due to rapidly growing mycobacteria. These organisms are resistant to antituberculous agents other than amikacin but are variably susceptible to several other antibiotics. Clarithromycin has dramatically changed the approach to therapy for infection with these organisms, as it inhibits all rapidly growing mycobacteria—except for 20 percent of *M. fortuitum* strains and most *Mycobacterium smegmatis* strains—at concentrations of ≤4 μg/mL. Other drugs with good activity include amikacin (which inhibits 80 to 100 percent of strains), cefoxitin (80 percent of *M. abscessus* and *M. fortuitum* strains), doxycycline (50 percent of *M. fortuitum* strains), imipenem (100 percent of *M. fortuitum* strains, 70 percent of *M. chelonae* strains, and 70 percent of *M. abscessus* strains), the fluorinated quinolones ciprofloxacin and ofloxacin (100 percent of *M. fortuitum* strains), and sulfonamides (90 percent of *M. fortuitum* strains).

Mycobacterium marinum *M. marinum*, a photochromogen, is typically susceptible to minocycline, rifampin, ethambutol, clarithromycin, and trimethoprim-sulfamethoxazole and is resistant to isoniazid.

Mycobacterium haemophilum Infection due to *M. haemophilum* occurs most commonly as disseminated disease in immunocompromised patients with and without AIDS. This organism can cause bone and joint infection and skin infection. Isolates typically show in vitro resistance to most drugs but may be susceptible to rifampin, rifabutin, quinolones, and clarithromycin.

Mycobacterium xenopi In the United States, *M. xenopi* most often causes nosocomial infections; these infections most commonly occur in the environment of the hospital's hot-water system. In one study from Brooklyn, New York, *M. xenopi* was the second most common pathogenic nontuberculous mycobacterial species; of the 86 hospitalized patients from whom it was isolated, 41 percent were HIV-positive. Drug therapy for *M. xenopi* infection is difficult because in vitro sensitivity tests do not reliably predict clinical results. *M. xenopi* is often resistant to first-line antituberculous agents but susceptible to the newer macrolides, quinolones, streptomycin, and ethionamide.

Mycobacterium genavense *M. genavense* is a newly recognized organism that grows only in liquid media, such as Bactec 12B or 13A. This organism almost exclusively infects AIDS patients, causing disseminated disease and being isolated from blood, bone marrow, liver, lymph node, spleen, and intestinal cultures. The in vitro susceptibility profile of *M. genavense* has not been well established. Some isolates are susceptible to amikacin, clarithromycin, ofloxacin, rifampin, and rifabutin.

BIBLIOGRAPHY

AD HOC COMMITTEE OF THE SCIENTIFIC ASSEMBLY ON MICROBIOLOGY, TUBERCULOSIS, AND PULMONARY INFECTIONS: Treatment of tuberculosis and tuberculosis infection in adults and children. Am J Respir Crit Care Med 149:1359, 1994

Antimycobacterial drugs, in *Drug Evaluations Annual 1995*. Chicago, American Medical Association, pp 1685–1725

BOBROWITZ D: Ethambutol in tuberculous meningitis. Chest 61:629, 1972

BROGDEN RN, FITTON A: Rifabutin: A review of its antimicrobial activity, pharmacokinetic properties and therapeutic efficacy. Drugs 47:983, 1994

Clinical update: Impact of HIV protease inhibitors on the treatment of HIV-infected tuberculosis patients with rifampin. Morb Mort Week Rep 45:921, 1996

GELBER RH: Chemotherapy of lepromatous leprosy: Recent developments and prospects for the future. Eur J Clin Microbiol Infect Dis 13:942, 1994

GOBLE M et al: Treatment of 171 patients with pulmonary tuberculosis resistant to isoniazid and rifampin. N Engl J Med 328:527, 1993

GONZALES-MONTANER LJ: Rifabutin for the treatment of newly diagnosed pulmonary tuberculosis: A multinational, randomized, comparative study versus rifampicin. Tubercle Lung Dis 75:341, 1994

GRANGE JM et al: Clinically significant drug interactions with antituberculosis agents. Drug Saf 11:242, 1994

HAVLIR DV et al: Prophylaxis against disseminated *Mycobacterium avium* complex with weekly azithromycin, daily rifabutin, or both. N Engl J Med 335:392, 1996

KOPANOFF DE et al: Isoniazid-related hepatitis. Am Rev Respir Dis 117:991, 1978

LEIBOLD JE: The ocular toxicity of ethambutol and its relation to dose. Ann NY Acad Sci 135:904, 1966

MUSSER JM: Antimicrobial agent resistance in mycobacteria: Molecular genetic insights. Clin Microbiol Rev 8:496, 1995

NIGHTINGALE SD et al: Two controlled trials of rifabutin prophylaxis against *Mycobacterium avium* complex infection in AIDS. N Engl J Med 329:828, 1993

PIERCE M et al: A randomized trial of clarithromycin as prophylaxis against disseminated *Mycobacterium avium* complex infection in patients with advanced acquired immunodeficiency syndrome. N Engl J Med 335:384, 1996

REYNOLDS JEF (ed): *Martindale, the Extra Pharmacopoeia,* 30th ed. London, The Pharmaceutical Press, 1993

SHAFRAN SD et al: A comparison of two regimens for the treatment of *Mycobacterium avium* complex bacteremia in AIDS: Rifabutin, ethambutol, and clarithromycin versus rifampin, ethambutol, clofazimine, and ciprofloxacin. N Engl J Med 335:377, 1996

STARKE JR et al: Medical progress: Resurgence of tuberculosis in children. J Pediatr 120:839, 1992

UNDERLIED CB: Antimycobacterial agents: In vitro susceptibility testing, spectrums of activity, mechanism of action and resistance, and assays for activity in biological fluid, in *Antibiotics in Laboratory Medicine*, 3d ed, V Lorian (ed). Baltimore, Williams & Wilkins, 1991, pp 134–197

WOLINSKY E: Nontuberculous mycobacteria and associated diseases. Am Rev Respir Dis 119:107, 1979

171 *Mario C. Raviglione, Richard J. O'Brien*

TUBERCULOSIS

DEFINITION Tuberculosis is caused by bacteria belonging to the *Mycobacterium tuberculosis* complex. The disease usually affects the lungs, although in up to one-third of cases other organs are involved. If properly treated, tuberculosis caused by drug-susceptible strains is curable in virtually all cases. If untreated, the disease may be fatal within 5 years in more than half of cases. Transmission usually takes place through the airborne spread of droplet nuclei produced by patients with infectious pulmonary tuberculosis.

HISTORY That tuberculosis is one of the oldest diseases known to affect humanity has been proved by the finding of tuberculous spinal disease in Egyptian mummies. The Greeks called the disease *phthisis* ("consumption"), emphasizing the dramatic aspect of general wasting associated with chronic untreated cases. During the industrial revolution and the period of related urbanization in the seventeenth and eighteenth centuries, tuberculosis became a problem of epidemic proportions in Europe, causing at least 20 percent of all deaths in England and Wales in 1650. In the eastern part of the United States, the annual mortality rate from tuberculosis in the early nineteenth century was approximately 400 per 100,000 population.

The infectious etiology of tuberculosis was debated until Robert Koch's discovery of the tubercle bacillus in 1882. Improvement of socioeconomic conditions and isolation of infectious patients in sanatoria had a favorable impact on the epidemiology of tuberculosis in the first half of the twentieth century. In Europe and the United States, mortality rates began to decrease decades before the introduction of antimycobacterial drugs in the middle of the century.

ETIOLOGIC AGENT Mycobacteria belong to the family Mycobacteriaceae and the order Actinomycetales. Of the pathogenic species belonging to the *M. tuberculosis* complex, the most frequent and important agent of human disease is *M. tuberculosis* itself. Closely related organisms that also infect humans include *Mycobacterium bovis* (the bovine tubercle bacillus, once an important cause of tuberculosis transmitted by unpasteurized milk and currently the cause of a small percentage of cases in developing countries) and *Mycobacterium africanum* (isolated in a small proportion of cases in West and Central Africa). In addition, *M. tuberculosis* is related to various other human pathogens belonging to the genus *Mycobacterium*, such as the agent of leprosy (*Mycobacterium leprae*; see Chap. 172) and mycobacteria other than tuberculosis or nontuberculous mycobacteria (see Chap. 173); some of the latter organisms are becoming increasingly important opportunistic pathogens.

M. tuberculosis is a rod-shaped, non-spore-forming, thin aerobic bacterium measuring about 0.5 μm by 3 μm. Mycobacteria, including *M. tuberculosis*, do not stain readily and are often neutral on Gram's staining. However, once stained, the bacilli cannot be decolorized by acid alcohol, a characteristic justifying their classification as acid-fast bacilli (AFB). Acid fastness is due mainly to the organisms' high content of mycolic acids, long-chain cross-linked fatty acids, and other cell-wall lipids. Microorganisms other than mycobacteria that display some acid fastness include species of *Nocardia* and *Rhodococcus*, *Legionella micdadei*, and the protozoa *Isospora* and *Cryptosporidium*. In the mycobacterial cell wall, lipids (e.g., mycolic acids) are linked to underlying arabinogalactan and peptidoglycan. This structure is responsible for the very low permeability of the cell wall and thus for the ineffectiveness of most antibiotics against the organism. In addition, lipids such as acylated trehaloses, or "cord factors," may play a role in the virulence of *M. tuberculosis* by inducing cytokine-mediated events. Another molecule in the mycobacterial cell wall, lipoarabinomannan, is involved in the pathogen-host interaction and facilitates the survival of *M. tuberculosis* within macrophages. The several proteins characteristic of *M. tuberculosis* include those in purified protein derivative (PPD) tuberculin, a mixture of non-species-specific molecules in an extract from a culture filtrate.

EPIDEMIOLOGY Approximately 3.8 million new cases of tuberculosis (all forms, pulmonary and extrapulmonary), 90 percent of them from developing countries, were reported annually to the World Health Organization in the early 1990s. However, because of a low level of case detection and poor reporting in many national programs, reported cases represent only a fraction of the total. It is estimated that 8.8 million cases of tuberculosis occurred worldwide in 1995, 95 percent of them in developing countries of Asia (5.5 million), Africa (1.5 million), the Middle East (745,000), and Latin America (600,000). It is also estimated that nearly 3 million deaths from tuberculosis occurred in 1995, 98 percent of them in developing countries.

Beginning in the mid-1980s in many industrialized countries, the number of tuberculosis case notifications, which had been falling steadily, stabilized or even began to increase. This phenomenon was first noted in the United States but was soon observed in many European countries as well. In the United States in 1995, 22,813 cases of tuberculosis (8.7 cases per 100,000 population) were reported to the Centers for Disease Control and Prevention; this figure represented an increase of 2.8 percent over the lowest-ever number of cases reported (22,201 in 1985). A number of factors—most notably infection due to human immunodeficiency virus (HIV); immigration from countries with high prevalences of tuberculosis; and social problems such as poverty, homelessness, and drug abuse—have been implicated in the increasing rates of tuberculosis in this country. In some areas (e.g., New York City), deterioration in the public health system and dismantling of tuberculosis management services have also contributed to the worsening situation. In the United States, tuberculosis is uncommon among young adults of European descent, who have only rarely been exposed to *M. tuberculosis* infection during recent decades. In contrast, because of a high risk in the past, the prevalence of *M. tuberculosis* infection is relatively high among the elderly Caucasian population, who remain at increased risk of developing active tuberculosis. Tuberculosis in this nation is a disease of young adult members of the HIV-infected, immigrant, and disadvantaged/marginalized populations. Similarly, in Europe, tuberculosis has reemerged as an important public health problem, mainly as a result of cases among immigrants from high-prevalence countries.

In developing countries of Africa and Asia, tuberculosis trends over the past several decades are not entirely clear. However, in sub-Saharan African countries with reliable reporting systems, the recent spread of the HIV epidemic has been accompanied by doubling or tripling of the number of reported cases of tuberculosis during a period as short as 10 years. At the same time, the growing number of young adults with *M. tuberculosis* infection has fueled the rates of active tuberculosis in many developing countries. If the tuberculosis-control situation worldwide remains as it is now, 90 million new cases and 30 million deaths due to tuberculosis are expected during the 1990s.

From Exposure to Infection *M. tuberculosis* is most commonly transmitted from a patient with infectious pulmonary tuberculosis to other persons by droplet nuclei, which are aerosolized by coughing, sneezing, or speaking. The tiny droplets dry rapidly; the smallest (<5 to 10 μm in diameter) may remain suspended in the air for several hours and may gain direct access to the terminal air passages. There may be as many as 3000 infectious nuclei per cough. In the past, a frequent source of infection was raw milk containing *M. bovis* from tuberculous cows. Other routes of transmission of tubercle bacilli, such as through the skin or the placenta, are uncommon and of no epidemiologic significance.

The probability of contact with a source case of *M. tuberculosis* infection, the intimacy and duration of that contact, the degree of infectiousness of the case, and the environment of the contact are all important determinants of transmission. Several studies of close contacts have clearly demonstrated that tuberculosis patients whose sputum contains AFB visible by microscopy play the greatest role in the spread of infection. These patients have cavitary pulmonary disease or tuberculosis of the respiratory tract (endobronchial or laryngeal tuberculosis) and produce sputa containing as many as 10^5 AFB/mL. Patients with sputum smear–negative/culture-positive tuberculosis are much less infectious, and those with culture-negative pulmonary disease and extrapulmonary tuberculosis are essentially noninfectious. Crowding in poorly ventilated rooms is one of the most important factors in the transmission of tubercle bacilli, since it increases the intensity of contact with a case.

In short, the risk of acquiring *M. tuberculosis* infection is determined mainly by exogenous factors. Because of delays in seeking care and in diagnosis, an estimated two or three contacts will usually be infected by each AFB-positive case before detection.

From Infection to Disease Unlike the risk of acquiring infection with *M. tuberculosis*, the risk of developing disease after being infected depends largely on endogenous factors, such as the individual's innate susceptibility to disease and level of function of cell-mediated immunity. Clinical illness directly following infection is classified as *primary tuberculosis* and is common among children up to 4 years of age. Although this form is often severe and disseminated, it is usually not transmissible. When infection is acquired later in life, the chance is greater that the immune system will contain it, at least temporarily. The majority of infected individuals who will ultimately develop tuberculosis do so within the first year or two after infection. Dormant bacilli, however, may persist for years before being reactivated to produce *secondary tuberculosis*, which is often infectious. Overall, it is estimated that about 10 percent of infected persons will eventually develop active tuberculosis. *Reinfection* of a previously infected individual, which is probably common in areas with high rates of tuberculosis transmission, may also favor the development of disease. Restriction fragment length polymorphism (RFLP) is an analytical tool by which the results of standard epidemiologic investigations can be confirmed. RFLP yields a unique and stable strain-specific pattern of nucleic acid bands of variable sizes after digestion with restriction enzymes (a "fingerprint"). Analysis and comparison of fingerprints from various strains of *M. tuberculosis* have suggested that up to one-third of cases of active tuberculosis in U.S. inner-city communities are due to recent transmission rather than to reactivation of latent infection.

As implied above, age is an important determinant of the risk of disease after infection. Among infected persons, the incidence of tuberculosis is highest during late adolescence and early adulthood; the reasons are unclear. The incidence among women peaks at 25 to 34 years of age. In this age group rates among women are usually higher than those among men, while at older ages the opposite is true. The risk may increase in the elderly, possibly because of waning immunity.

A variety of diseases favor the development of active tuberculosis. The most potent risk factor for tuberculosis among infected individuals is clearly HIV coinfection, which suppresses cellular immunity. The risk that latent *M. tuberculosis* infection will proceed to active disease is directly related to the patient's degree of immunosuppression. In a recent study of HIV-infected, PPD-positive persons, this risk varied from 2.6 to 13.3 cases per 100 person-years and depended upon the CD4 + cell count. The risk of developing tuberculosis is several times higher among HIV-infected than among HIV-uninfected hosts. Other conditions known to increase the risk of active tuberculosis among persons infected with tubercle bacilli include silicosis; lymphoma, leukemia, and other malignant neoplasms; hemophilia; chronic renal failure and hemodialysis; insulin-dependent diabetes mellitus; immunosuppressive treatment; and conditions associated with malnutrition, such as gastrectomy and jejunoileal bypass surgery. Moreover, the presence of old, self-healed, fibrotic tuberculous lesions constitutes a serious risk of active disease.

NATURAL HISTORY OF DISEASE Studies conducted in various countries before the advent of chemotherapy clearly showed that untreated tuberculosis is often fatal. About one-third of patients died within 1 year after diagnosis and one-half within 5 years. Five-year mortality among sputum smear–positive cases was 65 percent. Of the survivors at 5 years, about 60 percent had undergone spontaneous remission, while the remainder were still excreting tubercle bacilli.

The introduction of effective chemotherapy has markedly affected the natural history of tuberculosis. With proper treatment, patients have a good chance of being cured. However, improper use of antituberculosis drugs, while reducing mortality, may also result in large numbers of chronic infectious cases, often with drug-resistant bacilli.

PATHOGENESIS AND IMMUNITY The interaction of *M. tuberculosis* with the human host begins when droplet nuclei containing microorganisms from infectious patients are inhaled. While the majority of inhaled bacilli are trapped in the upper airways and expelled by ciliated mucosal cells, a fraction (usually fewer than 10 percent) reach the alveoli. There, nonspecifically activated alveolar macrophages ingest the bacilli. The balance between the bactericidal activity of the macrophage and the virulence of the bacillus is probably linked to the bacterium's lipid-rich cell wall and to its glycolipid capsule, which confers resistance to complement and free radicals of the phagocyte. The number of invading bacilli is also important.

Several observations suggest that genetic factors also play a key role in innate nonimmune resistance to infection with *M. tuberculosis*. The existence of this resistance is suggested by the differing degrees of susceptibility to tuberculosis in different populations. In mice, an allele called *bcg* appears to be responsible for resistance to bacille Calmette-Guérin (BCG). The protein product of the *bcg* gene, designated Nramp (natural resistance–associated macrophage protein), seems to regulate resistance and susceptibility to *M. tuberculosis* infection through macrophages. The existence of a human homologue of Nramp remains to be investigated.

In the initial stage of host-bacterium interaction, either the hosts macrophages contain bacillary multiplication by producing proteolytic enzymes and cytokines or the bacilli begin to multiply. If the bacilli multiply, their growth quickly kills the macrophage, which lyses. Nonactivated monocytes attracted from the bloodstream to the site by various chemotactic factors ingest the bacilli released from the lysed macrophages. These initial stages of infection are usually asymptomatic.

Two to four weeks after infection, two additional host responses to *M. tuberculosis* develop: a tissue-damaging response and a macrophage-activating response. The *tissue-damaging response* is the result of a delayed-type hypersensitivity (DTH) reaction to various bacillary antigens; it destroys nonactivated macrophages that contain multiplying bacilli. The *macrophage-activating response* is a cell-mediated phenomenon resulting in the activation of macrophages that are capable of killing and digesting tubercle bacilli. Although both of these responses can inhibit mycobacterial growth, it is the balance between the two that determines the form of tuberculosis that will develop subsequently.

With the development of specific immunity and the accumulation of large numbers of activated macrophages at the site of the primary lesion, granulomatous lesions (*tubercles*) are formed. These lesions consist of lymphocytes and activated macrophages, such as epithelioid cells and giant cells. Initially, the newly developed tissue-damaging response is the only event capable of limiting mycobacterial growth within macrophages. This response, mediated by various bacterial products, not only destroys macrophages but also produces early solid necrosis in the center of the tubercle. Although *M. tuberculosis* can survive, its growth is inhibited within this necrotic environment by low oxygen tension, low pH, and other factors. At this point, some lesions may heal by fibrosis and calcification, while others undergo further evolution.

Cell-mediated immunity is critical at this early stage. In the majority of infected individuals, local macrophages are activated when bacillary antigens processed by macrophages stimulate T lymphocytes to release interferon γ (IFNγ) and other lymphokines. These activated cells aggregate around the lesion's center and effectively neutralize tubercle bacilli without causing further tissue destruction. In the central part of the lesion, the necrotic material assumes the aspect of soft cheese (caseous necrosis). Even when healing takes place, viable bacilli may remain dormant within macrophages or in the necrotic material for years or even throughout the patient's lifetime. These "healed" lesions in the lung parenchyma and hilar lymph nodes may later undergo calcification (*Ranke complex*).

In a minority of cases, the macrophage-activating response is weak, and mycobacterial growth can be inhibited only by intensified DTH reactions, which lead to tissue destruction. The lesion tends to enlarge further, and the surrounding tissue is progressively damaged. At the center of the lesion, the caseous material liquefies. Bronchial walls as well as blood vessels are invaded and destroyed, and cavities are formed. The liquefied caseous material, containing large numbers of bacilli, is drained through bronchi. Within the cavity walls, tubercle bacilli can now multiply well and can spread into the airways and the environment through expectorated sputum.

In the early stages of infection, bacilli are usually transported by macrophages to regional lymph nodes, from which they disseminate widely to many organs and tissues. The resulting lesions may undergo the same evolution as those in the lungs, although most tend to heal. In young children with poor natural immunity, hematogenous dissemination may result in fatal miliary tuberculosis or tuberculous meningitis.

Cell-mediated immunity confers partial protection against *M. tuberculosis*, while humoral immunity has no defined role in protection. Two types of cells are essential: macrophages, which directly phagocytize tubercle bacilli, and T lymphocytes, which induce protection through the production of lymphokines.

After infection with *M. tuberculosis*, alveolar macrophages secrete a number of cytokines: interleukin (IL) 1 contributes to fever; IL-6 contributes to hyperglobulinemia; and tumor necrosis factor α (TNFα) contributes to the killing of mycobacteria, the formation of granulomas, and a number of systemic effects, such as fever and weight loss. Macrophages are also critical in processing and presenting antigens to T lymphocytes; the result is a proliferation of CD4+ lymphocytes, which are crucial to the host's defense against *M. tuberculosis*. Qualitative and quantitative defects of CD4+ T cells explain the inability of HIV-infected individuals to contain mycobacterial proliferation. CD4+ lymphocytes are important producers of IFNγ, whose role in tuberculosis is probably to stimulate macrophages to produce TNFα and 1,25-dihydroxyvitamin D—both effective mycobacterial inhibitors. After stimulation with IFNγ and TNFα, macrophages may release nitric oxide, which is essential for their bactericidal activity. Among CD4+ cells, two subpopulations, Th1 and Th2 cells, produce different cytokines whose interplay may determine the host's response to mycobacteria. Gamma-delta cells also appear to participate in the host's response to infection.

M. tuberculosis possesses various protein antigens. Some are present in the cytoplasm and cell wall; others are secreted. That the latter are more important in eliciting a T lymphocyte response is suggested by experiments documenting the appearance of protective immunity in animals only after immunization with live, protein-secreting mycobacteria. Among the antigens with a potential protective role are the 30- and 32-kDa molecules of the BCG85 complex, which may mediate the adhesion and invasion of bacilli, and the 10-kDa antigen (BCG-a), which stimulates the proliferation of lymphocytes. The 65-kDa heat-shock protein, previously believed to be of importance in immunity, is now recognized as a weak antigen.

Coincident with the appearance of immunity, DTH to *M. tuberculosis* develops. This abnormal host reactivity is revealed by the PPD skin test, currently the only test that reliably detects *M. tuberculosis* infection in persons without symptoms. The cellular mechanisms responsible for PPD reactivity are related mainly to previously sensitized CD4+ lymphocytes, which are attracted to the skin-test site. There, they proliferate and produce cytokines.

In 1891, Robert Koch discovered components of *M. tuberculosis* in a concentrated liquid culture medium. Subsequently named "old tuberculin" (OT), this material was initially believed to be useful in the treatment of tuberculosis (although this idea was later disproved). It soon became clear that OT was capable of eliciting a skin reaction when injected subcutaneously into patients with tuberculosis. In 1932, Seibert and Munday purified this product by ammonium sulfate precipitation. The result was an active protein fraction known as tuberculin

purified protein derivative. However, the complexity and diversity of the constituents of PPD rendered its standardization difficult. PPD-S, developed by Seibert and Glenn in 1941, was chosen as the international standard. Later, the World Health Organization and UNICEF sponsored large-scale production of a master batch of PPD, termed *RT23*, and made it available for general use. The greatest limitation of PPD is its lack of mycobacterial species specificity, a property that is due to the large number of proteins in this product that are highly conserved in the various species of mycobacteria.

While DTH is associated with protective immunity (PPD-positive persons being less susceptible to a new *M. tuberculosis* infection than PPD-negative persons), it by no means guarantees protection against reactivation. In fact, severe cases of active tuberculosis are often accompanied by strongly positive skin-test reactions.

CLINICAL MANIFESTATIONS   Tuberculosis is usually classified as pulmonary or extrapulmonary. Before the recognition of HIV infection, more than 80 percent of all cases of tuberculosis were limited to the lungs. However, up to two-thirds of HIV-infected patients with tuberculosis may have both pulmonary and extrapulmonary disease or extrapulmonary disease alone.

Pulmonary Tuberculosis   Pulmonary tuberculosis can be categorized as primary or postprimary (secondary).

Primary disease   Primary pulmonary tuberculosis results from an initial infection with tubercle bacilli. In areas of high tuberculosis prevalence, this form of disease is often seen in children and is frequently localized to the middle and lower lung zones. The lesion forming after infection is usually peripheral and accompanied by hilar or paratracheal lymphadenopathy, which may not be detectable on chest radiography. In the majority of cases, the lesion heals spontaneously and may later be evident as a small calcified nodule (*Ghon lesion*).

In children with impaired immunity, such as those with malnutrition or HIV infection, primary pulmonary tuberculosis may progress rapidly to clinical illness. The initial lesion increases in size and can evolve in different ways. Pleural effusion, a frequent finding, results from the penetration of bacilli into the pleural space from an adjacent subpleural focus. In the majority of cases, the effusion resolves spontaneously, although tuberculous empyema may ensue in the presence of severe multibacillary pulmonary disease. In severe cases, the primary site rapidly enlarges, its central portion undergoes necrosis, and acute cavitation develops (progressive primary tuberculosis). Tuberculosis in young children is almost invariably accompanied by hilar or mediastinal lymphadenopathy due to the spread of bacilli from the lung parenchyma through lymphatic vessels. Enlarged lymph nodes may compress bronchi, causing obstruction and subsequent segmental or lobar collapse. Partial obstruction may cause obstructive emphysema, and bronchiectasis may also develop. Hematogenous dissemination, which is common and is often asymptomatic, may result in the most severe manifestations of primary *M. tuberculosis* infection. Bacilli reach the bloodstream from the pulmonary lesion or the lymph nodes and disseminate into various organs, where they may produce granulomatous lesions. Although healing frequently takes place, immunocompromised subjects (e.g., persons with HIV infection and those recovering from measles) may develop miliary tuberculosis and/or tuberculous meningitis.

Postprimary disease   Also called adult-type, reactivation, or secondary tuberculosis, postprimary disease results from endogenous reactivation of latent infection and is usually localized to the apical and posterior segments of the upper lobes, where the high oxygen concentration favors mycobacterial growth. In addition, the superior segments of the lower lobes are frequently involved. The extent of lung parenchymal involvement varies greatly, from small infiltrates to extensive cavitary disease. With cavity formation, liquefied necrotic contents ultimately are discharged into the airways, resulting in satellite lesions within the lungs that may in turn undergo cavitation. Massive involvement of pulmonary segments or lobes, with coalescence of lesions, produces tuberculous pneumonia. While up to one-third of untreated patients reportedly succumb to severe pulmonary tuberculosis within a few weeks or months after onset, others undergo a process of spontaneous remission or proceed along a chronic, progressively debilitating course ("consumption"). Under these circumstances, some pulmonary lesions become fibrotic and may later calcify, but cavities persist in other parts of the lungs. Individuals with such chronic disease continue to discharge tubercle bacilli into the environment. Most patients have a definite clinical response to treatment, with defervescence, decreasing cough, weight gain, and a general improvement in well-being within several weeks.

Early in the course of disease, symptoms and signs are often nonspecific and insidious, consisting mainly of fever and night sweats, weight loss, anorexia, general malaise, and weakness. However, in the majority of cases, cough eventually develops—perhaps initially nonproductive and subsequently accompanied by the production of purulent sputum. Blood streaking of the sputum is frequently documented. Massive hemoptysis may ensue as a consequence of the erosion of a fully patent vessel located in the wall of a cavity. Hemoptysis, however, may also result from rupture of a dilated vessel in a cavity (Rasmussen's aneurysm) or from aspergilloma formation in an old cavity. Pleuritic chest pain sometimes develops in patients with subpleural parenchymal lesions but can also be the consequence of muscle strain due to persistent coughing. Extensive disease may produce dyspnea and (occasionally) adult respiratory distress syndrome (ARDS).

Physical findings are of limited use in pulmonary tuberculosis. Many patients have no abnormalities detectable by chest examination, while others have detectable rales in the involved areas during inspiration, especially after coughing. Occasionally, rhonchi due to partial bronchial obstruction and classical amphoric breath sounds in areas with large cavities may be heard. Systemic features include fever (often low-grade and intermittent) and wasting. In some cases, pallor and finger clubbing develop. The most common hematologic findings are mild anemia and leukocytosis. Hyponatremia due to the syndrome of inappropriate secretion of antidiuretic hormone (SIADH) has also been found.

Extrapulmonary Tuberculosis In order of frequency, the extrapulmonary sites most commonly involved in tuberculosis are the lymph nodes, pleura, genitourinary tract, bones and joints, meninges, and peritoneum. However, virtually all organ systems may be affected. As a result of hematogenous dissemination in HIV-infected individuals, extrapulmonary tuberculosis is seen more commonly today than in the past.

Pleural tuberculosis Involvement of the pleura is common in primary tuberculosis and results from penetration by a few tubercle bacilli into the pleural space. Depending on the extent of reactivity, the effusion may be small, remain unnoticed, and resolve spontaneously or may be sufficiently large to cause symptoms such as fever, pleuritic chest pain, and dyspnea. Physical findings are those of pleural effusion: dullness to percussion and absence of breath sounds. A chest radiograph reveals the effusion and, in no more than one-third of cases, also shows a parenchymal lesion. Thoracentesis is required to ascertain the nature of the effusion. The fluid is straw colored and at times hemorrhagic; it is an exudate with a protein concentration more than 50 percent of that in serum, a normal to low glucose concentration, a pH that is generally <7.2, and detectable white blood cells (usually 500 to 2500/mL). Neutrophils may predominate in the early stage, while mononuclear cells are the typical finding later. Mesothelial cells are generally rare or absent. AFB are very rarely seen on direct smear, but cultures may be positive for *M. tuberculosis* in up to one-third of cases. Needle biopsy of the pleura is often required for diagnosis and reveals granulomas and/or yields a positive culture in up to 70 percent of cases. This form of pleural tuberculosis responds well to chemotherapy and may resolve spontaneously.

Tuberculous empyema is a less common complication of pulmonary tuberculosis. It is usually the result of the rupture of a cavity, with delivery of a large number of organisms into the pleural space, or of a bronchopleural fistula from a pulmonary lesion. A chest radiograph may show pyopneumothorax with an air-fluid level. The effusion is purulent and thick and contains large numbers of lymphocytes. An acid-fast smear of pleural fluid is often found to be positive when examined by microscopy, as is culture of the pleural fluid. Surgical drainage is usually required as an adjunct to chemotherapy. Tuberculous empyema may result in severe pleural fibrosis and restrictive lung disease.

Tuberculosis of the upper airways Nearly always a complication of advanced cavitary pulmonary tuberculosis, tuberculosis of the upper airways may involve the larynx, pharynx, and epiglottis. Symptoms include hoarseness and dysphagia in addition to chronic productive cough. Findings depend on the site of involvement, and ulcerations may be seen on laryngoscopy. Acid-fast smear of the sputum is often positive, but biopsy may be necessary in some cases to establish the diagnosis. Cancer may have similar features but is usually painless.

Lymph-node tuberculosis (tuberculous lymphadenitis) One of the commonest presentations of extrapulmonary tuberculosis (being documented in more than 25 percent of cases), lymph-node disease is particularly frequent among HIV-infected patients. In the United States, children and women (particularly non-Caucasians) also seem to be especially susceptible. Lymph-node tuberculosis presents as painless swelling of the lymph nodes, most commonly at cervical and supraclavicular sites. Lymph nodes are usually discrete in early disease but may be inflamed and have a fistulous tract draining caseous material. Systemic symptoms are usually limited to HIV-infected patients, and concomitant lung disease may or may not be present. The diagnosis is established by fine-needle aspiration or surgical biopsy. AFB are seen in up to 50 percent of cases, cultures are positive in 70 to 80 percent, and histologic examination shows granulomatous lesions. Among HIV-infected patients, granulomas usually are not seen. Differential diagnosis includes a variety of infectious conditions as well as neoplastic diseases such as lymphomas or metastatic carcinomas (see Chap. 61).

Pericardial tuberculosis (tuberculous pericarditis) Due to direct progression of a primary focus within the pericardium, to reactivation of a latent focus, or to rupture of an adjacent lymph node, pericardial tuberculosis has often been a disease of the elderly in countries with low tuberculosis prevalence but develops frequently in HIV-infected patients. The onset may be subacute, although an acute presentation, with fever, dull retrosternal pain, and a friction rub, is possible. An effusion eventually develops in many cases; cardiovascular symptoms and signs of cardiac tamponade may ultimately appear (see Chap. 240). The effusion, detectable on chest radiography, is exudative in nature, with a high count of leukocytes (predominantly mononuclear cells). Hemorrhagic effusion is frequent. Culture of the fluid reveals *M. tuberculosis* in about 30 percent of cases, while biopsy has a higher yield. Without treatment, pericardial tuberculosis is usually fatal. Even with treatment, complications may develop, including chronic constrictive pericarditis with thickening of the pericardium, fibrosis, and sometimes calcification, which may be visible on a chest radiograph. A short course of glucocorticoids may prevent constriction.

Genitourinary tuberculosis Genitourinary tuberculosis accounts for about 15 percent of all extrapulmonary cases, may involve any portion of the genitourinary tract, and is usually due to hematogenous seeding following primary infection. Local symptoms predominate. Urinary frequency, dysuria, hematuria, and flank pain are common presentations. However, patients may be asymptomatic and the disease discovered only after severe destructive lesions of the kidneys have developed. Urinalysis gives abnormal results in 90 percent of cases, revealing pyuria and hematuria. The documentation of culture-negative pyuria in acidic urine raises the suspicion of tuberculosis. An intravenous pyelogram helps in diagnosis. Culture of three morning urine specimens yields a definitive diagnosis in nearly 90 percent of cases.

Genital tuberculosis is diagnosed more commonly in females than in males. In females, it affects the fallopian tubes and the endometrium and may cause infertility, pelvic pain, and menstrual abnormalities. Diagnosis requires biopsy or culture of specimens obtained by dilatation and curettage. In males, tuberculosis preferentially affects the epididymis, producing a slightly tender mass that may drain externally through a fistulous tract; orchitis and prostatitis may also develop. In almost half of cases of genitourinary tuberculosis, urinary tract disease is also present. Genitourinary tuberculosis responds well to chemotherapy.

Skeletal tuberculosis In early series of cases of extrapulmonary tuberculosis, disease of the bones and joints was responsible for 8 to

9 percent of cases. Today, rates are lower since skeletal tuberculosis is only infrequently described among HIV-infected patients. In bone and joint disease, pathogenesis is related to reactivation of hematogenous foci or to spread from adjacent paravertebral lymph nodes. Weight-bearing joints (spine, hips, and knees—in that order) are affected most commonly. Spinal tuberculosis (Pott's disease or tuberculous spondylitis) often involves two or more adjacent vertebral bodies. While the upper thoracic spine is the most common site of spinal tuberculosis in children, the lower thoracic and upper lumbar vertebrae are usually affected in adults. From the anterior superior or inferior angle of the vertebral body, the lesion reaches the adjacent body, also destroying the intervertebral disk. With advanced disease, collapse of vertebral bodies results in kyphosis (*gibbus*). A paravertebral "cold" abscess may also form. In the upper spine, this abscess may track to the chest wall as a mass; in the lower spine, it may reach the inguinal ligaments or present as a psoas abscess. Computed tomography (CT) or magnetic resonance imaging (MRI) reveals the characteristic lesion and suggests its etiology, although the differential diagnosis includes other infections and tumors. Aspiration of the abscess or bone biopsy confirms the tuberculous etiology, as cultures are usually positive and histologic findings highly typical. A catastrophic complication of Pott's disease is paraplegia, which is usually due to an abscess or a lesion compressing the spinal cord. Paraparesis due to a large abscess is a medical emergency and requires abscess drainage. Tuberculosis of the hip joints causes pain and limping; tuberculosis of the knee produces pain and swelling and sometimes follows trauma. If the disease goes unrecognized, the joints may be destroyed. Skeletal tuberculosis responds to chemotherapy, but severe cases may require surgery.

Gastrointestinal tuberculosis Any portion of the gastrointestinal tract may be affected by tuberculosis. Various pathogenetic mechanisms are involved: swallowing of sputum with direct seeding, hematogenous spread, or (rarely) ingestion of milk from cows affected by bovine tuberculosis. The terminal ileum and the cecum are the sites most commonly involved. Abdominal pain, at times similar to that associated with appendicitis, diarrhea, obstruction, hematochezia, and a palpable mass in the abdomen, are common findings at presentation. Fever, weight loss, and night sweats are also frequent. With intestinal-wall involvement, ulcerations and fistulae may simulate Crohn's disease. Anal fistulae should prompt an evaluation for rectal tuberculosis. As surgery is required in most cases, the diagnosis can be established by histologic examination and culture of specimens obtained intraoperatively.

Tuberculous peritonitis follows either the direct spread of tubercle bacilli from ruptured lymph nodes and intraabdominal organs or hematogenous seeding. Nonspecific abdominal pain, fever, and ascites should raise the suspicion of tuberculous peritonitis. The coexistence of cirrhosis (see Chap. 298) in patients with tuberculous peritonitis complicates the diagnosis. In tuberculous peritonitis, paracentesis reveals an exudative fluid with a high protein content and leukocytosis that is usually lymphocytic (although neutrophils occasionally predominate). The yield of direct smear and culture is relatively low; culture of a large volume of ascitic fluid can increase the yield, but peritoneal biopsy is often needed to establish the diagnosis.

Miliary or disseminated tuberculosis Miliary tuberculosis is due to hematogenous spread of tubercle bacilli. While in children it is often the consequence of a recent primary infection, in adults it may be due to either recent infection or reactivation of old disseminated foci. Lesions are usually yellowish granulomas 1 to 2 mm in diameter that resemble millet seeds (thus the term *miliary*, coined by nineteenth-century pathologists).

Clinical manifestations are nonspecific and protean, depending on the predominant site of involvement. Fever, night sweats, anorexia, weakness, and weight loss are presenting symptoms in the majority of cases. At times, patients have a cough and other respiratory symptoms due to pulmonary involvement as well as abdominal symptoms. Physical findings include hepatomegaly, splenomegaly, and lymphadenopathy. Eye examination may reveal choroidal tubercles, which are

pathognomonic of miliary tuberculosis, in up to 30 percent of cases. Meningismus occurs in fewer than 10 percent of cases.

A high index of suspicion is required for the diagnosis of miliary tuberculosis. Frequently, chest radiography reveals a miliary reticulonodular pattern (more easily seen on underpenetrated film), although no radiographic abnormality may be evident early in the course and among HIV-infected patients. Other radiologic findings include large infiltrates, interstitial infiltrates (especially in HIV-infected patients), and pleural effusion. A sputum smear is negative in 80 percent of cases. Anemia with leukopenia or leukocytosis with neutrophilia may be documented, and disseminated intravascular coagulation has been reported. Elevation of alkaline phosphatase levels and other abnormal values in liver function tests are detected in patients with severe hepatic involvement. The PPD test may be negative in up to half of cases, but reactivity may be restored during chemotherapy. Bronchoalveolar lavage and transbronchial biopsy are more likely to permit bacteriologic confirmation, and granulomas are evident in liver or bone-marrow biopsy specimens from many patients. If it goes unrecognized, miliary tuberculosis is lethal; with proper treatment, however, it is amenable to cure.

A rare presentation seen in the elderly is *cryptic miliary tuberculosis*, which has a chronic course characterized by mild intermittent fever, anemia, and—ultimately—meningeal involvement preceding death. An acute septicemic form, *nonreactive miliary tuberculosis*, occurs very rarely and is due to massive hematogenous dissemination of tubercle bacilli. Pancytopenia is common in this form of disease, which is rapidly fatal. At postmortem examination, multiple necrotic but nongranulomatous ("nonreactive") lesions are detected.

Tuberculous meningitis and tuberculoma Tuberculosis of the central nervous system accounts for about 5 percent of extrapulmonary cases. It is seen most often in young children but also develops in adults, especially those who are infected with HIV. Tuberculous meningitis results from the hematogenous spread of primary or postprimary pulmonary disease or from the rupture of a subependymal tubercle into the subarachnoid space. In more than half of cases, evidence of old pulmonary lesions or a miliary pattern is found on chest radiography. The disease may present subtly as headache and mental changes or acutely as confusion, lethargy, altered sensorium, and neck rigidity. Typically, the disease evolves over 1 or 2 weeks—a course longer than that of bacterial meningitis. Paresis of cranial nerves (ocular nerves in particular) is a frequent finding, and the involvement of cerebral arteries may produce focal ischemia. Hydrocephalus is common. Lumbar puncture is the cornerstone of diagnosis. In general, examination of the cerebrospinal fluid (CSF) reveals a high leukocyte count (usually with a predominance of lymphocytes but often with a predominance of neutrophils in the early stage), a protein content of 1 to 8 g/L (100 to 800 mg/dL), and a low glucose concentration; however, any of these three parameters can be within the normal range. AFB are seen on direct smear of CSF sediment in only 20 percent of cases, but repeated lumbar punctures increase the yield. Culture of CSF is diagnostic in up to 80 percent of cases. Imaging studies (CT and MRI) may show hydrocephalus and abnormal enhancement of basal cisterns or ependyma. If unrecognized, tuberculous meningitis is uniformly fatal. This disease responds to chemotherapy; however, neurologic sequelae are documented in 25 percent of treated cases, in most of which the diagnosis has been delayed. Glucocorticoids are a useful adjunct to chemotherapy, especially in cases with cerebral edema or high CSF protein levels.

Tuberculoma, an uncommon manifestation of tuberculosis, presents as one or more space-occupying lesions and usually causes seizures and focal signs. CT or MRI reveals contrast-enhanced ring lesions, but biopsy is necessary to establish the diagnosis.

Less common extrapulmonary forms Tuberculosis may cause chorioretinitis, uveitis, panophthalmitis, and painful hypersensitivity-related phlyctenular conjunctivitis. Tuberculous otitis is rare and presents as hearing loss, otorrhea, and tympanic membrane perforation. In the nasopharynx, tuberculosis may simulate Wegener's granulomatosis. Cutaneous manifestations of tuberculosis include primary infection due to direct inoculation, abscesses and chronic ulcers, scrofuloderma, lupus vulgaris, miliary lesions, and erythema nodosum. Adrenal tuberculosis is a manifestation of advanced disease presenting as signs of adrenal insufficiency. Finally, congenital tuberculosis results from transplacental spread of tubercle bacilli to the fetus or from ingestion of contaminated amniotic fluid. This rare disease affects the liver, spleen, lymph nodes, and various other organs.

HIV-Associated Tuberculosis Tuberculosis is an important opportunistic disease among HIV-infected persons worldwide. In developing countries of Africa, Southeast Asia, and Latin America, an estimated 8.5 million persons were coinfected as of the middle of 1996. In the United States, coinfection with HIV and *M. tuberculosis* is common in certain segments of the population, including drug users and some minorities. A person with skin test–documented *M. tuberculosis* infection who acquires HIV infection has a 3 to 15 percent annual risk of developing active tuberculosis.

The association between tuberculosis and HIV is supported by other epidemiologic observations. First, HIV seropositivity is several times higher among patients with tuberculosis than among the general population: in New York City the rate is nearly 50 percent, and in African countries it reaches 60 to 70 percent. Second, marked increases in numbers of tuberculosis cases have been reported at locations hard hit by the HIV epidemic, such as Zambia, Tanzania, Malawi, northern Thailand, and New York City. Globally, the proportion of tuberculosis cases associated with HIV infection is growing rapidly and may reach 14 percent by the year 2000.

HIV directly attacks the critical immune mechanisms involved in protection against tuberculosis. Tuberculosis can appear at any stage of HIV infection, but its presentation varies with the stage. When cell-mediated immunity is only partially compromised, pulmonary tuberculosis presents as a typical pattern of upper lobe infiltrates and cavitation, without significant lymphadenopathy or pleural effusion. In late stages of HIV infection, a primary tuberculosis–like pattern, with diffuse interstitial or miliary infiltrates, little or no cavitation, and intrathoracic lymphadenopathy, is more common. Overall, sputum smears may be positive less frequently among tuberculosis patients with HIV infection than among those without; thus the diagnosis of tuberculosis may be unusually difficult, especially in view of the variety of HIV-related pulmonary conditions mimicking tuberculosis.

As has been mentioned, extrapulmonary tuberculosis is common among HIV-infected patients. In various series studied in the United States and many developing countries, extrapulmonary tuberculosis—alone or in association with pulmonary disease—has been documented in 40 to 60 percent of all cases. The most common forms are lymph nodal, disseminated, pleural, and pericardial. Mycobacteremia and meningitis are also frequent, particularly in advanced HIV disease.

The diagnosis of tuberculosis in HIV-infected patients may be difficult not only because of the increased frequency of sputum-smear negativity (up to 40 percent in culture-proven pulmonary cases) but also because of atypical radiographic findings, a lack of classic granuloma formation in the late stages, and negative results in PPD skin tests. Delays in treatment may prove fatal. The response to short-course chemotherapy is similar to that in HIV-seronegative patients. However, adverse effects may be more pronounced, including severe or even fatal skin reactions to amithiozone (thiacetazone).

DIAGNOSIS The key to the diagnosis of tuberculosis is a high index of suspicion. Diagnosis is not difficult with a high-risk patient—e.g., a homeless alcoholic who presents with typical symptoms and a classic chest radiograph showing upper lobe infiltrates with cavities. On the other hand, the diagnosis can easily be missed in an elderly nursing-home resident or a teenager with a focal infiltrate.

Often, the diagnosis is first entertained when the chest radiograph of a patient being evaluated for respiratory symptoms is abnormal. If the patient has no complicating medical conditions that favor immunosuppression, the chest radiograph may show the typical picture of upper lobe infiltrates with cavitation. The longer the delay between the onset of symptoms and the diagnosis, the more likely is the finding of cavitary disease. On the other hand, immunosuppressed patients, including those with HIV infection, may have "atypical" findings on chest radiography—e.g., lower zone infiltrates without cavity formation.

AFB Microscopy A presumptive diagnosis is commonly based on the finding of AFB upon microscopic examination of a diagnostic specimen such as a smear of expectorated sputum or of tissue (for example, a lymph node biopsy). Most modern laboratories processing large numbers of diagnostic specimens use auramine-rhodamine staining and fluorescence microscopy. The more traditional method—light microscopy of specimens stained with Kinyoun or Ziehl-Neelsen basic fuchsin dyes—is satisfactory, although more time-consuming. For patients with suspected pulmonary tuberculosis, three sputum specimens, preferably collected early in the morning, should be submitted to the laboratory for AFB smear and mycobacteriology culture. If tissue is obtained, it is critical that the portion of the specimen intended for culture not be put in formaldehyde.

Mycobacterial Culture Definitive diagnosis is dependent on the isolation and identification of *M. tuberculosis* from a diagnostic specimen—in most cases, a sputum specimen obtained from a patient with a productive cough. Specimens may be inoculated onto egg- or agar-based medium (e.g., Löwenstein-Jensen or Middlebrook 7H10) and incubated at 37°C under 5% CO_2. Because most species of mycobacteria, including *M. tuberculosis*, are slow growing, 4 to 8 weeks may be required for growth to be detected. Although *M. tuberculosis* may be presumptively identified on the basis of growth time and colony pigmentation and morphology, a variety of biochemical tests have traditionally been used to speciate mycobacterial isolates. In today's laboratories, the use of liquid media with radiometric growth detection (e.g., BACTEC-460) and the identification of isolates by nucleic acid probes have replaced the traditional methods of isolation on solid media and identification by biochemical tests. These new methods have decreased the time required for isolation and speciation to 2 to 3 weeks.

Radiographic Procedures As noted above, the initial suspicion of pulmonary tuberculosis is often based on abnormal chest radiograph findings in a patient with respiratory symptoms. Although the "classic" picture is that of upper lobe disease with infiltrates and cavities, virtually any radiographic pattern—from a normal film or a solitary pulmonary nodule to diffuse alveolar infiltrates in a patient with ARDS—may be seen. In the era of AIDS, no radiographic pattern can be considered pathognomonic.

PPD Skin Testing Skin testing with PPD is most widely used in screening for *M. tuberculosis* infection (see below). The test is of limited value in the diagnosis of active tuberculosis because of its low sensitivity and specificity. False-negative reactions are common in immunosuppressed patients and in those with overwhelming tuberculosis. Positive reactions are sometimes obtained when patients have been infected with *M. tuberculosis* but do not have active disease and when persons have been sensitized by nontuberculous mycobacteria (see Chap. 173) or BCG vaccination. Although BCG vaccine is not commonly used in the United States, many immigrants will have received it. In the absence of a history of BCG vaccination, a positive skin test may provide additional support for the diagnosis of tuberculosis in culture-negative cases.

Drug Susceptibility Testing In general, the initial isolate of *M. tuberculosis* should be tested for susceptibility to the primary drugs used for treatment: isoniazid, rifampin, ethambutol, pyrazinamide, and streptomycin. In addition, drug susceptibility tests are mandatory when patients fail to respond to initial therapy or experience a relapse after the completion of treatment (see below). Susceptibility testing may be conducted directly (with the clinical specimen) or indirectly (with mycobacterial cultures) on solid or liquid medium. Results are obtained most rapidly by direct susceptibility testing on liquid medium, with an average reporting time of 3 weeks. With indirect testing on solid media, results may not be available for 8 weeks or longer.

Additional Diagnostic Procedures Other diagnostic tests may be used when pulmonary tuberculosis is suspected. Sputum induction by ultrasonic nebulization of hypertonic saline may be useful for patients unable to produce a sputum specimen spontaneously. Frequently, patients with radiographic abnormalities that are consistent with other diagnoses (e.g., bronchogenic carcinoma) undergo fiberoptic bronchoscopy with bronchial brushings or transbronchial biopsy of the lesion. Bronchoalveolar lavage of a lung segment containing an abnormality may also be performed. In all cases, it is essential that specimens be submitted for AFB smear and mycobacterial culture. For the diagnosis of primary pulmonary tuberculosis in children, who often do not expectorate sputum, specimens from early-morning gastric lavage may yield positive cultures.

Invasive diagnostic procedures are also indicated for patients with suspected extrapulmonary tuberculosis. In addition to specimens of involved sites (e.g., CSF for tuberculous meningitis, pleural fluid and biopsy samples for pleural disease), bone marrow and liver biopsy and culture have a good diagnostic yield in disseminated (miliary) tuberculosis. Blood from HIV-infected patients with suspected tuberculosis should be cultured.

In some cases, cultures will be negative, and a clinical diagnosis of tuberculosis will be supported by consistent epidemiologic evidence (e.g., a history of close contact with an infectious patient), a positive PPD skin test, and a compatible clinical and radiographic response to treatment. In the United States and other industrialized countries with low rates of tuberculosis, a significant percentage of patients with abnormal chest radiographs and sputum positive for AFB may have pulmonary disease due to organisms of the *Mycobacterium avium* complex (MAC) or *Mycobacterium kansasii* (see Chap. 173). Factors favoring the diagnosis of nontuberculous mycobacterial disease over tuberculosis include an absence of risk factors for tuberculosis, a negative PPD skin test, and underlying chronic obstructive pulmonary disease.

Patients with HIV-associated tuberculosis pose several diagnostic problems, as noted above in the description of clinical manifestations. Moreover, HIV-infected patients with sputum culture–positive and AFB-positive tuberculosis may present with a normal chest radiograph. Thus, in a patient with HIV infection, the finding of a normal chest radiograph does not rule out the diagnosis of pulmonary tuberculosis. An additional consideration is that, among relatively severely immunosuppressed AIDS patients in Europe and North America, MAC disease is more common than tuberculosis, usually presenting as a disseminated condition without pulmonary parenchymal involvement.

Adjunctive Diagnostic Tests A number of methods have been proposed as adjuncts to standard laboratory diagnosis. The most thoroughly investigated is serologic diagnosis based on detection of antibody to a variety of mycobacterial antigens. However, tests with most of the target antigens have a low predictive value when used in a population with a presumably low probability of disease. Tests aimed at detection of mycobacterial antigen by serologic methods have generally not been sufficiently sensitive to be useful. More promising are tests using biochemical and other methods to detect molecules that may be present in small amounts in diagnostic specimens. One example of a test that may be of some use, though its performance is presently limited to research laboratories, is the detection of tuberculostearic acid by gas-liquid chromatography in CSF from patients with tuberculous meningitis.

One of the most promising diagnostic techniques involves the amplification and detection of specific segments of DNA by polymerase chain reaction (PCR). The early problem with false-positive reactions due to amplicon contamination appears to have been solved. However, lingering problems with the preparation of specimens, particularly sputum specimens, have limited the sensitivity of the method. PCR may be most useful for the diagnosis of paucibacillary forms of pulmonary tuberculosis or extrapulmonary disease. Because of significant commercial interest, it is expected that the use of PCR in the diagnosis of tuberculosis will ultimately become established as technical problems are solved.

℞ TREATMENT

Chemotherapy for tuberculosis became possible with the discovery of streptomycin in the mid-1940s. Randomized clinical trials clearly indicated that the administration of streptomycin to patients with chronic tuberculosis reduced mortality and led to cure in a number of cases. However, monotherapy with streptomycin was frequently associated with the development of resistance to streptomycin and the attendant failure of treatment. With the discovery of para-aminosalicylic acid (PAS) and isoniazid, it became axiomatic that cure of tuberculosis required the concomitant administration of at least two agents to which the organism was susceptible. Furthermore, early clinical trials demonstrated that a long period of treatment—i.e., 12 to 24 months—was required to prevent the recurrence of tuberculosis.

The introduction of rifampin in the early 1970s heralded the era of effective short-course chemotherapy, with a treatment duration of less than 12 months. The discovery that pyrazinamide, which was first used in the 1950s, augmented the potency of isoniazid/rifampin regimens led to the use of a 6-month course of this triple-drug regimen as standard therapy.

Drugs Five major drugs are considered the first-line agents for the treatment of tuberculosis (see Chap. 170 for a detailed discussion): isoniazid, rifampin, pyrazinamide, ethambutol, and streptomycin (Table 171-1). The first four, which are usually given orally, are well absorbed, with peak serum levels at 2 to 4 h and nearly complete elimination within 24 h. These agents are recommended on the basis of their bactericidal activity (ability to rapidly reduce the number of viable organisms), their sterilizing activity (ability to kill all bacilli and thus sterilize the affected organ, measured in terms of the ability to prevent relapses), and their low rate of induction of drug resistance.

Because of a lower degree of efficacy and a higher degree of intolerability and toxicity, a number of second-line drugs are used only for the treatment of patients with tuberculosis resistant to first-line drugs. Included in this group are the injectable drugs kanamycin, amikacin, and capreomycin and the oral agents ethionamide, cycloserine, and PAS. Recently, quinolone antibiotics have been added to the list; although ofloxacin is generally recommended, sparfloxacin and levofloxacin have been more active in experimental studies. Other second-line drugs include clofazimine, amithiozone (thiacetazone, widely used with isoniazid in less wealthy countries but not marketed in North America or Europe), and amoxicillin/clavulanic acid. Long-acting rifamycin derivatives are also being evaluated for the treatment of tuberculosis, including rifabutin, which is used for prophylaxis against MAC disease in AIDS patients and is probably active against some tubercle bacilli with low-level resistance to rifampin, and rifapentine, which may be effective when given only once weekly.

Regimens Short-course regimens are divided into an initial or bactericidal phase and a continuation or sterilizing phase. During the initial phase, the majority of the tubercle bacilli are killed, symptoms

Table 171-1

Recommended Drugs and Dosages for the Initial Treatment of Tuberculosis in Adults*

Drug	Dosage	
	Daily	**Thrice Weekly†**
Isoniazid	5 mg/kg, max. 300 mg	15 mg/kg, max. 900 mg
Rifampin	10 mg/kg, max. 600 mg	10 mg/kg, max. 600 mg
Pyrazinamide	15–30 mg/kg, max. 2 g	50–70 mg/kg, max. 3 g
Ethambutol	15–25 mg/kg	25–30 mg/kg
Streptomycin	15 mg/kg, max. 1 g	25–30 mg/kg, max. 1.5 g

* Dosages for children are similar, except that some authorities recommend higher doses of isoniazid (10–20 mg/kg daily; 20–40 mg/kg intermittent) and rifampin (10–20 mg/kg).

† Dosages for twice-weekly administration are the same except for pyrazinamide (maximum, 4 g/d) and ethambutol (50 mg/kg).

SOURCE: Based on recommendations of the American Thoracic Society and the Centers for Disease Control and Prevention, 1994.

resolve, and the patient becomes noninfectious. The continuation phase is required to eliminate semidormant "persisters."

The treatment regimen of choice for virtually all forms of tuberculosis in both adults and children consists of a 2-month initial phase of isoniazid, rifampin, and pyrazinamide followed by a 4-month continuation phase of isoniazid and rifampin (Table 171-2). Except for patients who seem unlikely on epidemiologic grounds to be initially infected with a drug-resistant strain, ethambutol (or streptomycin) should be included in the regimen for the first 2 months or until the results of drug susceptibility testing become available. Treatment is most commonly given daily throughout the course, although intermittent regimens (either three times weekly throughout the course or a daily initial phase followed by twice-weekly treatment during the continuation phase) produce equivalent results. For patients with sputum culture–negative pulmonary tuberculosis, the duration of treatment may be reduced to a total of 4 months. Pyridoxine (10 to 25 mg/d) should be added to the regimen given to persons at high risk of vitamin deficiency (e.g., alcoholics; malnourished persons; pregnant and lactating women; and patients with conditions such as chronic renal failure, diabetes, and HIV infection or AIDS, which are also associated with neuropathy).

Patients' lack of adherence to treatment regimens is recognized worldwide as the most important impediment to cure. Moreover, the mycobacterial strains infecting patients who do not adhere to the prescribed regimen are especially likely to develop acquired drug resistance. Both patient- and provider-related factors may affect compliance. Patient-related factors include a lack of belief that the illness is significant and/or that treatment will have a beneficial effect; the existence of concomitant medical conditions (notably substance abuse); lack of social support; and poverty, with attendant joblessness and homelessness. Provider-related factors that may promote compliance include the education and encouragement of patients, the offering of convenient clinic hours, and the provision of incentives such as bus tokens.

In addition to specific measures addressing noncompliance, two other strategic approaches are used: direct observation of treatment and provision of drugs in combined formulations. Because it is difficult to predict which patients will adhere to the recommended treatment, all patients should have their therapy directly supervised, especially during the intensive phase. In the United States, personnel to supervise therapy are usually available through tuberculosis control programs of local public health departments. Supervision increases the proportion of patients completing treatment and greatly lessens the chances of relapse and acquired drug resistance. Combination products (isoniazid/rifampin and isoniazid/rifampin/pyrazinamide) are available and are strongly recommended as a means of minimizing the likelihood of prescription error and of the development of drug resistance (as the result of treatment with only one agent). In some formulations of these combination products, the bioavailability of rifampin has been found to be substandard. In North America and Europe, regulatory authorities ensure that combination products are of good quality; however, this type of monitoring cannot be assumed to take place in less affluent countries. Alternative regimens for patients who exhibit drug intolerance or adverse reactions are listed in Table 171-2.

Monitoring of the Response to Treatment Bacteriologic evaluation is the preferred method of monitoring the response to treatment for tuberculosis. Patients with pulmonary disease should have their sputum examined monthly until cultures become negative. With the recommended 6-month regimen, more than 80 percent of patients will have negative sputum cultures at the end of the second month of treatment. By the end of the third month, virtually all patients should be culture-negative. In some patients, especially those with extensive cavitary disease and large numbers of organisms, AFB smear conversion may follow culture conversion. This phenomenon is presumably due to the expectoration and microscopic visualization of dead bacilli. When a patient's sputum cultures remain positive at or beyond 3 months, treatment failure and drug resistance should be suspected (see below). A sputum specimen should be collected at the end of treatment to document cure. If mycobacterial cultures are not practical, then monitoring by AFB smear examination should be undertaken at 2, 5, and 6 months. Smears positive after 5 months should be considered indicative of treatment failure.

Bacteriologic monitoring of patients with extrapulmonary tuberculosis is more difficult and often is not feasible. In these cases, the response to treatment must be assessed clinically.

Monitoring of the response to treatment by serial chest radiographs is not recommended. Radiographic changes may lag behind bacteriologic response and are not highly sensitive. However, a chest radiograph at the end of treatment may be useful for comparative purposes should the patient develop symptoms of recurrent tuberculosis. After the completion of treatment, neither follow-up sputum examination nor chest radiography is recommended. However, patients should be instructed to report promptly for medical assessment should they develop any symptoms consistent with recurrent tuberculosis.

During treatment, patients should be monitored for drug toxicity. The most common adverse reaction of significance is hepatitis. Pa-

Table 171-2

Recommended Regimens for the Treatment of Tuberculosis

	Initial Phase		Continuation Phase	
Indication	Duration, Months	Drugs	Duration, Months	Drugs
New smear- or culture-positive case	2	HRZE*	4	HR*
New culture-negative case	2	HRZE*	2	HR*
Intolerance to H	2	RZE	7	RE
Intolerance to R	2	HES (±Z)	16	HE
Intolerance to Z	2	HRE	7	HR
Pregnancy	2	HRE	7	HR
Failure and relapse†	—	—	—	—
Standard retreatment (susceptibility testing unavailable)	3	HRZES‡	5	HRE
Resistance to H + R	Throughout (12–18)	ZE + O + S (or another injectable agent§)	t—	—
Resistance to all first-line drugs	Throughout (24)	1 injectable agent§ + 3 of these 4: ethionamide, cycloserine, PAS, O	—	—

* All drugs can be given daily or intermittently (three times weekly throughout or twice weekly after the initial phase of daily therapy).
† Regimen is tailored according to the results of drug susceptibility tests.
‡ Streptomycin treatment should be discontinued after 2 months.
§ Amikacin, kanamycin, or capreomycin. Treatment with all of these agents should be discontinued after 2 to 6 months, depending upon the patient's tolerance and response.

NOTE: H, isoniazid; R, rifampin; Z, pyrazinamide; E, ethambutol; S, streptomycin; O, ofloxacin; PAS, para-aminosalicylic acid.

tients should be carefully educated about the signs and symptoms of drug-induced hepatitis (e.g., dark urine, loss of appetite) and should be instructed to discontinue treatment promptly and see their health care provider should these symptoms occur. Although biochemical monitoring is not routinely recommended, all adult patients should undergo baseline assessment of liver function (e.g., measurement of levels of hepatic aminotransferases and serum bilirubin). Older patients, those with histories of hepatic disease, and those using alcohol daily should be monitored especially closely, with repeated measurements of aminotransferases, during the initial phase of treatment. Up to 20 percent of patients have small increases in aspartate aminotransferase (up to three times the upper limit of normal) that are accompanied by no symptoms and are of no consequence. For patients with symptomatic hepatitis and those with marked elevations in aspartate aminotransferase, treatment should be stopped and drugs reintroduced one at a time after liver function has returned to normal.

Hypersensitivity reactions usually require the discontinuation of administration of all drugs and rechallenge to determine which agent is the culprit. Because of the variety of regimens available, it is usually not necessary—although it is possible—to desensitize patients. Hyperuricemia and arthralgia caused by pyrazinamide can usually be managed by the administration of acetylsalicylic acid; however, pyrazinamide treatment should be stopped if the patient develops gouty arthritis. Individuals who develop autoimmune thrombocytopenia secondary to rifampin therapy should not receive the drug thereafter. Similarly, the occurrence of optic neuritis with ethambutol and the development of eighth-nerve damage with streptomycin are indications for permanent discontinuation of these respective drugs. Other common manifestations of drug intolerance, such as pruritus and gastrointestinal upset, can generally be managed without the interruption of therapy.

Treatment Failure and Relapse As stated above, treatment failure should be suspected when a patient's sputum cultures remain positive after 3 months or when AFB smears remain positive after 5 months. In the management of such patients, it is imperative that the current isolate be tested for susceptibility to first- and second-line agents. When the results of susceptibility testing are expected to become available within several weeks, changes in the regimen can be postponed until that time. However, if the patient's clinical condition is deteriorating, an earlier change in regimen may be indicated. A cardinal rule in the latter situation is always to add more than one drug at a time to a failing regimen: at least two and preferably three drugs that have never been used should be added. The patient may continue to take isoniazid and rifampin along with these new agents pending the results of susceptibility tests.

The mycobacterial strains infecting patients who experience a relapse after apparently successful treatment are less likely to have acquired drug resistance (see below) than are strains from patients in whom treatment has failed. However, if the regimen administered initially does not contain rifampin (and thus is not a short-course regimen), the probability of isoniazid resistance is high. Acquired resistance is uncommon among strains from patients who relapse after completing a short course of therapy. However, it is prudent to begin the treatment of all relapses with all five first-line drugs pending the results of susceptibility testing. In less affluent countries and other settings where facilities for culture and drug susceptibility testing are not available, a standard regimen should be used in all instances of relapse and treatment failure (Table 171-2).

Drug-Resistant Tuberculosis Strains of *M. tuberculosis* resistant to individual drugs arise by spontaneous point mutations in the mycobacterial genome, which occur at low but predictable rates. Because there is no cross-resistance among the commonly used drugs, the probability that a strain will be resistant to two drugs is the product of the probabilities of resistance to each drug and thus is low. The development of drug-resistant tuberculosis is invariably

the result of monotherapy—i.e., the failure of the health care provider to prescribe at least two drugs to which tubercle bacilli are susceptible or of the patient to take properly prescribed therapy.

Drug-resistant tuberculosis may be either primary or acquired. *Primary* drug resistance is that in a strain infecting a patient who has not previously been treated. *Acquired* resistance develops during the course of treatment with an inappropriate regimen. In North America and Europe, rates of primary resistance are generally low, and isoniazid resistance is most common. Much attention has been focused on disease due to isoniazid/rifampin-resistant or multidrug-resistant (MDR) tuberculosis. As noted above, drug-resistant tuberculosis can be prevented by adherence to the principles of sound therapy: the inclusion of at least two bactericidal drugs to which the organism is susceptible (in practice, four drugs are commonly given in the initial phase) and the verification that patients complete the prescribed course.

Although the 6-month regimen described in Table 171-2 is highly effective for patients with initial isoniazid-resistant disease, it is prudent to extend treatment to 9 months and to include ethambutol throughout. For disease with high-level isoniazid resistance, isoniazid probably does not contribute to a successful outcome and can be dropped from the regimen. MDR tuberculosis is more difficult to manage than is disease caused by a drug-susceptible organism, especially because resistance to other first-line drugs as well as to isoniazid and rifampin is common. For strains resistant to isoniazid and rifampin, combinations of ethambutol, pyrazinamide, and streptomycin (or, for those with streptomycin resistance as well, another injectable agent such as amikacin), given for 12 to 18 months and for at least 9 months after sputum culture conversion, may be effective. Many authorities would add ofloxacin to this regimen. For patients with bacilli resistant to all of the first-line agents, cure may be attained with a combination of three drugs chosen from ethionamide, cycloserine, PAS, and ofloxacin plus one drug chosen from amikacin, kanamycin, and capreomyin (Table 171-2). The optimal duration of therapy for MDR tuberculosis is not known; however, patients are commonly treated for up to 24 months. Because the management of patients with MDR tuberculosis is complicated by both social and medical factors, care of these patients should be restricted to specialists and tuberculosis control programs. For patients with localized disease and sufficient pulmonary reserve, lobectomy or pneumonectomy can lead to cure.

Special Clinical Situations Although comparative clinical trials of treatment for extrapulmonary tuberculosis are limited, the available evidence indicates that all forms of disease can be treated with the 6-month regimen recommended for patients with pulmonary disease. However, the American Academy of Pediatrics recommends that children with bone and joint tuberculosis, tuberculous meningitis, or miliary tuberculosis receive a minimum of 12 months of treatment.

Treatment for tuberculosis may be complicated by underlying medical problems that require special consideration. As a rule, patients with chronic renal failure should not receive aminoglycosides and should receive ethambutol only if serum levels can be monitored. Isoniazid, rifampin, and pyrazinamide may be given in the usual doses in cases of mild to moderate renal failure, but the dosages of isoniazid and pyrazinamide should be reduced for all patients with severe renal failure except those undergoing hemodialysis. Patients with hepatic disease pose a special problem because of the hepatotoxicity of isoniazid, rifampin, and pyrazinamide. Patients with severe hepatic disease may be treated with ethambutol and streptomycin and, if required, with isoniazid and rifampin under close supervision. The use of pyrazinamide by patients with liver failure should be avoided. Silicotuberculosis necessitates the extension of therapy by at least 2 months. Finally, patients with HIV infection or AIDS appear to respond well to standard 6-month therapy, although treatment may need to be prolonged if the response is suboptimal.

The regimen of choice for pregnant women is 9 months of treatment with isoniazid and rifampin supplemented by ethambutol for the first 2 months. When required, pyrazinamide may be given, although there are no data concerning its safety in pregnancy. Streptomycin is contraindicated because it is known to cause eighth-cranial-nerve damage in the fetus. Treatment for tuberculosis is not a contraindication to breast feeding; most of the drugs administered will be present in small quantities in breast milk, albeit at concentrations far too low to provide any therapeutic or prophylactic benefit to the child.

PREVENTION By far the best way to prevent tuberculosis is the rapid diagnosis of infectious cases with appropriate treatment until cure. Additional strategies include BCG vaccination and preventive chemotherapy.

BCG Vaccination BCG was derived from an attenuated strain of *M. bovis* and was first administered to humans in 1921. Many BCG vaccines are available worldwide; all are derived from the original strain, but the vaccines vary in efficacy. In fact, estimates of efficacy from randomized, placebo-controlled trials have ranged from 80 percent to nil. A similar range of efficacy was found in recent observational studies (case-control, historical cohort, and cross-sectional studies) in areas where infants are vaccinated at birth. These studies also found higher rates of efficacy in the protection of infants and young children from relatively serious forms of tuberculosis, such as tuberculous meningitis and miliary tuberculosis.

BCG vaccine is safe and rarely causes serious complications. The local tissue response begins 2 to 3 weeks after vaccination, with scar formation and healing within 3 months. Side effects—most commonly, ulceration at the vaccination site and regional lymphadenitis—occur in 1 to 10 percent of vaccinated persons. Some vaccine strains have caused osteomyelitis in approximately one case per million doses administered. Disseminated BCG infection and death have occurred in 1 to 10 cases per 10 million doses administered, although this problem is restricted almost exclusively to persons with impaired immunity, such as those with HIV infection. BCG vaccination induces PPD reactivity. The presence or size of PPD skin-test reactions after vaccination does not predict the degree of protection afforded.

BCG vaccine is recommended for routine use at birth in countries with high tuberculosis prevalences. However, because of the low risk of transmission of tuberculosis in the United States and the unreliable protection afforded by BCG, the vaccine has never been recommended for general use in the United States. Currently, vaccination is recommended only for PPD-negative infants and children who are at high risk of intimate and prolonged exposure to patients with MDR tuberculosis and who cannot take prophylactic isoniazid and for infants and children in groups in which the rate of new *M. tuberculosis* infections exceeds 1 percent per year.

Preventive Chemotherapy A major component of tuberculosis control in the United States involves the administration of isoniazid to persons with latent tuberculosis and a high risk of active disease. This intervention is based on the results of a large number of randomized, placebo-controlled clinical trials demonstrating that a 6- to 12-month course of isoniazid reduces the risk of active tuberculosis in infected people by 90 percent or more. In the absence of reinfection, the protective effect is believed to be lifelong. More recently, limited clinical trials have also shown that isoniazid prophylaxis reduces rates of tuberculosis among persons with HIV infection.

In most cases, candidates for prophylaxis (Table 171-3) are identified by PPD skin testing of high-risk groups of individuals. For skin testing, 5 tuberculin units of polysorbate-stabilized PPD should be injected intradermally into the volar surface of the forearm (Mantoux method). Multipuncture tests, which may be useful for screening large populations, are not recommended for this purpose; any positive reaction to a multipuncture test must be confirmed by Mantoux testing. Reactions are read at 48 to 72 h as the transverse diameter in millimeters of induration; the diameter of erythema is not considered. In some persons, PPD reactivity wanes with time but can be recalled by a second skin test administered 1 week or more after the first (i.e., two-step testing). For persons undergoing periodic PPD skin testing, such as health care workers and individuals admitted to long-term-care institutions, a repeat test in instances of an initially negative result

Table 171-3

Recommendations for Isoniazid Prophylaxis

Risk Group	Tuberculin Reaction, mm	Duration of Treatment, months
HIV-infected persons	≥5*	12
Close contacts of tuberculosis patients	≥5†	6 (9 for children)
Persons with fibrotic lesions on chest radiography	≥5	12
Recently infected persons	≥10	6
Persons with high-risk medical conditions‡	≥10	6–12
High-risk group, <35 years of age§	≥10	6
Low-risk group, <35 years of age	≥15	6

* Anergic HIV-infected persons with an estimated risk of *M. tuberculosis* infection of 10 percent may also be considered candidates.
† Tuberculin-negative contacts, especially children, should receive prophylaxis for 2 or 3 months after contact ends and should then be retested with PPD. Those whose results remain negative should discontinue prophylaxis.
‡ Includes diabetes mellitus, prolonged therapy with systemic glucocorticoids, other immunosuppressive therapy, some hematologic and reticuloendothelial diseases, injection drug use (with HIV seronegativity), end-stage renal disease, and clinical situations associated with rapid weight loss.
§ Includes persons born in high-prevalence countries, members of medically underserved low-income populations, and residents of long-term-care facilities.
SOURCE: Based on recommendations of the American Thoracic Society and the Centers for Disease Control and Prevention, 1994.

may preclude the misclassification of persons with boosted reactions as PPD converters.

The cutoff for a positive skin test (and thus for prophylaxis) is related both to the probability that the reaction represents true infection and to the likelihood that the individual, if truly infected, will develop tuberculosis. Thus positive reactions for close contacts of infectious cases, persons with HIV infection, and previously untreated persons whose chest radiograph is consistent with healed tuberculosis are defined as an area of induration ≥5 mm in diameter. A 10-mm cutoff is used to define positive reactions in most other at-risk persons. For persons with a very low risk of developing tuberculosis if infected, a cutoff of 15 mm is used.

Some PPD-negative individuals are also candidates for prophylaxis. Infants and children who have come into contact with infectious cases should be given prophylactic isoniazid and should have a repeat skin test 2 or 3 months after contact ends. Those whose test results remain negative should discontinue prophylaxis. HIV-infected persons who have a negative skin test and are at increased risk of tuberculosis may receive prophylaxis if they are found to be anergic on testing with other DTH antigens, such as *Candida* and mumps. Finally, some authorities recommend that all HIV-infected contacts of infectious cases be considered candidates for prophylaxis.

Isoniazid is administered in a dose of 5 mg/kg per day (up to 300 mg) for 6 to 12 months; the longer course is recommended for persons with HIV infection and for those with abnormal chest radiographs. On the basis of cost-benefit analyses, the shorter period is recommended for individuals in other categories. However, the American Academy of Pediatrics recommends that children receive a 9-month course of therapy. When supervised prophylaxis is desirable and feasible, isoniazid may be given at a dose of 15 mg/kg (up to 900 mg) twice weekly.

Contraindications to isoniazid prophylaxis include the presence of active liver disease. Since the major adverse reaction to this drug is hepatitis, persons at increased risk of toxicity (e.g., those aged 35 years or older, those consuming alcohol daily, and those with a history of liver disease) should undergo baseline and then monthly assessment of liver function during treatment. All patients should be carefully educated about hepatitis and instructed to discontinue use of the drug immediately should any symptoms develop. Moreover, patients should be seen and questioned about adverse reactions monthly during therapy and should be given no more than 1 month's supply of drug at each visit.

It may be more difficult to ensure compliance with a prophylactic regimen than with a therapeutic regimen for active tuberculosis. If family members of active cases are being treated, compliance and monitoring may be easier. For high-risk patients (such as HIV-infected injection-drug users) and persons who are institutionalized, twice-weekly supervised therapy may be useful. As in active cases, the provision of incentives may also be helpful.

BASICS OF CONTROL   The highest priority in any tuberculosis control program is the prompt detection of cases and the provision of directly observed short-course chemotherapy to all tuberculosis patients, with emphasis on the cure of sputum smear–positive cases. In addition, in low-prevalence countries with adequate resources, screening of high-risk groups (such as immigrants from high-prevalence countries and HIV-seropositive persons) is recommended. Identification of active cases of tuberculosis should be followed by treatment and that of PPD positivity in high-risk persons by prophylaxis. Contact investigation is also an important component of efficient tuberculosis control. In the United States, a great deal of attention has been given to the transmission of tuberculosis (particularly in association with HIV infection) in institutional settings such as hospitals, homeless shelters, and prisons. Measures to limit such transmission include respiratory isolation of persons with suspected tuberculosis until they are proven to be noninfectious (i.e., by sputum AFB smear negativity), proper ventilation in rooms of patients with infectious tuberculosis, use of ultraviolet lights in areas of increased risk of tuberculosis transmission, and periodic screening of personnel who may come into contact with known or unsuspected cases of tuberculosis. In the past, radiographic surveys, especially those conducted with portable equipment and miniature films, were advocated for case-finding. Today, however, the prevalence of tuberculosis in industrialized countries is sufficiently low that "mass miniature radiography" is not cost-effective.

In high-prevalence countries, tuberculosis control programs should be based on the following key elements: (1) case detection, predominantly through passive case-finding (e.g., microscopic examination of sputum from patients who present spontaneously to health care facilities with cough of more than 3 weeks' duration); (2) administration of standard short-course chemotherapy to all sputum smear–positive patients under proper case-management conditions—namely, supervised administration of drugs; (3) establishment and maintenance of a system of regular drug supply; and (4) establishment and maintenance of an effective system for patient evaluation and program management. This system should allow an analysis of treatment outcomes (e.g., cure, completion of treatment without proof of cure, death, treatment failure, and default) in all cases registered.

BIBLIOGRAPHY

AMERICAN THORACIC SOCIETY AND CENTERS FOR DISEASE CONTROL: Control of tuberculosis in the United States. Am Rev Respir Dis 146:1623, 1992
————: Treatment of tuberculosis and tuberculosis infection in adults and children. Am J Respir Crit Care Med 149:1359, 1994
ANTONUCCI G et al: Risk factors for tuberculosis in HIV-infected persons. A prospective cohort study. JAMA 274:143, 1995
BLOOM BR (ed): Tuberculosis. Pathogenesis, Protection, and Control. Washington, DC, American Society for Microbiology, 1994
CANTWELL MF et al: Epidemiology of tuberculosis in the United States, 1985 through 1992. JAMA 272:535, 1994
CENTERS FOR DISEASE CONTROL: Guidelines for preventing the transmission of tuberculosis in health-care settings, with special focus on HIV-related issues. Morb Mortal Week Rep 39(RR-17):1, 1990
CROFTON J et al: Clinical Tuberculosis. London, Macmillan Education, 1992
FINE PEM: Bacille Calmette-Guérin vaccines: A rough guide. Clin Infect Dis 20:11, 1995
HOPEWELL PC: Impact of human immunodeficiency virus infection on the epidemiology, clinical features, management, and control of tuberculosis. Clin Infect Dis 15:540, 1992
ISEMAN MD: Treatment of multidrug-resistant tuberculosis. N Engl J Med 329:784, 1993
MITCHISON DA: The action of antituberculosis drugs in short-course chemotherapy. Tubercle 66:219, 1985
O'BRIEN RJ: Preventive therapy for tuberculosis, in Clinical Tuberculosis, PDO Davies (ed). London, Chapman & Hall, 1994, pp 279–295
RAVIGLIONE MC et al: Global epidemiology of tuberculosis. Morbidity and mortality of a worldwide epidemic. JAMA 273:220, 1995
REICHMAN LB, HERSHFIELD ES (eds): Tuberculosis. A Comprehensive International Approach. New York, Mercel Dekker, 1993
SMALL PM et al: The epidemiology of tuberculosis in San Francisco: A population-based study using conventional and molecular methods. N Engl J Med 330:1703, 1994
SUMARTOJO E: When tuberculosis treatment fails. A social behavioral account of patient adherence. Am Rev Respir Dis 147:1311, 1993
STYBLO K: Epidemiology of tuberculosis, in Selected Papers, vol 24. The Hague, Royal Netherlands Tuberculosis Association, 1993
WORLD HEALTH ORGANIZATION: Treatment of Tuberculosis. Guidelines for National Programmes. Geneva, WHO, 1993

172   *Richard A. Miller*

LEPROSY (HANSEN'S DISEASE)

DEFINITION AND ETIOLOGY   Leprosy (Hansen's disease) is a chronic granulomatous infection of humans that attacks superficial tissues, especially the skin and peripheral nerves. *Mycobacterium leprae*, the causal agent, is an acid-fast rod assigned to the family Mycobacteriaceae on the basis of morphologic, biochemical, antigenic, and genetic similarities to other mycobacteria. Although it has not been cultivated in artificial media or tissue culture, *M. leprae* can be propagated in armadillos and in the footpads of mice. The bacillus multiplies exceedingly slowly, with an estimated optimal doubling time of 11 to 13 days during logarithmic growth in mouse footpads. The mouse model has been used extensively for the study of antileprosy drugs, and the high bacterial yield from armadillos has been crucial for immunologic and genetic studies. The genome of *M. leprae* has been completely mapped, and the genes for the major protein antigens have been cloned and sequenced.

The cellular components of *M. leprae* that are responsible for its pathogenicity and ability to survive within the host are poorly understood. The best-characterized virulence factor is phenolic glycolipid I, a prominent surface lipid specific to *M. leprae*. Phenolic glycolipid I can bind to complement component C3, which in turn mediates phagocytosis of the bacterium by mononuclear phagocytes via CR1, CR3, and CR4 receptors on their cell surfaces. Once the bacterium is inside the phagocyte, phenolic glycolipid I helps to protect it from oxidative killing by chemically scavenging hydroxyl radicals and superoxide anions.

EPIDEMIOLOGY   The number of leprosy cases worldwide has dropped dramatically in the past decade, from an estimated 10 to 12 million cases to 1.8 million cases. The explanation for this decline is controversial and undoubtedly multifactorial. Possible contributing factors include improved case detection, use of short-course multidrug therapeutic regimens, expanded bacillus Calmette-Guérin (BCG) vaccination programs, and increasing global urbanization. Leprosy remains largely a disease of the rural poor. In 1995, five countries— India, Brazil, Bangladesh, Indonesia, and Myanmar—accounted for 76 percent of the estimated number of cases in the world.

The distribution of infected individuals within countries is very nonhomogeneous. In some locales, 20 percent of the population is affected. The distribution of cases across the spectrum of leprosy also varies among countries, with lepromatous disease predominating in some countries, such as Mexico, and tuberculoid disease in others, such as India. Ninety percent of the cases diagnosed in the United States in the past two decades have occurred in immigrants from leprosy-endemic countries. Indigenous transmission takes place primarily in Hawaii, the Pacific Island territories, and (sporadically) along the Gulf Coast. The incidence of leprosy in the United States has fallen from a peak of 360 cases in 1985 (associated with an influx of immigrants from Southeast Asia) to an average of 150 cases per year.

Leprosy can present in persons of any age, although cases in infants less than 1 year of age are extremely rare. The age-specific incidence peaks during childhood in most developing countries; up to 20 percent of cases occur in children under 10. The sex ratio of leprosy presenting during childhood is 1:1, but males predominate by a 2:1 ratio among adult patients.

It is humbling to realize how little is known about the modes of transmission and acquisition of leprosy, given that the communicable nature of the infection has been recognized for millennia and that the etiologic agent was identified over 100 years ago. Direct human-to-human transmission is believed to be responsible for most cases of leprosy, although a history of exposure can be elicited from fewer than half of all patients. Animal reservoirs exist among feral armadillos and possibly among nonhuman primates, but in only a few human cases has zoonotic transmission been implicated. Detection of *M. leprae* in hematophagous insects and of phenolic glycolipid I in soil has led to speculation about environmental acquisition of infection. Among close family contacts of untreated lepromatous patients, the risk of disease is increased by approximately eightfold, and the attack rate can be as high as 10 percent. Development of clinical disease in contacts of tuberculoid patients is less common, although immunologic tests suggest that most of these contacts have been sensitized to *M. leprae*. The site of entry remains a matter of conjecture but is probably either the skin or the mucosa of the upper respiratory tract. The chief portal of exit is thought to be the nasal mucosa of untreated lepromatous patients.

The incubation period is frequently 3 to 5 years but has been reported to range from 6 months to several decades.

PATHOGENESIS The early events following the entry of *M. leprae* into the body have not been described in humans. The bacilli are surrounded by a dense, nearly inert lipid capsule; produce no exotoxins; and engender little inflammatory response. Immunologic and epidemiologic studies suggest that only a small fraction (possibly 10 to 20 percent) of the persons infected develop signs of indeterminate leprosy and that only about 50 percent of those with indeterminate disease experience a progression to full-blown clinical leprosy.

The intensity of the specific cell-mediated immune response to *M. leprae* correlates with the clinical and histologic disease class. Individuals with polar tuberculoid disease have an intense cellular response to *M. leprae* and a low bacillary load, whereas patients with lepromatous leprosy have no detectable cellular immunity to the leprosy bacillus. There is evidence from family studies that specific HLA-associated genes may be linked to different classes of disease. HLA-DR2 is inherited preferentially by children with polar tuberculoid disease, whereas HLA-MT1 and HLA-DQ1 are associated with polar lepromatous disease. The antigenic epitopes recognized by some of these major histocompatibility complex (MHC) molecules have been identified. The effect of the HLA-associated genes is limited to an influence on the type of leprosy that develops; there is no association between HLA haplotypes and overall susceptibility to leprosy.

The defect in cell-mediated immunity in lepromatous patients is extremely specific. These individuals do not suffer increased morbidity following infection by pathogens such as viruses, protozoa, or fungi, for which cellular immunity is important, and they are not at increased risk of neoplasia. In lepromatous leprosy, cells of the monocyte-macrophage family become engorged with *M. leprae* and are unable to kill or digest the organisms. However, when studied in vitro, monocytes from these patients respond normally to cytokines and display normal phagocytic and microbicidal activity. Patients with lepromatous leprosy have been shown to have an increased number of circulating CD8 + ("suppressor") lymphocytes that can be specifically activated by *M. leprae* antigens, and the lymphocytes present in their cutaneous granulomas are almost exclusively CD8 + . In contrast, CD4 + 4B4 + ("helper") cells predominate among the T cells in the cutaneous lesions of tuberculoid patients. In addition to these differences in lesional T cell populations, local cytokine production in lepromatous lesions is distinctly different from that in tuberculoid lesions. Lesions of tuberculoid leprosy characteristically have a predominant Th1 cytokine response, with high levels of production of interleukin (IL) 2, interferon γ (IFNγ), and IL-12. In contrast, IL-4 and IL-10 are dominant in lepromatous lesions, consistent with a Th2-like response. These observations have led to renewed interest in adjunctive therapy with immunomodulatory agents and may be crucial for vaccine development.

Intense bacillemia is very common in lepromatous leprosy, and organisms can often be seen in stained smears of peripheral blood or buffy coats; however, high fever and signs of systemic toxicity are absent. Even in the most advanced cases, destructive lesions are limited to the skin, peripheral nerves, anterior portions of the eyes, upper respiratory passages above the larynx, testes, and structures of the hands and feet. One feature common to these sites is that they are all usually several degrees cooler than 37°C. Two sites of preferential involvement are the ulnar nerves near the elbow and the peroneal nerves where they pass around the head of the fibula; above and below these areas, where these nerves take deeper courses, they are less severely involved. In patients with lepromatous leprosy, collections of bacilli are also found in the liver, spleen, and bone marrow, but no visceral organ system dysfunction has been associated with the presence of these bacilli.

CLINICAL AND HISTOPATHOLOGIC MANIFESTATIONS The variable immune response to infection with *M. leprae* results in a wide spectrum of histologic and clinical manifestations. Since there is a strong concordance between clinical findings and dermal histopathology, they will be discussed together.

Early or Indeterminate Leprosy The first signs of leprosy are usually cutaneous. The lesions of indeterminate leprosy are very subtle and are most commonly diagnosed during the examination of contacts of known leprosy patients. One or more hypopigmented or hyperpigmented macules or plaques may be seen. Often an anesthetic or paresthetic patch is the first symptom noted by the patient, but skin involvement can be found on careful examination. Sensation is often relatively preserved in these early lesions, particularly those on the face. The lesions may clear spontaneously in a year or two, but specific treatment is recommended.

Tuberculoid Leprosy The initial lesion of tuberculoid leprosy, one of the "poles" of the clinical and immunologic spectrum, is often a hypopigmented macule that is sharply demarcated and hypesthetic. Later the lesions enlarge by peripheral spread, and the margins become elevated and circinate or gyrate (Fig. 172-1). The central area in turn becomes atrophic and depressed. Fully developed lesions are densely anesthetic and have lost the normal skin organs (sweat glands and hair follicles). The lesions are single or few in number. Nerve involvement occurs early, and the superficial nerves leading from the lesions may

FIGURE 172-1 Tuberculoid leprosy. The large, solitary lesion has a raised, indurated border. The central clear area of the lesion is hypesthetic, with thinning of the dermis and loss of dermal structures such as sweat glands and hair follicles.

be enlarged. The larger peripheral nerves (especially the ulnar, peroneal, and greater auricular nerves and those closest to the skin lesion) may be palpably and visibly enlarged. The patient may experience severe neuritic pain. Neural involvement leads to muscle atrophy, especially of the small muscles of the hand. Contractures of the hand and foot are frequent. Trauma, especially from burns and splinters and from excessive pressure, leads to secondary infection of the hands and to plantar ulcers. Later, resorption and loss of phalanges may supervene. When the facial nerves are involved, there may be lagophthalmos, exposure keratitis, and corneal ulceration leading to blindness.

The histologic picture consists of noncaseating granulomas comprising lymphocytes, epithelioid cells, and perhaps giant cells; bacilli are frequently absent or difficult to demonstrate.

Lepromatous Leprosy   Lepromatous leprosy is the other polar form. Cutaneous involvement is extensive and roughly bilaterally symmetric across the midline of the host. Individual skin lesions are highly variable and can include macules, nodules, plaques, or papules. The borders of the lesions are ill defined, and the centers of raised lesions are indurated and convex (rather than concave, as in tuberculoid disease). There is diffuse infiltration of the dermis between discrete lesions, and apparently normal skin usually contains bacilli demonstrable by staining. The sites of predilection are the face (cheeks, nose, brows), ears, wrists, elbows, buttocks, and knees. At times, involvement with infiltration and little or no nodulation may progress so subtly that the disease goes unnoticed. Loss of the lateral portions of the eyebrows is common. Much later the skin of the face and forehead becomes thickened and corrugated (leonine facies), and the earlobes become pendulous.

Nasal "stuffiness," epistaxis, and obstructed breathing are common early symptoms. Complete nasal obstruction, laryngitis, and hoarseness also develop. Septal perforation and nasal collapse lead to saddlenose. Invasion of the anterior portion of the eye can result in keratitis and iridocyclitis. Painless inguinal and axillary lymphadenopathy occurs. In men, infiltration and scarring of the testes lead to sterility. Gynecomastia is common.

Involvement of the major nerve trunks is less prominent in the lepromatous than in the tuberculoid form, but diffuse hypesthesia involving the peripheral portions of the extremities is common in advanced disease. Pathologic studies reveal that the peripheral nerves are heavily infected but often better preserved than in the tuberculoid form.

Histologic examination detects a diffuse granulomatous reaction with macrophages, large foam (Virchow or lepra) cells, and many intracellular bacilli, frequently in spheroidal masses (globi). Epithelioid cells and giant cells are not found.

Borderline Leprosy   The borderline portion of the leprosy spectrum lies between the tuberculoid and lepromatous poles and is usually subdivided into borderline tuberculoid, borderline (or dimorphous), and borderline lepromatous classes. Classification within the borderline region of the spectrum is less precise than at the poles. Lesions tend to increase in number and heterogeneity but decrease in individual size as the lepromatous pole is approached. The skin lesions of borderline tuberculoid leprosy generally resemble those of tuberculoid disease but are more numerous and have less well-defined borders. Involvement of multiple peripheral nerve trunks is more common than in polar tuberculoid disease.

Increasing variability in the appearance of the skin lesions is characteristic of borderline leprosy. Papules and plaques may coexist with macular lesions. Anesthesia is less prominent than in tuberculoid disease. The earlobes may be slightly thickened, but the eyebrows and nasal regions are spared. Skin lesions become even more numerous in borderline lepromatous disease, but the distribution lacks the bilateral symmetry typical of polar lepromatous disease (Fig. 172-2).

The histopathology of the granulomas in borderline leprosy changes from an epithelioid cell predominance in borderline tuberculoid disease to a macrophage predominance as the lepromatous pole

FIGURE 172-2   Borderline lepromatous leprosy. Multiple macules, papules, and nodules have an asymmetric distribution. Individual lesions are small but may become confluent.

is approached. The presence and number of lymphocytes are variable and correlate poorly with disease class. Bacilli are present in large numbers in the skin granulomas of borderline and borderline lepromatous patients. For this reason, these categories of disease, together with polar lepromatous leprosy, are referred to as *multibacillary leprosy*. The borderline tuberculoid, polar tuberculoid, and indeterminate classes are grouped together as *paucibacillary leprosy*.

The borderline disease states are unstable and may shift toward the lepromatous form in the untreated patient or toward the tuberculoid pole during treatment. Change of either polar type to the other is exceedingly rare.

In all forms of leprosy, peripheral nerve involvement is a constant feature. In any histologic section, involvement of nerves tends to be more severe than involvement of other tissues. Much of the neural destruction appears to result from the granulomatous reaction of the host rather than from an innate neurotoxic property of the bacillus. Albeit uncommonly, neural involvement can occur in the absence of cutaneous lesions (pure neural leprosy).

REACTIONAL STATES   The general course of leprosy is indolent but may be interrupted by two types of reaction. Both reactions can occur in untreated patients but more often emerge as complications of chemotherapy.

Erythema Nodosum Leprosum   Erythema nodosum leprosum (ENL), or type 2 lepra reaction, develops in lepromatous and borderline lepromatous patients, most frequently in the latter half of the initial year of treatment. Tender, inflamed subcutaneous nodules develop, usually in crops. Each nodule lasts a week or two, but new crops may continue to appear. Thus ENL may last only a week or two or may persist for long periods. Fever, lymphadenopathy, and arthralgias can accompany severe ENL. Histologically, ENL is characterized by polymorphonuclear leukocyte infiltration and deposits of IgG and complement, resembling an Arthus reaction. The precise factors responsible for initiating attacks of ENL are unclear, but in vitro and in vivo data have established the central roles of IFNγ and tumor necrosis factor α (TNFα) in producing the observed clinical and immunologic abnormalities. In one study, exogenous IFNγ induced ENL in 6 of 10 lepromatous patients, probably through increased secretion of TNFα by activated monocytes. Patients with ENL often have elevated serum levels of TNFα, and the alleviation of ENL by thalidomide is mediated through specific inhibition of TNFα production.

Reversal Reaction   The reversal reaction, or type 1 lepra reaction, can complicate all three borderline categories. Existing skin lesions develop erythema and swelling, and new lesions may appear. An early influx of lymphocytes into existing lesions is followed by edema and a shift toward tuberculoid histology. Cellular immunity increases. Reversal reactions can be differentiated from disease progression or relapse by mouse inoculations to test bacillary viability and by histologic studies. *Downgrading reactions*, which clinically mimic reversal reactions, are most common in untreated patients and in women during the third trimester of pregnancy. Skin biopsies reveal a shift toward lepromatous histology and reflect a decrease in cellular immunity.

COMPLICATIONS   Leprosy is probably the most frequent cause of crippling of the hand in the world (Fig. 172-3). Trauma and secondary chronic infections can lead to loss of digits or distal extremities. Blindness is also common.

The *Lucio phenomenon*, characterized by arteritis, is limited to patients with diffuse, infiltrative, nonnodular lepromatous disease. Severe cases clinically resemble other forms of necrotizing vasculitis and are associated with a high mortality rate.

Secondary amyloidosis is a complication of severe lepromatous disease, especially that complicated by chronic ENL.

Leprosy and Human Immunodeficiency Virus (HIV) Infection   Surprisingly, given the experience with other mycobacterial diseases and the intricate immune response to *M. leprae*, concurrent infection with HIV appears to have little effect on the clinical manifestations or natural history of leprosy. Anecdotal reports suggest that the relapse rate after completion of therapy for paucibacillary disease may be slightly higher than usual among HIV-infected patients. In addition, HIV-positive patients with early or subclinical leprosy may be more likely to develop overt disease. Concurrent leprosy also may accelerate the course of HIV disease.

DIAGNOSIS   The demonstration of acid-fast bacilli in skin smears made by the scraped-incision method is strong evidence for leprosy, but in tuberculoid disease bacilli may not be demonstrable. Wherever possible, a skin biopsy specimen from the affected area should be sent to a pathologist knowledgeable in leprosy. The histologic involvement of peripheral nerves is pathognomonic, even in the absence of bacilli. Work is underway on the development of tests using genetic probes for the rapid identification and speciation of mycobacteria in clinical specimens, but current polymerase chain reaction (PCR) technology offers little improvement in sensitivity over conventional microscopy.

Hematologic and blood chemistry tests are of little help in establishing the diagnosis. Lepromatous patients frequently have mild anemia, an elevated erythrocyte sedimentation rate, and hyperglobulinemia. Between 10 and 20 percent of lepromatous patients have low-titer false-positive serologic tests for syphilis or autoantibodies directed against nuclear or cellular antigens.

Lepromin is a suspension of killed *M. leprae* prepared from heavily infected human or armadillo tissue. Intradermal injection elicits, somewhat variably, a tuberculin-like reaction at 48 h (the Fernandez reaction) and, more consistently, a papular reaction at 3 to 4 weeks (the Mitsuda reaction). The Mitsuda reaction is usually positive in tuberculoid patients and is always negative in lepromatous patients. However, because it is also positive in nearly all healthy adults, even those residing in areas free of endemic leprosy, it has no diagnostic value. Lepromin is not commercially available.

A specific serodiagnostic test for leprosy has been developed. Based on the detection of antibody to phenolic glycolipid I, this assay has a sensitivity of over 95 percent in polar lepromatous disease and about 30 percent in tuberculoid disease. The apparent correlation of the level of antibody with the bacillary load explains the high false-negative rate in polar tuberculoid disease. Despite this limitation, the near 100 percent specificity of this assay makes it potentially useful as a means of confirming the diagnosis of leprosy and as an epidemiologic tool for studying disease incubation and transmission.

The differential diagnosis includes lupus erythematosus, lupus vulgaris, sarcoidosis, yaws, dermal leishmaniasis, and a host of more mundane skin diseases. The skin lesions of leprosy, especially of turberculoid disease, are characterized by hypesthesia, and peripheral nerve involvement can always be demonstrated. Peripheral neuropathy from other causes and syringomyelia may be confused with leprosy, although skin involvement is not a feature of these other diseases. The combination of a chronic skin disease and peripheral nerve involvement should always lead to the consideration of leprosy.

℞ **TREATMENT**

The management of leprosy involves a broad multidisciplinary approach, including consultative services such as orthopedic surgery, ophthalmology, and physical therapy in addition to antimicrobial chemotherapy.

Specific Chemotherapy   *Dapsone* (4,4′-diaminodiphenylsulfone, DDS, diphenylsulfone), a folate antagonist, is the mainstay of therapy. The daily dosage is 50 to 100 mg in adults. Dapsone is very inexpensive, is safe in pregnancy, and has a long serum half-life of about 24 h that allows once-daily administration. Major side effects, which are relatively uncommon, include hemolysis, agranulocytosis, hepatitis, and potentially fatal exfoliative dermatitis. In lepromatous disease, enough bacilli are killed during the first 10 to 12 weeks of dapsone monotherapy to render mouse footpad inoculations negative. However, in this form of the disease, nonviable bacilli disappear slowly and may be found in the tissues for 5 to 10 years. Moreover, a few viable bacilli (persisters) may survive in the tissues for many years and cause a relapse if treatment is discontinued.

Years of dapsone monotherapy have led to the emergence of dapsone-resistant strains of *M. leprae*. Secondary resistance, which develops in 2 to 30 percent of lepromatous patients receiving dapsone monotherapy, presents as a clinical and bacteriologic relapse after several years of apparently successful regular therapy. Primary dapsone resistance in previously untreated patients has complicated empiric therapy in many parts of the world but remains uncommon (present in fewer than 3 percent of cases) in the United States. To counteract this problem, the World Health Organization (WHO) recommended in 1982 that defined-duration, multiple-drug therapy be administered to all leprosy patients. The results of multiple-drug therapy have exceeded expectations. The epidemic of dapsone resistance has been aborted, and active-case loads have fallen as patients have been declared cured.

Rifampin is the most rapidly mycobactericidal drug known for use against *M. leprae*. The viability of skin bacilli falls to undetect-

FIGURE 172-3   Borderline tuberculoid leprosy. Bilateral claw hand deformities result from ulnar and median nerve damage. Note the severe loss of muscle tissue in the forearms secondary to neuropathic and disuse atrophy.

able levels within 5 days after a single 1500-mg dose of oral rifampin. The usual dosage is 600 mg/d. The high cost of rifampin has limited its use in the developing world and has led to regimens in which it is given at a dosage of 600 or 900 mg once per month. Many leprologists prefer to treat with daily or twice-weekly rifampin if cost is not a crucial issue. Rare cases of rifampin-resistant *M. leprae* have been reported. Rifampin has not been approved for the intermittent treatment of leprosy by the Food and Drug Administration.

Clofazimine, a compound derived from a phenazine dye, is highly lipophilic and accumulates in the skin, the gastrointestinal tract, and macrophages and monocytes. It is usually given in a dosage of 50 to 200 mg/d and has an apparent half-life of over 70 days. Its major toxicity is restricted to the skin and the intestinal tract. The reddish skin pigmentation (often accompanied by ichthyosis) that is associated with clofazimine use is unacceptable to many light-skinned patients and can lead to poor compliance. The agent's intestinal toxicity is dose-related and is reflected in diarrhea and cramping abdominal pain. Clofazimine is not safe for use during pregnancy.

The several older agents with limited activity against *M. leprae* include ethionamide, prothionamide, thiambutosine, and amithiozone. All these drugs have significant toxicities, and none has yet been approved for the treatment of leprosy by the Food and Drug Administration. An extremely important and exciting development in the past few years has been the identification of several new antimicrobials with impressive activity against *M. leprae*. The most promising agents are minocycline, ofloxacin, and clarithromycin. These agents exhibit less bactericidal activity against *M. leprae* than does rifampin but are more active than dapsone or clofazimine. Combinations of these newer drugs will be important for the treatment of the rare cases of disease caused by rifampin-resistant *M. leprae*. Again, none of these drugs has yet been approved for the treatment of leprosy by the Food and Drug Administration.

Therapy for multibacillary disease should consist of three drugs, usually dapsone, rifampin, and clofazimine. If the organism is known to be dapsone-sensitive, the combination of dapsone and rifampin may be adequate for borderline and borderline lepromatous cases, but the likelihood of secondary dapsone resistance makes the addition of a third drug advisable in lepromatous disease. Objective measures of the response to therapy, including skin scrapings and biopsies, should be monitored and therapy continued at least until morphologically intact bacilli are consistently absent and the inflammatory cell infiltrate has resolved. The optimal duration of therapy is unknown, but a minimum of 2 years is recommended by WHO. An approach commonly used in the United States is to administer two or three drugs for the first 3 to 5 years and then to institute lifelong dapsone therapy.

Therapeutic regimens containing two drugs, usually dapsone and rifampin, are adequate for paucibacillary leprosy. WHO recommends a 6-month course and reports an annual failure rate after completion of only 0.1 percent. Standard practice in the United States is to use dapsone and rifampin for the first 6 to 12 months (depending on the clinical response) and then to use dapsone alone to complete a total of 24 months of therapy.

Evidence of clinical improvement should be visible by the second or third month of treatment. The clinical response to therapy may be obscured by intercurrent reactional states, but the disease stops progressing and the skin lesions gradually improve. Recovery from neurologic impairment is limited.

On the basis of promising results from preliminary studies, WHO is currently planning a large-scale trial comparing the combination of rifampin and ofloxacin with the conventional regimen of dapsone, rifampin, and clofazimine for the treatment of multibacillary disease. It is hoped that the duration of treatment can be shortened from the current minimum of 24 months to less than 6 months. Long-term follow-up is essential for the evaluation of all new regimens, as relapses continue to occur for more than 8 years after the completion of therapy with the dapsone/rifampin/clofazimine regimen.

Treatment of Reactional States Mild ENL is managed with antipyretics and anti-inflammatory agents. Severe cases can be rapidly controlled with high dosages of prednisone (60 to 120 mg/d). Antimicrobial therapy should be continued, since glucocorticoid therapy promotes the viability of *M. leprae* in mice not given antileprosy drugs. Rifampin enhances the metabolism of glucocorticoids by the liver, necessitating the administration of larger doses to achieve a given therapeutic effect. Thalidomide is the most effective drug for ENL. The usual initial dosage of 200 mg twice a day can be gradually tapered to a maintenance dosage of 50 to 100 mg/d for patients with chronic ENL. Thalidomide is absolutely contraindicated in women of childbearing age because of its teratogenicity but has proved relatively free of major side effects in other leprosy patients. This drug has not been approved by the Food and Drug Administration but is available through the Hansen's Disease Center, Carville, Louisiana, as an investigational agent. Clofazimine has anti-inflammatory properties as well as antimycobacterial activity and can be valuable in the treatment of chronic ENL; however, because it takes at least 3 to 4 weeks for clofazimine to reach effective levels, this drug is of little use in acute attacks. Other anti-inflammatory agents, including chloroquine, cyclosporine, and cytotoxic drugs, have been used in difficult cases; in general, these unusual situations should be managed in consultation with a leprosy specialist.

Reversal reactions are often acute and can lead to rapid and irreversible neurologic damage. Mild episodes may be managed with nonsteroidal anti-inflammatory agents, but glucocorticoids are essential in severe reversal reactions. Prolonged maintenance therapy is often necessary. Reversal reactions do not respond to thalidomide.

Other Measures Many of the deformities and disabilities of leprosy are preventable. Plantar ulcers, which are very common, may be prevented by rigid-soled footwear or walking plaster casts, and contractures of the hand may be prevented by physical therapy and application of casts. Reconstructive surgery is sometimes helpful. Nerve and tendon transplants and release of contractures can give patients more functional ability. All patients should undergo a thorough ophthalmologic examination, as up to 48 percent may have evidence of sight-threatening ocular complications. Vocational retraining is often necessary for those with permanent disability. Plastic surgery for facial deformities facilitates the acceptance of patients in society. The psychological trauma that historically resulted from prolonged segregation is now minimized by home therapy in virtually all cases.

CONTROL Case finding and chemotherapy form the present basis for the control of leprosy. Because infectiousness can be quickly suppressed with chemotherapy, early detection of cases is important. In endemic countries, early detection requires the establishment of local clinics or traveling teams. Family members and other close contacts of cases need to be examined regularly for leprosy. A benefit of the short (6- to 24-month) WHO-recommended multidrug treatment regimens is that patients can be certified as disease-free much sooner than was possible with dapsone monotherapy. Thus leprosy case workers can devote more effort to contact screening and case detection. In the United States, patients are eligible for treatment by the Public Health Service, and special clinics are located in several major cities. The risk of transmission—even by untreated patients—is very low, and no unusual infection-control precautions are required when patients are hospitalized. Chemoprophylaxis with dapsone may be effective, but contact screening by yearly physical examinations is preferred to empiric therapy in most situations. Vaccination with BCG appears to be more effective against leprosy than it is against tuberculosis. For unclear reasons, the vaccine's efficacy against leprosy has ranged widely (from 20 to 80 percent) in different trials. Several new vaccines are undergoing field trials, but preliminary results have failed to show significant improvement over BCG.

BIBLIOGRAPHY

BLAKE LA et al: Environmental nonhuman sources of leprosy. Rev Infect Dis 9:562, 1987

Cambau E et al: Multidrug-resistance to dapsone, rifampicin, and ofloxacin in *Mycobacterium leprae*. Lancet 349:103, 1997

Dana M et al: Ocular manifestations of leprosy in a noninstitutionalized community in the United States. Arch Ophthalmol 112:626, 1994

Editorial: Serological tests for leprosy. Lancet 1:533, 1986

Goodless DR et al: Reactional states in Hansen's disease: Practical aspects of emergency management. South Med J 84:237, 1991

Grosset J: Progress in the chemotherapy of leprosy. Int J Lepr Other Mycobact Dis 62:268, 1994

Hastings RC (ed): *Leprosy*. New York, Churchill Livingstone, 1985

Jacobson R: The face of leprosy in the United States today. Arch Dermatol 126:1627, 1990

Karonga Prevention Trial Group: Randomized controlled trial of single BCG, repeated BCG, or combined BCG and killed *Mycobacterium leprae* vaccine for prevention of leprosy and tuberculosis in Malawi. Lancet 348:17, 1996

Miko TL et al: Damage and regeneration of peripheral nerves in advanced treated leprosy. Lancet 342:521, 1993

Miller RA: Leprosy and AIDS. Int J Lepr Other Mycobact Dis 59:639, 1991

Noorden SK: Eliminating leprosy as a public health problem; why the optimism is justified. Int J Lepr Other Mycobact Dis 63:559, 1995

Ponnighaus JM et al: Efficacy of BCG vaccine against leprosy and tuberculosis in northern Malawi. Lancet 339:636, 1992

Sampaio EP et al: Influence of thalidomide on the clinical and immunologic manifestations of erythema nodosum leprosum. J Infec Dis 168:408, 1993

Yamamura M et al: Defining protective responses to pathogens: Cytokine profiles in leprosy lesions. Science 254:277, 1991

| 173 | *Bernard Hirschel* |

INFECTIONS DUE TO NONTUBERCULOUS MYCOBACTERIA

Mycobacteria are slightly curved or straight, rod-shaped or coccoid bacilli traditionally identified by the property of acid-fastness: once stained, the organisms are not easily decolorized, even with acid-alcohol, because of the composition of their cell walls. The genetic relation of mycobacteria with one another is evidenced by their ribosomal RNA sequence homology, which can be used for diagnostic purposes.

Because of the overwhelming clinical importance of tuberculosis, mycobacteriologists have distinguished the *Mycobacterium tuberculosis* complex (consisting of *M. tuberculosis*, *M. bovis*, and *M. africanum*) from all other mycobacteria. Except for *Mycobacterium leprae* (see Chap. 172), the other mycobacteria are referred to as atypical mycobacteria, mycobacteria other than tuberculosis (MOTT), or nontuberculous mycobacteria (NTM). The isolation of NTM—or the lack thereof—from an individual patient or laboratory specimen must be interpreted with the following facts in mind:

1. Some NTM require special media and/or growth conditions. The laboratory must be alerted and cultures for acid-fast bacilli requested if the diagnosis of these infections is not to be missed.
2. NTM grow slowly. Even the so-called rapid growers take 3 to 7 days to form visible colonies on solid media, whereas slow-growing mycobacteria take weeks or do not grow at all on artificial media.
3. The slow growth of mycobacteria complicates antibiotic susceptibility testing. During prolonged incubation, antibiotics may be degraded and disappear from the culture medium. Long delays reduce the clinical usefulness of whatever results are eventually obtained.
4. Data on in vitro susceptibility correlate poorly with clinical results. For example, clarithromycin, azithromycin, and clofazimine are highly and variably concentrated in tissues; consequently, the concentrations necessary for determining resistance are difficult to establish in vitro. Sensitivity testing, based on achievable serum levels, would have predicted that these drugs would have little efficacy in vivo; in fact, the opposite is true, both in animal models and in humans.

5. In contrast to *M. tuberculosis*, NTM are ubiquitous in the environment. Therefore, isolation of NTM from a site that is not normally sterile (such as sputum, urine, skin, or feces) does not constitute proof of disease. In Switzerland between 1983 and 1988, for example, only 23 of 513 human immunodeficiency virus (HIV)–negative patients with NTM isolates had clinically significant disease. Clusters of unusual isolates are more likely to suggest contamination—e.g., from tap water or bronchoscopy equipment—than to represent an epidemic of disease.

The original method for the classification of NTM, developed between 1950 and 1980, depends on speed of growth, morphology, and pigmentation of colonies on solid media as well as biochemical reactions. Although reliable and inexpensive, these procedures take a long time; a period of 12 weeks is often required for definitive identification. Of course, such delayed results are of little use in the care of patients.

The isolation of NTM from blood cultures requires the use of a special medium for lysis-centrifugation or radiometric broth culture. The lysis-centrifugation method (lysis of blood cells followed by centrifugation and plating of the pellet with the bacteria on solid medium) permits quantification of bacteremia; however, some mycobacteria (e.g., *M. genavense*) do not grow well on solid medium and will not be detected by this method. Culture in liquid broth, such as that used in the radiometric Bactec system, shortens the time needed to identify a positive culture but also precludes the study of colonial morphology and pigmentation. Molecular probes are now used for rapid identification of the most important species (*M. avium*, *M. intracellulare*, *M. gordonae*, *M. kansasii*, and the *M. tuberculosis* complex) in a positive culture; a color is produced upon hybridization of the probe to specific sequences of the mycobacterial ribosome.

Twenty years ago, the field of mycobacteriology was something of a backwater. Tuberculosis was incorrectly perceived as a disappearing problem, and NTM were causing only rare and chronic diseases. AIDS, however, has brought mycobacterial infections to the forefront of clinical medicine once more. HIV and *M. tuberculosis* make a volatile mixture, and disseminated infections with NTM are extremely frequent in the advanced stages of AIDS (see Chap. 308). In this setting, it is fortunate that new molecular techniques based on DNA amplification promise to accelerate diagnosis, identify common sources of infection, and reveal new types of NTM, while new antibiotics, such as the macrolides, the rifamycins, and the fluoroquinolones, offer improved options for treatment and prevention.

DISSEMINATED NTM INFECTIONS IN AIDS AND OTHER IMMUNODEFICIENCIES

ETIOLOGY   The majority of mycobacterial infections in immunocompromised hosts are caused by organisms belonging to the group referred to as the *M. avium* complex (MAC). This group has always been considered to include *M. avium* and *M. intracellulare* (designated by the abbreviation *MAI*) and in the past encompassed *M. scrofulaceum* as well (hence the abbreviation *MAIS*). With the development and marketing of diagnostic probes that distinguish *M. avium* from *M. intracellulare*, it has become clear that the vast majority of disseminated "MAC" infections in AIDS are actually caused by *M. avium*. Thus, from a microbiologic standpoint, this designation is now obsolete. However, it is still used in clinical practice and will be employed in that context herein.

M. genavense causes systemic infections similar to those caused by MAC organisms. It is difficult to estimate the relative frequencies of *M. genavense* and MAC infections because *M. genavense* does not grow well in culture and may therefore be missed in some instances. However, in a series of nearly 200 disseminated NTM infections from Switzerland, 13 percent of cases were due to *M. genavense*. Other NTM, including *M. xenopi*, *M. simiae*, *M. scrofulaceum*, *M. malmoense*, and *M. celatum*, may also be involved in such cases. In addition, AIDS patients with localized NTM diseases often have positive blood cultures (e.g., patients with skin disease due to *M. haemophilum* or with lung disease due to *M. kansasii*).

EPIDEMIOLOGY AND HOST FACTORS Because gastrointestinal symptoms often predominate in NTM infection and because the intestinal submucosa is intensely involved, ingestion seems logical as a primary route of infection. Many environments and animals teem with NTM (especially MAC organisms), including swamps in the southeastern United States, swine almost everywhere, piped water in New England and in Finland, and soil from potted plants in San Francisco. Birds are frequently infected with *M. genavense*. Skin-test data and humoral antibody patterns point to widespread exposure to NTM. However, a direct connection of the environment to the patient is often lacking, and it is not always clear whether strains found in the environment are pathogenic in humans. In an exhaustive study of dietary factors, patients with NTM were found to have consumed more hard cheese than controls without NTM, but no NTM could be found in samples of cheese. At present, the epidemiologic evidence is not strong enough to serve as a basis for dietary recommendations in persons at high risk of NTM infection. There is no evidence for nosocomial spread of NTM from patient to patient; however, hospital hot-water systems have been suspected as the source of isolated clusters of cases. Whereas regional variations in the environmental frequency of NTM are striking, it is difficult to correlate these variations with the frequency of NTM infection among HIV-infected patients.

Disseminated infections with NTM occur almost exclusively in severely immunosuppressed patients, usually those with AIDS. Rarely, such infections are found in patients immunosuppressed for other reasons, including transplant recipients and patients with any of several ill-defined congenital immunodeficiencies, leukemia (in particular, hairy-cell leukemia), or lymphoma. Finally, rare cases of dissemination occur in immunocompetent patients who have extensive pulmonary disease.

In patients with AIDS, the risk of NTM infection correlates well with the degree of depletion of CD4 lymphocytes. For example, among patients with fewer than 10 CD4 lymphocytes per microliter, the actuarial probability of having a blood culture positive for NTM reaches 40 percent after 1 year. NTM may ultimately infect most such patients unless they first die for another reason. In the early 1990s, because prophylaxis of *Pneumocystis carinii* pneumonia was so successful, more patients survived to develop NTM infection. It remains to be proven whether prophylaxis of NTM infection with rifabutin or clarithromycin will alleviate this problem, although studies have found these drugs to be effective in reducing the risk of disseminated MAC infection.

DIAGNOSIS Blood cultures on special media are the cornerstone of the diagnosis of NTM infection, both in patients with organ involvement and in those without. In most symptomatic patients, the intensity of mycobacteremia is such that most or all blood cultures are positive. Therefore, the performance of multiple, repetitive cultures at short intervals is not worthwhile. Rather, in clinical practice, two or three blood cultures are sufficient. In one study, the results of prospective cultures varied, and these variations (positive followed by negative or vice versa) were unrelated to symptom status. As mentioned above, liquid cultures (e.g., the Bactec system) are likely to become positive earlier (within 7 to 14 days) and are therefore preferred to cultures on solid medium. In patients infected with *M. genavense* or *M. xenopi* and in patients being treated for MAC infection, the interval to culture positivity may be much longer. In rare cases, organ involvement in NTM infection may be found to be widespread at autopsy despite multiple negative blood cultures during life.

Because the liver and bone marrow are often involved in disseminated NTM infection, the bacteria may be visible in acid-fast–stained biopsy samples from these sites. Presumptive diagnosis by examination of a biopsied liver specimen saves time. The yield has been as high as 50 percent in patients with clearly abnormal values in liver function tests. However, the yield of this method has been disappointing in patients with suspected NTM infection, negative blood cultures, and normal or nearly normal results in liver function tests.

CLINICAL MANIFESTATIONS Disseminated infection with NTM is essentially a disease of advanced immunodeficiency. In HIV-infected patients, the median CD4 lymphocyte count at the time of diagnosis is around 10/μL. Certainly, other diagnoses should be considered first when a patient with symptoms suggestive of NTM infection has more than 100 CD4 cells per microliter. Prospective monthly blood cultures have shown that NTM bacteremia often causes few or no symptoms. In clinical practice, however, cultures are not performed if the patient is asymptomatic.

Disseminated NTM infection should be suspected on the basis of prolonged fever (sometimes of varying intensity—particularly at first—and accompanied by night sweats) and weight loss. Signs of abdominal involvement that may be evident on computed tomography or ultrasonography include enlargement of the liver and spleen and swelling of abdominal lymph nodes, which may result in diarrhea and/or abdominal pain. Anemia and leukopenia are frequently documented; although it is tempting to relate these abnormalities to infection of bone marrow by NTM, multiple factors are usually involved.

In short, the clinical picture of infection with NTM is not distinctive. Many other conditions, including abdominal lymphoma, the HIV wasting syndrome, *Salmonella* or *Campylobacter* infection, cryptosporidiosis, or microsporidiosis, may mimic (and coexist with) disseminated NTM infection. As stated earlier, suspicion of such infection should prompt a request for blood cultures.

℞ TREATMENT

Compared with *M. tuberculosis*, NTM are of low virulence. NTM tend to affect severely immunosuppressed patients, who usually have many other medical problems. Treatment is complex and frequently needs to be continued indefinitely since the eradication of NTM is difficult and relies on the use of multiple drugs with numerous adverse effects. At the beginning of the AIDS era, many physicians and activists took a dim view of drug therapy for NTM infection. The pendulum has now swung the other way, for the following reasons:

1. Patients with AIDS and disseminated NTM infection do not survive as long as comparable patients without NTM infection. Moreover, among those AIDS patients with disseminated NTM infection, treatment is associated with longer survival. Although not proof of a cause-and-effect relation (without randomization, it is always possible that untreated patients are sicker than treated patients at the time of diagnosis), such indirect evidence can guide clinical practice until data from prospective studies become available.
2. In many cases, symptoms are dramatically alleviated after the initiation of treatment. Some of this improvement (e.g., a decrease in fatigue and an increase in energy) may be difficult to quantify but is nonetheless of great importance to the patient.
3. Newer drugs exhibit increased activity against NTM both in vitro and in vivo.

The drugs used for the treatment of disseminated NTM infection are different from those used against tuberculosis (see Chap. 170). In particular, isoniazid has little effect on MAC organisms. The best method for antibiotic sensitivity testing of NTM is controversial, and the question of what relation—if any—exists between in vitro resistance and treatment failure remains unanswered. From the clinician's viewpoint, growth inhibition in liquid (Bactec) cultures is preferred to other methods of sensitivity testing because the results become available within 7 days.

The agents most active against MAC organisms are the macrolides clarithromycin and azithromycin. Both of these drugs are well absorbed from the gastrointestinal tract and well concentrated in macrophages and tissues, where their levels exceed those in plasma by more than 10-fold. Given alone, either drug can render blood cultures negative in a substantial proportion of cases. However, resistance (due to a single point mutation in the gene coding for the large ribosomal subunit) invariably develops, and NTM reappears in the bloodstream.

A majority of MAC strains are sensitive to ethambutol, ciprofloxacin, clofazimine, amikacin, rifampin, and rifabutin; that is, the concentrations of these drugs attainable in serum are inhibitory in vitro. However, none of these drugs consistently reduces the intensity of mycobacteremia when used alone. Trials to identify the best drug combination are ongoing. In the meantime, the following suggestions for therapy are made:

1. Include either clarithromycin (500 mg bid) or azithromycin (500 mg/d) in all regimens unless the mycobacterial strain is known to be resistant to these drugs in broth culture.
2. Include ethambutol (15 to 25 mg/kg per day) in treatment regimens. Most MAC strains are sensitive to this drug, and studies of immunosuppressed mice with disseminated MAC infection have documented excellent activity in vivo.
3. Add a third oral drug to the regimen: rifabutin (300 mg/d; higher doses—600 mg/d—have caused uveitis in up to 40 percent of patients when the drug is used together with clarithromycin), clofazimine (100 mg/d), rifampin (600 mg/d), or ciprofloxacin (500 mg bid). On the basis of in vitro data, results in experimental animals, and findings in one clinical trial, rifabutin is preferred. The rifamycins stimulate cytochrome P450 enzymes in the liver; drug interactions occur frequently (see Chap. 170). Compliance is an important issue in the treatment of patients with advanced immunodeficiency, who must ingest many drugs.
4. The inclusion of intravenous amikacin in multidrug regimens has not conferred additional benefit. Nonetheless, this drug may be useful in certain cases—for example, when resistance to clarithromycin develops or when severe gastrointestinal symptoms interfere with oral therapy. In addition, amikacin may prevent the emergence of resistance to clarithromycin when the two drugs are used concurrently.

It is not clear how long therapy needs to be administered. Older regimens did not eradicate MAC, and many experts recommended lifelong treatment. Unfortunately, multidrug regimens are often poorly tolerated. In patients whose symptoms have lessened, whose blood cultures have become negative, and who desire to simplify their regimen, it is currently considered reasonable to cut back to two drugs (usually clarithromycin and ethambutol) after 3 months.

In vitro and in experimental animals, cytokines such as interleukin 12, granulocyte-macrophage colony-stimulating factor, and interferon γ act synergistically with antibiotics against MAC. In a small-scale pilot trial including seven HIV-negative patients, interferon γ was beneficial.

Encapsulation of many drugs into liposomes enhances their effect in animal models because both liposomes and MAC are ingested by macrophages. Relevant data from studies of humans are still scarce, however. Disseminated infections caused by NTM other than MAC have been too rare for therapy to be evaluated in controlled trials. The presently recommended treatment for these infections is the same as that for disseminated MAC infections (Table 173-1). In particular, *M. genavense* seems to be sensitive to clarithromycin and rifabutin.

Table 173-1

The Most Important Nontuberculous Mycobacteria

Mycobacterial Species	Disseminated Infections	Localized Infections			Contaminant/ Commensal	Recommended Therapy	Percentage of Strains
		Lung	Lymphadenitis	Skin and Soft Tissue			
M. abscessus	—	—	—	Typical, linked to surgery	Typical	Debridement; clarithromycin, clofazimine, amikacin	<1
M. avium	Typical in AIDS with CD4 count of <50/μL; rare in other immunodeficiencies	See *M. intracellulare*	In children (rare)	In disseminated infection (rare)	Typical in sputum and feces	Clarithromycin,* ethambutol, rifabutin	30–50
M. celatum	AIDS (rare)	Rare	—	—	—	See *M. avium*	<1
M. chelonae	Rare	—	—	Typical, linked to surgery	Typical	See *M. abscessus*	<1
M. fortuitum	Rare	Rare	—	Typical	Typical	Amikacin, ciprofloxacin, sulfonamides, clofazimine, clarithromycin	1
M. genavense	Typical in AIDS	—	Rare	—	—	See *M. avium*	5
M. gordonae	Rare	—	—	Rare	Typical	—	10–30
M. haemophilum	Typical in AIDS and other immunodeficiencies	—	—	Typical, in AIDS	—	See *M. avium*	<1
M. intracellulare	See *M. avium*	Cavities in CF or COPD† Lingular infection in normal hosts	In children (rare)	See *M. avium*	Possible in sputum	See *M. avium*	4–8
M. kansasii	In AIDS (rare)	Typical, resembling tuberculosis	Rare	Rare	Possible in sputum	Rifampin, isoniazid, ethambutol, clarithromycin, sulfonamides	2–4
M. malmoense	Rare	Rare	—	—	—	See *M. avium*	1–4
M. marinum	Rare	—	—	Typical	—	Trimethoprim-sulfamethoxazole‡	1
M. scrofulaceum	Rare	Rare	Typical	—	—	See *M. avium*	1
M. simiae	In AIDS (rare)	Rare	—	—	Possible	See *M. avium*	1
M. szulgai	—	Rare	—	Typical	—	Rifampin, isoniazid, ethambutol	<1
M. xenopi	Rare	Rare	—	—	Typical	See *M. avium*	10–20

* Or azithromycin.
† CF, cystic fibrosis; COPD, chronic obstructive pulmonary disease.
‡ Or minocycline.
SOURCE: Data are from J Clin Microbiol 31:1882, 1993 (335 strains) and the Mycobacteriology Laboratory of the University Hospital in Geneva (1993–1994, 313 strains, Dr. P. Rohner).

PREVENTION As has been discussed, disseminated infection with MAC occurs almost exclusively in persons severely immunocompromised by HIV infection. Prophylaxis with rifabutin (300 mg/d), clarithromycin (500 mg once or twice daily), or azithromycin (1200 mg weekly) decreases the incidence of positive blood cultures by about 60 percent in patients with fewer than 200 CD4 lymphocytes per microliter. Patients receiving prophylaxis have also had less fever, experienced less fatigue, and survived longer than patients not receiving prophylaxis. Although breakthrough bacteremia involving resistant organisms is a concern, this condition has not developed with rifabutin prophylaxis and is rare with clarithromycin. Prophylaxis should therefore be considered for patients with fewer than 100 CD4 cells/μL. Some physicians are more restrictive in their indications and treat only those patients with fewer than 75 or 50 CD4 cells/μL; their rationale is that most disseminated MAC infections occur at very low CD4 counts, that prophylaxis is expensive (e.g., the cost of drugs to prevent one case of MAC infection is 50- to 100-fold greater than the cost of drugs to prevent a single case of *P. carinii* pneumonia), and that MAC prophylaxis heightens the potential for adverse reactions and drug interactions.

LOCALIZED INFECTIONS DUE TO NTM

PULMONARY DISEASE **Etiology** The NTM most frequently causing pulmonary infections are *M. intracellulare*, *M. avium*, and *M. kansasii*. Many other species, such as *M. xenopi* and *M. malmoense*, can also be involved in these infections. Identification of the specific pathogen is important in the choice among the various therapeutic strategies. For example, *M. kansasii* responds to antituberculosis drugs, including isoniazid.

Epidemiology and Host Factors As has already been noted, NTM are ubiquitous in the environment, but their pathogenicity is low. Preexisting lung disease (e.g., chronic obstructive airway disease, cancer, previous tuberculosis, bronchiectasis, cystic fibrosis, and silicosis, with cavities and bronchiectases) is the main predisposing factor for pulmonary disease due to NTM.

Anecdotal evidence suggests that the proportion of patients without underlying lung pathology who are developing pulmonary disease due to NTM is increasing. These patients are usually elderly; many are women with pectus excavatum or scoliosis. In the latter elderly women, the lingula and the right middle lobes are particularly involved. Somewhat whimsically, the disease in these patients has been called "Lady Windermere syndrome" after the main character in Oscar Wilde's play *Lady Windermere's Fan*, who went to extremes to refrain from coughing.

The significance of isolation of NTM from the airways of AIDS patients merits special discussion. *M. avium* only rarely causes significant pulmonary disease in AIDS; its isolation from sputum in the absence of radiographic changes is usually without clinical significance (except that in patients with fewer than 50 CD4 lymphocytes per microliter it may signal an increased likelihood of positive blood cultures in the future). In contrast, the isolation of *M. kansasii* from the lung is clinically significant: this organism causes a disease—often predominant in the upper lobes—that resembles pulmonary tuberculosis, with fever, cough, infiltrates, and cavities.

Clinical Manifestations Most patients with pulmonary NTM infection present with chronic cough, low-grade fever, and malaise; some present with hemoptysis. These symptoms may be masked by those of the underlying disease process. AIDS patients with pulmonary *M. kansasii* infection may develop severe symptoms mimicking pulmonary tuberculosis.

Diagnosis In contrast to the isolation of *M. tuberculosis*, of which even a single colony—whatever its origin—is clinically significant, the isolation of NTM from the sputum never in itself proves the existence of disease. NTM are frequently commensals and colonize both diseased and normal airways. Because treatment of NTM infection is compli-

cated, it is important that the diagnosis be certain. The American Thoracic Society has formulated the following minimal guidelines for the diagnosis of pulmonary NTM disease: "evidence, such as an infiltrate visible on a chest roentgenogram, of disease, the cause of which has not been determined by careful clinical and laboratory studies, and . . . isolation of multiple colonies of the same strain of mycobacteria repeatedly, usually in the absence of other pathogens." For patients who have pulmonary infiltrates but not cavities, these criteria may not be specific enough; some patients are found to have cleared NTM after a 1-month trial of bronchial hygiene alone (inhalation of saline and bronchodilators to induce cough and sputum production). The detection by computed tomography of bronchiectases and nodular infiltrates in the same lobe may be particularly suggestive of NTM infection.

℞ TREATMENT

Lung disease due to NTM may be managed by follow-up without treatment, by resection, or by drug therapy. No randomized trial has determined which is the best option. In retrospectively analyzed case series, patients undergoing surgery have had a better outcome than those treated only with drugs. However, selection bias has probably influenced these results since patients with extensive lung disease are poor candidates for surgery.

Patients with minimal disease (in particular, HIV-infected patients with NTM in sputum or bronchoalveolar lavage fluid but little evidence of lung damage) do not need treatment at all. Likewise, NTM disease may present as a solitary pulmonary nodule that, once resected (to confirm or exclude a diagnosis of cancer), requires no further drug treatment.

Most other patients with pulmonary NTM disease are treated with antimicrobials; in addition, they may or may not undergo surgery. The drugs available for the treatment of infection with *M. avium* or *M. intracellulare* have already been discussed. The regimens recommended for disseminated MAC infection are preferred, although large doses of clarithromycin are often poorly tolerated by elderly patients. *M. intracellulare* may be easier to treat and eradicate than *M. avium*. In two small open studies, single-agent treatment with clarithromycin (500 mg bid) led to improvements detected by chest radiography and sputum culture.

Indications for surgery are difficult to establish but include a disappointing response to antibiotics, the presence of localized disease, and the absence of contraindications (especially impaired respiratory functions). Ideally, drug treatment should begin before surgery and should render the sputum negative by the time of the operation.

In contrast to MAC organisms, *M. kansasii* is predictably sensitive to antituberculosis agents. Treatment should consist of isoniazid (300 mg/d), rifampin (600 mg/d), and ethambutol (15 to 25 mg/kg per day), whether or not the patient is infected with HIV; the optimal duration of therapy is unknown, but most patients have been treated for 18 to 24 months. Recent data suggest that 12 months may suffice. Sulfamethoxazole is recommended for the occasional patient whose infection relapses after *M. kansasii* becomes resistant to rifampin.

LYMPHADENITIS NTM are among the causes of localized lymphadenitis. This disease occurs mostly in children between the ages of 1 and 5 years. Painless swelling of one node or a group of nodes usually affects the anterior cervical chain. Nodes may rapidly increase in size, with the formation of fistulas to the skin. *M. scrofulaceum* or MAC organisms most commonly cause NTM lymphadenitis, although many other species may be involved. Once tuberculosis has been excluded, the treatment of choice is excision without chemotherapy. When excision is dangerous because of proximity to the facial nerve, aspiration combined with chemotherapy may be effective.

SKIN DISEASE DUE TO NTM **Swimming-Pool and Fish-Tank Granuloma** Between 1 week and 2 months (usually 2 to 3 weeks) after contact with contaminated tropical fish tanks, swimming pools, or saltwater fish, a small violet nodule or pustule may appear at a site of minor trauma. This lesion may evolve to form a crusted ulcer or small abscess or may remain warty. Lesions are multiple and disseminated on occasion—particularly, but not exclusively, in immunosuppressed patients. The causative organism is *M. marinum.* The patient's clinical history, combined with the isolation of *M. marinum* after biopsy and culture, establishes the diagnosis. Lesions often heal spontaneously. In cases of persistence or dissemination, rifampin (300 to 600 mg/d) in combination with ethambutol (15 to 25 mg/kg per day), trimethoprim-sulfamethoxazole (160/800 mg/bid), or minocycline (100 mg/d) may be tried for a period of at least 3 months. Very rarely, a similar clinical picture is produced by *M. gordonae*, a frequently isolated but usually nonpathogenic species.

Buruli Ulcer In many tropical areas throughout the world, *M. ulcerans* may cause an itching nodule on the arms or legs, which then breaks down to form a shallow ulcer of variable size. The course of this condition is usually prolonged. *M. ulcerans* is difficult to culture; plates need to be incubated at low temperature. Excision constitutes the usual therapy. Treatment with rifampin, clofazimine, or trimethoprim-sulfamethoxazole has met with variable success.

NTM Skin Disease in Patients with AIDS and Other Deficits of Cell-Mediated Immunity MAC organisms, which frequently cause disseminated disease with positive blood cultures in AIDS, also are rarely associated with heterogeneous skin manifestations, such as nodules, ulcers, areas of erythema, pustules, abscesses, or panniculitis. Skin biopsies and blood cultures establish the diagnosis.

In contrast to MAC organisms, *M. haemophilum* has a tendency to involve the skin, bones, joints, and lungs, although most patients also have positive blood cultures. Skin lesions are nodular, may ulcerate, and are disseminated. In the absence of specific data, treatment should follow the guidelines for MAC infection.

NTM INFECTIONS OF SOFT TISSUE, TENDONS, BONES, AND JOINTS Infections Linked to Injections and Surgery Occasionally, mycobacteria are isolated from nodular skin lesions of hospitalized patients, particularly those who are immunosuppressed; in some instances there is associated lymphatic spread. Many cases are linked to injection; diabetic patients are at especially high risk. In ophthalmology, mycobacteria may cause keratitis and corneal ulceration after surgery or injury. Epidemics of mycobacterial infection following cardiac surgery have been linked to contaminated ice packs and contaminated porcine heart valves. These infections are usually due to *M. fortuitum, M. chelonae,* or *M. abscessus,* which are referred to collectively as the *M. fortuitum* complex. These are the so-called rapidly growing mycobacteria: colonies on solid medium appear 3 to 7 days after inoculation. As organisms may fail to grow at 37°C, incubation at 30 to 33°C is recommended. These mycobacteria are notoriously resistant to most antituberculosis drugs. Debridement is best combined with administration of two or three of the antibiotics mentioned in Table 173-1.

Infections of Tendons, Joints, and Bones In rare cases, mycobacteria invade deep tissues after direct inoculation, via contiguous spread from superficial sites of infection, or through the bloodstream. MAC organisms and *M. ulcerans* are most often cited in these instances. *M. szulgai* seems to be involved particularly frequently in olecranon bursitis.

BIBLIOGRAPHY

Diagnosis and treatment of disease caused by nontuberculous mycobacteria. Am Rev Respir Dis 142:940, 1990

HOOVER DR et al: Clinical manifestations of AIDS in the era of *Pneumocystis* prophylaxis. Multicenter AIDS Cohort Study. N Engl J Med 329:1922, 1993

HORSBURGH CR: *Mycobacterium avium* complex infection in the acquired immunodeficiency syndrome. N Engl J Med 324:1332, 1991

ISEMAN MD: *Mycobacterium avium* complex and the normal host: The other side of the coin. N Engl J Med 321:896, 1989

NOLTE FS, METCHOCK B: Mycobacteria, in *Manual of Clinical Microbiology*, 7th ed, PR Murray et al (eds). Washington, ASM Press, 1995, pp 400–437

WOLINSKY E: Mycobacterial lymphadenitis in children: A prospective study of 105 nontuberculous cases with long-term follow-up. Clin Infect Dis 20:954, 1995

SECTION 9

SPIROCHETAL DISEASES

174

Sheila A. Lukehart, King K. Holmes

SYPHILIS

DEFINITION Syphilis, a chronic systemic infection caused by *Treponema pallidum* subspecies *pallidum*, is usually sexually transmitted and is characterized by episodes of active disease interrupted by periods of latency. After an incubation period averaging 3 weeks, a primary lesion appears, often associated with regional lymphadenopathy. A secondary bacteremic stage, associated with generalized mucocutaneous lesions and generalized lymphadenopathy, is followed by a latent period of subclinical infection lasting many years. In about one-third of untreated cases, the tertiary stage is characterized by progressive destructive mucocutaneous, musculoskeletal, or parenchymal lesions; aortitis; or symptomatic central nervous system (CNS) disease.

ETIOLOGY Schaudinn and Hoffman discovered *T. pallidum* in syphilitic material in 1905. *T. pallidum* is one of the many spiral-shaped microorganisms that propel themselves by spinning around their longitudinal axis. The Spirochaetales include three genera that are pathogenic for humans and for a variety of other animals: *Leptospira*, whose species cause human leptospirosis; *Borrelia*, including *Borrelia recurrentis* and *Borrelia vincentii*, which cause relapsing fever and Vincent's angina, respectively, as well as *Borrelia burgdorferi*, the causative agent of Lyme disease; and *Treponema*, whose members are responsible for the diseases known as treponematoses. The genus *Treponema* includes *T. pallidum* subspecies *pallidum* (hereafter called *T. pallidum*), which causes venereal syphilis; *T. pallidum* subspecies *pertenue*, which causes yaws; *T. pallidum* subspecies *endemicum*, which causes endemic syphilis or bejel; and *Treponema carateum*, which causes pinta (see Chap. 175). Other *Treponema* species found in the human mouth, genital mucosa, and gastrointestinal tract have no proven pathogenic role. These spirochetes can be confused with *T. pallidum* on dark-field examination. Riviere and coworkers have described a new oral treponeme that is very closely related to *T. pallidum* antigenically and is significantly associated with periodontitis and acute necrotizing ulcerative gingivitis. Its etiologic role in these gum diseases is unknown.

T. pallidum, a thin, delicate organism with 6 to 14 spirals and tapered ends, measures 6 to 15 μm in total length and 0.2 μm in width. The cytoplasm is surrounded by a trilaminar cytoplasmic membrane, which in turn is surrounded by a delicate peptidoglycan layer providing some structural rigidity. This layer is surrounded by a lipid-rich outer membrane that contains relatively few integral membrane proteins, although a putative surface-exposed porin molecule was recently described. Six endoflagella wind around the cell body in a space between the inner cell wall and the outer membrane and may be the elements responsible for motility. None of the four pathogenic treponemes has yet been cultured in vitro in quantity, and no convincing genetic, morphologic, serologic, or metabolic differences among them has been discerned. They are distinguished primarily according

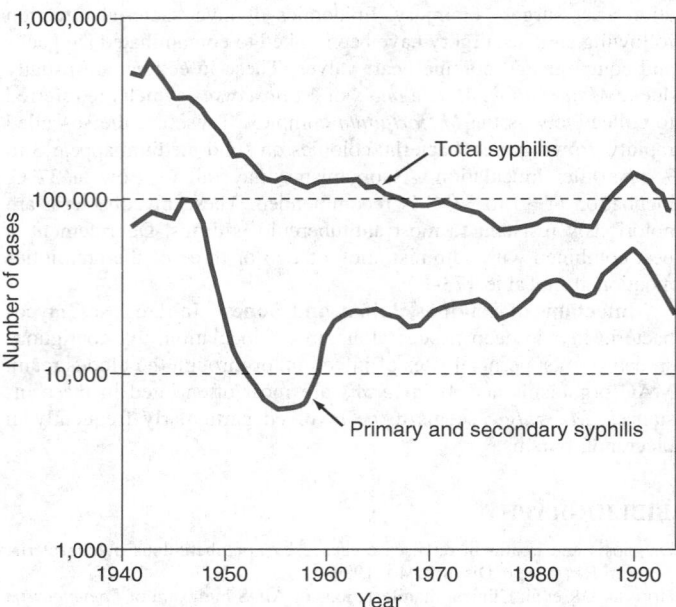

FIGURE 174-1 Number of cases of total syphilis and primary and secondary syphilis reported annually in the United States, 1940–1994. (*Data from the Centers for Disease Control and Prevention.*)

to the clinical syndrome they produce. The only known natural host for *T. pallidum* is the human. *T. pallidum* can infect many mammals, but only humans, higher apes, and a few laboratory animals regularly develop syphilitic lesions. Virulent strains of *T. pallidum* are grown and maintained in rabbits.

EPIDEMIOLOGY Nearly all cases of syphilis are acquired by sexual contact with infectious lesions (i.e., the chancre, mucous patch, skin rash, or condyloma latum). Less common modes of transmission include nonsexual personal contact and infection in utero or following blood transfusions.

The total number of cases of syphilis reported annually in the United States (Fig. 174-1) fell steadily from 575,593 in 1943 to a low of 64,621 in 1987—an 88 percent decrease—but then increased to

134,255 in 1990. The number of new cases of infectious syphilis reached a peak in 1947 and then fell to approximately 6000 in 1956; since then, a rather steady increase in infectious syphilis has been punctuated by four cycles of 7 to 10 years, each with a rapid rise and fall in incidence (with peaks in 1965, 1975, 1982, and 1990). Since 1990, the number of reported cases of infectious syphilis has again declined by more than 50 percent. In 1994, there were 20,627 reported cases of primary and secondary syphilis and 32,012 cases of early latent syphilis.

The populations at highest risk for acquiring syphilis have changed. Between 1977 and 1982, approximately half of all patients with early syphilis in the United States were homosexual or bisexual men. Largely because of changing sexual practices in this population due to the AIDS epidemic, this proportion has decreased. The most recent epidemic of syphilis predominantly involved black heterosexual men and women (Fig. 174-2) and occurred largely in urban areas, where infectious syphilis has been significantly correlated with the exchange of sex for "crack" cocaine. The incidence of syphilis peaks at 15 to 34 years of age. The reported incidence of syphilis is much higher among blacks than in other ethnic groups and is higher in urban than in rural areas. In addition, there is a striking concentration of cases in the southeastern United States.

The incidence of congenital syphilis roughly parallels that of infectious syphilis in females. The number of reported cases of congenital syphilis in infants ≤1 year of age was lowest (107 cases) in 1978, when infectious syphilis was most prevalent among homosexual and bisexual men. The dramatic increase in the incidence of primary and secondary syphilis among women from 1986 to 1990 resulted in a proportionate increase in the number of infants born with congenital syphilis—to 3275 infants in 1991. It is important to note, however, that the case definition for congenital syphilis was broadened in 1989 and now includes all live or stillborn infants delivered to women with untreated or inadequately treated syphilis at delivery.

Approximately one of every two individuals named as sexual contacts of persons with infectious syphilis becomes infected. Many sexual contacts will already have developed manifestations of syphilis when they are first seen, and about 30 percent of apparently uninfected contacts who are examined within 30 days of exposure actually have incubating infection and will later develop infectious syphilis if not treated. Thus, the identification and "epidemiologic" treatment of all recently exposed sexual contacts constitute an important aspect of syphilis control. Also important is the identification of infected persons by serologic testing of pregnant women, persons admitted to hospitals, military inductees, and persons undergoing examination in physicians' offices. Still controversial are laws and regulations requiring routine premarital serologic testing for syphilis, where—though national data are not available—the yield is undoubtedly lower.

NATURAL COURSE AND PATHOGENESIS OF UNTREATED SYPHILIS *T. pallidum* rapidly penetrates intact mucous membranes or microscopic abrasions in skin and within a few hours enters the lymphatics and blood to produce systemic infection and metastatic foci long before the appearance of a primary lesion. Blood from a patient with incubating or early syphilis is infectious. The generation time of *T. pallidum* during early active disease in vivo is estimated to be 30 to 33 h, and the incubation period of syphilis is inversely proportional to the number of organisms inoculated. The concentration of treponemes generally reaches at least 10^7 per gram of tissue before the appearance of a clinical lesion. Experimental infection

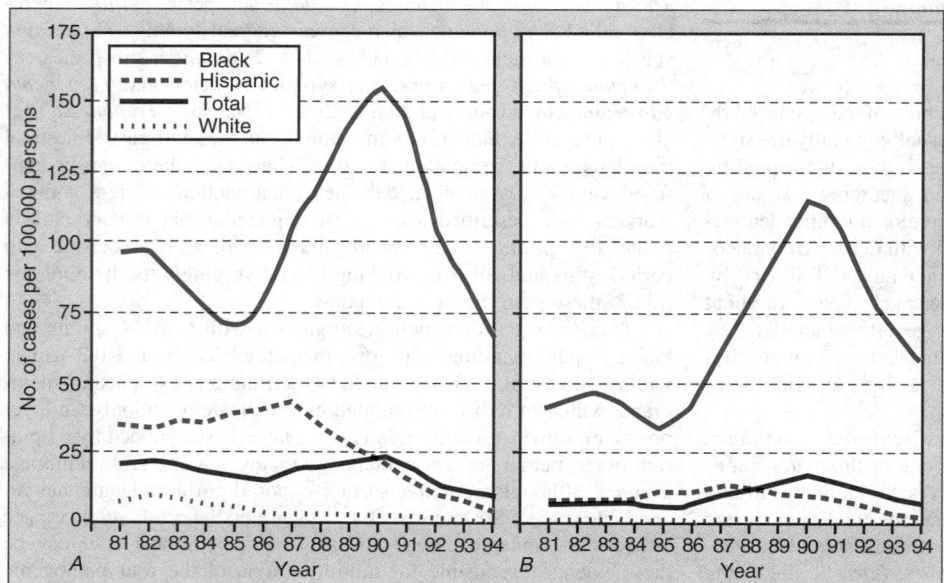

FIGURE 174-2 Rates of primary and secondary syphilis among (*A*) men and (*B*) women in the United States, by ethnic origin, 1981–1994. (*Data from the Centers for Disease Control and Prevention.*)

of rabbits or humans with very few treponemes leads to a discernible lesion only after several weeks, although histopathologic changes are evident earlier. In contrast, intradermal injection of 10^6 organisms usually produces a lesion within 72 h. On the basis of intradermal injection of graded doses of *T. pallidum* into eight volunteers, the 50 percent infectious dose was calculated to be 57 organisms. The median incubation period in humans (about 21 days) suggests an average inoculum of 500 to 1000 infectious organisms for naturally acquired disease. The incubation period (from inoculation until the primary lesion becomes discernible) rarely exceeds 6 weeks. Subcurative therapy during the incubation period may delay the onset of the primary lesion, but it is not certain that such treatment reduces the probability that symptomatic disease will ultimately develop.

The primary lesion appears at the site of inoculation, usually persists for 2 to 6 weeks, and then heals spontaneously. Histopathologic examination of primary lesions shows perivascular infiltration, chiefly by lymphocytes (including CD8 + and CD4 + cells), plasma cells, and macrophages, with capillary endothelial proliferation and subsequent obliteration of small blood vessels. The CD4 + infiltration displays a T_H1-type cytokine profile consistent with the activation of macrophages. At this time *T. pallidum* is demonstrable in the chancre in spaces between epithelial cells; within invaginations or phagosomes of epithelial cells, fibroblasts, plasma cells, and the endothelial cells of small capillaries; within lymphatic channels; and in the regional lymph nodes. Phagocytosis of organisms by activated macrophages ultimately causes their destruction, which results in spontaneous resolution of the chancre.

The generalized parenchymal, constitutional, and mucocutaneous manifestations of secondary syphilis usually appear about 6 to 8 weeks after healing of the chancre, although 15 percent of patients with secondary syphilis still have persisting or healing chancres. In other patients, secondary lesions may appear several months after the chancre has healed, and some patients may enter the latent stage without ever recognizing secondary lesions. The histopathologic features of secondary maculopapular skin lesions are hyperkeratosis of the epidermis, capillary proliferation with endothelial swelling in the superficial corium, and dermal papillae with transmigration of polymorphonuclear leukocytes and, in the deeper corium, perivascular infiltration by monocytes, plasma cells, and lymphocytes. Treponemes are found in many tissues, including the aqueous humor of the eye and the cerebrospinal fluid (CSF). Invasion of the CNS by *T. pallidum* occurs during the first weeks or months of infection, and CSF abnormalities are detected in as many as 40 percent of patients during the secondary stage. Clinical hepatitis and immune complex–induced membranous glomerulonephritis are relatively rare but recognized manifestations of secondary syphilis; liver function tests may yield abnormal results in up to a quarter of patients with early syphilis. Generalized nontender lymphadenopathy is noted in 85 percent of patients with secondary syphilis. The paradoxical appearance of secondary manifestations despite high titers of antibody (including immobilizing antibody) to *T. pallidum* is unexplained. Secondary lesions subside within 2 to 6 weeks, and the infection enters the latent stage, which is detectable only by serologic testing. In the preantibiotic era, up to 25 percent of untreated patients experienced one or more subsequent generalized or localized mucocutaneous relapses during the first 2 to 4 years after infection. Since 50 percent of such infectious relapses occur during the first year, identification and examination of sexual contacts are most important for patients with syphilis of less than 1 year's duration. Recurrent generalized rash is now rare.

In the preantibiotic era, about one-third of patients with untreated latent syphilis developed clinically apparent tertiary disease; today, in industrialized countries, specific treatment and coincidental therapy of early and latent syphilis have all but eliminated tertiary disease except for sporadic cases of neurosyphilis in persons infected with human immunodeficiency virus (HIV). In the past, the most common type of tertiary disease was the gumma, a usually benign granulomatous lesion. Today, gummas are very uncommon. Tertiary lesions are caused by obliterative small-vessel endarteritis, usually involving the vasa vasorum of the ascending aorta and less often involving the CNS.

Asymptomatic CNS involvement is demonstrable in up to 25 percent of patients with late latent syphilis. The factors that contribute to the development and progression of tertiary disease are unknown.

The course of untreated syphilis was studied retrospectively in a group of nearly 2000 patients with primary or secondary syphilis diagnosed clinically (the Oslo Study, 1891–1951); prospectively in 431 black men with seropositive latent syphilis of 3 or more years' duration (the notorious Tuskegee Study, 1932–1972); and retrospectively in a review of 198 autopsies of patients with untreated syphilis (the Rosahn Study, 1917–1942).

In the Oslo Study, 24 percent of patients developed relapsing secondary lesions within 4 years, and 28 percent eventually developed one or more manifestations of tertiary syphilis. Cardiovascular syphilis, including aortitis, was detected in 10 percent of patients, none of whom had been infected before age 15; 7 percent of patients developed symptomatic neurosyphilis, and 16 percent developed benign tertiary syphilis (gummas of the skin, mucous membranes, and skeleton). Syphilis was the primary cause of death in 15 percent of men and 8 percent of women. Cardiovascular syphilis was documented in 35 percent of men and 22 percent of women who eventually came to autopsy. In general, serious late complications were nearly twice as common among men as among women.

The Tuskegee Study showed that the death rate among untreated black men with syphilis (25 to 50 years old) was 17 percent higher than that among uninfected subjects and that 30 percent of all deaths were attributable to cardiovascular or CNS syphilis. The ethical issues eventually raised by this study, begun in the preantibiotic era but continuing into the early 1970s, had a major influence on the development of current guidelines for human medical experimentation, and the history of the study may still contribute to a reluctance of some African-Americans to participate as subjects in clinical research. By far the most important factor in increased mortality was cardiovascular syphilis. Anatomic evidence of aortitis was found in 40 to 60 percent of autopsied subjects with syphilis (versus 15 percent of control subjects), while CNS syphilis was found in only 4 percent. Rates of hypertension were also higher among the infected subjects.

These studies each showed that about one-third of patients with untreated syphilis develop clinical or pathologic evidence of tertiary syphilis, that about one-fourth die as a direct result of tertiary syphilis, and that there is additional excess mortality not directly attributable to tertiary syphilis.

MANIFESTATIONS **Primary Syphilis** The typical primary chancre usually begins as a single painless papule that rapidly becomes eroded and usually becomes indurated, with a characteristic cartilaginous consistency on palpation of the edge and base of the ulcer (Fig. 174-3). In heterosexual men the chancre is usually located on the

FIGURE 174-3 Primary syphilitic chancre on the penis. (*From E Stoltz: Sexually Transmitted Diseases. Rotterdam, Boehringer Ingelheim, 1977.*)

penis, whereas in homosexual men it is often found in the anal canal or rectum, in the mouth, or on the external genitalia. In women, common primary sites are the cervix and labia. Consequently, primary syphilis goes unrecognized in women and homosexual men more often than in heterosexual men.

Atypical primary lesions are common. The clinical appearance depends on the number of treponemes inoculated and on the immunologic status of the patient. A large inoculum produces a dark-field–positive ulcerative lesion in nonimmune volunteers but may produce a small dark-field–negative papule, an asymptomatic but seropositive latent infection, or no response at all in individuals with a history of syphilis. A small inoculum may produce only a papular lesion, even in nonimmune individuals. Therefore, syphilis should be considered even in the evaluation of trivial or atypical dark-field–negative genital lesions. The genital lesions that most commonly must be differentiated from those of primary syphilis include traumatic superinfected lesions, lesions of herpes simplex virus infection (see Chap. 184), and lesions of chancroid (see Chap. 152). *Primary genital herpes* may produce inguinal adenopathy, but the nodes are tender and the lesions consist of multiple painful vesicles, which later ulcerate and often are accompanied by systemic symptoms, including fever. *Recurrent genital herpes* typically begins with a unilateral cluster of painful vesicles, usually without associated adenopathy. *Chancroid* produces painful, superficial, exudative, nonindurated ulcers, more often multiple than in syphilis; adenopathy is common, can be either unilateral or bilateral, is tender, and may be suppurative.

Regional lymphadenopathy usually accompanies the primary syphilitic lesion, appearing within 1 week of the onset of the lesion. The nodes are firm, nonsuppurative, and painless. Inguinal lymphadenopathy is bilateral and may occur with anal as well as with external genital chancres, since lymphatic drainage of the anus involves inguinal nodes. Rectal chancres result in perirectal lymphadenopathy, while chancres of the cervix and vagina result in iliac or perirectal adenopathy. The chancre generally heals within 4 to 6 weeks (range, 2 to 12 weeks), but lymphadenopathy may persist for months.

Secondary Syphilis The protean manifestations of the secondary stage usually include localized or diffuse symmetric mucocutaneous lesions and generalized nontender lymphadenopathy. The healing primary chancre is still present in 15 percent of cases. The skin rash consists of macular, papular, papulosquamous, and occasionally pustular syphilides; often more than one form is present simultaneously. The eruption may be very subtle. Approximately 25 percent of patients with a discernible rash of secondary syphilis may be unaware that they have dermatologic manifestations. Initial lesions are bilaterally symmetric, pale red or pink, nonpruritic, discrete, round macules that measure 5 to 10 mm in diameter and are distributed on the trunk and

FIGURE 174-5 Secondary syphilitic rash on the palm and sole. [*From R Roddy, in Gynecology and Obstetrics, JW Sciarra (ed). New York, Harper & Row, 1985.*]

proximal extremities (Fig. 174-4). After several days or weeks, red papular lesions 3 to 10 mm in diameter also appear. These lesions, which may progress to necrotic lesions (resembling pustules) in association with increasing endarteritis and perivascular mononuclear infiltration, are distributed widely, frequently involve the palms and soles (Fig. 174-5), and may occur on the face and scalp. Tiny papular *follicular syphilides* involving hair follicles may result in patchy alopecia (alopecia areata), with loss of scalp hair, eyebrows, or beard in up to 5 percent of cases. Progressive endarteritis obliterans and ischemia result in superficial scaling of papules (*papulosquamous syphilides*) and eventually may lead to central necrosis (*pustular syphilides*).

In warm, moist, intertriginous areas, including the perianal area, vulva, scrotum, inner thighs, axillae, and skin under pendulous breasts, papules can enlarge and become eroded to produce broad, moist, pink or gray-white, highly infectious lesions called *condylomata lata*; these lesions develop in 10 percent of patients with secondary syphilis. Superficial mucosal erosions, called *mucous patches*, occur in 10 to 15 percent of patients and may involve the lips, oral mucosa, tongue (Fig. 174-6), palate, pharynx, vulva and vagina, glans penis, or inner prepuce. The typical mucous patch is a painless silver-gray erosion surrounded by a red periphery. During relapses of secondary syphilis, condylomata lata are particularly common, and skin lesions tend to be asymmetrically distributed and more infiltrated, resembling skin

FIGURE 174-4 Maculopapular rash of secondary syphilis. (*From E Stoltz: Sexually Transmitted Diseases. Rotterdam, Boehringer Ingelheim, 1977.*)

FIGURE 174-6 Mucous patches on the tongue of a patient with secondary syphilis. [*From R Roddy, in Sexually Transmitted Diseases, 2d ed. KK Holmes et al (eds). New York, McGraw-Hill, 1990.*]

lesions of late syphilis. These characteristics may reflect increasing cellular immunity.

Constitutional symptoms that may accompany or precede secondary syphilis include sore throat (15 to 30 percent), fever (5 to 8 percent), weight loss (2 to 20 percent), malaise (25 percent), anorexia (2 to 10 percent), headache (10 percent), and meningismus (5 percent). *Acute meningitis* occurs in only 1 to 2 percent of cases, but numbers of cells and levels of protein in CSF are increased in 30 percent of cases or more. *T. pallidum* has been recovered from CSF during primary and secondary syphilis in 30 percent of cases; this finding is often but not always associated with other CSF abnormalities.

Less common complications of secondary syphilis include hepatitis, nephropathy, gastrointestinal involvement (hypertrophic gastritis, patchy proctitis, ulcerative colitis, or a rectosigmoid mass), arthritis, and periostitis. Ocular findings that suggest secondary syphilis include otherwise unexplained pupillary abnormalities, optic neuritis, and a retinitis pigmentosa syndrome as well as the classic iritis (especially granulomatous iritis) or uveitis. The diagnosis of secondary syphilis is often considered only after the patient fails to respond to steroid therapy. Anterior uveitis has been reported in 5 to 10 percent of patients with secondary syphilis, and *T. pallidum* has been demonstrated in the aqueous humor from these patients. *Syphilitic hepatitis* is distinguished by an unusually high serum level of alkaline phosphatase and by a nonspecific histologic appearance that is unlike that of viral hepatitis and includes moderate inflammation with polymorphonuclear leukocytes and lymphocytes, some hepatocellular damage, and no cholestasis. *Renal involvement* produces proteinuria associated with an acute nephrotic syndrome (or rarely with hemorrhagic glomerulonephritis) and is characterized by subepithelial electron-dense deposits and glomerular immune complexes—findings suggesting immune-complex glomerulonephritis.

Latent Syphilis Positive reaginic and specific treponemal antibody tests for syphilis, together with a normal CSF examination and the absence of clinical manifestations of syphilis, indicate a diagnosis of latent syphilis. The diagnosis is often suspected on the basis of a history of primary or secondary lesions, a history of exposure to syphilis, or the delivery of an infant with congenital syphilis. A previous negative serologic test or a history of lesions or exposure may help establish the duration of latent infection. *Early latent* syphilis encompasses the first year after infection, while *late latent* syphilis (beginning 1 year or longer after infection in the untreated patient) is associated with relative immunity to infectious relapse and with increasing resistance to reinfection. *T. pallidum* may still seed the bloodstream intermittently during this stage. Pregnant women with latent syphilis may infect the fetus in utero. Moreover, syphilis has been transmitted through the transfusion of blood from patients with latent syphilis of many years' duration. It was previously thought that untreated late latent syphilis had three possible outcomes: (1) it could persist throughout the lifetime of the infected individual, (2) it could end in the development of late syphilis, or (3) it could end with the spontaneous cure of infection, with reversion of serologic tests to negative. It is now apparent, however, that the more sensitive treponemal antibody tests rarely, if ever, become negative without treatment. About 70 percent of untreated patients with latent syphilis never develop clinically evident late syphilis, but the occurrence of spontaneous cure is in doubt.

Late Syphilis The slowly progressive inflammatory disease leading to tertiary manifestations begins early during the pathogenesis of syphilis, although these manifestations may not become clinically apparent for years. Early syphilitic aortitis becomes evident soon after secondary lesions subside, and patients who develop CSF abnormalities during the early stages of syphilis appear to be at highest risk of late neurologic complications.

Asymptomatic neurosyphilis CNS syphilis represents a continuum comprising early invasion, usually within the first weeks or months of infection, and asymptomatic involvement, which may or may not lead to neurologic manifestations. Traditionally, the diagnosis of asymptomatic neurosyphilis has been made in patients who no longer have manifestations of primary or secondary syphilis, who lack

neurologic symptoms and signs, and who have certain CSF abnormalities. Such abnormalities are found in up to one-quarter of patients with untreated late latent syphilis, and it is these patients who are known to be at risk for neurologic complications. However, in early syphilis, *T. pallidum* can be isolated from CSF even in the absence of other CSF abnormalities. In approximately 40 percent of patients with primary or secondary syphilis, *T. pallidum* can be isolated from the CSF and/or abnormalities of the CSF consistent with asymptomatic neurosyphilis can develop. Although the therapeutic implications of these findings in early syphilis are uncertain, it seems appropriate to conclude that even patients with early syphilis who have such findings do indeed have asymptomatic neurosyphilis. In patients with untreated asymptomatic neurosyphilis, the overall cumulative probability of progression to clinical neurosyphilis is about 20 percent in the first 10 years but increases with time; the likelihood is highest among patients with the greatest degree of pleocytosis or protein elevation. Patients with untreated latent syphilis and normal CSF probably run no risk of subsequently developing neurosyphilis.

Symptomatic neurosyphilis Although mixed features are common, the major clinical categories of symptomatic neurosyphilis include meningeal, meningovascular, and parenchymatous syphilis. The last category includes general paresis and tabes dorsalis. The interval from infection to onset of symptoms is a few months to 20 years for meningeal syphilis (usually less than a year) and for meningovascular syphilis (average, 7 years), 20 years for general paresis, and 25 to 30 years for tabes dorsalis. However, symptomatic neurosyphilis, particularly in the antibiotic era, often presents not as a classic picture but rather as mixed and subtle or incomplete syndromes.

Meningeal syphilis may involve either the brain or the spinal cord, and patients may present with headache, nausea, vomiting, neck stiffness, cranial nerve palsies, seizures, and changes in mental status. *Meningovascular syphilis* reflects diffuse inflammation of the pia and arachnoid together with evidence of focal or widespread arterial involvement of small, medium, or large vessels. The most common presentation is a stroke syndrome involving the middle cerebral artery of a relatively young adult; however, unlike the usual thrombotic or embolic stroke syndrome of sudden onset, meningovascular syphilis often becomes manifest after a subacute encephalitic prodrome, with headaches, vertigo, insomnia, and psychological abnormalities, which is followed by a gradually progressive vascular syndrome.

The manifestations of *general paresis* reflect widespread parenchymal damage and include abnormalities corresponding to the mnemonic *paresis*: *p*ersonality, *a*ffect, *r*eflexes (hyperactive), *e*ye (e.g., Argyll Robertson pupils), *s*ensorium (illusions, delusions, hallucinations), *i*ntellect (a decrease in recent memory and in the capacity for orientation, calculations, judgment, and insight), and *s*peech. *Tabes dorsalis* presents as symptoms and signs of demyelination of the posterior columns, dorsal roots, and dorsal root ganglia. Symptoms include ataxic wide-based gait and footslap; paresthesias; bladder disturbances; impotence; areflexia; and loss of position, deep pain, and temperature sensations. Trophic joint degeneration (Charcot's joints) and perforating ulceration of the feet can result from loss of pain sensation. The small, irregular Argyll Robertson pupil, a feature of both tabes dorsalis and paresis, reacts to accommodation but not to light. *Optic atrophy* also occurs frequently in association with tabes.

Cardiovascular syphilis Cardiovascular manifestations are attributable to endarteritis obliterans of the vasa vasorum, which provide the blood supply to large vessels. This condition produces medial necrosis with destruction of elastic tissue, particularly in the ascending and transverse segments of the aortic arch, resulting in uncomplicated aortitis, aortic regurgitation, saccular aneurysm, or coronary ostial stenosis. Symptoms appear from 10 to 40 years after infection. Cardiovascular complications occur more often and at an earlier age among men than among women and may be more common among blacks than among whites. In the preantibiotic era, symptomatic cardiovascular complications developed in about 10 percent of persons with late untreated syphilis, and aortic regurgitation was two to four times as common as aneurysm. However, syphilitic aortitis was demonstrated at autopsy in about one-half of black men with untreated syphilis.

Linear calcification of the ascending aorta on chest x-ray films suggests asymptomatic syphilitic aortitis, as arteriosclerosis seldom produces this sign. Aortic dilation and a tambour quality to the sound of aortic closure are unreliable signs of aortitis. Syphilitic aneurysms—usually saccular, occasionally fusiform—do not lead to dissection. Approximately 1 in 10 aortic aneurysms of syphilitic origin involve the abdominal aorta, but these aneurysms tend to occur above the renal arteries, whereas arteriosclerotic abdominal aneurysms usually are found below the renal arteries. With increasing age, the nervous system is also affected in up to 40 percent of patients with cardiovascular syphilis.

Late lesions of the eyes   Iritis associated with pain, photophobia, and dimness of vision or chorioretinitis occurs not only during secondary syphilis but also as a relatively common manifestation of late syphilis. Adhesions of the iris to the anterior lens may produce a fixed pupil, not to be confused with Argyll Robertson pupil.

Late benign syphilis (gumma)   Gummas may be multiple or diffuse but are usually solitary lesions that range from microscopic size to several centimeters in diameter. From a histologic perspective, gummas consist of a granulomatous inflammation with a central area of necrosis surrounded by mononuclear, epithelioid, and fibroblastic cells, occasional giant cells, and perivasculitis. Although rarely demonstrated microscopically, *T. pallidum* has reportedly been recovered from these lesions. The most commonly involved sites include the skin and skeletal system, the mouth and upper respiratory tract, the larynx, the liver, and the stomach; however, any organ may be involved. Gummas of the skin produce painless and indurated nodular, papulosquamous, or ulcerative lesions that form characteristic circles or arcs, with peripheral hyperpigmentation. Gummas are usually indolent and may heal spontaneously with scarring, but they may also be explosive in onset and are often destructive. These lesions may resemble those of many other chronic granulomatous conditions, including tuberculosis and sarcoidosis, leprosy, and deep fungal infections. Skeletal gummas most frequently involve the long bones of the legs, although any bone may be affected. Trauma may predispose a specific site to involvement. Presenting symptoms usually include focal pain and tenderness. Radiographic abnormalities with advanced gummas of bone include periostitis or destructive or sclerosing osteitis. Upper respiratory gummas can lead to perforation of the nasal septum or palate. Gummatous hepatitis may produce epigastric pain and tenderness as well as low-grade fever and may be associated with splenomegaly and anemia.

The histopathology and extensive tissue necrosis associated with gummas suggest delayed hypersensitivity to *T. pallidum*. Certain individuals appear to develop an exaggerated delayed-hypersensitivity response to *T. pallidum*, which presumably is mediated by sensitized T lymphocytes and macrophages. Since the histologic changes may be suggestive but are nonspecific, the diagnosis of late benign syphilis is confirmed by serologic testing and by therapeutic trial. Treatment with penicillin results in rapid healing of active gummatous lesions.

Congenital Syphilis   Transmission of *T. pallidum* from a syphilitic woman to her fetus across the placenta may occur at any stage of pregnancy, but the lesions of congenital syphilis generally develop after the fourth month of gestation, when fetal immunologic competence begins to develop. This timing suggests that the pathogenesis of congenital syphilis depends on the immune response of the host rather than on a direct toxic effect of *T. pallidum*. The risk of infection of the fetus during untreated early maternal syphilis is estimated to be 75 to 95 percent, decreasing to about 35 percent for maternal syphilis of longer than 2 years' duration; some risk of fetal infection apparently continues throughout late latent maternal syphilis. Adequate treatment of the mother before the 16th week of pregnancy should prevent fetal damage. Untreated maternal infection may result in a

rate of fetal loss of up to 40 percent (with stillbirth more common than abortion because of the late onset of fetal pathology), prematurity, neonatal death, or nonfatal congenital syphilis. In one series of mothers with untreated syphilis of less than 2 years' duration, 21 percent aborted or had a stillbirth, 13 percent gave birth to infants who died within 2 months, 43 percent had infants with syphilis who were still alive at 2 months, and 23 percent had nonsyphilitic infants. Among infants born alive, only fulminant congenital syphilis is clinically apparent at birth, and these babies have a very poor prognosis. The most common clinical problem is the healthy-appearing baby born to a mother with a positive serologic test. Routine serologic testing in early pregnancy is considered cost-effective in virtually all populations, even in areas with a low prenatal prevalence of syphilis. To ensure prompt treatment, rapid plasma reagin (RPR) screening should be performed on site when pregnancy is detected in a woman who may prove noncompliant. Where the prevalence of syphilis is high and when the patient is at high risk, syphilis serology should be repeated in the third trimester and at delivery.

The manifestations of congenital syphilis can be divided into three types according to their timing: (1) early manifestations, which appear within the first 2 years of life (often between 2 and 10 weeks of age), are infectious, and resemble the manifestations of severe secondary syphilis in the adult; (2) late manifestations, which appear after 2 years and are noninfectious; and (3) residual stigmata. The earliest sign of congenital syphilis is usually rhinitis ("snuffles"), which is soon followed by other mucocutaneous lesions. These may include bullae (syphilitic pemphigus), vesicles, superficial desquamation, petechiae, and (later) papulosquamous lesions, mucous patches, and condylomata lata. The most common early manifestations are osteochondritis and osteitis (particularly involving the metaphyses of long bones), which progress in severity during the first 6 months of life and then spontaneously subside, and periostitis, which continues to progress after the first 6 months. Hepatosplenomegaly, lymphadenopathy, anemia, jaundice, thrombocytopenia, and leukocytosis are common. The anemia is usually hypoproliferative but may be hemolytic. The nephrotic syndrome in early congenital syphilis, as in adult secondary syphilis, represents immune complex–induced glomerulonephritis. A compilation of clinical presentations of congenital syphilis in nine studies involving a total of 212 infants included abnormal bone radiographs (61 percent), hepatomegaly (51 percent), splenomegaly (49 percent), petechiae (41 percent), other skin rashes (35 percent), anemia (34 percent), lymphadenopathy (32 percent), jaundice (30 percent), pseudoparalysis (28 percent), and snuffles (23 percent).

Neonatal congenital syphilis must be differentiated from other generalized congenital infections, including rubella, cytomegalovirus or herpes simplex virus infection, and toxoplasmosis, as well as from erythroblastosis fetalis. Neonatal death is usually due to pulmonary hemorrhage, secondary bacterial infection, or severe hepatitis. Pathologic findings include interstitial and perivascular inflammation followed by variable fibroblastic proliferation (with involvement of the skin, bones, liver, kidneys, pancreas, spleen, lungs, and intestines) and by extramedullary hematopoiesis.

Late congenital syphilis is defined as congenital syphilis that remains untreated after 2 years of age. In perhaps 60 percent of cases, the infection remains subclinical; the clinical spectrum in the remainder of cases differs in certain respects from that of acquired late syphilis in the adult. For example, cardiovascular syphilis rarely develops in late congenital syphilis, whereas interstitial keratitis is much more common and occurs between the ages of 5 and 25. Other manifestations associated with interstitial keratitis are eighth-nerve deafness and recurrent arthropathy. Bilateral knee effusions are known as *Clutton's joints*. Examination of CSF discloses asymptomatic neurosyphilis in about one-third of untreated patients without other late clinical manifestations; moreover, clinical neurosyphilis occurs in one-quarter of individuals over 6 years of age who have untreated congenital syphilis. The clinical manifestations of congenital neurosyphilis correspond to those of adult neurosyphilis. Gummatous periostitis occurs between the ages of 5 and 20 and, as in nonvenereal endemic childhood syphilis, tends to cause destructive lesions of the palate and nasal septum.

Characteristic stigmata include *Hutchinson's teeth*—centrally notched, widely spaced, peg-shaped upper central incisors—and "mulberry" molars—sixth-year molars with multiple, poorly developed cusps. The abnormal facies of congenital syphilis includes frontal bossing, saddle nose, and poorly developed maxillae. Saber shins, characterized by anterior tibial bowing, are rare. *Rhagades* are linear scars at the angles of the mouth and nose that are caused by secondary bacterial infection of the early facial eruption. Other stigmata include unexplained nerve deafness, old chorioretinitis, optic atrophy, and corneal opacities due to past interstitial keratitis.

LABORATORY EXAMINATIONS Dark-Field Examination Technique Dark-field examination is essential in evaluating moist cutaneous lesions, such as the chancre of primary syphilis or the condylomata lata of secondary syphilis. The surface of the suspected ulcerated lesion should be cleaned with saline and gauze and then gently abraded further with dry gauze, taking care not to induce bleeding. The lesion is then squeezed to express a serous transudate, a drop of which is picked up on the surface of a glass slide. A drop of saline (without bacteriostatic additives) may be mixed with the transudate if necessary, and this preparation is then covered with a coverslip and examined immediately for *T. pallidum* with a dark-field or phase-contrast microscope by an experienced individual. The identification of a single characteristic motile organism by a trained observer is sufficient for diagnosis. Examination of oral lesions and anal ulcers by this method is not recommended, as it is difficult to differentiate *T. pallidum* from other spirochetes that may be present. A single negative examination does not exclude the possibility of syphilis, since at least 10^4 treponemes per microliter of transudate must be present to be seen; furthermore, prior use of topical antiseptic or cleansing by the patient may confuse the results and therefore should be avoided. Ideally, the dark-field examination should be repeated on three successive days before being considered negative.

Direct Immunofluorescence Most syphilis is diagnosed in the offices of private physicians, where dark-field microscopy is not available; alternative methods for the identification of *T. pallidum* in exudate are needed. The direct fluorescent antibody *T. pallidum* (DFA-TP) test, available at central laboratories, uses fluorescein-conjugated polyclonal antitreponemal antibody for the detection of *T. pallidum* in fixed smears prepared from suspect lesions. A refinement of this technique uses a monoclonal antibody specific to the pathogenic treponemes but is not yet commercially available. The polymerase chain reaction is currently being evaluated for the detection of *T. pallidum* and other genital ulcer pathogens.

Demonstration of *T. pallidum* in Tissue It is often necessary to demonstrate *T. pallidum* in tissue when clinical or histopathologic features suggest the diagnosis of syphilis. Although the organism can be found in tissue with appropriate silver stains, these results should be interpreted with caution because artifacts resembling *T. pallidum* are often seen. Treponemes can be demonstrated more reliably in tissue by immunofluorescent or immunohistochemical methods using specific monoclonal or polyclonal antibodies to *T. pallidum*.

Serologic Tests for Syphilis The profusion of serologic tests for syphilis causes much unnecessary confusion. Syphilitic infection produces two types of antibodies—antilipid "reaginic" antibody and specific antitreponemal antibody—that are measured by the nontreponemal and treponemal tests, respectively (Table 174-1). Both types of tests are reactive in persons with any treponemal infection, including yaws, pinta, and endemic syphilis.

The nontreponemal antibodies produced in syphilis contain both IgG and IgM directed against a cardiolipin-lecithin-cholesterol antigen complex. The term *reagin* is unfortunate, since the unrelated IgE antibody involved in certain allergic phenomena is also known as reagin. The most widely used nontreponemal or reagin antibody tests for syphilis are the RPR test, which can be automated (ART); the Venereal Disease Research Laboratory (VDRL) slide test; and the toluidine red unheated serum test (TRUST). Less frequently used nontreponemal tests include the unheated serum reagin (USR) test and the reagin screen test (RST). In these tests, antibody is detected by the microscopic (VDRL and USR tests) or macroscopic (RPR test,

Table 174-1

Common Serologic Tests for Syphilis

Nontreponemal (reagin) tests	
Microscopic flocculation	Venereal Disease Research Laboratory (VDRL) test
Macroscopic flocculation	Rapid plasma reagin (RPR) test
	Toluidine red unheated serum test (TRUST)
Treponemal tests	
Immunofluorescence	Fluorescent treponemal antibody–absorbed (FTA-ABS) test; 19S IgM FTA-ABS test
Hemagglutination	*T. pallidum* hemagglutination assay (MHA-TP, TPHA)

TRUST, and RST) flocculation of the antigen suspension (see Table 174-1). New ELISA-based methods are being evaluated.

The RPR test is often more expensive than the VDRL test, but it is easier to perform and uses unheated serum; it is the test of choice for rapid serologic diagnosis in a clinic or office setting. The VDRL test, however, remains the standard for use with CSF.

The RPR and VDRL tests are equally sensitive and may be used for initial screening or for quantitation of serum antibody. The titer reflects the activity of the disease. A fourfold or greater rise in titer may be seen during the evolution of early syphilis. VDRL titers usually reach 1:32 or higher in secondary syphilis. A persistent fall of two dilutions (fourfold) or greater following treatment of early syphilis provides essential evidence of an adequate response to therapy. VDRL titers do not correspond directly to RPR titers, and sequential quantitative testing (as for response to therapy) must employ a single test.

There are two standard treponemal tests: the fluorescent treponemal antibody–absorbed (FTA-ABS) test and the microhemagglutination assay for antibodies to *T. pallidum* (MHA-TP). Another hemagglutination test, the *T. pallidum* hemagglutination (TPHA) test, is widely used in Europe but is not available in the United States. Both the hemagglutination and the FTA-ABS tests are very specific and, when used for confirmation of positive reaginic antibody tests, have a very high positive predictive value for the diagnosis of syphilis. However, even these tests give false-positive results at rates as high as 1 to 2 percent when used for the screening of normal populations. The *T. pallidum* immobilization (TPI) test, in which live *T. pallidum* organisms are immobilized by immune serum plus complement, is the most specific treponemal test but is more laborious than other methods and, in the United States, is available only in research laboratories.

The relative sensitivities of the VDRL test, the FTA-ABS test, and MHA-TP in the various stages of syphilis are shown in Table 174-2. The nontreponemal tests are nonreactive in about one-quarter of patients presenting with primary or late syphilis. In early primary syphilis, the detection of antibody can be maximized either by the performance of an FTA-ABS test or simply by repetition of a VDRL test after 1 to 2 weeks if the initial VDRL result is negative. However, a reagin antibody test alone is not sufficient for the detection of late

Table 174-2

Sensitivity of Serodiagnostic Tests in Untreated Syphilis

Test*	Mean Percentage Positive (Range) at Indicated Stage of Disease†			
	Primary	Secondary	Latent	Tertiary
VDRL	78 (74–87)	100	95 (88–100)	71 (37–94)
FTA-ABS	84 (70–100)	100	100	96
MHA-TP	76 (69–90)	100	100	94

* The specificity for each of these tests is 97 to 99 percent.
† In CDC studies.
SOURCE: Modified from Larsen et al.

symptomatic syphilis; the more sensitive FTA-ABS test should be performed routinely in suspected late syphilis. The hemagglutination tests may be less sensitive than the reagin tests in primary syphilis but are as sensitive as the FTA-ABS test in other stages. All treponemal and nontreponemal tests are reactive during secondary syphilis, and a nonreactive result virtually excludes syphilis in a patient with otherwise compatible mucocutaneous lesions. (Fewer than 1 percent of patients with secondary syphilis have a VDRL test that is nonreactive or weakly reactive with undiluted serum but is positive at higher serum dilutions—the *prozone* phenomenon.) While the nontreponemal tests will become nonreactive or will be reactive in lower titers following therapy for early syphilis, the treponemal tests often remain reactive after therapy and therefore are not helpful in determining the infection status of persons with past syphilis.

The presence of specific IgM antibody has been proposed as a marker for active syphilis, with the claim that IgM disappears following adequate therapy. However, because the rate at which IgM declines after therapy is quite variable from patient to patient, the use of this criterion for cure is not recommended. A new 19S IgM FTA-ABS test for syphilis has been approved by the Centers for Disease Control and Prevention (CDC) for the evaluation of infants with suspected congenital syphilis.

False-Positive Serologic Tests for Syphilis Because the antigen used in nontreponemal tests is found in other tissues, the tests may be reactive in persons without treponemal infection, although rarely do titers exceed 1:8 in such patients. In a population selected for screening because of clinical suspicion, history of exposure, or increased risk for sexually transmitted infections, fewer than 1 percent of reactive tests are falsely positive. False-positive reagin tests are classified as acute if they become negative within 6 months and as chronic if they persist for 6 months or longer. Pregnancy is often mentioned as a cause of false-positive reactivity. However, a number of studies have shown a very low rate of false-positive results among pregnant women, and a reactive VDRL or RPR test in such patients should be pursued aggressively. The high rates of false-positive reactivity reported several decades ago among patients with leprosy, infectious mononucleosis, and miscellaneous other infections were obtained mostly in studies with early lipoidal tests. The modern VDRL and RPR tests are 97 to 99 percent specific, and false-positive reactions are now limited largely to those conditions listed in Table 174-3. Reagin tests yield false-positive results in up to 25 percent of intravenous narcotic addicts. False positivity is also common among persons with autoimmune disorders. The prevalence of false-positive reagin tests increases with advancing age; 10 percent of people over 70 years of age have false-positive reactions. In the patient with a false-positive reagin test, syphilis is excluded by a nonreactive treponemal test.

For practical purposes, most clinicians need to be familiar with the three uses of serologic tests for syphilis: (1) testing of large numbers of sera for screening or diagnostic purposes (e.g., the RPR or VDRL test), (2) quantitative measurement of the reagin antibody titer to assess the clinical activity of syphilis or to monitor the response to therapy (e.g., the VDRL or RPR test), and (3) confirmation of the diagnosis of syphilis in a patient with a positive reagin antibody test or with a suspected clinical diagnosis of syphilis (e.g., the FTA-ABS test or MHA-TP).

Evaluation for Asymptomatic Neurosyphilis Asymptomatic involvement of the CNS is detected by examination of CSF for pleocytosis, increased protein concentration, and VDRL activity. CSF abnormalities can be demonstrated in up to 40 percent of cases of primary or secondary syphilis and in 25 percent of cases of latent syphilis. *T. pallidum* has been recovered by rabbit inoculation from up to 30 percent of patients with primary or secondary syphilis but rarely from those with latent syphilis. The demonstration of *T. pallidum* in CSF is often associated with other CSF abnormalities; however, organisms can be recovered from patients with otherwise normal CSF. Before the advent of penicillin, the risk of developing clinical neurosyphilis was roughly proportional to the intensity of CSF changes in early syphilis. CSF examination is essential in the evaluation of any seropositive patient with neurologic signs and symptoms and is recommended for all patients with untreated syphilis of unknown duration or of greater than 1 year's duration. The possibility of asymptomatic neurosyphilis in some patients with early disease is not addressed by these recommendations. Because standard therapy with penicillin G benzathine (benzathine benzylpenicillin) for early syphilis fails to result in treponemicidal levels in the CSF, some experts advise lumbar puncture in secondary and early latent syphilis, with follow-up examinations for patients with abnormalities.

The CSF VDRL test is highly specific if the fluid is not contaminated with blood. This test is relatively insensitive, however, and may be nonreactive even in cases of progressive symptomatic neurosyphilis. The degree of sensitivity is highest in meningovascular syphilis and paresis and is lower in asymptomatic neurosyphilis and tabes dorsalis. Measures of intrathecal antitreponemal IgM or IgG have proved to be insensitive. The unabsorbed FTA test on CSF is reactive far more often than the CSF VDRL test in all stages of syphilis, but FTA reactivity may reflect passive transfer of serum antibody into the CSF. A nonreactive CSF FTA test, however, may be used to rule out neurosyphilis. Even in the absence of confirmatory CSF examination, a therapeutic trial of penicillin in doses adequate for neurosyphilis is warranted in any patient with a positive serum treponemal antibody test who also has neurologic findings consistent with neurosyphilis.

Evaluation for Syphilis in Patients Infected with HIV Because persons at highest risk for syphilis (inner-city populations, homosexually active men, and people in many developing countries) are also at increased risk for HIV infection, these two infections are frequently found in the same patient. There is evidence that syphilis and other genital-ulcer diseases may be important risk factors for the acquisition and transmission of HIV infection.

The manifestations of syphilis may be altered in patients with concurrent HIV infection, and multiple cases of neurologic relapse following standard therapy have been reported in HIV-infected patients. *T. pallidum* has been isolated from the CSF of several patients after therapy for early syphilis with penicillin G benzathine. A recent multicenter U.S. study of early syphilis found similar therapeutic responses in persons with and without concurrent HIV infection, although the study lacked sufficient statistical power to exclude an effect of HIV and 41 percent of subjects were lost to follow-up. This investigation confirmed the high rate of CNS invasion in early syphilis and the persistence of *T. pallidum* after standard therapy: 11 of 43 HIV-infected patients and 21 of 88 HIV-uninfected patients had *T. pallidum* detectable in CSF before therapy; 7 of the 35 patients who underwent lumbar puncture after therapy (some HIV-infected and others uninfected) still had *T. pallidum* detectable in CSF.

Table 174-3

Causes of False-Positive Reactions in Nontreponemal Serologic Tests for Syphilis

Cause	Rate of False-Positive Reactions, %*
ACUTE FALSE-POSITIVE REACTION (<6 MONTHS)	
Recent viral illness or immunization	1–2
Genital herpes	4.4
Human immunodeficiency virus infection	1–4
Mycoplasma pneumoniae infection	1–2
Malaria	11
Parenteral drug use	20–25
CHRONIC FALSE-POSITIVE REACTION (≥6 MONTHS)	
Aging	9–11
Autoimmune disorders	1–20
Systemic lupus erythematosus	11–20
Rheumatoid arthritis	5
Parenteral drug use	20–25

* Data were collected from a variety of published reports.

The frequency of unusual clinical and laboratory manifestations of syphilis among patients coinfected with HIV is unknown. Such changes may be dependent on the stage of HIV infection and the degree of immunosuppression. There is no clear evidence that the sensitivity of serologic tests for syphilis or the serologic response to therapy in the vast majority of HIV-infected patients with early syphilis differs from the corresponding findings in patients not infected with HIV. Interpretation of serologic results should be the same for the two groups.

The evaluation of all syphilis patients should include serologic testing for HIV, with the patient's consent. Conversely, persons with newly diagnosed HIV infection should be tested for syphilis. Currently, some authorities, persuaded by reports of the persistence of *T. pallidum* in the CSF of HIV-infected persons after standard penicillin benzathine therapy for early syphilis, recommend examination of CSF for evidence of neurosyphilis for all coinfected patients, regardless of the clinical stage of syphilis, with treatment for neurosyphilis if CSF abnormalities are found or if CSF examination is not performed. Others do not recommend routine CSF examination for HIV-coinfected patients with early syphilis and believe that standard therapy is sufficient. Serologic testing after treatment is important for all patients with syphilis, particularly those also infected with HIV.

TREATMENT

Treatment of Acquired Syphilis Penicillin G is the drug of choice for all stages of syphilis. *T. pallidum* is killed by very low concentrations of penicillin G, although a long period of exposure to penicillin is required because of the unusually slow rate of multiplication of the organism. The efficacy of penicillin for syphilis remains undiminished after 50 years of use. Other antibiotics effective in syphilis include the tetracyclines, erythromycin, and the cephalosporins. Aminoglycosides and spectinomycin inhibit *T. pallidum* only in very large doses, and the sulfonamides and the quinolones are inactive.

Serum levels of penicillin G of 0.03 μg/mL or more for at least 7 days are considered necessary for the cure of early syphilis. Recurrence rates for a given regimen increase as infection progresses from incubating to seronegative primary to seropositive primary to secondary to late syphilis. Therefore, it is probable but unproven that a longer duration of therapy is required to effect cure as the infection progresses. For these reasons, some authorities use more prolonged penicillin therapy than that recommended by the U.S. Public Health Service when treating secondary, latent, or late syphilis.

The treatment regimens recommended for syphilis are summarized in Table 174-4 and are described in more detail below.

EARLY SYPHILIS Preventive (abortive, "epidemiologic") treatment is recommended for seronegative individuals without signs of syphilis who have been exposed to infectious syphilis within the previous 3 months. Before treatment is given, every effort should be made to establish a diagnosis by examination and serologic testing. *The regimens recommended for prevention are the same as those recommended for early syphilis.*

Penicillin G benzathine is the most widely used agent for the treatment of early syphilis (including primary, secondary, and early latent syphilis),

although it is more painful on injection than penicillin G procaine. A single dose of 2.4 million units cures more than 95 percent of cases of primary syphilis. Because the drug's efficacy in secondary syphilis may be slightly lower, some physicians administer a second dose of 2.4 million units 1 week after the initial dose at this stage of disease. Clinical relapse can follow treatment with penicillin G benzathine in patients with both HIV infection and early syphilis. Examination of CSF from HIV-seropositive individuals with syphilis of any stage is recommended by some experts. Furthermore, treatment with regimens effective against neurosyphilis has been proposed by some authorities for all HIV-seropositive individuals with syphilis of any stage.

For penicillin-allergic patients with early syphilis, a 2-week course of therapy with doxycycline or tetracycline is recommended. These regimens appear to be effective, although no well-controlled studies have been performed, and poor compliance may be problematic. Although ceftriaxone and azithromycin have shown activity against *T. pallidum* in animals, human trials have not been of sufficient scope to permit the recommendation of either drug for any stage of syphilis.

LATE LATENT AND LATE SYPHILIS Lumbar puncture should be performed in the evaluation of latent syphilis of more than 1 year's duration, in suspected neurosyphilis, and in late complications other than symptomatic neurosyphilis (since asymptomatic neurosyphilis may coexist with other late complications). In older asymptomatic seropositive individuals, the yield of lumbar puncture is relatively low. CSF examination is most clearly indicated in the following situations: neurologic signs or symptoms, treatment failure, a serum reagin titer of ≥1:32, HIV antibody positivity, other evidence of active syphilis (e.g., aortitis, gumma, visual or hearing changes), or plans to administer nonpenicillin therapy. The recommended treatment for late latent syphilis with normal CSF, for cardiovascular syphilis, and for late benign syphilis (gumma) is penicillin G benza-

Table 174-4

Recommendations for the Treatment of Syphilis*

Stage of Syphilis	Patients without Penicillin Allergy	Patients with Confirmed Penicillin Allergy
Primary, secondary, or early latent	Penicillin G benzathine (single dose of 2.4 million units IM, 1.2 million units in each buttock)	Tetracycline hydrochloride (500 mg PO qid) or doxycycline (100 mg PO bid) for 2 weeks
Late latent (or latent of uncertain duration), cardiovascular, or benign tertiary	Lumbar puncture CSF normal: Penicillin G benzathine (2.4 million units IM weekly for 3 weeks) CSF abnormal: treat as neurosyphilis	Lumbar puncture CSF normal: tetracycline hydrochloride (500 mg PO qid) or doxycycline (100 mg PO bid) for 4 weeks CSF abnormal: treat as neurosyphilis
Neurosyphilis† (asymptomatic or symptomatic)	Aqueous penicillin G (12–24 million units/d IV, given in divided doses every 4 h) for 10–14 days *or* Aqueous penicillin G procaine (2.4 million units/d IM) plus oral probenecid (500 mg qid), both for 10–14 days	Desensitization and treatment with penicillin if allergy is confirmed by skin testing
Syphilis in pregnancy	According to stage	Desensitization and treatment with penicillin if allergy is confirmed by skin testing

* See text for discussion of syphilis therapy in HIV-infected individuals.

† Some authorities recommend following these regimens with three doses of 2.4 million units of penicillin G benzathine, given IM 1 week apart. Penicillin G benzathine alone has given inferior results when used for the treatment of neurosyphilis. Drugs other than penicillin are not recommended. Many patients who give a history of penicillin allergy prove negative when skin-tested for immediate hypersensitivity to penicillin and can be given aqueous crystalline penicillin G for CNS syphilis under close supervision in the hospital.

SOURCE: These recommendations are modified from those issued by the Centers for Disease Control and Prevention in 1993.

thine, 2.4 million units intramuscularly once a week for 3 successive weeks (7.2 million units total). Doxycycline or tetracycline (given for 1 month) offers an untested alternative for penicillin-allergic patients with latent or late syphilis and normal CSF. If CSF abnormalities are found, the patient should be treated for neurosyphilis.

No studies of penicillin G benzathine for cardiovascular syphilis have been reported, and the efficacy of penicillin therapy in any form for this condition has not been proven. The response of cardiovascular syphilis to penicillin is seldom dramatic because aortic aneurysm and aortic regurgitation cannot be reversed by antibiotic treatment, although further progression of these lesions may be arrested. In contrast, the response of benign tertiary syphilis and of meningovascular syphilis to penicillin G is usually impressive. The response of parenchymal neurosyphilis has been variable. In Hahn's 1959 cooperative study of the treatment of 1086 general paretics with penicillin, the frequency of clinical improvement or termination of progression ranged from 38 percent among persons with severe involvement to 81 percent among those with mild involvement. Tabes dorsalis or optic atrophy responds less often. In general, treatment of inactive neurosyphilis in which neurologic damage has already been done may produce no clinical change, and retreatment of such cases is not warranted. However, the persistence of CSF pleocytosis or its recurrence after an initial response to treatment indicates continuing active infection, which should respond to additional treatment. The CDC's 1993 treatment guidelines for neurosyphilis are presented in Table 174-4. Penicillin G benzathine, given in total doses of up to 7.2 million units to adults or 50,000 units per kilogram to infants, does not produce detectable concentrations of penicillin G in CSF, and asymptomatic neurosyphilis may relapse in up to one-quarter of adults treated with 2.4 million units. Therefore, the use of penicillin G benzathine alone for the treatment of neurosyphilis is not recommended. On the other hand, administration of intravenous penicillin G in doses of 12 million units or more per day for 10 days or longer is thought to ensure treponemicidal concentrations of penicillin G in CSF and occasionally cures infection in patients who fail to respond to other therapy.

Several recent publications have reported neurologic relapse after high-dose intravenous penicillin therapy for neurosyphilis in HIV-infected patients. No alternative therapies have been explored, but careful follow-up is essential, and retreatment is warranted in such patients.

No data support the use of antibiotics other than penicillin G for the treatment of neurosyphilis; however, some of the third-generation cephalosporins may deserve further evaluation. In patients with penicillin allergy demonstrated by skin testing, desensitization may be the best course (see Chap. 126).

MANAGEMENT OF SYPHILIS IN PREGNANCY Every pregnant woman should undergo a nontreponemal test at her first prenatal visit, and women at high risk of exposure should have a repeat test in the third trimester and at delivery. In the pregnant patient with presumed syphilis (evidenced by a reactive serology, with or without clinical manifestations) and with no history of treatment for syphilis, expeditious evaluation and initiation of treatment are essential. Therapy should be administered according to the stage of the disease, as for nonpregnant patients. Patients should be warned of the risk of a Jarisch-Herxheimer reaction, which may be associated with mild premature contractions but rarely results in premature delivery.

Penicillin is the only recommended therapy for syphilis in pregnancy. If the patient has a well-documented penicillin allergy that is confirmed by the demonstration of an immediate wheal-and-flare response to skin testing with penicilloyl polylysine or penicillin G minor-determinant mixture, desensitization and penicillin treatment should be undertaken in a hospital according to the 1993 sexually transmitted diseases treatment guidelines issued by the CDC. After treatment, a quantitative reagin test should be repeated monthly throughout pregnancy. Treated women whose titers rise fourfold or

who do not show a fourfold decrease in titer in a 3-month period should be retreated.

Evaluation and Management of Congenital Syphilis Newborn infants of mothers with reactive VDRL or FTA-ABS tests may themselves have reactive tests, whether or not they have become infected, because of transplacental transfer of maternal IgG antibody. Rising or persistent titers indicate infection, and the infant should be treated. Neonatal IgM antibody can be detected in cord or neonatal serum with the 19S IgM FTA-ABS test, in which IgM is enriched by column chromatography (which removes IgG) and is detected by fluorescein-labeled anti-human IgM. This test avoids the specificity and sensitivity problems associated with earlier versions of the IgM FTA-ABS test. Alternatively, monthly quantitative reagin tests may be performed on asymptomatic infants born to women treated adequately with penicillin during pregnancy.

If the seropositive mother has received inadequate penicillin treatment or therapy with a drug other than penicillin, if her treatment status is unknown, or if the infant may be difficult to follow, the infant should be treated at birth. It is unwise to require proof of diagnosis before treatment in such cases. The CSF should be examined to obtain baseline values before treatment. Penicillin is the only recommended drug for syphilis in infants. The penicillin dosage used for the treatment of the patient with late congenital syphilis is calculated in the same way as that used in the infant, until dosage based on weight reaches that used for adult neurosyphilis. Specific recommendations for the treatment of infants are included in the CDC's 1993 guidelines.

Jarisch-Herxheimer Reaction A dramatic though usually mild reaction consisting of fever (average temperature elevation, 1.5°C), chills, myalgias, headache, tachycardia, increased respiratory rate, increased circulating neutrophil count (average total white blood cell count, 12,500/μL), and vasodilation with mild hypotension may follow the initiation of treatment for syphilis. This reaction occurs in approximately 50 percent of patients with primary syphilis, 90 percent of those with secondary syphilis, and 25 percent of those with early latent syphilis. The onset comes within 2 h of treatment, the temperature peaks at about 7 h, and defervescence takes place within 12 to 24 h. The reaction is more delayed in neurosyphilis, with fever peaking after 12 to 14 h. In patients with secondary syphilis, erythema and edema of the mucocutaneous lesions increase; occasionally, subclinical or early mucocutaneous lesions may first become apparent during the reaction. The pathogenesis of this reaction is undefined, although recent studies have demonstrated the induction of inflammatory mediators such as tumor necrosis factors by treponemal lipoproteins. Patients should be warned to expect such symptoms, which can be managed by bed rest and aspirin. Adjunctive steroid therapy has not been shown to prevent the Jarisch-Herxheimer reaction in syphilis and is not recommended.

Follow-Up Evaluation of Responses to Therapy The response of early syphilis to treatment should be determined by monitoring of the quantitative VDRL or RPR titer 1, 3, 6, and 12 months after treatment. More frequent serologic examination (1, 2, 3, 6, 9, and 12 months) is recommended for patients concurrently infected with HIV. Because the FTA-ABS and hemagglutination tests remain positive in most patients treated for seropositive early syphilis, these tests are not useful in following the response to therapy. After successful treatment of seropositive first-episode primary or secondary syphilis, the VDRL titer progressively declines, becoming negative by 12 months in 40 to 75 percent of seropositive primary cases and in 20 to 40 percent of secondary cases. Two years after treatment for first-episode primary syphilis, at least 60 percent of patients have a negative VDRL test, although 25 to 58 percent of patients with secondary disease and a higher proportion of those treated for early latent syphilis maintain low reagin titers. Patients with a history of syphilis have less rapid declines in titer and are less likely to become VDRL- or RPR-negative. If the VDRL test becomes negative or if VDRL titers drop to a fixed low value within 1 or 2 years, lumbar puncture is unnecessary since the CSF examination is almost invariably normal and there is little risk of subsequent neurosyphilis.

However, if a VDRL titer of 1:8 or more fails to fall at least fourfold within 12 months, if the VDRL titer rises fourfold, or if clinical symptoms persist or recur, retreatment is indicated. Every effort should be made to differentiate treatment failure from reinfection, and the CSF should be examined. Patients in whom treatment failure is suspected, especially those with abnormal CSF, should be treated as described for neurosyphilis. If the patient remains seropositive but asymptomatic after such retreatment, no further therapy is necessary. Patients treated for late latent syphilis frequently have low VDRL titers before therapy and may not have a fourfold drop after therapy with penicillin; about half of these patients remain seropositive (with low titers) for years after therapy. Retreatment is not warranted unless the titer rises or signs and symptoms of syphilis appear.

The activity of neurosyphilis correlates best with the degree of CSF pleocytosis. Changes in the CSF cell count and, to a lesser extent, in the CSF protein concentration provide the most sensitive index of response to treatment. CSF should be examined every 3 to 6 months for 3 years after the treatment of asymptomatic or symptomatic neurosyphilis or until CSF findings return to normal. An elevated CSF cell count falls to $\leq 10/\mu L$ in 3 to 12 months in 95 percent of adequately treated cases and becomes normal in all cases within 2 to 4 years. Elevated levels of CSF protein fall more slowly, and the CSF reagin titer declines gradually over a period of several years. Some evidence suggests that serum and CSF parameters may normalize more slowly in HIV-infected patients with neurosyphilis than in persons not infected with HIV.

Persistence of Treponemal Forms The persistence of *T. pallidum* in the aqueous humor, CSF, lymph nodes, brain, inflamed temporal arteries, and other tissues after "adequate" penicillin treatment has been suggested by dark-field microscopy, immunofluorescent antibody and silver staining techniques, rabbit inoculation, and polymerase chain reaction. Because the data on persisting treponemes are scanty, no modification of the treatment recommendations seems warranted for HIV-uninfected persons. Adherence to recommendations regarding CSF examination before the selection of therapy should minimize the possibility that *T. pallidum* will persist in the CSF.

IMMUNITY TO AND PREVENTION OF SYPHILIS About 30 to 50 percent of contacts of patients with primary and secondary syphilis become infected, but the actual risk of infection from a single exposure is probably much lower. The rate of development of acquired resistance to *T. pallidum* after natural or experimental infection is related to the amount of the antigenic stimulus, which depends on both the size of the infecting inoculum and the duration of infection before treatment. The role of serum antibody in conferring immunity to syphilis remains controversial. Reagin (VDRL) antibody is not protective, although it is opsonic for *T. pallidum*. Passively administered antibody prevents or delays the appearance of clinical manifestations of syphilis in the rabbit model; it does not prevent infection. Cellular immunity is considered to be of major importance in the healing of early lesions and the control of syphilitic infection. The cellular infiltration of early lesions predominantly involves T lymphocytes and macrophages; specifically sensitized T lymphocytes develop early in the course of infection in humans and experimentally infected rabbits. The cytokine milieu of primary and secondary lesions is of the T_H1 type, consistent with the clearance of organisms by activated macrophages. Specific antibody enhances phagocytosis and is required for macrophage-mediated killing of *T. pallidum*.

Inability to cultivate pathogenic treponemes in vitro has hindered the analysis of treponemal antigens. Attempts to induce immunity to syphilis by vaccination have shown limited promise, although repeated injection of rabbits with gamma-irradiated motile strains has conferred immunity to rechallenge. The outer membrane of *T. pallidum* contains few integral membrane proteins, although the first surface-exposed antigen, a porin molecule, has recently been identified. Many of the major antigens are lipoproteins, which are probably associated via their lipid tail with the inner membrane, projecting into the periplasmic space. None of these identified antigens has been shown to induce

protective immunity. Until a practical and effective vaccine is developed, the prevention of syphilis will depend on the use of condoms and on the detection and treatment of infectious cases.

BIBLIOGRAPHY

BERRY CD et al: Neurologic relapse after benzathine penicillin therapy for secondary syphilis in a patient with HIV infection. N Engl J Med 316:1587, 1987

BLANCO DR et al: Porin activity and sequence analysis of a 31-kilodalton *Treponema pallidum* subsp. *pallidum* rare outer membrane protein (Tromp 1). J Bacteriol 177:3556, 1995

CENTERS FOR DISEASE CONTROL: Guidelines for the prevention and control of congenital syphilis. Morb Mort Week Rep 37(S-1):1, 1988

CENTERS FOR DISEASE CONTROL AND PREVENTION: Summary of notifiable disease 1993. Morb Mort Week Rep 42(53):1, 1993

———: 1993 sexually transmitted diseases treatment guidelines. Morb Mort Week Rep 42(RR-14):1, 1993

DOWELL ME et al: Response of latent syphilis or neurosyphilis to ceftriaxone therapy in persons infected with human immunodeficiency virus. Am J Med 93:481, 1992

GORDON SM et al: The response of symptomatic neurosyphilis to high-dose intravenous pencillin G in patients with human immunodeficiency virus infection. N Engl J Med 331:1469, 1994

KATZ DA et al: Neurosyphilis in acquired immunodeficiency syndrome. Arch Neurol 46:895, 1989

LARSEN SA et al: Laboratory diagnosis and interpretation of tests for syphilis. Clin Microbiol Rev 8:1, 1995

LUKEHART SA et al: Invasion of the central nervous system by *Treponema pallidum*: Implications for diagnosis and treatment. Ann Intern Med 109:855, 1988

MARRA CM et al: Resolution of serum and cerebrospinal fluid abnormalities after treatment of neurosyphilis: Influence of concomitant human immunodeficiency virus infection. Sex Transm Dis 23:184, 1996

McLEISH WM et al: The ocular manifestations of syphilis in the human immunodeficiency virus type 1–infected host. Ophthalmology 97:196, 1990

MOHR JA et al: Neurosyphilis and penicillin in cerebrospinal fluid. JAMA 236:2208, 1976

MUSHER DM et al: Effect of human immunodeficiency virus infection on the course of syphilis and on the response to treatment. Ann Intern Med 113:872, 1990

RADOLF JD et al: Outer membrane ultrastructure explains the limited antigenicity of virulent *Treponema pallidum*. Proc Natl Acad Sci USA 86:2051, 1989

ROMANOWSKI B et al: Serologic response to treatment of infectious syphilis. Ann Intern Med 114:1005, 1991

SIMON RP: Neurosyphilis. Arch Neurol 42:606, 1985

THOMAS JC et al: Syphilis in the South: Rural rates surpass urban rates in North Carolina. Am J Public Health 85:1119, 1995

THOMAS SB: The Tuskegee syphilis study, 1932 to 1972: Implications for HIV education and AIDS risk education programs in the black community. Am J Public Health 81:1498, 1991

VAN VOORHIS WC et al: Primary and secondary syphilis lesions contain mRNA for T_H1 cytokines. J Infect Dis 173:491, 1996

WENDEL GD et al: Penicillin allergy and desensitization in serious infections during pregnancy. N Engl J Med 312:1229, 1985

175 | *Peter L. Perine*

ENDEMIC TREPONEMATOSES

GENERAL CONSIDERATIONS Nonvenereal treponematoses occur in less developed areas of the world. Yaws, pinta, and endemic syphilis are distinguished from venereal syphilis solely by clinical and epidemiologic features since they are caused by treponemes with no demonstrated significant morphologic or genetic differences from *Treponema pallidum*. The etiologic agents of endemic syphilis and yaws are generally held to be identical to *T. pallidum* and have been designated as *T. pallidum* ssp. *endemicum* and ssp. *pertenue*, respectively. Pinta is caused by *Treponema carateum* and involves the skin alone; yaws affects skin and bones; and endemic syphilis involves the skin, bones, and mucous membranes. Each disease tends to progress by stages, but these are neither as distinct nor as predictable as in venereal syphilis. Congenital infections and cardiovascular and central nervous system involvement occur rarely, if ever, in the nonvenereal treponematoses but are common in venereal syphilis. It is unclear whether the clinical and epidemiologic differences among yaws, pinta, endemic syphilis, and venereal syphilis are determined by environmental and host factors alone or are also attributable in part to undefined biologic differences among the causal treponemes. The relationships among the treponematoses are summarized in Table 175-1.

EPIDEMIOLOGY Treponemal antibodies are demonstrable in some proportion of nonhuman primates in regions of Africa where human yaws and endemic syphilis are common. Pathogenic treponemes have been found in skin lesions and lymph nodes of seropositive animals; these treponemes have produced yawslike lesions in susceptible monkeys and hamsters. No epidemiologic evidence indicates that these treponemes play a significant role in the epidemiology of yaws in humans.

Yaws and endemic syphilis are diseases of young children. Yaws occurs throughout the world between the tropics of Cancer and Capricorn in humid, warm environments. Transmission of yaws among children is favored by scanty clothing, poor hygiene, and frequent skin trauma. Spread occurs by direct contact with infected lesions and perhaps by passive transfer of treponemes by insects. Endemic syphilis occurs in arid subtropical or temperate climates in Africa, the eastern Mediterranean, the Arabian peninsula, and central Asia. It is not found in the western hemisphere. Skin-to-skin transmission is less important than in yaws; instead, infection of mucous membranes results from direct mouth-to-mouth contact or from contaminated fomites, such as shared drinking or eating utensils.

Although cutaneous pigmentary changes resembling late stages of pinta occur in yaws and endemic syphilis, pinta is a separate, more benign disease that occurs only in the western hemisphere. The onset is typically later than in yaws or endemic syphilis, usually between 10 and 20 years of age. Pinta is not highly contagious, and its mode of transmission is not well defined.

The WHO/UNICEF-assisted mass campaigns for eradication of endemic nonvenereal treponematoses from 1948 to 1969 were unusually successful. More than 160 million people were examined in 46 countries, and approximately 50 million cases, contacts, and latent infections were treated. The impact of this program was remarkable. The prevalence of active yaws lesions was reduced from over 20 percent to less than 1 percent in many rural areas. In Bosnia, endemic syphilis was eradicated—the only example of eradication of an endemic treponematosis.

Relaxation of active surveillance efforts since the mass campaigns has led to a resurgence of yaws, particularly in Africa. Yaws has not been eradicated in any large area. A large reservoir of yaws remains in West Africa and encompasses the Ivory Coast, Ghana, Togo, Benin, and the pygmies of Zaire and the Central African Republic. Yaws is also prevalent in Indonesia; Papua, New Guinea; and the Solomon Islands of the western Pacific. The Sahelian African nations of Mali, Niger, Burkina Faso, and Senegal have endemic syphilis prevalence rates of 10 to 15 percent in some areas. These rates exceed those reported before the mass treatment campaigns. Seroreactivity and late manifestations of endemic syphilis persist among nomads in Saudi Arabia. The resurgence of yaws and endemic syphilis led to a new yaws campaign in Ghana in 1980, and other national campaigns are planned to control resurgent yaws and endemic syphilis in Africa.

Antitreponemal and reaginic seroreactivity has been detected in a small percentage of children without clinical disease born after the mass campaigns in some areas (e.g., Nigeria, New Guinea, and Bosnia). This reactivity may represent attenuated or asymptomatic infection or may simply reflect the decrease in the predictive value of serologic tests (i.e., in the probability that disease is present if the test is positive) when the prevalence of disease is sharply reduced.

In the Americas, foci of yaws persist in Haiti; Dominica, St. Lucia, and St. Vincent; Peru, Colombia, and Ecuador; a few areas of Brazil; and Guyana and Surinam. Pinta is confined to Central America and northern South America, where it appears to have receded to remote Indian villages. Its prevalence today is probably less than 1 percent of that 20 years ago.

BIOLOGIC RELATIONSHIPS Specific humoral antibodies to *T. pallidum* are produced in individuals with yaws, pinta, or endemic syphilis, but the time of appearance of antibodies after the onset of infections is variable. The fluorescent treponemal antibody absorption (FTA-ABS) test, the *T. pallidum* hemagglutination (TPHA) test, and the *T. pallidum* immobilization (TPI) test cannot differentiate among the treponematoses.

In addition to the clinical and epidemiologic differences among the treponematoses in humans, the range of susceptible animal hosts and some manifestations of experimental infection are different. In particular, *T. carateum* has produced an infection in chimpanzees that resembles pinta, but attempts to infect other experimental animals have been unsuccessful. Individuals who have had yaws or pinta are considered relatively immune to syphilis, and persons with active pinta or syphilis cannot be superinfected with *T. pallidum* ssp. *pertenue* by experimental inoculation.

CLINICAL MANIFESTATIONS Yaws Also known as *pian*, *framboesia*, or *bouba*, yaws is a chronic infectious disease of childhood caused by *T. pallidum* ssp. *pertenue*. The disease is characterized by the development of one or more initial skin lesions and then of relapsing, nondestructive secondary lesions of

Table 175-1

Etiology, Epidemiology, and Clinical Manifestations of the Treponematoses

| Feature | Finding in Indicated Disease | | | |
	Venereal Syphilis	Endemic Syphilis	Yaws	Pinta
Organism	*T. pallidum* ssp. *pallidum*	*T. pallidum* ssp. *endemicum*	*T. pallidum* ssp. *pertenue*	*T. carateum*
Transmission	Sexual, transplacental*	Household contacts: mouth-to-mouth or via shared drinking/eating utensils	Skin-to-skin; insect vector?	Skin-to-skin; insect vector?
Usual age	Adulthood	Early childhood	Early childhood	Adolescence
Primary lesion	Cutaneous ulcer (chancre)	Rarely seen	Framboesioma (raspberry), or "mother yaw"	Nonulcerating papule with satellites
Secondary lesion	Mucocutaneous lesions; occasional periostitis	Florid mucocutaneous lesions (mucous patch, split papule, condyloma latum); osteoperiostitis	Cutaneous papulosquamous lesions; osteoperiostitis	Pintides
Tertiary	Gummas, cardiovascular and CNS lues	Destructive cutaneous osteoarticular gummas	Destructive cutaneous osteoarticular gummas	Dyschromic, achromic macules

* Since the nonvenereal treponematoses are usually acquired in childhood and treponemal bacteremia ceases with time, only in adult-onset venereal syphilis is there any likelihood that a mother will give birth to an infected child.

skin and bones. In the late stages, destructive lesions of skin, bones, and joints occur.

The incubation period following experimental inoculation of the causative organism into susceptible human beings is 3 to 4 weeks. Disruption of the skin by insect bites, abrasions, or injuries promotes the acquisition of natural infection from infected contacts, most likely by fingers contaminated directly or indirectly with material from early yaws lesions. The initial early lesion is a single papule, which is usually located on a leg. The lesion enlarges and becomes papillomatous (Fig. 175-1). This lesion, known as a *framboesioma* (raspberry) or "mother yaw," becomes superficially eroded and covered by a thin yellow crust of serous exudate containing *T. pallidum* ssp. *pertenue*. Erythema and induration do not occur. The lesion is mildly pruritic, and regional lymphadenopathy develops. The initial lesion usually heals in 6 months. As a result of treponemal bacteremia and autoinoculation, a generalized secondary eruption of similar lesions appears either before or after the initial lesion has healed and is most extensive on the exposed surfaces of the body. These early cutaneous lesions of yaws have a variety of forms, including desquamative macular and papular as well as papillomatous types. Painful papillomata on the soles of the feet result in a crablike gait referred to as "crab yaws." Early lesions are infectious and heal slowly. They may result in scarring, hyperpigmentation, or depigmentation; the pigmentary changes resemble those seen in pinta. Histologic findings include mononuclear cell infiltration, acanthosis, hyperkeratosis, and many treponemes.

Other manifestations of early yaws include lymphadenopathy and nocturnal bone pain and polydactylitis due to periostitis. Fever and other constitutional symptoms are rare unless lesions become secondarily infected. Infectious cutaneous relapses are characteristic during the first 5 years after infection. Late yaws lesions occur in about 10 percent of cases, starting 5 years or more after infection, and differ histologically from early lesions in that they exhibit endarteritis. Late lesions include gummas of the skin and long bones, particularly of the legs; hyperkeratoses of the soles and palms; osteitis; periostitis; juxtaarticular fibromatous nodes; and hydrarthrosis.

Late lesions of yaws are characteristically extensive and usually destructive. Destruction of the nose, maxilla, palate, and pharynx, termed *gangosa* or *rhinopharyngitis mutilans*, occurs in late yaws as well as in leprosy and leishmaniasis. Hypertrophic paranasal maxillary osteitis produces distinctive facies known as *goundou*.

The clinical features of yaws have become less reliable for diagnosis as the prevalence of yaws has decreased. Thus the use of easily performed serologic tests, such as the rapid plasma reagin (RPR) card test, has become necessary. *T. pallidum* ssp. *pertenue* can be demonstrated by dark-field examination in early cutaneous lesions but should not be confused with other spirochetes found in tropical ulcers. The serum reagin antibody tests become positive after 1 month, and the FTA-ABS test is also positive.

FIGURE 175-1 Squamous micropapules of early yaws with papillomas in the axilla and scapular area.

Endemic Syphilis Endemic syphilis (also called *bejel, siti, dichuchwa, njovera,* and *skerljevo*) is a chronic nonvenereal treponemal infection of childhood characterized by early mucous membrane or mucocutaneous lesions, a latent period of indeterminate duration, and late complications including gummas of bone and skin. The causative organism, *T. pallidum* ssp. *endemicum*, is indistinguishable from *T. pallidum* ssp. *pallidum*. Endemic syphilis differs from congenital syphilis in that dental changes, interstitial keratitis, and neurosyphilis rarely, if ever, occur. Cardiovascular complications are considered rare in both endemic and congenital syphilis.

Primary cutaneous lesions are infrequent and, when present, are extragenital. The earliest manifestation of endemic syphilis is usually an intraoral mucous patch or mucocutaneous lesion resembling the split papules or condylomata of secondary syphilis. Periostitis is common. Regional lymphadenopathy occurs, but generalized lymphadenopathy is unusual. Treponemes are abundant in the moist early lesions and in aspirates from regional lymph nodes. After a variable latent period, late lesions may develop. These lesions, which are the most frequent clinical manifestations, resemble the lesions of late benign syphilis and include osseous or cutaneous gummas. Destructive gummas, osteitis, and gangosa are more common than in late yaws. Gummas develop on the nipples of mothers who have previously had endemic syphilis and who breast-feed infants with oral lesions. Both early and late forms of endemic syphilis thus may coexist in the same family. The tertiary lesions of endemic syphilis sometimes result from repeated exposure of a previously sensitized host to reinfection.

Pinta Also known as *mal del pinto, carate, azul,* or *purupuru,* pinta is an infectious disease of the skin caused by *T. carateum.* This disease has three cutaneous stages characterized by marked changes in the skin color, does not involve osseous tissue or viscera, and causes no disability other than that associated with cosmetic disfigurement.

The initial lesion is a small papule that appears 7 to 30 days after exposure and is located most often on the extremities, face, neck, or buttocks. It slowly increases in size by peripheral extension and by coalescence with smaller satellite papules. Regional lymphadenopathy occurs. A secondary eruption not associated with generalized lymphadenopathy appears 1 month to 1 year after the appearance of the initial lesion. The secondary lesions are termed *pintides*, may be numerous, and evolve into a psoriatic or circinate configuration. Pintides are initially red but become deeply pigmented, turning a slate-blue color after an interval whose length is related to exposure to sun. Pigmentation changes occur most rapidly on the exposed parts of the body. Tertiary pigmented lesions are known as *dyschromic macules* and contain treponemes that are located principally in the epidermis in older lesions. Histologic study reveals deposition of pigment in the dermis, with decreased melanin in the basal cell layer. Within 3 months to a year, most of the pintides show varying degrees of depigmentation, becoming brown and finally white and giving the skin a mottled appearance. The porcelain-white achromic lesions represent the "late" stage of the disease, in which the epidermis is atrophic and melanocytes and melanin are absent. *T. carateum* can be demonstrated in transudates from initial, early secondary, or dyschromic lesions. Reaginic and antitreponemal antibody tests are positive but may take four times longer to become positive in pinta than in venereal syphilis.

℞ TREATMENT

Treatment is similar for all the endemic treponematoses. Intramuscular administration of 2.4 million units of benzathine penicillin G to adults and of half this dose to children results in rapid resolution of lesions and prevents recurrence. A regimen of procaine penicillin G in oil and 2% aluminum monostearate (PAM) has been used extensively. When patients are allergic to penicillin, tetracycline hydrochloride in a dose similar to that used for infectious syphilis (see Chap. 174) is effective. In areas where fewer than 5 percent of the population have active disease, cases are managed on an individual basis, and all contacts of infected persons are treated with antibiotics.

PREVENTION Although the nonvenereal treponematoses are less amenable to eradication than smallpox, the resurgence of yaws has led some authorities to suggest that selective epidemiologic control, like that used in smallpox eradication, be applied to yaws control. This strategy emphasizes ongoing active surveillance, investigation of outbreaks, and treatment of active cases and their contacts rather than mass treatment. There is concern that the epidemiology and course of yaws and endemic syphilis will be adversely affected by the human immunodeficiency virus (HIV) pandemic in Africa and Asia. It is feared that, in HIV-infected individuals, cutaneous lesions may last longer, may more easily become secondarily infected, and may serve as a portal for nonvenereal transmission of HIV.

BIBLIOGRAPHY

BURKE JP et al (eds): International symposium on yaws and other endemic treponematoses. Rev Infect Dis 7:S217, 1985

ENGELKENS HJH et al: Endemic treponematosis. Int J Dermatol 30:77, 1991

GUTHE T: Clinical, serological and epidemiological features of framboesia tropica (yaws) and its control in rural communities. Acta Dermatol Venereol 49:343, 1969

KOFF AB, ROSEN T: Nonvenereal treponematoses: Yaws, endemic syphilis, and pinta. J Am Acad Dermatol 29:519, 1993

NOORDHOEK GT, VAN EMBDEN JDA: Yaws, an endemic treponematosis reconsidered in the HIV era. Eur J Clin Microbiol Infect Dis 10:4, 1991

MEHEUS A, ANTAL GM: Endemic treponematoses: Not yet eradicated. World Health Stat Q 45:228, 1992

PERINE PL et al: *Handbook of Endemic Treponematoses.* Geneva, World Health Organization, 1984

Treponematoses Research: Report of a WHO Scientific Group, WHO Technical Report Series 674, 1982

176	*Peter Speelman*

LEPTOSPIROSIS

Leptospirosis is an infectious disease caused by pathogenic leptospires and is characterized by a broad spectrum of clinical manifestations, varying from inapparent infection to fulminant, fatal disease. In its mild form, leptospirosis may present as an influenza-like illness with headache and myalgias. Severe leptospirosis, characterized by jaundice, renal dysfunction, and hemorrhagic diathesis, is referred to as *Weil's syndrome.*

ETIOLOGIC AGENTS Leptospires are spirochetes belonging to the order Spirochaetales and the family Leptospiraceae. Traditionally, the genus *Leptospira* comprised two species: the pathogenic *L. interrogans* and the free-living *L. biflexa.* Although seven species of pathogenic leptospires are now recognized on the basis of their DNA relatedness, it is more practical clinically and epidemiologically to use a classification based on serologic differences. The pathogenic leptospires are divided into serovars according to their antigenic composition. More than 200 serovars make up the 23 serogroups.

Leptospires are coiled, thin, highly motile organisms with hooked ends and two periplasmic flagella, which enable the organisms to burrow into tissue. These organisms are 6 to 20 μm long and about 0.1 μm wide; they stain poorly but can be seen microscopically by dark-field examination and after silver impregnation staining. Leptospires require special media and conditions for growth; it may take weeks for cultures to become positive.

EPIDEMIOLOGY Leptospirosis is a zoonosis with a worldwide distribution that affects at least 160 mammalian species. Rodents, especially rats, are the most important reservoir, although dogs, other wild mammals, fish, and birds may also harbor these microorganisms. Leptospires establish a symbiotic relationship with their host and can persist in the renal tubules for years. Some serovars are associated with particular animals—e.g., icterohaemorrhagiae/copenhageni with rats, grippotyphosa with voles, hardjo with cattle, canicola with dogs, and pomona with pigs.

Transmission of leptospires may follow direct contact with urine, blood, or tissue from an infected animal or exposure to a contaminated environment; human-to-human transmission is rare. Since leptospires are excreted in the urine and can survive in water for many months, water is an important vehicle in their transmission. Leptospirosis occurs most commonly in the tropics because the climate as well as the sometimes poor working and hygienic conditions favor the pathogen's survival.

Humans are not commonly infected with leptospires. However, in the United States, the 40 to 120 cases reported annually to the Centers for Disease Control and Prevention certainly represent a significant underestimation of the total number. Certain occupational groups are at especially high risk; included are veterinarians, agricultural workers, sewage workers, slaughterhouse employees, and workers in the fishing industry. Such individuals may acquire leptospirosis through direct exposure to or contact with contaminated water and soil.

In western countries, recreational exposure and domestic-animal contact are also prominent sources of leptospirosis. Recreational water use, such as canoeing, windsurfing, swimming, and waterskiing, place persons at risk for leptospirosis. Sometimes the infection is acquired during travel abroad. In a recent study in the Netherlands, 14 percent of patients with confirmed leptospirosis had acquired the infection while traveling in tropical countries, mostly in Southeast Asia. Transmission via laboratory accidents has been reported but is rare. Occasionally, leptospirosis develops after unanticipated immersion in contaminated water (e.g., in an automobile accident). Most cases occur in men, with a peak incidence during the summer and fall in western countries and during the rainy season in the tropics.

PATHOGENESIS The pathogenesis of leptospirosis is incompletely understood. Leptospires may enter the host through abrasions in the skin or through intact mucous membranes, especially the conjunctiva and the lining of the oro- and nasopharynx. Drinking of contaminated water may introduce leptospires through the mouth, throat, or esophagus. After entry of the organisms, leptospiremia develops, with subsequent spread to all organs. Multiplication takes place in blood and in tissues, and leptospires can be isolated from blood and cerebrospinal fluid (CSF) during the first 4 to 10 days of illness. It is not clear why the presence of leptospires in the CSF does not cause damage. An important role for a toxin in the pathogenesis of the disease has been suggested but not proved.

Leptospire-inflicted damage to the capillary endothelium results in vasculitis, which is responsible for the most important manifestations of the disease. Although leptospires mainly infect the kidneys and liver, any organ may be affected. In the kidney, leptospires migrate to the interstitium, renal tubules, and tubular lumen, causing interstitial nephritis and tubular necrosis. Hypovolemia due to dehydration or altered capillary permeability may contribute to the development of renal failure. In the liver, centrilobular necrosis with proliferation of Kupffer cells may be found. However, severe hepatocellular necrosis is not a feature of leptospirosis. Pulmonary involvement is the result of hemorrhage and not of inflammation. Invasion of skeletal muscle by leptospires results in swelling, vacuolation of the myofibrils, and focal necrosis. In severe leptospirosis, vasculitis may ultimately impair the microcirculation and increase capillary permeability, resulting in fluid leakage and hypovolemia.

When antibodies are formed, leptospires are eliminated from all sites in the host except the eye, the proximal renal tubules, and perhaps the brain, where they may persist for weeks or months. The persistence of leptospires in the aqueous humor occasionally causes chronic or recurrent uveitis. The systemic immune response is effective in eliminating the organism but may also produce symptomatic inflammatory reactions. A rise in antibody titer coincides with the development of meningitis; this association suggests that an immunologic mechanism is responsible.

After the start of antimicrobial treatment for leptospirosis, a Jarisch-Herxheimer reaction similar to that seen in other spirochetal diseases may develop. Although frequently described in older publications, this reaction seems to be a rare event in leptospirosis and is certainly less frequent in this infection than in other spirochetal diseases.

CLINICAL MANIFESTATIONS Serologic evidence of past inapparent infection is found in 15 to 40 percent of persons who have been exposed but have not become ill. In symptomatic cases of leptospirosis, clinical manifestations vary from mild to serious or even fatal. More than 90 percent of symptomatic persons have the relatively mild and usually anicteric form of leptospirosis, with or without meningitis. Severe leptospirosis with profound jaundice (Weil's syndrome) develops in 5 to 10 percent of infected individuals.

The incubation period is usually 1 to 2 weeks but ranges from 2 to 26 days. Typically, an acute leptospiremic phase is followed by an immune leptospiruric phase. The distinction between the first and second phases is not always clear, and milder cases do not always include the second phase.

Anicteric Leptospirosis Leptospirosis may present as an acute influenza-like illness, with fever, chills, severe headache, nausea, vomiting, and myalgias. Muscle pain, which especially affects the calves, back, and abdomen, is an important feature of leptospiral infection. Less common features include sore throat and rash. The patient usually has an intense headache (frontal or retroorbital) and sometimes develops photophobia. Mental confusion may be evident. Pulmonary involvement, manifested in most cases by cough and chest pain and in a few cases by hemoptysis, is not uncommon.

The most common finding on physical examination is fever with conjunctival suffusion. Less common findings include muscle tenderness, lymphadenopathy, pharyngeal injection, rash, hepatomegaly, and splenomegaly. The rash may be macular, maculopapular, erythematous, urticarial, or hemorrhagic. Mild jaundice may be present.

Most patients become asymptomatic within 1 week. After an interval of 1 to 3 days, the illness recurs in a number of cases. The start of this second (immune) phase coincides with the development of antibodies. Symptoms are more variable than during the first (leptospiremic) phase. Usually the symptoms last for only a few days, but occasionally they persist for weeks. Often the fever is less pronounced and the myalgias are less severe than in the leptospiremic phase. An important event during the immune phase is the development of aseptic meningitis. Although no more than 15 percent of all patients have symptoms and signs of meningitis, many patients may have CSF pleocytosis. Meningeal symptoms usually disappear within a few days but may persist for weeks. Similarly, pleocytosis generally disappears within 2 weeks but occasionally persists for months. Iritis, iridocyclitis, and chorioretinitis—late complications that may persist for years—can become apparent as early as the third week but often present several months after the initial illness.

Severe Leptospirosis (Weil's Syndrome) Weil's syndrome, the most severe form of leptospirosis, is characterized by jaundice, renal dysfunction, hemorrhagic diathesis, and high mortality. This syndrome is frequently but not exclusively associated with infection due to serovar icterohaemorrhagiae/copenhageni. The onset of illness is no different from that of less severe leptospirosis; however, after 4 to 9 days, jaundice as well as renal and vascular dysfunction generally develop. Although some degree of defervescence may be noted after the first week of illness, a biphasic disease pattern like that seen in anicteric leptospirosis is lacking. The jaundice of Weil's syndrome, which can be profound and give an orange cast to the skin, is usually not associated with severe hepatic necrosis. Death is rarely due to liver failure. Hepatomegaly and tenderness in the right upper quadrant are usually detected. Splenomegaly is found in 20 percent of cases.

Renal failure may develop, often during the second week of illness. Hypovolemia and decreased renal perfusion contribute to the development of acute tubular necrosis with oliguria or anuria. Dialysis is sometimes required, although a fair number of cases can be managed without dialysis. Renal function may be completely regained.

Pulmonary involvement occurs frequently, resulting in cough, dyspnea, chest pain, and blood-stained sputum and sometimes in hemoptysis or even respiratory failure. Hemorrhagic manifestations are seen in Weil's syndrome: epistaxis, petechiae, purpura, and ecchymo-

ses are found commonly, while severe gastrointestinal bleeding and adrenal or subarachnoid hemorrhage are detected rarely.

Rhabdomyolysis, hemolysis, myocarditis, pericarditis, congestive heart failure, cardiogenic shock, adult respiratory distress syndrome, and multiorgan failure have all been described during severe leptospirosis.

LABORATORY AND RADIOLOGIC FINDINGS The kidneys are invariably involved in leptospirosis. Related findings range from urinary sediment changes (leukocytes, erythrocytes, and hyaline or granular casts) and mild proteinuria in anicteric leptospirosis to renal failure and azotemia in severe disease.

The erythrocyte sedimentation rate is usually elevated. In anicteric leptospirosis, peripheral leukocyte counts range from 3000 to 26,000/μL, with a left shift; in Weil's syndrome, leukocytosis is often marked. Mild thrombocytopenia occurs in up to 50 percent of patients and is associated with renal failure.

In contrast to patients with acute viral hepatitis, those with leptospirosis typically have elevated serum levels of bilirubin and alkaline phosphatase as well as mild increases (up to 200 U/L) in serum levels of aminotransferases. In Weil's syndrome, the prothrombin time may be prolonged but can be corrected with vitamin K. Levels of creatine phosphokinase, which are elevated in up to 50 percent of patients with leptospirosis during the first week of illness, may help to differentiate this infection from viral hepatitis.

When a meningeal reaction develops, polymorphonuclear leukocytes predominate initially and the number of mononuclear cells increases later. The protein concentration in the CSF may be elevated; CSF glucose levels are normal.

In severe leptospirosis, pulmonary radiographic abnormalities are more common than would be expected on the basis of physical examination. These abnormalities most frequently develop 3 to 9 days after the onset of illness. The most common radiographic finding is a patchy alveolar pattern that corresponds to scattered alveolar hemorrhage. Radiographic abnormalities most often affect the lower lobes in the periphery of the lung fields.

DIAGNOSIS A definite diagnosis of leptospirosis is based either on isolation of the organism from the patient or on seroconversion or a rise in antibody titer in the microscopic agglutination test (MAT). For a presumptive diagnosis of leptospirosis, an antibody titer of ≥1:100 in the MAT or a positive macroscopic slide agglutination test in the presence of a compatible clinical illness is required. Antibodies generally do not reach detectable levels until the second week of illness. The antibody response can be affected by early treatment.

The macroscopic slide agglutination test with killed antigen is useful for screening but is not specific. The MAT, which uses a battery of live leptospiral strains, and the enzyme-linked immunosorbent assay (ELISA), which uses a broadly reacting antigen, are the standard serologic procedures. These tests usually are available only in specialized laboratories and are used for the determination of the antibody titer and for the tentative identification of the serovar involved (thus the importance of using antigens representative of the serovars prevalent in the particular geographic area). Since cross-reactions occur frequently, however, it is often impossible to identify the infecting serovar. Serologic testing cannot be used as the basis for a decision about whether to start treatment.

In addition to the MAT and the ELISA, various other tests with diagnostic value have been developed. Some tests, such as an indirect hemagglutination test, a microcapsule agglutination test, and an IgM ELISA, are commercially available. Recently, dot-ELISA, gold immunoblot, and polymerase chain reaction techniques have been developed, but these techniques are not yet used for routine diagnosis.

Leptospires can be isolated from blood and/or CSF during the first 10 days of illness and from urine for several weeks beginning at around 1 week. Sometimes urine cultures remain positive for months or years after the start of illness. For isolation of leptospires from body fluids or tissues, Ellinghausen-McCullough-Johnson-Harris (EMJH) medium is useful; other possibilities are Fletcher medium and Korthoff medium. Specimens can be mailed to a reference laboratory for culture since leptospires remain viable in anticoagulated blood for up to 11 days. Isolation of leptospires is important since it is the only way the infecting serovar can be correctly identified. Dark-field examination of blood or urine frequently results in misdiagnosis and should not be used.

DIFFERENTIAL DIAGNOSIS Leptospirosis should be differentiated from other febrile illnesses associated with headache and muscle pain, such as malaria, enteric fever, viral hepatitis, dengue, Hantavirus infections, and rickettsial diseases. In light of the strong similarity in epidemiology and clinical presentation between leptospirosis and Hantavirus infections and given the reported occurrence of dual infections, it is advisable to conduct serologic testing for Hantavirus in cases of suspected leptospirosis. When patients have a flulike disease with disproportionately severe myalgia or aseptic meningitis, a diagnosis of leptospirosis should be considered.

 TREATMENT
The effect of antimicrobial therapy for the mild febrile form of leptospirosis is controversial, but such treatment is indicated for more severe forms. Treatment should be initiated as early as possible; nevertheless, contrary to previous reports, treatment started after the first 4 days of illness is effective.

For severe cases of leptospirosis, intravenous administration of penicillin G, amoxicillin, ampicillin, or erythromycin is recommended (Table 176-1). In milder cases, oral treatment with tetracycline, doxycycline, ampicillin, or amoxicillin should be considered. Although several other antibiotics, including newer cephalosporins, are highly active against leptospires in vitro, no clinical experience has yet been gained with these drugs.

In rare cases, a Jarisch-Herxheimer reaction develops within hours after the start of antimicrobial therapy (see "Pathogenesis" above). The only effective mode of management of this reaction is supportive. Patients with severe leptospirosis and renal failure may require dialysis. Those with Weil's syndrome may need transfusions of whole blood and/or platelets. Intensive care may be necessary.

Most patients with leptospirosis recover. Mortality is highest among patients who are elderly and those who have Weil's syndrome. Leptospirosis during pregnancy is associated with high fetal mortality. Long-term follow-up of patients with renal failure and hepatic dysfunction has documented good recovery of renal and hepatic function.

PREVENTION Individuals who may be exposed to leptospires through their occupations or their involvement in recreational water

Table 176-1

Treatment and Chemoprophylaxis of Leptospirosis

Purpose of Drug Administration	Regimen
Treatment	
Mild leptospirosis	Doxycycline, 100 mg orally bid
	or
	Ampicillin, 500–750 mg orally qid
	or
	Amoxicillin, 500 mg orally qid
Moderate/severe leptospirosis	Penicillin G, 1.5 million units IV qid
	or
	Ampicillin, 1 g IV qid
	or
	Amoxicillin, 1 g IV qid
	or
	Erythromycin, 500 mg IV qid
Chemoprophylaxis	Doxycycline, 200 mg orally once a week

NOTE: All regimens used for treatment are administered for 7 days.

activities should be informed about the risks. Measures for controlling leptospirosis include avoidance of exposure to urine and tissues from infected animals, vaccination of animals, and rodent control. The animal vaccine used in a given area should contain the serovars known to be present in that area. Unfortunately, some vaccinated animals still excrete leptospires in their urine. Vaccination of humans against a specific serovar prevalent in an area has been undertaken in some European and Asian countries and has proved effective. Chemoprophylaxis with doxycycline (200 mg once a week) has appeared to be efficacious in military personnel but is indicated only in rare instances of sustained short-term exposure.

BIBLIOGRAPHY

FARR RW: Leptospirosis. Clin Infect Dis 21:1, 1995
FEIGIN RD, ANDERSON DC: Human leptospirosis. Crit Rev Clin Lab Sci 5:413, 1975
MCCLAIN JBL et al: Doxycycline therapy for leptospirosis. Ann Intern Med 100:696, 1984
O'NEILL KM et al: Pulmonary manifestations of leptospirosis. Rev Infect Dis 13:705, 1991
SHAKED Y et al: Leptospirosis in pregnancy and its effect on the fetus: Case report and review. J Infect Dis 17:241, 1993
VAN CREVEL R et al: Leptospirosis in travelers. Clin Infect Dis 19:132, 1994
WATT G et al: Placebo-controlled trial of intravenous penicillin for severe and late leptospirosis. Lancet 1:433, 1988
———— et al: Skeletal and cardiac muscle involvement in severe, late leptospirosis. J Infect Dis 162:266, 1990

177 *David T. Dennis, Grant L. Campbell*

RELAPSING FEVER

DEFINITION The term *relapsing fever* describes two distinct borrelial disease entities: louse-borne relapsing fever (LBRF) and tick-borne relapsing fever (TBRF). Both are characterized by recurrent acute episodes of spirochetemia and fever alternating with spirochetal clearance and apyrexia.

ETIOLOGY A clinical and epidemiologic distinction between LBRF and similar fevers of different etiology, such as typhus fever, was made in Scotland in the mid-nineteenth century. Spirochetes were first seen in the blood of patients with relapsing fever by Obermeier in Germany in 1868, and spirochete-infected blood was shown to be infectious shortly thereafter. The worldwide distribution of relapsing spirochetal fevers was recognized in the early part of the twentieth century, and the causative agents were shown to be transmitted by lice and ticks. Relapsing-fever spirochetes were described as borreliae belonging to the family Spirochaetaceae. *Borrelia recurrentis* was identified as the cause of LBRF, and strains of borreliae causing TBRF were identified and named, often according to the species of *Ornithodoros* tick responsible for their transmission (Table 177-1).

Relapsing-fever borreliae are gram-negative helical bacteria that average 0.2 to 0.5 μm in width and 5 to 20 μm in length. They comprise an outer membrane, an intermediate peptidoglycan layer, and an inner cytoplasmic membrane, which encloses the protoplasmic cylinder. Periplasmic flagella (15 to 20 at each end of the bacterium) are situated beneath the outer membrane. Relapsing-fever borreliae are slow-growing and microaerophilic; they grow best at 30 to 35°C. TBRF spirochetes grow well in a modification of Kelly's medium, Barbour-Stoenner-Kelly (BSK) medium; LBRF spirochetes are more fastidious in the laboratory and grow poorly on artificial medium.

Relapsing-fever borreliae are distinguished by remarkable antigenic variability and strain heterogeneity. New *Borrelia* serotypes spontaneously emerge at a high rate, resulting from a unique process of DNA rearrangement within genes located on linear plasmids. These genes code for variable major proteins (VMPs) located on the spirochete's outer-membrane surface. This antigenic variation, generated by sequential expression of previously silent *vmp* genes for serotype-specific VMPs, allows the borreliae to escape the immune response of the host and results in the relapse phenomenon characteristic of infection with these organisms.

EPIDEMIOLOGY Louse-Borne Relapsing Fever Body lice (*Pediculus humanus* var. *corporis*) become infected with *B. recurrentis* by feeding on spirochetemic humans, the only reservoirs of infection. In lice, *B. recurrentis* spirochetes are found almost exclusively in the hemolymph; humans acquire infection when infected body lice are crushed and their fluids contaminate mucous membranes or bite wounds or other breaks in the skin (such as abrasions caused by scratching of pruritic louse bites). Louse-borne spirochetes are transmitted neither by the bite of a louse (anterior station transmission) nor by inoculation of louse feces (posterior station transmission). Lice have a short life span, feed at frequent intervals, and survive only a few days off the human host. Louse infestation of patients and the environmental circumstances of exposure are easily identified. Persons of all ages and both sexes are equally susceptible to infection.

LBRF has severely affected military and civilian populations disrupted by war and other disasters. During the Industrial Revolution, the disease was common among slum dwellers, prisoners, and other impoverished and overcrowded groups in Great Britain and Europe. Outbreaks occurred in the mid-nineteenth century in Philadelphia and other east coast cities and in the mining camps of the western United States. LBRF and louse-borne typhus were epidemic in eastern Europe and in Russia in the early part of the twentieth century. During the Second World War, LBRF spilled out of Ethiopia and spread across the Sudan to West Africa, causing many thousands of cases and deaths. Most recently, outbreaks of LBRF have occurred in northeastern Africa among refugees fleeing war and famine. LBRF has disappeared over large regions of the world as improvements have been made in standards of living, sanitation, and hygiene; it is now an important endemic disease only in northeastern Africa, especially the highlands of Ethiopia, where an estimated 10,000 cases occur annually. In Ethiopia, the disease affects mostly homeless men crowded together in unhygienic circumstances, especially during the cool rainy season, when it is more difficult for them to change and wash their clothing. LBRF does not pose a significant risk to tourists or other casual visitors but can be acquired from lice by persons (such as relief workers) in intimate contact with those affected as well as through accidental needle stick or mucocutaneous contact with infected blood.

Tick-Borne Relapsing Fever Soft ticks (Argasidae, *Ornithodoros* spp.) transmit TBRF. The ticks become infected by feeding on spirochetemic mammalian hosts. Except for *Borrelia duttoni* (a prominent cause of TBRF in sub-Saharan Africa), TBRF borreliae are zoonotic disease agents found naturally in rodents (rats, mice, chipmunks, and squirrels) and in lagomorphs (rabbits and hares). In ticks, TBRF borreliae invade all tissues, including the salivary glands and the ovaries. The spirochetes are transmitted to humans and animals via saliva and coxal fluid when the tick feeds. Infection in ticks is transmitted vertically from one stage to the next; in some tick species, infection is transmitted transovarially over several generations. Soft ticks are hardy and can survive for 10 years or more with only an occasional blood meal. These ticks feed painlessly, relatively quickly (for 20 to 45 minutes), and usually at night while

hosts are sleeping; thus patients with TBRF are often unaware of tick exposures.

TBRF borreliae are widely distributed throughout the world. TBRF is most highly endemic in sub-Saharan Africa but is also found in countries of the Mediterranean littoral, Middle Eastern states, southern Russia, the Indian subcontinent, and China. In the United States, this disease occurs west of the Mississippi River, especially in mountainous areas, where *B. hermsii* is the causative agent. TBRF is reported at low frequency throughout Latin America. The disease typically occurs sporadically or in small—often familial—clusters. Infected soft ticks may cause repeated infections among persons living or sleeping in the same dwelling. In sub-Saharan Africa, *O. moubata*, the vector of *B. duttoni*, infests native huts and rest houses, hiding in crevices of floors and walls during the day and emerging at night to feed on sleeping inhabitants. In the United States, *B. hermsii* infections most often occur during spring and summer months in mountain cabins. Infections of humans are sometimes precipitated by the disappearance of rodents (e.g., as a result of epizootic plague) that nest in foundations, wall spaces, and attics and that serve as the usual maintenance hosts for *O. hermsi* ticks. Outbreaks caused by *B. hermsii* have recently taken place among persons staying in rustic cabins along the north rim of the Grand Canyon and in the mountains of California, Idaho, and Colorado. Rodent-infested caves in southwestern states are associated with occasional cases of human infection with *B. turicatae*.

PATHOGENESIS AND PATHOLOGY In humans, relapsing-fever borreliae penetrate the skin or mucous membranes, multiply in the blood, and circulate in great numbers during febrile periods. The organisms also may be found in the liver, spleen, central nervous

Table 177-1

Characteristics and Distribution of Louse-Borne and Tick-Borne Borreliae

Borrelia Species	Arthropod Vector	Animal Reservoir	Distribution	Type(s) of Relapsing Fever
B. recurrentis*	Pediculus humanus var. corporis	Humans	Worldwide	Louse-borne, epidemic
B. duttoni	Ornithodoros moubata	Humans	Central, eastern, southern Africa	East African tick-borne, endemic
B. hispanica	O. erraticus (large variety)	Rodents	Spain, Portugal, Morocco, Algeria, Tunisia	Hispano-African tick-borne
B. crocidurae, B. merionesi, B. microti, B. dipodilli	O. erraticus (small variety)	Rodents	Morocco, Libya, Egypt, Iran, Turkey, Senegal, Kenya	North African tick-borne
B. persica	O. tholozani†	Rodents	From western China and Kashmir to Iraq and Egypt, former USSR, India	Asiatic-African tick-borne
B. caucasica	O. verrucosus	Rodents	Caucasus to Iraq	Caucasian tick-borne
B. latyschewii	O. tartakovskyi	Rodents	Iran, Central Asia	Caucasian tick-borne
B. hermsii	O. hermsi	Rodents	Western United States	American tick-borne
B. turicatae	O. turicata	Rodents	Southwestern United States	American tick-borne
B. parkeri	O. parkeri	Rodents	Western United States	American tick-borne
B. mazzotti	O. talaje‡	Rodents	Southern United States, Mexico, Central and South America	American tick-borne
B. venezuelensis	O. rudis§	Rodents	Central and South America	American tick-borne

* Synonyms: *B. obermeyeri*, *B. novyi*.
† Synonyms: *O. papillipes*, *O. crossi*?
‡ Synonym: *O. dugesi*?
§ Synonym: *O. venezuelensis*.

SOURCE: From Burgdorfer and Schwan.

system, bone marrow, and other tissues and may be sequestered at these sites during periods of remission. The severity of disease is positively related to spirochete density in the blood; however, the role of borreliae in causing the systemic manifestations of relapsing fever is incompletely understood. Even though the pathophysiologic manifestations of the disease resemble responses to endotoxin, and although plasma from some patients with relapsing fever coagulates *Limulus* amebocyte lysates, borreliae and other spirochetes have not been shown to contain endotoxin. Infection with *B. recurrentis* does, however, activate protein mediators of inflammation, such as Hageman factor, prekallikrein, and proteins of the complement system; further, a spirochetal heat-stable pyrogenic factor stimulates mononuclear phagocytes to express increased amounts of leukocyte pyrogen and thromboplastin.

The Jarisch-Herxheimer reaction in LBRF patients is associated with a release of various cytokines into the plasma, including tumor necrosis factor, interleukin 6, interleukin 8, and C-reactive protein. These mediators of inflammation and fever most likely underlie many manifestations of relapsing fever, especially the complex series of pathophysiologic events that occur while spirochetes are being cleared rapidly from the blood, either during a spontaneous crisis or in response to antibiotic treatment. Meptazinol, a partial opioid agonist, diminishes the Jarisch-Herxheimer reaction in LBRF; this effect may indicate an exhaustion of endogenous opioids.

Findings at autopsy of relapsing-fever patients most often include enlargement of the liver and spleen and variable edema and swelling of other organs, such as the brain, lungs, and kidneys. On microscopic examination, the spleen is congested and contains multiple microabscesses of mononuclear cells that replace the white pulp, the myocardium displays diffuse histiocytic inflammation and interstitial edema, and the liver has areas of midzonal necrosis. Petechial hemorrhages are commonly evident over the surfaces of the meninges, pleura, heart, spleen, liver, kidneys, and mesentery. Subcapsular and parenchymal hemorrhagic infarcts of the spleen, heart, liver, and brain are sometimes grossly visible. Icterus is a common finding in severe and fatal cases of relapsing fever.

CLINICAL MANIFESTATIONS The clinical manifestations of LBRF and TBRF are similar. The mean incubation period is 7 days (range, 2 to 18 days), and the onset of illness is sudden, with fever, headache, shaking chills, sweats, myalgias, and arthralgias. The arthralgia of relapsing fever can be severe, involving small and large joints, but there is no evidence of arthritis. Dizziness, nausea, and vomiting are common. Sleep may be difficult and is sometimes accompanied by disturbing dreams. The patient is coherent but withdrawn, thirsty, and disinterested in food and other outside stimuli. The fever is high from the first (with a usual temperature of ≥40°C), is most often irregular in pattern, and is sometimes accompanied by delirium. Patients become progressively prostrate as the disease advances. The pulse is rapid and the patient is mildly tachypneic. Meningism may be found. The conjunctivae are often injected, and the patient usually exhibits photophobia. The sclerae are sometimes icteric, most commonly in the later stages of illness. The mucous membranes are often dry, and the patient is mildly dehydrated. Scattered petechiae develop on the trunk, extremities, and mucous membranes in one-third or more of LBRF patients and in fewer TBRF patients. A nonproductive cough is common, but chest sounds are usually normal; pleuritic pain and an accompanying pleuritic rub are sometimes noted. Cardiac findings are compatible with a high-output state; tachycardia and summation gallop are common. Upper quadrant abdominal tenderness and slight or moderate enlargement of the spleen and liver frequently characterize the acute phase of illness.

Epistaxis and blood-tinged sputum are common complications; clinically apparent gastrointestinal and central nervous system hemorrhage occur infrequently. Other complications of variable incidence include iridocyclitis, meningitis, coma, isolated cranial-nerve palsy, pneumonitis, myocarditis, and rupture of the spleen. Infection during pregnancy can result in spontaneous abortion, stillbirth, or neonatal infection. Life-threatening complications are unusual in otherwise healthy persons, especially if the illness is diagnosed and treated early.

Without treatment, symptoms intensify over a 2- to 7-day period (average, 5 days in LBRF and 3 days in TBRF), ending in a spontaneous crisis during which spirochetes disappear from the circulation. Treatment with one of the rapidly acting antibiotics, such as erythromycin, a tetracycline, or chloramphenicol, regularly precipitates a Jarisch-Herxheimer reaction within 1 to 4 h. This reaction is indistinguishable from the spontaneous crisis; its severity is positively correlated with the density of spirochetes in the blood at the time of treatment. In the first phase of the crisis or reaction (the *chill phase*), rigors and rising fever are accompanied by an increasing metabolic rate, alveolar hyperventilation, high cardiac output, increasing peripheral vascular resistance, and decreased pulmonary arterial pressure. The body temperature commonly rises to 41.5°C or higher. This high fever is accompanied often by agitation and confusion and sometimes by delirium. Fever can be partially controlled by the use of a cooling blanket and ice packs and by sponging of the patient with tepid water and alcohol. The chill phase terminates after 10 to 30 min, giving way to a *flush phase* characterized by a fall in body temperature, drenching sweats, and sometimes (more commonly in LBRF) a potentially dangerous fall in systemic arterial pressure and rise in pulmonary arterial pressure. Although cardiac output is maintained at high levels, the effective circulating blood volume decreases as peripheral vascular resistance falls. Vital signs must be monitored carefully during this period of the reaction, which usually lasts 8 h or less. Clinical and electrocardiographic evidence of myocarditis and myocardial dysfunction includes a prolonged QT$_c$ interval, a third heart sound (S$_3$), elevated central venous pressure, arterial hypotension, and pulmonary edema.

The crisis is followed by a period of exhaustion, sleep, and a rapid and uneventful recovery. Not uncommonly, in the first week of convalescence, patients experience 1 or 2 days of mild fever unassociated with detectable spirochetemia. In untreated cases, spirochetemia and symptoms may recur after a period of several days or weeks (average interval to first relapse, 9 days in LBRF and 7 days in TBRF). Only one or two relapses characteristically occur in untreated LBRF, while as many as 10 (average, three) can occur in untreated TBRF. In most cases, the illness becomes shorter and milder and the afebrile intervals longer with each relapse. Because of the great antigenic variation among *Borrelia* strains, infection does not confer protective immunity, and repeated infections of the same individual have been recorded.

Diseases that should be considered in the differential diagnosis of relapsing fever or that may complicate relapsing fever include typhus fever, typhoid, nontyphoid salmonellosis, malaria, dengue and other arboviral illnesses, tuberculosis, and leptospirosis. In the United States, the geographic distribution of Colorado tick fever overlaps that of TBRF, and the two diseases have similar manifestations early in their courses.

LABORATORY FINDINGS AND DIAGNOSIS The diagnosis of relapsing fever is confirmed most easily by the detection of spirochetes in blood, bone marrow aspirates, or cerebrospinal fluid. Motile spirochetes can be seen when fresh blood is examined by darkfield microscopy, and fixed organisms are clearly visible in Wright-, Giemsa-, or acridine orange-stained preparations of thin or dehemoglobinized thick smears of peripheral blood or buffy-coat preparations (Fig. 177-1). Organisms are found in blood taken during periods of fever preceding the crisis; smears from 70 percent or more of LBRF patients and from fewer TBRF patients are positive. In reference laboratories, relapsing-fever spirochetes are cultured from blood by the inoculation of BSK medium or by the intraperitoneal inoculation of immature laboratory mice. The detection of agglutinins against *Proteus* OX-K (Weil-Felix reaction) in convalescent-phase serum supports the diagnosis. Serum antibodies to *Borrelia* can be detected by enzyme immunoassays, but these tests are unstandardized and subject to insensitivity due to antigenic variations among strains. Serologic cross-reactions occur with other spirochetes, including *Borrelia burgdorferi*, the agent of Lyme disease, and *Treponema pallidum*.

FIGURE 177-1 Blood smear (dehemoglobinized thick film) from a patient with louse-borne relapsing fever, showing multiple spirochetes (Wright's stain, × 600).

Other laboratory findings in relapsing fever are generally nonspecific. The leukocyte count is normal or moderately elevated, with an unremarkable cell differential. Serum bilirubin levels are generally only slightly elevated. Thrombocytopenia (mean platelet count about 50,000/μL) is evident in LBRF patients at admission and rebounds during early convalescence. Prothrombin and partial thromboplastin times are moderately prolonged during acute illness, as are standardized bleeding times. Fibrinogen concentrations in the blood are normal, and fibrinolysis is mild or absent. Results of the Rumpel-Leede tourniquet test are negative, despite the presence of petechiae.

℞ TREATMENT

Relapsing-fever borreliae are exquisitely sensitive to antibiotics. Treatment with erythromycin, a tetracycline, chloramphenicol, or penicillin produces rapid clearance of spirochetes and a remission of symptoms (Table 177-2). For children less than 9 years of age and for pregnant women, erythromycin and penicillin are the preferred drugs. The use of delayed-release intramuscular penicillin may prolong or delay the clearance of spirochetes and attenuate the accompanying Jarisch-Herxheimer reaction, but this response is not predictable; furthermore, single-dose penicillin treatment sometimes results in relapse of spirochetemia and symptoms. Although a single dose of erythromycin, a tetracycline, or chloramphenicol is highly effective in the treatment of LBRF, less is known about the efficacy of single-dose treatment of TBRF. Empirical treatment of TBRF for 7 days is therefore recommended to reduce the risk of persisting or

relapsing borreliosis. Glucocorticoids and nonsteroidal anti-inflammatory agents do not prevent or significantly modify the cardiopulmonary disturbances of the Jarisch-Herxheimer reaction, although hydrocortisone and acetaminophen given at the same time as antibiotics reduce peak body temperature. Close monitoring of fluid balance, arterial and venous pressures, and myocardial function is advised in supportive management of the Jarisch-Herxheimer reaction in LBRF patients. The management of patients with myocardial dysfunction requires caution in the administration of intravenous fluids and, in some cases, rapid digitalization. Bleeding is not controlled by heparin, and clinical studies do not suggest that disseminated intravascular coagulopathy is important. Vitamin K and other soluble vitamins are sometimes given to counter dietary deficiencies in LBRF patients. Because postural hypotension is often pronounced during the acute phase of relapsing fever and in the early stage of recovery, patients should be assisted when arising from bed.

Untreated LBRF has a high case-fatality rate, especially in persons in otherwise poor health, such as those in famine-affected populations. The fatality rate among treated persons is usually less than 5 percent. In general, TBRF is a milder disease than LBRF: the spontaneous crisis and the Jarisch-Herxheimer reactions are less pronounced and the case-fatality rates are lower for TBRF than for LBRF.

PREVENTION AND CONTROL LBRF can be prevented by elimination of circumstances that promote louse infestation (crowding, poverty, homelessness), by use of personal hygienic practices that eliminate or reduce numbers of body lice (bathing, washing clothes, changing clothes at frequent intervals), and by application of acaricides to clothing. Secondary complications and the spread of infection can be prevented by early case detection and treatment. Historically, outbreaks of LBRF have been controlled by mass delousing. In situations like those in refugee camps, individuals, their clothes, and their bedding should be deloused with appropriate acaricides, such as lindane (1% dust), malathion (1% dust), or pyrethrins; in addition, provisions should be made for washing and changing of clothing. Impregnation of clothing with permethrin, a residual acaricide, can provide long-term protection against infestation. In outbreaks of fever that involve louse-infested populations, empirical single-dose treatment with doxycycline will be effective against typhus as well as LBRF. *B. recurrentis* has a fragile life cycle and is eradicable.

TBRF can be prevented by the avoidance of rodent- and tick-infested dwellings and infested natural sites in areas endemic for relapsing fever. Limiting rodent access to the foundations and attics of homes and vacation cabins and eliminating harborage for rodents in and around these dwellings reduce the potential for tick exposure. Rodents and rodent nests should be removed from infested buildings and their surroundings. Tick harborages of infested buildings or other circumscribed sites, such as rodent burrows and nests in hollow logs surrounding dwellings and in rodent-infested caves, can be chemically treated by pest-control specialists using various acaricides, such as carbaryl, diazinon, chlorpyrifos, pyrethrins, and malathion. Persons who enter tick-infested sites can protect themselves by wearing clothing that denies ticks access to the skin, by applying repellents to exposed skin and to clothing, and by applying an acaricide containing permethrin to clothing. Reporting of suspected cases of relapsing fever to public health authorities is important so that an epidemiologic investigation and control measures can be initiated promptly.

BIBLIOGRAPHY

BARBOUR AG: Antigenic variation of relapsing fever *Borrelia* species. Annu Rev Microbiol 44:155, 1990

BURGDORFER W, SCHWAN TG: *Borrelia*, in *Manual of Clinical Microbiology* 6, PR Murray et al (eds). Washington, DC, American Society for Microbiology, 1995, pp 626–635

Table 177-2

Antibiotic Treatment of Louse-Borne and Tick-Borne Relapsing Fever in Adults

Medication	Louse-Borne Relapsing Fever (Single Dose)	Tick-Borne Relapsing Fever (7-Day Schedule)
Oral		
Erythromycin	500 mg	500 mg q 6 h
Tetracycline	500 mg	500 mg q 6 h
Doxycycline	100 mg	100 mg q12 h
Chloramphenicol	500 mg	500 mg q 6 h
Parenteral*		
Erythromycin	500 mg	500 mg q 6 h
Tetracycline	250 mg	250 mg q 6 h
Doxycycline	100 mg	100 mg q 12 h
Chloramphenicol	500 mg	500 mg q 6 h
Penicillin G (procaine)	600,000 IU	600,000 IU daily

* For tick-borne relapsing fever, parenteral therapy is used only until oral treatment is tolerated.

FEKADE D et al: Prevention of Jarisch-Herxheimer reactions by treatment with antibodies against tumor necrosis factor α. N Engl J Med 335:311, 1996

HORTON JM, BLASER MJ: The spectrum of relapsing fever in the Rocky Mountains. Arch Intern Med 145:871, 1985

PERINE PL, TEKLU B: Antibiotic treatment of louse-borne relapsing fever in Ethiopia: A report of 377 cases. Am J Trop Med Hyg 32:1096, 1983

SPACH DH et al: Tick-borne diseases in the United States. N Engl J Med 329:936, 1993

| 178 | *Allen C. Steere* |

LYME BORRELIOSIS

DEFINITION Lyme borreliosis, a tick-transmitted spirochetal illness, usually begins with a characteristic expanding skin lesion, erythema migrans (EM; stage 1, localized infection). After several days or weeks, the spirochete may spread hematogenously to many different sites (stage 2, disseminated infection). Possible manifestations of disseminated infection include secondary annular skin lesions, meningitis, cranial or peripheral neuritis, carditis, atrioventricular nodal block, or migratory musculoskeletal pain. Months to years later (usually after periods of latent infection), intermittent or chronic arthritis, chronic encephalopathy or polyneuropathy, or acrodermatitis may develop (stage 3, persistent infection). Most patients experience early symptoms of the illness during the summer, but the infection may not become symptomatic until it progresses to stage 2 or 3. Despite regional variations, the basic stages of the illness are similar worldwide.

ETIOLOGIC AGENT *Borrelia burgdorferi*, the causative agent of the disease, is a fastidious, microaerophilic bacterium that grows best at 33°C in a complex liquid medium called Barbour, Stoenner, Kelly (BSK) medium. Culture of the spirochete from clinical specimens (except for biopsy samples of skin at sites of EM or acrodermatitis) has been difficult. Three groups of *B. burgdorferi* organisms, together referred to as *B. burgdorferi sensu lato*, have been identified, and more groups surely exist. To date, most North American strains have belonged to the first group, *B. burgdorferi sensu stricto*. Although all three of the identified groups have been found in Europe and Asia, most isolates there have been strains of group 2 (*B. garinii*) or group 3 (*B. afzelii*). These differences may well account for the clinical variations in the disease in different geographic regions.

EPIDEMIOLOGY The distribution of Lyme borreliosis correlates closely with the geographic ranges of certain ixodid ticks—*Ixodes dammini* (also called *I. scapularis*), *I. pacificus*, *I. ricinus*, and *I. persulcatus*. *I. dammini* is the principal vector in the northeastern United States from Massachusetts to Maryland and in the midwestern states of Wisconsin and Minnesota. Surveys in these regions have documented infection in at least 20 percent of *I. dammini* ticks; most cases of Lyme disease in the United States have occurred in these areas. *I. pacificus* is the vector in the western states of California and Oregon. The disease is acquired throughout Europe (from Great Britain to Scandinavia to European Russia), where *I. ricinus* is the vector, and in Asian Russia, China, and Japan, where *I. persulcatus* is the vector. These ticks transmit other diseases that may have similar symptoms. In the United States, *I. dammini* also transmits babesiosis and ehrlichiosis; in Europe and Asia, *I. ricinus* and *I. persulcatus* also transmit tick-borne encephalitis.

The *Ixodes* ticks have different animal hosts. For *I. dammini*, the white-footed mouse is the preferred host of the immature larval and nymphal ticks. It is critical that both of the tick's immature stages feed on the same host, because the life cycle of the spirochete depends on horizontal transmission: in early summer from infected nymphs to mice and in late summer from infected mice to larvae, which then molt to become the infected nymphs that will begin the cycle again the following year. White-tailed deer, which are not involved in the

life cycle of the spirochete, are the preferred host for *I. dammini*'s adult stage and seem to be critical to the survival of the tick.

Lyme disease is now the most common vector-borne infection in the United States, with more than 50,000 cases reported to the Centers for Disease Control and Prevention (CDC) during the past 10 years. Cases have been reported in 47 states, but the life cycle of *B. burgdorferi* has been identified in only 19 states. As already mentioned, most new cases have their onset during the summer months. Cases have occurred in association with hiking, camping, or hunting trips and with residence in wooded or rural areas. Persons of all ages and both sexes are affected.

PATHOGENESIS After injection into the skin, *B. burgdorferi* may migrate outward, producing EM, and may spread hematogenously to other organs. Spread within the host is probably facilitated through binding to the spirochete's surface by human plasminogen and urokinase-type plasminogen activator, which activates plasmin, a potent protease. The spirochete can adhere to many types of mammalian cells; it binds specifically to certain ubiquitous host integrin receptors in the extracellular matrix, to vitronectin and fibronectin, and to matrix glycosaminoglycans. *B. burgdorferi* seems to have a particular tropism for tissues of the skin, nervous system, and joints, from all of which it has been cultured, seen in histologic sections, or (more commonly) detected (via its DNA) by the polymerase chain reaction (PCR). These findings and the response of all stages of the disease to antibiotic therapy suggest that the organism persists in affected tissues throughout the illness, but the mechanisms of persistent infection are not yet clear.

The immune response in Lyme disease develops gradually. After the first several weeks of infection, mononuclear cells generally exhibit heightened responsiveness to *B. burgdorferi* antigens, and evidence of B-cell hyperactivity is found, including elevated total serum IgM levels, cryoprecipitates, and circulating immune complexes. Titers of specific IgM antibody to *B. burgdorferi* peak between the third and sixth week after disease onset. The specific IgG response develops gradually over months, with response to an increasing array of 12 or more spirochetal polypeptides and maximal expansion during the period of arthritis. The spirochete is a potent inducer of proinflammatory cytokines, including tumor necrosis factor α and interleukin 1β. Histologic examination of all affected tissues reveals an infiltration of lymphocytes and plasma cells with some degree of vascular damage (including mild vasculitis or hypervascular occlusion), suggesting that the spirochete may have been present in or around blood vessels.

CLINICAL MANIFESTATIONS **Early Infection: Stage 1 (Localized Infection)** After an incubation period of 3 to 32 days, EM, which occurs at the site of the tick bite, usually begins as a red macule or papule that expands slowly to form a large annular lesion, most often with a bright red outer border and partial central clearing. Because of the small size of ixodid ticks, most patients do not remember the preceding tick bite. The center of the lesion sometimes becomes intensely erythematous and indurated, vesicular, or necrotic. In other instances, the expanding lesion remains an even, intense red; several red rings are found within an outside ring; or the central area turns blue before the lesion clears. Although EM can be located anywhere, the thigh, groin, and axilla are particularly common sites. The lesion is warm but not often painful. Perhaps as many as 25 percent of patients do not exhibit this characteristic skin manifestation.

Early Infection: Stage 2 (Disseminated Infection) Within days or weeks after the onset of EM, the organism often spreads hematogenously to many sites. In these cases patients frequently develop secondary annular skin lesions similar in appearance to the initial lesion. Skin involvement is frequently accompanied by severe headache, mild stiffness of the neck, fever, chills, migratory musculoskeletal pain, arthralgias, and profound malaise and fatigue. Less common manifestations include generalized lymphadenopathy or splenomegaly, hepatitis, sore throat, nonproductive cough, conjunctivitis, iritis, or testicular swelling. Except for fatigue and lethargy, which are often constant, the early signs and symptoms of Lyme disease are typically intermittent and changing. Even in untreated patients, the early symptoms usually become less severe or disappear within several weeks.

Symptoms suggestive of meningeal irritation may develop early in Lyme disease when EM is present but usually are not associated with cerebrospinal fluid (CSF) pleocytosis or an objective neurologic deficit. After several weeks or months, about 15 percent of untreated patients develop frank neurologic abnormalities, including meningitis, subtle encephalitic signs, cranial neuritis (including bilateral facial palsy), motor or sensory radiculoneuropathy, mononeuritis multiplex, or myelitis—alone or in various combinations. In the United States, the usual pattern consists of fluctuating symptoms of meningitis accompanied by facial palsy and peripheral radiculoneuropathy. Lymphocytic pleocytosis (about 100 cells per microliter) is found in CSF, often along with elevated protein levels and normal or slightly low glucose concentrations. In Europe and Asia, the first neurologic sign is characteristically radicular pain, which is followed by the development of CSF pleocytosis (called Bannwarth's syndrome), but meningeal or encephalitic signs are frequently absent. These early neurologic abnormalities usually resolve completely within months, but chronic neurologic disease may occur later.

Within several weeks after the onset of illness, about 8 percent of patients develop cardiac involvement. The most common abnormality is a fluctuating degree of atrioventricular block (first-degree, Wenckebach, or complete heart block). Some patients have more diffuse cardiac involvement, including electrocardiographic changes indicative of acute myopericarditis, left ventricular dysfunction evident on radionuclide scans, or (in rare cases) cardiomegaly or pancarditis. Cardiac involvement usually lasts for only a few weeks but may recur. One case of chronic cardiomyopathy caused by *B. burgdorferi* has been reported.

During this stage, musculoskeletal pain is common. The typical pattern consists of migratory pain in joints, tendons, bursae, muscles, or bones (usually without joint swelling) lasting for hours or days and affecting one or two locations at a time.

Late Infection: Stage 3 (Persistent Infection) Months after the onset of infection, about 60 percent of patients in the United States who have received no antibiotic treatment develop frank arthritis. The typical pattern comprises intermittent attacks of oligoarticular arthritis in large joints (especially the knees), lasting for weeks to months in a given joint. Small joints and periarticular sites also may be affected, primarily during early attacks. The number of patients who continue to have recurrent attacks decreases each year. However, in a small percentage of cases, involvement of large joints—usually one or both knees—becomes chronic and may lead to erosion of cartilage and bone. These patients have a higher frequency of the class II major histocompatibility complex allele HLA-DR4 than patients with brief Lyme arthritis or normal control subjects.

White cell counts in joint fluid range from 500 to 110,000/μL (average, 25,000/μL); most of these cells are polymorphonuclear leukocytes. Tests for rheumatoid factor or antinuclear antibodies usually give negative results. Examination of synovial biopsy samples reveals fibrin deposits, villous hypertrophy, vascular proliferation, microangiopathic lesions, and a heavy infiltration of lymphocytes and plasma cells.

Although less common, chronic neurologic involvement may also become apparent months or years after the onset of infection, sometimes following long periods of latent infection. The most common form of chronic central nervous system involvement is subtle encephalopathy affecting memory, mood, or sleep and often accompanied by axonal polyneuropathy manifested as either distal paresthesias or spinal radicular pain. Patients with encephalopathy frequently have evidence of memory impairment in neuropsychological tests and abnormal results in CSF analyses. In cases with polyneuropathy, electromyography generally shows extensive abnormalities of proximal and distal nerve segments. Encephalomyelitis or leukoencephalitis, a rare manifestation of Lyme borreliosis, is a severe neurologic disorder that may include spastic parapareses, upper motor-neuron bladder dysfunction, and lesions in the periventricular white matter. The prolonged course of chronic neuroborreliosis following periods of latent infection is reminiscent of tertiary neurosyphilis.

Acrodermatitis chronica atrophicans, the late skin manifestation of the disorder, has been associated primarily with *B. afzelii* infection in Europe and Asia. It has been observed primarily in elderly women. The skin lesions, which are usually found on the acral surface of an arm or leg, begin insidiously with reddish-violaceous discoloration; they become sclerotic or atrophic over a period of years.

DIAGNOSIS Lyme disease is usually diagnosed by the recognition of a characteristic clinical picture with serologic confirmation. Although serologic testing may yield negative results during the first several weeks of infection, most patients have a positive antibody response to *B. burgdorferi* after that time. The limitation of serologic tests is that they do not clearly distinguish between active and inactive infection. Patients with previous Lyme disease—particularly in cases progressing to late stages—often remain seropositive for years, even after adequate antibiotic treatment. In addition, some patients are seropositive because of asymptomatic infection. If these individuals subsequently develop another illness, the positive serologic test for Lyme disease may cause diagnostic confusion. On the other hand, a few patients who receive inadequate antibiotic therapy during the first several weeks of infection develop subtle joint or neurologic symptoms but are seronegative. The important point is that seronegative Lyme disease is usually a mild, attenuated illness.

For serologic analysis in Lyme disease, the CDC recommends a two-step approach in which samples are first tested by ELISA and equivocal or positive results are then tested by western blotting. During the first month of infection, both IgM and IgG responses to the spirochete should be determined, preferably in both acute- and convalescent-phase serum samples. Approximately 20 to 30 percent of patients have a positive response detectable in acute-phase samples, whereas about 70 to 80 percent have a positive response during convalescence (2 to 4 weeks later). After that time, the great majority of patients continue to have a positive IgG antibody response, and a single test (that for IgG) is usually sufficient. In persons with illness of longer than 1 month's duration, a positive IgM test result alone is likely to be false-positive. According to current criteria adopted by the CDC, an IgM western blot is considered positive if two of the following three bands are present: 23, 39, and 41 kDa. However, the combination of the 23- and 41-kDa bands may still represent a false-positive result. An IgG blot is considered positive if 5 of the following 10 bands are present: 18, 23, 28, 30, 39, 41, 45, 58, 66, and 93 kDa.

Because serologic tests do not distinguish between active and inactive infection, tests that detect the spirochete directly are being researched. *B. burgdorferi* may be cultured from skin lesions of patients with the disorder, but its culture from other sites has been a low-yield proposition. Detection of spirochetal DNA by PCR may serve as a substitute for culture in cases of Lyme arthritis. In a recent study, *B. burgdorferi* DNA was detected in synovial fluid samples from 75 (85 percent) of 88 patients and in none of 64 control samples. However, the sensitivity of PCR determinations in CSF from patients with neuroborreliosis has not been as high. The role of PCR in the detection of *B. burgdorferi* DNA from blood or urine samples is not yet clear.

DIFFERENTIAL DIAGNOSIS The most common problem in diagnosis is to distinguish late Lyme disease from chronic fatigue syndrome or fibromyalgia. This difficulty is compounded by the fact that a small percentage of patients develop these chronic pain or fatigue syndromes in association with or soon after Lyme disease. Compared with Lyme disease, chronic fatigue syndrome (see Chap. 384) or fibromyalgia tends to produce more generalized and disabling symptoms, including marked fatigue, severe headache, diffuse musculoskeletal pain, multiple symmetric tender points in characteristic locations, pain and stiffness in many joints, diffuse dysesthesias, difficulty with concentration, and sleep disturbances. Patients with chronic fatigue syndrome or fibromyalgia lack evidence of joint inflammation; they have normal results in neurologic tests; and they usually have a greater degree of anxiety and depression than patients with chronic neuroborreliosis.

℞ TREATMENT

As outlined in the algorithm in Fig. 178-1, the various manifestations of Lyme disease can usually be treated successfully with orally administered antibiotics; the exceptions are objective neurologic abnormalities, which seem to require intravenous therapy. For early Lyme disease, doxycycline (100 mg twice a day) is effective in men and in nonpregnant women. An advantage of this regimen is that it is also effective against the agent of human granulocytic ehrlichiosis, which is transmitted by the same tick that transmits the Lyme disease agent. Amoxicillin (500 mg three times a day), cefuroxime axetil (500 mg twice a day), and erythromycin (250 mg four times a day) or its congeners are second-, third-, and fourth-choice alternatives, respectively. In children, amoxicillin is effective (50 mg/kg per day, but not more than 2 g/d) in divided doses; in cases of penicillin allergy, cefuroxime axetil or erythromycin may be used. For patients with infection localized to the skin, a 10-day course of therapy is generally sufficient; in contrast, for patients with disseminated infection, a 20- to 30-day course is recommended. Approximately 15 percent of patients experience a Jarisch-Herxheimer-like reaction during the first 24 h of therapy.

These oral antibiotic regimens, when given for 30 to 60 days, are effective for the treatment of Lyme arthritis. However, the response to therapy may be slow. A small percentage of patients with arthritis, particularly those with the HLA-DR4 allele and an immune response to the OspA or OspB protein of the spirochete, do not respond to antimicrobial therapy. Treatment with anti-inflammatory agents or synovectomy may be successful in such cases.

For objective neurologic abnormalities (with the possible exception of facial palsy alone), parenteral antibiotic therapy seems to be necessary. Intravenous ceftriaxone (2 g/d for 4 weeks) is most commonly used for this purpose, but intravenous cefotaxime (2 g three times a day) or intravenous penicillin G (20 million units per day in divided doses) for the same duration may also be effective. In patients with high-degree atrioventricular block or a PR interval of greater than 0.3 s, intravenous therapy for at least part of the course and cardiac monitoring are recommended. In patients with complete heart block or congestive heart failure, glucocorticoids may be of benefit if antimicrobial therapy alone does not result in improvement within 24 h.

It is unclear how and whether asymptomatic infection should be treated, but patients with such infection are often given a course of oral antibiotics. The appropriate treatment for Lyme disease during pregnancy is also unclear. Because the risk of maternal-fetal transmission seems to be very low, standard therapy for the documented stage and manifestation of the illness may be sufficient. Relapse may follow the use of any of the antibiotic regimens for Lyme disease, and a second course of therapy may be necessary. On the other hand, in patients who develop chronic fatigue syndrome or fibromyalgia after Lyme disease, further antibiotic therapy does not seem to be of benefit.

The risk of infection with *B. burgdorferi* after a recognized tick bite is so low that antibiotic prophylaxis is not routinely indicated. However, if the tick is engorged, if follow-up is difficult, or if the patient is quite anxious, therapy with amoxicillin or doxycycline for 10 days is likely to prevent Lyme disease. A vaccine for Lyme disease is currently being tested but is not yet available.

PROGNOSIS The response to treatment is best early in the disease. Later treatment of Lyme borreliosis is still effective, but convalescence may be longer. Eventually, most patients recover with minimal or no residual deficit.

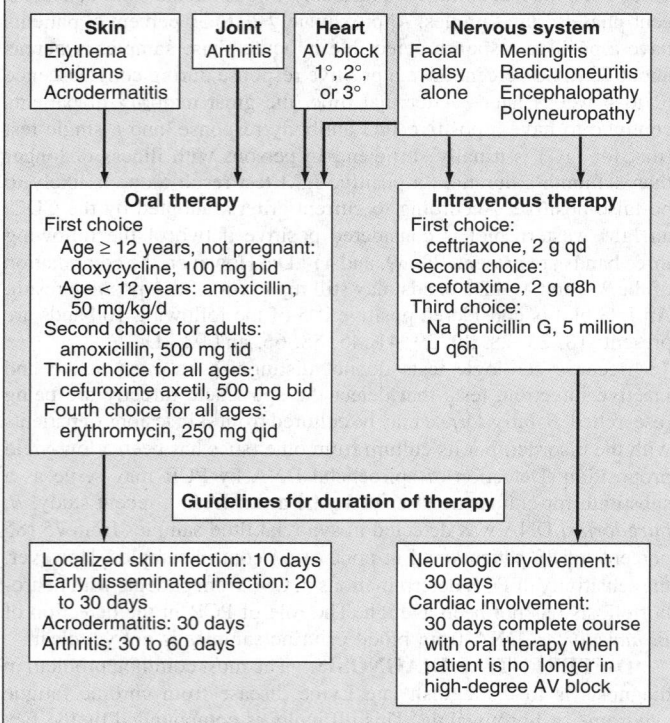

FIGURE 178-1 Algorithm for the treatment of the various acute or chronic manifestations of Lyme borreliosis. Relapse may occur with any of these regimens, and a second course of treatment may be necessary. AV, atrioventricular.

BIBLIOGRAPHY

BARBOUR AG, HAYES SF: Biology of *Borrelia* species. Microbiol Rev 50:381, 1986

DRESSLER F et al: Western blotting in the serodiagnosis of Lyme disease. J Infect Dis 167:392, 1993

LOGIGIAN EL et al: Chronic neurologic manifestations of Lyme disease. N Engl J Med 323:1438, 1990

LUFT BJ et al: Azithromycin compared with amoxicillin in the treatment of erythema migrans. Ann Intern Med 124:785, 1996

MCALISTER HF et al: Lyme carditis: An important cause of reversible heart block. Ann Intern Med 110:339, 1989

NOCTON JJ et al: Detection of *Borrelia burgdorferi* DNA by polymerase chain reaction in synovial fluid in Lyme arthritis. N Engl J Med 330:229, 1994

PACHNER AR, STEERE AC: The triad of neurologic manifestations of Lyme disease: Meningitis, cranial neuritis, and radiculoneuritis. Neurology 35:47, 1985

RAHN DW, MALAWISTA SE: Lyme disease: Recommendations for diagnosis and treatment. Ann Intern Med 114:472, 1991

SAINT GIRONS I et al: Molecular biology of *Borrelia*, bacteria with linear replicons. Microbiology 140:1803, 1994

————: Lyme disease. N Engl J Med 321:586, 1989

———— et al: The early clinical manifestations of Lyme disease. Ann Intern Med 99:76, 1983

———— et al: The clinical evolution of Lyme arthritis. Ann Intern Med 107:725, 1987

———— et al: Treatment of Lyme arthritis. Arthritis Rheum 37:878, 1994

179 | *David Walker, Didier Raoult, Philippe Brouqui,*
Thomas Marrie

RICKETTSIAL DISEASES

The rickettsiae make up a family of gram-negative coccobacilli and short bacilli that grow strictly in eukaryotic cells. Characteristics of these organisms include their intracellular localization and persistence. The rickettsiae move through mammalian reservoirs; they are transmitted by insect vectors. Except for louse-borne typhus, humans are incidental hosts. Only *Coxiella burnetii* (the agent of Q fever) is able to survive for an extended period outside of the reservoir or vector. Clinical infections with rickettsiae can be classified into five general groups: (1) tick- and gamasid mite-borne spotted fever group (SFG) rickettsial diseases; (2) flea- and louse-borne typhus group rickettsial diseases; (3) chigger-borne scrub typhus; (4) ehrlichioses; and (5) Q fever.

TICK- AND MITE-BORNE SPOTTED FEVERS

ROCKY MOUNTAIN SPOTTED FEVER Rocky Mountain spotted fever (RMSF), a severe rickettsial disease, is caused by *Rickettsia rickettsii*, the prototype SFG organism. *R. rickettsii* has two major immunodominant surface-exposed proteins, OmpA and OmpB, which have species-specific conformational epitopes. OmpA functions as an adhesin for the host cell; OmpB, the most abundant outer-membrane protein, shares genetic sequences and limited antigens with typhus group rickettsiae. This small (0.3 μm by 1.0 μm) bacillus has a typical gram-negative cell wall structure (see Chap. 139); its lipopolysaccharide shares antigens mainly within the SFG and, in the quantities found in human infections, is not a potent endotoxin.

RMSF has been documented in 48 states and in Canada, Mexico, Costa Rica, Panama, Colombia, and Brazil. It is transmitted by *Dermacentor variabilis*, the American dog tick, in the eastern two-thirds of the United States and California; by *Dermacentor andersoni*, the Rocky Mountain wood tick, in the western United States; by *Rhipicephalus sanguineus* in Mexico; and by *Amblyomma cajennense* in Mexico and Central and South America. Although it is maintained principally by transovarian transmission from one generation of ticks to the next, *R. rickettsii* can be acquired by uninfected ticks through the ingestion of a blood meal from rickettsemic small mammals.

Humans become infected during the active season of the vector tick species. In northern areas, cases occur mainly in the spring; in warmer southern states, most cases occur from May to September, although some cases are reported in the winter. Four percent of *D. variabilis* ticks carry rickettsiae, the vast majority of which are nonpathogenic species such as *Rickettsia montana* and *Rickettsia bellii*. The likelihood of an individual tick's containing *R. rickettsii* is slight. From 1986 to 1992, approximately 600 cases of RMSF were reported annually. This number is probably an underestimate, since the diagnosis is difficult and reporting is incomplete. The incidence of infection is highest among 5- to 9-year-old children. In the preantibiotic era, the mortality rate was 20 to 25 percent; it still runs around 5 percent, primarily because of delayed diagnosis and delayed treatment. The case-fatality ratio is higher for males than for females and increases with each decade of life above age 20.

Pathogenesis *R. rickettsii* organisms are inoculated into the dermis along with secretions of the tick's salivary glands after ≥6 h of feeding. Rickettsiae spread throughout the body by the lymphatics and the bloodstream, attach via OmpA to the endothelial cell membrane, and induce their own engulfment. Once intracellularly located, they escape rapidly from the phagosome, replicate in the cytosol by binary fission, and spread from cell to cell, propelled by polar polymerization of the host cell's actin (Fig. 179-1). After an incubation period of approximately 1 week (range, 3 to 12 days; the length is

FIGURE 179-1 A spotted fever group rickettsia (r) in the cytosol of a cultured endothelial cell demonstrates a prominent actin tail (arrows), the source of the propulsive force that permits intracellular motion and intercellular spread. Bar = 0.5 μm. (*Courtesy of Dr. Vsevolod L. Popov.*)

dependent on the size of the rickettsial inoculum), numerous foci of contiguous, heavily infected endothelial cells that are extensive enough to manifest as injury develop. *R. rickettsii* is more invasive than other rickettsiae, routinely spreading to infect vascular smooth-muscle cells. Damage to these cells results in increased vascular permeability, edema, the development of a host mononuclear-cell tissue response, and hemorrhage.

Although occlusive thrombosis and ischemic necrosis are often cited as the pathologic basis for tissue and organ injury in RMSF, it is in fact increased vascular permeability, with resulting edema, hypovolemia, and ischemia, that is responsible. Indeed, immunohistologic studies of severely infected humans and animals have demonstrated numerous zones of infected endothelium, only a small proportion of which contain thrombi. The thrombi are usually located to one side of the lumen, which is not occluded. These hemostatic plugs appear to be an appropriate host response rather than a pathogenic process. Consumption of platelets may result in thrombocytopenia in up to half of infected patients, but disseminated intravascular coagulation with hypofibrinogenemia is rare in RMSF. Activation of platelets, generation of thrombin, and activation of the fibrinolytic system all appear to be homeostatic physiologic responses to endothelial injury.

Clinical Manifestations Early in the illness, when medical attention usually is first sought, RMSF is difficult to distinguish from many self-limiting viral illnesses. During the first 3 days, fever, headache, malaise, myalgia, nausea, vomiting, and anorexia are the most frequent symptoms. The untreated illness progresses insidiously as vascular infection and injury advance. In one large series, only one-third of patients were diagnosed with presumptive RMSF early in the clinical course and were treated appropriately as outpatients. All too often, RMSF is recognized only when its late severe manifestations, developing at the end of the first week or in the second week of illness in patients without appropriate treatment, prompt admission to the intensive care unit.

The progressive nature of the infection is clearly manifested in the skin. Rash is evident in 14 percent of patients on the first day of illness and in 49 percent during the first 3 days. Despite widespread hematogenous dissemination of rickettsiae to the skin during the incubation period, vascular injury usually makes its appearance between the third and the fifth febrile day as macules up to 5 mm in diameter on the wrists and ankles. Subsequently, similar lesions develop on the remainder of the extremities and the trunk. The pink foci of vasodilation become leaky, with local edema and conversion to maculopapules that blanch on compression. Later, more severe vascular damage results in frank hemorrhage at the center of the maculopapule, creating a petechia that does not disappear upon compression. Effective treatment may delay or abort this sequence of events. In fact, rash does not appear until day 6 or afterward in 20 percent of cases and does not develop at all in around 10 percent of cases, including some patients with severe visceral lesions that result in death. Overall, petechiae occur in about half of cases, developing on or after day 6 in most. Involvement of the palms and soles, often considered diagnostically important, usually occurs relatively late in the course (after day 5 in 43 percent of cases) and does not occur at all in many cases.

The systemic and pulmonary microcirculations are the target of the vascular changes induced by intracellular rickettsial infection, and clinical manifestations reflect the ensuing damage. Widespread increases in vascular permeability result in edema, decreased plasma volume, hypoalbuminemia, reduced serum oncotic pressure, and prerenal azotemia. Hypotension is reported in 17 percent of cases. Extensive infection of the pulmonary microcirculation is associated with noncardiogenic pulmonary edema in the face of normal or near-normal left ventricular function. True cardiac involvement is most frequently manifested as dysrhythmia, which is detected in up to 16 percent of cases. Pulmonary involvement with severe respiratory distress, often requiring mechanical ventilation, is frequently a prominent factor in fatal cases. In one series, 9 of 10 RMSF patients who required mechanical ventilation died.

Central nervous system involvement is the other important clinical feature of RMSF. Encephalitis due to vascular injury, presenting as confusion or lethargy, is apparent in 25 percent of cases. Progressively more severe encephalitis manifests as stupor or delirium, ataxia, coma, and seizures. Numerous other neurologic abnormalities have been seen, including cranial nerve palsies, hearing loss, severe vertigo, nystagmus, dysarthria, aphasia, unilateral corticospinal signs, ankle clonus, extensor toe signs, hyperreflexia, spasticity, fasciculations, athetosis, neurogenic bladder, hemiplegia, paraplegia, and complete paralysis. Meningoencephalitis results in cerebrospinal fluid (CSF) pleocytosis in about one-third of cases; usually there are 10 to 100 cells per microliter with a mononuclear predominance, but occasionally there are more than 100 cells per microliter with a polymorphonuclear predominance. The protein concentration in CSF may be increased, but the glucose concentration is usually normal.

Renal failure, a result of hypoperfusion of the kidneys, occurs in the more severely ill patients with RMSF. Hypovolemia and hypotension cause a reduction in the glomerular filtration rate and prerenal azotemia; these abnormalities are often reversible with rehydration. In the most severe cases, shock results in acute tubular necrosis–induced renal failure, which may require hemodialysis.

Hepatic injury is manifested in 38 percent of cases as mildly or moderately increased serum aminotransferase concentrations owing to focal necrosis of hepatocytes, but hepatic failure does not occur. An elevated serum bilirubin concentration and frank jaundice are sometimes found and are probably consequences of both hemolysis and hepatocyte injury. Many patients develop gastrointestinal symptoms, including abdominal pain, nausea, vomiting, and diarrhea.

Bleeding is a potentially life-threatening effect of severe vascular damage. Anemia develops in 30 percent of cases and may be severe enough to require transfusions of red blood cells. Blood is detected in the stools or vomitus of 10 percent of patients, and death has followed massive upper gastrointestinal hemorrhage.

Other characteristic findings include a normal white blood cell count with increased numbers of immature myeloid cells and increased plasma concentrations of proteins of the acute-phase response (C-reactive protein, fibrinogen, ferritin, and others). Hyponatremia is reported in 56 percent of cases and is due to the inappropriate secretion of antidiuretic hormone in response to the hypovolemic state. Skeletal muscle injury, clinically manifested as myositis, has been documented in several individual cases by the detection of marked elevations in

serum creatine kinase levels or of histopathologic evidence of vascular injury in skeletal muscle and multifocal rhabdomyonecrosis. Ocular involvement includes conjunctivitis in 30 percent of cases and retinal vein engorgement, flame hemorrhages, arterial occlusion, and papilledema with normal CSF pressure in some instances.

In untreated cases, death usually occurs within 2 weeks after the onset of illness. A rare presentation, fulminant RMSF, is fatal within 5 days after onset. This fulminant presentation has been associated with RMSF in black males with a glucose-6-phosphate dehydrogenase deficiency and is believed to be related to an undefined effect of hemolysis on the rickettsial infection. Although survivors of RMSF usually appear to return to their previous state of health, patients who have been severely ill may sustain permanent sequelae, including neurologic deficits, and may need to have gangrenous extremities amputated.

Diagnosis The diagnosis of RMSF during the acute stage is more difficult than is generally appreciated. Clinical and epidemiologic considerations are more important than a laboratory diagnosis early in the illness. The most important epidemiologic factor is a history of exposure within 12 days before onset to a potentially tick-infested environment during a season of possible tick activity. However, only 60 percent of patients actually recall being bitten by a tick during the incubation period.

The differential diagnosis for early clinical manifestations of RMSF (fever, headache, and myalgia without a rash) includes influenza, enterovirus infection, infectious mononucleosis, viral hepatitis, leptospirosis, typhoid fever, gram-negative or gram-positive bacterial sepsis, and other rickettsial diseases. Enterocolitis may be suggested by nausea, vomiting, and abdominal pain; a prominence of abdominal tenderness has resulted in exploratory laparotomy. Central nervous system infection, including bacterial and viral meningoencephalitis, should be considered in the presence of seizures, coma, neurologic signs, and CSF abnormalities. Cough, pulmonary signs, and chest roentgenographic opacities may lead to the diagnostic consideration of bronchitis or pneumonia.

During the first 3 days of illness, only 3 percent of patients exhibit the classic triad of fever, rash, and history of tick exposure. When a rash appears, a diagnosis of RMSF should certainly be considered. However, many other illnesses considered in the differential diagnosis may also be associated with a rash, including rubeola, rubella, meningococcemia, disseminated gonococcal infection, secondary syphilis, toxic shock syndrome, drug hypersensitivity, idiopathic thrombocytopenic purpura, thrombotic thrombocytopenic purpura, Kawasaki syndrome, and immune complex vasculitis. The converse is also true: Any person in an endemic area with a provisional diagnosis of one of the above illnesses may have RMSF.

Serologic tests for RMSF are usually negative at the time of presentation for medical care, and treatment should not be delayed while a positive serologic result is awaited. The most common laboratory test for confirmation of the diagnosis is the indirect immunofluorescence assay. Between 7 and 10 days after the onset of illness, a diagnostic titer of ≥64 is usually detectable. Latex agglutination and a solid-state enzyme immunoassay are also available commercially. Latex agglutination usually yields a diagnostic titer of ≥128 at 1 week after onset.

The sensitivity and specificity of the indirect immunofluorescence assay are 94 to 100 percent and 100 percent, respectively; the latex agglutination test has a sensitivity of 71 to 94 percent and a specificity of 96 to 99 percent. The performance of the solid-state immunoassay has not been reported. The historically significant, but insensitive and nonspecific, Weil-Felix *Proteus vulgaris* OX-19 and OX-2 agglutination tests are unreliable and should not be used. Weil and Felix found that serum from a patient convalescing from typhus agglutinated a *Proteus* isolate (which they designated X-2) from the patient's urine. These researchers also found that another strain of *Proteus*, X-19, was similarly agglutinated but to a much higher titer. Because the X-2 and X-19 antigens were determined to be part of the heat-stable somatic or O antigen, these strains have commonly been referred to as OX strains. In 1934, Castaneda showed that *Proteus vulgaris* OX-19 and

Rickettsia prowazekii shared antigens. By studies with *Proteus* strains OX-19 and OX-2 as well as a third *Proteus* strain (OX-K, which was agglutinated by serum from patients with tsutsugamushi fever, or scrub typhus), it was possible to diagnose spotted fever, in which all three strains were agglutinated; scrub typhus, in which only strain OX-K was agglutinated; and epidemic (murine) typhus, in which only strain OX-19 was agglutinated. With the development of more specific tests, however, the Weil-Felix test has been abandoned. The test's rate of false positivity is about 20 percent, and it is insensitive.

The only diagnostic test that is useful during the acute illness is immunohistologic examination (immunofluorescence or immunoenzyme staining) of a cutaneous biopsy of a rash lesion for *R. rickettsii*. Examination of a 3-mm punch biopsy of such a lesion is 70 percent sensitive and 100 percent specific. Except in the preterminal stage, polymerase chain reaction (PCR) amplification and detection of *R. rickettsii* DNA in peripheral blood is an insensitive approach, since rickettsiae are present in large quantities in heavily infected foci of endothelial cells but in relatively low quantities in the circulation. Cultivation of rickettsiae in cell culture is technically feasible but is seldom undertaken because of biohazard and technologic concerns.

℞ TREATMENT

The drug of choice for the treatment of adults with RMSF is doxycycline, except for patients who are pregnant or are allergic to the drug. Because tetracyclines are known to stain the teeth of young children (<9 years old), their use by these children and by pregnant women may raise concern. Although perhaps not as effective, chloramphenicol has been used successfully for the treatment of RMSF and is recommended for use by pregnant women and perhaps by young children. Doxycycline is administered orally (or, in the presence of coma or vomiting, intravenously) at a dosage of 200 mg/d in two divided doses. Other regimens include oral tetracycline (25 to 50 mg/kg per day) in four divided doses or chloramphenicol (50 to 75 mg/kg per day) in four divided doses. The most seriously ill patients are managed in intensive care units, with careful administration of fluids to achieve optimal tissue perfusion without precipitating noncardiogenic pulmonary edema. In some severely ill patients, hypoxemia requires intubation and mechanical ventilation; oliguric or anuric acute renal failure requires hemodialysis; seizures necessitate the use of antiseizure medication; anemia or severe hemorrhage necessitates transfusions of packed red blood cells; and bleeding with severe thrombocytopenia necessitates platelet transfusions. Heparin is not a useful component of treatment, and there is no evidence that glucocorticoids, although frequently administered, affect the outcome of RMSF.

Prevention   Avoidance of tick bites is the only available preventive approach. Protective clothing and tick repellents, which could reduce the risk, are seldom actually used. After possible exposure to ticks, it is wise to inspect the body once or twice a day and remove ticks before they inoculate rickettsiae.

MEDITERRANEAN SPOTTED FEVER (BOUTONNEUSE FEVER) AND OTHER SPOTTED FEVERS   The etiologic agent of *Mediterranean spotted fever*, *Rickettsia conorii*, is prevalent in southern Europe (below the 45th parallel), all of Africa, and southwestern and south-central Asia. *Rhipicephalus sanguineus*, the brown dog tick, is the vector and reservoir. The names for this disease vary with the region in which it occurs; examples include *Mediterranean spotted fever* (also known as *boutonneuse fever*), *Kenya tick typhus*, *Indian tick typhus*, *Israeli spotted fever*, and *Astrakhan spotted fever*. Whatever the designation, the clinical manifestations are similar, characteristically including high fever, rash, and—in most geographic locales—an inoculation eschar (tâche noire) at the site of the tick bite. A clinically severe form of the disease, associated with a 50 percent mortality rate, has been observed in patients with diabetes, alcoholism, or heart failure.

A strain that has been referred to as *Rickettsia africae* is prevalent among *Amblyomma* ticks in central, eastern, and southern Africa. *R. africae* causes *African tick-bite fever*, which appears to be milder than classic Mediterranean spotted fever, with 2 to 5 days of fever and a tâche noire. *Rickettsia japonica* causes *Japanese* or *Oriental spotted fever*. Patients present with fever, a cutaneous eruption, and an inoculation eschar.

In Australia, two spotted fevers have been described. *Queensland tick typhus* is due to *Rickettsia australis* and is transmitted by *Ixodes holocyclus*. The skin rash in this disease is usually maculopapular but is sometimes vesicular, and there is an inoculation eschar. The spotted fever observed on *Flinders Island* (near Tasmania) is due to *Rickettsia honei*.

The diagnosis of these other tick-borne spotted fevers is based on clinical and epidemiologic findings and is confirmed by isolation of rickettsiae (by techniques not available in most laboratories) or by serology (Table 179-1). In an endemic area, patients presenting with fever, rash, and/or a skin lesion consisting of a black necrotic area or a crust surrounded by erythema should be considered to have one of these rickettsial spotted fevers. Treatment is outlined in Table 179-1.

RICKETTSIALPOX   Rickettsialpox was first described in 1946 by a general practitioner in New York City and soon afterwards was shown to be caused by a distinct rickettsial species, *Rickettsia akari*. This species is isolated from mice and their mites (*Liponyssoides sanguineus*), which maintain the organisms by transovarian transmission. *R. akari* shares lipopolysaccharide antigens with other members of the SFG.

More than 100 cases of rickettsialpox were diagnosed annually in the northeastern United States in the late 1940s and 1950s, and outbreaks occurred in the Ukraine in the 1950s. However, few cases are diagnosed currently. Recently, a culture-confirmed case of rickettsialpox was documented in southern Europe. This case was initially misdiagnosed as Mediterranean spotted fever on the basis of the development of serum antibodies cross-reactive with *R. conorii*. Recent cases of rickettsialpox have also been reported in Arizona, Utah, and Ohio.

In rickettsialpox, a papule forms at the site of the mite-bite inoculation of rickettsiae. The lesion develops a central vesicle that becomes a 1- to 2.5-cm painless black crusted eschar surrounded by an erythematous halo. Enlargement of the lymph nodes draining the region of the eschar is typical. After a 10-day incubation period, during which the eschar and regional lymphadenopathy frequently go unnoticed, the onset of illness is marked by malaise, chills, fever, headache, and myalgia. A macular rash appears 2 to 6 days later and evolves sequentially into papules, vesicles, and crusts that heal without scarring. In some cases the rash remains macular or maculopapular. Some patients suffer nausea, vomiting, abdominal pain, cough, conjunctivitis, or photophobia.

The diagnosis and treatment of rickettsialpox are summarized in Table 179-1. Untreated rickettsialpox is not fatal, with fever lasting 6 to 10 days.

FLEA- AND LOUSE-BORNE RICKETTSIAL DISEASES

ENDEMIC (MURINE) TYPHUS (FLEA-BORNE)   Murine typhus was postulated to be a distinct disease, with rats as the reservoir and fleas as the vector, by Maxcy in 1926. Dyer isolated *Rickettsia typhi* from rats and fleas in 1931. By the end of World War II, murine typhus was known to be a global disease. Recently, a novel typhus-group *Rickettsia* has been shown by Azad and coworkers to be maintained transovarially in cat fleas and to cause human infection. This flea-transmitted typhus-group species shares epitopes of the surface protein homologous to SFG rickettsial OmpB and of lipopolysaccharide, but it totally lacks OmpA. Clear differences between the genes for the 17-kDa lipoprotein citrate synthase and 16S rRNA indicate that *R. typhi* and the novel cat-flea rickettsia are separate species. This novel organism, designated *Rickettsia felis* (previously called the ELB agent), has been found in 4 percent of cat fleas and in 33 percent of opossums collected in the vicinity of human murine typhus cases in southern Texas.

Epidemiology *R. typhi* is maintained in mammalian host/flea cycles, with rats (*Rattus rattus* and *Rattus norvegicus*) and the Oriental rat flea (*Xenopsylla cheopis*) as the classic zoonotic niche. Fleas acquire *R. typhi* from rickettsemic rats and carry the organisms for the rest of their lives. Nonimmune rats and humans are infected when rickettsia-laden flea feces are "scratched" into pruritic bite lesions; less frequently, the flea bite itself transmits the organisms. Yet another possible route of transmission is the inhalation of aerosols of flea feces. Infected rats appear healthy, although they are rickettsemic for approximately 2 weeks.

Currently, fewer than 100 cases of endemic typhus are reported annually in the United States. These cases occur mainly in southern Texas and in southern California—locations where the classic rat/flea cycle is absent and a cycle involving the opossum and the cat flea (*Ctenocephalides felis*) is prominent. Although *X. cheopis* fleas are inefficient at the transovarian maintenance of *R. felis*, cat fleas are highly effective at the transovarian transmission of this organism, whose natural occurrence has been detected in fleas in California, Texas, and Oklahoma. *R. felis*–infected opossums and cat fleas as well as a case of human infection were reported from Corpus Christi, Texas, in the same environment where humans, opossums, and cat fleas are infected with *R. typhi*. Cases of endemic typhus occur year-round, mainly in warm (often coastal) areas. The peak prevalence in southern Texas is from April through June and elsewhere is during the warm months of summer and early fall. Although patients seldom recall a fleabite or exposure to fleas, exposure to animals such as cats, opossums, raccoons, skunks, and rats is reported by nearly 40 percent of those who are questioned.

Clinical Manifestations The incubation period of experimental murine typhus in volunteers averages 11 days, with a range of 8 to 16 days. Close observation during this period reveals prodromal symptoms of headache, myalgia, arthralgia, nausea, and malaise developing 1 to 3 days before the abrupt onset of chills and fever. Nearly all patients experience nausea and vomiting early in the illness.

The duration of untreated illness averages 12 days (range, 9 to 18 days). Rash is present in only 13 percent of patients at the time of presentation for medical care (about 4 days after the onset of symptoms), appearing an average of 2 days later in half of the remaining patients and never appearing in the other half. The initial macular rash is often detected by careful inspection of the axilla or the inner surface of the arm. Subsequently, the rash becomes maculopapular, involving the trunk more often than the extremities; it is seldom petechial and rarely involves the face, palms, or soles. A rash is detected in only 20 percent of patients with dark brown or black skin.

Pulmonary involvement is frequently prominent in murine typhus. Thirty-five percent of patients have a hacking, nonproductive cough, and 23 percent of those who undergo chest radiography are found to have pulmonary densities due to interstitial pneumonia, pulmonary edema, and pleural effusions. Bibasilar rales are the most common pulmonary sign. Less commonly observed symptoms and signs include abdominal pain, confusion, stupor, seizures, ataxia, coma, and jaundice. Laboratory studies frequently reveal anemia and leukopenia early in the course and leukocytosis late in the course, thrombocytopenia, hyponatremia, hypoalbuminemia, mildly increased serum levels of hepatic aminotransferases, and prerenal azotemia. Complications may include respiratory failure requiring intubation and mechanical ventilation, hematemesis, cerebral hemorrhage, and hemolysis (in patients with glucose-6-phosphate dehydrogenase deficiency and in those with some hemoglobinopathies). The illness is severe enough to necessitate the admission of 10 percent of hospitalized patients to an intensive care unit. A greater degree of severity is generally associated with old age, underlying disease, and treatment with a sulfa drug; the case-fatality rate in these situations is 1 percent. In a study of children with murine typhus, 50 percent suffered only nocturnal fevers, feeling well enough for active daytime play.

Diagnosis and Treatment See Table 179-1.

EPIDEMIC TYPHUS (LOUSE-BORNE) Epidemic typhus due to infection with *R. prowazekii* is transmitted by the human body louse (*Pediculus humanus corporis*), which lives in clothes and is

Table 179-1

Laboratory Diagnosis and Treatment of Selected Rickettsial Diseases

Disease(s)	Laboratory Diagnosis	Treatment
Mediterranean spotted fever Japanese or Oriental spotted fever Queensland tick typhus Flinders Island spotted fever	Isolation of rickettsiae, shell-vial culture; serology, IFA* (IgM, ≥1:64; or IgG, ≥1:128); PCR amplification of DNA from tissue specimens (especially for *R. japonica*)	Doxycycline (100 mg bid PO for 1–5 days) *or* Ciprofloxacin (750 mg bid PO for 5 days) *or* Chloramphenicol (500 mg qid PO for 7–10 days) *or* (in pregnancy) Josamycin† (3 g/d PO for 5 days)
Rickettsialpox	IFA: seroconversion to a titer of ≥1:64 or a single titer of ≥1:128; cross-absorption to eliminate antibodies to shared antigens necessary for a specific diagnosis of the spotted fever rickettsial species	Doxycycline (100 mg bid PO for 1–5 days) *or* Ciprofloxacin (750 mg bid PO for 5 days) *or* Chloramphenicol (500 mg qid PO for 7–10 days) *or* (in pregnancy) Josamycin† (3 g/d PO for 5 days)
Endemic (murine) typhus	IFA: fourfold rise to a titer of ≥1:64 or a single titer of ≥1:128; immunohistology: skin biopsy; PCR amplification of *R. typhi* or *R. felis* DNA from blood; dot ELISA* and immunoperoxidase methods also available	Doxycycline (100 mg bid PO for 7–15 days) *or* Chloramphenicol (500 mg qid PO for 7–15 days)
Epidemic typhus	IFA: titer of ≥1:128; necessary to use clinical and epidemiologic data to distinguish among louse-borne epidemic typhus, flying-squirrel typhus, and Brill-Zinsser disease	Doxycycline (200 mg PO as a single dose or until patient is afebrile for 24 h)
Scrub typhus	IFA: titer of ≥1:200; PCR amplification of *Orientia tsutsugamushi* DNA from blood of febrile patients	Doxycycline (100 mg bid PO for 7–15 days) or chloramphenicol (500 mg qid PO for 7–15 days; for children, 150 mg/kg per day for 5 days); azithromycin more effective than doxycycline in vitro against both doxycycline-susceptible and -resistant strains of *O. tsutsugamushi*

* IFA, indirect immunofluorescence assay; ELISA, enzyme-linked immunosorbent assay.
† Not approved by the Food and Drug Administration.

found in conditions of poor hygiene. The infected louse defecates during its blood meal, and the patient autoinoculates the organisms by scratching. Since the louse does not pass the organism to its offspring, the disease usually is spread from person to person by the louse-borne route. This epidemic form of typhus is associated with poverty, cold weather, war, and disasters and is currently prevalent in mountainous areas of Africa, South America, and Asia. In the United States, sporadic cases are transmitted by flying-squirrel fleas.

Brill-Zinsser disease is a recrudescent, mild form of epidemic typhus occurring years after the acute disease, probably as a result of immunosuppression or old age. Nathan Brill first identified recrudescent typhus in New York in 1898. In 1923, Hans Zinsser noted that more than 90 percent of patients with recrudescent typhus had emigrated from typhus-endemic areas of Europe. Strains of *R. prowazekii* indistinguishable from classic strains were isolated from patients with recrudescent typhus. Furthermore, *R. prowazekii* was isolated from the lymph nodes of patients undergoing elective surgery who had had typhus years earlier. Thus, the typhus rickettsiae can remain dormant for years and can reactivate with waning immunity.

Clinical Manifestations   After an incubation period of 1 week, the onset of illness is abrupt, with prostration, severe headache, and rapidly rising temperatures of 38.8 to 40.0°C (102 to 104°F). A rash begins on the upper trunk by the fifth day of fever and later becomes generalized, involving all of the body except the face, palms, and soles. Initially, this rash is macular; without treatment, it becomes maculopapular, petechial, and confluent. Photophobia, with considerable conjunctival injection and eye pain, is frequent. The tongue may be dry, brown, and furred. Skin necrosis and gangrene of the digits have been noted in severe cases. Untreated disease is fatal in up to 40 percent of cases, with outcome depending primarily on the condition of the host. Patients with untreated infections develop renal insufficiency and multivisceral involvement, with prominent neurologic manifestations in 12 percent of cases. North American *R. prowazekii* infection transmitted by flying-squirrel ectoparasites is a much milder illness than epidemic louse-borne typhus—whether because of host-related factors (e.g., health status) or organism-related factors (e.g., virulence). Brill-Zinsser disease is similar to epidemic typhus in terms of symptoms but is usually a milder illness.

Diagnosis and Treatment   See Table 179-1.

CHIGGER-BORNE SCRUB TYPHUS

The etiologic agent of scrub typhus is a small, obligately intracellular bacterium of the family Rickettsiaceae that differs substantially from other family members in its genetic and cell-wall composition; for example, this organism lacks lipopolysaccharide and peptidoglycan. Consequently, it has been classified as a species in a separate genus, *Orientia tsutsugamushi*.

O. tsutsugamushi is maintained in nature by transovarian transmission in trombiculid mites, mainly of the genus *Leptotrombidium*. After hatching, infected mite larvae (the only stage that feeds on an animal host) inoculate organisms into the skin while feeding. Scrub typhus is found in environments that harbor the infected chiggers, particularly areas of heavy scrub vegetation—e.g., where forest is regrowing after being cleared and along riverbanks. Human infections occur during the wet season, when the mites lay their eggs. The disease is endemic in eastern and southern Asia, northern Australia, and islands of the western Pacific Ocean. Scrub typhus is also found in tropical areas of India, Sri Lanka, and Bangladesh; in temperate areas of Japan, Korea, far-eastern Russia, Tadzhikistan, and the Himalayan Mountains; and in nontropical areas of China. Those infected include indigenous rural workers, residents of suburban areas, and Westerners visiting endemic areas for military, business, or recreational purposes. Infections are more prevalent than the number of clinical diagnoses would suggest: in some areas more than 3 percent of the population is infected or reinfected each month. (Immunity wanes over 1 to 3 years.)

Clinical Manifestations   The illness resulting from scrub typhus varies in severity from mild and self-limiting to fatal. After an incuba-

tion period of 6 to 21 days (usually 8 to 10 days), the onset of disease is characterized by fever, headache, myalgia, cough, and gastrointestinal symptoms. Some patients develop no further signs or symptoms and recover spontaneously after a few days. The classic case description includes an eschar at the site of chigger feeding, regional lymphadenopathy, and a maculopapular rash—signs that are seldom observed in indigenous patients. Fewer than 50 percent of western patients develop eschars; fewer than 40 percent develop a rash on day 4 to 6 of illness. Severe cases typically include prominent encephalitis and interstitial pneumonia as key features of vascular injury. Severe illness in persons deficient in glucose-6-phosphate dehydrogenase has been accompanied by hemolysis. The case-fatality rate for untreated classic cases is 7 percent; however, the figure would probably be lower if all relatively mild cases (which are underdiagnosed) were included.

Diagnosis and Treatment   See Table 179-1.

EHRLICHIOSES

Two members of the genus *Ehrlichia* have emerged as etiologic agents of life-threatening human disease in the United States. *Ehrlichia chaffeensis*, which targets mainly macrophages and monocytes, causes human monocytic ehrlichiosis; an *Ehrlichia equi*–like organism causes human granulocytic ehrlichiosis (Table 179-2). Ehrlichiae are small, gram-negative, obligately intracellular bacteria that grow as microcolonies in phagosomes (Fig. 179-2). The appearance of the cytoplasmic inclusion, a vacuolar cluster of Giemsa-stained ehrlichiae in phagocytes, accounts for its name, *morula*, the Latin word for mulberry.

Ehrlichiae were discovered by veterinary scientists: *Anaplasma marginale* in 1910, *Cowdria ruminantium* in 1925, *Ehrlichia canis* in 1935, and *Ehrlichia phagocytophila* in 1940. The veterinary investigation of ehrlichiae was further stimulated by an outbreak of fatal canine ehrlichiosis among military dogs during the Vietnam War and by the recognition of equine monocytic ehrlichiosis along the Potomac River in 1979. The agent of a human disease resembling infectious mononucleosis was isolated in Japan in 1953 and was subsequently designated as *Ehrlichia sennetsu*.

The taxonomy of *Ehrlichia* is being resolved by the tools of molecular phylogeny. Present knowledge suggests that three separate genetic clusters may represent three different genera. *E. chaffeensis* belongs among other tick-borne organisms, such as *E. canis* and *C. ruminantium*. The human granulocytic ehrlichiae fit into another genogroup of tick-borne bacteria that includes *E. equi*, *E. phagocytophila*, and *A. marginale*. *E. sennetsu* belongs to the group of organisms that parasitize fish-infesting flukes. This fish helminth occupies an interesting evolutionary niche as far from those of the human ehrlichial pathogens found in the United States as their substantial genetic divergence would suggest. The

Table 179-2

Comparison of Two Human Ehrlichioses: Human Monocytic Ehrlichiosis (HME) and Human Granulocytic Ehrlichiosis (HGE)

Feature	HME	HGE
Etiologic agent	*E. chaffeensis*	*E. equi*–like organism
Tick vector(s)	*Amblyomma americanum, Dermacentor variabilis* (dog tick)	*Ixodes scapularis* (deer tick), *I. ricinus*
Seasonality	April through September	Year-round; peak May through July
Major target cell	Monocyte	Granulocyte
Morulae seen	Rarely	Frequently
Antigen used in IFA*	*E. chaffeensis*	*E. equi*
Diagnostic titer	Fourfold rise or single titer of ≥1:128; cutoff for negative titer, 1:64	Fourfold rise; cutoff for negative titer, 1:80
Treatment of choice	Doxycycline	Doxycycline
Mortality	2–3%	5%

* IFA, indirect immunofluorescence assay.

FIGURE 179-2 *Ehrlichia chaffeensis* microcolonies (morulae) within cytoplasmic vacuoles manifest as two morphologic forms: reticulate cells (r) and dense-core cells (d). Bar = 1 μm. *(Courtesy of Dr. Vsevolod L. Popov.)*

ecologic niche of the tick-borne *Ehrlichia* species involves a persistently infected mammalian reservoir from which immature ticks acquire organisms that are maintained during stage-to-stage molting (but not transovarially) and are transmitted by tick bite.

HUMAN MONOCYTIC EHRLICHIOSIS Epidemiology Hundreds of cases of *E. chaffeensis* infection have been documented serologically in 30 states, mostly in the south-central, southeastern, and mid-Atlantic regions, as well as in Europe and Africa. The Lone Star tick (*Amblyomma americanum*) is the major vector, and the white-tailed deer is an important reservoir host. Most patients recall tick bites or exposures during the 3 weeks before the onset of illness; usually these events take place during the season of greatest tick activity—i.e., from April to September, with a peak from May through July. Human monocytic ehrlichiosis (HME) is most common in rural areas. The median age of patients is 44 years (older than for RMSF), and 75 percent of patients are male.

Clinical Manifestations After the tick-bite inoculation of *E. chaffeensis* and a median incubation period of 9 days, only one-third of persons who seroconvert actually become ill. However, in documented cases, the illness lasts for a median of 23 days; 62 percent of patients are hospitalized, and 2 to 3 percent die. The clinical signs and symptoms, which do not point to a specific diagnosis, include fever (97 percent), headache (81 percent), myalgia (68 percent), anorexia (66 percent), nausea (48 percent), vomiting (37 percent), rash (6 percent at onset, 25 percent during the first week, and 36 percent overall), cough (26 percent), pharyngitis (26 percent), diarrhea (25 percent), lymphadenopathy (25 percent), abdominal pain (22 percent), and confusion (20 percent). Severe illness may be manifested as respiratory insufficiency (in some cases with pulmonary infiltrates); neurologic involvement, with seizures, coma, CSF pleocytosis (including the presence of ehrlichiae); acute renal failure; gastrointestinal hemorrhage; and opportunistic fungal or viral infection. Laboratory abnormalities that are indicative of multisystem illness and are often diagnostically useful include thrombocytopenia, leukopenia (absolute lymphopenia and/or neutropenia), and elevated levels of serum aspartate and alanine aminotransferases. The bone marrow is usually hyperplastic and contains noncaseating granulomas. *Ehrlichia*-containing monocytes are seldom seen in the peripheral blood, but macrophages with ehrlichial morular inclusions have been demonstrated in bone marrow, spleen, liver, lymph node, lung, kidney, and CSF.

Diagnosis Clinical suspicion, based on fever and exposure to ticks in an endemic area during the prior 3 weeks, is essential to the diagnosis of HME. The finding of leukopenia and thrombocytopenia supports a presumptive diagnosis and the institution of empirical treatment with doxycycline. Serologic confirmation of the diagnosis is generally possible during convalescence, when antibodies to *E. chaffeensis* antigens are detected by indirect immunofluorescence assay at a titer of ≥64. Laboratory diagnosis during the acute stage of illness can be established by PCR amplification of *E. chaffeensis* DNA from blood.

℞ TREATMENT

Tetracycline drugs such as doxycycline (100 mg twice daily) have been shown to shorten the course of HME. However, no controlled trials of antimicrobial therapy have been conducted. Moreover, the required duration of administration of doxycycline is not known. Retrospective analysis has revealed that the administration of doxycycline markedly reduces the likelihood that an outpatient will require hospitalization and significantly shortens the duration of illness in a hospitalized patient. Although chloramphenicol also appears to shorten the course of illness, some patients do not respond to treatment with this agent, and *E. chaffeensis* is resistant to chloramphenicol in cell culture. Persistent ehrlichial infection has been documented after treatment with tetracycline and chloramphenicol.

HME is prevented by the avoidance of tick bite in endemic areas. Valuable precautions include the wearing of protective clothing; the use of tick repellent; and careful, frequent checking of the body, with prompt removal of ticks.

Ehrlichial infection is most likely controlled by a combination of cell-mediated and humoral immune mechanisms. Successful treatment is followed by an unusual rebound lymphocytosis of predominantly γ/δ T lymphocytes.

HUMAN GRANULOCYTIC EHRLICHIOSIS Epidemiology As of 1995, approximately 150 cases of human granulocytic ehrlichiosis (HGE) had been documented in 11 states, mostly in the upper midwestern and northeastern regions, with a distribution similar to that of Lyme disease. Since the first report of a series of cases of HGE by Bakken and colleagues in 1994, the frequency of its recognition has increased rapidly, but its geographic limits still are not known precisely. Most cases have been diagnosed within the range of various *Ixodes ricinus*–complex ticks, particularly *Ixodes scapularis (dammini)*, but some cases have been found in the range of southern-type *I. scapularis, Ixodes pacificus* (in the far-western states), and *I. ricinus* (in Europe). Agents of HGE have been detected in *I. scapularis (dammini)* in the upper Midwest and the Northeast as well as in the blood of deer in the upper Midwest and California and of horses and dogs in the upper Midwest, the Northeast, and Sweden. A role for rodents and deer in maintaining HGE in nature is suspected but not yet defined.

The agent of HGE is virtually indistinguishable from *E. equi*, which is transmitted to horses by *I. pacificus* in California, or from *E. phagocytophila*, which is transmitted to deer, cattle, and sheep by *I. ricinus* in Europe. Indeed, transfusion of human blood containing the agent of HGE into horses causes typical equine granulocytic ehrlichiosis and confers protective immunity against subsequent challenge with *E. equi*. The HGE agent, *E. equi*, and *E. phagocytophila* may in fact be different strains of a single species.

The incidence of HGE peaks in June and July, but the disease occurs throughout the year in conjunction with human exposure to *Ixodes* ticks. HGE predominantly affects males (79 percent of cases) and older persons (median age, 58 years).

Clinical Manifestations After a median incubation period of 8 days, patients with HGE usually suffer a flulike illness with fever (100 percent), chills (98 percent), malaise (98 percent), headache (85 percent), nausea (39 percent), and vomiting (34 percent). Some patients develop a cough (29 percent) or confusion (17 percent)—generally later in the course. Rash and seizures are rare. Patients frequently develop thrombocytopenia, leukopenia, anemia, and elevated serum aminotransferase concentrations. Bone marrow examination has demonstrated hypercellularity or normal marrow. Severe disease affects elderly patients in particular; however, children are also susceptible to the infection. The illness as presently recognized has a moderate to severe course unless treated early. The natural history of untreated HGE in adults is a 3- to 11-week illness with a possibly fatal outcome. One child who was not treated with an antiehrlichial drug was febrile for a shorter period (10 days). Overall, 56 percent of cases have required hospitalization, 7 percent have resulted in admission to an intensive care unit, and 5 percent have ended in death. Autopsies in fatal cases of HGE have revealed opportunistic fungal pneumonia due to *Aspergillus fumigatus*, *Cryptococcus neoformans*, or *Candida albicans*. This finding suggests compromised host defenses, similar to the defective function of neutrophils and of T and B lymphocytes documented in sheep infected with *E. phagocytophila*. Coinfection with the agent of HGE and *Borrelia burgdorferi* or *Babesia microti*—which are transmitted by the same vector, *I. scapularis (dammini)*—probably occurs on occasion. Serologic studies have demonstrated antibodies to the agent of HGE in substantial portions of patients with Lyme disease, and both this agent and *B. burgdorferi* have been found in individual ticks. It is possible that microbial interactions in this situation lead to more severe disease than infection with a single agent.

Diagnosis HGE should be suspected clinically when patients from an endemic area have a flulike febrile illness and have been exposed to an environment infested with *I. scapularis*, *I. pacificus*, or *I. ricinus* ticks. The detection of thrombocytopenia should increase the level of suspicion. Thorough examination of a peripheral-blood smear reveals neutrophils containing *Ehrlichia*-filled vacuoles in many but by no means all cases. PCR based upon primers specific for 16S rDNA sequences of the *E. phagocytophila* genogroup is diagnostically sensitive when performed under optimal laboratory conditions. Serodiagnosis by indirect immunofluorescence assay, with *E. equi*–infected equine neutrophils as antigen, is highly sensitive but is useful mainly for retrospective documentation of seroconversion to a titer of 80 or greater during convalescence.

℞ **TREATMENT**

Doxycycline is an effective therapeutic drug. Of 35 HGE patients treated with doxycycline, 94 percent defervesced within 24 to 48 h. One patient who did not receive doxycycline had the agent of HGE detected by PCR in the blood on day 28 of illness.

Like HME, HGE is prevented by avoidance of tick bite and prompt removal of attached ticks.

Q FEVER

Q fever results from infection with *Coxiella burnetii*. This small gram-negative microorganism (0.2 μm × 0.7 μm) exists in two antigenic forms: phase I and phase II. When *C. burnetii* is passaged in cell cultures or embryonated eggs, its lipopolysaccharide undergoes changes that result in an antigenic shift called *phase variation*. In humans and other animals, the organism exists in the phase I form, which is extremely infectious. Passage in cell culture or embryonated eggs results in a shift to the phase II form, which is avirulent. The ability of *C. burnetii* to form spores allows it to survive in harsh environments. Indeed, it can survive for more than 40 months in skim milk at room temperature and is readily recovered from soil up to 1 month after contamination. Three different plasmids have been described in various isolates of *C. burnetii*.

Q fever encompasses two broad clinical syndromes: acute and chronic infection. It is likely that the host's immune response (rather than characteristics of the infecting strain) determines whether or not chronic Q fever develops.

Epidemiology Q fever is a zoonosis. The primary sources of human infection are infected cattle, sheep, and goats. However, infected cats, rabbits, and dogs have also been shown to transmit *C. burnetii* to humans. The extensive wildlife reservoir for *C. burnetii* includes mammals, birds, and ticks. In the infected female mammal, *C. burnetii* localizes to the uterus and the mammary glands; infection is reactivated during pregnancy, and high concentrations of *C. burnetii* are found in the placenta. At parturition, *C. burnetii* is dispersed as

an aerosol, and infection follows inhalation of these organisms by a susceptible host. Infected female animals shed the organism in milk for weeks or months after parturition. In rare instances, human-to-human transmission has followed childbirth by an infected woman or autopsy on an infected patient. *C. burnetii* has been transmitted via blood transfusion. It is evident that the persons at risk for Q fever include abattoir workers, veterinarians, and others who vocationally or avocationally come into contact with infected animals. Exposure to infected newborn animals or to infected products of conception poses the highest risk. Sexual transmission has been demonstrated experimentally in mice, as has transmission during artificial insemination in cattle. Whether *C. burnetii* is sexually transmitted in humans is not yet known. While the experimental evidence on this point is contradictory, the ingestion of contaminated milk in some areas is probably a major route of infection.

Infections due to *C. burnetii* occur in most countries. Indeed, the only areas known to be free of *C. burnetii* are New Zealand and Antarctica. The primary manifestation of acute Q fever differs from place to place. In Nova Scotia (Canada) it is pneumonia, while in Marseille (France) it is granulomatous hepatitis. In the Basque country of Spain, both pneumonia and granulomatous hepatitis occur. It has been suggested that these differences may reflect the route of infection—i.e., that the ingestion of contaminated milk results in hepatitis while the inhalation of contaminated aerosols results in pneumonia.

Clinical Manifestations The incubation period for *acute Q fever* ranges from 3 to 30 days. The clinical presentations include flu-like syndromes, prolonged fever, pneumonia, hepatitis, pericarditis, myocarditis, meningoencephalitis, and infection during pregnancy. The symptoms of acute Q fever are nonspecific; common among them are fever, extreme fatigue, and severe headache. Other symptoms include chills, sweats, nausea, vomiting, and diarrhea, which occur in 5 to 20 percent of patients. Cough develops in about half of all patients with Q fever pneumonia. Neurologic manifestations of acute Q fever are uncommon. However, in one outbreak in the West Midlands of the United Kingdom, 23 percent of 102 patients had neurologic signs and symptoms as the major manifestation of acute Q fever. A nonspecific skin rash may be evident in some patients. The white blood cell count is usually normal. Thrombocytopenia is present in about 25 percent of patients, and reactive thrombocytosis (with platelet counts of up to 1 million/μL [1×10^{12}/L]) frequently develops during recovery. This thrombocytosis may account for cases of deep-vein thrombophlebitis complicating acute Q fever in some series. Uncommon manifestations of acute Q fever include optic neuritis, extrapyramidal neurologic disease, Guillain-Barré syndrome, inappropriate secretion of antidiuretic hormone, epididymitis, orchitis, priapism, hemolytic anemia, mediastinal lymphadenopathy mimicking lymphoma, pancreatitis, erythema nodosum, and mesenteric panniculitis. Chest radiography may show an opacity that is indistinguishable from those seen in pneumonia of other causes. Multiple rounded opacities are common. In the appropriate epidemiologic setting, these opacities are highly suggestive of Q fever pneumonia; however, right-sided endocarditis resulting in septic pulmonary emboli can produce the same radiographic appearance.

Chronic Q fever almost always implies endocarditis. This infection usually occurs in patients with previous valvular heart disease, immunosuppression, or chronic renal insufficiency. Fever is usually absent or, if present, is low grade. Patients may have nonspecific symptoms for up to 1 year before diagnosis. Valvular vegetations have been seen in only 12 percent of patients with transthoracic echocardiograms, but the rate of detection may be higher with the use of transesophageal echocardiography. A high index of suspicion is necessary for a correct diagnosis. All patients with valvular heart disease and an unexplained purpuric eruption, renal insufficiency, stroke, and/or progressive heart failure should be tested for *C. burnetii* infection. Patients with chronic Q fever have hepatomegaly and/or splenomegaly. These two findings, especially in combination with positive rheumatoid factor, high erythrocyte sedimentation rate, high C-reactive protein level, and/or increased gamma globulin concentrations, suggest this diagnosis. Other manifestations of chronic Q fever include infection of vascular prostheses, aneurysms, and bone.

Diagnosis *C. burnetii* can be isolated from buffy-coat blood samples or tissue specimens by a shell-vial technique; however, most laboratories are not currently permitted to attempt the isolation of *C. burnetii*, since it is considered highly infectious. PCR can be used to amplify *C. burnetii* DNA from tissue or biopsy specimens. This technique can also be used on paraffin-embedded tissues. Serology, however, is the most commonly used diagnostic tool. Three techniques are available: complement fixation, indirect immunofluorescence, and enzyme-linked immunosorbent assay. Indirect immunofluorescence is sensitive and specific and is the method of choice. Rheumatoid factor should be absorbed from the specimen before testing. An IgG titer of ≥1:800 to phase I antigen is suggestive of chronic Q fever. In almost all instances of chronic Q fever, the phase I antibody titer is much higher than the phase II antibody titer. The reverse is true in acute Q fever. In addition, in acute Q fever, it is usually possible to demonstrate a fourfold rise in titer between acute- and convalescent-phase samples.

R̄x **TREATMENT**

Treatment of acute Q fever with doxycycline (100 mg twice daily for 14 days) is usually successful. Quinolones are also effective. Treatment of chronic Q fever should include at least two antibiotics active against *C. burnetii*. The combination of rifampin and doxycycline has been used with success. Doxycycline should be given as 100 mg twice daily and rifampin as 300 mg once daily. The optimal duration of antibiotic therapy for chronic Q fever remains undetermined. We recommend a minimum of 3 years of treatment. Therapy should be discontinued only if the phase I IgA antibody titer is ≤1:50 and the phase I IgG titer is ≤1:200. Another therapeutic option under investigation is the combination of doxycycline (100 mg twice daily) with hydroxychloroquine (600 mg once daily). In vitro, the addition of hydroxychloroquine at a concentration of 1 mg/mL renders doxycycline bactericidal for *C. burnetii*. A vaccine has been shown to be effective in preventing Q fever in abattoir workers in Australia.

BIBLIOGRAPHY

ARCHIBALD LK, SEXTON DJ: Long-term sequelae of Rocky Mountain spotted fever. Clin Infect Dis 20:1122, 1995

AZAD AF: Epidemiology of murine typhus. Annu Rev Entomol 35:553, 1990
——— et al: Genetic characterization and transovarial transmission of a typhus-like rickettsia found in cat fleas. Proc Natl Acad Sci USA 89:43, 1992

BAKKEN JS et al: Human granulocytic ehrlichiosis in the upper midwest United States. A new species emerging? JAMA 272:212, 1994

BROUQUI P, RAOULT D: In vitro antibiotic susceptibility of the newly recognized agent of ehrlichiosis in humans, *Ehrlichia chaffeensis*. Antimicrob Agents Chemother 36:2799, 1992

DALTON MJ et al: National surveillance for Rocky Mountain spotted fever, 1981–1982: Epidemiologic summary and evaluation of risk factors for fatal outcome. Am J Trop Med Hyg 52:405, 1995

DAWSON JE et al: Isolation and characterization of an *Ehrlichia* sp. from a patient diagnosed with human ehrlichiosis. J Clin Microbiol 29:2741, 1991

DUMLER JS et al: Clinical and laboratory features of murine typhus in south Texas, 1980 through 1987. JAMA 266:1365, 1991

FICHTENBAUM CJ et al: Ehrlichiosis presenting as a life-threatening illness with features of the toxic shock syndrome. Am J Med 95:351, 1993

FISHBEIN DB et al: Human ehrlichiosis in the United States, 1985 to 1990. Ann Intern Med 120:736, 1994

HELMICK CG et al: Rocky Mountain spotted fever: Clinical, laboratory, and epidemiological features of 262 cases. J Infect Dis 150:480, 1984

HIGGINS JA et al: *Rickettsia felis*: A new species of pathogenic rickettsia isolated from cat fleas. J Clin Microbiol 34:671, 1996

KASS EM et al: Rickettsial pox in a New York City hospital, 1980–1989. N Engl J Med 331:1612, 1994

MARRIE TJ: Q fever, in *Q Fever*, vol 1, TJ Marrie (ed). Boca Raton, FL, CRC Press, 1990

O'CONNOR LF et al: A cluster of murine typhus cases in Western Australia. Med J Aust 165:24, 1996

RAOULT D, DRANCOURT M: Antimicrobial therapy of rickettsial diseases. Antimicrob Agents Chemother 35:2457, 1991

RATNASAMY N et al: Central nervous system manifestations of human ehrlichiosis. Clin Infect Dis 23:314, 1996

RIKIHISA Y: The tribe *Ehrlichieae* and ehrlichial diseases. Clin Microbiol Rev 4:286, 1991

SCHRIEFER ME et al: Identification of a novel rickettsial infection in a patient diagnosed with murine typhus. J Clin Microbiol 32:949, 1994

SILPAPOJAKUL K et al: Murine typhus in Thailand: Clinical features, diagnosis and treatment. Q J Med 86:43, 1993

STRICKMAN D et al: *In vitro* effectiveness of azithromycin against doxycycline-resistant and -susceptible strains of *Rickettsia tsutsugamushi*, etiologic agent of scrub typhus. Antimicrob Agents Chemother 39:2406, 1995

WALKER DH et al: Fulminant Rocky Mountain spotted fever. Its pathologic characteristics associated with glucose-6-phosphate dehydrogenase deficiency. Arch Pathol Lab Med 107:121, 1983

YEVICH SJ et al: Seroepidemiology of infections due to spotted fever group *Rickettsia* and *Ehrlichia* species in military personnel exposed in areas of the United States where such infections are endemic. J Infect Dis 171:1266, 1995

180 *Gail H. Cassell, Gregory C. Gray, K. B. Waites*

MYCOPLASMA INFECTIONS

Mycoplasmas are the smallest free-living microorganisms and are commonly found in plants, animals, and humans. Individual cells range in diameter from 100 to 300 nm. Many of the biologic properties of mycoplasmas, including resistance to β-lactam antibiotics and marked cellular pleomorphism, stem from the lack of a cell wall. The extremely small size of the mycoplasmal genome severely limits the organism's biosynthetic capabilities, helps explain the complex nutritional requirements for its cultivation, and necessitates a parasitic or saprophytic existence. Mycoplasmas most commonly colonize mucosal surfaces and typically cause chronic inflammatory diseases of the respiratory tract, urogenital tract, and joints of a wide variety of animal species. Fourteen mycoplasmal species are known to occur in humans, some only rarely. *Mycoplasma orale* and *Mycoplasma salivarium* are common oral commensals. *Mycoplasma pneumoniae* is a common cause of pneumonia in all age groups. Both *Ureaplasma urealyticum* and *Mycoplasma hominis* often colonize the genitourinary tract of normal asymptomatic individuals but are important opportunistic pathogens in adults and newborn infants. *Mycoplasma genitalium*, *Mycoplasma fermentans*, and *Mycoplasma penetrans* have been detected in the respiratory and genitourinary tracts and warrant further attention as potential causes of human disease. However, these species have been described relatively recently, and detailed information concerning their true ecologic niche is lacking. They appear to be even more fastidious than other *Mycoplasma* species found in humans.

MECHANISMS OF PATHOGENICITY

Adhesion to host cells is a prerequisite for mycoplasmal colonization and for infection. *M. pneumoniae* adheres and attaches by a complex and multifactorial process requiring a number of accessory proteins; adhesion is followed by induction of ciliostasis. Factors involved in the adherence of *U. urealyticum* and *M. hominis* have not been characterized. While most mycoplasmas reside attached to the cell surface, intracellular localization of *M. fermentans*, *M. penetrans*, and (to a limited extent) *M. pneumoniae* has now been documented. This intracellular localization can protect mycoplasmas from antibodies and antibiotics, contributing to the chronicity of disease and to the difficulties encountered in cultivation of the organisms on artificial media.

The pathogenic properties of *U. urealyticum* and *M. hominis* have not been elucidated. However, surface antigens of both organisms undergo variation at a high rate that may be related to mycoplasmal persistence at invasive sites. One important property of *M. hominis* is its ability to metabolize arginine and thus to release large, potentially cytotoxic amounts of ammonia. *M. pneumoniae* and *M. hominis* produce hydrogen peroxide, which is also thought to play a role in cell injury.

Ureaplasmas differ from all other genera within the class Mollicutes in that they possess urease activity. Like other prokaryotes that have urease activity, *U. urealyticum* can induce urinary calculi. Ureaplasmas—but not *M. hominis* or *M. pneumoniae*—exhibit specific protease activity through which they can degrade human IgA1 but not IgA2; this activity is believed to be a virulence factor.

M. pneumoniae, like many other species of mycoplasmas, can nonspecifically stimulate B lymphocytes and—to a lesser extent—T lymphocytes. Certain individuals infected with *M. pneumoniae* develop autoantibodies, including those reactive with brain, heart, and muscle; erythrocyte I antigen; intermediate filaments; and mitotic spindles of dividing cells. Infection with *M. pneumoniae* may evoke IgM autoantibodies that agglutinate human erythrocytes at 4°C (cold agglutinins). This effect sometimes causes complications. *M. pneumoniae* uses specific long-chain sialooligosaccharides at the host-cell surface as receptors. These sialooligosaccharides contain I antigen in their backbones and are richly expressed at the primary site of infection—the ciliated bronchial epithelium—and on erythrocytes. The autoantibodies to I antigen are directed to cell membrane receptors and may be triggered by an autoimmunogenic mycoplasma-receptor complex in which the lipid-rich microorganism serves as an adjuvant. Cold agglutinins are thought to contribute to the anemia often seen in *M. pneumoniae*–infected patients. With the exception of cold agglutinins, the role of immunologic factors in *M. pneumoniae*–induced disease is unknown.

MYCOPLASMA PNEUMONIAE

EPIDEMIOLOGY Approximately 10 to 20 percent of all pneumonias are due to *M. pneumoniae*. This organism is a common cause of tracheobronchitis and other respiratory syndromes such as bronchiolitis and pharyngitis. Symptoms can persist for weeks or months. *M. pneumoniae* is spread by aerosol from person to person. However, in contrast to that of other respiratory infections, person-to-person spread of mycoplasmal infections by aerosols is slow, even among family members. The incubation period is 1 to 3 weeks long. In large urban areas, *M. pneumoniae* infection appears to be endemic and occurs throughout the year. Epidemics can occur every 3 to 7 years.

M. pneumoniae was previously thought to be rare among children under 5 years of age and to cause only acute, self-limited respiratory disease. However, recent studies indicate that the incidence may actually be highest among 3 and 4 year olds and that the rate of hospitalization for *M. pneumoniae* pneumonia among children under 5 is high. Recent studies of adults (mean age, 62 years) have indicated that *M. pneumoniae* accounts for as many as 15 percent of cases of community-acquired pneumonia in this age group. Prospective studies of adults (mean age, 56 years) requiring hospitalization for community-acquired pneumonia have confirmed that up to 18 percent of these cases are caused by *M. pneumoniae*. The common misconception that *M. pneumoniae* disease is rare among the very young and among older adults has led to a failure of physicians even to consider this condition in the differential diagnosis.

CLINICAL MANIFESTATIONS Although *M. pneumoniae* is best known as the primary cause of "walking" or "atypical" pneumonia, the clinical syndrome for which it is most frequently responsible is tracheobronchitis, often accompanied by upper respiratory tract symptoms. Typical complaints include sore throat, headache, chills, coryza, and general malaise. The throat may be erythematous, but cervical adenopathy is uncommon. Myringitis and otitis sometimes develop. Severe mycoplasmal respiratory disease has been thought to be uncommon, yet recent reports suggest that the disease spectrum is wider than was previously thought and that severe pulmonary involvement is possible in otherwise healthy children and adults of all ages. Lung abscesses, pneumatoceles, extensive lobar consolidation, respiratory distress, and pleural effusion may develop. Small effusions are found in 20 percent of cases. *M. pneumoniae* is sometimes isolated from the pleural fluid in relatively severe cases.

EXTRAPULMONARY COMPLICATIONS Meningoencephalitis, aseptic meningitis, encephalitis, ascending paralysis, and transverse myelitis have been reported. Some cases with neurologic complications are fatal. Recovery from neurologic dysfunction is often slow, and some patients are left with a permanent neurologic deficit. The initial failure of investigators to demonstrate direct invasion of the central nervous system (CNS) by mycoplasmas and the fact that many reported cases were diagnosed solely on the basis of serologic testing led many investigators to regard the association of *M. pneumoniae* infection with CNS disease as rather tenuous. However, CNS infection has now been documented by polymerase chain reaction and cultural isolation of *M. pneumoniae* from cerebrospinal fluid and from brain tissue obtained at autopsy in the absence of other infectious agents and other identifiable causes of clinical manifestations. As already mentioned, *M. pneumoniae* frequently evokes cold agglutinins. A positive Coombs test and detection of reticulocytosis suggest that subclinical anemia may be common. Other complications include hemolytic anemia, paroxysmal cold hemoglobinuria, Raynaud's phenomenon, disseminated intravascular coagulation, thrombocytopenia, and renal failure.

Cardiac involvement is generally thought to be rare, but the true incidence is unknown. Myocardial dysfunction is often associated with hemolytic anemia and may mimic infarction. Myopericarditis, hemopericardium, congestive heart failure, and complete heart block have been reported, and marked electrocardiographic changes may be evident without cardiac symptoms. *M. pneumoniae* has been isolated in pure culture from pericardial fluid and cardiac tissue.

Mucocutaneous lesions are found in approximately 25 percent of *M. pneumoniae* infections. Erythematous maculopapular and vesicular exanthems are most common. Half of patients with mucocutaneous lesions also have ulcerative stomatitis and conjunctivitis. In many cases, throat and bulla-fluid cultures are positive for *M. pneumoniae*.

M. pneumoniae infection occasionally is associated with joint manifestations, including arthritis. Illnesses suggestive of rheumatic fever have been described. About 25 percent of cases of *M. pneumoniae* infection include nausea, vomiting, and/or diarrhea.

DIAGNOSIS The possibility of *M. pneumoniae* infection should be considered in patients of any age who have respiratory manifestations. Although complications appear to be uncommon, their true incidence may have been underestimated. Because of the mistaken impression that severe pneumonia and extrapulmonary complications are inconsistent with *M. pneumoniae* disease, this etiology often is not included in the differential diagnosis. Extrapulmonary manifestations usually begin 1 to 21 days after respiratory symptoms. However, some patients have no history of respiratory symptoms, and others report only upper respiratory illness. Extrapulmonary manifestations have been reported in all age groups.

Routine laboratory tests usually yield normal results. About one-fourth of all patients with mycoplasmal pneumonia develop leukocytosis, and one-third have an elevated erythrocyte sedimentation rate. Chest radiographs of patients with mycoplasmal pneumonia may reveal diffuse reticulonodular or interstitial infiltrates, usually located in the lower lobes and often appearing as streaks radiating from the hilus to the base. Lung involvement tends to be unilateral but can be bilateral. Clinical, radiologic, and laboratory findings in *M. pneumoniae* infections are sufficiently indistinct to serve as a basis for an accurate diagnosis. *Chlamydia pneumoniae*, *Chlamydia psittaci*, *Streptococcus pneumoniae*, *Haemophilus influenzae*, *Moraxella catarrhalis*, *Francisella tularensis*, *Bordetella pertussis*, *Coxiella burnetii*, *Legionella* species, and several viruses (including adenoviruses) can produce infections that are clinically indistinguishable from *M. pneumoniae* infection and may in fact occur simultaneously with mycoplasmal infections. Although a cold agglutinin response is not specific for *M. pneumoniae* and is detected in ≤50 percent of cases, it suggests the diagnosis, is easy to document, and may be evident within the first week of infection. To detect this response, the patient's serum is mixed with type O erythrocytes, the mixture is incubated at 0°C for several minutes, and the presence or absence of hemagglutination is noted. A titer of 1:32 is suggestive of infection with *M. pneumoniae*. A rapid bedside test can also be performed: A 1-mL volume of the patient's blood is drawn into a tube containing anticoagulant. The tube is cooled in wet ice or in a standard refrigerator for 3 to 4 min, and the contents are examined for hemagglutination.

At present, no rapid diagnostic methods for the detection of *M. pneumoniae* in clinical specimens are commercially available. In addition, culture services often are not readily available, a positive result takes time to obtain, and the collection of proper diagnostic specimens in some types of respiratory infections is impractical. Therefore, serologic tests are most commonly used to confirm *M. pneumoniae* infection. The enzyme-linked immunosorbent assay is the preferred serologic method. Definitive diagnosis requires seroconversion documented by paired specimens obtained 2 to 4 weeks apart. Although single-titer IgM assays purported to detect current infection have recently become commercially available, it is not clear how long IgM persists after acute infection, and as many as 50 percent of adults may not mount a detectable IgM response. Conversely, some children may not mount an IgG response. Therefore, reliance on a single serologic test could be clinically misleading, and paired assays for both IgM and IgG are recommended. While complement fixation is acceptable, this technique is not satisfactory for the detection of IgG and is also rather insensitive.

℞ TREATMENT

Orally administered erythromycin (250 to 500 mg every 6 h for adults, 20 to 50 mg/kg daily in three or four doses for children) is the drug of choice for mycoplasmal respiratory infections, although tetracycline (250 to 500 mg every 6 h) or doxycycline (100 mg every 12 h) are suitable alternatives for older children and adults. Clindamycin is active in vitro but may not be active in vivo and should not be considered a first-line agent. Fluoroquinolones such as ciprofloxacin (500 mg every 12 h) exhibit some antimycoplasmal activity in vitro but not nearly as much as the macrolides and tetracyclines; therefore, fluoroquinolones should not be used when alternatives are available. Newer agents such as clarithromycin (500 mg every 12 h for adults, 15 mg/kg daily in two doses for children) and azithromycin[1] (500 mg on day 1, then 250 mg daily) are highly effective in vitro against *M. pneumoniae* at concentrations equivalent to or lower than those of erythromycin, demonstrate similar clinical efficacy, and are available as pediatric suspensions. Moreover, they are better tolerated, cause fewer gastrointestinal side effects, and have a longer half-life that allows less frequent administration. Like that of erythromycin, the administration of clarithromycin may cause an increase in serum theophylline concentrations. Because mycoplasmas are slow-growing organisms, it is logical to expect infections to respond better to longer courses of treatment than might be offered for other types of infections. Therefore, a 14- to 21-day course of oral therapy with most agents is appropriate.

In addition to antimicrobials, preparations such as cough suppressants, antipyretics, and analgesics should be given as needed to relieve headache and other systemic symptoms caused by *M. pneumoniae* infection. Since most extrapulmonary manifestations are diagnosed late in the course of disease, the benefit of early or prolonged treatment in preventing them or diminishing their severity is unknown.

---

[1] This drug has not been approved by the Food and Drug Administration for use against *M. pneumoniae*.

EPIDEMIOLOGY Genital mycoplasmas may be found throughout the lower urogenital tract of asymptomatic women. In addition, mycoplasmas have been isolated from the urine, the semen, and the distal urethra of asymptomatic men. *U. urealyticum* is detected in the vagina of 40 to 80 percent of sexually mature, asymptomatic women and *M. hominis* in 21 to 53 percent; the incidence of each is somewhat lower in males.

Both ureaplasmas and *M. hominis* can be isolated from amniotic fluid in the presence of intact membranes as early as 12 to 20 weeks of gestation. Up to 14 percent of the isolates of *U. urealyticum* and up to 30 percent of the isolates of *M. hominis* from endotracheal aspirates collected at birth from infants whose birth weight is <2500 g are from infants born by cesarean section to women with intact membranes. These figures indicate that in utero acquisition is rather common, at least among preterm infants. *U. urealyticum* and *M. hominis* can be acquired in utero either by an ascending route secondary to colonization of the mother's genital tract or transplacentally from the mother's blood. Both organisms have been isolated from maternal and umbilical-cord blood. The rate of vertical transmission of *U. urealyticum* and *M. hominis* among infants ranges from 18 to 55 percent. Rates of colonization among healthy full-term infants decline after 3 months of age. Fewer than 10 percent of older children and sexually inexperienced adults are colonized with either ureaplasmas or *M. hominis*.

DISEASES OF THE GENITOURINARY TRACT OF ADULTS Three conditions of the urinary tract definitively shown to be caused by mycoplasmas are urethritis due to *U. urealyticum* in males, urinary calculi due to *U. urealyticum*, and pyelonephritis due to *M. hominis*. Although the exact proportion of cases for which it is responsible is unknown, *M. hominis* is considered to be a cause of pelvic inflammatory disease (PID). Inoculation of *M. hominis* into fallopian tubes of monkeys induces parametritis and salpingitis within 3 days, and inoculation of human fallopian tube explants produces ciliostasis; the organism has been isolated in pure cultures from the fallopian tubes of approximately 8 percent of women with salpingitis diagnosed by laparoscopy; the figure for women without lesions is zero. *M. hominis* is sometimes isolated from the endometrium. In addition, a role for this organism in cases of PID associated with neither *Neisseria gonorrhoeae* nor *Chlamydia trachomatis* is supported by significant increases in specific antibody. While *U. urealyticum* can be isolated directly from affected fallopian tubes, it is usually found in the presence of other known pathogens.

Given that *M. hominis* is a cause of salpingitis, it is reasonable to assume that severe tubal infections with this organism can lead to occlusion and infertility. However, prospective studies are needed to prove this point. Although the possibility that *U. urealyticum* plays a role in involuntary infertility in humans was first raised more than 20 years ago, the association remains speculative.

PERINATAL MORBIDITY AND MORTALITY *U. urealyticum* is a common cause of histologic chorioamnionitis. Individual case reports provide compelling evidence that, in at least some individuals, *U. urealyticum* alone causes spontaneous abortion and premature birth. Rates of placental isolation of ureaplasmas are inversely related to infants' gestational age and birth weight. *M. hominis* also commonly invades the chorioamnion and amniotic fluid but is rarely found in the absence of other organisms, particularly ureaplasmas. Therefore, it is unclear whether *M. hominis* alone causes histologic chorioamnionitis or clinical amnionitis.

U. urealyticum is the single most common organism isolated from the CNS and lower respiratory tract of newborn infants, particularly those delivered prematurely and weighing <1000 g. The isolation of the organism in pure culture from pleural fluid, lung biopsy, and lung tissue obtained at autopsy from infants with pneumonia, along with the production of similar histologic lesions in lungs of newborn mice and prematurely born nonhuman primates with these isolates, proves that this organism can cause pneumonia in newborn infants. Ureaplasmal pneumonia may play a role in the development of chronic lung disease. While the occurrence of clinically significant hydrocephalus and meningitis is variable in CNS infections with *U. urealyticum* and *M. hominis*, it is clear that in some cases the organisms cause these conditions. *M. hominis* is also a cause of septicemia, pneumonia, pericarditis, adenitis, and abscesses of the subcutaneous tissue in newborn infants.

EXTRAGENITAL INFECTIONS IN CHILDREN AND ADULTS While *U. urealyticum* and *M. hominis* typically remain localized in the lower genital tract, both organisms can cause extragenital infections. Infections at extragenital sites have been reported in patients of both sexes and a broad range of ages (14 to 76 years). Disseminated infection has been reported in otherwise healthy hosts, but most infections follow genitourinary manipulation or trauma of the genitourinary tract or develop in individuals with underlying immunosuppression.

The ability of *M. hominis* to infect surgical wounds or sites of trauma is well documented. Heart-lung transplant recipients commonly develop sternal wound infections due to *M. hominis*, with associated mediastinitis and empyema. *M. hominis* has been identified in cases of meningitis following trauma and in brain abscesses of immunocompromised patients. In addition, *M. hominis* has been reported as a cause of lower respiratory tract infection and pneumonia in immunosuppressed and other compromised patients. *U. urealyticum* is the predominant cause of sinopulmonary disease and progressive lung failure in agammaglobulinemic patients. Both *U. urealyticum* and *M. hominis* have been isolated from pericardial fluid and/or pericardial tissue of patients with large pericardial effusions requiring surgical drainage. Prosthetic valve endocarditis and persistent and fatal bloodstream infection due to *M. hominis* have been reported. Peritonitis following organ transplantation and renal dialysis can also result from *M. hominis* infection. Both *M. hominis* and *U. urealyticum* are common causes of postpartum bacteremia, endometritis, and cesarean wound infection. *M. hominis* has also been associated with postpartum pneumonia and arthritis.

Approximately 20 percent of individuals with agammaglobulinemia develop joint inflammation; evidence suggests that mycoplasmas may be responsible for the majority of cases. Furthermore, both *U. urealyticum* and *M. hominis* can cause arthritis in other types of immunosuppressed or otherwise compromised patients (i.e., those with prosthetic joints). In most reported cases, the arthritis has been persistent, lasting from several months to more than 1 year. Aggressive, erosive arthritis can progress despite anti-inflammatory therapy and gamma globulin replacement. Osteomyelitis has been reported in association with invasive infection with both *U. urealyticum* and *M. hominis*.

DIAGNOSIS *M. hominis* and *U. urealyticum* grow more rapidly than *M. pneumoniae* in culture and can be detected in 2 to 5 days. While commercial media are available for the culture of genital mycoplasmas, no commercial serologic assays or rapid detection tests are available for routine diagnosis.

℞ **TREATMENT**

Oral tetracyclines, given for at least 7 days in the same doses used for mycoplasmal respiratory infections, have historically been the drugs of choice for the treatment of urogenital infections due to *M. hominis*; however, 20 to 40 percent of clinical isolates are now resistant to these agents. Clindamycin (150 to 450 mg every 6 h for adults, 10 to 40 mg/kg daily in three or four doses for children) is an alternative agent for the treatment of tetracycline-resistant *M. hominis* infection. Either erythromycin or tetracyclines can be used in therapy for *U. urealyticum* infections, but tetracycline resistance occurs in 10 to 15 percent of clinical isolates. The activity of quinolones is not affected by tetracycline resistance caused by the tetM transposon. Ciprofloxacin is generally less active than ofloxacin in vitro against either agent. A 7-day course of oral ofloxacin (200 to 400 mg every 12 h for adults) appears to be adequate for urethritis, but studies of this regimen have focused on *C. trachomatis* rather than on *U. urealyticum*. A single (1-g) dose of azithromycin is

approved for treatment of urethritis due to *C. trachomatis* and has been shown to work as well clinically as 7 days of doxycycline therapy in persons with infection due to *U. urealyticum*. *M. hominis* is resistant to macrolides.

Infections in immunocompromised hosts may be caused by resistant organisms refractory to antimicrobial therapy and may require prolonged administration of a combination of intravenous antimicrobials, intravenous immunoglobulin, and/or antisera prepared specifically against the infecting species. Despite aggressive therapy, relapses are likely. No specific treatment guidelines for neonates with systemic mycoplasmal or ureaplasmal infections have been established, and no controlled trials of clinical efficacy have been conducted. However, appropriately modified dosages of the same drugs used for older children have been used successfully in numerous reported cases in neonates.

BIBLIOGRAPHY

CASSELL GH et al: *Ureaplasma urealyticum* intrauterine infection: Role in prematurity and disease in the newborn. Clin Microbiol Rev 6:69, 1993
———: The changing role of mycoplasmas in respiratory disease and AIDS. Clin Infect Dis 17(Suppl):S1, 1993
——— et al: Genital mycoplasmal infections, in *Current Pediatric Therapy*, FD Burg et al (eds). Orlando, Saunders, 1995, p 673
CHAN ED, WELSH CH: Fulminant *Mycoplasma pneumoniae* pneumonia. West J Med 162:133, 1995

181 *Walter E. Stamm*

CHLAMYDIAL INFECTIONS

The genus *Chlamydia* contains three species that infect humans: *Chlamydia psittaci*, *Chlamydia trachomatis*, and *Chlamydia pneumoniae* (formerly the TWAR agent). *C. psittaci* is widely distributed in nature, producing genital, conjunctival, intestinal, or respiratory infections in many mammalian and avian species. Genital infections with *C. psittaci* have been well characterized in several species and cause complications such as abortion and infertility. Although mammalian strains of *C. psittaci* are not known to infect humans, avian strains occasionally do so, causing pneumonia and the systemic illness known as psittacosis.

C. pneumoniae is a fastidious chlamydial species that appears to be a frequent cause of upper respiratory tract infection and pneumonia, primarily in children and young adults, and is a cause of recurrent respiratory infections in older adults. No animal reservoir has been identified for *C. pneumoniae*; it appears to be a human pathogen spread via the respiratory route through close personal contact. To date, all strains of *C. pneumoniae* studied have been serologically homologous.

C. trachomatis is exclusively a human pathogen and was identified as the cause of trachoma in the 1940s. Since then, *C. trachomatis* has been recognized as a major cause of sexually transmitted and perinatal infection.

Chlamydiae are obligate intracellular parasites. They possess both DNA and RNA, have a cell wall and ribosomes similar to those of gram-negative bacteria, and are inhibited by antibiotics such as tetracycline. Chlamydiae are classified as bacteria belonging to their own order (Chlamydiales).

A unique feature of all chlamydiae is their complex reproductive cycle. Two forms of the microorganism—the extracellular elementary body and the intracellular reticulate body—participate in this cycle. The elementary body is adapted for extracellular survival and is the infective form transmitted from one person to another. Elementary bodies attach to susceptible target cells (usually columnar or transitional epithelial cells) and enter the cells within a phagosome. Within 8 h, the elementary bodies reorganize into reticulate bodies. These forms are adapted to intracellular survival and multiplication. They undergo binary fission, eventually producing numerous replicates contained within the membrane-bound "inclusion body," which occupies much of the infected host cell. Chlamydial inclusions resist lysosomal fusion until late in the developmental cycle. After 24 h, the reticulate bodies condense and form elementary bodies still contained within the inclusion. The inclusion then ruptures, releasing elementary bodies from the cell to initiate infection of adjacent cells.

Recent studies using monoclonal antibodies to and nucleotide sequencing of the major outer-membrane protein have delineated at least 20 serotypes of *C. trachomatis*. According to the serovar classification system of Wang and Grayston, strains associated with trachoma have generally been those of the A, B, Ba, and C serovars, while serovars D through K have largely been associated with sexually transmitted and perinatally acquired infections. Serovars L$_1$, L$_2$, and L$_3$ produce lymphogranuloma venereum (LGV) and hemorrhagic proctocolitis. The LGV strains demonstrate unique biologic behavior in that they are more invasive than the other serovars, produce disease in lymphatic tissue, grow readily in cell culture systems and macrophages, and are fatal when inoculated intracerebrally into mice and monkeys. Non-LGV strains of *C. trachomatis* characteristically produce superficial infections involving the columnar epithelium of the eye, genitalia, and respiratory tract.

C. trachomatis has been reported as an infrequent cause of endocarditis, peritonitis, pleuritis, and possibly periappendicitis and may occasionally cause respiratory infections in older children and adults. Immunosuppressed patients with pneumonia have had, in some cases, either serologic or cultural evidence of *C. trachomatis* infection, but more data are necessary to define the role of *Chlamydia* in these patients.

SEXUALLY TRANSMITTED AND PERINATAL INFECTIONS DUE TO *C. TRACHOMATIS*

SPECTRUM OF *C. TRACHOMATIS* GENITAL INFECTIONS Genital infections caused by *C. trachomatis* represent the most common bacterial sexually transmitted diseases (STDs) in the United States. An estimated 4 million cases occur each year. In adults the clinical spectrum of sexually transmitted *C. trachomatis* infections parallels the spectrum of gonococcal infections (Table 181-1). Chlamydial and gonococcal infections have been associated with urethritis, proctitis, and conjunctivitis in both sexes; with epididymitis in men; and with mucopurulent cervicitis (MPC), acute salpingitis, bartholinitis, and the Fitz-Hugh–Curtis syndrome (perihepatitis) in women. Moreover, both types of infection can be associated with systemic complications, particularly arthritis. In general, however, chlamydial infections produce fewer symptoms and signs than corresponding gonococcal infections at the same anatomic site; in fact, the former are often totally asymptomatic. Increasing evidence suggests that many chlamydial infections of the genital tract, especially in women, persist for months without producing symptoms. Simultaneous infection with *C. trachomatis* often occurs in women with cervical gonococcal infection and in heterosexual men with gonococcal urethritis.

EPIDEMIOLOGY Infections due to *C. trachomatis* have now been made reportable in many states, and national incidence data show steadily rising numbers of reported infections, undoubtedly reflecting both increased testing and increased reporting. The annual occurrence of nongonococcal urethritis (NGU) has been measured through surveys of diagnoses made by physicians in private practice and has been used as a surrogate measure of trends in chlamydial infection. The incidence of NGU increased dramatically during the 1960s and 1970s, a period when chlamydiae caused 30 to 50 percent of such cases. Even as the incidence of gonococcal urethritis fell during the 1980s, the incidence of NGU stabilized in the United States, probably reflecting the relative lack of implementation of programs to control chlamydial infections. More recently, the implementation of such programs in some regions has been associated with a decline in the proportion of NGU cases

Table 181-1

Clinical Parallels Between Sexually Transmitted Infections due to *Neisseria gonorrhoeae* and *Chlamydia trachomatis*

	Clinical Syndrome Caused by	
Site of Infection	*N. gonorrhoeae*	*C. trachomatis*
MEN		
Urethra	Urethritis	Nongonococcal or post-gonococcal urethritis
Epididymis	Epididymitis	Epididymitis
Rectum	Proctitis	Proctitis
Conjunctiva	Conjunctivitis	Conjunctivitis
Systemic	Disseminated gonococcal infection	Reiter's syndrome
WOMEN		
Urethra	Acute urethral syndrome	Acute urethral syndrome
Bartholin's gland	Bartholinitis	Bartholinitis
Cervix	Cervicitis	Cervicitis
Rectum	Proctitis	Proctitis
Endometrium	Endometritis	Endometritis
Fallopian tube	Salpingitis	Salpingitis
Conjunctiva	Conjunctivitis	Conjunctivitis
Liver capsule	Perihepatitis	Perihepatitis
Systemic	Disseminated gonococcal infection	Reiter's syndrome

caused by chlamydiae; thus trends in NGU may now be less reliable as a surrogate for trends in the incidence of chlamydial infection.

The age of peak incidence of genital *C. trachomatis* infections, as of other sexually transmitted infections, is the late teens and early twenties. The prevalence of chlamydial urethral infection among young men is 3 to 5 percent for those seen in general medical settings, over 10 percent for asymptomatic soldiers undergoing routine physical examination, and 15 to 20 percent for heterosexual men seen in STD clinics. In areas where chlamydial control programs have been implemented, prevalence may be markedly reduced. In short, prevalence varies widely with the population group studied and with the geographic locale. Urethral chlamydial infection is less common among homosexual than among heterosexual men, but rectal infections occur in homosexual men who practice receptive anorectal intercourse without condoms. The ratio of chlamydial to gonococcal urethritis is highest for heterosexual men and for those with high socioeconomic status and is lowest for homosexual men and indigent populations.

The prevalence of cervical infection among women is approximately 5 percent for asymptomatic college students and prenatal patients in the United States, over 10 percent for women seen in family planning clinics, and over 20 percent for women seen in STD clinics. As in men, prevalence varies substantially by geographic locale. In the United States, the prevalence of *C. trachomatis* in the cervix of pregnant women is 5 to 10 times higher than that of *Neisseria gonorrhoeae*. The prevalence of genital infection with either agent is highest among individuals who are single, non-Caucasian, and between ages 18 and 24. Oral contraceptive use and the presence of cervical ectopy also confer an increased risk of chlamydial infection. The proportion of infections that are asymptomatic appears to be higher for *C. trachomatis* than for *N. gonorrhoeae*, and symptomatic *C. trachomatis* infections are clinically less severe. It is suspected that mild or asymptomatic chlamydial infections of the fallopian tubes may nonetheless cause ongoing tubal damage and infertility. Furthermore, because the total number of *C. trachomatis* infections exceeds the total number of *N. gonorrhoeae* infections in industrialized countries, the total morbidity caused by *C. trachomatis* genital infections in these countries equals or exceeds that caused by *N. gonorrhoeae*. The prevalence of *C. trachomatis* is higher than that of *N. gonorrhoeae* in industrialized countries, in part because measures such as treatment of sex partners and routine cultures for case detection in asymptomatic individuals have been applied much more effectively to the control of gonorrhea than to the control of *C. trachomatis* infection.

CHAPTER 181
Chlamydial Infections **1057**

CLINICAL MANIFESTATIONS **Nongonococcal and Post-gonococcal Urethritis** NGU is a diagnosis of exclusion that is applied to men with symptoms and/or signs of urethritis who do not have gonorrhea. Postgonococcal urethritis (PGU) refers to nongonococcal urethritis developing in men 2 to 3 weeks after treatment of gonococcal urethritis with single doses of agents such as amoxicillin or cephalosporins that lack sufficient activity against chlamydiae. Since current treatment for gonorrhea also includes tetracycline, doxycycline, or azithromycin for concomitant chlamydial infection, both the incidence of PGU and the causative role of chlamydiae in this syndrome have declined. *C. trachomatis* causes 20 to 40 percent of the cases of NGU and PGU in heterosexual men but is less commonly isolated from homosexual men with these syndromes. The cause of most of the remaining cases is uncertain, although considerable evidence suggests that *Ureaplasma urealyticum* causes many of these infections, while *Trichomonas vaginalis* and herpes simplex virus (HSV) cause some cases of NGU.

NGU is diagnosed by documentation of a leukocytic urethral exudate and by exclusion of gonorrhea by Gram's staining or culture. *C. trachomatis* urethritis is generally less severe than gonococcal urethritis, although in an individual patient these two forms of urethritis cannot be reliably differentiated solely on clinical grounds. Symptoms include urethral discharge, dysuria (often whitish and mucoid rather than frankly purulent), and urethral itching. Physical examination may reveal meatal erythema and tenderness and a urethral exudate that is often demonstrable only by stripping of the urethra. At least one-third of males with *C. trachomatis* urethral infection have no demonstrable signs or symptoms of urethritis. Asymptomatic chlamydial urethritis has been demonstrated in 5 to 10 percent of sexually active adolescent males screened in teen clinics. Such patients frequently have first-glass pyuria ($\geq$15 leukocytes per 400$\times$ microscopic field in the sediment of first-voided urine), a positive leukocyte esterase test, or an increased number of leukocytes on Gram-stained smear prepared from a urogenital swab inserted 1 to 2 cm into the anterior urethra. For the enumeration of leukocytes, the smear is first scanned at low power to identify areas of the slide containing the highest concentration of leukocytes. These areas are then examined under oil immersion (1000$\times$). An average of four or more leukocytes in at least three of five 1000$\times$ (oil-immersion) fields is indicative of urethritis and correlates with the recovery of *C. trachomatis*. To differentiate between true urethritis and functional symptoms among symptomatic patients or to make a presumptive diagnosis of *C. trachomatis* infection in asymptomatic men (e.g., male patients in STD clinics, sex partners of women with nongonococcal salpingitis or MPC, fathers of children with inclusion conjunctivitis), the examination of an endourethral specimen for increased leukocytes is useful if specific diagnostic tests for chlamydiae are not available. Alternatively, noninvasive screening for urethritis can be accomplished by testing of a first-void urine sample for pyuria, either by microscopy or by the leukocyte esterase test. Urine can also be directly tested for chlamydiae or gonococci by DNA amplification methods, as described below.

Epididymitis *C. trachomatis* is the major cause of epididymitis in sexually active heterosexual men under 35 years of age, accounting for about 70 percent of cases. *N. gonorrhoeae* causes most of the remaining cases, and some men have simultaneous infections with both pathogens, usually accompanied by asymptomatic urethritis as defined above. In homosexual men, sexually transmitted coliform infection acquired via rectal intercourse may cause epididymitis. Coliform bacteria and *Pseudomonas aeruginosa*, usually in association with preceding urologic instrumentation or surgery, are the most common causes of epididymitis in men over 35. Men with epididymitis typically present with unilateral scrotal pain, fever, and epididymal tenderness or swelling on examination. The illness may be mild enough to treat on an outpatient basis or severe enough to require hospitalization. Testicular torsion should be excluded promptly by radionuclide scan, Doppler flow study, or surgical exploration in a teenager or young adult who presents with acute unilateral testicular pain without urethritis. The possibility of testicular tumor or chronic infection (e.g.,

tuberculosis) should be excluded when a patient with unilateral intrascrotal pain and swelling does not respond to appropriate antimicrobial therapy.

Reiter's Syndrome Reiter's syndrome consists of conjunctivitis, urethritis (or cervicitis in females), arthritis, and characteristic mucocutaneous lesions (see Chap. 317). *C. trachomatis* has been recovered from the urethra of up to 70 percent of men with untreated nondiarrheal Reiter's syndrome and associated urethritis. In the absence of overt urethritis, it is important to exclude subclinical urethritis in the men in whom this diagnosis is suspected.

The pathogenesis of Reiter's syndrome remains obscure. However, since more than 80 percent of affected patients have the HLA-B27 phenotype and since other mucosal infections (with *Salmonella*, *Shigella*, or *Campylobacter*, for example) produce an identical syndrome, chlamydial infection is thought to initiate an aberrant and hyperactive immune response that produces inflammation at the involved target organs in these genetically predisposed individuals. Evidence of exaggerated cell-mediated and humoral immune responses to chlamydial antigens in Reiter's syndrome supports this hypothesis. The presumptive demonstration of chlamydial elementary bodies and chlamydial DNA in the joint fluid and synovial tissue of patients with Reiter's syndrome suggests that chlamydiae may actually spread from genital to joint tissues in these patients, perhaps in macrophages.

Proctitis *C. trachomatis* strains of either the genital immunotypes D through K or the LGV immunotypes cause proctitis in homosexual men who practice receptive anorectal intercourse. In the United States, the vast majority of cases are due to immunotypes D through K and present either as asymptomatic infection or as mild proctitis not unlike gonococcal proctitis. These infections may develop in heterosexual women as well. Patients present with mild rectal pain, mucous discharge, tenesmus, and (occasionally) bleeding. Nearly all have neutrophils in their rectal Gram's stain. Anoscopy in these non-LGV cases of chlamydial proctitis reveals mild, patchy mucosal friability and mucopurulent discharge, and the disease process is limited to the distal rectum. LGV strains produce more severe ulcerative proctitis or proctocolitis that can be confused clinically with HSV proctitis (severe rectal pain, bleeding, discharge, and tenesmus) and that histologically resembles Crohn's disease in that giant cell formation and granulomas can be seen (see Chap. 286). In the United States, these cases occur almost exclusively in homosexual men.

Mucopurulent Cervicitis Although many women with *C. trachomatis* infection of the cervix have no symptoms or signs, a careful speculum examination reveals evidence of MPC in 30 to 50 percent of cases. As is discussed more fully in Chap. 130, MPC is associated with yellow mucopurulent discharge from the endocervical columnar epithelium and with $\geq$20 neutrophils per 1000$\times$ microscopic field within strands of cervical mucus on a thinly smeared, Gram-stained preparation of endocervical exudate. Other characteristic findings include edema of the zone of cervical ectopy and a propensity of the mucosa to bleed on minor trauma—e.g., when specimens are collected with a swab. A pap smear shows increased numbers of neutrophils as well as a characteristic pattern of mononuclear inflammatory cells, including plasma cells, transformed lymphocytes, and histiocytes. Cervical biopsy shows a predominantly mononuclear cell infiltrate of the subepithelial stroma, often with follicular cervicitis.

Pelvic Inflammatory Disease (PID) *C. trachomatis* plays an important causative role in salpingitis. Infection with *C. trachomatis* has been demonstrated in laparoscopically verified salpingitis, the organism has been recovered from the fallopian tubes in the absence of other pathogens, and serologic evidence of recent *C. trachomatis* infection has been found in women with PID. In the United States, *C. trachomatis* has been identified in the fallopian tubes or endometrium of up to 50 percent of women with PID, and its role as an important etiologic agent in this syndrome is well accepted.

PID occurs via ascending intraluminal spread of *C. trachomatis* from the lower genital tract. MPC is thus followed by endometritis, endosalpingitis, and finally pelvic peritonitis. Evidence of MPC is usually found in women with laparoscopically verified salpingitis. Similarly, endometritis, demonstrated by endometrial biopsy showing plasma cell infiltration of the endometrial epithelium, is documented in most women with laparoscopically verified chlamydial (or gonococcal) salpingitis. Chlamydial endometritis also can occur in the absence of clinical evidence of salpingitis: approximately 40 to 50 percent of women with MPC have plasma cell endometritis. Histologic evidence of endometritis has been correlated with an "endometritis syndrome" consisting of vaginal bleeding, lower abdominal pain, and uterine tenderness in the absence of adnexal tenderness. It is not known what proportion of women who have chlamydial endometritis without adnexal tenderness also have salpingitis. However, chlamydial salpingitis may produce milder symptoms than does gonococcal salpingitis and may be associated with less marked adnexal tenderness. Mild adnexal or uterine tenderness in sexually active women with cervicitis suggests PID.

Infertility associated with fallopian-tube scarring has been strongly linked to antecedent *C. trachomatis* infection in serologic studies. Since many infertile women with tubal scarring and antichlamydial antibody have no history of PID, it appears that subclinical tubal infection ("silent salpingitis") may produce scarring. Ectopic pregnancy, which occurs in more than 70,000 women in the United States annually, is also thought to be related to *Chlamydia*-induced tubal scarring in many cases. While the pathogenesis of *Chlamydia*-induced tubal scarring remains poorly understood, antibodies to the chlamydial 60-kDa heat-shock protein have been correlated with tubal infertility, ectopic pregnancy, and Fitz-Hugh–Curtis syndrome (see below). Thus this antigen may initiate an immune-mediated process that ultimately damages the fallopian tube. Host genetic susceptibility, as defined by HLA type, may also play an important role.

Perihepatitis, or the Fitz-Hugh–Curtis syndrome, was originally described as a complication of gonococcal PID. However, cultural and/or serologic evidence of *C. trachomatis* infection is found in three-quarters of women with this syndrome. *C. trachomatis* has also been cultured from exudate on the hepatic capsule in laparoscopically verified cases. This syndrome should be suspected whenever a young, sexually active woman presents with an illness resembling cholecystitis (fever and right upper quadrant pain of subacute or acute onset). Symptoms and signs of salpingitis may be minimal. High titers of antibodies to *C. trachomatis* are generally present.

Urethral Syndrome in Women   In the absence of infection with uropathogens such as coliforms or *Staphylococcus saprophyticus*, *C. trachomatis* is the pathogen most commonly isolated from college women with dysuria, frequency, and pyuria (see Chap. 131). *Chlamydia* also can be isolated from the urethra of women without symptoms of urethritis, and up to 25 percent of female STD clinic patients with chlamydial urogenital infection have cultures positive for *C. trachomatis* from the urethra only.

***C. trachomatis* Infection in Pregnancy**   *C. trachomatis* in pregnancy has been associated in some studies (but not in others) with premature delivery and with postpartum endometritis. Whether these complications are in part attributable to *C. trachomatis* is not clear.

PERINATAL INFECTIONS: INCLUSION CONJUNCTIVITIS AND PNEUMONIA   Epidemiology   Studies in the United States have demonstrated that 5 to 25 percent of pregnant women have *C. trachomatis* infections of the cervix. In these studies, approximately one-half to two-thirds of children exposed during birth have acquired *C. trachomatis* infection. Roughly half of the infected infants (or 25 percent of the group exposed) have developed clinical evidence of inclusion conjunctivitis. In addition to infecting the eye, *C. trachomatis* has been isolated frequently and persistently from the nasopharynx, rectum, and vagina of infants, occasionally for periods exceeding 1 year in the absence of treatment. Pneumonia develops in about 10 percent of children infected perinatally, and otitis media may in some cases result from perinatally acquired chlamydial infection.

Inclusion Conjunctivitis of the Newborn (Neonatal Chlamydial Conjunctivitis)   Neonatal chlamydial conjunctivitis has an acute onset and often produces a profuse mucopurulent discharge. In the newborn, chlamydial conjunctivitis generally has a longer incubation period than gonococcal conjunctivitis (usually 5 to 14 days vs. 1 to 3 days); however, this guideline is not reliable for the diagnosis of individual cases, and in any event it is impossible to differentiate chlamydial conjunctivitis from other forms of neonatal bacterial conjunctivitis on clinical grounds; instead, laboratory diagnosis is required. Besides *C. trachomatis* and *N. gonorrhoeae*, the other important infectious causes of conjunctivitis in newborns include *Haemophilus influenzae*, *Streptococcus pneumoniae*, and HSV. Inclusions within epithelial cells are often detected in Giemsa-stained conjunctival smears, but these smears are less sensitive than cultures or antigen detection tests. Gram-stained smears may show gonococci or occasional small gram-negative coccobacilli in *Haemophilus* conjunctivitis, but smears should be accompanied by cultures for these agents. Very rarely, a trachoma-like eye disease occurs in children who have chlamydial infection and who live in areas that do not have endemic trachoma. Since concomitant pharyngeal infection is often present, neonatal chlamydial conjunctivitis should be treated with oral antimicrobials in order to prevent chlamydial pneumonia.

Infant Pneumonia   *C. trachomatis* causes a distinctive pneumonia syndrome in infants. Recent epidemiologic studies have linked chlamydial pulmonary infection in infants with increased occurrence of subacute lung disease (bronchitis, asthma, wheezing) in later childhood.

LYMPHOGRANULOMA VENEREUM   Definition   LGV is a sexually transmitted infection caused by *C. trachomatis* strains of the L_1, L_2, and L_3 serovars. In the United States, most cases are caused by L_2 organisms. Acute LGV in heterosexual men is characterized by a transient primary genital lesion followed by multilocular suppurative regional lymphadenopathy. Women, homosexual men, and—in occasional instances—heterosexual men may develop hemorrhagic proctitis with regional lymphadenitis. Acute LGV is almost always associated with systemic symptoms such as fever and leukocytosis but is rarely associated with systemic complications such as meningoencephalitis. After a latent period of years, late complications include genital elephantiasis due to lymphatic involvement; strictures; and fistulas of the penis, urethra, and rectum.

Epidemiology   LGV is usually sexually transmitted, but occasional transmission by nonsexual personal contact, fomites, or laboratory accidents has been documented. Laboratory work involving the creation of aerosols of LGV organisms (e.g., sonication, homogenization) must be conducted only with appropriate measures for biologic containment.

The peak incidence of LGV corresponds to the age of greatest sexual activity: the second and third decades of life. The worldwide incidence of LGV is falling, but the disease is still endemic and a major cause of morbidity in Asia, Africa, South America, and parts of the Caribbean. In the Bahamas, an apparent outbreak of LGV has been described in association with a concurrent increase in heterosexual infection with human immunodeficiency virus. However, only 235 cases were reported in the United States in 1994.

The frequency of infection following exposure is believed to be much lower than that for gonorrhea and syphilis. Early manifestations are recognized far more often in men than in women, who usually present with late complications. In the United States, where the reported male-to-female ratio of cases is 3.4:1, most cases have involved homosexually active men and persons returning from abroad (travelers, sailors, and military personnel). The main reservoir of infection, although it has not been directly demonstrated, is presumed to be asymptomatically infected individuals.

Clinical Manifestations   In heterosexuals, a *primary genital lesion* develops from 3 days to 3 weeks after exposure. It is a small, painless vesicle or nonindurated ulcer or papule located on the penis in men and on the labia, posterior vagina, or fourchette in women. The primary lesion is noticed by fewer than one-third of men with LGV and only rarely by women. It heals in a few days without scarring and, even when noticed, usually is recognized as LGV only in retrospect. LGV strains of *C. trachomatis* have occasionally been recovered from genital ulcers and from the urethra of men and the endocervix of women who present with inguinal adenopathy; these areas may be the primary site of infection in some cases.

In women and homosexual men, *primary anal* or *rectal infection* develops after receptive anorectal intercourse. In women, rectal infection with LGV (or non-LGV) strains of *C. trachomatis* presumably can also arise by the contiguous spread of infected secretions along the perineum (as in rectal gonococcal infections in women) or perhaps by spread to the rectum via the pelvic lymphatics.

From the site of the primary urethral, genital, anal, or rectal infection, the organism spreads via the regional lymphatics. Penile, vulvar, or anal infection can lead to inguinal and femoral lymphadenitis. Rectal infection produces hypogastric and deep iliac lymphadenitis. Upper vaginal or cervical infection results in enlargement of the obturator and iliac nodes.

The most common presenting picture in heterosexual men is the *inguinal syndrome*, which is characterized by painful inguinal lymphadenopathy beginning 2 to 6 weeks after presumed exposure; in rare instances, the onset comes after a few months. The inguinal adenopathy is unilateral in two-thirds of cases, and palpable enlargement of the iliac and femoral nodes is often evident on the same side as the enlarged inguinal nodes. The nodes are initially discrete, but progressive periadenitis results in a matted mass of nodes that becomes fluctuant and suppurative. The overlying skin becomes fixed, inflamed, and thin and finally develops multiple draining fistulas. Extensive enlargement of chains of inguinal nodes above and below the inguinal ligament ("the sign of the groove") is not specific and, although not uncommon, is documented in only a minority of cases. On histologic examination, infected nodes are initially found to have characteristic small stellate abscesses surrounded by histiocytes. These abscesses coalesce to form large, necrotic, suppurative foci. Spontaneous healing usually takes place after several months; inguinal scars or granulomatous masses of various sizes persist for life. Massive pelvic lymphadenopathy in women or homosexual men may lead to exploratory laparotomy.

As cultures and serologic tests for *C. trachomatis* are being used more often, increasing numbers of cases of LGV proctitis are being recognized in homosexual men. Such patients present with anorectal pain and mucopurulent, bloody rectal discharge. Although these patients may complain of diarrhea, they are often referring not to diarrhea but rather to frequent, painful, unsuccessful attempts at defecation (tenesmus). Sigmoidoscopy reveals ulcerative proctitis or proctocolitis, with purulent exudate and mucosal bleeding. The histopathologic findings in the rectal mucosa include granulomas with giant cells, along with crypt abscesses and extensive inflammation. These clinical, sigmoidoscopic, and histopathologic findings may closely resemble those of Crohn's disease of the rectum.

Constitutional symptoms are common during the stage of regional lymphadenopathy and, in cases of proctitis, may include fever, chills, headache, meningismus, anorexia, myalgias, and arthralgias. These findings in the presence of lymphadenopathy sometimes are mistakenly interpreted as representing malignant lymphoma. Other systemic complications are infrequent but include arthritis with sterile effusion, aseptic meningitis, meningoencephalitis, conjunctivitis, hepatitis, and erythema nodosum. Chlamydiae have been recovered from the cerebrospinal fluid and in one case were isolated from the blood of a patient with severe constitutional symptoms—a result indicating the dissemination of infection. Laboratory-acquired infections suspected of being due to the inhalation of aerosols have been associated with mediastinal lymphadenitis, pneumonitis, and pleural effusion.

Complications of untreated anorectal infection include perirectal abscess; fistula in ano; and rectovaginal, rectovesical, and ischiorectal fistulas. Secondary bacterial infection probably contributes to these complications. Rectal stricture is a late complication of anorectal infection and usually develops 2 to 6 cm from the anal orifice—i.e., at a site within reach on digital rectal examination. Proximal extension of the stricture for several centimeters may lead to a mistaken clinical and radiographic diagnosis of carcinoma.

A small percentage of cases of LGV in men present as chronic progressive infiltrative, ulcerative, or fistular lesions of the penis, urethra, or scrotum. Associated lymphatic obstruction may produce elephantiasis. When urethral stricture occurs, it usually involves the posterior urethra and causes incontinence or difficulty with urination.

APPROACH TO THE DIAGNOSIS AND TREATMENT OF *C. TRACHOMATIS* GENITAL INFECTIONS

Four types of laboratory procedure are available to confirm *C. trachomatis* infection: direct microscopic examination of tissue scrapings for typical intracytoplasmic inclusions or elementary bodies; isolation of the organism in cell culture; detection of chlamydial antigens or nucleic acid by immunologic or hybridization methods; and detection of antibody in serum or in local secretions.

Except in conjunctivitis, direct microscopic examination of Giemsa-stained cell scrapings for typical inclusions has an unacceptably low degree of sensitivity, and false-positive interpretations by inexperienced observers are common. Even for conjunctivitis, this approach has been replaced by direct fluorescent antibody staining of conjunctival smears to identify chlamydial elementary bodies (see below).

Cell culture techniques for isolation of *C. trachomatis* are available in most large medical centers but not in other clinical settings. In addition to limited availability, other disadvantages of cell culture include its low and variable level of sensitivity (60 to 80 percent), its requirement for rigorous transport conditions, and its high cost and technically demanding nature. Therefore, nonculture alternatives utilizing antigen detection or nucleic acid hybridization have been developed. In the immunofluorescent slide test, potentially infected genital or ocular secretions are smeared onto a slide, fixed, and stained with fluorescein-conjugated monoclonal antibody specific for chlamydial antigens. The observation of fluorescing elementary bodies confirms the diagnosis. Compared with culture, this test is 70 to 85 percent sensitive, and it is quite specific when used for confirmation of urethral, cervical, or ocular infection in high-risk patients with suspected *C. trachomatis* infection. The sensitivity and specificity of the test depend directly upon the skill of the microscopist. The apparently lower sensitivity of the test in low-risk populations, along with its relatively labor-intensive nature, limits its value as a screening tool.

Enzyme-linked immunosorbent assay (ELISA) techniques for the detection of chlamydial antigens provide another alternative to culture. The reported sensitivity and specificity of these tests for genital infections (as compared with culture) have been 60 to 80 percent and 97 to 99 percent, respectively, in high-risk populations. Sensitivities have generally been higher in cervical infection and lower in urethritis among males. Like the direct fluorescent antibody slide test, the ELISA is less accurate in low-prevalence populations. ELISAs are better suited to screening than is direct immunofluorescence because large numbers of specimens can easily be processed.

Assays using nucleic acid probes have also been developed for chlamydial diagnosis. One such test uses DNA-RNA hybridization and appears to be approximately equal to the best ELISAs in terms of sensitivity and specificity. Recently, nucleic acid probes have been developed for use in amplification assays such as ligase chain reaction and polymerase chain reaction (PCR). These tests are now the most sensitive chlamydial diagnostic methods available, being the first nonculture assays actually to surpass culture itself in sensitivity. The ability of these tests to detect chlamydial genes in urine with a high degree of sensitivity and specificity allows their use with urine specimens rather than with conventional urethral and cervical swabs. The use of urine specimens is particularly appealing for public-health chlamydial screening programs.

Serologic tests are of limited usefulness in the diagnosis of chlamydial oculogenital infections. The complement fixation (CF) test with heat-stable, genus-specific antigen has been used with some success to diagnose LGV but is insensitive in infections due to non-LGV strains of *C. trachomatis*. The microimmunofluorescence (micro-IF) test with *C. trachomatis* antigens is more sensitive but is generally available only in research laboratories. The test measures antibodies by serovar specificity and by immunoglobulin class (IgM, IgG, IgA, secretory IgA) in both serum and local secretions. Serologic diagnosis by the micro-IF test may be useful in infant pneumonia (in which high-titer IgM antibody and/or fourfold rises in titer are often demonstrated), in chlamydial salpingitis (especially Fitz-Hugh–Curtis syndrome), and in LGV.

Table 181-2 summarizes the diagnostic tests of choice for patients with suspected chlamydial infection. With few exceptions, the most suitable method for diagnosis is demonstration of the agent by either cell culture or one of the newer nonculture techniques. Selection of the most appropriate of these tests often depends upon local availability and expertise. However, it is clear that, in most settings and for most purposes, sensitivity and specificity will be greatest with nucleic acid amplification techniques. For patients to whom medicolegal considera-

tions may apply (victims of sexual or child abuse), cultures or nucleic acid amplification methods should always be used. Since *C. trachomatis* is an intracellular pathogen, adequate specimens for chlamydial diagnostic testing must include epithelial cells. Cultures or nonculture tests of pus are less often positive. In urethritis, a thin-shafted urogenital swab should be inserted at least 2 cm into the urethra to obtain an appropriate specimen. Although cultures of urine for chlamydiae are less sensitive than urethral cultures, recent studies suggest that nucleic acid amplification testing of a first-void urine specimen from men is a more sensitive and less painful diagnostic alternative to the more invasive urethral swab–based tests. The first 30 mL of voided urine should be collected for testing. When a cervical sample is collected, the external os should first be cleaned of debris and purulent material; a plastic-shafted swab should then be inserted into the cervix, rotated slowly several times, and withdrawn. For the diagnosis of infections in women, testing of a first-void urine specimen by nucleic acid amplification methods is at least as sensitive as testing of a cervical swab. When conjunctival specimens are sought, the epithelium should be swabbed to remove cells rather than just purulent material. All specimens for chlamydial culture should be placed immediately into transport medium and then either refrigerated (if they will reach the labora-

Table 181-2

Diagnostic Tests for *Chlamydia trachomatis* Infection

Infection	Suggestive Signs/Symptoms	Presumptive Diagnosis*	Confirmatory Test of Choice
MEN			
NGU, PGU	Discharge, dysuria	Gram's stain with >4 neutrophils per oil-immersion field; no gonococci	Urethral culture or nonculture test for *C. trachomatis*; urine PCR or LCR for *C. trachomatis*
Epididymitis	Unilateral intrascrotal swelling, pain, tenderness; fever; NGU	Gram's stain with >4 neutrophils per oil-immersion field; no gonococci; urinalysis with pyuria	Urethral culture or nonculture test for *C. trachomatis*; urine PCR or LCR for *C. trachomatis*
WOMEN			
Cervicitis	Mucopurulent cervical discharge, bleeding and edema of the zone of cervical ectopy	Cervical Gram's stain with ≥20 neutrophils per oil-immersion field in cervical mucus	Cervical culture or nonculture test for *C. trachomatis*; urine PCR or LCR for *C. trachomatis*
Salpingitis	Lower abdominal pain, cervical motion tenderness, adnexal tenderness or masses	*C. trachomatis* always potentially present in salpingitis	Cervical culture or nonculture test for *C. trachomatis*; urine PCR or LCR for *C. trachomatis*
Urethritis	Dysuria and frequency without urgency or hematuria	MPC; sterile pyuria; negative routine urine culture	Urethral and cervical cultures or nonculture test for *C. trachomatis*; urine PCR or LCR for *C. trachomatis*
ADULTS OF EITHER SEX			
Proctitis	Rectal pain, discharge, tenesmus, bleeding; history of receptive anorectal intercourse	Negative gonococcal culture and Gram's stain; at least 1 neutrophil per oil-immersion field in rectal Gram's stain	Rectal culture or direct immunofluorescence test for *C. trachomatis*
Reiter's syndrome	NGU, arthritis, conjunctivitis, typical skin lesions	Gram's stain with >4 neutrophils per oil-immersion field; lack of gonococci indicative of NGU	Urethral culture or nonculture test for *C. trachomatis*
LGV	Regional adenopathy, primary lesion, proctitis, systemic symptoms	None	Isolation of LGV strain from node or rectum, occasionally from urethra or cervix; LGV CF titer, ≥1:64; micro-IF titer, ≥1:512
NEONATES			
Conjunctivitis	Purulent conjunctival discharge 6 to 18 days postdelivery	Negative culture and Gram's stain for gonococci, *Haemophilus* species, pneumococci, staphylococci	Conjunctival culture or nonculture test for *C. trachomatis*; Giemsa-stained scraping of conjunctival material capable of providing more rapid diagnosis but less sensitive
Infant pneumonia	Afebrile, staccato cough, diffuse rales, bilateral hyperinflation, interstitial infiltrates	None	Chlamydial culture of sputum, pharynx, eye, rectum; micro-IF antibody to *C. trachomatis*— fourfold change in IgG or IgM antibody titer

* A presumptive diagnosis of chlamydial infection is often made in the syndromes listed when gonococci are not found. A positive test for *Neisseria gonorrhoeae* does not exclude the involvement of *C. trachomatis*, which often is present in patients with gonorrhea.

NOTE: CF, complement-fixing; LCR, ligase chain reaction; LGV, lymphogranuloma venereum; micro-IF, microimmunofluorescence; MPC, mucopurulent cervicitis; NGU, nongonococcal urethritis; PCR, polymerase chain reaction; PGU, postgonococcal urethritis.

tory within 12 to 18 h) or frozen at −70°C (if longer storage is anticipated). A major advantage of the nonculture diagnostic techniques is their less rigid transport requirements; neither refrigeration nor rapid transport is needed.

From a public health viewpoint, the most effective use of chlamydial diagnostic testing has not been established and varies with the clinical population, local resources, and laboratory expertise. The Centers for Disease Control and Prevention have recommended empiric treatment (without diagnostic testing if resources are not available for testing) of selected high-risk groups. These include men with NGU or sexually transmitted epididymitis; women with MPC or PID; asymptomatic sex partners of patients with these syndromes; women and heterosexual men with gonorrhea (because of the high proportion of these patients who also have *C. trachomatis* infection); and sexual contacts of men or women with gonorrhea. However, diagnostic testing (in addition to empiric therapy) offers several potential benefits in the management of these patients, including confirmation of infection and support of the clinical diagnosis (especially in women with MPC or PID), enhancement of sex-partner referral and compliance with drug therapy, determination of prognosis, and education of physicians regarding the correlation of signs and symptoms with culture results. Since chlamydial diagnostic testing has become more widely available, its use for specific diagnosis in such patients should be promoted. From a public health perspective, high priority should be given to the screening of asymptomatic high-risk women who would not otherwise receive treatment for presumptive chlamydial infection, especially those seen in high-risk settings (e.g., STD clinics or abortion clinics) and those with a high-risk profile (e.g., sexually active and ≤21 years of age, new sex partner within the preceding 2 months, or more than one current sex partner). Similar screening programs should be used to detect and treat asymptomatic urethritis in high-risk adolescent males. Screening programs of this type have been associated with reductions in the prevalence of chlamydial infection and of the complications of chlamydial infection, such as PID.

ANTIMICROBIAL SUSCEPTIBILITY In laboratory tests that evaluate the growth of chlamydiae in cell cultures, the tetracyclines, erythromycin, rifampin, certain fluoroquinolones (especially ofloxacin), and the new macrolide azithromycin are all highly active against these organisms. Sulfonamides and clindamycin are also active against *C. trachomatis*, but to a lesser degree. Penicillin and ampicillin suppress chlamydial multiplication but do not eradicate the organism in vitro. The cephalosporins appear to be relatively ineffective against *C. trachomatis*. Streptomycin, gentamicin, neomycin, kanamycin, vancomycin, ristocetin, spectinomycin, and nystatin are not effective at concentrations inhibitory for most bacteria and fungi. There does not appear to be much strain-to-strain variation in susceptibility to antibiotics, and no clinically significant antimicrobial resistance in chlamydiae has been described. Thus antimicrobial susceptibility testing is not needed in the routine management of patients with chlamydial infection.

℞ TREATMENT

Until the introduction of azithromycin, chlamydial infections could not be eradicated by single-dose or short-term antimicrobial regimens. In most situations in adults, 7 days of treatment with doxycycline or tetracycline should be given for uncomplicated genital infections, but a 2-week course of therapy is recommended for complicated chlamydial infections (e.g., PID, epididymitis) and at least a 3-week course for LGV. Failure of treatment of genital infections with a tetracycline usually indicates poor compliance or reinfection rather than the involvement of a drug-resistant strain.

Therapy for *C. trachomatis* urethritis is more effective than therapy for nonchlamydial NGU. *C. trachomatis* is eradicated from the urethra by treatment with tetracycline hydrochloride (500 mg qid for 7 days) or doxycycline (100 mg by mouth bid for 7 days). An effective alternative regimen is erythromycin at a dose of 500 mg qid for 7 days.

Eradication of *C. trachomatis* from the cervix by tetracycline, doxycycline, and erythromycin, given at similar doses and for similar

durations, has been demonstrated. Erythromycin base (500 mg qid for 10 to 14 days) is the regimen of choice for pregnant women with *C. trachomatis* infection. Amoxicillin (500 mg tid for 10 days) has also been used successfully in pregnant women. Tetracycline hydrochloride (500 mg qid) or doxycycline (100 mg bid) for 14 days produces clinical and microbiologic cure of epididymitis and PID associated with *C. trachomatis* infection, but in this situation tetracycline should always be used together with a drug that is highly effective against gonorrhea.

Two other antimicrobial agents can be used for the treatment of uncomplicated chlamydial genital infections in men and women. Ofloxacin (300 mg orally bid for 7 days) is as effective as doxycycline for the treatment of chlamydial infection and appears to be safe and well tolerated. It cannot be used in pregnancy. Azithromycin, a macrolide, is highly active against *C. trachomatis*, exhibits prolonged bioavailability, and is concentrated intracellularly. In comparative trials, a 1-g single dose of azithromycin has been as effective as 7 days of doxycycline for uncomplicated chlamydial infection. Azithromycin causes fewer adverse gastrointestinal reactions than do older macrolides like erythromycin. Both ofloxacin and azithromycin offer alternatives for treatment that may be of value in selected patients who are allergic to or intolerant of tetracyclines and erythromycin, but they are considerably more expensive than these standard regimens. The single-dose regimen of azithromycin has great appeal for the treatment of patients with uncomplicated chlamydial infection (especially those without symptoms and those with a likelihood of poor compliance) and of sexual partners of infected patients. Although not approved by the U.S. Food and Drug Administration, the 1-g single-dose regimen of azithromycin has been safe and effective in the treatment of pregnant women.

Treatment of Sex Partners The continued high prevalence of chlamydial infections in most parts of the United States is due primarily to the failure to diagnose—and therefore treat—patients with symptomatic or asymptomatic infection and their sex partners. Patients with NGU, epididymitis, Reiter's syndrome, or MPC sometimes are not treated with antimicrobials, and their sex partners are treated even less often. *C. trachomatis* urethral or cervical infection has been well documented in a high proportion of the sex partners of patients with NGU, epididymitis, Reiter's syndrome, salpingitis, or endocervicitis. If possible, confirmatory laboratory tests for *Chlamydia* should be undertaken in these individuals, but even those without evidence of clinical disease who have recently been exposed to proven or possible chlamydial infection (for example, NGU) should be offered therapy.

Treatment of Neonates and Infants In neonates with conjunctivitis or infants with pneumonia, erythromycin ethylsuccinate or estolate can be given orally in a dose of 50 mg/kg per day, preferably as 12.25 mg/kg qid, for 2 weeks. Careful attention must be given to compliance with therapy—a frequent problem. Relapses of eye infection are common following treatment with topical erythromycin or tetracycline ophthalmic ointment and may also occur after oral erythromycin therapy. Thus follow-up cultures should be performed after treatment. Both parents should be examined for *C. trachomatis* infection and, if diagnostic testing is not readily available, should be treated with doxycycline or azithromycin.

PREVENTION Efforts to develop a vaccine for chlamydial infection have not yet been successful. Early diagnosis and treatment shorten the duration of infectiousness of the carrier and therefore constitute primary prevention of chlamydial infection. By the early 1990s, one of the 10 regions of the United States (Region X, the Pacific Northwest) had formally undertaken a chlamydial control program involving widespread testing. Approximately 500,000 tests per year were conducted in 150 family planning clinics throughout the region in women meeting the criteria for high risk. Within 5 years, the prevalence of chlamydial infection had fallen from 10 percent to 5 percent. While other regions of the United States have now initiated similar programs, many family planning and STD clinics still do not offer chlamydial testing. The availability of highly sensitive and specific diagnostic tests that can be done with urine specimens and of single-dose therapy makes it feasible to mount an effective chlamydial control program nationwide.

TRACHOMA AND ADULT INCLUSION CONJUNCTIVITIS

DEFINITION   Trachoma is a chronic conjunctivitis associated with infection by *C. trachomatis* serovar A, B, Ba, or C. It has been responsible for an estimated 20 million cases of blindness throughout the world and remains an important cause of preventable blindness. Inclusion conjunctivitis is an acute ocular infection caused by sexually transmitted *C. trachomatis* strains (usually serovars D through K) in adults exposed to infected genital secretions and in their newborn offspring.

EPIDEMIOLOGY   Epidemiologically, two types of eye disease are caused by *C. trachomatis*. In trachoma-endemic areas where the classic eye disease is seen, transmission is from eye to eye via hands, flies, towels, and other fomites and usually involves serovar A, B, Ba, or C. In nonendemic areas, organisms of serovars D through K can be transmitted from the genital tract to the eye, usually causing only the inclusion conjunctivitis syndrome, occasionally with keratitis. Rarely, the eye disease acquired in this way progresses, with the development of pannus and scars similar to those seen in endemic trachoma. These cases may be referred to as paratrachoma to differentiate them epidemiologically from eye-to-eye-transmitted endemic trachoma.

The worldwide incidence and severity of trachoma have decreased dramatically during the past 35 years, mainly as a result of improving hygienic and economic conditions. Endemic trachoma is still the major cause of preventable blindness in northern Africa, sub-Saharan Africa, the Middle East, and parts of Asia. The endemic disease is transmitted primarily through close personal contact, particularly among young children in rural communities with limited water supplies. In endemic areas, trachoma is associated with repeated exposure and reinfection, but the infection can also be latent. In the United States a mild form of endemic trachoma still occurs in Mexican Americans as well as in immigrants from areas where trachoma is endemic. Acute relapse of old trachoma occasionally follows treatment with cortisone eye ointment or develops in very old persons who were exposed in their youth.

CLINICAL MANIFESTATIONS   Both endemic trachoma and adult inclusion conjunctivitis present initially as a conjunctivitis characterized by small lymphoid follicles in the conjunctiva. In regions with hyperendemic classic blinding trachoma, the disease usually starts insidiously before the age of 2 years. Reinfection is common and probably contributes to the pathogenesis of trachoma. Studies using PCR techniques indicate that chlamydial DNA is often present in the ocular secretions of patients with trachoma, even in the absence of positive cultures. Thus persistent infection may be more common than was previously thought.

The cornea becomes involved, with inflammatory leukocytic infiltrations and superficial vascularization (pannus formation). As the inflammation continues, conjunctival scarring eventually distorts the eyelids, causing them to turn inward so that the inturned lashes constantly abrade the eyeball (trichiasis and entropion); eventually the corneal epithelium is abraded and may ulcerate, with subsequent corneal scarring and blindness. Destruction of the conjunctival goblet cells, lacrimal ducts, and lacrimal gland may produce a "dry-eye" syndrome, with resultant corneal opacity due to drying (xerosis) or secondary bacterial corneal ulcers.

Communities with blinding trachoma often experience seasonal epidemics of conjunctivitis due to *H. influenzae* that contribute to the intensity of the inflammatory process. In such areas the active infectious process usually resolves spontaneously in affected persons between 10 and 15 years of age, but the conjunctival scars continue to shrink, producing trichiasis and entropion and subsequent corneal scarring in adults. In areas with milder and less prevalent disease, the process may be much slower, with active disease continuing into adulthood; blindness is rare in these cases.

Eye infection with genital *C. trachomatis* strains in sexually active young adults presents as the acute onset of unilateral follicular conjunctivitis and preauricular lymphadenopathy similar to that seen in acute adenovirus or herpesvirus conjunctivitis. If untreated, the disease may persist for 6 weeks to 2 years. It is frequently associated with corneal inflammation in the form of discrete opacities ("infiltrates"), punctate epithelial erosions, and minor degrees of superficial corneal vascularization. Very rarely, conjunctival scarring and eyelid distortion occur, particularly in patients treated for many months with topical glucocorticoids. Recurrent eye infections develop most often in patients whose sexual consorts are not treated with antimicrobials.

DIAGNOSIS   The clinical diagnosis of classic trachoma can be made if two of the following signs are present:

1. Lymphoid follicles on the upper tarsal conjunctiva
2. Typical conjunctival scarring
3. Vascular pannus
4. Limbal follicles or their sequelae, Herbert's pits

The clinical diagnosis of endemic trachoma should be confirmed by laboratory tests in children with more marked degrees of inflammation. Intracytoplasmic chlamydial inclusions are found in 10 to 60 percent of Giemsa-stained conjunctival smears in such populations, but isolation in cell cultures, newer antigen detection testing, or chlamydial PCR is more sensitive. Follicular conjunctivitis in adult Europeans or Americans living in trachomatous regions is rarely due to trachoma.

Sporadic cases of adult inclusion conjunctivitis must be differentiated from keratoconjunctivitis due to adenovirus or HSV and from bacterial conjunctivitis during the first 15 days after onset; later, they must be distinguished from other forms of chronic follicular conjunctivitis. Demonstration of chlamydiae by Giemsa- or immunofluorescent-stained smears, by isolation in cell cultures, or by newer nonculture tests constitutes definitive evidence of infection. Genital examination and tests for genital chlamydial infection are indicated. Serum antibody does not constitute evidence of chlamydial eye infection since many sexually active adults have acquired serum antibody from genital infection.

DIFFERENTIAL DIAGNOSIS OF CONJUNCTIVITIS AND KERATOCONJUNCTIVITIS   The eye and its adnexa may be infected during the course of many cutaneous and systemic viral diseases. Sometimes these ocular infections produce minor manifestations, such as the transient loss of accommodation in dengue and the milder forms of conjunctivitis in systemic adenovirus infections. Other virus infections, however, such as herpes simplex (see Chap. 184), herpes zoster (see Chap. 185), measles (see Chap. 196), and vaccinia (see Chap. 188), occasionally produce serious and permanent visual loss. In addition, congenital infections are an important cause of blindness, particularly rubella, which leads to cataracts and microphthalmos; cytomegalic inclusion disease with retinal involvement; and syphilis with interstitial keratitis or optic neuritis. Among the viral infections limited to the outer eye and manifested as follicular conjunctivitis are epidemic keratoconjunctivitis, herpes simplex keratoconjunctivitis, Newcastle disease virus conjunctivitis, and acute hemorrhagic conjunctivitis.

R̶x̶ **TREATMENT**
Public health control programs for endemic trachoma have consisted of the mass application of tetracycline or erythromycin ointment to the eyes of all children in affected communities for 21 to 60 days or on an intermittent schedule. These programs also include surgical correction of inturned eyelids by a mobile surgical team that visits each locale. Single-dose azithromycin therapy offers an alternative method of mass antibiotic treatment for trachoma of young children and pregnant women that is now being evaluated.

Adult inclusion conjunctivitis responds well to treatment with full doses of systemic tetracycline or erythromycin for 3 weeks. Treatment of all sexual consorts of the patient simultaneously is also necessary to prevent ocular reinfection and to avoid genital disease due to chlamydial infection. Topical antibiotic treatment is not required for patients who receive systemic antibiotics.

PREVENTION Efforts to develop a trachoma vaccine have not yet been successful. General hygienic measures associated with improved living standards are effective in the elimination of endemic trachoma. An adequate water supply for personal cleanliness may be a key factor. In some areas the reduction of numbers of flies in the household is important.

PSITTACOSIS

DEFINITION Psittacosis is primarily an infectious disease of birds that is caused by *C. psittaci*. Transmission of infection from birds to humans results in a febrile illness characterized by pneumonitis and systemic manifestations. Inapparent infections or mild influenza-like illnesses may also occur. The term *ornithosis* is sometimes applied to infections contracted from birds other than parrots or parakeets, but *psittacosis* is the preferred generic term for all forms of the disease.

EPIDEMIOLOGY Almost any avian species can harbor *C. psittaci*. Psittacine birds (parrots, parakeets, budgerigars) are most commonly infected, but human cases have been traced to contact with pigeons, ducks, turkeys, chickens, and many other birds. Psittacosis may be considered an occupational disease of pet-shop owners, poultry workers, pigeon fanciers, taxidermists, veterinarians, and zoo attendants. During the past 20 years, there has been an increase in incidence, with cases and outbreaks occurring primarily among employees of poultry-processing plants. It is suspected that many cases go undiagnosed and unreported. The disease appears to be especially common in England, where budgerigars are popular household pets and where restrictions on the importation of these birds have been eased.

The agent is present in nasal secretions, excreta, tissues, and feathers of infected birds. Although the disease can be fatal, infected birds frequently show only minor evidence of illness, such as ruffled feathers, lethargy, and anorexia. Asymptomatic avian carriers are common, and complete recovery may be followed by continued shedding of the organism for many months.

Psittacosis is almost always transmitted to humans by the respiratory route. On rare occasions the disease may be acquired from the bite of a pet bird. Prolonged contact is not essential for transmission of the disease; a few minutes spent in an environment previously occupied by an infected bird has resulted in human infection. The severity of the disease in humans bears no apparent relationship to closeness or duration of contact, although sick birds are more likely to transmit infection than healthy ones. A psittacosis-like agent has been transmitted among hospital personnel, with severe and sometimes fatal infections. There is evidence that these "human" strains are more virulent than avian organisms. There is no record of infection acquired by the ingestion of poultry products.

PATHOGENESIS The psittacosis agent gains entrance to the body through the upper part of the respiratory tract, spreads via the bloodstream, and eventually localizes in the pulmonary alveoli and in the reticuloendothelial cells of the spleen and liver. Invasion of the lung probably takes place by way of the bloodstream rather than by direct extension from the upper air passages. A lymphocytic inflammatory response occurs on both the interstitial and the respiratory surfaces of the alveoli as well as in the perivascular spaces. The alveolar walls and interstitial tissues of the lung are thickened, edematous, necrotic, and occasionally hemorrhagic. Histologic examination of the affected areas reveals alveolar spaces filled with fluid, erythrocytes, and lymphocytes. The picture is not pathognomonic of psittacosis unless macrophages containing characteristic cytoplasmic inclusion bodies [Levinthal-Coles-Lillie (LCL) bodies] can be identified. The respiratory epithelium of the bronchi and bronchioles usually remains intact.

CLINICAL MANIFESTATIONS The clinical manifestations and course of psittacosis are extremely variable. After an incubation period of 7 to 14 days or longer, the disease may start abruptly with shaking chills and fever, with temperatures ranging as high as 40.5°C (105°F); however, the onset is often gradual, with fever increasing over a 3- to 4-day period. Headache is almost always a prominent symptom; it is usually diffuse and excruciating and is often the patient's chief complaint.

Many patients present with a dry hacking cough that is usually nonproductive, but small amounts of mucoid or bloody sputum may be raised as the disease progresses. Cough may begin early in the course of the disease or as late as 5 days after the onset of fever. Chest pain, pleurisy with effusion, or a friction rub may all occur but are rare. Pericarditis and myocarditis have been reported. Most patients have a normal or slightly increased respiratory rate; marked dyspnea with cyanosis occurs only in severe psittacosis with extensive pulmonary involvement. In psittacosis, as in most nonbacterial pneumonias, the physical signs of pneumonitis tend to be less prominent than symptoms and x-ray findings would suggest. The initial examination may reveal fine sibilant rales, or clinical evidence of pneumonia may be completely lacking. Rales usually become audible and more numerous as the illness progresses. Signs of frank pulmonary consolidation are usually absent. Symptoms of upper respiratory tract infection are not prominent, although mild sore throat, pharyngitis, and cervical adenopathy are often documented; on occasion, the last may be the only manifestation of illness. Epistaxis is encountered early in the course of nearly one-fourth of cases. Photophobia is also a common complaint.

Patients often report generalized myalgia, and spasm and stiffness of the muscles of the back and neck may lead to an erroneous diagnosis of meningitis. Lethargy, mental depression, agitation, insomnia, and disorientation have been prominent features of the illness in some epidemics but not in others; delirium and stupor develop near the end of the first week in severe cases. Occasional patients are comatose when first seen, and the diagnosis of psittacosis may be elusive in these cases. Gastrointestinal problems such as abdominal pain, nausea, vomiting, or diarrhea are noted in some cases; constipation and abdominal distention sometimes occur as late complications. Icterus, the result of severe hepatic involvement, is a rare and ominous finding. A faint macular rash (Horder's spots) simulating the rose spots of typhoid fever has been described.

Patients without cough or other clinical evidence of respiratory involvement present with fever of unknown origin (see Chap. 125). The pulse rate is slow in relation to the fever. When splenomegaly is noted in a patient with acute pneumonitis, psittacosis should be considered; the reported incidence of splenomegaly in this disease ranges from 10 to 70 percent. Nontender hepatic enlargement also occurs, but jaundice is rare. Thrombophlebitis is not unusual during convalescence; indeed, pulmonary infarction is sometimes a late complication and may be fatal.

In untreated cases of psittacosis, sustained or mildly remittent fever persists for 10 days to 3 weeks or occasionally for as long as 3 months. Over this period, the respiratory manifestations gradually abate. Psittacosis contracted from parrots or parakeets is more likely to be a severe, prolonged illness than infection acquired from pigeons or barnyard fowl. Relapses occur but are rare. Occasional patients develop endocarditis, and *C. psittaci* infection should be considered in cases of culture-negative endocarditis. Secondary bacterial infections are uncommon. Immunity to reinfection is probably permanent.

LABORATORY FINDINGS The chest x-ray in psittacosis is nonspecific and may show pneumonic lesions that are usually patchy in appearance but can be hazy, diffuse, homogeneous, lobar, atelectatic, wedge-shaped, nodular, or miliary. The white blood cell count is normal or moderately decreased in the acute phase of the disease but may rise in convalescence. The erythrocyte sedimentation rate frequently is not elevated. Transient proteinuria is common. The cerebrospinal fluid sometimes contains a few mononuclear cells but is otherwise normal. Despite hepatomegaly, the results of liver function tests are generally normal or mildly elevated.

The diagnosis can be confirmed only by isolation of the causative microorganism or by serologic studies. The agent is present in the blood during the acute phase of the disease and in the bronchial secretions for weeks or sometimes years after infection, but it is difficult to isolate. Further, the organism is hazardous to work with in the laboratory, and most clinical laboratories do not offer culture for *C. psittaci*. Thus psittacosis is most readily diagnosed by the demonstration of a rising titer of CF antibody in the serum of a patient with a compatible clinical syndrome. Both an acute-phase and a convalescent-phase specimen should always be tested. *C. trachomatis*, *C. psittaci*, and *C. pneumoniae* all share a genus-specific "group" antigen, which is the basis of the CF test. Thus acute infections with *C. trachomatis* or *C. pneumoniae* can also produce titer rises in the CF test. However, these three species have different major outer-membrane proteins that are the principal antigens in the micro-IF test. If there is doubt as to the interpretation of the CF test, the micro-IF test can be used to differentiate among them. The prompt initiation of treatment with tetracycline has been shown to delay an antibody rise in convalescence for several weeks or months.

DIFFERENTIAL DIAGNOSIS A history of exposure to birds may be the only clinical basis for differentiating psittacosis from a variety of infectious and noninfectious febrile disorders. The list of pulmonary diseases that may be confused with psittacosis includes *Mycoplasma* pneumonia, *C. pneumoniae* pneumonia, legionellosis, viral pneumonia, Q fever, coccidioidomycosis, tuberculosis, enterovirus infection, carcinoma of the lung with bronchial obstruction, and common bacterial pneumonias. In the early stages, before pneumonitis appears, psittacosis may be mistaken for influenza, typhoid fever, miliary tuberculosis, or infectious mononucleosis.

℞ TREATMENT

The tetracyclines are consistently effective in the treatment of psittacosis. Defervescence and alleviation of symptoms usually take place within 24 to 48 h after the institution of therapy with 2 g daily in four divided doses. To avoid relapse, treatment should probably be continued for at least 7 to 14 days after defervescence. In severe cases, hospitalization and pulmonary intensive care may be indicated. Sulfonamides are not active against *C. psittaci*. Erythromycin can be used in patients allergic to or intolerant of tetracyclines.

C. PNEUMONIAE INFECTIONS

A third chlamydial species, *C. pneumoniae*, has been described in the past decade. *C. pneumoniae* can be distinguished from the other two species on the basis of DNA hybridization and restriction endonuclease analyses. Although *C. pneumoniae* can be grown in a variety of cell cultures, it is considerably more difficult to culture than other chlamydiae, especially from clinical specimens. HL cells appear to be the most effective cell line for isolation of *C. pneumoniae*.

Knowledge of the epidemiology of *C. pneumoniae* infections has been derived primarily from serologic studies. Infections begin to occur in late childhood, achieve peak incidence in young adults, but continue throughout adult life. Seroprevalence in the many adult populations that have been tested throughout the world exceeds 40 percent—a figure suggesting that *C. pneumoniae* infections are ubiquitous. Secondary episodes (reinfections) appear to occur in older adults throughout life. In Scandinavia, *C. pneumoniae* produces epidemics of pneumonia and respiratory illness followed by periods of infrequent infection. The incidence of infections outside of epidemics remains poorly defined. Transmission appears to be from person to person, probably primarily in schools and family units.

The clinical spectrum of *C. pneumoniae* infection includes acute pharyngitis, sinusitis, bronchitis, and pneumonitis, primarily in young adults. The clinical manifestations of primary infection appear to be more severe and prolonged than those of reinfection. The pneumonitis resembles that of *Mycoplasma pneumoniae* pneumonia in that leukocytosis is frequently lacking and patients often have prominent antecedent upper respiratory tract symptoms, fever, nonproductive cough, a mild to moderate degree of illness, minimal findings on chest auscultation, and small segmental infiltrates on chest x-ray. In elderly patients, pneumonia due to *C. pneumoniae* can be especially severe and may necessitate hospitalization and respiratory support.

Epidemiologic studies have demonstrated an association between serologic evidence of *C. pneumoniae* infection and atherosclerotic disease of the coronary and other arteries. In addition, *C. pneumoniae* has been identified in atherosclerotic plaques by electron microscopy, DNA hybridization, and immunocytochemistry. The clinical significance of these findings is not yet clear.

Diagnosis of *C. pneumoniae* infection is currently difficult because cell culture techniques are not available for routine clinical use and nonculture tests using antigen detection methods or DNA probes have not been developed. Acute- and convalescent-phase sera can be tested for chlamydial CF antibody to make a retrospective diagnosis. However, this test does not distinguish *C. pneumoniae* infection from infection due to *C. trachomatis* or *C. psittaci*. Although controlled treatment trials have not been conducted, *C. pneumoniae* is inhibited in vitro by erythromycin and tetracycline. Recommended therapy consists of 2 g per day of either agent for 10 to 14 days.

BIBLIOGRAPHY

Bauwens JE et al: Diagnosis of *Chlamydia trachomatis* urethritis in men by polymerase chain reaction assay of first catch urine. J Clin Microbiol 31:3013, 1993

Cates W Jr, Wasserheit JN: Genital chlamydial infections: Epidemiology and reproductive sequelae. Am J Obstet Gynecol 164:1771, 1991

Centers for Disease Control and Prevention: Recommendations for the prevention and management of *Chlamydia trachomatis* infections, 1993. Morb Mortal Week Rep 42(RR-12):1, 1993

Coults II et al: Clinical and radiographic features of psittacosis infection. Thorax 40:530, 1985

Grayston JT: Infections caused by *Chlamydia pneumoniae*, strain TWAR. Clin Infect Dis 15:757, 1992

——— et al: A new *Chlamydia psittaci* strain, TWAR, isolated in acute respiratory tract infections. N Engl J Med 315:161, 1986

Holmes KK: Lower genital tract infections in women: Cystitis, urethritis, vulvovaginitis, and cervicitis, in *Sexually Transmitted Diseases*, 2d ed, KK Holmes et al (eds). New York, McGraw-Hill, 1990

Lee HH et al: Diagnosis of *Chlamydia trachomatis* genitourinary infection in women by ligase chain reaction assay of urine. Lancet 345:213, 1995

Martin DH et al: A controlled trial of a single dose of azithromycin for the treatment of chlamydial urethritis and cervicitis. N Engl J Med 327:921, 1992

Rettig PJ: Perinatal infections with *Chlamydia trachomatis*. Clin Perinatol 15:321, 1988

Schachter J, Stamm WE: Chlamydia, in *Manual of Clinical Microbiology*, PR Murray et al (eds). Washington, DC, ASM Press, 1995

——— et al: Experience with the routine use of erythromycin for chlamydial infections in pregnancy. N Engl J Med 314:276, 1986

Scholes D et al: Prevention of pelvic inflammatory disease by screening for cervical chlamydial infection. N Engl J Med 334:1362, 1996

Soper D: Pelvic inflammatory disease. Infect Dis Clin North Am 8:821, 1994

Stamm WE: Towards control of sexually transmitted chlamydial infections. Ann Intern Med 119:432, 1993

———, Holmes KK: *Chlamydia trachomatis* infections in adults, in *Sexually Transmitted Diseases*, 2d ed, KK Holmes et al (eds). New York, McGraw-Hill, 1990

——— et al: Azithromycin for empirical treatment of the nongonococcal urethritis syndrome in men. A randomized double-blind study. JAMA 274:545, 1995

——— et al: *Chlamydia trachomatis* urethral infections in men. Prevalence, risk factors, and clinical manifestations. Ann Intern Med 100:47, 1984

Stergachis A et al: Selective screening for *Chlamydia trachomatis* infections in a primary care population of women. Am J Epidemiol 138:143, 1993

Weinstock H et al: *Chlamydia trachomatis* infections. Infect Dis Clin North Am 8:797, 1994

182   *Fred Wang, Elliott Kieff*

MEDICAL VIROLOGY

HISTORICAL PERSPECTIVE

Although descriptions of poxvirus and herpesvirus infections extend back to antiquity, the field of virology is barely 100 years old. In contrast, bacteriology was developing rapidly through much of the second half of the nineteenth century. By the end of the nineteenth century, many types of bacteria could be grown on media and could be identified in cultures and in tissues by light microscopy; growth media could be sterilized by passage through porcelain filters; and Henle and Koch had written postulates for establishing the bacterial etiology of disease. In 1892, Ivanofsky in Russia showed that the infectious agent of mosaic tobacco-leaf disease was not a bacterium because it passed through a porcelain filter. Over the next 20 years, several animal infections were shown to be caused by filterable agents, and the term *virus* began to be applied to these agents. From the 1920s through the 1950s, research on bacterial, plant, and animal (including human) viral infections of cells, tissues, organs, and organisms led to improved techniques for the culture of cells and viruses in vitro. Improved culture techniques made it feasible to study the biochemical and genetic properties of viruses. Viruses came to be recognized as genetically simple tools for learning about fundamental biologic and biochemical processes in cells, tissues, organs, and animals, including humans.

DEFINING A VIRUS

Viruses consist of a nucleic acid surrounded by one or more proteins. Some viruses also have an outer-membrane envelope. Viruses differ from other replicating organisms in that they do not have ribosomes or enzymes for high-energy phosphate generation or for protein, carbohydrate, or lipid metabolism. Viruses are obligate intracellular parasites—that is, they require cells in order to replicate. Typically, viral nucleic acids encode proteins necessary for replicating and packaging the nucleic acids into new viral particles.

Viruses differ from viroids, prions, and virusoids. *Virusoids* are nucleic acids that depend on helper viruses to package the nucleic acids into virus-like particles. *Viroids* are simply molecules of naked, cyclical, mostly double-stranded, small RNAs and are restricted to plants. *Prions* are abnormal cellular proteins that can spread from cell to cell and effect changes in normal cellular proteins, thereby disrupting cellular function and propagating themselves. Prions have been implicated in neurodegenerative conditions such as Creutzfeldt-Jakob disease, kuru, and Gerstmann-Sträussler syndrome. Recently, prions have also been implicated in the putative human transmission of bovine spongiform encephalopathy.

VIRAL STRUCTURE

Viruses have from a few to 200 genes. These genes may be embodied in a single-strand or double-strand DNA genome or in a single-strand sense, a single-strand or segmented antisense, or a double-strand segmented RNA genome. Sense-strand RNA genomes can be translated directly into protein. Sense and antisense genomes are also referred to as positive-strand and negative-strand genomes, respectively. The viral nucleic acid is usually associated with one or more virus-encoded nucleoproteins in the core of the viral particle. The viral nucleic acid is almost always enclosed in a protein shell called a capsid. Because of the limited genetic complexity of viruses, their capsids are usually composed of multimers of identical capsomers. Capsomers are in turn composed of one or a few proteins. The capsomers assemble into capsids with icosahedral or helical symmetry. Icosahedral structures

approximate spheres but have two-, three-, and fivefold axes of symmetry, while helical structures have only a twofold axis of symmetry. Capsids filled with nucleic acid are called nucleocapsids. Many human viruses have a simple nucleocapsid structure; others are more complex and have an outer envelope that is derived from membranes of the infected cell. The membrane that composes the viral envelope has been modified by the insertion of virus-encoded glycoproteins. Enveloped viruses frequently have matrix or tegument proteins that fill the space between the nucleocapsid and the envelope. In general, enveloped viruses are sensitive to solvents and nonionic detergents that can disrupt the envelope, while viruses that consist only of nucleocapsids are usually more resistant. The schematic diagram of a herpesvirus shown in Fig. 182-1 illustrates the components of a complicated DNA virus. Prototypical pathogenic human viruses are listed in Table 182-1. The relative sizes and structures of typical pathogenic human viruses are shown in Fig. 182-2.

TAXONOMY OF PATHOGENIC HUMAN VIRUSES

As is apparent from Table 182-1 and Fig. 182-2, the classification of viruses into orders and families is based on nucleic acid composition, nucleocapsid size and symmetry, and envelopment status. Viruses of a single family have similar types of genomes and are morphologically similar in electron micrographs. Further subclassification into genus is dependent on similarities in epidemiology and biologic effects and on the degree of colinear nucleic acid sequence homology. In general, each human virus has a common name related to its pathologic effects or the circumstances of its discovery and a formal species name assigned by the International Committee on Taxonomy of Viruses (http://www.ncbi.nlm.nih.gov/ICTV). The latter designation consists of the name of the host followed by the family or genus of the virus and a number. This dual terminology has created a confusing situation in which viruses are referred to and referenced by either name—e.g., varicella-zoster virus (VZV) or human herpesvirus type 3.

VIRAL INFECTION IN VITRO

STAGES OF INFECTION   At the cellular level, viral infection proceeds in stages: (1) viral interactions at the cell surface, (2) viral gene expression and replication, and (3) viral assembly and egress.

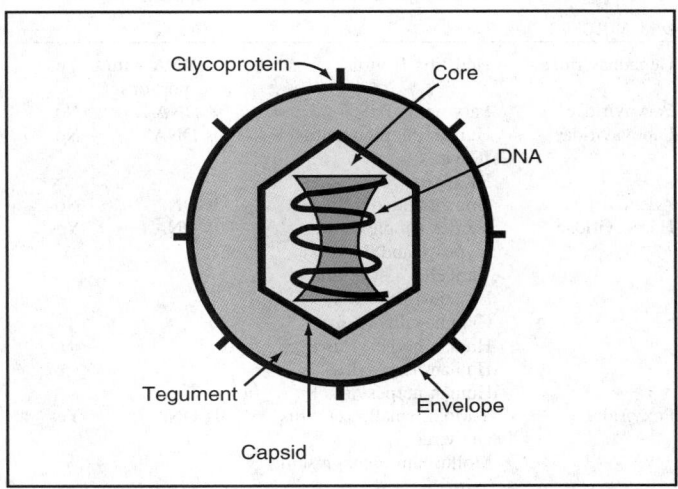

FIGURE 182-1 Schematic diagram of an enveloped herpesvirus with an icosahedral nucleocapsid. The approximate respective dimensions of the nucleocapsid and the enveloped particles are 100 μm and 180 μm. The capsid is composed of 162 capsomeres: 150 with sixfold and 12 with fivefold axes of symmetry.

Table 182-1

Virus Families Pathogenic for Humans

Family	Representative Viruses	Type of RNA/DNA	Lipid Envelope
RNA VIRUSES			
Picornaviridae	Poliovirus	(+) RNA	No
	Coxsackievirus		
	Echovirus		
	Enterovirus		
	Rhinovirus		
	Hepatitis A virus		
Caliciviridae	Norwalk agent	(+) RNA	No
	Hepatitis E virus		
Togaviridae	Rubella virus	(+) RNA	Yes
	Eastern equine encephalitis virus		
	Western equine encephalitis virus		
Flaviviridae	Yellow fever virus	(+) RNA	Yes
	Dengue virus		
	St. Louis encephalitis virus		
	Hepatitis C virus		
	Hepatitis G virus		
Coronaviridae	Coronavirus	(+) RNA	Yes
Rhabdoviridae	Rabies virus	(−) RNA	Yes
	Vesicular stomatitis virus		
Filoviridae	Marburg virus	(−) RNA	Yes
	Ebola virus		
Paramyxoviridae	Parainfluenza virus	(−) RNA	Yes
	Respiratory syncytial virus		
	Newcastle disease virus		
	Mumps virus		
	Rubeola (measles) virus		
Orthomyxoviridae	Influenza A, B, and C viruses	(−) RNA, 8 segments	Yes
Bunyaviridae	Hantavirus	(−) RNA, 3 circular segments	Yes
	California encephalitis virus		
	Sandfly fever virus		
Arenaviridae	Lymphocytic choriomeningitis virus	(−) RNA, 2 circular segments	Yes
	Lassa fever virus		
	South American hemorrhagic fever virus		
Reoviridae	Rotavirus	ds RNA, 10–12 segments	No
	Reovirus		
	Colorado tick fever virus		
DNA VIRUSES			
Hepadnaviridae	Hepatitis B virus	ds DNA with ss portions	Yes
Parvoviridae	Parvovirus B19	ss DNA	No
Papovaviridae	Human papillomavirus	ds DNA	No
	JC virus		
	BK virus		
Adenoviridae	Human adenovirus	ds DNA	No
Herpesviridae	Herpes simplex virus types 1 and 2*	ds DNA	Yes
	Varicella-zoster virus†		
	Epstein-Barr virus‡		
	Cytomegalovirus§		
	Human herpesvirus 6		
	Human herpesvirus 7		
	Human herpesvirus 8		
Poxviridae	Variola (smallpox) virus	ds DNA	Yes
	Orf virus		
	Molluscum contagiosum virus		

* Also called human herpesvirus (HHV) 1 and 2, respectively.
† Also called HHV-3.
‡ Also called HHV-4.
§ Also called HHV-5.
ABBREVIATIONS: ds, double-strand; ss, single-strand.

Viral Interactions at the Cell Surface First, virus adsorbs to a receptor on the cell surface. Adsorption is the consequence of a molecular interaction of a viral surface protein with a molecule on the cell's plasma membrane. For example, a poliovirus capsid protein binds to a cell plasma-membrane protein of the immunoglobulin super-family type; a rhinovirus capsid protein binds to intracellular adhesion molecule 1; an echovirus capsid protein binds to an integrin; the influenza virus envelope hemagglutinin protein binds to sialic acid; the envelope glycoprotein of human immunodeficiency virus (HIV) binds to CD4 and to chemokine receptors; the herpes simplex virus (HSV) envelope glycoproteins bind to heparan sulfate and to a tumor necrosis factor receptor; and an Epstein-Barr virus (EBV) glycoprotein binds to the B lymphocyte complement receptor CD21. Adsorption characteristically proceeds almost as well at 4°C as at 37°C, and adsorbed virus can still be neutralized by antibody.

After adsorption, viruses penetrate through or fuse with the cell membrane and are uncoated as they enter the cytoplasm. Penetration and uncoating as well as subsequent steps in viral replication depend on the cell's energy metabolism and on biochemical changes in the cell's plasma membrane and cytoskeleton. Therefore, penetration proceeds slowly at temperatures below 37°C. The process of penetration is frequently initiated by the interaction of viral surface proteins with cellular receptors during adsorption. The viral protein that engages the receptor is displayed on the surace of the virus in at least several copies. Similarly, the cell's plasma membrane has at least several and usually hundreds of receptor molecules. The interaction of virus with its receptors usually induces receptor aggregation at the site of viral adsorption. Receptor aggregation triggers signaling events in the cytoplasm and active changes in the plasma membrane. The cell usually perceives that the receptor has encountered its "normal ligand." Frequently, the aggregated receptor is internalized through an endocytic process that involves clathrin-coated pits. The virus is thereby brought into endosomes in the cytoplasm. Endocytosis is important in the entry of viruses as diverse as picornaviruses, influenza viruses, adenoviruses, and herpesviruses. In many instances, further fusion of the virus with the endosomal membrane is dependent on lowering of the endosomal pH. The effect of pH on viral penetration has been well studied in the case of influenza virus. Influenza hemagglutinin mediates adsorption, receptor aggregation, and endocytosis. In low-pH endosomes, changes in the conformation of the hemagglutinin expose amphipathic domains that interact chemically with the cell membrane and initiate the fusion of the viral and cellular membranes. Little is known about the biochemical details of the fusion and uncoating processes for most viral capsids or envelopes. The end result of fusion is the mixture of viral envelope lipids and proteins with the lipids and proteins of cell membranes. In the case of complex viruses, viral surface proteins other than the protein that mediates adsorption may mediate fusion with the cell membrane. For some viruses, there is evidence of different receptors or membrane-fusion partners on different tissues or on different surfaces of polarized epithelial cells.

Viral Gene Expression and Replication As a result of the interaction of viruses with their receptors and subsequent steps in uncoating, viral nucleic acids and associated viral proteins are released into the cell's cytoplasm. Viral nucleic acid and virion structural proteins must be synthesized, and the nucleic acid and proteins must be assembled into progeny virions. Most viruses differentially regulate the transcription of their messenger RNAs (mRNAs), which are then translated into proteins. Most RNA viruses replicate their nucleic acid and assemble entirely in the cytoplasm, while most DNA viruses replicate their nucleic acid and assemble into nucleocapsid complexes in the nucleus.

Positive-strand RNA viruses Genomic RNA from positive-strand RNA viruses is released into the cytoplasm without associated enzymes. The recognition and association of cell ribosomes with an internal ribosome entry sequence in the viral genomic RNA permit the translation of a polyprotein that is a fusion of many or all of the viral proteins. The viral RNA polymerase and other viral proteins are cleaved from the polyprotein by protease components of the polyprotein. Antigenomic RNA is then transcribed from the genomic RNA

Positive-strand RNA viruses

	Picornaviridae	Caliciviridae	Togaviridae	Flaviviridae	Coronaviridae
Genome size (kb)	7.2–8.4	8	12	10	16–21
Envelope	No	No	Yes	Yes	Yes
Capsid symmetry	Icosahedral	Icosahedral	Icosahedral	Icosahedral?	Helical

Negative-strand RNA viruses

	Rhabdoviridae	Filoviridae	Paramyxoviridae
Genome size (kb)	13–16	13	16–20
Envelope	Yes	Yes	Yes
Capsid symmetry	Helical	Helical	Helical

Segmented negative-strand RNA viruses

Segmented double-strand RNA viruses

	Orthomyxoviridae	Bunyaviridae	Arenaviridae	Reoviridae
Genome size (kb)	14	13–21	10–14	16–27
Envelope	Yes	Yes	Yes	No
Capsid symmetry	Helical	Helical	Helical	Icosahedral

Retroviruses

	Retroviridae
Genome size (kb)	3–9
Envelope	Yes
Capsid symmetry	Icosahedral

DNA viruses

	Parvoviridae	Papovaviridae	Adenoviridae	Herpesviridae	Poxviridae
Genome size (kb)	5	5–9	36–38	100–250	240
Envelope	No	No	No	Yes	Yes
Capsid symmetry	Icosahedral	Icosahedral	Icosahedral	Icosahedral	Complex

100 nm

FIGURE 182-2 Schematic diagrams of the major virus families including species that infect humans. The viruses are grouped by genome type and are drawn approximately to scale. Key: |———|, 100 nm.

template. Positive-strand genomes and mRNAs are next transcribed from the antigenomic RNA by the viral RNA polymerase. Positive-strand genomic RNA is encapsidated in the cytoplasm.

Negative-strand RNA viruses Negative-strand RNA virus genomes are released into the cytoplasm with an associated RNA polymerase. Most negative-strand RNA viruses replicate entirely in the cytoplasm. The RNA polymerase transcribes mRNAs as well as full-length antigenomic RNA, which is the template for replication of genomic RNA. The mRNAs encode for RNA polymerase and accessory factors as well as for viral structural proteins. Influenza virus is an unusual segmented negative-strand RNA virus that transcribes its mRNAs and antigenomic RNA in the cell's nucleus. The infecting RNA segments must make their way to the nucleus with their associ-

ated RNA polymerase and accessory proteins. The nuclear localization of influenza RNA permits the use of two cell-nuclear processes: (1) the incorporation of cell mRNA cap sequences to enhance ribosomal recognition and translational initiation of viral mRNAs, and (2) the splicing of some influenza virus mRNAs. Negative-strand RNA viruses, including influenza virus, assemble in the cytoplasm.

DNA viruses Most DNA viruses except for poxviruses must get to the cell's nucleus for their DNA to be transcribed by cellular RNA polymerase II. Except for a few viral proteins that contribute to transcriptional regulation, DNA viruses depend on the cell for mRNA synthesis and processing. Herpesvirus nucleocapsids are released into the cytoplasm along with tegument proteins. The complex is then transported along microtubules to nuclear pores, and the DNA is released into the nucleus along with a viral tegument protein that can activate transcription of viral immediate-early genes. Immediate-early genes require only a component of the viral tegument and preexisting cellular transcription factors to be actively transcribed. In herpesvirus infections, immediate-early proteins are stringently required to turn on viral early-gene transcription. Other DNA viruses do not depend absolutely on the immediate-early transactivators encoded from the viral genome for early-gene transcription. Most early genes encode proteins that are necessary for viral DNA synthesis and for the turn-on of late-gene transcription. Late genes encode mostly viral structural proteins or viral proteins necessary for the assembly and egress of the virus from the infected cell. Late-gene transcription is continuously dependent on DNA replication. Therefore, inhibitors of DNA replication also stop late-gene transcription.

Each DNA virus family uses unique mechanisms for replicating its DNA. Herpesvirus DNAs are linear in the virion but circularize in the infected cell. The circular viral genome is replicated into linear concatemers through a "rolling-circle" mechanism. Herpesviruses encode their own polymerase and several enzymes that increase the pool of nucleotide precursors. Adenovirus genomes are linear in the virion and are replicated into complementary linear copies by a virus-encoded DNA polymerase and an initiator protein complex. The double-strand circular papovavirus genomes are replicated into progeny circular DNA molecules by cellular DNA replication enzymes. A single viral early protein contributes to the initiation of viral DNA replication. The early papovavirus proteins stimulate cellular DNA synthesis, thus facilitating viral DNA replication. Occasionally, papovaviruses (e.g., papillomaviruses) integrate into the host chromosome; overexpression of viral proteins and excessive stimulation of cellular growth result. Sometimes the consequence is the development of malignancies such as cervical cancer (see "Role of Persistent Viral Infections in Human Cancers" below).

Poxviruses are unique among the DNA viruses in replicating entirely in the cytoplasm. Pox virions have virus-encoded transcription factors and an RNA polymerase as well as enzymes for RNA capping and polyadenylation. Poxvirus DNA also has a unique structure. The two strands of the double-strand linear DNA are covalently linked at the ends so that the genome is also a covalently closed single-strand circle. In addition, there are inverted repeats at the ends of the DNA. During DNA replication, the genome is cleaved within the terminal inverted repeat, and the inverted repeats self-prime complementary-strand synthesis by the virus-encoded DNA polymerase. Like herpesviruses, poxviruses encode several enzymes that increase nucleotide levels and thus facilitate viral DNA synthesis.

Viruses with both RNA and DNA genomes Retroviruses, lentiviruses, and hepatitis B virus are not purely RNA or DNA viruses.

Retroviruses and lentiviruses are enveloped RNA viruses with diploid sense-strand genomes and associated reverse transcriptase and integrase enzymes. Retroviruses and lentiviruses differ from all other viruses in that they reverse-transcribe themselves into partially duplicated double-strand DNA copies and then routinely integrate into the host genome as part of their replication strategy. Viral mRNAs and genomic RNAs are then transcribed from a single integrated proviral promoter. Remnants of simple retroviral DNA in the human genome suggest the possibility of replication-competent simple human retroviruses, but little other evidence supports their existence. Human T cell leukemia virus (HTLV) types I and II are more complicated retroviruses that are endemic in specific human populations, where they cause tropical spastic paraparesis and adult T cell leukemia. HTLV transcripts include both the full-length genomic transcripts characteristic of all retroviruses (encoding Gag, polymerase/integrase, and envelope glycoprotein) and spliced transcripts (encoding Tax and Rex, which are regulators of transcription and RNA processing). HIV types 1 and 2 are full-fledged lentiviruses that cause AIDS and a milder immunodeficiency syndrome; these viruses have a larger number of spliced viral transcripts that encode the regulatory proteins Tat, Rev, Nef, Vpr, Vpu, and Vif. All of the viral transcripts and proteins are

usually expressed in HTLV- or HIV-infected cells. Retroviruses and lentiviruses assemble near the plasma membrane. The nucleocapsid is composed of two copies of a full genomic transcript, cellular transfer RNA, and proteins cleaved from the viral Gag protein. The nucleocapsid is enveloped at sites in the plasma membrane that have been modified by viral glycoprotein insertion.

Hepatitis B virus is an enveloped virus with an incomplete double-strand circular DNA genome. On entry into the cytoplasm, virion polymerase completes DNA synthesis; the covalently closed circular genome resides in the nucleus. Viral mRNAs are transcribed from the closed circular viral episome by cellular RNA polymerase II. A capped and polyadenylated, full-genome-length, terminally redundant transcript is packaged into viral core particles in the cytoplasm of infected cells. This RNA is associated with the viral polymerase, which has reverse transcriptase activity and converts the full-length, terminally redundant, core-particle, encapsidated RNA genome into partially double-strand DNA.

Viral Assembly and Egress As viral nucleic acid and structural proteins are synthesized, nucleic acid and proteins begin to assemble. The assembly and egress of mature infectious virus mark the end of the eclipse phase of infection, during which infectious virus cannot be recovered from the infected cell. Nucleic acids from RNA viruses and poxviruses assemble into nucleocapsids in the cytoplasm. For all DNA viruses except poxviruses, viral DNA assembles into nucleocapsids in the nucleus. In general, the capsid proteins of viruses with icosahedral nucleocapsids can self-assemble into densely packed and highly ordered capsid structures. Viral nucleic acid or nucleoprotein complex then enters or spools into the assembled capsid. In contrast, helical nucleocapsids frequently appear to assemble around the nucleic acid, which contributes to capsid organization.

Viruses must egress from the infected cell and not bind back to its plasma membrane. In many cases, enveloped viruses simply egress and acquire their envelope by budding through the cell's plasma membrane. Excess viral membrane protein is synthesized to saturate cell receptors and facilitate viral envelopment. Other viruses encode membrane proteins with enzymatic activity for receptor destruction. Influenza virus, for example, encodes a glycoprotein with neuraminidase activity, which destroys sialic acid on the infected cell's plasma membrane. Herpesvirus nucleocapsids acquire their initial envelope by budding through the nuclear membrane. Enveloped herpesviruses are released from the cell either by maturation in cytoplasmic vesicles, which fuse with the plasma membrane and release the virus by exocytosis, or by "de-envelopment" and release of the nucleocapsid into the cytoplasm and "re-envelopment" at the plasma membrane. In most instances, nonenveloped nucleocapsid viruses appear to depend on the death and dissolution of the infected cell for their release.

FIDELITY OF VIRAL REPLICATION While cells grow by doubling their genome and dividing, viral replication typically results in the release of 10 to 1000 infectious progeny and of many more partially assembled genomes and structures. Replication can alter the viral genomic sequence by various mechanisms. In general, viral nucleic acid replication is more error-prone than cellular nucleic acid replication. For RNA viruses and retroviruses, RNA polymerase and reverse transcriptase are intrinsically more error-prone than DNA polymerases. These errors can lead to the emergence of mutant viral strains capable of evading immune-system recognition or resisting the action of antiviral drugs. For DNA viruses, errors are probably due to less adequate postreplication repair (proofreading) in the virus-infected cell. Other mechanisms for introducing change into viral nucleic acid sequences include reassortment of segmented RNA genomes, as in influenza viruses, and recombination of homologous nucleic acid sequences between related viral strains. Defective viruses, consisting of empty nucleocapsids or viruses with deletions or rearrangements of the viral genome, are produced frequently by many viruses but are of uncertain pathophysiologic significance. For most viruses, there are 5 to 10 times more mature-appearing viral particles than fully infectious virions.

OTHER VIRAL GENES Many RNA and DNA viruses also have genes encoding proteins that are not directly involved in replication or packaging of the viral nucleic acid, in virion assembly, or in regulation of the transcription of viral genes involved in those processes. Many of these genes have provided important insights into normal cell biology and may play a role during viral infection of humans. Most of these proteins fall into four classes: (1) proteins that directly or indirectly alter cell growth; (2) proteins that inhibit cellular DNA, RNA, or protein synthesis so that viral mRNA can be efficiently transcribed or translated; (3) proteins that promote the cell's survival or inhibit apoptosis so that progeny virus can mature and escape from the infected cell; and (4) proteins that downregulate host inflammatory or immune responses so that viral infection can proceed in the infected patient. As the basic processes of viral replication have become better understood, contemporary virology has focused increasingly on these more sophisticated issues of cellular and organismal biology.

HOST RANGE The cell types in which a virus can replicate define the host range for that virus. For the most part, the host-range limitations of a virus are defined by specific cell-surface proteins required for its adsorption or penetration. Another common basis for host-range limitation involves transcription. DNA viruses depend not only on cellular RNA polymerase II and the basal components of the cellular transcription complex but also on activated components and transcriptional accessory factors, both of which differ among differentiated tissues; among cells at various phases of the cell cycle; and among resting, G_0, and cycling cells.

The concept of host range needs to be modified in the cases of papovaviruses and herpesviruses. Some cell types may be permissive for infection with these viruses and nonpermissive or partially permissive for their replication. A papovavirus or herpesvirus may persist in a latent state in a cell that is nonpermissive for its replication. Human papillomaviruses infect cells of the basal layer of the skin but replicate only when the cells further differentiate into keratinocytes. HSV infects cells of the dorsal root ganglia but cannot replicate in these cells until they are stimulated by fever, skin injury, or psychic trauma, all of which somehow turn on transcription of the viral immediate-early genes in previously latently infected neurons. EBV, another herpesvirus, establishes latency in B lymphocytes, in which it initially expresses proteins that cause the proliferation of the latently infected cells. This virus also expresses a protein that prevents lymphocytes from becoming activated and turning on viral replication in response to src-family kinase-mediated signal transduction events. This blockade must be bypassed when the lymphocytes traffic near the oropharyngeal epithelium so that these cells can become permissive for viral replication and the virus can be released into saliva to complete its life cycle in humans.

VIRAL CYTOPATHIC EFFECTS AND INHIBITION OF APOPTOSIS The replication of almost all viruses has adverse effects on the infected cell, inhibiting cellular synthesis of DNA, RNA, or proteins. This inhibitory effect probably stems from the viruses' need to prevent or limit the induction of interferon and to replicate rapidly and efficiently, thereby gaining a foothold before an effective host immune response is mounted. Most commonly, viruses specifically inhibit host protein synthesis by attacking a component of the translational initiation complex—frequently, a component that is not required for efficient translation of viral RNAs. Poliovirus protease 2A, for example, cleaves a cellular component of the complex that ordinarily facilitates translation of cellular mRNAs by interacting with their 5′ cap structure. Poliovirus RNA is efficiently translated without a 5′ cap since it has an internal ribosome entry sequence. Influenza virus inhibits the processing of mRNA by snatching 5′ cap structures from nascent cellular RNAs and using them as primers in the synthesis of viral mRNA. HSV has a virion tegument protein that inhibits cellular mRNA translation.

A frequent corollary of the inhibition of cellular macromolecular synthesis is the induction of apoptosis. While this event may be important for the release of virions (particularly in the case of nonenveloped viruses), viruses have also acquired genes or parts of genes that enable them to forestall infected-cell apoptosis. Some adenoviruses and some herpesviruses encode analogues of the cellular protein Bc12, which inhibits apoptosis in lymphocytes. In addition, some papillo-maviruses and adenoviruses have proteins that counteract the action of p53 in inducing cell-cycle arrest and apoptosis in virus-infected cells.

VIRAL INFECTION IN VIVO

The capsid and envelope of a virus enable the genome to escape degradation, to spread from cell to cell, and to spread among humans or to humans from other animals, including insects. Most common viral infections are spread by inhalation of aerosolized particles, by ingestion of contaminated water or food, or by direct contact. In all of these situations, infection begins on an epithelial or mucosal surface and spreads along it or from it to deeper tissues. Infection may then spread through the body via the bloodstream, lymphatics, or neural circuits. Parenteral inoculation also serves to transmit some viral infections among humans or from animals (including insects) to humans.

PRIMARY INFECTION The duration of primary (first-episode) viral infection usually varies from several days to several weeks. During this period, the concentration of virus at sites of infection rises and then falls, usually to unmeasurable levels. The rate at which the intensity of viral infection rises and falls at a given site depends on the accessibility of that organ or tissue to both the virus and systemic immune effectors, the intrinsic ability of the virus to replicate at that site, and endogenous nonspecific and specific resistance. Typically, infections with enterovirus, mumps virus, measles virus, rubella virus, rotavirus, influenza virus, adenovirus, HSV, and VZV are cleared from almost all sites within 3 to 4 weeks. Some of these viruses can alter or evade the immune response; primary infection then lasts for several months. Characteristically extending beyond several weeks are primary infections due to hepatitis virus (B, C, or D), EBV, cytomegalovirus (CMV), HIV, papillomavirus, and molluscum contagiosum virus. Primary infection with CMV may last for several months, and that with HIV, papillomavirus, or molluscum contagiosum virus may last even longer.

Disease manifestations usually arise as a consequence of viral replication at a specific site but do not necessarily correlate with levels of replication at that site. For example, the clinical manifestations of limited infection with poliovirus, enterovirus, rabies virus, measles virus, mumps virus, or HSV in neural cells are severe relative to the level of viral replication at mucosal surfaces. Similarly, severe morbidity may be associated with fetal infections with rubella virus or CMV.

Primary infections are cleared by specific and nonspecific immune responses. Thereafter, an immunocompetent person is usually immune to the disease manifestations of reinfection by the same virus. Immunity does not prevent transient surface colonization on reexposure to virus.

PERSISTENT AND LATENT INFECTIONS Relatively few viruses cause persistent or latent infections. Hepatitis B and C viruses, rabies virus, measles virus, HIV, HTLV, papovaviruses, herpesviruses, and some poxviruses are notable exceptions. In part, RNA viruses can escape immune destruction because their genomes can change over time during the infection of an individual. Hepatitis C virus and HIV undergo significant evolution during the course of primary and persistent infection in individual patients. Double-strand DNA replication is less error-prone, and DNA viruses appear not to change significantly during their persistence in humans. Papovaviruses and herpesviruses persist by establishing long-term latency in some cells. In the latent state, the viruses are mostly hidden from the normal immune response. When reactivated at epithelial surfaces, papovaviruses and herpesviruses are shed intermittently or continuously at a low level by healthy humans. The continued production of these viruses by humans despite an immune response that is adequate to suppress most or all manifestations of disease creates a continuous supply of these viruses and permits viral spread to children and to susceptible adults, ensuring viral perpetuation in human populations.

Molluscum contagiosum virus is a poxvirus causing a proliferative and hypertrophic wart-like disease that can persist for several months or years. The hypertrophic nature of other poxvirus infections has been attributed to viral homologues of cellular growth factors, including an epidermal growth factor homologue. However, the DNA sequence of molluscum contagiosum virus shows no homology to known epidermal or fibroblast growth factors. The DNA sequence does reveal a chemokine homologue that is likely to block inflammatory responses and a class I major histocompatibility analogue that may block cytotoxic T lymphocyte attack.

ROLE OF PERSISTENT VIRAL INFECTIONS IN HUMAN CANCERS Estimates of the fraction of human malignancies that result directly from viral infection range from 10 to 20 percent. Most hepatocellular carcinomas are presumed to be caused by infection with hepatitis B or C virus, almost all cervical carcinomas by infection with "high-risk" strains of genital papillomavirus, all anaplastic nasopharyngeal carcinomas by infection with EBV, and most adult cutaneous T cell lymphomas/leukemias by infection with HTLV-I. The presumption of a causal relationship between the hepatitis viruses and hepatocellular carcinoma is based on epidemiologic data and on studies with experimental models, which indicate that chronic liver injury attributable to these viruses can cause hepatocellular cancer in rodents. Hepatitis B viral DNA can integrate into cellular DNA, and this integration can contribute to oncogenicity. For cervical cancer, nasopharyngeal carcinoma, and adult T cell leukemia, the corresponding presumptions are based on epidemiologic data, the universal presence of viral DNA in tumor cells, the ability of the viruses to transform human cells in culture, and the pathophysiologic links between specific viral genes expressed in premalignant or malignant cells and cell-transforming effects in various assays in vitro. EBV has been implicated in lymphoproliferative diseases in immunosuppressed patients, in some B and T lymphocyte malignancies, in some gastric cancers, in muscle tumors in AIDS patients, and in a significant fraction of cases of Hodgkin's disease. Specific EBV genes and gene products have been genetically and pathophysiologically linked to effects on cell growth. Recent evidence suggests that a newly identified herpesvirus may cause Kaposi's sarcoma. Formal proof of the viral etiology of these malignancies will most likely come from efforts to prevent or intervene in infections with the putative oncogenic human viruses.

RESISTANCE TO VIRAL INFECTIONS Resistance to viral infection is initially provided by factors that are not specific for individual viruses. Physical protection is afforded by the cornified layers of the skin and by mucous secretions that continuously sweep over mucosal surfaces. Once the first cell is infected, interferons become important as local resistance factors. Viral infection may also cause the release of other cytokines from infected cells. Viral protein epitopes expressed on the cell surface in the context of histocompatibility proteins can attract T cells with appropriate receptors. Cytokines, inflammatory agents, and antigens released by virus-induced cell death attract inflammatory cells, granulocytes, natural killer cells, and lymphocytes to the site of initial infection. Interferons and natural killer cells are particularly important in containing viral infection for the first several days. Granulocytes and macrophages also are important in the phagocytosis and degradation of viruses, particularly after the onset of an antibody response.

Near the end of the first week or the beginning of the second week after infection, several responses can be detected: a virus-specific antibody response; a virus-specific, histocompatibility leukocyte antigen (HLA) class II–restricted, CD4+ helper T lymphocyte response; and a virus-specific, HLA class I–restricted, CD8+ cytotoxic T lymphocyte response. The magnitude of these responses, which are important in rapid recovery, typically increases over the second and third weeks of infection. Also between the second and third weeks, the antibody isotype usually changes from IgM to IgG, and virus-specific IgA antibody may be detected at mucosal surfaces. Antibody may neutralize virus directly by binding to its surface and preventing its adsorption or penetration. Complement usually enhances virus neutralization. Antibody and complement can also lyse virus-infected cells that express viral proteins on their surface. A cell infected with an enveloped virus usually expresses viral glycoprotein components of the envelope on its surface. Thus, the infected cell is rendered subject to destruction by antibodies to the glycoprotein and complement.

The antibody response and the CD4+ and CD8+ T lymphocyte responses tend to persist for several months after primary infection. Antibody-producing lymphocytes persist in small numbers as memory cells and begin to proliferate rapidly in response to reexposure, providing an early barrier to reinfection with the same virus. Immunologic memory for T cell responses appears to be less long lived, and redevelopment of T cell immunity may take longer than secondary antibody responses, particularly when many years have elapsed between primary infection and reexposure. Some viruses have genes that alter the normal host response. Examples of viral genes that hinder host resistance include adenoviral VA RNAs, which prevent interferon from shutting off protein synthesis in adenovirus-infected cells; adenoviral E1A protein, which inhibits interferon responsiveness at specific promoters; adenoviral E3 proteins, which prevent cytolysis induced by tumor necrosis factor and block class I antigen synthesis by the infected cell; and herpes simplex viral ICP47 and cytomegaloviral US11, which block class I antigen presentation. Clearly, many viruses have evolved to include genes that inhibit interferon, natural killer, and CD8+ cytotoxic cell effects. The adoption of these strategies by viruses highlights the importance of these host resistance factors in containing viral infection and also highlights the redundancy in host resistance. Even when viruses block one or several effectors of host resistance, infection can still be contained in the vast majority of immunocompetent hosts.

Much has been written about the role of specific aspects of the host immune response in containment of specific viral infections. Certainly, T lymphocyte disorders are particularly associated with relatively severe primary and reactivated herpesvirus infections, and antibody responses are important in resistance to many RNA virus infections. However, that antibody responses are also important in resistance to herpesvirus infections is evidenced by the utility of immunoglobulin therapy in herpesvirus infections. In addition, T lymphocyte responses are important in resistance to RNA virus infections; this importance is exemplified by the presence of cytotoxic T cells specific for influenza virus nucleoprotein. Redundancy in host resistance allows interferon, natural killer cell, B lymphocyte, or T lymphocyte responses to compensate in most instances for a deficiency in one of these host resistance factors.

Redundancy in host resistance has its price. Clearly, aspects of the host response contribute to the pathophysiologic manifestations of viral infection. Inflammation at sites of infection is essential to an effective local response but also contributes to local and systemic symptoms and local cell death. The systemic immune balance can be altered by viral infection, and the change can result in an immune attack on neural or other cells. The notion has been put forward that some of these aberrant responses may be due in part to cross-reactivity between viral and cellular antigens. While such effects can be demonstrated in experimental models, their role in the autoimmune manifestations of primary or recurrent human viral infections is uncertain.

INTERFERONS All human cells can synthesize interferon α or β in response to viral infection. The induction of an interferon response is usually due to the presence of double-strand viral RNA, which can be made by both RNA and DNA viruses. Interferon γ is not directly related to interferons α and β and is produced mainly by natural killer cells and by immune T lymphocytes responding to interleukin 12. Interferons α and β bind to the interferon α receptor, while interferon γ binds to a different but related receptor. Both receptors signal through receptor-associated JAK kinases and other cytoplasmic proteins, including STAT proteins. These proteins are tyrosine phosphorylated by JAK kinases, translocate to the nucleus, and transactivate promoters for specific cellular genes. Three types of antiviral effect are induced by interferon at the transcriptional level. The first involves the induction of 2′-5′ oligo(A) synthetases, which require double-strand RNA for activation. Activated synthetase polymerizes oligo(A) and thereby activates RNAse L, which in turn degrades single-strand RNA. The second effect involves the induction of PKR, a serine and threonine kinase that is also activated by double-strand RNA. PKR phosphorylates and negatively regulates the translational initiation factor eIF2 α, shutting down protein synthesis in the infected cell. The third effect entails the induction of Mx proteins, a family of GTPases that are particularly important in inhibiting the replication of influenza virus and vesicular stomatitis virus. None of these effects of interferons are specifically directed against the virus; infected-cell synthesis of RNA and proteins is inhibited globally. Interferon probably results in the death of the infected cell.

ANTIVIRAL AGENTS Twenty-five years ago, the field of clinically useful antiviral agents was limited to amantadine prophylaxis of influenza A virus infection. The synthesis of acycloguanosine and the discovery of its utility for the treatment of severe herpesvirus infections led to antiviral drug discovery programs at every major pharmaceutical company. Recent areas of focus include viral kinases, proteases, RNA polymerases, and polymerase accessory factors. The identification of HIV as the causative agent of AIDS led to worldwide efforts to develop antiretroviral drugs and renewed efforts to develop agents that would be effective against other viral infections in AIDS patients. The current status of clinically useful antivirals is summarized in Chap. 183.

Augmentation of the normal immune response by passive transfer of immunoglobulins or virus-specific T cells can be an effective mode of antiviral therapy. Human immunoglobulin enriched with antibodies to VZV is used to prevent disease in exposed susceptible individuals and to ameliorate disease in immunodeficient patients. Moreover, immunoglobulins are useful for prophylaxis of hepatitis and rabies virus infection and of CMV disease in transplant recipients; immunoglobulin administration appears to have a role in the treatment of parvovirus-induced aplastic anemia. Cellular immunotherapy effectively prevents and treats diseases induced by CMV and EBV in transplant recipients. In this instance, the number of virus-specific T cells is expanded in vitro, and the cells are readministered later, when the patient is at high risk for untoward consequences of viral infection.

DIAGNOSTIC VIROLOGY A wide variety of methods are now used to diagnose viral infection, but serology and viral isolation in tissue culture continue to form the backbone of diagnostic virology. Acute- and convalescent-phase sera with rising titers of antibody to virus-specific antigens and a shift from IgM to IgG antibodies are generally accepted as findings diagnostic of acute viral infection. Traditionally, virus-specific antibodies have been detected by hemadsorption, hemagglutination, or indirect immunofluorescence. Immunofluorescence assays use fixed virus-infected cells as a target for serum antibodies. Hemadsorption and hemagglutination assays measure the ability of serum antibodies to the hemagglutinin proteins of RNA viruses to inhibit virus-induced adsorption or agglutination of red cells. Serologic diagnosis is based on a greater than fourfold rise in IgG antibody concentration when acute- and convalescent-phase sera are analyzed at the same time. A simultaneous fall in IgM antibody confirms recent primary viral infection.

Immunofluorescence, hemadsorption, and hemagglutination assays are labor intensive and are being replaced by enzyme-linked immunoassays (ELISAs). ELISAs generally use specific viral proteins purified from virus-infected cells or produced by recombinant DNA technology. These viral antigens are attached to a solid phase, where they can be incubated with serum; washed to eliminate nonspecific antibodies; and allowed to react with an enzyme-linked reagent to detect either human IgG or IgM antibody specifically adhering to the viral antigen on the solid phase. The amount of antibody is then quantitated by the intensity of a color reaction mediated by the linked enzyme. ELISAs can be automated and can be more sensitive than immunofluorescence, hemagglutination, or hemadsorption assays.

Western blots measure antibody to multiple viral proteins simultaneously. The proteins are separated by size and transferred to an inert membrane, where they are incubated with serum antibodies. Western blots have an internal specificity control in that the level of reactivity for viral proteins can be compared with that for cellular proteins in

the same sample. Although western blots are useful for confirmatory testing, they require individual evaluation and are inherently difficult to quantitate.

The isolation of virus in tissue culture depends on the infection of susceptible cells and amplification through viral replication in infected cells. Viruses growing in tissue culture are frequently identified by their effect on the tissue culture, as detected under light microscopy. For example, HSV produces a typical cytopathic effect in rabbit kidney cells within 3 days. Other viral cytopathic effects may not be as definitively diagnostic and may require confirmation by staining with virus-specific monoclonal antibodies. Viruses growing in tissue culture can also be identified by hemadsorption, by interference (e.g., rubella virus–infected cells resist lysis induced by echoviral infection), or by electron microscopy (assuming that the specimen has altered cellular morphology detectable by ordinary light microscopy).

The efficiency and speed with which viruses are identified can be enhanced if short-term culture is combined with immune detection. With shell vials of tissue-culture cells growing on a coverslip, viral infection can be detected by staining with a monoclonal antibody to a specific viral protein expressed early in viral replication. Thus, virus-infected cells can be detected within hours or days of inoculation—i.e., before the several rounds of replication that would be required to produce a visible cytopathic effect.

The sensitivity of viral isolation is highly dependent on the collection of specimens from the appropriate site and their rapid transport in the appropriate medium to the virology laboratory. Rapid transport ensures viral viability and limits bacterial and fungal overgrowth. Lipid-enveloped viruses are generally much more sensitive than nonenveloped viruses to the effects of freezing and thawing. The most appropriate site for culture depends on the pathogenesis of the virus in question. Nasopharyngeal, tracheal, or endobronchial aspirates are most appropriate for the identification of respiratory viruses; sputum cultures generally are not appropriate because bacterial contamination and viscosity threaten tissue-culture cell viability. Aspirates of vesicular fluid are useful for the isolation of HSV and VZV. Nasopharyngeal aspirates and stool specimens may be useful in instances of fever and rash in which enteroviral infection is suspected. Adenoviruses can be cultured from the urine of patients with hemorrhagic cystitis. CMV can frequently be isolated from cultures of urine or the buffy-coat portion of peripheral blood. Material obtained by biopsy can be cultured effectively when viruses infect major organs—e.g., in herpesviral encephalitis or adenoviral pneumonia. Unlike serologic testing, the isolation of a virus does not establish the time of primary infection. Many viruses persistently or intermittently colonize normal human mucosal surfaces. Saliva is not infrequently positive for herpesviruses, and 1 percent of normal urine samples are positive for CMV. Isolations from blood, cerebrospinal fluid, or biopsy specimens are more likely to be diagnostic of significant viral infection.

Another method aimed at increasing the speed of viral diagnosis is direct antigen testing. Virus-infected cells obtained directly from the patient are detected by staining with virus-specific monoclonal antibodies; for example, epithelial cells obtained by nasopharyngeal aspiration can be stained with a variety of monoclonal antibodies to respiratory viruses. The Tzanck preparation used to detect multinucleated giant cells in lesions induced by HSV or VZV was the predecessor for these direct antigen tests, which can be enhanced by the use of monoclonal antibodies specific for HSV or VZV. Similarly, monoclonal antibodies can be applied to histopathology specimens to identify virus-infected cells.

Advances in nucleic acid technology may revolutionize diagnostic virology. Because of the speed and sensitivity of tests that directly amplify minute amounts of viral nucleic acids present in clinical specimens, detection no longer depends on viable virus and viral replication. For example, amplification and detection of nucleic acids of HSV leaking into the cerebrospinal fluid of patients with HSV encephalitis can be more sensitive than culture of HSV from cerebrospinal fluid.

The extreme sensitivity of these tests can also be problematic: trivial amounts of contamination can lead to false-positive results. Before their application in clinical diagnostic practice, these methods must be standardized and their clinical utility systematically evaluated.

Recent studies suggest that the progression of AIDS and the clinically significant emergence of drug-resistant variants can be detected by quantitative viral-load measurements based on the polymerase chain reaction. Thus, the Food and Drug Administration has approved nucleic acid tests to quantify HIV load. The usefulness of these tests in the cost-effective management of patients remains to be maximized.

IMMUNIZATION (See also Chap. 122) The development of viral vaccines is among the outstanding accomplishments of twentieth-century science. The scourge of smallpox has been eradicated, and the eradication of poliovirus infection may soon follow. Rabies and measles can be contained or eradicated. The excess mortality due to influenza epidemics can be eliminated, and the threat of influenza pandemics is now minimal. Widespread use of hepatitis B virus vaccination has dramatically lessened the frequency of acute and chronic hepatitis and is expected to lead to a dramatic decrease in the incidence of hepatocellular carcinoma. The ease with which some viruses are attenuated in tissue culture has facilitated widespread immunization against rubella, measles, mumps, and chickenpox and reduction of their attendant morbidity. Recombinant DNA–based strategies will make it possible to prevent severe infections with many other viruses through the use of purified proteins or genetically engineered live-virus vaccines. Unfortunately, there are limits to these prospects. The evolutionary divergence of HIV and hepatitis C virus appears to preclude the development of highy effective immunogens for the prevention of infection with these agents. However, modestly effective immunogens may prove useful against exposure to very low doses of even these pathogens.

BIBLIOGRAPHY

ALKHATIB G et al: CC CKR5: A Rantes, MIP-1α, MIP-1β receptor as a fusion cofactor for macrophage-tropic HIV-1. Science 272:1955, 1996

FIELDS BN et al (eds): *Virology*, 3d ed. New York, Raven Press, 1996

LAKEMAN FD, WHITLEY RJ: Diagnosis of herpes simplex encephalitis: Application of polymerase chain reaction to cerebrospinal fluid from brain-biopsied patients and correlation with disease. National Institute of Allergy and Infectious Diseases Collaborative Antiviral Study Group. J Infect Dis 172:1641, 1995

MCFADDEN G (ed): *Viroreceptors, Virokines, and Related Immune Modulators Encoded by DNA Viruses*. Austin, TX, Landes, 1995

MONTGOMERY R et al: Herpes simplex virus-1 entry into cells mediated by a novel member of the TNF/NGF receptor family. Cell 87:427, 1996

SAAG MS et al: HIV viral load markers in clinical practice. Nat Med 2:625, 1996

SENKEVICH T et al: Genome sequence of a human tumorigenic poxvirus: Prediction of specific host response-evasion genes. Science 273:813, 1996

TELLING G et al: Evidence for the conformation of the pathologic isoform of the prion protein enciphering and propagating prion diversity. Science 274:2079, 1996

WIEDBRAUK DL, JOHNSTON SLG: *Manual of Clinical Virology*. New York, Raven, 1993

183 *Raphael Dolin*

ANTIVIRAL CHEMOTHERAPY

The use of antiviral compounds for chemotherapy and chemoprophylaxis of viral diseases is a new development in the field of infectious diseases, particularly relative to the more than 50 years of experience with antibacterial agents. The principles that underlie the use of antiviral compounds have been modeled after those successfully employed in the treatment of bacterial infections, as outlined in Chap. 140. However, application of these principles to antiviral chemotherapy and chemoprophylaxis presents a number of unique problems.

First, antiviral compounds must possess a high degree of selectivity because of the biologic properties of viruses. Bacteria can replicate extracellularly and have evolved metabolic and structural features that differ considerably from those of mammalian cells. In contrast, viruses must replicate intracellularly and often employ host cell enzymes, macromolecules, and organelles for the synthesis of virus particles. Therefore, safe and effective antiviral compounds must be able to discriminate with a high degree of efficiency between cellular and virus-specific functions. Inhibitors of virus replication that lack this selectivity are likely to be too toxic for clinical use.

Second, because of the nature of virus replication, the in vitro sensitivity of virus isolates to antiviral compounds must be evaluated in a complex culture system consisting of living cells (e.g., tissue culture). The results from such assay systems vary widely according to the type of tissue culture cells employed and the conditions of assay. Furthermore, the precise relationship between the in vitro sensitivity of an isolate and the outcome of antiviral therapy has not been well worked out for many viral infections.

Third, information regarding the pharmacokinetics of some antiviral compounds, particularly in diverse clinical settings, is limited, particularly when compared with that available for antibacterial agents. Assays to determine concentrations of antivirals, particularly of active moieties within cells, are not widely available. There are few guidelines with which to adjust dosage levels in order to maximize antiviral activity and minimize toxicity. Therefore, clinical use of antiviral compounds must be accompanied by particular vigilance for unanticipated adverse effects or toxicity.

Fourth, it is clear that highly complex host defense systems play critical roles in the course of viral infections. The presence or absence of preexisting immunity and the ability to mount humoral and/or cell-mediated immune responses are especially important determinants in the outcome of viral infections. The state of host defenses and their interactions with antiviral compounds need to be considered when antivirals are utilized or evaluated.

Finally, as with antibacterial agents, the optimal use of antiviral compounds requires that a specific and timely diagnosis be made. For some viral infections, such as herpes zoster, the clinical manifestations are so characteristic that a diagnosis can be made on clinical grounds alone. For other viral infections, such as influenza A, epidemiologic information (e.g., the documentation of a community-wide outbreak) can be used to make a presumptive diagnosis with a high degree of accuracy. However, for most other viral infections, including herpes simplex encephalitis, cytomegalovirus infections other than retinitis, and acute viral gastroenteritis, diagnosis on clinical grounds alone cannot be accomplished with certainty. For such infections, rapid noninvasive viral diagnostic techniques are sorely needed. Considerable progress has been made in recent years in the development of such tests for a number of viral infections.

Despite these complexities, the efficacy of a number of antiviral compounds has been clearly established in rigorously conducted and controlled studies. The compounds that are currently licensed or are likely to be licensed in the immediate future for clinical use are discussed below and summarized in Table 183-1.

ANTIVIRAL DRUGS

AMANTADINE AND RIMANTADINE Amantadine (1-adamantanamine hydrochloride) and the closely related compound rimantadine (α-methyl-1-adamantanemethylamine hydrochloride) are primary symmetric amines with antiviral activity limited to influenza A viruses, whose replication they inhibit by interfering with the uncoating of virus after infection of the cell. This interference is attributable to the agents' interaction with the influenza A M2 matrix protein, during which the ion channel function of M2 is inhibited. A substitution of a single amino acid in the M2 protein can result in a virus that is resistant to amantadine and rimantadine.

Amantadine and rimantadine have been demonstrated to be effective in the prophylaxis of influenza A in large-scale studies of young adults and in less extensive studies of children and elderly subjects.

Table 183-1

Antiviral Chemotherapy and Chemoprophylaxis

Infection	Drug	Route	Dosage	Comment
Influenza A				
Prophylaxis	Amantadine or rimantadine	Oral	Adults: 200 mg/d for period at risk Children ≤9 yrs: 5 mg/kg per day (maximum, 150 mg/d)	Therapy must continue for duration of outbreak. Dosage should be reduced (more for amantadine) in patients with renal failure and the elderly. Drugs can be administered along with vaccine.
Treatment	Amantadine or rimantadine	Oral	As above for 5–7 days	Both drugs are effective in uncomplicated influenza. Neither has been thoroughly studied in complicated cases (e.g., pneumonia). Rimantadine is not approved for the treatment of children.
RSV infection	Ribavirin	Small-particle aerosol	Administered continuously from reservoir containing 20 mg/mL for 3–6 days	Ribavirin is used for treatment of infants and young children hospitalized with RSV pneumonia and bronchiolitis.
CMV retinitis in immunocompromised host	Ganciclovir	IV	5 mg/kg bid for 14–21 days; then 5 mg/kg per day as maintenance dose	Both drugs are licensed for treatment of CMV retinitis in immunosuppressed patients, including those with AIDS. They are also used for colitis, pneumonia, or "wasting" syndromes associated with CMV and for prevention of CMV disease in transplant recipients. Foscarnet is not myelosuppressive and is active against acyclovir- and ganciclovir-resistant herpesviruses.
		Oral	1 g tid as maintenance dose	
	Foscarnet	IV	60 mg/kg q 8 h for 14–21 days; then 90–120 mg/kg per day as maintenance dose	
HIV infection	Zidovudine (ZDV)	Oral IV	200 mg q 8 h 1–2 mg/kg q 4 h	ZDV is licensed for treatment of patients with HIV infection and CD4 counts of <500/μL. The optimal time to initiate therapy is controversial. Administration during pregnancy, during delivery, and to newborns reduces rates of perinatal HIV transmission. Higher doses are preferred for AIDS-related dementia.
	Didanosine (ddI)	Oral	125–200 mg (tablets) bid	ddI is licensed for treatment of HIV-infected patients who are intolerant of or failing to respond to ZDV. Clinical benefit is evident when patients are switched from ZDV to ddI, even if they have been stable on the former.
	Zalcitabine (ddC)	Oral	0.75 mg q 8 h	ddC is licensed for use in combination with ZDV in patients with advanced HIV infection who are not responding to ZDV alone. ddC appears inferior to ZDV as monotherapy in patients with advanced disease (median CD4 count, 89/μL). Combination of ZDV and ddC is superior to ZDV alone in patients with less advanced disease (median CD4 count, 354/μL).
	Stavudine (d4T)	Oral	30–40 mg bid	Stavudine is licensed for treatment of patients with advanced HIV infection who are intolerant of or failing to respond to approved therapy. Patients with CD4 counts of 50–500/μL with ≥6 mo of ZDV therapy benefit from a switch to stavudine.
	Lamivudine (3TC)	Oral	150 mg bid	3TC is used in combination with ZDV or d4T in patients with HIV infection and clinical or immunologic disease progression. 3TC retards the emergence of phenotypic resistance to ZDV.
	Saquinavir	Oral	600 mg tid	This protease inhibitor is approved for combination therapy with nucleoside analogues in advanced HIV infection, is well tolerated, has a low level of oral bioavailability, and should be taken within 2 h of a meal; it is subject to important drug interactions via the P450 system.

(continued)

Table 183-1—*(Continued)*

Antiviral Chemotherapy and Chemoprophylaxis

Infection	Drug	Route	Dosage	Comment
HIV infection (continued)	Indinavir	Oral	800 mg q 8 h	This protease inhibitor is approved for antiretroviral therapy in HIV infection. The drug is associated with hyperbilirubinemia and nephrolithiasis. It should be taken on an empty stomach. Indinavir is subject to important interactions via the P450 system.
	Ritonavir	Oral	600 mg bid	This protease inhibitor is approved for antiretroviral therapy in HIV infection. In advanced disease, ritonavir is associated with improved survival and delayed disease progression. Because of frequent gastrointestinal intolerance, the drug should be taken with meals. It is subject to important drug interactions via the P450 system.
Varicella Immunocompetent host	Acyclovir	Oral	20 mg/kg (maximum, 800 mg) 4 or 5 times daily for 5 days	Treatment confers modest clinical benefit when administered within 24 h of onset of rash.
Immunocompromised host	Acyclovir Vidarabine	IV IV	500 mg/m^2 q 8 h for 7 days 10 mg/kg per day as 12-h infusion for 5 days	No studies have compared IV acyclovir with vidarabine for varicella. Limited data from placebo-controlled studies suggest similar effects for the two drugs.
Herpes simplex encephalitis	Acyclovir	IV	10 mg/kg q 8 h for 10 days	Acyclovir is the drug of choice on the basis of comparative trials with vidarabine. Results are optimal when therapy is initiated early.
	Vidarabine	IV	15 mg/kg per day as continuous infusion over 12 h for 10 days	Drug must be given as dilute solution. Therapy can result in substantial fluid load.
Neonatal herpes simplex	Vidarabine	IV	30 mg/kg per day as continuous infusion over 12 h for 14–21 days	Vidarabine and acyclovir are equivalent in clinical efficacy. Serious morbidity is frequent despite therapy.
	Acyclovir	IV	10 mg/kg q 8 h for 14–21 days	
Genital herpes simplex Primary (treatment)	Acyclovir	IV	5 mg/kg q 8 h for 5–10 days	The IV route is preferred for infections severe enough to warrant hospitalization or with neurologic complications.
		Oral	200 mg 5 times daily for 10 days	This is the preferred route for patients whose condition does not warrant hospitalization. Adequate hydration must be maintained.
		Topical	5% ointment; 4–6 applications daily for 7–10 days	Topical use—largely supplanted by oral therapy—may obviate systemic administration to pregnant women. Systemic symptoms and untreated areas are not affected.
Recurrent Treatment	Acyclovir	Oral	200 mg 5 times daily for 5 days	Clinical effect is modest and is enhanced if therapy is initiated early. Treatment does not affect recurrence rates.
	Famciclovir Valacyclovir	Oral Oral	125 mg bid for 5 days 500 mg bid for 5 days	
Suppression	Acyclovir	Oral	400 mg bid for ≥12 mo	Suppressive therapy is recommended only for patients with at least 6–10 recurrences per year. "Breakthrough" occasionally takes place, and asymptomatic shedding of virus occurs. Need for suppressive therapy should be reevaluated after 1 year
Mucocutaneous herpes simplex in immunocompromised host Treatment	Acyclovir	IV Oral Topical	250 mg/m^2 q 8 h for 7 days 400 mg 5 times daily for 10 days 5% ointment; 4–6 applications daily for 7 days or until healed	Choice of intravenous or oral route depends on severity of infection and patient's ability to take oral medication. Oral or IV treatment has supplanted topical therapy except for small, easily accessible lesions.

(continued)

Table 183-1—(Continued)

Antiviral Chemotherapy and Chemoprophylaxis

Infection	Drug	Route	Dosage	Comment
	Vidarabine	IV	10 mg/kg per day for 7 days as 12-h infusion	Efficacy has been demonstrated in HSV-1 infections and in patients older than 40. Vidarabine appears to be less useful than acyclovir in this setting.
Prevention of recurrences during intense immunosuppression	Acyclovir	Oral IV	200 mg qid 5 mg/kg q 12 h	Acyclovir is administered during periods when intense immunosuppression is expected—e.g., during antitumor chemotherapy or after transplantation. After therapy is discontinued, lesions recur.
Herpes simplex keratitis	Trifluridine	Topical	1 drop of 1% ophthalmic solution q 2 h while awake (maximum, 9 drops daily)	Therapy should be undertaken in consultation with an ophthalmologist.
	Vidarabine	Topical	0.5-in ribbon of 3% ophthalmic ointment 5 times daily	
Herpes zoster				
Immunocompromised host	Acyclovir Vidarabine	IV IV	500 mg/m² q 8 h for 7 days 10 mg/kg per day as 12-h infusion for 5 days	Both drugs are effective in localized zoster, particularly when given early; acyclovir appears to be more effective. Studies of treatment of disseminated zoster are under way. High-dose oral acyclovir (4 g/d) is also used for herpes zoster in these patients.
Immunocompetent host	Valacyclovir	Oral	1 g tid for 7 days	Valacyclovir may be more effective than acyclovir for relief of pain; otherwise, it has a similar effect on cutaneous lesions and should be given within 72 h of onset of rash.
	Famciclovir	Oral	500 mg q 8 h for 7 days	Duration of postherpetic neuralgia is shorter than with placebo. Famciclovir showed overall efficacy similar to that of acyclovir in a comparative trial. It should be given ≤72 h after onset of rash.
	Acyclovir	Oral	800 mg 5 times daily for 7–10 days	Acyclovir causes faster resolution of skin lesions than placebo and provides some relief of acute symptoms if given within 72 h of onset of rash.
Herpes zoster ophthalmicus	Acyclovir	Oral	600 mg 5 times daily for 10 days	Treatment reduces ocular complications, including ocular keratitis and uveitis.
Condyloma acuminatum	Interferon α2b	Intralesional	1 million units per wart (maximum of 5) thrice weekly for 3 weeks	Intralesional treatment frequently results in regression of warts, but lesions often recur. Parenteral administration may be useful if lesions are numerous.
	Interferon αn3	Intralesional	250,000 units per wart (maximum of 10) twice weekly for up to 8 weeks	
Chronic hepatitis, non-A, non-B/C	Interferon α2b	SC or IM	3 million units thrice weekly for 24 weeks	Serum alanine aminotransferase values return to normal in 40–50% of cases but relapse in half when treatment is stopped. Optimal duration and regimens are being studied.
Chronic hepatitis B	Interferon α2b	SC or IM	5 million units daily for 16 weeks	Hepatitis B **e** antigen and DNA are eliminated in 33–37% of cases. Histopathologic improvement is also evident.

NOTE: CMV, cytomegalovirus; HIV, human immunodeficiency virus; HSV, herpes simplex virus; RSV, respiratory syncytial virus.

In such studies, efficacy rates of 55 to 80 percent in the prevention of influenza-like illness were noted, and even higher rates were reported when virus-specific attack rates were calculated. Amantadine and rimantadine also have been demonstrated to be effective in the treatment of influenza A infection in studies involving predominantly young adults and, to a lesser extent, children. Administration of these compounds within 24 to 72 h after the onset of illness has resulted in a reduction of the duration of signs and symptoms by approximately 50 percent from that in a placebo-treated group. The effect on signs and symptoms of illness has been demonstrated to be superior to that of commonly used antipyretic-analgesics. Only anecdotal reports are available concerning the efficacy of amantadine or rimantadine in the prevention or treatment of complications of influenza (e.g., pneumonia).

Amantadine and rimantadine are available only in oral formulations and are ordinarily administered to adults once or twice daily in a dose of 100 to 200 mg/d. Despite their structural similarities, the pharmacokinetics of the two compounds are different. Amantadine is not metabolized and is excreted almost entirely by the kidney, with a half-life of 12 to 17 h and peak plasma concentrations of 0.4 µg/mL. Rimantadine is extensively metabolized to hydroxylated derivatives and has a half-life of 30 h. Only 30 to 40 percent of an orally administered dose is recovered in the urine. The peak plasma levels of rimantadine are approximately half those of amantadine, but rimantadine is concentrated in respiratory secretions to a greater extent than amantadine. For prophylaxis, the compounds must be administered daily for the period at risk (i.e., the peak duration of the outbreak).

For therapy, amantadine or rimantadine is generally administered for 5 to 7 days.

Although these compounds are generally well tolerated, 5 to 10 percent of amantadine recipients experience mild central nervous system side effects consisting primarily of dizziness, anxiety, insomnia, and difficulty in concentrating. These effects are rapidly reversible upon cessation of the drug's administration. At a dose of 200 mg/d, rimantadine is better tolerated than amantadine; in a large-scale study of young adults, adverse effects were no more frequent among rimantadine recipients than among placebo recipients. Seizures and worsening of congestive heart failure also have been reported in patients treated with amantadine, although a causal relationship has not been established. The dosage of amantadine should be reduced to 100 mg/d or less in patients with renal insufficiency [i.e., a creatinine clearance (CrCl) rate of <50 mL/min] and in the elderly. A rimantadine dose of 100 mg/d should be used for patients with a CrCl of <10 mL/min and in the elderly. Resistance to amantadine and rimantadine can be induced readily in vitro. The emergence and probable transmission of virus resistant to these drugs also have been noted in vivo after their use for the treatment of children or adults. In the United States, both amantadine and rimantadine are approved for the prophylaxis and treatment of influenza A in adults and for prophylaxis in children. Amantadine is also approved for the treatment of influenza A in children.

RIBAVIRIN   Ribavirin is a synthetic nucleoside analogue that inhibits a wide range of RNA and DNA viruses. The mechanism of action of ribavirin is not completely defined and may be different for different groups of viruses. Ribavirin-5′-monophosphate blocks the conversion of inosine-5′-monophosphate to xanthosine-5′-monophosphate and interferes with the synthesis of guanine nucleotides as well as that of both RNA and DNA. Ribavirin-5′-monophosphate also inhibits capping of virus-specific messenger RNA in certain viral systems. In studies demonstrating the effectiveness of ribavirin, the compound has been administered as a small-particle aerosol. It has been used to treat respiratory syncytial virus (RSV) infections in infants and—less extensively—to treat parainfluenza virus infections in children and influenza A and B virus infections in young adults. In infants with RSV infection who were given ribavirin by continuous aerosol for 3 to 6 days, illness and lower respiratory tract signs resolved more rapidly and arterial oxygen desaturation was less pronounced than in placebo-treated groups. Ribavirin has also had a beneficial clinical effect in infants with RSV infection who require mechanical ventilation. Aerosolized ribavirin has been administered to older children and adults with severe RSV and parainfluenza virus infections (including immunosuppressed patients), but the benefit of this treatment, if any, is unclear. Orally administered ribavirin has not been effective in the treatment of influenza A virus infections. Intravenous or oral ribavirin has reduced mortality among patients with Lassa fever; it has been particularly effective in this regard when given within the first 6 days of illness. Intravenous ribavirin has been reported to be of clinical benefit in the treatment of hemorrhagic fever with renal syndrome caused by Hantaan virus and as therapy for Argentinian hemorrhagic fever. Moreover, oral ribavirin has been recommended for the treatment and prophylaxis of Congo-Crimean hemorrhagic fever. Intravenous ribavirin is being evaluated as therapy for the hemorrhagic fever with pulmonary syndrome caused by newly described hantaviruses in the United States.

Large doses of ribavirin administered orally (800 to 1000 mg/d) have been associated with reversible hematopoietic toxicity, but this effect has not been observed with aerosolized ribavirin, apparently because little drug is absorbed systemically. Aerosolized administration of ribavirin is generally well tolerated but occasionally is associated with bronchospasm, rash, or conjunctival irritation. Aerosolized ribavirin has been licensed for treatment of RSV infection in infants and should be administered under close supervision—particularly in the setting of mechanical ventilation, where precipitation of the drug

is possible. Health care workers exposed to the drug have experienced minor toxicity, including eye and respiratory tract irritation. Because ribavirin is mutagenic, teratogenic, and embryotoxic, its use is generally contraindicated in pregnancy. Its administration as an aerosol poses a risk to pregnant health care workers.

ACYCLOVIR AND VALACYCLOVIR   Acyclovir, or 9-[(2-hydroxyethoxy)methyl]guanine, is a highly potent and selective inhibitor of the replication of certain herpesviruses, including herpes simplex virus (HSV) types 1 and 2 (HSV-1 and HSV-2), varicella-zoster virus (VZV), and Epstein-Barr virus (EBV). It is relatively ineffective in the treatment of human cytomegalovirus (CMV) infections. Valacyclovir, the L-valyl ester of acyclovir, is almost entirely converted to acyclovir after oral administration.

The high degree of selectivity of acyclovir is related to its mechanism of action, which requires that the compound first be phosphorylated to acyclovir monophosphate. This phosphorylation occurs efficiently in herpesvirus-infected cells by means of a virus-coded thymidine kinase. In uninfected mammalian cells, little phosphorylation of acyclovir occurs, and the drug is therefore concentrated in herpesvirus-infected cells. Acyclovir monophosphate is subsequently converted by host cell kinases to a triphosphate that is a potent inhibitor of virus-induced DNA polymerase but has relatively little effect on host cell DNA polymerase. Acyclovir triphosphate also can be incorporated into viral DNA, with early chain termination.

Acyclovir is available in intravenous, oral, and topical forms. Intravenous acyclovir is markedly effective in the treatment of mucocutaneous HSV infections in immunocompromised hosts, reducing time to healing, duration of pain, and virus shedding. When administered prophylactically during periods of intense immunosuppression (e.g., related to chemotherapy for leukemia or transplantation) and before the development of lesions, intravenous acyclovir reduces the frequency of HSV-associated disease. After prophylaxis is discontinued, HSV lesions recur. Intravenous acyclovir is also effective in the treatment of HSV encephalitis; two comparative trials have indicated that acyclovir is more effective than vidarabine for this indication (see below). Because VZV is generally less sensitive to acyclovir than is HSV, higher doses of acyclovir must be used to treat VZV infections. In immunocompromised patients with herpes zoster, intravenous acyclovir reduces the frequency of cutaneous dissemination and visceral complications and—in one comparative trial—was more effective than vidarabine. Acyclovir, administered orally at doses of 800 mg five times a day, had a modest beneficial effect on localized herpes zoster lesions in both immunocompromised and immunocompetent patients. The overall effect of acyclovir on postherpetic neuralgia is unclear and is being evaluated further in large-scale collaborative trials. A comparative study of acyclovir (800 mg orally five times daily) and valacyclovir (1 g orally three times daily) in immunocompetent patients with herpes zoster indicated that the latter drug may be more effective in eliciting the resolution of zoster-associated pain. Orally administered acyclovir (600 mg five times a day) reduced complications of herpes zoster ophthalmicus in a placebo-controlled trial.

In normal children with chickenpox, acyclovir—administered at 20 mg/kg four times a day, up to a maximum of 800 mg four times a day, within 24 h of the onset of rash—resulted in a modest overall clinical benefit. Intravenous acyclovir also has been reported to be effective in the treatment of immunocompromised children with chickenpox.

The most widespread use of acyclovir is in the treatment of genital HSV infections. Both intravenous and oral formulations have shortened the duration of symptoms, reduced virus shedding, and accelerated healing when employed for the treatment of primary genital HSV infections. Oral acyclovir has also had a modest effect on recurrent genital HSV infections. However, the failure of treatment of either primary or recurrent disease to reduce the frequency of subsequent recurrences has indicated that acyclovir is ineffective in eliminating latent infection. Chronic administration of oral acyclovir for periods of 1 to 6 years has been shown to reduce the frequency of recurrences markedly during therapy; once the drug is discontinued, lesions recur. In AIDS patients, chronic or intermittent administration of acyclovir has been associated with the development of HSV and VZV strains resistant to the action of the drug and with clinical failures. The most common mechanism of resistance is a deficiency of the virus-induced thymidine kinase. Patients with HSV or VZV infections resistant to acyclovir have frequently responded to foscarnet.

With the availability of the oral and intravenous forms, there are few indications for topical acyclovir, although treatment with this formulation has been modestly beneficial in primary genital HSV infections and in mucocutaneous HSV infections in immunocompromised hosts.

Overall, acyclovir is remarkably well tolerated and is generally free of toxicity. The most frequently encountered form of toxicity is renal dysfunction, particularly after rapid intravenous administration or with inadequate hydration. Central nervous system changes, including lethargy and tremors, are occasionally reported, primarily in immunosuppressed patients. However, whether these changes are related to acyclovir, to concurrent administration of other therapy, or to underlying infection remains unclear. Acyclovir is excreted primarily unmetabolized by the kidney, via both glomerular filtration and tubular secretion. Approximately 15 percent of a dose of acyclovir is metabolized to 9-[(carboxymethoxy)methyl]guanine or other minor metabolites. Reduction in dosage is indicated in patients with a CrCl of less than 50 mL/min per 1.73 m^2. The half-life of acyclovir is approximately 3 h in normal adults, and the peak plasma concentration after a 1-h infusion of a dose of 5 mg/kg is 9.8 μg/mL. Approximately 22 percent of an orally administered acyclovir dose is absorbed, and peak plasma concentrations of 0.3 to 0.9 μg/mL are attained after administration of a 200-mg dose. Acyclovir penetrates relatively well into the cerebrospinal fluid (CSF), with concentrations approaching half of those found in plasma.

Acyclovir causes chromosomal breakage at high doses, but its administration to pregnant women has not been associated with fetal abnormalities. Nonetheless, the potential risks and benefits of acyclovir should be carefully assessed before the drug is used in pregnancy.

Valacyclovir exhibits three to five times greater bioavailability than acyclovir. The concentration-time curve for valacyclovir, given as 1 g orally three times daily, is similar to that for acyclovir, given as 5 mg/kg intravenously every 8 h. The safety profiles of valacyclovir and acyclovir are similar, although thrombotic thrombocytopenic purpura/hemolytic-uremic syndrome has been reported in immunocompromised patients who have received high doses of valacyclovir. Valacyclovir is approved for the treatment of herpes zoster and recurrent genital HSV infections in immunocompetent adults. It is being studied for use against other herpesvirus infections in various clinical settings.

GANCICLOVIR   An analogue of acyclovir, ganciclovir, or 9-[(1,3-dihydroxy-2-propoxy)methyl]guanine, is active against HSV and VZV and is markedly more active than acyclovir against CMV. Ganciclovir triphosphate inhibits CMV DNA polymerase and can be incorporated into CMV DNA, whose elongation it eventually terminates. In HSV- and VZV-infected cells, ganciclovir is phosphorylated by virus-encoded thymidine kinases; in CMV-infected cells, it is phosphorylated by a viral kinase encoded by the UL97 gene. Ganciclovir triphosphate is present in 10-fold higher concentrations in CMV-infected cells than in uninfected cells. Ganciclovir is approved for the treatment of CMV retinitis in immunosuppressed patients and for the prevention of CMV disease in transplant recipients. It is widely used for the treatment of other CMV-associated syndromes, including pneumonia, esophagogastrointestinal infections, hepatitis, and "wasting" illness.

Ganciclovir is available for intravenous or oral administration. Because its oral bioavailability is low (5 to 9 percent), relatively large doses (1 g orally three times daily) need to be administered by this route. Oral bioavailability is enhanced if the drug is administered with food, as recommended. The serum half-life of ganciclovir is 3.5 h after intravenous administration and 4.8 h after oral administration. The drug is excreted primarily by the kidney in unmetabolized form, and its dosage should be reduced in cases of renal failure. The most commonly employed dosage for initial therapy—5 mg/kg intravenously every 12 h for 14 to 21 days—is followed by a maintenance dose of 5 mg/kg intravenously per day or 5 times per week, possibly for as long as immunosuppression persists. Oral ganciclovir is approved as an alternative to the intravenous preparation in maintenance therapy for CMV retinitis, where it appears to be somewhat less effective although more convenient than intravenous therapy. Intraocular ganciclovir, given by either intravitreal injection or intraocular implantation, has also been used to treat CMV retinitis. The use of oral ganciclovir as prophylaxis against CMV disease in AIDS patients is currently being evaluated.

The administration of ganciclovir has been associated with profound bone marrow suppression, particularly neutropenia, which significantly limits the drug's use in many patients. Bone marrow toxicity is potentiated when other bone marrow suppressants, such as zidovudine, are used concomitantly.

Resistance has been noted in CMV isolates obtained after therapy with ganciclovir, especially in patients with AIDS. Such resistance may develop through a mutation in either the viral UL97 gene or the viral DNA polymerase. Ganciclovir-resistant isolates are usually sensitive to foscarnet (see below).

FAMCICLOVIR AND PENCICLOVIR   Famciclovir is the diacetyl, 6-deoxyester of the guanosine analogue penciclovir (9-[4-hydroxy-3-hydroxymethylbut-1-yl]guanine). Famciclovir is well absorbed orally, with a bioavailability of 77 percent, and is rapidly converted by deacetylation and oxidation to penciclovir. Penciclovir's spectrum of activity and mechanism of action are similar to those of acyclovir. Penciclovir is phosphorylated initially by a virus-encoded thymidine kinase and subsequently by cellular kinases to penciclovir triphosphate, which inhibits HSV-1, HSV-2, and VZV DNA polymerases as well as hepatitis B virus. The serum half-life of penciclovir is 2 h, but the intracellular half-life of penciclovir triphosphate is 7 to 20 h—markedly longer than that of acyclovir triphosphate. Penciclovir is eliminated primarily in the urine by both glomerular filtration and tubular secretion. The recommended dosage interval (every 8 h) should be adjusted for renal insufficiency.

Two trials involving immunocompetent adults with herpes zoster showed that famciclovir was superior to placebo in eliciting the resolution of skin lesions and virus shedding and in shortening the duration of postherpetic neuralgia; moreover, it was least as effective as acyclovir administered orally at a dose of 800 mg five times daily. Famciclovir was well tolerated, with occasional headache, nausea, and diarrhea reported in frequencies similar to those among placebo recipients. The administration of high doses of famciclovir for 2 years was associated with an increased incidence of mammary adenocarcinomas in female rats, but the clinical significance of this effect is unknown.

Famciclovir is approved for the treatment of herpes zoster and recurrent genital HSV infections in immunocompetent adults. It is being studied for the treatment of herpes zoster in immunocompromised patients and of other HSV infections in various clinical settings.

FOSCARNET   Foscarnet (phosphonoformic acid) is a pyrophosphate-containing compound that potently inhibits herpesviruses, including CMV. This drug inhibits DNA polymerases at the pyrophosphate binding site at concentrations that have relatively little effect on cellular polymerases. Foscarnet does not require phosphorylation to exert its antiviral activity and is therefore active against HSV and VZV isolates that are resistant to acyclovir because of deficiencies in thymidine kinase as well as against most ganciclovir-resistant strains of CMV. Foscarnet also inhibits the reverse transcriptase of human immunodeficiency virus (HIV) and is active against HIV in vivo.

Foscarnet is poorly soluble and must be administered intravenously via an infusion pump in a dilute solution over 1 to 2 h. The plasma half-life of foscarnet is 3 to 5 h and increases with decreasing renal function, since the drug is eliminated primarily by the kidneys. It has been estimated that 10 to 28 percent of a dose may be deposited in bone, where it can persist for months. The most common initial dosage of foscarnet—60 mg/kg every 8 h for 14 to 21 days—is followed by a maintenance dose of 90 to 120 mg/kg once a day.

Foscarnet is licensed for the treatment of CMV retinitis in patients with AIDS. In a comparative clinical trial, the drug appeared to be about as efficacious as ganciclovir against CMV retinitis but was associated with a longer survival period, possibly because of its anti-HIV activity. Intraocular foscarnet has been used to treat CMV retinitis. Foscarnet also has been employed to treat acyclovir-resistant HSV and VZV infections as well as ganciclovir-resistant CMV infections, although resistance to foscarnet has been reported in CMV isolated during therapy.

The major form of toxicity associated with foscarnet is renal impairment. Thus renal function should be monitored closely, particularly during the initial phase of therapy. Since foscarnet binds divalent metal ions, hypocalcemia, hypomagnesemia, hypokalemia, and hypo- or hyperphosphatemia can develop. Saline hydration and slow infusion appear to protect the patient against nephrotoxicity and electrolyte disturbances. Although hematologic abnormalities have been documented (most commonly anemia), foscarnet is not generally myelosuppressive and may be administered concomitantly with myelosuppressive medications such as zidovudine.

IDOXURIDINE Idoxuridine (IUdR) inhibits the replication of herpesviruses and poxviruses. It was formerly used systemically to treat herpesvirus infections, but, because of associated toxicity and lack of proven efficacy, its systemic use has largely been abandoned. Topical IUdR is effective in the treatment of HSV keratitis, particularly in superficial infections, but has been supplanted by topically applied trifluridine and vidarabine (see below).

TRIFLURIDINE Trifluridine (5-trifluoromethyl-2'-deoxyuridine) is a pyrimidine nucleoside active against HSV-1, HSV-2, and CMV. Trifluridine monophosphate irreversibly inhibits thymidilate synthetase, and trifluridine triphosphate inhibits viral and, to a lesser extent, cellular DNA polymerases. Because of systemic toxicity, its use is limited to topical therapy. Trifluridine is approved for treatment of HSV keratitis, for which trials have shown that it is more effective than topical IUdR but similarly effective to topical vidarabine. The drug has benefited some patients with HSV keratitis who have failed to respond to IUdR or vidarabine. Topical application of trifluridine to acyclovir-resistant HSV mucocutaneous infections has also been beneficial in some cases.

VIDARABINE Vidarabine (9-β-D-arabinofuranosyladenine) is a purine nucleoside analogue with activity against HSV-1, HSV-2, VZV, and EBV. Vidarabine inhibits viral DNA synthesis through its 5'-triphosphorylated metabolite, although the precise molecular mechanisms of action are not completely understood. For systemic administration, vidarabine is available only as an intravenous preparation with poor solubility and is administered as a constant 12-h infusion; thus a substantial fluid load can result. At doses of 10 to 15 mg/kg per day vidarabine is generally well tolerated, but at somewhat higher doses (20 mg/kg per day) the drug has been associated with hematopoietic side effects, including anemia, leukopenia, and thrombocytopenia. Neurotoxicity has also been reported, particularly at high dosages and in patients with hepatic or renal insufficiency.

Vidarabine is clinically effective against varicella and mucocutaneous HSV infections in immunocompromised patients but has been supplanted by acyclovir because of the latter drug's ease of administration. Vidarabine has been ineffective in the treatment of acyclovir-resistant HSV infections in AIDS patients. In comparative trials, vidarabine was as effective as acyclovir in the treatment of neonatal HSV infections but was less effective than acyclovir in the treatment of herpes simplex encephalitis. A 3% vidarabine ophthalmic ointment is effective in the treatment of HSV keratitis.

OTHER ANTIVIRAL DRUGS Sorivudine (BV-ARA-U) is a nucleoside analogue that potently inhibits VZV. It is also active against HSV-1 and EBV but not against HSV-2 or CMV. Sorivudine triphosphate inhibits viral DNA synthesis and is concentrated in virus-infected cells. It is well absorbed when given orally and is generally well tolerated. Administration of high doses (75 to 750 times the weight-adjusted human dose) has been associated with hepatic and testicular neoplasms in rodents. Sorivudine appears to be promising as therapy for VZV infections and is currently undergoing clinical trials for the treatment of herpes zoster in immunosuppressed patients and of varicella in immunocompromised adults.

Cidofovir is a phosphonomethylether derivative of cytosine that is highly active against CMV, including some ganciclovir- and foscarnet-resistant strains. This agent is administered intravenously and is cleared largely by the kidney, with a serum half-life of 2.6 h. Concomitant administration with probenecid markedly prolongs the half-life of cidofovir and protects recipients against the major form of toxicity elicited by the drug (nephrotoxicity). The intracellular half-life of cidofovir diphosphate—17 to 30 h—is the basis for its infrequent administration (once a week or once every other week). Cidofovir is currently being evaluated for the treatment of CMV retinitis in patients with AIDS.

ANTIRETROVIRAL DRUGS

ZIDOVUDINE Zidovudine (ZDV), also known as azidothymidine (AZT), inhibits the replication of HIV-1 and HIV-2 through competitive inhibition of HIV reverse transcriptase (by ZDV triphosphate) and through chain termination of viral DNA synthesis. ZDV is usually administered orally, although an intravenous formulation is available as well. The plasma half-life of ZDV is approximately 1 h, and 90 percent of a dose is recovered in the urine, mostly as the glucuronide metabolite.

In 1987 a large-scale placebo-controlled trial involving patients with AIDS or advanced symptomatic HIV-associated disease demonstrated that administration of ZDV was associated with prolonged survival and with decreases in the frequency and severity of opportunistic infections. Subsequently, ZDV was shown to be beneficial in placebo-controlled trials involving patients with less advanced HIV disease, including persons with early symptomatic disease and asymptomatic patients with CD4 counts of ≤500/mL. However, the optimal point for initiation of ZDV therapy (i.e., during symptomatic or asymptomatic infection) remains controversial, and the use of this agent alone is inferior to its use in combination with various other antiretrovirals, according to recent trials. A recent study showed that the rate of perinatal transmission of HIV-1 was reduced by two-thirds when ZDV was administered at 14 to 34 weeks of pregnancy to women who had CD4 counts of >200/μL and who had received less than 6 months of previous antiretroviral therapy. In that study, ZDV was also administered intrapartum and subsequently was given to the newborn for 6 weeks.

The clinical benefits of ZDV monotherapy appear to wane after a variable period and often last for no more than 12 to 18 months in patients with advanced disease. The full explanation for this diminishing effect is unclear but may be related to the high frequency of resistance to ZDV among HIV-1 isolates from patients with advanced disease who have received the drug for 6 months or more. The development of resistance appears to be less frequent in asymptomatic patients and in patients with less advanced disease. ZDV resistance is associated with specific amino acid substitutions in the HIV reverse transcriptase through mutations at codons 41, 67, 70, 215, and 219. Strategies for the use of ZDV in combination with other agents are designed in part to decrease or otherwise modify the emergence of such resistant viruses.

The most frequently employed dosage of ZDV is 200 mg by mouth every 8 h, and comparative dosage studies indicate that total daily doses of 500 to 600 mg are as effective as and less toxic than the higher doses previously recommended. The major toxicities of ZDV are hematopoietic—most often anemia and granulocytopenia, which occur more frequently in patients with more advanced HIV disease. Nausea, headache, and malaise are also encountered frequently, and ZDV-related skeletal and cardiac myopathies can occur. Severe steatosis and lactic acidosis have been described with ZDV as well as with other nucleoside analogues.

DIDANOSINE Didanosine (ddI) is a nucleoside analogue with activity against HIV-1 and HIV-2. It is an inhibitor of the HIV reverse transcriptase and also can act as a chain terminator for viral DNA elongation. ddI is phosphorylated and converted to ddATP, which is the active antiviral moiety. ddI is active in vitro against most HIV isolates that are resistant to ZDV. Resistance to ddI has been described and is associated with mutations at position 74 (and, to a lesser extent, at positions 135 and 184) in the reverse transcriptase.

Because ddI is given orally and is highly acid labile, it must be administered with buffers against stomach acidity. These buffers are incorporated into the powder or tablet preparations. ddI is 20 to 25 percent more bioavailable in tablets than in powder. The plasma half-life of ddI is 1.5 h, and approximately 50 percent of a dose is cleared by renal mechanisms. The intracellular half-life of ddATP is considerably longer (8 to 24 h) and provides the rationale for the recommended dosing schedule of every 12 h.

ddI was licensed originally on the basis of its favorable effects on "surrogate markers" of HIV disease (CD4 cell counts and p24 antigen concentrations) for use in patients who were intolerant of or failing to respond clinically or immunologically to treatment with ZDV. Subsequently, controlled studies have shown that switching such patients from ZDV to ddI monotherapy confers a clear clinical benefit, as does switching some patients to ddI who otherwise appear to be clinically stable on ZDV. Comparisons of ddI and ZDV as initial monotherapy in HIV disease have yielded conflicting results: ddI was superior to ZDV in a population with somewhat less advanced disease (median CD4 cell count, 354/μL), while ZDV appeared to be more effective in a population with more advanced disease (median CD4 count, 130/μL). ddI is also being evaluated as part of various two- and three-drug combinations.

The major toxicities encountered in the use of ddI have been pancreatitis and peripheral neuropathy. Overall rates of pancreatitis among recipients of ddI have been estimated at 5 to 9 percent, with rates at the upper end of this range among patients with advanced HIV disease. Most cases are mild to moderate in severity, but fatal cases have occurred rarely. Painful peripheral neuropathy, primarily involving the lower extremities, may develop and is generally reversible if it is recognized early and if drug administration is stopped. Medications or other factors that can cause pancreatitis or peripheral neuropathy should be avoided by patients who are taking ddI. ddI has not been associated with consistent hematopoietic toxicity; in fact, hemoglobin levels and white blood cell and platelet counts frequently improve during ddI therapy. Thus ddI may be particularly useful when hematopoietic suppression—either from drugs or from underlying diseases—is present or anticipated.

ZALCITABINE Zalcitabine (ddC) is a nucleoside analogue that potently inhibits HIV-1 and HIV-2. The triphosphate of ddC (ddCTP) inhibits HIV reverse transcriptase activity and also acts as a chain terminator. ddC is administered orally, has a plasma half-life of 1.2 h, and is excreted primarily by the kidney. A study comparing ddC with ZDV in patients who had received ZDV for less than 3 months showed that ddC was less effective. Most of the interest in ddC has centered on its use for combination therapy. Because combinations of ZDV and ddC had beneficial effects on CD4 cell counts and p24 antigen concentrations, ddC was licensed for use with ZDV in patients failing to respond clinically or immunologically to ZDV alone. Recently, large-scale trials have indicated a greater clinical benefit of combinations of ZDV plus ddC than of ZDV alone, particularly in patients with less advanced HIV disease. Evaluations of other two- and three-drug combinations including ddC are under way.

The major toxicities of ddC are dose-related peripheral neuropathy and aphthous stomatitis. Hematologic toxicity, as manifested by anemia and neutropenia, has not been a particular problem. Resistance to ddC has been reported and involves substitutions in the reverse transcriptase at positions 65 and 69.

STAVUDINE Stavudine (d4T) is a thymidine nucleoside analogue active against HIV-1 and HIV-2. It is phosphorylated by cellular kinases to stavudine triphosphate, which inhibits HIV reverse transcriptase and also causes DNA chain termination. Stavudine's relatively limited ability to inhibit cellular thymidine metabolism may account for its relative lack of toxicity in certain cell systems, such

as human bone marrow progenitor cells. Stavudine is well absorbed orally, with a plasma half-life of approximately 1 h; stavudine triphosphate has an intracellular half-life of 3.5 h. Forty percent of a dose is eliminated by renal mechanisms, and dose reductions are recommended for patients with a CrCl of ≤50 mL/min.

Stavudine has been licensed for use in patients with advanced HIV infection who are intolerant of or are failing to respond to approved therapies. This licensure was based on studies in which the drug's administration was associated with improvement in CD4 cell counts and p24 antigen concentrations. Recently, other studies have indicated that patients who are clinically stable after 6 months or more of therapy with ZDV, with CD4 counts between 50 and 500 cells/μL, benefit clinically from being changed to stavudine rather than continuing on ZDV. Stavudine is also being studied as part of various combination regimens. The recommended dose of stavudine (given orally) is 40 mg twice daily for patients weighing ≥60 kg and 30 mg twice daily for patients weighing <60 kg.

Stavudine is generally well tolerated. The major form of toxicity associated with its use is painful peripheral neuropathy. The development of resistance to this agent in vivo has been difficult to characterize, although resistance after serial passage in vitro has been associated with mutations at positions 50 and 75 in the reverse transcriptase.

OTHER ANTIRETROVIRAL AGENTS Lamivudine (3TC) is another nucleoside analogue inhibitor of reverse transcriptase that is active against HIV-1 and HIV-2. Although well tolerated, it has been relatively unimpressive as monotherapy; moreover, resistance has emerged rapidly in association with mutation at position 184. However, when lamivudine is administered in combination with ZDV, the development of this mutation suppresses phenotypic resistance to ZDV. Clinical trials of ZDV/lamivudine combinations have revealed sustained beneficial effects on CD4 counts and virus loads. The clinical effects of these combinations are being studied.

Nonnucleoside reverse transcriptase inhibitors (nevirapine, delavirdine) are also being evaluated in clinical trials. These drugs are active against HIV-1 but not HIV-2. They are generally well tolerated, with rash as the most troublesome side effect. The rapid development of resistance has been noted during monotherapy; thus the role of these agents is likely to be in combination therapy with other antiretrovirals.

Among the most promising antiretrovirals are the protease inhibitors, including saquinavir, indinavir, and ritonavir. These potent inhibitors of HIV-1 and HIV-2, which have recently been approved by the FDA, interfere with the cleavage of the polyprotein product of viral mRNA. The development of these drugs has been hampered by problems with bioavailability and their other pharmacokinetic properties. Clinical trials of protease inhibitors have shown impressive improvement in CD4 counts and decreases in viral load markers, but viral resistance has emerged after variable periods. Large-scale trials with clinical endpoints are under way to evaluate therapy with these drugs, either singly or in combination with other antiretroviral drugs.

INTERFERONS

From the earliest descriptions of interferon, considerable interest has existed in its application to the prophylaxis and/or treatment of viral infections. Interferons are cytokines that exhibit a broad spectrum of antiviral activities as well as immunomodulating and antiproliferative properties. Early studies with human leukocyte interferon demonstrated an effect in the prophylaxis of experimentally induced rhinovirus infections in humans and in the treatment of VZV infections in immunosuppressed patients. DNA recombinant technology has made available highly purified α, β, and γ interferons that have been evaluated in a variety of viral infections. Results of such trials have confirmed the effectiveness of intranasally administered interferon in the prophylaxis of rhinovirus infections, although its use has been associated with nasal mucosal irritation. Studies have also demonstrated a beneficial effect of intralesionally or systemically administered interferons on genital warts. The effect of systemic administration consists primarily of a reduction in the size of lesions, and this mode of therapy may be useful in individuals who have numerous warts that cannot easily be treated by individual intralesional injection. However, lesions frequently recur after intralesional or systemic interferon therapy is discontinued.

Interferons have undergone extensive study in the treatment of chronic hepatitis B virus (HBV) infection. The administration of interferon α2b (5 million units daily for 16 weeks) to patients with stable chronic HBV infection resulted in loss of markers of HBV replication, such as hepatitis B **e** antigen (HBeAg) and HBV DNA, in 33 to 37 percent of cases; 10 to 20 percent of patients also became negative for hepatitis B surface antigen. In more than 80 percent of patients who lose HBeAg and HBV DNA markers, serum aminotransferases return to normal levels, and both short- and long-term improvements in liver histopathology have been described. Predictors of a favorable response to therapy include low pretherapy levels of HBV DNA, high pretherapy serum levels of alanine aminotransferase (ALT), a short duration of chronic HBV infection, and active liver histopathology. Adverse effects of the above dose of interferon are common and include fever, chills, myalgia, fatigue, neurotoxicity (primarily manifested as somnolence and confusion), and leukopenia. Approximately 25 percent of patients receiving a daily dose of 5 million units will require dose reduction, but fewer than 5 percent will require discontinuation of therapy.

Several interferon preparations, including α2a, α2b, and αL (lymphoblastoid), have been studied as therapy for chronic non-A, non-B/C hepatitis infections. A variety of regimens have been employed, of which the most common are 1 million and 3 million units three times per week for 6 months. A complete response, defined as a return to normal serum ALT values at the end of treatment, has been documented in approximately 40 percent of patients. In addition, liver biopsies have shown decreases in lobular and periportal inflammation. However, relapse has occurred in at least half of all cases upon discontinuation of therapy. Relapses have generally responded quickly to retreatment. Additional clinical studies aimed at developing more effective regimens and defining prognostic variables in this patient population are under way. A recent study of patients with chronic hepatitis D showed that interferon α2a (9 million units three times per week for 48 weeks) resulted in reversion of ALT values to normal, loss of hepatitis D viral RNA, and histologic improvement in approximately 50 percent of cases. However, relapse was common after treatment was discontinued.

Interferon is licensed in the United States for the treatment of chronic HBV infection (α2b), chronic hepatitis non-A, non-B/C infection (α2b), condyloma acuminatum (α2b, αn3), hairy-cell leukemia (α2a, α2b), and Kaposi's sarcoma (α2a, α2b). Interferon γ (γ1b) is licensed for the treatment of chronic granulomatous disease.

BIBLIOGRAPHY

BEUTNER KR et al: Valacyclovir compared with acyclovir for improved therapy for herpes zoster in immunocompetent adults. Antimicrob Agents Chemother 39:1546, 1995

CONNOR EM et al: Reduction of maternal-infant transmission of human immunodeficiency virus type 1 with zidovudine treatment. N Engl J Med 331:1173, 1994

DOLIN R et al: A controlled trial of amantadine and rimantadine in the prophylaxis of influenza A infection. N Engl J Med 307:580, 1982

FISCHL M et al: The efficacy of azidothymidine (AZT) in the treatment of patients with AIDS and AIDS-related complex; a double-blind placebo-controlled trial. N Engl J Med 317:185, 1987

HALL CB et al: Aerosolized ribavirin treatment of infants with respiratory syncytial viral infection: A randomized double-blind study. N Engl J Med 308:1443, 1983

KAHN JO et al: A controlled trial comparing continued zidovudine with didanosine in human immunodeficiency virus infection. N Engl J Med 327:581, 1992

PERILLO RP et al: A randomized, controlled trial of interferon alfa-2b, alone and after prednisone withdrawal, in the treatment of chronic hepatitis B infection. N Engl J Med 323:295, 1990

REICHMAN RC et al: Treatment of condyloma acuminatum with three different interferons administered intralesionally: A double-blind, placebo-controlled trial. Ann Intern Med 108:675, 1988

STUDIES OF THE OCULAR COMPLICATIONS OF AIDS RESEARCH GROUP: Mortality in patients with the acquired immunodeficiency syndrome treated with either foscarnet or ganciclovir for cytomegalovirus retinitis. N Engl J Med 326:213, 1992

WHITLEY RJ et al: Herpes simplex encephalitis: Adenine arabinoside versus acyclovir therapies. N Engl J Med 314:144, 1986

SECTION 12
DNA VIRUSES

---

184   *Lawrence Corey*

HERPES SIMPLEX VIRUSES

DEFINITION Herpes simplex viruses (HSV-1, HSV-2; *Herpesvirus hominis*) produce a variety of infections involving mucocutaneous surfaces, the central nervous system (CNS), and—on occasion—visceral organs. The advent of effective chemotherapy for HSV infections has made prompt recognition of these syndromes even more clinically important than in the past. A related virus, herpes B, is enzootic in some monkey species but has caused rare cases of fatal infection in humans following contact with infected animals.

ETIOLOGIC AGENT The genome of HSV is a linear, double-stranded DNA molecule (molecular weight about 100×10^6) that encodes more than 70 gene products. The genomic structures of the two HSV subtypes are similar, and the overall sequence homology between HSV-1 and HSV-2 is about 50 percent. The homologous sequences are distributed over the entire genome map, and most of the polypeptides specified by one viral type are antigenically related to polypeptides of the other viral type. Many type-specific regions unique to HSV-1 and HSV-2 proteins do exist, however, and many of these regions appear to be important in host immunity. Restriction endonuclease analysis of viral DNA can be used to distinguish between the two subtypes and among strains of each subtype. The variability of nucleotide sequences from clinical strains of HSV-1 and HSV-2 is such that HSV isolates obtained from two individuals can be differentiated by restriction enzyme patterns unless the isolates are from epidemiologically related sources, such as sexual partners, mother-infant pairs, or victims of a common-source outbreak.

The viral genome is packaged in a regular icosahedral protein shell (capsid) composed of 162 capsomers. The outer covering of the virus is a lipid-containing membrane (envelope) derived from modified cell membrane and acquired as the DNA-containing capsid buds through the inner nuclear membrane of the host cell. Between the capsid and lipid bilayer of the envelope is the tegument. Viral replication has both nuclear and cytoplasmic phases. The initial steps of replication include attachment, fusion between the viral envelope and the cell membrane to liberate the nucleocapsid into the cytoplasm of the cell, and disassembly of the nucleocapsid to release the viral DNA. Replication of HSV is highly regulated. Following fusion of the virion envelope with the host cell membrane, several viral proteins are released from the HSV virion. Some shut off host protein synthesis (by increasing cellular RNA degradation), while others "turn on" transcription of early genes of HSV replication. These early gene products, designated α *genes,* are required for synthesis of the subsequent polypeptide group, the β polypeptides, many of which are regulatory proteins and enzymes required for DNA replication. Most current antiviral drugs interfere with β proteins, such as the viral DNA polymerase enzyme. The third (γ) class of HSV genes requires viral DNA replication for expression and constitutes most of the structural proteins specified by the virus.

Following replication of the viral genome and synthesis of structural proteins, nucleocapsids are assembled in the nucleus of the cell. Envelopment occurs as the nucleocapsids bud through the inner nuclear membrane into the perinuclear space. In some cells, viral replication in the nucleus forms two types of inclusion bodies: type A basophilic Feulgen-positive bodies that contain viral DNA and an eosinophilic inclusion body that is devoid of viral nucleic acid or protein and represents a "scar" of viral infection. Virions are then transported via the endoplasmic reticulum and the Golgi apparatus to the cell surface.

HSV infection of some neuronal cells does not result in cell death. Instead, viral genomes are maintained by the cell in a repressed state compatible with survival and normal activities of the cell, a condition called *latency*. Latency is associated with transcription of only a limited number of virus-encoded proteins. Subsequently, activation of the viral genome may occur, resulting in the normal pattern of regulated viral gene expression, replication, and release of HSV. The release of virus from the neuron and its subsequent entry into epithelial cells result in viral replication. This process is termed *reactivation*. Whereas infectious virus rarely can be recovered from sensory or autonomic nervous system ganglia dissected from cadavers, maintenance and growth of the neural cells in tissue culture result in production of infectious virions (*explantation*) and in subsequent permissive infection of susceptible cells (*cocultivation*). The fact that HSV replication was first detected in neurons during reactivation in vitro suggested that the neuron harbors the latent virus in vivo. Viral DNA and RNA have since been found in neural tissue at times when infectious virus cannot be isolated. Two RNA "latency-associated" transcripts that overlap the immediate early (α) gene products, called ICP-O, are found in abundance in the nuclei of latently infected neurons. These latency-associated transcripts code proteins in an antisense direction. Deletion mutants of this region that can become latent have been made. However, the efficiency of their later reactivation is reduced; thus, the antisense transcripts may play a role in maintaining rather than in establishing latency. At present, the molecular mechanisms of the latency of HSV-1 and HSV-2 are not well understood, and strategies to interrupt latency or to maintain molecular latency in neurons are not available.

PATHOGENESIS Exposure to HSV at mucosal surfaces or abraded skin sites permits entry of the virus and initiation of its replication in cells of the epidermis and dermis. Initial HSV infection is often subclinical—i.e., without clinically apparent lesions. Both clinical acquisition and subclinical acquisition are associated with sufficient viral replication to permit infection of either sensory or autonomic nerve endings. Upon entry into the neuronal cell, the virus—or, more likely, the nucleocapsid—is transported intraaxonally to the nerve cell bodies in ganglia. In humans, the interval from inoculation of virus in peripheral tissue to spread to the ganglia is unknown. During the initial phase of infection, viral replication occurs in ganglia and contiguous neural tissue. Virus then spreads to other mucosal skin surfaces through centrifugal migration of infectious virions via peripheral sensory nerves. This mode of spread helps explain the large surface area involved, the high frequency of new lesions distant from the initial crop of vesicles that is characteristic in patients with primary genital or oral-labial HSV infection, and the recovery of virus from neural tissue distant from neurons innervating the inoculation site. Contiguous spread of locally inoculated virus also may take place and allow further mucosal extension of disease.

After the resolution of primary disease, infectious HSV can no longer be recovered in the ganglia. However, viral DNA can be found in 10 to 50 percent of ganglion cells in the anatomic region of the initial infection. Only about 1 percent of such cells express latency-associated transcripts of RNA detectable by current techniques. The mechanisms by which various stimuli cause the reactivation of HSV

infection are unknown. Ultraviolet light, immunosuppression, and trauma to the skin or ganglia are associated with reactivation.

Analysis of the DNA from sequentially isolated strains of HSV or from isolates from multiple infected ganglia in any one individual has revealed identical restriction endonuclease patterns in most persons. Occasionally (most frequently in immunocompromised persons), multiple strains of the same viral subtype are detected in one individual. This finding suggests that exogenous infection with different strains of the same subtype is possible although very uncommon.

IMMUNITY Host responses to infection with HSV influence the acquisition of disease, the severity of infection, resistance to the development of latency, the maintenance of latency, and the frequency of recurrences. Both antibody-mediated and cell-mediated reactions are clinically important. Immunocompromised patients with defects in cell-mediated immunity experience more severe and more extensive HSV infections than those with deficits in humoral immunity, such as agammaglobulinemia. Experimental ablation of lymphocytes indicates that T cells play a major role in preventing lethal disseminated disease, although antibodies help reduce virus titers in neural tissue. Some aspects of the pathogenesis of HSV disease also may be related to the host immune response (e.g., stromal opacities associated with recurrent herpetic keratitis). The surface viral glycoproteins have been shown to be antigens recognized by antibodies mediating neutralization and immune-mediated cytolysis (antibody-dependent cell-mediated cytotoxicity). Monoclonal antibodies specific for each of the known viral glycoproteins have, in experimental infections, conferred protection against subsequent neurologic disease or ganglionic latency. Multiple cell populations, including natural killer cells, macrophages, a variety of T lymphocytes, and lymphokines generated by these cells, play a role in host defenses against HSV infections. In animals, passive transfer of primed lymphocytes confers protection from subsequent challenge. Maximum protection usually requires the activation of multiple T cell subpopulations, including cytotoxic T cells and T cells responsible for delayed hypersensitivity. The latter cells may confer protection by the antigen-stimulated release of lymphokines (e.g., interferons), which may have a direct antiviral effect or may activate other nonspecific effector cells. The HSV virion contains a gene called unique long gene no. 12 (UL-12) that can bind to the cellular transporter-activating protein TAP-1 and reduce the ability of this protein to bind HSV peptides to HLA class I. Thus, the virus may reduce the classic MHC class I expression of the cytotoxic T cell response to itself. This may be an important mechanism for the frequent reactivation of HSV.

EPIDEMIOLOGY Seroepidemiologic studies have documented HSV infections worldwide. Much of the humoral immune response to HSV is to type-common antigenic determinants. Serologic assays with whole-virus antigen preparations, such as complement fixation, neutralization, indirect immunofluorescence, passive hemagglutination, radioimmunoassay, and enzyme-linked immunosorbent assay, do not reliably distinguish between the two viral subtypes. Serologic assays that identify antibodies to type-specific surface proteins of the two subtypes have been developed. These assays, which are based on the demonstration of antibodies to type-specific epitopes of the virus, can reliably distinguish between the human antibody responses to HSV-1 and HSV-2. The most commonly used assays are those which measure antibodies to glycoprotein G of HSV-1 (gG1) and HSV-2 (gG2). A western blot assay that can detect several HSV type-specific proteins can also be used.

Infection with HSV-1 is acquired more frequently and earlier than infection with HSV-2. More than 90 percent of adults have antibodies to HSV-1 by the fifth decade of life. In populations of low socioeconomic status, most persons acquire HSV-1 infection before the third decade of life.

Antibodies to HSV-2 are not detected routinely until puberty. Antibody prevalence rates correlate with past sexual activity and vary greatly among different population groups. Recent serosurveys indicate that nearly 22 percent of the U.S. population has antibodies to

HSV-2—a 30 percent increase in the past 12 years. In most routine obstetric and family planning clinics, 25 percent of women have HSV-2 antibodies, although only 10 percent report a history of genital lesions. As many as 50 percent of heterosexual adults attending sexually transmitted disease clinics have antibodies to HSV-2. Antibody prevalence rates average about 5 percent higher among women than among men. The large reservoir of unidentified carriers of HSV-2 and the frequent asymptomatic reactivation of virus from the genital tract have fostered the continued spread of genital herpes throughout the world. HSV-2 infection has been shown to be an independent risk factor for the acquisition and transmission of infection with human immunodeficiency virus (HIV) type 1. Among coinfected persons, HIV-1 virions can be shed from herpetic lesions of the genital region. This shedding may facilitate the spread of HIV via sexual contact.

HSV infections occur throughout the year. The incubation period ranges from 1 to 26 days (median, 6 to 8 days). Transmission can result from contact with persons with active ulcerative lesions or with persons without clinical manifestations of infection who are shedding HSV or on whose mucosal surfaces the virus is replicating. Asymptomatic salivary excretion of HSV-1 by 2 to 9 percent of adults and 5 to 8 percent of children has been reported. Subclinical shedding of HSV-2 by both men and women infected with this virus has been detected on an average of 2 to 3 percent of days.

The frequency of subclinical reactivation varies greatly among individuals. Twenty percent of women seropositive for HSV-2 may subclinically shed culture-detected virus on >8 percent of days. Recently, polymerase chain reaction (PCR)–based systems have detected HSV-2 shedding on mucosal surfaces of immunocompetent young adults on 15 to 40 percent of days. These data indicate that subclinical reactivation of HSV on mucosal surfaces is more common than has been appreciated. The implication is that most seropositive persons are potential transmitters of the infection. Such data are supported by the continued rise in the seroprevalence of HSV infection worldwide.

CLINICAL SPECTRUM HSV has been isolated from nearly all visceral or mucocutaneous sites. The clinical manifestations and course of HSV infection depend on the anatomic site involved, the age and immune status of the host, and the antigenic type of the virus. First episodes of HSV disease, especially primary infections (i.e., first infections with either HSV-1 or HSV-2 in which the host lacks HSV antibodies in acute-phase serum), are frequently accompanied by systemic signs and symptoms, involve both mucosal and extramucosal sites, and have a longer duration of symptoms, a longer duration of virus isolation from lesions, and a higher rate of complications than recurrent episodes of disease. Both viral subtypes can cause genital and oral-facial infections, and the infections caused by the two subtypes are clinically indistinguishable. However, the frequency of reactivation of infection is influenced by anatomic site and virus type. Genital HSV-2 infection is twice as likely to reactivate and recurs 8 to 10 times more frequently than genital HSV-1 infection. Conversely, oral-labial HSV-1 infection recurs more frequently than oral-labial HSV-2 infection.

Oral-Facial Infections Gingivostomatitis and pharyngitis are the most frequent clinical manifestations of first-episode HSV-1 infection, while recurrent herpes labialis is the most frequent clinical manifestation of reactivation HSV infection. HSV pharyngitis and gingivostomatitis usually result from primary infection and are most commonly seen in children and young adults. Clinical symptoms and signs, which include fever, malaise, myalgias, inability to eat, irritability, and cervical adenopathy, may last from 3 to 14 days. Lesions may involve the hard and soft palate, gingiva, tongue, lip, and facial area. HSV-1 or HSV-2 infection of the pharynx usually results in exudative or ulcerative lesions of the posterior pharynx and/or tonsillar pillars. Lesions of the tongue, buccal mucosa, or gingiva may occur later in the course in one-third of cases. Fever lasting from 2 to 7 days and cervical adenopathy are common. It can be difficult to differentiate HSV pharyngitis clinically from bacterial pharyngitis, *Mycoplasma*

pneumoniae infections, and pharyngeal ulcerations of noninfectious etiologies (e.g., Stevens-Johnson syndrome). No substantial evidence suggests that reactivation oral-labial HSV infection is associated with symptomatic recurrent pharyngitis.

Reactivation of HSV from the trigeminal ganglia may be associated with asymptomatic virus excretion in the saliva, development of intraoral mucosal ulcerations, or herpetic ulcerations on the vermilion border of the lip or external facial skin. About 50 to 70 percent of seropositive patients undergoing trigeminal nerve root decompression and 10 to 15 percent of those undergoing dental extraction develop oral-labial HSV infection a median of 3 days after these procedures.

In immunosuppressed patients, infection may extend into mucosal and deep cutaneous layers. Friability, necrosis, bleeding, severe pain, and inability to eat or drink may result. The lesions of HSV mucositis are clinically similar to mucosal lesions caused by cytotoxic drug therapy, trauma, or fungal or bacterial infections. Persistent ulcerative HSV infections are among the most common infections in patients with AIDS. HSV and *Candida* infections often occur concurrently. Systemic acyclovir therapy speeds the rate of healing and relieves the pain of mucosal HSV infections in immunosuppressed patients. Patients with atopic eczema also may develop severe oral-facial HSV infections (eczema herpeticum), which may rapidly come to involve extensive areas of skin and occasionally disseminate to visceral organs. Extensive eczema herpeticum has resolved promptly with the administration of intravenous acyclovir. Erythema multiforme (EM) also may be associated with HSV infections; some evidence suggests that HSV infection is the precipitating event in about 75 percent of cases of cutaneous EM. HSV antigen has been demonstrated both in circulatory immune complexes and in skin lesion biopsy samples from these patients. Patients with severe HSV-associated EM are candidates for chronic suppressive oral antiviral therapy.

HSV-1 has recently been implicated in the etiology of Bell's palsy (flaccid paralysis of the mandibular portion of the facial nerve). Whether antiviral chemotherapy can alter the course of this infection is unclear.

Genital Infections First-episode primary genital herpes is characterized by fever, headache, malaise, and myalgias. Pain, itching, dysuria, vaginal and urethral discharge, and tender inguinal lymphadenopathy are the predominant local symptoms. Widely spaced bilateral lesions of the external genitalia are characteristic. Lesions may be present in varying stages, including vesicles, pustules, or painful erythematous ulcers. The cervix and urethra are involved in more than 80 percent of women with first-episode infections. First episodes of genital herpes in patients who have had prior HSV-1 infection are associated with less frequent systemic symptoms and faster healing than primary genital herpes. The clinical courses of acute first-episode genital herpes among patients with HSV-1 and HSV-2 infections are similar. However, the recurrence rates of genital disease differ with the viral subtype: the 12-month recurrence rates among patients with first-episode HSV-2 and HSV-1 infections are ~90 percent and 55 percent, respectively (median number of recurrences, 4 and <1, respectively). Recurrence rates for genital HSV-2 infections vary greatly among individuals and over time within the same individual. HSV has been isolated from the urethra and urine of men and women without external genital lesions. A clear mucoid discharge and dysuria are characteristics of symptomatic HSV urethritis. HSV has been isolated from the urethra of 5 percent of women with the dysuria-frequency syndrome. Occasionally, HSV genital tract disease is manifested by endometritis and salpingitis in women and by prostatitis in men.

Both HSV-1 and HSV-2 can cause symptomatic or asymptomatic rectal and perianal infections. HSV proctitis is usually associated with rectal intercourse. However, subclinical perianal shedding of HSV is detected both in heterosexual men and in women who report no rectal intercourse. This phenomenon is due to the establishment of latency in the sacral dermatome from prior genital tract infection, with subsequent reactivation in epithelial cells in the perianal region. Such reactivations are often subclinical. Symptoms of HSV proctitis include anorectal pain, anorectal discharge, tenesmus, and constipation. Sigmoidoscopy reveals ulcerative lesions of the distal 10 cm of the rectal mucosa. Rectal biopsies show mucosal ulceration, necrosis, polymorphonuclear and lymphocytic infiltration of the lamina propria, and (in occasional cases) multinucleated intranuclear inclusion–bearing cells. Perianal herpetic lesions are also found in immunosuppressed patients receiving cytotoxic therapy. Extensive perianal herpetic lesions and/or HSV proctitis is common among patients with HIV infection.

Herpetic Whitlow Herpetic whitlow—HSV infection of the finger—may occur as a complication of primary oral or genital herpes by inoculation of virus via a break in the epidermal surface or by direct introduction of virus into the hand through occupational or some other type of exposure. Clinical signs and symptoms include the abrupt onset of edema, erythema, and localized tenderness of the infected finger. Vesicular or pustular lesions of the fingertip that are indistinguishable from lesions of pyogenic bacterial infection are seen. Fever, lymphadenitis, and epitrochlear and axillary lymphadenopathy are common. The infection may recur. Prompt diagnosis (to avoid unnecessary and potentially exacerbating surgical therapy and/or transmission) is essential. Antiviral chemotherapy (to speed the healing of the process) is usually recommended (see below).

Herpes Gladiatorum HSV may infect almost any area of skin. Mucocutaneous HSV infections of the thorax, ears, face, and hands have been described among wrestlers. Transmission of these infections is facilitated by trauma to the skin sustained during wrestling. Prompt diagnosis and therapy are required to contain the spread of this infection.

Eye Infections HSV infection of the eye is the most frequent cause of corneal blindness in the United States. HSV keratitis presents with an acute onset of pain, blurring of vision, chemosis, conjunctivitis, and characteristic dendritic lesions of the cornea. Use of topical glucocorticoids may exacerbate symptoms and lead to involvement of deep structures of the eye. Debridement, topical antiviral treatment, and/or interferon therapy hastens healing. However, recurrences are common, and the deeper structures of the eye may sustain immunopathologic injury. Chorioretinitis, usually a manifestation of disseminated HSV infection, may occur in neonates or in patients with HIV infection. HSV and varicella-zoster virus can cause acute necrotizing retinitis as an uncommon but severe manifestation.

Central and Peripheral Nervous System Infections HSV is the most commonly identified cause of acute, sporadic viral encephalitis in the United States, accounting for 10 to 20 percent of all cases. The estimated incidence is about 2.3 cases per million persons per year. Cases are distributed throughout the year, and the age distribution appears to be biphasic, with peaks at 5 to 30 and >50 years of age. Subtype 1 virus causes more than 95 percent of cases of HSV encephalitis.

The pathogenesis of HSV encephalitis varies. In children and young adults, primary HSV infection may result in encephalitis; presumably, exogenously acquired virus enters the CNS by neurotropic spread from the periphery via the olfactory bulb. However, most adults with HSV encephalitis have clinical or serologic evidence of mucocutaneous HSV-1 infection prior to the onset of the CNS symptoms. In about 25 percent of the cases examined, the HSV-1 strains from the oropharynx and brain tissue of the same patient differ; thus some cases may result from reinfection with another strain of HSV-1 that reaches the CNS. Two theories have been proposed to explain the development of actively replicating HSV in localized areas of the CNS in persons whose ganglionic and CNS isolates are similar. Reactivation of latent HSV-1 infection in trigeminal or autonomic nerve roots may be associated with extension of virus into the CNS via nerves innervating the middle cranial fossa. HSV DNA has been demonstrated by DNA hybridization in brain tissue obtained at autopsy—even from healthy adults. Thus, reactivation of long-standing latent CNS infection may be another mechanism for the development of HSV encephalitis.

The clinical hallmark of HSV encephalitis has been the acute onset of fever and focal neurologic (especially temporal-lobe) symptoms. Differentiation of HSV encephalitis from other viral encephalitides, as well as from other focal infections and noninfectious processes, is difficult. The most sensitive noninvasive method for early diagnosis

of HSV encephalitis is the demonstration of HSV DNA in cerebrospinal fluid (CSF) by PCR. Although titers of CSF and serum antibodies to HSV increase in most cases of HSV encephalitis, they rarely do so earlier than 10 days into the illness and therefore, while useful retrospectively, are generally not helpful in establishing an early clinical diagnosis. Demonstration of HSV antigen, HSV DNA, or HSV replication in brain tissue obtained by biopsy is highly sensitive and has a low complication rate; examination of such tissue also provides the best opportunity to identify alternative, potentially treatable causes of encephalitis. Antiviral chemotherapy reduces the rate of death from HSV encephalitis. Intravenous acyclovir is more effective than vidarabine. Even with therapy, however, neurologic sequelae are frequent, especially in persons over 35 years of age. Most authorities recommend the administration of intravenous acyclovir to patients with presumed HSV encephalitis until the diagnosis is confirmed or an alternative diagnosis is made.

HSV has been isolated from the CSF of 0.5 to 3 percent of patients presenting to the hospital with aseptic meningitis. HSV meningitis, which is usually seen in association with primary genital HSV infection, is an acute, self-limited disease manifested by headache, fever, and mild photophobia and lasting from 2 to 7 days. Lymphocytic pleocytosis in the CSF is characteristic. Neurologic sequelae of HSV meningitis are rare. HSV is the most commonly identified cause of recurrent lymphocytic meningitis (Mollaret's meningitis). Demonstration of HSV antibodies in CSF or persistence of HSV DNA in CSF can establish the diagnosis. Daily administration of antiviral therapy aimed at reducing the likelihood of clinical HSV reactivation has been successful in such cases.

Autonomic nervous system dysfunction, especially of the sacral region, has been reported in association with both HSV and varicella-zoster virus infections. Numbness, tingling of the buttocks or perineal areas, urinary retention, constipation, CSF pleocytosis, and (in males) impotence may occur. Symptoms appear to resolve slowly over days to weeks. Occasionally, hypesthesia and/or weakness of the lower extremities may persist for many months. Rarely, transverse myelitis manifested by a rapidly progressive symmetric paralysis of the lower extremities or a Guillain-Barré syndrome may follow HSV infection. Similarly, peripheral nervous system involvement (Bell's palsy) or cranial polyneuritis also may be related to reactivation of HSV-1 infection. Transitory hypesthesia of the area of skin innervated by the trigeminal nerve and vestibular system dysfunction as measured by electronystagmography are the predominant signs of disease. Studies to determine whether antiviral chemotherapy may abort these signs or reduce their frequency and severity are unavailable.

Visceral Infections HSV infection of visceral organs usually results from viremia, and multiple-organ involvement is common. Occasionally, however, the clinical manifestations of HSV infection involve only the esophagus, lung, or liver. HSV esophagitis may result from direct extension of oral-pharyngeal HSV infection into the esophagus or may occur de novo by reactivation and spread of HSV to the esophageal mucosa via the vagus nerve. The predominant symptoms of HSV esophagitis are odynophagia, dysphagia, substernal pain, and weight loss. There are multiple oval ulcerations on an erythematous base with or without a patchy white pseudomembrane. The distal esophagus is most commonly involved. With extensive disease, diffuse friability may spread to the entire esophagus. Neither endoscopic nor barium examination can differentiate HSV esophagitis from *Candida* esophagitis or from esophageal ulcerations due to thermal injury, radiation, or corrosives. Endoscopically obtained secretions for cytologic examination and culture provide the most useful material for diagnosis. Systemic antiviral chemotherapy usually reduces symptoms and heals esophageal ulcerations.

HSV pneumonitis is uncommon except in severely immunosuppressed patients and may result from extension of herpetic tracheobronchitis into lung parenchyma. Focal necrotizing pneumonitis usually ensues. Hematogenous dissemination of virus from sites of oral or genital mucocutaneous disease also may occur and produce bilateral interstitial pneumonitis. Bacterial, fungal, and parasitic pathogens are commonly present in HSV pneumonitis. The mortality rate from untreated HSV pneumonia in immunosuppressed patients is high (>80 percent). HSV also has been isolated from the lower respiratory tract of persons with adult respiratory distress syndrome (ARDS). However, the relationship between the isolation of HSV and the pathogenesis of ARDS is unclear.

HSV is an uncommon cause of hepatitis in immunocompetent patients. HSV infection of the liver is associated with fever, abrupt elevations of bilirubin and the serum aminotransferases, and leukopenia (<4000 white blood cells per microliter). Disseminated intravascular coagulation also may develop.

Other reported complications of HSV infection include monarticular arthritis, adrenal necrosis, idiopathic thrombocytopenia, and glomerulonephritis. Disseminated HSV infection in immunocompetent patients is rare. In immunocompromised, burned, or malnourished patients, HSV occasionally disseminates to other visceral organs, such as the adrenal glands, pancreas, small and large intestines, and bone marrow. Rarely, primary HSV infection in pregnancy disseminates and may be associated with the death of both mother and fetus. This uncommon event is usually associated with the acquisition of primary infection in the third trimester.

Neonatal HSV Infection Neonates (infants <6 weeks of age) have the highest frequency of visceral and/or CNS infection of any HSV-infected patient population. If not treated, neonatal herpes undergoes dissemination or develops into CNS infection in >70 percent of cases. Without therapy, the overall rate of death from neonatal herpes is 65 percent; fewer than 10 percent of neonates with CNS infection develop normally. While skin lesions are the most commonly recognized features of disease, many infants do not develop lesions until well into the course of disease. Of the 70 percent of neonatal HSV infections caused by HSV-2, almost all result from contact with infected genital secretions at the time of delivery. However, congenitally infected infants have been reported. Usually these infants are born to mothers who have acquired primary HSV infection during pregnancy. In most series, 30 percent of neonatal HSV infections are due to HSV-1. Most of these cases are associated with the maternal acquisition of primary genital HSV-1 late in pregnancy and the consequent contact of the infant with infectious genital secretions at birth. Neonatal HSV-1 infections may also be acquired through postnatal contact with immediate family members who have symptomatic or asymptomatic oral-labial HSV-1 infection or through nosocomial transmission within the hospital. Antiviral chemotherapy has reduced the rate of death from neonatal herpes to 25 percent. However, the rate of morbidity, especially in infants with HSV-2 infection involving the CNS, is still very high.

DIAGNOSIS Both clinical and laboratory criteria are useful for establishing the diagnosis of HSV infections. A clinical diagnosis can be made accurately when characteristic multiple vesicular lesions on an erythematous base are present. However, it is increasingly being recognized that herpetic ulcerations may clinically resemble skin ulcerations of other etiologies. Mucosal HSV infections may also present as urethritis or pharyngitis without cutaneous lesions. Thus, laboratory studies to confirm the diagnosis and to guide therapy are recommended. Staining of scrapings from the base of the lesions with Wright's, Giemsa's (Tzanck preparation), or Papanicolaou's stain demonstrates characteristic giant cells or intranuclear inclusions of herpesvirus infection. These cytologic techniques are often useful as quick office procedures to confirm the diagnosis. Limitations of the cytologic method are that it does not differentiate between HSV and varicella-zoster virus infections, that it is relatively insensitive, and that the correct identification of giant cells requires experience.

HSV infection is best confirmed in the laboratory by isolation of virus in tissue culture or by demonstration of HSV antigens or DNA in scrapings from lesions. HSV causes a discernible cytopathic effect in a variety of cell culture systems, and most specimens can be identified within 48 to 96 h after inoculation. Spin-amplified culture with subsequent staining for HSV antigen has shortened the time needed to identify HSV to less than 24 h. The sensitivity of viral isolation depends on the stage of lesions (with higher sensitivity in vesicular than in ulcerative lesions), on whether the patient has a first or a recurrent episode of the disease (with higher sensitivity in first than in recurrent episodes), and on whether the sample is from an immunosuppressed or an immunocompetent patient (with more antigen in immunosuppressed patients). Antigen detection procedures have approached viral isolation in terms of sensitivity in detecting HSV in genital or oral-labial lesions; however, antigen detection appears to be only about 50 percent as sensitive as viral isolation for the identification of HSV in cervical or salivary secretions of asymptomatic patients. PCR techniques appear to be more sensitive for HSV than viral isolation, especially for the diagnosis of CNS infections and for the detection of HSV as a cause of late-stage ulcerative lesions. Laboratory confirmation permits subtyping of the virus; information on subtype may be useful epidemiologically and may help to predict the frequency of reactivation after first-episode oral-labial or genital HSV infection.

Acute- and convalescent-phase serum can be useful in demonstrating seroconversion during primary HSV-1 or HSV-2 infection. However, only 5 percent of patients with recurrent mucocutaneous HSV infections have a fourfold or greater rise in titer of antibody to HSV in the interval between the collection of the first and second samples. Serologic assays, especially type-specific assays, should be used to identify asymptomatic carriers of HSV-1 or HSV-2 infection.

Several studies have shown that persons seropositive for HSV-2 to whom the clinical manifestations of HSV have been explained are able to identify symptomatic reactivations. Individuals seropositive for HSV-2 should be told about the high frequency of subclinical reactivation in mucosal surfaces not visible to the eye (e.g., cervix, urethra, perianal skin) or in microscopic ulcerations that may not be clinically symptomatic. Transmission of infection during such episodes is well established.

℞ TREATMENT

Many aspects of mucocutaneous and visceral HSV infections are amenable to antiviral chemotherapy. For mucocutaneous infections, acyclovir and its congeners famciclovir and valacyclovir have been the mainstay of therapy. Several antiviral agents are available for topical use in HSV eye infections: idoxuridine, trifluorothymidine, topical vidarabine, and (recently) cidofovir. For HSV encephalitis and neonatal herpes, intravenous acyclovir is the treatment of choice.

Several compounds have been developed that are effective in the treatment of HSV infections. To date, all work by inhibiting HSV DNA polymerase. One class of drugs, typified by the drug acyclovir, is made up of substrates for the HSV enzyme thymidine kinase. Acyclovir, ganciclovir, famciclovir, and valacyclovir are all selectively phosphorylated to the monophosphate form in virus-infected cells. Cellular enzymes convert the monophosphate form of the drug to the triphosphate, which is then incorporated into the viral DNA chain.

Acyclovir is the best-studied and most frequently used agent for the treatment of HSV infections. Famciclovir, the oral formulation of penciclovir, is also clinically effective in the treatment of a variety of HSV-1 and HSV-2 infections. Currently, no intravenous preparation of penciclovir is available. Thus, for serious HSV infections, acyclovir is the current standard of treatment. Valacyclovir is a valyl ester of acyclovir that has greater bioavailability than acyclovir. Ganciclovir has activity against both HSV-1 and HSV-2; however, as it is more toxic than acyclovir, valacyclovir, and famciclovir, it is generally not recommended for the treatment of HSV infections.

Acyclovir has been shown to be effective in shortening the duration of symptoms and lesions of mucocutaneous HSV infections in immunocompromised patients (Table 184-1). Intravenous and oral acyclovir also prevents reactivation of HSV in seropositive immunocompromised patients during induction chemotherapy for acute leukemia or in the period immediately following bone marrow

Mucocutaneous HSV infections

Infections in immunosuppressed patients

Acute symptomatic first or recurrent episodes: IV acyclovir (5 mg/kg q 8 h) or oral acyclovir (400 mg qid for 7–10 days) relieves pain and speeds healing. With localized external lesions, 5% topical acyclovir ointment applied 4–6 times daily may be beneficial.

Suppression of reactivation disease: IV acyclovir (5 mg/kg q 8 h) or oral acyclovir (400 mg 3–5 times per day) prevents recurrences during high-risk periods, e.g., the immediate posttransplantation period. In HIV-infected persons, oral famciclovir (500 mg bid) reduces rates of HSV-1 and HSV-2 reactivation.

Genital herpes

First episodes: Oral acyclovir (200 mg 5 times per day or 400 mg tid) is given. Oral valacyclovir (1000 mg bid) or famciclovir (250 mg bid) for 10–14 days is effective. IV acyclovir (5 mg/kg q 8 h for 5 days) is given for severe disease or neurologic complications such as aseptic meningitis.

Symptomatic recurrent genital herpes: Oral acyclovir (200 mg 5 times per day for 5 days), valacyclovir (500 mg bid), or famciclovir (125 mg bid) is effective in shortening lesion duration and viral excretion time.

Suppression of recurrent genital herpes: Oral acyclovir (200-mg capsules bid or tid, 400 mg bid, or 800 mg qd), famciclovir (250 mg bid), or valacyclovir (500 mg bid, or 1000 mg qd) prevents symptomatic reactivation.

Oral-labial HSV infections

First episode: Oral acyclovir (200 mg) is given 4 or 5 times per day.

Recurrent episodes: Topical penciclovir cream is effective in speeding the healing of oral-labial HSV. Topical acyclovir cream is licensed in Europe. The ointment formulation of acyclovir available in the U.S. has no clinical benefit. Oral acyclovir has minimal benefit.

Suppression of reactivation of oral-labial HSV: Oral acyclovir (400 mg bid), if started before exposure and continued for the duration of exposure (usually 5–10 days), will prevent reactivation of recurrent oral-labial HSV infection associated with severe sun exposure.

Herpetic whitlow: Oral acyclovir (200 mg) is given 5 times daily for 7–10 days.

HSV proctitis: Oral acyclovir (400 mg 5 times per day) is useful in shortening the course of infection. In immunosuppressed patients or in patients with severe infection, IV acyclovir (5 mg/kg q 8 h) may be useful.

Herpetic eye infections: In acute keratitis, topical trifluorothymidine, vidarabine, idoxuridine, acyclovir, and interferon are all beneficial. Debridement may be required; topical steroids may worsen disease.

CNS HSV infections

HSV encephalitis: Intravenous acyclovir (10 mg/kg q 8 h; 30 mg/kg per day) for 10 days is preferred.

HSV aseptic meningitis: No studies of systemic antiviral chemotherapy exist. If therapy is to be given IV, acyclovir (15–30 mg/kg per day) should be used.

Autonomic radiculopathy: No studies are available.

Neonatal HSV infections: Acyclovir (45–60 mg/kg per day) is given. Neonates appear to tolerate this high dose of acyclovir. The recommended duration of treatment is 21 days.

Visceral HSV infections

HSV esophagitis: Systemic acyclovir (15 mg/kg per day) should be considered. In some patients with milder forms of immunosuppression, oral therapy with valacyclovir or famciclovir is effective.

HSV pneumonitis: No controlled studies exist. Systemic acyclovir (15 mg/kg per day) should be considered.

Disseminated HSV infections: No controlled studies exist. Intravenous acyclovir nevertheless should be tried. No definite evidence indicates that therapy will decrease the risk of death.

Erythema multiforme associated with HSV: Anecdotal observations suggest that oral acyclovir (400 mg bid or tid) will suppress erythema multiforme.

Infections due to acyclovir-resistant HSV: Foscarnet (40 mg/kg IV q 8 h) should be given until lesions heal. The optimal duration of therapy and the usefulness of its continuation to suppress lesions are unclear. Some patients may benefit from cutaneous application of trifluorothymidine or 5% cidofovir gel. Trials of systemic cidofovir are under way.

transplantation. Famciclovir is currently under study and is also likely to be effective.

Oral acyclovir, famciclovir, and valacyclovir have been shown to speed the healing and resolution of symptoms in first and recurrent episodes of genital HSV-1 and HSV-2 infections. Chronic daily

suppressive therapy reduces the frequency of reactivation disease among patients with frequent genital herpes.

Intravenous acyclovir (30 mg/kg per day, given as a 10 mg/kg infusion over 1 h at 8-h intervals) is effective in reducing the rates of death and morbidity from HSV encephalitis. Early initiation of therapy is a critical factor in outcome. The major side effect associated with intravenous acyclovir is transient renal insufficiency, usually due to crystallization of the compound in the renal parenchyma. This adverse reaction can be avoided if the medication is given slowly over 1 h and the patient is well hydrated. Because CSF levels of acyclovir average only 30 to 50 percent of plasma levels, the dosage of acyclovir used for treatment of CNS infection (30 mg/kg per day) is double that used for treatment of mucocutaneous or visceral disease (15 mg/kg per day).

Acyclovir-resistant strains of HSV are being identified with increasing frequency, especially in HIV-infected persons. Almost all clinically significant acyclovir resistance has been seen in immunocompromised patients. Most acyclovir-resistant strains of HSV have an altered substrate specificity for phosphorylating acyclovir. Thus, cross-resistance to famciclovir is usually found. Occasionally, an isolate with altered thymidine kinase (TK) specificity will arise and will be sensitive to famciclovir but not to acyclovir. In some patients infected with TK-deficient virus, higher doses of acyclovir are associated with clearing of lesions. In others, clinical disease progresses despite high-dose therapy. Isolation of HSV from persisting lesions despite adequate dosages and blood levels of acyclovir should raise the suspicion of acyclovir resistance. Therapy with the antiviral drug foscarnet is useful (see Chap. 183). Because of its toxicity and cost, this drug is usually reserved for patients with extensive mucocutaneous infections. Cidofovir is a nucleotide analogue and exists as a phosphonate or monophosphate form. Most TK-deficient strains of HSV are sensitive to cidofovir. Cidofovir ointment has been shown to speed healing of acyclovir-resistant lesions. Clinical trials of systemic cidofovir are under way.

PREVENTION The large reservoir of persons with asymptomatic HSV-1 and HSV-2 infections indicates that the success of efforts to control HSV disease through suppressive antiviral chemotherapy and/or educational programs will be limited. Rather, control of HSV infection will require the prevention of infection—a goal most likely to be attained by vaccination. Several candidate vaccines are under investigation, and the prevention of HSV infection has been assigned a high public health priority.

Barrier forms of contraception, especially condoms, decrease the likelihood of transmission of HSV infection, especially during periods of asymptomatic viral excretion. However, when lesions are present, HSV infection may be transmitted by skin-to-skin contact despite the use of a condom. Nevertheless, the available data suggest that consistent condom use is an effective means of reducing the risk of genital HSV-2 transmission. Prevention of neonatal HSV requires the prevention of acquisition of HSV in the third trimester of pregnancy.

BIBLIOGRAPHY

ASHLEY R et al: Inability of enzyme immunoassays to accurately discriminate between infections with herpes simplex virus types 1 and 2. Ann Intern Med 115:520, 1991

BENEDETTI J et al: Recurrence rates in genital herpes after symptomatic first episode infection. Ann Intern Med 121:847, 1994

BROWN ZA et al: Neonatal herpes simplex virus infection in relation to asymptomatic maternal infection at the time of labor. N Engl J Med 324:1247, 1991

COREY L, SPEAR P: Infections with herpes simplex viruses. N Engl J Med 314:686, 1986

ERLICH KS et al: Acyclovir-resistant herpes simplex virus infections in patients with the acquired immunodeficiency syndrome. N Engl J Med 320:293, 1989

HOOK EW et al: Herpes simplex virus infection as a risk factor for human immunodeficiency virus infection in heterosexuals. J Infect Dis 165:251, 1992

LALEZARI JP et al: Treatment with intravenous (S)-1-[3-hydroxy-2-(phosphonylmethoxy)propyl]-cytosine of acyclovir-resistant mucocutaneous infection with herpes simplex virus in a patient with AIDS. J Infect Dis 170:570, 1994

MERTZ GJ et al: Risk factors for the sexual transmission of genital herpes. Ann Intern Med 116:197, 1992

OLIVER L et al: Seroprevalence of herpes simplex virus infections in a family medicine clinic. Arch Fam Med 4:228, 1995

PERRY CM, WAGSTAFF AJ: Famciclovir. A review of its pharmacological properties and therapeutic efficacy in herpesvirus infections. Drugs 50:396, 1995

SAFRIN S et al: A controlled trial comparing foscarnet with vidarabine for acyclovir-resistant mucocutaneous herpes simplex in the acquired immunodeficiency syndrome. N Engl J Med 325:551, 1991

STEWART JA et al: Herpesvirus infections in persons infected with human immunodeficiency virus. Clin Infect Dis 21(Suppl 1):S114, 1995

STONE KM, WHITTINGTON WL: Treatment of genital herpes. Rev Infect Dis 12:S610, 1990

TEDDER DG et al: Herpes simplex virus infection as a cause of benign recurrent lymphocytic meningitis. Ann Intern Med 121:334, 1994

WALD A et al: Suppression of subclinical shedding of herpes simplex virus type 2 with acyclovir. Ann Intern Med 124:8, 1996

WHITLEY RJ, GNANN JW JR: Acyclovir: A decade later. N Engl J Med 327:782, 1992; 328:671, 1993

————, LAKEMAN F: Herpes simplex virus infections of the central nervous system: Therapeutic and diagnostic considerations. Clin Infect Dis 20:414, 1995

---

185   *Richard J. Whitley*

VARICELLA-ZOSTER VIRUS INFECTIONS

DEFINITION Varicella-zoster virus (VZV) causes two distinct clinical entities: varicella, or chickenpox, and herpes zoster, or shingles. Chickenpox, a ubiquitous and extremely contagious infection, is usually a benign illness of childhood characterized by an exanthematous vesicular rash. With reactivation of latent VZV (which is most common after the sixth decade of life), herpes zoster presents as a dermatomal vesicular rash, usually associated with severe pain.

ETIOLOGY A clinical association between varicella and herpes zoster has been recognized for nearly 100 years. Early in the twentieth century, similarities in the histopathologic features of skin lesions resulting from varicella and herpes zoster were demonstrated. Viral isolates from patients with chickenpox and herpes zoster produced similar alterations in tissue culture—specifically, the appearance of eosinophilic intranuclear inclusions and multinucleated giant cells; these results suggested that the viruses were biologically similar. Restriction endonuclease analyses of viral DNA from a patient with chickenpox who subsequently developed herpes zoster verified the molecular identity of the two viruses responsible for these different clinical presentations.

VZV is a member of the herpesvirus family, sharing with other members such structural characteristics as a lipid envelope surrounding a nucleocapsid with icosahedral symmetry, a total diameter of approximately 150 to 200 nm, and centrally located double-stranded DNA with a molecular weight of approximately 80 million.

PATHOGENESIS AND PATHOLOGY **Primary Infection** Transmission is most likely to take place by the respiratory route; the subsequent localized replication of the virus at an undefined site (presumably the nasopharynx) leads to seeding of the reticuloendothelial system and ultimately to the development of viremia. Viremia in patients with chickenpox is reflected in the diffuse and scattered nature of the skin lesions and can be verified in selected cases by the recovery of VZV from the blood. Vesicles involve the corium and dermis, with degenerative changes characterized by ballooning, the presence of multinucleated giant cells, and eosinophilic intranuclear inclusions. Infection may involve localized blood vessels of the skin, resulting in necrosis and epidermal hemorrhage. With the evolution of disease, the vesicular fluid becomes cloudy because of the recruitment of polymorphonuclear leukocytes and the presence of degenerated cells and fibrin. Ultimately, the vesicles either rupture and release their fluid (which includes infectious virus) or are gradually reabsorbed.

Recurrent Infection The mechanism of reactivation of VZV that results in herpes zoster is unknown. It is presumed that the virus infects the dorsal root ganglia during chickenpox, where it remains latent until reactivated. Histopathologic examination of representative dorsal root ganglia during active herpes zoster demonstrates hemorrhage, edema, and lymphocytic infiltration.

Active replication of VZV in other organs, such as the lung or the brain, can occur during either chickenpox or herpes zoster but is uncommon in the immunocompetent host. Pulmonary involvement is characterized by interstitial pneumonitis, multinucleated giant cell formation, intranuclear inclusions, and pulmonary hemorrhage. Central nervous system (CNS) infection leads to histopathologic evidence of perivascular cuffing similar to that encountered in measles and other viral encephalitides. Focal hemorrhagic necrosis of the brain, characteristic of herpes simplex virus encephalitis, is uncommon in VZV infection.

EPIDEMIOLOGY AND CLINICAL MANIFESTATIONS **Chickenpox** Humans are the only known reservoir for VZV. Chickenpox is highly contagious, with an attack rate of at least 90 percent among susceptible (seronegative) individuals. Individuals of both sexes and all races are infected equally often. The virus is endemic in the population at large; however, it becomes epidemic among susceptible individuals during seasonal peaks—namely, late winter and early spring in the temperate zone. Children between the ages of 5 and 9 are most commonly affected and account for 50 percent of all cases. Most other cases involve children aged 1 to 4 and those aged 10 to 14. Approximately 10 percent of the population of the United States over the age of 15 is susceptible to infection.

The incubation period of chickenpox ranges between 10 and 21 days but is usually between 14 and 17 days. Secondary attack rates in susceptible siblings within a household are between 70 and 90 percent. Patients are infectious approximately 48 h prior to the onset of the vesicular rash, during the period of vesicle formation (which generally lasts 4 to 5 days), and until all vesicles are crusted.

Clinically, chickenpox presents as a rash, low-grade fever, and malaise, although a few patients develop a prodrome 1 to 2 days before onset of the exanthem. In the immunocompetent patient, this is usually a benign illness that is associated with lassitude and with body temperatures of 37.8 to 39.4°C (100 to 103°F) of 3 to 5 days' duration. The skin lesions—the hallmark of the infection—include maculopapules, vesicles, and scabs in various stages of evolution. These lesions, which evolve from maculopapules to vesicles over hours to days, appear on the trunk and face and rapidly spread to involve other areas of the body. Most are small and have an erythematous base with a diameter of 5 to 10 mm. Successive crops appear over a 2- to 4-day period. Lesions also can be found on the mucosa of the pharynx and/or the vagina. Their severity varies from one individual to another. Some individuals have very few lesions, while others have as many as 2000. Younger children tend to have fewer vesicles than older individuals. Secondary and tertiary cases within families are associated with a relatively large number of vesicles. Immunocompromised individuals—both children and adults, particularly those with leukemia—have lesions (often with a hemorrhagic base) that are more numerous and take longer to heal than those of immunocompetent patients. Immunocompromised individuals are also at greater risk for visceral complications, which occur in 30 to 50 percent of cases and are fatal 15 percent of the time.

The most common infectious complication of varicella is secondary bacterial superinfection of the skin, which is usually caused by *Streptococcus pyogenes* or *Staphylococcus aureus*. This complication may result from excoriation of skin lesions after scratching. Gram's staining of skin lesions should help clarify the etiology of unusually erythematous and pustulated lesions.

The most common extracutaneous site of involvement in children is the CNS. The syndrome of acute cerebellar ataxia and meningeal irritation generally appears around 21 days after the onset of the rash and rarely develops in the preeruptive phase. The cerebrospinal fluid (CSF) contains lymphocytes and elevated levels of protein. CNS involvement is a benign complication of VZV infection in children and generally does not require hospitalization. Aseptic meningitis, encephalitis, transverse myelitis, Guillain-Barré syndrome, and Reye's syndrome also can occur. Encephalitis is reported in 0.1 to 0.2 percent of children with chickenpox. Other than supportive care, no specific therapy is available for patients with CNS involvement.

Varicella pneumonia is the most serious complication following chickenpox, developing more commonly in adults (up to 20 percent of cases) than in children. It usually has its onset 3 to 5 days into the illness and is associated with tachypnea, cough, dyspnea, and fever. Cyanosis, pleuritic chest pain, and hemoptysis are frequent. Roentgenographic evidence of disease consists of nodular infiltrates and interstitial pneumonitis. Resolution of pneumonitis parallels improvement of the skin rash; however, patients may have persistent fever and compromised pulmonary function for weeks.

Other complications of chickenpox include myocarditis, corneal lesions, nephritis, arthritis, bleeding diatheses, acute glomerulonephritis, and hepatitis. Hepatic involvement, distinct from Reye's syndrome and usually asymptomatic, is common in chickenpox and is usually characterized by elevated levels of liver enzymes, particularly aspartate and alanine aminotransferases.

Perinatal varicella is associated with a high mortality rate when maternal disease develops within 5 days before delivery or within 48 h thereafter. Because the newborn does not receive protective transplacental antibodies and has an immature immune system, the illness may be unusually severe. The reported mortality rate has been as high as 30 percent in this group. Congenital varicella, with clinical manifestations of limb hypoplasia, cicatricial skin lesions, and microcephaly at birth, is extremely uncommon.

Herpes Zoster   Herpes zoster, a sporadic disease, is the consequence of reactivation of latent VZV from the dorsal root ganglia. Most patients have no history of recent exposure to other individuals with VZV infection. Herpes zoster occurs at all ages, but its incidence is highest (5 to 10 cases per 1000 persons) among individuals in the sixth through the eighth decades of life. It has been suggested that approximately 2 percent of patients with herpes zoster will develop a second episode of infection.

Herpes zoster, also called shingles, is characterized by a unilateral vesicular eruption within a dermatome, often associated with severe pain. The dermatomes from T3 to L3 are most frequently involved. If the ophthalmic branch of the trigeminal nerve is involved, zoster ophthalmicus results. The factors responsible for the reactivation of VZV are not known. In children reactivation is usually benign, whereas in adults it can be debilitating. The continuum of pain from onset to resolution is known as *zoster-associated pain*. The onset of disease is heralded by pain within the dermatome that may precede lesions by 48 to 72 h; an erythematous maculopapular rash evolves rapidly into vesicular lesions. In the normal host, these lesions may remain few in number and continue to form only for a period of 3 to 5 days. The total duration of disease is generally between 7 and 10 days; however, it may take as long as 2 to 4 weeks for the skin to return to normal. In a few patients, characteristic localization of pain to a dermatome with serologic evidence of herpes zoster has been reported in the absence of skin lesions. When branches of the trigeminal nerve are involved, lesions may appear on the face, in the mouth, in the eye, or on the tongue. In Ramsay Hunt syndrome, pain and vesicles appear in the external auditory canal, and patients lose their sense of taste in the anterior two-thirds of the tongue while developing ipsilateral facial palsy. The geniculate ganglion of the sensory branch of the facial nerve is involved.

The most debilitating complication of herpes zoster, in both the normal and the immunocompromised host, is pain associated with

acute neuritis and postherpetic neuralgia. Postherpetic neuralgia is uncommon in young individuals; however, at least 50 percent of patients over age 50 with zoster report some degree of pain in the involved dermatome months after the resolution of cutaneous disease. Changes in sensation in the dermatome, resulting in either hypo- or hyperesthesia, are common.

CNS involvement may follow localized herpes zoster. Many patients without signs of meningeal irritation have CSF pleocytosis and moderately elevated levels of CSF protein. Symptomatic meningoencephalitis is characterized by headache, fever, photophobia, meningitis, and vomiting. A rare manifestation of CNS involvement is granulomatous angiitis with contralateral hemiplegia, which can be diagnosed by cerebral arteriography. Other neurologic manifestations include transverse myelitis with or without motor paralysis.

Like chickenpox, herpes zoster is more severe in the immunocompromised host than in the normal individual. Lesions continue to form for over a week, and scabbing is not complete in most cases until 3 weeks into the illness. Patients with Hodgkin's disease and non-Hodgkin's lymphoma are at greatest risk for progressive herpes zoster. Cutaneous dissemination develops in about 40 percent of these patients. Among patients with cutaneous dissemination, the risk of pneumonitis, meningoencephalitis, hepatitis, and other serious complications is increased by 5 to 10 percent. However, even in immunocompromised patients, disseminated zoster is rarely fatal.

Patients who have received a bone marrow transplant are at particularly high risk of VZV infection. Thirty percent of cases of posttransplantation VZV infection occur within 1 year (50 percent of these within 9 months); 45 percent of the patients involved have cutaneous or visceral dissemination. The mortality rate in this situation is 10 percent. Postherpetic neuralgia, scarring, and bacterial superinfection are especially frequent in VZV infections occurring within 9 months of transplantation. Among infected patients, concomitant graft-versus-host disease increases the chance of dissemination and/or death.

DIFFERENTIAL DIAGNOSIS   The diagnosis of chickenpox is not difficult. The characteristic rash and a history of recent exposure should lead to a prompt diagnosis. Other viral infections that can mimic chickenpox include disseminated herpes simplex virus infection in patients with atopic dermatitis and the disseminated vesiculopapular lesions sometimes associated with coxsackievirus infection, echovirus infection, or atypical measles. However, these rashes are more commonly morbilliform with a hemorrhagic component rather than vesicular or vesiculopustular. Rickettsialpox can be confused with chickenpox; however, it can be distinguished easily by detection of the "herald spot" at the site of the mite bite and the development of a more pronounced headache. Serologic testing is useful in differentiating rickettsialpox from varicella.

Unilateral vesicular lesions in a dermatomal pattern should lead rapidly to the diagnosis of herpes zoster, although the occurrence of shingles without a rash has been reported. Both herpes simplex virus infections and coxsackievirus infections can cause dermatomal vesicular lesions. Supportive diagnostic virology and fluorescent staining of skin scrapings with monoclonal antibodies are helpful in ensuring the proper diagnosis. In the prodromal stage of herpes zoster, the diagnosis can be exceedingly difficult and may be made only after lesions have appeared or by retrospective serologic assessment.

LABORATORY FINDINGS   Unequivocal confirmation of the diagnosis is possible only through the isolation of VZV in susceptible tissue-culture cell lines, by the demonstration of seroconversion, or by the demonstration of a fourfold or greater rise in antibody titer between convalescent- and acute-phase serum specimens. A rapid impression can be obtained by a Tzanck smear, with scraping of the base of the lesions in an attempt to demonstrate multinucleated giant cells, although the sensitivity of this method is low. Polymerase chain reaction technology for the detection of viral DNA in vesicular fluid is available in some diagnostic laboratories. Direct immunofluorescent staining of cells from the lesion base or detection of viral antigens by other assays (such as the immunoperoxidase assay) is also useful, although these tests are not commercially available. The most frequently employed serologic tools for assessing host response are the immunofluorescent detection of antibodies to VZV membrane antigens, the fluorescent antibody to membrane antigen (FAMA) test, immune adherence hemagglutination, and enzyme-linked immunosorbent assay (ELISA). The FAMA test and the ELISA appear to be the most sensitive.

PROPHYLAXIS While chickenpox in the otherwise healthy host is relatively benign, it can cause morbidity and death. Furthermore, the parents of a child with chickenpox often lose a significant amount of time from work. Recently, a live attenuated varicella vaccine was licensed for administration to all immunocompetent children.

The immunocompromised individual is at significant risk for developing progressive varicella; modalities of prevention include passive immunization or experimental administration of the same live attenuated vaccine used in the immunocompetent child. Immune prophylaxis can consist of the administration of specific zoster immune globulin (ZIG) derived from patients with herpes zoster, varicella-zoster immune globulin (VZIG), or the intravenous formulation of zoster immune plasma (ZIP). Both ZIG and VZIG should be given within 96 h (preferably within 72 h) of exposure to ensure efficacy. It is likely that ZIP can be given somewhat later. Indications for the administration of VZIG are summarized in Table 185-1.

Clinical trials in Japan and the United States have demonstrated the efficacy of live attenuated VZV vaccine (OKA) in both immunocompetent and immunocompromised hosts. This live attenuated vaccine may be licensed in the United States in the near future.

℞ TREATMENT

Medical management of chickenpox in the immunologically normal host is directed toward the prevention of avoidable complications. Obviously, good hygiene includes daily bathing and soaks. Secondary bacterial infection of the skin can be avoided by meticulous skin care, particularly with close cropping of fingernails. Pruritus can be decreased with topical dressings or the administration of antipruritic drugs. Tepid water baths and wet compresses are better than drying lotions for the relief of itching. Aluminum acetate soaks for the management of herpes zoster can be both soothing and cleansing. Administration of aspirin to children with chickenpox should be avoided because of the association of aspirin derivatives with the development of Reye's syndrome. Acyclovir therapy (800 mg by mouth five times daily for 5 to 7 days) is recommended for adoles-cents and adults with chickenpox of ≤24 h duration. Acyclovir therapy for children <12 years of age may likewise be of benefit if initiated early in the disease (<24 h) at a dose of 20 mg/kg every 6 h.

Patients with herpes zoster benefit from oral acyclovir therapy, as evidenced by accelerated healing of lesions and resolution of zoster-associated pain. The dosage is 800 mg/d for 7 to 10 days. Recently, two new drugs have been licensed for the treatment of herpes zoster (see Chap. 183). Famciclovir, the prodrug of penciclovir, is at least as effective as acyclovir and perhaps more so. One recent study showed twofold faster resolution of postherpetic neuralgia in famciclovir-treated patients with zoster than in recipients of placebo. The dose is 500 mg by mouth three times daily for 7 to 10 days. Valacyclovir, the prodrug of acyclovir, accelerates healing and resolution of zoster-associated pain more promptly than acyclovir. The dose is 1 g by mouth three times daily for 7 to 10 days. Both of these new drugs offer the advantage of a lower dosing frequency.

Both chickenpox and herpes zoster in the immunocompromised host should be treated with intravenous acyclovir, which reduces the occurrence of visceral complications but has no effect on healing of skin lesions or pain. The dose is 10 to 12.5 mg/kg every 8 h for 7 days. These treatment recommendations apply to immunocompromised patients with disseminated herpes zoster as well. Oral acyclovir therapy is not recommended for the treatment of VZV infections in immunocompromised patients. Concomitant with the administration of intravenous acyclovir, it is desirable to attempt to wean these patients from immunosuppressive treatment.

Patients with varicella pneumonia may require removal of bronchial secretions and ventilatory support. Persons with zoster ophthalmicus should be referred immediately to an ophthalmologist. Therapy for this condition consists of the administration of analgesics for severe pain and the use of atropine. Acyclovir will accelerate healing.

The management of acute neuritis and/or postherpetic neuralgia can be particularly difficult. In addition to the judicious use of analgesics, ranging from nonnarcotics to narcotic derivatives, drugs such as amitriptyline hydrochloride and fluphenazine hydrochloride have been reported to be beneficial for pain relief. In one study, glucocorticoid therapy administered early in the course of localized herpes zoster significantly accelerated such quality-of-life improvements as a return to usual activity and termination of analgesia. The dose of prednisone administered orally was 60 mg/d on days 1 through 7, 30 mg/d on days 8 through 14, and 15 mg/d on days 15 through 21. This regimen is appropriate only for relatively healthy elderly persons who have moderate or severe pain. Patients with osteoporosis, diabetes mellitus, glycosuria, or hypertension may not be appropriate candidates. Glucocorticoids should not be used without concomitant antiviral therapy.

Table 185-1

Recommendations for VZIG Administration

Exposure criteria
  A. Both exposure to person with chickenpox or zoster as:
    1. Continuous household contact
    2. Playmate for >1 h indoors
    3. Hospital contact (same room or prolonged face-to-face)
    4. Mother (see C below)
  B. And time elapsed ≤96 h (preferably ≤72 h)

Candidates (provided they have significant exposure) include
  A. Immunocompromised susceptible children
  B. Immunocompetent susceptible adolescents (≥15 years old) and adults, especially pregnant women
  C. Newborn infants of mothers with onset of chickenpox <5 days before or <2 days after delivery
  D. Hospitalized premature infants
    1. ≥28 weeks of gestation when mother has no history of chickenpox
    2. <28 weeks of gestation and/or birth weight of ≤1000 g, regardless of maternal history

SOURCE: Adapted from American Academy of Pediatrics, in Red Book, Report of the Committee on Infectious Diseases, G Peter (ed), Elk Grove Village, IL, American Academy of Pediatrics, 1994.

BIBLIOGRAPHY

BALFOUR HH JR et al: Acyclovir treatment of varicella in otherwise healthy adolescents. J Pediatr 120:627, 1992

BEUTNER KR et al: Valacyclovir compared with acyclovir for improved therapy for herpes zoster in immunocompetent adults. Antimicrob Agents Chemother 39:1547, 1995

BRUNELL PA et al: Prevention of varicella by zoster immune globulin. N Engl J Med 280:1191, 1969

DUNKLE LM et al: A controlled trial of acyclovir for chickenpox in normal children. N Engl J Med 325:1539, 1991

ESSMAN V et al: Prednisone does not prevent postherpetic neuralgia. Lancet 2:126, 1987

GERSHON AA et al: Live attenuated varicella vaccine. JAMA 252:355, 1984

HOPE-SIMPSON RE: The nature of herpes zoster: A long-term study and a new hypothesis. Proc R Soc Med 58:9, 1965

LOCKSLEY RM et al: Infection with varicella-zoster virus after marrow transplantation. J Infect Dis 152:1172, 1985

PROBER CG et al: Acyclovir therapy of chickenpox in immunosuppressed children—a collaborative study. J Pediatr 101:622, 1982

SHEPP D et al: Treatment of varicella-zoster virus in severely immunocompromised patients: A randomized comparison of acyclovir and vidarabine. N Engl J Med 314:208, 1987

TYRING S et al: Famciclovir for the treatment of acute herpes zoster. Effects on acute disease and postherpetic neuralgia: A randomized, double-blind, placebo-controlled trial. Ann Intern Med 123:89, 1995

WEIBEL RE et al: Live attenuated varicella virus vaccine: Efficacy trial in healthy children. N Engl J Med 310:1409, 1984

WELLER TH: Varicella and herpes zoster: Changing concepts of the natural history, control, and importance of a not-so-benign virus. N Engl J Med 309:1362, 1983

WHITLEY RJ et al: Early vidarabine therapy to control the complications of herpes zoster in immunosuppressed patients. N Engl J Med 307:971, 1982

——— et al: Vidarabine therapy of varicella in immunosuppressed patients. J Pediatr 1:125, 1982

——— et al: Varicella-zoster virus infections, in Antiviral Agents and Viral Diseases of Man, GJ Galasso et al (eds). New York, Raven, 1984, vol 2, pp 517–542

——— et al: Disseminated herpes zoster in the immunocompromised host: A comparative trial of acyclovir and vidarabine. J Infect Dis 165:450, 1992

——— et al: Acyclovir with and without prednisone for the treatment of herpes zoster: A randomized, placebo-controlled trial. Ann Intern Med 125:376, 1996

WOOD MJ et al: A randomized trial of acyclovir for 7 days or 21 days with and without prednisolone for treatment of acute herpes zoster. N Engl J Med 330:896, 1994

ZAIA JA et al: Evaluation of varicella-zoster immune globulin: Protection of immunosuppressed children after household exposure to varicella. J Infect Dis 147:737, 1983

186 *Jeffrey I. Cohen*

EPSTEIN-BARR VIRUS INFECTIONS, INCLUDING INFECTIOUS MONONUCLEOSIS

DEFINITION Epstein-Barr virus (EBV) is the cause of heterophile-positive infectious mononucleosis (IM), which is characterized by fever, sore throat, lymphadenopathy, and atypical lymphocytosis. EBV is also associated with several human tumors, including nasopharyngeal carcinoma, Burkitt's lymphoma, Hodgkin's disease, and—in patients with immunodeficiencies (including AIDS)—B-cell lymphoma. The virus, initially discovered in Burkitt's lymphoma cells, is a member of the family Herpesviridae. The viral genome consists of a linear, double-stranded DNA core surrounded by an icosahedral nucleocapsid and by the viral envelope, which contains glycoproteins. The two types of EBV that are widely prevalent in nature are not distinguished by conventional serologic tests.

EPIDEMIOLOGY EBV infections occur worldwide. These infections are most common in early childhood, with a second peak during late adolescence. By adulthood, more than 90 percent of individuals have been infected and have antibodies to the virus. IM is usually a disease of young adults. In lower socioeconomic groups and in areas of the world with lower standards of hygiene (e.g., developing countries), EBV tends to infect children at an early age, and symptomatic IM is uncommon. In areas with higher standards of hygiene (e.g., the United States), infection with EBV is often delayed until adulthood, and IM is more prevalent.

EBV is spread by contact with oral secretions. The virus is frequently transmitted from adults to infants and among young adults by transfer of saliva during kissing. Transmission by less intimate contact is rare. EBV has been transmitted by blood transfusion and by bone marrow transplantation. While earlier studies suggested that 20 percent of asymptomatic seropositive individuals shed the virus in oropharyngeal secretions, more sensitive studies suggest a figure of more than 90 percent, with up to one-fourth of seropositive persons secreting virus on most days. Rates of virus shedding are especially high among patients with IM and among immunosuppressed patients.

PATHOGENESIS EBV is transmitted by salivary secretions, usually from asymptomatic persons shedding the virus. The virus infects the epithelium of the oropharynx and the salivary glands and is shed from these cells. While B cells may become infected after contact with epithelial cells, recent studies suggest that lymphocytes in the tonsillar crypts can be infected directly. The virus then spreads through the bloodstream and disseminates throughout the body. The proliferation and expansion of EBV-infected B cells along with reactive T cells during IM result in enlargement of lymphoid tissue. During the acute phase of IM, about 1 in every 1000 B cells in the peripheral blood is infected by EBV, while after recovery, about 1 in every million B cells is infected. Recent data suggest that the B cell, not the epithelial cell, is the reservoir for EBV in the body: Shedding of EBV from the oropharynx stops but the virus persists in B cells when patients are treated with acyclovir.

The EBV receptor (CD21), present on the surface of B cells and epithelial cells, is also the receptor for the C3d component of complement. EBV infection of epithelial cells results in replication of the virus, with the production of virions. When B cells are infected by EBV in vitro, they become transformed and can proliferate indefinitely. During latent infection of B cells, only the EBV nuclear antigens (EBNAs), latent membrane proteins, and small EBV RNAs are expressed in vitro. EBV-transformed B cells secrete immunoglobulin; only a small fraction of cells produce virus.

Acute infection with EBV is accompanied by polyclonal activation of B cells, and antibodies are made to both host-cell and viral proteins. During the first week of infection, the number of T cells increases. Moreover, the percentage of CD4+ T cells decreases, while the percentage of CD8+ T cells increases; the result is an inverted CD4+/CD8+ ratio. Cellular immunity is more important than humoral immunity in controlling EBV infection. In the initial phase of infection, suppressor T cells, natural killer cells, and nonspecific cytotoxic T cells are important in controlling the proliferation of EBV-infected B cells. Levels of markers of T-cell activation and serum interferon γ are elevated. Later in infection, HLA-restricted cytotoxic T cells that can recognize EBNAs and latent membrane proteins and can destroy EBV-infected cells are generated. Recent studies have shown that one of the late genes expressed during EBV replication, *BCRF1*, exhibits a high degree of amino acid homology with interleukin 10 and can inhibit the production of interferon γ by mononuclear cells in vitro.

If T-cell immunity is compromised, EBV-infected B cells may begin to proliferate. When EBV is associated with lymphoma, its mechanisms of B-cell stimulation are diverse and, in general, EBV-induced proliferation is one step in a multistep process of neoplastic transformation.

CLINICAL MANIFESTATIONS Most EBV infections in infants and young children either are asymptomatic or present as mild pharyngitis with or without tonsillitis. In contrast, up to 75 percent of infections in adolescents present as IM.

Signs and Symptoms The incubation period for IM in young adults is about 4 to 6 weeks. A prodrome of fatigue, malaise, and myalgia may last for 1 to 2 weeks before the onset of fever, sore throat, and lymphadenopathy. Fever is usually low-grade and is most common in the first 2 weeks of the illness; however, it may persist for over a month. Common signs and symptoms are listed along with their frequencies in Table 186-1. Lymphadenopathy and pharyngitis are most prominent during the first 2 weeks of the illness, while splenomegaly is more prominent during the second and third weeks. Lymphadenopathy most often affects the posterior cervical nodes but may be generalized. Enlarged lymph nodes are frequently tender and symmetrical but are not fixed in place. Pharyngitis, often the most prominent sign, can be accompanied by enlargement of the tonsils with an exudate resembling that of streptococcal pharyngitis. A morbilliform or papular rash, usually on the arms or trunk, develops in about 5 percent of cases. Most patients treated with ampicillin develop a macular rash; this rash is not predictive of future adverse reactions to penicillins. Erythema nodosum and erythema multiforme have also been described (see Chap. 57). Most patients have symptoms for 2 to 4 weeks, but malaise and difficulty concentrating can persist for months.

Symptomatic IM is uncommon in infants and young children. IM in the elderly presents relatively often as nonspecific symptoms, including prolonged fever, fatigue, myalgia, and malaise; in contrast,

Table 186-1

Signs and Symptoms of Infectious Mononucleosis

Manifestation	Median Percentage of Patients (Range)
SYMPTOMS	
Sore throat	75 (50–87)
Malaise	47 (42–76)
Headache	38 (22–67)
Abdominal pain, nausea, or vomiting	17 (5–25)
Chills	10 (9–11)
SIGNS	
Lymphadenopathy	95 (83–100)
Fever	93 (60–100)
Pharyngitis or tonsillitis	82 (68–90)
Splenomegaly	51 (43–64)
Hepatomegaly	11 (6–15)
Rash	10 (0–25)
Periorbital edema	13 (2–34)
Palatal enanthem	7 (3–13)
Jaundice	5 (2–10)

pharyngitis, lymphadenopathy, splenomegaly, and atypical lymphocytes are relatively rare in elderly patients.

Laboratory Findings The white blood cell count is usually elevated and peaks at 10,000 to 20,000/µL during the second or third week of illness. Lymphocytosis is usually demonstrable, with more than 10 percent atypical lymphocytes. The latter cells are enlarged lymphocytes that have abundant cytoplasm, vacuoles, and indentations of the cell membrane. CD8 + cells predominate among the atypical lymphocytes. Low-grade neutropenia and thrombocytopenia are common during the first month of illness. Liver function is abnormal in more than 90 percent of cases. Serum levels of aminotransferases and alkaline phosphatase are usually mildly elevated; the serum concentration of bilirubin is elevated in about 40 percent of cases.

Complications Most cases of IM are self-limited. Deaths are very rare and most often are due to central nervous system (CNS) complications, splenic rupture, upper airway obstruction, or bacterial superinfection.

CNS complications usually develop during the first 2 weeks of EBV infection; in some patients, especially children, they are the only clinical manifestations of IM. Heterophile antibodies and atypical lymphocytes may be absent. Meningitis and encephalitis are the most common neurologic abnormalities, and patients may present with headache, meningismus, or cerebellar ataxia; acute hemiplegia and psychosis have also been described. The cerebrospinal fluid (CSF) contains mainly lymphocytes, with occasional atypical lymphocytes. Most cases resolve without neurologic sequelae. Acute EBV infection has also been associated with cranial nerve palsies (especially ones involving cranial nerve VII), Guillain-Barré syndrome, acute transverse myelitis, and peripheral neuritis.

Autoimmune hemolytic anemia occurs in about 2 percent of cases during the first 2 weeks. In most cases the anemia is Coombs'-test positive, with cold agglutinins directed against the i red blood cell antigen. Most patients with hemolysis have mild anemia that lasts for 1 or 2 months, but some patients have severe disease with hemoglobinuria and jaundice. Nonspecific antibody responses may also include rheumatoid factor, antinuclear antibodies, anti-smooth muscle antibodies, antiplatelet antibodies, and cryoglobulins. IM has been associated with red-cell aplasia, severe granulocytopenia, pancytopenia, and hemophagocytic syndrome. The spleen ruptures in fewer than 0.5 percent of cases. Splenic rupture is more common among males than among females and may be manifest as abdominal pain, referred shoulder pain, or hemodynamic compromise.

Hypertrophy of lymphoid tissue in the tonsils or adenoids can result in upper airway obstruction, as can inflammation and edema of the epiglottis, pharynx, or uvula. About 10 percent of patients with IM develop streptococcal pharyngitis after their initial sore throat resolves.

Other rare complications associated with acute EBV infection include hepatitis (which can be fulminant), myocarditis or pericarditis with electrocardiographic changes, pneumonia with pleural effusion, interstitial nephritis, and vasculitis.

OTHER DISEASES ASSOCIATED WITH EBV INFECTION EBV-associated lymphoproliferative disease has been described in patients with congenital or acquired immunodeficiency, including those with ataxia-telangiectasia, severe combined immunodeficiency, or AIDS; recipients of bone marrow transplants; and recipients of organ transplants who are receiving immunosuppressive drugs (especially cyclosporine). Proliferating EBV-infected B cells infiltrate lymph nodes and multiple organs, and patients present with fever and lymphadenopathy or gastrointestinal symptoms. Pathologic studies show B-cell hyperplasia or poly- or monoclonal lymphoma. The X-linked lymphoproliferative syndrome (Duncan's disease) is a recessive disorder of young boys who have a normal response to childhood infections but develop fatal lymphoproliferative disorders after infection with EBV. Most patients with this syndrome die of acute IM; others develop hypogammaglobulinemia, malignant B-cell lymphomas, aplastic anemia, or agranulocytosis. IM has also proved fatal to some patients with no obvious preexisting immune abnormality.

Oral hairy leukoplakia is an early manifestation of infection with human immunodeficiency virus (HIV) in adults (see Chap. 308). Most patients present with raised, white corrugated lesions on the tongue (and occasionally on the buccal mucosa) that contain EBV DNA. Children infected with HIV can develop lymphoid interstitial pneumonitis; EBV DNA is often found in lung tissue from these patients.

Patients with the chronic fatigue syndrome may have titers of antibody to EBV that are elevated but are not significantly different from those in healthy EBV-seropositive adults. While some patients have malaise and fatigue that persists for weeks or months after IM, persistent EBV infection is not a cause of the chronic fatigue syndrome. Chronic active EBV infection is very rare and is distinct from the chronic fatigue syndrome. The affected patients have an illness lasting more than 6 months with markedly elevated titers of antibody to EBV and evidence of organ involvement, including hepatosplenomegaly, lymphadenopathy, and pneumonitis, uveitis, or neurologic disease.

EBV is associated with several malignancies. About 15 percent of cases of Burkitt's lymphoma in the United States and about 90 percent of those in Africa are associated with EBV (see Chap. 113). African patients with Burkitt's lymphoma have high levels of antibody to EBV, and their tumor tissue usually contains viral DNA. Anaplastic nasopharyngeal carcinoma is uniformly associated with EBV; the affected tissues contain viral DNA and antigens. Patients with nasopharyngeal carcinoma often have elevated titers of antibody to EBV (see Chap. 89).

EBV has been associated with Hodgkin's disease, especially the mixed-cellularity type (see Chap. 113). Patients with Hodgkin's disease often have elevated titers of antibody to EBV, and in about half of cases viral DNA and antigens are found in Reed-Sternberg cells. In some cases, EBV DNA has been detected in tonsillar carcinoma, angioimmunoblastic lymphadenopathy, angiocentric immunoproliferative lesions, T-cell lymphoma, thymoma, gastric carcinoma, and CNS lymphoma tissues from patients with no underlying immunodeficiency. Recent studies have demonstrated viral DNA in leiomyosarcomas from AIDS patients and in smooth muscle tumors from organ transplant recipients. Virtually all CNS lymphomas in AIDS patients are associated with EBV.

DIAGNOSIS **Serologic Testing** The heterophile test is used for the diagnosis of IM in children and adults (Table 186-2). Heterophile antibody is an IgM antibody that does not bind EBV proteins. In the test for this antibody, human serum is absorbed with guinea pig kidney, and the heterophile titer is defined as the greatest serum dilution that agglutinates sheep, horse, or cow erythrocytes. A titer of 40-fold or greater is diagnostic of acute EBV infection in a patient who has symptoms compatible with IM and atypical lymphocytes. Tests for heterophile antibodies are positive in 40 percent of patients with IM during the first week of illness and in 80 to 90 percent during the third week. Therefore, repeated testing may be necessary, especially if the initial test is performed early. Tests usually remain positive for 3 months after the onset of illness, but heterophile antibodies can persist for up to 1 year. These antibodies usually are not detectable in children less than 5 years of age, in the elderly, or in patients presenting with symptoms not typical of IM. The commercially available monospot test for heterophile antibodies is somewhat more sensitive than the classic heterophile test. False-positive results in the monospot test are more common in children and in patients with other viral infections.

EBV-specific antibody testing is used for patients with suspected acute EBV infection who lack heterophile antibodies and for patients with atypical infections. Serologic tests are particularly useful in young children, who often do not develop heterophile antibodies. Titers of IgM and IgG antibodies to viral capsid antigen (VCA) are elevated in the serum of more than 90 percent of patients at the onset of disease. IgM antibody to VCA is useful for the diagnosis of acute IM because it is present at elevated titers only during the first 2 months of the disease; in contrast, IgG antibody to VCA is often used to assess exposure to EBV in the past because it persists for life.

Antibodies to early antigens (EAs) are found either in a diffuse pattern in the nucleus and cytoplasm of infected cells (EA-D antibody) or restricted to the cytoplasm (EA-R antibody). These antibodies are detectable 3 to 4 weeks after the onset of symptoms in patients with IM. About 70 percent of individuals with IM, especially those with relatively severe disease, have EA-D antibodies during the course of their illness. These antibodies usually persist for only 3 to 6 months. Levels of EA-D antibodies are also elevated in patients with nasopharyngeal carcinoma or chronic active EBV infection. EA-R antibodies are only occasionally detected in patients with IM but are often found at elevated titers in patients with African Burkitt's lymphoma or chronic active EBV infection.

IgA antibodies to EBV antigens have proved useful for the identification of patients with nasopharyngeal carcinoma and of persons at high risk for the disease. Seroconversion to EBNA positivity is also useful for the diagnosis of acute infection with EBV. Antibodies to EBNA are detectable relatively late (3 to 6 weeks after the onset of symptoms) in nearly all cases of acute EBV infection and persist for the lifetime of the patient. These antibodies may be lacking in immunodeficient patients and in those with chronic active EBV infection.

Other Studies Detection of EBV DNA, RNA, or proteins has been valuable in demonstrating the association of the virus with various malignancies. The polymerase chain reaction has been used to detect EBV DNA in the CSF of some AIDS patients with lymphomas and to monitor the amount of EBV DNA in the blood of patients with lymphoproliferative disease. Culture of EBV from throat washings or blood is not helpful in the diagnosis of acute infection, since EBV commonly persists in the oropharynx and in B cells for the lifetime of the infected individual.

Differential Diagnosis The differential diagnosis of IM and atypical lymphocytosis includes acute infection with cytomegalovirus, *Toxoplasma*, HIV, human herpesvirus 6, and hepatitis virus as well as drug hypersensitivity reactions. Cytomegalovirus is the most common cause of heterophile-negative mononucleosis, usually involves older patients, and is associated with a lower frequency of sore throat, splenomegaly, and lymphadenopathy than IM due to EBV. Other diseases that share some of the features of IM include rubella, acute infectious lymphocytosis in children, and lymphoma or leukemia.

Table 186-2

Serologic Features of EBV-Associated Diseases

| | | Result in Indicated Test* | | | | |
| | | Anti-VCA | | Anti-EA | | |
Condition	Heterophile	IgM	IgG	EA-D	EA-R	Anti-EBNA
Acute infectious mononucleosis	+	+	+ +	+	−	−
Convalescence	±	−	+	−	±	+
Past infection	−	−	+	−	−	+
Reactivation with immunodeficiency	−	−	+ +	+	+	±
Burkitt's lymphoma	−	−	+ + +	±	+ +	+
Nasopharyngeal carcinoma	−	−	+ + +	+ +	±	+

* VCA, viral capsid antigen; EA, early antigen; EA-D antibody, antibody to early antigen, diffuse pattern in nucleus and cytoplasm of infected cells; EA-R antibody, antibody to early antigen, restricted to the cytoplasm; and EBNA, Epstein-Barr nuclear antigen.

SOURCE: Adapted from Okano.

℞ TREATMENT

Therapy for IM consists of supportive measures, with rest and analgesia. Excessive physical activity during the first month should be avoided to reduce the possibility of splenic rupture. If splenic rupture occurs, splenectomy is required. Glucocorticoid therapy is not indicated for uncomplicated IM and in fact may predispose to bacterial superinfection. Prednisone (40 to 60 mg/d for 2 to 3 days, with subsequent tapering of the dose over 1 to 2 weeks) have been used for the prevention of airway obstruction in patients with severe tonsillar hypertrophy, for autoimmune hemolytic anemia, and for severe thrombocytopenia. These agents have also been used in a few selected patients with severe malaise and fever and in patients with severe CNS or cardiac disease.

Acyclovir has had no significant clinical impact on IM in controlled trials. However, at a dosage of 400 to 800 mg five times daily, it has been effective for the treatment of oral hairy leukoplakia (despite common relapses) and some cases of chronic active EBV disease. Acyclovir generally has not been beneficial for patients with lymphoproliferative syndromes. When possible, therapy for EBV lymphoproliferative disease should be directed toward the reduction of immunosuppressive medication. New therapies, including the use of interferon α and the infusion of donor T cells or EBV-specific cytotoxic T cells, are being studied.

The isolation of patients with IM is unnecessary. Vaccines directed against the major EBV glycoprotein have been effective in animal studies and are currently undergoing small-scale clinical trials.

BIBLIOGRAPHY

COHEN JI: Epstein-Barr virus lymphoproliferative disease associated with acquired immunodeficiency. Medicine 70:137, 1991

HESLOP HE et al: Long-term restoration of immunity against Epstein-Barr virus infection by adoptive transfer of gene-modified virus-specific T lymphocytes. Nat Med 2:551, 1996

KHANNA R et al: Immune regulation in Epstein-Barr virus-associated diseases. Microbiol Rev 59:387, 1995

OKANO M et al: Epstein-Barr virus and human diseases: Recent advances in diagnosis. Clin Microbiol Rev 1:300, 1988

PAPADOPOULOS EB et al: Infusions of donor leukocytes to treat Epstein-Barr virus-associated lymphoproliferative disorders after allogeneic bone marrow transplantation. N Engl J Med 330:1185, 1994

PATHMANATHAN R et al: Clonal proliferations of cells infected with Epstein-Barr virus in preinvasive lesions related to nasopharyngeal carcinoma. N Engl J Med 333:693, 1995

RICKINSON AB, KIEFF E: Epstein-Barr virus, in *Fields Virology,* 3d ed, BN Fields et al (eds). Philadelphia, Lippincott-Raven, 1996

SCHLOSSBERG D (ed): *Infectious Mononucleosis,* 2d ed. New York, Springer-Verlag, 1989

STRAUS SE et al: Epstein-Barr virus infections: Biology, pathogenesis, and management. Ann Intern Med 118:45, 1993

VAN DER HORST C et al: Lack of effect of peroral acyclovir for the treatment of infectious mononucleosis. J Infect Dis 164:788, 1991

187   *Martin S. Hirsch*

CYTOMEGALOVIRUS AND HUMAN HERPESVIRUS TYPES 6, 7, AND 8

CYTOMEGALOVIRUS

DEFINITION Cytomegalovirus (CMV), which was initially isolated from patients with congenital cytomegalic inclusion disease, is now recognized as an important pathogen in all age groups. In addition to inducing severe birth defects, CMV causes a wide spectrum of disorders in older children and adults, ranging from an asymptomatic, subclinical infection to a mononucleosis syndrome in healthy individuals to disseminated disease in immunocompromised patients. Human CMV is one of several related species-specific viruses that cause similar diseases in various animals. All are associated with the production of characteristic enlarged cells—hence the name *cytomegalovirus*.

CMV is a member of the beta herpesvirus group and has double-stranded DNA, a protein capsid, and a lipoprotein envelope. Like other members of the herpesvirus group, CMV demonstrates icosahedral symmetry, replicates in the cell nucleus, and can cause either a lytic and productive or a latent infection. CMV can be distinguished from other herpesviruses by certain biologic properties, such as host range and type of cytopathology induced. Viral replication is associated with the production of large intranuclear inclusions and smaller cytoplasmic inclusions. The virus appears to replicate in a variety of cell types in vivo; in tissue culture it grows preferentially in fibroblasts. Although there is little evidence that CMV is oncogenic in vivo, the virus does transform fibroblasts in rare instances, and genomic transforming fragments have been identified.

EPIDEMIOLOGY CMV has a worldwide distribution. Approximately 1 percent of newborns in the United States are infected with CMV, and the percentage is higher in many less developed countries. Communal living and poor personal hygiene facilitate early spread. Perinatal and early childhood infections are common. Virus may be present in milk, saliva, feces, and urine. Transmission of CMV has been identified among young children in day-care centers and has been traced from infected toddler to pregnant mother to developing fetus. When an infected child introduces CMV into a household, 50 percent of susceptible family members seroconvert within 6 months.

The virus is not readily spread by casual contact but requires repeated or prolonged intimate exposure for transmission. In late ado-lescence and young adulthood, CMV is often transmitted sexually, and asymptomatic viral carriage in semen or cervical secretions is common. CMV antibody is present at detectable levels in nearly 100 percent of female prostitutes and sexually active homosexual men. Sexually active adults may harbor several strains of CMV simultaneously. Transfusion of whole blood or certain blood products containing viable leukocytes also may transmit CMV, with a frequency of 0.14 to 10 percent per unit transfused.

Once infected, an individual probably carries the virus for life. The infection usually remains latent. However, CMV reactivation syndromes develop frequently when T lymphocyte–mediated immunity is compromised—for example, after organ transplantation or in association with lymphoid neoplasms and certain acquired immunodeficiencies (in particular, infection with human immunodeficiency virus or HIV; see Chap. 308). Most primary CMV infections in organ transplant recipients result from transmission of the virus in the graft itself. In CMV-seronegative transplant recipients, infection results from reactivation of latent virus or, less commonly, from reinfection by a new strain of CMV.

PATHOGENESIS Congenital CMV infection can result from either primary or reactivation infection of the mother. However, clinical disease in the fetus or newborn is almost exclusively related to primary maternal infection (Table 187-1). The factors determining the severity of congenital infection are unknown; a deficient capacity to produce precipitating antibodies and to mount T cell responses to CMV is associated with relatively severe disease.

Primary infection in late childhood or adulthood is often associated with a vigorous T lymphocyte response that may contribute to the development of a mononucleosis syndrome similar to that observed following Epstein-Barr virus infection (see Chap. 186). The hallmark of such infection is the appearance of atypical lymphocytes in the peripheral blood; these cells are predominantly activated CD8+ T lymphocytes. Polyclonal activation of B cells by the virus contributes to the development of rheumatoid factors and other autoantibodies during CMV mononucleosis.

Once acquired by symptomatic or asymptomatic primary infection, CMV persists indefinitely in tissues of the host. The sites of persistent or latent infection are unclear but probably include multiple cell types and various organs. Transmission following blood transfusion or organ transplantation is due to silent infections in these tissues. Autopsy studies suggest that salivary glands and bowel also may be areas of latent infection.

If the host's T cell responses become compromised by disease or by iatrogenic immunosuppression, latent virus can be reactivated to cause a variety of syndromes. Chronic antigenic stimulation in the presence of immunosuppression (for example, following tissue transplantation) appears to be an ideal setting for CMV activation and CMV-induced disease. Certain particularly potent suppressants of T cell immunity, such as antithymocyte globulin, are associated with a high rate of clinical CMV syndromes, which may follow either primary or reactivation infection. CMV may itself contribute to further T lymphocyte hyporesponsiveness, which often precedes superinfection with other opportunistic pathogens, such as *Pneumocystis carinii*. CMV and *P. carinii* are frequently found together in immunosuppressed patients with severe interstitial pneumonia. CMV may function as a cofactor to activate latent HIV infection.

PATHOLOGY Cytomegalic cells in vivo (presumed to be infected epithelial cells) are two to four times larger than surrounding cells and often contain an 8- to 10-μm intranuclear inclusion that is eccentrically placed and is surrounded by a clear halo, producing an

Table 187-1

CMV in the Immunocompromised Host

Population	Risk Factors	Principal Syndromes	Treatment	Prevention
Fetus	Primary maternal infection/early pregnancy	Cytomegalic inclusion disease	None	Avoidance of exposure
Organ transplant recipient	Seropositive donor, seronegative recipient; intensive immunosuppression, particularly with antilymphocyte globulins, cyclosporine	Febrile leukopenia; pneumonia; gastrointestinal disease	Ganciclovir	Donor matching; CMV immunoglobulin; ganciclovir or high-dose acyclovir
Bone marrow transplant recipient	Graft-vs.-host disease; older age; seropositive recipient; viremia	Pneumonia; gastrointestinal disease	Ganciclovir plus CMV immunoglobulin	Ganciclovir or high-dose acyclovir
Person with AIDS	<100 CD4+ cells per microliter; CMV seropositivity	Retinitis; gastrointestinal disease; neurologic disease	Foscarnet or ganciclovir	Trials under way; oral ganciclovir?

"owl's eye" appearance. Smaller granular cytoplasmic inclusions are demonstrated occasionally. Cytomegalic cells are found in a wide variety of organs, including salivary gland, lung, liver, kidney, intestine, pancreas, adrenal gland, and the central nervous system.

The cellular inflammatory response to infection consists of plasma cells, lymphocytes, and monocyte-macrophages. Granulomatous reactions occasionally develop, particularly in the liver. Immunopathologic reactions may contribute to CMV disease. Immune complexes have been detected in infected infants, sometimes in association with CMV-related glomerulopathies. Immune-complex glomerulopathy has been observed in some CMV-infected patients after renal transplantation.

CLINICAL MANIFESTATIONS Congenital CMV Infection Fetal infections range from inapparent to severe and disseminated. Cytomegalic inclusion disease develops in approximately 5 percent of infected fetuses and is seen almost exclusively in infants born to mothers who develop primary infections during pregnancy. Petechiae, hepatosplenomegaly, and jaundice are the most common presenting features (60 to 80 percent of cases). Microcephaly with or without cerebral calcifications, intrauterine growth retardation, and prematurity are reported in 30 to 50 percent of cases. Inguinal hernias and chorioretinitis are less common. Laboratory abnormalities, in decreasing order of frequency, include a serum IgM level of >0.20 g/L (>20 mg/dL), atypical lymphocytosis, elevated concentrations of liver aminotransferases, thrombocytopenia, hyperbilirubinemia, and a cerebrospinal fluid protein level of >0.20 g/L (>20 mg/dL). The prognosis for severely infected infants is poor; the mortality rate is 20 to 30 percent, and few of the patients who survive escape intellectual or hearing difficulties in later years. The differential diagnosis of cytomegalic inclusion disease in infants includes syphilis, rubella, toxoplasmosis, infection with herpes simplex virus or enterovirus, and bacterial sepsis.

Most congenital CMV infections are clinically inapparent at birth. Between 5 and 25 percent of asymptomatically infected infants develop significant psychomotor, hearing, ocular, or dental abnormalities over the next several years.

Perinatal CMV Infection The newborn may acquire CMV at the time of delivery by passage through an infected birth canal or by postnatal contact with maternal milk or other secretions. Approximately 40 to 60 percent of infants who are breast-fed for longer than 1 month by seropositive mothers become infected. Iatrogenic transmission also can result from neonatal blood transfusion. Screening of blood products before they are transfused into low-birth-weight seronegative infants or into seronegative pregnant women decreases the risk of infection.

The great majority of infants infected at or after delivery remain asymptomatic. However, protracted interstitial pneumonitis has been associated with perinatally acquired CMV infection, particularly in premature infants, and occasionally has been accompanied by infection with *Chlamydia trachomatis*, *P. carinii*, or *Ureaplasma urealyticum*. Poor weight gain, adenopathy, rash, hepatitis, anemia, and atypical lymphocytosis also may be found, and CMV excretion often persists for months or years.

CMV Mononucleosis The most common clinical manifestation of CMV infection in normal hosts beyond the neonatal period is a heterophil antibody–negative mononucleosis syndrome. This manifestation may develop spontaneously or may follow the transfusion of leukocyte-containing blood products. Although the syndrome occurs at all ages, it most often involves sexually active young adults. Incubation periods range from 20 to 60 days, and the illness generally lasts for 2 to 6 weeks. Prolonged high fevers, sometimes accompanied by chills, profound fatigue, and malaise, characterize this disorder. Myalgias, headache, and splenomegaly are frequent, but in CMV mononucleosis (as opposed to infectious mononucleosis caused by Epstein-Barr virus), exudative pharyngitis and cervical lymphadenopathy are rare. Occasional patients develop rubelliform rashes, often after exposure to ampicillin. Less commonly observed are interstitial or segmental pneumonia, myocarditis, pleuritis, arthritis, and encephalitis. In rare cases, Guillain-Barré syndrome complicates CMV mononucleosis. The characteristic laboratory abnormality is relative lymphocytosis in periph-

eral blood, with more than 10 percent atypical lymphocytes. Total leukocyte counts may be low, normal, or markedly elevated. Although significant jaundice is uncommon, serum aminotransferase and alkaline phosphatase levels are often moderately elevated. Heterophil antibodies are absent; however, transient immunologic abnormalities are common and may include the presence of cryoglobulins, rheumatoid factors, cold agglutinins, and antinuclear antibodies. Hemolytic anemia, thrombocytopenia, and granulocytopenia complicate recovery in rare instances.

Most patients recover without sequelae, although postviral asthenia may persist for months. The excretion of CMV in urine, genital secretions, and/or saliva often continues for months or years. Rare patients have recurrent episodes of fever and malaise, sometimes associated with autonomic nervous system dysfunction (e.g., attacks of sweating or flushing).

CMV Infection in the Immunocompromised Host (See also Table 187-1) CMV appears to be the most common and important viral pathogen complicating organ transplantation. In recipients of kidney, heart, lung, and liver transplants, CMV induces a variety of syndromes, including fever and leukopenia, hepatitis, pneumonitis, esophagitis, gastritis, colitis, and retinitis. The period of maximal risk is between 1 and 4 months after transplantation, although retinitis may be a later complication. The risk of disease appears to be greater after primary infection than after reactivation. In addition, molecular studies indicate that seropositive transplant recipients are susceptible to reinfection with donor-derived, genotypically variant CMV, and such infection often results in disease. Reactivation infection, although frequent, is less likely than primary infection to be important clinically. Clinical disease is related to various factors (see Table 187-1), such as the degree of immunosuppression; patients receiving certain immunosuppressive agents, such as antithymocyte globulin, appear to be more likely to have severe infections than those receiving other agents, such as cyclosporine. The transplanted organ is particularly vulnerable as a target for CMV infection; thus, there is a tendency for CMV hepatitis to follow liver transplantation and for CMV pneumonitis to follow lung transplantation.

CMV pneumonia occurs in nearly 15 to 20 percent of bone marrow transplant recipients, with a case-fatality rate of 84 to 88 percent. The risk is greatest between 5 and 13 weeks after transplantation, and the several risk factors identified include certain types of immunosuppressive therapy, acute graft-versus-host disease, older age, viremia, and seropositivity before transplantation.

CMV is recognized as an important pathogen in patients with AIDS (see Chap. 308). In fact, CMV infection is nearly universal in these patients and often causes retinitis or disseminated disease, contributing to death. CMV-associated clinical syndromes occur predominantly when peripheral-blood CD4+ cell counts fall below 50 to 100/μL. CMV-induced immunosuppression probably contributes to the T lymphocyte deficiency initiated by the etiologic retrovirus.

Syndromes produced by CMV in the immunocompromised host often begin with prolonged fever, malaise, anorexia, fatigue, night sweats, and arthralgias or myalgias. Liver function abnormalities, leukopenia, thrombocytopenia, and atypical lymphocytosis may be observed during these episodes. The development of tachypnea, hypoxia, and unproductive cough signals respiratory involvement. Radiologic examination of the lung often demonstrates bilateral interstitial or reticulonodular infiltrates, which begin in the periphery of the lower lobes and spread centrally and superiorly; localized segmental, nodular, or alveolar patterns are less common. The differential diagnosis includes infection with *P. carinii*; infections due to other viral, bacterial, or fungal pathogens; pulmonary hemorrhage; and injury secondary to irradiation or to treatment with cytotoxic drugs.

Gastrointestinal CMV involvement may be localized or extensive and almost exclusively affects compromised hosts. Ulcers of the esophagus, stomach, small intestine, or colon may result in bleeding or perforation. CMV infection may lead to exacerbations of underlying ulcerative colitis. Hepatitis occurs frequently, particularly following liver transplantation, and CMV-associated acalculous cholecystitis and adrenalitis have been described.

CMV rarely causes meningoencephalitis in otherwise healthy individuals. Two forms of CMV encephalitis are seen in patients with AIDS. One resembles HIV encephalitis and presents as progressive dementia; the other is a ventriculoencephalitis characterized by cranial-nerve deficits, nystagmus, disorientation, lethargy, and ventriculomegaly. In immunocompromised patients, CMV also can cause subacute progressive polyradiculopathy, which is often reversible if recognized and treated promptly.

CMV retinitis is an important cause of blindness in immunocompromised patients, particularly patients with AIDS. Early lesions consist of small, opaque, white areas of granular retinal necrosis that spread in a centrifugal manner and are later accompanied by hemorrhages, vessel sheathing, and retinal edema (see **Plate III-1**). CMV retinopathy must be distinguished from that due to other conditions, including toxoplasmosis, candidiasis, and herpes simplex virus infection.

Fatal CMV infections often are associated with persistent viremia and the involvement of multiple organ systems. Progressive pulmonary infiltrates, pancytopenia, hyperamylasemia, and hypotension are characteristic features that are frequently found in conjunction with a terminal bacterial, fungal, or protozoan superinfection. Extensive adrenal necrosis with CMV inclusions is often documented at autopsy, as is CMV involvement of many other organs.

DIAGNOSIS The diagnosis of CMV infection usually cannot be made reliably on clinical grounds alone. Isolation of the virus from appropriate clinical specimens, together with demonstration of a fourfold or greater rise in antibody titers or persistently elevated antibody titers, is the preferred diagnostic approach. Virus excretion or viremia is readily detected by culture of appropriate specimens on human fibroblast monolayers. If viral titers are high, as is frequently the case in congenital disseminated infection or in patients with AIDS, characteristic cytopathic effects may be detected within a few days. However, in some situations—such as CMV mononucleosis—viral titers are low, and cytopathic effects may take several weeks to appear. Many laboratories expedite diagnosis by using an overnight tissue-culture method (shell vial assay) involving centrifugation and an immunocytochemical detection technique employing monoclonal antibodies to an immediate-early CMV antigen. Isolation of virus from urine or saliva does not, by itself, constitute proof of acute infection, since excretion from these sites may continue for months or years after illness. Detection of CMV viremia is a better predictor of acute infection. Detection of CMV immediate-early antigens (pp65) or DNA in peripheral-blood leukocytes may hasten the diagnosis of CMV disease in certain populations, including organ transplant recipients and persons with AIDS. Such assays may yield a positive result several days earlier than culture methods. The detection of CMV DNA in cerebrospinal fluid by the polymerase chain reaction is useful in the diagnosis of CMV encephalitis or polyradiculopathy.

A variety of serologic assays [complement fixation, immunofluorescence, indirect hemagglutination, enzyme-linked immunosorbent assay (ELISA)] are available to detect increases in titers of antibody to CMV antigens. An increased antibody level may not be detectable for up to 4 weeks after primary infection, and titers often remain high for years after infection. For this reason, single-sample antibody determinations are of no value in assessing the acuteness of infection. Detection of CMV-specific IgM is sometimes useful in the diagnosis of recent or active infection; circulating rheumatoid factors may result in occasional false-positive IgM tests.

℞ TREATMENT

Several prophylactic measures are useful for the prevention of CMV infection in patients at high risk. The use of blood from seronegative donors or of blood that has been frozen, thawed, and deglycerolized greatly decreases the rate of transfusion-associated transmission of CMV. Similarly, matching of organ or bone marrow transplants by CMV serology, using only organs from seronegative donors for seronegative recipients, reduces rates of primary infection following transplantation. Both live attenuated (Towne strain) and CMV subunit vaccines have been evaluated, but neither is close to approval for general use.

CMV immune globulin has been reported to reduce rates of occurrence of CMV-associated syndromes and fungal or parasitic superinfections among seronegative renal transplant recipients. Similar studies in bone marrow transplant recipients have produced conflicting results. Prophylactic acyclovir has been demonstrated to reduce CMV infection and disease in certain seronegative renal transplant recipients; acyclovir is not effective in the treatment of active CMV disease, however.

Ganciclovir (dihydroxypropoxymethylguanine, DHPG) is a guanosine derivative that has considerably more activity against CMV than its congener acyclovir. After intracellular conversion by a viral phosphotransferase encoded by CMV gene region UL97, ganciclovir triphosphate is a selective inhibitor of CMV DNA polymerase. Several clinical studies have indicated response rates of 70 to 90 percent among patients with AIDS given ganciclovir for the treatment of CMV retinitis or colitis. In bone marrow transplant recipients with CMV pneumonia, ganciclovir is less effective when given alone, but it elicits a favorable clinical response 50 to 70 percent of the time when it is combined with CMV immune globulin. Prophylactic or suppressive ganciclovir may be useful in high-risk bone marrow or organ transplant recipients (e.g., those who are CMV-seropositive before transplantation or who are CMV culture–positive afterward). In many patients with AIDS and CMV disease, clinical and virologic relapses occur promptly if treatment with ganciclovir is discontinued. Therefore, prolonged maintenance regimens are recommended. Resistance to ganciclovir is common among patients treated for more than 3 months and is usually related to mutations in the CMV UL97 gene.

Ganciclovir therapy for CMV retinitis consists of a 14- to 21-day induction course (5 mg/kg intravenously twice a day) followed by a prolonged intravenous or oral maintenance regimen. For parenteral maintenance, the dose is 5 mg/kg daily or 6 mg/kg 5 days per week. Peripheral-blood neutropenia develops in 16 to 29 percent of treated patients but is often ameliorated by granulocyte or granulocyte-macrophage colony-stimulating factor. Oral ganciclovir at a high dose (3 g/d) can also be used for maintenance, although the blood levels achieved are insufficient for acute induction regimens. Although progression (as assessed by funduscopy) is more rapid with oral than with intravenous ganciclovir maintenance (mean time to progression, 68 vs. 96 days; $p = 0.03$), the ease of administration and reduced toxicity of the oral preparation may make it an acceptable alternative for some patients. The use of oral ganciclovir as prophylaxis in high-risk AIDS patients (i.e., those with CD4+ cell counts of $<100/\mu L$) has been studied in two placebo-controlled trials, with somewhat contradictory results.

Foscarnet (sodium phosphonoformate) also acts against CMV infection by inhibiting viral DNA polymerase. Because this agent does not require phosphorylation to be active, it is also effective against ganciclovir-resistant CMV isolates. A comparative trial of foscarnet and ganciclovir in 234 patients with AIDS and CMV retinitis demonstrated equivalent activity against retinitis but longer survival (12.6 vs. 8.5 months) in the foscarnet group. Although the reasons for the latter difference are unclear, the antiretroviral activity of foscarnet and the greater use of zidovudine by foscarnet recipients are strong possibilities. Foscarnet is less well tolerated than ganciclovir and causes considerable toxicity, including renal dysfunction, hypomagnesemia, hypokalemia, hypocalcemia, genital ulcers, dysuria, nausea, and paresthesia. Moreover, foscarnet administration requires the use of an infusion pump and close clinical monitoring. With aggressive hydration and dose adjustments for renal dysfunction, the toxicity of foscarnet can be reduced. The use of foscarnet should be avoided when a saline load cannot be tolerated (e.g., in cardiomyopathy). The approved induction regimen is 60 mg/kg every

8 h for 2 weeks, although 90 mg/kg every 12 h is equally effective and no more toxic. Maintenance infusions should deliver 90 to 120 mg/kg once daily; no oral preparation is available. Foscarnet-resistant viruses may emerge during extended therapy.

Ganciclovir has recently been administered via a slow-release pellet sutured into the eye. Although this intraocular device provides good local protection, contralateral eye disease and disseminated disease are not affected, and early retinal detachment is possible. A combination of intraocular and systemic therapy is being studied, as are combinations of ganciclovir and foscarnet. New drugs are being investigated, and one, cidofovir (also known as HPMPC), is available through expanded-access programs.

HUMAN HERPESVIRUS TYPES 6, 7, AND 8

Human herpesvirus (HHV) type 6 was first isolated in 1986 from peripheral-blood leukocytes of six persons with various lymphoproliferative disorders. Although initially thought to be B-lymphotropic and thus designated *human B-lymphotropic virus*, HHV-6 is clearly primarily T-lymphotropic. The virus has a worldwide distribution, and two genetically distinct variants (HHV-6A and HHV-6B) are now recognized.

Infection with HHV-6 frequently develops during infancy as maternal antibody wanes. Although HHV-6A has not yet been associated with disease, HHV-6B can cause exanthem subitum (roseola infantum), a common illness characterized by fever with subsequent rash. HHV-6B is also a major cause of febrile seizures without rash during infancy. In older age groups, HHV-6B has been associated with mononucleosis syndromes, focal encephalitis, and (in immunocompromised hosts) pneumonitis and disseminated disease. As many as 80 percent of adults are seropositive for HHV-6. The virus may be transmitted by saliva and possibly by genital secretions. There is no established treatment or vaccine.

HHV-7 was isolated in 1990 from T lymphocytes from the peripheral blood of a healthy 26-year-old man. Other isolates have since been obtained. It appears that the virus is frequently acquired during childhood and is frequently present in the saliva of healthy adults. No human disease has yet been definitively linked to HHV-7, although some cases of exanthem subitum have been associated with HHV-7 infection.

Unique herpesvirus-like DNA sequences were reported during 1994 and 1995 in tissues derived from Kaposi's sarcoma and body cavity–based lymphoma occurring in patients with AIDS. These sequences are partially homologous to the DNA of Epstein-Barr virus and herpesvirus saimiri of squirrel monkeys. When subjected to representational-difference analyses, more than 90 percent of Kaposi's sarcoma tissue samples were found to contain these sequences, whereas appropriate control tissues did not. The same herpesvirus-like DNA sequences have been reported in Kaposi's sarcoma tissue from non-AIDS patients, in a subgroup of AIDS-related B-cell body cavity–based lymphomas, in certain brain tumors, and in some proliferative skin lesions of organ transplant recipients. Approximately 15 percent of non-Kaposi's-sarcoma tissue specimens from patients with AIDS contain these sequences, which have also been found in semen from both AIDS and non-AIDS patients. Because of the uniqueness of these sequences, some authors have tentatively called the virus from which they come HHV-8. Its role in Kaposi's sarcoma and other diseases remains to be established. The recent isolation of HHV-8 in cell culture should help define its role in disease by making diagnostic techniques more reliable.

BIBLIOGRAPHY

AKASHI K et al: Severe infectious mononucleosis-like syndrome and primary human herpesvirus 6 infection in an adult. N Engl J Med 329:168, 1993

BALFOUR HH et al: A randomized, placebo-controlled trial of oral acyclovir for the prevention of cytomegalovirus disease in recipients of renal allografts. N Engl J Med 320:1381, 1989

BOWDEN RA et al: Cytomegalovirus (CMV)–specific intravenous immunoglobulin for the prevention of primary CMV infection and disease after marrow transplant. J Infect Dis 164:483, 1991

BUHLES WC et al: Ganciclovir treatment of life- or sight-threatening cytomegalovirus infection: Experience in 314 immunocompromised patients. Rev Infect Dis 10:S495, 1988

CESARMAN E et al: Kaposi's sarcoma–associated herpesvirus-like DNA sequences in AIDS-related body-cavity based lymphomas. N Engl J Med 332:1186, 1995

CHANG Y et al: Identification of herpesvirus-like DNA sequences in AIDS-associated Kaposi's sarcoma. Science 266:1865, 1994

DREW WL et al: Oral ganciclovir as maintenance treatment for cytomegalovirus retinitis in patients with AIDS. N Engl J Med 333:615, 1995

HIRSCH MS: The treatment of cytomegalovirus in AIDS: More than meets the eye. N Engl J Med 326:262, 1992

HO M: *Cytomegalovirus: Biology and Infection*, 2d ed. New York, Plenum Press, 1991

JABS DA: Controversies in the treatment of cytomegalovirus retinitis: Foscarnet versus ganciclovir. Infect Agents Dis 4:131, 1995

LEACH CT et al: Human herpesvirus 6 infection of the female genital tract. J Infect Dis 169:1281, 1994

MANEZ R et al: Time to detection of cytomegalovirus (CMV) DNA in blood leukocytes is a predictor for the development of CMV disease in CMV-seronegative recipients of allografts from CMV-seropositive donors following liver transplantation. J Infect Dis 173:1072, 1996

McCUTCHAN JA: Cytomegalovirus infections of the nervous system in patients with AIDS. Clin Infect Dis 20:747, 1995

MERIGAN TC et al: A controlled trial of ganciclovir to prevent cytomegalovirus disease after heart transplantation. N Engl J Med 326:1182, 1992

MONINI P et al: Kaposi's sarcoma–associated herpesvirus DNA sequences in prostate tissue and human semen. N Engl J Med 334:1168, 1996

ONORATO IM et al: Epidemiology of cytomegaloviral infections: Recommendations for prevention and control. Rev Infect Dis 7:479, 1985

PASS RF et al: Young children as a probable source of maternal and congenital cytomegalovirus infection. N Engl J Med 316:1366, 1987

RENNE R et al: Lytic growth of Kaposi's sarcoma–associated herpesvirus (human herpesvirus 8) in culture. Nature Med 2:342, 1996

SMYTH RL et al: Cytomegalovirus infection in heart-lung transplant recipients: Risk factors, clinical associations, and response to treatment. J Infect Dis 164:1045, 1991

SNYDMAN DR et al: Use of cytomegalovirus immune globulin to prevent cytomegalovirus disease in renal transplant recipients. N Engl J Med 317:1049, 1987

STUDIES OF OCULAR COMPLICATIONS OF AIDS RESEARCH GROUP, AIDS CLINICAL TRIALS GROUP: Mortality in patients with the acquired immunodeficiency syndrome treated with either foscarnet or ganciclovir for cytomegalovirus retinitis. N Engl J Med 326:213, 1992

———: Combination foscarnet and ganciclovir therapy vs monotherapy for the treatment of relapsed cytomegalovirus retinitis in patients with AIDS. The cytomegalovirus retreatment trial. Arch Ophthalmol 114:23, 1996

WYATT LS et al: Human herpesvirus 7 is a constitutive inhabitant of adult human saliva. J Virol 66:3206, 1992

188 *Fred Wang*

SMALLPOX, VACCINIA, AND OTHER POXVIRUSES

Poxviruses are characterized by a brick-shaped morphology and a large double-stranded DNA genome. These are the only DNA viruses that replicate in cytoplasm, where accumulated viral particles form eosinophilic inclusions, or Guarnieri bodies, visible by light microscopy. Poxviruses associated with human disease include variola, vaccinia, and molluscum contagiosum viruses as well as other agents that cause zoonotic infections (the most important being monkeypox virus).

SMALLPOX

The last case of endemic smallpox was reported in 1977 from Somalia. In 1980 the World Health Organization officially declared that smallpox had been eliminated worldwide as a result of a global vaccination and ocular vaccinia resulting from inadvertent inoculation but is of no value for the treatment of postinfectious encephalitis.

and eradication program. Several features contributed to this unique accomplishment, including (1) universal interest in eliminating this costly disease with high morbidity and mortality, (2) the infection's long incubation period and low level of communicability, (3) the ease of diagnosis of skin lesions by characteristic histology or antigen detection, (4) the fact that humans were the sole reservoir of the infection, (5) the absence of a carrier state, and (6) the availability of an effective live-virus vaccine that could readily be delivered to less developed countries because of its resistance to chemicals, temperature changes, and drying. The only known remaining repositories of smallpox virus are two research laboratories (located in the United States and Russia, respectively), and the issue of whether these last samples should be maintained or destroyed remains controversial. However, there is currently a moratorium on destroying the virus before 1999.

Before the eradication of smallpox, variola virus existed as two related strains: *variola major* (smallpox), with a case-mortality rate of 20 to 50 percent, and *variola minor* (alastrim), which caused a clinically milder form of smallpox with a mortality of less than 1 percent. Smallpox was a relatively noncontagious disease whose transmission required close contact. Fever and macular rash appeared after an average incubation period of 12 days, with a progression to typical vesicular and pustular lesions over 1 to 2 weeks.

VACCINIA

The origin of vaccinia virus—the virus used for vaccination against smallpox—is uncertain, but it was probably derived from cowpox virus, variola virus, or a hybrid of the two. It is now a laboratory virus with no natural host. Experience has proven the effectiveness of live vaccinia-virus vaccine, although its efficacy and safety have not been established in controlled studies. Percutaneous administration of vaccinia virus vaccine results in protective cellular and humoral immune responses in more than 95 percent of primary vaccinees. Formation of a pustule and scab at the site of inoculation is indicative of immunity; because immunity wanes after 10 to 20 years, revaccination every 10 years is recommended for continued protection. Routine smallpox vaccination was discontinued in 1971 and has not been required for international travel since 1982. However, the development of recombinant vaccinia viruses for potential use in vaccines against other infectious agents or as immunotherapy against malignant diseases has led to the recommendation that laboratory and health care employees working directly with vaccinia virus vectors be considered for vaccination. Selected groups that may be exposed to poxviruses (e.g., some military personnel and individuals who work with animals) are also vaccinated.

The most frequent adverse complication of vaccination is inadvertent inoculation (usually autoinoculation) at other sites. More serious complications, which are more common among primary vaccinees and infants than among revaccinees and adults, include (1) generalized vaccinia in otherwise healthy individuals, which is generally self-limited; (2) eczema vaccinatum, which consists of disseminated cutaneous lesions in highly susceptible patients with eczema or other chronic skin diseases and is occasionally severe or even fatal; (3) progressive vaccinia (vaccinia necrosum), which is a severe, potentially fatal illness occurring in patients with immunodeficiency, whether congenital, acquired (e.g., via leukemia or lymphoma), iatrogenic (e.g., via chemotherapy or glucocorticoid treatment), or human immunodeficiency virus (HIV)–induced; and (4) postinfectious encephalitis, which is rare (3 cases per million primary vaccinees) but can be fatal in 15 to 25 percent of cases and can leave 25 percent of patients with permanent neurologic sequelae. Since vaccinees can transmit vaccinia virus to susceptible individuals, vaccination is contraindicated if the proposed recipient or his/her household contacts have eczema, are immunocompromised, or are pregnant. Vaccinia immune globulin (0.6 mL/kg) derived from the plasma of vaccinated persons may be useful for the treatment of severe generalized vaccinia, eczema vaccinatum, progressive vaccinia,

MOLLUSCUM CONTAGIOSUM

Molluscum contagiosum is generally a benign disease characterized by pearly, flesh-colored, umbilicated skin lesions 2 to 5 mm in diameter. The infection can be transmitted by close contact, including sexual intercourse. Lesions typically occur in the genital region but can be found anywhere on the body except the palms and the soles. In most cases the disease is self-limited and has no systemic complications. Molluscum contagiosum develops especially often in association with the advanced stages of HIV infection, with a prevalence of 5 to 18 percent among HIV-infected patients (see Chap. 308). The disease is often more generalized, severe, and persistent in AIDS patients than in other groups, frequently involving the face and upper body. Extensive molluscum contagiosum has also been reported in conjunction with other types of immunodeficiency.

The diagnosis of molluscum contagiosum can be made by histologic demonstration of cytoplasmic eosinophilic inclusions characteristic of poxvirus replication. This poorly characterized virus cannot be propagated in vitro, but electron microscopy and molecular studies can be used for its identification.

There is no specific systemic treatment for molluscum contagiosum, but a variety of techniques for physical ablation have been used.

MONKEYPOX VIRUS AND OTHER POXVIRUSES

Monkeypox virus naturally infects nonhuman primates in the tropical rain forests of western and central Africa and can infect humans who come into direct contact with infected animals. Human disease is rare and is characterized by a vesicular rash similar to that of variola. The disease is occasionally fatal, especially to young children and individuals who have not received smallpox vaccine.

Other poxviruses can cause localized vesicular lesions when humans come into direct contact with infected animals. These viruses include cowpox virus (cows, rodents); milkers' node virus (cows); buffalopox virus (buffaloes); bovine papular stomatitis virus (cows); and orf virus, which is also known as contagious pustular dermatitis virus (sheep, goats).

BIBLIOGRAPHY

BREMAN JG, ARITA I: The confirmation and maintenance of smallpox eradication. N Engl J Med 303:1263, 1980
JEZEK Z et al: Human monkeypox: Clinical features of 282 patients. J Infect Dis 156:293, 1987
JOKLIK WK et al: Why the smallpox virus stocks should not be destroyed. Science 262:1225, 1993
MAHY BW et al: The remaining stocks of smallpox virus should be destroyed. Science 262:1223, 1993
MOSS B: Vaccinia virus: A tool for research and vaccine development. Science 252:1662, 1991
SCHWARTZ JJ, MYSKOWSKI PL: Molluscum contagiosum in patients with human immunodeficiency virus infection. A review of twenty-seven patients. J Am Acad Dermatol 27:583, 1992
Vaccinia (smallpox) vaccine. Recommendations of the Immunization Practices Advisory Committee (ACIP). Morb Mortal Week Rep 40:1, 1991

189 Neil R. Blacklow

PARVOVIRUS

DEFINITION The parvovirus group includes several species-specific viruses of animals. One parvovirus, designated B19, is known to be a human pathogen. B19 is a small (diameter, 20 to 25 nm), icosahedral, nonenveloped, single-stranded DNA virus with an outer capsid formed by two structural proteins. Individual virus particles contain DNA strands of positive or negative polarity. The virus is stable and retains infectivity after incubation at 60°C for 16 h. It has failed to grow in conventional cell culture lines and animal model systems but does replicate in vitro in erythroid progenitor cells derived from human bone marrow, umbilical cord, peripheral blood, or fetal liver sources.

During the 1980s, it was discovered that B19 causes a variety of disorders ranging from erythema infectiosum and acute arthropathy in otherwise healthy hosts to transient aplastic crisis and chronic anemia in compromised patients to fetal infection manifested by death or hydrops fetalis. Many of the severe manifestations of B19 viremia relate to the propensity of the virus to infect and lyse erythroid precursor cells in the bone marrow. The name B19 is derived from the code number of the human serum in which the virus was discovered.

PATHOGENESIS Two studies of adult volunteers have provided a basis for understanding the pathogenesis of B19 infection, which has two phases. The first phase is characterized by viremia that develops approximately 6 days after intranasal inoculation of B19 into susceptible individuals who lack serum antibodies to the virus. The viremia lasts about 1 week; its clearance is correlated with the development of IgM antibodies to B19, which remain detectable for up to a few months. IgG antibodies develop several days later and persist indefinitely. Nonspecific systemic symptoms lasting 2 or 3 days occur early during the viremic phase; these symptoms include headache, malaise, myalgia, fever, chills, and pruritus and are accompanied by reticulocytopenia and excretion of the virus from the respiratory tract. Several days after the onset of symptoms, a clinically insignificant decline in hemoglobin concentration is noted; the decreased level is maintained for 7 to 10 days, during which time examination of bone marrow samples reveals a marked depletion of erythroid precursor cells. Transient mild lymphopenia, neutropenia, and a drop in platelet count also may be found. A second phase of illness begins around 17 or 18 days after virus inoculation (after the clearance of viremia, the cessation of viral shedding in throat secretions, and the resolution of reticulocytopenia). This illness mimics erythema infectiosum in adults, with 2 or 3 days of fine maculopapular rash accompanied by arthralgias and arthritis that last another 1 or 2 days. This phase occurs in the presence of rising serum titers of antibody to B19.

The studies just described indicate that B19 disease in the otherwise *healthy host*, manifested by self-limited erythema infectiosum and/or arthropathy, is almost certainly an immune-complex disorder. This concept is supported by the induction of erythema infectiosum through the infusion of immunoglobulins into chronically viremic patients. In contrast, B19 disease in the *compromised host* (chronic hemolytic disease or immunodeficiency syndromes) is often serious, resulting from the destruction by B19 of erythroid precursor cells. Normal hosts can tolerate 7 to 10 days of shutoff of erythropoiesis; however, patients with hemolytic disease who require increased production of erythrocytes do not tolerate erythroid cell destruction and thus usually develop severe transient aplastic crisis. Patients who are immunodeficient may fail to clear B19 viremia, the results being persistent infection of red blood cells and chronic severe anemia. The fetus requires a higher level of red cell production than do adults and has an immature immune system; both these factors could explain B19-induced hydrops fetalis.

B19 binds specifically to a cellular receptor, erythrocyte P antigen; this specific binding explains the tropism of B19 for erythroid progenitor cells, particularly pronormoblasts and normoblasts. The few persons who lack P antigen cannot be infected with B19.

EPIDEMIOLOGY Although B19 infections occur year-round, they appear most commonly as outbreaks of erythema infectiosum in schools during winter and spring months. Between 20 and 60 percent of children in outbreaks are symptomatic, and many are asymptomatically infected. Seroepidemiologic studies indicate that approximately half of adults possess serum antibodies to B19. Antibody prevalence (reflecting prior exposure and probable immunity to the virus) rises rapidly between the ages of 5 and 18 years and continues to increase with age—a pattern probably indicating ongoing exposure during adulthood. B19 can be detected in throat swabbings, respiratory tract secretions, and serum, and its detection at these sites probably correlates with infectiousness. Thus, patients with transient aplastic crisis are highly infectious. Their infectivity has been firmly documented as the source of one well-defined nosocomial outbreak of erythema infectiosum among nurses. In contrast, individuals with erythema infectiosum are much less infectious. The usual route of viral transmission under natural conditions is unknown but may be respiratory or through direct contact. B19 can be transmitted during therapy with clotting factor concentrate, even after exposure to steam or dry heat.

CLINICAL MANIFESTATIONS **Erythema Infectiosum** Erythema infectiosum is the most common manifestation of B19 infection and occurs predominantly in children. This entity is also called *fifth disease* because it was classified in the late nineteenth century as the fifth in a series of six exanthems of childhood. Normally a mild illness, erythema infectiosum typically presents as a facial rash with a "slapped-cheek" appearance that is sometimes preceded by low-grade fever. The rash may develop quickly on the arms and legs and usually has a lacy, reticular, erythematous appearance. The trunk, palms, and soles are less commonly involved. Occasionally, the rash appears with maculopapular, morbilliform, vesicular, purpuric, or pruritic characteristics. The typical rash resolves in about a week but can recur intermittently for several weeks, particularly after stress, exercise, exposure to sunlight, bathing, or change in environmental temperature. Arthralgia and arthritis are uncommon among children but are frequent among adults, in whom the rash is often absent or nonspecific, with a lack of the characteristic facial erythema.

Arthropathy B19 infection in adults most commonly presents as acute arthralgias and arthritis, sometimes accompanied by rash. The arthritis is characteristically symmetric and peripheral, involving the wrists, hands, and knees most frequently. It normally resolves in about 3 weeks and is nondestructive. However, a small percentage of patients have arthritis persisting for months or even (in rare cases) for years. It is not known whether these individuals have persistent infection or an abnormal immune response to the virus. Several case reports have suggested a link—as yet unproven—between B19 and idiopathic thrombocytopenic purpura, virus-associated hemophagocytic syndrome with pancytopenia, Lyme-like arthritis, recurrent paresthesia, fibromyalgia, systemic lupus erythematosus, and vasculitis (including polyarteritis nodosa, Wegener's granulomatosis, and Kawasaki disease).

Transient Aplastic Crisis B19 infection is the cause in most instances of transient aplastic crisis developing suddenly in patients with chronic hemolytic disease. Nearly all hemolytic conditions can be affected by B19 infection, including sickle cell disease, erythrocyte enzyme deficiencies, hereditary spherocytosis, thalassemias, paroxysmal nocturnal hemoglobinuria, and autoimmune hemolysis. B19-induced aplastic crisis also can occur in the setting of acute blood loss. Patients present with weakness, lethargy, pallor, and severe anemia, a syndrome often preceded by a few days of nonspecific symptoms. These patients have intense reticulocytopenia lasting 7 to 10 days, and their bone marrow contains no erythroid precursor cells despite a normal myeloid series. Transient aplastic crisis can produce life-threatening anemia and may require urgent transfusion therapy. Unlike patients with erythema infectiosum or arthropathy, those with transient aplastic crisis are viremic and can readily transmit B19 infection to other people.

Chronic Anemia in Immunodeficient Patients Immunodeficient patients may be unable to eliminate B19 infection, probably because they cannot produce adequate levels of virus-specific IgG antibodies. The result is persistent infection with destruction of erythroid precursor cells in the bone marrow and chronic transfusion-dependent anemia. This condition has been described in patients with immunodeficiency related to infection with human immunodeficiency virus, congenital immunodeficiencies, and acute lymphocytic leukemia during maintenance chemotherapy as well as in recipients of bone marrow transplants. In addition, some cases of idiopathic pure red-cell aplasia probably are caused by persistent B19 infection. B19-induced chronic anemia may be the presenting finding of an otherwise unrecognized immunodeficiency. Chronic anemia may fluctuate in intensity over time and may be cured or controlled by immunoglobulin therapy. Both the spectrum of immunodeficiencies associated with B19-induced chronic anemia and the frequency of the association remain to be determined.

Fetal and Congenital Infection   Maternal B19 infections usually do not adversely affect the fetus. More often than not, in fact, the fetus remains uninfected. Therefore, couples in which the pregnant woman is infected should be counseled as to the relatively low risk of fetal infection. It is estimated that fewer than 10 percent of maternal B19 infections lead to fetal death; when fetal death does occur, it is usually attributable to the development of nonimmune hydrops fetalis, wherein the fetus succumbs to severe anemia and congestive heart failure. B19 can be detected in fetal tissues, with predominant infection of erythroblasts. Pregnant women with known exposure to B19 should have their serum monitored for IgM antibodies to the virus and for elevated levels of alpha fetoprotein; ultrasonic examinations of the fetus for hydrops should also be conducted. Some hydropic fetuses survive B19 infection and appear normal at delivery. Rarely, fetal infection with hydrops results in congenital anemia and hypogammaglobulinemia that is unresponsive to immunoglobulin therapy.

DIAGNOSIS   Diagnosis most commonly relies on measurements of B19-specific IgM and IgG antibodies, which can be detected with commercially available immunoassay kits. The virus, its DNA, or its antigens are also detected in the serum or infected tissues of some patients. Acute infection can be proven by B19-compatible symptoms and the presence of IgM antibodies or virus itself, whereas past infection is documented by IgG antibodies. Individuals with erythema infectiosum and acute arthropathy usually have IgM antibodies without detectable virus in serum. Those with transient aplastic crisis may have IgM antibodies but typically possess high titers of virus and its DNA in serum; the bone marrow of these patients shows characteristic giant pronormoblasts and hypoplasia. Immunodeficient patients with anemia often lack readily detectable antibodies but have viral particles and DNA in serum. Fetal infection may be recognized by hydrops fetalis and the presence of B19 DNA in amniotic fluid or fetal blood in association with maternal IgM antibodies to B19.

℞ TREATMENT

Erythema infectiosum usually requires no treatment; the same is true for many cases of arthropathy. More severe cases of arthritis, particularly those involving chronic symptoms, can be treated with nonsteroidal anti-inflammatory agents. Transient aplastic crisis is usually treated with erythrocyte transfusions. In immunodeficient anemic patients, B19 infection should be treated with commercial intravenous immunoglobulin, which is known to contain IgG antibodies to B19. This therapy controls and may cure B19 infection. Prophylaxis of B19 infection with immunoglobulin should be considered for patients with chronic hemolysis or immunodeficiency and for pregnant women. The risk of infection for these persons may be reduced by hand washing before eating or after contact with respiratory or other secretions when B19 is known to be present in a community. Patients with transient aplastic crisis or chronic B19 infection (but not those with erythema infectiosum or arthropathy) pose a serious risk for nosocomial transmission of infection. They should be hospitalized in a private room with contact and respiratory isolation precautions. It is not known whether pre- or postexposure administration of immunoglobulin prevents infection. No vaccine for B19 is currently available; however, a baculovirus-infected insect cell line that expresses noninfectious immunogenic B19 capsid proteins is being evaluated as a vaccine candidate.

BIBLIOGRAPHY

ANDERSON LJ: Human parvoviruses. J Infect Dis 161:603, 1990

ANDERSON MJ et al: Experimental parvoviral infection in humans. J Infect Dis 152:257, 1985

BANSAL GP et al: Candidate recombinant vaccine for human B19 parvovirus. J Infect Dis 167:1034, 1993

BELL LM et al: Human parvovirus B19 infection among hospital staff members after contact with infected patients. N Engl J Med 321:485, 1989

BROWN KE et al: Congenital anemia after transplacental B19 parvovirus infection. Lancet 343:895, 1994

———— et al: Resistance to parvovirus B19 infection due to lack of virus receptor (erythrocyte P antigen). N Engl J Med 330:1192, 1994

BRUU AL, NORDBO SA: Evaluation of five commercial tests for detection of immunoglobulin M antibodies to human parvovirus B19. J Clin Microbiol 33:1363, 1995

CENTERS FOR DISEASE CONTROL: Risks associated with human parvovirus B19 infection. Morb Mort Week Rep 38:81, 1989

FINKEL TH et al: Chronic parvovirus B19 infection and systemic necrotising vasculitis: Opportunistic infection or aetiological agent? Lancet 343:1255, 1994

FRICKHOFEN N et al: Persistent B19 parvovirus infection in patients infected with human immunodeficiency virus type 1 (HIV-1): A treatable cause of anemia in AIDS. Ann Intern Med 113:926, 1990

HARRIS JW: Parvovirus B19 for the hematologist. Am J Hematol 39:119, 1992

KURTZMAN G et al: Pure red-cell aplasia of 10 years' duration due to persistent parvovirus B19 infection and its cure with immunoglobulin therapy. N Engl J Med 321:519, 1989

MOREY AL et al: Clinical and histopathological features of parvovirus B19 infection in the human fetus. Br J Obstet Gynaecol 99:566, 1992

NAIDES SJ et al: Rheumatologic manifestations of human parvovirus B19 infection in adults: Initial two-year clinical experience. Arthritis Rheum 33:1297, 1990

PLUMMER FA et al: An erythema infectiosum–like illness caused by human parvovirus infection. N Engl J Med 313:74, 1985

RODIS JF et al: Management and outcomes of pregnancies complicated by human B19 parvovirus infections: A prospective study. Am J Obstet Gynecol 163:1168, 1990

190   *Richard C. Reichman*

HUMAN PAPILLOMAVIRUS INFECTIONS

DEFINITION   Human papillomaviruses (HPVs) selectively infect the epithelium of the skin and mucous membranes. These infections may be asymptomatic, produce warts, or be associated with a variety of benign and malignant neoplasias.

ETIOLOGIC AGENT   Papillomaviruses are members of the *Papillomavirus* genus of the family Papovaviridae. They are nonenveloped, measure 50 to 55 nm in diameter, have icosahedral capsids composed of 72 capsomeres, and contain a double-stranded circular DNA genome of about 7900 base pairs. The genomic organization of all papillomaviruses is similar and consists of an early (E) region, a late (L) region, and a long-control region (LCR). Oncogenic HPV types can immortalize human keratinocytes, and this activity has been mapped to products of early genes E6 and E7. E6 protein mediates the degradation of the p53 tumor suppressor protein, and E7 protein binds the retinoblastoma gene product. The E1 and E2 proteins modulate viral DNA replication and regulate gene expression. The L1 gene codes for the major capsid protein, which makes up 80 percent of the virion mass. L2 codes for a minor capsid protein. Type-specific conformational antigenic determinants are located on the virion surface. Papillomavirus types are distinguished from one another by the degree of nucleic acid sequence homology. Distinct types share fewer than 90 percent of their DNA sequences in L1. More than 70 types of HPV are recognized, and individual types are associated with specific clinical manifestations (Table 190-1). HPVs are species-specific and have not been propagated in tissue culture or in common experimental animals. However, HPV types 1, 6, 11, and 16 have been produced in human tissues implanted in immunodeficient mice.

EPIDEMIOLOGY   There are few good studies of the incidence or prevalence of warts in well-defined human populations. Common warts (verruca vulgaris) are found in as many as 25 percent of some groups and are most prevalent among young children. Plantar warts

Table 190-1

CHAPTER 190
Human Papillomavirus Infections   **1099**

Correlation of Human Papillomavirus Type with Disease

Disease	Associated HPV Types
Plantar warts	1,* 2,* 4, 63
Common warts	1,* 2,* 4, 26, 27, 29, 41,† 57, 65, 77
Common warts of meat handlers	1, 2,* 3, 4, 7,* 10, 28
Flat warts	3,* 10,* 27, 38, 41,† 49, 75, 76
Intermediate warts	10,* 26, 28
Epidermodysplasia verruciformis	2,* 3,* 5,*† 8,*† 9,* 10,* 12,* 14,*† 15,* 17,*† 19, 20,† 21, 22, 23, 24, 25, 36, 37, 38,† 47, 50
Condyloma acuminatum	6,* 11,* 30,† 42, 43, 44, 45,† 51,† 54, 55, 70
Intraepithelial neoplasias	
Unspecified	30,† 34, 39,† 40, 53, 57, 59, 61, 62, 64, 66,† 67, 68, 69, 70, 71, 74
Low-grade	6,* 11,* 16,† 18,† 31,† 33,† 35,† 42, 43, 44, 45,† 51,† 52†
High-grade	6, 11, 16,*† 18,*† 31,† 33,† 35,† 39,† 42, 44, 45,† 51,† 52,† 56,† 58,† 66†
Bowen's disease	16,*† 31,† 34
Bowenoid papulosis	16,*† 34, 39,† 42, 45,† 55
Cervical carcinoma	16,*† 18,*† 31,† 33,† 35,† 39,† 45,† 51,† 52,† 56,† 58,† 66†
Laryngeal papillomas	6,* 11*
Focal epithelial hyperplasia of Heck	13,* 32*
Conjunctival papillomas	6,* 11,* 16*†
Others	6, 11, 16,† 30,† 33,† 36, 37, 38,† 41,† 48,† 60, 72, 73

* Most common associations.
† High malignant potential.

(verruca plantaris) are also widely prevalent; they occur most often among adolescents and young adults. Condyloma acuminatum (which manifests as anogenital warts) is one of the most common sexually transmitted diseases in the United States. HPV infection of the uterine cervix produces the squamous-cell abnormalities most frequently detected on Papanicolaou smears.

Most genital HPV infections are transmitted through direct contact with infectious lesions. Both direct contact and fomites play a role in transmission of cutaneous nongenital warts. Minor trauma at the site of inoculation may facilitate transmission. Recurrent respiratory papillomatosis in young children is an uncommon disease that is acquired from maternal genital tract infection; in adults orogenital sexual contact may transmit the disease.

HPV infection has been strongly associated with the development of dysplasia and cancer of the uterine cervix. More than 90 percent of cervical cancers contain DNA of oncogenic (high-risk) HPV types, such as 16, 18, and 31. HPV DNA is also present in the precursor lesions of cervical cancer, known as cervical intraepithelial neoplasias. Such lesions containing DNA of oncogenic HPV types are more likely to progress than those associated with low-risk types, such as 6 and 11. HPV DNA is transcribed in tumor tissues, and many epidemiologic studies have confirmed a relation between HPV infection (with or without cofactors) and the development of cervical cancer. Infection with specific HPV types has also been associated with squamous cell carcinomas and dysplasias of the penis, anus, vagina, and vulva. In patients with epidermodysplasia verruciformis, squamous cell cancers develop frequently at sites infected with specific HPV types, including 5 and 8.

Recent serologic studies employing virus-like particles as antigens have demonstrated a modest prevalence of antibodies among patients with HPV genital tract infections.

CLINICAL MANIFESTATIONS The clinical manifestations of HPV infection depend on the location of the lesions and the type

of virus. Common warts usually occur on the hands as flesh-colored to brown, exophytic, hyperkeratotic papules. Plantar warts may be quite painful; they can be differentiated from calluses by paring of the surface to reveal thrombosed capillaries. Flat warts (verruca plana) are most common among children and occur on the face, neck, chest, and flexor surfaces of the forearms and legs.

Anogenital warts develop on the skin and mucosal surfaces of the external genitalia and perianal areas. In men, warts are found most frequently at the frenum or coronal sulcus but may affect any part of the penis. They occur commonly at the urethral meatus and may extend proximally. Perianal warts are common among homosexual men but develop in heterosexual men as well. In women, warts appear first at the posterior introitus and adjacent labia. They then spread to other parts of the vulva and commonly involve the vagina and cervix. These lesions may be present without external warts. The differential diagnosis of anogenital warts includes condylomata lata of secondary syphilis, molluscum contagiosum, hirsutoid papillomatosis (pearly penile papules), fibroepitheliomas, and a variety of benign and malignant mucocutaneous neoplasms. Respiratory papillomatosis in young children may be life-threatening and presents as hoarseness, stridor, or respiratory distress. The disease in adults is usually mild.

Immunosuppressed patients, particularly those undergoing organ transplantation, often develop pityriasis versicolor–like lesions, from which DNA of several HPV types has been extracted. Occasionally, such lesions appear to undergo malignant transformation. Patients infected with human immunodeficiency virus (HIV) frequently have severe clinical manifestations of HPV infection and appear to be at unusually high risk for cervical and anal malignancies. HPV disease in patients with HIV infection is difficult to treat and often recurs.

Epidermodysplasia verruciformis is a rare autosomal recessive disease characterized by the inability to control HPV infection. Patients are often infected with unusual HPV types and frequently develop cutaneous squamous cell malignancies, particularly in sun-exposed areas. The lesions resemble flat warts or macules similar to those of pityriasis versicolor.

The complications of warts include itching and occasionally bleeding. In rare cases warts become secondarily infected with bacteria or fungi. Large masses of warts may cause mechanical problems, such as obstruction of the birth canal. Dysplasias of the uterine cervix are generally asymptomatic until frank carcinoma develops.

PATHOGENESIS The incubation period of HPV disease is usually 3 to 4 months, with a range of 1 month to 2 years. All types of squamous epithelium can be infected by HPV, and the gross and histologic appearances of individual lesions vary with the site of infection and the type of virus. The replication of HPV begins with the infection of basal cells. As cellular differentiation proceeds, HPV DNA replicates and is transcribed. Ultimately, virions are assembled in the nucleus and released when keratinocytes are shed. This process is associated with proliferation of all epidermal layers except the basal layer and produces acanthosis, parakeratosis, and hyperkeratosis. Koilocytes, large round cells with pyknotic nuclei, appear in the granular layer. Histologically normal epithelium may contain HPV DNA, and residual DNA after treatment can be associated with recurrent disease.

Episomal HPV DNA is present in the nuclei of infected cells in benign lesions caused by the virus. However, in severe dysplasias and cancers, HPV DNA is generally integrated, with disruption of the E1/E2 open reading frames. This disruption leads to upregulation of E6 and E7 and subsequent interference with cellular tumor suppressor proteins.

Host defense responses to HPV infection are incompletely understood, and immune correlates of protection from infection and resolution of disease have not been established. Because patients with defects in cell-mediated immune responses, including transplant recipients and patients with HIV infection, frequently develop severe HPV disease, such responses are probably important for the control of virus replication. Histologic studies demonstrating an epidermal lymphomonocytic infiltrate in resolving warts suggest that local immunity may be of particular importance in the resolution of disease. HPV infection can also elicit a serologic response, and antibodies to the viral capsid have been found in sera from patients with anogenital warts, cutaneous warts, and respiratory papillomatosis. Antibodies to E-region proteins, most notably E7, have been detected among patients with cervical carcinoma. Vaccine studies in animals have shown that the production of neutralizing antibodies can be associated with protection from papillomavirus infection.

DIAGNOSIS Most warts that are visible to the naked eye can be diagnosed correctly by history and physical examination alone. The use of a colposcope is invaluable in assessing vaginal and cervical lesions and is helpful in the diagnosis of oral and cutaneous HPV disease as well. Papanicolaou smears prepared from cervical scrapings often show cytologic evidence of HPV infection. Persistent or atypical lesions should be biopsied and examined by routine histologic methods. The most sensitive and specific methods of virologic diagnosis entail the use of techniques such as the polymerase chain reaction or the hybrid capture assay to detect HPV nucleic acids and to identify specific virus types. Serologic techniques to diagnose HPV infection are in the early stages of development and are not yet widely available.

℞ **TREATMENT**

Decisions regarding the initiation of therapy should be made with the knowledge that currently available modes of treatment are not completely effective and some have significant side effects. In addition, treatment may be expensive, and many HPV lesions resolve spontaneously. Frequently used therapies include cryosurgery, application of caustic agents, electrodesiccation, surgical excision, and ablation with a laser. Topical antimetabolites such as 5-fluorouracil also have been used. Both failure and recurrence have been well documented with all of these methods of treatment. Cryosurgery is the initial treatment of choice for condyloma acuminatum. Topically applied podophyllum preparations as well as podofilox may also be used. Various interferon preparations have been employed with modest success in the treatment of respiratory papillomatosis and condyloma acuminatum. A topically applied interferon inducer, imiquimod, appears to be of benefit in the treatment of condyloma

acuminatum. The diagnosis and management of anogenital dysplasias and of internal anogenital warts require special skills and resources, and patients with such lesions should be referred to a qualified specialist.

No effective methods for the prevention of HPV infections are available at present other than the avoidance of contact with infectious lesions. Barrier methods of contraception may be helpful in preventing the transmission of condyloma acuminatum and other HPV-associated diseases of the genital tract. Vaccine preparations including virus-like particles have shown promise in the prevention of papillomavirus infection and disease in some animal models.

BIBLIOGRAPHY

BONNEZ W et al: A randomized, double-blind, placebo-controlled trial of systemically administered alpha-, beta-, or gamma-interferon in combination with cryotherapy for the treatment of condyloma acuminatum. J Infect Dis 171:1081, 1995
———— et al: Current and future approaches to the treatment of condylomata acuminata (anogenital warts), in *Principles and Practice of Infectious Diseases Updates*, GL Mandell et al (eds). New York, Churchill Livingstone, 1996, vol 4, no 2
BOSCH FX et al: Prevalence of human papillomavirus in cervical cancer: A worldwide perspective. J Natl Cancer Inst 87:796, 1995
CARTER JJ et al: Use of human papillomavirus type 6 capsids to detect antibodies in people with genital warts. J Infect Dis 172:11, 1995
HO GYF et al: Persistent genital human papillomavirus infection as a risk factor for persistent cervical dysplasia. J Natl Cancer Inst 87:1365, 1995
KJAER SK et al: Human papillomavirus—the most significant risk determinant of cervical intraepithelial neoplasia. Int J Cancer 65:601, 1996
ORTH G, ZUR HAUSEN H: General features: Infections of the anogenital tract, in *Encyclopedia of Virology*. 1994, pp 1013–1026
REICHMAN RC, BONNEZ W: Papillomaviruses, in *Mandell, Douglas and Bennett's Principles and Practice of Infectious Diseases*, 4th ed, GL Mandell et al (eds). New York, Churchill Livingstone, 1995
ROSE RC et al: Human papillomavirus type 11 (HPV-11) virus-like particles (VLPs) induce the formation of neutralizing antibodies and detect genital HPV-specific antibodies in human sera. J Gen Virol 75:2075, 1994
SCHIFFMAN MH: Epidemiology of cervical human papillomavirus infections. Curr Top Microbiol Immunol 186:55, 1994
————, BRINTON LA: The epidemiology of cervical carcinogenesis. Cancer 76:1888, 1995
SUZICH JA et al: Systemic immunization with papillomavirus L1 protein completely prevents the development of viral mucosal papillomas. Proc Natl Acad Sci USA 92:11553, 1995

Section 13

DNA AND RNA RESPIRATORY VIRUSES

191 *Raphael Dolin*

COMMON VIRAL RESPIRATORY INFECTIONS

GENERAL CONSIDERATIONS Acute viral respiratory illnesses are among the most common of human diseases, accounting for one-half or more of all acute illnesses. The incidence of acute respiratory disease in the United States is from 3 to 5.6 cases per person per year. The rates are highest among children under 1 year old (6.1 to 8.3 cases per year) and remain high until age 6, when a progressive decrease begins. Adults have 3 to 4 cases per person per year. Morbidity from acute respiratory illnesses accounts for 30 to 50 percent of time lost from work by adults and for 60 to 80 percent of time lost from school by children.

It has been estimated that two-thirds to three-fourths of cases of acute respiratory illnesses are caused by viruses. More than 200 antigenically distinct viruses from 8 different genera have been reported to cause acute respiratory illness, and it is likely that additional

agents will be described in the future. The vast majority of these viral infections involve the upper respiratory tract, but lower respiratory tract disease can also develop, particularly in younger age groups and in certain epidemiologic settings.

The illnesses caused by respiratory viruses traditionally have been divided into multiple distinct syndromes, such as the "common cold," pharyngitis, croup (laryngotracheobronchitis), tracheitis, bronchiolitis, bronchitis, and pneumonia. Each of these general categories of illnesses has a certain epidemiologic and clinical profile; for example, croup occurs exclusively in very young children and has a characteristic clinical course. Some types of respiratory illnesses are more likely to be associated with certain viruses (e.g., the common cold with rhinoviruses), while others occupy characteristic epidemiologic niches (e.g., adenovirus infections in military recruits). The syndromes most commonly associated with infections with the major respiratory virus groups are summarized in Table 191-1. Most respiratory viruses clearly have the potential to cause more than one type of respiratory illness, and frequently features of several types of illness are found in the same patient. Moreover, the clinical illnesses induced by these viruses are rarely sufficiently distinctive to permit an etiologic diagnosis on

Table 191-1

CHAPTER 191
Common Viral Respiratory Infections **1101**

Illnesses Associated with Respiratory Viruses

Virus	Frequency of Respiratory Syndromes		
	Most Frequent	Occasional	Infrequent
Rhinoviruses	Common cold	Exacerbation of chronic bronchitis and asthma	Pneumonia in children
Coronaviruses	Common cold	Exacerbation of chronic bronchitis and asthma	Pneumonia and bronchiolitis
Respiratory syncytial virus	Pneumonia and bronchiolitis in young children	Common cold in adults	Pneumonia in elderly and immunosuppressed patients
Parainfluenza viruses	Croup and lower respiratory tract disease in young children	Pharyngitis and common cold	Tracheobronchitis in adults; lower respiratory tract disease in immunosuppressed patients
Adenoviruses	Common cold and pharyngitis in children	Outbreaks of acute respiratory disease in military recruits*	Pneumonia in children; lower respiratory tract and disseminated disease in immunosuppressed patients
Influenza A viruses	Influenza-like illness†	Pneumonia and excess mortality in high-risk patients	Pneumonia in healthy individuals
Influenza B viruses	Influenza-like illness†	Rhinitis and pharyngitis alone	Pneumonia
Enteroviruses	Acute undifferentiated febrile illnesses‡	Rhinitis and pharyngitis	Pneumonia
Herpes simplex viruses	Gingivostomatitis in children; pharyngotonsillitis in adults	Tracheitis and pneumonia in immunocompromised patients	Disseminated infection in immunocompromised patients

* Serotypes 4 and 7.
† Fever, cough, myalgia, malaise.
‡ May or may not have a respiratory component.

clinical grounds alone, although the epidemiologic setting increases the likelihood that one group of viruses rather than another is involved. In general, laboratory methods must be relied on to establish a specific viral diagnosis.

This chapter reviews viral infections caused by five of the major groups of respiratory viruses: rhinoviruses, coronaviruses, respiratory syncytial viruses, parainfluenza viruses, and adenoviruses. Influenza viruses, which are a major cause of mortality as well as morbidity, are reviewed in Chap. 193. Herpesviruses, which occasionally cause pharyngitis and which also cause lower respiratory tract disease in immunosuppressed patients, are reviewed in Chap. 184. Enteroviruses, which account for occasional respiratory illnesses during the summer months, are reviewed in Chap. 195.

RHINOVIRUS INFECTIONS

ETIOLOGIC AGENT Rhinoviruses are members of the Picornaviridae family, small (15 to 30 nm) nonenveloped viruses that contain a single-stranded RNA genome. In contrast to other members of the picornavirus family, such as enteroviruses, rhinoviruses are acid-labile and are almost completely inactivated at pH 3 or lower. Rhinoviruses grow preferentially at 33 to 34°C—the temperature of the human nasal passages—rather than at the higher temperature (37°C) of the lower respiratory tract. One hundred distinct serotypes and one subtype of rhinovirus are recognized.

EPIDEMIOLOGY Rhinoviruses are a major cause of the common cold and have been isolated from 15 to 40 percent of adults with common cold–like illnesses. Overall rates of infection with rhinoviruses are higher among infants and young children and decrease with increasing age. Rhinovirus infections occur throughout the year, with seasonal peaks in early fall and spring in temperate climates. Rhinovirus infections are most often introduced into families by preschool or grade-school children younger than 6 years old. Between 25 and 70 percent of initial illnesses in family settings are followed by secondary cases, with the highest attack rates among the youngest siblings at home. Attack rates also increase with family size.

Rhinoviruses appear to spread via direct contact with infected secretions, usually respiratory droplets. In some studies of volunteers, transmission was most efficient by hand-to-hand contact, with subsequent self-inoculation of the conjunctival or nasal mucosa. In other studies, transmission by large- or small-particle aerosol was demonstrated. Virus also can be recovered from plastic surfaces inoculated 1 to 3 h previously; this observation suggests that environmental surfaces contribute to transmission. In studies of married couples in which neither partner had detectable serum antibody, transmission was associated with prolonged contact (122 h or more) during a 7-day period. Transmission was infrequent unless virus was recoverable from the donor's hands and nasal mucosa, at least 1000 $TCID_{50}$ of virus was present in nasal washes from the donor, and the donor was at least moderately symptomatic with the "cold." Despite anecdotal observations, exposure to cold temperatures, fatigue, or sleep deprivation has not been associated with increased rates of rhinovirus-induced illness in volunteers.

Infection with rhinoviruses is worldwide in distribution. By the time they reach adulthood, nearly all individuals have neutralizing antibodies to multiple serotypes, although the prevalence of antibody to any one serotype varies widely. Multiple serotypes circulate simultaneously, and generally no single serotype or group of serotypes has been more prevalent than the others.

PATHOGENESIS Rhinoviruses infect cells via attachment to specific cellular receptors; the major group of such receptors has been identified as intercellular adhesion molecule 1 (ICAM-1). Relatively limited information is available on the histopathology and pathogenesis of acute rhinovirus infections in humans. Examination of biopsy specimens obtained during experimentally induced and naturally occurring illness indicates that the nasal mucosa is edematous, is often hyperemic, and—during acute illness—is covered by a mucoid discharge. There is a mild infiltrate with inflammatory cells, including neutrophils, lymphocytes, plasma cells, and eosinophils. Mucus-secreting glands in the submucosa appear hyperactive; the nasal turbinates are engorged, a condition that may lead to obstruction of nearby openings of sinus cavities.

The incubation period for rhinovirus illness is short, generally 1 or 2 days. Virus shedding coincides with the onset of illness or may begin shortly before symptoms develop. The mechanisms of immunity to rhinovirus are not well worked out. In some studies, the presence of homotypic antibody has been associated with significantly reduced rates of subsequent infection and illness, but data conflict regarding the relative importance of serum and local antibody in protection from rhinovirus infection.

CLINICAL MANIFESTATIONS The most common clinical manifestations of rhinovirus infections are those of the common cold. Initially, illness begins with rhinorrhea and sneezing accompanied by nasal congestion. The throat is frequently sore, and in some cases sore throat is the initial complaint. Systemic signs and symptoms, such as malaise and headache, are mild or absent, and fever is unusual. Illness generally lasts for 4 to 9 days and resolves spontaneously without sequelae. In children, bronchitis, bronchiolitis, and bronchopneumonia have been reported; nevertheless, it appears that rhinoviruses are not major causes of lower respiratory tract disease in children. Rhinoviruses also may cause exacerbations of asthma and chronic pulmonary disease in adults. The vast majority of rhinovirus infections resolve without sequelae, but complications related to obstruction of the eustachian tubes or sinus ostia, including otitis media or acute sinusitis, can develop.

DIAGNOSIS   Although rhinoviruses are the most frequently recognized cause of the common cold, similar illnesses are caused by a variety of other viruses, and the etiologic diagnosis cannot be made on clinical grounds alone. Rather, rhinovirus infection is diagnosed by isolation of the virus from nasal washes or nasal secretions in tissue culture. In practice, this procedure is rarely undertaken because of the benign, self-limited nature of the illness. Given the many serotypes of rhinovirus, diagnosis by serum antibody tests is currently impractical. Likewise, common laboratory tests, such as white cell count and sedimentation rate, are not helpful.

℞ TREATMENT

Rhinovirus infections are generally mild and self-limited, so treatment is not necessary. Some patients may benefit from the use of analgesics and nasal decongestants, and reduction of activity is prudent in instances of significant discomfort or fatigability. Antibacterial agents should be used only if bacterial complications such as otitis media or sinusitis develop. Specific antiviral therapy is not available. Application of interferon sprays intranasally has been effective in the prophylaxis of rhinovirus infections but is also associated with local irritation of the nasal mucosa. Prevention of rhinovirus infection by antibodies directed against rhinovirus receptors or by the soluble purified receptors themselves is under study. Experimental vaccines to certain rhinovirus serotypes have been prepared, but their utility is questionable because of the myriad serotypes and the uncertainty regarding mechanisms of immunity. Thorough hand washing, environmental decontamination, and protection against autoinoculation may help to reduce rates of transmission of infection.

CORONAVIRUS INFECTIONS

ETIOLOGIC AGENT   Coronaviruses are pleomorphic, single-stranded RNA viruses that measure 80 to 160 nm in diameter. The name derives from the crownlike appearance produced by the club-shaped projections that stud the viral envelope. Three antigenically distinct coronavirus subgroups, designated B814, 229E, and OC43, have been isolated from humans. Coronaviruses are fastidious and are difficult to culture in vitro. Some strains will grow only in human tracheal organ cultures rather than in tissue culture.

EPIDEMIOLOGY   Only limited seroepidemiologic studies of coronavirus infections have been conducted. Seroprevalence studies of two strains, 229E and OC43, have demonstrated the presence of serum antibodies at rates ranging from 12 percent to more than 80 percent in various populations. Overall, coronaviruses account for 10 to 20 percent of common colds. Coronavirus infections appear to be particularly prevalent in late fall, winter, and early spring—an interval when rhinovirus infections are less common. A cyclical pattern has been suggested for outbreaks of infection with strains OC43 and 229E, with outbreaks occurring every 2 to 4 years.

CLINICAL FEATURES   The clinical features of illness caused by coronaviruses are similar to those of illness caused by rhinoviruses. In studies of volunteers, the mean incubation period of illness induced by coronaviruses (3 days) is somewhat longer than that of illness caused by rhinoviruses, and the duration of illness is somewhat shorter (mean, 6 to 7 days). In some studies, the amount of nasal discharge was somewhat greater in colds induced by coronaviruses than in those

induced by rhinoviruses. Coronaviruses have been recovered from infants with pneumonia and from military recruits with lower respiratory tract disease and have been associated with worsening of chronic bronchitis. However, the overall significance of coronaviruses in lower respiratory tract disease in humans remains unclear.

℞ TREATMENT

The approach to the treatment of common colds caused by coronaviruses is similar to that discussed above for rhinovirus-induced illnesses. Because of uncertainty regarding the number and relative importance of coronavirus subgroups and the mechanisms of immunity, vaccines against coronaviruses have not been developed.

RESPIRATORY SYNCYTIAL VIRUS INFECTIONS

ETIOLOGIC AGENT   Respiratory syncytial virus (RSV) is a member of the Paramyxoviridae family and comprises the genus *Pneumovirus*. RSV, an enveloped virus approximately 150 to 300 nm in diameter, is so named because its replication leads to the fusion of neighboring cells into large multinucleated syncytia. The single-stranded RNA genome codes for 10 virus-specific proteins. Viral RNA is contained in a helical nucleocapsid surrounded by a lipid envelope bearing two glycoproteins: the G protein, by which the virus attaches to cells, and the F (fusion) protein, which facilitates entry of the virus into the cell by fusing host and viral membranes. RSV was once considered to be of a single antigenic type, but two distinct groups (A and B) and multiple subtypes within each group have now been described. The epidemiologic and clinical significance of subtype differences is being investigated.

EPIDEMIOLOGY   RSV is the major respiratory pathogen of young children and the foremost cause of lower respiratory disease in infants. Infection with RSV is seen throughout the world in annual epidemics that occur in late fall, winter, or spring and that last up to 5 months. The virus is rarely encountered during the summer. Rates of illness are highest among infants between 1 and 6 months of age, peaking between 2 and 3 months of age. The attack rates among susceptible infants and children are extraordinarily high, approaching 100 percent in settings such as day-care centers where large numbers of susceptible infants are present. RSV accounts for 20 to 25 percent of hospital admissions of young infants and children for pneumonia and for up to 75 percent of cases of bronchiolitis in this age group. It has been estimated that more than half of infants who are at risk will become infected during an RSV epidemic.

In older children and adults, reinfection with RSV is frequent but disease is milder than in infancy. A common cold–like syndrome is the illness most commonly associated with RSV infection in adults. Severe lower respiratory tract disease with pneumonitis can occur in elderly (often institutionalized) adults and in patients with immuno-compromising disorders or treatment, including recipients of bone-marrow and solid-organ transplants. RSV is also an important nosocomial pathogen; during an outbreak; it can infect pediatric patients and up to 25 to 50 percent of the staff on pediatric wards. The spread of virus among families is efficient: up to 40 percent of siblings may become infected when RSV is introduced into the family setting.

RSV is transmitted primarily by close contact with contaminated fingers or fomites and by self-inoculation of the conjunctiva or anterior nares. Virus also may be spread by coarse aerosols produced by coughing or sneezing, but it is inefficiently spread by fine-particle aerosols. The incubation period of illness is approximately 4 to 6 days, and virus shedding may last for 2 weeks or longer in children and for shorter periods of time in adults.

PATHOGENESIS   Little is known about the histopathology of minor RSV infection. Severe bronchiolitis or pneumonia is characterized by necrosis of the bronchiolar epithelium and a peribronchiolar infiltrate of lymphocytes and mononuclear cells. Interalveolar thickening and filling of alveolar spaces with fluid can also be found. The characteristics of the immune response to RSV are not well elucidated. Because reinfection occurs frequently and is often associated with illness, the immunity that develops after single episodes of infection obviously is not complete or long-lasting. However, the cumulative effect of multiple reinfections is to temper subsequent disease and to provide some temporary measure of protection against infection. Studies of experimentally induced disease in healthy volunteers indicate that the presence of nasal IgA neutralizing antibody correlates more closely with protection than does the presence of serum antibody. Studies in infants, however, suggest that maternally acquired antibody provides some protection from lower respiratory tract disease, although illness can be severe even in infants who have moderate levels of maternally derived serum antibody. The relatively severe disease observed in immunosuppressed patients and experimental animal models indicates that cell-mediated immunity is an important mechanism of host defense against RSV.

CLINICAL MANIFESTATIONS RSV infection leads to a wide spectrum of respiratory illnesses. In infants, 25 to 40 percent of infections result in lower respiratory tract involvement, including pneumonia, bronchiolitis, and tracheobronchitis. In this age group, illness begins most frequently with rhinorrhea, low-grade fever, and mild systemic symptoms, often accompanied by cough and wheezing. Most patients recover gradually over 1 to 2 weeks. In more severe illness, tachypnea and dyspnea develop, and eventually frank hypoxia, cyanosis, and apnea can ensue. Physical examination may reveal diffuse wheezing, rhonchi, and rales. Chest radiography shows hyperexpansion, peribronchial thickening, and variable infiltrates ranging from diffuse interstitial infiltrates to segmental or lobar consolidation. Illness may be particularly severe in children born prematurely and in those with congenital cardiac disease, bronchopulmonary dysplasia, nephrotic syndrome, or immunosuppression. One study documented a 37 percent mortality rate for infants with RSV pneumonia and congenital cardiac disease.

In adults, the most common symptoms of RSV infection are those of the common cold, with rhinorrhea, sore throat, and cough. Illness is occasionally associated with moderate systemic symptoms such as malaise, headache, and fever. RSV also has been reported to cause lower respiratory tract disease with fever in adults, including severe pneumonia in the elderly. RSV pneumonia can be a significant cause of morbidity and mortality in patients (particularly children) undergoing bone-marrow and solid-organ transplantation.

LABORATORY FINDINGS AND DIAGNOSIS The diagnosis of RSV infection can be suspected on the basis of a suggestive epidemiologic setting—that is, severe illness among infants during an outbreak of RSV in the community. Infections in older children and adults cannot be differentiated with certainty from those caused by other respiratory viruses. The specific diagnosis is established by isolation of RSV from respiratory secretions, including sputum, throat swabs, or nasopharyngeal washes. Virus is detected in tissue culture and is identified specifically through immunologic reactions detected by immunofluorescence, enzyme-linked immunosorbent assay (ELISA), or other techniques. Immunofluorescence microscopy of nasal scrapings or washings provides a rapid diagnosis. Serologic tests that depend on fourfold or greater rises in complement-fixing or neutralizing antibody titers are useful for diagnosis in older children and adults but are less sensitive in children under 4 months of age. ELISA is more sensitive than complement-fixation or neutralization tests in the detection of serum antibody. Serologic diagnosis requires comparison of acute- and convalescent-phase serum specimens and is therefore not useful during acute illness.

℞ TREATMENT

Treatment of upper respiratory tract RSV infection is aimed primarily at the alleviation of symptoms and is similar to that for other viral infections of the upper respiratory tract. For lower respiratory tract infections, respiratory therapy, including hydration, suctioning of secretions, and administration of humidified oxygen and antibronchospastic agents, is given as needed. In severe hypoxia, intubation and ventilatory assistance may be required. Studies of infants with RSV infection who were given aerosolized ribavirin, a nucleoside analogue active in vitro against RSV, have demonstrated a beneficial effect on the resolution of lower respiratory tract illness, including alleviation of blood-gas abnormalities. No similar studies have been performed in adults with RSV pneumonitis, and the benefit of ribavirin in these patients is unknown. Immunoglobulins with high titers of antibodies to RSV conferred protection against severe lower respiratory tract disease when administered to infants at high risk for complications of RSV infection in a multicenter trial. This approach is undergoing further study.

Considerable interest exists in the development of vaccines against RSV. Inactivated whole-virus vaccines have been ineffective; in one study, they actually potentiated the disease in infants. Other approaches include immunization with purified F and G surface glycoproteins of RSV or generation of stable, live attenuated virus vaccines. In settings such as pediatric wards where rates of transmission are high, barrier methods for the protection of hands and conjunctivae may be useful in reducing the spread of virus.

PARAINFLUENZA VIRUS INFECTIONS

ETIOLOGIC AGENT Parainfluenza viruses are members of the Paramyxoviridae family and comprise the genus *Paramyxovirus*. Parainfluenza viruses are 150 to 250 nm in diameter, are enveloped, and contain a single-stranded RNA genome. The envelope is studded with two glycoproteins: one possessing both hemagglutinin and neuraminidase activity and the other containing fusion activity. The viral RNA genome is enclosed in a helical nucleocapsid and codes for seven or eight virus-specific proteins. All four distinct serotypes of parainfluenza viruses share certain antigens with other members of the Paramyxoviridae family, including mumps and Newcastle disease viruses.

EPIDEMIOLOGY Parainfluenza viruses are distributed throughout the world, although infection with type 4 (subtypes 4A and 4B) has been reported less widely, probably because type 4 is more difficult to grow in tissue culture. Infection is acquired in early childhood, so that by 8 years of age most children have antibodies to serotypes 1, 2, and 3. Types 1 and 2 cause epidemics during the fall, primarily in odd-numbered years. Type 3 infection has been detected during all seasons of the year, but epidemics have occurred annually in the spring.

The contribution of parainfluenza infections to respiratory disease varies with both the location and the year. In studies conducted in the United States, parainfluenza virus infections accounted for 4.3 to 22 percent of respiratory illnesses in children. In adults, parainfluenza infections are generally mild and account for fewer than 5 percent of respiratory illnesses. The major importance of parainfluenza viruses is as a cause of respiratory illness in young children, in whom they rank second only to RSV as causes of lower respiratory tract illness. Parainfluenza virus type 1 is the most frequent cause of croup (laryngotracheobronchitis) in children, while serotype 2 causes similar, although generally less severe, disease. Type 3 is an important cause of bronchiolitis and pneumonia in infants, while illnesses associated with type 4 have generally been mild. Unlike types 1 and 2, type 3 frequently causes illness during the first month of life, while passively acquired maternal antibody is still present. Parainfluenza viruses are spread through infected respiratory secretions, primarily by person-to-person contact and/or by large droplets. The incubation period has varied from 3 to 6 days in experimental infections but may be somewhat shorter for naturally occurring disease in children.

PATHOGENESIS Immunity to parainfluenza viruses is incompletely understood, but evidence suggests that immunity to infections with serotypes 1 and 2 is mediated by local IgA antibodies in the respiratory tract. Passively acquired serum neutralizing antibodies also confer some protection against infection with types 1, 2, and—to a lesser degree—3. Studies in experimental animal models and in immunosuppressed patients suggest that cell-mediated immunity may also be important in parainfluenza virus infections.

CLINICAL MANIFESTATIONS Parainfluenza virus infections occur most frequently among children, in whom initial infection with serotype 1, 2, or 3 is associated with an acute febrile illness 50 to 80 percent of the time. Children may present with coryza, sore throat, hoarseness, and cough that may or may not be croupy. In severe croup, fever persists, with worsening coryza and sore throat. A brassy or barking cough may progress to frank stridor. Most children recover over the next 1 or 2 days, although progressive airway obstruction and hypoxia ensue occasionally. If bronchiolitis or pneumonia develops, progressive cough accompanied by wheezing, tachypnea, and intercostal retractions may occur. In this setting, sputum production increases modestly. Physical examination shows nasopharyngeal discharge and oropharyngeal injection, along with rhonchi, wheezes, or coarse breath sounds. Chest x-rays can show air trapping and occasionally interstitial infiltrates.

In older children and adults, parainfluenza infections tend to be milder, presenting most frequently as a common cold or as hoarseness, with or without cough. Lower respiratory tract involvement in older children and adults is uncommon, but tracheobronchitis in adults has been reported. Severe, prolonged, and even fatal parainfluenza infection has been reported in children and adults with severe immunosuppression, including bone-marrow and solid-organ transplant recipients.

LABORATORY FINDINGS AND DIAGNOSIS Like other respiratory viral diseases, the clinical syndromes caused by parainfluenza viruses (with the possible exception of croup in young children) are not sufficiently distinctive to be diagnosed on clinical grounds alone. A specific diagnosis is established by detection of virus in respiratory tract secretions, throat swabs, or nasopharyngeal washings. Virus is detected by growth in tissue culture, either by hemagglutination or by a cytopathic effect, or by immunofluorescence of viral antigens in exfoliated cells from the respiratory tract. Serologic diagnosis is based on a fourfold or greater rise in antibody titer, as detected by hemagglutination inhibition or by complement-fixation or neutralization tests in acute- and convalescent-phase specimens. However, as frequent heterotypic responses occur among the parainfluenza serotypes, the serotype causing illness often cannot be identified by serologic techniques alone.

Acute epiglottitis caused by *Haemophilus influenzae* type b must be differentiated from viral croup. Influenza A virus also is a common cause of croup during epidemic periods.

℞ **TREATMENT**

For upper respiratory tract illness, symptoms can be treated as discussed for other viral respiratory tract illnesses. If complications such as sinusitis, otitis, or superimposed bacterial bronchitis develop, appropriate antibiotics should be administered. Mild cases of croup should be treated with bed rest and moist air generated by vaporizers. More severe cases require hospitalization and close observation for the development of respiratory distress. If acute respiratory distress develops, humidified oxygen and intermittent racemic epinephrine are usually administered. High-dose systemic glucocorticoids also may be of benefit. No specific antiviral therapy is available, although ribavirin is active against parainfluenza viruses in vitro and is being evaluated clinically. Effective vaccines against parainfluenza viruses have not been developed.

ADENOVIRUS INFECTIONS

ETIOLOGIC AGENT Adenoviruses are complex DNA viruses that measure 70 to 80 nm in diameter. Human adenoviruses belong to the genus *Mastadenovirus*, which includes at least 47 serotypes. Adenoviruses have a characteristic morphology consisting of an icosahedral shell composed of 20 equilateral triangular faces and 12 vertices. The protein coat (capsid) consists of hexon subunits with group-specific and type-specific antigenic determinants and penton subunits at each vertex primarily containing group-specific antigens. A fiber with a knob at the end projects from each penton; this fiber contains type-specific and some group-specific antigens. Human adenoviruses have been divided into six subgenera (A through F) on the basis of the homology of DNA genomes and other properties. The adenovirus genome is a linear double-stranded DNA that codes for structural and nonstructural polypeptides. The replicative cycle of adenovirus may result either in lytic infection of cells or in the establishment of a latent infection (primarily involving lymphoid cells). Some adenovirus types can induce oncogenic transformation, and tumor formation has been observed in rodents; however, despite intensive investigation, adenoviruses have not been associated with tumors in humans.

EPIDEMIOLOGY Adenovirus infections most frequently affect infants and children. Infections occur throughout the year but are most common from fall to spring. Adenoviruses account for 3 to 5 percent of acute respiratory infections in children but for fewer than 2 percent of respiratory illnesses in civilian adults. Nearly 100 percent of adults have serum antibody to multiple serotypes—a finding indicating that infection is common in childhood. Types 1, 2, 3, and 5 are the most frequent isolates from children. Certain adenovirus serotypes—particularly 4 and 7 but also 3, 14, and 21—are associated with outbreaks of acute respiratory disease in military recruits in winter and spring. Adenovirus infection can be transmitted by inhalation of aerosolized virus, by inoculation of virus into conjunctival sacs, and probably by the fecal-oral route as well. Type-specific antibody generally develops after infection and is associated with protection against infection with the same serotype.

CLINICAL MANIFESTATIONS In children, adenoviruses cause a variety of clinical syndromes. The most common is an acute upper respiratory tract infection, with prominent rhinitis. On occasion, lower respiratory tract disease, including bronchiolitis and pneumonia, also develops. Adenoviruses, particularly types 3 and 7, cause pharyngoconjunctival fever, a characteristic acute febrile illness of children that occurs in outbreaks, most often in summer camps. The syndrome is marked by bilateral conjunctivitis in which the bulbar and palpebral conjunctivae have a granular appearance. Low-grade fever is frequently present for the first 3 to 5 days, and rhinitis, sore throat, and cervical adenopathy develop. The illness generally lasts for 1 to 2 weeks and resolves spontaneously. Febrile pharyngitis without conjunctivitis also has been associated with adenovirus infection. Adenoviruses have been isolated from cases of whooping cough with or without *Bordetella pertussis;* the significance of adenovirus in that disease is unknown.

In adults, the most frequently reported illness has been acute respiratory disease caused by adenovirus types 4 and 7 in military recruits. This illness is marked by a prominent sore throat and the gradual onset of fever, which often reaches 39°C on the second or third day of illness. Cough is almost always present, and coryza and regional lymphadenopathy are frequently seen. Physical examination may show pharyngeal edema, injection, and tonsillar enlargement with little or no exudate. If pneumonia has developed, auscultation and x-ray of the chest may indicate areas of patchy infiltration.

Adenoviruses have been associated with a number of non–respiratory tract diseases, including acute diarrheal illness caused by adenovirus types 40 and 41 in young children and hemorrhagic cystitis caused by adenoviruses 11 and 21. Epidemic keratoconjunctivitis, caused most frequently by adenovirus types 8, 19, and 37, has been associated with contaminated common sources such as ophthalmic solutions and roller towels. Adenoviruses also have been implicated in disseminated disease and pneumonia in immunosuppressed patients, including patients with AIDS and recipients of solid-organ or bone-marrow transplants.

LABORATORY FINDINGS AND DIAGNOSIS Adenovirus infection should be suspected in the epidemiologic setting of acute respiratory disease and in certain of the clinical syndromes (such as pharyngoconjunctival fever or epidemic keratoconjunctivitis) in which outbreaks of characteristic illnesses occur. In most cases, however, illnesses caused by adenovirus infection cannot be differentiated from those caused by a number of other viral respiratory agents and *Mycoplasma pneumoniae.* A definitive diagnosis of adenovirus infection is established by culture or detection of the virus from sites such as the conjunctiva and oropharynx or from sputum, urine, or stool. Virus may be detected in tissue culture by cytopathic changes and specifically identified by immunofluorescence or other immunologic techniques. Adenovirus types 40 and 41, which have been associated with diarrheal disease in children, require special tissue-culture cells for isolation, and these serotypes are most commonly detected by direct ELISA of stool. Serum antibody rises can be demonstrated by complement-fixation or neutralization tests, ELISA, or radioimmunoassay. Hemagglutination inhibition tests also may be done for those adenoviruses that hemagglutinate red cells.

℞ TREATMENT

Only symptom-based treatment and supportive therapy are available for adenovirus infections, and no clinically useful antiviral compounds have been identified. Live vaccines have been developed against adenovirus types 4 and 7 and are widely used to control illness in military recruits. These vaccines consist of live, unattenuated virus administered in enteric-coated capsules. Infection of the gastrointestinal tract with types 4 and 7 does not cause disease but stimulates local and systemic antibodies that are protective against subsequent acute respiratory disease due to those serotypes. Vaccines prepared from purified subunits of adenovirus are being investigated.

BIBLIOGRAPHY

RHINOVIRUSES

GWALTNEY JM: Rhinoviruses, in *Principles and Practice of Infectious Diseases*, 4th ed, GF Mandell et al (eds). New York, Churchill Livingstone, 1995, pp 1656–1663

McKINLAY MA et al: Treatment of the picornavirus common cold by inhibitors of viral uncoating and attachment. Annu Rev Microbiol 46:635, 1992

ROSSMAN MG et al: Structure of a human common cold virus and functional relationships to other picornaviruses. Nature 317:145, 1985

TYRRELL DAJ: Common colds. Intervirology 25:177, 1986

CORONAVIRUSES

LARSON HE et al: Isolation of rhinoviruses and coronaviruses from 38 colds in adults. J Med Virol 5:221, 1980

McINTOSH K: Coronaviruses, in *Virology*, 3d ed, BN Fields (ed). New York, Raven, 1995, pp 1095–1103

MONTO AS: Medical reviews, coronaviruses. Yale J Biol Med 47:234, 1974

RESPIRATORY SYNCYTIAL VIRUS

ANDERSON LJ et al: Multicenter study of strains of respiratory syncytial virus. J Infect Dis 163:687, 1991

CHANOCK RM et al: Serious respiratory tract disease caused by respiratory syncytial virus: Prospects for improved therapy and effective immunization. Pediatrics 90:137, 1992

ENGLUND JA et al: Respiratory syncytial virus infection in immunocompromised adults. Ann Intern Med 109:203, 1988

GLEZEN WP et al: Risk of primary infection and reinfection with respiratory syncytial virus. Am J Dis Child 140:543, 1986

HALL CB et al: Aerosolized ribavirin treatment of infants with respiratory syncytial viral infection. A randomized double blind study. N Engl J Med 308:1443, 1983

HENDERSON FW et al: Respiratory syncytial virus infections, reinfections and immunity. N Engl J Med 300:530, 1979

PARAINFLUENZA VIRUSES

DENNY FW et al: Croup: An 11 year study in a pediatric practice. Pediatrics 71:871, 1983

HEILMAN CA: Respiratory syncytial and parainfluenza viruses. J Infect Dis 161:402, 1990

WRIGHT PF: Parainfluenzaviruses, in *Textbook of Human Virology*, 2d ed, RB Belshe (ed). St. Louis, Mosby, 1991, pp 342–350

ADENOVIRUSES

BAUM SG: Adenoviruses, in *Principles and Practice of Infectious Diseases*, 4th ed, G Mandell et al (eds). New York, Churchill Livingstone, 1995, pp 1382–1387

FOX JP et al: The Seattle virus watch. VII. Observations of adenovirus infections. Am J Epidemiol 105:362, 1977

HIERHOLZER JC: Adenoviruses in the immunocompromised host. Clin Microbiol Rev 5:262, 1992

ROSE HM et al: Adenoviral infection in military recruits. Arch Environ Health 21:356, 1970

SECTION 14
RNA VIRUSES

192   *Anthony S. Fauci, Dan L. Longo*

THE HUMAN RETROVIRUSES

The retroviruses, which make up a large family (Retroviridae), infect mainly vertebrates. They have a unique replication cycle whereby their genetic information is encoded by RNA rather than DNA. Retroviruses contain an RNA-dependent DNA polymerase (a reverse transcriptase) that directs the synthesis of a DNA form of the viral genome after infection of a host cell. The designation *retrovirus* denotes that information in the form of RNA is transcribed into DNA in the host cell—a sequence that overturned a central dogma of molecular biology: that information passes unidirectionally from DNA to RNA to protein. Interest in this class of viruses was stimulated by the pioneering studies of Peyton Rous, who in 1911 identified an agent that was transmissible and filterable (that is, smaller than a cell) and that produced sarcoma in chickens, and by those of Ludwig Gross, who in the 1950s demonstrated a viral etiology for murine leukemia. The observation that RNA was the source of genetic information in the causative agents of these and other animal tumors led to a number of paradigm-shifting biologic insights regarding not only the direction of genetic-information passage but also the viral etiology of certain cancers and the concept of oncogenes as normal host genes scavenged and altered by a viral vector.

The family Retroviridae includes three subfamilies (Table 192-1): Oncovirinae, of which human T-cell lymphotropic virus (HTLV) type I is the most important in humans; Lentivirinae, of which human immunodeficiency virus (HIV) is the most important in humans; and Spumavirinae, the "foamy" viruses, named for the pathologic appearance of infected cells. A number of spumaviruses have been isolated from humans; however, they are not associated with any known disease and therefore are not discussed further in this chapter.

The wide variety of interactions of a retrovirus with its host range from completely benign events (e.g., silent carriage of endogenous retroviral sequences in the germ-line genome of many animal species) to rapidly fatal infections (e.g., exogenous infection with an oncogenic virus such as Rous sarcoma virus in chickens). The ability of retroviruses to acquire and alter the structure and function of host cell sequences has revolutionized our understanding of molecular carcinogenesis. The viruses can insert into the germ-line genome of the host cell and behave as a transposable or movable genetic element. They can activate or inactivate genes near the site of integration into the genome. They can rapidly alter their own genome by recombination and mutation under selective environmental stimuli.

Most human viral diseases occur as a consequence of either tissue destruction by the virus itself or the host's response to the virus. Although these mechanisms are operative in retroviral infections, retroviruses have additional mechanisms of inducing disease, including the malignant transformation of an infected cell and the induction of an immunodeficiency state that leads to opportunistic diseases (infections and neoplasms).

STRUCTURE AND LIFE CYCLE Despite the wide range of biologic consequences of retroviral infection, all retroviruses are similar in structure, genome organization, and mode of replication. Retroviruses are 70 to 130 nm in diameter and have a lipid-containing envelope surrounding an icosahedral capsid with a dense inner core. The core contains two identical copies of the single-stranded RNA genome (rendering retroviruses diploid). The RNA molecules are 8 to 10 kb long and are complexed with reverse transcriptase and tRNA. Other viral proteins, such as integrase, are also components of the virion particle. The RNA has features usually found in mRNA: a cap site at the 5′ end of the molecule, which is important in the initiation of mRNA translation, and a polyadenylation site at the 3′ end, a feature that seems to influence mRNA turnover (i.e., messages with shorter polyA tails turn over faster than messages with longer polyA tails). However, the retroviral RNA is not translated; instead it is transcribed into DNA. The DNA form of the retroviral genome is called a *provirus*.

The replication cycle of retroviruses proceeds in two phases (Fig. 192-1). In the first phase, the virus enters the cytoplasm after binding to a specific cell-surface receptor; the viral RNA and reverse transcriptase synthesize a double-stranded DNA version of the RNA template; and the provirus moves into the nucleus and integrates into the host cell genome. This proviral integration is permanent. Although some animal retroviruses integrate into a single specific site of the host genome in every infected cell, the four known pathogenic human retroviruses (HLTV-I, HTLV-II, HIV-1, and HIV-2) integrate randomly. This first phase of replication depends entirely on gene products in the virus. The second phase includes the synthesis and processing of viral genomes, mRNAs, and proteins using host cell machinery, often under the influence of viral gene products. Virions are assembled and released from the cell by budding from the membrane; host cell membrane proteins are frequently incorporated into the envelope of the virus. Proviral integration occurs during the S phase of the cell cycle; thus, in general, nondividing cells are resistant to retroviral infection. Only the lentiviruses are able to infect nondividing cells. Once a host is infected, it is infected for life.

Retroviral genomes include both coding and noncoding sequences (Fig. 192-2). In general, noncoding sequences are important recognition signals for DNA or RNA synthesis or processing events and are located in the 5′ and 3′ terminal regions of the genome. All retroviral genomes are terminally redundant, containing identical sequences

called long terminal repeats (LTRs). The ends of the retroviral genome differ slightly in sequence from the integrated retroviral DNA. In the latter, the LTR sequences are repeated in both the 5′ and the 3′ terminus of the virus. The LTRs contain sequences involved in initiating the expression of the viral proteins, the integration of the provirus, and the polyadenylation of viral RNAs. The primer binding site, which is critical for the initiation of reverse transcription, and the viral packaging sequences are located outside the LTR sequences. The coding regions include the *gag* (group-specific antigen, core protein), *pol* (RNA-dependent DNA polymerase), and *env* (envelope) genes. The *gag* gene encodes a precursor polyprotein that is cleaved to form three to five capsid proteins; a fraction of the Gag precursor proteins also contain a protease responsible for cleaving the Gag and Pol polyproteins. A Gag-Pol polyprotein gives rise to the protease that is responsible for cleaving the Gag-Pol polyprotein. The *pol* gene encodes three proteins: the reverse transcriptase, the integrase, and the protease. The reverse transcriptase functions to copy the viral RNA into the double-stranded DNA provirus, which can attach to the host cell DNA via the action of integrase. The protease functions to cleave the Gag-Pol polyprotein into smaller protein products. The *env* gene encodes the envelope glycoproteins: one protein that binds to specific surface receptors and determines what cell types can be infected and a smaller transmembrane protein that anchors the complex to the envelope. The cartoon in Fig. 192-3 shows how the retroviral gene products make up the virus structure.

HTLVs have a region between *env* and the 3′ LTR that encodes at least two proteins in overlapping reading frames; Tax, a 40-kD protein that does not bind to DNA but induces the expression of host cell transcription factors that alter host cell gene expression; and Rex, a 27-kD protein that regulates the expression of viral mRNAs. These two proteins are produced from messages that are similar but that are spliced differently from overlapping but distinct exons.

The lentiviruses in general, and HIV-1 and -2 in particular, contain a larger genome than other pathogenic retroviruses; the size of this genome is related to the presence of an untranslated region between *pol* and *env* that encodes portions of several proteins, varying with the reading frame into which the mRNA is spliced. Tat is a 14-kD protein that augments the expression of virus from the LTR. The Rev protein regulates RNA splicing and/or RNA transport in HIV-1 and may function in a manner similar to the Rex protein of HTLV. The Nef protein appears to down-regulate CD4, the cellular receptor for HIV; to alter host T-cell activation pathways; and to enhance viral infectivity. The Vif protein is necessary for the proper assembly of the HIV nucleoprotein core in many types of cells; without Vif, proviral DNA is not efficiently produced in these infected cells. Vpr, Vpu (HIV-1 only), and Vpx (HIV-2 only) are viral proteins encoded by translation of the same message in different reading frames. As noted above, oncogenic retroviruses depend on cell proliferation for their replication; lentiviruses can infect nondividing cells, largely owing to effects mediated by Vpr. Vpr appears to facilitate transport of the provirus into the nucleus and can induce other cellular changes, such as G2 growth arrest and differentiation of some target cells. Vpx is structurally related to Vpr, but its functions are not fully defined. Vpu promotes the degradation of CD4 in the endoplasmic reticulum and stimulates the release of virions from infected cells.

Retroviruses can be either exogenously acquired by infection with a virion capable of replication or transmitted in the germ line as endogenous virus. Endogenous retroviruses are often replication-defective. The human genome contains endogenous retroviral se-

Table 192-1

Classification of Retroviruses: the Family Retroviridae

Subfamily	Group*	Example	Feature
Oncovirinae (oncogenic viruses)	Avian leukosis	Rous sarcoma virus	Contains *src* oncogene
	Mammalian C-type	Abelson leukemia virus	Contains *abl* oncogene
	B-type	Murine mammary tumor virus	Can be endogenous or exogenous
	D-type	Mason-Pfizer monkey virus	—
	HTLV-BLV	HTLV-I	Causes T-cell lymphoma and neurologic disease
Lentivirinae (slow viruses)	—	HIV-1, HIV-2	Causes AIDS
		Visna virus	Causes lung and brain diseases in sheep
		Feline immunodeficiency virus	Causes immunodeficiency in cats
Spumavirinae (foamy viruses)	—	Simian foamy virus, human foamy virus	Causes no known disease

Abbreviations: HTLV, human T-lymphotropic virus; BLV, bovine leukemia virus; HIV, human immunodeficiency virus.
* The Oncovirinae were originally grouped into types A–D on the basis of morphologic features (size, core location, budding) under electron microscopy; however, this system has been replaced by groupings based on relationships of genome structure and sequence.

quences, but there are no known replication-competent endogenous retroviruses in humans.

In general, viruses that contain only the *gag*, *pol*, and *env* genes either are not pathogenic or take a long time to induce disease because the pathogenesis of neoplastic transformation relies on the chance integration of the provirus at a spot in the genome that will result in the expression of a cellular gene (proto-oncogene) that becomes transforming by virtue of its unregulated expression. For example, avian leukosis virus causes B-cell leukemia by inducing the expression of *myc*. Some retroviruses possess captured and altered cellular genes near their integration site, and these viral oncogenes are capable of transforming the infected host cell. Viruses that have oncogenes often have lost a portion of their genome that is required for replication. Such viruses need helper viruses to reproduce, a feature that may explain why these acute transforming retroviruses are rare in nature. All human retroviruses identified to date are exogenous and are not acutely transforming (that is, they lack a transforming oncogene).

These remarkable properties of retroviruses have led to experimental efforts to use them as vectors to insert specific genes into particular cell types, a process known as *gene therapy* or *gene transfer*. The process could be used to repair a genetic defect or to introduce a new property that could be used therapeutically; for example, it could be possible to insert a gene (e.g., thymidine kinase) that would make a tumor cell susceptible to killing by a drug (e.g., ganciclovir). One source of concern about the use of retroviral vectors in humans is that replication-competent viruses might rescue endogenous retroviral replication, with unpredictable results. This concern is not merely hypothetical: The detection of proteins encoded by endogenous retroviral sequences on the surface of cancer cells implies that the genetic events leading to the cancer were able to activate the synthesis of these usually silent genes.

HUMAN T-CELL LYMPHOTROPIC VIRUS

HTLV-I was isolated in 1980 from a T-cell lymphoma cell line from a patient originally thought to have cutaneous T-cell lymphoma. Later it became clear that the patient had a distinct form of lymphoma (originally reported in Japan) called adult T-cell leukemia/lymphoma (ATL). Serologic data have determined that HTLV-I is the cause of at least two important diseases: ATL and tropical spastic paraparesis, also called HTLV-I–associated myelopathy (HAM).

Two years after the isolation of HTLV-I, HTLV-II was isolated from a patient with an unusual form of hairy cell leukemia that affected T cells. Although early epidemiologic studies of HTLV-II failed to reveal a consistent disease association, more recent studies suggest an association of HTLV-II with human disease (see "Associated Diseases"

under "Features of HTLV-II Infection" below), particularly among injection drug users.

BIOLOGY AND MOLECULAR BIOLOGY   Because the biology of HTLV-I and that of HTLV-II are similar and because these viruses are generally grouped together, the following discussion will focus on HTLV-I.

The cellular receptor for HTLV-I has not yet been identified, but it maps to chromosome 17. Generally, only T cells are productively infected, but infection of B cells and other cell types is occasionally detected. The most common outcome of HTLV-I infection is latent

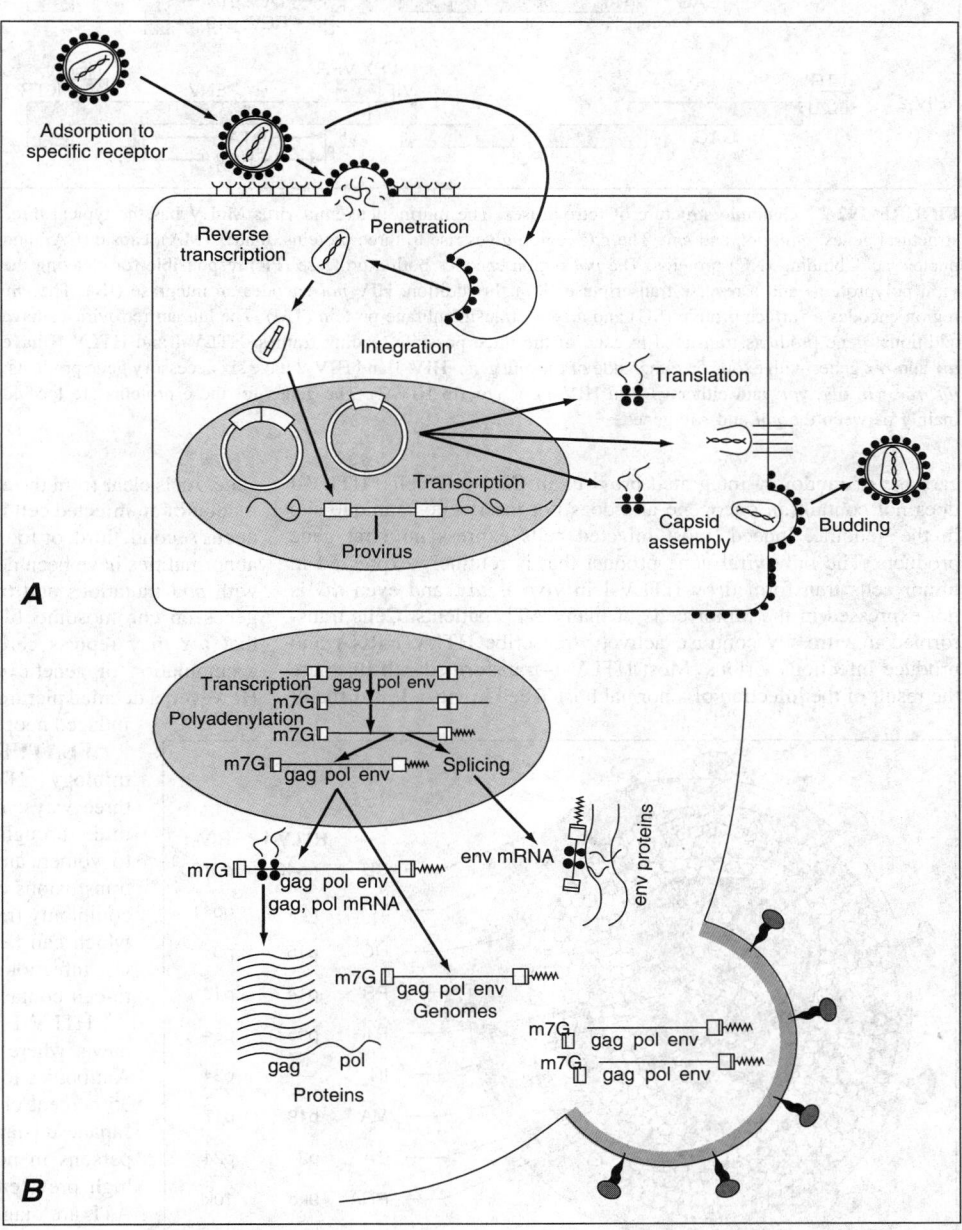

FIGURE 192-1   The life cycle of retroviruses. *A.* Overview of virus replication. The retrovirus enters a target cell by binding to a specific cell-surface receptor; once the virus is internalized, its RNA is released from the nucleocapsid and is reverse-transcribed into proviral DNA. The provirus is inserted into the genome and then transcribed into RNA; the RNA is translated; and virions assemble and are extruded from the cell membrane by budding. *B.* Overview of retroviral gene expression. The provirus is transcribed, capped, and polyadenylated. Viral RNA molecules then have one of three fates: They are exported to the cytoplasm, where they are packaged as the viral RNA in infectious viral particles; they are spliced to form the message for the envelope polyprotein; or they are translated into Gag and Pol proteins. Most of the messages for the Pol protein fail to initiate Pol translation because of a stop codon before its initiation; however, in a fraction of the messages, the stop codon is missed and the Pol proteins are translated. (*Modified from Coffin.*)

FIGURE 192-2 Genomic structure of retroviruses. The murine leukemia virus MuLV has the typical three structural genes: *gag*, *pol*, and *env*. The *gag* region gives rise to three proteins: matrix (MA), capsid (CA), and nucleic acid–binding (NC) proteins. The *pol* region encodes both a protease (PR) responsible for cleaving the viral polyproteins and a reverse transcriptase (RT). In addition, HIV *pol* encodes an integrase (IN). The *env* region encodes a surface protein (SU) and a small transmembrane protein (TM). The human retroviruses have additional gene products translated in each of the three possible reading frames. HTLV-I and HTLV-II have *tax* and *rex* genes with exons on either side of the *env* gene. HIV-1 and HIV-2 have six accessory gene products: *tat*, *rev*, *vif*, *nef*, *vpr*, and either *vpu* (in HIV-1) or *vpx* (in HIV-2). The genes for these proteins are located mainly between the *pol* and *env* genes.

carriage of randomly integrated provirus in CD4+ T cells. HTLV-I does not contain an oncogene and does not insert into a unique site in the genome. Indeed, most infected cells express no viral gene products. The only viral gene product that is routinely expressed in tumor cells transformed by HTLV-I in vivo is *tax*, and even *tax* is not expressed in the tumor cells of many ATL patients. Cells transformed in vitro, by contrast, actively transcribe HTLV-I RNA and produce infectious virions. Most HTLV-I–transformed cell lines are the result of the infection of a normal host T cell in vitro. It is difficult to establish cell lines derived from authentic ATL cells.

Although *tax* does not itself bind to DNA, it does induce the expression of a wide range of host-cell gene products, including transcription factors (especially *c-rel*, *ets*-1 and -2, and members of the *fos/jun* family), cytokines [e.g., interleukin (IL) 2, granulocyte-macrophage colony-stimulating factor, and tumor necrosis factor (TNF)], and membrane proteins and receptors [major histocompatibility (MHC) molecules and IL-2 receptor α]. The genes activated by *tax* are generally controlled by transcription factors of the *c-rel* and cyclic AMP response element binding (CREB) protein families. It is unclear how this induction of host gene expression leads to neoplastic transformation. Induction of a cytokine-autocrine loop has been proposed; however, IL-2 is not the crucial cytokine. The involvement of IL-4 and IL-7 has been proposed, and the newly identified cytokine IL-15 may play a role.

In light of the irregular expression of *tax* in ATL cells, it has been suggested that *tax* is important in the early phases of transformation but is not essential for the maintenance of the transformed state. As is clear from the epidemiology of HTLV-I infection, transformation of an infected cell is a rare event and may depend on heterogeneous second, third, or fourth genetic hits. No consistent chromosomal abnormalities have been described in ATL; however, individual cases with *p53* mutations and translocations involving the T-cell receptor genes on chromosome 14 have been reported. Recent data suggest that *tax* may repress certain DNA repair enzymes, permitting the accumulation of genetic damage that would normally be repaired. However, a detailed picture of the molecular pathogenesis of HTLV-I–induced neoplasia is not yet available.

FEATURES OF HTLV-I INFECTION **Epidemiology** HTLV-I infection is transmitted in at least three ways: from mother to child, especially in breast milk; through sexual activity, more commonly from men to women; and through the blood—i.e., via contaminated transfusions or contaminated needles. The virus is most commonly transmitted perinatally. Compared with HIV, which can be transmitted in cell-free form, HTLV-I is less infectious, and its transmission usually requires cell-to-cell contact.

HTLV-I is endemic in southwestern Japan and Okinawa, where more than 1 million persons are infected. Antibodies to HTLV-I are present in the serum of up to 35 percent of Okinawans, 10 percent of residents of the Japanese island of Kyushu, and fewer than 1 percent of persons in nonendemic regions of Japan. Despite this high prevalence of infection, only about 500 cases of ATL are diagnosed in this area each year. Other clusters of infection have been noted in other areas of the Orient, such as Taiwan; in the Caribbean basin, including northeastern South America; in central Africa; in Italy; in Israel; in the Arctic; and in the southeastern part of the United States.

Although early epidemiologic studies indicated an increasing seroprevalence of HTLV-I among injection drug users, more recent investigations with the use of confirmatory serologic assays that reliably distinguish between HTLV-I and HTLV-II indicate that the vast

	HTLV-I	HIV-1
SU	gp46	gp120
TM	p21	gp41
NC	p15	p6
PR	p14	p10
RT	p95	p64
IN	—	p34
MA	p19	p17
CA	p24	p24
RNA	9kb	10kb

FIGURE 192-3 Schematic structure of human retroviruses. The surface glycoprotein (SU) is responsible for binding to receptors of host cells. The transmembrane protein (TM) anchors SU to the virus. NC is a nucleic acid–binding protein found in association with the viral RNA. A protease (PR) cleaves the polyproteins encoded by the *gag*, *pol*, and *env* genes into their functional components. RT is reverse transcriptase, and IN is an integrase present in some retroviruses (e.g., HIV-1) that facilitates insertion of the provirus into the host genome. MA is a Gag protein closely associated with the lipid of the envelope. The capsid protein (CA) forms the major internal structure of the virus, the core shell.

majority of HTLV infections among injection drug users are, in fact, due to HTLV-II (see below). The development of ATL is rare among persons infected by blood products; however, about 20 percent of patients with HAM acquire HTLV-I from contaminated blood.

A progressive spastic or ataxic myelopathy that develops in an individual who is HTLV-I positive (i.e., who has serum antibodies to HTLV-I) is likely to be due to direct nervous system infection with the virus; a similar disorder may result from infection with HIV or HTLV-II. In rare instances, patients with HAM are seronegative but have detectable antibody to HTLV-I in the cerebrospinal fluid (CSF).

The cumulative lifetime risk of developing ATL is 2 to 5 percent among HTLV-I–infected patients; a similar risk is projected for HAM. The distribution of the two diseases overlaps the distribution of HTLV-I, with more than 95 percent of affected patients showing serologic evidence of HTLV-I infection. The latent period between infection and the emergence of disease is 20 to 30 years for ATL. For HAM, the median latency period is about 3.3 years; the interval is usually shorter (one case occurred within 4 months of a contaminated transfusion) but can also be as long as 20 to 30 years.

Associated Diseases *Adult T-cell leukemia/lymphoma* Four clinical types of HTLV-I–induced neoplasia have been described: acute, lymphomatous, chronic, and smoldering. All of these tumors are monoclonal proliferations of CD4 + post-thymic T cells with clonal proviral integrations and clonal T-cell receptor gene rearrangements.

About 60 percent of patients who develop malignancy have classic *acute* ATL, which is characterized by a short clinical prodrome (~2 weeks between the first symptoms and the diagnosis) and an aggressive natural history (median survival period, 6 months). The clinical picture is dominated by rapidly progressive skin lesions, pulmonary involvement, hypercalcemia, and lymphocytosis with cells containing lobulated or "cloven-hoof" nuclei (see the Atlas of Hematology in this volume). The malignant cells have monoclonal proviral integrations and express CD4, CD3, and CD25 (low-affinity IL-2 receptors) on their surface. Serum levels of CD25 can be used as a tumor marker. Anemia and thrombocytopenia are rare. The skin lesions may be difficult to distinguish from those in mycosis fungoides. Lytic bone lesions, which are common, do not contain tumor cells but rather are composed of osteolytic cells, usually without osteoblastic activity. Despite the leukemic picture, bone marrow involvement is patchy in most cases.

The hypercalcemia of ATL is multifactorial; the tumor cells produce osteoclast-activating factors (TNFα, IL-1, lymphotoxin) and can also produce a parathyroid hormone–like molecule. The affected patients have an underlying immunodeficiency that makes them susceptible to opportunistic infections similar to those seen in patients with AIDS (see Chap. 308). The pathogenesis of the immunodeficiency is unclear. Pulmonary infiltrates in ATL patients reflect leukemic infiltration half the time and opportunistic infections with organisms such as *Pneumocystis carinii* and other fungi the other half. Gastrointestinal symptoms are nearly always related to opportunistic infection. Serum concentrations of lactate dehydrogenase (LDH) and alkaline phosphatase are often elevated. About 10 percent of patients have leptomeningeal involvement leading to weakness, altered mental status, paresthesias, and/or headache. Unlike other forms of central nervous system (CNS) lymphoma, ATL may be accompanied by normal CSF protein levels. The diagnosis depends on finding ATL cells in the CSF (see Chap. 113).

The *lymphomatous* type of ATL occurs in about 20 percent of patients and is similar to the acute form in its natural history and clinical course, except that circulating abnormal cells are rare and lymphadenopathy is evident. The histology of the lymphoma, which can fit any of five diagnostic types usually used for lymphoma classification, does not influence the natural history. In general, the diagnosis is suspected on the basis of the patient's birthplace and the presence of skin lesions and hypercalcemia. The diagnosis is confirmed by the detection of antibodies to HTLV-I in serum.

Patients with the *chronic* form of ATL generally have normal serum levels of calcium and LDH and no involvement of the CNS, bone, or gastrointestinal tract. The median duration of survival for these patients is 2 years. In some cases, chronic ATL progresses to the acute form of the disease.

No more than 5 percent of patients have the *smoldering* form of ATL. In this form, the malignant cells have monoclonal proviral integration; fewer than 5 percent of peripheral-blood cells exhibit typical morphologic abnormalities; hypercalcemia, adenopathy, and hepatosplenomegaly do not develop; the CNS, the bones, and the gastrointestinal tract are not involved; and skin and pulmonary lesions may be present. The median survival period of this small subset of patients appears to be 5 years or longer.

HTLV-I–associated myelopathy (tropical spastic paraparesis) In contrast to ATL, in which there is a slight predominance of male patients, HAM affects females disproportionately. HAM resembles multiple sclerosis in certain ways (see Chap. 373). The onset is insidious. Symptoms include weakness or stiffness in one or both legs, back pain, and urinary incontinence. Sensory changes are usually mild, but peripheral neuropathy may develop. The disease generally takes the form of slowly progressive and unremitting thoracic myelopathy; one-third of patients are bedridden within 10 years of diagnosis, and one-half are unable to walk unassisted by this point. Patients display spastic paraparesis or paraplegia with hyperreflexia, ankle clonus, and extensor plantar responses. Cognitive function is usually spared; cranial nerve abnormalities are unusual.

Magnetic resonance imaging (MRI) reveals lesions in both the white matter and the paraventricular regions of the brain as well as in the spinal cord. Pathologic examination of the spinal cord shows symmetrical degeneration of the lateral columns, including the corticospinal tracts; some cases involve the posterior columns as well. The spinal meninges and cord parenchyma contain an inflammatory infiltrate with myelin destruction.

HTLV-I usually is not found in cells of the CNS, but it may be detected in a small population of lymphocytes present in the CSF. In general, HTLV-I replication is greater in HAM than in ATL, and patients with HAM have a stronger immune response to the virus. Antibodies to HTLV-I are present in the serum and appear to be produced in the CSF of HAM patients, where titers are often higher than in the serum. It has been proposed that the pathophysiology of HAM involves the induction of autoimmune destruction of neural cells by T cells with specificity for viral components such as Tax or Env proteins. One theory is that susceptibility to HAM may be related to the presence of human leukocyte antigen (HLA) alleles capable of presenting viral antigens in a fashion that leads to autoimmunity. There are insufficient data at present to confirm such an HLA association.

Other putative HTLV-I–related diseases In areas where HTLV-I is endemic, diverse inflammatory and autoimmune diseases have been attributed to the virus, including uveitis, dermatitis, pneumonitis, rheumatoid arthritis, and polymyositis. However, a causal relationship between HTLV-I and these illnesses has not been rigorously established.

Prevention of Disease The principles of prevention of HTLV-I–induced disease are clear. Women in endemic areas should not breast-feed their children, and blood donors should be screened for serum antibodies to HTLV-I. As in the prevention of HIV infection, the practice of safe sex and the avoidance of needle sharing are important. Conscientious adherence to these principles should have an enormous impact on the prevalence of HTLV-I infection.

℞ TREATMENT

For the small number of patients who develop HTLV-I–related disease, therapies are not curative. In patients with the acute and lymphomatous types of ATL, the disease progresses rapidly. Hypercalcemia is generally controlled by glucocorticoid administration and cytotoxic therapy directed against the neoplasm. The tumor is highly responsive to combination chemotherapy that is employed against other forms of lymphoma; however, patients are susceptible to overwhelming bacterial and opportunistic infections, and ATL relapses within 4 to 10 months after remission in most patients. The combination of interferon α and zidovudine reportedly elicits responses in a substantial fraction of patients with less toxicity than the usual lymphoma regimens. Survival may be extended by this treatment. Because viral replication is not clearly associated with ATL progression, zidovudine is probably effective through its cytotoxic effects (as a chain-terminating thymidine analogue) rather than its antiviral effects. An experimental approach using an yttrium 90–labeled antibody to the IL-2 receptor appears promising but is not widely available. Patients with the chronic or smoldering form of ATL may be managed with an expectant approach: Treat any infections, and watch and wait for signs of progression to acute disease.

Patients with HAM may obtain some benefit from the use of glucocorticoids to reduce inflammation. Antiretroviral regimens have not been effective. In one study, danazol (200 mg tid) produced significant neurologic improvement in five of six treated patients, with resolution of urinary incontinence in two cases, decreased spasticity in three, and the restoration of the ability to walk after confinement to a wheelchair in two. Physical therapy and rehabilitation are important components of management.

FEATURES OF HTLV-II INFECTION **Epidemiology** HTLV-II is endemic in certain Native American tribes. It is generally considered to be a New World virus that was brought from Asia to the Americas 10,000 to 40,000 years ago during the migration of infected populations across the Bering land bridge.

The mode of transmission of HTLV-II is probably the same as that of HTLV-I (see above). HTLV-II may be less readily transmitted sexually than HTLV-I.

Because of their biologic similarity and the previous lack of distinguishing serologic assays, HTLV-I and HTLV-II were often grouped together in seroepidemiologic studies. This practice led to the incorrect conclusion that HTLV-I was becoming quite prevalent among injection drug users in the United States. Studies of large cohorts of injection drug users with serologic assays that reliably distinguish HTLV-I from HTLV-II indicate that the vast majority of HTLV-positive subjects are infected with HTLV-II. The seroprevalence of HTLV in a cohort of 7841 injection drug users from drug treatment centers in Baltimore, Chicago, Los Angeles, New Jersey (Asbury Park and Trenton), New York City (Brooklyn and Harlem), Philadelphia, and San Antonio was 20.9 percent, with more than 97 percent of cases due to HTLV-II. The seroprevalence of HTLV-II was higher in the Southwest and the Midwest than in the Northeast. In contrast, the seroprevalence of HIV-1 was higher in the Northeast than in the Southwest or the Midwest. Approximately 3 percent of the cohort members were infected with both HTLV-II and HIV-1. The seroprevalence of HTLV-II increased linearly with age, as did that of HTLV-I in other studies. Women were significantly more likely to be infected with HTLV-II than were men; the virus is thought to be more efficiently transmitted from male to female than from female to male.

Associated Diseases Although HTLV-II was isolated from a patient with a T-cell variant of hairy cell leukemia, this virus has not been consistently associated with a particular disease and in fact has been thought of as "a virus searching for a disease." However, evidence is accumulating that HTLV-II may play a role in certain neurologic, hematologic, and dermatologic diseases. These data require confirmation, particularly in light of the previous confusion regarding the relative prevalences of HTLV-I and HTLV-II among injection drug users.

Prevention Given current information on the prevalence of HTLV-II among injection drug users in the United States, the impact of preventive measures could be substantial. Avoidance of needle sharing, safe-sex practices, screening of blood (by assays for HTLV-I, which also detect HTLV-II), and avoidance of breast-feeding by infected women are important principles in the prevention of spread of HTLV-II.

HUMAN IMMUNODEFICIENCY VIRUS (See Chap. 308)

HIV-1 and HIV-2 are members of the lentivirus subfamily of Retroviridae and are the only lentiviruses known to infect humans. The lentiviruses are slow-acting by comparison with viruses that cause acute infection (e.g., influenza virus) but not by comparison with other retroviruses. The features of acute primary infection with HIV resemble those of more classic acute infections. The characteristic chronicity of HIV disease is consistent with the designation *lentivirus*. HIV is discussed in considerable detail in Chap. 308. The following brief discussion focuses on those aspects of HIV that distinguish it from the other human retroviruses.

BIOLOGY AND MOLECULAR BIOLOGY Unlike HTLV-I and HTLV-II, which are oncogenic viruses that transform cells in culture, HIV-1 and HIV-2 are cytopathic in culture. The primary receptor for HIV is the CD4 molecule, which is present predominantly on the surface of a subset of T lymphocytes but also on monocytes. These two types of cell are thus the major targets of HIV infection. Other cell types express CD4 and are variably susceptible to HIV infection (see Chap. 308). In addition to CD4, other cell-surface molecules—referred to as *coreceptors*—function as accessory receptors in target cells that express CD4. In this regard, it has been demonstrated that certain cell-surface molecules that belong to the seven transmembrane G protein–coupled family of receptors serve as coreceptors for different strains of HIV-1. The molecule termed *fusin* is the coreceptor for T cell–tropic strains of HIV-1 (such as strain IIIB), while the β-chemokine receptor CCCKR5 is the coreceptor for macrophage-tropic strains of HIV-1 (such as strain Ba-L) (see Chap. 308). Certain cell-surface markers clearly enhance infection of CD4 + cells by HIV; these include Fc receptors (FcRs) or complement (C') receptors. The binding of virus by antibody may lead to increased efficiency of infection of FcR-positive cells, and the formation of immune complexes of HIV, antibody, and C' may lead to increased efficiency of infection of cells expressing C' receptors. It is still unclear whether FcRs and C' receptors can mediate infection independently of CD4. Finally, certain receptors may function as primary receptors in HIV infection of CD4 − cells. For example, the glycolipid galactosyl ceramide (galactocerebroside, GalC) is one candidate cell-surface receptor for the infection of CD4 − glial and neuroblastoma cells. Once the virus binds to the target cell, fusion with the cell membrane occurs via the gp41 molecule of the viral envelope, and the HIV genomic RNA is uncoated and internalized. HIV then proceeds with its life cycle as outlined in Fig. 192-1.

HIV has little sequence homology with the HTLVs; however, these viruses have some important similarities in genomic makeup. Both groups have flanking LTRs as well as the *gag*, *pol*, and *env* structural genes. The HIV equivalents of the HTLV *rex* and *tax* genes are *rev* and *tat*. However, HIV also possesses several auxiliary genes, including *nef*, *vpr*, *vpu* (HIV-1 only), and *vpx* (HIV-2 only) (see "Structure and Life Cycle" above). The LTRs of HIV include conventional regulatory sequences, such as the polyadenylation signal sequence and the TATA promoter sequence. The binding sites for both cellular and viral transcription factors have been mapped to the U3 and R regions of the LTR. Three functional domains in the U3 and R regions have been described: (1) a modulatory element that includes binding sites for activation protein 1 (AP-1), nuclear factor κB (NFκB), nuclear factor of activated T cells (NFAT), upstream stimulatory factor, and T-cell factor 1α; (2) a core promoter element that contains three binding sites for SP1 and the TATA sequence; and (3) a transactivator response (TAR) element that contains binding sites for both cellular and viral factors, including the viral Tat protein.

All of these factors may exert either positive or negative effects on viral RNA transcription. For example, the SP1, TATA, and TAR sequences as well as NFκB exert a positive effect on viral transcription. In contrast, some *upstream* sequences in the LTR exert negative effects on viral transcription and thus are designated the *negative regulatory element*. Stimulation of the initiation of transcription depends strictly on the presence of these factors in their active forms. Factors that exert a positive effect on viral transcription are abundant in activated cells; thus, the stimulation of viral RNA transcription depends on the state of activation of the target cells.

The mRNA species that are transcribed as a result of the binding of these factors to HIV LTR are multiply spliced (containing the viral LTR and the major viral regulatory genes *tat*, *rev*, and *nef*), singly spliced (containing the *env* coding sequences), or unspliced (containing the *gag-pol* sequences). Multiply spliced mRNA enters the cytoplasm, where it is translated. Tat is responsible for the upregulation of expression of all the other HIV genes, particularly *rev*. The principal function of the Rev protein is to allow for the cytoplasmic expression of the singly spliced and unspliced HIV mRNAs. In the absence of Rev, these mRNAs remain sequestered in the nucleus, where they ultimately are either degraded or multiply spliced. Accumulation of the Rev protein promotes the production of viral mRNAs that encode for structural proteins. The Rev protein interacts with the Rev responsive element (RRE); Rev-RRE binding is thought to mediate nuclear export and translation of unspliced or singly spliced mRNAs, resulting in the production of structural proteins such as Gag, Gag-Pol, and Env as well as of enzymatic proteins required for the creation of virus particles (Fig. 192-1). Virions are assembled at the inner surface of the plasma membrane of the infected cell; this process is regulated by the Gag polyprotein. The viral RNA contains a packaging sequence critical to the efficient incorporation of genomic RNA into virions. Assembly, budding, and maturation of virions take place in the absence of the envelope glycoprotein. Incorporation of the envelope protein occurs on the outer surface of the plasma membrane during the budding process. Once virus particles are released from the cell surface, Gag and Gag-Pol polyproteins are cleaved by viral protease.

MOLECULAR HETEROGENEITY Molecular analysis of various HIV isolates reveals variation over many parts of the viral genome. For example, the coding sequences of the viral envelope protein can differ by only a few percent or by as much as 50 percent. The percentage of actual envelope-protein sequence differences can be even greater. These changes tend to cluster in hypervariable regions. One such region, V3, is a target for neutralizing antibodies and contains recognition sites for T-cell responses. Variability in this region is probably due to selective pressure from the host's immune system. The extraordinary variability within HIV-1 contrasts markedly with the relative genetic stability of HTLV-I and HTLV-II. On the basis of this molecular heterogeneity, HIV-1 isolates have been categorized into two *groups*: group M, which is responsible for most of the infections in the world, and group O, which is a relatively rare outlier group currently found in Cameroon, Gabon, and France. The M group comprises eight sequence *subtypes* or *clades*, designed A through H. Subtype A viruses are most common worldwide, while subtype B viruses are found only in the United States. Phylogenetic-tree analysis and the distribution of various HIV-1 subtypes throughout the world are discussed in Chap. 308.

EPIDEMIOLOGY HIV is spread by sexual contact, contaminated blood or blood products, contaminated injection equipment, intrapartum and perinatal mother-child contact, and breast-feeding (see Chap. 308). HIV has caused a global pandemic, with the number of infected individuals worldwide estimated at approximately 20 million in 1996. The predominant mode of transmission around the world—particularly prominent in developing countries—is by heterosexual contact with an infected individual. Although heterosexual spread is increasing in frequency in developed countries, homosexual contact and injection drug use remain the predominant modes of transmission in the United States. Intrapartum/perinatal transmission from a mother to a fetus or an infant is a major source of infection in developing countries and is becoming more important in developed countries as rates of heterosexual spread rise.

HIV-1 is the predominant agent of HIV infection worldwide. HIV-2 is prominent in West Africa; moreover, it is now being documented in other regions of Africa as well as in Western Europe, in South America (particularly Brazil), and—to a much lesser extent—in Canada and the United States.

ASSOCIATED DISEASES HIV disease is characterized by progressive immunodeficiency associated with quantitative depletion and qualitative defects in CD4+ T cells. Advanced HIV disease is referred to as the acquired immunodeficiency syndrome, or AIDS. When the CD4+ T-cell count falls below a certain critical level, usually 200/μL, the infected individual becomes highly susceptible to a number of opportunistic infections and neoplasms. These conditions are AIDS-defining illnesses; diminution of the CD4+ T-cell count to <200/μL, even if the individual is asymptomatic, still constitutes a diagnosis of AIDS. Compared with HIV-1, HIV-2 is believed to cause disease that is more indolent and that evolves to the advanced stages over a longer period. HIV-1 causes neurologic disease in a high proportion of patients. This form of disease may be manifested as AIDS dementia complex, aseptic meningitis, myelopathy, peripheral neuropathy, and/or myopathy. A number of organ-specific abnormalities are also associated with HIV infection.

PREVENTION Strategies for the prevention of HIV infection are similar to those for the prevention of HTLV infection (see above and Chap. 308). → *The treatment of HIV infection and its complications is discussed in detail in Chap. 308.*

BIBLIOGRAPHY

BARRE-SINOUSSI F et al: Isolation of a T-lymphotropic retrovirus from a patient at risk for acquired immune deficiency syndrome (AIDS). Science 220:868, 1983

BRIGGS NC et al: Seroprevalence of human T cell lymphotropic virus type II infection, with or without human immunodeficiency virus type I coinfection, among US intravenous drug users. J Infect Dis 172:51, 1995

COFFIN JM: Retroviridae and their replication, in *Fields Virology*, BN Fields, DM Knipe (eds). New York, Raven Press, 1990, p 1437

FAUCI AS: Multifactorial nature of human immunodeficiency virus disease: Implications for therapy. Science 262:1011, 1993

FRANCHINI G: Molecular mechanisms of human T-cell leukemia/lymphotropic virus type I infection. Blood 86:3619, 1995

GALLO RC: Human retroviruses in the second decade: A personal perspective. Nature Med 1:753, 1995

―――― et al: Frequent detection and isolation of cytopathic retroviruses (HTLV-III) from patients with AIDS and at risk for AIDS. Science 224:500, 1984

GILL PS et al: Treatment of adult T-cell leukemia-lymphoma with a combination of interferon alpha and zidovudine. N Engl J Med 332:1744, 1995

HARRINGTON WJ Jr et al: Tropical spastic paraparesis/HTLV-I-associated myelopathy (TSP/HAM): Treatment with an anabolic steroid danazol. AIDS Res Hum Retroviruses 7:1031, 1991

HOLLSBERG P, HAFLER DA: Pathogenesis of diseases induced by human lymphotropic virus type I infection. N Engl J Med 328:1173, 1993

KORBER BTM et al: Mutational trends in V3 loop protein sequences observed in different genetic lineages of human immunodeficiency virus type I. J Virol 68:6730, 1994

MYERS G: HIV: Between past and future. AIDS Res Hum Retroviruses 10:1317, 1994

PANTALEO G et al: The role of lymphoid organs in the pathogenesis of HIV infection. Semin Immunol 5:157, 1993

――――, FAUCI AS: The acquired immunodeficiency syndrome (AIDS), in *Handbook of Experimental Immunology*, LA Herzenberg et al (eds). Oxford, Blackwell Scientific, 1996

POIESZ BJ et al: Detection and isolation of type C retrovirus particles from fresh and cultured lymphocytes of a patient with cutaneous T-cell lymphoma. Proc Natl Acad Sci USA 77:7415, 1980

TRONO D: HIV accessory proteins: Leading roles for the supporting cast. Cell 82:189, 1996

URBA WJ, LONGO DL: The clinical spectrum of human retroviral-induced diseases. Cancer Res 45:4637, 1985

―――― et al: Adult T-cell leukemia/lymphoma, in *Clinical Oncology*, MD Abeloff et al (eds). New York, Churchill Livingstone, 1995, p 2173

WALDMANN TA: The multichain interleukin-2 receptor: A target for immunotherapy. Ann Intern Med 116:148, 1992

ZEHENDER G et al: High prevalence of human T-cell lymphotropic virus type II infection in patients affected by human immunodeficiency virus type I–associated predominantly sensory polyneuropathy. J Infect Dis 172:1595, 1995

193 *Raphael Dolin*

INFLUENZA

DEFINITION Influenza is an acute respiratory illness caused by infection with influenza viruses. The illness affects the upper and/or lower respiratory tract and is often accompanied by systemic signs and symptoms such as fever, headache, myalgia, and weakness. Outbreaks of illness of variable extent and severity occur nearly every winter. Such outbreaks result in significant morbidity in the general population and in increased mortality rates among certain high-risk patients, mainly as a result of pulmonary complications.

ETIOLOGIC AGENT Influenza viruses are members of the Orthomyxoviridae family. Influenza A and B viruses constitute one genus, and influenza C viruses make up the other. The designation of influenza viruses as type A, B, or C is based on antigenic characteristics of the nucleoprotein (NP) and matrix (M) protein antigens. Influenza A viruses are further subdivided (subtyped) on the basis of the surface hemagglutinin (H) and neuraminidase (N) antigens (see below); individual strains are designated according to the site of origin, isolate number, year of isolation, and subtype—for example, influenza A/Johannesburg/33/94 (H3N2). Influenza B and C viruses are similarly designated, but H and N antigens from these viruses do not receive subtype designations, since intratypic variations in these antigens are less extensive in these viruses.

Most of the information on the molecular biology of influenza viruses has come from studies of influenza A viruses, and less is known about the replicative cycle of influenza B and C viruses. Morphologically, influenza viruses A, B, and C are similar. The virions are irregularly shaped spherical particles, 80 to 120 nm in diameter, and have a lipid envelope from the surface of which the H and N glycoproteins project (Fig. 193-1). The hemagglutinin is the site by which virus binds to cell receptors, whereas the neuraminidase degrades the receptor and probably plays a role in the release of virus from infected cells after replication has taken place. Antibodies to the H antigen are the major determinants of immunity to influenza virus, while those to the N antigen limit viral spread and contribute to reduction of the infection. The inner surface of the lipid envelope contains the M proteins M1 and M2, the functions of which are incompletely understood but which may be involved in virus assembly and in stabilization of the lipid envelope. The virion also contains the NP antigen, which is associated with the viral genome, as well as three polymerase (P) proteins that are essential for transcription and synthesis of viral RNA. Two nonstructural (NS) proteins of unknown function are also present in infected cells.

The genome of influenza A virus consists of eight single-stranded RNA segments, which code for the structural and nonstructural proteins. Because the genome is segmented, the opportunity for reassortment of genes during infection is high, and reassortment occurs frequently during infection of cells with more than one influenza A virus.

EPIDEMIOLOGY Influenza outbreaks are recorded virtually every year, although their extent and severity vary widely. Localized outbreaks take place at variable intervals, usually every 1 to 3 years. Global epidemics or pandemics have occurred approximately every 10 to 15 years since the 1918–1919 pandemic (Table 193-1).

The most extensive and severe outbreaks are caused by influenza A viruses. In part, this predominance is a result of the remarkable propensity of the H and N antigens of influenza A virus to undergo periodic antigenic variation. Major antigenic variations are referred to as *antigenic shifts*, which may be associated with pandemics and are restricted to influenza A viruses. Minor variations are called *antigenic drifts*. These antigenic changes may involve the hemagglutinin alone or both the hemagglutinin and the neuraminidase. In human infections, three major antigenic subtypes of hemagglutinins (H1, H2, and H3) and two of neuraminidases (N1 and N2) have been recognized. The hemagglutinins formerly designated as H0 and Hsw1 are now classified as variants of H1. An example of an antigenic shift involving both the hemagglutinin and the neuraminidase is that of 1957, when the predominant influenza A virus subtype shifted from H1N1 to H2N2; this shift resulted in a severe pandemic, with an estimated 70,000 excess deaths (i.e., deaths in excess of the number expected without an influenza epidemic) in the United States alone. In 1968, an antigenic shift involving only the hemagglutinin occurred (H2N2 to H3N2); the subsequent pandemic was less severe than that of 1957. In 1977, an H1N1 virus emerged and caused a pandemic that primarily affected younger individuals (i.e., those born after 1957). As can be seen in Table 193-1, H1N1 viruses circulated from 1918 to 1956; thus, individuals born prior to 1957 would be expected to have some degree of immunity to H1N1 viruses. During most outbreaks of influenza A, a single subtype has circulated at a time. However, since 1977, H1N1 and H3N2 viruses have circulated simultaneously, resulting in outbreaks of varying severity. In some outbreaks, influenza B viruses have also circulated simultaneously with influenza A viruses.

The origin of pandemic strains is unknown. Given the marked differences between the primary structures of the hemagglutinins of different subtypes of influenza A viruses (H1, H2, and H3), it seems unlikely that antigenic shifts result from spontaneous mutations in the hemagglutinin gene. Because the segmented genome of influenza viruses may result in high rates of reassortment, it has been suggested that pandemic strains may emerge by reassortment of genes between human and animal viruses. Influenza B viruses do not have an animal reservoir and do not undergo antigenic shifts, although they do undergo antigenic drift.

Pandemics provide the most dramatic evidence of the impact of influenza. However, illnesses that occur between pandemics account for greater total mortality and morbidity, albeit over a longer period. From 1972 to 1991, interpandemic illness was associated with 20,000

FIGURE 193-1 An electron micrograph of influenza virus (×143,000). (*From R Dolin, Am Fam Phys 14:74, 1976.*)

Table 193-1

Emergence of Antigenic Subtypes of Influenza A Virus Associated with Pandemic or Epidemic Disease

Year	Subtype	Extent of Outbreak
1889–90	H2N8*	Severe pandemic
1900–03	H3N8*	?Moderate epidemic
1918–19	H1N1† (formerly HswN1)	Severe pandemic
1933–35	H1N1† (formerly H0N1)	Mild epidemic
1946–47	H1N1	Mild epidemic
1957–58	H2N2	Severe pandemic
1968–69	H3N2	Moderate pandemic
1977–78‡	H1N1	Mild pandemic

* As determined by retrospective serologic survey of individuals alive during those years ("seroarcheology").

† Hemagglutinins formerly designated as Hsw and H0 are now classified as variants of H1.

‡ From this time until the present (1995–96), no new antigenic subtypes of influenza A virus have emerged. Rather, viruses of the H1N1 and H3N2 subtypes have circulated either in alternating years or concurrently.

or more excess deaths during each of 10 epidemics in the United States; more than 40,000 influenza-associated deaths occurred in each of three of these epidemics. Influenza A viruses that circulate between pandemics demonstrate antigenic drifts in the H antigen. These antigenic drifts apparently result from point mutations involving the RNA segment that codes for the hemagglutinin. Epidemiologically significant strains—that is, those with the potential to cause widespread outbreaks—exhibit changes in amino acids in at least two of the major antigenic sites in the hemagglutinin molecule. Since two point mutations are unlikely to occur simultaneously, it is believed that antigenic drifts result from point mutations occurring sequentially during the spread of virus from person to person. Antigenic drifts have been reported nearly annually since 1977 for H1N1 viruses and since 1968 for H3N2 viruses.

Influenza A epidemics begin abruptly, peak over a 2- to 3-week period, generally last for 2 to 3 months, and often subside almost as rapidly as they began. The first indication of influenza activity in a community is an increase in the number of children with febrile respiratory illnesses who present for medical attention. This increase is followed by increases in rates of influenza-like illnesses among adults and eventually by an increase in hospital admissions for patients with pneumonia, worsening of congestive heart failure, and exacerbations of chronic pulmonary disease. Rates of absence from work and school also rise at this time. An increase in the number of deaths caused by pneumonia and influenza is generally a late observation in an outbreak. Attack rates have been highly variable from outbreak to outbreak but most commonly are in the range of 10 to 20 percent of the general population. During the pandemic of 1957, it was estimated that the attack rate of clinical influenza exceeded 50 percent in urban populations and that an additional 25 percent or more of individuals in these populations may have been subclinically infected with influenza A virus. Among institutionalized populations and in semiclosed settings with a large number of susceptible individuals, even higher attack rates have been reported.

Epidemics of influenza occur almost exclusively during the winter months in the Northern and Southern Hemispheres. It is highly unusual to detect influenza A virus at other times, although serologic rises or even outbreaks have been noted rarely during warm-weather months. Where or how influenza A virus persists between outbreaks is unknown. It is possible that influenza A viruses are maintained in the human population on a worldwide basis by person-to-person transmission and that large population clusters support a low level of interepidemic transmission. Alternatively, human strains may persist in animal reservoirs. Convincing evidence to support either explanation is not available. In the modern era, rapid transportation may contribute to the transmission of viruses among widespread geographic locales.

The factors that result in the inception and termination of outbreaks of influenza are incompletely understood. A major determinant of the extent and severity of an outbreak is the level of immunity in the population at risk. With the emergence of an antigenically novel influenza virus to which little or no antibody is present in a community, extensive outbreaks may occur. When the absence of antibody is worldwide, epidemic disease may spread around the globe, resulting in a pandemic. Such pandemic waves can continue for several years, until immunity in the population reaches a high level. In the years following pandemic influenza, antigenic drifts among influenza viruses result in outbreaks of variable severity in populations with high levels of immunity to the pandemic strain that circulated earlier. This situation persists until another antigenically novel pandemic strain emerges. On the other hand, outbreaks sometimes end despite the persistence of a large pool of susceptible individuals in the population.

Occasionally, the emergence of a significantly different antigenic variant will result only in a localized outbreak. The swine influenza outbreak of 1976 in the United States, caused by an A/H1N1 virus antigenically similar to the virus that circulated in 1918–1919 (see Table 193-1), may be an example, although this outbreak may have represented simply the introduction of a swine influenza virus into a crowded human population without spread beyond that setting. It also has been suggested that certain viruses, such as recently circulating

A/H1N1 strains, may be intrinsically less virulent and cause less severe disease than other variants, even in immunologically virgin subjects. If so, then other undefined factors besides the level of preexisting immunity must play a role in the epidemiology of influenza.

Influenza B virus causes outbreaks that are generally less extensive and are associated with less severe disease than those caused by influenza A virus. The hemagglutinin and neuraminidase of influenza B virus undergo less frequent and less extensive variation than those of influenza A viruses; this characteristic may account, in part, for the lesser extent of disease. Influenza B outbreaks are seen most frequently in schools and military camps, although outbreaks in institutions in which elderly individuals reside also have been noted on occasion. The most serious complication of influenza B virus infection is Reye's syndrome (see Chap. 300). Influenza C virus has been only infrequently associated with human disease, although the wide prevalence of serum antibody to this virus indicates that asymptomatic infection may be common.

The morbidity and mortality caused by influenza outbreaks continue to be substantial. Most individuals who die in this setting have underlying diseases that place them at high risk for complications of influenza. Excess hospitalizations for adults with high-risk medical conditions have reached rates of 800 per 100,000 during recent outbreaks of influenza. The most prominent high-risk conditions are chronic cardiac and pulmonary diseases as well as old age. Mortality among individuals with chronic metabolic, renal, and certain immunosuppressive diseases has also been high, although lower than that among patients with chronic cardiopulmonary diseases. The morbidity attributable to influenza in the general population is considerable. For each of three outbreaks in the United States that were studied during the 1960s, it has been estimated that direct and indirect economic costs ranged from 1.5 to 3.5 billion dollars; today such costs would obviously be much greater.

PATHOGENESIS The initial event in influenza is infection of the respiratory epithelium with influenza virus acquired from respiratory secretions of acutely infected individuals. In all likelihood, transmission occurs via aerosols generated by coughs and sneezes, although hand-to-hand contact, other personal contact, and even fomite transmission may take place. Experimental evidence suggests that infection by a small-particle aerosol (particle diameter, less than 10 μm) is more efficient than that by larger droplets. Initially, viral infection involves the ciliated columnar epithelial cells, but it also may involve other respiratory tract cells, including alveolar cells, mucous gland cells, and macrophages. In infected cells, virus replicates within 4 to 6 h, after which infectious virus is released to infect adjacent or nearby cells. In this way, infection spreads from a few foci to a large number of respiratory cells over several hours. In experimentally induced infection, the incubation period of illness has ranged from 18 to 72 h, depending on the size of the virus inoculum. Histopathologic study reveals degenerative changes, including granulation, vacuolization, swelling, and pyknotic nuclei, in infected ciliated cells. The cells eventually become necrotic and desquamate; in some areas, previously columnar epithelium is replaced by flattened and metaplastic epithelial cells. The severity of illness is correlated with the quantity of virus shed in secretions; thus, the degree of viral replication itself may be an important mechanism in the pathogenesis of illness. Despite the frequent development of systemic signs and symptoms such as fever, headache, and myalgias, influenza virus has only rarely been detected in extrapulmonary sites (including the bloodstream), and the pathogenesis of systemic symptoms in influenza remains unknown.

The host response to influenza infections involves a complex interplay of humoral antibody, local antibody, cell-mediated immunity, interferon, and other host defenses. Serum antibody responses, which can be detected by the second week after primary infection, are measured by a variety of techniques: hemagglutination inhibition (HAI), complement fixation (CF), neutralization, enzyme-linked immunosorbent assay (ELISA), and antineuraminidase antibody assay. Antibodies directed against the hemagglutinin appear to be the most important mediators of immunity; in several studies, HAI titers of 40 or greater have been associated with protection from infection. Secretory antibodies produced in the respiratory tract are predominantly of the IgA class and also play a major role in protection against infection. Secretory antibody neutralization titers of 4 or higher also have been associated with protection. A variety of cell-mediated immune responses, both antigen-specific and non-antigen-specific, can be detected early after infection, depending on the prior immunity of the host. These responses include T-cell proliferative, T-cell cytotoxic, and natural killer cell activity. Interferons have been detected in respiratory secretions shortly after the shedding of virus has begun, and rises in interferon titers coincide with decreases in virus shedding.

The host defense factors responsible for cessation of virus shedding and resolution of illness have not been defined specifically. Virus shedding generally stops within 2 to 5 days after symptoms first appear, at a time when serum and local antibody responses often are not detectable by conventional techniques (although antibody rises may be detected earlier by use of highly sensitive techniques, particularly in individuals with previous immunity to the virus). It has been suggested that interferon, cell-mediated immune responses, and/or nonspecific inflammatory responses are important in the resolution of illness.

MANIFESTATIONS Influenza has been most frequently described as an illness characterized by the abrupt onset of systemic symptoms, such as headache, feverishness, chills, myalgia, or malaise, and accompanying respiratory tract signs, particularly cough and sore throat. In many cases, the onset is so abrupt that patients can recall the precise time they became ill. A typical case of naturally occurring influenza is depicted in Fig. 193-2. However, the spectrum of clinical presentations is wide, ranging from a mild, afebrile respiratory illness similar to the common cold (with either gradual or abrupt onset) to severe prostration with relatively few respiratory signs and symptoms. In most of the cases that come to a physician's attention, the patient has a fever, with temperatures of 38 to 41°C. A rapid temperature rise within the first 24 h of illness is generally followed by a gradual defervescence over a 2- to 3-day period, although, on occasion, fever may last for as long as a week. Patients report a feverish feeling and

FIGURE 193-2 Clinical characteristics of a naturally occurring case of influenza A in an otherwise healthy 28-year-old man. (*From R Dolin, Am Fam Phys 14:74, 1976.*)

chilliness, but true rigors are rare. Headache, either generalized or frontal, is often particularly troublesome. Myalgias may involve any part of the body but are most common in the legs and lumbosacral area. Arthralgias also may develop.

Respiratory complaints often become more prominent as systemic symptoms subside. Many patients have a sore throat or persistent cough, which may last for a week or more and which is often accompanied by substernal discomfort. Ocular signs and symptoms include pain on motion of the eyes, photophobia, and burning of the eyes.

Physical findings are usually minimal in cases of uncomplicated influenza. Early in the illness, the patient appears flushed and the skin is hot and dry, although diaphoresis and mottled extremities are sometimes evident, particularly in older patients. Examination of the pharynx may yield surprisingly unremarkable results despite a severe sore throat, but injection of the mucous membranes and postnasal discharge are apparent in some cases. Mild cervical lymphadenopathy may be noted, particularly in younger individuals. The results of chest examination are largely negative in uncomplicated influenza, although rhonchi, wheezes, and scattered rales have been reported with variable frequency in different outbreaks. Frank dyspnea, hyperpnea, cyanosis, diffuse rales, and signs of consolidation are indicative of pulmonary complications. Patients with apparently uncomplicated influenza have been reported to have a variety of mild ventilatory defects and increased alveolar-capillary diffusion gradients; thus, subclinical pulmonary involvement may be more frequent than is appreciated.

In uncomplicated influenza, the acute illness generally resolves over a 2- to 5-day period, and most patients have largely recovered in 1 week. In a significant minority (particularly the elderly), however, symptoms of weakness or lassitude (postinfluenzal asthenia) may persist for several weeks and may prove troublesome for persons who wish to resume their full level of activity promptly. The pathogenetic basis for this asthenia is unknown, although pulmonary function abnormalities may persist for several weeks after uncomplicated influenza.

COMPLICATIONS OF INFLUENZA The most common complication of influenza is pneumonia: "primary" influenza viral pneumonia, secondary bacterial pneumonia, or mixed viral and bacterial pneumonia. Primary influenza viral pneumonia is the least common but most severe of the pneumonic complications. It presents as acute influenza that does not resolve but instead progresses relentlessly, with persistent fever, dyspnea, and eventual cyanosis. Sputum production is generally scanty, but the sputum can contain blood. Few physical signs may be evident early in the illness. In more advanced cases, diffuse rales may be noted, and chest x-ray findings consistent with diffuse interstitial infiltrates and/or acute respiratory distress syndrome may be present. In such cases, arterial blood-gas determinations show marked hypoxia. Viral cultures of respiratory secretions and lung parenchyma, particularly if samples are taken early in illness, yield high titers of virus. In fatal cases of primary viral pneumonia, histopathologic examination reveals a marked inflammatory reaction in the alveolar septa, with edema and infiltration with lymphocytes, macrophages, occasional plasma cells, and variable numbers of neutrophils. Fibrin thrombi in alveolar capillaries, along with necrosis and hemorrhage, also have been noted. Eosinophilic hyaline membranes can be found lining alveoli and alveolar ducts.

Primary influenza viral pneumonia has a predilection for individuals with cardiac disease, particularly those with mitral stenosis, but also has been reported in otherwise healthy young adults as well as in older individuals with chronic pulmonary disorders. In some epidemics of influenza (notably those of 1918 and 1957), pregnancy increased the risk of primary influenza pneumonia.

Secondary bacterial pneumonia follows acute influenza. Improvement of the patient's condition over 2 to 3 days is followed by a reappearance of fever along with clinical signs and symptoms of bacterial pneumonia, including cough, production of purulent sputum, and physical and x-ray signs of consolidation. The most common bacterial pathogens in this setting are *Streptococcus pneumoniae*, *Staphylococcus aureus*, and *Haemophilus influenzae*—organisms that can colonize the nasopharynx and that cause infection in the wake of changes in bronchopulmonary defenses. The etiology can often be determined by Gram's staining and culture of an appropriately obtained sputum specimen. Secondary bacterial pneumonia occurs most frequently in high-risk individuals with chronic pulmonary and cardiac disease and in elderly individuals. Patients with secondary bacterial pneumonia often respond to antibiotic therapy when it is instituted promptly.

Perhaps the most common of the pneumonic complications during outbreaks of influenza is mixed viral and bacterial pneumonia. The clinical course of this complication includes features of both primary and secondary pneumonia. Patients may experience a gradual progression of their acute illness or may show transient improvement followed by clinical exacerbation, with eventual manifestation of the clinical features of bacterial pneumonia. Sputum cultures may contain both influenza A virus and one of the bacterial pathogens described above. Patchy infiltrates or areas of consolidation may be detected by physical examination and chest x-ray. Patients with mixed viral and bacterial pneumonia generally have less widespread involvement of the lung than those with primary viral pneumonia, and their bacterial infections may respond to appropriate antibiotics. Mixed viral and bacterial pneumonia occurs primarily in patients with chronic cardiovascular and pulmonary diseases.

Other pulmonary complications associated with influenza include worsening of chronic obstructive pulmonary disease and exacerbation of chronic bronchitis and asthma. In children, influenza infection may present as croup.

In addition to the pulmonary complications of influenza, a number of extrapulmonary complications may occur. These include *Reye's syndrome*, a serious complication in children that is associated with influenza B and to a lesser extent with influenza A virus infection as well as with varicella-zoster virus infection. An epidemiologic association between Reye's syndrome and aspirin therapy for the antecedent viral infection has been noted, and the incidence of Reye's syndrome has decreased markedly with widespread warnings regarding the use of aspirin by children with acute viral respiratory infections. → *A detailed description of Reye's syndrome is found in Chap. 300.*

Myositis, rhabdomyolysis, and myoglobinuria are occasional complications of influenza infection. Although myalgias are exceedingly common in influenza, true myositis is rare. Patients with acute myositis have exquisite tenderness of the affected muscles, most commonly in the legs, and may not be able to tolerate even the slightest pressure, such as the touch of bedsheets. In the most severe cases, there is frank swelling and bogginess of muscles. Serum levels of creatine phosphokinase and aldolase are markedly elevated, and an occasional patient has developed renal failure from myoglobinuria. The pathogenesis of influenza-associated myositis is also unclear, although the presence of influenza virus in affected muscles has been reported.

Myocarditis and pericarditis were reported in association with influenza virus infection during the 1918–1919 pandemic; these reports were based largely on histopathologic findings, and these complications have been reported only infrequently since that time. Electrocardiographic changes during acute influenza are common among patients who have cardiac disease but have been ascribed most often to exacerbations of the underlying cardiac disease rather than to direct involvement of the myocardium with influenza virus.

Central nervous system (CNS) diseases, including encephalitis, transverse myelitis, and Guillain-Barré syndrome, have been reported during influenza. The etiologic relationship of influenza virus to such CNS illnesses remains unestablished. Toxic shock syndrome caused by *S. aureus* infection following acute influenza infection has also been reported (see Chap. 142).

In addition to complications involving the specific organ systems described above, influenza outbreaks include a number of cases in which elderly and other high-risk individuals develop influenza and subsequently experience a gradual deterioration of underlying cardiovascular, pulmonary, or renal function—changes that occasionally are irreversible and lead to death. These fatalities contribute to the overall excess mortality associated with influenza A outbreaks.

LABORATORY FINDINGS AND DIAGNOSIS Laboratory diagnosis is accomplished during acute influenza by isolation of the virus from throat swabs, nasopharyngeal washes, or sputum. Virus usually is detected in tissue culture or less commonly is found in the amniotic cavity of chick embryos within 48 to 72 h after inoculation. Viral antigens may be detected somewhat earlier by immunodiagnostic techniques in tissue culture or directly in exfoliated nasopharyngeal cells obtained by washings, although currently the latter method is less sensitive than isolation of virus in tissue culture. The type of influenza virus (A or B) may be determined by either immunofluorescence or HAI techniques, and the hemagglutinin subtype of influenza A virus (H1, H2, or H3) may be identified by HAI with use of subtype-specific antisera. Serologic methods for diagnosis require comparison of antibody titers in sera obtained during the acute illness with those in sera obtained 10 to 14 days after the onset of illness and are useful primarily in retrospect. Fourfold or greater titer rises as detected by HAI or CF or significant rises as measured by ELISA are diagnostic of acute infection. CF tests are generally less sensitive than other serologic techniques but, as they detect type-specific antigens, they may be particularly useful when subtype-specific reagents are not available.

Other laboratory tests are generally not helpful in making a specific diagnosis of influenza virus infection. Leukocyte counts are variable, frequently being low early in illness and normal or slightly elevated later. Severe leukopenia has been described in overwhelming viral or bacterial infection, while leukocytosis with more than 15,000 cells per microliter raises the suspicion of secondary bacterial infection.

DIFFERENTIAL DIAGNOSIS On clinical grounds alone, an individual case of influenza may be difficult to differentiate from an acute respiratory illness caused by any of a variety of respiratory viruses or by *Mycoplasma pneumoniae*. Severe streptococcal pharyngitis or early bacterial pneumonia may mimic acute influenza, although bacterial pneumonias generally do not run a self-limited course. Purulent sputum in which a bacterial pathogen can be detected by Gram's staining is an important diagnostic feature in bacterial pneumonia. The fact that influenza occurs in characteristic outbreaks during the winter months may facilitate a clinical diagnosis. When local health authorities indicate that influenza is present in the community, an acute febrile respiratory illness can be attributed to influenza with a high degree of certainty, particularly if the typical features of abrupt onset and systemic symptoms are present.

℞ **TREATMENT**

In uncomplicated cases of influenza, therapy with either acetaminophen or salicylates for the relief of headache, myalgia, and fever may be considered, but the use of salicylates should be avoided in children below 18 years of age because of the possible association of salicylates with Reye's syndrome. Since cough is ordinarily self-limited, treatment with cough suppressants generally is not indicated, although codeine-containing compounds may be employed if the cough is particularly troublesome. Patients should be advised to rest and maintain hydration during acute illness and should return to full activity only gradually after the illness has resolved, particularly if the illness has been severe.

Specific antiviral therapy in the form of amantadine and rimantadine is available for influenza A. These drugs are active only against influenza A viruses and have been licensed for the prophylaxis and therapy of influenza A virus infections in the United States. If begun within 48 h of the onset of illness, treatment with amantadine or rimantadine reduces the duration of systemic and respiratory symptoms of influenza by approximately 50 percent. In some studies, these drugs have been shown to be superior to antipyretic-analgesics in this regard. From 5 to 10 percent of individuals who receive amantadine will experience mild CNS side effects, primarily jitteriness, anxiety, insomnia, or difficulty in concentrating. These side effects disappear promptly upon cessation of the drug. Rimantadine appears to be equally efficacious and is associated with less frequent CNS side effects than is amantadine. In adults, the usual dose of amantadine or rimantadine is 200 mg/d for 3 to 7 days. Since both drugs are excreted via the kidney, the dose should be reduced to 100 mg/d or less in elderly patients and patients with renal insufficiency. Rimantadine has not been approved for the treatment of influenza A in children. Ribavirin, a nucleoside analogue with activity against a variety of viral agents, has been reported to be effective against both influenza A and influenza B virus infections when administered as an aerosol, although it is relatively ineffective when administered orally.

Studies demonstrating the therapeutic efficacy of antiviral compounds in influenza have almost exclusively included young adults with uncomplicated disease; it is not known whether such compounds are effective in the treatment of complications such as influenza pneumonia. Therapy for primary influenza pneumonia is directed at maintaining oxygenation and is most appropriately undertaken in an intensive care unit, with aggressive respiratory and hemodynamic support as needed. Bypass membrane oxygenators have been employed in this setting with variable results. When an acute respiratory distress syndrome develops, fluids must be administered cautiously, with close monitoring of blood gases and hemodynamic function.

Antibacterial drugs should be reserved for the therapy of bacterial complications of acute influenza, such as secondary bacterial pneumonia. The choice of antibiotics should be guided by Gram's staining and culture of appropriate specimens of respiratory secretions, such as sputum or transtracheal aspirates. If the etiology of a case of bacterial pneumonia is unclear from an examination of respiratory secretions, empirical antibiotics effective against the most common bacterial pathogens in this setting (*S. pneumoniae, S. aureus,* and *H. influenzae*) should be selected (see Chaps. 141, 142, and 152).

PROPHYLAXIS The major public health measure for prevention of influenza has been the use of inactivated influenza vaccines derived from influenza A and B viruses that circulated during the previous influenza season. If the vaccine virus and the currently circulating viruses are closely related, 50 to 80 percent protection against influenza would be expected. Presently available vaccines have been highly purified and are associated with few reactions. Up to 5 percent of individuals experience low-grade fever and mild systemic symptoms 8 to 24 h after vaccination, and up to one-third develop mild redness or tenderness at the vaccination site. Since the vaccine is produced in eggs, individuals with true hypersensitivity to egg products either should be desensitized or should not be vaccinated. Although the 1976 swine influenza vaccine appears to have been associated with an increased frequency of Guillain-Barré syndrome, influenza vaccines administered since 1976 generally have not been. Possible exceptions were noted during 1990–1991 in 18- to 64-year-old vaccinees and during 1993–1994 among vaccine recipients. However, the risk of this syndrome following influenza outweighs the potential risk associated with vaccination. Live attenuated ("cold-adapted") influenza A vaccines also have been developed and appear to be promising in ongoing studies in adults and children. Such vaccines are administered intranasally and stimulate local antibody production more efficiently than conventional inactivated vaccines.

The U.S. Public Health Service recommends influenza vaccination for any individual older than 6 months of age who is at an increased risk for complications of influenza. Included are individuals with chronic cardiovascular or pulmonary disorders (including asthma) and residents of nursing homes and other chronic-care facilities. Other populations for whom the vaccine is recommended include healthy individuals over 65 years of age and individuals who have required regular medical attention for diabetes mellitus, renal disease, hemoglobinopathies, or immunosuppression. Individuals who provide care for high-risk patients or who come into frequent contact with such patients, including household members, also should receive vaccine to reduce the likelihood of transmission of infection. Since commercially available vaccines are inactivated ("killed"), they may be administered

safely to immunocompromised patients. Influenza vaccination is not associated with exacerbations of chronic nervous-system diseases such as multiple sclerosis. Vaccine should be administered early in the autumn before influenza outbreaks occur and should be repeated annually to maintain immunity against the most current influenza virus strains.

Studies have shown amantadine and rimantadine to be 70 to 100 percent effective in the prophylaxis of illness associated with influenza A virus infection. Such prophylaxis is most likely to be used for high-risk individuals who have not received influenza vaccine or in a situation where the vaccines previously administered are relatively ineffective because of antigenic changes in the circulating virus. During an outbreak, amantadine can be administered simultaneously with inactivated vaccine, since it will not interfere with an immune response to the vaccine. In fact, there is evidence that the protective effects of amantadine and vaccine may be additive. Amantadine has also been employed to control nosocomial outbreaks of influenza A. For prophylaxis, administration of amantadine or rimantadine should be instituted promptly when influenza A activity is detected and must be continued daily for the duration of the outbreak. The dosage most frequently employed has been 200 mg/d for adults, but the dose of amantadine should be reduced for patients with renal insufficiency and for the elderly. Viruses resistant to both amantadine and rimantadine can emerge quickly after therapy with these drugs, and the possible transmission of these resistant viruses has been reported.

BIBLIOGRAPHY

CENTERS FOR DISEASE CONTROL: Prevention and control of influenza. Morb Mort Week Rep 45(RR–5):1, 1996

DOLIN R et al: A controlled trial of amantadine and rimantadine in the prophylaxis of influenza A infection. N Engl J Med 307:580, 1982

GLEZEN WP: Serious morbidity and mortality associated with influenza epidemics. Epidemiol Rev 4:25, 1982

GROSS PA et al: Association of influenza immunization with reduction in mortality in an elderly population: A prospective study. Arch Intern Med 148:562, 1988

MURPHY BR, WEBSTER RG: Orthomyxoviruses, in *Virology*, 3d ed, BN Fields (ed). New York, Raven Press, 1995, pp 1091-1152

YINNON AM, DOLIN R: Using antivirals to fight influenza. J Respir Dis 12:1146, 1991

---

194 *Harry B. Greenberg*

VIRAL GASTROENTERITIS

In less developed countries, acute infectious diarrheal disease is a leading cause of morbidity in all age groups and of mortality in infants and young children. In developed countries, acute diarrheal illness remains an important cause of morbidity among both children and adults. Two distinct groups of viruses—the rotaviruses and the enteric caliciviruses, such as Norwalk virus—as well as a variety of bacterial pathogens (see Chap. 128) have emerged as important etiologic agents of gastroenteritis. The rotaviruses are primarily pathogens of young children. The Norwalk and related enteric caliciviruses affect adults as well as children.

ROTAVIRUS Classification and Characterization Rotaviruses are members of the Reoviridae family. The rotavirus virion consists of a 100-nm triple-shelled icosahedral capsid surrounding a genome composed of 11 segments of double-stranded RNA. The virus has two surface proteins, both of which are involved with viral neutralization. Because rotaviruses have a segmented genome, they are capable of undergoing gene reassortment at high frequency. The role of gene reassortment in generating rotavirus antigenic diversity is not known. In humans, rotavirus infection is characterized by replication that is localized almost exclusively in the small intestinal epithelial cells.

Epidemiology Rotavirus infection occurs worldwide. By the age of 3 years, virtually every individual has been infected by rotaviruses at least once. In areas with a temperate climate, rotavirus infection is seasonal, occurring in the cooler winter months. In the United States, the annual seasonal rotavirus epidemic tends to spread from west to east, starting in California and ending in New England. In tropical areas, rotavirus infection tends to occur throughout the year, with some increase in incidence during the cooler rainy season.

Rotaviruses are the single most important cause of severe dehydrating diarrhea in infants and young children (under age 3) in both developed and less developed countries and account for 30 to 50 percent of all cases of diarrhea requiring hospitalization or intensive rehydration therapy. Although severe rotavirus infections are confined primarily to infants and small children, these agents are frequently associated with diarrhea in adults, particularly family members of affected infants, geriatric patients, and immunocompromised hosts. They account for up to 10 percent of cases of traveler's diarrhea (see Chap. 128). Rotaviruses also may be responsible for occasional cases of acute and chronic diarrhea in patients with AIDS.

The majority of rotavirus infections are subclinical or cause mild gastrointestinal illnesses that do not require hospitalization. Subclinical infections in neonates have been shown to protect these children against severe rotavirus gastroenteritis for up to 3 years.

At least nine distinct serotypes of human rotavirus have been described, but only four types are commonly encountered. The relationship of the frequency of infection with these serotypes to host immune status is unclear. A large variety of mammalian and avian species can be infected by rotavirus, but it appears that these animal rotavirus strains do not cause disease in humans very frequently. Rotaviruses are shed in very large numbers (up to 10^{10} particles per gram of feces) in the stool; it is presumed that transmission occurs via fecal-oral spread.

Pathophysiology Rotavirus infects and kills the mature villus tip cells of the small intestine. The mature epithelial cells are replaced by immature absorptive cells that cannot absorb carbohydrates or other nutrients efficiently. Rotavirus infection leads to osmotic diarrhea due to nutrient malabsorption. Changes in intracellular cyclic adenosine monophosphate or guanosine monophosphate are not involved in the etiology of rotavirus diarrhea.

Manifestations The manifestations of rotavirus infection range from subclinical infections through mild diarrhea to severe, occasionally fatal illness. Most information concerning the signs and symptoms of rotavirus infection has been derived from studies of hospitalized young children. The onset of illness is usually abrupt. More than 80 percent of affected children develop vomiting followed by diarrhea. About one-third of hospitalized children have a temperature of greater than 39°C (102.2°F). Gastrointestinal symptoms usually last between 2 and 6 days. Mucus is commonly found in the stool, but white and red blood cells are present in fewer than 15 percent of cases.

Rotavirus infection frequently occurs in conjunction with respiratory tract symptoms, but there is little evidence to indicate that rotavirus replicates in the respiratory tract. Rotavirus infection has been observed in association with a wide variety of other clinical syndromes, including sudden infant death syndrome, Reye's syndrome, encephalitis, aseptic meningitis, pneumonia, exanthema subitum, Kawasaki's syndrome, necrotizing enterocolitis, intussusception, Schönlein-Henoch purpura, hemolytic-uremic syndrome, disseminated intravascular coagulation, and Crohn's disease. The etiologic relationship between these clinical syndromes and rotavirus infection is probably coincidental rather than causal. Rotavirus infection may be especially severe, and even fatal, in immunocompromised children.

Clinical Immunity Relative immunity to rotavirus illness is acquired following infection early in childhood. Immunity is not complete, and adults with low levels of antibody can be symptomatically infected. Local humoral immunity appears to be the critical determinant in protection, and cellular immune mechanisms appear to be involved as well.

Diagnosis Because rotavirus is shed in large amounts in the stool, detection is relatively easy. A variety of specific commercial immunoassays are available to detect rotavirus antigen in fecal specimens. DNA probe diagnosis also appears to be sensitive and specific. There are no pathognomonic signs or symptoms of rotavirus infection,

but this infection is more frequently associated with severe dehydration than are infections caused by other enteric bacterial or viral pathogens.

 TREATMENT Despite the fact that rotavirus diarrhea is caused by intestinal epithelial-cell lysis and death, it can be adequately treated by standard oral rehydration therapy. Only rarely is intravenous rehydration required. Since rotavirus infections have persisted in developed countries with advanced sanitation facilities and widely available clean water, it is unlikely that these infections will be preventable by hygienic measures alone. Progress with a number of candidate live attenuated vaccines suggests that prevention through vaccination may be feasible in the near future.

NORWALK AND RELATED ENTERIC CALICIVIRUSES

Classification and Characterization A variety of round 27- to 32-nm particles, some with clearly defined ultrastructure, have been identified in the stools of individuals with acute nonbacterial gastroenteritis. These agents have been difficult to classify because they are shed in the stool in small amounts for only a few days, and they have not been adapted to cell culture or to animal models. The Norwalk virus is the most extensively studied and best characterized member of this group of agents, which also includes such serologically distinct viruses as the Hawaii agent, the Snow Mountain agent, the W-Ditchling agent, and a number of agents described as calicivirus-like. The Norwalk virus and the Snow Mountain virus have a protein structure similar to that of typical caliciviruses. Recently, the genomes of Norwalk virus and several related viruses have been cloned and sequenced. The genomes are plus-stranded RNA molecules of approximately 7.5 kilobases. The genomic organization of Norwalk virus is similar to that of other members of the calicivirus family.

Epidemiology Norwalk infection occurs year-round and is common. More than 70 percent of adults in both developed and less developed countries have antibodies to this virus. Antibody acquisition occurs at a younger age among children in less developed countries than among those in developed areas; this observation is consistent with the presumption that Norwalk virus is spread by the fecal-oral route. In developed countries, the virus is responsible for approximately one-third of all epidemics of nonbacterial gastroenteritis. Norwalk virus has been incriminated in a variety of food-borne epidemics, and transmission vehicles have included oysters, green salad, and chocolate icing. The virus is a common cause of waterborne epidemics of gastroenteritis and has been shown to be the etiologic agent in nursing home, cruise ship, and institutional (summer camp and school) outbreaks. Norwalk virus is also responsible for a small proportion of cases of traveler's diarrhea. The role of Norwalk-like virus infection in childhood diarrhea is currently under investigation.

In less developed countries, the role of Norwalk-like virus infection in the etiology of diarrhea has not been thoroughly investigated. Preliminary studies indicate that Norwalk virus can cause mild diarrhea in young children, but it does not appear to cause severe illness in infants in either developed or less developed countries. The other serologically distinct calicivirus-like gastroenteritis agents must be studied in more detail before their epidemiology can be distinguished from that of Norwalk virus. It appears, however, that some human caliciviruses, especially those with well-defined ultrastructure, are primarily pathogens of young children rather than adults.

Pathophysiology Following infection with Norwalk or Hawaii virus, the proximal small intestinal architecture is altered, with villus shortening, crypt hyperplasia, and infiltration of the lamina propria by polymorphonuclear and mononuclear cells. No changes are observed in the stomach or colon. The cells in which viral replication occurs have not been identified. The histologic alterations are accompanied by mild steatorrhea, carbohydrate malabsorption, and decreased levels of some brush border enzymes. No changes in adenylate cyclase activity have been observed.

Manifestations Norwalk illness has an incubation period of between 18 and 72 h. Disease is characterized by the abrupt onset of nausea and abdominal cramps followed by vomiting and/or diarrhea. Vomiting is reported more frequently for children than for adults. Low-grade fever [above 37.5°C (99.5°F)] develops in about half of affected individuals. Headache, myalgias, and abdominal pain are common. The white blood cell count is normal; rarely, there is leukocytosis with relative lymphopenia. Red and white cells are not found in the stool. The illness is usually mild and self-limited, lasting 24 to 48 h.

Clinical Immunity Most people do not develop long-term resistance (i.e., resistance lasting 2 years or more) to Norwalk reinfection. In volunteers challenged with Norwalk agent, there is a paradoxical relationship between the level of antibody to Norwalk virus and susceptibility to illness: Low levels of Norwalk antibody in the serum and intestine are associated with clinical resistance to illness. It appears, therefore, that immune mechanisms are not the primary determinants of protection from Norwalk virus.

Diagnosis, Treatment, and Prevention Enzyme-linked immunosorbent assays and polymerase chain reaction–based assays have recently been developed for Norwalk virus and several other 27- to 30-nm gastroenteritis agents. Because Norwalk illness is acute and self-limited, treatment is not usually required. In the rare case of severe vomiting or diarrhea, oral or intravenous rehydration is indicated. Because long-term immunity to Norwalk illness does not usually follow natural infection, the role of vaccination is unclear.

MISCELLANEOUS ENTERIC VIRAL PATHOGENS Enteric adenoviruses are a minor cause of diarrheal illness in infants and children, accounting for 10 percent of cases. These viruses differ from other adenovirus strains in a variety of ways, including neutralization serotype, restriction endonuclease digestion pattern, and ability to grow in tissue culture. The role of enteric adenovirus illness in adults or in persons in less developed countries is not known.

Several strains of antigenically distinct rotaviruses, presently called atypical rotaviruses or groups B and C rotaviruses, have been identified as the cause of occasional episodes of diarrhea in humans and animals.

Preliminary epidemiologic studies have indicated that astroviruses are a relatively frequent cause of mild to moderate diarrhea in young children in developed and less developed countries, accounting for about half as much illness as group A rotaviruses. Astroviruses are 27 to 32 nm in diameter, have a characteristic icosahedral ultrastructure, and contain a plus-stranded RNA genome with a size of approximately 7.0 kilobases and a unique genomic organization. At least seven distinct serotypes have been identified. The recent availability of sensitive and specific diagnostic assays should facilitate more complete assessment of the importance of these agents. Preliminary studies indicate that astroviruses are a common cause of diarrhea in immunocompromised hosts, such as bone marrow transplant recipients and patients with AIDS.

Coronaviruses are frequent causes of diarrheal disease in a variety of animals. Several investigators, using electron microscopy, have identified putative coronavirus-like particles in the stools of patients with diarrhea. In most cases, however, these particles do not have the typical morphologic features of coronaviruses and may represent bacterial breakdown products or cellular fragments.

BIBLIOGRAPHY

Bernstein DI: Evaluation of rhesus rotavirus monovalent and tetravalent reassortant vaccines in U.S. children. JAMA 273:1191, 1995

Blacklow NR, Greenberg HB: Viral gastroenteritis. N Engl J Med 325:252, 1991

Glass RI et al: Rotavirus vaccines: Success by reassortment. Science 265:1389, 1994

Grohmann GS et al: Enteric viruses and diarrhea in HIV-infected patients. N Engl J Med 329:14, 1993

Jiang X et al: Sequence and genomic organization of Norwalk virus. Virology 195:51, 1993

Lewis TL et al: Analysis of astrovirus serotype 1 RNA, identification of viral RNA-dependent RNA polymerase motif and expression of a viral structural protein. J Virol 68:77, 1994

Okhuysen PC: Viral shedding and fecal IgA after Norwalk virus infection. J Infect Dis 171:566, 1995

195 *Jeffrey I. Cohen*

ENTEROVIRUSES AND REOVIRUSES

ENTEROVIRUSES

CLASSIFICATION AND CHARACTERIZATION Enteroviruses are so named because of their ability to multiply in the gastrointestinal tract. Despite their name, these viruses are not a prominent cause of gastroenteritis. Members of the picornavirus (Spanish *pico*, "a little bit" + RNA + virus) family, enteroviruses encompass 67 human serotypes: 3 serotypes of poliovirus, 23 serotypes of coxsackievirus A, 6 serotypes of coxsackievirus B, 31 serotypes of echovirus, and enteroviruses 68 through 71.

Human enteroviruses contain a single-stranded RNA genome that is translated to form a polyprotein; this polyprotein is cleaved into 11 different proteins. The RNA is surrounded by an icosahedral capsid comprising four viral proteins (VP1 through VP4). VP1 is the predominant target of neutralizing antibody. The three-dimensional structure of poliovirus has been determined by x-ray diffraction; a deep cleft on the surface is thought to contain the site of attachment to the cellular receptor. The receptor for poliovirus is a member of the immunoglobulin superfamily, the receptor for echovirus types 1 and 8 is VLA-2 integrin, and the receptor for enterovirus 7 is CD55, or decay-accelerating factor. Poliovirus infection is limited to primates, primarily because of the ability of these cells to express the poliovirus receptor. While cultured mouse cells cannot be infected with the virus, expression of the receptor in transgenic mice allows these animals to become infected with poliovirus and to develop central nervous system (CNS) disease. Several enterovirus genomes have been cloned, and cDNA copies of these genomes are infectious in cultured cells. Construction of recombinant viruses containing portions of virulent and attenuated genomes from these cDNAs has allowed mapping of viral sequences that are responsible for attenuation of the live oral poliovirus vaccines.

Enteroviruses have no lipid envelope and are stable in acidic environments, including the stomach. These viruses are resistant to inactivation by standard disinfectants (e.g., alcohol, detergents) and can persist for days at room temperature.

PATHOGENESIS AND IMMUNITY Much of what is known about the pathogenesis of enteroviruses has been derived from studies of poliovirus infection. After ingestion, poliovirus is thought to infect epithelial cells in the mucosa of the gastrointestinal tract and then to spread to and replicate in the submucosal lymphoid tissue of the tonsils and Peyer's patches. The virus next spreads to the regional lymph nodes, enters the bloodstream during the first (minor) viremic phase, and replicates in organs of the reticuloendothelial system. In some cases poliovirus again infects the bloodstream (major viremia) and then replicates further in various tissues, sometimes causing symptomatic disease. It is uncertain whether poliovirus reaches the CNS during viremia or whether it also spreads via peripheral nerves. Since viremia precedes the onset of neurologic disease in humans and in experimentally infected chimpanzees, it has been assumed that the virus enters the CNS via the bloodstream. Recent studies demonstrating the poliovirus receptor in the end-plate region of muscle at the neuromuscular junction suggest that if the virus enters the muscle during viremia, it could travel across the neuromuscular junction up the axon to the anterior horn cells. Studies of monkeys or transgenic mice expressing the poliovirus receptor show that, after intramuscular injection, poliovirus does not reach the spinal cord if the sciatic nerve is cut. Taken together, these findings suggest that poliovirus can spread directly from muscle to the CNS by neural pathways.

Poliovirus can usually be cultured from the blood 3 to 5 days after infection, before the development of neutralizing antibodies. While viral replication at secondary sites begins to slow 1 week after infection, it continues in the gastrointestinal tract. Poliovirus is shed from the oropharynx for up to 3 weeks after infection and from the gastrointestinal tract for as long as 8 weeks; immunodeficient patients can shed poliovirus for very long periods. During replication in the gastrointestinal tract, attenuated oral poliovirus can mutate, reverting to a more neurovirulent phenotype within a few days. The clinical significance of this increased neurovirulence is unknown.

Humoral and secretory immunity in the gastrointestinal tract is important for the control of enterovirus infections. Enteroviruses induce specific IgM, which usually persists for less than 6 months, and specific IgG, which persists for life. Neutralizing antibody generally confers lifelong protection against subsequent disease caused by the same serotype but does not prevent infection or virus shedding. Enteroviruses also induce cellular immunity, but the importance of this mechanism in limiting infection is uncertain. Patients with impaired cellular immunity are not known to develop unusually severe disease when infected with enteroviruses. In contrast, the severe infections in patients with agammaglobulinemia emphasize the importance of humoral immunity in controlling enterovirus infections. IgA antibodies are important in reducing poliovirus replication in and shedding from the gastrointestinal tract. Breast milk contains IgA specific for enteroviruses and can protect humans from infection.

EPIDEMIOLOGY   Enteroviruses have a worldwide distribution. More than 50 percent of nonpoliovirus enterovirus infections and more than 90 percent of poliovirus infections are subclinical. When symptoms do develop, they are usually nonspecific and occur in conjunction with fever and sometimes with upper respiratory tract manifestations; only a minority of infections are associated with specific clinical syndromes. The incubation period for most enterovirus infections ranges from 2 to 14 days but usually is less than a week.

Enterovirus infection is more common in socioeconomically disadvantaged areas, especially in those where conditions are crowded and in tropical areas where hygiene is poor. Infection is most common among infants and young children; serious illness develops most often during the first few days of life and in older children and adults. In developing countries, where children are infected at an early age, poliovirus infection has less often been associated with paralysis; in countries with better hygiene, older children and adults are more likely to be seronegative, become infected, and develop paralysis. The acquisition of maternal antibody reduces the risk of symptomatic infection in neonates. Young children are the most frequent shedders of enteroviruses and are usually the index cases in family outbreaks. In temperate climates enterovirus infections occur most often in the summer and fall; no seasonal pattern is apparent in the tropics.

Most enteroviruses are transmitted primarily by the fecal-oral route from fecally contaminated fingers or inanimate objects. Patients are most infectious shortly before and after the onset of symptomatic disease, when virus is present in the stool and throat. The ingestion of virus-contaminated food or water can also cause disease. Certain enteroviruses (such as enterovirus 70, which causes acute hemorrhagic conjunctivitis) can be transmitted by direct inoculation from the fingers to the eye. Airborne transmission is important for some viruses that cause respiratory tract disease, such as coxsackievirus A21. Enteroviruses can be transmitted across the placenta from mother to fetus, causing severe disease in the newborn. The transmission of enteroviruses through blood transfusions or insect bites has not been documented. Nosocomial spread of coxsackievirus and echovirus has taken place in hospital nurseries.

DIAGNOSIS   Isolation of enterovirus in cell culture is the most common procedure for the diagnosis of infection. While cultures of stool, nasopharyngeal, or throat samples from patients with enterovirus diseases are often positive, isolation of the virus from these sites does not prove that it is directly associated with disease because these sites are frequently colonized for weeks in patients with subclinical infections. Isolation of virus from the throat is more likely to be associated with disease than isolation from the stool since virus is shed for shorter periods from the throat. Cultures of cerebrospinal fluid (CSF), serum, fluid from body cavities, or tissues are positive less frequently, but a positive result is indicative of disease caused by enterovirus. In some cases the virus can be isolated only from the blood or only from the CSF; therefore, it is important to culture multiple sites. Cultures are more likely to be positive early than later in the course of infection. Most human enteroviruses can be detected within a week after inoculation of cell cultures. Cultures may be negative because of the presence of neutralizing antibody, lack of susceptibility of the cells used, or inappropriate handling of the specimen. Coxsackievirus A may require inoculation into special cell-culture lines or into suckling mice.

Identification of the serotype of an enterovirus is useful primarily for epidemiologic studies and, with a few exceptions, has little clinical utility. It is important to identify serious infections with enterovirus during epidemics and to distinguish the vaccine strain of poliovirus from the other enteroviruses in the throat or in the feces. Stool and throat samples for culture as well as acute- and convalescent-phase serum specimens should be obtained from all patients with suspected poliomyelitis. In the absence of a positive CSF culture, a positive culture of stool obtained within the first 2 weeks after the onset of symptoms is most often used to confirm the diagnosis of poliomyelitis. If poliovirus is isolated, it should be sent to the Centers for Disease Control and Prevention (CDC) in Atlanta for identification as a wild-type or a vaccine virus.

The polymerase chain reaction (PCR) has been used to amplify viral nucleic acid from CSF, serum, and tissues. The high degree of homology among the different enterovirus serotypes at the 5′ end of the genome allows the detection of most (more than 92 percent) of the human serotypes with a single pair of PCR primers. With the proper controls, PCR of the CSF is highly sensitive ($\geq$95 percent) and specific (nearly 100 percent) and is more rapid and probably more sensitive than culture. PCR may be particularly helpful for the diagnosis and follow-up of enterovirus disease in immunodeficient patients receiving immunoglobulin therapy, whose viral cultures may be negative. Antigen detection and hybridization of enterovirus sequences in human tissues with a specific probe are additional options, but these techniques are generally less sensitive than PCR.

Serologic diagnosis of enterovirus infection is limited by the large number of serotypes and the lack of a common antigen. Demonstration of seroconversion may be useful in rare cases for confirmation of culture results, but serologic testing is usually limited to epidemiologic studies. Serum should be collected and frozen soon after the onset of disease and again about 4 weeks later. Measurement of neutralizing titers is the most accurate method for antibody determination; measurement of complement-fixation titers is usually less sensitive. Titers of virus-specific IgM are elevated in both acute and chronic infection.

℞ **TREATMENT**

Most enterovirus infections are mild and resolve spontaneously; however, intensive supportive care may be needed for cardiac, hepatic, or CNS disease. Intravenous, intrathecal, or intraventricular immunoglobulin has been used with apparent success for the treatment of chronic enterovirus meningoencephalitis and dermatomyositis in patients with hypo- or agammaglobulinemia. The disease may stabilize or resolve during therapy; however, some patients decline inexorably despite therapy. Intravenous administration of immunoglobulin with high titers of antibody to the infecting virus has been successful in the treatment of some cases of life-threatening neonatal infection; neonates with such infection may not have maternally acquired antibody. In a recent trial involving neonates with enterovirus infections, immunoglobulin containing very high titers of antibody to the infecting virus reduced rates of viremia; however, no substantial clinical benefit was apparent. The ability of the study to detect a difference in outcome was limited by the small number of patients included. While antiviral agents that inhibit the growth of enterovirus in vitro and in animal models have been developed, these drugs have not yet undergone clinical trials. Glucocorticoids are contraindicated.

Good hand-washing practices and the use of gowns and gloves are important in limiting nosocomial transmission of enteroviruses during epidemics. Enteric precautions are indicated for 7 days after the onset of enterovirus infections.

POLIOVIRUS

MANIFESTATIONS Most infections with poliovirus are asymptomatic. After an incubation period of 3 to 6 days, about 5 percent of patients present with a minor illness (abortive poliomyelitis) manifested by fever, malaise, sore throat, anorexia, myalgias, and headache. This condition usually resolves in 3 days. About 1 percent of patients present with aseptic meningitis (nonparalytic poliomyelitis). Examination of CSF reveals lymphocytic pleocytosis, a normal glucose level, and a normal or slightly elevated protein level; CSF polymorphonuclear leukocytes may be present early. In some patients, especially children, malaise and fever precede the onset of aseptic meningitis.

The least common presentation is that of paralytic disease. After one or several days, signs of aseptic meningitis are followed by severe back, neck, and muscle pain and by the rapid or gradual development of motor weakness. In some cases the disease appears to be biphasic, with aseptic meningitis followed first by apparent recovery but then (1 or 2 days later) by the return of fever and the development of paralysis; this form is more common among children than among adults. Weakness is generally asymmetric, is proximal more than distal, and may involve the legs (most commonly); the arms; or the abdominal, thoracic, or bulbar muscles. Paralysis develops during the febrile phase of the illness and usually does not progress after defervescence. Urinary retention may also occur. Examination reveals weakness, fasciculations, decreased muscle tone, and reduced or absent reflexes in affected areas. Transient hyperreflexia sometimes precedes the loss of reflexes. Patients frequently report sensory symptoms, but objective sensory testing usually yields normal results. Bulbar paralysis leads to dysphagia, difficulty in handling secretions, or dysphonia. Respiratory insufficiency due to aspiration, involvement of the respiratory center in the medulla, or paralysis of the phrenic or intercostal nerves may occur, and severe medullary involvement may lead to circulatory collapse. Most patients with paralysis recover some function weeks to months after infection. About two-thirds of patients have residual neurologic sequelae.

Paralytic disease is more common among older individuals, pregnant women, and persons exercising strenuously or undergoing trauma at the time of CNS symptoms. Tonsillectomy predisposes to bulbar poliomyelitis, and intramuscular injections increase the risk of paralysis in the involved limb(s).

At present, the only cases of poliomyelitis in the United States are due to live poliovirus vaccine; 5 to 10 such cases are reported each year. About half of these cases occur in vaccine recipients; vaccine-induced disease is most frequent among infants after the first dose. The median interval from vaccination to the onset of symptoms is 3 weeks. Most of the other cases develop in close contacts of these patients—usually persons over 20 years old who have not received a full course of vaccine. About 5 percent of the cases of poliomyelitis associated with vaccine occur in members of the community who have had no known direct contact with vaccinees. About 15 percent of all cases of vaccine-associated poliomyelitis involve immunodeficient children or adults, most of whom have hypo- or agammaglobulinemia. In these patients the median interval between vaccination and the onset of symptoms is 6 weeks, but disease can develop up to 6 months after vaccination. The risk of developing poliomyelitis after oral vaccination

is estimated at 1 case per 2.5 million doses administered. The risk of developing paralytic disease after oral vaccination is about 2000 times higher among immunodeficient patients than among immunocompetent children.

The postpolio syndrome presents as a new onset of weakness, fatigue, fasciculations, and pain with additional atrophy of the muscle group involved during the initial paralytic disease 20 to 30 years earlier. The onset is insidious, and weakness occasionally extends to muscles that were not involved during the initial illness. The prognosis is generally good; progression to further weakness is usually slow, with plateau periods that range from 1 to 10 years. The syndrome is thought to be due to progressive dysfunction and loss of motor neurons that compensated for the neurons lost during the original infection and not to persistent or reactivated poliovirus infection.

PREVENTION AND ERADICATION (See also Chap. 122) After a peak of 57,879 cases of poliomyelitis in the United States in 1952, the introduction of inactivated vaccine in 1955 and of oral vaccine in 1961 ultimately eradicated disease due to wild-type poliovirus in the western hemisphere. Such disease has not been documented in the United States since 1979, when cases occurred among religious groups who had declined immunization. In the western hemisphere, paralysis due to wild-type poliovirus was last documented in 1991.

In 1988 the World Health Organization adopted a resolution to eradicate poliomyelitis by the year 2000. From 1985 to 1994, the number of cases worldwide decreased by 84 percent, with 6241 cases reported from 51 countries in 1994. More than 70 percent of cases worldwide were from the Indian subcontinent; outbreaks of poliomyelitis in Europe and North America have been traced to cases imported from this region. Poliomyelitis still occurs in sub-Saharan Africa and in parts of Asia (including several republics of the former Soviet Union) and is a source of concern for unimmunized or partially immunized travelers to these regions. Clearly, global eradication of polio is necessary to eliminate the risk of importation of wild-type virus. Outbreaks are thought to have been facilitated by suboptimal rates of vaccination, isolated pockets of unvaccinated children, poor sanitation and crowding, improper vaccine-storage conditions, and a reduced level of response to one of the serotypes in the vaccine.

For the development of live oral poliovirus vaccine (OPV) containing all three serotypes, wild-type virus was attenuated by passage in monkey kidney cell cultures. OPV strains differ from the wild-type strain in a limited number of nucleotide changes (i.e., fewer than 60). Multiple doses are required to ensure infection and development of immunity to all three serotypes. OPV is given at 2, 4, and 6 to 18 months and at 4 to 6 years of age. While intramuscular injections of other vaccines (live or attenuated) can be given concurrently with OPV, unnecessary intramuscular injections should be avoided during the first month after vaccination because of the risk of vaccine-associated paralysis.

Inactivated poliovirus vaccine is generated by formalin inactivation of the three serotypes of live poliovirus. Since 1988 an enhanced–potency inactivated poliovirus vaccine (IPV-e) has been available in the United States. IPV-e is recommended for adults because of the slightly greater risk of paralysis with OPV in adults than in children. Either children or adults immunized with IPV-e should receive three doses; children should receive a fourth dose when entering school. Current indications and contraindications for OPV and IPV-e are listed in Table 195-1.

The efficacy of OPV after three doses is estimated to be nearly 100 percent. OPV and IPV-e induce antibodies that persist for at least 5 years. Both vaccines induce IgG and IgA antibodies. Compared with recipients of IPV-e, recipients of OPV shed less virus and less frequently develop reinfection with wild-type virus after exposure to poliovirus. Although IPV-e is safe and efficacious, OPV has been used for routine immunization in the United States because of its ease of administration, lower cost, and induction of intestinal immunity resulting in a reduction in the risk of community transmission of wild-type virus. While OPV has been the vaccine of choice for childhood immunization in the United States, the CDC recommended in late

1996 that children receive a sequential schedule of two doses of IPV-e followed by two doses of OPV. A four-dose schedule of either IPV-e or OPV is an acceptable option and may be preferred in certain circumstances. Vaccination with the sequential regimen is expected to reduce the number of cases of vaccine-associated poliomyelitis by 50 to 75 percent.

COXSACKIEVIRUS, ECHOVIRUS, AND OTHER ENTEROVIRUSES

An estimated 5 to 10 million cases of symptomatic enterovirus disease occur in the United States each year. Enteroviruses are the major cause of aseptic meningitis and nonspecific febrile illnesses of neonates. Certain clinical syndromes are more likely to be caused by certain serotypes (Table 195-2), but there is much overlap. From 1970 to 1983, 70 percent of enterovirus infections were caused by only 10 of the 67 human serotypes. Echoviruses 9 and 11 alone accounted for 24 percent of recognized enterovirus infections; echoviruses 4, 6, and 30 and coxsackieviruses A9 and B2 through B5 accounted for 46 percent.

Nonspecific Febrile Illness (Summer Grippe) The most common clinical manifestation of enterovirus infection is a nonspecific febrile illness. After an incubation period of 3 to 6 days, patients present with an acute onset of fever, malaise, and headache. Many cases include upper respiratory symptoms, and some cases include nausea and vomiting. Symptoms often last for 3 to 4 days, and most cases resolve in a week. While infections with other respiratory viruses occur more often from late fall to early spring, enterovirus febrile illness frequently occurs in the summer.

Generalized Disease of the Newborn Most serious enterovirus infections in infants develop during the first week of life, although severe disease can occur up to 3 months of age. Neonates often present with an illness resembling bacterial sepsis, with fever, irritability, and lethargy. Laboratory abnormalities include leukocytosis with a left shift, thrombocytopenia, elevated values in liver function tests, and CSF pleocytosis. The illness can be complicated by myocarditis and hypotension, fulminant hepatitis and disseminated intravascular coagulation, meningitis or meningoencephalitis, or pneumonia. It may be difficult to distinguish enterovirus infection from bacterial sepsis, although a history of a recent virus-like illness in the mother provides a clue.

Aseptic Meningitis and Encephalitis Enteroviruses are the cause of up to 90 percent of cases of aseptic meningitis in children and young adults in which an etiologic agent can be identified. Patients with aseptic meningitis typically present with an acute onset of fever, chills, headache, photophobia, and pain on eye movement. Nausea and vomiting are also common. Examination reveals meningismus without localizing neurologic signs; drowsiness or irritability may also be apparent. In some cases, a febrile illness may be reported that remits but returns several days later in conjunction with signs of meningitis. Other systemic manifestations may pro-

Table 195-1

Indications for and Contraindications to Poliovirus Vaccination

INDICATIONS FOR IMMUNIZATION WITH ORAL POLIOVIRUS VACCINE (OPV)

1. Normal infants and children undergoing routine immunization*
2. Unimmunized or partially immunized children at imminent risk of exposure to poliovirus
3. Adults at future risk of exposure to poliomyelitis who have in the past received one or more doses of OPV or IPV(-e)

INDICATIONS FOR IMMUNIZATION WITH ENHANCED-POTENCY INACTIVATED POLIOVIRUS VACCINE (IPV-e)

1. Normal infants, children, or adults undergoing routine immunization*
2. Immunodeficient persons, including those infected with human immunodeficiency virus (HIV), who are unimmunized or partially immunized
3. Household contacts of an HIV-infected or otherwise immunodeficient person
4. Partially immunized or unimmunized adults in households (or other close contacts) of children receiving OPV, provided that timely immunization of the child can be ensured
5. Adults at future risk of exposure to poliomyelitis who have been partially immunized with IPV(-e) or OPV or have received a primary series of IPV(-e)†
6. Individuals refusing OPV vaccination

CONTRAINDICATIONS TO IMMUNIZATION

1. Pregnant women should not receive OPV or IPV-e unless immediate protection is needed.
2. Immunodeficient patients (e.g., those with AIDS, hypogammaglobulinemia, or generalized malignancy and recipients of immunosuppressive therapy) should not receive OPV.
3. Household contacts of immunodeficient persons should not receive OPV.
4. Families with a history of immunodeficient children should not receive OPV until the immune status of all family members is documented and immunodeficiency is excluded.

* A sequential schedule of two doses of IPV-e followed by two doses of OPV is now recommended by the CDC for infants and children (see text for details and options).
† OPV is also acceptable.
SOURCE: Modified from 1994 Redbook, Report of the Committee on Infectious Diseases.

vide clues to an enteroviral cause, including pharyngitis and cough, diarrhea, myalgias, rash, pleurodynia, myocarditis, and herpangina. Examination of the CSF invariably reveals pleocytosis; early in the course, polymorphonuclear leukocytes may be present or even predominate, raising the possibility of bacterial or other nonviral causes of meningitis. Partially treated bacterial meningitis may be particularly difficult to exclude in some instances. A useful rule is that the CSF cell count in enteroviral meningitis shows a shift to lymphocytic predominance within 24 h of presentation, and the total count generally does not exceed 1000 cells/μL. Additional CSF findings consist of a normal glucose content and a normal or only slightly elevated (by ≤100 mg/mL) level of protein. Enteroviruses and mumps virus may produce a similar picture of meningitis with orchitis; a low CSF glucose level suggests mumps, whereas a normal CSF glucose level and transient CSF polymorphonuclear pleocytosis suggest enterovirus infection. Symptoms ordinarily resolve within a week, although CSF abnormalities can persist for several weeks. Neurologic sequelae are rare, and most patients have an excellent prognosis. Enteroviral encephalitis is much less common than enteroviral aseptic meningitis. Occasional highly inflammatory cases of enteroviral meningitis may be complicated by a mild form of encephalitis that is recognized on the basis of progressive lethargy, disorientation, and sometimes seizures. Less

Table 195-2

Manifestations Commonly Associated with Enterovirus Serotypes

	Serotype(s) of Indicated Virus	
Manifestation	Coxsackievirus	Echovirus (E) and Enterovirus (Ent)
Aseptic meningitis	A2, 4, 7, 9, 10; B1-5	E4, 6, 7, 9, 11, 16, 18, 30, 33; Ent70, 71
Exanthem	A4, 5, 9, 10, 16; B1, 3-5	E4-7, 9, 11, 16-19, 25, 30; Ent71
Generalized disease of the newborn	B2-5	E4-6, 9, 11, 14, 16, 19
Hand-foot-and-mouth disease	A5, 7, 9, 10, 16; B2, 5	Ent71
Herpangina	A1-10, 16, 22; B1-5	E6, 9, 11, 16, 17, 22, 25
Myocarditis, pericarditis	A4, 9, 16; B1-5	E6, 9, 11, 22
Paralysis	A4, 7, 9; B1-5	E2, 4, 6, 9, 11, 30; Ent70, 71
Pleurodynia	A1, 2, 4, 6, 9, 10, 16; B1-6	E1-3, 6–9, 11, 12, 14, 16, 19, 23–25, 30
Pneumonia	A9, 16; B1-5	E6, 7, 9, 11, 12, 19, 20, 30; Ent68, 71

commonly, severe primary encephalitis may develop. It is estimated that 10 to 20 percent of cases of viral encephalitis are due to enteroviruses. Immunocompetent patients generally have a good prognosis.

Patients with hypo- or agammaglobulinemia or severe combined immunodeficiency may develop chronic meningitis or encephalitis; about half of these patients have a dermatomyositis-like syndrome, with peripheral edema, rash, and myositis. They may also have chronic hepatitis. Patients may develop neurologic disease while receiving gamma globulin replacement therapy. Echoviruses (especially echovirus 11) are the most common pathogens in this situation.

Paralytic disease due to enteroviruses other than poliovirus occurs sporadically and is usually less severe than poliomyelitis. Most cases are due to enterovirus 70 or 71 or to coxsackievirus A7. Guillain-Barré syndrome is also associated with enterovirus infection. While some studies have suggested a link between enteroviruses and the chronic fatigue syndrome, most recent studies have not demonstrated such an association.

Pleurodynia (Bornholm Disease) Patients with pleurodynia present with an acute onset of fever and spasms of pleuritic chest or upper abdominal pain. Chest pain is more frequent in adults, and abdominal pain is more common in children. Paroxysms of severe, knifelike pain usually last 15 to 30 min and are associated with diaphoresis and tachypnea. Fever peaks within an hour after the onset of paroxysms and subsides when pain resolves. The involved muscles are tender to palpation, and a pleural rub may be detected. The white blood cell count and chest x-ray are usually normal. Most cases are due to coxsackievirus B and occur during epidemics. Symptoms resolve in a few days, and recurrences are rare. Treatment includes the administration of nonsteroidal anti-inflammatory agents or the application of heat to the affected muscles.

Myocarditis and Pericarditis Enteroviruses are estimated to cause up to one-third of cases of acute myocarditis. Coxsackievirus B and its RNA have been detected in pericardial fluid and myocardial tissue in some cases of acute myocarditis and pericarditis. Most cases of enteroviral myocarditis or pericarditis occur in newborns, adolescents, or young adults. More than two-thirds of patients are male. Patients often present with an upper respiratory tract infection that is followed by fever, chest pain, dyspnea, arrhythmias, and occasionally heart failure. A pericardial friction rub is documented in half of cases, and the electrocardiogram shows ST segment elevations or ST- and T-wave abnormalities. Serum levels of myocardial enzymes are often elevated. Neonates commonly have severe disease, while most older children and adults recover completely. Up to 10 percent of cases progress to chronic dilated cardiomyopathy. Chronic constrictive pericarditis may also be a sequela.

Exanthems Enterovirus infection is the leading cause of exanthems in children in the summer and fall. While exanthems are associated with many enteroviruses, certain types have been linked to specific syndromes. Echoviruses 9 and 16 have frequently been associated with exanthem and fever. Rashes may be discrete (rubelliform) or confluent (morbilliform), beginning on the face and spreading to the trunk and extremities. Echovirus 9 is the most common cause of rubelliform rash. Unlike the rash of rubella, the enteroviral rash occurs in the summer and is not associated with lymphadenopathy. Roseola-like rashes develop after defervescence, with macules and papules on the face and trunk. The Boston exanthem, caused by echovirus 16, is a roseola-like rash that often affects multiple members of a family. A variety of other rashes have been described, including erythema multiforme and vesicular, urticarial, petechial, or purpuric lesions. Enanthems also occur, including lesions that resemble the Koplik's spots seen with measles.

Hand-Foot-and-Mouth Disease After an incubation period of 4 to 6 days, patients with hand-foot-and-mouth disease present with fever, anorexia, and malaise; these manifestations are followed by the development of sore throat and vesicles on the buccal mucosa and often on the tongue and then by the appearance of tender vesicular

lesions on the dorsum of the hands, sometimes with involvement of the palms. The vesicles may form bullae and quickly ulcerate. About one-third of patients also have lesions on the palate, uvula, or tonsillar pillars, and one-third have a rash on the feet (including the soles) or on the buttocks. The disease is highly infectious, with attack rates of close to 100 percent among young children. The lesions usually resolve in 1 week. Most cases are due to coxsackievirus A16.

Herpangina Herpangina is usually caused by coxsackievirus A and presents as acute-onset fever, sore throat, dysphagia, and grayish-white papulovesicular lesions on an erythematous base that ulcerate. The lesions can persist for weeks; are present on the soft palate, anterior pillars of the tonsils, and uvula; and are concentrated in the posterior portion of the mouth. In contrast to herpes stomatitis, enteroviral herpangina is not associated with gingivitis. Acute lymphonodular pharyngitis associated with coxsackievirus A10 presents as white or yellow nodules surrounded by erythema in the posterior oropharynx. The lesions do not ulcerate.

Acute Hemorrhagic Conjunctivitis Patients with acute hemorrhagic conjunctivitis present with an acute onset of severe eye pain, blurred vision, photophobia, and watery discharge from the eye. Examination reveals edema, chemosis, and subconjunctival hemorrhage and often documents punctate keratitis and conjunctival follicles as well. Preauricular adenopathy is often found. Epidemics and nosocomial spread have been associated with enterovirus 70 and coxsackievirus A24. Systemic symptoms, including headache and fever, develop in 20 percent of cases, and recovery is usually complete in 10 days. The sudden onset and short duration of the illness help to distinguish acute hemorrhagic conjunctivitis from other ocular infections such as those due to adenovirus and *Chlamydia*. Paralysis has been associated with some cases of acute hemorrhagic conjunctivitis due to enterovirus 70 during epidemics.

Other Manifestations Enteroviruses are an infrequent cause of childhood pneumonia and the common cold. Coxsackievirus B has been isolated at autopsy from the pancreas of a few children presenting with insulin-dependent diabetes mellitus; however, most attempts to isolate the virus have been unsuccessful. Other diseases that have been associated with enterovirus infection include bronchitis, bronchiolitis, croup, infectious lymphocytosis, polymyositis, acute arthritis, and acute nephritis.

REOVIRUSES

Reoviruses are double-stranded RNA viruses encompassing three serotypes. Serologic studies indicate that most humans are infected with reoviruses during childhood; however, it has been difficult to establish a definite link of reovirus infection with a particular disease. It is likely that most infections either are asymptomatic or cause very mild disease. One outbreak of reovirus infection in children resulted in minor upper respiratory tract symptoms. Reovirus is considered a rare cause of mild gastroenteritis in infants and children. Speculation regarding an association of reovirus type 3 with idiopathic neonatal hepatitis and extrahepatic biliary atresia is based on a higher prevalence of antibody to reovirus in some of these patients and detection of virus in the porta hepatis in one case.

BIBLIOGRAPHY

ABZUG MJ et al: Neonatal enterovirus infection: Virology, serology, and effects of intravenous immune globulin. Clin Infect Dis 20:1201, 1995
CHEN RT et al: Seroprevalence of antibody against poliovirus in inner-city preschool children: Implications for vaccination policy in the United States. JAMA 275:1639, 1996
COCHI SL et al (eds): Global poliomyelitis eradication initiative; status report. J Infect Dis 175(Suppl 1):S1–S292, 1997
DALAKAS MC et al (eds): The postpolio syndrome: Advances in the pathogenesis and treatment. Ann NY Acad Sci 753:1, 1995
FADEN H: Long-term immunity to poliovirus in children immunized with live attenuated and enhanced-potency inactivated trivalent poliovirus vaccines. J Infect Dis 168:452, 1993
——— et al: Comparative evaluation of immunization with live attenuated and enhanced-potency inactivated trivalent poliovirus vaccines in childhood: Systemic and local immune responses. J Infect Dis 162:1291, 1990

IKEDA RM et al: Pleurodynia among football players at a high school. JAMA 270:2205, 1993

McKINNEY R et al: Chronic enteroviral meningoencephalitis in agammaglobu-linemic patients. Rev Infect Dis 9:334, 1987

ROTBART HA (ed): *Human Enterovirus Infections.* Washington, DC, ASM Press, 1995

STREBEL PM et al: Epidemiology of poliomyelitis in the United States one decade after the last reported case of indigenous wild virus–associated disease. Clin Infect Dis 14:568, 1992

——— et al: Intramuscular injections within 30 days of immunization with oral poliovirus vaccine—a risk factor for vaccine-associated paralytic poliomyelitis. N Engl J Med 332:500, 1995

196 *Anne Gershon*

MEASLES (RUBEOLA)

DEFINITION Measles (rubeola) is a highly contagious, acute, exanthematous respiratory disease with a characteristic clinical picture and pathognomonic enanthem. A successful live attenuated measles vaccine became available in 1963 in the United States and elsewhere, and measles is now an unusual disease in most developed countries where this vaccine is widely used. However, measles continues to occur sporadically in mini-epidemics in the United States, and major epidemics in developing nations make this disease a persistent cause of childhood morbidity and mortality.

ETIOLOGIC AGENT Measles virus is a member of the genus *Morbillivirus* and the family Paramyxoviridae. It is closely related to the viruses causing canine and porcine distemper, rinderpest of cattle, and *peste des petits ruminants* of goats and sheep. There is only one antigenic type, and the genome has been sequenced. Measles virions are pleomorphic spherical structures having a diameter of 100 to 250 nm and consisting of six proteins. The inner capsid is composed of a coiled helix of RNA and three proteins, and the outer envelope consists of a matrix protein bearing two types of short surface-glyco-protein projections or peplomers. One peplomer is a conical hemagglu-tinin (H) and the other a dumbbell-shaped fusion (F) protein.

EPIDEMIOLOGY Measles has a worldwide distribution; humans are the only natural hosts although other primates can be experimentally infected. During the prevaccination era in the United States, measles epidemics occurred every 2 to 5 years in the winter and spring. In an epidemic year, roughly half a million measles cases were reported; 99 percent of adults had serologic evidence of previous measles infection. After the live attenuated vaccine became available, the number of cases reported to the Centers for Disease Control and Prevention (CDC) fell, with a nadir of 1497 cases in 1983. More recently, after an upsurge to more than 27,000 cases (with 89 deaths) in 1990, the disease was once more brought under control (with only 312 cases reported to the CDC in 1993), in part through the routine administration of two doses of vaccine. The foremost reason for the resurgence of measles was failure to immunize infants and young children, especially in inner-city areas. Primary vaccine failure (documented in about 5 percent of individuals) and secondary vaccine failure or waning immunity accounted for some cases. In recent years the majority of cases of measles have involved preschool children. Mortality is highest among children under 2 years of age and among adults. Patients with impaired cell-mediated immunity are at especially high risk for severe or even fatal measles. The measles-associated mortality rate in the United States is about 0.3 percent; in developing countries, mortality frequently exceeds 1 percent and sometimes approaches 10 percent.

Measles virus is transmitted by respiratory secretions, predominantly through exposure to aerosols but also through direct contact with larger droplets. Patients are contagious from 1 or 2 days before the onset of symptoms until 4 days after the appearance of the rash. Infectivity peaks during the prodromal phase. The mean intervals from infection to onset of symptoms and to appearance of rash are 10 and 14 days, respectively.

PATHOGENESIS AND PATHOLOGY Measles virus invades the respiratory epithelium and spreads via the bloodstream to the reticuloendothelial system, from which it infects all types of white blood cells, thereby establishing infection of the skin, respiratory tract, and other organs. Both viremia and viruria develop. Multinucleated giant cells with inclusion bodies in the nucleus and cytoplasm (War-thin-Finkeldey cells) are found in respiratory and lymphoid tissues and are pathognomonic for measles. Direct invasion of T lymphocytes may play a role in the temporary depression of cellular immunity that accompanies and transiently follows measles. Infection of the entire respiratory tract accounts for the characteristic cough and coryza of measles and for the less frequent manifestations of croup, bronchiolitis, and pneumonia. Generalized damage to the respiratory tract, with resultant loss of cilia, predisposes to secondary bacterial infections such as pneumonia and otitis media.

Specific antibodies are not detectable before the onset of rash. Cellular immunity (consisting of cytotoxic T cells and possibly natural killer cells) plays a prominent role in host defense, and patients who are deficient in cellular immunity are at high risk for severe measles. Children with isolated agammaglobulinemia are not at increased risk. Immune reactions to the virus in the endothelial cells of dermal capillaries play a substantial role in the development of Koplik's spots (the pathognomonic enanthem) as well as in that of rash; in immunodeficient hosts, measles may be severe despite the absence of these manifestations. Measles antigens have been demonstrated in involved skin during early stages of the illness.

Pathologic changes in measles encephalitis include focal hemorrhage, congestion, and perivascular demyelination. Measles virus is rarely isolated from cerebrospinal fluid (CSF) in cases of encephalitis, which are thought to be due to the interaction of virus-infected cells with local cellular immune factors.

CLINICAL MANIFESTATIONS Measles begins with a 2- to 4-day respiratory prodrome of malaise, cough, coryza, conjunctivitis with lacrimation, nasal discharge, and increasing fever [with temperatures as high as 40.6°C (105°F), probably reflecting secondary viremia]. At this stage of the illness, in which the rash has not yet developed, influenza may be suspected. Just before the onset of the rash, Koplik's spots appear as 1- to 2-mm blue-white spots on a bright red background. Without adequate illumination for examination, they may be overlooked. Koplik's spots are typically located on the buccal mucosa alongside the second molars and may be extensive; they are not associated with any other infectious disease. The spots wane after the onset of rash and soon disappear. The entire buccal and inner labial mucosa may be inflamed, and the lips may be reddened.

The characteristic erythematous, nonpruritic, maculopapular rash of measles begins at the hairline and behind the ears, spreads down the trunk and limbs to include the palms and soles, and often becomes confluent. At this time, the patient is at the most severe point of the illness. By the fourth day, the rash begins to fade in the order in which it appeared. Brownish discoloration of the skin and desquamation may occur later. Fever usually resolves by the fourth or fifth day after the onset of rash; prolonged fever suggests a complication of measles. Lymphadenopathy, diarrhea, vomiting, and splenomegaly are common features. The chest x-ray may be abnormal, even in uncomplicated measles, because of the propensity of this virus to invade the respiratory tract. The entire illness usually lasts about 10 days. The disease tends to be more severe in adults than in children, with higher fever, more prominent rash, and a higher incidence of complications.

Milder forms of the illness with less intense symptoms and a milder rash, termed *modified measles*, may occur in individuals with preexisting partial immunity induced by active or passive vaccination. These patients include infants under 1 year of age who retain some proportion of passively acquired maternal antibodies. On occasion, individuals with a history of immunization may develop modified measles.

COMPLICATIONS The complications of measles can conveniently be divided into three groups, according to the site involved:

the respiratory tract, the central nervous system (CNS), and the gastrointestinal tract. Respiratory tract involvement, manifested as laryngitis, croup, or bronchitis, occurs in the majority of cases of uncomplicated measles. In young children, otitis media is the most common complication. Pneumonia is a frequent reason for hospitalization, especially of adults. The pneumonia is of viral origin in the majority of cases, but secondary bacterial infection (most commonly caused by streptococci, pneumococci, or staphylococci) also takes place with some frequency. Primary giant cell (Hecht's) pneumonia is most often documented in immunocompromised and/or malnourished patients.

Encephalographic abnormalities in the absence of symptoms of CNS disease are extremely frequent in measles. Symptomatic CNS disease, with fever, headache, drowsiness, coma, and/or seizures, occurs in about 1 case in 1000. Symptoms usually begin within days after the onset of rash but occasionally appear for the first time several weeks later. About 10 percent of patients do not survive acute measles encephalitis; a significant percentage of surviving patients develop permanent sequelae, such as mental retardation or epilepsy. Most cases appear to result from an immune-mediated response to myelin proteins (postinfectious encephalomyelitis) and not directly from viral infection of the CNS (see Chap. 376). Rarely, transverse myelitis follows measles. Immunocompromised patients are at risk for progressive fatal encephalitis 1 to 6 months after measles; in some cases, even though prior measles has not been recognized, the virus is identified at autopsy. Subacute sclerosing panencephalitis (SSPE)—a protracted, chronic, extremely rare form of measles encephalitis—sometimes follows measles and is particularly common among children who have measles before the age of 2 years (see Chap. 379). SSPE has virtually disappeared in the United States as a result of widespread vaccination. Typically, progressive dementia evolves over several months. SSPE is thought to be due to a complex interaction of the host with defective measles virus. It is associated with extremely high levels of antibodies to measles virus in the blood and CSF.

Gastrointestinal complications of measles include gastroenteritis, hepatitis, appendicitis, ileocolitis, and mesenteric adenitis. It is not uncommon to detect high levels of alanine and aspartate aminotransferases in the absence of gastrointestinal signs such as jaundice.

Other, rare complications include myocarditis, glomerulonephritis, and postinfectious thrombocytopenic purpura. Measles can exacerbate preexisting tuberculosis, presumably through depression of cellular immunity induced by the virus. Natural measles and immunization against measles can result in tuberculin skin-test anergy lasting for about 1 month.

ATYPICAL MEASLES An atypical form of measles has been reported in individuals who received formalin-inactivated measles vaccine (used in the United States from 1963 through 1967 and in Canada until 1970) and subsequently were exposed to measles virus. After a several-day prodrome of fever, myalgia, and headache, the rash appears. Unlike the rash of typical measles, that of atypical measles begins peripherally and moves centrally; it can be urticarial, maculopapular, hemorrhagic, and/or vesicular. Fever is usually high and is accompanied by edema of the extremities, interstitial pulmonary infiltrates, hepatitis, and (on occasion) pleural effusion. The differential diagnosis often includes Rocky Mountain spotted fever, Henoch-Schönlein purpura, meningococcemia, drug allergy, toxic shock syndrome, and varicella. Despite the severity of atypical measles, patients invariably recover after a convalescence that may be prolonged. Measles virus is not isolated from these patients, and they do not spread the virus to others. This disease is believed to be due to hypersensitivity to measles virus induced by the inactivated vaccine. Formalin inactivation destroys the antigenicity of the F protein, antibodies to which are important in preventing spread of the virus from one cell to another. The role of cellular immunity in this process is unknown. Extremely high convalescent titers of antibody to measles virus (e.g., 1:1,000,000) are diagnostic of atypical measles. To prevent this syndrome, adults who received formalin-inactivated measles vaccine should be reimmu-

nized with at least one dose of live attenuated measles vaccine. Since inactivated measles vaccine has not been available for more than 25 years, atypical measles has now virtually disappeared.

MEASLES IN THE IMMUNOCOMPROMISED HOST Patients with defects in cell-mediated immunity are at risk for severe protracted and fatal measles. Included in this category are patients with congenital cellular immune defects or malignancy, recipients of immunosuppressive therapy, or persons infected with human immunodeficiency virus (HIV). In these patients, measles may not be accompanied by a rash. Complications are primary measles (giant cell) pneumonia, progressive encephalitis beginning weeks to months after initial infection, and (in HIV-infected patients) progression to AIDS.

MEASLES IN ADULTS Measles is naturally a disease of childhood and, like many other viral infections, is more severe in adults than in children. About 3 percent of young adults with measles develop primary viral pneumonia and require hospitalization. Hepatitis and bronchospasm are more common among adults with measles than among children, and the rash is more severe and more confluent in adults. Bacterial superinfection is more common among adults, more than one-third of whom develop respiratory complications such as otitis media, sinusitis, and pneumonia. Adults may develop measles because they were never immunized or (more rarely) because their vaccine-induced immunity has waned. Very low titers of antibody to measles virus have been associated with lack of protection.

LABORATORY FINDINGS Lymphopenia and neutropenia are common in measles and may be due to invasion of leukocytes by the virus, with subsequent cell death. Leukocytosis may herald a bacterial superinfection. Patients with measles encephalitis usually have an elevated protein concentration in CSF as well as lymphocytosis. A specific diagnosis of measles can be made quickly by immunofluorescent staining of a smear of respiratory secretions for measles antigen; monoclonal antibodies conjugated to fluorescein are commercially available for this purpose. Secretions can also be examined microscopically for multinucleated giant cells. Measles virus can be isolated from respiratory secretions or urine and rapidly identified in tissue culture with fluorescein-labeled monoclonal antibodies. A number of serologic tests are available for the diagnosis of measles; however, a serologic diagnosis cannot necessarily be made quickly since both acute- and convalescent-phase sera are usually tested, ideally at the same time. The older hemagglutination inhibition test has been replaced by enzyme immunoassay (EIA), which is more sensitive and simpler to perform. EIA can be used to measure specific IgM and thus to diagnose measles on the basis of an acute-phase serum sample alone. Specific IgM antibodies are detectable within 1 to 2 days after the appearance of rash, and the IgG titer rises significantly after 10 days. As already mentioned, atypical measles and SSPE are associated with extremely high titers of antibody.

DIFFERENTIAL DIAGNOSIS Classic measles—with Koplik's spots, cough, coryza, conjunctivitis, and a rash beginning on the head—is easily diagnosed on clinical grounds. Modified measles is more difficult to diagnose clinically since one or more characteristic signs may be lacking. The differential diagnosis of measles includes Kawasaki's syndrome, scarlet fever, infectious mononucleosis, toxoplasmosis, drug eruption, and *Mycoplasma pneumoniae* infection. Most of these conditions can be identified by either culture or serologic assay. In the differential diagnosis of measles, attention should be paid to the current epidemiology of the disease in the community and to the patient's history of measles vaccination and foreign travel.

PREVENTION The development of live attenuated measles vaccine by Enders and his colleagues was a milestone in American medicine. This vaccine, used in the United States for the routine immunization of children since 1963, induces seroconversion in about 95 percent of recipients and probably confers lifelong protection. Waning immunity to measles after immunization has been documented only on rare occasions. For the past 25 years, measles vaccine has been available as the combination vaccine of measles-mumps-rubella (MMR); this combination MMR vaccine should be administered to children between the ages of 12 and 15 months. (Vaccination at 12 months is preferred for infants whose mothers were immunized against measles in childhood. These mothers have lower antibody titers than women who have had natural measles, and their infants correspondingly have transplacental antibodies of lower titer and shorter duration.) A second dose of MMR vaccine is recommended at 4 to 5 years of age (CDC) or at 12 years of age (American Academy of Pediatrics). This policy was developed in the late 1980s in response to measles outbreaks in the United States. Since the institution of the two-dose regimen and the increased effort to immunize all children, measles has again become an unusual disease in the United States. Regional guidelines that reflect the current local epidemiology of measles should be followed.

Older susceptible persons should also be immunized. Individuals should be considered susceptible to measles unless they have documentation of physician-diagnosed measles or of the receipt of two doses of vaccine, have laboratory evidence of measles immunity, or were born before 1957. Rarely, individuals born before 1957 develop measles, and those who are at risk of exposure to measles (e.g., health workers, teachers, and international travelers) should be tested for measles antibody and immunized if necessary. Approximately 10 percent of healthy vaccinees develop a fever, with temperatures up to 39.4°C (103°F), 5 to 7 days after vaccination; this fever lasts 1 to 5 days and is accompanied by a transient rash. Individuals previously immunized only with killed vaccine are considered susceptible and should receive at least one dose—and preferably two doses—of MMR vaccine. Transient adverse reactions in these individuals include fever, malaise, and redness and swelling at the injection site.

Children with asymptomatic HIV infection should receive MMR vaccine. Strong consideration should also be given to the vaccination of symptomatic HIV-infected children because of the severity of measles in this group and the lack of reported problems following vaccination. Measles vaccine is contraindicated for persons with impaired cell-mediated immunity, for pregnant women, and for persons with a history of anaphylaxis due to egg protein or neomycin. Minor illnesses, with or without fever and a history of convulsions, are not contraindications to vaccination. Vaccination should be deferred for 6 to 11 months after the receipt of immune globulin or of blood products containing antibodies and for at least 3 months after the discontinuation of immunosuppressive treatment. Vaccine failures have been ascribed to faulty storage of the preparation used, immunization of infants with preexisting (maternally derived) antibodies, and simultaneous administration of measles vaccine and immune globulin.

Children and adults who are susceptible to measles and are exposed to the disease should receive postexposure prophylaxis. Standard immune globulin, given intramuscularly within 6 days of exposure, can exert a protective or modifying effect; the earlier it is given, the better the outcome. The dose is 0.25 mL/kg for healthy persons and 0.5 mL/kg for immunocompromised persons, with a maximum dose of 15 mL. Immune globulin is particularly strongly indicated for susceptible household contacts, especially those less than 1 year of age, and for immunocompromised persons. HIV-infected persons should be given immune globulin after exposure, regardless of immune status and whether or not they are receiving intravenous immunoglobulin. Vaccination within 72 h of exposure may also provide protection against clinical measles, but this strategy is contraindicated as postexposure prophylaxis for immunocompromised individuals. Vaccine and immune globulin should not be given concurrently.

℞ **TREATMENT**
Therapy for measles is largely supportive and symptom-based. Patients with otitis media and pneumonia should be given standard antibiotics. Patients with encephalitis need supportive care, including observation for increased intracranial pressure. Controlled trials suggest clinical benefit from high doses of vitamin A in severe or potentially severe measles, especially in children under the age of 2 years. A dose of 50,000 IU is used for infants aged 1 to 6 months, 100,000 IU for infants aged 7 to 12 months, and 200,000 IU for children over 1 year. A single dose is administered on two consecutive days. Transient vomiting and headache may be associated with the administration of vitamin A. Ribavirin is effective against measles virus in vitro and may be considered for use in immunocompromised individuals.

BIBLIOGRAPHY

EBERHART-PHILLIPS JE et al: Measles in pregnancy: A descriptive study of 58 cases. Obstet Gynecol 82:797, 1993

FORNI AL et al: Severe measles pneumonitis in adults: Evaluation of clinical characteristics and therapy with intravenous ribavirin. Clin Infect Dis 19:454, 1994

GREMILLION DH et al: Measles pneumonia in young adults. An analysis of 106 cases. Am J Med 71:539, 1981

HUSSEY GD et al: A randomized, controlled trial of vitamin A in children with severe measles. N Engl J Med 323:160, 1990

KAPLAN LJ et al: Severe measles in immunocompromised patients. JAMA 267:1237, 1992

LA BOCCETTA AC et al: Measles encephalitis. Report of 61 cases. Am J Dis Child 107:247, 1964

MARKOWITZ LE et al: Duration of live measles vaccine–induced immunity. Pediatr Infect Dis J 9:101, 1990

PELTOLA H et al: The elimination of indigenous measles, mumps, and rubella from Finland by a 12-year, two-dose vaccination program. N Engl J Med 331:1397, 1994

SMARON MF et al: Diagnosis of measles by fluorescent antibody and culture of nasopharyngeal secretions. J Virol Methods 33:223, 1991

TAKAHASHI H et al: Detection and comparison of viral antigens in measles and rubella rashes. Clin Infect Dis 22:36, 1996

WATSON BM et al: Safety and immunogenicity of a combined live attenuated measles, mumps, rubella, and varicella vaccine (MMR(II)V) in children. J Infect Dis 173:731, 1996

197 *Anne Gershon*

RUBELLA (GERMAN MEASLES)

DEFINITION Rubella is an acute viral infection of children and adults that characteristically includes rash, fever, and lymphadenopathy and has a broad spectrum of other possible manifestations. However, a high percentage of rubella infections in both children and adults are subclinical. In addition, the illness can resemble a mild attack of measles (rubeola) and can cause arthritis, especially in adults. Rubella during pregnancy can lead to fetal infection, with the production of a significant constellation of malformations (*congenital rubella syndrome*) in a high proportion of infected fetuses.

ETIOLOGIC AGENT Rubella virus, a togavirus, is closely related to the alphaviruses. Unlike these agents, however, it does not require a vector for transmission. Moreover, there is no RNA sequence homology between rubella virus and the alphaviruses.

The rubella virion is composed of an inner helical capsid of RNA and protein that is surrounded by a lipid-containing envelope with a diameter of about 60 nm. The structural proteins associated with rubella virus are E1 and E2 (transmembrane envelope glycoproteins) and C (the capsid protein that surrounds the viral RNA).

EPIDEMIOLOGY In the United States during the prevaccine era, rubella was most common in the spring and most often affected school-age children; only 80 to 90 percent of adults were immune; and major epidemics occurred every 6 to 9 years. In 1968, 18,269 cases of rubella were reported in the United States, with 30 cases of congenital rubella syndrome. Since the introduction of live attenuated rubella vaccine in 1969, there have been no epidemics; limited outbreaks have been reported in settings where susceptible individuals come into close contact with one another (e.g., schools and workplaces). In 1994, only 227 cases of postnatally acquired rubella—most of them in young adults—and 7 cases of congenital rubella syndrome were reported to the Centers for Disease Control and Prevention (CDC).

Whether symptomatic or subclinical, rubella is contagious, albeit less so than measles. Its incubation period is 18 days on average, with a range of 12 to 23 days. The virus, which is spread in droplets shed in respiratory secretions, infects the respiratory tract and then the bloodstream. In postnatally acquired infections, rubella virus is shed during the prodromal phase of the illness, and shedding from the pharynx can continue for about a week after onset. Despite high titers of specific neutralizing antibodies, infants with congenital rubella may excrete rubella virus from the respiratory tract and in the urine until the age of 2 years. This excretion raises important issues related to infection control in hospital and day-care settings. Persons recently immunized with live attenuated rubella vaccine do not transmit the vaccine virus to others, although low titers of rubella virus may be detected transiently in the pharynx.

After an attack of rubella, specific antibodies and cell-mediated immunity develop and probably play a significant role in protection against future disease. Although asymptomatic reinfection is rarely if ever associated with viremia, it is common upon reexposure to the virus. Rubella virus has been cultured from respiratory secretions during reinfection. Fetal infection may occur during maternal reinfection but is acknowledged to be extremely rare because of the absence of maternal viremia under these circumstances. Viremia following reinfection of individuals immunized against rubella is also rare. Thus the current level of congenital rubella in the United States is exceedingly low.

PATHOGENESIS AND PATHOLOGY Little is known about the microscopic pathology of postnatally acquired rubella since the disease is invariably self-limited. Like that of measles, the rash of rubella is immunologically mediated; its onset coincides with the development of specific antibodies. Viremia can be demonstrated for about a week before and ends within a few days after the onset of rash.

The cause of the damage to cells and organs in congenital rubella is not well understood. Proposed mechanisms of fetal damage include mitotic arrest of cells, tissue necrosis without inflammation, and chromosomal damage. The growth of the fetus may be retarded. Other findings may include decreased numbers of megakaryocytes in the bone marrow, extramedullary hematopoiesis, and interstitial pneumonia.

CLINICAL MANIFESTATIONS **Postnatally Acquired Rubella** Infection acquired after birth usually results in an extremely mild or subclinical illness. A prodromal phase is uncommon in children; adults may have more severe disease, with a brief prodrome of malaise, fever, and anorexia. The foremost symptoms of postnatally acquired rubella include posterior auricular, cervical, and suboccipital lymphadenopathy; fever; and rash. The rash often begins on the face and spreads down the body. It is maculopapular but not confluent, is sometimes accompanied by mild coryza and conjunctivitis, and generally lasts for 3 to 5 days. A petechial enanthem on the soft palate, designated *Forschheimer spots*, may occur but is not specific for rubella. Fever may be absent entirely or may be present for only several days in the early phase of the illness.

Complications of postnatally acquired rubella are uncommon; bacterial superinfection is rare. One particularly troublesome complication is seen almost exclusively in women: arthritis, most frequently involving the fingers, wrists, and/or knees, develops as the rash is appearing and may take several weeks to resolve. Chronic arthritis resulting from rubella is extremely rare. Rubella virus has been isolated from joint fluid during acute rubella arthritis and from peripheral blood in chronic rubella arthritis.

Another complication of postnatally acquired rubella is hemorrhage due to both thrombocytopenia and vascular damage, which occurs in 1 of every 3000 patients. Thrombocytopenia may last for weeks or months; it can have long-term consequences if there is bleeding into organs such as the eye or the brain.

Both children and adults may develop encephalitis after rubella; the incidence is about five times lower than that of encephalitis following measles. Adults are more likely than children to develop encephalitis; the mortality rate from this complication is 20 to 50 percent. Mild hepatitis is an unusual complication. Immunosuppressed patients are not at increased risk for rubella as they are for measles.

Congenital Rubella Maternal infection in early pregnancy can lead to fetal infection, with resultant congenital rubella. The classic signs of congenital rubella are cataract, heart disease, and deafness, but a myriad of other defects have been reported. These abnormalities include signs and symptoms that are transient, such as low birth weight, thrombocytopenia, hepatosplenomegaly, jaundice, and pneumonia; those that are permanent, such as deafness, pulmonic stenosis, patent ductus arteriosus, glaucoma, and cataract; and those that are developmental, such as mental retardation, diabetes mellitus, and behavioral disorders.

The most important factor in the pathogenicity of rubella virus for the fetus is gestational age at the time of infection. Maternal infection during the first trimester leads to fetal infection in about 50 percent of cases; maternal infection early in the second trimester leads to fetal infection in about one-third of cases. Fetal malformations not only are more common after maternal infection in the first trimester but also tend to be more severe and to involve more organ systems. While a fetus infected in the fourth week of gestation may develop many problems, one infected later (e.g., in the 20th week) may have isolated deafness as the only symptom.

DIAGNOSIS Since postnatally acquired rubella is such a mild disease and since many cases are subclinical, diagnosis on clinical grounds can be difficult. Other diseases that may mimic rubella include toxoplasmosis, scarlet fever, modified measles, roseola, fifth disease (erythema infectiosum due to parvovirus B19), and enteroviral infection. Routine laboratory tests usually reveal leukopenia and atypical lymphocytes.

The isolation of rubella virus in cell cultures of throat samples, urine, or other secretions is difficult and expensive but is sometimes undertaken. This technique is most useful when congenital rubella is suspected. A laboratory diagnosis is more often made serologically. The most commonly used test is an enzyme-linked immunosorbent assay (ELISA) for IgG and IgM antibodies. Acute rubella is diagnosed by the documentation of a fourfold or greater rise in the titer of IgG antibodies in paired acute- and convalescent-phase serum specimens or by the detection of rubella-specific IgM antibodies in one serum specimen. However, false-negative and -positive IgM reactions are sometimes obtained. Moreover, true-positive IgM reactions can be obtained in both primary infection and reinfection. Congenital rubella is diagnosed by the isolation of rubella virus, the detection of IgM antibodies in a single serum sample, and/or the documentation of either the persistence of rubella antibodies in serum beyond 1 year of age or a rising antibody titer anytime during infancy in an unvaccinated child. Biopsied tissues and/or blood and cerebrospinal fluid have also been used for the demonstration of rubella antigens with monoclonal antibodies and for the detection of rubella RNA by in situ hybridization and polymerase chain reaction.

PREVENTION Live attenuated rubella vaccine was licensed in 1969, 7 years after the virus was first isolated in culture. This vaccine was developed as a strategy to prevent congenital rubella by ensuring that very few pregnant women would be susceptible and that there would be little circulating wild-type virus. Rubella vaccine induces seroconversion in more than 95 percent of recipients. Since its licensure, there have been no major epidemics in the United States, and the number of cases has declined by 98 percent. The last large-scale epidemic of rubella in the United States took place in 1964 and 1965; this epidemic resulted in the birth of tens of thousands of infants with the congenital rubella syndrome. The vaccine currently licensed in the United States, RA 27/3, is propagated in human diploid cells and is more immunogenic (particularly with regard to the stimulation of secretory immunity) than previously licensed vaccines. The present vaccination strategy, developed in part when measles was not being adequately controlled, is to immunize all infants at 12 to 15 months of age with measles-mumps-rubella (MMR) vaccine and to administer a second dose during childhood. Rubella vaccine may also be administered to anyone who is thought to be susceptible to the infection and is not pregnant; it is particularly important that hospital workers of either sex be immune to rubella so that nosocomial transmission is avoided. While there has been little change in the prevalence of immunity to rubella among women of childbearing age (about 80 percent), the incidence of congenital rubella is extremely low—about 10 cases annually. It is likely that, although antibody may be undetectable years after immunization, protection against infection—possibly due to cell-mediated immunity—is the rule. At present, there is little if any evidence of significant waning of clinically important immunity to rubella with time.

On occasion, rubella vaccine may cause arthralgia or arthritis, especially in young women. Very rarely, rubella vaccination results in chronic arthritis; however, even cases of frank arthritis in vaccinees are self-limited, lasting only about 1 week.

After investigation of a series of more than 400 women who were inadvertently immunized during pregnancy and who carried their infants to term, the CDC has concluded that vaccine-type rubella virus either does not cause the congenital rubella syndrome at all or does so at an incidence too low to be detected. Nonetheless, rubella vaccine is contraindicated for use in pregnant women, and it is recommended that pregnancy be avoided for at least 3 months after rubella vaccination. It is acceptable for rubella-susceptible children whose mothers are also susceptible to be immunized, since vaccinated individuals do not shed rubella virus or transmit it to susceptible individuals. Although it is recommended that rubella vaccine not be given to immunosuppressed persons, the vaccine is given to children infected with human immunodeficiency virus. No adverse effects of rubella vaccine have been reported in immunocompromised patients.

℞ **TREATMENT**
There is no specific therapy for rubella. At one time, immune globulin was used in an effort to prevent congenital rubella when pregnant women became infected. However, since administration of immune globulin did not prevent maternal viremia, this approach was discarded. Treatment is given for symptoms such as fever, arthralgia, and arthritis.

BIBLIOGRAPHY

BOSMA TJ et al: Use of PCR for prenatal and postnatal diagnosis of congenital rubella. J Clin Microbiol 33:2881, 1995

CHANTLER JK et al: Persistent rubella virus infection associated with chronic arthritis in children. N Engl J Med 313:1117, 1985

CUSI MG et al: Serological evidence of reinfection among vaccinees during rubella outbreak. Lancet 336:1071, 1991

GREGG NM: Congenital cataract following German measles in the mother. Trans Ophthalmol Soc Aust 3:35, 1941

HERRMANN KL: Available rubella serologic tests. Rev Infect Dis 7:S108, 1985

HORSTMANN D et al: Persistence of vaccine-induced immune responses to rubella: Rev Infect Dis 7:S80, 1985

MELLINGER AK et al: High incidence of congenital rubella syndrome after a rubella outbreak. Pediatr Infect Dis J 14:573, 1995

SKENDZEL LP: Rubella immunity: Defining the level of protective antibody. Am J Clin Pathol 106:170, 1996

SMITH CA et al: Rubella virus and arthritis. Rheum Dis Clin North Am 13:810, 1987

TOWNSEND JJ et al: Progressive rubella panencephalitis: Late onset after congenital rubella. N Engl J Med 292:990, 1975

WEIBEL RE, BENOR DE: Chronic arthropathy and musculoskeletal symptoms associated with rubella vaccines: A review of 124 claims submitted to the National Vaccine Injury Compensation Program. Arthritis Rheum 39:1529, 1996

198 *Anne Gershon*

MUMPS

DEFINITION Mumps is an acute, systemic, communicable viral infection whose most distinctive feature is swelling of one or both parotid glands. Involvement of other salivary glands, the meninges, the pancreas, and the gonads is also common.

ETIOLOGIC AGENT Mumps virus, a paramyxovirus, is pleomorphic and has a diameter ranging from 100 to 600 nm. The virion is composed of RNA and five proteins. The RNA is surrounded by an envelope with glycoprotein projections. There are two envelope glycoproteins—a hemagglutinin-neuraminidase (HN) and a hemolysis cell fusion antigen (F)—as well as a matrix envelope protein (M). There are two internal components: a nucleocapsid protein (NP) and an RNA polymerase protein. There is only one antigenic type of mumps virus.

EPIDEMIOLOGY After the introduction of mumps vaccine in 1967, the incidence of clinical mumps declined significantly in the United States. In 1968 (before widespread immunization), 152,209 cases of mumps were reported in this country. The 1537 cases reported in 1994 represent a reduction in the number of cases by >99 percent from prevaccine levels; this is the lowest number of cases ever reported in a year. Before widespread vaccination, the incidence of mumps was highest in the winter and spring, with epidemics every 2 to 5 years. At that time mumps was principally a disease of childhood, although today more than 50 percent of cases occur in young adults. Epidemics tended to occur in confined populations, such as those in schools and the military services.

The incubation period of mumps generally ranges from 14 to 18 days, with extremes of 7 and 23 days. However, because a contact may be shedding virus before the onset of clinical disease or (like one-third of patients) may have subclinical infection, the incubation period in individual cases is often uncertain. One attack of mumps usually confers lifelong immunity. Long-term immunity is also associated with immunization.

PATHOGENESIS Mumps virus is transmitted by droplet nuclei, saliva, and fomites. Replication of the virus in the epithelium of the upper respiratory tract leads to viremia, which is followed by infection of glandular tissues and/or the central nervous system (CNS).

Little is known of the pathology of mumps since the disease is rarely fatal. The affected glands contain perivascular and interstitial mononuclear cell infiltrates with prominent edema. Necrosis of acinar and epithelial duct cells is evident in the salivary glands and in the germinal epithelium of the seminiferous tubules.

CLINICAL MANIFESTATIONS The prodrome of mumps consists of fever, malaise, myalgia, and anorexia. Parotitis, if it develops, usually does so within the next 24 h but may be delayed for as long as a week; it is generally bilateral, although the onset on the two sides may not be synchronous and at times only one side is affected. The submaxillary and sublingual glands are involved less often than the parotid and are almost never involved alone. Swelling of the parotid is accompanied by tenderness and obliteration of the space between the ear lobe and the angle of the mandible. The patient frequently reports an earache and finds it difficult to eat, swallow, or talk. Glandular swelling increases for a few days and then gradually subsides, disappearing within a week. The orifice of Stensen's duct is commonly red and swollen. Presternal pitting edema has been described in about 5 percent of mumps cases, often in association with submandibular adenitis.

Other than parotitis, orchitis is the most common manifestation of mumps among postpubertal males, developing in about 20 percent of cases. The testis is painful and tender and is enlarged to several times its normal size; accompanying fever is common. Later, testicular atrophy develops in half of the affected men. Since orchitis is bilateral in fewer than 15 percent of cases, sterility after mumps is rare. Oophoritis in women—far less common than orchitis in men—may cause lower abdominal pain but does not lead to sterility.

Aseptic meningitis, which may develop before, during, after, or in the absence of parotitis, is a common manifestation of mumps in both children and adults. Symptoms include stiff neck, headache, and drowsiness. Pleocytosis of the cerebrospinal fluid (CSF), with up to 1000 cells/μL, may develop in up to 50 percent of cases of clinical mumps, but clinical signs of meningeal irritation are documented in only 5 to 25 percent of cases. Within the first 24 h, polymorphonuclear leukocytes may predominate in CSF, but by the second day nearly all the cells are lymphocytes. The glucose level in CSF may be abnormally low, and this finding may arouse suspicion of bacterial meningitis. Aseptic meningitis due to mumps without parotitis is indistinguishable clinically from that caused by other viruses. Mumps meningitis is almost invariably self-limited, although cranial nerve palsies have occasionally led to permanent sequelae, particularly deafness. More rarely, mumps virus may cause encephalitis, which presents as high fever with marked changes in the level of consciousness and frequently results in permanent sequelae in survivors. Other CNS problems occasionally associated with mumps include cerebellar ataxia, facial palsy, transverse myelitis, Guillain-Barré syndrome, and aqueductal stenosis leading to hydrocephalus.

Mumps pancreatitis, which may present as abdominal pain, is difficult to diagnose because an elevated serum amylase level can be associated with either parotitis or pancreatitis. Other unusual complications of mumps include myocarditis, mastitis, thyroiditis, nephritis, arthritis, and thrombocytopenic purpura. An excessive number of spontaneous abortions is associated with gestational mumps when the disease occurs during the first trimester. Mumps in pregnancy does not lead to premature birth or fetal malformations.

DIFFERENTIAL DIAGNOSIS   The diagnosis of mumps is made easily in patients with acute bilateral parotitis and a history of recent exposure. When parotitis is unilateral or absent or when sites other than the parotid gland are involved, laboratory diagnosis is required (see below).

The myriad causes of bilateral parotid swelling other than mumps virus include infection with other viruses, such as parainfluenza virus type 3, coxsackieviruses, and influenza A virus; metabolic diseases, such as diabetes mellitus and uremia; and drugs, such as phenylbutazone and thiouracil. Unilateral parotid swelling can result from a tumor, a cyst, or a ductal obstruction due to stones or strictures. Other conditions associated with chronic parotid swelling include sarcoidosis, Sjögren's syndrome, and infection with human immunodeficiency virus (HIV). Suppurative parotitis, usually caused by *Staphylococcus aureus*, is most often unilateral.

Other entities should be considered when manifestations consistent with mumps appear in organs other than the parotid. Testicular torsion may produce a painful scrotal mass resembling that seen in mumps orchitis. Other viruses (e.g., enteroviruses) may cause aseptic meningitis that is clinically indistinguishable from that due to mumps virus.

LABORATORY DIAGNOSIS   Mumps virus is readily isolated after inoculation of appropriate clinical specimens into a variety of host systems, such as rhesus monkey kidney cells and human embryonic lung fibroblasts. The virus can be rapidly identified by the use of cells grown in shell vials and of fluorescein-labeled monoclonal antibodies. Mumps virus may be recovered from saliva, throat, and urine during the first few days of illness and from the CSF of patients with mumps meningitis. Shedding of virus in the urine may persist for as long as 2 weeks. No particular peripheral blood cell count is characteristic of mumps.

Highly sensitive enzyme-linked immunosorbent assays (ELISA) are useful for diagnosis of mumps and for determination of susceptibility to the disease. Acute mumps can be diagnosed either by the examination of acute- and convalescent-phase sera for a significant increase in antibody titer or by the demonstration of specific IgM in one serum specimen. Use of a skin-test antigen to assess immunity to mumps has been replaced by serologic testing.

℞ **TREATMENT**

Therapy for parotitis and other manifestations of mumps is symptom-based. The administration of analgesics and the application of warm or cold compresses to the parotid area may be helpful. Mumps immune globulin is of no value in the prophylaxis or treatment of established disease. Testicular pain may be minimized by the local application of cold compresses and gentle support for the scrotum. Anesthetic blocks may also be used. Neither the administration of

glucocorticoids nor incision of the tunica albuginea is of proven value for the treatment of severe orchitis. Anecdotal information on a small number of patients with orchitis suggests that administration of interferon α may be helpful.

PREVENTION   Live attenuated mumps vaccine (Jeryl Lynn strain) induces antibodies that protect against infection in more than 95 percent of cases. The subcutaneously administered vaccine may be given to children older than 1 year but is not recommended for younger infants because of the potential for interference by passive maternal antibodies. Mumps vaccine is usually administered as part of the measles-mumps-rubella (MMR) vaccine at the age of 15 months and again later in childhood. This MMR vaccine is also recommended for susceptible older children, adolescents, and adults, particularly adolescent males who have not had mumps. For these patients, either MMR or monovalent mumps vaccine may be given; two doses are preferred. Inadvertent immunization of individuals who are already immune is not associated with significant adverse reactions. Mumps vaccine is not recommended for pregnant women, for patients receiving glucocorticoids, or for other immunocompromised hosts. However, children with HIV infection can safely be immunized against mumps; MMR vaccine is usually used for this purpose.

BIBLIOGRAPHY

BROWN E et al: The Urabe AM9 mumps vaccine is a mixture of viruses differing at amino acid 335 of the hemagglutinin-neuraminidase gene with one form associated with disease. J Infect Dis 174:619, 1996

CENTERS FOR DISEASE CONTROL: Update on adult immunization: Recommendations of the Immunization Practices Advisory Committee (ACIP). Morb Mort Week Rep 40:22, 1991

———: Mumps surveillance—United States. Morb Mort Week Rep 44:1, 1995

CHAUDARY S et al: Fulminant mumps myocarditis. Ann Intern Med 110:569, 1989

GUT JP et al: Symptomatic mumps reinfections. J Med Virol 45:17, 1995

HAREL L et al: Mumps arthritis in children. Pediatr Infect Dis J 9:928, 1990

HERSH BS et al: Mumps outbreak in a highly vaccinated population. J Pediatr 119:187, 1991

LYON RP et al: Mumps epididymo-orchitis: Treatment by anesthetic block of the spermatic cord. JAMA 196:736, 1966

MCDONALD JC et al: Clinical and epidemiologic features of mumps encephalitis and possible causes of vaccine-related disease. Pediatr Infect Dis J 8:751, 1989

RUTHER U et al: Successful interferon-alpha 2 therapy for a patient with acute mumps orchitis. Eur Urol 27:174, 1995

199   *Lawrence Corey*

RABIES VIRUS AND OTHER RHABDOVIRUSES

RABIES VIRUS

DEFINITION   Rabies is an acute viral disease of the central nervous system (CNS) that affects all mammals and that is transmitted by infected secretions, usually saliva. Most exposures to rabies are through the bite of an infected animal, but on occasion contact with a virus-containing aerosol or the ingestion or transplantation of infected tissues may initiate the disease process.

ETIOLOGY   The rabies virus is a bullet-shaped, enveloped, single-stranded RNA virus that is 75 to 80 nm in diameter and belongs to the rhabdovirus family. Within this family is the genus *Lyssavirus*, which includes the group of agents causing rabies in humans and other animals. Placement of a particular virus within the genus *Lyssavirus* is based on similarities in neutralization of prototype antisera, a feature related to the viruses' surface glycoprotein structure. The envelope glycoproteins are arranged in knoblike structures that cover the surface of the virion. The viral glycoproteins bind to acetylcholine receptors, contribute to the neurovirulence of rabies virus, elicit neutralizing and hemagglutination-inhibiting antibodies, and stimulate cytotoxic T cell immunity. The nucleocapsid antigen induces a complement-fixing antibody as well as T helper cell reactivity. Neutralizing antibodies to the surface glycoproteins appear to be protective. Most of the neutralizing antibodies appear to be directed at conformational epitopes of the viral envelope glycoprotein. The antibodies to rabies virus used in diagnostic immunofluorescence assays are generally directed against the nucleocapsid antigens. Isolates of rabies virus from different animal species and locales differ in their antigenic and biologic properties. These variations may account for differences in virulence between isolates. Interferon is induced by rabies virus, particularly in those tissues with high virus concentrations, and may play some role in retarding progressive infection.

EPIDEMIOLOGY Rabies is found in animals in all regions of the world except Australasia and Antarctica. Rabies exists in two epidemiologic forms: *urban*, propagated chiefly by unimmunized domestic dogs and/or cats, and *sylvatic*, propagated by skunks, foxes, raccoons, mongooses, wolves, and bats. Infection in domestic animals usually represents a "spillover" from sylvatic reservoirs of infection, and human beings can be infected in either an urban or a sylvatic setting. Hence human infection tends to occur in locales where rabies is enzootic or epizootic, where there is a large population of unimmunized domestic animals, and where human contact with the outdoors is common. While only about 1000 rabies deaths are reported to the World Health Organization each year, the worldwide incidence of rabies is estimated at more than 30,000 cases per year. Southeast Asia, the Philippines, Africa, the Indian subcontinent, and tropical South America are areas where the disease is especially common. In some endemic areas, 1 to 2 percent of autopsies yield evidence of rabies. Increased spread of terrestrial rabies (i.e., rabies in animals that walk on the ground rather than rabies in animals that fly) and increased travel to countries where urban rabies exists have made the recognition of clinical rabies and its prevention of increasing importance. During the 1980s and 1990s, there has been continued spread of focal epidemics of terrestrial rabies within the United States and Europe. Antigenic analyses have shown that these epidemics arise from the introduction of particular viral strains within the wildlife population and the rapid dissemination of this variant within the animal populace. In the United States, human rabies is exceedingly rare, and most cases now originate either from animal bites in countries where canine rabies is endemic or from exposure to bats.

In most areas of the world, the dog is the most important vector of rabies virus for humans. However, the wolf (in eastern Europe and Arctic regions), the mongoose (in South Africa and the Caribbean), the fox (in western Europe), and the vampire bat (in Latin America) also may be prominent vectors. In the United States, feline rabies is now reported more frequently than canine rabies; thus the vaccination of domestic cats is extremely important. Rodents and lagomorphs are rarely infected with rabies virus. Although rabies in wildlife is common throughout both the developed and the undeveloped world, most cases of postexposure prophylaxis are associated with domesticated animals such as dogs and cats. Several cases of human-to-human transmission of rabies through corneal transplantation also have been documented.

PATHOGENESIS The first event in rabies is the introduction of live virus through the epidermis or onto a mucous membrane. Initial viral replication appears to occur within striated muscle cells at the site of inoculation. The peripheral nervous system is exposed at the neuromuscular and/or neurotendinous spindles of unmyelinated sensory nerve cell endings. The virus then spreads centripetally up the nerve to the CNS, probably via peripheral nerve axoplasm, at a rate of approximately 3 mm/h. Viremia has been documented in experimental conditions but is thought not to play a role in naturally acquired disease. Once the virus reaches the CNS, it replicates almost exclusively within the gray matter and then passes centrifugally along autonomic nerves to other tissues—the salivary glands, adrenal medulla, kidneys, lungs, liver, skeletal muscles, skin, and heart. Passage of the virus into the salivary glands and viral replication in mucinogenic acinar cells facilitate further transmission via infected saliva. The incubation period of rabies is exceedingly variable, ranging from 7 days to over 1 year (mean,

1 to 2 months) and apparently depending on the amount of virus introduced, the amount of tissue involved, host defense mechanisms, and the actual distance that the virus has to travel from the site of inoculation to the CNS. Rates of infection and mortality are highest from bites on the face, intermediate from bites on the hands and arms, and lowest from bites on the legs. Cases of human rabies with an extended incubation period (2 to 7 years) have been reported, but they are rare. Host immune responses and viral strains also influence disease expression.

The neuropathology of rabies resembles that of other viral diseases of the CNS: hyperemia, varying degrees of chromatolysis, nuclear pyknosis, and neuronophagia of the nerve cells; infiltration by lymphocytes and plasma cells of the Virchow-Robin space; microglial infiltration; and parenchymal areas of nerve cell destruction. In experimental animal models, adenohypophyseal infection with rabies virus, with reduction in growth hormone and vasopressin release, is common. The most characteristic pathologic finding of rabies in the CNS is the formation of cytoplasmic inclusions called *Negri bodies* within neurons. Each eosinophilic mass measures approximately 10 nm and is made up of a finely fibrillar matrix and rabies virus particles. Negri bodies are distributed throughout the brain, particularly in Ammon's horn, the cerebral cortex, the brainstem, the hypothalamus, the Purkinje cells of the cerebellum, and the dorsal spinal ganglia. Negri bodies are not demonstrated in at least 20 percent of cases of rabies, and their absence from brain material does not rule out the diagnosis.

CLINICAL MANIFESTATIONS The clinical manifestations of rabies can be divided into four stages: (1) a nonspecific prodrome, (2) an acute encephalitis similar to other viral encephalitides, (3) a profound dysfunction of brainstem centers that produces the classic features of rabies encephalitis, and (4) death or—in rare cases—recovery.

The prodromal period usually lasts 1 to 4 days and is marked by fever, headache, malaise, myalgias, increased fatigability, anorexia, nausea and vomiting, sore throat, and a nonproductive cough. The prodromal symptom suggestive of rabies is the complaint of paresthesia and/or fasciculations at or around the site of inoculation of virus. These sensations, which may be related to the multiplication of virus in the dorsal root ganglion of the sensory nerve supplying the area of the bite, are reported by 50 to 80 percent of patients.

The encephalitic phase is usually ushered in by periods of excessive motor activity, excitation, and agitation. Confusion, hallucinations, combativeness, bizarre aberrations of thought, muscle spasms, meningismus, opisthotonic posturing, seizures, and focal paralysis soon appear. Characteristically, the periods of mental aberration are interspersed with completely lucid periods, but as the disease progresses the lucid periods get shorter until the patient lapses into coma. Hyperesthesia, with excessive sensitivity to bright light, loud noise, touch, and even gentle breezes, is very common. On physical examination, the temperature may be found to be as high as 40.6°C (105°F). Abnormalities of the autonomic nervous system include dilated irregular pupils, increased lacrimation, salivation, perspiration, and postural hypotension. Evidence of upper motor neuron paralysis, with weakness, increased deep tendon reflexes, and extensor plantar responses, is the rule. Paralysis of the vocal cords is common.

The manifestations of brainstem dysfunction begin shortly after the onset of the encephalitic phase. Cranial nerve involvement causes diplopia, facial palsies, optic neuritis, and the characteristic difficulty with deglutition. The combination of excessive salivation and difficulty in swallowing produces the traditional picture of "foaming at the mouth." Hydrophobia, the painful, violent, involuntary contraction of the diaphragmatic, accessory respiratory, pharyngeal, and laryngeal muscles initiated by swallowing liquids, is seen in about 50 percent of cases. Involvement of the amygdaloid nucleus may result in priapism and spontaneous ejaculation. The patient lapses into coma, and involvement of the respiratory center produces an apneic death. The prominence of early brainstem dysfunction distinguishes rabies from other viral encephalitides and accounts for the rapid downhill course. The median period of survival after the onset of symptoms is 4 days, with a maximum of 20 days, unless artificial supportive measures are instituted.

If intensive respiratory support is used, a number of late complications may appear. These include inappropriate secretion of antidiuretic hormone, diabetes insipidus, cardiac arrhythmias, vascular instability, adult respiratory distress syndrome, gastrointestinal bleeding, thrombocytopenia, and paralytic ileus. Recovery is very rare and, when it occurs, gradual.

Rabies may also present as an ascending paralysis resembling the Landry/Guillain-Barré syndrome (dumb rabies, *rage tranquille*). Initially, this clinical pattern was reported most frequently among persons bitten by vampire bats who were given postexposure rabies prophylaxis. Paralytic rabies also occurs in Southeast Asia among persons with canine exposures.

The difficulty of diagnosing rabies associated with ascending paralysis is illustrated by two cases of person-to-person transmission of the virus by tissue transplantation. Corneal transplants from two donors who died of presumed Landry/Guillain-Barré syndrome produced clinical rabies in and caused the deaths of the recipients. Retrospective pathologic examinations of the brains of both recipients demonstrated Negri bodies, and rabies virus was subsequently isolated from each donor's frozen eye.

LABORATORY FINDINGS   Early in the disease, hemoglobin values and routine blood chemistry results are normal; abnormalities develop as hypothalamic dysfunction, gastrointestinal bleeding, and other complications ensue. The peripheral white blood cell count is usually slightly elevated (12,000 to 17,000/μL) but may be normal or as high as 30,000/μL.

As in any viral infection, the specific diagnosis of rabies depends on (1) the isolation of virus from infected secretions [saliva or—rarely—cerebrospinal fluid (CSF)] or tissue (brain), (2) the serologic demonstration of acute infection, (3) the detection of viral antigen in infected tissue (e.g., corneal impression smears, skin biopsies, or brain), or (4) the detection of viral nucleic acid (RNA) by polymerase chain reaction (PCR). Samples of brain obtained either on postmortem examination or at brain biopsy should be subjected to (1) mouse inoculation studies for virus isolation, (2) fluorescent antibody (FA) staining for viral antigen, and (3) histologic and/or electron-microscopic examination for Negri bodies or reverse transcription PCR for detection of rabies virus RNA. While mouse inoculation studies for virus isolation and direct FA staining for viral antigen are quite reliable and sensitive, "autosterilization" may occur and these tests may be negative if the patient's life has been prolonged and high levels of neutralizing antibody are present in serum and CSF. The use of FA staining of skin biopsies, corneal impression smears, and saliva to obtain evidence of rabies antigen has been helpful in diagnosing rabies during life. Confirmation of these findings, either serologically or by demonstration of virus or of viral antigen or RNA in the brain, should be sought.

If the patient has not been immunized against rabies, a fourfold rise in titer of neutralizing antibody to rabies virus in serial serum samples is diagnostic. If the patient has been vaccinated, a clue to the diagnosis may be obtained from the absolute titers of serum neutralizing antibody and the presence of neutralizing antibody in CSF. Postexposure rabies prophylaxis rarely produces CSF neutralizing antibody to rabies virus. If present after prophylaxis, it is usually found at a low titer (<1:64), whereas CSF titers in human rabies may vary from 1:200 to 1:160,000.

DIFFERENTIAL DIAGNOSIS   There is little to distinguish rabies from other viral encephalitides. The most helpful clue to the diagnosis is a history of exposure. Other problems to be considered in the differential diagnosis include hysterical reactions to animal bites (pseudohydrophobia), Landry/Guillain-Barré syndrome, poliomyelitis, and allergic encephalomyelitis developing in response to rabies vaccine. The latter is most common after the use of nerve tissue–derived vaccine and usually begins 1 to 4 weeks after vaccination.

℞ TREATMENT

Each year more than 1 million Americans are bitten by animals. In each instance, a decision must be made whether to initiate postexposure rabies prophylaxis. In this decision, the following considerations apply: (1) whether the individual came into physical contact with saliva or another substance likely to contain rabies virus, (2) whether rabies is known or suspected in the species and area associated with the exposure (e.g., all persons within the continental United States bitten by a bat that escapes should receive postexposure prophylaxis), and (3) the circumstances surrounding the exposure (e.g., whether the bite was provoked or unprovoked). A guide for postexposure rabies prophylaxis is provided in Fig. 199-1.

If rabies is known or suspected to be present in the animal species involved in a human exposure, the implicated animal should be captured if possible. Any wild animal involved in a rabies exposure; any ill, unvaccinated, or stray domestic animal involved in a rabies exposure; and any animal inflicting an unprovoked bite, exhibiting abnormal behavior, or suspected of being rabid should be humanely killed. The animal's head should be sent immediately to an appropriate laboratory for rabies FA examination. If examination of the brain by the FA technique gives negative results, it can be assumed that the saliva contains no virus, and the exposed person need not be treated. Persons exposed to wild animals that subsequently escape, that are capable of carrying rabies (bats, skunks, coyotes, foxes, raccoons, etc.), and that inhabit an area where rabies is known or suspected to be present should undergo both passive and active immunization against rabies (see below).

In an area in which feline or canine rabies is not prevalent, a healthy biting dog or cat can be confined and observed for 10 days. If it becomes ill or behaves abnormally during the observation period,

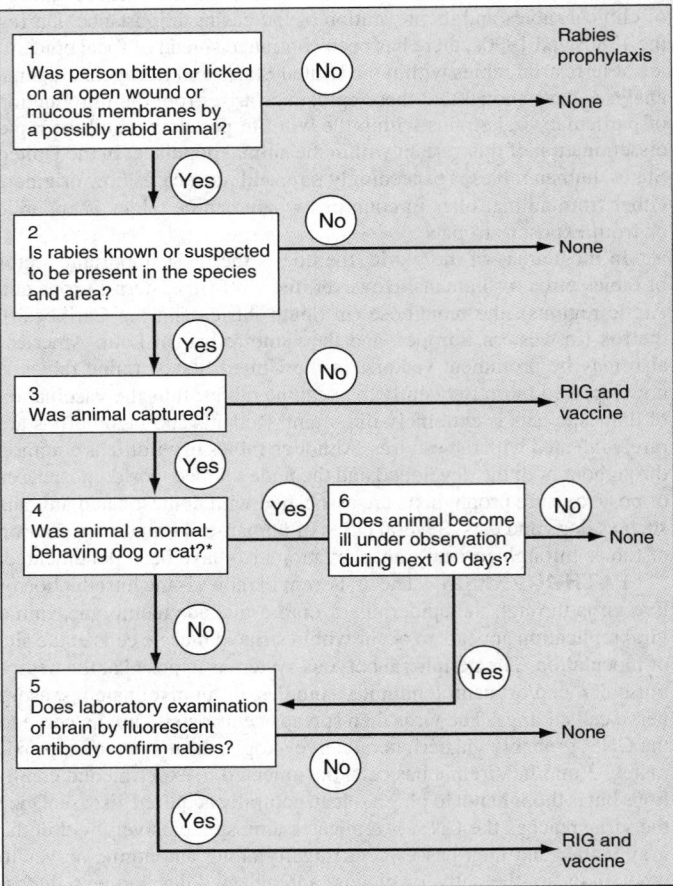

FIGURE 199-1   Postexposure rabies prophylaxis algorithm. *Instances of exposure to livestock or to normal-behaving, unvaccinated dogs or cats should be considered individually, and local and state public health officials should be consulted.

the animal should be killed for FA examination. Experimental and epidemiologic evidence suggests that animals that remain healthy for 10 days after a bite will not have transmitted rabies virus at the time of the bite. In areas of high endemicity for canine rabies, immediate examination of the animal's brain, especially in the case of a severe bite, may be warranted.

PREVENTION **Postexposure Prophylaxis** Postexposure prophylaxis of rabies includes local treatment of the wound and the administration of rabies vaccine together with antirabies immunoglobulin.

1. *Local wound therapy.* Local treatment of the bite wound is an important component of rabies prevention. The wound should be scrubbed with soap and then flushed with water. Both mechanical cleansing and chemical cleansing are important. Quaternary ammonium compounds such as 1 to 4% benzalkonium chloride or 1% cetrimonium bromide are useful because they inactivate the rabies virus. However, 0.1% benzalkonium solutions are less effective than 20% soap solutions. Usually tetanus toxoid and antibiotics should be administered.
2. *Passive immunization with antirabies antiserum of either equine or human origin.* Human rabies immune globulin (HRIG) is preferred because equine antiserum may cause serum sickness. Fifty percent of the total dose of 20 units per kilogram for HRIG and 40 units per kilogram for equine antiserum is given by local infiltration of the wound, and the rest is administered intramuscularly into the gluteal region.
3. *Active immunization with antirabies vaccine.* In the developed world, human diploid cell vaccine (HDCV) is the recommended rabies vaccine. In the United States, two products are licensed. One vaccine contains the Pitman-Moure strain of virus (Pasteur-Mérieux: Imovax), which is grown on human diploid cell cultures and inactivated with β-propiolactone. The other vaccine, rabies vaccine absorbed (RVA), is distributed by the Biologics Products Program of the Michigan Department of Public Health and is prepared from the Kissling strain of virus adapted to fetal rhesus lung diploid cells and adjuvanted with alum. The two vaccines are considered equally efficacious and safe but are expensive because the viral yield from diploid cells is limited. Severe reactions to HDCV are uncommon. Immediate hypersensitivity responses such as urticaria have been reported in approximately 1 of every 650 recipients. Systemic reactions such as fever, headache, and nausea are generally mild and are reported in 1 to 4 percent of recipients. Local reactions such as swelling, erythema, and induration at the injection site occur in 15 to 20 percent of vaccinees.

In the developing world, several other effective rabies vaccines have been licensed and used extensively. They include vaccines made in chick embryonic cells, primary hamster cells, Vero cells, and duck embryonic cells. These preparations appear to be safe, immunogenic, and effective for postexposure prophylaxis.

Five 1-mL doses of HDCV are given intramuscularly, preferably in the deltoid or anterolateral thigh area; the first dose is administered as soon as possible after exposure and should be accompanied by an injection of HRIG into the gluteal and local wound areas. The five doses of HDCV should be administered within 28 days on the following schedule: days 0, 3, 7, 14, and 28. The World Health Organization also recommends 21- and 90-day courses.

The combination of HRIG and HDCV elicits high titers of neutralizing antibodies in almost all recipients. Only rarely has this regimen proved unsuccessful in preventing the development of rabies. Administration of vaccine alone appears to be associated with a higher failure rate than use of the combination, especially in severe bite exposures. Because of cost, postexposure prophylaxis consisting of intradermal injections of rabies vaccine is being used increasingly in the developing world. The combination of HRIG plus 0.1-mL intradermal doses of HDCV at eight sites on day 0, four sites on day 7, and one site on days 28 and 91 produces good antibody responses and

has had excellent clinical results. Alternatively, the World Health Organization has approved a regimen of two 0.1-mL doses at two intradermal sites on days 0, 3, and 7 and a 0.1-mL intradermal injection at a single site on days 21 and 90.

Preexposure Prophylaxis Individuals at high risk of contact with rabies virus, including veterinarians, cave explorers, laboratory workers, and animal handlers, should receive preexposure prophylaxis with rabies vaccine. HDCV is the preferred preparation for preexposure prophylaxis; three 1-mL intramuscular or three 0.1-mL intradermal injections on days 0, 7, and 21 or 28 should be administered. RVA should not be used intradermally. The neutralizing antibody titer should be checked after vaccination. Concomitant chloroquine administration interferes with the antibody response to rabies vaccine. Depending on the level of risk, serologic testing should be done at 2- to 6-year intervals. When neutralizing titers fall below 1:5, booster doses should be given. Booster doses may be administered as a single 1-mL intramuscular or 0.1-mL intradermal injection. Postexposure prophylaxis in individuals previously given preexposure prophylaxis consists of two intramuscular doses of HDCV on days 0 and 3. HRIG is not given in these situations.

Booster doses of HDCV are associated with fever, headache, muscle aches, and joint pains in about 20 percent of recipients. Up to 6 percent of persons receiving intramuscular booster doses of HDCV develop an immune complex–like reaction characterized by urticaria, arthritis, nausea, vomiting, and occasionally angioedema. These reactions are self-limited and appear to be associated with the presence of β-propiolactone-altered human serum albumin in the vaccine and the development of IgE antibodies to this antigen. Persons who work in high-risk areas should undergo periodic measurement of antibodies, and booster doses are recommended for those with low antibody titers. Those at very low risk may elect not to receive routine booster doses but rather to undergo active immunization should any substantive exposure take place.

MOKOLA VIRUS

Mokola virus was first isolated from wild shrews captured in Nigeria and was subsequently shown to be related morphologically and serologically to rabies virus. However, neither of the two reported cases of human disease (both in children) had the classic clinical features of rabies. One patient had a nonfatal illness characterized by fever, pharyngitis, and convulsions; Mokola virus was recovered from CSF. In the second patient, fever with cough and vomiting was followed within several days by drowsiness, confusion, and generalized flaccid weakness. The CSF was normal. The patient progressed to deep coma and died within 10 days of onset. Mokola virus was isolated from the brain, and examination of histopathologic sections revealed finely granular cytoplasmic inclusions that were distinguishable from Negri bodies in many neurons.

VESICULAR STOMATITIS VIRUS

Vesicular stomatitis is a viral illness of animals that occasionally affects humans. It presents as an acute, self-limited, influenza-like disease. The disease in animals is found in the United States and South America and affects chiefly domestic cattle, horses, swine, wild deer, raccoons, skunks, and bobcats.

In animals, vesicular stomatitis is characterized by the development of vesicles on the oral mucosa, particularly the tongue; the udders; and the heels. The mode of spread is probably by direct contact; however, epidemics tend to occur in warm weather, and isolation of the virus from *Phlebotomus* sandflies in Panama and *Aedes* species in New Mexico suggests that these insects may be vectors. Two distinct serotypes, New Jersey and Indiana, have been recognized, and most outbreaks in North America have been attributed to the New Jersey strain. Vesicular stomatitis is most common among laboratory workers.

In one report, three-fourths of laboratory personnel handling experimentally infected animals or manipulating the virus developed neutralizing antibodies. The disease is also transmissible, however, under natural conditions among workers having direct contact with infected animals, especially cattle. An incubation period ranging from 1 to 6 days is followed by the sudden onset of fever [with temperatures of up to 40°C (104°F)], chills, profuse sweating, myalgias, malaise, headache, and pain on ocular movement. One-third to one-half of patients have a sore throat and cervical and/or submandibular adenopathy. Small raised vesicular lesions may appear on the buccal mucosa. Conjunctivitis and coryza are evident in about 20 percent of cases. Occasionally, small subcorneal, intraepithelial vesicles appear on the fingers, usually in association with direct inoculation of the virus. Symptoms generally last 3 to 4 days, but occasionally the course is diphasic. Inapparent infection is common: among laboratory workers with serologic evidence of infection, only about one-half reported symptoms. In some areas of Panama, 17 to 35 percent of the population have neutralizing antibodies to vesicular stomatitis virus.

The differential diagnosis includes hand-foot-and-mouth disease, herpangina, primary herpetic pharyngitis and other mucocutaneous syndromes, and influenza. The virus is not commonly isolated from patients. However, a rise in titer of complement-fixation and/or neutralizing antibody to vesicular stomatitis virus between acute- and convalescent-phase sera helps to confirm the diagnosis. Treatment is nonspecific.

BIBLIOGRAPHY

Fishbein DB, Robinson LE: Current concepts. Rabies. N Engl J Med 329:1632, 1993

Immunization Practices Advisory Committee (ACIP): Rabies prevention, United States, 1991. Morb Mort Week Rep 40(RR-3): 1, 1991

Javadi MA et al: Transmission of rabies by corneal graft. Cornea 15:431, 1996

Lopez RA et al: Outbreak of human rabies in the Peruvian jungle. Lancet 339:408, 1992

Sacramento D et al: PCR technique as an alternative method for diagnosis and molecular epidemiology of rabies virus. Mol Cell Probes 5:229, 1991

Smith JS: New aspects of rabies with emphasis on epidemiology, diagnosis, and prevention of the disease in the United States. Clin Microbiol Rev 9:166, 1996

Warrell MJ: Human deaths from cryptic bat rabies in the USA. Lancet 346:65, 1993

WHO Expert Committee: Report on Rabies, technical report series no. 824. Geneva, World Health Organization, 1992

Wilde H et al: Rabies in Thailand 1990. Rev Infect Dis 17:644, 1991

——— et al: Heterologous antisera and antivenins are essential biologicals: Perspectives on a worldwide crisis. Ann Intern Med 125:233, 1996

200   C. J. Peters

INFECTIONS CAUSED BY ARTHROPOD- AND RODENT-BORNE VIRUSES

Most viral infections that come to medical attention in office or hospital practice in the developed countries are caused by viruses that can be latent in the human host, such as the herpesviruses, or by viruses that are continuously transmitted among humans, such as measles virus, influenza virus, and human immunodeficiency virus. However, some other viruses are transmitted in nature without regard to humans and only incidentally infect and produce disease in humans; in addition, a few agents are regularly spread among humans by arthropods. Most of these viruses either are maintained by arthropods or chronically infect rodents. Obviously, the mode of transmission is not a rational basis for taxonomic classification. Indeed, zoonotic viruses from at least seven virus families act as significant human pathogens (Table

200-1). The virus families differ fundamentally from one another in terms of morphology, replication mechanisms, and genetics. Information on a virus's membership in a family or genus is enlightening with regard to maintenance strategies, sensitivity to antivirals, and some aspects of pathogenesis but does not necessarily predict which clinical syndromes—if any—the virus will cause in humans.

FAMILIES OF ARTHROPOD- AND RODENT-BORNE VIRUSES   The Arenaviridae The Arenaviridae are spherical, 110- to 130-nm particles that bud from the cell's plasma membrane and utilize ambisense RNA genomes with two segments for replication. There are two main phylogenetic branches of Arenaviridae: the old world viruses, such as Lassa fever and lymphocytic choriomeningitis viruses, and the new world viruses, including those causing the South American hemorrhagic fevers (HFs). Arenaviruses persist in nature by chronically infecting rodents with a striking one-virus–one-rodent species relationship. These rodent infections result in long-term virus excretion and perhaps in lifelong viremia; vertical infection is common with some arenaviruses. Humans become infected through the inhalation of aerosols containing arenaviruses, which are then deposited in the terminal air passages, and probably also through close contact with rodents and their excreta, which results in the contamination of mucous membranes or breaks in the skin.

The Bunyaviridae   The family Bunyaviridae includes four medically significant genera. All of these spherical viruses have three negative-sense RNA segments maturing into 90- to 120-nm particles in the Golgi complex and exiting the cell by exocytosis. Viruses of the genus *Bunyavirus* are largely mosquito borne and have a viremic vertebrate intermediate host; many are also transovarially transmitted in their specific mosquito host. One serologic group also uses biting midges as vectors. Sandflies or mosquitoes are the vectors for the genus *Phlebovirus* (named after phlebotomus fever or sandfly fever, the best-known disease associated with the genus), while ticks serve as vectors for the genus *Nairovirus*. Viruses of both of these genera are also associated with vertical transmission in the arthropod host and with horizontal spread through viremic vertebrate hosts. The genus *Hantavirus* is unique among the Bunyaviridae in that it is not transmitted by arthropods but is maintained in nature by rodent hosts that chronically shed virus. Like the arenaviruses, the hantaviruses usually display striking virus-rodent species specificity. As far as is known, however, the hantaviruses do not cause chronic viremia in their rodent host and are transmitted only horizontally from rodent to rodent.

Other Families   The Flaviviridae are positive-sense, single-stranded RNA viruses that form particles of 40 to 50 nm in the endoplasmic reticulum. The flaviviruses discussed here are from the genus *Flavivirus* and make up two phylogenetically and antigenically distinct divisions transmitted among vertebrates by mosquitoes and ticks, respectively. The mosquito-borne viruses fall into phylogenetic groups that include yellow fever viruses, the four dengue viruses, and the encephalitis viruses, while the tick-borne group encompasses a geographically varied spectrum of species, some of which are responsible for encephalitis or for hemorrhagic disease with encephalitis. The Reoviridae are double-stranded RNA viruses with multisegmented genomes. These 80-nm particles are the only viruses discussed in this chapter that do not have a lipid envelope and thus are insensitive to detergents. The Togaviridae have a single positive strand RNA genome and bud particles of approximately 60 to 70 nm from the plasma membrane. The togaviruses discussed here are all members of the genus *Alphavirus* and are transmitted among vertebrates by mosquitoes in their natural cycle. Alphaviruses are divided phylogenetically into two groups: one seems to have developed in the new world, and the other is associated primarily with the old world. → *The Filoviridae and the Rhabdoviridae are discussed in Chaps. 201 and 199, respectively.*

PROMINENT FEATURES OF ARTHROPOD- AND RODENT-BORNE VIRUSES   Although this chapter discusses the major features of selected arthropod- and rodent-borne viruses, it does not deal with more than 500 other distinct recognized zoonotic viruses, about one-fourth of which infect humans. Zoonotic viruses are undergoing genetic evolution, "new" zoonotic viruses are being discovered, and the epidemiology of zoonotic viruses is continuing to evolve through environmental changes affecting vectors, reservoirs, and humans. These zoonotic viruses are most numerous in the tropics but are also found in temperate and frigid climates. Their distribution and seasonal activity may be variable and often depend largely on ecologic conditions such as rainfall and temperature, which in turn affect the density of vectors and reservoirs and the development of infection therein.

Maintenance and Transmission Arthropod-borne viruses infect their vectors after the ingestion of a blood meal from a viremic vertebrate. The vectors then develop chronic, systemic infection as the viruses penetrate the gut and spread throughout the body. The viruses eventually reach the salivary glands during a period that is referred to as *extrinsic incubation* and that typically lasts 1 to 3 weeks in mosquitoes. At this point an arthropod is competent to continue the chain of transmission by infecting another vertebrate when a subsequent blood meal is taken. The arthropod generally is unharmed by the infection, and the natural vertebrate partner usually has only transient viremia with no overt disease. An alternative mechanism for virus maintenance in its arthropod host is transovarial transmission, which is most common among members of the family Bunyaviridae.

Rodent-borne viruses such as the hantaviruses and arenaviruses are maintained in nature by chronic infection transmitted between rodents. As in arthropod-borne virus cycles, there is usually a high degree of rodent-virus specificity, and there is no overt disease in the reservoir/vector.

Epidemiology The distribution of arthropod- and rodent-borne viruses is restricted by the areas inhabited by their reservoir/vectors and provides an important clue in the differential diagnosis. Table 200-2 shows the approximate geographic distribution of the most important of these viruses. Members of each family, each genus, and even each serologically related group usually occur in each area but may not be pathogenic in all areas or may not be a commonly recognized cause of disease in all areas and so may not be included in the table. Although there is generally no overt disease in the vertebrate reservoirs, disease in nonhuman target species may be a useful diagnostic clue, and serologic testing of selected animals may be a useful way to monitor virus circulation.

Most of these diseases are acquired in a rural setting; a few have urban vectors. Seoul, sandfly fever, and Oropouche viruses are examples of urban viruses, but the most notable are yellow fever, dengue, and chikungunya viruses, which are transmitted between humans with the mosquito *Aedes aegypti* as a principal or alternate vector. A history of mosquito bite has little diagnostic significance in the individual; a

Table 200-1

Major Zoonotic Virus Families and Some Characteristics of Typical Members

Family	Genus or Group	Syndrome(s): Typical Viruses	Maintenance Strategy
Arenaviridae	Old world complex	FM, E: Lymphocytic choriomeningitis virus HF: Lassa fever virus	Chronic infection of rodents, often with persistent viremia; vertical transmission common
	New world or Tacaribe complex	HF: South American HF viruses (Machupo, Junin, Guanarito, Sabia)	Chronic infection of rodents, sometimes with persistent viremia; vertical infection may occur
Bunyaviridae	*Bunyavirus*	E: California serogroup viruses (La Crosse, Jamestown Canyon, California encephalitis)	Mosquito-vertebrate cycle; transovarial transmission in mosquito common
		FM: Bunyamwera, group C, Tahyna viruses	
		FM: Oropouche virus	Transmitted by *Culicoides*
	Phlebovirus	FM: Sandfly fever, Toscana viruses FM: Punta Toro virus	Sandfly transmission between vertebrates, with prominent transovarial component in sandfly
		HF, FM, E: Rift Valley fever virus	Mosquito-vertebrate transmission, with transovarial component in mosquito
	Nairovirus	HF: Crimean Congo HF virus	Tick-vertebrate, with transovarial transmission in tick
	Hantavirus	HF: Hantaan, Dobrava, Puumala viruses	Rodent reservoir; chronic virus shedding, but chronic viremia unknown
		HF: Sin Nombre and related hantaviruses	Sigmodontine rodent reservoir
Filoviridae*		HF: Marburg virus, Ebola viruses (4 subtypes)	Unknown
Flaviviridae	*Flavivirus* (mosquito-borne)	HF: Yellow fever virus FM, HF: Dengue viruses (4 subtypes) E: St. Louis, Japanese, West Nile, and Murray Valley encephalitis viruses; Rocio viruses	Mosquito-vertebrate
	Flavivirus (tick-borne)	E: Central European tick-borne encephalitis, Russian spring-summer encephalitis, Powassan viruses HF: Omsk HF, Kyasanur Forest disease viruses	Tick-vertebrate
Reoviridae	*Coltivirus*	FM, E: Colorado tick fever virus	Tick-vertebrate
	Orbivirus	FM, E: Orungo, Kemerova viruses	Arthropod-vertebrate
Rhabdoviridae†	*Vesiculovirus*	FM: Vesicular stomatitis virus (Indiana, New Jersey); Chandipura, Piry viruses	Sandfly-vertebrate, with prominent transovarial component in sandfly
Togaviridae	*Alphavirus*	AR: Sindbis, chikungunya, Mayaro, Ross River, Barmah Forest viruses	Mosquito-vertebrate
		E: Eastern, western, and Venezuelan equine encephalitis viruses	

* The Filoviridae are discussed in Chap. 201.
† The Rhabdoviridae are discussed in Chap. 199.

NOTE: Abbreviations refer to the disease syndrome most commonly associated with the virus: FM, fever and myalgia; AR, arthritis and rash; E, encephalitis; HF, hemorrhagic fever.

history of tick-bite is more diagnostically specific. Rodent exposure is often reported by persons infected with an arenavirus or a hantavirus but again has little specificity. Indeed, aerosols may infect persons who have no recollection of having even seen rodents.

Syndromes Human disease caused by arthropod- and rodent-borne viruses is often subclinical. The spectrum of possible responses to infection is wide, and our knowledge of the outcome of most of these infections is limited. The usual disease syndromes associated with these viruses have been grouped into four categories: fever and myalgia, arthritis and rash, encephalitis, and hemorrhagic fever. Although for the purposes of this discussion most viruses have been placed in a single group, the categories often overlap. For example, West Nile and Venezuelan equine encephalitis viruses are discussed as encephalitis viruses, but during epidemics they may cause many cases of milder syndromes and relatively uncommon cases of encephalitis. Similarly, Rift Valley fever virus is best known as a cause of HF, but the attack rates for febrile disease are far higher, and encephalitis is occasionally seen as well. Lymphocytic choriomeningitis (LCM) virus is classified as a cause of fever and myalgia because this syndrome is its most common disease manifestation and, even when central nervous system (CNS) disease occurs, it is usually preceded by fever and myalgia. Dengue virus infection is considered as a cause of fever and myalgia (dengue fever) because this is by far the most common manifestation worldwide and is the syndrome most likely to be seen in the United States; however, dengue HF is also discussed in the HF section because of its complicated pathogenesis and importance in pediatric practice in certain areas of the world.

Diagnosis Laboratory diagnosis is required in any given case, although epidemics occasionally provide clinical and epidemiologic clues on which an educated guess as to etiology can be based. For most arthropod- and rodent-borne viruses, acute-phase serum samples (collected within 3 or 4 days of onset) have yielded isolates, and paired sera have been used to demonstrate rising antibody titers by a variety of tests. Intensive efforts to develop rapid tests for HF have resulted in an antigen-detection enzyme-linked immunosorbent assay (ELISA)

and an IgM-capture ELISA that can provide a diagnosis based on a single serum sample within a few hours and are particularly useful in severe cases. More sensitive reverse transcription polymerase chain reaction (RT-PCR) tests may yield diagnoses based on samples without detectable antigen and may also provide useful genetic information about the virus. Preliminary data suggest that similar tests applied to some fever-myalgia syndromes would give positive results if developed further. Hantavirus infections differ from others discussed here in that severe acute disease is immunopathologic; patients present with serum IgM that serves as the basis for a sensitive and specific test. Every ELISA must include a control incorporating a negative antigen with each serum sample tested; the frequent failure to include such a control has resulted in numerous false-positive results in diagnostic tests.

At the time of diagnosis, patients with encephalitis generally are no longer viremic or antigenemic and usually do not have virus in cerebrospinal fluid (CSF). In this situation, the value of serologic methods is being validated. IgM capture is increasingly being used for the testing of serum and CSF. IgG ELISA or classic serology is useful in the evaluation of past exposure to the viruses, many of which circulate in areas with a minimal medical infrastructure and sometimes cause mild or subclinical infection.

The remainder of this chapter offers general descriptions of the broad syndromes caused by arthropod- and rodent-borne viruses and then addresses specific differences between diseases. It is important to remember that most of the diseases under consideration have not been studied in detail with modern medical approaches and thus available data may be incomplete or biased.

FEVER AND MYALGIA

Fever and myalgia constitute the syndrome most commonly associated with zoonotic virus infection. Many of the numerous viruses belonging to the families listed in Table 200-1 probably cause this syndrome, but several viruses have been selected for inclusion in the table because of their prominent associations with the syndrome and their biomedical importance.

The syndrome typically begins with the abrupt onset of fever, chills, intense myalgia, and malaise. Patients may also report joint

Table 200-2

Geographic Distribution of Some Important and Commonly Encountered Human Zoonotic Viral Diseases

Area	Arenaviridae	Bunyaviridae	Flaviviridae	Rhabdoviridae	Togaviridae
North America	Lymphocytic choriomeningitis	La Crosse, Jamestown Canyon, California encephalitis; hantavirus (pulmonary syndrome)	St. Louis, Powassan encephalitis; dengue	Vesicular stomatitis	Eastern, western equine encephalitis
South America	Bolivian, Argentine, Venezuelan, and Brazilian HF; lymphocytic choriomeningitis	Oropouche, group C, Punta Toro infection; hantavirus pulmonary syndrome	Yellow fever, dengue, Rocio virus infection	Vesicular stomatitis, Piry virus infection	Mayaro virus infection, Venezuelan equine encephalitis
Europe	Lymphocytic choriomeningitis	Tahyna, Toscana, sandfly fever, HF with renal syndrome	West Nile, Central European tick-borne, Russian spring-summer encephalitis	—	Sindbis virus infection
Middle East	—	Sandfly fever, Crimean Congo HF	West Nile encephalitis, dengue	—	—
Eastern Asia	—	Sandfly fever; Hantaan, Seoul virus infection	Dengue; Japanese, Russian spring-summer encephalitis; Omsk HF	Chandipura virus infection	—
Southwestern Asia	—	Sandfly fever, Crimean Congo HF	West Nile, Japanese encephalitis; dengue; Kyasanur Forest disease	—	Chikungunya
Southeast Asia	—	Seoul virus infection	Japanese encephalitis, dengue	—	Chikungunya
Africa	Lassa fever	Bunyamwera virus infection, Rift Valley fever	Yellow fever, dengue	—	Sindbis virus infection, chikungunya
Australia	—	—	Murray Valley encephalitis, dengue	—	Ross River, Barmah Forest virus infection

NOTE: HF, hemorrhagic fever.

pains, but no true arthritis is detectable. Anorexia is characteristic and may be accompanied by nausea or even vomiting. Headache is common and may be severe, with photophobia and retroorbital pain. Physical findings are minimal and usually are confined to conjunctival injection with pain on palpation of muscles or the epigastrium. The duration of symptoms is quite variable but generally is 2 to 5 days, with a biphasic course in some instances. The spectrum of disease varies from subclinical to temporarily incapacitating.

Less constant findings include a maculopapular rash. Epistaxis may occur but does not necessarily indicate a bleeding diathesis. A minority of the cases caused by some viruses are known or suspected to include aseptic meningitis, but this diagnosis is difficult in remote areas, given the patients' photophobia and myalgia as well as the lack of opportunity to examine the CSF. Although pharyngitis may be noted or radiographic evidence of pulmonary infiltrates found in some cases, these viruses are not primary respiratory pathogens. The differential diagnosis includes anicteric leptospirosis, rickettsial diseases, and the early stages of other syndromes discussed in this chapter. These diseases are often described as "flulike," but the usual absence of cough and coryza makes influenza an unlikely confounder except at the earliest stages.

Complete recovery is generally the outcome in this syndrome, although prolonged asthenia and nonspecific symptoms have been described in some cases, particularly after infection with LCM or dengue virus. Treatment is supportive, with aspirin avoided because of the potential for exacerbated bleeding and Reye's syndrome. Efforts at prevention are best based on vector control, which, however, may be expensive or impossible. For mosquito control, destruction of breeding sites is generally the most economically and environmentally sound approach; spraying to kill adult mosquitoes and thus to reduce their numbers transiently may have a preventive role in selected settings but has not been notably effective in the past. Measures taken by the individual to avoid the vector can be valuable. Avoiding the vector's habitat and times of peak activity, preventing the vector from entering dwellings by using screens or other barriers, judiciously applying arthropod repellents such as diethyltoluamide (DEET) to the skin, and wearing permethrin-impregnated clothing are all possible approaches, depending on the vector and its habits.

LYMPHOCYTIC CHORIOMENINGITIS LCM is transmitted from the common house mouse (*Mus musculus*) to humans by aerosols of excreta and secreta. LCM virus, an arenavirus, is maintained in the mouse mainly by vertical transmission from infected dams. The vertically infected mouse remains viremic for life, with high concentrations of virus in all tissues. Infected colonies of pet hamsters have also served as a link to humans. LCM virus is widely used in immunology laboratories as a model of T cell function and can silently infect cell cultures and passaged tumor lines, resulting in infections among scientists and animal caretakers. Patients with LCM may have a history of residence in rodent-infested housing or other exposure to rodents. An antibody prevalence of about 5 to 10 percent has been reported in the United States, Argentina, and endemic areas of Germany.

LCM differs from the general syndrome of fever and myalgia in that its onset is gradual. Among the conditions occasionally associated with LCM are orchitis, transient alopecia, arthritis, pharyngitis, cough, and maculopapular rash. An estimated one-fourth of patients or fewer suffer a febrile phase of 3 to 6 days and then, after a brief remission, develop renewed fever accompanied by severe headache, nausea and vomiting, and meningeal signs lasting for about a week. These patients virtually always recover fully, as do the uncommon patients with clear-cut signs of encephalitis. Recovery may be delayed by transient hydrocephalus.

During the initial febrile phase, leukopenia and thrombocytopenia are common and virus can usually be isolated from blood. During the CNS phase of the illness, virus may be found in the CSF, but antibodies are present in blood. The pathogenesis of LCM is thought to resemble that following direct intracranial inoculation of the virus into adult mice; the onset of the immune response leads to T cell–mediated immunopathologic meningitis. During the meningeal phase, CSF

mononuclear-cell counts range from the hundreds to the low thousands per microliter, and hypoglycorrhachia is found in one-third of cases. The IgM-capture ELISA of serum and CSF is usually positive; recently, RT-PCR assays have been developed for application to CSF.

Infection with LCM virus should be suspected in acutely ill febrile patients with marked leukopenia and thrombocytopenia. In cases of aseptic meningitis, the well-marked febrile prodrome, adult age, autumn seasonality, low CSF glucose levels, or mononuclear cell counts exceeding 1000/μL all should raise a suspicion of this viral infection.

In pregnant women, LCM virus infection may lead to fetal invasion with consequent congenital hydrocephalus and chorioretinitis. Since the maternal infection may be mild, consisting of only a short febrile illness, antibodies to the virus should be sought in both the mother and the fetus in suspicious circumstances.

BUNYAMWERA VIRUS INFECTION The mosquito-transmitted Bunyamwera serogroup viruses are found on every continent except Australia and Antarctica. Bunyamwera virus and its close relative Ilesha virus commonly cause febrile disease in Africa. Other related viruses are implicated in such disease in Southeast Asia (Batai virus), Europe (Calovo virus), and South America (Wyeomyia virus). In North America, Cache Valley virus has been implicated in febrile human disease and in rare instances of more serious systemic illness; the presence of serum antibodies to this virus may be associated with congenital malformations. In Central America, the closely related Fort Sherman virus causes the fever-myalgia syndrome.

GROUP C VIRUS INFECTION The group C viruses include at least 11 agents transmitted by mosquitoes in neotropical forests. These agents are among the most common causes of arboviral infection in humans entering American jungles and cause acute febrile disease.

TAHYNA VIRUS INFECTION This California-serogroup virus (see discussion of California encephalitis below) occurs in central and western Europe, and related viruses are emerging in Russia. The significance of Tahyna virus in human health has been well studied only in the Czech and Slovak Republics; there, the virus was found to be a prominent cause of febrile disease, in some cases causing pharyngitis, pulmonary syndromes, and aseptic meningitis. The potential for arboviruses to be unexpectedly involved in such cases in areas of high mosquito prevalence needs to be kept in mind.

OROPOUCHE FEVER Oropouche virus is transmitted in Central and South America by a biting midge, *Culicoides paraensis*, which often breeds to high density in cacao husks and other vegetable detritus found in towns and cities. Explosive epidemics involving thousands of cases have been reported from several towns in Brazil and Peru. Rash and aseptic meningitis have been detected in a number of cases.

SANDFLY FEVER The sandfly *Phlebotomus papatasi* transmits sandfly fever. Female sandflies may be infected by the oral route as they take a blood meal and may transmit the virus to offspring when they lay their eggs after a second blood meal. This prominent transovarial pattern was the first to be recognized among dipterans and complicates virus control. The former designation for sandfly fever, "3-day fever," instructively describes the brief, debilitating course associated with this essentially benign infection. There is neither a rash nor CNS involvement, and complete recovery is the rule.

Sandfly fever is found in the circum-Mediterranean area, extending to the east through the Balkans into China as well as into the Middle East and southwestern Asia. The vector is found in both rural and urban settings and is known for its small size, which enables it to penetrate standard mosquito screens and netting, and for its short flight range. Epidemics have been described in the wake of natural disasters and wars. In parts of Europe, sandfly populations and virus transmission were greatly reduced by the extensive residual spraying conducted after World War II to control malaria, and the prevalence continues to decline. A common pattern of disease in endemic areas consists of high attack rates among travelers and military personnel with little or no disease in the local population, who are protected after childhood infection. In addition to the two well-characterized, non-cross-protective Sicilian and Naples virus species, more than 30 related phleboviruses are transmitted by sandflies and mosquitoes, but most are of unknown significance in terms of human health.

TOSCANA VIRUS DISEASE Toscana virus is a *Phlebovirus* (family Bunyaviridae) transmitted primarily by the circum-Mediterranean sandfly *Phlebotomus perniciosus*. The vertebrate amplifying host, if one exists, is unknown. Toscana virus infection is common during the summer among rural residents and vacationers; a number of cases have been identified in travelers returning to Germany and Scandinavia. The disease may manifest as an uncomplicated febrile illness but is often associated with aseptic meningitis, with virus isolated from the CSF.

PUNTA TORO VIRUS DISEASE Of the several phleboviruses that are associated with new world sandflies and infect humans, Punta Toro virus is the best known. The disease caused by this virus is clinically similar to but epidemiologically different from that caused by the Naples or Sicilian sandfly fever viruses. Punta Toro virus infections are sporadic and are acquired in the tropical forest, where the vectors rest on tree buttresses. Epidemics have not been reported, but antibody prevalences among inhabitants of villages in the endemic areas indicate a cumulative lifetime exposure rate of more than 50 percent.

DENGUE FEVER All four distinct dengue viruses (dengue 1–4) have *A. aegypti* as their principal vector, and all cause a similar clinical syndrome. In rare cases, second infection with a serotype of dengue virus different from that involved in the primary infection leads to dengue HF with severe shock (see below). Sporadic cases are seen in the settings of endemic transmission and epidemic disease. Year-round transmission between latitudes 25°N and 25°S has been established, and seasonal forays of the viruses to points as far north as Philadelphia are thought to have taken place in the United States. With increasing spread of the vector mosquito throughout the tropics and subtropics, large areas of the world have become vulnerable to the introduction of dengue viruses, particularly through air travel by infected humans, and both dengue fever and the related dengue HF are becoming increasingly common. Conditions favorable to dengue transmission exist in the southern United States, and bursts of dengue fever activity are to be expected in this region, particularly along the Mexican border, where water may be stored in containers and *A. aegypti* numbers may therefore be greatest: this mosquito, which also is an efficient vector of the yellow fever and chikungunya viruses, typically breeds near human habitation, using relatively fresh water from sources such as water jars, vases, discarded containers, coconut husks, and old tires. *A. aegypti* usually inhabits dwellings and bites during the day.

After an incubation period of 2 to 7 days, the typical patient experiences the sudden onset of fever, headache, retroorbital pain, and back pain along with the severe myalgia that gave rise to the colloquial designation "break-bone fever." There is often a macular rash on the first day as well as adenopathy, palatal vesicles, and scleral injection. The illness may last a week, with additional symptoms usually including anorexia, nausea or vomiting, marked cutaneous hypersensitivity, and—near the time of defervescence—a maculopapular rash beginning on the trunk and spreading to the extremities and the face. Epistaxis and scattered petechiae are often noted in uncomplicated dengue, and preexisting gastrointestinal lesions may bleed during the acute illness.

Laboratory findings include leukopenia, thrombocytopenia, and, in many cases, serum aminotransferase elevations. The diagnosis is made by IgM ELISA or paired serology during recovery or by antigen-detection ELISA or RT-PCR during the acute phase. Virus is readily isolated from blood in the acute phase if mosquito inoculation or mosquito cell culture is used.

COLORADO TICK FEVER Several hundred cases of Colorado tick fever are reported annually in the United States. The infection is acquired between March and November through the bite of an infected *Dermacentor andersoni* tick in mountainous western regions at altitudes of 1200 to 3000 m (4000 to 10,000 ft). Small mammals serve as the amplifying host. The most common presentation consists of fever and myalgia; meningoencephalitis is not uncommon, and hemorrhagic disease, pericarditis, myocarditis, orchitis, and pulmonary presentations are also reported. Rash develops in a substantial minority of cases. The disease usually lasts 7 to 10 days and is often biphasic. The most important differential diagnostic considerations since the turn of the century have been Rocky Mountain spotted fever and tularemia.

Infection of erythroblasts and other marrow cells by Colorado tick fever virus results in the appearance and persistence (for several weeks) of erythrocytes containing the virus. This feature, detected in smears stained by immunofluorescence, can be diagnostically helpful. The clinical laboratory detects leukopenia and thrombocytopenia.

ORBIVIRUS INFECTION The orbiviruses encompass many human and veterinary pathogens. For example, Orungo virus is widely transmitted by mosquitoes in tropical Africa and causes febrile disease in humans. The Kemerova complex includes the Kemerova, Lipovnik, and Tribec viruses of Russia and central Europe; these viruses are transmitted by ticks and are associated with febrile and neurologic disease.

VESICULAR STOMATITIS See Chap. 199.

ENCEPHALITIS

Arboviral encephalitis is a seasonal disease, commonly occurring in the warmer months. Its incidence varies markedly with time and place, depending on ecologic factors. The causative viruses differ markedly in terms of case-infection ratio (i.e., the ratio of clinical to subclinical infection), mortality, and residua (Table 200-3). Humans are not an important amplifier of these viruses.

All the viral encephalitides discussed in this section have a similar pathogenesis as far as is known. An infected arthropod ingests a blood meal from a human and infects the host. The initial period of viremia is thought to originate most commonly from the lymphoid system. Viremia leads to CNS invasion, presumably through infection of olfactory neuroepithelium with passage through the cribiform plate or through infection of brain capillaries and multifocal entry into the CNS. During the viremic phase, there may be little or no recognized disease except in the case of tick-borne flaviviral encephalitis, in which there may be a clearly delineated phase of fever and systemic illness. The disease process in the CNS arises partly from direct neuronal infection and subsequent damage and partly from edema, inflammation, and other indirect effects. The usual pathologic picture is one of focal necrosis of neurons, inflammatory glial nodules, and perivascular lymphoid cuffing; the severity and distribution of these abnormalities vary with the infecting virus. Involved areas display the "luxury perfusion" phenomenon, with normal or increased total blood flow and low oxygen extraction.

The typical patient presents with a prodrome of nonspecific constitutional symptoms, including fever, abdominal pain, vertigo, sore throat, and respiratory symptoms. Headache, meningeal signs, photophobia, and vomiting follow quickly. Involvement of deeper structures may be signaled by lethargy, somnolence, and intellectual deficit (as disclosed by the mental status examination or failure at serial 7 subtraction); more severely affected patients will be obviously disoriented and may be comatose. Tremors, loss of abdominal reflexes, cranial nerve palsies, hemiparesis, monoparesis, difficulty in swallowing, and frontal lobe signs are all common. Convulsions and focal signs may be evident early or may appear during the course of the disease. Some patients present with an abrupt onset of fever, convulsions, and other signs of CNS involvement. The results of human infection range from no significant symptoms through febrile headache to aseptic meningitis and finally to full-blown encephalitis; the proportions and severity of these manifestations vary with the infecting virus.

The acute encephalitis usually lasts from a few days to as long as 2 to 3 weeks, but recovery may be slow, with weeks or months required for the return of maximal recoupable function. Common complaints during recovery include difficulty concentrating, fatigability, tremors, and personality changes. The acute illness requires management of a comatose patient who may have intracranial pressure elevations, inappropriate secretion of antidiuretic hormone, respiratory failure, and convulsions. There is no specific therapy for these viral encephalitides. The only practical preventive measures are vector management and personal protection against the arthropod transmitting the virus; for Japanese encephalitis or tick-borne encephalitis, vaccination should be considered in certain circumstances (see relevant sections below).

The diagnosis of arboviral encephalitis depends on the careful evaluation of a febrile patient with CNS disease, with rapid identification of treatable herpes simplex encephalitis, ruling out of brain abscess, exclusion of bacterial meningitis by serial CSF examination, and performance of laboratory studies to define the viral etiology. Leptospirosis and neurosyphilis should also be considered. The CSF examination usually shows a modest cell count—in the tens or hundreds or perhaps a few thousand. Early in the process, a significant proportion of these cells may be polymorphonuclear leukocytes, but usually there is a mononuclear cell predominance. CSF glucose levels are usually normal. There are exceptions to this pattern of findings. In eastern equine encephalitis, for example, polymorphonuclear leukocytes may predominate during the first 72 h of disease and hypoglycorrhachia may be detected. In LCM, lymphocyte counts may be in the thousands, and the glucose concentration may be diminished. Experience with imaging studies is still evolving; clearly, however,

both computed tomography (CT) and magnetic resonance imaging (MRI) may be normal except for evidence of preexisting conditions or sometimes may suggest diffuse edema. Several patients with eastern equine encephalitis have had focal abnormalities, and individuals with severe Japanese encephalitis have presented with bilateral thalamic lesions that have often been hemorrhagic. Electroencephalography usually shows diffuse abnormalities and is not directly helpful.

A humoral immune response is usually detectable at or near the onset of disease. Both serum and CSF should be examined for IgM antibodies. Virus generally cannot be isolated from blood or CSF, although Japanese encephalitis virus has been recovered from CSF in severe cases. Virus can be obtained from and viral antigen is present in brain tissue, although its distribution may be focal.

CALIFORNIA, LA CROSSE, AND JAMESTOWN CANYON VIRUS ENCEPHALITIS The isolation of California encephalitis virus established the California serogroup of viruses as a cause of encephalitis, and its use as a diagnostic antigen led to the description of many cases of "California encephalitis." In fact, however, this virus has been implicated in only a few cases of encephalitis, and the serologically related La Crosse virus is the major cause of encephalitis among viruses in the California serogroup. "California encephalitis"

Table 200-3

Prominent Features of Arboviral Encephalitis

Virus	Natural Cycle	Incubation Period, Days	Annual No. of Cases	Case-to-Infection Ratio	Age of Cases	Case-Mortality Rate, %	Residua
La Crosse	*Aedes triseriatus*–chipmunk (transovarial component in mosquito also important)	~3–7	70 (U.S.)	<1:1000	<15 years	<0.5	Recurrent seizures in ~10%; severe deficits in rare cases; decreased school performance and behavioral change suspected in small proportion
St. Louis	*Culex tarsalis, Culex pipiens, Culex quinquefasciatus*–birds	4–21	85 (hundreds to thousands in epidemic years) (U.S.)	<1:200	Milder cases in the young; more severe cases in adults >40 years old, particularly the elderly	7	Common in the elderly
Japanese	*Culex tritaeniorhyncus*–birds	5–15	>25,000	1:200–300	All ages; children in highly endemic areas	20–50	Common (approximately half of cases); may be severe
West Nile	*Culex* mosquitoes–birds	3–6	?	Very low	Mainly the elderly and children	—	Uncommon
Central European	*Ixodes ricinus*–rodents, insectivores	7–14	Thousands	1:12	All ages; milder in children	1–5	20%
Russian spring-summer	*Ixodes persulcatus*–rodents, insectivores	7–14	Hundreds	—	All ages; milder in children	20	Approximately half of cases; often severe; limb-girdle paralysis
Powassan	*Ixodes cookei*–wild mammals	~10	~1 (U.S.)	—	All ages; some predilection for children	~10	Common (approximately half of cases)
Eastern equine	*Culiseta melanura*–birds	~5–10	5 (U.S.)	1:40 adult 1:17 child	All ages; predilection for children	50–75	Common
Western equine	*Culex tarsalis*–birds	~5–10	~20 (U.S.)	1:1000 adult 1:50 child 1:1 infant	All ages; predilection for children <2 years old (increased mortality in elderly)	3–7	Common only among infants < 1 year old
Venezuelan equine (epidemic)	Unknown (multiple mosquito species and horses in epidemics)	1–5	?	1:250 adult 1:25 child (approximate)	All ages; predilection for children	~10	—

due to La Crosse virus infection is most commonly reported from the upper Midwest but is also found in other areas of the central and eastern United States, most often in West Virginia, North Carolina, and Georgia. The serogroup includes 13 other viruses, some of which may also be involved in human disease that is misattributed because of the complexity of the group's serology; these viruses include the Jamestown Canyon, snowshoe hare, Inkoo, and Trivittatus viruses, all of which have *Aedes* mosquitoes as their vector and all of which have a strong element of transovarial transmission in their natural cycles.

The mosquito vector of La Crosse virus is *Aedes triseriatus*. In addition to a prominent transovarial component of transmission, a mosquito can also become infected through feeding on viremic chipmunks and other mammals as well as through venereal transmission from another mosquito. The mosquito breeds in sites such as tree holes and abandoned tires and bites during daylight hours; these findings correlate with the risk factors for cases: recreation in forested areas, residence at the forest's edge, and the presence of abandoned tires around the home. Intensive environmental modification based on these findings has reduced the incidence of disease in a highly endemic area in the Midwest. Most cases occur from July through September. The recently introduced Asian tiger mosquito, *Aedes albopictus*, efficiently transmits the virus to mice and also transmits the agent transovarially in the laboratory; the possible impact of this aggressive anthropophilic mosquito, which has the capacity to urbanize, on transmission to humans is of concern.

An antibody prevalence of ≥20 percent in endemic areas indicates that infection is common, but CNS disease has been recognized primarily in children <15 years of age. The illness varies from a picture of aseptic meningitis accompanied by confusion to severe and occasionally fatal encephalitis. Although there may be prodromal symptoms, the onset of CNS disease is sudden, with fever, headache, and lethargy often joined by nausea and vomiting, convulsions (in one-half of patients), and coma (in one-third of patients). Focal seizures, hemiparesis, tremor, aphasia, chorea, Babinski's sign, and other evidence of significant neurologic dysfunction are common, but residua are not. Perhaps 10 percent of patients have recurrent seizures in the succeeding months. Other serious sequelae are rare, although a decrease in scholastic standing has been reported and mild personality change has occasionally been suggested. Treatment is supportive over a 1- to 2-week acute phase during which status epilepticus, cerebral edema, and inappropriate secretion of antidiuretic hormone are important concerns.

The blood leukocyte count is commonly elevated, sometimes reaching levels of >20,000/μL, and there is usually a left shift. CSF cell counts are typically 30 to 500/μL with a mononuclear cell predominance (although 25 to 90 percent of cells are polymorphonuclear in some cases). The protein level is normal or slightly increased, and the glucose level is normal. Specific virologic diagnosis based on IgM-capture assays of serum and CSF is efficient. The only human anatomic site from which virus has been isolated is the brain.

Jamestown Canyon virus has been implicated in several cases of encephalitis in adults; in these cases the disease was usually associated with a significant respiratory illness at onset. Human infection with this virus has been documented in New York, Wisconsin, Ohio, Michigan, Ontario, and other areas of North America where the vector mosquito, *Aedes stimulans*, feeds on its main host, the white-tailed deer.

ST. LOUIS ENCEPHALITIS St. Louis encephalitis virus is transmitted between *Culex* mosquitoes and birds. This virus causes low-level endemic infection among rural residents of the western and central United States, where *Culex tarsalis* is the vector (see western equine encephalitis below), but the more urbanized mosquito species *Culex pipiens* and *Culex quinquefasciatus* have been responsible for epidemics resulting in hundreds or even thousands of cases in cities of the central and eastern United States. Most cases occur in June through October. The urban mosquitoes breed in accumulations of stagnant water and sewage with high organic content and readily bite humans in and around houses. The elimination of open sewers and

trash-filled drainage systems is expensive and may not be possible, but screening of houses and implementation of personal protective measures against the dusk-biting vectors may be an effective approach for individuals. The rural vector is most active at dusk and outdoors; its bites can be avoided by modification of activities and use of repellents.

Disease severity increases with age: infections that result in aseptic meningitis or mild encephalitis are concentrated in children and young adults, while severe and fatal cases primarily affect the elderly. Infection rates are similar in all age groups; thus the greater susceptibility of older persons to disease is a biologic consequence of aging. The disease has an abrupt onset, sometimes following a prodrome, and begins with fever, lethargy, confusion, and headache. In addition, nuchal rigidity, hypotonia, hyperreflexia, myoclonus, and tremor are common. Severe cases can include cranial nerve palsies, hemiparesis, and convulsions. Patients often complain of dysuria and may have viral antigen in urine as well as pyuria. The overall mortality is generally around 7 percent but may reach 20 percent among patients over the age of 60. Recovery is slow. Emotional lability, difficulties in concentration and memory, asthenia, and tremor are commonly prolonged in older patients.

The CSF of patients infected with St. Louis encephalitis virus usually contains tens to hundreds of cells, with a lymphocytic predominance and a normal glucose level. Leukocytosis with a left shift is often documented.

JAPANESE ENCEPHALITIS Japanese encephalitis virus is found throughout Asia, including far eastern Russia, Japan, China, India, Pakistan, and Southeast Asia, and causes occasional epidemics on western Pacific islands. Recently, the virus has been detected in the Torres Strait islands near the Australian mainland. This flavivirus is particularly common in areas where irrigated rice fields attract the natural avian vertebrate hosts and provide abundant breeding sites for mosquitoes such as *Culex tritaeniorhyncus*, which transmit the virus to humans. Additional amplification by pigs, which suffer abortion, and horses, which develop encephalitis, may be significant as well. Vaccination of these additional amplifying hosts can reduce the transmission of the virus. An effective, formalin-inactivated vaccine purified from mouse brain is produced in Japan and licensed for human use in the United States. It is given on days 0, 7, and 30 or—with some sacrifice in serum neutralizing titer—on days 0, 7, and 14. Vaccination is indicated for summer travelers to rural Asia, where the risk of clinical disease may be 0.05 to 2.1/10,000 per week. The severe and often fatal disease reported in expatriates must be balanced against the 0.1 to 1 percent chance of a late systemic or cutaneous allergic reaction. These reactions are rarely fatal but may be severe and have been known to begin 1 to 9 days after vaccination, with associated pruritus, urticaria, and angioedema. Live attenuated vaccines are being used in China but are not recommended in the United States at this time.

WEST NILE VIRUS INFECTION West Nile virus is transmitted among wild birds by *Culex* mosquitoes in Africa, the Middle East, southern Europe, and Asia. It is a frequent cause of febrile disease without CNS involvement, but it occasionally causes aseptic meningitis and severe encephalitis; these serious infections are particularly common among children and the elderly. In 1996, West Nile or a closely related virus caused more than 300 cases of CNS disease, with 10 percent mortality, in the Danube flood plains, including Bucharest. The febrile-myalgic syndrome caused by West Nile virus is distinguished from other such syndromes by the frequent appearance of a maculopapular rash concentrated on the trunk and lymphadenopathy. Headache, ocular pain, sore throat, nausea and vomiting, and arthralgia (but not arthritis) are common accompaniments. In addition, the virus has been implicated in severe and fatal hepatic necrosis in Central Africa.

West Nile virus falls into the same phylogenetic group of flaviviruses as St. Louis and Japanese encephalitis viruses, as do Murray Valley and Rocio viruses. The latter two viruses are both maintained in mosquitoes and birds and produce a clinical picture resembling that of Japanese encephalitis. Murray Valley virus has caused occasional epidemics and sporadic cases in Australia. Rocio virus caused recurrent epidemics in a focal area of Brazil in 1975 to 1977 and then virtually disappeared.

CENTRAL EUROPEAN TICK-BORNE ENCEPHALITIS AND RUSSIAN SPRING-SUMMER ENCEPHALITIS A spectrum of tick-borne flaviviruses has been identified across the Eurasian land mass. Many are known mainly as agricultural pathogens (e.g., louping ill virus in the United Kingdom). From Scandinavia to the Urals, central European tick-borne encephalitis is transmitted by *Ixodes ricinus*. Human cases occur between April and October, with a peak in June and July. A related and more virulent virus is that of Russian spring-summer encephalitis, which is associated with *Ixodes persulcatus* and is distributed from Europe across the Urals to the Pacific Ocean. The ticks transmit the disease primarily in the spring and early summer, with a lower rate of transmission later in summer. Small mammals are the vertebrate amplifiers for both viruses. The risk varies by geographic area and can be highly localized within a given area; human cases usually follow outdoor activities or consumption of raw milk from infected goats or other infected animals.

After an incubation period of 7 to 14 days or perhaps longer, the central European viruses classically result in a febrile-myalgic phase that lasts for 2 to 4 days and is thought to correlate with viremia. A subsequent remission for several days is followed by the recurrence of fever and the onset of meningeal signs. The CNS phase varies from mild aseptic meningitis, which is more common among younger patients, to severe encephalitis with coma, convulsions, tremors, and motor signs lasting for 7 to 10 days before improvement begins. Spinal and medullary involvement can lead to typical limb-girdle paralysis and to respiratory paralysis. Most patients recover, only a minority with significant deficits. Infections with the far eastern viruses generally run a more abrupt course. The encephalitic syndrome caused by these viruses sometimes begins without a remission and has more severe manifestations than the central European syndrome. Mortality is high, and major sequelae—most notably, lower motor neuron paralyses of the proximal muscles of the extremities, trunk, and neck—are common.

In the early stage of the illness, virus may be isolated from the blood. In the CNS phase, IgM antibodies are detectable in serum and/or CSF. Thrombocytopenia sometimes develops during the initial febrile illness, which resembles the early hemorrhagic phase of some other tick-borne flaviviral infections, such as Kyasanur Forest disease. Other tick-borne flaviviruses are less common causes of encephalitis, including louping ill virus in the United Kingdom and Powassan virus (see below).

There is no specific therapy for infection with these viruses. However, effective alum-adjuvanted, formalin-inactivated vaccines are produced in Austria, Germany, and Russia. Two doses of the Austrian vaccine separated by an interval of 1 to 3 months appear to be effective in the field, and antibody responses are similar when vaccine is given on days 0 and 14. Other vaccines have elicited similar neutralizing antibody titers. Since rare cases of postvaccination Guillain-Barré syndrome have been reported, vaccination should be reserved for persons likely to experience rural exposure in an endemic area during the season of transmission. Cross-neutralization for the central European and far eastern strains has been established, but there are no published field studies on cross-protection of formalin-inactivated vaccines. Because 0.2 to 4 percent of ticks in endemic areas may be infected, tick bites raise the issue of immunoglobulin prophylaxis. Prompt administration of high-titered specific preparations should probably be undertaken, although no controlled data are available to prove the efficacy of this measure. Immunoglobulin should not be administered late because of the risk of antibody-mediated enhancement.

POWASSAN ENCEPHALITIS Powassan virus is a member of the tick-borne encephalitis virus complex and is transmitted by *Ixodes cookei* among small mammals in eastern Canada and the United States, where it has been responsible for 20 recognized cases of human disease. Other ticks may transmit the virus in a wider geographic area, and there is some concern that *Ixodes dammini*, a competent vector in the laboratory, may become involved as it becomes more prominent in the United States. Patients with Powassan encephalitis—often children—present in May through December after outdoor exposure and an incubation period thought to be about 1 week. Powassan encephalitis is severe, and sequelae are common.

EASTERN EQUINE ENCEPHALITIS Eastern equine encephalitis is found primarily within endemic swampy foci along the eastern coast of the United States, with a few inland foci as far removed as Michigan. Human cases present from June through October, when the bird–*Culiseta* mosquito cycle spills over into other mosquito species such as *Aedes sollicitans*, or *Aedes vexans*, which are more likely to bite mammals. There is concern over the potential role of the introduced anthropophilic mosquito species *A. albopictus*, which has been found to be naturally infected and is an effective vector in the laboratory. Horses are a common target for the virus; if not vaccinated, they serve as a harbinger of human disease but probably do not play a significant role in amplification of the virus.

Eastern equine encephalitis is one of the most destructive of the arboviral conditions, with a brusque onset, rapid progression, high mortality, and frequent residua. This severity is reflected in the extensive necrotic lesions and polymorphonuclear infiltrates found at postmortem examination of the brain and the acute polymorphonuclear CSF pleocytosis often occurring during the first 1 to 3 days of disease. In addition, leukocytosis with a left shift is a common feature. A formalin-inactivated vaccine has been used to protect laboratory workers but is not generally available or applicable.

WESTERN EQUINE ENCEPHALITIS The primary maintenance cycle for western equine encephalitis virus in the United States is between *C. tarsalis* and birds, principally sparrows and finches. Equines and humans become infected, and both species suffer encephalitis without amplifying the virus in nature. St. Louis encephalitis is transmitted in a similar cycle in the same region but causes human disease about a month earlier than the period (July through October) in which western equine encephalitis virus is active. Large epidemics of western equine encephalitis took place in the western and central United States and Canada during the 1930s to 1950s, but in recent years the disease has been uncommon. There were 41 reported cases in the United States in 1987, but only 4 reported cases from 1988 to 1995. This decline in incidence may reflect in part the integrated approach to mosquito management that has been employed in irrigation projects and the increasing use of agricultural pesticides; it almost certainly reflects the increased tendency for humans to be indoors behind closed windows at dusk, the peak period of biting by the major vector.

Western equine encephalitis virus causes a typical diffuse viral encephalitis with an increased attack rate and increased morbidity in the young, particularly children under 2 years of age. In addition, mortality is high among the young and the very elderly. One-third of individuals who have convulsions during the acute illness have subsequent seizure activity. Infants under 1 year of age—particularly those in the first months of life—are at serious risk of motor and intellectual damage. Twice as many males as females develop clinical encephalitis after 5 to 9 years of age; this difference may be related to greater outdoor exposure of boys to the vector but is also likely to be due in part to biologic differences. A formalin-inactivated vaccine has been used to protect laboratory workers but is not generally available or applicable.

VENEZUELAN EQUINE ENCEPHALITIS There are six known types of virus in the Venezuelan equine encephalitis complex. An important distinction is between the "epizootic" viruses (subtypes IAB and IC) and the "enzootic" viruses (subtypes ID to IF and types II to VI). The epizootic viruses have an unknown natural cycle but periodically cause extensive epidemics in equines and humans in the Americas. These epidemics rely on the high-level viremia in horses and mules that results in the infection of several species of mosquitoes, which in turn infect humans and perpetuate virus transmission. Humans also have high-level viremia but probably are not important in virus transmission. Enzootic viruses are found primarily in humid tropical forest habitats and are maintained between *Culex* mosquitoes and rodents; these viruses cause human disease but are not pathogenic for horses and do not cause epizootics.

Epizootics of Venezuelan equine encephalitis occurred repeatedly in Venezuela, Colombia, Ecuador, Peru, and other South American countries at intervals of 10 years or less from the 1930s until 1969, when a massive epizootic spread throughout Central America and Mexico, reaching southern Texas in 1972. Genetic sequencing of the virus from the 1969 to 1972 outbreak suggested that it originated from residual "un-inactivated" virus in veterinary vaccines. The outbreak was terminated in Texas with the use of a live attenuated vaccine (TC-83) originally developed for human use by the U.S. Army; this virus was then used for further production of inactivated veterinary vaccines. No further epizootic disease was definitely identified until 1993 to 1995, when additional epizootics took place in Mexico, Colombia, and Venezuela. The viruses involved in these epizootics as well as previously epizootic subtype IC viruses have been shown to be close phylogenetic relatives of known enzootic subtype ID viruses. This finding suggests that active evolution and selection of epizootic viruses are under way in northern South America.

During epizootics, extensive human infection is the rule, with clinical disease in 10 to 60 percent of infected individuals. Most infections result in notable acute febrile disease, while relatively few result in encephalitis. A low rate of CNS invasion is supported by the absence of encephalitis among the many infections resulting from exposure to aerosols in the laboratory or from vaccine accidents. The most recent epizootic of Venezuelan equine encephalitis occurred in Colombia and Venezuela in 1995; of the more than 85,000 clinical cases, 4 percent (with a higher proportion among children than adults) included neurologic symptoms and 300 ended in death.

Enzootic strains of Venezuelan equine encephalitis virus are common causes of acute febrile disease, particularly in areas such as the Florida Everglades and the humid Atlantic coast of Central America. Encephalitis has been documented only in the Florida infections; the three cases were caused by type II enzootic virus, also called *Everglades virus*. All three patients had preexisting cerebral disease. Extrapolation from the rate of genetic change suggests that Everglades virus was introduced into Florida less than 200 years ago and that it is most closely related to the ID subtypes that appear to have given evolutionary rise to the epizootic strains active in South America.

The prevention of epizootic Venezuelan equine encephalitis depends on vaccination of horses with the attenuated TC-83 vaccine or with an inactivated vaccine prepared from that strain. Humans can be protected with similar vaccines, but the use of such products is restricted to laboratory personnel because of reactogenicity and limited availability. In addition, wild-type vaccine and perhaps TC-83 vaccine are thought to have some degree of fetal pathogenicity. Enzootic viruses are antigenically somewhat different from epizootic viruses, and protection against the former with vaccines prepared from the latter is relatively ineffective.

ARTHRITIS AND RASH

True arthritis is a common accompaniment of several viral diseases, such as rubella (caused by a non-alphavirus togavirus), parvovirus B19 infection, and hepatitis B; it is an occasional accompaniment of infection due to mumps virus, enteroviruses, herpesviruses, and adenoviruses. It is not generally appreciated that the alphaviruses are also common causes of arthritis. In fact, the alphaviruses discussed below all cause acute febrile diseases accompanied by the development of true arthritis and a maculopapular rash. Rheumatic involvement includes arthralgia alone, periarticular swelling, and (less commonly) joint effusions. Most of these diseases are less severe and have fewer articular manifestations in children than in adults. In temperate climates, these are summer diseases. No specific therapy or licensed vaccines for these viral diseases yet exist.

SINDBIS VIRUS INFECTION Sindbis virus is transmitted among birds by mosquitoes. Infections with the northern European strains of this virus (which cause, for example, Pogosta disease in Fin-

land, Karelian fever in the new independent states of the former Soviet Union, and Okelbo disease in Sweden) and with the genetically related southern African strains are particularly likely to result in the arthritis-rash syndrome. Exposure to a rural environment is commonly associated with this infection, which has an incubation period of less than 1 week.

The disease begins with rash and arthralgia. Constitutional symptoms are not marked, and fever is modest or lacking altogether. The rash, which lasts about a week, begins on the trunk, spreads to the extremities, and evolves from macules to papules that often vesiculate. The arthritis of this condition is multiarticular, migratory, and incapacitating, with resolution of the acute phase in a few days. Wrists, ankles, phalangeal joints, knees, elbows, and—to a much lesser extent—proximal and axial joints are involved. Persistence of joint pains and occasionally of arthritis is a major problem and may go on for months or even years despite a lack of deformity.

CHIKUNGUNYA VIRUS INFECTION It is likely that chikungunya virus ("that which bends up") is of African origin and is maintained among nonhuman primates on that continent by *Aedes* mosquitoes of the subgenus *Stegomyia* in a fashion similar to yellow fever virus. Like that flavivirus, chikungunya virus is readily transmitted among humans in urban areas by *A. aegypti*. The *A. aegypti*–chikungunya virus transmission cycle has also been introduced into Asia, where it poses a prominent health problem. The disease is endemic in rural areas of Africa, and intermittent epidemics take place in towns and cities of Africa and Asia. Chikungunya is one more reason (in addition to dengue and yellow fever) that *A. aegypti* must be controlled.

Full-blown disease is most common among adults, in whom the clinical picture may be dramatic. The brusque onset follows an incubation period of 2 to 3 days. Fever and severe arthralgia are accompanied by chills and constitutional symptoms such as headache, photophobia, conjunctival injection, anorexia, nausea, and abdominal pain. Migratory polyarthritis mainly affects the small joints of the hands, wrists, ankles, and feet, with lesser involvement of the larger joints. Rash may appear at the outset or several days into the illness; its development often coincides with defervescence, which takes place around day 2 or day 3 of disease. The rash is most intense on the trunk and limbs and may desquamate. Petechiae are occasionally seen, and epistaxis is not uncommon, but this virus is not a regular cause of the HF syndrome, even in children. A few patients develop leukopenia. Elevated levels of aspartate aminotransferase (AST) and C-reactive protein have been described, as have mildly decreased platelet counts. Recovery may require weeks. Some older patients continue to suffer from stiffness, joint pain, and recurrent effusions for several years; this persistence may be especially common in HLA-B27 patients. A live attenuated investigational vaccine has been developed but requires further testing.

A related virus, O'nyong-nyong, caused a major epidemic of arthritis and rash involving at least 2 million people as it moved across eastern and central Africa in the 1960s. After its mysterious emergence, the virus virtually disappeared, leaving only occasional evidence of its persistence in Kenya until a resurgence of activity in 1997.

MAYARO FEVER Mayaro virus is maintained in the forests of the Americas by *Haemagogus* mosquitoes and nonhuman primates. It causes a frequent endemic and sometimes epidemic infection of humans and appears to cause a syndrome resembling chikungunya.

EPIDEMIC POLYARTHRITIS (ROSS RIVER VIRUS INFECTION) Ross River virus has caused epidemics of distinctive clinical disease in Australia since the turn of the century and continues to be responsible for thousands of cases in rural and suburban areas annually. The virus is transmitted by *Aedes vigilax* and other mosquitoes, and its persistence is thought to involve transovarial transmission. No definitive vertebrate host has been identified, but several mammalian species, including wallabies, have been suggested. Endemic transmission has also been documented in New Guinea, and in 1979 the virus swept through the eastern Pacific Islands, causing hundreds of thousands of illnesses. The virus was carried from island to island by infected humans and was believed to have been transmitted among humans by *Aedes polynesiensis* and *A. aegypti*.

The incubation period is 7 to 11 days long, and the onset of illness is sudden, with joint pain usually ushering in the disease. The rash generally develops coincidentally or follows shortly but in some cases precedes joint pains by several days. Constitutional symptoms such as low-grade fever, asthenia, myalgia, headache, and nausea are not prominent and indeed are absent in many cases. Most patients are incapacitated for considerable periods by joint involvement, which interferes with sleeping, walking, and grasping. Wrist, ankle, metacarpophalangeal, interphalangeal, and knee joints are the most commonly involved, although toes, shoulders, and elbows may be affected with some frequency. Periarticular swelling and tenosynovitis are common, and one-third of patients have true arthritis. Only half of all arthritis patients can resume normal activities within 4 weeks, and 10 percent still must limit their activity at 3 months. Occasional patients are symptomatic for 1 to 3 years but without progressive arthropathy. Aspirin and nonsteroidal anti-inflammatory drugs are effective for the treatment of symptoms.

Clinical laboratory values are normal or variable in Ross River virus infection. Tests for rheumatoid factor and antinuclear antibodies are negative, and the erythrocyte sedimentation rate is acutely elevated. Joint fluid contains 1000 to 60,000 mononuclear cells per microliter, and Ross River virus antigen is demonstrable in macrophages. IgM antibodies are particularly valuable in the diagnosis of this infection. The isolation of the virus from blood by mosquito inoculation or mosquito cell culture is possible early in the illness. Because of the great economic importance of annual epidemics in Australia, an inactivated vaccine is being developed and has been found to be protective in mice.

Perhaps because of the high level of current interest in arboviruses in general and in Ross River virus in particular, other arthritogenic arboviruses have been identified in Australia, including Gan Gan virus, a member of the family Bunyaviridae; Kokobera virus, a flavivirus; and Barmah Forest virus, an alphavirus. The last virus is a common cause of infection and must be differentiated from Ross River virus by specific testing.

HEMORRHAGIC FEVERS

The viral HF syndrome is a constellation of findings based on vascular instability and decreased vascular integrity. An assault, direct or indirect, on the microvasculature leads to increased permeability and (particularly when platelet function is decreased) to actual disruption and local hemorrhage. Blood pressure is decreased, and in severe cases shock supervenes. Cutaneous flushing and conjunctival suffusion are examples of common, observable abnormalities in the control of local circulation. The hemorrhage is inconstant and is thought in most cases to be an indication of widespread vascular damage rather than a life-threatening loss of blood volume. Disseminated intravascular coagulation is occasionally found in any severely ill patient with HF but is thought to occur regularly only in the early phases of HF with renal syndrome, Crimean Congo HF, and perhaps some cases of filovirus HF. In some viral HF syndromes, specific organs may be particularly impaired, such as the kidney in HF with renal syndrome, the lung in hantavirus pulmonary syndrome, or the liver in yellow fever, but in all these diseases the generalized circulatory disturbance is critically important.

The pathogenesis of HF is poorly understood and varies among the viruses regularly implicated in the syndrome, which number more than a dozen. In some cases direct damage to the vascular system or even to parenchymal cells of target organs is important, whereas in others soluble mediators are thought to play the major role. The acute phase in most cases of HF is associated with ongoing virus replication and viremia. Exceptions are the hantavirus diseases and dengue HF/dengue shock syndrome (DHF/DSS), in which the immune response plays a major pathogenic role.

The HF syndromes all begin with fever and myalgia, usually of abrupt onset. Within a few days the patient presents for medical attention because of increasing prostration that is often accompanied by severe headache, dizziness, photophobia, hyperesthesia, abdominal or chest pain, anorexia, nausea or vomiting, and other gastrointestinal

disturbances. Initial examination often reveals only an acutely ill patient with conjunctival suffusion, tenderness to palpation of muscles or abdomen, and borderline hypotension or postural hypotension, perhaps with tachycardia. Petechiae (often best visualized in the axillae), flushing of the head and thorax, periorbital edema, and proteinuria are common. Levels of AST are usually elevated at presentation or within a day or two thereafter. Hemoconcentration from vascular leakage, which is usually evident, is most marked in hantavirus diseases and in DHF/DSS. The seriously ill patient progresses to more severe symptoms and develops shock and other findings typical of the causative virus. Shock, multifocal bleeding, and CNS involvement (encephalopathy, coma, convulsions) are all poor prognostic signs.

One of the major diagnostic clues is travel to an endemic area within the incubation period for a given syndrome (Table 200-4). Except for Seoul, dengue, and yellow fever virus infections, which have urban vectors, travel to a rural setting is especially suggestive of a diagnosis of HF.

Early recognition is important because of the need for virus-specific therapy and supportive measures, including prompt, atraumatic hospitalization; judicious fluid therapy that takes into account the patient's increased capillary permeability; use of pressors to maintain blood pressure at levels that will support renal perfusion; treatment of the relatively common secondary bacterial infections; replacement of clotting factors and platelets as indicated; and the usual precautionary measures used in the treatment of patients with hemorrhagic diatheses. Disseminated intravascular coagulation should be treated only if clear laboratory evidence of its existence is found and if laboratory monitoring of therapy is feasible; there is no proven benefit of such therapy. The available evidence suggests that HF patients have a decreased cardiac output and will respond poorly to fluid loading as it is often practiced in the treatment of shock associated with bacterial sepsis. Specific therapy is available for several of the HF syndromes. In addition, several diseases considered in the differential diagnosis—malaria, shigellosis, typhoid, leptospirosis, and rickettsial disease—are treatable and potentially lethal. Strict barrier nursing and other precautions against infection of medical staff and visitors are indicated in HF except that due to hantaviruses, yellow fever, Rift Valley fever, and dengue.

LASSA FEVER Lassa virus is known to cause disease in Nigeria, Sierra Leone, Guinea, and Liberia. This virus and its relatives exist elsewhere in Africa, but their health significance is unknown. Like other arenaviruses, Lassa virus is spread to humans by small-particle aerosols from chronically infected rodents and may be acquired during the capture or eating of these animals; it can also be transmitted by person-to-person contact. The virus is often present in urine during convalescence and is suspected to be present in seminal fluid early in recovery. Nosocomial spread has occurred but is uncommon if proper sterile parenteral techniques are used. People of all ages and both sexes are affected; the incidence of disease is highest in the dry season, but transmission takes place year-round. In countries where Lassa virus is endemic, Lassa fever can be a prominent cause of febrile disease. For example, in one hospital in Sierra Leone, laboratory-confirmed Lassa fever is consistently responsible for one-fifth of admissions to the medical wards. There are probably tens of thousands of Lassa fever cases annually in West Africa alone.

The average case has a gradual onset (among the HF agents, only the arenaviruses are typically associated with a gradual onset) that gives way to more severe constitutional symptoms and prostration. Bleeding is seen in only about 15 to 30 percent of cases. A maculopapular rash is often noted in light-skinned Lassa patients. Effusions are common, and male-dominant pericarditis may develop late. The fetal death rate is 92 percent in the last trimester, when maternal mortality is also increased from the usual 15 percent to 30 percent; these figures suggest that interruption of the pregnancy of infected women should be considered. White blood cell counts are normal or slightly elevated, and platelet counts are normal or somewhat low. Deafness coincides with clinical improvement in about 20 percent of cases and is permanent and bilateral in some. Reinfection may occur but has not been associated with severe disease.

High-level viremia or a high serum concentration of AST predicts a fatal outcome. Thus patients with an AST level of >150 IU/mL should be treated with intravenous ribavirin. This antiviral nucleoside analogue appears to be effective in reducing mortality from rates among retrospective controls, and its only major side effect is reversible anemia that usually does not require transfusion. The drug should be given by slow intravenous infusion in a dose of 32 mg/kg; this dose should be followed by 16 mg/kg q 6 h for 4 days and then by 8 mg/kg q 8 h for 6 days.

SOUTH AMERICAN HF SYNDROMES (ARGENTINE, BOLIVIAN, VENEZUELAN, AND BRAZILIAN) These diseases are similar to one another clinically, but their epidemiology differs with the habits of their rodent reservoirs and the interactions of these animals with humans (Table 200-4). Person-to-person or nosocomial transmission is rare but has occurred.

The basic disease resembles Lassa fever with two marked differences. First, thrombocytopenia—often marked—is the rule, and bleeding is quite common. Second, CNS dysfunction is much more common than in Lassa fever and is often manifest by marked confusion, tremors of the arms and tongue, and cerebellar signs. Some cases follow a predominantly neurologic course, with a poor prognosis. The clinical laboratory is helpful in diagnosis since thrombocytopenia, leukopenia, and proteinuria are typical findings.

Argentine HF is readily treated with convalescent-phase plasma given within the first 8 days of illness. In the absence of passive antibody therapy, intravenous ribavirin in the dose recommended for Lassa fever is likely to be effective in all the South American HF syndromes. The transmission of the disease from men convalescing from Argentine HF to their wives suggests the need for counseling of arenavirus HF patients concerning the avoidance of intimate contacts for several weeks after recovery. A safe, effective, live attenuated vaccine exists for Argentine HF. In experimental animals, this vaccine is cross-protective against the Bolivian HF virus.

RIFT VALLEY FEVER This mosquito-borne virus is also a pathogen of domestic animals such as sheep, cattle, and goats. It is maintained in nature by transovarial transmission in floodwater *Aedes* mosquitoes and presumably in a vertebrate amplifier. Epizootics and epidemics occur when sheep or cattle become infected during particularly heavy rains; developing high-level viremia, these animals infect many different species of mosquitoes. Remote sensing via satellite can detect the ecologic changes associated with high rainfall that predict the likelihood of Rift Valley fever transmission; it can also detect the special depressions from which the floodwater *Aedes* mosquito vectors emerge. In addition, the virus is infectious when transmitted by contact with blood or aerosols from domestic animals or their abortuses. The slaughtered meat is not infectious. The natural range of Rift Valley fever virus is confined to sub-Saharan Africa, but the virus has recently been found in Madagascar and has been introduced into Egypt twice, with extensive epidemics occurring on both occasions (1977 to 1979 and 1993 to 1995). Neither person-to-person nor nosocomial transmission has been documented.

Table 200-4

Viral Hemorrhagic Fever (HF) Syndromes and Their Distribution

Disease	Incubation Period, Days	Case-Infection Ratio	Case-Mortality Rate, %	Geographic Range	Target Population
Lassa fever	5–16	Mild infections probably common	15	West Africa	All ages, both sexes
South American HF	7–14	Most infections (more than half) result in disease	15–30	Selected rural areas of Bolivia, Argentina, Venezuela, and Brazil	Bolivia: Men in countryside; all ages, both sexes in villages. Argentina: All ages, both sexes; excess exposure and disease in men. Venezuela: All ages, both sexes
Rift Valley fever	2–5	~1:100 (most infections result in fever and myalgia)	~50	Sub-Saharan Africa, Madagascar, Egypt	All ages, both sexes; more often diagnosed in men; preexisting liver disease may predispose
Crimean Congo HF	3–12	1:5 or higher	15–30	Africa, Middle East, Balkans, southern region of former Soviet Union, western China	All ages, both sexes; men more exposed in some settings
HF with renal syndrome	9–35	>3:4, Hantaan; 1:20, Puumala	5–15, Hantaan; <1, Puumala	Worldwide, depending on rodent reservoir	Excess of male patients (partly due to greater exposure); mainly adults
Hantavirus pulmonary syndrome	~7–28	Very high	40–50	Americas	Excess of male patients due to some occupational exposure; mainly adults
Marburg or Ebola HF	3–16	High	25–90	Sub-Saharan Africa	All ages, both sexes; children less exposed
Yellow fever	3–6	1:2–1:20	20	Africa, South America	All ages, both sexes; adults more exposed in jungle setting; preexisting flavivirus immunity may cross-protect
Dengue HF/dengue shock syndrome	2–7	1:10,000, nonimmune; 1:100, heterologous immune	<1 with supportive treatment	Tropics and subtropics worldwide	Predominantly children; previous heterologous dengue infection predisposes to HF
Kyasanur Forest/Omsk HF	3–8	Variable	0.5–10	Mysore State, India/western Siberia	Variable

Rift Valley fever virus is unusual in that it causes at least four different clinical syndromes. Most infections are manifested as the febrile-myalgic syndrome. A small proportion result in HF with especially prominent liver involvement. Perhaps 10 percent of otherwise mild infections lead to retinal vasculitis; funduscopic examination reveals edema, hemorrhages, and infarction, and some patients permanently lose partial vision. A small proportion of cases (<1 in 200) are followed by typical viral encephalitis. One of the complicated syndromes does not appear to predispose to another.

There is no proven therapy for any of the syndromes described above. The sensitivity of animal models of Rift Valley fever to antibody or ribavirin therapy suggests that either could be given intravenously to persons with HF. Both retinal disease and encephalitis occur after the acute febrile syndrome has ended and serum neutralizing antibody has developed—events suggesting that only supportive care need be given. Epidemic disease is best prevented by vaccination of livestock. The established ability of this virus to propagate after an introduction into Egypt suggests that other potentially receptive areas, including the United States, should have a response ready to use in such an eventuality. It seems likely that this disease, like Venezuelan equine encephalitis, can be controlled only with adequate stocks of an effective live attenuated vaccine, and there are no such global stocks. A formalin-inactivated vaccine confers immunity on humans, but quantities are limited and three injections are required; this vaccine is recommended for exposed laboratory workers and for veterinarians working in sub-Saharan Africa.

CRIMEAN CONGO HF This severe HF syndrome has a wide geographic distribution, potentially being found wherever ticks of the genus *Hyalomma* occur (see Table 200-4). The propensity of these ticks to feed on domestic livestock and certain wild mammals means that veterinary serosurveys are the most effective mechanism for the surveillance of virus circulation in a region. Human infection is acquired via a tick bite or during the crushing of infected ticks. Domestic animals do not become ill but do develop viremia; thus there is danger of infection at the time of slaughter and for a brief interval thereafter (through contact with hides or carcasses). A recent epidemic was associated with slaughter of tick-infested ostriches in South Africa. Nosocomial epidemics are common and are usually related to extensive blood exposure or needle sticks.

Although generally similar to other HF syndromes, Crimean Congo HF causes extensive liver damage, resulting in jaundice in some cases. Clinical laboratory values indicate disseminated intravascular coagulation and show elevations in AST, creatine phosphokinase, and bilirubin. Patients with fatal cases generally have more marked changes even in the early days of illness and also develop leukocytosis rather than leukopenia. Thrombocytopenia is also more marked and develops earlier in cases with a fatal outcome.

No controlled trials have been performed with intravenous ribavirin, but clinical experience and retrospective comparison of patients with ominous clinical laboratory values suggest that ribavirin is efficacious and should be given. No human or veterinary vaccines are recommended.

HF WITH RENAL SYNDROME This disease, the first to be identified as an HF, is widely distributed over Europe and Asia; the major causative viruses and their rodent reservoirs on these two continents are Puumala virus (bank vole, *Clethrionomys glareolus*) and Hantaan virus (striped field mouse, *Apodemus agrarius*), respectively. Other potential causative viruses exist, including Dobrava virus (yellow-necked field mouse, *Apodemus flavicollus*), which causes severe HF with renal syndrome in the Balkans. Seoul virus is associated with the Norway or sewer rat, *Rattus norvegicus*, and has a worldwide distribution through the migration of the rodent; it is associated with mild or moderate HF with renal syndrome in Asia, but in many areas of the world the human disease has been difficult to identify. Most cases occur in rural residents or vacationers; the exception is Seoul virus disease, which may be acquired in an urban or rural setting or from contaminated laboratory rat colonies. Classic Hantaan disease in Korea (Korean HF) and in rural China (epidemic HF) is most common in spring and fall and is related to rodent density and agricul-

tural practices. Human infection is acquired primarily through aerosols of rodent urine, although virus is also present in saliva and feces. Patients with hantavirus diseases are not infectious. HF with renal syndrome is the most important form of HF today, with more than 100,000 cases of severe disease in Asia annually and milder Puumala infections numbering in the thousands as well.

Severe cases of HF with renal syndrome caused by Hantaan virus evolve in identifiable stages: the febrile stage with myalgia, lasting 3 to 4 days; the hypotensive stage, often associated with shock and lasting from a few hours to 48 h; the oliguric stage with renal failure, lasting 3 to 10 days; and the polyuric stage with diuresis and hyposthenuria.

The *febrile period* is initiated by the abrupt onset of fever, headache, severe myalgia, thirst, anorexia, and often nausea and vomiting. Photophobia, retroorbital pain, and pain on ocular movement are common, and the vision may become blurred with ciliary body inflammation. Flushing over the face, the V area of the neck, and the back are characteristic, as are pharyngeal injection, periorbital edema, and conjunctival suffusion. Petechiae often develop in areas of pressure, the conjunctivae, and the axillae. Back pain and tenderness to percussion at the costovertebral angle reflect massive retroperitoneal edema. Laboratory evidence of mild to moderate disseminated intravascular coagulation is present. Other laboratory findings include proteinuria and an active urinary sediment.

The *hypotensive phase* is ushered in by falling blood pressure and sometimes by shock. The relative bradycardia typical of the febrile phase is replaced by tachycardia. Kinin activation is marked. The rising hematocrit reflects increasing vascular leakage. Leukocytosis with a left shift develops, and thrombocytopenia continues. Atypical lymphocytes—which in fact are activated CD8+ and to a lesser extent CD4+ T cells—circulate. Proteinuria is marked, and the urine's specific gravity falls to 1.010. The renal circulation is congested and compromised from local and systemic circulatory changes resulting in necrosis of tubules, particularly at the corticomedullary junction, and oliguria.

During the *oliguric phase*, hemorrhagic tendencies continue, probably in large part because of uremic bleeding defects. The oliguria persists for 3 to 10 days before renal function returns and marks the onset of the *polyuric stage*, which carries the danger of dehydration and electrolyte abnormalities.

Mild cases of HF with renal syndrome may be much less stereotyped. The presentation may include only fever, gastrointestinal abnormalities, and transient oliguria followed by hyposthenuria.

HF with renal syndrome should be suspected in patients with rural exposure in an endemic area. Prompt recognition of the disease will permit rapid hospitalization and expectant management of shock and renal failure. Useful clinical laboratory parameters include leukocytosis, which may be leukemoid and is associated with a left shift; thrombocytopenia; and proteinuria. Mainstays of therapy are the management of shock, reliance on pressors, modest crystalloid infusion, intravenous use of human serum albumin, and treatment of renal failure with prompt dialysis for the usual indications. Hydration may result in pulmonary edema, and hypertension should be avoided because of the possibility of intracranial hemorrhage. Use of intravenous ribavirin has reduced mortality and morbidity in severe cases provided treatment is begun within the first 4 days of illness. The case-mortality rate may be as high as 15 percent among unrecognized cases but with proper therapy should be <5 percent. Sequelae have not been definitely established, but there is a correlation in the United States between chronic hypertensive renal failure and the presence of antibodies to Seoul virus.

Infections with Puumala virus, the most common cause of HF with renal syndrome in Europe, result in a much attenuated picture but the same general presentation. The syndrome may be referred to by its former name, *nephropathia epidemica*. Bleeding manifestations are found in only 10 percent of cases, hypotension rather than shock is usually seen, and oliguria is present in only about half of patients. The dominant features may be fever, abdominal pain, proteinuria, mild oliguria, and sometimes blurred vision or glaucoma followed by polyuria and hyposthenuria in recovery. Mortality is <1 percent.

The diagnosis is readily made by IgM-capture ELISA, which should be positive at admission or within 24 to 48 h thereafter. The isolation of virus is difficult, but RT-PCR of a blood clot collected early in the clinical course or of tissues obtained postmortem will give positive results. Such testing is undertaken only if definitive identification of the infecting viral species is required.

HANTAVIRUS PULMONARY SYNDROME Hantavirus pulmonary syndrome was discovered in 1993, but retrospective identification of cases by immunohistochemistry (1978) and serology (1959) support the idea that it is a recently discovered rather than a truly new disease. The causative viruses are hantaviruses of a distinct phylogenetic lineage that is associated with the rodent subfamily Sigmodontinae. Sin Nombre virus chronically infects the deer mouse (*Peromyscus maniculatus*) and is the most important virus causing hantavirus pulmonary syndrome in the United States. In the southern states, the disease is also caused by a Sin Nombre virus variant from the white-footed mouse (*Peromyscus leucopus*), by Black Creek Canal virus (*Sigmodon hispidus*, the cotton rat), and by Bayou virus (*Oryzomys palustris*, the rice rat). Viruses such as Andes virus are responsible for cases of hantavirus pulmonary syndrome in Argentina, Brazil, Chile, and Paraguay. The disease is linked to rodent exposure and particularly affects rural residents living in dwellings permeable to rodent entry or working at occupations that pose a risk of rodent exposure. Each rodent species has its own particular habits; in the case of the deer mouse, these behaviors include living in and around human habitation.

The disease begins with a prodrome of about 3 to 4 days (range, 1 to 11 days) comprising fever, myalgia, malaise, and often gastrointestinal disturbances such as nausea, vomiting, and abdominal pain. Dizziness is common and vertigo occasional. Severe prodromal symptoms sometimes bring some individuals to medical attention, but patients more commonly present as the pulmonary phase begins. Typically, there is slightly lowered blood pressure, tachycardia, tachypnea, mild hypoxemia, and early radiographic signs of pulmonary edema. Physical findings in the chest are often surprisingly scant. The conjunctival and cutaneous signs of vascular involvement seen in other types of HF are absent. During the next few hours, decompensation may progress rapidly to severe hypoxemia and respiratory failure. Most patients surviving the first 48 h of hospitalization are extubated and discharged within a few days, with no apparent residua.

Management during the first few hours after presentation is critical. The goal is to prevent severe hypoxemia by oxygen therapy and, if needed, intubation and intensive respiratory management. During this period, hypotension and shock with increasing hematocrit invite aggressive fluid administration, but this intervention should be undertaken with great caution. Because of low cardiac output and increased pulmonary vascular permeability, shock should be managed expectantly with pressors and modest infusion of fluid guided by the pulmonary capillary wedge pressure. Mild cases can be managed by frequent monitoring and oxygen administration without intubation. Many patients require intubation to manage hypoxemia and also develop shock. Mortality remains at about 40 percent with good management. The antiviral drug ribavirin inhibits the virus in vitro and is undergoing clinical trials for efficacy but did not have a marked effect on patients treated in an open-label study.

During the prodrome, the differential diagnosis of hantavirus pulmonary infection is difficult, but by the time of presentation or within 24 h thereafter, a number of helpful clinical features become apparent. Cough is not usually present at the outset but may develop later. Interstitial edema is evident on the chest x-ray. Later, bilateral alveolar edema with a central distribution develops in the setting of a normal-sized heart; occasionally, the edema is initially unilateral. Pleural effusions are often visualized. Thrombocytopenia, circulating atypical lymphocytes, and a left shift (often with leukocytosis) are almost always evident. Hemoconcentration, proteinuria, and hypoalbuminemia should also be sought. Although thrombocytopenia virtually always develops and prolongation of the partial thromboplastin time is the rule, clinical evidence for coagulopathy or laboratory indications of disseminated intravascular coagulation are found in only a minority of cases, usually in severely ill patients. These patients also have acidosis and elevated serum levels of lactate. Mildly increased values in renal function tests are common, but patients with severe cases often have markedly elevated concentrations of serum creatinine; some of the viruses other than Sin Nombre virus have been associated with more kidney involvement, but few such cases have been studied. The differential diagnosis includes abdominal surgical conditions and pyelonephritis as well as rickettsial disease, sepsis, meningococcemia, plague, tularemia, influenza, and relapsing fever.

A specific diagnosis is best made by IgM testing of acute-phase serum, which has yielded a positive result even in the prodrome. Tests using a Sin Nombre virus antigen detect the related hantaviruses causing the pulmonary syndrome in the Americas. Occasionally, heterologous viruses will react only in the IgG ELISA, but this finding is highly suspicious given the very low seroprevalence of these viruses in normal populations. RT-PCR is usually positive when used to test blood clots obtained in the first 7 to 9 days of illness as well as tissues; this test is useful in identifying the infecting virus in areas outside the home range of the deer mouse and in atypical cases.

YELLOW FEVER Yellow fever virus caused major epidemics in the Americas, Africa, and Europe before the discovery of mosquito transmission in 1900 led to its control through attacks on its urban vector, *A. aegypti*. Only then was it found that a jungle cycle also existed in Africa, involving other *Aedes* mosquitoes and monkeys, and that colonization of the new world with *A. aegypti*, originally an African species, had established urban yellow fever as well as an independent sylvatic yellow fever cycle in American jungles involving *Haemagogus* mosquitoes and new world monkeys. Today, urban yellow fever transmission occurs only in some African cities, but the threat exists in the great cities of South America, where reinfestation by *A. aegypti* has taken place and dengue transmission by the same mosquito is common. As late as 1905, New Orleans suffered more than 3000 cases with 452 deaths from "yellow jack." Despite the existence of a highly effective and safe vaccine, several hundred jungle yellow fever cases occur annually in South America, and thousands of jungle and urban cases occur each year in Africa.

Yellow fever is a typical HF accompanied by prominent hepatic necrosis. A period of viremia, typically lasting 3 or 4 days, is followed by a period of "intoxication." During the latter phase in severe cases, the characteristic jaundice, hemorrhages, black vomit, anuria, and terminal delirium occur, perhaps related in part to extensive hepatic involvement. Blood leukocyte counts may be normal or reduced and are often high in terminal stages. Albuminuria is usually noted and may be marked; as renal function fails in terminal or severe cases, the level of blood urea nitrogen rises proportionally. Abnormalities detected in liver function tests range from modest elevations of AST levels in mild cases to severe derangement.

Urban yellow fever can be prevented by the control of *A. aegypti*. The continuing sylvatic cycle requires vaccination of all visitors to areas of potential transmission. Reactions to vaccine are minimal; immunity is provided within 10 days and lasts for at least 10 years. An egg allergy dictates caution in vaccine administration. Although there are no documented harmful effects of the vaccine on the fetus, pregnant women should be immunized only if they are definitely at risk of yellow fever exposure. Since vaccination has been associated with several cases of encephalitis in children under 6 months of age, it should be delayed until after 12 months of age unless the risk of exposure is very high. Timely information on changes in yellow fever distribution and yellow fever vaccine requirements can be obtained from Health Information for Travelers, Centers for Disease Control and Prevention, Atlanta, GA 30333; by fax request (404-332-4565; document number 220022#); by phone (404-332-4559); or on the World-Wide Web at http://www.cdc.gov.

DENGUE HEMORRHAGIC FEVER/DENGUE SHOCK SYNDROME   A syndrome of HF noted in the 1950s among children in the Philippines and Southeast Asia was soon associated with dengue virus infections, particularly those occurring against a background of previous exposure to another serotype. The transient heterotypic protection after dengue virus infection is replaced within several weeks by the potential for heterotypic infection resulting in typical dengue fever (see above) or—uncommonly—for enhanced disease (secondary DHF/DSS). In rare instances, primary dengue infections lead to an HF syndrome, but much less is known about pathogenesis in this situation. In the past 20 years, *A. aegypti* has progressively reinvaded Latin America and other areas, and frequent travel by infected individuals has introduced multiple strains of dengue virus from many geographic areas. Thus the pattern of hyperendemic transmission of multiple dengue serotypes has now been established in the Americas and the Caribbean and has led to the emergence of DHF/DSS as a major problem there as well. Millions of dengue infections, including many thousands of cases of DHF/DSS, occur annually. The severe syndrome is unlikely to be seen in U.S. citizens since few children have the dengue antibodies that can trigger the pathogenetic cascade when a second infection is acquired.

Macrophage/monocyte infection is central to the pathogenesis of dengue fever and to the origin of DHF/DSS. Previous infection with a heterologous dengue-virus serotype may result in the production of nonprotective antiviral antibodies that nevertheless bind to the virion's surface and through interaction with the Fc receptor focus secondary dengue viruses on the target cell, the result being enhanced infection. The host is also primed for a secondary antibody response when viral antigens are released and immune complexes lead to activation of the classic complement pathway, with consequent phlogistic effects. Cross-reactivity at the T cell level results in the release of physiologically active cytokines, including interferon γ and tumor necrosis factor alpha. The induction of vascular permeability and shock depends on multiple factors, including the following:

1. *Presence of enhancing and nonneutralizing antibodies*—Transplacental maternal antibody may be present in infants <9 months old, or antibody elicited by previous heterologous dengue infection may be present in older individuals.
2. *Age*—Susceptibility to DHF/DSS drops considerably after 12 years of age.
3. *Sex*—Females are more often affected than males.
4. *Race*—Caucasians are more often affected than blacks.
5. *Nutritional status*—Malnutrition is protective.
6. *Sequence of infection*—For example, serotype 1 followed by serotype 2 is more dangerous than serotype 4 followed by serotype 2.
7. *Infecting serotype*—Type 2 is apparently more dangerous than other serotypes.

In addition, there is considerable variation among strains of a given serotype, with Southeast Asian serotype 2 strains having more potential to cause DHF/DSS than others.

Dengue HF is identified by the detection of bleeding tendencies (tourniquet test, petechiae) or overt bleeding in the absence of underlying causes such as preexisting gastrointestinal lesions. Dengue shock syndrome, usually accompanied by hemorrhagic signs, is much more serious and results from increased vascular permeability leading to shock. In mild DHF/DSS, restlessness, lethargy, thrombocytopenia (<100,000/μL), and hemoconcentration are detected 2 to 5 days after the onset of typical dengue fever, often at the time of defervescence. The maculopapular rash that often develops in dengue fever may also appear in DHF/DSS. In more severe cases, frank shock is apparent, with low pulse pressure, cyanosis, hepatomegaly, pleural effusions, ascites, and in some cases severe ecchymoses and gastrointestinal bleeding. The period of shock lasts only 1 or 2 days, and most patients respond promptly to close monitoring, oxygen administration, and infusion of crystalloid or—in severe cases—colloid. The mortality rates reported vary greatly with case ascertainment and the quality of treatment; however, most DHF/DSS patients respond well to supportive therapy, and overall mortality in an experienced center in the tropics is probably as low as 1 percent.

A virologic diagnosis can be made by the usual means, although multiple flavivirus infections lead to a broad immune response to several members of the group, and this situation may result in a lack of virus specificity of the IgM and IgG immune responses. A secondary antibody response can be sought with tests against several flavivirus antigens to demonstrate the characteristic wide spectrum of reactivity.

The key to control of both dengue fever and DHF/DSS is the control of *A. aegypti*, which also reduces the risk of urban yellow fever and chikungunya virus circulation. Control efforts have been handicapped by the presence of nondegradable tires and long-lived plastic containers in trash repositories, insecticide resistance, urban poverty, and an inability of the public health community to mobilize the populace to respond to the need to eliminate mosquito breeding sites. Live attenuated dengue vaccines are in the late stages of development and have produced promising results in early tests. Whether vaccines can provide safe, durable immunity to an immunopathologic disease such as DHF/DSS in endemic areas is an issue that will have to be tested, but it is hoped that vaccination will reduce transmission to negligible levels.

KYASANUR FOREST DISEASE AND OMSK HEMORRHAGIC FEVER   Kyasanur Forest virus and Omsk HF virus are geographically restricted, tick-borne flaviviruses that cause a syndrome of viral HF during a wave of viremia and that may also enter the CNS to cause subsequent viral encephalitis (see discussion of tick-borne encephalitis above). There is no therapy for these infections, but an inactivated vaccine has been used in India against Kyasanur Forest disease. A new and related virus isolate has been obtained from butchers with HF in the Middle East; the implication is that there are more agents in this group.

FILOVIRUS HEMORRHAGIC FEVER   → *See Chap. 201.*

BIBLIOGRAPHY

ZOONOTIC VIRUSES

CALISHER CH: Medically important arboviruses of the United States and Canada. Clin Microbiol Rev 7:89, 1994
KARABATSOS N: *International Catalogue of Arboviruses, Including Certain Other Viruses of Vertebrates*, 3d ed. San Antonio, TX, American Society of Tropical Medicine and Hygiene, 1985
MONATH TP (ed): *The Arboviruses: Epidemiology and Ecology*, vols I–V. Boca Raton, FL, CRC Press, 1988
TSAI TF: Arboviral infections in the US. Infect Dis Clin North Am 5:73, 1991
VASCONCELOS PFC et al: Clinical and ecoepidemiological situation of human arboviruses in Brazilian Amazonia. Ciencia e Cultura 44:117, 1992

HEMORRHAGIC FEVERS

CENTERS FOR DISEASE CONTROL AND PREVENTION: Management of patients with suspected viral hemorrhagic fever. Morb Mort Week Rep 37(S-3):1, 1988
———: Update: Management of patients with suspected viral hemorrhagic fever—United States. Morb Mort Week Rep 44:475, 1995
PETERS CJ et al: Management of patients infected with high-hazard viruses. Arch Virol 11(Suppl):141, 1996
———: Pathogenesis of viral hemorrhagic fevers, in *Viral Pathogenesis*, N Nathanson et al (eds). Philadelphia, Lippincott-Raven, 1996
——— et al: Viral hemorrhagic fevers, in *Atlas of Infectious Diseases*, vol 8, R Fekety (ed). Philadelphia, Current Medicine, 1997, pp 10.1–10.26
SMORODINTSEV AA et al: *Virus Hemorrhagic Fevers*. Jerusalem, Israel Program for Scientific Translations, 1964, 245 pp
ZAKI SR, PETERS CJ: Viral hemorrhagic fevers, in *The Pathology of Infectious Diseases*, DH Connor et al (eds). Stamford, CT, Appleton & Lange, 1997 pp 347–346

ARENAVIRUSES

BARRY M et al: Treatment of a laboratory-acquired Sabiá virus infection. N Engl J Med 333:294, 1995
ENRIA D, MAIZTEGUI JI: Antiviral treatment of Argentine hemorrhagic fever. Antiviral Res 23:23, 1994
JOHNSON KM et al: Hemorrhagic fevers of Southeast Asia and South America: A comparative appraisal. Prog Med Virol 9:105, 1967

———— et al: Clinical virology of Lassa fever in hospitalized patients. J Infect Dis 155:456, 1987

LARSEN PD et al: Hydrocephalus complicating lymphocytic choriomeningitis infection. Pediatr Infect Dis J 12:628, 1993

McCORMICK JB et al: A case-control study of the clinical diagnosis and course of Lassa fever. J Infect Dis 155:445, 1987

MOLINAS FC et al: Hemostasis and the complement system in Argentine hemorrhagic fever. Rev Infect Dis 11(Suppl 4):762, 1989

PETERS CJ: Arenaviruses, in *Clinical Virology*, DD Richman et al (eds). New York, Churchill Livingstone, 1997, pp 973–996

———— et al: Hemorrhagic fever in Cochabamba, Bolivia, 1971. Am J Epidemiol 99:425, 1974

SALAS R et al: Venezuelan hemorrhagic fever. Lancet 338:1033, 1991

BUNYAVIRIDAE

ANTONIADIS A et al: Direct genetic detection of Dobrava virus in Greek and Albanian haemorrhagic fever with renal syndrome (HFRS) patients. J Infect Dis 174:407, 1996

BRUNO P et al: The protean manifestations of hemorrhagic fever with renal syndrome. A retrospective review of 26 cases from Korea. Ann Intern Med 113:385, 1990

DUCHIN JS et al: Hantavirus pulmonary syndrome: A clinical description of 17 patients with a newly recognized disease. N Engl J Med 330:949, 1994

HUGGINS JW et al: Prospective, double-blind, concurrent, placebo controlled clinical trial of intravenous ribavirin therapy of hemorrhagic fever with renal syndrome. J Infect Dis 164:1119, 1991

KETAI LH et al: Hantavirus pulmonary syndrome (HPS): Radiographic findings in 16 patients. Radiology 191:665, 1994

KHAN AS et al: Hantavirus pulmonary syndrome: The first 100 U.S. cases. J Infect Dis 173:1297, 1996

LAUGHLIN LW et al: Epidemic Rift Valley fever in Egypt: Observations of the spectrum of human illness. Trans R Soc Trop Med Hyg 73:630, 1979

PETERS CJ, LeDuc JW: Bunyaviruses, phleboviruses, and related viruses, in *Textbook of Human Virology*, 2d ed, R Belshe (ed). St Louis, Mosby Year Book, 1991, pp 571–614

————, LINTHICUM KJ: Rift Valley fever, in *Handbook Series of Zoonoses, Section B: Viral Zoonoses*, 2d ed, GW Beran (ed). Boca Raton, FL, CRC Press, 1994, pp 125–138

SEXTON DJ et al: Life-threatening Cache Valley virus infection. N Engl J Med 336:547, 1997

SWANEPOEL R et al: Epidemiologic and clinical features of Crimean-Congo hemorrhagic fever in South Africa. Am J Trop Med Hyg 6:120, 1987

———— et al: The clinical pathology of Crimean-Congo hemorrhagic fever. Rev Infect Dis 11(Suppl 4):S794, 1989

SYMPOSIUM ON EPIDEMIC HEMORRHAGIC FEVER(May, 1954). Am J Med 16:1–617, 1954

ZAKI SR: Hantavirus-associated diseases, in *The Pathology of Infectious Diseases*, DH Connor et al (eds). Stamford, CT, Appleton & Lange, 1997

———— et al: Hantavirus pulmonary syndrome: Pathogenesis of an emerging infectious disease. Am J Pathol 146:552, 1995

FILOVIRUSES

CENTERS FOR DISEASE CONTROL AND PREVENTION: Update: Outbreak of Ebola viral hemorrhagic fever—Zaire, 1995. Morb Mort Week Rep 44:468, 1995

MARTINI GA, SIEGERT R (eds): *Marburg Virus Disease*. Berlin, Springer-Verlag, 1971

PETERS CJ et al: Filoviruses, in *Fields Virology*, 3d ed, BN Fields et al (eds). Philadelphia, Lippincott-Raven, 1996

WHO/INTERNATIONAL STUDY TEAM: Ebola hemorrhagic fever in Sudan, 1976. Bull World Health Organ 56:247, 1978

WORLD HEALTH ORGANIZATION: Ebola haemorrhagic fever in Zaire, 1976. Report of an international commission. Bull World Health Organ 56:271, 1978

FLAVIVIRUSES

BARROS MLB, BOECKEN G: Jungle yellow fever in the central Amazon. Lancet 348:969, 1996

HALSTEAD SB: Dengue and dengue hemorrhagic fever, in *Textbook of Pediatric Infectious Disease*, R Feigin and JD Cherry (eds). Philadelphia, Saunders, 1987, pp 1510–1521

————: Antibody, macrophages, dengue virus infection, shock, and hemorrhage: A pathogenic cascade. Rev Infect Dis 11(Suppl 4):S830, 1989

————, O'ROURKE EJ: Dengue viruses and mononuclear phagocytes. I. Infection enhancement by non-neutralizing antibody. J Exp Med 146:201, 1977

KERR JA: The clinical aspects and diagnosis of yellow fever, in *Yellow Fever*, GR Strode (ed). New York, McGraw-Hill, 1951, pp 385–425

KURANE I et al: Immunopathologic mechanisms of dengue hemorrhagic fever and dengue shock syndrome. Arch Virol 9:59, 1994

LUBY JP: St. Louis encephalitis, Rocio encephalitis, and West Nile fever, in *Kass Handbook of Infectious Diseases. Exotic Viral Infections*, JS Porterfield (ed). New York, Chapman and Hall, 1995, pp 183–202

MONATH TP, HEINZ FX: Flaviviruses, in *Fields Virology*, 3d ed, BN Fields et al (eds). Philadelphia, Lippincott-Raven, 1996, pp 961–1034

SABIN AB: Research on dengue during World War II. Am J Trop Med Hyg 1:30, 1952

TSAI T, YU XX: Japanese encephalitis vaccines, in *Vaccines*, 2d ed, SW Plotkin and E Mortimer (eds). Philadelphia, WB Saunders, 1994, pp 671–713

WALDVOGEL K et al: Severe tick-borne encephalitis following passive immunization. Eur J Pediatr 155:775, 1996

REOVIRUSES

EMMONS RW: Colorado tick fever, in *Handbook Series of Zoonoses, Section B: Viral Zoonoses, vol 1*, GW Beran (ed). Boca Raton, FL, CRC Press, 1981, pp 113–124

MONATH TP, GUIRAKHOO F: Orbiviruses and coltiviruses, in *Fields Virology*, 3d ed, BN Fields et al (eds). Philadelphia, Lippincott-Raven, 1996, pp 1735–1766

RHABDOVIRUSES

REIF JS: Vesicular stomatitis, in *Handbook Series of Zoonoses, Section B: Viral Zoonoses*, vol 1, 2d ed, GW Beran (ed). Boca Raton, FL, CRC Press, 1995, pp 113–124

TOGAVIRUSES

FRASER JRE: Epidemic polyarthritis and Ross River virus disease. Clin Rheum Dis 12:369, 1986

JOHNSTON RE, PETERS CJ: Alphaviruses, in *Fields Virology*, 3d ed, BN Fields et al (eds). Philadelphia, Lippincott-Raven, 1996, pp 843–898

MACKENZIE JS: Mosquito-borne viruses and epidemic polyarthritis. Med J Aust 164:90, 1996

NIKLASSON B: Sindbis and Sindbis-like viruses, in *The Arboviruses: Epidemiology and Ecology*, vol IV, TP Monath (ed). Boca Raton, FL, CRC Press, 1988, pp 167–176

PHILLIPS DA et al: Clinical and subclinical Barmah Forest virus infection in Queensland. Med J Aust 152:463, 1990

PINHEIRO FP et al: An outbreak of Mayaro virus disease in Belterra, Brazil. I. Clinical and virological findings. Am J Trop Med Hyg 30:674, 1981

RIVAS F et al: Epidemic Venezuelan equine encephalitis in La Guajira, Colombia, 1995. J Infect Dis 1997

ROBINSON MC: An epidemic of virus disease in Southern Province Tanganyika Territory, in 1952–53. I. Clinical features. Trans R Soc Trop Med Hyg 49:28, 1955

201 *Lawrence Corey*

MARBURG AND EBOLA VIRUSES (FILOVIRIDAE)

DEFINITION Both Marburg virus and Ebola virus cause an acute systemic febrile illness associated with high mortality. This illness is characterized by the abrupt onset of headache, myalgias, pharyngitis, rash, and hemorrhagic manifestations. Person-to-person and nosocomial contact may lead to secondary cases and intermittent outbreaks of infection.

ETIOLOGY The family Filoviridae includes two former members of the family Rhabdoviridae: Marburg virus, a unique agent with only one known subtype, and Ebola virus, which is antigenically distinct from Marburg virus and has three known subtypes. The Ebola virus subtypes (Zaire, Sudan, and Reston) have common as well as unique epitopes. The Reston subtype appears to be attenuated in its pathogenicity for humans. Antigenic and genomic analyses of the surface glycoprotein of the Sudan strains isolated from 1976 to 1979 appear identical; this finding is indicative of stability in the antigenic structure of the subtypes of Ebola virus. Both Ebola virus and Marburg virus can be isolated in a variety of cell culture systems, including vervet monkey kidney (Vero) cells. The virion contains one copy of linear, negative-sense, single-stranded RNA with a helical nucleocapsid and a lipid envelope derived from the host cell plasma membrane. Structurally, the virus appears as an 80- to 100-nm elongated filamentous particle with surface projections or peplomers. The viral genome is approximately 19 kb and codes for seven gene products. The surface glycoprotein makes up the surface spikes, mediates viral entry, and is highly glycosylated—a characteristic that may contribute to the rather low levels of neutralizing antibodies detected in infected individuals. Two matrix proteins called VP40 and VP24 appear to be involved in viral budding and uncoating. The viral nucleocapsid is composed of a major nucleoprotein and a minor protein (VP30). As in other negative-stranded RNA viruses, the virion contains an RNA polymerase protein. In infected cells, both Ebola virus and Marburg virus produce a nonstructural secreted glycoprotein that may play a role in interference with the host's immune responses. The viruses are stable and remain infectious for prolonged periods at room temperature. They are destroyed by heat (60°C, 30 min) and lipid solvents. Both viruses are biosafety level 4 pathogens and require maximal biologic containment facilities.

EPIDEMIOLOGY Marburg virus was first identified in Germany in 1967. The virus was isolated from laboratory workers exposed to African Green monkeys (*Cercopithecus aethiops*) that had been imported from Uganda. Virus was isolated from the blood and tissue of these monkeys and of several laboratory workers. Of the 25 cases of primary Marburg infection, 7 ended in death. Most of 6 secondary cases appeared to be related to accidental needle sticks or abrasions. Secondary spread to the wife of one patient was documented. Marburg virus was demonstrated in semen of the source contact despite the presence of circulating antibody. This secondary case is believed to have been acquired through sexual intercourse. Since this outbreak, isolated cases of Marburg infection have been reported, usually involving persons on the African continent.

In 1976, epidemics of severe hemorrhagic fever occurred simultaneously in Zaire and Sudan. Among 550 cases, there were more than 470 deaths. Ebola virus was isolated in both locations. Epidemic spread took place through close person-to-person contact and injections from reused needles. Both epidemics ended with the institution of strict quarantine procedures.

In 1989, numerous deaths from hemorrhagic fever among quarantined primates were noted in a primate import quarantine facility in Reston, Virginia. Ebola virus (Reston strain) was isolated from cynomolgus macaques from the Philippines and Indonesia that were being kept at the facility. Four employees were infected; none died.

In May 1995, an epidemic of hemorrhagic fever occurred in Kikwit, Zaire, resulting in 250 clinically identified cases and 80 percent mortality. Again, person-to-person spread within households and in hospitals facilitated secondary spread. During the outbreak, Ebola virus was isolated from sweat glands of symptomatic patients; thus contact with patients' perspiration may have facilitated the spread of the agent. Strict quarantine measures arrested the epidemic.

Despite extensive investigations, the reservoirs for the filoviruses are unknown. The viruses appear to be zoonotic, but all attempts to define the natural reservoir of infection have yielded unconvincing results. These viruses' similarity to Lassa virus suggests their persistence in an unidentified mammalian host. Whether subclinical filovirus infections occur in humans is still controversial.

PATHOLOGY Both Marburg virus and Ebola virus appear to be "pantropic"; viral replication takes place in almost all organs, including lymphoid tissue, liver, spleen, pancreas, adrenals, thyroid, kidneys, testes, skin, and brain. Focal necrosis of liver, lymphatic organs, kidneys, testes, and ovaries is common. In the liver, eosinophilic cytoplasmic bodies resembling the Councilman bodies of yellow fever have been noted. The lungs may exhibit interstitial pneumonitis as well as vascular lesions indicative of endarteritis in small arterioles. Neuropathologic changes consist of multiple small hemorrhagic infarcts with glial proliferation. The pathophysiology of the hemorrhagic manifestations of infection is unclear. Viral infection of endothelial cells, with in situ fibrin depletion, may be a factor. Inflammatory mediators of the "sepsis syndrome" may also play a role.

CLINICAL MANIFESTATIONS After an incubation period of 3 to 9 days, patients develop frontal and temporal headache, malaise, myalgias (especially in the lumbar area), nausea, and vomiting. Fever—with temperatures of 39.4 to 40°C (103 to 104°F)—is characteristic, and about half of all patients have conjunctivitis. Between 1 and 3 days after onset, watery diarrhea (often severe), lethargy, and a change in mentation are noted. An enanthem of the palate and tonsils and cervical lymphadenopathy also may become apparent during the first week of illness. The most reliable clinical feature is the appearance of a nonpruritic maculopapular rash, which begins on the fifth to seventh day on the face and neck and spreads centrifugally to the extremities. A fine desquamation of the affected skin, especially on the palms and soles, appears 4 to 5 days later. Hemorrhagic manifestations, including gastrointestinal, renal, vaginal, and/or conjunctival hemorrhages, generally develop between days 5 and 7 of disease.

During the first week, the temperature remains around 40°C (104°F), falling by lysis during the second week only to increase again between days 12 and 14. Other clinical signs apparent in the second week of disease include splenomegaly, hepatomegaly, facial edema, and scrotal or labial reddening. Complications include orchitis, which may lead to testicular atrophy; myocarditis, with irregular pulse and electrocardiographic abnormalities; and pancreatitis. Patients who die usually do so on the eighth to sixteenth days of illness. Recovery is often protracted over a 3- to 4-week period, during which loss of hair, intermittent abdominal pain, poor appetite, and prolonged psychotic disturbances have been noted. Late sequelae, including transverse myelitis and uveitis, have been reported. Marburg virus has been isolated from the anterior eye chamber and semen nearly 3 months after onset of disease.

LABORATORY FINDINGS Abnormalities in granulocyte function are found in filovirus infection. Leukopenia is detected as early as the first day, with leukocyte counts as low as 1000/μL and neutrophilia by the fourth day. Subsequently, atypical lymphocytes as well as neutrophils exhibiting the Pelger-Huët anomaly may appear. Thrombocytopenia develops early and is most marked (often with fewer than 10,000 cells/μL) between days 6 and 12. Fatal cases may include evidence of disseminated intravascular coagulation. Hypoproteinemia, proteinuria, and azotemia may develop. Elevations in aspartate and alanine aminotransferases are usual. Lumbar puncture may yield normal findings or reveal minimal pleocytosis. The erythrocyte sedimentation rate is usually low.

DIAGNOSIS The characteristic clinical course and epidemiologic features of filovirus infections form the basis for the diagnosis. Specific diagnosis requires isolation of the virus or detection of serologic evidence of infection in paired serum samples. In fatal filovirus infections, there is high-titer viremia and little evidence of a host immune response. Viremia coincides with the febrile stage of disease; virus has been isolated from tissue as well as from urine, semen, and throat and rectal swabs. *Attempts to isolate virus must be made only in specialized high-security laboratories.* Gamma irradiation is the most common way to inactivate virus. Staining for viral antigens and assays based on the reverse transcription polymerase chain reaction have been useful when conducted in specialized laboratories. Specimens should be sent to the Centers for Disease Control and Prevention, Atlanta, Georgia; the Central Public Health Laboratory, Colindale, London, England; or the National Institute of Virology, Sandringham, Republic of South Africa. Since person-to-person transmission is the means by which outbreaks are propagated, all patients should be managed under conditions of strict barrier isolation, and all specimens should be handled and shipped with extreme care according to World Health Organization guidelines.

℞ **TREATMENT**
Other than supportive care, no definitive treatment for filovirus infection is available. The administration of convalescent-phase serum from recovered patients has been proposed but has not been systematically evaluated. In any event, such serum is rarely available.

In vitro, neither Marburg virus nor Ebola virus is inhibited by the antiviral drug ribavirin.

BIBLIOGRAPHY

CENTERS FOR DISEASE CONTROL: Management of patients with suspected viral hemorrhagic fever. Morb Mort Week Rep 37(Suppl 3):1, 1988

ELLIOT LH et al: Improved specificity of testing methods for filovirus antibody. J Virol Methods 43:85, 1993

FISHER HOCH SP et al: Pathogenic potential of filovirus. J Infect Dis 166:753, 1992

GEISBERT TW et al: Differentiation of filoviruses by electron microscopy. Virus Res 39:129, 1995

JAAX NK et al: Lethal experimental infection of rhesus monkey with Ebola-Zaire (Mayinga) virus by the oral and conjunctival route of exposure. Arch Pathol Lab Med 120:140, 1996

PETERS CJ et al: Filoviruses as emerging pathogens. Semin Virol 5:147, 1994

SECTION 15

FUNGAL INFECTIONS

202   *John E. Bennett*

DIAGNOSIS AND TREATMENT OF FUNGAL INFECTIONS

MYCOLOGY FUNDAMENTALS

Fungi can appear microscopically as either rounded, budding forms (yeastlike organisms) or hyphae (molds). Yeastlike colonies are smooth, while mold colonies are fuzzy; fungi that grow as yeasts include species of *Candida* and *Cryptococcus*, while fungi that grow as molds include species of *Aspergillus*, *Rhizopus*, and dermatophytes (ringworm fungi). The fungi that cause histoplasmosis, blastomycosis, sporotrichosis, coccidioidomycosis, and paracoccidioidomycosis are called *dimorphic* ("having two forms") because they are rounded in tissue but grow like molds when cultured at room temperature. *Candida* species other than *Candida glabrata* appear in tissue as both budding yeasts and tubular elements called *pseudohyphae*.

Some fungi described in this text are given two different names. For example, *Histoplasma capsulatum* is also called *Ajellomyces capsulatus*, the latter being the name for the "perfect state." The diagnostic laboratory rarely sees a fungus growing in the perfect state and therefore does not use this name. One of the exceptions is *Scedosporium apiospermum*, which may be seen in the perfect state and is then called *Pseudallescheria boydii*. The reader is referred to standard textbooks of medical mycology for an explanation of the perfect state.

Most fungi that are pathogenic for humans are saprophytes in nature; they cause infection when airborne spores reach the lung or paranasal sinus or when hyphae or spores are accidentally inoculated into the skin or cornea. Acquisition of infection from another person or an animal has been reported in the case of ringworm but is very rare in other mycoses. Thus, hospitalized patients with fungal infections do not require special isolation. Most fungi infect hosts preferentially by one route and only infrequently by other routes. For example, the agents of ringworm, pityriasis versicolor, and piedra infect the epidermis and its appendages. Sporotrichosis and mycetoma usually arise from subcutaneous inoculation. Inhalation is the route of inoculation for the agents of most deep mycoses. Ingestion of fungi rarely causes infection; *Candida albicans*, a normal commensal in the mouth and intestine, reaches deeper tissues only when mucosal or cutaneous barriers are breached by disease, surgery, trauma, or catheterization. Histoplasmosis, blastomycosis, coccidioidomycosis, and paracoccidioidomycosis have been called "endemic" mycoses to emphasize their restricted geographic distribution. Some fungi, such as *Aspergillus*, are said to be opportunists in that they usually infect hosts with compromised immunity. This distinction is relative, not absolute.

Immunity after exposure to fungi may confer partial protection against reinfection. Residents of areas in which mycoses are endemic are less subject to infection than are newcomers. Predisposing factors are helpful in defining host defense. Immunoglobulin deficiencies do not appear to predispose to any mycosis, whereas neutropenia is common among patients who develop invasive aspergillosis or deep candidiasis. Cell-mediated immunity appears to be of paramount importance in most other deep mycoses.

DIAGNOSIS

Many fungi can be identified to the genus or even the species level by microscopic examination of smears or biopsy specimens. Calcofluor white staining with fluorescence microscopy is a sensitive technique for smears of sputum, bronchoalveolar lavage fluid, or pus. India ink smear remains the method of choice for detecting cryptococci in cerebrospinal fluid (CSF). Smears of vaginal or oral lesions for *Candida* pseudohyphae can be prepared by wet mounting or Gram's staining. For histopathology slides, Gomori methenamine silver and a neutral counterstain are preferred.

The method used has a marked effect on the rapidity and sensitivity of blood cultures for fungi, except in the case of *Candida* species, which are relatively easy to grow. For most other fungi, concentration of the blood by lysis centrifugation and culture on solid medium constitute the optimal technique. Commercially available nucleic acid hybridization techniques can speed the identification of slow-growing molds, such as *H. capsulatum* and *Coccidioides immitis*. Serology has limited value, but testing of serum or CSF for cryptococcal antigen or antibody to *C. immitis* can be diagnostic. Skin testing with fungal antigens is not useful in detecting active infection.

ANTIFUNGAL THERAPY

TOPICAL AGENTS   Imidazoles and Triazoles These synthetic compounds act by inhibiting ergosterol synthesis in the fungal cell wall and, when given topically, may cause direct damage to the fungal cytoplasmic membrane. The imidazoles available for cutaneous application include clotrimazole, econazole, ketoconazole, sulconazole, oxiconazole, and miconazole. Vaginal formulations include four imidazoles (miconazole, clotrimazole, tioconazole, and butoconazole) and one triazole (terconazole). Miconazole lotion and vaginal preparations of both miconazole and clotrimazole are available without prescription. As yet, no substantial differences in the efficacy of or local intolerance to the various topical azoles have become apparent. All are effective in the treatment of cutaneous candidiasis, tinea (pityriasis) versicolor, and mild to moderately severe ringworm of the glabrous skin. Vaginal formulations are effective for vulvovaginal candidiasis. Clotrimazole is poorly absorbed from the gastrointestinal tract, but the oral troche is useful as a topical treatment for oral and esophageal candidiasis.

Polyene Macrolide Antibiotics These broad-spectrum antifungal agents combine with sterol in the fungal cytoplasmic membrane, increasing membrane permeability. Topically, they are not active against ringworm but are effective against candidiasis of the skin and mucous membranes. Nystatin suspension is effective in oral thrush, and vaginal troches are effective in vulvovaginal candidiasis. Both nystatin and amphotericin B are available in topical preparations for cutaneous candidiasis.

Other Topical Antifungals Ciclopirox olamine, haloprogin, terbinafine, and naftifine have the same clinical spectrum among the cutaneous mycoses as the imidazoles. Tolnaftate and undecylenic acid are effective against ringworm but not candidiasis. Keratolytic agents, such as salicylic acid, are helpful as accessory drugs for some hyperkeratotic skin lesions.

SYSTEMIC ANTIFUNGALS **Griseofulvin** Griseofulvin is a useful drug in the treatment of certain kinds of ringworm; however, it is ineffective in the treatment of candidiasis. The microcrystalline and ultramicrocrystalline preparations differ in dose but not in efficacy. Absorption of both is enhanced when the drug is ingested with fat-containing foods. Griseofulvin interacts with phenobarbital and coumarin-type anticoagulants.

Terbinafine Oral terbinafine (250 mg once daily) is at least as effective as itraconazole and more effective than griseofulvin in onychomycosis and ringworm. Gastrointestinal distress is the most common side effect. Rash, hepatitis, and pancytopenia have occurred, but serious adverse effects have been uncommon. Terbinafine decreases cyclosporine levels. Cimetidine increases and rifampin decreases terbinafine levels in blood.

Imidazoles and Triazoles *Ketoconazole* Absorption of ketoconazole is variable among individuals, is not affected by food, and is poor in patients with AIDS and those taking cimetidine or other H_2 blocking agents. Simultaneous administration of antacids also can impair the absorption of ketoconazole. Its metabolism is chiefly hepatic, but substantial liver disease has only a minimal effect on its concentrations in plasma. Ketoconazole plasma levels are decreased in patients taking rifampin and also in some taking isoniazid. Ketoconazole administration can elevate cyclosporine and cisapride levels in blood, can increase the likelihood of terfenadine or astemizole cardiotoxicity, and occasionally can enhance the anticoagulant effect of warfarin. The drug is contraindicated during pregnancy and, because it appears in breast milk, during breast-feeding. Neither renal disease nor hemodialysis affects the metabolism of ketoconazole.

The most common toxicities of ketoconazole are dose-related nausea, anorexia, and occasionally vomiting. Hepatotoxicity is idiosyncratic and usually mild (manifesting as transiently elevated levels of aminotransferases) but, in rare instances, can be serious and fatal. Several dose-related, temporary endocrine effects have been observed: decreased adrenal cortical reserve; gynecomastia; a decrease in serum testosterone level, libido, and potency in males; and menstrual irregularity in females. Pruritus or rash also may occur.

Ketoconazole is effective in blastomycosis, histoplasmosis, paracoccidioidomycosis, chronic mucocutaneous candidiasis, esophageal candidiasis, and some forms of disseminated coccidioidomycosis and pseudallescheriasis. The usual adult dose is 400 mg once daily. Partial improvement may follow ketoconazole treatment of cutaneous sporotrichosis and chromoblastomycosis. Although vulvovaginal candidiasis, ringworm, and tinea versicolor are responsive to the drug, the toxicity of oral ketoconazole makes topical imidazoles or other drugs preferable for these indications.

Itraconazole This triazole analogue of ketoconazole is superior to the parent compound in safety and efficacy. Hormonal suppression and hepatotoxicity are less marked with itraconazole than with ketoconazole. Clinical indications for the use of itraconazole include all those cited for ketoconazole but also extend to selected cases of onychomycosis, sporotrichosis, cryptococcosis, and aspergillosis. The drug is marketed as 100-mg capsules. No parenteral formulation is available. The usual dose is 200 mg once or twice a day by mouth with food (to enhance absorption). Itraconazole is metabolized in the liver, and its hydroxy metabolite retains antifungal activity. Concurrent therapy with rifampin, carbamazepine, and H_2 receptor antagonists or phenytoin decreases itraconazole blood levels. Cardiotoxicity due to digoxin, terfenadine, or astemizole and nephrotoxicity due to cyclosporine may occur during concomitant itraconazole therapy. Itraconazole inhibits the metabolism of tacrolimus, midazolam, triazolam, oral hypoglycemic agents, and cisapride. Its use during pregnancy is contraindicated.

Fluconazole This triazole can be administered in tablet form, as a suspension, or as an intravenous infusion. With a half-life of about 31 h, fluconazole can be given once a day. Its bioavailability when given by the oral route is excellent and is unimpaired by lack of gastric acid or the presence of food. Fluconazole therapy can elevate blood

levels of phenytoin, cyclosporine, warfarin, rifabutin, and sulfonylureas. Approximately 80 percent of the drug is excreted unchanged in the urine. Patients with creatinine clearance rates of 21 to 50 mL/min and 11 to 20 mL/min should have their fluconazole doses reduced by 50 and 75 percent, respectively. The drug penetrates the CSF and other body fluids very well.

Nausea and abdominal distress are the most common forms of dose-limiting fluconazole toxicity. An allergic rash may develop and is particularly common among patients infected with human immunodeficiency virus (HIV). Fatal cases of Stevens-Johnson syndrome have been described in the HIV-infected population. Alopecia commonly follows prolonged administration of ≥400 mg daily but resolves when therapy is discontinued. Rare cases of anaphylaxis, hepatic necrosis, and neutropenia have been described.

Fluconazole is a useful drug in the treatment of adults with oropharyngeal and esophageal candidiasis. A single 150-mg tablet is effective in vulvovaginal candidiasis. Catheter-acquired candidemia in the immunocompetent host responds to 400 mg of fluconazole daily in conjunction with the removal of the infected catheter. Fluconazole is also effective in initial and maintenance therapy for cryptococcal meningitis in patients with AIDS, although most of these patients should initially receive a 2-week course of intravenous amphotericin B. Patients with coccidioidal meningitis can often be given fluconazole rather than intrathecal amphotericin B as maintenance therapy.

The incidence of deep candidiasis among recipients of allogeneic bone marrow transplants can be reduced by the administration of fluconazole (400 mg daily) for 75 days after initiation of the transplantation-preparative regimen. Prophylaxis in other neutropenic patients has not appeared useful. Fluconazole (200 mg daily) reduced the incidence of cryptococcosis and mucosal candidiasis among AIDS patients whose CD4+ cell counts were <200/μL and was particularly effective among those with counts of <50/μL. However, this regimen is not recommended because it does not reduce mortality, is expensive, and can lead to drug resistance.

Fluconazole is less effective than itraconazole in blastomycosis, histoplasmosis, and sporotrichosis. The drug is not active in aspergillosis or mucormycosis.

Amphotericin B A colloidal preparation of the polyene drug amphotericin B is available for intravenous or intrathecal administration. In-line filters with a 0.22-μm pore diameter may trap some of the colloid. The catabolism of amphotericin B is extremely slow and is not influenced by renal failure, hepatic failure, or hemodialysis. The drug's penetration into CSF and vitreous humor is poor; however, the concentrations in pleural, peritoneal, and articular exudates are adequate for many mycoses. Histoplasmosis, blastomycosis, paracoccidioidomycosis, candidiasis, and cryptococcosis are the most responsive mycoses; coccidioidomycosis, extraarticular sporotrichosis, aspergillosis, and mucormycosis are less responsive; and chromoblastomycosis, mycetoma, and pseudallescheriasis respond little, if at all. The usual course is 0.5 to 0.7 mg/kg daily for 8 to 10 weeks. Infusions are generally given in 5% dextrose over 2 to 4 h.

Initial doses of amphotericin B occasionally cause marked febrile reactions that may be poorly tolerated by adult patients with limited cardiac or pulmonary function. It may be prudent to give such patients an initial 1-mg test dose followed by rapidly escalating doses, depending on tolerance. Premedication with aspirin or acetaminophen or the addition of hydrocortisone (25 mg) to the infusion decreases chills and fever. Azotemia during treatment is usual, the extent depending on the daily dose. Saline infusions have been advocated to reduce azotemia. Permanent loss of renal function is related to the total dose of amphotericin B; this condition is generally noted in adults who have received more than 3 g. Other side effects include anemia, hypokalemia, renal tubular acidosis, nausea, anorexia, weight loss, phlebitis, and occasionally hypomagnesemia. Intrathecal amphotericin B has been used in coccidioidal meningitis and refractory cryptococcal meningitis, although this therapy is associated with considerable toxicity.

Newer formulations of intravenous amphotericin B have been marketed overseas and are in the process of becoming commercially available in the United States: amphotericin B lipid complex (ABLC), amphotericin B colloidal dispersion (ABCD), and a liposomal formulation (AmBisome). At doses two to five times higher than those used with the deoxycholate preparation, the nephrotoxicity of all three newer formulations has been minimal. Chills and hypokalemia have been reported with the latter two. No comparative efficacy trials have been conducted, and the indications for these more expensive formulations remain unknown. On the basis of uncontrolled trials, ABLC is marketed in the United States for the narrow indication of refractory aspergillosis; the recommended dose is 5 mg/kg daily. The deoxycholate formulation of amphotericin B has also been mixed with the intravenous lipid used for parenteral nutrition; the nephrotoxicity of this combination appears to be less than that of the deoxycholate formulation alone, but the effect of this mixing on antifungal efficacy remains to be determined.

Flucytosine Flucytosine (5-fluorocytosine) is a synthetic oral drug useful in cryptococcosis, candidiasis, and chromoblastomycosis. Within the fungal cell, flucytosine is converted to the antimetabolite 5-fluorouracil. Drug resistance appears rather rapidly when flucytosine is used alone. For this reason, the drug is generally used in combination with amphotericin B. The usual dose of flucytosine is 25 to 37.5 mg/kg every 6 h. Flucytosine is well absorbed from the gastrointestinal tract. The drug penetrates well into the CSF and is excreted unchanged in the urine. Even modest reductions in renal function may elevate flucytosine blood levels into the toxic range (≥100 to 125 μg/mL). Elevated levels are associated with a significant incidence of neutropenia and thrombocytopenia and also seem to predispose to colitis, the other major toxic effect of this drug. Hepatotoxicity is idiosyncratic and uncommon. An allergic rash may develop.

BIBLIOGRAPHY

GENERAL

Kwon-Chung KJ, Bennett JE: *Medical Mycology.* Philadelphia, Lea & Febiger, 1992

THERAPY

Bennett JE: Antifungal agents, in *Mandell, Douglas and Bennett's Principles and Practice of Infectious Diseases*, 4th ed, GL Mandell et al (eds). New York, Churchill Livingstone, 1995, pp 401–410

Bowden RA et al: Phase 1 study of amphotericin B colloidal dispersion for the treatment of invasive fungal infections after bone marrow transplant. J Infect Dis 173:1208, 1996

Lazar JD, Hilligoss DM: The clinical pharmacology of fluconazole. Semin Oncol 17:14, 1990

Powderly WG et al: A randomized trial comparing fluconazole with clotrimazole troches for the prevention of fungal infections in patients with advanced human immunodeficiency virus infection. N Engl J Med 332:700, 1995

Slavin MA et al: Efficacy and safety of fluconazole prophylaxis for fungal infections after marrow transplantation—a prospective, randomized, double-blind trial. J Infect Dis 171:1545, 1995

Tucker RM et al: Adverse events associated with itraconazole in 189 patients on chronic therapy. J Antimicrob Chemother 26:561, 1991

203   *John E. Bennett*

HISTOPLASMOSIS

ETIOLOGIC AGENT *Histoplasma capsulatum* is a dimorphic fungus that grows as a mold in nature or on Sabouraud's agar at room temperature. Hyphae bear both large and small spores, which are used for identification. Nucleic acid hybridization can also be used to identify the organism in culture. *H. capsulatum* grows as a small budding yeast in host tissue and on enriched agar, such as blood cysteine glucose, at 37°C. Despite its name, the fungus is unencapsulated. Coculture of isolates with opposite mating types can produce the perfect state called *Ajellomyces capsulatus.* (The reader is referred to standard textbooks of medical mycology for an explanation of the perfect state.)

EPIDEMIOLOGY Infection with *H. capsulatum* has been encountered in many areas of the world but is much more frequent in certain areas. Within the United States, infection is most common in the southeastern, mid-Atlantic, and central states. Endemicity is probably contingent on the availability of proper conditions in nature for growth of the fungus. *H. capsulatum* prefers moist surface soil, particularly soil enriched by droppings of certain birds and bats. The fungus has been isolated repeatedly from such sites, and many case clusters have occurred 5 to 18 days after the exposure of groups of people to dust, while (for example) raking, cleaning dirt-floored chicken coops, bulldozing, or cave exploring. Skin-test reactivity in many endemic areas indicates that 80 percent or more of residents over age 16 have been exposed.

PATHOGENESIS AND PATHOLOGY Microconidia, or small spores, of *H. capsulatum* are small enough to reach the alveoli on inhalation and are transformed there to budding forms. With time, an intense granulomatous reaction occurs. Caseation necrosis or calcification may mimic tuberculosis. In children, the primary infection usually heals completely but may leave spotty calcification in the hilar nodes or lung. Transient dissemination may leave calcified granulomas in the spleen. In adults, a rounded mass of scar tissue, with or without central calcification, may remain in the lung. This mass has been called a *histoplasmoma.* Previous exposure is thought to confer some protection against reinfection, but infection in persons with prior positive skin tests clearly has occurred.

In a small proportion of patients, histoplasmosis becomes a progressive, potentially fatal infection. The disease occurs either as chronic fibrocavitary pneumonia or, less commonly, as disseminated infection. Patients with either form lack a history of acute primary pulmonary histoplasmosis. Chronic pulmonary infection favors otherwise healthy males over the age of 40. A history of cigarette use is elicited from nearly all patients with chronic progressive pulmonary histoplasmosis. An acute, rapidly fatal course is most likely to be encountered among young children and immunosuppressed patients, including those with AIDS. A more chronic but equally lethal disseminated infection is more common among previously healthy adults.

CLINICAL MANIFESTATIONS The vast majority of infections are either asymptomatic or mild, and the diagnosis is elusive. Cough, fever, malaise, and chest x-ray findings of hilar adenopathy with or without one or more areas of pneumonitis are typical features. Erythema nodosum and erythema multiforme have been reported in a few outbreaks. Hilar adenopathy may cause temporary compression of the right-middle-lobe bronchus in children and young adults. Subacute pericarditis may develop, probably by extension from contiguous lymph nodes. Rarely, hilar nodes undergo a caseous, granulomatous reaction with perinodal fibrosis. Mediastinal structures become encased by progressive fibrosis, and compression of the pulmonary veins, superior vena cava, pulmonary arteries, and esophagus may take place over many years. Late in mediastinal disease, only rare nonviable *Histoplasma* cells can be found in caseous residua of lymph nodes.

Chronic pulmonary histoplasmosis is characterized by a gradual onset (over weeks or months) of increasing productive cough, weight loss, and sometimes night sweats. Chest x-ray reveals uni- or bilateral fibronodular apical infiltrates. Approximately one-third of cases stabilize or improve spontaneously early in the course. The remainder progress insidiously. Retraction and cavitation of the upper lobes occur, with spread to the apex of the lower lobes and other areas of the lung. Emphysema and bulla formation further compromise pulmonary function. Death from cor pulmonale, bacterial pneumonia, or histoplasmosis occurs after months or years.

Acute disseminated histoplasmosis may be mistaken for miliary tuberculosis (see Chap. 171). Common findings include fever, emaciation, hepatosplenomegaly, lymphadenopathy, jaundice, anemia, leukopenia, and thrombocytopenia. All these features may be noted in chronic dissemination as well, but chronic disease tends to be more localized. Indurated ulcers of the mouth, tongue, nose, or larynx are reported in about one-fourth of cases. Other focal findings include granulomatous hepatitis, Addison's disease, gastrointestinal ulceration, endocarditis, and chronic meningitis. Chest x-ray abnormalities are evident in half of cases and characteristically consist of discrete nodules or a miliary pattern.

The presumed *ocular histoplasmosis* syndrome is a distinct clinical form of uveitis. Although a positive histoplasmin skin test is a requisite for diagnosis, none of the patients involved has had active histoplasmosis.

Infection with *H. capsulatum* var. *duboisii* is rare outside of Africa. The yeast form is larger in tissue than that of *H. capsulatum* var. *capsulatum*. Clinical manifestations resemble those of blastomycosis more than those of histoplasmosis in that skin and bone lesions are very common.

DIAGNOSIS Culture of the etiologic organism is the preferred method for diagnosis of histoplasmosis but is often difficult. Blood cultures are best done by the lysis-centrifugation technique, with plates held at 30°C for at least 2 weeks. Approximately 15 mL of blood should be cultured from adults. Routine blood cultures in broth are generally unsuitable. Cultures of bone marrow, mucosal lesions, liver, and bronchoalveolar lavage fluid are diagnostically useful in disseminated histoplasmosis. Sputum culture is the preferred method for the diagnosis of chronic pulmonary histoplasmosis. However, growth may require 2 to 4 weeks to become visible, and other organisms may overgrow the plate. Diagnosis based on Giemsa-stained smears of blood or bronchoalveolar lavage fluid or on methenamine silver staining of infected lung, bone marrow, lymph node, or mucosal lesions requires considerable expertise, though these techniques yield results rapidly and provide specimens that can easily be sent to a referral laboratory. Organisms may be very scanty in lesions with marked caseous necrosis. A radioactive assay for *Histoplasma* antigen in blood or urine is commercially available and is useful both for diagnosis and for monitoring of the response to therapy in AIDS patients with disseminated infection. Tests for antibody to *H. capsulatum* have been of limited value. Histoplasmin skin testing has proven useful in epidemiologic studies but not in clinical diagnosis.

℞ **TREATMENT**

Acute pulmonary histoplasmosis requires no therapy. Patients with mediastinal fibrosis may benefit from surgery, but their ultimate prognosis is poor. All patients with disseminated or chronic fibronodular pulmonary histoplasmosis should receive chemotherapy. Intravenous amphotericin B (0.6 mg/kg daily) is the drug of choice for the initial treatment of patients who are severely ill or immunosuppressed or whose infection involves the central nervous system; the regimen can be changed to itraconazole (200 mg twice daily) once clinical improvement is evident in these patients. For AIDS patients with disseminated histoplasmosis who are known to have blood levels of itraconazole (measured by bioassay) of at least 2 μg/mL, the dose can be decreased to 200 mg once daily after 10 weeks. Maintenance therapy with itraconazole is continued for life in AIDS patients.

Immunocompetent patients can initially be given itraconazole (200 mg twice daily) and are generally treated for 6 to 12 months. Ketoconazole (400 to 800 mg once daily) can be used instead of itraconazole for the treatment of immunocompetent patients without central nervous system disease when the lower cost is more important than the higher complication rate. Alternatively, immunocompetent patients can be given a 10-week course of amphotericin B (0.5 mg/kg daily).

Whatever drug is administered, relapse is not rare, particularly among patients who are immunocompromised or have endocarditis.

BIBLIOGRAPHY

GOODWIN RA et al: Histoplasmosis in normal hosts. Medicine 60:231, 1981
RAYMOND LW et al: Scars without wounds: Spectrum of delayed manifestations of histoplasmosis outside of the endemic area. Crit Rev Diagn Imaging 14:37, 1980

WHEAT JL et al: Disseminated histoplasmosis in the acquired immune deficiency syndrome: Clinical findings, diagnosis and treatment, and review of the literature. Medicine 69:361, 1990
——: Endemic mycoses in AIDS: A clinical review. Clin Microbiol Rev 8:146, 1995
—— et al: Itraconazole treatment of disseminated histoplasmosis in patients with the acquired immunodeficiency syndrome. Am J Med 98:336, 1995

204 *John E. Bennett*

COCCIDIOIDOMYCOSIS

ETIOLOGIC AGENT *Coccidioides immitis* has two forms, growing as a white fluffy mold on most culture media but as a nonbudding spherical form (a spherule) in host tissue or under specialized conditions. The organism reproduces in host tissue by forming small endospores within mature spherules. After rupture of the spherule, the released endospores enlarge, become spherules, and repeat the cycle. The fungus is identified by its appearance and by the formation of thick-walled, barrel-shaped spores, called *arthrospores*, in the hyphae of the mold form.

EPIDEMIOLOGY, PATHOGENESIS, AND PATHOLOGY *C. immitis* is a soil saprophyte found in certain arid regions of the United States, Mexico, Central America, and South America. Within the United States, most cases of infection with *C. immitis* are acquired in California, Arizona, and western Texas. A few cases are acquired by exposure to fomites from endemic areas (e.g., in cotton bales).

Infection in humans and animals results from inhalation of windborne arthrospores from soil sites. This primary pulmonary infection is symptomatic in only 40 percent of cases, with symptoms ranging from a mild influenza-like illness to severe pneumonia. Mild self-limited infections may come to medical attention because of case clusters or hypersensitivity reactions: erythema nodosum, erythema multiforme, toxic erythema, arthralgia, arthritis, conjunctivitis, or episcleritis. Case clusters occur 10 to 14 days after a group of susceptible individuals is exposed to dust in an endemic area through such activities as unearthing Indian relics, rock hunting, participating in military maneuvers, or doing construction work. Windstorms can carry spores to adjacent nonendemic areas and cause case clusters. The usual course of primary pneumonia is complete healing, although an area of pneumonitis (detected on radiographs) may heal by the formation of a coinlike lesion called a *coccidioidoma*. Less commonly, a single thin-walled cavity remains as a chronic sequela in the area of consolidation. The consolidation may persist as chronic pneumonia or progress to fibronodular cavitary disease.

Pleural effusion may be the only manifestation of primary infection. Spontaneous healing of this form is common.

An uncommon but dreaded complication of coccidioidomycosis is dissemination beyond the lung and hilar lymph nodes. Dissemination is especially frequent among blacks, Filipinos, Native Americans, Mexican-Americans, pregnant women, and immunosuppressed patients, including those with AIDS.

C. immitis incites a chronic granulomatous reaction in host tissue, often with caseation necrosis. Lung and hilar node lesions may show calcification. Both IgM and IgG antibodies to *C. immitis* are induced by infection, but neither type of antibody appears to be protective. The amount of specific IgG antibody is a rough measure of the antigenic mass (i.e., of the intensity of infection), and a high titer is a poor prognostic sign. Appearance of delayed hypersensitivity to antigens of *C. immitis* is most common in clinical forms of disease with a good prognosis, such as self-limited primary pulmonary disease. In skin tests for *Coccidioides* antigens about half of patients with disseminated disease have negative results that portend a poor outcome.

CLINICAL MANIFESTATIONS Symptomatic primary pulmonary infection is manifested by fever, cough, chest pain, malaise, and sometimes the hypersensitivity reactions listed above. Chest radiographs may show an infiltrate, hilar adenopathy, or pleural effusion. Mild peripheral-blood eosinophilia may be found. Spontaneous improvement begins after several days to 2 weeks of illness and usually culminates in complete recovery.

The symptoms of a chronic thin-walled cavity include cough or hemoptysis in half of cases; the other half are asymptomatic. Chronic progressive pulmonary coccidioidomycosis causes cough, sputum production, variable degrees of fever, and weight loss. The first indications of dissemination usually appear during primary infection. Reactivation with dissemination in later years occurs occasionally, especially if Hodgkin's disease, non-Hodgkin's lymphoma, renal transplantation, AIDS, or immunosuppression of some other etiology has supervened. Dissemination should be suspected when fever, malaise, hilar or paratracheal lymphadenopathy, elevated sedimentation rate, and high complement fixation titers signal abnormal persistence in patients with primary pulmonary coccidioidomycosis. With time, lesions appear in the bone, skin, subcutaneous tissue, meninges, joints, and other sites. Chronic meningitis may be the only presenting manifestation of disseminated coccidioidomycosis. Cultures and smears of cerebrospinal fluid (CSF) are most often negative, but antibody is usually detectable in CSF by complement fixation. Skin lesions are indolent and maculopapular; soft tissue and bony lesions contain pus and may present as a draining sinus. Without treatment, disseminated coccidioidomycosis progresses to death over weeks to years.

DIAGNOSIS When coccidioidomycosis is suspected, sputum, urine, and pus should be examined for *C. immitis* by wet smear and culture. *The laboratory request should indicate clearly that coccidioidomycosis is suspected, because the mold form must be handled with extreme care to prevent infection of laboratory personnel.* On biopsy, smaller spherules must be distinguished from nonbudding forms of *Blastomyces* and *Cryptococcus*, but the appearance of the mature spherule is diagnostic.

Serologic tests are very helpful in the diagnosis of coccidioidomycosis. Latex agglutination and agar gel diffusion tests are useful in screening sera for antibody to *Coccidioides*. The complement fixation test is used for CSF determinations and for the confirmation and quantitation of serum antibody detected by screening tests. The number of cases with a positive complement fixation test depends on the severity of disease and on the laboratory performing the test. Positive tests are least common among patients with solitary pulmonary cavities or primary pulmonary infection, while sera from patients with disseminated disease in multiple organs are nearly all positive. Seroconversion is helpful in primary pulmonary coccidioidomycosis but may not occur for up to 8 weeks after onset. A positive complement fixation test of unconcentrated CSF is diagnostic of meningitis. Rarely, a parameningeal focus causes a positive complement fixation test of CSF.

Conversion of the skin test from negative to positive (≥ 5 mm of induration at 24 or 48 h) with either coccidioidin or spherulin, the two commercially available antigens, may take place between days 3 and 21 of symptoms in primary pulmonary coccidioidomycosis. Skin testing can be helpful in epidemiologic studies, such as investigations of case clusters or the definition of endemic areas. The utility of skin testing as a diagnostic tool is limited by the persistence of positive tests resulting from remote exposures to *Coccidioides* and by the frequency of negative skin tests among patients with either thin-walled cavities or disseminated coccidioidomycosis.

℞ **TREATMENT**

Primary pulmonary coccidioidomycosis usually resolves spontaneously. Some physicians give a few weeks of treatment with intravenous amphotericin B or itraconazole to patients with unusually severe or protracted primary infection in the hope of aborting disseminated or chronic pulmonary disease.

Patients with severe or rapidly progressing disseminated coccidioidomycosis are first given intravenous amphotericin B at a dose of 0.5 to 0.7 mg/kg daily. Patients whose condition improves after 2 to 3 months of treatment with amphotericin B or who have more indolent disseminated infection are given ketoconazole (400 mg/d), itraconazole (200 mg twice daily), or fluconazole (400 to 600 mg/d). These oral agents are useful for long-term suppression of infection, and treatment should be continued for years. Patients with coccidioidal meningitis usually are initially given fluconazole (400 to 800 mg/d) but may require intrathecal amphotericin B. Hydrocephalus is a frequent complication of uncontrolled meningitis. Surgical debridement of bone lesions or drainage of abscesses can be helpful. The prognosis for ultimate cure of disseminated coccidioidomycosis is guarded.

Resection of chronic progressive pulmonary lesions is a helpful adjunct to chemotherapy when infection is confined to the lung and to one lobe. A single thin-walled cavity tends to close spontaneously and ordinarily is not resected. Such a cavity responds poorly to chemotherapy.

BIBLIOGRAPHY

FISH DG et al: Coccidioidomycosis during human immunodeficiency virus infection. A review of 77 patients. Medicine 69:384, 1990

GRAYBILL JR et al: Itraconazole treatment of coccidioidomycosis. Am J Med 89:282, 1990

PEREZ JA et al: Fluconazole therapy in coccidioidal meningitis maintained with intrathecal amphotericin B. Arch Intern Med 155:1665, 1995

STEVENS DA: Coccidioidomycosis. N Engl J Med 332:1077, 1995

VINCENT T et al: The natural history of coccidioidal meningitis: VA-Armed Forces Cooperative Studies, 1955–58. Clin Infect Dis 16:247, 1993

205 *John E. Bennett*

BLASTOMYCOSIS

ETIOLOGIC AGENT *Blastomyces dermatitidis* is a dimorphic fungus that grows at room temperature as a white or tan mold but grows within the host or at 37°C as budding, round yeastlike cells. The fungus can be identified on the basis of its appearance, its dimorphism, the small spores borne on hyphae of the mold form, or the results of nucleic acid hybridization. When isolates of the two opposite mating types are grown close together on special culture medium, such as yeast extract or soil extract agar, sporulating structures that characterize the perfect state, called *Ajellomyces dermatitidis*, appear. (The reader is referred to standard textbooks of medical mycology for an explanation of the perfect state.)

EPIDEMIOLOGY The infection is restricted by geography and age. Blastomycosis is uncommon in any locality, but most cases occur in the southeastern, central, and mid-Atlantic areas of the United States, with occasional cases in other localities in the United States and Canada. Cases have also been encountered in Africa, Mexico, Central America, and (rarely) South America. Most patients are between 20 and 69 years old. The male-to-female ratio is about 10:1. There is no occupational predisposition to the development of blastomycosis.

PATHOGENESIS AND PATHOLOGY Infection with *B. dermatitidis* appears to be acquired by inhalation of the fungus from soil, decomposed vegetation, or rotting wood. Several case clusters have resulted from participation in recreational activities in wooded areas along waterways. Infection is not transmissible from person to person. The initial pulmonary infection may either heal spontaneously or become chronic. Spread to other portions of the lung, cavitation, or endobronchial lesions may be found in chronic cases. Whether or not the lung lesion resolves spontaneously, infection commonly spreads hematogenously to the skin, subcutaneous tissue, bone, prostate, epididymis, or mucosa of the nose, mouth, or larynx. Less commonly, infection spreads to the brain, meninges, liver, lymph nodes, or spleen. Dissemination may not be evident for weeks or years after the appearance of the lung lesion. Progressive infection is only rarely attributable to an underlying disease or to immunosuppressive treatment. The inflammatory response includes lymphocytes, giant cells, and neutrophils. Pseudoepitheliomatous hyperplasia may be striking and may lead to a mistaken diagnosis of squamous cell carcinoma.

CLINICAL MANIFESTATIONS A few patients have acute, self-limited pneumonia. Fever, productive cough, myalgia, and malaise usually resolve within a month. Pulmonary infiltrates clear slowly as *B. dermatitidis* disappears from the sputum.

In the vast majority of cases, blastomycosis has an indolent onset and a chronically progressive course. Fever, cough, weight loss, lassitude, skin lesions, and chest ache are common. Skin lesions favor exposed areas and enlarge over many weeks from pimples to well-circumscribed, verrucous, crusted, or ulcerated lesions. Pain and regional lymphadenopathy are minimal. Large chronic lesions may undergo central healing with scarring and contracture. Mucous membrane lesions resemble squamous cell carcinoma. Chest x-ray findings are abnormal in two-thirds of cases, with one or more pneumonic or nodular infiltrates. Calcification, hilar adenopathy, and large pleural effusions are rare. Osteolytic lesions may be found in nearly any bone and present as a cold abscess or a draining sinus. Extension to a contiguous joint may cause indolent swelling, pain, and restricted motion. Prostatic and epididymal lesions clinically resemble those of tuberculosis.

DIAGNOSIS The diagnosis of blastomycosis is made by demonstration of the fungus in a culture of sputum, pus, or urine. An expert can diagnose blastomycosis on the basis of the appearance of the organism in wet smear or histopathologic section. The fungus may be visible in a sputum cytology smear but is easily overlooked.

℞ TREATMENT

A few patients have developed only transitory lung lesions, but no guidelines are known to distinguish these patients from those whose disease will progress locally or disseminate. Therefore, every patient should receive treatment. Intravenous amphotericin B is the drug of choice for patients with rapidly progressive infections, severe illness, or meningitis. Skin and noncavitary lung lesions should be treated for about 8 to 10 weeks. The recommended total dose for an adult is about 2.0 g. Cavitary lung disease or infection extending beyond the lung and skin should be treated for about 10 to 12 weeks with 2.5 g or more.

Itraconazole (200 mg twice daily with food) is the drug of choice for the treatment of patients who have indolent nonmeningeal blastomycosis of mild to moderate severity and who take the drug reliably. Ketoconazole (400 to 800 mg daily) is an effective alternative agent. Therapy with either itraconazole or ketoconazole is continued for 6 to 12 months.

The mortality rate in appropriately treated cases is 15 percent or less.

BIBLIOGRAPHY

BAUMGARDNER DJ et al: Epidemiology of blastomycosis in a region of high endemicity in north-central Wisconsin. Clin Infect Dis 15:629, 1992

BRADSHER RW: Blastomycosis: Fungal infections of the lung. Update 1989. Semin Respir Infect 5:105, 1990

MANGINO JE, PAPPAS PG: Itraconazole for the treatment of histoplasmosis and blastomycosis. Int J Antimicrob Agents 5:219, 1995

PAPPAS PG et al: Blastomycosis in immunocompromised patients. Medicine 72:311, 1993

206 *John E. Bennett*

CRYPTOCOCCOSIS

ETIOLOGIC AGENT Cryptococcosis is an infection caused by the yeastlike fungus *Cryptococcus neoformans*. This fungus reproduces by budding and forms round, yeastlike cells. Within the host and on certain culture media, a large polysaccharide capsule surrounds each yeast cell. The fungus grows well in smooth, creamy-white colonies on Sabouraud's or other simple media at 20 to 37°C. Certain culture media for ringworm contain cycloheximide, which inhibits the growth of *C. neoformans*. Identification of the organism is based on gross and microscopic appearance, biochemical test results, and growth at 37°C. The results of nucleic acid hybridization or the formation of brown pigment on Niger seed agar can also be used for identification.

The fungus has four capsular serotypes, designated A, B, C, and D. There are also two mating types. Coculture of opposite mating types creates a transient diploid state called *Filobasidiella neoformans* var. *neoformans* for serotypes A and D and *Filobasidiella neoformans* var. *bacillispora* for serotypes B and C. Organisms not cultured under mating conditions are designated *C. neoformans* var. *neoformans* for serotypes A and D and *C. neoformans* var. *gattii* for serotypes B and C; a simple color medium distinguishes the two varieties.

EPIDEMIOLOGY Weathered pigeon droppings commonly contain serotype A or D (*C. neoformans* var. *neoformans*). *C. neoformans* var. *gattii* has been isolated from the litter around eucalyptus trees of the species *Eucalyptus camaldulensis* and *Eucalyptus tereticornis*. The latter isolates have so far typed as serotype B. The distribution of these eucalyptus species in Australia corresponds to the distribution of infections due to *C. neoformans* var. *gattii* in that country. The high prevalence of these trees in other subtropical climates has been postulated to explain the relative restriction of such infections to warm climates.

Cryptococcosis due to *C. neoformans* var. *neoformans* is a common complication of late infection with human immunodeficiency virus (HIV), having occurred in 6.2% of the 274,150 AIDS patients reported to the Centers for Disease Control and Prevention as of September 1993. Patients who have undergone solid-organ transplantation or glucocorticoid therapy and those with sarcoidosis are also at increased risk for infections with *C. neoformans* var. *neoformans*. Almost all such infections are caused by serotype A, although serotype D occurs in up to 20 percent of cases in Western Europe. Infections with var. *gattii* have been rare among AIDS patients and other immunocompromised patients, even in subtropical climates, where var. *gattii* infection occurs in previously healthy individuals.

Animals, particularly cats, can acquire cryptococcosis but have not transmitted the infection to other animals or to humans. The source from which humans acquire the infection is unknown, with the rare exception of cases acquired through a transplanted cornea, kidney, or other solid organ. Cryptococcosis is rare before puberty.

PATHOGENESIS AND PATHOLOGY Infection is thought to be acquired by inhalation of fungus into the lungs. Pulmonary infection has a tendency toward spontaneous resolution and is frequently asymptomatic. Silent hematogenous spread to the brain leads to clusters of cryptococci in the perivascular areas of cortical gray matter, in the basal ganglia, and, to a lesser extent, in other areas of the central nervous system. The inflammatory response around these foci is usually scant. In the more chronic cases, a dense basilar arachnoiditis is typical. Lung lesions are characterized by intense granulomatous inflammation. Cryptococci are best seen in tissue by staining with methenamine silver or periodic acid–Schiff. Although a strongly positive result upon mucicarmine staining of tissue is diagnostic, staining varies from intense to absent.

CLINICAL MANIFESTATIONS Most patients have *meningoencephalitis* at the time of diagnosis. This form of the infection is invariably fatal without appropriate therapy; death occurs any time from 2 weeks to several years after the onset of symptoms. Early manifestations include headache, nausea, staggering gait, dementia, irritability, confusion, and blurred vision. Both fever and nuchal rigidity are often mild or lacking. Papilledema is evident in one-third of cases at the time of diagnosis. Cranial nerve palsies, typically asymmetric, occur in about one-fourth of cases. Other lateralized signs are rare. With progression of the infection, deepening coma and signs of brainstem compression appear. Autopsy often reveals cerebral edema in more acute cases and hydrocephalus in more chronic cases.

Pulmonary cryptococcosis causes chest pain in about 40 percent of patients and cough in 20 percent. The chest x-ray shows one or more dense infiltrates, which are often well circumscribed. Cavitation, pleural effusions, and hilar adenopathy are infrequent. Calcification is not evident, and fibrotic stranding is rarely noticeable.

Ten percent of patients with cryptococcosis have skin lesions, and the vast majority of patients with skin lesions have disseminated infection. One or a few asymptomatic tiny papular lesions appear and slowly enlarge; and they display a tendency toward central softening leading to ulceration. Osteolytic lesions occur in 4 percent of cases and usually present as a cold abscess. Rare manifestations of cryptococcosis include prostatitis, endophthalmitis, hepatitis, pericarditis, endocarditis, and renal abscess.

DIAGNOSIS Fever and headache in a patient with AIDS or with risk factors for HIV infection suggest the possibility of cryptococcosis, toxoplasmosis, or central nervous system lymphoma. Evidence of a focal lesion on magnetic resonance imaging is unusual in cryptococcosis. Most cryptococcal cerebral mass lesions occur in patients infected with *C. neoformans* var. *gattii* who also have meningitis. In patients without AIDS, meningitis due to *C. neoformans* resembles that due to *Mycobacterium tuberculosis*, *Histoplasma capsulatum*, *Coccidioides immitis*, or metastatic cancer. Lumbar puncture is the single most useful diagnostic test. An india ink smear of centrifuged cerebrospinal fluid (CSF) sediment reveals encapsulated yeast in more than half of cases, although artifacts can cause confusion. In patients without AIDS, levels of glucose in CSF are reduced in half of all cases; protein levels are usually increased; and lymphocytic pleocytosis is usually found. CSF abnormalities are less pronounced in patients with AIDS, though india ink smear is more often positive.

Approximately 90 percent of patients with cryptococcal meningoencephalitis, including all those with a positive CSF smear, have capsular antigen detectable in CSF or serum by latex agglutination. An enzyme immunoassay for cryptococcal antigen is also available. Occasional false-positive results in the above tests make culture the definitive diagnostic test. *C. neoformans* is often present in urine from patients with meningoencephalitis. Fungemia occurs in 10 to 30 percent of patients and is particularly common among AIDS patients.

Pulmonary cryptococcosis mimics malignancy with regard to radiographic findings and symptoms. Sputum culture is positive in only 10 percent of cases, and serum antigen tests are positive in only one-third. Occasionally, *C. neoformans* appears in one or more sputum specimens as an endobronchial saprophyte. Biopsy is usually required for diagnosis.

Cutaneous cryptococcosis may be mistaken for a comedo, basal cell carcinoma, or sarcoidosis. In AIDS patients, skin lesions may be numerous and are sometimes mistaken for molluscum contagiosum. Biopsy reveals myriad cryptococci. Osseous cryptococcosis resembles tuberculosis.

TREATMENT

Patients with AIDS and cryptococcosis are treated initially with intravenous amphotericin B (with or without flucytosine) and later with fluconazole. During active infection, fluconazole (400 mg) is given once daily. After infection is controlled, treatment with a smaller dose of fluconazole (200 mg daily) is continued indefinitely. Itraconazole is less effective than fluconazole for maintenance therapy.

In patients without AIDS, cryptococcosis may be treated with amphotericin B alone or in combination with flucytosine. Amphotericin B is given in a dose of 0.5 to 0.7 mg/kg per day when used alone and in a dose of 0.3 to 0.5 mg/kg per day when used in combination with flucytosine. Flucytosine is given initially in a dose of 25 to 37.5 mg/kg every 6 h to patients with normal renal function. Although nomograms are available for adjusting flucytosine dosage in the presence of reduced renal function, the best way to prevent toxicity is to measure serum levels frequently and to maintain them between 50 and 100 µg/mL.

The duration of therapy in patients without AIDS is based on the results of lumbar punctures, which are best done weekly until culture conversion is clearly demonstrated. Six weeks of therapy may be adequate for patients whose CSF (2 to 4 mL) is cultured weekly and remains sterile for at least 4 weeks, whose india ink smear has become negative, and whose CSF glucose level is normal. Declining titers of cryptococcal antigen in CSF offer some assurance of therapeutic success; in contrast, serum antigen titers, while useful in diagnosis, have not proven useful in evaluation of the response to therapy. Approximately 50 to 70 percent of cases of cryptococcosis in non-AIDS patients are cured.

Hydrocephalus may be the presenting manifestation or a later complication of cryptococcosis. Blindness, dementia, and personality change are among the other sequelae. Daily lumbar puncture or CSF shunting has been advocated—in the hope of averting permanent blindness—for patients with marked cerebral edema who have incipient blurred vision.

Patients with extraneural cryptococcosis most often require treatment with intravenous amphotericin B, with or without flucytosine. Observation or excision of lesions may suffice for some patients who have previously been healthy; who have a single focus in lung, skin, or bone; and who have no cryptococci in CSF, urine, or blood. No guidelines are yet available for the use of fluconazole in non-AIDS patients. For reasons presented elsewhere (see Chap. 202), fluconazole is not recommended for the prevention of cryptococcosis in AIDS patients.

BIBLIOGRAPHY

MEYOHAS M-C et al: Pulmonary cryptococcosis: Localized and disseminated infections in 27 patients with AIDS. Clin Infect Dis 21:628, 1995
MURAKAWA GJ et al: Cutaneous *Cryptococcus* infection and AIDS: Report of 12 cases and review of the literature. Arch Dermatol 132:545, 1996
PINNER RW et al: Prospects for preventing cryptococcosis in persons infected with human immunodeficiency virus. Clin Infect Dis 21:S103, 1995
POWDERLY WG et al: Measurement of cryptococcal antigen in serum and cerebrospinal fluid: Value in the management of AIDS-associated cryptococcal meningitis. Clin Infect Dis 18:789, 1994
REX JR et al: Catastrophic visual loss due to *Cryptococcus neoformans* meningitis. Medicine 72:207, 1993
SPEED B, DUNT D: Clinical and host differences between infections with the two varieties of *Cryptococcus neoformans*. Clin Infect Dis 21:28, 1995
WHITE M et al: Cryptococcal meningitis: Outcome in patients with AIDS and patients with neoplastic disease. J Infect Dis 165:690, 1992

207 *John E. Bennett*

CANDIDIASIS

ETIOLOGIC AGENTS *Candida albicans* is the most common cause of candidiasis, but *Candida tropicalis*, *Candida parapsilosis*, *Candida guilliermondii*, *Candida glabrata*, *Candida krusei*, and a few other species can cause deep candidiasis that is sometimes fatal. *C. parapsilosis* is particularly notable for its ability to cause endocarditis. *C. tropicalis* accounts for about one-third of the cases of deep candidiasis in neutropenic patients.

All *Candida* species pathogenic for humans are also encountered as commensals of humans, particularly in the mouth, stool, and vagina. These species grow rapidly at 25 to 37°C on simple media as oval, budding cells. In special culture media and in tissue, hyphae or elongated branching structures called *pseudohyphae* are formed. *C. glabrata*, formerly called *Torulopsis glabrata*, differs from other members of the genus in that it forms no true hyphae or pseudohyphae in vitro or in infected tissue. *C. albicans* can be identified presumptively by its ability to form germ tubes in serum or by the formation of thick-walled large spores called *chlamydospores*. Final identification of all species requires biochemical tests.

PATHOGENESIS Candidiasis is often preceded by increased colonization of the mouth, vagina, and stool with *Candida* due to broad-spectrum antibiotic therapy. Additional local and systemic factors favor infection. Oropharyngeal thrush is particularly likely to occur in neonates and in patients with diabetes mellitus, human immunodeficiency virus (HIV) infection, or dentures. Vulvovaginal candidiasis is especially common in the third trimester of pregnancy. *Candida* from the perineum can enter the urinary tract via an indwelling bladder catheter. Cutaneous candidiasis most often involves macerated skin, such as that in the diapered area of infants, under pendulous breasts, or on hands constantly in water or covered by occlusive gloves. *Candida* can pass from the colonized surface into deep tissue when the integrity of the mucosa or skin is violated, as, for example, by perforation of the gastrointestinal tract through trauma, surgery, or peptic ulceration or by mucosal damage due to cytotoxic agents used for cancer chemotherapy. Although *Candida* is not normally a resident of the skin, secretions from the mouth, rectum, or vagina as well as drainage from surgical wounds or tracheostomy sites can contaminate the hub or skin site of a catheter in an umbilical or central vein, and this contamination can lead to severe *Candida* sepsis. Intravenous drug abuse or third-degree burns can also provide a skin portal for *Candida* that can lead to deep candidiasis. Once *Candida* has passed the integumentary barrier, very low birth weight (in neonates) and neutropenia or glucocorticoid therapy (in any patient) markedly decrease host defense. Hematogenous seeding is particularly evident in the retina, kidney, spleen, and liver.

CLINICAL MANIFESTATIONS *Oral thrush* presents as discrete and confluent adherent white plaques on the oral and pharyngeal mucosa, particularly in the mouth and on the tongue. These lesions are usually painless, but fissuring at the corners of the mouth can be painful. Unexplained oropharyngeal thrush raises the possibility of HIV infection. Oral thrush is common in acute HIV infection and becomes increasingly common as the CD4+ cell count falls. At CD4+ counts below 50/μL, esophageal thrush also becomes common. HIV infection appears not to be an independent risk factor for vulvovaginal thrush.

Cutaneous candidiasis presents as red macerated intertriginous areas, paronychia, balanitis, or pruritus ani. Candidiasis of the perineal and scrotal skin may be accompanied by discrete pustular lesions on the inner aspects of the thighs. *Chronic mucocutaneous candidiasis* or *Candida granuloma* typically presents as circumscribed hyperkeratotic skin lesions, crumbling dystrophic nails, partial alopecia in areas of scalp lesions, and both oral and vaginal thrush. Systemic infection is very rare, but disfigurement of the face and hands can be severe. Other findings may include chronic epidermophytosis, dental dysplasia, and hypofunction of the parathyroid, adrenal, or thyroid gland. A variety of defects in T cell function have been described in these patients. Vulvovaginal thrush causes pruritus, discharge, and sometimes pain on intercourse or urination. Speculum examination reveals an inflamed mucosa and a thin exudate, often with white curds.

Esophageal candidiasis is often asymptomatic but can cause substernal pain or a sense of obstruction on swallowing. Most lesions are in the distal third of the esophagus and appear on endoscopy as areas of redness and edema, focal white patches, or ulcers. Biopsy or brushing is required for the diagnosis and detection of concomitant infections, particularly herpes simplex in patients with hematologic malignancies and cytomegalovirus infection in AIDS patients. Esophagraphy is diagnostically insensitive but may reveal spasm or mucosal irregularities. *Candida* esophagitis can cause bleeding and impaired alimentation. Hematogenous dissemination from the esophagus probably occurs in some neutropenic patients but is rarely reported in HIV-infected patients.

Candida can cause cystitis, pyelitis, or renal papillary necrosis in an obstructed urinary tract. When a colonized urinary tract is operated on or instrumented, candidemia may result. However, most patients with *Candida* cultured from the urine simply have bladder colonization from a Foley catheter or a sizable volume of residual urine. Contamination of a voided midstream specimen by vaginal *Candida* is also common.

Hematogenous seeding can cause a wide spectrum of illnesses, ranging from septic shock to fever alone; the etiology of these conditions becomes clear later, when focal abscesses develop in multiple organs. Retinal lesions are visible on funduscopy within 2 weeks and

should be sought in all patients with candidemia. Blurred vision, scotoma, or ocular pain may not be noted for weeks, especially by obtunded or sedated patients. The earliest lesions are retinal exudates, unilateral in half of cases. Extension of lesions leads to vitreitis, vitreal abscess, retinal detachment, and hypopyon. Most cases with ocular involvement have occurred in nonneutropenic patients. In contrast, so-called hepatosplenic candidiasis is usually recognized in patients with acute leukemia who are recovering from profound neutropenia. This entity, better called *chronic disseminated candidiasis*, originates from intestinal seeding of the portal and venous circulation. Fever, modestly elevated serum concentrations of alkaline phosphatase, and multiple small abscesses evident on ultrasonography, magnetic resonance imaging, or computed tomography of the liver, spleen, or kidney suggest the diagnosis. During acute candidemia in neutropenic patients, small erythematous papules may appear anywhere on the skin. If the patient does not expire promptly from disseminated candidiasis, the lesions will develop a necrotic center. Painful muscle lesions may also be found. Punch biopsy of a skin lesion helps distinguish this extremely grave condition from *Malassezia* furunculosis, a similar-appearing but benign condition that can involve the cape area of the chest or the extremities of a sweaty febrile patient.

Hematogenous seeding in the neutropenic patient is occasionally visible radiologically as tiny pulmonary nodules. *Candida* pneumonia, apart from hematogenous candidiasis, is very rare. Organisms seeding a native or prosthetic cardiac valve originate principally from central venous catheters; occasionally, valvular seeding is encountered in intravenous drug abusers. Emboli to large arteries, such as the iliac or femoral artery, are characteristic. Intravenous injection of impure brown heroin has caused a clinical syndrome consisting of *Candida* endophthalmitis and purulent folliculitis, sometimes accompanied by vertebral osteomyelitis. This diffuse folliculitis favors hairy areas, including the scalp and the area under the beard.

Candida can cause indolent arthritis, most commonly of the knee, in patients who have received glucocorticoid injections into the joint, in patients who are immunosuppressed, and in low-birth-weight neonates. Prosthetic joints may become infected during implantation. Scanty growth of *Candida* from joint fluid can cause the laboratory to incorrectly dismiss the organism as a contaminant.

Hematogenous dissemination can lead to brain abscess or chronic meningitis. Diagnosis of infections of ventriculoperitoneal shunts is difficult because symptoms are indolent and cultures of lumbar fluid are usually sterile.

DIAGNOSIS Demonstration of pseudohyphae on wet smear with confirmation by culture is the procedure of choice for diagnosing superficial candidiasis. Scrapings for the smear may be obtained from skin, nails, and oral and vaginal mucosa. Culture alone is not diagnostic; however, recovery of *Candida* species from multiple superficial sites in immunosuppressed patients may portend visceral invasion.

Deeper lesions due to *Candida* may be diagnosed by histologic section of biopsy specimens or by culture of cerebrospinal fluid, blood, joint fluid, or surgical specimens. Blood cultures are useful in the diagnosis of *Candida* endocarditis and intravenous catheter–induced sepsis but are positive less often in other forms of disseminated disease. Serologic tests for antibody or antigen are not useful.

℞ **TREATMENT**
Cutaneous candidiasis of macerated areas responds to measures that reduce moisture and chafing plus topical application of an antifungal agent in a nonocclusive base. Nystatin powder or a cream containing ciclopirox or an azole is useful. Clotrimazole, miconazole, econazole, ketoconazole, sulconazole, and oxiconazole are available as creams or lotions. *Candida* vulvovaginitis responds better to an azole than to nystatin suppositories. There is little difference in efficacy among miconazole, clotrimazole, tioconazole, butoconazole, and terconazole vaginal formulations. Systemic treatment of *Candida* vulvovaginitis with a single 150-mg capsule of fluconazole is more convenient

than topical treatment but also poses a higher risk of adverse effects. Clotrimazole troches, used five times a day, are more effective in oral and esophageal candidiasis than nystatin suspension. Ketoconazole (200 to 400 mg daily) or itraconazole (200 mg daily) is also useful in *Candida* esophagitis, but many patients absorb the drugs poorly because they are receiving H$_2$ receptor antagonists or have AIDS. In AIDS patients, fluconazole (100 to 200 mg daily) is the most effective azole for oral and esophageal candidiasis.

Management of recurrent oropharyngeal candidiasis in the HIV-infected patient presents special problems. Patients with CD4 + cell counts below 100/μL who have received prolonged fluconazole therapy are at risk of developing azole resistance, requiring an increased dose to mount a response, relapsing early, and eventually failing to respond well to any dose of fluconazole. Therapy with itraconazole, ketoconazole, or clotrimazole at this point results in only transient or no improvement. The increasing azole resistance in this population suggests that HIV-infected patients with oropharyngeal candidiasis should be treated for each individual episode and that only when episodes become intolerably frequent should weekly or daily preventive therapy be given and even then at the lowest dose required to maintain remission. In contrast, AIDS patients with *Candida* esophagitis are so prone to relapse that preventive therapy with fluconazole is recommended for all proven cases. Most HIV-infected patients with azole-resistant oropharyngeal candidiasis also have esophagitis. Nearly all patients with azole-resistant oropharyngeal or esophageal candidiasis respond to intravenous amphotericin B (0.3 to 0.5 mg/kg daily) but relapse promptly after the completion of therapy.

Bladder thrush responds to bladder irrigations with amphotericin B (50 μg/mL for 5 days). If no bladder catheter is in place, oral fluconazole can be used to control candiduria. In all forms of superficial candidiasis, relapse after successful treatment is common unless the underlying factor can be eliminated.

Intravenous amphotericin B is the drug of choice in disseminated candidiasis. The drug is usually given at a dosage of 0.5 to 0.7 mg/kg daily. In patients with no contraindication to the use of flucytosine, administration of that drug at a dosage of 100 to 150 mg/kg per day along with amphotericin B (0.3 to 0.5 mg/kg per day) is an effective alternative. Fluconazole in an adult dose of 100 mg daily is probably the drug of choice for chronic mucocutaneous candidiasis.

Candida isolated from a culture of a properly obtained blood sample should be considered significant; true false-positives are rare. All patients with *Candida* cultured from peripheral blood should receive intravenous amphotericin B to treat acute infection and prevent late sequelae. In immunocompetent patients with intravenous catheter-acquired *C. albicans* fungemia, the catheter should be removed in conjunction with the administration of either fluconazole (400 mg daily) or amphotericin B (0.5 mg/kg daily). Patients with suppurative phlebitis of a peripheral vein should have the infected portion of the vein excised. Therapy for candidemia is continued for 2 weeks after the patient becomes afebrile. The *Candida* species involved should be considered in choosing between fluconazole and amphotericin B. *C. krusei* causes about 1 percent of all cases of candidemia but is resistant to fluconazole in vitro. *C. glabrata* exhibits an intermediate level of susceptibility to fluconazole, but too few cases have been studied to determine whether candidemia involving that species will respond as well to fluconazole as to amphotericin B. Strains of *Candida lusitaniae* resistant to amphotericin B but susceptible to azoles have been encountered. In every case of candidemia, a funduscopic examination for endophthalmitis should be undertaken, and therapy should be continued until retinal lesions have resolved. Intravenous amphotericin B, with or without flucytosine, is the preferred treatment for *Candida* endophthalmitis, although cures have been reported with fluconazole. Pars plana vitrectomy may facilitate diagnosis and cure when a *Candida* vitreous abscess is present. Leaving amphotericin B in the vitreous cavity at the end of the vitrectomy procedure should be considered.

Injection of amphotericin B into an infected joint, pleural cavity, or peritoneum is rarely indicated. Removal of prostheses, including prosthetic joints, cardiac valves, peritoneal dialysis catheters, and central venous catheters, is usually essential. Collections of pus, such as those in the postoperative abdomen, need to be drained surgically or by percutaneous, computed tomography–guided catheterization; an exception relates to the numerous small abscesses in liver, spleen, or kidney in chronic disseminated candidiasis, which cannot be drained effectively and require prolonged antifungal therapy. In general, treatment should continue until the patient with chronic disseminated candidiasis has been afebrile and nonneutropenic for at least 2 weeks. Defects may persist on imaging studies long after cure. Relapse during another episode of neutropenia is common unless the patient is receiving amphotericin B. Repeat cytotoxic therapy or even bone marrow transplantation can be undertaken in patients with prior chronic disseminated candidiasis, but amphotericin B should be given prophylactically during neutropenia.

Fluconazole can decrease the incidence of deep candidiasis in recipients of allogeneic bone marrow transplants when 400 mg is given daily until engraftment. Although the incidence of superficial candidiasis is also decreased by fluconazole prophylaxis, superficial infection can be readily detected and treated. Aspergillosis is not prevented by prophylactic fluconazole. Studies of leukemic and other neutropenic patients have found no beneficial effect of prophylactic fluconazole. Empirical administration of fluconazole to febrile neutropenic patients not responding to broad-spectrum antibacterial agents is not currently recommended.

The role of newer formulations of amphotericin B in the treatment of deep candidiasis or in empirical therapy is under study.

BIBLIOGRAPHY

Akler MA et al: Use of fluconazole in the treatment of candidal endophthalmitis. Clin Infect Dis 20:657, 1995

Anaissie E et al: Fluconazole therapy for chronic disseminated candidiasis in patients with leukemia and prior amphotericin B therapy. Am J Med 91:142, 1991

Laine L et al: Fluconazole compared with ketoconazole for the treatment of candida esophagitis in AIDS. Ann Intern Med 117:655, 1992

Lecciones JA et al: Vascular catheter-associated fungemia in patients with cancer: Analysis of 155 episodes. Clin Infect Dis 14:875, 1992

Odds FC: *Candida and Candidosis.* Philadelphia, Saunders, 1988

Rex JR et al: A randomized trial comparing fluconazole with amphotericin B for the treatment of candidemia in patients without neutropenia. N Engl J Med 331:1324, 1994

Slavin MA et al: Efficacy and safety of fluconazole prophylaxis for fungal infections after marrow transplantation—a prospective, randomized, double-blind study. J Infect Dis 171:1545, 1995

Thaler M et al: Hepatic candidiasis in cancer patients: The evolving picture of the syndrome. Ann Intern Med 198:88, 1988

Tosti A et al: Treatment of dermatophyte nail infections: An open randomized study comparing intermittent terbinafine with continuous terbinafine treatment and intermittent itraconazole therapy. J Am Acad Dermatol 34:595, 1996

White A, Goetz MB: Azole-resistant *Candida albicans:* Report of two cases of resistance to fluconazole and review. Clin Infect Dis 19:687, 1994

Wingard JR: Importance of *Candida* species other than *C. albicans* as pathogens in oncology patients. Clin Infect Dis 20:115, 1995

Winston DJ et al: Fluconazole prophylaxis of fungal infections in patients with acute leukemia. Ann Intern Med 118:495, 1993

208 *John E. Bennett*

ASPERGILLOSIS

ETIOLOGIC AGENTS *Aspergillus fumigatus* is the most common cause of aspergillosis, but *Aspergillus flavus, Aspergillus niger,* and several other species can also cause disease. *Aspergillus* is a mold with septate hyphae about 2 to 4 μm in diameter. The fungus is identified by its gross and microscopic appearance in culture.

PATHOGENESIS AND PATHOLOGY   All the common species of *Aspergillus* that cause disease in humans are ubiquitous in the environment, growing on dead leaves, stored grain, compost piles, hay, and other decaying vegetation. Inhalation of *Aspergillus* spores must be extremely common, but disease is rare. Invasion of lung tissue is confined almost entirely to immunosuppressed patients, in roughly 90 percent of whom two of the following three conditions will be operative: a granulocyte count in peripheral blood of <500/μL, treatment with supraphysiologic doses of adrenal glucocorticoids, and a history of treatment with cytotoxic drugs such as cyclosporine. Invasive aspergillosis is an occasional complication of AIDS. *Aspergillus* infection is characterized by hyphal invasion of blood vessels, thrombosis, necrosis, and hemorrhagic infarction. Chronic granulomatous disease of childhood also predisposes to invasive pulmonary aspergillosis, but in that situation the inflammatory response is granulomatous and blood vessel invasion is rare.

Massive inhalation of *Aspergillus* spores by healthy persons can lead to acute, diffuse, self-limited pneumonitis. Epithelioid granulomas with giant cells and central pyogenic areas containing hyphae are detected in these cases. Spontaneous recovery taking several weeks is the usual course.

Aspergillus can colonize the damaged bronchial tree, pulmonary cysts, or cavities of patients with underlying lung disease. Balls of hyphae within cysts or cavities (aspergillomas), usually in the upper lobe, may reach several centimeters in diameter and may be visible on chest x-ray. Tissue invasion does not occur. The term *allergic bronchopulmonary aspergillosis* denotes the condition of patients with preexisting asthma who have eosinophilia, IgE antibody to *Aspergillus*, and fleeting pulmonary infiltrates from bronchial plugging (see Chap. 253).

CLINICAL MANIFESTATIONS   *Endobronchial saprophytic pulmonary aspergillosis* presents as chronic productive cough, often with hemoptysis, in a patient with prior chronic lung disease, such as tuberculosis, sarcoidosis, bronchiectasis, or histoplasmosis. *Aspergillus* may be spread from its endocavitary or endobronchial site to the pleura during the course of bacterial lung abscess or surgery. Patients reported to have chronic necrotizing *Aspergillus* pneumonia appear in most instances to have had saprophytic endobronchial colonization and a pulmonary process attributable to another disease, with or without superimposed bacterial infections. Patients with chronic pneumonia and *Aspergillus* in the sputum should be assumed to have either pneumonia of a different etiology (e.g., histoplasmosis) or *Aspergillus* pneumonia with underlying immunosuppression [e.g., chronic granulomatous disease or infection with human immunodeficiency virus (HIV)].

Invasive aspergillosis in the immunocompromised host presents as an acute, rapidly progressive, densely consolidated pulmonary infiltrate and is most common among patients with acute leukemia and recipients of tissue transplants. Infection progresses by direct extension across tissue planes and by hematogenous dissemination to lung, brain, and other organs. Computed tomography (CT) has been helpful in identifying early lung infiltrates and, as neutrophil counts rise, in defining central areas of cavitation. *Aspergillus* may invade immunosuppressed patients through the skin at a site of minor trauma or through the upper airway mucosa. Early lesions in the nose should be sought in neutropenic patients with fever and minimal epistaxis. Scarlet-red patches of the mucosa rapidly become necrotic and white, then black. Rapid extension into the adjacent paranasal sinus, orbit, or face is usual, with or without the appearance of lung lesions.

Aspergillus sinusitis in immunocompetent patients may take two forms. A ball of hyphae may form in a chronically obstructed paranasal sinus, without tissue invasion. Much less commonly, a chronic, fibrosing granulomatous inflammation associated with *Aspergillus* hyphae within tissue may begin in the sinus and spread slowly to the orbit and the brain. *Aspergillus* is a cause of allergic fungal sinusitis, dark-walled fungi (e.g., *Cladosporium, Alternaria*) being more common in this setting. Patients usually have a history of chronic allergic rhinitis, sometimes with nasal polyps, but are otherwise healthy, presenting with painless proptosis, nasal obstruction, or dull aching pain. On CT or magnetic resonance imaging, a solid soft tissue mass pushing out the lateral wall of the ethmoid sinus or the medial wall of the maxillary sinus may be detected. On sinus exploration, the mucosa is found to be thickened and inflamed but intact. Within the sinus cavity, sticky mucopus with strands of neutrophils, eosinophils, Charcot-Leyden crystals, and occasional hyphae can be found.

Aspergillosis in HIV-infected patients most commonly involves the lung, presenting as fever, cough, and dyspnea. Typically, the CD4 cell count is below 50/μL. Roughly half of these patients have neutropenia or have recently been treated with glucocorticoids. Bilateral diffuse or focal pulmonary infiltrates with a tendency to cavitate constitute the most common radiologic manifestation. Well-localized, white, necrotic pseudomembranes full of hyphae or ulcers may develop in the trachea or the major bronchi. Progression of bronchitis to pneumonia is usual, but hematogenous dissemination is uncommon. Either allergic or invasive *Aspergillus* sinusitis can occur in HIV-infected patients; the allergic form can develop even at CD4 cell counts above 50/μL.

The growth of *Aspergillus* on cerumen and detritus within the external auditory canal is termed *otomycosis*. Trauma to the cornea may cause *Aspergillus* keratitis. Endophthalmitis follows the introduction of *Aspergillus* into the globe by trauma or surgery. *Aspergillus* may infect intracardiac or intravascular prostheses.

DIAGNOSIS   The repeated isolation of *Aspergillus* from sputum or the demonstration of hyphae in sputum or bronchoalveolar lavage fluid suggests endobronchial colonization or infection. Even a single isolation of *Aspergillus* from the sputum of a neutropenic patient with pneumonia, particularly a child or a nonsmoker, suggests the diagnosis of invasive aspergillosis. In patients with advanced AIDS, fever, and cough, the isolation of *Aspergillus* from respiratory secretions raises the possibility of aspergillosis and thus should prompt bronchoscopy. Fungus ball of the lung is usually detectable by chest x-ray. IgG antibody to *Aspergillus* antigens is demonstrable in the serum of many colonized patients and of virtually all patients with fungus ball.

Biopsy is usually required for the diagnosis of invasive aspergillosis of the lung, nose, paranasal sinus, bronchi, or sites of dissemination. Blood cultures are rarely positive, even in patients with infected cardiac valves (native or prosthetic). *Aspergillus* hyphae can be identified presumptively by histology, but culture is required for confirmation and for determination of the species. Only culture can reliably distinguish aspergillosis from pseudallescheriasis; drug therapy for these two diseases differs.

℞ **TREATMENT**

Patients with severe hemoptysis due to fungus ball of the lung may benefit from lobectomy. Poor pulmonary function in residual lung and dense pleural adhesions around the lesion can complicate the resection. Systemic chemotherapy is of no value in endobronchial or endocavitary aspergillosis.

Treatment with intravenous amphotericin B (1.0 to 1.5 mg/kg daily) has resulted in the arrest or cure of invasive aspergillosis when immunosuppression is not severe. Itraconazole (200 mg bid) is useful in some less immunosuppressed patients with indolent or slowly progressive invasive aspergillosis. Surgery is the only treatment needed for fungus ball of the sinus and for allergic fungal sinusitis. Antifungal therapy has little effect on either entity if used alone, but chronic suppressive therapy has been begun postoperatively for relapse of allergic fungal sinusitis. The prognosis for cure of invasive aspergillosis in the paranasal sinus is very poor when the patient has profound and unremitting neutropenia. The prognosis is better in less immunosuppressed patients.

BIBLIOGRAPHY

DENNING DW, STEVENS DA: Antifungal and surgical treatment of invasive aspergillosis: Review of 2121 published cases. Rev Infect Dis 12:1147, 1990

LOGAN PM et al: Invasive aspergillosis of the airways: Radiographic, CT and pathologic findings. Radiology 193:383, 1994

LOTHLOLARY O et al: Invasive aspergillosis in patients with acquired immuno-
deficiency syndrome: Report of 33 cases. Am J Med 95:177, 1993
SHIRAKUSA T et al: Surgical treatment of pulmonary aspergilloma and
Aspergillus empyema. Ann Thorac Surg 48:779, 1989
TALBOT GH et al: Invasive *Aspergillus* rhinosinusitis in patients with acute
leukemia. Rev Infect Dis 13:219, 1991

209   *John E. Bennett*

MUCORMYCOSIS

ETIOLOGIC AGENTS   Species of *Rhizopus*, *Rhizomucor*, and
Cunninghamella are most the common causes of mucormycosis, but
species of *Apophysomyces*, *Saksenaea*, *Mucor*, and *Absidia* also are
occasionally responsible for this infection. The organism in tissue is
composed of broad, rarely septate hyphae of uneven diameter (diameter
ranging from 6 to 50 μm). The organisms are inexplicably difficult
to grow from infected tissue. When growth does take place, it is rapid
and profuse on most media at room temperature. Identification is based
on the gross and microscopic appearance of the mold.

Zygomycosis is a term that includes mucormycosis and ento-
mophthoramycosis. The latter is a tropical infection of the subcutaneous tissue or paranasal sinuses caused by species of *Basidiobolus*
or *Conidiobolus*.

EPIDEMIOLOGY AND PATHOLOGY *Rhizopus* and
Rhizomucor species are ubiquitous, appearing on decaying vegetation,
dung, and foods of high sugar content. Mucormycosis is uncommon
and is largely confined to patients with serious preexisting diseases.
Mucormycosis originating in the paranasal sinuses and nose predominantly affects patients with poorly controlled diabetes mellitus. Patients
who have undergone organ transplantation, who have a hematologic
malignancy, or who are receiving long-term deferoxamine therapy are
predisposed to mucormycosis of either sinus or lung. Gastrointestinal
mucormycosis occurs in a variety of conditions, including uremia,
severe malnutrition, and diarrheal diseases. The infection is acquired
from nature, with no person-to-person spread. In all forms of mucormycosis, vascular invasion by hyphae is a prominent feature. Ischemic
or hemorrhagic necrosis is the foremost histologic finding.

CLINICAL MANIFESTATIONS   Mucormycosis originating
in the nose and paranasal sinuses produces a characteristic clinical
picture. Low-grade fever, dull sinus pain, and sometimes nasal congestion or a thin, bloody nasal discharge are followed in a few days by
double vision, increasing fever, and obtundation. Examination reveals
a unilateral generalized reduction of ocular motion, chemosis, and
proptosis. The nasal turbinates on the involved side may be dusky red
or necrotic. A sharply delineated area of necrosis, strictly respecting
the midline, may appear in the hard palate. The skin of the cheek may
become inflamed. Fungal invasion of the globe or ophthalmic artery
leads to blindness. Opacification of one or more sinuses is detected
by computed tomography (CT) or by magnetic resonance imaging
(MRI). Carotid arteriography may show invasion or obstruction of the
carotid siphon. Coma is due to direct invasion of the frontal lobe.
Early symptoms mimic those of bacterial sinusitis. Clouding of the
sensorium may be attributed to diabetic acidosis. Cavernous sinus
thrombosis may be considered when orbital invasion occurs. Without
treatment, the patient may die after an interval ranging from a few
days to a few weeks.

Pulmonary mucormycosis manifests as progressive severe pneumonia accompanied by high fever and toxicity. The necrotic center
of large infiltrates may cavitate. Hematogenous spread to other areas
of the lung, as well as to the brain and other organs, is common.
Survival beyond 2 weeks is unusual. Gastrointestinal invasion presents
as one or more ulcers that tend to perforate. Hematogenous dissemina-

tion can originate from the gastrointestinal tract, lung, or paranasal
sinuses. Sometimes no portal of entry can be found.

DIAGNOSIS   CT or MRI is very helpful in assessing the extent
of sinusitis before surgery and in evaluating the patient afterward. CT
is better for detecting bony erosion; MRI better visualizes extension
into the frontal lobe or carotid artery in the siphon. Lesions of the
lung and craniofacial structures are best diagnosed by biopsy and
histologic section. Cultural confirmation should be attempted. Wet
smear of crushed tissue can provide a rapid diagnosis. Cultures of blood
and cerebrospinal fluid are negative. Smear and culture of sputum may
be positive during cavitation of a lung lesion.

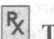 **TREATMENT**
Regulation of diabetes mellitus and a decrease in the dose of immuno-
suppressive drugs facilitate the treatment of mucormycosis. Extensive debridement of craniofacial lesions appears to be very important.
Orbital exenteration may be required. Intravenous amphotericin B
is clearly of value in craniofacial mucormycosis and should be
employed in the other forms of mucormycosis as well. The maximal
tolerated doses are given until progression is halted. With the deoxycholate formulation, 1 to 1.5 mg/kg daily is indicated. Therapy is
continued for a total of 10 to 12 weeks. Azoles are of no value.
Appropriate management results in cure of about half of craniofacial
infections. The survival of patients with pulmonary, gastrointestinal,
or disseminated mucormycosis is rare.

BIBLIOGRAPHY

BOELAERT JR: Mucormycosis (zygomycosis): Is there news for the clinician?
J Infect 28:S1, 1994
GALETTA SL et al: Rhinocerebral mucormycosis: Management and survival
after carotid occlusion. Ann Neurol 28:103, 1990
INGRAM CW et al: Disseminated zygomycosis: Report of four cases and review.
Rev Infect Dis 11:741, 1989
SINGH N et al: Invasive gastrointestinal zygomycosis in a liver transplant
recipient: Case report and review of zygomycosis in solid-organ transplant
recipients. Clin Infect Dis 20:617, 1995
TEDDER M et al: Pulmonary mucormycosis: Results of medical and surgical
therapy. Ann Thorac Surg 57:1044, 1994

210   *John E. Bennett*

MISCELLANEOUS MYCOSES AND *PROTOTHECA* INFECTIONS

CHROMOBLASTOMYCOSIS   This chronic subcutaneous
mycosis, rarely seen in the United States, presents as a verrucoid,
ulcerated, or crusted skin lesion. The disease follows the introduction
of any of several fungi into subcutaneous tissue by thorns or bits of
vegetation. The infection spreads over ensuing months and years to
contiguous tissue, causing few symptoms. The appearance of thick-
walled, dark-colored, rounded forms ("copper pennies") in tissue is
diagnostic. No satisfactory treatment is available.

DERMATOPHYTOSIS   **Definition**   Dermatophytosis, also
known as ringworm or tinea, is a chronic fungal infection of the skin,
hair, or nails.

Etiology   Species of *Trichophyton*, *Microsporum*, and *Epidermophyton* are called *dermatophytes*. These organisms grow in and remain
confined to the keratinous structures of the body. Other mycoses, such
as candidiasis, pityriasis versicolor, and tinea nigra, sometimes include
fungal invasion of keratinous structures but traditionally are not called
dermatophytoses.

Pathology and Pathogenesis   Dermatophyte species are referred
to as *anthropophilic*, *zoophilic*, or *geophilic*, depending on whether
their usual reservoir in nature appears to be humans, animals, or soil,
respectively. The infectivity of organisms from all these sources is
low, and outbreaks are largely confined to occasional clusters of cases

of scalp infection in children. Acquisition of a dermatophytosis appears to be favored by minor trauma, maceration, and poor hygiene of the skin. Infection does not seem to confer solid immunity: Repeated infection with the same species is common, particularly with anthropophilic species. The infrequency of scalp infection among adults has been attributed to local factors rather than immunity.

Invasion of the stratum corneum by dermatophytes may cause inflammation that is either mild or (particularly with zoophilic fungi) intense. Shedding of the stratum corneum is increased by inflammation. To the extent that fungal growth cannot keep up with shedding, inflammation may help terminate infection. Conversely, infection is probably favored when shedding is reduced by treatment with glucocorticoids and cytotoxic drugs. Antifungal drugs interfere with the ability of fungal growth to keep up with shedding.

Clinical Manifestations   The disease varies with the site of infection and the fungal species involved. Foot infection (athlete's foot, tinea pedis) may present as fissuring of the toe webs, scaling of the plantar surfaces, or vesicles around the toe webs and soles. Interdigital lesions may be pruritic or, when bacterial superinfection occurs, may be painful. Hand infection is less common but resembles foot infection.

Scalp dermatophytosis (tinea capitis) is characterized by areas of alopecia and scaling. In so-called endothrix infection, the hair shaft breaks off at the skin surface, leaving the hairs visible as black dots in the scalp. Some forms of scalp infection include an area of intense boggy suppuration called a *kerion*.

Dermatophytosis of the glabrous skin (tinea corporis) presents as circumscribed lesions with a wide variety of appearances, including scales, vesicles, and pustules. Inflammation may be minimal or intense. Central healing of less inflamed lesions may take place. The serpiginous border of inflammation is the source of the name *ringworm*.

Dermatophytosis of the bearded area (tinea barbae) appears as a pustular folliculitis. Onychomycosis (tinea unguium) presents as a white discoloration of the nails or as thickening, chalkiness, and crumbling of the nails. Peeling and fissuring of paronychial nail folds or keratotic debris under the nail edge also may be evident.

Diagnosis   Discolored hairs, scales, and keratotic debris under infected nails should be collected for KOH smear and culture. In the scraping of skin lesions, a drop of water on the skin site may keep the removed scales from flying off and thus may aid in their collection. Culture is important in distinguishing dermatophytes from *Candida* and fungal saprophytes growing in keratinaceous debris.

℞ TREATMENT

Noninflammatory lesions of the trunk, groin, hands, and feet usually respond to twice-daily applications of clotrimazole, miconazole, ketoconazole, econazole, naftifine, terbinafine, or ciclopirox olamine cream. Hyperkeratotic lesions of the palms and soles respond slowly to these agents and may benefit from Whitfield's ointment initially to thin the keratin. Ointment should not be used between the toes, in the groin, or in the gluteal crease because maceration promotes bacterial infection.

Ringworm that is moderately severe, that is unresponsive to topical therapy, or that involves the scalp, nails, or bearded area should be treated systemically. The drug of choice is griseofulvin. Either 500 mg of the microcrystalline form or 375 mg of the ultramicrocrystalline form is given once daily or divided into two doses and given with meals. Double this amount has been recommended for refractory infections. Treatment must be continued until all infected keratin is gone. Cutting of infected hair and cleansing of interdigital webs can expedite cure. Secondary bacterial infection of the foot may require soaks or antibacterial agents. The likelihood of relapse of dermatophyte foot infections may be decreased by keeping the feet clean and dry. Griseofulvin-resistant cases may respond to itraconazole (200 mg once daily). Onychomycosis responds poorly to griseofulvin but may respond to itraconazole. Terbinafine (250 mg orally) is at least as effective as itraconazole in onychomycosis and ringworm, but the comparative safety of the two drugs is unclear.

Onychomycosis, which most often is due to *Trichophyton rubrum*, must be treated systemically until all infected portions of the nails grow out and are trimmed off. Deformed nails may grow more slowly than usual. Treatment should continue for at least 3 months. Cultures and smears can be helpful in determining the appropriate time to end therapy. Relapse is common.

PROTOTHECOSIS   *Prototheca* species are ubiquitous achlorophyllic algae that enter the skin through trauma or surgery and cause localized infections in the olecranon bursa, skin, subcutaneous tissue, tendon sheaths, or deeper tissue. Diagnosis is based on culture or histopathologic demonstration of sporangia with endospores in tissue. Surgical debridement and treatment with intravenous amphotericin B are useful.

FUSARIOSIS   *Fusarium* species can cause localized or hematogenously disseminated infection. Almost all patients with the latter have had hematopoietic malignancy and neutropenia. Abrupt onset of fever, sometimes with myalgia, is followed by distinctive skin lesions in two-thirds of cases. The lesions resemble ecthyma gangrenosum, tend to be multiple, progressively expand in size, and favor the extremities. A portal of infection is not usually apparent. Blood cultures have been positive in 59 percent of cases. Amphotericin B is probably the drug of choice for the treatment of fusariosis, but recovery depends on the diminution of neutropenia.

***MALASSEZIA* INFECTION (PITYRIASIS)**   *Malassezia furfur* is part of the normal flora of the human skin but can cause tinea (pityriasis) versicolor or catheter-acquired sepsis. Tinea versicolor appears as asymptomatic, well-delineated, hyperpigmented or hypopigmented macules centered on the upper trunk and upper arms. Confluent lesions may cover large areas, making the border difficult to find. A fine "branny" scale or folliculitis is sometimes visible. When examined microscopically by KOH mount, skin sections are seen to contain characteristic round and elongated cells. On inspection with Wood's light, lesions either do not fluoresce or appear yellow-green. Erythrasma resembles tinea versicolor but is characterized by grampositive bacilli on smear and coral-red fluorescence. Azole creams are effective for the treatment of small areas of tinea versicolor; however, the application of selenium sulfide shampoo (Selsun) for 10 min daily, followed by showering to remove the shampoo, is more practical for large areas. Oral ketoconazole or itraconazole is also effective. Catheter-acquired sepsis due to *M. furfur* develops in patients (particularly neonates) receiving intravenous lipid. The organism requires special culture conditions for growth, and the infection is cured by catheter removal.

MYCETOMA   **Etiology**   *Actinomycetoma* refers to infection by actinomycetes of the genera *Nocardia*, *Nocardiopsis*, *Streptomyces*, and *Actinomadura*. *Eumycetoma* is caused by true fungi of many different genera. The predominant agent varies with the locality.

Pathogenesis and Pathology   The pathogens live in the soil and enter the skin through minor trauma. The most common site of infection is the foot. The infection runs a relentless course over many years, with destruction of contiguous bone and fascia. Grains are found in purulent foci surrounded by fibrosis and a mononuclear cell inflammatory response.

Clinical Manifestations   *Mycetoma* is a chronic suppurative infection originating in subcutaneous tissue and characterized by the presence of grains, which are tightly clumped colonies of the causative agent. The infected site is characterized by painless swelling, woody induration, and sinus tracts that discharge pus intermittently. Systemic symptoms do not develop, and spread to distant sites in the body does not take place.

Diagnosis   Although the clinical picture is characteristic, mycetoma is sometimes confused with chronic osteomyelitis or botryomycosis. The diagnosis requires demonstration of grains in pus from the draining sinus or in biopsy sections. Many histologic sections may need to be examined to locate a grain.

℞ TREATMENT

Actinomycetoma may respond to prolonged combination chemotherapy—e.g., with streptomycin and either dapsone or trimethoprimsulfamethoxazole. Eumycetoma rarely responds to chemotherapy; some cases caused by *Madurella mycetomatis* have appeared to respond to ketoconazole or itraconazole.

PARACOCCIDIOIDOMYCOSIS **Etiology** Formerly called *South American blastomycosis*, this mycosis is caused by *Paracoccidioides brasiliensis*. A dimorphic fungus, *P. brasiliensis* grows as a budding yeast in tissue but may be grown as either a yeast or a mold on culture medium. The organism is identified by its gross and microscopic appearance. A superficial resemblance to *Blastomyces dermatitidis* may cause misdiagnosis.

Pathogenesis and Pathology Infection is thought to be acquired by inhalation of spores from environmental sources, but the organism's reservoir in nature remains obscure. Pulmonary infection produces few symptoms initially. Hematogenous spread to the mucous membranes of the mouth and nose, the lymph nodes, and other sites causes patients to seek medical attention. In fatal cases, the infection spreads to the adrenals, the gastrointestinal tract, and many other viscera.

Clinical Manifestations Common signs include indurated ulcers of the mouth, oropharynx, larynx, and nose; enlarged and draining lymph nodes; lesions of the skin and genitalia; and productive cough, weight loss, dyspnea, and sometimes fever. Paracoccidioidomycosis is acquired only in South America, Central America, and Mexico, but its extreme indolence may delay its recognition until many years after the patient has left the endemic area. Chest radiography most often shows bilateral patchy pneumonia.

Diagnosis Cultures of sputum, pus, and mucosal lesions are often diagnostic. The diagnosis can be made by smear or histologic section, although confirmation by culture is preferable. Serologic tests are useful in suggesting the diagnosis and monitoring the response to therapy.

℞ TREATMENT

Relatively mild cases of paracoccidioidomycosis may be cured by 1 year of treatment with oral ketoconazole or itraconazole (200 to 400 mg daily). More advanced cases are treated with intravenous amphotericin B followed by itraconazole.

PHAEOHYPHOMYCOSIS This is the name given to infections caused by fungi with dark-walled hyphae, excluding those given conventional names like chromoblastomycosis. Although an extraordinary variety of fungi and clinical syndromes are encompassed by this definition, most patients have brain abscess, subcutaneous abscess, or allergic fungal sinusitis. Most of the brain abscesses are due to *Cladosporium trichoides* and occur in previously healthy persons. Subcutaneous abscesses are usually single, arise at the site of minor trauma, and occur in both immunosuppressed and immunocompetent individuals.

Allergic fungal sinusitis develops in patients with allergic rhinitis and presents as an expanding mucoid mass in one or more paranasal sinuses. The tenacious mucus contains eosinophils, Charcot-Leyden crystals, and occasional hyphae. Surgical excision of phaeohyphomycotic lesions is important; the response to antifungal therapy is often unsatisfactory.

PSEUDALLESCHERIASIS **Etiology** Also called *Petriellidium boydii*, *Pseudallescheria boydii* is a mold frequently found in soil. When the fungus is isolated in the imperfect state, it is called *Scedosporium apiospermum*. (The reader is referred to standard textbooks of medical mycology for an explanation of the perfect and imperfect states.)

Pathogenesis and Pathology Wind-borne spores of *P. boydii*, arising from the soil, are the presumed source of infection. The fungus grows as a mold within tissue, causing necrosis and abscess formation.

Clinical Manifestations *P. boydii* resembles *Aspergillus* in its ability to colonize the endobronchial tree, to form fungus balls in the lungs or paranasal sinuses, and to invade the cornea or globe of the eye, the soft tissues, the joints, or the bones following trauma or surgery and in its propensity to invade the lungs and paranasal sinuses of immunosuppressed hosts, including AIDS patients. Hyphae of *P. boydii* in tissue may be difficult to distinguish from those of *Aspergillus*. Infection with *P. boydii* is much less common than that with *Aspergillus*. Nevertheless *P. boydii* is the single most common cause of mycetoma in the United States. Intravascular hyphae, a hallmark of invasive aspergillosis, are also found in pseudallescheriasis. Near-drowning in polluted water has led to severe *P. boydii* pneumonia, often with dissemination and fatal brain abscesses.

Diagnosis Demonstration of hyphae in tissue and culture confirmation are required for diagnosis.

℞ TREATMENT

Therapy with intravenous miconazole, itraconazole, or ketoconazole is recommended, but the response to all drugs has been poor.

Scedosporium prolificans, a fungus closely related to *P. boydii*, has caused infections in bones, joints, or soft tissue, usually following trauma. These infections have responded to surgical debridement. Disseminated infection with *S. prolificans* in immunosuppressed patients has been fatal. The response to treatment with all antifungal agents has been poor.

SPOROTRICHOSIS **Etiology** *Sporothrix schenckii* lives as a saprophyte on plants in many areas of the world. In nature and on culture at room temperature the fungus grows as a mold, but within host tissue or at 37°C on enriched media it grows as a budding yeast. It is identified by its appearance in mold and yeast forms.

Pathogenesis and Pathology Infection results from the inoculation of *S. schenckii* into subcutaneous tissue via minor trauma. Nursery workers, florists, and gardeners acquire the illness from roses, sphagnum moss, and other plants. Infection may be limited to the site of inoculation (plaque sporotrichosis) or extend along proximal lymphatic channels (lymphangitic sporotrichosis). Spread beyond an extremity—the usual site of infection—is rare, and hematogenous dissemination from the skin remains unproven. The portal for osteoarticular, pulmonary, and other extracutaneous forms of sporotrichosis is unknown but is likely the lung.

Untreated sporotrichosis shows little evidence of self-healing and is capable of chronicity. The inflammatory response includes both the clustering of neutrophils and a marked granulomatous response with epithelioid cells and giant cells.

Clinical Manifestations In lymphangitic sporotrichosis, by far the most common manifestation, a nearly painless red papule forms at the site of inoculation. Over the next several weeks, similar nodules form along proximal lymphatic channels. The nodules intermittently discharge small amounts of pus. Ulceration may occur. The proximal extension of these lesions, often with skip areas, is quite distinctive but may be mimicked by lesions of *Nocardia brasiliensis*, *Mycobacterium marinum*, or (in rare cases) *Leishmania braziliensis* or *Mycobacterium kansasii*.

Plaque sporotrichosis manifests as a nontender red maculopapular granuloma confined to the site of inoculation. Osteoarticular sporotrichosis presents as mono- or polyarticular arthritis of indolent onset and progression over months or years, involving the elbows, knees, wrists, ankles, and (rarely) smaller joints of the extremities. Periarticular bone develops areas of demineralization detectable on x-ray, and draining sinuses may appear over joints and bursae. Hematogenous spread to the skin may take place during polyarticular disease, but none of the skin lesions shows lymphangitic spread. Immunosuppression, including advanced infection with human immunodeficiency virus, predisposes to hematogenous spread. Pulmonary sporotrichosis usually presents as a single chronic cavitary upper-lobe lung lesion. Chronic meningitis can develop in the absence of skin or lung lesions. *S. schenckii* is difficult to recover from cerebrospinal fluid.

Diagnosis Culture of pus, joint fluid, sputum, or skin biopsy specimen is the preferred method of diagnosis. The appearance of *S. schenckii* in tissue is quite variable. In skin lesions, the organisms are hard to find.

℞ **TREATMENT**

Cutaneous sporotrichosis can be cured with a saturated solution of potassium iodide given orally in increasing divided daily doses up to 4.5 to 9 mL/d for adults, as tolerated. Gastrointestinal disturbance or acneiform rash over the cape area and face is common, but therapy should be continued for 1 month after the resolution of all lesions. Itraconazole (100 to 200 mg daily) is an effective and better-tolerated alternative. Extracutaneous sporotrichosis rarely responds to iodides, but more than half of cases have been cured by prolonged courses of intravenous amphotericin B. Itraconazole (200 mg once or twice daily) is effective in some cases of extracutaneous sporotrichosis.

TRICHOSPOROSIS *Trichosporon beigelii* causes asymptomatic small white concretions on hair shafts, a condition called *white piedra*, but can also cause hematogenously disseminated infection in neutropenic patients (mostly those with leukemia). Multiple erythematous or purpuric papules accompany the fungemia. The lesions can evolve into large, tense hemorrhagic bullae. Blood cultures are usually positive. Prosthetic-valve endocarditis due to *T. beigelii* has been well described. Intravenous amphotericin B is the drug of choice for the treatment of *T. beigelii* infection.

BIBLIOGRAPHY

AMMARI LK et al: Catheter-related *Fusarium solani* fungemia and pulmonary infection in a patient with leukemia in remission. Clin Infect Dis 16:148, 1993

ARENAS R et al: Open randomized comparison of itraconazole versus terbinafine in onychomycosis. Int J Dermatol 34:138, 1995

BARBER GR et al: Catheter-related *Malassezia furfur* fungemia in immunocompromised patients. Am J Med 95:365, 1993

BOYD AS et al: Cutaneous manifestations of *Prototheca* infections. J Am Acad Dermatol 32:758, 1995

HAY RJ et al: Mycetoma. J Med Vet Mycol 30(Suppl 1):41, 1992

IACOVIELLO VR: Protothecosis complicating prolonged endotracheal intubation: Case report and literature review. Clin Infect Dis 15:959, 1992

MARCON MJ, POWELL DA: Human infections due to *Malassezia* spp. Clin Microbiol Rev 5:101, 1992

MARTINO P et al: Clinical patterns of *Fusarium* infections in immunocompromised patients. J Infect 28(Suppl 1):7, 1994

MEYER RD et al: Fungal sinusitis in patients with AIDS: Report of 4 cases and review of the literature. Medicine 73:69, 1994

NARANJO MS et al: Treatment of paracoccidioidomycosis with itraconazole. J Med Vet Mycol 28:67, 1990

NIELSEN K et al: Disseminated *Scedosporium prolificans* infection in an immunocompromised adolescent. Pediatr Infect Dis J 12:882, 1993

RABODONIRINA M et al: *Fusarium* infections in immunocompromised patients: Case reports and literature review. Eur J Clin Microbiol Infect Dis 13:153, 1994

RESTREPO A: Treatment of tropical mycoses. J Am Acad Dermatol 31:S91, 1994

RUXIN TA et al: *Pseudallescheria boydii* in an immunocompromised host: Successful treatment with debridement and itraconazole. Arch Dermatol 132:382, 1996

SUPPARATPINYO K et al: *Penicillium marneffei* infection in patients infected with human immunodeficiency virus. Clin Infect Dis 14:871, 1992

VARTIVARIAN SE et al: Emerging fungal pathogens in immunocompromised patients: Classification, diagnosis, and management. Clin Infect Dis 17:487, 1993

WINN RE et al: Systemic sporotrichosis treated with itraconazole. Clin Infect Dis 17:210, 1993

WOOLRICH A et al: Cutaneous protothecosis and AIDS. J Am Acad Dermatol 31:920, 1994

211 *Peter D. Walzer*

PNEUMOCYSTIS CARINII INFECTION

DEFINITION AND DESCRIPTION *Pneumocystis carinii* is an opportunistic pathogen whose natural habitat is the lung. The organism is an important cause of pneumonia in the compromised host.

The taxonomy of *P. carinii* has long been controversial; however, recent studies favor its placement in the fungal kingdom. Analysis of gene sequences of ribosomal RNA, mitochondrial proteins, and major enzymes (thymidylate synthase, dihydrofolate reductase) has demonstrated that *P. carinii* is more closely related to fungi than to protozoa. Moreover, biochemical studies have suggested that the cell wall of *P. carinii* contains glucans; drugs that inhibit 1,3-β-glucan synthesis in fungi are highly active against *P. carinii* in animal models. On the basis of this information, *P. carinii* is now considered a fungus in this textbook.

Study of the basic biology of *P. carinii* has been severely hampered by the lack of a reliable in vitro cultivation system. Major developmental stages of the organism include the small (1- to 4-μm) pleomorphic trophozoite or trophic form; the 5- to 8-μm cyst, which has a thick cell wall and contains up to eight intracystic bodies; and the precyst, an intermediate stage. The life cycle of *P. carinii* probably involves asexual replication by the trophic form and sexual reproduction by the cyst, which ends in release of the intracystic bodies; an intracellular stage has not been identified. Ultrastructurally, *P. carinii* has a primitive organelle system, but little is known about its metabolism.

P. carinii contains two prominent antigen groups. The 95- to 140-kDa major surface glycoprotein complex represents a family of proteins encoded by multiple genes. This complex plays a central role in the host-parasite relationship in *P. carinii* infection. The antigen facilitates the adherence of *P. carinii* to lung cells, contains protective epitopes, and is capable of antigenic variation. The other antigen, which migrates as a band of 35 to 55 kDa, is the most common antigen recognized by the host and thus may serve as a marker of infection.

EPIDEMIOLOGY *P. carinii* has a worldwide distribution among humans and has been found in a variety of animals. The organisms found in these hosts are morphologically identical, but molecular and antigenic data indicate that species and/or strain differences exist. Data about the fungal nature of *P. carinii* raise intriguing questions about previously undescribed developmental stages and environmental sources of the organism. Serologic surveys indicate that most healthy children have been exposed to the organism by 3 to 4 years of age. Animal model experiments have demonstrated that *P. carinii* is transmitted by the airborne route. Person-to-person transmission has been suggested by the occurrence of outbreaks of pneumocystosis among institutionalized debilitated infants and in hospitals caring for immunosuppressed patients. On the basis of animal studies, the incubation period is thought to be 4 to 8 weeks.

PATHOGENESIS AND PATHOLOGY *P. carinii* pneumonia occurs in the following hosts: premature, malnourished infants; children with primary immunodeficiency diseases; patients receiving immunosuppressive therapy (particularly glucocorticoids) for cancer, organ transplantation, and other disorders; and people with AIDS. The frequency of pneumocystosis among patients infected with human immunodeficiency virus (HIV) far exceeds that among other immunocompromised hosts. Despite the increased recognition of *P. carinii* and the wider use of chemoprophylaxis against it, the organism remains a leading cause of opportunistic infection and death among AIDS patients in industrialized countries.

Impaired cellular immunity is the major host factor that predisposes to pneumocystosis, although defects in B cell function also play a role. The importance of CD4 + cells in protection from *P. carinii* infection has been shown by studies correlating the risk of pneumocystosis in HIV-infected patients with CD4+ cell counts and by adoptive transfer experiments in animal models. Exposure to *P. carinii* stimulates a potent immune response, and experimental studies have shown that the cytokines tumor necrosis factor α and interleukin 1 play an important role in early host defenses against the organism. It has long been thought that *P. carinii* pneumonia develops by reactivation of latent infection, yet recent molecular evidence suggests that at least some episodes of the disease represent new bouts of infection.

Within the lung, *P. carinii* attaches firmly to the alveolar type I pneumocyte. This process is mediated by several factors, including extracellular proteins (fibronectin) and the mannose receptor. As the host's immune system becomes compromised, *P. carinii* organisms propagate slowly and gradually fill alveoli. These events are accompanied by an increase in alveolar-capillary permeability, a fall in surfactant phospholipids, a rise in surfactant proteins A and D, and damage to the type I cell.

On lung sections stained with hematoxylin and eosin, the alveoli are filled with a typical foamy, vacuolated exudate. Severe disease may include interstitial edema, fibrosis, and hyaline membrane formation. The host inflammatory changes usually consist of hypertrophy of alveolar type II cells, a typical reparative response, and a mild mononuclear cell interstitial infiltrate. Malnourished infants display an intense plasma cell infiltrate that gave the disease its early name: interstitial plasma cell pneumonia.

CLINICAL FEATURES Patients with *P. carinii* pneumonia develop dyspnea, fever, and nonproductive cough. Symptoms in non-AIDS patients often begin after the glucocorticoid dose has been tapered and typically last 1 to 2 weeks. AIDS patients are usually ill for several weeks or longer and have relatively subtle manifestations. However, the clinical picture in individual patients is quite variable, and a high index of suspicion and elicitation of a careful history are key factors in early detection.

Physical findings include tachypnea, tachycardia, and cyanosis, but lung auscultation reveals few abnormalities. The white blood cell count is variable and is usually governed by the patient's underlying disease. Assessment of arterial blood gases demonstrates hypoxia, an increased alveolar-arterial oxygen gradient ($PA_{O_2} - Pa_{O_2}$), and respiratory alkalosis. There also may be changes in pulmonary function test values (diffusing capacity) and increased uptake with nuclear imaging techniques (gallium scan). Elevated serum concentrations of lactate dehydrogenase (LDH) have been reported; they probably reflect lung parenchymal damage but are not specific to *P. carinii* infection. In general, laboratory abnormalities are less severe in AIDS patients than in those without AIDS.

The classic findings on chest radiography consist of bilateral diffuse infiltrates beginning in the perihilar regions, but a variety of atypical manifestations (nodular densities, cavitary lesions) have also been reported. Patients who receive aerosolized pentamidine have an increased frequency of upper-lobe infiltrates and pneumothorax. Early in the course of pneumocystosis, the chest radiograph may be normal.

Although *P. carinii* usually remains confined to the lungs, cases of disseminated infection have occurred in both AIDS and non-AIDS patients. Estimates of the frequency of extrapulmonary pneumocystosis have ranged from <1 to 3 percent. One risk factor in HIV-infected patients appears to be the administration of aerosolized pentamidine. The most common sites of extrapulmonary involvement are the lymph nodes (40 to 50 percent of cases); next in frequency are the spleen, liver, and bone marrow (30 to 40 percent). Other common sites include the gastrointestinal and genitourinary tracts, adrenal and thyroid glands, heart, pancreas, eyes, ears, and skin. Clinical manifestations range from incidental findings at autopsy to specific organ involvement (low-density lesions in the spleen on computed tomography, cotton-wool spots on the retina). Histopathologic examination reveals the presence of *P. carinii* and the characteristic associated foamy material. Treatment for the extrapulmonary forms of pneumocystosis is the same as that for pneumonia.

DIAGNOSIS Since the clinical picture of *P. carinii* infection can be produced by many other infectious and noninfectious agents, the diagnosis must be based on specific identification of the organism. A definitive diagnosis is made by histopathologic staining. Traditional stains have included reagents such as methenamine silver, toluidine blue, and cresyl echt violet, which selectively stain the wall of *P. carinii* cysts, and reagents such as Wright-Giemsa, which stain the nuclei of all developmental stages. Immunofluorescence with monoclonal antibodies is more sensitive than traditional staining but is also more expensive. Other reagents include nonspecific fluorochrome stains (calcofluor white) and Papanicolaou's stain. Selection of staining techniques is largely a matter of personal preference; frequently, more than one reagent is used to make the diagnosis. Molecular probes and the polymerase chain reaction offer promise in the diagnosis of *P. carinii* infection, but little progress has been made with culture or with antigen and antibody detection techniques.

Successful diagnosis of pneumocystosis requires an aggressive approach to the collection of proper specimens. In general, the yield from different diagnostic procedures is higher in AIDS patients than in non-AIDS patients, probably because of the higher organism burden in people with AIDS. In recent years, sputum induction has gained popularity as a simple, noninvasive technique; this procedure requires trained and dedicated personnel, and its success has varied at different institutions. Fiberoptic bronchoscopy with bronchoalveolar lavage (BAL), which is more sensitive and invasive than sputum induction, remains the mainstay of *P. carinii* diagnosis. This procedure provides information about the organism burden, the host inflammatory response, and the presence of other opportunistic infections. Transbronchial biopsy and open lung biopsy, which are the most invasive procedures, are reserved for situations in which a diagnosis cannot be made by lavage.

COURSE AND PROGNOSIS In the typical case of untreated *P. carinii* pneumonia, progressive respiratory embarrassment leads to death. Therapy is most effective when instituted early in the course of the disease, before there is extensive alveolar damage. The most widely used prognostic indicators have been the arterial oxygen pressure and the alveolar-arterial oxygen gradient. Other factors that may influence survival include the organism burden, percentage of neutrophils in BAL fluid, chest radiographic abnormalities, serum LDH and albumin levels, and the expertise of the hospital in caring for AIDS patients. Concurrent pulmonary infections also complicate management, but the presence of cytomegalovirus does not usually affect the outcome of pneumocystosis.

℞ TREATMENT

Trimethoprim-sulfamethoxazole (TMP-SMZ), which acts by inhibiting folic acid synthesis, is considered the drug of choice for all forms of pneumocystosis. TMP-SMZ is administered orally or intravenously at a dosage of 15 to 20 mg of TMP/kg per day and 75 to 100 mg of SMZ/kg per day in three or four divided doses. This agent is well tolerated by non-AIDS patients, but more than half of AIDS patients experience serious adverse reactions, including fever, rash, neutropenia, thrombocytopenia, hepatitis, and hyperkalemia.

The other major drug used to treat *P. carinii* pneumonia is pentamidine isethionate. Although pentamidine has been available for many years, its mode of action against *P. carinii* is unclear. Pentamidine is given as a single dose of 4 mg/kg per day by slow intravenous infusion. Pentamidine is about as effective as TMP-SMZ but is toxic for almost all recipients. Its principal adverse effects are hypotension, cardiac arrhythmia, dysglycemia, azotemia, electrolyte changes, and neutropenia.

Several regimens have been developed for patients in whom therapy with TMP-SMZ or pentamidine is unsuccessful or intolerable. TMP plus dapsone, clindamycin plus primaquine, and atovaquone are less toxic oral regimens that are used in mild to moderate pneumocystosis. Parenteral trimetrexate has been used in severe disease.

Treatment of *P. carinii* pneumonia should be continued for 14 days in non-AIDS patients and for 21 days in persons with AIDS.

Since AIDS patients respond more slowly than non-AIDS patients, it is prudent to wait at least 7 days before concluding that therapy has failed. The addition of drugs to an existing regimen is no more effective than switching regimens and may increase the risk of toxicity.

There is increasing evidence that the host's inflammatory or immune response contributes to lung damage in *P. carinii* pneumonia, but the mechanisms involved are poorly understood. Several studies have shown that the administration of glucocorticoids to AIDS patients with moderate to severe pneumocystosis (a P_{O_2} of ≤ 70 mmHg or a $PA_{O_2} - Pa_{O_2}$ of ≥ 35 mmHg) can prevent the early deterioration in respiratory function that frequently occurs after antimicrobial therapy and can improve the rate of survival. The administration of steroids should be started early in the course of the illness (usually when antimicrobial drugs are begun) for maximal benefit; the recommended regimen is 40 mg of prednisone orally twice daily, with tapering to a dose of 20 mg/d over a 3-week period. This regimen has generally proven to be safe despite concern about its effects on other opportunistic infections and Kaposi's sarcoma. The use of steroids as adjunctive therapy in non-AIDS patients remains to be evaluated.

Other important measures include the maintenance of oxygenation, nutrition, and electrolyte balance. Admission to the intensive care unit and mechanical ventilation (if instituted promptly) can improve the survival rate for patients who develop respiratory failure.

PREVENTION Primary prophylaxis is indicated for HIV-infected patients at high risk of developing pneumocystosis—that is, those who have CD4+ cell counts of $<200/\mu L$, unexplained fever [$>37.8°C$ ($>100°F$)] for ≥ 2 weeks, or a history of oropharyngeal candidiasis. Guidelines for the administration of primary prophylaxis to other immunocompromised hosts are less clear. Secondary prophylaxis is indicated for all patients who have recovered from *P. carinii* pneumonia. Among AIDS patients, the risk of recurrent episodes of pneumocystosis is high and lifelong; among non-AIDS patients, the risk is lower and exists for as long as the immunosuppressive condition persists.

One double-strength tablet of TMP-SMZ (160 mg of TMP, 800 mg of SMZ) per day is the prophylactic regimen of choice. The major limitation of TMP-SMZ is the high frequency of adverse reactions among HIV-infected patients. Recommended alternative regimens include TMP-SMZ at a reduced dose or frequency; dapsone alone; dapsone, pyrimethamine, and leucovorin; and aerosolized pentamidine (administered in a Respirgard II nebulizer).

Although there are no specific recommendations for preventing the spread of *P. carinii* in health care facilities, it seems prudent to prevent direct contact between patients with pneumocystosis and other susceptible hosts.

BIBLIOGRAPHY

BAUGHMAN RP: Current methods of diagnosis, in *Pneumocystis carinii Pneumonia*, P Walzer (ed). New York, Dekker, 1994, pp 381–401

BENNETT CL et al: The learning curve for AIDS-related *Pneumocystis carinii* pneumonia: Experience from 3981 cases in Veterans Affairs Hospitals 1987–1991. J Acquir Immun Defic Syndr Hum Retrovirol 8:373, 1995

CARTWRIGHT CP et al: Development and evaluation of a rapid and simple procedure for detection of *Pneumocystis carinii* by PCR. J Clin Microbiol 32:1634, 1994

HOFFMAN OA et al: *Pneumocystis carinii* stimulates tumor necrosis factor alpha release from alveolar macrophages through a beta-glucan-mediated mechanism. J Immunol 150:3932, 1993

HUGHES W et al: Comparison of atovaquone (566C80) with trimethoprim-sulfamethoxazole for the treatment of *Pneumocystis carinii* pneumonia in patients with AIDS. N Engl J Med 328:1521, 1993

KEELY SP et al: Genetic variation among *Pneumocystis carinii hominis* isolates in recurrent pneumocystosis. J Infect Dis 172:595, 1995

MASUR H: Drug therapy: Prevention and treatment of pneumocystis pneumonia. N Engl J Med 327:1853, 1992

NATIONAL INSTITUTES OF HEALTH—UNIVERSITY OF CALIFORNIA EXPERT PANEL FOR CORTICOSTEROIDS AS ADJUNCTIVE THERAPY FOR PNEUMOCYSTIS PNEUMONIA: Consensus statement on the use of corticosteroids as adjunctive therapy for pneumocystis pneumonia in the acquired immunodeficiency syndrome. N Engl J Med 323:1500, 1990

PEGLOW SL et al: Serologic responses to *Pneumocystis carinii* in health and disease. J Infect Dis 161:296, 1990

PHAIR J et al: The risk of *Pneumocystis carinii* pneumonia among men infected with human immunodeficiency virus type 1. N Engl J Med 322:161, 1990

SATTLER FR et al: Comparison of trimetrexate with leucovorin versus trimethoprim-sulfamethoxazole for moderate-to-severe episodes of *Pneumocystis carinii* pneumonia in patients with AIDS: A prospective, controlled multicenter investigation of the AIDS Clinical Trials Group protocol 029/031. J Infect Dis 170:165, 1994

SMULIAN AG et al: Analysis of *Pneumocystis carinii* organism burden, viability and antigens in bronchoalveolar lavage fluid in AIDS patients with pneumocystosis: Correlation with disease severity. AIDS 8:1555, 1994

STERNBERG RI et al: *Pneumocystis carinii* alters surfactant protein A concentrations in bronchoalveolar lavage fluid. J Lab Clin Med 125:462, 1995

TELZAK EE et al: Extrapulmonary *Pneumocystis carinii* infections. Rev Infect Dis 12:380, 1990

THEUS SA et al: Adoptive transfer of lymphocytes sensitized to the major surface glycoprotein of *Pneumocystis carinii* confers protection in the rat. J Clin Invest 95:2587, 1995

US PUBLIC HEALTH SERVICE/INFECTIOUS DISEASES SOCIETY OF AMERICA: Guidelines for the prevention of opportunistic infections in persons infected with human immunodeficiency virus: A summary. Morb Mort Week Rep 44(RR-8):1, 1995

WADA M et al: Antigenic variation by positional control of major surface glycoprotein gene expression in *Pneumocystis carinii*. J Infect Dis 171:1563, 1995

WALZER PD: *Pneumocystis carinii:* Recent advances in basic biology and their clinical application. AIDS 7:1293, 1993

SECTION 16
PROTOZOAL AND HELMINTHIC INFECTIONS: GENERAL CONSIDERATIONS

212	*Peter F. Weller*

APPROACH TO THE PATIENT WITH PARASITIC INFECTION

Because of the diversity of parasitic organisms that may infect humans, a range of factors are germane to an assessment of the possible parasitic etiology of a patient's disease. These factors include issues related to the patient's history, immune status, and presenting clinical and laboratory characteristics, especially eosinophilia. Complementing historical and immunologic information, a full clinical evaluation and laboratory testing provide additional data to direct the assessment for parasitic infection. The specific tests required, ranging from standard blood biochemical assays to imaging of selected organs, are dictated by the nature of the patient's illness. Additional diagnostic testing for parasitic infections (Chap. 213) completes the evaluation.

HISTORY Geographic History The history can provide valuable information about potential exposures to parasitic infections. A history of travel to, residence or work in, or immigration from areas of the world in which various parasites not endemic in the United States are encountered offers a clue to possible parasitic etiologies of a patient's disease. Some parasitic infections may become manifest early after a traveler's return home; paramount among these in terms of preventable mortality is malaria. If a patient has been in a region of the world where malaria is endemic (even only briefly, as in an airport layover), fever mandates a consideration of malaria, whether or not malaria chemoprophylaxis has been used. Falciparum malaria, which in a nonimmune patient may progress rapidly to serious and even life-threatening consequences (Chap. 216), is a potential medical emergency and must be considered at the initial evaluation, even if symptoms and fever patterns are suggestive of less specific flulike or gastrointestinal illness. Rarely, malaria transmission has been reported within the United States.

For patients with a history of recent travel, the onset of gastrointestinal symptoms only after return suggests protozoal diseases characterized by a 1- to 2-week delay between acquisition and appearance of symptoms—notably, giardiasis and cryptosporidiosis (Chap. 220). Gastrointestinal symptoms lasting longer than a week also suggest protozoan etiologies, including giardiasis, amebiasis, and cyclosporiasis. For patients who have traveled less recently, information on the specific countries and the types of regions (urban or rural) visited and on the nature and duration of the visit, whether for general tourism or for activities related to specific occupations, is helpful in concert with presenting clinical features and hematologic and other laboratory findings. Diseases that may become manifest only some years after an individual leaves an endemic region include schistosomiasis, some forms of filariasis, strongyloidiasis, echinococcosis, and cysticercosis.

For the illnesses of patients who have never left the United States, various parasitic etiologies should be considered, depending on the presenting disease. Trichomoniasis, trichinosis, strongyloidiasis, giardiasis, cryptosporidiosis, cyclosporiasis, echinococcosis, and pinworm are among the parasitic infections endemic in settings within the United States. Diseases that are more frequent where there is fecal contamination of soil or other environmental sites include hookworm, ascariasis, trichuriasis, amebiasis, and strongyloidiasis; dermal exposure, as by walking barefoot on soil contaminated with parasitic larvae, predisposes to the acquisition of cutaneous larva migrans, hookworm, and strongyloides by residents of such an area as well as by travelers.

Dietary History If more than one patient develops similar symptoms in a given situation, common-source waterborne diseases (giardiasis, cryptosporidiosis, cyclosporiasis) should be considered. These infections are more likely to be acquired from surface water supplies, ranging from mountain streams to municipal reservoirs. Likewise, attention to dietary history may be helpful. Trichinosis should be considered when the patient may have consumed contaminated pork, bear, walrus, or other meat from carnivores. Ingestion of undercooked fish predisposes to anisakiasis and to infection with other fish-dwelling nematodes, tapeworms (*Diphyllobothrium latum*), or flukes (*Nanophyetus salmincola*). Ingestion of snails or of produce contaminated with land snails can lead to infection with *Angiostrongylus cantonensis* (eosinophilic meningitis; Chap. 221). Ingestion of more exotic animal foodstuffs, including snakes, can result in the transmission of gnathostomiasis (Chap. 221). For children with a propensity for pica, ingestion of soil containing *Toxocara* eggs may lead to visceral larva migrans. Rarely, eosinophilic meningitis due to *Baylisascaris procyonis* has also been described. Consumption of ground-grown vegetables, including those shipped in from distant fields contaminated with human feces, provides an opportunity for the ingestion of nematode eggs of *Ascaris lumbricoides* or *Trichuris trichiura*.

Other Exposure Histories An antecedent blood transfusion raises the possibility of malaria (especially that due to *Plasmodium malariae* or *Plasmodium falciparum*), babesiosis, or Chagas' disease. A history of wading or swimming in fresh water is germane to the acquisition of schistosomiasis or avian schistosome dermatitis. Fresh water may be a source of infection with free-living amebae, and these protozoa may cause ocular infections, especially in persons wearing contact lenses. Arthropod vector–borne parasitic infections include malaria and lymphatic filariasis (carried by mosquitoes) and babesiosis (carried by ticks); the latter is transmitted in some regions of the United States.

Residence in an institutional setting where fecal-oral hygiene may be imperfect raises the possibility of giardiasis, cryptosporidiosis, or strongyloidiasis. Child-care centers provide opportunities for young children and their family members to acquire giardiasis, cryptosporidiosis, and pinworm infections. Trichomoniasis is transmitted sexually; giardiasis, cryptosporidiosis, amebiasis, and strongyloidiasis can be transmitted during anal intercourse or oral-anal contact.

IMMUNE STATUS The patient's immune status is relevant in determining which parasitic infections need to be considered. In patients infected with human immunodeficiency virus type 1, especially those with depressed CD4+ lymphocyte counts, specific protozoan diseases may develop opportunistically. These infections include toxoplasmosis, isosporiasis, cyclosporiasis, cryptosporidiosis, visceral leishmaniasis, American trypanosomiasis, microsporidiosis, and infections with free-living amebae (*Acanthamoeba* and related genera). In individuals infected with human T-lymphotropic virus type 1, strongyloidiasis is a prominent consideration. Patients who are asplenic are at risk not only for overwhelming infections due to encapsulated bacteria but also for fulminant infections caused by intraerythrocytic protozoa, including malaria and babesiosis. Patients with hypogammaglobulinemia or cystic fibrosis may develop refractory giardiasis. In patients developing symptoms of enterocolitis while receiving glucocorticoids, the possibility of an exacerbation of unsuspected strongyloidiasis or amebic colitis should be considered.

EOSINOPHILIA The role of eosinophilia in the evaluation for parasitic infection is worth mentioning. Eosinophilia offers a hematologic clue to the presence of some parasites. Only two protozoan parasites have been associated with eosinophilia: *Isospora belli* and, on occasion, *Dientamoeba fragilis*. In the latter instance, eosinophilia may be due in part to concomitant infection with pinworms. Thus the detection of eosinophilia generally mandates a consideration of the multicellular helminthic parasites that characteristically elicit this abnormality. (Helminth-elicited eosinophilia, however, may be suppressed by glucocorticoid therapy or by intercurrent bacterial or viral infections.) The magnitude of eosinophilia tends to correlate with the extent of tissue invasion by helminths. Marked blood eosinophilia (more than 3000 eosinophils per microliter) develops during the early transpulmonary migration of intestinal nematodes, including *Ascaris* and hookworms, at a time when eggs (whose presence confirms the diagnosis) have not yet been produced in the intestinal tract. Eosinophilia is also marked in the early stages of fluke infections, including schistosomiasis (Katayama fever), paragonimiasis, clonorchiasis, and fascioliasis; during the stage of muscle invasion in trichinosis; during tissue migration of adult worms in loiasis and gnathostomiasis; and with heavy infections in visceral larva migrans. Eosinophilia persisting for more than a year may be indicative of hookworm infection, strongyloidiasis, visceral larva migrans (especially in children), filarial infection (including onchocerciasis, loiasis, and tropical pulmonary eosinophilia), fluke infections (including schistosomiasis, fascioliasis, clonorchiasis, and paragonimiasis), and cysticercosis. Leakage of fluids from echinococcal cysts can cause intermittent increases in eosinophilia. Eosinophilia sometimes provides the only clue to the presence of helminthic infection and should prompt an evaluation for such infection. Serologic testing for schistosomiasis, filariasis, visceral larva migrans, and strongyloidiasis will be helpful in an assessment for some of the diseases most likely to elicit eosinophilia. Serologic evaluation for strongyloidiasis is especially important since autoinfection may permit persistence of the organisms for decades and put the patient at risk for disseminated disease if immunosuppressive glucocorticoids are later administered for any reason.

BIBLIOGRAPHY

GYORKOS TW et al: Seroepidemiology of *Strongyloides* infection in the Southeast Asian refugee population in Canada. Am J Epidemiol 132:257, 1990

——— et al: Intestinal parasite infection in the Kampuchean refugee population 6 years after resettlement in Canada. J Infect Dis 166:413, 1992

KAPPUS KD et al: Intestinal parasitism in the United States: Update on a continuing problem. Am J Trop Med Hyg 50:705, 1994

LIBMAN MD et al: Screening for schistosomiasis, filariasis, and strongyloidiasis among expatriates returning from the tropics. Clin Infect Dis 17:353, 1993

MANNHEIMER SB, SOAVE R: Protozoal infections in patients with AIDS. Cryptosporidiosis, isosporiasis, cyclosporiasis, and microsporidiosis. Infect Dis Clin North Am 8:483, 1994

PRATLONG F et al: Leishmania–human immunodeficiency virus coinfection in the Mediterranean basin: Isoenzymatic characterization of 100 isolates of the Leishmania infantum complex. J Infect Dis 172:323, 1995

SELIK RM et al: Trends in infectious diseases and cancers among persons dying of HIV infection in the United States from 1987 to 1992. Ann Intern Med 123:933, 1995

SUN T: Current topics in protozoal diseases. Am J Clin Pathol 102:16, 1994

SVENSON JE et al: Imported malaria. Clinical presentation and examination of symptomatic travelers. Arch Intern Med 155:861, 1995

WELLER PF: Eosinophilia in travelers. Med Clin North Am 76:1413, 1992

213 · Charles E. Davis

LABORATORY DIAGNOSIS OF PARASITIC INFECTIONS

The cornerstone for the diagnosis of parasitic infections is a thorough history of the patient's illness. Epidemiologic aspects of the illness are especially important because the risks of acquiring many parasites are closely related to occupation, recreation, or travel to areas of high endemicity. Without a basic knowledge of the epidemiology and life cycles of the major parasites, it is difficult to approach the diagnosis of parasitic infections systematically. Accordingly, the medical classi-

Table 213-1

Flatworm Infections

Parasite	Geographic Distribution	Life-Cycle Hosts Intermediate (Transmission)	Life-Cycle Hosts Definitive	Parasite Stage	Diagnosis Body Fluid or Tissue	Diagnosis Serologic Tests	Diagnosis Other
TAPEWORMS (CESTODES)							
Intestinal tapeworms							
Taenia saginata (beef tapeworm)	Worldwide	Beef	Humans	Ova, segments	Feces	—	Motile segments
Hymenolepis nana (dwarf tapeworm)	Worldwide	Grain beetles	Humans, mice*	Ova	Feces	—	—
Diphyllobothrium latum (fish tapeworm)	Worldwide	Copepods–fish‡	Humans, other mammals	Ova, segments	Feces	—	Megaloblastic anemia in 1%
Taenia solium† (pork tapeworm)	Worldwide	Swine	Humans	Ova, segments	Feces	WB	Especially Mexico, Central and South America, Africa
Somatic tapeworms							
Echinococcus granulosus (hydatid disease)	Sheep-raising and hunting areas	Sheep, camels, humans, others	Dogs	Hydatid	Lung, liver	WB	Chest radiography, CT, MRI
Echinococcus multilocularis (hydatid disease)	Subarctic areas	Rodents, humans	Foxes, dogs, cats	Hydatid	Liver		May resemble cholangiocellular carcinoma
Taenia solium† (pork tapeworm)	Worldwide	Swine, humans	Humans	Cysticercus	Muscles, CNS	WB	CT, MRI, radiography
FLUKES (TREMATODES)							
Intestinal flukes							
Fasciolopsis buski	China, India	Snails–water chestnuts	Humans	Ova	Feces	—	—
Heterophyes heterophyes	Far East, India	Snails–fish	Humans	Ova	Feces	—	—
Metagonimus yokogawai	Focal in Europe and North Africa	Snails–fish	Humans	Ova	Feces	—	—
Liver flukes							
Clonorchis sinensis	China, Southeast Asia	Snails–fish	Humans	Ova	Feces, bile	—	Recurrent bacterial cholangitis
Fasciola hepatica	Sheep-raising areas	Snails–watercress	Humans, sheep	Ova	Feces, bile	—	Cirrhosis, portal hypertension
Lung flukes							
Paragonimus spp.	Orient, Africa, South America	Snails–crabs/crayfish	Humans, other mammals	Adults, ova	Lung, sputum, CNS	WB	Chest radiography, CT, MRI
Blood flukes							
Schistosoma mansoni	Africa, Central and South America, West Indies	Snails	Humans	Ova, adults	Feces	EIA, WB	Rectal snips, liver biopsy
Schistosoma haematobium	Africa	Snails	Humans	Ova, adults	Urine	EIA, WB	Liver, urine, or bladder biopsy
Schistosoma japonicum	Far East	Snails	Humans	Ova, adults	Feces	EIA, WB	Liver biopsy

* Larvae also can mature in intestinal villi of humans and mice.

† *T. solium* can cause either intestinal infections or cysticercosis. Its ova are identical to those of *T. saginata*; scolices and segments of the two species differ.

‡ When there are two intermediate hosts, the first is separated from the second by a dash. Definitive hosts are infected by the second intermediate host.

NOTE: WB, western blot; CT, computed tomography; MRI, magnetic resonance imaging; CNS, central nervous system; EIA, enzyme immunoassay. Serologic tests listed in Tables 213-1, 213-2, and 213-3 are available from the Centers for Disease Control and Prevention, Atlanta, GA.

fication of important human parasites in this chapter emphasizes their geographic distribution, their transmission, and the anatomic location and stages of their life cycle in humans. The text and tables are intended to serve as a guide to the correct diagnostic procedures for the major parasitic infections and to direct the reader to other chapters that contain more comprehensive information about each infection. Tables 213-1, 213-2, and 213-3 summarize the geographic distributions, the anatomic locations, and the laboratory methods employed for the diagnosis of flatworm, roundworm, and protozoal infections, respectively.

In addition to selecting the correct diagnostic procedures, physicians must counsel their patients to ensure that specimens are collected properly and arrive at the laboratory promptly. For example, the diagnosis of bancroftian filariasis is unlikely to be confirmed by laboratory personnel unless blood is drawn near midnight, when the nocturnal

microfilariae are active. Laboratory personnel and surgical pathologists should be notified in advance when a parasitic infection is suspected. Continuing interaction with the laboratory staff and the surgical pathologists increases the likelihood that parasites in body fluids or biopsy specimens will be examined carefully by the most capable individuals.

INTESTINAL PARASITES Most helminths and protozoa exit the body in the fecal stream. The patient or the patient's attendant should be instructed to collect feces in a clean cardboard container and to record the time of collection on the container. Contamination with water, which could contain free-living protozoa, or with urine should be avoided. Fecal samples should be collected before ingestion of barium or other contrast agents for radiologic procedures and before treatment with antidiarrheal agents and antacids, because these substances change the consistency of the feces and interfere with microscopic detection of parasites. Because of the cyclic shedding of most parasites in the feces, a minimum of three samples collected on alternate days should be examined. When delays in transport to the laboratory are unavoidable or specimens must be shipped by mail, fecal

Table 213-2

Roundworm Infections

Parasite	Geographic Distribution	Intermediate (Transmission)	Definitive	Parasite Stage	Body Fluid or Tissue	Serologic Tests	Other
INTESTINAL ROUNDWORMS							
Enterobius vermicularis (pinworm)	Temperate and tropical zones	Fecal-oral	Humans	Ova	Perianal skin	—	"Scotch tape" test
Trichuris trichiura (whipworm)	Temperate and tropical zones	Soil, fecal-oral	Humans	Ova	Feces	—	Rectal prolapse
Ascaris lumbricoides (roundworm of humans)	Temperate and tropical zones	Soil, fecal-oral	Humans	Ova	Feces	—	Sx of pulmonary migration
Ancylostoma duodenale (Old World hookworm)	Eurasia, Africa, Pacific	Soil→skin	Humans	Ova/larvae	Feces	—	Sx of pulmonary migration, anemia
Necator americanus (New World hookworm)	U.S., Africa, worldwide	Soil→skin	Humans	Ova/larvae	Feces	—	Sx of pulmonary migration, anemia
Strongyloides stercoralis (strongyloidiasis)	Moist tropics and subtropics	Soil→skin	Humans	Larvae	Feces, sputum, duodenal fluid	EIA	Dissemination in immunodeficiency
TISSUE ROUNDWORMS							
Trichinella spiralis (trichinosis)	Worldwide	Swine/humans	Swine/humans	Larvae	Muscle	BF, EIA	Muscle biopsy
Wuchereria bancrofti (filariasis)	Coastal areas in tropics and subtropics	Mosquitoes	Humans	Microfilariae	Blood, lymph nodes	—	Nocturnal periodicity*
Brugia malayi (filariasis)	Asia, Indian subcontinent	Mosquitoes	Humans	Microfilariae	Blood	—	Nocturnal
Loa loa (African eye worm)	West and Central Africa	Mango flies (*Chrysops*)	Humans	Microfilariae	Blood	—	May be visible in eye, diurnal
Onchocerca volvulus (river blindness)	Africa, Mexico, Central and South America	Blackflies	Humans	Adults/larvae	Skin/eye	—	Examine nodules or skin snips
Dracunculus medinensis (guinea worm)	Orient, Africa, West Indies, Brazil	Cyclops	Humans	Adults/larvae	Skin	—	May be visible in lesion
LARVA MIGRANS SYNDROMES							
Ancylostoma braziliense (creeping eruption)	Tropical and temperate zones	Soil→skin	Dogs/cats, humans	Larvae	Skin	—	Dog and cat hookworm
Toxocara canis and *cati* (visceral larva migrans)	Tropical and temperate zones	Soil, fecal-oral	Dogs/cats, humans	Larvae	Viscera, CNS, eye	EIA†	Also caused by roundworms of other species

* Blood should be drawn at midnight, except for infection acquired in the South Pacific.
† The presence of hemagglutinins is a useful clue.
NOTE: BF, bentonite flocculation; Sx, signs/symptoms; EIA, enzyme immunoassay; CNS, central nervous system.

samples should be kept in polyvinyl alcohol to preserve protozoal trophozoites. Refrigeration also will preserve trophozoites for a few hours and protozoal cysts and helminthic ova for several days.

Analysis of fecal samples consists of both a macroscopic and a microscopic examination. Watery or loose stools are more likely to contain protozoal trophozoites, but protozoal cysts and all stages of helminths may be found in formed feces. If adult worms or tapeworm segments are observed, they should be transported promptly to the laboratory or washed and preserved in fixative for later examination. The only tapeworm with motile segments is *Taenia saginata*, the beef tapeworm, which patients will sometimes bring to the physician.

Motility is an important distinguishing characteristic, because the ova of *T. saginata* and *Taenia solium*, the cause of cysticercosis, are morphologically indistinguishable.

Microscopic examination of feces (Table 213-4) is not complete until direct wet mounts have been evaluated and concentration techniques as well as permanent stains have been applied. Before accepting a report of negativity for ova and parasites as final, the physician should insist that the laboratory undertake each of these procedures.

Table 213-3

Protozoal Infections

Parasite	Geographic Distribution	Life-Cycle Hosts Intermediate (Transmission)	Definitive	Parasite Stage	Body Fluid or Tissue	Serologic Tests	Other
INTESTINAL PROTOZOANS							
Entamoeba histolytica (amebiasis)	Worldwide, especially tropics	Fecal-oral	Humans	Troph, cyst	Feces, liver	ID, EIA, IHA, antigen detection	Ultrasound, liver CT
Giardia lamblia (giardiasis)	Worldwide	Fecal-oral	Humans	Troph, cyst	Feces	Antigen detection	String test
Isospora belli	Worldwide	Fecal-oral	Humans	Oocyst	Feces	—	Acid-fast
Cryptosporidium	Worldwide	Fecal-oral	Humans, other animals	Oocyst	Feces	Antigen detection	Acid-fast, biopsy, PCR
Enterocytozoon bieneusi (microsporidiosis)	Worldwide?	?	Animals, humans	Spore	Feces	—	Modified trichrome, biopsy, PCR
FREE-LIVING AMEBAS							
Naegleria	Worldwide	Warm water	Humans	Troph, cyst	CNS, nares	—	Biopsy, nasal swab
Acanthamoeba	Worldwide	Soil, water	Humans	Troph, cyst	CNS, skin, cornea	—	Biopsy, scrapings
BLOOD AND TISSUE PROTOZOANS							
Plasmodium spp. (malaria)	Subtropics and tropics	Mosquitoes	Humans	Asexual	Blood	Little use	PCR
Babesia microti (babesiosis)	U.S., especially New England	Ticks	Rodents, humans	Asexual	Blood	IIF	Animal spp. in asplenia
Trypanosoma rhodesiense (African sleeping sickness)	Sub-Saharan East Africa	Tsetse flies	Humans, herbivores	Tryp	Blood, CSF	Card agglutination, IIF*	Also chancre, lymph nodes
Trypanosoma gambiense (African sleeping sickness)	Sub-Saharan West Africa	Tsetse flies	Humans, swine	Tryp	Blood, CSF	Card agglutination, IIF*	Also chancre, lymph nodes
Trypanosoma cruzi (Chagas' disease)	Mexico→ South America	Reduviid bugs (triatomes)	Humans, dogs, wild animals	Amastigote, tryp	Multiple organs/ blood	CF, IIF, EIA	Reactivation in immunosuppression
Leishmania tropica, etc.	Widespread in tropics and subtropics	Sandflies (*Phlebotomus*)	Humans, dogs, rodents	Amastigote	Skin	IFA†	Biopsy, scraping, culture
Leishmania braziliensis (mucocutaneous)	Mexico→ South America	Sandflies (*Lutzomyia*)	Humans, dogs, rodents	Amastigote	Skin, mucous membranes	IFA†	Biopsy, scraping, culture
Leishmania donovani (kala-azar)	Widespread in tropics and subtropics	Sandflies (*Phlebotomus*)	Humans, dogs, wild animals	Amastigote	RE system	IFA†	Biopsy, culture
Toxoplasma gondii (toxoplasmosis)	Worldwide	Humans, other mammals	Cats	Cyst, troph	CNS, eye, muscles, other	EIA, IIF	Reactivation in immunosuppression

* Card agglutination provided to endemic countries by the World Health Organization; IIF available intermittently—contact the WHO or the CDC.
† Limited specificity. Most sensitive for *L. donovani* (kala-azar).

NOTE: ID, immunodiffusion by commercial kit (not available from the CDC); IHA, indirect hemagglutination; CT, computed tomography; CF, complement fixation; troph, trophozoite; tryp, trypomastigote form; IIF, indirect immunofluorescence; RE, reticuloendothelial; PCR, polymerase chain reaction; EIA, enzyme immunoassay.

Table 213-4

Laboratory Diagnosis of Parasites Found in Feces*

Parasites and Fecal Stages	Alternative Diagnostic Procedures
TAPEWORMS (CESTODES)	
Taenia saginata ova and segments	Perianal "Scotch tape" test for ova
Hymenolepis nana ova	None
Diphyllobothrium ova and segments	None
Taenia solium ova and segments	Brain biopsy for neurocysticercosis; serology
FLUKES (TREMATODES)	
Fasciolopsis buski ova	None
Heterophyes heterophyes ova	None
Metagonimus yokogawai ova	None
Clonorchis (Opisthorchis) sinensis ova	Examination of bile for ova and adults in cholangitis
Fasciola hepatica ova	Examination of bile for ova and adults in cholangitis
Paragonimus spp. ova	Sputum; biopsy of lung or brain for ova; serology
Schistosoma ova	Rectal snips (especially for *S. mansoni*), urine (*S. haematobium*), liver biopsy and serology for all
ROUNDWORMS	
Enterobius vermicularis ova and adults	Perianal "Scotch tape" test for ova and adults
Trichuris trichiura ova	None
Ascaris lumbricoides ova and adults	Examination of sputum for larvae in lung disease
Hookworm ova and occasional larvae	Examination of sputum for larvae in lung disease
Strongyloides larvae	Duodenal aspirate or jejunal biopsy; sputum or lung biopsy for filariform larvae in disseminated disease; serology
Capillaria philippinensis ova†	None
PROTOZOANS	
Entamoeba histolytica trophozoites and cysts	Liver biopsy for trophozoites; serology
Giardia lamblia trophozoites and cysts	Duodenal aspirate or jejunal biopsy‡
Isospora belli oocysts	Duodenal aspirate or jejunal biopsy‡
Cryptosporidium oocysts	Duodenal aspirate or jejunal biopsy‡
Enterocytozoon bieneusi spores	Duodenal aspirate or jejunal biopsy‡

* Stains and concentration techniques are discussed in the text.
† Can be confused with *Trichuris trichiura*.
‡ Commercial string test or Crosby capsule are satisfactory; *Isospora* and *Cryptosporidium* are acid-fast.

Some intestinal parasites are more readily detected in material other than feces. For example, use of the string test (or one of its commercial substitutes) to sample duodenal contents is sometimes necessary to detect *Giardia lamblia*, *Cryptosporidium*, and *Strongyloides* larvae. Use of the "Scotch tape" technique to detect pinworm ova on the perianal skin sometimes also reveals ova of *T. saginata* deposited perianally when the motile segments disintegrate (see Table 213-4).

Two routine solutions are used to make wet mounts for the identification of the various life stages of helminths and protozoa: physiologic saline for trophozoites, cysts, ova, and larvae and dilute iodine solution for protozoal cysts and ova. Iodine solution must never be used to examine specimens for trophozoites because it kills the parasites and thus eliminates their characteristic motility.

The two most common concentration procedures for detecting small numbers of cysts and ova are formalin-ether sedimentation and zinc sulfate flotation. The formalin-ether technique is preferable, because all parasites sediment but not all float. Slides permanently stained for trophozoites should be prepared before concentration. Additional slides stained for cysts and ova may be made from the concentrate.

In many instances, especially in the differentiation of *Entamoeba histolytica* from other amebas, identification of parasites from wet mounts or concentrates must be considered tentative. Permanently stained smears allow study of the cellular detail necessary for definitive identification. The iron-hematoxylin stain is excellent for critical work, but the trichrome stain, which can be completed in 1 h, is a satisfactory alternative that also stains parasites in specimens preserved in polyvinyl alcohol fixative.

BLOOD AND TISSUE PARASITES Invasion of tissue by protozoa and helminths renders the choice of diagnostic techniques more difficult. For example, physicians must understand that aspiration of an amebic liver abscess rarely reveals *E. histolytica* because the trophozoites are located primarily in the abscess wall. They must remember that the urine sediment offers the best opportunity to detect *Schistosoma haematobium* in the Ethiopian youngster or the American traveler who returns from Africa with hematuria (Table 213-5). Tables 213-1, 213-2, and 213-3, which offer a quick guide to the geographic distribution and anatomic locations of the major tissue parasites, should help the physician to select the appropriate body fluid or biopsy site for microscopic examination. Tables 213-5, 213-6, and 213-7 provide additional information about the identification of parasites in samples from specific anatomic locations. The laboratory procedures for detection of parasites in other body fluids are similar to those used in the examination of feces. The physician should insist on wet mounts, concentration techniques, and permanent stains for all body fluids. The trichrome or iron-hematoxylin stains are satisfactory for all tissue helminths in body fluids other than blood, but microfilarial worms and blood protozoa are more easily visualized when stained with Giemsa or Wright's stain.

The most common parasites detected in Giemsa-stained blood smears are the plasmodia, microfilariae, and African trypanosomes

Table 213-5

Identification of Parasites in Blood and Other Body Fluids

Body Fluid, Parasite	Enrichment/Stain	Culture Technique
BLOOD		
Plasmodium spp.	Thick and thin smears/ Giemsa or Wright's	Not useful for diagnosis
Leishmania spp.	Buffy coat/Giemsa	Media available from CDC
African trypanosomes*	Buffy coat, anion column/wet mount and Giemsa	Mouse or rat inoculation†
Trypanosoma cruzi‡	As for African species	As above and xenodiagnosis
Toxoplasma gondii	Buffy coat/Giemsa	Fibroblast cell lines
Microfilariae§	Nucleopore filtration/ wet mount and Giemsa	None
URINE¶		
Schistosoma haematobium	Centrifugation/wet mount	None
Microfilariae (in chyluria)	As for blood	None
SPINAL FLUID		
African trypanosomes	Centrifugation, anion column/wet mount and Giemsa	As for blood
Naegleria fowleri	Centrifugation/wet mount and Giemsa or trichrome	Nonnutrient agar overlaid with *Escherichia coli*

* *Trypanosoma rhodesiense* and *T. gambiense*.
† Inject mice intraperitoneally with 0.2 mL of whole heparinized blood (0.5 mL for rats). After 5 days, tail blood should be checked daily for trypanosomes as described above.
‡ Detectable in blood by conventional techniques only during acute disease. Xenodiagnosis is successful in about 50 percent of patients with chronic Chagas' disease.
§ Day (1000–1400 h) and night (2200–0200 h) blood should be drawn to maximize the chance of detecting *Wuchereria* (nocturnal except for Pacific strains), *Brugia* (nocturnal), and *Loa loa* (diurnal).
¶ *Trichomonas vaginalis* is often detectable in urine, but examination of vaginal secretions is probably the preferable technique.

(see Table 213-5). Most patients with Chagas' disease present in the chronic phase, when *Trypanosoma cruzi* is no longer microscopically detectable in blood smears. Wet mounts are sometimes more sensitive than stained smears for the detection of microfilariae and African trypanosomes because these active parasites cause noticeable movement of the erythrocytes in the microscopic field. Nuclepore filtration of blood facilitates the detection of microfilariae. The intracellular amastigote forms of *Leishmania* spp. and *T. cruzi* can sometimes be visualized in stained smears of peripheral blood, but aspirates of the bone marrow, liver, and spleen are the best sources for microscopic detection and culture of *Leishmania* in kala-azar and of *T. cruzi* in chronic Chagas' disease.

The diagnosis of malaria and the critical distinction among the various *Plasmodium* species are made by microscopic examination of stained thick and thin blood films (see Table 213-6). Most malariologists prefer Giemsa stain because of its overall high quality, suitability for staining of both thick and thin smears, and stability in tropical climates. Wright's stain can produce high-quality thin smears and is widely used in the Americas, but it deteriorates rapidly in the tropics because its methanol base is highly hygroscopic. Specimens of capillary or venous blood should be obtained every 4 to 12 h until a diagnosis is established. The thin smear is made on clean slides exactly like a blood film for a white blood cell differential. The thick film is made by placing one drop of blood on the slide and stirring it in a circular motion to a diameter of about 2 cm. The erythrocytes in the

Table 213-6

Differential Diagnosis of *Plasmodium* Species in Blood Smears

Feature	P. falciparum	P. vivax	P. malariae	P. ovale
FEATURE OF RED CELLS				
Size	All sizes	Large (young)	Small (old)	Large (young)
Shape	Round; may be crenated	Round or oval	Round	Round or pear-shaped, fimbriated
Stippling	Maurer's clefts: large, red (up to 20)	Schüffner's dots: numerous, small, red	None	Schüffner's dots
FEATURE OF PARASITE				
Ring trophozoites	Thread-like, multiple infections, double chromatin dots, accolé forms*	Thicker	Compact	Compact
Mature trophozoites	Absent	Ameboid, may fill cell	More regular, smaller band forms†	Less ameboid and smaller than those of *P. vivax*
Schizonts	Absent	12 to 24 merozoites	8 to 12 merozoites, often rosetted around pigment	8 to 12 merozoites
Gametocytes	Banana-shaped, central chromatin (female) or diffuse (male)	Round, fills cell, pigment often central	Round, large, coarse pigment	Smaller and oval, but similar to those of *P. vivax*
DIAGNOSTIC KEYS				
	Gametocyte, multiple rings, double chromatin dots, accolé forms, heavy infections	Schizont, large RBCs, ameboid forms	Schizont, small RBCs, band forms	Schizont and large RBCs, pear-shaped, fimbriated RBCs

* At periphery of RBCs; may be flattened into rod shape.
† Stretch across RBCs, but not banana-shaped.
NOTE: RBCs, red blood cells.

Table 213-7

Minor Procedures for Diagnosis of Parasitic Infections

Procedure	Parasite(s) and Stage
Skin snips: Lift skin with a needle and excise about 1 mg to a depth of 0.5 mm from several sites. Weigh each sample, place it in 0.5 mL of saline for 4 h, and examine wet mounts and Giemsa stains of the saline either directly or after filtration. Count microfilariae.*	*Onchocerca volvulus* and *Mansonella streptocerca* microfilariae
Biopsies of subcutaneous nodules: Stain routine histopathologic sections and impression smears with Giemsa.	*Loa loa* adults and *O. volvulus* adults and microfilariae
Muscle biopsies: Excise about 1.0 g of deltoid or gastrocnemius muscle and squash between two glass slides for direct microscopic examination.	*Trichinella spiralis* larvae (and perhaps *Taenia solium* cysticerci)
Rectal snips: From four areas of mucosa take 2-mg snips, tease onto a glass slide, and flatten with a second slide before examining directly at 10×. Preparations may be fixed in alcohol or stained.	*Schistosoma* ova of all species, but especially *S. mansoni*
Aspirate of chancre or lymph node†: Aspirate center with 18-gauge needle, place a drop on a slide, and examine for motile forms. An otherwise insufficient volume of material may be stained with Giemsa.	*Trypanosoma gambiense* and *Trypanosoma rhodesiense* trypomastigotes
Corneal scrapings: Obtain sample from ophthalmologist for immediate Giemsa staining and culture on nutrient agar overlaid with *Escherichia coli*.	*Acanthamoeba* species trophozoites or cysts
Swabs, aspirates, or punch biopsies of skin lesions: Obtain specimen from margin of lesion for Giemsa staining of impression smears and section and culture on special media from CDC.	Cutaneous and mucocutaneous species of *Leishmania*

* Counts of >100/mg are associated with significant risk of complications.
† Lymph node aspiration is contraindicated in some infections and should be used judiciously.

thick film are lysed with water, but the thin film is fixed in methanol to preserve erythrocyte morphology.

Although most tissue parasites stain with the traditional hematoxylin and eosin, surgical biopsy specimens should also be stained with appropriate special stains. The surgical pathologist who is accustomed to applying silver stains for *Pneumocystis carinii* to induced sputum and transbronchial biopsies may have to be reminded to examine wet mounts and iron-hematoxylin–stained preparations of pulmonary specimens for helminthic ova and *E. histolytica*. The clinician also should be able to advise the surgeon and pathologist about optimal techniques for the identification of parasites in specimens obtained by certain specialized minor procedures (see Table 213-7). For example, the excision of skin snips for the diagnosis of onchocerciasis, the collection of rectal snips for the diagnosis of schistosomiasis, and punch biopsy of skin lesions for the identification and culture of cutaneous and mucocutaneous species of *Leishmania* are simple procedures, but the diagnosis can be missed if the specimens are improperly obtained or processed.

NONSPECIFIC TESTS Eosinophilia is a common accompaniment of infections with most of the tissue helminths; absolute numbers of eosinophils may be high in trichinosis and the migratory phases of filariasis (Table 213-8). Intestinal helminths provoke eosinophilia only during pulmonary migration of the larval stages. Eosinophilia is not a manifestation of protozoal infections, with the possible exceptions of those due to *Isospora* and *Dientamoeba fragilis*.

Like the hypochromic, microcytic anemia of heavy hookworm infections, other nonspecific laboratory abnormalities may suggest parasitic infection in patients with appropriate geographic and/or environmental exposures. Biochemical evidence of cirrhosis or an abnor-

mal urine sediment in an African immigrant certainly raises the possibility of schistosomiasis, and anemia and thrombocytopenia in a febrile traveler or immigrant are among the hallmarks of malaria. Computed tomography and magnetic resonance imaging also contribute to the diagnosis of infections with many tissue parasites and have become invaluable adjuncts in the diagnosis of neurocysticercosis and cerebral toxoplasmosis.

ANTIBODY AND ANTIGEN DETECTION As shown in Table 213-9, there are useful antibody assays for many of the important tissue parasites. The antibody assays listed in Table 213-9 are available from the Centers for Disease Control and Prevention (CDC) in Atlanta. The results of most serologic tests not listed in the tables and not offered by the CDC should be interpreted with caution.

The value of antibody assays is limited in the case of the filarial worms and plasmodia. The detection of antibody to plasmodia is primarily an epidemiologic tool and is of limited use for establishing the diagnosis of malaria in individual patients. Filarial antigens crossreact with those from other nematodes, and antibody assays do not distinguish between past and current infection. In contrast, a negative result in an American or European traveler virtually rules out the diagnosis of bancroftian or brugian filariasis. Promising assays for filarial antigens in lymphatic filariasis are not yet available in commercial kits or from the CDC.

Despite these specific limitations, the restricted geographic distribution of many of the tropical parasites increases the usefulness of antibody detection as a means of establishing diagnoses in travelers from industrialized countries. On the other hand, a large proportion of the world has been exposed to *Toxoplasma gondii*, and the presence of IgG antibody does not constitute proof of active disease.

Fewer antibody assays are available for the diagnosis of infection with intestinal parasites. Problems of cross-reactivity and lack of efficient cultivation techniques, along with the ability to establish diagnoses without invasive procedures, have discouraged intensive investigation of these methods. *E. histolytica* is the major exception. The availability of sensitive, specific serologic tests is an invaluable aid in the diagnosis of amebiasis. Commercial kits for the detection of

Table 213-8

Parasites Frequently Associated with Eosinophilia*

Parasite	Comment
TAPEWORMS (CESTODES)	
Echinococcus granulosus	When hydatid cyst leaks
Taenia solium	During muscle encystation and in CSF with neurocysticercosis
FLUKES (TREMATODES)	
Paragonimus spp.	Uniformly high in acute stage
Fasciola hepatica	May be high in acute stage
Clonorchis (Opisthorchis) sinensis	Variable
Schistosoma mansoni	50% of infected travelers
Schistosoma haematobium	25% of infected travelers
Schistosoma japonicum	Up to 6000/µL in acute infection
ROUNDWORMS	
Ascaris lumbricoides	During larval migration
Hookworm species	During larval migration
Strongyloides stercoralis	Profound during migration and early years of infection
Trichinella spiralis	Up to 7000/µL
Filarial species†	Varies but can reach 5000 to 8000/µL
Toxocara spp.	>3000/µL
Ancylostoma braziliense	With extensive cutaneous eruption
Gnathostoma spinigerum	In visceral larva migrans and eosinophilic meningitis
Angiostrongylus cantonensis	In eosinophilic meningitis
Angiostrongylus costaricensis	During larval migration in mesenteric vessels
POSSIBLE PROTOZOAL CAUSES	
Isospora belli	A few reports of profound eosinophilia
Dientamoeba fragilis	Possible pathogenicity and eosinophilia

* Virtually every helminth has been associated with eosinophilia. This table includes both common and uncommon parasites that frequently elicit eosinophilia during infection.
† *Wuchereria bancrofti, Brugia* spp., *Loa loa*, and *Onchocerca volvulus*.

Table 213-9

Serologic and Molecular Tests for Parasitic Infections

Parasite, Infection	Antibody	Antigen or DNA/RNA
TAPEWORMS		
Echinococcosis	WB, IHA	
Cysticercosis	WB	
FLUKES		
Paragonimiasis	WB	
Schistosomiasis	EIA, WB	
ROUNDWORMS		
Strongyloidiasis	EIA	
Trichinellosis	BF, EIA	
Toxocariasis	EIA	
PROTOZOANS		
Amebiasis	IHA, EIA	EIA
Giardiasis		EIA, IIF, DFA
Cryptosporidiosis		IIF, EIA, DFA, PCR
Malaria (all species)	IIF*	PCR
Babesiosis (*B. microti*)	IIF	
Chagas' disease	IIF, CF, EIA	
Leishmaniasis	IIF, CF	
Toxoplasmosis	IIF (IgM), EIA	
Microsporidiosis		PCR

* Of use primarily for screening blood donors.

NOTE: BF, bentonite flocculation; CF, complement fixation; EIA, enzyme immunoassay; WB, western blot; IHA, indirect hemagglutination; IIF, indirect immunofluorescence; DFA, direct fluorescent antibody; PCR, polymerase chain reaction. All antibody tests listed are available from the CDC. Antigen and parasite detection kits are available commercially. The PCRs listed are those currently available from the CDC.

antigen by enzyme-linked immunosorbent assay (ELISA) or of whole organisms by fluorescent antibody assay are now available for several protozoan parasites (Table 213-9).

MOLECULAR TECHNIQUES DNA hybridization with probes that are repeated many times in the genome of a specific parasite and amplification of a specific DNA fragment by the polymerase chain reaction (PCR) are promising techniques for the diagnosis of infections with parasites and other infectious agents. Although molecular techniques for the detection of many parasites are already being used in insect vectors, animal models, and human trials, few are available for routine use in patients at this time. The only available commercial kit is that for the identification of *Trichomonas vaginalis* by hybridization of secretions from vaginal swabs with synthetic oligonucleotide probes. Currently, the CDC will perform PCR for microsporidia and cryptosporidia on frozen stool, on stool fixed in potassium dichromate, and on biopsy specimens fixed in methanol or ethanol and for plasmodia (identification or speciation) on blood treated with EDTA or blotted on filter paper (Table 213-9).

BIBLIOGRAPHY

DESPOMMIER DD, KARAPELEU JW: *Parasite Life Cycles.* New York, Springer-Verlag, 1987

FLECK SL, MOODY AH: *Diagnostic Techniques in Medical Parasitology.* London, Wright, 1988

GARCIA LS et al: Diagnosis of parasitic infections: Collection, processing, and examination of specimens, in *Manual of Clinical Microbiology*, 6th ed, PR Murray et al (eds). Washington, DC, ASM Press, 1995, pp 1145–1158

GUTIERREZ V, LITTLE MD (eds): *Clinics in Laboratory Medicine: Diagnosis of Important Parasitic Diseases.* Philadelphia, Saunders, 1991, vol 11

PEARSON RD, DE QUEIROZ SOUSA A: Clinical spectrum of leishmaniasis. Clin Infect Dis 22:1, 1996

TOMECKI KJ (ed): *Dermatologic Clinics, Systemic Mycoses and Parasitic Diseases.* Philadelphia, Saunders, 1989, vol 7

WEBER R et al: Improved light-microscopical detection of microsporidia spores in stool and duodenal aspirates. N Engl J Med 326:161, 1992

WEISS JB: DNA probes and PCR for diagnosis of parasitic infections. Clin Microbiol Rev 8:113, 1995

WELLER PF: Eosinophilia in travelers. Med Clin North Am 76:1413, 1992

WILSON M et al: Diagnosis of parasitic infections: Immunologic and molecular methods, in *Manual of Clinical Microbiology*, 6th ed, PR Murray et al (eds). Washington, DC, ASM Press, 1995, pp 1159–1170

214 | *Leo X. Liu, Peter F. Weller*

THERAPY FOR PARASITIC INFECTIONS

Chemotherapy for parasitic diseases is beset with potential problems. Knowledge of the fundamental biology and metabolism of eukaryotic parasites is still rudimentary. Many essential antiparasitic drugs, such as chloroquine and diethylcarbamazine, have been used for decades without a full understanding of their mechanisms of action. For a disease such as falciparum malaria, which causes tremendous suffering and mortality worldwide, the emergence of drug resistance poses an urgent problem. Because most parasitic infections primarily affect populations in poor developing countries, commercial incentives to develop and market antiparasitic drugs are limited.

Nevertheless, the introduction in recent years of several new agents, such as mefloquine, praziquantel, albendazole, and ivermectin, has led to improved therapy for several parasitic infections. Table 214-1 summarizes drug therapy for the more common parasitic diseases. Information regarding the indications, adverse effects, and contraindications for selected drugs is presented below. Drugs considered investigational by the Food and Drug Administration (FDA) for a given parasitic indication are marked with an asterisk (*). Other drugs, marked with a dagger (†), may not be generally available in the United States but can be obtained through the Centers for Disease Control and Prevention Drug Service, Atlanta, GA 30333 (telephone 404-639-3670). Antiparasitic drug treatment to be used for children and pregnant women or in certain unusual circumstances is detailed in the references.

Albendazole* This benzimidazole derivative is active against a variety of helminthic parasites but is still available only directly from the manufacturer (Smith Kline–Beecham). Albendazole is the drug of choice for the medical treatment of hydatid cysts and is also useful as an adjunct to surgical therapy. It is effective for cysticercosis, is promising for many intestinal and tissue nematode infections, and is less toxic than the older benzimidazoles. Adverse reactions to albendazole include occasional diarrhea and abdominal pain, and its use during pregnancy is contraindicated.

Benznidazole* This nitroimidazole derivative, not presently available in the United States, can ameliorate the course of acute Chagas' disease. Frequent side effects include rashes, nausea, and peripheral neuritis.

Bithionol† This drug is used for the treatment of fascioliasis and paragonimiasis. Adverse cutaneous and gastrointestinal reactions are common.

Chloroguanide* This pyrimidine derivative (also known as proguanil) is active against the preerythrocytic intrahepatic forms of *Plasmodium falciparum* and possibly *Plasmodium vivax*. Its use is largely limited to malaria prophylaxis (in combination with chloroquine) in parts of Africa where chloroquine-resistant *P. falciparum* is not yet widely prevalent. However, foci of resistance to chloroguanide exist in many regions, and clinical failures with this agent are common. Chloroguanide is not licensed in the United States but is sold in Canada, Europe, and Africa.

Chloroquine This mainstay of oral antimalarial therapy is a 4-aminoquinolone that rapidly kills schizonts and gametocytes of *P. vivax, Plasmodium ovale, Plasmodium malariae*, and susceptible strains of *P. falciparum*. Unfortunately, in many areas *P. falciparum* is resistant to chloroquine, and in Oceania resistance has emerged in *P. vivax*. Chloroquine is still effective for the treatment and prophylaxis of malaria in areas where resistance is not yet established. If chloroquine phosphate is not available, hydroxychloroquine sulfate (more commonly used as an antiarthritic agent) can be used effectively; 400 mg of the latter is equivalent to 500 mg of the former. Chloroquine is safe in children and pregnant women. Side effects may include abdominal discomfort, headache, and dizziness.

Diethylcarbamazine This piperazine derivative remains the drug of choice for lymphatic filariasis, despite adverse reactions. The mechanism of action of diethylcarbamazine is unclear, but the drug is microfilaricidal in vivo. Adverse reactions are generally proportional to the microfilarial burden and include fever, headache, dizziness, and transient exacerbation of lymphangitis. In patients with onchocerciasis, the drug elicits prominent pruritus and ocular and constitutional symptoms (the Mazzotti reaction) and thus has been supplanted by ivermectin. Diethylcarbamazine is effective for treatment and prophylaxis of *Loa loa* infection and has been used for visceral larva migrans. The drug is not commercially available in the United States; limited amounts may be obtained from the manufacturer (Wyeth-Ayerst).

Diloxanide Furoate† This amebicidal agent is poorly absorbed and is active only against luminal amebas. Its mode of action is unknown. Mild side effects include flatulence and gastrointestinal discomfort.

Eflornithine Commonly known as difluoromethylornithine or DFMO, this drug is effective in both hemolymphatic and central nervous system stages of *Trypanosoma brucei gambiense* infection (African trypanosomiasis). Eflornithine is available in the United States only from the manufacturer (Merrell Dow). It acts by irreversible inhibition of the trypanosomal ornithine decarboxylase, although *Trypanosoma brucei rhodesiense* is relatively insensitive to its effects. Adverse reactions—diarrhea, anemia, and leukopenia—are frequent but reversible.

Furazolidone This nitrofuran derivative is used as an alternative drug for the treatment of giardiasis. Unlike other drugs used for this

Table 214-1

Treatment of Parasitic Infections*

Infection (Etiologic Agent)	Treatment of Choice	Alternative Regimen
Amebiasis (*Entamoeba histolytica*)		
Asymptomatic infection	Diloxanide furoate 500 mg tid for 10 days	Iodoquinol 650 mg tid for 20 days, *or* paromomycin 25–30 mg/kg/d in 3 doses for 7 days
Mild to moderate disease	Metronidazole 750 mg tid for 10 days followed by iodoquinol 650 mg tid for 20 days	Tinidazole 2 g/d followed by iodoquinol as above
Severe intestinal disease	Metronidazole as above followed by iodoquinol as above	Tinidazole 600 mg bid or 800 mg tid for 5 days followed by iodoquinol as above
Hepatic abscess	Metronidazole as above for 5 days followed by iodoquinol as above	Tinidazole 600 mg bid or 800 mg tid for 5 days followed by iodoquinol as above
Amebic meningoencephalitis (*Naegleria*)	Amphotericin B 1 mg/kg/d IV for uncertain duration	—
Angiostrongyliasis		
Angiostrongylus cantonensis	Supportive therapy and glucocorticoids as needed	—
Angiostrongylus costaricensis	Thiabendazole 75 mg/kg/d in 3 doses for 3 days (max 3 g/d)	Mebendazole 200–400 mg tid for 10 days
Anisakiasis (*Anisakis*)	Surgical or endoscopic removal	—
Ascariasis (*Ascaris lumbricoides*)	Mebendazole 100 mg bid for 3 days, *or* piperazine 75 mg/kg (max 3.5 g) for 2 days	Pyrantel pamoate 11 mg/kg (max 1 g), *or* albendazole 400 mg once
Babesiosis (*Babesia*)	Clindamycin 1.2 g bid IV *or* 600 mg tid PO for 7 days plus quinine 650 mg tid PO for 7 days	
Balantidiasis (*Balantidium coli*)	Tetracycline 500 mg qid for 10 days	Metronidazole 750 mg tid for 5 days
Capillariasis (*Capillaria philippinensis*)	Mebendazole 200 mg bid for 20 days	Albendazole 200 mg bid for 10 days, *or* thiabendazole 25 mg/kg/d in 2 doses for 30 days
Cryptosporidiosis (*Cryptosporidium*)	No effective specific therapy; self-limited in normal hosts; paromomycin 500–750 mg qid possibly effective in some HIV-infected patients	—
Cutaneous larva migrans, or "creeping eruption" (hookworms, usually *Ancylostoma braziliense*)	Thiabendazole 10% suspension topically qid, *or* 25 mg/kg for 2–5 days	Ivermectin 150–200 μg/kg once, *or* albendazole 200 mg bid for 3 days
Cyclosporiasis (*Cyclospora cayetanensis*)	Trimethoprim-sulfamethoxazole 160/800 mg bid for 7 days	—
Cysticercosis (*Cysticercus cellulosae*)	Praziquantel 50 mg/kg/d in 3 doses for 15 days, *or* albendazole 15 mg/kg/d in 3 doses for 8–28 days, repeated as necessary, with concurrent glucocorticoids for CNS disease	Surgery
Dracunculiasis (*Dracunculus medinensis*)	Metronidazole 250 mg tid for 10 days plus worm removal	Thiabendazole 50–75 mg/kg/d in 2 doses for 3 days plus worm removal
Echinococcosis		
Echinococcus granulosus (hydatid cyst)	Surgical excision if possible and albendazole 400 mg bid for 20 days, repeated as necessary	—
Echinococcus multilocularis	Surgical excision	—
Enterobiasis (*Enterobius vermicularis*, pinworm)	Pyrantel pamoate 11 mg/kg once (max 1 g), *or* mebendazole 100 mg once, *or* albendazole 400 mg once; each repeated after 2 weeks	—
Filariasis		
Lymphatic filariasis (*Wuchereria bancrofti*, *Brugia malayi*)	Diethylcarbamazine Day 1: 50 mg PO Day 2: 50 mg tid Day 3: 100 mg tid Days 4–21: 6 mg/kg/d in 3 doses	—
Loiasis (*Loa loa*)	Diethylcarbamazine Day 1: 50 mg PO Day 2: 50 mg tid Day 3: 100 mg tid Days 4–21: 9 mg/kg/d in 3 doses	—
Mansonelliasis		
Mansonella ozzardi	Ivermectin 150 μg/kg single dose	—
M. perstans	Mebendazole 100 mg bid for 30 days	—
M. streptocerca	Diethylcarbamazine as for lymphatic filariasis	—
Tropical pulmonary eosinophilia	Diethylcarbamazine 6 mg/kg/d in 3 doses for 21 days	—
Onchocerciasis (*Onchocerca volvulus*)	Ivermectin 150 μg/kg once, repeated every 3–12 months	—

(continued)

Table 214-1 (Continued)

Treatment of Parasitic Infections*

Infection (Etiologic Agent)	Treatment of Choice	Alternative Regimen
Fluke infections		
Liver flukes (*Clonorchis sinensis; Opisthorchis viverrini*)	Praziquantel 75 mg/kg/d in 3 doses for 1 day	—
Sheep liver fluke (*Fasciola hepatica*)	Bithionol 30–50 mg/kg on alternate days for 10–15 doses	—
Intestinal flukes (*Fasciolopsis buski, Heterophyes heterophyes, Metagonimus yokogawai*)	Praziquantel 75 mg/kg/d in 3 doses for 1 day	—
Lung fluke (*Paragonimus westermani*)	Praziquantel 75 mg/kg/d in 3 doses for 2 days	Bithionol 30–50 mg/kg on alternate days for 10–15 doses
Giardiasis (*Giardia lamblia*)	Metronidazole 250 mg tid for 5 days	Tinidazole 2 g once, *or* paromomycin 25–30 mg/kg/d in 3 doses for 7 days, *or* furazolidone 100 mg qid for 7–10 days
Gnathostomiasis (*Gnathostoma spinigerum*)	Surgical removal plus albendazole 400–800 mg/d for 21 days	—
Hookworm (*Ancylostoma duodenale, Necator americanus*)	Mebendazole 100 mg bid for 3 days, *or* pyrantel pamoate 11 mg/kg (max 1 g) for 3 days	Albendazole 400 mg once
Isosporiasis (*Isospora belli*)	Trimethoprim-sulfamethoxazole 160/800 mg qid for 10 days, then bid for 3 weeks	Pyrimethamine 50–75 mg once daily for 3 weeks
Leishmaniasis: cutaneous, mucocutaneous, or visceral (*Leishmania braziliensis, L. mexicana, L. tropica, L. major, L. donovani*)	Stibogluconate sodium 20 mg/kg/d (max 800 mg/d) IV or IM for 20–28 days, *or* meglumine antimonate 20 mg/kg/d for 20–28 days; may be repeated or continued until response is demonstrated	Amphotericin B 0.25–1 mg/kg by slow infusion daily or every 2 days for up to 8 weeks, *or* pentamidine isethionate 2–4 mg/kg/d IM up to 15 doses
Malaria (*Plasmodium falciparum, P. ovale, P. vivax, P. malariae*)		
Treatment		
All except chloroquine-resistant *P. falciparum*		
Oral	Chloroquine phosphate 600 mg base (1 g), then 300 mg base (500 mg) at 6, 24, and 48 h	—
Parenteral	Quinidine gluconate 10 mg/kg loading dose (max 600 mg) over 1 h followed by continuous infusion of 0.02 mg/kg/min for 3 days maximum	—
Followed by (for *P. vivax* and *P. ovale* only)	Primaquine phosphate 15 mg base (26.3 mg)/d for 14 days or 45 mg base (79 mg)/wk for 8 weeks	—
Chloroquine-resistant *P. falciparum*		
Oral	Quinine sulfate 650 mg tid for 3 days plus pyrimethamine-sulfadoxine 3 tablets at once on last day of quinine, *or* plus tetracycline 250 mg qid for 7 days, *or* plus clindamycin 900 mg tid for 3 days	Mefloquine 750 mg followed by 500 mg 6–8 h later, *or* halofantrine 500 mg q6h for 3 doses, repeated in 1 week
Parenteral	Quinidine gluconate as above	—
Prophylaxis		
Chloroquine-sensitive areas	Chloroquine phosphate 300 mg base (500 mg salt) given PO once a week beginning 1 week before and continuing for 4 weeks after last exposure	—
Chloroquine-resistant areas	Mefloquine 250 mg given PO once a week and continuing for 4 weeks after last exposure, *or* doxycycline 100 mg/d during exposure and for 4 weeks afterward	Chloroquine phosphate as in chloroquine-sensitive areas plus pyrimethamine-sulfadoxine for presumptive treatment *or* plus proguanil† 200 mg/d in sub-Saharan Africa during exposure and for 4 weeks afterward
Schistosomiasis		
Schistosoma mansoni	Praziquantel 40 mg/kg/d in 2 doses for 1 day	Oxamniquine 15 mg/kg once; 30 mg/kg once in East Africa; 30 mg/kg once daily for 2 days in Egypt and South Africa
S. haematobium	Praziquantel 40 mg/kg/d in 2 doses for 1 day	—
S. japonicum, S. mekongi	Praziquantel 60 mg/kg/d in 3 doses for 1 day	—
Strongyloidiasis		
(*Strongyloides stercoralis*)	Thiabendazole 50 mg/kg/d in 2 doses (max 3 g/d) for 2 days; for disseminated disease, continue for 7 days (or longer if host is immunocompromised)	Ivermectin 200 μg/kg/d for 1–2 days, *or* albendazole 400 mg once daily for 3 days

(continued)

Table 214-1 *(Continued)*

Treatment of Parasitic Infections*

Infection (Etiologic Agent)	Treatment of Choice	Alternative Regimen
Tapeworm intestinal infections		
Diphyllobothrium latum—fish; *Taenia saginata*—beef; *T. solium*—pork; *Dipylidium caninum*—dog	Praziquantel 10–20 mg/kg once	—
Hymenolepis nana (dwarf tapeworm)	Praziquantel 25 mg/kg once	—
Toxoplasmosis		
(*Toxoplasma gondii*)	Pyrimethamine 25–100 mg/d plus sulfadiazine 1–1.5 g qid plus folinic acid 10 mg/d for 3–4 weeks	Clindamycin 1.8–2.4 g/d in divided doses plus pyrimethamine 25–100 mg/d plus folinic acid 10 mg/d for 3–4 weeks; *or* spiramycin 3–4 g/d in pregnancy continued until delivery
Trichinosis		
(*Trichinella spiralis*)	Glucocorticoids (for severe symptoms) plus mebendazole 200–400 mg tid for 3 days, then 400–500 mg tid for 10 days	—
Trichomoniasis		
(*Trichomonas vaginalis*)	Metronidazole 2 g once or 250 mg tid PO for 7 days, *or* tinidazole 2 g once	—
Trichostrongyliasis		
(*Trichostrongylus*)	Pyrantel pamoate 11 mg/kg once (max 1 g)	Mebendazole 100 mg bid for 3 days, *or* albendazole 400 mg once
Trichuriasis		
(*Trichuris trichiura*, whipworm)	Mebendazole 100 mg bid for 3 days, *or* albendazole 400 mg once	—
Trypanosomiasis		
Trypanosoma cruzi (Chagas' disease)	Nifurtimox 8–10 mg/kg/d PO in 4 doses for 120 days	Benznidazole 5–7 mg/kg/d for 30–120 days
T. brucei gambiense, *T. brucei rhodesiense* (sleeping sickness)		
Hemolymphatic stage	Suramin test dose of 100–200 mg IV, then 1 g IV on days 1, 3, 7, 14, 21; *or* eflornithine 100 mg/kg qid for 14 days, then 300 mg/kg/d PO for 3–4 weeks	Pentamidine isethionate 4 mg/kg/d IM for 10 days
Late stage with CNS involvement	Melarsoprol 2–3.6 mg/kg/d IV for 3 days, after 1 week 3.6 mg/kg/d IV for 3 days, repeated after 10–21 days; *or* eflornithine 100 mg/kg qid for 14 days, then 300 mg/kg/d PO for 3–4 weeks	Tryparsamide 30 mg/kg (max 2 g) IV q5d to total of 12 injections, sometimes repeated after 1 month; plus suramin 10 mg/kg IV q5d to total of 12 injections, sometimes repeated after 1 month
Visceral larva migrans		
(*Toxocara cani* or *T. cati*, toxocariasis)	Supportive therapy and glucocorticoids	Diethylcarbamazine 2 mg/kg tid for 7–10 days, *or* mebendazole 100–200 mg bid for 5 days, *or* albendazole 400 mg bid for 3–5 days

* For information on the treatment of infection due to *Pneumocystis carinii*, formerly considered a parasite but now classified as a fungus, see Chap. 211.
† Chloroguanide.

purpose, furazolidone is not bitter and is available in a liquid form useful for administration to young children. Nausea, vomiting, and allergic reactions occur. The drug is a monoamine oxidase (MAO) inhibitor and produces a disulfiram-like reaction when taken with alcohol.

Halofantrine This oral antimalarial drug has been used as an alternative for the treatment of malaria due to chloroquine-resistant *P. falciparum*. Adverse effects include abdominal pain, diarrhea, and pruritus. Halofantrine should not be used in pregnancy. Because this agent causes dose-related lengthening of the PR and QT_c intervals and has caused first-degree atrioventricular block, it should not be given to patients with cardiac conduction defects. Cardiac monitoring during treatment is advisable.

Iodoquinol This halogenated oxyquinolone is used for the treatment of noninvasive amebiasis and *Dientamoeba fragilis* infection and as an alternative agent for *Balantidium coli* infection. Adverse effects are uncommon, but optic neuritis has developed with prolonged use of excessively high doses.

Ivermectin† This semisynthetic derivative of avermectin is now the drug of choice for *Onchocerca volvulus* infections. A single oral dose of ivermectin is active against microfilariae but has no effect on adult worms. The agent's mechanism of action has not been conclusively identified. Ivermectin also is active against a range of intestinal nematodes and is being investigated for the treatment of lymphatic filariasis. The drug is safe and well tolerated in children and adults, but its safety in pregnancy has not been specifically investigated.

Mebendazole This benzimidazole derivative is effective against a spectrum of intestinal and tissue nematodes, including *Ascaris*, *Ancylostoma*, *Necator*, *Enterobius*, and *Trichuris*, and is an investigational drug for use against *Capillaria*. Benzimidazoles may act by binding β-tubulin to disrupt microtubule formation and glucose uptake. Side effects include mild abdominal pain and diarrhea. Benzimidazoles can be teratogenic in experimental animals and so are avoided during pregnancy.

Mefloquine This antimalarial agent is active against the blood stages of all malarial species and the schizonts of *P. falciparum*. A 4-aminoquinolone derivative, mefloquine is the preferred agent for the prophylaxis and oral treatment of chloroquine-resistant malaria. Adverse effects are generally dose-related and include nausea and dizziness and (more rarely) vomiting, diarrhea, psychosis, and seizures. Because it has been associated with sinus bradycardia, mefloquine is contraindicated in persons taking beta-adrenoreceptor and calcium-channel blocking agents and should not be given concurrently with quinine or quinidine. Resistance to mefloquine has been documented in *P. falciparum* in parts of Southeast Asia and Africa and poses a growing problem. Since its safety in pregnancy has not been established, mefloquine should not be given to pregnant women.

Melarsoprol† This organic arsenical compound is used only to treat late-stage African trypanosomiasis involving the central nervous system. Only after intravenous administration does enough drug enter the cerebrospinal fluid to kill the trypanosomes. Severe adverse effects are common and include myocarditis, encephalopathy, and the Jarisch-Herxheimer reaction.

Metronidazole This 5-nitroimidazole exhibits potent activity against anaerobic bacteria and several protozoa, including *Entamoeba histolytica, Giardia lamblia, Trichomonas vaginalis,* and *B. coli.* Metronidazole is the drug of choice for the treatment of giardiasis (although it is not FDA approved for this indication) and for the initial treatment of invasive amebiasis. It is generally well tolerated, but mild abdominal pain, headache, nausea, and a persistent metallic taste are common. The drug is teratogenic in animals and should be avoided in early pregnancy. Because it produces a disulfiram-like reaction, abstinence from alcohol during treatment is advisable.

Nifurtimox† This synthetic nitrofuran compound is active in acute *Trypanosoma cruzi* infection. Response rates are variable, and the drug has little effect in chronic Chagas' disease. Adverse reactions, including nausea, vomiting, insomnia, headache, vertigo, tremor, paresthesias, and convulsions, are common and dose-dependent.

Oxamniquine This tetrahydroquinolone derivative is used as an alternative agent for the treatment of *Schistosoma mansoni* infection. Higher doses are needed in Egypt and South Africa than elsewhere, and resistant strains have been encountered. Oxamniquine is well tolerated, with occasional side effects including headache, dizziness, drowsiness, and gastrointestinal disturbances. It should not be used in pregnancy.

Paromomycin This orally administered, poorly absorbed aminoglycoside is used as an alternative agent for the treatment of noninvasive amebiasis. Paromomycin also has been used in lieu of metronidazole to treat amebiasis and giardiasis in pregnant women, although it has not been approved for this purpose.

Pentamidine Isethionate This stable aromatic diamine compound is active against several protozoal pathogens, including *Leishmania* spp. and *T. brucei gambiense.* Its mechanism of action remains uncertain. Adverse reactions to parenteral pentamidine are common and include reversible nephrotoxicity, acute hypotension, pancreatitis, hypoglycemia, cardiac arrhythmias, blood dyscrasias, and sterile abscesses at the injection site.

Piperazine This inexpensive drug, widely used in developing countries for the treatment of ascariasis and enterobiasis, is an anticholinergic agent that paralyzes worms, allowing them to be flushed out by peristalsis. Intestinal disturbances, hypersensitivity reactions, and dizziness are occasional adverse reactions. Piperazine and pyrantel pamoate have antagonistic modes of action and should not be administered together.

Praziquantel This agent is the drug of choice for most trematode (fluke) and many cestode infections. Its mechanism of action is unknown. In schistosomes, however, it causes paralysis and tegumental disruption, which may permit a synergistic host immune response. Praziquantel is highly active against all human schistosome parasites, intestinal tapeworms, cysticerci, and other flukes exclusive of *Fasciola hepatica.* Side effects include headache, dizziness, drowsiness, and abdominal discomfort. Use of higher doses and adjunctive treatment with anti-inflammatory glucocorticoids are recommended for neurocysticercosis.

Primaquine This 8-aminoquinolone derivative is the only standard drug active against the intrahepatic hypnozoite forms of malarial species and is used for the radical cure of *P. vivax* and *P. ovale* malaria following schizonticidal therapy. It is also an effective gametocidal agent. A potent oxidant, primaquine causes acute hemolysis in the presence of glucose-6-phosphate dehydrogenase deficiency, and at-risk patients should be screened before such therapy is instituted. Use of primaquine is contraindicated during pregnancy.

Pyrantel This well-tolerated pyrimidine derivative acts against intestinal nematodes by inducing neuromuscular paralysis in the worms, which allows them to be expelled. A single dose is usually curative for ascariasis, enterobiasis, and trichostrongyliasis, but several doses are recommended for hookworm infection. Pyrantel is safe for use in pregnancy.

Pyrimethamine-Sulfonamides Pyrimethamine combined with sulfadiazine is used in the treatment of toxoplasmosis. The high doses required for this indication often result in significant folate deficiency,

necessitating folinic acid replacement. Abdominal symptoms and rashes are also common. Pyrimethamine combined with sulfadoxine is active against most strains of *P. falciparum,* although drug resistance has become increasingly widespread. As an adjunct to quinine, pyrimethamine-sulfadoxine is still useful in the oral treatment of chloroquine-resistant *P. falciparum* malaria but is no longer recommended for malaria prophylaxis because of occasional severe or even fatal skin hypersensitivity reactions and hepatitis.

Quinine and Quinidine These cinchona alkaloids have re-emerged as first-line drugs for the treatment of falciparum malaria because of widespread chloroquine resistance. Quinine in combination with a second active drug (to reduce the likelihood of recurrence) is recommended as oral therapy for *P. falciparum* malaria. For severe infections requiring intravenous therapy, only quinidine gluconate (which is at least as effective as parenteral quinine) is available in the United States. Cardiac monitoring during quinidine infusion is mandatory, and oral quinine should be substituted as soon as the patient is able to take it. Both quinine and quinidine can cause hypoglycemia. Symptoms of cinchonism, including tinnitus, headache, visual disturbances, nausea, and abdominal pain, often develop with treatment but are rarely grounds for discontinuing the drug. Oral quinine also is used with clindamycin to treat babesiosis.

Spiramycin This agent provides an alternative to antifolates in the treatment of toxoplasmosis, particularly for pregnant women, in whom it is safe.

Stibogluconate Sodium† (Sodium Antimony Gluconate)† This pentavalent antimonial parenteral solution is the drug of choice for all forms of leishmaniasis. Its mechanism of action is unknown. Adverse effects include muscle pain, joint stiffness, nausea, vomiting, and (less commonly) rash and cardiac or hepatic toxicity. Meglumine antimonate, another pentavalent antimonial drug, is used in many French- and Spanish-speaking countries.

Suramin† This complex derivative of urea is the drug of choice for the treatment of early African trypanosomiasis. It must be given intravenously and is excreted very slowly. Adverse effects are common, can be severe, and include vomiting, pruritus, urticaria, paresthesias, photophobia, peripheral neuropathy, anaphylaxis, and renal damage.

Tetracycline and Doxycycline Tetracycline is effective against *B. coli* and *D. fragilis* and is also used as an adjunct to quinine in the treatment of chloroquine-resistant falciparum malaria. Doxycycline (in once-daily form) may be used for chemoprophylaxis of chloroquine-resistant falciparum malaria. Tooth staining in children and photosensitivity are potential hazards.

Thiabendazole This older benzimidazole derivative is active against a variety of nematode parasites, but frequent and severe side effects limit its primary systemic use in the treatment of strongyloidiasis. These adverse reactions include dizziness, nausea, vomiting, drowsiness, pruritus, headache, neuropsychiatric disturbances, hepatitis, and hypersensitivity reactions (e.g., Stevens-Johnson syndrome). A topical suspension of thiabendazole is used for cutaneous larva migrans.

Tinidazole* This nitroimidazole is available only outside the United States for the treatment of amebiasis, giardiasis, and vaginal trichomoniasis. Tinidazole appears to be more effective and better tolerated than metronidazole.

Trimethoprim-Sulfamethoxazole This antifolate combination is active in *Cyclospora cayetanensis* and *Isospora belli* infections. Adverse effects are predominantly due to the sulfamethoxazole component and include skin, liver, and bone marrow toxicity.

BIBLIOGRAPHY

ABRAMOWICZ M (ed): Drugs for parasitic infections. Med Lett Drugs Ther 37:99, 1995

LIU LX, WELLER PF: An update on antiparasitic drugs. N Engl J Med 334:1178, 1996

WORLD HEALTH ORGANIZATION: *Model Prescribing Information: Drugs Used in Parasitic Diseases,* 2d ed. Geneva, WHO, 1995

215 *Sharon L. Reed*

AMEBIASIS AND INFECTION WITH FREE-LIVING AMEBAS

AMEBIASIS

DEFINITION Amebiasis is an infection with the intestinal protozoan *Entamoeba histolytica*. About 90 percent of infections are asymptomatic, and the remaining 10 percent produce a spectrum of clinical syndromes ranging from dysentery to abscesses of the liver or other organs.

LIFE CYCLE AND TRANSMISSION *E. histolytica* is acquired by ingestion of viable cysts from fecally contaminated water, food, or hands. Food-borne exposure is most prevalent and is particularly likely when food handlers are shedding cysts or food is being grown with feces-contaminated soil, fertilizer, or water. Less common means of transmission include contaminated water, oral and anal sexual practices, and—in rare instances—direct rectal inoculation through colonic irrigation devices. Motile trophozoites are released from cysts in the small intestine and, in most patients, remain as harmless commensals in the large bowel. After encystation, infectious cysts are shed in the stool and can survive for several weeks in a moist environment. In some patients, the trophozoites invade either the bowel mucosa, causing symptomatic colitis, or the bloodstream, causing distant abscesses of the liver, lungs, or brain. The trophozoites may not encyst in patients with active dysentery, and motile hematophagous trophozoites are frequently present in fresh stools. Trophozoites are rapidly killed by exposure to air or stomach acid, however, and therefore cannot cause infection.

EPIDEMIOLOGY About 10 percent of the world's population is infected with *E. histolytica*; amebiasis is the third most common cause of death from parasitic disease (after schistosomiasis and malaria). Areas of highest incidence (due to inadequate sanitation and crowding) include most developing countries in the tropics, particularly Mexico, India, and nations of Central and South America, tropical Asia, and Africa. The main groups at risk in developed countries are travelers, recent immigrants, homosexual men, and inmates of institutions.

All *E. histolytica* trophozoites and cysts are morphologically identical, but the wide spectrum of clinical disease is caused in part by infection with two different species of *Entamoeba*. Isolates of *E. histolytica* from patients with invasive amebiasis have unique isoenzymes, surface antigens, DNA markers, and virulence properties and now are classified as a separate species from the noninvasive species *Entamoeba dispar*.

Most asymptomatic carriers, including homosexual men and AIDS patients, harbor nonpathogenic strains and have self-limited infections. These findings suggest that nonpathogenic strains (i.e., *E. dispar*) are incapable of causing invasive disease, since *Cryptosporidium* and *Isospora belli*, which also cause only self-limited illnesses in immunocompetent people, cause devastating diarrhea in AIDS patients. However, host factors play a role as well: Some patients infected with strains shown (by isoenzyme patterns) to be pathogenic do not develop invasive amebiasis but rather remain asymptomatic. In one study, 10 percent of asymptomatic patients who were colonized with pathogenic strains went on to develop amebic colitis, while the rest remained asymptomatic and cleared the infection within 1 year.

PATHOGENESIS AND PATHOLOGY Both trophozoites (Fig. 215-1) and cysts (Fig. 215-2) are found in the intestinal lumen, but only trophozoites invade tissue. The trophozoite is 20 to 60 μm in diameter and contains vacuoles and a nucleus with a characteristic central karyosome. In animals, depletion of intestinal mucus, diffuse inflammation, and disruption of the epithelial barrier occur before

FIGURE 215-1 Trophozoite of *E. histolytica* demonstrating a single nucleus with a central, dotlike karyosome (trichrome stain).

trophozoites actually come into contact with the colonic mucosa. Trophozoites attach to colonic mucus and epithelial cells by a galactose-inhibitable lectin. The earliest intestinal lesions are microulcerations of the mucosa of the cecum, sigmoid colon, or rectum that release erythrocytes, inflammatory cells, and epithelial cells. Proctoscopy reveals small ulcers with heaped up margins and normal intervening mucosa. Submucosal extension of ulcerations under viable-appearing surface mucosa causes the classic "flask-shaped" ulcer containing trophozoites at the margins of dead and viable tissues. Although neutrophilic infiltrates may accompany the early lesions in animals, human intestinal infection is marked by a paucity of inflammatory cells, probably in part because of the killing of neutrophils by trophozoites. Treated ulcers characteristically heal with little or no scarring. Occasionally, however, full-thickness necrosis and perforation occur.

Rarely, intestinal infection results in the formation of a mass lesion, or ameboma, in the bowel lumen. The overlying mucosa is usually thin and ulcerated, while other layers of the wall are thickened, edematous, and hemorrhagic, resulting in exuberant formation of granulation tissue with little fibrous-tissue response.

A number of virulence factors have been linked to the ability of amebas to invade through the interglandular epithelium. One is an extracellular cysteine proteinase that degrades collagen, elastin, secre-

FIGURE 215-2 Cyst of *E. histolytica* showing three of the four nuclei (trichrome stain).

tory IgA, and the anaphylatoxins C3a and C5a. Other enzymes may disrupt glycoprotein bonds between mucosal epithelial cells in the gut. Amebas can lyse neutrophils, monocytes, lymphocytes, and cells of colonic and hepatic cell lines. The cytolytic effect of amebas appears to require direct contact with target cells and may be linked to the release of phospholipase A and pore-forming peptides.

Liver abscesses are always preceded by intestinal colonization, which may be asymptomatic. Blood vessels may be compromised early by lysis of the wall and thrombus formation. Trophozoites invade veins to reach the liver through the portal venous system. Pathogenic isolates are resistant to complement-mediated lysis, a property critical to survival in the bloodstream. In contrast, nonpathogenic strains are rapidly lysed by complement and are thus restricted to the bowel lumen. Inoculation of amebas into the portal system of hamsters results in an acute cellular infiltrate consisting predominantly of neutrophils. Later, the neutrophils are lysed by contact with amebas, and the release of neutrophil toxins may contribute to necrosis of hepatocytes. The liver parenchyma is replaced by necrotic material that is surrounded by a thin rim of congested liver tissue. The necrotic contents of a liver abscess are classically described as "anchovy paste," although the fluid is variable in color and is composed of bacteriologically sterile granular debris with few or no cells. Amebas, if seen, tend to be found only near the capsule of the abscess.

Clinical infection does not induce immunity to recurrent colonization with *E. histolytica*, but repeated episodes of colitis or liver abscess are unusual. Antibody is not protective; titers correlate with the length of illness rather than with the severity of disease. Studies of animals suggest that cell-mediated immunity may be important for protection, although patients with AIDS appear not to be predisposed to more severe disease.

CLINICAL SYNDROMES Intestinal Amebiasis The most common type of amebic infection is asymptomatic cyst passage. Even in highly endemic areas, most patients harbor nonpathogenic strains.

Symptomatic amebic colitis develops 2 to 6 weeks after the ingestion of infectious cysts. Lower abdominal pain and mild diarrhea develop gradually and are followed by malaise, weight loss, and diffuse lower abdominal or back pain. Cecal involvement may mimic acute appendicitis. Patients with full-blown dysentery may pass 10 to 12 stools per day. The stools contain little fecal material and consist mainly of blood and mucus. In contrast to those with bacterial diarrhea, fewer than 40 percent of patients with amebic dysentery are febrile. Virtually all patients have heme-positive stools.

More fulminant intestinal infection, with severe abdominal pain, high fever, and profuse diarrhea, is rare and occurs predominantly in children. Patients may develop toxic megacolon, in which there is severe bowel dilation with intramural air. Patients receiving glucocorticoids are at risk for severe amebiasis. Uncommonly, patients develop a chronic form of amebic colitis, which can be confused with inflammatory bowel disease. The positive association between severe amebiasis complications and steroid therapy emphasizes the importance of excluding amebiasis in any case in which inflammatory bowel disease is suspected. Amebomas are inflammatory mass lesions that develop owing to chronic intestinal forms of amebiasis. An occasional patient presents only with an asymptomatic or tender abdominal mass caused by an ameboma, which is easily confused with cancer on barium studies. A positive serologic test or biopsy can prevent unnecessary surgery in this setting. The syndrome of postamebic colitis—persistent diarrhea following documented cure of amebic colitis—is controversial; no evidence of recurrent amebic infection can be found, and re-treatment usually has no effect.

Amebic Liver Abscess Extraintestinal infection by *E. histolytica* most often involves the liver. Of travelers who develop an amebic liver abscess after leaving an endemic area, 95 percent do so within 5 months. Young patients with an amebic liver abscess are more likely than older patients to present in the acute phase with prominent symptoms of less than 10 days' duration. Most patients are febrile and have right upper quadrant pain, which may be dull or pleuritic in nature and radiate to the shoulder. Point tenderness over the liver and right-sided pleural effusion are common. Jaundice is rare. Although

the initial site of infection is the colon, fewer than one-third of patients with an amebic abscess have active diarrhea. Older patients from endemic areas are more likely to have a subacute course lasting 6 months, with weight loss and hepatomegaly. About one-third of patients with chronic presentations are febrile. Thus, the clinical diagnosis of an amebic liver abscess may be difficult to establish because the symptoms and signs are often nonspecific. Since 10 to 15 percent of patients present only with fever, amebic liver abscess must be considered in the differential diagnosis of fever of unknown origin.

Complications of Amebic Liver Abscess Pleuropulmonary involvement, which is reported in 20 to 30 percent of patients, is the most frequent complication of amebic liver abscess. Manifestations include sterile effusions, contiguous spread from the liver, and rupture into the pleural space. Sterile effusions and contiguous spread usually resolve with medical therapy, but frank rupture into the pleural space requires drainage. A hepatobronchial fistula may cause cough productive of large amounts of necrotic material that may contain amebas. This dramatic complication carries a good prognosis. Abscesses that rupture into the peritoneum may present as an indolent leak or an acute abdomen and require both percutaneous catheter drainage and medical therapy. Rupture into the pericardium, usually from abscesses of the left lobe of the liver, carries the gravest prognosis; it can occur during medical therapy and requires surgical drainage.

Other Extraintestinal Sites The genitourinary tract may become involved by direct extension of amebiasis from the colon or by hematogenous spread of the infection. Painful genital ulcers, characterized by a punched-out appearance and profuse discharge, may develop secondary to extension from either the intestine or the liver. Both these conditions respond well to medical therapy. Cerebral involvement has been reported in fewer than 0.1 percent of patients in large clinical series. Symptoms and prognosis depend on the size and location of the lesion.

DIAGNOSTIC TESTS Laboratory Diagnosis Stool examinations, serologic tests, and noninvasive imaging of the liver are the most important procedures in the diagnosis of amebiasis. Fecal findings suggestive of amebic colitis include a positive test for heme, a paucity of neutrophils, and the presence of Charcot-Leyden crystal protein (double pyramid-shaped crystals normally found in the cytoplasm of eosinophils). The definitive diagnosis of amebic colitis is made by the demonstration of hematophagous trophozoites of *E. histolytica* (Fig. 215-1). Because trophozoites are killed rapidly by water, drying, or barium, it is important to examine at least three fresh stool specimens. Examination of a combination of wet mounts, iodine-stained concentrates, and trichrome-stained preparations of fresh stool and concentrates for cysts (Fig. 215-2) or trophozoites (Fig. 215-1) confirms the diagnosis in 75 to 95 percent of cases. Cultures of amebas are more sensitive but are not routinely available. If stool examinations are negative, sigmoidoscopy with biopsy of the edge of ulcers may increase the yield, but this procedure is dangerous during fulminant colitis because of the risk of perforation. Trophozoites in a biopsy specimen from a colonic mass confirm the diagnosis of ameboma, but trophozoites are rare in liver aspirates. Accurate diagnosis requires experience, since trophozoites may be confused with neutrophils and the cysts must be differentiated morphologically from *Entamoeba hartmanni*, *Entamoeba coli*, and *Endolimax nana*, which do not cause clinical disease and do not warrant therapy. Unfortunately, the cysts of pathogenic strains of *E. histolytica* cannot be distinguished microscopically from those of nonpathogenic strains. Future diagnostic tests will focus on the detection of antigens with monoclonal antibodies or DNA amplification as a means of differentiating *E. histolytica* from *E. dispar*.

Serology is an important addition to the methods used for the parasitologic diagnosis of invasive amebiasis. Kits for the performance of counterimmunodiffusion assays, agar gel diffusion assays, and ELISAs are commercially available, and the results of these tests are positive in more than 90 percent of patients with colitis, amebomas, or liver abscess. Positive results in conjunction with the appropriate clinical syndrome suggest active disease because serologic findings usually revert to negative within 6 to 12 months. Even in highly endemic areas such as South Africa, fewer than 10 percent of asymptomatic people have a positive amebic serology. The interpretation of the indirect hemagglutination test is more difficult because titers may remain positive for as long as 10 years. Up to 10 percent of patients with acute amebic liver abscess may have negative serologic findings; in suspected cases with an initially negative result, testing should be repeated in a week. In contrast to carriers of nonpathogenic strains, most asymptomatic carriers of pathogenic strains develop antibodies. Thus, serologic tests are helpful in assessing the risk of invasive amebiasis in asymptomatic, cyst-passing individuals in nonendemic areas. Serologic tests also should be performed in patients with ulcerative colitis before the institution of steroid therapy to prevent the development of severe colitis or toxic megacolon owing to unsuspected amebiasis.

Routine hematology and chemistry tests are usually not very helpful in the diagnosis of invasive amebiasis. About three-fourths of patients with an amebic liver abscess have leukocytosis (>10,000 cells per microliter); this condition is particularly likely if symptoms are acute or complications have developed. Invasive amebiasis does not elicit eosinophilia. Anemia, if present, is usually multifactorial. Even with large liver abscesses, liver enzyme levels are normal or minimally elevated. The alkaline phosphatase level is most often elevated and may remain so for months. Aminotransferase elevations suggest acute disease or a complication.

Radiographic Studies   Radiographic barium studies are potentially dangerous in acute amebic colitis. Amebomas are usually identified first by a barium enema, but biopsy is necessary for differentiation from carcinoma.

Newer radiographic techniques have improved the detection of amebic liver abscesses. Liver scans, ultrasonography, computed tomography (Fig. 215-3), and magnetic resonance imaging are all useful for detection of the round or oval hypoechoic cyst. More than 80 percent of patients who have had symptoms for more than 10 days have a single abscess of the right lobe of the liver. Approximately 50 percent of patients who have had symptoms for less than 10 days have multiple abscesses. Findings associated with complications include large abscesses (>10 cm) in the superior part of the right lobe, which may rupture into the pleural space; multiple lesions, which must be differentiated from pyogenic abscesses; and lesions of the left lobe, which may rupture into the pericardium. Because abscesses resolve slowly and may increase in size in patients who are responding clinically to therapy, frequent follow-up ultrasonography may prove confusing. Complete resolution of a liver abscess within 6 months can be anticipated in two-thirds of patients, but 10 percent may have persistent abnormalities for a year.

DIFFERENTIAL DIAGNOSIS   The differential diagnosis of intestinal amebiasis includes bacterial diarrheas caused by *Campylobacter*; enteroinvasive *Escherichia coli*; and *Shigella*, *Salmonella*, and *Vibrio* species. Although the typical patient with amebic colitis has less prominent fever than in these conditions and heme-positive stools with few neutrophils, correct diagnosis requires bacterial cultures, microscopic examination of stools, and amebic serologic testing. As has already been mentioned, amebiasis must be ruled out in any patient thought to have inflammatory bowel disease.

Because of the variety of presenting signs and symptoms, amebic liver abscess can easily be confused with pulmonary or gallbladder disease or with any febrile illness with few localizing signs, such as malaria or typhoid fever. The diagnosis should be considered in members of high-risk groups who have recently traveled outside the United States and in inmates of institutions. Once radiographic studies have identified an abscess in the liver, the most important differential diagnosis is between amebic and pyogenic abscess. Patients with pyogenic abscess typically are older and have a history of underlying bowel disease or recent surgery. Amebic serology is helpful, but aspiration of the abscess, with Gram staining and culture of the material, may be required for differentiation of the two diseases.

℞ **TREATMENT**

Intestinal Disease   The drugs used to treat amebiasis can be classified according to their primary site of action. Luminal amebicides are poorly absorbed and reach high concentrations in the bowel, but their activity is limited to cysts and trophozoites close to the mucosa. Three luminal drugs are available in the United States: iodoquinol, paromomycin, and diloxanide furoate (Table 215-1). Indications for the use of luminal agents include eradication of cysts in patients with colitis or a liver abscess and treatment of asymptomatic carriers. Until probes are available for differentiating nonpathogenic from pathogenic cysts, it is prudent to treat asymptomatic individuals who pass cysts.

Tissue amebicides reach high concentrations in the blood and tissue after oral or parenteral administration. The development of nitroimidazole compounds, especially metronidazole, was a major advance in the treatment of invasive amebiasis. Patients with amebic colitis should be treated with intravenous or oral metronidazole (750 mg three times daily for 10 days). Side effects include nausea, vomiting, abdominal discomfort, and a disulfiram-like reaction.

Table 215-1

Drug Therapy for Amebiasis

Drug	Dosage
ASYMPTOMATIC CARRIER (LUMINAL AGENTS)	
Iodoquinol (650-mg tablets)	650 mg tid for 20 days
Diloxanide furoate* (500-mg tablets)	500 mg tid for 10 days
Paromomycin (250-mg tablets)	500 mg tid for 10 days
ACUTE COLITIS	
Metronidazole (250- or 500-mg tablets) *plus* Luminal agent as above	750 mg PO or IV tid for 5 to 10 days
AMEBIC LIVER ABSCESS	
Metronidazole	750 mg PO or IV tid for 5 to 10 days
Tinidazole†	2 g PO
Ornidazole† *plus* Luminal agent as above	2 g PO

* Available only through the Centers for Disease Control and Prevention at telephone number (404) 639-3356.
† Not available in the United States.

FIGURE 215-3   Abdominal computed tomography scan of a large amebic abscess of the left lobe of the liver. (*Courtesy of the Department of Radiology, UCSD Medical Center, San Diego.*)

Other imidazole compounds, such as tinidazole and ornidazole, are as effective but are not available in the United States. All patients should also receive a full course of therapy with a luminal agent, since metronidazole does not eradicate cysts. Resistance to metronidazole has not been identified. Relapses are not uncommon and probably represent reinfection or failure to eradicate amebas from the bowel because of an inadequate dosage or duration of therapy.

Amebic Liver Abscess Metronidazole is the drug of choice for amebic liver abscess. The usefulness of nitroimidazoles in single-dose or abbreviated regimens is important in endemic areas where access to hospitalization is limited. With early diagnosis and therapy, mortality from uncomplicated amebic liver abscess is less than 1 percent. The second-line therapeutic agents emetine and chloroquine should be avoided if possible because of the potential cardiovascular and gastrointestinal side effects of the former and the higher relapse rates with the latter. There is no evidence that combined therapy with two drugs is more effective than the single-drug regimen. Studies of South Africans with liver abscesses demonstrated that 72 percent of patients without intestinal symptoms were colonized asymptomatically with pathogenic strains; thus, all treatment regimens should include a luminal agent to eradicate cysts and prevent further transmission. Amebic liver abscess recurs rarely.

Aspiration of Liver Abscesses More than 90 percent of patients respond dramatically to metronidazole therapy with decreases in both pain and fever within 72 h. Indications for aspiration of liver abscesses are (1) the need to rule out a pyogenic abscess, particularly in patients with multiple lesions; (2) the failure to respond clinically in 3 to 5 days; (3) the threat of imminent rupture; and (4) the prevention of rupture of left-lobe abscesses into the pericardium. There is no evidence that aspiration, even of large abscesses (up to 10 cm), accelerates healing. Percutaneous drainage may be successful even if the liver abscess has already ruptured. Surgery should be reserved for instances of bowel perforation and rupture into the pericardium.

PREVENTION Amebic infection is spread by ingestion of food or water contaminated with cysts. Since an asymptomatic carrier may excrete up to 15 million cysts per day, prevention of infection requires adequate sanitation and eradication of cyst carriage. In high-risk areas, infection can be minimized by the avoidance of unpeeled fruits and vegetables and the use of bottled water. Because cysts are resistant to readily attainable levels of chlorine, disinfection by iodination (tetraglycine hydroperiodide) is recommended. There is no effective prophylaxis.

INFECTION WITH FREE-LIVING AMEBAS

EPIDEMIOLOGY Free-living amebas of the genera *Acanthamoeba* and *Naegleria* are distributed throughout the world and have been isolated from a wide variety of fresh and brackish water, including that from lakes, taps, hot springs, swimming pools, and heating and air-conditioning units, and even from the nasal passages of healthy children. Encystation may protect the protozoa from desiccation and food deprivation. The persistence of *Legionella pneumophila* in water supplies may be attributable in part to chronic infection of free-living amebas, particularly *Naegleria*.

NAEGLERIA INFECTIONS Altogether, more than 100 cases of primary amebic meningoencephalitis from *Naegleria fowleri* have been reported. Infection follows the aspiration of water contaminated with trophozoites or cysts or the inhalation of contaminated dust, leading to invasion of the olfactory neuroepithelium. After an incubation period of 2 to 15 days, severe headache, high fever, nausea, vomiting, and meningismus develop. Photophobia and palsies of the third, fourth, and sixth cranial nerves are common. Rapid progression to seizures and coma may follow, and most patients die within a week. Infection is most common in otherwise healthy children or young adults, who often report recent swimming in lakes or heated swimming pools.

Diagnosis depends on the detection of motile trophozoites in wet mounts of fresh spinal fluid. Other laboratory findings resemble those

for fulminant bacterial meningitis, with elevated intracranial pressure, high white blood cell counts (up to 20,000 cells per microliter), and elevated protein concentrations and low glucose levels in cerebrospinal fluid. The diagnosis should be considered in any patient who has purulent meningitis without evidence of bacteria on Gram staining, antigen detection assay, and culture. The prognosis is uniformly poor. Only four survivors, treated with high-dose amphotericin B and rifampin, have been reported. Antibodies to *Naegleria* spp. have been detected in normal adults; serologic testing is not useful in the diagnosis of acute infection.

ACANTHAMOEBA INFECTIONS **Granulomatous Amebic Encephalitis** Infection with *Acanthamoeba* species follows a more indolent course and occurs typically in chronically ill or debilitated patients. Risk factors include lymphoproliferative disorders, chemotherapy, glucocorticoid therapy, lupus erythematosus, and AIDS. Infection usually reaches the central nervous system hematogenously from a primary focus in the sinuses, skin, or lungs. In the central nervous system, the onset is insidious, and the syndrome often mimics a space-occupying lesion. Altered mental status, headache, and stiff neck may be accompanied by focal findings such as cranial nerve palsies, ataxia, and hemiparesis. Cutaneous ulcers or hard nodules containing amebas were detected in 8 of the 13 AIDS patients with disseminated *Acanthamoeba* infection described so far in the United States.

Examination of the cerebrospinal fluid for trophozoites may be diagnostically helpful, but lumbar puncture may be contraindicated because of increased intracerebral pressure. Computed tomography frequently reveals cortical and subcortical lesions of decreased density consistent with embolic infarcts. In other patients, multiple enhancing lesions with edema may mimic the computed tomographic appearance of toxoplasmosis. Demonstration of the trophozoites and cysts of *Acanthamoeba* on wet mounts or in biopsy specimens establishes the diagnosis. Culture on nonnutrient agar plates seeded with *Escherichia coli* may also be helpful. Fluorescein-labeled antiserum is available from the Centers for Disease Control and Prevention (CDC) for the detection of protozoa in biopsy specimens. At least nine cases of granulomatous amebic encephalitis have been reported in patients with AIDS, in whom the disease may have an accelerated course, with survival for only 3 to 40 days, because of their difficulty in forming granulomas. Although studies in animals suggest that rifampin may be useful, the infection is almost uniformly fatal. A similar syndrome may be caused by a leptomyxid ameba.

Keratitis The incidence of keratitis caused by *Acanthamoeba* has increased in the past 15 years; more than 250 infections have been reported to the CDC. The first of these infections to be recognized were associated with trauma to the eye and exposure to contaminated

FIGURE 215-4 Double-walled cyst of *Acanthamoeba castellani*, as seen by phase-contrast microscopy. *[From DJ Krogstad et al, in Manual of Clinical Microbiology, 5th ed, A Balows et al (eds), Washington, DC, American Society for Microbiology, 1991.]*

water. At present, most infections are linked to extended-wear contact lenses. Risk factors include the use of homemade saline, the wearing of lenses while swimming, and inadequate disinfection. Since contact lenses presumably cause microscopic trauma, the early corneal findings may be nonspecific. The first symptoms usually include tearing and the painful sensation of a foreign body. Once infection is established, progression is rapid; the characteristic clinical sign is an annular, paracentral corneal ring representing a corneal abscess. Deeper corneal invasion and loss of vision may follow.

The differential diagnosis includes bacterial, mycobacterial, and herpetic infection. The irregular polygonal cysts of *Acanthamoeba* (Fig. 215-4) may be identified in corneal scrapings or biopsy material, and trophozoites can be grown on special media. Cysts are resistant to available drugs, and the results of medical therapy have been disappointing. Some reports have suggested partial responses to propamidine isethionate eyedrops. Severe infections usually require keratoplasty.

BIBLIOGRAPHY

AMEBIASIS

ALLASON-JONES E et al: *Entamoeba histolytica* as a commensal intestinal parasite in homosexual men. N Engl J Med 315:353, 1986

CLARK CG, DIAMOND LS: Ribosomal RNA genes of "pathogenic" and "nonpathogenic" *Entamoeba histolytica* are distinct. Mol Biochem Parasitol 49:297, 1991

IRUSEN EM et al: Asymptomatic intestinal colonization by pathogenic *Entamoeba histolytica* in amebic liver abscess: Prevalence, response to therapy, and pathogenic potential. Clin Infect Dis 14:889, 1992

KATZENSTEIN D et al: New concepts of amebic liver abscess derived from hepatic imaging, serodiagnosis, and hepatic enzymes in 67 consecutive cases in San Diego. Medicine 61:237, 1982

LIEPPE M et al: Cytolytic and antibacterial activity of synthetic peptides derived from amoebapore, the pore-forming peptide of *Entamoeba histolytica*. Proc Natl Acad Sci USA 91:1440, 1994

McCOY JJ et al: Adherence and cytotoxicity of *Entamoeba histolytica*, or how lectins let parasites stick around. Infect Immun 62:3045, 1994

McKERROW JH: Pathogenesis in amebiasis: Is it genetic or acquired? Infect Agents Dis 1:11, 1992

PETRI WA: Amebiasis and the *Entamoeba histolytica* Gal/GalNAc lectin: From bench to bedside. J Invest Med 44:24, 1996

———: Recent advances in amebiasis. CRC Crit Rev Clin Lab Sci 33:1, 1996

RAVDIN JI: Amebiasis. Clin Infect Dis 20:1453, 1995

REED SL et al: Cloning of a virulence factor of *Entamoeba histolytica*. Pathogenic strains possess a unique cysteine proteinase gene. J Clin Invest 91:1532, 1993

——— et al: *Entamoeba histolytica* infection and AIDS. Am J Med 90:269, 1991

STANLEY SL: Progress toward an amebiasis vaccine. Parasitol Today 12:7, 1996

THOMPSON JE et al: Amebic liver abscess: A therapeutic approach. Rev Infect Dis 7:171, 1985

ACANTHAMOEBA AND *NAEGLERIA*

LARKIN DFP: *Acanthamoeba* keratitis. Int Ophthalmol Clin 31:163, 1991

MA P et al: *Naegleria* and *Acanthamoeba* infections: Review. Rev Infect Dis 12:490, 1990

MARTINEZ AJ, VISVESVARA GS: Laboratory diagnosis of pathogenic freeliving amoebas: *Naegleria, Acanthamoeba,* and *Leptomyxid.* Clin Lab Med 11:861, 1991

SISON JP et al: Disseminated acanthamoeba infection in patients with AIDS: Case reports and review. Clin Infect Dis 20:1207, 1995

MALARIA AND OTHER DISEASES CAUSED BY RED BLOOD CELL PARASITES

MALARIA

Malaria is a protozoan disease transmitted by the bite of infected *Anopheles* mosquitoes. It is the most important of the parasitic diseases of humans, affecting more than 500 million people and causing between 1 and 3 million deaths each year. Malaria has now been eradicated from North America, Europe, and Russia but, despite enormous control efforts, has resurged in many parts of the tropics. Added to this resurgence are the increasing problems of drug resistance of the parasite and insecticide resistance of the vectors. Malaria remains today, as it has been for centuries, a heavy burden on tropical communities and a danger to travelers.

ETIOLOGY AND PATHOGENESIS Four species of the genus *Plasmodium* cause nearly all infections in humans (although rare infections involve species normally affecting other primates). These are *Plasmodium vivax, Plasmodium ovale, Plasmodium malariae,* and *Plasmodium falciparum* (Table 216-1). Almost all deaths are caused by falciparum malaria. Human infection begins when a female anopheline mosquito inoculates plasmodial sporozoites from its salivary gland during a blood meal (Fig. 216-1). These microscopic motile forms of the malarial parasite are carried rapidly via the bloodstream to the liver, where they invade hepatic parenchymal cells and begin a period of asexual reproduction. By this amplification process (known as intrahepatic or preerythrocytic schizogony or merogony), a single sporozoite eventually produces thousands of daughter merozoites. The swollen liver cell eventually bursts, discharging motile merozoites into the bloodstream; at this point the symptomatic stage of the infection begins. In *P. vivax* and *P. ovale* infections, a proportion of the intrahepatic forms do not divide immediately but remain dormant for months to years before reproduction begins. These dormant forms, or hypnozoites, are the cause of the relapses that characterize infection with these two species.

After entry into the bloodstream, merozoites rapidly invade erythrocytes and become trophozoites. Attachment is mediated via a specific erythrocyte surface receptor. In the case of *P. vivax*, this receptor is related to the Duffy blood-group antigen Fy^a or Fy^b. Most West Africans and people with origins in that region carry the Duffy-negative FyFy phenotype and are therefore resistant to *P. vivax* malaria. During the early stage of intraerythrocytic development, the small "ring forms" of the four parasitic species appear similar under light microscopy. As the trophozoites enlarge, species-specific characteristics become evident, pigment becomes visible, and the parasite assumes an irregular or ameboid shape. By the end of the 48-h intraerythrocytic life cycle (72 h for *P. malariae*), the parasite has consumed nearly all the hemoglobin and grown to occupy most of the red cell. Multiple nuclear divisions take place (schizogony or merogony), and the red cell ruptures to release 6 to 30 daughter merozoites, each capable of invading a new red cell and repeating the cycle. The disease in human beings is caused by the direct effects of red cell invasion and destruction by the asexual parasite and the host's reaction. During this process, some parasites develop into morphologically distinct sexual forms (gametocytes, still within the erythrocytes), which are long-lived.

After being ingested in the blood meal of a biting female anopheline mosquito, the male and female gametocytes form a zygote in the insect's midgut. This zygote matures into an ookinete, which penetrates and encysts in the mosquito's gut wall. The resulting oocyst expands by asexual division until it bursts to liberate myriad motile sporozoites, which then migrate in the hemolymph to the salivary gland of the mosquito to await inoculation into another human at the next feeding.

EPIDEMIOLOGY Malaria occurs throughout most of the tropical regions of the world. *P. falciparum* predominates in Africa, New Guinea, and Haiti; *P. vivax* is more common in Central America and the Indian subcontinent. The prevalence of these two species is approximately equal in South America, eastern Asia, and Oceania. *P.malariae* is found in most endemic areas, especially throughout sub-Saharan Africa, but is much less common. *P. ovale* is relatively unusual outside Africa.

The epidemiology of malaria is complex and may vary considerably even within relatively small geographic areas. Endemicity is traditionally defined in terms of palpable-spleen rates in children 2 to 9 years of age as hypoendemic (<10 percent), mesoendemic (11 to 50 percent), hyperendemic (51 to 75 percent), and holoendemic (>75 percent). In holo- and hyperendemic areas—e.g., certain regions of tropical Africa or coastal New Guinea, where there is intense *P. falciparum* transmission (up to one human bite per infected mosquito per day)—people are infected repeatedly throughout their lives. Here, morbidity and mortality during childhood are considerable. Immunity against disease is hard won, but by adulthood malarial infections are largely asymptomatic. This situation is termed *stable transmission*. In areas where transmission is low, erratic, or focal, full protective immunity is not acquired, and symptomatic disease may occur at all ages. This situation is termed *unstable transmission*. Even in areas with stable transmission, there is often an increased incidence coinciding with increased mosquito breeding during the rainy season. Malaria behaves like an epidemic disease in some areas, such as in northern India, Sri Lanka, Southeast Asia, Ethiopia, southern Africa, and Madagascar. An epidemic can develop when there are changes in environmental, economic, or social conditions, such as heavy rains following drought or migrations (usually of refugees or workers) from a nonmalarious region to an area of high transmission. This situation usually results in considerable mortality among all age groups.

The principal determinants of the epidemiology of malaria are the number (density), the human-biting habits, and the longevity of the anopheline mosquito vectors. More specifically, the transmission of malaria is directly proportional to the density of the vector, the square of the number of human bites per day per mosquito, and the tenth power of the probability of the mosquito's surviving for 1 day. In other words, the most effective mosquito vectors are those (such as *Anopheles gambiae* in western Africa) that occur in high densities, bite humans frequently, and are long-lived. Mosquito longevity is particularly important, because the portion of the parasite's life cycle that takes place within the mosquito—from gametocyte ingestion to subsequent inoculation—lasts for a minimum of 7 days (depending on ambient temperature); thus, to transmit malaria, the mosquito must survive for longer than 7 days. The entomologic inoculation rate—the number of sporozoite-positive mosquito bites per year—is the most common measure of malarial transmission and varies from <1 in some parts of Latin America and Southeast Asia to >300 in parts of tropical Africa.

ERYTHROCYTE CHANGES IN MALARIA After invading an erythrocyte, the growing parasite progressively consumes and degrades intracellular proteins, principally hemoglobin; the parasite also alters the red cell membrane by changing its transport properties, exposing cryptic surface antigens, and inserting new parasite-derived proteins. The red cell becomes more irregular in shape, more antigenic, and less deformable.

In *P. falciparum* infections, membrane protuberances appear on

Table 216-1

Characteristics of *Plasmodium* Species Infecting Humans

Characteristic	Finding for Indicated Species			
	P. falciparum	*P. vivax*	*P. ovale*	*P. malariae*
Duration of intra-hepatic phase (days)	5.5	8	9	15
Number of merozoites released per infected hepatocyte	30,000	10,000	15,000	15,000
Duration of erythrocytic cycle (hours)	48	48	50	72
Red cell preference	Younger cells (but can invade cells of all ages)	Reticulocytes	Reticulocytes	Older cells
Morphology	Usually only ring forms;* banana-shaped gametocytes	Irregularly shaped large rings and trophozoites; enlarged erythrocytes; Schüffner's dots	Infected erythrocytes, enlarged and oval; Schüffner's dots	Band or rectangular forms of trophozoites common
Pigment color	Black	Yellow-brown	Dark brown	Brown-black
Ability to cause relapses	No	Yes	Yes	No

* Parasitemia sometimes exceeds 2 percent with multiple infections of a single erythrocyte.

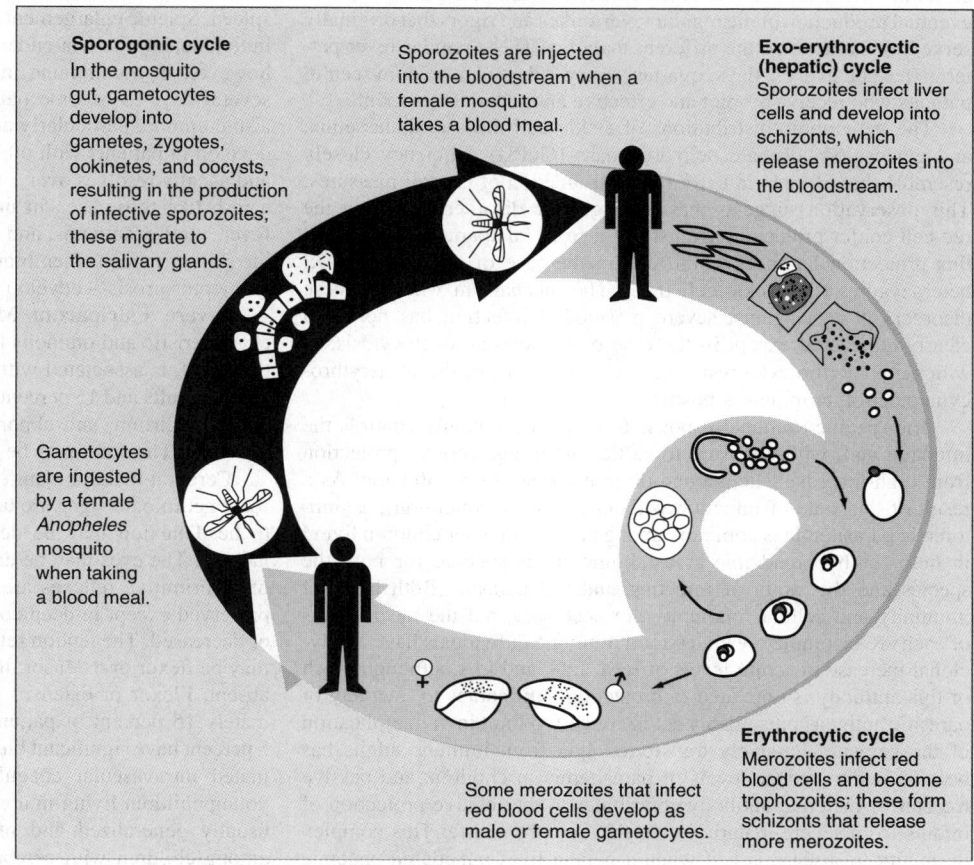

Sporogonic cycle
In the mosquito gut, gametocytes develop into gametes, zygotes, ookinetes, and oocysts, resulting in the production of infective sporozoites; these migrate to the salivary glands.

Sporozoites are injected into the bloodstream when a female mosquito takes a blood meal.

Exo-erythrocytic (hepatic) cycle
Sporozoites infect liver cells and develop into schizonts, which release merozoites into the bloodstream.

Gametocytes are ingested by a female *Anopheles* mosquito when taking a blood meal.

Some merozoites that infect red blood cells develop as male or female gametocytes.

Erythrocytic cycle
Merozoites infect red blood cells and become trophozoites; these form schizonts that release more merozoites.

FIGURE 216-1 The malaria transmission cycle.

the erythrocyte's surface in the second 24 h of the asexual cycle. These "knobs" extrude a high-molecular-weight, antigenically variant, strain-specific, adhesive protein that mediates attachment to receptors on venular and capillary endothelium—an event termed *cytoadherence*. Thus the infected erythrocytes sequester inside the small blood vessels. At the same stage, these *P. falciparum*–infected red cells may also adhere to uninfected red cells to form rosettes. The processes of cytoadherence and rosetting are central to the pathogenesis of falciparum malaria. They result in the sequestration of red cells containing mature forms of the parasite in vital organs (particularly the brain and heart), where they interfere with microcirculatory flow and metabolism. Sequestered parasites continue to develop out of reach of the principal host defense mechanism: splenic processing and filtration. As a consequence, only the younger ring forms of the asexual parasites are seen in the peripheral blood in falciparum malaria, and the level of peripheral parasitemia underestimates the true number of parasites within the body.

In the other three "benign" malarias, sequestration does not occur, and all stages of the parasite's development are evident on peripheral blood smears. Whereas *P. vivax*, *P. ovale*, and *P. malariae* show a marked predilection for either old red cells or reticulocytes and produce a level of parasitemia seldom exceeding 2 percent, *P. falciparum* can invade erythrocytes of all ages and may be associated with very high levels of parasitemia.

HOST RESPONSE   Initially, the host responds to plasmodial infection by activating nonspecific defense mechanisms. Splenic immunologic and filtrative clearance functions are augmented in malaria, and the removal of both parasitized and uninfected erythrocytes is accelerated. The parasitized cells escaping splenic removal are destroyed when the schizont ruptures. The material released induces the activation of macrophages and the release of proinflammatory mononuclear cell–derived cytokines, which cause fever and exert other pathologic effects. Temperatures of 40°C are schizonticidal; in untreated infections, the effect of such temperatures is to synchronize the parasitic cycle with eventual production of the regular fever spikes and rigors that originally served to characterize the different malarias. These regular fever patterns (tertian, every 2 days; quartan, every 3 days) are seldom seen in patients who receive prompt and effective antimalarial treatment.

The geographic distributions of sickle cell disease, thalassemia, and glucose-6-phosphate dehydrogenase (G6PD) deficiency closely resemble that of malaria before the introduction of control measures. This observation suggests that these genetic disorders affecting the red cell confer protection against death from falciparum malaria, and this protection has been confirmed in the case of hemoglobin A/S heterozygotes (the sickle cell trait). The mechanism whereby these disorders protect against severe plasmodial infection has not been clearly elucidated except in the case of Melanesian ovalocytosis, in which rigid erythrocytes resist merozoite invasion and the intraerythrocytic electrolyte milieu is hostile.

The specific immune response to malaria eventually controls the infection and, with exposure to sufficient strains, confers protection from high-level parasitemia and disease but not from infection. As a result of this state of infection without illness (premunition), asymptomatic parasitemia is common among adults and older children living in holo- or hyperendemic areas. Immunity is specific for both the species and the strain of infecting malarial parasite. Both humoral immunity and cellular immunity are necessary, but the mechanisms of each are incompletely understood. Immune individuals have a polyclonal increase in serum levels of IgM, IgG, and IgA, although much of this antibody is unrelated to protection. Antibodies to a variety of parasitic antigens presumably act in concert to limit in vivo replication of the parasite. Passively transferred IgG from immune adults has been shown to reduce levels of parasitemia in children, and passive transfer of maternal antibody contributes to the relative protection of infants from severe malaria in the first months of life. This complex immunity to disease is lost when a person lives outside an endemic area for several months or longer.

Several factors retard the development of cellular immunity. These factors include the absence of major histocompatibility antigens on the surface of infected red cells, which precludes direct T cell recognition; malaria antigen–specific immune unresponsiveness; and the enormous strain diversity of malarial parasites along with the ability of the parasites to express immunodominant variant antigens on the erythrocyte surface that change during the period of infection. Strain diversity also has an impact on the heterogeneity of the humoral antibody response. Immunity to all strains is never achieved. Parasites may persist in the blood for months (or, in the case of *P. malariae*, for many years) if treatment is not given. The complexity of the immune response in malaria, the sophistication of the parasites' evasion mechanisms, and the lack of a good in vitro correlate with clinical immunity have all slowed progress toward an effective vaccine.

CLINICAL FEATURES   The first symptoms of malaria are nonspecific; the lack of a sense of well-being, headache, fatigue, abdominal discomfort, and muscle aches followed by fever are all similar to the symptoms of a minor viral illness. In some instances, a prominence of headache, chest pain, abdominal pain, arthralgia, myalgia, or diarrhea may suggest another diagnosis. Although headache may be severe in malaria, there is no neck stiffness or photophobia resembling that in meningitis. While myalgia may be prominent, it is not usually as severe as in dengue fever, and the muscles are not tender as in leptospirosis or typhus. Nausea, vomiting, and orthostatic hypotension are common. The classic malarial paroxysms, in which fever spikes, chills, and rigors occur at regular intervals, suggest infection with *P. vivax* or *P. ovale*. The fever is irregular at first (that of falciparum malaria may never become regular); the temperature of nonimmune individuals and children often rises above 40°C in conjunction with tachycardia and sometimes delirium. Although childhood febrile convulsions may occur with any of the malarias, generalized seizures are specifically associated with falciparum malaria and may herald the development of cerebral disease. Many clinical abnormalities have been described in acute malaria, but most patients with uncomplicated infections have few abnormal physical findings other than fever, malaise, mild anemia, and (in some cases) a palpable spleen. Splenic enlargement is very common among otherwise-healthy individuals in malaria-endemic areas and reflects repeated infections; however, in nonimmune individuals with malaria, the spleen takes several days to become palpable. Slight enlargement of the liver is also common, particularly among young children. Mild jaundice may develop in patients with otherwise-uncomplicated falciparum malaria and usually resolves over 1 to 3 weeks. Malaria is not associated with a rash like those seen in meningococcal septicemia, typhus, enteric fever, viral exanthems, and drug reactions. Petechial hemorrhages in the skin or mucous membranes—features of viral hemorrhagic fevers and leptospirosis—develop only rarely in severe falciparum malaria.

Severe Falciparum Malaria   *Cerebral malaria*   Coma is a characteristic and ominous feature of falciparum malaria and, despite treatment, is associated with death rates of approximately 20 percent among adults and 15 percent among children. Lesser degrees of obtundation, delirium, and abnormal behavior should also be taken very seriously. The onset may be gradual or sudden following a convulsion.

Cerebral malaria manifests as diffuse symmetric encephalopathy; focal neurologic signs are unusual. Although some passive resistance to head flexion may be detected, signs of meningeal irritation are lacking. The eyes may be divergent and a pout reflex is common, but other primitive reflexes are usually absent. The corneal reflexes are preserved except in deep coma. Muscle tone may be either increased or decreased. The tendon reflexes are variable, and the plantar reflexes may be flexor or extensor; the abdominal and cremasteric reflexes are absent. Flexor or extensor posturing may be documented. Approximately 15 percent of patients have retinal hemorrhages. Fewer than 5 percent have significant bleeding or other clinical evidence of disseminated intravascular coagulation. Anemia is also common among young children living in areas with stable transmission. Convulsions, usually generalized and often repeated, are common, particularly among children with cerebral malaria. Whereas adults rarely suffer neurologic sequelae, approximately 10 percent of children surviving cerebral malaria—especially those with hypoglycemia, severe anemia, repeated seizures, and deep coma—have some residual neurologic deficit when they regain consciousness.

Hypoglycemia   An important and common complication of severe malaria, hypoglycemia is associated with a poor prognosis and is particularly problematic in children and pregnant women. Hypoglycemia in malaria results from a failure of hepatic gluconeogenesis and an increase in the consumption of glucose by both host and parasite. To compound the situation, quinine and quinidine, the drugs of choice for the treatment of severe chloroquine-resistant malaria, are powerful stimulants of pancreatic insulin secretion. Hyperinsulinemic hypoglycemia is especially troublesome in pregnant women receiving quinine treatment. In severe disease, the clinical diagnosis of hypoglycemia is difficult as the usual physical signs (sweating, gooseflesh, tachycardia) are absent and the neurologic impairment caused by hypoglycemia cannot be distinguished from that caused by malaria.

Lactic acidosis   Lactic acidosis commonly coexists with hypoglycemia in patients with malaria. Anaerobic glycolysis occurs in tissues where sequestered parasitized erythrocytes interfere with microcirculatory flow; lactate production by the parasites combines with a failure of hepatic lactate clearance to cause lactic acidosis. The prognosis of lactic acidosis is poor; acidotic breathing, a sign of poor prognosis in severe malaria, is usually followed by circulatory failure refractory to volume expansion or to treatment with inotropic drugs or by respiratory arrest.

Noncardiogenic pulmonary edema   Adults with severe falciparum malaria may develop noncardiogenic pulmonary edema even after several days of antimalarial therapy. The pathogenesis of this variant of the adult respiratory distress syndrome is unclear. Mortality is over 80 percent. This condition can be aggravated by overly vigorous administration of intravenous fluid.

Renal impairment   Renal impairment is common among adults with severe falciparum malaria but rare among children. The pathogenesis of renal failure is unclear but may be related to parasitized-erythrocyte sequestration interfering with renal microcirculatory flow and regional metabolism. Clinically and pathologically, this syndrome resembles acute tubular necrosis. Renal cortical necrosis never develops. Mortality in the initial phase of hypercatabolic acute renal failure is high; in survivors, urine flow resumes in a median of 4 days, and serum creatinine levels return to normal in a mean of 17 days (see Chap. 270). Dialysis considerably enhances the likelihood of a patient's survival.

Hematologic abnormalities   Anemia results from accelerated red cell destruction and removal by the spleen in conjunction with ineffective erythropoiesis. In severe malaria in nonimmune individuals and in areas with unstable transmission, anemia can develop rapidly and transfusion is often required. In many areas of Africa, children may develop severe anemia due to repeated malarial infections. This is a common consequence of continued infection resulting from treatment with chloroquine (or other drugs) to which the parasites are resistant.

Slight coagulation abnormalities are common in falciparum malaria, and mild thrombocytopenia is usual. Fewer than 5 percent of patients with cerebral malaria have significant bleeding with evidence of disseminated intravascular coagulation. Hematemesis, presumably from stress ulceration or acute gastric erosions, may also occur.

Other complications   Aspiration pneumonia following convulsions is an important cause of death in cerebral malaria. Malaria predisposes to bacterial superinfection, possibly through its effect on immune responsiveness. Chest infections and catheter-induced urinary tract infections are common among patients who are unconscious for more than 3 days. Spontaneous gram-negative septicemia develops occasionally in severe malaria, and *Salmonella* septicemia has been associated with *P. falciparum* infections in endemic areas.

Malaria in Pregnancy   Falciparum malaria is an important cause of fetal death. In hyper- and holoendemic areas, malaria in primigravida and secundigravida is associated with low birth weight. In general, infected mothers remain asymptomatic despite intense parasitization of the placenta due to sequestration of parasitized erythrocytes in the placental microcirculation.

In areas with unstable transmission of malaria, pregnant women are prone to severe infections and are particularly vulnerable to high-level parasitemia with anemia, hypoglycemia, and acute pulmonary edema. Fetal distress, premature labor, and stillbirth or low birth weight are common results. Congenital malaria occurs in fewer than 5 percent of newborns whose mothers are infected and is related directly to the parasitic density in maternal blood and in the placenta.

Malaria in Children   Most of the estimated 1 to 3 million persons who die of falciparum malaria each year are young African children. Convulsions, coma, hypoglycemia, metabolic acidosis, and severe anemia are relatively common among children with severe malaria, whereas deep jaundice, acute renal failure, and acute pulmonary edema are unusual. In general, children tolerate the antimalarial drugs well and respond rapidly to treatment.

Transfusion Malaria   Malaria can be transmitted by blood transfusion, needle-stick injury, sharing of needles by infected drug addicts, or organ transplantation. The incubation period in these settings is often short because there is no preerythrocytic stage of development. The clinical features and management of these cases are the same as for naturally acquired infections, although falciparum malaria tends to be especially severe in drug addicts. Radical chemotherapy with primaquine is unnecessary for *P. vivax* and *P. ovale* infections.

CHRONIC COMPLICATIONS OF MALARIA   **Tropical Splenomegaly (Hyperreactive Malarial Splenomegaly)**   Chronic or repeated malarial infections produce hypergammaglobulinemia; normochromic, normocytic anemia; and—in certain situations—splenomegaly. Some residents of malaria-endemic areas in tropical Africa and Asia exhibit an abnormal immunologic response to repeated infections that is characterized by massive splenomegaly, hepatomegaly, marked elevations in serum titers of IgM and malarial antibody, hepatic sinusoidal lymphocytosis, and (in Africa) peripheral (B cell) lymphocytosis. This syndrome has been associated with the production of cytotoxic IgM antibodies to suppressor (CD8 +) lymphocytes, which leads to uninhibited B cell production of IgM and the formation of cryoglobulins (IgM aggregates and immune complexes). This immunologic process stimulates reticuloendothelial hyperplasia and clearance activity and eventually produces splenomegaly. Patients with hyperreactive malarial splenomegaly (HMS) present with an abdominal mass or a dragging sensation in the abdomen and occasional sharp abdominal pains suggesting perisplenitis. Anemia and some degree of pancytopenia are usually evident, but in many cases malarial parasites cannot be found in peripheral blood smears. Vulnerability to respiratory and skin infections is increased; many patients die of overwhelming sepsis. Persons with HMS who are living in endemic areas should receive antimalarial chemoprophylaxis; the results are usually good. In nonendemic areas, treatment is advised. In some cases refractory to therapy, clonal lymphoproliferation may develop and then evolve into a malignant lymphoproliferative disorder.

Quartan Malarial Nephropathy   Chronic or repeated infections with *P. malariae* may cause soluble immune-complex injury to the renal glomeruli, resulting in the nephrotic syndrome. Other, unidentified factors must contribute to this process since only a very small proportion of infected patients develop renal disease. The histologic appearance is that of focal or segmental glomerulonephritis with splitting of the capillary basement membrane. Subendothelial dense deposits are seen on electron microscopy, and immunofluorescence reveals deposits of complement and immunoglobulins; in samples of renal tissue from children, *P. malariae* antigens are often visible. A coarse-granular pattern of basement membrane immunofluorescent deposits (predominantly IgG3) with selective proteinuria carries a better prognosis than a fine-granular, predominantly IgG2 pattern with nonselective proteinuria. Quartan nephropathy usually responds poorly to treatment with either antimalarial agents or glucocorticoids and cytotoxic drugs.

Burkitt's Lymphoma and Epstein-Barr Virus Infection   It is possible that malaria-related immunosuppression provokes infection with lymphoma viruses. Burkitt's lymphoma is strongly associated with Epstein-Barr virus. The prevalence of this childhood tumor is high in malarious areas of Africa.

DIAGNOSIS   Demonstration of the Parasite   The diagnosis of malaria rests on the demonstration of asexual forms of the parasite in peripheral blood smears subjected to Romanovsky staining. Giemsa at pH 7.2 is preferred; Wright's, Field's, or Leishman's stain can also be used. Both thin and thick blood smears should be examined.

The thin blood smear should be air-dried rapidly, fixed in anhydrous methanol, and stained, and the red cells in the tail of the film should then be examined under oil immersion. The level of parasitemia is expressed as the number of parasitized erythrocytes among 1000 cells, and this figure is then converted to the number of parasitized erythrocytes per microliter. A simple, sensitive, and specific diagnostic stick test that detects *P. falciparum* histidine-rich protein 2 in finger-prick blood samples has recently been introduced, and nucleic acid–based assays are being developed. The relation between parasitemia and prognosis is complex; in general, patients with more than 10^5 parasites per microliter are at increased risk of dying, but nonimmune patients may die with much lower counts. In severe malaria, a poor prognosis is indicated by a predominance of more mature *P. falciparum* parasites (i.e., more than 20 percent of parasites with visible pigment) or circulating schizonts in the peripheral blood film or by the presence of phagocytosed malarial pigment in more than 5 percent of neutrophils.

The thick blood film should be of uneven thickness. The smear should be dried thoroughly and stained without fixing. As many layers of erythrocytes overlie one another and are lysed during the staining procedure, the thick film has the advantage of concentrating the parasites (by 20- to 40-fold compared with a thin blood film) and thus increasing diagnostic sensitivity. Both parasites and white cells are counted, and the number of parasites per unit volume is calculated from the total leukocyte count. A minimum of 200 white cells should be counted. Interpretation of thick films requires some experience because artifacts are common. Before a thick smear is judged to be negative, 100 to 200 fields should be examined under oil immersion. Phagocytosed malarial pigment is sometimes seen inside peripheral blood monocytes or polymorphonuclear leukocytes and may provide a clue to recent infection if malarial parasites are not detectable. After the clearance of the parasites, malarial pigment is often evident for several days in peripheral blood phagocytes, bone marrow aspirates, or smears of fluid expressed after intradermal puncture. Staining of parasites with the fluorescent dye acridine orange allows more rapid diagnosis of cases in which the level of parasitemia is low.

Laboratory Findings   Normochromic, normocytic anemia is usually documented. The leukocyte count is generally low to normal, although it may be raised in very severe infections. The erythrocyte sedimentation rate, degree of plasma viscosity, and level of C-reactive protein are high. The platelet count is usually reduced to about 10^5 per microliter. Severe infections may be accompanied by prolonged prothrombin and partial thromboplastin times and by especially severe thrombocytopenia. Levels of antithrombin III are reduced even in mild infection. In uncomplicated malaria, plasma concentrations of electrolytes, blood urea nitrogen, and creatinine are usually normal. Findings in severe malaria may include metabolic acidosis, with low plasma concentrations of glucose, sodium, bicarbonate, calcium, phosphate, and albumin together with elevations in lactate, blood urea nitrogen, creatinine, urate, muscle and liver enzymes, and conjugated and unconjugated bilirubin. Hypergammaglobulinemia is usual in immune and semi-immune subjects, and urinalysis generally gives normal results. In adults and children with cerebral malaria, the mean opening pressure at lumbar puncture is about 160 mm of cerebrospinal fluid; the cerebrospinal fluid usually is normal or has a slightly elevated total protein level [<1.0 g/L (100 mg/dL)].

PREVENTION   In most of the tropics, the eradication of malaria is not feasible because of the widespread distribution of *Anopheles*

breeding sites, the great number of infected persons, and inadequacies in resources, infrastructure, and control programs. Where possible, the disease is contained by judicious use of insecticides to kill the mosquito vector, rapid diagnosis and appropriate patient management, and administration of chemoprophylaxis to high-risk groups. Despite massive investment in efforts to develop a malaria vaccine, no safe, effective, long-lasting vaccine is likely to be available for general use in the near future (see Chap. 122).

Personal Protection Against Malaria   Simple measures to reduce the frequency of mosquito bites in malarious areas are very important. These measures include the avoidance of exposure to mosquitoes at their peak feeding times (usually dusk and dawn) and the use of insect repellents, suitable clothing, and insecticide-impregnated bed nets. Widespread use of bed nets, particularly those treated with permethrin (a residual pyrethroid), often reduces the incidence of malaria and has recently been shown to reduce mortality in western and eastern Africa.

Chemoprophylaxis (See Table 216-2)   Few areas of therapeutics are as controversial as antimalarial drug prophylaxis. Recommendations for prophylaxis depend on a knowledge of local patterns of plasmodial drug sensitivity and the likelihood of acquiring malarial infection. Chemoprophylaxis is never entirely reliable, and malaria should always be considered in the differential diagnosis of fever in patients who have traveled to endemic areas, even if they are taking prophylactic antimalarial drugs.

All pregnant women at risk should receive prophylaxis. In addition, antimalarial prophylaxis should be considered for children between the ages of 3 months and 4 years in areas where malaria causes high childhood mortality. However, such prophylaxis may not be logistically feasible in many countries. Children born to nonimmune mothers in endemic areas (usually expatriates moving to these areas) should receive prophylaxis from birth.

Travelers should start taking antimalarial drugs at least 1 week before departure so that any untoward reactions can be detected and therapeutic antimalarial blood concentrations will be present when needed. Antimalarial prophylaxis should continue for 4 weeks after the traveler has left the endemic area.

Mefloquine has become the antimalarial prophylactic agent of choice for much of the tropics because it is usually effective against multidrug-resistant falciparum malaria and is reasonably well tolerated. Nausea, dizziness, muzziness, disturbed sleep patterns, and dysphoria are relatively common. Approximately 1 in every 10,000 recipients develops an acute reversible neuropsychiatric reaction manifest by confusion, psychosis, convulsions, or encephalopathy. In recent studies in Africa, mefloquine prophylaxis was found to be effective and safe during pregnancy.

Daily administration of doxycycline is an effective alternative to mefloquine that also exhibits some causal (preerythrocytic) prophylactic activity. It is generally well tolerated but may cause vulvovaginal thrush, diarrhea, and photosensitivity and cannot be used by children less than 8 years old or by pregnant women. Recent studies indicate that daily primaquine is effective for prophylaxis of *P. falciparum* and *P. vivax* malaria; further confirmatory studies are needed.

Chloroquine remains the drug of choice for the prevention of infection with drug-sensitive *P. falciparum* and with the other human malarial species (although chloroquine resistance in *P. vivax* has been reported recently from parts of eastern Asia and Oceania). This agent is generally well tolerated, although some patients are unable to take the drug because of dysphoria, headache, or—in dark-skinned patients—pruritus. (A concomitant filarial infection may provoke or aggravate chloroquine-induced pruritus.) Chloroquine is considered safe in pregnancy. With chronic administration over more than 5 years, a characteristic dose-related retinopathy may develop, but this condition is rare at the doses used for antimalarial prophylaxis. Idiosyncratic or allergic reactions are likewise rare. Skeletal and cardiac myopathy are rare and much more likely at the high doses used in the treatment of rheumatoid arthritis. Neuropsychiatric reactions and skin rashes are unusual. Amodiaquine, a related aminoquinoline, is associated with a high risk of agranulocytosis (approximately 1:2000) and is not recommended.

Table 216-2

Prophylaxis and Self-Treatment for Malaria

Drug	Usage	Adult Dosage	Child Dosage
Prophylaxis			
Mefloquine	Used in areas where chloroquine-resistant malaria has been reported	228 mg of base (250 mg of salt) orally, once/week*	<15 kg: 4.6 mg of base/kg (5 mg of salt/kg) 15–19 kg: ¼ tablet/week 20–30 kg: ½ tablet/week 31–45 kg: ¾ tablet/week >45 kg: 1 tablet/week
Doxycycline	Used as alternative to mefloquine	100 mg orally, once/day	>8 years of age: 2 mg/kg per day orally; maximum dose, 100 mg/d
Chloroquine	Used in areas where chloroquine-resistant malaria has *not* been reported	300 mg of base (500 mg of salt) orally, once/week	5 mg of base/kg (8.3 mg of salt/kg) orally, once/week; maximum dose, 300 mg of base
Proguanil (not available in U.S.)	Used simultaneously *with* chloroquine as alternative to mefloquine or doxycycline	200 mg orally, once/day, in combination with weekly chloroquine	<2 years: 50 mg/d 2–6 years: 100 mg/d 7–10 years: 150 mg/d >10 years: 200 mg/d
Primaquine	Used for travelers only after testing for G6PD deficiency; postexposure prevention for relapsing malaria	15 mg of base (26.3 mg of salt) orally, once/day for 14 days	0.3 mg of base/kg (0.5 mg of salt/kg) orally, once/day for 14 days
Self-treatment			
Pyrimethamine-sulfadoxine†	In areas with chloroquine-resistant malaria, should be carried during travel by persons taking mefloquine or doxycycline	3 tablets (75 mg of pyrimethamine and 1500 mg of sulfadoxine) orally, as a single dose	5–10 kg: ½ tablet 11–20 kg: 1 tablet 21–30 kg: 1½ tablets 31–45 kg: 2 tablets >45 kg: 3 tablets

* Tablets manufactured outside the United States may contain 250 mg of base.
† Regimen is used for treatment only.

In the past, the dihydrofolate reductase inhibitors pyrimethamine and proguanil (chloroguanide) have been administered widely, but resistant strains of both *P. falciparum* and *P. vivax* have limited their use. Whereas antimalarial quinolines such as chloroquine act on the erythrocyte stage of parasitic development, the dihydrofolate reductase inhibitors also inhibit preerythrocytic growth in the liver and development in the mosquito. Proguanil is safe and well tolerated, although mouth ulceration occurs in 8 percent of persons using this drug; it is considered the safest agent for antimalarial prophylaxis in pregnancy. The prophylactic use of the combination of pyrimethamine and sulfadoxine is not recommended because of an unacceptable incidence of severe toxicity, principally exfoliative dermatitis and other skin rashes, agranulocytosis, hepatitis, and pulmonary eosinophilia. The combination of pyrimethamine with dapsone (0.2/1.5 mg/kg weekly; 25/200 mg maximum) is a second-line drug available in some countries and can be used in areas with chloroquine-resistant *P. falciparum*. This combination is generally well tolerated; however, resistance is increasing, and dapsone may cause methemoglobinemia and allergic reactions and (at higher doses) may pose a significant risk of agranulocytosis.

Because of the increasing spread and intensity of plasmodial resistance to chloroquine in Africa and other areas of the world (Fig. 216-2), the Centers for Disease Control and Prevention, which recommends a weekly dose of mefloquine for all travelers, maintains an updated 24-h malaria information audiotape that can be accessed by touch-tone telephone (404-332-4555) and an interactive international travel information service that responds by fax (404-332-4565).

℞ TREATMENT

When a patient in or from a malarious area presents with fever, a blood smear should be prepared and examined to confirm the diagnosis and identify the species of infecting parasite. Patients with severe malaria or those unable to take oral drugs should receive parenteral antimalarial therapy. If there is any doubt about the resistance status of the infecting organism, then quinine or quinidine should be given. Several drugs are available for oral treatment, and the choice of drug depends on the likely sensitivity of the infecting parasites. Despite recent evidence of chloroquine resistance in *P. vivax* from Oceania, chloroquine remains the treatment of choice for the benign human malarias. Characteristics of various antimalarial agents are shown in Table 216-3, and regimens of drugs approved

FIGURE 216-2 Worldwide distribution of malaria and drug-resistant *Plasmodium falciparum*, 1996.

⬚ Chloroquine-resistant malaria   ● Chloroquine-sensitive malaria   ○ Multiple drug-resistant malaria

Table 216-3

Properties of Antimalarial Drugs

Drug(s)	Pharmacokinetic Properties	Antimalarial Activity	Minor Toxicity	Major Toxicity

Quinine, quinidine	Good oral and IM absorption; Cl and V_d reduced, but plasma protein binding (principally to ∝1 acid glycoprotein) increased (90%) in malaria; $t_{1/2}$: 16 h in malaria, 11 h in healthy persons	Acts mainly on trophozoite blood stage; kills gametocytes of *P. vivax*, *P. ovale*, and *P. malariae*; no action on liver stages	*Common:*
			  Cinchonism: tinnitus, high-tone hearing loss, nausea, vomiting, dysphoria, postural hypotension; ECG QT_c interval prolongation
			Rare:
			  Diarrhea, visual disturbance, rashes
			Note:
			  Bitter taste
				Common:
				  Hypoglycemia
				Rare:
				  Hypotension, blindness, deafness, cardiac arrhythmias, thrombocytopenia, hemolysis, hemolytic-uremic syndrome, cholestatic hepatitis, neuromuscular paralysis
				Note:
				  Quinidine more cardiotoxic

Chloroquine	Good oral absorption, very rapid IM and SC absorption; complex pharmacokinetics; enormous Cl and V_d (unaffected by malaria); blood concentration profile determined by distribution processes in malaria; $t_{1/2}$: 1–2 months	As for quinine but more rapid	*Common:*
			  Nausea, dysphoria, pruritus in dark-skinned patients, postural hypotension
			Rare:
			  Accommodation difficulties, rash
			Note:
			  Bitter taste, well tolerated
				Acute:
				  Hypotensive shock (parenteral), cardiac arrhythmias, neuropsychiatric reactions
				Chronic:
				  Retinopathy (cumulative dose, >100 g), skeletal and cardiac myopathy

Mefloquine	Adequate oral absorption; no parenteral preparation; $t_{1/2}$: 14–20 days (shorter in malaria)	As for quinine	Nausea, giddiness, dysphoria, confusion, sleeplessness, nightmares	Neuropsychiatric reactions, convulsions, encephalopathy
Tetracycline, doxycycline*	Excellent absorption; $t_{1/2}$: 8 h for tetracycline, 18 h for doxycycline	Weak antimalarial activity; should not be used alone for treatment	Gastrointestinal intolerance, deposition in growing bones and teeth, photosensitivity, moniliasis, benign intracranial hypertension	Renal failure in patients with impaired renal function (tetracycline)
Halofantrine†	Highly variable absorption; $t_{1/2}$: 1–3 days (active desbutyl metabolite $t_{1/2}$: 2–7 days)	As for quinine but more rapid	Diarrhea	Prolonged ECG QT_c interval, AV conduction delay, cardiac arrhythmias
Artemisinin and derivatives (artemether, artesunate)	Good oral absorption, variable absorption of IM artemether; artesunate and artemether biotransformed to active metabolite dyhydroartemisinin; all drugs eliminated rapidly	Broader stage specificity and more rapid than other drugs; no action on liver stages	Reduction in reticulocyte count; fever	Neurotoxicity reported in animals, but no evidence in humans
Pyrimethamine	Good oral absorption, variable IM absorption; $t_{1/2}$: 4 days	For blood stages, acts mainly on mature forms; causal prophylactic	Well tolerated	Megaloblastic anemia, pancytopenia, pulmonary infiltration
Proguanil (chloroguanide)	Good oral absorption; biotransformed to active metabolite cycloguanil; $t_{1/2}$: 16 h	Causal prophylactic; not used for treatment	Well tolerated, with mouth ulcers and rare alopecia	Megaloblastic anemia in renal failure
Primaquine	Complete oral absorption; active compound not known; $t_{1/2}$: 7 h	Radical cure; some activity against blood-stage infection, used to eradicate exoerythrocytic (hepatic) forms of *P. vivax* and *P. ovale* and to prevent relapses; kills gametocytes of *P. falciparum*	Nausea, vomiting, diarrhea, abdominal pain, hemolysis, methemoglobinemia	Massive hemolysis in subjects with severe G6PD deficiency

* Tetracycline and doxycycline should not be given to pregnant women or to children <8 years of age.
† Halofantrine should not be used by patients with long ECG QT_c intervals or known conduction disturbances or by those taking drugs that may affect ventricular repolarization—e.g., quinidine, quinine, mefloquine, chloroquine, neuroleptics, tricyclic antidepressants, terfenadine, or astemizole.
NOTE: Cl, systemic clearance; V_d, total apparent volume of distribution; IM, intramuscular; SC, subcutaneous; ECG, electrocardiogram.

by the U.S. Food and Drug Administration are detailed in Table 216-4.

Severe Malaria The antiarrhythmic quinidine gluconate is as effective as quinine and, as it is more readily available, has replaced quinine for the treatment of malaria in the United States. The administration of quinidine must be closely monitored if dysrrhythmias and hypotension are to be avoided. Total plasma levels in excess of 8 μg/mL, a QT_c interval of greater than 0.6 s, or QRS widening beyond 25 percent of baseline are indications for slowing infusion rates. If arrhythmia or saline-unresponsive hypotension develops, treatment with this drug should be discontinued. Quinine is safer than quinidine, and cardiovascular monitoring is not required except when the recipient has cardiac disease. In some areas, the Chinese drugs derived from artemisinin (artemether and artesunate) have become first-line treatments for severe malaria. These agents are rapidly effective against multidrug-resistant falciparum malaria and appear to be safe. They are not available in the United States.

Severe falciparum malaria constitutes a medical emergency requiring intensive nursing care and careful management. The patient should be weighed and, if comatose, placed on his or her side and given a single parenteral dose of phenobarbital (5 to 20 mg/kg) to prevent convulsions. Frequent evaluation of the patient's condition is essential. Ancillary drugs such as high-dose glucocorticoids, urea, heparin, and dextran are of no value. The choice of antimalarial drug depends on a knowledge of the prevailing sensitivity of *P. falciparum* to antimalarials. If there is any doubt, quinine or quinidine should be given. Because the systemic clearance and apparent volume of distribution of these alkaloids are markedly reduced and plasma protein binding is increased in severe malaria, the blood concentrations attained with a given dose are higher. The optimal therapeutic range for quinine in severe malaria is not known with certainty, but total plasma concentrations between 8 and 20 μg/mL are effective and do not cause serious toxicity. An initial loading dose should be given so that therapeutic concentrations are reached as soon as possible. If the patient remains seriously ill or in acute renal failure for more than 2 days, the maintenance doses should be reduced by 30 to 50 percent to prevent toxic accumulation of the drugs. The initial doses should never be reduced. If chloroquine is given, dose reduction is unnecessary even in renal failure. Provided that it can be performed safely, exchange transfusion is indicated for patients with high-level parasitemia (>15 percent) and vital organ dysfunction. Exchange transfusion should be considered for severely ill patients with a level of parasitemia between 5 and 15 percent.

When the patient is unconscious, the blood glucose level should be measured every 4 to 6 h, and values below 2.2 mmol/L (40 mg/dL) should prompt treatment with intravenous dextrose. All patients treated with intravenous quinine or quinidine should receive a continuous infusion of 5 to 10% dextrose. The parasite count and hematocrit level should be measured every 6 to 12 h. Anemia develops rapidly; if the hematocrit level falls below 20 percent, then whole blood (preferably fresh) or packed cells should be transfused slowly, with careful attention to circulatory status and judicious use of small doses of a diuretic to prevent fluid overload. Exchange transfusion should be strongly considered for patients with a high level of parasitemia (>10 percent) and altered mental status. Renal function should be checked daily. Management of fluid balance is difficult in severe malaria because of the thin dividing line between overhydration (leading to pulmonary edema) and underhydration (contributing to renal impairment). If necessary, pulmonary artery occlusion pressures should be measured and maintained in the low-normal range. As soon as the patient can take fluids, oral therapy should be substituted for parenteral treatment.

Uncomplicated Malaria   Infections due to *P. vivax*, *P. malariae*, *P. ovale*, and known sensitive strains of *P. falciparum* should be treated with oral chloroquine (25 mg of base/kg). In Africa, chloroquine-resistant strains are usually sensitive to sulfadoxine-pyrimethamine. Where there is resistance to the latter combination as well, either quinine plus tetracycline/doxycycline or mefloquine should be used; tetracycline and doxycycline cannot be given to pregnant women or to children <8 years of age. Oral quinine is extremely bitter and regularly produces cinchonism, a complex of symptoms comprising tinnitus, high-tone deafness, nausea, vomiting, and dysphoria. Compliance is poor with the required 5- to 7-day regimens of this drug. Mefloquine can be given at a dosage of 25 mg/kg (15 mg/kg followed 8 to 12 h later by 10 mg/kg). Although significant resistance to mefloquine has been documented in Thailand, Burma, Vietnam, and Cambodia, this agent usually is effective against multidrug-resistant strains of *P. falciparum*.

Patients should be monitored for vomiting for 1 h after the administration of any oral antimalarial drug. Symptom-based treatment, with tepid sponging and acetaminophen administration, lowers fever and thereby reduces the patient's propensity to vomit these drugs. Minor central nervous system reactions (nausea, dizziness, sleep disturbances) are common. The incidence of serious adverse neuropsychiatric reactions to mefloquine treatment is approximately 1 in 1000. All the antimalarial quinolines (chloroquine, mefloquine, and quinine) exacerbate the orthostatic hypotension associated with malaria, and all are tolerated better by children than by adults. Pregnant women, young children, patients unable to tolerate oral

Table 216-4

Recommended Therapeutic Doses of Antimalarial Drugs

Drug	Uncomplicated Malaria (Oral)	Severe Malaria* (Parenteral)
Chloroquine	10 mg of base/kg followed by 10 mg/kg at 24 h and 5 mg/kg at 48 h *or* by 5 mg/kg at 12, 24, and 36 h (total dose, 25 mg/kg); for *P. vivax* or *P. ovale*, primaquine (0.25 mg of base/kg/d for 14 days†) added for radical cure	10 mg of base/kg by constant-rate infusion over 8 h followed by 15 mg/kg over 24 h *or* by 3.5 mg of base/kg by IM or SC injection every 6 h (total dose, 25 mg/kg)
Sulfadoxine/pyrimethamine	20/1 mg/kg, single oral dose (3 tablets for adults)	—
Mefloquine	For semi-immunes, 15 mg of base/kg as a single dose; in areas with mefloquine resistance or for nonimmunes, 15 mg/kg followed 8–12 h later by second dose of 10 mg/kg;	—
Quinine	10 mg of salt/kg q 8 h for 7 days combined with tetracycline‡ (4 mg/kg qid) or doxycycline (3 mg/kg once daily) for 7 days	20 mg of salt/kg by IV infusion over 4 h§ followed by 10 mg/kg over 2–8 h every 8 h
Quinidine gluconate	—	10 mg of base/kg by constant-rate infusion over 1–2 h followed by 0.02 mg/kg per min, with ECG monitoring¶
Artesunate	In combination with 25 mg of mefloquine/kg, 10–12 mg/kg given in divided doses over 3–5 days (e.g., 4 mg/kg for 3 days or 4 mg/kg followed by 1.5 mg/kg per day for 4 days); if used alone, same dose divided over 7 days (usually 4 mg/kg initially followed by 2 mg/kg on days 2 and 3 followed by 1 mg/kg on days 4–7)	2.4 mg/kg IV or IM stat followed by 1.2 mg/kg at 12 and 24 h and then daily
Artemether	Same regimen as for artesunate	3.2 mg/kg IM stat followed by 1.6 mg/kg/d

* Oral treatment should be substituted for parenteral therapy as soon as the patient can take tablets by mouth.
† In Oceania and Southeast Asia, the dose should be 0.33 to 0.5 mg of base/kg. This regimen should not be used in patients with severe variants of G6PD deficiency.
‡ Neither tetracycline nor doxycycline should be given to pregnant women or to children <8 years old.
§ Alternatively, infusion of 7 mg of salt/kg over 30 minutes can be followed by 10 mg of salt/kg over 4 h.
¶ Some authorities recommend a lower dose of intravenous quinine: 6.2 mg of base/kg over 1–2 h followed by 0.0125 mg/kg per min.

NOTE: In severe malaria, quinine or quinidine should be used if there is any doubt about infecting strain's sensitivity to chloroquine. IM, intramuscular; SC, subcutaneous; IV, intravenous; ECG, electrocardiogram.

therapy, and nonimmune subjects (e.g., travelers) with suspected malaria should be hospitalized. If there is any doubt as to the identity of the infecting malarial species, treatment for falciparum malaria should be given. A negative blood smear does not rule out malaria; thick blood films should be checked 1 and 2 days later to exclude the diagnosis. Nonimmune subjects with malaria should have daily parasite counts performed until negative thick films indicate clearance of the parasite. If the level of parasitemia does not fall below 25 percent of the admission value in 48 h or if parasitemia has not cleared by 7 days (and compliance is assumed), drug resistance is likely and the regimen should be changed. Quinine (or quinidine) and tetracycline should be reserved for multidrug-resistant infections, but if falciparum malaria has been contracted in an area of known drug sensitivity, then treatment with chloroquine, sulfadoxine-pyrimethamine, or mefloquine is preferable because these agents are better tolerated and simpler to administer.

Primaquine (0.3 mg of base/kg; 15 mg of base, adult dose) should be given daily for 14 days to patients with *P. vivax* or *P. ovale* infections after laboratory tests for G6PD deficiency have proved negative. A dose of 22.5 to 30 mg is recommended for infections acquired in Southeast Asia and Oceania. If the patient has a mild variant of G6PD deficiency, primaquine can be given in a dose of 0.6 mg of base/kg (45 mg maximum) weekly for 8 weeks.

COMPLICATIONS **Acute Renal Failure** If the level of blood urea nitrogen or creatinine rises despite adequate rehydration, fluid administration should be restricted to prevent volume overload. The indications for dialysis are the same as those in other forms of hypercatabolic acute renal failure (see Chap. 270). Even with adequate peritoneal dialysis, secondary bacterial infections are common in the tropics, and hemodialysis or hemofiltration is preferable. Some patients will pass small volumes of urine sufficient to allow control of fluid balance; these cases can be managed conservatively if other indications for dialysis do not arise. Renal function usually improves within days, but full recovery may take weeks.

Other Complications Patients who develop spontaneous bleeding should be given fresh blood and intravenous vitamin K. Convulsions should be treated with intravenous or rectal benzodiazepines. Aspiration pneumonia should be suspected in any unconscious patient with convulsions, particularly with persistent hyperventilation. Intravenous antimicrobial agents and oxygen should be administered, and pulmonary toilet should be undertaken. Systemic *Salmonella* infections are common in African children with falciparum malaria. Hypoglycemia or gram-negative septicemia should be suspected when any patient suddenly deteriorates for no obvious reason while receiving antimalarial treatment.

BABESIOSIS

Babesiosis is a protozoan disease of animals that is transmitted by ticks; humans are infected incidentally and initially develop a nonspecific febrile illness. *Babesia* organisms enter red blood cells and resemble malarial parasites morphologically, thus posing a diagnostic problem.

ETIOLOGY AND NATURAL CYCLE Of the more than 100 species of *Babesia*, *Babesia microti* and *Babesia divergens* are the two that cause most human infections. Ixodid (or hard-bodied) ticks, in particular *Ixodes dammini* (*Ixodes scapularis*) and *Ixodes ricinus*, are the vectors of the parasite. Ticks ingest *Babesia* while feeding, and the parasite multiplies within the tick's gut wall. The organisms then spread to the salivary glands; their inoculation into a vertebrate host by a tick larva, nymph, or adult completes the cycle of transmission. Asexual reproduction of *Babesia* within red blood cells produces two or four parasites.

EPIDEMIOLOGY While *Babesia* infections in wild and domestic animals are distributed globally, almost all *B. microti* infections

in the United States occur along the northeastern coast, including Nantucket Island and Martha's Vineyard in Massachusetts, Long Island and Shelter Island in New York, and the nearby mainland, including Connecticut. Cases also have been reported from Wisconsin. *Babesia* isolates from patients in the states of Washington and California have been characterized recently as WA 1, a category that is genetically and antigenically distinct from *B. microti*. A strain isolated in Missouri differs from these isolates, suggesting that babesiosis may be an "emerging infection." The deer tick, *I. dammini*, is the vector associated with *B. microti*.

Transfusions are another source of babesiosis. In several transfusion-associated cases, no parasites were detected in blood donors, but serologic testing of their blood for *Babesia* gave positive results.

Infections with *B. divergens* have occurred sporadically in previously splenectomized patients in several countries in Europe. *I. ricinus* is probably the vector in these cases, as it is for the transmission of this organism among cattle. The infected persons were predisposed to illness by their asplenic status.

I. dammini feeds on rodents as a larva and a nymph and on deer as an adult; nymphs are abundant during the spring and summer and feed on humans readily. In some endemic areas, the seroprevalence in the human population may be greater than 2 percent. This figure indicates that asymptomatic infection is more frequent than is generally thought.

CLINICAL PRESENTATION The incubation period for *B. microti* infection is about 1 to 4 weeks. Immunosuppressed patients, splenectomized individuals, and the elderly have the most severe illness. The clinical presentation varies widely; symptoms and signs include a gradual onset of irregular fever, chills, sweating, muscle pain, and fatigue. Mild hepatosplenomegaly and mild hemolytic anemia may develop. The level of parasitemia may exceed 10 percent. The illness may continue for weeks or months.

Patients infected with *B. divergens* have a more severe illness, with a rapid onset of chills, fever, nausea, vomiting, and hemolytic anemia progressing to jaundice, hemoglobinemia, and renal failure. *B. divergens* infections are often fatal.

DIAGNOSIS Whether or not they have a history of exposure to ticks or tick bites, febrile persons living in endemic areas should have Giemsa-stained thick and thin blood films examined for small intraerythrocytic parasites. *B. microti* appears as a small ring form resembling *P. falciparum*. Unlike infection with *Plasmodium*, however, that with *Babesia* does not cause the production of pigment in parasites, nor are schizonts or gametocytes formed. Dividing within red blood cells, *B. microti* can form four daughter parasites attached by strands of cytoplasm; these "tetrad" forms are seen infrequently in human blood films but are a distinguishing feature. An indirect immunofluorescence antibody test is useful for the diagnosis of infection with *B. microti* but does not replace the blood smear. The serum antibody titer rises 2 to 4 weeks after the onset of illness and then wanes over 6 to 12 months; cross-reactions can occur with other species of *Babesia* and with *Plasmodium*. About half of patients infected with *B. microti* have antibody to *Borrelia burgdorferi*, the agent of Lyme disease (Chap. 178); this figure varies with the geographic area. The occurrence of mixed infections is not surprising since both organisms are transmitted by *I. dammini*. Intraperitoneal inoculation of blood from patients with babesiosis into hamsters or gerbils results in detectable parasitemia within 2 to 4 weeks.

℞ TREATMENT

B. microti infections in patients with intact spleens are generally self-limiting without treatment. Treatment with the combination of quinine sulfate (650 mg of salt orally, three times daily) and clindamycin (600 mg orally, three times daily; or 1.2 g parenterally, twice daily) for 7 to 10 days is effective in some cases but may not eliminate parasites. The pediatric dose is 20 to 40 mg/kg per day for quinine sulfate and 25 mg/kg per day for clindamycin, both in three doses given over 7 to 10 days. Atovaquone suspension (750 mg twice daily) plus azithromycin (500 to 1000 mg/d) may be effective when quinine and clindamycin fail. Symptoms may persist for months with or without treatment, although there are no permanent sequelae. More severe infections with high-level *B. microti* parasitemia in asplenic patients have been successfully treated with exchange transfusions in addition to quinine and clindamycin.

BIBLIOGRAPHY

BAIRD JK et al: Primaquine for prophylaxis against malaria among nonimmune transmigrants in Irian Jaya, Indonesia. Am J Trop Med Hyg 52:479, 1995

BOUSTANI MR, GELFAND JA: Babesiosis. Clin Infect Dis 22:611, 1996

BREMAN JG, STEKETEE RW: Malaria, in *Maxcy-Rosenau-Last Public Health and Preventive Medicine,* 13th ed, JM Last, RB Wallace (eds). Norwalk, CT, Appleton & Lange, 1992, pp 240–253

CENTERS FOR DISEASE CONTROL AND PREVENTION: *Health Information for International Travelers.* HHS publication no. (CDC) 96-8280. Washington, U.S. Department of Health and Human Services, 1996

GARNHAM PCC: Malaria parasites of man: Life cycles and morphology (excluding ultrastructure) in malaria, in *Principles and Practice of Malariology,* WH Wernsdorfer, I McGregor (eds). Edinburgh, Churchill Livingstone, 1988, pp 61–96

HERWALDT BL et al: Babesiosis in Wisconsin: A potentially fatal disease. Am J Trop Med Hyg 53:146, 1995

KITCHEN SF: Symptomatology: General considerations and falciparum malaria, in *Malariology,* vol 2, MF Boyd (ed). Philadelphia, Saunders, 1949, pp 996–1016

MOLINEAUX L, GRAMICCIA G: *The Garki Project. Research on the Epidemiology and Control of Malaria in the Sudan Savannah of West Africa.* Geneva, World Health Organization, 1980

PASLOSKE BL, HOWARD RJ: Malaria, the red cell and the endothelium. Annu Rev Med 45:283, 1994

PERSING DH et al: Infection with a *Babesia*-like organism in northern California. N Engl J Med 332:298, 1995

SHANKS GD: Malaria prevention and prophylaxis, in *Balliere's Clinical Infectious Diseases,* vol 2-2, G Pasvol (ed). London, Balliere Tindall, 1995, pp 331–349

SPITZ S: Pathology of acute falciparum malaria. Milit Med 99:555, 1946

STEKETEE RW et al: Malaria treatment and prevention in pregnancy: The indications for use and adverse events associated with use of chloroquine or mefloquine. Am J Trop Med Hyg 55(Suppl 1):50, 1996

WHITE NJ: The treatment of malaria. N Engl J Med 335:800, 1996

———, Ho M: The pathophysiology of malaria. Adv Parasitol 31:84, 1992

WORLD HEALTH ORGANIZATION, DIVISION OF CONTROL OF TROPICAL DISEASES:Severe and complicated malaria. Trans R Soc Trop Med Hyg 84(Suppl 2):1, 1990

---

217 *Barbara L. Herwaldt*

LEISHMANIASIS

DEFINITION The term *leishmaniases* refers collectively to various clinical syndromes that are caused by obligate intracellular protozoa of the genus *Leishmania* (order Kinetoplastida). Leishmaniasis is endemic in diverse ecologic settings in the tropics and subtropics, ranging from deserts to rain forests and from rural to periurban areas. It typically is a vector-borne zoonosis, with rodents, small mammals, and canines as common reservoir hosts and humans as incidental hosts. In humans, visceral, cutaneous, and mucosal leishmaniases result from infection of macrophages throughout the mononuclear-phagocyte system, in the skin, and in the naso-oropharyngeal mucosae, respectively. The age range of infected persons depends on such factors as the duration of leishmaniasis endemicity in the specific geographic area, sandfly behavior (e.g., whether the sandfly species typically is intra- or extradomiciliary), and host behavior and immunity. Current challenges in this field include the emergence of leishmaniasis in new geographic areas and host populations [e.g., visceral leishmaniasis in civil war–affected southern Sudan and in persons infected with human immunodeficiency virus (HIV)] and the need for field-applicable, rapid diagnostic tests; efficacious, safe, inexpensive, and short-course oral treatment regimens; and effective and affordable control measures and immunoprophylactic agents.

ETIOLOGY Visceral leishmaniasis is typically but not exclusively caused by organisms of the *Leishmania donovani* complex (Table 217-1); Old World cutaneous leishmaniasis by *Leishmania tropica, Leishmania major,* and *Leishmania aethiopica*; New World (or American) cutaneous leishmaniasis by organisms of the *Leishmania mexicana* complex and the species now commonly placed in the subgenus *Viannia* (*Leishmania braziliensis, Leishmania guyanensis, Leishmania panamensis,* and *Leishmania peruviana*); and mucosal leishmaniasis by some organisms in the latter group.

Because all of the leishmanial parasites associated with human disease are morphologically similar, their identification and classification can be challenging. Information on factors such as setting of acquisition (epidemiologic and geographic) and clinical manifestations is valuable; however, this information does not serve to classify the organisms taxonomically since these factors are quite variable. Thus, data on the intrinsic characteristics of the parasites are needed. To this end, the biochemical characteristics of *Leishmania* have been studied by techniques such as isoenzyme analysis, the genetic characteristics by methods including kinetoplast-DNA hybridization, and the immunologic characteristics by approaches such as monoclonal antibody specificity determination and excreted-factor serotyping.

LIFE CYCLE Leishmaniasis is transmitted by the bite of female phlebotomine sandflies [genus *Phlebotomus* (Old World) or *Lutzomyia* (New World)]. As the flies attempt to feed, they regurgitate the parasite's flagellated promastigote stage into the skin of mammalian hosts. The saliva of *Lutzomyia longipalpis* sandflies, which transmit *Leishmania chagasi* infection, contains an erythema-producing peptide (maxadilan) that may enhance the infectivity of promastigotes and influence the course of infection. Promastigotes attach to receptors on macrophages, are phagocytized, and transform within phagolysosomes into the nonflagellated amastigote stage, which multiplies by binary fission. After rupture of infected macrophages, amastigotes are phagocytized by other macrophages. If ingested by feeding sandflies, amastigotes transform back into promastigotes, which require at least 7 days to become infective.

IMMUNOLOGY Advances in the understanding of the immunology of leishmaniasis have made this parasitic disease the paradigm for studies of the T cell subsets and cytokines that govern resistance and susceptibility to intracellular pathogens. The paradigm is best demonstrated in murine leishmaniasis. In inbred mice, the nature of the T cell response determines the outcome of *L. major* infection: T helper type 1 (Th1) cells, which produce interferon γ and interleukin (IL) 2, are involved in cell-mediated immunity and resistance (the healing phenotype), whereas T helper type 2 (Th2) cells, which produce IL-4, IL-5, and IL-10, confer susceptibility (the nonhealing phenotype).

Not all aspects of leishmaniasis in mice, whose susceptibility to leishmanial infection is genetically determined, apply to human infection, for which the genetic determinants have yet to be identified. However, a consistent principle is that healing and resistance to reinfection are associated with expanding numbers of *Leishmania*-specific Th1 cells, production of interferon γ, and activation of macrophages to kill intracellular amastigotes. Whereas IL-12 promotes the development of Th1 responses, factors such as IL-4 and transforming growth factor β (murine leishmaniasis) and IL-10 (human visceral leishmaniasis) suppress their development. In murine macrophages, nitrogen oxides mediate intracellular killing, which occurs by nonoxidative mechanisms.

DIAGNOSIS Definitive diagnosis of leishmaniasis requires demonstration of the parasite. To identify amastigotes by light-microscopic examination, the specimen obtained from an infected site (e.g., thin smear, histologic section) should be stained with Giemsa or another Romanovsky stain and presumptive amastigotes (2 to 4 μm in diameter) examined under oil immersion for the presence of a nucleus and a rod-shaped kinetoplast; the latter is a specialized mitochondrial structure that contains extranuclear DNA. Other means of parasitologic confirmation include in vitro culture (e.g., on Novy-MacNeal-Nicolle medium), inoculation into animals (e.g., golden hamsters, BALB/c mice), and use of molecular techniques (e.g., polymerase chain reaction). The parasites can be identified to the species level by isoenzyme analysis of cultured promastigotes or by use of monoclonal antibodies or DNA probes.

Indirect immunologic methods for diagnosis include serologic assays (e.g., indirect immunofluorescence antibody testing) and tests for *Leishmania*-specific cell-mediated immunity (e.g., skin testing for delayed-type hypersensitivity reactions). The usefulness of such methods depends on the clinical syndrome (see, for example, the section on diagnosis of visceral leishmaniasis). However, traditional serologic assays do not reliably distinguish past from current infection, and no leishmanin skin-test preparation has yet been approved for use in the United States.

℞ TREATMENT

For decades, the pentavalent antimonial (Sb^v) compounds sodium stibogluconate (Pentostam; Wellcome Foundation, United Kingdom; 100 mg of Sb^v/mL) and meglumine antimonate (Glucantime; Rhône Poulenc, France; 85 mg of Sb^v/mL) have been the mainstay of therapy for leishmaniasis. The Centers for Disease Control and Prevention (CDC) in Atlanta makes sodium stibogluconate available to U.S.-licensed physicians through the CDC Drug Service (404-639-3670) under an investigational new-drug protocol. The CDC generally recommends a daily parenteral (either intravenous or intramuscular) dose of 20 mg of Sb^v/kg, with a duration of therapy of 20 consecutive days for cutaneous leishmaniasis and 28 consecutive days for visceral and mucosal leishmaniasis. Alternative Sb^v regimens (e.g., longer or shorter courses) may have merit in some circumstances. Toxicity (manifested, for example, as myalgia, arthralgia, fatigue, hepatotoxicity, chemical pancreatitis, or electrocardiographic abnormalities) becomes increasingly common as the course of treatment progresses but usually does not limit therapy and is reversible.

Amphotericin B and pentamidine are the traditional parenteral alternatives to Sb^v but are generally considered more toxic. Amphotericin B elicits reactions such as fever, chills, hypotension, nephrotoxicity, hypokalemia, and anemia, while pentamidine can cause hypotension, hypoglycemia, diabetes, vomiting, and pain at the injection site. Many other agents have been advocated as alternatives or adjuncts to Sb^v, often on the basis of suboptimal data; even the results of well-conducted clinical trials may not be generalizable to the treatment of patients in other settings, particularly patients infected with other leishmanial species or strains. Even in the absence of a consensus about if, when, or how to use other agents, it is important to consider whether the patient's illness could result in substantial morbidity or in death and therefore requires expeditious treatment with a regimen that usually is highly effective.

PREVENTION AND CONTROL The transmission of *Leishmania* species is typically focal, with local "hot spots." This pattern is due in part to the characteristics of sandflies, whose flight is noiseless and limited in range; because of their short, hopping flight style, they usually remain within a few hundred meters of their breeding site. They rest in dark, moist places and are found in habitats ranging from deserts to rain forests; peridomestic sandflies rest in debris or rubble near buildings.

Personal protective measures include the avoidance of outdoor activities when sandflies are most active (dusk to dawn); the use of mechanical barriers such as screens and bed-nets that keep out sandflies, which are about one-third the size of mosquitoes; the wearing of protective clothing; and the application of insect repellent to exposed skin. Impregnation of clothing, bed-nets, and screens with permethrin may also be useful, as may spraying of dwellings with residual-action insecticide. Vaccine strategies are being investigated. Treatment of human cases is an effective control measure only where humans are the primary reservoirs of infection. Vector control and elimination of reservoir hosts (e.g., domestic dogs) may be useful in some settings—for example, where transmission is intra- or peridomiciliary.

VISCERAL LEISHMANIASIS Visceral leishmaniasis, which has been reported in 47 countries and continues to be epidemic in eastern India, has emerged in new geographic areas (e.g., southern Sudan, where persons of all ages have been affected), in new settings (e.g., suburban areas in northeastern Brazil, where most cases have occurred in children <10 years of age), and among new host populations (e.g., HIV-infected persons). The causative leishmanial species typically are species of the *L. donovani* complex (Table 217-1); *Leishmania amazonensis* in Latin America and *L. tropica* in the Old World also can cause visceral infection. The organisms can be transmitted not only by sandflies but also congenitally and parenterally (e.g., via blood transfusion or sharing of needles). Infection begins in macrophages at the inoculation site (e.g., in dermal macrophages at the site of a sandfly bite) and disseminates

Table 217-1

Major *Leishmania* Species That Cause Disease in Humans

Species*	Clinical Syndrome†	Geographic Distribution
SUBGENUS *LEISHMANIA*		
L. donovani complex		
L. donovani	VL (PKDL, OWCL)	China, Indian subcontinent, southwestern Asia, Ethiopia, Kenya, Sudan; possibly sporadic in sub-Saharan Africa
L. infantum	VL (OWCL)	China, central and southwestern Asia, Middle East, southern Europe, North Africa, Ethiopia, Sudan; sporadic in sub-Saharan Africa
L. chagasi	VL (NWCL)	Central and South America
L. mexicana complex		
L. mexicana	NWCL (DCL)	Texas, Mexico, Central and South America
L. amazonensis	NWCL (ML, DCL, VL)	Panama and South America
L. tropica	OWCL (VL)‡	Central Asia, India, southwestern Asia, Middle East, Turkey, Greece, North Africa, Ethiopia, Kenya, Namibia
L. major	OWCL§	Central Asia, India, southwestern Asia, Middle East, Turkey, North Africa, Sahel region of north-central Africa, Ethiopia, Sudan, Kenya
L. aethiopica	OWCL (DCL)	Ethiopia, Kenya
SUBGENUS *VIANNIA*		
L. (V.) braziliensis	NWCL (ML)	Central and South America
L. (V.) guyanensis	NWCL (ML)	South America
L. (V.) panamensis	NWCL (ML)	Central America, Venezuela, Colombia, Ecuador, Peru
L. (V.) peruviana	NWCL¶	Peru (western slopes of Andes)

* Other species besides those listed here have been reported to infect humans. The taxonomy of the *Leishmania* species has not been finalized.

† Abbreviations: VL, visceral leishmaniasis; PKDL, post–kala-azar dermal leishmaniasis; OWCL, Old World cutaneous leishmaniasis; NWCL, New World (American) cutaneous leishmaniasis; DCL, diffuse cutaneous leishmaniasis; ML, mucosal leishmaniasis. Clinical syndromes less frequently associated with the various species are shown in parentheses.

‡ *L. tropica* also causes leishmaniasis recidivans and viscerotropic leishmaniasis.

§ *L. major*–like organisms also cause New World cutaneous leishmaniasis.

¶ The cutaneous leishmaniasis syndrome caused by this species is called *uta*.

throughout the mononuclear-phagocyte system in the context of both specific (i.e., to leishmanial antigens) and nonspecific (e.g., to tuberculin) anergy.

Manifestations Visceral infection can remain subclinical or can become symptomatic, with an acute, subacute, or chronic course. In some settings, inapparent infections far outnumber clinically apparent ones; malnutrition is a risk factor for the development of disease. The incubation period usually ranges from weeks to months but can be as long as years. Whereas the general term *visceral leishmaniasis* covers a broad spectrum of severity and manifestations, the term *kala-azar* (Hindi for "black fever," indicating that the skin can turn gray) generally conjures up the classic image of profoundly cachectic, febrile patients who are heavily parasitized and have life-threatening disease. Splenomegaly (with the spleen most often soft and nontender) typically is more impressive than hepatomegaly, and the spleen can in fact be massive; both splenomegaly and hepatomegaly in visceral leishmaniasis result from reticuloendothelial cell hyperplasia. Peripheral lymphadenopathy is common in some geographic areas, including Sudan.

The abnormal laboratory findings associated with advanced disease include pancytopenia—anemia, leukopenia (neutropenia, marked eosinopenia, relative lymphocytosis and monocytosis), and thrombocytopenia—as well as hypergammaglobulinemia (chiefly involving IgG, from polyclonal B cell activation) and hypoalbuminemia. Causes of anemia can include bone-marrow infiltration, hypersplenism, autoimmune hemolysis, and bleeding.

Some patients develop post–kala-azar dermal leishmaniasis. This syndrome is manifested by skin lesions (including pigmented or depigmented macules, papules, nodules, and patches) that typically are most prominent on the face. These lesions can develop during or within a few months after therapy (e.g., in East Africa) or years after therapy (e.g., in India). Visceral infection can relapse. Persons with persistent skin lesions can serve as reservoirs of infection.

So-called *viscerotropic leishmaniasis* caused by *L. tropica*, which typically is dermotropic, has been recognized among U.S. soldiers who participated in Operation Desert Storm in the Persian Gulf. The affected persons have had light parasite burdens and either no symptoms or nonspecific symptoms such as fatigue, fever, and gastrointestinal problems.

Diagnosis Parasitologic diagnosis of visceral leishmaniasis is accomplished by demonstration of the parasite on stained slides or in cultures of a tissue aspirate or a biopsy specimen (e.g., of spleen, liver, bone marrow, or lymph node). The diagnostic yield is highest for splenic aspiration (specifically, as high as 98 percent for splenic aspirates vs. <90 percent for other specimens), but this procedure can cause hemorrhage. Patients who have kala-azar typically carry a relatively heavy parasite burden; develop high titers of antibody to *Leishmania* (diagnostically useful but not protective); and have undetectable *Leishmania*-specific cell-mediated immunity (with leishmanin skin-test reactivity as well as lymphocyte proliferation and interferon γ responses to leishmanial antigens noted only after recovery). In contrast, viscerotropic leishmaniasis can be difficult to diagnose because of a light parasite burden and a minimal antibody response.

The differential diagnosis of visceral leishmaniasis includes other tropical infectious diseases that cause fever or organomegaly (e.g., typhoid fever, miliary tuberculosis, brucellosis, malaria with tropical splenomegaly syndrome, and schistosomiasis) as well as diseases such as leukemia and lymphoma. Post–kala-azar dermal leishmaniasis should be differentiated from syphilis, yaws, and leprosy.

℞ **TREATMENT**
Because classic cases of kala-azar generally are fatal if not appropriately treated, highly effective therapy is essential, as is close monitoring for bleeding and intercurrent infectious conditions such as pneumonia and diarrhea. In general, use of a pentavalent antimonial agent (i.e., 20 mg of Sb^v/kg given intravenously or intramuscularly once daily for 28 consecutive days) still constitutes first-line therapy. However, parasite-related factors such as apparent primary drug resistance and host characteristics such as coinfection with HIV can complicate treatment so that prolonged Sb^v administration or use of an alternative or adjunctive agent may be indicated (see below).

Typically, patients feel better and become afebrile during the first week of treatment. Abnormal laboratory findings and splenomegaly improve during therapy but may take weeks or months to resolve; the reappearance of eosinophils in the leukocyte differential count is a good sign. The best indicator of permanent cure is freedom from clinical relapse during at least 6 months of follow-up. Repeat tissue sampling is indicated if the patient's status is in question. The results of repeat tissue sampling must be interpreted with caution: the persistence of some parasites is not necessarily a poor prognostic indicator, whereas the apparent absence of parasites does not ensure that the patient will not relapse. The possibility of HIV coinfection should be considered if the patient does not respond to therapy or repeatedly relapses.

In India, where unresponsiveness to Sb^v therapy is becoming increasingly problematic, amphotericin B (0.5 to 1.0 mg/kg daily or every other day, given intravenously for a total dose of 7 to 20 mg/kg) has been found to be a highly effective, though potentially toxic, alternative. Pentamidine (2 to 4 mg/kg daily or every other day, given intravenously or intramuscularly for at least 15 doses) is reasonably effective but may need to be administered in prolonged courses that are associated with toxicity. Formulations of liposomal amphotericin B may prove highly effective and less toxic: liposomes passively target amphotericin away from the kidneys to macrophage-rich organs.

Various parenteral agents have been advocated as adjuncts to accelerate or improve the response to Sb^v therapy. The aminoglycoside aminosidine (12 to 15 mg/kg per day, intravenously or intramuscularly), which is the chemical equivalent of paromomycin, is an effective adjunct but is not available in the United States. Cytokine immunotherapy with subcutaneous injections of recombinant interferon γ or granulocyte macrophage colony-stimulating factor, both of which activate macrophages, also shows promise as an adjunctive measure. The oral agents allopurinol and ketoconazole have been used as adjuncts, but, because of the highly variable results obtained, their use cannot be generally recommended.

Visceral Leishmaniasis in HIV-Infected Persons Visceral leishmaniasis is becoming an important opportunistic infection among persons infected with HIV-1 in geographic areas in which both infections are endemic. To date, most coinfections have been reported from southern Europe, where *Leishmania infantum* is endemic and visceral leishmaniasis is no longer primarily a disease of young children. In HIV-infected patients, even relatively avirulent leishmanial strains can disseminate to the viscera. Clinical leishmaniasis in patients with HIV infection can represent newly acquired or reactivated infection; most coinfected patients who have clinically evident leishmaniasis have fewer than 200 CD4 lymphocytes per microliter. A better understanding of the interaction of these two infections is needed.

A diagnosis of visceral leishmaniasis should be considered for HIV-infected patients who have ever been in leishmaniasis-endemic areas and who have such manifestations as unexplained fever, organomegaly, anemia, or pancytopenia. Coinfected patients can develop unusual manifestations of visceral leishmaniasis, in part because of atypical localization of the parasite (e.g., in the gastrointestinal tract).

The diagnostic sensitivity of classic serologic methods is lower in coinfected than in immunocompetent patients (about 50 percent vs. >90 percent). On the other hand, parasitologic diagnosis by noninvasive means is easier in the case of coinfected patients; parasites are more commonly found in the circulating blood monocytes of these patients, and sensitivities are about 50 percent for a Giemsa-stained peripheral-blood smear and 70 to 75 percent for a stained or cultured buffy-coat preparation. Invasive methods of parasitologic diagnosis (e.g., microscopic examination or culture of a bone-marrow aspirate) typically are highly sensitive, especially for previously untreated patients, who commonly have heavy parasite burdens.

Coinfected patients may initially respond well to antileishmanial therapy, albeit with more drug toxicity than is experienced by most immunocompetent persons. However, coinfected patients commonly have a chronic or relapsing course, seemingly irrespective of the drug regimens used for induction and suppression therapy. Comparative clinical trials of candidate drug regimens are urgently needed.

CUTANEOUS LEISHMANIASIS Cutaneous leishmaniasis, which has been reported from 61 countries, has traditionally been classified as New World (American) or Old World. Local names for New World disease include *chiclero ulcer*, *pian bois* (bush yaws), and *uta*; those for Old World disease include *oriental sore*, *bouton d'orient*, *Aleppo boil*, and *Baghdad sore*. In the Americas, the leishmaniasis-endemic area extends from southern Texas to northern Argentina; in many affected regions, most cases occur in men who have forest-related occupational exposures. The etiologic agents typically are those of the *L. mexicana* complex and the *Viannia* group (Table 217-1) but also include *L. major*–like organisms and *L. chagasi*. Old World cutaneous leishmaniasis is caused by *L. tropica*, *L. major*, and *L. aethiopica* as well as by *L. infantum* and *L. donovani*.

Clinical Manifestations Although the incubation period for clinically evident disease typically ranges from weeks to months, local trauma can activate latent infection. The first clinical manifestation is usually a papule at the site of the sandfly bite but is sometimes regional lymphadenopathy (sometimes bubonic) in *L. (V.) braziliensis* infection. Most skin lesions evolve from papular to nodular to ulcerative, with a central depression (which can be several centimeters in diameter) surrounded by a raised indurated border; some lesions persist as nodules or plaques. Multiple primary lesions, satellite lesions, regional adenopathy, sporotrichosis-like subcutaneous nodules, lesion pain or pruritus, and secondary bacterial infection are variably present. The infecting species, the location of the lesion, and the host's immune response are major determinants of the clinical manifestations and chronicity of untreated lesions. For example, in the New World, lesions caused by *L. mexicana* tend to be smaller and less chronic than those caused by *L. (V.) braziliensis*; in the Old World, *L. major* tends to cause "wet" exudative lesions that are less chronic than the "dry" lesions with central crusting that are caused by *L. tropica*. The spontaneous resolution of lesions, which may require weeks, months, or even years, does not preclude reactivation or reinfection.

The polyparasitic and oligoparasitic ends of the spectrum of cutaneous leishmaniasis are respectively represented by the rare syndromes of diffuse cutaneous leishmaniasis (DCL) and leishmaniasis recidivans, both of which are notoriously difficult to treat. DCL, caused by *L. aethiopica* (Old World) or by the *L. mexicana* complex (New World), develops in the context of *Leishmania*-specific anergy and is manifested by chronic, nonulcerative skin lesions; on histopathologic examination of samples of these lesions, abundant parasites but few lymphocytes are noted. Leishmaniasis recidivans, a hyperergic variant with scarce parasites, is usually caused by *L. tropica* and manifested by a chronic solitary lesion on the cheek that expands slowly despite central healing.

Diagnosis Dermal scrapings of debrided ulcerative lesions are useful for histologic examination, aspirates of skin lesions and lymph nodes for in vitro culture, and biopsy specimens for both examination and culture. Although examination of histologic sections of biopsy specimens can help exclude other diagnoses, amastigotes appear larger and are more easily recognizable on Giemsa-stained thin smears (e.g., smears of dermal scrapings, touch preparations of biopsy specimens). As lesions age, amastigotes become more scarce and parasitologic confirmation becomes more difficult.

Serologic testing is an insensitive means for diagnosing cutaneous leishmaniasis; antibody titers are at most minimally elevated except in patients who have DCL. In contrast, leishmanin skin-test reactivity usually is evident or develops in persons who have simple cutaneous or recidivans leishmaniasis but not in those who have DCL.

Cutaneous leishmaniasis is frequently confused with tropical, traumatic, and venous-stasis ulcers; foreign-body reactions; superinfected insect bites; impetigo; fungal infections (e.g., sporotrichosis); myco-

bacterial infections; and other diseases (e.g., sarcoidosis, neoplasms). DCL and leishmaniasis recidivans must be differentiated from lepromatous leprosy and lupus vulgaris, respectively.

℞ TREATMENT

In decisions about whether and how to treat cutaneous leishmaniasis, the possibility of mucosal dissemination should be considered, as should lesion location (the cosmetic implications), number, size, evolution, and chronicity. When optimal efficacy is important, Sb^v therapy is recommended. In general, a regimen of 20 mg of Sb^v/kg (intravenous or intramuscular) should be given once daily for 20 consecutive days; lower daily doses or shorter courses may have merit in some situations. The clinical response begins with lesion flattening and continues after the end of therapy, whereas relapse typically is manifested by clinical reactivation at the margin of the lesion.

A study in Colombia showed that pentamidine (3 mg/kg intramuscularly, every other day for four doses) is an effective parenteral alternative to Sb^v. The oral agents that are currently available—most notably, the imidazoles ketoconazole (adult dosage, 600 mg/d for 28 days) and itraconazole (adult dosage, 200 mg twice daily for 28 days); allopurinol; and dapsone—probably are modestly active at best and are effective only against some leishmanial species/strains. Adjunctive immunotherapy remains highly experimental but may be useful in DCL.

Unless used in an adjunctive role, local or topical therapy should be considered only for the treatment of infection that does not have the potential for dissemination (e.g., for relatively benign lesions caused by *L. mexicana* or *L. major*). Examples of local approaches include the application of an ointment containing paromomycin and methylbenzethonium chloride (not licensed in the United States), the intralesional administration of Sb^v (not an approved use of drug obtained through the CDC), heat therapy, and cryotherapy. Excisional biopsy poses a substantial risk for relapse and is not recommended.

MUCOSAL LEISHMANIASIS Leishmanial infection of the naso-oropharyngeal mucosae is a relatively rare but potentially disfiguring metastatic complication of cutaneous leishmaniasis. Mucosal disease develops despite antileishmanial cell-mediated immunity and most commonly is caused by organisms of the *Viannia* group [typically *L. (V.) braziliensis* but also *L. (V.) panamensis* and *L. (V.) guyanensis*]. Although mucosal disease usually becomes clinically evident within several years after the healing of the original cutaneous lesions, cutaneous and mucosal lesions can exist simultaneously or can appear decades apart. Typically, the original cutaneous lesions in these cases were not treated or were inadequately treated.

Mucosal involvement generally is manifested first by persistent unusual nasal symptoms (e.g., epistaxis), with erythema and edema of the nasal mucosae, and then by progressive, ulcerative, naso-oropharyngeal destruction. Supportive laboratory data (e.g., a positive serologic test) are useful, but the scarcity of amastigotes makes parasitologic confirmation difficult. The differential diagnosis includes sarcoidosis, neoplasms, midline granuloma, rhinoscleroma, paracoccidioidomycosis, histoplasmosis, syphilis, and tertiary yaws.

Pentavalent antimonial therapy (20 mg of Sb^v/kg per day, given intravenously or intramuscularly for 28 days) is moderately effective for mild mucosal disease, whereas advanced disease may not respond to such therapy or may relapse repeatedly. Therapy with amphotericin B is the best alternative currently available. Patients who develop signs of respiratory compromise during therapy may benefit from concomitant steroid treatment.

BIBLIOGRAPHY

BERMAN JD: Human leishmaniasis: Clinical, diagnostic, and chemotherapeutic developments in the last 10 years. Clin Infect Dis 24:684, 1997

DAVIDSON RN et al: Liposomal amphotericin B (AmBisome) in Mediterranean visceral leishmaniasis: A multi-centre trial. Q J Med 87:75, 1994

GRIMALDI G, TESH RB: Leishmaniases of the New World: Current concepts and implications for future research. Clin Microbiol Rev 6:230, 1993

HERWALDT BL, BERMAN JD: Recommendations for treating leishmaniasis with sodium stibogluconate (Pentostam) and review of pertinent clinical studies. Am J Trop Med Hyg 46:296, 1992

——— et al: The natural history of cutaneous leishmaniasis in Guatemala. J Infect Dis 165:518, 1992

——— et al: American cutaneous leishmaniasis in U.S. travelers. Ann Intern Med 118:779, 1993

HO JL et al: Cytokines in the treatment of leishmaniasis: From studies of immunopathology to patient therapy. Biotherapy 7:223, 1994

KALTER DC: Laboratory tests for the diagnosis and evaluation of leishmaniasis. Dermatol Clin 12:37, 1994

MAGILL AJ: Epidemiology of the leishmaniases. Dermatol Clin 13:505, 1995

——— et al: Visceral infection caused by *Leishmania tropica* in veterans of Operation Desert Storm. N Engl J Med 328:1383, 1993

PEARSON RD, DE QUEIROZ SOUSA A: Clinical spectrum of leishmaniasis. Clin Infect Dis 22:1, 1996

ROSENTHAL E et al: Visceral leishmaniasis and HIV-1 co-infection in southern France. Trans R Soc Trop Med Hyg 89:159, 1995

SEAMAN J et al: Epidemic visceral leishmaniasis in southern Sudan: Treatment of severely debilitated patients under wartime conditions and with limited resources. Ann Intern Med 124:664, 1996

WORLD HEALTH ORGANIZATION: Control of the leishmaniases. Technical Report Series 793. Geneva, World Health Organization, 1990

218

Louis V. Kirchhoff

TRYPANOSOMIASIS

CHAGAS' DISEASE

DEFINITION Chagas' disease, or American trypanosomiasis, is a zoonosis caused by the protozoan parasite *Trypanosoma cruzi*. Acute Chagas' disease is usually a mild febrile illness that results from initial infection with the organism. After spontaneous resolution of the acute illness, most infected persons remain for life in the indeterminate phase of chronic Chagas' disease, which is characterized by subpatent parasitemia, easily detectable antibodies to *T. cruzi*, and an absence of symptoms. In a minority of chronically infected patients, cardiac and gastrointestinal lesions develop that can result in serious morbidity and even death.

LIFE CYCLE AND TRANSMISSION *T. cruzi* is transmitted among its mammalian hosts by hematophagous triatomine insects, or reduviid bugs. The insects become infected by sucking blood from animals or humans who have circulating parasites. Ingested organisms multiply in the gut of the reduviids, and infective forms are discharged with the feces at the time of subsequent blood meals. Transmission to a second vertebrate host occurs when breaks in the skin, mucous membranes, or conjunctivae become contaminated with bug feces that contain infective parasites. *T. cruzi* also can be transmitted by the transfusion of blood donated by infected persons, from mother to fetus, and in laboratory accidents.

PATHOLOGY An indurated inflammatory lesion called a *chagoma* often appears at the site of the parasite's entry. Local histologic changes include the presence of parasites within leukocytes and cells of subcutaneous tissues and the development of interstitial edema, lymphocytic infiltration, and reactive hyperplasia of adjacent lymph nodes. After dissemination of the organisms through the lymphatics and the bloodstream, muscles (including the myocardium) may become heavily parasitized. The characteristic pseudocysts seen in sections of infected tissues are intracellular aggregates of multiplying parasites.

The pathogenesis of chronic Chagas' disease is poorly understood. The heart is the organ most commonly affected, and changes include biventricular enlargement, thinning of the ventricular walls, apical aneurysms, and mural thrombi. Widespread lymphocytic infiltration, diffuse interstitial fibrosis, and atrophy of myocardial cells are often demonstrated, but parasites are rarely seen in myocardial tissue. Conduction-system involvement often affects the right branch and the left anterior branch of the bundle of His. In chronic Chagas' disease of the gastrointestinal tract (megadisease), the esophagus and colon may ex-

hibit varying degrees of dilatation. On microscopic examination, focal inflammatory lesions with lymphocytic infiltration are seen, and the number of neurons in the myenteric plexus may be markedly reduced.

EPIDEMIOLOGY *T. cruzi* is found only in the Americas. Wild and domestic mammals harboring *T. cruzi* and infected reduviids are found in spotty distributions from the southern United States to southern Argentina. Humans become involved in the cycle of transmission when infected vectors take up residence in the primitive wood, adobe, and stone houses common in much of Latin America. Thus, human *T. cruzi* infection is a health problem primarily among the poor in rural areas of Central and South America. Most new *T. cruzi* infections in rural settings occur in children, but the incidence is unknown because most cases go undiagnosed. Thousands of individuals also become infected every year through blood transfusions in urban areas. Currently, it is estimated that 16 to 18 million people, more than a third of whom live in Brazil, are chronically infected with *T. cruzi*. Chronic Chagas' disease is a major cause of morbidity and mortality in many Latin American countries, including Mexico, since many chronically infected persons eventually develop symptomatic cardiac lesions or gastrointestinal disease.

Acute Chagas' disease is rare in the United States. Four cases of autochthonous transmission have been described, and three instances of transmission by blood transfusion have recently been reported. In addition, between 1971 and 1992, seven laboratory-acquired infections and nine imported cases of acute Chagas' disease were reported to the Centers for Disease Control and Prevention (CDC). In contrast, the prevalence of chronic *T. cruzi* infections in the United States has increased considerably in recent years. Since the mid-1970s, enormous numbers of Central Americans have emigrated to the United States. In one study conducted in Washington, D.C., 5 percent of Salvadoran and Nicaraguan immigrants were found to have chronic *T. cruzi* infections. Estimates based on the latter study and on a small number of studies done in U.S. blood banks put the total number of infected immigrants now living here at more than 50,000. The presence of these carriers of *T. cruzi* creates a substantial risk of transmission by blood transfusion, as is evidenced by the occurrence of the three transfusion-associated cases just cited.

CLINICAL COURSE The first signs of acute Chagas' disease develop at least 1 week after invasion by the parasites. When the organisms have entered through a break in the skin, an indurated area of erythema and swelling (the chagoma), accompanied by local lymphadenopathy, may appear. Romaña's sign—the classic finding in acute Chagas' disease, which consists of unilateral painless edema of the palpebrae and periocular tissues—can result when the conjunctiva is the portal of entry. These initial local signs are followed by malaise, fever, anorexia, and edema of the face and lower extremities. Generalized lymphadenopathy and mild hepatosplenomegaly may appear. Severe myocarditis develops rarely; most deaths in acute Chagas' disease are due to heart failure. Neurologic signs are not common, but meningoencephalitis has been reported. The acute symptoms resolve spontaneously in virtually all patients, who then enter the asymptomatic or indeterminate phase of chronic *T. cruzi* infection.

Symptomatic chronic Chagas' disease becomes apparent years or even decades after the initial infection. The heart is commonly involved, and symptoms are caused by rhythm disturbances, cardiomyopathy, and thromboembolism. Right bundle-branch block is the most common electrocardiographic abnormality, but other types of atrioventricular block, premature ventricular contractions, and tachy- and bradyarrhythmias are seen frequently. Cardiomyopathy often results in right-sided or biventricular heart failure. Embolization of mural thrombi to the brain or other areas may take place. Patients with megaesophagus suffer from dysphagia, odynophagia, chest pain, and regurgitation. Aspiration can occur, especially during sleep, and repeated episodes of aspiration pneumonitis are common. Weight loss, cachexia, and pulmonary infection can result in death. Patients with megacolon are plagued by abdominal pain and chronic constipation, and advanced megacolon can cause obstruction, volvulus, septicemia, and death.

DIAGNOSIS The diagnosis of acute Chagas' disease requires the detection of parasites. Microscopic examination of fresh anticoagulated blood or of the buffy coat is the simplest way to see the motile organisms. Parasites also can be seen in Giemsa-stained thin and thick blood smears. When repeated attempts to visualize the organisms are unsuccessful, mouse inoculation and culture of blood in specialized media should be performed. As a last resort, xenodiagnosis should be attempted. In this technique, uninfected reduviid bugs are allowed to feed on the patient's blood. Approximately 30 days after the blood meal, the intestinal contents of the bugs are examined for parasites. When done properly, this method is positive in virtually all cases of acute Chagas' disease and in approximately half of chronic infections. Since early treatment of acute Chagas' disease is extremely important, however, the decision to initiate therapy for *T. cruzi* infection despite negative wet preparations and smears must be made on clinical and epidemiologic grounds before the results of these indirect methods become available. Serologic testing is of limited usefulness in diagnosing acute Chagas' disease.

The diagnosis of chronic Chagas' disease is made by the detection of antibodies that bind to *T. cruzi* antigens. Demonstration of the parasite is not of primary importance. Several highly sensitive serologic tests for the detection of antibodies to *T. cruzi* are used widely in Latin America, including complement-fixation and immunofluorescence tests and enzyme-linked immunosorbent assay (ELISA). However, a persistent problem with these conventional assays is the occurrence of false-positive reactions, typically with sera from patients who have other parasitic infections or autoimmune diseases. For this reason, it is generally recommended that positivity in one assay be confirmed by two other tests and that well-characterized positive and negative comparison sera be included in each run. A highly sensitive and specific method for detecting antibodies to *T. cruzi* [approved by the Clinical Laboratory Improvement Amendment (CLIA) and available in the author's laboratory] employs immunoprecipitation of radiolabeled *T. cruzi* antigens and electrophoresis. Serodiagnostic assays that employ recombinant *T. cruzi* proteins as target antigens are being developed, as are tests based on the amplification of *T. cruzi* DNA sequences by polymerase chain reaction. However, these tests are not yet available for general use.

℞ **TREATMENT**

Therapy for Chagas' disease is unsatisfactory. Nifurtimox is the only drug active against *T. cruzi* that is available in the United States. In acute Chagas' disease, nifurtimox markedly reduces the duration of symptoms and parasitemia and decreases mortality. Nevertheless, its efficacy at eradicating parasites is low. Limited studies have shown that only approximately 50 percent of acute infections are cured parasitologically by a full course of treatment. Despite its limitations, nifurtimox treatment should be initiated as early as possible in acute Chagas' disease. Moreover, when laboratory accidents occur in which it appears likely that *T. cruzi* infection could become established, nifurtimox therapy should be initiated without waiting for clinical or parasitologic indications of infection.

The usefulness of nifurtimox in individuals with indeterminate-phase or symptomatic chronic Chagas' disease has not been established. No evidence suggests that patients in the indeterminate phase are less likely to develop symptomatic disease after treatment with nifurtimox, nor has this agent been shown to have any effect on symptomatic chronic disease. Moreover, posttreatment xenodiagnoses are positive in a large proportion of chronically infected patients given this drug. Hence there is no indication for nifurtimox treatment of chronic *T. cruzi* infections.

Common adverse effects of nifurtimox include abdominal pain, anorexia, nausea, vomiting, and weight loss. Neurologic reactions to the drug may include restlessness, disorientation, insomnia, twitching, paresthesia, polyneuritis, and seizures. These symptoms usually disappear when the dosage is reduced or treatment is discontinued. The recommended daily dosage is 8 to 10 mg/kg for adults, 12.5 to 15 mg/kg for adolescents, and 15 to 20 mg/kg for children 1 to 10 years of age. The drug should be given orally in four divided doses each day, and therapy should be continued for 90 to 120 days. Nifurtimox is available from the Drug Service of the CDC in Atlanta, Georgia (telephone number, 770-639-3670).

Benznidazole is a second agent used to treat Chagas' disease. Its efficacy is similar to that of nifurtimox, and its adverse effects include peripheral neuropathy, rash, and granulocytopenia. The recommended oral dosage is 5 mg/kg per day for 60 days. Benznidazole is used widely in Latin America but is not available in the United States. In a recent poll, many Brazilian authorities on Chagas' disease indicated that they would treat patients in the indeterminate phase of the illness with benznidazole. It has not been shown, however, that such treatment reduces the likelihood of symptomatic disease. None of those polled favored using the drug for the treatment of symptomatic chronic Chagas' disease.

Recent studies have shown that allopurinol is not useful for the treatment of chronic *T. cruzi* infections. Studies in mice have shown that recombinant interferon γ decreases the duration and severity of acute *T. cruzi* infection; however, its usefulness in persons with acute Chagas' disease has not been evaluated systematically.

Patients who develop cardiac and/or gastrointestinal disease in association with *T. cruzi* infection should be referred to appropriate subspecialists for further evaluation and treatment.

PREVENTION Since drug therapy is unsatisfactory and vaccines are not available, the control of *T. cruzi* transmission in endemic countries must depend on reduction of domiciliary vector populations by spraying of insecticides and improvement of housing. In addition, in endemic areas, programs for the screening of donated blood for *T. cruzi* need to be expanded and improved to reduce rates of transmission by transfusion. Tourists traveling in endemic areas should avoid sleeping in dilapidated houses outside urban areas. Mosquito nets and insect repellent will provide additional protection.

In the United States, blood donations should not be accepted from immigrants from regions in which Chagas' disease is endemic, unless serologic assays indicate that the donor is not infected with *T. cruzi*. Moreover, all immigrants from endemic regions should be screened for serologic evidence of infection with the parasite. Identification of infected individuals in this group is important not only in preventing transmission by blood transfusion but also in prompting physicians who care for these patients to undertake appropriate diagnostic monitoring and supportive therapy when indicated. Laboratory personnel should wear gloves and eye protection when working with *T. cruzi* and infected vectors. Patients with end-stage chagasic cardiopathies should not undergo cardiac transplantation because the immunosuppression required after surgery often leads to reactivation of *T. cruzi* infection, with serious consequences and even death.

SLEEPING SICKNESS

DEFINITION Sleeping sickness, or African trypanosomiasis, is caused by flagellated protozoan parasites that belong to the *Trypanosoma brucei* complex and are transmitted to humans by tsetse flies. In untreated patients, the trypanosomes first cause a febrile illness that is followed months or years later by progressive neurologic impairment and death.

THE PARASITES AND THEIR TRANSMISSION The East African (*rhodesiense*) and the West African (*gambiense*) forms of sleeping sickness are caused, respectively, by two trypanosome subspecies: *T. brucei rhodesiense* and *T. brucei gambiense*. These subspecies are morphologically indistinguishable but cause illnesses that are epidemiologically and clinically distinct. The parasites are transmitted by blood-sucking tsetse flies of the genus *Glossina*. The insects acquire the infection when they ingest blood from infected mammalian hosts. After many cycles of multiplication in the midgut of the vector, the parasites migrate to the salivary glands. Their transmission takes place when they are inoculated during a subsequent blood meal. The injected trypanosomes multiply in the blood and other extracellular spaces and evade immune destruction in mammalian hosts for long periods by undergoing antigenic variation, a process by which the antigenic structure of their surface coat of glycoproteins changes periodically.

PATHOGENESIS AND PATHOLOGY A self-limited inflammatory lesion (trypanosomal chancre) may appear a week or so after the bite of an infected tsetse fly. A systemic febrile illness then evolves as the parasites are disseminated through the lymphatics and bloodstream. Systemic African trypanosomiasis without central nervous system (CNS) involvement is generally referred to as *stage I disease*. In this stage, widespread lymphadenopathy and splenomegaly reflect marked lymphocytic and histiocytic proliferation and invasion of morular cells, which are plasmacytes that may be involved in the production of IgM. Endarteritis, with perivascular infiltration of both parasites and lymphocytes, may develop in lymph nodes and spleen. Myocarditis develops frequently in patients with stage I disease and is especially common in *T. b. rhodesiense* infections.

Hematologic manifestations that accompany stage I trypanosomiasis include moderate leukocytosis, thrombocytopenia, and anemia. High levels of immunoglobulins, consisting primarily of polyclonal IgM, are a constant feature, and heterophile antibodies, antibodies to DNA, and rheumatoid factor are often detected. High levels of antigen-antibody complexes may play a role in the tissue damage and increased vascular permeability that facilitate dissemination of the parasites.

Stage II trypanosomiasis involves invasion of the CNS. The presence of trypanosomes in perivascular areas is accompanied by intense infiltration of mononuclear cells. Abnormalities in cerebrospinal fluid (CSF) include increased pressure, elevated total protein concentration, and pleocytosis. In addition, trypanosomes are frequently found in CSF.

EPIDEMIOLOGY The trypanosomes that cause sleeping sickness are found only in Africa. Approximately 20,000 new cases are reported each year, but this number is surely an underestimate of the true incidence. Humans are the only reservoir of *T. b. gambiense*, which occurs in widely distributed foci in tropical rain forests of Central and West Africa. Gambiense trypanosomiasis is primarily a problem in rural populations; tourists rarely become infected. Trypano-tolerant antelope species in savanna and woodland areas of Central and East Africa are the principal reservoir of *T. b. rhodesiense*. Cattle also can become infected but generally succumb to the parasite. Since risk results for the most part from contact with tsetse flies that feed on wild animals, humans acquire *T. b. rhodesiense* infection only incidentally, usually while working in areas where infected game and vectors are present. In addition, occasional cases occur among visitors to game parks in East Africa. During the past two decades, 16 cases of imported African trypanosomiasis have been reported to the CDC, most of which were caused by *T. b. rhodesiense*.

CLINICAL COURSE A painful trypanosomal chancre appears in some patients at the site of inoculation of the parasite. Hematogenous and lymphatic dissemination (stage I disease) is marked by the onset of fever. Typically, bouts of high temperatures lasting several days are separated by afebrile periods. Lymphadenopathy is prominent in *T. b. gambiense* trypanosomiasis. The nodes are discrete, movable, rubbery, and nontender. Cervical nodes are often visible, and enlargement of the nodes of the posterior cervical triangle, or Winterbottom's sign, is a classic finding. Pruritus is frequent, and a circinate rash is often present. Inconstant findings include malaise, headache, arthralgias, weight loss, edema, hepatosplenomegaly, and tachycardia.

CNS invasion (stage II disease) is characterized by the insidious development of protean neurologic manifestations that are accompanied by progressive abnormalities in the CSF. A picture of progressive indifference and daytime somnolence develops (hence the designation "sleeping sickness"), sometimes alternating with restlessness and insomnia at night. A listless gaze accompanies a loss of spontaneity, and speech may become halting and indistinct. Extrapyramidal signs may include choreiform movements, tremors, and fasciculations. Ataxia is frequent, and the patient may appear to have Parkinson's

disease, with a shuffling gait, hypertonia, and tremors. In the final phase, progressive neurologic impairment ends in coma and death.

The most striking difference between the West African and East African trypanosomiases is that the latter illness tends to follow a more acute course. Typically, in tourists, systemic signs of infection, such as fever, malaise, and headache, appear before the end of the trip or shortly after the return home. Persistent tachycardia unrelated to fever is common early in the course of *T. b. rhodesiense* trypanosomiasis, and death may result from arrhythmias and congestive heart failure before CNS disease develops. In general, untreated East African trypanosomiasis leads to death in a matter of weeks to months, often without a clear distinction between the hemolymphatic and CNS stages.

DIAGNOSIS A definitive diagnosis of African trypanosomiasis requires detection of the parasite. If a chancre is present, fluid should be expressed and examined directly by light microscopy for the highly motile trypanosomes. The fluid also should be fixed and stained with Giemsa stain. Material obtained by needle aspiration of lymph nodes early in the course of the illness should be examined similarly. Examination of wet preparations and Giemsa-stained thin and thick films of serial blood samples is also useful. If parasites are not found by these methods, the buffy coat from 10 to 15 mL of anticoagulated blood or the pellet obtained by centrifugation of the eluate from 25 to 50 mL of blood passed through a DEAE-cellulose column should be examined. Trypanosomes may be seen in material aspirated from the bone marrow; the aspirate can be inoculated into liquid culture medium, as can blood, buffy coat, lymph node aspirates, and CSF. Finally, *T. b. rhodesiense* infection can be detected by inoculation of these specimens into mice or rats, which results in patent parasitemia in a week or two. Although this method is highly sensitive for the detection of *T. b. rhodesiense*, it unfortunately does not detect *T. b. gambiense* because of host specificity.

It is essential to examine CSF from all patients in whom African trypanosomiasis is suspected. An increase in the CSF cell count is the first abnormality to be detected; increases in opening pressure and in levels of total protein and IgM develop later. Trypanosomes may be seen in the sediment of centrifuged CSF. Any CSF abnormality in a patient in whom trypanosomes have been found at other sites must be viewed as pathognomonic for CNS involvement and thus must prompt specific treatment for CNS disease.

A number of serologic assays are available to aid in the diagnosis of African trypanosomiasis, but their variable sensitivity and specificity mandate that decisions about treatment be based on demonstration of the parasite. These tests are of value for epidemiologic surveys.

℞ TREATMENT

The drugs traditionally used for treatment of African trypanosomiasis are suramin, pentamidine, and organic arsenicals. An addition to this list is eflornithine (difluoromethylornithine), which was approved by the U.S. Food and Drug Administration (FDA) in November 1990 for the treatment of West African trypanosomiasis. In the United States these drugs can be obtained from the CDC. Therapy for African trypanosomiasis must be individualized on the basis of the infecting organism (*T. b. gambiense* or *T. b. rhodesiense*), the presence or absence of CNS disease, adverse reactions, and (occasionally) drug resistance. The choices of drugs for the treatment of African trypanosomiasis are summarized as follows.

Stage I (normal CSF) West African trypanosomiasis (*T. b. gambiense*) should be treated with either suramin or eflornithine. Pentamidine can be used as an alternative drug. Stage II West African trypanosomiasis (abnormal CSF) should be treated with eflornithine.

Stage I East African trypanosomiasis (*T. b. rhodesiense*) should be treated with suramin, and pentamidine can be used as an alternative drug. Since suramin and pentamidine do not penetrate the CNS well and since eflornithine has variable efficacy against *T. b. rhodesiense*, stage II East African trypanosomiasis should be treated with melarsoprol. Patients who cannot tolerate the latter drug should be treated with tryparsamide plus suramin.

Suramin is highly effective against stage I disease. However, it can cause serious adverse effects and must be administered under the close supervision of a physician. A 100- to 200-mg intravenous test dose should be administered to detect hypersensitivity. The dosage for adults is 1 g intravenously on days 1, 3, 7, 14, and 21. The regimen for children is 20 mg/kg (maximum, 1 g) intravenously on days 1, 3, 7, 14, and 21. The drug is given by slow intravenous infusion of a freshly prepared 10% aqueous solution. Approximately 1 patient in 20,000 has an immediate, severe, and potentially fatal reaction to the drug, developing nausea, vomiting, shock, and seizures. Less severe reactions include fever, photophobia, pruritus, arthralgias, and skin eruptions. Renal damage is the most common important adverse effect of suramin. Transient proteinuria often appears during treatment. A urinalysis should be undertaken before each dose, and treatment should be discontinued if proteinuria increases or if casts and red cells appear in the sediment. Suramin should not be given to patients with renal insufficiency.

Eflornithine is highly effective for treatment of both stages of West African trypanosomiasis. In the trials on which the FDA based its approval, this agent cured more than 90 percent of 600 patients with stage II disease. The recommended treatment schedule is 400 mg/kg per day intravenously in four divided doses for 2 weeks followed by 300 mg/kg per day orally for 3 to 4 weeks. Adverse reactions include diarrhea, anemia, thrombocytopenia, seizures, and hearing loss. The efficacy of eflornithine in *T. b. rhodesiense* infection has not been determined. The high dosage and long duration of therapy required are disadvantages that may make widespread use of eflornithine difficult.

Pentamidine is the alternative drug for patients with stage I African trypanosomiasis, although some *T. b. rhodesiense* infections are unresponsive to this agent. The dose for both adults and children is 4 mg/kg per day intramuscularly or intravenously for 10 days. Frequent, immediate adverse reactions include nausea, vomiting, tachycardia, and hypotension. These reactions are usually transient and do not warrant cessation of therapy. Other adverse reactions include nephrotoxicity, abnormal liver function tests, neutropenia, rashes, hypoglycemia, and sterile abscesses.

The arsenical melarsoprol is the drug of choice for the treatment of East African trypanosomiasis with CNS involvement. Melarsoprol cures both stages of the disease and therefore is also indicated for the treatment of stage I disease in patients who fail to respond to or cannot tolerate suramin and/or pentamidine. However, because of its relatively high toxicity, melarsoprol is never the first choice for the treatment of stage I disease. The drug should be given to adults in three courses of 3 days each. The dosage is 2 to 3.6 mg/kg per day intravenously in three divided doses for 3 days followed 1 week later by 3.6 mg/kg per day, also in three divided doses and for 3 days. The latter course is repeated 10 to 21 days later. In debilitated patients, suramin is administered for 2 to 4 days before therapy with melarsoprol is initiated. An 18-mg initial dose of the latter drug, followed by progressive increases to the standard dose, has been recommended. For children, a total of 18 to 25 mg/kg should be given over 1 month. A starting dose of 0.36 mg/kg intravenously should be increased gradually to a maximum of 3.6 mg/kg at 1- to 5-day intervals, for a total of 9 or 10 doses.

Melarsoprol is highly toxic and should be administered with great care. The incidence of reactive encephalopathy has been reported to be as high as 18 percent in some series. Clinical manifestations of reactive encephalopathy include high fever, headache, tremor, impaired speech, seizures, and even coma and death. Treatment with melarsoprol should be discontinued at the first sign of encephalopathy but may be restarted cautiously at small doses a few days after signs have resolved. Extravasation of the drug results in intense local reactions. Vomiting, abdominal pain, nephrotoxicity, and myocardial damage can occur.

The treatment of patients with stage II East African disease who cannot tolerate melarsoprol is problematic. The combination of the arsenical tryparsamide and suramin is one possible approach, but its efficacy is limited because suramin does not penetrate the CNS well and tryparsamide is much less effective against *T. b. rhodesiense* than it is against *T. b. gambiense*. The schedule for tryparsamide therapy is 30 mg/kg (maximum 2 g) in a single intravenous dose every 5 days for a total of 12 doses; that for suramin treatment is 10 mg/kg intravenously every 5 days, also for a total of 12 injections. Tryparsamide can cause encephalopathy, fever, vomiting, abdominal pain, rash, tinnitus, and a variety of ocular symptoms. Alternatively, eflornithine can be administered as outlined above to patients who cannot tolerate melarsoprol, but, as noted, its effectiveness against *T. b. rhodesiense* is variable.

PREVENTION The trypanosomiases pose complex public-health and epizootic problems in Africa. Considerable progress has been made in some areas through control programs that focus on eradication of vectors and drug treatment of infected humans, but there is no consensus on the best approach to solving the overall problem. Individuals can reduce their risk of acquiring trypanosomiasis by avoiding areas known to harbor infected insects, by wearing protective clothing, and by using insect repellent. Chemoprophylaxis is not recommended, and no vaccine is available to prevent transmission of the parasites.

BIBLIOGRAPHY

CHAGAS' DISEASE

BOCCHI EA: Long-term follow-up after heart transplantation in Chagas' disease. Transplant Proc 25:1329, 1993

HAGAR JM, RAHIMTOOLA SH: Chagas' heart disease in the United States. N Engl J Med 325:763, 1991

KIRCHHOFF LV: Is *Trypanosoma cruzi* a new threat to our blood supply? Ann Intern Med 111:773, 1989

———: American trypanosomiasis (Chagas' disease): A persistent problem in Latin America now affects the United States. N Engl J Med 329:639, 1993

——— et al: American trypanosomiasis (Chagas' disease) in Central American immigrants. Am J Med 82:915, 1987

——— et al: Increased specificity of serodiagnosis of Chagas' disease by detection of antibody to the 72- and 90-kilodalton glycoproteins of *Trypanosoma cruzi*. J Infect Dis 155:561, 1987

———: American trypanosomiasis (Chagas' disease). Gastroenterol Clin North Am 25:517, 1996

OCHS DE et al: Postmortem diagnosis of autochthonous acute chagasic myocarditis by PCR amplification of a species-specific DNA sequence of *Trypanosoma cruzi*. Am J Trop Med Hyg 54:526, 1996

SALAZAR SCHETTINO PM et al: Chagas disease in Mexico. Parasitol Today 4:348, 1988

SCHMUNIS GA: *Trypanosoma cruzi*, the etiologic agent of Chagas' disease: Status in the blood supply in endemic and nonendemic countries. Transfusion 31:547, 1991

SLEEPING SICKNESS

BRYAN RT et al: African trypanosomiasis in American travelers: A 20 year review, in *International Travel Medicine*, R Steffen (ed). Berlin, Springer-Verlag, 1990

JORDAN AM: *Trypanosomiasis Control and African Rural Development*. London, Longman, 1986

MILORD F et al: Efficacy and toxicity of eflornithine for treatment of *Trypanosoma brucei gambiense* sleeping sickness. Trans R Soc Trop Med Hyg 87:652, 1992

PEPIN J, MILORD F: The treatment of African trypanosomiasis. Adv Parasitol 33:1, 1994

POLTERA AA: Pathology of human African trypanosomiasis with reference to experimental African trypanosomiasis and infections of the central nervous system. Br Med Bull 41:169, 1985

VANHAMME L, PAYS E: Control of gene expression in trypanosomes. Microbiol Rev 59:223, 1995

VICKERMAN K: Developmental cycles and biology of pathogenic trypanosomes. Br Med Bull 41:105, 1985

TOXOPLASMA INFECTION

DEFINITION　Toxoplasmosis is the disease caused by infection with the obligate intracellular parasite *Toxoplasma gondii*. Acute infection acquired after birth is asymptomatic but frequently results in the chronic persistence of cysts within the tissues of the host. Both acute and chronic toxoplasmosis are conditions in which the parasite is responsible for the development of clinically evident disease, including lymphadenopathy, encephalitis, myocarditis, and pneumonitis. Congenital toxoplasmosis is an infection of newborns that results from the transplacental passage of parasites from an infected mother to the fetus. These infants usually are asymptomatic at birth but later manifest a wide range of signs and symptoms, including chorioretinitis, strabismus, epilepsy, and psychomotor retardation.

ETIOLOGY　*T. gondii* is an intracellular coccidian that infects both birds and mammals. There are two distinct stages in the life cycle of *T. gondii*: the nonfeline and feline stages. In the nonfeline stage, tissue cysts that contain bradyzoites or sporulated oocysts are ingested by an intermediate host (e.g., a human, mouse, sheep, or pig). The cyst is rapidly digested by the acidic-pH gastric secretions. Bradyzoites or sporozoites are released, enter the small-intestinal epithelium, and transform into rapidly dividing tachyzoites. The tachyzoites are able to infect and replicate in all mammalian cells except red blood cells. Once attached to the host cell, the parasite penetrates the cell and forms a parasitophorous vacuole within which it divides. Parasite replication continues until the number of parasites within the cell approaches a critical mass and the cell ruptures, releasing parasites that infect adjoining cells.

As a result of this process, an infected organ soon shows evidence of cytopathology. Most of the tachyzoites are eliminated by means of humoral and cell-mediated immune responses of the host. Tissue cysts containing many bradyzoites develop 7 to 10 days after the systemic tachyzoite infection. These tissue cysts occur in a variety of host organs but are found principally within the central nervous system (CNS) and muscle, where they may exist for the lifetime of the host. The development of this chronic stage completes the nonfeline portion of the life cycle. Active infection in the immunocompromised host is most likely due to the spontaneous release of encysted parasites that undergo rapid transformation into tachyzoites within the CNS.

The principal stage in the life cycle of the parasite takes place in the cat (the definitive host) and its prey. The parasite's sexual phase is defined by the formation of oocysts within the feline host. This enteroepithelial cycle begins with the ingestion of the bradyzoite tissue cysts and culminates after several intermediate stages in the production of gametes. Gamete fusion produces a zygote, which envelops itself in a rigid wall and is secreted in the feces as an unsporulated oocyst. After 2 to 3 days of exposure to air at ambient temperature, the noninfectious oocyst sporulates to produce eight sporozoite progeny. The sporulated oocyst can be ingested by an intermediate host, such as a person emptying a cat's litter box, a pig rummaging in a barnyard, or perhaps a mouse. It is in the intermediate host that the parasite completes its life cycle.

EPIDEMIOLOGY　*T. gondii* is able to infect a wide range of mammals and birds. Its seroprevalence is dependent on the locale and the age of the population. Generally, hot arid climatic conditions are associated with a low prevalence of infection. In the United States and most European countries, the prevalence of seroconversion increases with age and exposure. For example, in the United States, 5 to 30 percent of individuals 10 to 19 years old and 10 to 67 percent of those over the age of 50 years show serologic evidence of exposure; seroprevalence increases by approximately 1 percent per year. In Central America, France, Turkey, and Brazil, the seroprevalence is much higher, approaching 90 percent by age 40.

ORAL TRANSMISSION　The principal source of human *Toxoplasma* infection remains uncertain. Transmission usually takes place by the oral route and can be attributable to ingestion of either sporulated oocysts from contaminated soil or bradyzoites from undercooked meat. During acute feline infection, a cat may excrete as many as 100 million parasites per day. These very stable sporozoite-containing oocysts are highly infectious and may remain viable for many years in the soil. Humans infected during a well-documented outbreak of oocyst-transmitted infection develop stage-specific antibodies to the oocyst/sporozoite.

Children and adults also can acquire infection from tissue cysts containing bradyzoites. The ingestion of a single cyst is all that is required for human infection. Undercooking or insufficient freezing of meat is an important source of infection in the developed world. In the United States, 10 to 20 percent of lamb products and 25 to 35 percent of pork products show evidence of cysts that contain bradyzoites. The incidence in beef is much lower—perhaps as low as 1 percent. Direct ingestion of bradyzoite cysts in these various meat products leads to acute infection.

In addition to oral transmission, direct transmission of the parasite by blood or organ products during transplantation takes place at a low incidence. Viable parasites can be cultured from refrigerated anticoagulated blood, which may be a source of infection in individuals receiving blood transfusions. *T. gondii* infection also has been reported in kidney and heart transplant recipients who were uninfected before transplantation.

TRANSPLACENTAL TRANSMISSION　About one-third of all women infected with *T. gondii* during pregnancy transmit the parasite to the fetus; the remainder give birth to normal, uninfected babies. Of the various factors that influence fetal outcome, gestational age at the time of infection is the most critical. Few data support a role for recrudescent maternal infection as the source of congenital disease. Thus women who are seropositive before pregnancy usually are protected against acute infection and do not give birth to congenitally infected neonates.

The following general guidelines can be used to evaluate congenital infection. There is essentially no risk if the mother is infected 6 months or more before conception. If infection is acquired less than 6 months before conception, the likelihood of transplacental infection increases as the interval between infection and conception decreases. In pregnancy, if the mother becomes infected during the first trimester, the incidence of transplacental infection is lowest (about 15 percent), but the disease in the neonate is most severe. If maternal infection occurs during the third trimester, the incidence of transplacental infection is greatest (65 percent), but the infant is usually asymptomatic at birth. Recent evidence, however, suggests that infected infants who are normal at birth may have a higher incidence of learning disabilities and chronic neurologic sequelae than uninfected children. Only a small proportion (20 percent) of women infected with *T. gondii* develop clinical signs of infection. Often the diagnosis is first appreciated when routine postconception serologic tests show evidence of specific antibody.

PATHOGENESIS　Upon the ingestion by the host of either tissue cysts containing bradyzoites or oocysts containing sporozoites, the parasites are released from the cysts by a digestive process. Bradyzoites are resistant to the effect of pepsin and quickly invade and multiply within the gastrointestinal tract of the host. Within enterocytes, the parasites undergo morphologic transformation, giving rise to invasive tachyzoites. These tachyzoites are able to induce host secretory immunity, as evidenced by increased levels of parasite-specific IgA. The parasites are disseminated to a variety of organs, particularly lymphatic tissue, skeletal muscle, myocardium, retina, placenta, and (most frequently) the CNS. In these organs, the parasite infects host cells, replicates, and invades the adjoining cells. In this fashion, the hallmarks of the infection develop: cell death and focal necrosis surrounded by an acute inflammatory response.

In the normal immune host, both the humoral and the cellular immune responses are important in controlling infection. Tachyzoites are sequestered by a variety of immune mechanisms, including induction of parasiticidal antibody, activation of macrophages, production of interferon γ (IFNγ), and stimulation of cytotoxic T lymphocytes of the CD8 + phenotype. These antigen-specific lymphocytes are capable of killing both extracellular parasites and target cells infected with parasites. As tachyzoites are cleared from the acutely infected host, tissue cysts containing bradyzoites begin to appear, usually within the CNS and the retina. A number of immune factors, including altered antibody levels within the CNS, IFNγ, and CD4 + and CD8 + T cells, modulate the normal host immune response.

In the immunocompromised or fetal host, the immune factors necessary to control the spread of tachyzoite infection are lacking. This altered immune state gives rise to a progression of focal destruction that results in organ failure (i.e., necrotizing encephalitis, pneumonia, and myocarditis).

Persistence of infection with cysts containing bradyzoites is common in the normal host. This lifelong infection usually remains subclinical. Although bradyzoites are in a slow metabolic phase, cysts do degenerate and rupture within the CNS. This degenerative process, with the development of new bradyzoite-containing cysts, is the most likely stimulus for the persistence of antibody titers in the normal host. Degeneration of these cysts is the most probable source of recrudescent infection in immunocompromised individuals.

PATHOLOGY Cell death and focal necrosis due to replicating tachyzoites induce an intense mononuclear inflammatory response in any tissue or cell type infected. Tachyzoites rarely can be visualized by routine histopathologic staining of these inflammatory lesions. However, immunofluorescence staining with parasite antigen–specific antibodies can reveal either the organism itself or evidence of antigen. In contrast to this inflammatory process caused by tachyzoites, bradyzoite-containing cysts cause inflammation only at the early stages of development, and even this inflammation may be a response to the presence of tachyzoite antigens. Once the cysts reach maturity, the inflammatory process can no longer be detected, and the cysts remain immunologically quiescent within the brain matrix until they rupture.

Lymph Nodes During acute infection, lymph node biopsy demonstrates characteristic findings, including follicular hyperplasia and irregular clusters of tissue macrophages with eosinophilic cytoplasm. Granulomas rarely are evident in these specimens. Although tachyzoites are not usually visible, they can be sought either by subinoculation of infected tissue into mice, with resultant disease, or by the polymerase chain reaction (PCR). PCR amplification of DNA fragments representing either p30 (SAG-1) or p22 (SAG-2) antigen has been shown to be an effective and sensitive assay for establishing infection of lymph node tissue by tachyzoites.

Eyes In the eye, infiltrates of monocytes, lymphocytes, and plasma cells may produce uni- or multifocal lesions. Granulomatous lesions and retinochoroiditis can be observed in the posterior chamber following acute necrotizing retinitis. Other ocular complications of infection include iridocyclitis, cataracts, and glaucoma.

Central Nervous System During CNS involvement, both focal and diffuse meningoencephalitis can be documented, with evidence of necrosis and microglial nodules. Necrotizing encephalitis in the patient without AIDS is characterized by small diffuse lesions with perivascular cuffing in contiguous areas. In the AIDS population, polymorphonuclear leukocytes may be present in addition to monocytes, lymphocytes, and plasma cells. Cysts containing bradyzoites frequently are found contiguous with the necrotic tissue border. In the mouse model, parasite DNA has been detected by PCR amplification in association with reactivation of CNS toxoplasmosis.

Lungs Among patients with AIDS who die of toxoplasmosis, 40 to 70 percent have involvement of the heart and lung. Interstitial pneumonitis can develop in the neonate and the immunocompromised patient. Thickened and edematous alveolar septa infiltrated with mononuclear and plasma cells are apparent. This inflammation may extend to the endothelial walls. Tachyzoites and bradyzoite-containing cysts have been observed within the alveolar membrane. Superimposed bronchopneumonia can be caused by other microbial agents.

Heart Cysts and aggregates of parasites in cardiac muscle tissue are evident in patients with AIDS who die of toxoplasmosis. Focal necrosis surrounded by inflammatory cells is associated with hyaline necrosis and disrupted myocardial cells. Pericarditis is associated with toxoplasmosis in some patients.

Other Sites Pathologic changes during disseminated infection are similar to those described for the lymph nodes, eyes, and CNS. In patients with AIDS, the skeletal muscle, pancreas, stomach, and kidneys can be involved, with necrosis, invasion by inflammatory cells, and (rarely) the presence of tachyzoites detectable by routine staining. Large necrotic lesions may cause direct tissue destruction. In addition, secondary effects from acute infection of these various organs, including pancreatitis, myositis, and glomerulonephritis, have been reported.

HOST IMMUNE RESPONSE Acute *Toxoplasma* infection evokes a cascade of protective immune responses in the normal host. *Toxoplasma* enters the host at the gut mucosal level and evokes the production of IgA antibody. This isotype, which constitutes more than 80 percent of all antibody in the mucosa, has now been shown to be a potentially important modulator of protection and indicator of infection. Titers of serum IgA antibody directed at p30 (SAG-1) have been shown to be a useful marker of congenital and acute toxoplasmosis. Milk-whey IgA from acutely infected mothers contains a high titer of antibody to *T. gondii* and is able to block infection of enterocytes in vitro. The predominant parasite antigen recognized by the whey IgA is p30. In mice, IgA intestinal secretions directed at the parasite are abundant and are associated with the induction of mucosal T cells.

If the parasite evades the host mucosal response, both humoral immunity and cellular immunity are evoked. *T. gondii* rapidly induces detectable levels of both IgM and IgG antibodies in serum. Monoclonal gammopathy of the IgG class can occur in congenitally infected infants. IgM levels may be increased in the newborn with congenital infection. The polyclonal IgG antibodies evoked by infection are parasiticidal in vitro in the presence of serum complement and are the basis for the Sabin-Feldman dye test. However, cell-mediated immunity is the major protective response evoked by the parasite during host infection. Macrophages are activated following phagocytosis of antibody-opsonized parasites. This activation can lead to death of the parasite by either an oxygen-dependent or an oxygen-independent process. Recent studies demonstrate that if the parasite is not phagocytosed and enters the macrophage by active penetration, it continues to replicate. In addition, T cells are activated by a variety of parasite antigens. These antigens can be either membrane-associated or cytoplasmic. The CD4 + and CD8 + T cell responses are antigen-specific and further stimulate the production of a variety of important lymphokines that expand the T cell and natural killer cell repertoire. IFNγ is an important factor in eliciting host immune protection against *Toxoplasma* infection. T cells exhibiting both T_{H1} (associated with IFNγ production) and T_{H2} [associated with interleukin (IL) 4 production] have been isolated from seropositive individuals. CD8 + cells appear critical to host immunity. In humans, prolonged alteration in T cell subpopulations is associated with *T. gondii* infection. Both asymptomatic patients and those with active infection may show a depression in the ratio of CD4 + to CD8 + lymphocytes. This shift may be correlated with a disease syndrome but is not necessarily correlated with disease outcome. Human T cell clones of both the CD4 + and the CD8 + phenotypes are cytolytic against parasite-infected macrophages. These T cell clones produce cytokines that are "microbistatic." IL-12 and perhaps IL-7 and IL-15 appear to be important during acute infection, upregulating the production of IFNγ. Recent studies suggest that the effect of IFNγ may be paradoxical, with stimulation of a host downregulatory response as well.

In patients with AIDS, both the humoral response and the cellular response to *T. gondii* are altered. Although infection in the patient with AIDS is believed to be recrudescent, determination of antibody titers is not helpful in establishing reactivation. Because of the severe depletion in CD4 + T cells, quite frequently there is no observed increase in antibody titer during exacerbation of infection. T cells from AIDS patients with reactivation of toxoplasmosis fail to secrete both INFγ and IL-2. This alteration in the production of these critical immune cytokines contributes to the persistence of infection. *Toxoplasma* infection frequently develops late in the course of AIDS, when the loss of T cell–dependent protective mechanisms, particularly CD8 + T cells, becomes most pronounced.

CLINICAL MANIFESTATIONS In the person whose immune system is intact, acute toxoplasmosis is usually asymptomatic and self-limited. This condition can go unrecognized in 80 to 90 percent of adults and children with acquired infection. The asymptomatic nature of this infection makes diagnosis difficult in mothers infected during pregnancy. In contrast, the wide range of clinical manifestations in congenitally infected children includes severe neurologic complications such as hydrocephalus, microcephaly, mental retardation, and retinochoroiditis. If prenatal infection is severe, multiorgan failure and subsequent intrauterine fetal death can occur. In children and adults, chronic infection can persist throughout life, with little consequence to the immunocompetent host.

Toxoplasmosis in the Immunocompetent Person The most common manifestation of acute toxoplasmosis is cervical lymphadenopathy. The nodes may be single or multiple, are usually nontender, are discrete, and vary in firmness. Lymphadenopathy also may be found in suboccipital, supraclavicular, inguinal, and mediastinal areas. Generalized lymphadenopathy occurs in 20 to 30 percent of symptomatic patients. Between 20 and 40 percent of patients with lymphadenopathy also have headache, malaise, fatigue, and fever (usually with a temperature of <40°C). A smaller proportion of symptomatic individuals have myalgia, sore throat, abdominal pain, maculopapular rash, meningoencephalitis, and confusion. Rare complications associated with infection in the normal immune host include pneumonia, myocarditis, encephalopathy, pericarditis, and polymyositis. Symptoms associated with acute infection usually resolve within several weeks, although the lymphadenopathy may persist for some months. In a recent epidemic, toxoplasmosis was diagnosed correctly in only 3 of the 25 patients who consulted physicians. If toxoplasmosis is considered in the differential diagnosis, routine laboratory and serologic screening should be performed before node biopsy.

The results of routine laboratory studies are usually unremarkable except for minimal lymphocytosis, an elevated sedimentation rate, and a nominal increase in liver aminotransferases. Evaluation of cerebrospinal fluid (CSF) in cases with evidence of encephalopathy or meningoencephalitis shows an elevation of intracranial pressure, mononuclear pleocytosis (10 to 50 cells/mL), a slight increase in protein concentration, and (occasionally) an increase in the gamma globulin level. PCR amplification of the *Toxoplasma* DNA target sequence in the CSF may be beneficial. The CSF of chronically infected individuals is normal.

Ocular Infection Infection with *T. gondii* is estimated to cause 35 percent of all cases of chorioretinitis in the United States and Europe. Most ocular involvement is believed to be due to congenital infection, with a very low incidence following acquired infection. Individuals with AIDS also can develop debilitating chorioretinitis. A variety of ocular manifestations are documented, including blurred vision, scotoma, photophobia, and eye pain. Macular involvement occurs with loss of central vision, and nystagmus is secondary to poor fixation. Involvement of the extraocular muscles may lead to disorders of convergence and to strabismus. Ophthalmologic examination should be undertaken in newborns with suspected congenital infection. As the inflammation resolves, vision improves, but episodic flare-ups of chorioretinitis, which progressively destroy retinal tissue and lead to glaucoma, are common.

The ophthalmologic examination reveals yellow-white, cotton-like patches with indistinct margins of hyperemia. As the lesions age, white plaques with distinct borders and black spots within the retinal pigment become more apparent. Lesions usually are located near the posterior pole of the retina; they may be single but are more commonly multiple. Congenital lesions may be unilateral or bilateral and show evidence of massive chorioretinal degeneration with extensive fibrosis. Surrounding these areas of involvement are a normal retina and vasculature. In patients with AIDS, retinal lesions are often large with diffuse necrosis of the retina and include both free tachyzoites and cysts containing bradyzoites.

Infection of the Immunocompromised Person Patients with AIDS and those receiving immunosuppressive therapy for lymphoproliferative disorders are at greatest risk for developing acute toxoplasmosis. This predilection may be due either to reactivation of latent infection or to acquisition of parasites from exogenous sources such as blood or transplanted organs. In individuals with AIDS, more than 95 percent of cases of *Toxoplasma* encephalitis are believed to be due to recrudescent infection. In most of these cases, encephalitis develops when the CD4 + cell count falls below 100 cells/µL. In the immunocompromised individual, the disease may be rapidly fatal if untreated. Thus accurate diagnosis and initiation of appropriate therapy are necessary to prevent fulminant infection.

Toxoplasmosis is a principal opportunistic infection of the CNS in persons with AIDS. Although geographic origin may be related to frequency of infection, it has no correlation with the severity of disease in the immunocompromised host. Individuals with AIDS who are seropositive for *T. gondii* are at a very high risk for developing encephalitis. In the United States, about one-third of the 15 to 40 percent of adult patients with AIDS who are latently infected with the parasite develop *Toxoplasma* encephalitis.

The signs and symptoms of acute toxoplasmosis in the immunocompromised patient are principally within the CNS. More than 50 percent of patients with clinical manifestations have intracerebral involvement. Clinical findings at the time of presentation can range from nonfocal to focal dysfunction. These findings include encephalopathy, meningoencephalitis, and mass lesions. Patients may present with altered mental status (75 percent), fever (10 to 72 percent), seizures (33 percent), headaches (56 percent), and focal neurologic findings (60 percent), including motor deficits, cranial nerve palsies, movement disorders, dysmetria, visual-field loss, and aphasia. Patients who present with evidence of diffuse cortical dysfunction develop evidence of focal neurologic disease as the infection progresses. This altered condition is due not only to the necrotizing encephalitis caused by direct invasion of the parasite but also to secondary effects, including vasculitis, edema, and hemorrhage. The onset of infection can range from an insidious process over several weeks to an acute confusional state with fulminant focal deficits, including hemiparesis, hemiplegia, visual-field defects, localized headache, and focal seizures.

Although lesions can occur anywhere within the CNS, the areas most involved appear to be the brainstem, basal ganglia, pituitary gland, and corticomedullary junction. Brainstem involvement gives rise to a variety of neurologic dysfunctions, including cranial nerve palsy, dysmetria, and ataxia. With basal ganglionic infection, patients may develop hydrocephalus, choreiform movements, and choreoathetosis. Because *Toxoplasma* usually causes encephalitis, meningeal involvement is uncommon, and thus CSF findings may be unremarkable or may include a modest increase in cell count and in protein—but not glucose—concentration.

Cerebral toxoplasmosis needs to be differentiated from other opportunistic infections or tumors within the CNS of those afflicted with AIDS. The differential diagnosis includes herpes simplex encephalitis, cryptococcal meningitis, progressive multifocal leukoencephalopathy, and primary CNS lymphoma. Involvement of the pituitary gland can give rise to panhypopituitarism and hyponatremia from inappropriate secretion of vasopressin (antidiuretic hormone). AIDS-dementia complex may present as cognitive impairment, attention loss, and altered memory. Brain biopsy in those patients who have been treated for *Toxoplasma* encephalitis but who continue to exhibit neurologic dysfunction often fails to identify organisms.

Autopsies of patients infected with *Toxoplasma* have demonstrated multiple organ involvement with or without CNS disease. The organs infected include the lungs, gastrointestinal tract, pancreas, skin, eyes, heart, and liver. *Toxoplasma* pneumonia can occur and can be confused with *Pneumocystis carinii* infection. Respiratory involvement usually presents as dyspnea, fever, and a nonproductive cough and may rapidly progress to acute respiratory failure with hemoptysis, metabolic acidosis, hypotension, and (occasionally) disseminated intravascular coagulation. Histopathologic studies demonstrate necrosis and a mixed cellular infiltrate. The presence of organisms is a helpful diagnostic indicator, but organisms can also be found in healthy tissue. Most commonly, myocardial infection is asymptomatic. However, infection of the heart can be associated with cardiac tamponade or biventricular failure. As discussed previously, ocular involvement can occur without concomitant encephalitis. This infection should be distinguished from chorioretinitis caused by cytomegalovirus, which is usually more hemorrhagic in character. Toxoplasmic retinochoroiditis may be a prodrome to the development of encephalitis.

A presumptive clinical diagnosis of toxoplasmic encephalitis in patients with AIDS is based on clinical presentation, history of exposure as evidenced by positive serology, and radiologic evaluation. When these criteria are used, the predictive value is as high as 80 percent. More than 97 percent of patients with AIDS and toxoplasmosis have IgG antibody to the parasite in their sera. IgM serum antibody is usually not demonstrable. Intrathecal antibody to *T. gondii* may be present. Neuroradiologic evaluation should include double-dose contrast computed tomography (CT) of the head. By this test, single and frequently multiple contrast-enhancing lesions (<2 cm) may be identified. Magnetic resonance imaging (MRI) usually demonstrates multiple lesions and provides a more sensitive evaluation of the efficacy of therapy than does CT. Patients with primary CNS lymphoma are four times more likely than patients with *Toxoplasma* encephalitis to have solitary lesions on an MRI scan. A therapeutic trial of anti-*Toxoplasma* medications frequently is used to assess the diagnosis. Recent studies have shown that treatment of presumptive *Toxoplasma* encephalitis with pyrimethamine/clindamycin results in quantifiable clinical improvement in more than 50 percent of patients by day 3. By day 7, more than 90 percent of treated patients show evidence of improvement. In contrast, if patients fail to respond or have lymphoma, clinical signs and symptoms worsen by day 7. Patients in this category require brain biopsy with or without a change in therapy. This procedure can now be performed by a stereotactic CT-guided method that reduces the potential for complications. Brain biopsy for *T. gondii* identifies organisms in 50 to 75 percent of cases. More recent studies indicate that PCR amplification of target genes significantly increases the sensitivity of detection of parasites.

Congenital Toxoplasmosis   Between 400 and 4000 infants born each year in the United States are affected by congenital toxoplasmosis. Infection of the placenta leads to hematogenous infection of the fetus. As has already been stated, the proportion of fetuses that becomes infected increases but the clinical severity of the infection declines as gestation proceeds. Persistence of the parasite can ultimately result in reactivation and further damage decades later. Factors associated with relatively severe disabilities include delayed diagnosis and initiation of therapy, neonatal hypoxia and hypoglycemia, profound visual impairment, uncorrected hydrocephalus, and increased intracranial pressure. If treated appropriately, upwards of 70 percent of children have normal developmental, neurologic, and ophthalmologic findings at follow-up evaluations. Treatment for 1 year with pyrimethamine and sulfonamide is tolerated with minimal toxicity (see below).

DIAGNOSIS   Tissue and Body Fluid   The diagnosis of acute toxoplasmosis can be made by isolation of the parasite from either blood or other body fluids after subinoculation of the body fluid into the peritoneal cavity of mice. Mice should be tested for organisms in the peritoneal fluid 6 to 10 days after inoculation. If no parasites are found in the mouse's peritoneal fluid, its anti-*Toxoplasma* serum titer can be evaluated 4 to 6 weeks after inoculation. Isolation of *T. gondii* from the patient's body fluids reflects acute infection, whereas isolation from biopsied tissue is an indication only of the presence of tissue cysts and should not be misinterpreted as acute toxoplasmosis. Persistent parasitemia in patients with latent, asymptomatic infection is rare.

Histologic examination of lymph nodes may suggest the characteristic changes described above. Demonstration of tachyzoites in lymph nodes establishes the diagnosis of acute toxoplasmosis. As with subinoculation into mice, demonstration of cysts containing bradyzoites in histologic specimens confirms prior infection with *T. gondii* but is nondiagnostic for acute infection.

Serology   The preceding procedures have great diagnostic value but are limited by difficulties encountered either in the growth of parasites in vivo or in the identification of tachyzoites by histochemical methods. Serologic testing has become the routine method of diagnosis. A wide range of serologic tests that can be used to measure antibody to *T. gondii* are available commercially. The reader is referred to the excellent review of the various tests by Remington and McLeod.

Diagnosis of acute infection with *T. gondii* can be established by detection of the simultaneous presence of IgG and IgM antibody to *Toxoplasma* in serum. The presence of circulating IgA favors the diagnosis of an acute infection. The Sabin-Feldman dye test, the indirect fluorescent antibody test, and the enzyme-linked immunosorbent assay (ELISA) all satisfactorily measure circulating IgG antibody to *Toxoplasma*. Positive IgG titers (>1:10) can be detected as early as 2 to 3 weeks after infection. These titers usually peak at 6 to 8 weeks and decline slowly to a new baseline level that persists for life. It is necessary to measure the serum IgM titer in concert with the IgG titer to better establish the time of infection. The methods currently available for this determination are the double-sandwich IgM-ELISA and the IgM-immunosorbent assay (IgM-ISAGA). Both of these assays are specific and sensitive, and their use precludes the false-positive results associated with rheumatoid factor and antinuclear antibody. The double-sandwich IgA-ELISA is more sensitive than the IgM-ELISA for detecting congenital infection in the fetus and newborn.

The Immunocompetent Adult or Child   For the patient who presents with lymphadenopathy only, a positive IgM titer is an indication of acute infection—and an indication for therapy, if that is clinically warranted (see "Treatment" below). The serum IgM titer should be determined again in 3 weeks. An elevation in the IgG titer without an increase in the IgM titer suggests that infection is present but that it is not acute. If there is a borderline increase in either IgG or IgM, the titers should be assessed again in 3 to 4 weeks.

Ocular Toxoplasmosis   Because of the congenital nature of ocular toxoplasmosis, the serum antibody titer may not correlate with the presence of active lesions in the fundus. In general, a positive IgG titer (measured in undiluted serum if necessary) in conjunction with typical lesions establishes the diagnosis. If lesions are atypical and the titer is in the low-positive range, the diagnosis is presumptive.

The Immunocompromised Host   As discussed above, in patients with AIDS, the presence of IgG and radiologic findings consistent with toxoplasmosis are grounds for a presumptive diagnosis. Attempts to evaluate rising IgG titers or to determine whether IgM is present are not productive. Serologic evidence of infection virtually always precedes the development of *Toxoplasma* encephalitis. It is therefore important to determine the *Toxoplasma* antibody status of all patients infected with human immunodeficiency virus (HIV). Antibody titers may range from negative to 1:1024 in patients with AIDS and *Toxoplasma* encephalitis. Fewer than 3 percent of patients have no demonstrable antibody to *Toxoplasma* at the time of diagnosis. Determination of the intrathecal antibody titer may be useful in identifying prior infection. PCR amplification of genetic material of the parasite found in the CSF may prove diagnostically beneficial in the future.

Patients with toxoplasmic encephalitis have focal or multifocal abnormalities demonstrable by CT or MRI. These findings are not pathognomonic of *Toxoplasma* infection since 40 percent of CNS lymphomas are multifocal and 50 percent are ring-enhancing. Lesions on CT scan are multiple and are located in both hemispheres, with the basal ganglia and corticomedullary junction most commonly involved. A CT scan may underestimate the degree of inflammation during early disease. Double-dose contrast enhancement may increase the sensitivity of diagnosis. For both MRI and CT scans, the rate of false-negative results is approximately 10 percent. The finding of a single lesion on an MRI scan increases the suspicion of primary lymphoma and strengthens the argument for the performance of a brain biopsy. MRI should be performed if the CT scan shows only a single lesion. CT and MRI scans are important for assessment of the response to therapy. As in other conditions, the radiologic response may lag behind the clinical response. Resolution of lesions may take from 3 weeks to 6 months. Some patients show clinical improvement despite worsening radiographic findings.

A presumptive diagnosis of *Toxoplasma* encephalitis should prompt the immediate initiation of therapy. Patients should be monitored for neurologic deterioration during the first 7 days of treatment. After this time, therapy should result in stabilization or improvement in clinical status. After 3 weeks, repeat radiologic studies should detect improvement. If glucocorticoids have been administered, radiologic studies should be repeated at the time of discontinuation to determine whether an exacerbation of disease has occurred. If the patient's clinical condition becomes worse, performance of a biopsy must be strongly considered.

Diagnosis of Congenital Infection The issue of concern when a pregnant woman has evidence of recent *T. gondii* infection is obviously whether the fetus is infected. PCR of the amniotic fluid to detect the B1 gene of the parasite has replaced fetal blood sampling. However, the definitive test for congenital infection is the direct inoculation of placental tissue or of newborn blood or CSF into susceptible mice. Serologic diagnosis is based on the persistence of IgG antibody or a positive IgM titer after the first week of life (a time frame that excludes placental leak). The IgG determination should be repeated every 2 months. An increase in IgM beyond the first week of life is indicative of acute infection. However, up to 25 percent of infected newborns may be seronegative and have normal routine physical examinations. Thus assessment of the eye and the brain, with ophthalmologic testing, CSF evaluation, and radiologic studies, is important in establishing the diagnosis.

℞ TREATMENT

Immunologically competent adults and older children who have only lymphadenopathy do not require specific therapy unless they have persistent and severe symptoms. Patients with ocular toxoplasmosis should be treated for 1 month with pyrimethamine plus either sulfadiazine or clindamycin. A large percentage of patients with chorioretinitis improve clinically with treatment.

Patients with AIDS should be treated for acute toxoplasmosis. Current therapeutic protocols are directed at folate metabolism, protein synthesis, or nucleic acid synthesis of the parasite. Pyrimethamine and trimethoprim inhibit the enzyme dihydrofolate reductase. Inhibitors of protein synthesis, including clindamycin, chlortetracycline, and azithromycin, affect growth of the parasite. Inhibitors of purine synthesis, such as arprinocid, may prove to be important. Atovaquone, which blocks pyrimidine salvage, has demonstrated activity against both *T. gondii* and *P. carinii*.

In the immunocompromised patient, toxoplasmosis is rapidly fatal if untreated. The mainstay of treatment for *Toxoplasma* encephalitis is a combination regimen. Pyrimethamine and sulfadiazine administered together block folic acid metabolism and successfully reduce the parasite burden. Leucovorin (calcium folinate) is given as an adjunct to prevent the bone marrow toxicity associated with pyrimethamine. Both pyrimethamine and sulfadiazine cross the blood-brain barrier. A prominent consequence of dual therapy is the high incidence of associated toxicity (40 percent). Rash may develop during the first 3 weeks in up to 20 percent of patients but does not preclude the use of this combination. Other complications include hematologic effects, crystalluria, hematuria, radiolucent renal stones, and nephrotoxicity. During therapy, serum levels of these drugs may be erratic, but such fluctuations have not been correlated with these complications.

The current regimen consists of pyrimethamine (a 200-mg loading dose followed by 50 to 75 mg/d) plus sulfadiazine (4 to 6 g/d in four divided doses). In addition, the administration of leucovorin (10 to 15 mg/d for 6 weeks) is required. These agents are active only against the tachyzoite stage of the parasite. Thus, after patients complete the initial course (lasting 4 to 6 weeks or until radiologic improvement is documented), they must receive lifelong suppressive therapy with pyrimethamine (25 to 50 mg/d) and sulfadiazine (2 to 4 g/d). If sulfadiazine cannot be tolerated, a combination of pyrimethamine (75 mg/d) plus clindamycin (450 mg tid) can be used. It is possible that pyrimethamine (50 to 75 mg/d) is sufficient for chronic suppressive therapy. Congenitally infected neonates are treated with daily oral pyrimethamine (0.5 to 1 mg/kg) and sulfadiazine (100 mg/kg) for 1 year. In addition, therapy with spiramycin (100 mg/kg per day) plus prednisone (1 mg/kg per day) has been shown to be efficacious for congenital infection.

Alternative therapies have been established because of the toxicity associated with the long-term antimicrobial therapy necessary for many individuals infected with *T. gondii*. Dapsone (diaminodiphenyl sulfone), with its longer serum half-life and decreased toxicity, is an effective alternative to sulfadiazine. Spiramycin, which has been used in Europe to treat pregnant women, reduces transplacental transmission. However, spiramycin has been ineffective as primary prophylaxis in patients with AIDS. Clindamycin is well absorbed from the gastrointestinal tract, and serum levels peak 1 to 2 h after administration. The combination of oral pyrimethamine (25 to 75 mg/d) plus intravenous clindamycin (1200 to 4800 mg/d) is effective for patients with AIDS who have *Toxoplasma* encephalitis. Toxic effects of clindamycin include nausea, vomiting, neutropenia, rash, and pseudomembranous colitis. Other macrolides that have been evaluated include roxithromycin, clarithromycin, and azithromycin. A combination of pyrimethamine and clarithromycin appears to be effective. Evidence suggests that the macrolides are not beneficial by themselves. Atovaquone (750 mg tid or qid) is an optional agent for the treatment of individuals who are intolerant of other agents. Glucocorticoids can be used to treat intracerebral edema, but their benefit has not yet been established. It is difficult to assess the benefit of glucocorticoids when they are administered in conjunction with anti-*Toxoplasma* medication. Anticonvulsants are sometimes necessary for the treatment of seizures, but attention should be given to the potential interaction between sulfadiazine and phenytoin. A regimen of trimethoprim-sulfamethoxazole or dapsone plus pyrimethamine with leucovorin may prevent the development of *Toxoplasma* encephalitis in individuals infected with HIV who are seropositive for *T. gondii* after their CD4+ T lymphocyte count falls to 100/μL.

PREVENTION The chances of primary infection with *Toxoplasma* can be reduced by not eating undercooked meat and by avoiding oocyst-contaminated material (i.e., a cat's litter box). Meat should be heated to 60°C or frozen to kill cysts. Hands should be washed thoroughly after work in the garden, and all fruits and vegetables should be washed. Blood intended for transfusion into *Toxoplasma*-seronegative immunocompromised individuals should be screened for antibody to *T. gondii*. Although such serologic screening is not routinely performed, seronegative women should be screened for evidence of infection several times during pregnancy if they are exposed to environmental conditions that put them at risk for infection with *T. gondii*. HIV-positive individuals should closely adhere to these preventive measures.

BIBLIOGRAPHY

CHANNON JY, KASPER LH: *Toxoplasma gondii*–induced immune suppression by human peripheral blood monocytes: Role of gamma interferon. Infect Immun 64:1181, 1996

FADUL CE et al: Survival of immunoglobulin G–opsonized *Toxoplasma gondii* in nonadherent human monocytes. Infect Immun 63:4290, 1995

KASPER LH, BOOTHROYD JC: *T. gondii* and toxoplasmosis, in *Immunology and Molecular Biology of Parasitic Infections*, 3d ed, KS Warren, N Agabian (eds). Oxford, Blackwell Scientific, 1993

LUFT BJ, REMINGTON JS: Toxoplasmic encephalitis in AIDS. Clin Infect Dis 15:211, 1992

McAULEY J et al: Early and longitudinal evaluations of treated infants and children with congenital toxoplasmosis. Clin Infect Dis 18:38, 1994

PODZAMCZER D et al: Intermittent trimethoprim-sulfamethoxazole compared with dapsone-pyrimethamine for the simultaneous primary prophylaxis of *Pneumocystis* pneumonia and toxoplasmosis in patients infected with HIV. Ann Intern Med 122:755, 1995

Prophylaxis for *Toxoplasma* encephalitis. Infect Dis Alert 11:164, 1992

REMINGTON JS et al: Toxoplasmosis, in *Infectious Diseases of the Fetus and Newborn Infant*, 4th ed, JS Remington, JO Klein (eds). Philadelphia, Saunders, 1994

———, McLEOD R: Toxoplasmosis, in *Infectious Diseases in Medicine and Surgery*, J Bartlett et al (eds). Philadelphia, Saunders, 1992

RICHARDS FO JR et al: Preventing toxoplasmic encephalitis in persons infected with human immunodeficiency virus. Clin Infect Dis 19:S49, 1995

WONG S-Y et al: AIDS-associated toxoplasmosis, in *The Medical Management of AIDS*, 4th ed, MA Sande, PA Volberding (eds). Philadelphia, Saunders, 1994

220 Theodore E. Nash, Peter F. Weller

PROTOZOAL INTESTINAL INFECTIONS AND TRICHOMONIASIS

PROTOZOAL INFECTIONS

GIARDIASIS *Giardia lamblia* is a cosmopolitan protozoal parasite that inhabits the small intestines of humans and other mammals. Giardiasis is one of the most common parasitic diseases worldwide and causes both endemic and epidemic intestinal disease and diarrhea.

Life Cycle and Epidemiology Infection follows the ingestion of the environmentally hardy cysts, which excyst in the small intestine, releasing trophozoites that multiply by binary fission, occasionally to enormous numbers. *Giardia* remains a pathogen of the proximal small bowel and does not disseminate hematogenously. Trophozoites remain free in the lumen or attach to the mucosal epithelium by means of a ventral sucking disk. As a trophozoite encounters altered conditions, it forms a morphologically distinct cyst, which is the stage of the parasite usually found in the feces. Trophozoites may be present and even predominate in loose or watery stools, but it is the resistant cyst that survives outside the body and is responsible for transmission. Cysts do not tolerate heating, desiccation, or continued exposure to feces but do remain viable for months in cold fresh water. The number of cysts excreted varies widely but can approach 10^7 per gram of stool.

Giardia infections are common in both developed and developing countries. Ingestion of as few as 10 cysts is sufficient to cause infection in humans. Because cysts are infectious when excreted or shortly thereafter, person-to-person transmission occurs where fecal hygiene is poor. Giardiasis, as a symptomatic or an asymptomatic infection, is especially prevalent in day-care centers; person-to-person spread also takes place in other institutional settings with poor fecal hygiene and during homosexual contact. If food is contaminated with *Giardia* cysts after cooking or preparation, food-borne transmission can occur. Waterborne transmission accounts for episodic infections (e.g., in campers and other travelers) and for massive epidemics in metropolitan areas. Surface water, ranging from mountain streams to large municipal reservoirs, can become contaminated with fecally derived *Giardia* cysts; outmoded water systems are subject to cross-contamination from leaking sewer lines. The efficacy of water as a means of transmission is enhanced by the small infectious inoculum of *Giardia*, the prolonged survival of cysts in cold water, and the resistance of cysts to killing by routine chlorination methods that are adequate for controlling bacteria. Viable cysts can be eradicated from water by either boiling or filtration. In the United States, *Giardia* is the agent most commonly identified in waterborne epidemics of gastroenteritis, and cross-sectional studies

in selected populations show prevalences from a few tenths of a percent to 50 percent or higher. In developing countries, *Giardia* infections can be extremely common, with cumulative rates close to 100 percent by 2 years of age and prevalences of 20 to 30 percent or higher among adults.

The importance of animal reservoirs as sources of infection for humans is unclear. *Giardia* parasites morphologically similar to those in humans are found in a large number of mammals, including beavers from reservoirs implicated in epidemics, dogs, cats, and ruminants. Although the high degree of isolate heterogeneity noted in humans is consistent with infections originating from different animal sources, animals have not been directly established as sources of human infection.

Giardiasis, like cryptosporidiosis, creates a significant economic burden because of the costs incurred in the installation of water filtration systems required to prevent waterborne epidemics, in the management of epidemics that involve large communities, and in the evaluation and treatment of endemic infections. In the United States, giardiasis results in about the same number of hospitalizations as shigellosis.

Pathophysiology The reasons why some, but not all, infected patients develop clinical manifestations and the mechanisms by which *Giardia* causes alterations in small-bowel function are largely unknown. While trophozoites adhere to the epithelium, they do not cause invasive or locally destructive alterations. The development of lactose intolerance and significant malabsorption in a minority of infected adults and children are clinical signs of the loss of brush border enzyme activities. In most infections the morphology of the bowel is unaltered, but in a few—usually in chronically infected, symptomatic patients—the histopathologic findings (including flattened villi) and the clinical manifestations resemble those of tropical sprue and gluten-sensitive enteropathy. The pathogenesis of diarrhea in giardiasis is not known.

The natural history of *Giardia* infection is not well defined and varies markedly. Infections may be aborted, transient, recurrent, or chronic. Parasite as well as host factors may be important in determining the course of infection and disease. Both cellular and humoral responses develop in human infections, but their precise roles in the control of infection and/or disease are unknown. Because patients with hypogammaglobulinemia commonly suffer from prolonged, severe infections that are poorly responsive to treatment, humoral immune responses appear to be important. The greater susceptibility of the young than of the old and of newly exposed persons than of chronically exposed populations also suggests that at least partial protective immunity may develop. Although no strains of the parasite that are clearly nonpathogenic have been identified, *Giardia* isolates vary biochemically and biologically. The marked biochemical differences among some isolates may help account for the different courses of infection noted in experimentally infected humans and animals. The surface of trophozoites is covered by a family of related cysteine-rich proteins that undergo surface antigenic variation and may contribute to prolonged and/or repeated infections.

Clinical Manifestations Disease manifestations of giardiasis range from asymptomatic carriage to fulminant diarrhea and malabsorption. Most infected persons are asymptomatic, but in epidemics the proportion of symptomatic cases may be higher. Symptoms may develop suddenly or gradually. In persons with acute giardiasis, symptoms develop after an incubation period that lasts at least 5 to 6 days and usually 1 to 3 weeks. Prominent early symptoms include diarrhea, abdominal pain, bloating, belching, flatus, nausea, and vomiting. Although diarrhea is common, upper intestinal manifestations such as nausea, vomiting, bloating, and abdominal pain may predominate. The duration of acute giardiasis is usually in excess of 1 week, although diarrhea often subsides. Individuals with chronic giardiasis may present with or without having experienced an antecedent acute symptomatic episode. Diarrhea is not necessarily prominent, but increased flatus, loose stools, sulfurous burping, and (in some instances) weight loss occur. Symptoms may be continual or episodic and can persist for years. Some persons who have relatively mild symptoms for long periods recognize the extent of their discomfort only in retrospect.

Fever, the presence of blood and/or mucus in the stools, and other signs and symptoms of colitis are uncommon and suggest a different diagnosis or a concomitant illness. Symptoms tend to be intermittent yet recurring and gradually debilitating, in contrast with the acute disabling symptoms associated with many enteric bacterial infections. Because of the less severe illness and the propensity for chronic infections, patients may seek medical advice late in the course of the illness; however, disease can be severe, resulting in malabsorption, weight loss, growth retardation, dehydration, and (in rare cases) death. A number of extraintestinal manifestations have been described, such as urticaria, anterior uveitis, and arthritis; whether these are caused by giardiasis or concomitant processes is unclear.

Giardiasis can be life-threatening in patients with hypogamma-globulinemia and is typically difficult to treat and eradicate. *Giardia* infections can complicate other preexisting intestinal diseases, such as cystic fibrosis. Although *Giardia* can cause enteric illness in patients with AIDS, neither the course of infection nor the response to treatment differs for patients with and without AIDS.

Diagnosis Giardiasis is diagnosed by the identification of cysts in the feces or of trophozoites in the feces or small intestines. Cysts are oval, measure 8 to 12 μm $\times$ 7 to 10 μm, and characteristically contain four nuclei. Trophozoites are pear-shaped, dorsally convex, flattened parasites with two nuclei and four pairs of flagella. The diagnosis is sometimes difficult to establish. Direct examination of fresh or properly preserved stools as well as concentration methods should be used. Because cyst excretion is variable and may be undetectable at times, repeated examination of stool, sampling of duodenal fluid, and biopsy of the small intestine may be required to detect the parasite. Tests for parasitic antigen in stool, now commercially available, are as sensitive and specific as good microscopic examinations and easier to perform. All of these methods occasionally yield false-negative results.

℞ TREATMENT

Cure rates with metronidazole (250 mg tid for 5 days) are usually higher than 80 percent; those with furazolidone (100 mg qid for 7 to 10 days) are somewhat lower. The latter agent is frequently used to treat children because it is available as a palatable elixir that is not bitter. Quinacrine, the first effective drug for the treatment of giardiasis, is no longer available.

Patients in whom initial treatment fails can be re-treated with a longer course. Almost all patients respond to therapy and are cured, although some with chronic giardiasis experience delayed resolution of symptoms after eradication of *Giardia*. Those who remain infected after repeated treatments should be evaluated for reinfection through family members, close personal contacts, and environmental sources as well as for hypogammaglobulinemia. In cases refractory to multiple treatment courses, prolonged therapy with metronidazole (750 mg tid for 21 days) has been successful. Tinidazole, not available in the United States, is considered more effective than metronidazole or quinacrine. When children attending day-care centers infect an entire family, treatment of all infected family members, including asymptomatic carriers, may be required to prevent reinfection. Paromomycin, an oral aminoglycoside that is not well absorbed, can be given to symptomatic pregnant women, although the experience accumulated thus far is not a sufficient basis on which to judge how often this agent either eradicates infection or ameliorates symptoms.

Prevention Although *Giardia* is extremely infectious, disease can be prevented by the exclusive consumption of noncontaminated food and water. Cooking food adequately and boiling or filtering potentially contaminated water prevent infection.

CRYPTOSPORIDIOSIS The coccidian parasite *Cryptosporidium* is now known to cause diarrheal disease in immunocompetent human hosts and to be especially common among persons with AIDS or other forms of immunodeficiency.

Life Cycle and Epidemiology Cryptosporidiosis is acquired by the consumption of oocysts, which excyst to liberate sporozoites that in turn enter and infect intestinal epithelial cells. The parasite's further development involves both asexual and sexual cycles, which produce forms capable of infecting other epithelial cells and of generating oocysts that are passed in the feces. *Cryptosporidium* spp. infect a number of animals and can spread from infected animals to humans. Since oocysts are infectious when passed in feces, person-to-person transmission takes place in day-care centers and among household contacts and medical providers. As with giardiasis, waterborne transmission accounts for infections in travelers and for common-source epidemics. Oocysts are quite hardy and resist killing by routine chlorination.

Pathophysiology Although intestinal epithelial cells harbor the parasite in an intracellular vacuole, the means by which secretory diarrhea is elicited remain uncertain. No characteristic pathologic changes are found by biopsy. The distribution of infection can be spotty within the principal site of infection, the small bowel. In some cases, cryptosporidia are found in the pharynx, stomach, and large bowel; they have been recovered from the respiratory tract, although the pathogenicity of the infection for human respiratory epithelium has not been determined. Involvement of the biliary tract can cause papillary stenosis, sclerosing cholangitis, or cholecystitis.

Clinical Manifestations Asymptomatic infections can occur in both immunocompetent and immunocompromised hosts. In immunocompetent persons, symptoms develop after an incubation period of about a week and consist principally of watery nonbloody diarrhea, at times in conjunction with abdominal pain, nausea, anorexia, fever, and/or weight loss. In these hosts, the illness usually subsides after 1 to 2 weeks, whereas in immunocompromised hosts, especially those with AIDS, diarrhea can be chronic, persistent, and remarkably profuse, causing clinically significant fluid and electrolyte depletion. Stool volumes may range from 1 to 25 L/d. Weight loss, wasting, and abdominal pain may be severe. Biliary tract involvement can manifest as midepigastric or right upper quadrant pain.

Diagnosis Evaluation usually starts with fecal examination for small oocysts, which are 4 to 5 μm in diameter and are smaller than the fecal stages of most other parasites. Detection is enhanced by evaluation of stools (obtained on multiple days) by several techniques, including modified acid-fast and direct immunofluorescent stains and enzyme immunoassays. If low numbers of oocysts are being excreted, Sheather's coverslip flotation method concentrates them for examination. Cryptosporidia also can be identified by light and electron microscopy at the apical surfaces of intestinal epithelium from biopsy specimens of the small bowel and, less frequently, the large bowel.

℞ TREATMENT

To date, no chemotherapeutic agents effective against *Cryptosporidium* have been identified, although paromomycin (500 to 750 mg qid) may be partially effective for some patients infected with human immunodeficiency virus (HIV). Treatment includes supportive care with replacement of fluids and electrolytes and administration of antidiarrheal agents. Biliary tract obstruction may require papillotomy or T-tube placement. Prevention requires minimizing exposure to infectious oocysts in human or animal feces.

ISOSPORIASIS The coccidian parasite *Isospora belli* causes human intestinal disease. Infection is acquired by the consumption of oocysts, after which the parasite invades intestinal epithelial cells and undergoes both sexual and asexual cycles of development. Oocysts excreted in stool are not immediately infectious but must undergo further maturation. Although *I. belli* infects many animals, little is known about the epidemiology or prevalence of this parasite in humans. It appears to be more common in tropical and subtropical countries. Acute infections can begin abruptly with fever, abdominal pain, and watery nonbloody diarrhea and may last for weeks or months. In patients who have AIDS or are immunocompromised for other reasons, infections often are not self-limited but rather resemble cryptosporidiosis, with chronic, profuse watery diarrhea. Eosinophilia, which is not found in other enteric protozoan infections, may be detectable. The diagnosis is usually made by detection of the large (~25-μm) oocysts in stool by modified acid-fast staining. Oocyst excretion may be low-level and intermittent; if repeated stool examinations are unrevealing, sampling of duodenal contents by aspiration or a string test (Enterotest) or small-bowel biopsy (often with electron-microscopic examination) may be necessary.

In contrast to cryptosporidiosis, isosporiasis responds to chemotherapy. Trimethoprim-sulfamethoxazole (160/800 mg qid for 10 days and then bid for 3 weeks) has been effective; for patients intolerant of sulfonamides, pyrimethamine (50 to 75 mg/day) can be used. Relapses can occur in persons with AIDS and necessitate maintenance therapy with trimethoprim-sulfamethoxazole (160/800 mg three times a week) or combined sulfadoxine (500 mg) and pyrimethamine (25 mg) once weekly.

CYCLOSPORIASIS Coccidian parasites of the genus *Cyclospora* have been identified as the causative organisms in diarrheal illness formerly ascribed to blue-green algal or *Cyanobacteria*-like forms. This parasite is globally distributed: illness due to *Cyclospora cayetanensis* has been reported in the United States, Asia, Africa, Latin America, and Europe. The epidemiology of this parasite has not yet been fully defined, but waterborne transmission has been recognized as one means of its acquisition. The incubation period may be as brief as a day or two. The full spectrum of illness attributable to *Cyclospora* has not been delineated. Some patients may harbor the infection without symptoms, but many with cyclosporiasis have diarrhea, flulike symptoms, and flatulence and burping. The illness can be self-limited, can wax and wane, or (in many cases) can involve prolonged diarrhea, anorexia, and upper gastrointestinal symptoms, with sustained fatigue and weight loss in some instances. Diarrheal illness may persist for longer than a month. *Cyclospora* can cause enteric illness in patients infected with HIV, albeit at an unknown frequency.

The parasite is detectable in epithelial cells of small-bowel biopsy samples and elicits secretory diarrhea by an unknown means. The absence of fecal blood and leukocytes indicates that disease due to *Cyclospora* is not caused by destruction of the small-bowel mucosa. The diagnosis can be made by detection of spherical 8- to 10-μm oocysts in the stool. These refractile oocysts are variably acid-fast and are fluorescent when viewed with ultraviolet light microscopy. Cyclosporiasis should be considered in the differential diagnosis of prolonged diarrhea, with or without a history of travel by the patient to other countries.

Cyclosporiasis is effectively treated with trimethoprim-sulfamethoxazole (160/800 mg bid for 7 days). Patients infected with HIV, however, may experience relapses after such treatment and thus may require longer-term suppressive maintenance therapy.

MICROSPORIDIOSIS Microsporidia are obligate intracellular spore-forming protozoa that infect many animals and recently have been recognized as causing disease in humans, especially as opportunistic pathogens in AIDS. Microsporidia are members of a distinct phylum, Microspora, which contains dozens of genera and hundreds of species. The various microsporidia are differentiated by their developmental life cycles, by ultrastructural features, and (more recently) by molecular taxonomy based on ribosomal RNA. The organisms' complex life cycles result in the production of infectious spores. Currently, six genera of microsporidia—*Encephalitozoon*, *Pleistophora*, *Nosema*, *Vittaforma*, *Septata*, and *Enterocytozoon*—are recognized as causes of human disease; a seventh genus—*Microsporidium*, which includes organisms of uncertain taxonomic status—also causes disease in humans. Though some microsporidia are probably prevalent causes of self-limited or asymptomatic infections in immunocompetent patients, little is known of how microsporidiosis is acquired.

Microsporidiosis is most common among patients with AIDS, less common among patients with other types of immunocompromise, and rare among immunocompetent hosts. In patients with AIDS, intestinal infections with *Enterocytozoon bieneusi* and *Encephalitozoon* (formerly *Septata*) *intestinalis* are increasingly recognized to contribute to chronic diarrhea and wasting; these infections are found in 10 to 40 percent of patients with chronic diarrhea. Both organisms have been found in the biliary tracts of patients with cholecystitis. *E. intestinalis* may also disseminate to cause fever, diarrhea, sinusitis, cholangitis, and bronchiolitis. In patients with AIDS, *Encephalitozoon hellem* has caused superficial keratoconjunctivitis as well as sinusitis, respiratory tract disease, and disseminated infection. Myositis due to *Pleistophora* has been documented in two patients. *Nosema*, *Vittaforma*, and *Microsporidium* have caused stromal keratitis associated with trauma in immunocompetent patients.

Microsporidia are small gram-positive organisms with mature spores measuring 0.5 to 2 μm × 1 to 4 μm. Diagnosis of microsporidial infections in tissue often requires electron microscopy, although intracellular spores can be visualized by light microscopy with hematoxylin and eosin, Giemsa, or tissue Gram's stains. For the diagnosis of intestinal microsporidiosis, chromotrope 2R-based staining and Uvitex 2B or calcofluor fluorescent staining reveal spores in smears of feces or duodenal aspirates. Definitive therapies for microsporidial infections remain to be established. For superficial keratoconjunctivitis due to *E. hellem*, topical therapy with fumagillin suspension has shown promise (see Chap. 213). For enteric infections with *E. bieneusi* and *E. intestinalis* in HIV-infected patients, therapy with albendazole may be efficacious (see Chap. 213).

OTHER INTESTINAL PROTOZOA **Balantidiasis** *Balantidium coli* is a large ciliated protozoal parasite that can produce a spectrum of large-intestinal disease analogous to amebiasis. The parasite is widely distributed in the world. Since it infects pigs, cases in humans are more common where pigs are raised; in Muslim countries, rodents may be important carriers. Infective cysts can be transmitted from person to person and through water, but many cases are due to the ingestion of cysts derived from porcine feces in association with slaughtering, with use of pig feces for fertilizer, or with contamination of water supplies by pig feces.

Ingested cysts liberate trophozoites, which reside and replicate in the large bowel. Many patients remain asymptomatic, but some have persisting intermittent diarrhea, and a few develop more fulminant dysentery. In symptomatic individuals, the pathology in the bowel—both gross and microscopic—is similar to that seen in amebiasis, with varying degrees of mucosal invasion, focal necrosis, and ulceration. Balantidiasis, unlike amebiasis, does not spread hematogenously to other organs. The diagnosis is usually made by detection of the trophozoite stage in stool or sampled colonic tissue. Tetracycline (500 mg qid for 10 days) is an effective therapeutic agent.

***Blastocystis hominis* Infection** *Blastocystis hominis,* long considered a nonpathogenic yeast, is believed by some to be a protozoan capable of causing intestinal disease, although its taxonomy and inherent pathogenicity remain uncertain. Some patients who pass *B. hominis* in their stools are asymptomatic, whereas others have diarrhea and associated intestinal symptoms. Diligent evaluation reveals other potential bacterial, viral, or protozoal causes of diarrhea in some but not all patients with symptoms. Because the pathogenicity of *B. hominis* is uncertain and because therapy for *Blastocystis* infection is neither specific nor uniformly effective, patients with prominent intestinal symptoms should be fully evaluated for other infectious causes of diarrhea. If diarrheal symptoms associated with *Blastocystis* are prominent, either metronidazole (750 mg tid for 10 days) or iodoquinol (650 mg tid for 20 days) can be used.

***Dientamoeba fragilis* Infection** *Dientamoeba fragilis* is unique among intestinal protozoa in that it has a trophozoite stage but not a cyst stage. How trophozoites survive to transmit infection is not known, but the unusually high prevalence of *D. fragilis* infection among persons with pinworm infection raises the possibility that eggs or larvae of *Enterobius* facilitate the transmission of *D. fragilis*. When symptoms develop in *D. fragilis* infection, they are generally mild and include intermittent diarrhea, abdominal pain, and anorexia. The diagnosis is made by the detection of trophozoites in stool, but the lability of these forms accounts for the greater yield when fecal samples are preserved immediately after collection. Since fecal excretion rates vary, examination of several samples obtained on alternate days increases the rate of detection. Iodoquinol (650 mg tid for 20 days), paromomycin (25 to 30 mg/kg per day in three doses for 7 days), or tetracycline (500 mg qid for 10 days) is appropriate for treatment.

Sarcosporidiosis Various *Sarcocystis* spp. of coccidian parasites are widely distributed agents of infection in numerous animals. These parasites have an obligatory cycle of development involving two hosts. Sexual reproduction occurs in the intestine, with sporocysts passed in the feces; asexual multiplication leads to the development of muscle cysts. Humans can develop intestinal infections—albeit apparently infrequently—by ingesting muscle-stage cysts in undercooked pork or beef. While the full spectrum of the intestinal disease is not defined, a diarrheal illness can ensue, and sporocysts are found in the stool. Alternatively, ingestion of fecally derived sporocysts can lead to the development of cysts in striated or cardiac muscle. Some patients experience muscle pain and swelling, but the frequency and nature of symptoms elicited by muscle involvement are not clear, and these cysts, measuring 100 to 325 μm, also have been found incidentally in muscle specimens. Muscle-stage infections are not followed by further spread in humans. No specific therapy exists for either intestinal or muscle-stage *Sarcocystis* infections in humans.

TRICHOMONIASIS

Various species of trichomonads can be found in the mouth (in association with periodontitis) and occasionally in the gastrointestinal tract. *Trichomonas vaginalis*—one of the most prevalent protozoal parasites in the United States—is a pathogen of the genitourinary tract and a major cause of symptomatic vaginitis.

Life Cycle and Epidemiology *T. vaginalis* is a pear-shaped, actively motile organism that measures about 10 by 7 μm, replicates by binary fission, and inhabits the lower genital tract of females and the urethra and prostate of males. In the United States, it accounts for about 3 million infections per year in women. While the organism can survive for a few hours in moist environments and could be acquired by direct contact, person-to-person venereal transmission accounts for virtually all cases of trichomoniasis. Its prevalence is greatest among persons with multiple sexual partners and among those with other sexually transmitted diseases.

Clinical Manifestations Most men infected with *T. vaginalis* are asymptomatic, although some develop urethritis and a few have epididymitis or prostatitis. In contrast, infection in women, which has an incubation period of 5 to 28 days, is usually symptomatic and manifests with malodorous vaginal discharge (often yellow), vulvar erythema and itching, dysuria or urinary frequency (in 30 to 50 percent of cases), and dyspareunia. These manifestations, however, do not clearly distinguish trichomoniasis from other types of infectious vaginitis.

Diagnosis Detection of motile trichomonads by microscopy of wet mounts of vaginal or prostatic secretions has been the conventional means of diagnosis. Although such microscopy provides an immediate diagnosis, its sensitivity for the detection of *T. vaginalis* is only about 50 to 60 percent in routine evaluations of vaginal secretions. Direct immunofluorescent antibody staining is more sensitive (70 to 90 percent) than wet-mount examinations. *T. vaginalis* can be recovered from the urethra of both males and females and is detectable in males after prostatic massage. Culture of the parasite is the most sensitive means of detection; however, the facilities for culture are not generally available, and detection of the organism takes 3 to 7 days.

℞ **TREATMENT**

Metronidazole is the mainstay of treatment and may be given either as a single 2-g dose or as 250 mg tid for 7 days. It is important that all sexual partners be treated concurrently to prevent reinfection,

especially from asymptomatic males. Alternatives to metronidazole for treatment during pregnancy are not readily available, although use of 100-mg clotrimazole vaginal suppositories nightly for 2 weeks may cure some infections in pregnant women. Reinfection often accounts for apparent treatment failures, but strains of *T. vaginalis* exhibiting high-level resistance to metronidazole have been encountered. Treatment of these resistant infections with higher oral doses, parenteral doses, or concurrent oral and vaginal doses of metronidazole has been successful.

BIBLIOGRAPHY

GENERAL

KAPPUS KD et al: Intestinal parasitism in the United States: Update on a continuing problem. Am J Trop Med Hyg 50:705, 1994
MANNHEIMER SB, SOAVE R: Protozoal infections in patients with AIDS. Cryptosporidiosis, isosporiasis, cyclosporiasis, and microsporidiosis. Infect Dis Clin North Am 8:483, 1994

GIARDIASIS

LENGERICH EJ et al: Severe giardiasis in the United States. Clin Infect Dis 18:760, 1994
OVERTURF GD: Endemic giardiasis in the United States—role of the daycare center. Clin Infect Dis 18:764, 1994
THOMPSON RCA et al: *Giardia: From Molecules to Disease*. Wallingford, UK, CAB International, 1994

CRYPTOSPORIDIOSIS

DUPONT HL et al: The infectivity of *Cryptosporidium parvum* in healthy volunteers. N Engl J Med 332:855, 1995
GOODGAME RW et al: Intestinal function and injury in acquired immunodeficiency syndrome–related cryptosporidiosis. Gastroenterology 108:1075, 1995
WHITE AC JR et al: Paromomycin for cryptosporidiosis in AIDS: A prospective, double-blind trial. J Infect Dis 170:419, 1994

CYCLOSPORIASIS

CENTERS FOR DISEASE CONTROL AND PREVENTION: Outbreaks of *Cyclospora cayetanensis*—United States, 1996. Morb Mort Week Rep 45:549, 1996
HOGE CW et al: Placebo-controlled trial of co-trimoxazole for cyclospora infections among travellers and foreign residents in Nepal. Lancet 345:691, 1995
HUANG P et al: The first reported outbreak of diarrheal illness associated with *Cyclospora* in the United States. Ann Intern Med 123:409, 1995
PAPE JW et al: *Cyclospora* infection in adults infected with HIV. Clinical manifestations, treatment, and prophylaxis. Ann Intern Med 121:654, 1994

MICROSPORIDIOSIS

MOLINA JM et al: Disseminated microsporidiosis due to *Septata intestinalis* in patients with AIDS: Clinical features and response to albendazole therapy. J Infect Dis 171:245, 1995
WEBER R, BRYAN RT: Microsporidial infections in immunodeficient and immunocompetent patients. Clin Infect Dis 19:517, 1994
——— et al: Human microsporidial infections. Clin Microbiol Rev 7:426, 1994
WEISS LM: . . . And now microsporidiosis. Ann Intern Med 123:954, 1995

OTHER INTESTINAL PROTOZOA

PREISS U et al: On the clinical importance of *Dientamoeba fragilis* infections in childhood. J Hyg Epidemiol Microbiol Immunol 35:27, 1991

TRICHOMONIASIS

HEINE P, MCGREGOR JA: *Trichomonas vaginalis:* A reemerging pathogen. Clin Obstet Gynecol 36:137, 1993
KRIEGER JN: Trichomoniasis in men: Old issues and new data. Sex Transm Dis 22:83, 1995

221   *Leo X. Liu, Peter F. Weller*

TRICHINOSIS AND INFECTIONS WITH OTHER TISSUE NEMATODES

Nematodes are elongated, symmetric roundworms and constitute one of the largest phyla in the animal kingdom. Most nematode species are free-living, but some have evolved into parasites of plants and animals, including humans. Parasitic nematodes of medical significance may be broadly classified as intestinal or tissue nematodes, but such a classification system is imprecise. This chapter covers trichinosis, visceral and ocular larva migrans, cutaneous larva migrans, cerebral angiostrongyliasis, and gnathostomiasis. All are zoonotic infections caused by incidental exposure to infectious nematodes. The clinical symptoms of these infections are due largely to invasive larval stages that (except in the case of *Trichinella*) do not reach maturity in humans.

TRICHINOSIS   Trichinosis develops after the ingestion of meat containing cysts of *Trichinella*—for example, pork or meat from a carnivore. While most infections are mild and asymptomatic, heavy infections can cause severe enteritis, periorbital edema, myositis, and (infrequently) death.

Life Cycle and Epidemiology   Five species of *Trichinella* are now recognized as causes of infection in humans. Two species are distributed worldwide: *Trichinella spiralis*, which is found in a great variety of carnivorous and omnivorous animals, and *Trichinella pseudospiralis*, which is found in mammals and birds. *Trichinella nativa* is present in Arctic regions and infects bears; *Trichinella nelsoni* is found in equatorial Africa, where it is common among felid predators and scavengers such as hyenas and bush pigs; and *Trichinella bitovi* is found in temperate areas of Europe and western Asia among carnivores but not among domestic swine.

After the consumption of trichinous meat by the host, encysted larvae are liberated by digestive acid and pepsin. The larvae invade the small-bowel mucosa and mature rapidly into adult worms. After about 1 week, female worms release newborn larvae that migrate via the circulation to striated muscle. The larvae of all species except *T. pseudospiralis* then encyst by inducing a radical transformation in the muscle cell architecture. Although host immune responses may help to expel the adult worms, they have little effect on the muscle-dwelling larvae.

Human trichinosis is most often caused by the ingestion of infected pork products and thus can occur in almost any location where the meat of domestic or wild swine is eaten. Human trichinosis also may be acquired from the meat of other animals, including dogs (in parts of Asia and Africa), horses (in Italy and France), and bears and walruses (in northern regions). Although cattle (being herbivores) are not natural hosts of *Trichinella*, beef has been implicated in outbreaks when contaminated or adulterated with trichinous pork. Laws that prohibit the feeding of uncooked garbage to pigs have greatly reduced the transmission of trichinosis in the United States. About 50 to 100 cases of trichinosis are reported annually in this country, but most mild cases probably remain undiagnosed. Recent U.S. outbreaks have been attributable to undercooked ethnic pork dishes, homemade and commercial sausage, wild boar meat, and walrus meat.

Pathogenesis and Clinical Features   Clinical symptoms of trichinosis arise from the successive phases of parasite enteric invasion, larval migration, and muscle encystment. Most light infections (those with fewer than 10 larvae per gram of muscle) are asymptomatic, whereas heavy infections (which can involve more than 50 larvae per gram of muscle) can be life-threatening. Invasion of the gut by large numbers of parasites occasionally provokes diarrhea during the first week after infection. Abdominal pain, constipation, nausea, or vomiting also may be prominent. The prolonged and fulminant diarrhea noted with Arctic trichinosis probably reflects a response to repeated infection.

Symptoms due to larval migration and muscle invasion begin to appear in the second week after infection. The migrating *Trichinella* larvae provoke a marked local and systemic hypersensitivity reaction, with fever and hypereosinophilia. Periorbital and facial edema is common, as are hemorrhages in the subconjunctivae, retina, and nail beds ("splinter" hemorrhages). A maculopapular rash, headache, cough, dyspnea, or dysphagia sometimes develops. Myocarditis with tachyarrhythmias or heart failure—and, less commonly, encephalitis or pneumonitis—may develop and accounts for most deaths of patients with trichinosis.

Upon onset of larval encystment in muscle 2 to 3 weeks after infection, symptoms of myositis with myalgias, muscle edema, and weakness develop, usually overlapping with the inflammatory reactions to migrating larvae. The most commonly involved muscle groups include the extraocular muscles; the biceps; and the muscles of the jaw, neck, lower back, and diaphragm. Peaking about 3 weeks after infection, symptoms subside only gradually during a prolonged convalescence.

Laboratory Findings and Diagnosis   Blood eosinophilia develops in more than 90 percent of patients with symptomatic trichinosis and may peak at a level of greater than 50 percent between 2 and 4 weeks after infection. Serum levels of IgE and muscle enzymes, including creatine phosphokinase, lactate dehydrogenase, and aspartate aminotransferase, are elevated in most symptomatic patients. Patients should be questioned thoroughly about their consumption of pork or wild-animal meat and about illness in other individuals who ate the same meat. A presumptive clinical diagnosis can be based on fevers, eosinophilia, periorbital edema, and myalgias after a suspect meal. A rise in the titer of parasite-specific antibody (assayed by the bentonite flocculation test), which usually does not occur until after the third week of infection, confirms the diagnosis. Alternatively, a definitive diagnosis requires surgical biopsy of at least 1 g of involved muscle; the yields are highest near tendon insertions. The fresh muscle tissue should be compressed between glass slides and examined microscopically, because larvae may be overlooked by examination of routine histopathologic sections alone.

℞ TREATMENT

Current anthelmintic drugs are ineffective against *Trichinella* larvae in muscle. Fortunately, most lightly infected patients recover uneventfully with bed rest, antipyretics, and analgesics. Glucocorticoids like prednisone (1 mg/kg daily for 5 days) are beneficial for severe myositis and myocarditis. Mebendazole, like thiabendazole, appears to be active against enteric stages of the parasite, but its efficacy against encysted larvae has not been conclusively demonstrated.

Prevention   Larvae may be killed by cooking pork until it is no longer pink or by freezing it at $-15°C$ for 3 weeks. However, Arctic *T. nativa* larvae in walrus or bear meat are relatively resistant and may remain viable despite freezing.

VISCERAL AND OCULAR LARVA MIGRANS   Visceral larva migrans is a syndrome caused by nematodes that are normally parasitic for nonhuman host species. In humans, the nematode larvae do not typically develop into adult worms but instead migrate through host tissues and elicit eosinophilic inflammation. The most common form of visceral larva migrans is toxocariasis due to larvae of the canine ascarid *Toxocara canis* or, less commonly, the feline ascarid *Toxocara cati*. Rare cases with eosinophilic meningoencephalitis have been caused by the raccoon ascarid *Baylisascaris procyonis*.

Life Cycle and Epidemiology   The canine roundworm *T. canis* is distributed among dogs worldwide. Ingestion of infective eggs by dogs is followed by liberation of *Toxocara* larvae, which penetrate the gut wall and migrate intravascularly into the canine liver, muscle, and other tissues, where most remain in a developmentally arrested state. During pregnancy, some larvae resume migration in bitches and infect puppies prenatally (via transplacental transmission) or after birth (via suckling). Thus, in lactating bitches and puppies, larvae return to the intestinal tract and develop into adult worms, which produce eggs that are released in the feces. Humans acquire toxocariasis mainly by eating soil contaminated by puppy feces containing infective *T. canis* eggs. Visceral larva migrans is most common among children who habitually eat dirt, but most toxocaral infections are subclinical. Reported rates of *Toxocara* seropositivity range from 2 percent in an unselected American population to greater than 20 percent among kindergarten children in the United States and England.

Pathogenesis and Clinical Features Clinical disease most commonly afflicts preschool children. After humans ingest *Toxocara* eggs, the larvae hatch and penetrate the intestinal mucosa, from which they are carried by the circulation to a wide variety of organs and tissues. The larvae invade the liver, lungs, central nervous system, and other sites, releasing toxic products and provoking intense local eosinophilic granulomatous responses. The degree of clinical illness depends on larval number and tissue distribution, reinfection, and host immune responses. Most light infections are asymptomatic and may be manifest only by blood eosinophilia. Characteristic symptoms of visceral larva migrans include fever, malaise, anorexia and weight loss, cough, wheezing, and rashes. Hepatosplenomegaly is common. These features are often accompanied by extraordinary peripheral eosinophilia, which may approach 90 percent. Uncommonly, seizures or behavioral disorders develop. The rare deaths in this disease are due to severe neurologic, pneumonic, or myocardial involvement.

Diagnosis In addition to prominent eosinophilia, leukocytosis and hypergammaglobulinemia are usually evident. Transient pulmonary infiltrates are apparent on chest x-rays of about half of patients with symptoms of pneumonitis. The clinical diagnosis can be confirmed by an enzyme-linked immunosorbent assay for toxocaral antibodies. Stool examination, while important in the evaluation of unexplained eosinophilia, is worthless for toxocariasis, since the larvae do not develop into egg-producing adults in humans.

The ocular form of the larva migrans syndrome occurs when *Toxocara* larvae invade the eye. An eosinophilic granulomatous mass, most commonly in the posterior pole of the retina, develops around the entrapped larva. The retinal lesion can mimic retinoblastoma in appearance, and mistaken diagnosis of the latter condition can lead to unnecessary enucleation. The spectrum of eye involvement also includes endophthalmitis, uveitis, and chorioretinitis. Unilateral visual disturbances, strabismus, and eye pain are the most common presenting symptoms. In contrast to visceral larva migrans, ocular toxocariasis usually develops in older children or young adults with no history of pica; these patients seldom have eosinophilia or visceral manifestations.

℞ TREATMENT

The vast majority of *Toxocara* infections are self-limited and resolve without specific therapy. In patients with severe myocardial, central nervous system, or pulmonary involvement, glucocorticoids may be employed to reduce inflammatory complications. Available anthelmintic drugs, including diethylcarbamazine, mebendazole, and albendazole, have not been shown conclusively to alter the course of larva migrans. Control measures include prohibiting dog excreta in public parks and playgrounds, deworming dogs, and preventing pica in children. Treatment of ocular disease is unsatisfactory, and the role of glucocorticoids or anthelmintic drugs in management is controversial.

CUTANEOUS LARVA MIGRANS Cutaneous larva migrans ("creeping eruption") is a serpiginous skin eruption caused by burrowing larvae of animal hookworms, usually the dog and cat hookworm *Ancylostoma braziliense*. The larvae hatch from eggs passed in dog and cat feces and mature in the soil. Humans become infected after skin contact with soil in areas frequented by dogs and cats, such as areas underneath house porches or scrub vegetation. Cutaneous larva migrans is especially prevalent among children and in regions with warm humid climates, including the southeastern United States.

After larvae penetrate the skin, erythematous lesions form along the tortuous tracts of their migration through the dermal-epidermal junction; the larvae advance several centimeters in a day. The intensely pruritic lesions may occur anywhere on the body and can be numerous if the patient has lain on the ground. Vesicles and bullae may form later. The animal hookworm larvae do not mature in humans and, without treatment, will die out after several weeks, with resolution of skin lesions. The diagnosis is made readily on clinical grounds, and a skin biopsy only rarely yields diagnostic parasite material. Symptoms can be alleviated by thiabendazole administered orally (25 mg/kg bid) or topically (10% aqueous or petroleum jelly suspension) for 2 to 5 days, by ivermectin (150 to 200 μg/kg one time), or by albendazole (200 mg bid for 2 days).

***ANGIOSTRONGYLUS CANTONENSIS* INFECTION** *Angiostrongylus cantonensis*, the rat lungworm, is the most common cause of human eosinophilic meningitis.

Life Cycle and Epidemiology This infection occurs principally in Southeast Asia and the Pacific Basin. *A. cantonensis* larvae produced by adult worms in the rat lung migrate to the gastrointestinal tract and are expelled with the feces. They develop into infective larvae within land snails and slugs. Humans acquire the infection by ingesting raw infected mollusks; vegetables contaminated by mollusk slime; or crabs, freshwater shrimp, and certain marine fish that have themselves eaten infected mollusks. The larvae then migrate to the brain.

Pathogenesis and Clinical Features The parasites eventually die in the central nervous system, but not before initiating pathologic consequences that, in heavy infections, can result in permanent neurologic sequelae or death. Migrating larvae cause proteolytic damage and marked local eosinophilic inflammation and hemorrhage, with subsequent necrosis and granuloma formation around dying worms. Clinical symptoms develop between 2 and 35 days after the ingestion of larvae. Patients usually present with an insidious or abrupt excruciating frontal, occipital, or bitemporal headache. Neck stiffness, nausea and vomiting, and paresthesias are also common. Fever, cranial and extraocular nerve palsies, seizures, paralysis, and lethargy are uncommon.

Laboratory Findings Examination of the cerebrospinal fluid is mandatory in suspected cases and usually reveals an elevated opening pressure, a white blood cell count of 150 to 2000/μL, and an eosinophilic pleocytosis of >20 percent. The protein concentration is usually elevated and the glucose level normal. The motile larvae of *A. cantonensis* are only rarely seen in the cerebrospinal fluid. Peripheral-blood eosinophilia may be mild. The diagnosis is generally based on the clinical presentation of eosinophilic meningitis together with a compatible epidemiologic history.

℞ TREATMENT

Specific chemotherapy has not been shown to be of benefit in angiostrongyliasis; larvicidal agents may actually exacerbate inflammatory brain lesions. Management consists of supportive measures, including the administration of analgesics, sedatives, and—in severe cases—glucocorticoids. In most patients, cerebral angiostrongyliasis has a self-limited course, and recovery is complete. The infection may be prevented by adequately cooking snails, crabs, and prawns and inspecting vegetables for mollusk infestation. Other parasitic causes of eosinophilic meningitis in endemic areas may include gnathostomiasis, paragonimiasis, schistosomiasis, and neurocysticercosis.

GNATHOSTOMIASIS Infection of human tissues with larvae of *Gnathostoma spinigerum* can cause eosinophilic meningoencephalitis, migratory cutaneous swellings, or invasive masses of the eye and visceral organs.

Life Cycle and Epidemiology Human gnathostomiasis is endemic in Southeast Asia and parts of China and Japan. In nature, the mature adult worms parasitize the gastrointestinal tract of dogs and cats. First-stage larvae hatch from eggs passed into water and are ingested by *Cyclops* species (water fleas). Infective third-stage larvae develop in the flesh of many animal species (including fish, frogs, eels, snakes, chickens, and ducks) that have eaten either infected *Cyclops* or another infected second intermediate host. Humans typically acquire the infection by eating raw or undercooked fish or poultry. The raw fish dishes of *somfak* in Thailand and *sashimi* in Japan account for most cases of human gnathostomiasis. Some cases in Thailand result from the local practice of applying frog or snake flesh as a poultice.

Pathogenesis and Clinical Features Clinical symptoms are due to the aberrant migration of a single larva into cutaneous, visceral, neural, or ocular tissues. After invasion, larval migration may cause local inflammation, with pain, cough, or hematuria accompanied by fever and eosinophilia. Painful, itchy, migratory swellings may develop in the skin, particularly in the distal extremities or periorbital area. Cutaneous swellings usually last about a week but often recur intermittently over many years. Larval invasion of the eye can provoke a sight-threatening inflammatory response. Finally, invasion of the central nervous system results in eosinophilic meningitis with myeloencephalitis, a serious complication due to ascending larval migration along a large nerve track. Patients characteristically present with agonizing radicular pain and paresthesias in the trunk or a limb, which are followed shortly by paraplegia. Cerebral involvement, with focal hemorrhages and tissue destruction, is often fatal.

Diagnosis and Treatment Cutaneous migratory swellings with marked peripheral eosinophilia, supported by an appropriate geographic and dietary history, generally constitute an adequate basis for a clinical diagnosis of gnathostomiasis. However, patients may present with ocular or cerebrospinal involvement without antecedent cutaneous swellings. In the latter case, eosinophilic pleocytosis will be demonstrable (usually along with hemorrhagic or xanthochromic cerebrospinal fluid), but worms will almost never be recovered from the cerebrospinal fluid. Surgical removal of the parasite from subcutaneous or ocular tissue, though rarely feasible, is both diagnostic and therapeutic. Albendazole (400 to 800 mg daily for 21 days) may be helpful. At present, cerebrospinal involvement is managed with supportive measures and generally with a course of glucocorticoids. Gnathostomiasis can be prevented by adequate cooking of fish and poultry in endemic areas.

BIBLIOGRAPHY

ANDREWS JR et al: *Trichinella pseudospiralis* in humans: Description of a case and its treatment. Trans R Soc Trop Med Hyg 88:200, 1994

DAVIES HD et al: Creeping eruption. A review of clinical presentation and management of 60 cases presenting to a tropical disease unit. Arch Dermatol 129:588, 1993

GILLESPIE SH et al: The spectrum of ocular toxocariasis. Eye 7:415, 1993

GLICKMAN LT, MAGNAVAL JF: Zoonotic roundworm infections. Infect Dis Clin North Am 7:717, 1993

HOTEZ PJ: Visceral and ocular larva migrans. Semin Neurol 13:175, 1993

JELINEK T et al: Cutaneous larva migrans in travelers: Synopsis of histories, symptoms, and treatment of 98 patients. Clin Infect Dis 19:1062, 1994

LANDRY SM et al: Trichinosis: Common source outbreak related to commercial pork. South Med J 85:428, 1992

LEWIS JM, MAIZELS RM (eds): *Toxocara and Toxocariasis: Clinical, Epidemiological, and Molecular Perspectives.* London, Institute of Biology, 1993

LIU LX, WELLER PF: Antiparasitic drugs. N Engl J Med 334:1178, 1996

MACLEAN JD et al: Epidemiologic and serologic definition of primary and secondary trichinosis in the Arctic. J Infect Dis 165:908, 1992

MAGNAVAL JF: Comparative efficacy of diethylcarbamazine and mebendazole for the treatment of human toxocariasis. Parasitology 110:529, 1995

MURRELL KD, BRUSCHI F: Clinical trichinellosis. Prog Clin Parasitol 4:117, 1994

WELLER PF, LIU LX: Eosinophilic meningitis. Semin Neurol 13:161, 1993

222 *Leo X. Liu, Peter F. Weller*

INTESTINAL NEMATODES

More than a billion people worldwide are infected with one or more species of intestinal nematodes. Table 222-1 summarizes biologic and clinical features of infections due to the major intestinal parasitic nematodes. These parasites are most common in regions with poor fecal sanitation, particularly in developing countries in the tropics and subtropics but also in the United States. Although nematode infections are not usually fatal, they contribute to malnutrition and diminished work capacity. Humans may on occasion be infected with nematode parasites that ordinarily infect animals; these zoonotic infections include trichostrongyliasis, anisakiasis, capillariasis, and abdominal angiostrongyliasis.

Intestinal nematodes are roundworms; they range in length from 1 mm to many centimeters when mature (see Table 222-1). Their life cycles are complex and highly varied; some species, including *Strongyloides stercoralis* and *Enterobius vermicularis*, can be transmitted directly from person to person, while others, such as *Ascaris lumbricoides*, *Necator americanus*, and *Ancylostoma duodenale*, require a soil phase for development. Because most helminthic parasites do not self-replicate, the acquisition of a heavy burden of adult worms requires repeated exposure to the parasite in its infectious stage, whether larva or egg. Hence, clinical disease, as opposed to asymptomatic infection, generally develops only with prolonged residence in an endemic area. Eosinophilia and elevated serum IgE levels are features of many helminthic infections and, when unexplained, should always prompt a search for occult helminthiasis. Significant protective immunity to intestinal nematodes appears not to develop in humans, although mechanisms of parasite immune evasion and host immune responses to these infections have not been elucidated in detail.

ASCARIASIS *A. lumbricoides* is the largest intestinal nematode parasite of humans, reaching up to 40 cm in length. An estimated 1 billion people are infected worldwide. Most infected individuals have low worm burdens and are asymptomatic. Clinical disease arises from pulmonary hypersensitivity and intestinal complications.

Life Cycle Adult worms live in the lumen of the small intestine. Mature female *Ascaris* worms are extraordinarily fecund, each producing up to 240,000 eggs a day, which pass with the feces. Ascarid eggs, which are remarkably resistant to environmental stresses, become infective after several weeks of maturation in the soil and can remain infective for years. After infective eggs are swallowed, larvae hatched in the intestine invade the mucosa, migrate via the circulation to the lungs, break into the alveoli, ascend the bronchial tree, and return via swallowing to the small intestine, where they develop into adult worms. Between 2 and 3 months elapse between initial infection and egg production. The adult worms live for approximately 1 to 2 years.

Epidemiology *Ascaris* is widely distributed in tropical and subtropical regions as well as in other humid areas, including the rural southeastern United States. Transmission typically occurs via fecally contaminated soil and is due either to a lack of sanitary facilities or to the use of human manure ("night soil") as fertilizer. With their propensity for hand-to-mouth fecal carriage, younger children in impoverished rural areas are most affected. Infection outside endemic areas, though uncommon, can occur via eggs borne on transported vegetables.

Clinical Features During the lung phase of larval migration, about 9 to 12 days after egg ingestion, patients may develop an irritating nonproductive cough and burning substernal discomfort that is aggravated by coughing or deep inspiration. Dyspnea and blood-tinged sputum are less common. Fever is usually reported, with temperatures sometimes exceeding 38.5°C. Eosinophilia develops during this symptomatic phase and subsides slowly over weeks. Chest x-rays may reveal evidence of eosinophilic pneumonitis (Loeffler's syndrome), with round or oval infiltrates a few millimeters to several centimeters in size. These infiltrates may be transient and intermittent, clearing after several weeks. Where there is seasonal transmission of the parasite, seasonal pneumonitis with eosinophilia may develop in previously infected and sensitized hosts.

In established infections, adult worms in the small intestine usually cause no symptoms. In heavy infections, particularly in children, a large bolus of entangled worms can cause pain and small-bowel obstruction, sometimes complicated by perforation, intussusception, or volvulus. Single worms may cause disease when they migrate into aberrant sites. A large worm can enter and occlude the biliary tree, causing biliary colic, cholecystitis, cholangitis, pancreatitis, and (rarely) intrahepatic abscesses. Migration of an adult worm up the esophagus can provoke coughing and oral expulsion of the worm. In highly endemic areas, intestinal and biliary ascariasis can rival acute appendicitis and gallstones as causes of surgical acute abdomen.

Laboratory Findings Most cases of ascariasis can be diagnosed by the microscopic detection of characteristic mamillated *Ascaris* eggs (65 by 45 μm) in fecal samples. Occasionally, patients present after passing an adult worm—identifiable by its large size and smooth cream-colored surface—in the stool or through the mouth or nose. During the early transpulmonary migratory phase, when eosinophilic pneumonitis occurs, larvae can be found in sputum or gastric aspirates before diagnostic eggs appear in the stool. The eosinophilia that is prominent during this early stage usually decreases to minimal levels in established infection. The large adult worms may be visualized, occasionally serendipitously, on contrast studies of the gastrointestinal tract. A plain abdominal film may reveal masses of worms in gas-filled loops of bowel in patients with intestinal obstruction. Pancreaticobiliary worms can be detected by ultrasound and endoscopic retrograde cholangiopancreatography; the latter method also has been used to extract biliary *Ascaris* worms.

℞ TREATMENT

Ascariasis should always be treated to prevent potentially serious complications. Mebendazole or albendazole (which is not yet approved by the Food and Drug Administration) is effective. These benzimidazoles are contraindicated in pregnancy and in heavy infections, in which they may provoke ectopic migration. Pyrantel pamoate and piperazine citrate are safe in pregnancy. Mild diarrhea and abdominal pain are uncommon side effects of these agents. Partial intestinal obstruction should be managed with nasogastric suction, intravenous fluid administration, and instillation of piperazine through the nasogastric tube, but complete obstruction and its severe complications require immediate surgical intervention.

HOOKWORM One-fourth of the world's population is infected with one of the two hookworm species (*A. duodenale* and *N. americanus*). Most infected individuals are asymptomatic. Hookworm disease develops from a combination of factors—a heavy worm burden, a prolonged duration of infection, and an inadequate iron intake—and results in iron-deficiency anemia and, on occasion, hypoproteinemia.

Life Cycle Adult hookworms, which are about 1 cm long, use buccal teeth (*Ancylostoma*) or cutting plates (*Necator*) to attach to the small-bowel mucosa and suck blood (0.2 mL/day per *Ancylostoma* adult) and interstitial fluid. The adult hookworms produce thousands of eggs daily. The eggs are deposited with feces in soil, where rhabditiform larvae hatch and develop over a 1-week period into infectious filariform larvae. Infective larvae penetrate the skin and reach the

---

Table 222-1

Major Human Intestinal Parasitic Nematodes

Feature	Parasitic Nematode				
	Ascaris lumbricoides (Roundworm)	*Necator americanus, Ancylostoma duodenale* (Hookworm)	*Strongyloides stercoralis*	*Trichuris trichiura* (Whipworm)	*Enterobius vermicularis* (Pinworm)
Global prevalence in humans (millions)	1000	900	50	500	300
Endemic areas	Worldwide	Hot, humid regions	Hot, humid regions	Worldwide	Worldwide
Infective stage	Egg	Filariform larva	Filariform larva	Egg	Egg
Route of infection	Oral	Percutaneous	Percutaneous or autoinfection	Oral	Oral
Gastrointestinal location of worms	Jejunal lumen	Jejunal mucosa	Small-bowel mucosa	Cecum, colonic mucosa	Cecum, appendix
Adult worm size	15–40 cm	7–12 mm	2 mm	30–50 mm	8–13 mm (female)
Pulmonary passage of larvae	Yes	Yes	Yes	No	No
Incubation period* (days)	60–75	40–100	17–28	70–90	35–45
Longevity	1 y	*N. americanus*: 2–5 y *A. duodenale*: 6–8 y	Decades (owing to autoinfection)	5 y	2 months
Fecundity (eggs/day/ worm)	240,000	*N. americanus*: 4000–10,000 *A. duodenale*: 10,000–25,000	5000–10,000	3000–7000	2000
Principal symptoms	Rarely gastrointestinal or biliary obstruction	Iron-deficiency anemia in heavy infection	Gastrointestinal symptoms; malabsorption or sepsis in hyperinfection	Gastrointestinal symptoms, anemia	Perianal pruritus
Diagnostic stage	Eggs in stool	Eggs in fresh stool, larvae in old stool	Larvae in stool or duodenal aspirate; sputum in hyperinfection	Eggs in stool	Eggs from perianal skin on cellulose acetate tape
Treatment	Mebendazole Albendazole† Pyrantel pamoate Piperazine citrate	Mebendazole Pyrantel pamoate Albendazole†	Thiabendazole Albendazole† Ivermectin†	Mebendazole Albendazole†	Mebendazole Pyrantel pamoate Albendazole†

* Time from infection to egg production by mature female worm.
† Not approved by the Food and Drug Administration.

lungs by way of the bloodstream. There they invade alveoli and ascend the airways before being swallowed and reaching the small intestine. The prepatent period from skin invasion to appearance of eggs in the feces is about 6 to 8 weeks, but it may be longer with *A. duodenale*. Larvae of *A. duodenale*, if swallowed, can survive and develop directly in the intestinal mucosa. Adult hookworms may survive over a decade but usually live about 6 to 8 years for *A. duodenale* and 2 to 5 years for *N. americanus*.

Epidemiology *A. duodenale* is prevalent in southern Europe, North Africa, and northern Asia, and *N. americanus* is the predominant species in the western hemisphere and equatorial Africa. The two species overlap in many tropical regions, particularly Southeast Asia. In most areas, older children have the greatest incidence and intensity of hookworm infection. In rural areas where fields are fertilized with night soil, older working adults also may be heavily affected.

Clinical Features Most hookworm infections are asymptomatic. Infective larvae may provoke pruritic maculopapular dermatitis ("ground itch") at the site of skin penetration as well as serpiginous tracts of subcutaneous migration (similar to cutaneous larva migrans) in previously sensitized hosts. Larvae migrating through the lungs occasionally cause mild transient pneumonitis, but this condition develops less frequently in hookworm infection than in ascariasis. In the early intestinal phase, infected persons may develop epigastric pain (often with postprandial accentuation), inflammatory diarrhea, or other abdominal symptoms accompanied by eosinophilia. The major consequence of chronic hookworm infection is iron deficiency. Symptoms are minimal if iron intake is adequate, but marginally nourished individuals develop symptoms of progressive iron-deficiency anemia and hypoproteinemia, including weakness, shortness of breath, and skin depigmentation. Intercurrent infections may precipitate frank cardiac failure. Changes in the intestinal mucosa are minimal, and malabsorption is uncommon.

Laboratory Findings The diagnosis is established by the finding of characteristic 40- by 60-μm oval hookworm eggs in the feces. Stool-concentration procedures may be required to detect light infections. Eggs of the two species are indistinguishable. In a stool sample that is not fresh, the eggs may have hatched to release rhabditiform larvae, which need to be differentiated from those of *S. stercoralis*. Hypochromic microcytic anemia, occasionally with eosinophilia or hypoalbuminemia, is characteristic of hookworm disease.

℞ TREATMENT

Hookworms can be eradicated with several safe and highly effective anthelmintic drugs, including mebendazole and pyrantel pamoate (see Chap. 214). Mild iron-deficiency anemia often can be treated with oral iron alone. Severe hookworm disease with protein loss and malabsorption necessitates nutritional support and oral iron replacement along with deworming.

Ancylostoma caninum This parasite, the canine hookworm, has been identified as a cause of human eosinophilic enteritis, especially in northeastern Australia. In this zoonotic infection, adult hookworms attach to the small intestine (where they may be visualized by endoscopy) and elicit abdominal pain and intense local eosinophilia. Treatment with mebendazole (100 mg twice daily for 3 days) is effective.

STRONGYLOIDIASIS *S. stercoralis* is distinguished by a capacity, unusual among helminths, to replicate in the human host. This capacity permits ongoing cycles of autoinfection due to internal production of infective larvae. Strongyloidiasis can thus persist for decades without further exposure of the host to exogenous infective larvae. In immunocompromised hosts, large numbers of invasive *Strongyloides* larvae can disseminate widely and can be fatal.

Life Cycle In addition to a parasitic cycle of development, *Strongyloides* can undergo a free-living cycle of development in the soil. This adaptability facilitates the parasite's survival in the absence of mammalian hosts. Rhabditiform larvae passed in feces can transform into infectious filariform larvae either directly or after a free-living phase of development. Humans acquire strongyloidiasis when filariform larvae in fecally contaminated soil penetrate the skin or mucous membranes. The larvae then travel through the bloodstream to the lungs, where they break into the alveolar spaces, ascend the bronchial tree, are swallowed, and thereby reach the small intestine. There the larvae mature into adult worms that penetrate the mucosa of the proximal small bowel. The minute (2-mm-long) parasitic adult female worms reproduce by parthenogenesis; parasitic adult males do not exist. Eggs hatch locally in the intestinal mucosa, releasing rhabditiform larvae that migrate to the lumen and pass with the feces into soil. Alternatively, rhabditiform larvae in the bowel can develop directly into filariform larvae that penetrate the colonic wall or perianal skin and enter the circulation to repeat the migration that establishes ongoing internal reinfection. This autoinfection cycle allows strongyloidiasis to persist for decades after the host has left an endemic area.

Epidemiology *S. stercoralis* is spottily distributed in tropical areas and other hot, humid regions and is particularly common in Southeast Asia, sub-Saharan Africa, and Brazil. In the United States, the parasite is endemic in parts of the South and is found in residents of mental institutions who practice poor hygiene and in immigrants and military veterans who have lived in endemic areas abroad.

Clinical Features In uncomplicated strongyloidiasis, many patients are asymptomatic or have mild cutaneous and/or abdominal symptoms. Recurrent urticaria, often involving the buttocks and wrists, is the most common cutaneous manifestation. Migrating larvae can elicit a pathognomonic serpiginous eruption, *larva currens* ("running larva")—a pruritic, raised, erythematous lesion that advances as rapidly as 10 cm/h along the course of larval migration. Adult parasites burrow into the duodenojejunal mucosa and can cause abdominal (usually midepigastric) pain, which resembles peptic ulcer pain except that it is aggravated by food ingestion. Nausea, diarrhea, gastrointestinal bleeding, mild chronic colitis, and weight loss can occur. Pulmonary symptoms are rare in uncomplicated strongyloidiasis. Eosinophilia is common, with levels fluctuating over time.

The ongoing autoinfection cycle of strongyloidiasis is normally contained by unknown factors of the host's immune system. Abrogation of host immunity after immunosuppressive therapy or with concomitant malignancy or malnutrition leads to hyperinfection, with the generation of large numbers of filariform larvae. Colitis, enteritis, or malabsorption may develop. In disseminated strongyloidiasis, larvae may invade not only gastrointestinal tissues and the lungs but also the central nervous system, peritoneum, liver, and kidney. Moreover, bacteremia may develop due to the entry of enteric flora through disrupted mucosal barriers. Gram-negative sepsis, pneumonia, or meningitis may complicate or dominate the clinical course. Eosinophilia is often absent in severely infected patients. Disseminated strongyloidiasis, particularly in patients with unsuspected infection who are given immunosuppressive drugs, can be fatal. Strongyloidiasis is a frequent complication of infection with human T cell lymphotropic virus type I, but disseminated strongyloidiasis is not common among patients infected with human immunodeficiency virus.

Diagnosis In uncomplicated strongyloidiasis, the finding of rhabditiform larvae in feces is diagnostic. The eggs are almost never detectable because they hatch in the intestine. Rhabditiform larvae are 200 to 250 μm long, with a short buccal cavity that distinguishes them from hookworm rhabditiform larvae. Single stool examinations will detect only about one-third of uncomplicated infections, in which few larvae are passed. Serial examinations or use of the Baermann concentration method improves the sensitivity of stool diagnosis. If the result of stool examination is negative, *Strongyloides* can be assayed by sampling of the duodenojejunal contents by aspiration, biopsy, or the Enterotest string method. An enzyme-linked immunosorbent assay for antibodies to excretory-secretory antigens of *Strongyloides* is a sensitive method of diagnosing uncomplicated infections. In disseminated strongyloidiasis, filariform larvae (550 μm long) should be sought in stool as well as in samples obtained from sites of potential larval migration, including sputum, bronchoalveolar lavage fluid, or surgical drainage fluid.

℞ TREATMENT

Even in the asymptomatic state, strongyloidiasis must be treated because of the potential for fatal hyperinfection. Thiabendazole (25 mg/kg bid) is generally administered for 2 days, but in disseminated strongyloidiasis, treatment should be extended for at least 5 to 7 days or until the parasites are eradicated. Common adverse effects of thiabendazole include nausea, vomiting, diarrhea, dizziness, and neuropsychiatric disturbances. Because thiabendazole is not uniformly effective, stool examinations, eosinophil counts, and monitoring of clinical symptoms should be continued after treatment. Albendazole and ivermectin are newer drugs effective in the treatment of intestinal disease, but, to date, efficacy in disseminated strongyloidiasis has been demonstrated only for thiabendazole.

Strongyloides fülleborni This unusual species, which has been encountered in Africa and Papua, New Guinea, is thought to be transmitted from person to person and via maternal milk. *S. fülleborni* releases membranous sacs filled with eggs into the stool. Most commonly affected are infants and young children, who present with abdominal distention, respiratory distress, vomiting, or diarrhea.

TRICHURIASIS Most infections with the whipworm *Trichuris trichiura* are asymptomatic, but heavy infections may cause gastrointestinal symptoms. Like the other soil-transmitted helminths, whipworm is distributed globally in the tropics and subtropics and is most common among poor children.

Life Cycle A broad posterior section and a thin anterior portion give *Trichuris* its characteristic whiplike shape. The adult worms reside in the colon and cecum, the anterior portions threaded into the superficial mucosa. Thousands of eggs laid daily by adult female worms pass via the feces and mature in the soil. After ingestion, infective eggs hatch in the duodenum, releasing larvae that mature before migrating to the large bowel. The entire cycle takes about 3 months, and adult worms may live for several years.

Clinical Features Tissue reactions to whipworms are mild. Most infected individuals have no symptoms or eosinophilia. Heavy infections may result in abdominal pain, anorexia, and bloody or mucoid diarrhea resembling inflammatory bowel disease. Rectal prolapse can result from massive infections in children, who often suffer from malnourishment and other diarrheal illnesses. Moderately heavy whipworm burdens also contribute to growth retardation.

Diagnosis and Treatment The characteristic 50- by 20-μm lemon-shaped whipworm eggs are readily detected on stool examination. Adult worms, which are 3 to 5 cm long, occasionally can be seen on proctoscopy. Mebendazole is safe and effective for treatment (see Chap. 214).

ENTEROBIASIS (PINWORM) *E. vermicularis* is more common in temperate countries than in the tropics. More than 40 million Americans, particularly schoolchildren, are estimated to be infected with pinworms.

Life Cycle and Epidemiology *Enterobius* adult worms are about 1 cm long and dwell in the bowel lumen. The gravid female worm migrates nocturnally out into the perianal region and releases up to 10,000 immature eggs. The eggs become infective within hours and are transmitted via hand-to-mouth passage. The larvae hatch and mature entirely within the intestine. This life cycle takes about 1 month, and adult worms survive for about 2 months. Self-infection results from perianal scratching and transport of infective eggs on the hands or under the nails to the mouth. Owing to the ease of person-to-person spread, pinworm infections are common among family members and institutionalized populations.

Clinical Features Most pinworm infections are asymptomatic. Perianal pruritus is the cardinal symptom. The itching is often worse at night owing to the nocturnal migration of the female worms, and it may lead to excoriation and bacterial superinfection. Heavy infections have been claimed to cause abdominal pain and weight loss. On rare occasions, pinworms invade the female genital tract, causing vulvovaginitis and pelvic or peritoneal granulomas. Eosinophilia or elevated levels of serum IgE are rare.

Diagnosis Since pinworm eggs are not usually released in the bowel, the diagnosis cannot be made by looking for eggs in the feces. Instead, eggs deposited in the perianal region are detected by the application of clear cellulose acetate tape to the perianal region in the morning. After the tape is transferred to a microscope slide, low-power examination will reveal the characteristic pinworm eggs, which are oval, measure 55 by 25 μm, and are flattened along one side.

℞ TREATMENT

All affected individuals should be given a dose of mebendazole or pyrantel pamoate, with treatment repeated after 10 to 14 days (see Chap. 214). Treatment of household members is also advocated to eliminate asymptomatic reservoirs of potential reinfection.

TRICHOSTRONGYLIASIS *Trichostrongylus* species that are normally parasites of herbivorous animals occasionally infect humans, particularly in Asia and Africa. This parasite has been termed *pseudohookworm* because of similarities to the hookworms in life cycle and egg morphology. Humans acquire the infection by accidentally ingesting *Trichostrongylus* larvae on contaminated leafy vegetables. The larvae do not migrate in humans but mature directly into adult worms in the small bowel. These worms ingest far less blood than hookworms; most infected people are asymptomatic, but heavy infections may give rise to mild anemia and eosinophilia. *Trichostrongylus* eggs encountered on stool examination resemble those of hookworms but are larger (85 by 115 μm). Appropriate treatment consists of mebendazole (see Chap. 214).

ANISAKIASIS Anisakiasis is a gastrointestinal infection caused by the accidental ingestion in uncooked saltwater fish of nematode larvae belonging to the family Anisakidae. The incidence of anisakiasis in the United States has increased as a result of the growing popularity of raw fish dishes. Most cases occur in Japan, the Netherlands, and Chile, where raw fish—sushi, pickled green herring, and seviche, respectively—are national culinary staples. Anisakid nematodes parasitize large sea mammals such as whales, dolphins, and seals. As part of a complex parasitic life cycle involving marine food chains, infectious larvae migrate to the musculature of a variety of fish. Both *Anisakis simplex* and *Pseudoterranova decipiens* have been implicated in human anisakiasis, but an identical gastric syndrome may be caused by the red larvae of eustrongylid parasites of fish-eating birds. When humans consume infected raw fish, live larvae may be coughed up within 48 h. Alternatively, larvae may immediately penetrate the mucosa of the stomach. Within hours, violent upper abdominal pain accompanied by nausea and occasionally vomiting ensues, mimicking an acute abdomen. The diagnosis can be established by direct visualization on upper endoscopy, outlining of the worm by contrast radiographic studies, or histopathologic examination of extracted tissue. In experienced hands, the first technique is preferable because extraction of the burrowing larvae by endoscopic technique is curative. In addition, larvae may pass to the small bowel, where they penetrate the mucosa and provoke a vigorous eosinophilic granulomatous response. Symptoms may appear 1 or 2 weeks after the infective meal, with intermittent abdominal pain, diarrhea, nausea, and fever resembling the manifestations of Crohn's disease. The diagnosis may be suggested by barium studies and confirmed by curative surgical resection of a granuloma in which the worm is embedded. Anisakid eggs will not be found in the stool, since the larvae do not mature in humans. Anisakid larvae in saltwater fish are killed by cooking to 60°C, freezing at −20°C for 3 days, or commercial blast freezing, but not usually by salting, marinating, or cold smoking.

CAPILLARIASIS Intestinal capillariasis is caused by ingestion of raw fish infected with *Capillaria philippinensis*. Subsequent autoinfection can lead to a severe wasting syndrome. The disease occurs in the Philippines and Thailand and, on occasion, elsewhere in Asia. The natural cycle of *C. philippinensis* involves fish from fresh and brackish water. When humans eat infected raw fish, the larvae mature in the intestine into adult worms, which produce invasive larvae that cause intestinal inflammation and villus loss. Capillariasis has an insidious onset with nonspecific abdominal pain and watery diarrhea. If untreated, progressive autoinfection can lead to protein-losing enteropathy and severe malabsorption and ultimately to death from cachexia, cardiac failure, or superinfection. The diagnosis is established by identification of the characteristic peanut-shaped (20- by 40-μm) eggs on stool examination. Severely ill patients require hospitalization and supportive therapy in addition to prolonged anthelmintic treatment with mebendazole or albendazole (see Chap. 214).

ABDOMINAL ANGIOSTRONGYLIASIS Abdominal angiostrongyliasis is found in Latin America and Africa. The zoonotic parasite *Angiostrongylus costaricensis* causes eosinophilic ileocolitis after the ingestion of contaminated vegetation. *A. costaricensis* normally parasitizes the cotton rat and other rodents, with slugs and snails serving as intermediate hosts. Humans become infected by accidentally ingesting infective larvae in mollusk slime deposited on fruits and vegetables; children are at highest risk. The larvae penetrate the gut wall and migrate to the mesenteric artery, where they develop into adult worms. Eggs deposited in the gut wall provoke an intense eosinophilic granulomatous reaction, and adult worms may cause mesenteric arteritis, thrombosis, or frank bowel infarction. Symptoms may mimic those of appendicitis, including abdominal pain and tenderness, fever, vomiting, and a palpable mass in the right iliac fossa. Leukocytosis and eosinophilia are prominent. A barium enema may reveal ileocecal filling defects, but a definitive diagnosis is usually made surgically with partial bowel resection. Pathologic study reveals a thickened bowel wall with eosinophilic granulomas surrounding the *Angiostrongylus* eggs. In nonsurgical cases, the diagnosis rests solely on clinical grounds because larvae and eggs cannot be detected in the stool. Medical therapy for abdominal angiostrongyliasis is of uncertain efficacy. Careful observation and surgical resection for severe symptoms are the mainstays of treatment.

BIBLIOGRAPHY

Ash LR, Orihel TC: *Atlas of Human Parasitology*, 3d ed. Chicago, ASCP Press, 1990

Cooper ES, Bundy DAP: Trichuris is not trivial. Parasitol Today 4:301, 1988

Croese J et al: Human enteric infection with canine hookworms. Ann Intern Med 120:369, 1994

Cross JH: Intestinal capillariasis. Clin Microbiol Rev 5:120, 1992

Duarte Z et al: Abdominal angiostrongyliasis in Nicaragua: A clinico-pathological study on a series of 12 case reports. Ann Parasitol Hum Comp 66:259, 1991

Genta RM et al: Strongyloidiasis in US veterans of the Vietnam and other wars. JAMA 258:49, 1987

Gyorkos TW et al: Intestinal parasite infection in the Kampuchean refugee population 6 years after resettlement in Canada. J Infect Dis 166:413, 1992

Haque AK et al: Pathogenesis of human strongyloidiasis: Autopsy and quantitative parasitological analysis. Mod Pathol 7:276, 1994

Hotez PJ, Pritchard DI: Hookworm infection. Sci Am 272:68, 1995

Khuroo MS et al: Hepatobiliary and pancreatic ascariasis in India. Lancet 335:1503, 1990

Liu LX, Weller PF: Strongyloidiasis and other intestinal nematode infections. Infect Dis Clin North Am 7:655, 1993

Ochoa B: Surgical complications of ascariasis. World J Surg 15:222, 1991

Schad GA, Warren KS (eds): *Hookworm Disease: Current Status and New Directions*. London, Taylor and Francis, 1990

Schantz PM: The dangers of eating raw fish. N Engl J Med 320:1143, 1989 [Editorial]

Thomas B. Nutman, Peter F. Weller

FILARIASIS AND RELATED INFECTIONS (LOIASIS, ONCHOCERCIASIS, AND DRACUNCULIASIS)

Filarial worms are nematodes that dwell in the subcutaneous tissues and the lymphatics. Eight filarial species infect humans (Table 223-1); of these, four—*Wuchereria bancrofti*, *Brugia malayi*, *Onchocerca volvulus*, and *Loa loa*—are responsible for most serious filarial infections. Filarial parasites, which infect an estimated 140 million persons worldwide, are transmitted by specific species of mosquitoes or other arthropods and have a complex life cycle including infective larval stages that are carried by insects and adult worms that reside in either lymphatic or subcutaneous tissues of humans. The offspring of adults are microfilariae, which, depending on their species, are 200 to 250 μm long and 5 to 7 μm wide, may or may not be enveloped in a loose sheath, and either circulate in the blood or migrate through the skin (see Table 223-1). To complete the life cycle, microfilariae are ingested by the arthropod vector and develop over 1 to 2 weeks into new infective larvae. Adult worms live for many years, whereas microfilariae survive from 3 to 36 months.

Usually, infection is established only with repeated and prolonged exposures to infective larvae. Since the clinical manifestations of filarial diseases develop relatively slowly, these infections should be considered chronic diseases with possible long-term debilitating effects. In terms of the nature, severity, and timing of clinical manifestations, patients with filariasis who are native to endemic areas and undergo lifelong exposure may differ significantly from those who are travelers or who have recently moved to these areas. Characteristically, the disease is more acute and intense in newly exposed individuals than in natives of endemic areas.

LYMPHATIC FILARIASIS

Lymphatic filariasis is caused by *W. bancrofti*, *B. malayi*, or *Brugia timori*. The threadlike adult parasites reside in lymphatic channels or lymph nodes, where they may remain viable for more than two decades.

EPIDEMIOLOGY *W. bancrofti*, the most widely distributed human filarial parasite, affects an estimated 80 million people and is found throughout the tropics and subtropics, including Asia and the Pacific Islands, Africa, areas of South America, and the Caribbean basin. Humans are the only definitive host for the parasite. Generally, the subperiodic form is found only in the Pacific Islands; elsewhere, *W. bancrofti* is nocturnally periodic. (Nocturnally periodic forms of microfilariae are scarce in peripheral blood by day and increase at night, whereas subperiodic forms are present in peripheral blood at all times and reach maximal levels in the afternoon.) Natural vectors for *W. bancrofti* are *Culex fatigans* mosquitoes in urban settings and anopheline or aedean mosquitoes in rural areas.

Brugian filariasis due to *B. malayi* occurs primarily in China, India, Indonesia, Korea, Japan, Malaysia, and the Philippines. *B. malayi* also has two forms distinguished by the periodicity of microfilaremia. The more common nocturnal form is transmitted in areas of coastal rice fields, while the subperiodic form is found in forests. *B. malayi* naturally infects cats as well as humans. *B. timori* exists only on islands of the Indonesian archipelago.

PATHOLOGY The principal pathologic changes result from inflammatory damage to the lymphatics, which is caused by adult worms and not by microfilariae. Adult worms live in afferent lymphatics or sinuses of lymph nodes and cause lymphatic dilatation and thickening of the vessel walls. The infiltration of plasma cells, eosinophils, and macrophages in and around the infected vessels, along with endothelial and connective tissue proliferation, leads to tortuosity of the lymphatics and damaged or incompetent lymph valves. Lymphedema and chronic-stasis changes with hard or brawny edema develop in the overlying skin. These consequences of filariasis are due both to direct effects of the worms and to the immune response of the host to the parasite. These immune responses are believed to cause the granulomatous and proliferative processes that precede total lymphatic obstruction. It is thought that the vessel remains patent as long as the worm remains viable, and that death of the worm leads to enhanced granulomatous reaction and fibrosis. Lymphatic obstruction results, and, despite collateralization of the lymphatics, lymphatic function is compromised.

CLINICAL FEATURES The common manifestations of lymphatic filariasis are asymptomatic microfilaremia, hydrocele, lymphatic inflammation, and lymphatic obstruction. Asymptomatic microfilaremia is found in most infected individuals who are clinically well. Infected males frequently develop disease in the scrotum, primarily because of the presence of adult worms in the lymphatics of the spermatic cord. Hydrocele may develop and, in advanced stages, may evolve into scrotal elephantiasis. Acute lymphangitis and lymphadenitis with high fever ("filarial fevers") are often accompanied by shaking chills and transient local edema. Episodes can recur frequently and usually abate spontaneously after 7 to 10 days. The lymphangitis characteristically develops in a retrograde or descending fashion, extending peripherally from the draining node where the parasite presumably resides. Regional lymph nodes are often enlarged, and the entire lymphatic channel can become indurated and inflamed. Concomitant local thrombophlebitis can develop. In brugian filariasis, a local abscess may form over a lymphatic tract and rupture. Lymphadenitis and lymphangitis involve both the upper and the lower extremities in bancroftian and brugian filariasis, but genital lymphatic involvement develops almost exclusively in relation to *W. bancrofti* infection. Genital involvement can be manifested by funiculitis, epididymitis, and scrotal pain and tenderness.

If lymphatic damage progresses to lymphatic obstruction, the permanent changes associated with elephantiasis may ensue. Brawny edema follows early pitting edema. With thickening of subcutaneous tissues come hyperkeratosis, fissuring of the skin, and hyperplastic changes. Bacterial superinfection of the poorly vascularized tissues is common. In bancroftian filariasis, scrotal lymphedema can develop. If the retroperitoneal lymphatics become obstructed, increased pressure leads to the rupture of renal lymphatics and the development of chyluria, which is usually intermittent and most prominent in the morning.

The clinical manifestations of filarial infections in travelers or transmigrants who have recently entered an endemic region are distinctive. Given a sufficient number of bites by infected vectors, usually over a 3- to 6-month period, recently exposed patients can develop acute lymphatic or scrotal inflammation with or without urticaria and localized angioedema. Lymphadenitis of epitrochlear, axillary, femoral, or inguinal lymph nodes is often followed by retrogradely evolving lymphangitis. Acute attacks are short-lived and, in contrast to filarial fevers in patients native to endemic areas, are usually not accompanied by fever. With prolonged exposure to infected mosquitoes, these attacks, if untreated, become more severe and lead to permanent lymphatic inflammation and obstruction.

DIAGNOSIS A definitive diagnosis can be made only by detection of the parasites and hence can be difficult. Adult worms localized in lymphatic vessels or nodes are largely inaccessible. Microfilariae can be found in blood, in hydrocele fluid, or (occasionally) in other body fluids. Such fluids can be examined microscopically, either directly or—for greater sensitivity—after concentration of the parasites by the passage of fluid through a polycarbonate cylindrical pore filter (pore size, 3 μm) or by the centrifugation of fluid fixed in 2% formalin (Knott's concentration technique). The timing of blood collection is critical and should be based on the periodicity of the microfilariae in the endemic region involved. Many infected individuals do not have microfilaremia, and definitive diagnosis in such cases can be difficult; in some instances, the diagnosis must be made on clinical grounds. In acute episodes, lymphatic filariasis must be distinguished from thrombophlebitis, infection, and trauma. Retrogradely evolving lymphangitis is a characteristic feature that helps distinguish filarial lymphangitis from typically ascending bacterial lymphangitis. Chronic filarial lymphedema must be distinguished from the lymphedema of malignancy, postoperative scarring, trauma, chronic edematous states, and congenital lymphatic-system abnormalities.

Eosinophilia and elevations of serum concentrations of IgE and antifilarial antibody support the diagnosis of lymphatic filariasis. There is, however, extensive cross-reactivity between filarial antigens and antigens of other helminths, including the common intestinal roundworms; thus, interpretations of serologic findings can be difficult. In addition, residents of endemic areas can become sensitized to filarial antigens through exposure to infected mosquitoes without having patent filarial infections.

Assays for circulating antigens of *W. bancrofti* permit the diagnosis of microfilaremic and cryptic (amicrofilaremic) infection. Polymerase

Table 223-1

Characteristics of the Filariae

Organism	Periodicity	Distribution	Vector	Location of Adult	Microfilarial Location	Sheath
Wuchereria bancrofti	Nocturnal	Cosmopolitan areas worldwide, including South America and Africa	*Culex* (mosquitoes)	Lymphatic tissue	Blood	+
		Mainly India	*Anopheles* (mosquitoes)			
		China, Indonesia	*Aedes* (mosquitoes)			
	Subperiodic	Eastern Pacific	*Aedes* (mosquitoes)	Lymphatic tissue	Blood	+
Brugia malayi	Nocturnal	Southeast Asia, Indonesia, India	*Mansonia, Anopheles* (mosquitoes)	Lymphatic tissue	Blood	+
	Subperiodic	Indonesia, Southeast Asia	*Coquilletidia, Mansonia* (mosquitoes)	Lymphatic tissue	Blood	+
Brugia timori	Nocturnal	Indonesia	*Anopheles* (mosquitoes)	Lymphatic tissue	Blood	+
Loa loa	Diurnal	West and Central Africa	*Chrysops* (deerflies)	Subcutaneous tissue	Blood	+
Onchocerca volvulus	None	South and Central America, Africa	*Simulium* (blackflies)	Subcutaneous tissue	Skin, eye	−
Mansonella ozzardi	None	South and Central America	*Culicoides* (midges)	Undetermined site	Blood	−
		Caribbean	*Simulium* (blackflies)			
Mansonella perstans	None	South and Central America, Africa	*Culicoides* (midges)	Body cavities, mesentery, perirenal tissue	Blood	−
Mansonella streptocerca	None	West and Central Africa	*Culicoides* (midges)	Subcutaneous tissue	Skin	−

chain reaction–based assays for DNA of *W. bancrofti* and *B. malayi* in blood have also been developed.

Evaluation of lymphatic function with lymphoscintigraphy can provide useful information in cases of lymphatic filariasis. The procedure involves the intradermal or subcutaneous injection of ^{99}Tc-labeled albumin or ^{99}Tc-labeled dextran [although the latter is not approved by the Food and Drug Administration (FDA)] and subsequent sequential imaging with a gamma camera. In males with suspected lymphatic filariasis, examination of the scrotum by ultrasonography may reveal nodules or lymphatic dilatation. The use of high-frequency (7.5- to 10-MHz) transducers and Doppler techniques may reveal motile worms within the scrotal lymphatics.

℞ TREATMENT

Treatment for lymphatic filariasis is currently limited to diethylcarbamazine (DEC) given at 6 mg/kg per day in either single or divided doses for 2 to 3 weeks. This regimen clears microfilariae from the blood and has a limited but definite effect on adult parasites. If at least some adult parasites survive, as is often the case, microfilaremia along with clinical symptoms can recur within months after therapy. There is some evidence that several courses of DEC or chronic administration of low-dose DEC may effect a cure. Ivermectin, a drug active in onchocerciasis, has been used in trials of therapy for lymphatic filariasis; in a single dose (although not approved by the FDA), it appears to be as effective as DEC at clearing microfilariae. Side effects of treatment with DEC (or ivermectin) include fever, chills, arthralgia, headaches, nausea, and vomiting. Both the development and the severity of these reactions, which may reflect an acute response to the antigens released by dying parasites, are related directly to the number of microfilariae circulating in the blood. These side effects can be avoided either by the initial use of a small dose of DEC, with an increase to a full dose over a few days, or by premedication of the patient with glucocorticoids.

Treatment of chronic lymphatic obstruction is difficult but may be helpful. Elevation of the infected limb, use of elastic stockings, and local foot care eliminate some of the associated symptoms. Surgical decompression with a nodovenous shunt may provide relief for severely affected limbs. Hydroceles can be drained or managed surgically. The management of filarial chyluria is unsatisfactory; neither surgical intervention nor sclerosis of infected lymphatics is effective.

PREVENTION Avoidance of mosquito bites usually is not feasible for residents of endemic areas, but visitors should use insect repellent and mosquito nets. DEC can kill developing filarial larvae and is useful as a prophylactic agent, although the optimal regimen for prophylaxis has not been ascertained. Mass treatment with DEC may reduce community levels of microfilariae so as to interrupt vector-borne transmission among humans.

TROPICAL PULMONARY EOSINOPHILIA

Tropical pulmonary eosinophilia (TPE) is a distinct syndrome that develops in some individuals infected with lymphatic filarial species. This syndrome affects males and females at a ratio of 4:1, often during the third decade of life. The majority of cases have been reported from India, Pakistan, Sri Lanka, Brazil, and Southeast Asia.

CLINICAL FEATURES The main features include a history of residence in filarial endemic regions, paroxysmal cough and wheezing that are usually nocturnal (and probably related to the nocturnal periodicity of microfilariae), weight loss, low-grade fever, adenopathy, and pronounced blood eosinophilia (>3000 eosinophils/μL). Chest x-rays may be normal but generally show increased bronchovascular markings; diffuse miliary lesions or mottled opacities may be present in the middle and lower lung fields. Tests of pulmonary function show restrictive abnormalities in most cases and obstructive defects in half.

Total serum IgE levels (10,000 to 100,000 ng/mL) and antifilarial antibody titers are characteristically elevated.

PATHOLOGY In TPE there is rapid clearance of microfilariae and parasite antigens from the bloodstream by the lungs, and the clinical symptoms result from allergic and inflammatory reactions elicited by the cleared parasites. In some subjects, trapping of microfilariae in other reticuloendothelial organs can cause hepatomegaly, splenomegaly, or lymphadenopathy. A prominent, eosinophil-enriched, intraalveolar infiltrate is often reported. In the absence of successful treatment, interstitial fibrosis can lead to progressive pulmonary damage.

DIFFERENTIAL DIAGNOSIS TPE must be distinguished from asthma, Löffler's syndrome, allergic bronchopulmonary aspergillosis, allergic granulomatosis with angiitis (Churg-Strauss syndrome), the systemic vasculitides (most notably periarteritis nodosa and Wegener's granulomatosis), chronic eosinophilic pneumonia, and the idiopathic hypereosinophilic syndrome. In addition to a geographic history of filarial exposure, useful features for distinguishing TPE include wheezing that is solely nocturnal, very high levels of antifilarial antibodies, and a rapid initial response to treatment with DEC.

℞ TREATMENT

DEC is used at a dosage of 4 to 6 mg/kg of body weight per day for 14 days. Symptoms usually resolve within 3 to 7 days after the initiation of therapy. Relapse, which occurs in approximately 12 to 25 percent of cases (sometimes after an interval of years), requires retreatment.

ONCHOCERCIASIS

Onchocerciasis ("river blindness") is caused by the filarial nematode *O. volvulus*, which infects an estimated 13 million individuals. The majority of individuals infected with *O. volvulus* live in the equatorial region of Africa extending from the Atlantic coast to the Red Sea. About 70,000 persons are infected in Guatemala and Mexico, with smaller foci in Venezuela, Colombia, Brazil, Ecuador, Yemen, and Saudi Arabia. Onchocerciasis is the second leading cause of infectious blindness worldwide.

ETIOLOGY AND EPIDEMIOLOGY Infection in humans begins with the deposition of infective larvae on the skin by the bite of an infected blackfly. The larvae develop into adults, which are typically found in subcutaneous nodules. About 7 months to 3 years after infection, the gravid female releases microfilariae that migrate out of the nodule and throughout the tissues, concentrating in the dermis. Infection is transmitted to other persons when a female fly ingests microfilariae from the host's skin and these microfilariae then develop into infective larvae. Adult *O. volvulus* females and males are about 40 to 60 cm and 3 to 6 cm in length, respectively. The life span of adults can be as long as 18 years, with an average of approximately 9 years. Because the blackfly vector breeds along free-flowing rivers and streams (particularly in rapids) and generally restricts its flight to an area within several kilometers of these breeding sites, both biting and disease transmission are most intense in these locations.

PATHOLOGY Onchocerciasis affects primarily the skin, eyes, and lymph nodes. In contrast to that in lymphatic filariasis, the damage in onchocerciasis is elicited by microfilariae and not by adults. In the skin, there are mild but chronic inflammatory changes that can result in loss of elastic fibers, atrophy, and fibrosis. The subcutaneous nodules, or onchocercomata, consist primarily of fibrous tissues surrounding the adult worm, often with a peripheral ring of inflammatory cells. In the eye, neovascularization and corneal scarring lead to corneal opacities and blindness. Inflammation in the anterior and posterior chambers frequently results in anterior uveitis, chorioretinitis, and optic atrophy. Although punctate opacities are due to an inflammatory reaction surrounding dead or dying microfilariae, the pathogenesis of most manifestations of onchocerciasis is still unclear.

CLINICAL FEATURES Skin Pruritus and rash are the most frequent manifestations of onchocerciasis. The pruritus can be incapacitating; the rash is typically a papular eruption that is generalized rather than localized to a particular region of the body. Long-term infection results in exaggerated and premature wrinkling of the skin, loss of elastic fibers, and epidermal atrophy that can lead to loose, redundant skin and hypo- or hyperpigmentation. Localized eczematoid dermatitis can cause hyperkeratosis, scaling, and pigmentary changes. Such lesions are often seen in the lower extremities but can be distributed more extensively.

Onchocercomata These subcutaneous nodules, which can be palpable and/or visible, contain the adult worm. In African patients, they are common over the coccyx and sacrum, the trochanter of the femur, the lateral anterior crest, and other bony prominences; in Latin American patients, they tend to develop preferentially in the upper part of the body, particularly on the head, neck, and shoulders. Nodules vary in size and characteristically are firm and not tender. It has been estimated that, for every palpable nodule, there are four deeper nonpalpable ones.

Ocular Tissue Visual impairment is the most serious complication of onchocerciasis and usually affects only those persons with moderate or heavy infections. Lesions may develop in all parts of the eye. The most common early finding is conjunctivitis with photophobia. In the cornea, punctate keratitis—consisting of acute inflammatory reactions surrounding dying microfilariae manifested as "snowflake" opacities—is frequent in younger patients and resolves without apparent complications. Sclerosing keratitis occurs in approximately 5 percent of persons infected with savannah strains and 1 percent of those infected with forest strains and is the leading cause of onchocercal blindness in Africa. Anterior uveitis and iridocyclitis develop in about 5 percent of infected persons in Africa. In Latin America, complications of the anterior uveal tract (pupillary deformity) may cause secondary glaucoma. Characteristic chorioretinal lesions develop as a result of atrophy and hyperpigmentation of the retinal pigment epithelium and the choriopapillaris. Constriction of the visual field and frank optic atrophy may occur.

Lymph Nodes Mild to moderate lymphadenopathy is frequent, particularly in the inguinal and femoral areas, where the enlarged nodes may hang down in response to gravity ("hanging groin"), sometimes predisposing to inguinal and femoral hernias.

Systemic Manifestations Some heavily infected individuals develop cachexia with loss of adipose tissue and muscle mass. Among adults who become blind, there is a three- to fourfold increase in the mortality rate.

DIAGNOSIS Definitive diagnosis depends on the detection of an adult worm in an excised nodule or, more commonly, of microfilariae in a skin snip. Skin snips are obtained with a corneal-scleral punch, which collects a blood-free skin biopsy sample extending to just below the epidermis, or by lifting of the skin with the tip of a needle and excision of a small (1- to 3-mm) piece with a sterile scalpel blade. The biopsy tissue is incubated in tissue culture medium or in saline on a glass slide or flat-bottomed microtiter plate. After incubation for 2 to 4 h (or occasionally overnight in light infections), microfilariae emergent from the skin can be visualized by low-power microscopy.

℞ **TREATMENT**

The main goals of therapy are to prevent the development of irreversible lesions and to alleviate symptoms. Surgical excision is recommended when nodules are located on the head, because of the proximity of microfilaria-producing adult worms to the eye, but chemotherapy is the mainstay of management. Ivermectin, a semisynthetic macrocyclic lactone active against microfilariae, is the first-line agent for the treatment of onchocerciasis. It is given orally in a single dose of 150 μg/kg, either yearly or semiannually. After treatment, most individuals have few or no reactions. Pruritus, cutaneous edema, and/or maculopapular rash occurs in approximately 1 to 10 percent of treated individuals. Contraindications to treatment include pregnancy, breast feeding, central nervous system (CNS) disorders that may increase the penetration of ivermectin into the CNS (e.g., meningitis), and an age of less than 5 years. Although ivermectin treatment results in a marked drop in microfilarial density,

its effect may last for only 6 months. Suramin, a potent but potentially toxic macrofilaricidal agent, is recommended only if total cure is necessary. Because of the drug's nephrotoxicity, renal function must be monitored closely during treatment.

PREVENTION Vector control has been beneficial in highly endemic areas in which breeding sites are vulnerable to insecticide spraying, but most areas endemic for onchocerciasis are not suited to this type of control. While persons working in fly-infested areas can minimize the number of bites they sustain by wearing protective garments, this approach is not feasible for the large majority of individuals in endemic foci. No drug has been shown to prevent infection with *O. volvulus*.

LOIASIS

ETIOLOGY AND EPIDEMIOLOGY Loiasis is caused by *L. loa* (the African eye worm), which is present in the rain forests of West and Central Africa. Adult parasites (females, 50 to 70 mm long and 0.5 mm wide; males, 25 to 35 mm long and 0.25 mm wide) live in subcutaneous tissues; microfilariae circulate in the blood with a diurnal periodicity that peaks between 12:00 noon and 2:00 P.M.

CLINICAL FEATURES Manifestations of loiasis in natives of endemic areas may differ from those in temporary residents or visitors. Among the indigenous population, loiasis is often an asymptomatic infection with microfilaremia. Infection may be recognized only after subconjunctival migration of an adult worm or may be manifested by episodic Calabar swellings, evanescent localized areas of angioedema and erythema developing on the extremities and less frequently at other sites. Nephropathy, encephalopathy, and cardiomyopathy are rare. In patients who are not residents of endemic areas, allergic symptoms predominate, episodes of Calabar swelling tend to be more frequent and debilitating, microfilaremia is rare, and eosinophilia and increased levels of antifilarial antibodies are characteristic.

PATHOLOGY The pathogenesis of the manifestations of loiasis is poorly understood. Calabar swellings are thought to result from a hypersensitivity reaction to the adult worm.

DIAGNOSIS Definitive diagnosis of loiasis requires the detection of microfilariae in the peripheral blood or the isolation of the adult worm from the eye or from a subcutaneous biopsy specimen from a site of swelling developing after treatment. In practice, the diagnosis must often be based on a characteristic history and clinical presentation, blood eosinophilia, and elevated levels of antifilarial antibodies, particularly in travelers to the endemic region, who are usually amicrofilaremic. Other clinical findings in the latter individuals include hypergammaglobulinemia, elevated levels of serum IgE, and elevated leukocyte and eosinophil counts.

℞ **TREATMENT**

DEC (8 to 10 mg/kg per day for 21 days) is effective against both the adult and the microfilarial forms of *L. loa*, but multiple courses are frequently necessary before the disease resolves completely. In cases of heavy microfilaremia, allergic or other inflammatory reactions can take place during treatment, including CNS involvement with coma and encephalitis. Heavy infections are treated initially with low doses of DEC (0.5 mg/kg per day) and glucocorticoids (40 to 60 mg of prednisone per day). If antifilarial treatment has no adverse effects, the prednisone dose can be rapidly tapered and the dose of DEC gradually increased to 8 to 10 mg/kg per day.

Albendazole and ivermectin (although not FDA-approved) have been shown to be effective in reducing microfilarial loads. DEC (300 mg weekly) is an effective prophylactic regimen for loiasis.

STREPTOCERCIASIS

Mansonella streptocerca, found mainly in the tropical forest belt of Africa from Ghana to Zaire, is transmitted by biting midges. The major clinical manifestations involve the skin and include pruritus, papular rashes, and pigmentation changes. Many infected individuals have inguinal adenopathy, although most are asymptomatic. The diagnosis is made by detection of the characteristic microfilariae in skin snips. DEC (6 mg/kg per day in divided doses for 14 to 21 days) is effective in killing both microfilariae and adult worms. As in onchocerciasis, treatment is sometimes accompanied by urticaria, arthralgias, myalgias, headaches, and abdominal discomfort.

MANSONELLA PERSTANS INFECTION

Mansonella perstans, distributed across the center of Africa and in northeastern South America, is transmitted by midges. Adult worms reside in serous cavities—pericardial, pleural, and peritoneal—as well as in the mesentery and the perirenal and retroperitoneal tissues. Microfilariae circulate in the blood without periodicity. The clinical and pathologic features of the infection are poorly defined. Most patients appear to be asymptomatic, but manifestations may include transient angioedema and pruritus of the arms, face, or other parts of the body (analogous to the Calabar swellings of loiasis), fever, headache, arthralgias, and right upper quadrant pain. Occasionally, pericarditis and hepatitis occur. The diagnosis is based on the demonstration of microfilariae in blood or serosal effusions. Perstans filariasis is often associated with peripheral-blood eosinophilia and antifilarial antibody elevations. Although DEC (8 to 10 mg/kg per day for 21 days) is the standard therapeutic agent, there is little evidence that it is effective. Cure is evidenced by the disappearance of symptoms and eosinophilia; multiple courses of therapy are usually required. Mebendazole (100 mg twice daily for 30 days) has been reported to be effective.

MANSONELLA OZZARDI INFECTION

The distribution of *Mansonella ozzardi* is restricted to Central and South America and certain Caribbean islands. Adult worms are rarely recovered from humans. Microfilariae circulate in the blood without periodicity. Although this organism has often been considered nonpathogenic, headache, articular pain, fever, pulmonary symptoms, adenopathy, hepatomegaly, pruritus, and eosinophilia have been ascribed to *M. ozzardi* infection. Diagnosis is made by the detection of microfilariae in peripheral blood. No drug has been proved to be effective for therapy; ivermectin was effective in a single case report.

DRACUNCULIASIS (GUINEA WORM INFECTION)

ETIOLOGY AND EPIDEMIOLOGY Dracunculiasis, caused by *Dracunculus medinensis*, is a parasitic infection whose incidence has declined dramatically because of global eradication efforts. Current estimates suggest that there are only 100,000 cases worldwide, the majority in Sudan and West Africa (particularly Nigeria and Niger). Humans acquire this infection when they ingest water containing infective larvae derived from *Cyclops*, a crustacean that is the intermediate host. Larvae penetrate the stomach or intestinal wall, mate, and mature. The adult male probably dies; the female *Dracunculus* develops over a year and migrates to subcutaneous tissues, usually in the lower extremity. As the thin female *Dracunculus*, ranging in length from 300 cm to 1 m, approaches the skin, a blister forms that, over days, breaks down and forms an ulcer. When the blister opens, large numbers of motile, rhabditiform larvae can be released into stagnant water; ingestion by *Cyclops* completes the life cycle.

CLINICAL FEATURES Few or no clinical manifestations of dracunculiasis are evident until just before the blister forms, when

there is an onset of fever and generalized allergic symptoms, including periorbital edema, wheezing, and urticaria. The emergence of the worm is associated with local pain and swelling. When the blister ruptures (usually as a result of immersion in water), the adult worm releases larva-rich fluid, and this release is associated with a relief of symptoms. The shallow ulcer surrounding the emerging adult worm heals over weeks to months. Such ulcers, however, can become secondarily infected, the result being cellulitis, local inflammation, abscess formation, or (uncommonly) tetanus. Occasionally, the adult worm does not emerge but becomes encapsulated and calcified.

DIAGNOSIS The diagnosis is based on the findings developing with the emergence of the adult worm, as described above.

 TREATMENT
Gradual extraction of the worm by winding of a few centimeters on a stick each day remains the common and effective practice. Worms may be excised surgically. The administration of thiabendazole (25 mg/kg twice daily for 3 days) or metronidazole (250 mg three times daily for 10 days) may relieve symptoms but has no proven activity against the worm.

PREVENTION Prevention, which remains the only real control measure, depends on the provision of safe drinking water.

ZOONOTIC FILARIAL INFECTIONS

Dirofilariae that affect primarily dogs, cats, and raccoons and *Brugia* parasites that affect small mammals occasionally infect humans incidentally. Because humans are an abnormal host, the parasites never develop fully. Pulmonary dirofilarial infection caused by the canine heartworm *Dirofilaria immitis* generally presents in humans as a solitary pulmonary nodule. Chest pain, hemoptysis, and cough are uncommon. Infections with *Dirofilaria repens* (from dogs) or *Dirofilaria tenuis* (from raccoons) can cause local subcutaneous nodules in humans. Zoonotic *Brugia* infection can produce isolated lymph node enlargement. Eosinophilia levels and antifilarial antibody titers are not commonly elevated. Excisional biopsy is both diagnostic and curative; these infections usually do not respond to chemotherapy.

BIBLIOGRAPHY

ADOLPH PE et al: Diagnosis and treatment of *Acanthocheilonema perstans* filariasis. Am J Trop Med Hyg 11:76, 1962

AMARAL F et al: Live adult worms detected by ultrasonography in human bancroftian filariasis. Am J Trop Med Hyg 50:753, 1994

CENTERS FOR DISEASE CONTROL AND PREVENTION: Progress toward global eradication of dracunculiasis. Morb Mort Week Rep 44:875, 1995

EBERHARD ML, LAMMIE PJ: Laboratory diagnosis of filariasis. Clin Lab Med 11:977, 1991

FREEDMAN DO et al: Lymphoscintigraphic analysis of lymphatic abnormalities in symptomatic and asymptomatic human filariasis. J Infect Dis 170:927, 1994

KLION AD et al: Loiasis in endemic and non-endemic populations: Immunologically mediated differences in clinical presentation. J Infect Dis 163:1318, 1991

MARINKELLE CJ, GERMAN E: Mansonelliasis in the Comisaria del Vaupes of Colombia. Trop Geogr Med 22:101, 1970

MEYERS WM et al: Human streptocerciasis: A clinicopathologic study of 40 Africans (Zairians) including identification of the adult filaria. Am J Trop Med Hyg 21:528, 1972

OTTESEN EA: Filarial infections. Infect Dis Clin North Am 7:619, 1993

———, NUTMAN TB: Tropical pulmonary eosinophilia. Annu Rev Med 43:417, 1992

RO JY et al: Pulmonary dirofilariasis: The great imitator of primary or metastatic lung tumor. A clinicopathologic analysis of seven cases and a review of the literature. Hum Pathol 20:69, 1989

WHO EXPERT COMMITTEE ON FILARIASIS: Lymphatic filariasis: Diagnosis and pathogenesis. Bull WHO 71(2):135, 1993

WHO EXPERT COMMITTEE ON ONCHOCERCIASIS: Onchocerciasis and its control: Fourth report. Technical Report Series No. 852, Geneva, WHO, 1995

SCHISTOSOMIASIS AND OTHER TREMATODE INFECTIONS

The trematodes (flukes) that commonly infect humans live in the intestines, biliary tract, lungs, and venules of the intestines or genitourinary tract. Except in the case of the intestinal schistosomes, which cause a unique type of liver fibrosis, disease is limited primarily to the organs where the parasites reside. The pathophysiology of disease differs among the trematodes. Schistosomiasis is the best understood, and some of the factors important in disease development in this infection appear to apply to infections caused by many of the other trematodes. In endemic areas, large proportions of the population are infected but asymptomatic; the disease is mostly limited to heavily infected persons. Distinct acute and chronic syndromes are recognizable, as are predictable pathologic changes over time. Eosinophilia and fever are common findings in acute disease. Because many of these parasites follow complicated migration routes and/or are poorly adapted to survival in a human host, infections in ectopic locations are an important cause of morbidity.

LIFE CYCLE AND EPIDEMIOLOGY Infections in humans are limited to digenetic trematodes—i.e., those that reproduce sexually and produce eggs in mammalian definitive hosts and reproduce asexually in snails. After eggs reach water, they either hatch immediately or mature before releasing a free-swimming *miracidium*, which seeks out the appropriate intermediate snail host or is ingested by the snail. After a number of cycles of multiplication in the snail, free-swimming *cercariae* are released and, depending on the species, can (1) infect the definitive host; (2) seek out a second intermediate host, such as a fish or crustacean; or (3) encyst on vegetation. The encysted cercaria, or *metacercaria*, is a dormant, relatively resistant form that infects the host following ingestion. With the exception of schistosomes, most trematodes are flat, leaf-shaped parasites that vary in length from 1 mm to 7 cm. They possess two grasping organs called *suckers* and lack a body cavity. The gut usually lacks an anus, and digested food is regurgitated through the oral opening. The surfaces of trematodes are covered by a syncytium of cells, or tegument, through which nutrients are absorbed.

Schistosomes differ in a number of important ways from the other trematodes that infect humans. Most trematodes are hermaphroditic, but the sexes are separate in the schistosomes, and completion of the sexual cycle requires the presence of male and female worms. The adult schistosomes reside in the bloodstream, whereas the other trematodes dwell in the liver, lung, or intestines. In schistosomiasis, humans are infected by free-swimming cercariae that invade the skin; in contrast, in the other trematode infections, humans are infected after ingestion. The eggs of hermaphroditic trematodes possess a characteristic operculum, or caplike structure. The morphology of schistosome ova differs from that of other trematode ova, as described below.

A large number of trematodes can infect humans. With the exception of some species of schistosomes, most trematodes have domestic or wild animals as definitive hosts, and humans are accidentally infected. In highly endemic situations or under particularly advantageous circumstances, humans are able to maintain the life cycle in the absence of the usual definitive host. Some infections are rare or occur in populations in limited geographic areas, while others affect large numbers of persons over extensive areas or produce recognizable syndromes.

DIAGNOSIS A pertinent history is important in the diagnosis of trematode infections. Persons from endemic areas; travelers who are exposed to fresh water or who ingest undercooked fish, crustacea, or potentially contaminated vegetation; and others who ingest locally obtained but potentially contaminated vegetation such as watercress or undercooked, pickled, or smoked fish can be infected. Eosinophilia is common in acute invasive trematode infections. The definitive diagnosis is established by the demonstration of eggs in stool or sputum or by biopsy of the affected tissue. Serologic tests are available for schistosomiasis, fascioliasis, and paragonimiasis; a positive test is indicative of infection. Serologic tests for other trematode infections may be available in endemic areas or research laboratories.

℞ TREATMENT

Since disease is associated primarily with heavy trematode infection, one of the goals of therapy is to reduce the worm burden to below the level associated with disease. This goal is particularly pertinent in the treatment and prevention of disease in large populations. A number of studies of schistosomiasis and liver fluke infection have demonstrated that treatment does in fact lower the intensity of infection (which is roughly reflected by the number of ova excreted) and result in a marked decrease in disease prevalence. On occasion, a small number of parasites can cause significant disease either by lodging in a strategic location in the tissue that is normally involved (e.g., in the ureter for *Schistosoma haematobium*) or by localizing ectopically [e.g., in the central nervous system (CNS) for *Schistoma* and *Paragonimus*]. Since these complications do not appear to be related to the intensity of infection, elimination of every parasite is a reasonable goal. The pathophysiology of other complications, such as bladder cancer in *S. haematobium* infections and cholangiocarcinoma in liver fluke infections, is unclear; thus, complete elimination of the infection is appropriate. In short, the goals of treatment depend on the person or population involved and the risk of subsequent disease.

Praziquantel is the drug of choice for the treatment of most trematode infections except fascioliasis. Although less costly, other available therapies are inconvenient, have greater side effects, or are experimental. The efficacy of treatment is assessed in most instances by the disappearance of viable ova and/or by the improvement of relevant clinical parameters. Assessment should take place after enough time has passed for ova to have cleared from the tissues or excreta and after damaged worms that were not killed have had a chance to recover, but before reinfection has occurred. Low-level residual infections are not uncommon; patients with such infections can be re-treated if necessary.

SCHISTOSOMIASIS

Three major schistosome species—*Schistosoma mansoni*, *S. haematobium*, and *Schistosoma japonicum*—and a number of less prevalent species infect humans. Both *S. mansoni* and *S. japonicum* adults reside in the venules of the intestine, and the major disease manifestations of these parasites are hepatic. *S. mansoni* is found in parts of South America (Brazil, Venezuela, and Surinam), some Caribbean islands, Africa, and the Middle East, while infections with *S. japonicum* occur in the Far East, mostly in China and the Philippines. *S. haematobium* adults are found mostly in the venules of the urinary tract and cause lesions primarily of the ureters and bladder. Infections with this species occur in Africa and the Middle East. Of lesser importance are *Schistosoma mekongi*, a parasite related to *S. japonicum* that is found along the Mekong River in Indochina, and *Schistosoma intercalatum*, a species found in certain areas of central West Africa. Worldwide, as many as 200 million persons may be infected with schistosomes, and infection of entire communities is common. However, most infected persons experience few or no signs and symptoms, and only a small minority develop significant disease.

LIFE CYCLE The schistosome species infecting humans all share the same basic life cycle but are unique in ways that account for some of the variation in clinical and pathologic findings. Important differences include the length of time before egg laying begins (prepatent period), the location of the adult worms, the number of eggs produced by each pair of worms, the response by the host to the ova, and the eventual fate of retained eggs. The morphology of the parasites and the types of intermediate host snail are also distinct.

Humans become infected after contact with water containing the infective stage of the parasite, which is called a *cercaria*; this microscopic form possesses a forked tail, used for swimming, and a head, which is the anlage of the worm. With the help of secreted enzymes, cercariae penetrate the unbroken skin and transform into *schistoso-mules*, or developing schistosomes. After 2 to 3 days, the schistoso-mules migrate to the lungs and then to the portal vein, probably by an intravascular route. In the portal vein, the maturing male and female schistosomes pair. They then migrate to the venules of the mesentery, bladder, or ureters (depending on the species of schistosome), and begin to deposit eggs. The time spent in migration and maturation differs. *S. mansoni* and *S. japonicum* begin depositing eggs around 4 to 5 weeks after infection, while egg deposition begins after 2 to 3 months for *S. haematobium*. Adult worms are about 1 to 2 cm long and migrate in the blood vessels without eliciting a local inflammatory reaction. Adult worms do not multiply in humans, and immunosup-pressive therapy does not result in increased numbers of worms.

Once released, eggs are either retained in the tissues at the site of deposition or swept back, mostly to the liver. In the case of the intestinal schistosomes, this transport occurs via the venous portal system. Eggs are deposited mainly in the bladder and ureters by *S. haematobium*. Some of the mature schistosome ova are extruded into the lumen of the intestines, bladder, or ureters. After contact with water they hatch, releasing a miracidium. This free-swimming ciliated stage seeks out the proper intermediate snail vector and burrows into its soft tissues. After 1 to 2 months (depending on the species), the miracidium develops into a primary and then a secondary sporocyst, which, after further development, begins releasing cercariae into the surrounding water. Thousands of cercariae can be released daily from each infected snail. Therefore, one miracidium produces many cercar-iae, and this arrangement amplifies the number of infective parasites and the risk of infection. Cercariae are most infectious immediately after shedding and are no longer viable 48 h after release, so storage of water for 48 h before contact prevents exposure and infection.

Unlike most other trematodes, schistosomes are of two sexes, but this characteristic is evident only in the adult stage. Ova are laid only when males and females infect the same individual.

PATHOPHYSIOLOGY A number of factors govern the dis-ease manifestations of schistosomiasis. These include the duration and intensity of infection, the location of egg deposition, host genetics, concurrent infections, and other still undefined factors.

In individuals from endemic areas, initial infection goes unnoticed. There are a number of possible reasons for the lack of symptoms, including age at initial exposure; manner of exposure; and transfer of antigens, antibodies, and anti-idiotypes from the mother to the fetus. In contrast, in visitors to endemic areas, initial infection with schisto-somes commonly results in an acute febrile illness (Katayama fever, or acute schistosomiasis), which most likely is a manifestation of the immune response to the developing schistosomes and eggs. These individuals mount a vigorous hypersensitivity response that becomes modulated; they develop elevated levels of eosinophils and immune complexes; and they display a marked reaction to schistosome anti-gens, which may be measured by lymphocyte blastogenesis. Despite ongoing infection, symptoms subside, as do blastogenic responses to schistosome antigens but not to unrelated antigens such as purified protein derivative of tuberculin. The exudative acute granulomatous response to schistosome eggs is also modulated.

A major factor in the development of disease in humans is the worm burden of the host, which determines the number of eggs produced. The inflammatory and fibrotic response to these eggs accounts for most of the morbidity and mortality associated with schistosomiasis. Factors that limit the survival of the parasite will also limit the development of disease. Immunity exists in experimental animals. In human schisto-some infections, protective immunity also is thought to develop, be-cause reinfection rates are reduced in previously treated adults despite continuing water contact. In the first few days after infection, the schistosomule is relatively susceptible to immune attack. A number of systems employing antibody and/or eosinophils, neutrophils, macro-

phages, and complement have been used to kill schistosomules in vitro. However, as the schistosomules mature, they become refractory to these immune responses. In addition, schistosomes coat their tegument with host proteins and evade recognition by the host. Antibodies that block effective killing also may enhance parasite survival. Schistoso-mule and adult worm antigens have been defined in the hope of devel-oping vaccines; the administration of murine monoclonal antibodies to some of these antigens has reduced worm burdens in challenge infections by about 50 percent, and immunization of rodents with a number of defined antigens has produced similar levels of protection. Successful vaccination with anti-idiotypes also has been reported.

Schistosome eggs elicit a granulomatous response that is best understood in *S. mansoni* infections. The host becomes sensitized to the egg proteins by a T cell–mediated mechanism that induces a larger granuloma. However, with continued infection, the granuloma decreases in size. The mechanisms involved in the induction of granu-lomas, the immune sensitization that results in an increase in granuloma size, and the immune modulation that leads to a decrease in granuloma size are areas of intense investigation. Studies suggest that granuloma-tous responses to *S. mansoni* eggs are T_H2-dependent. Administration of interleukin 12—a potent stimulator of the T_H1 response and suppres-sor of the T_H2 response—at the same time as egg sensitization signifi-cantly reduces granuloma formation and subsequent egg-induced fibro-sis after challenge infection by replacing the usually predominant T_H2 response to *S. mansoni* eggs with a T_H1 response. This approach offers the promise of controlling disease manifestations by preventing the potentially harmful inflammatory and fibrotic response to eggs. Serum factors, including the anti-idiotypic network, also modulate immune responses. The regulation of granulomas due to *S. japonicum* eggs differs from that of granulomas from *S. mansoni* eggs.

Both eggs and granulomas release factors that induce fibroblast proliferation in vitro. The early cellular response induced by granu-lomas is followed by fibrosis in vivo; however, liver fibrosis in humans probably involves more than simple fusion of fibrotic granulomas. After years of continued infection, some heavily infected individuals develop end-stage fibrotic lesions, mainly portal fibrosis (Symmers' fibrosis); esophageal varices and splenomegaly often follow in *S. mansoni*, *S. japonicum*, and *S. mekongi* infections, and fibrosis of the ureters and bladder frequently follows in *S. haematobium* infections. After the development of portal fibrosis, eggs are shunted to the lungs via portal-systemic collateral veins, resulting in cor pulmonale in about 15 percent of patients with Symmers' fibrosis. Immune complexes shunted to the systemic circulation cause glomerulonephritis.

Host genetic factors have been found to influence the development of Symmers' fibrosis, although there is no general agreement as to which are important. Moreover, even schistosomes of the same species are genetically diverse, as has been shown by endonuclease restriction analysis, but the effect of this diversity on disease in humans is un-known.

CLINICAL SYNDROMES (See Table 224-1) **Acute Schisto-somiasis** Acute schistosomiasis, or Katayama fever, follows initial exposure and infection with *S. mansoni* or *S. japonicum*. It rarely follows infection with *S. haematobium*. Acute schistosomiasis is sel-dom recognized in endemic populations but rather is noted primarily in visitors to endemic areas. Immediately after exposure, patients frequently complain of intense transient itching. From 2 to 6 weeks or longer after exposure, the patient may complain of a variety of symptoms, including fever, chills, headache, hives or angioedema, weakness, weight loss, nonproductive cough, abdominal pain, and diarrhea. Sometimes symptoms abate but return with increased inten-sity about the time egg laying commences. These symptoms gradually diminish but may last as long as 2 to 3 months. Other newly infected individuals may be asymptomatic or have only minimal symptoms. In these individuals, the diagnosis is established only after further evaluation prompted by suggestive laboratory test results or exposure history. More severe symptoms occur with heavier infections, but light infections may cause severe illness. CNS lesions may develop during acute schistosome infection. The diagnosis of acute schistosomiasis is suggested by the clinical findings and the presence of eosinophilia,

Clinical Manifestations of Disease due to Various *Schistosoma* Species*

Manifestation	S. mansoni	S. japonicum	S. haematobium
Acute toxemic schistosomiasis	+	+	+
Chronic asymptomatic schistosomiasis	+	+	+
Hepatosplenic schistosomiasis	+	+	0
Cor pulmonale	+	+	±
Glomerulonephritis (clinically significant)	+	+	0†
Colonic polyposis	+	+	±
Ectopic lesions			
Brain	±	+	±
Spinal cord	+	±	+
Skin	+	+	+
Chronic cystitis and ureteritis	0	0	+
Mass lesions, bladder and ureters	0	0	+
Bladder cancer	0	0	+
Association with *Salmonella*	+	+	+
Prolonged fever	+	+	+
Urinary carrier state	?	?	+
Swimmers' itch‡	+	+	+

* +, recognized complications of infections by this species; ±, findings much less prominent in individuals infected by this species; 0, complications not present in infections by this species.
† Except with associated *Salmonella* infections.
‡ Usually from schistosomes that do not infect humans.

with values sometimes greater than 50 percent. Leukocytosis, increased levels of immune complexes, and elevated concentrations of IgM, IgG, and IgE are found commonly. Although it has been suggested that immune complexes play a role in the pathophysiology of acute schistosomiasis, glomerulonephritis and vasculitis have not been reported. The specific diagnosis can be established, even before the shedding of ova, by the detection of antibodies to adult schistosome gut antigens or, after egg excretion (5 to 6 weeks after exposure), by appropriate serologic testing and the finding of eggs in the stool or a rectal biopsy sample. Clinically, acute schistosomiasis is frequently misdiagnosed as typhoid fever; in fact, it can be confused with any prolonged febrile illness. Although patients seem to tolerate chemotherapy well, it is unclear whether therapy shortens the course of disease or decreases symptoms. Glucocorticoids may be useful, but their usefulness has not been demonstrated in controlled studies.

Liver Fibrosis The most important complication of intestinal schistosome infection is the development of periportal or Symmers' fibrosis and portal hypertension (hepatosplenic schistosomiasis). This finding is pathognomonic in *S. mansoni, S. japonicum,* and *S. mekongi* infections, but it has been studied best in *S. mansoni* infections, where it normally develops after 10 to 15 years of prolonged exposure and infection. The liver may be enlarged, although in many cases it is small, firm, and nodular, and the left lobe is characteristically prominent. Macroscopic examination shows finger-sized bands of fibrosis ("pipe-stem" fibrosis) encompassing the large portal tracts. The portal venous tracts are replaced with fibrous tissue; this situation sometimes leads to presinusoidal blockage, portal hypertension, splenomegaly, and esophageal and gastric varices. The intrahepatic pressure is normal. Hepatic function is generally well preserved, and patients commonly present with hematemesis and/or signs and symptoms of splenomegaly. Ascites, hepatic coma, edema, spider angiomas, gynecomastia, and other signs of liver failure occur less frequently than in alcoholic and postnecrotic cirrhosis. Despite repeated episodes of hematemesis, patients may do reasonably well.

In the past, the diagnosis of periportal fibrosis required a wedge biopsy of the liver; needle biopsy specimens are frequently inadequate. Ultrasonograms of the liver show characteristic findings. The fibrotic bands appear as dense echogenic areas surrounding the portal vein and its tributaries. Studies comparing the effectiveness of wedge biopsy of the liver with ultrasonographic examination showed the latter technique to have both a specificity and a sensitivity of 100 percent. Ultrasonography should replace invasive biopsies as the method of choice for the diagnosis of hepatic schistosomiasis.

Ultrasonographic evaluation of *S. mansoni*–infected populations in the Sudan revealed a much higher prevalence of periportal fibrosis than could be identified by physical examination. As many as half the patients studied lacked palpable splenomegaly, and a majority did not give a history of hematemesis. Treatment resulted in regression of periportal fibrosis in some cases.

Patients with periportal fibrosis may not have schistosome eggs in the feces because of previous treatment and/or attrition of adult worms without subsequent reinfection. Since schistosome infections are practically universal in many populations, the mere presence of schistosome eggs in the feces does not establish the diagnosis of schistosomal periportal fibrosis; other liver diseases may be present. It is not clear whether splenectomy or shunting procedures, although used commonly, are beneficial. Mortality among patients with portal fibrosis has not been well studied, but in one group the rate was 8.2 percent after 3.6 years.

Glomerulonephritis and Pulmonary Hypertension These two complications develop almost exclusively in patients with periportal fibrosis and portal hypertension. Pulmonary hypertension appears to be due to obliteration of pulmonary arterioles by granulomatous inflammation induced by shunted and embolized schistosome eggs. This condition is most frequently recognized with *S. mansoni* and *S. japonicum* infections but is also seen with *S. haematobium.* The association of glomerulonephritis and schistosomiasis has been noted in humans and in experimentally infected animals. This complication is manifested clinically as proteinuria and/or renal failure. Schistosome-specific antibodies and antigens have been detected in the glomeruli of infected patients.

Other Complications Focal dense deposits of eggs of *S. mansoni* in the large intestine (and less commonly of *S. haematobium* and probably of *S. japonicum*) incite an exudative granulomatous response resulting in the formation of inflammatory polyps. Histologic study reveals that these polyps consist of masses of eggs, inflammatory cells, and fibrotic tissue. The major clinical presentation is bloody diarrhea, sometimes associated with protein-losing enteropathy and anemia. This type of involvement of the bowel is recognized primarily in Egypt and the Sudan. Gastrointestinal symptoms are not greater in most chronically infected patients than in control populations, although blood in the stool has been found more frequently in chronic infection in some studies. Granulomatous masses involving the bowel wall may mimic carcinoma of the bowel. With regard to CNS involvement, *S. mansoni* and *S. haematobium* show a predilection for the spinal cord, while the brain is involved more commonly in *S. japonicum* infections. An increased incidence of brain and/or spinal cord involvement has been noted in foreign visitors infected with *S. haematobium* via contact with water from Lake Malawi in southeastern Africa.

Patients infected with the three major species of schistosomes and subsequently infected with *Salmonella* may develop a prolonged intermittent febrile illness. In *S. haematobium* infections, prolonged excretion of *Salmonella* in the urine is common. In many cases, treatment of the *Salmonella* infection alone is not effective, and specific antischistosomal chemotherapy is also required. *Salmonella* may be protected from host immune responses by residence in the schistosome gut or by adherence to the surface of the schistosome.

SCHISTOSOMA MANSONI **Epidemiology and Manifestations** *S. mansoni* is found in South America, in certain Caribbean islands, in Africa, and in the Middle East. The prepatent period is about 4 to 5 weeks. The intermediate hosts are various species in the genus *Biomphalaria*.

Although infection is frequent and sometimes universal in endemic areas, the development of disease is relatively uncommon and depends on a number of factors, including the duration and intensity of infection. In endemic populations, chronic infections are usual, often lasting for decades, and disease manifestations develop in a predictable manner. For the most part, the initial infection of persons living in endemic areas goes unnoticed. Throughout the first decade of life, the intensity of infection—as measured by the number of eggs excreted in the feces—increases in endemic populations, and prevalence rates in this age group often approach 100 percent in highly endemic communities. Few, if any, symptoms are attributable to schistosomiasis during this time. The liver, particularly the left lobe, gradually enlarges and becomes firm. Between 10 and 15 years of age, some heavily infected persons develop splenomegaly, which partly reflects the presence of portal fibrosis and portal hypertension. At about the same time, the number of eggs in the feces decreases; there is evidence to suggest that immune factors as well as decreased water contact are responsible. During the next three decades of life, persons with portal fibrosis and hypertension may experience repeated bouts of hematemesis secondary to esophageal varices or symptoms secondary to a massively enlarged spleen. Because of prior chemotherapy, decreased exposure, or increased host immunity, it is not uncommon for patients with end-stage portal fibrosis to no longer excrete eggs. Adult schistosomes can survive for 20 years or more in the human host but usually live for 5 to 8 years. The prognosis and the potential for reversing complications of infection after appropriate chemotherapy depend on the stage of disease. Ultrasound examination indicates that some regression of periportal fibrosis follows chemotherapy, but in most individuals with advanced periportal fibrosis and clinical manifestations, regression does not occur. Glomerulonephritis and cor pulmonale secondary to schistosomiasis develop exclusively in patients with portal fibrosis. The CNS can become involved at any stage, whatever the intensity of infection.

Diagnosis The diagnosis of *S. mansoni* infection is established by identification of ova in the feces or tissues. The ova are 114 to 175 μm in length and 45 to 68 μm in width and have a prominent lateral spine. In light infections with fewer than 50 eggs per gram of feces, ova may not be detected in the stool without the use of techniques that sample large volumes. Even in light infections, ova can usually be detected in rectal biopsy specimens and are best identified by squashing a small amount of tissue between two glass slides and viewing the tissue microscopically.

Many serologic tests have been employed in the diagnosis of schistosomiasis. These tests are not standardized and differ in sensitivity and specificity. Most current tests have greater than 90 percent sensitivity, and a positive serologic test result is indicative of a present or past infection. An immunofluorescent antibody test employing sections of adult schistosomes to assess the presence of antibodies to schistosome gut antigens has been extremely useful in identifying recently infected persons or those with acute schistosomiasis. Recently, antigen detection assays have been developed that appear to be useful in diagnosing infections and determining treatment response.

TREATMENT

Because drugs used to treat schistosomiasis are relatively safe and effective, most persons with active infections should be treated. These patients carry live eggs that can be identified by microscopy (by an experienced parasitologist), by the presence of flame cells, or by the ability of the eggs to hatch after contact with water. In the past, because of the toxicity of older treatment regimens, chemotherapy was offered only to relatively heavily infected individuals, who were more likely to develop disease than those less intensely infected. However, even in light infections, there is the risk that complications will arise from ectopic location of the schistosome eggs (e.g., in the spinal cord). Relatively few ova may be excreted in schistosomiasis, and their detection therefore may not be easy. Infection may be suggested by a positive result in a serologic test. Because treatment of lightly infected persons with praziquantel is associated with few signs and symptoms, such treatment may be warranted if active infection is likely or cannot be reasonably ruled out. The effectiveness of treatment is evaluated by the cessation of egg excretion after 2 to 3 months. Some types of serologic tests revert to negative after treatment, but these tests are technically difficult to perform and are not generally available. Successful treatment is associated with a reduction of organomegaly and of periportal fibrosis and/or inflammation in some patients. These patients tend to be young people with less severe involvement.

Although a number of drugs are available for the treatment of *S. mansoni* infection, praziquantel and oxamniquine are the drugs of choice (Table 224-2). The two drugs are equally safe and effective in *S. mansoni* infections found in the Caribbean and South America. Because some strains of *S. mansoni* in Africa are relatively resistant to oxamniquine, praziquantel is the better drug. Both drugs can be used in patients with portal fibrosis. The side effects of praziquantel and oxamniquine are frequent but transient and mild. In the author's experience, many of the troublesome side effects associated with praziquantel treatment are the result of the host's response to the injured parasites or ova. Since the worms reside mostly in the intestines, these adverse effects are primarily intestinal and include abdominal pain, lethargy, diarrhea, and fever. In contrast, use of the same drug in the treatment of cysticercosis, in which the worms commonly reside in the CNS, causes symptoms related to the brain. The side effects of oxamniquine include dizziness, tiredness, nausea and vomiting, neuropsychiatric manifestations, and (in rare instances) convulsions.

***SCHISTOSOMA JAPONICUM* Epidemiology and Clinical Manifestations** *S. japonicum* is found in Southeast Asia and is an important health concern in areas of China and the Philippines. The intermediate hosts are amphibious snails of the genus *Oncomelania*. Besides humans, numerous other mammals, such as cattle and water

Table 224-2

Treatment of Schistosomiasis

Species	Drug	Total Dose* (mg/kg of Body Weight)	Regimen
S. haematobium	Praziquantel	40	Single dose or two doses of 20 mg/kg
	Metrifonate†	22.5–30	Single dose of 7.5 to 10 mg/kg given every other week × 3
S. mansoni			
Americas and Caribbean	Oxamniquine	15	Single dose with food
	Praziquantel	40	Single dose or two doses of 20 mg/kg 4 h apart with food
Africa and Middle East	Oxamniquine	60	15 mg/kg twice a day for 2 days with food
	Praziquantel	40	Single dose or two doses of 20 mg/kg 4 h apart with food
S. japonicum or *S. mekongi*	Praziquantel	60	20 mg/kg every 4 h with food

* All recommended drugs are given orally.

† Available from the Parasitic Diseases Division, Center for Infectious Diseases, Centers for Disease Control and Prevention, Atlanta, GA 30333.

buffalo, are naturally infected and serve as reservoirs of infection. The prepatent period is about 4 weeks.

The course of infection and clinical manifestations for *S. japonicum* are similar to those for *S. mansoni*, but the epidemiology and disease manifestations have been less well studied. Experimental infections with *S. japonicum* are more virulent than those with *S. mansoni*, probably because each *S. japonicum* worm pair produces 10 times as many eggs as each *S. mansoni* worm pair. The granulomas contain clusters of eggs, are larger than those caused by *S. mansoni*, and frequently show central necrosis. As in *S. mansoni* infections, periportal fibrosis is the major clinical manifestation. The other clinical syndromes described in *S. mansoni* infection also occur as complications of *S. japonicum* infection. However, there are some notable differences in disease manifestations, particularly CNS involvement. In acute schistosomiasis associated with *S. japonicum* infections, about 2 to 3 percent of patients experience CNS symptoms and signs that mimic acute encephalitis or a focal neurologic process. Computed tomography shows multiple enhancing lesions. In chronic infections, patients may present with focal lesions of the brain that mimic brain tumors. These lesions contain masses of eggs and granulomas. Uncontrolled studies suggest that treatment with antischistosomal drugs and glucocorticoids is effective.

Diagnosis The principles of diagnosis are similar to those used in *S. mansoni* infection and require the demonstration of the typical ova in the tissues or feces of infected individuals. The eggs are oval in shape, measure 70 to 100 μm by 50 to 65 μm, and have a vestigial spine. Old, calcified, dead eggs are commonly retained in the tissues for long periods and do not indicate active infection. Computed tomography shows a characteristic pattern of calcified eggs in the liver and intestine.

 TREATMENT
Most infected persons should be treated. The only safe and effective therapy for *S. japonicum* infections is praziquantel (see Table 224-2).

SCHISTOSOMA MEKONGI *S. mekongi* occurs in the Mekong River in Indochina (Laos, Cambodia, and Thailand). The intermediate host is an aquatic snail, *Tricula aperta*. The eggs are similar to those of *S. japonicum* but are slightly smaller (about 56 by 64 μm) and round. Dogs and human beings frequently are naturally infected. The prepatent period is about 5 weeks. The disease manifestations appear to be similar to those for *S. japonicum* but have not been fully documented. Praziquantel is effective therapy for this infection (see Table 224-2).

SCHISTOSOMA HAEMATOBIUM **Epidemiology and Clinical Manifestations** *S. haematobium* infections occur in extensive areas of Africa and in the Middle East. The intermediate hosts are of the genus *Bulinus*. The prepatent period is 2 to 3 months. Natural infection is primarily limited to human beings.

As in *S. mansoni* infection, the prevalence and intensity of *S. haematobium* infection among persons in endemic areas increase until 10 to 15 years of age. Thereafter, the intensity decreases markedly, while the prevalence rate falls moderately. Owing to the predilection of *S. haematobium* for the veins of the urinary tract, the signs and symptoms caused by the organism result from involvement of the ureters and bladder. In contrast to the asymptomatic period following initial infection with the intestinal schistosomes, dysuria and hematuria are frequently noted 2 to 3 months after *S. haematobium* infection. These findings may continue throughout the course of active infection. Initially, the eggs evoke an intense inflammatory and granulomatous response, which may cause anatomic and/or functional obstruction, hydroureter and hydronephrosis, and masses in the bladder or ureters. Cystoscopic examination may reveal friable masses extending into the bladder, ulceration, petechiae, and granulomas. These early lesions are reversible by antischistosomal chemotherapy. Eggs shed into the urine are usually easily demonstrable. As the infection progresses, the inflammatory component lessens, possibly owing to a modulating effect of the host's immune response, and fibrosis increases, most likely owing to the accumulation of many old and some new lesions. Later, most lesions consist of masses of dead and calcified eggs in

fibrous tissue. When the concentration of calcified eggs in the tissues is high enough, radiographic opacification of the affected areas of the urinary tract becomes evident. Fibrotic lesions that cause hydroureter and hydronephrosis are not reversible by antischistosomal chemotherapy. Renal failure occurs in a surprisingly small proportion of infected individuals.

Portal fibrosis and clinically significant glomerulonephritis are not complications of this infection, but passage of eggs into the lungs may result in pulmonary hypertension. Prolonged excretion of *Salmonella* in the urine and intermittent bacteremia are well documented. Urinary tract infections with other bacteria do not appear to be increased in frequency unless there is instrumentation of the urinary tract; however, they may be difficult to eradicate once established. CNS infection most commonly involves the spinal cord, as in *S. mansoni* infections. Although eggs of *S. haematobium* are frequently detected in the feces in low numbers and are often found in rectal biopsy specimens, intestinal polyposis is uncommon. In certain geographic areas, squamous cell cancer of the bladder is thought to be associated with *S. haematobium* infection and is a significant cause of morbidity and mortality.

Diagnosis The diagnosis of *S. haematobium* infection is established by demonstration of the characteristic eggs in the tissues or urine. These eggs measure 112 to 170 μm by 40 to 70 μm, have a prominent terminal spine, and are easily seen in the urine. An increased number of eggs is excreted around midday, and microscopic examination of a centrifuged urine specimen collected at this time usually reveals ova. In light infections, examination of increased volumes of urine is sometimes required. Gross or microscopic hematuria is common in endemic populations, and its presence always suggests the diagnosis in exposed individuals. Antibodies to *S. haematobium* can be detected with *S. mansoni* antigen preparations. Ultrasonographic examinations reveal anatomic alteration of the genitourinary tract.

 TREATMENT
Infected persons should be treated. Dead and calcified eggs are common in tissue, are often seen in urine specimens, and should be differentiated from viable eggs. Although a number of drugs have been used to treat *S. haematobium* infection, praziquantel is the treatment of choice (see Table 224-2). Metrifonate—a safe, orally administered agent—is also effective. Its major advantage is low cost, and its major disadvantage is that, to cure infection, it needs to be given in three doses 2 weeks apart.

SCHISTOSOMA INTERCALATUM *S. intercalatum* infection is limited to areas of West Africa. Eggs (140 to 240 μm by 50 to 85 μm) are found in the stool and have a terminal spine. Few symptoms are attributable to this infection, and no cases of portal fibrosis have been reported. Praziquantel is effective for treatment.

SCHISTOSOME DERMATITIS (SWIMMERS' ITCH) When cercariae penetrate the skin, they may provoke a reaction known as *schistosome dermatitis*. Symptoms develop most commonly after penetration by schistosomes that ordinarily infect birds or mammals other than humans. In previously unexposed persons, the initial invasion causes transient itching and occasionally urticaria followed by the development of macules within 24 h and papules after 24 h. Following repeated exposures, the signs and symptoms increase dramatically and occur earlier. Large, pruritic, erythematous papules and (uncommonly) vesicles develop within 24 h. The lesions are most intense 2 to 3 days following exposure and subside after a few days. These lesions represent a delayed hypersensitivity reaction to the invading schistosome. Nonhuman schistosomes do not develop fully in humans, and the signs and symptoms are limited to the skin. A similar dermatitis follows infection with human schistosomes.

Schistosome dermatitis develops after exposure to fresh water in many areas of the world but is particularly common in the north-central and western United States. Dermatitis following seawater exposure (clam diggers' itch) also has been described.

Treatment is based on symptoms. Since cercariae need some time to invade the skin (15 min or less), rapid removal of cercaria-containing droplets after water contact will decrease the intensity of exposure. Limiting the numbers of the intermediate host snail in areas frequented by humans can effectively control exposure.

CONTROL OF SCHISTOSOMIASIS Theoretically, schistosome infections can be controlled by a variety of methods, but the application of these control techniques has generally been only partially successful. Simple and effective health-education measures, such as the elimination of indiscriminate urination and defecation, are difficult to implement in endemic areas. The intermediate molluscan host can be eliminated by the use of molluscicides or the destruction of its habitat. Both methods require dedication of resources and personnel that often are not readily available. Mass chemotherapy of populations has been tried; the need for repeated treatments depends on the degree of reinfection. Some authorities advocate the treatment of persons likely to develop serious disease (e.g., those heavily infected). The methods employed will depend on the nature of the endemic area and the resources available.

OTHER TREMATODES

BILIARY DUCT–DWELLING TREMATODES: *CLONORCHIS SINENSIS, OPISTHORCHIS VIVERRINI, AND OPISTHORCHIS FELINEUS* These closely related trematodes commonly infect the human biliary system, have similar life cycles and routes of infection, appear to have similar pathophysiology and disease manifestations, and produce similar eggs. They are responsible for symptoms and signs related to obstruction of the biliary tract or pancreatic duct and are associated with an increased risk of cholangiocarcinoma. *C. sinensis* is endemic in China, Taiwan, Korea, Japan, and Vietnam; *O. viverrini* is found in Laos and Thailand; and *O. felineus* is found in parts of eastern Europe and the former U.S.S.R.

Life Cycle Humans become infected after ingesting metacercariae in poorly cooked, pickled, or smoked fish. The metacercariae excyst in the small intestine and migrate through the ampulla of Vater into the biliary ducts, where they mature in 3 to 4 weeks. Worms are 7 to 20 mm by 1.5 to 3 mm (depending on the species) and may live for 20 to 25 years (*C. sinensis*).

Pathophysiology Disease manifestations (mostly described for *O. viverrini* and *C. sinensis*) depend on the duration of infection, worm burden, and location of the parasites. Flukes reside mostly in small to medium-sized biliary ducts but at times are also found in the larger biliary ducts as well as the gallbladder. They do not invade the parenchyma of the liver, and most disease manifestations reflect direct or indirect effects of the adult trematodes on the biliary ducts. Their presence leads to adenomatous hyperplasia and varying amounts of periductal inflammation followed by periductal fibrosis. Diffuse and localized dilation of ducts due to obstruction by worms, stones, or strictures is frequently found. Remnants of parasites have been found in biliary stones. The number of persons with disease in a given population increases with the worm burden (thousands of flukes in heavy infections), and manifestations include the findings noted above as well as enlarged gallbladder, cholelithiasis, cholecystitis, and cholangiocarcinoma. The last is found with much greater frequency in *O. viverrini* and *C. sinensis* endemic areas and is an important cause of death. In heavy infections, flukes are also found in the pancreatic duct and may be associated with pancreatitis.

Clinical Manifestations Acute infections are infrequently recognized and are characterized by fever, eosinophilia, and hepatomegaly. In endemic areas, almost the entire population may be infected; however, most are lightly infected and asymptomatic. More heavily infected persons suffer vague constitutional complaints and symptoms associated with cholelithiasis and pancreatitis. The liver may be enlarged and tender. Ascending cholangitis is a serious complication. Cholangiocarcinomas usually are associated with proximal obstruction

and subsequent massive dilation of the biliary ducts. Ultrasonography reveals varying degrees of peripheral dilation of the biliary ducts without proximal obstruction. Biliary stones and flukes also may be noted ultrasonographically. Endoscopic cholangiopancreatography reveals ductal dilation, proliferation, irregularities, and blunting of the terminal branches in a majority of cases. Adult worms are visualized as multiple filling defects.

Diagnosis and Treatment Diagnosis is based on the clinical presentation and the detection of the characteristic ova in the feces or bile. Worms can be visualized by a number of techniques and are frequently noted at surgery. Eggs measure about 30 by 12 μm and are ovoid in shape. At the smaller end, an operculum—a sort of cap—appears to rest on a rim that protrudes slightly from the eggs. The other end is broader and has a median knob. The eggs of *C. sinensis* and *O. viverrini* are difficult to tell apart, but those of *O. felineus* are somewhat longer and thinner. The treatment of choice is praziquantel (25 mg/kg tid for 1 day).

LUNG-DWELLING TREMATODES: *PARAGONIMUS WESTERMANI* **AND RELATED SPECIES** More than 30 species of *Paragonimus* have been described, and a number of these infect humans. Adult flukes reside mainly in the lungs, but ectopic localization is relatively common. *P. westermani*, found in the Far East, is the most common species causing infection in humans. Others include *Paragonimus skrjabini (szechuanensis)* (China), *Paragonimus heterotrema* (Southeast Asia), *Paragonimus philippinensis* (Philippines), *Paragonimus mexicanus* (Central America and parts of South America), *Paragonimus africanus* (Nigeria and Cameroon), and *Paragonimus uterobilateralis* (Nigeria and other areas of West Africa). *Paragonimus kellicotti* is indigenous to the United States but has rarely been documented in humans.

Life Cycle Humans become infected primarily by ingesting poorly cooked or pickled crabs or crayfish. Metacercariae excyst in the duodenum and within 1 h pass through the intestinal wall into the peritoneal cavity. After 3 to 6 h they migrate into the abdominal wall and then through the diaphragm into the pleura and lung tissue, where they become encapsulated, usually in pairs or triplets. It takes 65 to 90 days for the flukes to develop fully, although symptoms may begin earlier. Eggs are shed around the worm and, with rupture of the contents of the encapsulated cyst into the bronchioles, are excreted in the sputum or swallowed and excreted in the feces. Adults measure 7.5 to 12 mm by 4 to 6 mm by 3.5 to 5 mm and may live for 20 years.

Pathophysiology Disease is caused by the inflammation and fibrosis elicited by the worms in the lungs or in ectopic locations. Manifestations depend on the duration of infection and probably on the intensity of infection, although the latter association is not well documented. Flukes and eggs initially elicit an acute inflammatory response, mostly consisting of eosinophils, which is followed by the formation of a fibrous capsule. In the lung parenchyma, the cysts rupture into the bronchioles, extruding blood, eggs, and inflammatory exudate. Pleura-based lesions cause eosinophilic empyemas that can be confused clinically with tuberculosis. Lesions in long-standing infections exhibit increased fibrosis and decreased inflammatory responses, and some eventually calcify. Not uncommonly, flukes are found in abnormal locations, including the pleura, abdominal wall, viscera, and brain, where they elicit inflammation and fibrosis. Brain involvement is a particularly serious complication. Although frequent and severe bacterial infections may be associated with paragonimiasis, this relationship has not been substantiated. Ectopic lesions of the abdominal wall and liver are hallmarks of *P. skrjabini* infections.

Clinical Manifestations Manifestations can be both acute and chronic. Acute disease is noted infrequently and may include fever, hepatosplenomegaly, cough, eosinophilia, pleural effusions, pulmonary abnormalities, pneumothorax, and signs and symptoms referable to ectopic locations. The findings in chronic infections often include cough, expectoration of rusty or pigmented sputum, and hemoptysis. Dyspnea, chest pain, fever, and constitutional symptoms are found less frequently. Chest x-ray findings are varied, nondiagnostic, and often confused with those of tuberculosis. Localized or multisegmental infiltrates, usually poorly defined, are most common, but nodular, cystic, cavitary, ring shadow patterns are also found. Other findings include pleural effusions, empyemas, pleural thickening, and calcification of lesions. In contrast to the findings in tuberculosis, apical lesions do not predominate, cavities are smooth and regular, and infiltrates are less well defined. Although lung involvement alone appears to cause little mortality, morbidity and mortality are significant with ectopic lesions. In one series, 30.7 and 8.4 percent of hospitalized patients had ectopic lesions and brain involvement, respectively. Both acute and chronic forms of brain involvement are recognized: the former associated with the sudden onset of neurologic symptoms, usually in the presence of pulmonary disease, and the latter most often associated with seizures and long-term deficits. "Soap bubble" calcifications are a characteristic x-ray pattern in chronic neuroparagonimiasis.

Diagnosis and Treatment The diagnosis is established by detection of the characteristic ova in stool or sputum. The golden-brown eggs are unembryonated and measure 80 to 118 μm by 48 to 60 μm. Concentration techniques may be needed for the detection of eggs in lightly infected patients. Serologic tests are available and may be particularly useful in lightly infected individuals or those with suspected ectopic lesions. In acute disease, eggs may not be detected until 2 to 3 months after exposure. Praziquantel is the treatment of choice at 25 mg/kg three times a day for 2 days. Bithionol is also effective but is more toxic.

LIVER-DWELLING TREMATODES: *FASCIOLA HEPATICA* Humans are infected accidentally with this parasite of sheep, cattle, and other ruminants. Acute manifestations consist of a combination of systemic symptoms and signs and manifestations directly referable to invasion of the liver. Chronic disease has many features indistinguishable from those caused by the other liver flukes.

Life Cycle Ruminants become infected after ingestion of metacercariae encysted on aquatic vegetation. Watercress is commonly implicated in human infections. Metacercariae excyst in the duodenum, pass through the intestine into the peritoneum, invade the liver through Glisson's capsule, and eventually reside in the biliary ducts. In humans, the flukes require at least 3 to 4 months to mature, but eggs may not be detected in stool. Adults are relatively large, measuring 30 by 13 mm. Infections occur worldwide in areas where sheep and cattle are raised, including Europe, Australia, and other developed countries. Endogenously acquired infections are rare in the continental United States but occur in Puerto Rico.

Pathophysiology The severity of infection depends on its intensity and duration and the responses of the host. Early manifestations are due to migration of the flukes through the tissues. Punctate hemorrhages, tracts, and nodules are seen on the surface of the liver and constitute points of entry, migration routes, and areas of encapsulated eosinophilic abscesses, respectively. Granulomatous reactions also occur around eggs themselves. In chronic infections, worms reside in the biliary system, and the anatomic changes caused by the worms generally resemble those caused by other liver flukes. However, intermittent obstruction of the biliary passages by worms appears more common in fascioliasis and leads to periods of jaundice.

Clinical Findings Fever, hepatomegaly and/or abdominal pain, and eosinophilia are the hallmarks of acute fascioliasis, which usually begins within 2 to 3 months following ingestion. Nausea, diarrhea, cough, and urticaria are also frequent. Elevation of liver function values is inconstant, anemia is usually evident, and the erythrocyte sedimentation rate is commonly elevated. Untreated, the disease lasts from months to years, but the manifestations change and with time more closely resemble those of other liver fluke infections, including intermittent obstruction, gallbladder and biliary duct thickening, cholecystitis, lithiasis, and the development of strictures. Ectopic localization of flukes is also relatively common and leads to findings related to the invaded tissue. In contrast to the other liver flukes, *F. hepatica* has no apparent association with cholangiocarcinoma. Because exposure is sometimes long-standing, acute and chronic manifestations may occur at the same time. Computed tomography scans show multiple, hypodense, irregular lesions in the liver; ultrasonography sometimes fails to detect these lesions but is helpful in detecting resulting biliary duct pathology.

Diagnosis The presence of fever, eosinophilia, and hepatomegaly or liver pain in the proper clinical setting suggests the diagnosis. Definitive diagnosis is established by the detection of ova in the feces and/or by serologic tests. Ova may not be detected in the feces because the disease becomes manifest before patency, because the ova are unable to pass into the biliary system, or because the worms are in an ectopic location or there is a low level of excretion of ova. Therefore, stool concentration methods should be employed. The ova of *F. hepatica* are immature in the feces, measure 130 to 150 μm by 90 μm, and are indistinguishable from those of *Fasciolopsis buski* (see below).

℞ TREATMENT

Although praziquantel is effective for other trematodes, it does not appear to be very effective in *F. hepatica* infection, and bithionol at 30 to 50 mg/kg on alternate days for 10 to 15 doses is the treatment of choice. Infections also have been treated successfully with the experimental drugs triclabendazole and albendazole.

INTESTINE-DWELLING TREMATODES *Fasciolopsis buski* One of the largest parasites infecting humans, *F. buski* measures 20 to 70 mm by 8 to 20 mm by 0.5 to 3 mm and resides in the small intestine and occasionally in the colon or pylorus. Geographically, it is confined to the Far East. The adults attach to the intestinal epithelium, causing ulcerations and localized inflammation. Light infections are generally asymptomatic, but persons heavily infected have diarrhea, fever, and abdominal pain and may develop ascites, anasarca, and intestinal obstruction. The pathophysiology of *F. buski* infection has not been well studied. The diagnosis is established by the detection of ova (indistinguishable from those of *F. hepatica*) in the feces. The treatment of choice is praziquantel (25 mg/kg tid for 1 day).

Heterophyes heterophyes and *Metagonimus yokogawai* The major clinical manifestation of infection with both of these tiny (about 1 mm) intestine-dwelling parasites is diarrhea. Humans acquire infection after the ingestion of undercooked freshwater fish. *H. heterophyes* and *M. yokogawai* are found in the Far East, but the former is also common in the Nile Delta and is present in other areas of the Middle East. The worms attach to and at times burrow into the intestinal mucosa, eliciting inflammatory responses. Ova of *H. heterophyes* have been found in the heart and other organs and have reportedly caused clinically significant myocarditis. The diagnosis is established by the detection of ova in the feces; the ova of the two species are identical and resemble those of *C. sinensis* and related parasites. Praziquantel is the drug of choice (25 mg/kg tid for 1 day).

Nanophyetus salmincola This tiny small-intestine–dwelling trematode has recently infected humans in the Pacific Northwest. It was previously known to infect humans in eastern Siberia. Infections follow the ingestion of undercooked, smoked, or raw fish, usually salmon or trout. Symptoms vary from asymptomatic carriage to watery diarrhea, abdominal pain, bloating, and other gastrointestinal problems. Eosinophilia is found in most cases but is not universal. Unembryonated ova (64 to 97 μm by 34 to 55 μm) appear in the feces after 1 week but are excreted in low numbers so that concentration techniques are needed for detection. The treatment of choice is praziquantel (20 mg/kg tid for 1 day).

BIBLIOGRAPHY

Cheever AW: Infection versus disease and hypersensitivity versus immunity. Am J Pathol 142:699, 1993

Dragana J, Sher A: Initiation and regulation of CD4 + T-cell function in host-parasite models. Chem Immunol 63:51, 1996

Elkins DB et al: A high frequency of hepatobiliary disease and suspected cholangiocarcinoma associated with heavy *Opisthorchis viverrini* infection in a small community in northeast Thailand. Trans R Soc Trop Med Hyg 84:715, 1990

Fritsche TR et al: Praziquantel for treatment of human *Nanophyetus salmincola (Troglotrema salmincola)* infection. J Infect Dis 160:896, 1989

Gutierrez Y: *Diagnostic Pathology of Parasitic Infections with Clinical Correlations.* Philadelphia, Lea & Febiger, 1990

HAGAN P: Reinfection, exposure and immunity in human schistosomiasis. Parasitol Today 8:12, 1992

HOMEIDA M: Diagnosis of pathologically confirmed Symmers' periportal fibrosis by ultrasonography: A prospective blinded study. Am J Trop Med Hyg 39:86, 1988

———— et al: Morbidity associated with Schistosoma mansoni infection as determined by ultrasound: A study in Gezira, Sudan. Am J Trop Med Hyg 39:196, 1988

———— et al: Association of the therapeutic activity of praziquantel with the reversal of Symmers' fibrosis induced by Schistosoma mansoni. Am J Trop Med Hyg 45:360, 1991

NASH TE et al: Schistosome infections in humans: Perspective and recent findings. Ann Intern Med 97:740, 1982

SAAD AMA et al: Oesophageal varices in region of the Sudan endemic for Schistosoma mansoni. Br J Surg 78:1252, 1991

SINGH TS et al: Pulmonary paragonimiasis: Clinical features, diagnosis and treatment of 39 cases in Manipur. Trans R Soc Trop Med Hyg 80:967, 1986

SITHITHAWORN P et al: Quantitative post-mortem study of Opisthorchis viverrini in man in northeast Thailand. Trans R Soc Trop Med Hyg 85:765, 1991

TAKEYAMA N et al: Computed tomography findings of hepatic lesions in human fascioliasis: Report of two cases. Am J Gastroenterol 81:1078, 1986

WYNN TA: An IL-12-based vaccination method for preventing fibrosis induced by schistosome infection. Nature 376:594, 1995

YOKOGAWA M: Epidemiology and control of paragonimiasis, in Parasitic Diseases, EM Sasa (ed). Tokyo, International Medical Foundation of Japan, 1974, pp 137–149

| 225 | *Thomas B. Nutman, Peter F. Weller* |

CESTODES

Cestodes, or tapeworms, are segmented worms. The adults reside in the gastrointestinal tract, but the larvae can be found in almost any organ. Human tapeworm infections can be divided into two major clinical groups. In one group, humans are the definitive hosts, and the adult tapeworms live in the gastrointestinal tract (*Taenia saginata*, *Diphyllobothrium*, *Hymenolepis*, and *Dipylidium caninum*). In the other, humans are intermediate hosts, and larval-stage parasites are present in the tissues. Diseases in this category include echinococcosis, sparganosis, and coenurosis. For *Taenia solium*, the human may be either the definitive or the intermediate host.

The ribbon-shaped tapeworm attaches to the intestinal mucosa by means of sucking cups or grooves located on the head (scolex). Behind the scolex is a short, narrow neck from which proglottids (segments) form. As each proglottid matures, it is displaced further back from the neck by the formation of new, less mature segments. The progressively elongating chain of attached proglottids, called the *strobila*, constitutes the bulk of the tapeworm; it may consist of more than 1000 proglottids and may be several meters long. As each proglottid becomes gravid, eggs are released. Since eggs of the different *Taenia* species are morphologically identical, differences in the morphology of the scolex or proglottids provide the only basis for diagnostic identification to the species level. Most human tapeworms require at least one intermediate host for complete larval development. After ingestion by an intermediate host, an egg develops into a larval oncosphere capable of penetrating the intestinal mucosa. The oncosphere migrates to tissues and develops into an encysted form known as a *cysticercus* (single scolex), a *coenurus* (multiple scolices), or a *hydatid* (cyst with daughter cysts, each containing several scolices). Ingestion by the definitive host of tissues containing a cyst enables a scolex to develop into a tapeworm.

TAENIASIS SAGINATA The beef tapeworm *T. saginata* occurs in all countries where raw or undercooked beef is eaten. It is most prevalent in sub-Saharan African and Middle Eastern countries.

Etiology and Pathogenesis Humans are the only definitive host for the adult stage of *T. saginata*. This tapeworm, which can reach 3 to 8 m in length, inhabits the upper jejunum and has a scolex with four prominent suckers and 1000 to 2000 proglottids. Each gravid segment has 15 to 30 uterine branches (in contrast to 8 to 12 for *T. solium*). The eggs are indistinguishable from those of *T. solium*; each measures 30 to 40 μm and has a thick brown striated shell containing a fully developed embryo. Eggs deposited on vegetation can live for months to years until they are ingested by cattle or other herbivores. The embryo released after ingestion invades the intestinal wall and is carried to striated muscle (predominantly in the hind limbs, diaphragm, and tongue), where it transforms into a cysticercus. When ingested in raw or undercooked beef, this form can infect humans. After the cysticercus is ingested, it takes about 2 months for an adult worm to develop.

Clinical Manifestations Patients become aware of the infection most commonly by noting passage of proglottids in their feces. They may experience perianal discomfort when proglottids are discharged. Although usually minimal or mild, abdominal pain or discomfort, nausea, change in appetite, weakness, and weight loss can occur with *T. saginata* infection.

Diagnosis The diagnosis is made by the detection of eggs or proglottids in the stool as soon as about 3 months after infection. Eggs also may be present in the perianal area; thus, if proglottids or eggs are not found in the stool, the perianal region should be examined with use of a cellophane-tape swab (as in pinworm infection). The distinguishing of *T. saginata* from *T. solium* requires examination of mature proglottids or the scolex. Serologic tests are not helpful diagnostically. Eosinophilia and elevated levels of serum IgE may be detected.

℞ TREATMENT

A single dose of praziquantel (5 to 10 mg/kg) is highly effective for therapy.

Prevention The major means of preventing infection is the adequate cooking of beef; exposure to temperatures as low as 56°C for 5 min will destroy cysticerci. Refrigeration or salting for long periods or freezing at −10°C for 9 days also kills cysticerci in beef. General preventive measures include inspection of beef and proper disposal of human feces.

TAENIASIS SOLIUM AND CYSTICERCOSIS The pork tapeworm *T. solium* can cause two distinct forms of infection. The form that develops depends on whether humans are infected with adult tapeworms in the intestine or with larval forms in the tissues (cysticercosis). Humans are the only definitive hosts for *T. solium*; pigs are the usual intermediate hosts, although dogs, cats, and sheep may harbor the larval forms. *T. solium* exists worldwide but is most prevalent in Mexico, Africa, Southeast Asia, eastern Europe, and South America. Cysticercosis occurs in industrialized nations largely as a result of the immigration of infected persons from endemic areas.

Etiology and Pathogenesis The adult tapeworm generally resides in the upper jejunum. Its globular scolex attaches by both sucking disks and two rows of hooklets. Often only one adult worm is present, but that worm may live for up to 25 years. The tapeworm, usually about 3 meters in length, may have as many as 1000 proglottids, each of which produces up to 50,000 eggs. Groups of 3 to 5 proglottids generally are released and excreted into the feces, and the eggs in these proglottids are infective for both humans and animals. The eggs survive in the environment for several months. After ingestion by the intermediate host, eggs embryonate, penetrate the intestinal wall, and are carried to many tissues, with a predilection for striated muscle of the neck, tongue, and trunk. Within 60 to 90 days, the encysted larval stage develops. These cysticerci can survive for long periods. Humans acquire infections that lead to intestinal tapeworms by ingesting undercooked pork containing cysticerci. Infections that cause human cysticercosis follow the ingestion of *T. solium* eggs, usually from fecally contaminated food. Autoinfection may occur if an individual with an egg-producing tapeworm ingests eggs derived from his or her own feces or if eggs pass by reflux from the intestine into the stomach.

Clinical Manifestations Intestinal infections with *T. solium* may be asymptomatic. Epigastric discomfort, nausea, a sensation of hunger,

In cysticercosis, the clinical manifestations are entirely different. Since cysticerci can be found anywhere in the body (most commonly in the brain and the skeletal muscle), their location and size determine the clinical presentation. The manifestations of cysticercosis reflect two distinct processes: the local inflammatory response induced by the parasite and the local effect of the space-occupying lesions. Neurologic manifestations constitute the most common presentation. When inflammation surrounds lesions, seizures and focal neurologic deficits are frequent, and communicating and noncommunicating hydrocephalus and meningitis also can be seen. Generalized, focal, or Jacksonian seizures occur in most cases. Signs of increased intracranial pressure, including headache, nausea, vomiting, changes in vision, dizziness, ataxia, and confusion, often are present. Patients with hydrocephalus may develop papilledema and may experience alterations of mental status. The unusual racemose form of cyticercosis is characterized by grapelike clusters of proliferating larval membranes. This form typically occurs at the base of the brain or in the subarachnoid space and causes chronic meningitis and arachnoiditis. Communicating or noncommunicating hydrocephalus is common. The clinical presentation of neurocysticercosis therefore depends on the number, form, and location of cysticerci, the extent of cyst-associated inflammatory responses, and the duration of disease.

Diagnosis The diagnosis of intestinal *T. solium* infection is made by the detection of eggs or proglottids, as described for *T. saginata*. For cysticercosis, definitive diagnosis requires examination of the cysticercus in an involved tissue, but a diagnosis often can be based on clinical presentation in conjunction with compatible results in radiographic studies—especially computed tomography (CT) and magnetic resonance imaging (MRI)—and serologic tests.

For soft tissue involvement, plain films may reveal multiple calcified "puffed-rice" lesions. For cerebral cysticercosis, CT studies demonstrate parenchymal lesions of varying number and size that are either cystic or solid and may exhibit contrast enhancement. Some or many of the lesions seen by CT may be calcified; thus, multiple punctate calcifications are common findings in neurocysticercosis. Ventricular dilation may be demonstrable, but the CT finding of multiple calcified or noncalcified cystic lesions is strongly suggestive of cerebral cysticercosis. MRI detects cystic structures on T_1- and T_2-weighted images as well as high-intensity rims around cysts, particularly on T_2-weighted images. Use of gadolinium contrast enhances the sensitivity of MRI studies. Because CT is more sensitive in identifying calcified lesions and MRI is better at identifying small cystic lesions, both techniques are useful in evaluating neurocysticercosis.

Most patients with cerebral cysticercosis have cerebrospinal fluid (CSF) pleocytosis with a predominance of mononuclear cells. The glucose level is often decreased and the protein level elevated in CSF. Serologic tests of CSF and sera are helpful in establishing the diagnosis. Of the variety of serologic assays that have been used, many have been complicated by cross-reactivity with other tapeworm, filarial, and echinococcal infections. An immunoblotting technique has improved specificity to 98 percent, with sensitivities reaching 91 percent. Even with this technique, however, patients with single intracranial neurocysticercotic lesions may be seronegative.

℞ **TREATMENT**

Intestinal *T. solium* infection is treated with praziquantel, as specified for *T. saginata* infection. However, praziquantel can evoke an inflammatory response in the central nervous system if concomitant cryptic cysticercosis is present.

The management of cysticercosis can involve chemotherapy, surgery, and supportive medical treatment. Asymptomatic patients with calcified soft tissue or neural lesions generally require no treatment. For symptomatic patients with neurocysticercosis, both praziquantel (50 mg/kg per day in three doses for 15 days) and albendazole (15 mg/kg per day in three doses for 8 to 28 days) are effective. Because both agents provoke inflammatory responses around dying cysticerci, patients receiving either drug should be hospitalized and

given high doses of glucocorticoids during treatment. The efficacy of therapy can be monitored by radiographic imaging. The size of active lesions should decrease within 3 to 6 months. For ocular and spinal lesions, drug-induced inflammation may cause irreversible damage; thus, these lesions as well as those within the ventricles are best managed by surgical resection. Ventricular obstruction may require ventriculostomy or ventriculoperitoneal shunting. Not all neurologic deficits resolve after therapy, and some patients may require continued anticonvulsive treatment.

Prevention Measures for the prevention of intestinal *T. solium* infection consist of the application to pork of precautions similar to those described above for beef with regard to *T. saginata* infection. The prevention of cysticercosis involves minimizing the opportunities for ingestion of fecally derived eggs by means of good personal hygiene, effective fecal disposal, and treatment and prevention of human intestinal infections.

ECHINOCOCCOSIS Echinococcosis is an infection of humans caused by the larval stage of *Echinococcus granulosus*, *Echinococcus multilocularis*, or *Echinococcus vogeli*. *E. granulosus*, which produces unilocular cystic lesions, is prevalent in areas where livestock is raised in association with dogs. This tapeworm species is found in Australia, Argentina, Chile, Africa, eastern Europe, the Middle East, New Zealand, and the Mediterranean region, particularly Lebanon and Greece. *E. multilocularis*, which causes multilocular alveolar lesions that are locally invasive, is found in sub-Arctic or Arctic regions, including Canada, the United States, and northern Europe and Asia. *E. vogeli* causes polycystic hydatid disease and is found only in Central and South America. Like other cestodes, echinococcal species have both intermediate and definitive hosts. The definitive hosts are dogs that pass eggs in their feces. Cysts develop in the intermediate hosts—sheep, cattle, humans, goats, camels, and horses for *E. granulosus* and mice and other rodents for *E. multilocularis*—after the ingestion of eggs. When a dog ingests beef or lamb containing cysts, the life cycle is completed.

Etiology The small (5 mm long) adult *E. granulosus* worm, which lives for 5 to 20 months in the jejunum of dogs, has only three proglottids—one immature, one mature, and one gravid. The gravid segment splits to release eggs that are morphologically indistinguishable from *Taenia* eggs and are extremely hardy. After humans ingest the eggs, embryos escape from the eggs, penetrate the intestinal mucosa, enter the portal circulation, and are carried to various organs, most commonly the liver and lungs. Larvae develop into fluid-filled unilocular hydatid cysts that consist of an external membrane and an inner germinal layer. Daughter cysts develop from the inner aspect of the germinal layer, as do germinating cystic structures called *brood capsules*. New larvae, called *scolices*, develop in large numbers within the brood capsule. The cysts expand slowly over a period of years.

The life cycle of *E. multilocularis* is similar except that small rodents serve as the intermediate hosts. The cyst of *E. multilocularis*, however, is quite different in that the larval form remains in the proliferative phase, the hydatid cyst is always multilocular, and vesicles progressively invade the host tissue by peripheral extension of processes from the germinal layer.

Clinical Manifestations Slowly enlarging echinococcal cysts generally remain asymptomatic until their expanding size or their space-occupying effect in an involved organ elicits symptoms. The liver and the lungs are the most common sites of these cysts. Since a period of 5 to 20 years often elapses before cysts enlarge sufficiently to cause symptoms, they may be discovered incidentally on a routine x-ray or ultrasound study.

Patients with hepatic echinococcosis who are symptomatic most often present with abdominal pain or a palpable mass in the right upper quadrant. Compression of a bile duct or leakage of cyst fluid into the biliary tree may mimic recurrent cholelithiasis, and biliary obstruction can result in jaundice. Rupture of or episodic leakage from a hydatid cyst may produce fever, pruritus, urticaria, eosinophilia, or fatal anaphylaxis. Pulmonary hydatid cysts may rupture into the bronchial tree or peritoneal cavity and produce cough, chest pain, or hemoptysis. By spreading the multitudinous infectious scolices, the rupture of hydatid cysts leads to multifocal dissemination of new cyst-forming elements. Rupture can occur spontaneously or at surgery and in the latter instance is especially likely when a cyst is not recognized to be of echinococcal etiology. Cysts may involve any organ. Other presentations are due to the involvement of bone (invasion of the medullary cavity with slow bone erosion producing pathologic fractures), the central nervous system (space-occupying lesions), and the heart (conduction defects, pericarditis).

The cysts of *E. multilocularis* characteristically present as a slowly growing hepatic tumor, with progressive destruction of the liver and extension into vital structures. Patients commonly complain of upper quadrant and epigastric pain, and obstructive jaundice may be apparent. A minority of patients experience the metastasis of lesions to the lung and brain.

Diagnosis Radiographic and related imaging studies are important in detecting and evaluating echinococcal cysts. Plain films will define pulmonary cysts—usually as rounded irregular masses of uniform density—but may miss other cysts in other organs unless there is cyst wall calcification (as occurs in the liver). MRI, CT, and ultrasound reveal well-defined cysts with thick or thin walls. When older cysts contain a layer of hydatid sand that is rich in accumulated scolices, these imaging methods may detect this fluid layer of different density. However, the most pathognomonic finding, if demonstrable, is that of daughter cysts within the larger cyst. This finding, like eggshell or mural calcification on CT, is indicative of *E. granulosus* infection and helps to distinguish the cyst from carcinomas, bacterial or amebic liver abscesses, or hemangiomas. CT of alveolar hydatid cysts reveals indistinct solid masses with central necrosis and plaquelike calcifications.

A specific diagnosis can be made by the examination of aspirated fluids for scoliceal hooklets, but diagnostic aspiration is not conventionally recommended because of the risk of fluid leakage resulting in either dissemination of infection or anaphylactic reactions. However, CT-guided aspiration of hydatid cysts for diagnosis has been used successfully in some centers. Pretreatment with albendazole (a 1-month course) is believed to minimize biopsy complications. Serodiagnostic assays can be useful, although a negative test does not exclude the diagnosis of echinococcosis. While cysts in the liver are more likely to elicit positive antibody responses than those in the lungs, up to 50 percent of infected individuals may have negative serology. Detection of antibody to specific echinococcal antigens by immunoblotting has the highest degree of specificity, although false-positive findings may be obtained in cysticercosis.

℞ **TREATMENT**

Therapy for echinococcosis is based on considerations of the size, location, and manifestations of cysts and the overall health of the patient. Surgery, when feasible, is the principal definitive method of treatment; *E. granulosus* cysts are excised, or tissue containing *E. multilocularis* cysts is resected. Risks at surgery from leakage of fluid include anaphylaxis and dissemination of infectious scolices. The latter complication has been minimized by the instillation of scolicidal solutions such as hypertonic saline or ethanol, which may cause hypernatremia, intoxication, or sclerosing cholangitis. Albendazole, which has antiechinococcal activity, can be administered adjunctively in the perioperative period and may be useful for medical treatment of echinococcosis. While albendazole has shown efficacy, the exact role of chemotherapy, perhaps combined with percutaneous drainage, remains to be defined. As medical therapy, albendazole, given at a dose of 400 mg twice a day for 12 weeks, is most efficacious against hepatic and pulmonary cysts, although multiple courses may be necessary. Response to treatment is best assessed by repeated evaluation of cysts by CT or MRI, with particular attention to cyst size and consistency.

Prevention In endemic areas, echinococcosis can be prevented by administering praziquantel to infected dogs and by denying dogs access to butchering sites and to the offal of infected animals. Limitation of the number of stray dogs is helpful in reducing the prevalence of infection among humans.

HYMENOLEPIASIS NANA Infection with *Hymenolepis nana*, the dwarf tapeworm, is the most common of all the cestode infections. *H. nana* is endemic in both temperate and tropical regions of the world. Infection is spread by fecal/oral contamination and is common among institutionalized children.

Etiology and Pathogenesis *H. nana* is the only cestode of humans that does not require an intermediate host. Both the larval and adult phases take place in the human. The adult, the smallest tapeworm parasitizing humans, is about 2 cm long and dwells in the proximal ileum. Proglottids, which are quite small and are rarely seen in the stool, release spherical eggs 30 to 44 μm in diameter, each of which contains an oncosphere with six hooklets. The eggs are immediately infective and are unable to survive in the external environment for more than 10 days. *H. nana* also can be acquired by the ingestion of infected insects (especially larval meal-worms and larval fleas). When the egg is ingested by a new host, the oncosphere is freed and penetrates the intestinal villi, becoming a cysticercoid larva. Larvae migrate back into the intestinal lumen, attach to the mucosa, and mature over 10 to 12 days into adult worms. Eggs also may hatch before passing into the stool, causing internal autoinfection with increasing numbers of intestinal worms. Although the life span of adult *H. nana* is only about 4 to 10 weeks, the autoinfection cycle perpetuates the infection.

Clinical Manifestations *H. nana* infection, even with many intestinal worms, is usually asymptomatic. When infection is intense, anorexia, abdominal pain, and diarrhea develop.

Diagnosis Infection is diagnosed by the finding of eggs in the stool.

℞ **TREATMENT**

Praziquantel (25 mg/kg once) is the treatment of choice, since it acts against both the adult worms and the cysticercoids in the intestinal villi.

Prevention Good personal hygiene and improved sanitation can eradicate the disease. Epidemics have been controlled by mass chemotherapy coupled with improved hygiene.

HYMENOLEPIASIS DIMINUTA *Hymenolepis diminuta*, a cestode of rodents, occasionally infects small children, who ingest the adult worm in uncooked cereal foods contaminated by fleas and other insects in which larvae develop. Infection is usually asymptomatic and is diagnosed by the detection of eggs in the stool. Treatment with praziquantel results in cure in most cases.

DIPHYLLOBOTHRIASIS *Diphyllobothrium latum* and other *Diphyllobothrium* species are found in the lakes, rivers, and deltas of the northern hemisphere, Central Africa, and Chile.

Etiology and Pathogenesis The adult worm, the longest tapeworm (up to 25 m), attaches to the ileal and occasionally to the jejunal mucosa by its suckers, which are located on its elongated scolex. The adult worm has 3000 to 4000 proglottids, which release approximately 1 million eggs daily into the feces. If an egg reaches water, it hatches and releases a free-swimming embryo that can be eaten by small freshwater crustaceans (*Cyclops* or *Diaptomus* species). After an infected crustacean containing a developed procercoid is swallowed by a fish, the larva migrates into the fish's flesh and grows into a plerocercoid, or sparganum larva. Humans acquire the infection by ingesting infected raw fish. Within 3 to 5 weeks, the tapeworm matures into an adult in the human intestine.

Clinical Manifestations Most *D. latum* infections are asymptomatic, although manifestations may include transient abdominal discomfort, diarrhea, vomiting, weakness, and weight loss. Occasionally, infection can cause acute abdominal pain and intestinal obstruction; in rare cases cholangitis or cholecystitis may be produced by migrating proglottids. Because the tapeworm absorbs large quantities of vitamin B_{12} and interferes with ileal B_{12} absorption, vitamin B_{12} deficiency can develop. Up to 2 percent of infected patients, especially the elderly, have megaloblastic anemia resembling pernicious anemia and may exhibit neurologic sequelae of B_{12} deficiency.

Diagnosis The diagnosis is made readily by the detection of the characteristic eggs in the stool. The eggs possess a single shell with an operculum at one end and a knob at the other. Mild to moderate eosinophilia may be detected.

℞ **TREATMENT**

Praziquantel (5 to 10 mg/kg once) is highly effective. Parenteral vitamin B_{12} should be given if B_{12} deficiency is manifest.

Prevention Infection can be prevented by heating fish to 54°C for 5 min or by freezing it at −18°C for 24 h. Placing fish in brine with a high salt concentration for long periods kills the eggs.

DIPYLIDIASIS *Dipylidium caninum*, a common tapeworm of dogs and cats, may accidentally infect humans. Dogs, cats, and occasionally humans become infected by ingesting fleas harboring cysticercoids. Children are more likely to become infected than adults. Most infections are asymptomatic, but abdominal pain, diarrhea, anal pruritus, urticaria, and eosinophilia can occur. The diagnosis is made by the detection of proglottids in the stool. As in *D. latum* infection, therapy consists of praziquantel. Prevention requires anthelmintic treatment and flea control for pet dogs or cats.

SPARGANOSIS Humans can be infected by the sparganum, or plerocercoid larva, of a diphyllobothrid tapeworm of the genus *Spirometra*. Infection can be acquired by the consumption of water containing infected *Cyclops*; by the ingestion of infected snakes, birds,

or mammals; or by the application of infected flesh as poultices. The worm migrates slowly in tissues, and infection commonly presents as a subcutaneous swelling. Periorbital tissues can be involved, and ocular sparganosis may destroy the eye. Surgical excision is used to treat localized sparganosis.

COENUROSIS This rare infection of humans by the larval stage (coenurus) of the dog tapeworm *Taenia multiceps* or *Taenia serialis* results in a space-occupying cystic lesion. As in cysticercosis, involvement of the central nervous system and subcutaneous tissue is most common. Both definitive diagnosis and treatment require surgical excision of the lesion. Chemotherapeutic agents generally are not effective.

BIBLIOGRAPHY

Botero D et al: Taeniasis and cysticercosis. Infect Dis Clin North Am 7:683, 1993

Flisser A: Taeniasis and cysticercosis due to *Taenia solium*. Prog Clin Parasitol 4:77, 1994

Gil-Grande LA et al: Randomised controlled trial of efficacy of albendazole in intra-abdominal hydatid disease. Lancet 342:1269, 1993

Kammerer WS, Schantz PM: Echinococcal disease. Infect Dis Clin North Am 7:605, 1993

Schaefer JW, Khan MY: Echinococcosis (hydatid disease): Lessons from experience with 59 patients. Rev Infect Dis 13:243, 1991

Schantz PM, Kramer HJ: Larval cestode infections: Cysticercosis and echinococcosis. Curr Opin Infect Dis 8:342, 1995

Scharf D: Neurocysticercosis: Two hundred thirty eight cases from a California hospital. Arch Neurol 46:77, 1989

SECTION 1
DIAGNOSIS

226

Eugene Braunwald

APPROACH TO THE PATIENT WITH HEART DISEASE

The symptoms caused by heart disease result most commonly from myocardial ischemia, from disturbance of the contraction and/or relaxation of the myocardium, from obstruction to blood flow, or from an abnormal cardiac rhythm or rate. Ischemia is manifest most frequently as chest discomfort, while reduction of the pumping ability of the heart commonly leads to weakness and fatigability or, when severe, produces cyanosis, hypotension, syncope, and elevated intravascular pressure behind a failing ventricle; the latter results in abnormal fluid accumulation, which in turn leads to dyspnea, orthopnea, and systemic or pulmonary edema. Obstruction to blood flow, as in valvular stenosis, can cause symptoms resembling those resulting from congestive heart failure. Cardiac arrhythmias often develop suddenly, and the resulting signs and symptoms—palpitation, dyspnea, angina, hypotension, and syncope—generally occur abruptly and may disappear as rapidly as they develop.

A cardinal principle useful in the evaluation of the patient with suspected heart disease is that myocardial or coronary function that may be adequate at rest may be inadequate during exertion. Thus a history of chest discomfort and/or dyspnea that appears only during activity is characteristic of heart disease, while the opposite pattern, i.e., the appearance of these symptoms at rest and their remission during exertion, is rarely observed in patients with organic heart disease.

Patients with cardiocirculatory disease also may be asymptomatic, both at rest and during exertion, but may present an abnormal physical finding, such as a heart murmur, elevated arterial pressure, or an abnormality of the electrocardiogram (ECG) or of the cardiac silhouette on the chest roentgenogram. Patients may exhibit asymptomatic ischemia on an exercise stress test or an ambulatory ECG.

Diseases of the heart and circulation are so common and the laity is so well acquainted with the major symptoms resulting from these disorders that patients, and occasionally physicians, erroneously attribute many noncardiac complaints to cardiovascular disease. The combination of the widespread fear of heart disease with the deep-seated emotional connotations concerning this organ's function results in the frequent development of symptoms that mimic those of organic disease in persons with normal cardiovascular systems. The unraveling of symptoms and signs due to organic heart disease from those not directly related is an important and challenging task in these patients.

Dyspnea, one of the cardinal manifestations of diminished cardiac reserve, is not limited to heart disease but is also characteristic of conditions as diverse as pulmonary disease, marked obesity, and anxiety (Chap. 32). Similarly, chest discomfort may result from a variety of causes other than myocardial ischemia (Chap. 13). Whether heart disease is responsible for these symptoms can frequently be determined by carrying out a careful clinical examination. Noninvasive testing using electrocardiography at rest and during exercise (Chap. 228), echocardiography, roentgenography, and myocardial imaging usually provides important additional information to permit the correct interpretation of symptoms; more specialized invasive examinations (catheterization and angiography; Chap. 229) are occasionally necessary.

DIAGNOSIS   As outlined by the New York Heart Association, the elements of a complete cardiac diagnosis include consideration of

1. *The underlying etiology.* Is the disease congenital, infectious, hypertensive, or ischemic in origin?
2. *The anatomic abnormalities.* Which chambers are involved? Which valves are affected? Is there pericardial involvement? Has there been a myocardial infarction?
3. *The physiologic disturbances.* Is an arrhythmia present? Is there evidence of congestive heart failure or of myocardial ischemia?
4. *The extent of functional disability.* How strenuous is the physical activity required to elicit symptoms? The latter should be evaluated in the light of the intensity of therapy.

One example may serve to illustrate the importance of establishing a complete diagnosis. The identification of myocardial ischemia as the etiology of a patient's exertional chest discomfort is of great clinical importance. However, the recognition of ischemia is insufficient to formulate a therapeutic strategy or prognosis until the underlying anatomic abnormalities responsible for the myocardial ischemia, e.g., coronary atherosclerosis or aortic stenosis, are identified and a judgment made as to whether other physiologic disturbances that cause an imbalance between myocardial oxygen supply and demand, such as severe anemia, thyrotoxicosis, or supraventricular tachycardia, play a contributory role. In many instances, the extent of functional disability is a determinant of whether medical or interventional therapy is utilized.

The establishment of a correct and complete cardiac diagnosis often requires the use of six different methods of examination: (1) history, (2) physical examination (Chap. 227), (3) ECG (Chap. 228), (4) chest roentgenogram, (5) noninvasive graphic examinations (echocardiogram, radionuclide and other noninvasive imaging techniques), and occasionally (6) specialized invasive examinations, i.e., cardiac catheterization, angiocardiography, and coronary arteriography (Chap. 229). In order to be most effective, the results obtained from each of these six modalities should be analyzed independently of one another as well as with the information derived from the other methods clearly in mind. Only in this way can one avoid overlooking a subtle, though important, finding. For example, an ECG should be obtained in every patient suspected of having heart disease. It may provide the critical clue in establishing the correct diagnosis, e.g., the finding of a mild atrioventricular conduction disturbance in a patient with unexplained syncope, even when all other methods of examination reveal no abnormal findings, can be the clue that asystole might be the cause. On the other hand, when combined intelligently with the results of other methods of examination, the ECG may provide essential confirmatory data. Thus the knowledge that a patient has an apical diastolic rumbling murmur may direct particular attention to the P waves, and the recognition of left atrial enlargement electrocardiographically supports the suggestion that the murmur is caused by mitral stenosis. The diagnosis can be confirmed by echocardiography, a technique that can also determine the severity of the obstruction and its effects on cardiac function.

Family History   In obtaining the history of a patient with known or suspected cardiovascular disease, particular attention should be directed to the family history. Familial clustering is common in many forms of heart disease. Genetic transmission may occur, as in hypertrophic cardiomyopathy (Chap. 239), the Marfan syndrome (Chap. 348), and sudden death associated with a prolonged QT syndrome (Chap. 231). In patients with essential hypertension or coronary atherosclerosis, the genetic component may be less obvious but is also of considerable importance. Familial clustering of cardiovascular diseases may occur not only on a genetic basis but also may be related to familial dietary or behavior patterns, such as excessive ingestion of salt or calories or cigarette smoking.

Assessment of Functional Impairment When an attempt is made to determine the severity of functional impairment in a patient with heart disease, it is helpful to ascertain with as much precision as possible the level of activity and the rate at which it is performed before symptoms develop. Thus breathlessness that occurs after running up two long flights of stairs denotes far less functional impairment than similar symptoms occurring after taking a few steps on the level. Also, the degree of customary physical activity at work and during recreation should be considered. The development of two-flight dyspnea in a marathon runner may be far more significant than the development of one-flight dyspnea in a previously sedentary person. Similarly, the history must include a detailed consideration of the patient's therapeutic regimen. For example, the persistence or development of edema, breathlessness, and other manifestations of heart failure in a patient whose diet is rigidly restricted in sodium content and who is receiving optimal doses of diuretics is far more grave than the development of similar manifestations of heart failure in the absence of these measures. In an effort to determine the rate of progression of symptoms, and thereby of the severity of the underlying illness, it may be useful to ascertain what, if any, specific tasks the patient could carry out 1 year earlier which he or she cannot carry out now.

Electrocardiogram Although the ECG is an invaluable aspect of every cardiovascular examination, with the exception of the identification of arrhythmias and of many instances of acute myocardial infarction, it rarely permits establishment of a specific diagnosis. In the absence of other abnormal findings, electrocardiographic changes must not be overinterpreted. The range of normal electrocardiographic findings is wide, and the tracing can be affected significantly by many noncardiac factors, such as age, body habitus, and serum electrolyte concentrations.

Natural History The natural history of cardiovascular disease must be appreciated. Cardiovascular disorders often present acutely, as in a previously asymptomatic patient with extensive coronary atherosclerosis who develops an acute myocardial infarction or the previously asymptomatic patient with hypertrophic cardiomyopathy whose first clinical manifestation is syncope or even sudden death. However, in both instances, the alert physician may recognize the patient at risk of these complications long before they occur and can often take measures to prevent their occurrence. For example, the patient with acute myocardial infarction may well have had risk factors for atherosclerosis for many years. Had these been recognized, their elimination or reduction might have delayed or even prevented the infarction. Similarly, the patient with hypertrophic cardiomyopathy may have had the familial form of this disorder, and a careful family history might have led to an echocardiographic examination and the recognition of the condition long before the acute manifestations.

PITFALLS IN CARDIOVASCULAR MEDICINE Increasing subspecialization in internal medicine and the perfection of advanced diagnostic techniques in cardiology can lead to several undesirable consequences, which can be summarized as follows:

1. Failure by the *noncardiologist* to recognize cardiac manifestations of systemic illnesses. Examples of the latter are (a) the Down syndrome (associated with endocardial cushion defect); (b) bony abnormalities of the upper extremities (associated with atrial septal defect in the Holt-Oram syndrome); (c) muscular dystrophies (associated with cardiomyopathy); (d) hemochromatosis and glycogen storage disease (associated with myocardial infiltration and restrictive cardiomyopathy); (e) congenital deafness (associated with prolonged QT interval and serious cardiac arrhythmias); (f) Raynaud's disease (associated with primary pulmonary hypension and coronary vasospasm); (g) connective tissue disorders, i.e., the Marfan syndrome, Ehlers-Danlos and Hurler syndromes, and related disorders of mucopolysaccharide metabolism (aortic dilatation, prolapsed mitral valve, a variety of arterial abnormalities); (h) acromegaly (hypertension, accelerated coronary atherosclerosis, conduction defects, cardiomyopathy); (i) hyperthyroidism (heart failure, atrial fibrillation); (j) hypothyroidism (pericardial effusion, coronary artery disease); (k) rheumatoid arthritis (pericarditis, aortic valve disease); (l) scleroderma (cor pulmonale, myocardial fibrosis, pericarditis); (m) systemic lupus erythematosus (valvulitis, myocarditis, pericarditis); (n) sarcoidosis (arrhythmias, cardiomyopathy); and (o) exfoliative dermatitis (high-output heart failure). In patients with these and other systemic disorders a detailed clinical and noninvasive examination of the cardiovascular system should be carried out to identify cardiovascular involvement.

2. Failure by the cardiologist to recognize an underlying systemic illness, such as those listed above, among patients with a cardiac disorder. Patients known or suspected of having heart disease require a detailed general assessment and a search for the frequent *noncardiac* manifestations of systemic disorders with cardiovascular manifestations. For example, infective endocarditis should be considered in patients with known congenital or valvular heart disease with fever, anemia, or albuminuria. A cardiovascular abnormality may provide the clue critical to the recognition of some systemic disorders. For instance, in an elderly person, unexplained atrial fibrillation may provide the first clue to the diagnosis of thyrotoxicosis.

3. Overreliance on and overutilization of laboratory tests, particularly invasive techniques for the examination of the cardiovascular system. Catheterization of the right and left sides of the heart, selective angiography, and coronary arteriography (Chap. 229) provide precise diagnostic information under many circumstances. For example, they aid in establishing a specific anatomic diagnosis and in determining the physiologic consequences of the abnormalities in patients with chest pain of uncertain cause in whom ischemic heart disease is suspected, and in determining the functional significance of valvular abnormalities in patients with rheumatic heart disease being considered for surgical treatment. Although a great deal of attention has been lavished on these specialized examinations, it should be recognized that they serve to *supplement*, not *supplant*, a careful examination carried out by clinical and noninvasive techniques. Sometimes coronary arteriography is carried out in patients with chest pain suspected of having ischemic heart disease instead of taking a careful history; although coronary arteriography may establish whether the coronary arteries are obstructed, the results often do not provide a definite answer to the question of whether a patient's complaint of chest pain is clearly attributable to coronary arteriosclerosis. Catheterization of the left side of the heart is all too frequently employed to determine whether operative treatment of valvular disease is indicated, even before the patient has had a trial of medical therapy.

Despite the enormous value of these invasive tests it must not be overlooked that they entail some small risk to the patient, involve discomfort and substantial cost, and place a strain on existing medical facilities. Therefore, they should be carried out not as part of a "fishing expedition" or as evidence to the patient and the family that "everything is being done," but only if, after detailed clinical examination and assessment by noninvasive tests, the results of the invasive examination can be expected to modify or aid in the patient's management.

℞ **TREATMENT**

After a complete diagnosis has been established, a number of therapeutic options are usually available. Several examples may be used to demonstrate some of the principles of cardiovascular therapeutics:

1. In the absence of evidence of heart disease, a clear, definitive statement to that effect should be made and the patient should *not* be asked to return at intervals for repeated examinations. If

there is no evidence for disease, such continued attention may lead to the patient developing inappropriate anxiety and fixation on the heart.

2. If there is no evidence of cardiovascular disease but the patient has one or more risk factors for the development of ischemic heart disease (Chap. 242), a plan for their reduction should be developed and the patient should be retested at intervals to assess that he or she is complying and that these risk factors are in fact being reduced.

3. Asymptomatic or mildly symptomatic patients with valvular heart disease that is anatomically severe should be evaluated periodically, every 6 to 12 months, by clinical and noninvasive examinations. Early signs of deterioration of ventricular function can be detected in this manner and in appropriate patients may signify the need for cardiac catheterization and surgical treatment before the development of disabling symptoms, irreversible myocardial damage, and an excessive risk of surgical treatment (Chap. 237).

4. It is critical to establish clear criteria for deciding on the form of treatment (medical, angioplasty, or surgical revascularization) in patients with ischemic heart disease (Chap. 244). Mechanical revascularization represents a major therapeutic advance in the treatment of this most common form of heart disease, but operation has probably been employed too widely in the United States; the mere presence of angina pectoris and/or the demonstration of critical coronary arterial narrowing at angiography should not reflexly evoke a decision to treat the patient surgically or by angioplasty. Instead, these forms of treatment should be limited to those patients with ischemic heart disease in whom it has been demonstrated that these treatments are superior to medical treatment.

BIBLIOGRAPHY

BRAUNWALD E (ed): *Heart Disease*, 5th ed. Philadelphia, Saunders, 1997

CHRISTIE LG, CONTI CR: Systematic approach to the evaluation of angina-like chest pain. Am Heart J 102:897, 1981

CONSTANT J: *Bedside Cardiology*, 4th ed. Boston, Little, Brown, 1993

THE CRITERIA COMMITTEE OF THE NEW YORK HEART ASSOCIATION: *Nomenclature and Criteria for Diagnosis*, 9th ed. Boston, Little, Brown, 1994

HURST JW: *Cardiovascular Diagnosis: The Initial Examination*. St. Louis, Mosby, 1993

MARRIOTT HJL: *Bedside Cardiac Diagnosis*. Philadelphia, Lippincott, 1993

SCHMITT BP et al: The diagnostic usefulness of the history of the patient with dyspnea. J Gen Intern Med 1:386, 1986

SUTTON GC: Symptoms of heart disease, in *Diseases of the Heart*, DG Julian (ed). London, Balliere Tindall, 1989, pp 89–99

227 *Robert A. O'Rourke, Eugene Braunwald*

PHYSICAL EXAMINATION OF THE CARDIOVASCULAR SYSTEM

A meticulous physical examination is a low-cost method for assessing the cardiovascular system and often provides important information for the appropriate selection of additional tests. First, the general physical appearance should be evaluated. The patient may appear tired because of a chronic low cardiac output; the respiratory rate may be rapid in cases of pulmonary venous congestion. Central cyanosis, often associated with clubbing of the fingers and toes, indicates right-to-left cardiac or extracardiac shunting or inadequate oxygenation of blood by the lungs. Cyanosis in the distal extremities, cool skin, and increased sweating result from vasoconstriction in patients with severe heart failure (Chap. 36). Noncardiovascular details can be equally important. For example, the diagnosis of infective endocarditis is highly likely in patients with petechiae, Osler's nodes, and Janeway lesions (Chap. 126).

The blood pressure should be taken in both arms and with the patient supine and upright; the heart rate should be timed for 30 s. Orthostatic hypotension and tachycardia may indicate a reduced blood volume, while resting tachycardia may be due to heart failure.

Careful examination of the optic fundi is essential (Chap. 246), and the retinal vessels may show evidence of systemic hypertension, arteriosclerosis, or embolism. The latter may result from atherosclerosis in larger arteries (e.g., the carotid) or may represent a complication of valvular heart disease (e.g., endocarditis).

Palpation of the peripheral arterial pulses in the upper and lower extremities is necessary to define the adequacy of systemic blood flow and to detect the presence of occlusive arterial lesions. It is also important to examine both legs for evidence of edema, varicose veins, or thrombophlebitis (Chap. 248). The cardiovascular examination includes careful evaluation of both the carotid arterial and the jugular venous pulses, as well as deliberate precordial palpation and attentive cardiac auscultation.

ARTERIAL PRESSURE PULSE The normal central aortic pulse wave is characterized by a fairly rapid rise to a somewhat rounded peak (Fig. 227-1). The anacrotic shoulder, present on the ascending limb, occurs at the time of peak rate of aortic flow just before maximum pressure is reached. The less steep descending limb is interrupted by a sharp downward deflection, synchronous with aortic valve closure, called the *incisura*. As the pulse wave is transmitted peripherally, the initial upstroke becomes steeper, the anacrotic shoulder becomes less apparent, and the incisura is replaced by the smoother dicrotic notch. Accordingly, palpation of a peripheral arterial pulse (e.g., the radial pulse) frequently gives less information than examination of a more central pulse (e.g., the carotid pulse) regarding alterations in left ventricular ejection or aortic valve function. However, certain findings, such as the hyperkinetic pulse of aortic regurgitation or pulsus alternans, are more evident in peripheral arteries (Fig. 227-2). The carotid pulse is best examined with the sternocleidomastoid muscle relaxed and with the head rotated slightly toward the examiner. In palpating the brachial arterial pulse, the examiner can support the subject's relaxed elbow with the right arm while compressing the brachial pulse with the thumb. The usual technique is to compress the artery with the thumb or forefinger until the maximum pulse is sensed. Varying degrees of pressure should then be applied while concentrating on the

FIGURE 227-1 *A.* Schematic representation of electrocardiogram, aortic pressure pulse (AOP), phonocardiogram recorded at the apex, and apex cardiogram (ACG). On the phonocardiogram, S_1, S_2, S_3, and S_4 represent the first through fourth heart sounds; OS represents the opening snap of the mitral valve, which occurs coincident with the O point of the apex cardiogram. S_3 occurs coincident with the termination of the rapid-filling wave (RFW) of the ACG, while S_4 occurs coincident with the *a* wave of the ACG. *B.* Simultaneous recording of electrocardiogram, indirect carotid pulse (CP), phonocardiogram along the left sternal border (LSB), and indirect jugular venous pulse (JVP). ES, ejection sound; SC, systolic click.

separate phases of the pulse wave. This method, known as *trisection*, is useful for assessing the sharpness of the upstroke, systolic peak, and diastolic slope of the arterial pulse. In most normal persons, a dicrotic wave is not palpable.

A small weak pulse, *pulsus parvus*, is common in conditions with a diminished left ventricular stroke volume, a narrow pulse pressure, and increased peripheral vascular resistance (Fig. 227-2). A *hypokinetic* pulse may be due to hypovolemia, to left ventricular failure, to restrictive pericardial disease, or to mitral valve stenosis. In aortic valve stenosis, the delayed systolic peak, *pulsus tardus*, results from obstruction to left ventricular ejection. In contrast, a large, bounding (*hyperkinetic*) pulse is usually associated with an increased left ventricular stroke volume, a wide pulse pressure, and a decrease in peripheral vascular resistance. This pattern occurs characteristically in patients with an elevated stroke volume, as in complete heart block; with hyperkinetic circulation due to anxiety, anemia, exercise, or fever; or with a rapid runoff of blood from the arterial system (as caused by a patent ductus arteriosus or peripheral arteriovenous fistula). Patients with mitral regurgitation or a ventricular septal defect also may have a bounding pulse, since vigorous left ventricular ejection produces a rapid upstroke in the arterial pulse, even though the duration of systole and the forward stroke volume may be diminished. In aortic regurgitation, the rapidly rising, bounding arterial pulse results from an increased left ventricular stroke volume and an increased rate of ventricular ejection.

The *bisferiens pulse*, which has two systolic peaks, is characteristic of aortic regurgitation (with or without accompanying stenosis) and of hypertrophic cardiomyopathy (Chap. 239). In the latter condition, the pulse wave upstroke rises rapidly and forcefully, producing the first systolic peak ("percussion wave"). A brief decline in pressure follows because of the sudden decrease in the rate of left ventricular ejection during midsystole, when severe obstruction often develops. This pressure trough is followed by a smaller and more slowly rising positive pulse wave ("tidal wave") produced by continued ventricular ejection and by reflected waves from the periphery. The *dicrotic pulse* has two palpable waves, one in systole and one in diastole. It occurs most frequently in patients with a very low stroke volume, particularly in those with dilated cardiomyopathy.

Pulsus alternans is a pattern in which there is regular alteration of the pressure pulse amplitude, despite a regular rhythm (Fig. 227-2). It is due to alternating left ventricular contractile force, usually denotes severe impairment of left ventricular function, and commonly occurs in patients who also have a loud third heart sound. Pulsus

alternans also may occur during or following paroxysmal tachycardia or for several beats following a premature beat in patients without heart disease. In *pulsus bigeminus*, there is also a regular alteration of pressure pulse amplitude, but it is caused by a premature ventricular contraction that follows each regular beat. In *pulsus paradoxus*, the decrease in systolic arterial pressure that normally accompanies the reduction in arterial pulse amplitude during inspiration is accentuated. In patients with pericardial tamponade (Chap. 240), airway obstruction, or superior vena cava obstruction, the decrease in systolic arterial pressure frequently exceeds the normal decrease of 10 mmHg and the peripheral pulse may disappear completely during inspiration.

Simultaneous palpation of the radial and femoral arterial pulses, which normally are virtually coincident, is important to rule out aortic coarctation, in which the latter pulse is weakened and delayed (Chap. 235).

JUGULAR VENOUS PULSE (JVP)   The two main objectives of the examination of the neck veins are inspection of their waveform and estimation of the central venous pressure (CVP). In most patients, the right internal jugular vein is best for both purposes. Usually, the pulsation of the internal jugular vein is greatest when the trunk is inclined by less than 30°. In patients with elevated venous pressure, it may be necessary to elevate the trunk further, sometimes to as much as 90°. When the neck muscles are relaxed, shining a beam of light tangentially across the skin overlying the vein exposes the pulsations of the internal jugular vein. Simultaneous palpation of the left carotid artery aids the examiner in deciding which pulsations are venous and in relating the venous pulsations to their timing in the cardiac cycle.

The normal JVP reflects phasic pressure changes in the right atrium and consists of two or sometimes three positive waves and two negative troughs (Fig. 227-1). The positive presystolic *a* wave is produced by venous distention due to right atrial contraction and is the dominant wave in the JVP, particularly during inspiration. Large *a* waves indicate that the right atrium is contracting against an increased resistance (Fig. 227-3), such as occurs with tricuspid stenosis or more commonly with increased resistance to right ventricular filling (pulmonary hypertension or pulmonic stenosis). Large *a* waves also occur during arrhythmias whenever the right atrium contracts while the tricuspid valve is closed by right ventricular systole. Such "cannon" *a* waves may occur regularly (as during junctional rhythm) or irregularly (as in atrioventricular dissociation with ventricular tachycardia or complete heart block). The *a* wave is absent in patients with atrial fibrillation, and there is an increased delay between the *a* wave and the carotid arterial pulse in patients with first-degree atrioventricular block.

The *c* wave, often observed in the JVP, is a positive wave produced by the bulging of the tricuspid valve into the right atrium during right ventricular isovolumetric systole and by the impact of the carotid artery adjacent to the jugular vein. The *x* descent is due both to atrial relaxation and to the downward displacement of the tricuspid valve during ventricular systole. The *x* descent wave during systole is often accentuated in patients with constrictive pericarditis (Fig. 227-3), but this wave is reduced with right ventricular dilation and often is reversed

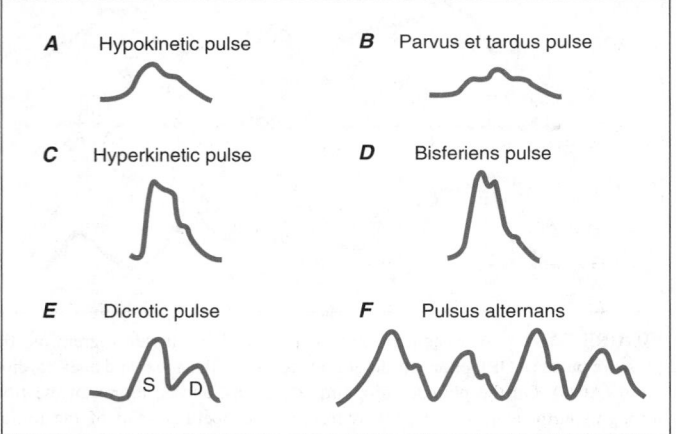

FIGURE 227-2   Schematic representation of arterial pulse waveforms that occur with alterations in cardiac hemodynamics, which may result from normal physiologic responses or may be due to cardiac disease. S, systole; D, diastole. [*Modified from RA O'Rourke, in The Heart, 7th ed, JW Hurst et al (eds). New York, McGraw-Hill, 1990, with permission.*]

FIGURE 227-3   Abnormal jugular venous pulse waveforms commonly present in patients with cardiac disease and/or arrhythmias. See text. [*Modified from RA O'Rourke, in The Heart, 7th ed, JW Hurst et al (eds). New York, McGraw-Hill, 1990, with permission.*]

in tricuspid regurgitation. The positive, late systolic v wave results from the increasing volume of blood in the right atrium during ventricular systole when the tricuspid valve is closed. Tricuspid regurgitation causes the v wave to be more prominent; when tricuspid regurgitation becomes severe, the combination of a prominent v wave and obliteration of the x descent results in a single large positive systolic wave. After the v wave peaks, the right atrial pressure falls because of the decreased bulging of the tricuspid valve into the right atrium as right ventricular pressure declines and the tricuspid valve opens (Fig. 227-3).

This negative descending limb—the y descent of the JVP—is produced mainly by the opening of the tricuspid valve and the subsequent rapid inflow of blood into the right ventricle. A rapid, deep y descent in early diastole occurs with severe tricuspid regurgitation. A venous pulse characterized by a sharp y descent, a deep y trough, and a rapid ascent to the baseline is seen in patients with constrictive pericarditis or with severe right-sided heart failure and a high venous pressure. A slow y descent in the JVP suggests an obstruction to right ventricular filling, as occurs with tricuspid stenosis or right atrial myxoma.

The right internal jugular is the best vein to use for accurate estimation of the central venous pressure. The sternal angle is used as the reference point, because the center of the right atrium lies approximately 5 cm below the sternal angle in the average patient, regardless of body position. The patient is examined at the optimal degree of trunk elevation for visualization of venous pulsations. The vertical distance between the top of the oscillating venous column and the level of the sternal angle is determined; generally it is less than 3 cm (3 cm + 5 cm = 8 cm blood). The most common cause of a high venous pressure is an elevated right ventricular diastolic pressure. In patients suspected of having right ventricular failure who have a normal CVP at rest, the abdominojugular reflux test may be helpful. The palm of the examiner's hand is placed over the abdomen, and firm pressure is applied for 10 s or more. In normal persons, this maneuver does not alter the jugular venous pressure significantly, but when right heart function is impaired, the upper level of venous pulsation usually increases. A positive abdominojugular test is best defined as an increase in JVP during 10 s of firm midabdominal compression followed by a rapid drop in pressure by 4 cm blood on release of the compression. The most common cause of a positive test is right-sided heart failure secondary to elevated left heart filling pressures. Also, abdominal compression may elicit the JVP pattern typical of tricuspid regurgitation when the resting pulse wave is normal. Kussmaul's sign—an increase rather than the normal decrease in the CVP during inspiration—is most often caused by severe right-sided heart failure; it is a frequent finding in patients with constrictive pericarditis or right ventricular infarction.

PRECORDIAL PALPATION The location, amplitude, duration, and direction of the cardiac impulse usually can be best appreciated with the fingertips. The normal left ventricular apex impulse is located at or medial to the left midclavicular line in the fourth or fifth intercostal space and is a tapping, early systolic outward thrust localized to a point not more than 3 cm in diameter. It is due primarily to recoil of the heart as blood is ejected and should be evaluated with the patient supine and in the left lateral position. Left ventricular hypertrophy results in exaggeration of the amplitude, duration, and often size of the normal left ventricular thrust. The impulse may be displaced laterally and downward into the sixth or seventh interspace, particularly in patients with a left ventricular volume load such as occurs in cases of aortic regurgitation or dilated cardiomyopathy.

Additional abnormal features that are detectable at the left ventricular apex include marked presystolic distention of the left ventricle, which is often accompanied by a fourth heart sound in patients with an excessive left ventricular pressure load or myocardial ischemia/infarction, and a prominent early diastolic rapid-filling wave, which is often accompanied by a third heart sound in patients with left ventricular failure or mitral valve regurgitation (Fig. 227-1). A double systolic apical impulse often is palpable in patients with hypertrophic cardiomyopathy.

Right ventricular hypertrophy often results in a sustained systolic lift at the lower left parasternal area, which starts in early systole and is synchronous with the left ventricular apical impulse.

Abnormal precordial pulsations occur during systole in patients with left ventricular dyssynergy due to ischemic heart disease or to diffuse myocardial disease from some other cause. These pulsations often occur in patients with a recent myocardial infarction and may be present in some patients only during episodes of anginal pain. They are most commonly felt in the left midprecordium one or two interspaces above and/or 1 to 2 cm medial to the left ventricular apex. A systolic bulge occurring in the region of the apex is difficult to distinguish from the impulse of left ventricular hypertrophy.

A left parasternal lift is present frequently in patients with severe mitral regurgitation. This pulsation occurs distinctly later than the left ventricular apical impulse, is synchronous with the v wave in the left atrial pressure curve, and is due to anterior displacement of the right ventricle by an enlarged, expanding left atrium. A similar impulse occurs to the right of the sternum in some patients with severe tricuspid regurgitation and a giant right atrium. Pulsation of the right sternoclavicular joint may indicate a right-sided aortic arch or aneurysmal dilation of the ascending aorta. Pulmonary artery pulsation is often visible and palpable in the second left intercostal space. While it may be normal in children or thin young adults, in others this pulsation usually denotes pulmonary hypertension, increased pulmonary blood flow, or poststenotic pulmonary artery dilation.

Thrills are palpable, low-frequency vibrations associated with heart murmurs. The systolic murmur of mitral regurgitation may be palpated at the cardiac apex. When the palm of the hand is placed over the precordium, the thrill of aortic stenosis crosses the palm toward the right side of the neck, while the thrill of pulmonic stenosis radiates more often to the left side of the neck. The thrill due to a ventricular septal defect is usually located in the third and fourth intercostal spaces near the left sternal border.

Percussion should be performed in each patient to identify normal or abnormal position of the heart, stomach, and liver. However, in patients with a normal cardiac situs, percussion adds little to careful inspection and palpation in the recognition of cardiac enlargement.

CARDIAC AUSCULTATION

To obtain the most information from cardiac auscultation, the observer should keep in mind several principles: (1) Auscultation should be performed in a quiet room to avoid the distracting noises of normal activity. (2) For optimal auscultation, attention must be focused on the phase of the cardiac cycle during which the auscultatory event is expected to occur. (3) The timing of a heart sound or murmur can be determined accurately from its relation to other observable events in the cardiac cycle—the carotid arterial pulse, the apical impulse, or the JVP. (4) To define the significance of a cardiac sound or murmur, it is often necessary to observe alterations in its timing or intensity during various physiologic and/or pharmacologic interventions (Table 227-1).

HEART SOUNDS The major components of heart sounds are vibrations associated with the abrupt acceleration or deceleration of blood in the cardiovascular system. Studies using simultaneous echocardiographic-phonocardiographic recordings indicate that the first and second heart sounds are produced primarily by the closure of the atrioventricular (AV) and semilunar valves and the events that accompany these closures. The intensity of the *first heart sound* (S_1) is influenced by (1) the position of the mitral leaflets at the onset of ventricular systole, (2) the rate of rise of the left ventricular pressure pulse, (3) the presence or absence of structural disease of the mitral valve, and (4) the amount of tissue, air, or fluid between the heart and the stethoscope. S_1 is louder if diastole is shortened because of tachycardia, if atrioventricular flow is increased because of high cardiac output or prolonged because of mitral stenosis, or if atrial contraction precedes ventricular contraction by an unusually short interval, reflected in a short PR interval. The loud S_1 in mitral stenosis usually signifies that the valve is pliable and that it remains open at the onset of isovolumetric contraction because of the elevated left atrial pressure. A reduction in the intensity of S_1 may be due to poor conduction of sound through the chest wall, a slow rise of the left ventricular pressure pulse, a long PR interval, or imperfect closure due to reduced valve substance, as in mitral regurgitation. S_1 is also soft when the anterior mitral leaflet is immobile because of rigidity and calcification, even in the presence of predominant mitral stenosis.

Splitting of the two high-pitched components of S_1 by 10 to 30 ms is a normal phenomenon (Fig. 227-1). The first component of S_1 is attributed to mitral valve closure, and the second to tricuspid valve closure. Widening of the S_1 is due most often to complete right bundle branch block and the resulting delay in onset of the right ventricular pressure pulse. Reversed splitting of the S_1, in which the mitral component follows the tricuspid component, may be present in patients with severe mitral stenosis, left atrial myxoma, and left bundle branch block.

Splitting of S_2 into audibly distinct aortic (A_2) and pulmonic (P_2) components occurs normally during inspiration, when the augmented inflow into the right ventricle increases its stroke volume and ejection period and thus delays closure of the pulmonic valve. P_2 is coincident with the incisura of the pulmonary artery pressure curve, which is separated from the right ventricular pressure tracing by an interval termed the "hangout time." The absolute value of this interval reflects the resistance to pulmonary blood flow and the impedance characteris-

tics of the pulmonary vascular bed. This interval is prolonged, and physiologic splitting of S_2 is accentuated, in conditions associated with right ventricular volume overload and a distensible pulmonary vascular bed. However, in patients with an increase in pulmonary vascular resistance, the hangout time is markedly reduced, and narrow splitting of S_2 is present. Splitting that persists with expiration (heard best at the pulmonic area or left sternal border) is usually abnormal when the patient is in the upright position. Such splitting may be due to many causes: delayed activation of the right ventricle (right bundle branch block); left ventricular ectopic beats; a left ventricular pacemaker; prolongation of right ventricular contraction with an increased right ventricular pressure load (pulmonary embolism or pulmonic stenosis); or delayed pulmonic valve closure because of right ventricular volume overload associated with right ventricular failure or diminished impedance of the pulmonary vascular bed and a prolonged hangout time (atrial septal defect).

In pulmonary hypertension, P_2 is increased in intensity, and splitting of the second heart sound may be diminished, normal, or accentuated, depending on the cause of the pulmonary hypertension, the pulmonary vascular resistance, and the presence or absence of right ventricular decompensation. Early aortic valve closure, occurring with mitral regurgitation or a ventricular septal defect, also may produce splitting that persists during expiration. It also may occur with constrictive pericarditis. In patients with an atrial septal defect, the proportion of right atrial filling contributed by the left atrium and the venae cavae varies reciprocally during the respiratory cycle, so that right atrial inflow remains relatively constant. Therefore, the volume and duration of right ventricular ejection are not significantly increased by inspiration, and there is little inspiratory exaggeration of the splitting of S_2. This phenomenon, termed *fixed splitting* of the second heart sound, is of considerable diagnostic value.

A delay in aortic valve closure causing P_2 to precede A_2 results in so-called reversed (paradoxic) splitting of S_2. Splitting is then maximal in expiration and decreases during inspiration with the normal delay of pulmonic valve closure. The most common causes of reversed splitting of S_2 are left bundle branch block and delayed excitation of the left ventricle from a right ventricular ectopic beat. Mechanical prolongation of left ventricular systole, resulting in reversed splitting of S_2, also may be caused by severe aortic outflow obstruction, a large aorta-to-pulmonary artery shunt, systolic hypertension, and ischemic heart disease or cardiomyopathy with left ventricular failure. P_2 is normally softer than A_2 in the second left intercostal space; a P_2 that is greater than A_2 in this area suggests pulmonary hypertension, except in patients with atrial septal defect.

The *third heart sound* (S_3) is a low-pitched sound produced in the ventricle 0.14 to 0.16 s after A_2, at the termination of rapid filling. This sound is frequent in normal children and in patients with high cardiac output. However, in patients over 40 years old, an S_3 usually indicates impairment of ventricular function, AV valve regurgitation, or other conditions that increase the rate or volume of ventricular filling. The left-sided S_3 is best heard with the bell piece of the stethoscope at the left ventricular apex during expiration and with the patient in the left lateral position. The right-sided S_3 is best heard at the left sternal border or just beneath the xiphoid and usually is louder with inspiration. Often it is accompanied by the systolic murmur of functional tricuspid regurgitation. Third heart sounds often disappear with treatment of heart failure.

An S_3 that is earlier (0.10 to 0.12 s after A_2) and higher-pitched than normal (a pericardial knock) often occurs in patients with constrictive pericarditis (Chap. 240); its presence depends on the restrictive effect of the adherent pericardium, which halts diastolic filling abruptly.

The *opening snap* (OS) is a brief, high-pitched, early diastolic sound which is usually due to stenosis of an AV valve, most often the mitral valve. It is generally heard best at the lower left sternal border and radiates well to the base of the heart. The A_2-OS interval is inversely related to the height of the mean left atrial pressure and ranges from 0.04 to 0.12 s. In the second intercostal space, an OS is often confused with P_2. However, careful auscultation will reveal both

---

Table 227-1

Effects of Physiologic and Pharmacologic Interventions on the Intensity of Heart Murmurs and Sounds*

Respiration Systolic murmurs due to TR or pulmonic blood flow through a normal or stenotic valve and diastolic murmurs of TS or PR generally increase with inspiration, as do right-sided S_3 and S_4. Left-sided murmurs and sounds usually are louder during expiration.

Valsalva maneuver Most murmurs decrease in length and intensity. Two exceptions are the systolic murmur of HCM, which usually becomes much louder, and that of MVP, which becomes longer and often louder. Following release of the Valsalva maneuver, right-sided murmurs tend to return to control intensity earlier than left-sided murmurs.

After VPB or AF Murmurs originating at normal or stenotic semilunar valves increase in the cardiac cycle following a VPB or in the cycle after a long cycle length in AF. By contrast, systolic murmurs due to AV valve regurgitation either do not change, diminish (papillary muscle dysfunction), or become shorter (MVP).

Positional changes With *standing,* most murmurs diminish, two exceptions being the murmur of HCM, which becomes louder, and that of MVP, which lengthens and often is intensified. With *squatting,* most murmurs become louder, but those of HCM and MVP usually soften and may disappear. Passive leg raising usually produces the same results.

Exercise Murmurs due to blood flow across normal or obstructed valves (e.g., PS, MS) become louder with both isotonic and submaximal isometric (handgrip) exercise. Murmurs of MR, VSD, and AR also increase with handgrip exercise. However, the murmur of HCM often decreases with near maximum handgrip exercise. Left-sided S_4 and S_3 are often accentuated by exercise, particularly when due to ischemic heart disease.

Pharmacologic interventions During the initial relative hypotension following amyl nitrite inhalation, murmurs of MR, VSD, and AR decrease, while murmurs of aortic stenosis or sclerosis increase. During the later tachycardia phase, murmurs of MS and right-sided lesions also increase. The response in MVP often is biphasic (first softer and then louder than control). The arterial constrictor phenylephrine tends to produce the opposite effects.

Transient arterial occlusion Transient external compression of both arms by bilateral cuff inflation to 20 mmHg over peak systolic pressure augments the murmurs of MR, VSD, and AR, but not murmurs due to other causes.

---

* TR, tricuspid regurgitation; TS, tricuspid stenosis; PR, pulmonic regurgitation; HCM, hypertrophic cardiomyopathy; MVP, mitral valve prolapse; PS, pulmonic stenosis; MS, mitral stenosis; MR, mitral regurgitation; VSD, ventricular septal defect; AR, aortic regurgitation; VPB, ventricular premature beat; and AF, atrial fibrillation.

components of S₂, followed by the OS. The OS of tricuspid stenosis occurs later in diastole than the mitral OS and is often overlooked in patients with more prominent mitral valve disease.

The *fourth heart sound* (S₄) is a low-pitched, presystolic sound produced in the ventricle during ventricular filling; it is associated with an effective atrial contraction and is heard best with the bell piece of the stethoscope. The sound is absent in patients with atrial fibrillation. The S₄ occurs when diminished ventricular compliance increases the resistance to ventricular filling, and it is present frequently in patients with systemic hypertension, aortic stenosis, hypertrophic cardiomyopathy, ischemic heart disease, and acute mitral regurgitation. Most patients with an acute myocardial infarction and sinus rhythm have an audible S₄. The fourth heart sound is frequently accompanied by visible and palpable presystolic distention of the left ventricle. It peaks in intensity at the left ventricular apex when the patient is in the left lateral position and is accentuated by mild isotonic or isometric exercise in the supine position. The right-sided S₄ is present in patients with right ventricular hypertrophy secondary to either pulmonic stenosis or pulmonary hypertension and frequently accompanies a prominent presystolic *a* wave in the JVP.

An S₄ frequently accompanies delayed AV conduction even in the absence of clinically detectable heart disease. The incidence of an audible S₄ increases with increasing age. Whether an audible S₄ in adults without other evidence of cardiac disease is abnormal remains controversial.

The *ejection sound* is a sharp, high-pitched event occurring in early systole and closely following the first heart sound. Ejection sounds occur in the presence of semilunar valve stenosis and in conditions associated with dilation of the aorta or pulmonary artery. The aortic ejection sound is usually heard best at the left ventricular apex and the second right intercostal space; the pulmonary ejection sound is strongest at the upper left sternal border. The latter, unlike most other right-sided acoustical events, is heard better during expiration.

Nonejection or *midsystolic clicks*, occurring with or without a late systolic murmur, often denote prolapse of one or both leaflets of the mitral valve (Chap. 237). They also may be caused by tricuspid valve prolapse. They probably result from chordae tendineae that are functionally unequal in length on either or both AV valves and are heard best along the lower left sternal border and at the left ventricular apex. Systolic clicks may be single or multiple, and they may occur at any time in systole but usually are later than the systolic ejection sound.

HEART MURMURS Cardiac murmurs result from vibrations set up in the bloodstream and the surrounding heart and great vessels as a result of turbulent blood flow, the formation of eddies, and cavitation (bubble formation as a result of sudden decrease in pressure).

The intensity (loudness) of murmurs may be graded from I to VI. A grade I murmur is so faint that it can be heard only with special effort; a grade IV murmur is commonly accompanied by a thrill; and a grade VI murmur is audible with the stethoscope removed from contact with the chest. The configuration of a murmur may be crescendo, decrescendo, crescendo-decrescendo (diamond-shaped), or plateau. The precise time of onset and time of cessation of a murmur depend on the instant in the cardiac cycle at which an adequate pressure difference between two chambers arises and disappears (Fig. 227-4).

The location on the chest wall where the murmur is best heard and the areas to which it radiates can be helpful in identifying the cardiac structure from which the murmur originates. For example, the murmur of aortic valve stenosis usually is loudest in the second right intercostal space and radiates to the carotid arteries. By contrast, the murmur of mitral regurgitation most often is loudest at the cardiac apex. It may radiate to the left sternal border and base of the heart when the posterior mitral leaflet is predominantly involved or to the axilla and back when the anterior leaflet is more severely affected. In the latter case, the regurgitant blood is directed toward the posterior left atrial wall.

Often it is difficult to classify a cardiac murmur with certainty on the basis of its timing, configuration, location, radiation, pitch, or intensity. However, by noting changes in the characteristics of the murmur during maneuvers that alter cardiac hemodynamics, the aus-

cultator often can identify its correct origin and significance (Table 227-1).

Accentuation of a murmur during inspiration (a maneuver that augments systemic venous return) implies that it originates on the right side of the circulation; expiratory exaggeration has less significance. Prolonged expiratory pressure against a closed glottis (i.e., the Valsalva maneuver) reduces the intensity of most murmurs by diminishing both right and left ventricular filling (i.e., ventricular preload). The systolic murmur associated with *hypertrophic cardiomyopathy* and the late systolic murmur due to *mitral valve prolapse* are exceptions and may be paradoxically accentuated during the Valsalva maneuver. Murmurs due to flow across a normal or obstructed semilunar valve increase in intensity in the cycle following a premature ventricular beat or a long RR interval in atrial fibrillation. In contrast, murmurs due to AV valve regurgitation or a ventricular septal defect do not change appreciably during the beat following a prolonged diastole. Standing, which decreases left ventricular volume, accentuates the murmur of hypertrophic cardiomyopathy and occasionally the murmur due to mitral valve prolapse. Squatting, which increases both venous return and systemic arterial resistance and thus ventricular afterload, increases most murmurs, except those due to hypertrophic cardiomyopathy and mitral regurgitation due to a prolapsed mitral valve, which often decrease. Sustained handgrip exercise, which increases systemic arterial pressure and heart rate, often accentuates the murmurs of mitral regurgitation, aortic regurgitation, and mitral stenosis but usually diminishes those due to aortic stenosis or hypertrophic cardiomyopathy. Pharmacologic interventions include inhalation of amyl nitrite, which reduces systemic arterial pressure and increases blood flow, thereby increasing the intensity of murmurs due to valvular stenosis while diminishing those due to aortic or mitral regurgitation (Table 227-1). Transient external arterial occlusion by the inflation of bilateral arm cuffs to 20 mmHg (2.66 kPa) above systolic blood pressure for 5 s usually intensifies murmurs due to left-sided regurgitant lesions; this method is applicable to almost all patients and does not require administration of any drug.

FIGURE 227-4 *A.* Schematic representation of ECG, aortic pressure (AOP), left ventricular pressure (LVP), and left atrial pressure (LAP). The shaded areas indicated a transvalvular pressure difference during systole. HSM, holosystolic murmur; MSM, midsystolic murmur. *B.* Graphic representation of ECG, aortic pressure (AOP), left ventricular pressure (LVP) and left atrial pressure (LAP) with shaded areas indicating transvalvular diastolic pressure difference. EDM, early diastolic murmur; PSM, presystolic murmur; MDM, middiastolic murmur.

Systolic Murmurs *Holosystolic (pansystolic) murmurs* are generated when there is flow between two chambers that have widely different pressures throughout systole, such as the left ventricle and either the left atrium or the right ventricle (Fig. 227-4). The pressure gradient occurs early in contraction and lasts until relaxation is almost complete. Therefore, holosystolic murmurs begin before aortic ejection, and at the area of maximal intensity they begin with S_1 and end after S_2. Holosystolic murmurs accompany mitral or tricuspid regurgitation, ventricular septal defect, and, under certain circumstances, aortopulmonary shunts. Although the typical high-pitched murmur of mitral regurgitation usually continues throughout systole, the shape of the murmur may vary considerably. The holosystolic murmurs of mitral regurgitation and ventricular septal defect are augmented by transient exercise and are diminished by lowering the left ventricular systolic pressure by inhalation of amyl nitrite. The murmur of tricuspid regurgitation associated with pulmonary hypertension is holosystolic and frequently increases during inspiration. Not all patients with mitral or tricuspid regurgitation or ventricular septal defect have holosystolic murmurs (Chap. 237). Often, a mild valvular regurgitant jet, detected by color flow Doppler techniques, is not associated with an audible murmur despite optimal auscultation. Such regurgitant jets usually do not indicate clinical heart disease.

Midsystolic murmurs, also called *systolic ejection murmurs*, which are often crescendo-decrescendo in shape, occur when blood is ejected across the aortic or pulmonic outflow tracts (Fig. 227-4). The murmur starts shortly after S_1, when the ventricular pressure becomes high enough to open the semilunar valve. As the velocity of ejection increases, the murmur gets stronger, and as ejection declines, it diminishes. The murmur ends before the ventricular pressure falls enough to permit closure of the aortic or pulmonic leaflets. When the semilunar valves are normal, an increased flow rate (as occurs in states of elevated cardiac output), ejection into a dilated vessel beyond the valve, or increased transmission of sound through a thin chest wall may be responsible for this murmur. Most benign, functional murmurs are midsystolic and originate from the pulmonary outflow tract. Valvular or subvalvular obstruction of either ventricle also may cause such a midsystolic murmur, the intensity being related to the flow rate.

The murmur of aortic stenosis is the prototype of the left-sided midsystolic murmur. The location and radiation of this murmur are influenced by the direction of the high-velocity jet within the aortic root. In *valvular aortic stenosis*, the murmur is usually maximal in the second right intercostal space, with radiation into the neck. In *supravalvular aortic stenosis*, the murmur is occasionally loudest even higher, with disproportionate radiation into the right carotid artery. In hypertrophic cardiomyopathy, the midsystolic murmur originates in the left ventricular cavity and is usually maximal at the lower left sternal edge and apex, with relatively little radiation to the carotids. When the aortic valve is immobile (calcified), the aortic closure sound (A_2) may be soft and inaudible so that the length and configuration of the murmur are difficult to determine. Midsystolic murmurs also occur in patients with mitral regurgitation or, less frequently, tricuspid regurgitation resulting from papillary muscle dysfunction. Such murmurs due to mitral regurgitation are often confused with those originating in the aorta, particularly in elderly patients.

The patient's age and the area of maximal intensity aid in determining the significance of midsystolic murmurs. Thus, in a young adult with a thin chest and a high velocity of blood flow, a faint or moderate midsystolic murmur heard only in the pulmonic area is usually without clinical significance, while a somewhat louder murmur in the aortic area may indicate congenital aortic stenosis. In elderly patients, pulmonic flow murmurs are rare, while aortic systolic murmurs are common and may be due to aortic dilation, to a significant degree of valvular aortic stenosis, or to nonstenotic deformity (sclerosis) of the aortic valve. Midsystolic aortic and pulmonic murmurs are intensified after amyl nitrite inhalation and during the cardiac cycle following a premature ventricular beat, while those due to mitral

regurgitation are unchanged or softer. Aortic systolic murmurs are diminished by interventions that increase aortic impedance, such as intravenous phenylephrine administration. Echocardiography or cardiac catheterization may be necessary to separate a prominent and exaggerated functional murmur from one due to congenital or acquired semilunar valve stenosis.

Early systolic murmurs begin with the first heart sound and end in midsystole. In *large ventricular septal defects with pulmonary hypertension*, the shunting at the end of systole may be small or absent, resulting in an early systolic murmur. A similar murmur may occur with very *small muscular ventricular septal defects,* the shunt being interrupted in late systole. An early systolic murmur is a feature of *tricuspid regurgitation occurring in the absence of pulmonary hypertension.* This lesion is common in narcotics abusers with infective endocarditis, in whom a tall regurgitant right atrial *v* wave reaches the level of the normal right ventricular pressure in late systole, confining the murmur to early systole. Patients with acute mitral regurgitation into a noncompliant left atrium and a large *v* wave often have a loud early systolic murmur that diminishes as the pressure gradient between the left ventricle and left atrium decreases in late systole (Chap. 237).

Late systolic murmurs are faint or moderately loud, high-pitched apical murmurs that start well after ejection and do not mask either heart sound. They are probably related to papillary muscle dysfunction caused by infarction or ischemia of these muscles or to their distortion by left ventricular dilation. They may appear only during angina but are common in patients with myocardial infarction or diffuse myocardial disease. Late systolic murmurs following midsystolic clicks are due to late systolic mitral regurgitation caused by prolapse of the mitral valve into the left atrium (Chap. 237).

Diastolic Murmurs *Early diastolic murmurs* (Fig. 227-4) begin with or shortly after S_2, as soon as the corresponding ventricular pressure falls enough below that in the aorta or pulmonary artery. The high-pitched murmurs of aortic regurgitation or of pulmonic regurgitation due to pulmonary hypertension are generally decrescendo, since there is a progressive decline in the volume or rate of regurgitation during diastole. Faint, high-pitched murmurs of aortic regurgitation are difficult to hear unless they are specifically sought by applying firm pressure with the diaphragm over the left midsternal border while the patient sits leaning forward and holds a breath in full expiration. The diastolic murmur of aortic regurgitation is enhanced by an acute elevation of the arterial pressure, such as occurs with handgrip exercise; it diminishes with a decrease in arterial pressure, as with amyl nitrite inhalation. The diastolic murmur of congenital pulmonic regurgitation without pulmonary hypertension is low- to medium-pitched. The onset of this murmur is delayed because the regurgitant flow is minimal at the onset of pulmonic valve closure when the reverse pressure gradient responsible for the regurgitation is negligible.

Middiastolic murmurs usually arise from the AV valves (Fig. 227-4), occur during early ventricular filling, and are due to disproportion between valve orifice size and flow rate. Such murmurs may be quite loud (grade III), despite only slight AV valve stenosis, when there is normal or increased blood flow. Conversely, the murmurs may be soft or even absent despite severe obstruction if the cardiac output is markedly reduced. When stenosis is marked, the diastolic murmur is prolonged, and the duration of the murmur is more reliable than its intensity as an index of the severity of valve obstruction.

The low-pitched, middiastolic murmur of mitral stenosis characteristically follows the OS. It should be specifically sought by placing the bell of the stethoscope at the site of the left ventricular impulse, which is best localized with the patient on the left side. Frequently, the murmur of mitral stenosis is present only at the left ventricular apex, and it may be increased in intensity by mild supine exercise or by inhalation of amyl nitrite. In tricuspid stenosis, the middiastolic murmur is localized to a relatively limited area along the left sternal edge and may be stronger during inspiration.

Middiastolic murmurs may be generated across the mitral valve in cases of mitral regurgitation, patent ductus arteriosus, or ventricular septal defect, and across the tricuspid valve in cases of tricuspid regurgitation or atrial septal defect. These murmurs are related to the torrential flow across an AV valve, usually follow an S_3, and tend to occur with large left-to-right shunts or severe AV valve regurgitation. A soft middiastolic murmur may sometimes be heard in patients with acute rheumatic fever (Carey-Coombs murmur). It has been attributed to inflammation of the mitral valve cusps or excessive left atrial blood flow as a consequence of mitral regurgitation.

In acute, severe aortic regurgitation, the left ventricular diastolic pressure may exceed the left atrial pressure, resulting in a middiastolic murmur due to "diastolic mitral regurgitation." In severe, chronic aortic regurgitation, a murmur is frequently present that may be either middiastolic or presystolic (Austin-Flint murmur). This murmur appears to originate at the anterior mitral valve leaflet when blood enters the left ventricle simultaneously from both the aortic root and the left atrium.

Presystolic murmurs begin during the period of ventricular filling that follows atrial contraction and therefore occur in sinus rhythm. They are usually due to AV valve stenosis and have the same quality as the middiastolic filling rumble, but they are usually crescendo, reaching peak intensity at the time of a loud S_1. The presystolic murmur corresponds to the AV valve gradient, which may be minimal until the moment of right or left atrial contraction. It is the presystolic murmur that is most characteristic of tricuspid stenosis and sinus rhythm. A right or left *atrial myxoma* may occasionally cause either middiastolic or presystolic murmurs that resemble the murmurs of mitral or tricuspid stenosis.

Continuous Murmurs These begin in systole, peak near S_2, and continue into all or part of diastole. These murmurs result from continuous flow due to a communication between high- and low-pressure areas which persists through the end of systole and the beginning of diastole. A *patent ductus arteriosus* causes a continuous murmur as long as the pressure in the pulmonary artery is much below that in the aorta. The murmur is intensified by elevation of the systemic arterial pressure and is reduced by amyl nitrite inhalation. When pulmonary hypertension is present, the diastolic portion may disappear, leaving the murmur confined to systole. A continuous murmur is uncommon in cases of aortopulmonary septal defect, as that malformation generally is associated with severe pulmonary hypertension. Surgically produced connections and the subclavian–pulmonary artery anastomosis result in murmurs similar to that of a patent ductus.

Continuous murmurs may result from congenital or acquired *systemic arteriovenous fistula*, *coronary arteriovenous fistula*, anomalous origin of the left coronary artery from the pulmonary artery, and communications between the *sinus of Valsalva and the right side of the heart*. Continuous murmurs also may occur in patients with a small atrial septal defect with a high left atrial pressure. Murmurs associated with *pulmonary arteriovenous fistulas* may be continuous but are usually only systolic. Continuous murmurs may also be due to disturbances of flow pattern in constricted systemic (e.g., renal) or pulmonary arteries when marked pressure differences between the two sides of the narrow segment persist; a continuous murmur in the back may be present in *coarctation of the aorta*; *pulmonary embolism* may cause continuous murmurs in partially occluded vessels.

In nonconstricted arteries, continuous murmurs may be due to rapid flow through a tortuous bed. Such murmurs typically occur within the bronchial arterial collateral circulation in cyanotic patients with severe pulmonary outflow obstruction. The "mammary souffle," an innocent murmur heard over the breasts during late pregnancy and in the early postpartum period, may be systolic or continuous. The innocent cervical venous hum is a continuous murmur usually audible over the medial aspect of the right supraclavicular fossa with the patient upright. The hum is usually louder during diastole and can be abolished instantaneously by digital compression of the ipsilateral internal jugular vein. Transmission of a loud venous hum to the area below the clavicles may result in a mistaken diagnosis of patent ductus arteriosus.

Pericardial Friction Rub These adventitious sounds may have presystolic, systolic, and early diastolic scratchy components, may be confused with a murmur or extracardiac sound when heard only in systole. It is best appreciated with the patient upright and leaning forward and may be accentuated during inspiration.

BIBLIOGRAPHY

CRAWFORD MH: *Examination of the Heart*, Part 2: *Inspection and Palpation of Venous and Arterial Pulses*. Chicago, American Heart Association, 1990

EILEN SD et al: Accuracy of precordial palpation for detecting increased left ventricular volume. Ann Intern Med 99:628, 1983

EWY GA: The abdominojugular test: Technique and hemodynamic correlates. Ann Intern Med 109:456, 1988

GREWE K et al: Differentiation of cardiac murmurs by auscultation. Curr Probl Cardiol 13(10):699, 1988

LEMBO NJ et al: Bedside diagnosis of systolic murmurs. N Engl J Med 318:1572, 1988

PERLOFF JK (ed): *Physical Examination of the Heart and Circulation*, 2d ed. Philadelphia, Saunders, 1990

———, BRAUNWALD E: Physical examination of the heart and circulation, in *Heart Disease*, 5th ed, E Braunwald (ed). Philadelphia, Saunders, 1997, pp 15–52

SHAVER JA: Cardiac auscultation: A cost-effective diagnostic skill. Curr Probl Cardiol 20(7):441, 1995

228 *Ary L. Goldberger*

ELECTROCARDIOGRAPHY

The electrocardiogram (ECG or EKG) is a graphic recording of electric potentials generated by the heart. The signals are detected by means of metal electrodes attached to the extremities and chest wall and are then amplified and recorded by the electrocardiograph. ECG *leads* actually display the instantaneous *differences* in potential between these electrodes.

The clinical utility of the ECG derives from its immediate availability as a noninvasive, inexpensive, and highly versatile test. In addition to its use in detecting arrhythmias, conduction disturbances, and myocardial ischemia, electrocardiography may reveal other findings related to life-threatening metabolic disturbances (e.g., hyperkalemia) or increased susceptibility to sudden cardiac death (e.g., QT prolongation syndromes). The advent of coronary thrombolysis or angioplasty in the early therapy of acute myocardial infarction (Chap. 243) has refocused particular attention on the sensitivity and specificity of ECG signs of myocardial ischemia.

ELECTROPHYSIOLOGY (See also Chaps. 230 and 231) Depolarization of the heart is the initiating event for cardiac contraction. The electric currents that spread through the heart are produced by three components: cardiac pacemaker cells, specialized conduction tissue, and the heart muscle itself. The ECG, however, records only the depolarization (stimulation) and repolarization (recovery) potentials generated by the atrial and ventricular myocardium. Under resting conditions, myocardial cells are *polarized*; that is, they carry an electric charge on their surface due to transmembrane ion concentration differences. The charge measured across atrial and ventricular cell membranes is about 90 mV, with the inside negative relative to the outside. When these cells are stimulated above a critical threshold potential, they rapidly depolarize and transiently reverse their membrane polarity. This depolarization process spreads in a wavelike manner through the atria and ventricles. The return of myocardial fibers to their original resting state occurs during repolarization.

The depolarization stimulus for the normal heartbeat originates in the *sinoatrial* (SA) *node* (Fig. 228-1) or *sinus node*, a collection of *pacemaker* cells. These cells fire spontaneously; that is, they exhibit *automaticity*. The first phase of cardiac electrical activation is the spread of the depolarization wave through the right and left atria, followed by atrial contraction. Next, the impulse stimulates pacemaker and specialized conduction tissues in the atrioventricular (AV) nodal and His-bundle areas; together, these two regions constitute the AV junction. The bundle of His bifurcates into two main branches, the right and left bundles, which rapidly transmit depolarization wavefronts to

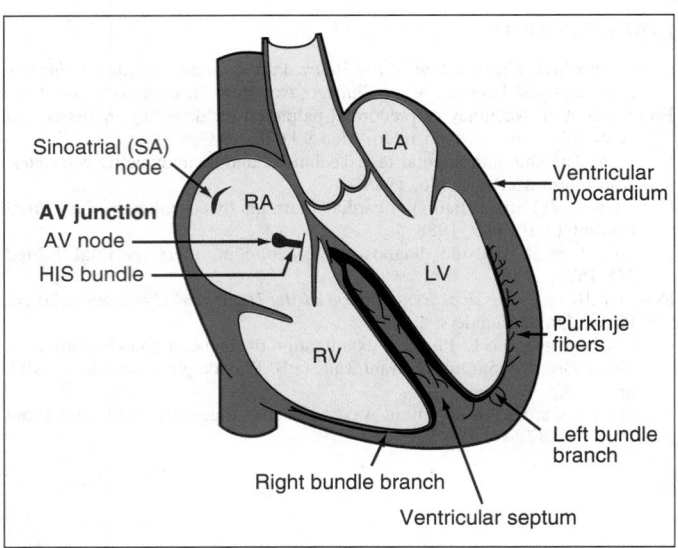

FIGURE 228-1 Schematic of the cardiac conduction system.

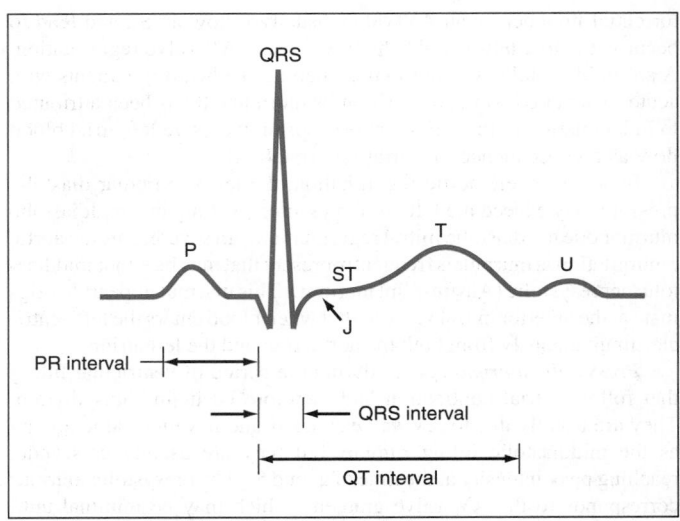

FIGURE 228-2 Basic ECG waveforms and intervals. Not shown is the R-R interval, the time between consecutive QRS complexes.

the right and left ventricular myocardium by way of Purkinje fibers. The main left bundle bifurcates into two primary subdivisions, a left anterior fascicle and a left posterior fascicle. The depolarization wavefronts then spread through the ventricular wall, from endocardium to epicardium, triggering ventricular contraction.

Since the cardiac depolarization and repolarization waves have direction and magnitude, they can be represented by vectors. *Vectorcardiograms* that measure and display these instantaneous potentials are no longer used much in clinical practice. However, the general principles of vector analysis remain fundamental to understanding the genesis of normal and pathologic ECG waveforms. Vector analysis illustrates a central concept of electrocardiography—that the ECG records the complex spatial and temporal summation of electrical potentials from multiple myocardial fibers conducted to the surface of the body. This principle accounts for inherent limitations in both ECG *sensitivity* (activity from certain cardiac regions may be canceled out or may be too weak to be recorded) and *specificity* (the same vectorial sum can result from either a selective gain or a loss of forces in opposite directions).

ECG WAVEFORMS AND INTERVALS The ECG waveforms are labeled alphabetically, beginning with the P wave, which represents atrial depolarization (Fig. 228-2). The QRS complex represents ventricular depolarization, and the ST-T-U complex (ST segment, T wave, and U wave) represents ventricular repolarization. The J point is the junction between the end of the QRS complex and the beginning of the ST segment. Atrial repolarization is usually too low in amplitude to be detected, but it may become apparent in such conditions as acute pericarditis or atrial infarction.

The QRS-T waveforms of the surface (extracellular) ECG correspond in a general way with the different phases of simultaneously obtained ventricular *action potentials*, the intracellular recordings from single myocardial fibers (Fig. 228-3) (see also Chap. 230). The rapid upstroke (phase 0) of the action potential corresponds to the onset of QRS. The plateau (phase 2) corresponds to the isoelectric ST segment, and active repolarization (phase 3) to the inscription of the T wave. Factors that decrease the slope of phase 0 by impairing the influx of Na$^+$ (e.g., drugs such as quinidine or procainamide, or hyperkalemia) tend to increase QRS duration. Conditions that prolong phase 2 (amiodarone, hypocalcemia) increase the QT interval. In contrast, shortening of ventricular repolarization (phase 2), as by digitalis or hypercalcemia, abbreviates the ST segment.

The electrocardiogram is ordinarily recorded on special graph paper which is divided into 1-mm^2 gridlike boxes (Fig. 228-4). Since

the ECG paper speed is generally 25 mm/s, the smallest (1 mm) horizontal divisions correspond to 0.04 s (40 ms), with heavier lines at intervals of 0.20 s (200 ms). Vertically, the ECG graph measures the amplitude of a given wave or deflection (1 mV = 10 mm with standard calibration; the voltage criteria for hypertrophy mentioned below are given in millimeters). There are four major ECG intervals: R-R, PR, QRS, and QT (Fig. 228-2). The heart rate (beats per minute) can be readily computed from the interbeat (R-R) interval by dividing the number of large (0.20 s) time units between consecutive R waves into 300 or the number of small (0.04 s) units into 1500. The PR interval (normally 120 to 200 ms) measures the time (normally 120 to 200 ms) between atrial and ventricular depolarization, which includes the physiologic delay imposed by stimulation of cells in the AV junction area. The QRS interval (normally 100 ms or less) reflects the duration of ventricular depolarization. The QT interval includes both ventricular depolarization and repolarization times and varies inversely with the heart rate. A rate-related ("corrected") QT interval, QT$_c$, can be calculated as QT/$\sqrt{\text{R-R}}$ and normally is ≤0.44 s.

The QRS complex is subdivided into specific deflections or waves. If the initial QRS deflection in a given lead is negative, it is termed a *Q wave*; the first positive deflection is termed an *R wave*. A negative deflection after an R wave is an *S wave*. Subsequent positive or negative waves are labeled R′ and S′, respectively. Lowercase letters (qrs)

FIGURE 228-3 The QRS-T cycle corresponds to different phases of the ventricular action potential as described in Chap. 230.

are used for waves of relatively small amplitude. An entirely negative QRS complex is termed a *QS wave*.

ECG LEADS The 12 conventional ECG leads record the difference in potential between electrodes placed on the surface of the body. These leads are divided into two groups; six extremity (limb) leads and six chest (precordial) leads. The extremity leads record potentials transmitted onto the *frontal plane* (Fig. 228-5*A*), and the chest leads record potentials transmitted onto the *horizontal plane* (Fig. 228-5*B*). The six extremity leads are further subdivided into three *bipolar* leads (I, II, and III) and three *unipolar* leads (aVR, aVL, and aVF). Each bipolar lead measures the difference in potential between electrodes at two extremities: lead I = left arm − right arm voltages; lead II = left leg − right arm; and lead III = left leg − left arm. The unipolar leads measure the voltage (V) at one locus relative to an electrode (called the *central terminal* or *indifferent electrode*) that has approximately zero potential. Thus, aVR = right arm, aVL = left arm, and aVF = left leg (foot). The lowercase *a* indicates that these unipolar potentials are electrically augmented by 50 percent. The right leg electrode functions as a ground. The spatial orientation and polarity of the six frontal plane leads is represented on the hexaxial diagram (Fig. 228-6).

The six chest leads (Fig. 228-7) are unipolar recordings obtained by electrodes in the following positions: lead V_1, fourth intercostal space, just to the right of the sternum; lead V_2, fourth intercostal space, just to the left of the sternum; lead V_3, midway between V_2 and V_4; lead V_4, midclavicular line, fifth intercostal space; lead V_5, anterior axillary line, same level as V_4; and lead V_6, midaxillary line, same level as V_4 and V_5.

Together, the frontal and horizontal plane electrodes provide a three-dimensional representation of cardiac electrical activity. Each lead can be likened to a different camera angle "looking" at the same events—atrial and ventricular depolarization and repolarization—from different spatial orientations. The conventional 12-lead ECG can be supplemented with additional leads under special circumstances. For example, right precordial leads V_3R, V_4R, etc. are useful in detecting evidence of acute right ventricular ischemia. Esophageal leads may reveal atrial activity not detectable on the surface ECG. Bedside telemetry units and ambulatory ECG (Holter) recordings usually employ only one or two modified leads, respectively. → *Intracardiac electrocardiography and electrophysiologic testing are discussed in Chaps. 230 and 231.*

The ECG leads are configured so that a positive (upright) deflection is recorded in a lead if a wave of depolarization spreads toward the positive pole of that lead, and a negative deflection if the wave spreads toward the negative pole. If the mean orientation of the depolarization vector is at right angles to a given lead axis, a biphasic (equally positive and negative) deflection will be recorded.

GENESIS OF THE NORMAL ECG

P WAVE The normal atrial depolarization vector is oriented downward and toward the subject's left, reflecting the spread of depolarization from the sinus node to the right and then the left atrial myocardium. Since this vector points toward the positive pole of lead II and toward

FIGURE 228-4 The ECG graph paper records the time (interval) between cardiac electrical events along the horizontal axis and their amplitude (voltage) along the vertical axis.

the negative pole of lead aVR, the normal P wave will be positive in lead II and negative in lead aVR. By contrast, activation of the atria from an ectopic pacemaker in the lower part of either atrium or in the AV junction region may produce retrograde P waves (negative in lead II, positive in lead aVR).

QRS COMPLEX Normal ventricular depolarization proceeds as a rapid, continuous spread of activation wavefronts. This complex process can be divided into two major, sequential phases, and each phase can be represented by a mean vector (Fig. 228-8). The first phase is depolarization of the interventricular septum from the left to the right (vector 1). The second results from the simultaneous depolarization of the main mass of the right and left ventricles; it is normally dominated by the more massive left ventricle, so that vector 2 points leftward and posteriorly. Therefore, a right precordial lead (V_1) will record this biphasic depolarization process with a small positive deflection (septal r wave) followed by a larger negative deflection (S wave). A left precordial lead, e.g., V_6, will record the same sequence with a small negative deflection (septal q wave) followed by a relatively tall positive deflection (R wave). Intermediate leads show a relative increase in R-wave amplitude (normal R-wave progression) and a decrease in S-wave amplitude progressing across the chest from the right to left. The precordial lead where the R and S waves are of approximately equal amplitude is referred to as the *transition zone* (usually V_3 or V_4) (Fig. 228-9).

The QRS pattern in the extremity leads may vary considerably from one normal subject to another depending on the *electrical axis* of the QRS, which describes the mean orientation of the QRS vector with reference to the six frontal plane leads. Normally, the QRS axis

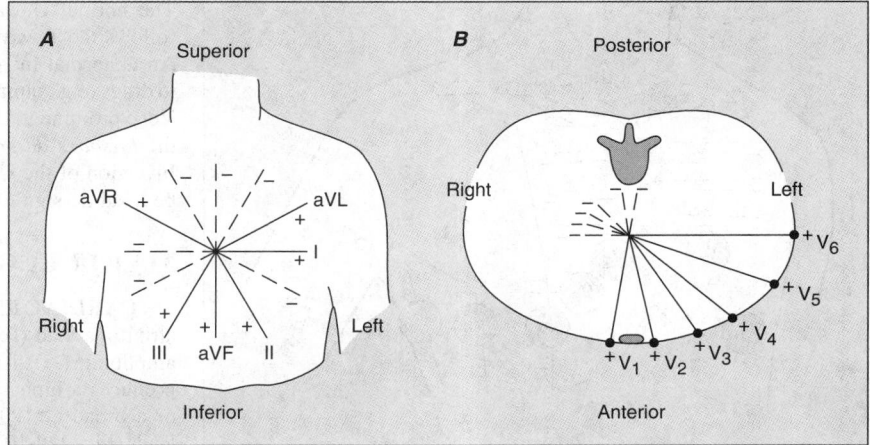

FIGURE 228-5 The six frontal plane (*A*) and six horizontal plane (*B*) leads provide a three-dimensional representation of cardiac electrical activity.

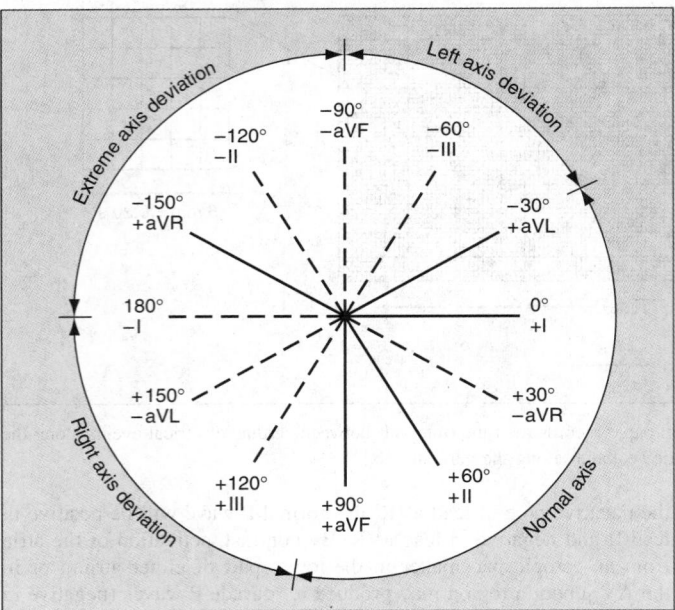

FIGURE 228-6 The frontal plane (extremity or limb) leads are represented on a hexaxial diagram. Each ECG lead has a specific spatial orientation and polarity. The positive pole of each lead axis (*solid line*) and negative pole (*hatched line*) are designated by their angular position relative to the positive pole of lead I (0°). The mean electrical axis of the QRS complex is measured with respect to this display.

ranges from −30° to +100° (Fig. 228-6). An axis more negative than −30° is referred to as *left axis deviation*, while an axis more positive than +100° is referred to as *right axis deviation*. Left axis deviation may occur as a normal variant but is more commonly associated with left ventricular hypertrophy, a block in the anterior fascicle of the left bundle system (left anterior fascicular block or hemiblock), or inferior myocardial infarction. Right axis deviation also may occur as a normal variant (particularly in children and young adults), as a spurious finding due to reversal of the left and right arm electrodes, or in conditions such as right ventricular overload (acute or chronic), infarction of the lateral wall of the left ventricle, dextrocardia, left pneumothorax, or left posterior fascicular block.

T WAVE AND U WAVE Normally, the mean T-wave vector is oriented roughly concordant with the mean QRS vector. Since depolarization and repolarization are electrically opposite processes,

FIGURE 228-7 The horizontal plane (chest or precordial) leads are obtained with electrodes in the locations shown.

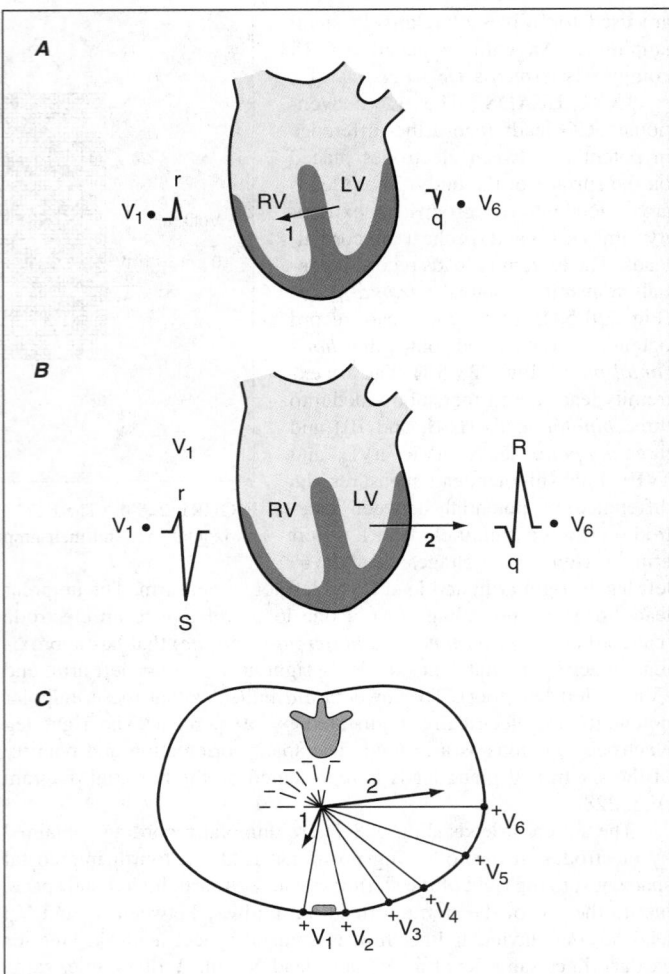

FIGURE 228-8 Ventricular depolarization can be divided into two major phases, each represented by a vector. *A.* The first phase (*arrow 1*) denotes depolarization of the ventricular septum, beginning on the left side and spreading to the right. This process is represented by a small "septal" r wave in lead V_1 and a small septal q wave in lead V_6. *B.* Simultaneous depolarization of the left and right ventricles (LV and RV) constitutes the second phase. Vector 2 is oriented to the left and posteriorly, reflecting the electrical predominance of the LV. *C.* Vectors (*arrows*) representing these two phases are shown in reference to the horizontal plane leads. (*After Goldberger and Goldberger.*)

this normal QRS−T-wave vector concordance indicates that repolarization must normally proceed in the reverse direction from depolarization (i.e., from epicardium to endocardium or from cardiac apex to base). The normal U wave is a small, rounded deflection (≤1 mm) that follows the T wave and usually has the same polarity as the T wave. An abnormal increase in U-wave amplitude is most commonly due to drugs (e.g., quinidine, procainamide, disopyramide) or hypokalemia. Very prominent U waves are a marker of increased susceptibility to the *torsades de pointes* type of ventricular tachycardia (Chap. 231). Inversion of the U wave in the precordial leads is abnormal and may be a subtle sign of ischemia.

MAJOR ECG ABNORMALITIES

CARDIAC ENLARGEMENT AND HYPERTROPHY Right atrial overload (acute or chronic) may lead to an increase in P-wave amplitude (≥2.5 mm) (Fig. 228-10). Left atrial overload typically produces a biphasic P wave in V_1 with a broad negative component or a broad (≥120 ms), often notched P wave in one or more limb leads (Fig. 228-10). This pattern also may occur with left atrial conduction delays in the absence of actual atrial enlargement, leading to the more general designation of *left atrial abnormality*.

Right ventricular hypertrophy due to a pressure load (as from pulmonic valve stenosis or pulmonary artery hypertension) is characterized by a relatively tall R wave in lead V_1 (R ≥ S wave), usually with right axis deviation (Fig. 228-11); alternatively, there may be a qR pattern in V_1 or V_3R. ST depression and T-wave inversion in the right to midprecordial leads are also often present. This so-called ventricular strain pattern is attributed to repolarization abnormalities in hypertrophied muscle. Right ventricular hypertrophy due to ostium secundum–type atrial septal defects, with the accompanying right ventricular volume overload, is commonly associated with an incomplete or complete right bundle branch block pattern with a rightward QRS axis.

Acute cor pulmonale due to pulmonary embolism (Chap. 261) for example, may be associated with a normal ECG or a variety of abnormalities. Sinus tachycardia is the most common arrhythmia, although other tachyarrhythmias, such as atrial fibrillation or flutter, may occur. The QRS axis may shift to the right, sometimes in concert with the so-called $S_1Q_3T_3$ pattern (prominence of the S wave in lead I, Q wave in lead III, with T-wave inversion in lead III). Acute right ventricular dilation also may be associated with poor R-wave progression and T-wave inversions in V_1 to V_4 (right ventricular "strain") simulating acute anterior infarction. A right ventricular conduction disturbance may appear.

Chronic cor pulmonale due to obstructive lung disease (Chap. 238) usually does not produce the classic ECG patterns of right ventricular hypertrophy noted above. Instead of tall right precordial R waves, chronic lung disease more typically is associated with small R waves in right to midprecordial leads (poor R-wave progression) due in part to downward displacement of the diaphragm and the heart. Low-voltage complexes are commonly present, owing to hyperaeration of the lungs.

A number of different voltage criteria for *left ventricular hypertrophy* (Fig. 228-11) have been proposed on the basis of the presence of tall left precordial R waves and deep right precordial S waves [e.g., $SV_1 + (RV_5 \text{ or } RV_6) \geq 35$ mm; or $(RV_5 \text{ or } RV_6) \geq 25$ mm]. Repolarization abnormalities (ST depression with T-wave inversions) also may appear (left ventricular "strain" pattern) in leads with prominent R waves. However, prominent precordial voltages may occur as a normal variant, especially in athletic or thin-chested individuals. Left ventricular hypertrophy may increase limb lead voltage (e.g., RaVL ≥ 11 to 13 mm, RaVF ≥ 20 mm; $R_I + S_{III} \geq 25$ mm) with or without increased precordial voltage. The presence of left atrial abnormality increases the likelihood of underlying left ventricular hypertrophy in cases with borderline voltage criteria. Left ventricular hypertrophy often progresses to incomplete or complete left bundle branch block. The sensitivity of conventional voltage criteria for left ventricular hypertrophy is decreased in obese persons and in women. ECG evidence for left ventricular hypertrophy is a major noninvasive marker of increased risk of cardiovascular morbidity and mortality, including sudden cardiac death. However, because of false-positive and false-negative diagnoses, the ECG is of limited utility in diagnosing atrial or ventricular enlargement. More definitive information is provided by echocardiography.

BUNDLE BRANCH BLOCKS Intrinsic impairment of conduction in either the right or left bundle system (intraventricular conduction disturbances) leads to prolongation of the QRS interval. With complete bundle branch blocks the QRS interval is ≥ 120 ms in duration; with incomplete blocks the QRS interval is between 100 and 120 ms. The QRS vector is usually oriented in the direction of the myocardial region where depolarization is delayed (Fig. 228-12). Thus,

FIGURE 228-9 Normal electrocardiogram from a healthy subject. Sinus rhythm is present with a heart rate of 75 beats per minute. PR interval is 0.16 s; QRS interval (duration) is 0.08 s; QT interval is 0.36 s; the mean QRS axis is about +70°. The precordial leads show normal R-wave progression with the transition zone (R wave = S wave) in lead V_3.

with right bundle branch block, the terminal QRS vector is oriented anteriorly and to the right (rSR′ in V_1 and qRS in V_6, typically). Left bundle branch block alters both early and later phases of ventricular depolarization. The major QRS vector is directed to the left and posteriorly. In addition, the normal early left-to-right pattern of septal activation is disrupted such that septal depolarization proceeds from right to left as well. As a result, left bundle branch block generates wide, predominantly negative (QS) complexes in lead V_1 and entirely positive (R) complexes in lead V_6. A pattern identical to that of left bundle branch block, preceded by a sharp spike, is seen in most cases of electronic right ventricular pacing because of the relative delay in left ventricular activation.

Bundle branch block may occur in a variety of conditions. In subjects without structural heart disease, right bundle branch block is

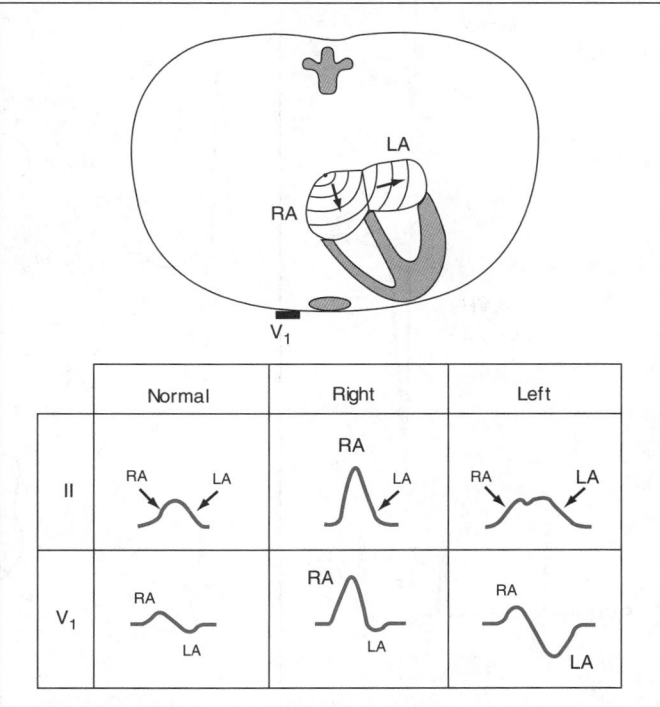

FIGURE 228-10 Right atrial (RA) overload may cause tall, peaked P waves in the limb or precordial leads. Left atrial (LA) abnormality may cause broad, often notched P waves in the limb leads and a biphasic P wave in lead V_1 with a prominent negative component representing delayed depolarization of the LA. *(After MK Park, WG Guntheroth: How to Read Pediatric ECGs, 2d ed. St. Louis, Mosby–Year Book, 1987.)*

seen more commonly than left bundle branch block. Right bundle branch block also occurs with heart disease, both congenital (e.g., atrial septal defect) and acquired (e.g., valvular, ischemic). Left bundle branch block is often a marker of one of four underlying conditions: ischemic heart disease, long-standing hypertension, severe aortic valve disease, and cardiomyopathy. Bundle branch blocks may be chronic or intermittent. A bundle branch block may be rate-related; for example, often it occurs when the heart rate exceeds some critical value.

Bundle branch blocks and depolarization abnormalities secondary to artificial pacemakers not only affect ventricular depolarization (QRS) but are also characteristically associated with *secondary repolarization* (ST-T) abnormalities. With bundle branch blocks, the T wave is typically opposite in polarity to the last deflection of the QRS (Fig. 228-12). This discordance of the QRS–T-wave vectors is caused by the altered sequence of repolarization that occurs secondary to altered depolarization. In contrast, *primary repolarization* abnormalities are independent of QRS changes and are related instead to actual alterations in the electrical properties of the myocardial fibers themselves (for example, in the resting membrane potential or action potential duration), not just to changes in the sequence of repolarization. Ischemia, electrolyte imbalance, and drugs such as digitalis all cause such primary ST–T-wave changes. Primary and secondary T-wave changes may coexist. For example, T-wave inversions in the right precordial leads with left bundle branch block or in the left precordial

leads with right bundle branch block may be important markers of underlying ischemia or other abnormalities.

Partial blocks ("hemiblocks") in the left bundle system (left anterior or posterior fascicular blocks) generally do not prolong the QRS duration substantially but instead are associated with shifts in the frontal plane QRS axis (leftward or rightward, respectively). More complex combinations of fascicular and bundle branch blocks may occur involving the left and right bundle system. Examples of *bifascicular block* include right bundle branch block and left posterior fascicular block, right bundle branch block with left anterior fascicular block, and complete left bundle branch block. Chronic bifascicular block in an asymptomatic individual is associated with a relatively low risk of progression to high-degree AV heart block. In contrast, new bifascicular block with acute anterior myocardial infarction carries a much greater risk of complete heart block. Alternation of right and left bundle branch block is a sign of *trifascicular disease*. However, the presence of a prolonged PR interval and bifascicular block does not necessarily indicate trifascicular involvement, since this combination may arise with AV node disease and bifascicular block. Intraventricular conduction delays also can be caused by extrinsic (toxic) factors that slow ventricular conduction, particularly hyperkalemia or drugs (type 1 antiarrhythmic agents, tricyclic antidepressants, phenothiazines).

Prolongation of QRS duration does not necessarily indicate a conduction delay but may be due to *preexcitation* of the ventricles via a bypass tract, as in the Wolff-Parkinson-White (WPW) syndrome (Fig. 231-10) and related variants. The diagnostic triad of WPW consists of a wide QRS complex associated with a relatively short PR interval and slurring of the initial part of the QRS (delta wave), the latter effect due to aberrant activation of ventricular myocardium. The presence of a bypass tract predisposes to reentrant supraventricular tachyarrhythmias (Chap. 231).

MYOCARDIAL ISCHEMIA AND INFARCTION (See also Chap. 243) The ECG is a cornerstone in the diagnosis of acute and chronic ischemic heart disease. The findings depend on several key factors: the nature of the process [reversible (i.e., ischemia) versus irreversible (i.e., infarction)], the duration (acute versus chronic), extent (transmural versus subendocardial), and localization (anterior versus inferoposterior), as well as the presence of other underlying abnormalities (ventricular hypertrophy, conduction defects).

Ischemia exerts complex time-dependent effects on the electrical properties of myocardial cells. Severe, acute ischemia lowers the resting membrane potential and shortens the duration of the action potential. Such changes cause a voltage gradient between normal and ischemic zones. As a consequence, current flows between these regions. These so-called currents of injury are represented on the surface ECG by deviation of the ST segment (Fig. 228-13). When the acute ischemia is *transmural*, the ST vector is usually shifted in the direction of the outer (epicardial) layers, producing ST elevations and sometimes, in the earliest stages of ischemia, tall, positive so-called hyperacute T waves over the ischemic zone. With ischemia confined primarily to the *subendocardium*, the ST vector typically shifts toward the subendocardium and ventricular cavity, so that overlying (e.g., anterior precordial) leads show ST-segment depression (with ST elevation in lead aVR). Multiple factors affect the amplitude of acute ischemic ST deviations. Profound ST elevation or depression in multiple leads usually indicates very severe ischemia. Complete

FIGURE 228-11 Left ventricular hypertrophy (LVH) increases the amplitude of electrical forces directed to the left and posteriorly. In addition, repolarization abnormalities may cause ST-segment depression and T-wave inversion in leads with a prominent R wave "strain" pattern. Right ventricular hypertrophy (RVH) may shift the QRS vector to the right; this effect usually is associated with an R, RS, or qR complex in lead V_1. T-wave inversions may be present in right precordial leads ("strain" pattern).

resolution of ST elevation promptly following thrombolytic therapy is a relatively specific, though not sensitive, marker of successful reperfusion.

The ECG leads are more helpful in localizing regions of Q wave than non-Q-wave ischemia. For example, acute anterior wall ischemia leading to Q-wave infarction is reflected by ST elevations or increased T-wave positivity (Fig. 228-14) in one or more of the precordial leads (V_1 to V_6) and leads I and aVL. Anteroseptal ischemia produces these changes in leads V_1 to V_3, apical or lateral ischemia in leads V_4 to V_6. Inferior wall ischemia produces changes in leads II, III, and aVF. Posterior wall ischemia may be indirectly recognized by *reciprocal* ST depressions in leads V_1 to V_3. Prominent reciprocal ST depressions in these leads also occur with certain inferior wall infarcts, particularly those with posterior or lateral wall extension. Right ventricular ischemia usually produces ST elevations in right-sided chest leads (Fig. 228-7). When ischemic ST elevations occur as the earliest sign of acute infarction, they are typically followed within a period ranging from hours to days by evolving T-wave inversions and often by Q waves occurring in the same lead distribution. (T-wave inversions due to evolving or chronic ischemia correlate with prolongation of repolarization and are often associated with QT lengthening.) Reversible transmural ischemia, for example, due to coronary vasospasm (Prinzmetal's variant angina), may cause transient ST-segment elevations without development of Q waves. Depending on the severity and duration of such ischemia, the ST elevations may either resolve completely in minutes or be followed by T-wave inversions that persist for hours or even days. Patients with ischemic chest pain who present with deep T-wave inversions in multiple precordial leads (e.g., V_1 to V_4) with or without cardiac enzyme elevations typically have severe obstruction in the left anterior descending coronary artery system (Fig. 228-15). In contrast, patients whose baseline ECG already shows abnormal T-wave inversions may develop T-wave normalization (pseudonormalization) during episodes of acute transmural ischemia.

FIGURE 228-13 Acute ischemia causes a current of injury. With predominant subendocardial ischemia (*A*), the resultant ST vector will be directed toward the inner layer of the affected ventricle and the ventricular cavity. Overlying leads therefore will record ST depression. With ischemia involving the outer ventricular layer (*B*) (transmural or epicardial injury), the ST vector will be directed outward. Overlying leads will record ST elevation.

With infarction, depolarization (QRS) changes often accompany repolarization (ST-T) abnormalities. Necrosis of sufficient myocardial tissue may lead to decreased R-wave amplitude or frank abnormal Q waves in the anterior or inferior leads (Fig. 228-16). Previously, abnormal Q waves were considered to be markers of transmural myocardial infarction, while subendocardial infarcts were thought not to produce Q waves. However, careful ECG-pathology correlative studies have indicated that transmural infarcts may occur without Q waves and that subendocardial (nontransmural) infarcts may sometimes be associated with Q waves. Therefore, infarcts are more appropriately classified

FIGURE 228-12 Comparison of typical QRS-T patterns in right bundle branch block (RBBB) and left bundle branch block (LBBB) with the normal pattern in leads V_1 and V_6. Note the secondary T-wave inversions (*arrows*) in leads with an rSR' complex with RBBB and in leads with a wide R wave with LBBB.

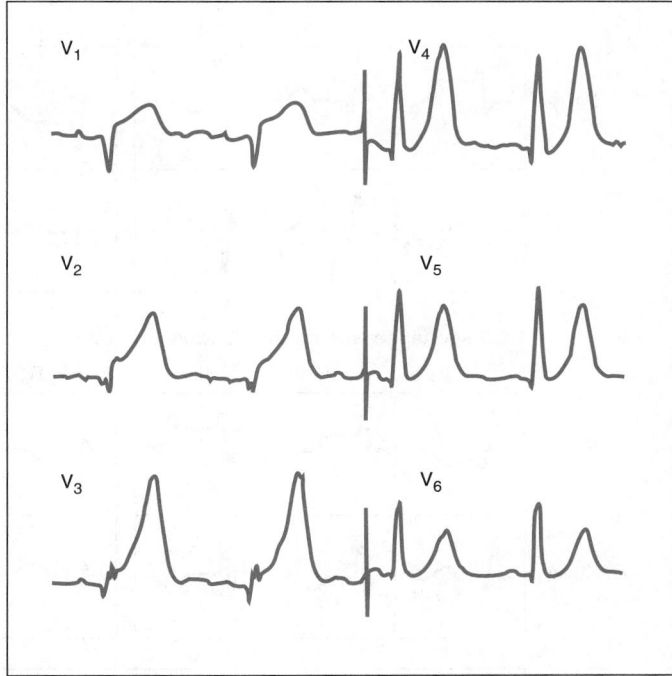

FIGURE 228-14 Hyperacute phase of anteroseptal myocardial infarction (MI). Note the tall positive T waves (V_2 to V_3) along with ST-segment elevations and Q waves (V_1 to V_3).

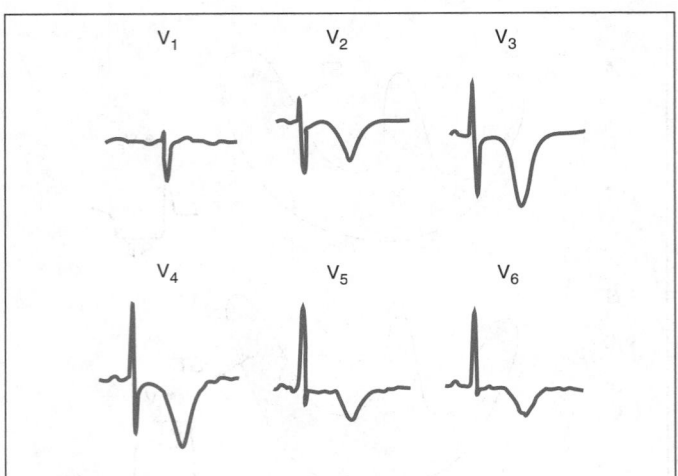

FIGURE 228-15 Severe anterior wall ischemia (with or without infarction) may cause prominent T-wave inversions in the precordial leads. This pattern is usually associated with a high-grade stenosis of the left anterior descending coronary artery.

as "Q-wave" or "non-Q-wave." The major acute ECG changes in syndromes of ischemic heart disease are schematically summarized in Fig. 228-17. Loss of depolarization forces due to posterior or lateral infarction may cause reciprocal increases in R-wave amplitude in leads V_1 and V_2 without diagnostic Q waves in any of the conventional leads. Atrial infarction may be associated with PR-segment deviations due to an atrial current of injury, changes in P-wave morphology, or atrial arrhythmias. In the weeks and months following infarction, these ECG changes may persist or begin to resolve. Complete normalization of the ECG following Q-wave infarction is uncommon but may occur, particularly with smaller infarcts. In contrast, ST-segment elevations that persist for several weeks or more after a Q-wave infarct usually

correlate with a severe underlying wall motion disorder (akinetic or dyskinetic zone), although not necessarily a frank ventricular aneurysm.

ECG changes due to ischemia may occur spontaneously or may be provoked by various exercise protocols (stress electrocardiography) (Chap. 244). In patients with severe ischemic heart disease, exercise testing is most likely to elicit signs of subendocardial ischemia (horizontal or downsloping ST depression in multiple leads). ST-segment elevation during exercise is most often observed after a Q-wave infarct. This repolarization change does not necessarily indicate active ischemia but correlates strongly with the presence of an underlying ventricular wall motion abnormality. However, in patients *without* prior infarction, transient ST-segment elevation with exercise is a reliable sign of transmural ischemia.

The ECG has important limitations in both sensitivity and specificity in the diagnosis of ischemic heart disease. Although a single normal ECG does not exclude ischemia or even acute infarction, a normal ECG *throughout* the course of an acute infarct is distinctly uncommon. Prolonged chest pain without diagnostic ECG changes, therefore, should always prompt a careful search for other noncoronary causes of chest pain (see Chap. 13). Furthermore, the diagnostic changes of acute or evolving ischemia are often masked by the presence of left bundle branch block, electronic ventricular pacemaker patterns, and WPW preexcitation. On the other hand, clinicians may overdiagnose ischemia or infarction based on the presence of ST-segment elevations or depressions, T-wave inversions, tall positive T waves, or Q waves *not* related to ischemic heart disease (pseudoinfarct patterns). For example, ST-segment elevations simulating ischemia may occur with acute pericarditis (Fig. 228-18) or myocarditis or as a normal variant ("early repolarization" pattern). Similarly, tall, positive T waves do not invariably represent hyperacute ischemic changes but also may be caused by normal variants, hyperkalemia, cerebrovascular injury, and left ventricular volume overload due to mitral or aortic regurgitation, among other causes. ST-segment elevations and tall, positive T waves are common findings in leads V_1 and V_2 in left bundle branch or left ventricular hypertrophy in the absence of ischemia. The differential diagnosis of Q waves (Table 228-1) includes physiologic or positional variants, ventricular hypertrophy, acute or chronic noncoronary myo-

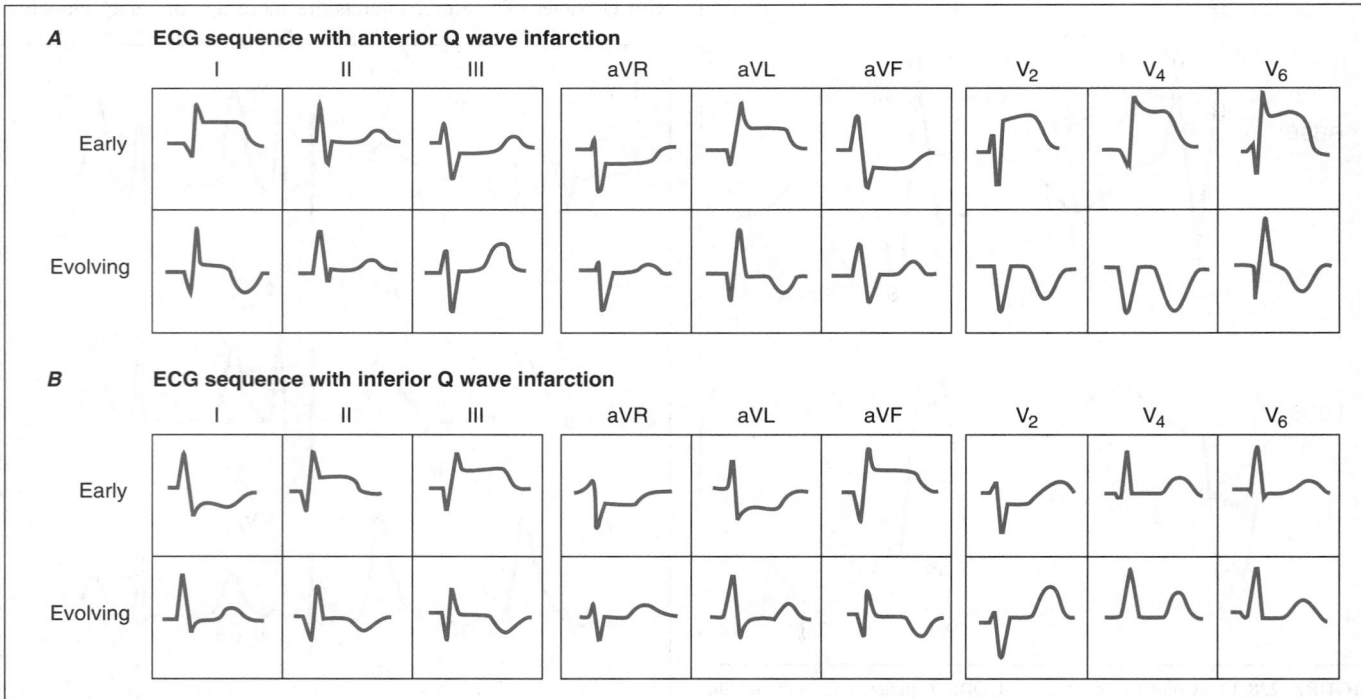

FIGURE 228-16 Sequence of depolarization and repolarization changes with (*A*) acute anterior and (*B*) acute inferior wall Q-wave infarctions. With anterior infarcts, ST elevation in leads I, aVL, and the precordial leads may be accom-

panied by reciprocal ST depressions in leads II, III, and aVF. Conversely, acute inferior (or posterior) infarcts may be associated with reciprocal ST depressions in leads V_1 to V_3. (*After Goldberger and Goldberger.*)

FIGURE 228-17 Variability of ECG patterns with acute myocardial ischemia. The ECG also may be normal or nonspecifically abnormal. Furthermore, these categorizations are not mutually exclusive. For example, a non-Q-wave infarct may evolve into a Q-wave infarct; ST elevations may be followed by a non-Q-wave infarct; or ST depressions and T-wave inversions may be followed by a Q-wave infarct. *(After Goldberger.)*

cardial injury, hypertrophic cardiomyopathy, and ventricular conduction disorders. Digitalis, ventricular hypertrophy, hypokalemia, and a variety of other factors may cause ST-segment depression mimicking subendocardial ischemia. Prominent T-wave inversion may occur with ventricular hypertrophy, cardiomyopathy, myocarditis, and cerebrovascular injury (particularly intracranial bleeds; Fig. 228-19), among many other conditions.

METABOLIC FACTORS AND DRUG EFFECTS A variety of metabolic and pharmacologic agents alter the ECG and, in particular, cause changes in repolarization (ST-T-U) and sometimes QRS prolongation. Certain life-threatening electrolyte disturbances may be diagnosed initially and monitored from the ECG. *Hyperkalemia* produces a sequence of changes usually beginning with narrowing and peaking (tenting) of the T waves. Further elevation of extracellular K^+ leads to AV conduction disturbances, diminution in P-wave amplitude, and

Table 228-1

Differential Diagnosis of Q Waves (with Selected Examples)

Physiologic or positional factors
1. Normal variant "septal" q waves
2. Normal variant Q waves in V_1 to V_2, aVL, III, and aVF
3. Left pneumothorax or dextrocardia: loss of lateral R-wave progression

Myocardial injury or infiltration
1. Acute processes: myocardial ischemia or infarction, myocarditis, hyperkalemia
2. Chronic processes: myocardial infarction, idiopathic cardiomyopathy, myocarditis, amyloid, tumor, sarcoid, scleroderma, Chagas' disease, echinococcus cyst

Ventricular hypertrophy/enlargement
1. Left ventricular (poor R-wave progression*)
2. Right ventricular (reversed R-wave progression† or poor R-wave progression, particularly with chronic obstructive lung disease)
3. Hypertrophic cardiomyopathy (may simulate anterior, inferior, posterior, or lateral infarcts)

Conduction abnormalities
1. Left bundle branch block (poor R-wave progression*)
2. Wolff-Parkinson-White patterns

---

* Small or absent R waves in the right to midprecordial leads.
† Progressive decrease in R-wave amplitude from V_1 to the mid- or lateral precordial leads.
SOURCE: After Goldberger

widening of the QRS interval. Severe hyperkalemia eventually causes cardiac arrest with a slow sinusoidal type of mechanism ("sine-wave" pattern) followed by asystole. *Hypokalemia* (Fig. 228-19) prolongs ventricular repolarization, often with prominent U waves. Prolongation of the QT interval (Fig. 228-19) is also seen with drugs that increase the duration of the ventricular action potential—type 1A antiarrhythmic agents and related drugs (e.g., quinidine, disopyramide, procainamide, tricyclic antidepressants, phenothiazines) and type III agents (amiodarone, sotalol). Marked QT prolongation, sometimes with deep, wide T-wave inversions, may occur with intracranial bleeds, particularly subarachnoid hemorrhage ("CVA T-wave" pattern) (Fig. 228-19). Systemic *hypothermia* (Fig. 228-19) also prolongs repolarization, usually with a distinctive convex elevation of the J point (Osborn wave). *Hypocalcemia* typically prolongs the QT interval (ST portion), while *hypercalcemia* shortens it (Fig. 228-20). Digitalis glycosides also shorten the QT interval, often with a characteristic "scooping" of the ST–T-wave complex (*digitalis effect*).

FIGURE 228-18 Acute pericarditis often produces diffuse ST-segment elevations (in this case in leads I, II, aVF, and V_2 to V_6) due to a ventricular current of injury. Note also the characteristic PR-segment deviation (opposite in polarity to the ST segment) due to a concomitant atrial injury current.

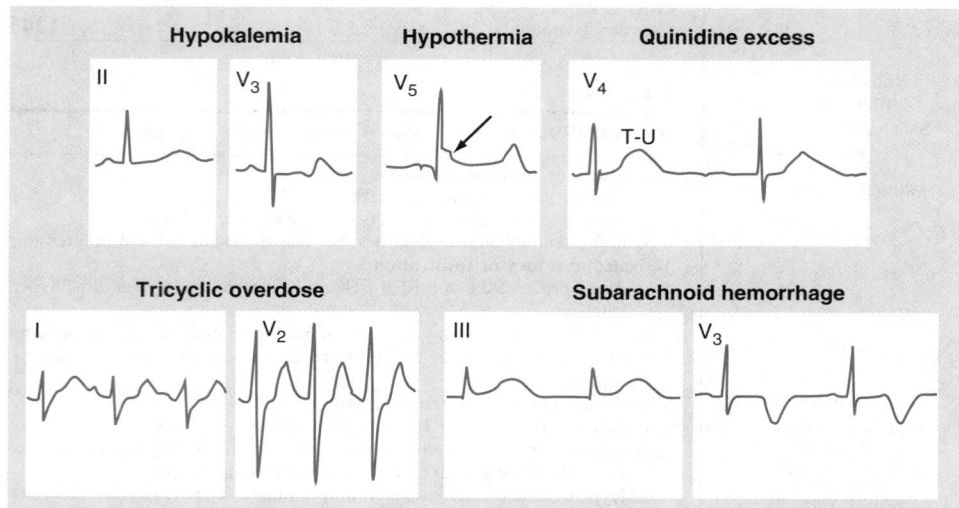

FIGURE 228-19 A variety of metabolic derangements, drug effects, and other factors may prolong ventricular repolarization with QT prolongation or prominent U waves. Repolarization prolongation, particularly if due to hypokalemia or pharmacologic agents, indicates increased susceptibility to torsades de pointes type ventricular tachycardia. Hypothermia is associated with a distinctive convex "hump" at the J point (Osborn wave, *arrow*). Note QRS and QT prolongation along with sinus tachycardia in the case of tricyclic antidepressant overdose.

Many other factors are associated with ECG changes, particularly alterations in ventricular repolarization. T-wave flattening, minimal T-wave inversions or slight ST-segment depression ("nonspecific ST–T-wave changes") may occur with a variety of electrolyte and acid-base disturbances, a variety of infectious processes, central nervous system disorders, endocrine abnormalities, many drugs, ischemia, hypoxia, and virtually any type of cardiopulmonary abnormality. While subtle ST–T-wave changes may be markers of ischemia, transient nonspecific repolarization changes also may occur following a meal or with postural (orthostatic) change, hyperventilation, or exercise in healthy individuals.

ELECTRICAL ALTERNANS Electrical alternans—a beat-to-beat alternation in one or more components of the ECG signal—is a common type of nonlinear cardiovascular response to a variety of perturbations. For example, total electrical alternans (P-QRS-T) with sinus tachycardia is a relatively specific sign of pericardial effusion, often with cardiac tamponade. The mechanism relates to a periodic swinging motion of the heart in the effusion at a frequency exactly one-half the heart rate. ST-T alternans is a sign of electrical instability and may precede ventricular fibrillation.

CLINICAL INTERPRETATION OF THE ECG

Accurate analysis of ECGs requires thoroughness and care. The patient's age, gender, and clinical status should always be taken into account. For example, T-wave inversions in leads V_1 to V_3 are more likely to represent a normal variant in a healthy young adult woman ("persistent juvenile T-wave pattern") than in an elderly man with chest discomfort. Similarly, the likelihood that ST-segment depression during exercise testing represents ischemia depends partly on the prior probability of coronary artery disease (Chap. 3).

Many mistakes in ECG interpretation are errors of omission. Therefore, a systematic approach is desirable. The following 14 points should be analyzed carefully in every ECG: (1) standardization (calibration) and technical features (including lead placement and artifacts), (2) heart rate, (3) rhythm, (4) PR interval, (5) QRS interval, (6) QT interval, (7) P waves, (8) QRS voltages, (9) mean QRS electrical axis, (10) precordial R-wave progression, (11) abnormal Q waves, (12) ST segments, (13) T waves, and (14) U waves.

Only after analyzing all these points should the interpretation be formulated. Where appropriate, important clinical correlates or inferences should be mentioned. For example, prolonged ventricular repolarization with prominent U waves should suggest hypokalemia or drug toxicity (e.g., due to quinidine or procainamide) (see Fig. 228-19). The combination of left atrial abnormality (enlargement) and signs of right ventricular hypertrophy suggests mitral stenosis. Low voltage with sinus tachycardia raises the possibility of pericardial tamponade or chronic obstructive lung disease. Sinus tachycardia with QRS and QT (U) prolongation suggests tricyclic antidepressant overdose (Fig. 228-19). Comparison with previous ECGs is essential. → *The diagnosis and management of specific cardiac arrhythmias and conduction disturbances are discussed in Chaps. 230 and 231.*

COMPUTERIZED ELECTROCARDIOGRAPHY Computerized ECG systems are increasingly used. Digital systems provide for convenient storage and immediate retrieval of thousands of ECG records. In recent years, computer programs for ECG analysis have become more reliable. However, despite these advances, computer interpretation of ECGs has important limitations. Incomplete or inaccurate readings are most likely with arrhythmias and complex abnormalities. Therefore, computerized interpretation (including measurements of basic ECG intervals) should not be accepted without careful physician review.

FIGURE 228-20 Prolongation of the Q-T interval (ST-segment portion) is typical of hypocalcemia. Hypercalcemia may cause abbreviation of the ST segment and shortening of the QT interval.

BIBLIOGRAPHY

FISCH C: Electrocardiography and vectorcardiography, in *Heart Disease: A Textbook of Cardiovascular Medicine*, 5th ed, E Braunwald (ed). Philadelphia, Saunders, 1997, pp 108–152

GOLDBERGER AL: *Myocardial Infarction: Electrocardiographic Differential Diagnosis*, 4th ed. St. Louis, Mosby–Year Book, 1991

———, GOLDBERGER E: *Clinical Electrocardiography: A Simplified Approach*, 5th ed. St. Louis, Mosby–Year Book, 1994

MACFARLAND PW, LAWRIE TDV: *Comprehensive Electrocardiography: Theory and Practice in Health and Disease*. New York, Pergamon Press, 1989

MIRVIS DM: *Electrocardiography: A Physiologic Approach*. St. Louis, Mosby–Year Book, 1993

DIAGNOSTIC CARDIAC CATHETERIZATION AND ANGIOGRAPHY

Cardiac catheterization and angiography remain the gold standard for the assessment of both anatomy and physiology of the heart and vasculature. After initial animal experimentation, cardiac catheterization was first applied to humans in 1929 by Werner Forssmann, who at age 25 performed a right heart catheterization on himself. Although Forssmann's primary goal was to develop a therapeutic technique for the direct delivery of drugs into the heart, the potential for using cardiac catheterization as a diagnostic tool was appreciated by others, especially André Cournand and Dickinson Richards in New York, who shared the Nobel Prize with Forssmann in 1956. Today, more than 1 million cardiac catheterization and angiographic procedures are performed each year for diagnostic purposes, therapeutic intervention, or both. This chapter deals with cardiac catheterization as a diagnostic tool.

INDICATIONS AND CONTRAINDICATIONS Cardiac catheterization is recommended when there is a need to confirm the presence of a clinically suspected condition, define its anatomic and physiologic severity, and determine whether important associated conditions are present. This need most commonly arises when a patient is experiencing significant or increasing symptoms of cardiac dysfunction or when objective measures (such as exercise testing or echocardiography) suggest that the patient is at high risk of rapid deterioration, myocardial infarction, or other adverse events.

While there is debate as to whether cardiac catheterization is necessary in all patients being considered for cardiac surgery, cardiac catheterization and coronary arteriography remain the only techniques capable of defining coronary anatomy with sufficient precision to provide the data for decisions regarding coronary surgery or balloon angioplasty. In patients with other forms of heart disease (e.g., dilated cardiomyopathy, valvular heart disease), cardiac catheterization can provide hemodynamic characterization essential for the design of an appropriate medical regimen as well as for an assessment of prognosis. In some instances, however, decisions regarding cardiac surgery can be made without cardiac catheterization and angiography. Examples of such instances include children with simple congenital heart disease (e.g., patent ductus arteriosus, atrial septal defect), for whom a definitive diagnosis can be established by clinical examination and noninvasive studies, especially echocardiography.

Relative contraindications to cardiac catheterization are listed in Table 229-1.

A history of *allergic reaction* to radiographic contrast agents, which may range from urticaria to frank anaphylactic reaction, is an important relative contraindication to cardiac catheterization; it necessitates appropriate pretreatment with glucocorticoids (prednisone, 20 to 40 mg every 6 h), conventional antihistamines (e.g., diphenhydra-mine, 25 mg every 6 h), and H_2 antagonists (cimetidine, 300 mg every 6 h), starting 18 to 24 h prior to the procedure. Alternatively, one of the newer nonionic contrast agents may be used with less risk of a severe allergic reaction. Despite these precautions, occasional individuals still develop anaphylactic reactions during radiographic contrast angiography, and intravenous epinephrine must be at hand to treat such instances.

COMPLICATIONS OF CARDIAC CATHETERIZATION Since cardiac catheterization is an invasive technique, it is not surprising that potential complications include death, myocardial infarction, stroke, perforation of the heart or great vessels, and local vascular problems. Table 229-2 lists those characteristics associated with increased risk of death from cardiac catheterization.

TECHNIQUES

Cardiac catheterization is performed with the patient in the fasting state and awake although sedated. Typical sedatives include diazepam (Valium, 5 to 10 mg orally) and diphenhydramine (Benadryl, 25 to 50 mg orally). Prophylactic antibiotics are not necessary. If patients have been anticoagulated chronically with warfarin, this agent must be discontinued at least 48 h prior to the procedure, and the prothrombin time must be less than 18 s if the study is to be done safely. Although cardiac catheterization used to be performed exclusively as an inpatient procedure, current practice is to perform most elective procedures on an outpatient basis.

The technique of cardiac catheterization involves either direct exposure of artery and vein (usually the brachial artery and vein in the antecubital fossa) or catheterization by a percutaneous approach (usually via the femoral artery and vein). Either technique can be used for right and/or left heart catheterization with coronary arteriography, but many procedures (e.g., intraaortic balloon pumping, mitral valve valvuloplasty, coronary atherectomy) require the femoral approach. For a procedure where either approach would be possible, the brachial approach has advantages in the patient with peripheral vascular disease involving the abdominal aorta and iliac or femoral arteries and suspected thrombosis of the femoral or iliac vein or inferior vena cava. Advantages of the percutaneous femoral approach are that arteriotomy and arterial repair are not required; the procedure can be performed repeatedly in the same patient at intervals; infection and thrombophlebitis at the catheterization site are quite rare, and no scar is left. At present, more than 85 percent of cardiac catheterizations are performed by the femoral route.

Table 229-1

Relative Contraindications to Cardiac Catheterization and Angiography

Uncontrolled ventricular irritability: increased risk of ventricular tachycardia and fibrillation during catheterization if ventricular irritability is uncontrolled
Uncorrected hypokalemia or digitalis toxicity
Uncorrected hypertension: predisposes to myocardial ischemia and/or heart failure during angiography
Intercurrent febrile illness
Decompensated heart failure: especially acute pulmonary edema, unless catheterization can be done with patient sitting up
Anticoagulated state: prothrombin time >18 s
Severe allergy to radiographic contrast agent
Severe renal insufficiency and/or anuria: unless dialysis is planned to remove fluid and radiographic contrast load

Table 229-2

Patient Characteristics Associated with Increased Mortality from Cardiac Catheterization

Age: Infants (<1 month old) and the elderly (>80 years old) are at increased risk of death during cardiac catheterization. Elderly women appear to be at higher risk than elderly men.
Functional class: Mortality in class IV patients is more than 10 times greater than in class I–II patients.
Severity of coronary obstruction: Mortality for patients with left main coronary artery disease is more than 10 times greater than in patients with one- or two-vessel disease.
Valvular heart disease: Especially when severe and combined with coronary disease, is associated with a higher risk of death at cardiac catheterization than coronary artery disease alone.
Left ventricular dysfunction: Mortality in patients with a left ventricular ejection fraction <30 percent is more than 10 times greater than in patients with an ejection fraction ≥50 percent.
Severe noncardiac disease: Patients with renal insufficiency, insulin-requiring diabetes, advanced cerebrovascular and/or peripheral vascular disease, or severe pulmonary insufficiency have an increased incidence of death and other major complications from cardiac catheterization.

RIGHT HEART CATHETERIZATION This procedure is most commonly performed under fluoroscopic guidance using a balloon flotation catheter, which is advanced from a suitable vein (femoral, brachial, subclavian, or internal jugular) into the superior vena cava, where blood is sampled for oximetry. The catheter is then positioned in the right atrium, where pressure is measured. The balloon is inflated with air or carbon dioxide and advanced sequentially into the right ventricle, pulmonary artery, and pulmonary artery wedge positions. Pressures are recorded in each position. After the wedge pressure is recorded, the balloon is deflated so that pulmonary artery pressure can be monitored and blood samples can be obtained for oximetry. With a thermistor-tipped balloon catheter, cardiac output can be measured using cold saline injection and a small computer (thermodilution technique). Comparison of oxygen saturations in the superior and inferior vena cava, chambers of the right heart, and pulmonary artery permits assessment of the presence of a left-to-right shunt at the atrial, ventricular, or pulmonary artery level, which will be manifested as an increase ("step-up") in oxygen saturation of blood as it traverses these vessels and chambers. As discussed below, measurements of the pulmonary artery and aortic oxygen content and oxygen consumption allow calculation of the cardiac output by the Fick principle as an alternative to use of thermodilution.

The experienced operator will be alert to abnormalities in the course of the catheter during its passage through the right heart chambers, which could indicate the presence of congenital heart disease. For example, the catheter may pass directly from the right to the left atrium through an atrial septal defect, may enter an anomalous pulmonary vein draining into the right atrium, or may pass from the pulmonary artery directly into the aorta through a patent ductus arteriosus.

LEFT HEART CATHETERIZATION When left heart catheterization is done from the *brachial approach*, surgical cut-down is performed in the right (or left) antecubital fossa, with exposure of the brachial artery. An arteriotomy is made, and an appropriate catheter (e.g., a Sones catheter) is advanced under fluoroscopic guidance to the central aorta, where pressure is measured and recorded. Next, the catheter is advanced in retrograde fashion across the aortic valve into the left ventricle, where pressure is measured. If a right heart catheter is in place, this is an appropriate time for simultaneous measurement and recording of left heart, right heart, and peripheral arterial pressures together with a determination of cardiac output by either thermodilution or the Fick principle. These measures allow assessment of possible pressure gradients across the mitral and aortic valves, and catheter pullback on the right side permits assessment of possible gradients across the pulmonic and tricuspid valves. Simultaneous measurement of pressures and cardiac output provides the data for calculation of systemic and pulmonary vascular resistances.

The *percutaneous femoral approach* to left heart catheterization involves puncture of the right (or left) femoral artery with a Seldinger needle, passage of a J-tipped guidewire retrogradely to the abdominal aorta under fluoroscopic guidance, and placement of an intraarterial sheath with a side arm port for flushing. An appropriate catheter (e.g., a pigtail catheter) is then advanced through this sheath and over the guidewire to the descending aorta, at which time the guidewire is removed and the catheter aspirated and flushed vigorously. Under pressure monitoring and fluoroscopic guidance, the catheter is advanced to the ascending aorta, where pressure is recorded simultaneously with peripheral arterial pressure. The subsequent steps in the procedure are identical to those listed for the brachial approach.

An additional method of left heart catheterization is the *transseptal approach*. This approach, which is not commonly employed today except for special diagnostic problems or for purposes of therapeutic intervention (especially mitral valvuloplasty), involves a controlled puncture of the interatrial septum from the right atrial side with a long stainless steel needle. Advancement of a Teflon catheter or sheath over the needle then allows catheterization of the left atrium and catheter passage across the mitral valve into the left ventricle. Rarely, direct catheterization of the left heart through the chest wall is necessary, by *left ventricular puncture* using a needle inserted into the cardiac apex.

CARDIAC ANGIOGRAPHY

Cardiac angiography involves injection of an iodine-based liquid radiopaque contrast agent into a specific cardiac chamber or vessel using either hand injection or power injection through an automated syringe. The contrast agents used today are classified as either high-osmolar or low-osmolar; the low-osmolar contrast agents (including true nonionic contrast agents and the ionic dimer ioxaglate) have a lesser myocardial depressant effect and produce fewer side effects (hypotension, nausea, bradycardia, or a sensation of marked warmth following injection) than earlier high-osmolar agents. They are, however, substantially more expensive than traditional high-osmolar ionic agents, so they are not used routinely in patients who are at low risk for complications with the less expensive high-osmolar contrast agents.

CORONARY ANGIOGRAPHY This common procedure involves the selective injection of a radiographic contrast agent into the coronary arteries. Placement of the catheter tip into the right and left coronary arteries is carried out under fluoroscopic guidance, and contrast agent is injected by hand during recording of the radiographic image. Each coronary artery is usually viewed in several projections to permit assessment of the severity of stenosis and to minimize the overlap of adjacent vessels. In addition to the detection of coronary artery stenoses, coronary angiography is useful for the detection of congenital abnormalities of the coronary circulation, coronary arteriovenous fistulas, and patency of coronary artery bypass grafts. Examples of normal and abnormal coronary anatomy are shown in Figs. 229-1 to 229-3.

LEFT VENTRICULOGRAPHY Injection of radiographic contrast material directly into the left ventricular cavity is an important part of routine left heart catheterization and yields important diagnostic information. A power injector is used to inject 30 to 45 mL of radiographic contrast material into the left ventricular chamber at a rate of 10 to 12 mL/s. Angiographic assessment of the left ventricular silhouette at end-diastole and end-systole permits calculation of the left ventricular chamber volumes and ejection fraction, as well as assessment of regional wall motion abnormalities. The normal left ventricle ejects 50 to 80 percent of its end-diastolic volume with each beat; i.e., its *ejection fraction* is 0.50 to 0.80. In adults, normal values for left ventricular volumes are, for end-diastolic volume, 72 ± 15 mL/m^2 (mean $\pm$ standard deviation) and, for end-systolic volume, 20 ± 8 mL/m^2. Regional abnormalities of wall motion are illustrated in Fig. 229-4 and include diminished inward motion of a myocardial segment (*hypokinesis*), absence of inward movement of a myocardial segment (*akinesis*), and paradoxical systolic expansion of a regional myocardial segment (*dyskinesis*).

Left ventriculography is usually performed in the right anterior oblique projection, which allows assessment of the mitral and aortic valves. Mitral regurgitation is easily visualized as the leakage of radiographic contrast material back into the left atrium during left ventricular systole. Its severity can be estimated qualitatively using a grading system of 1 + (mild; radiographic contrast material clears with each beat and never opacifies the entire left atrium) to 4 + (severe; opacification of the entire left atrium occurs within one beat, and contrast material can be seen refluxing into the pulmonary veins). The *regurgitant fraction* can be calculated by determining the total left ventricular stroke volume (left ventricular end-diastolic volume minus end-systolic volume), subtracting the forward stroke volume (determined by the Fick or indicator-dilution technique), and dividing by the total stroke volume. The cause of mitral regurgitation—for example, myxomatous degeneration of the mitral leaflets and chordal rupture—may sometimes be identified from the left ventricular cineangiogram. Mitral and aortic stenosis can be suspected when the speed and completeness with which the mitral and aortic leaflets open are reduced. Other clues include increased thickness of the mitral and aortic leaflets and the

FIGURE 229-1 Representation of coronary anatomy relative to the interventricular and atrioventricular valve planes. Coronary branches are indicated as L Main (left main), LAD (left anterior descending), D (diagonal), S (septal), CX (circumflex), OM (obtuse marginal), RCA (right coronary artery), CB (conus branch), SN (sinus node), AcM (acute marginal), PD (posterior descending, PL (posterolateral left ventricular). RAO, right anterior oblique, LAO, left anterior oblique. [*From DS Baim, W Grossman, in Cardiac Catheterization, Angiography, and Intervention, 5th ed, DS Baim, W Grossman (eds). Baltimore, Williams & Wilkins, 1996.*]

FIGURE 229-2 Coronary angiogram showing a right coronary artery (RCA) with a severe (95 percent) stenosis at its midpoint (*arrow*).

FIGURE 229-3 Coronary angiogram of a left coronary artery (LCA) with a tight stenosis in the proximal left anterior descending (LAD) artery (*black arrow*) immediately prior to the origin of a large septal branch. The circumflex artery (CX) has two moderately severe stenoses (*white arrows*).

presence and extent of leaflet calcification. These findings, however, are usually not useful in estimating the *severity* of physiologic stenosis.

Left ventriculography performed in the left anterior oblique projection permits detection of abnormal communications, such as a ventricular septal defect (Chap. 235). In the most common form of hypertrophic cardiomyopathy (Chap. 239) (idiopathic hypertrophic subaortic stenosis, IHSS), left ventriculography in this projection shows anterior motion of the anterior leaflet of the mitral valve during systole and bulging of the interventricular septum into the left ventricular cavity, especially in the subaortic region. Mural thrombi within the left ventricular chamber may be well visualized during left ventriculography. They occur most commonly in the left ventricular apex.

AORTOGRAPHY   Rapid injection of radiographic contrast material into the ascending aorta allows detection of abnormalities involving the aorta and aortic valve. It permits detection and qualitative

assessment of the severity of aortic regurgitation, which is recorded using a 1 + to 4 + scale, as for mitral regurgitation. Abnormal communications between the aorta and right side of the heart, such as a patent ductus arteriosus or ruptured aneurysm of a sinus of Valsalva, may be visualized. Aortography can permit identification of aortic aneurysm and of aortic dissection (Chap. 247) and may visualize an intimal flap within the aortic lumen.

PRESSURE MEASUREMENTS

Pressures within the cardiac chambers and great vessels are recorded routinely during cardiac catheterization and provide important information concerning the function of ventricular myocardium and cardiac valves. Normal values for pressures measured during cardiac catheterization are summarized in Table 229-3.

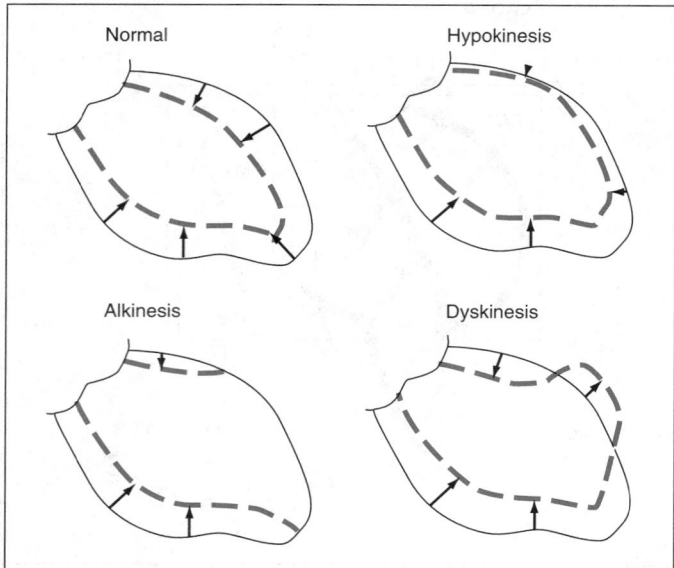

FIGURE 229-4 Diagrammatic representation of end-diastolic (*solid line*) and end-systolic (*dashed line*) silhouettes of left ventricular cineangiograms in various forms of localized wall motion disorder in patients with coronary heart disease. Normal wall motion is symmetric; a patient with *hypokinesis* exhibits reduced contraction, seen here over the anterior and apical surfaces; a patient with *akinesis* exhibits absent wall motion, seen here over the anteroapical surface; a patient with *dyskinesis* exhibits paradoxic bulging of a small portion of the anterior wall with systole.

Simultaneous measurement of pressures in the left ventricle, aorta, and left atrium (or pulmonary capillary wedge position) permits assessment of mitral and aortic valve function. As seen in Fig. 229-5, left ventricular and aortic pressures are essentially equal during systole, while left atrial (pulmonary capillary wedge) and left ventricular pressures are equal during diastole in the normal heart. If a pressure gradient is present between the left ventricle and aorta during systole, it may be due to obstruction at the level of the aortic valve (e.g., *calcific aortic stenosis*) or at the subaortic level (e.g., *hypertrophic*

Table 229-3

Normal Values for Hemodynamic Parameters

Pressures (mmHg)	
Systemic arterial	
Peak systolic/end-diastolic	100–140/60–90
Mean	70–105
Left ventricle	
Peak systolic/end-diastolic	100–140/3–12
Left atrium (or pulmonary capillary wedge)	
Mean	2–10
a wave	3–15
v wave	3–15
Pulmonary artery	
Peak systolic/end-diastolic	15–30/4–12
Mean	9–18
Right ventricle	
Peak systolic/end-diastolic	15–30/2–8
Right atrium	
Mean	2–8
a wave	2–10
v wave	2–10
Resistances [(dyn·s)/cm^5]	
Systemic vascular resistance	700–1600
Pulmonary vascular resistance	20–130
Cardiac index [(L/min)/m^2]	2.6–4.2
Oxygen consumption index [(L/min)/m^2]	110–150
Arteriovenous oxygen difference (mL/L)	30–50

FIGURE 229-5 Left ventricular (LV), radial artery, and pulmonary capillary wedge (PCW) pressures in a patient with normal cardiovascular function. Note the absence of a pressure gradient between the LV and radial artery in systole and between the LV and PCW in diastole.

obstructive cardiomyopathy). A pressure gradient between the left atrium (pulmonary capillary wedge pressure) and the left ventricle in diastole generally indicates *mitral stenosis*, although it also may be seen in rare conditions such as cor triatriatum and left atrial myxoma. An example of a large diastolic pressure gradient in a patient with mitral stenosis is seen in Fig. 229-6. As seen in Fig. 229-7, patients with significant mitral regurgitation may have a prominent *v* wave in the pulmonary capillary wedge pressure, which often increases substantially during modest exercise. Severe *aortic regurgitation* produces a widening of the aortic pulse pressure, with equilibration of aortic and left ventricular pressures in diastole (Fig. 229-8). Right-sided pressures exhibit a characteristic deformity in the presence of valvular heart disease affecting the tricuspid or pulmonic valves. In patients with severe *tricuspid regurgitation*, the right atrial pressure resembles the right ventricular pressure closely in appearance. Mean right atrial pressure and right ventricular end-diastolic pressure are both elevated in tricuspid regurgitation. In *tricuspid stenosis*, there is a pressure gradient between the right atrium and ventricle during diastole.

Characteristic deformities of right and left ventricular diastolic pressures occur in patients with *cardiac tamponade* or *pericardial constriction*. In both conditions there is equalization of left and right ventricular diastolic pressures. However, in constrictive pericarditis, nearly all ventricular filling occurs shortly after mitral and tricuspid valve opening; after this period of rapid filling, ventricular volumes cannot increase further owing to the constricting pericardium. This abnormality produces an abrupt early ventricular diastolic pressure rise with a mid- and late-ventricular pressure plateau, giving the so-called square root sign (Fig. 229-9). In contrast, in tamponade there is equalization of diastolic pressures with a gradual increase throughout diastole.

FIGURE 229-6 Pulmonary capillary wedge (PCW) and left ventricular (LV) pressure tracings in a 40-year-old woman with mitral stenosis. This patient also had systemic hypertension and significant elevation of her LV diastolic pressure. [*From BA Carabello, W Grossman, in Cardiac Catheterization, Angiography, and Intervention, 5th ed, DS Baim, W Grossman (eds). Baltimore, Williams & Wilkins, 1996.*]

Congestive heart failure due to myocardial contractile dysfunction is associated with characteristic alterations in the ventricular pressure waveforms seen at cardiac catheterization. Neither the rise nor the decline in isovolumic pressure is as steep as in the normal heart. The reduced slopes of pressure rise and decline are associated with an abbreviated ejection period, giving the left ventricular pressure tracing a triangular appearance (Fig. 229-10). Also, the pressure decline does not continue to zero, so the minimal left ventricular diastolic pressure may be elevated. This hemodynamic finding correlates with an increased ventricular end-systolic volume, which is a sign of depressed contractile function of the left ventricular myocardium.

MEASUREMENT OF FLOW

Systemic and pulmonary blood flows may be measured by either the Fick or the indicator-dilution method. In the normal heart, these flows are equal and constitute the *cardiac output*. Specialized techniques have made it possible to measure coronary artery blood flow (through the use of a catheter- or guidewire-tip-mounted Doppler flowmeter), coronary sinus blood flow (by the thermodilution technique), and renal, cerebral, and femoral blood flows as well.

Cardiac output is most commonly measured by the thermodilution technique, but the standard method, against which this technique and others are calibrated, remains the direct Fick oxygen method. In the direct Fick method, O_2 consumption is measured simultaneously with determination of the arteriovenous oxygen difference across the lungs. Fick's principle states that

$$Q \text{ (L/min)} = \frac{O_2 \text{ consumption (mL/min)}}{\text{arteriovenous oxygen difference (mL/L)}}$$

In order to compare individuals of different body weights and sizes, O_2 consumption and cardiac output (Q) are commonly divided by

FIGURE 229-7 Hemodynamic findings at rest and during exercise in a patient with mitral regurgitation. Left ventricular (LV), pulmonary capillary wedge (PCW), and radial artery pressure tracings are shown before (*left*) and during (*right*) the sixth minute of supine bicycle exercise. PCW mean pressure and *v* wave increase substantially with exercise. [*From BH Lorell, W Grossman, in Cardiac Catheterization, Angiography, and Intervention, 5th ed, DS Baim, W Grossman (eds). Baltimore, Williams & Wilkins, 1996.*]

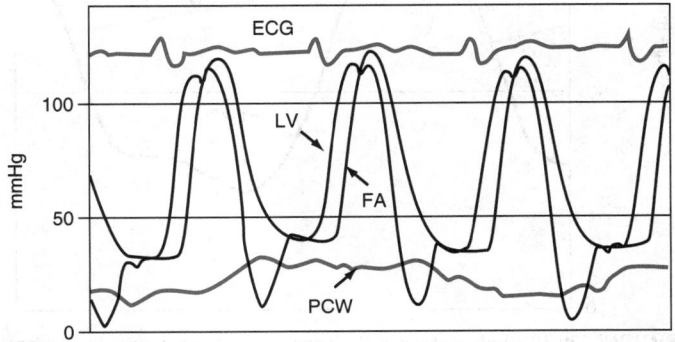

FIGURE 229-8 Severe aortic regurgitation. There is equilibration between the left ventricular (LV) and aortic or femoral artery (FA) pressures in diastole. Also, LV diastolic pressure exceeds pulmonary capillary wedge (PCW) pressure early in diastole, indicating premature closure of the mitral valve (a characteristic feature of severe aortic regurgitation). [*From W Grossman, in Cardiac Catheterization, Angiography, and Intervention, 5th ed, DS Baim, W Grossman (eds). Baltimore, Williams & Wilkins, 1996.*]

FIGURE 229-9 Left ventricular (LV), right ventricular (RV), and pulmonary capillary wedge (PCW) pressure tracings in a patient with severe constrictive pericarditis. Note the diastolic dip and plateau ("square root sign") pattern for left and right ventricular diastolic pressures (*left*). The wedge pressure (*right*) shows early systolic and early diastolic dips.

body surface area. Normal values for O_2 consumption and cardiac output are given in Table 229-3. Cardiac output is calculated by dividing O_2 consumption by the arteriovenous O_2 difference across the lungs (estimated pulmonary venous–pulmonary arterial O_2 content); this quantity actually provides a measure of *pulmonary blood flow* (Q_p). In patients with a left-to-right shunt at the atrial, ventricular, or pulmonary artery levels, pulmonary blood flow will exceed systemic blood flow. In such cases, systemic blood flow (Q_s) is calculated by dividing O_2 consumption by the systemic arteriovenous O_2 difference. The latter is calculated as the systemic arterial blood O_2 content minus

the mixed venous blood O_2 content as estimated using blood from the chamber immediately proximal to the level of the shunt. The Fick method is most dependable when the cardiac output is low and the arteriovenous oxygen difference is large.

For indicator-dilution measurement of cardiac output using the thermodilution technique, a thermistor is mounted on the tip of a balloon flotation catheter, and the catheter is advanced so that the balloon tip and thermistor are located in the pulmonary artery. Cold dextrose solution or saline is injected via a proximal port on the catheter into the vena cava or right atrium, and the change in temperature monitored at the thermistor is integrated electronically. This integral is inversely proportional to the volume flow rate past the thermistor, and if the temperatures of the injectate and pulmonary artery blood are measured, cardiac output (actually, pulmonary blood flow) can be calculated. In contrast to the Fick method, the indicator-dilution method is least reliable when the cardiac output is low.

Valve Areas and Resistances Using simultaneous measures of pressure and flow, the resistance to blood flow across the cardiac valves as well as the pulmonary and systemic arteriolar beds may be estimated. Valve areas are calculated using the Gorlin formula:

$$A = \frac{flow}{K\sqrt{\Delta P}}$$

where A = valve orifice area (cm^2), *flow* is the blood flow (mL/s) across the stenotic valve, ΔP is the mean pressure gradient (mmHg) during the period of blood flow, and K is a constant (44.3 for the aortic valve and 37.7 for the mitral valve).

The resistance to blood flow through the systemic vascular bed is

$$SVR = 80(MAP - RA)/SBF$$

where SVR is systemic vascular resistance [$(dyn·s)/cm^5$], MAP and RA are mean aortic and right atrial pressures (mmHg), 80 is a constant for converting to metric units, and SBF is systemic blood flow (L/min).

Resistance to blood flow through the pulmonary vascular bed is

$$PVR = 80(PA - PCW \text{ or } LA)/PBF$$

where PVR is pulmonary vascular resistance [$(dyn·s)/cm^5$]; PA, PCW, and LA are pulmonary artery, pulmonary capillary wedge, and left atrial mean pressures, respectively, (mmHg); and PBF is pulmonary blood flow (L/min). Normal values for pulmonary and systemic vascular resistances are given in Table 229-3.

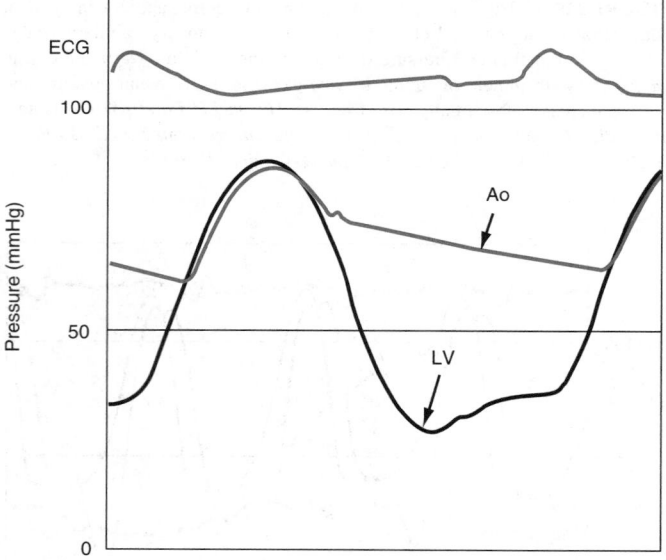

FIGURE 229-10 Left ventricular (LV) and aortic (Ao) pressures in a patient with advanced dilated cardiomyopathy. Marked slowing of the rates of left ventricular pressure rise and fall (impairment of contractility and relaxation) give the LV pressure pulse a triangular appearance. Also, the minimal value for left ventricular diastolic pressure is markedly elevated, suggesting an increased end-systolic volume and a reduced LV ejection fraction. [*From W Grossman, in Cardiac Catheterization, Angiography, and Intervention, 5th ed, DS Baim, W Grossman (eds). Baltimore, Williams & Wilkins, 1996.*]

BIBLIOGRAPHY

BAIM DS, GROSSMAN W (eds): *Cardiac Catheterization, Angiography, and Intervention*, 5th ed. Baltimore, Williams & Wilkins, 1996

DAVIDSON CJ et al: Cardiac catheterization, in *Heart Disease*, 5th ed, E Braunwald (ed). Philadelphia, Saunders, 1997, p 177

GODLEWSKI KJ et al: Interpretation of cardiac pathophysiology from pressure waveform analysis: Acute aortic insufficiency. Cathet Cardiovasc Diagn 28:244, 1993

JOHNSON LW, KRONE R: Cardiac catheterization 1991: A report of the Registry

of the Society for Cardiac Angiography and Interventions (SCA&I). Cathet Cardiovasc Diagn 28:219, 1993

KERN MJ et al: Interpretation of cardiac pathophysiology from pressure waveform analysis: Simultaneous left and right ventricular pressure measurements. Cathet Cardiovasc Diagn 28:51, 1993

SECTION 2
DISORDERS OF RHYTHM

Mark E. Josephson, Peter Zimetbaum,
Francis E. Marchlinski, Alfred E. Buxton

230

THE BRADYARRHYTHMIAS: DISORDERS OF SINUS NODE FUNCTION AND AV CONDUCTION DISTURBANCES

ANATOMY OF THE CONDUCTING SYSTEM   Under normal conditions, the pacemaker function of the heart resides in the sinoatrial (SA) node, which lies at the junction of the right atrium and superior vena cava. The SA node is approximately 1.5 cm long and 2 to 3 mm wide and is supplied by the sinus node artery, which arises from either the right coronary artery (60 percent) or the left circumflex coronary artery (40 percent). Once the impulse exits the sinus node and perinodal tissue, it traverses the atrium until it reaches the atrioventricular (AV) node. The blood supply of the AV node is derived from the posterior descending coronary artery (90 percent). The AV node lies at the base of the interatrial septum just above the tricuspid annulus and anterior to the coronary sinus. The electrophysiologic properties of the AV node result in slow conduction, which is responsible for the normal delay in AV conduction, i.e., the PR interval.

The bundle of His emerges from the AV node, enters the fibrous skeleton of the heart, and courses anteriorly across the membranous interventricular septum. It has a dual blood supply from the AV nodal artery and a branch of the anterior descending coronary artery. The branching (distal) portion of the bundle of His gives rise to a broad sheet of fibers that course over the left side of the interventricular septum to form the left bundle branch and a narrow cable-like structure on the right side that forms the right bundle branch. The arborization of both the right and left bundle branches gives rise to the distal His-Purkinje system, which ultimately extends throughout the endocardium of the right and left ventricles.

The sinus node, atrium, and AV node are significantly influenced by autonomic tone. Vagal influences depress automaticity of the sinus node, depress conduction, and prolong refractoriness in the tissue surrounding the sinus node; inhomogeneously decrease atrial refractoriness and slow atrial conduction; and prolong AV nodal conduction and refractoriness. Sympathetic influences exert the opposite effect.

ELECTROPHYSIOLOGIC PRINCIPLES

In the resting state, the interior of most cardiac cells, with the exception of the sinus and AV nodes, is approximately -80 to -90 mV, negative with respect to a reference extracellular electrode. The resting membrane potential is determined primarily by the concentration gradient of potassium across the cell membrane. Activation of cardiac cells results from movement of ions across the cell membrane, causing a transient depolarization known as the *action potential*. The ionic species responsible for the action potential varies among the cardiac

tissues, and the configuration of the action potential is therefore unique to each tissue (Fig. 230-1).

The action potential of the His-Purkinje system and ventricular myocardium has five phases (Fig. 230-2). The rapid depolarizing current (phase 0) is mainly determined by an influx of sodium into myocardial cells followed by a secondary (slower) influx of calcium which produces a slow inward current. The repolarization phases of the action potential (phases 1 to 3) are primarily related to outward flux of potassium. The resting membrane potential is phase 4.

The bradyarrhythmias result from abnormalities either of impulse formation, i.e., automaticity, or of conduction. *Automaticity*, which is normally observed in the sinus node, the specialized fibers of the His-Purkinje system, and some specialized atrial fibers, is the property of a cardiac cell that causes it to depolarize spontaneously during phase 4 of the action potential, leading to the generation of an impulse. To exhibit automaticity, the resting membrane potential must decrease spontaneously until threshold potential is reached and an all-or-none regenerative response occurs. The ionic currents producing spontaneous diastolic depolarization appear to involve the inward current of

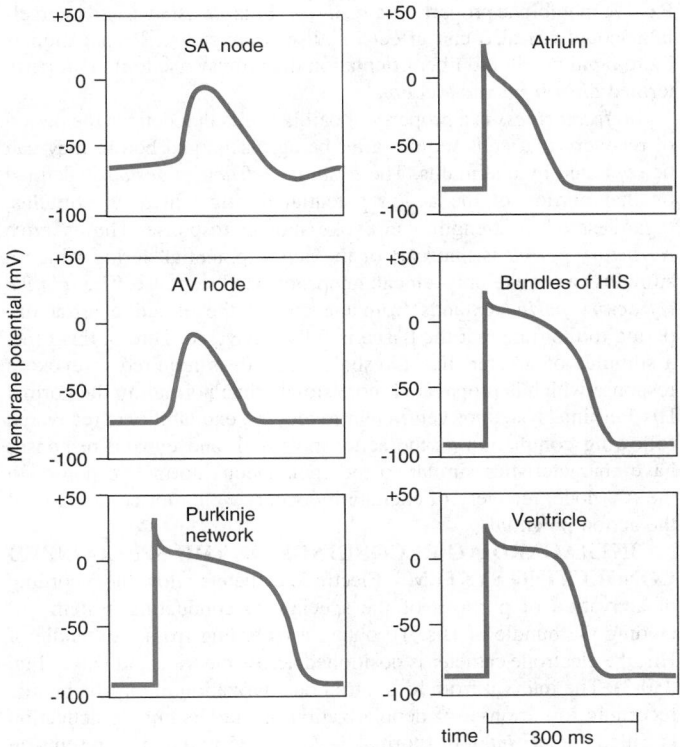

FIGURE 230-1   Action potential configurations in different regions of the mammalian heart. (*From AM Katz, Physiology of the Heart, New York, Raven, 1977.*)

FIGURE 230-2 Schematic representation of the action potential in normal ventricle depicting the direction, strength, and period of flow of the ionic currents underlying the action potential. The arrow's direction and size indicate whether current is inward- or outward-directed and the approximate current strength of the ion identified at the arrow's base. The horizontal position of the arrow corresponds to the same moment in the time course of action potential (see text). The five phases of the action potential are indicated by the numerals placed along the waveform. *(From Ten Eick et al, Prog Cardiovasc Dis 24(2):157, 1981, with permission.)*

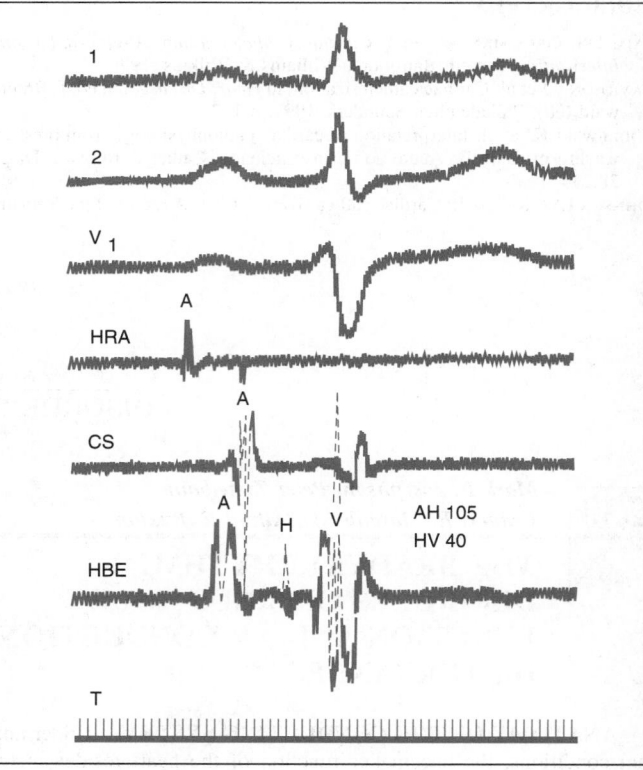

FIGURE 230-3 Normal intracardiac recording. Surface ECG leads I, II, and V_1 are displayed with intracardiac ECGs from the high right atrium (HRA), left atrium from the coronary sinus (CS), and AV junction to obtain a His bundle electrogram (HBE). T, time lines; A, atrial activation; H, His bundle activation; V, ventricular activation. Atrial activation begins in the high right atrium and spreads inferiorly to the low atrial septum, as recorded in the HBE, and the left atrium, as recorded in the CS. The AH and HV intervals represent AV nodal and His-Purkinje conduction times, respectively. Vertical lines = 0.10 s. *(From ME Josephson, SF Seides, Clinical Cardiac Electrophysiology: Techniques and Interpretations. Philadelphia, Lea & Febiger, 1979.)*

either sodium or calcium. The velocity of *conduction*, i.e., impulse propagation through cardiac tissues, depends on the magnitude of inward current, which is directly related to the rate of rise and amplitude of phase 0 of the action potential. The more positive the threshold potential and the slower the rate of depolarization toward threshold, the slower is the rate of rise of phase 0 of the action potential and the slower is the conduction velocity. Disease states or drugs may result in lower rates of rise of phase 0 at any given membrane potential. Passive membrane properties (e.g., intracellular resistance and intercellular coupling) also can affect impulse propagation. Propagation is more rapid parallel to fiber orientation than transverse to it, a property termed *anisotropic conduction*.

Refractoriness is a property of cardiac cells that defines the period of recovery that cells require after being discharged before they can be reexcited by a stimulus. The *absolute refractory period* is defined by that portion of the action potential during which no stimulus, regardless of its strength, can evoke another response. The *effective refractory period* is that part of the action potential during which a stimulus can evoke only a local, nonpropagated response. The *relative refractory period* extends from the end of the effective refractory period to the time that the tissue is fully recovered. During this time, a stimulus of greater than threshold strength is required to evoke a response which is propagated more slowly than normal. In the normal His-Purkinje system or ventricular myocytes, excitability is recovered following completion of the action potential, and evoked responses have characteristics similar to the spontaneous normal response. In the AV node, recovery of excitability occurs well after completion of the action potential.

INTRACARDIAC RECORDINGS OF THE SPECIALIZED CONDUCTING SYSTEM Electrode catheters allow the recording of activation of portions of the specialized conducting system, including the bundle of His. To obtain a recording from the bundle of His, the electrode catheter is positioned across the tricuspid valve (Fig. 230-3). The interval from local atrial depolarization in the His bundle recording to the onset of depolarization of the His bundle deflection is called the *AH interval* (normal = 60 to 125 ms) and represents an indirect method of assessing AV nodal conduction time. The interval from the beginning of the His bundle deflection to the earliest onset of ventricular activation, as measured from any of multiple-surface

electrocardiogram (ECG) leads or the intracardiac ventricular electrogram, is called the *HV interval* (normal = 35 to 55 ms) and represents conduction time through the His-Purkinje system. Electrode catheters can be positioned in the area of the sinus node to record high right atrial activity. Left atrial activity may be recorded directly via a catheter placed across a patent foramen ovale or indirectly using a catheter inserted into the coronary sinus. The atrial activation sequence may be "mapped," and sites of intra- and interatrial conduction abnormalities may be ascertained.

SINUS NODE DYSFUNCTION

The sinus node is normally the dominant cardiac pacemaker because its intrinsic discharge rate is the highest of all potential cardiac pacemakers. Its responsiveness to alterations in autonomic nervous system tone is responsible for the normal acceleration of heart rate during exercise and the slowing that occurs during rest and sleep. Increases in sinus rate normally result from an increase in sympathetic tone acting via beta-adrenergic receptors and/or a decrease in parasympathetic tone acting via muscarinic receptors. Slowing of the heart rate is normally due to opposite alterations. In adults, the normal sinus rate under basal conditions is 60 to 100 beats per minute. Sinus bradycardia is said to exist when the sinus rate is less than 60 beats per minute, and sinus tachycardia when it exceeds 100 beats per minute. However, there is wide variation among individuals, and rates less than 60 beats per minute do not necessarily indicate pathologic states. For example, trained athletes often exhibit resting rates under 50 beats per minute due to increases in vagal tone. Normal elderly individuals also may show marked sinus bradycardia at rest.

ETIOLOGY Sinus node dysfunction most often is found in the elderly as an isolated phenomenon. Although interruption of the blood supply to the sinus node may produce dysfunction, the correlation between obstruction of the sinus node artery and clinical evidence of sinus node dysfunction is poor. Specific disease states associated with sinus node dysfunction include senile amyloidosis and other conditions associated with infiltration of the atrial myocardium. Sinus bradycardia is associated with hypothyroidism, advanced liver disease, hypothermia, typhoid fever, and brucellosis; it occurs during episodes of hypervagotonia (vasovagal syncope), severe hypoxia, hypercapnia, acidemia, and acute hypertension. However, in most cases of sinus node dysfunction a specific cause cannot be identified.

MANIFESTATIONS Although marked ($\leq$50 beats per minute) sinus bradycardia may cause fatigue and other symptoms due to inadequate cardiac output, more commonly sinus node dysfunction is manifest as paroxysmal dizziness, presyncope, or syncope. These symptoms usually result from abrupt, prolonged sinus pauses caused by failure of sinus impulse formation (sinus arrest) or block of conduction of sinus impulses to the surrounding atrial tissue (sinus exit block). In either case, the ECG manifestation is a prolonged period ($>$3 s) of atrial asystole. In some patients, sinus node dysfunction is accompanied by abnormalities in AV conduction. In addition to the absence of atrial activity, lower pacemakers fail to emerge during the sinus pauses, resulting in periods of ventricular asystole and syncope. Occasionally, sinus node dysfunction is manifested by an inadequate acceleration in sinus rate in response to a stress such as exercise or fever. In some patients, sinus node dysfunction may become manifest only in the presence of certain cardioactive drugs: cardiac glycosides, beta-adrenergic blocking drugs, verapamil, quinidine, and other antiarrhythmic agents. These agents, which do not cause sinus node dysfunction in normal people, may unmask evidence of sinus node dysfunction in susceptible individuals.

The *sick sinus syndrome* refers to a combination of symptoms (dizziness, confusion, fatigue, syncope, and congestive heart failure) caused by sinus node dysfunction and manifested by marked sinus bradycardia, sinoatrial block, or sinus arrest. Because these symptoms are nonspecific, and because ECG manifestations of sinus node dysfunction are not infrequently intermittent, it may be difficult to prove that such symptoms are actually caused by sinus node dysfunction.

Atrial tachyarrhythmias such as atrial fibrillation, atrial flutter, or atrial tachycardia may be accompanied by sinus node dysfunction. The *bradycardia-tachycardia syndrome* refers to paroxysmal atrial arrhythmia that upon termination is followed by prolonged sinus pauses (Fig. 230-4) or in which there are alternating periods of tachyarrhythmia and bradyarrhythmia. Syncope or presyncope may result from failure of the sinus node to recover function following suppression of automaticity by atrial tachyarrhythmia.

DIAGNOSIS *First-degree sinoatrial exit block* denotes a prolonged conduction time from the sinus node to the surrounding atrial tissue. It cannot be recognized on a standard (surface) ECG but requires invasive intracardiac recordings (see below). *Second-degree sinoatrial exit block* denotes the intermittent failure of conduction of sinus impulses to the surrounding atrial tissue; it is manifested as the intermittent absence of P waves (Fig. 230-5). *Third-degree*, or *complete, sinoatrial block* is characterized by a lack of atrial activity or by the presence of an ectopic subsidiary atrial pacemaker. On the standard ECG it cannot be distinguished from sinus arrest, but direct intracardiac recordings of sinus node activity permit this distinction. The *bradycardia-tachycardia syndrome* is manifested on the standard ECG as tachyarrhythmias (see Fig. 230-4). Most often these are atrial flutter or fibrillation, although any tachycardia during which the atria are activated may cause overdrive suppression of the sinus node resulting in clinical appearance of this syndrome.

The most important step in the diagnosis is to correlate symptoms with ECG evidence of sinus node dysfunction. While ambulatory ECG (Holter) moni-

toring remains a mainstay in evaluating sinus node function, most episodes of syncope are paroxysmal and unpredictable. Single and even multiple 24-h Holter monitor recordings may fail to include a symptomatic episode. Therefore, noting the response to carotid sinus pressure and pharmacologic autonomic "denervation" of the heart is frequently helpful. Carotid sinus pressure is particularly useful in patients in whom paroxysmal dizziness or syncope is compatible with the hypersensitive carotid sinus syndrome (see Chap. 20). In such patients, the response can be dramatic, and sinus pauses in excess of 5 s may occur. Normally, a sinus pause of $\leq$3 s results from 5 s of unilateral carotid sinus massage. However, in elderly patients, pauses $>$3 s are common and do not necessarily signify a diagnostic response. In all individuals it is important to correlate symptoms with such ECG phenomena. The other noninvasive test of sinus node function involves the use of pharmacologic agents to manipulate the autonomic nervous system and assess the balance of parasympathetic and sympathetic activity on the sinus node. Physiologic or pharmacologic maneuvers that are vagomimetic (Valsalva maneuver or phenylephrine-induced hypertension), vagolytic (atropine), sympathomimetic (isoproterenol or hypotension by nitroprusside), or sympatholytic (beta-adrenergic blocking agents) can be utilized, singly and in combination. These studies are designed to test the response of the sinus node to autonomic stimulation and inhibition and thereby characterize the status of autonomic regulation of the sinus node. Abnormalities of the autonomic control of sinus function are particularly common in patients in whom asymptomatic sinus bradycardia is documented.

Intrinsic Heart Rate This is a manifestation of the primary activity of the sinus node, and its determination requires chemical autonomic blockade of the heart with a combination of atropine and a beta blocker. Normal values of intrinsic heart rate (in beats per minute) are calculated by the formula $118.1 - (0.57 \times \text{age})$. The use of autonomic blockade can separate patients with asymptomatic sinus bradycardia into a group with primary sinus node dysfunction (slow intrinsic heart rate) and a group with autonomic imbalance (normal intrinsic heart rate). Autonomic blockade is particularly useful when combined with invasive assessment of sinus node function (see Table 230-1). Autonomic blockade may depress conduction in patients with intrinsic disease of the conduction system and should be carried out only in a setting where arrhythmias can be monitored and treated rapidly.

Sinus Node Recovery Time Sinus node recovery time (SNRT) is evaluated by assessing the response of the sinus node to rapid atrial pacing (Fig. 230-6). When atrial pacing is discontinued, a pause, the *SNRT*, occurs prior to resumption of spontaneous sinus rhythm. When the SNRT is prolonged, the results of this test mimic the prolonged sinus pauses seen following termination of atrial tachyarrhythmias in the bradycardia-tachycardia syndrome (see Fig. 230-4). The SNRT is usually corrected for the spontaneous sinus rate and is normally less than 550 ms. In patients with symptomatic sinus node dysfunction, prolongation of the SNRT is often observed. Patients with abnormally slow intrinsic heart rates usually have an abnormal SNRT, while those with normal intrinsic heart rates have normal recovery times.

Sinoatrial Conduction Time Determination of the conduction time from the sinus node to the atrium allows for the differentiation of abnormalities of sinoatrial conduction from abnormalities of sinus impulse formation. The conduction time equals one-half the difference

FIGURE 230-4 Tachycardia-bradycardia syndrome. Rhythm strip of ECG lead II showing spontaneous cessation of supraventricular tachycardia followed by a 5.6-s pause prior to resumption of sinus activity. The patient was asymptomatic during supraventricular tachycardia, but the sinus pause caused severe light-headedness.

FIGURE 230-5 Second-degree sinoatrial exit block. Surface ECG denoting abrupt absence of P wave during sinus rhythm. Prior to the pause, the sinus rate is regular. The interval of the pause is exactly twice the basal sinus cycle length. The arrow marks the appropriate location for the absent P wave. SA exit block can be 2:1 as above or longer, as shown in Fig. 230-6.

FIGURE 230-6 Example of sinus node recovery time in a patient with symptomatic sinus node dysfunction. Cessation of atrial pacing at 150 beats per minute (cycle length 400 ms) results in a prolonged sinus pause (2.8 s). Surface ECG leads V_1 and V_6 are shown in addition to intracardiac recordings at the high right atrium (A), which demonstrates atrial pacing rate.

between the pause following termination of brief periods of pacing and the sinus cycle length. Alternatively, the sinus node electrogram can be recorded directly by a catheter electrode placed near the sinoatrial node, and direct measurement of sinoatrial conduction can be obtained.

EVALUATION The electrophysiologic investigation of sinus node dysfunction should be undertaken in patients who have had symptoms compatible with sinus node dysfunction and in whom no documentation of the arrhythmia responsible for these symptoms has been obtained by prolonged Holter monitoring. Asymptomatic patients with sinus bradycardia need *not* be tested, since no therapy is indicated. Similarly, symptomatic patients with ECG documentation of asystole, sinoatrial block or arrest, or the bradycardia-tachycardia syndrome do not require electrophysiologic tests for diagnosis. However, in symptomatic patients without documentation of an arrhythmia, electrophysiologic assessment of sinus node function can yield information that may be used to guide appropriate therapy.

The results of tests of sinus node function must be interpreted with caution. Sinus node dysfunction coexists frequently with other disorders such as AV conduction disturbances, which may cause symptoms such as syncope. Electrophysiologic evaluation of patients with symptoms such as undiagnosed syncope must not stop with the demonstration of abnormalities of sinus node dysfunction or carotid sinus hypersensitivity. Instead, complete evaluation, including His bundle recordings and programmed atrial and ventricular stimulation (see Chap. 231), is necessary to search for additional electrophysiologic abnormalities that could be responsible for symptoms.

Table 230-1

Electrophysiologic Evaluation of the Conduction System

SINUS NODE EVALUATION

1. Sinus node recovery time (SNRT): Amount of time required by the sinus node to recover from overdrive suppression. The SNRT is corrected for the mean sinus rate at baseline. The normal value is <550 ms.
2. Sinoatrial conduction time: Measured from the response of the sinus node to stimulated atrial premature depolarizations or by direct recording from a sinus node electrogram. The normal value is 45–125 ms.
3. Intrinsic heart rate (IHR): Heart rate measured after autonomic blockade with atropine (0.5–2.0 mg IV) and propranolol (1–4 μg/min IV). The normal IHR is calculated by the formula:
$$HR = 118.1 - (0.57 \times age)$$
An abnormally low value suggests sinus node dysfunction.

ATRIOVENTRICULAR CONDUCTION EVALUATION

1. Atrial activation times: Measurement of intraatrial conduction times. Prolonged activation times may be associated with atrial flutter or fibrillation.
2. Measurement of AH and HV intervals: Prolongation of AH interval (>125 ms) or prolongation of the HV interval (>55 ms) may help localize the site of delay.
3. Incremental atrial pacing: To determine the cycle length at which block occurs in the AV node and/or His-Purkinje system. Block below the His bundle at rates of <150 beats per minute portends the development of infra-His block.

TREATMENT

Permanent pacemakers (see p. 1258) are the mainstay of therapy for patients with symptomatic sinus node dysfunction. Patients with intermittent paroxysms of bradycardia or sinus arrest and with the cardioinhibitory form of the hypersensitive carotid sinus syndrome are usually adequately treated by demand ventricular pacemakers. These devices are reliable, relatively inexpensive, and suffice to prevent episodic symptoms due to abrupt bradycardia. Patients with symptomatic chronic sinus bradycardia or frequent prolonged episodes of sinus node dysfunction do better with dual-chamber pacemakers that preserve the normal AV activation sequence. Although theoretically an atrial demand pacemaker should be adequate for patients with sinus node dysfunction, the frequent accompaniment of dysfunction in other portions of the cardiac conduction system usually mandates placement of a pacemaker capable of ventricular pacing. Recent studies suggest that AV sequential pacing also may be useful in preventing atrial fibrillation, an important component of the bradycardia-tachycardia syndrome.

AV CONDUCTION DISTURBANCES

The specialized cardiac conducting system normally ensures synchronous conduction of each sinus impulse from the atria to the ventricles. Abnormalities of conduction of the sinus impulse to the ventricles may portend the development of heart block, which can ultimately lead to syncope or cardiac arrest. In order to evaluate the clinical significance of conduction abnormalities, the physician must assess (1) the site of conduction disturbance, (2) the risk of progression to complete block, and (3) the probability that a subsidiary escape rhythm arising distal to the site of block will be electrophysiologically and hemodynamically stable. This latter point is perhaps the most important, since the rate and stability of the escape pacemaker determine what symptoms result from heart block. The escape pacemaker following AV nodal block is usually in the His bundle, which generally has a stable rate of 40 to 60 beats per minute and is associated with a QRS complex of normal duration (in the absence of a preexisting intraventricular conduction defect). This contrasts with escape rhythms arising in the distal His-Purkinje system, which have lower intrinsic rates (25 to 45 beats per minute), manifest wide QRS complexes with prolonged duration, and are unstable. Although prolonged QRS complexes are invariable when the distal His-Purkinje pacemakers form the escape mechanism, wide QRS complexes also can coexist with AV nodal block and a His bundle rhythm. Therefore, QRS morphology alone may not be adequate to identify the site of block.

ETIOLOGY The AV node is supplied by the parasympathetic and sympathetic nervous systems and is sensitive to variations in autonomic tone. Chronic slowing of AV nodal conduction may be seen in highly trained athletes who have hypervagotonia at rest. A variety of diseases also can influence AV nodal conduction. These include acute processes such as myocardial infarction (particularly inferior), coronary spasm (usually of the right coronary artery), digitalis intoxication, excesses of beta and/or calcium blockers, acute infections such as viral myocarditis, acute rheumatic fever, infectious mononucle-

FIGURE 230-7 *A.* Mobitz type I second-degree AV block. Intracardiac recordings demonstrate that the PR prolongation (320, 615 ms) is localized to the AV node (AH 240, 535 ms, respectively). HBE, His bundle electrogram; A, atrium; H, His; V, ventricle. Time lines (T) = 100 ms. *(From ME Josephson, SF Seides, Clinical Cardiac Electrophysiology: Techniques and Interpretations. Philadelphia, Lea & Febiger, 1979.) B.* Mobitz type II second-degree AV block. Intracardiac recordings document block below the His bundle.

osis, and miscellaneous disorders such as Lyme disease, sarcoidosis, amyloidosis, and neoplasms, particularly cardiac mesotheliomas. AV nodal block also may be congenital.

Two degenerative diseases are commonly responsible for damage to the specialized conducting system and produce AV block usually associated with bundle branch block (see Chap. 228). In *Lev's disease*, there is calcification and sclerosis of the fibrous cardiac skeleton, which frequently involves the aortic and mitral valves, the central fibrous body, and the summit of the ventricular septum. *Lenegre's disease* appears to be a primary sclerodegenerative disease within the conducting system itself with no involvement of the myocardium or the fibrous skeleton of the heart. These two diseases are probably the most common causes of isolated chronic heart block in adults. Hypertension and aortic and/or mitral stenosis are specific disorders that either accelerate the degeneration of the conducting system or have a direct effect by calcification and fibrosis involving the conducting system.

First-degree AV block, more properly termed *prolonged AV conduction*, is characterized by a PR interval >0.20 s. Since the PR interval is determined by atrial, AV nodal, and His-Purkinje activation, delay in any one or more of these structures can contribute to a prolonged PR interval. In the presence of a QRS complex of normal duration, a PR interval >0.24 s almost invariably is due to a delay within the AV node. If the QRS is prolonged, delays may be present at any of the levels mentioned above. Delay within the His-Purkinje system is always accompanied by a prolonged QRS duration in addition to a prolonged PR interval. However, as indicated below, it is only with intracardiac recordings that the exact site of delay can be determined.

Second-degree heart block (intermittent AV block) is present when some atrial impulses fail to conduct to the ventricles. Mobitz type I second-degree AV block (AV Wenckebach block) is characterized by progressive PR interval prolongation prior to block of an atrial impulse (Fig. 230-7A). The pause hat follows is less than fully compensatory (i.e., is less than two normal sinus intervals), and the PR interval of the first

conducted impulse is shorter than the last conducted atrial impulse prior to the blocked P wave. This type of block is almost always localized to the AV node and associated with a normal QRS duration. It is seen most often as a transient abnormality with inferior wall infarction or with drug intoxication, particularly digitalis, beta blockers, and occasionally calcium channel antagonists. This type of block also can be observed in normal individuals with heightened vagal tone. Although Mobitz type I block can progress to complete heart block, this is uncommon, except in the setting of acute inferior wall myocardial infarction. Even when it does, however, the heart block is usually well tolerated because the escape pacemaker usually arises in the proximal His bundle and provides a stable rhythm. As a result, the presence of Mobitz type I second-degree AV block rarely mandates aggressive therapy. Therapeutic decisions depend on the ventricular response and the symptoms of the patient. If the ventricular rate is adequate and the patient is asymptomatic, observation is sufficient.

In Mobitz type II second-degree AV block, conduction fails suddenly and unexpectedly without a preceding change in PR intervals (Fig. 230-7B). It is generally due to disease of the His-Purkinje system and is most often associated with a prolonged QRS duration. It is important to recognize this type of block because it has a high incidence of progression to complete heart block with an unstable, slow, lower escape pacemaker. Therefore, pacemaker implantation is necessary in this condition. Mobitz type II block may occur in the setting of anteroseptal infarction or in the primary or secondary sclerodegenerative or calcific disorders of the fibrous skeleton of the heart. In so-called high-degree AV block there are periods of two or more consecutively blocked P waves, but intermittent conduction can be demonstrated. Block is usually in the His-Purkinje system, but simultaneous block in the AV node may also be present. Regardless of the site of origin of the escape rhythm, if it is slow and the patient is symptomatic, a cardiac pacemaker is mandatory.

Third-degree AV block is present when no atrial impulse propagates to the ventricles. If the QRS complex of the escape rhythm is of normal duration, occurs at a rate of 40 to 55 beats per minute, and increases with atropine or exercise, AV nodal block is probable. Congenital complete AV block is usually localized to the AV node (Fig. 230-8). If the block is within the His bundle, the escape pacemaker usually is less responsive to these perturbations. If the escape rhythm of the QRS is wide and associated with rates ≤40 beats per minute, block is usually localized in, or distal to, the His bundle and mandates a pacemaker, since the escape rhythm in this setting is unreliable. Some patients with infra-His bundle block are capable of retrograde conduction. In such patients, a "pacemaker syndrome" (see below) may develop if a simple ventricular pacemaker is used. Dual-chambered pacemakers eliminate this potential problem.

AV DISSOCIATION AV dissociation exists whenever the atria and ventricles are under the control of two separate pacemakers and, while present in complete AV block, can occur in the absence of a primary conduction disturbance. AV dissociation unrelated to heart block may occur under two circumstances: First, it may develop with an AV junctional rhythm in response to severe sinus bradycardia. When the sinus rate and the escape rate are similar and the P waves occur just before, in, or following the QRS complex, *isorhythmic AV dissociation* is said to be present. Treatment usually consists of removal of the offending cause of sinus bradycardia (i.e., discontinuation of digitalis, beta blockers, or calcium antagonists), accelerating the sinus

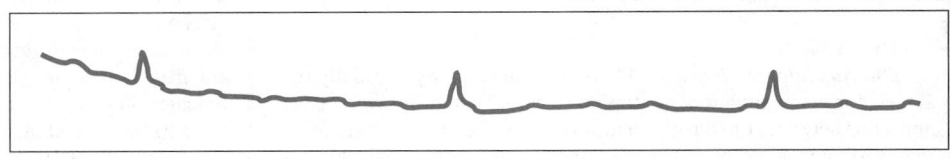

FIGURE 230-8 Third-degree AV block. Complete heart block with a narrow QRS. In this instance, the block was in the AV node.

node by vagolytic agents, or insertion of a pacemaker if the escape rhythm is slow and results in symptoms. Second, AV dissociation can be caused by an enhanced lower (junctional or ventricular) pacemaker that competes with normal sinus rhythm and frequently exceeds it. This has been called *interference AV dissociation* because the rapid lower pacemaker results in bombardment of the AV node in a retrograde fashion, rendering it refractory to the normal sinus impulses. Thus failure of antegrade conduction is a physiologic response in this circumstance. Interference dissociation commonly occurs during ventricular tachycardia, accelerated junctional or ventricular rhythms seen with digitalis intoxication, myocardial ischemia and/or infarction, or local irritation following cardiac surgery. The accelerated rhythm should be treated with either antiarrhythmic drugs (see Chap. 231), removal of an offending drug, or correction of the metabolic abnormality or ischemia.

INTRACARDIAC ELECTROCARDIOGRAPHIC RECORDINGS IN DIAGNOSIS AND MANAGEMENT The main therapeutic decision in patients with AV conduction disturbance is whether or not a permanent pacemaker is required, and a number of circumstances exist in which His bundle electrocardiography can be a useful diagnostic tool upon which to base this decision. It is unquestionable that patients with *symptomatic* second- or third-degree AV block should be paced, and therefore, these patients do not require electrophysiologic study. However, intracardiac ECG recordings can be useful in at least the following three groups of patients:

1. *Patients with syncope and bundle branch or bifascicular block without documentation of AV block.* In such patients, the demonstration of marked infra-His bundle conduction disturbances, i.e., a prolonged HV interval (>100 ms), may usually be taken as an indication of the need for the insertion of the permanent pacemaker. Complete electrophysiologic evaluation, including atrial and ventricular programmed stimulation, is indicated to help identify other possible cardiac etiologies for the syncope. Since the incidence of significant advanced AV block is low in *asymptomatic* patients who have bifascicular block, electrophysiologic evaluation or permanent pacemakers are not cost-effective. In this group, observation appears most reasonable.

2. *Patients with 2:1 atrioventricular conduction.* Intracardiac recordings are necessary to ascertain the site of the conduction disturbance because the typical ECG features of Mobitz type I or Mobitz type II block cannot be discerned during a 2:1 pattern of AV conduction on the surface ECG. Intracardiac recordings may demonstrate that AV nodal block, intra-His bundle block, infra-His bundle block, or combinations of block may be responsible. A surface ECG finding that suggests an infra-His bundle lesion is the presence of alternating bundle branch block associated with changing PR intervals. Intracardiac recordings in such patients confirm that the block is almost always in the His-Purkinje system. Increasing block with exercise or following atropine suggests intra- or infra-His block. The finding of infra- or intra-His bundle block in patients with asymptomatic second-degree AV block mandates pacemaker therapy because of the high likelihood of the development of symptomatic high-grade AV block and syncope.

3. *Asymptomatic patients with third-degree AV block.* In such patients, electrophysiologic studies may be useful in assessing the stability of the junctional pacemaker. Pacing is indicated when the His bundle escape pacemaker is shown to be unstable by an inadequate response to exercise, atropine, or isoproterenol or by a prolonged junctional recovery time following ventricular pacing.

℞ TREATMENT

Pharmacologic Therapy Pharmacologic therapy is usually reserved for acute situations. Atropine (0.5 to 2.0 mg intravenously) and isoproterenol (1 to 4 μg/min intravenously) are useful in increasing heart rate and decreasing symptoms in patients with sinus bradycardia or AV block localized to the AV node. They have an insignificant effect on lower pacemakers. In patients with neurovascular

syncope, beta blockers and disopyramide have been suggested as methods to depress left ventricular function and decrease mechanoreceptor-related reflexes. Mineralocorticoids, ephedrine, and theophylline also have been reported to be of benefit to occasional patients. Unfortunately, no controlled study has shown that any of these pharmacologic modalities works in a predictable fashion in all patients. Further work on delineating different mechanisms in different patient groups may allow us to apply pharmacologic agents more appropriately. Long-term therapy of bradyarrhythmias is best accomplished by pacemakers.

Pacemakers External energy sources can be used to stimulate the heart when disorders in impulse formation and/or transmission lead to symptomatic bradyarrhythmias. Pacer stimuli can be applied to the atria and/or ventricles. Indications for pacemaker insertion are listed in Table 230-2.

TEMPORARY PACING This is usually instituted to provide immediate stabilization prior to permanent pacemaker placement or to provide pacemaker support when a bradycardia is precipitated by what is presumed to be a transient event such as ischemia or drug toxicity. Temporary pacing is usually achieved by the transvenous insertion of an electrode catheter with the catheter positioned in the right ventricular apex and attached to an external generator. This procedure is associated with a small risk of cardiac perforation, infection at the insertion site, and thromboembolism; the risk of the latter two complications increases markedly if the pacing wire is left in place for more than 48 h. The development of an entirely external transthoracic cardiac pacing system may preclude the need for transvenous pacing in selected patients. However, occasional failure of ventricular capture and significant discomfort related to the large current required for effective transthoracic ventricular stimulation preclude the uniform use of this approach.

PERMANENT PACING This mode of pacing is instituted for persistent or intermittent symptomatic bradycardia not related to a self-limiting precipitating factor or for documented infranodal second- or third-degree AV block. Permanent pacing leads are usually inserted transvenously through the subclavian or cephalic vein with the leads positioned in the right atrial appendage for atrial pacing and the right ventricular apex for ventricular pacing. The leads are then attached to the pulse generator, which is inserted into a subcutaneous pocket below the clavicle. Epicardial lead placement is used when (1) transvenous access cannot be obtained, (2) the chest is already open, i.e., in the course of a cardiac operation, and (3) adequate endocardial lead placement cannot be achieved. Most pacemaker generators are powered by lithium batteries. The life expectancy of the generator is related to (1) voltage output required for capture, (2) requirement for incessant or intermittent pacing, and (3) number of cardiac chambers paced. Life expectancy of the simple ventricular demand pacemaker can exceed 10 years.

PACING CODE A code consisting of three to five letters has been developed for describing pacemaker type and function (Table 230-3). The first letter indicates the chamber(s) paced and is designated *V* for ventricular pacing, *A* for atrial pacing, or *D* for dual-chamber (both atrial and ventricular) pacing. The second letter indicates the chamber in which electrical activity is sensed and is also indicated by *A*, *V*, or *D*. An additional designation, *O*, has been used when pacemaker discharge is not dependent on a sensed electrical activity. The third letter refers to the response to a sensed electric signal. The letter *O* represents no response to an underlying electric signal, usually related to the absence of associated sensing function; *I* represents inhibition of pacing function; *T* represents triggering of pacing function; and *D* indicates a dual response, i.e., spontaneous atrial and ventricular activity inhibiting atrial and ventricular pacing and atrial activity triggering a ventricular response. Additional fourth and fifth letters of the pacing code have been recommended to indicate whether the pacemaker is programmable and has rate modulation (fourth) and whether special antitachycardia functions are available (i.e., antitachycardia pacing, *T*, and delivery of high- or low-energy shocks). In the fourth category, *M* represents multiprogrammability and *R* represents rate response ("physiologic") pacing.

Table 230-2

Indications for Permanent Pacing*

ACQUIRED AV BLOCK IN ADULTS

Class I

1. Complete heart block, permanent or intermittent, at any anatomic level, associated with any anatomic level, associated with any one of the following complications:
   a. Symptomatic bradycardia. In the presence of complete heart block, symptoms must be presumed to be due to the heart block unless proved to be otherwise.
   b. Congestive heart failure.
   c. Ectopic rhythms and other medical conditions that require drugs that suppress the automaticity of escape pacemakers and result in symptomatic bradycardia.
   d. Documented periods of asystole ≥ 3.0 s or any escape rate < 40 beats per minute in symptom-free patients.
   e. Confusional states that clear with temporary pacing.
   f. Post-AV junction ablation, myotonic dystrophy.
2. Second-degree AV block, permanent or intermittent, regardless of the type or the site of block, with symptomatic bradycardia.
3. Atrial fibrillation, atrial flutter, or rare cases of supraventricular tachycardia with complete heart block or advanced AV block, bradycardia, and any of the conditions described under a. The bradycardia must be related to digitalis or drugs known to impair AV conduction.

Class II

1. Asymptomatic complete heart block, permanent or intermittent, at any anatomic site, with ventricular rates of 40 beats per minute or faster.
2. Asymptomatic type II second-degree AV block, permanent or intermittent.
3. Asymptomatic type I second-degree AV block at infra-His or intra-His levels.

Class III

1. First-degree AV block.
2. Asymptomatic type I second-degree AV block at the supra-His (AV node) level.

AFTER MYOCARDIAL INFARCTION

Class I

1. Persistent advanced second-degree AV block or complete heart block after acute myocardial infarction with block in the His-Purkinje system (bilateral bundle branch block).
2. Transient advanced AV block and associated bundle branch block.

Class II

1. Persistent advanced block at the AV node.

Class III

1. Transient AV conduction disturbances in the absence of intraventricular conduction defects.
2. Transient AV block in the presence of isolated left anterior hemiblock.
3. Acquired left anterior hemiblock in the absence of AV block.
4. Persistent first-degree AV block in the presence of bundle branch block not demonstrated previously.

BIFASCICULAR AND TRIFASCICULAR BLOCK

Class I

1. Bifascicular block with intermittent complete heart block associated with symptomatic bradycardia.

2. Bifascicular or trifascicular block with intermittent type II second-degree AV block without symptoms attributable to the heart block.

Class II

1. Bifascicular or trifascicular block with syncope that is not proved to be due to complete heart block, but other possible causes for syncope are not identifiable.
2. Markedly prolonged HV (>100 ms).
3. Pacing-induced infra-His block.

Class III

1. Fascicular block without AV block or symptoms.
2. Fascicular block with first-degree AV block without symptoms.

SINUS NODE DYSFUNCTION

Class I

1. Sinus node dysfunction with documented symptomatic bradycardia. In some patients this will occur as a consequence of long-term (essential) drug therapy of a type and dose for which there are no acceptable alternatives.

Class II

1. Sinus node dysfunction, occurring spontaneously or as a result of necessary drug therapy, with heart rates < 40 beats per minute when a clear association between significant symptoms consistent with bradycardia and the actual presence of bradycardia has not been documented.

Class III

1. Sinus node dysfunction in asymptomatic patients, including those in whom substantial sinus bradycardia (heart rate < 40 beats per minute) is a consequence of long-term drug treatment.
2. Sinus node dysfunction in patients in whom symptoms suggestive of bradycardia are clearly documented not to be associated with a slow heart rate.

HYPERSENSITIVE CAROTID SINUS AND NEUROVASCULAR SYNDROMES

Class I

1. Recurrent syncope associated with clear, spontaneous events provoked by carotid sinus stimulation; minimal carotid sinus pressure induces asystole of >3 s duration in the absence of any medication that depresses the sinus node or AV conduction.

Class II

1. Recurrent syncope without clear, provocative events and with a hypersensitive cardioinhibitory response.
2. Syncope with associated bradycardia reproduced by a head-up tilt with or without isoproterenol or other forms of provocative maneuvers and in which a temporary pacemaker and a second provocative test can establish the likely benefits of a permanent pacemaker.

Class III

1. A hyperactive cardioinhibitory response to carotid sinus stimulation in the absence of symptoms.
2. Vague symptoms, such as dizziness, light-headedness, or both, with a hyperactive cardioinhibitory response to carotid sinus stimulation.
3. Recurrent syncope, light-headedness, or dizziness in the absence of a cardioinhibitory response.

* Class I: agreement that permanent pacemaker should be implanted. Class II: divergence of opinion regarding need for implantation. Class III: agreement that pacemaker is unnecessary.
SOURCE: LS Dreifus et al, with permission.

Table 230-3

The NASPE/BPEG Generic Pacemaker Code

Position Category	I Chamber(s) Paced	II Chamber(s) Sensed	III Response to Sensing	IV Programmability, Rate Modulation	V Antitachyarrhythmia Function(s)
	O, None	O, None	O, None	O, None	O, None
	A, Atrium	A, Atrium	T, Triggered	P, Simple programmable	P, pacing (antitachyarrhythmia)
	V, Ventricle	V, Ventricle	I, Inhibited	M, Multiprogrammable	S, Shock
	D, Dual (A + V)	D, Dual (A + V)	D, Dual (T + I)	C, Communicating	D, Dual (P + S)
				R, Rate modulation	
Manufacturer's designation	S, single (A or V)	S, (A or V)			

SOURCE: Zipes, DP: Cardiac pacemakers and antiarrhythmia devices, in *Heart Disease: A Textbook of Cardiovascular Medicine*, 5th ed, E Braunwald (ed). Philadelphia, Saunders, pp 705–741.

It follows from the described code that the standard VVIR (ventricular demand pacemaker) paces the ventricle, senses the ventricle, is inhibited by sensed spontaneous ventricular activity, and has rate modulation, while the DDDR pulse generator is capable of sensing and pacing both the atria and ventricles and has a dual response to the sensed atrial and ventricular activity as described above (Fig. 230-9). Both pacemakers have rate modulation (*R*). "Physiologic" pacemakers use sensors (muscular activity, respiratory rate, temperature, O_2 saturation, QT interval, etc.) as methods to allow the pacemaker to increase the heart rate in response to physiologic demands, i.e., exercise. These pacemakers are essential when chronotropic incompetence is present and an increase in heart rate is required to enhance physiologic performance. Studies have shown that such "physiologic" pacemakers improve exercise tolerance and relieve symptoms to a greater degree than fixed-rate pacemakers.

Selection of the appropriate pacemaker and pacing mode depends on the clinical condition and the type of bradyarrhythmia being treated. The two most common pacing mode selections are DDD and VVI. DDD provides AV sequential pacing, which is ideally suited for the relatively young and active patient who has intact sinus node function or intermittent dysfunction and high-grade persistent or intermittent AV block. The DDD mode will allow for physiologic atrial sensed and ventricular paced rates and improve exercise tolerance. AV synchrony and dual-chamber pacing also may be desirable in patients with borderline hemodynamic reserve who are dependent on atrial contribution to cardiac output and in those patients who develop the pacemaker syndrome (see below) in response to ventricular demand pacing.

Rate-responsive DDD (i.e., DDDR) pacing is indicated when chronotropic incompetence is present in a patient who requires AV synchrony. The DDD pacing mode is contraindicated in chronic atrial fibrillation or flutter, because rapid and irregular ventricular pacing will occur to the upper rate limit. In some cases this will produce a more rapid ventricular rate than the patient's own rate in the absence of a pacemaker. DDD pacemakers must either automatically

switch or be reprogrammed to the VVI mode. Almost all such pacemakers are now combined with some form of rate responsiveness so that when the device functions in the VVI mode, it also will respond to physiologic demands (VVIR).

Chronotropic insufficiency (i.e., the inability of the sinus rate to accelerate) is a contraindication for a DDD pacemaker, since such a pacemaker will act as a "fixed-rate" pacemaker at the programmed lower rate. In these situations, a rate-adaptive or "physiologic" pacemaker is indicated (VVIR or DDDR). In patients with impaired sinus node function or chronic atrial fibrillation, a sensor-driven, rate-adaptive pacemaker must be implanted. As mentioned earlier, these pacemakers automatically adjust ventricular pacing rates to a sensed indicator of exertion. The DDD pacing mode also may be contraindicated in patients with intermittent or persistent ventriculoatrial conduction, who may develop pacemaker-mediated tachycardia (see below).

PROGRAMMABILITY OF PACEMAKERS This allows for modification of pacing function after implantation and for adaptation to changes in clinical needs. Pacemaker programming is accomplished by activation of the programming head positioned over the implanted pulse generator after making the desired changes in programmable parameters (see Table 230-3). A radio frequency system is routinely used to communicate the program to the pacemaker. A high degree of sophistication is required to recognize the presence and causes of pacemaker malfunction and their treatment.

COMPLICATIONS Adverse effects of permanent pacing are usually associated with failure or malfunction of the pacing system. These problems are usually secondary to over- or undersensing, output failure, and/or lead fracture or displacement. Two other problems may occur. The *pacemaker syndrome* consists of fatigue, dizziness, syncope, and distressing pulsations in the neck and chest and can be associated with adverse hemodynamic effects. The pathophysiologic contributors to the pacemaker syndrome include (1) loss of atrial contribution to ventricular systole; (2) vasodepressor reflex initiated by cannon *a* waves, which are caused by atrial contractions against a closed tricuspid valve and observed in the jugular venous pulse (Chap. 227); and (3) systemic and pulmonary venous regurgitation due to atrial contraction against a closed AV valve. The symptoms associated with the pacemaker syndrome can be prevented by maintaining AV synchrony by dual-chamber pacing or, in the case of a ventricular demand pacemaker, by programming an escape rate 15 to 20 beats per minute below that of the paced rate (i.e., hysteresis). As a result of this programming, sinus activity and thus atrial contraction will be less likely to occur at the same time as ventricular pacing and ventricular contraction. The second major problem peculiar to dual-chamber pacemakers is the development of *pacemaker-mediated tachycardia*. In this instance, retrograde depolarization of the atria, resulting from a premature ventricular depolarization or a paced ventricular complex, is sensed and leads to subsequent triggering of ventricular pacing. This, in turn, can result in repetition of the phenomenon of ventriculoatrial conduction with the development of an endless-loop, pacemaker-mediated tachycardia. It may be corrected by reprogramming the atrial refractory period.

FIGURE 230-9 Normally functioning DDD pacemaker. All three panels show a lead II rhythm strip at 50 mm/s. The programmed lower rate is approximately 55 beats per minute. (*Top*) AV sequential pacing with a paced AV interval of 160 ms is shown for the first two complexes. A VPC occurs and is sensed, resetting the cycle. (*Middle*) The first beat is AV paced, but spontaneous sinus P waves and APC trigger a ventricular paced complex with a sensed P to QRS of 120 ms. (*Bottom*) After the first AV paced complex, a paced atrial complex conducts to the ventricle with a PR of 120 ms, inhibiting the ventricular pacemaker.

BIBLIOGRAPHY

BAROLD SS, ZIPES DP: Cardiac pacemakers and antiarrhythmia devices, in *Heart Disease: A Textbook of Cardiovascular Medicine,* 5th ed, E Braunwald (ed). Philadelphia, Saunders, 1997, p 705

———— et al: Electrocardiography of contemporary DDD pacemakers. Basic concepts: Upper rate response, retrograde ventriculoatrial conduction and differential diagnosis of pacemaker tachycardias, in *Electrical Therapy for Cardiac Arrhythmias: Pacing, Antitachycardia Devices, Catheter Ablation,* S Saksena, N Goldschlager (eds). Philadelphia, Saunders, 1990, p 225

BERNSTEIN AD et al: The NASPE/BPEG generic pacemaker code for antibradyarrhythmias and adaptive-rate pacing and antitachyarrhythmia devices. PACE 10:794, 1987

DREIFUS LS et al: Guidelines for implantation of cardiac pacemakers and antiarrhythmic devices: A report of the American College of Cardiology/ American Heart Association Task Force on Assessment of Diagnostic

Programmed lower rate

Programmed lower rate

Programmed lower rate

and Therapeutic Cardiovascular Procedures (Committee on Pacemaker Implantation). J Am Coll Cardiol 18:1, 1991

ELLENBOGEN KA et al: New insights into pacemaker syndrome gained from hemodynamic, humoral and vascular responses during ventriculo-atrial pacing. Am J Cardiol 65(1):53, 1990

HUANG SK et al: Carotid sinus hypersensitivity in patients with unexplained syncope: Clinical, electrophysiologic and long-term follow-up observations. Am Heart J 116:989, 1988

JOSEPHSON ME: Clinical Electrophysiology, 2d ed. Philadelphia, Lea and Febiger, 1993, chaps 4, 5, 6, 13

MENDES LA, DAVIDOFF R: Cardiogenic seizure with bradyarrhythmia: Documentation of the mechanism during asytole. Am Heart J 125:1786, 1993

MICHAËLSON M, JANZON A: Isolated congenital complete atrioventricular block in adult life. A prospective study. Circulation 92:442, 1995

REINOLD SL et al: Risk factors for the development of recurrent atrial fibrillation: Role of pacing and clinical variables. Am Heart J 129:1127, 1995

SRA JS et al: Comparison of cardiac pacing with drug therapy in the treatment of neurocardiogenic (vasovagal) syncope with bradycardia or asytole. N Engl J Med 328:1085, 1993

WALLER BF et al: Anatomy, histology and pathology of the cardiac conduction system: Part II. Clin Cardiol 16:347, 1993

231

Mark E. Josephson, Peter Zimetbaum, Alfred E. Buxton, Francis E. Marchlinski

THE TACHYARRHYTHMIAS

MECHANISMS OF TACHYARRHYTHMIAS

Tachyarrhythmias may be divided into disorders of impulse propagation and disorders of impulse formation. Disorders of impulse propagation (reentry) are generally considered to be the most common mechanism of sustained paroxysmal tachyarrhythmia. The requirements for initiating reentry include (1) electrophysiologic inhomogeneity (i.e., differences in conduction and/or refractoriness) in two or more regions of the heart connected with each other to form a potentially closed loop; (2) unidirectional block in one pathway; (3) slow conduction over an alternative pathway, allowing time for the initially blocked pathway to recover excitability; and (4) reexcitation of the initially blocked pathway to complete a loop of activation (Fig. 231-1). Repetitive circulation of the impulse over this loop can produce a sustained tachyarrhythmia. While anatomic obstacles may underlie reentry and provide an inexcitable center around which the impulse can circulate, they are not essential. Reentrant arrhythmias can be reproducibly initiated and terminated by premature complexes and rapid stimulation. The response of these arrhythmias to stimulation can help distinguish them from arrhythmias caused by triggered activity.

Disorders of impulse formation can be subdivided into tachyarrhythmias caused by enhanced automaticity and those caused by triggered activity. In addition to the sinus node, automatic pacemaker activity can be observed in specialized atrial fibers, fibers of the atrioventricular (AV) junction, and Purkinje fibers (see Chap. 230). Myocardial cells do not normally possess pacemaker activity. Enhancement of normal automaticity in latent pacemaker fibers or the development of abnormal automaticity due to partial depolarization of the resting membrane occurs as a consequence of a variety of pathophysiologic states, which include (1) increased endogenous or exogenous catecholamines, (2) electrolyte disturbances (e.g., hyperkalemia), (3) hypoxia or ischemia, (4) mechanical effects (e.g., stretch), and (5) drugs (e.g., digitalis). Tachycardia caused by automaticity cannot be started or stopped by pacing.

Rhythms due to *triggered activity* are events that do not occur spontaneously but require a change in cardiac frequency as a trigger. Triggered activity may be caused by early afterdepolarizations, which occur during phases 2 and 3 of the action potential, or delayed afterdepolarizations, which occur following completion of phase 3 of the action potential (see Fig. 230-2). Triggered activity has been observed in atrial, ventricular, and His-Purkinje tissue under conditions such as increased local catecholamine concentration, hyperkalemia, hypercal-

cemia, and digitalis intoxication (delayed afterdepolarizations) or during bradycardia, hypokalemia, or other situations prolonging action potential duration (early afterdepolarizations). All of these conditions produce an accumulation of intracellular calcium. With increasing amplitude of the afterdepolarizations, threshold can be reached and repetitive activity produced. The exact role of triggered activity in spontaneous clinical arrhythmias is unknown, but tachyarrhythmias associated with digitalis intoxication, accelerated idioventricular rhythm in acute infarction and/or reperfusion, and exercise-induced ventricular tachycardia (VT) are believed to be caused by triggered activity due to delayed afterdepolarizations. Torsades de pointes (polymorphic VT associated with long QT intervals) may be caused by triggered activity due to early afterdepolarizations.

The use of electrophysiologic studies, i.e., intracardiac recordings and programmed stimulation, has greatly expanded the understanding of the mechanisms of tachyarrhythmias. In addition to helping diagnose arrhythmias, these techniques may be of value in determining the most appropriate types of therapy because they allow the physician to observe the hemodynamic and symptomatic consequences of the arrhythmia in the presence or absence of therapy. Electrophysiologic studies of tachycardias require the positioning of multiple electrode catheters at critical areas within the heart. These electrodes must be capable of both stimulating and recording from multiple sites in the atria and/or ventricles.

PREMATURE COMPLEXES

ATRIAL PREMATURE COMPLEXES (APCs) APCs can be found on 24-h Holter monitoring in over 60 percent of normal adults. APCs are usually asymptomatic and benign, although at times they may be associated with palpitations. In susceptible patients, they can initiate paroxysmal supraventricular tachycardias. APCs may originate from any location in either atrium, and they are recognized on the electrocardiogram (ECG) as early P waves with a morphology that differs from the sinus P wave (Fig. 231-2A). While APCs usually conduct to the ventricles when they occur late in the cardiac cycle, early APCs may reach the AV conduction system while it is still in its relative refractory period, resulting in a conduction delay manifested by prolonged PR interval following the premature P wave (Fig. 231-2A). Very early APCs may even block in the AV node if this structure is encountered during its effective refractory period. APCs, whether conducted or not, are usually followed by a pause before a return to sinus activity. Most commonly, an APC enters and resets the sinus node, so the sum of the pre- and postextrasystolic PP intervals

FIGURE 231-1 Schema of reentry. Y branching of the Purkinje system to ventricular muscle is shown in panels *A* through *C*. The right limb (*grey area*) of the Purkinje system has a longer refractory period than the left. *A.* During a slow stimulated rate (S₁), conduction proceeds normally over both Purkinje fibers, resulting in collision in the ventricular muscle. *B.* An early premature stimulus (S₂) results in block in the Purkinje fiber on the right and slow conduction down the left. The impulse conducts through the ventricle and attempts to reenter the initial site of block but fails because this site has not fully recovered excitability. *C.* An earlier stimulus (S₃) again results in block on the left. The resulting slower propagation down the left fiber provides enough time for the initial site of block to recur and allows the impulse to conduct through it to produce a reentrant circuit.

is less than the sum of two sinus PP intervals (Fig. 231-2A). In this case, the pause is said to be less than fully compensatory. The QRS complex following most APCs is normal, although early APCs may be followed by aberrantly conducted QRS complexes due to the premature complex falling within the relative refractory period of the His-Purkinje system.

Since most APCs are asymptomatic, treatment is not required. When they cause palpitations or trigger paroxysmal supraventricular tachycardias (see below), treatment may be useful. Factors that precipitate APCs, such as alcohol, tobacco, or adrenergic stimulants, should be identified and eliminated, and in their absence, mild sedation or the use of a beta blocker may be tried.

AV JUNCTIONAL COMPLEXES The site of origin of these complexes is thought to be in the bundle of His, since the normal AV node in vivo possesses no automaticity. AV junctional complexes are less common than either atrial or ventricular premature complexes and are more often associated with cardiac disease or digitalis intoxication. Junctional premature impulses can conduct both antegradely to the ventricles and retrogradely to the atrium and, on rare occasions, may fail to conduct in either direction. Premature AV junctional complexes can be recognized by normal-appearing QRS complexes that are not preceded by a P wave. Retrograde P waves (inverted in leads II, III, and aVF) may be observed after the QRS complex.

While often asymptomatic, junctional premature complexes may be associated with palpitations and cause cannon *a* waves, which may result in distressing pulsations in the neck. When symptomatic, they should be treated like APCs.

VENTRICULAR PREMATURE COMPLEXES (VPCs) These are among the most common arrhythmias and occur in patients with and without heart disease. Of adult males, ≥60 percent will

exhibit VPCs during a 24-h Holter monitoring. In patients without heart disease, VPCs have not been shown to be associated with any increased incidence in mortality or morbidity. VPCs may occur in up to 80 percent of patients with previous myocardial infarction, and in this setting, if frequent (>10 per hour) and/or complex (occurring in couplets), they have been associated with increased mortality. However, cardiac mortality in such patients usually occurs in association with significantly impaired ventricular function. While frequent and complex ventricular ectopy is an independent risk factor, it is not as strong a risk factor as is impaired ventricular function. Moreover, even though ventricular tachycardia and/or fibrillation may be the basis for the sudden death in these patients, this does not a priori establish a cause-and-effect relation between spontaneous ectopy and life-threatening ventricular tachycardia or fibrillation. Very early cycle (R-on-T) VPCs have been stated by some to increase the risk of sudden death. Although this has been observed during acute ischemia and in the setting of QT prolongation, frequently, VT or fibrillation is precipitated by VPCs that occur after the T wave of the prior beat.

VPCs are recognized by wide (usually >0.14 s), bizarre QRS complexes that are not preceded by P waves (Fig. 231-3A). They may bear a relatively fixed relationship to the preceding sinus complex (i.e., fixed coupled VPCs). When fixed coupling is not present and the interval between VPCs has a common denominator, *ventricular parasystole* is said to be present (Fig. 231-4). Under these circumstances, the VPCs are a manifestation of abnormal automaticity of a protected ventricular focus. Because this focus is not penetrated by sinus impulses, it is not reset by them, and the interectopic intervals remain relatively fixed (≤120 ms variation of mean RR cycle length).

VPCs may occur singly; in patterns of bigeminy, in which every sinus beat is followed by a VPC; in trigeminy, in which two sinus beats are followed by a VPC; in quadrigeminy, etc. Two successive VPCs are termed *pairs* or *couplets*, while three or more consecutive VPCs are termed *ventricular tachycardia* when the rate exceeds 100 beats per minute. VPCs may have similar morphologies (monomorphic, or uniform) or different morphologies (polymorphic, or multiformed) (Fig. 231-3C).

Most commonly, VPCs are not conducted retrogradely to the atrium to reset the sinoatrial node. Thus they produce a fully compensatory pause; i.e., the interval between conducted sinus beats that bracket the VPC equals two basic RR intervals. Ventricular impulses also may manifest retrograde conduction to the atrium and cause inverted P waves in leads II, III, and aVF. This retrograde atrial activation can reset the sinus node, and the pause that results may therefore be less than compensatory. In many instances, the VPC will not be associated with retrograde ventriculoatrial (VA) conduction but may block retrogradely in the AV node. This renders the AV node refractory to the subsequent sinus beat and causes slowed conduction (i.e., prolonged PR interval) or block of the next sinus P wave. This prolonged PR interval is said to be a manifestation of concealed retrograde conduction of the ventricular impulse into the AV node. A VPC that does not produce any manifestation of retrograde concealed conduction and fails to influence the oncoming sinus impulse is termed an *interpolated VPC*.

VPCs can cause palpitations or neck pulsations secondary to either the occurrence of cannon *a* waves or the increased force of contraction due to postextrasystolic potentiation of ventricular contractility. Patients with frequent VPCs or bigeminy may rarely develop syncope or lightheadedness because the VPCs do not result in an adequate stroke volume and the cardiac output is reduced by the "halving" of the heart rate.

FIGURE 231-2 *A.* ECG lead II. Sinus rhythm with two atrial premature complexes (*arrows*). Note the difference in P-wave configuration between sinus and the premature atrial complexes. In addition, note that the PR interval of the premature complexes is prolonged, due to slowed conduction of the premature impulse through the AV conduction system. *B.* ECG lead V₁. Atrial tachycardia with varying degrees of AV block, typical of digitalis toxicity. *C.* ECG lead II. Atrial flutter. Note the characteristic sawtooth baseline seen in the inferior ECG leads during atrial flutter. Variable degrees of AV conduction block are present. *D.* ECG lead II. Atrial fibrillation. Note the irregular wavy baseline without discrete atrial activity. The ventricular response is irregularly irregular. *E.* ECG leads I, aVR, and V₁. Atrial fibrillation in a patient with Wolff-Parkinson-White syndrome. Note the extremely rapid, grossly irregular ventricular rate with wide, bizarre QRS complexes.

FIGURE 231-3 *A.* Single ventricular ectopy. During sinus rhythm, two premature ventricular complexes (*arrows*) occur. Note that the QRS configuration is bizarre, different from that during sinus rhythm. The premature ventricular complexes are not preceded by P waves. The QRS width of the premature complexes is approximately 160 ms. The pause surrounding the premature complexes is fully compensatory, the sinus beat after the premature complex occurring on time. *B.* A 5-beat run of nonsustained ventricular tachycardia having a uniform morphology. Although intraventricular conduction during sinus rhythm is slightly prolonged, during the run of ventricular tachycardia the QRS duration is further prolonged. Note that 2:1 VA conduction is present during ventricular tachycardia. Retrograde P waves are denoted by the arrows. *C.* Simultaneous recordings of ECG leads I, aVF, and V₁. A 4-beat run of polymorphic nonsustained ventricular tachycardia is demonstrated. No two consecutive QRS complexes are the same. Polymorphic VT is not associated with a prolonged QT interval in this case.

FIGURE 231-4 Ventricular parasystole. At varying sinus cycle lengths during exercise, interectopic intervals remain constant at 1620 to 1640 ms. However, the coupling intervals between sinus and ectopic complexes vary between 510 and 310 ms.

TREATMENT

In the absence of cardiac disease, isolated asymptomatic VPCs, regardless of configuration and frequency, need no treatment. When arrhythmias are symptomatic, the symptoms should first be addressed by either allaying the patient's anxiety or, if this is not successful, reducing the frequency of the VPCs with antiarrhythmic agents. Beta-adrenergic blockers may be successful in managing VPCs that occur primarily in the daytime or under stressful situations and in specific settings such as mitral valve prolapse and thyrotoxicosis. Class I antiarrhythmic agents may be tried should this be unsuccessful. In patients with cardiac disease, frequent VPCs are associated with an increased risk of sudden and nonsudden cardiac death, and many physicians have attempted to eliminate or reduce the frequency of these VPCs in an attempt to reduce this risk. However, the cause-and-effect relationship of the VPCs to fatal events has never been established. The ability of pharmacologic antiarrhythmic therapy guided by continuous ECG monitoring to reduce the risk of sudden death in patients with frequent (≥6 per minute) VPCs was tested by the Cardiac Arrhythmia Suppression Trial (CAST). This study compared mortality in patients whose ectopy was suppressed by one of three agents (encainide, flecainide, or moricizine) and then randomized to treat with either the "effective" drug or placebo. After a mean follow-up of 2 years, the study was discontinued because both the sudden death and overall mortality rate were significantly increased in patients receiving antiarrhythmic agents. This study has shown that in patients having the characteristics of the study population, abolition of ventricular ectopy by pharmacologic therapy cannot be used as a marker to define reduction of the risk of sudden death after myocardial infarction and, in fact, may increase mortality. Ongoing studies are examining the ability of more advanced techniques, such as electrophysiologic testing, to reduce the rate of sudden death in higher-risk patients, i.e., those with left ventricular ejection fractions of ≤40 and nonsustained VT (≥3 consecutive VPCs).

Antiarrhythmic agents also can produce the lethal arrhythmias that they are given to prevent (proarrhythmic effects). Thus therapy directed toward VPCs in the setting of chronic cardiac disease may result in an inappropriate and costly use of agents without proven efficacy and with potential side effects in many patients. The high incidence of side effects and the frequent exacerbation of arrhythmias caused by all antiarrhythmic drugs make it mandatory to monitor patients being treated with such agents.

In acute myocardial infarction, the greatest incidence of primary ventricular fibrillation occurs within the first 24 h (Chap. 243). Temporary prophylactic antiarrhythmic therapy with lidocaine or procainamide was formerly recommended for all patients with acute infarction, regardless of the presence or degree of spontaneous ectopy. However, failure to improve overall survival and drug toxicity have led most physicians to recommend prophylactic antiarrhythmic therapy only to young patients with complicated infarctions, where a favorable risk-benefit ratio may be obtained. Other studies have shown that intravenous beta blockers also may reduce the incidence of primary ventricular fibrillation.

TACHYCARDIAS

Tachycardias refer to arrhythmias with three or more complexes at rates exceeding 100 beats per minute; they occur more often in structurally diseased than in normal hearts. Those paroxysmal tachycardias that are initiated by APCs or VPCs are considered to be due to reentry, except some of the digitalis-induced tachyarrhythmias, which are probably due to triggered activity (see below).

If the patient is hemodynamically stable, an attempt should be made to determine the mechanism and origin of the tachycardia, since this will usually lead to an appropriate therapeutic decision. Information to be obtained from the ECG includes (1) the presence, frequency, morphology, and regularity of P waves and QRS complexes; (2) the relationship between atrial and ventricular activity; (3) a comparison of the QRS morphology during sinus rhythm and during the tachycardia; and (4) the response to carotid sinus massage or other vagal maneuvers. It is useful first to compare a 12-lead ECG during the tachycardia with one recorded during sinus rhythm. One also can utilize the electrodes situated at the end of a flexible pacing catheter inserted into the esophagus behind the left atrium to record atrial activity.

Observation of the jugular venous pulse can provide clues to the presence of atrial activity and its relationship to ventricular ectopy. Intermittent cannon *a* waves suggest AV dissociation, while persistent cannon *a* waves suggest 1:1 VA conduction. Flutter waves may be seen or no atrial activity may be apparent, as in the presence of atrial flutter and fibrillation, respectively. The arterial pulse also may manifest AV dissociation or atrial fibrillation by demonstrating variations in amplitude. A first heart sound of variable intensity during a regular rhythm also suggests AV dissociation or atrial fibrillation.

Carotid sinus pressure should only be applied while the patient is electrocardiographically monitored with resuscitative equipment available to manage the rare episode of asystole and/or ventricular fibrillation associated with this procedure. Carotid sinus massage should not be performed in patients with carotid arterial bruits. The patient should be positioned flat with the neck extended. Massage of one carotid bulb at a time should be performed by applying firm pressure just underneath the angle of the jaw for up to 5 s. Alternative vagomimetic maneuvers include the Valsalva maneuver, immersion of the face in cold water, and administration of 5 to 10 mg edrophonium.

SINUS TACHYCARDIA In the adult, sinus tachycardia is said to be present when the heart rate exceeds 100 beats per minute: sinus tachycardia rarely exceeds 200 beats per minute and is not a primary arrhythmia; instead, it represents a physiologic response to a variety of stresses, such as fever, volume depletion, anxiety, exercise, thyrotoxicosis, hypoxemia, hypotension, or congestive heart failure. Sinus tachycardia has a gradual onset and offset. The ECG demonstrates P waves with sinus contour preceding each QRS complex. Carotid sinus pressure usually produces modest slowing with a gradual return to the previous rate upon cessation. This contrasts with the response of paroxysmal supraventricular tachycardias, which may slow slightly and terminate abruptly.

℞ TREATMENT

Sinus tachycardia should not be treated as a primary arrhythmia, since it is almost always a physiologic response to a demand placed on the heart. As such, the therapy should be directed to the primary disorder. This may involve institution of digitalis and/or diuretics for heart failure and oxygen for hypoxemia, treatment of thyrotoxicosis, volume repletion, aspirin for fever, or tranquilizers for emotional upset.

ATRIAL FIBRILLATION (AF) This common arrhythmia may occur in paroxysmal and persistent forms. It may be seen in normal subjects, particularly during emotional stress or following surgery, exercise, or acute alcoholic intoxication. It also may occur in patients with heart or lung disease who develop acute hypoxia, hypercapnia, or metabolic or hemodynamic derangements. Persistent AF usually occurs in patients with cardiovascular disease, most commonly rheumatic heart disease, nonrheumatic mitral valve disease, hypertensive cardiovascular disease, chronic lung disease, atrial septal defect, and a variety of miscellaneous cardiac abnormalities. AF may be the presenting finding in thyrotoxicosis. So-called lone AF, which occurs in patients without underlying heart disease, is considered to represent the tachycardia phase of the tachycardia-bradycardia syndrome (p. 1255).

The morbidity associated with AF is related to (1) excessive ventricular rate, which in turn may lead to hypotension, pulmonary conges-

tion, or angina pectoris in susceptible individuals; (2) the pause following cessation of AF, which can cause syncope; (3) systemic embolization, which occurs most commonly in patients with rheumatic heart disease; (4) loss of the contribution of atrial contraction to cardiac output, which may cause fatigue; and (5) anxiety secondary to palpitations. In patients with severe cardiac dysfunction, particularly those with hypertrophied, noncompliant ventricles, the combination of the loss of the atrial contribution to ventricular filling and the abbreviated filling period due to the rapid ventricular rate in AF can produce marked hemodynamic instability, resulting in hypotension, syncope, or heart failure. In patients with mitral stenosis, in whom ventricular filling time is critical, development of AF with a rapid ventricular rate may precipitate pulmonary edema (see Chap. 237). AF may also cause a cardiomyopathy related to persistent rapid rates.

AF is characterized by disorganized atrial activity without discrete P waves on the surface ECG (Fig. 231-2*D*). Atrial activation is manifested by an undulating baseline or by more sharply inscribed atrial deflections of varying amplitude and frequency ranging from 350 to 600 beats per minute. The ventricular response is irregularly irregular. This results from the large number of atrial impulses that penetrate the AV node, making it partially refractory to subsequent impulses. This effect of nonconducted atrial impulses to influence the response to subsequent atrial impulses is termed *concealed conduction*. As a result, the ventricular response is relatively slow, considering the actual atrial rate. AF may convert to atrial flutter, especially in response to antiarrhythmic drugs like quinidine or flecainide. If AF converts to atrial flutter, which has a slower atrial rate, the effect of concealed conduction may be diminished, and a paradoxic increase in the ventricular response may occur. The main factor determining the rate of the ventricular response is the functional refractory period of the AV node or the most rapid paced rate at which 1:1 conduction through the AV node can be observed.

If, in the presence of AF, the ventricular rhythm becomes regular and slow (e.g., 30 to 60 beats per minute), complete heart block is suggested, and if the ventricular rhythm is regular and rapid (e.g., ≥100 beats per minute), a tachycardia arising in the AV junction or ventricle should be suspected. Digitalis intoxication is a common cause of both phenomena.

Patients with AF exhibit a loss of *a* waves in the jugular venous pulse and variable pulse pressures in the carotid arterial pulse. The first heart sound usually varies in intensity. On echocardiography, the left atrium is frequently enlarged, and in patients in whom the left atrial diameter exceeds 4.5 cm, it may not be possible to convert AF to sinus rhythm or to maintain the latter, despite therapy.

℞ TREATMENT

In acute AF, a precipitating factor such as fever, pneumonia, alcoholic intoxication, thyrotoxicosis, pulmonary emboli, congestive heart failure, or pericarditis should be sought. When such a factor is present, therapy should be directed toward the primary abnormality. If the patient's clinical status is severely compromised, electrical cardioversion is the treatment of choice. In the absence of severe cardiovascular compromise, slowing of ventricular rate becomes the initial therapeutic goal. This may be most rapidly accomplished with beta-adrenergic blockers and/or calcium channel antagonists. Both prolong the refractory period of the AV node and slow conduction within it. When catecholamine levels or sympathetic nervous system tone is likely to be elevated, beta blockers may be favored. Digitalis preparations are less effective, take longer to act, and are associated with more toxicity. Conversion to sinus rhythm may then be attempted, using quinidine-like (class IA) drugs or flecainide or other class IC drugs (Table 231-1). It is important to increase AV node refractoriness prior to administering such drugs because their vagolytic effect and their ability to convert AF to atrial flutter may reduce the concealed conduction and lead to an excessively rapid ventricular response. Beta-adrenergic blockers are especially useful in this regard. If medical therapy fails to convert AF in 24 h, electrical cardioversion is useful; it generally requires 100 to 200 W·s of energy. In situations where AF has been present for 48 to 72 h or

Table 231-1

CHAPTER 231
The Tachyarrhythmias   **1265**

Classification of Antiarrhythmic Drugs

Class I	Drugs that reduce maximal velocity of phase of depolarization (V_{max}) due to block of inward Na^+ current in tissue with fast response action potentials
	A $\downarrow$ V_{max} at all heart rates and $\uparrow$ action potential duration, e.g., quinidine, procainamide, disopyramide
	B Little effect at slow rates on V_{max} in normal tissue; $\downarrow$ V_{max} in partially depolarized cells with fast response action potentials Effects increased at faster rates No change or $\downarrow$ in action potential duration, e.g., lidocaine, phenytoin, tocainide, mexiletine
	C $\downarrow$ V_{max} at normal rates in normal tissue Minimal effect on action potential duration, e.g., flecainide, propafenone, moricizine
Class II	Antisympathetic agents, e.g., propranolol and other beta-adrenergic blockers: $\downarrow$ SA nodal automaticity, $\uparrow$ AV nodal refractoriness, and $\downarrow$ AV nodal conduction velocity
Class III	Agents that prolong action potential duration in tissue with fast-response action potentials, e.g., bretylium, amiodarone, sotalol
Class IV	Calcium (slow) channel blocking agents: $\downarrow$ conduction velocity and $\uparrow$ refractoriness in tissue with slow-response action potentials, e.g., verapamil, diltiazem

Drugs that cannot be classified by this schema:
  Digitalis
  Adenosine

---

more, anticoagulation should be started at least 2 weeks prior to and continued for 2 weeks following any attempt at cardioversion, either pharmacologic or electrical. Anticoagulation appears to decrease the incidence of systemic embolization associated with cardioversion. Some advocate the use of transesophageal echocardiography. In the absence of clot, cardioversion can be undertaken and anticoagulation started immediately. It is less likely for chronic AF to convert to or remain in sinus rhythm in the presence of long-standing rheumatic heart disease and/or when the atria are markedly enlarged. It is also unlikely for patients with lone AF to be converted to and maintained in sinus rhythm.

The goal of therapy in patients in whom AF cannot be converted to sinus rhythm is control of the ventricular response. This can usually be accomplished by digitalis, beta blockers, or calcium channel blockers singly or in combination. In occasional patients, the ventricular response cannot be controlled by pharmacologic therapy alone. In such patients, the creation of complete heart block by radiofrequency catheter ablation of the AV junction followed by permanent pacemaker implantation is appropriate. Surgical or direct-current catheter ablation of the AV junction is rarely required to achieve AV block.

If sinus rhythm is restored electrically or pharmacologically, quinidine or related agents as well as the class IC agents (e.g., flecainide) or amiodarone may be used to prevent recurrence. In patients in whom cardioversion is unsuccessful or in whom AF is likely to recur, it is probably wisest to allow the patient to remain in AF and to control the ventricular response with calcium antagonists, beta-adrenergic blockers, or digitalis glycosides. Since such patients are always at risk of systemic embolization, particularly in the presence of organic heart disease, chronic anticoagulation must be considered. Several studies have now demonstrated conclusively that the incidence of embolization in patients with AF not associated with valvular heart disease is reduced by chronic anticoagulation with warfarin-like agents. Aspirin also may be effective for this purpose, but the data supporting its use are less extensive.

ATRIAL FLUTTER This arrhythmia occurs most often in patients with organic heart disease. Flutter may be paroxysmal, in which case there is usually a precipitating factor, such as pericarditis or acute respiratory failure, or it may be persistent. Atrial flutter (as well as AF) is very common during the first week following open-heart surgery. Atrial flutter is usually less long-lived than is AF, although on occasion it may persist for months to years. Most commonly, if it

lasts for more than a week, atrial flutter will convert to AF. Systemic embolization is less common in atrial flutter than in AF.

Atrial flutter is characterized by an atrial rate between 250 and 350 beats per minute. Typically, the ventricular rate is half the atrial rate, i.e., approximately 150 beats per minute. If the atrial rate is slowed to <220 beats per minute by antiarrhythmic agents such as quinidine, which also possess vagolytic properties, the ventricular rate may rise suddenly because of the development of 1:1 AV conduction. Classically, flutter waves are seen as regular sawtooth-like atrial activity, most prominent in the inferior leads (Fig. 231-2C). When the ventricular response is regular and not a simple fraction of the atrial rate, complete AV block is present, which may be a manifestation of digitalis toxicity. Activation mapping suggests that atrial flutter is a form of atrial reentry localized to the right atrium.

℞ TREATMENT

The most effective treatment of atrial flutter is direct-current cardioversion, which can be accomplished at low energy (25 to 50 W·s) under mild sedation. Higher energies (100 to 200 W·s) are often used because they are less likely to cause *atrial fibrillation,* which not infrequently occurs following lower energy delivery. In patients who develop atrial flutter following open-heart surgery or recurrent flutter in the setting of acute myocardial infarction, particularly if they are being treated with digitalis, atrial pacing (using temporary pacing wires implanted at the time of operation or a pacing lead inserted into the atrium pervenously) at rates of 115 to 130 percent of the atrial flutter rate can usually convert the atrial flutter to sinus rhythm. Atrial pacing also may result in the conversion of atrial flutter to AF, which allows for easier control of the ventricular response. If immediate conversion of atrial flutter is not mandated by the patient's clinical status, the ventricular response should first be slowed by blocking the AV node with a beta blocker, calcium antagonist, or digitalis. Digitalis is the least effective and occasionally converts atrial flutter into AF. Once AV nodal conduction is slowed with any of these drugs, an attempt to convert flutter to sinus rhythm using a class I (A or C) agent or amiodarone should be made. Increasing doses of the drug selected are administered until the rhythm converts or side effects occur.

Quinidine, quinidine-like drugs, flecainide, propafenone, and amiodarone (Table 231-2) may be useful in preventing recurrences of both atrial flutter and atrial fibrillation.

PAROXYSMAL SUPRAVENTRICULAR TACHYCAR-DIAS (PSVT) In most cases, functional differences in conduction and refractoriness in the AV node or the presence of an AV bypass tract provide the substrate for the development of PSVT (previously termed *paroxysmal atrial tachycardia*). Electrophysiologic studies have demonstrated that reentry is responsible for the vast majority of cases of PSVT (Fig. 231-5). Reentry has been localized to the sinus node, atrium, AV node, or a macroreentrant circuit involving conduction in the antegrade direction through the AV node and retrograde through an AV bypass tract. Such a bypass tract also may conduct antegradely, in which case the Wolff-Parkinson-White (WPW) syndrome is said to be present. When the bypass tract manifests only retrograde conduction, it is termed a *concealed bypass tract* (Fig. 231-5B). In these cases, the QRS complex during sinus rhythm is normal. In the absence of the WPW syndrome, reentry through the AV node or through a concealed bypass tract makes up more than 90 percent of all PSVTs.

AV NODAL REENTRANT TACHYCARDIA There is no age or disease predisposition for the development of AV nodal reentrant tachycardia, the most common cause of supraventricular tachycardia. It is, however, more commonly observed in women. It usually presents as a regular narrow QRS complex tachycardia at rates of 120 to 250 beats per minute. APCs that initiate the arrhythmia are almost always associated with a prolonged PR interval. Retrograde P waves may be

Table 231-2

Drugs Used to Treat Cardiac Tachyarrhythmias

Drug	Sinus Node	Atrium and Ventricle	AV Node	His-Purkinje System	AV Bypass Tracts
ELECTROPHYSIOLOGIC EFFECTS					
Digoxin and other cardiac glycosides	NC; pts with sinus node disease may develop sinus exit block or arrest	Controversial	↑ ERP, ↓ conduction velocity, due to drug action and vagomimetic effects	NC	NC or ↓ ERP
Adenosine	↓ automaticity	Atrium: ↓ ERP Ventricle: no effect	↓ conduction velocity		
Quinidine (class IA)	NC; may suppress sinus node if node disease exists	↑ ERP; ↓ conduction velocity	↓ or NC in ERP; NC in conduction velocity	↓ automaticity; ↓ conduction velocity; ↑ ERP	↑ ERP may abolish all conduction
Procainamide (class IA)	NC	↑ ERP; ↓ conduction velocity	↓ or NC in ERP; ↓ or NC in conduction velocity	↓ automaticity; ↓ conduction velocity; ↑ ERP	↑ ERP may abolish conduction
Disopyramide (class IIA)	NC	↑ ERP; ↓ conduction velocity	↓ or NC in ERP; NC in conduction velocity	↓ automaticity; ↑ ERP; ↓ conduction velocity	↑ ERP may abolish conduction
Lidocaine (class IB)	NC	NC in ERP	NC or ↓ in ERP	NC or ↓ ERP	NC, ↓, or ↑ in ERP
Phenytoin (class IB)	NC	NC in ERP	NC or ↓ in ERP; NC or ↑ in conduction velocity	↓ in ERP; ↓ automaticity	
Tocainide (class IB)	NC	NC	NC	NC; ↓ automaticity	↑ ERP
Mexiletine (class IB)	NC; pts with sinus node disease may develop sinus arrest	NC	Variable and inconsistent effects on conduction and refractoriness	↑ ERP; NC or ↓ conduction velocity	
Flecainide (class IC)	NC; pts with sinus node disease may develop exit block or arrest	↓ conduction velocity; ↑ ERP	↓ conduction velocity; ↑ ERP	↓ conduction velocity	↓ conduction velocity; ↑ ERP; may abolish all conduction
Propafenone (class IC) (also beta blocker)	No significant effect	↓ conduction velocity; ↑ ERP	↓ in conduction velocity; ↑ ERP	↓ conduction velocity; ↑ ERP	↑ ERP
Moricizine (class IC)	No significant effect	Atrium: NC in ERP; ↓ conduction velocity Ventricle: slight increase in ERP; ↓ conduction velocity	↓ conduction velocity	↓ conduction velocity	
Propranolol, atenolol, metoprolol (class II)	↓ sinus rate; ↑ sinus node recovery time	NC	↑ ERP; ↓ conduction velocity	NC	NC
Bretylium (class III)	Initial increase in sinus rate, followed by decrease	↑ ERP	NC	NC	
Amiodarone (class III)	↓ sinus rate	↑ ERP	↑ ERP; ↓ conduction velocity	↑ ERP; ↓ conduction velocity	↑ ERP
Sotalol (class III) (also beta blocker)	↓ sinus rate	↑ ERP	↑ ERP; ↓ conduction velocity	↑ ERP	↑ ERP
Verapamil, diltiazem (class IV)	↓ sinus rate	NC	↑ ERP; ↓ conduction velocity	NC	NC

NOTE: NC, no change; ↑, increase; ↓, decrease; ERP, effective refractory period; AF, atrial fibrillation; VT, ventricular tachycardia; AV, atrioventricular; VF, ventricular fibrillation; SVT, supraventricular tachycardia; VPCs, ventricular premature complexes; CHF, congestive heart failure.

Table 231-2

Drugs Used to Treat Cardiac Tachyarrhythmias *(continued)*

Indications	Side Effects and Toxicity
CLINICAL EFFECTS	
Slowing of ventricular rate during AF, flutter, and other atrial tachycardias in the absence of preexcitation; slowing, termination and/or prevention of SVT due to AV nodal reentry and AV reentry utilizing bypass tracts; may terminate or prevent intraatrial reentrant tachycardias; ineffective in prevention of automatic atrial tachycardias	Atrial tachycardia, VT, AV nodal block, accelerated junctional rhythms, atrial and ventricular premature depolarizations, VT, VF, anorexia, nausea, vomiting, acceleration of ventricular rate during AF flutter in the presence of preexcitation causing VF
Acute termination of regular reentrant SVT involving the AV node	Transient atrial standstill following termination of SVT; transient hypotension
Atrial and ventricular extrasystoles; atrial and ventricular tachyarrhythmias; all types of SVT; control of ventricular rate in pts with preexcitation and AF and flutter	
Same as quinidine	Anorexia, nausea, vomiting, diarrhea, cinchonism, tinnitus, confusion, hearing and visual changes; thrombocytopenia, hemolytic anemia, rash, drug interactions, elevation of digoxin levels; phenytoin and phenobarbital will decrease quinidine levels; QT prolongation associated with polymorphic VT (torsades de pointes); conversion of nonsustained to sustained acceleration of ventricular response to atrial flutter and fibrillation
Same as quinidine	Anorexia, nausea, confusion, hallucinations, agranulocytosis, and lupus erythematosus–like syndrome; QT prolongation associated with polymorphic VT (torsades de pointes); marked elevations in the primary metabolic rate (NAPA); may be more likely to cause polymorphic VT; conversion of nonsustained to sustained VT; acceleration of ventricular response to atrial flutter and fibrillation
Same as quinidine	Anticholinergic actions, including dry mouth, blurred vision, urinary retention, hesitancy, constipation, narrow-angle glaucoma, congestive heart failure, especially in patients with abnormal ventricular function and QT prolongation associated with polymorphic VT (torsades de pointes)
VT and VF, especially during acute ischemia and myocardial infarction	Dizziness, paresthesias, confusion, delirium, seizures, coma; may depress sinus node in pts with underlying sinus node disease; may suppress escape foci in pts with complete heart block; congestive heart failure or liver disease increases risk of side effects
Tachyarrhythmias induced by digitalis; occasionally effective for ventricular tachyarrhythmias not induced by digitalis, alone or in combination with other antiarrhythmic agents; polymorphic VT associated with increased QT	Gingival hypertrophy, rash, blood dyscrasias, nystagmus, ataxia, stupor, coma, lupus erythematosus syndrome, lymph node hyperplasia, peripheral neuropathy, hypocalcemia, hyperglycemia, phlebitis, and hypotension during IV administration
VT, VF, frequent VPCs	Ataxia, tremor, paresthesias, light-headedness, nausea, rash, lupus erythematosus syndrome, pulmonary fibrosis, bone marrow suppression; may exacerbate heart failure in pts with ventricular dysfunction
Refractory atrial and ventricular tachyarrhythmias; SVT due to AV node reentry and AV bypass tracts	Nausea, vomiting, ataxia, tremor, gait disturbances, rash
Refractory atrial and ventricular tachyarrhythmias; SVT due to AV node reentry and AV bypass tracts	Refractory polymorphic VT without increased QT if dose is increased too rapidly or in pts with abnormal conduction system; sinus arrest in pts with normal sinus node function; nausea, dizziness, blurred vision; may precipitate heart failure in pts with ventricular dysfunction
Atrial tachyarrhythmias including AF, SVT (not approved by the FDA for therapy of these arrhythmias), ventricular tachycardias	May exacerbate arrhythmias (increase frequency, convert nonsustained to sustained tachycardias); negative inotropic actions may worsen CHF; beta-blocking activity may worsen asthma, AV block, visual blurring, dizziness, paresthesias, taste disturbances
Slowing of ventricular rate during AF, atrial flutter, and other atrial tachycardias in the absence of preexcitation; SVT due to AV nodal reentry, reentry utilizing bypass tracts; arrhythmias induced by exercise; arrhythmias occurring in the presence of hyperthyroidism; polymorphic VT associated with congenital long QT syndrome.	Sinus bradycardia, AV node block, congestive heart failure, bronchospasm, masking symptoms of hypoglycemia
Atrial and ventricular tachyarrhythmias (not FDA approved for atrial arrhythmias)	May exacerbate ventricular tachycardia; dizziness, nausea
Refractory VT and VF, especially due to acute ischemia	Initially, transient hypertension; subsequent hypotension increased in upright position; the hypotensive effect can be prevented by tricyclic drugs; nausea, vomiting
Refractory atrial and ventricular tachyarrhythmias; refractory SVT due to AV nodal reentry and AV reentry utilizing bypass tracts; not approved by FDA for atrial arrhythmias; atrial and ventricular extrasystoles and tachyarrhythmias (not yet approved by the FDA)	Marked sinus bradycardia, complete heart block; IV administration may cause hypotension; increased QT associated with polymorphic VT; increased T_4, hypo- and hyperthyroidism; peripheral neuropathy; proximal myopathy, pulmonary fibrosis; increased liver enzymes; hepatitis; blue-gray skin discoloration; corneal microdeposits; elevation of digoxin levels; potential of oral coagulants; exacerbation of CHF, polymorphic VT associated with QT prolongation
Slowing of ventricular rate during atrial fibrillation, atrial flutter, and other atrial tachycardias in the absence of preexcitation: SVT due to AV nodal reentry, reentry utilizing bypass tracts; idiopathic left ventricular tachycardia	Sinus bradycardia, AV node block, congestive heart failure, constipation, peripheral edema, drug interactions

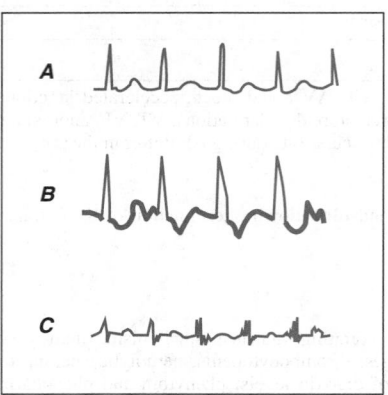

FIGURE 231-5 Examples of reentrant PSVT. *A.* AV nodal reentry. No P waves are visible. *B.* AV reentry using a concealed bypass tract. Inverted retrograde P waves are superimposed on the T wave. *C.* Intraatrial reentry. P waves precede the QRS complex.

absent, buried in the QRS complex, or appear as distortions at the terminal parts of the QRS complex (Fig. 231-5*A*).

AV nodal reentrant PSVT (Fig. 231-6) can be reproducibly initiated and terminated by appropriately timed atrial premature stimuli. The onset of the tachycardia is almost always associated with prolongation of the PR interval due to marked AV nodal conduction delay (prolonged AH interval) following the APC that is critical for the genesis of the arrhythmia. The sudden prolongation of the AH interval is consistent with the concept of dual AV nodal pathways: (1) a beta (fast) pathway, which exhibits rapid conduction and a long refractory period; and (2) an alpha (slow) pathway, which has a short refractory period but conducts slowly. During sinus rhythm, only conduction

over the fast pathway is manifest, resulting in a normal PR interval (see Fig. 231-6). Atrial extrastimuli at a critical coupling interval are blocked in the beta pathway because of its longer refractory period and are conducted slowly through the alpha pathway. If conduction down the alpha pathway is slow enough to allow the previously refractory beta pathway time to recover excitability, a single atrial echo or sustained tachycardia ensues. A critical balance between conduction velocity and refractoriness within the node is required to sustain AV nodal reentry. Retrograde atrial and antegrade ventricular activation occur simultaneously, explaining why P waves may not be apparent on the surface ECG.

Clinical Features AV nodal reentry may produce palpitations, syncope, and heart failure depending on the rate and duration of the arrhythmia and the presence and severity of any underlying heart disease. Hypotension and syncope may occur because of the sudden loss of the atrial contribution to ventricular filling; this also can lead to a marked increase in atrial pressure, acute pulmonary edema, and a reduction in ventricular filling. Simultaneous atrial and ventricular contraction produces cannon *a* waves with each heartbeat.

℞ **TREATMENT**

In patients without hypotension, vagal maneuvers, particularly carotid sinus massage, can terminate the arrhythmia in 80 percent of cases. If hypotension is present, raising the blood pressure by the cautious use of intravenous phenylephrine in 0.1-mg increments may terminate the arrhythmia alone or in combination with carotid sinus pressure. If these maneuvers are unsuccessful, verapamil (2.5 to 10 mg intravenously) or adenosine (6 to 12 mg intravenously) is the agent of choice. We prefer to use adenosine because of its extremely short half-life, lessening the consequences of any side effects. Beta blockers also may be used to slow or terminate the tachycardia but are agents of second choice. Digitalis glycosides have a slower onset of action and should *not* be used for acute therapy. When these drugs fail to terminate the tachycardia, or when the tachycardia is recurrent, atrial or ventricular pacing via a temporary pacemaker

FIGURE 231-6 Mechanism of AV nodal reentry: The atrium, AV node (AVN), and His bundle are shown schematically. The AV node is longitudinally dissociated into two pathways, with different functional properties. The alpha pathway conducts relatively slowly while the beta pathway conducts rapidly (see text). In each panel of this diagram, blue lines denote excitation in the AV node, which is manifest on the surface electrocardiogram, while black lines denote conduction, which is concealed and not apparent on the surface electrocardiogram. *A.* During sinus rhythm (NSR) the impulse from the atrium conducts down both pathways. However, only conduction over the fast (beta) pathway is manifest on the surface ECG, producing a normal PR interval of 0.16 s. *B.* An atrial premature depolarization (APD) blocks in the beta pathway.

The impulse conducts over the alpha pathway to the His bundle and ventricles, producing a PR interval of 0.24 s. Because the impulse is premature, conduction over the alpha pathway occurs more slowly than it would during sinus rhythm. *C.* A more premature atrial impulse blocks in the beta pathway, conducting with increased delay in the alpha pathway, producing a PR interval of 0.28 s. The impulse conducts retrogradely up the beta pathway producing a single atrial echo. Sustained reentry is prevented by subsequent block in the alpha pathway. *D.* A still more premature atrial impulse blocks initially in the beta pathway, conducting over the alpha pathway with increasing delay producing a PR interval of 0.36 s. Retrograde conduction occurs over the beta pathway and reentry occurs, producing a sustained tachycardia (SVT). *(After Josephson.)*

inserted pervenously may be used to terminate the arrhythmia. However, if severe ischemia and/or hypotension is caused by the tachycardia, dc cardioversion should be considered.

AV nodal reentry can usually be prevented by the use of drugs that act primarily on the antegrade slow pathway (such as digitalis, beta blockers, or calcium channel antagonists) or on the fast pathway (class IA or IC; see Table 231-2). We favor as initial therapy digitalis, beta blockers, or calcium channel antagonists because the risk-benefit ratio associated with treatment with these agents is more favorable than that of IA or IC agents. Drugs most likely to avert recurrences prevent induction of the arrhythmias by programmed stimulation. This technique utilizes temporary pacemaker catheters connected to a physiologic stimulator capable of variable rate pacing and stimulation with one or more precisely timed premature impulses. In symptomatic patients who require chronic therapy, radiofrequency catheter modification of the AV node should be considered. This technique can cure AV nodal reentry in >90 percent of cases and has been proven to be safe, although a 1 to 2 percent risk of AV block requiring a permanent pacemaker exists.

AV REENTRANT TACHYCARDIA PSVT due to AV reentry incorporates a concealed AV bypass tract as part of the tachycardia circuit. Thus the impulse passes antegradely from the atria through the AV node and His-Purkinje system to the ventricles and then retrogradely through the (concealed) bypass tract back to the atrium. Patients with this disorder manifest the same type of PSVT as do patients with the WPW syndrome (see below), but the bypass tract cannot conduct in an antegrade direction during sinus rhythm or other atrial tachyarrhythmias.

AV reentrant tachycardia can be initiated and terminated by either APCs or VPCs. Initiation of PSVT by a VPC is virtually diagnostic of AV reentry. Alternation of the QRS complexes occurs in approximately one-third of such tachycardias. Since atrial activation must follow ventricular activation during AV reentry, the P wave usually occurs after the QRS complex (see Fig. 231-5B).

Atrial activation mapping is of major value in evaluating the origin of these tachycardias. Most concealed bypass tracts are left-sided. Thus, during PSVT or during ventricular pacing, the earliest activation sequence is recorded in the left atrium, usually via a catheter in the coronary sinus (Fig. 231-7). This eccentric atrial activation is quite distinct from the normal retrograde activation sequence in which the earliest activation of the atria is in the area of the AV junction. The ability of a ventricular stimulus to conduct to the atrium at a time when the bundle of His is refractory and the termination of the tachycardia by a ventricular stimulus that does not reach the atrium are diagnostic of retrograde conduction over a concealed bypass tract.

℞ TREATMENT

This is similar to the treatment for AV nodal reentry tachycardia. Although pharmacologic agents may be used, patients who require chronic therapy should be considered candidates for radiofrequency catheter ablation of the bypass tract. This requires detailed electrophysiologic study to exclude other arrhythmias that may be responsible for patients' symptoms and to determine the location of the bypass tract(s). The efficacy of this procedure exceeds 90 percent, with minimal risks. In the remaining small number of patients failing catheter ablation, surgical ablation or pharmacologic therapy can be used.

SINUS NODE REENTRY AND OTHER ATRIAL TACHYCARDIAS Reentry in the region of the sinus node or within the atria is invariably initiated by APCs. These arrhythmias are less common than AV nodal or AV reentry and are more often associated with underlying cardiac disease. During sinus node reentry, the P-wave morphology is identical to that occurring in sinus rhythm, but the PR interval is prolonged. This is in contrast to sinus tachycardia, in which the PR interval tends to shorten. With intraatrial reentry, the P-wave configuration differs from that during sinus rhythm, and the PR interval is prolonged (see Fig. 231-5C).

℞ TREATMENT

Sinus node and atrial reentrant arrhythmias are managed like other reentrant PSVTs, except that catheter ablation is less successful because multiple foci may be present.

NONREENTRANT ATRIAL TACHYCARDIAS These may be a manifestation of digitalis intoxication or may be associated with severe pulmonary or cardiac disease, with hypokalemia, or with the administration of theophylline or adrenergic drugs. Multifocal atrial tachycardia (MAT) (Fig. 231-8) is particularly common following theophylline administration. By definition, MAT requires three or more consecutive P waves of different morphologies at rates greater than 100 beats per minute. MAT usually has an irregular ventricular rate because of varying AV conduction. There is a high incidence of atrial fibrillation (50 to 70 percent) in patients with MAT. Treatment should be directed at the underlying disorder. The digitalis-induced arrhythmias are caused by triggered activity. In such atrial tachycardias with AV block secondary to digitalis intoxication (see Fig. 231-2B), the atrial rate rarely exceeds 180 beats per minute, and typically 2:1 block is present. Atrial arrhythmias precipitated by digitalis usually can be treated by withdrawal of the drug.

Automatic atrial tachycardias not caused by digitalis are difficult to terminate, and in such cases the main goal of therapy should be to control the ventricular response, either by drugs that affect the AV node, such as digitalis, beta blockers, or calcium channel antagonists, or by ablation techniques. Catheter ablation and surgery have been employed to eradicate the arrhythmia's focus or create heart block for rate control.

FIGURE 231-7 Intracardiac recordings during supraventricular tachycardia using a left-sided AV bypass tract. Intracardiac recordings during sinus rhythm (NSR) and in supraventricular tachycardia (SVT) are shown. ECG leads I, aVF, and V₁ are displayed with electrograms from the high right atrium (HRA), coronary sinus (CS), His bundle (HBE), and right ventricle (RV). During NSR, the QRS complex and the AH and HV intervals are normal. During SVT the retrograde atrial activation sequence is abnormal. The earliest site of atrial activation is in the CS, which is followed by activation in the HBE and HRA. This activation sequence is diagnostic of a left-sided AV bypass tract conduction retrogradely from ventricle to atrium. *[From ME Josephson, in Update IV, Harrison's Principles of Internal Medicine, KJ Isselbacher et al (eds), New York, McGraw-Hill, 1983; used with permission.]*

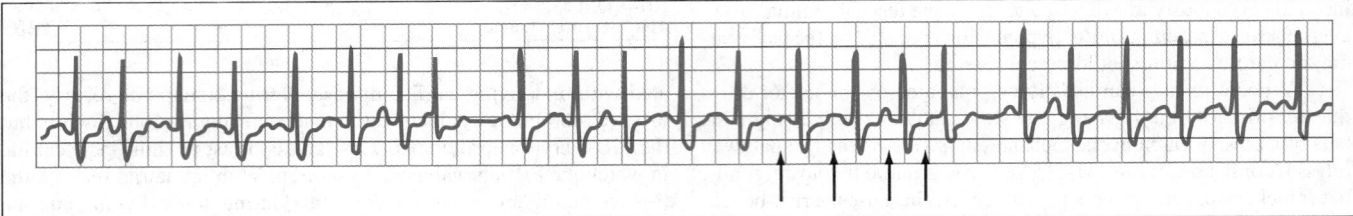

FIGURE 231-8 Multifocal atrial tachycardia. A lead I rhythm strip demonstrates a multifocal atrial tachycardia defined by ≥3 consecutive P waves of variable morphology and rate >100 beats per minute (*arrows*).

PREEXCITATION (WPW) SYNDROME The most frequently encountered type of ventricular preexcitation is that associated with AV bypass tracts. These connections are composed of strands of atrial-like muscle which may occur almost anywhere around the AV rings. The term *Wolff-Parkinson-White syndrome* is applied to patients with both preexcitation on the ECG and paroxysmal tachycardias. AV bypass tracts can be associated with certain congenital abnormalities, the most important of which is Ebstein's anomaly.

AV bypass tracts that conduct in an antegrade direction produce a typical ECG pattern of a short PR interval (<0.12 s), a slurred upstroke of the QRS complex (delta wave), and a wide QRS complex. This pattern results from a fusion of activation of the ventricles over both the bypass tract and the AV nodal His-Purkinje system (Fig. 231-9). The relative contribution of activation over each system determines the amount of preexcitation.

During PSVT in WPW, the impulse is usually conducted antegradely over the normal AV system and retrogradely through the bypass tract. The characteristics are identical to those described on p. 1265. Rarely (approximately 5 percent), tachycardias occurring in patients with WPW will exhibit a reverse pattern with antegrade conduction through the bypass tract and retrograde conduction through the normal AV system. This produces a tachycardia with a wide QRS complex in which the ventricles are totally activated by the bypass tract. Atrial flutter and AF also occur commonly in patients with WPW syndrome. Since the bypass tract does not have the same decremental conducting properties as the AV node, the ventricular responses during atrial flutter or fibrillation may be unusually rapid (see Fig. 231-2*E*) and may cause ventricular fibrillation (VF).

The goals of electrophysiologic evaluation in patients suspected of having the WPW syndrome are (1) to confirm the diagnosis, (2) to localize the bypass tract and determine how many bypass tracts are present, (3) to demonstrate the role of the bypass tract in the genesis of the arrhythmias, (4) to determine the potential for the development of possibly life-threatening rates during atrial flutter or fibrillation, and (5) to evaluate therapeutic options.

FIGURE 231-9 ECG in WPW syndrome. There is a short PR interval (0.11 s), a wide QRS complex (0.12 s), and slurring on the upstroke of the QRS produced by early ventricular activation over the bypass tract (delta wave, d in lead I). The negative delta waves in V_1 are diagnostic of a right-sided bypass tract. Note the Q wave (negative delta wave) in lead III, mimicking myocardial infarction.

℞ TREATMENT

Pharmacologic therapy is aimed at altering the electrophysiologic properties (i.e., refractoriness or conduction velocity) of one or more components of the reentrant circuit. This is most often accomplished by agents such as beta blockers or calcium channel blockers that slow conduction and increase refractoriness of the AV node or by agents such as quinidine or flecainide that slow conduction and increase refractoriness primarily in the bypass tract. Some drugs may affect multiple sites (Fig. 231-10).

Acute management of episodes of PSVT in patients with WPW syndrome is similar to that of PSVT in patients with concealed bypass tracts.

In patients with the WPW syndrome and AF, dc cardioversion should be carried out if there is a life-threatening, rapid ventricular response. Alternatively, lidocaine (3 to 5 mg/kg) or procainamide (15 mg/kg) administered intravenously over 15 to 20 min will usually slow the ventricular response. Caution should be employed when using digitalis or intravenous verapamil in patients with the WPW syndrome and AF, since these drugs can shorten the refractory period of the accessory pathway and can increase the ventricular rate, thereby placing the patient at increased risk for VF. Chronic oral therapy with verapamil is not associated with this risk. In addition to these drugs, beta-blocking agents are of no utility in controlling the ventricular response during AF when conduction proceeds over the bypass tract. Although atrial or ventricular pacing can almost always terminate PSVT in patients with the WPW syndrome, they can induce AF. As such, chronic pacemaker therapy is to be discouraged.

While surgical ablation of bypass tracts offers a permanent cure of supraventricular tachycardia (SVT) and most AFs associated with SVT, the advent of radiofrequency catheter ablation has virtually eliminated the need for surgery. Catheter ablation of bypass tracts is possible in more than 90 percent of patients and is the treatment of choice in patients with symptomatic arrhythmias. It is safer, more cost-effective, and just as successful as surgery. Nevertheless, surgical ablation may be required in the occasional patient in whom catheter ablation fails.

NONPAROXYSMAL JUNCTIONAL TACHYCARDIA

This rhythm usually results from conditions that produce enhanced automaticity or triggered activity in the AV junction and is most commonly due to digitalis intoxication, inferior wall myocardial infarction, myocarditis, endogenous or exogenous catecholamine excess, acute rheumatic fever, or aftereffects of valve surgery.

The onset of nonparoxysmal junctional tachycardia is usually gradual, with a "warm-up" period prior to stabilization of the rate, which can range from 70 to 150 beats per minute, faster rates usually being associated with digitalis intoxication. Nonparoxysmal junctional tachycardia is recognized by a QRS complex identical to that of sinus rhythm. The rate can be influenced by autonomic tone and can be increased by catecholamines, vagolytic agents, or exercise and slowed somewhat by carotid sinus pressure. When this rhythm is due to digitalis intoxication, it usually is associated with AV block and/or dissociation. Soon after cardiac surgery, retrograde conduction is more likely to be present because of the heightened sympathetic state.

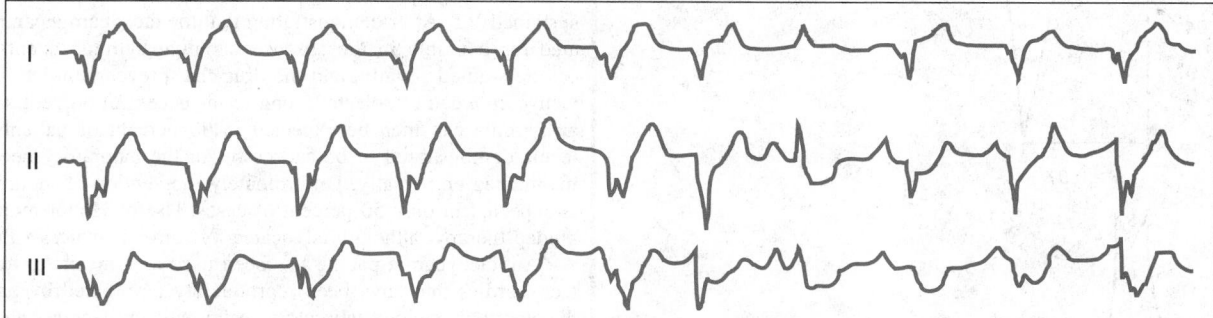

FIGURE 231-10 Site of action of antiarrhythmic agents in the WPW syndrome. The atrium, ventricle, antegrade conduction through the AV node (↓), retrograde conduction through the AV node (↑), and the bypass tract are shown. Drugs on the left affect antegrade AV nodal conduction. Type IA drugs on the upper right affect retrograde conduction over the node and antegrade conduction over the bypass tract. Drugs on the lower right affect conduction in both directions in the AV node and the bypass tract.

℞ TREATMENT

This is directed toward elimination of the underlying etiologic factors. Since digitalis is the most common cause of this rhythm, discontinuation of this drug is indicated. If the rhythm is associated with other serious manifestations of digitalis intoxication, such as ventricular or atrial irritability, active intervention with lidocaine or a beta blocker may be useful, and in some instances, use of digitalis antibodies (Fab fragments) should be considered. Cardioversion of this rhythm should not be attempted, particularly in the setting of digitalis intoxication. When AV conduction is intact, atrial pacing can capture and override the junctional focus and provide the AV synchrony necessary to maximize cardiac output. Nonparoxysmal junctional tachycardia usually is not a chronic, recurrent problem, and attention to the acute precipitating events can often resolve the tachycardia.

VENTRICULAR TACHYCARDIA *Sustained ventricular tachycardia* is defined as VT that persists for more than 30 s or requires termination because of hemodynamic collapse. VT generally accompanies some form of structural heart disease, most commonly chronic ischemic heart disease associated with a prior myocardial infarction. Sustained VT also may be associated with nonischemic cardiomyopathies, metabolic disorders, drug toxicity, or prolonged QT syndrome, and it occurs occasionally in the absence of heart disease or other predisposing factors. Nonsustained VT (three beats to 30 s) is also associated with cardiac disease but occurs in its absence more often than the sustained arrhythmia. While nonsustained VT usually does not produce symptoms, sustained VT is almost always symptomatic and is often associated with marked hemodynamic compromise and/or the development of myocardial

ischemia. A fixed anatomic substrate, not acute ischemia, is responsible for most recurrent episodes of sustained uniform VT. Acute ischemia appears to have little role in the genesis of sustained uniform VT associated with chronic infarction but may play a role in the degeneration of stable VT into VF or initiation of polymorphic VT. Most episodes of VF begin with VT.

The ECG diagnosis of VT is suggested by a wide-complex QRS tachycardia at a rate exceeding 100 beats per minute. The QRS configuration during any episode of VT may be uniform (monomorphic) (Fig. 231-3*B*), or it may vary from beat to beat (polymorphic) (Fig. 231-3*C*). *Bidirectional tachycardia* refers to VT that shows an alternation in QRS amplitude and axis. Typically this appears as a QRS with a right bundle branch block pattern with alternating superior (leftward) and inferior axes (rightward). While the rhythm is usually quite regular, slight irregularity may exist. Atrial activity may be dissociated from ventricular activity, or the atria may be depolarized retrogradely. The onset of the tachycardia is generally abrupt, but in nonparoxysmal tachycardias it can be gradual. Paroxysmal VT is usually initiated by a VPC.

It is important to distinguish supraventricular tachycardia with aberration of intraventricular conduction from VT because the clinical implications and management of these two arrhythmias are totally different. The most important clinical predictor of VT is the presence of structural heart disease. The observation of intermittent cannon *a* waves and varying first heart sounds suggests AV dissociation and is diagnostic of VT. In a majority of cases, the diagnosis can and should be made by close examination of the 12-lead ECG. Pharmacologic maneuvers, such as administration of intravenous verapamil or adenosine, can be hazardous and should be avoided. It is always useful to have a 12-lead ECG recorded during sinus rhythm for comparison with that during tachycardia. When the tracing obtained during sinus rhythm demonstrates the same morphologic features as those during the tachycardia, the diagnosis of PSVT with aberration is favored. An infarction pattern on the sinus rhythm tracing suggests the potential presence of the anatomic substrate necessary for VT. Characteristics of the 12-lead ECG during the tachycardia that suggest a ventricular origin for the arrhythmia are (1) a QRS complex >0.14 s in the absence of antiarrhythmic therapy, (2) AV dissociation (with or without fusion or captured beats) or variable retrograde conduction (Fig. 231-11), (3) a superior QRS axis in the presence of a right bundle branch block pattern, (4) concordance of the QRS pattern in all precordial leads (i.e., all positive or all negative deflections), and (5) other QRS patterns (morphology) with prolonged duration that are inconsistent with typical right or left bundle branch block patterns. (See Table 231-3 for a detailed synopsis of ECG criteria that favor the diagnosis of VT over SVT for wide complex tachycardia.) A wide, complex, bizarre tachycardia that is very irregular suggests AF with conduction over an AV bypass tract (see Fig. 231-2*E*). Similarly, a QRS complex in excess of 0.20 s is uncommon during VT in the absence of drug therapy and is more common with preexcitation. Intravenous verapamil

FIGURE 231-11 Ventricular tachycardia with AV dissociation. P waves are dissociated from the underlying wide complex rhythm and result in fusion and capture beats (complexes 7 and 8).

will stop most recalcitrant SVTs involving the AV junction, but it is rarely effective for VT. Because of this property, verapamil has been utilized to attempt to differentiate SVT with aberrant conduction from VT. However, this is extremely hazardous, since intravenous verapamil can precipitate cardiac arrest in patients with VT.

It has been possible to replicate sustained uniform VT in more than 95 percent of patients with this arrhythmia using programmed stimulation. In most patients the tachycardia is initiated with ventricular premature stimuli. A sustained monomorphic VT with a morphology identical to that of the spontaneous arrhythmia is the rule. The clinical significance of polymorphic VT initiated by programmed stimulation is not clear, since more aggressive stimulation (i.e., the use of three or four extrastimuli) can induce polymorphic VT and even VF in some normal subjects and in patients who have never had a clinical arrhythmia.

Sustained uniform VT can be terminated by programmed stimulation or rapid pacing in at least 75 percent of patients; the remainder require cardioversion. The ability to reproducibly initiate and terminate

Table 231-3

Wide Complex Tachycardia

ECG CRITERIA THAT FAVOR VENTRICULAR TACHYCARDIA

1. AV dissociation
2. QRS width: >0.14 s with RBBB configuration
   >0.16 s with LBBB configuration
3. QRS axis: left axis deviation with RBBB morphology
   extreme left axis deviation (northwest axis) with LBBB morphology
4. Concordance of QRS in precordial leads
5. Morphologic patterns of the QRS complex
   RBBB: mono- or biphasic complex in V_1
   RS (*only with left axis deviation*) or QS in V_6

LBBB: broad R wave in V_1 or V_2 ≥ 0.04 s
onset of QRS to nadir of S wave in V_1 or V_2 of ≥ 0.07 s
notched downslope of S wave in V_1 or V_2
Q wave in V_6

a sustained, uniform VT permits assessment of pharmacologic and electrical therapy of these arrhythmias.

The reproducible termination of VT by programmed stimulation permits evaluation of the effectiveness of antitachycardia pacemakers for long-term therapy of paroxysmal episodes of arrhythmia. Unfortunately, rapid pacing, the most effective form of therapy, can accelerate the tachycardia and/or produce VF. Therefore, antitachycardia pacing is a viable form of therapy only when the pacing device includes backup defibrillation capabilities.

Clinical Features   Symptoms resulting from VT depend on the ventricular rate, duration of the tachycardia, and presence and extent of underlying cardiac disease. When the tachycardia is rapid and associated with severe myocardial dysfunction and cerebrovascular disease, hypotension and syncope are common. However, the presence of hemodynamic stability does not preclude a diagnosis of VT. The rate, loss of the atrial contribution to ventricular filling, and abnormal sequence of ventricular activation are important factors producing a decreased cardiac output during VT.

The *prognosis* of VT depends on the underlying disease state. If sustained VT develops within the first 6 weeks following acute myocardial infarction, the prognosis is poor, with a 75 percent mortality rate at 1 year. Patients with nonsustained VT following myocardial infarction have a threefold greater risk of death than a comparable group of patients without this arrhythmia. However, a cause-and-effect relationship between the nonsustained tachycardia and subsequent sudden death has not been established. Patients without heart disease who have uniform VT have a good prognosis and have an extremely low risk of sudden death.

℞ **TREATMENT**

The risk-benefit ratio of treating each specific type of VT should be considered before beginning therapy. This is important because antiarrhythmic agents can produce or exacerbate the very arrhythmias that they are given to prevent. In general, patients with VT but without organic heart disease have a benign course; such patients with asymptomatic, nonsustained VT need not be treated because their prognosis will not be affected. An exception is the patient with congenital long QT syndrome. Such patients have recurrent polymorphic VT and a high mortality from sudden death if untreated. Patients with sustained VT in the absence of heart disease usually require therapy because the arrhythmia causes symptoms. These tachycardias may respond to beta blockers, verapamil, or class IA or IC or class III agents. In patients with VT and organic heart disease, if marked hemodynamic compromise is present or if there is evidence of ischemia, congestive heart failure, or central nervous system hypoperfusion, the rhythm should be promptly terminated by dc cardioversion (see below). If the patient with organic heart disease tolerates the VT well, pharmacologic therapy may be tried. Procainamide is probably the most effective agent for acute therapy. It may or may not terminate the tachycardia but almost always slows the rate. In stable patients in whom these drugs do not terminate the arrhythmia, a pacing catheter can be inserted pervenously into the right ventricular apex, and the tachycardia can be terminated by overdrive pacing.

Programmed stimulation is probably the most effective way to select the appropriate antiarrhythmic agent to prevent recurrent, sustained VT. After demonstrating that the tachycardia can be initiated reproducibly in the absence of antiarrhythmic agents, drugs can be studied serially, and the drug that prevents initiation of the tachycardia can be selected; long-term successful prevention of the arrhythmia can then be expected in 90 percent of patients. Drug levels demonstrated to be successful in the laboratory need to be maintained chronically. Unfortunately, prevention of inducible VT is expected in only 50 percent of cases. Use of Holter monitor for guided therapy, although advocated by some, is of less value.

Antitachycardia pacing has been used as a means to terminate tachycardias that have been reproducibly terminated by pacing in the electrophysiology laboratory. Automatic antitachycardia pacing devices are not used alone because pacing during VT may accelerate tachycardia, converting a stable arrhythmia into an unstable one and resulting in severe hemodynamic compromise. However, devices combining antitachycardia pacing with an implantable cardioverter/defibrillator (ICD) (see below) afford a "backup" means of terminating unstable arrhythmias.

The advent of endocardial catheter and intraoperative mapping led to the development of surgical techniques for the management of VT. Activation mapping permits localization of the site of origin of the arrhythmia. In centers in which expertise in mapping is available, operation has been successfully employed to cure tachycardias in the majority of patients in whom it has been undertaken. Even though most patients with VT and ischemic heart disease have markedly impaired left ventricular function and multivessel coronary artery disease, the operative mortality rate has ranged between 8 and 15 percent. Following operation, more than 90 percent of survivors are controlled either off (two-thirds of patients) or on (one-third) antiarrhythmic agents that were previously ineffective in controlling these rhythms.

Specific Types of VT *Torsades de pointes* ("twisting of the points") (Fig. 231-12) refers to VT characterized by polymorphic QRS complexes that change in amplitude and cycle length, giving the appearance of oscillations around the baseline. This rhythm is, by definition, associated with QT prolongation. The latter may result from electrolyte disturbances (particularly hypokalemia and hypomagnesemia), use of a variety of antiarrhythmic drugs (especially quinidine), phenothiazines and tricyclic antidepressants, liquid protein diets, intracranial events, and bradyarrhythmias, particularly third-degree AV block. It also may occur as an isolated idiopathic congenital or acquired anomaly.

The electrocardiographic hallmark is polymorphic VT preceded by marked QT prolongation, often in excess of 0.60 s. These patients often have multiple episodes of nonsustained polymorphic VT associated with recurrent syncope, but they also may develop VF and sudden cardiac death.

Therapy should be directed at removing the precipitating factors, i.e., correcting metabolic abnormalities and removing drugs that have induced the prolonged QT interval. In the setting of drug-induced torsades de pointes, atrial or ventricular overdrive pacing and the administration of magnesium also have been useful in terminating and preventing the arrhythmia. For patients with the congenital prolonged QT interval syndrome, beta-adrenergic blocking agents have been the mainstay of therapy; agents that shorten the QT interval also may be useful (e.g., phenytoin). Cervicothoracic sympathectomy has been proposed as a form of therapy for congenital prolonged QT syndrome, but it is not often effective as the sole therapy. Pacing in combination with beta blockers and sympathectomy is often required.

Polymorphic tachycardias associated with normal QT intervals in patients with ischemic heart disease that are initiated by "R-on-T" VPCs are probably caused by reentry, and their treatment is totally different. This is not true torsades de pointes. In such cases, class I or III agents may be the most effective form of therapy and should be administered in full antiarrhythmic doses. However, these arrhythmias also may result from acute, severe ischemia and will only respond to abolition of the ischemia, usually by revascularization.

Accelerated idioventricular rhythm This arrhythmia, also termed *slow VT*, with a rate that ranges from 60 to 120 beats per minute,

usually occurs in acute myocardial infarction, often during reperfusion. It also may be seen following cardiac operations; in patients with cardiomyopathy, rheumatic fever, or digitalis intoxication; as well as in patients with no evidence of heart disease. The rhythm is usually transient and rarely causes significant hemodynamic compromise or symptoms.

Treatment is rarely necessary and should usually be considered only if symptoms arise due to impaired hemodynamics, most commonly due to AV dissociation. In most cases, atropine can accelerate the sinus rate to overdrive the ventricular rhythm.

VENTRICULAR FLUTTER AND VENTRICULAR FIBRILLATION (VF) (See Fig. 231-13; see also Chap. 39)   These arrhythmias occur most often in patients with ischemic heart disease. They also occur following administration of antiarrhythmic drugs, particularly those which induce prolonged QT intervals and torsades de pointes (see above), in patients with severe hypoxia or ischemia, and in those with WPW who develop AF with an extremely rapid ventricular response (see p. 1270). Electrical accidents frequently cause cardiac arrest due to the development of VF. The onset of these arrhythmias is rapidly followed by loss of consciousness and, if untreated, death. Episodes of cardiac arrest recorded during Holter monitoring reveal that approximately three-fourths of the sudden deaths are due to VT or VF.

In patients with nonischemic VF, the onset usually begins with a short run of rapid VT, which is initiated by a relatively late coupled VPC. In patients with acute myocardial infarction or ischemia, however, VF is usually precipitated by a single early ventricular complex beat falling on the T wave (the vulnerable period), which produces a rapid VT that degenerates into VF (see Fig. 231-13).

The clinical setting in which VF occurs is important. Most patients who have primary VF within the first 48 h of the onset of acute infarction have a good long-term prognosis, with a very low rate of recurrence or sudden cardiac death. Their short-term mortality may, however, be slightly increased. In contrast, patients who experience VF unassociated with the development of acute myocardial infarction have a recurrence rate of 20 to 30 percent in the year following the event (see Chap. 39).

Ventricular flutter usually appears as a sine wave with a rate between 150 and 300 beats per minute. These oscillations make it impossible to assign a specific morphology to the arrhythmia and in some cases to distinguish it from rapid VT. VF is recognized by grossly irregular undulations of varying amplitudes, contours, and rates (see Fig. 231-13). Electrophysiologic studies have demonstrated that regardless of the apparent gross irregularity on the surface ECG, VF usually starts out with a rapid repetitive sequence of VT that ultimately breaks down into multiple wavelets of reentry.

Electrophysiologic studies have been useful in patients who have been resuscitated from cardiac arrest. Programmed stimulation has demonstrated that in approximately 70 percent of such patients one can reproducibly initiate a sustained VT. Treatment is discussed in Chap. 39.

QT–72

FIGURE 231-12   Torsades de pointes. Polymorphic VT is associated with a pause and QT at 0.72 s.

℞ TREATMENT

Pharmacologic Antiarrhythmic Therapy Prior to initiation of pharmacologic antiarrhythmic therapy, potential aggravating factors such as transient metabolic abnormalities, congestive heart failure, or acute ischemia must be corrected; in some cases this may suffice to control arrhythmias. In addition, the potential role of drugs as a cause or exacerbating factor in the development of the arrhythmia must be considered. It must be recognized that we do not have a good understanding of the effects of antiarrhythmic agents on the spontaneous onset of tachyarrhythmias. In some cases, they may facilitate the onset.

Antiarrhythmic drugs are used in three principal situations: (1) to terminate an acute arrhythmia, (2) to prevent recurrence of an arrhythmia, and (3) to prevent a life-threatening arrhythmia for which the patient is perceived to be at risk but which has never occurred. (The acute pharmacologic therapy of tachyarrhythmias is summarized in Table 231-4.)

Most currently available antiarrhythmic agents have a relatively low toxic/therapeutic ratio; all can exert proarrhythmic effects, and therefore they may exacerbate underlying arrhythmias. Serum levels can be determined for most currently available antiarrhythmic agents. Standards for therapeutic and toxic levels can serve only as a rough guide for selecting the appropriate dose in any individual patient. In the final analysis, the therapeutic level in a given patient is the concentration that achieves the desired antiarrhythmic effect, and the toxic level for each patient is the concentration at which undesirable side effects occur. Since many adverse effects are directly related to drug concentrations, the lowest serum level that achieves an effective antiarrhythmic response should be chosen.

In order to determine the therapeutic level for a patient, one must have a standard to judge drug efficacy. For a patient with an incessant arrhythmia, antiarrhythmic drugs may be administered empirically until the arrhythmia is suppressed. If a reproducible precipitating factor such as exercise can be identified, serial drug testing during such a provocative maneuver may be performed. Unfortunately, most arrhythmias are sporadic and occur unpredictably without identifiable precipitating factors. In these cases, if one waits to observe spontaneous recurrences on each antiarrhythmic drug, assessment of drug efficacy may require months. This type of assessment of efficacy may be adequate for arrhythmias that are not life-threatening. However, this mode of assessment is inadequate for arrhythmias that compromise hemodynamic stability, result in syncope, or cause cardiac arrest. In such cases, two methods for determination of arrhythmic drug efficacy have been utilized. The first, which consists of continuous ECG monitoring in the control state and then in the presence of antiarrhythmic drugs, has been used in order to determine the effect that each drug has on spontaneous atrial or ventricular ectopy. This method presupposes that the mechanism responsible for sustained arrhythmias is the same as that causing isolated premature depolarizations (which may or may not be true) and that therefore eradication of isolated ectopy will correlate with prevention of sustained arrhythmias. This method has a number of limitations. First, patients frequently show marked degrees of spontaneous variation in frequency of ectopy, which may mimic antiarrhythmic drug effects. Second, 25 to 30 percent of patients

with sustained ventricular arrhythmias such as VT or VF demonstrate only rare spontaneous ectopy. Finally, many patients demonstrate a dissociation between the effects of antiarrhythmic agents on spontaneous ectopy and the effects of the same agent on sustained arrhythmias.

An alternative method to assess drug efficacy is programmed stimulation. Numerous studies have demonstrated that most clinically occurring supraventricular and ventricular tachyarrhythmias may be reproducibly initiated and terminated safely using this technique. Studies are performed initially in a baseline state in the absence of antiarrhythmic drugs (Fig. 231-14). If the patient's clinical arrhythmia can be reproducibly initiated, then the ability of individual antiarrhythmic drugs to prevent reinduction of the arrhythmia can be assessed either after the drug is administered intravenously or after several days of oral loading in order to achieve a steady-state serum concentration. Use of this method assumes that (1) the induced and spontaneous arrhythmias are identical, and (2) prevention of induction of arrhythmias will correlate with prevention of recurrent spontaneous tachycardias on the same drug regimen. This technique has been validated in patients with a variety of reentrant PSVTs, VT, and VF. The technique is safe when carefully performed, the potential complications being those of any intravascular catheterization. Appropriate interpretation of the results of programmed stimulation is critically dependent on correlating the patient's spontaneous arrhythmias with those induced in the laboratory, with regard to rate and morphology, in order to be certain that the arrhythmia induced in the laboratory represents the same arrhythmia that occurred spontaneously and caused symptoms.

CLASSIFICATION OF ANTIARRHYTHMIC DRUGS A number of classifications of antiarrhythmic drugs have been proposed; the most frequently used is a modification of one proposed by Vaughan-Williams (see Table 231-1). This classification is based in part on the ability of antiarrhythmic drugs to modify the cardiac cellular (1) excitatory currents (Na^+ or Ca^{2+}), (2) action potential duration, and (3) automaticity (phase 4 depolarization). These effects of the drugs on isolated cardiac cells are thought to account for some of the antiarrhythmic properties of the drugs. Thus depression of excitatory currents by class I and class IV antiarrhythmics results in slowing of conduction velocity and may interrupt arrhythmias by blocking conduction in areas of marginal excitability, where conduction velocity is already slow. Class III antiarrhythmics allegedly exert their

Table 231-4

Acute Pharmacologic Therapy of Tachyarrhythmias

Arrhythmia	Drug
Atrial tachyarrhythmias (including AF and atrial flutter) in patients without preexcitation	Initially verapamil, diltiazem, or beta-blocking agent to control ventricular response, then procainamide or quinidine
Atrial tachyarrhythmias (including AF and atrial flutter) in patients with preexcitation	Procainamide
SVT with regular rate and narrow QRS complex	Adenosine
Sustained monomorphic VT	Verapamil Procainamide Lidocaine

NOTE: AF, atrial fibrillation; SVT, supraventricular tachycardia; VT, ventricular tachycardia.

FIGURE 231-13 Ventricular fibrillation. In a patient with coronary disease ventricular fibrillation is initiated by a VPC that produces a rapid polymorphic ventricular tachycardia which rapidly degenerates to ventricular fibrillation (note the undulating baseline with indistinguishable systole and diastole).

FIGURE 231-14 Selections of an effective antiarrhythmic drug for ventricular tachycardia by programmed stimulation. From top to bottom, the effects of programmed stimulation during the control state and following administration of several antiarrhythmic agents. During the control state two ventricular extrastimuli initiate the ventricular tachycardia at a rate of 230 per minute. Lidocaine, phenytoin, and disopyramide at the plasma levels shown failed to prevent induction of the tachycardia. Both procainamide and quinidine at the plasma levels shown prevented initiation of sustained tachycardia. Chronic oral quinidine therapy effectively prevented recurrences of the arrhythmia. *(From JA Kastor et al, N Engl J Med 304:1004, 1981; reprinted by permission.)*

action by increasing refractoriness through prolongation of the action potential duration. However, this classification has a number of limitations. The electrophysiologic effects of these drugs in vivo may differ from their effects on isolated cells. Also, the effects of heart rate and fiber geometry are not considered. Not all drugs (e.g., adenosine) fit into the classifications. Finally, some drugs (e.g., amiodarone) exhibit properties consistent with multiple classes. The uses and actions of currently available antiarrhythmic drugs are summarized in Tables 231-2 and 231-5.

Electrical Therapy of Tachyarrhythmias PACEMAKERS Cardiac pacing can be used to terminate and in selected cases prevent recurrent supraventricular and ventricular arrhythmias. Because many tachyarrhythmias appear to be due to a reentrant mechanism with the impulse traveling in a circuit, a properly timed paced impulse can penetrate and prematurely depolarize part of the circuit, rendering it refractory to the next circulating wavefront and thereby interrupting

the circus movement. Pacing therapy for arrhythmias is generally reserved for patients whose arrhythmias are refractory to drug therapy and who remain hemodynamically stable during the tachycardia. All forms of pacing therapy require repeated demonstration of their effectiveness and reliability in terminating the arrhythmias during electrophysiologic testing prior to implantation of the pacing device.

The type of pacing device and modality selected for arrhythmia termination depends on (1) the rate of the tachycardia (rates >160 beats per minute are rarely terminated by a single premature stimulus), (2) the type of arrhythmia (atrial flutter and VT are rarely terminated by single extrastimuli), and (3) concomitant drug therapy.

Because many tachycardias cannot be terminated by single premature stimuli, pacemakers have been developed that allow for multiple extrastimuli (burst pacing) to be introduced. In the current era, antitachycardia pacing is almost exclusively for ventricular arrhythmias because of the success of radiofrequency ablative therapy for supraventricular arrhythmias.

Cardiac pacing also has been used to prevent ventricular tachyarrhythmias. Polymorphic VT associated with a long QT interval and bradycardia (torsades de pointes, p. 1273) is most likely to respond. Pacing the atrium and/or ventricle at rates between 90 and 120 beats per minute appears to increase the homogeneity of electrical recovery and markedly reduces the propensity for a recurrence of arrhythmias.

Pacemakers may be self-contained or energized by an external radiofrequency source. The self-contained pacemaker may function automatically [i.e., it incorporates an arrhythmia recognition program (circuit)], or it may be activated by an external magnet. The major advantage of a fully automatic system is that there is no need for the patient to recognize the arrhythmia in order for termination to occur. The advantages of the externally activated system include (1) the decreased risk of unnecessary treatment because of faulty sensing, and (2) the opportunity to initiate monitoring at the time of attempted termination of arrhythmia. This type of monitoring is frequently helpful if pacing techniques are employed to terminate VT, given the risk of acceleration of the arrhythmia by pacing.

The limitations of pacing therapy are primarily related to (1) the changes in the characteristics of the arrhythmia over time such that programmed pacing parameters no longer terminate the tachycardia, (2) the risk of acceleration of the tachycardia with the development of AF when stimulating the atrium and the development of rapid VT and VF when stimulating the ventricles, and (3) inappropriate recognition of supraventricular tachyarrhythmias as ventricular tachycardias, leading to delivery of therapy unnecessarily, which can initiate VT or VF. Future pacing generators that can perform cardioversion and defibrillation will increase the applicability of pacing therapy for the treatment of arrhythmias (see below).

CARDIOVERSION AND DEFIBRILLATION Electrical cardioversion and defibrillation remain the most reliable methods for terminating arrhythmias. By depolarizing all or at least a large portion of excitable myocardium in a near homogeneous fashion, the electrical shock can interrupt reentrant arrhythmias. External cardioversion is routinely performed by placing two paddles 12 cm in diameter in firm contact with the chest wall, with one paddle usually located to the right of the sternum at the level of the second rib and the other in the left anterior axillary line in the fifth intercostal space. If the patient is conscious, a short-acting barbiturate to act as an anesthetic or an amnesic drug such as diazepam or medazolam should be administered to prevent patient discomfort. A person skilled in maintaining an airway should be present.

Energy is delivered synchronously with the QRS complex for all arrhythmias except ventricular flutter and VF, since asynchronous shocks can produce VF. The amount of energy used will vary with the type of tachycardia being treated. With the exception of AF,

SVTs can frequently be terminated with energy levels in the range of 25 to 50 W·s, while AF usually requires ≥100 W·s for termination. For terminating VT, energy levels ≥100 W·s should probably be employed. While energies as low as 25 W·s may be used successfully, they also have a higher incidence of producing VF or AF. At least 200 W·s of energy should be used for initial attempts at terminating VF. If the initial shock fails, all repeated attempts at defibrillation should be with the maximum energy that the defibrillator is capable of delivering (320 to 400 W·s).

Indications for cardioversion depend on the clinical setting and the patient's general condition. Any tachycardia (except sinus tachycardia) that produces hypotension, myocardial ischemia, or heart failure warrants consideration of prompt termination using external cardioversion. Arrhythmias that fail to terminate with pharmacologic therapy also may be terminated by electrical cardioversion. Transient bradycardias and supraventricular and ventricular irritability following cardioversion are common and usually do not warrant antiarrhythmic intervention.

IMPLANTED CARDIOVERSION/DEFIBRILLATION ICD devices have been developed that will promptly recognize and terminate life-threatening ventricular arrhythmias. These devices can deliver <1 to 40 W·s, the amount of which can be programmed. Current devices have antitachycardia pacing capabilities such that VT can be sensed and terminated without resorting to a painful shock. In such devices, high-energy shocks are reserved for hypotensive VT, acceleration of VT, or failure to terminate VT after a programmed

FIGURE 231-15 Normally functioning implantable defibrillators. A continuous Holter monitoring tracing is shown. On the top strip, a rapid polymorphic tachycardia is initiated which beats more uniformly. The automatic implantable cardioverter-defibrillator (AICD) senses the rhythm and delivers a shock which restores sinus rhythm.

Table 231-5

Dose, Serum Half-Life ($t_{1/2}$) Following Oral Administration, and Route of Metabolism of Drugs Used in Treatment of Arrhythmias

Drug	Mode of Administration	$t_{1/2}$ (Oral), h	Route of Metabolism
Digoxin	IV, 0.25–1.5 mg		Renal
	Oral, 0.75–1.5 mg loading dose over 12–24 h	36	
	Maintenance, 0.23–0.50 mg/d		
Propranolol	IV, 0.5–1 mg/min to total dose of 0.15–0.2 mg/kg		Hepatic
	Oral, 10–200 mg q 6 h	3–6	
Esmolol	IV, loading dose of 500 μg/kg/min for 1 min followed by maintenance infusion of 50 μg/kg/min for 4 min; if effect is inadequate, repeat load followed by maintenance of 100 μg/kg/min, up to a maximum maintenance of 200 μg/kg/min. $t_{1/2}$ I.V. = 9 min	NA	
Metoprolol	IV, load with 5–10 mg q 5 min for 3 doses, then 3 mg q 6 h	3–4	
	Oral, 25–100 mg bid		
Verapamil	IV, 2.5–10 mg over 1–2 min to total of 0.15 mg/kg		Hepatic
	Oral, 80–120 mg q 6–8 h	3–8	
Diltiazem	IV, load with 0.25 mg/kg over 2 min; if response is inadequate, repeat after 15 min with 0.35 mg over 2 min	NA	
	Maintenance dose is 10–15 mg/h		
	Oral, 180–360 mg qd or in divided dosages		
Quinidine	IV, 20 mg/min to total of 10–15 mg/kg		Hepatic: 80%
	Oral, 200–400 mg q 6 h	5–9	Renal: 20%
Procainamide	IV, 40–50 mg/min to total of 10–20 mg/kg		Hepatic: 50%
	Oral, 500–1000 mg q 4 h	3–5	Renal: 50%
Disopyramide	Oral, 100–300 mg q 6–8 h	8–9	Renal: 50%
			Hepatic: 50%
Lidocaine	IV, 20–50 mg/min to total of 5-mg/kg loading dose followed by 1–4 mg/kg	1–2	Hepatic: 100%
Phenytoin	IV, 20 mg/min total dose to 1000 mg		Hepatic
	Oral, 1000-mg loading over 24 h	18–36	
	Maintenance, 100–400 mg/d		
Tocainide	Oral, 400–600 mg q 8–12 h	10–17	Hepatic-renal
Bretylium	IV, 1–2 (mg/kg)/min to total of 5–10 mg/kg	8–14	Renal
	Maintenance, 0.5–2 mg/min		
Amiodarone	IV, 5–10 mg/kg		Unknown
	Oral, load 800–1400 mg/d for 1–2 weeks	Unknown	
	Maintenance, 100–600 mg/d		
Moricizine	Oral, 200–400 mg q 8 h	2–6	Hepatic
Propafenone	Oral, 450–900 mg q 8 h	5–8	Hepatic
Sotalol	Oral, 80–160 mg q 12 h for atrial fibrillation; up to 320 mg q 12 h for ventricular arrhythmias. Dose adjusted based on creatinine clearance	10–20	Renal: 90%
Adenosine	IV bolus, 6–12 mg	<10 s	
Mexiletine	Oral, 100–300 mg q 6–8 h	9–12	Hepatic: 100%
Flecainide	Oral, begin at 50–100 mg bid; increase by no more than 50 mg not more often than every 4 days to a maximum of 400 mg daily	7–23	Hepatic: 75%
			Renal: 25%

FIGURE 231-16 Radiofrequency ablation in Wolff-Parkinson-White syndrome. Leads I, II, III, V₁, V₂, and V₆ are shown. Preexcitation using a left lateral bypass tract is present in the final four complexes. Following the third complex, radiofrequency energy is applied. By the second beat, preexcitation is lost as the bypass tract is destroyed.

FIGURE 231-17 Radiofrequency ablation of idiopathic ventricular tachycardia in a patient with prior infarction. Leads I, II, and III are shown. Ventricular tachycardia with a right bundle branch block and left axis deviation is shown in a patient with a prior inferior wall infarction. Radiofrequency applied to the site of origin terminates the tachycardia.

duration (see Fig. 231-15). ICDs now can be implanted transvenously, and some are small enough to be implanted in a manner similar to pacemakers. Clinical trials testing the function of these devices in patients with drug-refractory ventricular arrhythmias have demonstrated survival from sudden death at 1 year ranging between 92 and 100 percent. Currently, ICDs should be considered for patients with VT that is not hemodynamically tolerated. They are also indicated for patients with cardiac arrest whose arrhythmias are refractory to drug therapy or in whom there are no good endpoints to assess drug efficacy.

The most frequent problem with the device has been its inappropriate discharge in the absence of sustained ventricular arrhythmias. Additional potential problems include an increase in defibrillation threshold and decrease in tachycardia rates below the rate cut-off of the device in response to many antiarrhythmic drugs. Permanently implanted ventricular pacemakers may interfere with the device's ability to sense VF. This can be avoided by using committed bipolar pacing systems. Diagnostic features of newer, all-in-one devices are able to identify the probable cause of an ICD discharge (e.g., AF, SVT, fractured lead) and to adjust pharmacologic therapy or reprogram the device to avoid such inappropriate shocks. These newer devices have the capability to take a "second look" prior to shock delivery and thus may abort delivery for self-terminating arrhythmias. In addition, the range of candidates suitable for implantation will be expanded because the newer devices have the capability of shock therapy for patients whose arrhythmias do not cause loss of consciousness.

ABLATIVE THERAPY FOR ARRHYTHMIAS Catheter-based mapping techniques have provided a nonoperative approach to the identification and cure of a variety of arrhythmias. In fact, catheter ablation techniques are now the procedures of choice for symptomatic patients with (1) concealed or manifest (WPW) bypass tracts, (2) AV nodal reentrant SVT, (3) typical atrial flutter, and (4) poorly controlled ventricular responses to atrial arrhythmias, most commonly AF. Successful ablation of bypass tracts and modifications of the AV node by radiofrequency energy are extremely successful and cost-effective and are the procedure of choice for patients with recurrent episodes (Fig. 231-16). The creation of AV block with implantation of a pacemaker is the method of choice in managing patients with AF and poorly controlled ventricular response. Idiopathic VTs (Fig. 231-17) that are associated with coronary artery disease are also amenable to ablation but the result is somewhat less successful.

Surgical therapy is now relegated to cases of sustained VT associated with coronary artery disease when operative intervention is needed for coronary bypass surgery and/or aneurysmectomy or VT associated with specific structural abnormalities (e.g., idiopathic left ventricle aneurysm, s/p surgery for tetralogy of Fallot). It also may be undertaken for the unusual instances of failed catheter ablation for SVTs associated with bypass tracts.

BIBLIOGRAPHY

ALMENDRAL J et al: The importance of antitachycardia pacing for patients presenting with ventricular tachycardia. Pacing Clin Electrophysiol 16:535, 1993

BAROLD SS, ZIPES DP: Cardiac pacemakers and antiarrhythmic devices, in *Heart Disease: A Textbook of Cardiovascular Medicine,* 5th ed, E Braunwald (ed). Philadelphia, Saunders, 1997, pp 705–741

BRUGADA J et al: The complexity of mechanisms in ventricular tachycardia. Pacing Clin Electrophysiol 16:680, 1993

CALKINS H et al: Diagnosis and cure of the Wolff-Parkinson-White syndrome or paroxysmal supraventricular tachycardias during a single electrophysiologic test. N Engl J Med 324:1612, 1991

COX JL: Surgical management of cardiac arrhythmias, in *Cardiac Pacing and Electrophysiology,* N El-Sherif, P Samet (eds). Philadelphia, Saunders, 1991, p 436

DREIFUS LS: Guidelines for implantation of cardiac pacemakers and antiarrhythmic devices: A report of the American College of Cardiology/American Heart Association Task Force on Assessment of Diagnostic and Therapeutic Cardiovascular Procedures (Committee on Pacemaker Implantation). J Am Coll Cardiol 18:1, 1991

ECHT DS et al: Mortality and morbidity in patients receiving encainide, flecainide, or placebo: The Cardiac Arrhythmia Suppression Trial (CAST). N Engl J Med 324:781, 1991

GUARDIAN MULTICENTER INVESTIGATORS GROUP: Long term multicenter experience with a second-generation implantable pacemaker-defibrillator in patients with malignant ventricular tachyarrhythmias. J Am Coll Cardiol 19:490, 1992

GUIRAUDON GM et al: Surgery for atrial flutter, atrial fibrillation, and atrial tachycardia, in *Cardiac Electrophysiology: From Cell to Bedside*, DP Zipes, J Jalife (eds). Philadelphia, Saunders, 1990, p 915

JACKMAN WM et al: Catheter ablation of accessory atrioventricular pathways (Wolff-Parkinson-White syndrome) by radiofrequency current. N Engl J Med 324:1605, 1991

JOSEPHSON ME: *Clinical Cardiac Electrophysiology*, 2d ed. Philadelphia, Lea & Febiger, 1993

KADISH A, GOLDBERGER J: Ablative therapy for atrioventricular nodal reentry arrhythmias. Prog Cardiovasc Dis 37:273, 1995

KIM YH et al: Nonpharmacologic therapies in patients with ventricular tachyarrhythmias. Catheter ablation and ventricular tachycardia surgery. Cardiol Clin 11:85, 1993

KUTALEK SP, DREIFUS LS: Implantable cardioverter-defibrillators. Adv Intern Med 38:421, 1993

PLUMB VJ: Catheter ablation of the accessory pathways of Wolff-Parkinson-White syndrome and its variants. Prog Cardiovasc Dis 37:295, 1995

PRITCHETT ELC: Management of atrial fibrillation. N Engl J Med 326:1264, 1991

RODEN DM: Treatment of cardiovascular diseases: Arrhythmias, in *Clinical Pharmacology: Basic Principles in Therapeutics*, KL Melmon et al (eds). New York, McGraw-Hill, 1992, pp 151–185

WYSE DG: Pharmacologic therapy in patients with ventricular tachyarrhythmias. Cardiol Clin 11:65, 1993

ZIPES DP: Specific arrhythmias: Diagnosis and treatment, in *Heart Disease: A Textbook of Cardiovascular Medicine*, 5th ed, E Braunwald (ed). Philadelphia, Saunders, 1997, p 640–704

———: Genesis of cardiac arrhythmias: Electrophysiological considerations, in *Heart Disease: A Textbook of Cardiovascular Medicine*, 5th ed, E Braunwald (ed). Philadelphia, Saunders, 1997, p 548–592

———: Management of cardiac arrhythmias: Pharmacological, electrical, and surgical techniques, in *Heart Disease: A Textbook of Cardiovascular Medicine*, 5th ed, E Braunwald (ed). Philadelphia, Saunders, 1997, p 593–639

SECTION 3

DISORDERS OF THE HEART

232   *Eugene Braunwald*

NORMAL AND ABNORMAL MYOCARDIAL FUNCTION

CELLULAR BASIS OF CARDIAC CONTRACTION

The *myocardium* is composed of individual striated muscle cells (fibers), normally 10 to 15 μm in diameter and 30 to 60 μm in length (Fig. 232-1*A*). Each fiber contains multiple cross-banded strands (myofibrils) that run the length of the fiber and are, in turn, composed of serially repeating structures, the sarcomeres. The cytoplasm between the myofibrils contains other cell constituents (Fig. 232-1*B*), such as the single centrally located nucleus, numerous mitochondria, and intracellular membrane system, the sarcoplasmic reticulum.

The *sarcomere*, the structural and functional unit of contraction, is delimited by two adjacent dark lines, the Z lines (Fig. 232-1*C*). The distance between Z lines varies with the degree of contraction or stretch of the muscle and ranges between 1.6 and 2.2 μm. Within the confines of the sarcomere are alternating light and dark bands, giving the myocardial fibers their striated appearance under the light microscope. At the center of the sarcomere is a dark band of constant length (1.5 μm), the A band, which is flanked by two lighter bands, the I bands, which are of variable length. The sarcomere of heart muscle, like that of skeletal muscle, is made up of two sets of interdigitating myofilaments (Fig. 232-1*D*). Thicker filaments, composed principally of the protein myosin, traverse and are limited to the A band. They are about 10 nm (100 Å) in diameter, with tapered ends, and measure 1.5 to 1.6 μm in length. Thinner filaments, composed primarily of actin, course from the Z line through the I band into the A band. They are approximately 5 nm (50 Å) in diameter and 1.0 μm in length. Thus there is overlapping of thick and thin filaments only within the A band, while the I band contains only thin filaments (Fig. 232-1*C*). On electron-microscopic examination, bridges may be seen to extend between the thick and thin filaments within the A band.

THE CONTRACTILE PROCESS   The sliding model for muscle rests on the fundamental observation that the thick and thin filaments are constant in overall length during both contraction and relaxation. With activation, repeated interactions take place at the bridges between the actin and myosin filaments, and the actin filaments are propelled further into the A band. In the process, the A band remains constant in length, whereas the I band shortens and the Z lines move toward one another.

The *myosin* molecule is a complex, asymmetric fibrous protein with a molecular weight of about 500,000; it has a rodlike portion that is about 150 nm (1500 Å) in length with a globular portion at its end. This globular portion of the myosin is the site of adenosine triphosphatase (ATPase) activity and also forms the bridges between the myosin and actin. In forming the thick myofilament, which is composed of 300 longitudinally stacked myosin molecules, the rodlike segments of the myosin molecules are laid down in an orderly, polarized manner, leaving the globular portions projecting outward so that they can interact with actin to generate force and shortening (Fig. 232-2). *Actin* has a molecular weight of 47,000. The thin filament is composed of a double helix of two chains of actin molecules wound about each other on a larger molecule, tropomyosin, which serves as a "backbone" to the thin filament. A group of these regulatory proteins, troponins C, I, and T, are spaced at regular intervals on this filament (Fig. 232-3). In contrast to myosin, actin has no intrinsic enzymatic activity, but it has the ability to combine reversibly with myosin in the presence of ATP and Mg^{2+}, which activates the myosin ATPase. In relaxed muscle this interaction is inhibited by tropomyosin. *Titin* is a large, flexible, myofibrillar protein that connects myosin to the Z line. Its stretching is believed to contribute to the elasticity of the heart.

During activation of the myocyte, Ca^{2+} becomes attached to troponin C, which results in a conformational change in the regulatory protein tropomyosin, which in turn exposes the actin cross-bridge interaction sites. Repetitive interaction between myosin heads and actin filaments is termed *cross-bridge cycling*, which results in sliding of the actin along the myosin filaments, ultimately causing muscle shortening and/or the development of tension. The splitting of ATP then dissociates the myosin cross-bridge from the actin. In the presence of ATP (Fig. 232-2), linkages between actin and myosin filaments are made and broken cyclically as long as sufficient Ca^{2+} is present; these linkages are broken when Ca^{2+} concentration falls below a critical level, and the troponin-tropomyosin complex once more prevents interactions between the myosin cross-bridges and the actin filaments. Ionic calcium is a principal mediator of the inotropic state of the heart; most positive inotropic drugs, including the digitalis glycosides, beta-adrenergic agonists, and phosphodiesterase inhibitors, act by increasing the concentrations of Ca^{2+} in the vicinity of the myofilaments. Cyclic AMP enhances the phosphorylation of troponin I, a protein that accelerates cardiac relaxation.

The *sarcoplasmic reticulum* (Fig. 232-1B) is a complex network of anastomosing intracellular channels that invests the myofibrils. It is less profuse in cardiac than in skeletal muscle. Its longitudinally disposed membrane-lined tubules are closely applied to the surfaces of individual sarcomeres but have no direct continuity with the outside of the cell. However, closely related to the sarcoplasmic reticulum, both structurally and functionally, are the transverse tubules or T system, formed by tubelike invaginations of the sarcolemma that extend into the myocardial fiber along the Z lines, i.e., the ends of the sarcomeres.

CARDIAC ACTIVATION
At rest, the cardiac cell is polarized; i.e., the interior has a negative charge relative to the outside of the cell, with a transmembrane potential of -80 to -100 mV (Chap. 230). The sarcolemma, which in the resting state is largely impermeable to Na^+, has a Na^+- and K^+- stimulating pump requiring ATP that extrudes Na^+ from the cell; the pump plays a critical role in establishing this resting potential. Thus, on the inside of the cell $[K^+]$ is relatively high and $[Na^+]$ is far lower, while in the extracellular milieu $[Na^+]$ is high and $[K^+]$ is low. At the same time, in the resting state, the extracellular $[Ca^{2+}]$ greatly exceeds the free intracellular $[Ca^{2+}]$.

During the plateau of the action potential (phase 2) there is a slow inward current that reflects primarily a movement of Ca^{2+} into the cell (Fig. 232-4), although the absolute quantity of Ca^{2+} that crosses the surface membrane is relatively small and itself appears to be incapable of bringing about full activation of the contractile apparatus. The depolarizing current not only extends across the surface of the cell but penetrates deeply into the cell by way of the ramifying T system; this current triggers the release of much larger quantities of Ca^{2+} from the sarcoplasmic reticulum, a process termed *regenerative release* of Ca^{2+}. This rise in intracellular Ca^{2+} is the key step in initiating myocyte contraction.

The Ca^{2+} released from the sarcoplasmic reticulum then diffuses toward the sarcomere and, as already described, combines with troponin C. By repressing this inhibitor of contraction, Ca^{2+} activates the myofilaments to produce contraction. During repolarization the

sarcoplasmic reticulum reaccumulates Ca^{2+} against a concentration gradient. This is an energy-requiring process that lowers the concentration of Ca^{2+} in the vicinity of the myofibrils to a level that inhibits the actin-myosin interaction responsible for contraction and in this manner leads to relaxation. Thus, the cell membrane, transverse tubules, and sarcoplasmic reticulum, with their ability to transmit an action potential, to release, and then to reaccumulate Ca^{2+}, appear to play a fundamental role in the rhythmic contraction and relaxation of heart muscle.

The ATP formed from substrate oxidation is the principal source of energy for almost all of the mechanical work of contraction performed by the myocardial cell. The high-energy phosphate stores in ATP are in equilibrium with those in the form of creatine phosphate.

FIGURE 232-1 Microscopic structure of heart muscle. *A.* Myocardium as seen under the light microscope. Branching of fibers is evident. Each fiber, or cell, contains a centrally located nucleus. *B.* Myocardial cell, reconstructed from electron micrographs. Each cell is composed of multiple parallel fibrils. Each fibril is composed of serially connected sarcomeres (N, nucleus). *C.* Sarcomere from a myofibril, with diagrammatic representation of myofilaments. Thick filaments (1.5 μm long, composed of myosin) form the A band, and thin filaments (1 μm long, composed primarily of actin) extend from the Z line through the I band into the A band. The overlapping of thick and thin filaments is seen only in the A band. *D.* Cross sections of the sarcomere indicate the specific lattice arrangements of the myofilaments. In the center of the sarcomere only the thick, or myosin, filaments arranged in a hexagonal array are seen. In the distal portions of the A band, both thick and thin, or actin, filaments are found, with each thick filament surrounded by six thin filaments. In the I band only thin filaments are present. *(From E Braunwald et al, Mechanisms of Contraction of the Normal and Failing Heart, Boston, Little, Brown, 1968.)*

muscle, which in turn is closely related to the ventricular end-diastolic volume.

The activity of myosin ATPase determines the rate of forming and breaking of the actin-myosin cross-bridges and ultimately the velocity of muscle contraction.

THE ROLE OF MUSCLE LENGTH In all striated muscle, including cardiac muscle, the force of contraction depends on initial muscle length. The sarcomere length associated with the most forceful contraction is approximately 2.2 μm. At this length the two sets of myofilaments of the sarcomere are situated so as to provide the greatest area for their interaction. The length of the sarcomere also appears to regulate the extent of activation of the contractile system, i.e., its sensitivity to Ca^{2+}. According to this concept, termed *length-dependent activation*, at the optimal sarcomere length of 2.2 μm the myofilament sensitivity to Ca^{2+} is maximal. When sarcomere length is increased to 3.65 μm, the thin filaments are entirely withdrawn from the A band, and no tension can be developed. Similarly, when the sarcomeres are shorter than 2.0 μm, the thin filaments bypass one another, doubly overlapping each other and so reducing both the sensitivity of the contractile sites to Ca^{2+} and the capacity for force development.

The relation between the initial length of the muscle fibers and the developed force is of prime importance for the function of heart muscle. This forms the basis of the Frank-Starling relation (Starling's law of the heart), which states that, within limits, the force of ventricular contraction is a function of the end-diastolic length of the cardiac

MYOCARDIAL MECHANICS

THE FORCE-VELOCITY CURVE The mechanical activity of all striated muscle may be expressed externally in two ways: shortening and the development of tension. Hill showed in skeletal muscle that the velocity of shortening is inversely related to the tension development, an expression of the so-called force-velocity relation, now recognized to be a fundamental property of muscle. Expressed simply, the greater the load the muscle is called upon to lift, the lower the velocity of shortening and vice versa. The force-velocity relation also applies to cardiac muscle. However, in this respect there is a basic difference between skeletal and cardiac muscle. Skeletal muscle fibers have a single, essentially fixed, force-velocity curve; i.e., at any given muscle length, force and velocity are always related to each other in the same manner. The contractile activity of skeletal muscle is controlled by varying the frequency of nerve impulses stimulating the muscle, and thereby the number of contractions of each fiber per unit of time, as well as by the recruitment of additional muscle fibers, i.e., motor units, while the contractile properties of each individual fiber, expressed in the force-velocity curve, remain constant. Although resting length also influences the characteristics of contraction, this variable remains essentially fixed in vivo because of the skeletal muscles' skeletal attachments. In contrast, the number of cardiac cells and within them the myofibrils and sarcomeres that become activated during each contraction is constant. However, the contractile activity of the myocardium is readily altered under physiologic conditions by changes in resting fiber length and by changes in the inotropic state, i.e., the contractility, both of which shift the myocardial force-velocity curve. Many neurohumoral influences affect contractility, but the most important influence is the adrenergic nervous system operating via its neurotransmitter, norepinephrine.

Cardiac muscle exhibits an inverse relation between the force against which it contracts, i.e., the afterload, and the extent and velocity of shortening. The myocardial force-velocity curve obtained in isolated heart muscle represents this inverse relation and can be used to describe myocardial performance.

VENTRICULAR EJECTION AND FILLING

Analysis of the heart as a pump has classically centered on the relation between the end-diastolic volume of the ventricle (which is related to the length of the muscle fibers) and its stroke volume (the Frank-Starling relation). The end-diastolic or "filling" pressure of the ventricle is sometimes used as a surrogate for the end-diastolic volume. In the heart-lung preparation the stroke volume within limits correlates directly with the diastolic fiber length (preload) and inversely with the arterial resistance (afterload), and the failing heart delivers a smaller-than-normal stroke volume from a normal or elevated end-diastolic volume. The relation between the ven-

FIGURE 232-2 Reaction mechanism of actomyosin ATPase, simplified to show four steps. In relaxed muscle (upper left), ATP bound to the myosin cross-bridge dissociates the thick and thin filaments. *Step 1:* Hydrolysis of myosin-bound ATP by the ATPase site on the myosin head transfers the chemical energy of the nucleotide to the activated cross-bridge (upper right). When cytosolic Ca^{2+} concentration is low, as in relaxed muscle, the reaction cannot proceed because tropomyosin and the troponin complex on the thin filament do not allow the active sites on actin to interact with the cross-bridges. Therefore, even though the cross-bridges are energized, they cannot interact with actin. *Step 2:* When Ca^{2+} binding to troponin C has exposed active sites on the thin filament, actin interacts with the myosin cross-bridges to form an active complex (lower right) in which the energy derived from ATP is retained in the actin-bound cross-bridge, whose orientation has not yet shifted. *Step 3:* The muscle contracts when ADP dissociates from the cross-bridge; this step leads to the formation of the low-energy rigor complex (lower left), in which the chemical energy derived from ATP hydrolysis has been expended to perform mechanical work (the "rowing" motion of the cross-bridge). *Step 4:* The muscle returns to its resting state, and the cycle ends when a new molecule of ATP binds to the rigor complex and dissociates the cross-bridge from the thin filament. This cycle continues until calcium is dissociated from troponin C in the thin filament, which causes the contractile proteins to return to the resting state with the cross-bridge in the energized state. *[From AM Katz, in WS Colucci (ed), Heart Failure: Cardiac Function and Dysfunction, in Atlas of Heart Diseases, vol 4, E Braunwald (series ed), Philadelphia, Current Medicine, 1995.]*

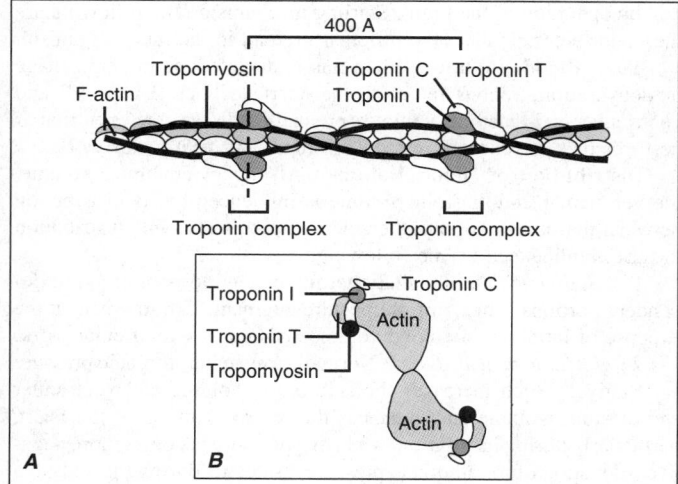

FIGURE 232-3 Structure of the thin filament. *A.* The "backbone" of the thin filament, seen in a longitudinal view, is F-actin, which contains two strands of actin monomers (light blue and white). Troponin complexes, made up of one molecule each of troponin C, troponin I, and troponin T, are distributed at approximately 400-Å intervals along the thin filament. Elongated tropomyosin molecules (solid) lie in the grooves between the two actin strands. *B.* A cross section of the thin filament at the level where the troponin complexes are located shows probable relationships between actin, tropomyosin, and the three components of the troponin complex. The strength of the bond linking troponin I and actin varies, depending on whether Ca^{2+} is bound to troponin C. *[From AM Katz: Molecular and cellular basis of contraction, in WS Colucci (ed): Heart Failure: Cardiac Function and Dysfunction, in E Braunwald (Series ed): Atlas of Heart Diseases, vol 4. Philadelphia, Current Medicine, 1995, p 1.5. Adapted from Katz. With permission of the publisher.]*

tricular end-diastolic pressure and the stroke work of the ventricle (the ventricular function curve) provides a useful definition of the level of the contractile, or inotropic, state of the ventricle. An increase in ventricular contractility is accompanied by a shift of the ventricular function curve upward and to the left [greater stroke work at any level of ventricular end-diastolic pressure (or volume), or lower end-diastolic pressure at any level of stroke work], while depression of contractility is characterized by a shift downward and to the right.

During the adrenergic stimulation of the myocardium accompanying exercise, relatively little change in ventricular end-diastolic volume occurs, while cardiac output, aortic flow velocity, stroke work, and the rate of ventricular pressure development are all augmented, sometimes greatly, reflecting an increase in myocardial contractility.

The important influence of the adrenergic neurotransmitter, norepinephrine (Chap. 70), on the mechanical properties of the myocardium has long been recognized. Direct stimulation of the cardiac adrenergic nerves augments ventricular function as a consequence of the release of norepinephrine from adrenergic nerve endings in the heart. Norepinephrine activates myocardial beta receptors and thereby increases the concentration of cyclic AMP (see Fig. 232-9, p. 1286). The latter, in turn, causes a more rapid, forceful contraction by phosphorylating the Ca^{2+} channel in the myocardial sarcolemma, thereby enhancing the influx of Ca^{2+} into the myocyte which, in turn, acts on the contractile apparatus, as described on p. 1279. The adrenergic effects are evidenced by tachycardia, a reduction in cardiac dimensions, increased velocity of ejection, and an enhanced rate of tension development.

ASSESSMENT OF CARDIAC FUNCTION Several techniques are available for defining impaired cardiac function in patients. With the patient at rest, the cardiac output and stroke volume may be depressed, but not uncommonly these variables are within normal limits, even in the presence of heart failure. A more sensitive index is the ejection fraction, i.e., the ratio of stroke volume to end-diastolic

volume (normal value $= 67 \pm 8$ percent), which may be estimated by radiocontrast or radionuclide angiography or echocardiography and which is frequently depressed in systolic heart failure even when the stroke volume itself is normal. Alternatively, the detection of abnormally elevated ventricular end-diastolic volumes (normal value $= 70 \pm 20$ mL/m²) in the presence of a normal or presumably normal stroke volume signifies impairment of left ventricular systolic function. A limitation of the measurement of cardiac output, ejection fraction, and ventricular volume in the assessment of cardiac function is that these variables are influenced strongly by ventricular loading conditions. Thus, a depressed ejection fraction and lowered cardiac output may be observed in patients with normal ventricular function but reduced preload, as occurs in hypovolemia, or with increased afterload, as occurs in acutely elevated arterial pressure.

The end-systolic left ventricular pressure-volume relationship is a particularly useful index of ventricular performance since it is independent of both preload and afterload. At any level of myocardial contractility, left ventricular end-systolic volume varies inversely with end-systolic pressure; as contractility declines, end-systolic volume (at any level of end-systolic pressure) rises. Noninvasive techniques, particularly echocardiography and radionuclide angiography, are of great value in the clinical assessment of myocardial function. They provide measurements of end-systolic volume (or end-systolic dimension) that can be related to systolic arterial pressure also determined noninvasively. In addition, they provide convenient measurements of ejection fraction and systolic shortening rate and allow measurement of ventricular filling (see below).

Exercise A useful technique for evaluating ventricular performance involves the measurement of the circulatory changes occurring during exercise. Thus, left ventricular performance may be estimated accurately by measuring the left ventricular end-diastolic pressure, cardiac output, and total-body O_2 consumption at rest and during exercise. In persons with normal cardiac function, the cardiac output rises by more than 500 mL/min for each 100-mL increase in minute O_2 consumption. The left ventricular end-diastolic pressure at rest is less than 12 mmHg and rises slightly, remains unchanged, or decreases slightly during exercise, while stroke volume usually rises, especially when exercise is carried out in the upright position. The failing left ventricle, on the other hand, is characterized by an elevation of end-diastolic pressure during exercise to above 12 mmHg, accompanied by either no change or a fall in stroke volume and a subnormal increase in cardiac output related to the increase in minute O_2 consumption. The overall performance of the cardiopulmonary system in delivering oxygen to the metabolizing tissue can be estimated by measuring the maximal O_2 consumption achieved during escalating treadmill exercise ($\dot{V}max_{O_2}$). Normal values exceed 20 mL/min per kilogram body weight, while values under 10 mL/min per kilogram represent severe impairment of function, usually seen in patients with severe heart failure and a poor prognosis.

The potential value of stressing the left ventricle in assessing its performance is emphasized by the fact that the normal range of left ventricular end-diastolic pressure, cardiac index, and ventricular stroke work in the resting state is wide, with values that frequently overlap those seen in patients with ventricular dysfunction. The response to stress may prove useful not only in the detection of the impairment of myocardial function but also in expressing the severity of such impairment quantitatively.

Diastolic Performance This important variable is best assessed by continuously measuring the flow velocity across the mitral valve using Doppler echocardiography. Normally, the flow velocity is more rapid in early diastole than during atrial systole; with impaired relaxation the rate of early diastolic filling declines, while the rate of presystolic filling rises. With severe impairment of filling the pattern is "pseudo-normalized" and early ventricular filling becomes more rapid as left atrial pressure upstream to the stiff left ventricle rises (Fig. 232-5).

CONTROL OF CARDIAC PERFORMANCE AND OUTPUT

The extent of shortening of mammalian heart muscle and, therefore, the stroke volume of the intact ventricle are determined by three influences: (1) the length of the muscle at the onset of contraction, i.e., the preload; (2) the inotropic state of the muscle, i.e., the position of its force-velocity-length relation; and (3) the tension that the muscle is called upon to develop during contraction, i.e., the afterload. Heart rate determines the cardiac output at any stroke volume as long as the other three influences are maintained. Ventricular filling is influenced by the extent and speed of myocardial relaxation, which in turn is determined by the rate of uptake of Ca^{2+} by the sarcoplasmic reticulum; the latter may be augmented by positive inotropic stimuli and reduced by ischemia. Filling may be impeded by the stiffness of the ventricular wall, which may be increased by ventricular hypertrophy and conditions that infiltrate the myocardium, or by an extrinsic constraint (e.g., pericardial compression).

VENTRICULAR END-DIASTOLIC VOLUME (PRE-LOAD) At any level of inotropic state and afterload, the performance of the myocardium is influenced profoundly by ventricular end-diastolic fiber length and therefore by diastolic ventricular volume, i.e., by operation of the Frank-Starling mechanism. The following are the major determinants of ventricular preload in the intact organism:

Total Blood Volume When this is depleted, as in hemorrhage or dehydration, venous return to the heart declines (Chap. 38) and ventricular end-diastolic volume (preload) falls, as does ventricular performance, as reflected in stroke volume and ventricular work.

Distribution of Blood Volume At any given blood volume, the ventricular end-diastolic volume is influenced by its distribution between the intra- and extrathoracic compartments. This distribution in turn is influenced by the following:

1. *Body position.* Gravitational forces tend to pool blood in dependent portions. Thus, upright posture augments extrathoracic at the expense of intrathoracic blood volume and reduces ventricular work.

2. *Intrathoracic pressure.* Normally, mean intrathoracic pressure is negative, which increases thoracic blood volume and ventricular end-diastolic volume and enhances the return of blood to the heart, particularly during inspiration, when this pressure becomes more negative. Elevation of intrathoracic pressure, as occurs during the Valsalva maneuver or prolonged bouts of coughing or with positive-pressure ventilation, tends to impede venous return, diminish intrathoracic blood volume, and ultimately reduce stroke volume and ventricular work.

3. *Intrapericardial pressure.* When this pressure is elevated, as in pericardial tamponade (Chap. 240), there is interference with cardiac filling, and the resultant reduction in ventricular diastolic volume reduces stroke volume and ventricular work.

FIGURE 232-4 Calcium fluxes that activate contraction are downhill, and those that cause relaxation are uphill. As depicted in heart muscle at rest, calcium channels in the sarcolemmal membrane are closed; intracellular calcium is stored in the sarcoplasmic reticulum. With excitation and membrane depolarization, voltage-sensitive sodium channels (not shown) and calcium channels in the sarcolemma open to allow rapid entry of extracellular sodium and calcium. Entry of calcium is believed to cause release of calcium from the sarcoplasmic reticulum that initiates contraction. Reuptake of calcium by the sarcoplasmic reticulum by an ATP-dependent calcium pump is essential for the heart to relax. Importantly, contraction is activated mainly by passive calcium fluxes from the sarcoplasmic reticulum. By contrast, during diastole calcium must be pumped out of the cytosol to accomplish relaxation. Energy also must be expended during diastole to restore sodium and calcium gradients across the sarcolemma, which provide for the depolarizing ionic currents that generate the action potential. Sodium transport is accomplished by the sarcolemmal sodium pump (Na^+, K^+-ATPase), which utilizes ATP to pump sodium out of the cell in exchange for potassium. The resultant sodium gradient is largely responsible for active transport of calcium out of the cell during relaxation, via sodium-calcium exchange. *[Reproduced by permission from AM Katz, VE Smith, Hosp Prac, 19(1):69, 1984. Illustration by Bunji Tagawa.]*

4. *Venous tone.* The venous system is not a simple system of passive conduits between the systemic capillary bed and the right atrium. Instead, the smooth muscle in the walls of the venules and veins responds to a variety of neural and humoral stimuli. Venoconstriction occurs during muscular exercise, deep respiration, fright, or marked hypotension, tending to diminish extrathoracic and to augment intrathoracic and intraventricular blood volumes and ventricular performance.

5. *The pumping action of skeletal muscle.* During muscular exercise the contracting skeletal muscles squeeze blood out of the venous bed and, with the aid of the venous valves, displace it centrally, thereby increasing intrathoracic blood volume, ventricular end-diastolic volume, and ventricular work.

Atrial Contraction Vigorous, appropriately timed atrial contraction augments ventricular filling and end-diastolic volume. The atrial contribution to ventricular filling, the so-called atrial kick, is of particular importance in patients with concentric ventricular hypertrophy, in whom the loss of atrial systole (as in atrial fibrillation) tends to reduce ventricular end-diastolic pressure and volume, ultimately lowering myocardial performance. The atrial contribution to ventricular filling may also be reduced by atrioventricular dissociation, prolongation or abbreviation of the P-R interval, and depression of the inotropic state of the atrium.

INOTROPIC STATE (MYOCARDIAL CONTRACTILITY) A number of factors determine

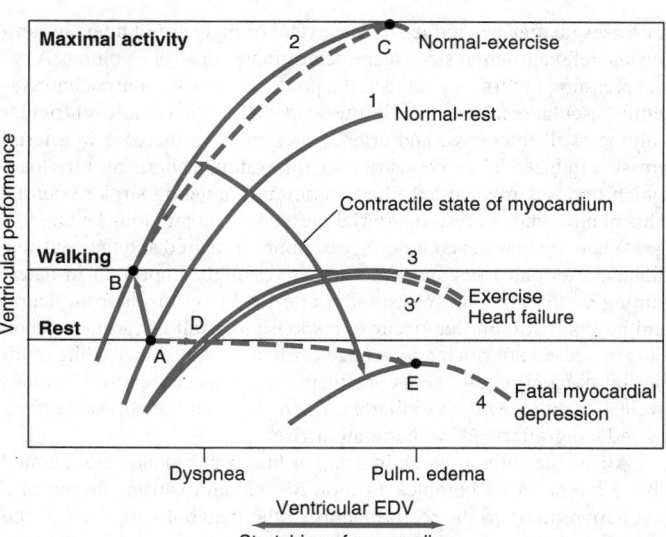

FIGURE 232-5 Patterns of left ventricular filling, as recorded by diastolic Doppler mitral flow velocities. In the normal pattern there is a large E wave and a small A wave. There are three abnormal patterns of mitral filling representing progressively worsening left ventricular diastolic performance. With "impaired relaxation" the E wave is less than the A wave. In the "pseudonormalized" pattern the E wave is larger than the A wave. In the "restricted" filling pattern E is much larger than A with a very short t_{dec}. *(From Little and Braunwald.)*

FIGURE 232-6 Diagram showing the interrelations among influences on ventricular end-diastolic volume (EDV) through stretching of the myocardium and the contractile state of the myocardium. Levels of ventricular EDV associated with filling pressures that result in dyspnea and pulmonary edema are shown on the abscissa. Levels of ventricular performance required when the subject is at rest, while walking, and during maximal activity are designated on the ordinate. The broken lines are the descending limbs of the ventricular-performance curves, which are rarely seen during life but which show the level of ventricular performance if end-diastolic volume could be elevated to very high levels. For further explanation see text. *(Modified from E Braunwald et al, Mechanisms of Contraction of the Normal and Failing Heart, Boston, Little, Brown, 1968.)*

the level of ventricular performance at any given ventricular end-diastolic volume, i.e., the position of the ventricular function curve (Fig. 232-6). These influences may be considered to operate by modifying myocardial force-velocity relations. In the final analysis, most of these influences act by altering the concentration of Ca^{2+} in the vicinity of the myofilaments, which in turn trigger cross-bridge cycling (p. 1279).

Adrenergic Nerve Activity (See also Chap. 70) The quantity of norepinephrine released by adrenergic nerve endings in the heart is determined by the adrenergic nerve impulse traffic; alterations in the frequency of these nerve impulses modify the quantity of norepinephrine released and acting on the beta-adrenergic receptors in the myocardium. This mechanism is the most important one that acutely modifies the myocardial contractility under physiologic conditions.

Circulating Catecholamines (See also Chap. 70) When it is stimulated by adrenergic nerve impulse, the adrenal medulla releases catecholamines, which, when they reach the heart, augment the inotropic state and the frequency of contraction.

The Force-Frequency Relation The position of the myocardial force-velocity curve also is influenced by the rate and rhythm of cardiac contraction; e.g., ventricular extrasystoles result in postextrasystolic potentiation, presumably by increasing the Ca^{2+} that enters the cardiac cell. The contractility of the normal (but not of the failing) heart is augmented by an increase in frequency.

Exogenously Administered Inotropic Agents Isoproterenol, dopamine, dobutamine, and other sympathomimetic agents, cardiac glycosides, calcium, amrinone, milrinone, and other phosphodiesterase inhibitors all improve the myocardial force-velocity relation and therefore may be used to stimulate ventricular performance.

Physiologic Depressants Included among these are severe myocardial hypoxia, ischemia, and acidosis. Acting either singly or in combination, these influences depress the myocardial force-velocity curve and left ventricular work at any given ventricular end-diastolic volume.

Pharmacologic Depressants These include procainamide, disopyramide, calcium antagonists such as verapamil, beta blockers, and large doses of barbiturates, alcohol, and general anesthetics as well as many other drugs.

Loss of Myocytes When a sufficiently large portion of ventricular myocardium becomes nonfunctional or necrotic, as occurs transiently during ischemia (Chap. 244) and permanently in myocardial infarction (Chap. 243), total ventricular performance at any given level of end-diastolic volume becomes depressed. Programmed cell death (apoptosis) can cause scattered loss of myocytes and, when

sufficiently widespread, can impair ventricular function and cause heart failure.

Intrinsic Myocardial Depression Although the fundamental mechanisms responsible for depression of myocardial contractility in most cases of chronic congestive heart failure secondary to prolonged ventricular overload or cardiomyopathy remain to be elucidated (p. 1287), it is now apparent that in this condition the inotropic state of individual surviving myocytes is depressed, and as a consequence the ventricular performance at any ventricular preload and afterload is lowered.

VENTRICULAR AFTERLOAD The stroke volume is ultimately a function of the extent of ventricular fiber shortening. In the intact heart, as in isolated cardiac muscle, extent (and velocity) of shortening of ventricular muscle fibers at any level of diastolic fiber length (preload) and myocardial inotropic state are inversely related to the afterload, i.e., the load that opposes shortening. In the intact heart the afterload may be defined as the tension or stress developed in the ventricular wall during ejection. Therefore, the afterload is determined by the aortic pressure as well as the volume and thickness of the ventricular cavity. Laplace's law indicates that the tension of the myocardial fiber is a function of the product of the intracavitary ventricular pressure and ventricular radius divided by the wall thickness. Therefore, at any given level of aortic pressure, the afterload faced by a dilated left ventricle of normal thickness is higher than that encountered by a ventricle of normal size. Conversely, at the same aortic pressure and ventricular diastolic volume, the afterload of a thick-walled ventricle is lower than of a thin-walled chamber. The aortic pressure is determined by the peripheral vascular resistance, the physical characteristics of the arterial tree, and the volume of blood it contains at the onset of ejection.

The critical role played by the ventricular afterload in cardiovascular regulation is shown in Fig. 232-7. As already noted, increases in both preload and contractility increase myocardial fiber shortening, while increases in afterload reduce it. The extent of myocardial fiber shortening and left ventricular size are the determinants of stroke volume. Arterial pressure, in turn, is related to the product of cardiac output and systemic vascular resistance, while afterload is a function of left ventricular volume, wall thickness, and arterial pressure. An increase in arterial pressure induced by vasoconstriction, for example, augments afterload, which opposes myocardial fiber shortening, reducing stroke volume. This in turn tends to restore arterial pressure to its previous level.

When myocardial contractility becomes impaired and the ventricle dilates, afterload rises and becomes increasingly important in determining cardiac output. Increases in afterload may result from neural and humoral stimuli that occur in response to a fall in cardiac output. This increased afterload may reduce cardiac output further while myocardial oxygen requirements are increased. This can cause a vicious cycle. Treatment with vasodilators (Chap. 233) has the opposite effect; by reducing afterload cardiac output rises.

All of the influences acting on cardiac performance enumerated above interact in a complex fashion to maintain cardiac output at a level appropriate to the requirements of the metabolizing tissues, and in a normal person interference with any one of these mechanisms may not influence the cardiac output. For example, a moderate reduction of blood volume *or* the loss of the atrial contribution to ventricular contraction can ordinarily be sustained without a reduction in the cardiac output at rest. Other factors, such as increases in the frequency of adrenergic nerve impulses to the heart and in heart rate, will, in a normal individual, serve as compensatory mechanisms, augment contractility, and sustain cardiac output. In individuals with normal hearts, the preload, which in turn is related to the volume of blood available for filling the heart, rather than the inotropic state of the myocardium or the afterload limits cardiac output. An improvement of myocardial contractility or the reduction of afterload with nitroprusside causes little elevation of the cardiac output in normal individuals. On the other hand, in the presence of congestive heart failure, the cardiac output usually is limited by the depression of myocardial contractility and a positive inotropic drug and/or reduction of afterload raises cardiac output (Chap. 233).

EXERCISE The hemodynamic changes that occur normally during exercise in the upright position are complex (Fig. 232-6). The hyperventilation, the pumping action of the exercising muscles, and the venoconstriction during exercise all tend to augment venous return and hence ventricular filling and preload. Simultaneously, the increase in the adrenergic nerve impulses to the myocardium, the increased concentration of circulating catecholamines, and the tachycardia that all occur during exercise combine to augment the contractile state of the myocardium (Fig. 232-6, curves 1 and 2) and lead to an elevation of stroke work and stroke volume, with no change or even a decrease of end-diastolic pressure and volume (Fig. 232-6, points A and B). Vasodilatation occurs in the exercising muscles, thus tending to counteract the marked increase in arterial pressure that would otherwise occur as cardiac output rises to levels as high as five times basal during maximal exercise. This vasodilatation ultimately allows the achievement of a greatly elevated cardiac output during exercise, at an arterial pressure only moderately higher than in the resting state.

THE FAILING HEART

Though heart failure may be readily described as a clinical syndrome, characterized by well-known symptoms and physical signs (Chap. 233), a precise physiologic or biochemical definition is far more difficult. However, from the clinical point of view, heart failure may be considered to be the condition in which *an abnormality of cardiac function is responsible for the inability of the heart to pump blood at a rate commensurate with the requirements of the metabolizing tissues and/or can do so only from an abnormally elevated ventricular diastolic volume.* Abnormalities during systole and/or diastole may be present in heart failure (Fig. 232-8). In so-called *systolic heart failure* (p. 1288), an impairment of myocardial contractility causes weakened systolic contraction, which leads, ultimately, to a reduction in stroke volume, inadequate ventricular emptying, cardiac dilatation, and often elevation of ventricular diastolic pressure. Idiopathic dilated cardiomyopathy (Chap. 239) is the prototype of systolic heart failure.

In *diastolic heart failure* (p. 1288) the principal abnormality is impaired relaxation and filling of the ventricle and leads to an elevation of ventricular diastolic pressure at any given diastolic volume. Failure of relaxation can be functional and transient, as during ischemia, while impaired ventricular filling can be caused by a stiffened, thickened ventricle (Fig. 232-5). Typical conditions in which diastolic failure occurs are restrictive cardiomyopathy secondary to infiltrative conditions, such as amyloidosis or hemochromatosis, as well as hypertrophic cardiomyopathy (Chap. 239). The concentric hypertrophy associated with chronic hypertension can also impair ventricular filling but rarely causes overt heart failure. In many patients with cardiac hypertrophy and dilatation, systolic and diastolic failure coexist; the ventricle both empties and fills abnormally. There may be cardiac dilatation, but the ventricle's pressure-volume relation is shifted, raising the ventricular diastolic pressure at any given volume.

Though a defect in myocardial contraction is characteristic of systolic heart failure, this defect may result from a primary abnormality in the heart muscle, as in cardiomyopathy, or it may be secondary to a chronic excessive work load as in hypertension or valvular heart disease. In ischemic heart disease systolic heart failure results from a loss in the quantity of normally contracting cells (secondary to myocardial infarction) or from transient loss of function in reversibly impaired myocardium.

It is important to distinguish heart failure from (1) states of circulatory insufficiency in which myocardial function is not primarily impaired, such as cardiac tamponade or hemorrhagic shock; (2) conditions in which there is circulatory congestion because of abnormal salt and water retention but in which there is no serious disturbance of the heart's function, such as in acute glomerulonephritis; and (3) conditions in which a normal myocardium is suddenly presented with a load that exceeds its capacity, such as accelerated hypertension or rupture of a valve cusp secondary to infective endocarditis.

ADAPTIVE MECHANISMS A number of mechanisms aid the heart faced with an increased hemodynamic burden, such as pressure or volume overload, or which has sustained loss of myocardium. These adaptive mechanisms include: (1) the Frank-Starling mechanism operating through an increase in preload (p. 1280); (2) the development of myocardial hypertrophy, which restores elevated ventricular wall stress to normal; (3) redistribution of a subnormal cardiac output away from the skin, skeletal muscle, and kidneys with maintenance of blood flow to vital organs such as the

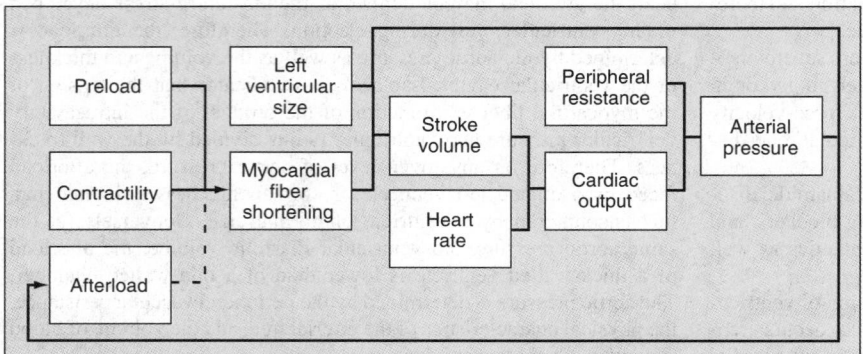

FIGURE 232-7 Scheme of interactions among various components that regulate cardiac activity. Solid lines indicate an augmenting effect; broken line represents an inhibiting effect. (*From E Braunwald, N Engl J Med 290:1124–1129, 1420–1425, 1974.*)

brain and the heart itself; and (4) neurohumoral adjustments, which tend to maintain arterial pressure and are discussed on p. 1283 and in Chap. 70.

The contractility of strips of myocardium removed from failing animal hearts has been shown to be depressed soon after the imposition of a pressure overload. The laying down of additional myofibrils (compensatory hypertrophy) often restores contractility to normal, but when the overload is maintained for prolonged periods, myocardial contractility again declines. Myocytes isolated from the left ventricles of patients with heart failure secondary to dilated cardiomyopathy exhibit reduced shortening.

The failing ventricle may still eject a normal or nearly normal stroke volume despite considerable depression of function through an increase in preload (end-diastolic volume), i.e., through the operation of the Frank-Starling mechanism. As outlined above (p. 1280), an increase in the initial volume of the ventricle is associated with stretching of the sarcomere, which increases the interaction between actin and myosin filaments and their sensitivity to Ca^{2+}.

BIOCHEMICAL ABNORMALITIES IN HEART FAILURE There is no unifying theory providing a biochemical basis for heart failure. The common forms of low-output heart failure, secondary to coronary atherosclerosis, hypertension, cardiomyopathy, and certain valvular and congenital lesions, are characterized by an absolute or a relative reduction in the external work delivered by the heart, although myocardial oxygen consumption remains normal or is only slightly lowered. Therefore, the external efficiency, i.e., the ratio of external work performed to energy consumed, is often depressed.

Alterations in Energy Metabolism When heart failure occurs in the presence of acute or chronic ischemia, it can be attributed to reduced myocardial energy supplies. However, in some forms of experimental and clinical heart failure without ischemia, myocardial energy stores in the form of creatine phosphate are decreased, as is the activity of the enzyme creatine kinase required for the shuttling of high-energy phosphate between creatine phosphate and adenosine diphosphate, suggesting that reductions in myocardial energy reserves may be responsible.

Alterations in Regulatory Proteins There is considerable evidence that changes in the regulatory proteins occur in chronic heart failure. These changes include a reduction of myosin ATPase activity, which could be caused by an alteration in the expression of troponin T and/or of myosin light kinase 2, two proteins that could be responsible for lowering the rate of interaction between myosin and actin myofilaments.

Abnormalities of Excitation-Contraction Coupling Substantial evidence supports the view that in many forms of heart failure the delivery of Ca^{2+} to the contractile sites is reduced, thereby impairing cardiac performance. However, the molecular basis of this abnormality, indeed the subcellular structures involved, i.e., the sarcolemma, T tubules, and/or sarcoplasmic reticulum, have yet to be defined. There is, however, evidence for a reduction in the messenger RNAs of the proteins regulating Ca^{2+} movements, including the sarcolemmal Ca^{2+} channels, as well as the Ca^{2+} release channels and the Ca^{2+} uptake pump, which play critical roles in the movement of Ca^{2+} between the sarcoplasmic reticulum and the cytoplasm and vice versa, respectively. Impaired expression of the genes encoding these proteins can impair both myocardial contraction and relaxation and thereby contribute to the development of diastolic heart failure. In addition, a reduction of Ca^{2+} release by the sarcoplasmic reticulum to the myofilaments can cause systolic heart failure.

NEUROHUMORAL ADJUSTMENTS A reduction in cardiac performance evokes a series of neurohumoral adjustments, which may be considered to be both adaptive and maladaptive. Although they are useful because they maintain arterial perfusion pressure in

the face of a reduction of cardiac output, they increase the hemodynamic burden and oxygen requirements of the failing ventricle.

The Renin-Angiotensin-Aldosterone System When cardiac output declines, the renin-angiotensin-aldosterone system (Chap. 332) is activated. Concentrations of circulating angiotensin II and aldosterone are both increased, the former contributing to excess vasoconstriction and the latter to the retention of salt and water. Patients with heart failure are usually improved by blocking this system with angiotensin-converting enzyme inhibitors, angiotensin II receptor blockers, and aldosterone antagonists (Chap. 233).

The Adrenergic Nervous System In patients with heart failure the levels of circulating norepinephrine may be markedly elevated, reflecting the increased activity of the adrenergic nervous system; indeed the prognosis varies inversely with the concentration. This increased activity of the adrenergic neurons supports ventricular contractility in congestive heart failure. Heart failure is intensified when large doses of beta-adrenergic blocking agents are administered to such patients. However, the chronic adrenergic stimulation in heart failure may also increase afterload by raising vascular resistance and cause arrhythmias and further myocardial damage directly. The latter may be further prevented by the cautious administration of gradually increasing doses of beta blockers (p. 1296).

The density of adrenergic receptors and concentration of cardiac norepinephrine are both reduced in chronic, severe heart failure. These changes are accompanied by a reduction in the activity of adenylate cyclase, which may lower the intracellular concentration of cyclic AMP. The latter in turn reduces the activation of protein kinase, the phosphorylation of Ca^{2+} channels, transarcolemmal Ca^{2+} entry, as well as the phosphorylation of phospholamban, a protein in the sarcoplasmic reticulum, thereby depressing the reuptake of Ca^{2+} by the latter (Fig.

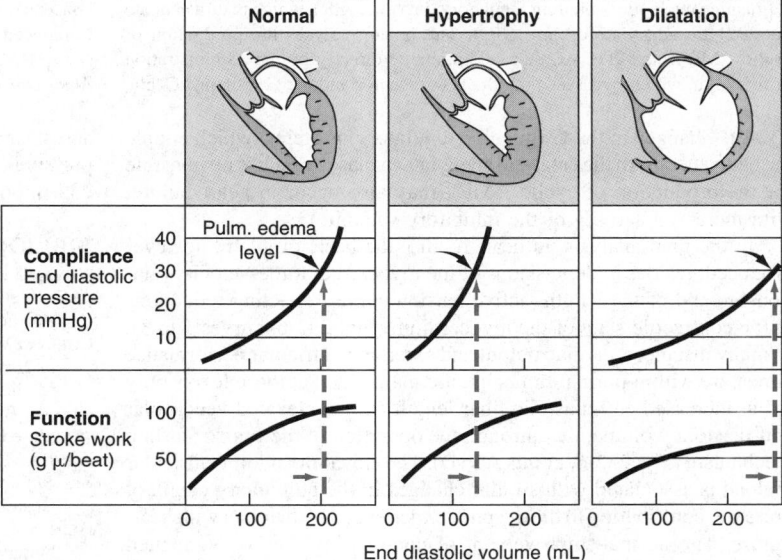

FIGURE 232-8 Relationship between left ventricular end-diastolic volume and (1) end-diastolic pressure (*top*), describing the *compliance* of the left ventricle, i.e., its *diastolic* properties; and (2) left ventricular stroke work (*bottom*), describing the ventricle's *systolic* function curve. The normal left ventricle (*left*) reaches an end-diastolic pressure of 30 mmHg (pulmonary edema level) when its end-diastolic volume is elevated to 200 mL. The concentrically hypertrophied left ventricle (*center*) exhibits normal systolic function since the relation between left ventricular end-diastolic volume and stroke work is unchanged, but there is "diastolic failure" in that end-diastolic pressure reaches pulmonary edema level (i.e., 30 mmHg) at a lower level than normal (i.e., 130 mL). The dilated ventricle (*right*) exhibits "systolic failure" in that the maximal stroke work and the stroke volume at any level of end-diastolic volume are depressed. The left ventricle displays increased diastolic compliance, i.e., distensibility, with a higher than normal end-diastolic volume (280 mL) required to reach the pulmonary edema level. (*Reprinted with permission from R Gorlin, Prim Cardiol 6:84, 1980.*)

FIGURE 232-9 Schematic representation of influences on intramyocardial Ca^{2+} concentration and excitation-contraction coupling. The action potential is associated with intracellular entry of Na^+ and the extrusion of K^+ (not shown) and the entry of Ca^{2+} (shown). The Na^+-Ca^{2+} exchanger depends on concentration gradients and does not require ATP. Not shown is the energy-dependent sarcolemmal Ca^{2+} pump which extrudes Ca^{2+} from the cell. Isoproterenol and norepinephrine, the latter shown intraneuronally, stimulate the beta-adrenergic receptor in the outer sarcolemma. The beta receptor is coupled to G (guanine nucleotide–binding regulatory) proteins (GR), which in turn activate the catalytic adenylate cyclase (AC). The latter catalyzes the production of cyclic AMP from ATP. AC can be stimulated directly by the administration of forskolin, which bypasses both the beta receptor and the G proteins. Cyclic AMP activates protein kinase, which in turn enhances the phosphorylation of the Ca^{2+} channel, increasing transarcolemmal Ca^{2+} influx. Activated protein kinase also phosphorylates phospholamban, which in its phosphorylated form enhances the uptake of Ca^{2+} by the sarcoplasmic tubular network. Phosphodiesterase catalyzes the breakdown of cyclic AMP to AMP while milrinone, caffeine, and isobutylmethylxanthine inhibit phosphodiesterase, thereby augmenting cyclic AMP concentration. Digoxin inhibits the Na^+, K^+-ATPase in the sarcolemma, inhibiting Na^+ efflux from and K^+ influx into the cell. As a consequence the intracellular Na^+ concentration falls and Na^+-Ca^{2+} exchange is reduced, thereby raising intracellular Ca^{2+}. P represents phosphorylation. *(From AMD Feldman et al: Circulation 75:331, 1987, with permission of the American Heart Association, Inc.)*

232-9). Changes in the G (guanine regulatory) proteins, which couple the beta receptor to the catalytic adenylate cyclase (which is responsible for the production of cyclic AMP), may also occur in heart failure, with increased activity of the inhibitory subunit.

In the final analysis, in heart failure, the basic problem, however produced, resides in depressions of the myocardial force-velocity relationship and of the length–active tension curve, reflecting reductions in the contractile state of the myocardium (Fig. 232-6, curves 1 to 3). In many instances, cardiac output and external ventricular performance at rest are within normal limits but are maintained at these levels only by an increased end-diastolic fiber length and an elevated ventricular end-diastolic volume, i.e., through the operation of the Frank-Starling mechanism (Fig. 232-6, points A to D). The elevation of left ventricular preload is associated with similar changes in the pulmonary capillary pressure, contributing to the dyspnea experienced by patients with heart failure. The normal improvement of contractility due to augmented adrenergic activity during exercise is attenuated or even prevented by norepinephrine depletion and downregulation of myocardial beta receptors, which occur in severe heart failure (Fig. 232-6, curves 3 and 3'). The factors that tend to augment ventricular filling during exercise in the normal individual push the failing myocardium along its flattened length–active tension curve, and although the left ventricle may perform somewhat better, this occurs only as a consequence of an inordinate elevation of ventricular end-diastolic volume and pressure and, therefore, of the pulmonary capillary pressure. The latter intensifies dyspnea and therefore plays an important role in limiting the intensity of exercise that the patient can perform. Left ventricular failure becomes fatal when the myocardial length–active tension curve is depressed (Fig. 232-6, curve 4) to the point at which cardiac performance fails to satisfy the requirements of the peripheral tissues even

at rest, and/or the left ventricular end-diastolic and pulmonary capillary pressures are elevated to levels that result in pulmonary edema (Fig. 232-6, point E).

BIBLIOGRAPHY

ANVERSA P et al: Myocyte death in heart failure. Curr Opin Cardiol 11:245, 1996

ARAI M et al: Sarcoplasmic reticulum gene expression in cardiac hypertrophy and heart failure. Circ Res 74:555, 1994

COLUCCI WS (ed): *Heart Failure: Cardiac Function and Dysfunction*, in *Atlas of Heart Diseases*, vol 4, E Braunwald (series ed). Philadelphia, Current Medicine, 1995

———, BRAUNWALD E: Pathophysiology of heart failure, in *Heart Disease*, 5th ed, E Braunwald (ed). Philadelphia, Saunders, 1997, pp 394–420

FORBES MS, SPERELAKIS N: Ultrastructure of mammalian cardiac muscle, in *Physiology and Pathophysiology of the Heart*, 3d ed, N Sperelakis (ed). Boston, Kluwer Academic, 1995, pp 1–35

HEIN S et al: Altered expression of titin and contractile proteins in failing human myocardium. J Mol Cell Biol 26:1291, 1994

KATZ AM: Heart failure, in *Physiology of the Heart*, 2d ed. New York, Raven Press, 1992, pp 638–668

LITTLE WC, BRAUNWALD E: Assessment of cardiac function, in *Heart Disease*, 5th ed, E Braunwald (ed). Philadelphia, Saunders, 1997, pp 421–444

OPIE LH: Mechanisms of cardiac contraction and relaxation, in *Heart Disease*, 5th ed, E Braunwald (ed). Philadelphia, Saunders, 1997, pp 360–393

REEVES JP: Cardiac sodium-calcium exchange system, in *Physiology and Pathophysiology of the Heart*, 3d ed, N Sperelakis (ed). Boston, Kluwer Academic, 1995, pp 309–318

SCHWARTZ K, MERCADIER J-J: Molecular and cellular biology of heart failure. Curr Opin Cardiol 11:227, 1996

SOLARO RJ et al: Regulatory proteins and diastolic relaxation, in *Diastolic Relaxation of the Heart*, BH Lorell, W Grossman (eds). Boston, Kluwer Academic, 1994, pp 43–53

WOLFF MR et al: Rate of tension development in cardiac muscle varies with level of activator calcium. Circ Res 76:154, 1995

HEART FAILURE

Heart failure is the pathophysiologic state in which an abnormality of *cardiac* function is responsible for the failure of the heart to pump blood at a rate commensurate with the requirements of the metabolizing tissues *and/or* can do so only from an abnormally elevated diastolic volume. Heart failure is frequently, but not always, caused by a defect in myocardial contraction, and then the term *myocardial failure* is appropriate. The latter may result from a primary abnormality in heart muscle, as occurs in the cardiomyopathies and in viral myocarditis (Chap. 239). Myocardial failure also may result from extramyocardial abnormalities, such as coronary atherosclerosis which leads to myocardial ischemia and infarction, as well as from abnormalities of the heart valves in which the heart muscle is damaged by the long-standing excessive hemodynamic burden imposed by the valvular abnormality, and/or by the rheumatic process (Chap. 236).

In other patients with heart failure, however, a similar clinical syndrome is present but without any detectable abnormality of *myocardial* function. In some of these patients the normal heart is suddenly presented with a mechanical load that exceeds its capacity, such as an acute hypertensive crisis, rupture of an aortic valve cusp, or massive pulmonary embolism. Heart failure, in the presence of normal myocardial function, also occurs in chronic conditions in which there is impairment of filling of the ventricles due to a mechanical abnormality such as tricuspid and/or mitral stenosis, constrictive pericarditis without myocardial involvement, endocardial fibrosis, and some forms of hypertrophic cardiomyopathy. In many patients with heart failure, particularly those with valvular or congenital heart disease, a combination of impaired myocardial function and mechanical abnormality exists.

Heart failure should be distinguished from (1) conditions in which there is circulatory congestion consequent to abnormal salt and water retention but in which there is no disturbance of cardiac function per se (the latter syndrome, termed the *congested state*, may result from the abnormal salt and water retention of renal failure or from excess parenteral administration of fluids and electrolytes) and (2) noncardiac causes of inadequate cardiac output, including shock due to hypovolemia and redistribution of blood volume (Chap. 38).

The ventricles respond to a chronically increased hemodynamic burden with the development of hypertrophy. With volume overload when the ventricle is called on to deliver an elevated cardiac output for prolonged periods, as in valvular regurgitation, it develops *eccentric hypertrophy,* i.e., cavity dilatation, with an increase in muscle mass so that the ratio between wall thickness and ventricular cavity size remains relatively constant. With chronic pressure overload, as in valvular aortic stenosis or untreated hypertension, it develops *concentric hypertrophy,* in which the ratio between wall thickness and ventricular cavity size increases. In both conditions, a stable hyperfunctioning state may exist for many years, but myocardial function may ultimately deteriorate, leading to heart failure. Heart failure represents a major public health problem in industrialized nations. It appears to be the only common cardiovascular condition that is increasing in prevalence and incidence. In the United States, heart failure is responsible for almost 1 million hospital admissions and 40,000 deaths annually. Since heart failure is more common in the elderly, its prevalence is likely to continue to increase as the population ages.

CAUSES OF HEART FAILURE

In evaluating patients with heart failure, it is important to identify not only the *underlying cause* of the heart disease but also the *precipitating cause* of heart failure. The cardiac abnormality produced by a congenital or acquired lesion such as valvular aortic stenosis may exist for many years and produce no clinical disability. Frequently, however, clinical manifestations of heart failure appear for the first time in the course of some acute disturbance that places an additional load on a myocardium that chronically is excessively burdened. The heart may be compensated but have little additional reserve, and the additional load imposed by a precipitating cause results in further deterioration of cardiac function. Identification of such precipitating causes is of critical importance because their prompt alleviation may be lifesaving. In the absence of underlying heart disease, these acute disturbances do not usually, by themselves, lead to heart failure.

PRECIPITATING CAUSES

1. *Infection.* Patients with pulmonary vascular congestion are also more susceptible to pulmonary infections; any infection may precipitate heart failure. The resulting fever, tachycardia, and hypoxemia and the increased metabolic demands may place a further burden on the overloaded, but compensated myocardium of a patient with chronic heart disease.

2. *Anemia.* In the presence of anemia, the oxygen needs of the metabolizing tissues can be met only by an increase in the cardiac output (Chap. 59). Although such an increase in cardiac output can be sustained by a normal heart, a diseased, overloaded, but otherwise compensated heart may be unable to augment sufficiently the volume of blood that it delivers to the periphery. In this manner, the combination of anemia and previously compensated heart disease can lead to inadequate oxygen delivery to the periphery and precipitate heart failure.

3. *Thyrotoxicosis and pregnancy.* As in anemia and fever, in thyrotoxicosis and pregnancy, adequate tissue perfusion requires an increased cardiac output. The development or intensification of heart failure may actually be one of the first clinical manifestations of hyperthyroidism in a patient with underlying heart disease that was previously compensated (Chap. 331). Similarly, heart failure not infrequently occurs for the first time during pregnancy in women with rheumatic valvular disease, in whom cardiac compensation may return following delivery.

4. *Arrhythmias.* In patients with compensated heart disease, arrhythmias are among the most frequent precipitating causes of heart failure. They exert a deleterious effect for a variety of reasons: (a) Tachyarrhythmias reduce the time period available for ventricular filling. In patients with ischemic heart disease, tachyarrhythmias also may cause ischemic myocardial dysfunction. (b) The dissociation between atrial and ventricular contractions characteristic of many arrhythmias results in the loss of the atrial booster pump mechanism, thereby raising atrial pressures. (c) In any arrhythmia associated with abnormal intraventricular conduction, myocardial performance may become further impaired because of the loss of normal synchronicity of ventricular contraction. (d) Marked bradycardia associated with complete atrioventricular block or other severe bradyarrhythmias reduces cardiac output unless stroke volume rises reciprocally; this compensatory response cannot occur with serious myocardial dysfunction even in the absence of heart failure.

5. *Rheumatic and other forms of myocarditis.* Acute rheumatic fever and a variety of other inflammatory or infectious processes affecting the myocardium may impair myocardial function in patients with or without preexisting heart disease (Chaps. 236 and 239).

6. *Infective endocarditis.* The additional valvular damage, anemia, fever, and myocarditis that often occur as a consequence of infective endocarditis may, singly or in concert, precipitate heart failure (Chap. 126).

7. *Physical, dietary, fluid, environmental, and emotional excesses.* The augmentation of sodium intake, the inappropriate discontinuation of medications to treat heart failure, blood transfusions, physical overexertion, excessive environmental heat or humidity, and emotional crises all may precipitate heart failure in patients with heart disease who were previously compensated.

8. *Systemic hypertension.* Rapid elevation of arterial pressure, as may occur in some instances of hypertension of renal origin or upon discontinuation of antihypertensive medication, may result in cardiac decompensation (Chap. 246).

9. *Myocardial infarction.* In patients with chronic but compensated ischemic heart disease, a fresh infarct, sometimes otherwise silent clinically, may further impair ventricular function and precipitate heart failure (Chap. 243).

10. *Pulmonary embolism.* Physically inactive patients with low cardiac output are at increased risk of developing thrombi in the veins of the lower extremities or the pelvis. Pulmonary emboli may result in further elevation of pulmonary arterial pressure, which in turn may produce or intensify ventricular failure. In the presence of pulmonary vascular congestion, such emboli also may cause pulmonary infarction (Chap. 261).

A systematic search for these precipitating causes should be made in every patient with the new development or recent intensification of heart failure, especially if it is refractory to the usual methods of therapy. If properly recognized, the precipitating cause of heart failure usually can be treated more effectively than the underlying cause. Therefore, the prognosis in patients with heart failure in whom a precipitating cause can be identified, treated, and eliminated is more favorable than it is in patients in whom the underlying disease process has advanced to the point of producing heart failure.

FORMS OF HEART FAILURE

Heart failure may be described as *systolic* or *diastolic*, *high-output* or *low-output*, *acute* or *chronic*, *right-sided* or *left-sided*, and *forward* or *backward*. These descriptors are often useful in a clinical setting, particularly early in the patient's course, but late in the course of chronic heart failure the differences between them often become blurred.

SYSTOLIC VERSUS DIASTOLIC FAILURE The distinction between these two forms of heart failure, described on p. 1284 and in Fig. 232-8, relates to whether the principal abnormality is the inability to contract normally and expel sufficient blood (systolic failure) or to relax and fill normally (diastolic failure). The major clinical manifestations of systolic failure relate to an inadequate cardiac output with weakness, fatigue, reduced exercise tolerance, and other symptoms of hypoperfusion, while in diastolic failure they relate principally to an elevation of filling pressures. In many patients, particularly those who have both ventricular hypertrophy *and* dilatation, abnormalities both of contraction and relaxation coexist.

Diastolic heart failure may be caused by increased resistance to ventricular inflow and reduced ventricular diastolic capacity (constrictive pericarditis and restrictive, hypertensive, and hypertrophic cardiomyopathy), impaired ventricular relaxation (acute myocardial ischemia, hypertrophic cardiomyopathy), and myocardial fibrosis and infiltration (dilated, chronic ischemic, and restrictive cardiomyopathy).

HIGH-OUTPUT VERSUS LOW-OUTPUT HEART FAILURE It is useful to classify patients with heart failure into those with a low cardiac output, i.e., *low-output heart failure*, and those with an elevated cardiac output, i.e., *high-output heart failure*. The former occurs secondary to ischemic heart disease, hypertension, dilated cardiomyopathy, and valvular and pericardial disease, while the latter is seen in patients with heart failure and hyperthyroidism, anemia, pregnancy, arteriovenous fistulas, beriberi, and Paget's disease. In clinical practice, however, low-output and high-output heart failure cannot always be readily distinguished. The normal range of cardiac output is wide [2.2 to 3.5 (L/min)/m²], and in many patients with so-called low-output heart failure the cardiac output may actually be just within the normal range at rest (although it is lower than it had been previously), but it fails to rise normally during exertion. On the other hand, in patients with so-called high-output heart failure the output may not exceed the upper limits of normal (although it would have been elevated had it been measured before heart failure supervened), but rather it may have fallen to the upper limit of normal. Regardless of the *absolute* level of the cardiac output, however, cardiac failure may be said to be present when the characteristic clinical manifestations described below are accompanied

by a depression of the curve relating ventricular end-diastolic volume to cardiac performance (see Fig. 232-6).

An integral physiologic component of *systolic* heart failure (p. 1284) is the delivery of an inadequate quantity of oxygen required by the metabolizing tissues. In the absence of peripheral shunting of blood, this is reflected in an abnormal widening of the normal arterial–mixed venous oxygen difference (35 to 50 mL/L in the basal state). In mild cases, such an abnormality may not be present at rest but becomes evident only during exertion or other hypermetabolic states. In patients with high cardiac output states, such as those associated with arteriovenous fistula or thyrotoxicosis, the arterial–mixed venous oxygen difference is normal or low. The mixed venous oxygen saturation is raised by the admixture of blood that has been diverted from the metabolizing tissues, and it may be presumed that even in these patients the delivery of oxygen to the latter is reduced despite the normal or even elevated mixed venous oxygen saturation. When heart failure occurs in such patients, the arterial–mixed venous oxygen difference, regardless of the absolute value, still exceeds the level that existed prior to the development of heart failure. Therefore, the cardiac output, though normal or even elevated, is lower than before heart failure supervened.

The mechanisms responsible for the development of heart failure in patients whose cardiac outputs are initially high are complex and depend on the underlying disease process. In most of these conditions the heart is called on to pump abnormally large quantities of blood in order to deliver the normal quota of oxygen to the metabolizing tissues. The burden placed on the myocardium by the increased flow load resembles that produced by chronic regurgitant valvular lesions. In addition, thyrotoxicosis and beriberi also may impair myocardial metabolism directly, while severe anemia may interfere with myocardial function by producing myocardial anoxia, especially in the presence of underlying obstructive artery disease.

ACUTE VERSUS CHRONIC HEART FAILURE The prototype of acute heart failure is the patient who is entirely well but who suddenly develops a large myocardial infarction or rupture of a cardiac valve. Chronic heart failure is typically observed in patients with dilated cardiomyopathy or multivalvular heart disease that develops or progresses slowly. Acute heart failure is usually largely systolic, and the sudden reduction in cardiac output often results in systemic hypotension without peripheral edema. In chronic heart failure, arterial pressure tends to be well maintained until very late in the course, but there is often accumulation of edema. Despite these obvious differences in clinical presentation, there is no fundamental distinction between acute and chronic heart failure. For example, intensive efforts to prevent expansion of blood volume by means of dietary sodium restriction and the administration of diuretics will frequently delay the development of exertional dyspnea and edema in patients with chronic valvular heart disease (i.e., it will mask the clinical manifestations of chronic heart failure) until an acute episode, such as an arrhythmia or infection, precipitates acute heart failure. Without intensive efforts to restrict blood volume, the same patients would have been considered to have been suffering from chronic heart failure, even though their underlying myocardial disease was no further advanced.

RIGHT-SIDED VERSUS LEFT-SIDED HEART FAILURE Many of the clinical manifestations of heart failure result from the accumulation of excess fluid behind either one or both ventricles (Chaps. 32 and 37). This fluid usually localizes upstream to (behind) the specific cardiac chamber that is initially affected. For example, patients in whom the left ventricle is mechanically overloaded (e.g., aortic stenosis) or weakened (e.g., postmyocardial infarction) develop dyspnea and orthopnea as a result of pulmonary congestion, a condition referred to as *left-sided heart failure*. In contrast, when the underlying abnormality affects the right ventricle primarily (e.g., valvular pulmonic stenosis or pulmonary hypertension secondary to pulmonary thromboembolism), symptoms resulting from pulmonary congestion such as orthopnea or paroxysmal nocturnal dyspnea are less common, and edema, congestive hepatomegaly, and systemic venous distention, i.e., clinical manifestations of *right-sided heart failure*, are more prominent. However, when heart failure has existed for months or years, such localization of excess fluid behind the failing ventricle may no longer exist. For example, patients with long-standing aortic valve disease or systemic hypertension may have ankle edema, congestive hepatomegaly, and systemic venous distention late in the course of their disease, even though the abnormal hemodynamic burden initially was placed on the left ventricle. This occurs in part because of the secondary pulmonary hypertension and resultant right-sided heart failure but also because of the retention of salt and water characteristic of all forms of heart failure (Chap. 37). The muscle bundles composing both ventricles are continuous, and both ventricles share a common wall, the interventricular septum. Also, biochemical changes that occur in heart failure and that may be involved in the impairment of myocardial function (Chap. 232), such as norepinephrine depletion and alterations in the activity of myosin ATPase, occur in the myocardium of *both* ventricles, regardless of the specific chamber on which the abnormal hemodynamic burden is placed initially.

BACKWARD VERSUS FORWARD HEART FAILURE For many years a controversy has revolved around the question of the mechanism of the clinical manifestations resulting from heart failure. The concept of *backward heart failure* contends that in heart failure, one or the other ventricle fails to discharge its contents or fails to fill normally. As a consequence, the pressures in the atrium and venous system behind the failing ventricle rise, and retention of sodium and water occurs as a consequence of the elevation of systemic venous and capillary pressures and the resultant transudation of fluid into the interstitial space (Chap. 37). In contrast, the proponents of the *forward heart failure* hypothesis maintain that the clinical manifestations of heart failure result directly from an inadequate discharge of blood into the arterial system. According to this concept, salt and water retention is a consequence of diminished renal perfusion and excessive proximal tubular sodium reabsorption and of excessive distal tubular reabsorption through activation of the renin-angiotensin-aldosterone system.

A rigid distinction between *backward* and *forward* heart failure (like a rigid distinction between right and left heart failure) is artificial, since both mechanisms appear to operate to varying extents in most patients with heart failure. However, the rate of onset of heart failure often influences the clinical manifestations. For example, when a large portion of the left ventricle is suddenly destroyed, as in myocardial infarction, although stroke volume and blood pressure are suddenly reduced (both manifestations of forward failure), the patient may succumb to acute pulmonary edema, a manifestation of backward failure. If the patient survives the acute insult, clinical manifestations resulting from a chronically depressed cardiac output, including the abnormal retention of fluid within the systemic vascular bed, may develop. Similarly, in the case of massive pulmonary embolism, the right ventricle may dilate and the systemic venous pressure may rise to high levels (backward failure), or the patient may develop shock secondary to low cardiac output (forward failure), but this low-output state may have to be maintained for some days before sodium and water retention sufficient to produce peripheral edema occurs.

REDISTRIBUTION OF CARDIAC OUTPUT The redistribution of cardiac output serves as an important compensatory mechanism when cardiac output is reduced. This redistribution is most marked when a patient with heart failure exercises, but as heart failure advances, redistribution occurs even in the basal state. Blood flow is redistributed so that the delivery of oxygen to vital organs, such as the brain and myocardium, is maintained at normal or near-normal levels, while flow to less critical areas, such as the cutaneous and muscular beds and viscera, is reduced. Vasoconstriction mediated by the adrenergic nervous system is largely responsible for this redistribution, which in turn may be responsible for many of the clinical manifestations of heart failure, such as fluid accumulation (reduction of renal flow), low-grade fever (reduction of cutaneous flow), and fatigue (reduction of muscle flow).

SALT AND WATER RETENTION (See also Chap. 37)

When the volume of blood pumped by the left ventricle into the systemic vascular bed is reduced, a complex sequence of adjustments occurs that ultimately results in the abnormal accumulation of fluid. On the one hand, many of the troubling clinical manifestations of heart failure are secondary to this excessive retention of fluid; on the other, this abnormal fluid accumulation and the expansion of blood volume that accompanies it also constitute an important compensatory mechanism that tends to maintain cardiac output and therefore perfusion of the vital organs. Except in the terminal stages of heart failure, the ventricle operates on an ascending, albeit depressed and flattened, function curve (Fig. 232-6), and the augmented ventricular end-diastolic volume and pressure characteristic of heart failure must be regarded as helping to maintain the reduced cardiac output, despite causing pulmonary and/or systemic venous congestion.

Congestive heart failure is also characterized by a complex series of neurohumoral adjustments. The activation of the adrenergic nervous system is discussed on p. 1285; there is also activation of the renin-angiotensin-aldosterone system and increased release of antidiuretic hormone. These influences elevate systemic vascular resistance and enhance sodium and water retention and potassium excretion. These actions are, to a minor extent, opposed by the release of atrial natriuretic peptide, which also occurs in congestive heart failure. Patients with severe heart failure may exhibit a reduced capacity to excrete a water load, which may result in dilutional hyponatremia. In the presence of heart failure, effective filling of the systemic arterial bed is reduced, a condition that initiates the renal and hormonal changes mentioned above.

The elevation of systemic venous pressure and the alterations of renal and adrenal function characteristic of heart failure vary in their relative importance in the production of edema in different patients with heart failure. The renin-angiotensin-aldosterone axis is activated most intensely by acute heart failure, and its activity tends to decline as heart failure becomes chronic. In patients with tricuspid valve disease or constrictive pericarditis, the elevated venous pressure and the transudation of fluid from systemic capillaries appear to play the dominant role in edema formation. On the other hand, severe edema may be present in patients with ischemic or hypertensive heart disease, in whom systemic venous pressure is within normal limits or is only minimally elevated. In such patients, the retention of salt and water is probably due primarily to a redistribution of cardiac output and a concomitant reduction in renal perfusion, as well as activation of the renin-angiotensin-aldosterone axis. Regardless of the mechanisms involved in fluid retention, untreated patients with chronic congestive heart failure have elevations of total blood volume, interstitial fluid volume, and body sodium. These abnormalities diminish after clinical compensation has been achieved by treatment.

CLINICAL MANIFESTATIONS OF HEART FAILURE

Dyspnea Respiratory distress that occurs as the result of increased effort in breathing is the most common symptom of heart failure (Chap. 32). In early heart failure, dyspnea is observed only during activity, when it may simply represent an aggravation of the breathlessness that occurs normally under these circumstances. As heart failure advances, however, dyspnea appears with progressively less strenuous activity. Ultimately, breathlessness is present even when the patient is at rest. The principal difference between exertional dyspnea in normal persons and in patients with heart failure is the degree of activity necessary to induce the symptom. Cardiac dyspnea is observed most frequently in patients with elevations of pulmonary venous and capillary pressures. Such patients usually have engorged pulmonary vessels and interstitial pulmonary edema, which may be evident on radiologic examination. This reduces the compliance of the lungs and thereby increases the work of the respiratory muscles required to inflate the lungs. The activation of receptors in the lungs results in the rapid, shallow breathing characteristic of cardiac dyspnea. The oxygen cost of breathing is increased by the excessive work of the respiratory muscles. This is coupled with the diminished delivery of oxygen to these muscles, which occurs as a consequence of the reduced cardiac output and which may contribute to fatigue of the respiratory muscles and the sensation of shortness of breath.

Orthopnea Dyspnea in the recumbent position is usually a later manifestation of heart failure than exertional dyspnea. Orthopnea occurs because of the redistribution of fluid from the abdomen and lower extremities into the chest causing an increase in the pulmonary capillary hydrostatic pressure, as well as elevation of the diaphragm accompanying supine posture. Patients with orthopnea must elevate their heads on several pillows at night and frequently awaken short of breath or coughing (the so-called nocturnal cough) if their heads slip off the pillows. The sensation of breathlessness usually is relieved by sitting upright, since this position reduces venous return and pulmonary capillary pressure, and many patients report that they find relief from sitting in front of an open window. In far-advanced heart failure, orthopnea may become so severe that patients cannot lie down at all and must spend the entire night in a sitting position. On the other hand, in other patients with long-standing, severe left ventricular failure, symptoms of pulmonary congestion may actually diminish with time as the function of the right ventricle becomes impaired.

Paroxysmal (Nocturnal) Dyspnea This term refers to attacks of severe shortness of breath and coughing that generally occur at night, usually awaken the patient from sleep, and may be quite frightening. Though simple orthopnea may be relieved by sitting upright at the side of the bed with legs dependent, in the patient with paroxysmal nocturnal dyspnea, coughing and wheezing often persist even in this position. The depression of the respiratory center during sleep may reduce ventilation sufficiently to lower arterial oxygen tension, particularly in patients with interstitial lung edema and reduced pulmonary compliance. Also, ventricular function may be further impaired at night because of reduced adrenergic stimulation of myocardial function. *Cardiac asthma* is closely related to paroxysmal nocturnal dyspnea and nocturnal cough and is characterized by wheezing secondary to bronchospasm—most prominent at night. *Acute pulmonary edema* (Chap. 32) is a severe form of cardiac asthma due to marked elevation of pulmonary capillary pressure leading to alveolar edema, associated with extreme shortness of breath, rales over the lung fields, and the transudation and expectoration of blood-tinged fluid. If not treated promptly, acute pulmonary edema may be fatal.

Cheyne-Stokes Respiration Also known as *periodic* or *cyclic respiration*, Cheyne-Stokes respiration is characterized by diminished sensitivity of the respiratory center to arterial P_{CO_2}. There is an apneic phase, during which the arterial P_{O_2} falls and the arterial P_{CO_2} rises. These changes in the arterial blood stimulate the depressed respiratory center, resulting in hyperventilation and hypocapnia, followed in turn by recurrence of apnea. Cheyne-Stokes respiration occurs most often in patients with cerebral atherosclerosis and other cerebral lesions, but the prolongation of the circulation time from the lung to the brain that occurs in heart failure, particularly in patients with hypertension and coronary artery disease and associated cerebral vascular disease, also appears to precipitate this form of breathing.

Fatigue, Weakness, and Abdominal Symptoms These nonspecific but common symptoms of heart failure are related to the reduction of perfusion of skeletal muscle. Exercise capacity is reduced by the limited ability of the failing heart to increase its output and deliver oxygen to the exercising muscle. Anorexia and nausea associated with abdominal pain and fullness are frequent complaints and may be related to the congested liver and portal venous system.

Cerebral Symptoms In severe heart failure, particularly in elderly patients with accompanying cerebral arteriosclerosis, reduced cerebral perfusion, and arterial hypoxemia, there may be alterations in the mental state characterized by confusion, difficulty in concentration, impairment of memory, headache, insomnia, and anxiety. *Nocturia* is common in heart failure and may contribute to insomnia.

PHYSICAL FINDINGS (See Chap. 227) In moderate heart failure, the patient appears to be in no distress at rest except that he or she may be uncomfortable when lying flat for more than a few minutes. In more severe heart failure, the pulse pressure may be diminished, reflecting a reduction in stroke volume, and occasionally, the diastolic arterial pressure is elevated as a consequence of generalized vasoconstriction. In acute heart failure, hypotension may be prominent. There may be cyanosis of the lips and nail beds and sinus tachycardia, and the patient may insist on sitting upright. *Systemic venous pressure* is often abnormally elevated in heart failure and may be recognized by observing the extent of distention of the jugular veins. In the early stages of heart failure, the venous pressure may be normal at rest but may become abnormally elevated during and immediately after exertion as well as with sustained pressure on the abdomen (positive abdominojugular reflux).

Third and fourth heart sounds are often audible but are not specific for heart failure, and *pulsus alternans*, i.e., a regular rhythm in which there is alternation of strong and weak cardiac contractions and therefore alternation in the strength of the peripheral pulses, may be present. Pulsus alternans, a sign of severe heart failure, may be detected by sphygmomanometry and in more severe instances by palpation; it frequently follows an extrasystole and is observed most commonly in patients with cardiomyopathy or hypertensive or ischemic heart disease.

Pulmonary Rales Moist, inspiratory, crepitant rales and dullness to percussion over the lung bases are common in patients with heart failure and elevated pulmonary venous and capillary pressures. In patients with pulmonary edema, rales may be heard widely over both lung fields; they are frequently coarse and sibilant and may be accompanied by expiratory wheezing. Rales may, however, be caused by many conditions other than left ventricular failure. Some patients with long-standing heart failure have no rales because of increased lymphatic drainage of alveolar fluid.

Cardiac Edema (See Chap. 37) This is usually dependent, occurring in the legs symmetrically, particularly in the pretibial region and ankles in ambulatory patients, in whom it is most prominent in the evening, and in the sacral region of individuals at bed rest. Pitting edema of the arms and face occurs rarely and then only late in the course of heart failure.

Hydrothorax and Ascites Pleural effusion in congestive heart failure results from the elevation of pleural capillary pressure and transudation of fluid into the pleural cavities. Since the pleural veins drain into *both* the systemic and pulmonary veins, hydrothorax occurs most commonly with marked elevation of pressure in both venous systems but also may be seen with marked elevation of pressure in either venous bed. It is more frequent in the right pleural cavity than in the left. *Ascites* also occurs as a consequence of transudation and results from increased pressure in the hepatic veins and the veins draining the peritoneum (Chap. 46). Marked ascites occurs most frequently in patients with tricuspid valve disease and constrictive pericarditis.

Congestive Hepatomegaly An enlarged, tender, pulsating liver also accompanies systemic venous hypertension and is observed not only in the same conditions in which ascites occurs but also in milder forms of heart failure from any cause. With prolonged, severe hepatomegaly, as in patients with tricuspid valve disease or chronic constrictive pericarditis, enlargement of the spleen, i.e., congestive splenomegaly, also may occur.

Jaundice This is a late finding in congestive heart failure and is associated with elevations of both the direct- and indirect-reacting bilirubin; it results from impairment of hepatic function secondary to hepatic congestion and the hepatocellular hypoxia associated with central lobular atrophy. Serum transaminase concentrations are frequently elevated. If hepatic congestion occurs acutely, the jaundice may be severe and the enzymes strikingly elevated.

Cardiac Cachexia With severe chronic heart failure there may be serious weight loss and cachexia because of (1) elevation of circulating concentrations of tumor necrosis factor; (2) elevation of the metabolic rate, which results in part from the extra work performed by the respiratory muscles, the increased oxygen needs of the hypertrophied heart, and/or the discomfort associated with severe heart failure; (3)

anorexia, nausea, and vomiting due to central causes, to digitalis intoxication, or to congestive hepatomegaly and abdominal fullness; (4) impairment of intestinal absorption due to congestion of the intestinal veins; and (5) rarely, in patients with particularly severe failure of the right side of the heart, protein-losing enteropathy.

Other Manifestations With reduction of blood flow, the extremities may be cold, pale, and diaphoretic. Urine flow is depressed, and the urine contains albumin and has a high specific gravity and a low concentration of sodium. In addition, prerenal azotemia may be present. In patients with long-standing severe heart failure, impotence and depression are common.

ROENTGENOGRAPHIC FINDINGS In addition to the enlargement of the particular chambers characteristic of the lesion responsible for heart failure, distention of pulmonary veins and redistribution to the apices is common in patients with heart failure and elevated pulmonary vascular pressures. Also, pleural effusions may be evident and associated with interlobar effusions.

DIFFERENTIAL DIAGNOSIS The diagnosis of congestive heart failure may be established by observing some combination of the clinical manifestations of heart failure described above, together with the findings characteristic of one of the etiologic forms of heart disease. Table 233-1 shows the Framingham criteria, which are useful in the diagnosis of heart failure. Since chronic heart failure is often associated with cardiac enlargement, the diagnosis should be questioned, but is by no means excluded, when all chambers are normal in size. Two-dimensional echocardiography is particularly useful in assessing the dimensions of each cardiac chamber. Heart failure may be difficult to distinguish from pulmonary disease, and the differential diagnosis is discussed in Chap. 32. Pulmonary embolism also presents many of the manifestations of heart failure, but hemoptysis, pleuritic chest pain, a right ventricular lift, and the characteristic mismatch between ventilation and perfusion on lung scan should point to this diagnosis (see Chap. 261).

Ankle edema may be due to varicose veins, cyclic edema, or gravitational effects (Chap. 37), but in these patients there is no jugular venous hypertension at rest or with pressure over the abdomen. Edema secondary to renal disease can usually be recognized by appropriate renal function tests and urinalysis and is rarely associated with elevation of venous pressure. Enlargement of the liver and ascites occur in patients with hepatic cirrhosis and also may be distinguished from heart failure by normal jugular venous pressure and absence of a positive abdominojugular reflux.

 TREATMENT

The treatment of heart failure may be divided logically into three components: (1) removal of the precipitating cause, (2) correction of the underlying cause, and (3) control of the congestive heart failure state. The first two are discussed in other chapters together with each specific disease entity or complication. An example is the treatment of pneumococcal pneumonia and acute heart failure (removal of the precipitating cause) followed by mitral valvotomy (correction of the underlying cause) in a patient with mitral stenosis. In many instances, surgical treatment will correct or at least alleviate the underlying cause. The third component of the treatment of heart failure, i.e., control of the congestive heart failure state, may, in turn, be divided into three categories: (1) reduction of cardiac work load, including both the preload and the afterload; (2) control of excessive retention of salt and water; and (3) enhancement of myocardial contractility. The vigor with which each of these measures is pursued in any individual patient should depend on the severity of heart failure. Following effective treatment, recurrence of the clinical manifestations of heart failure can often be prevented by continuing those measures that were originally effective.

While a simple rule for the treatment of all patients with heart failure cannot be formulated because of the varied etiologies, hemodynamic features, clinical manifestations, and severity of heart failure, insofar as the treatment of chronic congestive failure is concerned, the administration of an angiotensin-converting enzyme inhibitor (e.g., lisinopril 10 mg q.d.) has been shown to retard the development of heart failure and should be begun early in patients with cardiac dilatation and/or hypertrophy, even if they are asymptomatic. Then, as symptoms develop, simple measures such as moderate restriction of activity and sodium intake should be tried (Fig. 233-1). If these and the ACE inhibitor are insufficient, therapy with a combination of a diuretic, a vasodilator, and usually a digitalis glycoside is then begun. The next step is more rigorous restriction of salt intake and higher doses of loop diuretics, sometimes accompanied by other diuretics. If heart failure persists, hospitalization with rigid salt restriction, bed rest, intravenous vasodilators, and positive inotropic agents comes next. In some patients, the order in which these measures are applied may be altered.

Table 233-1

Framingham Criteria for Diagnosis of Congestive Heart Failure*

MAJOR CRITERIA

Paroxysmal nocturnal dyspnea
Neck vein distention
Rales
Cardiomegaly
Acute pulmonary edema
S_3 gallop
Increased venous pressure (>16 cmH$_2$O)
Positive hepatojugular reflux

MINOR CRITERIA

Extremity edema
Night cough
Dyspnea on exertion
Hepatomegaly
Pleural effusion
Vital capacity reduced by one-third from normal
Tachycardia (≥120 bpm)

MAJOR OR MINOR

Weight loss ≥4.5 kg over 5 days' treatment

* To establish a clinical diagnosis of congestive heart failure by these criteria, at least one major and two minor criteria are required.

SOURCE: KKL Ho et al, Circulation 88:107, 1993.

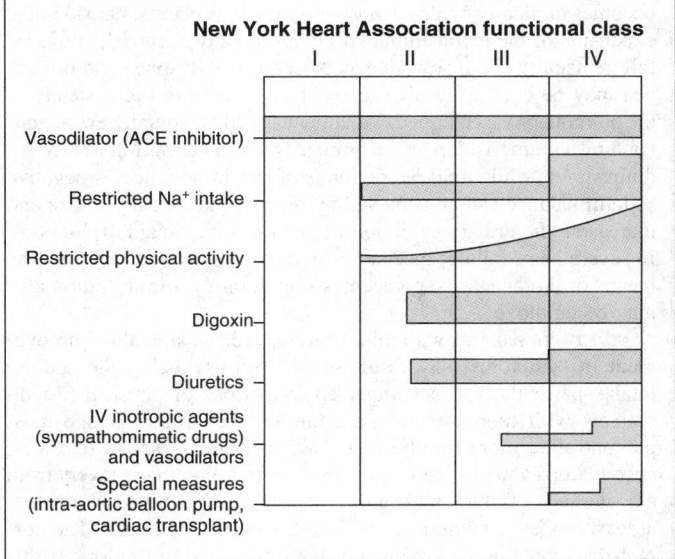

FIGURE 233-1 Overview of the treatment of heart failure. *[From RA Kelly, TW Smith: Treatment of stable heart failure: Digitalis and diuretics, in Heart Failure: Cardiac Function and Dysfunction, in WS Colucci (ed), Atlas of Heart Diseases, vol 4, E Braunwald (series ed), Philadelphia, Current Medicine, 1995.]*

Reduction of Cardiac Work Load This consists of reducing physical activity, instituting emotional rest, and reducing afterload. Modest restriction of physical activity in mild cases and rest in bed or in a chair in severe failure remain cornerstones in the treatment of heart failure. Meals should be small in quantity but perhaps more frequent, and every effort should be made to diminish the patient's anxiety; sometimes drugs such as diazepam (2 to 5 mg tid) for several days are useful. Physical and emotional rest tends to lower arterial pressure and reduce the load on the myocardium by diminishing the requirements for cardiac output. These influences act in concert to diminish the need for redistribution of the cardiac output, and in many patients, particularly those with mild heart failure, simple bed rest and mild sedation often result in an effective diuresis.

Rest should be maintained for 1 to 2 weeks in patients with overt congestive failure and should be continued for several days after the patient's condition has stabilized. The hazards of phlebothrombosis and pulmonary embolism which occur with bed rest may be reduced with anticoagulants, leg exercises, and elastic stockings. *Absolute* bed rest rarely is required or advisable, and the patient should be encouraged to sit in a chair and be given toilet privileges unless heart failure is extreme. Heavy sedation should be avoided, but small doses of tranquilizers may be helpful in calming the emotionally disturbed patient during the first few days of therapy and in permitting much-needed sleep. In patients with chronic, moderately severe heart failure, additional periods of bed rest on weekends frequently allow continuation of gainful employment. Following recovery from heart failure, the patient's activities should be assessed, and often, professional, community, and/or family responsibilities must be curtailed. Intermittent rest during the day (e.g., a scheduled 1-h nap or rest following lunch) and the avoidance of strenuous exertion are often helpful once compensation has been restored. Weight reduction by restriction of caloric intake in obese patients with heart failure also diminishes cardiac work load and is an essential component of the therapeutic program. Vasodilator therapy (p. 1293) may be considered a form of reduction of the cardiac work load. This form of therapy has been shown not only to ameliorate heart failure but also to retard its development in patients with left ventricular dysfunction.

Control of Excessive Fluid Many of the clinical manifestations of heart failure result from hypervolemia and expansion of the interstitial fluid volume. By the time fluid retention due to heart failure becomes clinically evident, most commonly as edema, considerable expansion of the extracellular space has already occurred, and heart failure usually is already advanced. Exertional dyspnea and orthopnea may be caused by displacement of fluid from the systemic to the pulmonary vascular bed. Treatment aimed at reducing extracellular fluid volume is dependent primarily on lowering total-body sodium stores, while fluid restriction is of less importance. A negative sodium balance can be achieved by reducing the dietary intake and increasing the urinary excretion of this ion with the aid of diuretics. In severe heart failure, mechanical removal of extracellular fluid by means of thoracentesis, paracentesis, and, rarely, ultrafiltration also may be employed.

DIET In patients with mild heart failure, considerable improvement in symptoms may result simply from reducing the sodium intake, particularly if accompanied by periods of physical rest. In patients with more severe heart failure, the sodium intake must be controlled more rigidly, and other measures, such as diuretics, vasodilators, and glycosides, are used. Even following recovery from a bout of heart failure, if the underlying cause has not been corrected, at least moderate sodium restriction should be maintained. The normal diet contains approximately 6 to 10 g sodium chloride; this intake can be reduced by half simply by excluding salt-rich foods and salt added at the table. Reduction of the ordinary dietary intake to approximately one-fourth of normal may be achieved if, in addition, all salt is omitted from cooking. In patients with severe heart

failure, in whom the daily sodium chloride intake should be reduced to between 500 and 1000 mg, milk, cheese, bread, cereals, canned vegetables and soups, some salted cuts of meat, and some fresh vegetables, including spinach, celery, and beets, must be eliminated. A variety of fresh fruit, green vegetables, specially processed breads and milk, and salt substitutes are permissible, but it is difficult to keep such diets palatable over the long term. Water intake may be ad libitum in all but the most severe forms of congestive heart failure. Late in the course of heart failure, dilutional hyponatremia may develop in patients who are unable to excrete a water load, sometimes because of excessive secretion of antidiuretic hormone. In such cases, water intake as well as sodium intake must be restricted.

Attention also must be directed to the caloric content of the diet. Calories should be restricted in obese patients with heart failure. On the other hand, in patients with severe heart failure and cardiac cachexia, an attempt must be made to maintain nutritional intake and to avoid caloric and vitamin deficiencies; nutritional supplements may be in order.

DIURETICS A variety of diuretic agents are available (Table 246-4, p. 1387), and in patients with mild heart failure, almost all are effective. However, in the more severe forms of heart failure, the selection of diuretics is more difficult, and abnormalities in serum electrolytes must be taken into account. Overtreatment must be avoided, since the resultant hypovolemia may reduce cardiac output, interfere with renal function, and produce profound weakness and lethargy. The following is a list of the most widely used diuretics:

1. *Thiazide diuretics.* These agents are used widely in clinical practice because of their effectiveness when administered orally. In patients with chronic heart failure of mild or moderate severity, the continued administration of a thiazide diuretic abolishes or diminishes the need for rigid dietary sodium restriction, although salty foods and table salt still should be avoided. Thiazides are well absorbed following oral administration; chlorothiazide and hydrochlorothiazide reach their peak action in 4 h, and diuresis persists for approximately 12 h. Thiazide diuretics reduce the reabsorption of sodium and chloride in the first half of the distal convoluted tubule and a portion of the cortical ascending limb of the loop of Henle, and water follows the unreabsorbed salt. Thiazides fail to increase free water clearance, and in some instances reduce it, supporting the hypothesis that these drugs inhibit selective reabsorption of sodium chloride in the distal cortical diluting segment, at a site where the urine is normally diluted (Chap. 269). This may result in the excretion of a hypertonic urine and may contribute to dilutional hyponatremia. As a consequence of increased delivery of sodium to the distal nephron, sodium-potassium ion exchange is enhanced, and kaliuresis results. In contrast to the loop diuretics, which enhance calcium excretion, the thiazides have the opposite effect. These drugs are effective and useful in the treatment of heart failure as long as the glomerular filtration rate exceeds approximately 50 percent of normal.

Chlorothiazide is administered in doses of up to 500 mg every 6 h. Many derivatives of this compound are available but differ principally in dosage and duration of action and therefore offer few, if any, significant advantages over the parent compound, except for chlorthalidone, which may be administered once daily. Potassium depletion and metabolic alkalosis (the latter due to increased H^+ secretion as a substitute for the depleted intracellular stores of potassium and increased proximal tubular reabsorption of filtered HCO_3^- when there is relative depletion of the extracellular fluid volume) are the chief adverse metabolic effects following prolonged administration of the thiazides, of metolazone, and of the loop diuretics. Hypokalemia may enhance seriously the dangers of digitalis intoxication, induce fatigue and lethargy, and may be prevented by the oral supplementation of potassium chloride. However, the solution is not palatable and may be hazardous in patients with renal failure. Therefore, to prevent potassium depletion in patients receiving thiazide diuretics, intermittent dosage schedules, e.g., omitting the diuretic every third day, and the addition of a potassium-retaining diuretic, such as a spironolactone or triamterene, may be preferable.

Other side effects of thiazides include reduction of the excretion of uric acid, which may lead to hyperuricemia, and a hyperglycemic effect, which rarely may precipitate hyperosmolar coma in the poorly regulated diabetic patient. Skin rashes, thrombocytopenia, and granulocytopenia also have been reported.

2. *Metolazone.* This quinethazone derivative has a site of action and potency similar to those of the thiazides but has been reported to be effective in the presence of moderate renal failure. The usual dose is 5 to 10 mg/d.

3. *Furosemide, bumetanide, ethacrynic acid, piretanide, and torsemide.* These "loop" diuretics are similar physiologically but differ chemically. These extremely powerful diuretics reversibly inhibit the reabsorption of sodium, potassium, and chloride in the thick ascending limb of Henle's loop, apparently by blocking a cotransport system in the luminal membrane. They may induce renal cortical vasodilatation and can produce rates of urine formation that may be as high as one-fourth of the glomerular filtration rate. While other diuretics lose their effectiveness as blood volume is restored to normal levels, the loop diuretics remain effective despite the elimination of excessive extracellular fluid volume. The major side effects of these agents are due to this marked diuretic potency, which on rare occasions may result in contraction of the plasma volume, circulatory collapse, reductions in the renal blood flow and glomerular filtration rate, and the development of prerenal azotemia. Metabolic alkalosis is produced by a large increase in the urinary excretion of chloride, hydrogen, and potassium ions. Hypokalemia (see discussion of thiazides, above) and hyponatremia may occur, and hyperuricemia and hyperglycemia are observed occasionally, as with thiazide diuretics. The reabsorption of free water is decreased.

All five drugs are readily absorbed orally and are excreted in the bile and urine. They are usually effective by mouth and intravenously. Weakness, nausea, and dizziness may complicate the administration of all loop diuretics; ethacrynic acid has been associated with transient or even permanent deafness as well as with skin rash and granulocytopenia.

These extremely effective diuretics are useful in all forms of heart failure, particularly in otherwise refractory heart failure and pulmonary edema. They have been shown to be effective in patients with hypoalbuminemia, hyponatremia, hypochloremia, hypokalemia, and reductions in the glomerular filtration rate and to produce a diuresis in patients in whom thiazide diuretics and aldosterone antagonists, alone and in combination, are ineffective.

In patients with refractory heart failure, the action of loop diuretics may be potentiated by intravenous administration and the addition of other diuretics, i.e., thiazides, carbonic anhydrase inhibitors, osmotic diuretics, and the potassium-sparing diuretics—spironolactone, triamterene, and amiloride. The latter agents act on the cortical collecting ducts, are relatively weak, and therefore are rarely indicated as sole agents. However, their potassium-sparing properties make them particularly useful in conjunction with the more potent kaliuretic agents, the loop diuretics, and thiazides. The potassium-sparing agents fall into two classes, as noted below.

4. *Aldosterone antagonists.* The 17-spironolactones resemble aldosterone structurally and act on the distal half of the convoluted tubule and the cortical portion of the collecting duct by competitive inhibition of aldosterone, thereby blocking the exchange between sodium and both potassium and hydrogen in the distal tubules and collecting ducts. These agents produce a sodium diuresis, and in contrast to the thiazides, ethacrynic acid, and furosemide, they result in potassium retention. Although secondary hyperaldosteronism exists in some patients with congestive heart failure, the spironolactones are effective even in patients in whom the serum aldosterone concentration is within normal limits. Aldactone A may be administered in doses of 25 to 100 mg three to four times daily by mouth. The maximal effect of this regimen is not observed for approximately 4 days. Spironolactones are most effective when administered in combination with thiazide and/or loop diuretics. The opposing action of these drugs on urine and serum potassium makes possible a sodium diuresis without either hyper- or hypokalemia when spirono-

lactone and one of these other agents are administered in combination. Also, since spironolactone, triamterene, and amiloride act on the distal tubule, they are particularly effective when used in combination with one of these other diuretics that act more proximally.

Spironolactone, triamterene, and amiloride should not be administered alone to patients with hyperkalemia, renal failure, or hyponatremia. Reported complications include nausea, epigastric distress, mental confusion, drowsiness, gynecomastia, and erythematous eruptions.

5. *Triamterene and amiloride.* These two drugs exert renal effects similar to those of the spironolactones; i.e., they block sodium reabsorption and secondarily inhibit potassium secretion in the distal tubules. However, their fundamental mechanism of action differs from that of the spironolactones, since they are active in adrenalectomized animals and their action does not depend on the presence of aldosterone. The effective dose of triamterene is 100 mg once or twice daily, and that of amiloride is 5 mg daily. Side effects include nausea, vomiting, diarrhea, headache, granulocytopenia, eosinophilia, and skin rash. Both triamterene and the chemically unrelated diuretic amiloride resemble Aldactone A in that their diuretic potency is not great, but they are effective in preventing the hypokalemia characteristic of the administration of thiazides, furosemide, and ethacrynic acid. A number of diuretic preparations contain a combination of a thiazide and either triamterene or amiloride in a single capsule. They may be useful in patients who develop hypokalemia with a thiazide but should not be used in patients with impaired renal function and/or hyperkalemia.

When making a *choice of diuretics,* orally administered thiazides and metolazone are the agents of choice in the treatment of chronic cardiac edema of mild to moderate degree in patients without hyperglycemia, hyperuricemia, or hypokalemia. Spironolactones, triamterene, and amiloride are not potent diuretics when used alone, but they potentiate other diuretics, particularly the thiazide and loop diuretics. However, in patients with heart failure and severe secondary hyperaldosteronism, spironolactone may be quite effective. Ethacrynic acid, bumetanide, and furosemide, given alone or with spironolactone or triamterene, are the agents of choice in patients with severe heart failure refractory to other diuretics. In very severe heart failure, the combination of a thiazide, a loop diuretic, and a potassium-sparing diuretic is required.

Vasodilator Therapy In many patients with heart failure, left ventricular afterload is increased as a consequence of the several neural and humoral influences that act to constrict the peripheral vascular bed. These include the previously mentioned increased activity of the adrenergic nervous system, elevation of circulating catecholamines, and activation of the renin-angiotensin system, and perhaps increased circulating antidiuretic hormone. In addition to the vasoconstriction, the ventricular end-diastolic and end-systolic volumes rise in systolic heart failure. As a consequence of the operation of Laplace's law, which relates myocardial wall tension to the product of intraventricular pressure and radius (both of which may become elevated in heart failure), the aortic impedance, i.e., the force that opposes left ventricular ejection, or the ventricular afterload, rises. Vasoconstriction is generally considered to be a useful compensatory mechanism that allows blood flow to vital organs to persist in the presence of hypovolemia and many forms of shock associated with reduction of the total cardiac output (Chap. 38). However, in the presence of impaired cardiac function, the increase in afterload may reduce cardiac output further.

As shown in Fig. 232-7 (p. 1284), afterload is a major determinant of cardiac function. When cardiac function is normal, a moderate elevation in afterload does not reduce stroke volume significantly, because the resultant increase in left ventricular end-diastolic volume, i.e., preload, can be tolerated easily. However, when myocardial systolic function is impaired, such an increase in preload evoked by an elevation of afterload may raise ventricular end-diastolic and pulmonary capillary pressures to levels that may produce severe pulmonary congestion or even pulmonary edema. In many patients with heart failure, the ventricle is already operating at the peak, flat portion of its Frank-Starling curve (Fig. 232-6 p. 1283), and any additional increase in aortic impedance (afterload) will reduce stroke volume. Conversely, a modest reduction of afterload has no significant effect on stroke volume in normal individuals, but in patients with heart failure it tends to restore hemodynamics to normal by elevating the stroke volume of the failing ventricle and reducing the elevated ventricular filling pressure.

The pharmacologic reduction of impedance to left ventricular ejection with vasodilator drugs represents an important adjunct in the management of heart failure. This approach may be particularly helpful but is by no means limited to patients with acute systolic heart failure due to myocardial infarction (Chap. 243), valvular regurgitation (Chap. 237), elevated systemic vascular resistance and/or arterial pressure, and marked cardiac dilatation. The reduction of afterload by means of a variety of vasodilators reduces left ventricular end-diastolic pressure, volume, and oxygen consumption while raising stroke volume and cardiac output and causing only modest reduction in aortic pressure. Vasodilators should, of course, not be used in patients with hypotension.

In patients with both acute and chronic heart failure secondary to ischemic heart disease, cardiomyopathy, or valvular regurgitation who are treated with vasodilators, cardiac output rises, the pulmonary wedge pressure falls, the signs and symptoms of heart failure are relieved, and a new steady state is achieved in which cardiac output is higher and afterload lower with no or only mild reduction of arterial pressure (Fig. 233-2). Furthermore, the reduction of an elevated left end-diastolic pressure may improve subendocardial perfusion, further improving myocardial contraction.

Vasodilator therapy is useful in the treatment of all forms of systolic heart failure, ranging from the mild-chronic to the severe-acute forms. Vasodilators are *not* useful in the management of isolated diastolic heart failure.

FIGURE 233-2 Effects of various vasodilators on the relationship between left ventricular end-diastolic pressure (LVEDP) and cardiac index or stroke volume in normal (N) and failing (F) hearts. H represents hydralazine or any other pure arterial dilator. It produces only a minimal increase in cardiac index in the normal individual (A′ → H′) or in the patient with heart failure with normal LVEDP (C → H″). In contrast, it elevates output in the patient with heart failure and elevated LVEDP (A → H). P represents a balanced vasodilator, such as sodium nitroprusside or an ACE inhibitor. It reduces filling pressure in all patients, elevates cardiac output in patients with heart failure and elevated LVEDP (A → P), lowers cardiac output in normal individuals (A′ → P′), and has little effect on cardiac output in heart failure patients with normal filling pressures (C → P″). *(From Smith et al, with permission.)*

The several available vasodilators vary in their hemodynamic effects, locus and duration of action, and mode of administration (Table 246-4, p. 1387). Some vasodilators, such as hydralazine, minoxidil, and the alpha-adrenergic blocking agents, such as prazosin, act predominantly on the arterial bed and primarily increase stroke volume; others, such as nitroglycerin and isosorbide dinitrate, act almost entirely on the venous side of the circulation. The latter agents cause pooling of blood in the venous bed and act primarily to reduce ventricular filling pressures. ACE inhibitors, prazosin, and sodium nitroprusside are "balanced vasodilators," i.e., they act on both the arterial and venous beds. Some agents, such as sodium nitroprusside, must be administered by continuous intravenous infusion; nitroglycerin requires administration in ointment patch or intravenous forms when a prolonged effect is desired; and isosorbide dinitrate is most effective when it is administered by the sublingual route.

The ideal vasodilator for the treatment of *acute* heart failure should have a rapid onset and brief duration of action when administered by intravenous infusion; sodium nitroprusside (0.1 to 3.0 μg/kg per minute) qualifies as such a drug, but its use requires careful monitoring of the arterial pressure and, if possible, of the pulmonary artery wedge pressure in an intensive care unit. For the treatment of chronic congestive heart failure, the agent should be effective on oral administration, and its action should persist for at least 6 h. ACE inhibitors (e.g., captopril, 10 to 50 mg tid) satisfy these requirements and have, quite properly, become the most useful and widely used vasodilators. It is advisable to commence therapy with very low doses, particularly in patients receiving diuretics, in order to avoid hypotension and gradually increase the dose.

Vasodilators are potent and effective in acutely improving the deranged hemodynamics of heart failure, and there is evidence in favor of a beneficial chronic effect as well. Studies with ACE inhibitors have demonstrated a favorable long-term reduction of symptoms and enhancement of exercise tolerance. Importantly, these drugs and, to a lesser extent, the combination of hydralazine and isosorbide dinitrate prolong survival of patients with heart failure. The administration of ACE inhibitors has been shown to prevent or retard the development of heart failure in patients with left ventricular dysfunction but without heart failure and to reduce long-term mortality when it is begun in such patients shortly after acute myocardial infarction. Direct acting vasodilators, such as hydralazine or minoxidil, may be useful when added to an ACE inhibitor in patients who have failed ACE inhibitor therapy.

Enhancement of Myocardial Contractility—Digitalis   The improvement of myocardial contractility by means of cardiac glycosides is useful in the control of heart failure.

Digoxin, which has a half-life of 1.6 days, is filtered in the glomeruli and secreted by the renal tubules; 85 percent is excreted in the urine. The ratio of digoxin clearance to endogenous creatinine clearance is 0.8, and the percentage of the body's total stores of digoxin lost per day can be calculated as $(14 \pm 0.2) \times$ creatinine clearance in milliliters per minute. Significant reductions of the glomerular filtration rate reduce the elimination of digoxin and, therefore, may prolong digoxin's effect, allowing it to accumulate to toxic levels if it is administered in patients with impaired renal function. The administration of most diuretics does not alter the excretion of digoxin significantly, but spironolactone can inhibit tubular secretion of digoxin, resulting in significant accumulation of the drug. In patients with normal renal function, a plateau concentration in the blood and tissue is reached after 5 days of daily maintenance treatment without a loading dose (see Fig. 68-2).

MECHANISM OF ACTION   The most important effect of digitalis on cardiac muscle is to shift its force-velocity relation upward (Chap. 232). This positive inotropic effect is exhibited in normal, nonfailing hypertrophied, and failing hearts. In the absence of heart failure, however, when cardiac output is not limited by cardiac contractility, the drug does not elevate the output.

Excitation-contraction coupling (p. 1279) is the membrane and intracellular process most likely involved in producing the positive inotropic effect of digitalis glycosides. These drugs inhibit transmembrane sodium and potassium movement by inhibition of the monovalent cation transport enzyme–coupled Na$^+$,K$^+$-ATPase. The latter, localized to the sarcolemma, appears to be the receptor for cardioactive glycosides, whose action results in an increase in intracellular sodium content; this, in turn, increases intracellular calcium concentration through a Na$^+$-Ca^{2+} exchange carrier mechanism. The increased myocardial uptake of calcium augments calcium released to the myofilaments during excitation and, therefore, invokes a positive inotropic response.

Cardiac glycosides also produce alterations in the electrical properties of both the contractile cells and the specialized automatic cells, leading to increased automaticity and ectopic impulse activity. The conduction velocity is slowed, which is conducive to the development of reentry. Thus the known electrophysiologic effects of digitalis glycosides are capable of explaining the development of the arrhythmias associated with digitalis intoxication, i.e., ventricular arrhythmias and ventricular fibrillation.

The glycosides also prolong the effective *refractory period* of the atrioventricular node, largely as a result of an enhanced vagal effect. This helps to explain the slowing of ventricular rate produced by digitalis in atrial flutter and fibrillation.

Digitalis slows the sinus rate usually only in the presence of heart failure, in part due to an effect on the central nervous system leading to withdrawal of sympathetic activity and increased vagal action.

In addition, the digitalis glycosides also exert an action on the peripheral vasculature, causing venous and arterial constriction in normal individuals and reflex dilatation resulting from withdrawal of sympathetic constrictor activity in patients with congestive heart failure.

USE IN HEART FAILURE Digitalis is particularly effective in patients with heart failure accompanied by atrial flutter and fibrillation and a rapid ventricular rate, who benefit from both slowing of the ventricular rate and the positive inotropic effect. Although digitalis does not improve survival in patients with sinus rhythm and left ventricular systolic failure, it reduces the need for hospitalization for heart failure in such patients. By stimulating myocardial contractility moderately, digitalis improves ventricular emptying; i.e., it increases cardiac output, augments the ejection fraction, promotes diuresis, and reduces the elevated diastolic pressure and volume and end-systolic volume of the failing ventricle with consequent reduction of symptoms resulting from pulmonary vascular congestion and elevated systemic venous pressure. It is most beneficial in patients in whom ventricular contractility is impaired secondary to chronic ischemic heart disease or when hypertensive, valvular, or congenital heart disease imposes an excessive volume or pressure load. It is of relatively little value in most forms of cardiomyopathy, myocarditis, beriberi with heart failure, mitral stenosis, thyrotoxicosis (all with sinus rhythm), chronic constrictive pericarditis (Chap. 240), and any form of diastolic heart failure (p. 1288).

DIGITALIS INTOXICATION Digitalis intoxication is a serious and potentially fatal complication. The lethal dose of most glycosides is approximately 5 to 10 times the minimal effective dose and only about twice the dose that leads to minor toxic manifestations. Advanced age, acute myocardial infarction or ischemia, hypoxemia, magnesium depletion, renal insufficiency, hypercalcemia, electrical cardioversion, and hypothyroidism all may reduce tolerance to digitalis. The most common precipitating cause of digitalis intoxication, however, is depletion of potassium stores, which occurs often in patients with heart failure as a result of diuretic therapy and secondary hyperaldosteronism. Since it is not necessary for a patient to receive a maximally tolerated dose of digitalis to derive a beneficial effect, even small doses provide some therapeutic action; this point should be considered if these drugs are to be used in patients prone to toxicity, particularly the elderly.

Anorexia, nausea, and vomiting, which are among the earliest signs of digitalis intoxication, are caused by direct stimulation of centers in the medulla. The most frequent disturbance of cardiac rhythm is ventricular premature beats, bigeminy, ventricular tachycardia, and, rarely, ventricular fibrillation. Atrioventricular block of varying degrees of severity may occur. Nonparoxysmal atrial tachycardia with variable atrioventricular block is quite characteristic of digitalis intoxication. Sinus arrhythmia, sinoatrial block, sinus arrest, and atrioventricular junctional and multifocal ventricular tachycardia also may occur. Chronic digitalis intoxication may be insidious in onset and characterized by exacerbations of heart failure, weight loss, cachexia, neuralgias, gynecomastia, yellow vision, and delirium.

The administration of quinidine, verapamil, amiodarone, and propafenone to patients receiving digoxin raises the serum concentration of the latter by reducing both the renal and nonrenal elimination of digoxin and by reducing its volume of distribution. These drugs increase the propensity to digitalis intoxication, and the dose of digitalis should be reduced by half in patients receiving these drugs. Serum digoxin concentrations and electrocardiograms should be followed carefully when these drugs are administered to digitalized patients.

The radioimmunoassay for digoxin makes possible the correlation of serum glycoside levels with the presence of toxicity. In patients receiving standard maintenance doses of digoxin (0.125 to 0.375 mg daily) in whom no sign of intoxication is present, serum concentrations approximate 1 to 1.5 ng/mL. When signs of intoxication are present, serum levels of more than 2 ng/mL are often found. Since many factors other than the serum concentration determine digitalis intoxication, and since there is considerable overlap in serum glycoside concentrations in patients with and without toxicity, these levels cannot be used as a sole guide to digitalis dosage. However, when taken together with findings on the clinical examination and electrocardiogram, they add useful information to the clinical evaluations of digitalis intoxication. In addition, they will indicate whether a patient for whom the history of digitalis intake is in doubt has, in fact, been receiving the drug.

Treatment of digitalis intoxication When tachyarrhythmias result from digitalis intoxication, withdrawal of the drug and treatment with potassium, phenytoin, a beta-adrenoceptor blocker, or lidocaine are indicated. Potassium should be administered cautiously and by the oral route whenever possible if hypokalemia is present. *Potassium must not be employed in the presence of atrioventricular block or hyperkalemia.* Lidocaine is effective in the treatment of digitalis-induced ventricular tachyarrhythmias in the absence of preceding atrioventricular block. A cardiac pacemaker may be required in digitalis-induced atrioventricular block. Electrical conversion may be lifesaving in digitalis-induced ventricular fibrillation but is usually ineffective in other tachyarrhythmias secondary to digitalis intoxication. Quinidine and procainamide are of limited value in the treatment of digitalis intoxication. Fab fragments of purified, intact digitalis antibodies are a potentially lifesaving approach to the treatment of severe intoxication.

Sympathomimetic Amines (See also Chap. 70) Five sympathomimetic amines that act largely on beta-adrenergic receptors—norepinephrine, epinephrine, isoproterenol (isoprenaline), dopamine, and dobutamine—improve myocardial contractility in various forms of heart failure (Table 70-1, p. 437). The latter two agents appear to be most effective in the management of heart failure; they must be administered by constant intravenous infusion and are useful in patients with intractable heart failure, particularly those with a reversible component, such as exists in patients who have undergone cardiac surgery, and in some instances of myocardial infarction and shock or pulmonary edema. While they improve the hemodynamics in these conditions, it is not clear that they improve survival. Their administration should be accompanied by careful and continuous monitoring of the electrocardiogram, arterial pressure, and, if possible, pulmonary artery wedge pressure.

DOPAMINE(p. 1256) This naturally occurring immediate precursor of norepinephrine has a combination of actions that makes it particularly useful in the treatment of a variety of hypotensive states and congestive heart failure. At very low doses, i.e., 1 to 2 (μg/kg)/min, it dilates renal and mesenteric blood vessels through stimulation of specific dopaminergic receptors, thereby augmenting renal and mesenteric blood flow and sodium excretion. In the range of 2 to 10 (μg/kg)/min, dopamine stimulates myocardial beta receptors but induces relatively little tachycardia, while at higher doses it also stimulates alpha-adrenergic receptors and elevates arterial pressure.

DOBUTAMINE This synthetic catecholamine acts on beta$_1$, beta$_2$, and alpha receptors. It exerts a potent inotropic action, has only a modest cardioaccelerating effect, and lowers peripheral vascular resistance, but since it simultaneously raises cardiac output, it has little effect on systemic arterial pressure. Dobutamine, given in continuous infusions of 2.5 to 10 (μg/kg)/min, is useful in the treatment of acute heart failure without hypotension. Like the other sympathomimetic amines, it may be particularly valuable in the management of patients requiring relatively short-term inotropic support—up to 1 week—in conditions that are reversible, such as the cardiac depression that sometimes follows open-heart surgery, or in patients with acute heart failure who are being prepared for operation, including cardiac transplantation. Adverse effects include sinus tachycardia, tachyarrhythmias, and hypertension.

A major problem with all sympathomimetics is the loss of responsiveness, apparently due to "downregulation" of adrenergic receptors, which becomes evident within 8 h of continuous administration. This problem may be managed by intermittent therapy.

AMRINONE AND MILRINONE These bipyridines are noncatecholamine, nonglycoside agents that exert both positive inotropic and vasodilator actions by inhibiting a specific phosphodiesterase. They are suitable for intravenous use only; by simultaneously stimulating cardiac contractility and dilating the systemic vascular bed they reverse the major hemodynamic abnormalities associated with severe heart failure.

ANTICOAGULANTS Patients with advanced heart failure are at increased risk of pulmonary emboli secondary to venous thrombosis and to systemic emboli secondary to intracardiac thrombi. Patients with heart failure and additional risk factors such as atrial fibrillation, previous venous thrombosis, and pulmonary or systemic emboli should receive heparin followed by warfarin.

BETA-ADRENOCEPTOR BLOCKERS While large doses of beta-adrenergic receptor blockers can intensify heart failure, the administration of gradually escalating doses of drugs such as metoprolol, carvedilol, and bucindolol have been reported to improve the symptoms of heart failure and, in some patients, to improve left ventricular function and exercise tolerance and retard the progression of heart failure. In patients with moderately severe heart failure (classes II and III), the administration of 5 mg metoprolol bid, increasing over 6 weeks to a target dose of 50 to 75 mg bid may prove beneficial.[1]

Diastolic Heart Failure The major goal in the treatment of this condition is to eliminate or reduce the causes of diastolic dysfunction, such as ventricular hypertrophy, fibrosis, or ischemia. The second is to reduce pulmonary and/or systemic venous congestion, a major consequence of diastolic dysfunction (Table 233-2).

Management of Arrhythmias Premature ventricular contractions and episodes of asymptomatic ventricular tachycardia are common in advanced heart failure. Sudden death, presumably due to ventricular fibrillation, is responsible for about one-half of all deaths in this condition. (The remainder are due to failure of the cardiac pump.) The management of arrhythmias should commence with correction of electrolyte and acid-base disturbances (Chaps. 49 and 50), especially diuretic-induced hypokalemia, as well as digitalis

[1] Beta-adrenoceptor blockers have not been approved for the treatment of heart failure at the time of this writing.

Table 233-2

Management of Diastolic Dysfunction

Reduce the congestive state
  Salt restriction, diuretics, angiotensin-converting enzyme (ACE) inhibitors
  Dialysis or plasmapheresis
Maintain atrial contraction
  Direct-current or pharmacologic cardioversion
  Sequential atrioventricular pacing
Prevent tachycardia and promote bradycardia
  Beta blockers, calcium blockers
  Radiofrequency ablation and pacing
Treat and prevent myocardial ischemia
  Nitrates, beta blockers, calcium blockers
  Bypass surgery, angioplasty
Control hypertension and promote regression of hypertrophy
  Antihypertensive agents
Attenuate neurohormonal activation
  Beta blockers, ACE inhibitors
Prevent fibrosis and promote regression of fibrosis
  ACE inhibitors, spironolactone
  Anti-ischemic agents
Improve ventricular relaxation
  Beta-adrenergic agonists
  Systolic unloading
  Treat ischemia
  Calcium blockers (in hypertrophic cardiomyopathy)

SOURCE: WH Gaasch et al, Management of left ventricular diastolic dysfunction in *Cardiovascular Therapeutics*, TW Smith (ed), Philadelphia, Saunders, 1996

intoxication (p. 1295). Treatment with class I antiarrhythmics such as quinidine, procainamide, or flecainide (Chap. 231) is fraught with danger because these drugs are proarrhythmic in patients with heart failure. Amiodarone (p. 1295), on the other hand, is well tolerated and is the drug of choice for patients with atrial fibrillation and symptomatic tachyarrhythmia and perhaps for frequent, prolonged asymptomatic ventricular tachyarrhythmias as well. In patients who have been resuscitated from sudden death, the automatic implantable defibrillator may prevent recurrence and back-up pacing may prevent sudden death due to bradyarrhythmias. It is not yet clear whether these devices alter overall mortality or only the mode of death in patients with advanced heart failure.

Refractory Heart Failure When the response to ordinary treatment is inadequate, heart failure is considered to be refractory. Before assuming that this condition simply reflects advanced, perhaps preterminal, myocardial depression, careful consideration must be given to several possibilities: (1) an underlying and overlooked cause of the heart disease that may be amenable to specific surgical or medical therapy, such as silent aortic or mitral stenosis, infective endocarditis, hypertension, or thyrotoxicosis; (2) one or a combination of the precipitating causes of heart failure, such as pulmonary or urinary tract infection, recurrent pulmonary emboli, arterial hypoxemia, anemia, or arrhythmia; and (3) complications of overly vigorous therapy, such as digitalis intoxication, hypovolemia, or electrolyte imbalance.

Recognition and proper treatment of the aforementioned complications are likely to make the patient responsive to therapy again. Perhaps the most common complication results from overzealous treatment with diuretics. When administered too rapidly, these drugs can produce sudden hypovolemia before edema fluid can be mobilized to replace the loss of blood volume, the result being a shocklike state with evidence of systemic hypoperfusion in the presence of edema. The chronically excessively diuresed patient may have exchanged the hazards of pulmonary edema and the inconvenience of systemic edema for a persistently depressed cardiac output with its associated weakness, lethargy, prerenal azotemia, and sometimes cardiac cachexia. Temporarily easing salt restriction and diuretic administration may overcome this difficulty, but as heart failure worsens, this course of action may lead to increased pulmonary congestion, which is equally unacceptable.

Hyponatremia is a late manifestation of refractory heart failure. It, too, may be a complication of overaggressive diuresis leading to reduced glomerular filtration rate and decreased delivery of NaCl to the diluting sites in the distal tubule. Hyponatremia also may result from nonosmotic stimuli for the continued secretion of antidiuretic hormone. Therapy involves improvement of the cardiovascular status, if possible (sometimes requiring the administration of a sympathomimetic amine such as dopamine or dobutamine), as well as temporary cessation of diuretic therapy and restriction of oral water intake. Hypertonic saline is very rarely indicated because total-body sodium is usually elevated, not depressed, in heart failure.

The combination of an intravenously administered vasodilator, such as sodium nitroprusside, along with a potent sympathomimetic amine, such as dopamine or dobutamine, often results in an additive effect, raising cardiac output and lowering filling pressure. Intravenous amrinone or milrinone, sometimes accompanied by the administration of an ACE inhibitor, also may be useful in patients with refractory heart failure.

In hospitalized patients with refractory heart failure, therapy guided by hemodynamic measurements provided by a balloon flotation (Swan-Ganz) catheter may be helpful. The goal of manipulating diuretics, vasodilators, and inotropic agents is to achieve a pulmonary capillary wedge pressure of 15 to 18 mmHg, a right atrial pressure of 5 to 8 mmHg, a cardiac index > 2.2 (L/min)/m², and a systemic vascular resistance of 800 to 1200 dynes · s · cm⁻⁵. Once these values are achieved, the patient can usually be converted from intravenous to oral therapy.

CARDIAC TRANSPLANTATION When patients with heart failure become unresponsive to a combination of all the aforementioned therapeutic measures, are in New York Heart Association class IV, and are deemed unlikely to survive 1 year, they should be considered for cardiac transplantation (see Chap. 234).

Treatment of Acute Pulmonary Edema Pulmonary edema secondary to left ventricular failure or mitral stenosis is described in Chap. 32. It is life-threatening and must be considered a medical emergency. As is the case for the more chronic forms of heart failure, in the treatment of pulmonary edema, attention must be directed to identifying and removing any precipitating causes of decompensation, such as an arrhythmia or infection. However, because of the acute nature of the problem, a number of additional nonspecific measures are necessary. If it does not delay treatment unduly, recording pulmonary vascular pressures through a Swan-Ganz catheter and intraarterial pressure directly is advisable. The first six measures listed below are ordinarily applied simultaneously or nearly so.

1. Morphine is administered intravenously repetitively, as needed, in doses from 2 to 5 mg. This drug reduces anxiety, reduces adrenergic vasoconstrictor stimuli to the arteriolar and venous beds, and thereby helps to break a vicious cycle. Naloxone should be available in case respiratory depression occurs.
2. Because the alveolar edema interferes with oxygen diffusion, resulting in arterial hypoxemia, 100% oxygen should be administered, preferably under positive pressure. The latter increases intraalveolar pressure and therefore reduces transudation of fluid from the alveolar capillaries and impedes venous return to the thorax, reducing pulmonary capillary pressure.
3. The patient should be maintained in the sitting position, with the legs dangling along the side of the bed, if possible, which also tends to reduce venous return.
4. Intravenous loop diuretics, such as furosemide or ethacrynic acid (40 to 100 mg), or bumetanide (1 mg) will, by rapidly establishing a diuresis, reduce circulating blood volume and thereby hasten the relief of pulmonary edema. In addition, when given intravenously, furosemide also exerts a venodilator action, reduces venous return, and reduces pulmonary edema even before the diuresis commences.
5. Afterload reduction is achieved with intravenous sodium nitroprusside at 20 to 30 μg/min in patients whose systolic arterial pressures exceed 100 mmHg.
6. Inotropic support should be provided by dopamine or dobutamine as described on p. 1296. Patients with systolic heart failure

who are not receiving digitalis should receive 1.0 mg digoxin intravenously.
7. Sometimes, aminophylline (theophylline ethylenediamine), 240 to 480 mg intravenously, is effective in diminishing bronchoconstriction, increasing renal blood flow and sodium excretion, and augmenting myocardial contractility.
8. If the above-mentioned measures are not sufficient, rotating tourniquets should be applied to the extremities.

After these emergency therapeutic measures have been instituted and the precipitating factors treated, the diagnosis of the underlying cardiac disorder responsible for the pulmonary edema must be established if it is not already known. After stabilization of the patient's condition, a long-range strategy for prevention of future episodes of pulmonary edema must be established, and this may require surgical treatment.

PROGNOSIS

The prognosis in heart failure depends primarily on the nature of the underlying heart disease and on the presence or absence of a precipitating factor that can be treated. When one of the latter can be identified and removed, the outlook for immediate survival is far better than if heart failure occurs without any obvious precipitating cause. In the latter situation, survival usually ranges between 6 months and 4 years depending on the severity of the heart failure (Fig. 233-3). Also, the long-term prognosis for heart failure is most favorable when the underlying forms of heart disease can be treated. The prognosis also can be estimated by observing the response to treatment. When clinical improvement occurs with only modest dietary sodium restriction and small doses of diuretics, the outlook is far better than if, in addition to these measures, intensive diuretic therapy and vasodilators are necessary. Other factors that have been shown to be associated with a poor prognosis in heart failure include a severely depressed ejection fraction (<25 percent), a reduced maximal O_2 uptake [<15 (mL/kg)/min], the inability to walk on the level and at a normal pace for more than 3 min, reduced (<133 mEq/L) serum sodium concentration, reduced (<3 mEq/L) serum potassium concentration, elevated circulating atrial natriuretic peptide and norepinephrine concentrations, as well as frequent ventricular extrasystoles on Holter monitoring. A large fraction of patients with congestive heart failure die suddenly, presumably of ventricular fibrillation. Unfortunately, there is no evidence that this complication can be prevented by the administration of antiarrhythmic agents.

FIGURE 233-3 The natural history of congestive heart failure (CHF). Once left ventricular systolic dysfunction is present, it usually progresses, albeit not predictably. As left ventricular dysfunction progresses and symptoms increase, mortality rate increase and the process becomes inexorable. Myocyte loss and fibrosis become irreversible. An effective preventive measure must be introduced before onset or early in the course of progressive left ventricular dysfunction. *(From BM Massie and NH Shah, with permission.)*

BIBLIOGRAPHY

Cody RJ: Optimising ACE inhibitor therapy of congestive heart failure. Clin Pharmacokinet 24:59, 1993

Colucci WS (ed): *Heart Failure: Cardiac Function and Dysfunction*, in *Atlas of Heart Diseases*, vol 4, E Braunwald (series ed). Philadelphia, Current Medicine, 1995

——— et al: Clinical aspects of heart failure, in *Heart Disease*, 5th ed, E Braunwald (ed). Philadelphia, Saunders, 1996, pp 445–470

Francis GS et al: Neurohumoral activation in preclinical heart failure. Remodeling and the potential for intervention. Circulation 87 (Suppl 5):IV90, 1993

Groden DL: Vasodilator therapy for congestive heart failure. Lessons from mortality trials. Arch Intern Med 153:445, 1993

Kannel WB: Epidemiologic aspects of heart failure, in *Heart Failure: Current Concepts and Management*, Cardiology Clinics Series 7/1, KT Weber (ed). Philadelphia, Saunders, 1989

Kelly RA, Smith TW: Pharmacological treatment of heart failure, in *Goodman and Gilman's The Pharmacological Basis of Therapeutics*, 9th ed. New York, McGraw-Hill, 1996, pp 809–838

Kubo SH, Cohn JN: Long-term treatment of the ambulatory patient with heart failure, in *Cardiovascular Therapeutics*, TW Smith (ed). Philadelphia, Saunders, 1996, pp 210–231

Massie BM, Shah NH: The heart failure epidemic: Magnitude of the problem and potential mitigating approaches. Curr Opin Cardiol 11:221, 1996

Slatton ML, Eichorn EJ: β-blocker therapy for heart failure. Curr Opin Cardiol 11:263, 1996

Smith TW et al: Management of heart failure, in *Heart Disease*, 5th ed, E Braunwald (ed). Philadelphia, Saunders, 1997, pp 492–514

SOLVD Investigators: Effect of enalapril on survival in patients with reduced left ventricular ejection fractions and congestive heart failure. N Engl J Med 325:293, 1991

Stevenson LW, Colucci WS: Management of patients hospitalized with heart failure, in Cardiovascular Therapeutics, TW Smith (ed). Philadelphia, Saunders, 1996, pp 199–209

Swedberg K: Reduction in mortality by pharmacological therapy in congestive heart failure. Circulation 87 (Suppl 5):IV126, 1993

Wilcox CS: Diuretics, in *The Kidney*, 5th ed, BM Brenner, FC Rector Jr (eds). Philadelphia, Saunders, 1996, pp 2299–2330

| 234 | *John S. Schroeder* |

CARDIAC TRANSPLANTATION

Orthotopic allograft cadaver cardiac transplantation as a treatment for end-stage cardiac disease will achieve its thirtieth anniversary on December 7, 1997. On that day in 1967 Dr. Christiaan Barnard accomplished the first successful cardiac transplant in a human, quickly followed by Dr. Norman Shumway and Dr. Richard Lower at Stanford University. After an initial early wave of enthusiasm, the problems of immunosuppression slowed application of the procedure until the introduction of cyclosporine in 1980. A subsequent worldwide expansion of cardiac transplantation has resulted in approximately 2500 cardiac transplants per year, with further increases limited only by the donor supply. Current 1- and 5-year survival rates of 85 and 70 percent indicate that cardiac transplantation is the therapy of choice in patients with end-stage heart disease who are unlikely to survive the next 6 to 12 months.

INDICATIONS AND SELECTION OF CANDIDATES The limited donor supply and relatively high cost of cardiac transplantation have restricted it to patients most likely to survive and resume a functional life after transplantation. It is estimated that only 2000 potential donors in the United States, for a pool of at least 20,000 candidates based on current guidelines, become available yearly. Attempts to increase donor awareness in both physicians and the public are being made. Optimal candidates for this procedure are those who would be expected to return to a functional life if their hearts were replaced (Table 234-1). This requires a mentally vigorous, medically compliant person who has not suffered extensive other end-stage organ damage from cardiac failure, does not have other systemic disease

Table 234-1

Indications and Contraindications for Cardiac Transplantation

INDICATIONS

1. End-stage heart disease that limits prognosis for survival over 2 years or severely limits daily quality of life despite optimal medical and other surgical therapy
2. No secondary exclusion criteria
3. Suitable psychosocial profile and social support system
4. Suitable physiologic/chronologic age

EXCLUSION CRITERIA

1. Active infectious process
2. Recent pulmonary infarction
3. Insulin-requiring diabetes with evidence of end-organ damage
4. Irreversible pulmonary hypertension [pulmonary vascular resistance (PVR) poorly responsive to nitroprusside with PVR > 2 or pulmonary systolic pressure > 50 mmHg at peak dose or at mean arterial pressure of 65–70 mmHg]
5. Presence of circulating cytotoxic antibodies
6. Presence of active peptic ulcer disease
7. Active or recent malignancy
8. Presence of severe chronic obstructive pulmonary disease or chronic bronchitis
9. Substance or alcohol abuse
10. Presence of peripheral or cerebrovascular disease
11. Other systemic diseases that would jeopardize rehabilitation posttransplant

such as severe diabetes mellitus or collagen vascular disease, or is not positive for human immunodeficiency virus. Long-standing pulmonary hypertension or recurrent pulmonary emboli and infarction may result in irreversible pulmonary hypertension leading to intraoperative death. Several heart transplant centers have initiated cardiac transplantation for newborns with left ventricular hypoplasia, but long-term survival experience is still very limited.

Timing of the recommendation to undergo cardiac transplantation can be difficult and requires assessment of the patient's current disability, stability of course, and likelihood of surviving the next 6 to 12 months. Generally, left ventricular ejection fractions under 15 to 20 percent and presence of serious ventricular arrhythmias indicate a 1-year survival rate of 50 percent or less. Estimating prognosis remains very challenging. A maximal oxygen uptake during exercise (maximal $\dot{V}_{O_2}$) of <10 mL O_2 per kilogram per minute usually indicates poor likelihood of survival for 1 year and has been a criterion for transplant candidacy in some programs. Maximal $\dot{V}_{O_2}$ values between 10 and 14 mL O_2 per kilogram per minute are in a borderline range, with values >14 usually predicting good 1 to 2 year survival. The increasing acceptance of cardiac transplantation as a treatment modality for heart failure without a corresponding increase in donor availability has led to prolonged waiting times of as much as 2 years or more. This longer waiting time has led to more rigorous medical care of the patient awaiting transplant with meticulous monitoring of electrolytes, fluid status, and overall well-being. Aggressive therapy for congestive heart failure with high-dose angiotensin-converting enzyme inhibitors and beta blockers and meticulous monitoring of serum electrolytes and renal function have led to stabilization and many times some improvement in the functional status of patients awaiting a donor. This has led to as many as 30 to 40 percent of listed patients being placed "on hold" based on their improved status. Whether these patients can maintain their improved state or will subsequently deteriorate remains to be seen. Recurrent hospitalizations may be required. Patients may become dopamine/dobutamine-dependent to maintain adequate cardiac output. This dependency moves the patient to the highest ("status I") priority for a donor heart.

In addition to these pharmacologic bridges to transplantation, mechanical bridges are occasionally used where pharmacologic therapy is no longer effective. Three approaches are currently used. The first is intraaortic balloon pumping, which can increase cardiac output by 15 to 20 percent. The second is a left ventricular assist device (LVAD), which empties blood via a tube placed in the apex of the left ventricle and pumps it with an electrically driven "bellows-type" mechanism into the abdominal aorta. This approach is highly effective and has been used for several months with successful subsequent transplantation. Limitations include right ventricular failure and/or high pulmonary vascular resistance, since the LVAD does not "unload" the right ventricle. Blood clotting in the device remains a problem, in addition to the obvious problems of infection. Finally, total mechanical heart replacement is also applied in some transplant centers. This complete replacement circumvents the problem of right ventricular failure but is limited by the greater complexity of the device, which can lead to clotting and systemic emboli. Patients who underwent mechanical assistance *and* received a donor heart have 1-year survival statistics similar to those who went directly to transplantation.

Tissue cross-matching between donor and recipient has generally not been done because of difficulty in obtaining good matches and lack of correlation between match and outcome. Size, ABO matching, negative lymphocyte cross-match, and avoidance of a transplantation from a cytomegalovirus (CMV)-positive donor to a CMV-negative recipient are more important.

OPERATIVE PROCEDURE The surgeon removes the diseased heart but leaves the posterior wall of the right atrium in place and the superior and inferior venae cavae intact. The posterior wall of the left atrium is also left in situ with pulmonary veins intact. The donor heart is then removed in toto with the posterior wall of the right and left atria incised, which allows suturing of left atrial donor rim to recipient rim and right atrial donor rim to recipient rim, with anastomosis of the aorta and pulmonary artery.

IMMUNOSUPPRESSION AND REJECTION Controlling rejection while avoiding the adverse side effects of immunosuppressive agents is pivotal to successful transplantation. Rejection is characterized by perivascular infiltration of killer T lymphocytes, which migrate into the myocardium and cause cellular necrosis if not checked. Since early rejection can be silent, it is important to detect it before necrosis occurs. Immunologic monitoring of activated T lymphocytes in peripheral blood offers clues to the timing of a rejection process but has not been sufficiently reliable to dictate antirejection therapy. Therefore, repeated percutaneous transvenous right ventricular endomyocardial biopsies via the right internal jugular vein are required for histologic determination of the state of immunosuppression and rejection.

One widely used scheme for grading the stages of rejection is as follows: cannot rule out rejection, mild early rejection, moderate rejection, and severe rejection. Serial biopsies are taken every 1 to 2 weeks early after transplantation, with gradually widening intervals depending on the patient's course and rejection history. Prolongation of isovolumic relaxation time measured by echocardiography also may provide early clues to rejection.

Immunosuppressive therapy regimens vary but usually include triple therapy with cyclosporine, azathioprine, and prednisone. Prophylactic courses of monoclonal antibody OKT3 or antithymocyte globulin also may be given early after transplantation. Careful monitoring of the adverse side effects of these agents is extremely important because they include nephrotoxicity, bone marrow suppression, and opportunistic infections.

EARLY COURSE AND COMPLICATIONS It is rare for a cardiac transplant patient to have a completely uncomplicated postoperative course. In the immediate postoperative period, right-sided heart failure due to pulmonary vascular disease is most life-threatening. During the 2 to 3 weeks after transplantation, the patient is hospitalized with meticulous monitoring for evidence of rejection and infections, repeated percutaneous transvenous endomyocardial biopsies, and adjustment of immunosuppressive drugs. During the ensuing 4 to 6 weeks, infectious complications, including bacterial, viral, and protozoan infections, are common. A successful transplant program requires a highly aggressive and sophisticated approach to diagnosis and therapy of infections in the immunocompromised host. Depending on the degree of cardiac cachexia preoperatively, the patient is usually functional at 1 week and discharged from the hospital at 2 to 3 weeks if no major complication occurs.

The average first-year cost ranges from \$100,000 to \$150,000, depending on the need for repeated hospitalization and cardiac biopsies, and is occasionally much higher. Yearly costs for immunosuppressive agents range from \$5000 to \$10,000, in addition to the expense of medical surveillance for rejection or complications.

PHYSIOLOGY AND FUNCTION Since the allografted heart remains denervated, cardiac function differs from that of the innervated heart during both rest and exercise. The electrocardiogram of a recipient shows two P waves; the P wave of the recipient's heart reflects the residual sinus node and posterior walls of the remaining native atria but is dissociated from the QRS, since the depolarization impulse does not cross the suture line. Although it does not control donor heart rate, the recipient's sinus node remains innervated and under the influence of the autonomic nervous system. The donor sinus node controls the rate of the transplanted heart. The donor heart's P wave has a regular PR interval, reflecting conduction to the ventricles. Since the controlling sinus node is denervated, it maintains a heart rate of 100 to 110 beats per minute, and rate increase depends on alterations in chronotropic agents perfusing the sinus node. Partial reinnervation may occur in some patients late after transplantation. This is manifested primarily by the occurrence of angina-like symptoms in patients who have developed accelerated graft atherosclerosis (see below).

Ventricular function in response to isometric and isotonic exercise has been studied extensively. The early response to exercise is more dependent on the Frank-Starling mechanism and change in ventricular volume and filling pressure. As exercise proceeds and catecholamines are released with their positive inotropic and chronotropic effects, cardiac output begins to rise. The cardiac transplant recipient can achieve approximately 70 percent of the maximal cardiac output expected for his or her age, easily sufficient for the stresses of everyday life.

LATE COURSE AND COMPLICATIONS Although the rejection process partially subsides, lifelong administration of immunosuppressive drugs, albeit at lower doses, is still required and remains a hazard. Infectious complications and unsuspected rejection continue to occur, requiring ongoing surveillance and monitoring. Routine cardiac biopsies are performed at 3-month intervals to monitor for unsuspected early rejection. Acute rejection or infection predominates in the first year after transplantation. Chronic rejection (i.e., accelerated coronary vascular disease) becomes the most important cause of death after the first year. The process is a fibrointimal hyperplasia that can go undetected by coronary arteriography at first and then cause diffuse atherosclerotic changes. Risk factors for its development may include repeated rejection episodes and elevated lipid levels. CMV infections also have been associated with higher frequency of this disease. Angina is rare, and patients may present with sudden death or silent myocardial infarction. This diffuse accelerated vascular process affects both proximal and distal coronary vessels so that standard approaches, such as angioplasty or coronary artery bypass grafting, are not generally useful but occasionally are successful.

Uncontrolled trials with anticoagulation, aspirin, and improved immunosuppression with cyclosporine have done little to lower this frequency; 40 to 50 percent of patients show arteriographic evidence of coronary vascular disease 5 years after transplantation. Retransplantation has been employed for some patients with severe graft atherosclerosis, but it is limited by the scarcity of donors and poorer survival expectations after the second transplant. Diltiazem has been reported to reduce the severity and occurrence of this accelerated vascular process when started at the time of transplantation. Recently, pravastatin has been reported not only to lower lipid levels but to have a beneficial effect on rejection, 1-year survival, and incidence of coronary vasculopathy. The mechanism is under investigation.

In addition to the well-known hazards of long-term glucocorticoid usage, the immunosuppressed patient is at increased risk for neoplasia. An unusual form of lymphoma can occur frequently in extranodal locations, which is linked to prior Epstein-Barr viral infection. This lymphoma can be polyclonal or monoclonal, is associated with excessive immunosuppression, and may respond to simply lowering doses of cyclosporine and administration of acyclovir rather than requiring more aggressive chemo- or radiotherapy. Many cases regress fully and do not recur.

HEART-LUNG TRANSPLANTATION

Patients with congenital heart disease with Eisenmenger's complex (Chap. 235) or primary pulmonary hypertension (Chap. 260) are now considered for heart-lung transplantation. The surgical technique is similar to that for heart transplantation, except that the pulmonary venous attachments to the left atrium are left intact, and a tracheal anastomosis is required. The postoperative period is more complex, since the lungs may be rejected separately from the heart, requiring repeated endobronchoscopic biopsies when rejection is suspected. The immunosuppressive regimen is similar to that for heart transplants, except that glucocorticoids are avoided in the first 1 to 2 weeks to allow healing of the tracheal anastamosis. Long-term survival has in the past been limited by obliterative bronchiolitis due to chronic unrecognized rejection; survival rates have been approximately 60 percent at 1 year and 50 percent at 2 years but appear to be improving. Heart-lung transplants also have been applied to primary pulmonary hypertension, but more recent experience with single-lung transplants for these patients has been satisfactory, thus utilizing scarce donors more effectively. Single-lung transplants are also being applied increasingly for patients with advanced emphysema. Double-lung transplants for patients with cystic fibrosis also have become the operation of choice for this group. →*For further discussion, see Chap. 267.*

BIBLIOGRAPHY

CAREY NR: Diagnostic criteria of chronic rejetion in transplanted hearts. Transplant Proc 25:2026, 1993

GAO S-Z et al: Progressive coronary luminal narrowing after cardiac transplantation. Circulation 82(Suppl IV):IV-269, 1990

GRATTAN MT et al: Cytomegalovirus infection is associated with cardiac allograft rejection and atherosclerosis. JAMA 261:3561, 1989

HALLE AA 3RD et al: Coronary angioplasty, atherectomy and bypass surgery in cardiac transplant recipients. Int J Cardiol 49:119, 1995

KOBASHIGAWA JA et al: Effect of pravastatin on outcomes after cardiac transplantation. N Engl J Med 333:621, 1995

REEDY JE et al: Bridge to heart transplantation: Importance of patient selection. J Heart Transplant 9:475, 1990

REITZ B: Heart and heart-lung transplantation, in E Braunwald (ed). *Heart Disease*, 5th ed, Philadelphia, Saunders, 1997, p 515

SCHROEDER JS et al: A preliminary study of diltiazem in the prevention of coronary artery disease in heart-transplant recipients. N Engl J Med 328:30, 1993

TANIO JW, EISEN HJ: Medical aspects of cardiac transplantation. Hosp Pract 28:61, 1993

235	*William F. Friedman, John S. Child*

CONGENITAL HEART DISEASE IN THE ADULT

Congenital heart disease complicates approximately 1 percent of all live births. Substantial numbers of affected infants reach adulthood because of successful medical and/or surgical management, or because the alteration caused in cardiovascular physiology is well tolerated.

ETIOLOGY AND PREVENTION Congenital cardiovascular malformations are generally the result of aberrant embryonic development of a normal structure, or failure of such a structure to progress beyond an early stage of embryonic or fetal development. Malformations are due to complex multifactorial genetic and environmental causes. Recognized chromosomal aberrations and mutations of single genes account for fewer than 10 percent of all cardiac malformations (Table 235-1).

The presence of a cardiac malformation as one component of the multiple system involvement in Down's, Turner's, and the trisomy 13-15(D_1) and 17-18 (E) syndromes may be anticipated in occasional pregnancies by detection of abnormal chromosomes in fetal cells obtained from amniotic fluid or chorionic villus biopsy. Identification in such cells of the enzyme disorders characteristic of Hurler's syndrome, homocystinuria, or type II glycogen storage disease may also allow one to predict cardiac disease.

PATHOPHYSIOLOGY The anatomic and physiologic changes in the heart and circulation due to any specific congenital cardiocirculatory lesion are not static but rather progress from prenatal life to adulthood. Thus, malformations that are benign or escape detection in childhood may become clinically significant in the adult. For example, the functionally normal, congenitally bicuspid aortic valve may thicken and calcify with time, resulting in significant aortic stenosis; or the well-tolerated left-to-right shunt of an atrial septal defect may not result in cardiac decompensation, with or without pulmonary hypertension, until the fourth or fifth decade.

Pulmonary Hypertension This is a common companion of many congenital cardiac lesions, and the status of the pulmonary vascular bed is often the principal determinant of the clinical manifestations, the course, and the feasibility of surgical repair. Increases in pulmonary arterial pressure result from elevation of pulmonary blood flow and/or resistance, the latter due sometimes to an increase in vascular tone but usually the result of obstructive, obliterative structural changes within the pulmonary vascular bed. Because pulmonary vascular obstructive disease can be the determining factor in assessing the advisability of operation, it is important to quantify and compare pulmonary to systemic flows and resistances in patients with severe pulmonary hypertension. The causes of pulmonary vascular obstructive disease are unknown, although increased pulmonary blood flow, increased pulmonary arterial blood pressure, elevated pulmonary venous pressure, polycythemia, systemic hypoxemia, acidosis, and the bronchial circulation have been implicated. The designation *Eisenmenger syndrome* is applied to patients with a large communication between the two circulations at the aortopulmonary, ventricular, or atrial levels and bidirectional or predominantly right-to-left shunts because of high-resistance and obstructive pulmonary hypertension. No specific treatment has proved beneficial for obstructive pulmonary vascular disease, although single lung transplantation and intracardiac defect repair, or total heart-lung transplantation show promise (see Chaps. 234 and 267).

Erythrocytosis The chronic hypoxemia in cyanotic congenital heart disease results in *erythrocytosis* due to increased erythropoietin production (see Chap. 36). The commonly used term *polycythemia* is a misnomer because white cell counts are normal and platelet counts are normal to decreased. Cyanotic patients with erythrocytosis may have compensated or decompensated hematocrits. Compensated erythrocytosis with iron-replete equilibrium hematocrits rarely results in symptoms of hyperviscosity at hematocrits less than 65 percent and occasionally with hematocrits of 70 percent or more. Therapeutic phlebotomy is rarely required in compensated erythrocytosis. In contrast, patients with decompensated erythrocytosis fail to establish equilibrium with unstable, rising hematocrits and recurrent hyperviscosity symptoms. Therapeutic phlebotomy, a two-edged sword, allows temporary relief of symptoms but begets instability of the hematocrit and compounds the problem by iron depletion. Iron-deficiency symptoms are usually indistinguishable from those of hyperviscosity; progressive symptoms after recurrent phlebotomy are usually due to iron depletion with hypochromic microcytosis. Iron depletion results in a larger number of smaller (microcytic) hypochromic red cells that are less capable of carrying oxygen and less deformable in the microcirculation. Because these microcytes are less deformable in the microcirculation and there are more of them relative to the plasma volume, the viscosity is greater than for an equivalent hematocrit with fewer, larger, iron-replete, deformable cells. As such, iron-depleted erythrocytosis results in increasing symptoms due to decreased oxygen delivery to the tissues.

Table 235-1

Syndromes with Associated Cardiovascular Involvement

Syndrome	Major Cardiovascular Manifestations	Major Noncardiac Abnormalities
HERITABLE AND POSSIBLY HERITABLE		
Ellis–van Creveld	Single atrium or atrial septal defect	Chondrodystrophic dwarfism, nail dysplasia, polydactyly
TAR (thrombocytopenia-absent radius)	Atrial septal defect, tetralogy of Fallot	Radial aplasia or hypoplasia, thrombocytopenia
Holt-Oram	Atrial septal defect (other defects common)	Skeletal upper limb defect, hypoplasia of clavicles
Kartagener	Dextrocardia	Situs inversus, sinusitis, bronchiectasis
Laurence-Moon-Biedl	Variable defects	Retinal pigmentation, obesity, polydactyly
Noonan	Pulmonary valve dysplasia, cardiomyopathy (usually hypertrophic)	Webbed neck, pectus excavatum, cryptorchidism
Tuberous sclerosis	Rhabdomyoma, cardiomyopathy	Phakomatosis, bone lesions, hamartomatous skin lesions
Multiple lentigines (leopard) syndrome	Pulmonic stenosis	Basal cell nevi, broad facies, rib anomalies, deafness
Rubenstein-Taybi	Patent ductus arteriosus (others)	Broad thumbs and toes, hypoplastic maxilla, slanted palpebral fissures
Familial deafness	Arrhythmias, sudden death	Sensorineural deafness
Osler-Rendu-Weber	Arteriovenous fistulas (lung, liver, mucous membranes)	Multiple telangiectasia
Apert	Ventricular septal defect	Craniosynostosis, midfacial hypoplasia, syndactyly
Crouzon	Patent ductus arteriosus, aortic coarctation	Ptosis, craniosynostosis, maxillary hypoplasia
Hypertrophic cardiomypathy	Asymmetric septal hypertrophy	Family history of sudden death
Incontinentia pigmenti	Patent ductus arteriosus	Irregular pigmented skin lesions, patchy alopecia, hypodontia
Alagille (arteriohepatic dysplasia)	Peripheral pulmonic stenosis, pulmonic stenosis	Biliary hypoplasia, vertebral anomalies, prominent forehead, deep-set eyes
DiGeorge	Interrupted aortic arch, tetralogy of Fallot, truncus arteriosus	Thymic hypoplasia or aplasia, parathyroid aplasia or hypoplasia, ear anomalies
Friedreich's ataxia	Cardiomyopathy and conduction defects	Ataxia, speech defect, degeneration of spinal cord dorsal columns
Muscular dystrophy	Cardiomyopathy	Pseudohypertrophy of calf muscles, weakness of trunk and proximal limb muscles
Cystic fibrosis	Cor pulmonale	Pancreatic insufficiency, malabsorption, chronic lung disease
Sickle cell anemia	Cardiomyopathy, mitral regurgitation	Hemoglobin SS
Conradi-Hünermann	Ventricular septal defect, patent ductus arteriosus	Asymmetric limb shortness, early punctate mineralization, large skin pores
Cockayne	Accelerated atherosclerosis	Cachectic dwarfism, retinal pigment abnormalities, photosensitivity dermatitis
Progeria	Accelerated atherosclerosis	Premature aging, alopecia, atrophy of subcutaneous fat, skeletal hypoplasia
CONNECTIVE TISSUE DISORDERS		
Cutis laxa	Peripheral pulmonic stenosis	Generalized disruption of elastic fibers, diminished skin resilience, hernias
Ehlers-Danlos	Arterial dilatation and rupture, mitral regurgitation	Hyperextensible joints, hyperelastic and friable skin
Marfan	Aortic dilatation, aortic and mitral incompetence	Gracile habitus, arachnodactyly with hyperextensibility, lens subluxation
Osteogenesis imperfecta	Aortic incompetence	Fragile bones, blue sclera
Pseudoxanthoma elasticum	Peripheral and coronary arterial disease	Degeneration of elastic fibers in skin, retinal angioid streaks
INBORN ERRORS OF METABOLISM		
Pompe's disease	Glycogen storage disease of heart	Acid maltase deficiency, muscular weakness
Homocystinuria	Aortic and pulmonary arterial dilatation, intravascular thrombosis	Cystathionine synthetase deficiency, lens subluxation, osteoporosis
Mucopolysaccharidosis:		
Hurler, Hunter	Multivalvular and coronary and great artery disease, cardiomyopathy	Hurler: Deficiency of α-L-iduronidase, corneal clouding, coarse features, growth and mental retardation Hunter: Deficiency of sulfoiduronide sulfatase, coarse facies, clear cornea, growth and mental retardation
Morquio, Scheie, Maroteaux-Lamy	Aortic incompetence	Morquio: Deficiency of N-acetylhexosamine sulfate sulfatase, cloudy cornea, normal intelligence, severe bony changes involving vertebrae and epiphyses Scheie: Deficiency of α-L-iduronidase, cloudy cornea, normal intelligence, peculiar facies Maroteaux-Lamy: Deficiency of arylsulfatase B, cloudy cornea, osseous changes, normal intelligence

(continued)

Table 235-1

Syndromes with Associated Cardiovascular Involvement *(Continued)*

Syndrome	Major Cardiovascular Manifestations	Major Noncardiac Abnormalities
CHROMOSOMAL ABNORMALITIES		
Trisomy 21 (Down's syndrome)	Endocardial cushion defect, atrial or ventricular septal defect, tetralogy of Fallot	Hypotonia, hyperextensible joints, mongoloid facies, mental retardation
Trisomy 13 (D)	Ventricular septal defect, patent ductus arteriosus, double-outlet right ventricle	Single midline intracerebral ventricle with midfacial defects, polydactyly, nail changes, mental retardation
Trisomy 18 (E)	Congenital polyvalvular dysplasia, ventricular septal defect, patent ductus arteriosus	Clenched hand, short sternum, low-arch dermalridge pattern on fingertips, mental retardation
Cri-du-chat (short-arm deletion-5)	Ventricular septal defect	Cat cry, microcephaly, antimongoloid slant of palpebral fissures, mental retardation
XO (Turner)	Coarctation of aorta, bicuspid aortic valve	Short female, broad chest, lymphedema, webbed neck
XXXY and XXXXX	Patent ductus arteriosus	XXXY: hypogenitalism, mental retardation, radialulnar synostosis XXXXX: small hands, incurving of fifth fingers, mental retardation
SPORADIC DISORDERS		
VATER association	Ventricular septal defect	Vertebral anomalies, anal atresia, tracheo-esophageal fistula, radial and renal anomalies
CHARGE association	Tetralogy of Fallot (other defects common)	Colobomas, choanal atresia, mental and growth deficiency, genital and ear anomalies
Williams	Supravalvular aortic stenosis, peripheral pulmonic stenosis	Mental deficiency, "elfin" facies, loquacious personality, hoarse voice
Cornelia de Lange	Ventricular septal defect	Micromelia, synophrys, mental and growth deficiency
Shprintzen (velocardiofacial)	Ventricular septal defect, tetralogy of Fallot, right aortic arch	Cleft palate, prominent nose, slender hands, learning disability
Long QT (Jervell and Lange-Nielson, Romano-Ward)	Long QT interval, ventricular arrythmias	Family history of sudden death, congenital deafness (not in Romano-Ward)
TERATOGENIC DISORDERS		
Rubella	Patent ductus arteriosus, pulmonic valvular and/or arterial stenosis, atrial septal defect	Cataracts, deafness, microcephaly
Alcohol-induced	Ventricular septal defect (other defects)	Microcephaly, growth and mental deficiency, short palpebral fissures, smooth philtrum, thin upper lip
Phenytoin-induced	Pulmonic stenosis, aortic stenosis, coarctation, patent ductus arteriosus	Hypertelorism, growth and mental deficiency, short phalanges, bowed upper lip
Thalidomide-induced	Variable	Phocomelia
Lithium-induced	Ebstein's anomaly, tricuspid atresia	None

Hemostasis is abnormal in cyanotic congenital heart disease, due in part to the increased blood volume and engorged capillaries, abnormalities in platelet function and sensitivity to aspirin or nonsteroidal anti-inflammatory agents, and abnormalities of the extrinsic and intrinsic coagulation system. Oral contraceptives are contraindicated for cyanotic women because of the enhanced risk of vascular thrombosis.

The risk of stroke is greatest in children less than 4 years old with cyanotic heart disease and iron deficiency, often with dehydration as an aggravating cause. In contrast, adults with cyanotic congenital heart disease do not appear to be at increased risk for stroke, unless there are excessive, injudicious phlebotomies or inappropriate use of aspirin or anticoagulants.

Symptoms of hyperviscosity can be produced in any cyanotic patient with erythrocytosis if dehydration causes a reduction of plasma volume. Phlebotomy, when required for symptoms of hyperviscosity not due to dehydration or iron deficiency, is a simple outpatient removal of 500 mL of blood over 45 min with isovolumetric replacement with isotonic saline (5% dextrose if congestive heart failure exists). Acute phlebotomy without volume replacement is contraindicated. Iron repletion in decompensated iron-depleted erythrocytosis ameliorates irondeficiency symptoms but must be done gradually to avoid a sudden excessive rise in hematocrit and resultant hyperviscosity.

PREGNANCY The physiologic alterations during normal gestation (see Chap. 7) can create symptoms and physical findings that may be attributed erroneously to heart disease. Dyspnea due to progesterone and elevated diaphragms in association with peripheral edema and fatigability may be attributed inappropriately to heart failure. The jugular venous pulsations normally become more apparent after the twentieth week. Elevation of the diaphragms can cause basal rales (which disappear with deep breathing). Both ventricles are more easily palpated due to the normal increase in ventricular volumes and elevation of the diaphragm. Third heart sounds, already relatively frequent in normal nongravid young women, increase in frequency and intensity with pregnancy because of increased heart rate and volume of flow across the mitral and tricuspid valves. Midsystolic murmurs across the pulmonary outflow tract and supraclavicular systolic murmurs are caused by increased cardiac output. Venous hums and mammary souffles are usual during pregnancy.

These normal circulatory changes may impinge upon the woman's cardiac reserve. The mother is most at risk if she has a cardiovascular lesion associated with pulmonary vascular disease and pulmonary hypertension (e.g., Eisenmenger's physiology or mitral stenosis) or left ventricular outflow tract obstruction (e.g., aortic stenosis) but also risks death with any malformation that may cause heart failure or a hemodynamically important arrhythmia (Table 235-2). Women with aortic coarctation or Marfan's syndrome are at risk for aortic dissection. Patients with cyanotic heart disease, pulmonary hypertension, or Marfan's syndrome should not become pregnant; those with correctable lesions should be counseled about the risks of pregnancy with an uncorrected malformation versus repair and later pregnancy. The effect of pregnancy in postoperative patients depends upon the outcome of the repair including the presence and severity of residua, sequelae, or complications. Contraception is an important topic with such patients.

Table 235-2

CHAPTER 235
Congenital Heart Disease in the Adult   **1303**

Tolerance of Pregnancy by Patients with Various Congenital Cardiac Malformations

Well Tolerated	Intermediate Effect	Poorly Tolerated
NYHA class I	NYHA class II–III	NYHA class IV
Left-right shunts without PHTN	Repaired transposition of the great arteries	Right-left shunt, unrepaired cyanotic heart disease
Aortic or mitral valvular regurgitation (mild-moderate)	Fontan repairs	PHTN and/or pulmonary vascular disease (e.g., Eisenmenger's, "primary PHTN")
Pulmonic or tricuspid regurgitation (if low pressure, even severe)	Aortic or mitral stenosis (moderate)	Aortic or mitral stenosis (severe)
Pulmonic stenosis (mild-moderate)	Ebstein's anomaly	Pulmonic stenosis (severe)
Well-repaired tetralogy of Fallot		Marfan's or aortic coarctation

NOTE: NYHA, New York Heart Association; PHTN, pulmonary hypertension.

Tubal ligation should be considered in those in whom pregnancy is strictly contraindicated.

INFECTIVE ENDOCARDITIS (See also Chap. 126)   Routine antimicrobial prophylaxis is recommended for all patients with congenital heart disease and for the majority of patients after operative repair of the lesion, but it should be recognized that antibiotic prophylaxis is not uniformly effective. Nonetheless, it is recommended for all dental procedures, gastrointestinal and genitourinary surgery, and diagnostic procedures such as proctosigmoidoscopy and cystoscopy. The clinical and bacteriologic profile of infective endocarditis in patients with congenital heart disease has changed with the advent of intracardiac surgery and of prosthetic devices. Two major predisposing causes of infective endocarditis are a susceptible cardiovascular substrate and a source of bacteremia. Prophylaxis includes both chemotherapeutic (antimicrobial) and nonchemotherapeutic (hygienic) measures. Meticulous dental and skin care is required.

EXERCISE   Advice on athletics and exercise is governed by the nature of the exercise and by the type and severity of the congenital cardiovascular lesion. Patients with lesions characterized by left ventricular outflow tract obstruction, if more than mild to moderate, or pulmonary vascular disease risk syncope or even sudden death. In Fallot's tetralogy, isotonic exercise–induced decrease in systemic vascular resistance relative to the right ventricular outflow obstruction augments the right-to-left shunt, increases hypoxemia, and causes an increase in subjective breathlessness due to the response of the respiratory center to the changes in blood gases and pH.

INSURABILITY AND EMPLOYABILITY   Most patients with congenital heart disease must pay significantly more than standard life insurance rates, assuming their anomaly places them in a category that companies have determined is eligible for insurance. There is a paucity of actuarial survival data beyond adolescence for most cardiac lesions that have undergone operative repair. Accordingly, it is often difficult to convince insurance companies to offer insurance at reasonable cost to individual patients whose long-term prognosis is quite good.

Employment is affected by the patient's physical capacity relative to the type of job sought. Job discrimination exists, often because the employer is reluctant to accept health insurance responsibilities. Further, eligibility for some occupations is governed by public safety regulations, e.g., airline pilots, bus drivers.

SPECIFIC CARDIAC DEFECTS

Table 235-3 provides a classification of cardiac anomalies that recognizes the general categories of clinical presentation, functional consequences, and site of origin of congenital defects.

Categorizing the defect(s) in an individual patient requires an answer to a number of basic questions. Is the patient acyanotic or cyanotic? Is pulmonary arterial blood flow increased or not? Does the malformation originate in the left or right side of the heart? Which is the dominant ventricle? Is pulmonary hypertension present or not? With the above information as a foundation, using more refined diagnostic techniques such as transthoracic (precordial) and transesophageal echocardiography and Doppler imaging, magnetic resonance imaging, and/or hemodynamic study and angiocardiography leads to a precise anatomic and functional assessment.

ACYANOTIC CONGENITAL HEART DISEASE WITH A LEFT-TO-RIGHT SHUNT

ATRIAL SEPTAL DEFECT   This is a common cardiac anomaly in adults that occurs more frequently in females. The *sinus venosus* type occurs high in the atrial septum near the entry of the superior vena cava and is associated frequently with anomalous connection of pulmonary veins from the right lung to the junction of the superior vena cava and right atrium. *Ostium primum* anomalies are a form of atrioventricular septal defect that lie immediately adjacent to the atrioventricular valves, either of which may be deformed and incompetent. Ostium primum defects occur commonly in patients with Down's syndrome, although the more complex atrioventricular septal defects with a common atrioventricular valve and a posterior defect of the basal portion of the interventricular septum are more characteristic of this chromosomal defect. The most common atrial septal defect involves the fossa ovalis, is midseptal in location, and is of the *ostium secundum* type. This type of defect should not be confused with a *patent foramen ovale*. Anatomic obliteration of the foramen ovale ordinarily follows its functional closure soon after birth, but residual "probe patency" is a normal variant; atrial septal defect denotes a true deficiency of the atrial septum and implies functional and anatomic patency.

The magnitude of the left-to-right shunt through an atrial septal defect depends on the defect size, the diastolic properties of both ventricles, and the relative impedance in the pulmonary and systemic circulations. The left-to-right shunt causes diastolic overloading of the right ventricle and increased pulmonary blood flow.

Patients with atrial septal defect are usually asymptomatic in early life, although there may be some physical underdevelopment and an increased tendency for respiratory infections; cardiorespiratory symptoms occur in many older patients. Beyond the fourth decade, a significant number of patients develop atrial arrhythmias, pulmonary arterial hypertension, bidirectional and then right-to-left shunting of blood, and cardiac failure. Patients exposed to the chronic environmental hypoxia of high altitude tend to develop pulmonary hypertension at younger ages. In some older patients, left-to-right shunting across the defect increases as progressive systemic hypertension and/or coronary artery disease result in reduced compliance of the left ventricle.

Physical Examination   Examination usually reveals a prominent right ventricular cardiac impulse and palpable pulmonary artery pulsation. The first heart sound is normal or split, with accentuation of the tricuspid valve closure sound. Increased flow across the pulmonic valve is responsible for a midsystolic pulmonary ejection murmur. The second heart sound is widely split and is relatively fixed in relation to respiration. A middiastolic rumbling murmur, loudest at the fourth intercostal space and along the left sternal border, reflects increased flow across the tricuspid valve. In patients with ostium primum defects, an apical thrill and holosystolic murmur indicate associated mitral or tricuspid incompetence or a ventricular septal defect.

The physical findings are altered when an increase in the pulmonary vascular resistance results in diminution of the left-to-right shunt. Both the pulmonary and tricuspid murmurs decrease in intensity, the pulmonic component of the second heart sound and a systolic ejection sound are accentuated, the two components of the second heart sound may fuse, and a diastolic murmur of pulmonic regurgitation appears. Cyanosis and clubbing accompany the development of a right-to-left shunt.

In adults with an atrial septal defect and atrial fibrillation, the physical findings may be confused with the findings of mitral stenosis with pulmonary hypertension because the tricuspid flow murmur and widely split second heart sound may be mistakenly thought to represent the diastolic murmur of mitral stenosis and the mitral "opening snap," respectively.

Electrocardiogram In patients with an ostium secundum defect, the ECG usually shows right axis deviation and an rSr' pattern in the right precordial leads representing delayed posterobasal activation of the ventricular septum and enlargement of the right ventricular outflow tract. An ectopic atrial pacemaker or first-degree heart block occurs occasionally in patients with defects of the sinus venosus type. In patients with an ostium primum defect, the right ventricular conduction defect is characteristically accompanied by left axis deviation and by superior orientation and counterclockwise rotation of the QRS loop in the frontal plane. Varying degrees of right ventricular and right atrial hypertrophy may occur with each type of defect, depending on the height of the pulmonary artery pressure. *Chest roentgenograms* reveal enlargement of the right atrium and ventricle, dilatation of the pulmonary artery and its branches, and increased pulmonary vascular marking.

Echocardiogram This shows pulmonary arterial and right ventricular dilatation, and anterior systolic (paradoxical) or flat interventricular septal motion if a significant right ventricular volume overload is present. The defect may be visualized directly from subcostal, right parasternal, or apical echocardiographic windows. In most institutions, two-dimensional echocardiography, supplemented by conventional or color Doppler flow examination, has supplanted cardiac catheterization as the confirmatory test for atrial septal defect. Transesophageal echocardiography is indicated if the transthoracic echocardiogram is ambiguous, which is often the case with sinus venosus defects. Cardiac catheterization is then employed if inconsistencies exist in the clinical data, if significant pulmonary hypertension or associated malformations are suspected, or if coronary artery disease is a possibility.

℞ **TREATMENT**

Operative repair, ideally in children between 3 and 6 years of age, should be advised for all patients with uncomplicated atrial septal defects in whom there is significant left-to-right shunting, i.e., with pulmonary-to-systemic flow ratios exceeding approximately 2.0:1.0. Excellent results may be anticipated, at low risk, even in patients beyond 40 years of age in the absence of pulmonary hypertension. The defect is closed, usually with a patch of pericardium or of prosthetic material, with the patient on cardiopulmonary bypass. In patients with ostium primum defects, cleft, deformed, and incompetent valves often require repair. Intraoperative transesophageal echocardiography is used to monitor the surgical results of mitral valve repair. Operation should not be carried out in patients with small defects and trivial left-to-right shunts, or in those with severe pulmonary vascular disease without a significant left-to-right shunt.

Patients with atrial septal defect of the sinus venosus or ostium secundum types rarely die before the fifth decade. During the fifth and sixth decades the incidence of progressive symptoms, often leading to severe disability, increases substantially. Medical management should include prompt treatment of respiratory tract infections, antiarrhythmic medications for atrial fibrillation or supraventricular tachycardia, and the usual measures for hypertension, coronary disease, or heart failure (see Chap. 233), if these complications occur. The risk of infective endocarditis is quite low unless the defect is complicated by valvular regurgitation or has recently been repaired with a patch (see Chap. 126).

VENTRICULAR SEPTAL DEFECT Defects of the ventricular septum are common as isolated defects and as one component of a combination of anomalies. The opening is usually single and situated in the membranous portion of the septum. The functional disturbance is dependent primarily on its size and on the status of the pulmonary vascular bed, rather than on the location of the defect. Only small or moderate-size defects are usually seen initially in adulthood as the vast majority of patients with isolated large defects come to medical and, often, surgical attention very early in life.

A wide spectrum exists in the natural history of ventricular septal defect, ranging from spontaneous closure to congestive cardiac failure and death in early infancy. Within this spectrum is the possible development of pulmonary vascular obstruction, right ventricular outflow tract obstruction, aortic regurgitation, and infective endocarditis. Spontaneous closure is more common in patients born with a small ventricular septal defect and occurs in early childhood in most patients.

Patients with large ventricular septal defects and pulmonary hypertension are those at greatest risk for developing pulmonary vascular obstruction. Thus, large defects should be corrected surgically early in life when pulmonary vascular disease is still reversible or not yet developed. In patients with severe pulmonary vascular obstruction (Eisenmenger syndrome), symptoms in adult life consist of exertional dyspnea, chest pain, syncope, and hemoptysis. The right-to-left shunt leads to cyanosis, clubbing, and erythrocytosis. In all patients, the degree to which pulmonary vascular resistance is elevated before operation is a critical factor determining prognosis. If the pulmonary vascular resistance is one-third or less of the systemic value, progression of pulmonary vascular disease after operation is unusual. However, if a moderate to severe increase in pulmonary vascular resistance exists preoperatively, either no change or a progression of pulmonary vascular disease is common postoperatively.

Right ventricular outflow tract obstruction develops in approximately 5 to 10 percent of patients who present in infancy with a moderate to large left-to-right shunt. With time, as subvalvular right ventricular outflow tract obstruction progresses, the findings in these patients begin to resemble more closely those of the cyanotic tetralogy of Fallot.

In approximately 5 percent of patients, incompetence of the aortic valve results from insufficient cusp tissue or prolapse of the cusp through the interventricular defect; the aortic regurgitation then complicates and usually dominates the clinical course.

Two-dimensional *echocardiography* with conventional or color Doppler examination can usually define the number and location of defects in the ventricular septum and detect associated anomalies. Hemodynamic and angiographic study may be employed to assess the status of the pulmonary vascular bed and clarify details of the altered anatomy.

℞ **TREATMENT**

Surgery is not recommended for patients with normal pulmonary arterial pressures with small shunts (pulmonary-to-systemic flow ratios of less than 1.5 to 2.0:1.0). Operative correction is indicated when there is a moderate to large left-to-right shunt with a pulmonary-to-systemic flow ratio that exceeds 1.5:1.0 or 2.0:1.0, in the absence of prohibitively high levels of pulmonary vascular resistance.

PATENT DUCTUS ARTERIOSUS The ductus arteriosus is a vessel leading from the bifurcation of the pulmonary artery to the aorta just distal to the left subclavian artery. Normally, the vascular channel is open in the fetus but closes immediately after birth. The flow across the ductus is determined by the pressure and resistance relationships between the systemic and pulmonary circulations and by the cross-sectional area and length of the ductus. In most adults with this anomaly, pulmonary pressures are normal and a gradient and shunt from aorta to pulmonary artery persist throughout the cardiac cycle, resulting in a characteristic thrill and a continuous "machinery" murmur with a late systolic accentuation at the upper left sternal edge. In adults who were born with a large left-to-right shunt through the ductus arteriosus, pulmonary vascular obstruction (Eisenmenger syndrome) with pulmonary hypertension, right-to-left shunting, and cyanosis have usually developed. Severe pulmonary vascular disease results in reversal of flow through the ductus, unoxygenated blood is shunted to the descending aorta, and the toes, but not the fingers, become cyanotic and clubbed, a finding termed *differential cyanosis*. The leading causes of death in adults with patent ductus are cardiac failure and infective endocarditis; occasionally severe pulmonary vascular obstruction may cause aneurysmal dilatation, calcification, and rupture of the ductus.

tomatic patients. Doppler echocardiography demonstrates the site of drainage; if the site of origin is proximal, it may be detectable by two-dimensional echocardiography. Retrograde thoracic aortography

℞ **TREATMENT**

In the absence of severe pulmonary vascular disease and predominant left-to-right shunting of blood, the patent ductus should be surgically ligated or divided. Transcatheter closure is experimental, using coils, buttons, plugs, and umbrellas. Operation should be deferred for several months in patients treated successfully for infective endocarditis, because the ductus may remain somewhat edematous and friable.

AORTIC ROOT TO RIGHT HEART SHUNTS The three most common causes of aortic root to right heart shunts are congenital aneurysm of an aortic sinus of Valsalva with fistula, coronary arteriovenous fistula, and anomalous origin of the left coronary artery from the pulmonary trunk. *Aneurysm of an aortic sinus of Valsalva* consists of a separation or lack of fusion between the media of the aorta and the annulus fibrosis of the aortic valve. Rupture usually occurs in the third or fourth decade of life; most often the aorticocardiac fistula is between the right coronary cusp and the right ventricle, but occasionally, when the noncoronary cusp is involved, the fistula drains into the right atrium. Abrupt rupture causes chest pain, bounding pulses, a continuous murmur accentuated in diastole, and volume overload of the heart. Diagnosis is confirmed by two-dimensional and Doppler echocardiographic studies; cardiac catheterization quantifies the left-to-right shunt, and thoracic aortography visualizes the fistula. Medical management is directed at cardiac failure, arrhythmias, or endocarditis. At operation, the aneurysm is closed and amputated, and the aortic wall is reunited with the heart, either by direct suture or with a prosthesis.

Coronary arteriovenous fistula, an unusual anomaly, consists of a communication between a coronary artery and another cardiac chamber, usually the coronary sinus or right atrium or ventricle. The shunt is usually of small magnitude, and myocardial blood flow is not usually compromised. Potential complications include infective endocarditis, thrombus formation with occlusion or distal embolization, rupture of an aneurysmal fistula, and rarely, pulmonary hypertension and congestive failure. A loud, superficial, continuous murmur at the lower or midsternal border usually prompts a further evaluation of asymp-

Table 235-3

Classification of Congenital Heart Disease

ACYANOTIC WITH LEFT-TO-RIGHT SHUNT

I. Atrial level shunt
  A. Atrial septal defect
    1. Ostium primum
    2. Ostium secundum
    3. Sinus venosus
  B. Atrial septal defect with mitral stenosis (Lutembacher's syndrome)
  C. Partial anomalous pulmonary venous connection
II. Ventricular level shunt
  A. Ventricular septal defect
    1. Inlet septum
    2. Muscular septum
    3. Perimembranous septum
    4. Infundibular septum
  B. Ventricular septal defect with aortic regurgitation
  C. Ventricular septal defect with left ventricular to right atrial shunt

III. Aortic root to right heart shunt
  A. Ruptured sinus of Valsalva aneurysm
  B. Coronary arteriovenous fistula
  C. Anomalous origin of the left coronary artery from the pulmonary trunk
IV. Aortopulmonary level shunt
  A. Aortopulmonary window
  B. Patent ductus arteriosus
V. Multiple level shunts
  A. Complete common atrioventricular canal
  B. Ventricular septal defect with atrial septal defect
  C. Ventricular septal defect with patent ductus arteriosus

ACYANOTIC WITHOUT A SHUNT

I. Left heart malformations
  A. Congenital obstruction to left atrial inflow
    1. Pulmonary vein stenosis
    2. Mitral stenosis
    3. Cor triatriatum
  B. Mitral regurgitation
    1. Atrioventricular septal (endocardial cushion)
    2. Congenitally corrected transposition of the great arteries
    3. Anomalous origin of the left coronary artery from the pulmonary trunk
    4. Miscellaneous (double-orifice mitral valve, congenital perforations, accessory commissures with anomalous chordal insertion, congenitally short or absent chordae, cleft posterior leaflet, parachute mitral valve, etc.)
  C. Primary dilated endocardial fibroelastosis

  D. Aortic stenosis
    1. Discrete subvalvular
    2. Valvular
    3. Supravalvular
  E. Aortic valve regurgitation
  F. Coarctation of the aorta
II. Right heart malformations
  A. Acyanotic Ebstein's anomaly of the tricuspid valve
  B. Pulmonic stenosis
    1. Subinfundibular
    2. Infundibular
    3. Valvular
    4. Supravalvular (stenosis of pulmonary artery and its branches)
  C. Congenital pulmonary valve regurgitation
  D. Idiopathic dilatation of the pulmonary trunk

CYANOTIC

I. Increased pulmonary blood flow
  A. Complete transposition of the great arteries
  B. Double-outlet right ventricle of the Taussig-Bing type
  C. Truncus arteriosus
  D. Total anomalous pulmonary venous connection
  E. Single ventricle without pulmonic stenosis
  F. Common atrium
  G. Tetralogy of Fallot with pulmonary atresia and increased collateral arterial flow
  H. Tricuspid atresia with large ventricular septal defect and no pulmonic stenosis
  I. Hypoplastic left heart (aortic atresia, mitral atresia)

II. Normal or decreased pulmonary blood flow
  A. Tricuspid atresia
  B. Ebstein's anomaly with right-to-left atrial shunt
  C. Pulmonary atresia with intact ventricular septum
  D. Pulmonic stenosis or atresia with ventricular septal defect (tetralogy of Fallot)
  E. Pulmonic stenosis with right-to-left atrial shunt
  F. Complete transposition of the great arteries with pulmonic stenosis
  G. Double-outlet right ventricle with pulmonic stenosis
  H. Single ventricle with pulmonic stenosis
  I. Pulmonary arteriovenous fistula
  J. Vena caval to left atrial communication

OTHER

I. Congenitally corrected transposition of the great arteries
II. The cardiac malpositions
III. Congenital complete heart block

SOURCE: Modified from JK Perloff, *The Clinical Recognition of Congenital Heart Disease*, Philadelphia, Saunders, 1991.

or coronary arteriography permits identification of the size and anatomic features of the fistulous tract, which may be closed by suture obliteration.

The third anomaly causing a shunt from the aortic root to the right heart is *anomalous origin of the left coronary artery from the pulmonary artery*. Myocardial infarction and fibrosis commonly lead to death within the first year, though up to 20 percent of patients survive to adolescence and beyond without surgical correction. The diagnosis is supported by the electrocardiographic findings of an anterolateral myocardial infarction. Operative management of adults consists of coronary artery bypass with an internal mammary artery graft or saphenous vein–coronary artery graft.

ACYANOTIC CONGENITAL HEART DISEASE WITHOUT A SHUNT

CONGENITAL AORTIC STENOSIS Malformations that cause obstruction to left ventricular outflow include congenital valvular aortic stenosis, discrete subaortic stenosis, supravalvular aortic stenosis, and hypertrophic obstructive cardiomyopathy (Chap. 239).

Valvular Aortic Stenosis This malformation occurs three to four times more often in males than in females. The congenital bicuspid aortic valve, which is not necessarily stenotic, is one of the most common congenital malformations of the heart, although it may go undetected in early life. Because bicuspid valves may become stenotic with time or be the site of infective endocarditis, the lesion may be difficult to distinguish in adults from acquired rheumatic or degenerative calcific aortic stenosis.

The dynamics of blood flow associated with a congenitally deformed, rigid aortic valve commonly lead to thickening of the cusps and, in later life, to calcification. Hemodynamically significant obstruction causes concentric hypertrophy of the left ventricular wall and dilatation of the ascending aorta.

→ *The clinical manifestations and hemodynamic abnormalities are discussed in Chap. 237.*

Ⓡ **TREATMENT**

The medical management of congenital valvular aortic stenosis includes prophylaxis against infective endocarditis and, in patients with diminished cardiac reserve, the administration of digitalis and diuretics and sodium restriction while awaiting operation. If severe aortic stenosis is present, strenuous physical activity should be avoided even when the patient is asymptomatic, and participation in competitive sports should probably be restricted in patients with milder degrees of obstruction. Aortic valve replacement is indicated in adults with critical obstruction, an aortic valve area < 1.0 cm^2, and symptoms secondary to left ventricular dysfunction or myocardial ischemia or hemodynamic evidence of left ventricular dysfunction. In asymptomatic children or adolescents or young adults with critical aortic stenosis without valvular calcification or these features, aortic balloon valvuloplasty is often useful (Chap. 245). If surgery is contraindicated in older patients because of a complicating medical problem such as malignancy or renal or hepatic failure, balloon valvuloplasty may provide short-term improvement. It may serve as a bridge to aortic valve replacement in patients with severe heart failure.

Subaortic Stenosis The most common form of subaortic stenosis is the *idiopathic hypertrophic* variety, also termed *hypertrophic cardiomyopathy*, which is present at birth in about one-third of the patients and is discussed in Chap. 239. In contrast, both clinically and physiologically, the *discrete* form of subaortic stenosis resembles valvular aortic stenosis. The lesion usually consists of a membranous diaphragm or fibrous ring encircling the left ventricular outflow tract just beneath the base of the aortic valve. Echocardiography demonstrates the subaortic obstruction; Doppler studies show turbulence proximal to the aortic valve and also detect and quantify the pressure gradient and

severity of aortic regurgitation. Treatment consists of excision of the membrane or fibrous ridge.

Supravalvular Aortic Stenosis This anomaly consists of a localized or diffuse narrowing of the ascending aorta originating just above the level of the coronary arteries at the superior margin of the sinuses of Valsalva. In contrast to other forms of aortic stenosis, the coronary arteries are subjected to the elevated pressures that exist within the left ventricle and are often dilated and tortuous.

COARCTATION OF THE AORTA Narrowing or constriction of the lumen of the aorta may occur anywhere along its length but is most common distal to the origin of the left subclavian artery near the insertion of the ligamentum arteriosum. Coarctation occurs in about 7 percent of patients with congenital heart disease, is twice as common in males as in females, and is most frequent in patients with gonadal dysgenesis. Clinical manifestations depend on the site and extent of obstruction and the presence of associated cardiac anomalies, most commonly a bicuspid aortic valve. Aneurysmal arterial dilatation of the circle of Willis produces a high risk of sudden rupture and death.

Most children and young adults with isolated, discrete coarctation are asymptomatic. Headache, epistaxis, cold extremities, and claudication with exercise may occur, and attention is usually directed to the cardiovascular system when a heart murmur or hypertension in the upper extremities and absence, marked diminution, or delayed pulsations in the femoral arteries are detected on physical examination. Enlarged and pulsatile collateral vessels may be palpated in the intercostal spaces anteriorly, in the axillae, or posteriorly in the interscapular area. The upper extremities and thorax may be more developed than the lower extremities. A midsystolic murmur over the anterior part of the chest, back, and spinous processes may become continuous if the lumen is narrowed sufficiently to result in a high-velocity jet across the lesion throughout the cardiac cycle. Additional systolic and continuous murmurs over the lateral thoracic wall may reflect increased flow through dilated and tortuous collateral vessels. The electrocardiogram usually reveals left ventricular hypertrophy. Roentgenograms may show a dilated left subclavian artery high on the left mediastinal border and a dilated ascending aorta. Indentation of the aorta at the site of coarctation and pre- and poststenotic dilatation (the "3" sign) along the left paramediastinal shadow are almost pathognomonic. Notching of the ribs, an important radiographic sign, is due to erosion by dilated collateral vessels. Two-dimensional echocardiography from para- or suprasternal windows identifies the site and length of coarctation, while Doppler studies record and quantify the pressure gradient. Transesophageal echocardiography and magnetic resonance imaging or digital angiography allow visualization of the length and severity of the obstruction and the associated collateral arteries. In adults, cardiac catheterization is indicated primarily to evaluate the coronary arteries.

The chief hazards result from severe hypertension and include the development of cerebral aneurysms and hemorrhage, rupture of the aorta, left ventricular failure, and infective endocarditis.

Ⓡ **TREATMENT**

This is usually surgical; resection and end-to-end anastomosis or subclavian flap angioplasty are employed commonly, although it may be necessary to use a tubular graft, patch, or bypass conduit if the narrowed segment is long. Systemic hypertension postoperatively, in the absence of residual coarctation, appears to be related to the duration of preoperative hypertension. Postsurgical recoarctation may be successfully treated with percutaneous balloon dilatation.

PULMONARY STENOSIS WITH INTACT VENTRICULAR SEPTUM Obstruction to right ventricular outflow may be localized to the supravalvular, valvular, or subvalvular levels or occur at a combination of these sites. Multiple sites of narrowing of the peripheral pulmonary arteries are a feature of *rubella embryopathy* and may occur with both the familial and sporadic forms of supravalvular aortic stenosis. Valvular pulmonic stenosis is the most common form of isolated right ventricular obstruction.

The severity of the obstructing lesion, rather than the site of narrowing, is the most important determinant of the clinical course.

In the presence of a normal cardiac output, a peak systolic transvalvular pressure gradient between 50 and 80 mmHg is considered to be moderate stenosis; levels below and above that range are classified as mild and severe, respectively. Patients with mild pulmonic stenosis are generally asymptomatic and demonstrate little or no progression in the severity of obstruction with age. In patients with more significant stenosis, the severity may increase with time. Symptoms vary with the degree of obstruction. Fatigue, dyspnea, right ventricular failure, and syncope may limit the activity of older patients, in whom moderate or severe obstruction may prevent an augmentation of cardiac output with exercise. In patients with severe obstruction, the systolic pressure in the right ventricle may exceed that in the left ventricle, since the ventricular septum is intact. Right ventricular ejection is prolonged with moderate or severe stenosis, and the sound of pulmonary valve closure is delayed and soft. Right ventricular hypertrophy reduces the compliance of that chamber, and a forceful right atrial contraction is necessary to augment right ventricular filling. A fourth heart sound, prominent *a* waves in the jugular venous pulse, and, occasionally, presystolic pulsations of the liver reflect vigorous atrial contraction. The clinical diagnosis is supported by a right parasternal lift and harsh systolic ejection murmur and thrill at the upper left sternal border, typically preceded by a systolic ejection sound, if the obstruction is valvular. The holosystolic decrescendo murmur of tricuspid regurgitation may accompany severe pulmonic stenosis, especially in the presence of congestive heart failure. Cyanosis usually reflects right-to-left shunting through a patent foramen ovale or atrial septal defect. In patients with supravalvular or peripheral pulmonary arterial stenosis, the murmur is systolic or continuous and is best heard over the area of narrowing, with radiation to the peripheral lung fields.

The *electrocardiogram* may be helpful in assessing the degree of right ventricular obstruction. In mild cases, the electrocardiogram is often normal, whereas moderate and severe stenoses are associated with right axis deviation and right ventricular hypertrophy. A ventricular strain pattern, as well as high-amplitude P waves in leads II and V_1, indicating right atrial enlargement, is associated with severe stenosis. The chest roentgenogram with mild or moderate pulmonic stenosis often shows a heart of normal size and normal vascularity of the lungs. In the presence of valvular stenosis, poststenotic dilatation of the main and left pulmonary arteries may be evident. With severe obstruction and resultant right ventricular failure, right atrial and ventricular enlargement are generally evident. The pulmonary vascularity may be reduced with severe stenosis, right ventricular failure, and/or a right-to-left shunt at the atrial level. Two-dimensional *echocardiography* visualizes pulmonary valve morphology; the outflow tract pressure gradient can be estimated by Doppler ultrasonography.

 TREATMENT
The cardiac catheter technique of balloon valvuloplasty (Chap. 229) is usually effective. Direct surgical relief of moderate and severe obstruction may be accomplished at a low risk. Multiple stenoses of the peripheral pulmonary arteries are usually inoperable, but narrowing of a single branch or at the bifurcation of the main pulmonary trunk may be corrected.

CYANOTIC CONGENITAL HEART DISEASE WITH INCREASED PULMONARY BLOOD FLOW

COMPLETE TRANSPOSITION OF THE GREAT ARTERIES In this condition the aorta arises from the right ventricle to the right of and anterior to the pulmonary artery, which emerges from the left ventricle (Fig. 235-1, *left panel*). This results in two separate and parallel circulations, and some communication between them must exist after birth to sustain life. Most patients have an interatrial communication, two-thirds have a patent ductus arteriosus, and about one-third have an associated ventricular septal defect. Transposition is more common in males and accounts for approximately 10 percent of cyanotic heart disease.

FIGURE 235-1 Complete transposition of the great arteries is depicted in the left panel. The aorta arises from the right ventricle and the pulmonary artery from the left ventricle. The only mixing between the two circulations occurs across a patent foramen ovale. In the right panel, the tetralogy of Fallot cartoon illustrates the two most important anatomic findings, a large ventricular septal defect and right ventricular outflow tract obstruction. A right-to-left shunt is shown across the ventricular septum.

The course is determined by the degree of tissue hypoxia, the ability of each ventricle to sustain an increased work load in the presence of reduced coronary arterial oxygenation, the nature of the associated cardiovascular anomalies, and the status of the pulmonary vascular bed. Pulmonary vascular obstruction develops by 1 to 2 years of age in patients with an associated large ventricular septal defect or large patent ductus arteriosus in the absence of obstruction to left ventricular outflow.

 TREATMENT
The balloon or blade catheter or surgical creation or enlargement of an interatrial communication in the neonate is the simplest procedure for providing increased intracardiac mixing of systemic and pulmonary venous blood. Systemic–pulmonary artery anastomosis may be indicated in the patient with severe obstruction to left ventricular outflow and diminished pulmonary blood flow. Intracardiac repair may be accomplished by rearranging the venous returns so that the systemic venous blood is directed to the mitral valve and thence to the left ventricle and pulmonary artery, while the pulmonary venous blood is diverted through the tricuspid valve and right ventricle to the aorta (Mustard or Senning operation). Preferably, this malformation is corrected in infancy by transposing both coronary arteries to the posterior artery and transecting, contraposing, and anastomosing the aorta and pulmonary arteries (arterial switch operation). For those patients with a ventricular septal defect in whom it is necessary to bypass a severely obstructed left ventricular outflow tract, corrective operation employs an intracardiac ventricular baffle and extracardiac prosthetic conduit to replace the pulmonary artery (Rastelli procedure).

SINGLE VENTRICLE This is a family of complex lesions with both atrioventricular valves or a common atrioventricular valve opening to a single ventricular chamber. Associated anomalies include abnormal great artery positional relationships, pulmonic valvular or subvalvular stenosis, and subaortic stenosis.

Survival to adulthood depends upon a relatively normal pulmonary blood flow and good ventricular function. Modifications of the Fontan approach are generally applied to these patients with creation of a pathway(s) from the systemic veins to the pulmonary arteries.

CYANOTIC CONGENITAL HEART DISEASE WITH DECREASED PULMONARY BLOOD FLOW

TRICUSPID ATRESIA This malformation is characterized by atresia of the tricuspid valve, an interatrial communication, and, frequently, hypoplasia of the right ventricle and pulmonary artery. The clinical picture is usually dominated by severe cyanosis due to obligatory admixture of systemic and pulmonary venous blood in the left ventricle. The electrocardiogram characteristically shows right atrial enlargement, left axis deviation, and left ventricular hypertrophy.

Atrial septostomy and palliative operations to increase pulmonary blood flow, often by anastomosis of a systemic artery or vein to a pulmonary artery, may allow survival to the second or third decade. A Fontan atriopulmonary connection may then allow functional correction in those patients with normal or low pulmonary arterial resistance pressure and good left ventricular function.

EBSTEIN'S ANOMALY Characterized by a downward displacement of the tricuspid valve into the right ventricle, due to anomalous attachment of the tricuspid leaflets, the Ebstein tricuspid valve tissue is dysplastic and results in tricuspid regurgitation. The abnormally situated tricuspid orifice produces an "atrialized" portion of the right ventricle lying between the atrioventricular ring and the origin of the valve, which is continuous with the right atrial chamber. Often the right ventricle is hypoplastic. Although the clinical manifestations are variable, some patients come to initial attention because of progressive cyanosis from right-to-left atrial shunting, or symptoms due to tricuspid regurgitation and right ventricular dysfunction, or paroxysmal atrial tachyarrhythmias. Diagnostic findings by two-dimensional echocardiography include the abnormal positional relation between the tricuspid and mitral valves with apical displacement of the septal tricuspid leaflet. Tricuspid regurgitation is quantified by Doppler examination. Surgical approaches include prosthetic replacement of the tricuspid valve when the leaflets are tethered or repair of the native valve.

TETRALOGY OF FALLOT The four components of the tetralogy of Fallot are ventricular septal defect, obstruction to right ventricular outflow, aortic override (straddle) of the ventricular septal defect, and right ventricular hypertrophy (Fig. 235-1, right panel).

The severity of right ventricular outflow obstruction determines the clinical presentation. The severity of hypoplasia of the right ventricular outflow tract varies from mild to complete (pulmonary atresia). Pulmonary valve stenosis and supravalvular and peripheral pulmonary arterial obstruction may coexist; rarely there is unilateral absence of a pulmonary artery (usually the left). A right-sided aortic arch and descending aorta occur in about 25 percent of patients with tetralogy.

The relationship between the resistance to blood flow from the ventricles into the aorta and into the pulmonary vessels plays a major role in determining the hemodynamic and clinical picture. Thus, the severity of obstruction to right ventricular outflow is of fundamental significance. When the obstruction is severe, the pulmonary blood flow is reduced markedly, and a large volume of desaturated systemic venous blood is shunted from right to left across the ventricular septal defect. Severe cyanosis and erythrocytosis occur, and symptoms and sequelae of systemic hypoxemia are prominent. In many infants and children the obstruction is mild but progressive.

The *electrocardiogram* ordinarily shows right ventricular and, less often, right atrial hypertrophy. Radiologic examination characteristically reveals a normal-sized, boot-shaped heart (*coeur en sabot*) with prominence of the right ventricle and a concavity in the region of the pulmonary conus. The pulmonary vascular markings are typically diminished, and the aortic arch and knob may be on the right side. Two-dimensional echocardiography from the parasternal or subcostal windows demonstrates the malalignment of the ventricular septal defect and the subpulmonary stenosis. Selective angiocardiography with right ventricular injection provides architectural details of the right ventricular outflow tract, pulmonary valve and annulus, and caliber of the main branches of the pulmonary artery; coronary arteriography identifies the anatomy and course of the coronary arteries.

℞ TREATMENT

Factors that may complicate the treatment of patients with tetralogy of Fallot include infective endocarditis, paradoxic embolism, excessive erythrocytosis, coagulation defects, and cerebral infarction or abscess. Corrective operation is advisable at some point for almost all patients with this anomaly. Successful correction avoids progressive infundibular obstruction, delayed growth, and complications due to hypoxemia and excessive erythrocytosis. The size of the pulmonary arteries rather than the age or size of the infant or child is the most important determinant in establishing candidacy for primary repair. Pronounced hypoplasia of the pulmonary arteries is a relative contraindication for an early corrective surgical procedure. When this problem is present, a palliative operation, such as creation of a systemic arterial–pulmonary arterial shunt, is carried out and is usually followed by complete correction, which can be carried out at a lower risk later in childhood.

OTHER FORMS OF CONGENITAL HEART DISEASES

CONGENITALLY CORRECTED TRANSPOSITION The two fundamental anatomic abnormalities in this malformation are transposition of the ascending aorta and pulmonary trunk and inversion of the ventricles. This arrangement results in desaturated systemic venous blood passing from the right atrium through the mitral valve to the left ventricle and into the pulmonary trunk, whereas arterialized pulmonary venous blood flows from the left atrium through the tricuspid valve to the right ventricle and into the aorta. Thus, the circulation is corrected functionally. The clinical presentation, course, and prognosis of patients with congenitally corrected transposition vary depending on the nature and severity of any complicating intracardiac anomalies. Ebstein-type anomalies of the left-side tricuspid atrioventricular valve, ventricular septal defect, obstruction to outflow from the venous ventricle, and congenital heart block are often associated with corrected transposition. The diagnosis of the malformation and associated lesions can often be established by two-dimensional echocardiography and Doppler examination.

MALPOSITIONS OF THE HEART Positional anomalies refer to conditions in which the cardiac apex is in the right side of the chest (dextrocardia), or at the midline (mesocardia), or in which there is a normal location of the heart in the left side of the chest but abnormal position of the viscera (isolated levocardia). Knowledge of the position of the abdominal organs and of the branching pattern of the main stem bronchi is important in categorizing these malpositions. When dextrocardia occurs *without* situs inversus, when the *visceral situs is indeterminate*, or if *isolated levocardia* is present, associated, often complex, multiple cardiac anomalies are usually present. In contrast, mirror-image dextrocardia is usually observed with complete situs inversus, which occurs most frequently in individuals whose hearts are otherwise normal.

SURGICALLY MODIFIED CONGENITAL HEART DISEASE

Because of the enormous strides in cardiovascular surgical techniques that have occurred in the past 20 years, a large number of long-term survivors of corrective operations in infancy and childhood have reached adulthood. These patients are often challenging because of the diversity of anatomic, hemodynamic, and electrophysiologic residua and sequelae of cardiac operations.

The proper care of the survivor of operation for congenital heart disease requires that the clinician understand the details of the malformation prior to operation, pay meticulous attention to the details of the operative procedure, and recognize the postoperative residua (conditions left totally or partially uncorrected), sequelae (conditions

Table 235-4

CHAPTER 236
Rheumatic Fever

1309

Potential Late Postoperative Problems

Residual shunts
Residual ventricular outflow obstruction
Residual valvular anomalies
Systemic arterial hypertension
Pulmonary vascular obstruction
Arrhythmias and conduction defects
Myocardial dysfunction
Prosthetic valve malfunction
Prosthetic conduit obstruction
Infective endocarditis

caused by surgery), and the complications that may have resulted from the operation. With the exception of ligation and division of an uncomplicated patent ductus arteriosus, almost every other surgical repair of an anomaly leaves behind or causes some abnormality of the heart and circulation that may range from trivial to serious. Intraoperative transesophageal echocardiography assists in detecting unsuspected lesions, in monitoring the repair, and in verifying a satisfactory result or directing further repair. Thus, even with results that are considered clinically to be good to excellent, continued long-term postoperative follow-up is advisable.

Table 235-4 lists the categories of common late postoperative problems. Cardiac operations importantly involving the atria, such as closure of atrial septal defect, repair of total or partial anomalous pulmonary venous return, or venous switch corrections of complete transposition of the great arteries (the Mustard or Senning operations), may be followed years later by sinus node or atrioventricular node dysfunction or by atrial arrhythmias. Intraventricular surgery may also result in electrophysiologic consequences, including complete heart block necessitating pacemaker insertion to avoid sudden death. In addition, valvular problems may arise late after initial cardiac operation. An example is the progressive stenosis of an initially nonobstructive bicuspid aortic valve in the patient who underwent aortic coarctation repair. Such aortic valves may also be the site of infective endocarditis. After repair of the ostium primum atrial septal defect, the cleft mitral valve may become progressively incompetent. Tricuspid regurgitation may also be progressive in the postoperative patient with tetralogy of Fallot if right ventricular outflow tract obstruction was not relieved adequately at initial surgery. In many patients with surgically modified congenital heart disease, inadequate relief of an obstructive lesion, or a residual regurgitant lesion, or a residual shunt will cause or hasten the onset of clinical signs and symptoms of myocardial dysfunction. Despite a good hemodynamic repair, many patients with a subaortic right ventricle will develop right ventricular decompensation and signs of "left heart failure." In many patients, particularly those who were cyanotic for many years before operation, a preexisting compromise in ventricular performance is due to the original underlying malformation.

A final category of postoperative problems involves the use of prosthetic valves, patches, or conduits in the operative repair. The special risks include infective endocarditis, thrombus formation, and premature degeneration and calcification of the prosthetic materials. There are many patients in whom extracardiac conduits are required to correct the circulation functionally and often to carry blood to the lungs from the right atrium or right ventricle. These conduits may develop intraluminal obstruction and, if they include a prosthetic valve, it may show progressive calcification and thickening.

BIBLIOGRAPHY

CHILD JS: Echo-Doppler and color-flow imaging in congenital heart disease. Cardiol Clin 8:289, 1990
———, MARELLI AJ: The application of transesophageal echocardiography in the adult with congenital heart disease, in *Transesophageal Echocardiography*, G Maurer (ed). New York, McGraw-Hill, 1994, pp159–188
DAJANI AS et al: Prevention of bacterial endocarditis. Recommendations of the American Heart Association. JAMA 264:2919, 1990

FRIEDMAN WF: Congenital heart disease in infancy and childhood, in *Heart Disease*, 5th ed, E Braunwald (ed). Philadelphia, Saunders, 1997, pp 877–962
GRAHAM TP JR et al: Task Force 1: Congenital heart disease. 26th Bethesda Conference: Recommendations for determining eligibility for competition in athletes with cardiovascular abnormalities. J Am Coll Cardiol 24:845, 1994
HIRSCH R et al: Diagnosis in adolescents and adults with congenital heart disease. Prospective assessment of individual and combined roles of magnetic resonance imaging and transesophageal echocardiography. Circulation 90:2937, 1994
KONSTANTINIDES S et al: A comparison of surgical and medical therapy for atrial septal defect in adults. N Engl J Med 333:469, 1995
PERLOFF JK: Congenital heart disease and pregnancy. Clin Cardiol 17:579, 1994
———, CHILD JS: *Congenital Heart Disease in Adults*. Philadelphia, Saunders, 1991

236 *Edward L. Kaplan*

RHEUMATIC FEVER

Acute rheumatic fever is much less common at the close of the twentieth century than it was 50 years earlier. In the late 1940s, patients with rheumatic fever and rheumatic heart disease accounted for more than half of schoolchildren recognized to have cardiovascular problems in the United States. During the Second World War, there were more than 20,000 cases of acute rheumatic fever in U.S. Navy personnel alone. The incidence of rheumatic fever has declined remarkably in the industrialized countries of the world, where the disease has become rare. However, in many developing countries, which account for almost two-thirds of the world's population, streptococcal infections, rheumatic fever, and rheumatic heart disease remain a very significant public health problem. The magnitude of the problem in these countries today is similar to that in North America 50 years ago.

The decreased incidence of acute rheumatic fever and the low prevalence of rheumatic heart disease in industrialized countries have led many physicians and public health authorities to the incorrect conclusion that these conditions are no longer a problem. However, starting in the 1980s unexpected scattered outbreaks of acute rheumatic fever among both adults and children in North America have confirmed the capacity for this potentially serious illness to reappear and pose significant public health problems. Neither antimicrobial agents nor other public health measures have been totally effective in the control of rheumatic fever.

EPIDEMIOLOGY   The epidemiology of acute rheumatic fever is identical to that of group A streptococcal upper respiratory tract infections (Chap. 143). As is the case for streptococcal sore throat, acute rheumatic fever most often occurs in children; the peak age-related incidence is between 5 and 15 years. Most initial attacks in adults take place at the end of the second and beginning of the third decades of life. Rarely, initial attacks occur as late as the fourth decade and recurrent attacks may be seen even later; attacks have been documented in the fifth and sixth decades.

Epidemiologic risk factors classically associated with individual attacks and especially with outbreaks of acute rheumatic fever include lower standards of living, especially crowding; the disease has been more common among socially and economically disadvantaged populations. However, the outbreaks in the United States in the late 1980s and early 1990s cannot be explained entirely by these factors. The large Utah outbreak of almost 300 cases during 7 years affected patients in primarily middle-class families with ready access to medical care. Therefore, one can conclude that the organism itself as well as the degree of host/herd immunity to the prevalent serotypes in an affected community are equally important risk factors.

Studies have shown that approximately 3 percent of individuals with untreated group A streptococcal pharyngitis will develop rheumatic fever. The epidemiology of rheumatic fever is also influenced by the serotypes of group A streptococci present in a population. The concept of "rheumatogenecity" of specific strains is largely based upon epidemiologic evidence associating certain serotypes with rheumatic fever (serotypes 5, 6, 18, etc.). Mucoid or highly encapsulated strains have been associated with rheumatic fever.

PATHOGENESIS More than half a century ago the pioneering studies of Lancefield differentiated beta-hemolytic streptococci into several serologic groups. This ultimately led to the association of infection by the group A organism of the oropharynx (not of other sites) and the subsequent development of acute rheumatic fever. However, the mechanism(s) responsible for the development of rheumatic fever after an infection remains elusive. Historically, approaches to understanding the pathogenesis of rheumatic fever have been grouped into three major categories: (1) direct infection by the group A streptococcus, (2) a toxic effect of streptococcal extracellular products on the host tissues, and (3) an abnormal or dysfunctional immune response to one or more as yet unidentified somatic or extracellular antigens produced by all (or perhaps only by some) group A streptococci.

There is insufficient evidence to support direct infection of the heart as the inciting event. Additionally, while toxins such as streptolysin O and others have been postulated to be responsible for this sequel, there is relatively little convincing evidence at the present time. Major efforts have focused on an abnormal immune response by the human host to one or more group A streptococcal antigens. The hypothesis of "antigenic mimicry" between human and bacterial antigens has been studied extensively and has concentrated on two interactions. The first is the similarity between the group-specific carbohydrate of the group A streptococcus and the glycoprotein of heart valves; the second involves the molecular similarity between either streptococcal cell membrane or streptococcal M protein and sarcolemma or other moieties of the human myocardial cell. The possibility of a predisposing genetic influence in some individuals is one of the most tantalizing of the incompletely understood factors that might contribute to the susceptibility to rheumatic fever. The precise genetic factors influencing the attack rate have never been adequately defined. Observations have been described that support the concept that this nonsuppurative sequel to a group A streptococcal infection results from an abnormal immune response by the human host. Thus differences in immune responses to streptococcal extracellular antigens have been reported, with a unique surface marker on non-T lymphocytes of rheumatic fever patients.

DIAGNOSIS There is no specific laboratory test that can establish a diagnosis of rheumatic fever. The diagnosis, therefore, is a clinical one but requires supporting evidence from the clinical microbiology and clinical immunology laboratories. Because of the variety of signs and symptoms associated with the rheumatic fever syndrome, in 1944 Jones first proposed criteria to assist the clinician in standardizing the diagnosis of rheumatic fever. The most recent modification of the *Jones criteria* was published in 1992 by a Special Writing Group of the American Heart Association (Table 236-1).

There are five criteria termed *major* because they are most commonly found in patients with rheumatic fever: carditis, migratory polyarthritis, Sydenham's chorea, subcutaneous nodules, and erythema marginatum.

The *carditis* of acute rheumatic fever is a pancarditis involving the pericardium, myocardium, and endocardium. In most published series, between 40 and 60 percent of patients with acute rheumatic fever have evidence of carditis, which is characterized by one or more of the following: sinus tachycardia, the murmur of mitral regurgitation, an S₃ gallop, a pericardial friction rub, and cardiomegaly. The introduction of echocardiography has assisted in the identification of subtle abnormalities of the mitral valve, and these may be present in an additional 20 percent of patients who do not have an audible heart murmur. A prolonged PR interval and evidence of heart failure may be present as well.

Healing of the rheumatic valvulitis may cause fibrous thickening and adhesion, resulting in the most serious complication of rheumatic fever, i.e., valvular stenosis and/or regurgitation (Chap. 237). The mitral valve is involved most frequently, followed by the aortic valve. Even minor degrees of rheumatic valvular involvement can lead to susceptibilities to infective endocarditis (Chap. 126). Although rheumatic pericarditis can cause a serous effusion, fibrin deposits, and even pericardial calcification, it does not lead to constrictive pericarditis.

A *migratory polyarthritis* is present in as many as 75 percent of cases, most often affecting the ankles, wrists, knees, and elbows over a period of days. It usually does not affect the small joints of the hands or feet and seldom involves the hip joints. Since salicylates and other anti-inflammatory drugs usually cause prompt resolution of joint symptoms, it is important that the clinician *not* prescribe these medications until it is determined whether the arthritis is migratory. The arthritis of acute rheumatic fever is extremely painful. Pain can be controlled with codeine or similar analgesics until the diagnosis is established. The difference between arthralgia (joint pain) and arthritis (joint pain and swelling) must be understood. Too often, arthralgia is used (incorrectly) as a major criterion.

Sydenham's chorea occurs in fewer than 10 percent of patients with rheumatic fever. The latent period between the onset of the initiating streptococcal infection and the onset of Sydenham's chorea may be as long as several months. While differing from the other manifestations, this central nervous system disorder is a part of the rheumatic fever complex and should be managed as such. Many patients who appear to have only chorea may present several decades later with evidence of typical rheumatic valvular disease. There is no definitive laboratory test for establishing a diagnosis of Sydenham's chorea, and the diagnosis is one of exclusion. Patients with Sydenham's chorea should be given secondary prophylaxis for prevention of recurrent attacks, even if they do not appear to have rheumatic heart disease.

Subcutaneous nodules and *erythema marginatum* are rare major manifestations, usually present in fewer than 10 percent of cases. Subcutaneous nodules are found over extensor surfaces of joints, are seen most often in patients with long-standing rheumatic heart disease, and are extremely rare in patients experiencing an initial attack. Erythema marginatum is an uncommon manifestation. It is an evanescent macular eruption with rounded borders—usually concentrated on the trunk.

The *minor criteria* (Table 236-1) are nonspecific and may be present in many clinical conditions.

To fulfill the Jones criteria, either two major criteria, or one major criterion and two minor criteria, *plus* evidence of an antecedent streptococcal infection are required. The latter may be provided by recovery of the organism on culture or by evidence of an immune response to one of the commonly measured group A streptococcal antigens (e.g., anti-streptolysin O, anti-deoxyribonuclease B, anti-hyaluronidase). Since the accurate diagnosis of rheumatic fever has future medical

Table 236-1

The Jones Criteria for Rheumatic Fever, Updated 1992

Major Criteria	Minor Criteria
Carditis	Clinical
Migratory polyarthritis	Fever
Sydenham's chorea	Arthralgia
Subcutaneous nodules	Laboratory
Erythema marginatum	Elevated acute phase reactants
	Prolonged PR interval

plus

Supporting evidence of a recent group A streptococcal infection (e.g., positive throat culture or rapid antigen detection test; and/or elevated or increasing streptococcal antibody test)

SOURCE: Modified from the Special Writing Group of the American Heart Association.

and financial implications, the clinician is obligated to evaluate any patient completely until the suspected diagnosis is either established or excluded. Group A streptococcal pyoderma is *not* thought to predispose to rheumatic fever.

Both the clinical microbiology and the clinical immunology laboratories have important roles in confirming the diagnosis of rheumatic fever. An attempt should be made to recover the organism from a throat culture, although group A streptococci can be recovered from the upper respiratory tract of only 25 to 40 percent of patients. If a rapid antigen detection test is used but is negative, a confirmatory throat culture should be performed. It is helpful to obtain two or three cultures from the throat at the time the diagnosis is suspected but before initiating antibiotic therapy.

At least 80 percent of patients with acute rheumatic fever have an elevated anti-streptolysin O titer at presentation. If one employs two additional streptococcal antibody tests such as the anti-DNAse B or anti-hyaluronidase test, the percentage of patients who show evidence of a preceding group A streptococcal infection will rise to more than 95 percent. While an initially elevated titer is convincing, being able to demonstrate a rise in titer from the acute to the convalescent phase is a more reliable means of documenting the recent infection. If three antibody tests are done and there is no evidence of a preceding infection, the diagnosis must be seriously reconsidered.

℞ TREATMENT

There are two necessary therapeutic approaches to patients with acute rheumatic fever: anti-streptococcal therapy and therapy for the clinical manifestations of the disease. At the time of diagnosis, *all* patients with acute rheumatic fever should be treated as if they have a group A streptococcal infection, whether or not the organism is recovered by culture. In addition to the relatively large percentage of such patients who may have a negative throat culture at the time of diagnosis, others may have only a few organisms present in the throat. Conventional antibiotic treatment should be started immediately: a complete 10-day course in adults of either oral penicillin V (500 mg twice daily), or erythromycin (250 mg four times daily) for those with penicillin allergy. Many choose intramuscular benzathine penicillin G (a single intramuscular injection of 1.2 million units) for the treatment of the presumed streptococcal infection; this will also serve as the first prophylactic treatment for the prevention of recolonization of the upper respiratory tract in the future. Intramuscular benzathine penicillin G has been reported to result in a transient elevation of the sedimentation rate.

Following the initial anti-streptococcal therapy, secondary prophylaxis should be initiated to prevent subsequent colonization of the upper respiratory tract with group A streptococci. Recommendations of the American Heart Association and of the World Health Organization are for intramuscular injection of 1.2 million units of benzathine penicillin G every 4 weeks or for oral penicillin V (250 mg twice daily) or oral sulfadiazine (1.0 g daily). Recent studies have shown that in those individuals who are at high risk for recurrence of rheumatic fever, intramuscular benzathine penicillin G given every 3 weeks is more effective in reducing the risk of recurrence. Secondary prevention should not be discontinued in patients with rheumatic heart disease, those with a history of multiple attacks of rheumatic fever, or those within 10 years of an attack.

Medical therapy for the manifestations of rheumatic fever depends on the clinical status of the patient. For adult patients with the arthritis of rheumatic fever, salicylates in doses escalating to 2 g four times daily are very effective and will result in marked clinical improvement, often within 12 h. When this prompt relief does not occur, one should reexamine the original diagnosis. Salicylates may be given for 4 to 6 weeks and gradually tapered so as to prevent a rebound. The erythrocyte sedimentation rate is one method for determining the rate of taper for salicylates. Usually this requires at least 2 weeks. There are no conclusive data to support using nonsteroidal anti-inflammatory drugs for acute rheumatic fever. There is no indication for the use of glucocorticoids solely for the treatment of the arthritis of rheumatic fever.

Most experienced physicians believe that there is a role for glucocorticoids in patients with severe carditis accompanied by congestive heart failure. However, neither salicylates nor glucocorticoids influence the future development of valvular heart disease. In adults, prednisone can be started in doses as high as 30 mg four times daily in especially severe cases, and, as the patient improves, salicylates can be added during the tapering of the steroid dose; this may require 4 to 6 weeks.

In the presence of congestive heart failure, conventional medical measures (see Chap. 233) are indicated. In the past, patients with acute rheumatic fever were kept at complete bed rest for months. This is inappropriate unless there is a specific reason such as persistent active carditis or severe heart failure. Patients with arthritis will begin to feel better very soon after anti-inflammatory therapy is begun. They may be released from bed rest but should not resume full activity until signs of inflammatory process have abated and the acute-phase reactants have returned to normal.

BIBLIOGRAPHY

BISNO AL et al: Streptococcal infections that fail to cause recurrences of rheumatic fever. J Infect Dis 136:278, 1977

COMMITTEE ON RHEUMATIC FEVER, ENDOCARDITIS AND KAWASAKI DISEASE OF THE COUNCIL ON CARDIOVASCULAR DISEASE IN THE YOUNG OF THE AMERICAN HEART ASSOCIATION: Treatment of acute streptococcal pharyngitis and prevention of rheumatic fever: A statement for health professionals. Pediatrics 96:758, 1995

DAJANI A: Rheumatic fever, in *Heart Disease*, 5th ed, E Braunwald (ed). Philadelphia, Saunders, 1997, pp 1769–1775

KAPLAN EL: Global assessment of rheumatic fever and rheumatic heart disease at the close of the century. The influences and dynamics of population and pathogens: A failure to realize prevention? (The T. Duckett Jones Memorial Lecture.) Circulation 88:1964, 1993

————: The group A streptococcal upper respiratory tract carrier state: An enigma. J Pediatr 97:337, 1980

LUE HC et al: Long-term outcome of patients with rheumatic fever receinving benzathine penicillin G prophylaxis every three weeks versus every four weeks. J Pediatr 125:812, 1994

MARKOWITZ M, GORDIS L: *Rheumatic Fever*. Philadelphia, Saunders, 1972

SPECIAL WRITING GROUP OF THE COMMITTEE ON RHEUMATIC FEVER, ENDOCARDITIS AND KAWASAKI DISEASE OF THE COUNCIL ON CARDIOVASCULAR DISEASE IN THE YOUNG OF THE AMERICAN HEART ASSOCIATION: Guidelines for the diagnosis of rheumatic fever. Jones criteria, 1992 Update. JAMA 268:2069, 1992

VEASY GL et al: Persistence of acute rheumatic fever in the intermountain area of the United States. J Pediatr 24:9, 1994

237 *Eugene Braunwald*

VALVULAR HEART DISEASE

The role of physical examination in the evaluation of patients with valvular disease is also considered in Chap. 227; of electrocardiography in Chap. 228; of cardiac catheterization and angiography in Chap. 229; and of balloon valvuloplasty in Chap. 245.

MITRAL STENOSIS

ETIOLOGY AND PATHOLOGY Two-thirds of all patients with mitral stenosis (MS) are female. MS is generally rheumatic in origin; rarely, it is congenital. Pure or predominant MS occurs in approximately 40 percent of all patients with rheumatic heart disease. The valve leaflets are diffusely thickened by fibrous tissue and/or calcific deposits. The mitral commissures fuse, the chordae tendineae fuse and shorten, the valvular cusps become rigid, and these changes, in turn, lead to narrowing at the apex of the funnel-shaped valve. While the initial insult to the mitral valve is rheumatic, the later changes may be a nonspecific process resulting from trauma to the valve caused by altered flow patterns due to the initial deformity. Calcification of the stenotic mitral valve immobilizes the leaflets and narrows the orifice further. Thrombus formation and arterial embolization may arise from the calcific valve itself.

PATHOPHYSIOLOGY In normal adults the mitral valve orifice is 4 to 6 cm². In the presence of significant obstruction, i.e., when the orifice is less than approximately 2 cm², blood can flow from the left atrium to the left ventricle only if propelled by an abnormally elevated left atrioventricular pressure gradient (Fig. 229-6), the hemodynamic hallmark of MS. When the mitral valve opening is reduced to 1 cm², a left atrial pressure of approximately 25 mmHg is required to maintain a normal cardiac output. The elevated pulmonary venous and capillary pressures reduce pulmonary compliance, causing exertional dyspnea. The first bouts of dyspnea are usually precipitated by clinical events that increase the rate of blood flow across the mitral orifice, resulting in further elevation of the left atrial pressure (see below). In order to assess the severity of obstruction, both the transvalvular pressure gradient and flow rate must be measured (Chap. 229). The latter is dependent not only on the cardiac output but on the heart rate as well. An increase in heart rate shortens diastole proportionately more than systole and diminishes the time available for flow across the mitral valve. Therefore, at any given level of cardiac output, tachycardia augments the transvalvular gradient and elevates further the left atrial pressure. (Similar considerations apply to the tricuspid valve.)

The left ventricular diastolic pressure is normal in isolated MS; coexisting aortic valve disease, systemic hypertension, mitral regurgitation (MR), ischemic heart disease, and perhaps the residua of damage produced by rheumatic myocarditis are sometimes responsible for elevations that reflect impaired left ventricular function and/or reduced left ventricular compliance. Left ventricular dysfunction, as reflected in reduced ejection fraction, occurs in about one-fourth of patients with severe, chronic MS. This may be a consequence of prolonged reduction of preload and extension of the scarring from the valve into the adjacent myocardium. In pure MS and sinus rhythm, the elevated left atrial and pulmonary artery wedge pressures exhibit a prominent atrial contraction (*a* wave) and a gradual pressure decline after mitral valve opening (*y* descent). In severe MS and whenever the pulmonary vascular resistance is significantly increased, the pulmonary arterial pressure is elevated even when the patient is at rest, and in extreme cases it may approach the systemic arterial pressure. Further elevations of left atrial, pulmonary capillary, and pulmonary arterial pressures occur during exercise. When the pulmonary arterial systolic pressure exceeds approximately 50 mmHg in patients with MS, or for that matter with any lesion affecting the left side of the heart, the increased right ventricular afterload impedes the emptying of this chamber, and right ventricular end-diastolic pressure and volume usually rise.

Cardiac Output The hemodynamic response to mitral obstruction ranges from a normal cardiac output at rest and a high left atrioventricular pressure gradient to a reduced cardiac output and low transvalvular pressure gradient. In the majority of patients with moderate MS, the cardiac output is normal or almost so at rest but rises subnormally during exertion. In patients with severe MS, particularly those in whom the pulmonary vascular resistance is strikingly elevated, the cardiac output is subnormal at rest and may fail to rise or may even decline during activity. The depressed cardiac output in patients with MS is related primarily to the obstruction of the mitral orifice but also may be due to the impairment of the function of either ventricle.

Pulmonary Hypertension The clinical and hemodynamic features of MS are influenced importantly by the level of the pulmonary artery pressure. Pulmonary hypertension results from (1) the passive backward transmission of the elevated left atrial pressure; (2) pulmonary arteriolar constriction, which presumably is triggered by left atrial and pulmonary venous hypertension (reactive pulmonary hypertension); (3) interstitial edema in the walls of the small pulmonary vessels; and (4) organic obliterative changes in the pulmonary vascular bed.

Severe pulmonary hypertension results in tricuspid and pulmonary incompetence as well as right-sided heart failure. The changes in the pulmonary vascular bed also may be considered to exert a protective effect; the elevated precapillary resistance reduces the likelihood of symptoms of pulmonary congestion by reducing the surge of blood into the pulmonary capillary bed during activity which then dams up behind the stenotic mitral valve. However, this protection occurs at the expense of a reduced cardiac output.

SYMPTOMS AND COMPLICATIONS In temperate climates the latent period between the initial attack of rheumatic carditis (in the increasingly rare circumstances in which a history of one can be elicited) and the development of symptoms due to MS is generally on the order of two decades; most patients begin to experience disability in the fourth decade. Studies carried out prior to the development of mitral valvuloplasty revealed that once a patient with MS becomes seriously symptomatic, continuous progression of the disease to death usually occurs in 2 to 5 years. In economically deprived areas, particularly on the Indian subcontinent, in Central America, and the Middle East, MS tends to progress more rapidly and frequently causes serious symptoms before the age of 20 years. On the other hand, slowly progressive MS in the elderly is being recognized with increasing frequency in the United States and western Europe.

When valvular obstruction is mild, many of the physical signs of MS may be present in the absence of any symptoms. However, even in patients whose mitral orifices are large enough to accommodate a normal blood flow with only mild elevations of left atrial pressure, elevations of pulmonary capillary pressure leading to dyspnea and cough may be precipitated by extreme exertion, excitement, fever, severe anemia, paroxysmal tachycardia, sexual intercourse, pregnancy, and thyrotoxicosis. As stenosis progresses, lesser stresses precipitate dyspnea, and the patient becomes limited in his or her daily activities. Redistribution of blood from the dependent portions of the body to the lungs, which occurs when the recumbent position is assumed, leads to orthopnea and paroxysmal nocturnal dyspnea. *Pulmonary edema* develops when there is a sudden surge in flow across a markedly narrowed mitral orifice. When moderately severe MS has existed for several years, *atrial arrhythmias*—premature contractions, paroxysmal tachycardia, flutter, and fibrillation—occur with increasing frequency. The rapid ventricular rate associated with untreated or inadequately treated atrial fibrillation is frequently responsible for acute exacerbations of dyspnea. The development of permanent atrial fibrillation often marks a turning point in the patient's course and is generally associated with acceleration of the rate at which symptoms progress.

Hemoptysis (Chap. 33) results from rupture of pulmonary-bronchial venous connections secondary to pulmonary venous hypertension. It occurs most frequently in patients who have elevated left atrial pressures *without* markedly elevated pulmonary vascular resistances and is almost never fatal. True hemoptysis must be distinguished from the bloody sputum that occurs with pulmonary edema, pulmonary infarction, and bronchitis, three conditions that occur with increased frequency in the presence of MS.

As the condition progresses and the pulmonary vascular resistance rises or when tricuspid stenosis (TS) or tricuspid regurgitation (TR) develops, symptoms secondary to pulmonary congestion sometimes diminish, and the episodes of acute pulmonary edema and hemoptysis may become reduced in frequency and severity. Elevation of pulmonary vascular resistance further increases right ventricular systolic pressure, leading to right ventricular failure, fatigue, abdominal discomfort due to hepatic congestion, and edema.

Recurrent pulmonary emboli (Chap. 261), sometimes with infarction, are an important cause of morbidity and mortality late in the course of MS. *Pulmonary infections*, i.e., bronchitis, bronchopneumonia, and lobar pneumonia, commonly complicate untreated MS. *Infective endocarditis* is rare in *pure* MS but is not uncommon in patients with combined stenosis and regurgitation. *Chest pain* occurs in about 10 percent of patients with severe MS; it may be due to pulmonary hypertension or myocardial ischemia secondary to coronary atherosclerosis; often the cause cannot be discovered.

Pulmonary Changes In addition to the aforementioned changes in the pulmonary vascular bed, fibrous thickening of the walls of the alveoli and pulmonary capillaries occurs commonly in MS. The vital capacity, total lung capacity, maximal breathing capacity, and oxygen uptake per unit of ventilation are reduced (Chap. 250), and in patients with severe MS, the latter fails to rise normally during exertion. Pulmonary compliance falls further as pulmonary capillary pressure rises during exercise. In some patients, airway resistance is abnormally increased. These alterations in pulmonary mechanics contribute to an increase in the work of breathing and are responsible for dyspnea. The diffusing capacity may be reduced, particularly during exertion, as a result of structural changes in the diffusing surface and reduction of the pulmonary capillary blood volume. These changes in the lungs are due, in part, to increased transudation of fluid from the pulmonary capillaries into the interstitial and alveolar space. As in other conditions in which left atrial pressure is elevated, pulmonary blood flow in the erect position is displaced from the basal to the apical segments of the lung (Chap. 250). The increased capacity of the pulmonary lymphatic system to drain excess fluid retards the development of alveolar edema.

Thrombi and Emboli *Thrombi* may form in the left atria, particularly in the enlarged atrial appendages of patients with MS. If they *embolize*, they do so most commonly to the brain, kidneys, spleen, and extremities. Embolization occurs much more frequently in patients with atrial fibrillation or unstable rhythms, in older patients, and in those with a reduced cardiac output, and it is seen in patients with relatively mild, as well as in those with severe, obstruction. Thus systemic embolization may be the presenting complaint in otherwise asymptomatic patients with mild MS. At operation, thrombi are *not* found more frequently in the left atria of patients with a past history of embolization than in those without this complication, indicating that it is usually the freshly formed clots that dislodge. Patients who have had one or more systemic emboli have an increased predilection for further embolic episodes. Rarely, a large pedunculated thrombus or a free-floating clot may suddenly obstruct the stenotic mitral orifice. Such "ball valve" thrombi produce syncope, angina, and changing auscultatory signs with alterations in position, findings that resemble those produced by a left atrial myxoma (Chap. 241).

PHYSICAL FINDINGS (See also Chap. 227) **Inspection** In patients with severe MS, there may be a malar flush with pinched and blue facies. In patients with sinus rhythm who have severe pulmonary hypertension or associated TS, the jugular venous pulse reveals prominent *a* waves due to vigorous right atrial systole. When atrial fibrillation is present, the jugular pulse reveals only a single expansion during systole (*c-v* wave). The systemic arterial pressure is usually normal or slightly low.

Palpation A right ventricular tap along the left sternal border signifies an enlarged right ventricle. The first heart sound may be palpable in patients with pliable valve leaflets. In patients with pulmonary hypertension, the impact of pulmonary valve closure can usually be felt in the second and third left intercostal spaces just left of the sternum. A diastolic thrill is frequently present at the cardiac apex, particularly in the left lateral recumbent position.

Auscultation The first heart sound (S_1) is generally accentuated and snapping, and since the mitral valve does not close until the left ventricular pressure reaches the level of the elevated left atrial pressure, this sound is often slightly delayed, causing a prolonged Q-S_1 interval on phonocardiography, particularly in patients with severe stenosis. In patients with pulmonary hypertension, the pulmonary component of the second heart sound (P_2) is often accentuated, and the two components of the second heart sound are closely split. A pulmonary systolic ejection click may be heard in patients with severe pulmonary hypertension and marked dilatation of the pulmonary artery. The opening snap (OS) of the mitral valve is most readily audible in expiration at, or just medial to, the cardiac apex but also may be easily heard along the left sternal edge or at the base of the heart. This sound generally follows the sound of aortic valve closure (A_2) by 0.05 to 0.12 s; that is, it follows P_2. Since the OS occurs when the left ventricular pressure falls below the left atrial pressure, the time interval between A_2 closure and OS varies inversely with the severity of the

MS. The intensities of the OS and S_1 correlate with the mobility of the anterior mitral leaflet.

The OS is followed by a low-pitched, rumbling, diastolic murmur, heard best at the apex with the patient in the left lateral recumbent position. It is accentuated by exercise carried out just before auscultation and reduced during the strain of a Valsalva maneuver. In general, the duration of this murmur correlates with the severity of the stenosis. In patients with sinus rhythm, the murmur often reappears or becomes reaccentuated during atrial systole, as atrial contraction reelevates the rate of blood flow across the narrowed orifice. Soft (grade I or II/VI) systolic murmurs are commonly heard at the apex or along the left sternal border in patients with pure MS and do not necessarily signify the presence of MR. Hepatomegaly, ankle edema, ascites, and pleural effusion, particularly in the right pleural cavity, may occur in patients with right MS and right ventricular failure.

Associated Lesions With severe pulmonary hypertension, a pansystolic murmur produced by functional TR may be audible along the left sternal border. Characteristically, this murmur is accentuated by inspiration, diminishes during forced expiration (Carvallo's sign) or during performance of the Valsalva maneuver, and it should not be confused with the apical pansystolic murmur of MR, since management of the two valvular lesions is quite different.

The recognition of associated MR is of considerable clinical importance in patients with MS. A presystolic murmur and an accentuated S_1 speak against the presence of serious associated MR, but when the S_1 and/or the OS are soft or absent in a patient with mitral valve disease who also has an apical systolic murmur, it is likely that significant MR and/or serious calcification of the deformed mitral valve leaflets are present. A third heart sound at the apex often signifies that the MR is serious; this sound is generally duller, lower pitched, and follows the OS. Occasionally, in patients with pure MS, physical signs may falsely suggest MR. Thus, in the presence of severe pulmonary hypertension and right ventricular failure, a third heart sound may originate from the right ventricle. The enlarged right ventricle may rotate the heart in a clockwise direction and form the cardiac apex, giving the examiner the erroneous impression of left ventricular enlargement. Under these circumstances, the rumbling diastolic murmur and the other auscultatory features of MS become less prominent or may even disappear and be replaced by the systolic murmur of functional TR which is mistaken for MR. When cardiac output is markedly reduced in a patient with MS, the typical auscultatory findings, including the diastolic rumbling murmur, may not be detectable (silent MS), but they may reappear as compensation is restored. Associated TS also tends to obscure many of the physical signs of MS.

The Graham Steell murmur of pulmonary regurgitation, a high-pitched, diastolic, decrescendo blowing murmur along the left sternal border, results from dilatation of the pulmonary valve ring and occurs in patients with mitral valve disease and severe pulmonary hypertension. This murmur may be indistinguishable from the more common murmur produced by aortic regurgitation (AR), except that it is rarely audible at the second right intercostal space and may disappear following successful surgical treatment of the MS.

LABORATORY EXAMINATION **Electrocardiogram** In MS and sinus rhythm, the P wave usually suggests left atrial enlargement (Chap. 228). It may become tall and peaked in lead II and upright in lead V_1 when severe pulmonary hypertension or TS complicates MS and right atrial enlargement occurs. The QRS complex may be normal, even in patients with critical MS. However, with severe pulmonary hypertension, right axis deviation and right ventricular hypertrophy are often present. When the electrocardiogram shows left ventricular hypertrophy, it generally indicates that an additional lesion which places a significant burden on the left ventricle, such as MR, aortic valve disease, or hypertension, is present.

Echocardiogram The echocardiogram is the most sensitive and specific noninvasive method for diagnosing MS. Transthoracic two-dimensional color Doppler flow echocardiographic imaging and Doppler ultrasound provide critical information, including an estimate of the transvalvular gradient and of mitral orifice size, the presence and severity of accompanying MR, the extent of restriction of valve leaflets, their thickness, and the degree of distortion of the subvalvular apparatus. In addition, echocardiography provides an assessment of the size of the cardiac chambers, an estimation of the pulmonary artery pressure, and an indication of the presence and severity of associated TR and pulmonic regurgitation. Transesophageal echocardiography provides superior images and should be employed when transthoracic imaging is inadequate for guiding therapy.

Roentgenogram   The earliest changes are straightening of the left border of the cardiac silhouette, prominence of the main pulmonary arteries, dilatation of the upper lobe pulmonary veins, and backward displacement of the esophagus by an enlarged left atrium. In patients with mild or moderate MS, the heart is not grossly enlarged. In severe MS, however, all chambers and vessels upstream to the narrowed valve are prominent, including the atria, pulmonary arteries and veins, right ventricle, and superior vena cava. Kerley B lines are fine, dense, opaque, horizontal lines that are most prominent in the lower and midlung fields and that result from distention of interlobular septa and lymphatics with edema when the resting mean left atrial pressure exceeds approximately 20 mmHg. In patients who have had multiple hemoptyses, hemosiderin-containing macrophages fill the air spaces, and if they become confluent, they result in a fine, diffuse nodulation most prominent in the lower lung fields (pulmonary hemosiderosis).

DIFFERENTIAL DIAGNOSIS   Significant MR may be associated with a prominent diastolic murmur at the apex, but this murmur commences slightly later than in patients with MS, and there is often clear-cut evidence of left ventricular enlargement. An apical pansystolic murmur of at least grade III/VI intensity as well as a third heart sound should arouse the suspicion of significant associated regurgitation. Similarly, the apical middiastolic murmur associated with AR (Austin Flint murmur) may be mistaken for MS. TS, which occurs rarely in the absence of MS, may mask many of the clinical features of MS. Echocardiography is particularly useful in detecting MS in patients who have or are suspected of having other valve lesions and in defining the severity of the various lesions.

Primary pulmonary hypertension (Chap. 260) results in a number of the clinical and laboratory features observed in MS. It occurs most frequently in young women. The OS and diastolic rumbling murmur are absent, and the pulmonary artery wedge and left atrial pressures are normal, as is the size of the left atrium on echocardiography. *Atrial septal defect* (Chap. 235) also may be mistaken for MS; in both conditions there is often clinical, electrocardiographic, and roentgenographic evidence of right ventricular enlargement and accentuation of the pulmonary vascularity. The widely split S_2 of atrial septal defect may be confused with the mitral OS, and the diastolic flow murmur across the tricuspid valve may be mistaken for the mitral diastolic murmur. However, the absence of left atrial enlargement and of Kerley B lines and the demonstration of fixed splitting of S_2 favor atrial septal defect over MS.

Left atrial myxoma (Chap. 241) may obstruct left atrial emptying, causing dyspnea, a diastolic murmur, and hemodynamic changes resembling those of MS. However, patients with left atrial myxoma often demonstrate findings suggestive of a systemic disease, with weight loss, fever, anemia, systemic emboli, and elevated erythrocyte sedimentation rate and serum IgG concentration. Usually an OS is not audible, and the auscultatory findings frequently change with body position. The diagnosis can be established by demonstrating a characteristic echo-producing mass in the left atrium by two-dimensional echocardiography.

CARDIAC CATHETERIZATION AND ANGIOCARDIOGRAPHY   Left heart catheterization (Chap. 229) is helpful in deciding whether valvulotomy is necessary in the rare patient in whom it is difficult to estimate the severity of obstruction by noninvasive tests. It is helpful in assessing associated lesions such as aortic stenosis

(AS) and AR. Catheterization and coronary arteriography are not usually necessary to aid in the decision regarding surgery in younger patients with typical findings of severe obstruction on clinical examination and echocardiography. In males over 45 years and females over 55 years and younger patients with coronary risk factors, coronary angiography is usually advisable preoperatively, in order to detect patients with critical coronary obstructions that should be bypassed at the time of operation. Catheterization and left ventricular angiography are also indicated in most patients who have undergone previous mitral valve operations and who have redeveloped serious symptoms; in such patients, clinical assessment may be particularly difficult, and the hemodynamic studies allow determination of the severity of the lesion and intelligent planning of the reoperation.

℞ **TREATMENT**

In the asymptomatic adolescent with mitral valve disease, penicillin prophylaxis of beta-hemolytic streptococcal infections (Chap. 236) and prophylaxis for infective endocarditis (Chap. 126) are important. In symptomatic patients, some improvement usually occurs with restriction of sodium intake and maintenance doses of oral diuretics. Digitalis glycosides do not alter the hemodynamics and usually do not benefit patients with pure stenosis and sinus rhythm but are necessary for slowing the ventricular rate of patients with atrial fibrillation. Small doses of beta blockers (e.g., atenolol 25 to 50 mg/d) may be added when cardiac glycosides fail to control ventricular rate in patients with atrial fibrillation or flutter. Hemoptysis is treated by measures designed to diminish pulmonary venous pressure, including bed rest, the sitting position, salt restriction, and diuresis. Anticoagulants should be administered for at least 1 year in patients with MS who have suffered systemic and/or pulmonary embolization and continuously in those with atrial fibrillation.

If atrial fibrillation is of relatively recent origin in a patient whose MS is not severe enough to warrant surgical treatment or balloon valvuloplasty, reversion to sinus rhythm pharmacologically or by means of electrical countershock is indicated. Usually this should be undertaken following 3 weeks of anticoagulant treatment. Conversion to sinus rhythm is rarely helpful in patients with severe MS, particularly those in whom the left atrium is especially enlarged or in whom atrial fibrillation has been present for more than 1 year, since reversion to atrial fibrillation is common.

Mitral Valvulotomy   Unless there is a specific contraindication, mitral valvulotomy is indicated in the symptomatic patient with pure MS whose effective orifice is less than approximately 1.0 cm^2. Operation usually not only results in striking symptomatic and hemodynamic improvement but also prolongs survival. In uncomplicated cases, the surgical mortality rate should be less than 2 percent. However, there is no evidence that surgical treatment improves the prognosis of patients with slight or no functional impairment. Therefore, unless recurrent systemic embolization has occurred, valvulotomy is *not* recommended for patients who are entirely asymptomatic, regardless of hemodynamic findings. When there is little symptomatic improvement following valvulotomy, it is likely that the procedure was ineffective, that it induced MR, or that associated valvular or myocardial disease was present. The recurrence of symptoms several years after what appeared to be a satisfactory initial result is usually due to an inadequate valvulotomy, but progression of other valvular lesions, restenosis of the mitral valve, or some combination of these conditions also may be responsible. More than half of all patients undergoing mitral valvulotomy require reoperation by 10 years. In the *pregnant patient* with MS, valvulotomy should be carried out if pulmonary congestion occurs despite intensive medical treatment.

An "open" operation using cardiopulmonary bypass is usually preferable to closed commissurotomy. In addition to opening the valve commissures, it is important to loosen any subvalvular fusion of papillary muscles and chordae tendineae and to remove large deposits of calcium, thereby improving valvular function, and to remove atrial thrombi. In patients with significant associated MR, those in whom the valve has been severely distorted by previous operative manipulation, or those in whom the surgeon does not find it possible to improve valve function significantly, the valve may have to be replaced with a prosthesis. Since the operative mortality of replacement of the mitral valve is still approximately 4 percent, and since there are long-term complications of valve replacement, patients in whom preoperative evaluation suggests the possibility that replacement may be required should be operated on only if they have *critical* MS, i.e., an orifice <0.6 cm²/m² body surface area and are in the New York Heart Association class III, i.e., symptomatic with ordinary activity, despite optimal medical therapy. The overall 10-year survival of operative survivors following mitral valve replacement is approximately 65 percent. Long-term prognosis is worse in older patients and those with marked disability and striking depression of the cardiac index preoperatively.

Percutaneous Balloon Valvuloplasty This is an alternative to surgical mitral valvulotomy in patients with pure or predominant rheumatic MS. It is the procedure of choice in young patients without extensive valvular calcification, thickening, subvalvular deformity, or MR; in them the results are similar to those of surgical valvuloplasty. It is particularly useful in pregnant women but also may be used in older patients with severe valvular deformity who are poor operative candidates (Fig. 245-7).

MITRAL REGURGITATION

ETIOLOGY Chronic rheumatic heart disease is the cause of severe MR in about one-third of cases. In contrast to MS, rheumatic MR occurs more frequently in males. The rheumatic process produces rigidity, deformity, and retraction of the valve cusps and commissural fusion, as well as shortening, contraction, and fusion of the chordae tendineae. MR also may occur as a congenital anomaly (Chap. 235), most commonly as a defect of the endocardial cushions. MR may occur with fibrosis of a papillary muscle in patients with healed myocardial infarction as well as in patients with infarction involving the base of a papillary muscle. Transient regurgitation also may occur during periods of ischemia involving a papillary muscle or the adjacent myocardium and may accompany bouts of angina pectoris. MR may occur with marked left ventricular enlargement of any cause in which dilatation of the mitral annulus and lateral displacement of the papillary muscles interfere with coaptation of the valve leaflets. In hypertrophic cardiomyopathy, the anterior leaflet of the mitral valve is displaced anteriorly during systole, leading to regurgitation (Chap. 239). Calcification of the mitral annulus of unknown cause, presumably degenerative, which occurs most commonly in elderly women, also can be responsible for significant MR. The *prolapsing mitral valve leaflet syndrome* (see below) is another important cause of MR. *Acute* MR may occur secondary to infective endocarditis involving the valve or chordae tendineae, in acute myocardial infarction with rupture of a papillary muscle or one of its heads, as a consequence of trauma, or following apparently spontaneous chordal rupture.

Regardless of cause, severe MR is often progressive, since enlargement of the left atrium places tension on the posterior mitral leaflet, pulling it away from the mitral orifice and thereby aggravating the valvular dysfunction. Similarly, the dilatation of the left ventricle increases the regurgitation, which in turn enlarges further the left atrium and ventricle, causing chordal rupture and resulting in a vicious cycle; hence the aphorism, "mitral regurgitation begets mitral regurgitation."

PATHOPHYSIOLOGY The resistance to left ventricular emptying is reduced in patients with MR. As a consequence, the left ventricle is decompressed into the left atrium during ejection, and with the reduction in left ventricular size there is a rapid decline in left ventricular tension, i.e., a progressive reduction in left ventricular afterload. The initial compensation to acute MR consists of more complete systolic emptying of the left ventricle. However, left ventricular volume increases progressively as the severity of the regurgitation increases and the function of the left ventricle deteriorates. This is often accompanied by a depressed forward cardiac output. The regurgitant volume varies directly with the left ventricular systolic pressure and

the size of the regurgitant orifice; the latter, in turn, is influenced profoundly by the degree of left ventricular dilatation.

The *v* wave in the left atrial pressure pulse is usually prominent. During early diastole, as the distended left atrium suddenly empties, there is a particularly rapid *y* descent as long as there is no associated MS (Fig. 229-7). In chronic MR, there is often an increase in left ventricular compliance, so ventricular volume may be increased with little elevation in end-diastolic pressure. The effective (forward) cardiac output is usually reduced in seriously symptomatic patients. A brief, early diastolic atrioventricular pressure gradient may occur in patients with pure regurgitation as a result of the torrential flow of blood across a normal-sized mitral orifice.

The prompt appearance of contrast material in the left atrium following its injection into the left ventricle signifies the presence of MR. The regurgitant volume can be measured by determining the difference between the total left ventricular stroke volume estimated angiocardiographically and the effective forward stroke volume determined by the Fick method (Chap. 229). Qualitative, but clinically useful, estimates of the severity of regurgitation may be made by Doppler echocardiography, color Doppler flow echocardiographic imaging, and observation on cineangiograms of the degree of left atrial opacification following the injection of contrast material into the left ventricle.

The compliance, i.e., the pressure-volume relationship, of the left atrium and pulmonary venous bed affects the clinical picture. Patients with *normal or reduced compliance* usually have *acute* MR, little enlargement of the left atrium, but marked elevation of the left atrial pressure, particularly of the *v* wave. Pulmonary edema is common. Patients with a *marked increase in left atrial compliance* are the opposite end of the spectrum, having severe long-standing severe MR, marked enlargement of the left atrium, and normal or only slightly elevated left atrial and pulmonary artery pressures. These patients usually complain of severe fatigue and exhaustion secondary to a low cardiac output, while symptoms resulting from pulmonary congestion are less prominent; atrial fibrillation is almost invariably present. Most common are patients whose clinical and hemodynamic features are between those in the other two groups, with variable degrees of enlargement of the left atrium and with significant elevation of the left atrial pressure. Symptoms are secondary to both reduced cardiac output and pulmonary congestion.

SYMPTOMS Fatigue, exertional dyspnea, and orthopnea are the most prominent complaints in patients with chronic, severe MR. Hemoptysis and systemic embolism also occur less frequently in MR than in MS. Right-sided heart failure, with painful hepatic congestion, ankle edema, distended neck veins, ascites, and TR, may be observed in patients with MR who have associated pulmonary vascular disease and marked pulmonary hypertension. In patients with *acute*, severe MR, left ventricular failure with acute pulmonary edema and/or cardiovascular collapse is common.

PHYSICAL FINDINGS The arterial pressure is usually normal, and in severe MR the arterial pulse is often characterized by a sharp upstroke. The jugular venous pulse shows abnormally prominent *a* waves in patients with sinus rhythm and marked pulmonary hypertension and prominent *v* waves in those with accompanying severe TR.

Palpation A systolic thrill is often palpable at the cardiac apex, the left ventricle is hyperdynamic with a brisk systolic impulse and a palpable rapid-filling wave, and the apex beat is often displaced laterally. When the left atrium is markedly enlarged, it may extend anteriorly, and its expansion may be palpable along the sternal border late during ventricular systole, resembling a right ventricular lift. The combination of retraction of the left ventricle and expansion of the left atrium during systole may produce a characteristic rocking motion of the chest with each cardiac cycle. A right ventricular tap and the shock of pulmonary valve closure may be palpable in patients with marked pulmonary hypertension.

Auscultation The first heart sound is generally absent, soft, or buried in the systolic murmur; an accentuated mitral closure sound is useful in excluding severe regurgitation. In patients with severe MR, the aortic valve may close prematurely, resulting in wide splitting of the second heart sound. An OS indicates associated MS but does not exclude predominant regurgitation. A low-pitched third heart sound (S_3) occurring 0.12 to 0.17 s after the aortic valve closure sound, i.e. at the completion of the rapid-filling phase of the left ventricle, is believed to be caused by the sudden tensing of the papillary muscles, chordae tendineae, and valve leaflets and is an important auscultatory feature of severe MR. The absence of an S_3 indicates that if MR exists, it may not be severe. The S_3 may be followed, often after a brief interval, by a short, rumbling, diastolic murmur, even in the absence of MS. A fourth heart sound is often audible in patients with acute, severe MR of recent onset who are in sinus rhythm. A presystolic murmur is not ordinarily heard in patients with pure MR and sinus rhythm but is present when there is significant associated MS.

A systolic murmur of at least grade III/VI intensity, is the most characteristic auscultatory finding in severe MR. It is usually holosystolic (Chap. 227), but it may be decrescendo and cease in late systole in patients with acute, severe MR when the tall v wave in the left atrial pressure pulse reduces the late systolic left ventricular–atrial pressure gradient. In MR due to papillary muscle dysfunction or mitral valve prolapse (MVP), the systolic murmur commences in midsystole (see below). The systolic murmur is usually most prominent at the apex and radiates into the axilla. However, in patients with ruptured chordae tendineae or primary involvement of the posterior mitral leaflet, the regurgitant jet strikes the left atrial wall adjacent to the aortic root, and the systolic murmur is transmitted to the base of the heart and therefore may be confused with the murmur of aortic stenosis (AS). In patients with ruptured chordae tendineae the systolic murmur may have a cooing or "sea gull" quality; in patients with a flail leaflet the murmur may have a musical quality. The systolic murmur of MR is intensified by isometric strain but is reduced during the Valsalva maneuver.

LABORATORY EXAMINATION **Electrocardiogram** In patients with sinus rhythm there is evidence of left atrial enlargement, but right atrial enlargement also may be present when pulmonary hypertension is severe. Chronic, severe MR with left atrial enlargement is generally associated with atrial fibrillation. In many patients there is no clear-cut electrocardiographic evidence of enlargement of either ventricle. In others the signs of left ventricular hypertrophy are present.

Echocardiogram Doppler echocardiography and color Doppler flow imaging are the most accurate noninvasive techniques for the detection and estimation of MR. The left atrium is usually enlarged and/or exhibits increased pulsations; the left ventricle may be hyperdynamic. With ruptured chordae tendineae or a flail leaflet, coarse, erratic motion of the involved leaflets may be noted. Findings that help to determine the etiology of MR can often be identified. These include vegetations associated with infective endocarditis, incomplete coaptation of the anterior and posterior mitral leaflets, and annular calcification, as well as left ventricular dilatation, aneurysm, or dyskinesis. The echocardiogram in patients with MVP is described below.

Roentgenogram The left atrium and left ventricle are the dominant chambers; in chronic cases, the former may be massively enlarged and forms the right border of the cardiac silhouette. Pulmonary venous congestion, interstitial edema, and Kerley B lines are sometimes noted. Marked calcification of the mitral leaflets occurs commonly in patients with long-standing combined MR and MS. Calcification of the mitral annulus may be visualized. Contrast left ventriculography is useful in the quantification of MR.

℞ TREATMENT

Medical The nonsurgical management of MR is directed toward restricting those physical activities that regularly produce dyspnea and excessive fatigue, reducing sodium intake, and enhancing sodium excretion with the appropriate use of diuretics (Chap. 233). Vasodilators and digitalis glycosides increase the forward output of the failing left ventricle. Intravenous nitroprusside (Chap. 233) or nitroglycerin to reduce afterload and thereby the volume of regurgitant flow are useful in stabilizing patients with acute and/or severe MR. Angiotensin-converting enzyme (ACE) inhibitors are useful in chronic MR, as is hydralazine. The same considerations as in patients with MS apply to the reversion of atrial fibrillation to sinus rhythm. In the late stages of heart failure anticoagulants and leg binders are used to diminish the likelihood of venous thrombi and pulmonary emboli.

Surgical In the selection of patients for surgical treatment, the chronic, often slowly progressive nature of the disease must be balanced against the immediate risks and long-term uncertainties attendant on valve reconstruction or replacement. Patients with MR who are asymptomatic or who are limited only during strenuous exertion are not considered to be candidates for surgical treatment, since their condition may remain stable for many years. On the other hand, unless there are contraindications, surgical treatment should be offered to patients with severe MR whose limitations do not allow them to work full time or to perform normal household activities despite optimal medical management. Even in patients with mild symptoms, surgical treatment is indicated when left ventricular dysfunction is progressive, with left ventricular end-systolic volume (estimated angiographically) rising above 50 mL/m^2 and/or end-systolic cavity dimension on echocardiography rising above 45 mm/m^2. In patients with chronic heart failure, the risk of surgery rises sharply, the recovery of impaired left ventricular function is incomplete, and the long-term survival is reduced. However, conservative management has little to offer these patients, so operative treatment may be indicated even at an advanced stage of the disease, and occasionally, the clinical and hemodynamic improvement following surgical treatment in patients with advanced disease is dramatic. Though most patients who survive operation appear to be greatly improved, some degree of myocardial dysfunction may persist.

When surgical treatment is contemplated, right- and left-sided heart catheterization and left ventricular angiocardiography are generally indicated. These studies are helpful in confirming the presence of severe regurgitation and aid in the identification of patients with primary myocardial disease and relatively mild, functional MR, who usually do not benefit from operation. Hemodynamic studies are also helpful in detecting and assessing the severity of any associated valve lesions, which may have to be dealt with at the time of operation or which may limit the patient's ultimate improvement if they are left untreated. Coronary angiography identifies patients who require concomitant coronary revascularization.

Surgical treatment of MR, especially that caused by valves that are markedly deformed, with shrunken, calcified leaflets secondary to rheumatic fever, requires replacement of the valve with a prosthesis, although in an increasing fraction of patients, particularly those with severe annular dilatation, flail leaflets, MVP, ruptured chordae, or infective endocarditis, reconstruction of the mitral valve apparatus (mitral valvuloplasty) and/or mitral annuloplasty with an annuloplasty ring may be successful. Valve reconstruction should be carried out whenever feasible since the operative risk is about half (1 to 4 percent) of that associated with valve replacement. Also, reconstruction spares the patient the long-term adverse consequences of valve replacement (i.e., thromboembolic and hemorrhagic complications in the case of mechanical prostheses and late valve failure necessitating repeat valve replacement in the case of bioprostheses). In addition, by preserving the integrity of the papillary muscles and subvalvular apparatus, mitral valvuloplasty maintains left ventricular function.

MITRAL VALVE PROLAPSE

MVP, also variously termed the *systolic click-murmur syndrome*, *Barlow's syndrome*, *floppy-valve syndrome*, and *billowing mitral leaflet syndrome*, is a common, but highly variable, clinical syndrome resulting from diverse pathogenic mechanisms of the mitral valve apparatus. Among these are excessive or redundant mitral leaflet tissue, which is commonly involved with myxomatous degeneration and greatly increased concentration of acid mucopolysaccharide. It is a frequent finding in patients with heritable disorders of connective tissue, including the Marfan syndrome (Chap. 348), osteogenesis imperfecta, and the Ehler-Danlos syndrome. In most patients with MVP, however, myxomatous degeneration is confined to the mitral valve leaflets without other clinical or pathologic manifestations of disease; the posterior leaflet is usually more affected than the anterior, and the mitral valve annulus is often greatly dilated. In many patients, elongated redundant chordae tendineae cause or contribute to the regurgitation.

In the majority of patients with MVP, the cause is unknown, but in some it appears to be a genetically determined collagen tissue disorder. A reduction in the production of type III collagen has been incriminated, and electron microscopy has revealed fragmentation of collagen fibrils. MVP may be associated with thoracic skeletal deformities similar to but not as severe as those in Marfan's syndrome, including a high arched palate and alterations of the chest and thoracic spine. MVP also may occur as a sequel of acute rheumatic fever, in chronic rheumatic heart disease and following mitral valvulotomy, in ischemic heart disease, and in cardiomyopathies, as well as in 20 percent of patients with ostium secundum atrial septal defect.

MVP may lead to excessive stress on the papillary muscles, which in turn leads to dysfunction and ischemia of the papillary muscles and subjacent ventricular myocardium; rupture of chordae tendineae and progressive annular dilatation and calcification also contribute to valvular regurgitation, which then places more stress on the diseased mitral valve apparatus, thereby creating a vicious cycle. The electrocardiographic changes (see below) and ventricular arrhythmias appear to result from regional ventricular dysfunction related to increased stress placed on the papillary muscles.

CLINICAL FEATURES MVP is more common in females and has been noted in a wide age range but most commonly between the ages of 14 and 30 years. There is an increased familial incidence in some patients, suggesting an autosomal dominant form of inheritance. MVP encompasses a broad spectrum of severities, ranging from patients with only a systolic click and murmur and mild prolapse of the posterior leaflet of the mitral valve to those with severe MR due to chordal rupture and massive prolapse of both leaflets. In many patients, this condition progresses over years or decades.

Most patients are asymptomatic and remain so for their entire lives. Although severe MR is a relatively uncommon complication of MVP, the latter is now the most common cause of isolated *severe* MR in the United States. Arrhythmias, most commonly ventricular premature contractions and paroxysmal supraventricular and ventricular tachycardia, have been reported and may cause palpitations, lightheadedness, and syncope. Sudden death is a very rare complication. Many patients have chest pain that is difficult to evaluate. It is often substernal, prolonged, poorly related to exertion, and rarely resembles typical angina pectoris. Transient cerebral ischemic attacks secondary to emboli from the mitral valve due to endothelial disruption have been reported. Infective endocarditis may occur in patients with MR associated with MVP.

Auscultation The most important finding is the mid- or late (nonejection) systolic click, which occurs 0.14 s or more after the first heart sound and is thought to be generated by the sudden tensing of slack, elongated chordae tendineae or by the prolapsing mitral leaflet when it reaches its maximum excursion. Systolic clicks may be multiple and may be followed by a high-pitched late systolic crescendo-decrescendo murmur, occasionally "whooping" or "honking," which is heard best at the apex. The click and murmur occur earlier with standing, the Valsalva maneuver, or inhalation of amyl nitrate, interventions that decrease left ventricular volume, exaggerating the propensity of mitral leaflet prolapse. Conversely, squatting and isometric exercise, which increase left ventricular end-diastolic volume, diminish mitral prolapse, and the click-murmur complex is delayed and may even disappear. Some patients have a midsystolic click without the murmur; others have the murmur without a click.

LABORATORY EXAMINATION The *electrocardiogram* most commonly is normal but may show biphasic or inverted T waves in leads II, III, and aVF and occasionally supraventricular or ventricular premature contractions. *Two-dimensional echocardiography* is particularly useful in identifying the abnormal position and prolapse of the mitral valve leaflets; a useful echocardiographic definition of MVP is systolic displacement (in the parasternal view) of the mitral valve leaflets into the left atrium with coaptation superior to the plane of the mitral annulus. Thickening of the mitral valve leaflets identifies a subgroup of patients at higher risk of infective endocarditis and the development of severe MR. *Color-imaging* and *Doppler studies* are helpful in revealing and evaluating accompanying MR. *Angiocardiography* generally shows prolapse of the posterior and sometimes of both mitral valve leaflets and, rarely, severe MR.

℞ TREATMENT

The management of patients with MVP consists of reassurance of the asymptomatic patient without severe MR or arrhythmias, the prevention of infective endocarditis with antibiotic prophylaxis in patients with a systolic murmur and/or thickening of mitral valve leaflets on endocardiography and the relief of the atypical chest pain; beta blockers have been found to be helpful in this regard, although their use is empirical. Antiarrhythmic agents as dictated by electrophysiologic studies should be administered if symptomatic tachyarrhythmias have occurred. If the patient is symptomatic from severe MR, mitral valve repair (or rarely, replacement) is indicated. Antiplatelet aggregation agents such as aspirin should be given to patients with transient ischemic attacks, and if these are not effective, anticoagulants should be employed.

AORTIC STENOSIS

AS occurs in about one-fourth of all patients with chronic valvular heart disease; approximately 80 percent of adult patients with symptomatic valvular AS are male.

ETIOLOGY AS may be congenital in origin, it may be secondary to rheumatic inflammation of the aortic valve, or it may be due to degenerative calcification of the aortic cusps of unknown cause. The *congenitally affected valve* may already be stenotic at birth (see Chap. 235) and may become progressively more fibrotic, calcified, and stenotic. In others the valve may be congenitally deformed, usually bicuspid, without serious narrowing of the aortic orifice during childhood; its abnormal architecture makes its leaflets susceptible to otherwise ordinary hemodynamic stresses, which ultimately lead to valvular thickening, calcification, increased rigidity, and narrowing of the aortic orifice.

Rheumatic endocarditis of the aortic leaflets produces commissural fusion, resulting sometimes in a bicuspid valve. This, in turn, makes the leaflets more susceptible to trauma and ultimately leads to calcification and further narrowing. By the time the obstruction to left ventricular outflow causes serious clinical disability, the valve is usually a rigid calcified mass, and careful examination may make it difficult or even impossible to determine the etiology of the underlying process. Rheumatic AS is almost always associated with rheumatic involvement of the mitral valve. A rheumatic etiology is favored by a history of active rheumatic fever and by associated severe aortic regurgitation.

Idiopathic calcific AS (also known as senile, sclerotic, or sclerocalcific AS) is a common disorder in the elderly, and may be associated with fibrosis and fusion of the valve cusps; the pathologic process is considered to be a degenerative one—a "wear-and-tear" phenomenon. It may produce many of the characteristic systolic murmurs of AS. However, the valvular obstruction is usually relatively mild and of little, if any, hemodynamic significance; it may, on occasion, produce critical obstruction.

**OTHER FORMS OF OBSTRUCTION TO LEFT VENTRIC-
ULAR OUTFLOW**   Besides valvular AS, three other lesions may
be responsible for obstruction to left ventricular outflow.

1. *Hypertrophic cardiomyopathy.* This condition is characterized by
   marked hypertrophy of the left ventricle, involving in particular
   the interventricular septum of the left ventricular outflow tract,
   and may cause subaortic obstruction, as described in Chap. 239.
2. *Discrete congenital subvalvular AS.* This congenital anomaly is
   produced by either a membranous diaphragm or a fibrous ridge
   just below the aortic valve (Chap. 235).
3. *Supravalvular AS.* This uncommon congenital anomaly is produced by narrowing of the ascending aorta or by a fibrous diaphragm with a small opening just above the aortic valve (Chap.
   235).

PATHOPHYSIOLOGY   The obstruction to left ventricular outflow produces a systolic pressure gradient between the left ventricle
and aorta. When severe obstruction is suddenly produced experimentally, the left ventricle responds by dilatation and reduction of stroke
volume. However, in patients the obstruction may be present at birth
and/or increases gradually over the course of many years, and left
ventricular output is maintained by the presence of left ventricular
hypertrophy. This serves as a useful compensatory mechanism because
it reduces toward normal the systolic stress developed by each segment
of myocardium. A large transaortic valvular pressure gradient may
exist for many years without a reduction of cardiac output, left ventricular dilatation, or the development of symptoms; ultimately, these
changes occur.

A peak systolic pressure gradient exceeding 50 mmHg in the face
of a normal cardiac output or an effective aortic orifice less than
approximately 0.5 cm^2/m^2 of body surface area, i.e., less than approximately one-third of the normal orifice, is generally considered to
represent critical obstruction to left ventricular outflow. The left ventricular pressure pulse exhibits a rounded summit as the contraction
of this chamber becomes progressively more isometric. The elevated
left ventricular end-diastolic pressure observed in many patients with
severe AS does not necessarily signify the presence of left ventricular
dilatation or failure but may reflect diminished compliance of the
hypertrophied left ventricular wall.

A large *a* wave in the left atrial pressure pulse is usually present
in severe AS. Loss of an appropriately timed, vigorous atrial contraction, as occurs in atrial fibrillation or atrioventricular dissociation, may
result in a rapid aggravation of symptoms. Although the cardiac output
at rest is within normal limits in the majority of patients with severe
AS, it may fail to rise normally during exercise. Late in the course
the cardiac output and left ventricular–aortic pressure gradient decline,
and the mean left atrial, pulmonary artery wedge, pulmonary arterial,
and right ventricular pressures rise.

The hypertrophied left ventricular muscle mass elevates myocardial oxygen requirements. In addition, even in the absence of obstructive coronary artery disease, there may be interference with coronary
blood flow, because the pressure compressing the coronary arteries
exceeds the coronary perfusion pressure. Metabolic evidence of myocardial ischemia can be demonstrated in patients with AS both in the
presence and in the absence of coronary arterial narrowing.

A significant fraction of patients with rheumatic AS has associated
mitral valve disease. AS intensifies the severity of MR by increasing
the pressure driving blood from the left ventricle to the left atrium.

SYMPTOMS   AS is rarely of hemodynamic or clinical importance until the valve orifice has narrowed to approximately one-third
of normal, i.e., to 0.5 cm^2/m^2 in adults. Even critical AS may exist
for many years without producing any symptoms because of the ability
of the hypertrophied left ventricle to generate the elevated intraventricular pressures required for a normal stroke volume.

Most patients with pure or predominant AS have gradually increasing obstruction for years but do not become symptomatic until the

fifth to seventh decades. Exertional dyspnea, angina pectoris, and
syncope are the three cardinal symptoms. Often there is a history of
insidious progression of fatigue and dyspnea associated with gradual
curtailment of activities. *Dyspnea* results primarily from elevation of
the pulmonary capillary pressure; the latter is caused by elevations of
left atrial and left ventricular end-diastolic pressures secondary to
reduced compliance and/or left ventricular dilatation. *Angina pectoris*
usually develops somewhat later and reflects an imbalance between the
augmented myocardial oxygen requirements and reduced oxygen
availability; the former results from the increased myocardial mass
and intraventricular pressure, while the latter may result from accompanying coronary artery disease, which is not uncommon in patients
with AS, as well as from compression of the coronary vessels by the
hypertrophied myocardium. Therefore, angina may occur in severe AS
even without obstructive epicardial coronary artery disease. *Exertional
syncope* may result from a decline in arterial pressure caused by
vasodilatation in the exercising muscles and inadequate vasoconstriction in nonexercising muscles in the face of a fixed cardiac output or
from a sudden fall in cardiac output produced by an arrhythmia.

Since the cardiac output at rest is usually well maintained until
late in the course, marked fatigability, weakness, peripheral cyanosis,
and other clinical manifestations of a low cardiac output are usually not
prominent until this stage is reached. Orthopnea, paroxysmal nocturnal
dyspnea, and pulmonary edema, i.e., symptoms of left ventricular
failure, also occur only in the advanced stages of the disease. Severe
pulmonary hypertension leading to right ventricular failure and systemic venous hypertension, hepatomegaly, atrial fibrillation, and TR
are usually preterminal findings.

When AS and MS coexist, the reduction of cardiac output induced
by MS lowers the pressure gradient across the aortic valve and thereby
masks many of the clinical findings produced by AS. Left heart catheterization is helpful in defining the relative importance of each valvular abnormality.

PHYSICAL FINDINGS   The systemic arterial pressure is usually within normal limits. In the late stages, however, when stroke
volume declines, the systolic pressure may fall and the pulse pressure
narrow. Systemic hypertension is unusual in patients with marked AS,
and a basal systolic arterial pressure exceeding 200 mmHg practically
excludes severe narrowing of this valve. The peripheral arterial pulse,
as palpated in the carotid or brachial arteries, rises slowly to a delayed
sustained peak (pulsus parvus et tardus). In the elderly, the stiffening
of the arterial wall may mask this important physical sign. A palpable
double systolic arterial pulse, the so-called bisferiens pulse, excludes
pure or predominant AS and signifies dominant aortic regurgitation.
In the late stages of valvular AS, when the pulse pressure is reduced,
the pulse amplitude may be so small that the anacrotic nature of the
pulse and the delay in its upstroke may become difficult to appreciate.
In many patients the *a* wave in the jugular venous pulse is accentuated.
This results from the diminished distensibility of the right ventricular
cavity caused by the bulging, hypertrophied interventricular septum.

Palpation   The apex beat is usually active and displaced laterally,
reflecting the presence of left ventricular hypertrophy. A double apical
impulse may be appreciated, particularly with the patient in the left
lateral recumbent position; the first outward expansion occurs during
atrial systole and reflects the important contribution made by atrial
contraction to ventricular filling, while the second occurs during ventricular systole and usually is forceful and sustained during ejection.
The right ventricle is palpable when pulmonary hypertension develops
in the late stages. A systolic thrill is generally present at the base of
the heart, in the jugular notch, and along the carotid arteries, but
occasionally it is palpable only during expiration and with the patient
leaning forward. In patients who do not have marked pulmonary
emphysema, a thick chest wall, thoracic deformity, or heart failure,
the absence of a systolic thrill suggests that the AS is relatively mild.

Auscultation   The rhythm is generally regular until very late in
the course; at other times, atrial fibrillation should suggest the possibility of associated mitral valve disease. An early systolic ejection sound,
actually the OS of the aortic valve, is frequently audible in children
and adolescents with congenital *noncalcific* valvular AS. This sound

usually disappears when the valve becomes calcified and rigid. The sound of aortic valve closure also can be identified most frequently in patients with AS who have pliable valves, and calcification diminishes the intensity of this sound as well. As AS increases in severity, left ventricular systole may become prolonged so that the aortic valve closure sound no longer precedes the pulmonic valve closure sound, and the two components may become synchronous, or aortic valve closure may even follow pulmonic valve closure, causing paradoxic splitting of the second heart sound (Chap. 227). Frequently, a fourth heart sound is audible at the apex and reflects the presence of left ventricular hypertrophy and an elevated left ventricular end-diastolic pressure; a third heart sound generally occurs when the left ventricle dilates and fails.

The murmur of AS is characteristically an ejection systolic murmur that commences shortly after the first heart sound, increases in intensity to reach a peak toward the middle of ejection, and ends just before aortic valve closure (Chap. 227). It is usually low-pitched, rough, and rasping in character, loudest at the base of the heart, most commonly in the second right intercostal space. It is transmitted to the jugular notch and upward along the carotid arteries. Occasionally, it is transmitted downward and to the apex and may be confused with the systolic murmur of MR; the latter, however, is usually holosystolic. In almost all patients with severe obstruction, the murmur is at least grade III/VI. In patients with mild degrees of obstruction or in those with severe stenosis with heart failure in whom the stroke volume and therefore the transvalvular flow rate are reduced, the murmur may be relatively soft and brief.

LABORATORY EXAMINATION **Electrocardiogram** This reveals left ventricular hypertrophy in the majority of patients with severe AS (Chap. 228). In advanced cases, ST-segment depression and T-wave inversion (left ventricular "strain") in standard leads I and aVL and in the left precordial leads are evident. However, there is no close correlation between the electrocardiogram and the hemodynamic severity of obstruction, and the absence of electrocardiographic signs of left ventricular hypertrophy does not exclude severe obstruction. The presence of left atrial enlargement should suggest the possibility of associated mitral valve disease.

Echocardiogram The key findings are left ventricular hypertrophy and in patients with valvular calcification, multiple, bright, thick, echoes from within the aortic root. Eccentricity of the aortic valve cusps is characteristic of congenitally bicuspid valves. Transesophageal imaging displays the obstructed orifice. Left ventricular dilatation and reduced systolic shortening reflect impairment of left ventricular function. The transaortic valvular gradient can be estimated by Doppler echocardiography. Echocardiography is particularly useful for identifying valvular abnormalities such as MS and AR, which sometimes accompany AS, and for differentiating valvular from obstructive hypertrophic cardiomyopathy.

Roentgenogram The chest roentgenogram may show no or little overall cardiac enlargement for many years, since the development of concentric left ventricular hypertrophy is the initial response to obstruction to left ventricular outflow. Hypertrophy without dilatation may produce some rounding of the cardiac apex in the frontal projection and slight backward displacement in the lateral view; critical AS is often associated with poststenotic dilatation of the ascending aorta. Aortic calcification is usually readily apparent on fluoroscopic examination with an image intensifier or by echocardiography; *the absence of valvular calcification in an adult suggests that severe valvular AS is not present.* In later stages of the disease as the left ventricle dilates, there is increasing evidence of left ventricular enlargement, roentgenographic signs of pulmonary congestion, as well as enlargement of the left atrium, pulmonary artery, and right side of the heart.

Catheterization and Angiocardiography Catheterization of the left side of the heart and coronary arteriography should generally be carried out in patients suspected of having severe AS, particularly before a final decision concerning operative treatment is made. The goals are to (1) determine the severity of the aortic obstruction, often previously estimated by Doppler echocardiography; (2) assess the status of left ventricular function; and (3) determine the location of the left ventricular outflow obstruction. These investigations are especially indicated in the following:

1. Young, asymptomatic patients with noncalcific congenital AS (Chap. 235), in order to define the severity of obstruction to left ventricular outflow, since operation (which does not usually require aortic valve replacement) or balloon valvuloplasty may be indicated in them if severe AS is present, even in the absence of symptoms.
2. Patients in whom it is suspected that the obstruction to left ventricular outflow may not be at the aortic valve but rather in the sub- or supravalvular regions.
3. Patients with clinical signs of AS and symptoms of myocardial ischemia, in whom associated coronary artery disease is suspected. An effort should be made to determine whether AS or coronary atherosclerosis is primarily responsible for the symptoms, and coronary arteriography should be carried out in addition to catheterization of the left side of the heart.
4. Patients with multivalvular disease, in whom the role played by each valvular deformity should be defined to aid in the planning of definitive operative treatment.

NATURAL HISTORY Death in patients with severe AS occurs most commonly in the seventh and eighth decades. Based on data obtained at postmortem examination in patients *not treated surgically,* the average time to death after the onset of various symptoms was as follows: angina pectoris, 3 years; syncope, 3 years; dyspnea, 2 years; and congestive heart failure, 1.5 to 2 years. Moreover, in more than 80 percent of patients who died with AS, symptoms had existed for less than 4 years. Congestive heart failure was considered to be the cause of death in one-half to two-thirds of patients. Among adults dying with valvular AS, sudden death, which presumably results from an arrhythmia, occurred in 10 to 20 percent and at an average age of 60 years. However, the vast majority of sudden deaths occur in previously symptomatic patients.

℞ **TREATMENT**
All patients with moderate or severe AS require careful periodic follow-up. In patients with *severe* AS, strenuous physical activity should be avoided even in the asymptomatic stage. Digitalis glycosides, sodium restriction, and the cautious administration of diuretics are indicated in the treatment of congestive heart failure, but care must be taken to avoid volume depletion. While nitroglycerin is helpful in relieving angina pectoris, vasodilator therapy for heart failure is usually of little value and may, in fact, be harmful.

Surgical Treatment The most critical decision in the management of AS concerns the advisability of surgical treatment which, in the majority of adults with calcific AS and critical obstruction (aortic orifice <0.5 cm^2/m^2 body surface area), consists of valve replacement. In most instances, it is prudent to postpone operation in patients with severe calcific AS who are asymptomatic, since their future course is difficult to predict and they may continue to do well for many years. However, they should be followed carefully by clinical examination for the development of symptoms and by serial echocardiograms for evidence of deteriorating left ventricular function; operation is generally indicated in patients with severe AS and progressive left ventricular dysfunction, even if they are asymptomatic. In patients without heart failure, the operative risk of aortic valve replacement is approximately 4 percent.

When angina pectoris, syncope, or left ventricular decompensation develops in adults with severe valvular AS, the outlook, despite medical treatment, is very poor and can be improved significantly by replacement of the aortic valve. The operative risk in this group of patients (approximately 7 to 10 percent) is considerably lower than the risk incurred by nonoperative treatment; moreover, the symptomatic improvement in some survivors of operation has been remarkable. There is evidence that regression of left ventricular hypertrophy may occur following relief of obstruction.

Operation should, if possible, be carried out before frank left ventricular failure develops; at this late stage, the operative risk is high (15 to 20 percent), and evidence of myocardial disease may persist even when the operation is technically successful. Furthermore, long-term postoperative survival also correlates inversely with preoperative left ventricular dysfunction. Nonetheless, in view of the very poor prognosis of such patients when they are treated medically, there is usually little choice but to advise immediate surgical treatment. In patients in whom severe AS and coronary artery disease coexist, relief of the AS and revascularization of the myocardium by means of aortocoronary bypass grafting may result in striking clinical and hemodynamic improvement.

Since many patients with calcific AS are elderly, particular attention must be directed to the adequacy of hepatic, renal, and pulmonary function before valve replacement is recommended. The mortality rate depends to a substantial extent on the patient's preoperative clinical and hemodynamic state. The 10-year survival rate of patients with aortic valve replacement is approximately 60 percent. Approximately 15 percent of bioprosthetic valves evidence primary valve failure in 10 years, requiring re-replacement, and an approximately equal percentage of patients with mechanical prostheses develop significant hemorrhagic complications as a consequence of treatment with anticoagulants.

Percutaneous Balloon Aortic Valvuloplasty This procedure, described in Chap. 245, is an alternative to surgery in children and young adults with congenital AS. It is not commonly employed in elderly patients with severe calcific AS because of a high restenosis rate. Nonetheless, this procedure has been employed in patients who are too ill or frail to undergo operation, in patients with life-threatening AS and advanced extracardiac disease, and as a "bridge to surgery" in patients with severe left ventricular dysfunction.

AORTIC REGURGITATION

ETIOLOGY Approximately three-fourths of patients with pure or predominant AR are males; females predominate among patients with AR who have associated mitral valve disease. In approximately two-thirds of patients with AR the disease is rheumatic in origin, resulting in thickening, deformation, and shortening of the individual aortic valve cusps, changes that prevent their proper opening during systole and closure during diastole. A rheumatic origin is less common in patients with isolated AR. Acute AR also may result from infective endocarditis, which can develop on a valve previously affected by rheumatic disease, a congenitally deformed valve, or rarely a normal aortic valve, and perforate or erode one or more of the leaflets. Patients with discrete membranous subaortic stenosis often develop thickening of the aortic valve leaflets, which in turn leads to mild or moderate degrees of AR and makes these valves particularly susceptible to endocarditis. AR also may occur in patients with congenital bicuspid aortic valves. Prolapse of an aortic cusp, resulting in progressive chronic AR, occurs in approximately 15 percent of patients with ventricular septal defect (Chap. 235). Congenital fenestrations of the aortic valve occasionally produce mild AR. Although traumatic rupture of the aortic valve is an uncommon cause of acute AR, it does represent the most frequent serious lesion observed in patients surviving nonpenetrating cardiac injuries. In patients with AR due to primary valvular disease, dilatation of the aortic annulus may occur secondarily and intensify the regurgitation.

AR, both acute and chronic, also may be due entirely to marked aortic dilatation, i.e., aortic root disease, without primary involvement of the valve leaflets; widening of the aortic annulus and separation of the aortic leaflets are responsible for the AR. Syphilis and ankylosing rheumatoid spondylitis may be associated with cellular infiltration and scarring of the media of the thoracic aorta, leading to aortic dilatation,

aneurysm formation, and severe regurgitation. In syphilis of the aorta, the involvement of the intima may narrow the coronary ostia, which in turn may be responsible for myocardial ischemia. Cystic medial necrosis of the ascending aorta, which may or may not be associated with other manifestations of the Marfan syndrome, idiopathic dilatation of the aorta, osteogenesis imperfecta, and severe hypertension all may widen the aortic annulus and lead to progressive AR. Occasionally, AR is caused by retrograde dissection of the aorta involving the aortic annulus.

The coexistence of hemodynamically significant AS with AR usually excludes all the rarer forms of AR because it occurs almost exclusively in patients whose AR is on a rheumatic or congenital basis.

PATHOPHYSIOLOGY The total stroke volume ejected by the left ventricle (i.e., the sum of the effective forward stroke volume and the volume of blood that regurgitates back into the left ventricle) is increased in AR. In patients with wide-open (*free*) AR, the volume of regurgitant flow may equal the effective forward stroke volume. In contrast to MR, in which a fraction of the left ventricular stroke volume is delivered into the low-pressure left atrium, in AR the entire left ventricular stroke volume is ejected into a high-pressure zone, the aorta. An increase in the left ventricular end-diastolic volume (increased preload) constitutes the major hemodynamic compensation for AR. The dilatation of the left ventricle allows this chamber to eject a larger stroke volume without requiring any increase in the relative shortening of each myofibril. Therefore, severe AR may occur with a normal effective forward stroke volume and a normal ejection fraction [total (forward plus regurgitant) stroke volume/end-diastolic volume], together with an elevated left ventricular end-diastolic pressure and volume. However, through the operation of Laplace's law (which indicates that myocardial wall tension is the product of intracavitary pressure and left ventricular radius), left ventricular dilatation increases the left ventricular systolic tension required to develop any given level of systolic pressure. As left ventricular function deteriorates, the end-diastolic volume rises and the ejection fraction and forward stroke volume decline. Deterioration of left ventricular function often precedes the development of symptoms. Considerable thickening of the left ventricular wall also occurs with chronic AR, and at autopsy the hearts of these patients may be among the largest encountered, sometimes exceeding 1000 g in weight.

The reverse pressure gradient from aorta to left ventricle, which is responsible for the aortic regurgitant flow, falls progressively during diastole, accounting for the decrescendo nature of the diastolic murmur. Equilibration between aortic and left ventricular pressures may occur toward the end of diastole in patients with severe AR, particularly when the heart rate is slow, and the left ventricular end-diastolic pressure may be elevated, occasionally to extremely high levels (>40 mmHg). Rarely, in acute, severe AR, the left ventricular pressure exceeds the left atrial pressure toward the end of diastole (Fig. 229-8), and this reversed pressure gradient closes the mitral valve prematurely or causes diastolic MR.

In patients with severe AR, the effective forward cardiac output usually is normal or only slightly reduced at rest, but often it fails to rise normally during exertion. Early signs of left ventricular dysfunction include reductions in the fraction of systolic shortening and in the ejection fraction, determined by echocardiography or radionuclide or contrast angiography. In advanced stages there may be considerable elevation of the left atrial, pulmonary artery wedge, pulmonary arterial, and right ventricular pressures and lowering of the forward cardiac output at rest.

Myocardial ischemia may occur in patients with AR because myocardial oxygen requirements are elevated by both left ventricular dilatation and elevated left ventricular systolic tension. However, the major portion of coronary blood flow occurs during diastole, when arterial pressure is subnormal, thereby reducing coronary perfusion pressure. This combination of increased oxygen demand and reduced supply may cause myocardial ischemia.

HISTORY A family history may frequently be elicited from patients with AR associated with the Marfan syndrome. A history compatible with infective endocarditis may sometimes be elicited from patients with rheumatic or congenital involvement of the aortic valve, and the infection often precipitates or seriously aggravates preexisting symptoms. Ankylosing spondylitis is usually self-evident.

Patients with severe AR may remain asymptomatic for as long as 10 to 15 years.

In chronic, severe AR, uncomfortable awareness of the heartbeat, especially on lying down, may be an early complaint. Sinus tachycardia during exertion or with emotion or premature ventricular contractions may produce particularly uncomfortable palpitations, as well as head pounding. These complaints may persist for many years before the development of exertional dyspnea, usually the first symptom of diminished cardiac reserve. This is followed by orthopnea, paroxysmal nocturnal dyspnea, and excessive diaphoresis. Chest pain occurs frequently, even in younger patients, and it is not necessary to invoke the presence of coronary artery disease to explain this symptom in patients with severe AR. Anginal pain may develop at rest as well as during exertion. Nocturnal angina may be a particularly troublesome symptom, and it may be accompanied by marked diaphoresis. The anginal episodes can be prolonged and often do not respond satisfactorily to sublingual nitroglycerin. Systemic fluid accumulation, including congestive hepatomegaly, ankle edema, and ascites, may develop very late in the course of the disease.

In patients with acute, severe AR, as may occur in infective endocarditis or trauma, the left ventricle cannot dilate sufficiently to maintain stroke volume, and left ventricular diastolic pressure rises rapidly with associated elevations of left atrial and pulmonary capillary pressures. Pulmonary edema and/or cardiogenic shock may develop rapidly.

PHYSICAL FINDINGS Even prior to the examination of the heart of the patient with free AR, the jarring of the entire body and the bobbing motion of the head with each systole can be appreciated, and the abrupt distention and collapse of the larger arteries are easily visible. The examination should be directed toward the detection of conditions predisposing to AR, such as the Marfan syndrome, rheumatoid spondylitis, and ventricular septal defect.

Arterial Pulse A rapidly rising "water-hammer" pulse, which collapses suddenly as arterial pressure falls rapidly during late systole and diastole (Corrigan's pulse), and capillary pulsations, an alternate flushing and paling of the skin at the root of the nail while pressure is applied to the tip of the nail (Quincke's pulse), are characteristic of free AR. A booming, "pistol-shot" sound can be heard over the femoral arteries (Traube's sign), and a to-and-fro murmur (Duroziez's sign) is audible if the femoral artery is lightly compressed with a stethoscope.

The arterial pulse pressure is widened, with an elevation of the systolic pressure, sometimes to as high as 300 mmHg, and a depression of the diastolic pressure. The measurement of arterial diastolic pressure with a sphygmomanometer may be complicated by the fact that systolic sounds are frequently heard with the cuff completely deflated. However, the level of cuff pressure at the time of muffling of the Korotkoff sounds generally corresponds fairly closely to the true intraarterial diastolic pressure. The severity of AR does not always correlate directly with the arterial pulse pressure, and severe regurgitation may exist in patients with arterial pressures in the range of 140/60 mmHg. As the disease progresses and the left ventricular end-diastolic pressure rises markedly, the arterial diastolic pressure may actually rise also, since the aortic diastolic pressure cannot fall below the left ventricular end-diastolic pressure.

Palpation The apex beat is heaving and displaced laterally and inferiorly. The systolic expansion and diastolic retraction of the apex are prominent and contrast sharply with the sustained systolic thrust characteristic of severe AS. A diastolic thrill is often palpable along the left sternal border, and a prominent systolic thrill may be palpable in the jugular notch and transmitted upward along the carotid arteries. This thrill and the accompanying systolic murmur are due to the markedly increased blood flow across the aortic orifice and do not necessarily signify the coexistence of AS. In many patients with pure AR or with combined AS and AR, the carotid arterial pulse is bisferiens, i.e., with two systolic waves separated by a trough.

Auscultation In patients with severe AR, the aortic valve closure sound is usually diminished or absent. A third heart sound and systolic ejection sound are frequently audible, and occasionally, a fourth heart sound also may be heard. The murmur of AR is typically a high-pitched, blowing, decrescendo diastolic murmur, heard best in the third intercostal space along the left sternal border. In patients with mild regurgitation, this murmur is brief, but as the severity increases, the murmur generally becomes louder and longer, and in patients with free AR it is usually holodiastolic. When the murmur is soft, it can be heard best with the diaphragm of the stethoscope and with the patient sitting up, leaning forward, and with the breath held in forced expiration. In patients in whom the AR is caused by primary valvular disease, the diastolic murmur is usually louder along the left than the right sternal border. However, when the murmur is heard best along the right sternal border, it suggests that the AR is caused by aneurysmal dilatation of the aortic root. "Cooing" or musical diastolic murmurs suggest eversion of an aortic cusp vibrating in the regurgitant stream. Unless it is trivial in magnitude, the AR is usually accompanied by peripheral signs such as a widened pulse pressure or a collapsing pulse. On the other hand, with the Graham Steell murmur of pulmonary regurgitation, there usually is clinical evidence of severe pulmonary hypertension, including a loud and palpable pulmonary component of the second heart sound.

A midsystolic ejection murmur is frequently audible in AR. It is generally heard best at the base of the heart and is transmitted along the carotid vessels. This murmur may be quite loud without signifying obstruction; it is often higher pitched, shorter, and less rasping in quality than the ejection systolic murmur heard in patients with predominant AS. A third murmur frequently heard in patients with severe AR is the Austin Flint murmur, a soft, low-pitched, rumbling middiastolic bruit. It is probably produced by the displacement of the anterior leaflet of the mitral valve by the aortic regurgitant stream but does not appear to be associated with hemodynamically significant mitral obstruction. Both the Austin Flint murmur and the rumbling diastolic murmur of MS are loudest at the apex, but the murmur of MS is usually accompanied by a loud first heart sound and immediately follows the OS of the mitral valve, while the Austin Flint murmur is often shorter in duration than the murmur of MS; in patients with sinus rhythm the latter exhibits presystolic accentuation. The auscultatory features of AR are intensified by isometric exercise such as strenuous handgrip, which augments systemic resistance, and reduced by inhalation of amyl nitrite. A blowing holosystolic murmur at the apex, which is transmitted to the axilla, also may be heard in patients with AR who have marked left ventricular dilatation and functional MR.

In *acute*, severe AR, the elevation of left ventricular end-diastolic pressure may lead to early closure of the mitral valve, an associated middiastolic sound, a soft or absent S_1, a pulse pressure that is not particularly wide, and a soft, short diastolic murmur.

LABORATORY EXAMINATION Electrocardiogram In patients with mild AR, there may be no electrocardiographic abnormalities, but with severe, chronic AR, the electrocardiographic signs of left ventricular hypertrophy become manifest (Chap. 228). In addition, these patients frequently exhibit ST-segment depression and T-wave inversion in leads I, aVL, V_5, and V_6 ("left ventricular strain"). Left axis deviation and/or QRS prolongation denote diffuse myocardial disease, generally associated with patchy fibrosis, and usually signify a poor prognosis.

Echocardiogram This reveals increased systolic excursion of the posterior left ventricular wall; the extent and velocity of wall motion are normal or even supernormal, until myocardial contractility declines. A rapid, high-frequency fluttering of the anterior mitral leaflet produced by the impact of the aortic regurgitant jet is a characteristic finding. The echocardiogram is also useful in determining the cause of AR, by detecting dilatation of the aortic annulus. Thickening and failure of coaptation of the leaflets also may be noted. Color Doppler flow echocardiographic imaging is very sensitive in the detection of

AR, and Doppler echocardiography is helpful in assessing its severity. Serial two-dimensional echocardiography is valuable in evaluating left ventricular performance and in detecting progressive myocardial dysfunction.

Roentgenogram In severe chronic AR, the apex is displaced downward and to the left in the frontal projection, and frequently the cardiac shadow extends below the left diaphragm. Left ventricular enlargement also may be apparent in the left anterior oblique and lateral projections, in which the left ventricle is displaced posteriorly and encroaches on the spine. In patients in whom primary valvular disease is responsible for the AR, the ascending aorta and aortic knob may be moderately dilated. When AR is caused by primary disease of the aortic wall, aneurysmal dilatation of the aorta may be noted, and the aorta may fill the retrosternal space in the lateral view.

Cardiac Catheterization and Angiography These tests should be carried out to aid in the decision regarding surgical treatment. In addition to providing an accurate measurement of the magnitude of regurgitation and the status of left ventricular function, the condition of the coronary arterial bed may be evaluated.

R̶x̶ **TREATMENT**

Although operation constitutes the principal treatment of AR and should be carried out before the development of heart failure, the latter usually does respond initially to treatment with digitalis glycosides, salt restriction, diuretics, and vasodilators, especially ACE inhibitors. Digitalis also may be indicated in patients with severe regurgitation and dilated left ventricles without symptoms of frank left ventricular failure. Cardiac arrhythmias and infections are poorly tolerated in patients with free AR and must be treated promptly and vigorously. Although nitroglycerin and long-acting nitrates are not as helpful in relieving anginal pain as in patients with ischemic heart disease, they are worth a trial. Patients with syphilitic aortitis should receive a full course of penicillin therapy (Chap. 174).

Surgery In deciding on the advisability and proper timing of surgical treatment, two points should be kept in mind: (1) patients with chronic AR usually do not become symptomatic until *after* the development of myocardial dysfunction, and (2) surgical treatment often does not restore normal left ventricular function. Therefore, in patients with severe AR, careful clinical follow-up and noninvasive testing with echocardiography at approximately 6-month intervals are necessary if operation is to be undertaken at the optimal time, i.e., after the onset of left ventricular dysfunction but prior to the development of severe symptoms. Operation can be deferred as long as the patient remains asymptomatic *and* retains normal left ventricular function. In general, operation should be carried out even in asymptomatic patients with progressive left ventricular dysfunction and a left ventricular ejection fraction <50 percent, a left ventricular or end-systolic volume >55 mL/m^2, or end-systolic diameter >55 mm.

Replacement of the aortic valve with a suitable mechanical or tissue prosthesis is generally necessary in patients with rheumatic AR and in many patients with other forms of regurgitation. Rarely, when a leaflet has been perforated during an episode of infective endocarditis or torn from its attachments to the aortic annulus, surgical repair may be possible. When AR is due to aneurysmal dilatation of the annulus and ascending aorta rather than to primary valvular involvement, it may be possible to reduce the regurgitation by narrowing the annulus or by excising a portion of the aortic root without replacing the valve. More frequently, however, regurgitation can be eliminated only by replacing the aortic valve, excising the aneurysm responsible for the regurgitation, and replacing the latter with a graft. This formidable procedure entails a higher risk than aortic valve replacement alone.

As in patients with other valvular abnormalities, both the operative risk of aortic valve replacement and late mortality are largely dependent on the stage of the disease and on myocardial function

at the time of operation; patients with marked cardiac enlargement and prolonged left ventricular dysfunction experience an operative mortality of approximately 10 percent and a late mortality of approximately 5 percent per year despite a technically satisfactory operation. Nonetheless, because of the poor prognosis with medical management, even patients with left ventricular failure should be considered for operation.

ACUTE AORTIC REGURGITATION Infective endocarditis, aortic dissection, and trauma are the most common causes of severe, acute AR. Since the left ventricle has not had time to dilate, stroke volume declines and ventricular diastolic pressure rises markedly; the arterial pulse pressure is often not markedly widened, and the physical signs characteristic of severe chronic AR may be absent. Premature closure of the mitral valve is common and can be recognized by echocardiography. The first heart sound is soft or absent; the aortic diastolic murmur is characteristically brief. Patients present with pulmonary congestion and edema, as well as hypotension secondary to a low cardiac output. Acute, severe regurgitation requires prompt surgical treatment, which may be lifesaving.

TRICUSPID STENOSIS

TS, a relatively uncommon valvular lesion in North America and western Europe, is more common on the Indian subcontinent and in Latin America. It is generally rheumatic in origin and is more common in women than in men. It does not occur as an isolated lesion but is usually observed in association with MS. Hemodynamically significant TS occurs in 5 to 10 percent of patients with severe MS; rheumatic TS is commonly associated with some degree of regurgitation.

PATHOPHYSIOLOGY A diastolic pressure gradient between the right atrium and ventricle can be recorded with a double-lumen cardiac catheter. It is augmented when the transvalvular blood flow increases during inspiration and is reduced during expiration. A *mean* diastolic pressure gradient exceeding 4 mmHg is usually sufficient to elevate the mean right atrial pressure to levels that result in systemic venous congestion and, unless sodium intake has been restricted and diuretics administered, it is associated with ascites and edema. In patients with sinus rhythm, the right atrial *a* wave may be extremely tall and may even approach the level of the right ventricular systolic pressure. The resting cardiac output is usually depressed and fails to rise during exercise. The low cardiac output is responsible for the normal or only slightly elevated left atrial, pulmonary arterial, and right ventricular systolic pressures despite the presence of MS.

SYMPTOMS Since the development of MS generally precedes that of TS, many patients initially have symptoms of pulmonary congestion. Amelioration of the latter should raise the possibility that TS may be developing. Characteristically, patients complain of relatively little dyspnea for the degree of hepatomegaly, ascites, and edema that they present. Fatigue secondary to a low cardiac output and discomfort due to refractory edema, ascites, and marked hepatomegaly are common in patients with TS and/or regurgitation. In some patients, TS may be suspected for the first time when symptoms of right ventricular failure persist after an adequate mitral valvulotomy.

PHYSICAL FINDINGS Since TS usually occurs in the presence of other obvious valvular disease, the diagnosis may be missed unless it is specifically considered and searched for. Severe TS is associated with marked hepatic congestion, often resulting in cirrhosis, jaundice, serious malnutrition, anasarca, and ascites. Congestive hepatomegaly and, in cases of severe tricuspid valve disease, splenomegaly are present. The jugular veins are distended, and in patients with sinus rhythm there may be giant *a* waves. The *v* waves are less conspicuous, and since tricuspid obstruction impedes right atrial emptying during diastole, there is a slow *y* descent. In patients with sinus rhythm there may be prominent presystolic pulsations of the enlarged liver as well.

The right ventricle and the shock of pulmonic valve closure are usually not palpable. Indeed, a giant *a* wave in the jugular venous pulse without palpatory evidence of pulmonary hypertension or right ventricular enlargement should suggest the possibility of TS. On auscultation, the pulmonic closure sound is not accentuated, and occasionally, an OS of the tricuspid valve may be heard approximately 0.06 s after pulmonic valve closure. The diastolic murmur of TS has many of the qualities of the diastolic murmur of MS, and since TS almost always occurs in the presence of MS, the less common valvular lesion may be missed. However, the tricuspid murmur is generally heard best along the left lower sternal margin and over the xiphoid process and is most prominent during presystole in patients with sinus rhythm. The diastolic murmur is reduced in amplitude as the stethoscope is inched laterally, only to intensify or reappear as the mitral murmur at the apex. The murmur is augmented during inspiration, and it is reduced during expiration and particularly during the Valsalva maneuver, when tricuspid blood flow is reduced. This finding is often most easily elicited when the patient is in the erect position.

LABORATORY EXAMINATION The features of right atrial enlargement (Chap. 228) include tall, peaked P waves in lead II, as well as prominent, upright P waves in lead V$_1$. The *absence* of electrocardiographic evidence of right ventricular hypertrophy in a patient with right-sided heart failure who is believed to have MS should suggest associated tricuspid valve disease. The chest roentgenograms in patients with combined TS and MS show particular prominence of the right atrium and superior vena cava without much enlargement of the pulmonary artery and with less evidence of pulmonary vascular congestion than occurs in patients with isolated MS. On echocardiographic examination, the tricuspid valve is usually thickened; the transvalvular gradient can be estimated by Doppler echocardiography.

℞ TREATMENT

Patients with TS generally exhibit marked systemic venous congestion; intensive salt restriction and diuretic therapy are required during the preoperative period. Such a preparatory period may diminish hepatic congestion and thereby improve hepatic function sufficiently so that the risks of operation are diminished. Surgical treatment of the tricuspid valve is not ordinarily indicated at the time of mitral valve surgery in patients with *mild* TS. On the other hand, definitive surgical relief of the TS should be carried out, preferably at the time of mitral valvulotomy, in patients with moderate or severe TS who have mean diastolic pressure gradients exceeding approximately 5 mmHg and tricuspid orifices less than 1.5 to 2.0 cm^2. TS is almost always accompanied by significant TR. Open-heart operations utilizing cardiopulmonary bypass may permit substantial improvement of tricuspid valve function. If this cannot be accomplished, the tricuspid valve may have to be replaced with a prosthesis, preferably a tissue valve.

TRICUSPID REGURGITATION

Most commonly, TR is functional and secondary to marked dilatation of the right ventricle and the tricuspid annulus. Functional TR may complicate right ventricular enlargement of any cause, including inferior wall infarcts that involve the right ventricle, and it is commonly seen in the late stages of heart failure due to rheumatic or congenital heart disease with severe pulmonary hypertension, as well as in ischemic heart disease, cardiomyopathy, and cor pulmonale. It is in part reversible if pulmonary hypertension is relieved. Rheumatic fever may produce organic TR, often associated with TS. Infarction of right ventricular papillary muscles, tricuspid valve prolapse, carcinoid heart disease, endomyocardial fibrosis, infective endocarditis, and trauma all may produce TR. Less commonly, regurgitation results from congenitally deformed tricuspid valves, and it occurs with defects of the atrioventricular canal as well as with Ebstein's malformation of the tricuspid valve (Chap. 235).

As is the case for TS, the clinical features of TR result primarily from systemic venous congestion and reduction of cardiac output. With the onset of TR in patients with pulmonary hypertension, symptoms of pulmonary congestion diminish, but the clinical manifestations of right-sided heart failure become intensified. The neck veins are distended with prominent *v* waves, and marked hepatomegaly, ascites,

pleural effusions, edema, systolic pulsations of the liver, and positive hepatojugular reflux are common. A prominent right ventricular pulsation along the left parasternal region and a blowing holosystolic murmur along the lower left sternal margin, which may be intensified during inspiration and reduced during expiration or the Valsalva maneuver, are characteristic findings; atrial fibrillation is usually present.

The electrocardiogram usually shows changes characteristic of the lesion responsible for the enlargement of the right ventricle that leads to TR. Roentgenographic examination usually reveals enlargement of both the right atrium and ventricle. Echocardiography may be helpful by demonstrating right ventricular dilatation and prolapsing or flail tricuspid leaflets; the diagnosis of TR can be made by color flow echocardiography, and the severity estimated by Doppler examination. The latter is also useful in estimating pulmonary artery pressure.

In patients with severe TR, the cardiac output is usually markedly reduced, and the right atrial pressure pulse may exhibit no *x* descent during early systole but a prominent *c-v* wave with a rapid *y* descent. The mean right atrial and the right ventricular end-diastolic pressures are often elevated.

℞ TREATMENT

Isolated TR, without pulmonary hypertension, such as that occurring as a consequence of infective endocarditis or trauma, is usually well tolerated and does not require operation. Indeed, even total excision of an infected tricuspid valve is often well tolerated if the pulmonary artery pressure is normal. Treatment of the underlying cause of heart failure usually reduces the severity of functional TR. In patients with mitral valve disease and TR due to pulmonary hypertension and massive right ventricular enlargement, effective surgical correction of the mitral valvular abnormality results in lowering of the pulmonary vascular pressures and gradual reduction or disappearance of the TR without direct treatment of the tricuspid valve. However, recovery may be much more rapid in patients with severe secondary TR if, at the time of mitral valve replacement, tricuspid annuloplasty (generally with the insertion of a plastic ring) or, in the rare instance of severe organic tricuspid valve disease, tricuspid valve replacement is performed. Surgical treatment of the TR also should be carried out in patients with severe regurgitation secondary to deformity of the tricuspid valve due to rheumatic fever, particularly those *without* severe pulmonary hypertension.

PULMONIC VALVE DISEASE

The pulmonic valve is affected by rheumatic fever far less frequently than are the other valves, and it is uncommonly the seat of infective endocarditis. The most common acquired abnormality affecting the pulmonic valve is regurgitation secondary to dilatation of the pulmonic valve ring as a consequence of severe pulmonary hypertension. This produces the Graham Steell murmur, a high-pitched, decrescendo, diastolic blowing murmur along the left sternal border, which is difficult to differentiate from the far more common murmur produced by AR. It is usually of little hemodynamic significance; indeed, surgical removal or destruction of the pulmonic valve by infective endocarditis does not produce heart failure unless serious pulmonary hypertension is also present. The *carcinoid syndrome* may cause pulmonic stenosis and/or regurgitation. → *Congenital pulmonic stenosis* is discussed in Chap. 235.

VALVE REPLACEMENT

The results of replacement of any valve are dependent primarily on (1) the patient's myocardial function at the time of operation, (2) the technical abilities of the operative team and the quality of the postoperative care, and (3) the durability, hemodynamic characteristics, and thrombogenicity of the prosthesis. Increased operative mortality is associated with the degree of preoperative functional disability and pulmonary hypertension. Late complications of replacement of any valve, which fortunately are declining in incidence, include paravalvular leakage, thromboemboli, bleeding due to anticoagulants, mechanical dysfunction of the prosthesis, and infective endocarditis.

The considerations regarding the choice between a bioprosthetic (tissue) and artificial mechanical valve are similar in the mitral and aortic positions and in the treatment of stenotic, regurgitant, or mixed lesions. All patients who have undergone replacement of any valve with a mechanical prosthesis must be maintained permanently on anticoagulants. The primary advantage of bioprostheses over mechanical prostheses is the reduction of thromboembolic complications, and except for patients with chronic atrial fibrillation, few such instances have been associated with their use. The major disadvantage of bioprosthetic valves is their mechanical deterioration. This results in the need to replace the prosthesis in 30 percent of patients by 10 years and 50 percent by 15 years. Bioprostheses are ordinarily not used in younger patients (<35 years) because of accelerated deterioration but are particularly useful in the elderly (>70 years), in whom there is more concern about chronic anticoagulation than about long-term (>15 years) valve durability. These valves are also indicated in women who expect to become pregnant, as well as others in whom anticoagulation may be contraindicated. Alternative bioprostheses are homograft (allograft) aortic valves obtained from cadavers and cryopreserved, as well as pulmonary autograft transplanted into the aortic position. In patients without the above contraindications, particularly those under 65 years, a mechanical prosthesis may be preferable. Many surgeons now select the St. Jude prosthesis, a double-disk tilting prosthesis, for replacement of both aortic and mitral valves because of somewhat more favorable hemodynamic characteristics and a suggestion of lower thrombogenicity.

BIBLIOGRAPHY

ANTUNES MJ, FRANCO CG: Advances in surgical treatment of acquired valve disease. Curr Opin Cardiol 11:139, 1996

BLOOMFIELD P et al: Twelve year comparison of a Bjork-Shiley mechanical heart valve with porcine bioprostheses. N Engl J Med 324:573, 1991

BRAUNWALD E: Valvular heart disease, in *Heart Disease*, 5th ed, E Braunwald (ed). Philadelphia, Saunders, 1997, pp 1007–1076

DAVID TE: Update on mitral valve repair. Ann Thorac Surg 59:1257, 1995

ENRIQUEZ-SARANO M et al: Valve repair improves the outcome of surgery for mitral regurgitation: Multivariate analysis. Circulation 91:1022, 1995

FELDMAN T: Rheumatic heart disease. Curr Opin Cardiol 11:126, 1996

GAASCH WH, EISENHAUER AC: The management of mitral valve disease. Curr Opin Cardiol 11:114, 1996

——— et al: Managing asymptomatic patients with chronic mitral regurgitation. Chest 108:842, 1995

GRAY RJ, HELFANT RH: Timing of surgery for valvular heart disease. Cardiovasc Clin 23:209, 1993

HESS OM et al: Diastolic dysfunction in aortic stenosis. Circulation 87(Suppl 5):IV73, 1993

KIRKLIN JW, BARRATT-BOYES BG: Part III. Acquired valvular heart disease, in *Cardiac Surgery*, 2d ed, JW Kirklin, BG Barratt-Boyes (eds). New York, Wiley, 1993, p 425

LINDROOS M et al: Factors associated with calcific aortic valve degeneration in the elderly. Eur Heart J 15:865, 1994

RAHIMTOOLA S (ed): *Valvular Heart Disease*, in E Braunwald (series ed), *Atlas of Heart Diseases*, vol 11. Philadelphia, Current Medicine, 1996

REED D et al: Prediction of outcome after mitral valve replacement in patients with symptomatic chronic mitral regurgitation. Circulation 84:23, 1991

REYES VP et al: Percutaneous balloon valvuloplasty compared with open surgical commissurotomy for mitral stenosis. N Engl J Med 331:961, 1994

SLATE J et al: Comparison of cardiac catheterization and Doppler echocardiography in the decision to operate in aortic and mitral valve disease. J Am Coll Cardiol 17:1026, 1991

ZUPPIROLI A et al: Natural history of mitral valve prolapse. Am J Cardiol 75:1028, 1995

COR PULMONALE*

DEFINITIONS   *Cor pulmonale* is enlargement of the right ventricle secondary to diseases of the lung, thorax, or pulmonary circulation. It is sometimes accompanied by right ventricular failure, with an elevation of transmural right ventricular end-diastolic pressure. Approximately 20 percent of hospital admissions for heart failure are caused by right ventricular failure associated with cor pulmonale. More than half of the patients with chronic obstructive lung diseases (COLD) have cor pulmonale, and this condition constitutes between 5 and 10 percent of all adult heart diseases in the United States. Cor pulmonale constitutes a higher percentage of all forms of heart disease in countries where the incidence of obstructive lung disease is higher, such as the United Kingdom.

NORMAL FUNCTION OF THE PULMONARY CIRCULATION

The pulmonary circulation is interposed between the right and left ventricles for the purpose of gas exchange, the filtering out of particles, and the chemical modification of the blood, such as the conversion of angiotensin I to angiotensin II. Normally, flow through the pulmonary vascular bed depends not only on the pumping action of the right ventricle but also on respiratory movements and the contraction of the left ventricle. Respiratory motion facilitates pulmonary blood flow by aspirating blood into the thorax on inhalation; the blood is then propelled forward by the positive pressure of exhalation acting on a one-way valved system.

The stroke volume of the right ventricle, as of the left, is regulated by its preload, contractility, and afterload (Chap. 232). Since the right ventricle is a relatively thin, compliant reservoir, acute changes in venous return (e.g., an increase with inhalation and decline with exhalation) are accommodated with little change in transmural right ventricular pressure. However, the ability of the right ventricle to increase its systolic pressure is limited. Normally, the right ventricular afterload, which is closely related to the pulmonary artery pressure, is low. The pulmonary artery pressure normally rises slightly when blood is displaced into the chest at the start of exercise; on assuming recumbency; or with cold, anxiety, or pain. A driving pressure of only about 5 cmH$_2$O between the pulmonary artery (15 cmH$_2$O) and the left atrium (10 cmH$_2$O) normally propels the entire cardiac output of approximately 5 L/min at rest through the lungs, and only a modest increase in pressure is necessary to drive a flow of up to 25 L/min through the pulmonary capillary bed during maximal exercise.

The resistance of the pulmonary circulation (R), i.e., the pulmonary vascular resistance (p. 1252), is calculated as the intravascular driving pressure (DP), i.e., pulmonary artery pressure minus pulmonary venous or left atrial pressure, divided by the pulmonary blood flow rate ($\dot{Q}$). The caliber of a distensible vessel depends on its transmural pressure. R increases when vessels collapse, narrow, or lengthen, or when the viscosity of the blood increases.

$$R = Kl\mu/r^4$$

where K = constant; l = length; r = radius; and μ = viscosity. There is no single value of R that describes the pulmonary vascular bed because the relationship between driving pressure and flow is not linear; calculated R decreases with increasing pulmonary blood flow because pulmonary vessels are distended and collapsed vessels are recruited (Fig. 238-1).

PATHOPHYSIOLOGY   The severity of right ventricular enlargement in cor pulmonale is a function of the increase in afterload. When the pulmonary vascular resistance is elevated and relatively

---

* This chapter was co-authored by the late Dr. John Butler in the 13th edition.

FIGURE 238-1 Relationship between flow and driving pressure ("vascular resistance") in the pulmonary circulation. Note that it does not pass through zero at the origin since an opening pressure must be overcome before flow starts. Thus the calculated vascular resistance (reciprocal of relationship of flow to pressure, dashed lines) falls (1 → 2) as flow increases. *(After R Graham et al, J Appl Physiol 54:1277, 1983, with permission.)*

fixed, as in pulmonary vascular or severe parenchymal lung disease, an elevation in cardiac output as occurs with physical exertion can elevate pulmonary artery pressure markedly. Right ventricular afterload can be augmented when lung volume is enlarged, as in COLD, due to the compression of the alveolar capillaries and the lengthening of the pulmonary vessels. Right ventricular afterload can also increase when lung volume is reduced following extensive pulmonary resection, as well as in restrictive lung diseases in which pulmonary vessels are compressed and distorted. Right ventricular afterload rises with hypoxic pulmonary vasoconstriction caused by hypoxia or acidosis, which are important causes of pulmonary hypertension. Hypoxic vasoconstriction in regions of the lung affected by disease distributes blood flow to normally ventilated regions. Hypoxic vasoconstriction results from alveolar, rather than intravascular, hypoxia and is made worse by hypercarbia, probably because of the associated acidosis. When the hematocrit becomes markedly elevated with chronic hypoxemia, the increase in blood viscosity can aggravate the pulmonary hypertension. Chronic hypoxic pulmonary vasoconstriction may cause pulmonary vascular disease with endothelial swelling and medial hypertrophy (see below).

The elevation of right ventricular afterload responsible for cor pulmonale is caused principally by pulmonary vascular or parenchymal disease. The principal syndromes and their pathophysiologic mechanisms are summarized in Table 238-1.

PULMONARY VASCULAR DISEASES

In these conditions the right ventricular afterload is elevated as a consequence of the restriction to pulmonary blood flow. In cor pulmonale secondary to pulmonary vascular disease, pulmonary hypertension is usually more severe than in pulmonary parenchymal disease. Chronic cor pulmonale secondary to pulmonary vascular disease may result from repeated pulmonary emboli, pulmonary vasculitis, pulmonary vasoconstriction secondary to high altitude, congenital heart disease with left-to-right shunting (e.g., atrial or ventricular septal defect, patent ductus arteriosus; Chap. 235), as well as pulmonary venoocclusive disease. When the cause of elevated pulmonary vascular resistance responsible for cor pulmonale is unknown, the condition is referred to as *primary pulmonary hypertension* (Chap. 260).

COR PULMONALE DUE TO PULMONARY EMBOLI This condition is associated with two distinct syndromes.

Acute Cor Pulmonale It has been estimated that in the United States about 50,000 people die each year from pulmonary emboli (Chap. 261). Probably half die within the first hour from acute right heart failure due to massive or multiple emboli. A large embolic burden causes a sudden, low-output state resulting from the right ventricle's inability to generate the high pressure necessary to drive blood through the acutely compromised pulmonary vascular bed. Depression of cardiac output can also occur with a moderate-sized embolism if the pulmonary circulation has been critically compromised by previous pulmonary vascular or parenchymal disease. The right ventricle begins to fail when systolic pressure is suddenly forced to double, i.e., to exceed approximately 40 to 45 mmHg. Acute right ventricular failure secondary to pulmonary embolism is suggested by the history of the sudden onset of severe dyspnea and cardiovascular collapse in a patient with, or predisposed to, venous thrombosis.

Clinical manifestations The low cardiac output causes pallor, sweating, hypotension, and a rapid pulse of small amplitude. The neck

Table 238-1

Cor Pulmonale		
Mechanisms	**Responses**	**Characteristics**
PULMONARY VASCULAR DISEASES		
Emboli, large or multiple	Fall in cardiac output due to acute obstruction	Acute cor pulmonale Right ventricular distention Shock
Emboli, small; vasculitis; widespread lung damage (ARDS)	Pulmonary hypertension due to widespread hypoxia and microvascular obstruction	Subacute cor pulmonale Right ventricular distention Breathlessness and fever
Emboli, medium and recurrent; primary pulmonary hypertension; diet or drug vasopathy	Pulmonary hypertension due to vascular obstruction Low or normal cardiac output	Chronic cor pulmonale Right heart hypertrophy Breathlessness
RESPIRATORY DISEASES		
Obstructive Chronic bronchitis and emphysema; chronic asthma	Pulmonary hypertension due to hypoxia, vascular stretching and loss of vessels Heart beat impeded externally by lung hyperinflation Normal or high output	Chronic cor pulmonale "Blue bloater" or "Pink puffer" (see Chap. 258)
Restrictive 1. Intrinsic: interstitial fibrosis, lung resection	Hypertension due to hypoxia, vascular distortion and loss Normal or low output	Chronic cor pulmonale Breathlessness Hyperventilation
2. Extrinsic: obesity, myxedema, muscle weakness, kyphoscoliosis, upper airway obstruction, diminished respiratory drive, high altitude	Hypertension due to alveolar hypoxia Normal or high output	Chronic cor pulmonale Peripheral edema Hypoventilation

NOTE: ARDS, adult respiratory distress syndrome.

veins are distended and often exhibit the prominent *v* waves of tricuspid regurgitation. The liver may be pulsatile, distended, and tender. A systolic murmur of tricuspid regurgitation at the left sternal border may be accompanied by a presystolic (S_4) gallop sound. Arterial blood gas frequently shows hypoxemia due to ventilation/perfusion mismatching and a low Pa_{CO_2} due to hyperventilation.

℞ TREATMENT

If the cardiac output remains adequate to sustain the patient during the critical first 2 or 3 h, the natural lytic response usually results in fragmentation of the clot so that the patient survives. Although it has been shown that treatment with thrombolytic agents lyses clots more rapidly than does heparin (Chap. 261), this therapy is probably indicated only when blood flow is critically reduced and not improving. In acute cor pulmonale and in right ventricular failure due to acute right ventricular infarction, expansion of blood volume helps to maintain cardiac output. When hypoxic pulmonary vasoconstriction contributes to pulmonary hypertension, inhalation of 100% O_2 may help to reduce right ventricular afterload.

Chronic Cor Pulmonale Secondary to Pulmonary Vascular Disease   In contrast to acute, massive thromboembolism, when the elevation in pulmonary vascular resistance and the development of right ventricular hypertrophy develop gradually, higher pulmonary vascular pressures, sometimes even approaching systemic arterial levels, may be generated. Chronic cor pulmonale can be caused by recurrent, medium-sized emboli that fail to lyse, but organize and recanalize. Particles from intravenous drug abuse, parasites, or tumor tissue that embolizes into the pulmonary vascular bed also may cause persistent pulmonary hypertension. Chronic cor pulmonale also can be caused by *primary pulmonary hypertension* (Chap. 260) or any chronic widespread vasculitis, such as occurs in association with the collagen vascular disorders and that affects the pulmonary vascular bed, particularly the CREST syndrome (Chap. 314).

Clinical Manifestations   Breathlessness is a characteristic feature of pulmonary hypertension due to pulmonary vascular disease. It may be distressing during mild exertion or even at rest and is *not* relieved by sitting upright. An unproductive cough is another frequent complaint. Anterior chest pain, due to acute dilation of the root of the pulmonary artery or right ventricular ischemia, can occur. The elevation in systemic venous pressure can cause hepatomegaly and ankle edema.

Patients with pulmonary hypertension and consequent cor pulmonale often have tachypnea that is evident both on mild exertion and at rest and may even persist during sleep. Occasionally there is cyanosis due to arterial hypoxemia and low cardiac output. A right ventricular heave may be palpable along the left sternal border or in the epigastrium, and a high-pitched pulmonary ejection click may be audible to the left of the upper sternum. The second (pulmonary) component of the second heart sound is intensified and may be palpable; fixed splitting of the second heart sound may be present, and a right ventricular protodiastolic gallop (S_3), which increases during inspiration, may be present. A systolic murmur of tricuspid regurgitation, which is augmented by inspiration (p. 1323), is often audible; occasionally, a diastolic murmur of pulmonary regurgitation also is heard. Prominent *a* (and sometimes also *v*) waves in the jugular venous pulse are evident. The onset of right ventricular failure is reflected by an increase of venous pressure, the development of larger *v* waves associated with worse tricuspid regurgitation, a hepatojugular reflux, and a gallop rhythm with both third and fourth heart sounds. These physical findings of right ventricular failure can disappear rapidly when pulmonary artery pressure is suddenly reduced by relief of hypoxemia.

Hypocarbia due to alveolar hyperventilation is an important feature of chronic pulmonary hypertension secondary to pulmonary vascular disease. Usually there are no abnormalities on spirometry, but the ratio of dead space to tidal volume may be high, particularly when large-vessel obstruction is present. The diffusing capacity of the lung is reduced when a capillary vasculitis and/or loss of capillary blood volume is associated with pulmonary vascular disease. Typically, exercise causes a marked fall in Pa_{O_2}. The assessment of exercise capacity may be a useful way of following changes in the severity of pulmonary vascular disease in patients with chronic cor pulmonale, because exercise ability is limited by cardiac output and the latter, in turn, by the severity of the pulmonary vascular obstruction.

Laboratory Examination   On *radiologic examination* the pulmonary trunk and hilar vessels are enlarged. Widening of the hilum may be judged from the ratio of the distance between the start of the first divisions of the right and left main pulmonary arteries divided by the transverse diameter of the thorax; a ratio >0.36 suggests pulmonary hypertension. Another radiologic indicator of pulmonary hypertension is widening of the descending right pulmonary artery shadow, from a normal value of <16 mm to >20 mm. Ventilation and perfusion lung scans and systemic venography showing deep vein thrombosis are helpful in confirming the diagnosis of embolic pulmonary vascular disease. In the presence of severe pulmonary hypertension, the electrocardiogram (ECG) shows P pulmonale, right axis deviation, and right ventricular hypertrophy (Chap. 228).

Echocardiography allows measurement of the thickness of the right ventricular wall and can show enlargement of the right ventricular cavity in relation to the left. The interventricular septum may be displaced leftward. Right ventricular systolic pressure can be estimated from measurement of the peak tricuspid regurgitant flow and pulmonic regurgitant flow with Doppler echocardiography.

Magnetic resonance imaging is useful for measuring right ventricular mass, wall thickness, cavity volume, and ejection fraction.

Failure of the right ventricular ejection fraction (measured by radionuclide ventriculography) to increase on exercise appears to be a good indicator of pulmonary hypertension and/or intrinsic right ventricular dysfunction. Myocardial perfusion scintigraphy with thallium 201 or sestamibi is also useful for diagnosing cor pulmonale, since the hypertrophied right ventricle is visualized by these radionuclides. (Normally the right ventricle is not imaged because of the much greater uptake by the left ventricle.)

Cardiac catheterization is necessary for the precise measurement of pulmonary vascular pressures, the determination of pulmonary vascular resistance, and its response to oxygen and vasodilators. Catheterization is sometimes indicated in patients with cor pulmonale to exclude congenital and left heart diseases, and it allows pulmonary angiography to be carried out to confirm the nature of the pulmonary vascular obstruction. Measurements of pulmonary vascular pressures and flow should also be made during exercise to look for abnormal pressure increments or poor responses of cardiac output.

Lung biopsy can be useful in demonstrating vasculitis in some types of pulmonary vascular disease such as the collagen vascular diseases, rheumatoid arthritis, and Wegener's granulomatosis.

PARENCHYMAL PULMONARY DISEASES

Cor pulmonale may be caused by both obstructive and restrictive lung diseases, more frequently the former. In these conditions there are usually only modest elevations of pulmonary artery pressure. The development of cor pulmonale confers a poor prognosis on patients with respiratory disease; in patients with cor pulmonale and right ventricular failure, the 3-year survival is approximately 40 percent. Respiratory diseases causing cor pulmonale are often associated with distortions of the lung that affect the position of the heart, so that cardiac physical signs are altered.

CHRONIC OBSTRUCTIVE LUNG DISEASE (See Chap. 258)   This is the most common cause of chronic cor pulmonale. The enlargement of the right ventricle is attributed to the mild-to-moderate pulmonary hypertension that is common in severe obstructive bronchitis and emphysema. Pulmonary artery systolic pressure is typically in the range of 40 to 50 mmHg, far below the systemic levels that appear to be tolerated in patients with congenital heart disease and in those with primary pulmonary hypertension. Patients with cor pulmonale due to COLD usually have an advanced form of the disease with $FEV_1 < 1.0$ L (Chap. 250) and $Pa_{O_2} \le 60$ mmHg. Right ventricular failure secondary to COLD often occurs when there is "acute-on-chronic" respiratory failure with intensification of hypoxemia.

Pulmonary hypertension in COLD is due to the pulmonary vasoconstriction caused by the alveolar hypoxia, acidemia, and hypercarbia; by the mechanical effects of the high lung volume on the pulmonary vessels; by the loss of small vessels in the vascular bed in regions of emphysema and lung destruction; and sometimes by the increased cardiac output and blood viscosity caused by polycythemia secondary to hypoxia. Of these causes hypoxia is undoubtedly the most important. Pulmonary artery pressure rises further on exercise and often falls acutely on inspiration of 100% O_2. Cardiac output tends to be high in the absence of heart failure if hypoxia and hypercarbia are present. Because of the importance of hypoxic pulmonary vasoconstriction in causing pulmonary hypertension, the hypoventilating "blue bloater" with alveolar hypoxia and hypercarbia more frequently suffers from pulmonary hypertension and consequent cor pulmonale than does the emphysematous "pink puffer" without alveolar hypoxia. Ischemic left ventricular dysfunction is a frequent accompaniment since patients with cor pulmonale secondary to COLD usually have a history of heavy cigarette smoking, a major risk factor for ischemic heart disease. The elevation of pulmonary artery pressure may be secondary, in part, to the increase in left atrial pressure resulting from left-heart dysfunction. Almost half of all patients who die with cor pulmonale due to COLD also have left ventricular hypertrophy on postmortem examination.

Right ventricular failure often complicates cor pulmonale when patients with COLD develop ventilatory failure with hypoxia and hypercarbia. When there is a worsening of the airflow due to increasing airway obstruction, the resulting hypoxia and hypercarbia may increase cardiac output by their vasodilator effect on the systemic arteriolar bed. Hypoxic pulmonary vasoconstriction is intensified, and both supraventricular and ventricular arrhythmias may occur. The liver becomes palpable and tender because it is engorged and displaced downward by the low diaphragm; a hepatojugular reflux may be present.

An exacerbation of airway obstruction elevates intrathoracic pressure, which impedes venous return, raises jugular venous pressure, and may cause peripheral edema, even in the absence of heart failure. This elevation of venous pressure secondary to airway obstruction is *not* necessarily associated with an increase in the transmural right ventricular pressure, the hallmark of right ventricular failure. The venous hypertension due to airflow obstruction declines, sometimes very rapidly, with relief of the obstruction.

Pathology   In COLD right ventricular hypertrophy increases progressively. The main pulmonary arteries are enlarged, and the muscular pulmonary arteries show prominent longitudinal muscle, fibrosis, and elastic changes that continue into the arterioles, where the media becomes muscularized. The small vessels and capillaries are distorted or disappear in regions of lung hyperinflation.

Clinical Manifestations   A history of a productive cough and dyspnea, perhaps with wheezing, is frequently elicited. Breathlessness limits the patient's ability in the minor stresses of daily living. Frequently there is a history of emergency hospital admissions because of respiratory infection, sometimes necessitating mechanical ventilation. In breathing oxygen, there may be increasing somnolence or other symptoms of hypercarbia such as recurring headaches, confusion, and even vomiting which, when combined with blurred optic discs (also due to cerebral vasodilation), constitutes the "pseudo tumor cerebri" syndrome. Hypoxia due to hypoventilation is usually worse at night, particularly when severe snoring leads to obstructive apnea (Chap. 264).

Physical findings   Often there is nicotine staining of the fingers, a tell-tale sign reflecting many years of heavy cigarette smoking. The skin may be warm and the arterial pulse bounding in the high cardiac output state induced by hypoxia and hypercarbia. The distention of the chest due to the airflow obstruction and the rhonchi and wheezes secondary to chronic bronchitis usually make cardiac auscultation

difficult. A right-sided protodiastolic gallop sound (S_3) and a systolic murmur of tricuspid regurgitant may be audible. Signs of right-heart failure are, as discussed above, difficult to separate from those due to severe airflow obstruction. However, a sudden worsening of peripheral edema and rise of systemic venous pressure when atrial fibrillation occurs or when pulmonary infection supervenes are usually considered to be evidence of heart failure. This may be supported by the presence of a positive hepatojugular reflux. The distinction is important since patients can survive for years with the high systemic venous pressure and edema secondary to airflow obstruction but usually have a poor prognosis after right-heart failure develops.

Laboratory Examination   *Pulmonary function studies* show marked airflow obstruction with hypoxemia and hypercarbia. Exercise is limited by ventilatory rather than cardiac dysfunction until right ventricular failure develops. The *chest roentgenogram* reveals hyperinflation, which makes the degree of right-heart enlargement difficult to assess. The central pulmonary arteries are large, but the vessels are narrowed and disappear at the periphery, particularly in regions of the lungs that are markedly emphysematous. The ECG is relatively insensitive in demonstrating right-heart enlargement because the enlarged lungs are poor electrical conductors and the inspiratory position of the chest is associated with a vertically positioned heart. Arrhythmias, particularly atrial fibrillation and multifocal atrial tachycardia, are common.

Echocardiographic imaging is often difficult because of the air in the distended lungs, but it usually reveals an increased cross section of the right ventricular cavity and abnormal thickening of the right ventricular wall. Myocardial perfusion scintigraphy shows an abnormally high ratio of right-to-left ventricular uptake.

Right heart catheterization can be carried out at the bedside with a balloon-tipped, flow-directed, multilumen catheter fitted with thermocouples for measuring cardiac output by thermodilution (Chap. 229). The pulmonary artery wedge pressure is usually normal in patients at rest who have uncomplicated cor pulmonale. Cardiac catheterization may be useful in assessing the severity of the pulmonary hypertension and its response to respiring oxygen as well as left ventricular function. Pressure measurements during exercise study may be helpful, particularly in assessing the contribution of left-heart dysfunction to the clinical state.

℞ **TREATMENT**

First, medical management of the acute and/or chronic lung disease must be optimal (Chaps. 258 and 265). Alveolar hypoxia should be corrected by improving alveolar ventilation through relieving the airflow obstruction and by judiciously increasing the inspired O_2 concentration. Long-term O_2 therapy is helpful in patients with severe COLD and reduces pulmonary artery pressure and pulmonary vascular resistance. When the lung disease improves and pulmonary vasoconstriction secondary to the alveolar hypoxia and hypercarbia are corrected, tachypnea and the signs attributed to right-heart failure are relieved. Bronchodilators and antibiotics lessen the airflow obstruction, and diuretics relieve the edema. Loop diuretics must be used with care since they may cause a metabolic alkalosis and thereby blunt the respiratory drive. Digitalis should be used in the presence of overt right ventricular failure, and slow phlebotomy should be considered when the hematocrit exceeds 55 to 60 percent.

RESTRICTIVE LUNG DISEASES   Cor pulmonale in a variety of restrictive disorders affecting the lung (Chap. 259) is often associated with obliteration of the pulmonary vascular bed by lung destruction and fibrosis. Treatment of the underlying disorder and management of right ventricular failure, as described above, are indicated.

DISORDERS OF VENTILATION   A variety of disorders of the neuromuscular apparatus, diaphragm, and chest wall cause pulmonary hypertension and cor pulmonale secondary to chronic hypoxia and/or compression of pulmonary vessels. Disorders of ventilatory control, including the sleep apnea syndrome, and upper airways obstruction may be responsible for chronic hypoxia and secondary pulmonary hypertension, cor pulmonale, and, when the latter are severe, eventual right ventricular failure. Management of these patients consists of treating the underlying disorder, as discussed in Chaps. 263 and 264, the inhalation of oxygen, and the management of right ventricular failure with diuretics and digoxin.

BIBLIOGRAPHY

BRADLEY TD, PHILLIPSON EA: Central sleep apnea. Clin Chest Med 13:493, 1992

FERGUSON GT, CHERNIACK RM: Management of chronic obstructive pulmonary disease. N Engl J Med 328:1017, 1993

JAIN D, ZARET BJ: Assessment of right ventricular function. Role of nuclear imaging techniques. Cardiol Clin 10:23, 1992

KLINGER JR, HILL NS: Right ventricular dysfunction in chronic obstructive pulmonary disease: Evaluation and management. Chest 99:715, 1991

LOH E: Cor pulmonale, in *Cardiopulmonary Diseases and Cardiac Tumors*, S Goldhaber (ed), in *Atlas of Heart Diseases*, vol 3, E Braunwald (series ed). Philadelphia, Current Medicine, 1995, pp 1.1–1.24

MACNEE W: Pathophysiology of cor pulmonale in chronic obstructive pulmonary disease. Am J Respir Crit Care Med 150:833, 1994

PATTYNAMA PMT et al: Early diagnosis of cor pulmonale with MR imaging of the right ventricle. Radiology 182:375, 1992

SALVATERRA CG, RUBIN LJ: Investigation and management of pulmonary hypertension in chronic obstructive pulmonary disease. Am Rev Respir Dis 148:1414, 1993

WEITZENBLUM E et al: Benefit from long-term O$_2$ therapy in chronic obstructive pulmonary disease patients. Respiration 59(Suppl I):14, 1992

——— et al: Pulmonary hemodynamics in patients with chronic obstructive pulmonary disease before and during an episode of peripheral edema. Chest 105:1377, 1994

WIEDEMANN HP, MATTHAY RA: Cor pulmonale, in *Heart Disease*, 5th ed, E Braunwald (ed). Philadelphia, Saunders, 1997, pp 1604–1625

| 239 | *Joshua Wynne, Eugene Braunwald* |

THE CARDIOMYOPATHIES AND MYOCARDITIDES

The cardiomyopathies are diseases that involve the myocardium primarily and are not the result of hypertension or congenital, valvular, coronary, arterial, or pericardial abnormalities.* When the cardiomyopathies are classified on an etiologic basis, two fundamental forms are recognized: (1) a primary type, consisting of heart muscle disease of unknown cause, and (2) a secondary type, consisting of myocardial disease of known cause or associated with a disease involving other organ systems (Table 239-1). (In the World Health Organization classification, *specific cardiomyopathy* is used to describe heart muscle diseases associated with certain systemic or cardiac disorders; examples include hypertensive and metabolic cardiomyopathy. In many

---

* Diffuse myocardial fibrosis secondary to multiple myocardial scars produced by extensive coronary arterial narrowing and occlusion can impair left ventricular function and is frequently referred to as *ischemic cardiomyopathy*. This is a colloquial use of the term, however, and should be avoided; the term *cardiomyopathy* should be restricted to a condition *primarily* involving heart muscle. In so-called ischemic cardiomyopathy the *primary* involvement is of the coronary vessels.

cases it is not possible to arrive at a specific etiologic diagnosis, and thus it is often more desirable to classify the cardiomyopathies on the basis of differences in their pathophysiology and clinical presentation (Tables 239-2 and 239-3).

DILATED CARDIOMYOPATHY

Left and/or right ventricular systolic pump function is impaired, leading to cardiac enlargement and often producing symptoms of congestive heart failure. Mural thrombi are often present, particularly in the left ventricular apex. Histologic examination reveals extensive areas of interstitial and perivascular fibrosis. Myocyte necrosis and cellular infiltration may be present but are not prominent. [The prevalence of this condition appears to be increasing.] Although no cause is apparent in many cases, dilated cardiomyopathy probably is the end result of myocardial damage produced by a variety of toxic, metabolic, or infectious agents. Dilated cardiomyopathy may be the late sequel of acute viral myocarditis, possibly mediated through an immunologic mechanism. Although most commonly a disease of middle-aged men and more common in African-Americans, it may occur in any patient population. A reversible form of dilated cardiomyopathy may be found with alcohol abuse, pregnancy, selenium deficiency, hypophosphatemia, hypocalcemia, thyroid disease, cocaine use, and chronic uncontrolled tachycardia. Approximately 20 percent of patients have familial forms of the disease. The disease is genetically heterogeneous; autosomal dominant, autosomal recessive, and X-linked transmission have been documented. *Right ventricular dysplasia* is a unique cardiomyopathy marked by progressive replacement of the right ventricular wall with adipose tissue. Often associated with ventricular arrhythmias, the clinical course is variable but sudden death is a constant threat.

CLINICAL MANIFESTATIONS   Symptoms of left- and right-sided congestive failure, manifested by dyspnea on exertion, fatigue, orthopnea, paroxysmal nocturnal dyspnea, peripheral edema, and palpitations, develop gradually in most patients. Some patients have left ventricular dilatation for months or even years before becoming symp-

Table 239-1

Etiologic Classification of Cardiomyopathies

PRIMARY MYOCARDIAL INVOLVEMENT

Idiopathic (D,R,H)
Familial (D,H)
Eosinophilic endomyocardial disease (R)
Endomyocardial fibrosis (R)

SECONDARY MYOCARDIAL INVOLVEMENT

Infective (D)	Connective tissue disorders (D)
Viral myocarditis	Systemic lupus erythematosus
Bacterial myocarditis	Polyarteritis nodosa
Fungal myocarditis	Rheumatoid arthritis
Protozoal myocarditis	Progressive systemic sclerosis
Metazoal myocarditis	Dermatomyositis
Spirochetal	Infiltrations and granulomas (R,D)
Rickettsial	Amyloidosis
Metabolic (D)	Sarcoidosis
Familial storage disease (D,R)	Malignancy
Glycogen storage disease	Neuromuscular (D)
Mucopolysaccharidoses	Muscular dystrophy
Hemochromatosis	Myotonic dystrophy
Fabry's disease	Friedreich's ataxia (H,D)
Deficiency (D)	Sensitivity and toxic reactions (D)
Electrolytes	Alcohol
Nutritional	Radiation
	Drugs
	Peripartum heart disease (D)

NOTE: The principal clinical manifestation(s) of each etiologic grouping is denoted by D (dilated), R (restrictive), or H (hypertrophic) cardiomyopathy.

SOURCE: Adapted from the WHO/ISFC task force report on the definition and classification of cardiomyopathies, 1980.

Table 239-2

CHAPTER 239
The Cardiomyopathies and Myocarditides

1329

Clinical Classification of Cardiomyopathies

1. Dilated: Left and/or right ventricular enlargement, impaired systolic function, congestive heart failure, arrhythmias, emboli
2. Restrictive: Endomyocardial scarring or myocardial infiltration resulting in restriction to left and/or right ventricular filling
3. Hypertrophic: Disproportionate left ventricular hypertrophy, typically involving septum more than free wall, with or without an intraventricular systolic pressure gradient; usually of a nondilated left ventricular cavity

tomatic. Others develop symptoms after recovery from a viral infection. Although vague chest pain may be present, typical angina pectoris is unusual and suggests the presence of concomitant ischemic heart disease.

PHYSICAL EXAMINATION Variable degrees of cardiac enlargement and findings of congestive heart failure are noted. In patients with advanced disease, the pulse pressure is narrow and the jugular venous pressure is elevated. Third and fourth heart sounds are common, and mitral or tricuspid regurgitation may occur. Diastolic murmurs, valvular calcification, and severe hypertension reduce the likelihood of cardiomyopathy.

LABORATORY EXAMINATIONS The chest roentgenogram demonstrates enlargement of the cardiac silhouette due to left ventricular enlargement, although generalized cardiomegaly often is seen. The lung fields may demonstrate evidence of pulmonary venous hypertension and interstitial or alveolar edema. The electrocardiogram often shows sinus tachycardia or atrial fibrillation, ventricular arrhythmias, left atrial enlargement, diffuse nonspecific ST-T wave abnormalities, and sometimes intraventricular conduction defects. Echocardiography and radionuclide ventriculography show left ventricular dilatation, with normal or minimally thickened or thinned walls, and systolic dysfunction (reduced ejection fraction).

Cardiac catheterization usually is performed only to exclude ischemic heart disease. The left ventricular end-diastolic, left atrial, and pulmonary capillary wedge pressures usually are elevated; when failure of the right side of the heart supervenes, the right ventricular end-diastolic, right atrial, and central venous pressures also rise. Angiography reveals a dilated, diffusely hypokinetic left ventricle, often with some degree of mitral regurgitation; the coronary arteries are normal, thereby excluding so-called ischemic cardiomyopathy. Transvenous endomyocardial biopsy (Chap. 229) usually is not necessary, but may be helpful in excluding certain conditions such as myocardial infiltration by amyloid.

℞ **TREATMENT**
Most patients pursue an inexorably downhill course, and the majority, particularly those over 55 years of age, die within 2 years of the onset of symptoms. Spontaneous improvement or stabilization occurs in about a quarter of patients. Death is due to either congestive heart failure or ventricular tachy- or bradyarrhythmia; sudden death is a constant threat. Systemic embolization is common, and although the issue is controversial, all patients without contraindications should be considered for chronic anticoagulation. Strenuous exertion should be interdicted. Standard therapy of heart failure with salt restriction, diuretics, digitalis, and vasodilators may produce symptomatic improvement. Mortality

is reduced by angiotensin-converting enzyme inhibitors and the combination of hydralazine and isosorbide dinitrate. Some patients with dilated cardiomyopathy who have biopsy evidence of myocardial inflammation have been treated with immunosuppressive therapy, but long-term evidence of efficacy is lacking. Others have been treated cautiously with gradually increasing doses of beta-adrenergic blockers with apparent clinical benefit. Antiarrhythmic agents are best avoided for fear of proarrhythmic and other side effects, unless they are needed to treat symptomatic or serious arrhythmias. Implantation of an automatic internal defibrillator is useful in patients with malignant arrhythmias. In patients with advanced disease who are refractory to medical therapy, cardiac transplantation should be considered (Chap. 234).

ALCOHOLIC CARDIOMYOPATHY Individuals who consume large quantities of alcohol over many years may develop a clinical picture identical to idiopathic dilated cardiomyopathy; indeed, alcoholic cardiomyopathy is the major form of secondary dilated cardiomyopathy in the western world. Ceasing alcohol consumption before severe heart failure has developed may halt the progression or even reverse the course of this disease, unlike the idiopathic variety, which is marked by progressive deterioration. Alcoholic patients with advanced heart failure have a poor prognosis, particularly if they continue to drink; fewer than one-quarter survive 3 years. The key to the treatment of alcoholic cardiomyopathy is total and permanent abstinence. The toxic effect of alcohol on striated muscle often extends beyond the heart to cause myopathy in skeletal muscles. A second presentation of alcoholic cardiotoxicity may be found in individuals without overt heart failure and consists of recurrent supraventricular or ventricular tachyarrhythmias. Termed the *holiday heart syndrome*, it typically appears after a drinking binge; atrial fibrillation is seen most frequently, followed by atrial flutter and ventricular premature depolarizations. Other patients develop left ventricular hypertrophy, perhaps related to concomitant systemic hypertension; they may present with symptoms of pulmonary congestion due to abnormal diastolic stiffness (diminished compliance) of the left ventricle.

Table 239-3

Laboratory Evaluation of the Cardiomyopathies

	Dilated	Restrictive	Hypertrophic
Chest roentgenogram	Moderate to marked cardiac enlargement Pulmonary venous hypertension	Mild cardiac enlargement	Mild to moderate cardiac enlargement
Electrocardiogram	ST-segment and T-wave abnormalities	Low voltage, conduction defects	ST-segment and T-wave abnormalities Left ventricular hypertrophy Abnormal Q waves
Echocardiogram	Left ventricular dilatation and dysfunction	Increased left ventricular wall thickness Normal or mildly reduced systolic function	Asymmetric septal hypertrophy (ASH) Systolic anterior motion (SAM) of the mitral valve
Radionuclide studies	Left ventricular dilatation and dysfunction (RVG)	Normal or mildly reduced systolic function (RVG)	Vigorous systolic function (RVG) Perfusion defect (^{201}Tl)
Cardiac catheterization	Left ventricular dilatation and dysfunction Elevated left- and often right-sided filling pressures Diminished cardiac output	Normal or mildly reduced systolic function Elevated left- and right-sided filling pressures	Vigorous systolic function Dynamic left ventricular outflow obstruction Elevated left- and right-sided filling pressures

NOTE: RVG, radionuclide ventriculogram; ^{201}Tl, thallium 201.

PERIPARTUM CARDIOMYOPATHY Cardiac dilatation and congestive heart failure of unexplained cause may develop during the last trimester of pregnancy or within 6 months after delivery; most women develop symptoms in the month before or immediately after delivery. The cause of this disorder is unknown, but in some patients endomyocardial biopsy has shown evidence of a myocarditis. Necropsy shows cardiac enlargement, often with mural thrombi, along with histologic evidence of myocardial degeneration and fibrosis. The patient who develops peripartum cardiomyopathy typically is multiparous, African American, and over the age of 30, although the disease may be found in a wide spectrum of patients. The symptoms, signs, and treatment are similar to those in patients with idiopathic dilated cardiomyopathy. The mortality rate is quite variable but may be as high as 25 to 50 percent. The prognosis in these patients appears to be closely related to whether the heart size returns to normal after the first episode of congestive heart failure. If it does, subsequent pregnancies may sometimes be well tolerated; if the heart remains enlarged, however, further pregnancies frequently produce increasing myocardial damage, ultimately leading to refractory congestive heart failure and death. Those who recover should be encouraged to avoid further pregnancies, particularly if cardiomegaly persists.

NEUROMUSCULAR DISEASE (See also Chap. 383) Cardiac involvement is common in many of the muscular dystrophies. In *Duchenne's progressive muscular dystrophy*, myocardial involvement is most frequently indicated by a distinctive and unique electrocardiographic pattern consisting of tall R waves in right precordial leads with an R/S ratio greater than 1.0, often associated with deep Q waves in the limb and lateral precordial leads. These electrocardiographic abnormalities appear to result from selective transmural necrosis of the posterobasal left ventricle and associated papillary muscle. A variety of supraventricular and ventricular arrhythmias are frequently found. Rapidly progressive congestive heart failure may develop despite extended periods of apparent circulatory stability during which the only detectable abnormalities are in the electrocardiogram. *Myotonic dystrophy* is characterized by a variety of electrocardiographic abnormalities, especially disorders of impulse formation and particularly conduction, but other overt clinical evidence of heart disease is uncommon. Because of the abnormalities of impulse generation and conduction, syncope and sudden death are major hazards; in appropriate patients, insertion of a permanent pacemaker may be effective. In *limb-girdle dystrophy* and *fascioscapulohumeral dystrophy*, cardiac involvement is uncommon and seldom severe. Involvement of the heart is very common in *Friedreich's ataxia* (manifested by abnormal electrocardiographic or echocardiographic findings), with as many as half the patients developing cardiac symptoms. The electrocardiogram most commonly demonstrates ST-segment and T-wave abnormalities. The echocardiogram may demonstrate left ventricular hypertrophy, with either symmetric or asymmetric hypertrophy of the left ventricular septum compared with the free wall. Although morphologically similar to some cases of hypertrophic cardiomyopathy, cellular disarray is lacking.

DRUGS A variety of pharmacologic agents may damage the myocardium acutely, producing a pattern of inflammation (myocarditis), or they may lead to chronic damage of the type seen with idiopathic dilated cardiomyopathy. Certain drugs produce only electrocardiographic abnormalities, while others may precipitate fulminant congestive heart failure and death. The anthracycline derivatives, particularly *doxorubicin* (Adriamycin), are powerful antineoplastic agents that, when given in high doses (more than 550 mg/m^2 for doxorubicin), may produce fatal heart failure. The incidence of heart failure is related not only to the dose of the drug but also to the presence or absence of several risk factors (cardiac irradiation, age greater than 70 years, underlying heart disease, hypertension, treatment with cyclophosphamide); at any dose patients with these risk factors have an eight- to tenfold greater frequency of developing heart failure than do patients lacking them. Radionuclide ventriculography and endocardial biopsy may document preclinical deterioration of left ventricular function and allow appropriate dose adjustments; by so monitoring left ventricular function, it is often possible to continue doxorubicin even in patients at high risk for developing heart failure. Recent efforts to modify the dose schedule by giving the drug more slowly have further reduced the risk of cardiotoxicity.

Some patients with congestive heart failure, even those with severe depression of left ventricular function, have demonstrated recovery of cardiac function with aggressive management with digitalis, diuretics, and vasodilators. In others, late asymptomatic contractile dysfunction is common, even in those without initial cardiotoxicity. Children may demonstrate reduced myocardial hypertrophy and mass over time, presumably due to doxorubicin's inhibition of myocardial cell growth. High-dose *cyclophosphamide* may produce congestive heart failure acutely or within 2 weeks of administration; a characteristic histopathologic feature is myocardial edema and hemorrhagic necrosis. Rarely, patients treated with *5-fluorouracil* will develop chest pain and electrocardiographic changes of myocardial ischemia or infarction. Electrocardiographic changes and arrhythmias may result from treatment with tricyclic antidepressants, the phenothiazines, emetine, lithium, and various aerosol propellants. *Cocaine abuse* is associated with a variety of life-threatening cardiac complications, including sudden death, myocarditis, dilated cardiomyopathy, and acute myocardial infarction (resulting from coronary spasm and/or thrombosis with or without underlying coronary artery stenosis). Nitrates and calcium antagonists have been used as well to treat a variety of cocaine-induced cardiotoxicities; beta-adrenergic blockers should be avoided.

HYPERTROPHIC CARDIOMYOPATHY

This disease is characterized by left ventricular hypertrophy, typically of a nondilated chamber, without obvious cause such as hypertension or aortic stenosis. Two features of the disease have attracted the greatest attention: (1) heterogeneous left ventricular (LV) hypertrophy, often with preferential hypertrophy of the interventricular septum resulting in asymmetric septal hypertrophy (ASH); and (2) a dynamic left ventricular outflow tract pressure gradient, related to a narrowing of the subaortic area as a consequence of the midsystolic apposition of the anterior mitral valve leaflet against the hypertrophied septum, i.e., systolic anterior motion (SAM) of the mitral valve. Initial studies of this disease emphasized the dynamic "obstructive" features, and it has been termed *idiopathic hypertrophic subaortic stenosis* (IHSS), *hypertrophic obstructive cardiomyopathy* (HOCM), and *muscular subaortic stenosis*. It has become clear, however, that only about one-quarter of patients with hypertrophic cardiomyopathy demonstrate an outflow tract gradient. The ubiquitous pathophysiologic abnormality is not systolic but rather *diastolic* dysfunction (Chap. 232), characterized by increased stiffness of the hypertrophied muscle that results primarily from an abnormality in calcium handling with attendant intracellular calcium overload. This results in elevated diastolic filling pressures and is present despite a hyperdynamic left ventricle.

The pattern of hypertrophy is distinctive in hypertrophic cardiomyopathy and differs from that seen in secondary hypertrophy (as in hypertension). Most patients have striking regional variations in the extent of hypertrophy in different portions of the left ventricle, and the majority demonstrate a ventricular septum whose thickness is disproportionately increased when compared with the free wall. Other patients may demonstrate disproportionate involvement of the apex or left ventricular free wall; 10 percent or more of patients have concentric involvement of the ventricle. All, however, show a bizarre and disorganized arrangement of cardiac muscle cells in the septum, with disorganization of the myofibrillar architecture, whether or not a systolic intraventricular pressure gradient is present, along with a variable degree of myocardial fibrosis and thickening of the small intramural coronary arteries.

About half of all cases of hypertrophic cardiomyopathy have a positive family history compatible with autosomal-dominant transmission. About 40 percent of these are associated with mutations of the beta cardiac myosin heavy chain gene on chromosome 14, with certain mutations associated with more malignant prognoses. About 15 percent have a mutation of the cardiac troponin T gene, 10 percent a mutation of myosin binding protein L, and about 5 percent a mutation of the α tropomyosin gene. The remainder of familial cases presumably are due to mutations of other genes. Echocardiographic studies have confirmed that about one-third of the first-degree relatives (i.e., parents, siblings, and children) of patients with familial hypertrophic cardiomyopathy have evidence of the disease, although in many of these patients the extent of hypertrophy is mild, no outflow tract pressure gradient is present, and symptoms are not prominent. Since the hypertrophic characteristics may not be apparent in childhood and often appear first in adolescence, a single normal echocardiogram in a child does not entirely exclude the presence of the disease.

In contrast to the obstruction produced by a fixed narrowed orifice, such as valvular aortic stenosis, the pressure gradient in hypertrophic cardiomyopathy, when present, is dynamic and may change between examinations and even from beat to beat. Obstruction appears to result from further narrowing of an already small left ventricular outflow tract by SAM of the mitral valve against the hypertrophied septum. While SAM may be found in a variety of other conditions besides hypertrophic cardiomyopathy, it is *always* found when obstruction is present in hypertrophic cardiomyopathy. Three basic mechanisms are involved in the production of the dynamic pressure gradient: (1) increased left ventricular contractility, (2) decreased ventricular volume (preload), and (3) decreased aortic impedance and pressure (afterload). Interventions that increase myocardial contractility, such as exercise, isoproterenol, and digitalis glycosides, and those that reduce ventricular volume, such as the Valsalva maneuver, sudden standing, nitroglycerin, amyl nitrite, or tachycardia, all may cause an increase in the gradient and the murmur. Conversely, elevation of arterial pressure by phenylephrine, squatting, sustained handgrip, augmentation of venous return by passive leg raising, and expansion of the blood volume all increase ventricular volume and ameliorate the gradient and murmur.

CLINICAL FEATURES Many patients with hypertrophic cardiomyopathy are asymptomatic and may be relatives of patients with known disease. Unfortunately, the first clinical manifestation of the disease may be sudden death, frequently occurring in children and young adults, often during or after physical exertion. In symptomatic patients, the most common complaint is dyspnea, largely due to increased stiffness of the left ventricular walls, which impairs ventricular filling and leads to elevated left ventricular diastolic and left atrial pressures. Other symptoms include angina pectoris, fatigue, syncope, and near-syncope ("graying-out spells"). Symptoms are not related to the presence or severity of an outflow gradient. Most patients with gradients demonstrate a double or triple apical precordial impulse, a rapidly rising carotid arterial pulse, and a fourth heart sound. The hallmark of obstructive hypertrophic cardiomyopathy is a systolic murmur, which is typically harsh, diamond-shaped, and usually begins well after the first heart sound, since ejection is unimpeded early in systole. The murmur is best heard at the lower left sternal border as well as at the apex, where it is often more holosystolic and blowing in quality, no doubt due to the mitral regurgitation that usually accompanies obstructive hypertrophic cardiomyopathy.

LABORATORY EVALUATION The *electrocardiogram* commonly shows left ventricular hypertrophy and widespread, deep, broad Q waves that suggest an old myocardial infarction. Many patients demonstrate arrhythmias, both atrial (supraventricular tachycardia or atrial fibrillation) and ventricular (ventricular tachycardia), during ambulatory (Holter) monitoring. *Chest roentgenography* may be normal, although a mild to moderate increase in the cardiac silhouette is common. The mainstay of the diagnosis of hypertrophic cardiomyopathy is the *echocardiogram*, which demonstrates left ventricular hypertrophy, often with the septum 1.3 or more times the thickness of the high posterior left ventricular free wall. The septum may demonstrate an unusual ground glass appearance, probably related to its abnormal cellular architecture and myocardial fibrosis. SAM of the mitral valve is found in patients with pressure gradients. The left ventricular cavity typically is small in hypertrophic cardiomyopathy, with vigorous pos-

terior wall motion but reduced septal excursion. A rare form of hypertrophic cardiomyopathy, characterized by apical hypertrophy, is often associated with giant negative T waves on the electrocardiogram and a "spade-shaped" left ventricular cavity on angiography; it usually has a benign clinical course. *Radionuclide scintigraphy* with thallium 201 frequently reveals evidence of myocardial perfusion defects even in asymptomatic patients.

Although cardiac catheterization is not required to diagnose hypertrophic cardiomyopathy, the two typical *hemodynamic* features are an elevated left ventricular diastolic pressure due to diminished left ventricular compliance and, when obstruction is present, a systolic pressure gradient between the body of the left ventricle and the subaortic region. When a gradient is not present, it often can be induced by provocative maneuvers such as infusion of isoproterenol, inhalation of amyl nitrite, or the Valsalva maneuver.

℞ **TREATMENT**
Competitive sports and probably strenuous activity should be proscribed. Beta-adrenergic blockers often are used and may ameliorate angina pectoris and syncope in one-third to one-half of patients to some degree. Resting intraventricular pressure gradients usually are unchanged, although these drugs may limit the increase in the gradient that occurs during exercise. It is not known whether beta-adrenergic blockers offer any protection against sudden death. It is not established whether any antiarrhythmic agent, for that matter, is effective in this setting. However, amiodarone appears to be effective in reducing the frequency of supraventricular as well as life-threatening ventricular arrhythmias. Verapamil and diltiazem may reduce the stiffness of the ventricle, reduce the elevated diastolic pressures, increase exercise tolerance, and, in some instances, reduce the severity of outflow tract gradients, although adverse side effects occur in about one-quarter of patients. Disopyramide has been used in some patients to reduce left ventricular contractility and the outflow gradient. Dual-chamber permanent pacing recently has gained favor because it improves symptoms and reduces the outflow gradient in some patients with severe symptoms, presumably by altering the pattern of ventricular contraction. Infarction of the interventricular septum induced by ethanol injections into the septal artery has also been reported to reduce obstruction. The insertion of an implantable automatic defibrillator should be considered in patients surviving cardiac arrest and those with high-risk ventricular tachyarrhythmias. A surgical myotomy/myectomy of the hypertrophied septum may result in lasting symptomatic improvement in about three-quarters of operated patients, but the mortality of 3 to 5 percent limits the operation to severely symptomatic patients with large pressure gradients who are unresponsive to medical management. The effect of any of these therapies on the natural history is not clear. Digitalis, diuretics, nitrates, and beta-adrenergic agonists are best avoided if possible, particularly in patients with known left ventricular outflow tract pressure gradients.

PROGNOSIS The natural history of hypertrophic cardiomyopathy is variable, although many patients demonstrate an improvement or stabilization of symptoms with time. Atrial fibrillation is common late in the course of the disease; its onset may lead to an increase in symptoms, presumably due to loss of the atrial contribution to filling of the thickened ventricle. Infective endocarditis occurs in fewer than 10 percent of patients, and endocarditis prophylaxis is indicated, particularly in patients with resting obstruction and mitral regurgitation. Progression of hypertrophic cardiomyopathy to left ventricular dilatation and dysfunction without an outflow gradient has been reported but is unusual; in about 5 to 10 percent of patients, however, some degree of left ventricular systolic impairment, wall thinning, and chamber enlargement occurs over time. The major cause of mortality in hypertrophic cardiomyopathy is sudden death, which may occur in asymptomatic patients or interrupt an otherwise stable course in symptomatic ones. Predictors of sudden death include age less than 30 years, ventricular tachycardia on ambulatory monitoring, marked ventricular hypertrophy, syncope (especially in children), genetic mutations associated with an increased risk, and a family history of sudden death. There is no correlation between the risk of sudden death and the severity of symptoms or the presence or severity of an outflow tract pressure gradient. Since sudden death often occurs during or just after physical exertion, strenuous exercise should be avoided in all patients, regardless of symptoms. It is likely that most deaths, particularly those that are sudden, are due to ventricular arrhythmias.

RESTRICTIVE CARDIOMYOPATHY

The hallmark of the restrictive cardiomyopathies is abnormal diastolic function (Chap. 232); the ventricular walls are excessively rigid and impede ventricular filling. Myocardial fibrosis, hypertrophy, or infiltration due to a variety of causes is usually responsible. The infiltrative diseases, which represent important causes for secondary restrictive cardiomyopathy, also may show some impairment of systolic function. Myocardial involvement with *amyloid* is a common cause of secondary restrictive cardiomyopathy, although restriction is also seen in hemochromatosis, glycogen deposition, endomyocardial fibrosis, sarcoidosis, Fabry's disease, the eosinophilias, neoplastic infiltration, and myocardial fibrosis of diverse causes. In many of these conditions, particularly those with substantial concomitant endocardial involvement, partial obliteration of the ventricular cavity by fibrous tissue and thrombus contributes to the abnormally increased resistance to ventricular filling.

The inability of the ventricle to fill limits cardiac output and raises filling pressure. Therefore, exercise intolerance and dyspnea are usually the most prominent symptoms. As a result of persistently elevated venous pressure, these patients commonly have dependent edema, ascites, and an enlarged, tender liver. The jugular venous pressure is elevated and does not fall normally, or it may rise with inspiration (Kussmaul's sign). The heart sounds may be distant, and third and fourth heart sounds are common. In contrast to constrictive pericarditis, which the restrictive cardiomyopathies resemble in many respects, the apex impulse is usually easily palpable, and mitral regurgitation is more common. The electrocardiogram shows low-voltage, nonspecific ST-T-wave changes and various arrhythmias. Pericardial calcification on x-ray, which would suggest constrictive pericarditis, is absent. Echocardiography typically reveals symmetrically thickened left ventricular walls and normal or slightly reduced ventricular volumes and systolic function. Doppler recordings demonstrate accentuated early diastolic filling. Cardiac catheterization shows a decreased cardiac output, elevation of the right and left ventricular end-diastolic pressures and a dip-and-plateau configuration of the diastolic portion of the ventricular pressure pulse resembling that seen in constrictive pericarditis. As in the latter condition, the *x* and *y* descents of the atrial pressure pulse are prominent, resulting in a "W"-shaped pattern.

Differentiation from constrictive pericarditis may be difficult (Chaps. 229 and 240). This distinction is of importance because the latter condition is potentially curable by operation. Helpful in the differentiation of these two diseases are right ventricular transvenous endomyocardial biopsy (by revealing myocardial infiltration or fibrosis in restrictive cardiomyopathy) and computed tomography or magnetic resonance imaging (by demonstrating a thickened pericardium in constrictive pericarditis). Treatment usually is disappointing, except for hemochromatosis (where desferoxamine has been helpful in reducing myocardial iron content).

ENDOMYOCARDIAL FIBROSIS This is a progressive disease of unknown cause that occurs most commonly in children and young adults residing in tropical and subtropical Africa, particularly Uganda and Nigeria. Endomyocardial fibrosis is a frequent cause of heart failure in Africa, accounting for up to one-quarter of deaths due to heart disease. The condition is characterized by fibrous endocardial

lesions of the inflow portion of the right or left ventricle (or both) and often involves the atrioventricular valves, producing valvular regurgitation. The apex of the ventricles may be obliterated by a mass of thrombus and fibrous tissue. In some ways this disease resembles eosinophilic endomyocardial disease (see below), although they occur in quite different geographic areas and age groups and generally are felt to be different diseases.

The clinical picture depends on which ventricle and atrioventricular valve show predominant involvement; left-sided involvement results in symptoms of pulmonary congestion, while predominant right-sided disease presents features of a restrictive cardiomyopathy. Medical treatment is often disappointing, and surgical excision of the fibrotic endocardium and replacement of the involved atrioventricular valve have led to substantial symptomatic improvement in some patients.

EOSINOPHILIC ENDOMYOCARDIAL DISEASE Also called *Loeffler's endocarditis* and *fibroplastic endocarditis*, this disease appears to be a subcategory of the hypereosinophilic syndrome in which the heart is predominantly involved, with cardiac damage the apparent result of the toxic effects of eosinophilic proteins. Typically, the endocardium of either or both ventricles thickens markedly, with involvement of the underlying myocardium. Large mural thrombi may develop in either ventricle, thereby compromising the size of the ventricular cavity and serving as a source of pulmonary and systemic emboli. Hepatosplenomegaly and localized eosinophilic infiltration of other organs are usually present. Management with diuretics, afterload-reducing agents, and anticoagulation in conjunction with glucocorticoids and cytotoxic drugs (hydroxyurea in particular), appears to have improved survival substantially. Surgical treatment, as for endomyocardial fibrosis, may be helpful.

DIFFERENTIAL DIAGNOSIS Involvement of the heart is the most frequent cause of death in *primary amyloidosis* (Chap. 309), while clinically significant cardiac involvement is uncommon in the secondary form. Focal deposits of amyloid in elderly patients (*senile cardiac amyloidosis*) are common and usually clinically insignificant. Aspiration of abdominal fat or biopsy of the rectal mucosa, gingiva, liver, kidney, or myocardium permits the diagnosis to be made before death in over three-quarters of cases. The heart is firm, rubbery, and noncompliant, and four clinical presentations (alone or in combination) are seen: (1) diastolic dysfunction (restrictive cardiomyopathy), (2) systolic dysfunction, (3) arrhythmias, and (4) orthostatic hypotension. The two-dimensional echocardiogram may be helpful in making the diagnosis of amyloidosis and may show a thickened myocardial wall with a distinctive "speckled" appearance.

Hemochromatosis (Chap. 342) often is the result of multiple transfusions or a hemoglobinopathy; the familial (autosomal recessive) form should be suspected if cardiomyopathy occurs in the setting of diabetes mellitus, hepatic cirrhosis, and increased skin pigmentation. The diagnosis may be confirmed by endocardial biopsy. Phlebotomy may be of some benefit if employed early in the course of the disease. Continuous subcutaneous administration of deferoxamine may reduce body iron stores and result in clinical improvement.

Myocardial *sarcoidosis* (Chap. 320) is generally associated with other manifestations of systemic disease and may cause restrictive as well as congestive features, since cardiac infiltration by sarcoid granulomas results not only in increased stiffness of the myocardium but also in diminished systolic contractile function. A variety of arrhythmias, including atrioventricular block, have been noted. A common cardiac manifestation of systemic sarcoidosis is right heart overload due to pulmonary artery hypertension as a result of parenchymal pulmonary involvement. The *carcinoid syndrome* results in endocardial fibrosis and stenosis and/or regurgitation of the tricuspid and/or pulmonary valve (Chap. 237).

MYOCARDITIDES

Myocarditis, i.e., cardiac inflammation, is most commonly the result of an infectious process. Myocarditis also may result from a hypersensitivity to drugs or may be caused by radiation, chemicals, or physical agents. In an unknown number of cases, acute myocarditis progresses to chronic dilated cardiomyopathy. While almost every infectious agent is capable of producing myocarditis (Table 239-1), clinically significant acute myocarditis in the United States is caused most commonly by viruses, especially coxsackievirus B. The clinical manifestations range from an asymptomatic state, with the presence of myocarditis inferred only by the finding of transient electrocardiographic ST-T-wave abnormalities, to a fulminant condition with arrhythmias, heart failure, and death. In some patients myocarditis simulates acute myocardial infarction, with chest pain, electrocardiographic changes, and elevated serum levels of myocardial enzymes.

Physical examination usually is normal, although more severe cases may show a muffled first heart sound, along with a third heart sound and a murmur of mitral regurgitation. A pericardial friction rub may be audible in patients with associated pericarditis.

Though viral myocarditis is most often self-limited and without sequelae, severe involvement may recur, and it is likely that acute viral myocarditis occasionally progresses to a chronic form and to dilated cardiomyopathy. Patients with viral myocarditis often give a history of a preceding upper respiratory febrile illness, and viral nasopharyngitis or tonsillitis may be evident clinically. The isolation of virus from the stool, pharyngeal washings, or other body fluids and changes in specific antibody titers are helpful clinically.

Experimental studies suggest that exercise may be deleterious in patients with viral myocarditis, and strenuous activity should be proscribed until the electrocardiogram has returned to normal. Patients who develop congestive heart failure respond to the usual measures (digitalis, diuretics, salt restriction), but they appear to be unusually sensitive to digitalis. Arrhythmias are common and are occasionally difficult to manage. Deaths attributed to heart failure, tachyarrhythmias, and heart block have been reported, and it seems prudent to monitor the electrocardiogram of patients with arrhythmias, especially during the acute illness.

HUMAN IMMUNODEFICIENCY VIRUS (HIV) MYOCARDITIS (See also Chap. 308) Many HIV-infected patients have subclinical cardiac involvement, including pericardial effusion, right-sided chamber enlargement, and neoplastic involvement. Overt clinical involvement is seen in 10 percent of HIV patients, and the most common finding is left ventricular dysfunction that in some cases appears to be due to infiltration of the myocardium by the virus itself. In other patients the heart is affected by any of the various opportunistic infections common in AIDS, such as toxoplasmosis, as well as by cardiac metastases in Kaposi's sarcoma. The clinical manifestations of cardiac involvement may be incorrectly attributed to concurrent noncardiac problems such as pneumonia. This is unfortunate, since the dilated cardiomyopathy of HIV infection may respond at least transiently to standard therapy with digitalis, diuretics, and vasodilators.

BACTERIAL MYOCARDITIS Bacterial involvement of the heart is uncommon, but when it does occur, it is usually as a complication of bacterial endocarditis (typically due to *Staphylococcus aureus* and enterococci). Myocardial abscess formation may involve the valve rings and interventricular septum. *Diphtheritic myocarditis* develops in over one-quarter of the patients with diphtheria, is one of the most serious complications, and is the most common cause of death due to diphtheria (Chap. 144). Cardiac damage is due to the liberation of a toxin that inhibits protein synthesis and leads to a dilated, flabby, hypocontractile heart; the conducting system is frequently involved as well. Cardiomegaly and severe congestive heart failure typically appear after the first week of illness. Prompt therapy with antitoxin is crucial; antibiotic therapy is also indicated but is of less urgency.

CHAGAS' DISEASE Chagas' disease, caused by the protozoan *Trypanosoma cruzi* and transmitted by an insect vector (Chap. 218), produces an extensive myocarditis that typically becomes evident years after the initial infection. It is one of the most common causes of heart disease encountered in Central and South America; in rural endemic areas 20 to 75 percent of the population may be affected. An increasing number of cases are found in the United States as patients migrate from endemic areas. Although only about 1 percent of infected individuals have an acute illness, which may include acute myocarditis, upwards of one-third develop chronic myocardial damage many years later. The chronic form is characterized by dilatation of several cardiac chambers, fibrosis and thinning of the ventricular wall, aneurysm formation (especially at the left ventricular apex), and mural thrombi. Chronic progressive heart failure is the rule and is associated with poor survival. The electrocardiogram is abnormal in most patients with cardiac involvement and typically shows right bundle branch block and left anterior hemiblock which may progress to complete atrioventricular block. The *echocardiogram* may reveal a unique pattern of hypokinesis of the posterior left ventricular wall and relatively preserved septal motion. Ventricular arrhythmias are common and are seen especially during and after exertion; oral amiodarone appears to be particularly effective in treating ventricular tachyarrhythmias. The cause of death is either intractable congestive heart failure or an arrhythmia, with a minority of patients dying from embolic phenomena. Therapy is directed toward amelioration of the congestive heart failure and arrhythmias; progressive conduction system disease and heart block may require implantation of a pacemaker. Anticoagulation (if feasible) may reduce the risk of thromboembolism. Medical therapy often is unsatisfactory or unavailable (especially in poor rural areas), however, and a more promising tactic in endemic areas has been the institution of public health measures, particularly the use of insecticides to eliminate the vector.

GIANT CELL MYOCARDITIS This rare myocarditis of unknown cause is characterized by the presence of multinucleated giant cells in the myocardium. It usually causes rapidly fatal congestive heart failure and arrhythmia in young to middle-aged adults. At necropsy, the distinctive features include cardiac enlargement, ventricular thrombi, grossly visible serpiginous areas of myocardial necrosis in both ventricles, and microscopic evidence of giant cells within an extensive inflammatory infiltrate. The cause of giant cell myocarditis remains obscure, although it occurs in association with thymoma, systemic lupus erythematosus, and thyrotoxicosis. Although glucocorticoids usually are tried, no therapy has been shown conclusively to be efficacious.

LYME CARDITIS (See also Chap. 178) Lyme disease is caused by a tick-borne spirochete and is most common in the Northeast, upper Midwest and Pacific Coastal regions of the United States during the summer months. About 10 percent of patients develop symptomatic cardiac involvement, with atrioventricular nodal conduction abnormalities and their consequences, such as syncope. Concomitant myopericarditis is not uncommon, and mild asymptomatic left ventricular dysfunction may occur. Intravenous ceftriaxone or penicillin is used in all but the mildest forms of Lyme carditis, in which case oral amoxicillin or doxycycline is employed. Hospitalization with electrocardiographic monitoring is indicated in patients with second or third degree atrioventricular block. A temporary pacemaker may be needed for symptomatic heart block; the utility of glucocorticoids in reversing heart block is uncertain, but they are usually employed.

BIBLIOGRAPHY

ANAN R et al: Prognostic implications of novel beta cardiac myosin heavy chain gene mutations that cause familial hypertrophic cardiomyopathy. J Clin Invest 93:280, 1994

CANNON RO et al: Results of permanent dual-chamber pacing in symptomatic nonobstructive hypertrophic cardiomyopathy. Am J Cardiol 73:571, 1994

DEC GW, FUSTER V: Medical progress: Idiopathic dilated cardiomyopathy. N Engl J Med 331:1564, 1994

HAGAR JM, RAHIMTOOLA SH: Chagas' heart disease. Curr Probl Cardiol 20:827, 1995

HERSKOWITZ A et al: Myocarditis and cardiotropic viral infection associated with severe left ventricular dysfunction in late-stage infection with human immunodeficiency virus. J Am Coll Cardiol 24:1025, 1994

KASPER EK et al: The causes of dilated cardiomyopathy: A clinicopathologic review of 673 consecutive patients. J Am Coll Cardiol 23:586, 1994

KLONER RA, HALE S: Unraveling the complex effects of cocaine on the heart. Circulation 87:1046, 1993

KYLE RA: Amyloidosis. Circulation 91:1269, 1995

MARON BJ et al: 26th Bethesda conference: Recommendations for determining eligibility for competition in athletes with cardiovascular abnormalities. Task Force 3: Hypertrophic cardiomyopathy, myocarditis and other myopericardial diseases and mitral valve prolapse. J Am Coll Cardiol 24:880, 1994

MASON JW et al: A clinical trial of immunosuppressive therapy for myocarditis. N Engl J Med 333:269, 1995

MCKENNA WJ et al: Diagnosis of arrhythmogenic right ventricular dysplasia/cardiomyopathy. Task Force of the Working Group Myocardial and Pericardial Disease of the European Society of Cardiology and of the Scientific Council on Cardiomyopathies of the International Society and Federation of Cardiology. Br Heart J 71:215, 1994

NAKAO S et al: An atypical variant of Fabry's disease in men with left ventricular hypertrophy. N Engl J Med 333:288, 1995

O'CONNELL JB et al: Treatment of end stage dilated cardiomyopathy. Br Heart J 72:S52, 1994

RICHARDSON P et al: Report of the 1995 World Health Organization/International Society and Federation of Cardiology Task Force on the Definition and Classification of Cardiomyopathies. Circulation 93:841, 1996

ROBIOLIO PA et al: Carcinoid heart disease. Correlation of high serotonin levels with valvular abnormalities detected by cardiac catheterization and echocardiography. Circulation 92:790, 1995

SINGH SN et al: Amiodarone in patients with congestive heart failure and asymptomatic ventricular arrhythmia. N Engl J Med 333:77, 1995

STOCKINS BA et al: Prognosis in patients with diphtheric myocarditis and bradyarrhythmias: Assessment of results of ventricular pacing. Br Heart J 72:190, 1994

WATKINS H et al: Mutations in the genes for cardiac troponin T and α-tropomyosin in hypertrophic cardiomyopathy. N Engl J Med 332:1058, 1995

WYNNE J, BRAUNWALD E: The cardiomyopathies and myocarditides, in *Heart Disease*, 5th ed, E. Braunwald (ed). Philadelphia, Saunders, 1997, pp 1404–1463

240 *Eugene Braunwald*

PERICARDIAL DISEASE

NORMAL FUNCTIONS OF THE PERICARDIUM The visceral pericardium is a serous membrane that is separated by a small amount (15 to 50 mL) of fluid, an ultrafiltrate of plasma, from a fibrous sac, the parietal pericardium. The pericardium prevents sudden dilatation of the cardiac chambers during exercise and with hypervolemia. As the result of the development of a negative intrapericardial pressure during ejection, it facilitates atrial filling during ventricular systole. The pericardium also restricts the anatomic position of the heart, minimizes friction between the heart and surrounding structures, prevents displacement of the heart and kinking of the great vessels, and probably retards the spread of infections from the lungs and pleural cavities to the heart. Notwithstanding the foregoing, total absence of the pericardium does not produce obvious clinical disease. In partial left pericardial defects the main pulmonary artery and left atrium may bulge through the defect; very rarely, herniation and subsequent strangulation of the left atrium may cause sudden death.

ACUTE PERICARDITIS

Acute pericarditis, by far the most common pathologic process involving the pericardium, may be classified both clinically and etiologically (Table 240-1). Pain, a pericardial friction rub, electrocardiographic changes, and pericardial effusion with cardiac tamponade and paradoxic pulse are cardinal manifestations of many forms of acute pericarditis and will be considered prior to a discussion of the most common forms of the disorder.

Chest pain is an important but not invariable symptom in various forms of acute pericarditis (Chap. 13); it is usually present in the acute infectious types and in many of the forms presumed to be related to

hypersensitivity or autoimmunity. Pain is often absent in a slowly developing tuberculous, postirradiation, neoplastic, or uremic pericarditis. The pain of pericarditis is often severe. It is characteristically retrosternal and left precordial, referred to the back and the trapezius ridge. Often the pain is pleuritic consequent to accompanying pleural inflammation, i.e., sharp and aggravated by inspiration, coughing, and changes in body position, but sometimes it is a steady, constricting pain that radiates into either arm or both arms and resembles that of myocardial ischemia; therefore, confusion with myocardial infarction is common. Characteristically, however, the pericardial pain may be relieved by sitting up and leaning forward and is intensified by lying supine. There is often a pleural component, with aggravation of the pain with coughing and deep inspiration. The differentiation of acute myocardial infarction from acute pericarditis becomes perplexing when, with acute pericarditis, the serum transaminase and creatine kinase levels rise, presumably because of concomitant involvement of the epicardium. However, these enzyme elevations, if they occur,

Table 240-1

Classification of Pericarditis

CLINICAL CLASSIFICATION

 I. Acute pericarditis (<6 weeks)
    A. Fibrinous
    B. Effusive (serous or sanguineous)
 II. Subacute pericarditis (6 weeks to 6 months)
    A. Effusive-constrictive
    B. Constrictive
III. Chronic pericarditis (>6 months)
    A. Constrictive
    B. Effusive
    C. Adhesive (nonconstrictive)

ETIOLOGIC CLASSIFICATION

 I. Infectious pericarditis
    A. Viral (coxsackievirus A and B, echovirus, mumps, adenovirus, hepatitis, HIV)
    B. Pyogenic (pneumococcus, streptococcus, staphylococcus, *Neisseria*, *Legionella*)
    C. Tuberculous
    D. Fungal (histoplasmosis, coccidioidomycosis, *Candida*, blastomycosis)
    E. Other infections (syphilitic, parasitic)
 II. Noninfectious pericarditis
    A. Acute myocardial infarction
    B. Uremia
    C. Neoplasia
       1. Primary tumors (benign or malignant)
       2. Tumors metastatic to pericardium (lung and breast cancer, lymphoma, Hodgkin's disease)
    D. Myxedema
    E. Cholesterol
    F. Chylopericardium
    G. Trauma
       1. Penetrating chest wall
       2. Nonpenetrating
    H. Aortic dissection (with leakage into pericardial sac)
    I. Postirradiation
    J. Familial Mediterranean fever
    K. Familial pericarditis
       1. Mulibrey nanism*
    L. Acute idiopathic
III. Pericarditis presumably related to hypersensitivity or autoimmunity
    A. Rheumatic fever
    B. Collagen vascular disease (SLE, rheumatoid arthritis, scleroderma, acute rheumatic fever, Wegener's granulomatosis)
    C. Drug-induced (e.g., procainamide, hydralazine, phenytoin, isoniazide, doxorubicin)
    D. Postcardiac injury
       1. Postmyocardial infarction (Dressler's syndrome)
       2. Postpericardiotomy
       3. Posttraumatic

* An autosomal recessive syndrome, characterized by growth failure, muscle hypotonia, hepatomegaly, ocular changes, enlarged cerebral ventricles, mental retardation, and chronic constrictive pericarditis.

are quite modest, given the extensive electrocardiographic ST-segment elevation in pericarditis.

The *pericardial friction rub* is the most important physical sign; it may have up to three components per cardiac cycle and is high-pitched, scratching, and grating, as described in Chap. 227; it can sometimes be elicited only when firm pressure with the diaphragm of the stethoscope is applied to the chest wall at the left lower sternal border. It is heard most frequently during expiration with the patient in the sitting position. The rub is often inconstant and the loud to-and-fro leathery sound may disappear within a few hours, possibly to reappear the following day.

The *electrocardiogram* in acute pericarditis without massive effusion usually displays changes secondary to acute subepicardial inflammation (see Fig. 228-18, p. 1245). There is widespread elevation of the ST segments, involving two or three standard limb leads and V_2 to V_6, with reciprocal depressions only in aVR and sometimes V_1. Usually there are no significant changes in QRS complexes, except for some reduction in voltage in patients with large pericardial effusions. After several days, the ST segments return to normal, and only then do the T waves become inverted. In contrast, in acute myocardial infarction, reciprocal depression of ST segments is usually more prominent; QRS changes occur, particularly the development of Q waves, as well as notching and loss of the amplitude of R waves; and T-wave inversions usually occur within hours *before* the ST segments have become isoelectric. Sequential electrocardiograms are useful in distinguishing acute pericarditis from acute myocardial infarction. In the latter, elevated ST segments return to normal within hours. Early repolarization is a normal variant and also may cause widespread ST-segment elevation, most prominent in left precordial leads. However, in this condition the T waves are usually tall and the ST/T ratio is under 0.25, but it exceeds this number in acute pericarditis. Depression of the PQ segment (below the TP segment) also is common and reflects atrial involvement. With large pericardial effusions, the QRS voltage is reduced; atrial premature beats and atrial fibrillation are sometimes noted.

PERICARDIAL EFFUSION Usually associated with pain and/or the above-mentioned electrocardiographic changes characteristic of pericarditis and an enlargement of the cardiac silhouette, pericardial effusion is especially important clinically when it develops within a relatively short time, since it may lead to cardiac tamponade. Differentiation from cardiac enlargement may be difficult, but heart sounds tend to become faint; the friction rub may disappear or remain clearly audible, and the apex impulse may vanish, but sometimes it remains palpable albeit medial to the left border of cardiac dullness. The base of the left lung may be compressed by pericardial fluid, producing Ewart's sign, a patch of dullness beneath the angle of the left scapula. The chest roentgenogram may show a "water bottle" configuration of the cardiac silhouette, but it also may be normal or almost so. Lucent pericardial fat lines may be seen deep within the cardiopericardial silhouette. Fluoroscopic examination may show the ventricular pulsations to be diminished.

Diagnosis of Pericardial Effusion Echocardiography is the most effective diagnostic laboratory technique available, since it is sensitive, specific, simple, noninvasive, and may be performed at the bedside. The presence of pericardial fluid is recorded by two-dimensional transthoracic echocardiography as a relatively echo-free space between the posterior pericardium and left ventricular epicardium in patients with small effusions and a space between the anterior right ventricle and the parietal pericardium just beneath the anterior chest wall with larger effusions (Fig. 240-1). In patients with large effusions the heart may swing freely within the pericardial sac; when severe, the extent of this motion alternates and may be associated with electrical alternans. Echocardiography also allows localization and estimation of the quantity of pericardial fluid. When pericardial effusion causes tamponade, during inspiration right ventricular diameter increases while left ventricular diameter and mitral valve opening decrease. Often the right ventricular cavity is reduced, and there is late diastolic inward motion (collapse) of the right ventricular free wall and of the right atrium. Doppler ultrasound shows exaggerated

tricuspid and pulmonic flow with reciprocal changes in mitral flow during inspiration. The diagnosis of pericardial fluid or thickening may be confirmed by computed tomography (CT) or magnetic resonance imaging (MRI); these techniques may be superior to echocardiography in detecting loculated pericardial effusions.

When it is deemed desirable to remove pericardial fluid for diagnostic and/or therapeutic purposes, a needle attached to a properly grounded electrocardiographic lead is inserted into the pericardial space, usually through a subxiphoid approach, and, if possible, using echocardiographic control. Intrapericardial pressure should be measured before fluid is withdrawn. Pericardial effusion nearly always has the physical characteristics of an exudate. Bloody fluid is commonly due to tuberculosis or tumor but may also be found in the effusion of rheumatic fever; in post-cardiac injury and post-myocardial

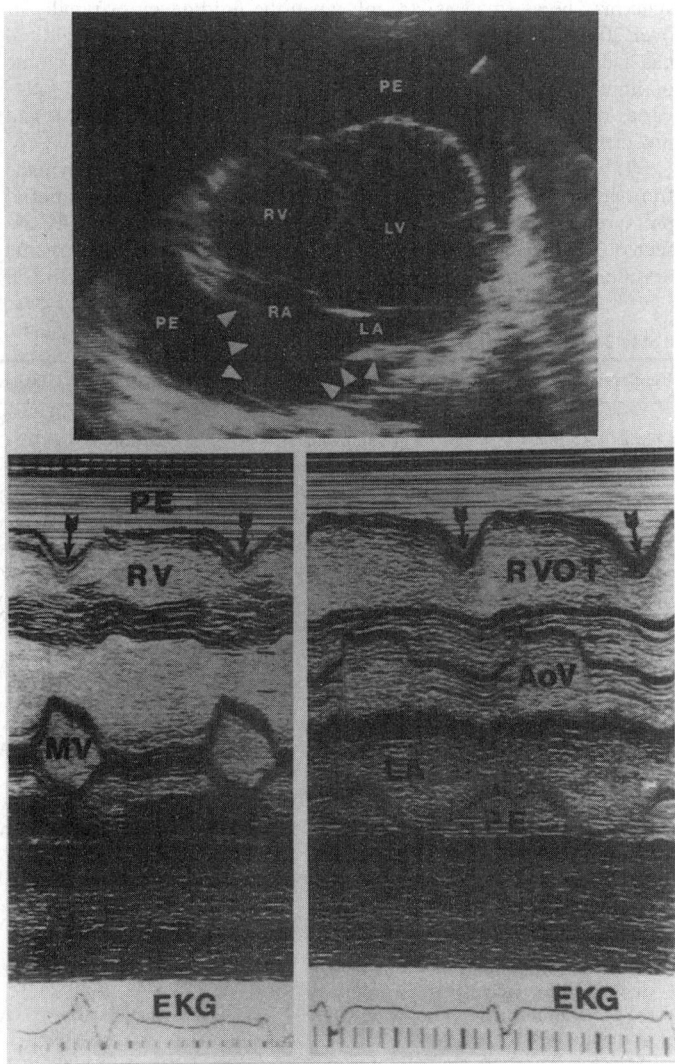

FIGURE 240-1 Two-dimensional (*upper panel*) and M-mode (*lower panels*) echocardiograms of a patient with a malignant pericardial effusion and cardiac tamponade. The two-dimensional image shows a large pericardial effusion (PE) adjacent to the borders of the right ventricle (RV), right atrium (RA), and left ventricle (LV). The effusion is sufficiently large that fluid is also present behind the left atrium (LA). Diastolic compression (white arrowheads) of both the right and left atria is present. The M-mode images also show striking diastolic compression (dark arrows) of the right ventricle during diastole when the mitral valve (MV) is open and compression of the right ventricular outflow tract (RVOT) in early to mid-diastole after aortic valve (AoV) closure. (*From Lorell, with permission.*)

infarction, especially following the administration of anticoagulants; and in uremic pericarditis.

CARDIAC TAMPONADE The accumulation of fluid in the pericardium in an amount sufficient to cause serious obstruction to the inflow of blood to the ventricles results in cardiac tamponade. This grave complication may be fatal if it is not recognized and treated promptly. The three most common causes of tamponade are neoplastic disease, idiopathic pericarditis, and uremia, but it also results from bleeding into the pericardial space either following cardiac operations and trauma (including cardiac perforation during diagnostic procedures) or from tuberculosis and hemopericardium; the latter may result when a patient with any form of acute pericarditis is treated with anticoagulants. The three principal features of tamponade are elevation of intracardiac pressures, limitation of ventricular filling, and reduction of cardiac output. The amount of fluid necessary to produce this critical state may be as small as 200 mL when the fluid develops rapidly or over 2000 mL in slowly developing effusions when the pericardium has had the opportunity to stretch and adapt to the increasing volume of fluid. The volume of fluid required to produce tamponade also varies directly with the thickness of the ventricular myocardium and inversely with the thickness of the parietal pericardium.

Table 240-2 lists the features that distinguish cardiac tamponade from constrictive pericarditis. The classic findings of falling arterial pressure, rising venous pressure, and faint heart sounds usually are seen only with severe, acute tamponade, as occurs with cardiac trauma or rupture. Tamponade may also develop more slowly, and the clinical manifestations resemble those of heart failure, including dyspnea, orthopnea, hepatic engorgement, and jugular venous hypertension. A high index of suspicion for cardiac tamponade is required, since, in many instances, no obvious cause for pericardial disease is apparent, and tamponade should be considered in any patient with hypotension and elevation of jugular venous pressure with a prominent *x* descent; in contrast to constrictive pericarditis, often the *y* descent is diminutive or absent. A positive Kussmaul sign (see below) is rare in cardiac tamponade, as is a pericardial knock. Their presence suggests that an organizing process and epicardial constriction are present in addition to effusion. A widening of the area of flatness to percussion across the anterior aspect of the chest wall, a paradoxical pulse (see below), relatively clear lung fields, diminished pulsations of the cardiac silhouette on fluoroscopy, enlargement of the cardiac silhouette (especially in subacute or chronic tamponade), reduction in amplitude of the QRS complexes, and *electrical alternans* of the P, QRS, and T waves should raise the suspicion of cardiac tamponade.

Since immediate treatment of tamponade may be lifesaving, prompt measures to establish the diagnosis by echocardiography should be undertaken. The right atrial pressure is elevated with prominence of the *x* but not of the *y* descent (Table 240-2). If measured, the pericardial pressure is also elevated and equal to the right atrial pressure. There is "equalization" of pressures, i.e., the pulmonary artery wedge is equal, or close, to right atrial, right ventricular, and pulmonary artery diastolic pressures. The "square root" sign in the ventricular pressure pulses and the prominent *y* descent in atrial and jugular venous pressure are characteristic of constrictive pericarditis (see below) and are rarely present in tamponade. In an emergency, pericardiocentesis may be carried out without cardiac catheterization but, whenever possible, after confirmation of the clinical diagnosis by echocardiography.

Paradoxical Pulse This important clue to the presence of cardiac tamponade consists of *a greater than normal (10 mmHg) inspiratory decline in systolic arterial pressure.* When severe, it may be detected by palpating weakness or disappearance of the arterial pulse during inspiration, but usually sphygmomanometric measurement of systolic pressure during slow respiration is required (Fig. 240-2).

Since both ventricles share a tight incompressible covering, i.e., the pericardial sac, in cardiac tamponade the inspiratory enlargement of the right ventricle compresses and reduces left ventricular volume substantially; leftward bulging of the interventricular septum further reduces the left ventricular cavity as the right ventricle enlarges during inspiration. Thus in cardiac tamponade the normal inspiratory augmentation of right ventricular volume causes an exaggerated reciprocal reduction in left ventricular volume. Also, respiratory distress increases the fluctuations in intrathoracic pressure, which exaggerates the mechanism just described. Right ventricular infarction (Chap. 243) may resemble cardiac tamponade with hypotension, elevated jugular venous pressure, an absent *y* descent in the jugular venous pulse, and occasionally pulsus paradoxus. The differences between these two conditions are shown in Table 240-2.

Paradoxical pulse, a hallmark of cardiac tamponade, occurs in only approxi-

Table 240-2

Features That Distinguish Constrictive Pericarditis From Similar Clinical Disorders

Characteristic	Tamponade	Constrictive Pericarditis	Restrictive Cardiomyopathy	RVMI*
Clinical				
Pulsus paradoxus	Common	Usually absent	Rare	Rare
Jugular veins				
Prominent *y* descent	Absent	Usually present	Rare	Rare
Prominent *x* descent	Present	Usually present	Present	Rare
Kussmaul's sign	Absent	Present	Absent	Absent
Third heart sound	Absent	Absent	Rare	May be present
Pericardial knock	Absent	Often present	Absent	Absent
Electrocardiogram				
Low ECG voltage	May be present	May be present	May be present	Absent
Electrical alternans	May be present	Absent	Absent	Absent
Echocardiography				
Thickened pericardium	Absent	Present	Absent	Absent
Pericardial calcification	Absent	Often present	Absent	Absent
Pericardial effusion	Present	Absent	Absent	Absent
RV size	Usually small	Usually normal	Usually normal	Enlarged
Myocardial thickness	Normal	Normal	Usually increased	Normal
Right atrial collapse and RVDC	Present	Absent	Absent	Absent
Increased early filling, ↑ mitral flow velocity	Absent	Present	Present	May be present
Exaggerated respiratory variation in flow velocity	Present	Present	Absent	Absent
CT/MRI				
Thickened/calcific pericardium	Absent	Present	Absent	Absent
Cardiac catheterization				
Equalization of diastolic procedures	Usually present	Usually present	Usually absent	Absent or present
Cardiac biopsy helpful?	No	No	Sometimes	No

* RV, right ventricle; RVMI, right ventricular myocardial infarction; RVDC, right ventricular diastolic collapse; ECG, electrocardiograph.

SOURCE: From GM Brockington et al, Cardiol Clin 8:645, 1990.

mately one-third of patients with constrictive pericarditis. Paradoxical pulse is not pathognomonic of pericardial disease because it may be observed in restrictive cardiomyopathies (Chap. 239) and in some cases of hypovolemic shock, chronic obstructive airways disease, and severe bronchial asthma.

Low-pressure tamponade refers to mild tamponade in which the intrapericardial pressure is increased from its slightly subatmospheric levels to +5 to +10 mmHg; in some instances hypovolemia coexists. As a consequence, the central venous pressure is normal or only slightly elevated while arterial pressure is unaffected. The patients are asymptomatic or complain of mild weakness and dyspnea. The diagnosis is aided by echocardiography, and both hemodynamic and clinical manifestations improve following pericardiocentesis.

℞ TREATMENT

The patient should be observed frequently for the development of an effusion; if a moderate or large effusion is already present, the patient should be hospitalized and watched for signs of tamponade. In the presence of an effusion, arterial and venous pressures and heart rate should be monitored or followed carefully and serial echocardiograms obtained. If manifestations of tamponade appear, pericardiocentesis must be carried out at once, since relief of the intrapericardial pressure may be lifesaving. A small catheter advanced over the needle inserted into the pericardial cavity may be left in place to allow draining of the pericardial space if fluid reaccumulates. When a *diagnostic* pericardiocentesis of a large effusion is carried out, an attempt should be made to remove as much fluid as possible.

VIRAL OR IDIOPATHIC FORM OF ACUTE PERICARDI-
TIS This disorder is frequent and may be confused with other, more serious illnesses. In some cases, an A or B coxsackievirus or the virus of influenza, echovirus type 8, mumps, herpes simplex, chickenpox, or adenovirus has been isolated from pericardial fluid and/or appropriate elevations in viral antibody titers have been noted; in many instances, acute pericarditis has occurred in association with illnesses of known viral origin and, presumably, was caused by the same agent. Commonly, there is an antecedent infection of the respiratory tract, but in many patients such an association is not evident and viral isolation and serologic studies are negative. Acute pericarditis occurs in patients infected with human immunodeficiency virus (HIV). Most frequently, a viral causation cannot be established, nor can it be excluded; the term *acute idiopathic pericarditis* is then appropriate.

Acute pericarditis occurs at all ages but is more frequent in young adults. Regardless of the specific cause, the clinical manifestations are similar. Pericarditis is often associated with pleural effusions and pneumonitis. The appearance of fever and precordial pain at about the same time, often 10 to 12 days after a presumed viral illness, constitutes an important feature in the differentiation of acute pericarditis from myocardial infarction, in which pain precedes fever. The constitutional symptoms are usually mild to moderate, but occasionally the initial symptoms are stormy, the temperature rising to 40°C. The disease ordinarily runs its course in a few days to 4 weeks, but one or more recurrences occur in about one-fourth of patients. Although accumulation of some pericardial fluid is common, tamponade is unusual, and constrictive pericarditis develops rarely. A pericardial friction rub is often audible. The ST-segment alterations in the electrocardiogram are usually transitory, but the abnormal T waves may persist for several years or indefinitely and be a source of confusion in persons without a clear history of pericarditis. Pleuritis and pneumoni-

tis frequently accompany pericarditis. The erythrocyte sedimentation rate is elevated; granulocytosis followed by lymphocytosis is common.

Viral or idiopathic pericarditis is usually self-limited and abates within 1 month. One or more episodes of recurrent pericarditis occur in up to one-fourth of patients. Constrictive pericarditis (p. 1339) is a rare complication.

℞ TREATMENT

There is no specific therapy, but bed rest and anti-inflammatory treatment with aspirin, if necessary up to 900 mg qid, may be given. If this is ineffective, one of the nonsteroidal anti-inflammatory agents, such as indomethacin (25 to 75 mg qid) or a glucocorticoid (e.g., prednisone, 20 to 80 mg daily) usually suppresses the clinical manifestations of the acute illness and may be useful in patients in whom the purulent and tuberculous forms of pericarditis have been excluded. Anticoagulants should be avoided. After the patient has been asymptomatic and afebrile for about a week, the dose of the anti-inflammatory agent is gradually tapered. When recurrences are multiple, frequent, disabling, and continue beyond 2 years, pericardiectomy may be effective in terminating the illness.

POST-CARDIAC INJURY SYNDROME An acute form of pericarditis may appear under a variety of circumstances that have one common feature: previous injury to the myocardium, with blood in the pericardial cavity. The syndrome has been observed when the injury has been induced in the course of a cardiac operation (postpericardiotomy syndrome). It may develop after cardiac trauma (Chap. 241), e.g., a stab wound, contusions after a nonpenetrating blow to the chest, or perforation of the heart with a catheter. Rarely, it follows myocardial infarction (Dressler's syndrome; Chap. 243).

The principal symptom is the pain of acute pericarditis, which usually develops 1 to 4 weeks following the cardiac injury but sometimes appears only after a lapse of months. Recurrences are common and may occur up to 2 years or more after the injury. Fever with temperature up to 40°C, pericarditis, pleuritis, and pneumonitis are the outstanding features, and the bout of illness usually subsides in 1 or 2 weeks. The pericarditis may be of the fibrinous variety, or it may be a pericardial effusion, which is often serosanguineous, rarely causes tamponade, and may be accompanied by arthralgias. Leukocytosis, an increased sedimentation rate, and electrocardiographic changes typical of acute pericarditis also may occur.

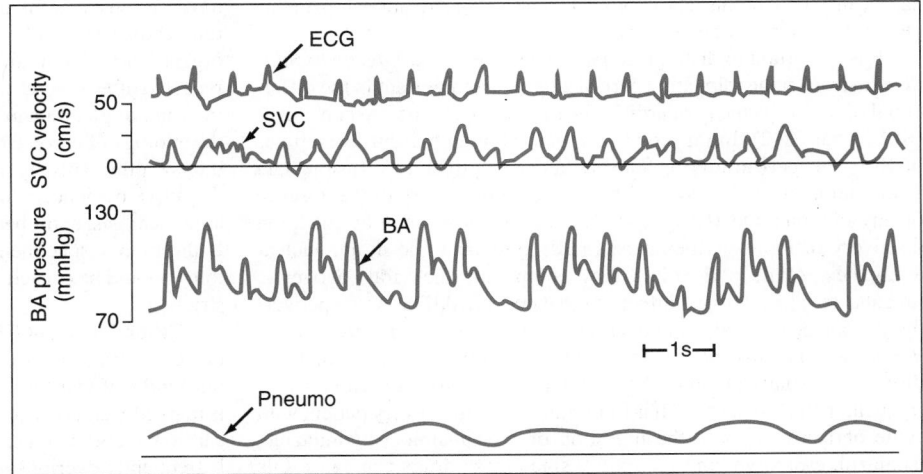

FIGURE 240-2 Simultaneous recording of electrocardiogram (ECG), blood flow velocity in the superior vena cava (SVC), brachial arterial pressure (BA), and the pneumogram (Pneumo) in a patient with cardiac compression and paradoxical pulse. A downward deflection of the pneumogram denotes inspiration, when SVC blood velocity rises and arterial pressure falls (paradoxical pulse). Arterial pressure is maintained during prolonged expiratory pause.

The mechanisms responsible for this syndrome have not been identified, but they are probably the result of a hypersensitivity reaction in which the antigen originates from injured myocardial tissue and/or pericardium; the suggested designation of *post-cardiac injury syndrome* for this group of disorders implies that they may have a common pathogenetic mechanism. Circulating autoantibodies to myocardium occur frequently, but their precise role has not been defined. Viral infection also may play an etiologic role, since antiviral antibodies are often elevated in patients who develop this syndrome following cardiac surgery.

The clinical picture of the post-cardiac injury syndrome mimics acute viral or acute idiopathic pericarditis. Moreover, it is possible that the recurrences that occur so frequently in the latter condition are not always caused by an exacerbation of the original (presumably viral) infection but that the original injury may have initiated the sequence of events that culminates in the post-cardiac injury syndrome.

Often no treatment is necessary aside from aspirin and analgesics. The management of pericardial effusion and tamponade has already been discussed. When the illness is followed by a series of disabling recurrences, therapy with a nonsteroidal anti-inflammatory agent or a glucocorticoid is usually effective.

DIFFERENTIAL DIAGNOSIS Since there is no specific test for *acute idiopathic pericarditis* the diagnosis is one of exclusion. Consequently, all other disorders that may be associated with acute fibrinous pericarditis must be considered. When associated with *acute myocardial infarction*, acute fibrinous pericarditis may be confused with acute viral or idiopathic pericarditis; this complication of infarction, described in Chap. 243, is characterized by the occurrence of fever, pain, and a friction rub in the first 4 days following the development of the infarct (to be distinguished from the pericarditis in Dressler's syndrome, which is a form of post-cardiac injury pericarditis and which occurs a week or two following myocardial infarction). Electrocardiographic abnormalities (such as the appearance of Q waves, brief ST-segment elevations with reciprocal changes, and earlier T-wave changes in myocardial infarction), the extent of the elevations of myocardial enzymes, and the total clinical picture are helpful in differentiating pericarditis from acute myocardial infarction. A common diagnostic error is mistaking acute viral or idiopathic pericarditis for acute myocardial infarction and vice versa.

Pericarditis secondary to post-cardiac injury is differentiated from acute idiopathic pericarditis chiefly by timing. If it occurs within a few weeks of a myocardial infarction or a chest blow, it may be justified to conclude that the two are probably related. If the infarct has been silent or the chest blow forgotten, the relationship to the pericarditis may not be recognized.

It is important to distinguish *pericarditis due to collagen vascular disease* from acute idiopathic pericarditis. Most important in the differential diagnosis is the pericarditis due to systemic lupus erythematosus (SLE; Chap. 312). In this condition, pain is often present; sometimes in SLE the pericarditis appears as an asymptomatic effusion, and rarely, tamponade develops. When pericarditis occurs in the absence of any obvious underlying disorder, the diagnosis may be made on discovery of lupus erythematosus (LE) cells or a rise in antinuclear antibodies. Acute pericarditis may complicate the viral, pyogenic, mycobacterial, and fungal infections that occur in AIDS. Acute pericarditis is an occasional complication of *rheumatoid arthritis*, *scleroderma*, and *polyarteritis nodosa*, but again, other evidence of these diseases is usually obvious. Asymptomatic pericardial effusion is also frequent in these disorders. It is important to question every patient with acute pericarditis about the ingestion of procainamide, hydralazine, isoniazid, cromolyn, and minoxidil, since these drugs can cause this syndrome.

The pericarditis of *acute rheumatic fever* is generally associated with evidence of severe pancarditis and with cardiac murmurs (Chap. 236). *Pyogenic (purulent) pericarditis* is usually secondary to cardiothoracic operations, immunosuppressive therapy, rupture of the esoph-

agus into the pericardial sac, or rupture of a ring abscess in a patient with infective endocarditis and with septicemia complicating aseptic pericarditis. It is accompanied by fever, chills, septicemia, and evidence of infection elsewhere. *Tuberculous pericarditis* (see Chap. 171) may present as an acute pericarditis, associated with fever, weight loss, and other clinical manifestations of active systemic tuberculosis; the diagnosis may be aided by a positive tuberculin test and evidence of pulmonary or mediastinal tuberculosis. Tubercle bacilli can be cultured from the pericardial space only infrequently, and a biopsy of the pericardium with bacteriologic and histologic examination may be required. Alternatively, tuberculous pericarditis may present as a chronic asymptomatic effusion, as subacute effusive-constrictive pericarditis (see below), or as frank chronic constrictive pericarditis (see below).

Uremic pericarditis (Chap. 271) occurs in up to one-third of patients with chronic uremia and is seen most frequently in patients undergoing chronic hemodialysis. It may be fibrinous and is generally associated with an effusion that may be sanguineous. A friction rub is common, but pain is usually absent. Treatment with an anti-inflammatory agent and intensification of hemodialysis is usually adequate. Occasionally, tamponade occurs and pericardiocentesis is required. When uremic pericarditis is recurrent, persistent, or very troubling, it may be necessary to perform pericardiectomy. Pericarditis due to *neoplastic diseases* results from extension or invasion of primary or metastatic tumors (most commonly carcinoma of the lung and breast, malignant melanoma, lymphoma, and leukemia) to the pericardium; pain, atrial arrhythmias, and tamponade are complications that occur occasionally. *Mediastinal irradiation* for neoplasm may cause acute pericarditis and/or chronic constrictive pericarditis after eradication of the tumor. Unusual causes of acute pericarditis include syphilis, fungal infection (histoplasmosis, blastomycosis, aspergillosis, and candidiasis), and parasitic infestation (amebiasis, toxoplasmosis, echinococcosis, trichinosis).

CHRONIC PERICARDIAL EFFUSIONS Chronic pericardial effusions are sometimes encountered in patients without an antecedent history of acute pericarditis. They may cause few symptoms per se, and their presence may be detected by finding an enlarged cardiac silhouette on chest roentgenogram.

Tuberculosis This is a common cause of chronic pericardial effusion, although less so in the United States than in other parts of the world (Chap. 171). The symptoms are often those of a chronic, systemic illness in a patient with pericardial effusion. It is important to bear this condition in mind when a middle-aged or elderly person with fever has enlargement of the cardiac silhouette of undetermined origin, with or without elevation of venous pressure. Weight loss, fever, and fatigability are sometimes observed. Inasmuch as treatment is quite effective, overlooking a tuberculous pericardial effusion may have serious consequences. A chest roentgenogram for pulmonary tuberculosis should be obtained, and a search for tuberculosis in other organs carried out; tuberculin skin tests should be performed and repeated after several weeks; and cultures and smears of gastric washings and of pleural and pericardial fluid should be obtained. Finally, if the etiology of chronic pericardial effusion is still obscure, a pericardial biopsy, preferably by a limited thoracotomy, should be performed. If definitive evidence is then still lacking but the specimen shows caseation necrosis, antituberculous chemotherapy is indicated (Chap. 171). If the biopsy specimen shows a thickened pericardium, pericardiectomy should be carried out in order to prevent the development of constriction.

Other Causes of Chronic Pericardial Effusion *Myxedema* may be responsible for a pericardial effusion that is sometimes massive but rarely, if ever, causes cardiac tamponade. The cardiac silhouette is markedly enlarged and an echocardiogram is necessary to distinguish cardiomegaly from pericardial effusion. The diagnosis of myxedema is frequently overlooked. It is important, therefore, to carry out appropriate tests for thyroid function (Chap. 331) as well as echocardiography in patients with an enlarged cardiac outline of undetermined origin. *Cholesterol pericardial disease* produces large pericardial effusions with a high cholesterol content, which may induce an inflammatory response and constrictive pericarditis.

Neoplasms, SLE, rheumatoid arthritis, mycotic infections, radiation therapy, pyogenic infections, severe chronic anemia, and chylopericardium also may cause chronic pericardial effusion and should be considered and specifically looked for in such patients.

Aspiration and analysis of the pericardial fluid are often helpful in diagnosis. In infections the organism can often be identified by smear or culture. Grossly sanguineous pericardial fluid results most commonly from a neoplasm, tuberculosis, uremia, or slow leakage from an aortic aneurysm.

CHRONIC CONSTRICTIVE PERICARDITIS

This disorder results when the healing of an acute fibrinous or serofibrinous pericarditis or a chronic pericardial effusion is followed by obliteration of the pericardial cavity with the formation of granulation tissue. This gradually contracts and forms a firm scar, encasing the heart and interfering with filling of the ventricles. In some reports, a high percentage of all cases has been of tuberculous origin. In the United States tuberculosis is now an infrequent cause. Chronic constrictive pericarditis also may follow purulent infection, trauma, cardiac operation of any type, mediastinal irradiation, histoplasmosis, neoplastic disease (especially breast cancer and lymphoma), acute viral or idiopathic pericarditis, rheumatoid arthritis, SLE, and chronic renal failure with uremia treated by chronic dialysis. In many patients the cause of the pericardial disease is undetermined, and in them an asymptomatic or forgotten bout of viral pericarditis, acute or idiopathic, may have been the inciting event. The heart also may be constricted and compressed by malignant tumors or organized blood clot in the pericardial cavity.

The basic physiologic abnormality in symptomatic patients with chronic constrictive pericarditis, as in those with cardiac tamponade, is the inability of the ventricles to fill because of the limitations imposed by the rigid, thickened pericardium or the tense pericardial fluid. In constrictive pericarditis, ventricular filling is unimpeded during early diastole but is reduced abruptly when the elastic limit of the pericardium is reached, while in cardiac tamponade, ventricular filling is impeded throughout diastole. In chronic constrictive pericarditis, stroke volume is reduced and the end-diastolic pressures in both ventricles and the mean pressures in the atria, pulmonic veins, and systemic veins are all elevated to about the same levels. Despite these hemodynamic changes, myocardial function may actually be normal or only slightly impaired; instead, the ventricles may be considered to be underloaded.

In constrictive pericarditis, the central venous and right and left atrial pressure pulses display an M-shaped contour, with prominent x and y descents; the y descent (absent or diminished in cardiac tamponade) is the most prominent deflection and is interrupted by a rapid rise in pressure during early diastole, when ventricular filling is impeded by the constricting pericardium. These characteristic changes are transmitted to the jugular veins, where they may be recognized by inspection. In constrictive pericarditis, both ventricular pressure pulses exhibit characteristic "square root" signs during diastole. These hemodynamic changes, although characteristic, are not pathognomonic of constrictive pericarditis but also may be observed in cardiomyopathies characterized by restriction of ventricular filling, as discussed in Chap. 239.

CLINICAL AND LABORATORY FINDINGS (See Table 240-2) Weakness, fatigue, weight loss, and anorexia are common. The patient often appears to be chronically ill with decreased skeletal muscle mass and a protuberant abdomen. Dyspnea, though absent or slight at rest, is usually present on exertion, and orthopnea is common, although not severe. However, attacks of acute left ventricular failure (acute pulmonary edema) practically never occur. The cervical veins are distended and may remain so even after intensive diuretic treatment, and venous pressure may fail to decline during inspiration (Kussmaul's sign). The pulse pressure is normal or reduced. In about one-third of the cases a paradoxical pulse can be detected. Congestive hepatomegaly is pronounced and may impair hepatic function; ascites is common and is usually more prominent than dependent edema. In about half of

patients the heart is normal in size; if it is enlarged, the enlargement is rarely extreme. The apical pulse is reduced in intensity, retracts in systole, and moves outward in diastole. The heart sounds may be distant; an early third heart sound, i.e., a pericardial knock, occurring 0.09 to 0.12 s after aortic valve closure that coincides with a sudden deceleration in ventricular filling, is often conspicuous, and murmurs are usually absent. The apex beat is poorly defined. Because of the high sustained venous pressure, congestive splenomegaly may make the spleen palpable. In the absence of infective endocarditis or tricuspid valve disease, splenomegaly in a patient with congestive heart failure should arouse suspicion of constrictive pericarditis. Protein-losing gastroenteropathy, due to impaired lymphatic drainage from the small intestine, and the nephrotic syndrome, or marked proteinuria or hypoalbuminemia, may complicate chronic constrictive pericarditis.

The *electrocardiogram* frequently displays low voltage of the QRS complex and diffuse flattening or inversion of the T waves. P mitrale may be present in patients with sinus rhythm; atrial fibrillation is present in about one-third of patients.

Systemic and/or pulmonary venous congestion is initially the result of impaired filling of the ventricles caused by the restrictive action of the inelastic pericardium. However, the fibrotic process may extend into the myocardium and cause myocardial scarring, and venous congestion may then be due to the combined effects of the myocardial and pericardial lesions. The interference with filling reduces the work of the heart, and perhaps this leads to myocardial atrophy. The latter probably accounts for the delayed beneficial effects of operative treatment observed in some patients with advanced disease.

Inasmuch as the usual physical signs of cardiac disease (murmurs, cardiac enlargement) may be inconspicuous or absent in chronic constrictive pericarditis, hepatic enlargement and dysfunction associated with intractable ascites may lead to a mistaken diagnosis of cirrhosis of the liver. This error can be avoided if the neck veins are inspected carefully in all patients with ascites and hepatomegaly. *Given a clinical picture resembling hepatic cirrhosis, but with the added feature of distended neck veins, careful search for calcification of the pericardium by chest roentgenography and echocardiography should be carried out and may disclose this curable or remediable form of heart disease.* Calcification occurs in only about one-half of these patients, usually in those with long-standing pericardial constriction. Most patients with chronic constrictive pericarditis show pericardial thickening on echocardiographic examination, and there is a distinctive pattern of transvalvular flow velocity on Doppler echocardiography. There is a reduction in blood flow velocity in the pulmonary veins and across the mitral valve during inspiration, with the opposite occurring during expiration. However, echocardiography cannot definitively exclude the diagnosis. MRI and CT scanning are more accurate than echocardiography in establishing or excluding the presence of a thickened pericardium. Pericardial thickening and even pericardial calcification, however, are not synonymous with constrictive pericarditis since they may occur without seriously impairing ventricular filling.

Prolonged hepatic congestion often leads to hypoalbuminemia, hyperbilirubinemia, and other abnormal tests of hepatocellular function.

DIFFERENTIAL DIAGNOSIS Like cor pulmonale (Chap. 238), chronic constrictive pericarditis may be associated with severe systemic venous hypertension but little pulmonary congestion; the heart usually is not enlarged, and a striking inspiratory fall in arterial pressure may be present. However, in cor pulmonale advanced parenchymal pulmonary disease is usually obvious and venous pressure *falls* during inspiration; i.e., Kussmaul's sign is negative. *Tricuspid stenosis* (p. 1322) also may simulate chronic constrictive pericarditis; congestive hepatomegaly, splenomegaly, ascites, and venous distention may be equally prominent, and the manifestations of left-sided heart failure may be inconspicuous. However, in tricuspid stenosis, the characteristic murmur, the almost universal coexistence of mitral stenosis, the absence of a paradoxical pulse, and the absence, in the jugular venous pulse, of the steep, deep *y* descent followed by a rapid ascent (manifested by the diastolic shock on palpation and its audible equivalent, the pericardial knock) facilitate the clinical differentiation.

Because constrictive pericarditis can be corrected surgically, it is important, though often difficult, to distinguish chronic constrictive pericarditis from restrictive cardiomyopathy (Chap. 239), which has a similar physiologic abnormality, i.e., restriction of ventricular filling. In many of these patients the ventricular wall is thickened on echocardiographic examination.

The features favoring the diagnosis of restrictive cardiomyopathy are a well-defined apex beat, enlargement of the heart, and pronounced orthopnea with attacks of acute left ventricular failure, left ventricular hypertrophy, gallop sounds (in place of a pericardial knock), bundle branch block, and in some cases abnormal Q waves on the electrocardiogram. At catheterization, patients with chronic constrictive pericarditis usually have left atrial or pulmonary arterial wedge pressure equaling right atrial pressure, the latter often exceeding 15 mmHg despite intensive medical treatment for heart failure. The pulmonary artery systolic pressure is often less than 50 mmHg, and the right ventricular end-diastolic pressure often reaches one-third of the systolic pressure. In contrast, in patients with restrictive cardiomyopathy, the left atrial usually exceeds the right atrial pressure by more than 5 mmHg, the mean right atrial pressure is often below 15 mmHg following intensive treatment with diuretics, the pulmonary artery systolic pressure often exceeds 50 mmHg, and the right ventricular end-diastolic pressure is usually less than one-third of the systolic pressure, while the cardiac output is markedly depressed. The volumes of both ventricles, as determined by angiography or echocardiography, are characteristically reduced or normal in constrictive pericarditis, and the ejection fractions are normal or almost so. The left ventricular end-diastolic volume also may be normal in some cardiomyopathies, but it is frequently elevated in others in which the ejection fraction is markedly reduced; the latter finding militates strongly against the diagnosis of constrictive pericarditis. The echocardiogram in chronic constrictive pericarditis characteristically shows pericardial thickening, i.e., a distinct echo posterior to the left ventricular wall, and paradoxical septal motion. The left ventricular wall moves sharply outward in early diastole and then remains flat. The definitive diagnosis of restrictive cardiomyopathy, when it is due to an infiltrative disease such as amyloidosis, can often be established by endomyocardial biopsy. CT scanning and MRI are very useful in distinguishing between restrictive cardiomyopathy and chronic constrictive pericarditis.

When a patient has progressive, disabling, and unresponsive congestive failure, and if he or she displays any of the features of constrictive heart disease, the most careful and detailed clinical and laboratory studies must be carried out in order to detect or exclude constrictive pericarditis, which is potentially a curable condition. Cardiac catheterization, angiocardiography, endomyocardial biopsy, and MRI may be required.

Occult Constrictive Disease Patients with this condition may have unexplained fatigue, dyspnea, and chest pain. No overt manifestations of pericardial disease are present, but following the rapid intravenous infusion of 1 L of saline solution, diastolic equilibration of intracardiac atrial and ventricular pressures found in overt constrictive pericarditis occur. Although symptomatic improvement may follow pericardiectomy, this procedure should not be carried out in asymptomatic persons.

℞ TREATMENT

Pericardial resection is the only definitive treatment of constrictive pericarditis, but dietary sodium restriction and diuretics are useful during preoperative preparation. The benefits derived from cardiac decortication are often striking, and the improvement, though slight at first, usually is progressive over a period of months. The risk of this operation depends on the extent of penetration of the myocardium by the calcific process, by the severity of myocardial atrophy, by the extent of secondary impairment of hepatic and/or renal function, and by the patient's general condition. Operative mortality is in the range of 5 to 15 percent; the patients with the most severe and/or advanced disease are at highest risk. Therefore, surgical treatment should be carried out relatively early in the course.

Many cases of constrictive pericarditis are of tuberculous origin. Antituberculous therapy during the phase of effusion may prevent the development of constriction, and such therapy should be carried out before and after operation if a tuberculous origin is suspected or cannot be excluded in a patient with chronic constrictive pericarditis (Chap. 171).

SUBACUTE EFFUSIVE-CONSTRICTIVE PERICARDITIS This form of pericardial disease is characterized by the combination of a tense effusion in the pericardial space and constriction of the heart by thickened pericardium. It shares a number of features both with chronic pericardial effusion (p. 1338) producing cardiac compression and with pericardial constriction. It may be caused by tuberculosis, multiple attacks of acute idiopathic pericarditis, radiation, traumatic pericarditis, uremia, and scleroderma. The heart is generally enlarged, and a paradoxical pulse and a prominent *x* descent (without a prominent *y* descent) are present in the atrial pressure pulse. Following pericardiocentesis, the physiologic findings may change from those of cardiac tamponade to those of pericardial constriction, with a "square root" sign in the ventricular pressure pulse and a prominent *y* descent in the atrial and jugular venous pressure pulses. Furthermore, the intrapericardial pressure and the central venous pressure may decline, but not to normal. In many patients the condition progresses to the chronic constrictive form of the disease. Wide excision of both the visceral and parietal pericardium is usually effective.

OTHER DISORDERS OF THE PERICARDIUM

Pericardial cysts appear as rounded or lobulated deformities of the cardiac silhouette, most commonly at the right cardiophrenic angle. They do not cause symptoms, and their major clinical significance lies in the possibility of confusion with a tumor, ventricular aneurysm, or massive cardiomegaly. *Tumors* involving the pericardium are most commonly secondary to malignant neoplasms originating in or invading the mediastinum, including carcinoma of the bronchus and breast, lymphoma, and melanoma. The most common *primary* malignant tumor is the mesothelioma. The usual clinical picture of malignant pericardial tumor is an insidiously developing, often bloody, pericardial effusion. Surgical exploration is required to establish a definitive diagnosis and to carry out definitive or, more commonly, palliative treatment.

BIBLIOGRAPHY

CUJEC B et al: Echocardiography in pericardial diseases, in *Marcus' Cardiac Imaging: A Companion to Braunwald's Heart Disease*, 2d ed, DJ Skorton et al (eds). Philadelphia, Saunders, 1996, pp 404–419

FOWLER NO: Tuberculous pericarditis. JAMA 266:99, 1991

HANCOCK EW: Subacute effusive-constrictive pericarditis. Circulation 43:183, 1971

KHAN AH: The postcardiac injury syndromes. Clin Cardiol 15:67, 1992

LORELL B: Pericardial diseases, in *Heart Disease*, 5th ed, E Braunwald (ed). Philadelphia, Saunders, 1997, pp 1478–1534

OH JK et al: Diagnostic role of Doppler echocardiography in constrictive pericarditis. J Am Coll Cardiol 23:154, 1994

SAGRISTA SAULEDA J et al: Purulent pericarditis: Review of a 20-year experience in a general hospital. J Am Coll Cardiol 22:1661, 1993

SHABETAI R: Treatment of pericardial disease, in *Cardiovascular Therapeutics: A Companion to Braunwald's Heart Disease*, TW Smith (ed). Philadelphia, Saunders, 1996, pp 742–750

SOLER-SOLER J: Massive chronic idiopathic pericardial effusion, in *Pericardial Disease: New Insights and Old Dilemmas*, J Soler-Soler et al (eds). Dordrecht, The Netherlands, Kluwer Academic, 1990, pp 153–165

STANFORD W, THOMPSON BH: Cardiac masses and pericardial disease: Imaging by electron-beam computed tomography, in *Marcus' Cardiac Imaging: A Companion to Braunwald's Heart Disease*, 2d ed, DJ Skorton et al (eds). Philadelphia, Saunders, 1996, pp 863–870

TIRILOMIS T et al: Pericardiectomy for chronic constrictive pericarditis: Risks and outcome. Eur J Cardiothorac Surg 8:487, 1994

VAITKUS PT, KUSSMAUL WG: Constrictive versus restrictive cardiomyopathy: A reappraisal and update of diagnostic criteria. Am Heart J 122:1431, 1991

——— et al: Treatment of malignant pericardial effusion. JAMA 272:59, 1994

Table 241-1

Relative Incidence of Primary Tumor of the Heart

Type	Percent
BENIGN	
Myxoma	30.5
Lipoma	10.5
Papillary fibroelastoma	9.9
Rhabdomyoma	8.5
Fibroma	4.0
Hemangioma	3.5
Teratoma	3.3
Mesothelioma of the AV node	2.8
Other benign tumors	2.1
Total	75.1
MALIGNANT	
Sarcomas	18.6
Lymphoma	1.6
Other malignant tumors	4.7
Total	24.9

SOURCE: Modified from HA McAllister, JJ Fenoglio, in Atlas of Tumor Pathology, Washington, Armed Forces Institute of Pathology, 1978, fasc 15, 2d series.

241

Wilson S. Colucci, Eugene Braunwald

CARDIAC TUMORS, CARDIAC MANIFESTATIONS OF SYSTEMIC DISEASES, AND TRAUMATIC CARDIAC INJURY

TUMORS OF THE HEART

PRIMARY TUMORS Primary tumors of the heart are rare and are often classified as "benign" histologically (Table 241-1). However, since all cardiac tumors have the potential for causing life-threatening complications, and many are now curable by surgery, it is important that this diagnosis be made whenever possible. Approximately three-quarters are *histologically* benign, and the remainder are malignant, in almost all cases sarcomas.

Clinical Presentation Cardiac tumors may present with a wide array of cardiac and noncardiac manifestations. There may be signs and symptoms of all the more common forms of heart disease, including chest pain, syncope, heart failure, murmurs, arrhythmias, conduction disturbances, and pericardial effusion or tamponade. The specific signs and symptoms produced are most closely related to the location of the tumor.

Myxoma Myxomas are the most common type of primary cardiac tumor for all age groups, accounting for one-third to one-half of all cases at postmortem and for approximately three-quarters of the tumors that are treated surgically. They occur at all ages and show no sex preference. Although the large majority of myxomas are sporadic, some are familial with autosomal dominant transmission or are part of a syndrome that involves a complex of abnormalities including lentigines or pigmented nevi, primary nodular adrenal cortical disease with or without Cushing's syndrome, myxomatous mammary fibroadenomas, testicular tumors, and/or pituitary adenomas with gigantism or acromegaly. Certain constellations of findings have been referred to as the *NAME syndrome* (nevi, atrial myxoma, myxoid neurofibroma, and ephelides) or the *LAMB syndrome* (lentigines, atrial myxoma, and blue nevi). Approximately 7 percent of cardiac myxomas are familial or part of the *syndrome myxoma* with complex abnormalities described above.

Most authorities consider myxoma to be a true neoplasm, while others have suggested that it is formed by organization of an intracardiac thrombus attached to the endocardium. The large majority of sporadic myxomas are solitary and located in the atria, particularly the left, where they arise from the interatrial septum in the vicinity of the fossa ovalis. Sporadic myxomas may also occur in the ventricles or may be found in multiple locations. In contrast to sporadic myxomas, familial or syndrome myxoma tumors tend to occur in younger individuals, are more often multiple in location, and are more likely to have postoperative recurrences, probably reflecting their multicentric nature (Table 241-2). Most are pedunculated on a fibrovascular stalk and average 4 to 8 cm in diameter. The most common clinical presentation resembles that of mitral valve disease, either stenosis as a result of tumor prolapse into the mitral orifice during diastole or regurgitation as a consequence of injury to the valve by tumor-induced trauma. Ventricular myxomas may cause outflow obstruction and may therefore mimic subaortic or subpulmonic stenosis.

The symptoms and signs of atrial myxomas are highly dependent on position, intermittent, and sudden in onset as a result of changes in tumor position with gravity. On auscultation, a characteristic low-pitched sound, termed a "tumor plop," is audible during early or middiastole and is thought to result from the tumor abruptly stopping as it strikes the ventricular wall. Myxomas may also present with peripheral or pulmonary emboli, or any of several noncardiac signs and symptoms including fever, weight loss, cachexia, malaise, arthralgia, rash, clubbing, Raynaud's phenomenon, hypergammaglobulinemia, anemia, polycythemia, leukocytosis, elevated erythrocyte sedimentation rate, thrombocytopenia, or thrombocytosis. Not surprisingly, myxomas are frequently misdiagnosed as endocarditis, collagen vascular disease, or noncardiac tumor.

Two-dimensional echocardiography is useful in the diagnosis of cardiac myxoma and allows determination of the site of tumor attachment and tumor size, important considerations in the planning of surgical excision. Computed tomography and particularly magnetic resonance imaging may provide important information regarding the size, shape, composition, and surface characteristics of the tumor. Because myxomas may be familial, echocardiographic screening of first-degree relatives is appropriate, particularly if the patient is young and has multiple tumors or other evidence of syndrome myxoma. While cardiac catheterization and angiography are often performed

Table 241-2

Comparison of Clinical Features of Sporadic Myxoma and Syndrome Myxoma

Feature	Sporadic	Syndrome
Age (year) (range)	56 (39–82)	25 (10–56)
Female/male ratio	2.7:1	1.8:1
Patients (no.)	70	44
Cardiac myxomas (no.)	72	103
Distributions of myxomas (%):		
Atrial/ventricular	100/0	87/13
Single/multiple	99/1	50/50
Biatrial	0	23
Recurrent	0	18
Freckling (%)	0	68
Noncardiac tumors (%)	0	57
Endocrine neoplasm (%)	0	30
Familial (%)	0	14

SOURCE: HJ Vidaillet et al, Br Heart J 57:247, 1987

prior to surgery, catheterization of the chamber from which the tumor originates is attended by the risk of dislodgment of tumor emboli. In many centers catheterization is no longer considered mandatory when adequate noninvasive information is available and other cardiac diseases (e.g., coronary artery disease) are not considered likely.

℞ TREATMENT

Surgical excision utilizing cardiopulmonary bypass is indicated and is generally curative. Myxomas recur in approximately 12 to 22 percent of familial cases and in about 1 to 2 percent of sporadic cases; tumor recurrence is most likely due to multifocal lesions in the former and inadequate resection in the latter.

Other Benign Tumors Cardiac *lipomas*, although relatively common, are usually incidental findings at postmortem examination and seldom result in symptoms. However, they may grow as large as 15 cm and present with symptoms due to mechanical interference with cardiac function, arrhythmias, or conduction disturbances, or as an abnormality of the cardiac silhouette on chest x-ray. *Papillary fibroelastomas*, similarly, are relatively common findings on cardiac valves or the adjacent endothelium at postmortem but seldom result in clinical symptoms. Occasionally, these growths may cause mechanical interference with valvular function. *Rhabdomyomas* and *fibromas*, the most frequent tumors in infants and children, most commonly occur in the ventricles, and therefore produce signs and symptoms by mechanical obstruction, which may mimic valvular stenosis, congestive heart failure, restrictive or hypertrophic cardiomyopathy, and pericardial constriction. Rhabdomyomas are probably hamartomatous growths, are multiple in about 90 percent of cases, and may be associated with tuberous sclerosis, adenoma sebaceum, and benign kidney tumors in approximately 30 percent of patients. Calcification of a cardiac tumor strongly suggests that it is a fibroma, although myxomas and sarcomas may also be calcified. *Hemangiomas* and *mesotheliomas* are generally small tumors, most often intramyocardial in location, and may cause atrioventricular conduction disturbances and even sudden death as a result of their propensity for location in the region of the AV node.

Sarcomas Cardiac sarcomas may be of several histologic types, but in general are characterized by a rapidly downhill course leading to the patient's death in weeks to months from the time of presentation as a result of hemodynamic compromise, local invasion, or distant metastases. Sarcomas commonly involve the right side of the heart, and because of their rapid growth, invasion of the pericardial space and obstruction of the cardiac chambers or venae cavae are common. Sarcomas also can occur on the left side of the heart and they may be mistaken for myxomas. At the time of presentation these tumors have often spread too extensively for surgical excision. While there are scattered reports of palliation with surgery, radiotherapy, and/or chemotherapy, the overall experience with cardiac sarcomas is poor. The one exception to this appears to be cardiac lymphosarcomas, which may respond to a combination of chemo- and radiotherapy.

TUMORS METASTATIC TO THE HEART Tumors metastatic to the heart are several times more common than primary tumors, and as the life expectancy of patients with various forms of malignant neoplasms is extended by more effective therapy, the frequency of cardiac metastases will also increase. Although cardiac metastases occur in 1 to 20 percent of all tumor types, the incidence is especially high in malignant melanoma and, to a somewhat lesser extent, in leukemia and lymphoma. In absolute numbers, cardiac metastases are most common in carcinoma of the breast and lung, reflecting the high incidence of these cancers. Cardiac metastases almost always occur in the setting of widespread primary disease, and most often there is either primary or metastatic disease elsewhere in the thoracic cavity. Nevertheless, occasionally a cardiac metastasis may be the initial presentation of a tumor elsewhere in the body.

Cardiac metastases reach the heart via the bloodstream, lymphatics, or direct invasion and generally are small, firm nodules; diffuse infil-

trations may also occur, especially with sarcomas or hematologic neoplasms. The pericardium is most often involved, followed by myocardial involvement of any chamber, and, rarely, by involvement of the endocardium or cardiac valves.

Cardiac metastases result in clinical manifestations only about 10 percent of the time, and rarely are they the cause of death. In most patients they are *not* the cause of the presenting clinical features but occur in the setting of a previously recognized malignant neoplasm. While cardiac metastases may present a large number of nonspecific signs and symptoms, the most common are dyspnea, signs of acute pericarditis, cardiac tamponade, a rapid increase in the cardiac silhouette on chest x-ray, the new onset of an ectopic tachyarrhythmia, AV block, and congestive heart failure. As with primary cardiac tumors, the clinical presentation is more closely related to the location and size of the tumor than to its histologic type. Many of these signs and symptoms may also occur with myocarditis, pericarditis, or cardiomyopathy resulting from radiotherapy or chemotherapy.

The electrocardiographic findings are entirely nonspecific and may include ST-T-wave changes, decreased QRS voltage, arrhythmias, and conduction disturbances. On chest roentgenography the cardiac silhouette is most often normal but may reveal a pericardial effusion or bizarre contour. Echocardiography is useful for the diagnosis of pericardial effusion and the visualization of larger metastases. Computed tomography, magnetic resonance imaging, and radionuclide imaging with gallium or thallium may provide useful anatomic information. Angiography may delineate discrete lesions, and pericardiocentesis can allow a specific cytologic diagnosis. Since most patients with cardiac metastases have widespread disease, therapy generally consists of pericardiocentesis when there is hemodynamic compromise and treatment directed at the primary tumor. The removal of a malignant effusion by pericardiocentesis, with or without concomitant instillation of a sclerosing agent (e.g., tetracycline), or placement of a pericardial window for drainage to the pleural space may palliate symptoms and delay or prevent reaccumulation of the effusion.

CARDIAC EFFECTS OF CANCER THERAPY → *See Chap. 239.*

CARDIOVASCULAR MANIFESTATIONS OF SYSTEMIC DISEASES

DIABETES MELLITUS (See Chap. 334) There is an increased incidence of large vessel atherosclerosis and myocardial infarction in patients with insulin- and non-insulin-dependent diabetes mellitus. Coronary artery disease is the most common cause of death in adults with diabetes mellitus. Diabetes mellitus is an independent risk factor for coronary artery disease, and the incidence of coronary artery disease is related to the duration of diabetes. In patients with diabetes mellitus, myocardial infarctions are not only more frequent but also tend to be larger in size and more likely to result in complications such as heart failure, shock, and death. Diabetic patients are more likely to have an abnormal or absent pain response to myocardial ischemia, probably as a result of generalized autonomic nervous system dysfunction. Ambulatory electrocardiographic monitoring has shown that up to 90 percent of the episodes of ischemia are silent in diabetic patients with coronary artery disease; the presentation of ischemia may be exertional or episodic dyspnea, flash pulmonary edema, arrhythmias, heart block, or syncope. Because coronary artery disease is more common in diabetics and often is not associated with typical anginal symptoms, the threshold for the diagnosis should be low, particularly when the duration of disease is long and other risk factors for coronary artery disease (e.g., hypertension, smoking, hyperlipidemia) are present. In such patients, exercise testing should be used to detect ischemia and to determine the need for cardiac catheterization and therapeutic interventions.

Diabetic patients may also have myocardial dysfunction characteristic of a restrictive cardiomyopathy in the absence of large-vessel coronary artery disease, with abnormal relaxation of the myocardium, and evidenced clinically by elevated left ventricular filling pressures. Histologically, these patients have interstitial fibrosis with increased amounts of collagen, glycoprotein, triglycerides, and cholesterol in the myocardial interstitium, and in some cases intimal thickening, hyaline deposition, and inflammatory changes have been observed in small intramural arteries. Diabetic patients have an increased risk of developing clinical heart failure, even after correction for the presence of coronary artery disease, hypertension, and obesity, and it is likely that diabetic cardiomyopathy contributes to excessive cardiovascular morbidity and mortality of these patients. There is some evidence that insulin therapy results in an amelioration of the myocardial dysfunction.

MALNUTRITION AND THIAMINE DEFICIENCY (BERIBERI) Malnutrition (See Chap. 74)   In patients whose intake of protein, calories, or both is severely deficient, the heart may become thin, pale, and flabby with myofibrillar atrophy and interstitial edema. The systolic pressure and cardiac output are low and the pulse pressure narrow. Generalized edema is common and is due to a combination of factors, including reduced serum oncotic pressure and myocardial dysfunction. Such profound states of malnutrition, termed *marasmus* in the case of caloric deficiency or *kwashiorkor* in the case of relative protein deficiency, are most common in underdeveloped countries. However, significant nutritional heart disease may also occur in developed nations, particularly in patients with chronic diseases such as AIDS, in the semistarvation that can occur in anorexia nervosa, or in patients with severe cardiac failure in whom gastrointestinal hypoperfusion and venous congestion may cause anorexia and malabsorption. Open-heart surgery poses an increased risk in such patients, who may benefit from preoperative intensive hyperalimentation. Deficient nutrients and minerals should be replaced gradually since rapid expansion of the intravascular space may stress the weakened heart and result in overt congestive heart failure.

Thiamine Deficiency (See Chap. 79)   In many cases, malnutrition is accompanied by thiamine deficiency, although this hypovitaminosis may also occur in the presence of an adequate protein and caloric intake, particularly in the Far East, where polished rice deficient in thiamine may be a major dietary component. Because of the widespread use of thiamine-enriched flour in western nations, this disease is seen primarily in alcoholics and food faddists. However, there is evidence that patients with chronic heart failure frequently have thiamine deficiency also, which can be quantified biochemically by the measurement of the erythrocyte thiamine-pyrophosphate effect (TPPE). A high TPPE, which indicates thiamine deficiency, has been found in 20 to 90 percent of patients with chronic heart failure. The basis for thiamine deficiency in these patients appears to be related to both reduced dietary intake and a diuretic-induced increase in the urinary excretion of thiamine. The acute administration of thiamine to such patients increases the left ventricular ejection fraction and the excretion of salt and water.

Clinically, there is usually evidence of generalized malnutrition, peripheral neuropathy, glossitis, and anemia. The characteristic cardiovascular syndrome is that of high-output heart failure with tachycardia, increased cardiac output, and often elevated filling pressures in the left and right sides of the heart. The major cause of the high-output state is vasomotor depression, the precise mechanism of which is not understood but which leads to a reduced systemic vascular resistance. The cardiac examination reveals a wide pulse pressure, tachycardia, a third heart sound, and, frequently, an apical systolic murmur. The electrocardiogram may show decreased voltage, a prolonged QT interval, and T-wave abnormalities; the chest x-ray generally shows a large heart with signs of congestive heart failure. The response to thiamine is often dramatic, with an increase in systemic vascular resistance, decrease in cardiac output, clearing of pulmonary congestion, and a reduction in heart size often occurring in 12 to 48 h. Although the response to digitalis and diuretics may be poor prior to thiamine therapy, these agents may be important *after* thiamine is given, since the left ventricle may not be capable of dealing with the increased workload presented by the return of vascular tone.

OBESITY (See Chap. 75)   Although not defined as a disease per se, severe obesity, particularly when it occurs in an upper-body distribution, is associated with an increase in cardiovascular morbidity and mortality, due in part to hypertension, glucose intolerance, and atherosclerotic coronary artery disease, all of which are more prevalent in obese patients. In addition, these patients have a distinct abnormality of the cardiovascular system characterized by increases in total and central blood volumes, cardiac output, and left ventricular filling pressure. It appears that cardiac output is elevated in order to help supply the metabolic needs of the excessive adipose tissue. Left ventricular filling pressure is often at the upper limits of normal and rises excessively with exercise. As a result of chronic volume overload, eccentric cardiac hypertrophy with cardiac dilatation and abnormal ventricular function may develop. Pathologically, there are left and, in some cases, right ventricular hypertrophy and generalized cardiac dilatation, which is not due simply to fatty infiltration of the myocardium. Although these patients may develop pulmonary congestion, peripheral edema, and exercise intolerance, these findings may be difficult to recognize in massively obese patients. Weight reduction is the most effective therapy and results in reduction in blood volume and in the return of cardiac output toward normal. However, rapid weight reduction may cause cardiac arrhythmias and sudden death due to electrolyte imbalance. Digitalis, sodium restriction, and diuretics may also be useful. This form of heart disease should be distinguished from the Pickwickian syndrome (Chap. 263), which may share several of the cardiovascular features but, in addition, frequently has components of central apnea, hypoxemia, pulmonary hypertension, and cor pulmonale.

THYROID DISEASE (See Chap. 331)   Thyroid hormone exerts a major influence on the cardiovascular system by a number of direct and indirect mechanisms, and not surprisingly, cardiovascular effects are prominent in both hypo- and hyperthyroidism. Thyroid hormone causes increases in total-body metabolism and oxygen consumption that indirectly place an increased workload on the heart. In addition, although the exact mechanism has not been defined, thyroid hormone exerts direct inotropic, chronotropic, and dromotropic effects that are similar to those seen with adrenergic stimulation (e.g., tachycardia, increased cardiac output). It has been shown that thyroid hormone increases the synthesis of myosin and of Na^+,K^+-ATPase, as well as the density of myocardial beta-adrenergic receptors.

Hyperthyroidism   Patients may present with palpitations, systolic hypertension, fatigue, or, in patients with underlying heart disease, angina or heart failure. Sinus tachycardia is found in about 40 percent of patients, and atrial fibrillation in about 15 percent. Other findings include a hyperactive precordium, a widened pulse pressure, an increase in the intensity of the first heart sound and the pulmonic component of the second heart sound, and a third heart sound. An increased incidence of mitral valve prolapse has been associated with hyperthyroidism, and in some cases there may be a midsystolic murmur heard best at the left sternal border with or without a systolic ejection click. A systolic scratchy sound, the *Means-Lerman scratch*, may occasionally be heard at the left second intercostal space during expiration and is thought to result from the rubbing of the hyperdynamic pericardium against the pleura. Elderly patients with hyperthyroidism, so-called apathetic hyperthyroidism, may present with only the cardiovascular manifestations of thyrotoxicosis, such as atrial fibrillation, which may be resistant to therapy until the hyperthyroidism is controlled. Angina pectoris and congestive heart failure are unusual unless there is coexistent underlying heart disease, and in many cases will resolve with therapy of the hyperthyroidism.

Hypothyroidism   There is a reduction in cardiac output, stroke volume, heart rate, blood pressure, and pulse pressure. In about one-third of patients there is a pericardial effusion which only rarely results in tamponade. Increased capillary permeability results in pleural and pericardial effusions. Other clinical signs include cardiomegaly, bradycardia, weak arterial pulses, and distant heart sounds. Although the signs and symptoms of myxedema may suggest the diagnosis of congestive heart failure, in the absence of other cardiac disease, myocardial failure is uncommon. The electrocardiogram generally shows sinus bradycardia and low voltage and may show prolongation of the QT interval, decreased P-wave voltage, prolonged AV conduction time, intraventricular conduction disturbances, and nonspecific ST-T-wave abnormalities. Chest x-ray may show cardiomegaly, often with a "water bottle" configuration, pleural effusions, and, in some cases, evidence of congestive heart failure. Pathologically, the heart is pale, dilated, and flabby, often with myofibrillar swelling, loss of striations, and interstitial fibrosis.

Patients with hypothyroidism frequently have elevations of cholesterol and triglycerides and severe atherosclerotic coronary artery disease. Prior to treatment with thyroid hormone, patients with hypothyroidism frequently do not have angina pectoris, presumably because of the low metabolic demands made by their condition. However, such patients, especially when elderly, are prone to angina and myocardial infarction during replacement of thyroid hormone, and this should always be done with care, starting with very low doses which are increased gradually.

MALIGNANT CARCINOID (See Chap. 95) These tumors elaborate a variety of vasoactive amines (e.g., serotonin), kinins, indoles, and other substances believed to be responsible for the diarrhea, flushing, and labile blood pressure seen in these patients. The cardiac lesions due to gastrointestinal carcinoids are almost exclusively in the right side of the heart and occur only when there are hepatic metastases, suggesting that the substance responsible for the cardiac lesions is inactivated by passage through the liver and lungs. Similar lesions occur in the left side of the heart when there is a right-to-left shunt or the tumor is located in the lungs. Fibrous plaques are found on the endothelium of the cardiac chambers, valves, and great vessels. These plaques, which result in distortion of the cardiac valves, consist of smooth-muscle cells embedded in a stroma of acid mucopolysaccharide and collagen and presumably result from healing of endothelial injury. The clinical syndrome is most often that of tricuspid regurgitation, pulmonic stenosis, or both. In some cases a high-output state may occur, presumably as a result of a decrease in systemic vascular resistance due to a vasoactive substance released by the tumor. Progression of the cardiac lesions does not appear to be affected by treatment with serotonin antagonists, and in some severely symptomatic patients valve replacement is indicated. Coronary artery spasm, presumably due to a circulating vasoactive substance, may occur in patients with carcinoid syndrome.

PHEOCHROMOCYTOMA (See Chap. 333) In addition to causing hypertension, which may be labile or sustained, the high circulating levels of catecholamines may also cause direct myocardial injury. Focal myocardial necrosis and inflammatory cell infiltration are seen in about 50 percent of patients who die with pheochromocytoma and may contribute to clinically significant left ventricular failure and pulmonary edema. Left ventricular function and congestive heart failure may resolve after removal of the tumor. In addition, hypertension results in left ventricular hypertrophy.

RHEUMATOID ARTHRITIS AND THE COLLAGEN VASCULAR DISEASES Rheumatoid Arthritis (See Chap. 313) There may be inflammation of any or all parts of the heart in patients with rheumatoid arthritis. *Pericarditis* is the most common cause of clinically apparent disease and may be found by echocardiography in 10 to 50 percent of all patients with rheumatoid arthritis, particularly those with subcutaneous nodules. However, only a small fraction of these patients have clinical evidence of pericarditis, which usually follows a benign course but occasionally may progress to cardiac tamponade or constrictive pericarditis. The pericardial fluid is generally an exudate, with decreased concentrations of complement and glucose and elevated cholesterol. Treatment is directed at the underlying rheumatoid arthritis and may include glucocorticoids. Pericardiectomy is usually required in cases of tamponade or persistent effusion. *Coronary arteritis* with intimal inflammation and edema is present in about 20 percent of cases but only rarely results in angina pectoris or myocardial infarction. The cardiac valves, most often the mitral and aortic, may be involved by inflammation and granuloma

formation that in some cases may cause clinically significant regurgitation due to valve deformity. Myocarditis rarely results in cardiac dysfunction.

Seronegative Arthropathies The seronegative arthropathies (Chaps. 317 and 325), ankylosing spondylitis, Reiter's syndrome, psoriatic arthritis, and the arthritides associated with ulcerative colitis and regional enteritis may be accompanied by a pancarditis and proximal aortitis; the latter may result in aortic regurgitation and may extend into the anterior mitral valve ring and/or AV node. Conduction disturbances are common, occurring in up to one-third of patients; they are more common in patients with aortic valve disease and appear to be associated with the presence of the HLA-B27 antigen. Both aortic regurgitation and AV block are more common in patients with peripheral joint involvement and long-standing disease; treatment with aortic valve replacement and permanent pacemaker placement may be required. Up to one-fifth of patients with peripheral joint involvement and disease for more than 30 years have significant aortic regurgitation. Occasionally, aortic regurgitation precedes the onset of arthritis, and, therefore, the diagnosis of a seronegative arthritis should be considered in young males with isolated aortic regurgitation.

Systemic Lupus Erythematosus (SLE) (See Chap. 312) Pericarditis is common, occurring in about two-thirds of patients, and generally pursues a benign course, although rarely tamponade or constriction may result. The characteristic *endocardial lesions* of SLE, described by Libman and Sacks, consist of wartlike lesions most often located at the angles of the AV valves or on the ventricular surface of the mitral valve. Hemodynamically important valvular regurgitation is rare. Patients with the antiphospholipid syndrome have a higher incidence of cardiovascular abnormalities including valvular disease (particularly regurgitant lesions), a variety of thrombotic disorders (venous and arterial thrombosis, thrombocytopenia, premature stroke), myocardial infarction, pulmonary hypertension, and cardiomyopathy. Myocarditis generally parallels the activity of the disease, and although common histologically, seldom results in clinical heart failure unless associated with hypertension. Although arteritis of large coronary arteries may rarely result in myocardial ischemia, there is also an increased frequency of coronary atherosclerosis that may be related to hypertension or glucocorticoid therapy.

TRAUMATIC HEART DISEASE

Cardiac damage may be due to both penetrating and nonpenetrating injuries. The most frequent cause of a *nonpenetrating injury* is impact of the chest against the steering wheel of an automobile. Serious injury of the heart may ensue even though no external sign of thoracic trauma is evident. Although the commonest injury is myocardial contusion, any structure of the heart may be affected by the trauma. If the valvular apparatus is ruptured, a loud heart murmur produced by valvular regurgitation may appear, followed by the development of rapidly progressive heart failure.

Myocardial contusion may cause arrhythmias, bundle branch block, or electrocardiographic abnormalities resembling those of infarction, and so it is important to bear trauma in mind as a cause of otherwise unexplained electrocardiographic changes. Similarly, myocardial contusion may produce positive radionuclide scans and regional impairment of ventricular function, as occurs in myocardial infarction (Chap. 243). Myocardial contusions are often not immediately appreciated. Increased serum creatine kinase (CK) MB levels may be seen in about 20 percent of patients, but false-positive MB elevations may be seen in the presence of massive injuries associated with large increases in total CK. Pericardial effusion may occur weeks or even months after the accident. In these cases, the pericardial effusion is a manifestation of the postcardiac injury syndrome, which resembles the postpericardiotomy syndrome (Chap. 240). The most serious consequence of nonpenetrating injury is rupture, either of the atria or of the ventricles. Although generally immediately fatal, survival of cardiac rupture has been reported in up to 40 percent of cases of patients who survived long enough to reach a specialized trauma center. Hemopericardium may also follow tearing of a pericardial vessel or coronary artery.

℞ TREATMENT

Acute myocardial failure resulting from rupture of a valve usually requires operative correction. The treatment of an uncomplicated myocardial contusion, with or without myocardial infarction, is similar to that for a myocardial infarction, except that anticoagulation is contraindicated, and should include monitoring for the development of complications such as arrhythmias and cardiac rupture (Chap. 243). Pericardial hemorrhage often leads to constriction, which must be treated by decortication.

Penetrating injuries of the heart, produced by bullets or stab wounds, usually result in immediate or very rapid death because of hemopericardium or massive hemorrhage. However, up to half of such patients may survive if they are resuscitated and/or survive long enough to reach a specialized trauma center. Another common cause of penetrating injuries is the fracture or dislodgment of an intravenous or intracardiac catheter or pacemaker lead. Immediate thoracotomy should be carried out if there is cardiac tamponade and/or shock, whether the trauma was penetrating or nonpenetrating. Pericardiocentesis may be helpful in patients with tamponade, but usually only as a holding maneuver. Patients who suffer penetrating injuries of the heart should be carefully examined several weeks after the event to rule out a ventricular septal defect or mitral regurgitation that may have gone undetected at the time of emergency surgery. Sometimes the patient survives the acute incident and presents with a cardiac murmur and congestive heart failure. A left-to-right shunt due to traumatic ventricular septal defect, aortopulmonary artery fistula, or coronary arteriovenous fistula may be suspected and confirmed by cardiac catheterization and angiocardiography. Operation is indicated if hemodynamically significant abnormalities are present or if a foreign body, e.g., a bullet, is lodged in the heart.

Rupture of the aorta is a common consequence of chest trauma. Indeed, rupture of the aorta at the isthmus or just above the aortic valve is the most common vascular deceleration injury. The clinical presentation is similar to that in aortic dissection (Chap. 247). The arterial pressure and pulse amplitude may be increased in the upper extremities and decreased in the lower extremities, and on chest roentgenogram there may be widening of the mediastinum. Occasionally, the rupture is limited by the aortic adventitia and results in a silent false aneurysm that may be discovered months or years after the injury. When great vessel rupture is due to a penetrating injury, there is usually a hemothorax and, less often, a hemopericardium. Hematoma formation may compress major vessels, and arteriovenous fistulae may be formed, sometimes resulting in high-output congestive heart failure.

BIBLIOGRAPHY

COBLYN JS, WEINBLATT M: Rheumatic diseases and the heart, in *Heart Disease*, 5th ed, E Braunwald (ed). Philadelphia, Saunders, 1997, p 1776

COHN PR, BRAUNWALD E: Traumatic heart disease, in *Heart Disease*, 5th ed, E Braunwald (ed). Philadelphia, Saunders, 1997, p 1535

COLUCCI WS, BRAUNWALD E: Primary tumors of the heart, in *Heart Disease*, 5th ed, E Braunwald (ed). Philadelphia, Saunders, 1997, p 394

DUFLOU J et al: Sudden death as a result of heart disease in morbid obesity. Am Heart J 130:306, 1995

HENDERSON VJ et al: Cardiac injuries: Analysis of an unselected series of 251 cases. J Trauma 36:341, 1994

IMPERATO-MCGINLEY J et al: Reversibility of catecholamine-induced cardiomyopathy in a child with a pheochromocytoma. N Engl J Med 316:793, 1987

KOISTINEN MJ et al: Asymptomatic coronary artery disease in diabetes: Relation to common risk factors, lipoproteins, apoproteins and apo E polymorphism. Acta Diabetol 31:210, 1994

LADENSON PW: Recognition and management of cardiovascular disease related to thyroid dysfunction. Am J Med 88:638, 1990

O'NEILL TW et al: The heart in ankylosing spondylitis. Ann Rheum Dis 51:705, 1992

REYNEN K: Cardiac myxomas. N Engl J Med 333:1610, 1995

ROBIOLIO PA: Carcinoid heart disease. Correlation of high serotonin levels with valvular abnormalities detected by cardiac catheterization and echocardiography. Circulation 92:790, 1995

ROLDAN C et al: Systemic lupus erythematosus valve disease by transesophageal echocardiography and the role of antiphospholipid antibodies. J Am Coll Cardiol 20:1127, 1992

SHAHIAN DM et al: Etiology and management of chronic valve disease in antiphospholipid antibody syndrome and systemic lupus erythematosus. J Card Surg 10:133, 1995

SHIMON I et al: Improved left ventricular function after thiamine supplementation in patients with congestive heart failure receiving long-term furosemide therapy. Am J Med 98:485, 1995

SMITH MK: Transesophageal echocardiography in the diagnosis of rupture of the aorta. N Engl J Med 332:356, 1995

UUSITUPA MI et al: Diabetic heart muscle disease. Ann Med 22:377, 1990

SECTION 4
VASCULAR DISEASE

---

242 *Peter Libby*

ATHEROSCLEROSIS

Atherosclerosis leads as a cause of death and disability in the developed world. The name, derived from Greek, refers to the thickening of the arterial intima (*sclerosis*, "hardening") and accumulation of lipid (*athere*, "gruel") that characterize the typical lesion. Despite our familiarity with this disease, some of its fundamental characteristics remain poorly recognized and understood. Although many generalized or systemic risk factors predispose to its development, this disease preferentially affects certain regions of the circulation. Atherosclerosis causes distinct clinical manifestations depending on the circulatory bed affected and the characteristics of individual lesions, which may be quite heterogeneous. Atherosclerosis of the coronary arteries commonly causes angina pectoris and myocardial infarction (Chaps. 243 and 244). Atherosclerosis of the arteries supplying the central nervous system frequently provokes transient cerebral ischemia and strokes (Chap. 366). In the peripheral circulation, atherosclerosis can cause intermittent claudication and gangrene and can jeopardize limb viability (Chap. 248). Involvement of the splanchnic circulation can cause mesenteric ischemia and bowel infarction. Atherosclerosis can affect the kidney directly (e.g., causing renal artery stenosis), and, in addition, the kidney is a frequent site of atheroembolic disease. Renal artery atherosclerosis can also contribute to the pathogenesis of hypertension, itself a risk factor for the development of atherosclerosis (Chap. 277).

Even in a given arterial bed, atherosclerosis tends to occur focally, typically in certain predisposed regions, while sparing adjacent segments. For example, in the coronary circulation, the proximal left anterior descending coronary artery has a particular predilection for developing atherosclerotic occlusive disease. Likewise, atherosclerosis preferentially affects the proximal portions of the renal arteries, and, in the cerebrovascular circulation, the carotid bifurcation. Other arteries, such as the internal mammary arteries, seldom harbor atherosclerotic lesions, even though they are close to commonly affected vessels and are similar to them structurally. Atherosclerotic lesions often form at branch points of arteries, which are regions of disturbed blood flow, suggesting that local fluid dynamic factors may contribute to the focal distribution of lesions.

Atherosclerosis develops focally in time as well as in space. Atherogenesis in humans typically occurs over many years, usually many decades. However, the growth of atherosclerotic plaques probably is discontinuous rather than smoothly linear, with periods of relative quiescence punctuated by episodes of rapid evolution. After a generally prolonged "silent" period, atherosclerosis may become clinically manifest. The clinical expressions of atherosclerosis may be chronic, as in the development of stable effort-induced angina pectoris or predictable and reproducible intermittent claudication. Alternatively, a much more dramatic acute clinical event, such as a myocardial infarction or cerebrovascular accident, may be the first manifestation of atherosclerosis. Other individuals never experience clinical manifestations of arterial disease, even though the presence of widespread atherosclerosis is demonstrated post mortem. Recently, understanding of the reasons why this disease can be stable, unstable, or clinically silent has advanced, as will be discussed below.

The way in which atherosclerosis affects an arterial segment also varies, an additional feature of the heterogeneity and complexity of this disease. Atheromas are usually thought of as stenotic lesions, causing flow limitation or arterial occlusion. However, atherosclerosis can also cause ectasia and development of aneurysmal disease with an increase in lumen caliber. This expression of atherosclerosis frequently occurs in the aorta, creating a predisposition to rupture or dissection rather than to stenosis or occlusion.

The heterogeneity of this disease and the diversity of its causes, natural histories, and clinical manifestations seem difficult to explain. However, contemporary research provides some fundamental pathobiologic principles that provide a basis for understanding this multifaceted process. To furnish a background for a clinical approach to patients with atherosclerotic disease, this chapter will consider the phases in the formation, progression, and complication of lesions. In particular, the chapter will emphasize emerging aspects of the biology of atherosclerosis that provide insight into its pathogenesis, in relation to the prevention or limitation of atherosclerosis and therapies for reducing its manifestations.

INITIATION OF ATHEROSCLEROSIS   Lipoprotein Accumulation and Modification   In normal human adults, the intimal layer of arteries contains some resident smooth muscle cells embedded in extracellular matrix and is covered with a monolayer of vascular endothelial cells (Fig. 242-1A). Taken together, experimental results in animals and studies of human atherosclerosis suggest that the "fatty streak" represents the initial lesion of atherosclerosis. The formation of these early lesions probably results from focal accumulation of lipoproteins in regions of the intimal layer of the artery (Fig. 242-2B). Lipoprotein particles transport lipids such as cholesterol and triglycerides in association with proteins and phospholipids that render the lipids soluble in blood. Low-density lipoprotein (LDL) particles, rich in cholesterol, are an example of an atherogenic lipoprotein (see Chap. 341). The accumulation of lipoprotein particles in the arterial intima during early atherogenesis may not result simply from an increase in the permeability or leakiness of the overlying endothelium. Rather, these lipoproteins may collect in the intima of arteries because they bind to constituents of the extracellular matrix, which increases their residence time in the arterial wall. Lipoproteins that accumulate in the extracellular space of the arterial intima often associate with proteoglycan molecules of the arterial extracellular matrix. At sites of lesion formation, the balance of different matrix constituents may vary in important ways. For example, of the three major classes of proteoglycans, a relative excess of heparan sulfate molecules in relation to keratan sulfate or chondroitin sulfate may promote the retention of lipoprotein particles by binding them and slowing their egress from nascent lesions.

Lipoprotein particles in the extracellular space of the intima, particularly those bound to matrix macromolecules, may undergo chemical modifications. Accumulating evidence supports a potentially pathogenic role for such modifications in atherogenesis. Two types of alterations are of particular interest in relation to how risk factors promote atherogenesis: oxidation and nonenzymatic glycation. Lipoproteins

FIGURE 242-1   Fatty Streak Formation. *A.* The normal artery. The normal artery consists of three layers. The intima, lined by a monolayer of endothelial cells in contact with the blood, contains smooth muscle cells embedded in extracellular matrix. The internal elastic lamina forms the border of the intima with the underlying tunica media. The media contains layers of smooth muscle cells invested with a collagen- and elastin-rich extracellular matrix. Elastic arteries such as the aorta contain concentric lamellae of smooth muscle cells sandwiched between dense bands of elastin. Muscular arteries have a looser organization of smooth muscle cells dispersed within the matrix. The external elastic lamina forms the border of the media with the adventitia. The adventitia contains nerves, some mast cells, and is the origin of the vasa vasorum which supply blood to the outer two-thirds of the tunica media. *B.* Accumulation of lipoprotein particles. Lipoprotein particles can accumulate in the intima of arteries, particularly when the ambient concentration is increased by hypercholesterolemic states. The lipoprotein particles often associate with constituents of the extracellular matrix, notably proteoglycans. Sequestration within the intima separates lipoproteins from some plasma antioxidants and can favor oxidative modification. Such modified lipoprotein particles may trigger a local inflammatory response responsible for signaling subsequent steps in lesion formation. *C.* Adhesion of leukocytes. In hypercholesterolemia, adhesion of mononuclear leukocytes to the luminal endothelium occurs early. The augmented expression of various adhesion molecules for leukocytes probably triggers this first step in the recruitment of white blood cells to the site of a nascent arterial lesion. *D.* Penetration of leukocytes. Once adherent, some white blood cells migrate into the intima. The directed migration of leukocytes probably depends on chemoattractant factors, including modified lipoprotein particles themselves and chemoattractant cytokines such as the chemokine macrophage chemoattractant protein 1 (MCP-1) produced by vascular wall cells in response to modified lipoproteins. *E.* Accumulation of leukocytes. Leukocytes resident in the evolving fatty streak can divide and exhibit augmented expression of receptors for modified lipoproteins (scavenger receptors). These mononuclear phagocytes imbibe lipids and transform into foam cells, whose cytoplasm is filled with lipid droplets. *F.* Formation of the fibrous cap and lipid core. As the fatty streak evolves into a more complicated atherosclerotic lesion, smooth muscle cells accumulate in the expanding intima and the amount of extracellular matrix increases. The fibrous cap, formed of extracellular matrix elaborated by the smooth muscle cells in the intima, characteristically overlies a lipid-rich core filled with macrophages. In addition to dividing, these core cells may die, releasing their lipid contents into the extracellular space.

Smooth
muscle
cells

Monocytes

T-lymphocyte

Macrophage

FIGURE 242-2 Plaque Rupture, Thrombosis, and Healing. *A.* Arterial remodeling during atherogenesis. During the first part of their history, atheromas often grow in an abluminal direction and do not encroach on the lumen. The compensatory enlargement of the artery in this phase accounts in part for the tendency of coronary arteriography to underestimate the degree of atherosclerosis. *B.* Focal inflammation characterizes unstable atherosclerotic plaques. Foci of inflammation often occur in atheromas. Analyses of lesions that have ruptured and caused fatal myocardial infarction characteristically show a prominent infiltration of macrophages and T lymphocytes. Both the leukocytes and the intrinsic vascular cells around points of plaque rupture show markers of inflammatory activation. *C.* Rupture of the plaque's fibrous cap causes thrombosis. A physical disruption of the atherosclerotic plaque (*c*) commonly causes arterial thrombosis by allowing blood coagulant factors to contact the thrombogenic collagen in the arterial extracellular matrix and tissue factors produced by macrophage-derived foam cells in the lipid core of the lesion. A site of plaque rupture thus serves as a nidus for thrombus formation. The normal artery wall has several fibrinolytic and antithrombotic mechanisms that tend to resist thrombosis and lyse clots that begin to form in situ. Such antithrombotic or thrombolytic molecules include thrombomodulin, tissue and urokinase-type plasminogen activators, heparan sulfate proteoglycans, prostacyclin, and nitric oxide. These mechanisms may prevail, or they may be overwhelmed, allowing the clot to propagate (as in *E*). *D.* Healing of a mural thrombus leads to lesion fibrosis and progression and luminal narrowing. Instances of thrombosis in which the thrombus undergoes lysis or is organized into a mural thrombus without occluding the vessel instances may be clinically silent. The subsequent thrombin-induced fibrosis and healing cause a fibroproliferative response that can lead to a more fibrous lesion. Specifically, local thrombin activation can stimulate smooth muscle proliferation. Proteins released from platelets, including platelet-derived growth factors and transforming growth factor β, may also augment collagen production by smooth muscle cells and modulate their growth. Thus, healing may can promote lesion fibrosis and luminal encroachment. Interestingly, such a sequence of events may convert an unstable atheroma with a thin, rupture-prone fibrous cap into a more stable fibrous plaque with a reinforced cap. Angioplasty of unstable coronary lesions may stabilize the lesions by a similar mechanisms. *E.* Plaque rupture with a propagated, occlusive thrombus can cause acute myocardial infarction. When a persistent, occlusive thrombus forms in a coronary artery, the consequences depend on the degree of existing collateral circulation. In a patient with chronic multivessel occlusive coronary artery disease, collateral channels have usually formed. In such circumstances, even a total arterial occlusion may cause no myocardial infarction or may cause an unexpectedly modest or "non-Q-wave" infarct. In the patient with less advanced disease who lacks substantial stenotic lesions, sudden plaque rupture and arterial occlusion commonly produce Q wave infarction.

sequestered from plasma antioxidants in the extracellular space of the intima may be particularly susceptible to oxidative modification. Oxidatively modified LDL, rather than being chemically homogenous, actually comprises a variable and incompletely defined mixture. Both the lipid and the protein moieties of these particles can participate in oxidative processes. Modifications of the lipids may include formation of hydroperoxides, lysophospholipids, oxysterols, and aldehydic breakdown products of fatty acids. Modifications of the apoprotein moieties may include breaks in the peptide backbone as well as derivatization of certain amino acid residues (typically the side chain amino group of lysine) with components of the oxidized lipids (9-hydroxynonenol or malondialdehyde). Considerable evidence supports the presence of such chemical entities in atherosclerotic lesions. In diabetics with sustained hyperglycemia, nonenzymatic glycation of apolipoproteins and other arterial proteins likely occurs and may likewise alter the function of these components and their propensity to accelerate atherogenesis. A good deal of experimental work suggests that both oxidatively modified and glycated lipoproteins or lipoprotein constituents can contribute to many of the subsequent cellular events of lesion development.

Leukocyte Recruitment and Foam-Cell Formation Recruitment of leukocytes is the second step in formation of the fatty streak (Fig. 242-1*C*). The main white blood cell types typically found in the evolving atheroma are cells of the mononuclear lineage—monocytes and lymphocytes. A number of adhesion molecules or receptors for leukocytes expressed on the surface of arterial endothelial cells likely participate in the recruitment of leukocytes to the nascent fatty streak. Adhesion molecules of particular interest in this regard include vascular cell adhesion molecule 1 (VCAM-1) and intercellular adhesion molecule 1 (ICAM-1) (members of the immunoglobulin superfamity) and P-selectin (a member of a distinct family of leukocyte receptors known as selectins). Lysophosphatidylcholine, a constituent of oxidatively modified LDL, can augment the expression of VCAM-1. This example illustrates how the accumulation of lipoproteins in the arterial intima may be linked to leukocyte recruitment and subsequent events in lesion formation.

Laminar shear forces, such as those present in most regions of normal arteries, can suppress the expression of leukocyte adhesion molecules such as VCAM-1. Sites where atherosclerotic lesions commonly form (e.g., branch points) often have disturbed laminar flow. Also, the laminar shear of normal blood flow augments the production by endothelial cells of nitric oxide (NO). In addition to its well-known vasodilator properties, this molecule, at the low levels constitutively produced by arterial endothelium, can act as a local anti-inflammatory autacoid, for example acting to limit local VCAM-1 expression. Thus, the normal endothelium, by secreting NO at a steady low level, can maintain vasodilation and resist the adhesion of leukocytes. Local disturbances in hemodynamic forces may influence such cellular mechanisms that protect against atherosclerotic lesion initiation and may help explain the focal distribution of atherosclerotic lesions.

Having adhered to the surface of the arterial endothelial cell by interacting with a receptor such as VCAM-1, the monocytes and lymphocytes penetrate the endothelial layer and take up residence in the intima (Fig. 242-1*D*). In addition to constituents of modified lipoproteins, cytokines (a class of protein mediators of inflammation) can regulate the expression of adhesion molecules involved in leukocyte recruitment. For example the cytokines interleukin (IL) 1 and tumor necrosis factor-α (TNFα) induce or augment the expression of VCAM-1 and ICAM-1 on endothelial cells. Since modified lipoproteins can induce cytokine release from vascular wall cells, this pathway may provide an additional link between the accumulation and modification of lipoproteins and leukocyte recruitment. The directed migration of leukocytes into the arterial wall may also result from the actions of modified lipoprotein. For example, in vitro assays suggest that oxidized LDL promotes the chemotaxis of leukocytes. Also, oxidatively modified lipoproteins can elicit the production by vascular wall cells of chemoattractant cytokines such as monocyte chemoattractant protein 1 (MCP-1).

Once resident in the intima, the mononuclear phagocytes differentiate into macrophages, which ultimately become lipid-laden foam cells (Fig. 242-1*E*–*F*). The transformation of mononuclear phagocytes into foam cells requires the uptake of lipoprotein particles by receptor-mediated endocytosis. One might suppose that the well-recognized LDL receptor would mediate this uptake. However, patients and animals that lack effective LDL receptors for genetic reasons (e.g., familial hypercholesterolemia) have abundant arterial lesions and extraarterial xanthomata rich in macrophage-derived foam cells. Also, exogenous cholesterol suppresses expression of the LDL receptor, so that under conditions of hypercholesterolemia the level of this receptor decreases. Alternative candidates for receptors that mediate the lipid loading of foam cells include the macrophage scavenger receptor that preferentially endocytose modified lipoproteins and other receptors for oxidized LDL or for beta very low density lipoprotein (VLDL), a type of lipoprotein abundant in certain hypercholesterolemic states (see Chap. 341). By imbibing lipids from the extracellular space, the mononuclear phagocytes may participate in clearing the lipoproteins accumulating in the developing lesion. Some lipid-laden macrophages may leave the artery wall, functioning to clear lipid from the artery. Lipid accumulation, and hence a tendency to form an atheroma, occurs if more lipid enters the artery wall than leaves it via mononuclear phagocytes or other pathways. Macrophages thus may play a vital role in the balance of lipid metabolism in the arterial wall during atherogenesis. Some foam cells in the expanding intimal lesion perish, perhaps by apoptosis (programmed cell death) and/or other means. The death of mononuclear phagocytes results in the formation of a lipid-rich *necrotic core* in the lesion, a feature characteristic of more complicated atherosclerotic plaques (Figs. 242-1*F* and 242-2*A*).

Like the vascular wall cells, macrophages taking up modified lipoproteins may produce cytokines and growth factors that elicit some of the further cellular events in lesion complication. A number of growth factors or cytokines elaborated by mononuclear phagocytes can stimulate smooth muscle cell proliferation and the production of extracellular matrix, which accumulates in atherosclerotic plaques. IL-1 and TNF-α are examples of cytokines that can induce local production of growth factors, incuding forms of platelet-derived growth factor and fibroblast growth factor, which may play a role in plaque evolution and complication. Other cytokines, particularly interferon γ derived from activated T cell lesions, can inhibit smooth muscle proliferation and the synthesis of interstitial forms of collagen. These examples illustrate how atherogenesis likely depends on a complex balance between mediators that can promote lesion formation and other pathways that can mitigate it.

Factors That Modulate Atheroma Initiation Elaboration of small molecules by activated mononuclear phagocytes and vascular wall cells in the evolving lesion may also modulate atherogenesis. Phagocytic leukocytes (as well as vascular endothelial and smooth muscle cells) can produce reactive oxygen species when appropriately stimulated. Such reactive oxygen species can modulate the growth of smooth muscle cells, activate inflammatory gene expression via the nuclear factor κB transcriptional control system, and annihilate nitric oxide radicals, decreasing the effect of NO. However, macrophages in the lesion may be activated to express the inducible form of the enzyme that synthesizes NO, known as inducible NO synthase. This high-capacity form of the enzyme can produce relatively large, potentially cytotoxic amounts of nitric oxide radicals. While the low concentrations of NO· produced by the constitutive NO synthase in endothelial cells may have beneficial effects, the higher levels produced by activated phagocytes may be deleterious.

Export by phagocytes may be one response to local lipid overload in the evolving lesion. Another mechanism—reverse cholesterol transport mediated by high-density lipoprotein (HDL)—may provide an independent pathway for removal of lipid from the atheroma. Multiple

observational studies have established a tight inverse relationship between the level of HDL cholesterol and the risk of coronary events. A higher level of HDL may explain in part why premenopausal women have less atherosclerosis than age-matched males. In various in vitro models, HDL can mediate net cholesterol removal from lipid-laden macrophages. Such reverse cholesterol transport may occur during human atherogenesis and may help to explain the protective effect against lesion formation provided by HDL.

Although clear evidence supports lipoprotein disorders as predisposing factors for atheroma formation, other etiologies may contribute to or modulate atherogenesis (Table 242-1). For example, hypertension is an independent risk factor for coronary events. Male gender and the postmenopausal state also augment the risk of developing coronary artery disease. As mentioned, premenopausal females have higher HDL levels than age-matched males. However, a favorable lipoprotein pattern only partially accounts for the protection against atherosclerosis conferred by the premenopausal state. Poorly understood direct effects of estrogens on the arterial wall may account for some of this benefit. Studies on the possible vasculoprotective effects of estrogen and the role of estrogen replacement therapy as an antiatherogenic strategy in postmenopausal women are in progress.

Diabetes mellitus accelerates atherogenesis. In addition to the well-known microvascular complications of diabetes, macrovascular disease such as atherosclerosis causes a great deal of excess mortality in the diabetic population (see Chap. 334). Diabetes-associated dyslipidemias strongly promote atherogenesis. In particular, the constellation of insulin resistance, high triglycerides, and low HDL, often accompanied by central adiposity and hypertension, that is common in type II diabetics seems to accelerate atherogenesis potently. As noted above, hyperglycemia may promote the nonenzymatic glycation of LDL. LDL modified in this manner, like oxidatively modified LDL, may signal many of the initial events in atherogenesis. Other lipoproteins, such as triglyceride-rich particles or lipoprotein (a), may also contribute to accelerated atherogenesis in diabetic individuals.

Lipoprotein (a) [Lp(a); it is often called "lipoprotein little a" to distinguish it from apolipoprotein AI] provides a potential link between hemostasis and blood lipids. The Lp(a) particle consists of an apoprotein (a) molecule bound by a sulfhydryl link to the apolipoprotein B moiety of an LDL particle. Apoprotein (a) has homology with plasminogen, and it may inhibit fibrinolysis by competing with plasminogen. Other risk factors for atherosclerosis related to blood clotting include elevated levels of fibrinogen or of plasminogen-activator inhibitor 1 (PAI-1), an inhibitor of fibrinolysis. Multiple studies have established a correlation between plasma fibrinogen levels and coronary risk. Synthesis of fibrinogen, an acute-phase reactant, increases in inflammatory states. Thus, hyperfibrinogenemia in patients with established atherosclerosis may be a secondary phenomenon but nonetheless may contribute to lesion evolution and thrombotic risk. Polymorphisms in the gene encoding PAI-1 may also correlate with manifestations of atherosclerosis. Yet another nonlipid risk factor for coronary events, elevated levels of homocysteine, may act by promoting thrombosis, although the pathophysiology of this association is uncertain.

The relationship between tobacco abuse and atherosclerosis also remains poorly understood. The rapid reduction in the risk of cardiac events that occurs after cessation of cigarette smoking implies that tobacco may promote thrombosis or some other determinant of plaque stability as well as the evolution of the atherosclerotic lesion itself. For example, tobacco smokers have elevated fibrinogen levels, a variable associated with increased atherosclerosis and acute cardiovascular events, as noted above. In other situations, antecedent inflammatory states may predispose to atherosclerosis. For example, the panarteritis caused by Kawasaki disease in childhood may promote development of vascular lesions in the arteries of adults (Chap. 319). Infectious agents continue to be proposed as instigators or potentiators of atherogenesis. Both viral and microbial pathogens have been invoked in this context (e.g., herpesviruses and *Chlamydia*). In some patients, immune or autoimmune reactions may contribute to atherogenesis. In the accelerated form of coronary arteriopathy that plagues heart transplant recipients (Chap. 234), immune factors may be important in pathogenesis. The roles of the immune response and of infectious diseases in usual atherosclerosis remain speculative.

Known genetic defects in lipoprotein metabolism account for only a fraction of the familial risk for coronary artery disease, so other genetic factors must also contribute. Mechanisms of disease susceptibility involving the arterial wall might account for some of the genetic predisposition to atherosclerosis not explained by lipoprotein disorders. Application of molecular genetic techniques should help to identify new polymorphisms linked to coronary risk and may eventually shed light on new pathophysiologic mechanisms.

ATHEROMA EVOLUTION AND COMPLICATION Involvement of Arterial Smooth Muscle Cells Although the fatty streak commonly precedes the development of a more advanced atherosclerotic plaque, not all fatty streaks progress to atheromas. Fatty streaks occur in populations not prone to late lesions (e.g., indigenous Africans). These findings raise several questions. Why do only some fatty streaks progress to fibrous lesions? By what mechanisms do fatty streaks evolve into more complex lesions? While accumulation of lipid-laden macrophages is the hallmark of the fatty streak, accumulation of fibrous tissue typifies the more advanced atherosclerotic lesion. The smooth muscle cell synthesizes most of the extracellular matrix of the complex atherosclerotic lesion. Thus, the arrival of smooth muscle cells and their elaboration of extracellular matrix is probably a critical transition, yielding a fibrofatty lesion in place of a simple accumulation of macrophage-derived foam cells.

Recent research has provided insight into the mechanisms that may trigger the migration and smooth muscle cells into the evolving intimal lesion, the proliferation of these cells in the lesion, and the accumulation of extracellular matrix. Cytokines and growth factors elicited by modified lipoproteins or other agents from both vascular wall cells and infiltrating leukocytes can modulate functions of the smooth muscle cell. For example, platelet-derived growth factors elaborated by activated endothelial cells can stimulate the migration of smooth muscle cells. This mechanism might induce smooth muscle cells resident in the tunica media to migrate into the intima (Fig. 242-1*F*). Various growth factors produced locally can stimulate the proliferation both of smooth muscle cells resident in the intima and of those that have migrated from the media. Transforming growth factor β, among other mediators, potently stimulates interstitial collagen production by smooth muscle cells. These mediators may arise not only from neighboring vascular cells or leukocytes (a paracrine pathway), but in some instances from the cell that responds to the factor (an autocrine pathway). Together, these alterations in smooth muscle cells, signaled by these local mediators, can hasten transformation of the fatty streak into a lesion richer in fibrous smooth muscle cells and extracellular matrix.

Traditionally atherosclerosis research has focused on the proliferation of smooth muscle cells. However, smooth muscle cells actually replicate rather slowly in complicated atherosclerotic lesions. Estimates of the rate of smooth muscle cell division at a given time in such lesions show a replicative rate below 1 percent. Such observations do not exclude bursts of proliferative activity at certain junctures in the history of an atheroma, perhaps in association with local thrombin generation due to microvascular hemorrhage or formation of a microthrombus at a site of localized endothelial denudation, as discussed below. On the other hand, cell death has been recognized as a component of atherogenesis since the time of Virchow in the mid-nineteenth century. Indeed, complex atheromas often have a primarily fibrous character, lacking the hyper-

cellular appearance of less advanced lesions and actually exhibiting a paucity of smooth muscle cells. This relative lack of smooth muscle cells in advanced atheromas may result from the ultimate predominance of cytostatic mediators such as transforming growth factor β or interferon γ, which can inhibit smooth muscle cell proliferation. Also, smooth muscle cells as well as macrophages in advanced atherosclerotic lesions can undergo apoptosis. Some of the same cytokines that activate atherogenic functions of vascular wall cells can also trigger apoptosis in these cells.

Factors That Modulate Atheroma Progression and Complication In addition to locally produced mediators and traditional atherogenic risk factors, signals related to blood coagulation and thrombosis likely contribute to atheroma evolution and complication. Current evidence suggests that fatty streak formation begins without frank denuding endothelial injury or desquamation. However, in advanced fatty streaks, microscopic breaches in the endothelium may occur. Microthrombi rich in platelets can form at such sites of limited endothelial denudation, owing to the exposure of the highly thrombogenic matrix of the underlying basement membrane. Activated platelets release numerous factors that can promote the fibrotic response. In addition to platelet derived growth factor and transforming growth factor β, low-molecular-weight mediators such as serotonin can also alter smooth muscle function. Most of these microthrombi probably resolve without clinical manifestations by a process of local fibrinolysis, resorption, and endothelial repair.

As atherosclerotic lesions advance, abundant plexi of microvessels develop in connection with the artery's vasa vasorum. These new microvascular networks may contribute to lesion complication in several ways. The vessels of these networks provide an abundant surface area for leukocyte trafficking and may serve as the portal by which white blood cells enter and leave the established atheroma. These microvessels may also be foci for intraplaque hemorrhage. Like the neovessels in the diabetic retina, plaque microvessels may be friable and likely to rupture and produce focal hemorrhage. Such a vascular leak would lead to thrombosis in situ and to the generation of thrombin from prothrombin. In addition to its role in blood coagulation, thrombin can modulate many aspects of vascular cell function; among other effects, it can stimulate the proliferation of and the release of cytokines from smooth muscle cells and the production of growth factors such as platelet-derived growth factors by endothelial cells. Atherosclerotic plaques often contain fibrin and hemosiderin, indications that

Table 242-1

Risk Factors for Atherosclerosis

Factor	Evidence for Causality	Modifiable	Comment
Hypercholesterolemia	Strong	Yes	
Low HDL level	Strong	Yes	Varies inversely with plasma triglyceride level
Hypertension	Strong	Yes	
Male gender	Strong	No	
Diabetes mellitus	Strong	Possibly	Effectiveness of stringent glycemic control uncertain
Family history of premature coronary artery disease	Strong	No	Premature onset before age 55 in first-degree relative
High lipoprotein (a) level	Strong	Modestly	Skewed distribution (see text)
Cigarette smoking	Good	Yes	
Post-menopausal state	Good	Possibly	Estrogen replacement therapy being evaluated
Hyperfibrinogenemia	Good	Possibly	Fibric acid derivatives may reduce
Hyperhomocysteinemia	Good	Yes	Some patients respond to folate supplementation
Physical inactivity	Good	Yes	
Obesity	Good	Yes	
Angiotensin converting enzyme polymorphism	Controversial	No	Homozygous deletion mutant associated with myocardial infarctions

episodes of intraplaque hemorrhage are an element in plaque complication.

Established atherosclerotic plaques also frequently accumulate calcium. Proteins specialized for binding calcium and usually associated with bone also occur in atherosclerotic lesions. For example, osteocalcin, osteopontin, and bone morphogenetic proteins localize in atherosclerotic plaques. In fact, complication of the atherosclerotic plaque recapitulates many aspects of bone formation.

Thus, during the evolution of the atherosclerotic plaque, a complex balance between entry and egress of lipoproteins and leukocytes, cell proliferation and cell death, extracellular matrix production and remodeling, as well as calcification and neovascularization contribute to lesion formation. Multiple and often competing signals trigger these various cellular events. There is a growing recognition of the links between atherogenic risk factors and the altered behavior of intrinsic vascular wall cells and infiltrating leukocytes that underlie the complex pathogenesis of these lesions.

CLINICAL SYNDROMES OF ATHEROSCLEROSIS Atherosclerotic lesions are ubiquitous in Western societies. Most atheromas produce no symptoms, and many never cause clinical manifestations. Numerous patients with diffuse atherosclerosis may succumb to unrelated illnesses without ever having experienced a clinically significant manifestation of atherosclerosis. What accounts for this variability in the clinical expression of atherosclerotic disease?

Arterial remodeling during atheroma formation represents a frequently overlooked but clinically important feature of lesion evolution. During the initial phases of atheroma development, the plaque usually grows in the direction away from the lumen (abluminally). Vessels affected by atherogenesis tend to increase in diameter, a type of vascular remodeling known as compensatory enlargement. Not until the plaque covers more than about 40 percent of the circumference of the internal elastic lamina does it begin to encroach on the arterial lumen. Thus, during much of its history, an atheroma will not cause stenosis that can limit blood flow.

Later in the history of the plaque, flow-limiting stenoses commonly form. Many such plaques manifest themselves by stable syndromes such as demand-induced angina pectoris or intermittent claudication in the extremities. In the coronary and other circulations, even occlusion due to atheroma does not invariably lead to infarction. The hypoxic stimulus of repeated bouts of ischemia characteristically induces the formation of collateral vessels in the myocardium, mitigating the consequences of an acute occlusion of an epicardial coronary artery. On the other hand, many lesions that cause acute or unstable atherosclerotic syndromes, particularly in the coronary circulation, may arise from atherosclerotic plaques that do not produce a flow-limiting stenosis. Such lesions may produce only minimal luminal irregularities on traditional angiograms and often do not meet the traditional criteria for "significance" by arteriography. The instability of such nonocclusive stenoses may explain why myocardial infarction is the first manifestation of coronary artery disease in about a third of all cases and why these patients report no prior history of angina pectoris, a syndrome usually caused by flow-limiting stenoses.

Pathologic studies afford considerable insight into the microanatomic reasons for the instability of plaques that are not critically stenotic. The culprit usually is a superficial erosion of the endothelium or a frank plaque rupture or fissure that gives rise to a thrombus. Such a thrombus may cause an episode of unstable angina pectoris or, if occlusive and relatively persistent, an acute myocardial infarction (Fig. 242-2E). In the case of carotid atheroma, a deeper ulceration that provides a nidus for formation of platelet thrombi may underlie the unstable syndromes that cause transient ischemic attacks.

Rupture of the plaque's fibrous cap permits coagulation factors in the blood to contact highly thrombogenic tissue factor, a procoagulant protein, expressed by macrophage foam cells in the plaque's lipid-rich core. If the ensuing thrombus is nonocclusive or transient, the episode of plaque disruption may not cause symptoms or may result

in ischemic symptoms such as rest angina (Fig. 242-2C). Occlusive thrombi that endure will often cause acute myocardial infarction, particularly in the absence of a well-developed collateral circulation supplying the affected territory. Repetitive episodes of plaque disruption and healing are one likely mechanism by which the fatty streak can evolve into a more complex fibrous lesion (Fig. 242-2D). The healing process in arteries, as in skin wounds, involves the laying down of new extracellular matrix and fibrosis.

Not all atheromas have the same propensity to rupture. Studies of the pathology of culprit lesions that have caused acute myocardial infarction show several characteristic features. These plaques tend to have a thin fibrous cap, a relatively large lipid core, and a high content of macrophages (Fig. 242-2A). Morphometric studies show that macrophages and T lymphocytes predominate at the site of plaque rupture (Fig. 242-2B) and that these sites contain relatively few smooth muscle cells. The cells that concentrate at sites of plaque rupture bear markers of inflammatory activation. The presence of the transplantation or histocompatibility antigen HLA-DR provides one convenient gauge of the degree of inflammation in cells in atheromas. Resting cells in normal arteries seldom express this transplantation antigen. However, macrophages and smooth muscle cells at sites of human coronary artery plaque disruption do bear it. Thus, the presence of macrophages and T cells positive for HLA-DR indicates an ongoing inflammatory response at sites of plaque rupture (Fig. 242-2B).

Inflammatory mediators may actually regulate processes that govern the integrity of the plaque's fibrous cap and hence its propensity to rupture. For example, the T cell–derived cytokine interferon γ, found in atherosclerotic plaques and required to induce the HLA-DR present at sites of rupture, can inhibit the growth and collagen synthesis of smooth muscle cells. Cytokines derived from activated macrophages, such as TNFα and IL-1 in addition to T cell–derived interferon γ, can elicit the expression of proteinases that can degrade the extracellular matrix of the plaque's fibrous cap. Thus, inflammatory mediators can both impair the collagen synthesis required for maintenance and repair of the fibrous cap and trigger degradation of extracellular matrix macromolecules, processes that should weaken the cap and enhance its vulnerability to rupture. In contrast, plaques with a dense extracellular matrix and relatively thick fibrous cap and without a substantial lipid core seem generally resistant to rupture and unlikely to provoke thrombosis (Fig. 242-2D).

PREVENTION AND TREATMENT OF ATHEROSCLEROSIS The prevention of atherosclerosis presents a long-term challenge to all health care professionals and to public health policy (Table 242-2). Both individual practitioners and organizations providing health care should strive to help patients to optimize their risk factor profile long before atherosclerotic disease becomes manifest. The care plan for all patients seen by physicians should include measures to assess and minimize cardiovascular risk. Physicians must counsel patients regarding the health risk of tobacco abuse and provide guidance regarding smoking cessation. Likewise, physicians should advise all patients about prudent dietary and exercise habits for maintaining ideal body weight. Obesity, particularly the male pattern of centripetal or visceral fat accumulation, can promote an atherogenic dyslipidemia characterized by elevated plasma triglycerides, low HDL levels, and glucose intolerance. Physicians should encourage their patients to take responsibility for modifiable risk factors. Conscientious counseling and patient education may delay or lessen the need for pharmacologic measures.

As part of an overall strategy for limiting atherosclerosis, hypertension should be controlled, by drug therapy if necessary (see Chap. 246). Most patients with diabetes mellitus die of atherosclerosis and its complications. It remains unproven that "tight" glycemic control can slow atherosclerosis and its complications in insulin-dependent diabetic patients. However, in view of the evidence that such strict euglycemia does favorably alter the development of microvascular complications of diabetes, special attention to glycemic control appears desirable for all such patients.

Lowering of Lipid Levels Current national guidelines recommend cholesterol screening in all adults (Table 242-3). They also recommend obtaining a fasting lipid profile (including total cholesterol, triglycerides, LDL cholesterol and HDL cholesterol) in all patients with known vascular disease and in those with several risk factors or elevated total cholesterol. Dietary measures, including specific consultation by health professionals with training in nutrition, should be offered to all patients with hyperlipidemia as defined by the National Cholesterol Education Project Adult Treatment Panel II. A "normal" total cholesterol level should not be taken as reassurance in an individual whose HDL cholesterol level is below 40 mg/dL or who has additional risk factors for coronary heart disease. Many patients with established atherosclerosis fall into this category. They should be particularly encouraged to adopt life-style measures such as diet and exercise programs aimed at increasing their levels of HDL cholesterol. In all patients with HDL cholesterol levels below 40 mg/dL, the physician must carefully weigh the potential adverse effects on HDL cholesterol levels of any medication. In particular, thiazide diuretics and beta-adrenergic blocking agents may adversely affect the lipid profile. Both of these classes of agents can raise triglycerides and lower HDL cholesterol, a point that should be borne in mind when selecting agents for long-term administration or with the goal of primary prevention in patients who have hypertension but no overt atherosclerosis. This concern about beta blockers should not discourage the practitioner from using these agents in appropriately selected survivors of acute myocardial infarction, however. Multiple well-designed clinical trials have established the efficacy of these agents in the prevention of cardiac death following myocardial infarction (Chap. 243).

The role of drug therapy in reducing the manifestations of atherosclerosis in asymptomatic patients with manifest vascular disease is incompletely defined. In asymptomatic patients with heterozygous familial hypercholesterolemia, the use of drugs to lower LDL levels reduces atherosclerosis in both men and women. The West of Scotland Study recently established that the use of pravastatin, a hydroxymethylglutaryl-coenzyme A (HMGCoA) inhibitor, to lower lipid levels reduced cardiac events and total mortality in a cohort of patients who had not had a myocardial infarction but who had cholesterol levels exceeding 250 mg/dL and elevated LDL levels.

Recent information also provides evidence for a benefit of drug therapy in patients with hypercholesterolemia and established coronary artery disease. The Scandinavian Simvastatin Survival Study showed a decrease in total mortality as well as in myocardial infarctions, cardiovascular death, and surgical or angioplastic revascularization procedures in patients with prior myocardial infarction treated with the HMGCoA inhibitor simvastatin. The incidence of cerebrovascular accidents also declined with simvastatin treatment in this cohort. No increase in noncardiac mortality occurred, providing reassurance that the excess noncardiac mortality encountered with some other forms of lipid-lowering therapy does not occur with HMGCoA reductase inhibitors over the period of study. Likewise, a meta-analysis of experience with controlled clinical trials of pravastatin shows a decrease in overall mortality and cardiovascular events. Even survivors of acute myocardial infarction with "average" cholesterol levels have reduced risk of recurrent coronary events when receiving an HMGCoA reductase inhibitor as shown by the recent Cholesterol and Recurrent Events (CARE) trial. Thus, it appears that effective lowering of LDL levels by treatment with an HMGCoA reductase inhibitor reduces cardiovascular morbidity and total mortality in patients with known coronary artery disease.

Curiously, it does not appear that lipid-lowering therapies exert their beneficial effects on cardiovascular events by causing a marked regression of obstructive coronary lesions (Table 242-4). Angiographi-cally monitored studies of lipid lowering have shown at best modest reductions in coronary artery stenoses over the duration of study, even though these studies all showed a resounding decrease in coronary events. These benefits may instead accrue from stabilization of atherosclerotic lesions. For example, the improved cholesterol balance resulting from a reduction in lipid levels may lead to a net egress of lipids from atherosclerotic lesions, resulting in a decrease in the proinflammatory aspects of lipid overloading discussed above. The beneficial effect on cardiovascular events of the lowering of LDL levels produced by HMGCoA reductase treatment seems to require 6 months to up to 2 years of treatment to appear. Improvement of vasomotor responses to endothelium-dependent vasodilators appears to be much more rapid, occurring in 6 months or less. The observations suggest that HMGCoA reductase inhibitors may act on the arteries of hypercholesterolemic individuals by two or more mechanisms. The more rapid effect on endothelium-dependent vasomotor responses could involve an increase in vascular nitric oxide production or a decrease in the production of superoxide anion, a molecule that inactivates nitric oxide, by lesional leukocytes or vascular cells. This effect on the endothelium or on periluminal cells follows the same time course as the reduction in plasma LDL cholesterol (weeks to months). The reduction in cardiovascular events may require removal of lipid and reduced activation of lesional macrophage foam cells from deeper in the lesions, processes that may require many months, perhaps accounting for the slower onset of the stabilizing effect of HMGCoA reductase treatment.

Table 242-2

Pharmacologic Treatment or Prevention of Atherosclerosis—Examples of the Evidence Base

Risk Factor	Treatment	Strength of Evidence for Effectiveness/Limitations of Therapy
High LDL level	Statins	Prevents coronary events, stroke; lowers total mortality in selected populations
High Lp(a) level	Nicotinic acid	May increase noncardiac mortality
High plasma triglyceride level	Fibric acid derivatives	May increase noncardiac mortality
Low HDL level	Nicotinic acid	Effective, but not proven to lower morbidity/mortality
Hypertension	Thiazide diuretics	Meta-analysis indicates reduced coronary events
Hyperglycemia	Insulin	Proven to reduce microvascular complications of diabetes; not yet proven to limit macrovascular disease
Hyperhomocysteinemia	Folic acid	Lowers homocysteine level in some individuals; not shown to influence atherosclerosis or its manifestations
High fibrinogen level	Fibric acid derivatives	May increase noncardiac mortality

Table 242-3

Treatment Decisions Based on LDL Cholesterol Level

Patient Category	LDL Cholesterol Level, mg/dL (mmol/L)	
	Initial	Goal
DIETARY THERAPY		
Without CHD and with fewer than two risk factors	≥160 (4.1)	<160 (4.1)
Without CHD and with two or more risk factors	≥130 (3.4)	<130 (3.4)
With CHD	>100 (2.6)	≤100 (2.6)
DRUG TREATMENT		
Without CHD and with fewer than two risk factors	≥190 (4.9)	<160 (4.1)
Without CHD and with two or more risk factors	≥160 (4.1)	<130 (3.4)
With CHD	≥130 (3.4)	≤100 (2.6)

ABBREVIATION: CHD, coronary heart disease

SOURCE: Summary of the second report of the National Cholesterol Education Program (NCEP) Expert Panel on Detection, Evaluation, and Treatment of High Blood Cholesterol in Adults (Adult Treatment Panel II). JAMA 269:3015, 1993.

Table 242-4

Summary of Results of Lipid-Lowering Trials

Study	Treatment Regimen	Regression, %	Reduction, Event, %
NHLBI	Diet + colestipol	7	33
CLAS-1	Diet + colestipol + niacin	16	25
POSCH	Partial ileal bypass + colestipol	14	35
FATS	Lovastatin or niacin + colestipol	39	80
CLAS-II	Diet + colestipol + niacin	18	43
STARS	Diet + colestipol	38	69
SCRIP	Diet + resin/niacin/lovastatin/fibrate	21	50

SOURCE: Adapted from BG Brown et al: Lipid lowering and plaque regression. New insights into prevention of plaque disruption and clinical events in coronary disease. Circulation 87:1781, 1993.

Large-scale clinical studies currently in progress should provide evidence regarding the utility of certain potential new avenues for antiatherosclerotic therapy. The treatments under evaluation include antioxidant vitamin supplementation as well as estrogen replacement therapy for postmenopausal women. Observational studies, small clinical trials, and evaluation of surrogates for disease, as well as current concepts of the biology of atherosclerosis, suggest that such therapies may prove beneficial. However their general use, particularly by lower-risk individuals, should await the results of rigorous prospective studies designed to define doses and appropriate patient groups and to evaluate the possibility of adverse or unwanted effects.

Estrogen Therapy The case of estrogen therapy illustrates some of the complexities encountered in formulating therapeutic strategies. In men, high-dose estrogen treatment causes an increase in mortality, probably owing to an increase in thromboembolic risk. In postmenopausal women, administration of estrogen either alone or combined with a progestin can improve biochemical variables associated with risk for coronary heart disease (lowering LDL levels, raising HDL levels, and lowering fibrinogen levels). Observational studies in women also indicate that estrogen replacement therapy has a beneficial effect in terms of cardiovascular events. However, unopposed estrogen replacement (i.e., without simultaneous progestin treatment) augments endometrial atypia and adenomatous changes. The balance between the possible increased risk of breast or uterine cancer and the cardiovascular benefit from this treatment remains uncertain. The variety of estrogen doses and dosage forms, and the inclusion of progestin cotherapy, complicates the design of controlled clinical trials aimed at monitoring clinical cardiovascular events. Such trials are underway, however, and their results should make it easier to formulate public health policy in this area. In the meantime, the practitioner must decide whether to recommend estrogen replacement therapy on the basis of an assessment of the balance of risks and benefits for individual patients in the light of their profiles of coronary risk factors, breast cancer, and personal preferences.

BIBLIOGRAPHY

BERLINER J et al: Atherosclerosis: Basic mechanisms—oxidation, inflammation, and genetics. Circulation 91:2488–2496, 1995

DAVIES MJ: A macro and micro view of coronary vascular insult in ischemic heart disease. Circulation 82:1138, 1990

FUSTER V: Mechanisms leading to myocardial infaction: Insights from vascular biology. Circulation 90:2126, 1994

LIBBY P: The molecular bases of the acute coronary syndromes. Circulation 91:2844, 1995

ROSS R: The pathogenesis of atherosclerosis: A perspective for the 1990s. Nature 362:801, 1993

STEINBERG D et al: Beyond cholesterol. Modifications of low-density lipoprotein that increase its atherogenicity. N Engl J Med 320:915, 1989

243

Elliott M. Antman, Eugene Braunwald

ACUTE MYOCARDIAL INFARCTION

Myocardial infarction is one of the most common diagnoses in hospitalized patients in industrialized countries. In the United States, approximately 1.5 million myocardial infarctions occur each year. The mortality rate with acute infarction is approximately 30 percent, with more than half of these deaths occurring before the stricken individual reaches the hospital. Although the mortality rate after admission for myocardial infarction has declined by about 30 percent over the last two decades, approximately 1 of every 25 patients who survives the initial hospitalization dies in the first year after myocardial infarction. Survival is markedly reduced in elderly patients (over age 65), whose mortality rate is 20 percent at 1 month and 35 percent at 1 year after infarction.

PATHOPHYSIOLOGY: ROLE OF ACUTE PLAQUE RUPTURE

Myocardial infarction generally occurs when there is an abrupt decrease in coronary blood flow following a thrombotic occlusion of a coronary artery previously narrowed by atherosclerosis. Slowly developing, high-grade coronary artery stenoses usually do not precipitate acute infarction because of the development of a rich collateral network over time. Instead, infarction occurs when a coronary artery thrombus develops rapidly at a site of vascular injury. This injury is produced or facilitated by factors such as cigarette smoking, hypertension, and lipid accumulation. In most cases, infarction occurs when an atherosclerotic plaque fissures, ruptures, or ulcerates and when conditions (local or systemic) favor thrombogenesis, so that a mural thrombus forms at the site of rupture and leads to coronary artery occlusion. Histologic studies indicate that the coronary plaques prone to rupture are those with a rich lipid core and a thin fibrous cap. After an initial platelet monolayer forms at the site of the ruptured plaque, a variety of agonists (collagen, ADP, epinephrine, serotonin) promote platelet activation. Following agonist stimulation, there is production and release of thromboxane A_2 (a compound capable of inducing vasoconstriction), further platelet activation, and potential resistance to thrombolysis.

In addition to generation of thromboxane A_2, activation of platelets by agonists promotes a conformational change in the glycoprotein IIbIIIa receptor. Once converted to its functional state, this receptor develops a high affinity for the sequence arginine-glycine-aspartic acid (called the RGD sequence) on the fibrinogen alpha chain and also for a dodecapeptide sequence on the fibrinogen gamma chain. Since fibrinogen is a multivalent molecule, it can bind to two different platelets simultaneously, resulting in platelet cross-linking and aggregation.

The coagulation cascade is activated on exposure of tissue factor in damaged endothelial cells at the site of the ruptured plaque. Factors VII and X are activated, ultimately leading to the conversion of prothrombin to thrombin, which then converts fibrinogen to fibrin. Fluid-phase and clot-bound thrombin participate in an autoamplification reaction leading to further activation of the coagulation cascade. The culprit coronary artery eventually becomes occluded by a thrombus containing platelet aggregates and fibrin strands.

In rare cases, infarction may be due to coronary artery occlusion caused by coronary emboli, congenital abnormalities, coronary spasm, and a wide variety of systemic—particularly inflammatory—diseases. Ultimately, the amount of myocardial damage caused by coronary occlusion depends on the territory supplied by the affected vessel, whether or not the vessel becomes totally occluded, native factors that can produce early spontaneous lysis of the occlusive thrombus, the quantity of blood supplied by collateral vessels to the affected tissue, and the demand for oxygen of the myocardium whose blood supply has been suddenly limited.

Patients at increased risk of developing acute myocardial infarction include those with unstable angina or Prinzmetal's variant angina (Chap. 244) and those with multiple coronary risk factors (Chap. 242). Less common underlying medical conditions predisposing patients to infarction include hypercoagulability, collagen vascular disease, cocaine abuse, and intracardiac thrombi or masses that can produce coronary emboli.

CLINICAL PRESENTATION

In roughly one-half of cases, a precipitating factor appears to be present prior to myocardial infarction, such as vigorous physical exercise, emotional stress, or a medical or surgical illness. Myocardial infarction may commence at any time of the day or night, but the frequency is highest in the morning within a few hours of awakening. This circadian peak may be due to a combination of an increase in sympathetic tone and an increased tendency to thrombosis between 6:00 A.M. and 12 noon. *Pain* is the most common presenting complaint in patients with myocardial infarction. In some instances, the discomfort may be severe enough to be described as the worst pain the patient has ever felt. The pain is deep and visceral; adjectives commonly used to describe it are *heavy*, *squeezing*, and *crushing*, although occasionally it is described as stabbing or burning (Chap. 13). It is similar in character to the discomfort of angina pectoris but usually is more severe and lasts longer. Typically the pain involves the central portion of the chest and/or the epigastrium, and on occasion it radiates to the arms. Less common sites of radiation include the abdomen, back, lower jaw, and neck. The frequent location of the pain beneath the xiphoid and patients' denial that they may be suffering a heart attack are chiefly responsible for the common mistaken impression of indigestion. The pain of myocardial infarction may radiate as high as the occipital area but not below the umbilicus. It is often accompanied by weakness, sweating, nausea, vomiting, anxiety, and a sense of impending doom. The discomfort may commence when the patient is at rest. When the pain begins during a period of exertion, it does not usually subside with cessation of activity, in contrast to angina pectoris.

Although pain is the most common presenting complaint, it is by no means always present. The incidence of painless infarcts is greater in patients with diabetes mellitus, and it increases with age. In the elderly, myocardial infarction may present as sudden-onset breathlessness, which may progress to pulmonary edema. Other less common presentations, with or without pain, include sudden loss of consciousness, a confusional state, a sensation of profound weakness, the appearance of an arrhythmia, evidence of peripheral embolism, or merely an unexplained drop in arterial pressure. The pain of myocardial infarction can simulate pain from acute pericarditis (Chap. 240), pulmonary embolism (Chap. 261), acute aortic dissection (Chap. 247), and costochondritis. These conditions should therefore be considered in the differential diagnosis.

PHYSICAL FINDINGS Most patients are anxious and restless, attempting unsuccessfully to relieve the pain by moving about in bed, altering their position, and stretching. Pallor associated with perspiration and coolness of the extremities occurs commonly. The combination of substernal chest pain persisting for more than 30 min and diaphoresis strongly suggests acute myocardial infarction. Although many patients have a normal pulse rate and blood pressure, within the first hour of infarction, about one-fourth of patients with anterior infarction have manifestations of sympathetic nervous system hyperactivity (tachycardia and/or hypertension), and up to one-half with inferior infarction show evidence of parasympathetic hyperactivity (bradycardia and/or hypotension).

The precordium is usually quiet, and the apical impulse may be difficult to palpate. In patients with anterior wall infarction, an abnormal systolic pulsation caused by dyskinetic bulging of infarcted myocardium may develop in the periapical area within the first days of the illness and then may resolve. Other physical signs of ventricular dysfunction that may be present include, in order of decreasing incidence, fourth (S_4) and third (S_3) heart sounds, decreased intensity of heart sounds, and, in more severe cases, paradoxical splitting of the

second heart sound (Chap. 227). A transient apical systolic murmur due to dysfunction of the mitral valve apparatus may be midsystolic or late systolic in timing. A pericardial friction rub is heard in many patients with transmural myocardial infarction at some time in the course of the disease, if they are examined frequently. The carotid pulse is often decreased in volume, reflecting reduced stroke volume. Jugular venous distention with clear lung fields should raise suspicion of right ventricular infarction. Temperature elevations up to 38°C may be observed during the first week after acute myocardial infarction; however, a temperature exceeding 38°C should prompt a search for other causes. The arterial pressure is variable; in most patients with transmural infarction, systolic pressure declines by approximately 10 to 15 mmHg from the preinfarction state.

LABORATORY FINDINGS

The laboratory tests of value in confirming the diagnosis of myocardial infarction may be divided into four groups: (1) the electrocardiogram (ECG), (2) serum cardiac markers, (3) cardiac imaging, and (4) nonspecific indexes of tissue necrosis and inflammation.

ELECTROCARDIOGRAM The *electrocardiographic manifestations* of acute myocardial infarction are described in Chap. 228. Transmural infarction is often present if the ECG demonstrates Q waves or loss of R waves; nontransmural infarction may be present if the electrocardiogram shows only transient ST-segment and T-wave changes. However, electrocardiographic-pathologic correlations are far from perfect and, therefore, a more rational nomenclature for designating electrocardiographic infarction is now commonly in use, with the terms *Q-wave* and *non-Q-wave infarction* replacing the terms *transmural* and *nontransmural infarction*, respectively.

Total occlusion of the infarct artery produces ST-segment elevation, and most such individuals ultimately evolve a Q-wave myocardial infarction. A small proportion may sustain only a non-Q wave myocardial infarction. When the obstructing thrombus is subtotally occlusive, obstruction is transient, or a rich collateral network is present, no ST-segment elevation is seen. Most such patients are diagnosed as having unstable angina, or, if a serum cardiac marker is detected, as having non-Q wave myocardial infarction. A minority of patients who present initially without ST-segment elevation may develop a Q-wave infarction. The presentations that constitute the spectrum ranging from unstable angina through non-Q-wave myocardial infarction to Q-wave myocardial infarction are called the *acute coronary syndromes* (Fig. 243-1).

SERUM CARDIAC MARKERS Certain proteins, called *serum cardiac markers*, are released into the blood in large quantities from necrotic heart muscle after myocardial infarction. The rate of liberation of specific proteins differs depending on their intracellular location and molecular weight, and the local blood and lymphatic flow. The temporal pattern of protein release is of diagnostic importance, but contemporary urgent reperfusion strategies necessitate making a decision (based largely on a combination of clinical and ECG findings) before the results of blood tests have returned from the central laboratory. Rapid whole-blood bedside assays for serum cardiac markers are now available and may facilitate management decisions, particularly in patients with nondiagnostic electrocardiograms.

Creatine phosphokinase (*CK*) rises within 4 to 8 h and generally returns to normal by 48 to 72 h. An important drawback of total CK measurement is its lack of specificity for myocardial infarction, as CK may be elevated with skeletal muscle trauma. A two- to threefold elevation of total CK may follow an intramuscular injection, for example. This ambiguity may lead to the erroneous diagnosis of myocardial infarction in a patient who has been given an intramuscular injection of a narcotic for chest pain of noncardiac origin. Other potential sources of total CK elevation worth noting are (1) muscular diseases, including muscular dystrophy, myopathies, and polymyositis; (2) electric cardioversion; (3) cardiac catheterization; (4) hypothyroidism; (5) stroke;

(6) surgery; and (7) skeletal muscle damage secondary to trauma, convulsions, and prolonged immobilization.

The MB isoenzyme of CK has the advantage total over CK that it is not present in significant concentrations in extracardiac tissue and therefore is considerably more specific. However, cardiac surgery, myocarditis, and electric cardioversion often result in elevated serum levels of the MB isoenzyme. A ratio (relative index) of CKMB mass:CK activity $\geq$ 2.5 percent suggests but is not diagnostic of a myocardial rather than skeletal muscle source for the CKMB elevation. This ratio is less useful when levels of total CK are high owing to skeletal muscle injury or when the total CK level is within the normal range but CKMB is elevated.

Rather than attempting to make the diagnosis of a myocardial infarction on the basis of a single measurement of CK and CKMB, clinicians should evaluate a series of measurements obtained over the first 24 h. Skeletal muscle release of CKMB typically produces a "plateau" pattern, whereas myocardial infarction produces a CKMB elevation that peaks at approximately 20 h after the onset of coronary occlusion. When released into the circulation, the myocardial form of CKMB (CKMB2) is acted on by the enzyme carboxypeptidase, which cleaves a lysine residue from the carboxy terminus to produce an isoform (CKMB1) with a different electrophoretic mobility. A CKMB2:CKMB1 ratio of >1.5 is highly sensitive for the diagnosis of myocardial infarction, particularly after 4 to 6 h have elapsed since coronary occlusion.

Cardiac-specific troponin T (cTnT) and *cardiac-specific troponin I (cTnI)* have different amino acid sequences than the skeletal muscle forms of these proteins. This difference has permitted the development of quantitative assays for cTnT and cTnI using highly specific monoclonal antibodies. Since cTnT and cTnI are not normally detectable in the blood of healthy individuals but may increase after myocardial infarction to levels over 20 times higher than the cutoff value (usually set only slightly above the noise level of the assay), measurement of cTnT or cTnI is of considerable diagnostic utility. These new serum cardiac markers are particularly valuable when there is clinical suspicion of either skeletal muscle injury or a small myocardial infarction that may be below the detection limit for CK and CKMB measurements. Levels of cTnI may remain elevated for 7 to 10 days after myocardial infarction, and cTnT levels may remain elevated for up to 10 to 14 days. Thus, measurement of cTnT or cTnI is preferable to measurement of lactate dehydrogenase (LDH) and its isoenzymes in patients with suspected myocardial infarction who come to medical attention more than 24 to 48 h after the onset of symptoms.

Myoglobin is released into the blood within only a few hours of the onset of myocardial infarction. Although myoglobin is one of the first serum cardiac markers that rises above the normal range after myocardial infarction, it lacks cardiac specificity, and it is rapidly excreted in the urine, so that blood levels return to the normal range within 24 h of the onset of infarction.

Many clinical centers have begun to use cTnT or cTnI rather than CKMB as the routine serum cardiac marker for diagnosis of myocardial infarction, although any of these analytes remains clinically acceptable. It is not cost-effective to measure both a cardiac-specific troponin and CKMB at all time points in every patient. However, in view of the prolonged elevation of cardiac-specific troponins (>1 week), episodes of recurrent ischemic discomfort and suspected recurrent myocardial infarction are more readily diagnosed with a serum cardiac marker that remains elevated in the blood more briefly, such as CKMB or myoglobin.

While it has long been recognized that the *total* quantity of protein released correlates with the size of the infarct, the *peak* protein concentration correlates only weakly with infarct size. Recanalization of a coronary artery occlusion (either spontaneously or by mechanical or pharmacologic means) in the early hours of myocardial infarction will cause earlier and higher peaking (at about 8 to 12 h after reperfusion) of serum cardiac markers.

Characteristic rises occur in serum cardiac markers in virtually all patients with clinically proven myocardial infarction. CK and CKMB levels generally do not rise in unstable angina. However, approximately one-third of patients who are considered to have unstable angina on the basis of a lack of CK or CKMB elevation have elevations of cTnT or cTnI, probably indicating the presence of microinfarction. The finding of an elevated cardiac-specific troponin level, even in the presence of normal CK and CKMB values, is indicative of an adverse prognosis, and such patients should be considered to have sustained myocardial infarction and managed as described below.

The *nonspecific reaction* to myocardial injury is associated with polymorphonuclear leukocytosis, which appears within a few hours after the onset of pain, persists for 3 to 7 days, and often reaches levels of 12,000 to 15,000 leukocytes per microliter. The erythrocyte sedimentation rate rises more slowly than the white blood cell count, peaking during the first week and sometimes remaining elevated for 1 or 2 weeks.

CARDIAC IMAGING   *Two-dimensional echocardiography* is the most frequently employed imaging modality in patients with acute myocardial infarction. Abnormalities of wall motion are almost universally present. Even when no ST-segment elevation is seen, echocardiographically detectable wall motion abnormalities may be observed. Although acute infarction cannot be distinguished from an old myocardial scar or from acute severe ischemia by echocardiography, the ease and safety of the procedure make its use appealing as a screening tool. In the emergency department setting, early detection of the presence or absence of wall motion abnormalities by echocardiography can aid in management decisions, such as whether or not thrombolytic agents should be administered. Echocardiographic estimation of left ventricular function is useful prognostically; detection of reduced function serves as an indication for therapy with an angiotensin converting enzyme inhibitor (see "Angiotensin Converting Enzyme Inhibitors," below). Echocardiography may also identify the presence of right ventricular infarction, ventricular aneurysm, pericardial effusion, and

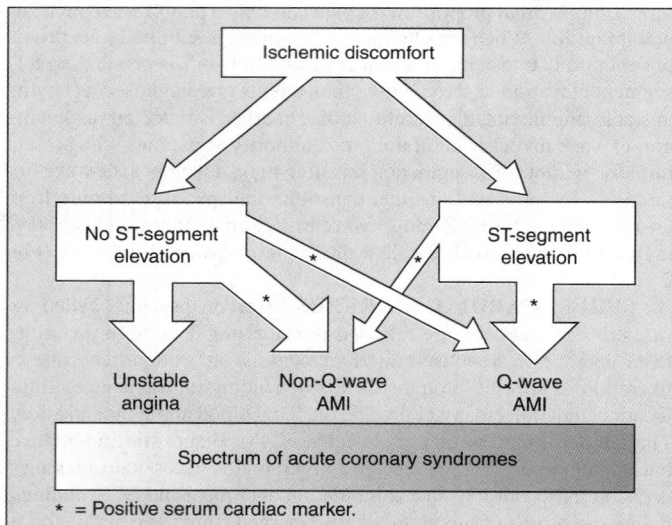

FIGURE 243-1 Acute coronary syndromes. Patients with ischemic discomfort may present with or without ST-segment elevation on the electrocardiogram. Of patients with ST-segment elevation, most (*large arrow*) ultimately develop a Q-wave acute myocardial infarction (AMI), while a minority (*small arrow*) develop a non-Q-wave AMI. Of the patients who present without ST-segment elevation, most (*large arrows*) are ultimately diagnosed as having either unstable angina or non-Q-wave AMI on the basis of the presence or absence of a cardiac marker such as CKMB detected in the serum; a minority of such patients ultimately develop a Q-wave AMI. The clinical conditions in the spectrum ranging from unstable angina through non-Q-wave AMI to Q-wave AMI are referred to as the acute coronary syndromes. [*From EM Antman, E Braunwald: Acute Myocardial Infarction, in Heart Disease, A Textbook of Cardiovascular Medicine, 5th ed, E Braunwald (ed). Philadelphia, Saunders, 1997.*]

left ventricular thrombus. In addition, Doppler echocardiography is useful in the detection and quantitation of a ventricular septal defect and mitral regurgitation, two serious complications of acute myocardial infarction.

Several radionuclide imaging techniques are available for evaluating patients with suspected acute myocardial infarction. However, these imaging modalities are used less often than echocardiography because they are more cumbersome and they a lack sensitivity and specificity in many clinical circumstances. Myocardial perfusion imaging with thallium 201 or technetium 99m sestamibi, which are distributed in proportion to myocardial blood flow and concentrated by viable myocardium, will reveal a defect ("cold spot") in most patients during the first few hours after development of a transmural infarct. However, although perfusion scanning is extremely *sensitive*, it cannot distinguish acute infarcts from chronic scars and thus is not *specific* for the diagnosis of *acute* myocardial infarction. Radionuclide ventriculography, carried out with ^{99m}Tc-labeled red blood cells, frequently demonstrates wall motion disorders and reduction in the ventricular ejection fraction in patients with acute myocardial infarction. While of value in assessing the hemodynamic consequences of infarction, and in aiding in the diagnosis of right ventricular infarction when the right ventricular ejection fraction is depressed, this technique is also quite nonspecific, as many cardiac abnormalities other than myocardial infarction alter the radionuclide ventriculogram.

MANAGEMENT

PREHOSPITAL CARE The prognosis in acute myocardial infarction is largely related to the occurrence of two general classes of complications: (1) electrical complications (arrhythmias) and (2) mechanical problems ("pump failure"). Most out-of-hospital deaths from myocardial infarction are due to the sudden development of ventricular fibrillation. The vast majority of deaths due to ventricular fibrillation occur within the first 24 h of the onset of symptoms, and, of these, over half occur in the first hour. Therefore, the major elements of prehospital care of patients with suspected acute myocardial infarction include (1) recognition of symptoms by the patient and prompt seeking of medical attention; (2) rapid deployment of an emergency medical team capable of performing resuscitative maneuvers, including defibrillation; and (3) expeditious transportation of the patient to a hospital facility that is continuously staffed by physicians and nurses skilled in managing arrhythmias, providing advanced cardiac life support, and initiating prompt reperfusion therapy. The biggest delay usually occurs not during transportation to the hospital but rather between the onset of pain and the patient's decision to call for help. This delay can best be reduced by education of the public by health care professionals concerning the significance of chest pain and the importance of seeking early medical attention. Increasingly, monitoring and treatment are carried out by trained personnel in the ambulance, further shortening the time between the onset of the infarction and appropriate treatment.

INITIAL MANAGEMENT IN THE EMERGENCY DEPARTMENT In the emergency department, the goals for the management of patients with suspected acute myocardial infarction include control of cardiac pain, rapid identification of patients who are candidates for urgent reperfusion therapy, triage of lower-risk patients to the appropriate location in the hospital, and avoidance of inappropriate discharge of patients with acute myocardial infarction. Many aspects of the treatment of acute myocardial infarction are initiated in the emergency department and then continued during the in-hospital phase of management.

Aspirin is now considered an essential element in the management of patients with suspected acute myocardial infarction and is effective across the entire spectrum of acute coronary syndromes (Fig. 243-1). Rapid inhibition of cyclooxygenase in platelets followed by a reduction of thromboxane A_2 levels is achieved by buccal absorption of a chewed 160 to 325 mg tablet in the emergency department. This measure should be followed by daily oral administration of aspirin in a dose of 160 to 325 mg.

Since patients with acute myocardial infarction may develop hypoxemia secondary to ventilation-perfusion abnormalities from left ventricular failure and intrinsic pulmonary disease, it has been a common practice to routinely administer *supplemental oxygen*, via the belief that an increase in the oxygen tension of the inspired air will protect the myocardium. In patients whose arterial oxygen saturation is normal as estimated by pulse oximetry or measured by an arterial blood gas specimen, supplemental oxygen is of limited clinical benefit and therefore is not cost-effective. However, when hypoxemia is demonstrated, oxygen should be administered by nasal prongs or face mask (2 to 4 L/min) for the first 6 to 12 h after infarction; the patient should then be reassessed to determine if there is a continued need for such treatment.

CONTROL OF PAIN *Morphine* is an extremely effective analgesic for the pain associated with myocardial infarction. However, it may reduce sympathetically mediated arteriolar and venous constriction, and the resulting venous pooling may reduce cardiac output and arterial pressure. This complication does not contraindicate morphine use. Hypotension associated with venous pooling usually responds promptly to elevation of the legs, but in some patients volume expansion with intravenous saline is required. The patient may experience diaphoresis and nausea, but these events usually pass and are replaced by a feeling of well-being associated with the relief of pain. Morphine also has a vagotonic effect and may cause bradycardia or advanced degrees of heart block, particularly in patients with posteroinferior infarction. These side effects usually respond to atropine (0.5 mg intravenously). Morphine is routinely administered by repetitive (every 5 min) intravenous injection of small doses (2 to 4 mg) rather than by the subcutaneous administration of a larger quantity, because absorption may be unpredictable by the latter route.

Before morphine is administered, sublingual *nitroglycerin* can be given safely to most patients with myocardial infarction. Up to three 0.4-mg doses should be administered at about 5-min intervals. In addition to diminishing or abolishing chest discomfort, nitroglycerin, once considered contraindicated in the setting of acute myocardial infarction, may be capable of both decreasing myocardial oxygen demand (by lowering preload) and increasing myocardial oxygen supply (by dilating infarct-related coronary vessels or collateral vessels). However, therapy with nitrates should be avoided in patients who present with low systolic arterial pressure (<100 mmHg) or in whom there is clinical suspicion of right ventricular infarction (inferior infarction on electrocardiogram, elevated jugular venous pressure, clear lungs, and hypotension). An idiosyncratic reaction to nitrates, consisting of sudden marked hypotension, sometimes occurs but can usually be reversed promptly by the rapid administration of intravenous atropine. In patients whose initially favorable response to sublingual nitroglycerin is followed by the return of chest pain, particularly if accompanied by other evidence of ongoing ischemia such as further ST-segment or T-wave shifts, the use of intravenous nitroglycerin should be considered.

Intravenous *beta blockers* are also useful in the control of the pain of acute myocardial infarction. These drugs have been shown to control pain effectively in some patients, presumably by diminishing myocardial oxygen demand and hence ischemia. More important, there is evidence that intravenous beta blockers reduce in-hospital mortality, particularly in high-risk patients (see "Beta-Adrenoceptor Blockers," below). A commonly employed regimen is metoprolol, 5 mg every 2 to 5 min for a total of three doses, provided the patient has a pulse greater than 60 beats per minute, systolic pressure greater than 100 mmHg, a PR interval of less than 0.24 sec, and rales that are no higher than 10 cm up from the diaphragm. Fifteen minutes after the last intravenous dose, an oral regimen is initiated of 50 mg every 6 h for 48 h followed by 100 mg every 12 h.

Unlike beta blockers, *calcium antagonists* are of little value in the acute setting, and there is evidence that they may be associated with an increased mortality risk.

MANAGEMENT STRATEGIES (Fig. 243-2) The primary tool for screening patients and making triage decisions is the initial 12-lead electrocardiogram. When ST-segment elevation of at least 1 mm is present in at least two contiguous leads, a patient should be considered a candidate for *reperfusion therapy* (Fig. 243-2A). If no contraindications are present (see "Contraindications and Complications," under "Thombolysis," below), thrombolytic therapy should ideally be initiated within 30 min. The process of selecting patients for thrombolysis versus primary percutaneous transluminal coronary angioplasty is discussed below. If the presenting electrocardiogram shows new or presumably new ST-segment depression and/or T-wave inversion, patients should be treated as though they are suffering from either unstable angina or non-Q-wave myocardial infarction (a distinction to be made on the basis of serial electrocardiograms and serum cardiac marker measurements). In the absence of ST-segment elevation, thrombolysis is not helpful, and evidence exists suggesting that it may be harmful. Pharmacotherapy for patients presenting without ST-segment elevation has not been studied as rigorously as that for patients who present with ST-segment elevation, but contemporary practice typically includes measures to control cardiac pain (as discussed above), aspirin, infusion of nitroglycerin, and either infusion of unfractionated heparin or subcutaneous administration of a low-molecular-weight heparin preparation. Further management recommendations for patients without ST segment elevation are outlined in Fig. 243-2B.

LIMITATION OF INFARCT SIZE The amount of myocardium that becomes necrotic owing to a coronary artery occlusion is determined by factors other than just the site of occlusion (Fig. 243-3). While the central zone of the infarct contains necrotic tissue that is irretrievably lost, the fate of the surrounding ischemic myocardium may be improved by timely restoration of coronary perfusion (Fig. 243-3, line B), reduction of myocardial oxygen demands, prevention of the accumulation of noxious metabolites, and blunting of the impact of mediators of reperfusion injury (e.g., calcium overload and oxygen-derived free radicals). Although up to one-third of patients with acute myocardial infarction may achieve spontaneous reperfusion of the infarct-related coronary artery and experience improved healing of infarcted tissue, it is now possible to minimize the infarct size by accelerating reperfusion either pharmacologically (by thrombolysis) or mechanically (by angioplasty). Protection of the ischemic myocardium by the maintenance of an optimal balance of myocardial oxygen through adequate pain control, treatment of congestive heart failure, and minimization of tachycardia and hypertension extends

FIGURE 243-2 Management strategies for patients with myocardial infarction. *A.* All patients suspected of having a Q-wave myocardial infarction (MI) (i.e., ST-segment elevation on ECG) should receive aspirin (ASA), beta blockers (in the absence of contraindications), and an antithrombin [particularly if tissue-type plasminogen activator (t-PA) is used for thrombolytic therapy]. Heparin is probably not required in patients receiving streptokinase (SK). Patients treated within 12 h who are eligible for thrombolytic therapy should expeditiously receive either t-PA or SK or be considered for primary percutaneous transluminal coronary angioplasty (PTCA). Immediate, primary PTCA is also to be considered when lytic therapy is contraindicated. Patients treated after 12 h should receive the initial medical therapy noted above and, on an individual basis, may be candidates for ACE inhibitors (particularly if left ventricular function is impaired). Further information is required to clarify the role of magnesium. *B.* All patients without ST elevation should be treated with an antithrombin and aspirin. Nitrates should be administered for recurrent episodes of angina. Adequate beta blockade should then be established; when that is not possible or contraindications exist, a calcium antagonist can be considered. Patients at high risk should be triaged to cardiac catheterization with plans for revascularization if clinically suitable, while patients who are clinically stable can be treated more conservatively with continued observation in the hospital and consideration of a stress test to screen for any provocable myocardial ischemia. (CABG, coronary artery bypass grafting; LV, left ventricular.) *[Modified from EM Antman: Overview of medical therapy, in RM Califf (ed): Acute Myocardial Infarction and Other Acute Ischemic Syndromes, in E Braunwald (Series ed): Atlas of Heart Diseases, vol. 8. Philadelphia, Current Medicine 1996.]*

the "window" of time for the salvage of myocardium by reperfusion strategies.

Glucocorticoids and nonsteroidal anti-inflammatory agents, with the exception of aspirin, should be avoided in the setting of acute myocardial infarction. They can impair infarct healing and increase the risk of myocardial rupture, and their use may result in a larger infarct scar. In addition, they can increase coronary vascular resistance, thereby potentially reducing flow to ischemic myocardium.

THROMBOLYSIS The thrombolytic agents tissue plasminogen activator (tPA), streptokinase, and anisoylated plasminogen streptokinase activator complex (APSAC) have been approved by the Food and Drug Administration for intravenous use in the setting of acute myocardial infarction. These drugs all act by promoting the conversion of plasminogen to plasmin, which subsequently lyses fibrin thrombi. Although considerable emphasis used to be placed on a distinction between more fibrin-specific agents, such as tPA, and non-fibrin-specific agents, such as streptokinase, it is now recognized that these differences are only relative, as some degree of systemic fibrinolysis occurs with tPA. The principal goal of thrombolysis is prompt restoration of coronary arterial patency. When assessed angiographically, flow in the culprit coronary artery is described by a simple qualitative scale called the TIMI grading system: grade 0 indicates complete occlusion of the infarct related artery; grade 1 indicates some penetration of the contrast material beyond the point of obstruction but without perfusion of the distal coronary bed; grade 2 indicates perfusion of the entire infarct vessel into the distal bed but with flow that is delayed compared with that of a normal artery; and grade 3 indicates full perfusion of the infarct vessel with normal flow. Early reports frequently lumped TIMI grades 2 and 3 under the general category of *patency*, but it is now recognized that grade 3 flow is the goal of reperfusion therapy, because full perfusion of the infarct-related coronary artery yields far better results in terms of infarct size, maintenance

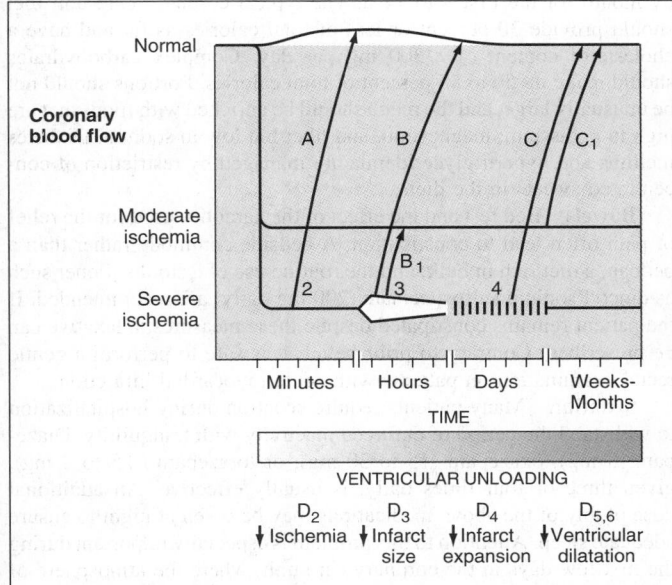

FIGURE 243-3 Therapeutic maneuvers in various stages of ischemia and infarction. Severely ischemic tissue (line 2) may be reperfused quickly with restoration of coronary blood flow to normal, thereby averting myocardial infarction (line A). Tissue undergoing infarction (3) may be reperfused, leading to sparing of myocardial tissue (line B) around a central core of necrotic myocardium. If only a moderate improvement in blood flow is achieved (B_1 = TIMI grade 1 or 2 flow), the myocardium may remain noncontractile although viable, i.e., hibernating. After completion of the infarct (4), late reperfusion (line C) may still be useful. Mechanical reperfusion of moderately ischemic myocardium (C_1) may restore the contractility of hibernating myocardium to normal. Ventricular unloading may be useful throughout the pre-infarct and post-infarct periods. Unloading may reduce ischemia (D_2), infarct size (D_3), infarct expansion (D_4), and ventricular dilation ($D_{5,6}$). (*From E Braunwald, MA Pfeffer, Am J Cardiol 68:4D, 1991.*)

of left ventricular function, and reduction of mortality over the short and long term.

Thrombolytic therapy can reduce the relative risk of in-hospital death by up to 50 percent when administered within the first hour of the onset of symptoms of myocardial infarction, and much of this benefit is maintained for 1 or more years. Appropriately employed thrombolytic therapy appears to reduce infarct size, limit left ventricular dysfunction, and reduce the incidence of serious complications such as septal rupture, cardiogenic shock, and malignant ventricular arrhythmias. Since myocardium can be salvaged only before it has been irreversibly injured, the timing of thrombolytic therapy is of extreme importance in achieving maximum benefit. While the upper time limit depends on specific factors in individual patients, it is clear that "every minute counts" and that patients treated within 1 to 3 h of the onset of symptoms generally benefit most. Although the reduction of mortality is more modest, benefit of therapy remains in many patients seen 3 to 6 h after the onset of infarction, and some benefit appears to be possible up to 12 h, especially if chest discomfort is still present and ST segments remain elevated in electrocardiographic leads that do not yet demonstrate new Q waves. In addition to the possibility of early treatment, clinical factors that favor proceeding with thrombolytic therapy include anterior wall injury, hemodynamically complicated infarction, and widespread ECG evidence of myocardial jeopardy. While younger patients (less than 65 years old) achieve a greater relative reduction in mortality rate than elderly patients, the higher absolute mortality rate (15 to 25 percent) in elderly patients results in similar absolute reductions in mortality rate (about 10 lives saved per 1000 patients treated with thrombolytics).

Intriguing data are accumulating to indicate that improved ventricular function and reduced mortality may also be achieved by *late coronary reperfusion* (Fig. 243-3, line C). The benefits of late reperfusion cannot be attributed to a reduction of infarct size but appear to result from improvement of tissue healing in the infarct zone with prevention of infarct expansion, enhancement of collateral flow, improvement of myocardial contractile performance, and reduction in the tendency to electrical instability. In addition, *hibernating myocardium* (i.e., poorly contractile myocardium in a zone that is supplied by a stenotic infarct-related coronary artery with slow antegrade perfusion, Chap. 244) may show improved contraction following angioplasty to increase coronary blood flow (Fig. 243-3, line C^1).

tPA is more effective than streptokinase at restoring full perfusion—i.e., TIMI grade 3 coronary flow—and has a small edge in improving survival as well. The current recommended regimen of tPA consists of a 15-mg bolus followed by 50 mg intravenously over the first 30 min, followed by 35 mg over the next 60 min. Streptokinase is administered as 1.5 million units intravenously over 1 h.

Contraindications and Complications Clear contraindications to the use of thrombolytic agents include a history of cerebrovascular hemorrhage at any time, a nonhemorrhagic stroke or other cerebrovascular event within the past year, marked hypertension (a reliably determined systolic arterial pressure greater than 180 mmHg and/or a diastolic pressure greater than 110 mmHg) at any time during the acute presentation, suspicion of aortic dissection, and active internal bleeding (excluding menses). While advanced age is associated with an increase in hemorrhagic complications, the benefit of thrombolytic therapy in the elderly appears to justify its use in most cases, particularly if no other contraindications are present and the amount of myocardium in jeopardy appears to be substantial.

Relative contraindications to thrombolytic therapy, which require careful assessment of the risk:benefit ratio, include current use of anticoagulants (international normalized ratio of >2 to 3), a recent (within 2 weeks) invasive or surgical procedure or prolonged (>10 min) cardiopulmonary resuscitation, known bleeding diasthesis, pregnancy, a hemorrhagic ophthalmic condition (e.g., hemorrhagic diabetic retinopathy), active peptic ulcer disease, and a history of severe hypertension that is currently adequately controlled. Because of the risk of an allergic reaction, patients should not receive streptokinase if that agent had been received within the preceding 5 days to 2 years.

Allergic reactions to streptokinase occur in approximately 2 percent of cases. While a minor degree of hypotension occurs in 4 to 10 percent of patients given these agents, marked hypotension occurs, though rarely, in association with severe allergic reactions.

Hemorrhage is the most frequent and potentially the most serious complication. Since bleeding episodes that require transfusion are more common when patients require invasive procedures, unnecessary venous or arterial interventions should be avoided in patients receiving thrombolytic agents. Hemorrhagic stroke is the most serious complication and occurs in approximately 0.5 to 0.7 percent of cases. This rate increases with advancing age, with patients older than 70 years experiencing roughly twice the rate of intracranial hemorrhage as those younger than 65 years. Large-scale intervention trials have suggested that the rate of intracranial hemorrhage with tPA is slightly higher than that seen with streptokinase.

Routine angiography after thrombolysis with the intent of performing angioplasty on underlying coronary artery stenoses in the culprit vessel is not recommended owing to higher rates of abrupt closure of the infarct-related coronary artery with a need for urgent coronary artery bypass surgery as well as a trend toward an increase in mortality rate. Instead, after thrombolytic therapy, cardiac catheterization and coronary angiography should be carried out if either (1) there is evidence of failure of reperfusion (persistent chest pain and ST-segment elevation beyond 90 min) in which case a *rescue angioplasty* should be considered, or (2) there is coronary artery reocclusion (reelevation of ST segments and/or recurrent chest pain) or recurrent ischemia develops (such as recurrent angina in the early hospital course or a positive exercise stress test prior to discharge), in which case an *elective angioplasty* should be considered. Coronary artery bypass surgery should be reserved for patients whose coronary anatomy is unsuited to angioplasty but in whom revascularization appears to be advisable because of extensive jeopardized myocardium or recurrent ischemia.

Primary Percutaneous Transluminal Coronary Angioplasty (See also Chap. 245) Primary percutaneous transluminal coronary angioplasty (PTCA) without preceding thrombolysis carried out on an emergency basis in the first few hours of infarction is also effective in restoring perfusion in acute myocardial infarction. It has the advantage of being applicable to patients who have contraindications to thrombolytic therapy but otherwise are considered appropriate candidates for reperfusion. It appears to be more effective than thrombolysis in opening occluded coronary arteries and, when performed by experienced operators in dedicated medical centers, is associated with a better short-term and long-term clinical outcome. Efforts are underway to determine whether the advantages of primary PTCA reported from organized research efforts can be replicated in routine clinical practice. However, this technique is expensive in terms of personnel and facilities, and its applicability is seriously limited by logistic considerations.

Subgroups of patients in whom direct PTCA may provide a special benefit over thrombolytic therapy include patients with cardiogenic shock and others at high risk because of advanced age (>70 years) or hemodynamic compromise (systolic arterial pressure >100 mmHg).

HOSPITAL PHASE MANAGEMENT

CORONARY CARE UNITS These units are routinely equipped with a system that permits continuous monitoring of the cardiac rhythm of *each* patient and hemodynamic monitoring in *selected* patients. Defibrillators, respirators, noninvasive transthoracic pacemakers, and facilities for introducing pacing catheters and flow-directed balloon-tipped catheters are also usually available. Equally important is the organization of a highly trained team of nurses who can recognize arrhythmias, adjust the dosage of antiarrhythmic, vasoactive, and anticoagulant drugs, and perform cardiac resuscitation, including electroshock, when necessary.

Patients should be admitted to a coronary care unit early in their illness when it is expected that they will derive benefit from the sophisticated and expensive care provided (e.g., adjustment of intravenous nitroglycerin infusion rate, hemodynamic monitoring, and initiation of afterload reduction for left ventricular failure). The availability of electrocardiographic monitoring and trained personnel outside the coronary care unit has made it possible to admit lower-risk patients (e.g., those not hemodynamically compromised and without active arrhythmias) to "intermediate care units."

The duration of stay in the coronary care unit is dictated by the ongoing need for intensive care. If a myocardial infarction has been ruled out (ideally within 8 to 12 h) and symptoms are controlled with oral therapy, patients may be transferred out of the coronary care unit. Also, patients who have a confirmed acute myocardial infarction but who are considered to be at low risk (no prior infarction and no persistent chest discomfort, congestive heart failure, hypotension, or cardiac arrhythmias) may be safely transferred out of the coronary care unit in 24 to 36 h.

Activity Factors that increase the work of the heart during the initial hours of infarction may increase the size of the infarct. Therefore, patients with acute infarction should be kept at bed rest for the first 12 h. However, in the absence of complications, patients should be encouraged, under supervision, to resume an upright posture by dangling their feet over the side of the bed and sitting in a chair within the first 24 h. This practice is both psychologically beneficial and usually results in a reduction in the pulmonary capillary wedge pressure. Provided no hypotension occurs, by the third day patients typically are ambulating in their room with increasing duration and frequency, and they may shower or stand at the sink to bathe. By day 4 to 5 after infarction, patients should be increasing their ambulation progressively to a goal of 600 feet at least three times a day.

Diet Because of the risk of emesis and aspiration soon after infarction, patients should receive either nothing or only clear liquids by mouth for the first 4 to 12 h. The typical coronary care unit diet should provide 30 percent or less of total calories as fat and have a cholesterol content of ≤300 mg per day. Complex carbohydrates should make up 50 to 55 percent of total calories. Portions should not be unusually large, and the menu should be enriched with foods that are high in potassium, magnesium, and fiber but low in sodium. Diabetes mellitus and hypertriglyceridemia are managed by restriction of concentrated sweets in the diet.

Bowels Bed rest and the effect of the narcotics used for the relief of pain often lead to constipation. A bedside commode rather than a bedpan, a diet rich in bulk, and the routine use of a stool softener such as dioctyl sodium sulfosuccinate (200 mg daily) are recommended. If the patient remains constipated despite these measures, a laxative can be prescribed. Contrary to prior belief, it is safe to perform a gentle rectal examination on patients with acute myocardial infarction.

Sedation Many patients require sedation during hospitalization to withstand the period of enforced inactivity with tranquillity. Diazepam (5 mg), oxazepam (15 to 30 mg), or lorazepam (0.5 to 2 mg), given three or four times daily, is usually effective. An additional dose of any of the above medications may be given at night to ensure adequate sleep. Attention to this problem is especially important during the first few days in the coronary care unit, where the atmosphere of 24-hour vigilance may interfere with the patient's sleep. However, sedation is no substitute for reassuring, quiet surroundings. It is to be noted that many drugs used in the coronary care unit, such as atropine, H_2 blockers, and narcotics, can produce delirium, particularly in the elderly. This effect should not be confused with agitation, and it is wise to conduct a thorough review of the patient's medications before arbitrarily prescribing additional doses of anxiolytics.

PHARMACOTHERAPY FOR ACUTE INFARCTION

ANTITHROMBOTIC AGENTS The use of antiplatelet and antithrombin therapy during the initial phase of myocardial infarction is based on extensive laboratory and clinical evidence that thrombosis plays an important role in the pathogenesis of acute infarction. The primary goal of treatment with antiplatelet and antithrombin agents is to establish and maintain patency of the infarct-related artery. A secondary goal is to reduce the patient's tendency to thrombosis and thus the likelihood of mural thrombus formation or deep venous thrombosis, either of which could result in pulmonary embolization. The degree to which antiplatelet and antithrombin therapy achieves these goals partly determines how effectively it reduces the risk of mortality from acute myocardial infarction.

As noted previously (see "Initial Management in the Emergency Department," above), the standard antiplatelet agent for patients with acute myocardial infarction is aspirin. The most compelling evidence for the benefits of antiplatelet therapy (mainly with aspirin) in acute myocardial infarction is found in the comprehensive overview by the Antiplatelet Trialists' Collaboration. Data from nearly 20,000 patients with acute myocardial infarction enrolled in nine randomized trials were pooled and revealed a reduction in the mortality rate from 11.7 percent in control patients to 9.3 percent in patients receiving antiplatelet agents. This corresponds to the prevention of 24 deaths for every 1000 patients treated. Similarly, 2 strokes and 12 recurrent infarctions are prevented for every 1000 patients treated with antiplatelet therapy.

The glycoprotein IIb/IIIa receptor is the focus of intense investigation by basic and clinical scientists. Because platelet-rich thrombi are more resistant to thrombolytic agents than platelet-poor thrombi and because platelet aggregates appear to play a role in reocclusion after initially successful thrombolysis, glycoprotein IIb/IIIa inhibition may facilitate thrombolysis and reduce the rate of reocclusion of reperfused vessels. Compounds have been developed that are capable of blocking the glycoprotein IIb/IIIa receptor. These drugs appear promising in the management of myocardial infarction patients undergoing angioplasty and may also prove useful in the medical management of patients both with and without ST segment elevation at presentation.

The standard antithrombin agent used in clinical practice is heparin. Despite numerous clinical trials, the precise role of heparin in patients treated with thrombolytic agents remains uncertain. The available data fail to show any convincing benefit of heparin with respect to either coronary arterial patency or mortality rate when heparin is added to a regimen of aspirin and a non-fibrin-specific thrombolytic agent such as streptokinase. Although not conclusively proven, it appears that the immediate administration of intravenous heparin, in addition to a regimen of aspirin and tPA, helps to facilitate thrombolysis and to establish and maintain patency of the infarct-related artery. This effect is achieved at the cost of an increased risk of bleeding. Most clinicians who use tPA also administer a bolus and infusion of heparin. Commonly employed heparin regimens include a bolus of 5000 units followed by a maintenance infusion of 1000 units per hour or a bolus of 70 units per kilogram followed by a maintenance infusion of 15 units per kilogram per hour. The activated partial thromboplastin time during maintenance therapy should be 1.5 to 2 times the control value.

For patients who do not receive thrombolytic therapy, the minimum antithrombin therapy consists of 7500 units of heparin subcutaneously every 12 h until the patient is ambulatory, to prevent deep venous thrombosis. If the patient is at an increased risk of systemic or pulmonary thromboembolism (i.e., if the patient has an anterior location of the infarction, severe left ventricular dysfunction, congestive heart failure, a history of embolism, two-dimensional echocardiographic evidence of mural thrombus, or atrial fibrillation), full intravenous heparin in the dose noted above should be initiated, followed by at least 3 months of warfarin therapy.

BETA-ADRENOCEPTOR BLOCKERS The benefits of beta blockers in patients with acute myocardial infarction can be divided into those that occur immediately when the drug is given acutely and those that accrue over the long term when the drug is given for secondary prevention following an index infarction. Acute intravenous beta blockade improves the myocardial oxygen supply-demand relationship, decreases pain, reduces infarct size, and decreases the incidence of serious ventricular arrhythmias. An overview of the data from 27,000 patients enrolled in nine randomized trials in the prethrombolytic era indicates that intravenous followed by oral beta blockade

is associated with a 15 percent relative reduction in mortality, nonfatal reinfarction, and nonfatal cardiac arrest. In patients who undergo thrombolysis soon after the onset of chest pain, no incremental mortality reduction is seen with beta blockers, but recurrent ischemia and reinfarction are reduced.

Beta blocker therapy after myocardial infarction thus is useful for most patients except those in whom it is specifically contraindicated (patients with heart failure or severely compromised left ventricular function, heart block, orthostatic hypotension, or a history of asthma) and perhaps those whose excellent long-term prognosis (defined as an expected mortality rate of less than 1 percent per year) markedly diminishes any potential benefit (patients with normal ventricular function, no complex ventricular ectopy, and no angina).

ANGIOTENSIN CONVERTING ENZYME INHIBITORS These drugs reduce mortality following myocardial infarction; the mortality benefits of angiotensin converting enzyme (ACE) inhibitors are additive to those achieved with aspirin and beta blockers. The maximum benefit is seen in high-risk patients (those who are elderly or have an anterior infarction, a prior infarction, and/or globally depressed left ventricular function) but there is also evidence suggesting that a short-term benefit occurs when ACE inhibitors are prescribed unselectively to all hemodynamically stable patients with infarction (i.e., those with a systolic pressure greater than 100 mmHg). The mechanism involves a reduction in ventricular remodeling after infarction (see "Ventricular Dysfunction," below) with a subsequent reduction in the risk of congestive heart failure. The rate of recurrent infarction also may be lower in patients treated chronically with ACE inhibitors after infarction.

ACE inhibitors should be prescribed within 24 h to all myocardial infarction patients with overt congestive heart failure as well as to hemodynamically stable patients with ST-segment elevation or left bundle branch block. There is little evidence to support the use of ACE inhibitors in myocardial infarction patients who present without ST-segment changes or only with ST-segment depression and without congestive heart failure. Prior to hospital discharge, left ventricular function should be assessed with an imaging study. ACE inhibition should be continued indefinitely in patients who have clinically evident congestive heart failure or in whom an imaging study shows a reduction in global left ventricular function or a large regional wall motion abnormality.

OTHER AGENTS Although the actual impact on mortality is slight (three to four lives saved per 1000 patients treated), *nitrates* (intravenous or oral) may be useful in the relief of pain associated with acute myocardial infarction. Favorable effects on the ischemic process and ventricular remodeling (see below) have led many physicians to routinely use intravenous nitroglycerin (5 to 10 μg/min initial dose and up to 200 μg/min as long as hemodynamic stability is maintained) for the first 24 to 48 h after the onset of infarction.

Results of multiple trials of different *calcium antagonists* have failed to establish a role for these agents in the treatment of most patients with myocardial infarction, in contrast to the more consistent data that exist for other drugs (e.g., beta blockers, aspirin, thrombolytic agents). The routine use of calcium antagonists cannot be recommended.

Intracellular *magnesium* levels are frequently reduced in patients with myocardial infarction, but this deficit is not adequately reflected in serum measurements, as magnesium is predominantly an intracellular ion, and less than 1 percent of the total body stores of magnesium are intravascular. Whether giving routine empirical supplemental infusions of magnesium to high-risk patients with myocardial infarction is beneficial remains an open question. At present, all patients should have a serum magnesium measurement on admission, and any demonstrated deficits should be corrected to minimize the risk of arrhythmias. There does not appear to be any benefit in the routine use of magnesium when it is administered late (greater than 6 h) or to patients with an uncomplicated infarction who have a low mortality risk.

COMPLICATIONS OF MYOCARDIAL INFARCTION AND THEIR TREATMENT

VENTRICULAR DYSFUNCTION Following myocardial infarction, the left ventricle undergoes a series of changes in shape, size, and thickness in both the infarcted and noninfarcted segments. This process is referred to as *ventricular remodeling* and generally precedes the development of clinically evident congestive heart failure in the months to years after infarction. Soon after myocardial infarction, the left ventricle begins to dilate. Acutely, this results from expansion of the infarct (i.e., slippage of muscle bundles, disruption of normal myocardial cells, and tissue loss within the necrotic zone, resulting in disproportionate thinning and elongation of the infarct zone). Later, lengthening of the noninfarcted segments occurs as well. The overall chamber enlargement that occurs is related to the size and location of the infarct, with greater dilation following infarction of the apex of the left ventricle and causing more marked hemodynamic impairment, more frequent heart failure, and a poorer prognosis. Progressive dilation and its clinical consequences may be ameliorated by therapy with ACE inhibitors and other vasodilators (e.g., nitrates) (Fig. 243-2). Thus, in patients with a lowered ejection fraction (less than 40 percent), regardless of whether or not heart failure is present, ACE inhibitors should be prescribed.

HEMODYNAMIC ASSESSMENT Pump failure is now the primary cause of in-hospital death from acute myocardial infarction. The extent of ischemic necrosis correlates well with the degree of pump failure and with mortality, both early (within 10 days of infarction) and later. The most common clinical signs are pulmonary rales and S_3 and S_4 gallop rhythms. Pulmonary congestion is also frequently seen on the chest roentgenogram. Elevation of left ventricular filling pressure and pulmonary artery pressure are the characteristic hemodynamic findings, but it should be appreciated that these findings may result from a reduction of ventricular compliance (diastolic failure) and/or a reduction of stroke volume with secondary cardiac dilation (systolic failure) (Chap. 232).

A classification originally proposed by Killip divides patients into four groups: class I, no signs of pulmonary or venous congestion; class II, moderate heart failure as evidenced by rales at the lung bases, S_3 gallop, tachypnea, or signs of failure of the right side of the heart, including venous and hepatic congestion; class III, severe heart failure, pulmonary edema; and class IV, shock with systolic pressure less than 90 mmHg and evidence of peripheral vasoconstriction, peripheral cyanosis, mental confusion, and oliguria. The expected hospital mortality rate of patients in these clinical classes when this classification was established in 1967 was as follows: class I, 0 to 5 percent; class II, 10 to 20 percent; class III, 35 to 45 percent; and class IV, 85 to 95 percent. With advances in management, the mortality rate has fallen, perhaps by as much as one-third to one-half, in each class.

Hemodynamic evidence of abnormal left ventricular function appears when contraction is seriously impaired in 20 to 25 percent of the left ventricle. Infarction of 40 percent or more of the left ventricle usually results in cardiogenic shock (see below). Positioning of a balloon flotation catheter in the pulmonary artery permits monitoring of left ventricular filling pressure; this technique is useful in patients who exhibit hypotension and/or clinical evidence of heart failure. Cardiac output can also be determined with a pulmonary artery catheter. With the addition of intraarterial pressure monitoring, systemic vascular resistance can be calculated as a guide to adjusting vasopressor and vasodilator therapy. Some patients with acute myocardial infarction have markedly elevated left ventricular filling pressures (>22 mmHg) and normal cardiac indexes [>2.6 and >3.6 L/(min/m²)], while others have relatively low filling pressures (<15 mmHg) and reduced cardiac indexes. The former patients usually benefit from diuresis, while the latter may respond to volume expansion by means of intravenous administration of colloid-containing solutions.

Hypovolemia This is an easily corrected condition that may contribute to the hypotension and vascular collapse associated with myocardial infarction in some patients. Hypovolemia may be secondary to previous diuretic use, to reduced fluid intake during the early stages of the illness, and/or to vomiting associated with pain or medications. Consequently, hypovolemia should be identified and corrected in patients with acute myocardial infarction and hypotension before more vigorous forms of therapy are embarked on. Central venous pressure reflects right rather than left ventricular filling pressure and is an inadequate guide for adjustment of blood volume, since left ventricular function is almost always affected much more adversely than right ventricular function in acute myocardial infarction. The optimal left ventricular filling or pulmonary artery wedge pressure may vary considerably among patients. Each patient's ideal level (generally approximately 20 mmHg) is reached by cautious fluid administration during careful monitoring of oxygenation and cardiac output. Eventually, the cardiac output plateaus and further increases in left ventricular filling pressure only increase congestive symptoms and decrease systemic oxygenation without raising arterial pressure.

℞ TREATMENT

The management of heart failure in association with myocardial infarction is similar to that of acute heart failure secondary to other forms of heart disease (avoidance of hypoxemia, diuresis, afterload reduction, inotropic support) (Chap. 233), except that the benefits of digitalis administration in acute myocardial infarction are unimpressive. On the other hand, diuretic agents are extremely effective, as they diminish pulmonary congestion in the presence of systolic and/or diastolic heart failure. A fall in left ventricular filling pressure and an improvement in orthopnea and dyspnea follow the intravenous administration of furosemide. This drug should be used with caution, however, as it can result in a massive diuresis with associated decrease in plasma volume, cardiac output, systemic blood pressure, and hence coronary perfusion. Nitrates in various forms may be used to decrease preload and congestive symptoms. Oral isosorbide dinitrate, topical nitroglycerin ointment, or intravenous nitroglycerin all have the advantage over a diuretic of lowering preload through venodilation without decreasing the total plasma volume. In addition, nitrates may improve ventricular compliance if ischemia is present, as ischemia causes an elevation of left ventricular filling pressure. The patient with pulmonary edema is treated as described in Chap. 233, but vasodilators must be used with caution to prevent serious hypotension. As noted earlier, ACE inhibitors are an ideal class of drugs for management of ventricular dysfunction following myocardial infarction, especially for the long term.

CARDIOGENIC SHOCK In recent years, efforts to reduce infarct size and prompt treatment of ongoing ischemia and other complications of myocardial infarction appear to have reduced the incidence of cardiogenic shock from 20 percent to about 7 percent. Only 10 percent of patients with this condition present with it on admission, while 90 percent develop it during hospitalization. Typically, patients who develop cardiogenic shock have severe multivessel coronary artery disease with evidence of "piecemeal" necrosis extending outward from the original infarct zone.

It is useful to consider cardiogenic shock as a form of severe left ventricular failure. This syndrome is characterized by marked hypotension with systolic arterial pressure of <80 mmHg and a marked reduction of cardiac index [<1.8 L/(min/m²)] in the face of an elevated left ventricular filling (pulmonary capillary wedge) pressure (>18 mmHg). Hypotension alone is not a basis for the diagnosis of cardiogenic shock, because many patients who make an uneventful recovery will have serious hypotension (systolic pressure of <80 mmHg) for several hours. Such patients often have low left ventricular filling pressures, and their hypotension usually resolves with the administration of intravenous fluids. In contrast to hypovolemic hypotension, cardiogenic shock is generally associated with a mortality rate of >70 percent; however, recent efforts to restore perfusion by coronary angioplasty or surgical revascularization suggest that this high mortality rate can be lowered by as much as one-half.

Risk factors for the in-hospital development of shock include advanced age, a depressed left ventricular ejection fraction on admission, a large infarct, previous myocardial infarction, and a history of diabetes mellitus. Patients with several of these risk factors should be considered for cardiac catheterization and mechanical reperfusion (by angioplasty or surgery) *before* the development of shock.

Pathophysiology of Severe Power Failure   A marked reduction in the quantity of contracting myocardium is the cause of cardiogenic shock in myocardial infarction. The initial insult reduces arterial pressure, and the reduction in coronary perfusion pressure and myocardial blood flow initiates a vicious cycle that further impairs myocardial function and may increase the size of the infarct. Arrhythmias and metabolic acidosis also contribute to this deterioration, because they are the result of inadequate perfusion. It is this positive feedback loop that accounts for the high mortality rate associated with the shock syndrome.

℞ TREATMENT

The physiology and ominous prognosis of this condition dictate that all patients with shock should, if possible, have continuous monitoring of arterial pressure and of left ventricular filling pressure (as reflected in the pulmonary capillary wedge pressure measured with a pulmonary artery balloon catheter) as well as frequent determinations of cardiac output. When pulmonary edema coexists, endotracheal intubation may be necessary to ensure oxygenation. The relief of pain is important, as some vasodepressor reflex activity may be a response to severe pain. However, narcotics should be used cautiously, in view of their propensity to lower arterial pressure. The primary objective of treatment is to maintain coronary perfusion by raising the arterial blood pressure with vasopressors (see below), intraaortic balloon counterpulsation, and manipulation of blood volume to a level that ensures an optimum left ventricular filling pressure (approximately 20 mmHg). The latter may require either infusion of crystalloid or diuresis.

In patients seen within the first 4 to 8 h of the onset of infarction, early reperfusion by PTCA (see "Primary Percutaneous Transluminal Coronary Angioplasty," above) may improve left ventricular function dramatically, thereby interrupting the cycle of hemodynamic deterioration.

Vasopressors   A variety of intravenous drugs may be used to augment arterial pressure and cardiac output in patients with cardiogenic shock. Unfortunately, all have important disadvantages or problems, and none has been shown to change the outcome in patients with established shock. *Isoproterenol* is a sympathomimetic amine that is now rarely used in the treatment of shock due to myocardial infarction. Although this agent increases contractility, it also produces peripheral vasodilation and increases heart rate. The resulting increase in myocardial oxygen consumption and reduction of coronary perfusion pressure may extend the area of ischemic injury. *Norepinephrine* (Chap. 70) is a potent alpha-adrenergic agent with powerful vasoconstrictor properties that also possesses beta-adrenergic activity and therefore enhances contractility. Because the increase in afterload and contractility associated with its use causes a marked increase in myocardial oxygen consumption, it should be reserved for desperate situations or for patients with cardiogenic shock and reduced systemic vascular resistance. It should be started at 2 to 4 μg/min. If pressure cannot be maintained with a dosage of 15 μg/min, it is unlikely that a further increase will be beneficial. *Dopamine* (Chap. 70) is useful in many patients with power failure. At low doses [2 to 10 μg/kg per min], the drug has positive chronotropic and inotropic effects as a consequence of beta receptor stimulation. At higher doses, a vasoconstrictor effect results from alpha receptor stimulation. At lower doses [≤2 μg/kg per min], dopamine also has the unique effect of dilating the renal and splanchnic vascular beds and apparently has little effect on myocardial oxygen consumption. Intravenous dopamine is started at an infusion rate of 2 to 5 μg/kg per min, and the dosage is increased every 2

to 5 min up to a maximum of 20 to 50 μg/kg per min. Systolic arterial blood pressure should be maintained at approximately 90 mmHg. *Dobutamine* is a synthetic sympathomimetic amine with positive inotropic action and minimal positive chronotropic or peripheral vasoconstrictive activity in the usual dosage range of 2.5 to 10 μg/kg per min. It should not be employed when a vasoconstrictor effect is required. However, in patients with less profound degrees of hypotension, dobutamine may be an extremely useful agent, particularly if positive chronotropy is to be avoided.

Amrinone and *milrinone* are positive inotropic agents without catecholamine structure or activity that act by inhibiting phosphodiesterase. These drugs resemble dobutamine in pharmacologic activity, although they have a more potent vasodilating action. For amrinone, an initial loading dose of 0.75 mg/kg is given over 2 to 3 min. If effective, it is followed by an infusion of 5 to 10 μg/kg per min. If necessary, the dose may then be increased up to 15 μg/kg per min for short periods. Milrinone is given as a loading dose of 50 μg/kg over 10 min followed by a maintenance infusion of 0.375 to 0.75 μg/kg per min.

Aortic Counterpulsation   In cardiogenic shock, mechanical assistance with an intraaortic balloon pumping system capable of augmenting both diastolic pressure and cardiac output may be helpful. A sausage-shaped balloon at the end of a catheter is introduced percutaneously into the aorta via the femoral artery, and the balloon is automatically inflated during early diastole, thereby augmenting coronary blood flow. The balloon collapses in early systole, thereby reducing the afterload against which left ventricular ejection takes place. Improvement in hemodynamic status has been observed with balloon pumping in a large number of patients. In the absence of early revascularization, however, long-term survival following this mode of therapy in patients with cardiogenic shock is still disappointing. The balloon counterpulsation system may best be reserved for patients whose condition merits mechanical (surgical or angioplastic) intervention (e.g., patients with continuing ischemia, ventricular septal rupture, or mitral regurgitation) and in whom a successful result is likely to reverse the cardiogenic shock. Intraaortic balloon pumping is contraindicated if aortic regurgitation is present or aortic dissection is suspected.

There is reason to believe that results of therapy for the shock syndrome secondary to myocardial infarction, while improving gradually as a result of meticulous attention to the details outlined above, will continue to be disappointing overall because a large fraction of patients with the syndrome have large areas of infarcted myocardium with severe, diffuse coronary atherosclerosis. There is suggestive evidence that dramatic results can be achieved with emergency revascularization surgery, or more commonly, coronary angioplasty. However, only a minority of patients developing cardiogenic shock have prompt access to these expensive techniques, and it is hoped that the widespread and early application of thrombolytic therapy will reduce the amount of myocardium that becomes necrotic and thereby reduce the incidence of this syndrome.

RIGHT VENTRICULAR INFARCTION   Approximately one-third of patients with inferoposterior infarction demonstrate at least a minor degree of right ventricular necrosis. An occasional patient with inferoposterior left ventricular infarction also has extensive right ventricular myocardial infarction, and rare patients present with infarction limited primarily to the right ventricle. Clinically significant right ventricular infarction causes signs of severe right ventricular failure (jugular venous distention, Kussmaul's sign, hepatomegaly) with or without hypotension. ST-segment elevations of the right-sided precordial electrocardiographic leads, particularly lead V_4R, are frequently present in the first 24 h in patients with right ventricular infarction. Two-dimensional echocardiography is helpful in determining the degree of right ventricular dysfunction. Catheterization of the right side of the heart often reveals a distinctive hemodynamic pattern resembling cardiac tamponade or constrictive pericarditis (steep right atrial "y" descent and an early diastolic dip and plateau in right ventricular waveforms) (Chap. 240). Therapy consists of volume expansion to maintain adequate right ventricular preload and efforts to improve left ventricular performance with attendant reduction in pulmonary capillary wedge and pulmonary arterial pressures.

MECHANICAL CAUSES OF HEART FAILURE **Free Wall Rupture** Myocardial rupture is a dramatic complication of myocardial infarction that is most likely to occur during the first week after the onset of symptoms; its frequency increases with the age of the patient. First infarction, a history of hypertension, no history of angina pectoris, and a relatively large Q-wave infarct are associated with a higher incidence of cardiac rupture. The clinical presentation typically is a sudden loss of pulse, blood pressure and consciousness while the electrocardiogram continues to show sinus rhythm (*apparent* electromechanical dissociation). The myocardium continues to contract, but forward flow is not maintained as blood escapes into the pericardium. Cardiac tamponade (Chap. 240) ensues, and closed-chest massage is ineffective. This condition is almost universally fatal, although dramatic cases of urgent pericardiotensis followed by successful surgical repair have been reported.

Ventricular Septal Defect The pathogenesis of perforation of the ventricular septum is similar to that of free wall rupture, but the chance of successful therapy is greater. Patients with ventricular septal rupture present with sudden, severe left ventricular failure in association with the appearance of a pansystolic murmur, often accompanied by a parasternal thrill. It is often impossible to differentiate this condition from rupture of a papillary muscle with resulting mitral regurgitation, and the presence in both conditions of a tall "v" wave in the pulmonary capillary wedge pressure further complicates the differentiation. The diagnosis of ventricular septal defect can be established by the demonstration of a left-to-right shunt (i.e., an oxygen step-up at the level of the right ventricle) by means of limited cardiac catheterization performed at the bedside using a flow-directed balloon catheter. Color flow doppler echocardiography can also be extremely useful for making this diagnosis at the bedside. A prolonged period of hemodynamic compromise may produce end-organ damage and other complications that can be avoided by early intervention, including nitroprusside infusion and intraaortic balloon counterpulsation.

The physiology of acute mitral regurgitation is similar to that of acute ventricular septal perforation in that the level of aortic systolic pressure partly determines the regurgitant volume, the principal difference being the chamber into which the regurgitant fraction is ejected. In septal perforation, a fraction of left ventricular output is ejected into the right ventricle. As in mitral regurgitation, lowering of the aortic systolic pressure by mechanical (intraaortic balloon counterpulsation) and/or pharmacologic (nitroglycerin or nitroprusside) means can decrease the hemodynamic compromise caused by perforation.

Mitral Regurgitation (See also Chap. 237) The reported incidence of apical systolic murmurs of mitral regurgitation during the first few days after the onset of a myocardial infarction varies widely (from 10 to 50 percent of patients) depending on the population studied and the acumen of the observers. Whether audible or angiographically demonstrated, mitral regurgitation is of hemodynamic importance in only a minority of these patients.

The most common cause of mitral regurgitation following myocardial infarction is dysfunction of the mitral valve due to ischemia or infarction. Left ventricular dilatation or alteration in the size or shape of the ventricle due to impaired contractility or to aneurysm formation causes disordered contraction of the papillary muscles. A papillary muscle, or, more commonly, the head of a papillary muscle, may rupture. Left ventricular function may deteriorate dramatically, with superimposition of severe mitral regurgitation. The major element in the differential diagnosis is perforation of the ventricular septum as discussed above. Surgical repair or replacement of the mitral valve may lead to dramatic improvement in patients in whom acute heart failure results primarily from severe mitral regurgitation due to papillary muscle rupture or dysfunction and in whom global ventricular function is relatively good.

If aortic systolic pressure is lowered in patients with mitral regurgitation, a greater fraction of the left ventricular output will be ejected antegradely, thus lessening the regurgitant fraction. To this end, both intraaortic balloon counterpulsation, which lowers the aortic systolic pressure mechanically, and the infusion of nitroglycerin or sodium nitroprusside, which reduce systemic vascular resistance, have been used with success in the interim management of patients with severe mitral regurgitation in the setting of acute myocardial infarction. Ideally, definitive operative treatment should be postponed until pulmonary congestion has cleared and the infarct has had time to heal. However, if the patient's hemodynamic and/or clinical condition does not improve or stabilize, surgical treatment should be undertaken, even in the acute stage.

ARRHYTHMIAS (See also Chaps. 230 and 231) The incidence of arrhythmias after myocardial infarction is higher in patients seen early after the onset of symptoms. The mechanisms responsible for infarction-related arrhythmias include autonomic nervous system imbalance, electrolyte disturbances, ischemia, and slowed conduction. An arrhythmia can usually be managed successfully if trained personnel and appropriate equipment are available when it develops. Since mortality from arrhythmia is greatest during the first few hours after infarction, it is obvious that the effectiveness of treatment relates directly to the speed with which patients come under medical observation. The prompt management of arrhythmias constitutes a significant advance in the treatment of myocardial infarction.

Ventricular Premature Beats Infrequent, sporadic ventricular premature depolarizations occur in almost all patients with infarction and do not require therapy. Whereas in the past, frequent, multifocal, or early diastolic ventricular extrasystoles (so-called warning arrhythmias) were routinely treated with antiarrhythmic drugs to reduce the risk of development of ventricular tachycardia and ventricular fibrillation, pharmacologic therapy is now reserved for patients with sustained ventricular arrhythmias. *Prophylactic antiarrhythmic therapy* (either intravenous lidocaine early or oral agents later) is *contraindicated* for ventricular premature beats in the absence of clinically important ventricular tachyarrhythmias, as such therapy may actually increase late mortality. Beta-adrenoceptor blocking agents are effective in abolishing ventricular ectopic activity in infarction patients and in the prevention of ventricular fibrillation. As described above (see "Beta-Adrenoceptor Blockers"), they should be used routinely in patients without contraindications. In addition, hypokalemia and hypomagnesemia are risk factors for ventricular fibrillation in patients with acute myocardial infarction; the serum potassium concentration should be adjusted to approximately 4.5 mmol/L and magnesium to about 2.0 mmol/L.

Ventricular Tachycardia and Fibrillation Within the first 24 h of myocardial infarction, ventricular tachycardia and fibrillation can occur without prior warning arrhythmias. The occurrence of ventricular fibrillation can be reduced by prophylactic administration of intravenous lidocaine. However, prophylactic use of lidocaine has not been shown to reduce overall mortality from acute myocardial infarction. In fact, in addition to causing possible noncardiac complications, lidocaine use may predispose to an excess risk of bradycardia and asystole. For these reasons, and with earlier treatment of active ischemia, more frequent use of beta-blocking agents, and the nearly universal success of electrical cardioversion or defibrillation, routine *prophylactic* antiarrhythmic drug therapy is no longer recommended. It should be reserved for patients who cannot reach a hospital or for those treated in hospitals that lack the constant presence in the coronary care unit of a physician or nurse trained in the recognition and treatment of ventricular fibrillation.

Sustained ventricular tachycardia that is well tolerated hemodynamically should be treated with an intravenous regimen of lidocaine [bolus of 1.0 to 1.5 mg/kg; infusion of 20 to 50 μg/kg per min], procainamide (bolus of 15 mg/kg over 20 to 30 min; infusion of 1 to 4 mg/min), or amiodarone (bolus of 75 to 150 mg over 10 to 15 min followed by infusion of 1.0 mg/min for 6 h and then 0.5 mg/min); if it does not stop promptly, electroversion should be used (Chap. 231). Electroshock (an unsynchronized discharge of 200 to 300 J) is used immediately in patients with ventricular fibrillation or when ventricular tachycardia causes hemodynamic deterioration. Ventricular tachycardia or fibrillation that is refractory to electroshock may be more responsive after treatment with epinephrine (1 mg intravenously or 10 mL of a 1:10,000 solution via the intracardiac route), bretylium (a 5-mg/kg bolus), or amiodarone (a 75 to 150-mg bolus).

Ventricular arrhythmias, including the unusual form of ventricular tachycardia known as *torsade de pointes* (Chap. 231), may occur in infarct patients as a consequence of other concurrent problems (such as hypoxia, hypokalemia, or other electrolyte disturbances) or of the toxic effects of an agent being administered to the patient (such as digoxin or quinidine). A search for such secondary causes should always be undertaken.

Although in-hospital mortality is increased, the long-term survival is good in patients who survive to hospital discharge after *primary* ventricular fibrillation, i.e., ventricular fibrillation that is a primary response to acute ischemia and is not associated with predisposing factors such as congestive heart failure, shock, bundle branch block, or ventricular aneurysm. This result is in sharp contrast to the poor prognosis for patients who develop ventricular fibrillation *secondary* to severe pump failure. In patients who develop ventricular tachycardia or ventricular fibrillation late in their hospital course (i.e., after the first 48 h), the mortality rate is increased both in hospital and during long-term follow-up. Such patients should be considered for electrophysiologic study (Chap. 231).

Accelerated Idioventricular Rhythm Accelerated idioventricular rhythm (AIVR, "slow ventricular tachycardia"), a ventricular rhythm with a rate of 60 to 100 beats per minute, occurs in 25 percent of patients with myocardial infarction. It often occurs transiently during thrombolytic therapy at the time of reperfusion. The rate of AIVR is usually similar to that of the sinus rhythm that precedes and follows it, and this similarity of rate plus the relatively minor hemodynamic effects make this rhythm more difficult to detect except by electrocardiographic monitoring. For the most part, AIVR is benign and does not presage the development of classic ventricular tachycardia. Most episodes of AIVR do not require treatment if the patient is monitored carefully, as degeneration into a more serious arrhythmia is rare, and, if it occurs, AIVR can generally be readily treated with a drug that increases the sinus rate (atropine).

Supraventricular Arrhythmias Sinus tachycardia is the most common type of supraventricular arrhythmia. If it occurs secondary to another cause (such as anemia, fever, heart failure, or a metabolic derangement), the primary problem should be treated first. However, if it appears to be due to sympathetic overstimulation, for example as part of a hyperdynamic state, then treatment with a beta blocker is indicated. Other common arrhythmias in this group are atrial flutter and atrial fibrillation, which are often secondary to left ventricular failure. Digoxin administration is usually the treatment of choice for supraventricular arrhythmias if heart failure is present. If heart failure is absent, beta blockers, verapamil, or diltiazem are suitable alternatives for controlling the ventricular rate, as they may also help control ischemia. If the abnormal rhythm persists for more than 2 h with a ventricular rate in excess of 120 beats per minute, or if tachycardia induces heart failure, shock, or ischemia (as manifested by recurrent pain or ECG changes), a synchronized electroshock (100 to 200 J) should be used.

Accelerated junctional rhythms have diverse causes but may be seen in patients with inferoposterior infarction. Digitalis excess must be ruled out as a cause. In some patients with severely compromised left ventricular function, the loss of appropriately timed atrial systole results in a marked decrease in cardiac output. Right atrial or coronary sinus pacing is indicated in such instances.

Sinus Bradycardia Treatment of sinus bradycardia is indicated if hemodynamic compromise results from the slow heart rate. Atropine is the most useful drug for increasing heart rate and should be given

intravenously in doses of 0.5 mg initially. If the rate remains below 50 to 60 beats per minute, additional doses of 0.2 mg, up to a total of 2.0 mg, may be given. Persistent bradycardia (<40 beats per minute) despite atropine may be treated with electrical pacing. Isoproterenol should be avoided.

Atrioventricular and Intraventricular Conduction Disturbances (See also Chap. 230) Both the in-hospital mortality rate and the post-discharge mortality rate of patients who have complete atrioventricular (AV) block in association with anterior infarction are markedly higher than those of patients who develop AV block with inferior infarction. This difference is related to the fact that heart block in inferior infarction is commonly a result of increased vagal tone and/or the release of adenosine and therefore is transient. In anterior wall infarction, heart block is usually related to ischemic malfunction of the conduction system, which commonly is associated with extensive myocardial necrosis.

Temporary electrical pacing provides an effective means of increasing the heart rate of patients with bradycardia due to AV block. However, acceleration of the heart rate may have only a limited impact on prognosis in patients with anterior wall infarction and complete heart block in whom the large size of the infarct is the major factor determining outcome. It should be carried out if it improves hemodynamics, however. Pacing does appear to be beneficial in patients with inferoposterior infarction who have complete heart block associated with heart failure, hypotension, marked bradycardia, or significant ventricular ectopic activity. A subgroup of these patients, those with right ventricular infarction, often respond poorly to ventricular pacing because of the loss of the atrial contribution to ventricular filling. In such patients, dual-chamber atrioventricular sequential pacing may be required.

External noninvasive pacing electrodes should be positioned in a "demand" mode for patients with sinus bradycardia (rate < 50 beats per minute) that is unresponsive to drug therapy, Mobitz II second-degree AV block, third-degree heart block, or bilateral bundle branch block (e.g., right bundle branch block plus left anterior fascicular block). Retrospective studies suggest that permanent pacing may reduce the long-term risk of sudden death due to bradyarrhythmias in the rare patient who develops combined persistent bifascicular and transient third-degree heart block during the acute phase of myocardial infarction.

OTHER COMPLICATIONS   Recurrent Chest Discomfort Recurrent angina develops in approximately 25 percent of patients hospitalized for acute myocardial infarction. This percentage is even higher in patients who undergo successful thrombolysis. Since recurrent or persistent ischemia often heralds *extension* of the original infarct or *reinfarction* in a new myocardial zone and is associated with a doubling of risk following acute myocardial infarction, patients with these symptoms should be considered for repeat thrombolysis or referred for prompt coronary arteriography and mechanical revascularization. Repeat administration of a thrombolytic agent is an alternative to early mechanical revascularization.

Pericarditis (See also Chap. 240) Pericardial friction rubs and/or pericardial pain are frequently encountered in patients with acute transmural myocardial infarction. This complication can usually be managed with aspirin (650 mg qid). It is important to diagnose the chest pain of pericarditis accurately, since failure to appreciate it may lead to the erroneous diagnosis of recurrent ischemic pain and/or infarct extension, with resulting inappropriate use of anticoagulants, nitrates, beta blockers, or coronary arteriography. Anticoagulants potentially could cause tamponade in the presence of acute pericarditis (as manifested by either pain or persistent rub), and therefore should not be used unless there is a compelling indication.

An infrequently occurring syndrome (post-myocardial infarction syndrome or Dressler's syndrome), characterized by fever and pleuropericardial chest pain, is thought to be due to an autoimmune pericarditis, pleuritis, and/or pneumonitis. It may begin from a few days to 6 weeks after myocardial infarction and usually responds promptly to therapy with salicylates.

Thromboembolism Clinically apparent thromboembolism complicates acute myocardial infarction in approximately 10 percent of cases, but embolic lesions are found in 20 percent of patients in necropsy series, suggesting that thromboembolism is often clinically silent. Thromboembolism is considered to be at least an important contributing cause of death in 25 percent of infarct patients who die following admission to the hospital. Arterial emboli originate from left ventricular mural thrombi, while most pulmonary emboli arise in the leg veins.

Thromboembolism typically occurs in association with large infarcts (especially anterior), heart failure, and a left ventricular thrombus detected by echocardiography. The incidence of arterial embolism from a clot originating in the ventricle at the site of an infarction is small but real. Two-dimensional echocardiography reveals left ventricular thrombi in about one-third of patients with anterior wall infarction but in few patients with inferior or posterior infarction. Arterial embolism often presents as a major complication, such as hemiparesis when the cerebral circulation is involved or hypertension if the renal circulation is compromised. When a thrombus has been clearly demonstrated by echocardiographic or other techniques or when a large area of regional wall motion abnormality is seen even in the absence of a detectable mural thrombus, systemic anticoagulation should be undertaken (in the absence of contraindications), as the incidence of embolic complications appears to be markedly lowered by such therapy. The appropriate duration of therapy is unknown, but 3 to 6 months is probably prudent.

Left Ventricular Aneurysm The term *ventricular aneurysm* is usually used to describe *dyskinesis* or local expansile paradoxical wall motion. Normally functioning myocardial fibers must shorten more if stroke volume and cardiac output are to be maintained in patients with ventricular aneurysm; if they cannot, overall ventricular function is impaired. True aneurysms are composed of scar tissue and neither predispose to nor are associated with cardiac rupture.

The complications of left ventricular aneurysm do not usually occur for weeks to months following myocardial infarction; they include congestive heart failure, arterial embolism, and ventricular arrhythmias. Apical aneurysms are the most common and the most easily detected by clinical examination. The physical finding of greatest value is a double, diffuse, or displaced apical impulse. Ventricular aneurysms are readily detected by two-dimensional echocardiography, which may also reveal a mural thrombus in an aneurysm.

Rarely, myocardial rupture may be contained by a local area of pericardium, along with organizing thrombus and hematoma. Over time, this *pseudoaneursym* enlarges, maintaining communication with the left ventricular cavity via a narrow neck. Because spontaneous rupture of a pseudoaneursym often occurs, this defect should be surgically repaired if recognized.

POSTINFARCTION RISK STRATIFICATION AND MANAGEMENT

Many clinical factors have been identified that are associated with an increase in cardiovascular risk following initial recovery from a myocardial infarction. Some of the most important factors include persistent ischemia (spontaneous or provoked), depressed left ventricular ejection fraction (less than 40 percent), rales above the lung bases on physical examination or congestion on chest radiograph, and symptomatic ventricular arrhythmias. Other features associated with increased risk include a history of previous myocardial infarction, age over 70 years, diabetes, prolonged sinus tachycardia, hypotension, the occurrence of ST-segment changes at rest without angina ("silent ischemia"), an abnormal signal-averaged electrocardiogram, nonpatency of the infarct-related coronary artery (if angiography is undertaken), and persistent advanced heart block or a new intraventricular

conduction abnormality on the electrocardiogram. Therapy must be individualized depending on the relative importance of the risk(s) present.

The goal of preventing reinfarction and death following recovery from myocardial infarction has led to strategies to evaluate risk following infarction. Early after infarction, this evaluation generally involves the use of noninvasive testing. In stable patients, submaximal exercise stress testing may be carried out prior to hospital discharge to detect residual ischemia and ventricular ectopy, and to provide the patient with a guideline for exercise in the early recovery period. Alternatively, or in addition, a maximal (symptom-limited) exercise stress test may be carried out 4 to 6 weeks after infarction. Evaluation of left ventricular function at rest and during exercise is usually warranted as well. Recognition of a depressed left ventricular ejection fraction by echocardiography or radionuclide ventriculography identifies patients who should receive ACE inhibitors (see "Angiotensin Converting Enzyme Inhibitors," above). Patients in whom angina is induced at relatively low workloads, those who have a large reversible defect on perfusion imaging or a depressed ejection fraction and demonstrable ischemia, and those in whom exercise provokes symptomatic ventricular arrhythmias should be considered at high risk for recurrent myocardial infarction or death from arrhythmia, and cardiac catheterization with coronary angiography and/or invasive electrophysiologic evaluation is advised.

Exercise tests also aid in formulating an individualized exercise prescription, which can be much more vigorous in patients who tolerate exercise without any of the above-mentioned adverse signs. Additionally, predischarge stress testing may provide an important psychological benefit, building the patient's confidence by demonstrating a reasonable exercise tolerance. Furthermore, particularly when no arrhythmias or signs of ischemia are identified, the patient benefits by the physician's reassurance that objective evidence suggests no immediate jeopardy.

In many hospitals a cardiac rehabilitation program with progressive exercise is initiated in the hospital and continued after discharge. Ideally, such programs should include an educational component that informs patients about their disease and its risk factors.

The usual duration of hospitalization for an uncomplicated myocardial infarction is 5 to 6 days. The remainder of the convalescent phase may be accomplished at home. During the first 2 weeks, the patient should be encouraged to increase activity by walking about the house and outdoors in good weather. Normal sexual activity may be resumed during this period. After 2 weeks, the physician must regulate the patient's activity on the basis of exercise tolerance. It is during this period of increasing activity that the patient may become aware of profound fatigue. Postural hypotension may still be a problem. Most patients will be able to return to work within 2 to 4 weeks.

SECONDARY PREVENTION OF INFARCTION

A variety of secondary preventive measures are at least partly responsible for the improvement in long-term mortality and morbidity following myocardial infarction. Long-term treatment with an antiplatelet agent following a myocardial infarction is associated with a 25 percent reduction in the risk of recurrent infarction, stroke, or cardiovascular mortality (36 fewer events for every 1000 patients treated). In addition, in patients taking aspirin chronically, myocardial infarctions tend to be smaller and are more likely to be non-Q-wave in nature. ACE inhibitors should be used indefinitely by patients with clinically evident heart failure, a moderate decrease in global ejection fraction, or a large regional wall motion abnormality to prevent late ventricular remodeling and recurrent ischemic events.

The chronic routine use of oral beta-adrenoceptor blockers for at least 2 years following acute myocardial infarction is supported by well-conducted placebo-controlled trials that have convincingly demonstrated reductions in the rates of total mortality, sudden death, and, in some instances, reinfarction. In contrast, calcium antagonists are not recommended for routine secondary prevention.

Evidence suggests that warfarin lowers late mortality and the incidence of reinfarction after an acute myocardial infarction. Since studies comparing aspirin and warfarin therapy separately or in combination have not yet been completed, most physicians use aspirin routinely in all patients without contraindications and add warfarin in patients at increased risk of embolism (see "Thromboembolism," above).

Finally, risk factors for *atherosclerosis* (Chap. 242) should be discussed with the patient, and, when possible, favorably modified. In particular, efforts should be made to ensure the cessation of smoking and the control of hypertension and hyperlipidemia (the target low-density lipoprotein level is less than 100 mg/dL). In addition, regular physical exercise and reduction of emotional stress should be encouraged. Hormone replacement therapy should be considered for postmenopausal women recovering from myocardial infarction, although the question of whether to use this modality may be complex given individual patient preferences and the small but finite risk of breast cancer.

BIBLIOGRAPHY

AMERICAN HEART ASSOCIATION: *Heart and Stroke Facts: 1995 Statistical Supplement.* Dallas, American Heart Association, 1995

ANTIPLATELET TRIALISTS' COLLABORATION: Collaborative overview of randomized trials of antiplatelet therapy. I: Prevention of death, myocardial infarction, and stroke by prolonged antiplatelet therapy in various categories of patients. BMJ 308:81, 1994

ANTMAN EM: Magnesium in acute MI. Timing is critical. Circulation 92:2367, 1995

————: Overview of medical therapy. In R Califf (ed): *Acute Myocardial Infarction and Other Acute Ischemic Syndromes,* in E Braunwald (Series ed): *Atlas of Heart Diseases,* vol. 8. Philadelphia, Current Medicine, 1996

———— et al: Evaluation of a rapid bedside assay for detection of serum cardiac troponin T. J Am Med Assoc 273:1279, 1995

CALIFF RM: Acute myocardial infarction. In *Cardiovascular Therapeutics,* TW Smith (ed). Philadelphia, Saunders, 1996, p 127

————, BENGTSON JR: Cardiogenic shock. N Engl J Med. 330:1724, 1994

COMMITTEE ON RADIONUCLIDE IMAGING: ACC/AHA Task Force Report: Guidelines for clinical use of cardiac radionuclide imaging. J Am Coll Cardiol 25:521, 1995

EPSTEIN AE et al: Mortality following ventricular arrhythmia suppression by encainide, flecainide, and moricizine after myocardial infarction. The original design concept of the Cardiac Arrhythmia Suppression Trial (CAST). J Am Med Assoc 270:2451, 1993

FALK E et al: Coronary plaque disruption. Circulation 92:657, 1995

FIBRINOLYTIC THERAPY TRIALISTS (FTT) COLLABORATIVE GROUP: Indications for fibrinolytic therapy in suspected acute myocardial infarction: Collaborative overview of early mortality and major morbidity results from all randomised trials of more than 1000 patients. Lancet 343:311, 1994

FUSTER V et al: The pathophysiology of coronary artery disease and the acute coronary syndromes. N Engl J Med. 326:242, 1992

GOLDMAN, L: Cost and quality of life: Thrombolysis and primary angioplasty. J Am Coll Cardiol 25:38S, 1995

JULIAN D, BRAUNWALD E (eds): *Management of Acute Myocardial Infarction,* London, Saunders, 1994

KINCH JW, RYAN TJ: Right ventricular infarction. N Engl J Med 330:1211, 1994

LIBBY P: Molecular basis of the acute coronary syndromes. Circulation 91:2844, 1995

MAGGIONI AP et al: Age-related increase in mortality among patients with first myocardial infarctions treated with thrombolysis. N Engl J Med 329:1442, 1993

MICHELS KB, YUSUF S: Does PTCA in acute myocardial infarction affect mortality and reinfarction rates? A quantitative verview (meta-analysis) of the randomized clinical trials. Circulation 91:476, 1995

NATIONAL HEART ATTACK ALERT PROGRAM COORDINATING COMMITEE—60 MINUTES TO TREATMENT WORKING GROUP: Emergency department: Rapid identification and treatment of patients with acute myocardial infarction. Ann Emerg Med. 23:311, 1994

PATRONO C: Aspirin as an antiplatelet drug. N Engl J Med 330:1287, 1994

PFEFFER JM et al: Angiotensin-converting enzyme inhibition and ventricular remodeling after myocardial infarction. Annu Rev Physiol 57:805, 1995

RAVKILDE J et al: Independent prognostic value of serum creatine kinase isoenzyme MB mass, cardiac troponin T and myosin light chain levels in suspected acute myocardial infarction. Analysis of 28 months of follow-up in 196 patients. J Am Coll Cardiol 25:574, 1995

ROGERS W et al: Treatment of myocardial infarction in the United States (1990 to 1993). Observations from the National Registry of Myocardial Infarction. Circulation 90:2103, 1994

RYAN TJ et al: Guidelines for the management of patients with acute myocardial infarction. A report of the American College of Cardiology/American Heart Association Task Force on Practice Guidelines. J Am Coll Cardiol 28:1328, 1996

THE GUSTO INVESTIGATORS: An international randomized trial comparing four thrombolytic strategies for acute myocardial infarction. N Engl J Med 329:673, 1993

THE TIMI IIIB INVESTIGATORS: Effects of tissue plasminogen activator and a comparison of early invasive and conservative strategies in unstable angina and non-Q-wave myocardial infarction: Results of the TIMI IIIB Trial. Circulation 89:1545, 1994

VAN BERGEN PFMM et al: Costs and effects of long-term oral anticoagulant treatment after myocardial infarction. J Am Med Assoc. 273: 925,1995

WEISMAN HF, HEALY B: Myocardial infarct expansion, infarct extension, and reinfarction: Pathophysiologic concepts. Prog Cardiovasc Dis 30:73, 1987

YUSUF S et al: Beta blockade during and after myocardial infarction: An overview of the randomized trials. Prog Cardiovasc Dis 27:335, 1985

244   *Andrew P. Selwyn, Eugene Braunwald*

ISCHEMIC HEART DISEASE

ETIOLOGY AND PATHOPHYSIOLOGY

Ischemia refers to a lack of oxygen due to inadequate perfusion, which results from an imbalance between oxygen supply and demand. The most common cause of myocardial ischemia is atherosclerotic disease of epicardial coronary arteries. Coronary artery disease (CAD) is the most common, serious, chronic, life-threatening illness in the United States, where more than 11 million persons have CAD. This condition causes more deaths, disability, and economic costs than many other illnesses.

By reducing the lumen of the coronary arteries, atherosclerosis causes an absolute decrease in myocardial perfusion in the basal state or limits appropriate increases in perfusion when the demand for flow is augmented. Coronary blood flow can also be limited by arterial thrombi, spasm, and rarely coronary emboli as well as by ostial narrowing due to luetic aortitis. Congenital abnormalities, such as anomalous origin of the left anterior descending coronary artery from the pulmonary artery, may cause myocardial ischemia and infarction in infancy, but this cause is very rare in adults. Myocardial ischemia can also occur if myocardial oxygen demands are abnormally increased, as in severe ventricular hypertrophy due to hypertension or aortic stenosis. The latter can present with angina that is indistinguishable from that caused by coronary atherosclerosis. A reduction in the oxygen-carrying capacity of the blood, as in extremely severe anemia or in the presence of carboxyhemoglobin, is a rare cause of myocardial ischemia. Not infrequently, two or more causes of ischemia will coexist, such as an increase in oxygen demand due to left ventricular hypertrophy and a reduction in oxygen supply secondary to coronary atherosclerosis. Often such a combination leads to clinical manifestations of ischemia.

Although the large epicardial coronary arteries are capable of constriction and relaxation, in healthy persons they serve largely as conduits and are referred to as *conductance vessels*, while the intramyocardial arterioles normally exhibit striking changes in tone and are therefore referred to as *resistance vessels*. Abnormal constriction or failure of normal dilation of the coronary resistance vessels also can cause ischemia. When it causes angina this condition is sometimes referred to as *microvascular angina*.

The normal coronary circulation is dominated and controlled by the heart's requirements for oxygen. This need is met by the ability of the coronary vascular bed to vary its resistance (and therefore blood flow) considerably while the myocardium extracts a high and relatively fixed percentage of oxygen (Chap. 13). Normally, intramyocardial resistance arterioles demonstrate an immense capacity for dilation. For example, the changing oxygen needs with exercise and emotional stress affect coronary vascular resistance and in this manner regulate the supply of oxygen and substrate (*metabolic regulation*). The coronary resistance vessels also adapt to physiologic alterations in blood pressure in order to maintain coronary blood flow at levels appropriate to myocardial needs (*autoregulation*).

CORONARY ATHEROSCLEROSIS (See also Chap. 242) Epicardial coronary arteries are a major site of atherosclerotic disease. The major risk factors for atherosclerosis [high plasma low-density lipoprotein (LDL), low plasma high-density lipoprotein (HDL), cigarette smoking, hypertension, and diabetes mellitus] are thought to disturb the normal functions of the vascular endothelium. Dysfunction of vascular endothelium and an abnormal interaction with blood monocytes and platelets lead to subintimal collections of abnormal fat, cells, and debris (i.e., atherosclerotic plaques), which develop at irregular rates in different segments of the epicardial coronary tree and lead eventually to segmental reductions in cross-sectional area. The relationship between pulsatile flow and luminal stenosis is complex, but experiments have shown that when a stenosis reduces the cross-sectional area by approximately 75 percent, a full range of increases in flow to meet increased myocardial demand is not possible. When the luminal area is reduced by more than approximately 80 percent, blood flow at rest may be reduced, and further minor decreases in the stenotic orifice can reduce coronary flow dramatically and cause myocardial ischemia.

Segmental atherosclerotic narrowing of epicardial coronary arteries is caused most commonly by the formation of a plaque, which is subject to fissuring, hemorrhage, and thrombosis. Any of these events can temporarily worsen the obstruction, reduce coronary blood flow, and cause clinical manifestations of myocardial ischemia, as described below. The location of the obstruction will influence the quantity of myocardium rendered ischemic and thus determine the severity of the clinical manifestations. Severe coronary narrowing and myocardial ischemia are frequently accompanied by the development of collateral vessels, especially when the narrowing develops gradually. When well developed, such vessels can provide sufficient blood flow to sustain the viability of the myocardium at rest but not during conditions of increased demand.

Once stenosis of a proximal epicardial artery has reduced the cross-sectional area by more than approximately 70 percent, the distal resistance vessels (when they function normally) dilate to reduce vascular resistance and maintain coronary blood flow. A pressure gradient develops across the proximal stenosis, and poststenotic pressure falls. When the resistance vessels are maximally dilated, myocardial blood flow becomes dependent on the pressure in the coronary artery distal to the obstruction. In these circumstances ischemia in the region perfused by the stenotic artery can be precipitated by increases in myocardial oxygen demands caused by physical activity, emotional stress, and/or tachycardia. Changes in the caliber of the stenosed coronary artery due to physiologic vasomotion, pathologic spasm, or small platelet plugs can all upset the critical balance between oxygen supply and demand and thus precipitate myocardial ischemia.

EFFECTS OF ISCHEMIA The inadequate oxygenation induced by coronary atherosclerosis may cause transient disturbances of the mechanical, biochemical, and electrical functions of the myocardium. The abrupt development of severe ischemia, as occurs with total or subtotal occlusion, is associated with almost instantaneous failure of normal muscle contraction and relaxation. The relatively poor perfusion of the subendocardium causes more intense ischemia of this portion of the wall. Ischemia of large portions of the ventricle will cause transient left ventricular failure, and if the papillary muscles are involved, mitral regurgitation can complicate this event. When ischemia is transient, it may be associated with angina pectoris; when

it is prolonged, it can lead to myocardial necrosis and scarring with or without the clinical picture of acute myocardial infarction (see Chap. 243). Coronary atherosclerosis is a focal process that usually causes nonuniform ischemia. Regional disturbances of ventricular contractility cause segmental bulging (dyskinesia), which can greatly reduce myocardial pump function.

Underlying these mechanical disturbances are a wide range of abnormalities in cell metabolism, function, and structure. When oxygenated, the normal myocardium metabolizes fatty acids and glucose to carbon dioxide and water. With severe oxygen deprivation, fatty acids cannot be oxidized, and glucose is broken down to lactate; intracellular pH is reduced, as are the myocardial stores of high-energy phosphates, adenosine triphosphate (ATP), and creatine phosphate. Impaired cell membrane function leads to potassium leakage and the uptake of sodium by myocytes. The severity and duration of the imbalance between myocardial oxygen supply and demand will determine whether the damage is reversible or whether it is permanent, with subsequent myocardial necrosis.

Ischemia also causes characteristic changes in the electrocardiogram (ECG) such as repolarization abnormalities, as evidenced by inversion of the T wave and, when more severe, by displacement of the ST segment (Chap. 228). Transient ST-segment depression often reflects subendocardial ischemia, while transient ST-segment elevation is thought to be caused by more severe transmural ischemia. Another important consequence of myocardial ischemia is electrical instability, which may lead to ventricular tachycardia or ventricular fibrillation (Chap. 231). Most patients who die suddenly from ischemic heart disease do so as a result of ischemia-induced malignant ventricular tachyarrhythmias (Chap. 39).

ASYMPTOMATIC VERSUS SYMPTOMATIC CORONARY ARTERY DISEASE Postmortem studies on accident victims and military casualties in western countries have shown that coronary atherosclerosis often begins to develop prior to age 20 and is widespread even among adults who were asymptomatic during life. When all age groups are considered, ischemic heart disease is the most common cause of death not only in men but also in women (Chap. 6). Exercise stress tests in asymptomatic persons may show evidence of silent myocardial ischemia, i.e., exercise-induced ECG changes not accompanied by angina; coronary angiographic studies of such persons may reveal obstructive CAD (p. 1374). Postmortem examination of patients with obstructive CAD without a history of any clinical manifestations of myocardial ischemia often shows macroscopic scars secondary to myocardial infarction in regions supplied by diseased coronary arteries. According to population studies, approximately 25 percent of patients who survive acute myocardial infarction may not reach medical attention, and these patients carry the same adverse prognosis as those who present with the classic clinical syndrome (Chap. 243). Sudden death may be unheralded and is a common presenting manifestation of ischemic heart disease (Chap. 39). Patients can also present with cardiomegaly and heart failure secondary to ischemic damage of the left ventricular myocardium that caused no symptoms prior to the development of heart failure; this condition is referred to as *ischemic cardiomyopathy*. In contrast to the asymptomatic phase of ischemic heart disease, the symptomatic phase is characterized by chest discomfort due to either angina pectoris or acute myocardial infarction (Chap. 243). Having entered the symptomatic phase, the patient may exhibit a stable or progressive course, revert to the asymptomatic stage, or suddenly die.

STABLE ANGINA PECTORIS

This episodic clinical syndrome is due to transient myocardial ischemia. Various diseases that cause myocardial ischemia as well as the numerous forms of discomfort with which it may be confused are discussed in Chap. 13. Males constitute approximately 70 percent of all patients with angina pectoris and an even greater fraction of those younger than 50 years of age.

HISTORY The typical patient with angina is a 50- to 60-year-old man or 65- to 75-year-old woman who seeks medical help for troublesome or frightening chest discomfort, usually described as heaviness, pressure, squeezing, smothering, or choking and only rarely as frank pain. When the patient is asked to localize the sensation, he or she will typically press on the sternum, sometimes with a clenched fist, to indicate a squeezing, central, substernal discomfort. This symptom is usually crescendo-decrescendo in nature and lasts 1 to 5 min. Angina can radiate to the left shoulder and to both arms and especially to the ulnar surfaces of the forearm and hand. It can also arise in or radiate to the back, neck, jaw, teeth, and epigastrium.

Although episodes of angina are typically caused by exertion (e.g., exercise, hurrying, or sexual activity) or emotion (e.g., stress, anger, fright, or frustration) and are relieved by rest, they may also occur at rest (see "Unstable Angina Pectoris," p. 1373) and at night while the patient is recumbent (angina decubitus). The patient may be awakened at night distressed by typical chest discomfort and dyspnea. The pathophysiology of nocturnal angina is analogous to that of paroxysmal nocturnal dyspnea (Chap. 233), i.e., the expansion of the intrathoracic blood volume that occurs with recumbency causes an increase in cardiac size and myocardial oxygen demand that lead to ischemia and transient left ventricular failure.

The threshold for the development of angina pectoris varies from person to person and may vary by time of day and emotional state. Many patients report a fixed threshold for angina, which occurs predictably at a certain level of activity. In these patients oxygen supply is fixed and ischemia is precipitated by an increase in myocardial oxygen demand. In other patients the threshold for angina may vary considerably within any given day and from day to day. In such patients variations in oxygen supply, most likely due to changes in coronary vascular tone, may play an important role. A patient may report symptoms upon minor exertion in the morning (a short walk or shaving) yet by midday may be capable of much greater effort without symptoms. Angina may be precipitated by unfamiliar tasks, a heavy meal, or exposure to cold.

Sharp, fleeting chest pain or prolonged, dull aches localized to the left submammary area are rarely due to myocardial ischemia. However, angina pectoris may be atypical in location and may not be strictly related to provoking factors. In addition, this symptom may exacerbate and remit over days, weeks, or months, and its occurrence can be seasonal.

Systematic questioning of the patient with suspected ischemic heart disease is important to uncover a positive family history of premature ischemic heart disease (under the age of 45 years in first-degree male relatives and under 55 in female relatives), diabetes, hyperlipidemia, hypertension, cigarette smoking, and other risk factors for coronary atherosclerosis.

PHYSICAL EXAMINATION The physical examination is often normal in the patient with stable angina. The general examination may reveal signs of risk factors associated with coronary atherosclerosis such as xanthelasma, xanthomas (Chap. 242), or diabetic skin lesions. There may also be signs of anemia, thyroid disease, and nicotine stains on the fingertips from cigarette smoking. Palpation can reveal thickened or absent peripheral arteries, signs of cardiac enlargement, and abnormal contraction of the cardiac impulse (left ventricular akinesia or dyskinesia). Examination of the fundi may reveal increased light reflexes and arteriovenous nicking as evidence of hypertension (Table 35-2), while auscultation can uncover arterial bruits, a third and/or fourth heart sound, and, if acute ischemia or previous infarction has impaired papillary muscle function, an apical systolic murmur due to mitral regurgitation. These auscultatory signs are best appreciated with the patient in the left decubitus position. Aortic stenosis, aortic regurgitation (Chap. 237), pulmonary hypertension, and hypertrophic cardiomyopathy (Chap. 239) must be excluded, since these disorders may cause angina even in the absence of coronary artery disease. Examination during an anginal attack is useful, since ischemia can cause transient left ventricular failure with the appearance of a third and/or fourth heart sound, a dyskinetic cardiac apex, mitral regurgitation, and even pulmonary edema.

LABORATORY EXAMINATION Although the diagnosis of ischemic heart disease can be made with confidence from a typical history, a number of simple laboratory tests can be helpful. The urine should be examined for evidence of diabetes mellitus and renal disease, since both these conditions may accelerate atherosclerosis. Similarly, examination of the blood should include measurements of lipids (cholesterol—total, low density, and high density), glucose, creatinine, hematocrit, and, if indicated based on the physical examination, thyroid function. A chest x-ray is important, since it may show the consequences of ischemic heart disease, i.e., cardiac enlargement, ventricular aneurysm, or signs of heart failure. Calcification of the coronary arteries can sometimes be identified on chest fluoroscopy. These signs can support the diagnosis of CAD and are important in assessing the degree of cardiac damage and the effects of treatment for heart failure.

Electrocardiogram A 12-lead ECG recorded at rest is normal in about half the patients with typical angina pectoris, but there may be signs of an old myocardial infarction (Chap. 228). Although repolarization abnormalities, i.e., T-wave and ST-segment changes and intraventricular conduction disturbances at rest, are suggestive of ischemic heart disease, they are nonspecific, since they can also occur in pericardial, myocardial, and valvular heart disease or with anxiety, changes in posture, drugs, or esophageal disease. Typical ST-segment and T-wave changes that accompany episodes of angina pectoris and disappear thereafter are more specific. The most characteristic changes include displacement of the ST segment that is similar in every way to that induced during a stress test (see below). The ST segment is usually depressed during angina but may be elevated—sometimes strikingly so—in Prinzmetal's angina.

Stress Testing The most widely used test in the diagnosis of ischemic heart disease involves recording the 12-lead ECG before, during, and after exercise on a treadmill or using a bicycle ergometer. The test consists of a standardized incremental increase in external workload while the patient's ECG, symptoms, and arm blood pressure are continuously monitored. Performance is usually symptom-limited, and the test is discontinued upon evidence of chest discomfort, severe shortness of breath, dizziness, fatigue, ST-segment depression of greater than 0.2 mV (2 mm), a fall in systolic blood pressure exceeding 10 mmHg, or the development of a ventricular tachyarrhythmia. This test seeks to discover any limitation in exercise performance and establish the relationship between chest discomfort and the typical ECG signs of myocardial ischemia. The ischemic ST-segment response is generally defined as flat depression of the ST segment of more than 0.1 mV below the baseline (i.e., the PR segment) and lasting longer than 0.08 s. This type of depression is designated "square wave" or "plateau" and is flat or downsloping (Fig. 244-1). Upsloping or junctional ST-segment changes are not considered characteristic of ischemia and do not constitute a positive test. Although T-wave abnormalities, conduction disturbances, and ventricular arrhythmias that develop during exercise should be noted, they are also not diagnostic. Negative exercise tests in which the target heart rate (85 percent of maximal heart rate for age and sex) is not achieved are considered to be nondiagnostic. When applying and interpreting ECG stress testing, one must first consider the probability that CAD exists in the patient or population under study (i.e., pretest probability). Overall, false-positive or -negative results can occur in 15 percent of cases. However, a positive result on exercise indicates that the likelihood of CAD is 98 percent in males over 50 years of age with a history of typical angina pectoris who develop chest discomfort during the test. The likelihood decreases progressively and significantly if the patient has atypical or no chest pain. The incidence of false-positive tests is significantly increased in asymptomatic men under the age of 40 or in premenopausal women with no risk factors for premature atherosclerosis (Bayes' theorem—Table 3-3). It is also increased in patients taking cardioactive drugs such as digitalis and quinidine, or in those with intraventricular conduction disturbances, resting abnormalities of the ST segment and the T wave, myocardial hypertrophy, or abnormal serum potassium levels. Obstructive disease limited to the circumflex coronary artery may result in a false-negative stress test since the posterior portion of the heart which this vessel supplies is not well represented on the surface 12-lead ECG. Since the overall sensitivity of exercise stress electrocardiography is only about 75 percent, a negative result does not exclude CAD, although it makes the likelihood of three-vessel or left main CAD extremely unlikely.

The physician should be present throughout the exercise test, and it is important to measure total duration of exercise, the times to the onset of ischemic ST-segment change and chest discomfort, the external work performed (generally expressed as a stage of exercise), and the internal cardiac work performed; the last is represented by the heart rate–blood pressure product. The depth of the ST-segment depression and the time needed for recovery of these ECG changes are also important. Because the risks of exercise testing are small but real—estimated at one fatality and two nonfatal complications per 10,000 tests—equipment for resuscitation should be available. Modified (heart rate–limited rather than symptom–limited) exercise tests can be performed safely in patients as early as 7 days after myocardial infarction.

The normal response to exercise includes a progressive increase in heart rate and blood pressure. Failure of the blood pressure to increase or an actual decrease in blood pressure with signs of ischemia during the test is an important adverse prognostic sign, since it may reflect ischemia-induced global left ventricular dysfunction. The presence of pain or severe (>0.2 mV) ST-segment depression at a low workload and ST-segment depression that persists for more than 5 min after the termination of exercise increases the specificity of the test and suggests severe ischemic heart disease and a high risk of further adverse events.

The information gained from an exercise test can be enhanced by stress myocardial perfusion imaging after the intravenous administration of a radioisotope such as thallium 201 or technetium 99m sestamibi during exercise (or a pharmacologic stress); the imaging is carried out both immediately after cessation of exercise and 4 h later (Fig. 244-2). Technetium 99m can also be used to label the blood pool for gated radioisotope angiography, which provides a measure of ventricular volume and ejection fraction at rest and during exercise. A reduction in ejection fraction during exercise is an important, albeit nonspecific, finding, and when present in CAD suggests the presence of severe ischemia and/or multivessel coronary disease.

An important fraction of patients who need noninvasive stress testing to identify myocardial ischemia and increased risk of coronary

events cannot exercise because of peripheral vascular or musculoskeletal disease. In these circumstances intravenous dipyridamole or adenosine can be used in place of exercise. The development of a transient perfusion defect with a tracer such as radioactive thallium or technetium 99m sestamibi is used to detect myocardial ischemia. Ambulatory monitoring of the ECG can assess myocardial ischemia as episodes of ST-segment depression. These techniques are sensitive and capable of identifying patients with ischemia who are at increased risk of coronary events.

Two-dimensional echocardiography of the left ventricle can assess both global and regional wall motion abnormalities due to myocardial infarction or persistent ischemia. Stress (exercise or dobutamine) echocardiography may cause the emergence of regions of akinesis or dyskinesis not present at rest. Stress echocardiography, like stress myocardial perfusion imaging, is more sensitive than exercise electrocardiography in the diagnosis of CAD.

Coronary Arteriography (See Chap. 229) This diagnostic method outlines the coronary anatomy and can be used to detect important evidence of coronary atherosclerosis or to exclude this condition. By this means, one can assess the severity of obstructive lesions and when combined with left ventricular angiocardiography can evaluate both global and regional function of the left ventricle.

Indications Coronary arteriography is indicated in (1) patients with chronic stable or unstable angina pectoris who are severely symptomatic despite medical therapy and who are being considered for revascularization, i.e., percutaneous transluminal coronary angioplasty (PTCA) or coronary artery bypass graft surgery; (2) patients with troublesome symptoms that present diagnostic difficulties in whom there is need to confirm or rule out the diagnosis of CAD; and (3) patients judged to be at high risk of sustaining coronary events based on signs of severe ischemia on noninvasive testing, regardless of the presence or severity of symptoms (see below).

Examples of other possible clinical situations include:

1. Patients with chest discomfort suggestive of angina pectoris but a negative exercise test who require a definitive diagnosis for guiding medical management, alleviating psychological stress, career or family planning, or insurance purposes.
2. Patients who have been admitted repeatedly to the hospital for suspected acute myocardial infarction but in whom this diagnosis

FIGURE 244-1 Lead V_4 at rest (*top*) and after 4½ min of exercise (*bottom*). There is 3 mm (0.3 mV) of horizontal ST-segment depression, indicating a positive test for ischemia. [*Modified from BR Chaitman Exercise Stress Testing, in E Braunwald (ed), Heart Disease, 5th ed, Philadelphia, Saunders, 1997, pp 153–176.*]

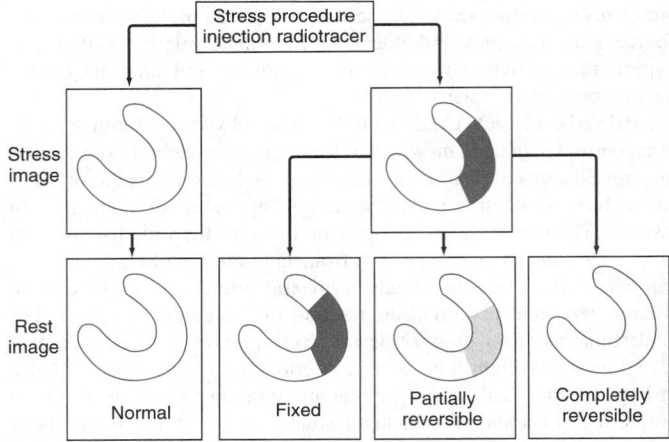

FIGURE 244-2 Interpretation of stress (exercise) and rest myocardial perfusion images. A normal image will show homogeneous accumulation of radiotracer on the exercise and rest (or delayed) image. An area with decreased uptake of the radiotracer (which appears as a darker area on a perfusion image) is referred to as a *defect*. A patient with a fixed perfusion defect will have an abnormal exercise image and an identical rest or delayed redistribution image (scarring). A partially reversible perfusion defect appears as an abnormal exercise image and an improved but still abnormal rest image (ischemia and scarring). A reversible perfusion defect appears as an abnormal exercise image and a normal rest or delayed image (ischemia). [*From FJ Wackers, in GA Beller (ed), Chronic Ischemic Heart Disease, in E Braunwald (series ed), Atlas of Heart Diseases, Philadelphia, Current Medicine, 1994.*]

has not been established and in whom the presence or absence of CAD should be determined.

3. Patients with careers that involve the safety of others (e.g., airline pilots) who have questionable symptoms, suspicious or positive noninvasive tests, and in whom there are reasonable doubts about the state of the coronary arteries.

4. Patients with aortic stenosis or hypertrophic cardiomyopathy and angina in whom the pain could be due to CAD.

5. Male patients aged 45 and females aged 55 years of age or older who will undergo valve replacement and who may or may not have clinical evidence of myocardial ischemia.

6. Patients who are at high risk after myocardial infarction because of the recurrence of angina, heart failure, frequent ventricular premature contractions, or signs of ischemia in the stress test.

7. Patients with angina pectoris, regardless of severity, in whom noninvasive testing reveals signs of severe ischemia.

PROGNOSIS

The principal prognostic indicators in patients with ischemic heart disease are the functional state of the left ventricle, the location and severity of coronary artery narrowing, and the severity or activity of myocardial ischemia. Angina pectoris of recent onset, unstable angina, angina that is unresponsive or poorly responsive to medical therapy or is accompanied by symptoms of congestive heart failure all indicate an increased risk for adverse coronary events. The same is true for the physical signs of heart failure, episodes of pulmonary edema, or for echocardiographic (or roentgenographic) evidence of cardiac enlargement. An abnormal resting ECG or positive evidence of myocardial ischemia during a stress test also indicate increased risk. Most importantly, the following signs during noninvasive testing indicate a high risk for coronary events: a strongly positive exercise test showing onset of myocardial ischemia at low workloads [$\geq$0.1 mV ST-segment depression in stage I (Bruce protocol) of the exercise test; $\geq$0.2 mV ST depression in any stage; ST depression for >5 min following the cessation of exercise; a decline in systolic pressure >10 mmHg during exercise; the development of ventricular tachyarrhythmias during exercise]; the development of large or multiple perfusion defects or increased lung uptake during stress radioisotope perfusion imaging; and a decrease in left ventricular ejection fraction during exercise on radionuclide ventriculography.

On cardiac catheterization, elevations in left ventricular end-diastolic pressure and ventricular volume and a reduced ejection fraction are the most important signs of left ventricular dysfunction and are associated with a poor prognosis. Patients with chest discomfort but normal left ventricular function and normal coronary arteries have an excellent prognosis. In patients with normal left ventricular function and mild angina but with critical stenoses ($\geq$70 percent luminal diameter) of one, two, or three epicardial coronary arteries, the 5-year mortality rates are approximately 2, 8, and 11 percent, respectively. Obstructive lesions of the proximal left anterior descending coronary artery are associated with a greater risk than are lesions of the right or left circumflex coronary artery, since the former vessel usually perfuses a greater quantity of myocardium. Critical stenosis of the left main coronary artery is associated with a mortality of about 15 percent per year.

With any degree of obstructive CAD, mortality is greatly increased when left ventricular function is impaired; conversely, at any level of left ventricular function, the prognosis is influenced importantly by the quantity of myocardium perfused by the critically obstructed vessels. Therefore, it is useful to collect all the evidence substantiating past myocardial damage (ECG and ventriculographic evidence of myocardial infarction), residual left ventricular function (ejection fraction), and risk of future damage from coronary events (extent of coronary disease and severity of ischemia defined by noninvasive stress testing). The larger the amount of established myocardial necrosis, the less the heart is able to withstand additional damage and the poorer the prognosis. All the above signs of past damage plus the risk of future damage should be considered indicators of risk.

The segmental atherosclerotic plaques in epicardial arteries go through phases of inflammatory cellular activity, degeneration, endothelial instability, abnormal vasomotion, platelet aggregation, and fissuring or hemorrhage. These factors can temporarily worsen the stenosis and cause abnormal reactivity of the vessel wall, thus exacerbating the manifestations of ischemia. The recent onset of symptoms, the appearance of severe ischemia during stress testing, and unstable angina pectoris (p. 1373) all reflect episodes of rapid progression in coronary lesions.

℞ TREATMENT

Each patient must be evaluated individually with respect to his or her expectations and goals, control of symptoms, and prevention of adverse clinical outcomes such as myocardial infarction and premature death. The degree of disability as well as the physical and emotional stress that precipitate angina must be carefully recorded in order to set treatment goals. Each management plan should consist of the following: (1) explanation and reassurance, (2) identification and treatment of aggravating conditions, (3) adaptation of activity, (4) treatment of risk factors that will decrease the occurrence of adverse coronary outcomes, (5) drug therapy for angina, and (6) consideration of mechanical revascularization.

Explanation and Reassurance Patients with ischemic heart disease need to understand their condition as best they can and to realize that a long and useful life is possible even though they suffer from angina pectoris or have experienced and recovered from an acute myocardial infarction. Offering case histories of persons in public life who have lived with coronary disease as well as results of national studies showing improved outcomes can be of great value when encouraging patients to resume or maintain activity and return to their occupation. A planned program of rehabilitation can encourage patients to lose weight, improve exercise tolerance, and control risk factors with more confidence.

Identification and Treatment of Aggravating Conditions A number of conditions that are not primarily cardiac in nature may either increase oxygen demand or decrease oxygen supply to the myocardium and may precipitate or exacerbate angina. In the former category, obesity, hypertension, and hyperthyroidism may be treated successfully in order to reduce the frequency of anginal attacks. Decreased myocardial oxygen supply may be due to reduced oxygenation of the blood (e.g., in pulmonary disease or, when carboxyhemoglobin is present, due to cigarette or cigar smoking) or decreased oxygen-carrying capacity (e.g., in anemia). Correction of these abnormalities, if present, may reduce or even eliminate anginal symptoms.

Adaptation of Activity Therapy of angina due to episodes of myocardial ischemia consists of eliminating the discrepancy between the demand of the heart muscle for oxygen and the ability of the coronary circulation to meet this demand. Most patients can be made to understand this fundamental concept and utilize it in the rational programming of activity. Many tasks that ordinarily evoke angina may be accomplished without symptoms simply by reducing the speed at which they are performed. Patients must appreciate the diurnal variation in their tolerance of certain activities and should reduce their energy requirements in the morning and immediately after meals. Sometimes it is helpful to alter the eating pattern, taking small and more frequent meals.

It may be necessary to recommend a change in employment or residence to avoid physical stress; however, with the exception of manual laborers, most patients with ischemic heart disease can usually continue to function merely by allowing more time to complete each task. In some patients, anger and frustration may be the most important factors precipitating myocardial ischemia. If these cannot be avoided, training in stress management may be useful. A treadmill exercise test to determine the approximate heart rate at which ischemic ECG changes or symptoms develop may be helpful in the development of a specific exercise program. Ambulatory recording of the ECG during daily activities may also be helpful in this regard.

Treatment of Risk Factors Although the treatment of risk factors was developed for the primary prevention of coronary atherosclerosis, there is growing evidence that it can reduce the occurrence of myocardial infarction and death both in subjects without clinical disease as well as those with a history of chronic angina or an acute coronary syndrome. A family history of premature coronary disease is an important indicator of increased risk and should trigger a search for treatable risk factors such as hyperlipidemia, hypertension, and diabetes. Obesity impairs the treatment of other risk factors, and when the patient is more than 30 percent above ideal body weight it increases the risk of adverse coronary events. In addition, obesity is often accompanied by two other risk factors—hypertension and hyperlipidemia. The treatment of obesity and these accompanying risk factors is an important component of any management plan.

Cigarette smoking accelerates coronary atherosclerosis in both sexes and at all ages and increases the risk of myocardial infarction and death. By increasing myocardial oxygen needs and reducing oxygen supply it aggravates angina. Smoking cessation studies have demonstrated important benefits with a significant decline in the occurrence of these adverse outcomes. The physician's message must be clear and strong and supported by programs that achieve and monitor abstinence. Hypertension (Chaps. 35 and 246) is associated with increased risk of adverse clinical events from coronary atherosclerosis as well as stroke. In addition, the left ventricular hypertrophy that results from sustained hypertension aggravates ischemia. There is evidence that long-term, effective treatment of hypertension can decrease the occurrence of adverse coronary events. Diabetes mellitus (Chap. 334) accelerates coronary and peripheral atherosclerosis and is frequently associated with dyslipidemias and increases in the risk of angina, myocardial infarction, and sudden coronary death. Strict control of diabetes is helpful in lowering the elevated levels of plasma LDL cholesterol and triglyceride in this condition.

The lowering of lipid levels is a critical aspect of the management of established CAD (see Chaps. 242 and 341). Patients with LDL cholesterol concentrations exceeding 3.2 mmol/L (125 mg/dL) should have these levels reduced. HMG-CoA reductase inhibitors (statins) are especially effective in this regard when they are added to a diet that restricts the intake of saturated fats. Two large clinical trials have shown that effective lowering of LDL cholesterol concentration can reduce the need for coronary revascularization as well as the occurrence of adverse events such as heart attack and death. Hypertriglyceridemia and low levels of HDL should be treated aggressively, as outlined in Chap. 341.

Physical conditioning usually improves the exercise tolerance of patients with angina and exerts substantial psychological benefits. It may also improve the chances of surviving a myocardial infarction. An exercise program within the limits of each patient's threshold for the development of angina pectoris should be encouraged.

RISK REDUCTION IN WOMEN WITH CAD The incidence of clinical CAD in premenopausal women is very low. However, following the menopause, the atherogenic risk factors increase (e.g., increased LDL, reduced HDL) and the rate of clinical coronary events accelerates to the levels observed in men. Women have not given up cigarette smoking as effectively as have men. Diabetes mellitus, which is more common in women, greatly increases the occurrence of clinical CAD and amplifies the deleterious effects of hypertension, hyperlipidemia, and smoking. The postmenopausal use of hormone replacement therapy (estrogen with or without a progestin) reduces adverse coronary outcomes but should not be given to patients at higher than usual risk of breast cancer. Cardiac catheterization and coronary revascularization are often applied more sparingly in women and at a later, and more severe, stage of the disease than in men. These factors likely explain the modest increase in complications. Although many of the clinical trials to date have not represented women adequately, the evidence is that when cholesterol lowering, beta blockers after myocardial infarction, and coronary artery bypass grafting are applied in the appropriate patient groups, women enjoy the same benefits of improved outcome as do men.

Drug Therapy The commonly used drugs for angina pectoris are summarized in Table 244-1.

NITRATES This valuable class of drugs in the management of angina pectoris acts by causing systemic venodilation, thereby reducing myocardial wall tension and oxygen requirements, as well as by dilating the epicardial coronary vessels and increasing blood flow in collateral vessels. The absorption of these agents is most rapid and complete through the mucous membranes. For this reason, nitroglycerin is administered sublingually in tablets of 0.4 or 0.6 mg. Patients with angina should be instructed to take the medication both to relieve angina and also in anticipation of stress (exercise or emotional) that is likely to induce an episode. The value of this prophylactic use of the drug cannot be overemphasized.

Table 244-1

Drugs Commonly Used for Angina Pectoris

Drug	Usual Dose	Side Effects	Contraindications
NITRATES			
Sublingual NTG	0.3–0.6 mg	Flushing, headache	Intolerance of side effects
Isosorbide dinitrate SR	80–120 mg	Flushing, headache, tolerance after 24 h	As above, worsening ischemia on withdrawal
Transdermal NTG	0.4–1.2 mg/h for 12–14 h	Flushing, headache, tolerance after 24 h	As above, worsening ischemia on withdrawal
Isosorbide-5-monitrate		Flushing, headache, tolerance after 24 h	As above, worsening ischemia on withdrawal
Oral	20–30 mg bid		
Oral SR	60–240 mg once daily		
BETA-ADRENOCEPTOR BLOCKING DRUGS			
Propranolol	20–80 mg qid	Depression, constipation, impotence, bronchospasm, heart failure, bradycardia	Asthma, AV conduction block, heart failure
Metoprolol	25–200 mg bid	As above	As above
Atenolol	50–150 mg once daily	As above	As above
CALCIUM CHANNEL BLOCKING DRUGS			
Nifedipine XL	30–90 mg once daily	Hypotension, flushing, edema, worsening angina	Hypotension, intolerance of side effects
Diltiazem SR	60–120 mg bid	Constipation, AV conduction block, worsening heart failure	AV conduction block, impaired LV function, bradycardia
Verapamil SR	180–240 mg once daily	Constipation, AV conduction block, worsening heart failure	AV conduction delay, impaired LV function, bradycardia
Amlodipine	5–10 mg once daily	Edema	Intolerance of side effects

NOTE: NTG, nitroglycerin; SR, slow release; XL, slow release preparation.

Headache and a pulsating feeling in the head are the most common side effects of nitroglycerin and fortunately only rarely become disturbing at the doses usually required to relieve or prevent angina. Nitroglycerin deteriorates with exposure to air, moisture, and sunlight, so that if the drug neither relieves discomfort or headache nor produces a slight sensation of burning at the sublingual site of absorption, the preparation may be inactive and a fresh supply should be obtained. If relief is not achieved after the first dose of nitroglycerin, a second or third dose may be given at 5-min intervals. If discomfort continues despite treatment, the patient should consult a physician or report promptly to a hospital emergency room for evaluation of possible unstable angina or acute myocardial infarction (Chap. 243).

Asking the patient with recently diagnosed angina pectoris to record the occurrence of pain as well as nitroglycerin consumption is often helpful to the physician attempting to tailor a management program. Such a diary may also be valuable for detecting changes in the frequency or severity of discomfort that may signify the development of unstable angina pectoris and/or herald an impending myocardial infarction.

None of the long-acting nitrates is as effective as sublingual nitroglycerin for the acute relief of angina. These preparations can be swallowed, chewed, or administered as a patch or paste by the transdermal route. They can provide effective plasma levels for up to 24 h, but the therapeutic response is highly variable. Different preparations and/or administration during the daytime should be tried only to prevent discomfort in the individual patient while avoiding side effects such as headache and dizziness. Individual dose titration is important in order to prevent side effects. Useful preparations include isosorbide dinitrate (10 to 60 mg PO bid or tid), nitroglycerin ointment (0.5 to 2.0 in. qid), or sustained-release transdermal patches (5 to 25 mg/d). Long-acting nitrates are relatively safe and can be used together with intermittent sublingual nitroglycerin to relieve discomfort and prevent attacks of angina. The nitrates likely bind to guanylate cyclase in vascular smooth muscle cells, oxidize sulfhydryl groups, and are converted to *S*-nitrosothiols. This leads to an increase in cyclic guanosine monophosphate which causes cell relaxation of vascular smooth muscle. Tolerance with loss of efficacy develops with 12 to 24 h of continuous exposure to all of the long-acting nitrates due to depletion of sulfhydryl groups and to counterregulatory alterations in intravascular fluid balance with fluid retention. In order to minimize the effects of tolerance, the minimum effective dose should be used and a minimum of 8 h each day kept free of the drug so as to restore any useful response(s).

BETA-ADRENOCEPTOR BLOCKADE (See also Chap. 70) These drugs represent an important component of the pharmacologic treatment of angina pectoris. They reduce myocardial oxygen demand by inhibiting the increases in heart rate and myocardial contractility caused by adrenergic activity. Beta blockade reduces these variables most strikingly during exercise while causing only small reductions in heart rate, cardiac output, and arterial pressure at rest. Propranolol is usually administered in an initial dose of 20 to 40 mg four times a day and is increased as tolerated to 320 mg per day in divided doses. Long-acting beta-blocking drugs (atenolol, 50 to 100 mg/d, and nadolol, 40 to 80 mg/d) offer the advantage of once-a-day dosage (Table 70-1). The therapeutic aims include relief of angina and ischemia. These drugs can also reduce mortality and reinfarction when given to patients after myocardial infarction. Side effects include fatigue, impotence, cold extremities, intermittent claudication, bradycardia, impaired atrioventricular conduction, left ventricular failure, bronchial asthma, and intensification of the hypoglycemia produced by oral hypoglycemic agents and insulin. Reducing the dose or even discontinuation of the drug may be necessary if these side effects develop and persist.

CALCIUM ANTAGONISTS Slow-release nifedipine (30 to 90 mg once daily), verapamil (80 to 120 mg tid), diltiazem (30 to 90 mg qid), amlodipine (2.5 to 10 mg daily) and other calcium antagonists are all coronary vasodilators that produce variable and dose-depen-

dent reductions in myocardial oxygen demand, contractility, and arterial pressure. These combined pharmacologic effects are advantageous and make these agents quite effective in the treatment of angina pectoris. Verapamil and diltiazem may produce symptomatic disturbances in cardiac conduction and bradyarrhythmias, exert negative inotropic actions, and are more likely to worsen left ventricular failure, particularly when used in combination with beta blockers in patients with left ventricular dysfunction. Although useful effects are usually achieved when calcium antagonists are combined with beta blockers and nitrates, careful individual titration of dose is essential with these potent combinations. Variant (Prinzmetal's) angina responds particularly well to calcium antagonists, supplemented when necessary by nitrates. Nifedipine as well as other calcium antagonists are now formulated as long-acting preparations including diltiazem (60 to 120 mg twice daily) and verapamil (180 to 240 mg once daily). Verapamil should not ordinarily be combined with beta-adrenoreceptor blocking drugs because of the combined effects on heart rate and contractility. Diltiazem can be combined with beta blockers with caution and only in patients with normal ventricular function and no conduction disturbances. Nifedipine or amlodipine and the beta blockers have complementary actions on coronary blood supply and myocardial oxygen demands. While the former decreases blood pressure and dilates coronary arteries, the latter slows heart rate and decreases contractility. Nifedipine and the other second-generation dihydropyridine calcium antagonists (nicardipine, isradipine, amlodipine, and felodipine) are potent vasodilators and useful in the simultaneous treatment of angina and hypertension. Short-acting dihydropyridines should be avoided in patients with acute coronary syndromes because of the risk of precipitating infarction, particularly in the absence of beta blockers.

TREATMENT OF ANGINA AND HEART FAILURE Transient left ventricular failure with angina can be controlled by the judicious use of nitrates, calcium antagonists, and even beta blockers. For patients with established congestive heart failure the increased left ventricular wall tension raises myocardial oxygen demand. Treatment of congestive heart failure with angiotensin-converting enzyme inhibitors, diuretics, and digitalis (Chap. 233) will decrease heart size, wall tension, and myocardial oxygen demands, which, in turn, will help to control angina and ischemia. Nocturnal angina can often be relieved by the treatment of heart failure; however, there is no benefit—and possibly aggravation of angina—when these drugs are used in patients with angina, a normal heart size and no evidence of heart failure. Nitrates are particularly useful and can simultaneously improve the disturbed hemodynamics of congestive heart failure by vasodilatation, thereby reducing preload, and relieve angina by preventing or reversing myocardial ischemia. There is some evidence that amlodipine is a calcium antagonist that is well tolerated by patients with left ventricular dysfunction and a valuable agent in the treatment of angina in patients with heart failure. The combination of congestive heart failure and angina in patients with CAD usually indicates a poor prognosis and warrants serious consideration of cardiac catheterization and mechanical revascularization, if possible (see p. 1373).

CHOICE BETWEEN BETA-ADRENERGIC RECEPTOR BLOCKADE AND CALCIUM ANTAGONISTS FOR INITIAL THERAPY Since beta blockers have been shown to improve life expectancy following myocardial infarction (p. 1359), they may be preferable in patients with chronic CAD. However, calcium antagonists are indicated in patients with the following: (1) angina and a history of asthma or chronic obstructive pulmonary disease; (2) sick-sinus syndrome or significant arteriovenous conduction disturbances; (3) Prinzmetal's angina; (4) symptomatic peripheral vascular disease; and (5) adverse reactions to beta blockers—depression, sexual disturbances, fatigue. Many patients with angina do well with a combination of a beta blocker and dihydropiridine calcium antagonist.

ASPIRIN Aspirin is an irreversible inhibitor of platelet cyclooxygenase activity and thereby interferes with platelet activation.

Chronic administration of 100 to 325 mg orally per day has been shown to reduce coronary events in asymptomatic adult men, patients with asymptomatic ischemia after myocardial infarction, patients with chronic stable angina, and patients who have survived unstable angina and myocardial infarction. Administration of this drug should be considered in all patients with CAD in the absence of side effects such as gastrointestinal bleeding, allergy, or dyspepsia.

CORONARY REVASCULARIZATION

While the basic management of patients with ischemic heart disease, which is a lifelong condition, is medical, as described above, many patients are improved by coronary revascularization procedures, as described below. These interventions should be employed in conjunction with but do not replace the continuing need to modify risk factors.

PERCUTANEOUS TRANSLUMINAL CORONARY ANGIOPLASTY AND RELATED CATHETER-BASED TECHNIQUES (See also Chap. 245) PTCA is a widely used method to achieve revascularization of the myocardium in patients with symptomatic ischemic heart disease and suitable stenoses of epicardial coronary arteries. Whereas patients with stenosis of the left main coronary artery and those with three-vessel CAD (especially with associated impaired left ventricular function) who require revascularization are best treated with coronary artery bypass surgery, PTCA is widely employed in patients with symptoms and evidence of ischemia due to stenoses of one or two vessels, and even selected patients with three-vessel disease, and may offer many advantages over surgery.

After a flexible guidewire is advanced into a coronary artery and across the stenosis to be dilated, a miniature balloon catheter is advanced over the guidewire and into the stenosis followed by repeated inflations until the stenosis is decreased or relieved. The development of a range of steerable guidewires, low-profile balloon catheters, and balloon catheters that also allow coronary flow during inflation have all helped to decrease complications, reach more distal lesions, and dilate more complex stenoses. In suitable stenoses affecting epicardial arteries that are ≥3 mm in diameter, a tubular metal stent can be expanded inside the dilated stenosis in order to achieve little or no residual stenosis, and to reduce the incidence of restenosis.

Indications and Patient Selection The most common clinical indication for PTCA is angina pectoris, stable or unstable, accompanied by evidence of ischemia in an exercise test. This symptom should be sufficiently severe to warrant the consideration of bypass graft surgery. PTCA is more effective than medical therapy for the relief of angina. The value of this procedure in reducing the occurrence of coronary death and myocardial infarction has not been established, and therefore it is not generally indicated in asymptomatic or mildly symptomatic patients. PTCA can be used to dilate stenoses in native coronary arteries as well as in bypass grafts in patients who have recurrent angina following coronary artery surgery. This is an important indication when the technical difficulties and the increased mortality that accompanies reoperation are considered. Angioplasty has also been carried out in patients with recent total occlusion (within 3 months) of a coronary artery and severe angina; in this group the primary success rate is decreased to approximately 50 percent.

Risks When coronary stenoses are discrete and symmetric, two and three vessels can be dilated in sequence. However, cautious case selection is essential in order to avoid a prohibitive risk of complications. Female gender, advanced age, stenoses with thrombus, left ventricular dysfunction, stenosis of an artery perfusing a large segment of myocardium without collaterals, long eccentric or irregular stenoses, and calcified plaques all increase the likelihood of complications but are not absolute contraindications, while left main coronary artery stenosis *is* an absolute contraindication. The major complications are usually due to dissection or thrombosis with vessel occlusion, uncontrolled ischemia, and ventricular failure. In experienced hands, the overall mortality rate should be less than 1 percent, the need for emergency coronary surgery less than 3 percent, and the occurrence of clinical myocardial infarction less than 5 percent of cases. Minor complications occur in 5 to 10 percent of patients and include occlusion of a branch of a coronary artery, release of CK-MB into the circulation, and complications of arterial catheterization.

Efficacy Primary success, i.e., adequate dilation (an increase in luminal diameter >20 percent and a residual diameter obstruction <50 percent) with relief of angina, is achieved in approximately 90 percent of cases. Recurrent stenosis of the dilated vessels occurs in 30 to 45 percent of cases within 6 months of the balloon procedure, and angina will recur within 6 to 12 months in 25 percent of cases. This recurrence of symptoms and restenosis is more common in patients with diabetes mellitus, unstable angina, incomplete dilation of the stenosis, dilation of the left anterior descending coronary artery, and stenoses containing thrombi. Dilation of arteries that are totally occluded and of stenotic or occluded vein grafts also exhibit a high incidence of restenosis. It is usual clinical practice to administer aspirin for months after the procedure. Although aspirin may help prevent acute coronary thrombosis during and immediately following PTCA, there are no controlled clinical trials that have demonstrated that these medications or any other can clearly reduce the incidence of restenosis. Successful deployment of a metal stent lowers the restenosis rate to 20 to 30 percent at 6 months but initially requires vigorous antiplatelet therapy (aspirin and Ticlopidine).

If patients do not develop restenosis or angina within the first year after angioplasty, the prognosis for maintaining improvement over the subsequent 4 years is excellent. If restenosis occurs, PTCA can be repeated with the same success and risk, but the likelihood of restenosis increases with the third or subsequent attempt.

Between 30 and 50 percent of patients with symptomatic CAD who require revascularization can be treated by PTCA and need not undergo coronary artery bypass surgery. Successful angioplasty is less invasive and expensive than coronary artery surgery, usually requires only 2 days in the hospital, and permits considerable savings in the initial cost of care; however, this economic benefit is greatly reduced over time because of the greater need for follow-up and for repeat procedures. Successful PTCA also allows earlier return to work and the resumption of an active life.

CORONARY ARTERY BYPASS GRAFTING In this procedure, a section of a vein (usually the saphenous) is used to form a connection between the aorta and the coronary artery distal to the obstructive lesion. Alternatively, anastomosis of one or both of the internal mammary arteries to the coronary artery distal to the obstructive lesion may be employed and is now preferred whenever possible.

Although some indications for coronary artery bypass surgery are controversial, certain areas of agreement exist:

1. The operation is relatively safe, with mortality rates less than 1 percent when the procedure is performed by an experienced surgical team in patients without serious comorbid disease and normal left ventricular function.
2. Intraoperative and postoperative mortality increases with the degree of ventricular dysfunction, comorbidities, age above 80 years, and surgical inexperience. The effectiveness and risk of coronary artery bypass grafting vary widely depending on case selection and the skill and experience of the surgical team, so that the latter must be taken into account when a patient is being considered as a candidate for this procedure.
3. *Occlusion of vein grafts* is observed in 10 to 20 percent during the first postoperative year and in approximately 2 percent per year during 5- to 7-year follow-up and 4 percent per year thereafter. Long-term patency rates are considerably higher for internal mammary artery implantations; in patients with left anterior descending coronary artery obstruction, survival is better when coronary bypass involves the internal mammary artery rather than a saphenous vein.
4. Angina is abolished or greatly reduced in approximately 90 percent of patients following complete revascularization. Although this is usually associated with graft patency and restoration of blood

flow, the pain may also have been alleviated as a result of infarction of the ischemic segment or a placebo effect. Within 3 years, angina recurs in about one-fourth of patients but is rarely severe.

5. Coronary artery bypass grafting does not appear to reduce the incidence of myocardial infarction in patients with chronic ischemic heart disease; perioperative myocardial infarction occurs in 5 to 10 percent of cases, but in most instances these infarcts are small.

6. Mortality is reduced by operation in patients with stenosis of the left main coronary artery as well as in patients with three-vessel CAD and impaired left ventricular function. However, there is no evidence that coronary artery bypass surgery improves survival in patients with one- or two-vessel disease who have chronic stable angina and normal left ventricular function or in patients with one-vessel disease and impaired left ventricular function. Evidence is conflicting concerning the effects of operation on survival in patients with impaired left ventricular function and obstructive disease of two coronary arteries, one of which is the proximal left anterior descending artery.

Indications for coronary artery bypass grafting are usually based on the severity of symptoms, coronary anatomy, and ventricular function. The ideal candidate is male, less than 75 years of age, has no other complicating disease, has troublesome or disabling symptoms that are not adequately controlled by medical therapy or does not tolerate medical therapy and wishes to lead a more active life, and has severe stenoses of several epicardial coronary arteries with objective evidence of myocardial ischemia as a cause of the chest discomfort. Great symptomatic benefit can be anticipated in such patients. When the patient has a disturbance of left ventricular function or critical obstructions in more than one major artery and in whom noninvasive testing shows a high risk of an adverse outcome (p. 1368), coronary artery bypass grafting may, in addition, prolong life.

Congestive heart failure and/or left ventricular dysfunction (ejection fraction <40 percent) are associated with a higher perioperative mortality and were once considered to be contraindications to coronary artery bypass grafting. However, it has now become clear that revascularization of chronically ischemic, noncontractile but viable (so-called hibernating) myocardium can improve left ventricular function and survival. Hibernating myocardium can be detected by positron emission tomographic (PET) scanning, which typically exhibits a mismatch between myocardial perfusion, which is reduced, and metabolism, an indicator of viability, which is sustained. Alternatively, the early or late uptake of thallium 201 in regions of myocardium that fail to contract on echocardiography or the conversion of noncontractile segments to contractile myocardium after low-dose intravenous dobutamine is a more practical approach for detecting hibernating myocardium in which function can be expected to improve by revascularization.

The Choice Between a Catheter-Based Technique and Coronary Bypass Surgery (See Table 244-2) A number of randomized trials have compared PTCA and coronary bypass surgery in patients with multivessel CAD who were suitable technically for both procedures. The occurrence of death or myocardial infarction has been found to be similar between both groups for up to 5 years. In patients with diabetes plus disease of two or more coronary arteries, bypass surgery results in significantly better outcomes and survival and should be the technique of choice. In addition, the recurrence of angina and stenosis and the need for additional revascularization was much higher in the angioplasty group (about 50 percent) than in the surgery group (about 10 percent). Based on these trials and observational studies, we now recommend that patients with an unacceptable level of angina despite optimal medical management should be considered for revascularization. Patients with single- or two-vessel disease with normal global left ventricular function and anatomically suitable lesions are ordinarily advised initially to undergo PTCA, coronary stenting, or other catheter-based procedure (Chap. 245). Patients with two- or three-vessel disease and impaired global left ventricular function (left ventricular ejection fraction <45 percent) or diabetes mellitus or those with lesions unsuitable for catheter-based procedures should

be considered for coronary bypass surgery as the initial method of revascularization.

UNSTABLE ANGINA PECTORIS

The following three patient groups may be said to have unstable angina pectoris: (1) patients with new onset (<2 months) angina that is severe and/or frequent (≥3 episodes per day); (2) patients with accelerating angina, i.e., those with chronic stable angina who develop angina that is distinctly more frequent, severe, prolonged, or precipitated by less exertion than previously; (3) those with angina at rest. Unstable angina may be primary, i.e., occur in the absence of an extracardiac condition that has intensified myocardial ischemia, or it may be precipitated by a condition extrinsic to the coronary vascular bed that has intensified myocardial ischemia, such as anemia, fever, infection, tachyarrhythmias, emotional stress, or hypoxemia. Unstable angina may also develop shortly after myocardial infarction. Unstable angina, particularly when it is characterized by rest pain with ST-segment changes on the ECG or occurs in the postinfarction state, is associated with a relatively high risk of death, myocardial (re)infarction, or intractable angina requiring revascularization. Patients with rest pain frequently develop a third or fourth heart sound during the episode and in some instances exhibit transient left ventricular failure.

When unstable angina is accompanied by objective ECG evidence of transient myocardial ischemia (ST-segment changes and/or T-wave inversions during episodes of chest pain), it is associated with critical stenoses in one or more major epicardial coronary arteries in about 85 percent of cases. The atherosclerotic lesions may have a complicated morphology, with evidence of superimposed thrombosis in approximately 25 to 60 percent of cases. Segmental spasm in the vicinity of atherosclerotic plaques may also play a role in the development of unstable angina. The prognosis is excellent with medical management (see below) in the minority of patients without critical or fixed coronary stenosis.

℞ TREATMENT

The patient with rest pain or severe angina developing after myocardial infarction should be admitted promptly to the hospital for observation, further diagnosis, and treatment. Concomitant conditions that

Table 244-2

Comparison of Revascularization Procedures in Multivessel Disease

Procedure	Advantages	Disadvantages
Percutaneous transluminal coronary angioplasty	Less invasive Shorter hospital stay Lower initial cost Easily repeated Effective in relieving symptoms	Restenosis High incidence of incomplete revascularization Relative inefficiency in patients with severe left ventricular dysfunction Uncertain long-term outcome (>10 years) Limited to specific anatomic subsets Poor outcome in diabetics with 2 plus coronary disease
Coronary artery bypass grafting	Effective in relieving symptoms Improved survival in certain subsets Ability to achieve complete revascularization Wider applicability	Cost Increased risk of a repeat procedure due to late graft closure Morbidity

SOURCE: Modified from DP Faxon, in GA Beller (ed), *Chronic Ischemic Heart Disease,* in E Braunwald (series ed), *Atlas of Heart Diseases,* Philadelphia, Current Medicine, 1994.

can intensify ischemia, such as uncontrolled tachycardia, hypertension and diabetes mellitus, cardiomegaly, heart failure, arrhythmias, thyrotoxicosis, and any acute febrile illness should be sought and treated. Acute myocardial infarction should be ruled out by means of serial ECGs and measurements of plasma cardiac enzyme activity.

Continuous ECG monitoring should be carried out, and the patients should receive reassurance and sedation. Thrombus formation frequently complicates this condition. Therefore, intravenous heparin should be given for 3 to 5 days to maintain the partial thromboplastin time at 2 to 2.5 times control, together with or followed by oral aspirin at a dose of 325 mg/d. A beta-adrenoceptor blocking drug should be administered with a calcium antagonist if necessary, but with caution and an awareness of the possible side effects discussed above. Dosages of these agents should be raised rapidly, but the patient must be observed carefully to avoid bradycardia, heart failure, and hypotension. Nitroglycerin should be given by the sublingual route as needed for symptoms. Intravenous nitroglycerin is quite effective, especially in patients with episodes of ischemia that are particularly severe or prolonged. It is begun at a dosage of 10 μg/min and is raised in 5-μg/min increments to a level at which chest pain is abolished but systolic arterial pressure is maintained or reduced only slightly and other side effects are avoided.

The majority of patients (approximately 80 percent) improve with such treatment over a 48-h period. However, the clinical outcome is highly variable. If angina and/or ECG evidence of ischemia do not diminish within 24 to 48 h of the comprehensive treatment described above in patients with no obvious contraindications for revascularization, then cardiac catheterization and coronary arteriography should be performed. If the anatomy is suitable, PTCA can be performed with surgical standby. PTCA in this condition, particularly in the presence of thrombus, is attended by a slightly increased risk of acute closure and ischemia. If angioplasty cannot be done, coronary artery bypass grafting should be considered to relieve symptoms and myocardial ischemia and as a means of preventing myocardial damage. The factors that influence the choice between catheter-based and surgical revascularization are similar to that in chronic stable angina.

If the patient's symptoms and signs are controlled on medical therapy, a diagnostic exercise ECG should be obtained near the time of hospital discharge. If there is evidence of severe myocardial ischemia and/or evidence of a high risk of coronary events (p. 1368), consideration should be given to catheterization and, depending on the findings, revascularization. It should be recognized that severe CAD is often present in patients with unstable angina who respond to medical therapy. Many patients in whom the unstable state is controlled are left with severe chronic stable angina and ultimately require mechanical revascularization.

PRINZMETAL'S VARIANT ANGINA This relatively uncommon form of unstable angina is characterized by recurrent, prolonged attacks of severe ischemia, caused by episodic focal spasm of an epicardial coronary artery. Approximately three-fourths of patients with Prinzmetal's angina exhibit a fixed obstruction within 1 cm of the site of spasm. Patients with this condition are often in their thirties and forties, i.e., younger than patients with unstable angina secondary to coronary atherosclerosis. Ischemic pain usually occurs at rest or awakens the patient from sleep and is characterized by multilead ST-segment elevation. The diagnosis may be confirmed by detecting transient spasm occurring spontaneously or following a provocative stimulus (intravenous ergonovine, intracoronary acetylcholine, hyperventilation) on coronary arteriography. While long-term survival is excellent, complications include episodes of disabling pain, myocardial infarction, serious ventricular arrhythmias, atrioventricular block, and, rarely, sudden death.

℞ TREATMENT

Management of the acute attack consists of multiple doses of sublingual nitroglycerin and short-acting nifedipine (10 to 30 mg); hypotension should be avoided. In chronic management, long-acting nitrates and calcium antagonists are useful. Beta-adrenergic blockers are of little value, while prazosin, a selective alpha-adrenoceptor blocker, may be useful. Occasionally, mechanical revascularization is helpful in patients with accompanying severe discrete obstructive lesions.

ASYMPTOMATIC (SILENT) ISCHEMIA

Obstructive CAD, acute myocardial infarction, and transient myocardial ischemia are frequently asymptomatic. During continuous ambulatory ECG monitoring, the majority of ambulatory patients with typical chronic stable angina are found to have objective evidence of myocardial ischemia (ST-segment depression) during episodes of chest discomfort while they are active outside the hospital, but many of these patients also appear to have more frequent episodes of asymptomatic ischemia. In addition, there is a large (but as yet unknown) number of totally asymptomatic people with severe coronary atherosclerosis who exhibit ST-segment changes during activity. Evidence of frequent episodes of ischemia (symptomatic and asymptomatic) during daily life appears to indicate an increased likelihood of adverse coronary events such as death and myocardial infarction. The widespread use of exercise ECG during routine examinations has also defined some of these heretofore unrecognized patients with asymptomatic CAD. Longitudinal studies have demonstrated an increased incidence of coronary events (sudden death, myocardial infarction, and angina) in asymptomatic patients with positive exercise tests. In addition, patients with asymptomatic ischemia after suffering a myocardial infarction are at far greater risk for a second coronary event. Patients who seek evaluation and who have asymptomatic ischemia should be subjected to a detailed noninvasive examination utilizing stress ECG and, if necessary, radionuclide scintigraphy.

℞ TREATMENT

The management of patients with asymptomatic ischemia must be individualized. Thus, the physician should consider the following: (1) the degree of positivity of the stress test, particularly the stage of exercise at which ECG signs of ischemia appear, the magnitude and number of the perfusion defect(s) on thallium scintigraphy, and the change in left ventricular ejection fraction which occurs on radionuclide ventriculography or ECG during ischemia and/or during exercise; (2) the ECG leads showing a positive response, with changes in the anterior precordial leads indicating a less favorable prognosis than changes in the inferior leads; and (3) the patient's age, occupation, and general medical condition. Most would agree that an asymptomatic 45-year-old commercial airline pilot with 0.4 mV ST-segment depression in leads V_1 to V_4 during mild exercise should undergo coronary arteriography, whereas the asymptomatic, sedentary 75-year-old retiree with 0.1 mV ST-segment depression in leads II and III during maximal activity need not. However, there is no consensus about the appropriate procedure in the large majority of patients for whom the situation is less extreme. Patients with evidence of severe ischemia on noninvasive testing (as outlined earlier) should undergo coronary arteriography. Asymptomatic patients with silent ischemia, three-vessel CAD, and impaired left ventricular function may be considered appropriate candidates for coronary artery bypass surgery.

The treatment of risk factors, particularly lipid lowering as described above, as well as aspirin and beta blockers have been shown to reduce events and improve outcomes in asymptomatic as well as symptomatic patients with ischemia and coronary disease. While the incidence of asymptomatic ischemia can be reduced by treatment with beta blockers, calcium channel antagonists, and long-acting nitrates, it is not clear whether this is necessary or desirable in patients who have not suffered a myocardial infarction. However, there is evidence that beta-adrenoceptor blockade begun

7 to 35 days after acute myocardial infarction improves survival (Chap. 243).

BIBLIOGRAPHY

THE BARI INVESTIGATORS: Comparison of coronary bypass surgery with angioplasty in patients with multivessel diseases. N Engl J Med 335:217, 1996

BERLINER JA et al: Atherosclerosis: Basic mechanisms, oxidation, inflammations, and genetics. Circulation 91:2488, 1995

BITTL JA: Advances in coronary angioplasty. N Engl J Med 335:1290, 1996

BRAUNWALD E et al: Diagnosing and managing unstable angina. Circulation 90:613, 1994

CALVIN JE et al: Risk stratification in unstable angina. Prospective validation of the Braunwald classification. JAMA 273:136, 1995

DIAMOND GA: Prior restraint: A Bayesian perspective on the optimization of technology utilization for diagnosis of coronary artery disease. Am J Cardiol 76:82, 1995

EAKERS ED: Cardiovascular disease in women. Circulation 88:1999, 1993

FARMER JA, GOTTO AM: Risk factors for coronary artery disease, in *Heart Disease*, 5th ed, E Braunwald (ed). Philadelphia, Saunders, 1997, pp 1126–1160

FISCHMAN DL et al: A randomized comparison of coronary stent placement and balloon angioplasty in the treatment of coronary artery disease. N Engl J Med 331:496, 1994

GERSH BJ et al: Chronic coronary artery disease, in *Heart Disease*, 5th ed, E Braunwald (ed). Philadelphia, Saunders, 1997, pp 1289–1365

HOLDRIGHT D et al: Comparison of the effect of heparin and aspirin versus aspirin alone on transient myocardial ischemia and in-hospital progress in patients with unstable angina. Am J Cardiol 24:39, 1994

KING SB et al: A randomized trial comparing angioplasty with coronary bypass surgery. N Engl J Med 331:1044, 1994

LEVINE GN et al: Cholesterol reduction in cardiovascular disease: Clinical benefits and possible mechanisms. N Engl J Med 332:512, 1995

MASERI A: *Ischemic Heart Disease*. New York, Churchill Livingstone, 1995

NYMAN I et al: Prevention of serious cardiac event by low-dose aspirin in patients with silent myocardial ischemia. Lancet 340:497, 1992

PAFFENBERGER RS JR: The association of changes in physical activity level and other life style characteristics with mortality among men. N Engl J Med 328:538, 1993

PARISI AF et al: A comparison of angioplasty with medical therapy in the treatment of single-vessel coronary artery disease. N Engl J Med 326:10, 1992

PATRONO C: Aspirin as an antiplatelet drug. N Engl J Med 330:1287, 1994

PEPI TRIAL WRITING GROUP: Effects of estrogen or estrogen/progestin regimens on heart disease risk factors in post menopausal women: The Post Menopausal Estrogen/Progestin Interventions (PEPI) Trial. JAMA 273:199, 1995

RYAN TJ et al: Special report: Guidelines for Percutaneous Transluminal Coronary Angioplasty. A report of the American Heart Association/American College of Cardiology Task Force on Assessment of Diagnostic and Therapeutic Cardiovascular Procedures. Circulation 88:2987, 1993

SCANDINAVIAN SIMVASTATIN SURVIVAL STUDY GROUP: Randomized trial of cholesterol lowering in 4444 patients with coronary heart disease: The Scandinavian Simvastatin Survival Study (4S). Lancet 344:1383, 1994

SELWYN AP et al: Pathophysiology of ischemia in patients with coronary artery disease. Prog Cardiovasc Dis 35:1, 1992

Table 245-1

Therapeutic Applications of Cardiac Catheterization

Treatment of coronary stenoses and occlusions
  Percutaneous transluminal coronary angioplasty (PTCA)
  Laser techniques
  Intravascular stents
  Atherectomy
Treatment of valvular stenoses
  Balloon valvuloplasty (aortic, mitral, pulmonic)
Treatment of congenital defects
  Atrial septostomy
  Umbrella closure of patent ductus arteriosus and defects in atrial or ventricular septum
  Coil closure of undesired collateral vessels

TREATMENT OF CORONARY STENOSES AND OCCLUSIONS WITH CORONARY ANGIOPLASTY

Percutaneous transluminal coronary angioplasty (PTCA) is an important form of therapy for coronary artery disease (see Chap. 244). More than 400,000 PTCA procedures are performed each year in the United States, exceeding the number of coronary bypass operations. Since PTCA is performed using local anesthesia, during a short (1- to 3-day) hospitalization, its use in suitable patients can greatly decrease expense and recovery time compared to coronary bypass surgery, although the procedure-related mortality of elective PTCA (0.4 to 1.0 percent), is similar to that of elective coronary bypass surgery.

INDICATIONS   The main indication for PTCA is the presence of one or more coronary stenoses that are approachable by balloon catheters and that are thought to be responsible for a clinical syndrome warranting revascularization (Fig. 245-1). Moreover, the risks and benefits of revascularization by PTCA should compare favorably with those of conventional surgery. Significant left main stenosis and multivessel disease in which vessels supplying significant areas of viable myocardium are not approachable by PTCA (owing to chronic total occlusion or other unfavorable anatomic features) constitute relative contraindications to PTCA if surgery is technically possible. Randomized trials comparing PTCA to bypass surgery in patients with multivessel coronary artery disease suggest that, while the two procedures have equivalent in-hospital and 3- to 5-year mortalities, more PTCA patients (40 to 50 percent versus 7 to 10 percent) will require a second revascularization procedure (generally a repeat PTCA to treat restenosis) to maintain an equivalent level of symptom relief.

For most patients, the clinical syndrome being treated is moderately severe, chronic, stable angina that persists despite medical antian-

---

| **245** | *Donald S. Baim, William Grossman* |

CORONARY ANGIOPLASTY AND OTHER THERAPEUTIC APPLICATIONS OF CARDIAC CATHETERIZATION

The development of catheter-based therapies for the treatment of cardiovascular disease has led to creation of the field known as *interventional cardiology*. In current practice, interventional cardiology provides a safe and effective alternative to conventional surgery for many patients with ischemic, valvular, and congenital heart disease (Table 245-1).

FIGURE 245-1   Right coronary angioplasty in a patient with unstable angina. The lesion is shown before (*left panel*) and after (*right panel*) inflation of the PTCA balloon catheter.

ginal therapy. Approximately 15 percent of current PTCA patients, however, have only mild anginal symptoms despite suitable coronary anatomy and objective evidence of ischemia (i.e., an abnormal exercise test). At the other extreme, many patients have more pressing indications for PTCA, including unstable angina or even acute myocardial infarction (with or without prior thrombolytic therapy).

As the clinical indications for PTCA have broadened, so have its anatomic capabilities. Thus, PTCA no longer is restricted to proximal, discrete, subtotal, concentric, noncalcified lesions, as was the case initially. Angioplasty catheters with smaller deflated profiles, controlled by highly steerable guidewires, can now be advanced successfully across severe stenoses located virtually anywhere in the coronary tree. These balloon catheters tolerate inflation pressures up to 20 atm, adequate to dilate even calcific lesions. Totally occluded coronary arteries (particularly ones that have been occluded for less than 6 months) can be crossed and dilated effectively, although the success rate remains somewhat lower than for subtotal lesions (i.e., 60 percent versus 90 percent for subtotal stenotic lesions). In addition to lesions in the native coronary tree, obstructions in saphenous vein or internal mammary artery bypass grafts also can be dilated successfully to treat postbypass angina. If multiple lesions are responsible for the clinical syndrome, most or all such lesions can generally be dilated during a single procedure.

RESULTS The current PTCA success rate (for dilating a target stenosis by >50 percent of its original diameter without producing an associated complication) exceeds 90 percent. About half the failures result from inability to cross the target lesion with the guidewire or balloon catheter, particularly when that target lesion is a chronic total occlusion. The remaining failures are due to excessive local dissection (separation of coronary artery intima from media) resulting from attempted dilatation. While some local dissection is present in virtually all successful PTCA procedures, more extensive dissection (particularly in association with local thrombus formation or vasospasm) can lead to abrupt closure of the dilated segment soon after withdrawal of the balloon catheter. Routine use of vasodilators (nitrates and calcium channel antagonists), anticoagulation (heparin, 10,000 to 15,000 units during the procedure), and antiplatelet therapy (acetylsalicylic acid, 325 mg/day starting at least 24 h prior to PTCA and continued for 3 to 6 months after the procedure) helps to prevent abrupt closure due to spasm and/or thrombus formation. Newer anti-thrombins (hirudin) or anti-platelet agents (blockers of IIb/IIIa receptors) may further reduce the incidence of ischemic complications within 72 h of PTCA. Closure due to dissection frequently can be reversed by repeat dilatation or, if that is unsuccessful, by the placement of a coronary stent (Fig. 245-2, and see below). When these measures fail, emergency bypass surgery may be necessary to restore blood flow and prevent myocardial infarction. While emergency bypass surgery is needed currently in only 1 to 2 percent of PTCA attempts, this potential difficulty means that angioplasty can be performed only in hospitals where immediate cardiac surgery is available.

FOLLOW-UP After successful PTCA of all "culprit" lesions, marked improvement or complete resolution of the presenting ischemic syndrome should be evident. In approximately 20 to 30 percent of patients, however, evidence of ischemia returns within 6 months, due to so-called restenosis of the dilated segment. This development appears to result from excessive local fibrointimal proliferation and vessel constriction triggered by adhesion of platelets to the freshly dilated surface. To date, despite considerable effort, no pharmacologic strategy has substantially reduced this restenosis rate. When recurrent ischemia develops more than 6 months after PTCA, it usually reflects progression of disease at another site, rather than restenosis. When repeat PTCA is used to treat either restenosis or disease progression, only about 10 percent of patients require bypass surgery during the 5 years following a successful PTCA procedure.

NEWER NONBALLOON TECHNIQUES While conventional balloon angioplasty offers unmatched anatomic versatility, the difficulty of using it for certain anatomic lesion types (e.g., calcified, eccentric, ostial, thrombus-containing, or bifurcation lesions) has fostered the development of a number of newer, nonballoon techniques. These techniques—which include stenting, atherectomy, and ablative laser treatment—moved from clinical investigation to routine clinical practice during the early 1990s and now account for 30 to 40 percent of coronary interventions in many centers. If used appropriately, these new techniques can improve the success, safety, and long-term results (restenosis rate) in lesion types that are difficult to treat using balloon techniques alone. Although most of these procedures cost more in terms of catheter expense, much of this cost can be recouped by the reduction in long-term expenses for the treatment of restenosis.

Stents These are metallic scaffolds that can be positioned in a diseased vessel segment to create a normal vessel lumen by resisting elastic recoil and obliterating any local dissection. By providing a larger acute lumen than does conventional balloon angioplasty, they can also reduce the incidence of subsequent restenosis by nearly one-third. The wire coil design was approved by the Food and Drug

FIGURE 245-2 Placement of coronary stent for dissection after angioplasty. *Left-hand panel*: A prominent filling defect (*curved arrow*) is visible at the site of attempted PTCA in the distal anastomosis of a saphenous vein graft to the circumflex. *Left center panel*: The coils of a Gianturco-Roubin stent are faintly visible (*arrows*). *Right center panel*: Angiogram following stent placement shows small filling defects (*arrows*) representing prolapse of dissected plaque between stent coils. *Right panel*: Following high-pressure postdilation, luminal appearance is near normal (*curved arrow*). The availability of coronary stents to manage actual and threatened abrupt closure has dramatically reduced the need for emergency bypass surgery in current angioplasty practice.

Administration (FDA) in 1993 for use in stabilizing actual or threatened abrupt closure, while the slotted tube design was approved in 1994 for elective treatment of native coronary lesions. In clinical practice, however, both stents have been used widely in other circumstances, including restenotic lesions and saphenous vein grafts (Fig. 245-3). Early experience suggested that these metallic implants were prone to thrombotic occlusion, either acute (<24 h) or subacute (1 to 14 days with a peak at 6 days), and that an aggressive anticoagulation regimen (aspirin, dipyridamole, low-molecular-weight dextran, and warfarin) was needed to prevent such thrombosis. This aggressive anticoagulant regimen led to longer hospitalization and an increased incidence of local vascular complications at the femoral arterial entry site. More recent data, however, suggest that many of these thrombotic complications were the result of incomplete stent expansion, and that more attention to full initial deployment allows the same stents to be used with only antiplatelet drugs (aspirin and ticlopidine) for anticoagulation and with more acceptable thrombosis and vascular complication rates (each <1 percent). On the basis of the overwhelming clinical success of these two early stents, more than a dozen second-generation designs (including stents that are easier to deliver or are coated with heparin or other bioactive agents) are now in clinical testing.

Atherectomy   While both balloon angioplasty and stenting enlarge the coronary lumen by displacing plaque, atherectomy catheters provide much of their lumen enlargement by removing plaque mass from the treated lesion. *Directional* atherectomy does so by using a special catheter with a windowed steel cylinder at its tip. Inflation of a low-pressure positioning balloon on the back of the cylinder presses plaque into the window, where it is cut and trapped by a spinning cup-shaped cutter (Fig. 245-4). This device was the first of the nonballoon technologies to reach clinical practice and it is still the treatment of choice for noncalcified lesions at the origin of the left anterior descending artery or at major coronary bifurcations. *Rotational* atherectomy uses burrs of various sizes (diameter 1.25 to 2.38 mm) that are coated

on their leading half with small diamond chips. The burr is spun at 160,000 to 180,000 rpm as it is advanced through a coronary lesion over a leading guidewire. The diamond chips grind through the obstructing plaque, pulverizing it into small (5 to 25 μm) particles, which pass through the distal coronary microcirculation. This device has emerged as an effective treatment for calcified, long (>20 mm), or ostial lesions; frequently it is followed by low-pressure balloon dilation and occasionally by stent placement (Fig. 245-5). *Extraction* atherectomy uses a combination of distal cutting blades rotating at low speed and continuous vacuum aspiration to remove coronary obstructions. The device has limited cutting efficiency, and its use is now confined to softer lesions (e.g., atherosclerotic saphenous vein grafts) or thrombotic lesions. Newer aspiration devices based on the Venturi effect may be able to remove clot more efficiently with less vessel disruption.

Lasers   Laser light [at wavelengths from the ultraviolet (308 nm) to the mid-infrared (2000 μm)] can be delivered to obstructing coronary plaques through small optical fibers bundled into flexible catheters whose outer diameter is between 1.2 and 2.0 mm. When these catheters are pulsed with laser energy as they are advanced through a coronary obstruction over a guidewire, they can ablate noncalcified coronary plaque by a combination of photoacoustic (blast), thermal, and photochemical effects. Although lasers have been used to treat ostial as well as diffuse coronary lesions, acceptance of the technique has been limited by the expense of the device and the fact that these lesions can be treated by other techniques, such as rotational atherectomy. Unique applications—such as use of a laser guidewire designed to cross total occlusions—may help entrench the technique. Earlier laser-thermal devices (in which a metal cap or the vessel wall was heated through a transparent angioplasty balloon) were tried but abandoned because of excessive vessel injury and late restenosis.

FIGURE 245-3   Stenting of a diseased saphenous vein graft. *Upper left*: Severe eccentric stenosis in an 8-year-old saphenous vein graft to the left anterior descending coronary artery. *Lower left*: Following balloon dilatation, significant stenosis persists owing to elastic recoil of the graft atherosclerotic plaque. *Upper right*: Further lumen enlargement following placement of a slotted-tube stent (*arrow*). *Lower right*: Diamond pattern is visible (*open arrow*) as contrast clears from the graft.

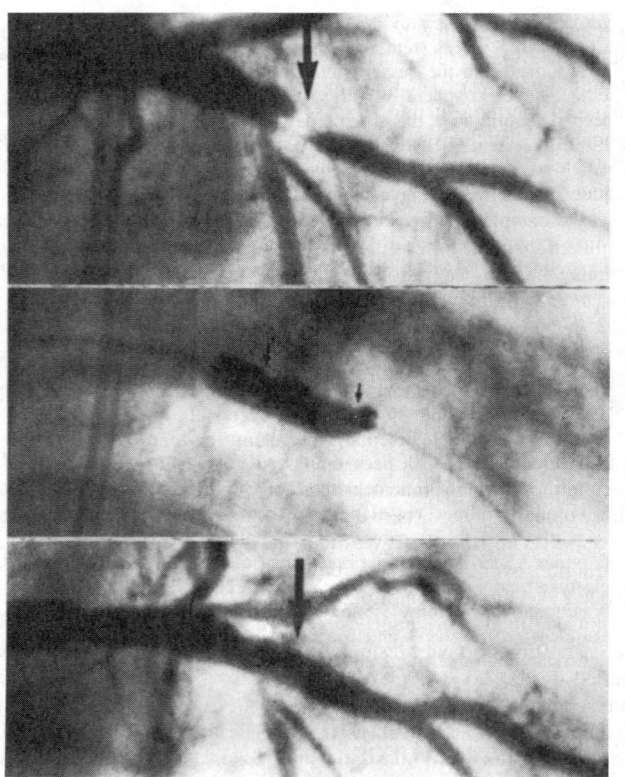

FIGURE 245-4 *Top*: Eccentric, ulcerated lesion in the mid-left anterior descending coronary artery. *Middle*: Lesion being treated by directional atherectomy. *Bottom*: the resulting large, smooth lumen.

TREATMENT OF VALVULAR STENOSIS: BALLOON VALVULOPLASTY

Once the efficacy of balloon dilatation for vascular stenoses was demonstrated, cardiologists treating both pediatric and adult patients applied the technique to the treatment of stenotic cardiac valves. The technique was used first for congenital pulmonic and aortic stenosis but has now been extended to acquired rheumatic and calcific stenoses of the mitral and aortic valves.

PULMONIC VALVULOPLASTY Although congenital pulmonic stenosis is mainly a pediatric disease, it is sometimes encountered in adults (see Chap. 235). Transvalvular pressure gradients of >50 mmHg may produce exertional symptoms or lead to progressive right ventricular hypertrophy or failure. Using a guidewire placed into the pulmonary artery from the femoral vein, one or more valvuloplasty balloons with a combined cross-sectional area as much as 20 percent larger than the pulmonic valve annulus are positioned within the stenotic valve and inflated with liquid contrast medium at pressures of 3 to 5 atm. This typically reduces the transvalvular gradient from 75 to 15 mmHg. Balloon pulmonary valvuloplasty now stands as the preferred therapy for this lesion.

MITRAL VALVULOPLASTY The main application of balloon mitral valvuloplasty is in patients with rheumatic mitral stenosis, in whom stenosis results primarily from commissural fusion with associated leaflet thickening. Such patients—who previously would have undergone open or closed surgical commissurotomy—are now treated almost exclusively by balloon valvuloplasty (Chap. 237). Patients with other kinds of problems (left atrial thrombus, mitral regurgitation, subvalvular disease, or leaflet thickening or rigidity) have less satisfactory results with either surgical commissurotomy or balloon valvuloplasty and are better treated by surgical valve replacement.

The usual approach to balloon mitral valvuloplasty involves transseptal puncture (right atrium to left atrium) followed by passage of a guidewire across the stenotic valve and into the left ventricle. One or more balloon catheters with a dilating area equivalent to a single 23-

FIGURE 245-5 Rotational atherectomy for a calcified lesion in the mid-left anterior descending coronary artery. *Upper left*: Calcified lesions such as this one (*arrow*) used to be treated by high-pressure balloon inflation, although that commonly resulted in severe local dissection. *Middle left*: In current practice, such lesions are generally treated by rotational atherectomy, shown here using a 2.0-mm diamond-chip–coated burr (*curved arrow*). *Lower left*: Following burr passage, much of the calcified lesion has been ablated (*arrow*). *Upper right*: After rotational atherectomy, inflation of the balloon at low pressure (4 atm) results in full balloon expansion. *Lower right*: Large, smooth lumen present after balloon postdilation.

to 30-mm diameter balloon are advanced over this guidewire and inflated within the stenotic valve. Alternatively, the newer Inoue balloon (Fig. 245-6) can be used to provide faster and more effective dilatation than is achieved with conventional cylindrical balloon designs. Successful dilatation separates fused commissures and enhances leaflet compliance, thus increasing the effective diastolic valve area from 0.9 to 2.0 cm² or more (Fig. 245-7). Although this opening is still restricted compared with the 3.5- to 5-cm² area of a normal mitral valve, it provides excellent symptomatic relief and is equivalent to or approaches the increase in orifice size resulting from surgical mitral commissurotomy or prosthetic mitral valve replacement.

The main complications of balloon mitral valvuloplasty relate to the potential for cardiac perforation during transseptal puncture (approximately 2 percent of patients) and the chance of systemic embolization (approximately 1 percent of patients) despite preprocedure echocardiographic exclusion of patients with left atrial thrombus.

AORTIC VALVULOPLASTY Balloon aortic valvuloplasty may be performed in children with congenital aortic stenosis and in adults with rheumatic or acquired calcific aortic stenosis. Some patients with rheumatic aortic stenosis have leaflet fusion, but the problem in acquired calcific aortic stenosis is due more to rigidity of the valve leaflets themselves. In the latter group of patients, balloon valvuloplasty fractures leaflet calcium (providing new hinge points along which the valve leaflets can open) and temporarily expands the aortic annulus.

The most common approach to balloon aortic valvuloplasty consists of femoral arterial puncture with retrograde passage of a guidewire and balloon (inflated diameter 18 to 23 mm) across the valve. Overdilatation of the valve annulus may cause leaflet avulsion and is generally avoided. Balloon aortic valvuloplasty typically increases the effective systolic valve area from 0.6 to 1.0 cm². The resulting valve area is still small compared with that of a normal aortic valve (3 to 4 cm²) or with the effective area of an inflated 20-mm balloon (3.1 cm²), but it does relieve symptoms at rest or during mild to moderate exertion in most patients with critical aortic stenosis. Unfortunately, the relatively small effective orifice achieved and the high incidence of valvular restenosis (up to 50 percent within 1 year after dilatation) make balloon aortic valvuloplasty most applicable as a temporary palliation for elderly patients who are poor risks for valve replacement or as a "bridge" to valve replacement.

TREATMENT OF CONGENITAL MALFORMATIONS

Pediatric interventional cardiologists have developed a number of innovative techniques to correct or palliate congenital cardiac lesions. Some were described above—balloon dilatation of stenotic pulmonary arteries, surgical stent placement, and balloon valvuloplasty—but others are unique to the pediatric population.

ATRIAL SEPTOSTOMY In certain patients with cyanotic congenital heart disease, such as some with transposition of the great vessels, it is desirable to produce or enlarge an atrial septal defect to facilitate passage of oxygenated blood into the right side of the heart. This can be achieved by passage of a balloon catheter from the right to left atrium across a patent foramen ovale, followed by forceful withdrawal of the inflated balloon. Alternatively, a catheter with a concealed blade can be passed across the septum. The blade can then

FIGURE 245-6 Inoue balloon for mitral valvuloplasty. Compared to earlier cylindrical balloons, the unique Inoue balloon permits fast and safe dilatation of stenotic mitral valves. *Upper left*: Transseptal puncture has been used to pass a coiled guidewire (*curved arrow*) and tapered dilator (*boxed arrow*) into the left atrium. *Lower left*: The deflated Inoue catheter is advanced into the left atrium over this guidewire (*open curved arrow*). *Upper right*: Partial inflation of the balloon helps it float across the mitral valve and into the left ventricle (1), whereupon it is pulled back against the mitral leaflets. *Middle right*: Further balloon inflation causes expansion of the proximal part of the balloon (2), trapping the mitral orifice between the proximal and distal portions of the balloon. *Lower right*: With the balloon thus anchored, full expansion of its central portion (3) effectively dilates the stenotic valve.

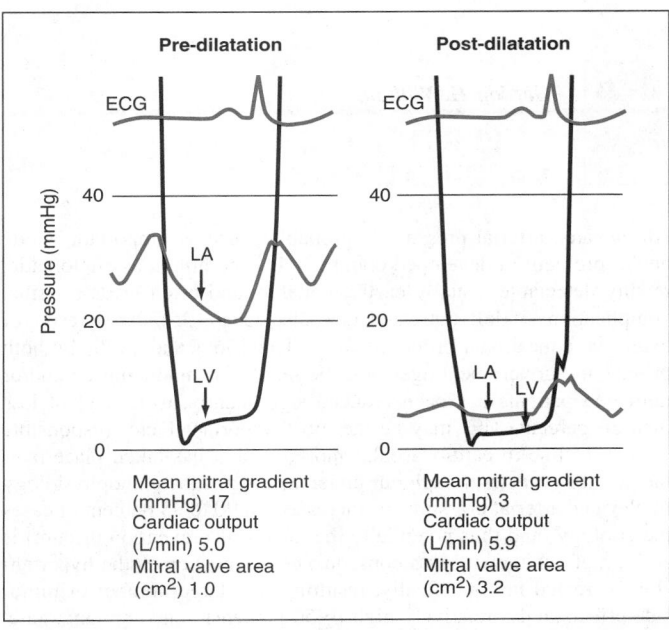

FIGURE 245-7 Hemodynamic results of mitral valvuloplasty in a 38-year-old woman with mitral stenosis. The transmitral gradient [from the left atrium (LA) to the left ventricle (LV)], cardiac output, and calculated mitral valve area are shown before (*left panel*) and after (*right panel*) balloon dilatation.

be deployed in the left atrium to incise the septum as the catheter is withdrawn. The resulting septal incision can be widened by conventional balloon septostomy.

CLOSURE OF UNDESIRED SHUNTS OR COLLATERAL VESSELS A variety of appliances have been developed to close undesired intracardiac shunts, including defects in the atrial or ventricular septum and patent ductus arteriosus. These devices resemble a double (back-to-back) umbrella, which can be folded into a cylinder for containment in a catheter. Under fluoroscopic guidance, the delivery catheter can be positioned across the target defect so that the umbrella can be deployed to block undesired flow.

Smaller vascular shunts can be closed using special coils. These coils can be placed in a catheter and delivered to the undesired vessel. Once in place, the coil interferes with blood flow and promotes local thrombotic occlusion of the target vessel.

BIBLIOGRAPHY

BAIM DS: Coronary angioplasty, in *Cardiac Catheterization, Angiography and Intervention*, 5th ed, D Baim, W Grossman (eds). Baltimore, Williams & Wilkins, 1996

BERMAN AD et al: Balloon valvuloplasty, in *Cardiac Catheterization, Angiography and Intervention*, 5th ed, D Baim, W Grossman (eds). Baltimore, Williams & Wilkins, 1996

DETRE K et al: Has improvement in PTCA intervention affected long-term prognosis? The NHLBI PTCA Registry experience. Circulation 91:2868, 1995

FISCHMAN DL et al: A randomized comparison of coronary stent placement and balloon angioplasty in the treatment of coronary artery disease. N Engl J Med 331:496, 1994

KING SB et al: A randomized trial comparing coronary angioplasty with bypass surgery. N Engl J Med 331:1044, 1994

PERRY SB et al: Pediatric interventions, in *Cardiac Catheterization, Angiography and Intervention*, 5th ed, D Baim, W Grossman (eds). Baltimore, Williams & Wilkins, 1996

RYAN TJ et al: Guidelines for percutaneous transluminal coronary angioplasty—a report of the ACC/AHA task force. J Am Coll Cardiol 22:2033, 1993

THE EPIC INVESTIGATORS: Use of a monoclonal antibody against the platelet glycoprotein IIb/IIIa receptor in high-risk coronary angioplasty. N Engl J Med 330:956, 1994

246 *Gordon H. Williams*

HYPERTENSIVE VASCULAR DISEASE

An elevated arterial pressure is probably the most important public health problem in developed countries. It is common, asymptomatic, readily detectable, usually easily treatable, and often leads to lethal complications if left untreated (see also Chap. 35). As a result of extensive educational programs in the late 1960s and 1970s by both private and government agencies, the number of undiagnosed and/or untreated patients has been reduced significantly, to a level of less than 20 percent. This may be the most important factor responsible for the decline in cardiovascular mortality that has taken place over the past 20 years. Although our understanding of the pathophysiology of elevated arterial pressure has increased, in 90 to 95 percent of cases the etiology (and thus potentially the means of prevention or cure) is still largely unknown. As a consequence, in most cases the hypertension is treated nonspecifically, resulting in a large number of minor side effects and a relatively high (~50 percent) noncompliance rate.

PREVALENCE The prevalence of hypertension depends on both the racial composition of the population studied and the criteria used to define the condition. In a white suburban population like that in the Framingham Study, nearly one-fifth of individuals have blood pressures greater than 160/95, while almost one-half have pressures greater than 140/90. An even higher prevalence has been documented in the nonwhite population. In females the prevalence is closely related to age, with a substantial increase occurring after age 50. This increase is presumably related to the hormonal changes of menopause. Thus, the ratio of hypertension frequency in women versus men increases from 0.6 to 0.7 at age 30 to 1.1 to 1.2 at age 65.

The prevalence of various forms of secondary hypertension depends on the nature of the population studied and on how extensive the evaluation is. There are no available data to define the frequency of secondary hypertension in the general population, although in middle-aged males it has been reported to be 6 percent. On the other hand, in referral centers where patients undergo an extensive evaluation, it has been reported to be as high as 35 percent. The various forms of hypertension are outlined in Table 246-1, and their relative frequencies are given in Table 246-2.

ESSENTIAL HYPERTENSION

Patients with arterial hypertension and no definable cause are said to have *primary*, *essential*, or *idiopathic hypertension*. Undoubtedly, the primary difficulty in uncovering the mechanism(s) responsible for the

Table 246-1

Classification of Arterial Hypertension

SYSTOLIC HYPERTENSION WITH WIDE PULSE PRESSURE

I. Decreased compliance of aorta (arteriosclerosis)
II. Increased stroke volume
    A. Aortic regurgitation
    B. Thyrotoxicosis
    C. Hyperkinetic heart syndrome
    D. Fever
    E. Arteriovenous fistula
    F. Patent ductus arteriosus

SYSTOLIC AND DIASTOLIC HYPERTENSION (INCREASED PERIPHERAL VASCULAR RESISTANCE)

I. Renal
    A. Chronic pyelonephritis
    B. Acute and chronic glomerulonephritis
    C. Polycystic renal disease
    D. Renovascular stenosis or renal infarction
    E. Most other severe renal diseases (arteriolar nephrosclerosis, diabetic nephropathy, etc.)
    F. Renin-producing tumors
II. Endocrine
    A. Oral contraceptives
    B. Adrenocortical hyperfunction
        1. Cushing's disease and syndrome
        2. Primary hyperaldosteronism
        3. Congenital or hereditary adrenogenital syndromes (17α-hydroxylase and 11β-hydroxylase defects)
    C. Pheochromocytoma
    D. Myxedema
    E. Acromegaly
III. Neurogenic
    A. Psychogenic
    B. Diencephalic syndrome
    C. Familial dysautonomia (Riley-Day)
    D. Polyneuritis (acute porphyria, lead poisoning)
    E. Increased intracranial pressure (acute)
    F. Spinal cord section (acute)
IV. Miscellaneous
    A. Coarctation of aorta
    B. Increased intravascular volume (excessive transfusion, polycythemia vera)
    C. Polyarteritis nodosa
    D. Hypercalcemia
    E. Medications, e.g., glucocorticoids, cyclosporine
V. Unknown etiology
    A. Essential hypertension (>90% of all cases of hypertension)
    B. Toxemia of pregnancy
    C. Acute intermittent porphyria

Table 246-2

CHAPTER 246
Hypertensive Vascular Disease **1381**

Prevalence of Various Forms of Hypertension in the General Population and in Specialized Referral Clinics*

Diagnosis	General Population, %	Specialty Clinic, %
Essential hypertension	92–94	65–85
Renal hypertension:		
Parenchymal	2–3	4–5
Renovascular	1–2	4–16
Endocrine hypertension:		
Primary aldosteronism	0.3	0.5–12
Cushing's syndrome	<0.1	0.2
Pheochromocytoma	<0.1	0.2
Oral contraceptive–induced	0.5–1	1–2
Miscellaneous	0.2	1

* Estimates based on a number of reports in the literature.

hypertension in these patients is attributable to the variety of systems that are involved in the regulation of arterial pressure—peripheral and/or central adrenergic, renal, hormonal, and vascular—and to the complexity of the interrelations of these systems. Several abnormalities have been described in patients with essential hypertension, often with a claim that one or more of them are primarily responsible for the hypertension. While it is still uncertain whether these individual abnormalities are primary or secondary, varying expressions of a single disease process or reflective of separate disease entities, the accumulating data increasingly support the latter hypothesis. Therefore, just as pneumonia is caused by a variety of infectious agents, even though the clinical picture observed may be similar, so essential hypertension likely has a number of distinct causes. Thus, the distinction between primary and secondary hypertension has become blurred, and the approach to both the diagnosis and therapy of hypertensive patients has been modified. For example, when a group of patients with essential hypertension is separated into a distinct subset (e.g., low-renin essential hypertension), the patients have not been reclassified as having a form of secondary hypertension but rather remain in the essential hypertensive group. In this chapter, individuals in whom a specific structural organ or gene defect is responsible for hypertension are defined as having a *secondary* form of hypertension. In contrast, individuals in whom generalized or functional abnormalities may be the cause of hypertension, even if the abnormalities are discrete, are defined as having *essential* hypertension.

HEREDITY Genetic factors have long been assumed to be important in the genesis of hypertension. Data supporting this view can be found in animal studies as well as in population studies in humans. One approach has been to assess the correlation of blood pressure in families (familial aggregation). From these studies, the minimum size of the genetic factor can be expressed by a correlation coefficient of approximately 0.2. However, the variation in the size of the genetic factor in different studies reemphasizes the probably heterogeneous nature of the essential hypertensive population. In addition, most studies support the concept that the inheritance is probably multifactorial or that a number of different genetic defects each have an elevated blood pressure as one of their phenotypic expressions. Finally, both monogenic defects (e.g., glucocorticoid-remediable aldosteronism and Liddle's syndrome), and susceptibility genes (e.g., the angiotensinogen gene) have now been reported which have as one of their consequences an increased arterial pressure (see below and Chap. 332).

ENVIRONMENT A number of environmental factors have been implicated in the development of hypertension, including salt intake, obesity, occupation, alcohol intake, family size, and crowding. These factors have all been assumed to be important in the increase in blood pressure with age in more affluent societies, in contrast to the decline in blood pressure with age in less affluent groups.

SALT SENSITIVITY The environmental factor that has received the greatest attention is salt intake. Even this factor illustrates the heterogeneous nature of the essential hypertensive population, in

that the blood pressure in only approximately 60 percent of hypertensives is particularly responsive to the level of sodium intake. The cause of this special sensitivity to salt varies, with primary aldosteronism, bilateral renal artery stenosis, renal parenchymal disease, and low-renin essential hypertension accounting for about half the patients. In the remainder, the pathophysiology is still uncertain, but postulated contributing factors include chloride intake, calcium intake, a generalized cellular membrane defect, insulin resistance, and "nonmodulation" (see below).

ROLE OF RENIN Renin is an enzyme secreted by the juxtaglomerular cell of the kidney and linked with aldosterone in a negative feedback loop (see Chap. 332). While a variety of factors can modify its rate of secretion, the primary determinant is the volume status of the individual, particularly as related to changes in dietary sodium intake. The end product of the action of renin on its substrate is the generation of the peptide angiotensin II. The response of target tissues to this peptide is uniquely determined by the prior dietary electrolyte intake. For example, sodium intake normally modulates adrenal and renal vascular responses to angiotensin II. With sodium restriction, adrenal responses are enhanced and the renal vascular responses reduced. Sodium loading has the opposite effect. The range of plasma renin activities observed in hypertensive subjects is broader than in normotensive individuals. In consequence, some hypertensive patients have been defined as having *low-renin* and others as having *high-renin* essential hypertension.

Low-Renin Essential Hypertension Approximately 20 percent of patients who by all other criteria have essential hypertension have suppressed plasma renin activity. This situation is more common in African-American than in white patients. Though these patients are not hypokalemic, they have been reported to have expanded extracellular fluid volumes, and it has been suggested but not proved that they have sodium retention and renin suppression due to excessive production of an unidentified mineralocorticoid. On the other hand, some studies have suggested that the adrenal cortex of some of these patients has an increased sensitivity to angiotensin II as the underlying mechanism. Not only does this hypothesis potentially explain their low plasma renin activity, it also suggests the cause of their hypertension. On a diet with a normal or high sodium content, aldosterone production will not be suppressed normally, leading to a mild degree of hyperaldosteronism with its resulting increased sodium retention, volume expansion, and increase in blood pressure. Since this altered sensitivity has been reported even in patients with normal-renin hypertension, it is likely that patients with low-renin hypertension are not a distinct subset but rather form part of a continuum of patients with essential hypertension.

Nonmodulating Essential Hypertension Another subset of hypertensive patients have an adrenal defect opposite to that observed in low-renin patients—a reduced adrenal response to sodium restriction. In these individuals, sodium intake does not modulate either adrenal or renal vascular responses to angiotensin II. Hypertensives in this subset have been termed *nonmodulators* because of the absence of the sodium-mediated modulation of target tissue responses to angiotensin II. These individuals make up 25 to 30 percent of the hypertensive population, have plasma renin activity levels that are normal to high if measured when the patient is on a low-salt diet, and have hypertension that is salt-sensitive because of a defect in the kidney's ability to excrete sodium appropriately. Furthermore, the abnormality appears to be genetically determined (associated with a certain allele of the angiotensinogen gene), and it can be corrected by the administration of a converting-enzyme inhibitor.

High-Renin Essential Hypertension Approximately 15 percent of patients with essential hypertension have plasma renin activity levels above the normal range. It has been suggested that plasma renin plays an important role in the pathogenesis of the elevated arterial pressure in these patients. However, most studies have found that saralasin (a substance that, like losartan, acts as a competitive antagonist of angiotensin II) significantly reduces blood pressure in less than half of these patients. This finding has led some investigators to postulate that the elevated renin levels and blood pressure may both be secondary to an increase in adrenergic system activity. It has been proposed that, in patients with angiotensin-dependent high-renin hypertension whose arterial pressures are lowered by an angiotensin II antagonist, the mechanism responsible for the increase in renin and, therefore, for the hypertension is the nonmodulating defect.

SODIUM ION VERSUS CHLORIDE OR CALCIUM Most studies assessing the role of salt in the hypertensive process have assumed that it is the sodium ion that is important. However, some investigators have suggested that the chloride ion may be equally important. This suggestion is based on the observation that feeding chloride-free sodium salts to salt-sensitive hypertensive animals fails to increase arterial pressure. Calcium also has been implicated in the pathogenesis of some forms of essential hypertension. A low calcium intake has been associated with an increase in blood pressure in epidemiologic studies; an increase in leukocyte cytosolic calcium levels has been reported in some hypertensives. Finally, calcium entry blockers are effective antihypertensive agents. Several studies have reported a potential link between the salt-sensitive forms of hypertension and calcium. It has been postulated that salt loading in combination with a defect in the kidney's ability to excrete salt may lead to a secondary increase in circulating natriuretic factors. One of these factors, the so-called digitalis-like natriuretic factor, inhibits ouabain-sensitive sodium-potassium ATPase and thereby leads to intracellular calcium accumulation and a hyperreactive vascular smooth muscle.

CELL MEMBRANE DEFECT Another postulated explanation for salt-sensitive hypertension is a generalized cell membrane defect. This hypothesis derives most of its data from studies on circulating blood elements, particularly red blood cells, in which abnormalities in the transport of sodium across the cell membrane have been documented. Since both increases and decreases in the activity of different transport systems have been reported, it is likely that some abnormalities are primary and some are secondary. It has been assumed that this abnormality in sodium transport reflects an undefined alteration in the cell membrane and that this defect occurs in many, perhaps all, cells of the body, particularly the vascular smooth muscle cells. The defect leads to an abnormal accumulation of calcium in vascular smooth muscle, resulting in a heightened vascular responsiveness to vasoconstrictor agents. This defect has been proposed to be present in 35 to 50 percent of essential hypertensive persons on the basis of studies using red cells. Other studies suggest that the abnormality in red cell sodium transport is not fixed but can be modified by environmental factors.

The common final pathway in all these hypotheses is an increase in cytosolic calcium resulting in increased vascular reactivity. However, as described above, several mechanisms might produce this calcium accumulation.

INSULIN RESISTANCE Insulin resistance and/or hyperinsulinemia have been suggested as being responsible for the increased arterial pressure in some patients with hypertension. While it is clear that a substantial fraction of the hypertensive population has insulin resistance and hyperinsulinemia, it is less certain that this is more than an association. Insulin resistance is common in patients with non-insulin-dependent diabetes mellitus (NIDDM) or obesity. Both obesity and NIDDM are more common in hypertensive than in normotensive subjects. However, several studies have found that hyperinsulinemia and insulin resistance are present even in lean hypertensive patients without NIDDM, suggesting that this relationship is more than a coincidence.

Hyperinsulinemia can increase arterial pressure by one or more of four mechanisms. An underlying assumption in each case is that some, but not all, of the target tissues of insulin are resistant to its effects. Specifically, tissues involved in glucose homeostasis are resistant (thereby producing the hyperinsulinemia), while tissues in-

volved in the hypertensive process are not. First, hyperinsulinemia produces renal sodium retention (at least acutely) and increases sympathetic activity. Either or both of these effects could lead to an increase in arterial pressure. Another mechanism is vascular smooth-muscle hypertrophy secondary to the mitogenic action of insulin. Finally, insulin also modifies ion transport across the cell membrane, thereby potentially increasing the cytosolic calcium levels of insulin-sensitive vascular or renal tissues. This mechanism would increase arterial pressure for reasons similar to those described above for the membrane-defect hypothesis. It is important to point out, however, that the role of insulin in controlling arterial pressure is only vaguely understood, and, therefore, its potential as a pathogenic factor in hypertension remains unclear.

Few of the features of hypertension discussed above remain constant in a given patient. Some may be a reflection of the current metabolic and hormonal status of the patient rather than a permanent feature of the disease process. For example, at one point a patient might have insulin resistance secondary to obesity, which could lead to sodium retention, intravascular volume expansion, and renin suppression. This patient would be labeled as having "low-renin essential hypertension." If the patient lost weight, however, the salt-retaining tendency would be reversed. If the blood pressure did not normalize, the patient might then have "normal or high-renin essential hypertension." Thus, the features reviewed above should not be considered mutually exclusive or permanent characteristics in a given patient with hypertension.

FACTORS THAT MODIFY THE COURSE OF ESSENTIAL HYPERTENSION Age, race, sex, smoking, alcohol intake, serum cholesterol, glucose intolerance, and weight may all alter the prognosis of this disease. The younger the patient when hypertension is first noted, the greater is the reduction in life expectancy if the hypertension is left untreated. In the United States, urban blacks have about twice the prevalence of hypertension as whites and more than four times the hypertension-induced morbidity rate. At all ages and in both white and nonwhite populations, females with hypertension fare better than males, and the prevalence of hypertension in premenopausal females is substantially less than that in age-matched males or postmenopausal women. Yet, compared with their normotensive counterparts, females with hypertension run the same relative risk of a morbid cardiovascular event as males do. Accelerated atherosclerosis is an invariable companion of hypertension. Thus, it is not surprising that independent risk factors associated with the development of atherosclerosis, such as an elevated serum cholesterol, glucose intolerance, and/or cigarette smoking, significantly enhance the effect of hypertension on mortality rate regardless of age, sex, or race (Chap. 242). There also is no question that a positive correlation exists between obesity and arterial pressure. A gain in weight is associated with an increased frequency of hypertension in subjects with normal blood pressure, and weight loss in obese subjects with hypertension lowers their arterial pressure and, if they are being treated for hypertension, the intensity of therapy required to keep them normotensive. Whether these changes are mediated by changes in insulin resistance is unknown.

NATURAL HISTORY Because essential hypertension is a heterogeneous disorder, variables other than the arterial pressure modify its course. Thus, the probability of developing a morbid cardiovascular event with a given arterial pressure may vary as much as 20-fold depending on whether associated risk factors are present (Table 246-3). Although exceptions have been reported, most untreated adults with hypertension will develop further increases in arterial pressure with time. Furthermore, it has been demonstrated from both actuarial data and experience in the era prior to effective therapy that untreated hypertension is associated with a shortening of life by 10 to 20 years, usually related to an acceleration of the atherosclerotic process, with the rate of acceleration in part related to the severity of the hypertension. Even individuals who have relatively mild disease—i.e., without evidence of end organ damage—that is left untreated for 7 to 10 years have a high risk of developing significant complications. Nearly 30 percent will exhibit atherosclerotic complications, and more than 50 percent will have end organ damage related to the hypertension itself,

Table 246-3

CHAPTER 246
Hypertensive Vascular Disease **1383**

Risk Factors for an Adverse Prognosis in Hypertension

Black race
Youth
Male sex
Persistent diastolic pressure >115 mmHg
Smoking
Diabetes mellitus
Hypercholesterolemia
Obesity
Excess alcohol intake
Evidence of end organ damage
    A. Cardiac
        1. Cardiac enlargement
        2. Electrocardiographic signs of ischemia or left ventricular strain
        3. Myocardial infarction
        4. Congestive heart failure
    B. Eyes
        1. Retinal exudates and hemorrhages
        2. Papilledema
    C. Renal: impaired renal function
    D. Nervous system: cerebrovascular accident

such as cardiomegaly, congestive heart failure, retinopathy, a cerebrovascular accident, and/or renal insufficiency. Thus, even in its mild forms, hypertension is a progressive and lethal disease if left untreated.

SECONDARY HYPERTENSION

As noted earlier, in only a small minority of patients with elevated arterial pressure can a specific cause be identified. Yet these patients should not be ignored for at least two reasons: (1) correction of the cause may cure their hypertension, and (2) these secondary forms of the disease may provide insight into the etiology of essential hypertension. Nearly all the secondary forms of hypertension are related to an alteration in hormone secretion and/or renal function and are discussed in detail in other chapters.

RENAL HYPERTENSION (See also Chap. 277) Hypertension produced by renal disease is the result of either (1) a derangement in the renal handling of sodium and fluids leading to volume expansion or (2) an alteration in renal secretion of vasoactive materials resulting in a systemic or local change in arteriolar tone. The main subdivisions of renal hypertension are renovascular hypertension, including preeclampsia and eclampsia, and renal parenchymal hypertension. A simple explanation for *renal vascular hypertension* is that decreased perfusion of renal tissue due to stenosis of a main or branch renal artery activates the renin-angiotensin system, described in Chap. 332. Circulating angiotensin II elevates arterial pressure by directly causing vasoconstriction, by stimulating aldosterone secretion with resulting sodium retention, and/or by stimulating the adrenergic nervous system. In practice, only about one-half of patients with renovascular hypertension have an absolute elevation in renin activity in peripheral plasma, although when renin measurements are referenced against an index of sodium balance, a much higher fraction have inappropriately high values.

Activation of the renin-angiotensin system also has been offered as an explanation for the hypertension in both acute and chronic *renal parenchymal disease*. In this formulation, the only difference between renovascular and renal parenchymal hypertension is that the decreased perfusion of renal tissue in the latter case results from inflammatory and fibrotic changes involving multiple small intrarenal vessels. There are enough differences between the two conditions, however, to suggest that other mechanisms are active in renal parenchymal disease. Specifically, (1) peripheral plasma renin activity is elevated far less frequently in renal parenchymal than in renovascular hypertension; (2) cardiac output is said to be normal in renal parenchymal hypertension (unless uremia and anemia are present) but slightly elevated in renovascular hypertension; (3) circulatory responses to tilting and to the Valsalva maneuver are exaggerated in the latter condition; and (4) blood volume tends to be high in patients with severe renal parenchy-

mal disease and low in patients with severe unilateral renovascular hypertension. Alternative explanations for the hypertension in renal parenchymal disease include the possibilities that the damaged kidneys (1) produce an unidentified vasopressor substance other than renin, (2) fail to produce a necessary humoral vasodilator substance (perhaps prostaglandin or bradykinin), (3) fail to inactivate circulating vasopressor substances, and/or (4) are ineffective in disposing of sodium. In the last case, the retained sodium would be responsible for the hypertension as outlined earlier. Although all these explanations, including participation of the renin-angiotensin system, probably have some validity in individual patients, the hypothesis involving sodium retention is particularly attractive. It is supported by the observation that those patients with chronic pyelonephritis or polycystic renal disease who are salt wasters do not develop hypertension and by the observation that removal of salt and water by dialysis or diuretics is effective in controlling arterial pressure in most patients with renal parenchymal disease.

A rare form of renal hypertension results from the excess secretion of renin by juxtaglomerular cell tumors or nephroblastomas. The initial presentation is similar to that of hyperaldosteronism, with hypertension, hypokalemia, and overproduction of aldosterone. However, in contrast to primary aldosteronism, peripheral renin activity is *elevated instead of subnormal*. This disease can be distinguished from other forms of secondary aldosteronism by the presence of normal renal function and unilateral increases in renal vein renin concentration without a renal artery lesion.

ENDOCRINE HYPERTENSION Adrenal Hypertension
Hypertension is a feature of a variety of adrenal cortical abnormalities. In *primary aldosteronism* (Chap. 332), there is a clear relationship between the aldosterone-induced sodium retention and the hypertension. Normal individuals given aldosterone develop hypertension only if they also ingest sodium. Since aldosterone causes sodium retention by stimulating renal tubular exchange of sodium for potassium, hypokalemia is a prominent feature in most patients with primary aldosteronism, and, therefore, the measurement of serum potassium provides a simple screening test. The effect of sodium retention and volume expansion in chronically suppressing plasma renin activity is critical for the definitive diagnosis. In most clinical situations, plasma renin activity and plasma or urinary aldosterone levels parallel each other, but in patients with primary aldosteronism, aldosterone levels are high and relatively fixed because of autonomous aldosterone secretion, whereas plasma renin activity levels are suppressed and respond sluggishly to sodium depletion. Primary aldosteronism may be secondary to either a tumor or bilateral adrenal hyperplasia. It is important to distinguish between these two conditions preoperatively, since usually the hypertension in the latter case is not modified by operation.

The sodium-retaining effect of large amounts of glucocorticoids (perhaps resulting in part from saturation of the 11β-hydroxysteroid hydrogenase enzyme system in the kidney by the increased concentration of cortisol) also offers an explanation for the hypertension in severe cases of Cushing's syndrome (Chap. 332). Moreover, increased production of mineralocorticoids also has been documented in some patients with Cushing's syndrome. However, the hypertension in many cases of Cushing's syndrome does not seem volume-dependent, leading investigators to speculate that it may be secondary to glucocorticoid-induced production of renin substrate (angiotensin-mediated hypertension). In the forms of the adrenogenital syndrome due to C-11 or C-17 hydroxylase deficiency (Chap. 332), deoxycorticosterone accounts for the sodium retention and the resulting hypertension, which is accompanied by suppression of plasma renin activity.

In patients with pheochromocytoma (Chap. 333), increased secretion of epinephrine and norepinephrine by a tumor (most often located in the adrenal medulla) causes excessive stimulation of adrenergic receptors, which results in peripheral vasoconstriction and cardiac stimulation. This diagnosis is confirmed by demonstrating increased urinary excretion of epinephrine and norepinephrine and/or their metabolites.

Acromegaly (See also Chap. 328) Hypertension, coronary atherosclerosis, and cardiac hypertrophy are frequent complications of this condition.

Hypercalcemia (See also Chap. 353) The hypertension which occurs in up to one-third of patients with hyperparathyroidism ordinarily can be attributed to renal parenchymal damage due to nephrolithiasis and nephrocalcinosis. However, increased calcium levels also can have a direct vasoconstrictive effect. In some cases, the hypertension disappears when the hypercalcemia is corrected. Thus, paradoxically, the increased serum calcium level in hyperparathyroidism raises blood pressure, while epidemiologic studies suggest that a high calcium intake lowers blood pressure. To further confuse the issue, calcium entry–blocking agents are effective antihypertensive agents. Additional studies are needed to resolve these seemingly conflicting observations.

Oral Contraceptives Several years ago, a common cause of endocrine hypertension was the use of estrogen-containing oral contraceptives. However, several recent studies suggest that this is no longer true, probably owing to the lower estrogen content of modern oral contraceptives. In patients receiving these agents who do become hypertensive, the mechanism is likely to be activation of the renin-angiotensin-aldosterone system. Thus, both volume (aldosterone) and vasoconstrictor (angiotensin II) factors are important. The estrogen component of oral contraceptive agents stimulates the hepatic synthesis of the renin substrate angiotensinogen, which in turn favors the increased production of angiotensin II and secondary aldosteronism. Some women taking oral contraceptives have increased plasma concentrations of angiotensin II and aldosterone with some increase in arterial pressure. However, only a small number actually have an increase in arterial pressure to a level greater than 140/90, and, in about half of these, the hypertension will remit within 6 months of stopping the drug.

Why some women taking oral contraceptives develop hypertension and others do not is unclear but may be related to (1) increased vascular sensitivity to angiotensin II, (2) the presence of mild renal disease, (3) familial factors (over one-half have a positive family history for hypertension), (4) age (hypertension is significantly more prevalent in women over age 35), (5) the estrogen content of the contraceptive, and/or (6) obesity. Indeed some investigators have suggested that the oral contraceptives are simply unmasking women with essential hypertension.

COARCTATION OF THE AORTA (See also Chap. 235) The hypertension associated with coarctation may be caused by the constriction itself or perhaps by the changes in the renal circulation, which result in an unusual form of renal arterial hypertension. The diagnosis of coarctation usually is evident from physical examination and routine x-ray findings.

EFFECTS OF HYPERTENSION

Patients with hypertension die prematurely; the most common cause of death is heart disease, with stroke and renal failure also frequent, particularly in patients with significant retinopathy.

EFFECTS ON THE HEART Cardiac compensation for the excessive workload imposed by increased systemic pressure is at first sustained by concentric left ventricular hypertrophy, characterized by an increase in wall thickness. Ultimately, the function of this chamber deteriorates, the cavity dilates, and the symptoms and signs of heart failure appear (Chap. 232). Angina pectoris also may occur because of the combination of accelerated coronary arterial disease and increased myocardial oxygen requirements as a consequence of the increased myocardial mass (Chap. 244). On physical examination, the heart is enlarged and has a prominent left ventricular impulse. The sound of

aortic closure is accentuated, and there may be a faint murmur of aortic regurgitation. Presystolic (atrial, fourth) heart sounds appear frequently in hypertensive heart disease, and a protodiastolic (ventricular, third) heart sound or summation gallop rhythm may be present. Electrocardiographic changes of left ventricular hypertrophy (Chap. 228) may occur, but the electrocardiogram substantially underestimates the frequency of cardiac hypertrophy compared with that observed with the echocardiogram. Evidence of ischemia or infarction may be observed late in the disease. Most deaths due to hypertension result from myocardial infarction or congestive heart failure.

NEUROLOGIC EFFECTS The neurologic effects of long-standing hypertension may be divided into retinal and central nervous system changes. Because the retina is the only tissue in which the arteries and arterioles can be examined directly, repeated ophthalmoscopic examination provides the opportunity to observe the progress of the vascular effects of hypertension (Table 35-2). The Keith-Wagener-Barker classification of the *retinal changes* in hypertension has provided a simple and excellent means for serial evaluation of hypertensive patients. Increasing severity of hypertension is associated with focal spasm and progressive general narrowing of the arterioles, as well as the appearance of hemorrhages, exudates, and papilledema. These retinal lesions often produce scotomata, blurred vision, and even blindness, especially when there is papilledema or hemorrhages of the macular area. Hypertensive lesions may develop acutely and, if therapy results in significant reduction of blood pressure, may show rapid resolution. Rarely, these lesions resolve without therapy. In contrast, retinal arteriolosclerosis results from endothelial and muscular proliferation, and it accurately reflects similar changes in other organs. Sclerotic changes do not develop as rapidly as hypertensive lesions, nor do they regress appreciably with therapy. As a consequence of increased wall thickness and rigidity, sclerotic arterioles distort and compress the veins where the two vessel types cross in their common fibrous sheath, and the reflected light streak from the arterioles is changed by the increased opacity of the vessel wall.

Central nervous system dysfunction also occurs frequently in patients with hypertension. Occipital headaches, most often occurring in the morning, are among the most prominent early symptoms of hypertension. Dizziness, light-headedness, vertigo, tinnitus, and dimmed vision or syncope also may be observed, but the more serious manifestations are due to vascular occlusion, hemorrhage, or encephalopathy (Chap. 366). The pathogeneses of the former two disorders are quite different. *Cerebral infarction* is secondary to the increased atherosclerosis observed in hypertensive patients, whereas *cerebral hemorrhage* is the result of both the elevated arterial pressure and the development of cerebral vascular microaneurysms (Charcot-Bouchard aneurysms). Only age and arterial pressure are known to influence the development of the microaneurysms. Thus, it is not surprising that arterial pressure shows a better association with cerebral hemorrhage than with either cerebral or myocardial infarction.

Hypertensive encephalopathy consists of the following symptom complex: severe hypertension, disordered consciousness, increased intracranial pressure, retinopathy with papilledema, and seizures. The pathogenesis is uncertain but probably is not related to arteriolar spasm or cerebral edema. Focal neurologic signs are infrequent and, if present, suggest that infarction, hemorrhage, or transient ischemic attacks are more likely diagnoses. Although some investigators have suggested that prompt lowering of arterial pressure in these patients may adversely affect cerebral blood flow, most studies indicate that this is not the case.

EFFECTS ON THE KIDNEY (See also Chap. 277) Arteriosclerotic lesions of the afferent and efferent arterioles and the glomerular capillary tufts are the most common renal vascular lesions in hypertension and result in a decreased glomerular filtration rate and tubular dysfunction. Proteinuria and microscopic hematuria occur because of glomerular lesions, and approximately 10 percent of the deaths caused by hypertension result from renal failure. Blood loss in hypertension occurs not only from renal lesions; epistaxis, hemoptysis, and metrorrhagia also occur frequently in these patients.

With Hypertension The detailed initial evaluation of the hypertensive patient is outlined in Chap. 35. It includes the critical elements of the history, physical examination, and basic laboratory investigation that aid in arriving at appropriate diagnostic and therapeutic decisions (see Table 35-2).

DIAGNOSIS OF SECONDARY HYPERTENSION Certain clues from the history, physical examination, and basic laboratory studies may suggest an unusual cause for the hypertension and dictate the need for special studies. For example, the abrupt onset of severe hypertension and/or the onset of hypertension of any severity under the age of 25 or after the age of 50 years should lead to laboratory tests to exclude renovascular hypertension and pheochromocytoma. A history of headaches, palpitations, anxiety attacks, unusual sweating, hyperglycemia, and weight loss also should lead to tests to exclude pheochromocytoma. The presence of an abdominal bruit should lead to a workup for renovascular hypertension, and the finding on physical examination of bilateral upper abdominal masses consistent with polycystic renal disease should lead to the performance of an abdominal ultrasound examination or intravenous pyelogram. An elevated creatinine or blood urea nitrogen level, associated with proteinuria and hematuria, should prompt a detailed workup for renal insufficiency (Chap. 269). Special studies for secondary hypertension are also indicated if there is therapeutic failure with the initial drug program. The specific diagnostic measures depend on the most likely causes of secondary hypertension.

Pheochromocytoma (See also Chap. 333) The easiest and best screening procedure for pheochromocytoma is the measurement of catecholamines or their metabolites in a 24-h urine sample collected while the patient is hypertensive. Measurement of plasma catecholamine levels also may be useful. These tests may be indicated even in patients who do not have episodic hypertension, since over half the patients with pheochromocytoma have fixed hypertension. Provocative tests are seldom, if ever, indicated, although occasionally a suppressive test may be useful.

Cushing's Syndrome (See also Chap. 332) A 24-h urine test for cortisol or the administration of 1 mg of dexamethasone at bedtime, followed by the measurement of plasma cortisol at 7 to 10 A.M., is the best test to screen for the presence of Cushing's syndrome. A urine cortisol level of less than 2750 nmol (100 μg) or suppression of the plasma cortisol level to below 140 nmol/L (5 μg/dL) effectively rules out Cushing's syndrome.

Renovascular Hypertension (See also Chap. 277) The standard screening test for renal vascular hypertension has been the rapid-sequence intravenous pyelogram (IVP). Features suggestive of renal ischemia include (1) unilateral delayed appearance and excretion of contrast material, (2) a difference in kidney size of greater than 1.5 cm, (3) an irregular renal silhouette, suggesting partial infarction or atrophy, (4) indentations on the ureter or renal pelvis, possibly due to dilated ureteral arteries (collateral notching), and (5) hyperconcentration of contrast medium in the collecting system of the smaller kidney. When these criteria are used, the false-positive rate is 11 percent and the false-negative rate 12 percent.

In many centers the IVP has been replaced by one or more of the following tests. (1) The digital subtraction angiogram has been received with considerable enthusiasm as a more precise screening test for renal vascular disease. Its ultimate place as a screening test is unclear, however, because of its relatively high cost and the need for an arterial rather than a venous injection. (2) The captopril-induced renogram takes advantage of the dependence of the renal vasculature on angiotensin II. Thus, when individuals with renal artery stenosis are given a converting-enzyme inhibitor (captopril) that reduces angiotensin II levels on the stenotic side, the result will be a renal blood flow pattern demonstrating a reduced uptake and delayed excretion as assessed by the isotope renogram. (3) Renal duplex ultrasound provides both an anatomic assessment (from B-mode imaging) and a functional assessment (from Doppler imaging) of the renal arteries. Thus, in theory, it should provide the most accurate noninvasive assessment. However, its precision is very dependent on the skill and expertise of the radiologist. Thus, in many centers, the converting enzyme inhibitor–induced renogram has displaced the IVP as the screening procedure of choice. The renal duplex ultrasound is favored in a few centers.

The definitive test for surgically correctable renal disease is the combination of a renal angiogram and renal vein renin determinations. The renal arteriogram both establishes the presence of a renal arterial lesion and aids in the determination of whether the lesion is due to atherosclerosis or to one of the fibrous or fibromuscular dysplasias. It does not, however, prove that the lesion is responsible for the hypertension, nor does it permit prediction of the chances of surgical cure. It must be noted (1) that renal artery stenosis is a frequent finding by angiography and at postmortem in normotensive individuals, and (2) that essential hypertension is a common condition and may occur in combination with renal arterial stenosis that is not responsible for the hypertension. Bilateral renal vein catheterization for measurement of plasma renin activity is therefore used to assess the functional significance of any lesion noted on arteriography. When one kidney is ischemic and the other is normal, all the renin released comes from the involved kidney. In the most straightforward situation, the ischemic kidney has a significantly higher venous plasma renin activity than the normal kidney, by a factor of 1.5 or more. Moreover, the renal venous blood draining the uninvolved kidney exhibits levels similar to those in the inferior vena cava below the entrance of the renal veins.

Significant benefit from operative correction may be anticipated in at least 80 percent of patients with the findings described above if care is taken to prepare the patient properly before renal vein blood sampling, i.e., by discontinuing renin-suppressing drugs, such as beta blockers, for at least 10 days; restricting the patient to a low sodium intake for 4 days; and/or giving a converting-enzyme inhibitor for 24 h. When obstructing lesions in the *branches* of the renal arteries are demonstrated by arteriography, an attempt to obtain blood samples from the main *branches* of the renal vein should be made in an effort to identify a localized intrarenal arterial lesion responsible for the hypertension.

Primary Aldosteronism (See also Chap. 332) These patients almost always exhibit hypokalemia. Diuretic therapy often complicates the picture when the hypokalemia is first observed and needs to be assessed. Given the presence of hypokalemia, the relation between plasma renin activity and the aldosterone level becomes the key to the diagnosis of primary aldosteronism. The aldosterone concentration or excretion rate is high and plasma renin activity is low in primary aldosteronism, and these levels are relatively unaffected by changes in sodium balance. A critical part of the evaluation after primary aldosteronism has been established is to determine whether disease is unilateral or bilateral, because surgical removal of the lesion usually reduces arterial pressure only in patients with unilateral disease.

Plasma Renin Activity Measurements Some studies have suggested that the plasma renin level should be measured in most hypertensive patients and related to a 24-h urine sodium excretion rate to assess whether high, low, or normal renin levels are present. It has been proposed that this information may be important for both therapeutic and prognostic reasons. However, as noted earlier, it is unclear, on the basis of the available data and treatment programs, that these random measurements are really useful except in patients with findings suggestive of renal vascular disease or mineralocorticoid excess in whom lateralizing renal vein renin levels or suppressed peripheral renin levels may be of diagnostic and/or therapeutic significance.

℞ **TREATMENT**

Indications for Therapy Virtually every patient with a diastolic arterial pressure that persistently exceeds 90 mmHg, or any patient over 65 years of age with a systolic arterial pressure over

160 mmHg, is a candidate for diagnostic studies and for subsequent treatment. Furthermore, at any given level of blood pressure elevation, the ultimate risk of developing hypertensive vascular complications is greater in men than in women and in younger than in older persons. It may be argued, then, that it is hard to justify producing the uncomfortable side effects of therapy in, for example, an asymptomatic woman over 70 years of age with a diastolic pressure of 90 mmHg. On the other hand, it is easy to justify side effects in a man of 30 with a diastolic pressure exceeding 110 mmHg because such a person may be expected to receive the greatest benefit from therapy. Fortunately, the choice of treatment is such that a satisfactory program to control arterial pressure with minimal side effects can be developed for most patients, particularly as more studies assessing the impact of specific therapeutic agents on the patient's quality of life are reported.

A reasonable guideline would be that all patients with a diastolic pressure repeatedly above 90 mmHg should be treated unless specific contraindications exist. Patients with isolated *systolic* hypertension (levels greater than 160 mmHg) also should be treated if they are over age 65. It is uncertain that individuals under age 65 who have isolated systolic hypertension will benefit from therapy until the results of a well-controlled, prospective study are completed. Patients with labile hypertension or isolated systolic hypertension who are not treated should have regular follow-up examinations at 6-month intervals because of the frequent development of progressive and/or sustained hypertension. Finally, if coronary artery disease or associated cardiovascular risks are present, then treatment of a patient with a lower blood pressure may be warranted. For example, patients with angina pectoris or diabetes mellitus with diastolic blood pressures between 85 and 90 mmHg may be candidates for antihypertensive therapy.

The identification of an operable form of secondary hypertension does not automatically mean that surgical treatment is indicated. The decision depends on the age and general health of the patient, the natural history of the lesion, and the response of the arterial pressure to drug therapy. In patients with renovascular hypertension, the feasibility of renal angioplasty, the advantages of surgical repair versus nephrectomy, and the degree of overall renal functional impairment must be considered. Age and general health are important in patients with renovascular hypertension due to arteriosclerosis, because there is no evidence that repair of the stenosis increases life expectancy in the elderly patient with other evidence of vascular disease. Knowledge of the natural history of the disease is especially important when making a decision in the case of a young patient with renal artery stenosis due to fibrous dysplasia. If the arteriographic appearance suggests that the stenosis is due to intimal or subadventitial fibroplasia, the lesion may be expected to progress, and operation or angioplasty is required. Medial fibroplasia, on the other hand, often remains stable, and operation or angioplasty may not be necessary if pressure can be controlled by drug therapy.

The decision regarding operation also should be considered carefully in patients with primary aldosteronism when neither abdominal computed tomography nor bilateral adrenal venography demonstrates a tumor, because such patients may prove to have multinodular hyperplasia. In that case, bilateral adrenalectomy would be required to eliminate the aldosterone excess, and, even then, hypertension would usually persist. If hypokalemia can be controlled by spironolactone or other drug therapy and arterial pressure lowered with antihypertensive agents, then it is reasonable to withhold operative treatment.

GENERAL MEASURES Nondrug therapeutic intervention is probably indicated in all patients with sustained hypertension and probably in most with labile hypertension. The general measures employed include (1) relief of stress, (2) dietary management, (3) regular aerobic exercise, (4) weight reduction (if needed), and (5) control of

other risk factors contributing to the development of arteriosclerosis. Relief of emotional and environmental stress is one of the reasons for the improvement in hypertension that occurs when a patient is hospitalized. Though it is usually impossible to extricate the hypertensive patient from all internal and external stresses, he or she should be advised to avoid unnecessary tensions. In rare instances, it may be appropriate to recommend a change of job or of life-style. It has been suggested that relaxation techniques also may lower arterial pressure. However, it is uncertain that these techniques alone have much long-term effect.

Dietary management has three aspects:

1. Because of the documented efficacy of sodium restriction and volume contraction in lowering blood pressure, patients previously were instructed to curtail sodium intake drastically. Some investigators have suggested that this is not necessary. They base their conclusion on two observations: (1) In many patients the blood pressure is not sensitive to the level of sodium intake, and (2) diuretics provide another method of decreasing body sodium stores in individuals whose blood pressure is sodium-sensitive. However, meta-analyses of previous diet studies have documented a 5-mmHg reduction in systolic pressure and a 2.6-mmHg reduction in diastolic pressure when sodium intake is reduced by approximately 75 mEq/day. In addition, several reports have documented that, while mild sodium restriction has little if any direct action on blood pressure, it significantly potentiates the efficacy of nearly all antihypertensive agents. Thus, by making it possible to control blood pressure with lower doses of drugs, sodium restriction leads to a reduction in side effects. In addition, it is quite clear that in some hypertensive patients, as noted above, the level of sodium intake does influence the blood pressure. Thus, since there is no apparent risk to mild sodium restriction, the most practical approach now is to advise mild dietary sodium restriction (up to 5 g NaCl per day), which can be achieved by eliminating all additions of salt to food that is prepared normally. Some studies also have reported a lowering of arterial pressure related to an *increase* in potassium and/or calcium intake. For example, in one meta-analysis, dietary potassium supplements of 50 to 120 mEq/day reduced blood pressure by about the same amount as salt restriction (by 6 mmHg systolic and 3.4 mmHg diastolic). While the advisability of these forms of dietary alteration is still controversial, the fact that a moderately high calcium intake (1.5 g elemental calcium daily) probably also reduces the extent of age-related osteoporosis, combined with the results of the potassium supplementation studies, indicate that they are probably useful adjuncts.

2. Caloric restriction should be urged for patients who are overweight. Some obese patients will show a significant reduction in blood pressure simply as a consequence of weight loss. In the Trial of Antihypertensive Interventions and Management (TAIM) study, weight reduction (average 4.4 kg over 6 months) lowered blood pressure by 2.5 mmHg.

3. A restriction in the intake of cholesterol and saturated fats is recommended, as this diet modification may diminish the incidence of arteriosclerotic complications. Reducing or eliminating alcohol intake is also beneficial. Regular exercise is indicated within the limits of the patient's cardiovascular status. Not only is exercise helpful in controlling weight, but also there is evidence that physical conditioning itself may lower arterial pressure. Isotonic exercises (jogging, swimming) are better than isometric exercises (weight lifting) since the latter, if anything, raises arterial pressure. The dietary management outlined above is aimed at the control of other risk factors. Probably the most significant additional step that could be taken in this area would be to convince the smoker to give up cigarettes.

DRUG THERAPY FOR HYPERTENSION (Table 246-4)

To make rational use of antihypertensive drugs, the sites and mechanisms of their action must be understood. In general, there are six classes of drugs: diuretics, antiadrenergic agents, vasodilators, calcium entry blockers, angiotensin-converting enzyme (ACE) inhibitors and angiotensin receptor antagonists.

Table 246-4

Drugs Used in Treatment of Hypertension—Listed According to Site of Action

Site of Action	Drug	Dosage	Indications	Contraindications/ Cautions	Frequent or Peculiar Side Effects
DIURETICS					
Renal tubule	Thiazides: e.g., hydrochlorothiazide	Depends on specific drug Oral: 12.5–25 mg daily or twice daily	Mild hypertension; as adjunct in treatment of moderate to severe hypertension	Diabetes mellitus, hyperuricemia, primary aldosteronism	Potassium depletion, hyperglycemia, hyperuricemia, hypercholesterolemia, dermatitis, purpura, depression, hypercalcemia
	Loop-acting: e.g., furosemide	Oral: 20–80 mg 2 or 3 times a day	Mild hypertension; as adjunct in severe or malignant hypertension, particularly with renal failure	Hyperuricemia, primary aldosteronism	Potassium depletion, hyperuricemia, hyperglycemia, hypocalcemia, blood dyscrasias, rash, nausea, vomiting, diarrhea
	Potassium-sparing: Spironolactone	Oral: 25 mg 2 to 4 times daily	Hypertension due to hypermineralocorticoidism; as adjunct to thiazide therapy	Renal failure	Hyperkalemia, diarrhea, gynecomastia, menstrual irregularities
	Triamterene	Oral: 50–100 mg 1 or 2 times daily			Hyperkalemia, nausea, vomiting, leg cramps, nephrolithiasis, GI disturbances
	Amiloride	Oral: 5–10 mg daily			
ANTIADRENERGIC AGENTS					
Central	Clonidine	Oral: 0.05–0.6 mg twice daily	Mild to moderate hypertension, renal disease with hypertension		Postural hypotension, drowsiness, dry mouth, rebound hypertension after abrupt withdrawal, insomnia
	Guanabenz	Oral: 4–16 mg twice daily			
	Guanfacine	Oral: 1–3 mg daily			
	Methyldopa (also acts by blocking sympathetic nerves)	Oral: 250–1000 mg twice daily IV: 250–1000 mg every 4–6 h (tolerance may develop)	Mild to moderate hypertension (oral), malignant hypertension (IV)	Pheochromocytoma, active hepatic disease (IV), during MAO inhibitor administration	Postural hypotension, sedation, fatigue, diarrhea, impaired ejaculation, fever, gynecomastia, lactation, positive Coombs' tests (occasionally associated with hemolysis), chronic hepatitis, acute ulcerative colitis, lupus-like syndrome
Autonomic ganglia	Trimethaphan	IV: 1–6 mg/min	Severe or malignant hypertension	Severe coronary artery disease, cerebrovascular insufficiency, diabetes mellitus (on hypoglycemic therapy), glaucoma, prostatism	Postural hypotension, visual symptoms, dry mouth, constipation, urinary retention, impotence
Nerve endings	Rauwolfia alkaloids: Reserpine	Oral: 0.05–0.25 mg daily	Mild to moderate hypertension in young patient	Pheochromocytoma, peptic ulcer, depression, during MAO inhibitor administration	Depression, nightmares, nasal congestion, dyspepsia, diarrhea, impotence
	Guanethidine Guanadrel	Oral: 10–150 mg daily Oral: 5–50 mg twice daily	Moderate to severe hypertension	Pheochromocytoma, severe coronary artery disease, cerebrovascular insufficiency, during MAO inhibitor administration	Postural hypotension, bradycardia, dry mouth, diarrhea, impaired ejaculation, fluid retention, asthma
Alpha receptors	Phentolamine	IV: 1–5 mg bolus	Suspected or proved pheochromocytoma	Severe coronary artery disease	Tachycardia, weakness, dizziness, flushing
	Phenoxybenzamine	Oral: 10–50 mg once or twice daily (tolerance may develop)	Proved pheochromocytoma		Postural hypotension, tachycardia, miosis, nasal congestion, dry mouth
	Prazosin	Oral: 1–10 mg twice daily	Mild to moderate hypertension	Use with caution in the elderly	Sudden syncope, headache, sedation, dizziness, tachycardia, anticholinergic effect, fluid retention
	Terazosin	Oral: 1–20 mg daily			
	Doxazosin	Oral: 1–8 mg daily			

(continued)

Table 246-4—(*Continued*)

Drugs Used in Treatment of Hypertension—Listed According to Site of Action

Site of Action	Drug	Dosage	Indications	Contraindications/ Cautions	Frequent or Peculiar Side Effects
Beta receptors	Propranolol	Oral: 10–120 mg 2 to 4 times daily	Mild to moderate hypertension (especially with evidence of hyperdynamic circulation); as adjunct to hydralazine therapy	Congestive heart failure, asthma, diabetes mellitus (on hypoglycemic therapy), during MAO inhibitor administration, COPD, sick sinus syndrome, 2d or 3d degree heart block	Dizziness, depression, bronchospasm, nausea, vomiting, diarrhea, constipation, heart failure, fatigue, Raynaud's phenomenon, hallucinations, hypertriglyceridemia, hypercholesterolemia, psoriasis; sudden withdrawal may precipitate angina or myocardial injury in patients with heart disease
	Metoprolol	Oral: 25–150 mg twice daily			
	Nadolol	Oral: 20–120 mg daily			
	Atenolol	Oral: 25–100 mg daily			
	Timolol	Oral: 5–15 mg twice daily			
	Betaxolol	Oral: 10–20 mg daily			
	Carteolol	Oral: 2.5–10 mg daily			
	Pindolol	Oral: 5–30 mg twice daily			Less resting bradycardia than other beta blockers
	Acebutolol	Oral: 200–600 mg twice daily			
Alpha/Beta receptor	Labetalol	Oral: 100–600 mg twice daily IV: 2 mg/min			Similar to beta blockers with more postural effects

VASODILATORS

Site of Action	Drug	Dosage	Indications	Contraindications/ Cautions	Frequent or Peculiar Side Effects
Vascular smooth muscle	Hydralazine	Oral: 10–75 mg 4 times daily IV or IM: 10–50 mg every 6 h (tolerance may develop)	As adjunct in treatment of moderate to severe hypertension (oral), malignant hypertension (IV or IM), renal disease with hypertension	Lupus erythematosus, severe coronary artery disease	Headache, tachycardia, angina pectoris, anorexia, nausea, vomiting, diarrhea, lupus-like syndrome, rash, fluid retention
	Minoxidil	Oral: 2.5–40 mg twice daily	Severe hypertension	Severe coronary artery disease	Tachycardia, aggravates angina, marked fluid retention, hair growth on face and body, coarsening of facial features, possible pericardial effusions
	Diazoxide	IV: 1–3 mg/kg up to 150 mg rapidly	Severe or malignant hypertension	Diabetes mellitus, hyperuricemia, congestive heart failure	Hyperglycemia, hyperuricemia, sodium retention
	Nitroprusside	IV: 0.5–8 (μg/kg)/min	Malignant hypertension		Apprehension, weakness, diaphoresis, nausea, vomiting, muscle twitching, cyanide toxicity

ANGIOTENSIN CONVERTING ENZYME INHIBITORS

Site of Action	Drug	Dosage	Indications	Contraindications/ Cautions	Frequent or Peculiar Side Effects
Converting enzyme	Captopril	Oral: 12.5–75 mg twice daily	Mild to severe hypertension, renal artery stenosis	Renal failure (reduction of dose), bilateral renal artery stenosis, pregnancy	Leukopenia, pancytopenia, hypotension, cough, angioedema, urticarial rash, fever, loss of taste, acute renal failure in bilateral renal artery stenosis, hyperkalemia
	Benazepril	Oral: 10–40 mg daily			Same as captopril, but little evidence for leukopenia, but perhaps increased frequency of cough and angioedema. All can be given once daily, but side effects are reduced if one-half dose is given twice daily. Fosinopril is excreted more in bile than the others.
	Enalapril	Oral: 2.5–40 mg daily			
	Enalaprilat	IV: 0.625–1.25 mg over 5 minutes every 6–8 h			
	Fosinopril	Oral: 10–40 mg daily			
	Lisinopril	Oral: 5–40 mg daily			
	Quinapril	Oral: 10–80 mg daily			
	Ramipril	Oral: 2.5–20 mg daily			

(*continued*)

Table 246-4—*(Continued)*

Drugs Used in Treatment of Hypertension—Listed According to Site of Action

Site of Action	Drug	Dosage	Indications	Contraindications/ Cautions	Frequent or Peculiar Side Effects
ANGIOTENSIN RECEPTOR ANTAGONISTS					
	Losartan	Oral: 25–50 mg once or twice daily	Mild to severe hypertension, renal artery stenosis	Pregnancy, bilateral renal artery stenosis	Hypotension, acute renal failure in bilateral renal artery stenosis, hyperkalemia
CALCIUM CHANNEL ANTAGONISTS					
Vascular smooth muscle	Nifedipine	Oral: 10–30 mg 4 times daily or as XL form 30–90 mg daily	Mild to moderate hypertension	Heart failure, 2d or 3d degree heart block	Tachycardia, flushing, gastrointestinal disturbances, hyperkalemia, edema, headache
	Amlodipine	Oral: 2.5–10 mg daily			
	Felodipine XL	Oral: 5–10 mg daily			
	Isradipine	Oral: 2.5–10 mg daily			
	Nicardipine	Oral: 20–40 mg 3 times daily			
	Benzothiazepines: Diltiazem	Oral: 30–90 mg 4 times daily or as CD form 180–300 mg daily	Mild to moderate hypertension	Heart failure, 2d or 3d degree heart block	Same as nifidepine, except no tachycardia or edema, but can cause heart block, constipation, and liver dysfunction
	Phenylalkylamine: Verapamil	Oral: 30–120 mg 4 times daily or as SR form 120–480 mg daily	Mild to moderate hypertension	Heart failure, 2d or 3d degree heart block	

DIURETICS (See also Chap. 233)   The thiazides are the most frequently used and most extensively investigated members of this group, and their early effect certainly is related to sodium diuresis and volume depletion. A reduction in peripheral vascular resistance also has been reported by some workers to be important in the long term. Traditionally, thiazide diuretics have formed the cornerstone of most therapeutic programs designed to lower arterial pressure, and they are usually effective within 3 to 4 days. Furthermore, they have been shown to reduce mortality and morbidity in long-term trials. However, in recent years there has been increasing resistance to their routine use, primarily because of their adverse metabolic effects, which include hypokalemia due to renal potassium loss, hyperuricemia due to uric acid retention, carbohydrate intolerance, and hyperlipidemia. The more potent loop-acting diuretics furosemide and bumetanide also have been shown to be antihypertensive, but they have been used less extensively for this indication, primarily because of their shorter duration of action. Spironolactone causes renal sodium loss by blocking the effect of mineralocorticoids, and, therefore, it may be more effective in patients whose mineralocorticoid levels are excessive, such as patients with primary or secondary aldosteronism. Although they do not compete directly with aldosterone, triamterene and amiloride act at the same site as spironolactone to impede sodium reabsorption. They are effective in the same situations as spironolactone, except that triamterene has little intrinsic antihypertensive effect. Their major disadvantage is that they can produce hyperkalemia, particularly in patients with impaired renal function. Any of these three potassium-sparing diuretics also can be given along with thiazide diuretics to minimize renal potassium loss.

ANTIADRENERGIC AGENTS (See also Chap. 70)   These drugs act at one or more sites—centrally on the vasomotor center, in peripheral neurons, where they modify catecholamine release, or in target tissues, where they block adrenergic receptor sites. Drugs that appear to have predominant *central actions* are *clonidine*, *methyldopa*, *guanabenz*, and *guanfacine*. These drugs and their metabolites are predominantly alpha-receptor agonists. Stimulation of alpha$_2$ receptors in the vasomotor centers of the brain *reduces* sympathetic outflow, thereby reducing arterial pressure. Usually a fall in cardiac output and heart rate also occurs, more commonly with clonidine and guanabenz, but the baroreceptor reflex is intact. Thus, postural symptoms are absent. However, rebound hypertension may occur rarely when these drugs, particularly clonidine and guanabenz, are stopped. This effect is probably secondary to an increase in norepinephrine release, which is inhibited by these agents owing their agonist effect on presynaptic alpha receptors.

Another class of antiadrenergic agents consists of the *ganglionic blocking drugs*, which are used infrequently now. Because of their side effects, ganglionic blocking agents are now usually reserved for the rapid lowering of arterial pressure by parenteral administration of the short-acting agent *trimethaphan* in patients with severe hypertension.

Various drugs act at *postganglionic adrenergic nerve endings*, but they are rarely used now because of their side effects. *Guanethidine* and its shorter-acting analogue guanadrel block the release of norepinephrine from adrenergic nerve endings. They usually reduce cardiac output and lower systolic more than diastolic blood pressure. They also produce a greater postural effect than the other drugs that act at the nerve endings, and orthostatic hypotension is a frequent side effect.

The last group of drugs affecting the adrenergic system are those that block the *peripheral adrenergic receptors*, alpha, beta, or both (see also Chap. 70).

Alpha-Adrenergic Receptor Blockers   *Phentolamine* and *phenoxybenzamine* block the action of norepinephrine at *alpha*-adrenergic receptor sites. These two compounds block both presynaptic (alpha$_2$) and postsynaptic (alpha$_1$) alpha receptors, and the former action accounts for the tolerance which develops. *Prazosin* is more effective because it selectively blocks only *postsynaptic alpha* receptors, i.e., alpha$_1$ receptors. Thus, presynaptic alpha activity remains, suppressing norepinephrine release, and tolerance occurs only infrequently. Accordingly, prazosin produces less tachycardia but more postural hypotension than direct-acting vasodilators, such as hydralazine, and rarely can produce substantial hypotension following the first dose.

Beta-Adrenergic Receptor Blockers (See also Chap. 244)   A number of effective *beta-adrenergic receptor blocking agents* are available that block sympathetic effects on the heart and should be most effective in reducing cardiac output and in lowering arterial pressure when there is increased cardiac sympathetic nerve activity. In addition, they block the adrenergic nerve–mediated release of renin from the renal juxtaglomerular cells, and this action may be an important component of their blood pressure–lowering action. Beta-adrenergic blockers are particularly useful when employed in conjunction with vascular smooth muscle relaxants, which tend to evoke a reflex increase in heart rate, and with diuretics, the administration of which often results in an elevation of circulating renin activity. In practice, beta blockers appear to be effective even when there is no evidence of increased sympathetic tone, with about one-half or more of all hypertensive patients showing a fall in pressure. Furthermore, like diuretics, they have been shown to reduce morbidity and mortality in long-term clinical trials. However, these agents can precipitate congestive heart failure and asthma in susceptible individuals, and they must be used with caution in diabetics receiving hypoglycemic therapy because they inhibit the usual sympathetic responses to hypoglycemia. Cardioselective beta-blocking agents (so-called beta$_1$ blockers: metoprolol, atenolol) have been developed and may be superior to nonselective beta blockers such as propranolol and timolol in patients with bronchospasm. Nadolol, a nonselective beta blocker, unlike other drugs of this class, is excreted unchanged in the urine and has a half-life of 14 to 20 h; only one dose a day is required. Atenolol also usually only needs to be given once a day. Pindolol and acebutolol are nonselective beta blockers that have partial agonist activity and, therefore, produce less bradycardia. Labetalol exerts both alpha- and beta-adrenergic blocking actions. Thus, it lowers arterial pressure not only by the same complex actions as do beta blockers but also directly by reducing systemic vascular resistance. Usually it has a more rapid onset of action but produces more postural symptoms and chronic sexual dysfunction than the other beta blockers.

VASODILATORS *Hydralazine* is the most versatile of the drugs that cause direct relaxation of vascular smooth muscle; it is effective both orally and parenterally, and acts mainly on arterial resistance rather than on venous capacitance vessels, as evidenced by lack of postural effects. Unfortunately, the effect of hydralazine on peripheral resistance is partly negated by a reflex increase in sympathetic discharge that raises heart rate and cardiac output. This response limits the usefulness of hydralazine, especially in patients with severe coronary artery disease. However, the efficacy of hydralazine can be increased if it is given in conjunction with a beta blocker or a drug such as methyldopa or clonidine, all of which block reflex sympathetic stimulation of the heart. A serious side effect of doses of hydralazine exceeding 300 mg/d has been the production of a lupus erythematosus–like syndrome.

Minoxidil is even more potent than hydralazine but unfortunately produces significant hypertrichosis and fluid retention and, therefore, is mainly limited to patients with severe hypertension and renal insufficiency.

Diazoxide, a thiazide derivative, is restricted in its application to acute situations. It is not a diuretic; in fact, it causes sodium retention. However, like other thiazides, it reduces carbohydrate tolerance. It must be given rapidly intravenously to guarantee an effect. It begins to act immediately to lower blood pressure, and its effects may last for several hours. *Nitroprusside* given intravenously also acts as a direct vasodilator, with onset and offset of actions that are almost immediate. *Nitroglycerin* is a third direct-acting vasodilator useful as an intravenous agent. These latter three drugs are useful only for the treatment of hypertensive emergencies (Table 246-5).

ACE INHIBITORS Drugs from several of the categories discussed above have been shown to possess an additional action resulting in inhibition of renin secretion. These include clonidine, reserpine, methyldopa, and beta blockers. A second group of drugs inhibit the enzyme converting angiotensin I into angiotensin II, the angiotensin converting enzyme (ACE). These agents are useful because they not only inhibit the generation of a potent vasoconstrictor (angiotensin II) but also may retard the degradation of a potent vasodilator (bradykinin), alter prostaglandin production (an effect most notable with captopril), and can modify the activity of the adrenergic nervous system. They are especially useful in renal or renovascular hypertension, as well as in accelerated and malignant hypertension. However, in patients with bilateral renal artery stenosis, rapid deterioration of renal function may occur. They are also as effective in mild, uncomplicated hypertension as beta blockers and thiazides—and probably have fewer side effects, particularly ones that adversely affect the patient's quality of life.

These drugs should be used with caution when the renin system is activated (for example, by severe heart failure, prior diuretic therapy, or substantial salt restriction) to avoid profound hypotension. Usually, diuretics are stopped 2 to 3 days before administration of an ACE inhibitor is begun and are added back later if needed.

ANGIOTENSIN RECEPTOR ANTAGONISTS These drugs have effects similar to those of ACE inhibitors. However, instead of blocking the production of angiotensin II, they competitively inhibit its binding to the angiotensin II AT$_1$ receptor subtype. Their utility and tolerability are similar to those of the ACE inhibitors, but they do not cause cough or angioedema.

CALCIUM CHANNEL ANTAGONISTS There are three subclasses of calcium channel antagonists: the phenylalkylamine derivatives (e.g., verapamil), the benzothiazepines (e.g., diltiazem), and the dihydropyridines (e.g., nifedipine). To date, there is only one therapeutic agent in each of the first two classes but a number of agents in the third class. All three subclasses modify calcium entry into cells by interacting with specific binding sites on the α$_1$ subunit of the L-type voltage-dependent calcium channel. Thus, since there are other calcium channels (e.g., the T and N types), the actions of these drugs only partially modify total calcium transport into cells. The relative specificity of each agent stems from the fact that each class has a unique binding site on the α$_1$ subunit, and these sites are variably

Table 246-5

Therapeutic Agents Used to Treat Malignant Hypertension

Drug	Route	Starting Dose	Onset	Peak	Duration	Oral Preparation Available
			Time Course of Action			
IMMEDIATE ONSET						
Nitroprusside	Continuous IV	0.25 μg/kg/min	<1 min	1–2 min	2–5 min	No
Trimethaphan	Continuous IV	0.5 mg/min	<1 min	1–2 min	2–5 min	No
Nitroglycerin	Continuous IV	5 μg/min	1–5 min	2–6 min	3–10 min	No
Diazoxide	IV bolus	50 mg q 5–10 min up to 600 mg	1–5 min	2–4 min	4–12 h	No
DELAYED ONSET						
Enalaprilat	IV	1.25 mg q 6 h	10–15 min	3–4 h	6–24 h	Yes
Hydralazine	IV, IM	5–10 mg q 20 min × 3	10–20 min	20–40 min	4–12 h	Yes
Labetalol	IV	20–80 mg q 10 min up to 300 mg	5 min	20–30 min	3–6 h	Yes
Nifedipine	Sublingual	10–20 mg	5–15 min	30–60 min	3–6 h	Yes

expressed in different tissues. Thus, while agents from all three subclasses cause vasodilation, usually only dihydropyridines produce reflex tachycardia. Diltiazem and verapamil can both slow atrioventricular conduction—a feature not observed with the dihydropyridines. While calcium channel antagonists are also useful in angina pectoris (see Chap. 244), because of their negative inotropic actions, they should be used with caution in hypertensive patients with heart failure. The short-acting dihydropyridines, such as nifedipine, should be used with caution for long-term therapy in hypertensive patients, since they have been reported to increase the incidence of acute coronary events. Verapamil, diltiazem, or long-acting dihydropyridines should be used instead.

APPROACH TO DRUG THERAPY (Fig. 246-1) The aim of drug therapy is to use the agents just described, alone or in combination, to return arterial pressure to normal levels with minimal side effects. Ideally, one would choose a therapeutic program that specifically corrects the underlying defect resulting in the elevated blood pressure—for example, treatment with spironolactone for patients with primary aldosteronism. As our knowledge of the mechanisms underlying the hypertension in individual patients increases, more specific drug programs will become available. Such programs presumably will result in normalization of blood pressure with fewer side effects. In the absence of this information, an empirical approach is used, which takes into consideration efficacy, safety, impact on the quality of life, compliance, ease of administration, and cost. When used in combination, drugs are chosen for their different sites of action. However, except for those patients with severe hypertension (average diastolic blood pressure >130 mmHg), in whom intensive therapy with several agents simultaneously usually is required, most patients should be treated *initially* with a single agent.

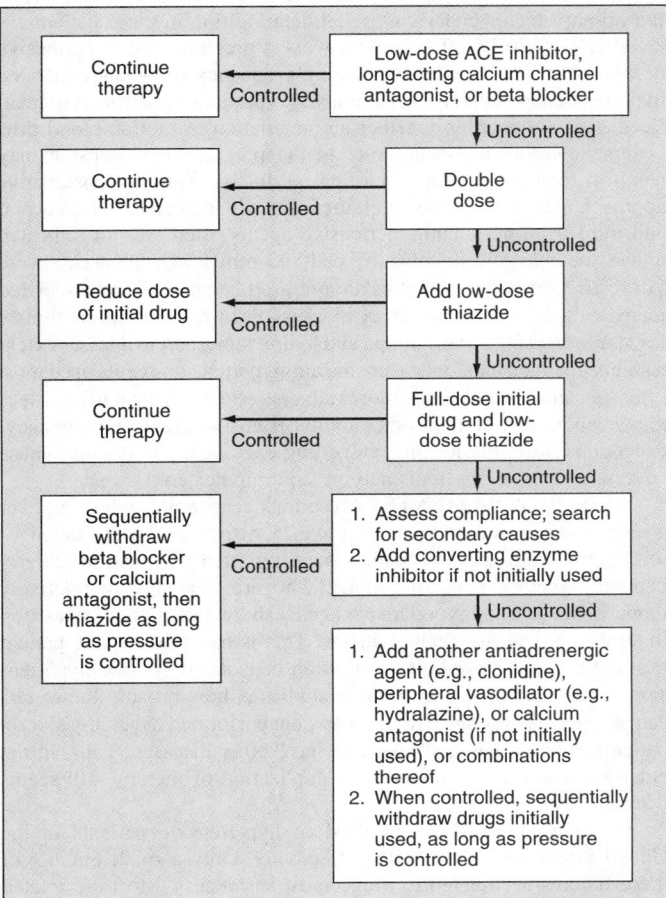

FIGURE 246-1 Schematic approach to the patient with hypertension for whom no specific form of therapy is known or available and who does not have volume expansion.

Since many effective antihypertensive agents are available, a number of useful therapeutic regimens have been developed, with the ideal program still unclear. Initial therapy with a diuretic or beta blocker has been the usual first approach, particularly as these are the only agents proven to reduce mortality. However, this practice does not mean that other effective antihypertensives would fail to have the same beneficial effect if used in similar trials. Thus, ACE inhibitors and calcium channel antagonists are also effective as first-line therapy, replacing the old stepped-care approach. The physician is therefore required to choose from four classes of agents for initial therapy, with little evidence that one is more effective than another. It has been suggested, and the author agrees, that an ACE inhibitor or some calcium channel antagonists be used first, because of their lower side effects, with a slight preference for ACE inhibitors because of their longer duration of action, potentially fewer adverse effects, and increased compliance rates. Angiotensin receptor antagonists may also be included, with the caution that their long-term efficacy and side effects are unknown. The choice of one drug over the others is empirical.

The schema outlined in Fig. 246-1 takes into account the presently available data on effectiveness, adverse reactions, compliance, impact on quality of life, and economic impact (including cost, usage of health care resources, and quality and quantity of work performance) in deciding when to use a given agent. This approach is applicable to all patients in whom an indication for a specific form of therapy is lacking. Because of its lower cost, low-dose thiazide therapy, e.g., 25 mg of hydrochlorothiazide (or its equivalent) daily, often has been the first choice. However, three major concerns with widespread thiazide usage have arisen: relatively poor compliance rates (approximately 80 percent), which probably reflect an adverse effect on the patient's quality of life, adverse metabolic effects (hypokalemia, hypomagnesemia, hyperglycemia, and hypercholesterolemia), and potentially an increased frequency of cardiac arrhythmias, including sudden death, probably secondary to the electrolyte disturbances. These concerns, coupled with the eight- to tenfold increase in cost associated with the frequent need for potassium supplementation or a potassium-sparing diuretic, have caused some to suggest that thiazides should play a more restricted role in initial antihypertensive therapy, being limited to individuals who have volume expansion. Thus, ACE inhibitors, beta blockers, and some calcium channel antagonists are probably the preferred agents for first-line therapy for hypertension, with beta blockers being particularly useful in patients with a hyperactive hemodynamic state, as in hypertension with an elevated heart rate.

Under any circumstances, the agent should be started at a low dose, e.g., 25 mg of atenolol, 25 mg of captopril, 5 mg of enalapril, or 120 mg of diltiazem (or their equivalents) in divided doses as needed (Table 246-4). If arterial pressure is lowered to less than 140/90 with any of these agents, no further therapy is indicated (see Fig. 246-1). If arterial pressure has not reached this level after 1 to 3 months, the next step is to double the dose of the primary agent. If hypertension still is not controlled, then 25 mg of hydrochlorothiazide (or its equivalent) per day should be added. Thiazides potentiate the action of ACE inhibitors and probably of beta blockers, and their antihypertensive effect is at least additive to that of calcium channel antagonists. Combining diuretics with ACE inhibitors is particularly appealing because the adverse metabolic effects of the thiazide will in part be ameliorated by the ACE inhibitor. Beta blockers and calcium antagonists do not have this advantage. Indeed, beta blockers and thiazides may actually potentiate each other's adverse effects, insofar as electrolyte alterations (hypokalemia) and metabolic actions (hypercholesterolemia) are concerned.

If therapy with two drugs does not achieve blood pressure control, the primary agent should be increased to full dose, e.g., 100 mg of captopril or atenolol, 20 mg of enalapril, or 360 mg of diltiazem. While doses larger than these can be used, it is probably advisable to switch to another medication rather than increase the dose further.

Occasionally, increasing the thiazide dose to the equivalent of 50 mg of hydrochlorothiazide daily may bring about control of the hypertension; however, thiazide doses higher than this are seldom, if ever, warranted because they almost invariably produce significant side effects. If the blood pressure is still not controlled, then a detailed search for a secondary cause of hypertension, as outlined above, is indicated. If none is found, then a dietary assessment often will reveal a high sodium intake. With reduction in salt intake to 5 g/d or less, blood pressure often is controlled. If the blood pressure is still not controlled, then the primary agent should be switched, maintaining the thiazide. Caution should be used if an ACE inhibitor was not the original agent, as administration of such an agent to a patient who already is taking a diuretic may lead to profound hypotension. If none of these changes produces better control of arterial pressure, then the combination of a calcium channel antagonist and an ACE inhibitor, or triple therapy, usually with a diuretic, ACE inhibitor, and hydralazine, may be effective.

If the blood pressure is controlled, then a stepwise reduction in the dose and/or withdrawal of some of the agents should be done to determine the minimal therapeutic program that will maintain the blood pressure at 140/90 mmHg or less.

Fewer than 5 percent of patients will still be hypertensive at this point. In them, one first should consider the reasons for therapeutic failure, as shown in Table 246-6. If none can be identified, then one of the other agents, such as one of the vasodilators listed in Table 246-4 (e.g., hydralazine) or an antiadrenergic agent (e.g., prazosin or clonidine) should be added. If blood pressure is controlled, previous drugs are withdrawn sequentially to determine the minimal therapeutic program that will maintain a normal blood pressure.

While the recommendations outlined above are satisfactory for a large majority of patients, it is important to use a flexible approach, because individual patients may respond differently to individual drugs and drug combinations. For those patients requiring multiple drugs, once the appropriate combination has been found, the use of a single formulation with the appropriate combination of drugs may simplify the regimen and thereby increase compliance. Every effort should be made to reduce the number of times each day the patients must interrupt their schedules for the medication. Pharmacologic treatment of essential hypertension is usually lifelong, and since most patients are asymptomatic, compliance with a complex regimen may be a serious problem, particularly if the therapeutic regimen has a negative impact on the quality of the patient's life. Finally, it is uncertain what level of arterial pressure should be accepted as representing adequate control. It is clear that reducing diastolic blood pressure to below 90 mmHg is appropriate and reduces morbidity and/or mortality. However, whether a reduction to a level below 85 mmHg is warranted, particularly in elderly patients, remains controversial.

Five groups of patients with hypertension require special consideration because of associated conditions. These groups are considered in the following sections.

RENAL DISEASE   Reduction of arterial pressure in hypertensive patients with impaired renal function is often accompanied initially

Table 246-6

Reasons for Poor Therapeutic Response in Patients with Hypertension

Inadequate patient compliance
Volume expansion
   Caused by excessive sodium intake
   Caused by nondiuretic antihypertensive agent
Excessive weight gain
Inadequate doses
Drug antagonism
Cold remedies
Sympathomimetics
Oral contraceptives (estrogens)
Adrenal steroids
Secondary forms of hypertension

by an increase in serum creatinine. This change does not represent further structural renal damage and should not deter the physician from continuing the therapy, since achievement of blood pressure control may eventually reduce the value toward normal. However, if serum creatinine increases in a patient treated with a converting-enzyme inhibitor, care needs to be exercised, because these patients may have bilateral renal artery disease. Their renal function will continue to deteriorate as long as the converting-enzyme inhibitor is given. Thus, converting-enzyme inhibitors should be used cautiously in patients with impaired renal function, and renal function should be assessed frequently (every 4 to 5 days) for the first 3 weeks. While converting-enzyme inhibitors are contraindicated in patients with bilateral renal artery stenosis, these are the drugs of choice in patients with unilateral renal artery stenosis and a normally functioning contralateral kidney, and probably also in patients with chronic renal failure with or without diabetes mellitus.

CORONARY ARTERY DISEASE   In these patients, who also may be taking cardiac glycosides, thiazides should be used judiciously, and a reduction in serum potassium levels should be watched for and, if found, should be corrected rapidly. Beta blockers should be withdrawn carefully, if at all, in these patients. Finally, calcium channel antagonists and converting-enzyme inhibitors may be useful in these patients because they minimize a number of potential adverse reactions that accompany the use of other therapeutic agents, particularly nonspecific vasodilators.

DIABETES MELLITUS   The diabetic patient with hypertension is particularly challenging to treat because many of the agents used to lower blood pressure can affect glucose metabolism adversely. Converting-enzyme inhibitors may be particularly useful in these individuals. They have no known adverse effects on glucose or lipid metabolism and minimize the development of diabetic nephropathy by reducing renal vascular resistance and renal perfusion pressure—the primary factor underlying renal deterioration in these patients.

PREGNANCY   The patient who is pregnant and hypertensive or who develops hypertension during pregnancy (pregnancy-induced hypertension, preeclampsia, eclampsia) is particularly difficult to treat. Because it is uncertain whether autoregulation of uterine blood flow occurs, lowering blood pressure in the pregnant hypertensive may result in reduced placental and fetal perfusion. Thus, a conservative approach to lowering blood pressure is usually indicated. In the second and third trimesters, antihypertensive agents often are not indicated unless the diastolic pressure exceeds 95 mmHg. In general, severe salt restriction and/or diuretics are not used because of the associated increase in fetal wastage. Beta blockers need to be used cautiously for similar reasons. Methyldopa and hydralazine, and to a lesser extent calcium channel antagonists, are the antihypertensive agents used most often, because they have no known adverse effects on the fetus. Little is known about the safety of other antihypertensive agents in pregnancy, except that nitroprusside and converting-enzyme inhibitors may cause adverse effects on the fetus and are contraindicated.

ELDERLY PATIENTS   Hypertensive patients who are over age 65, and particularly those over age 75, offer substantial challenges to the physician. Several studies have reported that healthy elderly patients, whether male or female, who are treated with relatively modest doses of antihypertensive agents show a substantial reduction in strokes and stroke-related deaths. This is true whether the patient has systolic and diastolic hypertension or isolated systolic hypertension. What is not clear from these studies is how broadly the results can be extrapolated, since the studies were performed in healthy elderly patients, while many such patients have other diseases. Thus, in the elderly hypertensive patient, individualization of therapy still seems warranted.

Probably fewer than one-third of hypertensive patients in the United States are being treated effectively. Only a small number of these failures are related to drug unresponsiveness. Most are related to (1) failure to detect hypertension, (2) failure to institute effective treatment of an asymptomatic hypertensive patient, and (3) failure of the asymptomatic hypertensive patient to adhere to therapy. To help with the latter problem, patients must be educated to continue treatment once an effective regimen has been identified. Side effects and inconveniences of treatment must be minimized or counteracted in order to obtain the patient's continued cooperation.

MALIGNANT HYPERTENSION

In addition to marked blood pressure elevation in association with papilledema and retinal hemorrhages and exudates, the full-blown picture of malignant hypertension may include manifestations of hypertensive encephalopathy, such as severe headache, vomiting, visual disturbances (including transient blindness), transient paralyses, convulsions, stupor, and coma. These manifestations have been attributed to spasm of cerebral vessels and to cerebral edema. In some patients who have died, multiple small thrombi have been found in the cerebral vessels. Cardiac decompensation and rapidly declining renal function are other critical features of malignant hypertension. Oliguria may, in fact, be the presenting feature. The vascular lesion characteristic of malignant hypertension is fibrinoid necrosis of the walls of small arteries and arterioles, and this development can be reversed by effective antihypertensive therapy.

The pathogenesis of malignant hypertension is unknown. However, at least two independent processes—dilation of cerebral arteries and generalized arteriolar fibrinoid necrosis—contribute to the associated signs and symptoms. The cerebral arteries dilate because the normal autoregulation of cerebral blood flow decompensates as a result of the markedly elevated arterial pressure. Cerebral blood flow therefore is excessive, producing the encephalopathy associated with malignant hypertension. Many patients also show evidence of a microangiopathic hemolytic anemia; this secondary phenomenon could contribute to the deterioration of renal function. Most patients also have elevated levels of peripheral plasma renin activity and increased aldosterone production, and these effects may be involved in causing vascular damage.

Perhaps less than 1 percent of hypertensive patients develop the malignant phase, which can occur in the course of both essential and secondary hypertension. Rarely, it is the first recognized manifestation of the blood pressure problem, and it is unusual for it to occur in patients under treatment. The average age at diagnosis is 40, and men are affected more often than women. Prior to the availability of effective therapy, the life expectancy after diagnosis of malignant hypertension was less than 2 years, with most deaths being due to renal failure, cerebral hemorrhage, or congestive heart failure. With the advent of effective antihypertensive therapy, at least half the patients survive for more than 5 years.

℞ TREATMENT

Malignant hypertension is a medical emergency that requires immediate therapy. However, it needs to be distinguished from severe hypertension, since overly aggressive therapy in malignant hypertension could result in a potentially hazardous reduction in myocardial and cerebral perfusion. The initial aims of therapy should be (1) correction of medical complications and (2) reduction of diastolic pressure by one-third, but not to a level below 95 mmHg. The drugs available for treatment of malignant hypertension can be divided into two groups on the basis of time of onset of action (see Table 246-5). Those in the first group act within a few minutes but are not satisfactory for long-term management. If the patient is having convulsions, and if arterial pressure must be reduced rapidly, then one from the immediate-acting group should be used.

The first three agents in this group require continuous infusion and close monitoring. *Nitroprusside* is given by continuous intravenous infusion at a dose of 0.25 to 8.0 μg/kg per min. It is probably the agent of choice in this condition, since it dilates both arterioles and veins. It has the advantage over the ganglionic blockers of not being associated with the development of tachyphylaxis and can be used for days with few side effects. The dosage must be controlled with an infusion pump. *Nitroglycerin* affects veins more than arterioles and is given by continuous infusion at a rate of 5 to 100 μg/min. It is particularly useful in the treatment of hypertension

following coronary bypass surgery, myocardial infarction, left ventricular failure, or unstable angina pectoris. *Diazoxide* is the easiest agent to administer, for no individual titration of dosage is required. However, it is probably less effective than the other agents. It primarily affects arteriolar and not venous tone. A dose of 50 to 150 mg is given rapidly intravenously, and the antihypertensive effect appears in 1 to 5 min. The same dose can be repeated in 5 to 10 min, if necessary, or when the pressure begins to rise, usually after several hours. The total dose should not exceed 600 mg/d. In an occasional patient, pressure may drop below normal levels after diazoxide administration. This drug should not be used in patients in whom aortic dissection or myocardial infarction is suspected. Because it can increase the force of myocardial contraction, often a beta blocker is given concomitantly. *Enalaprilat*, an intravenous form of the ACE inhibitor *enalapril*, also has proven effective, particularly in individuals with left heart failure. Finally, intravenous *labetalol* may be particularly useful in patients with a myocardial infarct or angina because it prevents an increase in heart rate. However, it may be ineffective in patients previously treated with beta blockers and is contraindicated in patients with heart failure, asthma, bradycardia, or heart block. It also may serve as an alternative therapy in patients with eclampsia who are unresponsive to hydralazine. *Trimethaphan*, a ganglionic blocker, is given at a rate of 0.5 to 5 mg/min. Currently, it is seldom used. It also dilates arterioles and veins. The patient should be in the sitting position, and the pressure should be monitored closely, preferably in an intensive care unit. Monitoring may be more complex than with nitroprusside, but trimethaphan may be the better therapy in acute aortic dissection.

Patients given any of these agents also should receive other medications effective for long-term control. Those in the second group in Table 246-5 require 30 min or more to produce their full effect, but they have the advantage of being satisfactory for subsequent oral administration and for long-term management of the patient's hypertension. If such a delay in the achievement of the full effect is acceptable, intravenous *hydralazine* is effective in many patients within 10 min; an effective protocol involves giving 10-mg doses intravenously every 10 to 15 min until the desired effect has been obtained or until a total of 50 mg has been administered. The total amount required for response may then be repeated intramuscularly or intravenously every 6 h. Hydralazine should be used with caution in patients with significant coronary artery disease and should be avoided in patients manifesting myocardial ischemia or aortic dissection. It is effective in preeclampsia. Sublingual *nifedipine* has been reported to be useful, although it may produce tachycardia.

Furosemide is an important adjunct to the therapy just discussed. Given either orally or intravenously, it serves to maintain sodium diuresis in the face of a falling arterial pressure and thus will speed recovery from encephalopathy and congestive heart failure as well as maintain the sensitivity to the primary antihypertensive drug. Digitalis (Chap. 233) also may be indicated if there is evidence of cardiac decompensation.

In patients with malignant hypertension in whom the existence of pheochromocytoma is suspected, urine should be collected for measurement of the products of catecholamine metabolism, and drugs that might release additional catecholamines, such as methyldopa, reserpine, and guanethidine, must be avoided. The parenteral drug of choice in these patients is phentolamine, administered with care to avoid a precipitous reduction in arterial pressure. There is hope even for patients who fail to respond sufficiently to any of the forms of therapy and who show progressive deterioration in renal function. In some, a period of peritoneal dialysis or hemodialysis to deplete extracellular fluid has resulted in better blood pressure control and eventual improvement in renal function. In other patients with refractory hypertension and renal failure who do not respond to volume depletion or hypotensive therapy, including minoxidil administration—particularly those with marked elevation of plasma renin activity—bilateral nephrectomy has resulted in amelioration of hypertension; subsequently, these patients have been maintained on chronic dialysis or have received renal homografts. However, bilateral nephrectomy should be avoided where possible because (1) the loss of renal erythropoietin will contribute to the associated anemia; (2) vitamin D metabolism may be adversely affected; and (3) all residual renal function will be lost.

BIBLIOGRAPHY

CALHOUN DA et al: Treatment of hypertensive crisis. N Engl J Med 323:1177, 1990

FRIES ED: The efficacy and safety of diuretics in treating hypertension. Ann Intern Med 122:223, 1995

FROHLICH ED et al: The heart in hypertension. N Engl J Med 327:998, 1992

HOLLENBERG NK, WILLIAMS GH: Abnormal renal function, sodium-volume homeostasis, and renin system behavior in normal-renin essential hypertension: The evolution of the non-modular concept, in JH Laragh et al (eds): *Hypertension. Pathophysiology, Diagnosis, and Management*, 2d ed. New York, Raven, 1995, vol 2, p 1837

INSUA JT et al: Drug treatment of hypertension in the elderly: A meta-analysis. Ann Intern Med 121:355, 1994

JAFFE LS, SEELY EW: The heterogeneity of the blood pressure response to hormonal contraceptives. Curr Opin Endo Diab 2:257, 1995

JOINT NATIONAL COMMITTEE ON DETECTION, EVALUATION AND TREATMENT OF HIGH BLOOD PRESSURE: The fifth report. Arch Intern Med 153:154, 1993

LEWIS EJ et al: The effect of angiotensin converting enzyme inhibition on diabetic nephropathy. N Engl J Med 329:1456, 1993

LIEBSON PR et al: Comparison of five antihypertensive monotherapies and placebo for change in left ventricular mass in patients receiving nutritional-hygienic therapy in the Treatment of Mild Hypertension Study (TOMHS). Circulation 91:698, 1995

MORTENSEN RM, WILLIAMS GH: Aldosterone action (physiology), in LJ De-Groot et al (eds): *Endocrinology*, 3d ed. Philadelphia, Saunders, 1994, p 1668

NALLY VJ et al: Diagnostic criteria of renovascular hypertension with captopril renography. A consensus statement. Am J Hypertension 4:749S, 1991

NATIONAL HIGH BLOOD PRESSURE EDUCATION PROGRAM WORKING GROUP: National High Blood Pressure Education Program Working Group report on hypertension in diabetes. Hypertension 23:145, 1994

PSATY BM et al: The risk of incident myocardial infarction associated with antihypertensive drug therapies. Circulation 91:925, 1995

SPEDDING M, PAOLETTI R: Classification of calcium channels and the sites of action of drugs modifying channel function. Pharmacol Rev 44:363, 1992

STERN N, TUCK ML: Mechanisms of hypertension in diabetes mellitus, in JH Laragh et al (eds): *Hypertension: Pathophysiology, Diagnosis and Management*. New York, Raven 1995, p 1698

SYSTOLIC HYPERTENSION IN THE ELDERLY PROGRAM COOPERATIVE RESEARCH GROUP: Implications of the Systolic Hypertension in the Elderly Program. Hypertension 21:335, 1993

WILLIAMS GH: Genetic approaches to understanding the pathophysiology of complex human traits. Kidney Int 46:1550, 1994

WILLIAMS GH: Quality of life considerations in therapeutic decision-making: Antihypertensive therapy as a model, in M Bergener et al (eds): *Aging, Health and Healing*. New York, Springer, 1995, p 257

247 *Victor J. Dzau, Mark A. Creager*

DISEASES OF THE AORTA

The aorta is the conduit through which the blood ejected from the left ventricle is delivered to the systemic arterial bed. In adults, its diameter is approximately 3 cm at the origin, 2.5 cm in the descending portion in the thorax, and 1.8 to 2 cm in the abdomen. The aortic wall consists of a thin intima composed of endothelium, subendothelial connective tissue, and an internal elastic lamina; a thick tunica media composed of smooth-muscle cells and extracellular matrix; and an adventitia composed primarily of connective tissue and enclosing the vasa vasorum and nervi vascularis. In addition to its conduit function, the

viscoelastic and compliant properties of the aorta also subserve a buffering function. The aorta is distended during systole to enable a portion of the stroke volume to be stored, and it recoils during diastole so that blood continues to flow to the periphery during diastole. Because of its continuous exposure to high pulsatile pressure and shear stress, the aorta is particularly prone to injury and disease resulting from mechanical trauma (Table 247-1). The aorta is also more prone to rupture than any other vessel, especially with the development of aneurysmal dilatation, since its wall tension, as governed by Laplace's law (i.e., proportional to the product of pressure and radius), is intrinsically high.

AORTIC ANEURYSM

An *aneurysm* is defined as a pathologic dilatation of a segment of a blood vessel. A *true aneurysm* involves all three layers of the vessel wall and is distinguished from a *pseudoaneurysm*, in which the intimal and medial layers are disrupted and the dilatation is lined by adventitia only and sometimes by perivascular clot. Aneurysms also may be classified according to their gross appearance. A *fusiform aneurysm* affects the entire circumference of a segment of the vessel, resulting in a diffusely dilated lesion. In contrast, a *saccular aneurysm* involves only a portion of the circumference, resulting in an outpouching of the vessel wall.

The most common pathologic condition associated with aortic aneurysm is atherosclerosis. It is controversial whether atherosclerosis itself actually causes aortic aneurysm or develops as a secondary event in the dilated aorta. Causality is implied by studies that have shown that many patients with aortic aneurysms have coexisting risk factors and atherosclerosis in other blood vessels. Familial clusterings of abdominal aortic aneurysms occur in 20 percent of patients, suggesting a hereditary basis of the disease. A mutation of the gene encoding type III procollagen has been implicated. Additional causes of aortic aneurysm include cystic medial necrosis; syphilis, tuberculosis, or other bacterial infections; Takayasu arteritis; giant cell arteritis; seronegative spondyloarthropathies; rheumatoid arthritis; and trauma. Congenital aortic aneurysms may be primary or associated with other anomalies, such as a bicuspid aortic valve or aortic coarctation.

Aortic aneurysms are also classified according to location, i.e., abdominal versus thoracic. Those in the abdominal aorta are almost always associated with atherosclerosis. Aneurysms of the ascending thoracic aorta are caused most often by cystic medial necrosis. Aneurysms of the descending thoracic aorta are *usually* contiguous with infradiaphragmatic aneurysms and, as with the latter, are associated with atherosclerosis.

Aortic aneurysms usually do not produce symptoms. However, as they expand, they may become painful. Compression or erosion of adjacent tissue by aneurysms also may cause symptoms. The formation of mural thrombi within the aneurysm may predispose to peripheral embolization. Occasionally, an aneurysm may leak, leading to extravasation of blood into the vessel wall and the periadventitial area and causing acute pain and local tenderness. This is usually a harbinger of rupture and represents a medical emergency. More often, acute rupture occurs without any prior warning, and this complication is always life-threatening.

Table 247-1

Diseases of the Aorta: Classification and Etiology

Aortic aneurysm	**Aortic occlusion**
Atherosclerosis	Atherosclerosis
Cystic medial necrosis	Thromboembolism
Syphilitic infection	**Aortitis**
Mycotic infection	Syphilitic aortitis
Rheumatic aortitis	Rheumatic aortitis
Trauma	Takayasu's arteritis and aortic arch
Aortic dissection	syndromes
Cystic medial necrosis	Giant cell arteritis
Systemic hypertension	
Atherosclerosis	

ATHEROSCLEROTIC ANEURYSMS Seventy-five percent of atherosclerotic aneurysms are located in the distal abdominal aorta below the renal arteries. An abdominal aneurysm commonly produces no symptoms and is usually detected on routine examination as a palpable, pulsatile, and nontender mass, or it is an incidental finding during an abdominal x-ray or ultrasound performed for other reasons. Some patients may complain of strong pulsations in the abdomen, others of lower back pain. Rarely, there is leakage of the aneurysm with severe pain and tenderness. Acute pain and hypotension occur with rupture of the aneurysm, requiring emergency operation.

Abdominal radiography may demonstrate the calcified outline of the aneurysm. However, about 25 percent of aneurysms are not calcified and cannot be visualized by plain x-ray. An abdominal ultrasound can delineate the transverse and longitudinal dimensions of an abdominal aortic aneurysm and may detect mural thrombus. Abdominal ultrasound is useful for serial documentation of aneurysm size and could be used to screen patients at risk for developing aortic aneurysms, such as those with affected siblings, peripheral atherosclerosis, or peripheral artery aneurysms. Abdominal aortography is used commonly for evaluating patients with aneurysm for surgery, but this procedure carries a small risk of complications, such as bleeding, allergic reactions, and atheroembolism. This technique is useful in documenting the extent of the aneurysm, especially its upper and lower limits, and the extent of associated atherosclerotic vascular disease. However, since the presence of mural clots may reduce the luminal size, aortography may underestimate the diameter of an aneurysm. Computed tomography (CT) with contrast and magnetic resonance imaging (MRI) are accurate noninvasive tests to determine the location and size of thoracic and abdominal aortic aneurysms and are becoming the gold standard for the detection and follow-up of aortic aneurysms.

Prognosis is related to both the size of the aneurysm and the severity of coexistent coronary artery and cerebral vascular diseases. The risk of rupture increases with the size of the aneurysm. The 5-year risk of rupture for aneurysms less than 5 cm in diameter is 1 to 2 percent, whereas it is 20 to 40 percent for aneurysms greater than 5 cm in diameter.

TREATMENT

Operative excision with replacement with a graft is indicated for abdominal aneurysms of any size that are expanding rapidly or that are associated with symptoms. For asymptomatic aneurysms, surgery is indicated if the diameter is greater than 6.5 cm. Operation may be recommended in patients with aneurysm diameters of 4 to 5 cm, except for patients with exceptionally high operative risk. Serial noninvasive follow-up of smaller (<5 cm) aneurysms is an alternative to immediate surgery. In surgical candidates, careful preoperative cardiac and general medical evaluations (followed by appropriate therapy of complicating conditions) are essential. Preexisting coronary artery disease, congestive heart failure, pulmonary disease, diabetes, and advanced age add to the risk of surgery. If clinically indicated, preoperative evaluation should identify high-risk coronary artery disease using an exercise stress test or dipyridamole thallium scanning. Noninvasive tests, such as stress or dobutamine echocardiography or ambulatory electrocardiographic monitoring for silent ischemia, are favored in some institutions. Perioperative management should include the placement of a Swan-Ganz catheter and arterial line to monitor and optimize left ventricular filling pressure, cardiac output, and arterial pressure, especially during clamping and declamping of aorta, as well as during the immediate postoperative period. With careful preoperative cardiac evaluation and postoperative care, which includes Swan-Ganz catheterization, operative mortality approximates 1 to 2 percent. Following acute rupture, the mortality of emergency operation is generally greater than 50 percent.

CYSTIC MEDIAL NECROSIS *Cystic medial necrosis* is the term used to describe the degeneration of collagen and elastic fibers in the tunica media of the aorta, as well as medial cell losses that are replaced by multiple clefts of mucoid material. Cystic medial necrosis

characteristically affects the proximal aorta, results in circumferential weakness and dilatation, and leads to the development of fusiform aneurysms involving the ascending aorta and the sinuses of Valsalva. This condition is particularly prevalent in patients with the Marfan syndrome and Ehlers-Danlos syndrome type IV (Chap. 348) but is also seen in pregnancy, hypertension, valvular heart disease, and sometimes as an isolated condition in patients without any other apparent disease. The clinical manifestations include expanding aneurysms, rupture, and aortic regurgitation.

TREATMENT

Because of this potential complication, the management of patients with Marfan's syndrome includes echocardiography to evaluate aortic root size, aortic valve regurgitation, and mitral and tricuspid prolapse and/or regurgitation. Patients with thoracic aortic aneurysms, and particularly Marfan patients with evidence of aortic root dilatation, should be given long-term beta-blocker therapy. Operative repair is indicated in patients with symptomatic thoracic aortic aneurysms and in those in whom the aortic root diameter exceeds 6 cm. In patients with Marfan's syndrome, thoracic aortic aneurysms >5 cm should be considered for repair. In pregnant Marfan patients with aortic root diameter <4 cm, beta-blockade therapy is indicated throughout pregnancy, with frequent surveillance of the aorta with echocardiography. Transluminal placement of endovascular stent grafts for treatment of descending thoracic aortic aneurysms is undergoing investigation.

MYCOTIC ANEURYSM This rare condition develops as the result of staphylococcal, streptococcal, or salmonella infections of the aorta, usually at an atherosclerotic plaque. Blood cultures are usually positive and reveal the nature of the infecting agent. The aneurysms are usually saccular. Treatment requires parenteral antibiotics and surgical excision.

TRAUMA Aortic rupture may develop following penetrating injury or blunt trauma. Horizontal deceleration injury may tear the aortic isthmus at the site of insertion of the ligamentum arteriosum. Other causes of aortic aneurysm, such as syphilitic infection and rheumatic vasculitides, are discussed below under "Aortitis."

AORTIC DISSECTION

Aortic dissection is caused by a circumferential or, less frequently, transverse tear of the intima. It usually occurs along the right lateral wall of the ascending aorta where the hydraulic shear stress is high. The initiating event is either a medial hemorrhage that dissects into and disrupts the intima or a primary intimal tear with secondary dissection into the media. Another common site is the descending thoracic aorta just below the ligamentum arteriosum. The pulsatile aortic flow then dissects along the elastic lamellar plates of the aorta and creates a false lumen. The dissection usually propagates distally down the descending aorta and into its major branches, but it also may propagate proximally. In some cases, a secondary distal intimal disruption occurs, resulting in the reentry of blood from the false to the true lumen.

There are at least two important pathologic and radiologic variants: intramural hematoma without an intimal flap and penetrating ulcer. The clinical picture and therapeutic management of intramural hematoma are similar to those for classic aortic dissection. On the other hand, penetrating ulcers are usually localized and not associated with extensive propagation. They are primarily found in the distal portion of the descending thoracic aorta and are associated with extensive atherosclerotic disease. The ulcer can erode beyond the intimal border, leading to medial hematoma, and may progress to false aneurysm formation or rupture.

DeBakey and coworkers classified aortic dissections as type I, in which an intimal tear occurs in the ascending aorta but which involves the descending aorta as well; type II, in which the dissection is limited

FIGURE 247-1 Classification of aortic dissections. Stanford classification: Top panels illustrate type A dissections that involve the ascending aorta independent of site of tear and distal extension; type B dissections (*bottom panels*) involve transverse and/or descending aorta without involvement of the ascending aorta. DeBakey classification: Type I dissection involves ascending to descending aorta (*top left*); type II dissection is limited to ascending or transverse aorta, without descending aorta (*top center + top right*); type III dissection involves descending aorta only (*bottom left*). [*From DC Miller, in Aortic Dissection, RM Doroghazi, EE Slater (eds), New York, McGraw-Hill, 1983, with permission.*]

to the ascending aorta; and type III, in which the intimal tear is located in the descending area with distal propagation of the dissection (Fig. 247-1). Another classification (Stanford) is that of type A, in which the dissection involves the ascending aorta (proximal dissection), and type B, in which it is limited to the descending aorta (distal dissection). From a management standpoint, classification into type A or B is more practical and useful, since DeBakey types I and II are managed in a similar manner.

The factors that predispose to aortic dissection include systemic hypertension, a coexisting condition in 70 percent of patients, and cystic medial necrosis. Aortic dissection is the major cause of morbidity and mortality in patients with the Marfan syndrome (Chap. 348). The incidence is also increased in patients with congenital aortic valve anomalies (e.g., bicuspid valve), in those with coarctation of the aorta, and in otherwise normal women during the third trimester of pregnancy.

CLINICAL MANIFESTATIONS The peak incidence is in the sixth and seventh decades. Men are more affected than women by a ratio of 2:1. The presentations of aortic dissection and its variants are the consequences of intimal tear, dissecting hematoma, occlusion of involved arteries, and compression of adjacent tissues. Acute aortic dissection presents with the sudden onset of pain (Chap. 13), which is often described as very severe and tearing and is associated with diaphoresis. The pain may be localized to the front or back of the chest, often the interscapular region, and typically migrates with propagation of the dissection. Other symptoms include syncope, dyspnea, and weakness. Physical findings may include hypertension or hypotension, loss of pulses, aortic regurgitation, pulmonary edema, and neuro-

logic findings due to carotid artery obstruction (hemiplegia, hemianesthesia) or spinal cord ischemia (paraplegia). Bowel ischemia, hematuria, and myocardial ischemia have all been observed. These clinical manifestations reflect complications resulting from the dissection occluding the major arteries. Furthermore, clinical manifestations may result from the compression of adjacent structures (e.g., superior cervical ganglia, superior vena cava, bronchus, esophagus) by the expanding dissection aneurysm and include Horner's syndrome, superior vena caval syndrome, hoarseness, dysphagia, and airway compromise. Hemopericardium and cardiac tamponade may complicate a type A lesion with retrograde dissection. Acute aortic regurgitation is an important and common (over 50 percent) complication of proximal dissection. This is the outcome of either a circumferential tear that widens the aortic root or a disruption of the annulus by dissecting hematoma that tears a leaflet(s) or displaces it below the line of closure. Signs of aortic regurgitation include bounding pulses, a wide pulse pressure, a diastolic murmur often radiating to the right sternal border, and evidence of congestive heart failure. The clinical manifestation depends on the severity of the regurgitation.

In dissections involving the ascending aorta, the chest x-ray often reveals a widened superior mediastinum. A pleural effusion (usually left-sided) also may be present. In dissections of the descending thoracic aorta, a widened mediastinum also may be observed on chest x-ray. In addition, the descending aorta may appear to be wider than the ascending portion. An electrocardiogram that shows no evidence of ischemia is helpful in distinguishing aortic dissection from myocardial infarction. Rarely, the dissection involves the right or left coronary ostium and causes acute myocardial infarction. The diagnosis of aortic dissection can be established by aortography or by the use of noninvasive techniques such as two-dimensional echocardiography, CT scan, or MRI. Aortography may be used to document the diagnosis; identify the entry point, the intimal flap, and the false and true lumina; and to establish the extent of dissection into the major arteries. Coronary angiography may be performed concomitantly in high-risk patients in the evaluation and preparation for surgery. The sensitivity of aortography is 70 percent for visualizing internal flap, 56 percent for the site of intimal tear, and 87 percent for false lumen. It is unable to recognize intramural hemorrhage. Transthoracic echocardiography can be performed simply and rapidly and has an overall sensitivity of 60 to 85 percent. For diagnosing proximal ascending aortic dissections, its sensitivity ranges from 80 to 100 percent; it is less useful for detecting dissection of the arch and descending thoracic aorta. Transesophageal echocardiography (Fig. 247-2) requires greater skill and patient cooperation but is very accurate in identifying dissections of the ascending and descending thoracic aorta, but not the arch, achieving 98 percent sensitivity and specificity. CT scan and MRI are each highly accurate in identifying the intimal flap and the extent of the dissection. They are useful in recognizing intramural hemorrhage and penetrating ul-

FIGURE 247-2 Aortic dissection. *Left.* Transesophageal echocardiogram of the ascending aorta demonstrating a freely mobile flap within the lumen of the vessel. Ao, aorta; La, left atrium; Fl, flap. *Right.* When color Doppler was superimposed on the image, the true lumen (*open arrow*) was easily separated from the false lumen (*solid arrow*).

cers. MRI also can detect blood flow, which may be useful in characterizing antegrade versus retrograde dissection. These noninvasive tests are now becoming the diagnostic procedures of choice. Their relative utility depends on the availability and expertise in individual institutions as well as on the hemodynamic stability of the patient, with CT and MRI obviously less suitable for more unstable patients.

℞ TREATMENT

Medical therapy should be initiated as soon as the diagnosis is considered. The patient should be admitted to an intensive care unit for monitoring hemodynamics and urine output. Unless hypotension is present, therapy should be aimed at reducing cardiac contractility and systemic arterial pressure, and thereby shear stress. For acute dissection, unless contraindicated, beta-adrenergic blockers should be administered via the parenteral route, using either intravenous propranolol, metoprolol, or the short-acting esmolol to achieve a heart rate of approximately 60 beats per minute. This should be accompanied by sodium nitroprusside infusion to lower systolic blood pressure to 120 mmHg or less. Recently, labetalol (p. 1388), a drug with both beta- and alpha-adrenergic blocking properties, also has been used as a parenteral agent in the acute therapy of dissection.

Trimethaphan, a ganglionic blocker, may be used if nitroprusside or labetalol cannot be employed. Experience with calcium antagonists is limited. Direct vasodilators, such as diazoxide and hydralazine, are contraindicated because these agents can increase hydraulic shear and may propagate dissection.

For ascending aortic dissection (type A), emergent or urgent surgical correction, which includes reconstruction of the aortic wall, is the preferred treatment. The overall in-hospital mortality rate after surgical treatment of patients with aortic dissection is reported to be 15 to 20 percent. The major causes of perioperative mortality and morbidity include myocardial infarction, paraplegia, renal failure, tamponade, hemorrhage, and sepsis. For uncomplicated and stable distal dissection (type B), medical therapy is the preferred treatment unless there is clinical evidence of propagation, compromise of major branches of the aorta, impending rupture, or continued pain. The in-hospital mortality rate of medically treated patients with type B dissection is 15 to 20 percent. Long-term therapy for patients with aortic dissection (with or without surgery) consists of the control of hypertension and reduction of cardiac contractility with the use of beta blockers plus other antihypertensive agents such as angiotensin-converting enzyme inhibitor or calcium antagonist. Patients with chronic type B dissection should be followed on an outpatient basis every 6 to 12 months by CT scan with contrast or MRI to detect propagation. Marfan patients are at high risk for postdissection complications. The long-term prognosis for patients with treated dissections is generally good with careful follow-up; the 10-year survival rate is approximately 60 percent.

AORTIC OCCLUSION

CHRONIC ARTERIOSCLEROTIC OCCLUSIVE DISEASE   Chronic occlusive disease usually involves the distal abdominal aorta below the renal arteries. Frequently the disease extends to the common iliac arteries, but it may spare the external iliac arteries. Because of the slowly progressive nature of the atherosclerotic process, the natural history of aortic occlusion is usually chronic and insidious. Claudication characteristically involves the lower back, buttocks, and thighs and may be associated with impotence in males (Leriche syndrome). The severity of the symptoms depends on the adequacy of collaterals. With sufficient collateral blood flow, a complete occlusion of the abdominal aorta may occur without the development of ischemic symptoms. The physical findings include absence of femoral and other distal pulses bilaterally and the detection of an audible bruit over the abdomen (usually at or below the umbilicus) and the common femoral arteries. Atrophic skin, loss of hair, and coolness of the lower extremities are usually observed. In advanced ischemia, rubor on dependency and pallor on elevation can be seen.

The diagnosis is usually established by the physical examination and noninvasive testing, including leg pressure measurements, Doppler velocity analysis, and pulse volume recordings. The anatomy may be defined by abdominal aortography prior to revascularization. Operative treatment is indicated in patients with debilitating symptoms and/or with the development of leg ischemia.

ACUTE OCCLUSION   Acute occlusion in the distal abdominal aorta represents a medical emergency because it threatens the viability of the lower extremities. It usually results from an occlusive embolus that almost always originates from the heart. Rarely, acute occlusion may occur as the result of in situ thrombosis in a preexisting severely narrowed segment of the aorta or plaque rupture and hemorrhage into such an area.

The clinical picture is one of acute ischemia of the lower extremities. Severe rest pain, coolness, and pallor of the lower extremities and the absence of distal pulses bilaterally are the usual manifestations. Diagnosis should be established rapidly by aortography. Emergency thrombectomy or revascularization is indicated.

AORTITIS

Aortitis frequently affects the ascending aorta and may result in aneurysmal dilatation and aortic regurgitation; it occasionally obstructs branch vessels of the aorta.

SYPHILITIC AORTITIS   This late manifestation of luetic infection (Chap. 174) usually affects the proximal ascending aorta, particularly the aortic root, resulting in aortic dilatation and aneurysm formation. Syphilitic aortitis may occasionally involve the aortic arch or the descending aorta. The aneurysms may be saccular or fusiform and are usually asymptomatic, but compression of and erosion into adjacent structures may result in symptoms; rupture also may occur.

The initial lesion is an obliterative endarteritis of the vasa vasorum, especially in the adventitia. This is an inflammatory response to the invasion of the adventitia by the spirochetes. Destruction of the aortic media occurs as the spirochetes spread into this layer, usually via the lymphatics accompanying the vasa vasorum. Destruction of collagen and elastic tissues leads to dilation of the aorta, scar formation, and calcification. These changes account for the characteristic radiographic appearance of a calcified ascending aortic aneurysm.

The disease typically presents as an incidental radiographic finding 15 to 30 years after initial infection. Symptoms may result from aortic regurgitation, narrowing of coronary ostia due to syphilitic aortitis, compression of adjacent structures (e.g., esophagus), or rupture. Diagnosis is established by a positive serologic test, i.e., VDRL or fluorescent treponemal antibody (see Chap. 174). Treatment includes penicillin and surgical excision and repair.

RHEUMATIC AORTITIS   Rheumatoid arthritis (Chap. 313), ankylosing spondylitis (Chap. 317), psoriatic arthritis (Chap. 325), Reiter's syndrome (Chap. 317), Behçet's syndrome (Chap. 318), relapsing polychondritis, and inflammatory bowel disorders may all be associated with aortitis involving the ascending aorta. The inflammatory lesions usually involve the ascending aorta and may extend to the sinuses of Valsalva, the mitral valve leaflets, and adjacent myocardium. The clinical manifestations are aneurysm, aortic regurgitation, and involvement of the cardiac conduction system.

TAKAYASU'S ARTERITIS AND OTHER AORTIC ARCH SYNDROMES   Inflammatory diseases of the aortic arch resulting in obstruction of the aorta and its major arteries characterize this major group of diseases. Takayasu's arteritis is also termed *pulseless disease* because of the frequent occlusion of the large arteries originating from the aorta. It also may involve the descending thoracic and abdominal aorta and occlude large branches such as the renal arteries. Aortic aneurysms may also occur. The pathology is a panarteritis with marked intimal hyperplasia, medial and adventitial thickening, and, in chronic form, fibrotic occlusion. The disease is most prevalent in young females of Asian descent. During the acute stage, fever, malaise, weight loss, and other systemic symptoms may be evident. An elevation of the erythrocyte sedimentation rate is common. The chronic stages of the disease present with symptoms related to large artery occlusion, such as upper extremity claudication, cerebral ischemia, and syncope. The chronic disease is intermittently active. Since the process is progressive and there is no definitive therapy, the prognosis is usually poor. Glucocorticoids and immunosuppressive agents have been reported to be effective in some patients during the acute phase. Occasionally, anticoagulation prevents thrombosis and complete occlusion of a large artery. Surgical bypass of a critically stenotic artery may be necessary.

GIANT CELL ARTERITIS (See Chap. 319)   Primarily large and medium-sized arteries are affected. The pathology is that of focal granulomatous lesions involving the entire arterial wall. It may be associated with polymyalgia rheumatica (Chap. 22). Obstruction of medium-sized arteries (e.g., temporal and ophthalmic arteries) and of major branches of the aorta and the development of aortitis and aortic regurgitation are some of the complications of the disease. High-dose glucocorticoid therapy may be effective when given early.

BIBLIOGRAPHY

CIGARROA JE et al: Diagnostic imaging in the evaluation of suspected aortic dissection: Old standards and new directions. N Engl J Med 328:35, 1993

CREAGER MA et al: Aneurysmal disease of the aorta and its branches, in *Vascular Medicine*, J Loscalzo et al (eds). Boston, Little, Brown, 1996, pp 907–925

ERNST CB: Abdominal aortic aneurysm. N Engl J Med 328:1167, 1993

EVANS JM et al: Increased incidence of aortic aneurysm and dissection in giant cell (temporal) arteritis. A population based study. Ann Intern Med 122:502, 1995

GUILMET D et al: Aortic dissection: Anatomic types and surgical approaches. J Cardiovasc Surg 34:23, 1993

ISSELBACHER EM et al: Diseases of the aorta, in *Heart Disease*, 5th ed, E Braunwald (ed). Philadelphia, Saunders, 1997, pp 1546–1581

KULVANIEMI H et al: Genetic causes of aortic aneurysms: Unlearning at least part of what the textbooks say. J Clin Invest 88:1441, 1991

NIENABER CA et al: The diagnosis of thoracic aortic dissection by noninvasive imaging procedures. N Engl J Med 328:1, 1993

———— et al: Intramural hemorrhage of the thoracic aorta. Diagnostic and therapeutic implications. Circulation 92:1465, 1995

O'GARA PT, DESANCTIS RN: Aortic dissection in vascular medicine. J Loscalzo et al (eds). Boston, Little, Brown, 1996, pp 927–950

SHORES J et al: Progression of aortic dilatation and the benefit of long-term beta-adrenergic blockade in Marfan's syndrome. N Engl J Med 330:1335, 1994

SPITTELL PC et al: Clinical features and differential diagnosis of aortic dissection: Experience with 236 cases (1980 through 1990). Mayo Clin Proc 68:642, 1993

248	*Mark A. Creager, Victor J. Dzau*

VASCULAR DISEASES OF THE EXTREMITIES

ARTERIAL DISORDERS

ATHEROSCLEROSIS OF THE EXTREMITIES   Atherosclerosis (arteriosclerosis obliterans) is the leading cause of occlusive arterial disease of the extremities in patients over 40 years old; the highest incidence occurs in the sixth and seventh decades of life. As in patients with atherosclerosis of the coronary and cerebral vasculature, there is an increased prevalence of peripheral atherosclerotic occlusive disease in individuals with hypertension, hypercholesterolemia, and diabetes mellitus and in cigarette smokers. Atherosclerosis of the extremities is seen most frequently in elderly males.

Pathology (See Chap. 242)   Segmental lesions causing stenosis or occlusion are usually localized in large and medium-sized vessels. The pathology of the lesions includes atherosclerotic plaques with calcium deposition, thinning of the media, patchy destruction of muscle and elastic fibers, fragmentation of the internal elastic lamina, and thrombi composed of platelets and fibrin. The primary sites of involvement are the abdominal aorta and iliac arteries (30 percent of symptomatic patients), the femoral and popliteal arteries (80 to 90 percent of patients), and the more distal vessels, including the tibial and peroneal arteries (40 to 50 percent of patients). Atherosclerotic lesions occur preferentially at arterial branch points, sites of increased turbulence, altered shear stress, and intimal injury. Involvement of the distal vasculature is most common in elderly individuals and patients with diabetes mellitus.

Clinical Evaluation   The most common *symptom* is intermittent claudication, which is defined as a pain, ache, cramp, numbness, or a sense of fatigue in the muscles; it occurs during exercise and is relieved by rest. The site of claudication is distal to the location of the occlusive lesion. For example, buttock, hip, and thigh discomfort occurs in patients with aortoiliac disease (Leriche syndrome), whereas calf claudication develops in patients with femoral-popliteal disease. Symptoms are far more common in the lower than in the upper extremities because of the higher incidence of obstructive lesions in the former region. In patients with severe arterial occlusive disease, rest pain may develop. Patients will complain of pain or a feeling of cold or numbness in the foot and toes. Frequently, these symptoms occur at night when the legs are in a "neutral" position and improve when the legs are in a dependent position. With severe ischemia, rest pain may be present.

Important *physical findings* of chronic arterial insufficiency include decreased or absent pulses distal to the obstruction, the presence of bruits over the narrowed artery, and muscle atrophy. With more severe disease, hair loss, thickened nails, smooth and shiny skin, reduced skin temperature, and pallor or cyanosis are frequent physical signs. In addition, ulcers or gangrene may occur. Elevation of the legs and repeated flexing of the calf muscles produce pallor of the soles of the feet, whereas rubor, secondary to reactive hyperemia, may develop when the legs are dependent. The time required for rubor to develop or for the veins in the foot to fill when the patient's legs are transferred from an elevated to a dependent position is related to the severity of the ischemia and the presence of collateral vessels. Patients with severe ischemia may develop peripheral edema because they keep their legs in a dependent position much of the time. Ischemic neuritis can result in numbness and hyporeflexia.

Noninvasive Testing   The history and physical examination are usually sufficient to establish the diagnosis of peripheral arterial occlusive disease. An objective assessment of the severity of disease is obtained by noninvasive techniques. These include digital pulse volume recordings, Doppler flow velocity waveform analysis, duplex ultrasonography (which combines B-mode imaging and pulse-wave Doppler examination), segmental pressure measurements, transcutaneous oximetry, stress testing (usually using a treadmill), and tests of reactive hyperemia. In the presence of significant arterial occlusive disease, the volume displacement in the leg is decreased with each pulse, and the Doppler velocity contour becomes progressively flatter. Duplex ultrasonography is often useful in detecting stenotic lesions in native arteries and bypass grafts.

Arterial pressure can be recorded noninvasively along the legs by serial placement of sphygmomanometric cuffs and use of a Doppler device to auscultate or record blood flow. Normally, blood pressure in the legs and arms is similar. Indeed, ankle pressure may be slightly higher than arm pressure due to pulse-wave reflection. In the presence of hemodynamically significant stenoses, the arterial pressure in the leg is decreased. Thus, if one were to obtain a ratio of the ankle and brachial artery pressures, it would be >1.0 in normal individuals and <1.0 in patients with occlusive disease. A ratio of <0.5 is consistent with severe ischemia.

Treadmill testing allows the physician to assess functional limitations objectively. Decline of the ankle-brachial systolic pressure ratio immediately after exercise may provide further support for the diagnosis of arterial occlusive disease in patients with equivocal symptoms and findings on examination. Exercise testing also allows simultaneous evaluation for the presence of coronary artery disease.

Contrast angiography should not be used for routine diagnostic testing but is performed prior to potential revascularization. It is useful in defining the anatomy to assist operative planning and is also indicated if nonsurgical interventions are being considered, such as percutaneous transluminal angioplasty or thrombolysis. Recent studies have suggested that magnetic resonance angiography has diagnostic accuracy comparable to that of contrast angiography.

Prognosis The natural history of patients with peripheral arterial occlusive disease is influenced primarily by the extent of coexisting coronary artery and cerebral vascular disease. Studies using coronary angiography have estimated that approximately one-half of patients with symptomatic peripheral arterial occlusive disease also have significant coronary artery disease. Life-table analysis has indicated that patients with claudication have a 70 percent 5-year and a 50 percent 10-year survival rate. Most deaths are either sudden or secondary to myocardial infarction. The likelihood of symptomatic progression of peripheral arterial occlusive disease appears less than the chance of succumbing to coronary artery disease. Approximately 70 percent of nondiabetic patients who present with mild to moderate claudication remain symptomatically stable. Improvement may occur in 10 to 15 percent of patients; deterioration is likely to occur in the remainder, with approximately 5 percent of the group ultimately undergoing amputation. The prognosis is worse in patients who continue to smoke cigarettes or who have diabetes mellitus.

℞ TREATMENT

Therapeutic options include supportive measures, pharmacologic treatment, nonoperative interventions, and surgery. Supportive measures include meticulous care of the feet, which should be kept clean and protected against excessive drying with moisturizing creams. Well-fitting and protective shoes are advised to reduce trauma. Sandals and shoes made of synthetic materials that do not "breathe" should be avoided. Elastic support hose should be avoided, as they reduce blood flow to the skin. In patients with ischemia at rest, shock blocks under the head of the bed together with a canopy over the feet may improve perfusion pressure and ameliorate some of the rest pain.

Treatment of associated factors that contribute to the development of atherosclerosis should be initiated. The importance of discontinuing cigarette smoking cannot be overemphasized. The physician must assume a major role in this life-style modification. It is important to control blood pressure in hypertensive patients but to avoid hypotensive levels. Treatment of hypercholesterolemia is advocated, although reduction in cholesterol levels has not been shown unequivocally to reverse peripheral atherosclerotic lesions. However, it has been shown to prevent or to slow progression of the disease and to improve survival in patients with coronary atherosclerosis. Patients with claudication also should be encouraged to exercise regularly and at progressively more strenuous levels. Supervised exercise training programs may improve muscle efficiency and prolong walking distance. Patients also should be advised to walk for 30 to 45 min daily, stopping at the onset of claudication and resting until the symptoms resolve before resuming ambulation. Other forms of exercise, such as bicycle riding and swimming, provide overall cardiovascular and psychological benefit and often are tolerated better than walking.

Pharmacologic Management This form of treatment of patients with peripheral arterial occlusive disease has not been as successful as the medical treatment of coronary artery disease (Chap. 244). In particular, vasodilators as a class have not proved to be beneficial. During exercise, peripheral vasodilation occurs normally distal to sites of significant arterial stenoses. As a result, perfusion pressure falls, often to levels less than that generated in the interstitial tissue by the exercising muscle. Drugs such as alpha-adrenergic blocking agents, calcium channel antagonists, papaverine, and other vasodilators have not been shown to be effective in patients with occlusive arterial disease. Pentoxifylline, a substituted xanthine derivative, has been reported to decrease blood viscosity and to increase red cell flexibility, thereby increasing blood flow to the microcircula-

tion and enhancing tissue oxygenation. Several placebo-controlled studies have reported that pentoxifylline increased the duration of exercise in patients with claudication, but its efficacy has not been confirmed in all clinical trials. Preliminary studies suggest that long-term parenteral administration of vasodilator prostaglandins decreases pain and facilitates healing of ulcers in patients with severe limb ischemia and improves walking distance in patients with claudication.

Platelet inhibitors, particularly aspirin, have been reported to decrease progression of atherosclerosis in patients with peripheral arterial occlusive disease. Aspirin also reduces the risk of adverse cardiovascular events in patients with peripheral atherosclerosis. Ticlopidine, a drug that inhibits platelet aggregation via its effect on ADP-dependent platelet-fibrinogen binding, also reduces cardiovascular morbidity and mortality in patients with claudication. The anticoagulants heparin and warfarin have not been shown to be effective in patients with chronic arterial occlusive disease but may be useful in acute arterial obstruction secondary to thrombosis or systemic embolism. Similarly, thrombolytic intervention using drugs such as streptokinase, urokinase, or recombinant tissue plasminogen activator may have a role in the treatment of acute thrombotic arterial occlusion but is not effective in patients with chronic arterial occlusion secondary to atherosclerosis.

Revascularization Revascularization procedures, including nonoperative as well as operative interventions, are usually reserved for patients with progressive, severe, or disabling symptoms and ischemia at rest, as well as for individuals who must be symptom-free because of their occupation. Angiography should be performed mainly in patients who are being considered for a revascularization procedure. Nonoperative interventions include percutaneous transluminal angioplasty (PTA), laser angioplasty, atherectomy, and stent placement (Chap. 245). PTA of the iliac artery is associated with a higher success rate than PTA of the femoral and popliteal arteries. Approximately 90 to 95 percent of iliac PTAs are initially successful, and the 3-year patency rate is in excess of 75 percent. Patency rates may be higher if a stent is placed in the iliac artery. The initial success rate for femoral-popliteal PTA is approximately 80 percent, with a 60 percent 3-year patency rate. Patency rates are influenced by the severity of pretreatment stenoses; the prognosis of total occlusive lesions is worse than that of nonocclusive stenotic lesions. Laser angioplasty usually is used in conjunction with PTA and results in similar patency rates. The efficacy of percutaneous atherectomy and stent placement is being addressed in clinical trials.

Several operative procedures are available for treating patients with aortoiliac and femoral-popliteal artery disease. The preferred operative procedure depends on the location and extent of the obstruction(s) and general medical condition of the patient. Operative procedures for aortoiliac disease include aortobifemoral bypass, axillofemoral bypass, femoral-femoral bypass, and aortoiliac endarterectomy. The most frequently used procedure is the aortobifemoral bypass using knitted Dacron grafts. Immediate graft patency approaches 99 percent, and 5- and 10-year graft patency in survivors is in excess of 90 and 80 percent, respectively. Operative complications include myocardial infarction and stroke, infection of the graft, peripheral embolization, and sexual dysfunction from interruption of autonomic nerves in the pelvis. Operative mortality ranges from 1 to 3 percent, mostly due to ischemic heart disease.

Operative therapy for femoral-popliteal artery disease includes in situ and reverse autogenous saphenous vein bypass grafts, placement of polytetrafluoroethylene (PTFE) or other synthetic grafts, and thromboendarterectomy. Operative mortality ranges from 1 to 3 percent. The long-term patency rate depends on the type of graft used, the location of the distal anastomosis, and the patency of runoff vessels beyond the anastomosis. Patency rates of femoral-popliteal saphenous vein bypass grafts at 1 year approach 90 percent and at 5 years, 70 to 80 percent. Five-year patency rates of infrapopliteal saphenous vein bypass grafts are 60 to 70 percent. In contrast, 5-year patency rates of infrapopliteal PTFE grafts are less than 30 percent. Lumbar sympathectomy alone or as an adjunct to aortofemoral reconstruction has fallen into disfavor.

Preoperative cardiac risk assessment may identify individuals especially likely to experience an adverse cardiac event during the perioperative period. Patients with angina, prior myocardial infarction, ventricular ectopy, or heart failure are among those at increased risk. Noninvasive tests, such as treadmill testing (if feasible), dipyridamole thallium or Sesta-MIBI scintigraphy, and ambulatory ischemia monitoring permit further stratification of patient risk. Patients with abnormal test results require close supervision and adjunctive management with antianginal medications. It is not known whether coronary angiography and coronary arterial revascularization reduce overall perioperative mortality in high-risk patients undergoing peripheral vascular surgery, but these procedures should be considered in patients suspected of having left main or three-vessel coronary artery disease.

FIBROMUSCULAR DYSPLASIA This is a hyperplastic disorder affecting medium-sized and small arteries. It occurs predominantly in females and usually involves renal and carotid arteries but can affect extremity vessels such as the iliac and subclavian arteries. The histologic classification includes intimal, medial, and periadventitial dysplasia. Medial dysplasia is the most common type and is characterized by hyperplasia of the media with or without fibrosis of the elastic membrane. It is identified angiographically by a "string of beads" appearance caused by thickened fibromuscular ridges contiguous with thin, less involved portions of the arterial wall. When limb vessels are involved, clinical manifestations are similar to those for atherosclerosis, including claudication and rest pain. PTA and surgical reconstruction have been beneficial in patients with debilitating symptoms or threatened limbs.

THROMBOANGIITIS OBLITERANS Thromboangiitis obliterans (Buerger's disease) is an inflammatory occlusive vascular disorder involving small and medium-sized arteries and veins in the distal upper and lower extremities. Cerebral, visceral, and coronary vessels also may be affected. This disorder develops most frequently in men under age 40. The prevalence is higher in Asians and individuals of eastern European descent. While the cause of thromboangiitis obliterans is not known, there is a definite relationship to cigarette smoking and an increased incidence of HLA-B5 and -A9 antigens in patients with this disorder.

In the initial stages of thromboangiitis obliterans, polymorphonuclear leukocytes infiltrate the walls of the small and medium-sized arteries and veins. The internal elastic lamina is preserved, and thrombus may develop in the vascular lumen. As the disease progresses, mononuclear cells, fibroblasts, and giant cells replace the neutrophils. Later stages are characterized by perivascular fibrosis and recanalization.

The clinical features of thromboangiitis obliterans often include a triad of claudication of the affected extremity, Raynaud's phenomenon (p. 1401), and migratory superficial vein thrombophlebitis. Claudication is usually confined to the lower calves and feet or the forearms and hands, because this disorder primarily affects distal vessels. In the presence of severe digital ischemia, trophic nail changes, painful ulcerations, and gangrene may develop at the tips of the fingers. The physical examination shows normal brachial and popliteal pulses but reduced or absent radial, ulnar, and/or tibial pulses. Arteriography is helpful in making the diagnosis. Smooth, tapering segmental lesions in the distal vessels are characteristic, as are collateral vessels at sites of vascular occlusion. Proximal atherosclerotic disease is usually absent. The diagnosis can be confirmed by excisional biopsy and pathologic examination of an involved vessel.

There is no specific treatment except abstention from tobacco. The prognosis is worse in individuals who continue to smoke, but results are discouraging even in those who do stop smoking. Arterial bypass of the larger vessels may be used in selected instances, as well as local debridement, depending on the symptoms and severity of ischemia. Antibiotics may be useful; anticoagulants and glucocorticoids are not helpful. If these measures fail, amputation may be required.

VASCULITIS Other vasculitides may affect the arteries supplying the upper and lower extremities. Takayasu's arteritis and giant cell (temporal) arteritis are discussed in Chap. 319.

ACUTE ARTERIAL OCCLUSION This results in the sudden cessation of blood flow to an extremity. The severity of ischemia and the viability of the extremity depend on the location and extent of the occlusion and the presence and subsequent development of collateral blood vessels. There are two principal causes of acute arterial occlusion: embolism and thrombus in situ.

The most common sources of arterial emboli are the heart, aorta, and large arteries. Cardiac disorders that cause thromboembolism include atrial fibrillation, both chronic and paroxysmal; acute myocardial infarction; ventricular aneurysm; cardiomyopathy; infectious and marantic endocarditis; prosthetic heart valves; and atrial myxoma. Emboli to the distal vessels also may originate from proximal sites of atherosclerosis and aneurysms of the aorta and large vessels. Less frequently, an arterial occlusion results paradoxically from a venous thrombus that has entered the systemic circulation via a patent foramen ovale or other septal defect. Arterial emboli tend to lodge at vessel bifurcations because the vessel caliber decreases at these sites; in the lower extremities, emboli lodge most frequently in the femoral artery, followed by the iliac artery, aorta, and popliteal and tibioperoneal arteries.

Acute arterial thrombosis in situ occurs most frequently in atherosclerotic vessels at the site of a stenosis or aneurysm and in arterial bypass grafts. Trauma to an artery also may result in the formation of an acute arterial thrombus. Arterial occlusion may complicate arterial punctures and placement of catheters. Less frequent causes include the thoracic outlet compression syndrome, which causes subclavian artery occlusion, and entrapment of the popliteal artery by abnormal placement of the medial head of the gastrocnemius muscle. Polycythemia and hypercoagulable disorders (Chaps. 111 and 119) are also associated with acute arterial thrombosis.

Clinical Features The symptoms of an acute arterial occlusion depend on the location, duration, and severity of the obstruction. Often, severe pain, paresthesia, numbness, and coldness develop in the involved extremity within 1 h. Paralysis may occur with severe and persistent ischemia. Physical findings include loss of pulses distal to the occlusion, cyanosis or pallor, mottling, decreased skin temperature, muscle stiffening, loss of sensation, weakness, and/or absent deep tendon reflexes. If acute arterial occlusion occurs in the presence of an adequate collateral circulation, as is often the case in acute graft occlusion, the symptoms and findings may be less impressive. In this situation, the patient complains about an abrupt decrease in the distance walked before claudication occurs or of modest pain and paresthesia. Pallor and coolness are evident, but sensory and motor functions are generally preserved. The diagnosis of acute arterial occlusion is usually apparent from the clinical presentation. Arteriography is useful for confirming the diagnosis and demonstrating the location and extent of occlusion.

℞ **TREATMENT**

Once the diagnosis is made, the patient should be anticoagulated with intravenous heparin to prevent propagation of the clot. In cases of severe ischemia of recent onset, and particularly when limb viability is jeopardized, immediate intervention to ensure reperfusion is indicated. Surgical thromboembolectomy or arterial bypass procedures are used to restore blood flow to the ischemic extremity promptly, particularly when a large proximal vessel is occluded.

Intraarterial thrombolytic therapy is effective when acute arterial occlusion is caused by a thrombus in an atherosclerotic vessel or arterial bypass graft. Thrombolytic therapy also may be indicated when the patient's overall condition contraindicates surgical intervention or when smaller distal vessels are occluded, thus preventing surgical access. Intraarterial streptokinase is administered as a bolus injection of 25,000 to 250,000 IU followed by a continuous infusion of 5000 to 15,000 IU/h. One approach for administering intraarterial urokinase is to give a bolus of 150,000 to 250,000 IU followed by 240,000 IU/h for 2 h, 120,000 IU/h for 2 h, and then 60,000 IU/h. Clinical trials are now in progress to assess the efficacy of intraarterial recombinant tissue plasminogen activator (tPA). Meticulous observation for hemorrhagic complications is required during intraarterial thrombolytic therapy.

If the limb is not in jeopardy, a more conservative approach that includes observation and administration of anticoagulants may be taken. Anticoagulation prevents recurrent embolism and reduces the likelihood of thrombus propagation. It can be initiated with intravenous heparin and followed by oral warfarin. Recommended dosages are the same as those used for deep vein thrombosis (see later). Emboli resulting from infectious endocarditis, the presence of prosthetic heart valves, or atrial myxoma often require surgical intervention to remove the cause.

ATHEROEMBOLISM Atheroembolism constitutes a subset of acute arterial occlusion. In this condition, multiple small deposits of fibrin, platelet, and cholesterol debris embolize from proximal atherosclerotic lesions or aneurysmal sites. Atheroembolism may occur after intraarterial procedures. Since the emboli tend to lodge in the small vessels of the muscle and skin and may not occlude the large vessels, distal pulses usually remain palpable. Patients complain of acute pain and tenderness at the site of embolization. Digital vascular occlusion may result in ischemia and the "blue toe" syndrome; digital necrosis and gangrene may develop. Localized areas of tenderness, pallor, and livedo reticularis (see below) occur at sites of emboli. Skin or muscle biopsy may demonstrate cholesterol crystals.

Ischemia resulting from atheroemboli is notoriously difficult to treat. Usually neither surgical revascularization procedures nor thrombolytic therapy is helpful because of the multiplicity, composition, and distal location of the emboli. Some evidence suggests that platelet inhibitors prevent atheroembolism. Surgical intervention to remove or bypass the atherosclerotic vessel or aneurysm that causes the recurrent atheroemboli may be necessary.

THORACIC OUTLET COMPRESSION SYNDROME This is a symptom complex resulting from compression of the neurovascular bundle (artery, vein, or nerves) at the thoracic outlet as it courses through the neck and shoulder. Cervical ribs, abnormalities of the scalenus anticus muscle, proximity of the clavicle to the first rib, or abnormal insertion of the pectoralis minor muscle may compress the subclavian artery and brachial plexus as these structures pass from the thorax to the arm. Patients may develop shoulder and arm pain, weakness, paresthesia, claudication, Raynaud's phenomenon, and even ischemic tissue loss and gangrene. Examination is often normal unless provocative maneuvers are performed. Occasionally, distal pulses are decreased or absent and digital cyanosis and ischemia may be evident. Tenderness may be present in the supraclavicular fossa. Abducting the affected arm by 90° and externally rotating the shoulder may precipitate symptoms. Several additional maneuvers are used to confirm the diagnosis of vascular compression and to suggest the location of the abnormality. These include the scalene maneuver (extension of the neck and rotation of the head to the side of the symptoms), the costoclavicular maneuver (posterior rotation of shoulders), and the hyperabduction maneuver (raising the arm 180°), which may cause subclavian bruits and loss of pulses in the arm. A chest x-ray will indicate the presence of cervical ribs. The electromyogram will be abnormal if the brachial plexus is involved.

℞ TREATMENT

Most patients can be managed conservatively. They should be advised to avoid the positions that cause symptoms. Many patients benefit from shoulder girdle exercises. Surgical procedures such as removal of the first rib or resection of the scalenus anticus muscle are necessary occasionally for relief of symptoms or treatment of ischemia.

ARTERIOVENOUS FISTULA Abnormal communications between an artery and a vein, bypassing the capillary bed, may be congenital or acquired. Congenital arteriovenous fistulas are the result of persistent embryonic vessels that fail to differentiate into arteries and veins; they may be associated with birthmarks, can be located in almost any organ of the body, and frequently occur in the extremities. Acquired arteriovenous fistulas are either created to provide vascular access for hemodialysis or occur as a result of a penetrating injury such as a gunshot or knife wound or as complications of arterial catheterization or surgical dissection. An infrequent cause of arteriovenous fistula is rupture of an arterial aneurysm into a vein.

The clinical features depend on the location and size of the fistula. Frequently, a pulsatile mass is palpable, and a thrill and bruit lasting throughout systole and diastole are present over the fistula. With long-standing fistulas, clinical manifestations of chronic venous insufficiency, including peripheral edema, large, tortuous varicose veins, and stasis pigmentation become apparent because of the high venous pressure. Evidence of ischemia may occur in the distal portion of the extremity. Skin temperature is higher over the arteriovenous fistula. Large arteriovenous fistulas may result in an increased cardiac output with consequent cardiomegaly and high-output heart failure (Chap. 233).

Diagnosis The diagnosis is often evident from the physical examination. Compression of a large arteriovenous fistula may cause reflex slowing of the heart rate (Nicoladoni-Branham sign). Arteriography can confirm the diagnosis and is useful in demonstrating the site and size of the arteriovenous fistula.

℞ TREATMENT

Management of arteriovenous fistulas may involve surgery, radiotherapy, or embolization. Congenital arteriovenous fistulas are often difficult to treat because the communications may be numerous and extensive, and new ones frequently develop after ligation of the most obvious ones. Many of these lesions are best treated conservatively using elastic support hose to reduce the consequences of venous hypertension. Occasionally, embolization with autologous material, such as fat or muscle, or with hemostatic agents, such as gelatin sponges or silicon spheres, is used to obliterate the fistula. Acquired arteriovenous fistulas are usually amenable to surgical treatment that involves division or excision of the fistula. Occasionally, autogenous or synthetic grafting is necessary to reestablish continuity of the artery and vein.

RAYNAUD'S PHENOMENON Raynaud's phenomenon is characterized by episodic digital ischemia, manifested clinically by the sequential development of digital blanching, cyanosis, and rubor of the fingers or toes following cold exposure and subsequent rewarming. Emotional stress also may precipitate Raynaud's phenomenon. The color changes are usually well demarcated and are confined to the fingers or toes. Typically, one or more digits will appear white when the patient is exposed to a cold environment or touches a cold object. The blanching, or pallor, represents the ischemic phase of the phenomenon and results from vasospasm of digital arteries. During the ischemic phase, capillaries and venules dilate, and cyanosis results from the deoxygenated blood that is present in these vessels. A sensation of cold or numbness or paresthesia of the digits often accompanies the phases of pallor and cyanosis.

With rewarming, the digital vasospasm resolves, and blood flow into the dilated arterioles and capillaries increases dramatically. This "reactive hyperemia" imparts a bright red color to the digits. In addition to rubor and warmth, patients often experience a throbbing, painful sensation during the hyperemic phase. Although the triphasic color response is typical of Raynaud's phenomenon, some patients may develop only pallor and cyanosis; others may experience only cyanosis.

Pathophysiology Raynaud originally proposed that cold-induced episodic digital ischemia was secondary to exaggerated reflex sympathetic vasoconstriction. This theory is supported by the fact that alpha-adrenergic blocking drugs as well as sympathectomy decrease the frequency and severity of Raynaud's phenomenon in some patients. An alternative hypothesis is that the digital vascular responsiveness to cold or to normal sympathetic stimuli is enhanced. It is also possible that normal reflex sympathetic vasoconstriction is superimposed on local digital vascular disease or that there is enhanced adrenergic neuroeffector activity.

Raynaud's phenomenon is broadly separated into two categories: the idiopathic variety, termed *Raynaud's disease*, and the secondary variety, which is associated with other disease states or known causes of vasospasm (Table 248-1).

Raynaud's Disease   This appellation is applied when the secondary causes of Raynaud's phenomenon have been excluded. Over 50 percent of patients with Raynaud's phenomenon have Raynaud's disease. Women are affected about five times more often than men, and the age of presentation is usually between 20 and 40 years. The fingers are involved more frequently than the toes. Initial episodes may involve only one or two fingertips, but subsequent attacks may involve the entire finger and may include all the fingers. The toes are affected in 40 percent of patients. Although vasospasm of the toes usually occurs in patients with symptoms in the fingers, it may happen alone. Rarely, the earlobes and the tip of the nose are involved. Raynaud's phenomenon occurs frequently in patients who also have migraine headaches or variant angina. These associations suggest that there may be a common predisposing cause for the vasospasm.

Results of physical examination often are entirely normal; the radial, ulnar, and pedal pulses are normal. The fingers and toes may be cool between attacks and may perspire excessively. Thickening and tightening of the digital subcutaneous tissue (sclerodactyly) develop in 10 percent of patients. Angiography of the digits for diagnostic purposes is not indicated.

In general, patients with Raynaud's disease appear to have the milder forms of Raynaud's phenomenon. Less than 1 percent of these patients lose a part of a digit. After the diagnosis is made, the disease spontaneously improves in approximately 15 percent of patients and progresses in about 30 percent.

Secondary Causes of Raynaud's Phenomenon   Raynaud's phenomenon occurs in 80 to 90 percent of patients with systemic sclerosis (scleroderma) and is the presenting symptom in 30 percent (Chap. 314). It may be the only symptom of scleroderma for many years. Abnormalities of the digital vessels may contribute to the development of Raynaud's phenomenon in this disorder. Ischemic fingertip ulcers may develop and progress to gangrene and autoamputation. About 20 percent of patients with systemic lupus erythematosus (SLE) have Raynaud's phenomenon (Chap. 312). Occasionally, persistent digital ischemia develops and may result in ulcers or gangrene. In most severe cases, the small vessels are occluded by a proliferative endarteritis.

Table 248-1

Classification of Raynaud's Phenomenon

Primary or idiopathic Raynaud's phenomenon: Raynaud's disease
Secondary Raynaud's phenomenon
  Collagen vascular diseases: scleroderma, systemic lupus erythematosus, rheumatoid arthritis, dermatomyositis, polymyositis
  Arterial occlusive diseases: atherosclerosis of the extremities, thromboangiitis obliterans, acute arterial occlusion, thoracic outlet syndrome
  Pulmonary hypertension
  Neurologic disorders: intervertebral disk disease, syringomyelia, spinal cord tumors, stroke, poliomyelitis, carpal tunnel syndrome
  Blood dyscrasias: cold agglutinins, cryoglobulinemia, cryofibrinogenemia, myeloproliferative disorders, Waldenström's macroglobulinemia
  Trauma: vibration injury, hammer hand syndrome, electric shock, cold injury, typing, piano playing
  Drugs: ergot derivatives, methysergide, beta-adrenergic receptor blockers, bleomycin, vinblastine, cisplatin

Raynaud's phenomenon occurs in about 30 percent of patients with dermatomyositis or polymyositis (Chap. 315). It frequently develops in patients with rheumatoid arthritis and may be related to the intimal proliferation that occurs in the digital arteries.

Atherosclerosis of the extremities is a frequent cause of Raynaud's phenomenon in men over age 50. Thromboangiitis obliterans is an uncommon cause of Raynaud's phenomenon but should be considered in young men, particularly in those who are cigarette smokers. The development of cold-induced pallor in these disorders may be confined to one or two digits of the involved extremity. Occasionally, Raynaud's phenomenon may follow acute occlusion of large and medium-sized arteries by a thrombus or embolus. Embolization of atheroembolic debris may cause digital ischemia. The latter situation often involves one or two digits and should not be confused with Raynaud's phenomenon. In patients with the thoracic outlet syndrome, Raynaud's phenomenon may result from diminished intravascular pressure, stimulation of sympathetic fibers in the brachial plexus, or a combination of both. Raynaud's phenomenon occurs in patients with primary pulmonary hypertension (Chap. 260); this is more than coincidental and may reflect a neurohumoral abnormality that affects both the pulmonary and digital circulations.

A variety of blood dyscrasias may be associated with Raynaud's phenomenon. Cold-induced precipitation of plasma proteins, hyperviscosity, and aggregation of red cells and platelets may occur in patients with cold agglutinins, cryoglobulinemia, or cryofibrinogenemia. Hyperviscosity syndromes that accompany myeloproliferative disorders and Waldenström's macroglobulinemia also should be considered in the initial evaluation of patients with Raynaud's phenomenon.

Raynaud's phenomenon occurs often in patients whose vocations require the use of vibrating hand tools, such as chain saws or jackhammers. The frequency of Raynaud's phenomenon also seems to be increased in pianists and typists. Electric shock injury to the hands or frostbite may lead to the later development of Raynaud's phenomenon.

Several drugs have been causally implicated in Raynaud's phenomenon. These include ergot preparations, methysergide, beta-adrenergic receptor antagonists, and the chemotherapeutic agents bleomycin, vinblastine, and cisplatin.

℞ TREATMENT

Most patients with Raynaud's phenomenon experience only mild and infrequent episodes. These patients need reassurance and should be instructed to dress warmly and avoid unnecessary cold exposure. In addition to gloves and mittens, patients should protect the trunk, head, and feet with warm clothing to prevent cold-induced reflex vasoconstriction. Tobacco use is contraindicated.

Drug treatment should be reserved for the severe cases. The calcium channel antagonists, especially nifedipine (10 to 30 mg tid) and diltiazem (30 to 90 mg tid), decrease the frequency and severity of Raynaud's phenomenon. Long-acting preparations of these drugs also may be effective. Adrenergic blocking agents, such as reserpine (0.25 to 0.5 mg qid), have been shown to increase nutritional blood flow to the fingers. Some, but not all, patients achieve satisfactory results with long-term reserpine therapy. Moreover, systemic use of this drug is limited by side effects of hypotension, nasal stuffiness, lethargy, and depression. The postsynaptic alpha$_1$-adrenergic antagonist prazosin (1 to 5 mg tid) has been used with favorable responses. Doxazosin and terazosin also may be effective. Other sympatholytic agents, such as methyldopa, guanethidine, and phenoxybenzamine, may be useful in some patients. Treatment with vasodilator prostaglandins is under investigation, and has been reported to improve symptoms in patients with scleroderma. Surgical sympathectomy is helpful in some patients who are unresponsive to medical therapy, but benefit is often transient.

ACROCYANOSIS   In this condition, there is arterial vasoconstriction and secondary dilation of the capillaries and venules with resulting persistent cyanosis of the hands and, less frequently, the feet. Cyanosis may be intensified by exposure to a cold environment. Women are affected much more frequently than men, and the age of onset is usually less than 30 years. Generally, patients are asymptomatic but seek medical attention because of the discoloration. Examination reveals normal pulses, peripheral cyanosis, and moist palms. Trophic skin changes and ulcerations do *not* occur. The disorder can be distinguished from Raynaud's phenomenon because it is persistent and not episodic, the discoloration extends proximally from the digits, and blanching does not occur. Ischemia secondary to arterial occlusive disease usually can be excluded by the presence of normal pulses. Central cyanosis and decreased arterial oxygen saturation are not present. Patients should be reassured and advised to dress warmly and avoid cold exposure. Pharmacologic intervention is not indicated.

LIVEDO RETICULARIS In this condition, localized areas of the extremities develop a mottled or netlike appearance of reddish to blue discoloration. The mottled appearance may be more prominent following cold exposure. The idiopathic form of this disorder occurs equally in men and women, and the most common age of onset is in the third decade. Patients with the idiopathic form usually are asymptomatic and seek attention for cosmetic reasons. Livedo reticularis also can occur following atheroembolism (see above). Rarely, skin ulcerations develop. Patients should be reassured and advised to avoid cold environments. No drug treatment is indicated.

PERNIO (CHILBLAINS) This is a vasculitic disorder associated with exposure to cold; acute forms have been described. Raised erythematous lesions develop on the lower part of the legs and feet in cold weather. These are associated with pruritus and a burning sensation, and they may blister and ulcerate. Pathologic examination demonstrates angiitis characterized by intimal proliferation and perivascular infiltration of mononuclear and polymorphonuclear leukocytes. Giant cells may be present in the subcutaneous tissue. Patients should avoid exposure to cold, and ulcers should be kept clean and protected with sterile dressings. Sympatholytic drugs may be effective in some patients.

ERYTHROMELALGIA (ERYTHERMALGIA) This disorder is characterized by burning pain and erythema of the extremities. The feet are involved more frequently than the hands, and males are affected more frequently than females. Erythromelalgia may occur at any age but is most common in middle age. It may be primary or secondary to disorders such as hypertension, polycythemia vera, essential thrombocytosis, or it may occur as an adverse effect of drugs such as nifedipine or bromocriptine. Patients complain of burning in the extremities that is precipitated by exposure to a warm environment and aggravated by a dependent position. The symptoms are relieved by exposing the affected area to cool air or water or by elevation. Erythromelalgia can be distinguished from ischemia secondary to arterial occlusive disorders and peripheral neuropathy because the peripheral pulses are present and the neurologic examination is normal. There is no specific treatment; aspirin may produce relief in patients with erythromelalgia secondary to myeloproliferative disease. Treatment of associated disorders in secondary erythromelalgia may be helpful.

FROSTBITE In this condition, tissue damage results from severe environmental cold exposure or from direct contact with a very cold object. Tissue injury results from both freezing and vasoconstriction. Frostbite usually affects the distal aspects of the extremities or exposed parts of the face, such as the ears, nose, chin, and cheeks. Superficial frostbite involves the skin and subcutaneous tissue. Patients experience pain or paresthesia, and the skin appears white and waxy. After rewarming, there is cyanosis and erythema, wheal and flare formation, edema, and superficial blisters. Deep frostbite involves muscle, nerves, and deeper blood vessels. It may result in edema of the hand or foot, vesicles and bullae, tissue necrosis, and gangrene.

Initial treatment is rewarming, performed in an environment where reexposure to freezing conditions will not occur. Rewarming is accomplished by immersion of the affected part in a water bath at temperatures of 40 to 44°C (104 to 111°F). Massage, application of ice water, and extreme heat are contraindicated. The injured area should be cleansed with soap or antiseptic and sterile dressings applied. Analgesics are often required during rewarming. Antibiotics are used if there is evidence of infection. The efficacy of sympathetic blocking drugs is not established. Following recovery, the affected extremity may exhibit increased sensitivity to cold.

VENOUS DISORDERS

Veins in the extremities can be broadly classified as either superficial or deep. In the lower extremity, the superficial venous system includes the greater and lesser saphenous veins and their tributaries. The deep veins of the leg accompany the major arteries. Perforating veins connect the superficial and deep systems at multiple locations. Bicuspid valves are present throughout the venous system to direct the flow of venous blood centrally.

VENOUS THROMBOSIS The presence of thrombus within a superficial or deep vein and the accompanying inflammatory response in the vessel wall is termed *venous thrombosis* or *thrombophlebitis*. Initially, the thrombus is composed principally of platelets and fibrin. Red cells become interspersed with fibrin, and the thrombus tends to propagate in the direction of blood flow. The inflammatory response in the vessel wall may be minimal or characterized by granulocyte infiltration, loss of endothelium, and edema.

The factors that predispose to venous thrombosis were initially described by Virchow in 1856 and include stasis, vascular damage, and hypercoagulability. Accordingly, a variety of clinical situations are associated with increased risk of venous thrombosis (Table 248-2). Venous thrombosis may occur in more than 50 percent of patients having orthopedic surgical procedures, particularly those involving the hip or knee, and in 10 to 40 percent of patients who undergo abdominal or thoracic operations. The prevalence of venous thrombosis is particularly high in patients with cancer of the pancreas, lungs, genitourinary tract, stomach, and breast. Approximately 10 to 20 percent of patients with idiopathic deep vein thrombosis have or develop clinically overt cancer; there is no consensus on whether these individuals should be subjected to intensive diagnostic workup to search for occult malignancy. Risk of thrombosis is increased following trauma, such as fractures of the spine, pelvis, femur, and tibia. Immobilization, regardless of the underlying disease, is a major predisposing cause of venous thrombosis. This fact may account for the relatively high incidence in patients with acute myocardial infarction or congestive heart failure. The incidence of venous thrombosis is increased during pregnancy, particularly in the third trimester and in the first month postpartum, and in individuals who use estrogens. A variety of clinical disorders that produce systemic hypercoagulability, including resistance to activated protein C (factor V Leiden); antithrombin III, protein C, and protein S deficiencies; antiphospholipid syndrome; systemic lupus erythematosus; myeloproliferative diseases; dysfibrinogenemia; and disseminated intravascular coagulation, may cause venous thrombosis. Venulitis occurring in thromboangiitis obliterans, Behçet's disease, and homocysteinuria also may cause venous thrombosis.

Table 248-2

Conditions Associated with an Increased Risk for Development of Venous Thrombosis

Surgery
  Orthopedic, thoracic, abdominal, and genitourinary procedures
Neoplasms
  Pancreas, lung, ovary, testes, urinary tract, breast, stomach
Trauma
  Fractures of spine, pelvis, femur, or tibia; spinal cord injuries
Immobilization
  Acute myocardial infarction, congestive heart failure, stroke, postoperative convalescence
Pregnancy
Estrogen use (for replacement or contraception)
Hypercoagulable states
  Resistance to activated protein C; deficiencies of antithrombin III, protein C, or protein S; antiphospholipid antibodies; myeloproliferative diseases; dysfibrinogenemia; disseminated intravascular coagulation
Venulitis
  Thromboangiitis obliterans, Behçet's disease, homocysteinuria
Previous deep vein thrombosis

DEEP VENOUS THROMBOSIS The most important consequences of this disorder are pulmonary embolism (Chap. 261) and the syndrome of chronic venous insufficiency. Deep thrombosis of the iliac, femoral, or popliteal veins is suggested by unilateral leg swelling, warmth, and erythema. Tenderness may be present along the course of the involved veins, and a cord may be palpable. There may be increased tissue turgor, distension of superficial veins, and the appearance of prominent venous collaterals. In some patients, deoxygenated hemoglobin in stagnant veins imparts a cyanotic hue to the limb, a condition called *phlegmasia cerulea dolens*. In markedly edematous legs, the interstitial tissue pressure may exceed the capillary perfusion pressure, causing pallor, a condition designated *phlegmasia alba dolens*.

The diagnosis of deep venous thrombosis of the calf is often difficult to make at the bedside. This is so because only one of multiple veins may be involved, allowing adequate venous return through the remaining patent vessels. The most common complaint is calf pain. Examination may reveal posterior calf tenderness, warmth, increased tissue turgor or modest swelling, and, rarely, a cord. Increased resistance or pain during dorsiflexion of the foot (Homans' sign) is an unreliable diagnostic sign.

Deep venous thrombosis occurs less frequently in the upper extremity than in the lower extremity, but the incidence is increasing because of greater utilization of indwelling central venous catheters. The clinical features and complications are similar to those described for the leg.

Diagnosis The noninvasive test used most often to diagnose deep venous thrombosis is duplex venous ultrasonography (B-mode, i.e., two-dimensional, imaging and pulse-wave Doppler interrogation). By imaging the deep veins, thrombus can be detected either by direct visualization or by inference when the vein does not collapse on compressive maneuvers. The Doppler ultrasound measures the velocity of blood flow in veins. This velocity is normally affected by respiration and by manual compression of the foot or calf. Flow abnormalities occur when deep venous obstruction is present. The positive predictive value of duplex venous ultrasonography approaches 95 percent for proximal deep vein thrombosis. In the calf, because calf veins are more difficult to visualize than proximal veins, the sensitivity of this technique is only 50 to 75 percent, although its specificity is 95 percent.

Impedance plethysmography measures changes in venous capacitance during physiologic maneuvers. Venous obstruction blunts the normal changes in venous capacitance that occur following inflation and deflation of a thigh cuff. The predictive value of this test for detecting occlusive thrombi in proximal veins is approximately 90 percent. However, it is much less sensitive for diagnosing deep venous thrombosis of the calves.

Magnetic resonance imaging is another noninvasive means to detect deep vein thrombosis. Its diagnostic accuracy for assessing proximal deep vein thrombosis is similar to that of duplex ultrasonography. It is useful in patients with suspected thrombosis of the superior and inferior venae cavae or pelvic veins.

Deep venous thrombosis also can be diagnosed by venography. Contrast medium is injected into a superficial vein of the foot and directed to the deep system by the application of tourniquets. The presence of a filling defect or absence of filling of the deep veins is required to make the diagnosis.

Deep vein thrombosis must be differentiated from a variety of disorders that cause unilateral leg pain or swelling, including muscle rupture, trauma, or hemorrhage; a ruptured popliteal cyst; and lymphedema. It may be difficult to distinguish swelling caused by the postphlebitic syndrome from that due to acute recurrent deep venous thrombosis. Leg pain also may result from nerve compression, arthritis, tendinitis, fractures, and arterial occlusive disorders. A careful history and physical examination can usually determine the cause of these symptoms.

℞ **TREATMENT**

Anticoagulants (See also Chap. 261) Prevention of pulmonary embolism is the most important reason for treating patients with deep vein thrombosis, since in the early stages the thrombus may be loose and poorly adherent to the vessel wall. Patients should be placed in bed, and the affected extremity should be elevated above the level of the heart until the edema and tenderness subside. Anticoagulants prevent thrombus propagation and allow the endogenous lytic system to operate. Heparin should be administered intravenously as an initial bolus of 7500 to 10,000 IU, followed by a continuous infusion of 1000 to 1500 IU/h. The rate of the heparin infusion should be adjusted so that the activated partial thromboplastin time (aPTT) is approximately twice the control value. Subcutaneous injection of heparin has been used as an alternative form of therapy. In less than 5 percent of patients, heparin therapy may cause thrombocytopenia. Infrequently, these patients develop arterial thrombosis and ischemia. Heparin treatment should be maintained for at least 5 to 7 days. Low-molecular-weight (4000 to 6000 daltons) heparins are reported to be as effective as or better than conventional, unfractionated heparin in preventing extension or recurrence of venous thrombosis. Depending on the specific preparation, low-molecular-weight heparin is administered subcutaneously, in fixed doses, once or twice daily. The incidence of thrombocytopenia is less with low-molecular-weight heparin than with conventional preparations. Warfarin is administered during the first week of treatment with heparin and may be started as early as the first day of heparin treatment if the aPTT is therapeutic. It is important to overlap heparin treatment with oral anticoagulant therapy for at least 4 to 5 days because the full anticoagulant effect of warfarin is delayed. The dose of warfarin should be adjusted to maintain the prothrombin time at an international normalized ratio (INR) of 2.0 to 3.0. The use of anticoagulants for isolated deep vein thrombosis of the calf is controversial. However, approximately 20 to 30 percent of calf thrombi propagate to the thigh, thereby increasing the risk of pulmonary embolism. Also, isolated calf vein thrombosis has been identified as a cause of embolic stroke via a patent foramen ovale.

Anticoagulant treatment is indicated for patients with proximal deep vein thrombosis, since pulmonary embolism may occur in approximately 50 percent of untreated individuals. The incidence of pulmonary embolism in patients presenting with deep calf vein thrombosis is 5 to 20 percent. Therefore, patients with calf vein thrombosis should either receive anticoagulants or be followed with serial noninvasive tests to determine whether proximal propagation has occurred. Anticoagulant treatment should be continued for 3 to 6 months for patients with acute idiopathic deep vein thrombosis and for those with a temporary risk factor for venous thrombosis to decrease the chance of recurrence. The duration of anticoagulant treatment for patients with calf vein thrombosis should be at least 6 weeks. The duration of treatment is indefinite for patients with recurrent deep vein thrombosis and for those in whom associated causes, such as malignancy or hypercoagulability, have not been eliminated. If treatment with anticoagulants is contraindicated because of a bleeding diathesis or risk of hemorrhage, protection from pulmonary embolism can be achieved by mechanically interrupting the flow of blood through the inferior vena cava. Inferior vena cava plication generally has been replaced by percutaneous insertion of a filter.

Thrombolytics Thrombolytic drugs such as streptokinase, urokinase, and tissue plasminogen activator also may be used, but there is no evidence that thrombolytic therapy is more effective than anticoagulants in preventing pulmonary embolism. However, early administration of thrombolytic drugs may accelerate clot lysis, preserve venous valves, and decrease the potential for developing postphlebitic syndrome.

Prophylaxis Prophylaxis should be considered in clinical situations where the risk of deep vein thrombosis is high. Low-dose heparin (5000 units 2 h prior to surgery and then 5000 units every 8 to 12 h postoperatively), warfarin, and external pneumatic compression are all useful. Low-dose heparin reduces the risk of deep vein thrombosis associated with thoracic and abdominal surgery and with prolonged bed rest. Low-molecular-weight heparins have been shown to prevent deep vein thrombosis in patients undergoing general or orthopedic surgery. They are said to be more effective than conventional heparin and to cause an equal or lower incidence of bleeding. Warfarin in a dose that yields a prothrombin time equivalent to an INR of 2.0 to 3.0 is effective in preventing deep vein thrombosis associated with bone fractures and orthopedic surgery. Warfarin is started the night before surgery and continued throughout the convalescent period. External pneumatic compression devices applied to the legs are used to prevent deep vein thrombosis when even low doses of heparin or warfarin might cause serious bleeding, as during neurosurgery or transurethral resection of the prostate.

SUPERFICIAL VEIN THROMBOSIS Thrombosis of the greater or lesser saphenous veins or their tributaries—i.e., superficial vein thrombosis—does not result in pulmonary embolism. It is associated with intravenous catheters and infusions, occurs in varicose veins, and may develop in association with deep vein thrombosis. Migrating superficial vein thrombosis is often a marker for a carcinoma and also may occur in patients with vasculitides, such as thromboangiitis obliterans. The clinical features of superficial vein thrombosis are easily distinguished from those of deep vein thrombosis. Patients complain of pain localized to the site of the thrombus. Examination reveals a reddened, warm, and tender cord extending along a superficial vein. The surrounding area may be red and edematous.

R̲x̲ **TREATMENT**
Treatment is primarily supportive. Initially, patients can be placed at bed rest with leg elevation and application of warm compresses. Nonsteroidal antiinflammatory drugs may provide analgesia but also may obscure clinical evidence of thrombus propagation. If a thrombosis of the greater saphenous vein develops in the thigh and extends toward the saphenofemoral vein junction, it is reasonable to consider anticoagulant therapy to prevent extension of the thrombus into the deep system and a possible pulmonary embolism.

VARICOSE VEINS Varicose veins are dilated, tortuous superficial veins that result from defective structure and function of the valves of the saphenous veins, from intrinsic weakness of the vein wall, from high intraluminal pressure, or, rarely, from arteriovenous fistulas. Varicose veins can be categorized as primary or secondary. Primary varicose veins originate in the superficial system and occur two to three times as frequently in women as in men. Approximately half of patients have a family history of varicose veins. Secondary varicose veins result from deep venous insufficiency and incompetent perforating veins or from deep venous occlusion causing enlargement of superficial veins that are serving as collaterals.

Patients with venous varicosities are often concerned about the cosmetic appearance of their legs. Symptoms consist of a dull ache or pressure sensation in the legs after prolonged standing; it is relieved with leg elevation. The legs feel heavy, and mild ankle edema develops occasionally. Extensive venous varicosities may cause skin ulcerations near the ankle. Superficial venous thrombosis may be a recurring problem, and, rarely, a varicosity ruptures and bleeds. Visual inspection of the legs in the dependent position usually confirms the presence of varicose veins.

Varicose veins usually can be treated with conservative measures. Symptoms often decrease when the legs are elevated periodically, when prolonged standing is avoided, and when elastic support hose are worn. External compression stockings provide a counterbalance to the hydrostatic pressure in the veins. Small symptomatic varicose veins can be treated with sclerotherapy, in which a sclerosing solution is injected into the involved varicose vein and a compression bandage is applied. Surgical therapy usually involves extensive ligation and stripping of the greater and lesser saphenous veins and should be reserved for patients who are very symptomatic, suffer recurrent superficial vein thrombosis, and/or develop skin ulceration. Surgical therapy also may be indicated for cosmetic reasons.

CHRONIC VENOUS INSUFFICIENCY Chronic venous insufficiency may result from deep vein thrombosis and/or valvular incompetence. Following deep vein thrombosis, the delicate valve leaflets become thickened and contracted so that they cannot prevent retrograde flow of blood; the vein becomes rigid and thick-walled. Although most veins recanalize after an episode of thrombosis, the large proximal veins may remain occluded. Secondary incompetence develops in distal valves because high pressures distend the vein and separate the leaflets. Primary deep venous valvular dysfunction also may occur without previous thrombosis. Patients with venous insufficiency often complain of a dull ache in the leg that worsens with prolonged standing and resolves with leg elevation. Examination demonstrates increased leg circumference, edema, and superficial varicose veins. Erythema, dermatitis, and hyperpigmentation develop along the distal aspect of the leg, and skin ulceration may occur near the medial and lateral malleoli. Cellulitis may be a recurring problem. Patients should be advised to avoid prolonged standing or sitting; frequent leg elevation is helpful. Graduated compression stockings should be worn during the day. These efforts should be intensified if skin ulcers develop. Ulcers should be treated with applications of wet to dry dressings and, occasionally, dilute topical antibiotic solutions. Commercially available dressings comprising antiseptic solutions and compressive bandages may be applied and should be changed weekly until healing occurs. Recurrent ulceration and severe edema may be treated by surgical interruption of incompetent communicating veins. Rarely, surgical valvuloplasty and bypass of venous occlusions are employed.

LYMPHATIC DISORDERS

Lymphatic capillaries are blind-ended tubes formed by a single layer of endothelial cells. The absent or widely fenestrated basement membrane of lymphatic capillaries allows access to interstitial proteins and particles. Lymphatic capillaries merge to form larger vessels which contain smooth muscle and are capable of vasomotion. Small and medium-sized lymphatic vessels empty into progressively larger channels, most of which drain into the thoracic duct. The lymphatic circulation is involved in the absorption of interstitial fluid and in the response to infection.

LYMPHEDEMA Lymphedema may be categorized as primary or secondary (Table 248-3). The prevalence of primary lymphedema is approximately 1 per 10,000 individuals. Primary lymphedema may be secondary to agenesis, hypoplasia, or obstruction of the lymphatic vessels. It may be associated with the Turner syndrome, the Noonan syndrome, the yellow nail syndrome, the intestinal lymphangiectasia syndrome, and lymphangiomyomatosis. Women are affected more frequently than men. There are three clinical subtypes: congenital lymphedema, which appears shortly after birth; lymphedema praecox, which has its onset at the time of puberty; and lymphedema tarda, which usually begins after age 35. Familial forms of congenital lymphedema (Milroy's disease) and lymphedema praecox (Meige's disease) may be inherited in an autosomal dominant manner with variable penetrance; autosomal or sex-linked recessive forms are less common.

Table 248-3

Causes of Lymphedema

Primary
   Congenital (includes Milroy's disease)
   Lymphedema praecox (includes Meige's disease)
   Lymphedema tarda
Secondary
   Recurrent lymphangitis
   Filariasis
   Tuberculosis
   Neoplasm
   Surgery
   Radiation therapy

Secondary lymphedema is an acquired condition resulting from damage to or obstruction of previously normal lymphatic channels (see Table 248-3). Recurrent episodes of bacterial lymphangitis, usually caused by streptococci, are a very common cause of lymphedema. The most common cause of secondary lymphedema worldwide is filariasis (Chap. 223). Tumors, such as prostate cancer and lymphoma, also can obstruct lymphatic vessels. Both surgery and radiation therapy for breast carcinoma may cause lymphedema of the upper extremity. Less common causes include tuberculosis, contact dermatitis, lymphogranuloma venereum, rheumatoid arthritis, pregnancy, and self-induced or factitious lymphedema following application of tourniquets.

Lymphedema is generally a painless condition, but patients may experience a chronic dull, heavy sensation in the leg, and most often they are concerned about the appearance of the leg. Lymphedema of the lower extremity, initially involving the foot, gradually progresses up the leg so that the entire limb becomes edematous. In the early stages, the edema is soft and pits easily with pressure. In the chronic stages, the limb has a woody texture, and the tissues become indurated and fibrotic. At this point the edema may no longer be pitting. The limb loses its normal contour, and the toes appear square. Lymphedema should be distinguished from other disorders that cause unilateral leg swelling, such as deep vein thrombosis and chronic venous insufficiency. In the latter condition, the edema is softer, and there is often evidence of a stasis dermatitis, hyperpigmentation, and superficial venous varicosities.

The evaluation of patients with lymphedema should include diagnostic studies to clarify the cause. Abdominal and pelvic ultrasound and computed tomography can be used to detect obstructing lesions such as neoplasms. Lymphoscintigraphy and lymphangiography are rarely indicated, but either can be used to confirm the diagnosis or to differentiate primary from secondary lymphedema. Lymphoscintigraphy involves the injection of radioactively labeled technetium-containing colloid into the distal subcutaneous tissue of the affected extremity. In lymphangiography, contrast material is injected into a distal lymphatic vessel that has been isolated and cannulated. In primary lymphedema, lymphatic channels are absent, hypoplastic, or ectatic. In secondary lymphedema, lymphatic channels usually are dilated, and it may be possible to determine the level of obstruction.

 TREATMENT

Patients with lymphedema of the lower extremities must be instructed to take meticulous care of their feet to prevent recurrent lymphangitis. Skin hygiene is important, and emollients can be used to prevent drying. Prophylactic antibiotics are often helpful, and fungal infection should be treated aggressively. Patients should be encouraged to participate in physical activity; frequent leg elevation can reduce the amount of edema. Patients can be fitted with graduated compression hose to reduce the amount of lymphedema that develops with upright posture. Occasionally, intermittent pneumatic compression devices can be applied at home to facilitate reduction of the edema. Diuretics are contraindicated and may cause depletion of intravascular volume and metabolic abnormalities. Recently, microsurgical lymphovenous anastomotic procedures have been performed to rechannel lymph flow from obstructed lymphatic vessels into the venous system.

BIBLIOGRAPHY

BROWSE NL: The diagnosis and management of primary lymphedema. J Vasc Surg 3:181, 1986

COFFMAN JD: *Raynaud's Phenomenon*. New York, Oxford University Press, 1989

CRIQUI MH et al: Mortality over a period of 10 years in patients with peripheral arterial disease. N Engl J Med 326:381, 1992

EUROPEAN WORKING GROUP ON CRITICAL LEG ISCHEMIA: Second European consensus document on chronic critical leg ischemia. Circulation 84:IV1, 1991

GARDNER AW, POEHLMAN ET: Exercise rehabilitation programs for the treatment of claudication pain. A meta-analysis. JAMA 274:975, 1995

GOLDHABER SZ: Thrombolysis in venous thromboembolism. An international perspective. Chest 94:176S, 1990

HIRSH J, HOAK J: Management of deep vein thrombosis and pulmonary embolism. A statement of health care professionals. Circulation 93:2212, 1996

ISNER JM, ROSENFIELD K: Redefining the treatment of peripheral artery disease. Role of percutaneous revascularization. Circulation 88:1534, 1993

LENSING AW et al: Treatments of deep venous thrombosis with low-molecular weight heparins. A meta-analysis. Arch Intern Med 155:601, 1995

LOSCALZO J et al: *Vascular Medicine*, 2d ed. Boston, Little, Brown, 1996

OLIN JW et al: The changing clinical spectrum of thromboangiitis obliterans. Circulation 82:IV3, 1990

PEARSON SD et al: A critical pathway to evaluate suspected deep vein thrombosis. Arch Intern Med 155:1773, 1995

RADACK K, WYDERSKI RJ: Conservative management of intermittent claudication. Ann Intern Med 113:135, 1990

SCHULMAN S et al: A comparison of six weeks with six months of oral anticoagulant therapy after a first episode of venous thromboembolism. N Engl J Med 332:1661, 1995

SMITH GD et al: Intermittent claudication, heart disease risk factor, and mortality: The Whitehall study. Circulation 82:1925, 1990

YOUNG JR et al: *Peripheral Vascular Diseases*. St. Louis, Mosby Year Book, 1996

PART NINE

DISORDERS OF THE RESPIRATORY SYSTEM

249

Jeffrey M. Drazen, Steven E. Weinberger

APPROACH TO THE PATIENT WITH DISEASE OF THE RESPIRATORY SYSTEM

Patients with disease of the respiratory system generally present because of symptoms, an abnormality on a chest radiograph, or both. A set of diagnostic possibilities often is suggested by the initial problems at presentation, including the particular symptom(s) and the appearance of any radiographic abnormalities. The differential diagnosis is then refined on the basis of additional information gleaned from physical examination, pulmonary function testing, additional imaging studies, and bronchoscopic examination. This chapter will consider the approach to the patient based on the major patterns of presentation, focusing on the history, the physical examination, and the chest radiograph. Pulmonary function testing is covered in Chap. 250, and other diagnostic studies are discussed in Chap. 251.

CLINICAL PRESENTATION

HISTORY Dyspnea (shortness of breath) and cough are the primary presenting symptoms for patients with respiratory system disease. Less common symptoms include hemoptysis (the coughing up of blood) and chest pain, often with a pleuritic quality.

Dyspnea (See also Chap. 32) When evaluating a patient with shortness of breath, one should first determine the time course over which the symptom has become manifest. Patients who were well previously and developed *acute* shortness of breath (over a period of hours to days) can have acute disease affecting the airways (an acute attack of asthma), the pulmonary parenchyma (acute pulmonary edema or an acute infectious process such as a bacterial pneumonia), the pleural space (a pneumothorax), or the pulmonary vasculature (a pulmonary embolus). A *subacute* presentation (over days to weeks) can suggest an exacerbation of preexisting airways disease (asthma or chronic bronchitis), a parenchymal infection or a noninfectious inflammatory process that proceeds at a relatively slow pace (*Pneumocystis carinii* pneumonia in a patient with AIDS, mycobacterial or fungal pneumonia, Wegener's granulomatosis, eosinophilic pneumonia, bronchiolitis obliterans with organizing pneumonia, and many others), neuromuscular disease (Guillain-Barré syndrome, myasthenia gravis), pleural disease (pleural effusion from a variety of possible causes), or chronic cardiac disease (congestive heart failure). A *chronic* presentation (over months to years) often indicates chronic obstructive lung disease, chronic interstitial lung disease, or chronic cardiac disease. Chronic diseases of airways (not only chronic obstructive lung disease but also asthma) are characterized by exacerbations and remissions. Patients often have periods when they are severely limited by shortness of breath, but these may be interspersed with periods in which symptoms are minimal or absent. In contrast, many of the diseases of pulmonary parenchyma are characterized by a slow but inexorable progression.

Other Respiratory Symptoms *Cough* (Chap. 33) indicates the presence of lung disease, but cough per se is not useful for the differential diagnosis. The presence of sputum accompanying the cough often suggests airway disease and may be seen in asthma, chronic bronchitis, or bronchiectasis.

Hemoptysis (Chap. 33) can originate from disease of the airways, the pulmonary parenchyma, or the vasculature. Diseases of the airways can be inflammatory (acute or chronic bronchitis, bronchiectasis, or cystic fibrosis) or neoplastic (bronchogenic carcinoma or bronchial carcinoid tumors). Parenchymal diseases causing hemoptysis may be either localized (pneumonia, lung abscess, tuberculosis, or infection with *Aspergillus*) or diffuse (Goodpasture's syndrome, idiopathic pulmonary hemosiderosis). Vascular diseases potentially associated with hemoptysis include pulmonary thromboembolic disease and pulmonary arteriovenous malformations.

Chest pain (Chap. 13) caused by diseases of the respiratory system usually originates from involvement of the parietal pleura. As a result, the pain is accentuated by respiratory motion and is often referred to as *pleuritic*. Common examples include primary pleural disorders, such as neoplasm or inflammatory disorders involving the pleura, or pulmonary parenchymal disorders that extend to the pleural surface, such as pneumonia or pulmonary infarction.

Additional Historical Information Information about risk factors for lung disease should be explicitly explored to assure a complete basis of historical data. A history of current and past smoking, especially of cigarettes, should be sought from all patients. The smoking history should include the number of years of smoking, the intensity (i.e., number of packs per day), and, if the patient no longer smokes, the interval since smoking cessation. The risk of lung cancer falls progressively with the interval following discontinuation of smoking, and loss of lung function above the expected age-related decline ceases with the discontinuation of smoking. Even though chronic obstructive lung disease and neoplasia are the two most important respiratory complications of smoking, other respiratory disorders (e.g., spontaneous pneumothorax, eosinophilic granuloma of the lung, and pulmonary hemorrhage with Goodpasture's syndrome) are also associated with smoking. A history of significant secondhand (passive) exposure to smoke, whether in the home or at the workplace, should also be sought as it may be a risk factor for neoplasia or an exacerbating factor for airways disease.

The patient may have been exposed to other inhaled agents associated with lung disease, which act either via direct toxicity or through immune mechanisms (Chaps. 253 and 254). Such exposures can be either occupational or avocational, indicating the importance of detailed occupational and personal histories, the latter stressing exposures related to hobbies or the home environment. Important agents include the inorganic dusts associated with pneumoconiosis (especially asbestos and silica dusts) and organic antigens associated with hypersensitivity pneumonitis (especially antigens from molds and animal proteins). Asthma often is exacerbated by exposure to environmental allergens (dust mites, pet dander, or cockroach allergens in the home or allergens in the outdoor environment such as pollen and ragweed) or may be caused by occupational exposures (diisocyanates). Exposure to particular infectious agents can be suggested by contacts with individuals with known respiratory infections (especially tuberculosis) or by residence in an area with endemic pathogens (histoplasmosis, coccidioidomycosis, blastomycosis).

A history of coexisting nonrespiratory disease or of risk factors for or previous treatment of such diseases should be sought, as they may predispose a patient to both infectious and noninfectious respiratory system complications. Common examples include systemic rheumatic diseases that are associated with pleural or parenchymal lung disease (Chap. 313), metastatic neoplastic disease in the lung, or impaired host defense mechanisms and secondary infection, which occurs in the case of hematologic and lymph node malignancies. Risk factors for AIDS should be sought, as the lungs not only are the most common site of AIDS-defining infection but also can be involved by nonfectious complications of AIDS (Chap. 308). Treatment of nonrespiratory disease can be associated with respiratory complications, either because of effects on host defense mechanisms (immunosuppressive agents, cancer chemotherapy) with resulting infection, or because of direct effects on the pulmonary parenchyma (cancer chemotherapy, radiation therapy, or treatment with other agents, such as amiodarone, that cause interstitial lung disease), or on the airways (beta-blocking agents causing airflow obstruction, angiotensin converting enzyme inhibitors causing cough) (Chap. 253).

Family history is important for evaluating diseases that have a genetic component. These include disorders such as cystic fibrosis, α_1-antitrypsin deficiency, and asthma.

PHYSICAL EXAMINATION   The general principles of inspection, palpation, percussion, and auscultation apply to the examination of the respiratory system. However, the physical examination should be directed not only toward ascertaining abnormalities of the lungs and thorax, but also toward recognizing other findings that may reflect underlying lung disease.

On *inspection*, the rate and pattern of breathing as well as the depth and symmetry of lung expansion are observed. Breathing that is unusually rapid, labored, or associated with the use of accessory muscles of respiration generally indicates either augmented respiratory demands or an increased work of breathing. Asymmetric expansion of the chest is usually due to an asymmetric process affecting the lungs, such as endobronchial obstruction of a large airway, unilateral parenchymal or pleural disease, or unilateral phrenic nerve paralysis. Visible abnormalities of the thoracic cage include kyphoscoliosis and ankylosing spondylitis, each of which can alter compliance of the thorax, increase the work of breathing, and cause dyspnea.

On *palpation*, the symmetry of lung expansion can be assessed, generally confirming the findings observed by inspection. Vibration produced by spoken sounds is transmitted to the chest wall and is assessed by the presence or absence and symmetry of tactile fremitus. Transmission of vibration is decreased or absent if pleural liquid is interposed between the lung and the chest wall, or if an endobronchial obstruction alters sound transmission. In contrast, transmitted vibration may increase over an area of underlying pulmonary consolidation.

The relative resonance or dullness of the tissue underlying the chest wall is assessed by *percussion*. The normal sound of underlying air-containing lung is resonant. In contrast, consolidated lung or a pleural effusion sounds dull, while air in the pleural space sounds hyperresonant.

On *auscultation* of the lungs, the examiner listens for both the quality and intensity of the breath sounds and for the presence of extra, or adventitious, sounds. Normal breath sounds heard through the stethoscope at the periphery of the lung are described as *vesicular breath sounds*, in which inspiration is louder and longer than expiration. If sound transmission is impaired by endobronchial obstruction or by air or liquid in the pleural space, breath sounds are weaker or absent. When sound transmission is improved through consolidated lung, the resulting *bronchial breath sounds* have a more tubular quality and a more pronounced expiratory phase. Sound transmission can also be assessed by listening to spoken or whispered sounds; when these are transmitted through consolidated lung, *bronchophony* and *whispered pectoriloquy*, respectively, are present. The sound of a spoken E becomes more like an A, though with a nasal or bleating quality, a finding that is termed *egophony*.

The primary adventitious (abnormal) sounds that can be heard include crackles (rales), wheezes, and rhonchi. *Crackles* represent the sound created when alveoli and small airways open or close during respiration, and often they are associated with interstitial lung disease, microatelectasis, or filling of alveoli by liquid. *Wheezes*, which are generally more prominent during expiration than inspiration, reflect the oscillation of airway walls that occurs when there is airflow limitation, as may be produced by bronchospasm, airway edema or collapse, or intraluminal obstruction by neoplasm or secretions. *Rhonchi* is the term applied to the sounds created when there is free liquid in the airway lumen; the viscous interaction between the free liquid and the moving air creates a low-pitched vibratory sound. Other adventitious sounds include pleural friction rubs and stridor. The gritty sound of a pleural friction rub indicates inflamed pleural surfaces rubbing against each other, often during both inspiratory and expiratory phases of the respiratory cycle. Stridor, which occurs primarily during inspiration, represents flow through a narrowed upper airway, as occurs in an infant with croup.

A summary of the patterns of physical findings on pulmonary examination in common types of respiratory system disease is shown in Table 249-1.

A meticulous *general physical examination* is mandatory in patients with disorders of the respiratory system. Enlarged lymph nodes in the cervical and supraclavicular regions should be sought. Disturbances of mentation or even coma occur in patients with acute carbon dioxide retention and hypoxemia. Telltale stains on the fingers point to heavy cigarette smoking; infected teeth and gums may occur in patients with aspiration pneumonitis and lung abscess.

Clubbing of the digits can be found in lung cancer, interstitial lung disease, and chronic infections in the thorax, such as bronchiectasis, lung abscess, and empyema. Clubbing can also be seen with congenital heart disease associated with right-to-left shunting and with

Table 249-1

Typical Chest Examination Findings in Selected Clinical Conditions

Condition	Percussion	Fremitus	Breath Sounds	Voice Transmission	Adventitious Sounds
Normal	Resonant	Normal	Vesicular (at lung bases)	Normal	Absent
Consolidation or atelectasis (with patent airway)	Dull	Increased	Bronchial	Bronchophony, whispered pectoriloquy, egophony	Crackles
Consolidation or atelectasis (with blocked airway)	Dull	Decreased	Decreased	Decreased	Absent
Asthma	Resonant	Normal	Vesicular	Normal	Wheezing
Interstitial lung disease	Resonant	Normal	Vesicular	Normal	Crackles
Emphysema	Hyperresonant	Decreased	Decreased	Decreased	Absent or wheezing
Pneumothorax	Hyperresonant	Decreased	Decreased	Decreased	Absent
Pleural effusion	Dull	Decreased	Decreased*	Decreased*	Absent or pleural friction rub

* May be altered by collapse of underlying lung, which will increase transmission of sound.

SOURCE: Adapted from Weinberger.

variety of chronic inflammatory or infectious diseases, such as inflammatory bowel disease and endocarditis. A number of systemic diseases, such as systemic lupus erythematosus, scleroderma, and rheumatoid arthritis, may be associated with pulmonary complications, even though their primary clinical manifestations and physical findings are not primarily related to the lungs. Conversely, other diseases that most affect the respiratory system, such as sarcoidosis, can have findings on physical examination not related to the respiratory system, including ocular findings (uveitis, conjunctival granulomas) and skin findings (erythema nodosum, cutaneous granulomas).

CHEST RADIOGRAPHY

Chest radiography is often the initial diagnostic study performed to evaluate patients with respiratory symptoms, but it can also provide the initial evidence of disease in patients who are free of symptoms. Perhaps the most common example of the latter situation is the finding of one or more nodules or masses when the radiograph is performed for a reason other than evaluation of respiratory symptoms.

A number of diagnostic possibilities are often suggested by the radiographic pattern. A localized region of opacification involving the air spaces is usually characterized as having an alveolar, an interstitial, or a nodular pattern. In contrast, increased radiolucency can be localized, as seen with a cyst or bulla, or generalized, as occurs with emphysema. The chest radiograph is also particularly useful for the detection of pleural disease, especially if manifested by the presence of air or liquid in the pleural space. An abnormal appearance of the hila and/or the mediastinum can suggest a mass or enlargement of lymph nodes.

A summary of representative diagnoses suggested by these common radiographic patterns is presented in Table 249-2.

Additional Diagnostic Evaluation   Further information for clarification of radiographic abnormalities is frequently obtained with computed tomographic scanning of the chest (see Chap. 251). This

Table 249-2

Major Respiratory Diagnoses with Common Chest Radiographic Patterns

Solitary circumscribed density—nodule (<6 cm) or mass (≥6 cm)
 Primary or metastatic neoplasm
 Localized infection (bacterial abscess, mycobacterial or fungal infection)
 Wegener's granulomatosis (one or several nodules)
 Rheumatoid nodule (one or several nodules)
 Vascular malformation
 Bronchogenic cyst
Localized opacification (infiltrate)
 Pneumonia (bacterial, atypical, mycobacterial, or fungal infection)
 Neoplasm
 Radiation pneumonitis
 Bronchiolitis obliterans with organizing pneumonia
 Bronchocentric granulomatosis
 Pulmonary infarction
Diffuse interstitial disease
 Idiopathic pulmonary fibrosis
 Pulmonary fibrosis with systemic rheumatic disease
 Sarcoidosis
 Drug-induced lung disease
 Pneumoconiosis
 Hypersensitivity pneumonitis
 Infection (*Pneumocystis*, viral pneumonia)
 Eosinophilic granuloma
Diffuse alveolar disease
 Cardiogenic pulmonary edema
 Acute respiratory distress syndrome
 Diffuse alveolar hemorrhage
 Infection (*Pneumocystis*, viral or bacterial pneumonia)
 Sarcoidosis
Diffuse nodular disease
 Metastatic neoplasm
 Hematogenous spread of infection (bacterial, mycobacterial, fungal)
 Pneumoconiosis
 Eosinophilic granuloma

technique is more sensitive than plain radiography in detecting subtle abnormalities, can suggest the presence of certain diseases based on the pattern of abnormality, and is very useful as a means of gathering quantitative information about specific radiographic findings. The use of other imaging studies, including magnetic resonance imaging, scintigraphic studies, ultrasound, and angiography, are discussed in Chap. 251.

Alteration in the function of the lungs as a result of respiratory system disease is assessed objectively by pulmonary function tests, and effects on gas exchange are evaluated by measurement of arterial blood gases or by oximetry (Chap. 250). As part of pulmonary function testing, quantitation of forced expiratory flow assesses the presence of obstructive physiology, which is consistent with diseases affecting the structure or function of the airways, such as asthma and chronic obstructive lung disease. Measurement of lung volumes assesses the presence of restrictive disorders, seen with diseases of the pulmonary parenchyma or respiratory pump and with space-occupying processes of the pleura.

Bronchoscopy is useful in some settings for visualizing abnormalities of the airways and for obtaining a variety of samples from either the airway or the pulmonary parenchyma (Chap. 251).

INTEGRATION OF THE PRESENTING CLINICAL PATTERN AND DIAGNOSTIC STUDIES

Patients with respiratory symptoms but a normal chest radiograph most commonly have diseases affecting the airways, such as asthma or chronic obstructive pulmonary disease. However, the latter diagnosis is also commonly associated with radiographic abnormalities, such as diaphragmatic flattening and attenuation of vascular markings. Other disorders of the respiratory system for which the chest radiograph is normal include disorders of the respiratory pump (either the chest wall or the neuromuscular apparatus controlling the chest wall) and occasionally interstitial lung disease. Chest examination and pulmonary function tests are generally helpful in sorting out these diagnostic possibilities. Obstructive diseases associated with a normal or relatively normal chest radiograph are often characterized by findings on physical examination and pulmonary function testing that are typical for these conditions. Similarly, diseases of the respiratory pump or interstitial diseases may also be suggested by findings on physical examination or by particular patterns of restrictive disease seen on pulmonary function testing.

When respiratory symptoms are accompanied by radiographic abnormalities, diseases of the pulmonary parenchyma or the pleura are usually present. Either diffuse or localized parenchymal lung disease is generally visualized well on the radiograph, and both air and liquid in the pleural space (pneumothorax and pleural effusion, respectively) are usually readily detected by radiography.

Radiographic findings in the absence of respiratory symptoms often indicate localized disease affecting the airways or the pulmonary parenchyma. One or more nodules or masses can suggest intrathoracic malignancy, but they also can be the manifestation of a current or previous infectious process. Patients with diffuse parenchymal lung disease present on radiographic examination may be free of symptoms, as is sometimes the case with pulmonary sarcoidosis.

In approaching the patient with pulmonary disease, consideration must be given to the observation that substantial changes in the relative incidence of disease affecting the respiratory system have taken place in the United States during the past three decades. The prevalence of chronic infectious disorders such as lung abscess and bronchiectasis has decreased. Tuberculosis declined only to undergo resurgence when two susceptible populations, patients with AIDS and immigrants from Southeast Asia, increased in number. Patients with chronic bronchitis and with emphysema now survive longer and form an increasing fraction of patients with chronic respiratory disease, as do patients with environmental lung disease and with drug-induced pulmonary disease. Modern intercontinental travel has increased the appearance in the western world of parasitic infestations of the lung. Also, the reduction of immune competence that occurs in patients with AIDS and in diabetics as well as in patients being treated for a variety of malignancies and those receiving immunosuppressive drugs has led to an increasing incidence of opportunistic infections of the lungs with a variety of microorganisms that were rarely pathogenic in the past.

BIBLIOGRAPHY

DeGowin R et al: *DeGowin & DeGowin's Diagnostic Examination*, 6th ed. New York, McGraw-Hill, 1994

Ebi-Kryston KL: Respiratory symptoms and pulmonary function as predictors of 10-year mortality from respiratory disease, cardiovascular disease, and all causes in the Whitehall Study. J Clin Epidemiol 41:251, 1988

Godden DJ et al: Outcome of wheeze in childhood. Symptoms and pulmonary function 25 years later. Am J Respir Crit Care Med 149:106, 1994

Weinberger SE: *Principles of Pulmonary Medicine*, 2d ed. Philadelphia, Saunders, 1992

Welty C et al: The relationship of airways responsiveness to cold air, cigarette smoking, and atopy to respiratory symptoms and pulmonary function in adults. Am Rev Respir Dis 130:198, 1984

250

Steven E. Weinberger, Jeffrey M. Drazen

DISTURBANCES OF RESPIRATORY FUNCTION

The respiratory system includes the lungs, the central nervous system (CNS), the chest wall (with the diaphragm and intercostal muscles), and the pulmonary circulation. The CNS controls the activity of the muscles of the chest wall, which constitute the pump of the respiratory system. Because these components of the respiratory system act in concert to achieve gas exchange, malfunction of an individual component or alteration of the relationships among components can lead to disturbances in function. In this chapter we consider three major aspects of disturbed respiratory function: (1) disturbances in ventilatory function, (2) disturbances in the pulmonary circulation, and (3) disturbances in gas exchange. Disorders relating to CNS control of ventilation are discussed in Chap. 263.

DISTURBANCES IN VENTILATORY FUNCTION

Ventilation is the process whereby the lungs replenish the gas in the alveoli. Measurements of ventilatory function in common diagnostic use consist of quantification of the gas volume contained in the lungs under certain circumstances and the rate at which gas can be expelled from the lungs. Two measurements of lung volume commonly used for respiratory diagnosis are total lung capacity (TLC) and residual volume (RV). The former is the volume of gas contained in the lungs after a maximal inspiration, whereas the latter is the volume of gas remaining in the lungs at the end of a maximal expiration. The volume of gas that is exhaled from the lungs in going from TLC to RV is called the *vital capacity* (VC) (Fig. 250-1).

Common clinical measurements of airflow are obtained from maneuvers in which the subject inspires to TLC and then forcibly exhales to RV. Three measurements are commonly made from a volume-time recording—i.e., a spirogram—obtained during such a forced expiratory maneuver: (1) the volume of gas exhaled during the first second of expiration (forced expiratory volume in 1 s, or FEV_1), (2) the total volume exhaled (forced vital capacity, or FVC), and (3) the average expiratory flow rate during the middle 50 percent of the vital capacity (forced expiratory flow between 25 and 75 percent of the

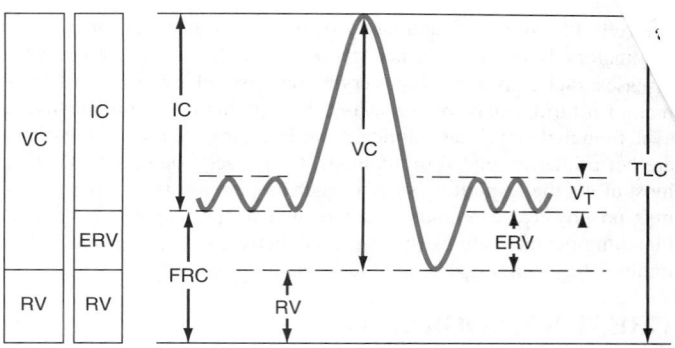

FIGURE 250-1 Lung volumes, shown by block diagrams *(left)* and by a spirographic tracing *(right)*. TLC, total lung capacity; VC, vital capacity; RV, residual volume; IC, inspiratory capacity; ERV, expiratory reserve volume; FRC, functional residual capacity; V_T, tidal volume. *(From Weinberger, with permission.)*

vital capacity, or $FEF_{25-75\%}$, also called the maximal midexpiratory flow rate, or MMFR) (Fig. 250-2).

PHYSIOLOGIC FEATURES The lungs are elastic structures, containing collagen and elastic fibers that resist expansion. For normal lungs to contain air, they must be distended either by a positive internal pressure—i.e., by a pressure in the airways and alveolar spaces—or by a negative external pressure—i.e., by a pressure outside the lung. The relationship between the volume of gas contained in the lungs and the distending pressure (the transpulmonary pressure, or P_{TP}, defined as internal pressure minus external pressure) is described by the pressure-volume curve of the lungs (Fig. 250-3A).

The chest wall is also an elastic structure, with properties similar to those of an expandable and compressible spring. The relationship between the volume enclosed by the chest wall and the distending pressure for the chest wall is described by the pressure-volume curve of the chest wall (Fig. 250-3B). For the chest wall to assume a volume different from its resting volume, the internal or external pressures acting on it must be altered.

At functional residual capacity (FRC), defined as the volume of gas in the lungs at the end of a normal exhalation, the lungs are partially inflated, so their elastic recoil exerts a force tending to empty the lungs. At the same time, chest wall volume is such that its elastic recoil promotes outward expansion. Functional residual capacity oc-

FIGURE 250-2 Spirographic tracings of forced expiration, comparing a normal tracing *(A)* and tracings in obstructive *(B)* and parenchymal restrictive *(C)* disease. Calculations of FVC, FEV_1, and $FEF_{25-75\%}$ are shown only for the normal tracing. Since there is no measure of absolute starting volume with spirometry, the curves are artificially positioned to show the relative starting lung volumes in the different conditions.

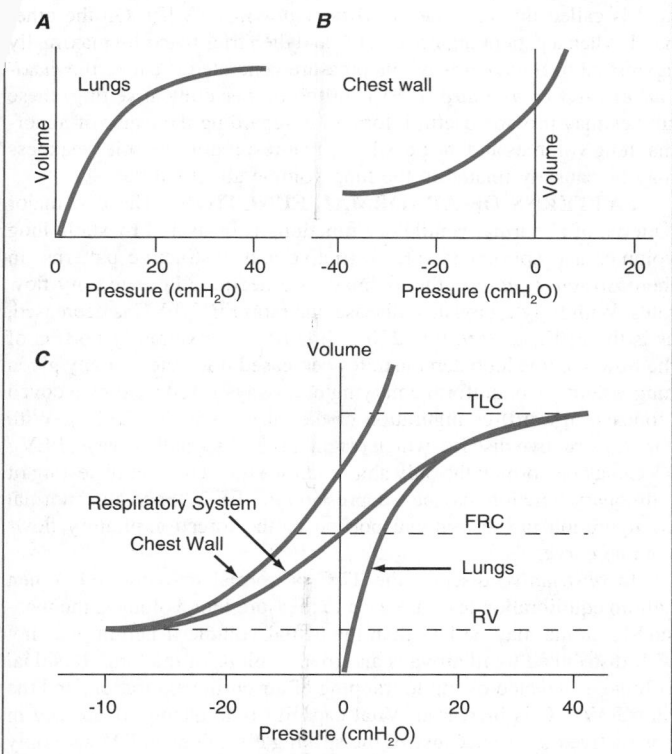

FIGURE 250-3 *A.* Pressure-volume curve of the lungs. *B.* Pressure-volume curve of the chest wall. *C.* Pressure-volume curve of the respiratory system, showing the superimposed component curves of the lungs and the chest wall. RV, residual volume; FRC, functional residual capacity; TLC, total lung capacity. *(From Weinberger, with permission.)*

curs at the lung volume at which the tendency of the lungs to contract is opposed by the equal and opposite tendency of the chest wall to expand (Fig. 250-3*C*).

For the lungs and the chest wall to achieve a volume other than the resting volume (FRC), either the pressures acting on them must be changed passively—for example, by a mechanical ventilator that delivers positive pressure to the airways and alveoli—or the respiratory muscles must actively oppose the tendency of the lungs and the chest wall to return to FRC. During inhalation to volumes above FRC, the inspiratory muscles actively overcome the tendency of the respiratory system to decrease volume back to FRC. During active exhalation to volumes below FRC, expiratory muscle activity must overcome the tendency of the respiratory system to increase volume back to FRC. At TLC, the maximal force applied by the inspiratory muscles to expand the lungs is opposed mainly by the inward recoil of the lungs. As a consequence, the major determinants of TLC are the stiffness of the lungs and inspiratory muscle strength. If the lungs become stiffer—i.e., less compliant—TLC is decreased. If the lungs become less stiff (more compliant), TLC is increased. If the inspiratory muscles are significantly weakened, they are less able to overcome the inward elastic recoil of the lungs, and TLC is lowered.

At RV, the force exerted by the expiratory muscles to decrease lung volume further is balanced by the outward recoil of the chest wall, which becomes extremely stiff at low lung volumes. Two factors influence the volume of gas contained in the lungs at RV. The first is the ability of the subject to exert a prolonged expiratory effort, which is related to muscle strength and the ability to overcome sensory stimuli from the chest wall. The second is the ability of the lungs to empty to a small volume. In normal lungs, as P_{TP} is lowered, lung volume decreases. In lungs with diseased airways, as P_{TP} is lowered, flow limitation or airway closure can limit the amount of gas that is expired. Consequently, either weak chest wall muscles or intrinsic airways disease can result in an elevation in measured RV.

Dynamic measurements of ventilatory function are made by having the subject inhale to TLC and then perform a forced expiration to RV. If a subject performs a series of such expiratory maneuvers using increasing muscular intensity, expiratory flow rates will increase until a certain level of effort is reached. Beyond this level, additional effort will not increase the forced expiratory flow rate; this phenomenon is known as the *effort independence* of forced expiratory flow. The physiologic mechanisms determining the flow rates during this effort-independent phase of forced expiratory flow have been shown to be the elastic recoil of the lung, the airflow resistance of the airways between the alveolar zone and the physical site of flow limitation, and the airway wall compliance at the site of flow limitation. Physical processes that decrease elastic recoil, increase airflow resistance, or increase airway wall compliance decrease the flow rate that can be achieved at any given lung volume. Conversely, processes that increase elastic recoil, decrease resistance, or stiffen airway walls increase the flow rate that can be achieved at any given lung volume.

MEASUREMENT OF VENTILATORY FUNCTION Ventilatory function is measured under static conditions for determination of lung volumes and under dynamic conditions for determination of forced expiratory flow rates. VC, expiratory reserve volume (ERV), and inspiratory capacity (IC) (see Fig. 250-1) are measured by having the patient breathe into and out of a spirometer, a device capable of measuring expired or inspired gas volume while plotting volume as a function of time. Other volumes—specifically, RV, FRC, and TLC—cannot be measured in this way because they include the volume of gas present in the lungs even after a maximal expiration. Two techniques are commonly used to measure these volumes: helium dilution and body plethysmography. In the helium dilution method, the subject repeatedly breathes in and out from a reservoir with a known volume of gas containing a trace amount of helium. The helium is diluted by the gas previously present in the lungs and is not absorbed into the pulmonary circulation. From knowledge of the reservoir volume and the initial and final helium concentrations, the volume of gas present in the lungs can be calculated. The helium dilution method may underestimate the volume of gas in the lungs if there are slowly communicating airspaces, such as bullae. In this situation, lung volumes can be more accurately measured with a body plethysmograph, a sealed box in which the patient sits while panting against a closed mouthpiece. Because there is no airflow into or out of the plethysmograph, the pressure changes in the thorax during panting cause compression and rarefaction of gas in the lungs and simultaneous rarefaction and compression of gas in the plethysmograph. By measuring the pressure changes in the plethysmograph and at the mouthpiece, the volume of gas in the thorax can be calculated using Boyle's law.

Lung volumes and measurements made during forced expiration are interpreted by comparing the values measured with the values expected given the age, height, sex, and race of the patient (see Appendix A). Regression curves have been constructed on the basis of data obtained from large numbers of normal, nonsmoking individuals without evidence of lung disease. Predicted values for a given patient can then be obtained by using the patient's age and height in the appropriate regression equation; different equations are used depending on the patient's race and gender. Because there is some variability among normal individuals, values between 80 and 120 percent of the predicted value have traditionally been considered normal. Increasingly, calculated percentiles are used in determining normality. Specifically, values of individual measurements falling below the fifth percentile are considered to be below normal.

The normal value for the ratio FEV_1/FVC is approximately 0.75 to 0.80, although this value does fall somewhat with advancing age. The $FEF_{25-75\%}$ is often considered a more sensitive measurement of early airflow obstruction, particularly in small airways. However, this measurement must be interpreted cautiously in patients with abnormally small lungs (low TLC and VC). These patients exhale less air during forced expiration, and the $FEF_{25-75\%}$ may appear abnormal rela-

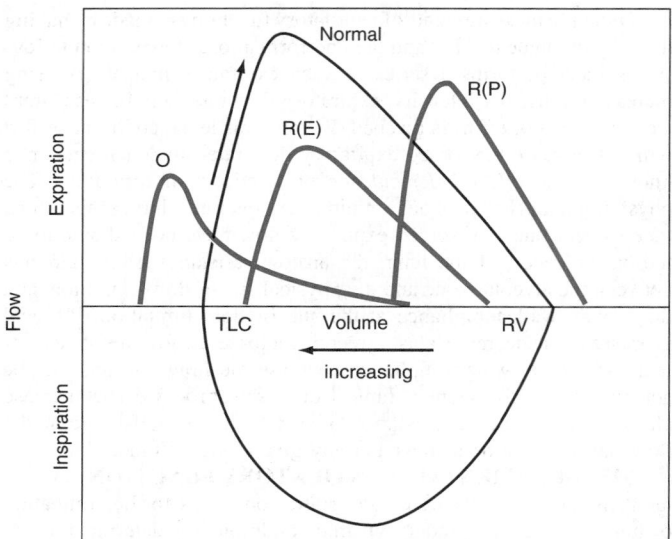

FIGURE 250-4 Flow-volume curves in different conditions: O, obstructive disease; R(P), parenchymal restrictive disease; R(E), extraparenchymal restrictive disease with limitation in inspiration and expiration. Forced expiration is plotted in all conditions; forced inspiration is shown only for the normal curve. TLC, total lung capacity; RV, residual volume. By convention, lung volume increases to the left on the abscissa. The arrow alongside the normal curve indicates the direction of expiration from TLC to RV.

tive to the usual predicted value, even though it is normal relative to the size of the patient's lungs.

It is also a common practice to plot expiratory flow rates against lung volume (rather than against time); the close linkage of flow rates to lung volumes produces a typical *flow-volume curve* (Fig. 250-4). In addition, the spirometric values mentioned above can be calculated from the flow-volume curve. Commonly, flow rates during a maximal inspiratory effort performed as rapidly as possible are plotted as well, making the flow-volume curve into a *flow-volume loop*. At TLC, before expiratory flow starts, the flow rate is zero; once forced expiration has begun, a high peak flow rate is rapidly achieved. As expiration continues and lung volume approaches RV, the flow rate falls progressively, in a nearly linear fashion as a function of lung volume for a person with normal lung function. During maximal inspiration from RV to TLC, inspiratory flow is most rapid at the midpoint of inspiration, so the inspiratory portion of the loop is U-shaped or saddle-shaped. The flow rates achieved during maximal expiration can be analyzed quantitatively by comparing the flow rates at specified lung volumes with the predicted values or qualitatively by analyzing the shape of the descending limb of the expiratory curve.

Assessing the strength of respiratory muscles is an additional part of the overall evaluation of some patients with respiratory dysfunction. When a patient exhales completely to RV and then tries to inspire

maximally against an occluded airway, the pressure that can be gⁿerated is called the *maximal inspiratory pressure* (MIP). On the oⁿ hand, when a patient inhales to TLC and then tries to expire maximaⁿ against an occluded airway, the pressure generated is called the *maxⁿmal expiratory pressure* (MEP). In the proper clinical setting, these studies may provide useful information regarding the cause of abnormal lung volumes and the possibility that respiratory muscle weakness may be causally related to the lung volume abnormalities.

PATTERNS OF ABNORMAL FUNCTION The two major patterns of abnormal ventilatory function, as measured by static lung volumes and spirometry, are restrictive and obstructive patterns. In the *obstructive pattern*, the hallmark is a decrease in expiratory flow rates. With fully established disease, the ratio FEV_1/FVC is decreased, as is the $FEF_{25-75\%}$ (see Fig. 250-2, line B). The expiratory portion of the flow-volume loop demonstrates decreased flow rates for any given lung volume. Nonuniform emptying of airways is reflected by a coved (concave upward) configuration of the curve (see Fig. 250-4). With early obstructive disease, which originates in the small airways, FEV_1/FVC may be normal; the only abnormalities noted on routine testing of pulmonary function may be a depression in $FEF_{25-75\%}$ and an abnormal configuration in the terminal portion of the forced expiratory flow-volume curve.

In *obstructive* disease, the TLC is normal or increased. When helium equilibration tests are used to measure lung volumes, the measured volume may be less than the actual volume if helium was not well distributed to all airways and to all regions of the lung. Residual volume is elevated owing to trapping of air during expiration, and the ratio RV/TLC is increased. Vital capacity is frequently decreased in obstructive disease because of the striking elevations in RV with only minor changes in TLC.

A *restrictive pattern* can be broadly divided into two subgroups, depending on the location of the pathology—pulmonary parenchymal and extraparenchymal. For extraparenchymal disease, dysfunction can be predominantly in inspiration or in both inspiration and expiration (Table 250-1). The hallmark of a restrictive pattern, found in all these subcategories, is a decrease in lung volumes, primarily TLC and VC. In pulmonary parenchymal disease, RV is also generally decreased, and forced expiratory flow rates are preserved. In fact, when FEV_1 is considered as a percentage of the FVC, the flow rates are often supranormal, i.e., disproportionately high relative to the size of the lungs (see Fig. 250-2, line C). The flow-volume curve may graphically demonstrate this disproportionate relationship between flow rates and lung volumes, since the expiratory portion of the curve appears relatively tall (preserved flow rates) but narrow (decreased lung volumes), as shown in Fig. 250-4.

In the extraparenchymal pattern characterized by *inspiratory dysfunction*, caused either by inspiratory muscle weakness or a stiff chest wall, inadequate distending forces are exerted on an otherwise normal lung. As a result, TLC values are less than predicted, RV is often not significantly affected, and expiratory flows are preserved. If inspiratory muscle weakness is the cause of this pattern, then MIP is decreased. In the extraparenchymal pattern characterized by *inspiratory and expiratory dysfunction*, the ability to expire to a normal RV is also limited, because of either expiratory muscle weakness or a deformed chest wall that is abnormally rigid at volumes below FRC. Consequently, RV is often elevated, unlike the pattern observed in the other restrictive subcategories. The ratio FEV_1/FVC is variable and depends on expiratory muscle strength. If expiratory muscle strength is significantly decreased, then MEP is decreased, the ability to expire rapidly is impaired, and FEV_1/FVC may be decreased even though there is no airflow obstruction. If expiratory muscle strength is normal but the chest wall is abnormally stiff below FRC, then FEV_1/FVC is normal or increased.

Table 250-1

Alterations in Ventilatory Function

	TLC	RV	VC	FEV₁/FVC	MIP	MEP
Obstructive	N to ↑	↑	↓	↓*	N	N
Restrictive						
Pulmonary parenchymal	↓	↓	↓	N to ↑	N	N
Extraparenchymal—inspiratory	↓	N to ↓	↓	N	↓/N†	N
Extraparenchymal—inspiratory + expiratory	↓	↑	↓	Variable	↓/N†	↓/N†

* Mild obstructive (small airways) disease may have FEF₍25-75%₎ with normal FEV₁/FVC.
† Reduced if due to respiratory muscle weakness; normal if due to chest wall stiffness.
NOTE: N = normal; for other abbreviations, see text.

Table 250-2

CHAPTER 250
Disturbances of Respiratory Function 1413

Common Respiratory Diseases by Diagnostic Categories

Obstructive

Asthma
Chronic obstructive lung disease (chronic bronchitis, emphysema)
Bronchiectasis
Cystic fibrosis
Bronchiolitis

Restrictive—Parenchymal

Sarcoidosis
Idiopathic pulmonary fibrosis
Pneumoconiosis
Drug- or radiation-induced interstitial lung disease

Restrictive—Extraparenchymal

Neuromuscular
  Diaphragmatic weakness/paralysis
  Myasthenia gravis*
  Guillain-Barré syndrome*
  Muscular dystrophies*
  Cervical spine injury*
Chest wall
  Kyphoscoliosis
  Obesity
  Ankylosing spondylitis*

* Can have inspiratory and expiratory limitation (see text).

CLINICAL CORRELATIONS Table 250-1 summarizes the expected alterations in ventilatory function as indicated by pulmonary function testing. One reason to establish a ventilatory diagnosis is to categorize the functional disorder. This information can be useful in diagnosis, as outlined in Table 250-2. Note that lung disease can be present without abnormal ventilatory function, but the presence of specific diagnostic findings is an aid in differential diagnosis.

DISTURBANCES IN THE PULMONARY CIRCULATION

PHYSIOLOGIC FEATURES The pulmonary vasculature must handle the entire output of the right ventricle, approximately 5 L/min in a normal adult at rest. The comparatively thin-walled vessels of the pulmonary arterial system provide relatively little resistance to flow and are capable of handling this large volume of blood at perfusion pressures that are low compared with those of the systemic circulation. The normal mean pulmonary artery pressure is 15 mmHg, as compared to approximately 95 mmHg for the normal mean aortic pressure. Regional blood flow in the lung is dependent on hydrostatic forces. In an upright person, pulmonary arterial pressure is lowest at the apex of the lung and highest at the lung base. As a result, in the upright position, perfusion is least at the apex and greatest at the base. When cardiac output increases, as occurs during exercise, the pulmonary vasculature is capable of recruiting previously unperfused vessels and distending underperfused vessels, thus responding to the increase in flow with a decrease in pulmonary vascular resistance. In consequence, the increase in mean pulmonary arterial pressure, even with a three- to fourfold increase in cardiac output, is small.

METHODS OF MEASUREMENT Assessment of circulatory function in the pulmonary vasculature depends on measuring pulmonary vascular pressures and cardiac output. Clinically, these measurements are commonly made in intensive care units capable of invasive monitoring and in cardiac catheterization laboratories. With a flow-directed pulmonary arterial (Swan-Ganz) catheter, pulmonary arterial and pulmonary capillary wedge pressures can be measured directly, and cardiac output can be obtained by the thermodilution method. Pulmonary vascular resistance can then be calculated according to the equation

$$PVR = 80(PAP - PCW)/CO$$

where PVR = pulmonary vascular resistance (dyn·s/cm^5); PAP = mean pulmonary arterial pressure (mmHg); PCW = pulmonary capillary wedge pressure (mmHg); and CO = cardiac output (L/min).

The normal value for pulmonary vascular resistance is approximately 50 to 150 dyn·s/cm^5.

MECHANISMS OF ABNORMAL FUNCTION (See also Chap. 260) Pulmonary vascular resistance may increase by a variety of mechanisms. Pulmonary arterial and arteriolar vasoconstriction is a prominent response to alveolar hypoxia. Pulmonary vascular resistance also increases if intraluminal thrombi or proliferation of smooth muscle in vessel walls diminishes the luminal cross-sectional area. If small pulmonary vessels are destroyed, either by scarring or by loss of alveolar walls, the total cross-sectional area of the pulmonary vascular bed diminishes, and pulmonary vascular resistance increases. When pulmonary vascular resistance is elevated, either pulmonary arterial pressure rises to maintain normal cardiac output or cardiac output falls if pulmonary arterial pressure does not increase.

CLINICAL CORRELATIONS Disturbances in the function of the pulmonary vasculature as a result of primary cardiac disease, either congenital heart disease or conditions that elevate left atrial pressure, such as mitral stenosis, are beyond the scope of this chapter and are discussed in Chaps. 235 and 237, respectively. Instead, the focus will be on the pulmonary vasculature as its function is affected by diseases primarily involving the respiratory system, including the pulmonary vessels themselves.

All diseases of the respiratory system causing hypoxemia are potentially capable of increasing pulmonary vascular resistance, since alveolar hypoxia is a very potent stimulus for pulmonary vasoconstriction. The more prolonged and intense the hypoxic stimulus, the more likely it is that a significant increase in pulmonary vascular resistance producing pulmonary hypertension will result. In practice, patients with hypoxemia caused by chronic obstructive lung disease, interstitial lung disease, chest wall disease, and the obesity hypoventilation–sleep apnea syndrome are particularly prone to developing pulmonary hypertension. If there are additional structural changes in the pulmonary vasculature secondary to the underlying process, these will increase the likelihood of developing pulmonary hypertension.

With diseases directly affecting the pulmonary vessels, a decrease in the cross-sectional area of the pulmonary vascular bed is primarily responsible for increased pulmonary vascular resistance, while hypoxemia generally plays a lesser role. In the case of recurrent pulmonary emboli, parts of the pulmonary arterial system are occluded by intraluminal thrombi originating in the systemic venous system. With primary pulmonary hypertension (Chap. 260) or with pulmonary vascular disease secondary to scleroderma, the small pulmonary arteries and arterioles are affected by a generalized obliterative process that narrows and occludes these vessels. Pulmonary vascular resistance increases, and significant pulmonary hypertension often results.

DISTURBANCES IN GAS EXCHANGE

PHYSIOLOGIC FEATURES The primary functions of the respiratory system are to remove the appropriate amount of CO_2 from blood entering the pulmonary circulation and to provide adequate O_2 to blood leaving the pulmonary circulation. For these functions to be carried out properly, there must be adequate provision of fresh air to the alveoli for delivery of O_2 and removal of CO_2 (ventilation), adequate circulation of blood through the pulmonary vasculature (perfusion), adequate movement of gas between alveoli and pulmonary capillaries (diffusion), and appropriate contact between alveolar gas and pulmonary capillary blood (ventilation-perfusion matching).

A normal individual at rest inspires approximately 12 to 16 times per minute, each breath having a tidal volume of approximately 500 mL. A portion (approximately 30 percent) of the fresh air inspired with each breath does not reach the alveoli but remains in the conducting airways of the lung. This component of each breath, which is not generally available for gas exchange, is called the *anatomic dead space component*. The remaining 70 percent reaches the alveolar zone, mixes rapidly with the gas already there, and can participate in gas exchange. In this example, the total ventilation each minute is approximately 7 L, composed of 2 L/min of dead space ventilation and 5 L/min of alveolar ventilation. In certain diseases, some alveoli are ventilated but not perfused, so that some ventilation in addition to the anatomic dead space component is wasted. If total dead space ventilation is increased but total minute ventilation is unchanged, then alveolar ventilation must fall correspondingly.

Gas exchange is dependent on alveolar ventilation rather than total minute ventilation, as outlined below. The partial pressure of CO_2 in arterial blood (Pa_{CO_2}) is directly proportional to the amount of CO_2 produced per minute ($\dot{V}_{CO_2}$) and inversely proportional to alveolar ventilation ($\dot{V}_A$), according to the relationship

$$Pa_{CO_2} = 0.863 \times \dot{V}_{CO_2}/\dot{V}_A$$

where $\dot{V}_{CO_2}$ is expressed in mL/min, $\dot{V}_A$ in L/min, and Pa_{CO_2} in mmHg. At fixed $\dot{V}_{CO_2}$, when alveolar ventilation increases, Pa_{CO_2} falls, and when alveolar ventilation decreases, Pa_{CO_2} rises. Maintaining a normal level of O_2 in the alveoli (and consequently in arterial blood) also depends on provision of adequate alveolar ventilation to replenish alveolar O_2. This principle will become more apparent from consideration of the alveolar gas equation below.

Diffusion of O_2 and CO_2   Both O_2 and CO_2 diffuse readily down their respective concentration gradients through the alveolar wall and pulmonary capillary endothelium. Under normal circumstances, this process is rapid, and equilibration of both gases is complete within one-third of the transit time of erythrocytes through the pulmonary capillary bed. Even in disease states in which diffusion of gases is impaired, the impairment is unlikely to be severe enough to prevent equilibration of CO_2 and O_2. Consequently, a diffusion abnormality rarely results in arterial hypoxemia at rest. If erythrocyte transit time in the pulmonary circulation is shortened, as occurs with exercise, and diffusion is impaired, then diffusion limitation may contribute to hypoxemia. Exercise testing can often demonstrate such physiologically significant abnormalities due to impaired diffusion. Even though diffusion limitation rarely makes a clinically significant contribution to resting hypoxemia, clinical measurements of what is known as *diffusing capacity* (see below) can be a useful measure of the integrity of the alveolar-capillary membrane.

Ventilation-Perfusion Matching   In addition to the absolute levels of alveolar ventilation and perfusion, gas exchange depends critically on the proper matching of ventilation and perfusion. The spectrum of possible ventilation-perfusion ($\dot{V}/\dot{Q}$) ratios in an alveolar-capillary unit ranges from zero, in which ventilation is totally absent and the unit behaves as a shunt, to infinity, in which perfusion is totally absent and the unit behaves as dead space. The P_{O_2} and P_{CO_2} of blood leaving each alveolar-capillary unit depend on the gas tension (of blood and air) entering that unit and on the particular $\dot{V}/\dot{Q}$ ratio of the unit. At one extreme, when an alveolar-capillary unit has a $\dot{V}/\dot{Q}$ ratio of 0 and behaves as a shunt, blood leaving the unit has the composition of mixed venous blood entering the pulmonary capillaries, i.e., $P\bar{v}_{O_2} \approx$ 40 mmHg and $P\bar{v}_{CO_2} \approx$ 46 mmHg. At the other extreme, when an alveolar-capillary unit has a high $\dot{V}/\dot{Q}$ ratio, it behaves almost like dead space, and the small amount of blood leaving the unit has partial pressures of O_2 and CO_2 ($P_{O_2} \approx$ 150 mmHg, $P_{CO_2} \approx$ 0 mmHg while breathing room air) approaching the composition of inspired gas.

In the ideal situation, all alveolar-capillary units have equal matching of ventilation and perfusion, i.e., a ratio of approximately 1 when each is expressed in L/min. However, even in the normal individual, some $\dot{V}/\dot{Q}$ mismatching is present, since there is normally a gradient of blood flow from the apices to the bases of the lungs. There is a similar gradient of ventilation from the apices to the bases, but it is less marked than the perfusion gradient. As a result, ventilation-perfu-

sion ratios are higher at the lung apices than at the lung bases. Therefore, blood coming from the apices has a higher P_{O_2} and lower P_{CO_2} than blood coming from the bases. The net P_{O_2} and P_{CO_2} of the blood mixture coming from all areas of the lung is a flow-weighted average of the individual components, which reflects both the relative amount of blood from each unit and the O_2 and CO_2 *content* of the blood coming from each unit. Because of the sigmoid shape of the oxyhemoglobin dissociation curve (see Fig. 107-1), it is important to distinguish between the partial pressure and the content of O_2 in blood. Hemoglobin is almost fully saturated at a P_{O_2} of 60 mmHg, and little additional O_2 is carried by hemoglobin even with a substantial elevation of P_{O_2} above 60 mmHg. On the other hand, significant O_2 desaturation of hemoglobin occurs once P_{O_2} falls below 60 mmHg and onto the steep descending limb of the curve. As a result, blood coming from regions of the lung with a high $\dot{V}/\dot{Q}$ ratio and a high P_{O_2} has only a small elevation in O_2 content and cannot compensate for blood coming from regions with a low $\dot{V}/\dot{Q}$ ratio and a low P_{O_2}, which has a significantly decreased O_2 content. Although $\dot{V}/\dot{Q}$ mismatching can influence P_{CO_2}, this effect is less marked and often is overcome by an increase in overall minute ventilation.

MEASUREMENT OF GAS EXCHANGE   Arterial Blood Gases   The most commonly used measures of gas exchange are the partial pressures of O_2 and CO_2 in arterial blood, i.e., Pa_{O_2} and Pa_{CO_2}, respectively. These partial pressures do not measure directly the quantity of O_2 and CO_2 in blood but rather the driving pressure for the gas in blood. The actual quantity or content of a gas in blood also depends on the solubility of the gas in plasma and the ability of any component of blood to react with or bind the gas of interest. Since hemoglobin is capable of binding large amounts of O_2, oxygenated hemoglobin is the primary form in which O_2 is transported in blood. The actual content of O_2 in blood therefore depends both on the hemoglobin concentration and on the Pa_{O_2}. The Pa_{O_2} determines what percentage of hemoglobin is saturated with O_2, based on the position on the oxyhemoglobin dissociation curve. Oxygen content in normal blood (at 37°C, pH 7.4) can be determined by adding the amount of O_2 dissolved in plasma to the amount bound to hemoglobin, according to the equation

$$O_2 \text{ content} = 1.34 \times [\text{hemoglobin}] \times \text{saturation} + 0.0031 \times P_{O_2}$$

since each gram of hemoglobin is capable of carrying 1.34 mL O_2 when fully saturated, and the amount of O_2 that can be dissolved in plasma is proportional to the P_{O_2}, with 0.0031 mL O_2 dissolved per deciliter of blood per mmHg P_{O_2}. In arterial blood, the amount of O_2 transported dissolved in plasma (approximately 0.3 mL O_2 per deciliter of blood) is trivial compared with the amount bound to hemoglobin (approximately 20 mL O_2 per deciliter of blood).

Most commonly, P_{O_2} is the measurement used to quantitate the adequacy of oxygenation of arterial blood. Direct measurement of O_2 saturation in arterial blood by oximetry is also important in selected clinical conditions. For example, in patients with carbon monoxide exposure, carbon monoxide preferentially displaces O_2 from hemoglobin, essentially making a portion of hemoglobin unavailable for binding to O_2. In this circumstance, carbon monoxide saturation is high and O_2 saturation is low, even though the driving pressure for O_2 to bind to hemoglobin, reflected by P_{O_2}, is normal. Measurement of O_2 saturation is also important for the determination of O_2 content when mixed venous blood is sampled from a pulmonary arterial catheter to calculate cardiac output by the Fick technique. In mixed venous blood, the P_{O_2} is normally about 40 mmHg, but small changes in P_{O_2} may reflect relatively large changes in O_2 saturation.

A useful calculation in the assessment of oxygenation is the alveolar-arterial O_2 difference ($PA_{O_2} - Pa_{O_2}$), commonly called the *alveolar-arterial O_2 gradient* (or A − a gradient). This calculation takes into account the fact that alveolar and, hence, arterial P_{O_2} can be expected to change depending on the level of alveolar ventilation, reflected by the arterial P_{CO_2}. When a patient hyperventilates and has a low P_{CO_2} in arterial blood and alveolar gas, alveolar and arterial P_{O_2} will rise; conversely, hypoventilation and a high P_{CO_2} are accompanied by a decrease in alveolar and arterial P_{O_2}. These changes in arterial P_{O_2} are independent of abnormalities in O_2 transfer at the alveolar-capillary level and reflect only the dependence of alveolar P_{O_2} on the level of alveolar ventilation.

In order to determine the alveolar-arterial O_2 difference, the alveolar P_{O_2} (PA_{O_2}) must first be calculated. The equation most commonly used for this purpose, a simplified form of the alveolar gas equation, is

$$PA_{O_2} = FI_{O_2} \times (P_B - P_{H_2O}) - Pa_{CO_2}/R$$

where FI_{O_2} = fractional concentration of inspired O_2 (≈ 0.21 when breathing room air); P_B = barometric pressure (approximately 760 mmHg at sea level); P_{H_2O} = water vapor pressure (47 mmHg when air is fully saturated at 37°C); and R = respiratory quotient (the ratio of CO_2 production to O_2 consumption, usually assumed to be 0.8). If the preceding values are substituted into the equation for the patient breathing air at sea level, the equation becomes

$$PA_{O_2} = 150 - 1.25 \times Pa_{CO_2}$$

The alveolar-arterial O_2 difference can then be calculated by subtracting measured Pa_{O_2} from calculated PA_{O_2}. In a healthy young person breathing room air, the $PA_{O_2} - Pa_{O_2}$ is normally less than 15 mmHg; this value increases with age and may be as high as 30 mmHg in elderly patients.

The adequacy of CO_2 elimination is measured by the partial pressure of CO_2 in arterial blood, i.e., Pa_{CO_2}. A more complete understanding of the mechanisms and chronicity of abnormal levels of P_{CO_2} also requires measurement of pH and/or bicarbonate (HCO_3^-), since P_{CO_2} and the patient's acid-base status are so closely intertwined (see Chap. 50).

Pulse Oximetry Because measurement of Pa_{O_2} requires arterial puncture and provides intermittent rather than continuous data about the patient's oxygenation, it is not ideal for close monitoring of unstable patients. Over the past several years, an alternative method for assessing oxygenation, pulse oximetry, has become readily available in many clinical settings. The pulse oximeter measures oxygen saturation (rather than Pa_{O_2}) using a probe usually clipped over a patient's finger. The device measures absorption of two wavelengths of light by hemoglobin in pulsatile, cutaneous arterial blood. Because of differential absorption of the two wavelengths of light by oxygenated and nonoxygenated hemoglobin, the percentage of hemoglobin that is saturated with oxygen, i.e., the Sa_{O_2}, can be calculated and displayed instantaneously.

Although the pulse oximeter has been a major advance in the noninvasive, continuous monitoring of oxygenation, there are several issues and potential problems concerning its use. First, the clinician must be aware of the relationship between oxygen saturation and tension as shown by the oxyhemoglobin dissociation curve (see Fig. 107–1). Because the curve becomes relatively flat above an arterial P_{O_2} of 60 mmHg (corresponding to Sa_{O_2} = 90 percent), the oximeter is relatively insensitive to changes in Pa_{O_2} above this level. In addition, the position of the curve and therefore the specific relationship between Pa_{O_2} and Sa_{O_2} may change depending on factors such as temperature, pH, and the erythrocyte concentration of 2,3-diphosphoglycerate (2,3-DPG). Second, when cutaneous perfusion is decreased, for example owing to low cardiac output or the use of vasoconstrictors, the signal from the oximeter may be less reliable or even unobtainable. Third, other forms of hemoglobin, such as carboxyhemoglobin and methemoglobin, are not distinguishable when only two wavelengths of light are used. The Sa_{O_2} values reported by the pulse oximeter are not reliable in the presence of significant amounts of either of these forms of hemoglobin. In contrast, the device used to measure oxygen saturation in samples of arterial blood, called the CO-oximeter, uses at least four wavelengths of light and is capable of distinguishing oxyhemoglobin, deoxygenated hemoglobin, carboxyhemoglobin, and methemoglobin. Finally, the clinician must remember that the often-used goal of $Sa_{O_2} \geq 90$ percent does not indicate anything about CO_2 elimination and therefore does not ensure a clinically acceptable P_{CO_2}.

Diffusing Capacity The ability of gas to diffuse across the alveolar-capillary membrane is ordinarily assessed by the diffusing capacity of the lung for carbon monoxide (DL_{CO}). In this test, a small concentra-

tion of carbon monoxide (0.3%) is inhaled, usually in a single breath that is held for approximately 10 s. The carbon monoxide is diluted by the gas already present in the alveoli and is also taken up by hemoglobin as the erythrocytes course through the pulmonary capillary system. The concentration of carbon monoxide in exhaled gas is measured, and DL_{CO} is calculated as the quantity of carbon monoxide absorbed per minute per mmHg pressure gradient from the alveoli to the pulmonary capillaries. The value obtained for DL_{CO} depends on the alveolar-capillary surface area available for gas exchange and on the pulmonary capillary blood volume. In addition, the thickness of the alveolar-capillary membrane, the degree of $\dot{V}/\dot{Q}$ mismatching, and the patient's hemoglobin level will affect the measurement. Because of this effect of hemoglobin levels on DL_{CO}, the measured DL_{CO} is frequently corrected to take the patient's hemoglobin level into account. The value for DL_{CO}, ideally corrected for hemoglobin, can then be compared with a predicted value, based either on age, height, and gender or on the alveolar volume (V_A) at which the value was obtained. Alternatively, the DL_{CO} can be divided by V_A and the resulting value for DL_{CO}/V_A compared with a predicted value.

Approach to the Patient

Arterial Blood Gases Hypoxemia is a common manifestation of a variety of diseases affecting the lungs or other parts of the respiratory system. The broad clinical problem of hypoxemia is often best characterized according to the underlying mechanism. The four basic mechanisms of hypoxemia are (1) a decrease in inspired P_{O_2}, (2) hypoventilation, (3) shunting, and (4) $\dot{V}/\dot{Q}$ mismatching. Hypoxemia due to decreased diffusion occurs only under selected clinical circumstances and is not usually included among the general categories of hypoxemia. Determining the underlying mechanism for hypoxemia depends on measurement of the Pa_{CO_2}, calculation of $PA_{O_2} - Pa_{O_2}$, and knowledge of the response to supplemental O_2. A flowchart summarizing the approach to the hypoxemic patient is given in Fig. 250-5.

A decrease in the inspired P_{O_2} and hypoventilation both cause hypoxemia by lowering PA_{O_2} and therefore Pa_{O_2}. In each case, gas exchange at the alveolar-capillary level occurs normally, and $PA_{O_2} - Pa_{O_2}$ is not elevated. Hypoxemia due to decreased inspired P_{O_2} can be diagnosed from knowledge of the clinical situation. Inspired P_{O_2} is lowered either because the patient is at a high altitude, where barometric pressure is low, or, much less commonly, because the patient is breathing a gas mixture containing less than 21% O_2. The hallmark of hypoventilation as a cause of hypoxemia is an elevation in Pa_{CO_2}. This is associated with an increase in PA_{CO_2} and a fall in PA_{O_2}. When hypoxemia is due purely to a low inspired P_{O_2} or to alveolar hypoventilation, $PA_{O_2} - Pa_{O_2}$ is normal. If $PA_{O_2} - Pa_{O_2}$ and Pa_{CO_2} are both elevated, then an additional mechanism, such as $\dot{V}/\dot{Q}$ mismatching or shunting, is contributing to hypoxemia.

Shunting is a cause of hypoxemia when desaturated blood effectively bypasses oxygenation at the alveolar-capillary level. This situation occurs either because a structural problem allows desaturated blood to bypass the normal site of gas exchange or because perfused alveoli are not ventilated. Shunting is associated with an elevation in the $PA_{O_2} - Pa_{O_2}$ value. When shunting is an important contributing factor to hypoxemia, the lowered Pa_{O_2} is relatively refractory to improvement by supplemental O_2.

Finally, the largest clinical category of hypoxemia is $\dot{V}/\dot{Q}$ mismatching. With $\dot{V}/\dot{Q}$ mismatching, regions with low $\dot{V}/\dot{Q}$ ratios contribute blood with a low P_{O_2} and a low O_2 content. Corresponding regions with high $\dot{V}/\dot{Q}$ ratios contribute blood with a high P_{O_2}. However, because blood is already almost fully saturated at a normal P_{O_2}, elevation of the P_{O_2} to a high value does not significantly increase O_2 saturation or content and therefore cannot compensate for the reduction of O_2 saturation and content in blood coming from regions with a low $\dot{V}/\dot{Q}$ ratio. When $\dot{V}/\dot{Q}$ mismatch is the primary cause of hypoxemia, $PA_{O_2} - Pa_{O_2}$ is elevated, and P_{CO_2} generally is normal. Supplemental O_2 corrects the hypoxemia by raising the P_{O_2} in blood coming from regions with a low $\dot{V}/\dot{Q}$ ratio; this response distinguishes hypoxemia due to $\dot{V}/\dot{Q}$ mismatching from that due to true shunt.

The essential mechanism underlying all cases of hypercapnia is alveolar ventilation that is inadequate for the amount of CO_2 produced. It is conceptually useful to characterize CO_2 retention further, based on a more detailed examination of the potential contributing factors. These include (1) increased CO_2 production, (2) decreased ventilatory drive ("won't breathe"), (3) malfunction of the respiratory pump or increased airways resistance, which makes it more difficult to sustain adequate ventilation ("can't breathe"), and (4) inefficiency of gas exchange (increased dead space or $\dot{V}/\dot{Q}$ mismatch) necessitating a compensatory increase in overall minute ventilation. In practice, more than one of these mechanisms is commonly responsible for hypercapnia, since increased minute ventilation is capable of compensating for increased CO_2 production and for inefficiencies of gas exchange.

Diffusing Capacity Although abnormalities in diffusion are rarely responsible for hypoxemia, clinical measurement of diffusing capacity is frequently used to assess the functional integrity of the alveolar-capillary membrane, which includes the pulmonary capillary bed. Diseases that affect solely the airways generally do not lower DL_{CO}, whereas diseases that affect the alveolar walls or the pulmonary capillary bed will have an effect on DL_{CO}. Even though DL_{CO} is a useful marker for assessing whether disease affecting the alveolar-capillary bed is present, an abnormal DL_{CO} does not necessarily imply that diffusion limitation is responsible for hypoxemia in a particular patient.

CLINICAL CORRELATIONS Useful clinical correlations can be made with the mechanisms underlying hypoxemia (see Fig. 250-5). A lowered inspired P_{O_2} contributes to hypoxemia if either the patient is at high altitude or if the concentration of inspired O_2 is less than 21%. The latter problem occurs if a patient receiving anesthesia or ventilatory support is inadvertently given a gas mixture to breathe containing less than 21% O_2 or if O_2 is consumed from the ambient gas, as can occur during smoke inhalation from a fire. The primary feature of hypoventilation as a cause of hypoxemia is an elevation in arterial P_{CO_2}. The clinical correlations with hypoventilation are discussed in Chap. 263.

Shunting as a cause of hypoxemia can reflect transfer of blood from the right to the left side of the heart without passage through the pulmonary circulation, as occurs with an intracardiac shunt. This problem is most common in the setting of cyanotic congenital heart disease, when an interatrial or interventricular septal defect is associated with pulmonary hypertension so that shunting is in the right-to-left rather than the left-to-right direction. Shunting of blood through the pulmonary parenchyma is most frequently due to disease causing absence of ventilation to perfused alveoli. This can occur if the alveoli are atelectatic or if they are filled with fluid, as in pulmonary edema (both cardiogenic and noncardiogenic) or with extensive intraalveolar exudation of fluid due to pneumonia. Less commonly, vascular anomalies with arteriovenous shunting in the lung can cause hypoxemia. These anomalies can be hereditary, as found with hereditary hemorrhagic telangiectasia (Osler-Rendu-Weber syndrome), or acquired, as in pulmonary vascular malformations secondary to hepatic cirrhosis, which are similar to the commonly recognized cutaneous vascular malformations ("spider hemangiomas").

Ventilation-perfusion mismatch is the most common cause of hypoxemia clinically. Most of the processes affecting either the airways or the pulmonary parenchyma are distributed unevenly throughout the lungs and do not necessarily affect ventilation and perfusion equally. Some areas of lung may have good perfusion and poor ventilation, whereas others may have poor perfusion and relatively good ventilation. Important examples of airways diseases in which $\dot{V}/\dot{Q}$ mismatch causes hypoxemia are asthma and chronic obstructive lung disease. Parenchymal lung diseases causing $\dot{V}/\dot{Q}$ mismatch and hypoxemia include interstitial lung disease and pneumonia.

Clinically important alterations in CO_2 elimination range from excessive ventilation and hypocapnia to inadequate CO_2 elimination and hypercapnia. These clinical problems are discussed in Chap. 263.

Diffusing Capacity Measurement of DL_{CO} may be useful for assessing disease affecting the alveolar-capillary bed or the pulmonary vasculature. In practice, three main categories of disease are associated with lowered DL_{CO}: interstitial lung disease, emphysema, and pulmonary vascular disease. With interstitial lung disease, scarring of alveolar-capillary units diminishes the area of the alveolar-capillary bed as well as pulmonary blood volume. With emphysema, alveolar walls are destroyed, so the surface area of the alveolar-capillary bed is again diminished. In patients with disease causing a decrease in the cross-sectional area and volume of the pulmonary vascular bed, such as

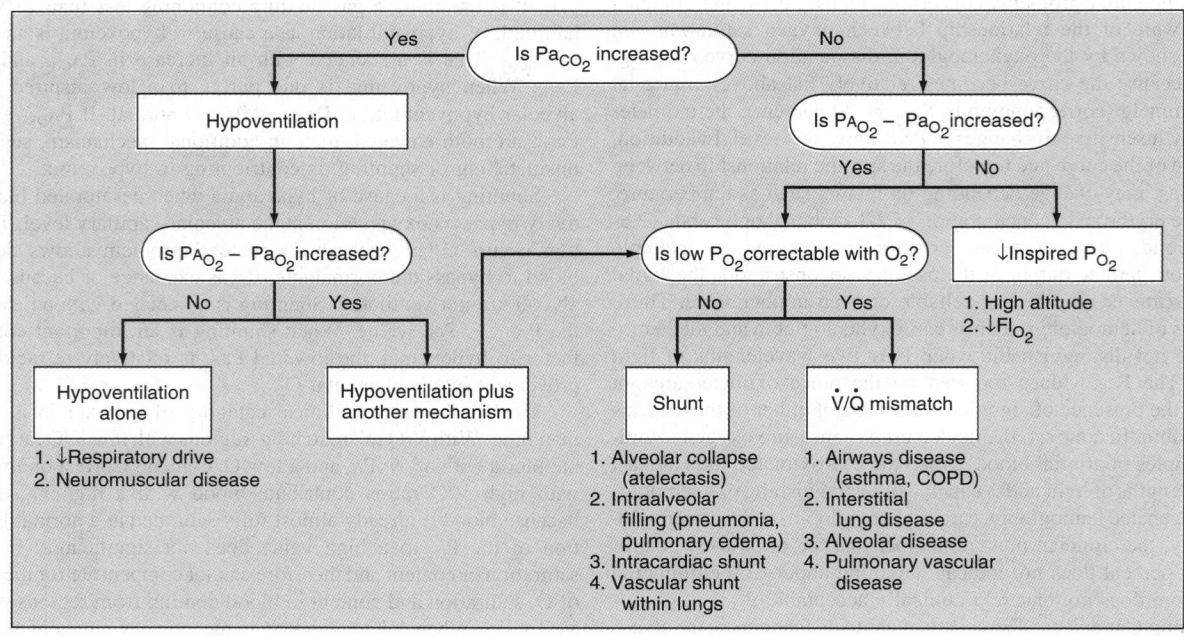

FIGURE 250-5 Flow diagram outlining the diagnostic approach to the patient with hypoxemia ($Pa_{O_2} < 80$ mmHg). $PA_{O_2} - Pa_{O_2}$ is usually < 15 mmHg for subjects ≤ 30 years old and increases by ~3 mmHg per decade after age 30.

recurrent pulmonary emboli or primary pulmonary hypertension, $D_{L_{CO}}$ is commonly diminished.

Diffusing capacity may be elevated if pulmonary blood volume is increased, as may be seen in congestive heart failure. However, once interstitial and alveolar edema ensue, the net $D_{L_{CO}}$ depends on the opposing influences of increased pulmonary capillary blood volume elevating $D_{L_{CO}}$ and pulmonary edema decreasing it. Finding an elevated $D_{L_{CO}}$ may be useful in the diagnosis of alveolar hemorrhage, as in Goodpasture's syndrome. Hemoglobin contained in erythrocytes in the alveolar lumen is capable of binding carbon monoxide, so the exhaled carbon monoxide concentration is diminished and the measured $D_{L_{CO}}$ is increased.

BIBLIOGRAPHY

AMERICAN THORACIC SOCIETY: Lung function testing: Selection of reference values and interpretative strategies. Am Rev Respir Dis 144:1202, 1991

CLARK JS et al: Noninvasive assessment of blood gases. Am Rev Respir Dis 145:220, 1992

CRAPO RO: Pulmonary-function testing. N Engl J Med 331:25, 1994

———, FORSTER RE II: Carbon monoxide diffusing capacity. Clin Chest Med 10:187, 1989

GIBSON GJ: Standardised lung function testing. Eur Respir J 6:155, 1993

QUANJER PH et al: Lung volumes and forced ventilatory flows. Report Working Party Standardization of Lung Function Tests, European Community for Steel and Coal. Official Statement of the European Respiratory Society. Eur Respir J [Suppl] 16:5, 1993

SOCIETY OF CRITICAL CARE MEDICINE: A model for technology assessment applied to pulse oximetry. Crit Care Med 21:615, 1993

WEINBERGER SE: *Principles of Pulmonary Medicine*, 2d ed. Philadelphia, Saunders, 1992

WEST JB: *Respiratory Physiology: The Essentials*, 5th ed. Baltimore, Williams & Wilkins, 1995

251 *Steven E. Weinberger, Jeffrey M. Drazen*

DIAGNOSTIC PROCEDURES IN RESPIRATORY DISEASE

The diagnostic modalities available for assessing the patient with suspected or known respiratory system disease include imaging studies and techniques for acquiring biologic specimens, some of which involve direct visualization of part of the respiratory system. Methods used to characterize the functional changes developing as a result of disease, including pulmonary function tests and measurements of gas exchange, are discussed in Chap. 250.

IMAGING STUDIES

ROUTINE RADIOGRAPHY Routine chest radiography, which generally includes both posteroanterior and lateral views, is an integral part of the diagnostic evaluation of diseases involving the pulmonary parenchyma, the pleura, and, to a lesser extent, the airways and the mediastinum. Common radiographic patterns and their clinical correlates are reviewed in Chap. 249. Lateral decubitus views are often useful for determining whether pleural abnormalities represent freely flowing fluid, whereas apical lordotic views can often visualize disease at the lung apices better than the standard posteroanterior view. Portable equipment, which is often used for acutely ill patients who either cannot be transported to a radiology suite or cannot stand up for posteroanterior and lateral views, generally yields just a single radiograph taken in the anteroposterior direction.

COMPUTED TOMOGRAPHY Computed tomography (CT) offers several advantages over routine chest radiography. First, the use of cross-sectional images often makes it possible to distinguish between densities that would be superimposed on plain radiographs. Second, CT is far better than routine radiographic studies at characterizing tissue density, distinguishing subtle differences in density between adjacent structures, and providing accurate size assessment of

lesions. As a result, CT is particularly valuable in assessing hilar and mediastinal disease (which is often poorly characterized by plain radiography), in identifying and characterizing disease adjacent to the chest wall or spine (including pleural disease), and in identifying areas of fat density or calcification in pulmonary nodules (Fig. 251-1). Its utility in the assessment of mediastinal disease has made CT an important tool in the staging of lung cancer (see Chap. 90), as an assessment of tumor involvement of mediastinal lymph nodes is critical to proper staging. With the additional use of contrast material, CT also makes it possible to distinguish vascular from nonvascular structures, particularly important in distinguishing lymph nodes and masses from vascular structures.

Helical CT scanning allows the collection of continuous data over a larger volume of lung during a single breath-holding maneuver than is possible with conventional CT. With high-resolution CT (HRCT), the thickness of individual cross-sectional images is approximately 1 to 2 mm, rather than the usual 10 mm, and the images are reconstructed using high-spatial-resolution algorithms. The detail that can be seen on HRCT scans allows better recognition of subtle parenchymal and airway disease, such as bronchiectasis, emphysema, and diffuse parenchymal disease (Fig. 251-2). Certain nearly pathognomonic patterns have now been recognized for many of the interstitial lung diseases, such as lymphangitic carcinoma, idiopathic pulmonary fibrosis, sarcoidosis, and eosinophilic granuloma; at present it is not yet clear in what settings these patterns will obviate the need for obtaining lung tissue.

MAGNETIC RESONANCE IMAGING The role of magnetic resonance imaging (MRI) in the evaluation of respiratory system disease is less well defined than that of CT. Because MRI generally provides a less detailed view of the pulmonary parenchyma as well as poorer spatial resolution, its usefulness in the evaluation of parenchymal lung disease is limited at present. However, MRI has advantages over CT in certain clinical settings. Because its images can be reconstructed in sagittal and coronal as well as transverse planes, MRI may be better for imaging abnormalities near the lung apex, the spine, and the thoracoabdominal junction. In addition, vascular structures can be distinguished from nonvascular structures without the need for contrast. Flowing blood does not produce a signal on MRI, so vessels appear as hollow tubular structures. This feature can be useful in determining whether abnormal hilar or mediastinal densities are vascular in origin and in defining aortic lesions such as aneurysms or dissection.

SCINTIGRAPHIC IMAGING Radioactive isotopes, administered by either intravenous or inhaled routes, allow the lungs to be imaged with a gamma camera. The most common use of such imaging is ventilation-perfusion lung scanning performed for evaluation of

FIGURE 251-1 CT scan demonstrating a mediastinal mass of heterogenous density. CT is superior to plain radiography for the detection of abnormal mediastinal densities and the distinction of masses from adjacent vascular structures.

FIGURE 251-2 High-resolution CT scan demonstrating pulmonary parenchyma with a heterogeneous appearance. Most of the parenchyma has a subtle "ground-glass" pattern of increased density, best recognized by comparison with the intervening areas of normal lung, which have irregular but well-defined borders. The ground-glass pattern in this patient was due to hypersensitivity pneumonitis.

pulmonary embolism. When injected intravenously, albumin macroaggregates labeled with technetium 99m become lodged in pulmonary capillaries; therefore, the distribution of the trapped radioisotope follows the distribution of blood flow. When inhaled, radiolabeled xenon gas can be used to demonstrate the distribution of ventilation. For example, pulmonary thromboembolism usually produces one or more regions of ventilation-perfusion mismatch—that is, regions in which there is a defect in perfusion that follows the distribution of a vessel and that is not accompanied by a corresponding defect in ventilation (see Chap. 261). Another common use of such radioisotope scans is in a patient with impaired lung function who is being considered for lung resection. The distribution of the isotope(s) can be used to assess the regional distribution of blood flow and ventilation, allowing the physician to estimate the level of postoperative lung function.

Another scintigraphic imaging technique, gallium imaging, has been of diagnostic value in patients with *Pneumocystis carinii* pneumonia and other opportunistic infections. Use of gallium imaging may provide clues to sort out the differential diagnosis of pulmonary infiltrates in immunosuppressed patients, especially patients with AIDS.

PULMONARY ANGIOGRAPHY The pulmonary arterial system can be visualized by pulmonary angiography, in which radiopaque contrast medium is injected through a catheter previously threaded into the pulmonary artery. When performed in cases of pulmonary embolism, pulmonary angiography demonstrates the consequences of an intravascular clot—either a defect in the lumen of a vessel (a "filling defect") or an abrupt termination ("cutoff") of the vessel. Other, less common indications for pulmonary angiography include visualization of a suspected pulmonary arteriovenous malformation and assessment of pulmonary arterial invasion by a neoplasm.

ULTRASOUND Because ultrasound energy is rapidly dissipated in air, ultrasound imaging is not useful for evaluation of the pulmonary parenchyma. However, it is helpful in the detection and localization of pleural liquid and is often used as a guide to placement of a needle for sampling of the liquid (i.e., for thoracentesis).

TECHNIQUES FOR OBTAINING BIOLOGIC SPECIMENS

COLLECTION OF SPUTUM Sputum can be collected either by spontaneous expectoration or after inhalation of an irritating aerosol, such as hypertonic saline. The latter method, called *sputum induction*,

is used routinely to obtain sputum for diagnostic studies. Knowledge of the appearance and quality of the sputum specimen obtained is especially important when one is interested in Gram's staining and culture. Because sputum consists mainly of secretions from the tracheobronchial tree rather than the upper airway, the finding of alveolar macrophages and other inflammatory cells is consistent with a lower respiratory tract origin of the sample, whereas the presence of squamous epithelial cells in a "sputum" sample indicates contamination by secretions from the upper airways.

Besides processing for routine bacterial pathogens by Gram's staining and culture, sputum can be processed for a variety of other pathogens, including staining and culture for mycobacteria or fungi, culture for viruses, and staining for *P. carinii*. In the specific case of sputum obtained for evaluation of *P. carinii* pneumonia in a patient infected with human immunodeficiency virus (HIV), for example, sputum should be collected by induction, rather than spontaneous expectoration, and an immunofluorescent stain should be used to detect the organisms. Cytologic staining of sputum for malignant cells, using the traditional Papanicolaou method, allows noninvasive evaluation for suspected lung cancer. Traditional stains and cultures are now also being supplemented in some cases by immunologic techniques and by molecular biologic methods, including the use of polymerase chain reaction amplification and DNA probes.

PERCUTANEOUS NEEDLE ASPIRATION A needle can be inserted through the chest wall into a pulmonary lesion for the purpose of aspirating material for analysis by cytologic or microbiologic techniques. The procedure is usually carried out under CT guidance, which assists in the positioning of the needle and assures that it is localized in the lesion. Although the potential risks of this procedure include intrapulmonary bleeding and creation of a pneumothorax with collapse of the underlying lung, the low risk of complication in experienced hands is usually worth the information obtained.

THORACENTESIS Sampling of pleural liquid by thoracentesis is commonly performed for diagnostic purposes or, in the case of a large effusion, for palliation of dyspnea. Diagnostic sampling, either by blind needle aspiration or after localization by ultrasound, allows the collection of liquid for microbiologic and cytologic studies. Analysis of the fluid obtained for its cellular composition and chemical constituents, including glucose, protein, and lactate dehydrogenase, allows the effusion to be classified as either exudative or transudative (Chap. 262). In some cases, particularly in the setting of possible tuberculous involvement of the pleura (tuberculous pleuritis), closed biopsy of the parietal pleura is also performed, using a cutting needle (either an Abrams or a Cope biopsy needle) to sample tissue for histopathologic examination and culture.

BRONCHOSCOPY Bronchoscopy is the process of direct visualization of the tracheobronchial tree. Bronchoscopy with a rigid bronchoscope is generally performed in an operating room on a patient under general anesthesia. The development of a flexible fiberoptic bronchoscope has revolutionized the diagnostic use of bronchoscopy. Although bronchoscopy is now performed almost exclusively with fiberoptic instruments, rigid bronchoscopes still have a role in selected circumstances, primarily because of their larger suction channel and the fact that the patient can be ventilated through the bronchoscope channel. These situations include the retrieval of a foreign body and the suctioning of a massive hemorrhage, for which the small suction channel of the bronchoscope may be insufficient.

Flexible Fiberoptic Bronchoscopy This is an outpatient procedure that is usually performed in an awake though sedated patient. The bronchoscope is passed through either the mouth or the nose, between the vocal cords, and into the trachea. The ability to flex the scope makes it possible to visualize virtually all airways to the level of subsegmental bronchi. The bronchoscopist is able to identify endobronchial pathology, including tumors, granulomas, bronchitis, foreign bodies, and sites of bleeding. Samples from airway lesions can be taken by several methods, including washing, brushing, and biopsy. Washing involves instillation of sterile saline through a channel of the bronchoscope and onto the surface of a lesion. A portion of the liquid is collected by suctioning through the bronchoscope, and the recovered material can be analyzed for cells (cytology) or organisms (by standard stains and cultures). Brushing or biopsy of the surface of the lesion, using a small brush or biopsy forceps at the end of a long cable inserted through a channel of the bronchoscope, allows recovery of cellular material or tissue for analysis by standard cytologic and histopathologic methods. The bronchoscope may provide the opportunity for treatment as well as diagnosis. For example, an aspirated foreign body may be retrieved with an instrument passed through the scope, and bleeding may be controlled with a balloon catheter similarly introduced.

The bronchoscope can be used to sample material not only from the regions that can be directly visualized (i.e., the airways) but also from the more distal pulmonary parenchyma. With the bronchoscope wedged into a subsegmental airway, aliquots of sterile saline can be instilled through the scope, allowing sampling of cells and organisms even from alveolar spaces. This procedure, called *bronchoalveolar lavage*, has been particularly useful for the recovery of organisms such as *P. carinii* in patients with HIV infection.

Brushing and biopsy of the distal lung parenchyma can also be performed using the same instruments that are used for endobronchial sampling. These instruments can be passed through the scope into small airways, where they penetrate the airway wall, allowing biopsy of peribronchial alveolar tissue. This procedure, called *transbronchial biopsy*, is used when there is either relatively diffuse disease or a localized lesion of adequate size. With the aid of fluoroscopic imaging, the bronchoscopist is able to determine not only whether and when the instrument is in the area of abnormality, but also the proximity of the instrument to the pleural surface. If the forceps are too close to the pleural surface, there is a risk of violating the visceral pleura and creating a pneumothorax; the other potential complication of transbronchial biopsy is pulmonary hemorrhage. The incidence of these complications is less than several percent.

A relatively new procedure involves use of a hollow-bore needle passed through the bronchoscope for sampling of tissue adjacent to the trachea or a large bronchus. The needle is passed through the airway wall, and cellular material can be aspirated from mass lesions or enlarged lymph nodes, generally in a search for malignant cells. This procedure can facilitate the staging of lung cancer by identifying mediastinal lymph node involvement and in some cases obviates the need for a more invasive procedure.

VIDEO-ASSISTED THORACIC SURGERY Recent advances in video technology have allowed the development of thoracoscopy, or video-assisted thoracic surgery (VATS), for the diagnosis and management of pleural as well as parenchymal lung disease. This procedure, done under general anesthesia, involves the passage of a rigid scope with a distal lens through a trocar inserted into the pleura. A high-quality image is shown on a monitor screen, allowing the operator to manipulate instruments passed into the pleural space through separate small intercostal incisions. With these instruments, the operator can biopsy lesions of the pleura under direct vision, which provides an obvious advantage over closed pleural biopsy. In addition, this procedure is now used commonly to biopsy peripheral lung tissue

or to remove peripheral nodules, for both diagnostic and therapeutic purposes. Because this procedure is much less invasive than the traditional thoracotomy performed for lung biopsy, it has largely supplanted "open lung biopsy."

THORACOTOMY Although frequently replaced by VATS, thoracotomy remains an option for the diagnostic sampling of lung tissue. It provides the largest amount of material, and it can be used to biopsy and/or excise lesions that are too deep or too close to vital structures for removal by VATS. The choice between VATS and thoracotomy needs to be made on a case-by-case basis, and the relative indications for each are still evolving as more experience is being gained with VATS.

MEDIASTINOSCOPY AND MEDIASTINOTOMY Tissue biopsy is often critical for the diagnosis of mediastinal masses or enlarged mediastinal lymph nodes. Although CT is useful for determining the size of mediastinal lymph nodes as part of the staging of lung cancer, confirmation that enlarged lymph nodes are actually involved with tumor generally requires biopsy and histopathologic examination. The two major procedures used to obtain specimens from masses or nodes in the mediastinum are mediastinoscopy (via a suprasternal approach) and mediastinotomy (via a parasternal approach). Both procedures are performed under general anesthesia by a qualified surgeon. In the case of suprasternal mediastinoscopy, a rigid mediastinoscope is inserted at the suprasternal notch and passed into the mediastinum along a pathway just anterior to the trachea. Tissue can be obtained with biopsy forceps passed through the scope, sampling masses or nodes that are in a paratracheal or pretracheal position. Left paratracheal and aortopulmonary lymph nodes are not accessible by this route and thus are commonly sampled by parasternal mediastinotomy (the Chamberlain procedure). This approach involves either a right or left parasternal incision and dissection directly down to a mass or node that requires biopsy.

BIBLIOGRAPHY

DICHTER JR et al: Approach to the immunocompromised host with pulmonary symptoms. Hematol Oncol Clin North Am 7:887, 1993

ETTINGER NA: Invasive diagnostic approaches to pulmonary infiltrates. Semin Respir Infect 8:168, 1993

HARRIS RJ et al: The diagnostic and therapeutic utility of thoracoscopy. A review. Chest 108:828, 1995

MCELVEIN RB: Procedures in the evaluation of chest disease. Clin Chest Med 13:1, 1992

MURRAY JF, NADEL JA: *Textbook of Respiratory Medicine*, 2d ed. Philadelphia, Saunders, 1994

NAIDICH DP et al: *Computed Tomography and Magnetic Resonance of the Thorax*, 2d ed. New York, Raven Press, 1991

WANG K-P, MEHTA AC: *Flexible Bronchoscopy*, Cambridge, MA, Blackwell, 1995

WEINBERGER SE: *Principles of Pulmonary Medicine*, 2d ed. Philadelphia, Saunders, 1992

SECTION 2

DISEASES OF THE RESPIRATORY SYSTEM

252 | *E. R. McFadden, Jr.*

ASTHMA

DEFINITION Asthma is a disease of airways that is characterized by increased responsiveness of the tracheobronchial tree to a multiplicity of stimuli. It is manifested physiologically by a widespread narrowing of the air passages, which may be relieved spontaneously

or as a result of therapy, and clinically by paroxysms of dyspnea, cough, and wheezing. Asthma is an episodic disease, acute exacerbations being interspersed with symptom-free periods. Typically, most attacks are short-lived, lasting minutes to hours, and clinically the patient seems to recover completely after an attack. However, there can be a phase in which the patient experiences some degree of airways obstruction daily. This phase can be mild, with or without superimposed severe episodes, or much more serious, with severe obstruction persisting for days or weeks, a condition known as *status asthmaticus*. In unusual circumstances, acute episodes can cause death.

PREVALENCE AND ETIOLOGY   Asthma is very common; it is estimated that 4 to 5 percent of the population of the United States is affected. Similar figures have been reported from other countries. Bronchial asthma occurs at all ages but predominantly in early life. About one-half of cases develop before age 10, and another third occur before age 40. In childhood, there is a 2:1 male/female preponderance, but the sex ratio equalizes by age 30.

From an etiologic standpoint, asthma is a heterogeneous disease. It is useful for epidemiologic and clinical purposes to classify asthma by the principal stimuli that incite or are associated with acute episodes. However, it is important to emphasize that this distinction may often be artificial, and the response of a given subclassification usually can be initiated by more than one type of stimulus. Further, the application of molecular and cell biologic techniques to asthma pathogenesis is also beginning to blur this type of classification. With these reservations in mind, one can describe two broad types of asthma: allergic and idiosyncratic.

Allergic asthma is often associated with a personal and/or family history of allergic diseases such as rhinitis, urticaria, and eczema, with positive wheal-and-flare skin reactions to intradermal injection of extracts of airborne antigens, with increased levels of IgE in the serum, and/or with a positive response to provocation tests involving the inhalation of specific antigen.

A significant fraction of asthmatic patients present with no personal or family history of allergy, with negative skin tests, and with normal serum levels of IgE, and therefore have disease that cannot be classified on the basis of defined immunologic mechanisms. These patients are said to have *idiosyncratic asthma*. Many develop a typical symptom complex upon contracting an upper respiratory illness. The initial insult may be little more than a common cold, but after several days the patient begins to develop paroxysms of wheezing and dyspnea that can last for days to months. These individuals should not be confused with persons in whom the symptoms of bronchospasm are superimposed on chronic bronchitis or bronchiectasis (Chaps. 256 and 258).

Many patients have disease that does not fit clearly into either of the preceding categories but instead falls into a mixed group with features of each. In general, asthma that has its onset in early life tends to have a strong allergic component, whereas asthma that develops late tends to be nonallergic or to have a mixed etiology.

PATHOGENESIS OF ASTHMA   The common denominator underlying the asthmatic diathesis is a nonspecific hyperirritability of the tracheobronchial tree. When airway reactivity is high, symptoms are more severe and persistent, and the amount of therapy required to control the patient's complaints is greater. In addition, the magnitude of diurnal fluctuations in lung function is greater, and the patient tends to awaken at night or in the early morning with breathlessness.

In both normal and asthmatic subjects, airway reactivity rises following viral infections of the respiratory tract and exposure to oxidant air pollutants such as ozone and nitrogen dioxide (but not sulfur dioxide). Viral infections have more profound consequences, and airway responsiveness may remain elevated for many weeks after a seemingly trivial upper respiratory tract infection. In contrast, airway reactivity remains high for only a few days after exposure to ozone. Allergens can cause airway responsiveness to rise within minutes and to remain elevated for weeks. If the dose of antigen is high enough, acute episodes of obstruction may occur daily for a prolonged period following a single exposure.

A number of causes have been postulated for the increased airway reactivity of asthma, but the basic mechanism remains unknown. The most popular hypothesis at present is that of airway inflammation. Increased numbers of mast cells, epithelial cells, neutrophils, eosinophils, and lymphocytes have been found in the bronchoalveolar lavage fluid of patients with asthma, as have a variety of mediators. An active inflammatory process is frequently observed in endobronchial biopsy specimens even from asymptomatic patients. The airways can be edematous and infiltrated with eosinophils, neutrophils, and lymphocytes, with or without thickening of the epithelial basement membrane. There may also be glandular hypertrophy. The most ubiquitous finding is a generalized increase in cellularity associated with an elevated capillary density. Occasionally, denudation of the epithelium may also be observed.

Although the translation of these histologic observations into a disease process is still incomplete, it is widely believed that the physiologic and clinical features of asthma derive from an interaction among the resident and infiltrating inflammatory cells in the airways and the surface epithelium. The cells thought to play important roles are mast cells, eosinophils, macrophages, neutrophils, and lymphocytes. The mediators released—histamine; bradykinin; the leukotrienes C, D, and E; platelet-activating factor; and prostaglandins (PGs) E_2, $F_2\alpha$, and D_2—produce an intense, immediate inflammatory reaction involving bronchoconstriction, vascular congestion, and edema formation. In addition to their ability to evoke prolonged contraction of airway smooth muscle and mucosal edema, the leukotrienes may also account for some of the other pathophysiologic features of asthma, such as increased mucus production and impaired mucociliary transport. This intense local event can then be followed by a more chronic one. The chemotactic factors elaborated (eosinophil and neutrophil chemotactic factors of anaphylaxis and leukotriene B_4) bring eosinophils, platelets, and polymorphonuclear leukocytes to the site of the reaction. These infiltrating cells as well as resident macrophages and the airway epithelium itself potentially are an additional source of mediators to enhance both the immediate and the cellular phase.

Like the mast cell in the early reaction, the eosinophil appears to play an important part in the infiltrative component. The granular proteins in this cell (major basic protein and eosinophilic cationic protein) are capable of destroying the airway epithelium, which then is sloughed into the bronchial lumen in the form of Creola bodies. Besides resulting in a loss of barrier and secretory function, such damage elicits the production of chemotactic cytokines, leading to further inflammation. In theory, it also can expose sensory nerve endings, thus initiating neurogenic inflammatory pathways. That, in turn, could convert a primary local event into a generalized reaction via a reflex mechanism.

T lymphocytes also appear to be important in the inflammatory response. These cells are present in increased numbers in asthmatic airways and produce cytokines that activate cell-mediated immunity, as well as humoral (IgE) immune responses. Furthermore, the T_H1 and T_H2 lymphocyte subtypes have functions that may influence the asthmatic response. The T_H1 cytokines interleukin (IL) 2 and interferon (IFN) γ can promote the growth and differentiation of B cells and the activation of macrophages, respectively. The T_H2 cytokine IL-4 and IL-5 stimulate B-cell growth and immunoglobulin secretion, and IL-5 promotes eosinophil proliferation, differentiation, and activation. It can also facilitate granule release from basophils.

The relative roles of each of these components in the production of heightened airway reactivity and clinical asthma has yet to be determined. It is unlikely that any one cell type or mediator accounts for every feature. For example, mast cell–derived mediators cannot explain the whole picture, for they have been found in the blood of individuals with mast cell–related diseases such as cold-induced and cholinergic-induced urticaria and in the airways of atopic nonasthmatics. Since these individuals had no lower respiratory illness or complaints, these alleged mediators of asthma would appear to need a unique background from which to exhibit their effects. Similarly, the inflammatory cells believed to be relevant to asthma are also found in the airways of atopic nonasthmatics, raising the possibility that they are merely nonspecific markers of atopy rather than specific indexes of asthma. Finally, therapeutic administration of IL-2 and granulocyte-macrophage colony stimulating factor to cancer patients results in eosinophilia with cell activation but not in asthma.

The stimuli that interact with airway responsiveness and incite acute episodes of asthma can be grouped into seven major categories:

allergenic, pharmacologic, environmental, occupational, infectious, exercise-related, and emotional.

Allergens Allergic asthma is dependent on an IgE response controlled by T and B lymphocytes and activated by the interaction of antigen with mast cell–bound IgE molecules. Most of the allergens that provoke asthma are airborne, and to induce a state of sensitivity they must be reasonably abundant for considerable periods of time. Once sensitization has occurred, however, the patient can exhibit exquisite responsivity, so that minute amounts of the offending agent can produce significant exacerbations of the disease. Immune mechanisms appear to be causally related to the development of asthma in 25 to 35 percent of all cases and to be contributory in perhaps another third. Higher prevalences have been suggested, but it is difficult to know how to interpret the data because of confounding factors. Allergic asthma is frequently seasonal, and it is most often observed in children and young adults. A nonseasonal form may result from allergy to feathers, animal danders, dust mites, molds, and other antigens that are present continuously in the environment. Exposure to antigen typically produces an immediate response in which airways obstruction develops in minutes and then resolves. In 30 to 50 percent of patients, a second wave of bronchoconstriction, the so-called late reaction, develops 6 to 10 h later. In a minority, only a late reaction occurs. It was formerly thought that the late reaction was essential to the development of the increase in airways reactivity that follows antigen exposure. Recent data show that not to be the case.

The mechanism by which an inhaled allergen provokes an acute episode of asthma depends in part on antigen-antibody interactions on the surface of pulmonary mast cells, with the subsequent generation and release of the mediators of immediate hypersensitivity. Current hypotheses hold that very small antigenic particles penetrate the lung's defenses and come in contact with mast cells that interdigitate with the epithelium at the luminal surface of the central airways. (No mechanism has yet been proposed that explains how antigen can contact the mast cells in the submucosa.) The subsequent elaboration of mediators and cytokines then produces the sequence outlined above.

Pharmacologic Stimuli The drugs most commonly associated with the induction of acute episodes of asthma are aspirin, coloring agents such as tartrazine, beta-adrenergic antagonists, and sulfiting agents. It is important to recognize drug-induced bronchial narrowing because its presence is often associated with great morbidity. Furthermore, death sometimes has followed the ingestion of aspirin (or other nonsteroidal anti-inflammatory agents) or beta-adrenergic antagonists. The typical aspirin-sensitive respiratory syndrome primarily affects adults, although the condition may be seen in childhood. This problem usually begins with perennial vasomotor rhinitis that is followed by a hyperplastic rhinosinusitis with nasal polyps. Progressive asthma then appears. On exposure to even very small quantities of aspirin, affected individuals typically develop ocular and nasal congestion and acute, often severe episodes of airways obstruction. The prevalence of aspirin sensitivity in asthmatic subjects varies from study to study, but many authorities feel that 10 percent is a reasonable figure. There is a great deal of cross reactivity between aspirin and other nonsteroidal anti-inflammatory compounds. Indomethacin, fenoprofen, naproxen, zomepirac sodium, ibuprofen, mefenamic acid, and phenylbutazone are particularly important in this regard. On the other hand, acetaminophen, sodium salicylate, choline salicylate, salicylamide, and propoxyphene are well tolerated. The exact frequency of cross reactivity to tartrazine and other dyes in aspirin-sensitive asthmatic subjects is also controversial; again, 10 percent is the commonly accepted figure. This peculiar complication of aspirin-sensitive asthma is particularly insidious, however, in that tartrazine and other potentially troublesome dyes are widely present in the environment and may be unknowingly ingested by sensitive patients.

Patients with aspirin sensitivity can be desensitized by daily administration of the drug. Following this form of therapy, cross tolerance also develops to other nonsteroidal anti-inflammatory agents. The mechanism by which aspirin and other such drugs produce bronchospasm has not yet been elucidated but may be related to aspirin-induced preferential generation of leukotrienes. Immediate hypersensi-

tivity does not seem to be involved. The availability of effective inhibitors of leukotriene synthesis or receptor activity should aid materially in the treatment of this problem.

Beta-adrenergic antagonists regularly obstruct the airways in asthmatics as well as in others with heightened airway reactivity and should be avoided by such individuals. Even the selective beta$_1$ agents have this propensity, particularly at higher doses. In fact, the local use of beta$_1$ blockers in the eye for the treatment of glaucoma has been associated with worsening asthma.

Sulfiting agents, such as potassium metabisulfite, potassium and sodium bisulfite, sodium sulfite, and sulfur dioxide, which are widely used in the food and pharmaceutical industries as sanitizing and preserving agents, also can produce acute airways obstruction in sensitive individuals. Exposure usually follows ingestion of food or beverages containing these compounds, e.g., salads, fresh fruit, potatoes, shellfish, and wine. Exacerbation of asthma has been reported following the use of sulfite-containing topical ophthalmic solutions, intravenous glucocorticoids, and some inhalational bronchodilator solutions. The incidence and mechanism of action of this phenomenon are unknown. When suspected, the diagnosis can be confirmed by either oral or inhalational provocations.

Environment and Air Pollution (See Chap. 254) Environmental causes of asthma are usually related to climatic conditions that promote the concentration of atmospheric pollutants and antigens. These conditions tend to develop in heavily industrial or densely populated urban areas and are frequently associated with thermal inversions or other situations creating stagnant air masses. In these circumstances, although the general population can develop respiratory symptoms, patients with asthma and other respiratory diseases tend to be more severely affected. The air pollutants known to have this effect are ozone, nitrogen dioxide, and sulfur dioxide. The last needs to be present in high concentrations and produces its greatest effects during periods of high ventilation. In some regions of North America, seasonal concentrations of airborne antigens such as pollen, can rise high enough to result in epidemics of asthma admissions to hospitals and an increase in the death rate. These events may be ameliorated by treating patients prophylactically with mast cell–stabilizing drugs before the allergy season begins.

Occupational Factors (See Chap. 254) Occupation-related asthma is a significant health problem, and acute and chronic airways obstruction has been reported to follow exposure to a large number of compounds used in many types of industrial processes. Bronchoconstriction can result from working with or being exposed to *metal salts* (e.g., platinum, chrome, and nickel), *wood and vegetable dusts* (e.g., those of oak, western red cedar, grain, flour, castor bean, green coffee bean, mako, gum acacia, karay gum, and tragacanth), *pharmaceutical agents* (e.g., antibiotics, piperazine, and cimetidine), *industrial chemicals and plastics* (e.g., toluene diisocyanate, phthalic acid anhydride, trimellitic anhydride, persulfates, ethylenediamine, *p*-phenylenediamine, and various dyes), *biologic enzymes* (e.g., laundry detergents and pancreatic enzymes), and *animal and insect dusts, serums, and secretions*. It is important to recognize that exposure to sensitizing chemicals, particularly those used in paints, solvents, and plastics, also can occur during leisure or non-work-related activities.

There seem to be three underlying mechanisms for this airways obstruction: (1) In some cases, the offending agent results in the formation of a specific IgE, and the cause seems immunologic (the immunologic reaction can be immediate, late, or dual); (2) in other cases, the substance causes a direct liberation of bronchoconstrictor substances; and (3) in other cases, the substance causes direct or reflex stimulation of the airways of either latent or frank asthmatics. In the case of asthmatic symptoms caused by occupational exposures that do not produce an immediate and dual immunologic reaction, patients give a characteristic cyclic history. They are well when they arrive at work, and symptoms develop toward the end of the shift, progress after the work site is left, and then regress. Absence from work during weekends or vacations brings about remission. Frequently, there are similar symptoms in fellow employees.

Infections Respiratory infections are the most common of the stimuli that evoke acute exacerbations of asthma. Well-controlled investigations have demonstrated that respiratory viruses and not bacteria or allergy are the major etiologic factors. In young children, the most important infectious agents are respiratory syncytial virus and parainfluenza virus. In older children and adults, rhinovirus and influenza virus predominate as pathogens. Simple colonization of the tracheobronchial tree is insufficient to evoke acute episodes of bronchospasm, and attacks of asthma occur only when symptoms of an ongoing respiratory tract infection are, or have been, present. The mechanism by which viruses induce exacerbations of asthma may be related to the production of T cell–derived cytokines that potentiate the infiltration of inflammatory cells into already susceptible airways.

Exercise Exercise is one of the most common precipitants of acute episodes of asthma. This stimulus differs from other naturally occurring provocations, such as antigens or viral infections, in that it does not evoke any long-term sequelae, nor does it change airway reactivity. Exercise probably provokes bronchospasm to some extent in every asthmatic patient, and in some it is the only trigger that produces symptoms. When such patients are followed for sufficient periods, however, they often develop recurring episodes of airway obstruction independent of exercise; thus, the onset of this problem frequently is the first manifestation of the full-blown asthmatic syndrome. There is a significant interaction between the ventilation produced by the exercise, the temperature, and the water content of the inspired air and the magnitude of the postexertional obstruction. Thus, for the same inspired air conditions, running will produce a more severe attack of asthma than will walking. Conversely, for a given task, the inhalation of cold air will markedly enhance the response, while warm, humid air will blunt or abolish it. Consequently, activities such as ice hockey, cross-country skiing, and ice skating are more provocative than is swimming in an indoor, heated pool. The mechanism by which exercise produces obstruction may be related to a thermally produced hyperemia and engorgement of the microvasculature of the bronchial wall and does not appear to involve smooth-muscle contraction.

Emotional Stress Abundant objective data demonstrate that psychological factors can interact with the asthmatic diathesis to worsen or ameliorate the disease process. The pathways and nature of the interactions are complex but have been shown to be operational to some extent in almost half the patients studied. Changes in airway caliber seem to be mediated through modification of vagal efferent activity, but endorphins also may play a role. The most frequently studied variable has been that of suggestion, and the weight of current evidence indicates that it can be quite important in selected asthmatics. When psychically responsive individuals are given the appropriate suggestion, they can actually decrease or increase the pharmacologic effects of adrenergic and cholinergic stimuli on their airways. The extent to which psychological factors participate in the induction and/ or continuation of any given acute exacerbation is not established but probably varies from patient to patient and in the same patient from episode to episode.

PATHOLOGY In a patient who has died of acute asthma, the most striking feature of the lungs at necropsy is their gross overdistention and failure to collapse when the pleural cavities are opened. When the lungs are cut, numerous gelatinous plugs of exudate are found in most of the bronchial branches down to the terminal bronchioles. Histologic examination shows hypertrophy of the bronchial smooth muscle, hyperplasia of mucosal and submucosal vessels, mucosal edema, denudation of the surface epithelium, pronounced thickening of the basement membrane, and eosinophilic infiltrates in the bronchial wall. In asthmatic patients who die from trauma and causes other than asthma itself, mucus casts, basement membrane thickening, and eosinophilic infiltrates are frequently observed. In both situations there

is an absence of any of the well-recognized forms of destructive emphysema. In a small proportion of asthmatics who die, the eosinophilic infiltration is replaced by neutrophils, and mucus plugging is conspicuously absent. The reasons for these differences are not yet clear.

PATHOPHYSIOLOGY The pathophysiologic hallmark of asthma is a reduction in airway diameter brought about by contraction of smooth muscle, vascular congestion, edema of the bronchial wall, and thick, tenacious secretions. The net result is an increase in airway resistance, a decrease in forced expiratory volumes and flow rates, hyperinflation of the lungs and thorax, increased work of breathing, alterations in respiratory muscle function, changes in elastic recoil, abnormal distribution of both ventilation and pulmonary blood flow with mismatched ratios, and altered arterial blood gas concentrations. Thus, although asthma is considered to be primarily a disease of airways, virtually all aspects of pulmonary function are compromised during an acute attack. In addition, in very symptomatic patients there frequently is electrocardiographic evidence of right ventricular hypertrophy and pulmonary hypertension. When a patient presents for therapy, his or her forced vital capacity tends to be ≤ 50 percent of normal. The 1-s forced expiratory volume (FEV_1) averages 30 percent or less of predicted, while the maximum and minimum midexpiratory flow rates are reduced to 20 percent or less of expected. In keeping with the alterations in mechanics, the associated air trapping is substantial. In acutely ill patients, residual volume (RV) frequently approaches 400 percent of normal, while functional residual capacity doubles. The patient tends to report that the attack has ended clinically when the RV has fallen to 200 percent of its predicted value and the FEV_1 reaches 50 percent of the predicted level.

Hypoxia is a universal finding during acute exacerbations, but frank ventilatory failure is relatively uncommon, being observed in 10 to 15 percent of patients presenting for therapy. Most asthmatics have hypocapnia and a respiratory alkalosis. In acutely ill patients, the finding of a normal arterial carbon dioxide tension tends to be associated with quite severe levels of obstruction. Consequently, when found in a symptomatic individual, it should be viewed as representing impending respiratory failure, and the patient should be treated accordingly. Equally, the presence of metabolic acidosis in the setting of acute asthma signifies severe obstruction. Usually, there are no clinical counterparts to the derangements in blood gases. Cyanosis is a very late sign. Hence, a dangerous level of hypoxia can go undetected. Likewise, signs attributable to carbon dioxide retention, such as sweating, tachycardia, and wide pulse pressure, or to acidosis, such as tachypnea, tend not to be of great value in predicting the presence of hypercapnia or hydrogen ion excess in individual patients, because they are too frequently seen in anxious patients with more moderate disease. Trying to judge the state of an acutely ill patient's ventilatory status on clinical grounds alone can be extremely hazardous, and clinical indicators should not be relied on with any confidence. Therefore, in patients with suspected alveolar hypoventilation, arterial blood gas tensions must be measured.

CLINICAL FEATURES The symptoms of asthma consist of a triad of dyspnea, cough, and wheezing, the last often being regarded as the *sine qua non*. In its most typical form, asthma is an episodic disease, and all three symptoms coexist. At the onset of an attack, patients experience a sense of constriction in the chest, often with a nonproductive cough. Respiration becomes audibly harsh, wheezing in both phases of respiration becomes prominent, expiration becomes prolonged, and patients frequently have tachypnea, tachycardia, and mild systolic hypertension. The lungs rapidly become overinflated, and the anteroposterior diameter of the thorax increases. If the attack is severe or prolonged, there may be a loss of adventitial breath sounds, and wheezing becomes very high pitched. Further, the accessory muscles become visibly active, and a paradoxical pulse often develops. These two signs have been found to be extremely valuable in indicating the severity of the obstruction. In the presence of either, pulmonary function tends to be significantly more impaired than in their absence. It is important to note that the development of a paradoxical pulse depends on the generation of large negative intrathoracic pressures.

Thus, if the patient's breathing is shallow, this sign and/or the use of accessory muscles could be absent even though obstruction is quite severe. The other signs and symptoms of asthma only imperfectly reflect the physiologic alterations that are present. Indeed, if the disappearance of subjective complaints or even of wheezing is used as the end point at which therapy for an acute attack is terminated, an enormous reservoir of residual disease will be missed.

The end of an episode is frequently marked by a cough that produces thick, stringy mucus, which often takes the form of casts of the distal airways (Curschmann's spirals) and, when examined microscopically, often shows eosinophils and Charcot-Leyden crystals. In extreme situations, wheezing may lessen markedly or even disappear, cough may become extremely ineffective, and the patient may begin a gasping type of respiratory pattern. These findings imply extensive mucus plugging and impending suffocation. Ventilatory assistance by mechanical means may be required. Atelectasis due to inspissated secretions occasionally occurs with asthmatic attacks. Other complications, such as spontaneous pneumothorax and/or pneumomediastinum, are rare.

Less typically, a patient with asthma may complain of intermittent episodes of nonproductive cough or exertional dyspnea. Unlike other asthmatics, when these patients are examined during symptomatic periods, they tend to have normal breath sounds but may wheeze after repeated forced exhalations and/or may show ventilatory impairments when tested in the laboratory. In the absence of both these signs, a bronchoprovocation test may be required to make the diagnosis.

DIFFERENTIAL DIAGNOSIS The differentiation of asthma from other diseases associated with dyspnea and wheezing is usually not difficult, particularly if the patient is seen during an acute episode. The physical findings and symptoms listed above and the history of periodic attacks are quite characteristic. A personal or family history of allergic diseases such as eczema, rhinitis, or urticaria is valuable contributory evidence. An extremely common feature of asthma is nocturnal awakening with dyspnea and/or wheezing. In fact, this phenomenon is so prevalent that its absence raises doubt about the diagnosis. *Upper airway obstruction by tumor* or *laryngeal edema* can occasionally be confused with asthma. Typically, a patient with such a condition will present with stridor, and the harsh respiratory sounds can be localized to the area of the trachea. Diffuse wheezing throughout both lung fields is usually absent. However, differentiation can sometimes be difficult, and indirect laryngoscopy or bronchoscopy may be required. Asthma-like symptoms have been described in patients with glottic dysfunction. These individuals narrow their glottis during inspiration and expiration, producing episodic attacks of severe airway obstruction. Occasionally carbon dioxide retention develops. However, unlike asthma, the arterial oxygen tension is well preserved, and the alveolar-arterial gradient for oxygen narrows during the episode, instead of widening as with lower airway obstruction. To establish the diagnosis of glottic dysfunction, the glottis should be examined when the patient is symptomatic. Normal findings at such a time exclude the diagnosis; normal findings during asymptomatic periods do not.

Persistent wheezing localized to one area of the chest in association with paroxysms of coughing indicates *endobronchial disease* such as foreign-body aspiration, a neoplasm, or bronchial stenosis.

The signs and symptoms of *acute left ventricular failure* occasionally mimic asthma, but the findings of moist basilar rales, gallop rhythms, blood-tinged sputum, and other signs of heart failure (Chap. 233) allow the appropriate diagnosis to be reached.

Recurrent episodes of bronchospasm can occur with *carcinoid tumors* (Chap. 95), *recurrent pulmonary emboli* (Chap. 261), and *chronic bronchitis* (Chap. 258). In chronic bronchitis there are no true symptom-free periods, and one can usually obtain a history of chronic cough and sputum production as a background upon which acute attacks of wheezing are superimposed. Recurrent emboli can be very difficult to separate from asthma. Frequently, patients with this condition will present with episodes of breathlessness, particularly on exertion, and they sometimes wheeze. Pulmonary function studies may show evidence of peripheral airway obstruction (Chap. 250); when these changes are present, lung scans also may be abnormal. The

therapeutic response to bronchodilators and to institution of anticoagulant therapy may be helpful, but pulmonary angiography may be necessary to establish the correct diagnosis.

Eosinophilic pneumonias (Chap. 253) are often associated with asthmatic symptoms, as are various chemical pneumonias and exposures to insecticides and cholinergic drugs. Bronchospasm occasionally is a manifestation of *systemic vasculitis* with pulmonary involvement.

DIAGNOSIS The diagnosis of asthma is established by demonstrating reversible airway obstruction. *Reversibility* is traditionally defined as a 15 percent or greater increase in FEV_1 following two puffs of a beta-adrenergic agonist. When the spirometry results are normal at presentation, the diagnosis can be made by showing heightened airway responsiveness to challenges with histamine, methacholine, or isocapnic hyperventilation of cold air. Once the diagnosis is confirmed, the course of the illness and the effectiveness of therapy can be followed by measuring peak expiratory flow rates (PEFRs) at home and/or the FEV_1 in the laboratory. Positive wheal-and-flare reactions to skin tests can be demonstrated to various allergens, but such findings do not necessarily correlate with the intrapulmonary events. Sputum and blood eosinophilia and measurement of serum IgE levels are also helpful but are not specific for asthma. Chest roentgenograms showing hyperinflation are also nondiagnostic.

℞ TREATMENT

Elimination of the causative agent(s) from the environment of an allergic asthmatic is the most successful means available for treating this condition (for details on avoidance, see Chap. 310). Desensitization or immunotherapy with extracts of the suspected allergens has enjoyed widespread favor, but controlled studies are limited and have not proved it to be highly effective.

Drug Treatment The available agents for treating asthma can be divided into two general categories: drugs that inhibit smooth muscle contraction (beta-adrenergic agonists, methylxanthines, and anticholinergics) and agents that prevent and/or reverse inflammation (glucocorticoids and mast cell–stabilizing agents). Inhibitors of mediator synthesis and mediator-receptor antagonists are currently undergoing clinical trials.

ADRENERGIC STIMULANTS The drugs in this category consist of the catecholamines, resorcinols, and saligenins. These agents are analogues and produce airway dilation through stimulation of beta-adrenergic receptors and activation of G proteins with the resultant formation of cyclic adenosine monophosphate (AMP). They also decrease release of mediators and improve mucociliary transport. The catecholamines in widespread clinical use are epinephrine, isoproterenol, isoetharine, rimiterol, and hexoprenaline. The last two are not available in the United States. As a group, these compounds are short-acting (30 to 90 min) and are effective only when administered by inhalational or parenteral routes. Epinephrine and isoproterenol are not beta$_2$-selective and have considerable chronotropic and inotropic cardiac effects. Epinephrine also has substantial alpha-stimulating effects. The usual dose is 0.3 to 0.5 mL of a 1:1000 solution administered subcutaneously. Isoproterenol is devoid of alpha activity and is the most potent agent of this group. It is usually administered in a 1:200 solution by inhalation. Isoetharine is the most beta$_2$-selective compound of this class, but it is a relatively weak bronchodilator. It is employed as an aerosol and supplied as a 1% solution. The pharmacologies of hexoprenaline and rimiterol are similar to that of isoetharine.

The commonly used resorcinols are metaproterenol, terbutaline, and fenoterol, and the most widely known saligenin is albuterol (salbutamol). With the exception of metaproterenol, these drugs are highly selective for the respiratory tract and virtually devoid of significant cardiac effects except at high doses. Their major side effect is tremor. They are active by all routes of administration, and because their chemical structures allow them to bypass the metabolic processes used to degrade the catecholamines, their effects are relatively long-lasting (4 to 6 h). Differences in potency and duration among agents can be eliminated by adjusting doses and/or administration schedules.

Inhalation is the preferred route of administration because it increases the bronchial selectivity of these drugs and allows maximal bronchodilation with fewer side effects. This is true not just in maintenance therapy but also during the treatment of severe acute obstruction. In the past it was fashionable to treat episodes of severe asthma with intravenous sympathomimetics such as isoproterenol. This approach no longer appears justifiable. Isoproterenol infusions clearly can induce myocardial damage, and even for the beta$_2$-selective agents such as terbutaline and albuterol, intravenous administration offers no advantages over the inhaled route.

Salmeterol, a very long-lasting (9 to 12 h) congener of albuterol, is now available in the United States. When given every 12 h, it is effective in providing sustained symptomatic relief. It is particularly helpful for conditions such as nocturnal and exercise-induced asthma. It is not recommended for the treatment of acute episodes because of its relatively slow onset of action (approximately 30 min), nor is it intended as a rescue drug for breakthrough symptoms. In addition, its long half life means that administration of extra doses can cause cumulative side effects.

METHYLXANTHINES   Theophylline and its various salts are medium-potency bronchodilators that work through an undefined mechanism. It was formerly thought that these drugs increased cyclic AMP by the inhibition of phosphodiesterase; however, the available evidence does not support this concept. The therapeutic plasma concentrations of theophylline traditionally have been thought to lie between 10 and 20 μg/mL. Some sources, however, recommend a lower target range between 5 and 15 μg/ml to avoid toxicity. The dose required to achieve the desired level varies widely from patient to patient owing to differences in the metabolism of the drug. Theophylline clearance, and thus the dosage requirement, is decreased substantially in neonates and the elderly and those with acute and chronic hepatic dysfunction, cardiac decompensation, and cor pulmonale. Clearance is also decreased during febrile illnesses. Clearance is increased in children. In addition, a number of important drug interactions can alter theophylline metabolism. Clearance falls with the concurrent use of erythromycin and other macrolide antibiotics, the quinolone antibiotics, and troleandomycin, allopurinol, cimetidine, and propranolol. It rises with use of cigarettes, marijuana, phenobarbital, phenytoin, or any other drug that has the capability of inducing hepatic microsomal enzymes.

For maintenance therapy, long-acting theophylline compounds are available and are usually given twice per day or once daily. The dose is adjusted on the basis of the clinical response with the aid of serum theophylline measurements. Single-dose administration in the evening reduces nocturnal symptoms and helps keep the patient complaint-free during the day. Aminophylline and theophylline are available for intravenous use. The recommendations for intravenous therapy in children aged 9 to 16 and in young adult smokers not currently receiving theophylline products are a loading dose of 6 mg/kg followed by an infusion of 1.0 mg/kg per hour for the next 12 h and then 0.8 mg/kg per hour thereafter. In nonsmoking adults, older patients, and those with cor pulmonale, congestive heart failure, and liver disease, the loading dose remains the same, but the maintenance dose is reduced to between 0.1 and 0.5 mg/kg per hour. In patients already receiving theophylline, the loading dose is frequently withheld or, in extreme situations, reduced to 0.5 mg/kg.

The most common side effects of theophylline are nervousness, nausea, vomiting, anorexia, and headache. At plasma levels greater than 30 μg/mL there is a risk of seizures and cardiac arrhythmias.

ANTICHOLINERGICS   Anticholinergic drugs such as atropine sulfate produce bronchodilation in patients with asthma, but their use is limited by systemic side effects. Nonabsorbable quaternary ammonium congeners (atropine methylnitrate and ipratropium bromide) have been found to be both effective and free of untoward effects. They may be of particular benefit for patients with coexistent heart disease, in whom use of methylxanthines and beta-adrenergic stimulants may be dangerous. There is some evidence that addition of anticholinergics may enhance the bronchodilation achieved by sympathomimetics, but the effect is not large. The major disadvantages of the anticholinergics are that they are slow to act (60 to 90 min may be required before peak bronchodilation is achieved) and they are only of modest potency.

GLUCOCORTICOIDS   Glucocorticoids are not bronchodilators, and their major use in asthma is in reducing airway inflammation. Systemic or oral steroids are most beneficial in acute illness when severe airway obstruction is not resolving or is worsening despite intense optimal bronchodilator therapy, and in chronic disease when there has been failure of a previously optimal regimen with frequent recurrences of symptoms of increasing severity.

The correct dose to use in acute situations is a matter of debate. The available data indicate that very high doses do not offer any advantage over more conventional amounts. In the United States, a usual starting dose is 40 to 60 mg of methylprednisolone intravenously every 6 h. Since intravenous and oral administration produce the same effects, prednisone, 60 mg every 6 h, can be substituted. Clinical impressions suggest that smaller quantities may work as effectively, but there are no confirmatory data. In the United Kingdom and elsewhere, acute asthma both in and out of hospital is frequently treated with doses of prednisolone ranging from 30 to 40 mg given once daily. It should be emphasized that the effects of steroids in acute asthma are not immediate and may not be seen for 6 h or more after the initial administration. Consequently, it is mandatory to continue vigorous bronchodilator therapy during this interval. Irrespective of the regimen chosen, it is important to appreciate that rapid tapering of glucocorticoids frequently results in recurrent obstruction. Most authorities recommend reducing the dose by one-half every third to fifth day following an acute episode. In situations in which it appears that continued steroid therapy will be needed, an alternate-day schedule should be instituted to minimize side effects. This is particularly important in children, since continuous corticosteroid administration interrupts growth. Long-acting preparations such as dexamethasone should not be used in this approach, for they defeat the purpose of alternate-day schedules by causing prolonged suppression of the pituitary-adrenal axis.

Several inhaled steroids of high topical potency are available and greatly facilitate the withdrawal of oral agents. They are also useful in reducing airways reactivity and as an alternative to oral glucocorticoids in situations where asthma symptoms are escalating. Some guidelines recommend starting aerosolized steroids in any patient whose disease is not controlled by inhaled bronchodilators. If symptoms are not eliminated at the standard dose, it has been suggested that the dose be increased twofold or more. While this course of action diminishes the need for oral glucocorticoids, it carries the risk of greater side effects. In addition to thrush and dysphonia, the increased systemic absorption that accompanies larger doses of inhaled steroids has been reported to produce adrenal suppression, cataract formation, decreased growth in children, interference with bone metabolism, and purpura. Many of the currently available inhaled steroid preparations require 2 to 4 weeks to produce a beneficial effect. Consequently, it is advisable to start a course of oral glucocorticoids simultaneously with the inhaled drug to facilitate symptom resolution. As the oral drugs are withdrawn, the improvements can be maintained via the inhaled route.

MAST CELL–STABILIZING AGENTS   Cromolyn sodium and nedocromil sodium do not influence airway tone. Their major therapeutic effect is to inhibit the degranulation of mast cells, thereby preventing the release of the chemical mediators of anaphylaxis.

Cromolyn and nedocromil, like the inhaled steroids, improve lung function and reduce symptoms and lower airway reactivity in asthmatics. They are most effective in atopic patients who have either seasonal disease or perennial airways stimulation. A therapeutic trial of two puffs four times daily for 4 to 6 weeks frequently is necessary before the beneficial effects of the drug appear. Unlike steroids, nedocromil and cromolyn, when given prophylactically, will block the acute obstructive effects of exposure to antigen, industrial chemicals, exercise, or cold air. With antigen, the late response is also abolished. Therefore, a patient who has intermittent exposure to either antigenic or nonantigenic stimuli that provoke acute episodes of asthma need not use these drugs continuously but instead can obtain protection by taking the drug only 15 to 20 min before contact with the precipitant.

MISCELLANEOUS AGENTS It has been suggested that steroid-dependent patients might benefit from the use of immunosuppressant agents such as methotrexate or gold salts. The effects of these agents on steroid dosage and disease activity are minor, and side effects can be considerable. Consequently, this form of treatment can only be viewed as experimental. Opiates, sedatives, and tranquilizers should be absolutely avoided in the acutely ill asthmatic because the risk of depressing alveolar ventilation is great, and respiratory arrest has been reported to occur shortly after their use. Admittedly, most individuals are anxious and frightened, but experience has shown that they can be calmed equally well by the physician's presence and reassurances. Beta-adrenergic blockers and parasympathetic agonists are contraindicated because they can cause marked deterioration in lung function.

Expectorants and mucolytic agents have enjoyed great vogue in the past, but they do not add significantly to the treatment of the acute or chronic phases of this disease. Mucolytic agents such as acetylcysteine may actually produce bronchospasm when administered to susceptible asthmatics. This effect can be overcome by aerosolizing them in solution with a beta-adrenergic agent. The use of intravenous fluids in the treatment of acute asthma also has been advocated. There is little evidence that this adjunct hastens recovery. Nonstandard bronchodilators, such as intravenous magnesium sulfate for the treatment of acute asthma attacks, are not yet warranted in clinical practice because of the controversy surrounding their efficacy.

SPECIAL INSTRUCTIONS The treatment of patients with asthma who have coexisting conditions such as heart disease or pregnancy does not differ materially from that outlined above. Therapy with inhaled beta$_2$-selective and anti-inflammatory agents is the mainstay. The lowest doses of adrenergics that produce the desired effects should be used.

FRAMEWORK FOR MANAGEMENT Emergency Situations

The most effective treatment for acute episodes of asthma is administration of aerosolized beta$_2$ agonists. These drugs provide three to four times more relief than intravenous aminophylline. In emergency situations, they can be given every 20 min by hand-held nebulizer for three doses. Thereafter, the frequency can be reduced to every 2 h until the attack has subsided. Aminophylline can be added to the regimen after the first hour in an attempt to speed resolution. Recent studies in a large series of patients demonstrate that beta$_2$ agonists alone terminate attacks in approximately two-thirds of patients, and that another 5 to 10 percent benefit from methylxanthine in combination with a sympathomimetic. The remainder have a poor acute response to all forms of therapy.

Acute episodes of bronchial asthma are one of the most common respiratory emergencies seen in the practice of medicine, and it is essential that the physician recognize which episodes of airway obstruction are life-threatening and which patients demand what level of care. These distinctions can be made readily by assessing selected clinical parameters in combination with measures of expiratory flow and gas exchange. The presence of a paradoxical pulse, use of accessory muscles, and marked hyperinflation of the thorax signify severe airways obstruction, and failure of these signs to remit promptly after aggressive therapy mandates objective monitoring of the patient using measurements of arterial blood gases and the peak expiratory flow rate (PEFR) or FEV$_1$.

In general, there is a direct correlation between the severity of the obstruction with which the patient presents and the time it takes to resolve it. Those individuals with the most impairment typically require the most extensive therapy for resolution. If the PEFR or FEV$_1$ is equal to or less than 20 percent of predicted on presentation and does not double within an hour of receiving the preceding therapy, the patient is likely to require extensive treatment including glucocorticoids before the obstruction dissipates. This group represents approximately 20 percent of all the patients who present for acute care. They generally require 24 h or more of inpatient treatment before becoming asymptomatic. In such individuals, if the clinical signs of a paradoxical pulse and accessory muscle use are diminishing, and/or if PEFR is increasing, there is no need to change medications or doses; the patient need only be followed. However, if the PEFR falls by more than 20 percent of its previous value or if the magnitude of the pulsus paradoxicus is increasing, serial measures of arterial blood gases are required, as well as a reconsideration of the therapeutic modalities being employed. If the patient has hypocarbia, one can afford to continue the current approaches a while longer. On the other hand, if the Pa$_{CO_2}$ is within the normal range or is elevated, the patient should be monitored in an intensive care setting, and therapy should be intensified to reverse or arrest the patient's respiratory failure.

Chronic Treatment The goal of chronic therapy is to achieve a stable, asymptomatic state with the best pulmonary function possible. A number of algorithms have been proposed to accomplish this task. The first step is to educate patients to function as partners in their management. The severity of the illness needs to be assessed and monitored with objective measures of lung function. Asthma triggers should be avoided or controlled, and plans should be made for both chronic management and treatment of exacerbations. Regular follow-up care is mandatory. With respect to pharmacologic interventions, in general, the simplest approach works best. Infrequent symptoms require only the use of an inhaled sympathomimetic on an "as needed" basis. When the disease worsens, as manifested by nocturnal awakenings and daytime symptoms, inhaled steroids and/or mast cell–stabilizing agents should be added. If symptoms do not abate, the dose of inhaled steroids can be increased. An upper limit has not yet been established, but side effects of glucocorticoid excess begin to appear more frequently when the dose exceeds 2.0 mg/d. Persistent asthma complaints can be treated with long-acting inhaled beta$_2$ agonists, sustained-release theophylline, and/or parasympatholytics. In patients with recurrent or perennial symptoms and unstable lung function, oral steroids in a single daily dose are added to the regimen. Once control is reached and sustained for several weeks, a step-down reduction in therapy should be undertaken, beginning with the most toxic drug, to find the minimum amount of medication required to keep the patient well. During this process, the PEFR should be monitored and medication adjustments should be based on objective changes in lung function as well as on the patient's symptoms.

PROGNOSIS AND CLINICAL COURSE The mortality rate from asthma is small. The most recent figures indicate fewer than 5000 deaths per year out of a population of approximately 10 million patients at risk. Death rates, however, appear to be rising in inner-city areas where there is limited availability of health care.

Information on the clinical course of asthma suggests a good prognosis for 50 to 80 percent of all patients, particularly those whose disease is mild and develops in childhood. The number of children who still have asthma 7 to 10 years after the initial diagnosis varies from 26 to 78 percent, averaging 46 percent; however, the percentage who continue to have severe disease is relatively low (6 to 19 percent).

Unlike other airway diseases such as chronic bronchitis, asthma is not progressive. Although there are reports of patients with asthma developing irreversible changes in lung function, these individuals frequently have comorbid stimuli such as cigarette smoking that could account for these findings. Even when untreated, asthmatics do not continuously move from mild to severe disease with time. Rather, their clinical course is characterized by exacerbations and remissions. Some studies suggest that spontaneous remissions occur in approximately 20 percent of those who develop the disease as adults and that 40 percent or so can be expected to experience improvement, with less frequent and severe attacks, as they grow older.

BIBLIOGRAPHY

AMERICAN THORACIC SOCIETY: Guidelines for the evaluation of impairment/ disability in patients with asthma. Am Rev Respir Dis 147:1056, 1993

AMERICAN THORACIC SOCIETY: Progress of the interface of inflammation and asthma. Am J Respir Crit Care Med 152:385, 1995

BURR ML: Epidemiology of asthma. Monogr Allergy 31:80, 1993

MCFADDEN ER JR: Evolving concepts in the pathogenesis and management of asthma. Adv Intern Med 39:357, 1994

MCFADDEN ER JR, GILBERT IA: Exercise-induced asthma. N Engl J Med 330:1362, 1994

MCFADDEN ER JR, HEJAL R: Asthma. Lancet 345:1215, 1995

MCFADDEN ER JR et al: Protocol therapy for acute asthma: Therapeutic benefits and cost savings. Am J Med 99:651, 1995

SHEFFER AL, TAGGART VS: The National Asthma Education Program. Expert panel report guidelines for the diagnosis and management of asthma. Med Care 31:MS20, 1993

SKORODIN MS: Pharmacotherapy for asthma and chronic obstructive pulmonary disease. Current thinking, practices, and controversies. Arch Intern Med 153:814, 1993

WARDLAW AJ: The role of air pollution in asthma. Clin Exp Allergy 23:81, 1993

253

Gary W. Hunninghake, Hal B. Richerson

HYPERSENSITIVITY PNEUMONITIS AND EOSINOPHILIC PNEUMONIAS

HYPERSENSITIVITY PNEUMONITIS

Hypersensitivity pneumonitis (HP), or extrinsic allergic alveolitis, is an immunologically induced inflammation of the lung parenchyma, involving alveolar walls and terminal airways, secondary to repeated inhalation of a variety of organic or other agents by a susceptible host. In contrast to many of the other interstitial lung diseases, etiologic agents of this interstitial and alveolar filling disease have been identified. The prevalence of HP is unknown but varies with the environmental exposure and the specific antigen involved. The prevalence of farmer's lung among Wisconsin dairy farmers has been reported as 4.2 per 1000. The diagnosis of HP requires a constellation of clinical, radiographic, physiologic, pathologic, and immunologic criteria, each of which is rarely pathognomonic alone, and the preferred treatment is avoidance of the causative antigen when practical.

ETIOLOGY Agents implicated as causes of HP include those listed in Table 253-1. Many cases of HP occurring in various occupations involve exposure to similar agents, particularly the thermophilic actinomycetes. Common sources of causative antigens are "moldy" hay, silage, or grain; pet birds; and heating, cooling, and humidification systems. Simple chemicals, such as isocyanates, may also cause hypersensitivity pneumonitis.

PATHOGENESIS The finding that precipitating antibodies against extracts of moldy hay were demonstrable in most patients with farmer's lung led to the early conclusion that HP was an immune-complex–mediated reaction. Subsequent investigations of HP in human beings and animal models provided evidence for the importance of cell-mediated hypersensitivity. The very early (acute) reaction is characterized by an increase in polymorphonuclear leukocytes in the alveoli and small airways. This early lesion is followed by an influx of mononuclear cells into the lung and the formation of granulomas that appear to be the result of a classic delayed (T cell mediated) hypersensitivity reaction to repeated inhalation of antigen and adjuvant-active materials.

Bronchoalveolar lavage (Chap. 251) in patients with HP consistently demonstrates an increase in T lymphocytes in lavage fluid (a finding that is also observed in patients with other granulomatous lung disorders). Patients with recent or continual exposure to antigen may have an increase in polymorphonuclear leukocytes in lavage fluid. Increased numbers of mast cells have also been reported. In most patients examined during recovery from acute disease, the T lymphocytes in lavage fluid are predominantly the CD8 + T cell subset. In patients with very recent exposure to antigen, however, the numbers of CD4 + T cells may increase in lavage fluid. Similar findings may be present in similarly exposed, asymptomatic individuals. These observations suggest that there is an active modulation of granuloma formation in the lung by immunoregulatory T cells and associated cytokines in this disorder.

CLINICAL PRESENTATION The *clinical picture* is that of an interstitial pneumonitis, although it varies from patient to patient and seems related to the frequency and intensity of exposure to the causative antigen and perhaps other host factors. The presentation can be *acute, subacute,* or *chronic.* In the *acute form,* symptoms such as cough, fever, chills, malaise, and dyspnea may occur 6 to 8 h after exposure to the antigen and usually clear within a few days if there is no further exposure to antigen. The *subacute form* often appears insidiously over a period of weeks marked by cough and dyspnea and may progress to cyanosis and severe dyspnea requiring hospitalization. In some patients, a subacute form of the disease may persist after an acute presentation of the disorder, especially if there is continued exposure to antigen. In most patients with the acute or subacute form of HP, the symptoms, signs, and other manifestations of HP disappear within days, weeks, or months if the causative agent is no longer inhaled. Transformation to a chronic form of the disease may occur in patients with continued antigen exposure, but the frequency of such progression is uncertain. The *chronic form* may also present as a gradually progressive interstitial disease associated with cough and exertional dyspnea without a prior history consistent with acute or subacute manifestations. Such a gradual onset frequently occurs with low-dose exposure to the antigen.

DIAGNOSIS Following acute exposure to antigen, neutrophilia and lymphopenia are frequently present. Eosinophilia is not a feature. All forms of the disease may be associated with elevations in erythrocyte sedimentation rate, C-reactive protein, rheumatoid factor, and serum immunoglobulins. Antinuclear antibodies are rarely present.

Examination for *serum precipitins* against suspected antigens, such as those listed in Table 253-1, is an important part of the diagnostic workup and should be performed on any patient with interstitial lung disease, especially if a suggestive exposure history is elicited. If found, precipitins indicate sufficient exposure to the causative agent for generation of an immunologic response. The diagnosis of HP is not established solely by the presence of precipitins, however, as precipitins are found in sera of many individuals exposed to appropriate antigens who demonstrate no other evidence of HP. False-negative results may occur because of poor-quality antigens or an inappropriate choice of antigens. Extraction of antigens from the suspected source may at times be helpful.

No specific or distinctive *chest roentgenogram* occurs in HP. It can be normal even in symptomatic patients. The acute or subacute phase may be associated with poorly defined, patchy, or diffuse infiltrates or with discrete, nodular infiltrates. In the chronic phase, the chest x-ray usually shows a diffuse reticulonodular infiltrate. Honeycombing may eventually develop as the condition progresses. Abnormalities rarely seen in HP include pleural effusion or thickening, and hilar adenopathy. High-resolution chest computed tomography (CT) has been reported to show a characteristic constellation of abnormalities, including (1) global lung involvement with increased lung density, (2) prominence of medium-sized bronchial walls, (3) patchy air space opacification with reticular and nodular patterns and midzone prominence, and (4) absence of hilar lymph node enlargement. No pathognomonic CT features of HP have been described.

Pulmonary function studies in all forms of HP typically show a restrictive pattern with loss of lung volumes, impaired diffusion capacity, decreased compliance, and an exercise-induced hypoxemia. A resting hypoxemia may be found. Functional abnormalities may gradually increase in severity or may occur rapidly following acute or subacute exposure to antigen.

Bronchoalveolar lavage is used in some centers to aid in diagnostic evaluation, and the characteristic features of the lavage fluid are described above.

Lung biopsy may be indicated in patients without sufficient other criteria to make a definitive diagnosis. The initial biopsy procedure is usually a transbronchial biopsy. In some patients, an open-lung biopsy may be necessary, as this procedure will provide adequate material for pathologic studies whereas transbronchial biopsy may not. Although the histopathology is distinctive, it may not be pathognomonic of HP. When the biopsy is taken during the active phase of disease, typical findings include an interstitial alveolar infiltrate consisting of plasma cells, lymphocytes, and occasional eosinophils and neutrophils, usually with accompanying granulomas. Interstitial fibrosis may be present but most often is mild in earlier stages of the disease. Some degree of bronchiolitis is found in about half the cases, whereas vasculitis is not a feature of the disorder. The triad of mononuclear bronchiolitis; interstitial infiltrates of lymphocytes and plasma cells; and single, nonnecrotizing, and randomly scattered parenchymal granulomas without mural vascular involvement is consistent with but not specific for HP.

The lack of standardized, nonirritating antigens and of proven controlled protocols makes *skin testing* and *inhalational challenge* useful only for research purposes. Similarly, *in vitro tests of cell-mediated (delayed) hypersensitivity* have not consistently been shown to correlate with clinical HP and have no place in the routine diagnostic workup.

In summary, the diagnosis in most cases is established by (1) consistent history, physical findings, pulmonary function tests, and chest x-ray; (2) exposure to a recognized antigen; and (3) finding an antibody to that antigen. In a few circumstances, bronchoalveolar lavage and/or lung biopsy may be needed. Provocation tests are research procedures and are not indicated.

DIFFERENTIAL DIAGNOSIS   Chronic HP may often be difficult to distinguish from a number of other interstitial lung disorders such as idiopathic pulmonary fibrosis, sarcoidosis, interstitial lung disease associated with a collagen vascular disorder, and drug-induced lung diseases. A negative history for use of relevant drugs and no evidence of a systemic disorder usually exclude the presence of drug-induced lung disease or a collagen vascular disorder. Bronchoalveolar lavage often shows predominance of neutrophils in idiopathic pulmonary fibrosis and a predominance of CD4+ lymphocytes in sarcoidosis. The diagnosis of sarcoidosis is also favored by hilar/paratracheal lymphadenopathy or evidence of multisystem involvement. In some patients, a lung biopsy may be required to differentiate chronic HP from other interstitial diseases.

Table 253-1

Selected Examples of Hypersensitivity Pneumonitis (HP)

Disease	Antigen	Source of Antigen
Bagassosis	Thermophilic actinomycetes*	"Moldy" bagasse (sugar cane)
Bird fancier's, breeder's, or handler's lung	Parakeet, budgerigar, pigeon, chicken, turkey proteins	Avian droppings or feathers
Cephalosporium HP	Contaminated basement (sewage)	*Cephalosporium*
Cheese washer's lung	*Penicillium casei*	Moldy cheese
Chemical worker's lung	Isocyanates	Polyurethane foam, varnishes, lacquer, foundry casting
Coffee worker's lung	Coffee bean dust	Coffee beans
Compost lung	*Aspergillus*	Compost
Detergent worker's disease	*Bacillus subtilis* enzymes	Detergent
Familial HP	*Bacillus subtilis*	Contaminated wood dust in walls
Farmer's lung	Thermophilic actinomycetes*	"Moldy" hay, grain, silage
Fish meal worker's lung	Fish meal dust	Fish meal
Furrier's lung	Animal fur dust	Animal pelts
Hot tub lung	*Cladosporium* sp.	Mold on ceiling
Humidifier or air-conditioner lung (ventilation pneumonitis)	*Aureobasidium pullulans* or other microorganisms	Contaminated water in humidification and forced-air air-conditioning systems
Japanese summer house HP	*Trichosporon cutaneum*	House dust? Bird droppings
Laboratory worker's HP	Male rat urine	Laboratory rat
Lycoperdonosis	*Lycoperdon* puffballs	Puffball spores
Malt worker's lung	*Aspergillus fumigatus* or *A. clavatus*	Moldy barley
Maple bark disease	*Cryptostroma corticale*	Maple bark
Miller's lung	*Sitophilus granarius* (wheat weevil)	Infested wheat flour
Mushroom worker's lung	Thermophilic actinomycetes,* other	Mushroom compost
Paulis HP	Paulis reagent	Laboratory reagent
Pituitary snuff taker's lung	Animal proteins	Heterologous pituitary snuff
Potato riddler's lung	Thermophilic actinomycetes,* *Aspergillus*	"Moldy" hay around potatoes
Sauna taker's lung	*Aureobasidium* sp., other	Contaminated sauna water
Sequoiosis	*Aureobasidium*, *Graphium* sp.	Redwood sawdust
Streptomyces albus HP	*Streptomyces albus*	Contaminated fertilizer
Suberosis	Cork dust mold	Cork dust
Tap water lung	Unknown	Contaminated tap water
Thatched roof disease	*Saccharomonospora viridis*	Dried grasses and leaves
Tobacco worker's disease	*Aspergillus* sp.	Mold on tobacco
Winegrower's lung	*Botrytis cinerea*	Mold on grapes
Wood trimmer's disease	*Rhizopus* sp., *Mucor* sp.	Contaminated wood trimmings
Woodman's disease	*Penicillium* sp.	Oak and maple trees
Woodworker's lung	Wood dust; *Alternaria*	Oak, cedar, and mahogany dusts; pine and spruce pulp

* Thermophilic actinomycetes species include *Micropolyspora faeni, Thermoactinomyces vulgaris, T. saccharrii, T. viridis,* and *T. candidus.*

The lung disease associated with acute or subacute HP may clinically resemble other disorders that present with systemic symptoms and recurrent pulmonary infiltrates, including the allergic bronchopulmonary mycoses and other eosinophilic pneumonias. Eosinophilic pneumonia is often associated with asthma and is typified by peripheral eosinophilia; neither of these is a feature of HP. Allergic bronchopulmonary aspergillosis (ABPA) is the most common example of the allergic bronchopulmonary mycoses and is sometimes confused with HP because of the presence of precipitating antibodies to *Aspergillus fumigatus*. ABPA is an obstructive rather than a restrictive lung disease, however, and is associated with allergic (atopic) asthma.

The term *organic dust toxic syndrome* (ODTS) has been applied to a condition that is more common than HP and is often mistaken for it; it follows heavy exposure to organic dusts and is characterized by transient fever and muscle aches, with or without respiratory symptoms. Serum precipitins are absent, and the chest x-ray is usually normal. Studies have shown no immunologic basis for ODTS. Endotoxin may be involved in its pathogenesis.

Massive exposure to moldy silage may result in a syndrome termed *pulmonary mycotoxicosis*, or *atypical farmer's lung*, with fever, chills, and cough and the presence of pulmonary infiltrates within a few hours of exposure. No previous sensitization is required, and precipitins are absent to *Aspergillus*, the suspected causative agent.

℞ **TREATMENT**

Because effective treatment depends largely on avoiding the antigen, identification of the causative agent and its source is essential. This is usually possible if the physician takes a careful environmental and occupational history or, if necessary, visits the patient's environment.

The simplest way to avoid the incriminated agent is to remove the patient from the environment or the source of the agent from the patient's environment. This recommendation cannot be taken lightly when it completely changes the life-style or livelihood of the patient. In many cases, however, the source of exposure (birds, humidifiers) can easily be removed. If occupational exposure is involved, an initial attempt can be made at antigen avoidance maneuvers least disruptive to the patient's livelihood, which usually means avoiding areas associated with heavy exposure and wearing an appropriate mask. This will not suffice for small-molecular-weight agents such as isocyanates, which require more elaborate respiratory systems. Pollen masks, personal dust respirators, air-stream helmets, and ventilated helmets with a supply of fresh air are increasingly efficient means of purifying inhaled air. If symptoms recur or physiologic abnormalities progress in spite of these measures, then more effective measures to avoid antigen exposure must be pursued.

Compromises with environmental control pertain primarily to the acute, recurrent, transient clinical form of HP and must be accompanied by careful follow-up. Subacute forms are ordinarily the result of a heavy, sustained exposure. The chronic form typically results from low-grade or recurrent exposure over many months to years, and the lung disease may already be partially irreversible. These patients are usually advised to avoid completely all possible contact with the offending agent, although follow-up studies of farmer's lung and bird fancier's lung have found resolution of the disease despite continued exposure in some patients.

Patients with the *acute*, recurrent form of HP usually recover without need for glucocorticoids. *Subacute* HP may be associated with severe symptoms and marked physiologic impairment and may continue to progress for several days despite hospitalization. Urgent establishment of the diagnosis and prompt institution of glucocorticoid treatment are indicated in such patients. Such therapy may also hasten recovery in patients with lesser involvement. Prednisone at a dosage of 1 mg/kg per day or its equivalent is continued for 7 to 14 days and then tapered over the ensuing 2 to 6 weeks at a rate that depends on the patient's clinical status.

Patients with *chronic* HP may gradually recover without therapy following environmental control. In many patients, however, a trial of prednisone may be useful to obtain maximal reversibility of the lung disease. Following initial prednisone therapy (1 mg/kg per day for 2 to 4 weeks), the drug is tapered to the lowest dosage that will maintain the functional status of the patient. Many patients will not require or benefit from long-term therapy if there is no further exposure to antigen. Available studies report no effect of glucocorticoid therapy on long-term prognosis of farmer's lung.

EOSINOPHILIC PNEUMONIAS

Eosinophilic pneumonias are composed of distinct individual syndromes characterized by eosinophilic pulmonary infiltrates and, commonly, peripheral blood eosinophilia. Since Loeffler's initial description of a transient, benign syndrome of migratory pulmonary infiltrates and peripheral blood eosinophilia of unknown cause, this group of disorders has been enlarged to include several diseases of both known and unknown etiology (Table 253-2). These diseases may be considered as putative hypersensitivity lung diseases but are not to be confused with HP (extrinsic allergic alveolitis), in which eosinophilia is not a feature.

When an eosinophilic pneumonia is associated with bronchial asthma, it is important to determine if the patient has extrinsic (allergic, atopic) asthma and has wheal-and-flare skin reactivity to *Aspergillus* or other relevant fungal antigens. If so, other criteria should be sought for diagnosis of allergic bronchopulmonary aspergillosis (ABPA) (Table 253-3) or other, rarer examples of allergic bronchopulmonary mycosis such as those caused by *Penicillium*, *Candida*, *Curvularia*, or *Helminthosporium* spp. *Aspergillus fumigatus* is the most common cause of ABPA, although other *Aspergillus* species have also been implicated. ABPA has been reported to complicate cystic fibrosis. The chest roentgenogram in ABPA may show transient, recurrent infiltrates or may suggest the presence of proximal bronchiectasis. High-resolution chest CT is a sensitive, noninvasive technique for the recognition of proximal bronchiectasis. The bronchial asthma of ABPA likely involves an IgE-mediated hypersensitivity, whereas the bronchiectasis associated with this disorder is thought to result from a deposition of immune complexes in proximal airways. Adequate treatment usually requires the long-term use of systemic glucocorticoids.

Tropical eosinophilia is usually caused by filarial infection; however, eosinophilic pneumonias also occur with other parasites such as *Ascaris*, *Ancyclostoma* sp., *Toxocara* sp., and *Strongyloides stercoralis*. Tropical eosinophilia due to *Wuchereria bancrofti* or *Wuchereria malayi* occurs most commonly in southern Asia, Africa, and South America, and is treated successfully with diethylcarbamazine.

Drug-induced eosinophilic pneumonias are exemplified by acute reactions to nitrofurantoin, which may begin 2 h to 10 days after nitrofurantoin is started, with symptoms of dry cough, fever, chills, and dyspnea; an eosinophilic pleural effusion accompanying patchy or diffuse pulmonary infiltrates may also occur. Other drugs associated with eosinophilic pneumonias include sulfonamides, penicillin, chlorpropamide, thiazides, tricyclic antidepressants, hydralazine, meph-

Table 253-2

Eosinophilic Pneumonias

ETIOLOGY KNOWN

Allergic bronchopulmonary mycoses
Parasitic infestations
Drug reactions
Eosinophilia-myalgia syndrome

IDIOPATHIC

Loeffler's syndrome
Acute eosinophilic pneumonia
Chronic eosinophilic pneumonia
Allergic granulomatosis of Churg and Strauss
Hypereosinophilic syndrome

Table 253-3

Diagnostic Features of Allergic Bronchopulmonary Aspergillosis (ABPA)

MAIN DIAGNOSTIC CRITERIA

Bronchial asthma
Pulmonary infiltrates
Peripheral eosinophilia ($>1000/\mu L$)
Immediate wheal-and-flare response to *Aspergillus fumigatus*
Serum precipitins to *A. fumigatus*
Elevated serum IgE
Central bronchiectasis

OTHER DIAGNOSTIC FEATURES

History of brownish plugs in sputum
Culture of *A. fumigatus* from sputum
Elevated IgE (and IgG) class antibodies specific for *A. fumigatus*

enesin, mecamylamine, nickel carbonyl vapor, gold salts, isoniazid, para-aminosalicylic acid, and others. Treatment consists of withdrawal of the incriminated drugs and the use of glucocorticoids, if necessary.

The eosinophilia-myalgia syndrome, caused by dietary supplements of L-tryptophan, is occasionally associated with pulmonary infiltrates.

The group of idiopathic eosinophilic pneumonias consists of diseases of varying severity. *Loeffler's syndrome* was originally reported as a benign, acute eosinophilic pneumonia of unknown cause characterized by migrating pulmonary infiltrates and minimal clinical manifestations. In some patients, these clinical characteristics may prove to be secondary to parasites or drugs. *Acute eosinophilic pneumonia* has been described recently as an idiopathic acute febrile illness of less than 7 days' duration with severe hypoxemia, pulmonary infiltrates, and no history of asthma. *Chronic eosinophilic pneumonia* presents with significant systemic symptoms including fever, chills, night sweats, cough, anorexia, and weight loss of several weeks' to months' duration. The chest x-ray classically shows peripheral infiltrates resembling a photographic negative of pulmonary edema. Some patients also have bronchial asthma of the intrinsic or nonallergic type. Dramatic clearing of symptoms and chest x-rays is often noted within 48 h after initiation of glucocorticoid therapy.

Allergic angiitis and granulomatosis of Churg and Strauss is a multisystem vasculitic disorder that frequently involves the skin, kidney, and nervous system in addition to the lung (Chap. 319). The disorder may occur at any age and favors persons with a history of bronchial asthma. The asthma often is progressive until the onset of fever and exaggerated eosinophilia, at which time the symptoms of asthma may ease. The illness may be fulminating and the prognosis grave unless treated aggressively with glucocorticoids and, at times, immunosuppressive therapy.

The *hypereosinophilic syndrome* is characterized by presence of over 1500 eosinophils per microliter of peripheral blood for 6 months or longer; lack of evidence for parasitic, allergic, or other known causes of eosinophilia; and signs or symptoms of multisystem organ dysfunction. Consistent features are blood and bone marrow eosinophilia with tissue infiltration by relatively mature eosinophils. The heart may be involved with tricuspid valve abnormalities or endomyocardial fibrosis and a restrictive, biventricular cardiomyopathy. Other organs affected typically include the lungs, liver, spleen, skin, and nervous system. Therapy of the disorder consists of glucocorticoids and/or hydroxyurea, plus therapy as needed for cardiac dysfunction, which is frequently responsible for much of the morbidity and mortality in this syndrome.

BIBLIOGRAPHY

HYPERSENSITIVITY PNEUMONITIS

DENIS M: Proinflammatory cytokines in hypersensitivity pneumonitis. Am J Respir Crit Care Med 151:164, 1995
GURNEY JW et al: Agricultural disorders of the lung. Radiographics 11:625, 1991

KOKKARINEN JI et al: Recovery of pulmonary function in farmer's lung. A five-year followup study. Am Rev Respir Dis 147:793, 1993
MARX JJ et al: Cohort studies of immunologic lung disease among Wisconsin dairy farmers. Am J Int Med 18:263, 1990
RICHERSON HB: Hypersensitivity pneumonitis, in *Organic Dusts: Exposure, Effects, and Prevention,* R Rylander, RR Jacobs (eds). Boca Raton, FL, CRC Press, 1994, pp 139–160
——— et al: Guidelines for the clinical evaluation of hypersensitivity pneumonitis. J Allergy Clin Immunol 84:839, 1989
ROSE C, KING TE: Controversies in hypersensitivity pneumonitis. Am Rev Respir Dis 145:1, 1992
SHARMA OP: Hypersensitivity pneumonitis. Dis-Mo 37:409, 1991

EOSINOPHILIC PNEUMONIA

BUCHEIT J et al: Acute eosinophilic pneumonia with respiratory failure: A new syndrome? Am Rev Respir Dis 145:716, 1992
FISESELMANN JF, RICHERSON HB: Respiratory diseases, in *Basic and Clinical Immunology,* 8th ed, DP Stites, AI Terr, TG Parslow (eds). Norwalk, CT, Appleton & Lange, 1994, pp 528–540
HAYAKAWA H et al: A clinical study of idiopathic eosinophilic pneumonia. Chest 105:1462, 1994
MROUEH S, SPOCK A: Allergic bronchopulmonary aspergillosis in patients with cystic fibrosis. Chest 105:32, 1994
PATTERSON R, GREENBERGER PA, ROBERTS ML (eds): *Allergic Bronchopulmonary Aspergillosis.* Providence, RI, OceanSide Pub, 1995
ROSENOW ECIII et al: Drug-induced pulmonary disease: An update. Chest 102:239, 1992

254   *Frank E. Speizer*

ENVIRONMENTAL LUNG DISEASES

This chapter provides perspectives on ways to assess pulmonary diseases for which environmental causes are suspected. This assessment is important because removal of the patient from a harmful environment is often the only intervention that might prevent further significant deterioration or lead to improvement in a patient's condition. Furthermore, the identification of an environment-associated disease in a single patient may lead to primary preventive strategies affecting other similarly exposed people who have not yet developed disease.

The exact magnitude of the problem is unknown, but there is no question that large numbers of people are at risk of developing serious respiratory disease as a result of occupational or environmental exposures. For example, recent estimates suggest that approximately 2.3 million workers in the United States have been exposed to crystalline silica or asbestos dust in mining and nonmining industries. Even if only 5 percent of these workers (a conservative estimate) are to suffer from respiratory disease as a result of their exposure, this figure represents more than 100,000 individuals.

Although industries are required to spend substantial amounts of capital in efforts to protect their workers, occupationally related respiratory diseases continue to occur. These diseases are often attributed to exposures in the past, at a time when we were not aware of the risk incurred and the need for worker protection to the degree that we are today.

HISTORY AND PHYSICAL EXAMINATION   The patient's history is of paramount importance in assessing any potential occupational or environmental exposure and the physician must ask the patient to describe a suspected environmental exposure in detail.

Inquiry into specific work practices should include questions about specific contaminants involved, the availability and use of personal respiratory protection devices, the size and ventilation of workspaces, and whether coworkers have similar complaints. In addition, the patient must be questioned about alternative sources for potentially toxic exposures, including hobbies or other environmental exposures at home. Short-term exposures to potential toxic agents in the distant past also must be considered (see Chap. 390).

Many people are aware of the potential hazards in their workplaces, and many states require that employees be informed about potentially hazardous exposures. These requirements include the provision of specific educational materials (including Material Safety Data Sheets), personal protective equipment and instructions in its use, and information on environmental control procedures. Reminders posted in the workplace may warn workers about hazardous substances. Protective clothing, lockers, and shower facilities may be considered necessary parts of the job. However, even in these more progressive industries, the introduction of new processes, particularly when related to the use of new chemical compounds, may change exposure significantly, and often only the employee on the production line is aware of the change. For the physician who regularly sees patients from a particular industry, a visit to the work site can be very instructive. Alternatively, physicians can request inspections by appropriate federal and/or state authorities.

The physical examination of patients with environment-related lung diseases may help to determine the nature and severity of the pulmonary condition. Unfortunately, the pulmonary response to most injurious agents is the development of a limited number of nonspecific physical signs. These findings do not point to the specific causative agent, and other types of information must be used to arrive at an etiologic diagnosis.

PULMONARY FUNCTION TESTS AND CHEST RADIOGRAPHY   Many mineral dusts produce characteristic alterations in the mechanics of breathing and lung volumes that clearly indicate a restrictive pattern (Chaps. 250 and 259). Exposures to a number of organic dusts or chemical agents capable of producing occupational asthma result in pronounced obstructive patterns of pulmonary dysfunction that may be reversible (Chap. 252). Measurement of change in forced expiratory volume (FEV_1) before and after a working shift can be used to detect an acute inflammatory or bronchoconstrictive response. An acute decrement of FEV_1 over the Monday work shift is a characteristic feature of cotton textile workers with byssinosis.

The chest radiograph is useful in detecting and monitoring the pulmonary response to mineral dusts. The International Labour Organization (ILO) International Classification of Radiographs of Pneumoconioses classifies chest radiographs according to the nature and size of opacities seen and the extent of involvement of the parenchyma. In general, opacities may be round or irregular, small (<10 mm in diameter) or large. They may be few in number, with visible normal lung markings, partially obscure normal markings, or totally obscure normal markings. Although useful for screening large numbers of workers, the ILO system lacks specificity and may over- or underestimate the functional impact of pneumoconiosis. With dusts causing rounded, regular opacities like those evident in coal worker's pneumoconiosis, the degree of involvement on the chest radiograph may be extensive, while pulmonary function may be only minimally impaired. In contrast, in pneumoconiosis causing linear, irregular opacities like those seen in asbestosis, the radiograph may lead to underestimation of the severity of the impairment. It is possible for a patient to have a history of exposure, a moderately reduced forced vital capacity (FVC), and a reduced diffusion capacity in asbestosis with a relatively normal chest radiograph. The radiographic findings of irregular or linear opacities are simply more difficult to separate from normal markings until relatively late in the disease. When shadows become large, the condition is termed *complicated pneumoconiosis*, sometimes called progressive massive fibrosis (PMF). For the individual patient with a history of exposure, conventional computed tomography (CT) and high-resolution computed tomography (HRCT) have improved the sensitivity of identifying diffuse parenchymal abnormalities of the lung. The procedures have been shown to provide earlier detection of silicosis and asbestosis.

Other diagnostic procedures of use in identifying environment-induced lung disease include evaluation of heavy metal concentrations

in urine (arsenic in smelter workers, cadmium in battery plant workers); bacteriologic studies (tuberculosis in medical care personnel, anthrax in wool sorters); fungal studies (coccidioidomycosis in southwestern farm workers, histoplasmosis in poultry or pigeon handlers); and serologic studies (psittacosis in pet shop workers or owners of sick birds, Q fever in tanners or slaughterhouse workers). Ultimately, a lung biopsy may be required both for morphologic diagnosis of the underlying pulmonary disease and for attempted identification of the specific etiologic agent.

MEASUREMENT OF EXPOSURE   If reliable environmental sampling data are available, this information should be used in assessing a patient's exposure. Since many of the chronic diseases result from exposure over many years, current environmental measurements should be combined with work histories to arrive at estimates of past exposure. Even in acute conditions, when monitoring of exposure may be possible, little may be known about the actual dose received by the lung. Most of the research on health effects of air pollutants (discussed later in this chapter) has relied on fixed-station monitoring of outdoor air, often at locations somewhat distant from the residences of the people being studied. In addition, most people spend less than 20 percent of their time outdoors. Therefore, outdoor measurements can be used only in a relative sense, and they cannot be relied on to estimate actual dose.

In situations where individual exposure to specific agents—either in a work setting or via ambient air pollutants—has been determined, transport of these agents through the airways may be an important factor affecting dose. Highly soluble gases such as sulfur dioxide are absorbed in the upper airway and presumably produce their effects by reflex response of sensitive neural fibrils in the trachea or larger airways. In contrast, nitrogen dioxide, which is less soluble, may reach the bronchioles and alveoli in sufficient quantities to result in an acute life-threatening disease in farmers exposed even briefly to the gas evolved from moldy hay in silos (silo-filler's disease).

Particle size and chemistry of air contaminants also must be considered. Particles above 10 to 15 μm in diameter, because of their settling velocities in air, do not penetrate beyond the upper airways. These larger particles are often referred to as "fugitive dusts" and include pollens, other windblown dusts, and dusts resulting from mechanical industrial processes. They have little or no role in chronic respiratory disease except perhaps as related to cancer (see below).

Particles below 10 μm in size are created by the burning of fossil fuels or high-temperature industrial processes resulting in condensation products from gases, fumes, or vapors. These particles are divided into two size fractions on the basis of their chemical characteristics. Particles of approximately 2.5 to 10 μm (coarse-mode fraction) contain crustal elements, such as silica, aluminum, and iron. These particles mostly deposit relatively high in the tracheobronchial tree. Particles of less than approximately 2.5 μm (fine-mode fraction or accumulation mode) contain sulfates, nitrates, and organic compounds. The fine-mode particles more often deposit in the terminal bronchioles and alveoli. The smallest particles, those less than 0.1 μm in size, remain in the airstream and deposit in the lung only on a random basis as they come into contact with the alveolar walls.

Besides the size characteristics of particles and the solubility of gases, the actual chemical composition, mechanical properties, and immunogenicity or infectivity of inhaled material determine in large part the nature of the diseases found among exposed persons.

OCCUPATIONAL EXPOSURES AND PULMONARY DISEASE

ASBESTOSIS   Except in localized regions with single industrial exposures, such as coal-mining or granite-quarrying regions, the most frequent inorganic dust–related chronic pulmonary diseases are associated with industries using *asbestiform fibers*. *Asbestos* is a generic term for several different mineral silicates, including chrysolite, amosite, anthophyllite, and crocidolite. Besides workers involved in the mining, milling, and manufacturing of asbestos products, workers in the building trades, including pipe fitters and boilermakers, were exposed to asbestos, which was widely used in construction because of its exceptional thermal and electric insulation properties. In addition, asbestos was used in the manufacture of fire-smothering blankets and safety garments, as filler for plastic materials, in cement and floor tiles, and in friction materials, such as brake and clutch linings.

Exposure to asbestos is not limited to persons who directly handle the material. Cases of asbestos-related diseases have been encountered in individuals with only moderate exposure, such as the painter or electrician who works alongside the insulation worker in a shipyard or the housewife who does no more than shake out and wash her husband's work clothes. Community exposure has probably resulted from the use of asbestos-containing material sprayed on steel girders in many large buildings as a safety feature to prevent buckling in case of fire.

Asbestos was first used extensively in the 1940s. Starting in 1975 it was mostly replaced with synthetic mineral fibers, such as fiberglass or slag wool. However, asbestos is still used in the manufacture of brake linings and remains as pipe and boiler insulation in hundreds of thousands of workplaces and homes. Despite current regulations mandating adequate training for any worker potentially exposed to asbestos, exposure probably continues among inexperienced demolition workers. The major health effects from exposure to asbestos are pulmonary fibrosis (asbestosis) and cancers of the respiratory tract, the pleura, and (in rare cases) the peritoneum.

Asbestosis is a diffuse interstitial fibrosing disease of the lung that is directly related to the intensity and duration of exposure. Except for its association with a history of exposure to asbestos (generally in a work setting), asbestosis resembles the other forms of diffuse interstitial fibrosis (Chap. 259). Usually, moderate to severe exposure has taken place for at least 10 years before the disease becomes manifest.

Physiologic studies reveal a restrictive pattern with a decrease in lung volumes. Flow rates are commonly reduced less than would be predicted on the basis of the volume reduction. An early sign of severe disease may be a reduction in diffusing capacity.

Pulmonary fibrosis may occur following sufficient exposure to any of the asbestiform fiber types. The fibrotic lesions do not appear to relate to either shape or chemical composition of any fiber type. During phagocytosis of the asbestos fiber, the membrane of the macrophage is damaged and this damage results in the release of lysosomes containing enzymes that may act to damage the lung parenchyma. The clinical manifestations are typical of those physical findings in any patient with pulmonary fibrosis (Chap. 259).

Diagnosis The chest radiograph can be used to detect a number of manifestations of asbestos exposure as well as to identify specific lesions. Past exposure is specifically indicated by pleural plaques, which are characterized by either thickening or calcification along the parietal pleura, particularly along the lower lung fields, the diaphragm, and the cardiac border. Without additional manifestations, pleural plaques imply only exposure, not pulmonary impairment. Benign pleural effusions may occur, particularly in patients with asbestosis, but are not necessarily restricted to those with overt disease. The fluid is sterile but may be a serous or blood-stained exudate and may occur bilaterally. The effusion may be slowly progressive or may resolve spontaneously.

The radiographic diagnosis of asbestosis depends on the presence of irregular or linear opacities, usually first noted in the lower lung fields and spreading into the middle and upper lung fields as the disease progresses. An indistinct heart border or a "ground glass" appearance in the lung fields is seen in some cases. As the fibrotic changes in the parenchyma begin to coalesce, the patient develops obliteration of entire acinar units, with eventual formation of the classical honey-combed lung, which appears on chest radiographs as coarse infiltrates with small (about 7- to 10-μm) air spaces. In cases in which the x-ray changes are less obvious, HRCT may show distinct changes of subpleural curvilinear lines 5 to 10 cm in length that appear to be parallel to the pleural surface; these alterations increase the positive predictive value of radiographic evidence from approximately 85 percent to about 100 percent.

In general, newly diagnosed cases will have resulted from exposure levels that were present many years before and, in spite of the patients' having left the industry, are attributable to that former exposure. Since the patient may be eligible for compensation within a specific time frame after the diagnosis of an asbestos-related disease is made, the physician making the diagnosis should be certain to inform the patient promptly. On occasion, the physician may have reason to suspect ongoing exposure from a patient's current job description or actual monitoring data. In such cases, federal or state health authorities may need to be notified. Present-day occupational safety and health regulations, if followed properly, protect workers from exposure.

Casual, nonoccupational exposure to undisturbed sources of asbestos-containing materials—e.g., in walls of schools or other buildings—represents little if any hazard to people who inhabit or work in such buildings. Because the association of smoking and asbestos exposure increases the risk of developing lung cancer (see below), it is extremely important to advise patients with a history of exposure to asbestos to stop smoking. No specific therapy is available in the management of patients with asbestosis. The supportive care is the same as that given to any patient with diffuse interstitial fibrosis from any cause.

Lung cancer (Chap. 90), either squamous cell carcinoma or adenocarcinoma, is the most frequent cancer associated with asbestos exposure. The excess frequency of lung cancer in asbestos workers is associated with a minimum lapse of 15 to 19 years between first exposure and development of the disease. Persons with more exposure are at greater risk of disease. In addition, there appears to be a significant multiplicative effect that leads to a far greater risk of lung cancer in persons who are cigarette smokers and have asbestos exposure than would be expected from the additive risk of each factor. To date, efforts to consider these high-risk individuals for special surveillance studies, including sputum cytologic examinations and repeated chest x-rays as frequently as every 4 to 6 months, have resulted in neither significant early detection nor prolonged survival once the lung cancer is found.

Mesotheliomas (Chap. 262), both pleural and peritoneal, are also associated with asbestos exposure. In contrast to lung cancers, these tumors do not appear to be associated with smoking. Relatively short-term asbestos exposures of 1 to 2 years or less occurring some 20 to 25 years in the past have been associated with the development of mesotheliomas (an observation that emphasizes the importance of obtaining a complete environmental exposure history). The risk for this type of tumor peaks 30 to 35 years after initial exposure. Although approximately 50 percent of mesotheliomas metastasize, the tumor generally is locally invasive, and death usually results from local extension. Most patients present with effusions that may obscure the underlying pleural tumor. In contrast to the findings in effusion due to other causes, because of the restriction placed on the chest wall, no shift of mediastinal structures toward the opposite side of the chest will be seen. The major diagnostic problem is differentiation from peripherally spreading pulmonary adenocarcinoma or from adenocarcinoma metastasized to pleura from an extrathoracic primary site. Although a needle biopsy may be diagnostic, an open biopsy is often necessary, and even the latter procedure may not provide a definitive diagnosis of the origin of the tumor.

Since epidemiologic studies have shown that more than 80 percent of mesotheliomas may be associated with asbestos exposure, documented mesothelioma in a worker with occupational exposure to asbestos may be compensable in many parts of the United States.

SILICOSIS In spite of the technical adequacy of existing protective equipment, *free silica* (SiO_2), or crystalline quartz, is still a major occupational hazard. In the United States, estimates of potential numbers of exposed workers range between 1.2 and 3 million people. The major occupational exposures include mining, stonecutting, employment in abrasive industries, foundry work, packing of silica flour, and quarrying, particularly of granite. Most often, progressive pulmonary fibrosis (silicosis) occurs in a dose-response fashion after many years of exposure.

Workers exposed through sandblasting in confined spaces, tunneling through rock with high quartz content (15 to 25 percent), or the manufacture of abrasive soaps may develop acute silicosis with as little as 10 months' exposure. The disease may be rapidly fatal in less than 2 years, despite the discontinuation of exposure. A radiographic picture of profuse miliary infiltration or consolidation is characteristic of acute silicosis.

In long-term, less intense exposure, small rounded opacities in the upper lobes, with retraction and hilar adenopathy, classically appear on the radiograph after 15 to 20 years. Calcification of hilar nodes may occur in as many as 20 percent of cases and produces the characteristic "eggshell" pattern. These changes may be preceded by or associated with a reticular pattern of irregular densities that are uniformly present throughout the upper lung zones.

The nodular fibrosis may be progressive in the absence of further exposure, with coalescence and formation of nonsegmental conglomerates of irregular masses in excess of 1 cm in diameter. These masses become quite large and are characteristic of PMF. Significant functional impairment with both restrictive and obstructive components may be associated with this form of silicosis. In the late stages of the disease, ventilatory failure may develop. In more subtle cases, CT may be helpful both in identifying nodules, which are preferentially located in the posterior aspect of the upper lobes, as well as in identifying larger opacities and more coalescence than might be noted on regular chest x-rays. Patients with silicosis are at greater risk of acquiring *Mycobacterium tuberculosis* infections (silicotuberculosis) and atypical mycobacterial infections. Because the frequency with which tuberculosis has been found at autopsy in patients with PMF exceeds considerably the frequency of premorbid diagnosis, treatment for tuberculosis is indicated in any patient with silicosis and a positive tuberculin test.

Other less hazardous silicates include Fuller's earth, kaolin, mica, diatomaceous earths, silica gel, soapstone, carbonate dusts, and cement dusts. The production of fibrosis in workers exposed to these agents is believed to be related to either the free silica content of these dusts or, for substances that contain no free silica, to the potentially large dust loads to which these workers may be exposed.

Other silicates, including *talc dusts*, may be contaminated with asbestos and/or free silica. Accidental exposure to significant quantities of talc may result in an acute syndrome with cough, cyanosis, and labored breathing (acute talcosis). Severe progressive fibrosis with respiratory failure may ensue within a few years. Far more common is the fibrosis and/or pleural or lung cancer associated with chronic exposure in rubber workers who use commercial talc as a lubricant in tire molds. Pure talc does not produce fibrosis; thus it is difficult to sort out whether the effects are due to the contamination of commercial talc by asbestos or by free silica.

COAL WORKER'S PNEUMOCONIOSIS (CWP)   *Coal dust* is associated with CWP, which has enormous social, economic, and medical significance in every nation in which coal mining is an important industry. Simple radiographically identified CWP is seen in 12 percent of all miners and in as many as 50 percent of anthracite miners with more than 20 years' work on the coal face. The prevalence of disease is lower in workers in bituminous coal mines. Since much western U.S. coal is bituminous, CWP is less prevalent in that region.

Much of the symptomatology associated with simple CWP appears to be similar and additive to the effects of cigarette smoking on the development of chronic bronchitis and obstructive lung disease (Chap. 258). In the early stages of simple CWP, radiographic abnormalities consist of small, irregular opacities (reticular pattern). With prolonged exposure, one sees small, rounded, regular opacities, 1 to 5 mm in diameter (nodular pattern). Calcification is generally not seen, although approximately 10 percent of older anthracite miners have calcified nodules.

Complicated CWP is manifested by the appearance on the chest radiograph of nodules ranging from 1 cm in diameter to the size of

an entire lobe, generally confined to the upper half of the lungs. This condition, considered a form of PMF, is accompanied by a significant reduction in diffusing capacity and is associated with premature mortality. In contrast to patients with silicosis, underground miners with simple CWP develop PMF at a rate of only 5 to 15 percent, depending on the type of coal.

The mechanism whereby PMF occurs in CWP is not fully understood. Several hypotheses have been proposed, including (1) sufficient free silica is present in the dust, (2) normal clearance mechanisms are unable to clear the excessive dust loads, (3) an interplay occurs between an intrinsic immunologic mechanism and the dust and/or damaged lung tissue, and (4) atypical reactions to *M. tuberculosis* occur. As previously described, PMF in silicosis is associated with prolonged duration and high intensity of exposure to free silica. Heavy exposure to carbon particles free of silica occurs in carbon black, graphite, and charcoal workers. The prolonged exposure of these workers may result in sufficient accumulation of carbon in the lung to produce PMF. The mechanism appears to relate to a breakdown of the clearance capacity of the airways.

Caplan's syndrome, which includes seropositive rheumatoid arthritis with characteristic PMF, is consistent with an immunopathologic mechanism. The syndrome was first described in coal miners but subsequently has been found in patients with a variety of pneumoconioses.

BERYLLIOSIS   Beryllium may produce an acute pneumonitis or, far more commonly, a chronic interstitial pneumonitis. Unless one inquires specifically about occupational exposures to beryllium in the manufacture of alloys, ceramics, high-technology electronics, and (before the 1950s) the production of fluorescent lights, one may miss entirely the etiologic relationship to an occupational exposure. Nonspecific pulmonary function tests may be normal or may indicate evidence of restrictive disease. Between 2 and 15 years of exposure, depending on its intensity, are required for the disease to become manifest. On open lung biopsy, granulomatous formation similar to that seen in sarcoidosis (Chap. 320) may make differentiation impossible unless tissue levels of beryllium are measured.

Rarely, other hard metals, including aluminum powders, chromium, cobalt, titanium dioxide, and tungsten, may produce an interstitial pneumonitis.

OTHER INORGANIC DUSTS   Other dusts are considered *nuisance dusts* because their major impact seems to be reduction in visibility and irritation of eyes, ears, nasal passages, and other mucous membranes. If they penetrate to the lower airways, these dusts do not affect the architecture of the terminal bronchioles or acinar spaces nor do they destroy collagen. Generally, clinical effects are reversible. Pulmonary function tests are usually normal unless another disease process coexists. If the dusts are radiodense, macular collections may produce striking radiographic pictures that are so characteristic that patients with a history of significant exposure are easily diagnosed as having the condition that bears the name reflecting the nature of the dust. Examples of radiodense dusts include iron and iron oxides from welding or silver finishing (*siderosis*); tin oxide used in metallurgy, color stabilization, printing, and the manufacture of porcelain, glass, and fabric (*stannosis*); and barium sulfate used as a catalyst for organic reactions, drilling mud components, and electroplating (*baritosis*). Other metal dusts producing similar radiodense pictures include *cerium dioxide* and *antimony salts*.

Most of the inorganic dusts discussed thus far are associated with the production of either dust macules or interstitial fibrotic changes in the lung. Another set of dusts (see Table 254-1), along with some of the dusts previously discussed, is associated with chronic mucous hypersecretion (chronic bronchitis), with or without reduction of expiratory flow rates. These conditions may be caused by cigarette smoking, and any effort to attribute some component of the disease to occupational and environmental exposures must take cigarette smoking into account. Most studies suggest an additive effect of dust exposure and smoking. The pattern of the effect is similar to that of cigarette smoking, suggesting that small airway inflammation may be the initial site of pathologic response in those cases as-

Table 254-1

CHAPTER 254
Environmental Lung Diseases **1433**

Selected Occupational Dusts Believed to be Associated with Mucous Hypersecretion and/or Obstructive Airway Disease and Other Respiratory Diseases*

Agent (Exposure)	Mucous Hypersecretion	Obstruction	Other Conditions†
INORGANIC DUSTS			
Antimony (storage batteries, solder, ceramics, glass, plastics)	X		P
Arsenic (manufacture of pesticides, pigments, glass, alloys)	X		C
Barium and compounds including BaO, BaSO₄, BaCO₃ (catalysts, drilling mud, electroplating)	X		P
Cadmium dust (electroplating, battery manufacture, welding, smelting, aluminum soldering)	X	X	P
Cement dust (construction trades, manufacture of cement blocks)	X	X	
Chromium and CrO₃, CrF₂ (corrosion inhibitor pigment, metallurgy, electroplating)	X		C
Coal dust (mining)	X		P
Coke oven emissions (retort house, coke ovens)	X	X	P, C
Graphite (steelmaking, lubricants, pencils, paints, stove polish)	X	X	P
Iron dust (steel and nonferrous foundry workers, welding)	X		P
Mica (insulation, roofing shingles, oil refining, rubber manufacturing)	X		P
Phosphorus, elemental chlorides, sulfides (manufacture of fireworks, agricultural chemicals, insecticides, pesticides)	X	X	
Rock dusts (miners, tunnelers, quarry workers)	X		P
Vanadium pentoxide (welding electrodes, additive to steel, by-product in ash from oil burning)	X	X	
ORGANIC DUSTS (see Chap. 253)			
Cotton dust, flax, hemp (manufacture of yarns for linen, rope, cotton; ginning, cottonseed crushing; waste fiber processing)	X	X	
Grain dusts (farmers, workers in grain elevators, barge and grain ship crew members)	X	X	
Moldy hay (farmers, other animal attendants)	X		HP

* The table excludes agents associated with asthma as the primary disease (see Chap. 252).
† Other conditions include hypersensitivity pneumonitis (HP), pneumoconiosis (P), and cancers (C).

NOTE: X indicates that mucous hypersecretion or obstruction is associated with exposure.

sociated with the development of obstructive lung disease. Cigarette smoke is usually the more noxious agent, and dust effects may be discernible only in nonsmokers.

ORGANIC DUSTS Some of the specific diseases associated with organic dusts are discussed in detail in the chapters on asthma (Chap. 252) and hypersensitivity pneumonitis (Chap. 253). Many of these diseases are named for the specific setting in which they are found, e.g., farmer's lung, malt worker's disease, or mushroom worker's disease. Occupational and other environmental exposures must be sought when these conditions are suspected. Often the temporal relation of symptoms to exposure furnishes the best evidence for the diagnosis. Three occupational groups are singled out for discussion because they represent the largest proportion of people affected by the diseases resulting from organic dusts.

Cotton Dust (Byssinosis) Estimates of the number of exposed persons in the United States vary, but probably over 800,000 persons are exposed occupationally to cotton, flax, or hemp in the production of yarns for cotton, linen, and rope making. Although this discussion focuses on cotton, the same syndrome—albeit somewhat less severe—has been reported in association with exposure to flax, hemp, and jute.

Exposure occurs throughout the manufacturing process but is most pronounced in those portions of the factory involved with the treatment of the cotton prior to spinning—i.e., blowing, mixing, and carding (straightening of fibers). Attempts to control dust levels by use of exhaust hoods, general increases in ventilation, and wetting procedures in some settings have been highly successful. However, respiratory protective equipment appears to be required during certain operations to prevent workers from being exposed to levels of dust that exceed the current U.S. cotton dust standard.

Byssinosis is characterized clinically as occasional (early stage) and then regular (late stage) chest tightness toward the end of the first day of the workweek ("Monday chest tightness"). In epidemiologic studies, depending on the level of exposure via the carding room air, up to 80 percent of employees may show a significant drop in their FEV_1 over the course of a Monday shift.

Initially the symptoms do not recur on subsequent days of the week. However, in 10 to 25 percent of workers, the disease may be progressive, with chest tightness recurring or persisting throughout the workweek. After more than 10 years of exposure, workers with recurrent symptoms are more likely to have an obstructive pattern on pulmonary function testing. These higher grades of impairment are seen in workers exposed both to high levels of dust and for greater durations. There is an additive effect of cotton dust exposure plus cigarette smoking. The highest grades of impairment are generally seen in smokers.

Treatment in the early stages of the disease is directed toward reversing the bronchospasm with bronchodilators; however, the chest tightness appears to relate, at least in part, to histamine release, and antihistamines have been shown to lessen the anticipated fall in FEV_1 the first day of the week. Clearly, reduction of dust exposure is of primary importance. All workers with persistent symptoms or significantly reduced levels of pulmonary function should be moved to areas of lower risk of exposure. Regular surveillance of pulmonary function in the industry has made it easier to identify affected persons. Persons with reduced pulmonary function, a personal history of respiratory allergy, and a history of continued cigarette smoking should be considered at increased risk of developing byssinosis in association with work in the cotton industry.

Grain Dust Although the exact number of workers at risk in the United States is not known, at least 500,000 people work in grain elevators, and over 2 million farmers are potentially exposed to grain dust. The presentation of disease in grain elevator employees or in workers in flour or feed mills is virtually identical to the characteristic findings in cigarette smokers, i.e., persistent cough, mucous hypersecretion, wheeze and dyspnea on exertion, and reduced FEV_1 and FEV_1/FVC ratio (Chap. 250).

Dust concentrations in grain elevators vary greatly but appear to be in excess of 10,000 μg/m³; approximately one-third of the particles, by weight, are in the respirable range. The effect of grain dust exposure is additive to that of cigarette smoking, with approximately 50 percent of workers who smoke having symptoms. Among nonsmoking grain elevator operators, approximately one-quarter have mucous hypersecretion, about five times the number that would be expected in unexposed nonsmokers. However, evidence of obstruction on pulmonary function studies is observed only in workers who smoke. It is not clear whether the reason is an enhancement of the cigarette smoking effect in exposed workers or a greater susceptibility of smokers to the effects of grain dust.

Farmer's Lung This condition results from exposure to moldy hay containing spores of thermophilic actinomycetes that produce a hypersensitivity pneumonitis (Chap. 253). There are few good population-based estimates of the frequency of occurrence of this condition in the United States. However, among farmers in Great Britain, the rate of disease ranges from approximately 10 to 50 per 1000. The prevalence of disease varies in association with rainfall, which determines the amount of fungal growth, and with differences in agricultural practices related to turning and stacking hay.

The patient with acute farmer's lung presents 4 to 8 h after exposure with fever, chills, malaise, cough, and dyspnea without wheezing. The history of exposure is obviously essential to distinguish this disease from influenza or pneumonia with similar symptoms. In the chronic form of the disease, the history of repeated attacks after similar exposure is important in differentiating this syndrome from other causes of patchy fibrosis (e.g., sarcoidosis).

A wide variety of other organic dusts are associated with the occurrence of hypersensitivity pneumonitis (Chap. 253). For those patients who present with hypersensitivity pneumonitis, specific and careful inquiry about occupations, hobbies, or other home environmental exposures will, in most cases, reveal the source of the etiologic agent.

ASSESSMENT OF DISABILITY Significant reduction of dust levels in coal mines has resulted from federal legislation, enacted in the United States in 1969, that requires that respirable dust levels in underground mines be reduced to less than 2000 μg/m³. This same legislation authorizes payment to coal miners (or their survivors) totally disabled by CWP. The criteria for disability from CWP remain unclear and arbitrary. It is critical that physicians involved in occupational lung disease claim cases be aware of detailed exposure histories of their patients, in terms of both occupational exposures and other environmental exposures (cigarette smoking). To assess disability properly may require input not only from physicians but also from experts in ergonomics and vocational rehabilitation, lawyers, and employer and employee representatives.

Most commonly, the patient presents with asthma, and it is the physician's task to decide whether the asthma is occupation-induced or work-aggravated asthma. The distinction is important not only because of the implications for disability compensation but also because the longer one is exposed to an inciting agent, the worse the prognosis for recovery from occupation-induced asthma. The clinical evaluation of such a patient requires adherence to a prescribed protocol that may include not only the components of the evaluation previously described but also rechallenge of the patient in a controlled setting or under a carefully monitored program in a work setting.

TOXIC CHEMICALS Exposure to toxic chemicals affecting the lung generally involves gases and vapors. A common accident is one in which the victim is trapped in a confined space where the chemicals have accumulated to toxic levels. In addition to the specific toxic effects of the chemical, the victim will often sustain considerable anoxia, which can play a dominant role in determining whether the individual survives.

Table 254-2 lists a variety of toxic agents that can produce acute and sometimes life-threatening reactions in the lung. All these agents in sufficient concentrations have been demonstrated, at least in animal

studies, to affect the lower airways and disrupt alveolar architecture, either acutely or as a result of chronic exposure. Some of these agents may be generated acutely in the environment. For example, when plastics burn, a number of compounds, including hydrogen cyanide and hydrochloric acid, may be formed and released. → *The effects and treatment of exposure to these toxic gases are discussed in Chap. 391.*

Firefighters and fire victims are at risk of *smoke inhalation*, a numerically important cause of acute cardiorespiratory failure. Smoke inhalation kills more fire victims than does thermal injury. Carbon monoxide poisoning with resulting significant hypoxemia can be life-threatening (Chap. 391). Firefighters may inappropriately use the "blackness" of the smoke to indicate the degree of incomplete combustion and thus of carbon monoxide elevation. The use of synthetic materials (plastic, polyurethanes), which, when burned, may release a variety of other toxic agents, must be considered when evaluating smoke inhalation victims. Exposed victims may suffer some degree of lower respiratory tract inflammation, similar to that seen with exposure to other irritant gases (e.g., chlorine). Severe cases may include pulmonary edema.

Firefighters and victims also may be exposed to large quantities of particulate smoke. Significant long-term effects are not clearly associated with this particulate exposure except as related to the production of irritating effects on the upper airways; however, increased airway responsiveness in firefighters with repeated episodes of smoke inhalation has been demonstrated.

Some agents used in the manufacture of synthetic materials such as plastics, polyurethanes, and other polymers have resulted in some workers' being sensitized to extremely low levels of *isocyanates*, *aromatic amines*, or *aldehydes*. Repeated exposure to these agents causes some workers to develop chronic cough and sputum production, asthma, or episodes of low-grade fever and malaise.

Exposure occurs by an unusual route in *polymer fume fever*. Polymers, notably fluorocarbons, which at normal temperatures produce no reaction, may be transmitted from a worker's hands to his or her cigarettes. As the cigarette burns, the polymer is volatilized, and the inhaled agent causes a characteristic syndrome of fever, chills, malaise, and occasionally mild wheezing. The same scenario applies when workers are exposed to heated polymers without cigarette use. The syndrome is obviously controlled by proper attention to hygiene in the workplace. A similar self-limited, influenza-like syndrome—*metal fume fever*—results from acute exposure to fumes or smoke of zinc, copper, magnesium, and other volatilized metals. The syndrome may begin several hours after work and resolves within 24 h, only to return on repeated exposure. A proper occupational history should make the diagnosis evident.

ENVIRONMENTAL RESPIRATORY CARCINOGENS Historically, it has been the astute clinician who has recognized a higher incidence of malignant tumors associated with certain environmental exposures. When these observations are linked to an occupational setting, they must be pursued by epidemiologic studies of relatively large groups of both current and former workers. Often the concentration and/or exact nature of the substances involved in the putative exposures cannot be determined. Rarely, the possibility that a substance can play an etiologic role in cancer is supported by observing that a few cases of a very rare tumor in a particular group represent "an epidemic." Examples are nasal sinus and lung cancer in nickel workers, angiosarcomas of the liver in vinyl chloride workers, and adenocarcinomas of the nose in woodworkers.

Only in those few cases in which animal studies have been carried out can one confirm that a given suspected agent is really a carcinogen. For example, bis(chloromethyl) ether (BCME) has been shown to produce tumors in animals and oat cell cancer of the lung in humans. In this particular case, BCME, used as a chemical intermediary in the manufacture of a number of organic compounds, was found to produce tumors in animals at about the same time as the substance was introduced into industry.

In addition to asbestos exposures, other occupational exposures associated with either proven or suspected respiratory carcinogens include those to acrylonitrile, arsenic compounds, beryllium (animal studies only), BCME, chromium, polycyclic hydrocarbons (through coke ovens), iron oxide, isopropyl oil (nasal sinuses), mustard gas, the various ores used to produce pure nickel, talc (possible asbestos contamination in both mining and milling), vinyl chloride, welding materials, wood used in woodworking (nasal cancer only), and uranium. The occurrence of excess cancers in uranium miners raises the possibility that a large number of workers are at risk by virtue of exposure to similar radiation hazards. This number includes not only workers involved in processing uranium but also workers exposed in underground mining operations where radon daughters may be emitted from rock formations.

GENERAL ENVIRONMENTAL EXPOSURES

AIR POLLUTION Dramatic and disastrous episodes of air pollution inversion have been documented in many industrialized centers in the world. Each of these episodes has been associated with excess acute mortality in the very old, the very young, and those with chronic cardiopulmonary diseases. The most dramatic event was the London fog of 1952, in which approximately 4000 excess deaths occurred over a 2-week period following 5 days of severe cold and dense fog. Similar episodes in the United States, although less dramatic in terms of total deaths, occurred in Donora, Pennsylvania, in 1948 and in New York City in the 1960s. In these episodes, which were generally associated with cold temperature and air stagnation, patients with underlying cardiopulmonary disease were most severely affected.

In addition to significant excess mortality during these episodes, a large number of people required medical care for cardiorespiratory complaints. Subsequent follow-up studies failed to implicate these

Table 254-2

Selected Common Toxic Chemical Agents Affecting the Lung

Agent(s)	Selected Exposures	Acute Effects from High or Accidental Exposure	Chronic Effects from Relatively Low Exposure
Acid fumes; H_2SO_4, HNO_3	Manufacture of fertilizers, chlorinated organic compounds, dyes, explosives, rubber products, metal etching, plastics	Mucous membrane irritation, followed by chemical pneumonitis 2–3 days later	Bronchitis and suggestion of mildly reduced pulmonary function in children with lifelong residential exposure to high levels; clinical significance unknown
Ammonia	Refrigeration; petroleum refining; manufacture of fertilizers, explosives, plastics, and other chemicals	Same as for acid fumes	Chronic bronchitis
Cyanides	Electroplating; extraction of gold or silver; manufacture of mirrors, fumigants, photo supplies	Increase in respiratory rate followed by respiratory arrest, lactic acidosis, pulmonary edema, death	No data
Diazomethane	Methylating agent for acid compounds; laboratory workers	Violent coughing, dyspnea, wheezing, pulmonary edema	No data
Formaldehyde	Manufacture of resins, leathers, rubber, metals, and woods; laboratory workers, embalmers; emission from urethane foam insulation	Same as for acid fumes	Cancers in one species; no data on humans
Halides (Cl, Br, F)	Bleaching in pulp, paper, textile industry; manufacture of chemical compounds; synthetic rubber, plastics, disinfectant, rocket fuel, gasoline	Mucous membrane irritation, pulmonary edema; possible reduced FVC 1–2 yrs after exposure	Dryness of mucous membrane, epistaxis, dental fluorosis, tracheobronchitis
Hydrogen sulfide	By-product of many industrial processes, oil, other petroleum processes and storage	Respiratory paralysis similar to cyanides	Conjunctival irritation, chronic bronchitis, recurrent pneumonitis
Isocyanates (TDI, HDI, MDI)	Production of polyurethane foams, plastics, adhesives, surface coatings	Mucous membrane irritation, dyspnea, cough, wheeze, pulmonary edema	Upper respiratory tract irritation, cough, asthma, allergic alveolitis
Nitrogen dioxide	Silage, metal etching, explosives, rocket fuels, welding, by-product of burning fossil fuels	Cough, dyspnea, pulmonary edema may be delayed 4–12 h; possible result from acute exposure: bronchiolitis obliterans in 2–6 wks	Emphysema in animals, ?chronic bronchitis
Ozone	Arc welding, flour bleaching, deodorizing, emissions from copying equipment, photochemical air pollutant	Mucous membrane irritant, pulmonary hemorrhage and edema, reduced pulmonary function transiently in children and adults exposed to summer haze	Chronic eye irritation
Phosgene	Organic compound, metallurgy, volatilization of chlorine-containing compounds	Delayed onset of bronchiolitis and pulmonary edema	Chronic bronchitis
Phthalic anhydride	Manufacture of resin esters, polyester resins, thermoactivated adhesives	Nasal irritation, cough	Asthma, chronic bronchitis
Sulfur dioxide	Manufacture of sulfuric acid, bleaches, coating of nonferrous metals, food processing, refrigerant, burning of fossil fuels, wood pulp industry	Mucous membrane irritant, epistaxis	?Chronic bronchitis

episodic disasters in the etiology of chronic respiratory disease in adults. On the other hand, many epidemiologic studies of both international and regional differences in the prevalences of chronic respiratory disease suggest that long-term exposures in polluted areas in the early to middle part of the twentieth century were associated with excess chronic respiratory disease.

In 1970, the U.S. government established air quality standards for several pollutants believed to be responsible for excess cardiorespiratory diseases. Primary standards regulated by the Environmental Protection Agency (EPA) designed to protect the public health with an adequate margin of safety exist for sulfur dioxide, particulates <10 μm in size, nitrogen dioxide, ozone, lead, and carbon monoxide. Standards for each of these pollutants are updated regularly through an extensive review process conducted by the EPA.

Pollutants are generated from both stationary sources (power plants and industrial complexes) and mobile sources (automobiles), and none of the pollutants occurs in isolation. Thus, except for the change in carboxyhemoglobin from carbon monoxide exposure, it becomes extremely difficult to relate any specific health effect to any single pollutant. Furthermore, pollutants may be changed by chemical reactions after being emitted. For example, reducing agents, such as sulfur dioxide and particulate matter from a power plant stack, may react in air to produce acid sulfates and aerosols, the precursors of acid rain, which can be transported long distances in the atmosphere. Oxidizing substances, such as oxides of nitrogen and oxidants from automobile exhaust, may react with sunlight to produce ozone. Although originally a problem confined to the southwestern part of the United States, in recent years, at least during the summertime, elevated ozone and acid aerosol levels have been documented throughout the United States. Both acute and chronic effects of these exposures are currently under investigation.

The symptoms and diseases associated with air pollution are the same as the nononcogenic conditions commonly associated with cigarette smoking. In addition, respiratory illness in early childhood has been associated with chronic exposure to only modestly elevated levels of SO_2 and respirable particles. Recent population-based studies comparing cities that have relatively high levels of particulate exposures with less polluted communities suggest excess morbidity and mortality from cardiorespiratory conditions in long-term residents of the former communities. This finding, in part, has led to greater emphasis on publicizing pollution alert levels. One can only advise individuals with significant cardiopulmonary impairment to stay indoors during periods when pollution exceeds current standards.

INDOOR EXPOSURE Because of increased concern about energy costs, efforts to become energy efficient have led to reduced air-exchange rates in indoor environments. The unintentional effect of these efforts has been to increase exposures to a variety of air contaminants heretofore not considered important.

Until relatively recently, little attention was given to the effects of *passive cigarette smoking*. Several studies have shown that the respirable particulate load in any household is directly proportional to the number of cigarette smokers living in the home. Increases in prevalence of respiratory illnesses and reduced levels of pulmonary function measured with simple spirometry have been found in children of smoking parents in a number of studies. Although a modest increase in the risk of lung cancer is found in the aggregate of studies, the long-term consequences in terms of nononcogenic respiratory diseases are unknown.

Radon gas is believed to be a risk factor for lung cancer. The main radon product (radon 222) is a gas that results from the decay series of uranium 238, with the immediate precursor being radium 226. The amount of radium in earth materials determines how much radon gas will be emitted. Outdoors, the concentrations are trivial. Indoors, levels are dependent on the ventilation rate and the size of the space into which the gas is emitted. Levels associated with excess lung cancer risk may be present in as many as 10 percent of the houses in the United States. When smokers reside in the household, the problem is potentially greater, since the molecular size of radon particles allows them to readily attach to smoke particles that are inhaled. Fortunately, technology is available for assessing and reducing the level of exposure.

Other indoor exposures associated with an increased risk of atopy and asthma include those to such specific recognized putative biologic agents as cockroach antigen, dust mites, and pet danders. Other indoor chemical agents include formaldehyde, perfumes, and latex particles. Of recent interest are the nonspecific responses associated with "tight-building syndrome," in which no particular agent has been implicated; the affected individuals suffer from a wide variety of complaints, including respiratory symptoms, that are relieved only by avoiding exposure in the building in question. The degree to which "smells" or other sensory stimuli are involved in the triggering of potentially incapacitating psychological or physical responses has yet to be determined, and the long-term consequences of such environmental exposures are as yet unknown.

PORTAL OF ENTRY The lung is a primary point of entry into the body for a number of toxic agents that affect other organ systems. For example, the lung is a route of entry for benzene (bone marrow), carbon disulfide (cardiovascular and nervous systems), cadmium (kidney), and metallic mercury (kidney, central nervous system). Thus, in any disease state of obscure origin, it is important to consider the possibility of inhaled environmental agents. Such consideration can sometimes furnish the clue needed to identify a specific external cause for a disorder that might otherwise be labeled "idiopathic."

BIBLIOGRAPHY

BALAAN MR et al: Clinical aspects of coal workers' pneumononiosis and silicosis. Occup Med 8:19, 1993

BECKLAKE MR et al: The relationship between acute and chronic airway responses to occupational exposures. Curr Pulmonol 9:25, 1988

BERRY G: Prediction of mesothelioma, lung cancer, and asbestosis in former Wittenoom asbestos workers. Br J Ind Med 48:793, 1991

CHAN-YEUNG M, MALO J-L: Occupational asthma. N Engl J Med 333: 107, 1995

COCHRANE AL, MOORE FA: A 20-year follow-up of men aged 55–64 including coal miners and foundry workers in Staveley. Br J Ind Med 37:226, 1980

Guidelines for the Use of International Labour Office Classification of Radiographs of Pneumoconiosis. Occupational Safety and Health Sciences 22 (Revised 1980). Geneva, ILO, 1980

LAPP NL, CASTRANOVA V: How silicosis and coal workers' pneumoconioses develop—a cellular assessment. Occup Med 8:35, 1993

LEONARD JF, TEMPLETON PA: Pulmonary imaging techniques in the diagnosis of occupational interstitial lung disease, in *Occupational Medicine: State of the Art Reviews*, vol 7, no 2, WS Beckett, R Bascon (eds). Philadelphia, Hanley and Belfus, 1992, pp 241–260

MULLOY KB et al: Use of chest radiographs in epidemiological investigations of pneumoconioses. Br J Ind Med 50:273, 1993

PARKES WR: *Occupational Lung Disorders*, 2d ed. London, Butterworth, 1982

ROGGLI VL et al: Asbestos fiber type in malignant mesothelioma: An analytical scanning electron microscopic study of 94 cases. Am J Ind Med 23:605, 1993

SAMET JM, SPENGLER JD: *Indoor Air Pollution: A Health Perspective*, Baltimore, The Johns Hopkins University, 1991, chaps 2 and 15

SCHENKER MB: Regulatory and policy issues, in *Occupational and Environmental Respiratory Disease*, P Harber et al: (eds). St Louis, Mosby Year Books, 1996, Chaps. 55–58

SHERSON D, LANDER F: Morbidity of pulmonary tuberculosis among silicotic and nonsilicotic foundry workers in Denmark. J Occup Med 32:110, 1990

PNEUMONIA, INCLUDING NECROTIZING PULMONARY INFECTIONS (LUNG ABSCESS)

Pneumonia is an infection of the pulmonary parenchyma. Various bacterial species, mycoplasmas, chlamydiae, rickettsiae, viruses, fungi, and parasites can cause pneumonia. Thus pneumonia is not a single disease but a group of specific infections, each with a different epidemiology, pathogenesis, clinical presentation, and clinical course. Identification of the etiologic microorganism is of primary importance, since this is the key to appropriate antimicrobial therapy. However, because of the serious nature of the infection, antimicrobial therapy generally needs to be started immediately, often before laboratory confirmation of the causative agent. The specific microbial etiology remains elusive in about one-third of cases—e.g., when no sputum is available for examination, blood cultures are sterile, and there is no pleural fluid. Serologic confirmation requires weeks because of the late formation of specific antibody.

Initial antimicrobial therapy is often empirical and is based on the setting in which the infection was acquired, the clinical presentation, patterns of abnormality on chest radiography, results of staining of sputum or other infected body fluids, and current patterns of susceptibility of the suspected pathogens to antimicrobial agents. After the etiologic agent is identified, specific antimicrobial therapy can be chosen.

DEFENSE MECHANISMS The lung is a complex structure composed of aggregates of units that are formed by the progressive branching of the airways. Approximately 80 percent of the cells lining the central airways are ciliated, pseudostratified, columnar epithelial cells; the percentage decreases in the peripheral airways. Each ciliated cell contains about 200 cilia that beat in coordinated waves about 1000 times per minute, with a fast forward stroke and a slower backward recovery. Ciliary motion is also coordinated between adjacent cells so that each wave is propagated toward the oropharynx. The cilia are covered by a liquid film that is about 5 to 10 μm thick and is composed of two layers. The outer, or gel, layer is viscous and traps deposited particles. The cilia beat in the less viscous inner, or sol, layer. During the forward stroke, the tips of the cilia just touch the viscous gel and propel it toward the oropharynx. During recovery, the cilia move entirely within the low-resistance sol layer. Ciliated cells are interspersed with mucus-secreting cells in the trachea and bronchi but not in the bronchioles.

The alveolar walls, from blood to air, consist of the endothelium that lines the network of anastomotic capillaries, the capillary basement membrane, the interstitial tissue, the alveolar basement membrane, the alveolar lining epithelial cells (either flattened type I pneumocytes that cover 95 percent of the alveolar surface or rounded, granular surfactant-producing type II pneumocytes), and epithelial lining fluid. The epithelial lining fluid contains surfactant, fibronectin, and immunoglobulin, which may opsonize or—in the presence of complement—lyse microbial pathogens deposited on the alveolar surface. Loosely attached to the lining cells or lying free within the lumen are the alveolar macrophages, lymphocytes, and a few polymorphonuclear leukocytes.

The lower respiratory tract is normally sterile, despite being adjacent to enormous numbers of microorganisms that reside in the oropharynx and being exposed to environmental microorganisms in inhaled air. This sterility is the result of efficient filtering and clearance mechanisms.

Infectious particles deposited on the squamous epithelium of distal nasal surfaces normally are removed by sneezing, while those deposited on the more proximal ciliated surfaces are swept posteriorly in the mucous lining into the nasopharynx, where they are swallowed or expectorated. Reflex closure of the glottis and cough protect the lower respiratory tract. Those particles deposited on the tracheobronchial surface are swept by ciliary motion toward the oropharynx.

Infectious particles that bypass defenses in the airways and are deposited on the alveolar surface are cleared by phagocytic cells and humoral factors. Alveolar macrophages are the major phagocytes in the lower respiratory tract. Some phagocytosed microorganisms are killed by the phagocyte's oxygen-dependent systems, lysosomal enzymes, and cationic proteins. Other microorganisms can evade microbicidal mechanisms and persist within the macrophage. For example, *Mycobacterium tuberculosis* persists within the lysosome, while *Legionella* resides within intracellular inclusions that fail to fuse with lysosomes. Intracellular pathogens can then be transported to the ciliated surfaces and into the oropharynx or via the lymphatics to regional lymph nodes. The alveolar macrophages process and present microbial antigens to the lymphocyte and also secrete cytokines (e.g., tumor necrosis factor and interleukin 1) that modulate the immune process in T and B lymphocytes. Cytokines facilitate the generation of an inflammatory response, activate alveolar macrophages, and recruit additional phagocytes and other immunologic factors from plasma. The inflammatory exudate is responsible for many of the local signs of pulmonary consolidation and the systemic manifestations of pneumonia, such as fever, chills, myalgias, and malaise.

TRANSMISSION Microbial pathogens enter the lung by one of several routes.

Aspiration of Organisms That Colonize the Oropharynx Most pulmonary pathogens originate in the oropharyngeal flora. Aspiration of these pathogens is the most common mechanism for the production of pneumonia. At various times during the year, healthy individuals transiently carry common pulmonary pathogens in the nasopharynx; these pathogens include *Streptococcus pneumoniae*, *Streptococcus pyogenes*, *Mycoplasma pneumoniae*, *Haemophilus influenzae*, and *Moraxella catarrhalis*. The sources of anaerobic pulmonary pathogens, such as *Porphyromonas gingivalis*, *Prevotella melaninogenica*, *Fusobacterium nucleatum*, *Actinomyces* spp., spirochetes, and anaerobic streptococci, are the gingival crevice and dental plaque, which contain more than 10^{11} colony-forming units (CFU) of microorganisms per gram. The frequency of aerobic gram-negative bacillary colonization of the oropharyngeal mucosa, which is unusual in healthy persons (<2 percent), increases with hospitalization, worsening debility, severe underlying illness, alcoholism, diabetes, and advanced age. This change may be a consequence of increased salivary proteolytic activity, which destroys fibronectin, a glycoprotein coating the surface of the mucosa. Fibronectin is the receptor for the normal gram-positive flora of the oropharynx. Loss of fibronectin exposes the receptors for aerobic gram-negative bacilli on the epithelial cell surface. The source of aerobic gram-negative bacilli may be the patient's own stomach (which can become colonized with these organisms as the result of an increase in gastric pH with atrophic gastritis or after the use of H_2-blocking agents or antacids), contaminated respiratory equipment, hands of health care workers, or contaminated food and water. Nasogastric tubes can facilitate the transfer of gastric bacteria to the pharynx.

About 50 percent of healthy adults aspirate oropharyngeal secretions into the lower respiratory tract during sleep. Aspiration occurs more frequently and may be more pronounced in individuals with an impaired level of consciousness (e.g., alcoholics; drug abusers; and patients who have had seizures, strokes, or general anesthesia), neurologic dysfunction of the oropharynx, and swallowing disorders or mechanical impediments (e.g., nasogastric or endotracheal tubes). Pneumonia due to anaerobes is an especially likely outcome if the aspirated material is large in volume or contains virulent components of the anaerobic microbial flora or foreign bodies, such as aspirated food or necrotic tissue. Impairment of the cough reflex increases the risk of pneumonia, as does mucociliary or alveolar macrophage dysfunction.

Inhalation of Infectious Aerosols Deposition of inhaled particles within the respiratory tract is determined primarily by particle diameter. Particles that are more than 10 μm in diameter are deposited mostly in the nose and upper airways. Particles that are less than 3 to 5 μm in diameter (also called *airborne droplet nuclei*) and that contain one or perhaps two microorganisms fail to settle out by gravity but rather remain suspended in the atmosphere for long periods unless removed by ventilation or by filtration in the lungs of the individual breathing the contaminated air. These infectious aerosols are small enough to bypass host defenses in the upper respiratory tract and airways. More particles are deposited in small bronchioles and alveoli as particle size decreases below 5 μm. One inhaled particle of appropriate size may be sufficient to reach the alveolus and initiate infection. The etiologies of pneumonia typically acquired by inhalation of infectious aerosols include tuberculosis, influenza, legionellosis, psittacosis, histoplasmosis, and Q fever.

Hematogenous Dissemination from an Extrapulmonary Site Infection, usually with *Staphylococcus aureus*, disseminates hematogenously to the lungs in patients (such as intravenous drug abusers) who have either right- or left-sided bacterial endocarditis and in patients with intravenous catheter infections. *Fusobacterium* infections of the retropharyngeal tissues (Lemierre's syndrome—i.e., retropharyngeal abscess and jugular venous thrombophlebitis) also disseminate to the lungs.

Direct Inoculation and Contiguous Spread Two additional routes of transmission of bacteria to the lungs are direct inoculation as a result of either tracheal intubation or stab wounds of the chest and contiguous spread from an adjacent site of infection.

PATHOLOGY The pneumonic process may involve primarily the interstitium or the alveoli. Involvement of an entire lobe is called *lobar pneumonia*. When the process is restricted to alveoli contiguous to bronchi, it is called *bronchopneumonia*. Confluent bronchopneumonia may be indistinguishable from lobar pneumonia. Cavities develop when necrotic lung tissue is discharged into communicating airways, resulting in either necrotizing pneumonia (multiple small cavities, each <2 cm in diameter, in one or more bronchopulmonary segments or lobes) or lung abscess (one or more cavities >2 cm in diameter). The classification of pneumonia is best based upon the causative microorganism rather than upon these anatomic characteristics (the criteria used in the past).

EPIDEMIOLOGY The patient's living circumstances, occupation, travel history, pet or animal exposure history, and contacts with other ill individuals as well as the physician's knowledge of the epidemic curve of community outbreaks provide useful clues to the microbial etiology of a given case of pneumonia (see Table 255-1).

The relative frequency of various pulmonary pathogens varies with the setting in which the infection was acquired—e.g., community, nursing home, or hospital. In patients hospitalized with community-acquired pneumonia, the most frequent pathogens are *S. pneumoniae*, *H. influenzae*, *Chlamydia pneumoniae*, and *Legionella pneumophila*. *M. pneumoniae*, which usually causes mild illness, is common among outpatients with community-acquired pneumonia. In contrast, enteric aerobic gram-negative bacilli and *Pseudomonas aeruginosa*, uncommon causes of community-acquired pneumonia, are estimated to account for more than 50 percent of cases of hospital-acquired pneumonia, while *S. aureus* is responsible for more than 10 percent. The relative frequencies of pathogens in pneumonia acquired in nursing homes fall somewhere between those of community- and hospital-acquired pneumonia. Enteric aerobic gram-negative bacilli and *P. aeruginosa* are more common among nursing home residents than among patients who acquire pneumonia in noninstitutional settings.

The season of the year and the geographic location are other predictors of etiology. The frequency of influenza virus as a cause of both community-acquired and institutionally acquired pneumonia increases during the winter months. Moreover, influenza virus infection causes an increase in the frequency of secondary bacterial pneumonia due to *S. pneumoniae*, *S. aureus*, and *H. influenzae*. Outbreaks of influenza in a community tend to be explosive and widespread, with many secondary cases resulting from the short incubation period of several days and the high degree of communicability. Legionellosis also occurs in explosive outbreaks when large numbers of susceptible people are exposed to an infectious aerosol; however, no secondary cases occur because of the low level of communicability of *L. pneumophila*. *Mycoplasma* can cause outbreaks, usually in relatively closed populations such as those at military bases, at colleges, or in households; however, because of its long incubation period (2 to 3 weeks) and its relatively low degree of communicability, *Mycoplasma* infection moves through the community slowly, affecting another person as the first is recovering. In communities where infection with human immunodeficiency virus (HIV) type 1 is endemic, *Pneumocystis carinii* and *M. tuberculosis* are more prominent causes of community-acquired pneumonia. Histoplasmosis, blastomycosis, and coccidioidomycosis are causes of pneumonia that have specific geographic distributions, and *Chlamydia psittaci* produces illness in bird handlers.

AGE AND COMORBIDITY Age is an important predictor of the infecting agent in pneumonia. *Chlamydia trachomatis* and respiratory syncytial virus are common among infants under 6 months of age; *H. influenzae* among children between 6 months and 5 years of age; *M. pneumoniae* and *C. pneumoniae* among young adults; and *H. influenzae*, *L. pneumophila*, and *M. catarrhalis* among elderly persons with chronic lung disease.

Oral anaerobes, frequently in combination with aerobic bacterial components of the human flora (e.g., viridans streptococci), are causes of community-acquired pneumonia and anaerobic lung abscess in patients who are prone to aspiration. Edentulous persons, who have lower numbers of oral anaerobes, are less likely to develop pneumonia due to anaerobes. When the etiology of community-acquired pneumonia in unselected hospitalized patients has been studied by methods that entail strict anaerobic bacteriology and that avoid contamination of lower respiratory tract secretions by the oral flora, anaerobic bacteria have been found to account for as many as 20 to 30 percent of cases. In hospital-acquired pneumonia, anaerobes are the pathogens—with or without aerobic copathogens—in about one-third of cases. However, the aerobic copathogens in hospital-acquired pneumonia are frequently virulent microorganisms in their own right (e.g., enteric aerobic gram-negative bacilli, *P. aeruginosa*, and *S. aureus*).

The patient's underlying disease may be characterized by specific immunologic or inflammatory defects that predispose to pneumonia due to specific pathogens (see Table 255-2). For example, patients who have severe hypogammaglobulinemia (<2.0 g/L) are at risk of infection with encapsulated bacteria such as *S. pneumoniae* and *H. influenzae*. HIV-infected patients also may exhibit ineffective antibody formation, which predisposes to infection with these encapsulated bacteria. Severe neutropenia (<500 neutrophils/μL) increases the risk of infections due to *P. aeruginosa*, Enterobacteriaceae, *S. aureus*, and (if neutropenia is prolonged) *Aspergillus*. The risk is unusually high for infections due to *M. tuberculosis* among HIV-infected patients

---

Table 255-1

Microbial Pathogens That Cause Pneumonia

Community-Acquired	Hospital-Acquired	HIV Infection–Associated
Mycoplasma pneumoniae	Enteric aerobic	*Pneumocystis carinii*
Streptococcus pneumoniae	gram-negative	*Mycobacterium*
Haemophilus influenzae	bacilli	*tuberculosis*
Chlamydia pneumoniae	*Pseudomonas*	*Streptococcus pneumoniae*
Legionella pneumophila	*aeruginosa*	*Haemophilus influenzae*
Oral anaerobes	*Staphylococcus*	
Moraxella catarrhalis	*aureus*	
Staphylococcus aureus	Oral anaerobes	
Nocardia spp.		
Viruses*		
Fungi†		
Mycobacterium		
tuberculosis		
Chlamydia psittaci		

* Influenza virus, cytomegalovirus, respiratory syncytial virus, measles virus, and varicella-zoster virus.
† *Histoplasma*, *Coccidioides*, and *Blastomyces* spp.

with circulating CD4 lymphocyte counts <500/L; for infections due to *P. carinii, Histoplasma capsulatum*, and *Crypcoccus neoformans* among those with CD4 counts <200/μL; and r infections due to *Mycobacterium avium-intracellulare* and cytnegalovirus among those with CD4 counts <50/μL. Long-term gcocorticoid therapy increases the risk of tuberculosis and nocardio:

CLINICAL MANIFESTATIONS   Cmmunity-Acquired Pneumonia
Community-acquired pneumonia s traditionally been thought to present as either of two syndromes: ttypical presentation and the atypical presentation. Although recent a suggest that these two syndromes may be less distinct than was on hought, the characteristics of the clinical presentation may neverth ss have some diagnostic value.

The "typical" pneumonia syndrome is charazized by the sudden onset of fever, cough productive of purulent tum, and in some cases pleuritic chest pain; signs of pulmonary cblidation (dullness, increased fremitus, egophony, bronchial breath ids, and rales) may be found on physical examination in areas of radaphic abnormality. The typical pneumonia syndrome is usually ca by the most common bacterial pathogen in community-acquire eumonia, *S. pneumoniae*, but can also be due to other bacterathogens, such as *H. influenzae* and mixed anaerobic and aerolomponents of the oral flora.

The "atypical" pneumonia syndrome is clterized by a more gradual onset, a dry cough, a prominence of extmonary symptoms (such as headache, myalgias, fatigue, sore th nausea, vomiting, and diarrhea), and abnormalities on chest radios despite minimal signs of pulmonary involvement (other than ran physical examination. Atypical pneumonia is classically prodvy *M. pneumoniae* but can also be caused by *L. pneumophila, C. poniae*, oral anaerobes, and *P. carinii* as well as by *S. pneumonia* he less frequently encountered pathogens *C. psittaci, Coxiella bu Francisella tularensis, H. capsulatum*, and *Coccidioides immitis* plasma pneumonia (see Chap. 180) may be complicated by ema multiforme, hemolytic anemia, bullous myringitis, encephad transverse myelitis. *Legionella* pneumonia (see Chap. 153) uently associated with deterioration in mental status, renal andc abnormalities, and marked hyponatremia; pneumonia due t apsulatum or *C. immitis* is often accompanied by erythema nodn *C. pneumoniae* pneumonia (see Chap. 181), sore throat, hoars nd wheezing are relatively common. The atypical pneumoni ome in patients whose behavioral history places them at risk o fection suggests *Pneumocystis* infection. These patients may h aurrent infections due to other opportunistic pathogens, such onary (and frequently extrapulmonary) tuberculosis, oral thr to *Candida albicans*, or extensive perineal ulcers due to her plex virus.

Certain viruses also produce pneumonia tually characterized by an atypical presentation—i.e., chills, v nonproductive cough, and predominance of extrapulmonary is. Primary viral

Table 255-2
Pulmonary Pathogens Associated with Specific Host Defenses

Defect	Pathogens
Severe hypogammaglobulinemia	Encapsulaa: *Streptococcus pneumon philus influenza*
Severe neutropenia	*Pseudomonosa, Enteroba Staphylococcus aureus, I*
Defective cell-mediated immunity CD4 lymphocyte count	
<500/μL	*Mycobactculosis*
<200/μL	*Pneumocy Histoplasma capsulato ccus neoform*
<50/μL	*Mycobact-intracellulare*, cytomeg
Long-term glucocorticoid therapy	*M. tubercrdia*

pneumonia can be caused by influenza virus infection (usually as part of a community outbreak in winter), by respiratory syncytial virus infection (in children and immunosuppressed individuals), by measles or varicella-zoster virus infection (accompanied by the characteristic rash), and by cytomegalovirus infection (in patients immunocompromised by HIV infection or by therapy given in association with organ transplantation). In addition, influenza, measles, and varicella can predispose to secondary bacterial pneumonia as a result of the destruction of the mucociliary barrier of the airways. Secondary bacterial infection may either follow the viral infection without interruption or be separated from the viral infection by several days of transient relief of symptoms. Bacterial infection may be heralded by sudden worsening of the patient's clinical condition, with persisting or renewed chills, fever, and cough productive of purulent sputum, possibly accompanied by pleuritic chest pain.

Patients with hematogenous *S. aureus* pneumonia may present with fever and dyspnea only. In these cases the inflammatory response is initially confined to the pulmonary interstitium. Cough, sputum production, and signs of pulmonary consolidation develop only after the infection extends into the bronchi. These patients are usually gravely ill, with intravascular infection as well as pneumonia, and may have signs of endocarditis (see Chap. 126).

Nocardiosis (see Chap. 167) is frequently complicated by metastasis of lesions to the skin and central nervous system. Signs of pulmonary consolidation, cough, and sputum production may be lacking in patients who are unable to mount an inflammatory response, such as those with agranulocytosis. The major manifestations in these patients may be limited to fever, tachypnea, agitation, and altered mental status. Elderly or severely ill patients may fail to develop fever.

Tuberculosis also produces an atypical presentation that is characterized by fever, night sweats, cough, and shortness of breath and sometimes by pleuritic chest pain and blood-streaked sputum. Several weeks usually elapse before the patient seeks medical attention because of the gradual worsening of these symptoms, by which time he or she will have lost considerable weight.

Nosocomial Pneumonia Patients with nosocomial pneumonia often pose a diagnostic challenge. The differential diagnosis of acute respiratory disease in critically ill, hospitalized patients is diverse and includes noninfectious entities, such as congestive heart failure, acute respiratory distress syndrome, preexisting lung disease, atelectasis, and oxygen- or drug-related toxicities, that may be difficult to distinguish clinically or radiologically from pneumonia. The usual criteria for nosocomial pneumonia, which include new or progressive pulmonary infiltrates, purulent tracheobronchial secretions, fever, and leukocytosis, are frequently unreliable in these patients, who often have preexisting pulmonary disease, endotracheal tubes that irritate the tracheal mucosa and may elicit an inflammatory exudate in respiratory secretions, or multiple other problems likely to produce fever and leukocytosis. Patients with nosocomial pneumonia complicating an underlying illness associated with significant neutropenia often have no purulent respiratory tract secretions or pulmonary infiltrates, and patients with nosocomial pneumonia complicating uremia or cirrhosis often remain afebrile. In addition, the patients at greatest risk for nosocomial pneumonia are most likely to be heavily colonized with potential pulmonary pathogens in the oropharyngeal or tracheobronchial mucosa; thus the presence of these organisms in gram-stained preparations or cultures of respiratory tract secretions does not necessarily confirm the diagnosis of pneumonia.

Aspiration Pneumonia and Anaerobic Lung Abscess Although the aspiration of oral anaerobes can initially lead to an infiltrative process, it ultimately results in putrid sputum, tissue necrosis, and pulmonary cavities. In about three-quarters of cases, the clinical course of an abscess of anaerobic, polymicrobial etiology is indolent and mimics that of pulmonary tuberculosis, with cough, shortness of breath, chills, fever, night sweats, weight loss, pleuritic chest pain, and blood-streaked sputum lasting for several weeks or more. In other patients the disease may present more acutely. Patients with anaerobic abscesses are usually prone to aspiration of oropharyngeal contents and have periodontal disease. One genus of oral anaerobes, *Actinomyces,* produces a chronic fibrotic necrotizing process that crosses tissue planes and may involve the pleural space, ribs, vertebrae, and subcutaneous tissue, with eventual discharge of sulfur granules (macroscopic bacterial masses) through the skin (empyema necessitatis).

DIAGNOSIS **Radiography** Chest radiographs can confirm the presence and location of the pulmonary infiltrate; assess the extent of the pulmonary infection; detect pleural involvement, pulmonary cavitation, or hilar lymphadenopathy; and gauge the response to antimicrobial therapy. However, chest radiographs may be normal when the patient is unable to mount an inflammatory response (e.g., in agranulocytosis) or is in the early stage of an infiltrative process (e.g., in hematogenous *S. aureus* pneumonia or in *Pneumocystis* pneumonia associated with AIDS).

The anatomic localization of the inflammatory process, as visualized in chest radiographs, occasionally has diagnostic implications. Most pulmonary pathogens produce focal lesions. A multicentric distribution suggests hematogenous infection, in which case the remote location of the primary infection (e.g., endocarditis or thrombophlebitis) should be sought. Hematogenous pneumonia, which results from septic embolization in patients with thrombophlebitis or right-sided endocarditis and from bacteremia in patients with left-sided endocarditis, appears on the chest radiograph as multiple areas of pulmonary infiltration that subsequently may cavitate. A diffuse distribution suggests the involvement of *P. carinii*, cytomegalovirus, measles virus, or varicella-zoster virus (with pneumonia due to the last two pathogens diagnosed by the characteristic accompanying rash). Pleurisy and hilar nodal enlargement are unusual with *Pneumocystis* and cytomegalovirus pneumonia; their presence suggests another etiology. Diffuse lesions in immunocompromised patients also suggest legionellosis, tuberculosis, histoplasmosis, *Mycoplasma* infection, or disseminated strongyloidiasis.

Oral anaerobes, *S. aureus*, *S. pneumoniae* serotype III, aerobic gram-negative bacilli, *M. tuberculosis*, and fungi as well as certain noninfectious conditions can produce tissue necrosis and pulmonary cavities (Table 255-3). In contrast, *H. influenzae*, *M. pneumoniae*, viruses, and most other serotypes of *S. pneumoniae* almost never cause cavities. Apical disease, with or without cavities, suggests reactivation tuberculosis. Anaerobic abscesses are located in dependent, poorly ventilated, and poorly draining bronchopulmonary segments and characteristically have air-fluid levels unlike the well-ventilated, well-drained upper-lobe cavities caused by *M. tuberculosis*, an obligate aerobe. Air-fluid levels may also be present in cavities due to pulmonary necrosis of other infectious etiologies. *Mucor* and *Aspergillus* invade blood vessels and cause pleura-based, wedge-shaped areas of pulmonary infarction; these infarcts may subsequently cavitate.

In the patient with an uncomplicated course, chest radiographs need not be repeated before discharge, since the resolution of infiltrates

---

Table 255-3

Causes of Pulmonary Cavities

INFECTIOUS

Bacteria: Oral anaerobes (*Bacteroides* spp., fusobacteria, *Actinomyces* spp., anaerobic and microaerophilic cocci), enteric aerobic gram-negative bacilli, *Pseudomonas aeruginosa*, *Legionella* spp., *Staphylococcus aureus*, *Streptococcus pneumoniae* serotype III, *Mycobacterium tuberculosis*, *Nocardia* spp.
Fungi: *Histoplasma capsulatum*, *Coccidioides immitis*, *Blastomyces* spp.

NONINFECTIOUS

Neoplasms, Wegener's granulomatosis, infarction, infected bullae and cysts

---

may take up to 6 weeks after initial presentation. However, patients who do not respond clinically, who have a pleural effusion on admission, who may have postobstructive pneumonia, or who are infected with certain pathogens (e.g., *S. aureus*, aerobic gram-negative bacilli, or oral anaerobes) need more intensive surveillance. At times, computed tomography may be especially helpful in distinguishing different processes—e.g., pleural effusion versus underlying pulmonary consolidation, hilar adenopathy versus pulmonary mass, and pulmonary abscess versus empyema with an air-fluid level.

Sputum Examination Examination of the sputum remains the mainstay of the evaluation of a patient with acute bacterial pneumonia. Unfortunately, expectorated material is frequently contaminated by potentially pathogenic bacteria that colonize the upper respiratory tract (and sometimes the lower respiratory tract) without actually causing disease. This contamination reduces the diagnostic specificity of any lower respiratory tract specimen. In addition, it has been estimated that the usual laboratory processing methods detect the pulmonary pathogen in fewer than 50 percent of expectorated sputum samples from patients with bacteremic *S. pneumoniae* pneumonia. This low sensitivity may be due to misidentification of the alpha-hemolytic colonies of *S. pneumoniae* as nonpathogenic alpha-hemolytic streptococci ("normal flora"), overgrowth of the cultures by hardier colonizing organisms, or loss of these fastidious organisms due to slow transport or improper processing. In addition, certain very common pulmonary pathogens, such as anaerobes, mycoplasmas, chlamydiae, *Pneumocystis*, mycobacteria, and legionellae, cannot be cultured by routine methods.

Since expectorated material is routinely contaminated by oral anaerobes, the diagnosis of anaerobic pulmonary infection is frequently tentative. Confirmation of such a diagnosis requires the culture of anaerobes from pulmonary secretions that are uncontaminated by oropharyngeal secretions which in turn requires the collection of pulmonary secretions by special techniques, such as transtracheal aspiration, transthoracic lung puncture, and protected brush via bronchoscopy. These procedures are invasive and usually are not used unless the patient fails to respond to empirical therapy.

Gram's staining of sputum specimens, screened initially under low-power magnification (10× objective and 10× eyepiece) to determine the degree of contamination with squamous epithelial cells, is of utmost diagnostic importance. In patients with the typical pneumonia syndrome who produce purulent sputum, the sensitivity and specificity of Gram's staining on minimally contaminated by upper respiratory tract secretion (polymorphonuclear leukocytes and <10 epithelial cells per lower field) in identifying the pathogen as *S. pneumoniae* are 62 percent, respectively. Gram's staining in this case is more specific and probably more sensitive than the accompanying sputum culture. A finding of mixed flora on Gram's staining of an uncontaminated specimen suggests an anaerobic infection. Acid-fast stain of sputum should be undertaken when mycobacterial infection is suspected. Examination by an experienced pathologist of Giemsa-stained expectorated respiratory secretions from patients with AIDS can satisfactory results in the diagnosis of *Pneumocystis* pneumonia; the sensitivity of sputum examination is enhanced by the use of monoclonal antibodies to *Pneumocystis* and is diminished by prior prophylactic use of inhaled pentamidine. Blastomycosis can be diagnosed by the examination of wet preparations of sputum. Sputum stained directly with fluorescent antibody can be examined for *Legionella*, but this test yields false-negative results relatively often. The sputum should also be cultured for *Legionella* on special media.

Expectorated sputum is easily collected from patients with a vigorous cough but scant in patients with an atypical syndrome, in the elderly persons with altered mental status. If the patient is not producing sputum and can cooperate, respiratory secretions should be induced with ultrasonic nebulization of 3% saline. An attempt to obtain respiratory secretions by passage of a catheter through the mouth rarely achieves the desired results in an alert patient arranged; usually the catheter can be found coiled in the oroph

In some cases that do not require the patient's hospitalization (see Table 255-4), an accurate microbial diagnosis may not be crucial, and empirical therapy can be started on the basis of clinical and epidemiologic evidence alone. This approach may also be appropriate for hospitalized patients who are not severely ill and who are unable to produce an induced sputum specimen. Use of invasive procedures to establish a microbial diagnosis carries risks that must be weighed against potential benefits. However, the decision to initiate empirical therapy without an evaluation of induced sputum should be undertaken with caution and, in the case of hospitalized patients, should always be accompanied by the culture of several blood samples. The ability to understand the cause of a poor response to empirical antimicrobial therapy (see Table 255-5) may be compromised by the lack of an initial sputum culture.

Invasive Procedures The sensitivities and specificities of the invasive procedures described below for obtaining pulmonary material vary with the type of immunocompromised patient, the type of pulmonary lesion, and the degree of prior exposure to therapeutic or prophylactic antimicrobial agents.

Transtracheal aspiration (TTA) Popular several decades ago, TTA is rarely performed today. Although the sensitivity of the procedure is high (approaching 90 percent), the specificity is low. The material obtained by TTA (from a catheter inserted through the cricothyroid cartilage and advanced toward the carina) is not contaminated by upper respiratory tract secretions but can contain organisms that colonize the tracheobronchial tree without necessarily causing pneumonia. Significant morbidity and even death have attended the use of TTA. Contraindicated in patients with a bleeding diathesis, TTA may cause infection at the puncture site and may lead to severe subcutaneous and mediastinal emphysema in patients who are coughing vigorously.

Percutaneous transthoracic lung puncture This procedure employs a skinny (small-gauge) needle that is advanced into the area of pulmonary consolidation with computed tomographic guidance. It requires that the patient cooperate, have good hemostasis, and be able to tolerate a possible associated pulmonary hemorrhage or pneumothorax. Patients on mechanical ventilation cannot undergo lung puncture because of the high incidence of complicating pneumothorax.

Fiberoptic bronchoscopy Fiberoptic bronchoscopy is safe and relatively well tolerated and has become the standard invasive procedure used to obtain lower respiratory tract secretions from seriously ill or immunocompromised patients with complex or progressive pneumonia. This technique provides a direct view of the lower airways. Specimens obtained by bronchoscopy should be subjected to Gram's, acid-fast, *Legionella* direct fluorescent antibody, and Gomori's methenamine silver staining and should be cultured for routine aerobic and anaerobic bacteria, *Legionella*, mycobacteria, and fungi. Samples are collected with a protected double-sheathed brush (PSB), by bronchoalveolar lavage (BAL), or by transbronchial biopsy (TBB) at the site of pulmonary consolidation. The PSB sample is usually contaminated by oropharyngeal flora; quantitative cultures of the 1 mL of sterile culture medium into which the brush is placed after withdrawal

Table 255-5

Factors Involved in Poor Response to Empirical Antimicrobial Therapy

Incorrect microbiologic diagnosis
Inappropriate antimicrobial agent or dosing regimen
Drug hypersensitivity or other adverse effect (e.g., *Clostridium difficile* colitis)
Infectious complication: empyema, metastatic spread, superinfection
Atelectasis, parapneumonic effusion, phlebitis
Poor host defenses (e.g., endobronchial obstruction, life-threatening comorbidity)

from the inner catheter must be performed to differentiate contamination (<1000 CFU/mL) from infection (≥1000 CFU/mL). The results of PSB are highly specific and highly sensitive, especially when the patient has not received antibiotics before culture. BAL is usually performed with 150 to 200 mL of sterile, nonbacteriostatic saline. When used to facilitate endoscopy, local anesthetic agents with antibacterial activity can lower the sensitivity of culture results. Quantitative bacteriologic evaluation of BAL fluid has given results similar to those obtained with the PSB technique. Gram's staining of the cytocentrifuged BAL fluid specimen can serve as an immediate guide in the selection of antimicrobial therapy to be administered while culture results are awaited.

Open-lung biopsy This procedure is most commonly needed when specimens obtained bronchoscopically from an immunocompromised patient with progressive pneumonia have been unrevealing. Limitations on the performance of an open-lung biopsy include hypoxemia and a bleeding diathesis, which may supervene while the physician is deciding whether to undertake this procedure. Results of an open-lung biopsy are considered diagnostic because of the large size of the tissue sample. The diagnostic yield of this procedure is greatest in focal lesions, whereas bronchoscopic evaluation is most useful in diffuse lesions.

Other Diagnostic Tests In the initial evaluation of a patient with pneumonia, at least two blood samples for culture should be obtained from different venipuncture sites; if empyema is a clinical consideration, diagnostic thoracentesis is indicated. Positive blood or pleural fluid culture is generally considered diagnostic of the etiology of pneumonia. However, bacteremia and empyema each occur in fewer than 10 to 30 percent of patients with pneumonia.

Serologic studies are sometimes helpful in defining the etiology of certain types of pneumonia, although serologic diagnosis, because it is often delayed by the need to demonstrate at least a fourfold rise in convalescent-phase antibody titer, is usually retrospective. A single IgM antibody titer of >1:16, a single IgG antibody titer of >1:128, or a fourfold or greater rise in the IgG titer obtained by indirect immunofluorescence is diagnostic of *M. pneumoniae* infection. A single IgM antibody titer of ≥1:20, a single IgG antibody titer of ≥1:128, or a fourfold or greater rise in the IgG titer obtained by micro-indirect immunofluorescence is diagnostic of *C. pneumoniae* infection. A single legionella antibody titer of ≥1:256 or a fourfold rise to a titer of ≥1:128 suggests acute legionellosis. A highly sensitive and specific urinary antigen test is available to detect *L. pneumophila* serogroup 1 in patients with pneumonia; this organism accounts for about 70 percent of cases of *L. pneumophila* infection.

DECISION TO HOSPITALIZE Use of hospital services is costly and at times poses a risk to the patient (e.g., the risk of nosocomial infections). Thus hospitalization must be justified by the patient's poor functional status or by an inadequate social-support system that would compromise care at home, poor prognostic factors, unstable vital signs, or the need for intensive nursing care or specialized diagnostic procedures. Guidelines for hospitalization are given in Table 255-4. Discharge from the hospital should be guided by similar considerations.

Table 255-4

Criteria for Hospitalization of Patients with Pneumonia

1. Elderly patient (>65 years of age)
2. Significant comorbidity (e.g., kidney, heart, or lung disease; diabetes mellitus; neoplasm; immunosuppression)
3. Leukopenia (<5000 white blood cells/μL) not attributable to a known condition
4. *Staphylococcus aureus*, gram-negative bacilli, or anaerobes as the suspected cause of pneumonia
5. Suppurative complications (e.g., empyema, arthritis, meningitis, endocarditis)
6. Failure of outpatient management
7. Inability to take oral medication
8. Tachypnea (>30/min); tachycardia (>140/min); hypotension (<90 mmHg systolic); hypoxemia (arterial P_{O_2}, <60 mmHg); acute alteration of mental status

TREATMENT

Community-Acquired Pneumonia: Outpatient Management Most cases of community-acquired pneumonia in otherwise-healthy adults do not require hospitalization. Since it is often impractical to make a microbial diagnosis in an office setting, the oral antimicrobial therapy administered is frequently empirical (see Table 255-6). The pathogen in such a situation is likely to be *M. pneumoniae*, *S. pneumoniae*, or *C. pneumoniae*. In older patients with underlying chronic respiratory disease, *L. pneumophila*, *H. influenzae*, or *M. catarrhalis* should also be considered. In patients at risk of aspiration, oral anaerobes may be involved. No oral regimen has a reliable spectrum encompassing all these pathogens (see Table 255-6). Whatever regimen is chosen, its antimicrobial activity should encompass *S. pneumoniae*, the most common cause of pneumonia. Increasing resistance among pneumococci to all available oral antimicrobial agents precludes the designation of any one agent as the clear drug of choice.

Strains of *S. pneumoniae* that have a minimal inhibitory concentration (MIC) of penicillin (as determined by the broth dilution method) of 0.1 to 1.0 µg/mL are considered to have intermediate-level resistance, while strains that have an MIC of >1.0 µg/mL are considered to have high-level resistance. The current, less time-consuming method to screen for penicillin resistance is the use of a 1-µg oxacillin disk in a disk diffusion assay. Penicillin resistance (i.e., an MIC of ≥0.1 µg/mL) is indicated by a zone of growth inhibition of ≤19 mm. A new method, the E-strip, which is as accurate as the MIC broth dilution technique and can be performed as rapidly as the oxacillin disk diffusion assay, may replace the oxacillin test in the future.

The resistance of *S. pneumoniae* to penicillin varies greatly with the source of the clinical sample tested (e.g., strains isolated from middle-ear fluid are most often resistant), the age of the patient (e.g., resistance is more frequent among children than among adults), the setting (e.g., resistance is more common in day-care centers and hospitals than in the community), the patient's socioeconomic status (the frequency of resistance is highest in samples from suburban and white patients), and the geographic region in which the specimen was collected. Caution must be exercised in the interpretation of surveys of antimicrobial resistance among pneumococci in the United States, which can be strongly affected by these types of sampling bias. In a national survey of clinical isolates from normally sterile body sites that was conducted by the Centers for Disease Control and Prevention (CDC) from October 1991 to September 1992, 6.6 percent of 544 isolates of *S. pneumoniae* were resistant to ≥0.1 µg of penicillin/mL and 1.3 percent were resistant to ≥2 µg/mL. However, in another national survey of the antimicrobial susceptibility of clinical isolates from respiratory tract sites in 1992 and 1993, 15 percent of 799 isolates (with a range of 4 to 50 percent in the various medical centers) displayed intermediate-level

penicillin resistance, and an additional 7 percent (with a range of 0 to 33 percent) were highly penicillin-resistant.

Penicillin-resistant strains can be expected to exhibit decreased susceptibility to oral cephalosporins as well as to other antimicrobial agents. In the CDC survey, 5.9 percent of isolates were resistant to erythromycin (MIC, ≥1 µg/mL), but erythromycin resistance has been reported in 10 to 20 percent of pneumococcal isolates from some centers in the United States. Erythromycin-resistant strains are also resistant to other macrolides, such as clarithromycin and azithromycin. Fewer than 5 percent of strains were resistant to tetracycline in the CDC survey. Resistance to all of these antibiotics currently is much more common in many other parts of the world than in the United States. The potential for increased resistance in the United States in the future deserves close scrutiny; such an increase would require changes in antibiotic recommendations.

Neither trimethoprim-sulfamethoxazole nor the fluoroquinolones should be considered options for empirical therapy. The former drug is not active against more than 10 percent of strains of *S. pneumoniae*, and the latter agents exhibit—at best—borderline activity against pneumococci in vitro.

Penicillin, ampicillin, or amoxicillin (e.g., 500 mg of amoxicillin every 8 h for 7 to 10 days) remains the drug of choice for the treatment of suspected pneumococcal pneumonia in the United States and is recommended for the treatment of community-acquired pneumonia with a "typical" presentation in young adult outpatients without preexisting disease. Erythromycin (500 mg every 6 h) or doxycycline (100 mg every 12 h) is another option.

In older patients or adult outpatients with preexisting respiratory disease and a "typical" presentation of community-acquired pneumonia (among whom β-lactamase-producing pathogens such as *H. influenzae* and *M. catarrhalis* are common), either amoxicillin plus the β-lactamase inhibitor clavulanic acid or doxycycline can be used. Erythromycin displays poor activity against *H. influenzae*; two new oral antibiotics related to erythromycin, azithromycin (a single dose of 500 mg on the first day and 250 mg once daily for 4 more days) and clarithromycin (500 mg twice daily for 7 to 10 days), show equal or greater potency against many lower respiratory pathogens and may elicit gastrointestinal intolerance less frequently. Although more costly than erythromycin, these new macrolides may replace the older drug as therapy for community-acquired pneumonia in outpatients if pneumococcal resistance to macrolides does not become a widespread problem.

Doxycycline and erythromycin are active against *M. pneumoniae* and *C. pneumoniae* and can be used in young adults with an atypical presentation in whom mild pneumonia due to these pathogens is suspected. Ciprofloxacin is also active against these pathogens but is inadequately active against the pneumococcus to justify empirical use in this situation. Although erythromycin is the drug of choice for the treatment of legionellosis, doxycycline, trimethoprim-sulfamethoxazole, and ciprofloxacin have been used successfully for this indication (according to anecdotal reports). The duration of therapy for *Mycoplasma* and *Legionella* infection is 2 to 3 weeks;

Table 255-6

Empirical Oral Antimicrobial Therapy for Outpatient Management of Community-Acquired Pneumonia

Pathogen	Value of Indicated Antimicrobial*						
	Penicillin G	Amoxicillin/ Clavulanate	Cefuroxime	Trimethoprim- Sulfamethoxazole	Doxycycline	Erythromycin	Ciprofloxacin
Streptococcus pneumoniae	+†	+†	+†	±	+	+†	±
Haemophilus influenzae	−	+	+	+	+	±‡	+
Moraxella catarrhalis	−	+	+	+	+	+	+
Anaerobes	±	+	±	−	−	−	−
Mycoplasma pneumoniae	−	−	−	−	+	+	+
Chlamydia pneumoniae	−	−	−	−	+	+	+
Legionella pneumophila	−	−	−	±	±	+	±

* +, effective; −, ineffective; ±, sometimes effective.

† Between 10 and 20 percent of strains have recently been reported to be resistant to β-lactams and macrolides in some locations in the United States.

‡ The new macrolides azithromycin and clarithromycin are more active against *H. influenzae* than erythromycin and are equally or more active against other respiratory pathogens.

the longer duration is frequently recommended to prevent relapse. The optimal duration of therapy for *C. pneumoniae* infection is unknown but probably is 2 to 3 weeks.

Pneumonia due to anaerobes can be treated with clindamycin (300 mg every 6 h or 450 mg every 8 h for 7 to 10 days), with amoxicillin (500 mg every 8 h) plus metronidazole (500 mg every 6 h), or with amoxicillin/clavulanic acid (500 mg every 8 h or 875 mg every 12 h). Metronidazole exhibits poor activity against microaerophilic gram-positive cocci and must be supplemented by a β-lactam agent that compensates for this deficit in coverage.

Community-Acquired Pneumonia: Inpatient Management Patients who have community-acquired pneumonia and are ill enough to be hospitalized (Table 255-4) must undergo prompt microbiologic evaluation, receiving empirical therapy based on Gram's staining of sputum and knowledge of the current antimicrobial sensitivities of the pulmonary pathogens in the local geographic area (Tables 255-7 and 255-8). Parenteral antimicrobial therapy in the hospitalized patient is usually mandatory. A lack of sputum production, an atypical clinical presentation, the presence of diffuse radiographic infiltrates, a rapidly progressive downhill course, and a poor response to prior empirical therapy are some of the indications for the use of invasive procedures to detect the pulmonary pathogen, especially in the immunocompromised patient. Although broad-spectrum antibacterial therapy should be started during a full evaluation in severely ill patients with rapidly progressing illness, these empirical regimens cannot encompass all the possible pathogens without unnecessary toxicity and expense. Indeed, in immunocompromised patients (including those with neutropenia or HIV infection), the number of microbial and noninfectious causes of pulmonary disease is large and increasing. Since failure to provide specific treatment can prove rapidly fatal, a diagnosis should be sought aggressively so that optimal therapy can be started promptly.

Penicillin or ampicillin remains the drug of choice for infection due to penicillin-susceptible pneumococci. Studies suggest that high-dose intravenous penicillin G (e.g., 10 to 20 million units daily), ampicillin (2 g every 6 h), ceftriaxone (1 or 2 g every 24 h), or cefotaxime (1 to 2 g every 6 h) constitutes adequate therapy for pneumonia due to strains exhibiting intermediate resistance to penicillin (MIC, 0.1 to 1 μg/mL). The effectiveness of high-dose intravenous penicillin against pneumonia due to highly resistant pneumococcal strains is unknown, but MICs of cefotaxime and ceftriaxone for these strains are usually lower than those of penicillin or ampicillin and most other β-lactam antibiotics. Ceftriaxone or cefotaxime may be effective when the MIC of penicillin is ≥1 μg/mL and those of ceftriaxone and cefotaxime are ≤2 μg/mL. However, highly cephalosporin-resistant strains have become a problem in certain geographic areas. Since all penicillin-resistant strains are sensitive to vancomycin, initial empirical therapy should include this antibiotic (1 g intravenously every 12 h) when the patient with pneumococcal pneumonia is severely ill, has significant comorbidity, and lives in a region where highly penicillin- or cephalosporin-resistant strains have become common.

Table 255-8

Dosage of Antimicrobial Agents for the Treatment of Pneumonia in Hospitalized Patients*

Drug	Dosage
Ampicillin/sulbactam	3 g IV q6h
Aztreonam	2 g IV q8h
Cefazolin	1–2 g IV q8h
Cefotaxime, ceftizoxime	1–2 g q8–12h
Ceftazidime	2 g IV q8h
Ceftriaxone	1–2 g IV q12–24h
Cefuroxime	750 mg IV q8h
Ciprofloxacin	400 mg IV or 750 mg PO q12h
Clindamycin	600–900 mg IV q8h
Erythromycin	0.5–1.0 g IV q6h
Gentamicin (or tobramycin)	5 mg/kg/d in 3 equally divided doses IV q8h
Imipenem	500 mg IV q6h
Metronidazole	500 mg IV or PO q6h
Nafcillin	2 g IV q4h
Penicillin G	1–3 million units IV q4–6h
Ticarcillin/clavulanate	3.1 g IV q4h
Vancomycin	1 g IV q12h

* Dosage must be modified for patients with renal failure. Guidelines on the duration of therapy for each pathogen are given in the text of this chapter and of chapters on specific infecting agents.

If the result of Gram's staining of sputum is not interpretable or not available, either (1) a third-generation cephalosporin plus metronidazole or (2) ampicillin plus sulbactam is generally an adequate empirical regimen; when *Legionella* or *Chlamydia* is the likely pathogen, erythromycin should be added to the regimen. Therapy can be switched from intravenous to oral agents to complete a 7- to 10-day course if the patient's clinical condition improves rapidly and if antimicrobial agents that are readily absorbed after oral administration and that reach tissue levels above the MIC are available. The presence of *S. aureus* or aerobic gram-negative bacilli or the development of suppurative complications requires a more prolonged course of therapy. Legionellosis should be treated with 1 g of erythromycin intravenously every 6 h for 3 weeks to prevent relapses; rifampin should be added to the regimen if the patient is critically ill. Anaerobic lung abscess should be treated with the regimens suggested for aspiration pneumonia until a chest radiograph (with radiography performed at 2-week intervals) is clear or shows only a small stable scar. Therapy is prolonged for 6 weeks or more to prevent relapse, although shorter courses are probably sufficient for most patients. Surgery is rarely required for lung abscess; indications for surgery include massive hemoptysis and suspected neoplasm. Supportive measures include the administration of supplemental oxygen and intravenous fluids, assistance in clearing secretions, fiberoptic bronchoscopy, and (if necessary) ventilatory support. Caution should be exercised in bronchoscopic drainage of large, fluid-filled

Table 255-7

Empirical Antimicrobial Therapy for the Management of Hospitalized Patients with Community-Acquired Pneumonia

Pathogen	Value of Indicated Antimicrobial*						
	Penicillin G	First-Generation Cephalosporin	Third-Generation Cephalosporin	Metronidazole	Trimethoprim-Sulfamethoxazole	Erythromycin	Ampicillin/Sulbactam
Streptococcus pneumoniae	+†	+†	+	−	±	+†	+
Staphylococcus aureus	−	+	+	−	+	−	+
Haemophilus influenzae	−	−	+	−	+	±	+
Moraxella catarrhalis	−	+	+	−	+	+	+
Anaerobic gram-positive cocci	+	+	+	+	−	−	+
Anaerobic gram-negative bacilli	−	−	−	+	−	−	+
Chlamydia pneumoniae	−	−	−	−	−	+	−
Legionella pneumophila	−	−	−	−	±	+	−

* +, effective; −, ineffective; ±, sometimes effective.

† Between 10 and 20 percent of strains have recently been reported to be resistant to β-lactams and macrolides in some locations in the United States.

lung abscesses because of the potential for sudden massive spillage of large collections of pus into the airways.

Patients with risk factors for HIV infection and an atypical pneumonia syndrome should be evaluated for *Pneumocystis* infection because of its frequency as an index diagnosis in HIV infection and its potential severity. Tuberculosis and other causes of atypical pneumonia must be excluded as part of the evaluation of these patients. Empirical therapy can consist of either trimethoprim-sulfamethoxazole (15 to 20 mg/kg of trimethoprim, given daily in four divided doses intravenously or by mouth) or pentamidine (3 to 4 mg/kg daily, given intravenously), and treatment is continued for 3 weeks in confirmed cases of *Pneumocystis* infection. Although some data suggest that trimethoprim-sulfamethoxazole is more effective than pentamidine, further studies directly comparing the two agents are needed. The frequency and severity of the adverse effects of the two drugs are generally thought to be equivalent. The addition of glucocorticoids (prednisone, 40 mg twice daily, with subsequent tapering of the dose) early in the course of *Pneumocystis* pneumonia in patients with an arterial P_{O_2} of <70 mmHg decreases the need for mechanical ventilation and improves the patient's chances of survival and functional status. Prophylaxis for recurrent *Pneumocystis* pneumonia must be started at the end of therapy.

Institutionally Acquired Pneumonia Pneumonia acquired in institutions such as nursing homes or hospitals is frequently caused by enteric aerobic gram-negative bacilli, *P. aeruginosa*, or *S. aureus*, with or without oral anaerobes. Again, the selection of empirical antimicrobial therapy should be guided by Gram's staining of sputum (see Tables 255-8 and 255-9) and knowledge of the prevalent nosocomial pathogens and their current in vitro antimicrobial sensitivity patterns in the institution involved. An aggressive diagnostic approach is needed in some circumstances, especially for the immunocompromised patient (as outlined above).

S. aureus acquired in some institutions is frequently methicillin-resistant. Such strains are resistant to all β-lactam antibiotics and may also be resistant to clindamycin, erythromycin, and the fluoroquinolones. Only vancomycin is predictably active against these

organisms, and this drug should be added to the empirical regimen when methicillin-resistant organisms may be involved in pneumonia.

When multiantibiotic resistance is a problem, pneumonia due to gram-negative bacilli in the institutionalized patient can be treated initially with a β-lactam active against *P. aeruginosa* (ceftazidime, piperacillin/tazobactam, ticarcillin/clavulanate, aztreonam, or imipenem) or a parenterally administered fluoroquinolone (ciprofloxacin or ofloxacin). Ticarcillin/clavulanate and piperacillin/tazobactam are preferred over other penicillins with activity against *P. aeruginosa* (e.g., ticarcillin or piperacillin alone), which are not sufficiently active against *Klebsiella pneumoniae*, a relatively common pathogen. However, if piperacillin/tazobactam is to be used for infection suspected to be due to *P. aeruginosa*, a higher dose (3.375 g every 4 h) than is recommended by the package insert is required; a lower dose contains less piperacillin than is needed to be effective against this organism. Ampicillin/sulbactam, the other parenterally administered β-lactam antibiotic/β-lactamase inhibitor combination, is not active against many nosocomial pathogens, such as *P. aeruginosa*, *Enterobacter* spp., and *Serratia* spp., and therefore is inappropriate as empirical therapy for nosocomial pneumonia.

In seriously ill patients, especially those infected with *P. aeruginosa*, use of a β-lactam/aminoglycoside combination for bactericidal synergy is prudent. Such combinations are also used to broaden the spectrum of antibacterial activity to cover the possibility of infection with resistant pathogens, to treat polymicrobial infection, and to prevent the emergence of antimicrobial resistance. Combinations of β-lactams or aminoglycosides with a fluoroquinolone are not expected to enhance the already-rapid bactericidal activity of the fluoroquinolone alone; nevertheless, they are expected to broaden the spectrum covered and perhaps prevent the emergence of resistance. A fluoroquinolone plus either a β-lactam or an aminoglycoside can be used in institutions where there is a relatively high expectation of infection with a fluoroquinolone-resistant nosocomial pathogen (e.g., *Acinetobacter calcoaceticus*) or with organisms in which resistance frequently emerges during therapy (e.g., *P. aeruginosa*).

Pneumonia due to possible coinfection with aerobic gram-negative bacilli and anaerobes, as reflected by a polymicrobial flora on Gram's staining of sputum, may usually be treated with any of the following regimens: (1) ceftazidime plus metronidazole or clindamycin, (2) aztreonam or a fluoroquinolone plus clindamycin, or (3) imipenem or ticarcillin/clavulanate. The regimens that include a β-lactam agent usually should also include an aminoglycoside (see Table 255-9).

The production of chromosomally encoded, inducible β-lactamases by some aerobic gram-negative bacilli, including *Serratia marcescens*, *Enterobacter cloacae*, *Citrobacter freundii*, *Morganella morganii*, *P. aeruginosa*, and *A. calcoaceticus*, has important implications for the treatment of nosocomial pneumonia in institutions where these organisms are common nosocomial pathogens. Antibiotic resistance in these pathogens has been attributed to two related mechanisms: inducible production of chromosomally encoded β-lactamases and selection of mutants that have lost a gene that controls expression of β-lactamase production. The control gene represses β-lactamase production in the absence of a β-lactam agent and allows β-lactamase production in the presence of a β-lactam agent. This group of organisms has a relatively high mutation rate for loss of this control gene, and the loss of the gene results in continuous production of large amounts of β-lactamase (stable derepression). The derepressed mutants are resistant to third-generation cephalosporins, aztreonam, and broad-spectrum penicillins. These chromosomally encoded, inducible β-lactamases are not inhibited by clavulanic acid or sulbactam.

Selection by the β-lactam antibiotic of the derepressed mutants present in the dense bacterial populations of infected pulmonary tissue at the initiation of antibiotic therapy apparently accounts for the emergence of resistance during therapy, which is especially problematic in severely compromised patients whose defective host defenses are unable to control the growth of a few resistant mutants. The only β-lactam agent that maintains activity against the dere-

Table 255-9

Empirical Antimicrobial Therapy, Based on Gram's Staining of Sputum, for Institutionally Acquired Pneumonia

Etiology	Regimen
Presumptive *Staphylococcus aureus*	Nafcillin or vancomycin*
Presumptive enteric aerobic gram-negative bacilli or *Pseudomonas aeruginosa*	1. Ceftazidime ± aminoglycoside 2. Ticarcillin/clavulanate ± aminoglycoside 3. Aztreonam ± aminoglycoside 4. Imipenem† ± aminoglycoside 5. Fluoroquinolone† ± aminoglycoside or β-lactam
Mixed flora	1. Ceftazidime + clindamycin (or metronidazole) ± aminoglycoside‡ 2. Ticarcillin/clavulanate or piperacillin/tazobactam ± aminoglycoside‡ 3. Aztreonam + clindamycin (or metronidazole§) ± aminoglycoside‡ 4. Imipenem† ± aminoglycoside‡ 5. Fluoroquinolone† + clindamycin (or metronidazole‡,§) ± aminoglycoside or β-lactam

* If methicillin-resistant *S. aureus* is known to exist in the institution, use vancomycin; otherwise, use an antistaphylococcal β-lactam such as nafcillin or cefazolin.
† Use when chromosomally encoded, inducible β-lactamase producers are endemic in the institution.
‡ Add vancomycin if methicillin-resistant *S. aureus* is present in the institution.
§ Metronidazole must be combined with vancomycin or another antimicrobial that covers microaerophilic and anaerobic gram-positive cocci.

pressed mutants is imipenem. Ciprofloxacin and aminoglycosides may also retain activity against these mutants. Trimethoprim-sulfamethoxazole may remain active against all of these gram-negative bacilli except *P. aeruginosa*, which is inherently resistant to this agent. Some clinicians have questioned the efficacy of aminoglycosides alone for the treatment of gram-negative bacillary pneumonia. The poor clinical efficacy of aminoglycosides has been attributed to the low levels attained in bronchial secretions and to a loss of antimicrobial activity due to the relative acidity of purulent secretions, the anaerobic conditions in infected lung, and (in the case of *P. aeruginosa*) the divalent cations calcium and magnesium. The nephrotoxicity and ototoxicity of aminoglycosides frequently lead to underdosing with these agents. These problems are compounded by unpredictable pharmacokinetics that necessitate measurement of serum levels of aminoglycosides. If multiantibiotic-resistant nosocomial organisms are likely to be pathogens in severely compromised patients, reliable empirical agents may be fluoroquinolones or imipenem—unless resistance to these drugs is also endemic in the institution. Up-to-date knowledge of the antimicrobial sensitivities of an institution's nosocomial pathogens and use of various preventive practices are mandatory.

Amantadine (200 mg/day for most adults and 100 mg/day for persons over 65 years of age) is effective for the prevention of influenza A virus infection in the unimmunized patient during an influenza A outbreak and for the treatment (for 5 to 7 days) of early influenza A virus infection. Ribavirin is effective for respiratory syncytial virus infection. Intravenous acyclovir (5 to 10 mg/kg every 8 h for 7 to 14 days) is appropriate for varicella pneumonia. Treatment of cytomegalovirus pneumonia has yielded unsatisfactory results, but intravenous immunoglobulin combined with ganciclovir may be effective in some instances.

PREVENTION The prevention of pneumonia involves either (1) decreasing the likelihood of encountering the pathogen or (2) strengthening the host's response once the pathogen is encountered. The former approach can include measures such as hand washing and glove use by persons who care for patients infected with contact-transmitted pathogens (e.g., aerobic gram-negative bacilli); use of face masks or negative-pressure isolation rooms for patients with pneumonia due to pathogens spread by the aerosol route (e.g., *M. tuberculosis*); prompt institution of effective chemotherapy for patients with contagious illnesses; and correction of conditions that facilitate aspiration. The latter approach includes the use of chemoprophylaxis or immunization for patients at risk. Chemoprophylaxis may be administered to patients who have encountered or are likely to encounter the pathogen before they become symptomatic (e.g., amantadine during a community outbreak of influenza A, isoniazid for tuberculosis, or trimethoprim-sulfamethoxazole for pneumocystosis) or to patients who are likely to have a recurrence following recovery from a symptomatic episode (e.g., trimethoprim-sulfamethoxazole for pneumocystosis in patients with HIV infection). Gastric acidity is a major factor that prevents colonization of the gastrointestinal tract by nosocomial gram-negative bacillary pathogens. To prevent stress ulceration, it is preferable to use sucralfate, which maintains gastric acidity, rather than H_2-blocking agents. Vaccines (see Chaps. 122, 141, and 152) are available for immunization against *S. pneumoniae*, *H. influenzae* type b, influenza viruses A and B, and measles virus. Influenza and pneumococcal vaccines are strongly recommended for individuals over 65 years of age and for persons of any age who are at risk of adverse consequences of influenza or pneumonia because of underlying conditions. Pneumococcal, haemophilus, and influenza vaccines are recommended for HIV-infected patients who are still capable of responding to a vaccine challenge. The currently available 23-valent pneumococcal vaccine covers 88 percent of the serotypes causing systemic disease as well as 8 percent of related serotypes. The increasing prevalence of multiantibiotic resistance among pneumococci makes pneumococcal immunization of high-risk individuals of utmost importance. Immune serum globulin is available for intravenous replacement therapy in those patients with congenital or acquired hypogammaglobulinemia.

The prevention of nosocomial pneumonia requires good infection control practices, judicious use of broad-spectrum antimicrobial agents, and maintenance of patients' gastric acidity.

BIBLIOGRAPHY

APPELBAUM PC: Antimicrobial resistance in *Streptococcus pneumoniae*: An overview. Clin Infect Dis 15:77, 1992

BARRY AL et al: In vitro activities of 12 orally administered antimicrobial agents against four species of bacterial respiratory pathogens from U.S. medical centers in 1992 and 1993. Antimicrob Agents Chemother 38:2419, 1994

BREIMAN RF et al: Emergence of drug-resistant pneumococcal infections in the United States. JAMA 271:1831, 1994

CRAVEN DE et al: Nosocomial pneumonia in the 1990s: Update of epidemiology and risk factors. Semin Respir Infect 5:157, 1990

FAIRCHOK MP et al: Carriage of penicillin-resistant pneumococci in a military population in Washington, DC: Risk factors and correlation with clinical isolates. Clin Infect Dis 22:966, 1996

FANG GD et al: New and emerging etiologies for community-acquired pneumonia with implications for therapy. Medicine 69:307, 1990

FINE MJ: Pneumonia in the elderly: The hospital admission and discharge decisions. Semin Respir Infect 65:303, 1990

HAHN DL et al: Association of *Chlamydia pneumoniae* (strain TWAR) infection with wheezing, asthmatic bronchitis and adult-onset asthma. JAMA 266:225, 1991

HOFFMAN J et al: The prevalence of drug-resistant *Streptococcus pneumoniae* in Atlanta. N Engl J Med 333:481, 1995

JACOBS MR: Treatment and diagnosis of infections caused by drug-resistant *Streptococcus pneumoniae*. Clin Infect Dis 15:119, 1992

LEVISON ME, BUSH L: Pharmacodynamics of antimicrobial agents. Bactericidal and postantibiotic effects. Infect Dis Clin North Am 3:415, 1989

——— et al: Clindamycin compared with penicillin for the treatment of anaerobic lung abscess. Ann Intern Med 98:466, 1983

LORBER B, SWENSON RM: Bacteriology of aspiration pneumonia, a prospective study of community and hospital acquired cases. Ann Intern Med 81:329, 1974

PALLARES R et al: Resistance to penicillin and cephalosporin and mortality from severe pneumococcal pneumonia in Barcelona, Spain. N Engl J Med 333:474, 1995

RIES K et al: Transtracheal aspiration in pulmonary infection. Arch Intern Med 133:453, 1974

RILEY RL: Airborne infection. Am J Med 57:466, 1974

SANDERS CC, SANDERS WE JR: Clinical significance of inducible beta-lactamase in gram-negative bacteria. Eur J Clin Microbiol 6:435, 1987

SHELHAMER JH et al: NIH Conference: Respiratory disease in the immunosuppressed patient. Ann Intern Med 117:415, 1992

STEINHOFF D et al: *Chlamydia pneumoniae* as a cause of community-acquired pneumonia in hospitalized patients in Berlin. Clin Infect Dis 22:958, 1996

THORNSBERRY C et al: Increased penicillin resistance in recent U.S. isolates of *Streptococcus pneumoniae*, in *Abstracts of the General Meeting of the American Society for Microbiology*. ASM, Washington, DC, 1992, abstract C-268

VERGHESE A, BERK SL: Bacterial pneumonia in the elderly. Medicine 62:271, 1982

WOODHEAD MA et al: Prospective study of the aetiology and outcome of pneumonia in the community. Lancet 1:671, 1987

256 *Steven E. Weinberger*

BRONCHIECTASIS

DEFINITION Bronchiectasis is an abnormal and permanent dilatation of bronchi. It may be either focal, involving airways supplying a limited region of pulmonary parenchyma, or diffuse, involving airways in a more widespread distribution. Although this definition is based on pathologic changes in the bronchi, diagnosis is often suggested by the clinical consequences of chronic or recurrent infection in the dilated airways and the associated secretions that pool within these airways.

PATHOLOGY The bronchial dilatation of bronchiectasis is associated with destructive and inflammatory changes in the walls of medium-sized airways, often at the level of segmental or subsegmental bronchi. The normal structural components of the wall, including cartilage, muscle, and elastic tissue, are destroyed and may be replaced by fibrous tissue. The dilated airways frequently contain pools of thick, purulent material, while more peripheral airways are often occluded by secretions or obliterated and replaced by fibrous tissue. Additional microscopic features include bronchial and peribronchial inflammation and fibrosis, ulceration of the bronchial wall, squamous metaplasia, and mucous gland hyperplasia. The parenchyma normally supplied by the affected airways is abnormal, containing varying combinations of fibrosis, emphysema, bronchopneumonia, and atelectasis. As a result of the inflammation, vascularity of the bronchial wall increases, with associated enlargement of the bronchial arteries and anastomoses between the bronchial and pulmonary arterial circulations.

Three different patterns of bronchiectasis were described by Reid in 1950. In *cylindrical bronchiectasis* the bronchi appear as uniformly dilated tubes that end abruptly at the point that smaller airways are obstructed by secretions. In *varicose bronchiectasis* the affected bronchi have an irregular or beaded pattern of dilatation resembling varicose veins. In *saccular (cystic) bronchiectasis* the bronchi have a ballooned appearance at the periphery, ending in blind sacs without recognizable bronchial structures distal to the sacs.

ETIOLOGY AND PATHOGENESIS Bronchiectasis is a consequence of inflammation and destruction of the structural components of the bronchial wall. Infection is the usual cause of the inflammation; microorganisms such as *Pseudomonas aeruginosa* and *Haemophilus influenzae* produce pigments, proteases, and other toxins that injure the respiratory epithelium and impair mucociliary clearance. The host inflammatory response induces epithelial injury, largely as a result of mediators released from neutrophils. As protection against infection is compromised, the dilated airways become more susceptible to colonization and growth of bacteria. Thus, a reinforcing cycle can result, with inflammation producing airway damage, impaired clearance of microorganisms, and further infection, which then completes the cycle by inciting more inflammation.

Infectious Causes A wide variety of infectious agents can initiate bronchiectasis. In the past, bronchiectasis during childhood was often a complication of measles or pertusis; these are now rare causes, as a result of effective immunization. At present, adenovirus and influenza virus are the main viruses that cause bronchiectasis in association with lower respiratory tract involvement. Although not as common as in the preantibiotic era, virulent bacterial infections, especially with potentially necrotizing organisms such as *Staphylococcus aureus*, *Klebsiella*, and anaerobes, remain important causes of bronchiectasis when antibiotic treatment of a pneumonia is not given or is significantly delayed. Bronchiectasis has been reported in patients with human immunodeficiency virus (HIV) infection, perhaps at least partly due to recurrent bacterial infection. Tuberculosis can produce bronchiectasis by a necrotizing effect on pulmonary parenchyma and airways and indirectly as a consequence of airway obstruction from bronchostenosis or extrinsic compression by lymph nodes. Nontuberculous mycobacteria are frequently associated with bronchiectasis, usually as secondary infections or colonizing organisms, though occasionally as primary pathogens. Mycoplasmal and necrotizing fungal infections are rare causes.

Impaired host defense mechanisms are often involved in the predisposition to recurrent infections. The major cause of localized impairment of host defenses is endobronchial obstruction. Bacteria and secretions cannot be cleared adequately from the obstructed airway, which develops recurrent or chronic infection. Although primary lung cancer is the most common cause of endobronchial obstruction, it is an infrequent cause of bronchiectasis, since either the involved area is removed surgically or the disease progresses before bronchiectasis becomes an important problem. Slowly growing endobronchial neo-

plasms such as carcinoid tumors are more commonly associated with bronchiectasis. Foreign body aspiration is another important cause of endobronchial obstruction, particularly in children. Airway obstruction can also result from bronchostenosis, from impacted secretions, or from extrinsic compression by enlarged lymph nodes.

Generalized impairment of pulmonary defense mechanisms occurs with immunoglobulin deficiency, primary ciliary disorders, or cystic fibrosis. Infections and bronchiectasis are therefore often more diffuse. With panhypogammaglobulinemia, the best described of the immunoglobulin disorders associated with recurrent infection and bronchiectasis, patients often also have a history of sinus or skin infections. Selective IgA deficiency can be associated with bronchiectasis, frequently with coexisting deficiency of IgG subclasses (especially IgG2 or IgG4).

The primary disorders associated with ciliary dysfunction are termed *primary ciliary dyskinesia*. Numerous defects are encompassed under this category, including structural abnormalities of the dynein arms, radial spokes, and microtubules. The cilia become dyskinetic, their coordinated, propulsive action is diminished, and bacterial clearance is impaired. The clinical effects include recurrent upper and lower respiratory tract infections, such as sinusitis, otitis media, and bronchiectasis. Because normal sperm motility also depends on proper ciliary function, males are generally infertile (see also Chap. 336). Approximately half of patients with primary ciliary dyskinesia fall into the subgroup of *Kartagener's syndrome*, in which situs inversus accompanies bronchiectasis and sinusitis. It has been hypothesized that ciliary motility is necessary for proper rotation of the viscera during embryogenesis, so that visceral rotation is random when normal ciliary motion is lost.

In cystic fibrosis (see Chap. 257), the tenacious secretions in the bronchi are associated with impaired bacterial clearance, resulting in colonization and recurrent infection with a variety of organisms, particularly mucoid strains of *P. aeruginosa* but also *S. aureus*, *H. influenzae*, *Escherichia coli*, and *P. cepacia*.

Noninfectious Causes Some cases of bronchiectasis are associated with exposure to a toxic substance that incites a severe inflammatory response. Examples include inhalation of a toxic gas such as ammonia or aspiration of acidic gastric contents, though the latter problem is often also complicated by aspiration of bacteria. An immune response in the airway may also trigger inflammation, destructive changes, and bronchial dilatation. This mechanism is presumably responsible at least in part for bronchiectasis with allergic bronchopulmonary aspergillosis (ABPA), which is due to an immune response to *Aspergillus* organisms that have colonized the airway (Chap. 253). Bronchiectasis accompanying ABPA often involves proximal airways and is associated with mucoid impaction. Bronchiectasis also occurs rarely in ulcerative colitis, rheumatoid arthritis, and Sjögren's syndrome, but it is not known whether an immune response triggers airway inflammation in these patients.

In α_1-antitrypsin deficiency, the usual respiratory complication is the early development of panacinar emphysema, but affected individuals may occasionally have bronchiectasis. In the *yellow nail syndrome*, which is due to hypoplastic lymphatics, the triad of lymphedema, pleural effusion, and yellow discoloration of the nails is accompanied by bronchiectasis in approximately 40 percent of patients.

CLINICAL MANIFESTATIONS Patients typically present with persistent or recurrent cough and purulent sputum production. Hemoptysis occurs in 50 to 70 percent of cases and can be due to bleeding from friable, inflamed airway mucosa. More significant, even massive bleeding is often a consequence of bleeding from hypertrophied bronchial arteries.

When a specific infectious episode initiates bronchiectasis, patients may describe a severe pneumonia followed by chronic cough and sputum production. Alternatively, patients without a dramatic initiating event often describe the insidious onset of symptoms. In some cases, patients are either asymptomatic or have a nonproductive cough, often associated with "dry" bronchiectasis in an upper lobe. Dyspnea or wheezing generally reflects either widespread bronchiectasis or underlying chronic obstructive pulmonary disease. With exacerbations of infection, the amount of sputum increases, the appearance becomes more purulent and often more bloody, and patients may become febrile. Such episodes may be due solely to exacerbations of the airway infection, but associated parenchymal infiltrates sometimes reflect an adjacent pneumonia.

Physical examination of the chest overlying an area of bronchiectasis is quite variable. Any combination of crackles, rhonchi, and wheezes may be heard, all of which reflect the damaged airways containing significant secretions. As with other types of chronic intrathoracic infection, clubbing may be present. Patients with severe, diffuse disease, particularly those with chronic hypoxemia, may have associated cor pulmonale and right ventricular failure. Amyloidosis can result from chronic infection and inflammation but is now seldom seen.

RADIOGRAPHIC AND LABORATORY FINDINGS

Though the chest radiograph is important in the evaluation of suspected bronchiectasis, the findings are often nonspecific. At one extreme, the radiograph may be normal with mild disease. Alternatively, patients with saccular bronchiectasis may have prominent cystic spaces, either with or without air-liquid levels, corresponding to the dilated airways. These may be difficult to distinguish from enlarged airspaces due to bullous emphysema or from regions of honeycombing in patients with severe interstitial lung disease. Other findings are due to dilated airways with thickened walls, which result from peribronchial inflammation. Because of decreased aeration and atelectasis of the associated pulmonary parenchyma, these dilated airways are often crowded together in parallel. When seen longitudinally, the airways appear as "tram tracks"; when seen in cross-section, they produce "ring shadows." Because the dilated airways may be filled with secretions, the lumen may appear dense rather than radiolucent, producing an opaque tubular or branched tubular structure.

Bronchography, which involves coating the airways with a radiopaque, iodinated lipid dye instilled through a catheter or bronchoscope, can provide excellent visualization of bronchiectatic airways. However, this technique has now been replaced by computed tomography (CT), which also provides an excellent view of dilated airways as seen in cross-sectional images (Fig. 256-1). With the advent of high-resolution CT scanning, in which the images are 1.0 to 1.5 mm thick, the sensitivity for detecting bronchiectasis has improved even further.

Examination of sputum often reveals an abundance of neutrophils and colonization or infection with a variety of possible organisms. Although common bacterial pathogens such as *Streptococcus pneumoniae* and *H. influenzae* may be present, a number of other organisms

are seen frequently. *P. aeruginosa* is particularly common and may be a clue to the presence of previously unsuspected bronchiectasis. Other organisms include *Staph. aureus*, anaerobes, and nontuberculous (atypical) mycobacteria. Appropriate staining and culturing of sputum often provides a guide to antibiotic therapy.

Additional evaluation is aimed at diagnosing the cause for the bronchiectasis. When bronchiectasis is focal, fiberoptic bronchoscopy may reveal an underlying endobronchial obstruction. In other cases, upper lobe involvement may be suggestive of either tuberculosis or ABPA. With more widespread disease, measurement of sweat chloride levels for cystic fibrosis, structural or functional assessment of nasal or bronchial cilia or sperm for primary ciliary dyskinesia, and quantitative assessment of immunoglobulins may explain recurrent airway infection. In an asthmatic person with proximal bronchiectasis or other historical features to suggest ABPA, skin testing, serology, and sputum culture for *Aspergillus* are helpful in confirming the diagnosis.

Pulmonary function tests may demonstrate airflow obstruction as a consequence of diffuse bronchiectasis or associated chronic obstructive lung disease. Bronchial hyperreactivity, e.g., to methacholine challenge, and some reversibility of the airflow obstruction with inhaled bronchodilators are relatively common for reasons not well defined. Other laboratory evaluation is often relatively nonspecific. For example, as a result of chronic infection within the thorax, patients may develop the normocytic, normochromic anemia of chronic disease.

℞ TREATMENT

Therapy has four major goals: (1) elimination of an identifiable underlying problem; (2) improved clearance of tracheobronchial secretions; (3) control of infection, particularly during acute exacerbations; and (4) reversal of airflow obstruction. Appropriate treatment should be instituted when a treatable cause is found, for example, treatment of hypogammaglobulinemia with immunoglobulin replacement, tuberculosis with antituberculous agents, and ABPA with glucocorticoids.

Secretions are typically copious and thick and contribute to the symptoms. Chest physical therapy with vibration, percussion, and postural drainage frequently helps patients with copious secretions. Mucolytic agents to thin secretions and allow better clearance are controversial. Aerosolized recombinant DNase, which decreases viscosity of sputum by breaking down DNA released from neutrophils, has been shown to improve pulmonary function in cystic fibrosis, but similar benefits have not been found with bronchiectasis due to other etiologies.

Chronic or recurrent bacterial infections cause much of the morbidity of bronchiectasis. Antibiotics have an important role in management, but which antibiotic should be given and the frequency and duration of administration are not well established. For patients with infrequent exacerbations characterized by an increase in quantity and purulence of the sputum, antibiotics are commonly used only during acute episodes. Although choice of an antibiotic may be guided by Gram's stain and culture of sputum, empiric coverage (e.g., with ampicillin, amoxicillin, trimethoprim-sulfamethoxazole, or cefaclor) is often given initially. When *P. aeruginosa* is present, oral therapy with a quinolone or parenteral therapy with an aminoglycoside or third-generation cephalosporin may be appropriate. In patients with chronic purulent sputum despite short courses of antibiotics, more prolonged courses, e.g., with oral amoxicillin or inhaled aminoglycosides, or intermittent but regular courses of single or rotating antibiotics have been used.

Bronchodilators to improve obstruction and aid clearance of secretions are particularly useful in patients with airway hyperreactivity and reversible airflow obstruction. Although surgical therapy was common in the past, more effective antibiotic and supportive therapy has largely replaced surgery. However, when bronchiectasis is localized and the morbidity is substantial despite adequate medical

FIGURE 256-1 Chest CT section demonstrating extensive bronchiectasis, best seen in the right middle lobe and the lingula. The airways are dilated, crowded, and surrounded by poorly aerated pulmonary parenchyma. The arrow marks an opacity that represents a mucous plug in a dilated, branching airway.

therapy, surgical resection of the involved region of lung should be considered.

Complications present additional treatment issues. When massive hemoptysis, often originating from the hypertrophied bronchial circulation, does not resolve with conservative therapy, including rest and antibiotics, therapeutic options are either surgical resection or bronchial arterial embolization (Chap. 33). Although resection may be successful if disease is localized, embolization is preferable with widespread disease. In patients with extensive disease, chronic hypoxemia and cor pulmonale may indicate the need for long-term supplemental oxygen. For selected patients who are disabled despite maximal therapy, lung transplantation is a therapeutic option.

BIBLIOGRAPHY

BARKER AF: Bronchiectasis. Semin Thorac Cardiovasc Surg 7:112, 1995

COLE PJ: Inflammation: A two-edged sword—the model of bronchiectasis. Eur J Respir Dis 69(Suppl 147):6, 1986

GREENSTONE M et al: Primary ciliary dyskinesia: Cytological and clinical features. Q J Med 67:405, 1988

HOLMES AH et al: Bronchiectasis in HIV disease. Q J Med 85:875, 1992

KANG EY et al: Bronchiectasis: Comparison of preoperative thin-section CT and pathologic findings in resected specimens. Radiology 195:649, 1995

MCGUINNESS G et al: Bronchiectasis: CT evaluation. Am J Roentgenol 160:253, 1993

SHADICK NA et al: Bronchiectasis. A late feature of severe rheumatoid arthritis. Medicine 73:161, 1994

TRUCKSIS M, SWARTZ MN: Bronchiectasis: A current view. Curr Clin Top Infect Dis 11:170, 1991

257

Richard C. Boucher

CYSTIC FIBROSIS

Cystic fibrosis (CF) is a monogenetic disorder that presents as a multisystem disease. The first signs and symptoms typically occur in childhood, but nearly 4 percent of patients are diagnosed as adults. Due to improvements in therapy, approximately 34 percent of patients reach adulthood and nearly 10 percent live past the age of 30. The average life span for both male and female CF patients is similar, ~28 years. Thus, CF is no longer only a pediatric disease, and internists must be prepared to recognize and treat its many complications. This disease is characterized by chronic airway infection that ultimately leads to bronchiectasis and bronchiolectasis, exocrine pancreatic insufficiency and intestinal dysfunction, abnormal sweat gland function, and urogenital dysfunction.

PATHOGENESIS Genetic Basis CF is an autosomal recessive disease resulting from mutations in a gene located on chromosome 7. The prevalence of CF varies with the ethnic origin of a population. CF is detected in approximately 1 in 3000 live births in the Caucasian population of North America and northern Europe, 1 in 17,000 live births of African-Americans, and 1 in 90,000 live births of the Asian population of Hawaii. The most common mutation in the CF gene (~70 percent of CF chromosomes) is a 3-base-pair deletion that results in an absence of phenylalanine at amino acid position 508 (ΔF_{508}) of the CF gene protein product, known as the CF transmembrane regulator (CFTR). The large number (>400) of relatively uncommon (<2 percent) mutations identified in the CF gene makes it difficult to use DNA diagnostic technologies for identifying heterozygotes in populations at large, and no simple physiologic measurements allow heterozygote detection.

CFTR Protein The CFTR protein is a single polypeptide chain containing 1480 amino acids that appears to function both as a cyclic AMP–regulated Cl^- channel and, as its name implies, as a regulator of other ion channels. The fully processed form of CFTR is found in the plasma membrane in normal epithelia (Fig. 257-1). Biochemical studies indicate that the ΔF_{508} mutation leads to improper processing and intracellular degradation of the CFTR protein. Thus, absence of CFTR at appropriate cellular sites is often part of the pathophysiology of CF. However, other mutations in the CF gene produce CFTR proteins that are fully processed but are nonfunctional or only partially functional at the appropriate cellular sites.

Epithelial Dysfunction The epithelia affected by CF exhibit different functions in their native state; i.e., some are volume-absorbing (airways and intestinal epithelia), some are salt-absorbing but not volume-absorbing (sweat duct), whereas others are volume-secretory (pancreas). Given this diverse array of native activities, it should not be surprising that CF produces very different effects on patterns of electrolyte and water transport. However, the unifying concept is that all affected tissues express abnormal ion transport function.

ORGAN-SPECIFIC PATHOPHYSIOLOGY Lung The diagnostic biophysical hallmark of CF is the raised transepithelial electric potential difference (PD) detected in airway epithelia. The transepithelial PD reflects components of both the rate of active ion transport and the resistance to ion flow of the superficial epithelium. CF airway epithelia exhibit both raised transport rates (Na^+) and decreased ion permeability (Cl^-) (Fig. 257-2). The Cl^- transport defect reflects at least in part the absence of cyclic AMP–dependent kinase and protein kinase C–regulated Cl^- transport that is mediated by the Cl^- channel functions of CFTR. An important observation is that there is an alternative Cl^- channel expressed in airway epithelia. This "alternative" Cl^- channel (Cl^-_a) is different from CFTR and is regulated by intracellular Ca^{2+} levels or by extracellular triphosphate nucleotides, e.g., uridine–adenine triphosphate (UTP), and perhaps by CFTR itself. This channel can substitute for CFTR with regard to net Cl^- transport and may be a potential therapeutic target.

Raised Na^+ absorption is a feature of CF airway epithelia. Na^+ transport abnormalities are not a widespread feature of the CF epithelial phenotype and appear confined to volume-absorbing epithelia. Recent studies demonstrate that the increased Na^+ transport reflects the absence of CFTR's tonic inhibitory regulatory function on Na^+ channel activity. It appears that CFTR inhibits Na^+ channel activity as a part of its general function to act as a "switch" that coordinates the balance between Na^+ absorption and Cl^- secretion.

The central hypothesis of CF airways pathophysiology has been that the abnormal Na^+ and Cl^- transport rates produce secretions that are dehydrated and poorly cleared. The unique predisposition of CF airways to chronic infection by *Staphylococcus aureus* and *Pseudomo-*

FIGURE 257-1 Cellular metabolism of the CFTR protein. In a normal cell (*left*), CFTR is synthesized in the rough endoplasmic reticulum (RER), glycosylated in the Golgi apparatus, and functions as a Cl^- channel and regulator of other ion channels when located in the plasma membrane. Two possible outcomes of mutations in the CF gene are shown (*right*). (1) If a mutation disturbs protein folding, e.g., the ΔF_{508} mutation, CFTR is degraded intracellularly so that no protein is transported to the plasma membrane. (2) With other mutations, the abnormal protein is processed and trafficks to the plasma membrane but functions abnormally at that site.

nas aeruginosa raises the issue that other as yet undefined abnormalities in airway surface liquid ionic composition also may contribute to the failure of lung defense.

Gastrointestinal Tract   The gastrointestinal effects of CF are diverse. In the exocrine pancreas, the absence of the CFTR Cl⁻ channel in the apical membrane of pancreatic ductal epithelia limits the function of an apical membrane $Cl^--HCO_3^-$ exchanger to secrete bicarbonate and Na^+ (by a passive process) into the duct. The failure to secrete $NaHCO_3$ and water leads to retention of enzymes in the pancreas and ultimately destruction of virtually all pancreatic tissue. The CF intestinal epithelium, because of the lack of Cl⁻ and water secretion, fails to flush the secreted mucins and other macromolecules from intestinal crypts. The diminished CFTR-mediated secretion of liquid may be exacerbated by excessive absorption of liquid, reflecting abnormalities of CFTR-mediated regulation of Na^+ absorption (both mediated by Na^+ channels and possibly other Na^+ transporters, e.g., Na^+-H^+ exchangers). Both dysfunctions lead to dessicated intralumenal contents and obstruction of both the small and large intestines. In the hepatobiliary system, defective hepatic ductal salt (Cl⁻) and water secretion causes retention of biliary secretions and focal biliary cirrhosis and bile duct proliferation in approximately 25 to 30 percent of CF patients. The inability of the CF gallbladder epithelium to secrete salt and water can lead to both chronic cholecystitis and cholelithiasis.

Sweat Gland   CF patients secrete nearly normal volumes of sweat in the sweat acinus. However, CF patients are not able to absorb NaCl from sweat as it moves through the sweat duct due to the inability to absorb Cl⁻ across the ductal epithelial cells.

DIAGNOSIS   Because of the large number of CF mutations, DNA analysis is not used for primary diagnosis. The diagnosis of CF rests on a combination of clinical criteria and analyses of sweat Cl⁻ values. The values for the Na^+ and Cl⁻ concentration in sweat vary with age, but typically in adults a Cl⁻ concentration of >70 mmol/L discriminates between CF patients and patients with other lung disease. Between 1 and 2 percent of patients with the clinical syndrome of CF have normal sweat Cl⁻ values. In most of these patients, the nasal transepithelial PD is raised into the diagnostic range for CF and sweat acini do not secrete in response to injected beta-adrenergic agonists. A single mutation of the CFTR gene, 3849 + 10 kb C→T, is associated with approximately 50 percent of CF patients with normal sweat Cl⁻ values.

It is likely that DNA analyses will be performed increasingly in CF patients. Comprehensive genotype-phenotype relationships have not yet been established sufficiently for prognosis. A relationship between ΔF_{508} homozygosity or other mutations and pancreatic insufficiency has been established, but no predictive relationship holds for ΔF_{508} homozygosity and lung disease.

CLINICAL FEATURES   Most CF patients present with signs and symptoms of the disease in childhood. Approximately 15 percent of patients present within the first 24 h of life with gastrointestinal obstruction, termed *meconium ileus*. Other common presentations within the first year or two of life include respiratory tract symptoms, most prominently cough and/or recurrent pulmonary infiltrates, and failure to thrive. A significant proportion of patients (~4 percent), however, are diagnosed after age 18.

Respiratory Tract   Upper respiratory tract disease is almost universal in CF patients. Chronic sinusitis is common in childhood and leads to nasal obstruction and rhinorrhea. The occurrence of nasal polyps approaches 25 percent and often requires surgery.

In the lower respiratory tract, the first symptom of CF is cough. With time, the cough becomes persistent and produces viscous, purulent, often greenish-colored sputum. Inevitably, periods of clinical stability are interrupted by "exacerbations," defined by increased cough, weight loss, increased sputum volume, and decrements in pulmonary function. These exacerbations require aggressive therapy, including frequent postural drainage and oral antibiotics, and often intravenous antibiotics (see below), with the goal being recovery of lost lung function. Over the course of years, the exacerbations become more frequent and the recovery of lost lung function less complete, leading to respiratory failure.

CF patients exhibit a characteristic sputum microbiology. *Haemophilus influenzae* and *S. aureus* are often the first organisms recovered from samples of lung secretions in newly diagnosed CF patients. *P. aeruginosa* is typically cultured from lower respiratory tract secretions thereafter. After repetitive antibiotic exposure, *P. aeruginosa*, often in a mucoid form, is usually the predominant organism recovered from sputum and may be present as several strains with different antibiotic sensitivities. *Burkholderia* (formerly *Pseudomonas*) *cepacia* has been recovered from CF sputum and is pathogenic. Patient-to-patient spread of certain strains of this organism indicates that infection control in the hospital should be practiced. Other gram-negative rods recovered from CF sputum include *Xanthomonas zylosoxida* and *P. gladioli*, and occasionally, mucoid forms of *Proteus*, *Escherichia coli*, and *Klebsiella*. Up to 50 percent of CF patients have *Aspergillus fumigatus* in their sputum, and up to 10 percent of these patients exhibit the syndrome of allergic bronchopulmonary aspergillosis. *Mycobacterium tuberculosis* is rare in CF patients. However, 10 to 20 percent of adult CF patients have sputum cultures positive for nontuberculous mycobacteria, and in some patients these microorganisms are associated with disease.

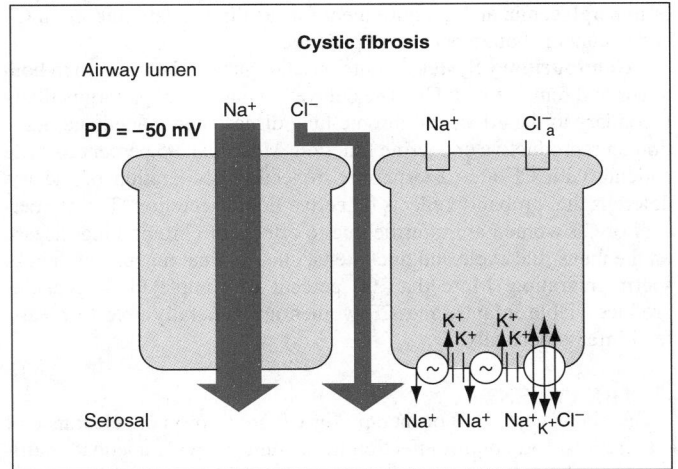

FIGURE 257-2   Comparison of ion transport properties of normal (*top*) and CF (*bottom*) airway epithelia. The vectors describe routes and magnitudes of Na^+ and Cl⁻ transport. The normal basal pattern for ion transport is absorption of Na^+ from the lumen via an amiloride-sensitive Na^+ channel. This process is accelerated in CF. The capacity to initiate cyclic cAMP–mediated Cl⁻ secretion is diminished in CF airway epithelia due to absence/dysfunction of the CFTR Cl⁻ channel. The accelerated Na^+ absorption in CF reflects the absence of CFTR inhibitory effects on Na^+ channels. Cl_a^-, alternative Cl⁻ channel; PD, potential difference; CFTR, cystic fibrosis transmembrane regulator.

The first lung function abnormalities observed in CF children, increased ratios of residual volume to total lung capacity, suggest that small airways disease is the first functional lung abnormality in CF. As the disease progresses, both reversible and irreversible changes in forced vital capacity (FVC) and forced expiratory volume (FEV_1) are noted. The reversible component reflects accumulation of intraluminal secretions and/or airway reactivity, which occurs in 40 to 60 percent of CF patients. The irreversible component reflects chronic destruction of the airway wall and bronchiolitis.

The earliest chest x-ray change in CF lungs is hyperinflation, reflecting small airways obstruction. Later, signs of luminal mucus impaction, bronchial cuffing, and finally, bronchiectasis, e.g., ring shadows, are noted. For reasons that are still unknown, the right upper lobe displays the earliest and most severe changes. Neither CT nor MRI scanning are routinely performed on CF patients.

CF pulmonary disease is associated with many intermittent complications. Pneumothorax is common (>10 percent of patients). The production of small amounts of blood in sputum is common in CF patients with advanced pulmonary disease and appears to be associated with lung infection. Massive hemoptysis is life-threatening and difficult to localize bronchoscopically. With advanced lung disease, digital clubbing becomes evident in virtually all patients with CF. As late events, respiratory failure and cor pulmonale are prominent features of CF.

Gastrointestinal Tract   The syndrome of meconium ileus in infants presents with abdominal distention, failure to pass stool, and emesis. The abdominal flat plate can be diagnostic, with small intestinal air fluid levels, a granular appearance representing meconium, and a small colon. In children and young adults, a syndrome termed *meconium ileus equivalent* or distal intestinal obstruction occurs. The syndrome presents with right lower quadrant pain, loss of appetite, occasionally emesis, and often a palpable mass. The syndrome can be confused with appendicitis, which occurs frequently in CF patients. The characteristic intestinal abnormalities are complicated by exocrine pancreatic insufficiency in more than 90 percent of CF patients. Insufficient pancreatic enzyme release yields the typical pattern of protein and fat malabsorption, with frequent, bulky, foul-smelling stools. Signs and symptoms of malabsorption of fat-soluble vitamins, including vitamins E and K, are also noted. Because pancreatic beta cells are typically spared, the appearance of hyperglycemia and a requirement for insulin is a late finding in CF and occurs in about 5 percent of patients.

Genitourinary System   Late onset of puberty is common in both males and females with CF. The delayed maturational pattern is likely secondary to the effects of chronic lung disease and inadequate nutrition on reproductive endocrine function. More than 95 percent of male patients with CF are azoospermic, reflecting obliteration of the vas deferens that probably reflects defective liquid secretion. Twenty percent of CF women are infertile due to effects of chronic lung disease on the menstrual cycle and thick, tenacious cervical mucus that blocks sperm migration. More than 90 percent of completed pregnancies produce viable infants, and CF women are generally able to breastfeed infants normally.

℞ **TREATMENT**

The major objectives of therapy for CF are to promote clearance of secretions and control infection in the lung, provide adequate nutrition, and prevent intestinal obstruction. Ultimately, gene therapy may be the treatment of choice.

Lung Disease   At present, the principal technique for clearing pulmonary secretions is a combination of breathing exercises and chest percussion. It should be stressed that regular use of these maneuvers is effective in preserving lung function. More than 95 percent of CF patients die of complications resulting from lung infection. Antibiotics are the principal agents available for treating lung infection, and their use should be guided by sputum culture results. Early intervention with antibiotics is useful, and long courses

of treatment are the rule. Because of increased total-body clearance and volume of distribution of antibiotics in CF patients, the required doses are higher for CF patients than for non-CF patients with similar chest infections.

Increased cough and mucus production are treated with antibiotics given by the oral route. Typical oral agents used to treat *Staphylococcus* include a semisynthetic penicillin or a cephalosporin. Oral ciprofloxacin may reduce pseudomonal bacterial counts and control symptoms. However, its clinical usefulness may be limited by rapid emergence of resistant organisms, and accordingly, courses should be intermittent (2 to 3 weeks) and not chronic. More severe exacerbations, or exacerbations associated with bacteria resistant to oral antibiotics, require intravenous antibiotics. Traditionally, intravenous therapy is given in the hospital, but outpatient intravenous antibiotic administration is gaining widespread acceptance. Usually, two drugs, often one of them an aminoglycoside, are used to treat *P. aeruginosa* to hinder emergence of resistant organisms. Drug dosage should be monitored so that levels for gentamicin or tobramycin peak at ranges of ~10 μg/mL and exhibit troughs of <2 μg/mL. Usually, a cephalosporin, e.g., ceftazadime, and/or a penicillin derivative is used as the second drug. Antibiotics directed at *Staphylococcus* and/or *H. influenzae* are added depending on the results of the culture. Aerosolization of antibiotics also may have an important role in treating CF lung infection. Large doses of aminoglycosides, e.g., 600 mg tobramycin twice daily, via aerosol are effective at delaying exacerbations. Aerosol administration also permits other drugs, e.g., colistin, to be utilized that are relatively ineffective by the intravenous route.

A number of pharmacologic agents for increasing mucus clearance are being tested. *N*-acetyl-cysteine, which solubilizes mucous glycoproteins, has not been shown to have clinically significant effects on mucus clearance and/or lung function. Recombinant human DNAse, however, degrades the concentrated DNA in CF sputum, decreases sputum viscosity, and increases airflow during short-term administration. Long-term (6 months) DNAse treatment also increases the time between pulmonary exacerbations, although mild adverse effects have been noted. Most patients receive a therapeutic trial of DNAse to test for efficacy, and a minority appear to demonstrate persistent objective benefits. Clinical trials of experimental drugs aimed at restoring salt and water content of secretions are underway. The combination of a sodium channel blocker (amiloride) to reduce excessive Na^+ absorption and UTP to initiate Cl^- secretion via non-CFTR-mediated Cl^- transport, although experimental, appears synergistic and promising.

Inhaled beta-adrenergic agonists can be useful to control airways constriction. They achieve a short-term increase in airflow, but long-term benefit has not been shown. Inhaled anticholinergics provide an alternative. Oral glucocorticoids are not first-line agents for controlling airways constriction and are of no use in improving the nonreversible component of lung function. Glucocorticoids may be useful for treating allergic bronchopulmonary aspergillosis.

The chronic damage to airway walls reflects to some degree the destructive activities of inflammatory enzymes generated in part by inflammatory cells. To date, specific therapies with antiproteases have not been successfully developed. However, a subset of adolescents with CF appears to benefit from long-term, high dose nonsteroidal (ibuprofen) therapy.

A number of pulmonary complications require acute interventions. Atelectasis is best treated with chest physiotherapy and antibiotic therapy. Pneumothoraces involving 10 percent or less of the lung can be observed without intervention. The use of chest tubes to expand collapsed, diseased lung often requires long periods of time, and sclerosing agents should be used with caution because of possible limitations for subsequent lung transplantation. Small-volume hemoptysis requires no specific therapy other than treatment of lung infection and assessment of coagulation and vitamin K status. If massive hemoptysis occurs, bronchial artery embolization can be successful. The most ominous complications of CF are respiratory failure and cor pulmonale. The most effective conventional therapy for these conditions is vigorous medical management of the lung disease and O_2 supplementation. Ultimately, the only effective treatment for respiratory failure in CF is lung transplantation. The 2-year survival for lung transplantation exceeds 60 percent, and deaths in transplant patients result principally from graft rejection, often involving obliterative bronchiolitis. The transplanted lungs do not develop a CF-specific phenotype.

Gastrointestinal Disease   Maintenance of adequate nutrition is critical for the health of the CF patient. Most (>90 percent) of CF patients benefit from pancreatic enzyme replacement. Capsules generally contain between 4000 and 24,000 units of lipase. The dose of enzymes (typically no more than 2000 units/kg per meal) should be adjusted on the basis of weight gain, abdominal symptomatology, and character of stools. Replacement of fat-soluble vitamins, particularly vitamins E and K, is usually required. Hyperglycemia most often becomes manifest in the adult. Principles for treating other causes of nonketotic hyperglycemia should be employed.

For treatment of acute obstruction due to meconium ileus equivalent, megalodiatrizoate or other hypertonic radiocontrast materials delivered by enema to the terminal ileum are utilized. For control of symptoms, adjustment of pancreatic enzymes and the supplementation of intake by salt solutions containing osmotically active agents, e.g., propyleneglycol, are utilized. Persistent symptoms may indicate a diagnosis of gastrointestinal malignancy, which is increased in incidence in CF patients. Hepatic and gallbladder complications are treated as for non-CF patients. End-stage liver disease can be treated by transplantation, which has a 2-year survival rate exceeding 50 percent.

Psychosocial Factors   CF imposes a tremendous burden on patients. Health insurance, career options, family planning, and life expectancy become major issues; thus, assisting patients with the psychosocial adjustments required by CF is critical.

BIBLIOGRAPHY

AITKEN ML, FIEL SB: Cystic fibrosis. Dis Mon 39:1, 1993

CHENG SH et al: Defective intracellular transport and processing of CFTR is the molecular basis of most cystic fibrosis. Cell 63:827, 1990

FITZSIMMONS SC: *CFF Patient Registry. 1994 Annual Report.* Bethesda, MD, Cystic Fibrosis Foundation, 1995

FUCHS HJ et al: Effect of aerosolized recombinant DNase on exacerbations of respiratory symptoms and on pulmonary function in patients with cystic fibrosis. The Pulmoenzyme Study Group. N Engl J Med 331:637, 1994

HARRIS A, ARGENT BE: The cystic fibrosis gene and its product CFTR. Semin Cell Biol 4:37, 1993

HIGHSMITH WE et al: A novel mutation in the cystic fibrosis gene in patients with pulmonary disease but normal sweat chloride concentrations. N Engl J Med 331:974, 1994

KONSTAN MW et al: Effect of high-dose ibuprofen in patients with cystic fibrosis. N Engl J Med 332:848, 1995

O'LOUGHLIN EV et al: Abnormal epithelial transport in cystic fibrosis jejunum. Am J Physiol 260:G758, 1991

RAMSEY BW et al: Efficacy of aerosolized tobramycin in patients with cystic fibrosis. N Engl J Med 328:1740, 1993

SFERRA TJ, COLLINS FS: The molecular biology of cystic fibrosis. Annu Rev Med 44:133, 1995

STUTTS MJ et al: CFTR as a cAMP-dependent regulator of sodium channels. Science 269:847, 1995

---

258   *Eric G. Honig, Roland H. Ingram, Jr.*

CHRONIC BRONCHITIS, EMPHYSEMA, AND AIRWAYS OBSTRUCTION

Chronic bronchitis and emphysema are two distinct processes, most often present in combination in patients with chronic airways obstruction. The diagnosis of chronic bronchitis is made by history, chronic airways obstruction is assessed physiologically, and emphysema can be diagnosed with certainty in most instances by high resolution CT scans or by histologic examination of sections of whole lung fixed at inflation. Although the relationships among clinical characteristics, physiologic derangements, and morphologic changes have been studied for many years, uniform clinical criteria are still not available.

DEFINITIONS   *Chronic bronchitis* is a condition associated with excessive tracheobronchial mucus production sufficient to cause cough with expectoration for at least 3 months of the year for more than 2 consecutive years. *Simple chronic bronchitis* describes a condition characterized by mucoid sputum production. *Chronic mucopurulent bronchitis* is characterized by persistent or recurrent purulence of sputum in the absence of localized suppurative diseases such as bronchiectasis. Since there may or may not be obstruction as assessed by the use of the forced expiratory vital capacity maneuver, *chronic bronchitis with obstruction* deserves a separate classification. There is a further subset of patients with chronic bronchitis and obstruction who experience severe dyspnea and wheezing in association with inhaled irritants or during acute respiratory infections. Such patients are said to have *chronic infective asthma* or *chronic asthmatic bronchitis*. Since there is considerable but not complete reversibility of airflow obstruction with bronchodilator treatment and abatement of inflammation, and since hyperresponsiveness of airways to nonspecific stimuli is seen in patients with chronic bronchitis with obstruction, confusion is possible between patients with this condition and those with asthma who may also have chronic airways obstruction (Chap. 252). The differentiation is based mainly on the history of the clinical illness. The patient with chronic bronchitis with obstruction has a long history of cough and sputum production with a later onset of wheezing, whereas the asthma patient with chronic obstruction gives a long history of wheezing with later onset of chronic productive cough.

Emphysema is defined as the permanent, abnormal distention of the air spaces distal to the terminal bronchiole with destruction of alveolar septa. *Chronic obstructive lung disease* is defined as a condition in which there is chronic obstruction to airflow due to chronic bronchitis and/or emphysema (see below). Although the degree of obstruction may be less when the patient is free from respiratory infection and may improve somewhat with bronchodilator drugs, significant obstruction is always present in patients with this condition.

PATHOLOGY   Chronic bronchitis is associated with hypertrophy of the mucus-producing glands found in the submucosa of large cartilaginous airways. Quantitation of this anatomic change, known as the Reid index, is based on the ratio of the thickness of the submucosal glands to that of the bronchial wall. In persons without a history of chronic bronchitis, the mean ratio is 0.44 ± 0.09, whereas in those with such a history the mean ratio is 0.52 ± 0.08. Although a low index is rarely associated with symptoms and a high index is commonly associated with symptoms during life, there is a great deal of overlap. Therefore, many persons will have morphologic changes in large airways without having had chronic bronchitis.

In lungs from patients with chronic obstructive lung disease which have been studied at postmortem, the major site of airflow obstruction has been shown to be in the small airways. Goblet cell hyperplasia, mucosal and submucosal inflammatory cells, edema, peribronchial fibrosis, intraluminal mucus plugs, and increased smooth muscle are characteristic findings in small airways.

The alveolar epithelium is both the target and the initiator of inflammation in chronic bronchitis. Bronchitic inflammation differs from the predominantly eosinophilic inflammation of asthma because of the predominance of neutrophils and the peribronchiolar location of fibrotic changes. It is the consequence of the actions of interleukin 8 and a variety of other chemotactic and proinflammatory cytokines and of colony stimulating factors released by airway epithelial cells in response to toxic, infectious, or inflammatory stimuli. Injured epithelium may also release reduced amounts of regulatory products such as angiotensin-converting enzyme or neutral endopeptidase. As with asthma, the strength of these inflammatory reactions correlates with bronchial reactivity. Sputum production is stimulated by increased exocytosis from secretory cells, lipid mediators, and inflammatory cell products, especially macrophage mucus secretagogue. Mucin gene expression is amplified by tumor necrosis factor α, and secretory cell hyperplasia is encouraged by the neutrophil enzymes elastase and cathepsin G.

Emphysema is classified according to the pattern of involvement of the gas-exchanging units (acini) of the lung distal to the terminal bronchiole. With *centriacinar emphysema*, the distention and destruction are mainly limited to the respiratory bronchioles with relatively less change peripherally in the acinus. Because of the large functional reserve in the lung, many units must be involved in order for overall dysfunction to be detectable. The centrally destroyed regions of the acinus have a high ventilation/perfusion ratio because the capillaries are missing, yet ventilation continues. This results in a deficit of perfusion relative to ventilation, while the peripheral portions of the acinus have crowded and small alveoli with intact, perfused capillaries giving a low ventilation/perfusion ratio. This results in a deficit of ventilation relative to blood flow, giving a high alveolar-arterial P_{O_2} difference $(P_{A_{O_2}} - Pa_{O_2})$ (Chap. 250). During normal aging, airspaces enlarge and alveolar ducts increase in diameter. These changes are extremely common in lungs from persons above age 50 and may be misidentified as emphysema.

Panacinar emphysema involves both the central and peripheral portions of the acinus, which results, if the process is extensive, in a reduction of the alveolar-capillary gas exchange surface and loss of elastic recoil properties. When emphysema is severe, it may be difficult to distinguish between the two types, which most often coexist in the same lung.

CONTRIBUTIONS TO PATHOGENESIS

SMOKING Cigarette smoking is the most commonly identified correlate with both chronic bronchitis during life and extent of emphysema at postmortem. Experimental studies have shown that prolonged cigarette smoking impairs ciliary movement, inhibits function of alveolar macrophages, and leads to hypertrophy and hyperplasia of mucus-secreting glands; massive exposure in dogs can produce emphysematous changes. It is probable that smoke also inhibits antiproteases and causes polymorphonuclear leukocytes to release proteolytic enzymes acutely. Inhaled cigarette smoke can produce an acute increase in airways resistance due to vagally mediated smooth-muscle constriction, presumably by way of stimulating submucosal irritant receptors. Increased airways responsiveness is associated with more rapid progression in patients with chronic airways obstruction. Obstruction of small airways is the earliest demonstrable mechanical defect in young cigarette smokers, and the obstruction may disappear completely after cessation of smoking. Although smoking cessation does not result in complete reversal of more pronounced obstruction, there is a significant slowing of the decline in lung function in all smokers who give up cigarettes. In effect, it is never too late to quit smoking cigarettes.

Passive exposure to tobacco smoke correlates with respiratory symptoms such as cough, wheeze, and sputum production. Not only is cigarette smoking the most common single factor leading to chronic airways obstruction, it also adds to the effects of every other contributory factor to be discussed below.

AIR POLLUTION The incidence and mortality rates of both chronic bronchitis and emphysema may be higher in heavily industrialized urban areas. Exacerbations of bronchitis are clearly related to periods of heavy pollution with sulfur dioxide (SO_2) and particulate matter. While nitrogen dioxide (NO_2) can produce small-airways obstruction (bronchiolitis) in experimental animals exposed to high concentrations, there are no data convincingly implicating NO_2, at even the highest pollutant levels, in the pathogenesis or worsening of airways obstruction in humans (Chap. 254).

OCCUPATION Chronic bronchitis is more prevalent in workers who engage in occupations exposing them to either inorganic or organic dusts or to noxious gases. Epidemiologic surveys have succeeded in demonstrating an accelerated decline in lung function in many such workers—e.g., workers in plastics plants exposed to toluene diisocyanate, and carding room workers in cotton mills (Chap. 254)—suggesting that their occupational exposure contributes to their future disability.

INFECTION Morbidity, mortality, and frequency of acute respiratory illnesses are higher in patients with chronic bronchitis. Many attempts have been made to relate these illnesses to infection with viruses, mycoplasmas, and bacteria. However, only the rhinovirus is found more often during exacerbations; that is to say, pathogenic bacteria, mycoplasmas, and viruses other than rhinovirus are found just as often between as during exacerbations. Epidemiologic studies, however, implicate acute respiratory illness as one of the major factors associated with the etiology as well as the progression of chronic airways obstruction. Cigarette smokers may either transitorily develop or worsen small-airways obstruction in association with even mild viral respiratory infections. There is also some evidence that severe viral pneumonia early in life may lead to chronic obstruction, predominantly in small airways.

FAMILIAL AND GENETIC FACTORS Familial aggregation of chronic bronchitis has been well demonstrated. Children of smoking parents may experience more frequent and severe respiratory illnesses and have a higher prevalence of chronic respiratory symptoms. In addition, nonsmokers who remain in the presence of cigarette smokers (passive smokers) have increased blood levels of carbon monoxide, which indicate that they are significantly exposed to smoke. Another well-documented form of indoor air pollution relates to the use of natural gas for cooking. The role of such pollution, however, remains controversial. Thus a part of the familial aggregation may be related to home air pollution. However, some studies of monozygotic twins have suggested some genetic predisposition to the development of chronic bronchitis independent of personal or familial smoking habits and other indoor air pollution. The exact genetic mode of transmission, if it exists at all, is uncertain.

Alpha$_1$-Antitrypsin Deficiency The protease inhibitor α_1-antitrypsin ($\alpha 1AT$) is an acute-phase reactant, and normally the serum levels rise in association with many inflammatory reactions and with estrogen administration. Either deficient or absent serum levels of $\alpha 1AT$ are found in some patients with the early onset of emphysema. By use of the techniques of acid starch gel and immunoelectrophoresis, genetic typing of the protease inhibitor types has been possible. Most members of the normal population have two M genes, designated as protease inhibitor type MM, and have serum $\alpha 1AT$ levels in excess of 2.5 g/L. Several genes are associated with alterations in levels of serum $\alpha 1AT$, but the most common ones associated with emphysema are the Z and S genes. Individuals who are homozygous ZZ or SS have serum levels often near 0 but always less than 0.5 g/L and develop severe panacinar emphysema in the third and fourth decades of life. The panacinar process predominates at the lung bases. Progressive dyspnea with minimal cough characterizes the clinical presentation, although chronic bronchitis is prominent in smokers. Given that α_1-protease inhibitors can be chemically synthesized or biologically produced in significant quantities and can be shown with intravenous infusion to restore the protease-antiprotease balance in liquid lavaged from the lungs of ZZ patients, it has been suggested that replacement therapy with $\alpha 1AT$ should be of value in preventing the development of emphysema in these patients. Since replacement therapy was available before efficacy had been assessed, a prospective, randomized trial has not been possible. Through a national registry, a natural history study is underway from which it might be possible to evaluate the effects of therapy if the treated and untreated groups turn out to be sufficiently comparable at entry.

The MZ and MS heterozygotes have intermediate levels of serum $\alpha 1AT$ (i.e., between 0.5 and 2.5 g/L); hence the genetic expression is that of an autosomal codominant allele. It is a matter of some controversy whether the heterozygous state is associated with lung function abnormalities. The matter is of some importance, since the heterozygous state is common, with incidence estimates varying between 5 and 14 percent of the general population.

The precise way in which antitrypsin deficiency produces emphysema is unclear. In addition to inhibition of trypsin, α1AT is an effective inhibitor of elastase and several other proteolytic enzymes. There is experimental evidence that the structural integrity of lung elastin depends on this antienzyme, which protects the lung from proteases released from leukocytes. It is tempting to speculate that recurrent inflammatory reactions related to infection and pollutants play some role in pathogenesis by calling forth leukocytes whose released proteases are uninhibited and are free to cause the damage.

The role of proteolytic enzymes in the induction of emphysema is not restricted to patients with α1AT deficiency. Evidence is accumulating that proteolytic enzymes derived from neutrophilic leukocytes and alveolar macrophages can produce emphysema even in subjects with normal circulating levels of antiproteases. It is possible that local concentrations of proteolytic enzymes may exceed the inhibitory capacity of antiproteases, that some proteases present are not susceptible to the available antiproteases, or that some of the proteolytic enzymes may be physically inaccessible to the antiprotease activity. The ultimate clinical utility of exogenously produced protease inhibitors currently under development will undoubtedly depend on which of the protease-antiprotease interactions predominates in the production of emphysema. Reduction of endogenous elastase release from leukocytes in the lung has been achieved by colchicine (0.6 mg/d orally) in a randomized, placebo-controlled trial in ex-smokers with chronic airways obstruction. Current smokers showed no such reductions. An assessment of the clinical efficacy of this inexpensive and nontoxic form of therapy in ex-smokers must await a large, prospective clinical trial.

PATHOPHYSIOLOGY Although both chronic bronchitis and emphysema can exist without evidence of obstruction, by the time a patient begins to experience dyspnea as a result of these processes, obstruction is always demonstrable. Although chronic bronchitis and emphysema are usually combined, one process may dominate over the other, and to the extent that inflammatory airways disease, secretions, and bronchospasm are present, there are therapeutic possibilities with some hope for improvement. Both chronic bronchitis and emphysema result in airways narrowing. In addition to the primary airways processes of chronic bronchitis, loss of elastic recoil of the lung in emphysema accounts for a decrease in airways caliber through loss of radial traction on airways. Narrowing of airways is often associated with both an increase in airways resistance and a diminution in maximal expiratory flow rates.

There are occasions in which a normal or only slightly elevated airways resistance is accompanied by low maximal expiratory flow rates. Under such circumstances, an increase in the dynamic collapsibility of intrathoracic airways during forced exhalation is a possible explanation. Also in this context, the elastic recoil pressure of the lung must be considered in a slightly different way. In addition to providing radial support to airways during quiet breathing, the elastic recoil properties of the lung serve as a major determinant of maximal expiratory flow rates. The static recoil pressure of the lung is the difference between alveolar and intrapleural pressure. During forced exhalations, when alveolar and intrapleural pressures are high, there are points in the airway at which bronchial pressure equals pleural pressure. Flow does not increase with higher pleural pressure after these points become fixed, so that the effective driving pressure between alveoli and such points is the elastic recoil pressure of the lung (Fig. 258-1). Hence maximal expiratory flow rates represent a complex and dynamic interplay between airways caliber, elastic recoil pressures, and collapsibility of airways. As a direct consequence of the altered pressure-airflow relationships, the work of breathing is increased in bronchitis and emphysema. Since flow-resistive work is flow rate–dependent, there is a disproportionate increase in the work of breathing with increased ventilation.

The designated subdivisions of the lung volume outlined in Chap. 250 are abnormal to varying degrees in both bronchitis and emphy-

sema. The residual volume (RV) and functional residual capacity (FRC) are almost always higher than normal. Since the normal FRC is the volume at which the inward recoil of the lung is balanced by the outward recoil of the chest wall, loss of elastic recoil of the lung results in a higher FRC. In addition, prolongation of expiration in association with obstruction would lead to a dynamic increase in FRC if inspiration is initiated before the respiratory system reaches its static balance point. Elevations of total lung capacity (TLC) are frequent. The exact cause is uncertain, but increases in TLC are often found in association with decreases in the elastic recoil of the lung. Although the vital capacity is frequently decreased, significant airways obstruction can be present with a normal to near-normal vital capacity.

Time constants for expiration are prolonged in all obstructive lung diseases because of increased airways resistance, increased lung compliance (e.g., emphysema), or a combination of both. When time constants are sufficiently prolonged, there may be insufficient time for expiration, even at normal respiratory rates, and the lungs may be unable to return to their mechanical equilibrium volume, FRC. The consequent progressive increase in lung volume moves tidal breathing to a higher, less compliant portion of the pressure-volume curve of the respiratory system and increases the work of breathing. The increased elastic recoil pressure associated with the higher end-tidal volume is

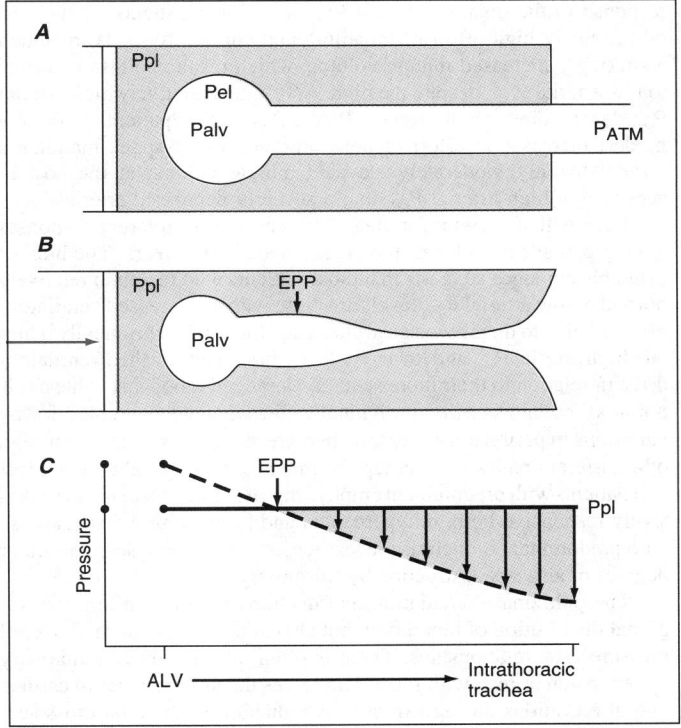

FIGURE 258-1 *A.* A schematic diagram of the lung and intrathoracic airways with no airflow. The alveolar pressure (Palv) is greater than pleural pressure (Ppl) by an amount equal to the elastic recoil pressure of the lung (Pel)—i.e., Palv is the algebraic sum of Ppl + Pel. With no airflow Palv equals atmospheric pressure (P$_{ATM}$), and for all of the intrathoracic airways, pressure outside is less than the pressure inside due to the Pel. *B.* The same schematic lung during forced exhalation when pleural pressure becomes quite positive (*arrow*). Palv is still greater than Ppl by an amount equal to Pel. However, there is a pressure drop along the airway associated with flow, and at some point Ppl equals local bronchial pressure (so-called equal pressure point, EPP). Mouthward from this point, Ppl exceeds local bronchial pressure and hence acts to compress the airways. *C.* Pressure within the airways from alveoli to the intrathoracic trachea is shown as a dashed line (---) and Ppl is shown as a constant (—). Therefore, the driving pressure from alveoli to EPP is equal to Pel, and a decrease in Pel (i.e., loss of elastic recoil) would mean a smaller driving pressure and smaller flow rates.

termed *intrinsic positive end-expiratory pressure (PEEP)*, or auto-PEEP (PEEPi), and represents an added threshold load that must be overcome to initiate the next inspiration. PEEPi is a common finding in patients with chronic airflow obstruction and contributes to their work of breathing and dyspnea. Hyperinflation contributes additionally to the discomfort associated with airflow obstruction by flattening the diaphragm and placing it at a mechanical disadvantage due to the length-tension relationship, the angle of diaphragmatic insertion with the lower ribs, and Laplace's law.

Maldistribution of inspired gas and blood flow is always present to some extent. When the mismatching is severe, impairment of gas exchange is reflected in abnormalities of arterial blood gases. There are regions of the lung with a deficit of perfusion in relation to ventilation that increase the wasted ventilation ratio (that is, V_d/V_t; Chap. 250). At a normal resting CO_2 production, the net effective alveolar ventilation, as reflected by the arterial P_{CO_2}, may be excessive, normal, or insufficient depending on the relationship of the overall minute volume to the wasted ventilation ratio. The net contribution of regions with perfusion in excess of ventilation can be assessed by either estimating or measuring the alveolar-arterial P_{O_2} difference (that is, $P_{A_{O_2}} - Pa_{O_2}$; Chap. 250). In chronic bronchitis and emphysema, there are increases in both wasted ventilation and wasted blood flow.

The clinical manifestations depend, in large part, on the ventilatory response to the disordered lung function. Some patients, at the cost of extremely high effort of breathing and chronic dyspnea, maintain a strikingly increased minute volume, which results both in a normal to low arterial P_{CO_2}, despite the high V_d/V_t, and a relatively high arterial P_{O_2}, despite the high difference, $P_{A_{O_2}} - Pa_{O_2}$. Other patients with only modest increases in effort of breathing and less dyspnea maintain a normal to only moderately elevated minute volume at the cost of accepting a high arterial P_{CO_2} and a severely depressed arterial P_{O_2}.

Factors that account for clear differences in ventilatory responses among patients have been studied and debated for years. The bulk of available evidence suggests that those patients who maintain relatively normal or low arterial P_{CO_2} levels are those with an increased ventilatory drive relative to their blood gas values, and those who chronically maintain high arterial P_{CO_2} and lower P_{O_2} levels have a diminished ventilatory drive in relation to their more severely deranged blood gas values. It is not at all certain whether individual differences are accounted for by variations in peripheral or central chemoreceptor sensitivity or through other afferent pathways. Perhaps of more immediate value is the fact that patients with predominant emphysema are either normally or excessively responsive both to hypercapnia and to exercise, whereas those with predominant bronchitis are less responsive to both, despite similar degrees of airways obstruction by spirometry.

The pulmonary circulation malfunctions not only in terms of regional distribution of blood flow but also in terms of abnormal overall pressure-flow relationships. There is often mild to severe pulmonary hypertension at rest, with further increases disproportionate to cardiac output elevations during exercise. A reduction in the total cross-sectional area of the pulmonary vascular bed can be attributed to anatomic changes and constriction of vascular smooth muscle in pulmonary arteries and arterioles as well as destruction of alveolar septa with loss of capillaries. Rarely does loss of capillaries alone lead to severe pulmonary hypertension with cor pulmonale, except as a near-terminal event (Chap. 238). Of more importance is the constriction of pulmonary vessels in response to alveolar hypoxia. The constriction is reversible upon increase in alveolar P_{O_2} with therapy. There is a synergism between hypoxia and acidosis that assumes importance during episodes of acute or chronic respiratory insufficiency. Chronic hypoxia leads not only to pulmonary vascular constriction but also to secondary erythrocytosis. The latter, although not proved to be a significant contributor to pulmonary hypertension, could add an unfavorable rheologic load. As discussed in Chap. 238, the chronic afterload on the right ventricle leads to hypertrophy and, in association with disordered blood gases, ultimately to failure.

CLINICAL-FUNCTIONAL CORRELATIONS Dyspnea and impairment of physical work capacity are characteristic only of severe to moderately severe airways obstruction. There is considerable variation among patients, and those with predominant emphysema have greater dyspnea and restriction of physical activity with lesser degrees of obstruction than those in whom chronic bronchitis predominates. The majority of patients have functionally mixed disease, usually experience exertional dyspnea when the forced expiratory volume in 1 s (FEV_1) falls below 50 percent of that predicted, and have dyspnea at rest when the FEV_1 is less than 25 percent of that predicted. In addition to dyspnea at rest, CO_2 retention and cor pulmonale frequently occur when the FEV_1 falls to 25 percent of that predicted. However, those with predominant bronchitis often have CO_2 retention and cor pulmonale with FEV_1 values above 25 percent of normal, in contrast to patients with predominant emphysema, whose FEV_1 usually falls well below that level before the onset of CO_2 retention and cor pulmonale. With a respiratory infection, small changes in the degree of obstruction can make a large difference in symptoms and gas exchange. Thus small therapeutic gains have rewarding results.

In general, the more severe the obstruction, the poorer the prognosis. Despite the general relationship, 20 to 30 percent of patients with severe obstruction and CO_2 retention will survive beyond 5 years.

CLINICAL SYNDROMES

The clinical presentation varies in severity from simple chronic bronchitis without disability to the severely disabled state with chronic respiratory failure. From a practical standpoint, it is well to consider that any symptom or any measurable abnormality may foreshadow the development of severe disabling disease; hence cessation of smoking and avoidance of environmental irritants and toxins are to be advised. However, the advice to modify behavior and life patterns is rarely taken, and most physicians are called on to categorize and treat patients with fully developed, chronic airways obstruction. Thus the approach taken here is to describe two polar opposite types of fully developed, chronic obstructive pulmonary disease with the realization that the majority of patients will have some features of both types. The salient features of each type are outlined in Table 258-1.

PREDOMINANT EMPHYSEMA These patients often give a long history of exertional dyspnea with minimal cough that is productive of only small amounts of mucoid sputum. Mucopurulent exacerba-

Table 258-1

Chronic Obstructive Lung Disease: Salient Features of the Two Types

	Predominant Emphysema	Predominant Bronchitis
Age at time of diagnosis, y	60±	50±
Dyspnea	Severe	Mild
Cough	After dyspnea starts	Before dyspnea starts
Sputum	Scanty, mucoid	Copious, purulent
Bronchial infections	Less frequent	More frequent
Respiratory insufficiency episodes	Often terminal	Repeated
Chest film	"Hyperinflation" ± bullous changes, small heart	Increased bronchovascular markings at bases, large heart
Chronic Pa_{CO_2}, mmHg	35–40	50–60
Chronic Pa_{O_2}, mmHg	65–75	45–60
Hematocrit, %	35–45	50–55
Pulmonary hypertension:		
Rest	None to mild	Moderate to severe
Exercise	Moderate	Worsens
Cor pulmonale	Rare, except terminally	Common
Elastic recoil	Severely decreased	Normal
Resistance	Normal to slight increase	High
Diffusing capacity	Decreased	Normal to slight decrease

tions in association with infections are not frequent. The body build is asthenic, with evidence of weight loss resulting from energy expenditure in excess of caloric intake. The patient appears distressed, with obvious use of accessory muscles of respiration which serve to lift the sternum in an anterosuperior direction with each inspiration. There is tachypnea with a relatively prolonged expiration through pursed lips, or expiration is begun with a grunting sound. While sitting, these patients often lean forward, extending the arms to brace themselves. The neck veins may be distended during expiration, yet they collapse briskly with inspiration. The lower intercostal spaces retract with each inspiration, and by palpation the lower lateral chest wall can be felt to move inward. The percussion note is hyperresonant, and by auscultation the breath sounds are diminished, with faint, high-pitched rhonchi heard toward the end of expiration. The cardiac impulse, if at all visible, is seen only in the xiphoid and subxiphoid regions, and cardiac dullness is either absent or severely reduced. By palpation there is frequently a sustained forward and downward right ventricular impulse in the subxiphoid region, and a presystolic gallop accentuated during inspiration is commonly heard.

The arterial P_{O_2} is often in the mid-70s (mmHg), and the P_{CO_2} is low to normal. Because of the maintained increase in minute volume and the maintenance of arterial P_{O_2} sufficient to nearly saturate hemoglobin, these patients have been referred to as "pink puffers." Their increased ventilatory drive probably accounts for their relatively preserved oxygenation and lack of hypercapnia; however, this increased drive with attendant increases in ventilation undoubtedly contributes to the severity of their dyspnea.

The TLC and RV are invariably increased, the vital capacity is low, and the maximal expiratory flow rates are diminished. The elastic recoil properties of the lung are severely impaired, and in direct proportion to this impairment, the capacity of the lung to transfer CO is lowered.

On radiographic examination the diaphragms are low and flattened, the bronchovascular shadows do not extend to the periphery of the lung, and the cardiac silhouette is lengthened and narrowed. These findings in association with a large retrosternal translucency on lateral chest radiographs are interpreted as hyperinflation, which correlates well with increases in TLC and loss of elastic recoil. Peripheral attenuation of bronchovascular markings and increased retrosternal lucency correlate best with subsequent postmortem demonstration of extensive and severe emphysema, predominantly of the panacinar type. Computed tomography (CT) has been shown to localize and quantitate emphysema. However, determining the localization of such regions most often is of little practical value, and the overall quantitative assessments from elastic recoil properties and CO transfer are just as good. Hence CT scans are not ordinarily employed for this purpose.

The patient with predominant emphysema is less prone to mucopurulent relapses than is the patient with predominant bronchitis, but such relapses frequently lead to severe respiratory failure and death. That is to say, right-sided heart failure and hypercapnic respiratory failure are often terminal events in those patients with predominant emphysema. In the absence of such relapses, the clinical course is characterized by severe and progressive dyspnea for which little can be done. The physician's role is to seek out and treat any factor that is possibly reversible and help the patient to avoid pollutants and infections.

PREDOMINANT BRONCHITIS The patient with predominant bronchitis usually has an impressive history of cough and sputum production for many years with an immodest history of cigarette smoking. Initially the cough is present only in the winter months, and the patient is apt to seek medical attention, if at all, only during the more severe of the frequent mucopurulent relapses. Over the years the cough progresses from hibernal to perennial, and mucopurulent relapses increase in frequency, duration, and severity. After beginning to experience exertional dyspnea, the patient often seeks medical help and will be found to have a severe degree of obstruction. Occasionally, such a patient will seek out a physician only after the onset of peripheral edema secondary to overt right ventricular failure. More rarely the initial medical contact is made by family members who present the

physician with a deeply cyanotic, edematous, and stuporous patient with acute respiratory insufficiency.

The patient with predominant bronchitis is often overweight and cyanotic. There is usually no apparent distress at rest, the respiratory rate is normal or only slightly increased, and there is no apparent usage of accessory muscles. The chest percussion note is normally resonant, and by auscultation one can usually hear coarse rhonchi and wheezes that change in location and intensity after a deep and productive cough. There may be a sustained heave along the lower left sternal border which indicates right ventricular hypertrophy. In the presence of right ventricular failure, there are often an early diastolic gallop and occasionally a holosystolic murmur, both of which are accentuated by inspiration. The latter finding is indicative of functional tricuspid regurgitation, which is frequently accompanied by neck vein distention characterized by large v waves and brisk y descents. With right ventricular failure, the cyanosis deepens and peripheral edema becomes prominent. Clubbing of the digits is unusual.

With or without right ventricular failure, the minute volume is only slightly increased due to an overall diminution in ventilatory drive which modulates the level of dyspnea. However, failure to increase minute volume greatly in the face of significant proportions of wasted ventilation and blood flow results in severely deranged arterial blood gases, with arterial P_{CO_2} values that are chronically increased to the range of the high 40s to low 50s (mmHg). The lowered P_{O_2} produces desaturation of hemoglobin, serves to stimulate erythropoiesis, and results in hypoxic pulmonary vasoconstriction. Desaturation and erythrocytosis combine to produce the cyanosis, and hypoxic pulmonary vasoconstriction accentuates the right-sided heart failure. Because of cyanosis and edema secondary to heart failure, such patients have been referred to as "blue bloaters." It has been proposed, with some supporting data, that one of the pathophysiologic events in blue bloaters is the occurrence of repeated episodes of severe nocturnal oxygen desaturation in association with episodes of sleep apnea or periods of worsening hypoventilation. Such sleep-related ventilatory events worsen the degree of pulmonary hypertension and secondary erythrocytosis.

The TLC is often normal, and there is a moderate elevation of RV. The vital capacity is mildly diminished, and maximal expiratory flow rates are invariably low. The elastic recoil properties of the lung are normal or only slightly impaired, and the capacity of the lung to transfer CO is either normal or minimally decreased.

There are no roentgenographic features that are definitive for chronic bronchitis. The two findings most commonly encountered are thickened bronchial walls manifested by tubular or "tramline" shadows, and a generalized increase in bronchovascular markings. In the presence of chronic pulmonary hypertension, the main pulmonary arterial segments enlarge and the cardiac silhouette may become more prominent due to right atrial and right ventricular chamber enlargement.

Despite well-planned management (see below), the patient with predominant bronchitis may experience many episodes of respiratory failure from which recovery is frequent with proper therapy (see later). The ability to recover from such repeated episodes in these patients is in striking contrast to the frequently fatal outcome of such events in those with predominant emphysema. Ultimately, the lungs at postmortem exhibit severe bronchitic changes in both large and small airways and only moderate emphysema, predominantly of the centriacinar variety.

The preceding syndromes—predominant emphysema and predominant bronchitis—are described as polar ends of a continuous spectrum of clinical features. Most patients have some characteristics of each syndrome. Recognizing and understanding the pathophysiologic bases for these aids in the planning of appropriate management strategies for each patient.

℞ TREATMENT

Intelligent management must be based on as complete knowledge as possible of the degree of obstruction, the extent of disability, and the relative reversibility of the patient's illness. To the extent that obstructive processes in the airways are contributory, there is a chance for treatment to be effective. Since emphysema is an irreversible process, prevention of progression and avoidance of acute insults constitute the main approach. History, physical examination, and chest radiographs should be supplemented by tests of lung function performed during a symptomatically stable period. Ideally, complete spirometry, plethysmographic lung volumes, transfer of CO, arterial blood gases, and lung elastic recoil properties should be measured. Spirometry and lung volumes should be remeasured after the administration of bronchodilators in order to assess the degree of acutely reversible airways obstruction. Failure to respond to a single bronchodilator agent at one point in time does not rule out the possibility of improvement with more prolonged administration of one or more of these agents and should not preclude their use. In instances in which the degree of exertional dyspnea appears to be disproportionately greater than the degree of obstruction, measurements of blood gases, minute volume, CO_2 production, and O_2 consumption during exercise are indicated in order to determine whether impaired lung function is sufficient to account for the symptoms. After the initial assessment, the physician has some idea of the relative emphasis to be placed on patient education, rehabilitative and preventive measures, and direct therapeutic interventions in management of the patient and the illness.

Smoking and the Environment Cessation of smoking is the only certain means of influencing the progression of the chronic obstructive airways syndromes, and although such behavior modification is most effective at early stages of the disease processes, it is effective in slowing the rate of decline in lung function, even when such function is severely compromised. The physician should always ask the patient about smoking, urge the patient to stop smoking, help the patient set a date to stop, and provide close follow-up support for the patient's efforts. Smoking cessation produces sustained reductions in the rate of the decline of FEV_1 that are greater in magnitude and more persistent than those achieved with bronchodilator therapy alone. Nicotine replacement therapy has been shown to be an effective modality in helping patients to stop smoking, producing average increments in abstinence rates of 10 to 15 percent over behavioral and educational programs without pharmacologic intervention. Benefits are greater for nicotine patches than for nicotine gum and are most marked in patients who are highly dependent upon nicotine. Nonetheless, 6 to 12 month abstinence rates for smoking cessation programs remain 20 to 25 percent in most reports. The best results have been achieved with highly motivated patients in dedicated smoking cessation clinics.

In patients in whom occupational or environmental exposures are thought to play a significant role, change of occupation or relocation of dwelling is advisable. The validity of such advice should be considered carefully, since the impact on both the patient and the family is likely to be great. A simple environmental change is that of eliminating aerosol sprays such as deodorants, hair sprays, and insecticides from the household. Hair sprays have been shown to produce acute airways responses even in normal subjects. Other preventive measures include yearly vaccination against the common or expected influenza virus strains. Patients need be given pneumococcal polysaccharide vaccine only once in a lifetime due to prolonged effectiveness of the immune response. However, if an earlier vaccine was used that contained only 14 capsular antigen types, revaccination with the current 23-valent vaccine is probably advisable.

Respiratory Infections Infections cannot be totally avoided, and the patient should be made aware that increasing purulence, viscosity, or volume of secretions signals the onset of an infection, which should be treated early. The most common pathogenic bacteria found are *Haemophilus influenzae*, *Streptococcus pneumoniae*, and *Moraxella catarrhalis*. As mentioned above, however, the role of

such bacteria is in question, since they are just as often isolated during periods of relative clinical quiescence. Nonetheless, an antibiotic effective against β-lactamase-producing organisms should be given for a 7- to 10-day course. It is practical to have the patient keep a 7- to 10-day supply of antibiotics at home and to begin treatment at the onset of symptoms. In Great Britain it is common practice to give continuous antibiotic therapy during winter months in order to prevent mucopurulent relapses. Although there is evidence that viruses are frequent causes of mucopurulent relapses, some clinical studies have shown that the standard antibiotic regimens decrease the duration and severity of infective episodes unrelated to culturable bacterial pathogens. The greatest benefits are seen in patients with more than four purulent exacerbations per year. Microscopic examination and culture of sputum are indicated if there are chills, fever, or chest pain or if purulence fails to respond to usually administered antibiotics.

Exercise and Nutrition Exercise programs, although not accompanied by measurable improvement in lung function, result in increased exercise tolerance and an improved sense of well-being. The improvement is usually task-specific, so most physicians advise walking in preference to the use of special apparatus, such as stationary bicycles. Arm exercise is poorly tolerated; the necessary muscles required for breathing are also recruited for the exercise task and hence are doing double duty.

If malnutrition (body weight less than 85 percent of ideal) is present, oral dietary supplements can result in improved muscle strength, less fatigability, and lessening of breathlessness. A carefully taken dietary history and elimination of other serious causes for low body weight and weight loss should precede the start of any major nutritional supplement effort. As with exercise programs, there is no direct and measurable effect on lung function from treating malnutrition, yet subjective relief and objective improvement in strength and exercise performance have been of great benefit in such patients.

Bronchodilator Drugs These are often quite helpful in alleviating symptoms, especially in patients who respond to them acutely in the laboratory. These drugs form three categories: the methylxanthines, sympathomimetics with strong beta₂-adrenergic-stimulating properties, and anticholinergics. The ethylene diamine salt of theophylline (aminophylline), the most commonly used methylxanthine, can be given orally or parenterally; in addition to bronchodilatation, it stimulates respiration and has cardiotonic and diuretic properties and may increase diaphragmatic contractility, especially in the setting of hypoxemia or muscle fatigue. Although it is a relatively weak bronchodilator and mechanical benefits are not consistently demonstrated, improved exercise performance and well-being are often seen. Oral theophylline preparations vary greatly in their intestinal release and rate of absorption. There is extreme variability in rates of absorption, degradation, and secretion among patients. Theophylline blood levels should be measured in those patients who, with standard doses, either fail to benefit or show signs of toxicity. Measurements at expected peak absorption and just before the subsequent dose will allow adjustment of dose. Blood levels between 10 and 15 mg/L should be maintained. Side effects such as insomnia and nervousness are frequent when levels are in the therapeutic range. Nausea, vomiting, tachyarrhythmias, and seizures are seen mainly when blood levels exceed 20 mg/L. Parenteral administration of theophylline is rarely indicated in the chronic obstructive syndromes, except during episodes of respiratory failure when agents cannot be given orally.

Selective beta₂-stimulating drugs such as albuterol, terbutaline, and metaproterenol can be given both orally and by aerosol with fewer cardiac side effects than are experienced with isoproterenol. Orally and parenterally administered beta₂ agonists are effective but are associated with greater tremulousness and cardiovascular side effects than result from inhaled agents. The latter can be most conveniently given in metered-dose inhalers at two to four puffs four to six times a day. Collecting chambers or spacers may improve the reliability of deposition of these agents. Anticholinergic agents such as atropine have been avoided in the past because of their tendency to desiccate secretions; however, ipratropium bromide, an anticholinergic agent in metered-dose inhaler form, is an effective bronchodilator in chronic bronchitic patients. It is considered by many to be the bronchodilator of choice for these patients.

Glucocorticoids   The use of systemic glucocorticoids is based on very little scientific data from properly controlled clinical trials. Since these agents have time- and dose-related side effects that vary from deleterious to catastrophic, the almost invariable subjective benefit must be supported by objective measurements. There is little room for doubt in the minds of physicians that some patients respond well, even dramatically, to these agents in both objective and subjective terms. The real problem is how to select those patients most likely to benefit. Eosinophilia in the sputum, rather than in the blood, appears in some instances to identify this subgroup in advance. However, the best guidelines are, first, to try these agents only after maximal bronchodilator and bronchopulmonary drainage measures have been tried without success; second, to begin prednisone at 30 mg once per day; third, to confirm the objective change in terms of spirometry and gas exchange, stopping these agents if no objective benefit is seen; and fourth, to decrease to the smallest dose that will maintain the improved level of function. Though some objective benefit has been shown in patients with bronchial hyperresponsiveness, the role, if any, of inhaled glucocorticoid agents for these patients, in contrast to asthmatic patients, has not been established in the syndromes with chronic obstruction.

Hypoxia and Erythrocytosis   When arterial hypoxia is persistent and severe (Pa_{O_2} of 55 to 60 mmHg) in association with cor pulmonale (see Chap. 238), erythrocytosis, and signs of right heart failure, continuous O_2 therapy is indicated. If the Pa_{O_2} is persistently <55 mmHg, with or without cor pulmonale, continuous O_2 supplementation also should be prescribed. The available data indicate that supplemental O_2 improves both exercise tolerance and neuropsychological function and alleviates pulmonary hypertension and right heart failure. In patients with severe hypoxemia, the need for hospitalization occurs less frequently and life span is lengthened by the use of supplemental O_2. Although long-term O_2 therapy has been shown to produce improvements in cognitive performance, quality of life, and exercise endurance, a survival benefit has not yet been demonstrated in those patients with less severe hypoxemia and who do not have cor pulmonale.

Since most patients with chronic airways obstruction, especially those with features of predominant bronchitis, can be shown to decrease their Pa_{O_2} values significantly during sleep, most prominently during the rapid eye movement phase, nocturnal O_2 administration has been suggested. While the rationale is clear and the results quite good, a cooperative clinical trial that compared nocturnal with continuous O_2 supplementation in severely hypoxic patients found that continuous O_2 administration was associated with a significantly lower mortality rate. Patients in both treatment groups experienced neuropsychological and hemodynamic benefits. Thus supplemental nocturnal O_2 is better than none, but continuous O_2 is better than nocturnal in such severely ill patients. Those patients not requiring continuous O_2 therapy may require supplementation during air travel. Even with modern pressurization, cabin altitudes may reach the equivalent of 8000 ft, at which the Pa_{O_2} may fall by 25 mmHg below that found at sea level. Hence O_2 supplementation during prolonged flights should be considered for patients with sea level Pa_{O_2} values in the mid-70s.

Secondary erythrocytosis with the hematocrit in excess of 50 percent is most easily viewed as a mechanism allowing greater O_2 delivery to compensate for the chronically lowered arterial P_{O_2}; hence improvement in oxygenation through improved lung function or by O_2 administration is the most physiologic means to reverse erythrocytosis. Since erythrocytosis results in elevation of blood viscosity at all shear rates, the proposal has been made that pulmonary vascular hypertension is aggravated by its presence. Although no study has demonstrated an objective improvement in hemodynamics, lung mechanics, or gas exchange at rest following phlebotomy, ventilatory and cardiovascular function during exercise improve. Some patients who complain of headaches and a sense of head fullness show a favorable subjective response to periodic phlebotomy when the hematocrit is in excess of 55 percent. In support of this subjective improvement is the demonstration that, following phlebotomy, cerebral blood flow, previously diminished, returns toward normal.

Other Measures   *Bronchopulmonary drainage* should be maintained in patients with hypersecretion. If the coughing mechanism is ineffective or if paroxysms of coughing are exhausting, postural drainage is often a useful adjunct. Although liquefaction of secretions by means of orally administered expectorants or aerosol delivery of mucolytic agents is an appealing idea, it has never been shown by properly designed trials to be more effective than simple maintenance of total-body hydration.

Intermittent positive-pressure breathing devices were formerly advocated for home management. The various rationales included diminution in the work of breathing, promotion of bronchopulmonary drainage, and more efficient delivery of bronchodilator drugs. The first of the rationales has been shown to have no basis in fact, and the goals of the last two have been shown to be as well accomplished by postural drainage and use of less elaborate aerosol generators. In fact, metered-dose inhalers, when used properly, are as effective as any powered nebulizer system. Hence the use of intermittent positive-pressure breathing devices and compressor-driven aerosol generators for home management cannot be justified.

Despite employing all the aforementioned measures, some patients remain severely incapacitated. For these patients, *lung transplantation* can return them to both a functional and comfortable state (see Chap. 267). Criteria for transplanting such patients are being evolved in the several centers performing this procedure. Medical directors of such programs should be consulted if the possibility of a lung transplant is being considered.

Surgical bullectomy may provide symptomatic relief in patients with large emphysematous bullae that are expanded by the greater retractive force exerted by the normal parenchyma. Benefit is seen only in patients who have stopped smoking, and long-term effects have not been clearly established. Thoracoscopic laser bullectomy procedures have recently been described. A favorable risk:benefit profile remains to be established for this procedure. Lung volume–reduction surgery has recently been reintroduced with the aim of improving elastic recoil by resecting multiple regions of overdistended lung in patients with diffuse, nonhomogeneous emphysema. The procedure is currently experimental and should be applied only within the confines of a well-designed clinical trial.

There are two therapeutic interventions well short of lung transplantation that have been proposed repeatedly by a few investigators and that remain extremely controversial. It cannot be denied that some supporting data exist; the counterintuitive nature of the interventions and the absence of controlled trials preclude their wide acceptance. These are (1) bilateral carotid body resection, and (2) periodic use of negative-pressure ventilation. The initial rationale for bilateral carotid body resection was to relieve dyspnea by diminishing the ventilatory responsiveness to hypoxemia and hypercapnia, which would present its own set of dangers. Several studies have shown improved lung mechanics and exercise performance after the procedure. Use of negative-pressure ventilation for periods up to 8 h/d for 2 consecutive days has been shown to improve gas exchange, muscle strength, and ventilatory responsiveness for several subsequent days. Negative-pressure ventilation is most effective in patients with hypercapnia and when care is taken to ensure that sufficient mechanical support is provided to truly rest the respiratory muscles. Patients who are unable to synchronize upper airway motor output with the negative-pressure ventilator have been reported to experience obstructive sleep apnea as a complication of this form of therapy.

ACUTE RESPIRATORY FAILURE IN PATIENTS WITH CHRONIC BRONCHITIS, EMPHYSEMA, AND AIRWAYS OBSTRUCTION

DIAGNOSIS Although it may be strongly suspected on clinical grounds, the firm diagnosis of acute respiratory failure in chronic airways obstruction is based on measurements of arterial blood gas (Pa_{O_2}, Pa_{CO_2}) and pH values that must be interpreted in relation to the patient's chronic status. Since many patients have chronically lowered Pa_{O_2} levels and increased Pa_{CO_2} values, the diagnosis is based on the degree of change from the usual state of the individual patient. With regard to oxygenation, an acute decrease in Pa_{O_2} from a usual mid-70 range to the low 60s (mmHg) is just as indicative of acute respiratory failure as is an acute drop from a chronic mid-50 range to the mid-40s (mmHg). Thus a drop in Pa_{O_2} equal to or greater than 10 to 15 mmHg indicates acute failure.

Since renal compensation for chronic hypercapnia results in adjustment of arterial pH to near-normal values, the acuteness of the increase in Pa_{CO_2} can often be judged by the pH, unless there is a concomitant metabolic acidemia. As a practical guide, any level of hypercapnia associated with an arterial pH value less than 7.30 should be considered as acute respiratory failure.

PRECIPITATING FACTORS Increases in volume, viscosity, and/or purulence of secretions, presumably due to infection of the tracheobronchial tree, are the most common antecedents of acute respiratory failure in chronic obstructive lung disease. Increasing airways obstruction with airways inflammation and secretion, especially in association with a relatively blunted ventilatory drive, leads to worsening hypoxia and increasing CO_2 retention. Agitation, insomnia, and increasing dyspnea with impending respiratory failure are occasionally treated, mistakenly, with either sedatives or narcotics, and these, too, may precipitate frank respiratory failure. In fact, depressant drugs that impair ventilatory drive should be avoided at all times in patients with severe chronic obstructive lung disease. Major episodes of air pollution also can lead to respiratory failure, and the physicians responsible for patients with severe bronchitis and emphysema should be alert to these environmental events.

Pneumonia, thromboembolism, left ventricular failure, and pneumothorax occasionally precipitate acute respiratory failure and are extremely difficult to detect unless considered and specifically sought. As a minimum, chest radiographs, electrocardiograms, and sputum examinations should be obtained in addition to arterial blood gas measurements in all patients with respiratory failure.

℞ TREATMENT

The management of acute respiratory failure consists of two simultaneous processes: (1) maintaining acceptable levels of oxygenation and ventilation, and (2) treatment of infection, removal of secretions, and reversal of any airways constriction present.

Control of Hypoxemia These patients need O_2 when they are severely hypoxic, and while fears of respiratory depression due to the removal of the hypoxic respiratory stimulus are realistic, O_2 must be used, yet in the smallest concentration possible, to give a Pa_{O_2} in the mid-50 range while the patient's Pa_{CO_2}, pH, and clinical status are carefully monitored. It is best to begin with only modest increases in $F_{I_{O_2}}$ to approximately 0.24 (cf. air at 0.21), which can be accomplished using nasal prongs with O_2 flows at 1 to 2 L/min or, more precisely, with the use of a 0.24 Venturi mask. These latter masks, based on Bernoulli's principle, deliver a fixed concentration of O_2 irrespective of the O_2 flow rate by entraining air in direct proportion to O_2 flow rate. They are high-flow masks (oxygen plus air entrained from the room), each designed for a specific $F_{I_{O_2}}$ (0.24, 0.28, 0.35, 0.40). Even small increases in Pa_{O_2} when starting from low levels result in significant increases in arterial oxygen content due to the shape of the oxygen-hemoglobin saturation curve over this range (Chap. 106).

With improved oxygenation some patients will increase their Pa_{CO_2} values. The standard explanation has been that this increase is due to the removal of the hypoxic drive to ventilation leading to further hypoventilation. While this is the most important mechanism, recent data indicate that worsening ventilation-perfusion relationships (Chap. 250) occur with O_2 treatment. This is attributed to reversal of hypoxic pulmonary arterial constriction in the more initially hypoxic, less well ventilated regions, which in turn leads to decreased perfusion of initially less hypoxic, better ventilated regions. The result is an increase in the wasted ventilation ratio (V_d/V_t; Chap. 250) leading to a smaller effective alveolar ventilation. In either case, the $F_{I_{O_2}}$ should be increased as little as possible to achieve a Pa_{O_2} in the mid-50 range. Some increase in Pa_{CO_2} can be expected and should not cause alarm if the patient is alert. The majority of patients can be managed in this conservative way with excellent results. However, occasionally, large increases in Pa_{CO_2} occur and lead to stupor and coma. This can be explained by CO_2-induced cerebral vascular dilatation with increased intracranial pressure, including the development of papilledema, combined with the effect of hypercapnia and hypoxia on cerebral function. Patients most at risk for O_2-induced CO_2 retention are those presenting with Pa_{O_2} below 50 mmHg and H^+ concentration greater than 55 nM (pH ~ 7.26). It must be emphasized that if stupor and coma supervene, stopping the administration of O_2 is the worst possible course of action. When CO_2 narcosis is present, respirations are sufficiently depressed from the CO_2 itself that the patient will no longer respond to the rapidly worsening hypoxia, and fatal arrhythmias, generalized seizures, and death may ensue.

ENDOTRACHEAL INTUBATION AND MECHANICAL VENTILATION These become necessary for patients who fail to respond to conservative management and who have hypercapnia with evidence of obtundation. Before committing to mechanical ventilation, the patient's wishes and expectations should be explored as carefully as circumstances permit. Where uncertainty exists, however, intubation should proceed. Ventilation may be withdrawn if it is later determined to be inappropriate or against the patient's wishes.

Noninvasive ventilation may be attempted as an alternative to endotracheal intubation. In the absence of anxiety, poor cooperation, impaired swallowing, severe hypoxemia, hemodynamic instability, or acute abdominal distress, the majority of patients with chronic airflow obstruction and acute respiratory failure can be successfully managed by continuous positive airway pressure or volume-controlled ventilation applied by face mask.

In any ventilated patient, the ventilator should be set to produce blood gases that support life while avoiding hyperinflation and barotrauma. Tidal volumes and respiratory rates should be kept as low as possible, and moderate degrees of hypercapnia may be tolerated. Once mechanical ventilation has been instituted, the tidal volume and frequency should be set to gradually decrease the Pa_{CO_2} only down to the chronically elevated level rather than to attempt to decrease it to or below a normal value. Since such patients have renal compensation for their chronic hypercapnia, Pa_{CO_2} values at or below the normal level result in significant alkalemia, which in turn can lead to severe tachyarrhythmias and generalized seizures.

Control of Infection, Bronchoconstriction, and Secretions As mentioned above, maintaining oxygenation and ventilation serves to buy time while secretion removal, bronchial dilatation, and treatment of infection are instituted. Removal of secretions is accomplished by urging the patient to cough or by passing suction catheters into the trachea which, in addition to removing secretions that are present, stimulate cough that brings more secretions up to the region of the catheter tip. The advantage, if any, from the use of mucolytic agents in this process has yet to be demonstrated. However, beta$_2$-adrenergic bronchodilating agents have been shown to increase the rate of transport of particles by the mucociliary blanket; thus, in addition to bronchodilatation, such agents should improve the clearance of airway secretions. Postural drainage and chest percussion are other often-used adjuncts that have been shown, especially when secretions are voluminous, to improve tracheobronchial clearance, to increase sputum volume beyond that produced by cough, and to reduce airways obstruction.

Bronchodilatation with beta$_2$-adrenergic agonists and/or anticholinergics by inhalation has assumed a prominent role in treatment of acute respiratory failure in chronic airways obstruction. The utility of adding oral or intravenous theophylline is controversial, but in addition to bronchodilatation, theophylline may improve bronchopulmonary clearance and may help induce diuresis and hemodynamic improvement when there is cor pulmonale with heart failure. Unless there is clearly an acute pneumonia, the use of antibiotics is more controversial in the setting of acute respiratory failure than in mucopurulent relapses without failure. Nonetheless, broad-spectrum antibiotics, if no single agent is suspected or isolated, or erythromycin, if legionellae or mycoplasmas are suspected, should be added to the regimen.

Management of Complications Complications arising in the course of treatment for acute respiratory failure are cardiac arrhythmias (most often multifocal supraventricular tachycardias), left ventricular failure, pulmonary emboli, and gastrointestinal hemorrhage from stress ulceration. *Cardiac arrhythmias* resulting from rapid decreases in oxygenation or increases in pH due to overventilation can be readily avoided. However, when giving multiple drugs having cardiotonic properties, the question always arises as to whether the arrhythmias are drug–related. Keeping serum theophylline levels in the 10 to 15 mg/L range and using relatively selective beta agonists, such as terbutaline or albuterol by inhalation, can minimize these effects.

Left ventricular failure, usually attributable to coronary atherosclerosis with acute myocardial infarction, systemic hypertension, or aortic valvular disease, is difficult to detect in the presence of cor pulmonale. Fortunately, improving lung function and oxygenation most often reverse the pulmonary hypertension and right ventricular failure (Chap. 238) and induce a brisk diuresis. If signs of congestive failure persist or worsen after providing adequate oxygenation, consideration must be given to left ventricular failure; an assessment in such patients is best made through echocardiography or radioventriculography, since the usual physical and radiographic findings are obscured in such patients. Only in the presence of adequate gas exchange and only with either the firm demonstration, or strong clinical suspicion, of left ventricular failure should digitalis be used. Diuretic agents should also be reserved for left ventricular failure. They almost invariably produce hypokalemic, hypochloremic metabolic alkalemia that results in depression of ventilatory drive and interference with removal from mechanical ventilatory support.

Pulmonary emboli are suspected to be common in the setting of acute respiratory failure and are difficult to detect, and signs of cor pulmonale fluctuate in concert with the degree of lung dysfunction. Although ventilation-perfusion scans of low and intermediate probability are frequent and are not diagnostically useful, high-probability scans are still unreliable in the presence of chronic airflow obstruction. Noninvasive evaluation of the lower extremities may be helpful in this setting. Low-dose heparin prophylaxis should be used to prevent pulmonary emboli.

Gastrointestinal hemorrhage in patients with chronic airflow obstruction and acute respiratory failure may be especially severe. Awareness of this complication enhances the ability to detect it and act quickly. Antacids, coating agents such as sucralfate, and/or H$_2$ blockers have been used to diminish the frequency.

Weaning from Mechanical Ventilation For those patients who have required mechanical ventilatory support, the process of removal from that support is largely empirical. Weaning should not be attempted until the patient is responsive and gas exchange and lung mechanics have been improved. Data such as a ratio of respiratory frequency to tidal volume less than 105, maximal voluntary inspiratory mouth pressures greater than 20 cmH$_2$O, vital capacity greater than 10 mL/kg of body weight, and spontaneous tidal volume greater than 5 mL/kg of body weight are reassuring. However, these indices carry an accuracy of only 70 to 80 percent, and many patients can be successfully removed from such support with lesser values than these.

Failure to maintain gas exchange after removal of mechanical ventilatory support can usually be explained. First on the list is the continued administration or persistence of sedative and tranquilizing drugs that may have been prescribed earlier for agitation. These should be discontinued, and time allowed for their metabolism. Second is the possibility that the endotracheal tube is of small bore and imposes a resistive load. If so, it should be replaced by a larger one. Third is worsening airways obstruction and accumulation of secretions; continued bronchial dilatation and airway suctioning avoid these. Fourth is a metabolic alkalemia, with or without diuretic therapy, that should be treated with potassium chloride. Fifth is having maintained, while on mechanical ventilation, a Pa$_{O_2}$ and Pa$_{CO_2}$ that are too high and too low, respectively. This can be avoided by using an F$_{I_{O_2}}$ just sufficient to keep the Pa$_{O_2}$ around 60 mmHg and using the assist mode with small enough tidal volumes to keep the Pa$_{CO_2}$ at the expected chronic level (i.e., that associated with a normal or slightly low arterial pH) before discontinuing mechanical support. Sixth is poor nutrition, hypokalemia, hypophosphatemia, or neuromuscular disease, making the patient too weak to maintain breathing or resulting in fatigue of the respiratory muscles. Nutrition, of course, is a longer range problem that should be anticipated, while hypokalemia is often handled along with the metabolic alkalemia. Hypophosphatemia can be addressed by specific parenteral repletion or by enteral administration of skim milk.

Muscle fatigue, especially diaphragmatic, has received a great deal of attention. From a practical standpoint, paradoxical (inward) movement of the upper abdomen with inspiration is the key clinical finding. Experimental evidence suggests that therapeutic levels of aminophylline or beta$_2$ agonists, such as fenoterol, reverse the manifestations of fatigue, but the role of respiratory stimulants continues to be debated, and the data to be inconclusive. In those patients with severely blunted ventilatory drive and improving lung function, stimulants may be tried cautiously. If there is severe metabolic alkalemia, acetazolamide can be tried as a stimulant while chloride replacement is being carried out. Medroxyprogesterone, a central stimulant, or almitrine, a peripheral chemoreceptor stimulant, appear to be safe and, in some instances, effective. Hypothyroidism is a metabolic condition with neuromuscular consequences and is difficult to detect in this clinical setting. Thus any prolonged and difficult weaning process should lead to the assessment of thyroid function.

PROGNOSIS

On the average, data collected on large populations demonstrate a slow and relentless diminution in ventilatory function in patients with chronic airways obstruction. Although slow, the decrement in function with time far exceeds the rate of change seen with normal aging. In general, the likelihood of episodes of acute respiratory failure increases when the FEV$_1$ falls below 25 percent of predicted normal values. Although the in-hospital mortality rate over the past 20 years averages 10 percent for a single episode and the 5-year survival rate after the initial episode of respiratory failure averages only 15 to 20 percent, the clinical syndrome is extremely important in determining both the short- and long-range prognosis. Pulmonary arterial pressure is a significant determinant of prognosis in patients with chronic airflow obstruction. As noted above, those patients with predominant emphysema have a poorer prognosis after the onset of respiratory failure than do those with predominant bronchitis. In either case, long-term O$_2$ treatment in those with severe hypoxemia results in prolongation of life and improvement in the quality of life.

VARIANTS OF EMPHYSEMA AND OBSTRUCTIVE AIRWAYS DISEASE

In addition to the centriacinar and panacinar forms of emphysema described above, other structural patterns have been described but are functionally less important. Often there is overdistention and alveolar septal destruction in lung regions surrounding scar tissue (paracicatricial or scar emphysema) or along the borders of the acinus (paraseptal emphysema). The latter form, when it occurs at the visceral pleural surface, may predispose to episodes of spontaneous pneumothorax (Chap. 262). Infants rarely develop a check valve mechanism in a lobar bronchus, which leads to rapid and life-threatening overdistention (congenital lobar emphysema).

Unilateral emphysema may be an incidental radiographic finding (Macleod's or Swyer-James's syndromes). Since, in this condition, the airways are normal in number and structure but the alveoli are reduced in number, this form of unilateral emphysema has been attributed to disease occurring before the age of 8 years when alveoli are normally increasing in number. Overdistention and alveolar septal destruction are not present, and so this condition does not fit the definition of true emphysema. Most often the pulmonary artery on the affected side is hypoplastic. Although usually an incidental finding, the affected lung may become repeatedly infected so that surgical excision may be indicated.

BULLOUS EMPHYSEMA Confluent air spaces with diameters in excess of 1 cm are occasionally congenital but most often are found in association with generalized emphysema or progressive fibrotic processes. Gradual increases in size of such air spaces (or bullae) result from traction applied by regions with better elastic recoil properties, and such regions lose volume as the bullae become enlarged. If disability is severe, if the bulla is extremely large, and if either lobar gas sampling or ventilation and perfusion scans demonstrate that sufficient function remains in the nonbullous regions, surgical excision of the bulla may lead to functional improvement. Usually, however, improvement is relatively transitory because other emphysematous regions gradually enlarge into bullae after surgery.

MISCELLANEOUS DIFFUSE OBSTRUCTIVE SYNDROMES *Bronchiolitis obliterans* is a term applied to widespread inflammatory and fibrotic obstruction of small airways. Initially this syndrome was thought to be restricted to those persons who had suffered severe viral infections in childhood, particularly those due to parainfluenza virus. However, recently this syndrome has also been described in adult patients with rheumatoid arthritis. The response to bronchodilator treatment is poor, as would be expected from the histopathologic findings, and fatal respiratory failure often ensues within 2 years. There have been reports suggesting a relationship between penicillamine therapy and the development of bronchiolitis obliterans in patients with rheumatoid arthritis; however, it is clear that this syndrome can develop in patients who have never received penicillamine.

A syndrome with similar histopathology has been described in recipients of autologous bone marrow transplants. Although most often interstitial pneumonitis and fibrosis are sequelae, it has been documented that some patients develop a bronchiolitis obliterans picture. It appears that the development of this process occurs most often in the setting of a chronic graft-versus-host syndrome; however, it is clear that diffuse airways obstruction has developed without evidence of this syndrome in bone marrow recipients.

Cystic fibrosis in the adult with chronic airways obstruction is discussed elsewhere (Chap. 257).

BIBLIOGRAPHY

ANTHONISEN NR et al: Effects of smoking intervention and the use of an inhaled anticholinergic bronchodilator on the rate of decline of FEV$_1$. The Lung Health Study. JAMA 272:1497, 1994

COOPER JD et al: Bilateral pneumectomy (volume reduction) for chronic obstructive pulmonary disease. J Thorac Cardiovasc Surg 109:106, 1995

FERGUSON GT, CHERNIACK RM: Management of chronic obstructive pulmonary disease. N Engl J Med 328:1017, 1993

JANSEN HM et al: Predisposing conditions to bacterial infection in chronic obstructive pulmonary disease. Am J Respir Crit Care Med 151:2073, 1995

LEUENBERGER P et al: Passive smoking exposure in adults and chronic respiratory symptoms (SAPALDIA study). Am J Respir Crit Care Med 150:1222, 1994

NINANE V et al: Intrinsic PEEP in patients with chronic obstructive pulmonary disease. Am Rev Respir Dis 148:1037, 1993

OSWALD-MAMMOSSER M et al: Prognostic factors in COPD patients receiving long-term oxygen therapy. Importance of pulmonary artery pressure. Chest 107:1193, 1995

RIES AL: Effects of pulmonary rehabilitation on physiologic and psychosocial outcomes in patients with chronic obstructive pulmonary disease. Ann Intern Med 122:823, 1995

SHELHAMER JH et al: Airway inflammation. Ann Intern Med 123:288, 1995

ST JOHN RC et al: Chronic obstructive pulmonary disease: Less common causes. An algorithm for the primary care physician. J Gen Intern Med 8:564, 1993

VAZ FRAGOSO CA, MILLER MA: Review of the clinical efficacy of theophylline in the treatment of chronic obstructive pulmonary disease. Am Rev Respir Dis 147:S40, 1993

259 *Herbert Y. Reynolds*

INTERSTITIAL LUNG DISEASES

The interstitial lung diseases (ILDs) represent a variety of conditions that involve the alveolar walls (septa), perialveolar tissue, and other contiguous supporting structures. The ILDs are nonmalignant and are not caused by any defined infectious agents. Although an acute phase of illness may occur, the onset is often insidious, and the disease is usually chronic in duration. The initial insult is injury to the epithelial surface causing inflammation in the air spaces and alveolar walls, creating an acute phase of intraluminal and mural alveolitis. If the disease is chronic and smoldering, inflammation will spread to adjacent portions of the interstitium and vasculature and eventually produce interstitial fibrosis. The resultant scarring and distortion of lung tissue leads to significant derangement of gas exchange and ventilatory function. Inflammation also can involve the conducting airways, and bronchiolitis obliterans associated with an organizing pneumonia is now part of the spectrum of an ILD.

Although diverse, this group of diseases has many features in common, including similarity of symptoms, comparable appearance of chest imaging studies, consistent alterations in pulmonary physiology, and typical histologic features. Lung pathology is usually confined to several general patterns, showing a mixture of alveolar inflammatory infiltrates and fibrotic/scarred areas with cystic, honeycomb spaces evident in advanced stages, often called *usual interstitial pneumonia*. Recently, diffuse, temporally uniform, single-time-appearing reactions have defied customary classifications and are considered as nonspecific interstitial pneumonia/fibrosis. However, ILDs have been difficult to classify because approximately 150 known individual diseases are characterized by some interstitial lung involvement, either as primary disease or as a significant part of a multiorgan process, as may occur in the collagen vascular diseases. The chest radiograph is of limited aid in classification because it can have a similar appearance in many of the ILDs as well as in other unrelated lung diseases; however, high-resolution computed tomography (HRCT) scanning of the chest has enhanced diagnostic accuracy. One useful approach for classification is to separate ILDs into two groups, those with known and unknown causes; each of these groups can be divided into subgroups according to the presence or absence of histologic evidence of granulomas in interstitial or vascular areas (Table 259-1). For each ILD there may be an acute phase, and there is usually a chronic one as well.

Among the ILDs of known cause, the largest group comprises occupational and environmental inhalant exposures; these include diseases due to inhalation of inorganic dusts (Chap. 254), organic dusts, and various irritative or noxious gases (Chap. 253). The number of ILDs of unknown cause is also very large. The major ones within this category are idiopathic pulmonary fibrosis (IPF), sarcoidosis, and the ILD often associated with collagen vascular disorders. ILD secondary to inorganic dust exposure usually can be recognized if the occupational history is pursued. For the myriad (see Table 259-1) of other diffuse ILDs, however, a precise diagnosis is obtained with difficulty, usually only after interpretation of an open-lung biopsy specimen; most of these diseases are relatively rare. The HRCT scan promises to improve diagnostic accuracy as further histologic-image correlations are perfected.

Although the initiating agent(s) or circumstances of the various ILDs may be multiple, and many are unknown, the immunopathogenic responses of lung tissue are limited, so the initial mechanisms of injury to the epithelial surface, the development of alveolitis, and the attempts at repair sometimes leading to fibrosis will have common features. IPF is discussed as the prototype ILD, since it is encountered relatively frequently and much of the recent research on mechanisms of inflammation and lung fibrosis has focused on this disease.

IDIOPATHIC PULMONARY FIBROSIS

Many patients who present with nonproductive cough, progressive dyspnea, a chest radiograph showing lower lung zone reticular or reticulonodular shadows, and pulmonary function tests showing a restrictive ventilatory pattern (Chap. 250) will be said to have IPF after the diagnostic evaluation is completed. This condition is also known as *cryptogenic fibrosing alveolitis*. Although the terms *idiopathic* and *cryptogenic* mean that the etiologic agent is unknown, this is not a nebulous "wastebasket" diagnosis or just a diagnosis of exclusion but rather a well-defined clinical entity.

IMMUNOPATHOGENESIS Several parts of the alveolar structure are affected in IPF, including the alveolar walls lined with

Table 259-1

Major Categories of Alveolar and Interstitial Inflammatory Lung Diseases

Known Cause	Unknown Cause
LUNG RESPONSE: ALVEOLITIS, INTERSTITIAL INFLAMMATION, AND FIBROSIS	
Asbestos	Idiopathic pulmonary fibrosis
Fumes, gases	Collagen vascular diseases
Drugs (antibiotics) and chemotherapy drugs	Systemic lupus erythematosus, rheumatoid arthritis, ankylosing spondylitis,
Radiation	systemic sclerosis, Sjögren's syndrome,
Aspiration pneumonia	polymyositis-dermatomyositis
Residual of adult respiratory distress syndrome	Pulmonary hemorrhage syndromes
	Goodpasture's syndrome, idiopathic pulmonary hemosiderosis
	Pulmonary alveolar proteinosis
	Lymphocytic infiltrative disorders (lymphocytic interstitial pneumonitis associated with collagen vascular diseases)
	Eosinophilic pneumonias
	Lymphangioleiomyomatosis
	Amyloidosis
	Inherited diseases
	Tuberous sclerosis, neurofibromatosis, Niemann-Pick disease, Gaucher's disease, Hermansky-Pudlak syndrome
	Gastrointestinal or liver diseases (Crohn's disease, primary biliary cirrhosis, chronic active hepatitis, ulcerative colitis)
	Graft vs. host disease (bone marrow transplantation)
LUNG RESPONSE: AS ABOVE BUT WITH GRANULOMA	
Hypersensitivity pneumonitis (organic dusts)	Sarcoidosis
Inorganic dusts: beryllium silica	Langerhans cell granulomatosis (eosinophilic granuloma)
	Granulomatous vasculitides
	Wegener's granulomatosis, allergic granulomatosis of Churg-Strauss, lymphomatoid granulomatosis
	Bronchocentric granulomatosis

type I squamous epithelial cells and type II pneumocytes and the interstitial supporting structure composed of mesenchymal cells (especially fibroblasts, myofibroblasts, occasional monocyte-macrophage cells, and lymphocytes), noncellular matrix of collagen, and various adhesive proteoglycans. The capillary endothelium also may be involved. The disease process does not affect the upper or conducting airways, but bronchiolitis of respiratory bronchioles may be present and alveolar units are always involved.

Normally, overlying or interspersed on the alveolar surface are a variety of immune cells, including alveolar macrophages, dendritic macrophages, lymphocytes, and inflammatory cells, such as polymorphonuclear leukocytes (PMNs) and eosinophils. The cellular content of normal bronchoalveolar lavage (BAL) fluid consists of approximately 80 percent alveolar macrophages, 10 percent lymphocytes (of which 70 percent are T lymphocytes), 1 to 5 percent B lymphocytes or plasma cells, 1 to 3 percent PMNs, and 1 percent eosinophils. In the lymphocyte population, the ratio of CD4 T helper and CD8 T suppressor/cytotoxic cells is about 1.5.

In the earliest, reversible forms of alveolar injury, "leakiness" of the alveolar type I cell layer and the adjacent capillary endothelial surface occurs, causing alveolar and interstitial edema and the formation of intraalveolar hyaline membranes. With persistence of the disease, increased alveolar-capillary permeability and desquamation of intraalveolar cells (alveolitis), mural inflammation, and interstitial fibrosis are present on biopsy. Histologically, the reaction can be patchy in distribution and various stages of development found. The presence and severity of the disease process are spotty in distribution; a continuum of inflammatory and fibrotic changes can be found throughout the affected lung. Fibrosis follows from an organization of inflammatory exudate within the airspaces in which fibroblasts beneath the type I epithelium proliferate and increase their production of fibronectin and collagen. Cicatrization can create cystic spaces.

Immunopathogenic mechanisms that interconnect the intraalveolar (luminal) and alveolar mural (septal) tissue with the interstitial space and capillary vascular areas are depicted in Fig. 259-1. Although the inciting agent or stimulus is unknown, it is likely an antigen that can initiate an immunoglobulin response. This is reflected by an increased ratio of IgG subclasses IgG1 and G3, an increased number of IgG-releasing cells, and perhaps the formation of immune complexes. Speculation continues that a microbial etiology, possibly viral, is probable for some cases of IPF.

This process is also reflected in the composition of cells and enzymes recovered in BAL fluid and in cellular components present in lung biopsy tissue. An increased number of macrophages, which are activated phagocytes capable of producing many cytokines that affect other lung cells, is a hallmark of the alveolitis. These macrophage cytokines or mediators can operate in two directions. First, through the production of chemokines, which include leukotriene B_4, interleukin (IL) 8, and tumor necrosis factor α, inflammatory cells such as PMNs and eosinophils are attracted into the alveoli. IPF lung macrophages express increased mRNA for IL-8, which roughly correlates with the percent of PMNs in BAL fluid. An increased percentage of PMNs (20 percent or more) and eosinophils (2 to 4 percent) in the profile of BAL cells is usual in IPF; eosinophil cationic protein is increased in BAL fluid. Lymphocytes are not usually increased, unless the IPF is part of a collagen vascular disease. Enzymes, such as collagenase, or oxidant radicals from inflammatory cells and histamine may cause local injury or alter the permeability of type I cells. Conversely, the antioxidant glutathione is deficient in the BAL fluid, further impairing neutralization of oxidants.

Second, macrophages are also capable of secreting substances that stimulate mesenchymal cells. For fibroblasts to replicate in the interstitium and in the alveolar walls, they must be primed to enter the G_1 phase of a growth cycle to proliferate. Several products from alveolar macrophages can participate in these steps. Platelet-derived growth factor B (PDGF-B) is a chemoattractant for mesenchymal cells and a stimulus for fibroblasts to change from resting cells to cells entering G_1. Although PDGF-B is not produced by normal monocytes or macrophages, alveolar macrophages obtained from patients with IPF make it abundantly. This is correlated with c-*sis*, a proto-oncogene that codes for the beta chain of PDGF-B, which is increased in IPF-derived macrophages. Interferon γ upregulates this gene activation. This mediator also acts as a chemoattractant and a growth factor for fibroblasts. Later in the fibroblast replication cycle, alveolar macrophage–derived insulin-like growth factors (IGF-1 and IGFBP-3) can accelerate proliferation. Transforming growth factor β, insulin, and other cellular or metabolic substances are needed in these growth-regulatory steps, also. Collagen peptides can be released locally, and N-terminal type III procollagen peptides have been found in BAL fluid. Surfactant protein A is reduced. Smooth-muscle cells also can proliferate. With continued activity of macrophages, fibrosis becomes more widespread and may involve the vasculature. Obliteration of functional alveolar structures occurs with scar tissue formation, and cystic areas develop from retraction of the terminal airways that once subtended the alveolar unit.

CLINICAL PRESENTATION **History** On average, patients are about 55 years old, although the range spans infancy to old age. Several family clusters have been reported, and it is possible that genetic factors may determine susceptibility to the disease. The first clinical manifestations of ILD or IPF are dyspnea, effort intolerance, and a dry cough without other obvious cause. A detailed work and environmental history is essential. For example, casual exposure to asbestos many years previously may provide a crucial clue to the etiology. Causes for hypersensitivity lung disease can be missed. Work-related compensation may influence complaints for some individuals.

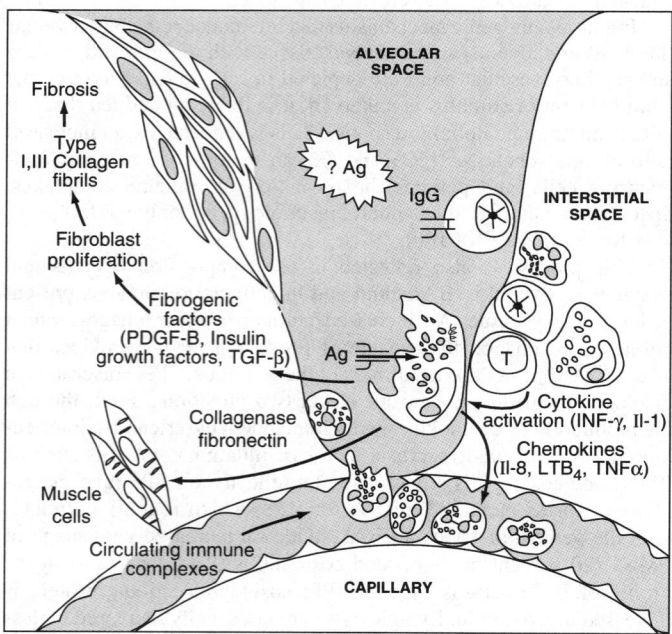

FIGURE 259-1 Immunologic mechanisms within the alveolar space, alveolar walls, and interstitium that can lead to inflammation and eventual fibrosis. The focus is the alveolar macrophage, which is activated, possibly by an immune complex and an as yet unidentified antigen (Ag). Through mediators, termed *chemokines*, the macrophage attracts PMNs and other cells from the circulation to the alveolar space, or it can initiate fibrogenesis with various mediators that can stimulate fibroblasts and muscle cells to proliferate. Interstitial fibrosis may result. Abbreviations: IL-8, interleukin 8; LTB₄, leukotriene B₄; TNF, tumor necrosis factor; INF-γ, interferon γ; IL-1, interleukin 1; TGF, transforming growth factor; PDGF-B, platelet-derived growth factor. (*After HY Reynolds, Chest 89:139, 1986.*)

Approximately one-third of patients can associate their awareness of dyspnea with the aftermath of a viral respiratory illness. Usually months or years elapse between the onset of exertional dyspnea and its progression perhaps to the point of breathlessness at rest. Dyspnea and frequent coughing are often accompanied by other constitutional symptoms such as fatigue, anorexia, weight loss, and arthralgias.

Physical Findings Initially, the physical examination may not be revealing, and auscultation of the chest may be normal. As the disease advances, dry crackles, or coarse crackles on inspiration, are usually heard at the lung bases. There may be tachypnea at rest, cyanosis, and clubbing of the fingers and toes, usually without hypertrophic osteoarthropathy. In later stages, cor pulmonale (Chap. 238) is evident, with findings of pulmonary hypertension, such as an accentuated pulmonic second sound or a right-sided lift, and eventually signs of right-sided heart failure. The right ventricular ejection fraction determined by radionuclide ventriculography is often depressed in the face of normal left ventricular performance.

LABORATORY AND DIAGNOSTIC TESTS **Imaging Studies** The chest radiograph usually reveals a pattern of diffuse reticular or reticulonodular markings, prominent in the lower lung zones. Several radiographic patterns on chest and HRCT scan can be seen that correlate roughly with the severity and duration of the disease. Early, a hazy "ground glass" appearance of the lower lung fields coincides with the stage of acute alveolitis. Later, curvilinear strands predominate and may coalesce into nodular infiltrates. With end-stage disease, the linear opacities are seen in all lung fields, the lung fields appear contracted, and ring-shaped opacities resulting from cystic and bronchiectatic changes are obvious, creating the *honey-combed* or *swiss cheese* appearance of the lung. HRCT patterns are helpful in monitoring disease activity also. Biopsy-proven forms of diffuse IPF occur occasionally in patients with normal chest radiographs (about 14 percent) despite significant exercise intolerance, abnormal pulmonary function tests (including a reduced diffusing capacity), and dry crackles. However, patients with biopsy-proven IPF may have no evidence of it on HRCT (found in only 3 of 25 patients, or 12 percent, in one study).

Laboratory Examination The erythrocyte sedimentation rate is usually elevated, circulating immune-complex titers and serum immunoglobulin levels may be increased, and cryoimmunoglobulins may be present. Serologic tests to screen for collagen vascular diseases are necessary to exclude these diagnoses. Although serum rheumatoid factor, antinuclear antibodies, depressed levels of complement, and other parameters of autoimmune diseases may be detected in approximately 10 percent of patients with IPF, the titers are generally quite low.

Lung Function Tests In patients with advanced disease, reductions in total lung capacity, vital capacity, and residual volume are found (Chap. 250). Usually, evidence of airway obstruction is minimal, and the FEV_1/FVC ratio is normal or increased. A restrictive ventilatory pattern is usually present, reflecting the stiff, noncompliant lungs characteristic of IPF and its common aftermath, fibrosis. There is usually resting arterial hypoxemia, but the carbon dioxide tension is normal or decreased. Blood pH is normal. The alveolar-arterial oxygen gradient during exercise is elevated, and exercise tolerance is reduced. The carbon monoxide diffusing capacity is usually reduced by 30 to 50 percent. Changes in these variables are useful in monitoring the course of the illness and in assessing the effectiveness of treatment. However, current or former cigarette smoking in IPF patients can alter lung function to misrepresent the extent of restriction and/or obstruction, if both emphysema and interstitial fibrosis are present. This has implications and raises caution for evaluating lung function in these patients.

Bronchoscopy Direct investigation of the airways by fiberoptic bronchoscopy is part of the evaluation, and four to six transbronchial biopsies are taken to obtain lung tissue for diagnosis. These provide a sufficient quantity of tissue for a definitive pathologic diagnosis in approximately one-fourth of all cases of IPF. In some diffuse granulomatous interstitial diseases, such as sarcoidosis (Chap. 320), transbronchial biopsy will yield a tissue diagnosis in about 80 percent of cases. Bronchoscopy also permits BAL, which gives useful information about cells and proteins in the airways that generally correlates with histologic changes in the interstitial and alveolar tissues. An analysis of BAL fluid and cells can reveal a number of changes in IPF.

Lung Biopsy The importance of an adequate sample of lung tissue to permit a full histologic evaluation, good microbial cultures, immunofluorescence and electron-microscopic studies, and analysis of inorganic substances cannot be overemphasized. Therefore, if a transbronchial biopsy does not yield sufficient tissue for a confident diagnosis, a thoracoscopic-guided or an open-lung biopsy should be considered. It is prudent to substantiate a tissue diagnosis before embarking on immunosuppressive therapy with its attendant complications.

DIAGNOSTIC APPROACH AND STAGING OF DISEASE ACTIVITY The importance of obtaining a thorough occupational and environmental history from the patient cannot be overemphasized. Also, a review of any prior chest films is usually helpful. Judging whether the lung disease is part of a multisystem process, related temporally to a new medication, or coincident with a change in neurologic status that would make aspiration and infection more likely are important in the differential diagnosis of ILD. Following the clinical examination, chest radiograph (or HRCT chest scan), pulmonary function tests [lung volumes, FEV_1/FVC, and diffusing capacity (Chap. 250)], and arterial blood gas determination measuring desaturation under exercising conditions, the functional disability from the lung disease can be estimated. However, a histologic analysis of lung tissue should be made before the disease is diagnosed definitively. Fiberoptic bronchoscopy is usually the first invasive procedure and is important for ruling out infection, malignancy, and other specific diseases. Although transbronchial biopsy has a lower diagnostic yield in IPF than in sarcoidosis and other granulomatous diseases, it is nevertheless a useful, low-risk procedure with a 20 to 30 percent success rate for obtaining an adequate sample for a confident pathologic diagnosis. BAL for cellular and protein analysis may be useful in judging the nature of alveolar inflammation and immunologic activity. However, the value of the periodic use of BAL analysis to monitor disease activity or its response to therapy has not been established. Use of gallium 67 lung scanning does not add more diagnostic accuracy or help with monitoring activity.

If the diagnosis is still in doubt after the bronchoscopy and related procedures, an imaged thorascopic or open-lung biopsy should be considered. The referring physician and the thoracic surgeon should cooperate in choosing the most representative areas of the lung for biopsy, and the proper microbial cultures and immunologic studies should be obtained.

℞ **TREATMENT**

Treatment is usually offered to patients with IPF, even to patients with advanced fibrotic disease. A trial of oral prednisone is begun in a dose of 1 mg/kg daily and continued for about 8 weeks. If lung disease shows objective improvement, the dose is tapered to a maintenance level of about 0.25 mg/kg for another 6 months or so. Should the disease not respond or be progressive, additional immunosuppression with cyclophosphamide should be considered. Cyclophosphamide is given at a dose of about 1.0 mg/kg daily (50 to 75 mg) with the patient continuing on a daily maintenance dose of oral prednisone (0.25 mg/kg). The dosages of cyclophosphamide may be increased as necessary by 50-mg increments at 7- to 10-day intervals. The objective is to reduce the white blood cell count to approximately half the normal baseline value, causing a distinct drop in the total blood lymphocyte count. However, a minimum count of 1000 PMNs/μL should be maintained. Alternatively, intravenous pulsed doses of cyclophosphamide given biweekly have been used with good success; 500 mg is given initially, and the dose can be increased in 100- to 200-mg increments to a total amount of 1.0 to 1.8 g and continued for a 12- to 18-month interval.

Use of high-dose, pulsed glucocorticoids does not offer special advantages over daily dosing. Azathioprine has been used in place of cyclophosphamide. Other agents such as penicillamine and cyclosporine have not been evaluated thoroughly. However, oral therapy with colchicine, which can inhibit macrophage-produced

fibroblast growth factors, given in a dose of 0.6 mg daily has been found to improve or permit a stable condition to occur in some patients; more testing of this therapy is indicated.

Several other measures may help respiratory function. It is imperative that patients discontinue cigarette smoking. Since there is frequently a marked drop in Pa_{O_2} with exercise, supplemental oxygen therapy may be useful, sometimes using transtracheal catheter oxygen delivery, which can reduce oxygen requirements and help with the logistics of supplying high-flow therapy. As the pulmonary vascular bed is destroyed by progressive fibrosis, pulmonary hypertension and cor pulmonale can develop; right-sided congestive heart failure can be difficult to control. Judicious use of diuretics is advised. Adequate oxygenation is probably the best treatment for right-sided heart failure (Chap. 238). Some patients also may develop obstruction to airflow and wheezing and coughing, which may respond to bronchodilators. Severe coughing episodes may require a narcotic-containing antitussive medication. Infection may occur during immunosuppressive therapy and should be treated promptly and aggressively. Prophylactic use of pneumococcal and influenza vaccines is indicated. If refractory disease limited to the chest is present, the possibility of lung transplantation should be considered. Success with single-lung transplantation for ILD makes this therapy a reality for some patients. Selection criteria, contraindications, and availability of organs must be discussed candidly with patients so as not to create unrealistic expectations.

INDIVIDUAL FORMS OF ILD

ILD ASSOCIATED WITH COLLAGEN VASCULAR DISORDERS In these diseases, various pulmonary structures can be affected, especially the pleura, so that ILD is but one manifestation of intrathoracic involvement and is often a minor part of the multiorgan process. The same is true for fibrosis.

Systemic Lupus Erythematosus (See Chap. 312) About half of patients with systemic lupus erythematosus ultimately develop overt lung disease. Pleuritis, pleural effusion(s), and acute pneumonitis from pulmonary capillaritis causing alveolar hemorrhage are the most frequent forms of lung disease, while a chronic, progressive ILD is uncommon. It is important to exclude pulmonary infection. Although pleuropulmonary involvement may not be evident clinically, pulmonary function testing, particularly the diffusing capacity for carbon monoxide, reveals abnormalities in many patients. A lymphocytic alveolitis may occur, which usually indicates a better response to immunosuppressive therapy.

Rheumatoid Arthritis (See Chap. 313) A variety of pulmonary manifestations can occur, including pleural disease (pleural effusion and subpleural nodules), parenchymal nodular infiltrates associated with pneumoconiosis in miners (Caplan's syndrome), and diffuse interstitial fibrosis. The ILD can develop before joint disease becomes evident, particularly in men, and is accompanied by high titers of rheumatoid factor. Bronchiolitis obliterans with organizing pneumonia has been reported. Patients with rheumatoid arthritis who are receiving treatment with methotrexate or gold may develop ILD that represents a drug hypersensitivity, which must be differentiated from a preexisting or developing ILD associated with the underlying disease. Penicillamine therapy in patients with rheumatoid arthritis has been implicated as a cause of bronchiolitis obliterans.

Ankylosing Spondylitis (See Chap. 317) Bilateral upper lobe fibrosis, which can be complicated by fibrocavitary disease, may develop late in the course.

Systemic Sclerosis (See Chap. 314) Radiographic evidence of lung involvement develops in a majority of patients, but its severity or progression is variable. Because distal esophageal motor dysfunction is present in many patients, reflux with regurgitation and chronic aspiration is common. Mast cells and their mediators in BAL fluid may be important in the alveolitis that develops. In addition, cutaneous scleroderma can involve the anterior chest wall and abdomen, causing restrictive lung function.

Sjögren's Syndrome (See Chap. 316) General dryness and lack of airways secretions cause the major problems of hoarseness, cough, and bronchitis. Presence of an ILD in these patients may signify a lymphocytic infiltrate in lung tissue, which can behave as a low-grade lymphoma. As small terminal airways can be affected with bronchiolitis obliterans, lung hyperinflation on pulmonary function testing may be a clue (high residual volume to total lung capacity ratio).

Polymyositis and Dermatomyositis (See Chap. 315) Although ILD is reported to occur in only 5 to 10 percent of patients, its presence is more common in the subgroup of patients with an anti-Jo-1 antibody that is directed to histidyl tRNA synthetase. Weakness of respiratory muscles contributing to aspiration pneumonitis is a common occurrence.

SYNDROMES OF ILD WITH PULMONARY HEMORRHAGE Recurrent hemoptysis, dyspnea, and hypoxemia in the presence of a chest radiographic pattern of diffuse alveolar opacities should raise the possibility of alveolar hemorrhage. An association between vasculitis involving the kidney (lung-renal syndromes) or other organ systems should be investigated. Alveolar hemorrhage occurs rarely in all collagen vascular disorders, but it is described most often with systemic lupus erythematosus. It can occur with systemic necrotizing vasculitis and is described as an initial presentation of Wegener's granulomatosis; with Behçet's disease, in which aneurysm formation and rupture of small muscular arteries are manifestations of necrotizing vasculitis; in allergic Churg-Strauss granulomatosis; in Henoch-Schönlein purpura syndrome; and in essential (mixed) cryoimmunoglobulinemia. Serologic tests for antinuclear antibody, anti-glomerular basement membrane antibody, and complement to document a vasculitis and immunologic disorder are the first steps, but renal biopsy and possibly lung biopsy may be required for a definitive diagnosis. Some specific syndromes in this category will be discussed next.

Goodpasture's Syndrome (See Chap. 275) Pulmonary hemorrhage and glomerulonephritis are the features of this disease in which most patients have autoantibodies to renal glomerular and lung alveolar basement membranes.

Idiopathic Pulmonary Hemosiderosis Diffuse alveolar hemorrhage can occur in the absence of other organ involvement or an obvious immunologic cause and is therefore a diagnosis of exclusion after considering the many causes of alveolar bleeding associated with collagen vascular and vasculitic diseases. A lung biopsy is usually necessary to document the lack of inflammatory injury in the lung tissues and to exclude other diseases with confidence. Children and young adults are usually affected. The clinical course can be variable, ranging from recurrent and fulminant with development of progressive interstitial fibrosis to minimal disease that may remit without sequelae. Glucocorticoid treatment is useful for control of bleeding acutely but is not a predictable long-term remedy for keeping the disease suppressed and preventing recurrence.

PULMONARY ALVEOLAR PROTEINOSIS Similar clinical symptoms and the general appearance of the chest radiograph, showing diffuse alveolar consolidation and/or nodular shadows typically radiating from the hilar regions, place pulmonary alveolar proteinosis (PAP) in the ILD category. Histologically, the alveoli are filled with granular material that stains with periodic acid Schiff reagent, but they exhibit no inflammation and have relatively normal septal structure. Strictly speaking, then, PAP is an intraalveolar process that resembles, but is not, an ILD. Because the proteinaceous response can be associated with inhaled dust exposure (silica and aluminum), malignancy, and chronic infection, termed *secondary PAP*, these disorders should be differentiated from primary PAP by lung biopsy. The intraalveolar material is a combination of surfactant phospholipid produced by type II pneumocytes, lactate dehydrogenase, and other proteins and immunoglobulins found in alveolar lining fluid. The macrophages exhibit large phagolysosomes that have diminished microbial killing capacity in vitro, but lung infections with unusual organisms are not frequent. Whole-lung lavage(s) provides relief to many patients with dyspnea and progressive deterioration of arterial oxygenation and also may provide long-term benefit.

LYMPHOCYTIC INFILTRATIVE DISORDERS This group of disorders features lymphocyte and plasma cell infiltration of the lung parenchyma; the disorders either are benign or can behave as low-grade lymphomas. Within the spectrum of chronic interstitial pneumonias, a subset has been described with lung histology that shows diffuse interstitial infiltration with lymphocytes and plasma cells. In some of these patients, an autoimmune disease or dysproteinemia exists. However, lymphocytic interstitial pneumonia is probably not a distinct entity, belongs within the IPF group, and can be associated with Sjögren's syndrome. Lymphocytic interstitial pneumonia has been reported in patients, particularly children, with AIDS.

Included among these disorders is immunoblastic lymphadenopathy, also termed *angioimmunoblastic lymphadenopathy*, which usually is a fulminant lymphoma-like disease that may have an element of ILD in some cases. *Lymphomatoid granulomatosis* can be included, but its granulomatous response also places it with the granulomatous ILDs (see Table 259-1).

EOSINOPHILIC PNEUMONIAS (See Chap. 253) These pneumonias encompass a spectrum of diseases in which lung hypersensitivity plays a role and in which a specific cause may or may not be identified. For example, with extrinsic asthma and exposure to fungal antigens, allergic bronchopulmonary mycosis can develop; filarial and other parasitic infections can cause tropical pulmonary eosinophilia; many common drugs can induce eosinophilic pneumonia. Chronic eosinophilic pneumonia has features that make it difficult to distinguish from IPF and other forms of progressive ILD. This disease, which more commonly affects older females, has several radiologic characteristics that are helpful in diagnosis: (1) a peripheral pattern of dense lung infiltrates that appear to cross anatomic lobar boundaries with sparing of the central lung regions, (2) regression but reappearance of infiltrates in the same lung locations, and (3) extreme sensitivity of the infiltrates (and disease symptoms) to modest doses of oral glucocorticoids. The diagnosis can be established by lung biopsy, which shows an eosinophilic inflammatory process. Many other lung diseases have eosinophilia and eosinophils found in lung tissue or in respiratory secretions, including asthma, IPF (as mentioned), and forms of granulomatous vasculitis.

LYMPHANGIOLEIOMYOMATOSIS Immature smooth-muscle cells can proliferate in lung tissue around and throughout bronchial, vascular, and lymphatic structures, causing local obstruction or creating constricting lesions that develop into cysts. Lymphatics and lymph nodes in other organs are also usually affected. Because this disorder occurs predominantly in females of reproductive age, an association between estrogens and the disease is probable. Pulmonary symptoms consist of dyspnea, cough, and hemoptysis; a more overt presentation occurs with spontaneous pneumothorax, which can be recurrent, or with chylous effusion. In addition, the chest radiograph shows reticulonodular shadows and small cystlike areas or honeycombing throughout the lung fields. In contrast to most forms of ILD, lung volumes are normal or increased, as is also the case with Langerhans cell granulomatosis (see below). Therapy for progressive lung disease has not been particularly effective. Pneumothoraces and effusions may require chemical or surgical pleurodesis. Treatment with hormone manipulation, including oophorectomy or tamoxifen, has not been helpful, but medroxyprogesterone acetate injections (400 to 800 mg per month intramuscularly for 1 year) have improved dyspnea in some patients and could be considered. Lung transplantation may be considered for some patients.

AMYLOIDOSIS (See Chap. 309) As part of primary systemic amyloidosis or a plasma cell dyscrasia, an ILD may occur from amyloid deposits in alveolar septa and associated blood vessels, producing dyspnea, radiographic findings of diffuse reticulonodular shadows, and restrictive pulmonary function.

INHERITED DISORDERS ASSOCIATED WITH ILD Pulmonary infiltrates and respiratory symptoms typical of mild ILD can develop in related family members and in several inherited diseases. These include the phacomatoses tuberous sclerosis and neurofibromatosis and the lysosomal storage diseases (Chap. 346), such as Niemann-Pick disease and Gaucher's disease. The *Hermansky Pudlak syndrome* is an autosomal recessive disorder in which granulomatous colitis and ILD may occur. It is characterized by oculocutaneous albinism, bleeding diathesis from platelet dysfunction, and the accumulation of a chromolipid, lipofuscin material in cells of the reticuloendothelial system. The pulmonary fibrosis is similar to IPF, but the alveolar macrophages may contain cytoplasmic ceroid-like inclusions.

GASTROINTESTINAL AND LIVER DISEASE Rarely, inflammatory bowel disease and chronic hepatitis may be associated with a mild form of ILD. Crohn's disease, which has a number of similarities with sarcoidosis, also may be accompanied by asymptomatic lymphocytic alveolitis. For some patients with cirrhosis or end-stage liver disease, findings that can suggest an ILD include dyspnea, hypoxemia, digital clubbing, and basilar interstitial markings on chest radiograph, which may in fact be pulmonary vascular dilatations. The dyspnea often occurs in the upright position (platypnea).

GRAFT-VERSUS-HOST DISEASE (See Chap. 116) Some degree of graft-versus-host disease, manifested by variably progressive obstructive lung function and obliterative bronchiolitis involving the terminal bronchioles, occurs in most patients receiving bone marrow transplantation and in between 20 and 50 percent of recipients of heart-lung or lung transplants. The syndrome occurs as an infection or part of an acute rejection episode, although there may be a more gradual, insidious onset of dry cough, mucositis, dyspnea, and airflow obstruction in the small airways, as demonstrated by pulmonary function testing. Chest radiographs reveal peribronchiolar infiltrates, and lung biopsy shows focal areas of interstitial infiltration with a mixture of lymphocytes and PMNs. The lesions are consistent with bronchiolitis; no vasculitis is present. Treatment includes increasing the doses of the immunosuppressive drugs together with bronchodilators and antibiotics. Infection, especially with a viral agent such as cytomegalovirus, is a common complication.

ILD WITH A GRANULOMATOUS RESPONSE IN LUNG TISSUE OR VASCULAR STRUCTURES Inhalation of organic dusts, which causes hypersensitivity pneumonitis, or of inorganic particles such as silica, which causes alveolitis and elicits a granulomatous inflammatory reaction leading to ILD, produces diseases of known etiology (see Table 259-1) that are discussed in Chaps. 253 and 254. Sarcoidosis (Chap. 320) is prominent among granulomatous diseases of *unknown cause* in which ILD is an important feature.

Langerhans Cell Granulomatosis (Eosinophilic Granuloma or Histiocytosis X) (See Chap. 61) This condition is being recognized with increasing frequency and may account for about 1 to 5 percent of ILD of unknown etiology. Previously, the proliferation of tissue macrophages (histiocytes) was thought to be characteristic of this disease that affects the lung, bones, and viscera. Now it is recognized that the precursor cell is the *dendritic cell*, which has potent stimulatory and accessory cell immune function, is normally found in the interstitium alveolar septal areas and in BAL fluid, and is distinctly different from a tissue macrophage. The dendritic cell can evolve into the Langerhans cell, characterized by a specific CD1a surface antigen that reacts with a monoclonal antibody identified as OKT_6. These cells have a low amount of autofluorescence and express L25, OK1a, RFD_1, and major histocompatibility complex class II antigens. Intracytoplasmic organelles that are called X bodies or Birbeck granules can be seen by electron microscopy. In Langerhans cell granulomatosis of the lung, 3 percent or more of the BAL cells may be so identified, which greatly exceeds the percentage found in other disorders. However, the Langerhans cells are not pathognomonic for this disease.

The pulmonary form of this disease occurs in young and middle-aged adults, usually males, and in those who use tobacco heavily; it may remain focal or involve one or several bony sites (long bones, spine, skull, or jaw). Occasionally, multifocal disease can affect the posterior pituitary gland, causing diabetes insipidus, a condition that is termed *Hand-Schüller-Christian disease*. In infants, *Letterer-Siwe disease* is a more fulminant visceral form of this disorder that mimics

a malignant lymphoma. In adults, the presenting symptoms and signs do not distinguish this disease from other forms of ILD unless signs of a bone lesion exist. Chest radiographs will show diffuse micronodular shadows and cystic spaces, sparing the costophrenic angles and preserving lung volume, as occurs in lymphangioleiomyomatosis. Pulmonary function tests may disclose a combination of obstructive and restrictive defects. As the disease progresses, greater airway obstruction may develop, and the chest radiograph can resemble that in advanced chronic obstructive lung disease.

℞ TREATMENT

This involves a mandatory cessation of tobacco use, which may cause the pulmonary disease to stabilize or regress. Glucocorticoids usually are not helpful. Penicillamine has been used in an attempt to prevent fibrosis, with variable success. Local bone lesions may require irradiation treatment. For patients with increasing symptoms of airway obstruction, supportive therapy and bronchodilators may be tried, but their success has been modest. Lung transplantation should be considered for certain patients.

Granulomatous Vasculitis (See Chap. 319) Certain forms of vasculitis, accompanied by a granulomatous response, can involve the respiratory tract as part of a multiorgan process or can occasionally be localized to the respiratory tract, as occurs with a predominantly pulmonary form of Wegener's granulomatosis in which glomerulonephritis may not be prominent. It is very important to differentiate these conditions from lymphomatoid granulomatosis. Allergic angiitis and the granulomatosis of Churg and Strauss are forms of granulomatous vasculitis affecting many organs but especially the lungs; a history of asthma and the presence of eosinophilia are distinguishing features.

Lymphomatoid Granulomatosis (See Chaps. 61 and 319) This involves primarily the lungs and less frequently the skin, central and peripheral nervous systems, and kidneys with an infiltration of lymphocytoid, plasma-like cells and macrophages creating a necrotic granulomatous inflammatory reaction, especially in or near blood vessels. The disease can progress as a lymphoproliferative disorder and evolve into malignant lymphoma in as many as 50 percent of patients. Treatment of lymphomatoid granulomatosis with glucocorticoids and cyclophosphamide may induce a remission, and if this occurs, subsequent relapse and development of lymphoma are not likely.

BRONCHOCENTRIC GRANULOMATOSIS In contrast to the necrotizing granulomatous reaction in lung vessels, i.e., angiocentric vasculitis, granulomatous destruction of bronchioles occurs in this condition. There is usually associated parenchymal inflammation causing ILD. Eosinophils can be present if asthma and hypersensitivity to fungal antigens within the bronchi have occurred. In other cases without these associated conditions, hypersensitivity to other microbial antigens is postulated. Bronchocentric granulomatosis must be differentiated from hypersensitivity pneumonitis caused by inhalation of organic dusts. → *For further discussion, see Chaps. 253 and 254.*

BIBLIOGRAPHY

BAUGHMAN RP, LOWER EE: Use of intermittent, intravenous cyclophosphamide for idiopathic pulmonary fibrosis. Chest 102:1090, 1992

EPLER GR et al: Bronchiolitis obliterans with organizing pneumonia. N Engl J Med 312:152, 1985

FUJIMOTO K et al: Eosinophil activation in patients with pulmonary fibrosis. Chest 108:48, 1995

HANSON D et al: Changes in pulmonary function test results after one year of therapy as predictors of survival in patients with idiopathic pulmonary fibrosis. Chest 108:305, 1995

HUNNINGHAKE GW, KALICA AR: Approaches to the treatment of pulmonary fibrosis. Am J Respir Crit Care Med 151:915, 1995

ORENS JB et al: The sensitivity of high-resolution CT in detecting idiopathic pulmonary fibrosis proved by open lung biopsy—a prospective study. Chest 108:109, 1995

PETERS SG et al: Colchicine in the treatment of pulmonary fibrosis. Chest 103:101, 1993

RAGHU G: Interstitial lung disease: A diagnostic approach (are CT scan and lung biopsy indicated in every patient?) Am J Respir Crit Care Med 151:909, 1995

REYNOLDS HY: Bronchoalveolar lavage. Am Rev Respir Dis 135:250, 1987

ALLEN JN, DAVIS WB: Eosinophilic lung diseases. Am J Respir Crit Care Med 150:1423, 1994

HELMERS R et al: Pulmonary manifestations associated with rheumatoid arthritis. Chest 100:235, 1991

HOFFMAN RM, ROGERS RM: Serum and lavage lactate dehydrogenase isoenzymes in pulmonary alveolar proteinosis. Am Rev Respir Dis 143:42, 1991

KITAICHI M et al: Pulmonary lymphangioleiomyomatosis: A report of 46 patients including a clinicopathologic study of prognostic factors. Am J Respir Crit Care Med 151:527, 1995

LAHDENSUO A, KORPELA M: Pulmonary findings in patients with primary Sjögren's syndrome. Chest 108:316, 1995

SCHWARZ MI et al: Pulmonary capillaritis and diffuse alveolar hemorrhage—a primary manifestation of polymyositis. Am J Respir Crit Care Med 151:2037, 1995

SOLER P et al: Pulmonary Langerhans' cell granulomatosis. Annu Rev Med 43:105, 1992

TROSHINSKY MB et al: Pulmonary function and gastroesophageal reflux in systemic sclerosis. Ann Intern Med 121:6, 1994

260 Stuart Rich

PRIMARY PULMONARY HYPERTENSION

Primary pulmonary hypertension is an uncommon disease characterized by increased pulmonary artery pressure and pulmonary vascular resistance without an obvious cause. The incidence has been estimated at approximately 2 cases per million. There is a female-to-male preponderance (1.7:1), with patients most commonly presenting in the third and fourth decades, although the age range is from infancy to greater than 60 years. Because the predominant symptom of primary pulmonary hypertension is dyspnea, which can have an insidious onset in an otherwise healthy person, the disease is typically diagnosed late in its course. By that time, the clinical and laboratory findings of severe pulmonary hypertension are usually present.

PATHOLOGY The histopathology of primary pulmonary hypertension is not pathognomonic for the disease but represents a pulmonary arteriopathy that is observed in pulmonary hypertension from a variety of causes. The most common patterns found are a plexogenic arteriopathy manifest by medial hypertrophy, concentric laminar intimal fibrosis, and plexiform lesions; and a thrombotic arteriopathy manifest by eccentric intimal fibrosis with medial hypertrophy, fibroelastic intimal pads in the arteries and arterioles, and scattered evidence of old recanalized thrombi appearing as fibrous webs. In most patients features of both patterns of vascular changes can be found.

The common pathogenetic denominator appears to be an undefined injury to the pulmonary vascular endothelium, which results in (1) an impaired ability to maintain a relaxed state of vasomotor tone, (2) intense medial hypertrophy and intimal proliferation that compromises the vascular lumen, and (3) a conversion to a procoagulant state within the pulmonary arteriolar bed that disposes to the development of in situ thrombosis. The types of vascular changes noted are likely determined by the nature of the injury to the pulmonary vascular endothelium and/or its duration, the patient's gender, and underlying genetic predisposition. The association of primary pulmonary hypertension with cirrhosis and portal hypertension, while statistically significant, remains unexplained.

Pulmonary venoocclusive disease is a rare and distinct pathologic entity, found in fewer than 10 percent of patients with primary pulmonary hypertension. Histologically, it is manifest by widespread intimal proliferation and fibrosis of the intrapulmonary veins and venules, occasionally extending to the arteriolar bed. The pulmonary venous obstruction explains the increased pulmonary capillary wedge pressure observed in patients with advanced disease. These patients may develop orthopnea that can mimic left ventricular failure.

Pulmonary capillary hemangiomatosis is also a very rare form of primary pulmonary hypertension. Histologically, it is characterized by infiltrating thin-walled blood vessels that are widespread throughout the pulmonary interstitium and walls of the pulmonary arteries and veins. These patients often have hemoptysis as a clinical feature.

ETIOLOGY The etiology of primary pulmonary hypertension remains unknown, although animal and human studies suggest an abnormality of the endothelial cell of the pulmonary arterial bed. In many individuals, a risk factor or "trigger" appears to influence pulmonary endothelial cell function, resulting in ineffective control of vasomotor tone, causing vasoconstriction, and platelet activation and thrombosis. Studies suggest that there is a release of growth factors and cytokines that act locally on the pulmonary arteriolar bed to induce vascular remodeling. Risk factors that have been linked to the development of unexplained pulmonary hypertension include essential hypertension, human immunodeficiency virus, portal hypertension, anorexigens, collagen vascular disease, and congenital shunts resulting in increased pulmonary blood flow.

A genetic basis for primary pulmonary hypertension appears likely. Familial primary pulmonary hypertension occurs in approximately 7 percent of cases, with the pattern of inheritance identified as autosomal dominant, with incomplete penetrance and genetic anticipation. The latter feature, which relates to offspring of subsequent generations manifesting the disease either at younger ages or by greater severity, is seen in other genetic diseases associated with a trinucleotide repeat expansion abnormality. The genetic basis of primary pulmonary hypertension may involve several genetic loci, with patients who present with sporadic disease possessing a genetic predisposition that becomes expressed following exposure to an external trigger or risk factor.

PATHOPHYSIOLOGY The underlying hemodynamic derangement in primary pulmonary hypertension is an increased resistance to pulmonary blood flow. Early in the disease there is a marked elevation in pulmonary artery pressure with relatively normal cardiac function. Over time the cardiac output becomes progressively reduced rather than the pulmonary artery pressure becoming progressively increased. Initially, the pulmonary arteries may respond to vasodilators, but as the disease progresses, the elevated pulmonary vascular resistance becomes fixed. The pulmonary capillary wedge pressure remains normal until the late stages, when it tends to rise in response to impaired diastolic filling of the left ventricle due to the altered configuration of the intraventricular septum. Eventually, as the right ventricle fails, the right atrial and right ventricular end-diastolic pressures rise in an attempt to compensate for the myocardial depression that has developed in response to chronic severe right ventricular pressure overload.

Pulmonary function is usually normal in primary pulmonary hypertension, although a mild restrictive pattern (see Chap. 250) is sometimes seen. Hypoxemia is common and is believed to be due to a mismatch between pulmonary ventilation and perfusion, magnified by a low cardiac output. Occasional patients with a patent foramen ovale may develop right-to-left shunting, which also can contribute to systemic arterial desaturation.

DIAGNOSIS A thorough diagnostic evaluation to look for all potential causes should be undertaken (see Fig. 260-1). The history usually reveals the gradual onset of shortness of breath with effort, progressing until the patient is dyspneic with minimal activity. The average duration from symptom onset until diagnosis is 2.5 years. Other common symptoms are fatigue, angina pectoris that likely represents right ventricular ischemia, syncope, near syncope, and peripheral edema.

The physical examination is characteristic. Increased jugular venous pressure, a reduced carotid pulse, and an easily palpable right ventricular lift are typical. Most patients have an increased pulmonic component of the second heart sound and right-sided third and fourth heart sounds. Tricuspid and pulmonic regurgitation and peripheral cyanosis and edema may be noted. Clubbing is not a feature.

The chest x-ray generally shows enlarged central pulmonary arteries and clear lung fields. The electrocardiogram usually reveals right axis deviation and right ventricular hypertrophy. The echocardiogram demonstrates right ventricular enlargement, a reduction in left ventricular cavity size, and abnormal septal configuration consistent with right ventricular pressure overload. Doppler studies have revealed a marked dependence on atrial systole for ventricular filling. Hypoxemia, hypocapnia, and an abnormal diffusing capacity for carbon monoxide are almost invariable findings. A mild restrictive pattern on pulmonary function is sometimes observed, but evidence of airways obstruction suggests a secondary etiology for the pulmonary hypertension. A perfusion lung scan may be normal or abnormal with multiple diffuse patchy filling defects of a nonsegmental nature and not suggestive of pulmonary thromboembolism. If the lung scan reveals perfusion defects of a segmental or subsegmental nature, a pulmonary angiogram must be done. Severe pulmonary hypertension in a patient with a high-probability lung scan should suggest a chronic process and *not* acute pulmonary embolism, since the nonconditioned right ventricle is unable to generate high systolic pressures acutely in the face of pulmonary thromboembolism. Chronic thromboembolic obstruction of the large pulmonary arteries (Chap. 261) can mimic primary pulmonary hyper-

tension but can be amenable to treatment with surgical thromboendarterectomy.

There is risk in performing pulmonary angiography in patients with primary pulmonary hypertension, and it is recommended that selective or subselective injections with small amounts of low-osmolar, nonionic contrast material be made following the pretreatment with 1 mg atropine to prevent vagally mediated bradycardia.

Cardiac catheterization is mandatory to characterize the disease and exclude an underlying cardiac shunt as the cause. The use of balloon-flotation catheters, especially those with removable guidewires, can facilitate right heart catheterization. A right-to-left shunt might be attributable to a patent foramen ovale, but any left-to-right shunting implies the presence of a congenital defect. Although it may be difficult to obtain, the pulmonary capillary wedge pressure is normal. If it is increased, left heart catheterization also should be performed to exclude mitral stenosis or increased left ventricular end-diastolic pressures as the cause of the pulmonary hypertension. Although the diagnostic evaluation of these patients can be hazardous, experience from a national multicenter study revealed no mortality or serious morbidity in more than 300 patients whose evaluation included pulmonary angiography and cardiac catheterization. It is not necessary to perform an open lung biopsy in these patients to make an accurate diagnosis.

On occasion a patient may have marked elevations in pulmonary artery pressure and a relatively mild disease that is known to cause pulmonary hypertension. It would be a mistake to characterize these patients as having primary pulmonary hypertension on the belief that the pulmonary hypertension is out of proportion to the underlying associated condition. Since the pulmonary vascular bed has variable vasoreactivity, these cases probably reflect an exaggerated pulmonary vasoconstrictive response to the associated condition. Thus severe pulmonary hypertension can coexist with mild chronic obstructive pulmonary disease, small intracardiac shunts, mild mitral stenosis, and even ischemic heart disease. The distinction, however, is important because the treatment of pulmonary hypertension should always be focused toward the underlying cause.

NATURAL HISTORY   The natural history of primary pulmonary hypertension is unknown because initially the disease is largely asymptomatic. Several older series have reported a mean survival of 2 to 3 years for patients from the time of diagnosis. Functional class is a strong predictor of survival, since patients who are functional classes II and III have a mean survival of 3.5 years compared with those who are functional class IV, in whom the mean survival is 6 months. The cause of death is usually right ventricular failure or sudden death; sudden death appears to be a late feature of the disease. Increased right atrial pressure above 15 mmHg and reduced cardiac index below 2 (L/min)/m² are hemodynamic predictors of a poor prognosis.

℞ TREATMENT
Because the pulmonary vascular resistance increases dramatically with exercise, patients should be cautioned against participating in activities that demand increased physical stress. The use of digoxin remains controversial, since no studies have documented a benefit or detriment. Diuretic therapy relieves dyspnea and peripheral edema and may be useful in reducing right ventricular volume overload in the presence of tricuspid regurgitation.

It is recommended that all patients in whom primary pulmonary hypertension is confirmed undergo acute drug testing with short-acting pulmonary vasodilators to determine the extent of pulmonary vasodilator reserve or reactivity (see Fig. 260-2). Intravenous adenosine, inhaled nitric oxide, and intravenous prostacyclin all appear to have similar effects in reducing pulmonary vascular resistance acutely with little effect on the systemic vascular bed. Adenosine is given as a constant infusion in doses of 50 (μg/kg)/min and increased every 2 min until side effects develop. Similarly, prosta-

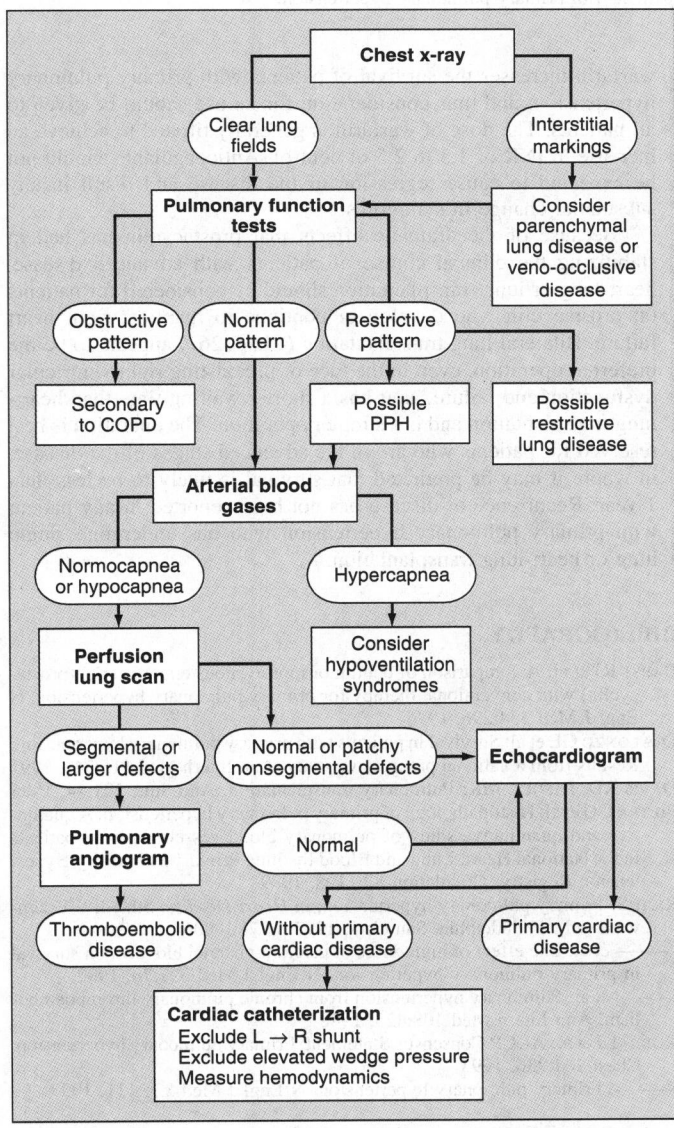

FIGURE 260-1   An algorithm for the workup of a patient with unexplained pulmonary hypertension. (*Adapted with permission from S Rich.*)

cyclin is given in doses of 2 (ng/kg)/min and increased every 30 min until side effects develop. Maximal physiologic effectiveness of the therapy is determined at the highest tolerated dose. Nitric oxide is generally administered via inhalation in 5 to 10 parts per million and increased every few minutes until no further effectiveness is obtained.

Patients who have substantial reductions in pulmonary vascular resistance from the short-acting vasodilators may be candidates to receive oral calcium channel blockers. These drugs must be administered under direct hemodynamic guidance in order to determine effectiveness and safety. Typically, patients will require high doses (e.g., nifedipine, 120 to 240 mg/d, or diltiazem, 540 to 900 mg/d,[1]). Patients who manifest significant reductions in mean pulmonary artery pressure and pulmonary vascular resistance should demonstrate improved symptoms, regression of right ventricular hypertrophy, and improved survival with chronic therapy. However, fewer than half the patients who are responsive to the short-acting vasodilators will respond to this regimen. It is unknown whether the response to calcium blockers depends on the histologic subtype, but the therapy appears to be more successful in patients who are diagnosed early and have less advanced disease.

Prostacyclin has recently been approved as a treatment of primary pulmonary hypertension for patients who are functional class III or IV and unresponsive to conventional therapy. Clinical trials have demonstrated that patients realize an improvement in symptoms and exercise tolerance and reduction in mortality. The drug can only be administered intravenously and requires placement of a permanent central venous catheter and continuous dose titration, as tolerance develops in all patients over a short period of time. The side effects of prostacyclin, which include flushing, jaw pain, and diarrhea, are generally tolerated by most patients. The major problems with this therapy have been infections related to the venous catheter, which requires close monitoring and diligence on behalf of the patient. Because of the complexity involved in managing patients on prostacyclin, it has been recommended that they be referred to centers with expertise in managing primary pulmonary hypertension for initiation of therapy.

None of the other classes of vasodilator drugs that have been investigated, including beta-adrenergic agonists, alpha-adrenergic blockers, smooth-muscle vasodilators, nitrates, and angiotensin-converting enzyme inhibitors, has shown similar sustained effectiveness.

The administration of vasodilators can have serious acute and chronic adverse effects. The most common response is a reduction in pulmonary vascular resistance, manifest by an increased cardiac output, without a reduction in the mean pulmonary artery pressure. This results in increased stroke work of the right ventricle, which can result in worsening of ventricular function and precipitate right ventricular failure over time. In addition, maintenance of adequate systemic blood pressure is crucial, since right ventricular coronary blood flow is already compromised due to the loss of the normal gradient for myocardial perfusion between the aorta and right ventricle. Vasodilator drugs can provoke acute right ventricular ischemia, and deaths have been reported. For these reasons, the pharmacologic evaluation of primary pulmonary hypertension should always be undertaken with direct monitoring of systemic and pulmonary arterial pressures and cardiac output.

Anticoagulant therapy also has been advocated based on the evidence that thrombosis in situ is common. One retrospective study and one prospective study have demonstrated that the anticoagulant

FIGURE 260-2 An algorithm for the evaluation and drug treatment of a patient with primary pulmonary hypertension.

warfarin increases the survival of patients with primary pulmonary hypertension, and thus consideration for its use should be given to all patients. The dose of warfarin is generally titrated to achieve an increase in INR of 1.5 to 2.5 of control. Anticoagulants should not be expected to cause regression of the disease and result in any substantial change in symptoms.

Because of the dramatic effects that prostacyclin has had in stabilizing the clinical course of patients with advanced disease, heart-lung or lung transplantation should be considered for patients on prostacyclin who develop or continue to manifest right heart failure. Bilateral lung transplantation (Chap. 267) appears to be the preferred operation, even in the face of preexisting right ventricular dysfunction and failure, as it has a shorter waiting time than heart-lung transplantation and is a simpler operation. The operation is best reserved for patients who are in the advanced stages of the disease, in whom it may be predicted that survival is likely to be less than 1 year. Recurrence of disease has not been reported in any patient with primary pulmonary hypertension who has undergone single lung or heart-lung transplantation.

BIBLIOGRAPHY

BARST RJ et al: A comparison of continuous intravenous epoprostenol (prostacyclin) with conventional therapy for primary pulmonary hypertension. N Engl J Med 334:296, 1996

D'ALONZO GE et al: Survival in patients with primary pulmonary hypertension: Results from a national prospective study. Ann Intern Med 115:343, 1991

DAVIS RD, PASQUE MK: Pulmonary transplantation. Ann Surg 221:14, 1995

PIETRA GG et al: Histopathology of primary pulmonary hypertension: A qualitative and quantitative study of pulmonary blood vessels from 58 patients in the National Heart, Lung and Blood Institute Primary Pulmonary Hypertension Registry. Circulation 80:1198, 1989

RICH S: Primary pulmonary hypertension, in *Heart Disease*, 5th ed, E Braunwald (ed). Philadelphia, Saunders, 1997 pp 780–806

——— et al: The effect of high doses of calcium-channel blockers on survival in primary pulmonary hypertension. N Engl J Med 327:76, 1992

——— et al: Pulmonary hypertension from chronic pulmonary thromboembolism. Ann Intern Med 108:425, 1988

RUBIN LJ et al: ACCP Consensus Statement. Primary pulmonary hypertension. Chest 104:236, 1993

———: Primary pulmonary hypertension. N Engl J Med 336:111, 1997

---

[1] These agents have not been approved for the treatment of primary pulmonary hypertension by the U.S. Food and Drug Administration.

PULMONARY THROMBOEMBOLISM

PATHOPHYSIOLOGY

Rudolf Virchow postulated more than a century ago that a triad of factors predisposed to venous thrombosis: (1) local trauma to the vessel wall, (2) hypercoagulability, and (3) stasis. We now believe that many patients who suffer pulmonary thromboembolism (PTE) have an underlying inherited predisposition that remains clinically silent until an acquired stressor occurs such as surgery, obesity, or pregnancy (Table 261-1).

FACTOR V LEIDEN The most frequent inherited predisposition to hypercoagulability is resistance to the endogenous anticoagulant protein, activated protein C. The phenotype of activated protein C resistance is associated with a single point mutation, designated *factor V Leiden*, in the factor V gene. This missense mutation—a single nucleotide substitution of adenine for guanine 1691—causes an amino acid substitution of glutamine for arginine at position 506.

The allelic frequency of this mutation is about 3 percent in healthy American male physicians participating in the Physicians' Health Study. However, the prevalence of the factor V mutation was three times higher among those physicians who subsequently developed venous thrombosis. Furthermore, after anticoagulation (for at least 3 months) was completed and discontinued, those participants with factor V Leiden had a much higher rate of recurrent venous thrombosis than those without. Factor V Leiden is more common than all other (identified) inherited hypercoagulable states combined, including deficiencies in protein C, protein S, antithrombin III, and disorders of plasminogen (Chap. 118).

EMBOLIZATION When venous thrombi become dislodged from their site of formation, they embolize to the pulmonary arterial circulation or, paradoxically, to the arterial circulation through a patent foramen ovale. About half of patients with pelvic vein thrombosis or proximal leg deep venous thrombosis (DVT) have PTE, which is usually asymptomatic. Isolated calf vein or upper extremity venous thromboses also pose a risk (albeit lower) of PTE. The small size of isolated calf vein thrombi does not necessarily render them benign; they can embolize through a patent foramen ovale and are the most common source of paradoxical embolism.

PHYSIOLOGY Pulmonary embolism can have the following effects:

1. *Increased pulmonary vascular resistance* due to vascular obstruction or neurohumoral agents including serotonin
2. *Impaired gas exchange* due to increased alveolar dead space from vascular obstruction and hypoxemia from alveolar hypoventilation in the nonobstructed lung, right-to-left shunting, and impaired carbon monoxide transfer due to loss of gas exchange surface
3. *Alveolar hyperventilation* due to reflex stimulation of irritant receptors
4. *Increased airway resistance* due to bronchoconstriction
5. *Decreased pulmonary compliance* due to lung edema, lung hemorrhage, and loss of surfactant.

Right Ventricular Dysfunction Progressive right heart failure is the usual immediate cause of death from PTE. As pulmonary vascular resistance increases, right ventricular wall tension rises and perpetuates further right ventricular dilatation and dysfunction. Consequently, the interventricular septum bulges into and compresses an intrinsically normal left ventricle. Increased right ventricular wall tension also compresses the right coronary artery and may precipitate myocardial ischemia and right ventricular infarction. Underfilling of the left ventricle may lead to a fall in left ventricular output and systemic arterial pressure, thereby provoking myocardial ischemia due to compromised coronary artery perfusion. Eventually, circulatory collapse and death may ensue.

DIAGNOSIS

The clinical setting can be immensely helpful in suggesting the diagnosis of PTE (Table 261-1).

CLINICAL SYDNDROMES Patients with *massive PTE* present with systemic arterial hypotension and usually have anatomically widespread thromboembolism. Primary therapy with thrombolysis or embolectomy offers the greatest chance of survival. Those with *moderate to large PTE* have right ventricular hypokinesis on echocardiography but normal systemic arterial pressure. There is increasing evidence that such patients may benefit from primary therapy to prevent recurrent embolism. Patients with *small to moderate PTE* have both normal right heart function and normal systemic arterial pressure. They have a good prognosis with either adequate anticoagulation or an inferior vena caval filter. The presence of *pulmonary infarction* usually indicates a small PTE, but one that is exquisitely painful, because it lodges near the innervation of pleural nerves.

Nonthrombotic pulmonary embolism may be easily overlooked. Possible etiologies include fat embolism after blunt trauma and long bone fractures, tumor embolism, or air embolism. Intravenous drug users may inject themselves with a wide array of substances, such as hair, talc, or cotton. *Amniotic fluid embolism* occurs when fetal membranes leak or tear at the placental margin. The pulmonary edema seen in this syndrome is probably due primarily to alveolar capillary leakage.

PTE-DVT RELATIONSHIP When considering PTE, the interviewer should always ask about prior PTE or DVT and about a family history of venous thromboembolism. The presence of confirmed DVT is usually an adequate surrogate for PTE. Therefore, symptoms and signs of DVT (Chap. 248) should also be sought when investigating the possibility of PTE.

SYMPTOMS AND SIGNS Dyspnea is the most frequent symptom of PTE, and tachypnea is its most frequent sign. Whereas dyspnea, syncope, hypotension, or cyanosis indicate a massive PTE, pleuritic pain, cough, or hemoptysis often suggest a small embolism located distally near the pleura. On *physical examination*, young and previously healthy individuals may simply appear anxious but otherwise seem deceptively well, even with an anatomically large PTE. They need not have "classic" signs such as tachycardia, low-grade fever, neck vein distention, or an accentuated pulmonic component of the second heart sound. Sometimes, a paradoxical bradycardia occurs.

In older patients who complain of vague chest discomfort, the diagnosis of PTE may not be apparent unless signs of right heart failure are present. Unfortunately, because acute coronary ischemic syndromes are so common, one may overlook the possibility of life-threatening PTE and may inadvertently discharge these patients from the hospital after the exclusion of myocardial infarction with serial cardiac enzyme measurements and electrocardiograms.

DIFFERENTIAL DIAGNOSIS The differential diagnosis of PTE is broad (Table 261-2). Although PTE is known as "the great masquerader," quite often another illness simulates PTE. For example, when the proposed diagnosis of PTE is supposedly confirmed with a combination of dyspnea, chest pain, and an abnormal lung scan, the correct diagnosis of pneumonia might become apparent 12 h later when an infiltrate blossoms on chest x-ray, purulent sputum is first produced, and high fever and shaking chills develop.

Table 261-1

Stressors That May Precipitate Pulmonary Thromboembolism

Surgery, trauma
Obesity
Oral contraceptives, pregnancy, postpartum
Cancer (sometimes occult) or cancer chemotherapy
Immobilization (stroke or intensive care unit patients)
Indwelling central venous catheter

Some patients have PTE and a coexisting illness such as pneumonia or heart failure. In such circumstances, clinical improvement will often fail to occur despite standard medical treatment of the concomitant illness. This situation can serve as a clinical clue to the possible coexistence of PTE.

NONIMAGING DIAGNOSTIC MODALITIES These are generally safer, less expensive, but also less specific than diagnostic modalities that employ imaging.

Blood Tests The quantitative *plasma D-dimer enzyme-linked immunosorbent assay (ELISA)* level is elevated (>500 ng/mL) in more than 90 percent of patients with PTE, reflecting plasmin's breakdown of fibrin and indicating endogenous (though clinically ineffective) thrombolysis. A qualitative latex agglutination D-dimer assay, which is more readily available and less expensive than an ELISA, can be obtained initially; if elevated, the ELISA will also be elevated. However, if the latex agglutination is normal, a D-dimer ELISA should be obtained, because the ELISA is much more sensitive than the latex agglutination D-dimer assay, which cannot be used to exclude PTE. The plasma D-dimer ELISA has a high negative predictive value and can be used to help exclude PTE. However, neither D-dimer assay is specific. Levels increase in patients with myocardial infarction, sepsis, or almost any systemic illness.

Data from the Prospective Investigation of Pulmonary Embolism Diagnosis (PIOPED) indicate that, contrary to classic teaching, *arterial blood gases* lack diagnostic utility for PTE. Among patients suspected of PTE, neither the room air arterial P_{O_2} nor calculation of the alveolar-arterial oxygen gradient can reliably differentiate or triage patients who actually have PTE at angiography.

Electrocardiogram Classic abnormalities include sinus tachycardia; new-onset atrial fibrillation or flutter; and an S wave in lead I, a Q wave in lead V_3, and an inverted T wave in lead V_3 (Chap. 228). Often, the QRS axis is greater than 90°. T-wave inversion in leads V_6 to V_4 reflects right ventricular strain.

NONINVASIVE IMAGING MODALITIES **Chest Roentgenography** A normal or near-normal chest x-ray in a dyspneic patient suggests PTE. Well-established abnormalities include focal oligemia (Westermark's sign), a peripheral wedged-shaped density above the diaphragm (Hampton's hump), or an enlarged right descending pulmonary artery.

Venous Ultrasonography Ultrasonography of the deep venous system relies upon loss of vein compressibility as the primary criterion for DVT. About one-third of patients with PTE have no imaging evidence of DVT. In these situations, the clot may have already embolized to the lung or is in the pelvic veins, where ultrasonography is usually inadequate. Therefore, the workup for PTE should continue if there is high clinical suspicion, despite a normal ultrasound examination.

The reliability of venous ultrasonography is well established for proximal leg DVT among *symptomatic* outpatients. However, ultrasonography is notoriously insensitive for DVT screening among *asymptomatic* inpatients. Consequently, the use of ultrasonography to screen for DVT in postoperative orthopedic surgery or neurosurgery patients will underestimate the frequency of proximal leg vein thrombosis.

Table 261-2

Differential Diagnosis of Pulmonary Thromboembolism

Myocardial infarction, unstable angina
Pneumonia, bronchitis, COPD exacerbation
Congestive heart failure
Asthma
Pericarditis
Primary pulmonary hypertension
Rib fracture, pneumothorax
Costochondritis, "musculoskeletal pain," anxiety

NOTE: COPD, chronic obstructive pulmonary disease.

Lung Scanning (See also Chap. 251) Lung scanning is the principal imaging test for the diagnosis of PTE. Small particulate aggregates of albumin labeled with a gamma-emitting radionuclide are injected intravenously and are trapped in the pulmonary capillary bed. A perfusion scan defect indicates absent or decreased blood flow, possibly due to PTE. Ventilation scans, obtained with radiolabeled inhaled gases such as xenon or krypton, improve the specificity of the perfusion scan. Abnormal ventilation scans indicate abnormal nonventilated lung, thereby providing possible explanations for perfusion defects other than acute PTE. A high probability scan for PTE is defined as having two or more segmental perfusion defects in the presence of normal ventilation.

Lung scanning is particularly useful if the results are normal or near-normal, or if there is a high probability for PTE. The diagnosis of PTE is very unlikely in patients with normal and near-normal scans but, in contrast, is about 90 percent certain in patients with high-probability scans. Unfortunately, fewer than half of patients with angiographically confirmed PTE have a high-probability scan. Importantly, as many as 40 percent of patients with high clinical suspicion for PTE and "low-probability" scans do, in fact, have PTE at angiography.

Echocardiography This technique is useful for rapid triage of acutely ill patients who may have PTE. Bedside echocardiography can usually reliably differentiate among illnesses that have radically different treatment, including acute myocardial infarction, pericardial tamponade, dissection of the aorta, and PTE complicated by right heart failure. Detection of right ventricular dysfunction due to PTE helps to stratify the risk, delineate the prognosis, and plan optical management.

INVASIVE DIAGNOSTIC MODALITIES **Pulmonary Angiography** Selective pulmonary angiography is the most specific examination available for establishing the definitive diagnosis of PTE and can detect emboli as small as 1 to 2 mm. A definitive diagnosis of PTE depends upon visualization of an intraluminal filling defect in more than one projection. Secondary signs of PTE include abrupt occlusion ("cut-off") of vessels; segmental oligemia or avascularity; a prolonged arterial phase with slow filling; or tortuous, tapering peripheral vessels.

Pulmonary angiography can be carried out safely among properly selected patients at hospitals that perform at least several studies per month. In PIOPED, the procedure resulted in death in five patients (0.5 percent), two of whom had severe heart failure prior to the procedure. Angiography is most useful when the clinical likelihood of PTE differs substantially from the lung scan result or when the lung scan is of intermediate probability for PTE.

Contrast Phlebography This technique has been mostly replaced by ultrasonography. Venography is costly, uncomfortable, and occasionally results in contrast allergy or contrast-induced phlebitis. Contrast phlebography is worthwhile when there is a discrepancy between the clinical suspicion and the ultrasound result, or if it is clinically important to screen asymptomatic postoperative or trauma patients at high risk for DVT. Phlebography is also useful for diagnosing isolated calf vein thrombosis or recurrent DVT.

INTEGRATED DIAGNOSTIC APPROACH We advocate an integrated diagnostic approach to streamline the workup of PTE (Fig. 261-1). This strategy combines the clinical likelihood of PTE with the results of noninvasive testing to determine whether pulmonary angiography is warranted.

℞ TREATMENT

Risk Stratification Anticoagulation with heparin and warfarin constitutes secondary prevention of recurrent PTE rather than primary therapy. Primary therapy (Table 261-3) consists of clot dissolution with thrombolysis or removal of PTE by embolectomy and is reserved for patients at high risk of death from right heart failure and for those at risk of recurrent PTE despite adequate anticoagulation. The echocardiogram has a pivotal role in risk stratification. Patients with right ventricular dysfunction on echocardiography may be appropriate candidates for primary therapy of PTE, even if normal systemic arterial pressure is preserved (Fig. 261-2).

Figure 261-1

High clinical suspicion

Lung scan

Normal: Stop W/U ← → High prob: Treat

Intermediate or low prob

Normal D–dimer: Stop W/U ← → High D–dimer: Pursue W/U

Leg U/S — PAgram — Echo

FIGURE 261-1 PTE diagnosis strategy. An integrated diagnostic approach. W/U, work up; U/S, ultrasound; PAgram, pulmonary arteriogram; ECHO, echocardiogram.

FIGURE 261-2 Acute PTE management: Risk stratification. RV, right ventricular; IVC, inferior vena cava.

When less than 30 percent of the lung scan is affected by PTE, then right ventricular function almost always remains normal. Such patients typically have good clinical outcomes with anticoagulation alone.

Adjunctive Therapy Important adjunctive measures include pain relief (especially with nonsteroidal anti-inflammatory agents), supplemental oxygenation, and psychological support. Dobutamine—a beta-adrenergic agonist with positive inotropic and pulmonary vasodilating effects—should be utilized to treat right heart failure and cardiogenic shock. In general, volume loading is ill advised because increased right ventricular dilatation can lead to even further reductions in left ventricular forward output.

Heparin Heparin binds to and accelerates the activity of antithrombin III, an enzyme that inhibits the coagulation factors thrombin (factor IIa), Xa, IXa, XIa, and XIIa. Heparin thus prevents additional thrombus formation and permits endogenous fibrinolytic mechanisms to lyse clot that has already formed. After 5 to 7 days of heparin, residual thrombus begins to stabilize in the endothelium of the vein or pulmonary artery. However, heparin does *not* directly dissolve thrombus that already exists.

DOSING Heparin administration can be instituted after major active bleeding has been excluded and after a rectal examination has been performed with testing for occult blood. The presence of occult blood does not preclude the use of heparin but indicates that the dose should be reduced. A typical bolus is 5000 to 10,000 units of unfractionated heparin followed by a continuous infusion of 1000 to 1500 units/h. An activated partial thromboplastin time that is at least twice the control value should provide a therapeutic level of heparin. Multiple nomograms (e.g., Raschke's) are available to assist in adjusting the infusion rate of heparin.

COMPLICATIONS The most important adverse effect of heparin is hemorrhage. For life-threatening or intracranial hemorrhage, protamine sulfate can be administered at the time heparin is discontinued.

Heparin-associated thrombocytopenia is usually of no clinical consequence. However, if the platelet count declines more than 50 percent from baseline, heparin should be discontinued. An ominous, immunologically mediated thrombocytopenia can promote platelet aggregation and destruction and may be associated with either thrombocytopenic bleeding or with life-threatening arterial ("white clot syndrome") and venous thrombosis.

Patients receiving prolonged heparin therapy may also develop osteopenia, osteoporosis, or pathologic bone fractures. Heparin-associated elevations in transaminase levels occur commonly but are rarely associated with clinical toxicity.

LOW-MOLECULAR-WEIGHT HEPARINS These fragments of unfractionated heparin exhibit less binding to plasma proteins and endothelial cells than does unfractionated heparin. They have a greater bioavailability, more predictable dose response, and longer half-life than unfractionated heparin. *Enoxaparin,* which has received Food and Drug Administration (FDA) approval for prophylaxis after total hip or knee replacement, has a lower rate of heparin-associated thrombocytopenia than does unfractionated heparin. *Dalteparin* has recently received FDA approval for once daily subcutaneous administration to prevent venous thromboembolism in patients undergoing general and pelvic surgery. Low-molecular-weight heparins have *not* received FDA approval for *treatment* of PTE or DVT.

Warfarin This is a vitamin K antagonist that prevents γ carboxylation activation of coagulation factors II, VII, IX, and X. The full effect of warfarin often requires 5 days, even if the prothrombin time, used for monitoring, becomes elevated more rapidly. When warfarin is initiated during an active thrombotic state, the levels of protein C and S decline, thus creating a thrombogenic potential. By overlapping heparin and warfarin for 5 days, the procoagulant effect of unopposed warfarin can be counteracted.

DOSING Warfarin is usually initiated in a dose of 7.5 to 10 mg. However, after several days, the dose usually needs to be reduced. Patients who are malnourished or who have received prolonged courses of antibiotics are probably deficient in vitamin K and should receive much smaller initial doses of warfarin, such as 2.5 mg. The prothrombin time should be reported according to the International Normalized Ratio (INR), not the prothrombin time ratio of the prothrombin time expressed in seconds (Chap. 119). The target INR should be approximately 3.0.

COMPLICATIONS As with heparin, bleeding is the most important and common complication associated with warfarin administration. Life-threatening bleeding can be treated with cryoprecipitate or fresh frozen plasma (usually 2 units) to achieve immediate hemostasis. For less serious bleeding, vitamin K may be administered, usually in an initial dose of 2.5 to 5 mg subcutaneously. This latter approach requires about 6 h to take effect and will help lower the INR toward the upper portion of the therapeutic range.

Warfarin induced skin necrosis is a rare complication that may be related to warfarin induced reduction of protein C. It is usually

Table 261-3

Primary Therapy for Pulmonary Thromboembolism

Classification	Specific Therapy
1. Medical	Thrombolysis (peripheral vein)
	Inotropic agents (e.g., dobutamine)
2. Catheter-based	Suction embolectomy
	Fragmentation and distal dispersion
	Mechanical pulverization
	Local, catheter-directed thrombolysis
	Balloon angioplasty (chronic)
3. Surgical	Embolectomy (acute)
	Thromboendarterectomy (chronic)

Table 261-4

Prevention of Pulmonary Thromboembolism

Condition	Strategy
Total hip or knee replacement; hip or pelvis fracture	Warfarin (Coumadin) (target INR 2.0–2.5) × 4–6 weeks
	Low-molecular-weight heparin × 5–14 d [e.g., enoxaparin (Lovenox), 30 mg SC twice daily]
	IPC ± warfarin (Coumadin)
Gynecologic cancer surgery	Warfarin (Coumadin) (target INR 2.0–2.5) ± IPC
	Unfractionated heparin, 5000 U q 8 h ± IPC
	Dalteparin (Fragmin) 2500 U once daily ± IPC
Urologic surgery	Warfarin (Coumadin) (target INR 2.0–2.5) ± IPC
Thoracic surgery	IPC *plus* unfractionated heparin, 5000 U q 8 h
High-risk general surgery (e.g., prior VTE, current cancer, or obesity)	IPC *or* graded-compression stockings *plus* unfractionated heparin, 5000 U q 8 h
	Dalteparin (Fragmin) 5000 U SC once daily
General, gynecologic, or urologic surgery (without prior VTE) for noncancerous conditions	Graded-compression stockings *plus* unfractionated heparin 5000 U q 12 h
	Dalteparin 2500 U SC once daily
	IPC alone
Neurosurgery, eye surgery, or other surgery when prophylactic anticoagulation is contraindicated	Graded-compression stockings ± IPC
Medical conditions	Graded-compression stockings ± heparin, 5000 U q 8–12 h
	IPC alone

NOTE: IPC, intermittent pneumatic compression; VTE, venous thromboembolism.

associated with administration of a high initial dose of warfarin during an acute thrombotic state in which heparin is withheld. During pregnancy, warfarin should be avoided if possible because of warfarin embryopathy, which is most common with exposure during the sixth through twelfth weeks of gestation. However, women can take warfarin postpartum and breast feed safely.

Duration of Anticoagulation After discontinuation of anticoagulation, the risk of recurrent PTE is surprisingly high. Schulman and colleagues found that after a 6-month course of anticoagulation, 14 percent of PTE patients suffered a recurrent venous thromboembolism within the ensuing 2 years. The recurrence rate was twice as high among patients who received only 6 weeks of anticoagulation. Patients with underlying cancer that is not cured or with massive obesity should probably be anticoagulated indefinitely. For other patients, it is reasonable to anticoagulate the first episode of isolated calf vein thrombosis for 3 months, proximal DVT for 6 months, and PTE for 1 year.

Inferior Vena Caval Filters When anticoagulation cannot be undertaken because of active bleeding, insertion of an inferior vena caval filter is usually necessary. Other indications include recurrent venous thrombosis despite adequate anticoagulation, prevention of recurrent PTE in patients with right heart failure who are not candidates for thrombolysis, or prophylaxis of extremely high risk patients. The Bird's Nest filter infrarenally or, if necessary, a Greenfield filter suprarenally are recommended.

Thrombolysis Thrombolytic therapy may rapidly reverse right heart failure and thus lead to a lower rate of death and recurrent PTE. Thrombolysis usually achieves the following: (1) dissolves much of the anatomically obstructing pulmonary arterial thrombus, (2) prevents the continued release of serotonin and other neurohu-

moral factors that might otherwise exacerbate pulmonary hypertension, and (3) dissolves much of the source of the thrombus in the pelvic or deep leg veins, thereby decreasing the likelihood of recurrent PTE.

The preferred thrombolytic regimen is 100 mg of recombinant tissue plasminogen activator administered as a continuous peripheral intravenous infusion over 2 h. Patients appear to respond to thrombolysis for up to 14 days after the PTE occurred.

Contraindications to thrombolysis include intracranial disease, recent surgery, or trauma. There is about a 1 percent risk of intracranial hemorrhage. Careful screening of patients for contraindications to thrombolysis is the best way to minimize bleeding risk.

Pulmonary Thromboendarterectomy Patients who develop chronic pulmonary hypertension due to prior PTE may become severely dyspneic at rest or with minimal exertion. They should be considered for pulmonary thromboendarterectomy which, if successful, can markedly reduce and at times even cure pulmonary hypertension.

Prevention Prevention of PTE is of paramount importance because it is both difficult to recognize and expensive to treat. Fortunately, effective mechanical and pharmacologic prophylaxis modalities are widely available and usually effective (Table 261-4).

BIBLIOGRAPHY

BERTINA RM et al: Mutation in blood coagulation factor V associated with resistance to activated protein C. Nature 369:64, 1994

BOUNAMEAUX H et al: Plasma measurement of D-dimer as diagnostic aid in suspected venous thromboembolism: An overview. Thromb Haemost 71:1, 1994

GOLDHABER SZ (ed): *Prevention of Venous Thromboembolism.* New York, Marcel Dekker, 1993

—— et al: Alteplase versus heparin in acute pulmonary embolism: Randomised trial assessing right-ventricular function and pulmonary perfusion. Lancet 341:507, 1993

—— (ed): Cardiopulmonary diseases and cardiac tumors, vol 3, in *Atlas of Heart Diseases,* E Braunwald (Series ed). Philadelphia, Current Medicine, 1995

——: Contemporary pulmonary embolism thrombolysis. Chest 107:45S, 1995

HIRSCH DR et al: A prospective study of deep venous thrombosis in medical intensive care unit patient. JAMA 274:335, 1995

LUALDI JC, GOLDHABER SZ: Right ventricular dysfunction after acute pulmonary embolism: Pathophysiologic factors, detection, and therapeutic implications. Am Heart J 130:1276, 1995

RASCHKE RA et al: The weight-based heparin dosing nomogram compared with a "standard care" nomogram: A randomized controlled trial. Ann Intern Med 119:874, 1993

RIDKER PM et al: Mutation in the gene coding for coagulation factor V and risks of future myocardial infarction, stroke, and venous thrombosis in apparently healthy men. N Engl J Med 332:912, 1995

SCHULMAN S et al: A comparison of six weeks with six months of oral anticoagulant therapy after a first episode of venous thromboembolism. N Engl J Med 332:1661, 1995

STEIN PD et al: Complications and validity of pulmonary angiography in acute pulmonary embolism. Circulation 85:462, 1992

—— et al: Arterial blood gas analysis in the assessment of suspected acute pulmonary embolism. Chest 109:78, 1996

262   *Richard W. Light*

DISORDERS OF THE PLEURA, MEDIASTINUM, AND DIAPHRAGM

DISORDERS OF THE PLEURA

PLEURAL EFFUSION The pleural space lies between the lung and chest wall and normally contains a very thin layer of fluid. This thin layer of liquid serves as a coupling system between the lung and chest wall. A pleural effusion is present when there is an excess quantity of fluid in the pleural space.

Etiology Pleural fluid accumulates when pleural fluid formation exceeds pleural fluid absorption. Normally, fluid enters the pleural space from the capillaries in the parietal pleura and is removed via the lymphatics situated in the parietal pleura. Fluid also can enter the pleural space from the interstitial spaces of the lung via the visceral pleura or from the peritoneal cavity via small holes in the diaphragm. The lymphatics have the capacity to absorb 20 times more fluid than is normally formed. Accordingly, a pleural effusion may develop when there is excess pleural fluid formation (from the parietal pleura, the interstitial spaces of the lung, or the peritoneal cavity) or when there is decreased fluid removal by the lymphatics.

Diagnostic Approach When a patient is found to have a pleural effusion, an effort should be made to determine the cause (Fig. 262-1). The first step is to determine whether the effusion is a transudate or an exudate. A *transudative* pleural effusion occurs when *systemic factors* that influence the formation and absorption of pleural fluid are

altered. The leading causes of transudative pleural effusions in the United States are left ventricular failure, pulmonary embolism, and cirrhosis. An *exudative* pleural effusion occurs when *local factors* that influence the formation and absorption of pleural fluid are altered. The leading causes of exudative pleural effusions are bacterial pneumonia, malignancy, viral infection, and pulmonary embolism. The primary reason to make this differentiation is that additional diagnostic procedures are indicated with exudative effusions to define the cause of the local disease.

Transudative and exudative pleural effusions are distinguished by measuring the lactate dehydrogenase (LDH) and protein levels in the pleural fluid. Exudative pleural effusions meet at least one of the following criteria, whereas transudative pleural effusions meet none.

1. Pleural fluid protein/serum protein >0.5
2. Pleural fluid LDH/serum LDH >0.6
3. Pleural fluid LDH more than two-thirds normal upper limit for serum

If a patient has an exudative pleural effusion, the following tests on the pleural fluid should be obtained: description of the fluid, glucose level, amylase level, differential cell count, microbiologic studies, and cytology.

Effusion due to Heart Failure The most common cause of pleural effusion is left ventricular failure. The effusion occurs because the increased amounts of fluid in the lung interstitial spaces exit in part across the visceral pleura. This overwhelms the capacity of the lymphatics in the parietal pleura to remove fluid. A diagnostic thoracentesis should be performed if the effusions are not bilateral and comparable in size, if the patient is febrile, or if the patient has pleuritic chest pain to verify that the patient has a transudative effusion. Otherwise the patient is best treated with diuretics. If the effusion persists despite diuretic therapy, a diagnostic thoracentesis should be performed. Diuretic therapy for a few days does not significantly change the biochemical characteristics of the pleural fluid.

Hepatic Hydrothorax Pleural effusions occur in approximately 5 percent of patients with cirrhosis and ascites. The predominant mechanism is the direct movement of peritoneal fluid through small holes in the diaphragm into the pleural space. The effusion is usually right-sided and frequently is large enough to produce severe dyspnea. If medical management does not control the ascites and the effusion, there are no good alternatives. Consideration can be given to inserting a peritoneal-venous shunt, thoracotomy with surgical repair of the leak, or tube thoracostomy with the injection of a sclerosing agent.

Parapneumonic Effusion Parapneumonic effusions are associated with bacterial pneumonia, lung abscess, or bronchiectasis and are probably the most common exudative pleural effusion in the United States. A *complicated parapneumonic effusion* requires tube thoracostomy for its resolution. *Empyema* refers to a grossly purulent effusion.

Patients with aerobic bacterial pneumonia and pleural effusion present with an acute febrile illness consisting of chest pain, sputum production, and leukocytosis. Patients with anaerobic infections present with a subacute illness with weight loss, a brisk leukocytosis, mild anemia, and a history of some factor that predisposes them to aspiration.

The possibility of a parapneumonic effusion should be considered whenever a patient with a bacterial pneumonia is initially evaluated. The presence of free pleural fluid can be demonstrated with a lateral decubitus radiograph. If the free fluid separates the lung from the chest wall by more than 10 mm on the decubitus radiograph, a diagnostic thoracentesis should be performed in order to determine whether or not a chest tube should be inserted. Any of the following is an indication for tube thoracostomy:

1. The presence of gross pus in the pleural space
2. Organisms visible on Gram stain of the pleural fluid
3. Pleural fluid glucose level of less than 50 mg/dL
4. Pleural fluid pH below 7.00 and 0.15 units lower than arterial pH

FIGURE 262-1 Approach to the diagnosis of pleural effusions; PF, pleural fluid.

There should be no delay in its performance because a free-flowing parapneumonic effusion can become loculated within a matter of hours.

If the pleural fluid is loculated and is not adequately drained with one chest tube, either streptokinase, 250,000 units, or urokinase, 100,000 units, should be injected intrapleurally to dissolve the fibrin membranes that create the loculations. If the pleural drainage is inadequate after the intrapleural thrombolytic therapy, either thoracoscopy with breakdown of adhesions or thoracotomy with decortication should be performed.

Effusion Secondary to Malignancy Malignant pleural effusions secondary to metastatic disease are the second most common type of exudative pleural effusion. The three tumors that cause approximately 75 percent of all malignant pleural effusions are lung carcinoma, breast carcinoma, and lymphoma. Most patients complain of dyspnea, which is frequently out of proportion to the size of the effusion. The pleural fluid is an exudate, and its glucose level may be reduced if the tumor burden in the pleural space is high.

The diagnosis is usually made via cytology of the pleural fluid. If the initial cytologic examination is negative, then a needle biopsy of the pleura with repeat cytology is indicated. If there is still no diagnosis, thoracoscopy is likely to provide the diagnosis if the patient has malignancy. At the time of thoracoscopy, talc or some similar agent should be instilled into the pleural space to effect a pleurodesis.

Patients with a malignant pleural effusion are treated symptomatically for the most part, since the presence of the effusion indicates disseminated disease and most malignancies associated with pleural effusion are not curable with chemotherapy. The only symptom that can be attributed to the effusion itself is dyspnea. If the patient's lifestyle is compromised by dyspnea, and if the dyspnea is relieved with a therapeutic thoracentesis, then one of the following procedures should be performed: (1) tube thoracostomy with the instillation of a sclerosing agent such as talc, 5 g in a slurry, or doxycycline, 500 mg, (2) thoracoscopy with pleural abrasion or the insufflation of talc, or (3) insertion of a pleuroperitoneal shunt.

Mesothelioma Malignant mesotheliomas are primary tumors that arise from the mesothelial cells that line the pleural cavities. Most are related to asbestos exposure. Patients with mesothelioma present with chest pain and shortness of breath. The chest radiograph reveals a pleural effusion, generalized pleural thickening, and a shrunken hemithorax. Thoracoscopy or open pleural biopsy is usually necessary to establish the diagnosis. Various treatment modalities, including radical surgery, chemotherapy, and radiation therapy, have been tried, but none has been proven to be more effective than symptomatic therapy. It is recommended that chest pain be treated with opiates and that shortness of breath be treated with oxygen and/or opiates.

Effusion Secondary to Pulmonary Embolization The diagnosis most commonly overlooked in the differential diagnosis of a patient with an undiagnosed pleural effusion is pulmonary embolism. Dyspnea is the most common symptom. The pleural fluid can be either transudative or exudative. The diagnosis is suggested by lung scanning and/or pulmonary arteriography (see Chap. 261). Treatment of the patient with a pleural effusion secondary to pulmonary embolism is the same as for any patient with pulmonary emboli. If the pleural effusion increases in size after anticoagulation, the patient probably has recurrent emboli or another complication such as a hemothorax or a pleural infection.

Tuberculous Pleuritis (See Chap. 171) In many parts of the world, the most common cause of an exudative pleural effusion is tuberculosis, but this is relatively uncommon in the United States. Tuberculous pleural effusions are thought to be due primarily to a hypersensitivity reaction to tuberculous protein in the pleural space. Patients with tuberculous pleuritis present with fever, weight loss, dyspnea, and/or pleuritic chest pain. The pleural fluid is an exudate with predominantly small lymphocytes. The diagnosis is usually established by the demonstration of granulomas on needle biopsy of the pleura. Adequate treatment consists of isoniazid, 300 mg/d, plus

rifampin, 600 mg/d, for 6 months. If the patient is suspected of having resistant organisms, ethambutol and pyrazinamide should also be included until the results of drug sensitivity tests are available.

Effusion Secondary to Viral Infection Viral infections are probably responsible for a sizable percentage of undiagnosed exudative pleural effusions. In many series, no diagnosis is established for approximately 20 percent of exudative effusions, and these effusions resolve spontaneously with no long-term residua. The importance of these effusions is that one should not be too aggressive in trying to establish a diagnosis for the undiagnosed effusion, particularly if the patient is improving clinically.

AIDS Pleural effusions are uncommon in such patients. The most common cause is Kaposi's sarcoma, followed by parapneumonic effusion. Other common causes are tuberculosis, cryptococcosis, and lymphoma. Pleural effusions are very uncommon with *Pneumocystis carinii* infection.

Chylothorax A chylothorax occurs when the thoracic duct is disrupted and chyle accumulates in the pleural space. The most common cause of chylothorax is trauma, but it also may result from tumors in the mediastinum. Patients with chylothorax present with dyspnea, and a large pleural effusion is present on the chest radiograph. Thoracentesis reveals milky fluid, and biochemical analysis reveals a triglyceride level that exceeds 110 mg/dL. Patients with chylothorax and no obvious trauma should have a lymphangiogram and a mediastinal computed tomographic (CT) scan to assess the mediastinum for lymph nodes. The treatment of choice for most chylothoraces is implantation of a pleuroperitoneal shunt. Patients with chylothoraces should not undergo prolonged tube thoracostomy with chest tube drainage because this will lead to malnutrition and immunologic incompetence.

Hemothorax When a diagnostic thoracentesis reveals bloody pleural fluid, a hematocrit should be obtained on the pleural fluid. If the hematocrit is greater than 50 percent that of the peripheral blood, the patient has a hemothorax. Most hemothoraces are the result of trauma; other causes include rupture of a blood vessel or tumor. Most patients with hemothorax should be treated with tube thoracostomy, which allows continuous quantification of bleeding. If the bleeding emanates from a laceration of the pleura, apposition of the two pleural surfaces is likely to stop the bleeding. If the pleural hemorrhage exceeds 200 mL/h, consideration should be given to thoracotomy.

Miscellaneous Causes of Pleural Effusion There are many other causes of pleural effusion (see Table 262-1). Key features of some of these conditions are as follows: If the pleural fluid amylase level is elevated, the diagnosis of esophageal rupture or pancreatic disease is likely. If the patient is febrile, has predominantly polymorphonuclear cells in the pleural fluid, and has no pulmonary parenchymal abnormalities, an intraabdominal abscess should be considered. The diagnosis of lupus pleuritis is best made by demonstrating an elevated antinuclear antibody (ANA) level in the pleural fluid. The diagnosis of an asbestos pleural effusion is one of exclusion. Benign ovarian tumors can produce ascites and a pleural effusion (Meigs' syndrome). Several drugs can cause pleural effusion, and the associated fluid is usually eosinophilic. Many pleural effusions follow from medical manipulations such as abdominal surgery, coronary artery bypass surgery, endoscopic variceal sclerotherapy, radiation therapy, liver or lung transplantation, or the intravascular insertion of central lines.

PNEUMOTHORAX Pneumothorax is the presence of gas in the pleural space. A *spontaneous pneumothorax* is one that occurs without antecedent trauma to the thorax. A *primary spontaneous pneumothorax* occurs in the absence of underlying lung disease, while a *secondary spontaneous pneumothorax* occurs in its presence. A *traumatic pneumothorax* results from penetrating or nonpenetrating chest injuries. A *tension pneumothorax* is a pneumothorax in which the pressure in the pleural space is positive throughout the respiratory cycle.

Primary Spontaneous Pneumothorax Primary spontaneous pneumothoraces are usually due to rupture of apical pleural blebs, small cystic spaces that lie within or immediately under the visceral pleura. Primary spontaneous pneumothoraces occur almost exclusively in smokers, which suggests that the patients indeed do have subclinical

Differential Diagnoses of Pleural Effusions

TRANSUDATIVE PLEURAL EFFUSIONS

1. Congestive heart failure
2. Cirrhosis
3. Nephrotic syndrome
4. Peritoneal dialysis
5. Superior vena cava obstruction
6. Myxedema
7. Pulmonary emboli
8. Urinothorax

EXUDATIVE PLEURAL EFFUSIONS

1. Neoplastic diseases
   a. Metastatic disease
   b. Mesothelioma
2. Infectious diseases
   a. Bacterial infections
   b. Tuberculosis
   c. Fungal infections
   d. Viral infections
   e. Parasitic infections
3. Pulmonary embolization
4. Gastrointestinal disease
   a. Esophageal perforation
   b. Pancreatic disease
   c. Intraabdominal abscesses
   d. Diaphragmatic hernia
   e. After abdominal surgery
   f. Endoscopic variceal sclerotherapy
   g. After liver transplant
5. Collagen-vascular diseases
   a. Rheumatoid pleuritis
   b. Systemic lupus erythematosus
   c. Drug-induced lupus
   d. Immunoblastic lymphadenopathy
   e. Sjögren's syndrome
   f. Wegener's granulomatosis
   g. Churg-Strauss syndrome
6. Post-cardiac injury syndrome
7. Asbestos exposure
8. Sarcoidosis
9. Uremia
10. Meigs' syndrome
11. Yellow nail syndrome
12. Drug-induced pleural disease
    a. Nitrofurantoin
    b. Dantrolene
    c. Methysergide
    d. Bromocriptine
    e. Procarbazine
    f. Amiodarone
13. Trapped lung
14. Radiation therapy
15. Electrical burns
16. Hemothorax
17. Iatrogenic injury
18. Ovarian hyperstimulation syndrome
19. Pericardial disease
20. Chylothorax

lung disease. Approximately one-half of patients with an initial primary spontaneous pneumothorax will have a recurrence. The initial recommended treatment for primary spontaneous pneumothorax is simple aspiration. If the lung does not expand with aspiration, or if the patient has a recurrent pneumothorax, tube thoracostomy with instillation of a sclerosing agent such as doxycycline is indicated. Thoracoscopy or thoracotomy with pleural abrasion is almost 100 percent successful in preventing recurrences.

Secondary Spontaneous Pneumothorax   Most secondary spontaneous pneumothoraces are due to chronic obstructive pulmonary disease, but pneumothoraces have been reported with virtually every lung disease. Pneumothorax in patients with lung disease is more life-threatening than it is in normal individuals because of the lack of pulmonary reserve in these patients. Nearly all patients with secondary spontaneous pneumothorax should be treated with tube thoracostomy and the instillation of a sclerosing agent such as doxycycline or talc. Patients with either primary or secondary spontaneous pneumothoraces who have a persistent air leak or an unexpanded lung after 5 days of tube thoracostomy should be subjected to thoracoscopy with bleb resection and pleural abrasion.

Traumatic Pneumothorax   Traumatic pneumothoraces can result from both penetrating and nonpenetrating chest trauma. Traumatic pneumothoraces should be treated with tube thoracostomy. If a hemo-pneumothorax is present, one chest tube should be placed in the superior part of the hemithorax to evacuate the air, and another should be placed in the inferior part of the hemithorax to remove the blood. Iatrogenic pneumothorax is a type of traumatic pneumothorax which is becoming more common. The leading causes are transthoracic needle aspiration, thoracentesis, and the insertion of central intravenous catheters. The treatment differs according to the degree of distress and can be observation, supplemental oxygen, aspiration, or tube thoracostomy.

Tension Pneumothorax   This condition usually occurs during mechanical ventilation or resuscitative efforts. The positive pleural pressure is life-threatening both because ventilation is severely compromised and because the positive pressure is transmitted to the medi-

astinum, which results in decreased venous return to the heart and reduced cardiac output.

Difficulty in ventilation during resuscitation or high peak inspiratory pressures during mechanical ventilation strongly suggest the diagnosis. The diagnosis is made by the finding of an enlarged hemithorax with no breath sounds and shift of the mediastinum to the contralateral side. Tension pneumothorax must be treated as a medical emergency. If the tension in the pleural space is not relieved, the patient is likely to die from inadequate cardiac output or marked hypoxemia. A large-bore needle should be inserted into the pleural space through the second anterior intercostal space. If large amounts of gas escape from the needle after insertion, the diagnosis is confirmed. The needle should be left in place until a thoracostomy tube can be inserted.

DISORDERS OF THE MEDIASTINUM

The mediastinum is the region between the pleural sacs. It is separated into three compartments. The *anterior mediastinum* extends from the sternum anteriorly to the pericardium and brachiocephalic vessels posteriorly. It contains the thymus gland, the anterior mediastinal lymph nodes, and the internal mammary arteries and veins. The *middle mediastinum* lies between the anterior and posterior mediastina and contains the heart; the ascending and transverse arches of the aorta; the venae cavae; the brachiocephalic arteries and veins; the phrenic nerves; the trachea, main bronchi, and their contiguous lymph nodes; and the pulmonary arteries and veins. The *posterior mediastinum* is bounded by the pericardium and trachea anteriorly and the vertebral column posteriorly. It contains the descending thoracic aorta, esophagus, thoracic duct, azygos and hemiazygos veins, and the posterior group of mediastinal lymph nodes.

MEDIASTINAL MASSES   The first step in evaluating a mediastinal mass lesion is to place it in one of the three mediastinal compartments, since each has different characteristic lesions. The most common lesions in the anterior mediastinum are thymomas, lymphomas, teratomatous neoplasms, and thyroid masses. The most common masses in the middle mediastinum are vascular masses, lymph node enlargement from metastases or granulomatous disease, and pleuro-pericardial and bronchogenic cysts. In the posterior mediastinum, neurogenic tumors, meningoceles, meningomyeloceles, gastroenteric cysts, and esophageal diverticula are commonly found.

CT scanning is the most valuable imaging technique for evaluating mediastinal masses and is the only imaging technique that should be done. Barium studies of the gastrointestinal tract are indicated in many patients with posterior mediastinal lesions, since hernias, diverticula, and achalasia are readily diagnosed in this manner. An iodine 131 nuclear medicine scan can efficiently establish the diagnosis of intrathoracic goiter.

A definite diagnosis can be obtained with mediastinoscopy or anterior mediastinotomy in many patients with masses in the anterior or middle mediastinal compartments. A diagnosis can be established without thoracotomy via percutaneous fine-needle aspiration biopsy of mediastinal masses in any of the mediastinal compartments. In many cases the diagnosis can be established and the mediastinal mass removed with video-assisted thoracoscopy.

ACUTE MEDIASTINITIS   Most cases of acute mediastinitis are either due to esophageal perforation or occur after median sternotomy for cardiac surgery. Patients with esophageal rupture are acutely ill with chest pain and dyspnea due to the mediastinal infection. The esophageal rupture can occur spontaneously or as a complication of esophagoscopy or the insertion of a Blakemore tube. Appropriate treatment is exploration of the mediastinum with primary repair of the esophageal tear and drainage of the pleural space and the mediastinum.

The incidence of mediastinitis following median sternotomy is 0.4 to 5.0 percent. Patients most commonly present with wound drainage. Other presentations include sepsis or a widened mediastinum. The diagnosis is usually established with mediastinal needle aspiration.

Treatment includes immediate drainage, debridement, and parenteral antibiotic therapy, but the mortality still exceeds 20 percent.

CHRONIC MEDIASTINITIS The spectrum of chronic mediastinitis ranges from granulomatous inflammation of the lymph nodes in the mediastinum to fibrosing mediastinitis. Most cases are due to tuberculosis or histoplasmosis, but sarcoidosis, silicosis, and other fungal diseases are at times causative. Patients with granulomatous mediastinitis are usually asymptomatic. Those with fibrosing mediastinitis usually have signs of compression of some mediastinal structure such as the superior vena cava or large airways, phrenic or recurrent laryngeal nerve paralysis, or obstruction of the pulmonary artery or proximal pulmonary veins. In most cases, mediastinal exploration is necessary to distinguish benign mediastinitis from malignant processes. Other than antituberculous therapy for tuberculous mediastinitis, no medical or surgical therapy has been demonstrated to be effective for mediastinal fibrosis.

PNEUMOMEDIASTINUM In this condition there is gas in the interstices of the mediastinum. The three main causes are (1) alveolar rupture with dissection of air into the mediastinum; (2) perforation or rupture of the esophagus, trachea, or main bronchi; and (3) dissection of air from the neck or the abdomen into the mediastinum. Typically, there is severe substernal chest pain with or without radiation into the neck and arms. The physical examination usually reveals subcutaneous emphysema in the suprasternal notch and *Hamman's sign*, which is a crunching or clicking noise synchronous with the heartbeat and best heard in the left lateral decubitus position. The diagnosis is confirmed with the chest radiograph. Usually no treatment is required, but the mediastinal air will be absorbed faster if the patient inspires high concentrations of oxygen. If mediastinal structures are compressed, the compression can be relieved with needle aspiration.

DISORDERS OF THE DIAPHRAGM

DIAPHRAGMATIC PARALYSIS The presence of bilateral diaphragmatic paralysis almost always causes severe morbidity in adults. The most common causes include high spinal cord injury, thoracic trauma (including cardiac surgery), multiple sclerosis, anterior horn disease, and muscular dystrophy. Most patients with severe diaphragmatic weakness present with hypercapnic respiratory failure, frequently complicated by cor pulmonale and right ventricular failure, atelectasis, and pneumonia.

The degree of diaphragmatic weakness is best quantitated by measuring transdiaphragmatic pressures. The treatment of choice is assisted ventilation for all or part of each day. This is best accomplished without tracheostomy using nasal intermittent positive airway pressure. If the nerve to the diaphragm is intact, diaphragmatic pacing may be a viable alternative. If the paralysis occurs during open heart surgery, recovery frequently occurs, but it may take 6 months or more.

Unilateral paralysis of the diaphragm is much more common than is bilateral paralysis. The most common cause is nerve invasion from malignancy, usually a bronchogenic carcinoma. If the patient does not have malignancy, then usually no cause for the paralysis is found. The diagnosis is suggested by finding an elevated hemidiaphragm on the chest roentgenogram. Confirmation is best established with the "sniff test." When a patient is observed with fluoroscopy while sniffing, the paralyzed diaphragm will move paradoxically upward due to the negative intrathoracic pressure. Patients with a unilateral paralyzed diaphragm are usually asymptomatic. Their vital capacity and total lung capacity are each reduced about 20 percent. If a patient has a mediastinal mass in conjunction with the diaphragmatic paralysis, further workup should be done. However, if the patient is asymptomatic with a normal chest radiograph, no invasive procedures are warranted.

BIBLIOGRAPHY

LIGHT RW: *Pleural Diseases.* Baltimore, Williams & Wilkins, 1995
———: Pleural diseases. Dis Mon 28:266, 1992
MULLER NL: Imaging of the pleura. Radiology 186:29, 1993
NAUNHEIM KS et al: Safety and efficacy of video-assisted thoracic surgical techniques for the treatment of spontaneous pneumothorax. J Thorac Cardiovasc Surg 109:1198, 1995
ROVIARO G et al: Videothoracoscopic excision of mediastinal masses: Indications and technique. Ann Thorac Surg 58:1679, 1994
WALKER-RENARD PB et al: Chemical pleurodesis for malignant pleural effusions. Ann Intern Med 120:56, 1994
WIENER-KRONISH JP, BROADDUS VC: Interrelationship of pleural and pulmonary interstitial liquid. Ann Rev Physiol 55:209, 1993

263 Eliot A. Phillipson

DISORDERS OF VENTILATION

HYPOVENTILATION

DEFINITION AND ETIOLOGY Alveolar hypoventilation exists by definition when arterial P_{CO_2} (Pa_{CO_2}) increases above the normal range of 37 to 43 mmHg, but in clinically important hypoventilation syndromes Pa_{CO_2} is generally in the range of 50 to 80 mmHg. Hypoventilation disorders can be acute or chronic. The acute disorders, which represent life-threatening emergencies, are discussed in Chap. 265; this chapter deals with chronic hypoventilation syndromes.

Chronic hypoventilation can result from numerous disease entities (Table 263-1), but in all cases the underlying mechanism involves a defect in either the metabolic respiratory control system, the respiratory neuromuscular system, or the ventilatory apparatus. Disorders associated with impaired respiratory drive, defects in the respiratory neuromuscular system, some chest wall disorders such as obesity, and upper airway obstruction produce an increase in Pa_{CO_2}, despite normal lungs,

Table 263-1

Chronic Hypoventilation Syndromes

Mechanism	Site of Defect	Disorder
Impaired respiratory drive	Peripheral and central chemoreceptors	Carotid body dysfunction, trauma Prolonged hypoxia Metabolic alkalosis
	Brainstem respiratory neurons	Bulbar poliomyelitis, encephalitis Brainstem infarction, hemorrhage, trauma Brainstem demyelination, degeneration Chronic drug administration Primary alveolar hypoventilation syndrome
Defective respiratory neuromuscular system	Spinal cord and peripheral nerves	High cervical trauma Poliomyelitis Motor neuron disease Peripheral neuropathy
	Respiratory muscles	Myasthenia gravis Muscular dystrophy Chronic myopathy
Impaired ventilatory apparatus	Chest wall	Kyphoscoliosis Fibrothorax Thoracoplasty Ankylosing spondylitis Obesity-hypoventilation
	Airways and lungs	Laryngeal and tracheal stenosis Obstructive sleep apnea Cystic fibrosis Chronic obstructive pulmonary disease

SOURCE: From Phillipson, with permission.

FIGURE 263-1 Physiologic and clinical features of alveolar hypoventilation. *(After Phillipson.)* Hb, hemoglobin; PA_{CO_2}, alveolar P_{CO_2}; PA_{O_2}, alveolar P_{O_2}.

PHYSIOLOGIC AND CLINICAL FEATURES Regardless of cause, the hallmark of all alveolar hypoventilation syndromes is an increase in alveolar P_{CO_2} (PA_{CO_2}) and therefore in Pa_{CO_2} (Fig. 263-1). The resulting respiratory acidosis eventually leads to a compensatory increase in plasma HCO_3^- concentration and a decrease in Cl^- concentration. The increase in PA_{CO_2} produces an obligatory decrease in PA_{O_2}, resulting in hypoxemia. If severe, the hypoxemia manifests clinically as cyanosis and can stimulate erythropoiesis and induce secondary polycythemia. The combination of chronic hypoxemia and hypercapnia also may induce pulmonary vasoconstriction, leading eventually to pulmonary hypertension, right ventricular hypertrophy, and congestive heart failure. The disturbances in arterial blood gases are typically magnified during sleep because of a further reduction in central respiratory drive. The resulting increased nocturnal hypercapnia may cause cerebral vasodilation leading to morning headache; sleep quality also may be severely impaired, resulting in morning fatigue, daytime somnolence, mental confusion, and intellectual impairment. Other clinical features associated with hypoventilation syndromes are related to the specific underlying disease (see Table 263-1).

DIAGNOSIS Investigation of the patient with chronic hypoventilation involves several laboratory tests that will usually localize the disorder to either the metabolic respiratory control system, the neuromuscular system, or the ventilatory apparatus (Fig. 263-2). Defects in the control system impair responses to chemical stimuli, including ventilatory, occlusion pressure, and diaphragmatic electromyographic (EMG) responses. During sleep, hypoventilation is usually more marked, and central apneas and hypopneas are common. However, because the behavioral respiratory control system (which is anatomically distinct from the metabolic control system), the neuromuscular system, and the ventilatory apparatus are intact, such patients can usually hyperventilate voluntarily, generate normal inspiratory and expiratory muscle pressures (PI_{max}, PE_{max}, respectively) against an occluded airway, generate normal lung volumes and flow rates on routine spirometry, and have normal respiratory system resistance and compli-

because of a reduction in overall minute volume of ventilation and hence in alveolar ventilation. In contrast, most disorders of the chest wall and disorders of the lower airways and lungs may produce an increase in Pa_{CO_2}, despite a normal or even increased minute volume of ventilation, because of severe ventilation-perfusion mismatching that results in net alveolar hypoventilation.

Several hypoventilation syndromes involve combined disturbances in two elements of the respiratory system. For example, patients with chronic obstructive pulmonary disease may hypoventilate not simply because of impaired ventilatory mechanics but also because of a reduced central respiratory drive, which can be inherent or secondary to a coexisting metabolic alkalosis (related to diuretic and steroid therapy).

Site of defect	Responses to CO₂, hypoxia Ventil. P.1 EMGdi			Sleep studies	Voluntary hyperventil.	PI_{max} PE_{max}	Volume flow rates	Resistance, compliance	(A-a) Po₂
Metabolic control system (chemoreceptors, brainstem integrating neurons)	↓	↓	↓	↑Hypoventil, central apneas	N	N	N	N	N
Respiratory neuromuscular system (brainstem motoneurons, spinal cord, respiratory nerves and muscles)	↓	↓	↓	↑Hypoventil, central apneas	↓	↓	↓	N	N
Ventilatory apparatus (chest wall, lungs, airways)	↓	N	N	Variable	↓	N	Abnormal	Abnormal	↑

FIGURE 263-2 Pattern of laboratory test results in alveolar hypoventilation syndromes, based on the site of defect. Ventil, ventilation; P.1, mouth pressure generated after 0.1 s of inspiration against an occluded airway; EMGdi, diaphragmatic EMG; PI_{max}, PE_{max}, maximum inspiratory or expiratory pressure that can be generated against an occluded airway; (A−a) P_{O_2}, alveolar-arterial P_{O_2} difference; N, normal. Defects in the metabolic control system impair central respiratory drive in response to chemical stimuli (CO_2 or hypoxia); therefore responses of EMGdi, P.1, and minute volume of ventilation are reduced and hypoventilation during sleep is aggravated. In contrast, tests of voluntary respiratory control, muscle strength, lung mechanics, and gas ex-

change [(A−a)P_{O_2}] are normal. Defects in the respiratory neuromuscular system impair muscle strength; therefore all tests dependent on muscular activity (voluntary or in response to metabolic stimuli) are abnormal, but lung resistance, lung compliance, and gas exchange are normal. Defects in the ventilatory apparatus usually impair gas exchange. Because resistance and compliance are also impaired, all tests dependent on ventilation (whether voluntary or in response to chemical stimuli) are abnormal; in contrast, tests of muscle activity or strength that do not involve airflow (that is, P.1, EMGdi, PI_{max}, PE_{max}) are normal. *(After Phillipson.)*

ance and a normal alveolar-arterial P_{O_2} [$(A - a)P_{O_2}$] difference. Patients with defects in the respiratory neuromuscular system also have impaired responses to chemical stimuli but in addition are unable to hyperventilate voluntarily or to generate normal static respiratory muscle pressures, lung volumes, and flow rates. However, at least in the early stages of the disease, the resistance and compliance of the respiratory system and the alveolar-arterial oxygen difference are normal.

In contrast to patients with disorders of the respiratory control or neuromuscular systems, patients with disorders of the chest wall, lungs, and airways typically demonstrate abnormalities of respiratory system resistance and compliance and have a widened $(A - a)P_{O_2}$. Because of the impaired mechanics of breathing, routine spirometric tests are abnormal, as is the ventilatory response to chemical stimuli. However, because the neuromuscular system is intact, tests that are independent of resistance and compliance are usually normal, including tests of respiratory muscle strength and of respiratory control that do not involve airflow.

℞ TREATMENT

The management of chronic hypoventilation must be individualized to the patient's particular disorder, circumstances, and needs and should include measures directed toward the underlying disease. Coexistent metabolic alkalosis should be corrected, including elevations of HCO_3^- that are inappropriately high for the degree of chronic hypercapnia. Administration of supplemental oxygen is effective in attenuating hypoxemia, polycythemia, and pulmonary hypertension, but can aggravate CO_2 retention and the associated neurologic symptoms. For this reason, supplemental oxygen must be prescribed judiciously and the results monitored carefully. Pharmacologic agents that stimulate respiration (particularly progesterone) are of benefit in some patients, but generally, results are disappointing.

Most patients with chronic hypoventilation related to impairment of respiratory drive or neuromuscular disease eventually require mechanical ventilatory assistance for effective management. When hypoventilation is severe, treatment may be required on a 24-h basis, but in most patients ventilatory assistance only during sleep produces dramatic clinical improvement and lowering of daytime Pa_{CO_2}. In patients with reduced respiratory drive but intact respiratory lower motor neurons, phrenic nerves, and respiratory muscles, diaphragmatic pacing through an implanted phrenic electrode can be very effective. However, for patients with defects in the respiratory nerves and muscles, electrophrenic pacing is contraindicated. Such patients can usually be managed effectively with either intermittent negative-pressure ventilation in a cuirass or intermittent positive-pressure ventilation delivered through a tracheostomy or nose mask. For patients who require ventilatory assistance only during sleep, positive-pressure ventilation through a nose mask is the preferred method because it obviates a tracheostomy and avoids the problem of upper airway occlusion that can arise in a negative-pressure ventilator.

Hypoventilation related to restrictive disorders of the chest wall (see Table 263-1) also can be managed effectively with nocturnal intermittent positive-pressure ventilation through a nose mask or tracheostomy. Nocturnal ventilatory assistance also has been advocated for patients with hypercapnic chronic obstructive lung disease as a means of alleviating possible chronic respiratory muscle fatigue, but the efficacy of such an approach is variable and often disappointing.

HYPOVENTILATION SYNDROMES

PRIMARY ALVEOLAR HYPOVENTILATION Primary alveolar hypoventilation (PAH) is a disorder of unknown cause characterized by chronic hypercapnia and hypoxemia in the absence of identifiable neuromuscular disease or mechanical ventilatory impairment. The disorder is thought to arise from a defect in the metabolic respiratory control system, but few neuropathologic studies have been re-

ported in such patients. Isolated PAH is relatively rare, and although it occurs in all age groups, the majority of reported cases have been in males aged 20 to 50 years. The disorder typically develops insidiously and often first comes to attention when severe respiratory depression follows administration of standard doses of sedatives or anesthetics. As the degree of hypoventilation increases, patients typically develop lethargy, fatigue, daytime somnolence, disturbed sleep, and morning headaches; eventually cyanosis, polycythemia, pulmonary hypertension, and congestive heart failure occur (see Fig. 263-1). Despite severe arterial blood gas derangements, dyspnea is uncommon, presumably because of impaired chemoreception and ventilatory drive. If left untreated, PAH is usually progressive over a period of months to years and ultimately fatal.

The key diagnostic finding in PAH is a chronic respiratory acidosis in the absence of respiratory muscle weakness or impaired ventilatory mechanics (see Fig. 263-2). Because patients can hyperventilate voluntarily and reduce Pa_{CO_2} to normal or even hypocapnic levels, hypercapnia may not be demonstrable in a single arterial blood sample, but the presence of an elevated plasma HCO_3^- level should draw attention to the underlying chronic disturbance. Despite normal ventilatory mechanics and respiratory muscle strength, ventilatory responses to chemical stimuli are reduced or absent (see Fig. 263-2), and breath-holding time may be markedly prolonged without any sensation of dyspnea.

Patients with PAH maintain rhythmic respiration when awake, although the level of ventilation is below normal. However, during sleep, when breathing is critically dependent on the metabolic control system, there is typically a further deterioration in ventilation with frequent episodes of central hypopnea or apnea, a disturbance that has been termed *Ondine's curse*.

PAH must be distinguished from other central hypoventilation syndromes that are secondary to underlying neurologic disease of the brainstem or chemoreceptors (see Table 263-1). This distinction requires a careful neurologic investigation for evidence of brainstem or autonomic disturbances. Unrecognized respiratory neuromuscular disorders, particularly those that produce diaphragmatic weakness, are often misdiagnosed as PAH. However, such disorders can usually be suspected on clinical grounds (see below) and can be confirmed by the finding of reduced voluntary hyperventilation, as well as PI_{max} and PE_{max}.

Some patients with PAH respond favorably to respiratory stimulant medications and to supplemental oxygen. However, the majority eventually require mechanical ventilatory assistance. Excellent long-term benefits can be achieved with diaphragmatic pacing by electrophrenic stimulation or with negative- or positive-pressure mechanical ventilation. The administration of such treatment only during sleep is sufficient in most patients.

RESPIRATORY NEUROMUSCULAR DISORDERS Several primary disorders of the spinal cord, peripheral respiratory nerves, and respiratory muscles produce a chronic hypoventilation syndrome (see Table 263-1). Hypoventilation usually develops gradually over a period of months to years and often first comes to attention when a relatively trivial increase in mechanical ventilatory load (such as mild airways obstruction) produces severe respiratory failure. In some of the disorders (such as motor neuron disease, myasthenia gravis, and muscular dystrophy), involvement of the respiratory nerves or muscles is usually a later feature of a more widespread disease. In other disorders, respiratory involvement can be an early or even isolated feature, and hence the underlying problem is often not suspected. Included in this category are the postpolio syndrome (a form of chronic respiratory insufficiency that develops 20 to 30 years following recovery from poliomyelitis), the myopathy associated with adult acid maltase deficiency, and idiopathic diaphragmatic paralysis.

Generally, respiratory neuromuscular disorders do not result in chronic hypoventilation unless there is significant weakness of the diaphragm. Distinguishing features of bilateral diaphragmatic weakness include orthopnea, paradoxical movement of the abdomen in the supine posture, and paradoxical diaphragmatic movement under fluoroscopy. However, the absence of these features does not exclude diaphragmatic weakness. Important laboratory features are a rapid deterioration of ventilation during a maximum voluntary ventilation maneuver and reduced PI_{max} and PE_{max} (see Fig. 263-2). More sophisticated investigations reveal reduced or absent transdiaphragmatic pressures, calculated from simultaneous measurement of esophageal and gastric pressures; reduced diaphragmatic EMG responses (recorded from an esophageal electrode) to transcutaneous phrenic nerve stimulation; and marked hypopnea and arterial oxygen desaturation during rapid eye movement sleep, when there is normally a physiologic inhibition of all nondiaphragmatic respiratory muscles and breathing becomes critically dependent on diaphragmatic activity.

The management of chronic alveolar hypoventilation due to respiratory neuromuscular disease involves treatment of the underlying disorder, where feasible, and mechanical ventilatory assistance as described for the primary alveolar hypoventilation syndrome. However, electrophrenic diaphragmatic pacing is contraindicated in these disorders, except for high cervical spinal cord lesions in which the phrenic lower motor neurons and nerves are intact.

OBESITY-HYPOVENTILATION SYNDROME Massive obesity represents a mechanical load to the respiratory system because the added weight on the rib cage and abdomen serves to reduce the compliance of the chest wall. As a result, the functional residual capacity (i.e., end-expiratory lung volume) is reduced, particularly in the recumbent posture. An important consequence of breathing at a low lung volume is that some airways, particularly those in the lung bases, may be closed throughout part or even all of each tidal breath, resulting in underventilation of the lung bases and widening of the $(A - a)P_{O_2}$. Nevertheless, in the majority of obese subjects, central respiratory drive is increased sufficiently to maintain a normal Pa_{CO_2}. However, a small proportion of obese subjects develop chronic hypercapnia, hypoxemia, and eventually polycythemia, pulmonary hypertension, and right-sided heart failure. Those patients who also develop daytime somnolence have been designated as having the *Pickwickian syndrome* (see Chap. 27). In many such patients, obstructive sleep apnea is a prominent feature, and even in those patients without sleep apnea, sleep-induced hypoventilation is an important element of the disorder and contributes to its progression. Most patients demonstrate a decrease in central respiratory drive, which may be inherent or acquired, and many have mild to moderate degrees of airflow obstruction, usually related to smoking. Based on these considerations, several therapeutic measures can be of considerable benefit, including weight loss, cessation of smoking, elimination of obstructive sleep apnea, and enhancement of respiratory drive by medications such as progesterone.

HYPERVENTILATION AND ITS SYNDROMES

DEFINITION AND ETIOLOGY Alveolar hyperventilation exists when Pa_{CO_2} decreases below the normal range of 37 to 43 mmHg. *Hyperventilation* is not synonymous with *hyperpnea*, which refers to an increased minute volume of ventilation without reference to Pa_{CO_2}. Although hyperventilation is frequently associated with dyspnea, patients who are hyperventilating do not necessarily complain of shortness of breath; and conversely, patients with dyspnea need not be hyperventilating.

Numerous disease entities can be associated with alveolar hyperventilation (Table 263-2), but in all cases the underlying mechanism involves an increase in respiratory drive that is mediated through either the behavioral or the metabolic respiratory control systems (Fig. 263-3). Thus hypoxemia drives ventilation by stimulating the peripheral chemoreceptors, and several pulmonary disorders and congestive heart failure drive ventilation by stimulating afferent vagal receptors in the lungs and airways. Low cardiac output and hypotension stimulate the peripheral chemoreceptors and inhibit the baroreceptors, both of which increase ventilation. Metabolic acidosis, a potent respiratory stimulant, excites both the peripheral and central chemoreceptors and increases the sensitivity of the peripheral chemoreceptors to coexistent hypoxemia. Hepatic failure also can produce hyperventilation, presumably as a result of metabolic stimuli acting on the peripheral and central chemoreceptors.

Table 263-2

Hyperventilation Syndromes

1. Hypoxemia
   a. High altitude
   b. Pulmonary disease
   c. Cardiac shunts
2. Pulmonary disorders
   a. Pneumonia
   b. Interstitial pneumonitis, fibrosis, edema
   c. Pulmonary emboli, vascular disease
   d. Bronchial asthma
   e. Pneumothorax
   f. Chest wall disorders
3. Cardiovascular disorders
   a. Congestive heart failure
   b. Hypotension
4. Metabolic disorders
   a. Acidosis (diabetic, renal, lactic)
   b. Hepatic failure
5. Neurologic and psychogenic disorders
   a. Psychogenic or anxiety hyperventilation
   b. Central nervous system infection, tumors
6. Drug-induced
   a. Salicylates
   b. Methylxanthine derivatives
   c. Beta-adrenergic agonists
   d. Progesterone
7. Miscellaneous
   a. Fever, sepsis
   b. Pain
   c. Pregnancy

Several neurologic and psychological disorders are thought to drive ventilation through the behavioral respiratory control system. Included in this category are psychogenic or anxiety hyperventilation and severe cerebrovascular insufficiency, which may interfere with the inhibitory influence normally exerted by cortical structures on the brainstem respiratory neurons. Rarely, disorders of the midbrain and hypothalamus induce hyperventilation, and it is conceivable that fever and sepsis also cause hyperventilation through effects on these structures. Several drugs cause hyperventilation by stimulating the central or peripheral chemoreceptors or by direct action on the brainstem respiratory neurons. Chronic hyperventilation is a normal feature of

FIGURE 263-3 Schematic diagram of the mechanisms involved in alveolar hyperventilation. *(From Slutsky and Phillipson.)*

pregnancy and results from the effects of progesterone and other hormones acting on the respiratory neurons.

PHYSIOLOGIC AND CLINICAL FEATURES   Because hyperventilation is associated with increased respiratory drive, muscle effort, and minute volume of ventilation, the most frequent symptom associated with hyperventilation is dyspnea. However, there is considerable discrepancy between the degree of hyperventilation, as measured by Pa_{CO_2}, and the degree of associated dyspnea. From a physiologic standpoint, hyperventilation is beneficial in patients who are hypoxemic, because the alveolar hypocapnia is associated with an increase in alveolar and arterial P_{O_2}. Conversely, hyperventilation can also be detrimental. In particular, the alkalemia associated with hypocapnia may produce neurologic symptoms, including dizziness, visual impairment, syncope, and seizure activity (secondary to cerebral vasoconstriction); parasthesias, carpopedal spasm, and tetany (secondary to decreased free serum calcium); and muscle weakness (secondary to hypophosphatemia). Severe alkalemia also can induce cardiac arrhythmias and evidence of myocardial ischemia. Patients with a primary respiratory alkalosis are also prone to periodic breathing and central sleep apnea (see Chap 264).

DIAGNOSIS   In most patients with a hyperventilation syndrome, the cause is readily apparent on the basis of history, physical examination, and knowledge of coexisting medical disorders (see Table 263-2). In patients in whom the cause is not clinically apparent, investigation begins with arterial blood gas analysis, which establishes the presence of alveolar hyperventilation (decreased Pa_{CO_2}) and its severity. Equally important is the arterial pH, which generally allows the disorder to be classified as either a primary respiratory alkalosis (elevated pH) or a primary metabolic acidosis (decreased pH). Also of importance is the Pa_{O_2} and calculation of the $(A-a)P_{O_2}$, since a widened alveolar-arterial oxygen difference suggests a pulmonary disorder as the underlying cause. The finding of a reduced plasma HCO_3^- level establishes the chronic nature of the disorder and points toward an organic cause. Measurements of ventilation and arterial or transcutaneous P_{CO_2} during sleep are very useful in suspected psychogenic hyperventilation, since such patients do not maintain the hyperventilation during sleep.

The disorders that most frequently give rise to unexplained hyperventilation are pulmonary vascular disease (particularly chronic or recurrent thromboembolism) and psychogenic or anxiety hyperventilation. Hyperventilation due to pulmonary vascular disease is associated with exertional dyspnea, a widened $(A-a)P_{O_2}$ and maintenance of hyperventilation during exercise. In contrast, patients with psychogenic hyperventilation typically complain of dyspnea at rest and not during mild exercise and of the need to sigh frequently. They are also more likely to complain of dizziness, sweating, palpitations, and paresthesias. During mild to moderate exercise, their hyperventilation tends to disappear and $(A-a)P_{O_2}$ is normal, but heart rate and cardiac output may be increased relative to metabolic rate.

℞ TREATMENT

Alveolar hyperventilation is usually of relatively minor clinical consequence and therefore is generally managed by appropriate treatment of the underlying cause. In the few patients in whom alkalemia is thought to be inducing significant cerebral vasoconstriction, paresthesia, tetany, or cardiac disturbances, inhalation of a low concentration of CO_2 can be very beneficial. For patients with disabling psychogenic hyperventilation, careful explanation of the basis of their symptoms can be reassuring and is often sufficient. Others have benefited from beta-adrenergic antagonists or an exercise program. Specific treatment for anxiety may also be indicated.

BIBLIOGRAPHY

CHERNIACK NS, LONGOBARDO GS: Abnormalities in respiratory rhythm, in *Handbook of Physiology*, section 3: *The Respiratory System*, vol 2, *Control of Breathing*, NS Cherniack, JG Widdicombe (eds). Bethesda, MD, Am Physiol Soc, 1986, pp 729–749

FANBURG BL, SICILIAN L (eds): Respiratory dysfunction in neuromuscular disease. Clin Chest Med 15:(4)607, 1994

MEYER TJ, HILL NS: Noninvasive positive pressure ventilation to treat respiratory failure. Ann Intern Med 120:760, 1994

PHILLIPSON EA: Hypoventilation syndromes, in *Textbook of Respiratory Medicine*, 2d ed, JF Murray, JA Nadel (eds). Philadelphia, Saunders, 1994, chap 83, pp 2291–2300

SLUTSKY AS, PHILLIPSON EA: Hyperventilation syndromes, in *Textbook of Respiratory Medicine*, JF Murray, JA Nadel (eds). Philadelphia, Saunders, 1994, chap 85, pp 2325–2332

264   *Eliot A. Phillipson*

SLEEP APNEA

DEFINITION AND CLASSIFICATION   *Sleep apnea* is defined as an intermittent cessation of airflow at the nose and mouth during sleep. By convention, apneas of at least 10 s duration have been considered important, but in most patients the apneas are 20 to 30 s in duration and may be as long as 2 to 3 min. *Sleep apnea syndrome* refers to a clinical disorder that arises from recurrent apneas during sleep. There is uncertainty as to the minimum number of apneas that should be considered clinically important, although by the time most patients come to attention they have at least 10 to 15 events per hour of sleep. The clinical importance of sleep apnea arises from the fact that it is one of the leading causes of excessive daytime sleepiness. Indeed, epidemiologic studies have established a prevalence of clinically important sleep apnea of at least 2 percent in middle-aged women and 4 percent in middle-aged men.

Sleep apneas have been classified into three types: central, obstructive, and mixed. In central sleep apnea (CSA) the neural drive to all the respiratory muscles is transiently abolished. In contrast, in obstructive sleep apnea (OSA) airflow ceases despite continuing respiratory drive because of occlusion of the oropharyngeal airway. Mixed apneas, which consist of a central apnea followed by an obstructive component, are a variant of OSA.

OBSTRUCTIVE SLEEP APNEA   Pathogenesis   The definitive event in OSA is occlusion of the upper airway usually at the level of the oropharynx (Fig. 264-1). The resulting apnea leads to progressive asphyxia until there is a brief arousal from sleep, whereupon airway patency is restored and airflow resumes. The patient then returns to sleep, and the sequence of events is repeated, often up to 400 to 500 times per night, resulting in marked fragmentation of sleep.

The immediate factor leading to collapse of the upper airway in OSA is the generation of a critical subatmospheric pressure during inspiration that exceeds the ability of the airway dilator and abductor muscles to maintain airway stability (see Fig. 264-1). Sleep plays a permissive but crucial role by reducing the activity of the muscles of the upper airways and the protective reflex response of the muscles to subatmospheric airway pressures. Alcohol is frequently an important cofactor because of its selective depressant influence on the upper airway muscles and on the arousal response that terminates each apnea. In most patients the patency of the airway is also compromised structurally and therefore predisposed to occlusion. In a minority of patients the structural compromise is due to obvious anatomic disturbances, such as adenotonsillar hypertrophy, retrognathia, and macroglossia. However, in the majority of patients the structural defect is simply a subtle reduction in airway size that can often be appreciated clinically as "pharyngeal crowding" and that can usually be demonstrated by imaging and acoustic reflection techniques. Obesity frequently contributes to the reduction in size of the upper airways, either by increasing fat deposition in the soft tissues of the pharynx or by compressing the pharynx by superficial fat masses in the neck. Snoring, a high-frequency vibration of the palatal and pharyngeal soft tissues that results from the decrease in size of the upper airway lumen, may aggravate the narrowing by producing edema of the soft tissues. More sophisticated studies also demonstrate a high airway compliance—

i.e., the airway is "floppy" and therefore prone to collapse. In some patients, a high upstream (i.e., nasal) resistance predisposes to collapse of the upper airway by increasing the subatmospheric pressure generated in the pharynx during inspiration as the strength of diaphragmatic contraction is increased to overcome airflow resistance in the nose.

Pathophysiologic and Clinical Features The narrowing of the upper airways during sleep, which predisposes to OSA, inevitably results in snoring. In most patients, snoring antedates the development of obstructive events by many years. However, the majority of snoring individuals do not have an OSA disorder. Although a few recent studies suggest that snoring per se may be associated with long-term health risks, definitive evidence in this regard is lacking. Hence, in the absence of other symptoms, snoring alone does not warrant an investigation for OSA but does call for preventive counselling, particularly with regard to weight gain and alcohol consumption.

The recurrent episodes of nocturnal asphyxia and of arousal from sleep that characterize OSA lead to a series of secondary physiologic events, which in turn give rise in some patients to the clinical complications of the syndrome (see Fig. 264-1). The most common manifestations are neuropsychiatric and behavioral disturbances that are thought to arise from the fragmentation of sleep and loss of slow-wave sleep induced by the recurrent arousal responses. Nocturnal cerebral hypoxia also may play an important role. The most pervasive manifestation is excessive daytime sleepiness. Initially, daytime sleepiness manifests under passive conditions, such as reading or watching television; but as the disorder progresses, sleepiness encroaches into all daily activities and can become disabling and dangerous. Several studies have demonstrated two to three times more motor vehicle accidents in patients with OSA compared with other drivers. Other related symptoms include intellectual impairment, memory loss, and personality disturbances. In men with OSA, impotence is a relatively frequent complaint.

The other major manifestations of OSA are cardiorespiratory in nature and are thought to arise from the recurrent episodes of nocturnal asphyxia (see Fig. 264-1). Many patients demonstrate a cyclical slowing of the heart during the apneas to 30 to 50 beats per minute, followed by a tachycardia of 90 to 120 beats per minute during the ventilatory phase. A small number of patients develop severe bradycardia with asystoles of 8- to 12-s duration or dangerous tachyarrhythmias,

including unsustained ventricular tachycardia. The presence of such arrhythmias has led to the notion that OSA may result in sudden death during sleep, but firm corroborative data are lacking. Unlike in healthy subjects, in patients with OSA systemic blood pressure fails to decrease during sleep. In fact, blood pressure typically rises abruptly at the termination of each obstructive event. Furthermore, several epidemiologic studies have implicated OSA as a risk factor for the development of systemic hypertension, myocardial ischemia and infarction, stroke, and premature death. However, because these studies were cross-sectional or retrospective in design, the natural history of OSA remains largely undefined. OSA also markedly aggravates left ventricular failure in patients with underlying heart disease. This complication is probably due to the combined effects of increased left ventricular afterload during each obstructive event, secondary to increased negative intrathoracic pressure (see Fig. 264-1), recurrent nocturnal hypoxemia, and chronically elevated sympathoadrenal activity. Treatment of OSA in such patients often results in dramatic improvement in left ventricular function. Finally, a small proportion of patients with OSA (<10 percent) develop pulmonary hypertension, right ventricular failure, polycythemia, and chronic hypercapnia and hypoxemia. All such patients have evidence of sustained daytime hypoxemia in addition to the nocturnal ventilatory disturbance, usually as a result of reduced ventilatory drive and/or diffuse airways obstruction. Most of these patients are obese and sleepy and are therefore said to have the *Pickwickian syndrome*.

Diagnosis Although OSA occurs at any age, and is more prevalent in women than was previously thought, the typical patient is a male aged 30 to 60 years who presents with a history of snoring, excessive daytime sleepiness, nocturnal choking or gasping, witnessed apneas during sleep, moderate obesity, and often mild to moderate hypertension. The diagnosis can often be confirmed by direct observation of the patient during sleep. However, the definitive investigation for suspected OSA is polysomnography, a detailed overnight sleep study that includes recording of (1) electrographic variables (electroencephalogram, electrooculogram, and submental electromyogram) that

FIGURE 264-1 The primary sequence of events, underlying mechanisms, physiologic responses, and clinical features of obstructive sleep apnea. (*From EA Phillipson, Med Clin North Am 23:2314, 1982.*)

permit the identification of sleep and its various stages, (2) ventilatory variables that permit the identification of apneas and their classification as central or obstructive, (3) arterial O_2 saturation by ear or finger oximetry, and (4) heart rate. Continuous measurement of transcutaneous P_{CO_2} (which reflects arterial P_{CO_2}) can also be very useful, particularly in patients with central sleep apnea. The key diagnostic finding in OSA is episodes of airflow cessation at the nose and mouth despite evidence of continuing respiratory effort.

Because polysomnography is a time-consuming and expensive test, there is considerable interest in the role of simplified, unattended, ambulatory sleep monitoring for the investigation of OSA that would allow the patient to be studied at home, rather than in the sleep laboratory. The most useful test in this context is the recording of arterial O_2 saturation by oximetry. However, the reliability of overnight oximetry in the diagnosis of OSA is dependent on the pretest probability of the disorder. In patients with a high pretest probability (based on a history of daytime sleepiness, habitual snoring, nocturnal choking or gasping, and witnessed apneas during sleep), overnight oximetry can be used to *confirm* the diagnosis by demonstrating recurrent episodes of arterial O_2 desaturation (at a rate of at least 10 to 15 events per hour). Such findings obviate the need for full polysomnography and allow initiation of treatment with nasal continuous positive airway pressure (CPAP) during sleep (see "Treatment"). However, negative results in a patient with a high clinical probability of OSA do not exclude the diagnosis but mandate that the patient proceed to polysomnography to investigate the cause of the daytime sleepiness. In contrast, when the pretest probability of OSA is low (such as the patient with only occasional snoring, few witnessed apneas, and no daytime sleepiness), the absence of arterial O_2 desaturation can be used to *exclude* the diagnosis and thereby obviate the need for full polysomnography.

Studies suggest that overnight oximetry can obviate the need for polysomnography in about one-third of clinic patients referred for consideration of OSA, either by *confirming* the diagnosis in patients with a *high* pretest probability of the disorder, or by *excluding* the diagnosis in patients with a *low* pretest probability. In the remaining two-thirds of patients with an intermediate pretest probability of OSA, overnight oximetry alone will not be definitive; hence such patients will require polysomnography.

℞ **TREATMENT**

Several approaches to treatment of OSA have been advocated, based on an understanding of the mechanisms underlying the disorder (Table 264-1). However, the majority of these treatment approaches has not been subjected to rigorous clinical trials. The specific choice of treatment depends largely on the severity of OSA. Mild to moderate OSA can often be managed effectively by modest weight reduc-

tion, avoidance of alcohol, improvement of nasal patency, and avoidance of sleeping in the supine posture. Intraoral appliances, designed to keep the mandible and tongue forward, may also be effective. In some patients with more severe OSA, tricyclic medications, particularly protriptyline (20 to 30 mg at bedtime), have been beneficial. The role of nocturnal supplemental oxygen in managing OSA is uncertain but is generally not satisfactory. The most widely used treatments in moderate to severe OSA are uvulopalatopharyngoplasty and nasal CPAP during sleep. Uvulopalatopharyngoplasty is a surgical procedure designed to increase the pharyngeal lumen by resecting redundant soft tissue. When applied to unselected patients with OSA, it produces long-term benefits in only about 50 percent. More recent attempts to select patients based on the specific site of upper airway occlusion have yielded a higher success rate. Nasal CPAP, which prevents upper airway occlusion by splinting the pharyngeal airway with a positive pressure delivered through a nose mask, is currently the most successful long-term approach to treatment, being well tolerated and effective in over 80 percent of patients, provided that they have received proper training. For the few patients with severe OSA in whom all other treatment approaches fail, tracheostomy provides immediate relief.

CENTRAL SLEEP APNEA Pathogenesis The definitive event in CSA is transient abolition of central drive to the ventilatory muscles. The resulting apnea leads to a primary sequence of events similar to those of OSA (see Fig. 264-1). Several underlying mechanisms can result in cessation of respiratory drive during sleep (Table 264-2). First are defects in the metabolic respiratory control system and respiratory neuromuscular apparatus. Such defects usually produce a chronic alveolar hypoventilation syndrome (in addition to CSA) that becomes more severe during sleep when the stimulatory effect of wakefulness on breathing is abolished. In contrast are CSA disorders that arise from transient instabilities in an otherwise intact respiratory control system. Common to all these disorders is a P_{CO_2} level during sleep that falls transiently below the critical P_{CO_2} required for respiratory rhythm generation. The most frequent instability of this type occurs at sleep onset, because the P_{CO_2} level of wakefulness is often lower than that required for rhythm generation in sleep; hence with loss of the stimulatory effect of wakefulness on breathing (referred to as the *waking neural drive*), an apnea develops at sleep onset until P_{CO_2} rises to the critical level (Fig. 264-2). However, if the central nervous system state fluctuates at sleep onset between "asleep" and "awake," a pattern of periodic breathing develops as respiration follows the changes in state. During each cycle, the waning phase of ventilation includes an hypopnea or outright central apnea (Cheyne-Stokes respiration). In most patients with CSA, the tendency to develop periodic breathing and central apneas during sleep is enhanced by some degree of chronic hyperventilation during wakefulness that drives the P_{CO_2}

Table 264-1

Management of Obstructive Sleep Apnea (OSA)

Mechanism	Mild to Moderate OSA	Moderate to Severe OSA
↑ Upper airway muscle tone	Avoidance of alcohol, sedatives	Tricyclics
↑ Upper airway lumen size	Weight reduction Avoidance of supine posture Oral prosthesis	Uvulopalatopharyngoplasty
↓ Upper airway subatmospheric pressure	Improved nasal patency	Nasal continuous positive airway pressure
Bypass occlusion		Tracheostomy

SOURCE: Phillipson, with permission.

Table 264-2

Mechanisms Underlying Central Sleep Apnea

Underlying Mechanism	Clinical Example
Defects in metabolic control system or respiratory muscles	Primary and secondary central alveolar hypoventilation syndromes Respiratory muscle weakness
Transient instabilities in central respiratory drive	Sleep onset Hyperventilation-induced hypocapnia Idiopathic Hypoxia (high altitude, pulmonary disease) Cardiovascular disease, pulmonary congestion CNS disease Prolonged circulation time
Inhibition of central respiratory drive by upper airway reflexes	Esophageal reflux Aspiration Upper airway collapse

SOURCE: Phillipson, with permission.

level below the threshold required for rhythm generation during sleep. Such hyperventilation is frequently idiopathic in nature. Hypoxia, whether due to high altitude or to underlying cardiorespiratory disease, also enhances the tendency to periodic breathing and CSA for the same reasons. Hyperventilation due to central nervous system disease or to lung congestion secondary to heart failure produces periodic breathing and CSA by a similar mechanism. Circulatory slowing secondary to cardiac failure also may induce ventilatory instability by prolonging the time lag between changes in blood gas values by ventilation and the detection of those changes by the peripheral and central chemoreceptors (Chap. 233). Consequently, the ventilatory system overshoots the mark before reversing direction, resulting in periodic breathing that frequently includes central apneas.

Pathophysiologic and Clinical Features Many healthy individuals demonstrate a small number of central apneas during sleep, particularly at sleep onset and in rapid eye movement sleep. These apneas are not associated with any physiologic or clinical disturbances. In patients with clinically important CSA, the primary sequence of events that characterizes the disorder leads to prominent physiologic and clinical consequences (see Fig. 264-1). In those patients whose CSA is a component of an alveolar hypoventilation syndrome, daytime hypercapnia and hypoxemia are usually evident, and the clinical picture is dominated by a history of recurrent respiratory failure, polycythemia, pulmonary hypertension, and right-sided heart failure. Complaints of sleeping poorly, morning headache, and daytime fatigue and sleepiness are also prominent. In contrast, in patients whose CSA results from an instability in respiratory drive, the clinical picture is dominated by features related to sleep disturbance, including recurrent nocturnal awakenings, morning fatigue, and daytime sleepiness.

Diagnosis Initially, many patients with CSA are suspected clinically of having OSA because of a history of snoring, sleep disturbance, and daytime sleepiness. However, obesity and hypertension are less prominent in CSA than in OSA. Definitive diagnosis of CSA requires a polysomnographic study, with the *key observation being recurrent apneas that are not accompanied by respiratory effort.* Measurements of transcutaneous P_{CO_2} are particularly useful in CSA. Those patients with a defect in respiratory control or neuromuscular function typically demonstrate an elevated P_{CO_2} that tends to increase progressively during the night, particularly during rapid eye movement sleep. In contrast, patients with instabilities in the respiratory control system typically demonstrate a mild degree of hypocapnia, which is an integral pathogenetic feature of their disorder (see above).

℞ TREATMENT

The management of patients whose CSA is a component of an alveolar hypoventilation syndrome is essentially the same as management of the underlying hypoventilation disorder (see Chap. 263). Management of patients whose CSA arises from an instability of respiratory drive is more problematic. Patients with hypoxemia usually respond favorably to nocturnal supplemental oxygen. Others have responded to acidification with acetazolamide, and recent reports indicate a good response to nasal CPAP (as for OSA). The mechanism by which CPAP abolishes central apneas probably involves a small increase in Pa_{CO_2} as a result of the added expiratory mechanical load. In patients whose CSA is secondary to congestive heart failure, CPAP is particularly effective in improving sleep quality and daytime cardiac function.

BIBLIOGRAPHY

DEEGAN PC, MCNICHOLAS WT: Pathophysiology of obstructive sleep apnoea. Eur Respir J 8:1161, 1995

NATIONAL COMMISSION ON SLEEP DISORDERS RESEARCH: *Wake up America: A National Sleep Alert.* Washington, DC, Government Printing Office, 1993

NAUGHTON MT et al: Treatment of congestive heart failure and Cheyne-Stokes respiration during sleep by continuous positive airway pressure. Am J Respir Crit Care Med 151:92, 1995

PHILLIPSON EA: Sleep disorders, in *Textbook of Respiratory Medicine,* 2d ed, JF Murray, JA Nadel (eds). Philadelphia, Saunders, 1994, chap 84, pp 2301–2324

———, BRADLEY TD (eds): Breathing disorders in sleep. Clin Chest Med 13:(3)383, 1992

YOUNG T et al: The occurrence of sleep-disordered breathing among middle-aged adults. N Engl J Med 328:1230, 1993

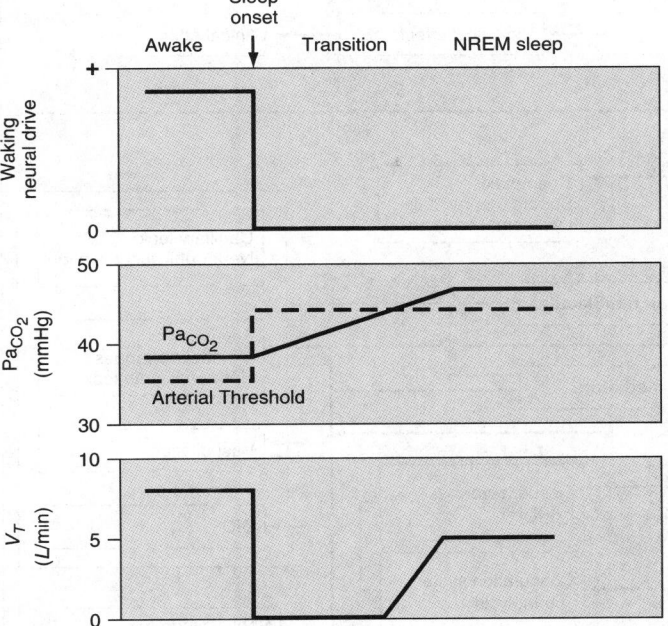

FIGURE 264-2 Schematic diagram of the mechanisms underlying central sleep apnea at sleep onset. With loss of the waking neural drive to breathing, the arterial threshold P_{CO_2} for rhythm generation increases above the Pa_{CO_2} present during wakefulness; hence tidal volume (V_T) falls to zero and apnea ensues until Pa_{CO_2} rises above the threshold for rhythm generation during sleep. NREM, non-rapid eye movement. *(From TD Bradley, EA Phillipson, Clin Chest Med 13:439, 1992.)*

265 *Eric G. Honig, Roland H. Ingram, Jr.*

ACUTE RESPIRATORY DISTRESS SYNDROME

The acute respiratory distress syndrome (ARDS; formerly known as the adult respiratory distress syndrome) is a condition characterized by acute hypoxemic respiratory failure due to pulmonary edema caused by increased permeability of the alveolar capillary barrier. ARDS represents the most serious manifestation of a spectrum of responses to acute lung injury (ALI); these responses occur as complications of a more widespread systemic response to acute inflammation or injury. Recent consensus groups have attempted to establish working definitions for ARDS and underlying systemic inflammatory states. ALI may be said to be present in the setting of severe hypoxemia of acute onset and bilateral diffuse opacities on a frontal chest radiograph when left atrial or pulmonary capillary hypertension have been excluded. ARDS is differentiated from ALI by the severity of the hypoxemia and is defined as a ratio of arterial P_{O_2} to inspired oxygen fraction (Pa_{O_2}/FI_{O_2}) $\leq$ 200 mmHg. ALI and ARDS should be viewed as the earliest and most recognizable manifestations of an infectious or inflammatory systemic disorder. The lung figures so prominently in systemic injury because it receives all of the cardiac output and because impairment of pulmonary function is readily apparent clinically.

ALI develops rapidly after a predisposing condition triggers a systemic inflammatory response, often within 90 min. Over half of all cases develop within 24 h of the underlying insult. ALI is most

Table 265-1

strongly associated with conditions that produce direct alveolar injury or indirect injury via the pulmonary capillary bed. These are listed in Table 265-1. The likelihood of ARDS varies with the precipitating causes, from a 13 percent risk associated with drug overdose to a 43 percent risk for patients with sepsis.

PATHOPHYSIOLOGY

ALI is the consequence of an unregulated overexpression of usual systemic inflammatory responses to infection and/or injury. Injury involves both the alveolar epithelium and the pulmonary capillary endothelium. The inciting event initiates a complex cascade of cellular and biochemical events outlined schematically in Fig. 265-1. These events may be thought of as occurring in three phases: *initiation*, in which the trigger event activates the cellular cascade; *amplification*, in which the effector cells are recruited and activated; and *injury*, i.e., expression of these events at the tissue level. Injury is produced by cellular events associated with neutrophils, macrophages, monocytes, and lymphocytes producing various cytokines, in turn producing cellular activation, chemotaxis, and adhesion. Activated cells produce a series of inflammatory mediators, including oxidants, proteases, kinins, growth factors, neuropeptides, activators of the complement cascade, intravascular coagulation, and fibrinolysis.

The pathophysiologic hallmark of ARDS is increased vascular permeability to proteins leaving the hydrostatic gradient unopposed so that even mild elevations in capillary pressures (due to increased intravenous liquid loads and cardiac dysfunction characteristic of sepsis) greatly increase interstitial and alveolar edema. This additive effect of permeability and hydrostatic factors is illustrated by the increased severity of disease involvement in dependent lung regions (Fig. 265-2). The increase in the ratio of lung tissue to gas in these lung zones causes alveolar closing pressures to exceed local transpulmonary pressures, leading to alveolar closure and collapse. The tendency to

Table 265-1

Conditions That May Lead to the Acute Respiratory Distress Syndrome

Direct injury to alveolar epithelium	Indirect lung injury
Aspiration	Sepsis syndrome
Diffuse infection	Severe nonthoracic trauma
Near-drowning	Hypertransfusion
Toxic inhalation	Cardiopulmonary bypass
Airway contusion	

alveolar collapse is further exaggerated by the quantitative reduction in surfactant synthesis due to injury to type II pneumocytes as well as to further abnormalities in the size, composition, and metabolism of the remaining surfactant pool. Although these atelectatic regions of the lung contribute to a reduction in the compliance of the lung as a whole, significant regions of nondependent lung have relatively normal mechanical and gas-exchanging properties. The burden of ventilation and gas exchange is shifted to these uninvolved lung regions; by analogy, the respiratory function of the adult patient must be provided by a pair of baby-sized lungs.

Because of the decreased compliance, large inspiratory pressures must be generated by the respiratory muscles, so the work of breathing is elevated. The large mechanical load may lead to fatigue of the muscles of breathing with resulting diminution in tidal volumes and worsening gas exchange. Both hypoxemia and the stimulation of receptors in the stiff lung parenchyma cause an increase in respiratory frequency, decrease in tidal volume, and deterioration in gas exchange.

Airways resistance may be increased because minute volume must be handled by a decreased number of ventilating airways and because of airway narrowing from excess liquid and bronchospasm. Pulmonary vascular resistance and pulmonary arterial pressures are also elevated, initially because of neurohumoral factors and later due to obstruction, obliteration, and remodeling. Gas exchange is characterized by low ventilation-perfusion ratios and extensive shunt accompanied by an elevated dead space. Shunt is due to atelectasis, alveolar collapse,

FIGURE 265-1 Multiple, simultaneous, and parallel pathways to sepsis and acute lung injury are shown. The complexity of the response and multiplicity of involved pathways present a formidable challenge to the design of effective pharmacotherapeutic approaches to sepsis and ARDS. LPS, lipopolysaccharide; LBP, LPS binding protein; DIC, disseminated intravascular coagulation; MOF, multiple organ failure. *[From MP Glauser et al, Clin Infect Dis 18(suppl 2):S205, 1994, with permission.]*

surfactant dysfunction, and attenuation of hypoxic vasoconstriction. Increase in dead space is caused by obstruction and obliteration of the pulmonary capillary bed.

PATHOLOGY   Pathologic changes in ARDS evolve over three distinct phases, and the lesions correlate with these phases much better than the underlying cause of lung injury since the lung has a limited number of ways in which it reacts to a wide variety of injuries. Grossly, the lungs are heavy and edematous, with regions of hemorrhage, atelectasis, and consolidation.

The acute exudative phase, covering the first 3 days after lung injury, is characterized by the formation of hyaline membranes composed of fibrin and other matrix proteins in alveolar ducts and airspaces. Epithelial cell injury is represented by extensive necrosis of type I pneumocytes and a denuded basement membrane that allows free entry of liquid and macromolecules into the airspaces. Endothelial injury becomes manifest as cellular edema and a widening of intercellular junctions. Thromboemboli and in situ thrombi are found within the vasculature. Over the next week, the alveolar exudate is either resolved or undergoes organization, i.e., the proliferative phase. Cuboidal type II cells and squamous epithelium cover denuded alveolar basement membranes. Fibroblasts begin to enter the hyaline membranes and to produce collagen. After 3 to 4 weeks, changes characteristic of the fibrotic phase are seen. Microcystic airspaces enlarge to form cystic and honeycomb changes in dependent lung. Airspaces and alveolar ducts undergo fibrosis, while peripheral bronchi become dilated. Fibrocellular intimal proliferation occurs in small muscular arteries, veins, and pulmonary lymphatics. Extensive remodeling of the pulmonary capillary bed occurs, as well as muscularization of acinar blood vessels.

CLINICAL CHARACTERISTICS   At the time of initial injury and for several hours thereafter, the patient may be free of respiratory symptoms or signs. The earliest sign often is an increase in respiratory frequency followed shortly by dyspnea. Arterial blood gas measurement in the earlier period will disclose a depressed P_{O_2} despite a decreased P_{CO_2}, so that the alveolar-arterial difference for oxygen (Chap. 250) is increased. At this early stage, administration of oxygen results in a significant increase in the Pa_{O_2}. The brisk rise in Pa_{O_2}

FIGURE 265-2   A standard posteroanterior chest radiograph from a patient with the acute respiratory distress syndrome secondary to a severe viral pneumonitis. Such a diffuse radiographic change is typical of all conditions listed in Table 265-1 when they are severe enough to cause acute hypoxemic respiratory failure. A similar radiographic picture is also seen in pulmonary edema due to left ventricular failure (Chap. 32). Often in such acutely ill patients, the radiograph must be taken with a portable unit and the film exposed from the anterior direction. Both the anteroposterior exposure and the failure to take a deep inspiration result in an apparent enlargement of the cardiac silhouette, which further obscures the reliable detection of left ventricular failure.

indicates that ventilation-perfusion mismatching and, possibly, diffusion impairment account for the widened alveolar-arterial P_{O_2} difference $[(A-a)P_{O_2}]$ initially. Physical examination may be unremarkable, although a few fine inspiratory rales may be audible. Radiographically, the lung fields may be clear or demonstrate only minimal and scattered interstitial infiltrates. With progression, the patient becomes cyanotic and increasingly dyspneic and tachypneic. Rales become more prominent and easily heard throughout both lung fields, along with regions of tubular breath sounds; the chest radiograph demonstrates diffuse, extensive bilateral interstitial and alveolar infiltrates (Fig. 265-2). At this point, hypoxemia cannot be corrected simply by increasing the oxygen concentration of the inspired gas, and mechanical ventilatory support must be started. Right-to-left shunting of blood through collapsed or filled alveoli becomes the major mechanism for arterial hypoxemia at this more advanced stage. In contrast to ventilation-perfusion mismatching and diffusion impairment, with right-to-left shunts the $(A-a)P_{O_2}$ remains high with breathing of pure oxygen. Positive end-expiratory pressure (PEEP) serves to increase lung volume, which in turn opens collapsed alveoli and decreases shunting. With further progression, and if mechanical ventilator and PEEP therapy are delayed, the combination of increasing tachypnea and decreasing tidal volumes results in alveolar hypoventilation, a rising P_{CO_2}, and worsening hypoxemia; these represent an ominous constellation of findings.

℞ TREATMENT

Supportive Management of Hypoxemia   The simplest method and the lowest inspired fraction of oxygen ($F_{I_{O_2}}$) should be used to achieve a Pa_{O_2} of 60 mmHg (O_2 saturation approximately 90%). Higher levels add little to oxygenation and introduce the risk of oxygen toxicity to the lung. The three main methods for delivering O_2, in order of increasing effectiveness, are soft nasal prongs, simple face masks, and face masks with inspiratory reservoir bags. It is reasonable to start with moderate flow rates (5 to 10 L/min of 100% O_2) and to monitor arterial blood gases, adjusting the flow rates and O_2 concentrations depending on results.

Mechanical Ventilatory Support   In the presence of ARDS, adequate oxygenation is usually not maintained with these less invasive measures. Endotracheal intubation is needed, and mechanical ventilatory support with a volume-cycled ventilator should be instituted (see Chap. 266). The rationale behind mechanical ventilatory support in a patient who is hyperventilating is not to increase ventilation but to increase mean lung volume, thereby opening previously closed airways and improving oxygenation. The goal of ventilation for ARDS is to provide physiologic support for gas exchange while avoiding adverse mechanical consequences of the intervention. Because of the heterogeneous involvement of the lung in ARDS, setting tidal volumes to accomplish this goal for the lung as a whole carries the risk of overdistending or rupturing less affected alveoli and producing extraalveolar air (barotrauma). The latter is best avoided by limiting alveolar distending pressures through the use of relatively small tidal volumes (approximately 6 to 10 mL/kg of lean body weight) with a respiratory frequency set to deliver a minute volume that produces a pH above 7.25 to 7.30. Because of the small volume of aerated lung, high frequencies may be needed to provide an adequate minute volume. Alveolar inflation pressure, or peak inflation pressure, should be kept as low as possible consistent with sufficient ventilation and oxygenation. Inspired oxygen fraction ($F_{I_{O_2}}$) is initially set at 1.0 and then decreased in steps to the lowest inspired fraction that will maintain a Pa_{O_2} of 60 mmHg.

If Pa_{O_2} cannot be maintained at 60 mmHg by an $F_{I_{O_2}}$ of 60% or less, PEEP may be added. PEEP improves oxygenation by elevating mean alveolar pressure, thereby recruiting atelectatic alveoli and preventing end-expiratory airway and alveolar closure. Because an adequate PEEP level for affected lung regions may overdistend uninvolved alveoli, PEEP should be added cautiously, starting at

5 cmH$_2$O and increasing in increments of 3 to 5 cmH$_2$O to a maximum of 15 cmH$_2$O. Because airway pressure is transmitted to the pleural space, cardiac output may be adversely affected. The optimal levels of PEEP are those associated with the greatest delivery of O$_2$ to the body; the latter is the product of cardiac output and arterial oxygen content.

It is desirable to minimize left atrial and left ventricular diastolic pressures. Small decrements in pulmonary capillary wedge pressure (PCWP) have been shown to produce significant decreases in extra-vascular lung water. However, caution must be exercised in reducing PCWP, since excessively vigorous diuresis, especially in the setting of PEEP, may reduce cardiac output and the perfusion of critical organs. During interventions that change intravascular volume, placement of a Swan-Ganz pulmonary arterial flotation catheter may be instructive in monitoring cardiac output and PCWP in order to assess the effects of therapeutic interventions. Mental status and urine output should also be followed closely. The development of a wide anion gap metabolic acidosis should alert the clinician to the possibility of lactic acidemia due to inadequate tissue perfusion. Insufficient intravascular volume can be identified by a decrease of arterial pressure with the addition of modest amounts of PEEP. For these patients, blood volume should be expanded as long as cardiac output increases in response to the infusion and PCWP does not rise above 12 mmHg. Where volume repletion is necessary, crystalloid solutions are preferable to colloids.

Recent reports have drawn attention to inhaled nitric oxide (NO) (5 to 80 parts per million) as a selective pulmonary vasodilator with therapeutic promise in ARDS (Chap. 71).

Mixed venous blood P$_{O_2}$ values have long been considered to indicate the adequacy of oxygen delivery relative to demand. A low value (e.g., <20 mmHg) surely indicates that there is tissue hypoxemia, irrespective of measured cardiac output and Pa$_{O_2}$. However, a high value does not exclude serious tissue hypoxia, especially in gram-negative septicemia, in which systemic low-resistance shunts can develop and leave several capillary beds underperfused.

In situations where maximal PEEP with an F$_{I_{O_2}}$ of 1.0 does not supply sufficient oxygen, placing the patient in the prone position has been found to be helpful. Maintaining supranormal systemic oxygen transport does not improve, and may actually worsen, survival in ARDS.

Management of Sepsis Causing ARDS (See also Chap. 124) Therapy of the underlying infectious/inflammatory state should proceed along two lines: (1) identify and treat any infectious process, and (2) attempt to control the unregulated immune response that drives the acute lung injury. A localized source of sepsis must be drained quickly. Although the surgical mortality is high, failure to drain a purulent focus leads to an almost uniformly fatal outcome.

Glucocorticoids have shown no benefit in early ARDS, except in the settings of meningococcemia in children and *Pneumocystis carinii* pneumonia. Preliminary data suggest that glucocorticoids may be of some benefit in the fibroproliferative stage of late ARDS.

COMPLICATIONS Measures used in the management of ARDS have the potential to cause significant complications. Oxygen toxicity, due to prolonged use of F$_{I_{O_2}}$ above 50%, and excessive hydration may cause worsening of pulmonary infiltrates. High ventilator tidal volumes and pressures may lead to barotrauma. Prolonged mechanical ventilation predisposes to nosocomial pneumonia. ARDS and its underlying disorders may lead to the development of bronchopleural fistula or disseminated intravascular coagulation. Pulmonary fibrosis, irreversible pulmonary hypertension, or multiple organ failure suggest a poor prognosis when they are seen in ARDS.

PROGNOSIS Since the initial description of ARDS in the literature in 1967, mortality has ranged from 50 to 70 percent, although it may now be declining with optimal therapy. Age greater than 65 years, the number of associated organ system failures, sepsis, and severe gas

exchange disturbances are negative prognostic factors, while patients with uncomplicated drug overdoses or aspiration have better outcomes. The majority of deaths in ARDS are due to nonrespiratory causes. Sepsis accounts for the majority of early deaths, and multiple organ failure is a prominent cause of late mortality.

In survivors with previously normal lung function, the long-term prognosis for recovery is excellent. Lung volumes and arterial blood gases have been shown to return to normal or near-normal levels within 6 months after respiratory failure. There are instances, however, when the fibrotic residua are sufficiently great that complete recovery is unlikely.

BIBLIOGRAPHY

BERNARD GR et al: The American-European consensus conference on ARDS: Definitions, mechanisms, relevant outcomes, and clinical trial coordination. Am J Respir Crit Care Med 149:818, 1994

HICKLING KG et al: Low mortality rate in ARDS using low-volume, pressure-limited ventilation with permissive hypercapnia: A prospective study. Crit Care Med 22:1568, 1994

HUDSON LD et al: Clinical risks for development of the acute respiratory distress syndrome. Am J Respir Crit Care Med 151:293, 1995

KOLLEF MH, SCHUSTER DP: The acute respiratory distress syndrome. N Engl J Med 332:27, 1995

LEWIS JF, JOBE AH: Surfactant and the adult respiratory distress syndrome. Am Rev Respir Dis 147:218, 1993

MCHUGH LG et al: Recovery of function in survivors of the acute respiratory distress syndrome. Am J Respir Crit Care Med 150:90, 1994

MILBERG JA et al: Improved survival of patients with acute respiratory distress syndrome (ARDS):1983–1993. JAMA 273:306, 1995

MITCHELL JP et al: Improved outcome based on fluid management in critically ill patients requiring pulmonary artery catheterization. Am Rev Respir Dis 145:990, 1992

ROSSAINT R et al: Inhaled nitric oxide for the adult respiratory distress syndrome. N Engl J Med 328:399, 1993

266　*Edward P. Ingenito, Jeffrey M. Drazen*

MECHANICAL VENTILATORY SUPPORT

Ventilators are specially designed pumps that can support the ventilatory function of the respiratory system and improve oxygenation through application of high oxygen content gas and positive pressure. They are a mainstay of physiologic supportive care and are used to stabilize patients with respiratory failure as the underlying disease process is definitively treated.

INDICATIONS FOR MECHANICAL VENTILATION

Respiratory failure is the primary indication for initiation of mechanical ventilation. There are two basic types of respiratory failure.

Hypoxemic respiratory failure most commonly results from pulmonary conditions such as severe pneumonia, pulmonary edema, pulmonary hemorrhage, and respiratory distress syndrome causing ventilation-perfusion (V/Q) mismatch and shunt. Hypoxemic respiratory failure is present when arterial oxygen saturations of less than 90 percent are observed despite an inspired oxygen fraction of greater than 0.6. The goal of ventilator treatment in this setting is to provide adequate arterial oxygen saturation.

Hypercarbic respiratory failure results from disease states causing either a decrease in minute ventilation or an increase in physiologic dead space such that, despite adequate total minute ventilation, alveolar ventilation is inadequate to meet metabolic demands. Common clinical conditions associated with hypercarbic respiratory failure include neuromuscular diseases, such as myasthenia gravis, ascending polyradiculopathy, and myopathies, as well as diseases that cause respiratory muscle fatigue due to increased workload, such as asthma, chronic obstructive pulmonary disease, and restrictive lung disease. *Acute* hypercarbic respiratory failure is present when arterial P_{CO_2} values exceed 50 mmHg and the arterial pH is below 7.30 (Chap. 50). *Chronic* hypercarbic respiratory failure is characterized by arterial P_{CO_2} values of greater than 50 mmHg and an arterial pH above 7.30.

Mechanical ventilation generally should be instituted in acute hypercarbic respiratory failure. In contrast, the decision to institute mechanical ventilation when components of both acute and chronic hypercarbic respiratory failure are present depends on blood gas parameters and clinical evaluation. In particular, if a patient is not in respiratory distress and is not mentally impaired by CO_2 accumulation, it is not mandatory to initiate mechanical ventilation while other forms of treatment are being administered. The goal of ventilator treatment in hypercarbic respiratory failure is to normalize arterial pH through changes in carbon dioxide tensions. In patients with severe obstructive or restrictive lung disease, elevation in airway pressures may limit tidal volumes to the extent that normalization of pH is not possible, a situation known as *permissive hypercapnia*. Hypoxemic and hypercarbic respiratory failure may coexist in a given individual; in such cases, the indications for and goals of mechanical ventilation are similar to those in these two individual entities.

Accepted therapeutic applications of mechanical ventilation include controlled hyperventilation to reduce cerebral blood flow in patients with increased intracranial pressure or to improve pulmonary hemodynamics in patients with postoperative pulmonary hypertension. Mechanical ventilation also has been used to reduce the work of breathing in patients with congestive heart failure, especially in the presence of myocardial ischemia. Ventilator support is also frequently used in conjunction with endotracheal intubation to prevent aspiration of gastric contents in otherwise unstable patients during gastric lavage for suspected drug overdose or during upper gastrointestinal endoscopy. In the critically ill patient, intubation and mechanical ventilation are indicated before essential diagnostic or therapeutic studies if it appears that respiratory failure may occur during these maneuvers.

PHYSIOLOGIC ASPECTS OF MECHANICAL VENTILATION

Most modern mechanical ventilators function by providing warmed and humidified gas to the airway opening in conformance with various specific volume, pressure, and time patterns. The ventilator serves as the energy source for inspiration, replacing the muscles of the diaphragm and chest wall. Expiration is passive, driven by the recoil of the lungs and chest wall; at the completion of inspiration, internal ventilator circuitry vents the airway to atmospheric pressure or a specified level of positive end-expiratory pressure (PEEP).

PEEP helps maintain alveolar patency in the presence of destabilizing factors and therefore reverses hypoxemia and atelectasis by improving matching of ventilation and perfusion ($\dot{V}/\dot{Q}$). PEEP levels between 0 and 5 cmH$_2$O are generally safe and effective; higher levels are recommended only in the management of significant refractory hypoxemia unresponsive to increments in inspired oxygen content up to an inspired oxygen content (F_{IO_2}) of 0.6.

ESTABLISHING AN AIRWAY   A cuffed endotracheal tube must be inserted to allow positive-pressure ventilators to deliver conditioned gas, at pressures above atmospheric pressure, to the lungs in a controlled fashion. If neuromuscular paralysis is to be induced during intubation, the use of agents whose mechanism of action includes depolarization at the neuromuscular junction, such as succinylcholine chloride, should be avoided in patients with renal failure, tumor lysis syndrome, crush injuries, or medical conditions associated with elevated serum potassium levels because these agents may elevate the serum potassium levels to potentially lethal levels. Opiates and benzodiazepines can have a deleterious effect on hemodynamics in patients with depressed cardiac function or low systemic vascular resistance and should be used cautiously in this setting. Morphine can promote histamine release from tissue mast cells and may worsen bronchospasm in patients with asthma; fentanyl, sufentanil, and alfentanil are acceptable alternatives to morphine. Ketamine may increase systemic arterial pressure as well as intracranial pressure and has been associated with dramatic hallucinatory responses; it should be used with caution in patients with hypertensive crisis, increased intracranial pressures, or a history of psychiatric disorders.

VENTILATOR MODE   This setting specifies the manner in which ventilator breaths are triggered, cycled, and limited; commonly used modes of mechanical ventilation are given in Table 266-1. The *trigger,* either an inspiratory effort or a time-based signal, defines what the ventilator senses to initiate an assisted cycle. *Cycle* refers to the factors that determine the end of inspiration. For example, in volume-cycled ventilation, inspiration ends when a specific tidal volume is delivered to the patient. Other types of cycling include pressure cycling, time cycling, and flow cycling. *Limiting factors* are operator-specified values, such as airway pressure, that are monitored by transducers internal to the ventilator circuit throughout the respiratory cycle; if the specified values are exceeded, inspiratory flow is immediately stopped and the ventilator circuit vented to atmospheric pressure or the specified PEEP.

Assist Control Mode Ventilation (ACMV)   An inspiratory cycle is initiated either by the patient's inspiratory effort or, if no patient effort is detected within a specified time window, by a timer signal within the ventilator. Every breath delivered consists of the operator-specified tidal volume. Ventilatory rate is determined either by the patient or by the operator-specified backup rate, whichever is of higher frequency (Fig. 266-1A). ACMV is the recommended mode for initiation of mechanical ventilation because it ensures a backup minute ventilation in the absence of an intact respiratory drive and allows for synchronization of the ventilator cycle with the patient's inspiratory effort.

Problems can arise when ACMV is used in patients with tachypnea due to nonrespiratory or nonmetabolic factors such as anxiety, pain, or airway irritation. Respiratory alkalemia may develop and trigger myoclonus or seizures. Dynamic hyperinflation (so-called auto-PEEP) may occur if the patient's respiratory mechanics are such that inadequate time is available for complete exhalation between inspiratory cycles. Auto-PEEP can limit venous return, decrease cardiac output, and increase airway pressures, predisposing to barotrauma. ACMV is not effective for weaning patients from mechanical ventilation because it provides full ventilator assistance on each patient-initiated breath.

Synchronized Intermittent Mandatory Ventilation (SIMV)   The major difference between SIMV and ACMV is that in the former the patient is allowed to breathe spontaneously, i.e., without ventilator assist, between delivered ventilator breaths. However, mandatory breaths are delivered in synchrony with the patient's inspiratory efforts at a frequency determined by the operator. If the patient fails to initiate a breath, the ventilator delivers a fixed-tidal-volume breath and resets the internal timer for the next inspiratory cycle (see Fig. 266-1B). SIMV differs from ACMV in that only the preset number of breaths is ventilator-assisted.

SIMV allows patients with an intact respiratory drive to exercise inspiratory muscles between assisted breaths. This characteristic makes SIMV a useful mode of ventilation for both supporting and weaning intubated patients. SIMV may be difficult to use in patients with tachypnea because they may attempt to exhale during the ventilator-programmed inspiratory cycle. When this occurs, the airway pressure may exceed the inspiratory pressure limit, the ventilator-assisted breath will be aborted, and minute volume may drop below that programmed by the operator. In this setting, if the tachypnea is in response to respiratory or metabolic acidosis, a change to ACMV will increase minute ventilation and help normalize the pH while the underlying process is further evaluated.

Continuous Positive Airway Pressure (CPAP)   This is not a true support-mode of ventilation, since all ventilation occurs through the patient's spontaneous efforts. The ventilator provides fresh gas to the breathing circuit with each inspiration and charges the circuit to a constant, operator-specified pressure that can range from 0 to 20 cmH_2O (see Fig. 266-1*C*). CPAP is used to assess extubation potential in patients who have been effectively weaned and are requiring little ventilator support and in patients with intact respiratory system function who require an endotracheal tube for airway protection.

Pressure-Control Ventilation (PCV) This form of ventilation is time triggered, time cycled, and pressure limited. During the inspiratory phase, a given pressure is imposed at the airway opening, and the pressure remains at this user-specified level throughout inspiration (Fig. 266-2*A*). Since inspiratory airway pressure is specified by the operator, tidal volume and inspiratory flow rate are *dependent* rather than *independent* variables and are not user specified. PCV is the preferred mode of ventilation for patients with documented barotrauma, since airway pressures can be limited, and for postoperative thoracic surgical patients, in whom the shear forces across a fresh suture line should be limited. When using PCV, minute ventilation and tidal volume must be monitored; minute ventilation is altered through changes in rate or in the pressure-control value.

The major practical limitation of PCV is patient-ventilator asynchrony related to its time-cycled and time-triggered characteristics. Since PCV requires that the patient passively accept ventilator breaths, most patients require heavy sedation to be maintained on this ventilatory mode, which may be hazardous in the hemodynamically unstable patient.

Pressure-Support Ventilation (PSV) This form of ventilation is patient triggered, flow cycled, and pressure limited; it is specifically designed for use in the weaning process. During PSV, the inspiratory phase is terminated when inspiratory airflow falls below a certain level; in most ventilators this flow rate cannot be adjusted by the operator. When PSV is used, patients receive ventilator assist only when the ventilator detects an inspiratory effort (see Fig. 266-2*B*). PSV also can be used in combination with SIMV to ensure volume-cycled backup for patients whose respiratory drive is depressed either spontaneously or as a result of various therapeutic maneuvers.

PSV is well tolerated by most patients who are being weaned: PSV parameters can be set in such a way as to provide full or nearly full ventilatory support and can be withdrawn slowly over a period of days in a systematic fashion to gradually load the respiratory muscles.

Proportional Assist Ventilation (PAV) This recently developed mode of ventilation provides pressure assist at the airway opening in proportion to *patient effort* rather than at a preset designated pressure level or tidal volume. The level of ventilator support continuously varies throughout the respiratory cycle and from one cycle to the next as patient effort changes. This unique approach to ventilator support is thought to improve patient-ventilator synchrony by matching the level of support to inspiratory effort. It may, therefore, lower airways pressures and improve respiratory muscle conditioning.

Since PAV is strictly patient triggered, it cannot be used to support patients who lack an intact respiratory drive. It is currently being studied as an alternative to PSV for weaning patients from mechanical ventilation.

Table 266-1

Clinical Characteristics of Commonly Used Modes of Mechanical Ventilation

Independent Variables (Set by User)	Dependent Variables (Monitored by User)	Trigger/Cycle Limit	Advantages	Disadvantages	Initial Settings
ASSIST CONTROL MODE VENTILATION (ACMV)					
F_{IO_2}	Peak airway pressure,	Patient/timer	Timer backup	Not useful for weaning	$F_{IO_2} = 1.0$*
Tidal volume	Pa_{O_2}, Pa_{CO_2}		Patient-vent synchrony	Potential for dangerous	$V_t = 10-15$
Ventilator rate	Mean airway pressure	Pressure limit	Patient controls minute	respiratory alkalosis	mL/kg
Level of PEEP	I/E ratio		ventilation		$f = 12-15$/min
Inspiratory flow pattern					PEEP = $0-5$
Peak inspiratory flow					cmH_2O
Pressure limit					Inspiratory flow = 60 L/min
SYNCHRONIZED INTERMITTENT MANDATORY VENTILATION (SIMV)					
Same as for ACMV	Same as for ACMV	Same as for ACMV	Timer backup useful for weaning	Potential dysynchrony	Same as for ACMV
CONTINUOUS POSITIVE AIRWAY PRESSURE (CPAP)					
F_{IO_2}	Tidal volume	No trigger	Allows assessment of	No backup	$F_{IO_2} = 0.5-1.0$*
Level of CPAP	Rate, flow pattern		spontaneous function		CPAP = $5-15$
	Airway pressure	Pressure limit	Helps prevent atelectasis		cmH_2O
	Pa_{O_2}, Pa_{CO_2}, I/E ratio				
PRESSURE-CONTROL VENTILATION (PCV)					
F_{IO_2}	Tidal volume	Timer/patient	System pressures regulated	Requires heavy sedation	$F_{IO_2} = 1.0$*
Inspiratory pressure level	Flow rate, pattern	Timer/pressure limit	Useful for barotrauma treatment		PC = $20-40$ cmH_2O
Ventilator rate	Minute ventilation;		Timer backup	Not useful for weaning	PEEP = $5-10$
Level of PEEP	Pa_{O_2}, Pa_{CO_2}				cmH_2O
Pressure limit					$f = 12-15$/min
I/E ratio					I/E = 0.7/1 $-$ 4/1
PRESSURE-SUPPORT VENTILATION (PSV)					
F_{IO_2}	Same as for PCV + I/E ratio	Inspiratory flow	Ensures synchrony	No timer backup	$F_{IO_2} = 0.5-1.0$*
Inspiratory pressure level		Pressure limit	Good for weaning		PS = $10-30$ cmH_2O
PEEP					5 cmH_2O usually the level used
Pressure limit					PEEP = $0-5$ cmH_2O

* F_{IO_2} is usually set to 1.0 initially, unless there is a specific clinical indication to minimize F_{IO_2}, such as history of chemotherapy with bleomycin. Once adequate oxygenation is documented by blood gas analysis, F_{IO_2} should be decreased in decrements of 0.1 to 0.2 as tolerated, until the lowest F_{IO_2} required for an Sa_{O_2} of greater than 90 percent is achieved.

ABBREVIATIONS: f, frequency; I/E, inspiration/expiration.

EXTRACORPOREAL MEMBRANE OXYGENATION (ECMO) This nonconventional mode of ventilator support employs a large surface area membrane system connected in series with the patient's circulation to exchange CO_2 and O_2. The lung functions primarily as a passive conduit with gas exchange occurring by diffusion across the membrane. ECMO was first examined in 1970 as an alterna-

tive to positive-pressure ventilation in the management of patients with acute respiratory distress syndrome (ARDS). Initial studies failed to demonstrate an improvement in survival among patients treated with ECMO. Although several uncontrolled trials have since suggested that ECMO does improve outcome among ARDS patients, a 1993 study comparing survival among ARDS patients treated with ECMO and conventional ventilator therapy showed no mortality difference but increased morbidity and hospital costs among ECMO-treated patients. Presently, use of ECMO among patients with ARDS is not recommended.

COMPLICATIONS OF MECHANICAL VENTILATION

Endotracheal intubation and positive-pressure mechanical ventilation have direct and indirect effects on several organ systems, including the lung and upper airways, the cardiovascular system, and the gastrointestinal system. Pulmonary complications include barotrauma, nosocomial pneumonia, oxygen toxicity, tracheal stenosis, and deconditioning of respiratory muscles. *Barotrauma,* which occurs when high pressures (i.e., greater than 50 cmH$_2$O) disrupt lung tissue, is clinically

FIGURE 266-1 *A.* Airway pressure and lung volume versus time profile during ACMV. Assisted breaths are triggered by the patient's effort. Controlled breaths are triggered by the ventilator timer. Every breath, whether triggered by the patient or by the timer, is a complete volume-cycled breath, with airway pressure as a dependent variable. The pressure limit is set above the peak inspiratory pressure. *B.* Airway pressure and lung volume versus time profiles during SIMV. Spontaneous breaths occur between patient-triggered assisted breaths and timer-triggered breaths. The tidal volume of the spontaneous breaths is determined by the patient's effort and lung impedance. Assisted and controlled breaths are volume cycled. *C.* Airway pressure and lung volume versus time profiles during CPAP. Breathing is spontaneous, and no ventilator assist is provided. The spontaneous profile is superimposed on an elevated mean airway pressure that the user specifies.

FIGURE 266-2 *A.* Airway pressure and lung volume versus time profiles during PCV. All breaths are timer triggered, timer cycled, and pressure limited. Peak airway pressure is set by the operator, and tidal volume is a dependent variable. The profiles shown here display the pressure limit as slightly higher than pressure-control level. This need not be the case, but it is appropriate to set the pressure limit only slightly above the pressure-control level when using this mode of ventilation for management of the patient with barotrauma. *B.* Airway pressure and airway flow versus time profiles during PSV. All breaths are patient triggered and flow cycled. Inspiration is cycled off when the inspiratory flow drops below a predetermined threshold internally set in the ventilator circuit. In the example shown, the pressure limit is slightly greater than the pressure-support level. Since each can be set independently, this need not be the case.

manifest by interstitial emphysema, pneumomediastinum, subcutaneous emphysema, or pneumothorax. Although the former conditions may resolve simply by reducing airway pressures, clinically significant pneumothorax, as indicated by hypoxemia, decreased lung compliance, and hemodynamic compromise, requires tube thoracostomy.

Patients intubated for longer than 72 h are at high risk for *nosocomial pneumonia* as a result of aspiration from the upper airways via small leaks around the endotracheal tube cuff; the most common organisms responsible for this condition are enteric gram-negative rods, *Staphylococcus aureus*, and anaerobic bacteria. Because the endotracheal tube and upper airways of patients on mechanical ventilation are commonly colonized with bacteria, the diagnosis of nosocomial pneumonia requires "protected brush" bronchoscopic sampling of airway secretions coupled with quantitative microbiologic techniques to differentiate colonization from infection.

Oxygen toxicity is a potential complication when an $F_{I_{O_2}}$ of 0.6 or greater is required for more than 72 h. The condition can be prevented in some cases through the use of PEEP to allow $F_{I_{O_2}}$ values below 0.6 to be used while primary therapy for the underlying condition is instituted. Although oxygen toxicity is thought to result from the effects of oxygen free radicals on the lung interstitium, the therapeutic use of antioxidants such as superoxide dismutase, catalase, selenium, and vitamin E remains experimental.

Hypotension resulting from elevated intrathoracic pressures with decreased venous return is almost always responsive to intravascular volume repletion. In patients judged to have hypotension together with respiratory failure on the basis of alveolar edema, hemodynamic monitoring with a pulmonary arterial catheter may be of value in optimizing oxygen delivery via manipulation of intravascular volume, $F_{I_{O_2}}$ and PEEP levels.

Gastrointestinal effects of positive-pressure ventilation include *stress ulceration* and *mild to moderate cholestasis*. It is common practice to provide prophylaxis with H_2-receptor antagonists or sucralfate for stress-related ulcers. Mild cholestasis (i.e., total bilirubin values ≤ 4.0) attributable to the effects of increased intrathoracic pressures on portal vein pressures is common and generally self-limited. Cholestasis of a more severe degree should not be attributed to a positive-pressure ventilation response and is more likely due to a primary hepatic process. Additional complications, including malnutrition, decubitus ulcers, muscle deconditioning, venous thrombosis, and depression, are common and require appropriate treatment.

WEANING FROM MECHANICAL VENTILATION

Removal of mechanical ventilator support requires that a number of criteria be met. Upper airway function must be intact for a patient to remain extubated but is difficult to assess in the intubated patient. Therefore, if a patient can breathe on his or her own through an endotracheal tube but develops stridor or recurrent aspiration once the tube is removed, upper airway dysfunction or an abnormal swallowing mechanism should be suspected and plans for achieving a stable airway developed. An intact cough when respiratory secretions are suctioned is a good indicator of a patient's ability to mobilize secretions. Respiratory drive and chest wall function are assessed by observation of respiratory rate, tidal volume, inspiratory pressure, and vital capacity. The weaning index, defined as the ratio of breathing frequency to tidal volume (breaths per minute per liter), has been shown to be both sensitive and specific for predicting the likelihood of successful extubation. When this ratio is less than 105 with the patient breathing without mechanical assistance through an endotracheal tube, successful extubation is likely. An inspiratory pressure of more than -30 cmH$_2$O and

a vital capacity of greater than 10 mL/kg are considered indicators of acceptable chest wall and diaphragm function. Alveolar ventilation is generally adequate when systemic arterial P_{CO_2} is less than or equal to 45 mmHg, and arterial oxygen saturations greater than 90 percent can be achieved with an $F_{I_{O_2}}$ of less than 0.5 and a PEEP of 5 cmH$_2$O or less. Although many patients may not meet all criteria for weaning, the likelihood that a patient will tolerate extubation without difficulty increases as more criteria are met.

Many approaches to weaning patients from ventilator support have been advocated. T-piece and CPAP weaning are best tolerated by patients who have undergone mechanical ventilation for brief periods and require little respiratory muscle reconditioning, while SIMV and PSV are best for patients who have been intubated for extended periods and require gradual respiratory-muscle reconditioning.

T-piece weaning involves brief spontaneous breathing trials with supplemental oxygen. These trials are usually initiated for 5 min/h followed by a 1-h interval of rest. T-piece trials are increased in 5- to 10-min increments until the patient can remain ventilator independent for periods of several hours. Extubation can then be attempted. CPAP weaning is similar to T-piece weaning except that trials of spontaneous breathing are conducted on the ventilator in CPAP mode.

Weaning by means of SIMV/IMV involves gradually tapering the mandatory backup rate in increments of 2 to 4 breaths per minute while monitoring blood gas parameters and respiratory rates. Rates of greater than 25 breaths per minute upon withdrawal of mandatory ventilator breaths generally indicate respiratory muscle fatigue and the need to combine periods of exercise with periods of rest. Exercise periods are gradually increased until a patient remains stable on SIMV at 4 breaths per minute or less without needing rest at higher SIMV rates. A CPAP or T-piece trial can then be attempted before planned extubation.

PSV, as described in detail above, is used primarily for weaning from mechanical ventilation. PSV is usually initiated at a level adequate for full ventilator support (PSV$_{max}$); i.e., PSV is set slightly below the peak inspiratory pressures the patient requires during volume-cycled ventilation. The level of pressure support is then gradually withdrawn in increments of 5 cmH$_2$O until a level is reached at which the respiratory rate increases to 25 breaths per minute. At this point, intermittent periods of higher-pressure support are alternated with periods of lower-pressure support to provide muscle reconditioning without causing diaphragmatic fatigue. Gradual withdrawal of PSV continues until the level of support is just adequate to overcome the resistance of the endotracheal tube (approximately 5 cmH$_2$O). At that point, support can be discontinued and the patient extubated.

BIBLIOGRAPHY

BOUCHARD L et al: Comparison of three methods of gradual withdrawal from ventilatory support during weaning from mechanical ventilation. Am J Respir Crit Care Med 150:896, 1994

COHN IL et al: Mechanical ventilation for the elderly patient in intensive care. Incremental changes and benefits. JAMA 269:1025, 1993

ESTEBAN A et al: A comparison of four methods of weaning patients from mechanical ventilation. N Engl J Med 332:345, 1995

HINSON JR, MARINI JJ: Principles of mechanical ventilator use in respiratory failure. Annu Rev Med 43:341, 1992

INGENITO EP, DRAZEN JM: Mechanical ventilators, in *Principles of Critical Care*, JB Hall, GA Schmidt, LDH Wood (eds). New York, McGraw-Hill, 1992, pp 142–154

MORRIS AH et al: Randomized clinical trial of pressure control inverse ratio ventilation and extracorporeal membrane oxygenation for adult respiratory distress syndrome. Am J Respir Crit Care Med 149:295, 1994

RANIERI VM et al: Physiologic effects of positive end expiratory pressure in patients with chronic obstructive pulmonary disease during acute ventilatory failure and controlled mechanical ventilation. Am Rev Respir Dis 147:5, 1993

YOUNES M: Proportional assist ventilation: A new approach to ventilatory support. Am Rev Respir Dis 145:114, 1992

LUNG TRANSPLANTATION

Lung transplantation for end-stage lung disease has been a therapeutic option since the 1980s. Several transplant options are available for carefully selected patients: unilateral lung transplant, bilateral lung transplant, heart-lung transplant, and living related lobar transplant. The first successful type of transplant was heart-lung, which was performed for a variety of indications in increasing numbers through 1989. Beginning in 1989, the numbers of both unilateral and bilateral lung transplants performed increased dramatically and greatly reduced the number of donor organs available for heart-lung procedures. By 1994, unilateral and bilateral lung transplants had plateaued, however, at around 500 and 400 per year respectively, and heart-lung procedures had dropped to approximately 100 per year. In late 1995, the Registry of the International Society for Heart and Lung Transplantation reported a cumulative total of 1708 heart-lung transplants. Unilateral and bilateral transplant recipients both have 1-year survivals of 67 percent and 3-year survivals of around 50 percent. Heart-lung recipient survivals are 56 percent at 1 year and less than 20 percent at 10 years. Among the unilateral transplant recipients, disease subcategories appear to affect early survival, with emphysema patients enjoying the best 1-year survival, approximately 75 percent, and pulmonary fibrosis patients experiencing the worst, at just over 60 percent. Data on survival of living related lobar recipients are not yet available.

INDICATIONS Emphysema, either smoking-induced or secondary to α_1-antitrypsin deficiency, has been the single largest indication for lung transplantation. This disease accounts for almost 60 percent of all single-lung transplants, more than 30 percent of all bilateral lung, and 9 percent of heart-lung transplants. Other major indications for single-lung transplantation include idiopathic pulmonary fibrosis, primary pulmonary hypertension, and a variety of other rarer diseases. Cystic fibrosis patients are the largest group of bilateral lung recipients, accounting for approximately 36 percent of the total, followed by emphysema patients and primary pulmonary hypertension patients. The major diagnoses among heart-lung recipients are primary and secondary pulmonary hypertension (60 percent of recipients) and cystic fibrosis (15 percent of recipients). With the widespread use of isolated unilateral and bilateral transplants, the indications for heart-lung transplant have become very circumscribed, so that most of these patients now have either concomitant left ventricular disease and end-stage lung disease or irreparable congenital heart disease with Eisenmenger's syndrome (Chap. 235). Patients receiving living related lobar donations have been either children or young adults, and most have suffered from cystic fibrosis. In the majority of living related donations, the recipient has received two lower lobes—one transplanted on the right, one on the left—taken from two separate donors.

Recipient Selection Because donor lungs are the scarcest of the common solid organs transplanted, patients with end-stage lung disease undergo extensive evaluation to select the best potential candidates. In general, good candidates have severe, progressive lung disease with a projected life span of less than 2 years. They must not be active smokers; the length of time of smoking abstinence required prior to consideration for transplant varies among programs but is usually at least 6 months. In addition, they should have no other systemic disease with significant end-organ damage that would impact on the posttransplant outcome. This includes significant coronary artery disease, renal insufficiency, hepatic disease, severe osteoporosis, or significant neurologic impairment. Other comorbid conditions such as previous malignancy, systemic illnesses, and chronic unresolved infections outside the lung may also preclude lung transplant. Considerations that are thought, though not proven, to enhance outcomes include ambulatory status, adequate nutrition, demonstrated motivation/compliance, and psychosocial stability.

In the early years of lung transplantation, patients with prior thoracic surgery were felt to have an unacceptably high risk of postoperative hemorrhage, and patients on glucocorticoids were felt to be at high risk of anastomotic healing complications. With improvements in surgical technique and refinements in early postoperative immunosuppressive management, potential candidates are now rarely rejected for either of these reasons provided the surgery has not been multiple or extensive and the glucocorticoid dose is less than 20 mg/d. Many programs use age cutoffs of between 55 and 65 years in selecting potential recipients. While these age limits are arbitrary, international registry data confirm that recipients older than age 60 have poorer survivals.

It is often difficult in the case of specific pulmonary diseases to determine when patients are within the transplant "window"—that is, have disease advanced enough to fit within the category of "end-stage" yet are not so ill that they will not survive the rigorous transplant operation or die during the long pretransplant waiting period. However, experience in evaluating patients and published longitudinal data has identified useful criteria for identifying appropriate candidates (Table 267-1). Emphysema patients and patients with Eisenmenger's physiology are the most difficult groups in which to predict life expectancy; patients with severe limitations even in activities of daily living may still have survivals at 3 to 5 years that are comparable to patients who have undergone transplantation. Thus, in many centers, the selection of emphysema candidates for transplantation involves not only projected survivals but also quality-of-life issues. Selecting patients with Eisenmenger's physiology is even more difficult. Survivals of patients waiting for at least a year for transplantation have been as good or better than the 1-year survival of similar transplanted patients. Clearly, this group of patients does not behave in the same way as primary pulmonary hypertensive patients, and more specific selection criteria are needed.

There are regional variations in waiting times for transplantation, and minor differences in the listing criteria for individual centers will reflect anticipated length of wait.

Selection of Transplant Procedure The only diseases that currently mandate a specific procedure are (1) irreparable congenital cardiac defects with Eisenmenger's syndrome, which requires heart-lung transplant; (2) advanced lung disease with concomitant left ventricular dysfunction, which requires heart-lung transplant; and (3) septic lung disease (e.g., cystic fibrosis), which requires bilateral lung transplant or bilobar related donor lung transplant to reduce the likelihood of lethal disseminated infection. In essentially all other diseases, single-lung transplantation can be performed with acceptable early and midterm results. Bilateral lung transplantation may be performed if there is anticipated difficulty in postoperative management, especially in pulmonary hypertension, significant bullous disease in emphysema, young age, surgeon preference, or as dictated by individual patient considerations. It is not yet known whether unilateral and

---

Table 267-1

Physiologic Guidelines for Determining Lung Transplant "Window"

Chronic obstructive pulmonary disease
    Postbronchodilator FEV_1 < 30 percent predicted
    Resting hypoxia (Pa_{O_2} < 55–60 mmHg) or hypercapnia
    Significant secondary pulmonary hypertension
    Severe limitation in activities of daily living
Cystic fibrosis
    Postbronchodilator FEV_1 < 30 percent predicted
    Resting hypoxia (Pa_{O_2} < 55 mmHg) or hypercapnia (Pa_{CO_2} > 50 mmHg)
    Increasing numbers of exacerbations, complications
Idiopathic pulmonary fibrosis
    Vital capacity or total lung capacity < 60 percent predicted
    Resting hypoxia
    Significant secondary pulmonary hypertension
Primary pulmonary hypertension
    New York Heart Association functional class III or IV
    Mean right atrial pressure > 10 mmHg
    Mean pulmonary arterial pressure > 50 mmHg
    Cardiac index < 2.5 (L/min)/m^2

bilateral lung transplant recipients will have similar long-term survivals and functional outcomes. However, most transplant physicians agree that maximizing the donor organ resource by performing unilateral transplants whenever possible is currently the optimum policy.

FUNCTIONAL OUTCOMES A variety of tests have been used to evaluate lung transplant outcomes including arterial blood gases, perfusion scans, pulmonary function studies, compliance measurements, and exercise studies. Arterial blood gases in both unilateral and bilateral lung recipients improve markedly by 3 months posttransplant. In both types of recipients, P_{CO_2} normalizes; in bilateral transplants, P_{O_2} also normalizes. Unilateral transplant recipients may continue to have mild hypoxemia but rarely require supplemental oxygen. Perfusion studies in unilateral transplant recipients have shown that by 3 months posttransplant the donor lung receives approximately 80 percent of the perfusion; this may be higher if the underlying diagnosis is pulmonary hypertension. Pulmonary function studies in patients receiving either one or two lungs reach their maximum values by between 3 and 12 months postoperatively. Unilateral lung recipients who had a preoperative diagnosis of pulmonary parenchymal disease reach 60 to 65 percent of the maximum predicted values of FVC and FEV$_1$. Bilateral lung recipients can reach normal predicted values but often have mild restriction. A moderate amount of restriction has been reported in heart-lung recipients, but this may reflect a policy of selecting relatively small donor lungs. Nongraded exercise tolerance (6-min walk test) is similar for all lung recipient groups and ranges between 600 and 700 m per 6 min. Bilateral lung transplant patients perform better on graded exercise studies (e.g., modified Bruce protocol) than do unilateral transplant patients, but both groups achieve only 40 to 60 percent of predicted maximums. The reason for this exercise limitation, particularly in bilateral recipients, is not clear. In most cases, the exercise limitation does not impact upon normal daily living, and patients report significant improvement in quality of life following lung transplantation.

POSTTRANSPLANT MANAGEMENT ISSUES **Acute Rejection** More than 75 percent of lung transplant recipients will experience at least one episode of acute rejection. Most episodes occur within the first 3 months, but acute rejection can occur up to several years posttransplant. Patients usually present primarily with dyspnea but can also have cough, fever, and malaise. Findings include rales, hypoxemia, deteriorating FVC and FEV$_1$, and, as the process advances, perihilar infiltrates on chest x-ray and leukocytosis. Often, however, if the patient presents early, the x-ray is unremarkable. The diagnosis is best made by transbronchial biopsy, which is sensitive and specific, and, especially in the early posttransplant period, it helps to rule out infections such as cytomegalovirus (CMV), which has a similar presentation. Most episodes respond to high-dose intravenous methylprednisolone. Up to 20 percent of asymptomatic patients will have at least one episode of acute rejection on surveillance transbronchial biopsy during the first 2 years posttransplant. It is not clear whether asymptomatic rejection requires therapy, since its impact on outcome is unknown. This uncertainty has led to varying practices among institutions concerning the use of surveillance bronchoscopy, which can be quite expensive.

Bronchiolitis Obliterans Bronchiolitis obliterans is the primary manifestation of chronic rejection in lung transplants. Some degree of bronchiolitis obliterans occurs in up to 50 percent of patients who survive at least 5 years and is the cause of death in more than one-fourth of long-term survivors. The only factors that clearly have been shown to predispose patients to the development of bronchiolitis obliterans are the number and severity of acute rejection episodes. The onset, usually at least 6 months posttransplant, is often subacute, with gradual onset of shortness of breath, viral-type symptoms, or malaise. It can be asymptomatic and detected incidentally by the insidious development of airflow obstruction on pulmonary function testing. Histology by transbronchial biopsy can confirm the diagnosis but is generally not very sensitive; therefore, a typical clinical picture with

airflow obstruction in the absence of any other etiology is now considered sufficient to document *bronchiolitis obliterans syndrome*. Patients developing this syndrome may have a rapidly progressive loss of lung function, but more often they have a gradual progressive fall in FEV$_1$ over months or years or have a sudden drop in FEV$_1$ with subsequent stabilization.

Unfortunately treatment, which is with augmented immunosuppression, is rarely successful in reversing obstructive changes but may slow the loss of function for variable periods of time.

Infections Infections are second only to rejection as a cause of morbidity in the lung transplant population and are the most common cause of mortality, accounting for a third of all deaths occurring both during and after the first 3 postoperative months. Infections are more common in the lung transplant recipient than in any other solid-organ recipient. The transplanted lung may be uniquely vulnerable to infection because of impaired mucociliary clearance, loss of cough reflex, and other poorly defined local factors. In addition, the donor lungs are often colonized with organisms that are transmitted directly to the recipient. Some series have reported that at least 60 percent of lung recipients experience an infectious episode requiring treatment. Most of the infections are pulmonary, either pneumonia or bronchitis, and most are bacterial or viral, though recently fungal infections, especially with *Aspergillus*, have been increasingly reported. Bacterial infections are caused most often by gram-negative bacilli or staphylococcal organisms. CMV infection with pneumonitis, as with all solid-organ transplants, remains a significant threat, especially in the highest risk group in which the donor is CMV serology–positive and the recipient is CMV serology–negative. Elaborate systems of antimicrobial prophylaxis, employed now by most centers, along with the increased experience of transplant physicians appear to have been effective in reducing the morbidity from the viral, bacterial, and *Pneumocystis carinii* organisms. Antifungal prophylaxis is also often used since invasive fungal infections have a high mortality rate. The two particularly high-risk periods for infection are in the first 3 post-operative months and late after transplant if the patient develops bronchiolitis obliterans. In the early posttransplant period, it may be very difficult to distinguish infection from rejection, and bronchoscopy with transbronchial biopsies and appropriate cultures are often required to make a diagnosis.

Late after transplant, many patients with bronchiolitis obliterans have an increased risk of bacterial infection. These patients often develop bronchiectasis, become chronically colonized with *Pseudomonas* organisms, and experience repeated episodes of *Pseudomonas* bronchitis or pneumonia.

Airway Complications Careful examination of posttransplant airways in the first few postoperative weeks reveals many small dehiscences, but approximately 15 percent of lung transplant recipients experience airway stenosis requiring either dilation, laser resection, or stenting. Other airway problems include impairment of the mucociliary clearance and the development of bronchial hyperreactivity by many patients. These changes may be due to denervation, ischemia, and low-grade chronic airway inflammation.

Immunosuppressive Complications These are common in lung transplant recipients. Nephrotoxicity, hypertension, and hyperlipidemia occur in the majority of patients treated with current immunosuppressive regimens; however, fewer than 5 percent develop renal failure requiring dialysis or renal transplant. Neurotoxicity, including strokes, coma, severe headaches, and seizures, occurs in up to 20 percent of patients, as does osteoporosis with vertebral compressions or other fractures. Lymphoproliferative disorders occur within the first year in approximately 5 percent of lung transplant recipients; many of these appear to be related to infection with Epstein-Barr virus. Late after transplant, there is an increased incidence of many types of carcinoma and non-Hodgkin's lymphoma.

Recurrence of Underlying Disease Recently, several episodes of recurrence of the underlying disease have been reported in patients undergoing lung transplantation. Several transplant centers have reported the recurrence of sarcoidosis in transplanted lungs, usually as a histologic diagnosis and not clinically apparent. There have also been case reports of recurrent lymphangioleiomyomatosis, giant cell interstitial pneumonitis, and panbronchiolitis. Presumably, α_1-antitrypsin deficiency–related emphysema (Chap. 258) will recur in susceptible patients if they survive long enough, but this has not yet been reported; α_1-antitrypsin replacement therapy is not universally employed in these patients. It must be made clear to all lung transplant recipients that permanent abstinence from smoking is necessary. The abnormal electrical potentials characteristic of cystic fibrosis epithelium (Chap. 257) do not develop in the normal lungs transplanted into cystic fibrosis patients.

BIBLIOGRAPHY

AMERICAN THORACIC SOCIETY: Lung transplantation. Report of the ATS workshop on lung transplantation. Am Rev Respir Dis 147:772, 1993

GROVER FL, ZAMORA MR (eds): Lung transplantation. Semin Resp Crit Care Med 17(2):1996

HOSENPUD JD et al: The Registry of the International Society for Heart and Lung Transplantation. Twelfth official report, 1995. J Heart Lung Transplant 14:805, 1995

PATTERSON GA (ed): Lung transplantation. Semin Thorac Cardiovasc Surg 4(2):1992

268 *Fredric L. Coe, Barry M. Brenner*

APPROACH TO THE PATIENT WITH DISEASES OF THE KIDNEYS AND URINARY TRACT

Diseases of the kidneys and urinary tract frequently give rise to consistent arrays or clusters of clinical signs, symptoms, and laboratory findings called *syndromes*. Syndromes are useful diagnostically because each has fewer causes than the individual clinical signs and symptoms it contains. For example, any injured capillary bed from glomerulus to urethral meatus can cause hematuria, but only glomerular injury also can cause heavy albuminuria and erythrocyte casts (Chap. 47), and only a few of the diseases that injure the glomerular capillaries enough to cause hematuria and proteinuria also cause a rapid fall in glomerular filtration rate. Routine clinical evaluation is often sufficient to suggest that a particular syndrome may be present (Table 268-1), but additional laboratory measurements beyond the routine, as well as radiologic and/or urologic evaluation and sequential clinical observations, are usually required to establish the diagnosis. This chapter presents the general features of the syndromes, lists the clinical and laboratory data required for their recognition, and outlines the diseases that cause them. Succeeding chapters describe the diseases and their treatment in detail.

ACUTE AND RAPIDLY PROGRESSIVE RENAL FAILURE

Whether the glomerular filtration rate (GFR) falls over days (acute renal failure; ARF) or weeks (rapidly progressive renal failure; RPRF) is a useful distinction, because the causes of these two syndromes are somewhat different (Table 268-1). For example, acute tubular necrosis, from sepsis, nephrotoxic materials, shock, or other cause (see Chap. 270), is the usual cause of ARF, whereas extracapillary proliferative (crescentic) glomerulonephritis, due to immunologic injury or to vasculitis, is an important cause of RPRF but not ARF (Chap. 274).

Proof for the existence of either syndrome requires serial determination of the GFR, blood urea nitrogen, or serum creatinine level. Anuria or oliguria (Chap. 47) strongly suggests ARF, since life cannot be sustained for long with such inadequate renal function. Symptoms and signs of uremia of recent onset suggest RPRF or ARF but also could result from chronic renal failure (CRF) that has only recently become life-threatening. Although edema, hypertension, and abnormalities of electrolytes and the urine sediment (Table 268-1) are frequent in both ARF and RPRF, they occur in other syndromes as well and are not specific.

Urinary obstruction, acute tubular necrosis, some forms of vasculitis, major renal vascular accidents, and endogenous and exogenous nephrotoxins are common causes of ARF. Vasculitis and crescentic glomerulonephritis are common causes of RPRF. Hemolytic-uremic syndrome, malignant nephrosclerosis, and essential mixed cryoimmunoglobulinemia occasionally present as RPRF. Idiopathic rapidly progressive glomerulonephritis—the prototype of a disease that produces RPRF—sometimes causes ARF. CRF may occur in some patients with diseases that typically cause ARF. Nevertheless, despite some variability of disease presentations, the finding of ARF or RPRF narrows the range of causes.

ACUTE NEPHRITIS

A number of diseases involve the glomeruli and, to a generally lesser extent, the tubules in an acute but transient inflammatory process, manifested clinically by acute reduction in GFR and salt and water retention. This process is called *glomerulonephritis*. Expansion of the extracellular volume, if marked, causes hypertension, pulmonary vascular congestion, and facial and peripheral

edema (Chap. 274). Since the causes of this syndrome all can damage the glomerular wall enough to permit red blood cells and plasma proteins to enter the urinary space and appear in the urine, gross or microscopic hematuria, red blood cell casts, and proteinuria are necessary for the diagnosis of acute glomerulonephritis, and their absence suggests other diagnoses. Acute glomerulonephritis is a transient inflammatory process, so its clinical and laboratory manifestations wax and wane over days to weeks. Many of the diseases that cause acute glomerulonephritis also cause ARF or RPRF. When acute glomerulonephritis is associated with RPRF, the term *rapidly progressive glomerulonephritis* is often applied as a clinical diagnosis, pending biopsy delineation of the precise disease process. Other diseases cause an acute but transitory inflammation of the tubules and interstitium (acute tubulointerstitial nephritis) but not of the glomerular capillaries. Hematuria, red blood cell casts, and reduction of GFR occur, as in acute glomerulonephritis, but proteinuria is less marked and, when present, consists mainly of low-molecular-weight proteins rather than albumin. Apart from the lesser proteinuria, tubulointerstitial nephritis may be manifested by increased urine leukocytes and especially urine eosinophils, as well as by peripheral blood eosinophilia.

Acute glomerulonephritis following infection with group A streptococci is the prototype of a disease that causes acute nephritis alone (Chap. 274). Immune complexes deposit in the subepithelial region of the glomerular capillary wall, between the basement membrane and the visceral epithelial cells that separate the membrane from the urinary space, and provoke an intense but transient inflammatory process. GFR falls but returns to normal within weeks to months in most patients. Deposition of immune complexes is also believed to be the cause of acute nephritis following other bacterial and viral infections and of lupus nephritis, membranoproliferative glomerulonephritis, Henoch-Schönlein purpura, and Berger's disease, i.e., IgA nephropathy. That the typical presentations of the last four diseases are chronic renal failure, nephrotic syndrome, and asymptomatic urinary abnormalities illustrates the weakness of relationships between pathogenesis and final clinical manifestations.

Renal biopsy is usually required for the evaluation of patients with acute nephritis, whether or not ARF or RPRF is also present. In patients with RPRF and glomerulonephritis (rapidly progressive glomerulonephritis), the usual histologic picture is that of proliferative glomerulonephritis, often with extracapillary crescent formation. However, this picture may also occur in patients without RPRF, and many other forms of histologic abnormality may be found in patients with acute glomerulonephritis. Thus, prediction of histopathology from clinical course is very uncertain. Prognosis and treatment are influenced strongly by the precise histologic and ultrastructural pattern, as well as the types of immune complexes and immunoglobulins deposited in the renal tissues. In patients with acute tubulointerstitial nephritis, inflammatory changes are prominent in the renal interstitium and evidence of tubule cell injury may be present, but glomerular abnormalities are often absent altogether.

CHRONIC RENAL FAILURE

CRF results from progressive and irreversible destruction of nephrons, regardless of cause (Chap. 271). This diagnosis implies that the GFR is known to have been reduced for at least 3 to 6 months (see Table 268-1). Often a gradual decline in GFR occurs over a period of years. Proof of chronicity is also provided by the demonstration of bilateral reduction of kidney size by scout film, ultrasonography, intravenous pyelography, or tomography. Other findings of long-standing renal failure, such as renal osteodystrophy or symptoms of uremia, also help to establish this syndrome. Several laboratory abnormalities are often regarded as reliable indicators of chronicity of renal disease, such as anemia, hyperphosphatemia, or hypocalcemia, but these are not specific (Chap. 269).

In contrast, the finding of broad casts in the urinary sediment (Chap. 47) is specific for CRF, the wide diameters of these casts reflecting the compensatory dilatation and hypertrophy of surviving nephrons. Proteinuria is a frequent but nonspecific finding, as is hematuria. Chronic obstructive uropathy, polycystic and medullary cystic diseases, analgesic nephropathy, and the inactive end stage of any chronic tubulointerstitial nephropathy are conditions in which the urine often contains little or no protein, cells, or casts even though nephron destruction has progressed to chronic renal failure.

When ARF occurs in the presence of CRF, the acute component must be evaluated as if CRF were not present, because the acute component is potentially reversible. In most instances, depletion of extracellular fluid volume is the cause of acute deterioration of renal function, but urinary tract obstruction, drug-induced nephrotoxicity, or exacerbation of underlying renal disease also may be responsible (Chap. 271).

NEPHROTIC SYNDROME This diagnosis previously implied that a patient excretes more than 3.5 g protein per 1.73 m^2 surface area per 24 h; the proteinuria consists mainly of albumin; and that the patient has reduced serum albumin, edema, and hyperlipidemia (Table 268-1). Massive proteinuria alone has now come to define the syndrome, since this finding connotes serious renal disease whether or not the protein losses lead to hypoalbuminemia, lipid disturbances, or edema (Chap. 47). Provided the proteins in the urine are not paraproteins readily excreted by the normal kidney (e.g., immunoglobulin

light chains in multiple myeloma), massive proteinuria is invariably a sign of injury to the glomeruli.

Common causes of the nephrotic syndrome include minimal change disease, idiopathic membranous glomerulopathy, focal and segmental glomerulosclerosis, and diabetic glomerulosclerosis (Chaps. 274 and 275). Because these diseases typically cause less inflammation than those that cause acute nephritis, the urine usually contains fewer cellular elements, and acute changes in GFR and urine volume are uncommon. Hematuria may occur in some forms of nephrotic syndrome, however, especially chronic membranoproliferative glomerulonephritis (Chap. 274). The presence of cellular or granular casts should suggest lupus nephritis (Chap. 275) or acute nephritis associated with massive proteinuria, such as essential mixed cryoimmunoglobulinemia, acute bacterial endocarditis, visceral sepsis, and Henoch-Schönlein purpura.

ASYMPTOMATIC URINARY ABNORMALITIES Mild microscopic hematuria, pyuria, and casts or less than 3.5 g protein per 1.73 m^2 surface area per 24 h may be present in the urine of a patient with no evidence of other nephrologic syndromes. By exclusion, these patients belong to the syndrome of asymptomatic urinary abnormalities. Isolated hematuria or proteinuria, or unexplained pyuria, are the most frequent abnormalities in this syndrome.

Isolated hematuria, without proteinuria or casts, may be the sole clue to the presence of neoplasm, stone, or infection (e.g., tuberculosis) in any part of the urinary tract (Chaps. 47, 96, 270, and 280). Isolated hematuria also may arise from renal papillae in analgesic and sickle cell nephropathies (Chaps. 276 and 277). Persistent isolated hematuria often requires intravenous pyelography, cystoscopy, and, occasionally,

Table 268-1

Initial Clinical and Laboratory Data Base for Defining Major Syndromes in Nephrology

Syndromes	Important Clues to Diagnosis	Findings that are Common	Location of Discussion of Diseases Causing Syndrome
Acute or rapidly progressive renal failure	Anuria Oliguria Documented recent decline in GFR	Hypertension, hematuria Proteinuria, pyuria Casts, edema	Chaps. 270, 274, 276, 277, 280
Acute nephritis	Hematuria, RBC casts Azotemia, oliguria Edema, hypertension	Proteinuria Pyuria Circulatory congestion	Chaps. 273, 274, 275
Chronic renal failure	Azotemia for >3 months Prolonged symptoms or signs of uremia Symptoms or signs of renal osteodystrophy Kidneys reduced in size bilaterally Broad casts in urinary sediment	Hematuria, proteinuria Casts, oliguria Polyuria, nocturia Edema, hypertension Electrolyte disorders	Chaps. 269, 271
Nephrotic syndrome	Proteinuria >3.5 g per 1.73 m^2 per 24 h Hypoalbuminemia Hyperlipidemia Lipiduria	Casts Edema	Chaps. 270, 275
Asymptomatic urinary abnormalities	Hematuria Proteinuria (below nephrotic range) Sterile pyuria, casts		Chap. 274
Urinary tract infection	Bacteriuria >10^5 colonies per milliliter Other infectious agent documented in urine Pyuria, leukocyte casts Frequency, urgency Bladder tenderness, flank tenderness	Hematuria Mild azotemia Mild proteinuria Fever	Chap. 131
Renal tubule defects	Electrolyte disorders Polyuria, nocturia Symptoms or signs of renal osteodystrophy Large kidneys Renal transport defects	Hematuria "Tubular" proteinuria Enuresis	Chaps. 276, 278
Hypertension	Systolic/diastolic hypertension	Proteinuria Casts Azotemia	Chaps. 38, 246, 277
Nephrolithiasis	Previous history of stone passage or removal Previous history of stone seen by x-ray Renal colic	Hematuria Pyuria Frequency, urgency	Chap. 279
Urinary tract obstruction	Azotemia, oliguria, anuria Polyuria, nocturia, urinary retention Slowing of urinary stream Large prostate, large kidneys Flank tenderness, full bladder after voiding	Hematuria Pyuria Enuresis, dysuria	Chap. 280

renal arteriography to identify the source of bleeding. *Nephronal hematuria*,
CHAPTER 268
Approach to the Patient with Diseases of the Kidneys and Urinary Tract **1497**

renal arteriography to identify the source of bleeding. *Nephronal hematuria*, in which casts contain red blood cells or hemoglobin pigment, indicates damage to the nephron (Chap. 47). It occurs without proteinuria, mainly in benign recurrent hematuria and Berger's disease (Chap. 274). *Nephronal hematuria and proteinuria* occur together in many renal diseases that may lead to chronic renal failure (Chap. 271). In general, the combination of nephronal hematuria and proteinuria suggests a worse prognosis than either alone.

Isolated proteinuria, without red blood cells or other formed elements in the urinary sediment, is characteristic of many renal diseases that manifest little or no inflammatory reaction within the glomeruli (e.g., diabetes mellitus, amyloidosis). Less than nephrotic-range proteinuria is common in mild forms of all the diseases that can cause overt nephrotic syndrome (Chaps. 274 and 275). "Tubular" proteinuria (Chap. 47) is the rule in cystinosis; in intoxication from cadmium, lead, or mercury; and in the peculiar Balkan nephropathy localized to a small region along the Danube River (Chap. 276).

Pyuria (leukocyturia) also may be a sole urinary abnormality and may reflect infection or inflammation of the lower urinary tract rather than parenchymal renal disease. Nevertheless, prominent pyuria can occur in any inflammatory disease of the kidneys, especially tubulointerstitial nephritis, lupus nephritis, pyelonephritis, and renal transplant rejection, but usually in association with mild proteinuria or hematuria. The finding of leukocyte casts (Chap. 47) establishes the kidney as the site of the inflammatory reaction.

Pyuria associated with urine that is sterile on *routine* bacteriologic culture presents a special problem. Causes of "sterile pyuria" include (1) recent bacterial urinary infection being treated with antibiotics, (2) glucocorticoid therapy, (3) acute febrile episodes, (4) cyclophosphamide administration, (5) pregnancy, (6) renal transplant rejection, (7) genitourinary trauma, (8) prostatitis and cystourethritis, and (9) all forms of tubulointerstitial nephritis. Leukocytes from vaginal secretions may contaminate the urine, so a midstream, clean-catch urine sample should be collected to substantiate a urinary origin. Pyuria associated with proteinuria, nephronal hematuria (Chap. 47), or casts usually signifies inflammatory disease of the renal glomeruli, tubules, interstitium, or microcirculation, and evaluation should focus not on the pyuria but on the nature of the renal disease.

Persistent sterile pyuria that cannot be ascribed to any of the foregoing causes has a narrow differential diagnosis. Unusual infections, such as tuberculosis, fungi, atypical mycobacteria, *Haemophilus influenzae*, anaerobic bacteria, fastidious bacteria that grow only on enriched media, and L forms, all must be sought. Intravenous pyelography may be needed to detect causes such as urinary tract calculi, papillary necrosis, and renal infiltration by lymphoma or myeloma cells. The latter is usually suspected because of other evidence of myeloma or lymphoma, for both rarely involve only the kidneys. If all tests are negative, cystoscopy may reveal cystitis or trigone inflammation.

URINARY TRACT INFECTION This syndrome is defined by the demonstration in urine of pathogenic organisms, either bacteria, tubercle bacilli, or fungi (Chap. 131). When urine is obtained for culture, the condition under which the urine is collected must minimize contamination from external surfaces. Women should void into a wide-mouthed sterile container after preliminary cleansing of the vulva with a moist, sterile gauze pledget. In men, midstream collection is usually adequate. Bacterial colony counts of 10^5 organisms per milliliter or greater in urine generally indicate urinary tract colonization and infection. Levels above 10^2 colonies per milliliter are sufficient to indicate infection in symptomatic patients (Table 268-1) and in urine samples obtained by suprapubic aspiration or bladder catheter. When the urinary tract is anatomically normal, *Escherichia coli* is the usual pathogen. After prolonged antibiotic treatment of persistent infections, particularly when urinary drainage is impaired or stones are present, *Klebsiella*, *Enterobacter*, and *Proteus* species predominate.

As discussed in Chap. 131, a positive urine culture need not imply that an organism is producing tissue inflammation or injury. In some patients, tissue effects may be trivial; in others, injury may occur even though symptoms or urinary abnormalities are not present at the time of evaluation. When bacteriuria is associated with tissue inflammation or injury, clinical manifestations usually depend on the site(s) involved. Dysuria, frequency, urgency, and suprapubic tenderness are common symptoms of bladder and urethral inflammation (Chap. 47 and Table 268-1). Prostatitis also leads to frequency, dysuria, and urgency, and the prostate may be boggy and tender on rectal examination. Flank pain, chills, fever, nausea and vomiting, hypotension from sepsis, and leukocyte casts all suggest true renal parenchymal infection, i.e., pyelonephritis; their absence, however, does not exclude pyelonephritis.

RENAL TUBULE DEFECTS This syndrome encompasses a large number of acquired and hereditary disorders, all of which tend to affect tubules more than glomeruli. Hereditary anatomic defects, including polycystic renal disease, medullary cystic disease, and medullary sponge kidney, are readily detected by ultrasonography or intravenous pyelography, which are usually performed because of hematuria, bacteriuria, flank pain, or unexplained azotemia (Chap. 278).

Defects in tubule transport functions, on the other hand, tend not to be associated with prominent renal anatomic defects and arise either as inherited traits (Chap. 278) or during the course of acquired renal disease (Chap. 276). In general, these functional defects impair secretion and/or reabsorption of electrolytes and organic solutes or limit urinary concentrating and diluting ability (see Table 268-1). Typical manifestations of such functional disturbances include polyuria and nocturia (Chap. 47), metabolic acidosis (Chap. 50), and various disorders of fluid and electrolyte balance (Chap. 49). Such defects are defined by direct physiologic measurements; their elucidation requires a sound understanding of normal renal physiology.

HYPERTENSION Hypertension implies that the average of a series of reliable blood pressure measurements exceeds 140 mmHg systolic or 90 mmHg diastolic (see Table 268-1). The pathogenetic mechanisms, clinical and laboratory manifestations, and therapeutic approaches are discussed in detail elsewhere (Chaps. 38 and 246). In addition, a number of renal complications of hypertension are reviewed in Chap. 277, as is the entity of renal artery stenosis, an infrequent but potentially curable cause of hypertension.

NEPHROLITHIASIS This syndrome is recognized with certainty when a stone is passed, visualized by x-ray, or removed at surgery or cystoscopy (see Table 268-1 and Chap. 279). Less certain, but suggestive, evidences of nephrolithiasis include renal colic; painful hematuria; or unexplained pyuria, dysuria, and urinary frequency (Chap. 47). Colic varies in its symptomatology but usually begins suddenly in one flank, radiates downward toward the groin, and is excruciatingly painful.

Most renal stones are composed of calcium, uric acid, cystine, or struvite (magnesium ammonium phosphate). All are radiopaque except for uric acid stones and are therefore visible by routine abdominal radiography. Uric acid stones appear as radiolucent filling defects and can be mistaken for tumor or blood clot.

URINARY TRACT OBSTRUCTION Documentation of the various structural or functional causes of urinary tract obstruction usually requires radiologic or surgical visualization. The most common initial evaluation at present is renal ultrasonography, although false-negative evaluations are not rare, especially when urine flow rate is low. The manifestations of obstruction, which initiate the search for its causes, are numerous (see Table 268-1) and are reviewed in Chap. 280. Anuria in an adult is almost always due to obstruction of bladder outflow. Less commonly, blockage of upper urinary drainage from both kidneys or from a solitary functioning kidney accounts for total or near-total cessation of urine flow. A large bladder after voiding is a sign of outflow obstruction, usually due to urethral stricture, tumor, stone, neurogenic causes, or prostatic hypertrophy. Nocturia, frequency and overflow incontinence, and slowing or hesitancy of micturition also suggest outflow obstruction (Chap. 47). Upper tract obstruction often produces few manifestations. When it is incomplete or unilateral, urine volume may be normal or even increased because of a loss of renal concentrating ability. Urinary stasis secondary to obstruction predisposes to recurrent urinary tract infection; chronic obstruction predisposes to progressive loss of renal function.

BIBLIOGRAPHY

KASISKE BL, KEANE WF: Laboratory assessment of renal disease. Clearance, urinalysis, and renal biopsy, in *The Kidney,* 5th ed, BM Brenner (ed). Philadelphia, Saunders, 1996, p 1137

ROSENBERG ME, HOSTETTER TH: Proteinuria, in *The Kidney,* DW Seldin, G Giebisch (eds). New York, Raven, 1992, p 3039

TISHER CC, CROKER BP: Indications for and interpretation of the renal biopsy. Evaluation by light, electron and immunofluorescence microscopy, in *Diseases of the Kidney,* RW Schrier, CW Gottschalk (eds). Boston, Little, Brown, 1993, p 485

---

269   *Barry M. Brenner, Harald S. Mackenzie*

DISTURBANCES OF RENAL FUNCTION

Near constancy of the composition of the internal environment, including the volume, tonicity, and compartmental distribution of the body fluids, is essential to survival. With day-to-day variations in the intake of food and water, preservation of the internal environment requires the excretion of these substances in amounts that balance the quantities ingested. Although losses from intestines, lungs, and skin contribute to this excretory capacity, the greatest responsibility for solute and water excretion is borne by the kidneys.

The kidneys regulate the composition and volume of the plasma water. This, in turn, determines the composition and volume of the entire *extracellular* fluid compartment. Through the continuous exchange of water and solutes across all cell membranes, the kidneys influence the *intracellular* fluid compartment as well. These functions are served by a variety of physiologic mechanisms that enable individuals to excrete excesses of water and nonmetabolized solutes contained in the diet, as well as the nonvolatile end products of nitrogen metabolism, such as urea and creatinine. Conversely, when faced with deficits of water or solute, excretion of water or specific solute(s) is curtailed via appropriate mechanisms for renal conservation, reducing the likelihood of volume or solute depletion. The purpose of this chapter is to review the excretory functions of the kidney and to examine how these functions are affected by chronic renal disease.

EFFECTS OF NEPHRON LOSS ON RENAL EXCRETORY MECHANISMS

The volume of urine excreted (averaging 1.5 L/day or roughly 1 mL/min) represents the sum of two large, directionally opposite processes—namely, *ultrafiltration* of 180 L/day or more of plasma water (or 125 mL/min) and *reabsorption* of more than 99 percent of this filtrate by transport processes in the renal tubules. Renal blood flow accounts for about 20 percent of resting cardiac output, yet the kidneys comprise only about 1 percent of total body weight. This disproportionate allocation of cardiac output, greatly exceeding blood flow per gram of brain, heart, or liver, is required for the process of ultrafiltration.

GLOMERULAR ULTRAFILTRATION   Urine production begins at the glomerulus where an ultrafiltrate of plasma is formed. The rate of glomerular ultrafiltration (glomerular filtration rate, GFR) is governed chiefly by forces favoring filtration on the one hand (hydraulic pressure in the glomerular capillaries) and forces opposing filtration on the other (the sum of hydraulic pressure in Bowman's space and colloid osmotic pressure in the glomerular capillaries). The rate of glomerular plasma flow and the total surface area of the glomerular capillaries are also determinants of glomerular filtration

rate. Decreased glomerular filtration rate can therefore be expected when (1) glomerular hydraulic pressure is reduced (as in circulatory shock); (2) tubule (hence Bowman's space) hydraulic pressure is elevated, as in urinary tract obstruction; (3) plasma colloid osmotic pressure rises to high levels (hemoconcentration due to severe volume depletion, myeloma, or other dysproteinemias); (4) renal, and hence glomerular, blood flow is reduced (severe hypovolemia, cardiac failure); (5) permeability is reduced (diffuse glomerular disease); or (6) filtration surface area is diminished, through focal or diffuse nephron loss in progressive renal failure.

The glomerular capillary wall is specially adapted to allow passage of extremely large volumes of water yet retain all but the smallest solute molecules. Molecules the size of inulin (approximately 5200 mol wt) pass freely across the glomerular filtration barrier, appearing at approximately the same concentration in Bowman's space as in plasma. The passage of solutes across the glomerular barrier decreases progressively with increasing molecular size such that, as the molecular weight of albumin is approached, most of the solute is retained in the plasma. Albumin, a polyanionic molecule in plasma, is further retarded at the glomerular filtration barrier by *electrostatic forces* imparted by negatively charged cell surface molecules on the epithelial foot processes that form the *filtration slits* and the *slit diaphragms.* With disruption of these structural and electrostatic barriers, as in many forms of glomerular injury (see Chaps. 273 to 275), large quantities of plasma proteins gain access to the glomerular filtrate.

Glomerular Adaptations to Nephron Loss   With loss of nephron mass, the remaining healthy (or least injured) nephrons tend to hypertrophy and take on an increased functional burden so that the overall loss of function is offset. For example, a patient with a unilateral nephrectomy loses one half of the nephron mass, resulting in a 50 percent reduction in GFR at the time of surgery. However, the GFR in the remaining kidney begins to increase after 1 or 2 weeks, and within several months GFR may rise to 80 percent of the preoperative value. This indicates that the GFR of the individual remaining nephrons has increased above normal. Increases in single-nephron GFR may be achieved by renal hemodynamic adjustments (increased glomerular plasma flow and increased glomerular capillary hydraulic pressure), which augment the forces driving ultrafiltration, and by glomerular hypertrophy, which increases the maximum surface area available for filtration. These structural adaptations are evident from the enlargement of glomeruli (and tubules) seen on histologic sections from people with single kidneys. Similar structural changes are observed in kidneys damaged by chronic disease processes; foci of hypertrophied glomeruli and tubules are interspersed with areas of atrophic or scarred parenchyma. Although direct measurements of single-nephron GFR cannot be made in humans, it is reasonable to assume that focal nephron enlargement in chronically diseased kidneys generally signifies focally increased single-nephron GFR, and that these adaptations represent compensatory adjustments for the effects of nephron loss through disease.

Glomerulotubular Balance   The close integration of glomerular and tubular functions (*glomerulotubular balance*) seen in chronic renal failure (CRF) supports the notion that progressive nephron obliteration is the usual mode of GFR reduction in CRF. Preservation of glomerulotubular balance until the terminal stages of CRF is fundamental to the *intact-nephron hypothesis,* which essentially states that as CRF advances, kidney function is supported by a diminishing pool of functioning (or hyperfunctioning) nephrons, rather than relatively constant numbers of nephrons, each with diminishing function. This concept has important implications for the mechanisms of disease progression in CRF. A considerable amount of evidence suggests that nephrons subjected to increased excretory burdens for prolonged periods actually sustain injury as a result of these adaptations: thus the cost of these compensatory adaptations to nephron loss may ultimately be relentless destruction of the remaining nephron pool.

The magnitude of the single-nephron *hyperfiltration* induced by loss of 50 percent of the total nephron mass usually has no serious adverse consequences, even when sustained over two to three decades. When more than 50 percent of the total nephron mass is lost, however, as in renal-sparing surgery for bilateral trauma or neoplasm or from a renal disease whose activity has abated, the remaining nephrons are forced to the limits of their compensatory capacity. While these adaptations achieve remarkable short-term success at offsetting the tendency for GFR to fall, over time, proteinuria and focal and segmental glomerulosclerosis develop, the more so where greater amounts of nephrons are lost or removed. As a result, a progressive decline in GFR ensues. Experimental study of the processes that advance glomerular injury show that the adverse long-term consequences of severe nephron deficits are invariably preceded by increases in glomerular capillary hydraulic pressure (glomerular capillary hypertension), glomerular hyperperfusion, and hypertrophy. Interventions directed against these adaptive responses can greatly ameliorate the subsequent development of renal failure. In particular, drugs (e.g., angiotensin-converting enzyme inhibitors) and other interventions (such as dietary protein restriction) that lower glomerular pressure can slow the rate of progression of experimental and human renal disease. Otherwise, more and more glomeruli cease to function through advancing glomerulosclerosis and disruption of tubule structure and function, leading eventually to total loss of GFR (i.e., end-stage renal disease). This *final common pathway* for chronic renal injury helps to explain the progressive nature of chronic renal failure resulting from many different kidney diseases.

Biologic Consequences of Sustained Reductions in GFR Although nephron loss can proceed, to some extent, without equivalent loss of GFR due to the compensatory mechanisms described above, determination of the total GFR of both kidneys remains the most reliable clinical index of overall excretory function. The effects of impaired GFR are to reduce the total rate of delivery of solute into the glomerular filtrate. When accompanied by comparably reduced rates of urinary excretion, *retention* and *accumulation* of the unexcreted solute occurs, resulting in increased concentrations of the substance in the plasma and other body fluids.

Figure 269-1 depicts the major types of response to impaired GFR. The degree of reduction in total GFR is plotted on the abscissa, expressed as a percentage of normal (100 percent). The renal handling of most solutes normally present in glomerular filtrate conforms to one of three patterns. Curve A describes the pattern with substances such as creatinine and urea that normally depend largely on glomerular filtration for urinary excretion; i.e., secretion contributes little to overall excretion. Therefore, as illustrated, gradual reductions in GFR are accompanied by progressive increases in plasma levels of creatinine, urea, and other substances normally excreted primarily by filtration.

The clinical course of CRF usually also approximates the pattern described by curve A. Patients with CRF usually pass from a long asymptomatic period of "compensation" to a more accelerated and clinically overt terminal phase. In other words, despite chronic injury leading to destruction of more than 50 percent of nephrons, plasma elevations of creatinine and urea may still lie within the normal limits for these substances. With further nephron loss and reduction in GFR, however, the limits of renal reserve are exceeded and continued accumulations of curve A–type solutes lead to abnormally elevated plasma concentrations (see Fig. 269-1). Because some of these retained solutes are thought to exert "toxic" effects on all organ systems, clinical manifestations of CRF may now become apparent. Consequently, in patients with substantial reductions in nephron mass but near-normal plasma creatinine, overt uremia may be precipitated by relatively modest additional decrements in GFR.

The accumulation of curve A–type solutes with chronic loss of renal function proceeds until external balance is restored, i.e., intake and/or production rates exactly match excretion rates. In the case of creatinine, for example, assuming a constant rate of creatinine production, a 50 percent reduction in GFR results in an approximate doubling of the plasma creatinine concentration. The latter restores the filtered load of creatinine (i.e., the product of GFR and plasma creatinine concentration) to normal, and the urinary excretion rate once again is equivalent to creatinine production. Since no alternative mechanisms exist for significantly augmenting creatinine excretion beyond this level, elimination of the retained creatinine is not possible and the plasma concentration remains twice normal. With further loss of GFR, elevations in plasma creatinine are compounded by loss of nephron excretory function and creatinine retained as the result of earlier nephron destruction (see Fig. 269-1). *In practice, so long as the net rates of acquisition and production (i.e., liver function and muscle mass) remain reasonably constant, the inverse relationship between plasma concentrations of solutes such as creatinine and urea and GFR is sufficiently reliable and predictable to serve as clinical indices of GFR.* However, where muscle mass is low or reduced by wasting, unremarkable plasma levels of creatinine may nevertheless belie substantial reductions in GFR.

In contrast to solutes of the curve A type, plasma levels of phosphate, urate, and potassium (K^+) and hydrogen (H^+) ions usually do not rise until the GFR falls to a small percentage of normal. With progressive renal failure this pattern of response (curve B in Fig. 269-1) reflects the participation of tubule transport mechanisms in the excretion of these substances. In other words, *as GFR declines, the tubules facilitate greater elimination of these substances, by enhancing secretion and/or by diminishing reabsorption, so that a greater fraction of the filtered load is excreted.* Plasma levels of curve B–type solutes, therefore, rise less than those of curve A because, with progressive reductions in GFR, *excretion rate per nephron* and therefore *fractional excretion* both increase. Eventually, however, with further loss of GFR, enhanced fractional excretion can no longer offset the reduction in net filtered load of these solutes and plasma levels rise (see Fig. 269-1). For urate, phosphate, and K^+, at least, increased fractional excretion serves to maintain normal plasma levels until GFR falls to less than one-fourth of normal.

Finally, for certain solutes, such as sodium chloride (NaCl), plasma concentrations remain normal throughout the course of CRF, despite unrestricted intake of these substances (curve C in Fig. 269-1). The compensatory mechanism required to achieve this represents a fundamental adaptation to chronic renal injury. To illustrate the magnitude of the adaptation involved, it is useful to compare the excretion of

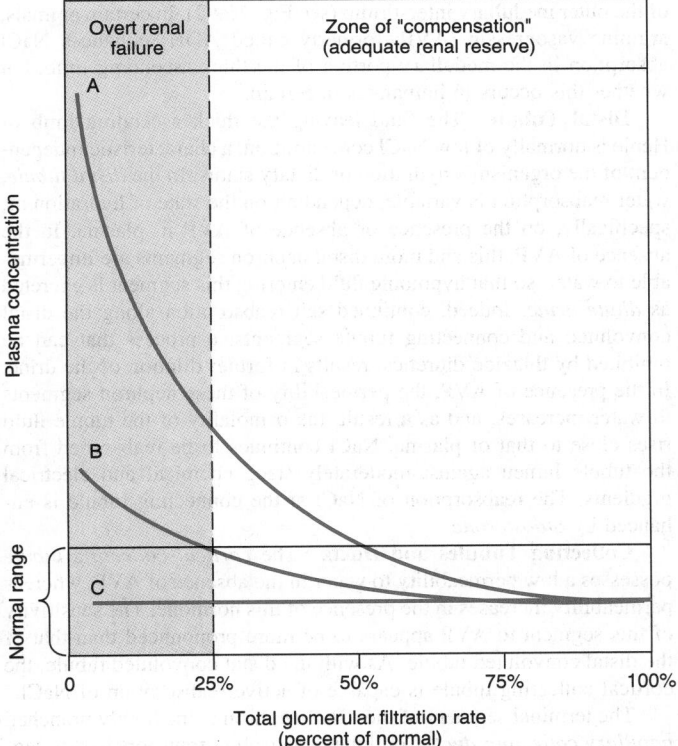

FIGURE 269-1 Representative patterns of adaptation for different types of solutes in body fluids in chronic renal failure. (*After NS Bricker et al, in Brenner, 1976.*)

sodium (Na⁺) in a normal individual (GFR of 125 mL/min) with that of a patient with advanced renal failure (GFR of 2 mL/min). Both individuals consume a diet containing 7 g/day of salt (120 mmol Na⁺). With a normal serum Na⁺ concentration of 140 mmol/L, external Na⁺ balance is achieved by excreting approximately 0.5 percent of the filtered load. By contrast, for external balance to be maintained in the patient with CRF, fractional excretion of Na⁺ must rise to 30 percent. In other words, *to maintain external Na⁺ balance, the same amount of Na⁺ must be excreted into the urine each day in the patient with CRF as in the normal individual.* Given the drastic reduction in GFR in CRF, external balance can only be maintained by large-magnitude adaptations in the reabsorptive processes in surviving tubules so that a progressively larger fraction of the filtered load escapes reabsorption and appears in the final urine. In short, *the rate of excretion of Na⁺ per surviving nephron increases in inverse proportion to the composite GFR in surviving nephrons.*

ADAPTATIONS IN TUBULE TRANSPORT MECHANISMS IN RESPONSE TO NEPHRON LOSS

Despite progressive nephron loss, many mechanisms that regulate renal solute and water balance differ only quantitatively, and not qualitatively, from those that operate normally. Thus, glomerulotubular balance is maintained. The most important of these mechanisms are considered below.

TUBULAR TRANSPORT OF SODIUM CHLORIDE AND WATER Most of the filtered water and sodium salts are reabsorbed by the tubules, leaving small and variable amounts, equivalent on average to the quantities ingested, to reach the final urine. About two-thirds of the glomerular ultrafiltrate is reabsorbed in the *proximal tubule* with little change in the osmolality or Na⁺ concentration of the unreabsorbed fraction (Fig. 269-2). In other words, fluid reabsorption in the proximal tubule is nearly *isosmotic* and is coupled to the active transport of Na⁺. Since chloride (Cl⁻) and bicarbonate (HCO₃⁻) are the primary anions in the extracellular fluid, they constitute the main solutes that accompany Na⁺ reabsorption in the renal tubules. In the earliest portion of the proximal tubule, bicarbonate is the principal anion that accompanies the reabsorption of Na⁺. This process occurs via a Na⁺/H⁺ exchanger at the luminal brush border and is dependent on the activity of carbonic anhydrase. Glucose, amino acids, and other organic solutes (e.g., lactate) are also extensively reabsorbed in the proximal tubule by cotransport mechanisms that link the cellular entry of these organic molecules with Na⁺. The coupling of water absorption (i.e., volume) with solute absorption appears to be dependent upon three processes. First, given the remarkably high water permeability of this segment, very small transepithelial osmolality differences, i.e., *luminal hypotonicity* of the order of 2 to 3 mosmol/L produced by solute absorption, could drive water absorption. Second, due to preferential absorption of HCO₃⁻ and organic solutes in the early portions of the proximal tubule, the concentrations of these substances decrease along the proximal tubule while that of chloride increases. Volume reabsorption would then occur if the diffusion of Na⁺ and Cl⁻ down their respective electrochemical gradients across the proximal tubule epithelium occurred more easily than the back-diffusion of sodium bicarbonate into the lumen, creating an *effective osmotic pressure gradient*. Finally, *lateral interstitial space hypertonicity* produced by differences in the rates at which solutes are transported into the spaces or exit them by diffusion may also contribute to the coupling of water and solute reabsorption.

Reabsorption of Fluid from Proximal Convoluted Tubules This is sensitive to *Starling forces*, i.e., the hydraulic and colloid osmotic (or oncotic) pressures across the walls of the peritubular capillaries. Because the plasma proteins in glomerular capillaries are concentrated by ultrafiltration, oncotic pressure rises markedly along the glomerular capillary network. This step-up in oncotic pressure is transmitted largely unchanged to the first branches of the peritubular capillaries via the efferent arterioles. These resistance vessels cause a substantial drop in hydraulic pressure, however, so that when the plasma reaches the peritubular capillaries, oncotic pressure greatly exceeds hydraulic pressure. The Starling forces are therefore oriented in an *uptake* mode, in contrast to their configuration at the glomerulus where hydraulic pressure exceeds oncotic pressure, favoring *filtration*. The extent to which oncotic pressure exceeds hydraulic pressure in the peritubular capillary network modulates the overall rate of fluid absorption by the peritubular capillaries. Therefore, when peritubular capillary oncotic pressure falls, or hydraulic pressure rises, uptake of fluid by these capillaries is reduced. As a result, fluid is retained in the interstitial space, tending to increase hydraulic pressure, ultimately retarding the egress of fluid from the lateral intercellular channels. Without an adequate route of drainage, fluid in the intercellular channels leaks back into the lumen, thereby *diminishing net fluid reabsorption* from this tubule segment. The opposite occurs in states where peritubular oncotic pressure is increased (increased filtration fraction) or hydraulic pressure is decreased (enhanced efferent arteriolar tone). Under these circumstances, peritubular capillary uptake of reabsorbate is augmented, leading ultimately to *enhanced net fluid reabsorption* by the proximal tubule. Although physical factors appear to be the major determinants of fluid reabsorption in the proximal tubule, hormones (e.g., angiotensin II) may also modulate fluid reabsorption directly, by enhancing luminal Na⁺ entry into proximal tubule cells via an apical Na⁺/H⁺ exchanger.

Thin Ascending Limb of Henle's Loop In contrast to the proximal tubule, active outward transport of Na has not been established for the *thin ascending limb of Henle's loop*. However, passive outward salt transport does occur, as indicated in Fig. 269-2. In the next nephron segment, the *medullary thick ascending limb of Henle*, the concentration of NaCl is reduced as fluid traverses this segment. Here Cl⁻ absorption occurs by an active process involving a furosemide-sensitive Na⁺:K⁺:2Cl⁻ cotransport mechanism in the luminal membrane, with one-half of Na⁺ absorption proceeding passively, driven by the lumen positive transepithelial voltage difference. Since the ascending limb of Henle is impermeable to water, net NaCl reabsorption generates hypotonic tubule fluid and gives rise to the high NaCl concentration of the outer medullary interstitium (see Fig. 269-2). In certain animals, arginine vasopressin (AVP; formerly called ADH) enhances NaCl absorption in the medullary portion of the thick ascending limb, but whether this occurs in humans is uncertain.

Distal Tubule The fluid leaving the thick ascending limb of Henle is normally of low NaCl concentration, a characteristic independent of the organism's hydration or dietary status. In the *distal tubule*, water reabsorption is variable, depending on the state of hydration or, specifically, on the presence or absence of AVP in plasma. In the absence of AVP, this and more distal nephron segments are impermeable to water, so that hypotonic fluid entering this segment is excreted as *dilute urine*. Indeed, continued salt reabsorption along the distal convoluted and connecting tubule segments, a process that can be inhibited by thiazide diuretics, results in further dilution of the urine. In the presence of AVP, the permeability of these nephron segments to water increases, and as a result, the osmolality of the tubule fluid rises close to that of plasma. NaCl continues to be reabsorbed from the tubule lumen against moderately steep chemical and electrical gradients. The reabsorption of NaCl at the connecting tubule is enhanced by *aldosterone*.

Collecting Tubules and Ducts The *cortical collecting tubule* possesses a low permeability to water in the absence of AVP, whereas permeability increases in the presence of this hormone. The sensitivity of this segment to AVP appears to be more pronounced than that of the distal convoluted tubule. As with the distal convoluted tubule, the cortical collecting tubule is capable of active reabsorption of NaCl.

The terminal segment of the distal nephron is the highly branched *papillary collecting duct*. Continued electrolyte transport in this segment results in the large ion concentration differences that normally exist between urine and plasma. As in the cortical collecting tubule, Na⁺ transport appears to be active, since reabsorption proceeds against sizeable electrochemical gradients. The rate of Na$^+$ transport in this segment depends on the load of Na$^+$ delivered from more proximal segments and is also affected by aldosterone. The permeability to water is also increased markedly in the presence of AVP.

EFFECTS OF NEPHRON LOSS ON SODIUM CHLORIDE TRANSPORT IN SURVIVING NEPHRONS

With progressive nephron loss, *maintenance of external balance for NaCl requires that fractional salt excretion increases as GFR decreases.* Several mechanisms contribute to this adaptive increase in fractional sodium excretion. With loss of functioning nephron units, peritubular capillary Starling forces are probably altered in directions that serve to reduce

proximal tubule reabsorption of NaCl and water. For example, a rise in peritubular capillary hydraulic pressure, which tends to inhibit net proximal fluid reabsorption, might be anticipated with systemic hypertension, a common feature of chronic renal failure. Similarly, reductions in peritubular capillary oncotic pressures may be anticipated due to reductions in both filtration fraction and hypoalbuminemia.

Aldosterone, which normally exerts a potent influence on tubule transport, probably does not figure prominently in reducing fractional

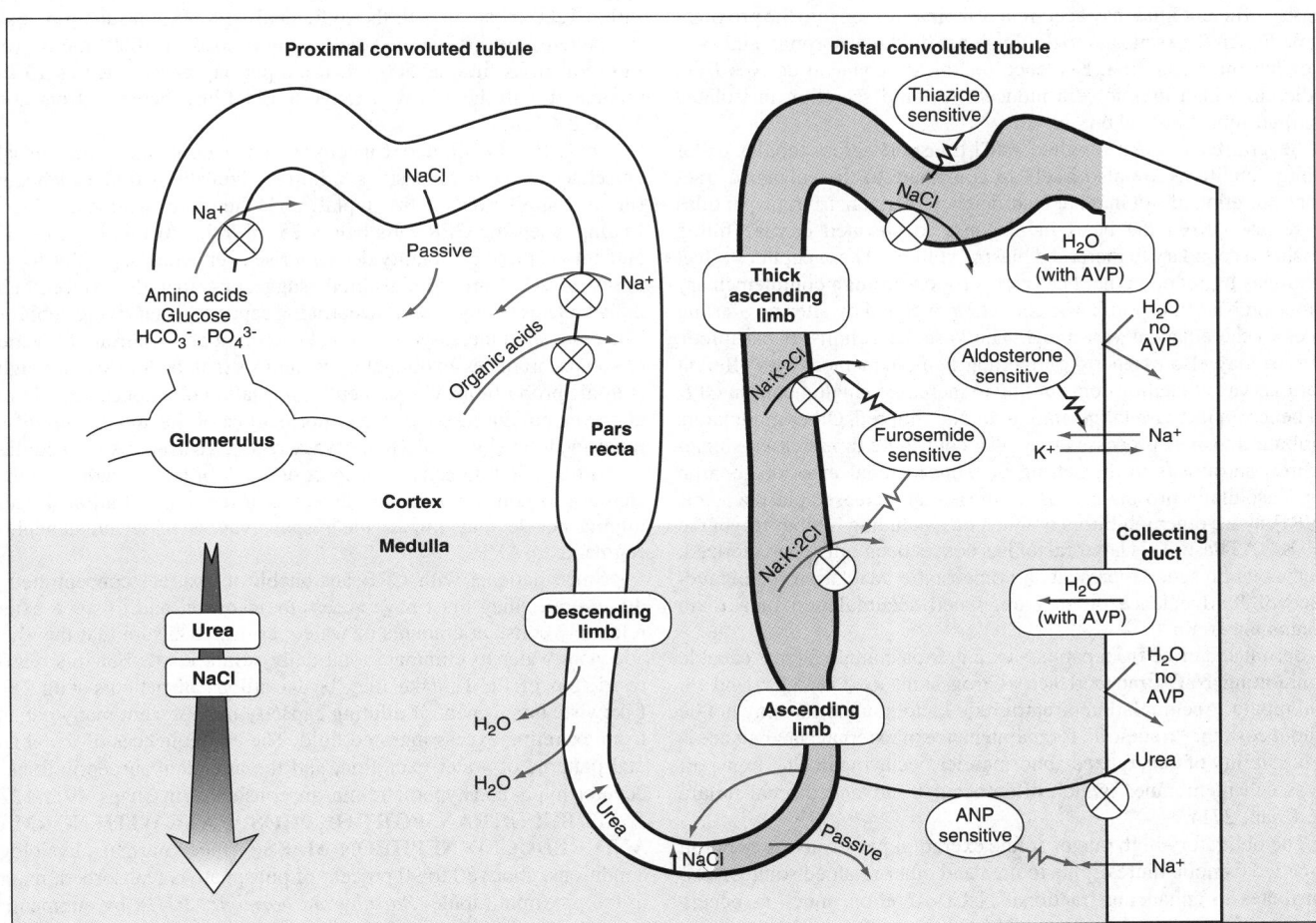

FIGURE 269-2 Transport functions of the various anatomic segments of the mammalian nephron. Fluid reabsorption across the proximal tubule is isosmotic and accounts for reabsorption of approximately two-thirds of the filtered Na$^+$ and H$_2$O. The major portions of the filtered HCO$_3^-$, amino acids, glucose, and phosphate are reabsorbed in the early proximal convoluted tubule. Reabsorption of glucose and amino acids is coupled to Na$^+$ transport and thereby generates a negative potential difference within the tubule lumen. At the same time, HCO$_3^-$ is reabsorbed by a nonelectrogenic mechanism, via H$^+$ secretion. The active transport of these solutes results in transepithelial concentration and effective osmotic pressure gradients promoting H$_2$O flow across the proximal tubule, into the peritubular capillaries. The rise in tubule fluid Cl$^-$ concentration is a necessary reciprocal consequence of the decreased luminal HCO$_3^-$ concentration. The resultant high concentration of Cl$^-$ becomes an important force for the outward passive transport of Cl$^-$ down its concentration gradient, resulting in a lumen-positive potential difference in the late proximal convoluted tubule. The pars recta of the proximal tubule is capable of active electrogenic transport of Na$^+$ independent of organic solute transport. Under normal conditions, approximately one-third of the glomerular filtrate enters the descending limb of Henle's loop. Because the thin descending limb is incapable of active outward NaCl transport and is characterized by low permeability to Na$^+$ but high H$_2$O permeability, H$_2$O is abstracted passively as the fluid approaches the bend of Henle's loop. Hypertonic fluid with a greater NaCl concentration but

lower urea concentration than the surrounding medullary interstitium thus enters the thin ascending limb of Henle, which is largely impermeable to H$_2$O and urea but highly permeable to NaCl. This permits passive outward diffusion of NaCl. Active Na:K:2Cl transport across the water-impermeable thick ascending limb of Henle allows for separation of solute and water. In consequence, tubule fluid becomes dilute and the medullary interstitium hypertonic.

Irrespective of the final osmolality of the urine, the fluid that enters the distal convoluted tubule is always hypoosmotic. This segment exhibits active Na$^+$ reabsorption. All but the terminal portion of the distal convoluted tubule is water-impermeable, even in the presence of AVP. Aldosterone exerts its effect in this segment by enhancing Na$^+$ reabsorption, which is variably coupled to K$^+$ and H$^+$ secretion. The cortical and papillary portions of the collecting duct are sites where AVP exerts its principal effect. The permeability of these segments to H$_2$O in the absence of AVP is very low but can be greatly enhanced in the presence of AVP. These segments are also characterized by active Na$^+$ reabsorption, which appears to depend on the presence of mineralocorticoid. In the absence of AVP, the collecting tubule is water-impermeable so that hypotonic tubule fluid courses through it. However, in the presence of AVP, water is avidly reabsorbed here, resulting in hypertonic final urine. Sites of action of furosemide and thiazide diuretics and of aldosterone and atrial natriuretic peptide (ANP) are shown.

Na$^+$ excretion, since aldosterone levels are seldom reduced in CRF. Furthermore, external Na$^+$ balance is preserved in bilaterally adrenalectomized dogs on fixed replacement doses of mineralocorticoid. Yet another factor contributing to the suppression of fractional NaCl reabsorption in CRF may relate to the retention of solutes as GFR declines. In addition to urea and creatinine, *organic acids* (including *hippurates*) also accumulate. These substances are normally excreted by both glomerular filtration and tubule secretion; the latter process involves a carrier-mediated organic transport system in proximal tubule cells. When GFR is reduced and plasma levels of these organic acids increase, sufficient fluid may accompany their secretion into the proximal tubule lumen (by osmosis) to diminish net fluid reabsorption and even favor net fluid secretion. Evidence for this mechanism derives from studies in which uremic sera induced net fluid secretion in isolated proximal tubules of rabbits in vitro.

Several factors that regulate NaCl transport across tubules under resting conditions are also likely to contribute to the enhanced fractional excretion of salt in renal insufficiency. Atrial natriuretic peptides are released from the heart in response to elevated cardiac filling pressures secondary to increased plasma volume. These peptides effect natriuresis by reducing net Na$^+$ reabsorption through complementary actions on Na$^+$ transport in the collecting duct and by altering Starling forces in the adjacent vasa recta. The vascular actions of natriuretic peptides may also extend to glomerular hemodynamics, with afferent arteriolar vasodilatation contributing to increased single-nephron GFR and hence an increase in the amount of Na$^+$ filtered. Other modulators of tubule transport processes may also contribute to increased single-nephron natriuresis in the setting of reduced renal mass or nephron loss. Vasodilator prostaglandins are present at increased plasma levels in CRF, as are other inhibitors of transport, including inhibitor(s) of the Na$^+$,K$^+$-ATPase. This latter factor has not yet been fully characterized; whether its presence represents a homeostatic adaptation for maintenance of fluid balance or an unregulated accumulation of a toxin remains uncertain.

Serum and urine from patients with uremia contain factors capable of inhibiting NaCl transport across frog skin, toad bladder, and rat renal tubule. Accumulation of natriuretic factors in uremia may not be without cost; the "trade-off" for maintenance of external Na$^+$ balance is the possibility of generalized abnormalities occurring in Na$^+$ transport across cell membranes, which often occur in advanced renal failure (see Chap. 271).

The obligatory high rate of solute excretion per surviving nephron (so-called osmotic diuresis due to urea and other retained solutes) also contributes to enhancing fractional NaCl excretion, much as occurs in normal individuals after the administration of mannitol or other nonreabsorbable solutes. Finally, certain forms of CRF are associated with unusually large losses of salt in the urine. These *salt-wasting nephropathies* include chronic pyelonephritis and other tubulointerstitial diseases (see Chap. 276) as well as polycystic and medullary cystic diseases. These disorders have in common greater destruction of medullary and tubulointerstitial, rather than cortical and glomerular, portions of the renal parenchyma. Preferential impairment of tubule reabsorptive function, rather than a primary reduction in glomerular filtration, may, therefore, underlie the salt-losing tendency in these disorders. Clinical derangements that alter renal handling of NaCl in CRF (including hypo- and hypervolemia, hypertension, etc.) are considered in Chap. 271.

EFFECTS OF NEPHRON LOSS ON WATER REABSORP-TION IN SURVIVING NEPHRONS As with NaCl, there is a progressive increase in the fractional excretion of water with advancing renal insufficiency so that external water balance can be maintained even with a total GFR of 5 mL/min or less. The adaptations of water handling by the diseased kidney are of importance in the defects in urinary concentration and dilution and hence the polyuria and nocturia and tendency to develop water overload encountered in CRF (see Chap. 47). To appreciate the mechanisms involved, the responses of

a normal and a uremic individual maintaining external water balance need to be considered. Assuming both individuals have the same dietary and fluid intakes, total solute and volume excretion in both should be identical as well. If the *obligatory solute load* to be excreted by each is 600 mmol/d (600 mosmol/d) and the urine osmolality is 300 mmol/kg water (300 mosmol/kg), a urine volume of 2 L/d will be required to excrete the total solute. If the GFR in normal and uremic individuals totals 180 and 4 L/d, respectively, urinary volume excretion of 2 L/d represents excretion of slightly more than 1 percent of the total glomerular filtrate in the normal subject compared with 50 percent in the uremic patient. Since the range of urine osmolalities that the diseased kidney can achieve [250 to 350 mmol/kg (250 to 350 mosmol/kg)] is narrower than in the normal kidney [40 to 1200 mmol/kg (40 to 1200 mosmol/kg)], the individual with normal function is able to excrete the obligatory daily solute load of 600 mmol (600 mosmol) in as little as 500 mL urine per day or as much as 15 L/d, compared with the narrower range in renal insufficiency, from about 1.7 to 2.4 L/d.

In CRF, the limited capacity to concentrate the urine usually correlates with other measures of impaired renal function. Isosthenuria (urine of similar osmolality to plasma) is therefore an almost universal finding when the GFR falls below 25 mL/min. At this level of GFR and below, urine osmolality does not rise even when supraphysiologic doses of AVP are administered, suggesting that the concentrating defect relates to impaired concentrating capacity in surviving nephrons. The associated increased fractional excretion per nephron of a variety of solutes produces an obligatory water loss (solute diuresis) at roughly isotonic proportions. Consequently, formation of a concentrated urine is prevented. Disease-induced abnormalities of the architecture of the renal medulla (loops of Henle, vasa recta), aberrations in medullary blood flow, and defective transport of NaCl in the ascending limb of Henle also contribute to this defect in urine concentration. Finally, uremia per se may impair the responsiveness of terminal nephron segments to AVP.

Since patients with CRF are unable to excrete concentrated or dilute urine, they must have access to adequate, and to some extent, relatively constant amounts of water per day to ensure that they have adequate water to eliminate total daily solute loads. For this reason, restriction of fluid intake may be hazardous in patients with CRF. Likewise, impairment of diluting capacity may prevent many patients from excreting excess ingested fluid. The consequences of the abnormal patterns of water excretion, and the attendant susceptibilities to develop hypo- and hypernatremia, are considered in Chaps. 49 and 271.

TUBULE TRANSPORT OF PHOSPHATE WITH NORMAL AND REDUCED NEPHRON MASS Under normal physiologic conditions, about 80 to 90 percent of phosphate is reabsorbed, mainly in the proximal tubule. *Parathyroid hormone (PTH)*, by augmenting phosphate excretion via inhibition of this proximal reabsorptive process (Chap. 353), plays a key role in phosphate homeostasis. When dietary phosphate intake increases, a *transient* rise in plasma phosphate concentration is usually observed. This results in a similarly transient reduction in the plasma ionized calcium level (due largely to deposition of calcium phosphate in bone), which is sensed by a specific receptor on parathyroid cells, stimulating PTH secretion. By enhancing fractional phosphate excretion, PTH restores external phosphate balance and normophosphatemia. This enables plasma ionized calcium levels to return to normal, thereby removing the stimulus to PTH release and restoring the phosphate control system to the original steady state.

With advancing renal failure and constant dietary intake of phosphate, external phosphate balance is achieved by progressive reduction in fractional phosphate reabsorption. Enhanced PTH secretion is an important determinant of this phosphaturic response. With succeeding decrements in total GFR, the amount of phosphate filtered by surviving glomeruli is reduced, leading to transient phosphate retention and, therefore, a rise (albeit small) in plasma phosphate concentration. This leads to a small, reciprocal decline in plasma levels of ionized calcium and a corresponding increase in PTH secretion. Although the phosphaturic response of surviving tubules to this elevation in circulating PTH restores plasma phosphate and calcium to normal levels (at least in the "compensated" stage of CRF described by curve B in Fig. 269-1), the new steady-state conditions are only achieved at the cost of *persistently elevated plasma PTH levels*. With progressive reductions in GFR, the process is repeated but at ever-increasing cost in terms of elevated PTH levels.

Alterations in Vitamin D Metabolism These alterations also contribute to elevated PTH levels in CRF. The kidney is normally the major site of *conversion of vitamin D to its active metabolites*. As discussed in Chap. 353, vitamin D, synthesized in skin or acquired in the diet, undergoes initial hydroxylation in the liver to form 25-hydroxyvitamin D [25(OH)D]. The kidney is the site of a second important conversion to 1,25-hydroxyvitamin D [1,25(OH$_2$)D]. This active form of vitamin D acts directly on the parathyroid gland to suppress PTH secretion as well as to enhance intestinal absorption of calcium and phosphate resorption and promote resorption of these ions from bone. In addition, 1,25(OH)D$_2$ probably opposes the phosphaturic actions of PTH in the renal tubule by augmenting, rather than diminishing, phosphate reabsorption. With advancing renal disease, nephron loss reduces the renal capacity for vitamin D hydroxylation; phosphate retention also impairs this reaction. Not only are the circulating levels of 1,25(OH)D$_2$ diminished in uremia, but the receptors that mediate its action at the parathyroid gland are also diminished. These two effects remove inhibitory influences on PTH secretion, leading to increased plasma PTH levels. Reduction in circulating 1,25(OH)D$_2$ levels, by suppressing intestinal calcium absorption, contributes to the development of the hypocalcemia and hyperparathyroidism of CRF (see Chap. 271).

Hyperparathyroidism in Chronic Renal Failure At least two additional processes are thought to contribute to hyperparathyroidism in CRF. One relates to resistance of bone to the calcemic effect of PTH in uremia. This resistance necessitates a higher level of PTH to demineralize bone and maintain the plasma calcium concentration. The other derives from the finding that reductions in renal mass impair the kidneys' capacity to degrade circulating PTH. Ultimately, however, phosphate conforms more to a curve $B-$ rather than a curve $C-$type pattern in Fig. 269-1, and phosphate retention occurs when the GFR falls below about 25 mL/min, signifying that these latter forms of adaptation play limited roles.

Since PTH exerts major effects on bone as well as renal tubules, the external balance of phosphate in CRF is achieved at the expense of elevated PTH levels, which, in turn, account for many of the bone changes of renal osteodystrophy (i.e., *secondary hyperparathyroidism*; see Fig. 271-1). In support of this *trade-off hypothesis*, when dietary phosphate intake is reduced in proportion to the reduction in GFR in animals with CRF, external balance of phosphate no longer requires augmentation of fractional phosphate excretion in surviving nephrons. Accordingly, circulating levels of PTH no longer rise, and the bone changes of secondary hyperparathyroidism are diminished, if not prevented.

HYDROGEN AND BICARBONATE TRANSPORT WITH NORMAL AND REDUCED RENAL MASS As discussed in Chap. 50, the pH of extracellular fluid is normally maintained within a narrow range (7.36 to 7.44) despite day-to-day fluctuations in the quantity of acids added to the extracellular fluid from dietary and metabolic sources (approximately 1 mmol H$^+$ per kilogram of body weight per day). These acids consume buffers from both extracellular and intracellular fluid, of which HCO$_3^-$ is the most important in the intracellular compartment. Such buffering minimizes changes in pH. Long-term effectiveness of the HCO$_3^-$ buffer system, however, requires mechanisms for replenishment, otherwise unrelenting acquisition of nonvolatile acids from dietary and metabolic sources would ultimately exhaust buffering capacity, culminating in fatal acidosis. The kidneys normally function to prevent this eventuality by *regenerating* bicarbonate, thereby maintaining plasma concentrations of HCO$_3^-$. In addition, the kidneys also *reclaim* HCO$_3^-$ in the glomerular ultrafiltrate. Reclamation of filtered HCO$_3^-$ takes place largely in the proximal tubule and, under normal circumstances, is virtually complete below a critical plasma HCO$_3^-$ concentration—the threshold concentration—which in humans is

normally about 26 mmol/L, identical to the concentration of HCO$_3^-$ in plasma. As a consequence, HCO$_3^-$ wastage is prevented. Alternatively, when plasma HCO$_3^-$ rises above this threshold, reabsorption becomes less complete, allowing escape of excess HCO$_3^-$ into the final urine, which restores the plasma HCO$_3^-$ towards normal levels. Despite complete reabsorption of HCO$_3^-$, metabolic acidosis would still ensue if HCO$_3^-$ consumed in buffering nonvolatile acids were not constantly regenerated.

The *reabsorption* of filtered HCO$_3^-$ occurs by the following mechanism. Filtered bicarbonate combines with H$^+$ secreted from proximal tubule cells, probably via a Na$^+$/H$^+$ exchanger, to form carbonic acid (H$_2$CO$_3$). Dehydration of carbonic acid under the influence of *luminal carbonic anhydrase* yields CO$_2$, which is free to diffuse from lumen to peritubular blood. In the proximal tubule cell, the OH$^-$ left behind by the H$^+$ secretion reacts with CO$_2$, under the influence of *intracellular carbonic anhydrase*, forming HCO$_3^-$. This ion is transported across the contraluminal proximal tubule cell membrane, via an electrogenic Na/HCO$_3^-$ cotransporter, to reenter the extracellular HCO$_3^-$ pool. The net result is *reclamation of a filtered bicarbonate ion*. Secreted H$^+$ is also free to react with nonbicarbonate buffers [e.g., phosphate or ammonia (NH$_4^+$)] in the tubule lumen, and hydrogen ions are excreted in these forms in the final urine. Again, the OH$^-$ left behind in the proximal tubule cell from H$^+$ secretion reacts with CO$_2$, forming bicarbonate—also representing *regeneration of an HCO$_3^-$ ion*.

Hydrogen ions in the urine are bound to filtered buffers (e.g., phosphate) in amounts equivalent to the amounts of alkali required to titrate the pH of the urine up to the pH of the blood (the so-called titratable acid). It is not usually possible to eliminate all the daily acid load in the form of titratable acid due to limits of urinary pH. Metabolism of glutamine by proximal tubule cells to yield ammonium (ammoniagenesis) serves as an additional mechanism for H$^+$ elimination and bicarbonate regeneration. Glutamine metabolism forms not only NH$_4^+$ (i.e., NH$_3$ plus H$^+$) but also HCO$_3^-$, which is transported across the proximal tubule (HCO$_3^-$ regeneration). The NH$_4^+$ must be excreted in the urine for this process to be effective in bicarbonate regeneration. The excretion of ammonium involves secretion by proximal tubule cells (possibly by the Na$^+$/H$^+$ exchanger as Na$^+$:NH$_4^+$), generation of high medullary interstitial NH$_4^+$ concentration by an elaborate countercurrent multiplication/exchange system, and finally, secretion of the interstitial NH$_4^+$ by the collecting duct by a combination of H$^+$ secretion and passive NH$_3$ diffusion. *Ammoniagenesis* is responsive to the acid-base needs of the individual. When faced with an acute acid burden and an increased need for HCO$_3^-$ regeneration, the rate of renal ammonia synthesis increases sharply.

The quantity of hydrogen ions excreted as titratable acid and NH$_4^+$ is equal to the quantity of HCO$_3^-$ regenerated in tubule cells and added to plasma. Under steady-state conditions, the net quantity of acid excreted into the urine (the sum of titratable acid and NH$_4^+$ less HCO$_3^-$) must equal the quantity of acid gained by the extracellular fluid from all sources. Metabolic acidosis and alkalosis result when this delicate balance is perturbed, the former the result of insufficient net acid excretion, and the latter due to excessive acid excretion.

Progressive loss of renal function usually causes little or no change in arterial pH, plasma bicarbonate concentration, or arterial carbon dioxide tension (P$_{CO_2}$) until GFR falls below 30 percent of normal. Thereafter, all three tend to decline as *metabolic acidosis* ensues. In general, the metabolic acidosis of CRF is not due to overproduction of acids but is rather a reflection of nephron loss, which limits the amount of NH$_3$ (and therefore also HCO$_3^-$) that can be generated. Although surviving nephrons appear to be capable of generating supranormal amounts of NH$_3$ *per nephron*, the diminished nephron population causes overall production to be reduced to an extent that is insufficient to permit sufficient buffering of H$^+$ in urine. As a result, although patients with CRF may be able to acidify their urine normally (i.e., urine pH as low as 4.5), the defect in NH$_3$ production limits daily net acid excretion to 30 to 40 mmol, or one-half to two-thirds the quantity of nonvolatile acid added to the extracellular fluid in the same time period. Metabolic acidosis resulting from this daily positive balance of H^+ is seldom florid in CRF of mild to moderate severity. Relative stability of plasma bicarbonate (albeit at reduced levels of 14 to 18 mmol/L) is maintained at the expense of buffering by bone. Because it contains large reserves of alkaline salts (calcium phosphate and calcium bicarbonate), bone constitutes a major reserve of buffering capacity. Dissolution of these buffers contributes to the osteodystrophy of CRF (see Fig. 271-1).

Although the acidosis of CRF is due to loss of tubule mass, it nevertheless depends to a large part on the level of GFR. When GFR is reduced to only a moderate extent (i.e., to about 50 percent of normal), retention of anions, principally sulfates and phosphates, is not pronounced. Therefore, as the plasma HCO_3^- falls owing to dysfunction or loss of tubules, retention of Cl^- by the kidneys leads to a *hyperchloremic acidosis*. At this stage *the anion gap is normal*. With further reductions in GFR and more pronounced azotemia, however, the retention of phosphates, sulfates, and other *unmeasured* anions ensues and plasma Cl^- falls to normal levels despite the reduction in plasma HCO_3^- concentration. *A moderate to large anion gap therefore develops.*

TUBULE POTASSIUM TRANSPORT WITH NORMAL AND REDUCED NEPHRON MASS As with H^+, the concentration of K^+ in extracellular fluid is normally maintained within a relatively narrow range, 4 to 5 mmol/L. Ninety-five percent or more of total-body K^+ is in the intracellular compartment, where the intracellular concentration is approximately 160 mmol/L. Normal individuals maintain external K^+ balance by excreting amounts into the urine that equal the intake, less the relatively small losses in stool and sweat. K^+ is freely filtered at the glomerulus, although the amount excreted usually represents no more than about 20 percent of the quantity filtered. The great bulk of the K^+ filtered is reabsorbed in the early portions of the nephron, about two-thirds in the proximal tubule, and an additional 20 to 25 percent in the loop of Henle. A K^+ *secretory process* operates in the distal tubule and terminal nephron segments. This process is largely dependent on Na^+ reabsorption and the accompanying lumen-negative voltage creating an electrical gradient across the tubule wall, favoring K^+ secretion into the lumen of the distal tubule and collecting duct.

The ability to maintain external K^+ balance and normal plasma K^+ concentration until relatively late in the course of CRF is a consequence primarily of a progressive increase in fractional excretion of K^+. Greatly enhanced rates of K^+ secretion occur in distal portions of surviving tubules. The augmented secretion rate of aldosterone contributes to enhanced tubule secretion of K^+. In addition, both the increased distal tubule flow rates in residual functioning nephrons due to the osmotic diuresis and enhanced luminal electronegativity created by the increased presence of highly impermeable anions such as phosphate and sulfate enhance K^+ secretion. Aldosterone also stimulates net entry of K^+ into the lumen of the colon, a mechanism known to be enhanced in CRF. → *More detailed discussions of abnormal K^+ homeostasis in acute and chronic forms of renal failure are given in Chaps. 270 and 271.*

BIBLIOGRAPHY

BRENNER BM: Nephron adaptation to renal injury or ablation. Am J Physiol 249:F324, 1985
——— et al: Diverse biological actions of atrial natriuretic peptides. Physiol Rev 70:665, 1990
———: *The Kidney*, 5th ed. Philadelphia, Saunders, 1996
FEINFELD DA, SHERWOOD LM: Parathyroid hormone and 1,25(OH)$_2$D$_3$ in chronic renal failure. Kidney Int 33:1049, 1988
KAJI D, KAHN T: Na$^+$-K$^+$ pump in chronic renal failure. Am J Physiol 252:F785, 1987
WARNOCK DG: Uremic acidosis. Kidney Int 34:278, 1988

270 Hugh R. Brady, Barry M. Brenner

ACUTE RENAL FAILURE

Acute renal failure (ARF) is a syndrome characterized by rapid decline in glomerular filtration rate (hours to weeks), retention of nitrogenous waste products, and perturbation of extracellular fluid volume and electrolyte and acid-base homeostasis. ARF complicates approximately 5 percent of hospital admissions and up to 30 percent of admissions to intensive care units. Oliguria (urine output <400 mL/d) is a frequent but not invariable clinical feature (~50 percent). ARF is usually asymptomatic and is diagnosed when biochemical screening of hospitalized patients reveals a recent increase in plasma urea and creatinine concentrations. It may complicate a wide range of diseases, which for purposes of diagnosis and management are conveniently divided into three categories: (1) diseases that cause renal hypoperfusion without compromising the integrity of renal parenchyma (*prerenal azotemia*, prerenal ARF) (~55 percent); (2) diseases that directly involve renal parenchyma (*renal azotemia*, intrinsic renal ARF) (~40 percent); and (3) diseases associated with urinary tract obstruction (*postrenal azotemia*, postrenal ARF) (~5 percent). Most ARF is reversible, the kidney being relatively unique among major organs in its ability to recover from almost complete loss of function. Nevertheless, ARF is associated with major in-hospital morbidity and mortality, in large part due to the serious nature of the illness that precipitated the ARF.

ETIOLOGY AND PATHOPHYSIOLOGY

PRERENAL AZOTEMIA (PRERENAL ARF) Prerenal azotemia is the most common form of ARF and represents a physiologic response to mild to moderate renal hypoperfusion. Prerenal azotemia is rapidly reversible upon restoration of renal blood flow and glomerular ultrafiltration pressure. Renal parenchymal tissue is not damaged; indeed, kidneys from individuals with prerenal azotemia function well when transplanted into recipients with normal cardiovascular function. More severe hypoperfusion may lead to ischemic injury of renal parenchyma and intrinsic renal azotemia. Thus, prerenal azotemia and ischemic ARF are part of a spectrum of manifestations of renal hypoperfusion. As shown in Table 270-1, prerenal azotemia can complicate any disease that induces hypovolemia, low cardiac output, systemic vasodilatation, or selective renal vasoconstriction.

Hypovolemia leads to a fall in mean systemic arterial pressure, which is detected as reduced stretch by arterial (e.g., carotid sinus) and cardiac baroreceptors. Activated baroreceptors trigger a coordinated series of neural and humoral responses designed to restore blood volume and arterial pressure. These include activation of the sympathetic nervous system and renin-angiotensin-aldosterone system and release of arginine vasopressin [AVP; formerly called antidiuretic hormone (ADH)]. Norepinephrine, angiotensin II, and AVP act in concert in an attempt to preserve cardiac and cerebral perfusion by stimulating vasoconstriction in relatively "nonessential" vascular beds such as the musculocutaneous and splanchnic circulations, inhibiting salt loss through sweat glands, stimulating thirst and salt appetite, and promoting renal salt and water retention. Glomerular perfusion, ultrafiltration pressure, and filtration rate are preserved during mild hypoperfusion through several compensatory mechanisms. Stretch receptors in afferent arterioles, in response to a reduction in perfusion pressure, trigger afferent arteriolar vasodilatation through a local myogenic reflex (autoregulation). Biosynthesis of vasodilator prostaglandins (e.g., prostacyclin, PGE_2) and possibly nitric oxide is also enhanced, and these compounds preferentially dilate afferent arterioles. In addition, angiotensin II induces preferential constriction of efferent arterioles. As a result, intraglomerular pressure is maintained, the fraction of plasma flowing through glomerular capillaries that is filtered is increased (filtration fraction), and glomerular filtration rate (GFR) is preserved. During states of more severe hypoperfusion, these compensatory responses are overwhelmed and GFR falls, leading to prerenal ARF.

Table 270-1

CHAPTER 270
Acute Renal Failure **1505**

Classification and Major Causes of Acute Renal Failure

PRERENAL AZOTEMIA

I. Hypovolemia
  A. Hemorrhage, burns, dehydration
  B. Gastrointestinal fluid loss: vomiting, surgical drainage, diarrhea
  C. Renal fluid loss: diuretics, osmotic diuresis (e.g., diabetes mellitus), hypoadrenalism
  D. Sequestration in extravascular space: pancreatitis, peritonitis, trauma, burns, severe hypoalbuminemia
II. Low cardiac output
  A. Diseases of myocardium, valves, and pericardium, arrhythmias, tamponade
  B. Other: pulmonary hypertension, massive pulmonary embolus, positive pressure mechanical ventilation
III. Altered renal systemic vascular resistance ratio
  A. Systemic vasodilatation: sepsis, antihypertensives, afterload reducers, anesthesia, anaphylaxis
  B. Renal vasoconstriction: hypercalcemia, norepinephrine, epinephrine, cyclosporine, amphotericin B
  C. Cirrhosis with ascites (hepatorenal syndrome)
IV. Renal hypoperfusion with impairment of renal autoregulatory responses
  Cyclooxygenase inhibitors, angiotensin-converting enzyme inhibitors
V. Hyperviscosity syndrome (rare)
  Multiple myeloma, macroglobulinemia, polycythemia

INTRINSIC RENAL AZOTEMIA

I. Renovascular obstruction (bilateral or unilateral with one functioning kidney)
  A. Renal artery obstruction: atherosclerotic plaque, thrombosis, embolism, dissecting aneurysm, vasculitis
  B. Renal vein obstruction: thrombosis, compression
II. Disease of glomeruli or renal microvasculature
  A. Glomerulonephritis and vasculitis
  B. Hemolytic uremic syndrome, thrombotic thrombocytopenic purpura, disseminated intravascular coagulation, toxemia of pregnancy, accelerated hypertension, radiation nephritis, systemic lupus erythematosus, scleroderma
III. Acute tubular necrosis
  A. Ischemia: as for prerenal azotemia (hypovolemia, low cardiac output, renal vasoconstriction, systemic vasodilatation), obstetric complications (abruptio placentae, postpartum hemorrhage)
  B. Toxins
    1. Exogenous: radiocontrast, cyclosporine, antibiotics (e.g., aminoglycosides), chemotherapy (e.g., cisplatin), organic solvents (e.g., ethylene glycol), acetaminophen, illegal abortifacients
    2. Endogenous: rhabdomyolysis, hemolysis, uric acid, oxalate, plasma cell dyscrasia (e.g., myeloma)
IV. Interstitial nephritis
  A. Allergic: antibiotics (e.g., β-lactams, sulfonamides, trimethoprim, rifampicin), nonsteroidal anti-inflammatory agents, diuretics, captopril
  B. Infection: bacterial (e.g., acute pyelonephritis, leptospirosis), viral (e.g., cytomegalovirus), fungal (e.g., candidiasis)
  C. Infiltration: lymphoma, leukemia, sarcoidosis
  D. Idiopathic
V. Intratubular deposition and obstruction
  Myeloma proteins, uric acid, oxalate, acyclovir, methotrexate, sulphonamides
VI. Renal allograft rejection

POSTRENAL AZOTEMIA (OBSTRUCTION)

I. Ureteric
  Calculi, blood clot, sloughed papillae, cancer, external compression (e.g., retroperitoneal fibrosis)
II. Bladder neck
  Neurogenic bladder, prostatic hypertrophy, calculi, cancer, blood clot
III. Urethra
  Stricture, congenital valve, phimosis

Autoregulatory dilatation of afferent arterioles is maximal at mean systemic arterial blood pressures of ~80 mmHg, and hypotension below this level is associated with a precipitous decline in GFR. Lesser degrees of hypotension may provoke prerenal azotemia in the elderly and in patients with diseases affecting the integrity of afferent arterioles

(e.g., hypertensive nephrosclerosis, diabetic vasculopathy). In addition, *drugs* that interfere with adaptive responses in the renal microcirculation may convert compensated renal hypoperfusion into overt prerenal azotemia or trigger progression of prerenal azotemia to ischemic ARF (see below). Pharmacologic inhibitors of either renal prostaglandin biosynthesis (*cyclooxygenase inhibitors*) or angiotensin-converting enzyme (ACE) activity (ACE inhibitors) are the major culprits and should be used judiciously in the setting of suspected renal hypoperfusion. *Nonsteroidal anti-inflammatory drugs*, which inhibit cyclooxygenases and prostaglandin biosynthesis, do not compromise GFR in healthy individuals but may precipitate prerenal azotemia in patients with volume depletion or in those with chronic renal insufficiency in whom GFR is maintained, in part, through prostaglandin-mediated hyperfiltration through the remaining functional nephrons. ACE inhibitors can also compromise GFR in subjects with renal hypoperfusion and should be used with special care in patients with bilateral renal artery stenosis or unilateral stenosis in a solitary functioning kidney. Glomerular perfusion and filtration may be exquisitely dependent on the actions of angiotensin II under the latter circumstances. Angiotensin II preserves glomerular filtration pressure distal to stenoses by elevating systemic arterial pressure and by triggering selective constriction of efferent arterioles. ACE inhibitors blunt these responses and precipitate ARF, usually reversible, in approximately ~30 percent of these patients.

Hepatorenal Syndrome This is a particularly aggressive form of ARF that frequently complicates hepatic failure due to advanced cirrhosis or other liver diseases, including malignancy, hepatic resection, and biliary obstruction. Intrarenal vasoconstriction and avid sodium retention are early sequelae of these diseases and may be detected before changes in systemic hemodynamics. Patients with advanced liver disease, portal hypertension, and ascites also have increased plasma volume but "effective" hypovolemia as a consequence of systemic vasodilatation and pooling of blood in the portal circulation. Azotemia typically develops slowly over weeks or months in parallel with deteriorating hepatic function but may accelerate dramatically following a variety of hemodynamic insults, including hemorrhage, paracentesis, and overzealous use of diuretics, vasodilators, or cyclooxygenase inhibitors. In full-blown hepatorenal syndrome, ARF progresses even after optimization of systemic hemodynamics and volume status and removal of nephrotoxins, probably as a result of ongoing intrarenal vasoconstriction, hypoperfusion, and ischemia triggered by a circulating or neural factor elaborated by the failing liver. Indeed, it must be remembered that patients with liver disease may develop other forms of ARF (e.g., sepsis, nephrotoxic medications), and a diagnosis of hepatorenal syndrome should be made only after exclusion of other possible reversible causes.

INTRINSIC RENAL AZOTEMIA (INTRINSIC RENAL ARF) Intrinsic renal azotemia can complicate many diverse diseases of the renal parenchyma. From a clinicopathologic viewpoint, it is useful to divide the causes of acute intrinsic renal azotemia into (1) diseases of large renal vessels, (2) diseases of the renal microcirculation and glomeruli, (3) ischemic and nephrotoxic ARF, and (4) tubulointerstitial diseases (Table 270-1). Most intrinsic renal azotemia is triggered by ischemia (ischemic ARF) or nephrotoxins (nephrotoxic ARF), insults that typically induce acute tubular necrosis (ATN). Accordingly, the terms ARF and ATN are usually used interchangeably in these settings. However, as many as 20 to 30 percent of patients with ischemic or nephrotoxic ARF do not have clinical (granular or tubular cell urinary casts) or morphologic evidence of tubular necrosis, underscoring the role of sublethal injury to tubular epithelium and injury to other renal cells (e.g., endothelial cells) in the pathophysiology of this syndrome.

Etiology and Pathophysiology of Ischemic ARF Prerenal azotemia and ischemic ARF are part of a spectrum of manifestations of renal hypoperfusion. Ischemic ARF differs from prerenal azotemia in that the hypoperfusion induces ischemic injury to renal cells, particularly tubular epithelium, and recovery typically takes 1 to 2 weeks after normalization of renal perfusion as it requires regeneration of tubular cells. In its most extreme form, ischemia leads to bilateral renal cortical necrosis and irreversible renal failure. Ischemic ARF occurs most frequently in patients undergoing major cardiovascular surgery or suffering severe trauma, hemorrhage, sepsis, and/or volume depletion (Table 270-1). Ischemic ARF can also complicate milder forms of true or "effective" hypovolemia if the latter occurs in the presence of other insults (e.g., nephrotoxins or sepsis) or in patients with compromised autoregulatory defense mechanisms or preexisting renal insufficiency.

The course of ischemic ARF is typically characterized by three phases: the initiation, maintenance, and recovery phases. The *initiation phase* (hours to days) is the initial period of renal hypoperfusion during which ischemic injury is evolving. GFR declines because (1) glomerular ultrafiltration pressure is reduced as a consequence of the fall in renal blood flow, (2) the flow of glomerular filtrate within

tubules is obstructed by casts comprising epithelial cells and necrotic debris derived from ischemic tubule epithelium, and (3) there is back-leak of glomerular filtrate through injured tubular epithelium (Fig. 270-1). Ischemic injury is most prominent in the terminal medullary portion of the proximal tubule (S_3 segment, pars recta) and the medullary portion of the thick ascending limb of the loop of Henle. Both segments have high rates of active (ATP-dependent) solute transport and oxygen consumption and are located in a zone of the kidney (the outer medulla) that is relatively ischemic, even under basal conditions, by virtue of the unique countercurrent arrangement of the medullary vasculature. Cellular ischemia results in a series of alterations in energetics, ion transport, and membrane integrity that ultimately lead to cell necrosis. These include depletion of ATP, inhibition of active sodium transport and transport of other solutes, impairment of cell volume regulation and cell swelling, cytoskeletal disruption and loss of cell polarity, accumulation of intracellular calcium, altered phospholipid metabolism, oxygen free radical formation, and peroxidation of membrane lipids. Importantly, renal injury can be limited by restoration of renal blood flow during this period.

The initiation phase is followed by a *maintenance phase* (typically 1 to 2 weeks) during which epithelial cell injury is established, GFR stabilizes at its nadir (typically 5 to 10 mL/min), urine output is lowest, and uremic complications arise (see below). The reasons why the GFR remains low during this phase, despite correction of systemic hemodynamics, are still being defined. Putative mechanisms include persistent intrarenal vasoconstriction and medullary ischemia triggered by dysregulated release of vasoactive mediators from injured endothelial cells (e.g., decreased nitric oxide, increased endothelin), congestion of medullary blood vessels, and reperfusion injury induced by reactive oxygen species and other mediators derived from leukocytes or renal parenchymal cells (Fig. 270-1). In addition, epithelial cell injury per se may contribute to persistent intrarenal vasoconstriction by a process termed *tubuloglomerular feedback*. Specialized epithelial cells in the macula densa region of distal tubules detect increases in distal salt (probably chloride) delivery that occur as a consequence of impaired reabsorption by more proximal nephron segments. Macula densa cells in turn stimulate constriction of adjacent afferent arterioles by a poorly defined mechanism and further compromise glomerular perfusion and filtration, thereby contributing to a vicious cycle. A *recovery phase* is characterized by tubule cell regeneration and a gradual return of GFR to or towards premorbid levels. The recovery phase may be complicated by marked diuresis diuretic phase due to excretion of retained salt and water and other solutes, continued use of diuretics, and/or delayed recovery of epithelial cell function (solute and water reabsorption) relative to glomerular filtration (see below).

Etiology and Pathophysiology of Nephrotoxic ARF Acute intrinsic renal azotemia can complicate exposure to many structurally diverse pharmaco-

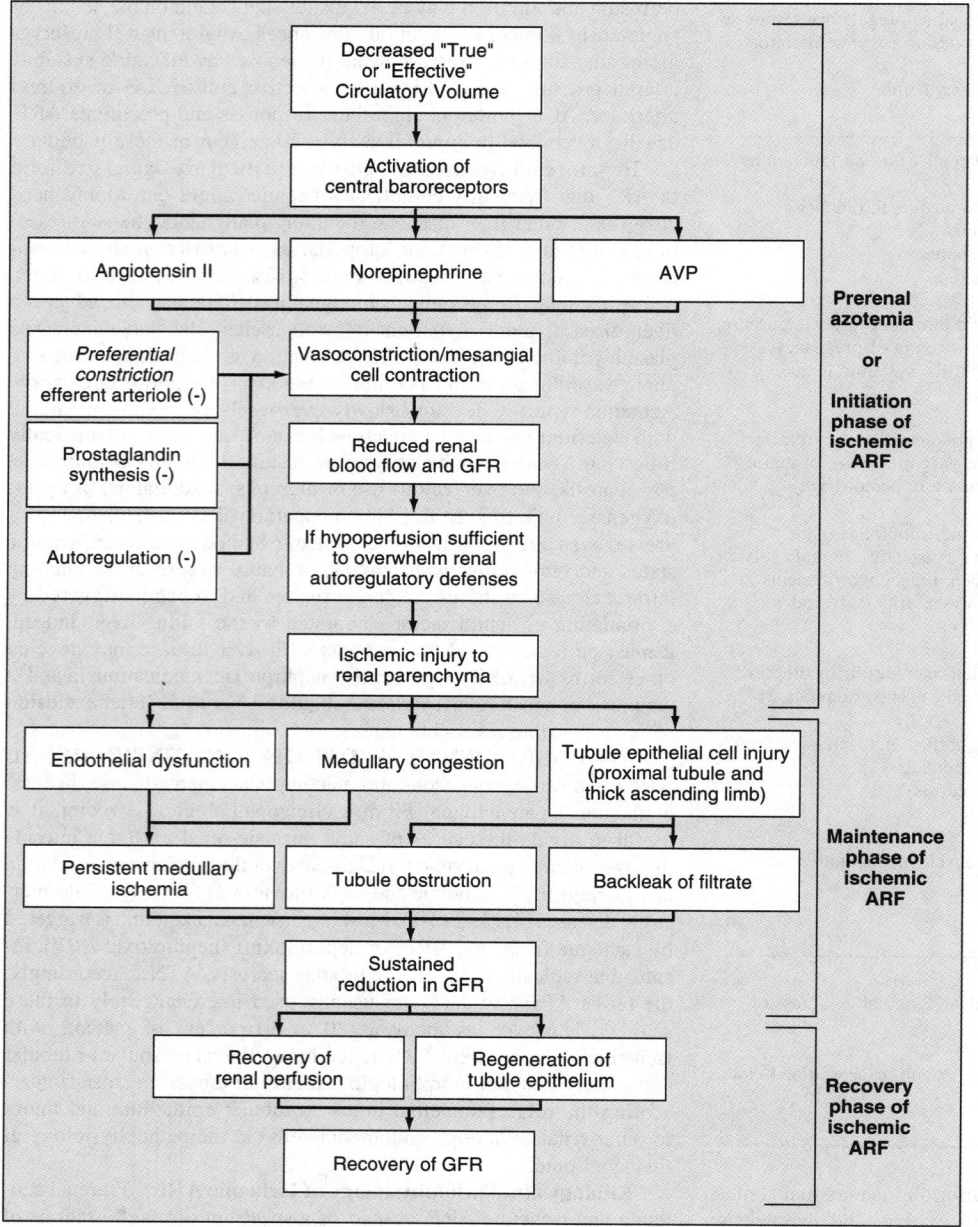

FIGURE 270-1 Overview of the pathophysiology of prerenal azotemia and ischemic ARF: A spectrum of manifestations of renal hypoperfusion (ARF, acute renal failure; AVP, arginine vasopressin; GFR, glomerular filtration rate.)

logic agents (Table 270-1). With most nephrotoxins, the incidence of ARF is increased in the elderly and in patients with preexisting chronic renal insufficiency, true or "effective" hypovolemia, or concomitant exposure to other toxins.

Intrarenal vasoconstriction is a pivotal event in ARF triggered by *radiocontrast agents* (contrast nephropathy) and *cyclosporine*. In keeping with this pathophysiology, both agents induce ARF that shares features with prerenal azotemia: namely, an acute fall in renal blood flow and GFR, a relatively benign urine sediment, and a low fractional excretion of sodium (see below). Severe cases may show clinical or pathologic evidence of ATN. Contrast nephropathy classically presents as an acute (onset within 24 to 28 h) but reversible (peak 3 to 5 days, resolution within 1 week) rise in blood urea nitrogen and creatinine and is most common in individuals with preexisting chronic renal insufficiency, diabetes mellitus, congestive heart failure, hypovolemia, or multiple myeloma. The syndrome appears to be dose-related, and its incidence is only slightly reduced in high-risk individuals by use of more expensive low osmolality, nonionic contrast agents. Endothelin, a potent vasoconstrictor peptide released from endothelial cells, is an important mediator of intrarenal vasoconstriction and mesangial cell contraction in this setting. Endothelin has also been implicated as an important mediator of cyclosporine-induced ARF.

Direct toxicity to tubule epithelial cells and/or intratubular obstruction are major pathophysiologic events in ARF induced by many antibiotics and anticancer drugs. Frequent offenders are the antimicrobial agents, such as acyclovir, foscarnet, aminoglycosides, amphotericin B, and pentamidine, and chemotherapeutic agents, such as cisplatin and ifosfamide. ARF complicates 10 to 30 percent of courses of *aminoglycoside antibiotics*, even in the presence of therapeutic levels. *Amphotericin B* causes dose-related ARF through intrarenal vasoconstriction and direct toxicity to proximal tubule epithelium. Cisplatin, like the aminoglycosides, is accumulated by proximal tubule cells and typically provokes ARF after 7 to 10 days of exposure by inducing mitochondrial injury, inhibition of ATPase activity and solute transport, and free radical–mediated injury to cell membranes.

The most common endogenous nephrotoxins are calcium, myoglobin, hemoglobin, urate, oxalate, and myeloma light chains. Hypercalcemia can compromise GFR, predominantly by inducing intrarenal vasoconstriction. Calcium phosphate deposition within the kidney may also contribute. Both *rhabdomyolysis* and *hemolysis* can induce ARF, particularly in hypovolemic or acidotic individuals. Myoglobinuric ARF complicates approximately 30 percent of cases of rhabdomyolysis. Common causes of the latter include traumatic crush injury, muscle ischemia, seizures, excessive exercise, heat stroke or malignant hyperthermia, alcoholism, and infectious or metabolic disorders. ARF due to hemolysis is relatively rare and is observed following massive blood transfusion reactions. It has been postulated that myoglobin and hemoglobin or other compounds released from muscle or red blood cells cause ARF via toxic effects on tubule epithelial cells or by inducing intratubular cast formation. Hypovolemia or acidosis may contribute to the pathogenesis of ARF in this setting by promoting intranephronal cast formation. In addition, both hemoglobin and myoglobin are potent inhibitors of nitric oxide bioactivity and may trigger intrarenal vasoconstriction and ischemia in patients with borderline renal hypoperfusion. The formation of intratubular casts containing filtered immunoglobulin light chains and other proteins, including Tamm-Horsfall protein produced by thick ascending limb cells, is the major trigger for ARF in patients with *multiple myeloma* (myeloma-cast nephropathy). Light chains may also be directly toxic to tubule epithelial cells. Intratubular obstruction may also be an important cause of ARF in patients with severe *hyperuricosuria* or *hyperoxaluria*. Acute uric acid nephropathy typically complicates treatment of lymphoproliferative or myeloproliferative disorders but occasionally occurs in other forms of primary or secondary hyperuricemia if the urine is concentrated.

Pathology of Ischemic and Nephrotoxic ARF The classic pathologic features of ischemic ARF are patchy and focal necrosis of tubule epithelium with detachment from its basement membrane and occlusion of tubule lumens with casts composed of intact or degener-

ating epithelial cells, cellular debris, Tamm-Horsfall mucoprotein, and pigments. Leukocyte accumulation is frequently observed in vasa recta; however, the glomeruli and renal vasculature are characteristically normal. Necrosis is most severe in the straight portion (pars recta) of proximal tubules but may also be prominent in the medullary thick ascending limb of the loop of Henle.

In nephrotoxic ARF, morphologic changes tend to be most prominent in both the convoluted and straight portions of proximal tubules. Tubule cell necrosis is less pronounced than in ischemic ARF.

Other Causes of Acute Intrinsic Renal Azotemia Patients with advanced atherosclerosis can develop ARF after manipulation of the aorta or renal arteries at surgery or angiography, following trauma, or, rarely, spontaneously due to embolization of cholesterol crystals to the renal vasculature (atheroembolic ARF). Cholesterol crystals lodge in small- and medium-sized arteries and incite a giant cell and fibrotic reaction in the vessel wall with narrowing or obstruction of the vessel lumen. Atheroembolic ARF is frequently irreversible. A myriad of structurally diverse pharmacologic agents induce ARF by triggering allergic interstitial nephritis, a disease characterized by infiltration of the tubulointerstitium by granulocytes (typically but not invariably eosinophils), macrophages, and/or lymphocytes and by interstitial edema. The most common offenders are antibiotics (e.g., penicillins, cephalosporins, trimethoprim, sulfonamides, rifampicin) and nonsteroidal anti-inflammatory drugs (Table 270-1).

POSTRENAL AZOTEMIA (See also Chap. 280) Urinary tract obstruction accounts for fewer than 5 percent of cases of ARF. Since one kidney has sufficient clearance capacity to excrete nitrogenous waste products, ARF from obstruction requires either obstruction to urine flow between the external urethral meatus and bladder neck, bilateral ureteric obstruction, or unilateral ureteric obstruction in a patient with one functioning kidney or preexisting chronic renal insufficiency. Bladder neck obstruction represents the most common cause of postrenal azotemia and is usually due to prostatic disease (e.g., hypertrophy, neoplasia, or infection), neurogenic bladder, or therapy with anticholinergic drugs. Less common causes of acute lower urinary tract obstruction include blood clots, calculi, and urethritis with spasm. Ureteric obstruction may result from intraluminal obstruction (e.g., calculi, blood clots, sloughed renal papillae), infiltration of the ureteric wall (e.g., neoplasia), or external compression (e.g., retroperitoneal fibrosis, neoplasia or abscess, inadvertent surgical ligature). During the early stages of obstruction (hours to days), continued glomerular filtration leads to increased intraluminal pressure upstream to the site of obstruction. As a result there are gradual distention of proximal ureter, renal pelvis, and calyces and a fall in GFR. Acute obstruction is initially associated with modest increase in renal blood flow, but arteriolar vasoconstriction soon supervenes, leading to a further decline in glomerular filtration.

CLINICAL FEATURES AND DIFFERENTIAL DIAGNOSIS

Patients presenting with azotemia should be assessed initially to determine if the decline in GFR is acute or chronic. An acute process is easily established if a review of laboratory records reveals a recent rise in blood urea and creatinine levels, but previous measurements are not always available. Findings that suggest chronic renal failure (Chap. 271) include anemia, neuropathy, and radiologic evidence of renal osteodystrophy or small scarred kidneys. However, it should be noted that anemia may also complicate ARF (see below), and renal size may be normal or increased in several chronic renal diseases (e.g., diabetic nephropathy, amyloidosis, polycystic kidney disease). Once a diagnosis of ARF has been established, several issues should be addressed promptly: (1) the identification of the cause of ARF, (2) the elimination of the triggering insult (e.g., nephrotoxin) and/or institution of disease-specific therapies, and (3) the prevention and management of uremic complications.

CLINICAL ASSESSMENT Clinical clues to *prerenal azotemia* are symptoms of thirst and orthostatic dizziness and physical evidence of orthostatic hypotension and tachycardia, reduced jugular venous pressure, decreased skin turgor, dry mucous membranes, and reduced axillary sweating. Case records should be reviewed for documentation of a progressive fall in urine output and body weight and treatment with cyclooxygenase or ACE inhibitors. Careful clinical examination may reveal stigmata of chronic liver disease and portal hypertension, advanced cardiac failure, sepsis, or other causes of "effective" hypovolemia (Table 270-1).

Intrinsic renal azotemia due to ischemia is likely following prolonged or severe renal hypoperfusion complicating hypovolemic or septic shock or following major surgery. The likelihood of ischemic ARF is increased further if ARF persists despite normalization of systemic hemodynamics. Diagnosis of nephrotoxic ARF requires careful review of the clinical data and pharmacy, nursing, and radiology records for evidence of recent exposure to nephrotoxic medications or radiocontrast agents or to endogenous toxins (e.g., myoglobin, hemoglobin, uric acid, myeloma protein, or elevated levels of serum calcium).

Although ischemic and nephrotoxic ARF account for more than 90 percent of cases of intrinsic renal azotemia, other renal parenchymal diseases must be considered (Table 270-2). Flank pain may be a prominent symptom following occlusion of a renal artery or vein and with other parenchymal diseases distending the renal capsule (e.g., severe glomerulonephritis or pyelonephritis). Subcutaneous nodules, livido reticularis, bright orange retinal arteriolar plaques, and digital ischemia, despite palpable pedal pulses, are clues to atheroembolization. ARF in association with oliguria, edema, hypertension, and an "active" urine sediment (nephritic syndrome) suggests acute glomerulonephritis or vasculitis. Malignant hypertension is a likely cause of ARF in patients with severe hypertension and evidence of hypertensive injury to other organs (e.g., left ventricular hypertrophy and failure, hypertensive retinopathy and papilledema, neurologic dysfunction). Fever, arthralgias, and a pruritic erythematous rash following exposure to a new drug suggest allergic interstitial nephritis, although systemic features of hypersensitivity are frequently absent.

Acute postrenal azotemia presents with suprapubic and flank pain due to distention of the bladder and of the renal collecting system and capsule, respectively. Colicky flank pain radiating to the groin suggests acute ureteric obstruction. Prostatic disease is likely if there is a history of nocturia, frequency, and hesitancy and enlargement or induration of the prostate on rectal examination. Neurogenic bladder should be suspected in patients receiving anticholinergic medications or with physical evidence of autonomic dysfunction. Definitive diagnosis of postrenal azotemia hinges on judicious use of radiologic investigations and rapid improvement in renal function following relief of obstruction.

URINALYSIS Anuria suggests complete urinary tract obstruction but may complicate severe cases of prerenal or intrinsic renal azotemia. Wide fluctuations in urine output raise the possibility of intermittent obstruction, whereas patients with partial urinary tract obstruction can present with polyuria due to impairment of urine concentrating mechanisms.

In prerenal azotemia, the sediment is characteristically acellular and contains transparent hyaline casts ("bland," "benign," "inactive" urine sediment). Hyaline casts are formed in concentrated urine from normal constitutents of urine—principally Tamm-Horsfall protein, which is secreted by epithelial cells of the loop of Henle. Postrenal azotemia may also present with an inactive sediment, although hematuria and pyuria are common in patients with intraluminal obstruction or prostatic disease. Pigmented "muddy brown" granular casts and casts containing tubule epithelial cells are characteristic of tubule necrosis and suggest ischemic or nephrotoxic ARF. They are usually found in association with microscopic hematuria and mild "tubular" proteinuria (<1 g/d); the latter reflects impaired reabsorption and processing of filtered proteins by injured proximal tubules. Casts are absent, however, in 20 to 30 percent of patients with ischemic or nephrotoxic ARF and are not a requisite for diagnosis. In general, red blood cell casts indicate glomerular injury or, less often, acute tubulointerstitial nephritis. White cell casts and nonpigmented granular casts suggest interstitial nephritis, whereas broad granular casts are characteristic of chronic renal disease and probably reflect interstitial fibrosis and dilatation of tubules. Eosinophiluria (>5 percent of urine leukocytes) is a common finding (~90 percent) in antibiotic-induced allergic interstitial nephritis when studied using Hansel's stain; however, lymphocytes may predominate in allergic interstitial nephritis induced by nonsteroidal anti-inflammatory drugs. Eosinophiluria is also a feature of atheroembolic ARF. Occasional uric acid crystals (pleomorphic in shape) are common in the concentrated urine of prerenal azotemia but suggest acute urate nephropathy if seen in abundance. Oxalate (envelope-shaped) and hippurate (needle-shaped) crystals raise the possibility of ethylene glycol ingestion and toxicity.

Increased urine protein excretion, but <1 g/d, is common in ATN due to failure of injured proximal tubules to reabsorb filtered protein and excretion of cellular debris ("tubular proteinuria"). Proteinuria of >1 g/d suggests injury to the glomerular ultrafiltration barrier ("glomerular proteinuria") or excretion of myeloma light chains. The latter are not detected by conventional dipsticks (which detect albumin) and must be sought by other means (e.g., sulfosalicylic acid test, immunoelectrophoresis). Heavy proteinuria is also a frequent finding (~80 percent) in patients who develop combined allergic interstitial nephritis and minimal change glomerulopathy when treated with cyclooxygenase inhibitors. A similar syndrome can be triggered by ampicillin, rifampicin, or interferon α. Hemoglobinuria or myoglobinuria should be suspected if urine is strongly positive for heme by dipstick, but contains few red cells, and if the supernatant of centrifuged urine is positive for free heme. Bilirubinuria may provide a clue to the presence of hepatorenal syndrome.

RENAL FAILURE INDICES Analysis of urine and blood biochemistry is particularly useful for distinguishing prerenal azotemia from ischemic or nephrotoxic intrinsic renal azotemia (Table 270-3). The fractional excretion of sodium (FeNa) is most useful in this regard. The FeNa relates sodium clearance to creatinine clearance. Sodium is reabsorbed avidly from glomerular filtrate in patients with prerenal azotemia, in an attempt to restore intravascular volume, but not in patients with ARF, as a result of tubular epithelial cell injury. In contrast, creatinine is not reabsorbed in either setting. Consequently, patients with prerenal azotemia typically have a FeNa of <1.0 percent (frequently <0.1 percent, whereas the FeNa in patients with ischemic or nephrotoxic ARF is usually >1.0 percent. The *renal failure index* (Table 270-3) provides comparable information, since clinical variations in serum sodium concentration are relatively small. *Urine sodium concentration* is a less sensitive index for distinguishing prerenal azotemia from ischemic and nephrotoxic ARF as values overlap between groups. Similarly, indices of urinary concentrating ability such as urine specific gravity, urine osmolality, urine to plasma urea ratio, and blood urea to creatinine ratio are of limited value in differential diagnosis.

Many caveats apply when interpreting biochemical renal failure indices. FeNa may be >1.0 percent in prerenal azotemia if patients are receiving diuretics or have bicarbonaturia (accompanied by sodium to maintain electroneutrality), preexisting chronic renal failure complicated by salt wasting, or adrenal insufficiency. In contrast, the FeNa is <1.0 percent in approximately 15 percent of patients with nonoliguric ischemic or nephrotoxic ARF. The FeNa is often <1.0 percent in ARF due to urinary tract obstruction, glomerulonephritis, and vascular diseases.

LABORATORY FINDINGS Serial measurements of serum creatinine can provide useful pointers to the cause of ARF. Prerenal azotemia is typified by fluctuating levels that parallel changes in hemodynamic function. Creatinine rises rapidly (within 24 to 48 h) in patients with ARF following renal ischemia, atheroembolization, and radiocontrast exposure. Peak creatinine levels are observed after 3 to 5 days with contrast nephropathy and return to baseline after 5 to 7 days. In contrast, creatinine levels typically peak later (7 to 10 days) in ischemic ARF and atheroembolic disease. The initial rise in serum creatinine is characteristically delayed until the second week of therapy

Table 270-2

Useful Clinical Features, Urinary Findings, and Confirmatory Tests in the Differential Diagnosis of Major Causes of Acute Azotemia

Cause of Acute Renal Failure	Suggestive Clinical Features	Typical Urinalysis	Some Confirmatory Tests
I. Prerenal Azotemia	Evidence of true volume depletion (thirst, postural or absolute hypotension and tachycardia, low jugular venous pressure, dry mucous membranes/axillae, weight loss, fluid output > input) or decreased "effective" circulatory volume (e.g., heart failure, liver failure), treatment with NSAIDs or ACE inhibitors	Hyaline casts FeNa <1% U_{Na} <10 mmol/L SG >1.018	Occasionally requires invasive hemodynamic monitoring; rapid resolution of ARF upon restoration of renal perfusion
II. Intrinsic renal azotemia			
A. Diseases involving large renal vessels			
1. Renal artery thrombosis	History of atrial fibrillation or recent myocardial infarct; flank or abdominal pain	Mild proteinuria Occasionally red cells	Elevated LDH with normal transaminases, renal arteriogram
2. Atheroembolism	Age usually > 50 years, recent manipulation of aorta, retinal plaques, subcutaneous nodules, palpable purpura, livedo reticularis, vasculopathy, hypertension	Often normal, eosinophiluria, rarely casts	Eosinophilia, hypocomplementemia, skin biopsy, renal biopsy
3. Renal vein thrombosis	Evidence of nephrotic syndrome or pulmonary embolism, flank pain	Proteinuria, hematuria	Inferior vena cavagram and selective renal venogram
B. Diseases of small vessels and glomeruli			
1. Glomerulonephritis/vasculitis	Compatible clinical history (e.g., recent infection) sinusitis, lung hemorrhage, skin rash or ulcers, arthralgias, new cardiac murmur, history of hepatitis B or C infection	Red cell or granular casts, red cells, white cells, mild proteinuria	Low C3, ANCA, anti-GBM Ab, ANA, ASO, anti-DNAse, cryoglobulins, blood cultures, renal biopsy
2. Hemolytic-uremic syndrome/thrombotic thrombocytopenic purpura	Compatible clinical history (e.g., recent gastrointestinal infection, cyclosporine, anovulants), fever, pallor, ecchymoses, neurologic abnormalities	May be normal, red cells, mild proteinuria, rarely red cell/granular casts	Anemia, thrombocytopenia, schistocytes on blood smear, increased LDH, renal biopsy
3. Malignant hypertension	Severe hypertension with headaches, cardiac failure, retinopathy, neurologic dysfunction, papilledema	Red cells, red cell casts, proteinuria	LVH by echocardiography/ECG, resolution of ARF with control of blood pressure
C. ARF mediated by ischemia or toxins (ATN)			
1. Ischemia	Recent hemorrhage, hypotension (e.g., cardiac arrest), surgery	Muddy brown granular or tubular epithelial cell casts FeNa >1% U_{Na} >20 mmol/L SG <1.015	Clinical assessment and urinalysis usually sufficient for diagnosis
2. Exogenous toxins	Recent radiocontrast study, nephrotoxic antibiotics or anticancer agents often coexistent with volume depletion, sepsis, or chronic renal insufficiency	Muddy brown granular or tubular epithelial cell casts FeNa >1% U_{Na} >20 mmol/L SG <1.015	Clinical assessment and urinalysis usually sufficient for diagnosis
3. Endogenous toxins	History suggestive of rhabdomyolysis (seizures, coma, ethanol abuse, trauma)	Urine supernatant positive for heme	Hyperkalemia, hyperphosphatemia, hypocalcemia, increased circulating myoglobin, MM, CPK and uric acid
	History suggestive of hemolysis (blood transfusion)	Urine supernatant pink and positive for heme	Hyperkalemia, hyperphosphatemia, hypocalcemia, hyperuricemia, pink plasma positive for hemoglobin
	History suggestive of tumor lysis (recent chemotherapy), myeloma (bone pain), or ethylene glycol ingestion	Urate crystals, dipstick-negative proteinuria, oxalate crystals, respectively	Hyperuricemia, hyperkalemia, hyperphosphatemia (for tumor lysis); circulating or urinary monoclonal spike (for myeloma); toxicology screen, acidosis, osmolal gap (for ethylene glycol)
D. Acute diseases of the tubulointerstitium			
1. Allergic interstitial nephritis	Recent ingestion of drug, and fever, rash, or arthralgias	White cell casts, white cells (frequently eosinphiluria) red cells, rarely red cell casts, proteinuria (occasionally nephrotic)	Systemic eosinophilia, skin biopsy of rash (leukocytoclastic vasculitis), renal biopsy
2. Acute bilateral pyelonephritis	Flank pain and tenderness, toxic, febrile	Leukocytes, proteinuria, red cells, bacteria	Urine and blood cultures
III. Postrenal azotemia	Abdominal or flank pain, palpable bladder	Frequently normal, hematuria if stones, hemorrhage, malignancy, or prostatic hypertrophy	Plain film, renal ultrasound, IVP, retrograde or anterograde pyelography, CT scan

NOTE: NSAIDs, nonsteroidal anti-inflammatory drugs; U_{Na}, urine sodium concentration; SG, specific gravity; LDH, lactate dehydrogenase; C3, complement component; ANCA, antineutrophil cytoplasmic autoantibody; GBM Ab, glomerular basement membrane antibody; ANA, antinuclear antibody; ASO, antistreptolysin O; LVH, left ventricular hypertrophy; ECG, electrocardiogram; CPK, creatine phosphokinase; IVP, intravenous pyelogram; CT, computed tomography.

SOURCE: Adapted with permission from HR Brady et al in *The Kidney*, 5th ed, BM Brenner (ed). Philadelphia, Saunders, 1996

Table 270-3

Urine Diagnostic Indices in Differentiation of Prerenal versus Intrinsic Renal Azotemia

Diagnostic Index	Typical Findings	
	Prerenal Azotemia	Intrinsic Renal Azotemia
Fractional excretion of sodium (%)* $$\frac{U_{Na} \times P_{Cr}}{P_{Na} \times U_{Cr}} \times 100$$	<1	>1
Urine sodium concentration (mmol/L)	<10	>20
Urine creatinine to plasma creatinine ratio	>40	>20
Urine urea nitrogen to plasma urea nitrogen ratio	>8	<3
Urine specific gravity	>1.018	<1.015
Urine osmolality (mosmol/kg H_2O)	>500	<300
Plasma BUN/creatinine ratio	>20	<10–15
Renal failure index* $$\frac{U_{Na}}{U_{Cr}/P_{Cr}}$$	<1	>1
Urinary sediment	Hyaline casts	Muddy brown granular casts

* Most sensitive indices

NOTE: U_{Na}, urine sodium concentration; P_{Cr}, plasma creatinine concentration; P_{Na}, plasma sodium concentration; U_{Cr}, urine creatinine concentration; BUN, blood urea nitrogen.

with many tubule epithelial cell toxins (e.g., aminoglycosides, cisplatin) and probably reflects the need for accumulation of these agents within cells before GFR falls.

Hyperkalemia, hyperphosphatemia, hypocalcemia, and elevations in serum uric acid and creatine kinase (MM isoenzyme) levels suggest a diagnosis of rhabdomyolysis. Hyperuricemia (>15 mg/dL) in association with hyperkalemia, hyperphosphatemia, and increased circulating levels of intracellular enzymes such as lactate dehydrogenase may indicate acute urate nephropathy and tumor lysis syndrome following cancer chemotherapy. A wide serum anion and osmolal gap (measured serum osmolality minus the serum osmolality calculated from serum sodium, glucose, and urea concentrations) indicate the presence of an unusual anion or osmole in the circulation and are clues to diagnosis of ethylene glycol or methanol ingestion. Severe anemia in the absence of hemorrhage raises the possibility of hemolysis, multiple myeloma, or thrombotic microangiopathy. Systemic eosinophilia suggests allergic interstitial nephritis but is also a feature of atheroembolic disease and polyarteritis nodosa.

RADIOLOGIC FINDINGS Imaging of the urinary tract by ultrasonography is useful to exclude obstructive uropathy. Computed tomography and magnetic resonance imaging are alternative imaging modalities. Whereas pelvicalyceal dilatation is usual with urinary tract obstruction (98 percent sensitivity), dilatation may be absent immediately following obstruction or in patients with ureteric encasement (e.g., retroperitoneal fibrosis, neoplasia). Retrograde or anterograde pyelography are more definitive investigations in complex cases and provide precise localization of the site of obstruction. Intravenous pyelography should be avoided as systemic radiocontrast may exacerbate ARF. A plain film of the abdomen, with tomography if necessary, is a valuable initial screening technique in patients with suspected nephrolithiasis. Doppler ultrasonography and magnetic resonance flow imaging appear promising for assessment of patency of renal arteries and veins in patients with suspected vascular obstruction; however, contrast angiography is usually required for definitive diagnosis.

RENAL BIOPSY Biopsy is reserved for patients in whom prerenal and postrenal failure have been excluded and the cause of intrinsic renal azotemia is unclear. Renal biopsy is particularly useful when clinical assessment and laboratory investigations suggest diagnoses other than ischemic or nephrotoxic injury that may respond to disease-specific therapy. Examples include glomerulonephritis, vasculitis, hemolytic-uremic syndrome, thrombotic thrombocytopenic purpura, and allergic interstitial nephritis.

COMPLICATIONS

ARF impairs renal excretion of sodium, potassium, and water and perturbs divalent cation homeostasis and urinary acidification mechanisms. As a result, ARF is frequently complicated by intravascular volume overload, hyponatremia, hyperkalemia, hyperphosphatemia, hypocalcemia, hypermagnesemia, and metabolic acidosis. In addition, patients are unable to excrete nitrogenous waste products and are prone to develop the uremic syndrome (Chap. 271). The speed of development and severity of these complications reflects the degree of renal impairment and catabolic state of the patient.

Expansion of extracellular fluid volume is an inevitable consequence of diminished salt and water excretion in oliguric or anuric individuals. Whereas milder forms are characterized by weight gain, bibasilar lung rales, raised jugular venous pressure, and dependent edema, continued volume expansion may precipitate life-threatening pulmonary edema. Hypervolemia may be particularly problematic in patients receiving multiple intravenous medications and enteral or parenteral nutrition. Excessive administration of free water either through ingestion or as hypotonic saline or isotonic dextrose solutions (dextrose being metabolized) can induce *hypoosmolality* and *hyponatremia*, which, if severe, lead to cerebral edema and neurologic abnormalities, including seizures.

Hyperkalemia is a frequent complication of ARF. Serum potassium typically rises by 0.5 mmol/L per day in oliguric and anuric patients due to impaired excretion of ingested or infused potassium and potassium released from injured tubular epithelium. Coexistent metabolic acidosis may exacerbate hyperkalemia by promoting potassium efflux from cells. Hyperkalemia may be particularly severe, even at the time of diagnosis, in patients with rhabdomyolysis, hemolysis, and tumor lysis syndrome. Mild hyperkalemia (<6.0 mmol/L) is usually asymptomatic. Higher levels are typically associated with electrocardiographic abnormalities (Chap. 228).

Metabolism of dietary protein yields between 50 and 100 mmol/d of fixed nonvolatile acids that are normally excreted by the kidneys. Consequently, ARF is typically complicated by *metabolic acidosis*, often with an increased serum anion gap (Chap. 50). Acidosis can be particularly severe when endogenous production of hydrogen ions is increased by other mechanisms (e.g., diabetic or fasting ketoacidosis; lactic acidosis complicating generalized tissue hypoperfusion, liver disease, or sepsis; metabolism of ethylene glycol or methanol).

Mild *hyperphosphatemia* is an almost invariable complication of ARF. Severe hyperphosphatemia may develop in highly catabolic patients or following rhabdomyolysis, hemolysis, or tumor lysis. Metastatic deposition of calcium phosphate can lead to *hypocalcemia*, particularly when the product of serum calcium (mg/dL) and phosphate (mg/dL) concentrations exceeds 70. Other factors that contribute to hypocalcemia include tissue resistance to the actions of parathyroid hormone and reduced levels of 1,25-dihydroxyvitamin D. Hypocalcemia is often asymptomatic but can cause perioral paresthesias, muscle cramps, seizures, hallucinations and confusion, and prolongation of the QT interval and nonspecific T-wave changes on electrocardiography (Chap. 354).

Anemia develops rapidly in ARF and is usually mild and multifactorial in origin. Contributing factors include impaired erythropoiesis, hemolysis, bleeding, hemodilution, and reduced red cell survival time. Prolongation of the *bleeding time* and *leukocytosis* are also common. Common contributors to the bleeding diathesis include mild thrombocytopenia, platelet dysfunction, and/or clotting factor abnormalities (e.g., factor VIII dysfunction), whereas leukocytosis usually reflects sepsis, a stress response, or other concurrent illness. *Infection* is a common and serious complication of ARF, occurring in 50 to 90 percent of cases and accounting for up to 75 percent of deaths. It is unclear whether patients with ARF have a clinically significant defect in host immune responses or whether the high incidence of infection reflects repeated breaches of mucocutaneous barriers (e.g., intravenous cannulae, mechanical ventilation, bladder catheterization). *Cardiac complications* of ARF include arrhythmias, myocardial infarction, and pulmonary embolism. Mild *gastrointestinal bleeding* is common (10 to 30 percent) and is usually due to stress ulceration of gastric or small intestinal mucosa.

Protracted periods of severe ARF are invariably associated with the development of the *uremic syndrome* (Chap. 271).

A vigorous diuresis can occur during the *recovery phase* of ARF (see above) and lead to intravascular volume depletion and delayed recovery of GFR by causing secondary prerenal azotemia. *Hypernatremia* can also complicate recovery if water losses via hypotonic urine are not replaced or if losses are inappropriately replaced by relatively hypertonic saline solutions. *Hypokalemia, hypomagnesemia, hypophosphatemia,* and *hypocalcemia* are less common metabolic complications during this period.

℞ TREATMENT

Prevention Because there are no specific therapies for treatment of ischemic or nephrotoxic ARF, prevention is of paramount importance. Many cases of ischemic ARF can be avoided by close attention to cardiovascular function and intravascular volume in high-risk patients. Indeed, aggressive restoration of intravascular volume has been shown to reduce the incidence of ARF dramatically after major surgery or trauma, burns, or cholera. The incidence of nephrotoxic ARF can be reduced by tailoring the dosage of potential nephrotoxins to body size and GFR; for example, reducing the dose or frequency of administration of drugs in patients with preexisting renal impairment. Adjusting drug dosage according to circulating drug levels also appears to limit renal injury in patients receiving aminoglycoside antibiotics or cyclosporine. Diuretics, cyclooxygenase inhibitors, ACE inhibitors, and other vasodilators should be used with caution in patients with suspected true or "effective" hypovolemia or renovascular disease as they may precipitate prerenal azotemia or convert the latter to ischemic ARF. Hypovolemia should be avoided in patients receiving nephrotoxic medications as renal hypoperfusion potentiates the toxicity of most nephrotoxins. Allopurinol and forced alkaline diuresis are useful in patients at high risk for acute urate nephropathy (e.g., cancer chemotherapy in hematologic malignancies) to limit uric acid generation and prevent precipitation of urate crystals in renal tubules. Forced alkaline diuresis may also prevent or attenuate ARF in patients receiving high-dose methotrexate or suffering from rhabdomyolysis. *N*-acetylcysteine limits acetaminophen-induced renal injury if given within 24 h of ingestion. Dimercaprol, a chelating agent, may prevent heavy metal nephrotoxicity. Ethanol inhibits ethylene glycol metabolism to oxalic acid and other toxic metabolites and is an important adjunct to hemodialysis in the emergency management of ethylene glycol intoxication. By inhibiting alcohol dehydrogenase, ethanol can also reduce the conversion of methanol to the highly toxic formic acid.

Specific Therapies By definition, *prerenal azotemia* is rapidly reversible upon correction of the primary hemodynamic abnormality, and *postrenal azotemia* resolves upon relief of obstruction. To date, there are no specific therapies for established intrinsic renal ARF due to ischemia or nephrotoxicity. Management of these disorders should focus on elimination of the causative hemodynamic abnormality or toxin, avoidance of additional insults, and prevention and treatment of complications. Specific treatment of other causes of intrinsic renal azotemia depends on the underlying pathology.

PRERENAL AZOTEMIA The composition of replacement fluids for treatment of prerenal azotemia due to hypovolemia must be tailored according to the composition of the lost fluid. Hypovolemia due to hemorrhage should be corrected with packed red blood cells in saline, whereas isotonic saline is usually appropriate replacement

for plasma loss (e.g., burns, pancreatitis). Urinary and gastrointestinal fluids can vary greatly in composition but are usually hypotonic. Hypotonic solutions (e.g., 0.45 percent saline) are usually recommended as initial replacement in patients with prerenal azotemia due to increased urinary or gastrointestinal fluid losses, although isotonic saline may be more appropriate in severe cases. Subsequent therapy should be based on measurements of the volume and ionic content of excreted or drained fluids. Serum potassium and acid-base status should be monitored carefully, and potassium and bicarbonate supplemented as appropriate. Cardiac failure may require aggressive management with positive inotropes, preload and afterload reducing agents, antiarrhythmic drugs, and mechanical aids such as intraaortic balloon pumps. Invasive hemodynamic monitoring may be required to guide therapy for complicated conditions in patients in whom clinical assessment of cardiovascular function and intravascular volume proves unreliable.

Fluid management may be particularly difficult in patients with cirrhosis complicated by ascites. In this setting, it is important to distinguish between full-blown hepatorenal syndrome (Chap. 299), which carries a grave prognosis, and reversible ARF due to "true" or "effective" hypovolemia by overzealous use of diuretics or sepsis (e.g., spontaneous bacterial peritonitis). The contribution of hypovolemia to ARF can be definitively assessed only by administration of a fluid challenge. Fluids should be administered slowly and titrated against jugular venous pressure and, if necessary, central venous and pulmonary capillary wedge pressure, abdominal girth, and urine output. Patients with a reversible prerenal component typically have an increase in urine output and fall in serum creatinine, whereas patients with hepatorenal syndrome do not and may suffer increased ascites formation and pulmonary edema if not monitored closely. Large volumes of ascitic fluid can usually be drained by paracentesis without deterioration in renal function if intravenous albumin is administered simultaneously. Indeed, "large-volume paracentesis" may afford an increase in GFR, possibly by lowering intraabdominal pressure and improving flow in renal veins. Shunting of ascitic fluid from the peritoneum to a central vein (peritoneojugular shunt, LeVeen or Denver shunts) is an alternative approach in refractory cases. This maneuver can also improve GFR and sodium excretion transiently, probably because the increase in central blood volume stimulates release of atrial natriuretic peptides and inhibits secretion of aldosterone and norepinephrine.

ACUTE INTRINSIC RENAL AZOTEMIA Many different approaches have been tested for their ability to attenuate injury or hasten recovery in *ischemic* and *nephrotoxic ARF*. Whereas many of these are beneficial in experimental models of ischemic or nephrotoxic ARF, they have either failed to confer consistent benefit or have proved too toxic for use in humans.

Acute renal failure due to *other intrinsic renal diseases* such as acute glomerulonephritis or vasculitis may respond to glucocorticoids, alkylating agents, and/or plasmapheresis, depending on the primary pathology. Glucocorticoids also hasten remission in some cases of allergic interstitial nephritis. Aggressive control of systemic arterial pressure is of paramount importance in limiting renal injury in malignant hypertensive nephrosclerosis, toxemia of pregnancy, and other vascular diseases. Hypertension and ARF due to scleroderma may be exquisitely sensitive to treatment with ACE inhibitors.

POSTRENAL AZOTEMIA Management of postrenal azotemia requires close collaboration between nephrologist, urologist, and radiologist. Obstruction of the urethra or bladder neck are usually managed initially by transurethral or suprapubic placement of a bladder catheter, which provides temporary relief while the obstructing lesion is identified and treated definitively. Similarly, ureteric obstruction may be treated initially by percutaneous catheterization of the dilated renal pelvis or ureter. Indeed, obstructing lesions can often be removed percutaneously (e.g., calculus, sloughed papilla) or bypassed by insertion of a ureteric stent (e.g., carcinoma). Most patients experience an appropriate diuresis for several days following relief of obstruction. Approximately 5 percent of patients develop a transient salt-wasting syndrome that may require administration of intravenous saline to maintain blood pressure.

Supportive Measures (Table 270-4) Following correction of hypovelemia, salt and water intake are tailored to match losses. *Hypervolemia* can usually be managed by restriction of salt and water intake and diuretics. Indeed, there is, as yet, no proven rationale for administration of diuretics in ARF except to treat this complication. High doses of loop-blocking diuretics such as furosemide (up to 200 to 400 mg intravenously) or bumetanide (up to 10 mg intravenously) may promote diuresis in patients who fail to respond to conventional doses. Subpressor doses of dopamine (1 to 5 μg/kg per min) are claimed to promote salt and water excretion by increasing renal blood flow and GFR and by inhibiting tubule sodium reabsorption; however, its efficacy has not been definitively established. Ultrafiltration or dialysis is used to treat severe hypervolemia when conservative measures fail. *Hyponatremia* and *hypoosmolality* can usually be controlled by restriction of free water intake. Conversely, *hypernatremia* is treated by administration of water or intravenous hypotonic saline or isotonic dextrose–containing solutions. The management of hyperkalemia is described in Chap. 49.

Metabolic acidosis is not treated unless serum bicarbonate concentration falls below 15 mmol/L or arterial pH falls below 7.2. More severe acidosis is corrected by oral or intravenous sodium bicarbonate. Initial rates of replacement are guided by estimates of bicarbonate deficit and adjusted thereafter according to serum levels (Chap. 50). Patients are monitored for complications of bicarbonate administration such as hypervolemia, metabolic alkalosis, hypocalcemia, and hypokalemia. From a practical point of view, most patients requiring sodium bicarbonate need emergency dialysis within days. *Hyperphosphatemia* is usually controlled by restriction of dietary phosphate and by oral aluminum hydroxide or calcium carbonate, which reduce gastrointestinal absorption of phosphate. *Hypocalcemia* does not usually require treatment unless severe, as may occur with rhabdomyolysis or pancreatitis or following administration of bicarbonate. *Hyperuricemia* is typically mild [<900 μmol/L (<15 mg/dL)] and does not require intervention.

The objective of *nutritional management* during the maintenance phase of ARF is to provide sufficient calories to avoid catabolism and starvation ketoacidosis, while minimizing production of nitrogenous waste. This is best achieved by restricting dietary protein to approximately 0.6 g/kg per day of protein of high biological value (i.e., rich in essential amino acids) and to provide most calories as carbohydrate (approximately 100 g daily). Nutritional management is easier in nonoliguric patients and following institution of dialysis. Vigorous parenteral hyperalimentation is claimed to improve prognosis; however, convincing benefit has yet to be demonstrated in controlled trials.

Anemia may necessitate blood transfusion or administration of recombinant human erythropoietin if severe or if recovery is delayed. Uremic bleeding usually responds to correction of anemia, administration of desmopressin or estrogens, or dialysis. Regular doses of antacids appear to reduce the incidence of *gastrointestinal hemorrhage* significantly and may be more effective in this regard than H₂ antagonists. Meticulous care of intravenous cannulae, bladder catheters, and other invasive devices is mandatory to avoid infections. Unfortunately, prophylactic antibiotics have not been shown to reduce the incidence of infection in these high-risk patients.

INDICATIONS AND MODALITIES OF DIALYSIS Dialysis replaces renal function until regeneration and repair restore renal function. Hemodialysis and peritoneal dialysis appear equally effective for management of ARF. Thus, the dialysis modality is chosen according to the needs of individual patients (e.g., peritoneal dialysis may be preferable if the patient is hemodynamically unstable, and hemodialysis after abdominal surgery involving the peritoneum), the expertise

Table 270-4

Management of Ischemic and Nephrotoxic Acute Renal Failure*

Management Issue	Therapy
REVERSE CAUSATIVE RENAL INSULT	
Ischemic ARF	Restore systemic hemodynamics and renal perfusion
Nephrotoxic ARF	Eliminate nephrotoxins
	Consider specific measures (e.g., forced alkaline diuresis, chelators: see text)
PREVENTION AND TREATMENT OF COMPLICATIONS	
Intravascular volume overload	Salt (1–2 g/d) and water (usually <1 L/d) restriction
	Diuretics (usually loop blockers ± thiazide)
	Ultrafiltration or dialysis
Hyponatremia	Restriction of enteral free water intake (<1 L/d)
	Avoid hypotonic intravenous solutions (including dextrose solutions)
Hyperkalemia	Restriction of dietary K⁺ intake (usually <40 mmol/d)
	Eliminate K⁺ supplements and K⁺-sparing diuretics
	Potassium-binding ion-exchange resins (e.g., sodium polystyrene sulphonate)
	Glucose (50 mL of 50% dextrose) and insulin (10 units regular)
	Sodium bicarbonate (usually 50–100 mmol)
	Calcium gluconate (10 mL of 10% solution over 5 min)
	Dialysis (versus low K⁺ dialysate)
Metabolic acidosis	Restriction of dietary protein (usually 0.6 g/kg per day of high biologic value)
	Sodium bicarbonate (maintain serum bicarbonate >15 mmol/L or arterial pH >7.2)
	Dialysis
Hyperphosphatemia	Restriction of dietary phosphate intake (usually <800 mg/d)
	Phosphate binding agents (calcium carbonate, aluminum hydroxide)
Hypocalcemia	Calcium carbonate (if symptomatic or if sodium bicarbonate to be administered)
	Calcium gluconate (10–20 mL of 10% solution)
Hypermagnesemia	Discontinue Mg²⁺-containing antacids
Hyperuricemia	Treatment usually not necessary [if <900 μmol/L (<15 mg/dL)]
Nutrition	Restriction of dietary protein (~0.6 g/kg per day)
	Carbohydrate (~100 g/d)
	Enteral or parenteral nutrition (if recovery prolonged or patient very catabolic)
Indications for dialysis	Clinical evidence (symptoms or signs) of uremia
	Intractable intravascular volume overload
	Hyperkalemia or severe acidosis resistant to conservative measures
	?Prophylactic dialysis when urea >100–150 mg/dL or creatinine >8–10 mg/dL
PRESCRIBING OF MEDICATIONS	
Choice of agents	Avoid other nephrotoxins, ACE inhibitors, cyclooxygenase inhibitors, and radiocontrast unless absolute indication and no alternative agent
Drug dosing	Adjust doses and frequency of administration for degree of renal impairment

* These are general recommendations and must be tailored to needs of individual patients.

of the nephrologist, and the facilities of the institution. Absolute indications for dialysis include symptoms or signs of the uremic syndrome and management of refractory hypervolemia, hyperkalemia, or acidosis. Many nephrologists also initiate dialysis empirically for blood urea levels of >100 mg/dL, even in the absence of clinical uremia; however, this approach has yet to be validated in controlled clinical trials. Nor is it clear whether intensive dialysis prescribed to maintain blood urea and creatinine below a certain level is beneficial. The latter are important issues since unnecessary or intensive hemodialysis can exacerbate ATN and delay renal recovery by triggering hypotension and repeated renal hypoperfusion.

Continuous arteriovenous hemodiafiltration (CAVH) and continuous venovenous hemodiafiltration (CVVH) are alternative hemodialysis techniques for treatment of ARF. They are generally reserved for patients in whom intermittent hemodialysis fails to control hypervolemia or uremia and for those who do not tolerate intermittent hemodialysis and in whom peritoneal dialysis is not possible. CAVH requires both arterial and venous access. The patient's own blood pressure generates an ultrafiltrate of plasma across a porous biocompatible dialysis membrane. A physiologic crystalloid solution is passed along the other side of the membrane to achieve diffusive clearance. CVVH, in contrast, requires only a double-lumen venous catheter as a blood pump generates ultrafiltration pressure across the dialysis membrane. These newer techniques have not been compared to conventional intermittent hemodialysis in prospective, adequately controlled trials. Such evaluations are needed given that continuous hemodialysis techniques require immobilization in bed, systemic anticoagulation, arterial cannulation (in CAVH), and prolonged exposure of blood to synthetic, albeit relatively biocompatible, dialysis membranes.

OUTCOME AND LONG-TERM PROGNOSIS

The mortality rate among patients with ARF approximates 50 percent and has changed little over the past 30 years. It should be stressed, however, that patients usually die from sequelae of the primary illness that induced ARF and not from ARF itself. Indeed, the kidney is one of the few organs whose function can be replaced artificially (i.e., by dialysis) for protracted periods of time. In agreement with this interpretation, mortality rates vary greatly depending on the cause of ARF: ~15 percent in obstetric patients, ~30 percent in toxin-related ARF, and ~60 percent following trauma or major surgery. Oliguria (~400 mL/d) at time of presentation and a rise in serum creatinine of greater than 3 mg/dL are associated with a poor prognosis and probably reflect the severity of renal injury and of the primary illness. Mortality rates are higher in older debilitated patients and in those with multiple organ failure. Most patients who survive an episode of ARF recover sufficient renal function to live normal lives. However, 50 percent have subclinical impairment of renal function or residual scarring on renal biopsy. Approximately 5 percent of patients never recover function and require long-term renal replacement with dialysis or transplantation. An additional 5 percent suffer progressive decline in GFR, following an initial recovery phase, probably due to hemodynamic stress and sclerosis of remnant glomeruli (see Chap. 273).

BIBLIOGRAPHY

BRADY HR et al: Acute renal failure, in *The Kidney*, 5th ed., BM Brenner (ed). Philadelphia, Saunders, 1996, pp 1200–1252

BRENNER BM, LAZARUS JM (eds): *Acute Renal Failure*, 3d ed. New York, Churchill Livingstone, 1993

LIEBERTHAL W, LEVINSKY NG: Acute clinical renal failure, in *The Kidney, Physiology and Pathophysiology*, 2d ed, DW Seldin, G Giebisch (eds). New York, Raven Press, 1992, p 3181

WEINBERG J: Pathogenetic mechanisms of ischemic acute renal failure, in *The Principles and Practice of Nephrology*, 2d ed, HR Jacobsen, et al (eds). Philadelphia, BC Decker, 1991, p 544

OLSEN S, SOLEZ K: Acute tubular necrosis and toxic renal injury, in *Renal Pathology with Clinical and Functional Correlations*, 2d ed, CC Tisher, BM Brenner (eds). Philadelphia, Lippincott, 1994, pp 769–809

271

J. Michael Lazarus, Barry M. Brenner

CHRONIC RENAL FAILURE

In contrast to the capacity of the kidneys to regain function following acute renal injury (see Chap. 270), renal injury of a more prolonged nature often leads to progressive and irreversible destruction of nephron mass. Such reduction of renal mass, in turn, causes structural and functional hypertrophy of surviving nephrons. As discussed in Chap. 269, this compensatory hypertrophy is due to adaptive hyperfiltration mediated by increases in glomerular capillary pressures and flows. Eventually, these adaptations prove maladaptive, in that they predispose to sclerosis of the residual glomerular population.

Glomerulonephritis, in its several forms, was the most common initiating cause of chronic renal failure (CRF) in the past. Possibly because of more aggressive treatment of glomerulonephritis, diabetes mellitus and hypertensive renal disease are now the leading causes of CRF (Fig. 271-1). Irrespective of cause, the eventual impact of severe reduction in nephron mass is an alteration in function of virtually every organ system in the body. *Uremia* is the term generally applied to the clinical syndrome that results from profound loss of renal function. Although the cause(s) of the syndrome remain unknown, the term *uremia* was adopted originally because of the presumption that the abnormalities result from retention in the blood of urea and other end products of metabolism normally excreted in the urine. Uremia involves more than renal excretory failure alone, however. A host of metabolic and endocrine functions normally subserved by the kidney are also impaired, and the inexorable course to renal failure often is accompanied by anemia, malnutrition, impaired metabolism of carbohydrates, fats, and proteins, and defective utilization of energy. Therefore, *uremia* refers to the constellation of signs and symptoms associated with CRF, irrespective of cause.

The severity of signs and symptoms of uremia vary from patient to patient, depending, at least in part, on the magnitude of the reduction in functioning renal mass and the rapidity with which renal function is lost. As discussed in Chap. 269, in the relatively early stage of CRF—i.e., when total glomerular filtration rate (GFR) is reduced to about 35 to 50 percent of normal—overall renal function is sufficient to keep the patient symptom-free, although renal reserve is diminished. At this stage, the biosynthetic, excretory, and other regulatory functions of the kidney are generally well maintained. Blood urea nitrogen and serum creatinine levels may be within the normal range or are only

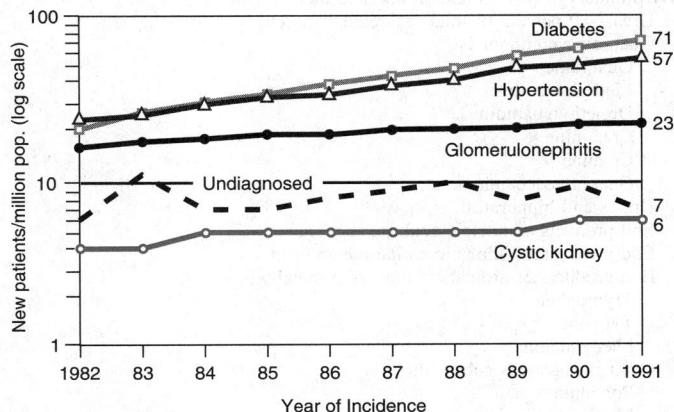

FIGURE 271-1 Incidence rates of treated end-stage renal disease (ESRD) per million population, by selected primary disease groups, 1982 through 1991. Rates are unadjusted. A semilog scale is used to show smaller rates. Rates do not include patients from Puerto Rico or U.S. Territories. Medicare patients only. *(From United States Renal Data System 1995 Annual Data Report. U.S. Department of Health and Human Services, Health Care Financing Administration.)*

slightly elevated and therefore serve as crude measures, at best, of the level of function (see Chap. 269). At a somewhat later stage in the course of CRF (GFR about 20 to 35 percent of normal), *azotemia* occurs, and initial manifestations of renal insufficiency usually appear. Although patients are still relatively asymptomatic, renal reserve is diminished sufficiently that sudden stress, such as intercurrent infection, urinary tract obstruction, dehydration, or administration of a nephrotoxic drug, may compromise renal function still further, inducing signs and symptoms of overt uremia. With further loss of nephron mass (GFR below approximately 20 percent of normal), the patient develops *overt renal failure*. Uremia may be viewed as the final stage in this inexorable process, when many or all of the untoward manifestations of CRF become evident clinically and biochemically.

PATHOPHYSIOLOGY AND BIOCHEMISTRY OF UREMIA

The finding that sera from patients with uremia exert toxic effects in a variety of biologic test systems has motivated an attempt to identify the responsible toxin(s). The most likely candidates as toxins in uremia are the byproducts of protein and amino acid metabolism. Unlike fats and carbohydrates, which are eventually metabolized to carbon dioxide and water—substances readily excreted even in uremic subjects via lungs and skin—the products of protein and amino acid metabolism depend primarily on the kidneys for excretion. A number of such products have been identified (Table 271-1). Nevertheless, the precise role of these substances in the pathogenesis of the uremic syndrome is unclear. As noted above, uremic symptoms correlate only in a rough and inconsistent way with concentrations of urea in blood. Although not the major cause of overt uremic toxicity, urea may contribute to some of the clinical abnormalities, including anorexia, malaise, vomiting, and headache. On the other hand, elevated levels of plasma *guanidinosuccinic acid*, by interfering with activation of platelet factor III by adenosine diphosphate (ADP), contribute to the impaired platelet function in CRF. *Creatinine* may cause adverse effects following conversion to metabolites such as sarcosine and methylguanidine. Nitrogenous compounds with a molecular mass of 500 to 12,000 daltons (so-called middle molecules) are also retained in CRF and similarly are believed to contribute to morbidity and mortality in

Table 271-1

Uremic "Toxins"

By-products of protein and amino acid metabolism
  Urea—80 percent of total (excreted nitrogen)
  Guanidino compounds
    Guanidine
    Methylguanidine
    Dimethylguanidine
    Creatinine
    Creatine
    Guanidinosuccinic acid
  Urates and hippurates
  End-products of nucleic acid metabolism
  End-products of aliphatic amine metabolism
  End-products of aromatic amino acid metabolism
    Tryptophan
    Tyrosine
    Phenylalanine
  Other nitrogenous substances
    Polyamines
    Myoinositol
    Phenols
    Benzoates
    Indoles
Advanced glycation end-products
Inhibitors of ligand-protein binding
Glucuronoconjugates and aglycones
Inhibitors of somatomedin and insulin action

uremic subjects. Decreased renal excretion is not the only reason why such middle-sized molecules, along with various cytokines and growth factors, accumulate in uremic plasma. The kidney normally catabolizes a number of circulating plasma proteins and polypeptides; with reduced renal mass, this capacity is impaired. Furthermore, plasma levels of many polypeptide hormones, including parathyroid hormone (PTH) insulin, glucagon, luteinizing hormone, and prolactin, rise with renal failure, often markedly, not only because of impaired renal catabolism but also because of enhanced glandular secretion. Of these, excessive PTH has been suggested to be an important uremic "toxin" because of its adverse effect of elevating cellular cytosolic calcium levels in several tissues and organs. The consequences of high circulating levels of PTH and other hormones in chronic renal failure are considered below.

EFFECTS OF UREMIA ON CELLULAR FUNCTIONS Alterations in the composition of intracellular and extracellular fluids in CRF are believed to be a consequence, at least in part, of defective ion transport across cell membranes, with retained uremic toxins possibly mediating these alterations in transmembrane ion transport. The integrity of the volume and composition of cells throughout the body depends to a large extent on the active transport of Na^+ out of the cell, the resulting intracellular fluid being relatively low in Na^+ and high in K^+, whereas the reverse is true for extracellular fluid. Active Na^+ transport is metabolically costly, accounting for a major fraction of basal energy utilization and oxygen consumption. The consequences of this efflux of Na^+ from cells include (1) the generation of a resting electrical potential difference across the cell membrane, with the cell interior electronegative relative to the cell exterior, and (2) a mechanism for enhancing the influx of K^+ into cells. In animals, deliberate inhibition of this active efflux of Na^+ across cell membranes leads to alterations in body composition and cell functions similar to those seen in the erythrocytes, leukocytes, skeletal muscle, and other tissues of uremic subjects. These include increased and decreased intracellular concentrations of Na^+ and K^+, respectively, and reduction in magnitude of the transmembrane voltage. In addition to these abnormalities in Na^+ and K^+ flux, inhibition of Ca^{2+} flux has also been demonstrated in uremic patients. These alterations are largely reversed by efficient hemodialysis and, for erythrocytes at least, are recreated when cells from normal subjects are incubated in uremic serum. Whether the uremic "toxins" that account for these derangements in cellular function represent abnormally retained products of metabolism or substances whose production is increased as a homeostatic response to renal insufficiency remains unknown. Increased levels of parathyroid and natriuretic hormones, examples of both such derangements, are discussed in this context in Chap. 269.

EFFECTS OF UREMIA ON WHOLE-BODY COMPOSITION What is the impact of the above-described disturbances of active transcellular ion transport on the organism as a whole? From the pathophysiologic considerations discussed previously, CRF is likely to lead to abnormally high intracellular Na^+ concentrations and hence to osmotically induced overhydration of cells, whereas these same cells are relatively deficient in K^+. With the development of malaise, anorexia, nausea, vomiting, and diarrhea, patients with CRF may eventually develop protein-calorie malnutrition and negative nitrogen balance, often with profound losses of lean body mass and fat deposits. Owing to the concomitant tendency for salt and water retention due to impaired excretion, these losses often go unnoticed until the late stages of CRF. Because a large fraction of the increase in total body water in uremia is the result of expansion of intracellular volume, extracellular volume also expands. With initiation of intermittent hemodialysis or renal transplantation, there is often an immediate loss of body weight, due primarily to correction of this overhydration. With successful transplantation, the initial diuresis is followed by a period of weight gain due to restoration of lean body mass and fat deposits to preillness levels. For patients on chronic dialysis, the anabolic response is often less dramatic, even when therapy is regarded as optimal, and involves mainly reaccumulation of fat deposits. The failure of lean body mass to return to normal with chronic dialysis may reflect alterations in the catabolic rate but more likely results from insufficient intake of calories and protein, which, in adequately dialyzed patients, should be maintained at levels of 150 kJ/kg (35 kcal/kg) and 1.2 to 1.4 g/kg of body weight per day, respectively.

Deficits in intracellular K^+ concentration in CRF may result from inadequate intake (poor diet or overzealous K^+ restriction by the physician), excessive losses (vomiting, diarrhea, diuretics), reduction of Na^+- and K^+-stimulated ATPase, or a combination of these. In addition to promoting losses of K^+ into urine (which may be substantial if urine volume remains relatively normal in uremic subjects), the high levels of plasma aldosterone often seen in CRF also may augment the net secretion of K^+ into the colon, thereby contributing to K^+ losses in stool or diarrheal fluids. Despite deficits in intracellular K^+, serum K^+ is usually normal or high in CRF, owing to metabolic acidosis, which induces an efflux of K^+ from cells. Uremic patients are also relatively resistant to the action of insulin (see below), which normally enhances K^+ uptake by skeletal muscle (see also Chap. 49).

EFFECTS OF UREMIA ON METABOLISM **Hypothermia** In animals, injections of urine, urea, or other retained toxic metabolites can induce hypothermia, and basal heat production diminishes soon after nephrectomy. Since active Na^+ transport across cell membranes accounts for a major proportion of basal energy production, the inverse relationship between body temperature and degree of azotemia is believed to be due, in part, to inhibition of the Na^+ pump by some retained toxin(s). Dialysis usually returns body temperature to normal.

Carbohydrate Metabolism The ability to metabolize glucose is impaired in most patients with CRF, as evidenced by a slowing of the rate at which the blood glucose level declines to normal after administration of a glucose load. Fasting blood sugar levels are usually normal or only slightly elevated. Severe hyperglycemia and/or ketosis due to uremia alone are not seen, and, therefore, the glucose intolerance of CRF usually does not require specific therapy (hence the term *azotemic pseudodiabetes*). Because insulin is removed from the plasma largely by renal cells, which degrade it intracellularly, circulating insulin levels in plasma are slightly to moderately increased in most fasting uremic subjects, and levels in excess of normal are usually demonstrable after a glucose load. However, the response to intravenous insulin in patients with CRF is impaired, and the rate of utilization of glucose by peripheral tissues is diminished. The glucose intolerance of uremia results largely from this peripheral resistance to the action of insulin. Other factors that may contribute to glucose intolerance include intracellular deficits of K^+, metabolic acidosis, and increased levels of glucagon, catecholamines, growth hormone, and prolactin as well as of the myriad of potentially toxic metabolites that are retained in CRF. Patients with true insulin-dependent diabetes often show a decrease in insulin requirement with progressive azotemia, which is due to the reduced uptake and catabolism of insulin by the kidney as well as to decreased caloric intake.

Nitrogen and Lipid Metabolism The altered state of metabolism in uremic patients leads to abnormal amino acid profiles. In addition to the hypercatabolism seen in uremia, the capacity to eliminate nitrogenous end products of protein catabolism is reduced, so CRF may be regarded as a state of protein intolerance. As noted earlier, the retention of end products of increased nitrogen metabolism is a major cause of organ dysfunction, leading to the signs and symptoms of uremia.

Hypertriglyceridemia, decreased plasma levels of high-density lipoprotein cholesterol, and increased plasma levels of lipoprotein a antigen [Lp(a)] are common in uremia, whereas cholesterol levels in plasma are usually near normal. Whether uremia accelerates triglyceride production by the liver and intestine is unknown. The enhancement of lipogenesis by insulin may contribute to increased triglyceride synthesis. In addition, the rate of removal of triglycerides from the circulation, which depends in large part on the enzyme lipoprotein lipase, is depressed in uremia, an effect not corrected appreciably by hemodialysis. The high incidence of premature atherosclerosis in patients on chronic dialysis (see "Cardiovascular and Pulmonary Abnormalities" below) may be related in part to these abnormalities in lipid metabolism.

Clinical Abnormalities in Uremia Chronic renal failure is associated with a constellation of signs and symptoms, which may or may not include reduced urine output but always include elevation in serum urea nitrogen and creatinine concentrations. As pointed out in Chap. 269, elevations of serum urea nitrogen and creatinine levels occur late in the course of renal failure. It can be difficult to differentiate acute from chronic renal failure. The usual hallmark of CRF is reduced kidney size as seen by ultrasound scanning or on an abdominal scout film or pyelogram. In the absence of small kidneys, renal biopsy may be necessary for diagnosis.

As noted earlier, CRF leads to disturbances in function of every organ system. The use of chronic dialysis reduces the incidence and severity of these disturbances, so that, where modern medicine is practiced, the overt and florid manifestations of uremia have largely disappeared. Unfortunately, as indicated in Table 271-2, even optimal dialysis therapy is not a panacea, because some disturbances resulting from impaired renal function fail to respond fully, while others continue to progress. Furthermore, as with many complex therapeutic modalities, dialysis may cause unique abnormalities not seen prior to initiation of therapy; these abnormalities should be viewed as complications of dialysis.

FLUID, ELECTROLYTE, AND ACID-BASE DISORDERS (See also Chaps. 49 and 50) **Sodium and Volume Homeostasis** In most patients with stable CRF, the total body contents of Na^+ and water are increased modestly, although expansion of the extracellular fluid (ECF) volume may not be apparent. With ingestion of excessive amounts of salt and water, however, control of excess volume becomes an important consideration. In general, excessive salt ingestion contributes to or aggravates congestive heart failure, hypertension, ascites, and edema. On the other hand, hyponatremia and weight gain are the consequence of excessive ingestion of water and in most patients are relatively mild or asymptomatic. In most predialysis patients, a daily intake of fluid equal in volume to the urine volume per day plus about 500 mL usually maintains the serum Na^+ concentration at normal levels. Patients on dialysis frequently demonstrate mild hyponatremia. Hypernatremia is relatively infrequent in CRF. In the edematous patient with CRF who is not on dialysis, diuretics and modest restriction of salt and water intake are the mainstays of therapy. In dialysis patients with volume expansion, management should include ultrafiltration and restriction of salt and water intake between dialyses. Patients with CRF have impaired renal mechanisms for conserving Na^+ and water (see Chap. 269). When an *extrarenal* cause for increased fluid loss is present (e.g., vomiting, diarrhea, fever), these patients are prone to volume depletion, leading to dry mucous membranes, dizziness, syncope, tachycardia, decreased filling of jugular veins, orthostatic hypotension, and eventual cardiovascular collapse. Depletion of extracellular fluid volume may result in deterioration of residual renal function and, in the previously stable and asymptomatic patient with mild CRF, signs and symptoms of overt uremia. Cautious fluid repletion usually restores extracellular and intravascular volumes to normal and often but not always restores renal function to prior levels.

Potassium Homeostasis Derangements in K^+ balance (see Chap. 49) are occasionally documented by laboratory analysis in patients with CRF but are rarely responsible for clinical symptoms unless the GFR is below 10 mL/min or unless an endogenous K^+ load (owing to hemolysis, trauma, infection) or an exogenous one (owing to administration of stored blood or K^+-containing medications) enters the system. Despite progression of renal failure, most patients maintain normal serum K^+ concentrations until the late stages of uremia. This ability to sustain K^+ balance in the face of advancing renal failure is due to adaptations in the renal distal tubules and colon, sites where aldosterone and other factors serve to enhance K^+ secretion.

Hyperkalemia Not surprisingly, oliguria or disruption of key adaptive mechanisms can lead to hyperkalemia and its potentially ominous effects on cardiac function. Antikaliuretic drugs such as spironolactone, triamterene, amiloride, trimethoprim, and pentamidine should be used with extreme caution in patients with CRF. Likewise, angiotensin converting enzyme inhibitors and beta blockers may cause or exacerbate hyperkalemia. In kidney transplant recipients, cyclosporine is another common cause of increased serum K^+. Hyperkalemia in CRF patients also may be induced by abrupt falls in blood pH, since acidosis is associated with efflux of K^+ from intracellular to extracellular fluids.

℞ TREATMENT

Correction of acidosis-induced hyperkalemia with sodium bicarbonate is the treatment of choice. This treatment is most often combined with the use of a loop diuretic, which not only enhances K^+ loss but also offsets the administered Na^+ load. Intravenous administration of insulin and dextrose, as well as administration of fludrocortisone and nebulized albuterol, are useful in lowering serum K^+ acutely, while the ion exchange resin sodium polystyrene sulfonate (Kayexalate) is the most effective agent in longer-term control of hyperkalemia. Oral administration of this agent may be accompanied by administration of a purgative, such as sorbitol, to expedite removal of the bound resin. However, sorbitol should not be used with rectal administration of sodium polystyrene sulfonate because of possible bowel dessication and perforation. When hyperkalemia persists in the absence of excessive K^+ intake, oliguria, or acute acidosis, the possibility of *hyporeninemic hypoaldosteronism* should be considered. Patients with this syndrome are often diabetic and have type 4 renal tubular acidosis (see Chap. 49).

Hypokalemia Hypokalemia is uncommon in most forms of CRF but may occur with poor dietary K^+ intake, usually in association with excessive diuretic therapy or gastrointestinal losses. When hypokalemia occurs as a result of primary K^+ wasting in urine, it may represent a solitary renal reabsorptive defect or, more commonly, may be associated with other solute transport abnormalities, as in Fanconi's syndrome, renal tubular acidosis, or other forms of hereditary or ac-

quired tubulointerstitial diseases. The clinical consequences and management of hypokalemia and hyperkalemia are discussed more fully in Chap. 49.

Metabolic Acidosis With advancing renal failure, total daily acid excretion and buffer production fall below the level needed to maintain external balance of hydrogen ions. Metabolic acidosis is the inevitable result, and the mechanisms involved are considered in Chap. 50. In most patients with stable renal insufficiency, administration of 20 to 30 mmol/d of sodium bicarbonate or sodium citrate corrects the acidosis. In response to a sudden acid challenge (whether from an endogenous or an exogenous source), however, patients with CRF are susceptible to severe acidosis, which requires more substantial quantities of alkali for correction. Administration of Na^+ must be carried out with careful attention to volume status and the potential need for diuretic agents. Also, citrate enhances aluminum absorption in the large bowel, and citrate-containing antacids should be avoided if aluminum-containing drugs are also administered.

BONE, PHOSPHATE, AND CALCIUM ABNORMALITIES (Fig. 271-2) *Renal osteodystrophy* and *metabolic bone disease* are terms that encompass a number of skeletal abnormalities, including osteomalacia, osteitis fibrosa cystica, and, in children, impaired bone growth. Many experts also include adynamic or aplastic bone disease, aluminum-induced osteomalacia, and dialysis-related amyloid bone disease, all of which are consequences of long-term dialysis. Adynamic or aplastic bone disease is a recently described condition that is detected primarily on bone biopsy, which reveals a reduction in osteoid as well as fibrosis. Aluminum-induced osteomalacia also involves low bone turnover but is related to aluminum deposition at the osteoid front. Accumulation of β_2-microglobulin amyloid leads to dialysis-related amyloidosis (DRA), which consists of carpal tunnel syndrome, tenosynovitis of the hands, shoulder arthropathy, bone cysts, cervical spondyloarthropathy, and cervical pseudotumors.

Although clinical symptoms of bone disease are present before dialysis in less than 10 percent of patients with advanced renal failure, radiologic and histologic abnormalities are observed in about 35 and 90 percent, respectively, of these patients. Secondary hyperparathyroidism and osteitis fibrosa cystica are more common

Table 271-2

Clinical Abnormalities in Uremia*

Fluid and electrolyte disturbances	Neuromuscular disturbances	Dermatologic disturbances
Volume expansion and contraction (I)	Fatigue (I)†	Pallor (I)†
Hypernatremia and hyponatremia (I)	Sleep disorders (P)	Hyperpigmentation (I, P, or D)
Hyperkalemia and hypokalemia (I)	Headache (I or P)	Pruritus (P)
Metabolic acidosis (I)	Impaired mentation (I)†	Ecchymoses (I)
Hyperphosphatemia (I)	Lethargy (I)†	Uremic frost (I)
Hypocalcemia (I)	Asterixis (I)	**Gastrointestinal disturbances**
Endocrine-metabolic disturbances	Muscular irritability (I)	Anorexia (I)
Secondary hyperparathyroidism (I or P)	Peripheral neuropathy (I or P)	Nausea and vomiting (I)
Aluminum-induced osteomalacia (D)	Restless legs syndrome (I or P)	Uremic fetor (I)
Vitamin D–deficient osteomalacia (I)	Paralysis (I or P)	Gastroenteritis (I)
Carbohydrate intolerance (I)	Myoclonus (I)	Peptic ulcer (I or P)
Hyperuricemia (I or P)	Seizures (I or P)	Gastrointestinal bleeding (I, P, or D)
Hypertriglyceridemia (P)	Coma (I)	Hepatitis (D)
Increased Lp(a) level (P)	Muscle cramps (D)	Idiopathic ascites (D)
Decreased high-density lipoprotein level (P)	Dialysis disequilibrium syndrome (D)	Peritonitis (D)
Protein-calorie malnutrition (I or P)	Dialysis dementia (D)	**Hematologic and immunologic disturbances**
Impaired growth and development (P)	Myopathy (P or D)	Normocytic, normochromic anemia (I)†
Infertility and sexual dysfunction (P)	**Cardiovascular and pulmonary disturbances**	Microcytic (aluminum-induced) anemia (D)
Amenorrhea (P)	Arterial hypertension (I or P)	Lymphocytopenia (P)
Hypothermia (I)	Congestive heart failure or pulmonary edema (I)	Bleeding diathesis (I or D)†
Dialysis-induced β_2-microglobulin amyloidosis	Pericarditis (I)	Increased susceptibility to infection (I or P)
	Cardiomyopathy (I or P)	Splenomegaly and hypersplenism (P)
	Uremic lung (I)	Leukopenia (D)
	Accelerated atherosclerosis (P or D)	Hypocomplementemia (D)
	Hypotension and arrhythmias (D)	

* Virtually all abnormalities in this table are completely reversed in time by successful renal transplantation. The response of these abnormalities to hemodialysis or peritoneal dialysis therapy is more variable. (I) denotes an abnormality that usually improves with an optimal program of dialysis and related therapy; (P) denotes one that tends to persist or even progress, despite an optimal program; (D) denotes one that develops only after initiation of dialysis therapy.
† Improves with dialysis and erythropoietin therapy.

in children than in adults and are especially common in patients with slowly progressive renal insufficiency. Radiologic examination of uremic patients not yet on dialysis can reveal three types of lesions: (1) changes analogous to those of nutritional rickets, namely, widened osteoid seams at the growth margins of bones (so-called renal rickets); (2) the bone changes of secondary hyperparathyroidism (osteitis fibrosa cystica), characterized by osteoclastic bone resorption and subperiosteal erosions, especially of the terminal phalanges, long bones, and distal ends of the clavicles; and (3) osteosclerosis, often best evidenced by enhanced bone density in the upper and lower margins of vertebrae, producing the so-called rugger jersey spine. In patients being treated with dialysis, aluminum-induced osteomalacia and adynamic bone disease are generally not detected on x-ray films and are diagnosed principally by bone biopsy. DRA occurs only after many years of dialysis, particularly in the elderly, and is characterized on x-ray films by cysts in the carpal bones and femoral neck. Amyloid tumoral masses may be best appreciated by ultrasound examination or computed tomography.

With osteitis fibrosa cystica, vitamin D–deficient and aluminum-induced osteomalacia, and DRA, patients are prone to spontaneous fractures, which are slow to heal. The ribs are most commonly involved in the case of osteitis fibrosa cystica. The femoral neck is a frequent site of aluminum-induced osteomalacia and DRA and is also prone to pathologic fractures. Bone pain, even in the absence of fractures, is common in all of the above disorders. In osteitis fibrosa cystica, a proximal myopathy often coexists, giving rise to gait abnormalities and to impairment of ambulation. Similar myopathy may also occur with amyloid arthropathy due to disease. In CRF, there is a tendency to extraosseous or metastatic calcification when the calcium-phosphorus product is very high (>70). Medium-sized blood vessels, the subcutaneous, articular, and periarticular tissues, the myocardium, the eyes, and the lungs are common sites of metastatic calcification.

℞ TREATMENT

Secondary hyperparathyroidism is best treated by reducing the serum phosphate concentration through the use of a phosphate-restricted diet as well as oral phosphate-binding agents. Calcium carbonate and calcium acetate are the preferred phosphate-binding agents, but in some circumstances a combination of aluminum hydroxide and calcium carbonate is necessary. Aluminum levels should be monitored, and citrate antacids, which enhance aluminum absorption, should be avoided. Dialysate calcium, calcium carbonate, calcium acetate, aluminum hydroxide, and calcitriol must be properly balanced to maintain the serum phosphorus concentration at approximately 1.4 mmol/L (4.5 mg/dL) and the serum calcium at approximately 2.5 mmol/L (10 mg/dL) in an attempt to suppress parathyroid hypertrophy, thus avoiding or reversing osteitis fibrosa cystica, osteomalacia, and myopathy. It is particularly important to keep the calcium-phosphorus product in the normal range to avoid metastatic calcification.

The recently described disorder of adynamic bone disease is thought to be secondary to overzealous treatment of secondary hyperparathyroidism. Therefore, suppression of PTH levels to less than 120 pg/mL in uremic patients may not be desirable. The incidence of aluminum-induced osteomalacia has been greatly reduced with the recognition of aluminum as the principal culprit. Therapy for this disorder is continued avoidance of aluminum with possible use of a chelating agent such as desferoxamine along with high-flux dialysis. At present, there is no good therapy for DRA; local physical therapy, corticosteroid injections and nonsteroidal anti-inflammatory agents constitute current options.

Other Solutes Uric acid retention is a common feature of CRF but rarely leads to symptomatic gout. Hypophosphatemia is usually a consequence of overzealous oral administration of phosphate-binding gels. Because serum magnesium levels tend to rise in CRF, magnesium-containing antacids and cathartics should be avoided.

CARDIOVASCULAR AND PULMONARY ABNORMALITIES

Fluid retention in uremia often results in congestive heart failure and/or pulmonary edema. A unique form of pulmonary congestion and edema may occur even in the absence of volume overload and is associated with normal or mildly elevated intracardiac and pulmonary capillary wedge pressures. This entity, characterized radiologically by peripheral vascular congestion giving rise to a "butterfly wing" distribution, is due to increased permeability of alveolar capillary membranes. This low-pressure pulmonary edema, as well as cardiopulmonary abnormalities associated with circulatory overload, usually respond promptly to vigorous dialysis.

Hypertension Hypertension is the most common complication of end-stage renal disease. When it is not found, the patient either has a salt-wasting form of renal disease (e.g., polycystic or medullary cystic disease, chronic tubulointerstitial disease, or papillary necrosis), is receiving antihypertensive therapy, or is volume-depleted, the last condition usually due to excessive gastrointestinal fluid losses or overzealous diuretic therapy. Since fluid overload is the major cause of hypertension in uremia, the normotensive state can usually be restored by aggressive ultrafiltration with dialysis. Nevertheless, because of hyperreninemia, some patients remain hypertensive despite rigorous salt and water restriction and ultrafiltration. Rarely, patients develop accelerated or malignant hypertension, manifested by markedly elevated systolic and diastolic pressures, extreme hyperreninemia, encephalopathy, seizures, retinal hemorrhages, and papilledema. Intravenous nitroprusside, labetolol, or enalaprilat, along with control of extracellular fluid volume, generally controls such hypertension. Subsequently, such patients usually require more than one oral antihypertensive drug. A high percentage of patients with CRF present with left ventricular hypertrophy or dilated cardiomyopathy. These changes are thought to be related to prolonged hypertension.

Pericarditis Retained metabolic toxins are thought to be the cause of uremic pericarditis. Once a common complication of CRF, pericarditis is now infrequent because of early initiation of dialysis.

FIGURE 271-2 Flowchart for the development of bone, phosphate, and calcium abnormalities in CRF.

The rare occurrence of pericarditis in the well-dialyzed patient is due to viral infection, systemic disease, transmural myocardial infarction, or cardiac surgery. The clinical presentation of pericarditis in uremic subjects is similar to that seen in nonuremic subjects (Chap. 240), except that effusions are usually hemorrhagic. Treatment with intensive dialysis is recommended, and systemic anticoagulation should be avoided to minimize the occurrence of hemorrhagic tamponade. Pericardiocentesis with intrapericardial instillation of air or glucocorticoids is usually effective for pericardial tamponade. Pericardiectomy should be considered only if more conservative measures fail.

Chronically dialyzed patients have a high incidence of accelerated atherosclerosis, leading to coronary, cerebral, and peripheral vascular disease. Causes for these complications include hypertension, hyperlipidemia, glucose intolerance, chronic high cardiac output, and metastatic vascular and myocardial calcification.

HEMATOLOGIC ABNORMALITIES Normochromic, Normocytic Anemia This abnormality occurs regularly and contributes to the symptomatology in CRF. Erythropoiesis is depressed in CRF, owing to the effects of retained toxins on bone marrow, to diminished biosynthesis of erythropoietin by the diseased kidney or, much less often, to the presence of erythropoietin inhibitors. The administration of recombinant human erythropoietin results in a dramatic increase in hematocrit and hemoglobin concentration, suggesting that a reduced level of serum erythropoietin is perhaps the most important of these factors. Hemolysis is a minor component of uremic anemia and, when present, is due to an extracorpuscular effect, since survival of erythrocytes from normal subjects is reduced when these cells are transfused into uremic patients, and erythrocytes from patients with CRF have relatively normal survival times when experimentally transfused into normal individuals. Such hemolysis usually disappears with institution of dialysis. Gastrointestinal blood loss (due to gastrointestinal lesions and abnormal platelet function) may contribute to anemia. Blood loss is exaggerated in hemodialysis patients because of the need for heparin during dialysis and the retention of blood in the dialyzer and associated tubing.

℞ **TREATMENT**

Administration of recombinant human erythropoietin is the treatment of choice for anemia in patients with advanced renal insufficiency, both before and after initiation of dialysis. Treatment should be instituted if the hematocrit is less than 30 percent. The improvements in cardiovascular function, mental status, and energy level that occur with an increase in hematocrit to approximately 34 to 38 percent enhance the quality of life. The starting dose is approximately 25 to 50 units per kilogram body weight three times per week, either subcutaneously or intravenously. Increases in dosage may be warranted after 8 to 12 weeks, with monitoring of the hematocrit every 2 to 4 weeks. Resistance to erythropoietin mandates a search for iron deficiency, aluminum-induced red blood cell microcytosis, marrow fibrosis from hyperparathyroidism, chronic inflammatory states, or primary hematologic diseases. In approximately 30 percent of patients receiving chronic erythropoietin therapy, the severity of hypertension is increased, perhaps for reasons related to increased production of endothelin. In most cases, routine antihypertensive drug therapy is effective.

Transfusions may contribute to suppression of erythropoiesis in CRF, and, because they increase the risk of hepatitis, hemosiderosis, and transplant sensitization, they should be avoided unless the anemia fails to respond to erythropoietin and the patient is symptomatic. Oral or parenteral iron therapy is indicated in patients with documented iron deficiency. Folic and ascorbic acids and the soluble B vitamins should be given to offset chronic losses of these substances via dialysis. Hemochromatosis has become an uncommon complication in dialysis patients since the advent of erythropoietin therapy.

Abnormal Hemostasis Abnormal hemostasis is also common in CRF and is characterized by a tendency to abnormal bleeding and bruising. Bleeding from surgical wounds and spontaneous bleeding into the gastrointestinal tract, pericardial sac, or intracranial vault (in the form of subdural hematoma or intracerebral hemorrhage) are of the greatest concern. Prolongation of bleeding time, decreased activity of platelet factor 3, abnormal platelet aggregation and adhesiveness, and impaired prothrombin consumption contribute to the clotting defects. The abnormality in platelet factor 3 correlates with increased plasma levels of guanidinosuccinic acid and can be corrected by dialysis. Prolongation of the bleeding time is common even in well-dialyzed patients. Abnormal bleeding times and coagulopathy in patients with renal failure may be reversed with desmopressin, cryoprecipitate, conjugated estrogens, and blood transfusions, as well as by the use of erythropoietin.

Enhanced Susceptibility to Infection Changes in leukocyte formation and function in uremia lead to enhanced susceptibility to infection. Lymphocytopenia and atrophy of lymphoid structures occur, whereas neutrophil production is relatively unimpaired. Nevertheless, the function of all leukocyte cell types may be affected adversely by uremic serum. Alterations in monocyte, lymphocyte, and neutrophil function cause impairment of acute inflammatory responses, decreased delayed hypersensitivity, and altered late immune function. There is a tendency for uremic patients to have less fever in response to infection, perhaps because of the effects of uremia on the hypothalamic temperature control center.

Leukocyte function also may be impaired in patients with CRF because of coexisting acidosis, hyperglycemia, protein-calorie malnutrition, and serum and tissue hyperosmolarity (due to azotemia). In patients receiving hemodialysis, leukocyte function is disturbed because of the effects of the bioincompatibility of various dialysis membranes (see Chap. 272). Activation of cytokine and complement cascades likewise occurs when blood comes in contact with dialysis membranes. These substances in turn alter inflammatory and immune responses of the uremic patient. Mucosal barriers to infection also may be defective, and, in dialysis patients, vascular and peritoneal access devices are common portals of entry for pathogens, especially staphylococci. Glucocorticoids and immunosuppressive drugs used for various renal diseases further increase the risk of infection.

NEUROMUSCULAR ABNORMALITIES Subtle disturbances of central nervous system function, including inability to concentrate, drowsiness, and insomnia, are among the early symptoms of uremia. Mild behavioral changes, loss of memory, and errors in judgment soon follow and may be associated with neuromuscular irritability, including hiccups, cramps, and fasciculations and twitching of muscles. Asterixis, myoclonus, and chorea are common in terminal uremia, as are stupor, seizures, and coma. Peripheral neuropathy is also common in advanced CRF. Initially, sensory nerves are involved more than motor nerves, the lower extremities more than the upper, and the distal portions of the extremities more than the proximal. The "restless legs syndrome" is characterized by ill-defined sensations of discomfort in the feet and lower legs and frequent leg movement. If dialysis is not instituted soon after onset of sensory abnormalities, motor involvement follows, including loss of deep tendon reflexes, weakness, peroneal nerve palsy (foot drop), and, eventually, flaccid quadriplegia. Accordingly, evidence of peripheral neuropathy is a firm indication for the initiation of dialysis or for transplantation. Many of the central nervous system and neuromuscular complications of advanced uremia resolve with dialysis, although nonspecific electroencephalographic abnormalities may persist (Table 271-2).

Two types of neurologic disturbances appear to be unique to patients on chronic dialysis. *Dialysis dementia* is seen in patients who have been on dialysis for many years and is characterized by speech dyspraxia, myoclonus, dementia, and eventually seizures and death. Aluminum intoxication is probably a major contributor to this syndrome, but other factors, such as viral infections, may play a role since only a small percent of patients with aluminum exposure develop the syndrome. *Dialysis disequilibrium*, which occurs during the first few dialyses in association with rapid reduction of blood urea levels, consists of nausea, vomiting, drowsiness, headache, and even convulsions. It has been attributed to cerebral edema and increased intracranial pressure due to the rapid (dialysis-induced) changes in pH and osmolality between extracellular and intracellular fluids.

GASTROINTESTINAL ABNORMALITIES Anorexia, hiccups, nausea, and vomiting are common early manifestations of uremia. Protein restriction is useful in diminishing nausea and vomiting late in the course of renal failure. However, protein restriction should not be implemented in patients with early signs of protein-calorie malnutrition. *Uremic fetor*, a uriniferous odor to the breath, derives from the breakdown of urea in saliva to ammonia and is often associated with an unpleasant metallic taste sensation. Mucosal ulcerations leading to blood loss can occur at any level of the gastrointestinal tract in the very late stages of CRF. Peptic ulcer disease is common in uremic patients. Whether this high incidence is related to altered gastric acidity, enhanced colonization by *Helicobacter pylori*, or hypersecretion of gastrin is unknown. Patients with CRF, particularly those with polycystic kidney disease, have an increased incidence of diverticulosis. Pancreatitis and angiodysplasia of the large bowel with chronic bleeding have been noted more commonly in dialysis patients. Hepatitis B antigenemia was very common in the past, but it is much less so now because of the implementation of universal precautions, the use of hepatitis B vaccine, and the diminished need for blood transfusions resulting from the introduction of erythropoietin. A higher incidence of hepatitis C virus antibody has been noted in patients receiving chronic hemodialysis. This infection does not seem to cause significant liver disease in most patients, but it is a definite concern in patients who subsequently undergo transplantation and immunosuppression, in whom the incidence of active chronic hepatitis and cirrhosis is much higher.

ENDOCRINE-METABOLIC DISTURBANCES Disturbances in parathyroid function, glucose tolerance, and insulin metabolism, as well as the lipid, protein-calorie, and other nutritional abnormalities of uremia, have already been considered. The functioning of the pituitary, thyroid, and adrenal is relatively normal, often despite abnormalities in circulating thyroxine, growth hormone, aldosterone, and cortisol levels. In women, estrogen levels are low, and amenorrhea and inability to carry pregnancies to term are common manifestations of uremia. While menses frequently reappear after chronic dialysis is initiated, successful pregnancies are rare. In men with CRF, including those receiving chronic dialysis, impotence, oligospermia, and germinal cell dysplasia are common, as are reduced plasma testosterone levels. Like growth, sexual maturation is often impaired in adolescent children, even among those receiving chronic dialysis.

DERMATOLOGIC ABNORMALITIES The skin may show evidence of anemia (pallor), defective hemostasis (ecchymoses and hematomas), calcium deposition and secondary hyperparathyroidism (pruritus, excoriations), dehydration (poor skin turgor, dry mucous membranes), and the general cutaneous consequences of protein-calorie malnutrition. A sallow, yellow cast may reflect the combined influences of anemia and retention of a variety of pigmented metabolites, or *urochromes*. In advanced uremia, the concentration of urea in sweat may be so high that, after evaporation, a fine white powder can be found on the skin surface—so-called uremic (urea) frost. Although many of these cutaneous abnormalities improve with dialysis, *uremic pruritus* is usually resistant to dialysis as well as to most systemic and topical therapies. Hemochromatosis causes a slate gray to bronze discoloration of the skin and is now uncommon in dialysis patients because of reduced transfusion requirements.

CONSERVATIVE MANAGEMENT OF PROGRESSIVE RENAL FAILURE

Treatment directed to specific organ system abnormalities has been discussed in the preceding paragraphs. Principles of dialysis and transplant therapy are discussed in Chap. 272. Conservative (nondialytic, nontransplant) therapy must be instituted early to control symptoms, minimize complications, prevent long-term sequelae, and slow the progression of renal insufficiency. The level of renal function should be ascertained periodically, and any reversible component that is present should be corrected. Prerenal factors, such as volume depletion, decreased cardiac output, and renal artery stenosis, and postrenal components, such as urethral or ureteric obstruction, may exacerbate chronic renal insufficiency and must be identified and corrected. Hypertension, urinary tract infections, nephrolithiasis, structural abnormalities of the urinary tract, and the forms of glomerulonephritis that respond to immunosuppressive therapy also should be treated aggressively. Preventive measures include avoidance of nephrotoxic drugs and radiocontrast agents in patients with compromised renal function. In patients with slowly progressive renal failure, urine output is usually well maintained.

As noted earlier, blood urea nitrogen and serum creatinine levels correlate only roughly with symptoms and are poor measures of GFR (see Chap. 269). The creatinine clearance (the product of the volume of urine produced per minute multiplied by the ratio of the concentration of creatinine in urine to the concentration of creatinine in plasma) tends to overestimate the GFR, while the calculated urea clearance often underestimates the GFR. By averaging simultaneously determined creatinine and urea clearances, a reasonably accurate estimation of GFR can be obtained. More exact measures of GFR can be obtained by isotope clearance techniques, which involve the injection of radioisotope and the accurate collection of urine specimens at timed intervals over a 2- to 4-h period. Of these methods, the iothalamate clearance is the most useful clinically.

Restriction of dietary sodium intake is important in the management of hypertension. As renal insufficiency progresses, foods rich in phosphate and potassium should also be restricted. Debate continues as to the clinical usefulness of lowering the protein content of the diet. The strongest evidence suggests that this measure is most effective if initiated early in the course of renal failure. Reduction of dietary protein content reduces anorexia, nausea, and vomiting late in uremia. If initiated early (while the GFR is > 40 to 50 mL/min), a low-protein diet (0.6 grams of protein per kilogram of body weight) may be effective in slowing the progression of renal disease.

The Modification of Diet in Renal Disease (MDRD) multicenter study sponsored by the U.S. National Institutes of Health/Health Care Financing Administration found that lowering the protein intake while the GFR was in the range of 25 to 55 mL/min was associated with a modest reduction in disease progression at 3 years of follow-up, especially in patients with proteinuria of >1 g per day. Because of the risk of malnutrition, aggressive reduction of dietary protein intake late in renal insufficiency should be discouraged if the patient's serum albumin concentration is below 3 g/dL or there is other evidence of malnutrition. The MDRD study demonstrated that the control of hypertension is as important as dietary protein restriction in slowing the progression of renal disease. The major finding of the MDRD study was that a decrease in blood pressure below a mean value of approximately 95 mmHg (i.e., 120/80) was effective in slowing progression of renal disease, again especially in patients with proteinuria of >1 g/d. Data from other studies, particularly in patients with early diabetic nephropathy, suggest a beneficial role for angiotensin converting enzyme (ACE) inhibitors in slowing progression of renal disease. Hyperkalemia and compromised renal function are complications of these drugs, especially in patients with bilateral renal artery stenosis (or unilateral stenosis in those with a solitary kidney). Combination therapy involving ACE inhibitors plus diuretics, alpha-adrenergic blockers, and/or beta-adrenergic blockers may be necessary to control hypertension as well as to delay progression to end-stage renal failure.

In more advanced uremia, it may be necessary to use sodium bicarbonate or calcium carbonate to correct metabolic acidosis and bicarbonate, dextrose-insulin combinations, or sodium-potassium exchange resins for treatment of hyperkalemia. Hypermagnesemia, hyperamylasemia, hypertriglyceridemia, and mild carbohydrate intolerance generally do not require or are not amenable to treatment.

Hyperuricemia should be treated with allopurinol (100 mg daily) only if gout develops. Treatment of anemia has been discussed above. Secondary hyperparathyroidism must be treated early to prevent bone disease. Vigorous use of phosphate-binding agents, calcium supplements, and vitamin D (dihydrotachysterol or calcitriol) to maintain the serum levels of calcium (9.5 to 10.5 mg/dL) and phosphorus (4.5 to 6.0 mg/dL) are often effective in suppressing parathyroid levels and preventing osteitis fibrosa and osteomalacia. However, the calcium-phosphorus product must be kept below 70 to avoid visceral, subcutaneous, joint and vascular calcifications.

Dietary restrictions of sodium, potassium, phosphate, and protein often prove unacceptable to patients. Consequently, when the complications of uremia worsen despite conservative management and malnutrition appears, dialysis and/or transplantation, along with an aggressive increase in calories and protein, should be instituted.

BIBLIOGRAPHY

ANDERSON S, BRENNER BM: Progressive renal disease: A disorder of adaptation. Q J Med 70:185, 1989

ATTMAN PO, ALAUPOVID P: Lipid abnormalities in chronic renal insufficiency. Kidney Int 39(Suppl 31):S16, 1991

CONVERSE RL JR et al: Sympathetic overactivity in patients with chronic renal failure. N Engl J Med 327:1912, 1992

ESCHBACH JW et al: Recombinant human erythropoietin in anemic patients with endstage renal disease: Results of phase III multicenter clinical trial. Ann Intern Med 111:992, 1989

FRASER CL, ARIEFF AF: Nervous system complications in uremia. Ann Intern Med 109:143, 1988

HAKIM RM, LAZARUS JM: Biochemical parameters in chronic renal failure. Am J Kidney Dis 11:238, 1988

KANG JY: The gastrointestinal tract in uremia. Digest Dis Sci 38:257, 1993

KLAHR S et al: The effects of dietary protein restriction and blood-pressure control on the progression of chronic renal disease. N Engl J Med 330:877, 1994

LEWIS EJ et al: The effect of angiotensin-converting-enzyme inhibition on diabetic nephropathy. N Engl J Med 329:1456, 1993

RITZ E, KOCH M: Morbidity and mortality due to hypertension in patients with renal failure. Am J Kidney Dis 21:113, 1993

ROSTAND SG et al: Cardiovascular complications in renal failure. J Am Soc Nephrol 2:1053, 1991

SHERRAD DJ et al: The spectrum of bone disease in end-stage renal failure—an evolving disorder. Kidney Int 43:436, 1993

272 *Charles B. Carpenter, J. Michael Lazarus*

DIALYSIS AND TRANSPLANTATION IN THE TREATMENT OF RENAL FAILURE

Over the past 30 years, dialysis and transplantation have prolonged the lives of thousands of patients with renal insufficiency. The approach to treatment in acute renal failure is different than in chronic renal failure because of the irreversible nature of the latter. Conservative medical management and dialysis are the mainstays of therapy for acute renal failure (Chap. 270). Obviously, transplantation is not a treatment for this group of patients.

The term *end-stage renal disease* (ESRD) is used by U.S. government agencies and has come to be synonymous with the late stages of chronic renal failure. Initially, patients with ESRD are managed with conservative therapy, but eventually they require hemodialysis, peritoneal dialysis, and/or transplantation. Because of limited success with each of these modalities, chronic renal failure should be approached with the concept of moving from one form of therapy to another as indicated by the degree of success and incidence of complications with each. Therapy for renal failure should *not* be initiated when the patient is totally asymptomatic; however, dialysis and/or

transplant should be started sufficiently early to prevent serious complications, as noted in Chaps. 270 and 271. Early dialysis is appropriate in patients with acute renal failure in whom resumption of renal function can be expected and in patients with chronic renal failure who have a good immunologic match with a related donor and are to be transplanted without prior long-term dialysis. In the remainder of patients, the clinical judgment to move from conservative treatment to dialysis or transplantation is determined by the patient's quality of life and whether or not the benefits of treatment outweigh the risks.

The correlation of uremic symptoms with renal function varies from patient to patient depending on the cause of renal disease (earlier onset of symptoms in subjects with diabetes mellitus), muscle mass (large, muscular patients tolerate high levels of azotemia), diet, nutritional status, and coexisting conditions. Therefore, it is ill-advised to assign a certain "usual" level of blood urea nitrogen, serum creatinine, or glomerular filtration rate to the need to start dialysis. In the United States, the Health Care Financing Administration has assigned levels of creatinine and creatinine clearance to qualify for reimbursement from Medicare for patients receiving dialysis. The creatinine must be greater than or equal to 8.0 mg/dL (700 μmol/L) and the creatinine clearance must be less than or equal to 10 mL/min (0.17 mL/s). The recently introduced regulations will undoubtedly affect physician practice. Treatment with dietary protein restriction and aggressive control of hypertension, as described in Chap. 271, may prolong the time before the need for dialysis and/or transplantation but should be carried out only if complications of such therapy, specifically malnutrition, do not occur.

DIALYSIS AND/OR TRANSPLANTATION

Selection of patients to receive dialysis and/or transplantation is a matter of some debate. Because of the reversible nature of acute renal failure, all patients with this diagnosis should be supported with dialysis, at least for some period of time, to allow return of renal function (see Chap. 270). In patients with irreversible or chronic renal failure, criteria for selection for transplantation are generally more stringent than those for dialysis (see below) and are guided by the possibility of complications related to immunosuppressive therapy. Table 272-1 lists considerations in the selection of recipients for a human renal allograft. Transplantation should be undertaken only when conservative treatment has failed, when there are no reversible elements in the renal failure, and when the patient is too ill to be maintained comfortably with the usual methods of treatment. However, morbidity is less if transplantation is performed before the patient is critically ill. Transplantation should not be utilized in an attempt to salvage patients, particularly the elderly, from failure to thrive on dialysis.

The recipient should be free of life-threatening extrarenal complications such as cancer, severe coronary artery disease, and cerebrovascular disease. Provided that diffuse vascular involvement is not present,

Table 272-1

Contraindications to Kidney Transplantation

ABSOLUTE CONTRAINDICATIONS

Reversible renal involvement
Ability of conservative measures to maintain useful life
Advanced forms of major extrarenal complications (cerebrovascular or coronary disease, neoplasia)
Active infection
Active glomerulonephritis
Previous sensitization to donor tissue

RELATIVE CONTRAINDICATIONS

Age
Presence of vesical or urethral abnormalities
Iliofemoral occlusive disease
Psychiatric problems
Oxalosis

diabetes mellitus is not a contraindication. Oxalosis may recur in relatively short order in a transplanted kidney and is generally a contraindication for transplantation. Although advanced age may be a limiting factor, it is advanced "physiologic" rather than chronologic age that contraindicates transplantation. In general, patients reach a "physiologic" limit at approximately age 60 to 65 years, when the incidence of complications due to glucocorticoids becomes much higher. Although abnormalities of the bladder and urethra present additional hazards, successful renal allografts have been placed in patients with these abnormalities by prior constitution of an artificial bladder (i.e., ileal conduit) into which the donor ureter is placed. Patients with any disease process that may be aggravated by glucocorticoids, cyclosporine, azathioprine, or other immunosuppressive agents or any patient with coexisting medical conditions so severe that the risks of operation and drug therapy are high should not be offered transplantation.

Criteria for treatment with hemodialysis or peritoneal dialysis are more liberal because dialysis has less morbidity than transplantation in older patients with the aforementioned medical complications. Because of the cost of these programs, some have suggested that entry be restricted in patients of advanced age. Such decisions, based on moral, social, and economic issues, continue to be debated. In general, in the United States and some other countries, nearly all patients are accepted for dialysis if they or their families desire prolongation of life. The physician should inform the patient of the likelihood of success and review the complications and untoward effects. The patient and family should be given an estimate of prognosis and expected quality of life. In most areas of the world, the cost of medical care for chronic renal failure is borne by government. In the United States, the mechanism of coverage is by Medicare, with all patients eligible regardless of age.

PREPARATION FOR THERAPY OF END-STAGE RENAL DISEASE While conservative measures are being carried out in patients with chronic renal failure (Chap. 271), it is important to prepare them with an intensive educational program, explaining the likelihood and timing of complete renal failure and the various forms of therapy available. The more knowledgeable patients are concerning hemodialysis, peritoneal dialysis, and transplantation, the easier and more appropriate will be their decisions at a later time. With hemodialysis, the major method of obtaining blood for treatment is from an arteriovenous fistula. Since these devices often take months to develop, prophylactic placement of a fistula in a patient opting for hemodialysis is important in minimizing future complications of circulatory access. For those who select peritoneal dialysis [continuous ambulatory peritoneal dialysis (CAPD) or continuous cyclic peritoneal dialysis (CCPD)], placement of the peritoneal catheter does not require prior preparation, and catheter placement and peritoneal dialysis can be instituted when uremic signs and symptoms develop. In those who may perform home dialysis or undergo transplantation, early education of family members for selection and preparation as a home dialysis helper or a related donor for transplantation should occur before the onset of symptomatic renal failure.

In patients who have a good antigenic match with a willing donor, transplantation without intervening hemodialysis or peritoneal dialysis should be considered. Approximately 25 percent of patients receiving renal transplants at our institution do so without having had prior dialysis. In considering related-donor transplantation, the risk of unilateral nephrectomy in the donor, including development of proteinuria and hypertension, should be considered by the family. As discussed below, the success rate of cadaver-donor transplantation has improved sufficiently that this form of therapy should be considered both by the patient and by potential donors. Early referral of patients to ESRD programs will allow education of the patient and family and preparation for an appropriate therapy. In recent years, unrelated living donors have become acceptable in most programs.

DIALYSIS

HEMODIALYSIS Hemodialysis employs the process of diffusion across a semipermeable membrane to remove unwanted substances from the blood while adding desirable components. A constant flow of blood on one side of the membrane and a cleansing solution (dialysate) on the other allow removal of waste products by diffusive and convective transport. By altering the composition of the dialysate, the method of exposure of blood and dialysate (geometry of the dialyzer), the type and surface area of dialysis membrane, and the frequency and duration of exposure (the dialysis prescription), patients without renal function can be maintained in a relatively healthy state.

Hemodialysis equipment consists of three components—the blood delivery system, the composition and delivery system of the dialysate, and the dialyzer itself (Fig. 272-1). Blood is pumped to the dialyzer by a roller pump through lines with appropriate equipment to measure flow and pressures within the system; blood flow should be approximately 300 to 450 mL/min. Negative hydrostatic pressure on the dialysate side of the system can be manipulated to achieve desirable fluid removal, so-called ultrafiltration. Dialysis membranes have differing ultrafiltration coefficients (i.e., mL removed per mmHg/min), the selection of which, along with the hydrostatic pressure changes, determines fluid removal. The dialysate is delivered to the dialyzer from a storage tank or proportioning system that manufactures dialysate on-line. In most systems, dialysate passes once across the membrane, countercurrent to blood flow at a rate of 500 mL/min. The composition of the dialysate is similar to normal plasma water but may be altered depending on need. The dialysate potassium is varied most often; the concentration of calcium, chloride, and bicarbonate generally remain unchanged in each dialysis unit. Sodium concentration may be varied during the course of dialysis (sodium modeling) in order to optimize fluid removal.

The principal dialyzer in use in the United States is the hollow fiber or capillary dialyzer, in which membrane material is spun into fine capillaries, thousands of which are packed into bundles with blood flowing through the capillaries while dialysate is circulated on the outside of the fiber bundle. The type of membrane and surface area (size) are determinants of ultrafiltration and clearance and are important in the immunologic (i.e., biocompatible) response by the patient. Cuprophan (Cupra-ammonium cellophane) and cellulose acetate are "tighter" membranes with less diffusive and ultrafiltration capabilities and less biocompatibility. Polyacrylnitrile, polymethylmethacrylate, polysulphon, and certain newer cellulose derivatives are porous (high flux) and more biocompatible but are more expensive.

With current dialysis techniques, most patients require between 9 and 12 h of dialysis per week, equally divided into several sessions. The time depends on body size, residual renal function, dietary intake, complicating illnesses, and degree of anabolism or catabolism. The dialysis duration, frequency of treatments, type and size of dialyzer, dialysate composition, and blood or dialysate flow may all be altered to accomplish specific needs (see Fig. 272-2).

Urea kinetic modeling is a technique to measure the delivered dose of dialysis. This may be determined by use of a pre- and postdialysis urea sample [urea reduction ratio (URR)] or by determining the KT/V (K = clearance, T = dialysis time, and V = volume of distribution of the patient), which is a dimensionless measure of treatment. An acceptable URR is 65 percent, which is equivalent to a KT/V of approximately 1.0 to 1.2. The development of bicarbonate dialysis, sodium modeling, and high-flux or ultraefficient membranes has resulted in the ability to reduce dialysis time. It is mandatory, however, that such decreases in dialysis time be monitored by one of the above measures of adequacy. Reduction of dialysis time without documentation of adequacy of treatment is associated with an increased mortality and morbidity.

In addition to hemodialysis, a new method of treatment has been developed for patients with acute renal failure. Slow continuous ultrafiltration, continuous arteriovenous hemodialysis (CAVHD), or continuous venovenous hemodialysis (CVVHD) are techniques that employ high-efficiency dialyzers with continuous treatment utilizing very low blood and dialysate flow rates. These therapies are useful in

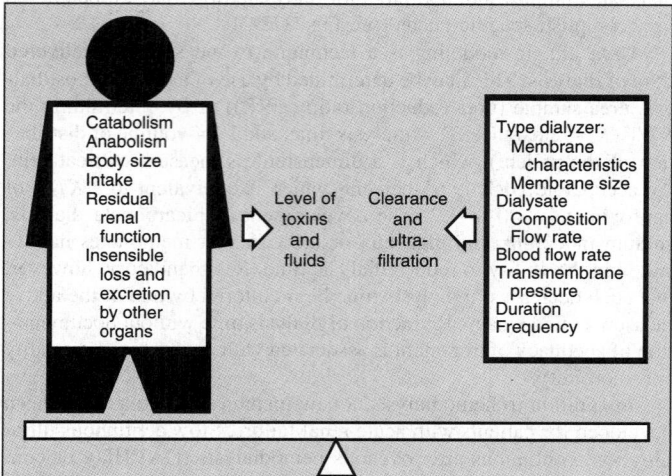

FIGURE 272-1 Schema for hemodialysis.

the unstable, acute renal failure patient and are often preferable to intermittent hemodialysis.

Complications of Hemodialysis Complications of chronic dialysis should be thought of as those related to unresolved uremia, direct complications of clearance and ultrafiltration, and complications created by long-term dialytic treatment. The persistent problems of uremia not corrected by dialysis are described in Chap. 271. Complications more directly related to the procedure include those related to access to the circulation or access to the peritoneal cavity, which are the Achilles' heel of dialysis treatment. Blood flows of 300 to 400 mL/min are necessary for hemodialysis. Blood from veins is inadequate,

and repeated puncture of a large artery is not feasible. Therefore, by surgically anastamosing a superficial artery and nearby vein, a fistula is created. If a native vein is not available because of fibrosis and atrophy due to prior needling, phlebitis, or other injury, a prosthetic vascular graft (extended polytetrafluoroethylene), bridging an artery and a nearby vein, may be utilized. Repeated cannulation of arteriovenous fistulas or graft fistulas with 14- to 16-gauge needles permits blood flow sufficient to carry out hemodialysis. Some patients require placement of a semipermanent indwelling internal jugular catheter when a fistula cannot be developed or is slow to develop. Unfortunately, thrombosis, infection, and aneurysm formation commonly occur in arteriovenous fistulas, particularly in the prosthetic types, and are the leading causes of hospital admission in these patients. There is a high incidence of septicemia and septic embolization associated with fistula infections and semipermanent internal jugular catheters; the most common infecting agent is *Staphylococcus aureus*. Peritoneal dialysis is performed through the placement of an indwelling peritoneal catheter. On occasion, these catheters become nonfunctional, but the more common complication is peritonitis, generally related to contamination of the system during exchange of peritoneal fluid.

The rapid flux in osmolality with hemodialysis may cause a disequilibrium syndrome consisting of confusion, clouding of consciousness, and seizures. In addition, rapid changes in electrolytes (particularly potassium) may lead to arrhythmia during dialysis. Hypotension during hemodialysis is due to many factors—the size of the extracorporeal circulation, degree of ultrafiltration, change in serum osmolality, presence of autonomic neuropathy, concomitant use of antihypertensive agents, removal of catecholamines, or alterations in body temperature due to the dialysate temperature. Careful estimation of the extracellular fluid to be removed and use of isolated ultrafiltration and higher dialysate sodium are helpful in preventing hypotension. The occurrence of dialysis dementia (a condition of decreasing mental function

FIGURE 272-2 Factors in the development of the uremic syndrome and considerations in its treatment.

with seizure activity and abnormal electroencephalogram), low-turnover osteomalacia, and microcytic anemia may be secondary to aluminum contamination of dialysate water or from high oral intake of aluminum hydroxide. These complications have nearly disappeared with awareness of the risk of aluminum exposure and its avoidance. An increased incidence of hepatitis B surface antigen (HBsAg) and hepatitis C virus (HCV) antigenemia are related to decreased immunology integrity and increased transfusions. Patients with chronic antigenemia are usually asymptomatic and have transient or mild derangement in liver function. The high rates of HCV infection and cytomegalovirus (CMV) infection do not have major impact on dialysis patients but do on patients who are subsequently transplanted. The use of recombinant human erythropoietin has reduced or eliminated the need for blood transfusion in hemodialysis patients (Chap. 271), thus reducing the risk of hepatitis and other bloodborne infections. In addition, the use of hepatitis vaccine has decreased the incidence of hepatitis B. Based on clinical experience and recommendations from the Centers for Disease Control and Prevention, only those patients with hepatitis B antigenemia need isolation. Strict compliance with universal precautions is absolutely essential in the dialysis unit, particularly because of patients with HCV and CMV and those who are positive for human immunodeficiency virus.

Mechanical and/or iatrogenic complications, such as hemolysis, air embolus, blood leaks, and contaminated dialysate, are less common with improved equipment. Membrane-induced adverse reactions may occur, as exemplified by complement-mediated leukopenia and hypoxemia. More prominent symptoms, such as back and chest pain, bronchospasm, and anaphylaxis, rarely occur from such reactions. Elaboration of cytokines, specifically interleukin (IL) 1, IL-6, and tumor necrosis factor, occur with exposure of blood to some dialysis membranes. Activation of the complement and cytokine systems likely plays a role in anorexia and hypercatabolism seen in hemodialysis patients. These cytokines also contribute, along with decreased excretion of β_2-microglobulin, to the development of dialysis-related amyloidosis—a syndrome consisting of carpal tunnel syndrome; destructive spondyloarthropathy; cervicooccipital pseudotumors; cyst formation in the femoral head and neck, carpal bones, and humoral head; scapulohumoral periarthritis; and increased visceral involvement with amyloidosis. Use of more biocompatible synthetic membranes (polycrilonitrile, polymethylmethacrylate, and polysulfone) rather than cellulosic-related membranes has been suggested to have a beneficial effect by reducing β_2-microglobulin production and increasing its removal. As mentioned earlier, these membranes are expensive. Reuse of such dialyzers, which occurs in approximately 70 to 75 percent of patients, makes their use feasible.

Heparin is necessary during the hemodialysis procedure to prevent clotting in the lines, but its use may lead to complications such as subdural hematoma and retroperitoneal, gastrointestinal, pericardial, and pleural hemorrhages. Recognition of the risks and modification of the dose of heparin reduce these complications.

The major cause of death in patients with ESRD receiving chronic hemodialysis or peritoneal dialysis is cardiovascular disease. Although this is not a direct complication of hemodialysis, it is probably related to inadequate treatment of hypertension, the persistence of hyperlipidemia in dialysis patients, and, in some cases, alterations in cardiovascular dynamics during the course of dialysis. In addition to aggressive removal of fluid, the appropriate use of antihypertensive agents may be necessary. One further major complication affecting morbidity and mortality in the dialysis population is malnutrition. Again, this is not directly related to the dialysis procedure except that the chronic exposure of the patient to dialysis may effect an increased catabolism and allow amino acid loss through the membrane. Recognition of amino acid loss, decreased protein and calorie intake, and hypercatabolism has led to the recommendation of more aggressive feeding of dialysis patients.

The potential for all of the above complications should cause the physician to evaluate the risk/benefit ratio of hemodialysis before proceeding with such treatment, particularly in the marginal patient. Advantages of hemodialysis are the relatively short treatment time

and minimal interruption of life-style between treatments. It is more efficient than peritoneal dialysis, allowing rapid changes in abnormal serum values. Hemodialysis can be performed in the home, but the patient requires an assistant during treatment.

PERITONEAL DIALYSIS Peritoneal dialysis, like hemodialysis, may be performed in various settings and with several techniques. In patients with acute renal failure, intermittent peritoneal dialysis (IPD) has largely been replaced by CAVHD or CAVVHD. Chronic peritoneal dialysis was attempted in the late 1940s but was impractical until the development of a permanent peritoneal catheter—the Tenckhoff catheter. Use of this indwelling catheter and closed continuous-cycle dialysate delivery equipment led to treatment protocols with which patients were treated two to three times per week for a total of 30 to 40 h IPD to achieve clearances and fluid removal similar to those of hemodialysis. In 1978, the concept of continuous peritoneal lavage with prolonged dwell times led to the development of CAPD, which differs from IPD in that patients instill fluid into the peritoneal cavity, seal the catheter, continue in an ambulatory mode, and every 4 to 6 h empty the peritoneal cavity and replace the dialysate. This technique generally utilizes 2 L of dialysate and obviates the need for dialysis equipment. Modification of the technique using a cyclic dialysate delivery device to exchange dialysate during the night with dwelling of fluid during the waking hours (CCPD) is more acceptable to some patients.

IPD performed in a center is not a practical approach due to high costs. CCPD may be performed at home (usually overnight), while CAPD can be performed anywhere. As with hemodialysis, the composition of the dialysate can be modified for individual needs. The major difference in peritoneal dialysate formulas is in the amount of dextrose used as an osmotic agent (1.5, 2.5, or 4.25 g/dL). Advantages of peritoneal dialysis are avoidance of heparinization and vascular surgery and a slower clearance rate (helpful for some cardiovascular patients). It is more amenable to self-treatment. Disadvantages include the longer treatment time with continuous involvement by the patient. It should not be used in patients with pulmonary disease or extensive abdominal adhesions due to surgery. Inadequate clearance may occur in patients with scleroderma, vasculitis, malignant hypertension or peritoneal fibrosis or in heavy patients (>70 kg) with no residual renal function.

Determination of adequacy of treatment by CAPD or CCPD is performed by measuring the clearance of creatinine and urea in a 24-h dialysate collection. The most common complication is peritonitis, including catheter tunnel infections. Protein loss leading to malnutrition is another major complication, while hypertriglyceridemia, hypercholesterolemia, obesity, and inguinal and abdominal hernias are rare complications. The average peritonitis rate is approximately one episode every 10 to 12 months. Tunnel infections are much less frequent but usually require the catheter to be removed, whereas peritonitis can be treated with intravenous or intraparenteral antibiotics with the catheter remaining in place.

TREATMENT OPTIONS AND SETTINGS An acutely ill or medically complicated patient will likely undergo dialysis in a hospital dialysis unit or intensive care unit, while stable patients are generally dialyzed as outpatients in free-standing facilities or at home. Most centers attempt to have patients participate in their own care, so-called self-care dialysis. Home dialysis (either hemodialysis or peritoneal) is preferable for many because of self-reliance and freedom from hospital and center schedules. Patient motivation is the primary factor in the selection of home hemodialysis or peritoneal dialysis. Dialysis in the hospital setting is most expensive, while home dialysis with a nonpaid family assistant or alone (peritoneal dialysis only) is marginally less expensive than satellite dialysis. Despite the absence of equipment, peritoneal dialysis is nearly as expensive as home hemodialysis because of the cost of dialysate and of hospitalizations related to complications of peritoneal dialysis.

In 1995, the total Medicare budget for ESRD (inpatient and outpatient care including hemodialysis, peritoneal dialysis, and transplantation and all other related medical expenses) was estimated by the Health Care Financing Administration to be $9.5 billion. The cost of the ESRD program has grown to be substantially greater than anticipated at its initiation in 1973. This large expenditure reflects an increasing number of recipients treated, not an increasing cost per patient, which, in fact, has been significantly reduced over the past 30 years.

RESULTS The mean age for patients undergoing hemodialysis and peritoneal dialysis is approximately 64 years. Of new patients entering ESRD therapy, approximately 35 to 50 percent are physically and psychologically suitable for transplantation. Not all of these patients opt for transplantation. Only those patients with living related and unrelated donors or those fortunate enough to match a cadaver donor undergo prompt transplantation. These patients are usually younger and healthier than those patients left behind on hemodialysis. The age of patients on dialysis continues to rise, partly because of an increase in acceptance of patients with age-related nephrosclerosis but also because of the selection process favoring transplantation in younger patients.

Approximately 10 to 20 percent of patients with chronic renal failure are totally rehabilitated by dialysis, and another 30 to 40 percent of nondiabetic patients may be rehabilitated to a functional status even if they are not employed. Twenty percent of patients reach a level of function not considered rehabilitated but are able to care for themselves. The remainder (approximately 20 percent) are totally dependent on support from others. Diabetic patients, who have rehabilitation and survival rates lower than those of nondiabetic patients, make up much of the latter two groups. Mortality rates vary, depending on the age of the patient and the disease process(es) involved. Yearly gross mortality rates of patients in the ESRD program in the United States have increased from a low of 20 percent in 1982 to approximately 24 percent in 1991, which has persisted. This increase in mortality may be due to case-mix factors, i.e., acceptance in recent years of older patients with a higher incidence of comorbid conditions such as diabetes mellitus, nephrosclerosis, coronary artery disease, peripheral vascular disease, and pulmonary and hepatic disease. Others have suggested that treatment has become inadequate for financial reasons. In recent years, measurement of both quality and quantity of dialysis treatment has been implemented, leading to increased treatment intensity in many programs. It is anticipated that this will have a favorable effect on mortality and morbidity. In patients less than 50 years of age with no complicating medical illnesses, mortality with hemodialysis, peritoneal dialysis, and transplantation remains below 3 to 5 percent per year.

TRANSPLANTATION

Transplantation of the human kidney is frequently the most effective treatment of advanced chronic renal failure. Worldwide, tens of thousands of such procedures have been performed. When azathioprine and prednisone were initially used as immunosuppressive drugs, the results with properly matched familial donors were superior to those with organs from cadaveric donors, namely, 75 to 90 percent compared with 50 to 60 percent graft survival rates at 1 year. During the 1970s and 1980s, the success rate at the 1-year mark for cadaveric transplants rose progressively. By the time cyclosporine was introduced in the early 1980s, cadaveric donor grafts had a 70 percent 1-year survival and were at the 80 to 85 percent level in the mid 1990s. After the first year, graft survival curves show an exponential decline in numbers of functioning grafts from which a half-life ($t_{1/2}$) in years is calculated. Mortality rates are less than 5 percent in the first year and lower thereafter. Occasionally, acute irreversible rejection may occur after many months of good function, especially if the patient neglects to take the immunosuppressive drugs. Most grafts, however, succumb at varying rates to a chronic vascular and interstitial obliterative process termed *chronic rejection*, although its pathogenesis is incompletely understood. Second and even third transplants can be performed, and the overall results show a 10 to 20 percent reduction in expected

survival compared with first transplants in those patients who rapidly rejected a prior transplant. Overall, transplantation returns the majority of patients to an improved life-style, as compared to patients on dialysis; however, careful prospective cohort studies have yet to be reported.

DONOR SELECTION Donors can be cadavers or volunteer living donors. The latter are usually family members selected to have at least partial compatibility for HLA antigens. Living volunteer donors should be normal on physical examination and of the same major ABO blood group, because crossing major blood group barriers prejudices survival of the allograft. It is possible, however, to transplant a kidney of a type O donor into an A, B, or AB recipient. Selective renal arteriography should be performed on donors to rule out the presence of multiple or abnormal renal arteries, because the surgical procedure is difficult and the ischemic time of the transplanted kidney long when vascular abnormalities exist. Cadaveric donors should be free of malignant neoplastic disease because of possible transmission to the recipient. Increased risk of graft failure exists when the donor is elderly or has renal failure and when the kidney has a prolonged period of ischemia and storage.

In the United States, there is a coordinated national system (United Network for Organ Sharing) of computerized information about and logistic support for the transportation of cadaver kidneys to suitable recipients. It is now possible to remove cadaver kidneys and to maintain them for over 48 h on cold pulsatile perfusion or simple flushing and cooling. This permits adequate time for typing, cross-matching, transportation, and selection problems to be solved.

TISSUE TYPING AND CLINICAL IMMUNOGENETICS Matching for antigens of the HLA major histocompatibility gene complex (Chap. 306) is the ideal criterion for selection of donors for renal allografts. Each mammalian species has a single chromosomal region that encodes the strong, or major, transplantation antigens, and this region on the human sixth chromosome is called *HLA*. HLA antigens have been classically defined by serologic techniques, but methods to define specific nucleotide sequences in genomic DNA are increasingly being used. Other antigens, called "minor," may nevertheless play crucial roles, especially the ABH(O) blood groups and endothelial antigens that are not shared with lymphocytes. Evidence for designation of HLA as the genetic region encoding major transplantation antigens comes from the success rate in living related donor renal and bone marrow transplantation, with superior results in HLA-identical sibling pairs. Nevertheless, 5 to 10 percent of HLA-identical renal allografts are rejected, often within the first weeks after transplantation. These failures represent states of prior sensitization to non-HLA antigens. Non-HLA antigens are relatively weak when initially encountered and are therefore suppressible by conventional immunosuppressive therapy. Once priming has occurred, however, secondary responses are much more refractory to treatment. ABO incompatibilities are hazardous because of the presence of natural anti-A and anti-B antibodies in recipients and the normal expression of A and B blood group substances on endothelium.

Living Donors When first-degree relatives are donors, graft survival rates at 1 year are slightly greater than those for cadaver grafts, with the exception of HLA-identical donors where 1-year results are approximately 95 percent. After the first year, the long-term survival rates as defined by the $t_{1/2}$ still favor the partially matched (one HLA haplotype) family donor over a randomly selected cadaver donor (Table 272-2). In addition, living donors provide the advantage of immediate availability. Waiting lists for cadaveric kidneys have grown faster than the available organ supply to the point where most new patients with end-stage renal disease wait for more than 3 years. In response to this increasing disparity between cadaver donor supply and patient demand, living unrelated volunteers, usually spouses or close friends, are being accepted as donors in increasing numbers. It is illegal in the United States to purchase organs for transplantation. The results of transplantation using living unrelated donors have been most satisfactory, with initial and long-term survival rates the same as for partial HLA-matched family donors and better than for partially matched cadaveric donors (Table 272-2).

Effect of HLA-A, B, DR Mismatching on Kidney Graft Survival*

Donor Mismatches	Half-Life of Graft Survival, years	10-Year Graft Survival, %
Living related donor (HLA-identical sib = no mismatches)	24.0	74
Cadaver (no mismatches for 6 antigens)	20.3	65
Living related donor (1 haplotype = 3 mismatches)	12.0	54
Living unrelated donor (average 4 mismatches)	12.0	54
Cadaver (overall)	9.0	40
Cadaver (1 or 2 mismatches)	10.4	45
Cadaver (3 or 4 mismatches)	8.4	38
Cadaver (5 or 6 mismatches)	7.7	34

* HLA antigens are codominantly inherited: each person has two A, two B, and two DR antigens, for a total of six.

Concern has been expressed regarding the potential risk to a volunteer kidney donor of premature renal failure after several years of increased blood flow and hyperfiltration per nephron in the remaining kidney. There are a few reports of the development of hypertension, proteinuria, and even lesions of focal segmental sclerosis in donors under long-term follow-up. Difficulties in donors followed for 20 or more years are unusual, however, and it may be that having a single kidney becomes significant only when another condition, such as hypertension, is superimposed. It is also desirable to consider the risk of development of type 1 diabetes mellitus in a family member who is a potential donor to a diabetic renal failure patient. Anti-insulin and anti-islet antibodies should be measured, and glucose tolerance tests should be performed in such donors to rule out a prediabetic state.

HLA Matching and Cadaveric Donors The question of whether matching of HLA antigens in unrelated donor-recipient pairs would approximate the high initial success rates and slow rates of subsequent graft loss with HLA-identical sib pairs could not be answered until the late 1980s when reliable class II histocompatibility (DR) typing became widely available. Now that pooled data on tens of thousands of cadaveric renal transplants from all over the world are available, the HLA-matching effect can be clearly seen, especially in the long-term $t_{1/2}$ half-life survival figures. It is shown in Fig. 272-3 that there is an overall beneficial effect of HLA matching in first cadaveric grafts. When compared with HLA-identical transplants, where the 1-year graft survival rate is 95 percent and the subsequent half-life is 25 years, one-HLA-haplotype–matched family donor transplants have 1-year survival rates of 85 percent with a 12-year half-life (Table 272-2). With increasing numbers of mismatches for cadaveric donors, the half-life decreases from 20 to 7.7 years. The survival rates at the 10-year mark are projected to range from 65 (zero mismatches) to 34 percent (six mismatches). Many centers now report 1-year graft survival rates in the 85 to 90 percent range for all renal transplants, possibly the result of heavy initial immunosuppression, but the subsequent half-lives are similar to those above. There is controversy regarding the value of cadaveric organ-sharing rules that are based entirely upon the numbers of HLA mismatches. Avoidance of mismatching for six antigens (Table 272-2) is a top priority in the United States, however, and 20 percent of kidneys are transplanted on this basis. Table 272-2 also shows the interaction of HLA matching and graft ischemia on results; namely, kidneys from HLA-incompatible spousal donors do better than those from similarly mismatched cadaver donors, suggesting that the additional ischemic injury of organ storage is important. When such a cadaveric donor is HLA-compatible, however, ischemia and storage do not impede the matching benefit.

Presensitization A positive cross match of recipient serum with donor T lymphocytes representing anti-HLA class I is usually predictive of an acute vasculitic event termed *hyperacute rejection*. Patients with anti-HLA antibodies can be safely transplanted if careful cross matching is performed. Patients sustained by dialysis often show fluctuating antibody titers and specificity patterns. At the time of assignment of a cadaveric kidney, cross matches are performed with more than one highly reactive serum, and the previously analyzed antibody specificities are also taken into account. Techniques for cross matching are not universally standardized; however, at least two techniques are employed in most laboratories. The minimal criterion for the cross match is avoidance of hyperacute rejection mediated by recipient antibodies to donor HLA class I antigens. Sensitive tests, such as the use of flow cytometry, can be useful for avoidance of accelerated, and often untreatable, early graft rejection in patients receiving second or third transplants. Donor T lymphocytes, which express only class I antigens, are used as targets for detection of anti-class I (HLA-A and -B) antibodies. Anti-class II (HLA-DR) antibodies do not contraindicate transplantation, unless present in high titer. B lymphocytes, expressing both class I and class II antigens are used in these assays. Non-HLA antigens restricted in expression to endothelium and sometimes monocytes have been described, but clinical relevance is not well established.

Blood Transfusions Exposure to leukocyte HLA antigens during transfusions was a major cause of sensitization that limited transplantation access and increased the risk of early graft rejection. In the 1970s, attempts to avoid all blood exposure in dialysed patients paradoxically increased the risk of graft rejection. The beneficial "transfusion effect" was never fully explained, and it almost disappeared in the 1980s as overall management of patients improved with the use of cyclosporine and more effective means of rejection treatment. Currently, with the use of erythropoietin the need for transfusion is much reduced. It has been noted, however, that nontransfused patients do have more rejection activity. Ongoing studies with HLA-typed blood donors indicate that transfusions are beneficial only when they are not completely mismatched for HLA, and in particular when there is one DR and one B antigen matched with the recipient.

IMMUNOLOGY OF REJECTION Knowledge of the immunology of tissue transplantation stems largely from animal experimentation. However, enough evidence has accumulated in humans to indicate that the mechanisms are similar, and not qualitatively different from those found in other areas of immunology (Chap. 305). Early

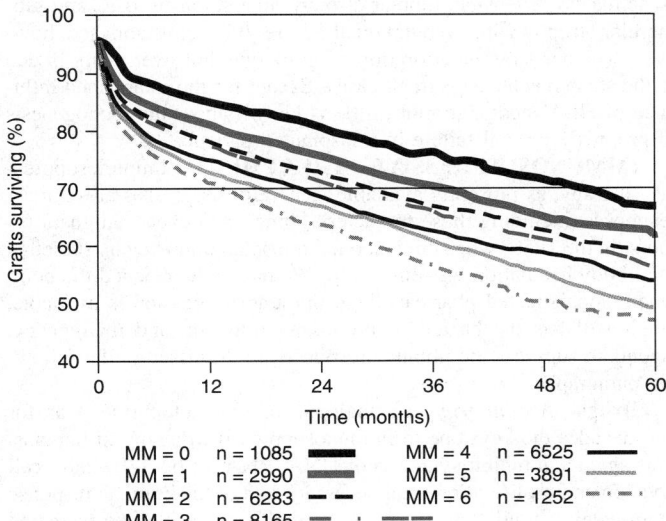

FIGURE 272-3 Survival of over 30,000 first cadaveric renal transplants over 5 years after transplantation. The transplants were performed in more than 200 centers around the world between 1982 and 1989. Cyclosporine was used in virtually all cases. The curves for each HLA matching grade are shown, according to the number of mismatches (MM) for HLA-A, -B, and -DR antigens. Since each individual has two genes for each locus, there is a potential for up to six mismatches. The overall effect of matching in this international Collaborative Transplant Study stratifies according to the mismatch grade (weighted regression, $p < 0.0001$) *(From Opelz.)*

rejection is associated with T lymphocytes having direct specificity against donor antigens. These may be cytotoxic cells (CD8+ or CD4+) or cells that mediate delayed hypersensitivity (CD4+); however, significant numbers of B lymphocytes, null cells, natural killer cells, and macrophages appear in the early infiltrate, and cells capable of mediating antibody-dependent cell-mediated cytotoxicity are also present (Fig. 272-4). Many of the B lymphocytes produce immunoglobulins. The spectrum of cellular and humoral response and graft injury is quite varied, depending on specific genetic differences between donor and recipient and states of presensitization. The greater the degree of presensitization, the more likely it is that one will find antibody-mediated vascular lesions. All the processes shown in Fig. 272-4 are possible, but their relative contribution varies from case to case. Monitoring of peripheral blood lymphocyte subsets utilizing monoclonal antibodies to functionally related surface molecules, such as CD4 (T helper cells) and CD8 (T suppressor/cytotoxic cells), has been related to the degree of rejection activity in some surveys. Since the principal role of the CD4 molecule is to promote interaction of T cells with class II HLA molecules on antigen-presenting cells, and similarly, CD8 interacts with class I HLA (see Chap. 305), it is not surprising that both types of T cells are usually present. Finally, the cytokine mediators of the cellular immune response [IL-1 to IL-4, IL-6, IL-10, IL-12, tumor necrosis factor (TNF), and interferon γ] are involved in the control and expression of the alloimmune rejection response. For example, T cell production of interferon γ causes increased expression of HLA antigens on endothelial cells. In normal immunobiology this effect may be to promote more efficient presentation of foreign antigen, while in transplantation it enhances the immunogenicity of the vascularized transplant. Also, IL-2, the major growth factor for expansion of effector T cells, is the product of a major subset of CD4 cells (Th1), while other CD4 cells (Th2) produce B cell growth factors, such as IL-4.

The failure of transplanted kidneys after several years of adequate function is said to be due to "chronic rejection." In such kidneys, the development of nephrosclerosis, with proliferation of the vascular intima of renal vessels, and intimal fibrosis, with marked decrease in the lumen of the vessels, takes place (Fig. 272-5). The result is renal ischemia, hypertension, tubular atrophy, interstitial fibrosis, and glomerular atrophy with eventual renal failure. It is not established, however, whether slow deterioration of graft function over years is due to the same mechanisms in all cases. Except for the established influence of HLA incompatibility, little is known about the pathogenesis of progressive renal failure in transplanted patients.

IMMUNOSUPPRESSIVE TREATMENT Immunosuppressive therapy, as presently available, generally suppresses all immune responses, including those to bacteria, fungi, and even malignant tumors. In the 1950s when clinical renal transplantation began, sublethal total-body irradiation was employed. We have now reached the point where sophisticated pharmacologic immunosuppression is available, but it still has the hazard of promoting infection and malignancy. Agents to suppress the immune response are discussed in the following paragraphs.

Drugs *Azathioprine*, an analogue of mercaptopurine, was for two decades the keystone to immunosuppressive therapy in humans. This agent can inhibit synthesis of DNA, RNA, or both. Because cell division and proliferation are a necessary part of the immune response to antigenic stimulation, suppression by this agent may be mediated by the inhibition of mitosis of immunologically competent lymphoid cells, interfering with synthesis of DNA. Alternatively, immunosuppression may be brought about by blocking the synthesis of RNA (possibly messenger RNA), inhibiting processing of antigens prior to lymphocyte stimulation. This drug has little effect in suppressing a secondary immune response, however. Therapy with azathioprine in doses of 1.5 to 2.0 mg/kg per day is generally added to cyclosporine as a means of decreasing the requirements for the latter. Because azathioprine is rapidly metabolized by the liver, its dosage need not

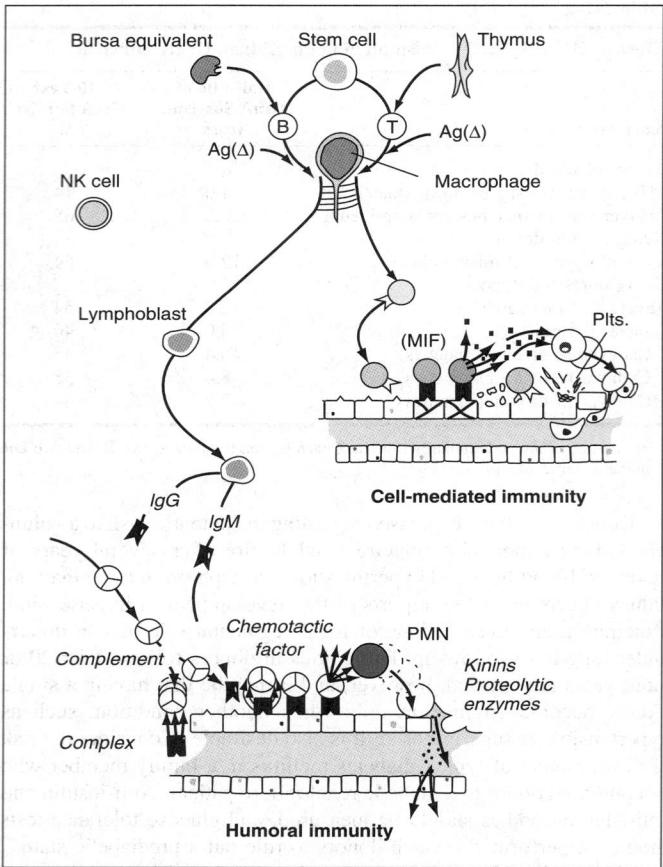

FIGURE 272-4 Overall scheme of the development of effector mechanisms in graft rejection. A set of bone marrow precursor stem cells is selected in the thymus gland to become mature thymus-derived (T) lymphocytes which are clonally determined to recognize non-self antigens (Δ) presented as fragments bound to self major histocompatibility molecules. These antigen-presenting structures are on the surfaces of macrophages, dendritic cells, and B lymphocytes. In transplantation, major histocompatibility antigens, such as HLA, may be recognized directly as the antigen-presenting molecules present in the grafted tissues or as fragments of donor HLA presented by recipient antigen-presenting cells. In avian species, but not in mammals, an anatomic site called the *bursa of Fabricius* provides the differentiating stimuli for maturation of B lymphocytes from bone marrow precursors. B lymphocytes with immunoglobulin receptors for a given antigen (Δ) proliferate and differentiate by a process of somatic mutation of immunoglobulin genes and selection by antigen for further growth. They begin to secrete IgM and, subsequently, IgG, IgE, and IgA. The response matures with help from T lymphocytes, which includes elaboration of the cytokines IL-4, IL-5, and IL-2. The proliferative phases of T and B lymphocyte response are illustrated by the lymphoblast.

Humoral immunity produces tissue injury following binding of immunoglobulins to tissue and, in particular, to the endothelium of a transplanted organ. Complement activation and chemotaxis of polymorphonuclear cells (PMN) are common in "hyperacute" rejection lesions when recipients have antidonor antibodies. Cell-mediated immunity is principally mediated by T lymphocytes bearing receptors for tissue antigens. These cells receive a major degree of help initially from macrophages that secrete the cytokines IL-6 and IL-1. Expanded populations of graft-specific T lymphocytes exert tissue damage by a delayed type hypersensitivity mechanism or by direct cytotoxic "killer" mechanisms. As noted in text, the T lymphocyte CD4 or CD8 phenotypes indicate whether the target antigens are HLA class II or class I, respectively.

The principal growth factor for T lymphocytes is an autocrine product, IL-2. Other T cell products include cytokines, such as interferon γ and tumor necrosis factor, which increase the pace of tissue injury. Activated macrophages can add nonspecifically to the inflammatory process. Natural killer cells (NK) play a minor role; however, they, along with other cells that bear receptors for the Fc portion of immunoglobulin, can provide cell-mediated target damage after fixation to IgG molecules previously bound to grafted cells (antibody-dependent cell-mediated cytotoxicity). Any of these mechanisms can result in vascular occlusion by platelet aggregation and thrombosis.

be varied directly in relation to renal function, even though renal failure results in retention of the metabolites of azathioprine. Some patients are unusually sensitive to this drug, particularly when renal function is compromised, and reduction in dosage is required because of leukopenia and occasionally thrombocytopenia. Excessive amounts of azathioprine also may cause jaundice, anemia, and alopecia. If it is essential to administer allopurinol concurrently, the azathioprine dose must be reduced, since inhibition of xanthine oxidase delays degradation. This combination is best avoided.

Mycophenolate mofetil is now used in place of azathioprine in many centers. It has a similar mode of action and a mild degree of gastrointestinal toxicity but produces minimal bone marrow suppression. Its advantage is its increased potency in preventing or reversing rejection.

Glucocorticoids are important adjuncts to immunosuppressive therapy. Of all the agents employed, prednisone has effects that are easiest to assess, and in large doses it is effective for the reversal of rejection. In general, 200 to 300 mg prednisone is given immediately prior to or at the time of transplantation, and the dosage is reduced to 30 mg within a week. The side effects of the glucocorticoids, particularly impairment of wound healing and predisposition to infection, make it desirable to taper the dose as rapidly as possible in the immediate postoperative period. Customarily, methylprednisolone, 0.5 to 1.0 g intravenously, is administered immediately upon diagnosis

of beginning rejection and continued once daily for 3 days. When the drug is effective, the results are usually apparent within 96 h. Such "pulse" doses are not effective in chronic rejection. Most patients whose renal function is stable after 6 months or a year do not require large doses of prednisone; maintenance doses of 10 to 15 mg/d are the rule. Many patients tolerate an alternate-day course of steroids without an increased risk of rejection.

A major effect of steroids is on the monocyte-macrophage system, preventing the release of IL-6 and IL-1. Lymphopenia after large doses of glucocorticoids is primarily due to sequestration of recirculating blood lymphocytes to lymphoid tissue.

Cyclosporine is a fungal peptide with potent immunosuppressive activity. It acts to block transcription of mRNA for IL-2 and other proinflammatory cytokines, thereby inhibiting T cell proliferation. Although it works alone, cyclosporine is more effective in conjunction with glucocorticoids. Since cyclosporine blocks production of IL-2 by T cells, its combination with steroids is expected to produce a double block in the macrophage → IL-6/IL-1 → T cell → IL-2 sequence. As noted, clinical results with tens of thousands of renal transplants have been impressive. Of its toxic effects (nephrotoxicity, hepatoxicity, hirsutism, tremor, gingival hyperplasia, diabetes), only nephrotoxicity presents a serious management problem and is further discussed below.

Tacrolimus (FK-506) is a fungal macrolide that has the same mode of action, and a similar side effect profile, as cyclosporine. De novo induction of diabetes mellitus is more common with tacrolimus. The drug is most useful in liver transplantation, for which it has received approval from the Food and Drug Administration, and may be tried as an alternative in renal patients whose rejections are poorly controlled by cyclosporine.

Sirolimus (previously called rapamycin) is another fungal macrolide, but has a different mode of action: namely, it inhibits T cell growth factor pathways, preventing the response to IL-2 and other cytokines. It shows some promise in clinical trials in combination with cyclosporine.

Antibodies to Lymphocytes When serum from animals made immune to host lymphocytes is injected into the recipient, a marked suppression of cellular immunity to the tissue graft results. The action on cell-mediated immunity is greater than on humoral immunity. A globulin fraction of serum [antilymphocyte globulin (ALG)] is the agent generally employed. For use in humans, peripheral human lymphocytes, thymocytes, or lymphocytes from spleens or thoracic duct fistulas have been injected into horses, rabbits, or goats to produce antilymphocyte serum, from which the globulin fraction is then separated. Although ALG or antithymocyte globulin (ATG) is unquestionably effective in prolonging grafts in animals, its efficacy in the transplantation of human tissue is less clear, since it varies from source to source. Heterologous antibody against defined T lymphocyte subsets, in the form of mouse antihuman monoclonal antibody, offers a more precise and standardized form of therapy. OKT3, at present, is the only such antibody in clinical use. It is directed to the CD3 molecules that form a portion of the T cell antigen-receptor complex; hence CD3 is expressed on all mature T cells. CD4 or CD8 molecules also form part of the fully activated cluster of molecules, and monoclonal antibodies to these offer the potential for more selective targeting of T cell subsets. Another approach to more selective therapy is to target the 55-kDa beta chain or the 70-kDa alpha chain of the IL-2 receptor, expressed only on T cells that have been recently activated. The problem with such mouse antibodies is the potential for developing human antimouse antibodies (HAMA), an event that limits the effective period of use. Clinical trials of genetically engineered "humanized" monoclonal antibodies are in progress. This approach offers the possibility of improved clearance and destruction of the targeted lymphocytes and reduced potential for development of HAMA.

CLINICAL COURSE AND MANAGEMENT OF THE RECIPIENT Bilateral nephrectomy at some point prior to transplantation is performed for a specific cause but not as a routine. Hypertension

FIGURE 272-5 Biopsy of the renal cadaveric allograft illustrating obliterative endarteritis. Loss of the media is associated with intimal thickening. The elastic tissue shows dissolution of the elastica. The evidence for arteritis with subsequent thrombosis is typically the gaps in the elastica and media. The intimal thickening probably represents organization of a thrombus formed in response to the arteritis. *[From GJ Dammin, JP Merrill, in Structural Basis for Renal Disease, EL Becker (ed), New York, Hoeber-Harper, 1968.]*

that is difficult to control or infection involving the end-stage kidneys are the two most common indications. Nephrectomized patients maintain a much lower hematocrit, but this is no longer considered a disadvantage because of the availability of recombinant erythropoietin. Nephrectomy per se does not appear to affect the survival of subsequent renal allografts.

Adequate hemodialysis should be performed within 48 h of surgery, and care should be taken that the serum potassium level is not markedly elevated so that intraoperative cardiac arrhythmias can be averted. The diuresis that commonly occurs postoperatively must be carefully monitored; in some instances it may be massive, reflecting the inability of ischemic tubules to regulate sodium and water excretion; with large diureses, massive potassium losses may occur. Most chronically uremic patients have some excess of extracellular fluid, and it is useful to maintain an expanded fluid volume in the immediate postoperative period. Acute tubular necrosis (ATN) may cause immediate oliguria or may follow an initial short period of graft function. ATN is most likely when cadaveric donors have been hypotensive or if the interval between cessation of blood flow and organ harvest (warm ischemic time) is more than a few minutes. Recovery usually occurs within 3 weeks, although periods as long as 6 weeks have been reported. Superimposition of rejection on ATN is common, and the differential diagnosis may be difficult without a graft biopsy. Cyclosporine therapy prolongs ATN, and some patients do not diurese until the dose is drastically reduced. Many centers avoid starting cyclosporine for the first several days, using ALG or a monoclonal antibody along with azathioprine and prednisone until renal function is established.

The Rejection Episode Early diagnosis of rejection allows prompt institution of therapy to preserve renal function and prevent irreversible damage. Clinical evidence of rejection is rarely characterized by fever, swelling, and tenderness over the allograft. Rejection may present only with a rise in serum creatinine, with or without a reduction in urine volume. The focus should be on ruling out other causes of functional deterioration.

Arteriography and radioactive iodohippurate sodium renograms of the transplanted kidney may be useful in ascertaining changes in the renal vasculature and in renal blood flow, even in the absence of urinary flow. Diagnostic ultrasound is the procedure of choice to rule out urinary obstruction or to confirm the presence of perirenal collections of urine, blood, or lymph. When renal function has been good initially, a rise in the serum creatinine level is the most sensitive and reliable indicator of possible rejection and may be the only sign.

Cyclosporine may cause deterioration in renal function in a manner similar to a rejection episode. In fact, rejection processes tend to be more indolent with cyclosporine, and the only way to make a diagnosis may be by renal biopsy. Cyclosporine has an afferent arteriolar constrictor effect on the kidney and, in addition, may produce permanent vascular and interstitial injury after sustained high-dose therapy. There is no universally accepted lesion(s) that makes a diagnosis of cyclosporine toxicity, although interstitial fibrosis, isometric tubular vacuolization, and thickening of arteriolar walls have been noted by some. Basically, if the biopsy does not reveal moderate and active cellular rejection activity, the serum creatinine will most likely respond to a reduction in cyclosporine dose. Blood levels of drug can be useful if very high or very low but do not correlate precisely with renal function. If rejection activity is present in the biopsy, appropriate therapy is indicated. The first rejection episode is usually treated with intravenous administration of methylprednisolone, 500 to 1000 mg daily for 3 days. Failure to respond is indication for antibody therapy, usually with OKT3.

OKT3 monoclonal antibody, given intravenously for 10 to 14 days, is effective in more than 90 percent of first rejections, and less so if methylprednisolone pulses have failed and in cases of severe recurrent rejection activity. A major problem with OKT3 is that severe systemic reactions may be produced during the first day or two of

therapy. Chills, fever, hypotension, and headache are the direct result of the antibody effects on the targeted T cells, most likely related to the known potential of OKT3 to activate T cells nonspecifically. If the antibody is administered to overhydrated oliguric patients, pulmonary edema may be induced. These reactions are not characteristic of other monoclonal antibodies, such as those to the IL-2 receptor. Recurrent or rebound rejection activity may require additional therapy. In such circumstances, methylprednisolone may be effective even though it failed initially. Second courses of OKT3 may be given in spite of HAMA generated in response to the first course if the titers are low and the human antibodies are not directed to the combining-site region (idiotype) of the OKT3.

Management Problems The usual clinical manifestations of infection in the posttransplant period are blunted by immunosuppressive therapy. The major toxic effect of azathioprine is bone marrow suppression, while cyclosporine has no marrow effects. They both may predispose to unusual opportunistic infections, however. The signs and symptoms of infection may be masked and distorted, and fever without obvious cause is common. Only after days or weeks will it become apparent that it has a viral or fungal origin. Bacterial infections are most common during the first month after transplantation. The importance of blood cultures in such patients cannot be overemphasized, because systemic infection without obvious foci is frequent, although wound infections with or without urinary fistulas are most common. Particularly ominous are rapidly occurring pulmonary lesions, which may result in death within 5 days of onset. When these become apparent, immunosuppressive agents should be discontinued, except for maintenance doses of prednisone. Aggressive diagnostic procedures, including transbronchial and open lung biopsy, are frequently indicated. In the case of *Pneumocystis carinii* (Chap. 211) infection, trimethoprim-sulfamethoxazole is the treatment of choice; amphotericin B has been used effectively in systemic fungal infections. Prophylaxis against *P. carinii* with daily, or alternate day, low-dose trimethoprim-sulfamethoxazole is very effective. Involvement of the oropharynx with *Candida* (Chap. 207) may be treated with local nystatin. Small doses (a total of 300 mg) of amphotericin given over a period of 2 weeks may be effective in refractory oral candidiasis. *Aspergillus* (Chap. 208), *Nocardia* (Chap. 167), and CMV (Chap. 187) infections also occur.

CMV is a common and dangerous infection in transplant recipients. It does not generally appear until the end of the first posttransplant month. Active CMV infection is sometimes associated, or occasionally confused, with rejection episodes. Patients at highest risk for severe CMV disease are those without anti-CMV antibodies who receive a graft from a CMV antibody–positive donor (15 percent mortality). Serial intravenous administration of high-titer CMV immune globulin is effective in reducing this risk. Prophylactic use of ganciclovir is an effective alternative. Treatment of active CMV disease with ganciclovir is always indicated. Many patients immune to CMV can activate the virus after heavy immunosuppression, such as with OKT3. Concurrent treatment with ganciclovir during OKT3 administration appears to be effective for prophylaxis of CMV activation. The complications of glucocorticoid therapy are well known and include gastrointestinal bleeding, impairment of wound healing, osteoporosis, diabetes mellitus, cataract formation, and hemorrhagic pancreatitis. The treatment of unexplained jaundice in transplant patients should include cessation of azathioprine or cyclosporine if hepatitis or drug toxicity is suspected. It is surprising that cessation of azathioprine or cyclosporine therapy in such circumstances often does not result in rejection of a graft, at least for several weeks. Antiplatelet agents and anticoagulants, although effective in theory, have not been successful in the prevention of the chronic vascular lesion. Persistent elevation of serum creatinine levels above 220 μmol/L (2.5 mg/dL) in patients on cyclosporine is an indication for dose reduction, particularly if cyclosporine blood levels are elevated. Some centers convert patients from cyclosporine to azathioprine after 6 to 12 months, but some patients have rejection episodes, and some of those lose their grafts. The alternative to conversion is to use lower doses of cyclosporine indefinitely. The risk of long-term cumulative toxicity to the kidney now seems to be low.

In general, minimal or no rejection during the first 6 months after transplantation is a predictor of safety in reducing immunosuppression therapy over subsequent months to years.

Despite the potential teratogenic effects of immunosuppressive agents, both women and men have become parents after transplantation. The incidence of congenital abnormalities in the offspring is not increased.

Glomerular Lesions   Glomerular lesions occur in 10 to 15 percent of allografts, even when the original disease was accidental removal of a solitary kidney. The pathogenesis is related to a chronic rejection process. In some cases the lesions resemble those of the original glomerular disease. In most instances, the recurrence of the original renal lesions represents no threat to the immediate prognosis, and a primary diagnosis of glomerulonephritis is rarely a contraindication to transplantation.

Malignancy   The incidence of tumors in patients on immunosuppressive therapy is 5 to 6 percent, or approximately 100 times greater than that in the general population of the same age range. The most common lesions are cancer of the skin and lips and carcinoma in situ of the cervix, as well as lymphomas, such as non-Hodgkin's lymphomas. The risks are increased in proportion to the total immunosuppressive load administered and time elapsed since transplantation.

Other Complications   *Hypercalcemia* after transplantation may indicate failure of hyperplastic parathyroid glands to regress. Aseptic necrosis of the head of the femur is probably due to preexisting hyperparathyroidism, with aggravation by glucocorticoid treatment. With improved management of calcium and phosphorus metabolism during chronic dialysis, the incidence of parathyroid-related complications has fallen dramatically.

Hypertension may be caused by (1) native kidneys; (2) rejection activity in the transplant; (3) renal artery stenosis, if an end-to-end anastomosis was constructed with an iliac artery branch; and (4) renal cyclosporine toxicity. The latter may improve with reduction in cyclosporine dose. Whereas angiotensin-converting enzyme inhibitors may be useful, calcium channel blockers are frequently more effective in cyclosporine-treated patients.

Chronic hepatitis, particularly when due to hepatitis B virus, can be a progressive, fatal disease over a decade or so. Patients who are persistently HBsAg-positive are at higher risk, according to some studies, but the presence of HCV is also a concern when one embarks on a course of immunosuppression in a transplant recipient.

Both chronic dialysis and renal transplant patients have a higher incidence of death from myocardial infarction and stroke than in the population at large, and this is particularly true in diabetic patients. Contributing factors are hypertension and hypertriglyceridemia. Increased low-density lipoprotein cholesterol and depressed high-density lipoprotein cholesterol concentrations may be exaggerated after transplantation and require treatment.

BIBLIOGRAPHY

CARPENTER CB: Long-term failure of renal transplants: Adding insult to injury. Kidney Int 48(suppl 50):40, 1995

DAUGIRDAS JT: Dialysis hypotension: A hemodynamic analysis. Kidney Int 39:233, 1991

DEPNER TA: Assessing adequacy of hemodialysis: Urea modeling. Kidney Int 45:1522, 1994

INSTITUTE OF MEDICINE SPECIAL REPORT: The Medicare end-stage renal disease program. N Engl J Med 324:1143, 1991

KEANE WF et al: Peritoneal dialysis–related peritonitis treatment recommendations, 1993 update. Perit Dial Int 13:14, 1993

MCKAY DB et al: Clinical aspects of renal transplantation, in *The Kidney*, 5th ed, B Brenner (ed). Philadelphia, Saunders, 1996, p 2602

MEHTA RL: Therapeutic alternatives in renal replacement for critically ill patients in acute renal failure. Semin Nephrol 14:64, 1994

OPELZ G: HLA matching should be utilized for improving kidney transplant success rates. Transplant Proc 23:46, 1991

OWEN WF JR et al: The urea reduction ratio and serum albumin concentration as predictors of mortality in patients undergoing hemodialysis. N Engl J Med 329:1001, 1993

PERKINS DL, CARPENTER CB: Immunobiology of transplantation, in *The Kidney*, 5th ed, B Brenner (ed). Philadelphia, Saunders, 1996, p 2576

SPRAGUE SM, POPOVTZER MM: Is β_2-microglobulin a mediator of bone disease? Kidney Int 47:1, 1995

TEEHAN B et al: Adequacy of continuous ambulatory peritoneal dialysis: Morbidity and mortality in chronic peritoneal dialysis. Am J Kidney Dis 24:990, 1994

TERASAKI PI, CECKA JM (eds): *Clinical Transplants 1994*. Los Angeles, UCLA Tissue Typing Laboratory, 1995

273   *Hugh R. Brady, Barry M. Brenner*

PATHOGENETIC MECHANISMS OF GLOMERULAR INJURY

The glomerulus is a modified capillary network that delivers an ultrafiltrate of plasma to Bowman's space, the most proximal portion of the renal tubule. Approximately 1.6 million glomeruli are present in two mature kidneys (range 0.5 to 2.4 million) and collectively produce 120 to 180 L of ultrafiltrate daily. Glomerular filtration rate (GFR) is dependent on glomerular blood flow, ultrafiltration pressure, and surface area. These parameters are tightly regulated through changes in afferent and efferent arteriolar tone (for blood flow and ultrafiltration pressure) and mesangial cell contractility (for filtration surface area). Arteriolar tone and mesangial cell contractility are, in turn, modulated by neurohumoral factors, local myenteric reflexes, and endothelium-derived vasoactive substances, such as nitric oxide, prostacyclin, and endothelins. In health, glomerular endothelium is also antithrombotic and antiadhesive for leukocytes and platelets, thereby preventing inappropriate vascular thrombosis and inflammation during the filtration process. Filtration of most plasma proteins and all blood cells is normally prevented as a consequence of the physiochemical and electrostatic charge characteristics of the glomerular filtration barrier, the latter composed of fenestrated glomerular endothelium, basement membrane, and the foot processes and slit diaphragms of visceral epithelial cells (podocytes). Parietal epithelium facilitates glomerular filtration by maintaining the integrity of Bowman's space. In keeping with the physiologic functions of the glomerulus outlined above, virtually all glomerular injury results in impairment of glomerular filtration or the inappropriate appearance of plasma proteins and blood cells in the urine.

CLINICOPATHOLOGIC CORRELATES IN GLOMERULAR DISEASE

The major glomerulopathies are described in Chap. 274, and major morphologic patterns of glomerular disease and their clinical features are summarized in Table 273-1. These clinicopathologic entities can be induced by a variety of different pathogenetic mechanisms. Thus, prompt diagnosis, optimal management, and accurate prognostication is a three-step process that requires (1) recognition of the presenting clinical syndrome, (2) delineation of the underlying morphologic pattern of glomerular injury, and (3) elucidation of the specific renal-limited or systemic disease that triggered glomerular dysfunction.

NOMENCLATURE   The terms *glomerulonephritis* and *glomerulopathy* are usually used interchangeably to denote glomerular injury, although some authorities reserve the former term for injury with evidence of inflammation such as leukocyte infiltration, antibody deposition, and complement activation. Glomerular diseases are classified as *primary* when the pathology is confined to the kidney and any systemic features are a direct consequence of glomerular dysfunction (e.g., pulmonary edema, hypertension, the uremic syndrome). Usually, but not always, the term primary is synonymous with *idiopathic*. Glomerular diseases are classified as *secondary* when part of a multisystem disorder. In general, *acute* refers to glomerular injury occurring

Table 273-1

Major Clinicopathologic Presentation of Glomerular Disease

Structural Pattern	Typical Clinical Presentation	Typical Pathology Findings	Most Common Etiologies*
Diffuse proliferative GN	Acute nephritic syndrome: Acute renal failure over days to weeks, hypertension, edema, oliguria, active urine sediment, subnephrotic proteinuria	Diffuse increase in cellularity of tufts of most glomeruli due to infiltration by neutrophils and monocytes, and proliferation of glomerular endothelial and mesangial cells.	Immune complex GN: idiopathic, postinfectious, SLE, SBE, cryoglobulinemia, Henoch-Schönlein purpura Pauci-immune GN and anti-GBM disease (crescentic GN common—see below)
Crescentic GN	Rapidly progressive glomerulonephritis (RPGN): Subacute renal failure over weeks to months, active urine sediment, variable amount of hypertension, edema, oliguria, and proteinuria	Majority of glomeruli contain areas of fibrinoid necrosis and crescents in Bowman's space, composed of proliferating parietal epithelial cells, infiltrating macrophages, and fibrin	Immune complex GN (as above) Pauci-immune GN: Wegener's granulomatosis, microscopic polyarteritis nodosa, renal-limited crescentic GN Anti-GBM disease (Goodpasture's syndrome if lung hemorrhage)
Focal proliferative GN	Mild to moderate glomerular inflammation: Active urine sediment and mild to moderate decline in GFR	Segmental areas of proliferation and necrosis in less than 50% of glomeruli, occasionally with crescent formation	Early and milder forms, or recovery phase of most diseases causing diffuse proliferative and crescentic GN IgA nephropathy/HSP
Mesangial proliferative GN	Chronic glomerular inflammation: Proteinuria, hematuria, hypertension, variable effect on GFR	Proliferation of mesangial cells and matrix	IgA nephropathy/HSP Early and milder forms, or recovery phases of most diseases causing diffuse proliferative and crescentic GN In association with minimal change glomerulopathy and FSGS
Membranoproliferative GN	Variable combination of nephritic and nephrotic features: Acute or subacute decline in GFR, active urine sediment, proteinuria often in nephrotic range	Diffuse proliferation of mesangial cells and infiltration of glomeruli by macrophages; increased mesangial matrix and thickening and reduplication of glomerular basement membrane	Immune complex GN (as for diffuse proliferative GN) In association with thrombotic microangiopathies (see below) In association with deposition diseases (see below) Postrenal or -marrow transplantation
Minimal change GN	Nephrotic syndrome: Proteinuria of >3–3.5 g/d, hypoalbuminemia, edema, hyperlipidemia, lipiduria, thrombotic diathesis, slow decline in GFR in 10–30%.	Light microscopy normal, but electron microscopy (EM) shows foot process effacement	Idiopathic In association with drug-induced interstitial nephritis, HIV infection, heroin, Hodgkin's and other lymphomas
Focal segmental glomerulosclerosis	Nephrotic syndrome: Proteinuria of >3–3.5 g/d, hypoalbuminemia, edema, hyperlipidemia, lipiduria, thrombotic diathesis, slow decline in GFR in 10–30%.	Segmental capillary collapse affecting <50% of glomeruli with entrapment of amorphous hyaline material. EM shows foot process effacement	Primary FSGS: idiopathic, HIV, heroin, lysosomal diseases, Charcot-Marie Tooth Secondary response to reduction in nephron number from any cause (hyperfiltration injury)
Nodular or global sclerosis	Proteinuria and chronic renal failure	Sclerosis of most glomeruli with interstitial fibrosis	Diabetic nephropathy Potential long-term consequence of most glomerulopathies listed above
Membranous GN	Nephrotic syndrome: Proteinuria of >3–3.5 g/d, hypoalbuminemia, edema, hyperlipidemia, lipiduria, thrombotic diathesis, slow decline in GFR in 10–30%	Diffuse thickening of the glomerular basement membrane with subepithelial projections ("spikes") around immune deposits	Idiopathic Infections (e.g., Hepatitis B & C, syphilis, schistosomiasis, malaria, leprosy) Drugs (e.g., gold, penicillamine, captopril) Autoimmune diseases (SLE, rheumatoid arthritis) Paraneoplastic
Deposition diseases	Combination of nephritic and nephrotic features: Renal failure over months to years, proteinuria, hematuria, and hypertension.	Mesangial expansion and thickening of glomerular capillary wall; variable cellular proliferation and crescent formation	Amyloid Cryoglobulinemia Light chain deposition disease Fibrillary/immunotactoid GN
Thrombotic microangiopathy	Acute or subacute renal failure: Variable degree of hypertension, edema and proteinuria, urine sediment usually contains red blood cells, but less activity than patients with nephritic syndrome or RPGN	Microthrombi in glomerular capillaries ± endothelial injury	Idiopathic In association with gastrointestinal infections, or drugs such as anovulants, mitomycin C Other diseases: SLE, scleroderma, toxemia, malignant hypertension
Nonimmune basement membrane abnormalities	Asymptomatic hematuria and variable renal failure	Alport's syndrome—mesangial hypercellularity with focal sclerosis and interstitial fibrosis; splintering of GBM on EM.	Alport's syndrome, Thin basement membrane disease, Nail patella syndrome, Lecithin–cholesterol acyltransferase deficiency

* Includes most common etiologies: For complete list, see Chap. 274.

NOTE: Diffuse, affecting ≥50% of glomeruli; focal, affecting <50% of glomeruli; global, affecting ≥50% of glomerular tuft; segmental, affecting <50% of glomerular tuft; GN, glomerulonephritis; FSGS, focal segmental glomerulosclerosis; HSP, Henoch-Schönlein purpura; SLE, systemic lupus erythematosus; HIV, human immunodeficiency virus; SBE, subacute bacterial endocarditis.

over days or weeks, *subacute* or *rapidly progressive* over weeks or a few months, and *chronic* over many months or years. Lesions are classified as *focal* or *diffuse* when they involve the minority (<50 percent) or majority (≥50 percent) of glomeruli, respectively. Lesions are termed *segmental* or *global* when they involve part of or almost all of the glomerular tuft, respectively. *Proliferative* is used to describe an increase in glomerular cell number, which can be due to infiltration by leukocytes or proliferation of resident glomerular cells. Proliferation of resident glomerular cells is classified as *intracapillary* or *endocapillary* when referring to endothelial or mesangial cells and *extracapillary* when referring to cells in Bowman's space. A *crescent* is a half-moon-shaped collection of cells in Bowman's space, usually composed of proliferating parietal epithelial cells and infiltrating monocytes. Because crescentic glomerulonephritis is often associated with renal failure that progresses rapidly over week to months, the clinical term *rapidly progressive glomerulonephritis* and pathologic term *crescentic glomerulonephritis* are often used interchangeably. The description *membranous* is applied to glomerulonephritis dominated by expansion of the glomerular basement membrane (GBM) by immune deposits. *Sclerosis* refers to an increase in the amount of homogeneous nonfibrillar extracellular material of the same ultrastructural appearance and chemical composition as GBM and mesangial matrix. This process is distinct from *fibrosis*, which involves deposition of collagens type I and III and is more commonly a consequence of healing of crescents or tubulointerstitial inflammation.

MAJOR CLINICOPATHOLOGIC ENTITIES Most glomerulopathies are still classified and named according to their morphologic features (Table 273-1). The major *inflammatory glomerulopathies* are focal proliferative glomerulonephritis (termed mesangial proliferative if the proliferating cells are predominantly mesangial cells), diffuse proliferative glomerulonephritis, and crescentic glomerulonephritis. These diseases typically present with a *nephritic-type* "active" urine sediment characterized by the presence of red blood cells, red blood cell casts, leukocytes, and *subnephrotic* proteinuria of <3 g/24 h. The severity of renal insufficiency varies in proportion to the degree of proliferation and necrosis.

The major morphologic patterns affecting the glomerular filtration barrier for proteins, namely the GBM and visceral epithelial cells, are membranous glomerulopathy, minimal change disease, and focal and segmental glomerulosclerosis. These entities typically present with *nephrotic-range* proteinuria of >3 g/24 h and the presence of few red blood cells, leukocytes, or cellular casts. As a consequence of the heavy proteinuria, nephrotic syndrome is associated with hypoalbuminemia, edema, hyperlipidemia, and lipiduria. Membranoproliferative glomerulonephritis, as the name suggests, is a hybrid lesion that presents with a combination of nephritic and nephrotic features.

The *glomerular deposition diseases* are a group of disorders characterized by prominent extravascular deposition of a paraprotein or fibrillar material. These diseases can also trigger nephritic-type and nephrotic-type responses (or a combination of both) and thus show marked clinical and morphologic overlap with the entities described above.

The *thrombotic microangiopathies* are a family of diseases in which the pathologic presentation is dominated by thrombi within the renal microvasculature, often leading to renal insufficiency.

MAJOR DETERMINANTS OF GLOMERULAR INJURY

Important determinants of the severity of glomerular injury include (1) the primary insult and the secondary mediator systems that it invokes, (2) the site of injury, and (3) the speed of onset, extent, and intensity of disease.

PRIMARY INSULT Glomeruli are susceptible to a variety of inflammatory, metabolic, hemodynamic, toxic, and infectious insults (Table 273-2). Most human glomerular disease is triggered by immune attack, diabetes mellitus, or hypertension. Diverse insults can induce similar clinicopathologic presentations, suggesting marked overlap among downstream molecular and cellular responses. For example, infections (e.g., streptococcal pharyngitis, bacterial endocarditis) and vasculitides (e.g., Henoch-Schönlein purpura, microscopic polyarteritis) can each trigger acute proliferative glomerulonephritis with the nephritic syndrome. Similarly, metabolic (e.g., diabetes mellitus) and deposition diseases (e.g., amyloid) can each induce glomerulosclerosis with nephrotic syndrome. An important corollary is that pharmacologic agents that inhibit common secondary mediator systems may prove effective in treating glomerular diseases of diverse etiologies (see below).

SITE OF INJURY The consequences of injury at different sites within the glomerulus can be predicted from the physiologic functions of the cells within the local milieu (Table 273-3). The major sequelae of injury to the *endothelium* and *subendothelial aspect of the GBM* are: (1) recruitment of leukocytes leading to inflammatory glomerulonephritis, (2) perturbed hemostasis leading to thrombotic microangiopathy, and (3) vasoconstriction and mesangial cell contraction leading to acute renal failure. It is usual for one of these phenotypes to dominate the presentation of specific diseases. *Mesangial* injury is usually immunologic in origin and, being more localized, induces less dramatic impairment of glomerular filtration. Patients typically present with

Table 273-2

Primary Mechanisms of Glomerular Injury

Mechanism of Injury	Some Renal Insults/Defects	Glomerular Disease
Immunologic*	Immunoglobulin†	Immune complex–mediated glomerulonephritis
	Cell-mediated injury†	Pauci-immune glomerulonephritis
	Cytokine (or other soluble factor)	Primary focal segmental glomerulosclerosis
	Persistent complement activation	Membranoproliferative glomerulonephritis (type II)
Metabolic*	Hyperglycemia†	Diabetic nephropathy
	Fabry's disease and sialidosis	Focal segmental glomerulosclerosis
Hemodynamic*	Systemic hypertension†	Hypertensive nephrosclerosis
	Intraglomerular hypertension†	Secondary focal segmental glomerulosclerosis
Toxic	E. coli–derived verotoxin	Thrombotic microangiopathy
	Therapeutic drugs (e.g., NSAIDs)	Minimal change disease
	Recreational drugs (heroin)	Focal segmental glomerulosclerosis
Deposition	Amyloid fibrils	Amyloid nephropathy
Infectious	Human immunodeficiency virus (HIV)	HIV nephropathy
	Subacute bacterial endocarditis	Immune complex glomerulonephritis
Inherited	Defect in gene for α5 chain of type IV collagen	Alport's syndrome
	Abnormally thin basement membrane	Thin basement membrane disease

* Most common categories.
† Most common insults within these categories.
NOTE: NSAIDs, nonsteroidal anti-inflammatory drugs.

asymptomatic abnormalities of the urinary sediment and mild renal insufficiency. Proteinuria dominates the clinical presentation of injury to *the subepithelial aspect of the GBM* and *visceral epithelial cells.* As with mesangial injury, GFR is often only mildly compromised in this setting. The classic pathologic manifestation of *parietal epithelial cell* injury is crescent formation. Crescents can be the dominant morphologic presentation of glomerular disease or complicate proliferative or membranous lesions.

SPEED OF ONSET, INTENSITY, AND EXTENT OF INJURY To illustrate the importance of the speed of onset, extent, and intensity of glomerular injury, it is instructive to compare acute postinfectious glomerulonephritis and IgA nephropathy, the latter being a more indolent disease of undetermined etiology. Postinfectious glomerulonephritis is characterized by rapid and extensive formation of immune complexes throughout the glomerular capillary wall, which often provokes acute renal failure with the classic hallmarks of acute inflammation: complement activation, leukocyte recruitment, lysosomal enzyme release, free radical generation, and perturbation of vascular tone and permeability. In contrast, IgA nephropathy is characterized by slow, but sustained, formation of immune complexes, largely confined to the mesangium; less dramatic activation of complement and other secondary mediator systems; and progressive renal insufficiency over 10 to 20 years.

IMMUNOLOGIC GLOMERULAR INJURY

Immune-mediated glomerulonephritis (see also Chaps. 274 and 275) accounts for a large fraction of acquired renal disease. The majority of cases are associated with the deposition of antibodies, often autoantibodies, within the glomerular tuft, indicating dysregulation of humoral immunity. Cellular immune mechanisms also contribute to the pathogenesis of antibody-mediated glomerulonephritis by modulating antibody production and through antibody-dependent cell cytotoxicity (see below). In addition, cellular immune mechanisms probably play a primary role in the pathophysiology of "pauci-immune" glomerulonephritides, notable for robust glomerular inflammation in the absence of immunoglobulin deposition.

ANTIBODY-MEDIATED INJURY (See Fig. 273-1) Most antibody-mediated glomerulonephritis in humans is initiated by reactivity of circulating antibodies with auto- or "planted" antigens. The major mechanisms of antibody deposition within the glomerulus are: (1) reactivity of circulating autoantibodies with intrinsic autoantigens that are components of normal glomerular parenchyma, (2) in situ formation of immune complexes through interaction of circulating antibodies and extrinsic antigens that have been planted within the glomerulus, and (3) intraglomerular trapping of immune complexes that have formed in the systemic circulation.

Generation of Nephritogenic Antibodies Exposure of the host to a foreign antigen (e.g., a prodromal infection) has been implicated as the trigger for the generation of nephritogenic autoantibodies in several forms of glomerulonephritis. Foreign antigens can provoke autoantibody formation through several mechanisms. First, a foreign

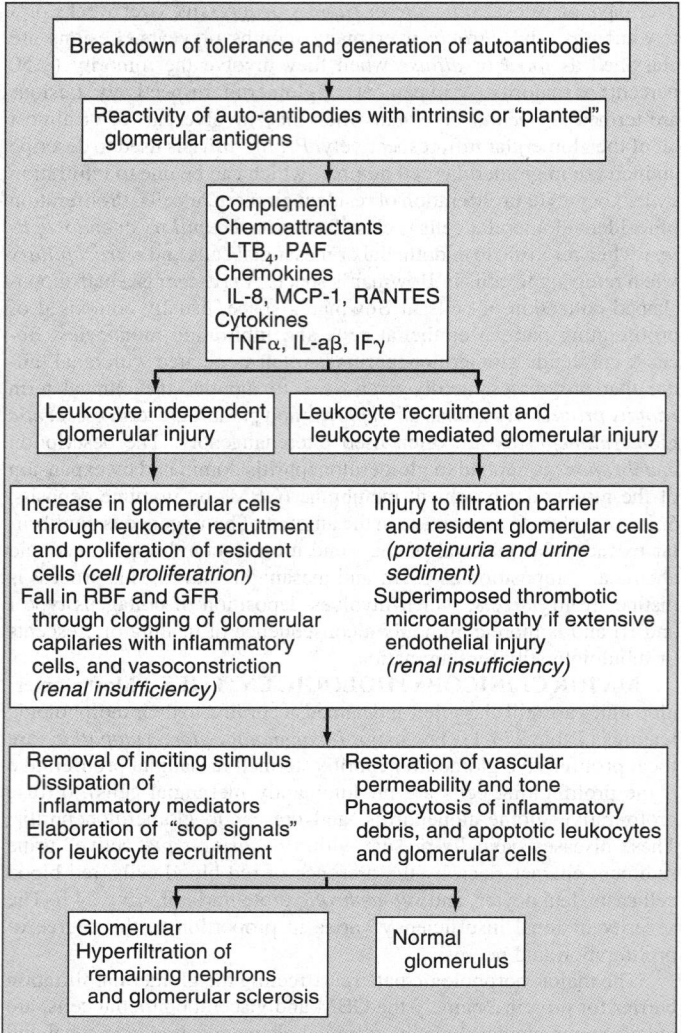

FIGURE 273-1 Mediator systems in acute immune complex–mediated glomerulonephritis: A paradigm of renal inflammation. Abbreviations: LTB$_4$, leukotriene B$_4$; PAF, platelet-activating factor; IL, interleukin; MCP-1, monocyte chemotactic peptide-1; TNFα, tumor necrosis factor alpha; IFγ, interferon-gamma; RBF, renal blood flow; GFR, glomerular filtration rate.

antigen, whose structure resembles that of a host glomerular antigen, may stimulate the production of autoantibodies that cross-react with the intrinsic glomerular antigen ("molecular mimickry"). Second, the foreign antigen may trigger aberrant expression of major histocompatibility complex class II molecules on glomerular cells which present previously "invisible" autoantigens to T lymphocytes and thereby generate an autoimmune response. Third, the foreign antigen can trigger polyclonal activation of B lymphocytes, some of which generate nephritogenic antibodies. Alternatively, individuals may suffer a breakdown of immune tolerance through other mechanisms

Table 273-3

Correlation between Site of Glomerular Injury and Clinicopathologic Presentation

Target of Injury	Physiologic Role	Response to Injury	Representative Glomerular Disease
Endothelial cell	Maintains glomerular perfusion	Vasoconstriction	Acute renal failure
	Prevents leukocyte adhesion	Leukocyte infiltration	Focal or diffuse proliferative GN
	Prevents platelet aggregation and clotting	Intravascular microthrombi	Thrombotic microangiopathies
Mesangial cell	Controls glomerular filtration surface area	Proliferation/increased matrix	Mesangioproliferative GN/glomerulosclerosis
Basement membrane	Prevents filtration of plasma proteins	Proteinuria	Membranous nephropathy
Visceral epithelial cell	Prevents filtration of plasma proteins	Proteinuria	Minimal change disease and FSGS
Parietal epithelial cell	Maintains Bowman's space	Crescent formation	Crescentic GN

NOTE: GN, glomerulonephritis; FSGS, focal segmental glomerulosclerosis.

(e.g., genetically programmed). Autoreactive B cells are usually deleted in the thymus during development (clonal deletion) or rendered anergic in peripheral lymphoid tissue (clonal anergy). Similar tolerogenic mechanisms exist for deleting or anergizing autoreactive T helper cells that modulate immunoglobulin production by autoreactive B cells. Perturbation of either of these tolerogenic mechanisms could drive immunoglobulin production in some forms of autoimmune glomerulonephritis. Indeed, defective clonal deletion of autoreactive T cells has been demonstrated in experimental lupus nephritis due to defective synthesis of Fas, a cell-surface receptor that modulates T cell deletion through apoptosis (programmed cell death) within the thymus.

Deposition of Nephritogenic Antibodies within the Glomerulus Anti-GBM antibody disease (p. 1539) is the classic nephritis initiated by interaction of autoantibody with intrinsic glomerular antigen. Afflicted patients have a circulating antibody directed at a 28-kDa antigen (Goodpasture antigen) located in the noncollagenous NC1 domain of the α3 chain of type IV collagen. This type of collagen is preferentially expressed in glomerular and pulmonary alveolar basement membranes. Autoantibodies against mesangial cell antigens have been detected in the serum of patients with IgA nephropathy, the most common form of glomerulonephritis in humans; however, the pathogenicity of these autoantibodies has yet to be defined. Poststreptococcal glomerulonephritis and lupus nephritis are examples of glomerulonephritides that are probably initiated by interaction of circulating antibodies with planted antigens. Several streptococcal antigens have been isolated from immune deposits of kidneys with poststreptococcal glomerulonephritis, including a 46-kDa nephritis strain–associated antigen and a 46-kDa cytoplasmic protein endostreptosin. In addition, patients with poststreptococcal glomerulonephritis can have circulating antibodies against laminin, type IV collagen, and heparan sulphate proteoglycans, suggesting that molecular mimicry may also contribute. Similar findings have been reported in experimental and human lupus nephritis. Here, circulating anti-DNA antibodies induce immune complex glomerulonephritis by reacting with DNA bound to GBM or with planted DNA-histone complexes (nucleosomes). Cryoglobulinemia, due to chronic hepatitis C infection, is an example of glomerulonephritis initiated by trapping of immune complexes. These patients have circulating and intraglomerular immune complexes composed of hepatitis C antigens, polyclonal antihepatitis C IgG, and a second antibody, usually a monoclonal IgM, directed against the IgG. In support of the pathogenicity of circulating cryoglobulins, their injection into laboratory mice induces glomerulonephritis with many of the hallmarks of human disease.

Site of Antibody Deposition The site of antibody deposition within the glomerulus is a critical determinant of the clinicopathologic presentation. Among the factors that determine the site of deposition are the avidity, affinity, and quantity of the antibody; the size, charge, and site of the antigen; the size of the immune complexes; the efficiency of the clearance mechanisms for immune complexes; and local hemodynamic factors. Relatively anionic antigens are repelled by the GBM, which is negatively charged, and tend to be trapped in the subendothelial cell space and mesangium. In contrast, relatively cationic antigens tend to permeate the GBM and deposit within the GBM or in the subepithelial space. Acute deposition of antibody in the subendothelial cell space or mesangium typically triggers a nephritic-type response characterized by rapid recruitment of leukocytes and platelets, probably because inflammatory mediators generated at these sites are strategically positioned to activate endothelial and hematogenous cells. Inflammation is more severe when antibody is deposited in the subendothelial space, as compared with mesangium, at least in part because the mesangium abuts only 25 to 33 percent of the capillary wall. Antibody deposition in the subepithelial cell space typically induces a nephrotic-type response characterized by proteinuria without a pronounced inflammatory cell infiltrate, probably because the immune complexes are shielded from circulating inflammatory cells by the GBM and because the large fluid flux from blood to Bowman's space minimizes back-diffusion of inflammatory mediators towards the endothelium and vascular lumen.

Recruitment of Inflammatory Cells Leukocytes and platelets are important mediators of injury in most forms of acute and subacute glomerulonephritis. Immunoglobulin can provoke recruitment of leukocytes through several mechanisms. Many antibody subclasses activate the complement cascade, and complement proteins such as C3a, C5a, and C5b-9 (membrane attack complex) are potent stimuli for leukocyte recruitment. Complement-independent mechanisms also contribute. Leukocytes express Fc receptors that can directly engage the Fc portion of immunoglobulin. Resident glomerular macrophages, endothelial cells, and mesangial cells also express Fc receptors, engagement of which can trigger release of an array of inflammatory mediators that promotes directed locomotion of leukocytes (chemotaxis), binding of leukocytes to inflamed endothelium through cell surface leukocyte adhesion molecules, and diapedesis of leukocytes to the extravascular space.

The mechanisms of platelet recruitment in glomerulonephritis are less well defined. Potential mechanisms include direct binding of platelet Fc receptors with immunoglobulin, and interactions of platelets with endothelium, collagen, and other components of exposed GBM, and to products of the coagulation cascade such as fibrin.

Mediators of Glomerular Injury *Nephritic-type antibody-mediated glomerular injury* is a vivid example of host defense gone awry. In normal host defense, leukocytes engulf microorganisms into phagosomes, which then fuse with intracellular lysosomes. Microorganisms are destroyed within phagolysosomes through the actions of free radicals, proteolytic enzymes, and other toxic molecules. This process facilitates killing with relative protection and preservation of host tissue. When host defense is inappropriately activated in autoimmune diseases, the inciting antigens are often fixed to (planted antigens) or are a component of host tissue (autoantigen). As a result, phagocytosis is less efficient ("frustrated phagocytosis"), and there is release of toxic moieties into the parenchyma where they destroy host cells and matrix components. In addition, cytotoxic T lymphocytes and natural killer cells can damage resident glomerular cells by releasing toxic compounds, such as perforins, a process that is facilitated by binding of these cytotoxic cells to glomerular cells through HLA molecules, Fc portions of immunoglobulin (antibody-dependent cell cytotoxicity), and other immune recognition systems. Platelets promote nephritic injury by promoting leukocyte recruitment and intrarenal vasoconstriction and by triggering microthrombi formation.

Leukocytes play a lesser role in *nephrotic-type antibody-mediated glomerular injury* (Chap. 274). Membranous glomerulopathy is the prototypic entity and is initiated by the formation of subepithelial immune complexes; these provoke production of "spikes" of new basement membrane that eventually encircle and incorporate the immune complexes into the GBM. The antigenic targets in human membranous glomerulopathy have not been determined. The frequent association with infections, malignancies, and drugs suggests involvement of planted antigens or molecular mimicry (see above); however, many cases may represent a true loss of tolerance against autoantigens.

CELL PROLIFERATION AND ACCUMULATION OF EXTRACELLULAR MATRIX A hallmark of the nephritic-type proliferative glomerulopathies is an increase in glomerular cell number. Initially, this hypercellularity is due predominantly to infiltration of the glomerular tuft by leukocytes. Subsequently, resident glomerular cells proliferate in response to growth factors (e.g., epidermal growth factor, platelet-derived growth factor, thrombospondin) released into the local inflammatory milieu. The proliferating cells are typically mesangial in mesangioproliferative glomerulonephritis, and both endothelial and mesangial cells in diffuse proliferative glomerulonephritis. The visceral epithelial cell is, for the most part, a terminally differentiated cell that does not proliferate rapidly, even when injured.

Whereas acute antibody-mediated glomerulonephritis typically induces acute diffuse proliferative glomerulonephritis and acute renal failure over days to weeks (nephritic syndrome), subacute immune injury often induces the formation of glomerular crescents and renal failure over weeks or a few months (termed *rapidly progressive glomerulonephritis*). As discussed above, crescents are extracapillary proliferations of cells in Bowman's space, composed of infiltrating monocytes, proliferating parietal epithelial cells, and fibrin.

Sustained immune complex deposition over months to years can provoke a marked increase in basement membrane or mesangial matrix production. Mild to moderate accumulation of matrix usually manifests as proteinuria due to disruption of the glomerular filtration barrier; however, in its most severe form, matrix accumulation causes glomerulosclerosis and chronic renal insufficiency.

RESOLUTION, REPAIR, AND SCARRING Glomerular inflammation can resolve with complete recovery of renal function or with a variable amount of scarring and chronic renal insufficiency. Acute poststreptococcal glomerulonephritis (p. 1537), for example, usually resolves spontaneously and fully in children, whereas adults are frequently left with residual renal impairment. The resolution process requires cessation of further antibody production and immune complex formation, removal of deposited and circulating immune complexes, inhibition of further recruitment of inflammatory cells, dissipation of the gradients of inflammatory mediators, restoration of normal endothelial adhesiveness and permeability, normalization of vascular tone, and clearance of infiltrating inflammatory cells and proliferating resident glomerular cells (Fig. 273-1).

Unfortunately, the resolution phase of most inflammatory glomerulopathies in adults terminates in glomerular scarring. This is particularly true in patients with crescentic glomerulopathies who may be left with end-stage renal failure requiring dialysis or transplantation. Transforming growth factor β (TGFβ), a cytokine, stimulates production of extracellular matrix by most glomerular cells, inhibits synthesis of tissue proteases that normally degrade matrix proteins, and is a potent stimulus for scar formation immediately following glomerular injury.

Moderate-to-severe glomerulonephritis is usually associated with a variable degree of tubulointerstitial inflammation and scarring in addition to glomerular injury. Indeed, the severity of tubulointerstitial injury usually correlates closely with long-term impairment of renal function. The pathogenesis of tubulointerstitial inflammation in this setting is unclear. Potential mechanisms include primary involvement of the tubulointerstitium in autoimmune disease and induction of tubulointerstitial inflammation by mediators, generated by diseased glomeruli, which diffuse into the tubulointerstitium via blood, tubular fluid, or the interstitial space.

OTHER MECHANISMS OF ANTIBODY-MEDIATED INJURY Several other autoantibodies have been implicated as mediators of renal injury in patients with glomerulonephritis.

Antineutrophil Cytoplasmic Antibodies (ANCA) Immunoglobulin is not detected in the glomerulus in approximately 40 percent of patients with rapidly progressive glomerulonephritis ("pauci-immune crescentic glomerulonephritis"). The majority of these patients have Wegener's granulomatosis, microscopic polyangiitis nodosa, or renal-limited crescentic glomerulonephritis and have autoantibodies against neutrophil cytoplasmic antigens in their circulation. ANCA stimulate cytokine-primed human neutrophils to generate reactive oxygen species and injure endothelium in vitro. These findings raise the possibility that ANCA may be pathogenetic in vivo in the presence of circulating cytokines, as may occur following a prodromal infection.

Antiendothelial Cell Antibodies Circulating antibodies against endothelial antigens have been reported in several inflammatory vasculitides and glomerulonephritides. Their titers tend to correlate with disease activity, and some activate endothelial cells and increase their adhesiveness for leukocytes, suggesting a pathogenetic role.

C3 Nephritic Factor Some patients with membranoproliferative glomerulonephritis (p. 1543) have large deposits of electron-dense material within the GBM that does not stain for immunoglobulin (dense deposit disease; membranoproliferative glomerulonephritis type II). Intriguingly, most of these patients have a circulating IgG, termed the *C3 nephritic factor*, directed at C3bBb (C3 convertase) of the alternative pathway of complement.

CELL-MEDIATED INJURY Although cell-mediated injury is as yet less well defined than antibody-mediated glomerular injury, T cells have also been implicated as independent mediators of glomerular injury and as modulators of the production of nephritogenic antibodies. T cells may be particularly important as initiators of injury in pauci-immune glomerulonephritis. T cells interact, through their cell surface T cell receptor/CD3 complex, with antigens presented in the groove of major histocompatibility complex molecules of resident glomerular endothelial, mesangial, and epithelial cells, a process that is facilitated by cell-cell adhesion and costimulatory molecules. Cytokines and other mediators released by activated T cells are potent stimuli for further leukocyte recruitment, cytotoxicity, and fibrogenesis. CD4 T lymphocytes are important recruiters of macrophages and trigger clonal expansion of autoreactive B cells; they also promote glomerular cell injury by CD8 cytotoxic T lymphocytes and natural killer cells and through antibody-dependent cell cytotoxicity. Soluble factors derived from T cells have also been implicated in the pathogenesis of proteinuria in minimal change disease and primary focal segmental glomerulosclerosis. Their identity and molecular characterization remain to be determined.

NONIMMUNOLOGIC GLOMERULAR INJURY

METABOLIC **Diabetic Nephropathy** (See also Chaps. 275 and 334) Nephropathy complicates approximately 30 percent and 20 percent of cases of type 1 and type 2 diabetes mellitus, respectively, and is characterized clinically by proteinuria and progressive renal insufficiency. The typical glomerular lesion is glomerulosclerosis due to thickening of the GBM and expansion of the mesangium with extracellular matrix. Factors implicated as triggers for increased matrix production in diabetic glomerulosclerosis include glomerular hypertension; the direct effects of hyperglycemia on mesangial cells; advanced glycosylation end-products that result from nonenzymatic glycation of proteins; growth factors such as growth hormone, insulin-like growth factor 1, and angiotensin II; cytokines such as TGFβ; hyperlipidemia; and cell sorbitol accumulation and myoinositol deficiency secondary to activation of the aldose reductase polyol pathway. Complementary clinical and laboratory approaches suggest a central role for hemodynamic factors. The GFR increases by 20 to 30 percent within months of the development of hyperglycemia due, in large part, to extracellular fluid volume expansion and resulting afferent arteriolar dilatation and increased glomerular ultrafiltration pressure.

The mechanism by which diabetes mellitus induces glomerular hyperfiltration is still being defined but appears to involve atrial natriuretic peptide. In this framework, glycosuria triggers increased reabsorption of glucose coupled to sodium in the proximal tubule, thereby increasing total-body sodium and extracellular fluid volume. As a compensatory response, atrial natriuretic peptide is released from cardiac myocytes and induces natriuresis by triggering afferent arteriolar dilatation and thereby increasing intraglomerular pressure and GFR. Whereas this compensatory response is appropriate in the short term, sustained glomerular hypertension provokes thickening of the GBM, increased mesangial matrix production, and glomerulosclerosis and disruption of barrier function. In keeping with a central role for intraglomerular pressure in the pathogenesis of diabetic nephropathy, angiotensin-converting enzyme inhibitors, which lower intraglomerular pressure, dramatically slow the progression of diabetic nephropathy, even in normotensive patients. It is likely that hemodynamic and metabolic factors act in concert to generate the final glomerulosclerotic phenotype in genetically predisposed patients.

Other Metabolic Diseases Several rare inherited lysosomal enzyme defects induce focal segmental glomerulosclerosis, probably by allowing accumulation of toxic metabolites in renal cells. *Fabry's disease* (α-galactosidase deficiency; Chap. 346) and *sialidosis* (N-acetylneuraminic acid hydrolase deficiency; Chap. 346) are the major culprits in this regard. Both tend to induce focal segmental or global glomerulosclerosis by preferentially affecting visceral epithelial cells, probably because these are terminally differentiated cells with a very slow replication rate. *Partial lipodystrophy* (Chap. 352) is a rare metabolic disorder characterized by lipoatrophy affecting the arms, neck, and chest, often with redistribution of fat to the hips and legs. Approximately one-third of patients develop glomerular disease, usually type II membranoproliferative glomerulopathy (dense deposit disease; see Chap. 274).

HEMODYNAMIC GLOMERULAR INJURY High intraglomerular pressure is a major cause of glomerular injury in humans and can result from systemic hypertension or a local change in glomerular hemodynamics (glomerular hypertension).

Systemic Hypertension (See also Chap. 246) Although the kidneys have evolved sophisticated mechanisms for autoregulating glomerular blood flow and pressure, marked or sustained increments in systemic blood pressure can overwhelm these compensatory systems and perturb glomerular morphology and function. In its most dramatic form, namely malignant hypertension, hemodynamic stress causes massive fibrinoid necrosis of afferent arterioles and glomeruli, thrombotic microangiopathy, acute renal failure, and a nephritic urinary sediment. Chronic sustained hypertension typically leads to arteriolar vasoconstriction and sclerosis, which, in turn, cause secondary atrophy and sclerosis of glomeruli and the tubulointerstitium. A variety of molecular signals appear to couple elevations in intravascular pressure to myointimal proliferation and eventually sclerosis of the vessel wall. These include growth factors such as angiotensin II, epidermal growth factor, and platelet-derived growth factor; cytokines such as TGFβ; and activation of stretch activated ion channels and early response genes.

Glomerular Hypertension The pathophysiology of diabetic nephropathy, discussed above, illustrates the importance of intraglomerular pressure as a stimulus for mesangial matrix production and glomerulosclerosis. Glomerular hypertension is also a key factor in the pathogenesis of the progressive glomerulosclerosis and renal failure that complicate the adaptive response of remnant nephrons to increased workload following loss of the other nephrons from any cause (see below). Importantly, these changes in glomerular hemodynamics and pressure appear to precede the development of systemic hypertension and are independent risk factors for glomerular injury.

TOXIC GLOMERULOPATHIES The renal microvasculature is a relatively uncommon site for toxic injury, by comparison with the tubular interstitium; however, there are a few important exceptions. Verotoxin, derived from *Escherichia coli* during bouts of infective diarrhea, is directly toxic to renal endothelium and induces the hemolytic-uremic syndrome. In this setting, verotoxin interacts with a specific cell membrane receptor, perturbs the antithrombotic phenotype of endothelium, and triggers the development of thrombotic microangiopathy. Irradiation, mitomycin, and anovulants can induce a similar syndrome through ill-defined mechanisms. Nonsteroidal anti-inflammatory drugs, rifampin, ampicillin, and interferon α can induce an unusual combination of acute renal failure with nephrotic syndrome. The characteristic pathologic correlates of this syndrome are allergic interstitial nephritis and fusion of the foot processes of the visceral epithelial cells, the latter accounting for the marked proteinuria. How these structurally diverse agents induce epithelial cell injury is unclear.

DEPOSITION DISEASES The glomerular deposition diseases are a group of diverse conditions in which abnormal proteins are deposited in glomeruli where they provoke an inflammatory reaction and/or glomerulosclerosis. The major glomerular deposition diseases are cryoglobulinemia, amyloidosis, light and heavy chain deposition disease, and fibrillary/immunotactoid glomerulopathy. *Cryoglobulins* (Chap. 319) are immunoglobulins that precipitate in the cold and can be composed of either monoclonal immunoglobulin, usually generated by a lymphoproliferative malignancy (type I); a mixture of polyclonal immunoglobulin (usually IgG) and monoclonal immunoglobulin (usually IgM) directed to epitopes on polyclonal IgG (type II); or a mixture of polyclonal antibodies, one or more having anti-IgG activity (type III). As discussed above, cryoglobulins can induce nephritic-type and nephrotic-type injury depending on the rapidity, severity, and site of immunoglobulin deposition. *Glomerular amyloidosis* (Chaps. 275 and 309) is one of the five most common causes of nephrotic syndrome

in adults and is characterized by extracellular deposition of amyloid fibrils composed, in part, of fragments of immunoglobulin light chains (AL amyloid) or serum amyloid A, the acute-phase reactant (AA amyloid). In light chain deposition diseases, intact immunoglobulin light chains, usually kappa, are deposited in a granular, rather than fibrillary, pattern. The composition of the deposits in *fibrillary/immunotactoid glomerulopathy* is still being defined and may also include immunoglobulin. These different types of deposits, in addition to directly disrupting glomerular architecture, provoke mesangial matrix production and glomerulosclerosis. Fibrillary/immunotactoid glomerulopathy can also present as acute or subacute glomerular inflammation. How these diverse deposits trigger glomerular matrix production and recruitment of inflammatory cells has yet to be determined.

INFECTIOUS CAUSES OF GLOMERULAR DISEASE Infectious organisms can induce glomerular disease through several different mechanisms: (1) by direct infection of renal cells, (2) by elaborating nephrotoxins such as *E. coli*–derived verotoxin, (3) by inciting intraglomerular deposition of immune complexes (e.g., postinfectious glomerulonephritis) or cryoglobulins (e.g., hepatitis B or C), and (4) by providing a chronic stimulus for amyloid fibril formation, as in AA amyloidosis. Direct infection of glomerular cells is a relatively rare mechanism of injury but has been implicated in the pathogenesis of nephropathy associated with human immunodeficiency virus. This entity is characterized histologically by focal segmental glomerulosclerosis, microcystic tubular dilatation, and interstitial fibrosis. Viral genome and p24 protein have been detected in glomerular and tubular cells in this disease, and infection of glomerular cells induces expression of TGFβ, a major stimulus for mesangial matrix production and sclerosis.

INHERITED GLOMERULAR DISEASES *Alport's syndrome* (hereditary nephritis; Chap. 275), the prototypical inherited glomerular disease, is usually transmitted as an X-linked dominant trait. Afflicted patients have a mutation in the COL4A5 gene that encodes the α5 chain of type IV collagen located on the X chromosome. As a result, the glomerular basement membrane is irregular with longitudinal layering, splitting, or thickening, and patients develop hematuria, progressive glomerulosclerosis, and renal failure. *Thin basement membrane disease* is another relatively common disorder of the GBM. In contrast to Alport's syndrome, this entity is usually inherited as an autosomal dominant or recessive trait and is benign. As the name suggests, the basement membrane is thin but otherwise ultrastructurally normal. Patients typically experience recurrent benign hematuria. The molecular basis for thin basement membrane disease has yet to be elucidated. Rarer hereditary glomerular diseases include *nail-patella syndrome* (osteoonychodysplasia), which is associated with a relatively benign mottling of the basement membrane with lucent rarefractions; *partial lipodystrophy*, which is associated with type II membranoproliferative glomerulonephritis (dense deposit disease); and *familial lecithin–cholesterol acyltransferase deficiency*, which is associated with distortion of the basement membrane by irregular rounded lucent zones, increased mesangial matrix production, and progressive sclerosis and renal insufficiency.

GLOMERULAR ADAPTATION TO NEPHRON LOSS

Nephron loss, from any cause, is followed by compensatory hyperfiltration in the remaining functional glomeruli. This adaptive response is appropriate in the short-term and maintains GFR. Over years, however, the hyperfiltering remnant nephrons develop focal and segmental glomerulosclerosis, and eventually global sclerosis, that manifests clinically as proteinuria, hypertension, and progressive renal insufficiency. Sustained glomerular capillary hypertension has been implicated as a major stimulus for glomerulosclerosis in this setting. Increased glomerular blood flow and ultrafiltration pressure are early findings in remnant nephrons in most experimental models in which the function of more

than 50 percent of nephron mass has been lost through surgical ablation, immunologic or toxic injury, or other mechanisms. Sustained
glomerular hypertension is thought to stimulate the accumulation of
extracellular matrix by perturbing the function of visceral epithelial and
mesangial cells, either directly or by increasing the flux of circulating
macromolecules through the glomerular capillary wall. As with most
forms of glomerulosclerosis, TGFβ may be an important regulator of
matrix accumulation in remnant nephrons. Angiotensin II, platelet-
derived growth factor, and endothelins are other potential modulators
of this process. Maneuvers that lower intraglomerular pressure, such
as low-protein diet or treatment with angiotensin-converting enzyme
inhibitors, slow the development of glomerulosclerosis and renal failure. Glomerular hypertrophy, intracapillary microthrombi, recruited
macrophages, and hyperlipidemia are other potential stimuli for glomerulosclerosis. Indeed, glomerular capillary hypertension and hypertrophy appear to be independent risk factors that could act synergistically to cause progressive renal insufficiency. Intriguingly, angiotensin
II may trigger TGFβ production in remnant nephrons, suggesting
that angiotensin-converting enzyme inhibitors may be renoprotective
through complementary effects on glomerular hemodynamics and matrix production.

BIBLIOGRAPHY

ADLER SG et al: Secondary glomerular diseases, in *The Kidney*, 5th ed, BM
    Brenner (ed). Philadelphia, Saunders, 1996, pp 1498–1596
BRADY HR: Leukocyte adhesion molecules and kidney diseases. Kidney Int
    45:1285, 1994
BRENNER BM: Hemodynamically mediated glomerular injury and the progres-
    sive nature of renal disease. Kidney Int 23:647, 1983
COTRAN R, RENNKE HG: Sites and the mechanisms of proteinuria. N Engl J
    Med 309:1050, 1983
COUSER WG: Mediation of glomerular injury. J Am Soc Nephrol 1:13, 1990
FALK RJ: ANCA-associated renal disease. Kidney Int 38:998, 1990
GLASSOCK RJ et al: Primary glomerular diseases, in *The Kidney*, 5th ed, BM
    Brenner (ed). Philadelphia, Saunders, 1996, pp 1392–1497
KELLY PT, HAPONIK EF: Goodpasture's syndrome: Molecular and clinical
    advances. Medicine (Baltimore) 73:171, 1994
MEYER TW et al: Nephron adaptation to renal injury, in *The Kidney*, 5th ed,
    BM Brenner (ed). Philadelphia, Saunders, 1995, pp 2011–2048
REES A: The immunogenetics of glomerulonephritis. Kidney Int 45:377, 1994
WILSON CB: Renal response to immunologic glomerular injury, in *The Kidney*,
    5th ed, BM Brenner (ed). Philadelphia, Saunders, 1996, pp 1253–1391

| **274** | *Hugh R. Brady, Yvonne M. O'Meara, Barry M. Brenner* |

THE MAJOR GLOMERULOPATHIES

Glomerular injury can arise from diverse renal-limited and systemic
diseases and is the major cause of end-stage renal disease (ESRD)
requiring dialysis and transplantation. In this chapter, we describe the
epidemiology, clinical presentations, pathology, and treatment of the
major glomerulopathies. We focus on the *primary glomerulopathies*,
glomerular diseases in which the pathologic process is confined to the
kidney and in which systemic features are a direct consequence of
impaired glomerular filtration (e.g., hypervolemia, hypertension, uremic syndrome). Considered here are the five major clinical presentations of glomerulopathy: acute nephritic syndrome, rapidly progressive
glomerulonephritis (RPGN), nephrotic syndrome, asymptomatic abnormalities of the urinary sediment (hematuria, proteinuria), and
chronic glomerulonephritis. Glomerulopathies associated with systemic diseases (*secondary glomerulopathies*) are discussed in Chap.
275. The nomenclature pertaining to the classification and clinicopathologic description of glomerular disease and the pathogenetic mechanisms of glomerular injury are reviewed in Chap. 273.

ACUTE NEPHRITIC SYNDROME AND RAPIDLY PROGRESSIVE GLOMERULONEPHRITIS

**CLINICAL FEATURES AND CLINICOPATHOLOGIC
CORRELATES**   The *acute nephritic syndrome* is the clinical correlate of acute glomerular inflammation. In its most dramatic form, the
acute nephritic syndrome is characterized by sudden onset (i.e., over
days to weeks) of *acute renal failure* and *oliguria* (<400 mL of urine
per day). Renal blood flow and glomerular filtration rate (GFR) fall as
a result of obstruction of the glomerular capillary lumen by infiltrating
inflammatory cells and proliferating resident glomerular cells. Renal
blood flow and GFR are further compromised by intrarenal vasoconstriction and mesangial cell contraction that result from local imbalances of vasoconstrictor (e.g., leukotrienes, platelet-activating factor,
thromboxanes, endothelins) and vasodilator substances (e.g., nitric
oxide, prostacyclin) within the renal microcirculation. *Extracellular
fluid volume expansion*, *edema*, and *hypertension* develop because of
impaired GFR and enhanced tubular reabsorption of salt and water.
As a result of injury to the glomerular capillary wall, urinalysis typically reveals *red blood cell casts*, dysmorphic red blood cells, leukocytes, and subnephrotic proteinuria of <3.5 g per 24 h ("nephritic
urinary sediment"). *Hematuria* is often macroscopic.

The classic pathologic correlate of the nephritic syndrome is *proliferative glomerulonephritis*. The proliferation of glomerular cells is
due initially to infiltration of the glomerular tuft by neutrophils and
monocytes and subsequently to proliferation of resident glomerular
endothelial and mesangial cells (endocapillary proliferation). In its
most severe form, the nephritic syndrome is associated with acute
inflammation of most glomeruli, i.e., *acute diffuse proliferative glomerulonephritis*. When less vigorous, fewer than 50 percent of glomeruli may be involved, i.e., *focal proliferative glomerulonephritis*. In
milder forms of nephritic injury, cellular proliferation may be confined
to the mesangium, i.e., *mesangioproliferative glomerulonephritis*.

RPGN is the clinical correlate of more *subacute glomerular inflammation*. Patients develop renal failure over weeks to months in
association with a nephritic urinary sediment, subnephrotic proteinuria
and variable oliguria, hypervolemia, edema, and hypertension. The
classic pathologic correlate of RPGN is crescent formation involving
most glomeruli (*crescentic glomerulonephritis*), crescents being half-
moon-shaped lesions in Bowman's space composed of proliferating
parietal epithelial cells and infiltrating monocytes (*extracapillary proliferation*). In practice, the clinical term *rapidly progressive glomerulonephritis* and the pathologic term *crescentic glomerulonephritis* are
often used interchangeably. In addition to classic crescentic glomerulonephritis, in which crescents dominate the glomerular pathology, crescents can also develop concomitantly with proliferative glomerulonephritis or as a complication of membranous glomerulopathy and other
more indolent forms of glomerular inflammation.

The acute nephritic syndrome and RPGN are part of a spectrum
of presentations of immunologically mediated proliferative glomerulonephritis. Studies of experimental models suggest that nephritic syndrome and diffuse proliferative glomerulonephritis represent an acute
immune response to a sudden large antigen load, whereas RPGN
and crescentic glomerulonephritis represent a more subacute immune
response to a smaller antigen load in presensitized individuals. At the
other end of the spectrum, chronic low-grade immune injury presents
with slowly progressive renal insufficiency or asymptomatic hematuria
in association with focal proliferative or mesangioproliferative glomerulonephritis. These more indolent forms of immune-mediated glomerulonephritis are discussed later in this chapter.

ETIOLOGY AND DIFFERENTIAL DIAGNOSIS   Acute nephritic syndrome and RPGN can result from renal-limited *primary*
glomerulopathy or *secondary* glomerulopathy complicating systemic
disease. Figure 274-1 highlights the histopathologic and serologic
features that help distinguish among the major causes of nephritic
syndrome and RPGN. In general, rapid diagnosis and prompt treatment
are critical to avoid the development of irreversible renal failure. Renal
biopsy remains the "gold standard" for diagnosis. *Immunofluorescence*

microscopy is particularly helpful and identifies three major patterns of deposition of immunoglobulin that define three broad diagnostic categories: (1) *granular* deposits of immunoglobulin, a hallmark of *immune-complex glomerulonephritis*; (2) *linear* deposition of immunoglobulin along the glomerular basement membrane (GBM), characteristic of *anti-GBM disease*; and (3) paucity or absence of immunoglobulin, typical of *pauci-immune glomerulonephritis* (Fig. 274-2). Most patients (>70 percent) with full-blown acute nephritic syndrome have immune-complex glomerulonephritis. Pauci-immune glomerulonephritis is less common in this setting (<30 percent) and anti-GBM disease is rare (<1 percent). Among patients with RPGN, immune-complex glomerulonephritis and pauci-immune glomerulonephritis are equally prevalent (~45 percent each), whereas anti-GBM disease again accounts for a minority of cases (<10 percent).

Three *serologic markers* often predict the immunofluorescence microscopy findings in nephritic syndrome and RPGN and may obviate the need for renal biopsy in classic cases. They are the serum C3 level and titers of anti-GBM antibody and antineutrophil cytoplasmic antibody (ANCA) (Fig. 274-1). As discussed in Chap. 273, the kidney is host to immune attack in immune-complex glomerulonephritis, most cases being initiated either by in situ formation of immune complexes or less commonly by glomerular trapping of circulating immune complexes. These patients typically have hypocomplementemia (low C3 and CH_{50} in 90 percent) and negative anti-GBM and ANCA serology. The glomerulus is the direct target of immune attack in anti-GBM disease, glomerular inflammation being initiated by an autoantibody directed at a 28-kDa autoantigen on the α3 chain of type IV collagen. Approximately 90 to 95 percent of patients with anti-GBM disease have circulating anti-GBM autoantibodies detectable by radioimmunoassay; serum complement levels are typically normal, and ANCA are usually not detected. The pathogenesis of pauci-immune glomerulonephritis is still being defined; however, most patients have circulating ANCA, implicating dysregulation of humoral immunity. The presence of mononuclear leukocytes in glomeruli and the paucity of glomerular immune deposits suggest that cellular mechanisms are also involved. Serum complement levels are typically normal, and anti-GBM titers are usually negative in ANCA-associated renal disease.

IMMUNE-COMPLEX GLOMERULONEPHRITIS

Immune-complex glomerulonephritis may (1) be idiopathic, (2) represent a response to a known antigenic stimulus (e.g., postinfectious glomerulonephritis), or (3) form part of a multisystem immune-complex disorder (e.g., lupus nephritis, Henoch-Schönlein purpura, cryoglobulinemia, bacterial endocarditis; Fig. 274-1). Here, we focus on *postinfectious glomerulonephritis*, the best characterized *primary* immune-complex glomerulonephritis. The major *secondary* immune-complex glomerulonephritides are discussed in Chap. 275. Nephritic syndrome and RPGN occasionally complicate two other primary glomerulopathies, namely, membranoproliferative glomerulonephritis (MPGN) and IgA nephropathy when there is a florid proliferative component. Because nephrotic syndrome and asymptomatic hematuria are more common presentations of MPGN

and IgA nephropathy, respectively, these glomerulopathies are discussed in later sections on nephrotic syndrome and asymptomatic urinary abnormalities.

POSTSTREPTOCOCCAL GLOMERULONEPHRITIS This is the prototypical postinfectious glomerulonephritis and a leading cause of acute nephritic syndrome. Most cases are sporadic, though the disease can occur as an epidemic. Glomerulonephritis develops, on average, 10 days after pharyngitis or 2 weeks after a skin infection (impetigo) with a nephritogenic strain of group A beta-hemolytic streptococcus. The known nephritic strains include M types 1, 2, 4, 12, 18, 25, 49, 55, 57, and 60. Immunity to these strains is type-specific and long-lasting, and repeated infection and nephritis are rare. Epidemic poststreptococcal glomerulonephritis is most commonly encountered in children of 2 to 6 years of age with pharyngitis during the winter months. This entity appears to be decreasing in frequency, possibly due to more widespread and prompt use of antibiotics. Poststreptococcal glomerulonephritis in association with cutaneous infections usually occurs in a setting of poor personal hygiene or streptococcal superinfection of another skin disease.

The classic clinical presentation of poststreptococcal glomerulonephritis is full-blown nephritic syndrome with oliguric acute renal failure; however, most patients have milder disease. Indeed, subclinical cases outnumber overt cases by four- to tenfold during epidemics.

FIGURE 274-1 Differential diagnosis of nephritic syndrome and rapidly progressive glomerulonephritis. Abbreviations: GN, glomerulonephritis; RPGN, rapidly progressive glomerulonephritis; MPGN, membranoproliferative glomerulonephritis; GBM, glomerular basement membrane; ANCA, antineutrophil cytoplasmic antibodies; Ig, immunoglobulin; C3, third component of complement; ASO, antistreptolysin O antibody titer; ADNAse, anti-deoxyribonuclease antibody titer; ANA, antinuclear antibody; anti-dsDNA, anti-double-stranded DNA antibody; HCV, hepatitis C virus; echo, echocardiogram; HSP, Henoch-Schönlein purpura; HUS, hemolytic-uremic syndrome; TTP, thrombotic thrombocytopenic purpura.
* Approximately 20% of patients with anti-GBM disease have ANCA, which may portend a better prognosis.
† Nephritic syndrome and RPGN are unusual presentations of IgA nephropathy and fibrillary GN.
‡ Atheroembolic renal disease may cause transient hypocomplementemia.
§ ANCA occasionally detected in association with lupus nephritis.

FIGURE 274-2 Typical findings on immunofluorescence microscopy of renal biopsy specimens from patients with anti-glomerular basement membrane antibody disease, immune-complex–mediated glomerulonephritis, and pauci-immune glomerulonephritis. Specimens in the upper and middle panels were stained for immunoglobulin and show the classical linear "ribbon-like" pattern of anti-GBM disease (*upper*) and granular pattern of immune-complex–mediated glomerulonephritis (*middle*). Immunoglobulin is sparse or absent in patients with pauci-immune glomerulonephritis; however, abundant fibrin is detected in crescents (*lower*). (*Micrographs courtesy of Dr. Helmut Rennke.*)

Patients with overt disease present with gross hematuria (red or "smoky" urine), headache, and generalized symptoms such as anorexia, nausea, vomiting, and malaise. Swelling of the renal capsule can cause flank or back pain. Physical examination reveals hypervolemia,

edema, and hypertension. The urinary sediment is nephritic, with dysmorphic red blood cells, red cell casts, leukocytes, occasionally leukocyte casts, and proteinuria. Fewer than 5 percent of patients develop nephrotic-range proteinuria. The latter may only manifest as acute nephritis resolves and renal blood flow and GFR recover. Coexistent rheumatic fever is extremely rare.

The serum creatinine is typically elevated at presentation [88 to 177 μmol/L (1 to 2 mg/dL)]. Serum C3 levels and CH_{50} are depressed within 2 weeks in ~90 percent of cases. C4 levels are characteristically normal, indicating activation of the alternate pathway of complement. Complement levels usually return to normal within 6 to 8 weeks. Persistently depressed levels after this period should suggest another cause, such as the presence of a C3 nephritic factor (see "Membrano-proliferative Glomerulonephritis"). The majority of patients (>75 percent) have transient hypergammaglobulinemia and mixed cryoglobulinemia. The antecedent streptococcal infection may still be evident or may have resolved either spontaneously or in response to antibiotic therapy. Most patients (>90 percent) have circulating antibodies against streptococcal exoenzymes such as antistreptolysin O (ASO), anti-deoxyribonuclease B (anti-DNAse B), antistreptokinase (ASKase), anti-nicotinyl adenine dinucleotidase (anti-NADase), and antihyaluronidase (AHase). ASO, anti-DNAse B, anti-NAD, and AHase are most useful after pharyngeal infection, whereas anti-DNAse B and AHase are more sensitive indices of streptococcal skin infection. Antibody titers tend to rise after 7 days, peak after 1 month, and return to normal levels after 3 to 4 months. These tests are relatively specific, with a false-positive rate of <5 percent. Early antibiotic therapy may prevent the development of an antibody response.

Acute poststreptococcal glomerulonephritis is usually diagnosed on clinical and serologic grounds, without resort to renal biopsy, especially in children with a typical antecedent history. The characteristic lesion on light microscopy is diffuse proliferative glomerulonephritis. Crescents are uncommon, and extraglomerular involvement is usually mild. Immunofluorescence microscopy reveals diffuse granular deposition of IgG and C3, giving rise to a "starry sky" appearance (Fig. 274-2). More extensive immunoglobulin deposition throughout the glomerular capillary wall ("garland pattern") is associated with a worse prognosis. The characteristic finding on electron microscopy is the presence of large electron-dense immune deposits in the subendothelial, subepithelial, and mesangial areas. It is likely that the acute inflammatory reaction is initiated, in large part, by the subendothelial and mesangial deposits, which activate complement and trigger leukocyte recruitment and glomerular injury. Subepithelial deposits may be more prominent on electron microscopy, however, probably because the subendothelial and mesangial deposits are scavenged more efficiently by invading phagocytes. Extensive subepithelial immune deposits, or "humps," tend to be associated with worse proteinuria, being juxtaposed to the glomerular filtration barrier for protein. → *The pathogenesis of immune-complex glomerulonephritis is discussed extensively in Chap. 273.*

In addition to poststreptococcal glomerulonephritis, the nephritic syndrome and RPGN can complicate acute immune-complex glomerulonephritis due to other viral, bacterial, fungal, and parasitic infections. Several warrant specific mention. Diffuse proliferative immune-complex glomerulonephritis is a well-described complication of acute and subacute bacterial endocarditis and is usually associated with hypocomplementemia. The glomerular lesion typically resolves following eradication of the cardiac infection. *Shunt nephritis* is a syndrome characterized by immune-complex glomerulonephritis secondary to infection of ventriculoatrial shunts inserted for treatment of childhood hydrocephalus. The most common offending organism is coagulase-negative staphylococcus. Renal impairment is usually mild and associated with hypocomplementemia. Nephrotic syndrome complicates 30 percent of cases. Acute proliferative glomerulonephritis can also complicate *chronic suppurative infections* and *visceral abscesses*. Patients typically present with a fever of unknown origin and an active urine sediment. Although immune deposits containing IgG an C3 are detected on renal biopsy, serum complement levels are usually normal.

TREATMENT

Treatment of poststreptococcal glomerulonephritis focuses on eliminating the streptococcal infection with antibiotics and providing supportive therapy until spontaneous resolution of glomerular inflammation occurs. Patients are usually confined to bed during the acute inflammatory phase. Diuretics and antihypertensive agents are employed to control extracellular fluid volume and blood pressure. Dialysis is rarely needed to control hypervolemia or the uremic syndrome. Poststreptococcal glomerulonephritis carries an excellent prognosis and rarely causes ESRD. Microscopic hematuria may persist for as long as 1 year after the acute episode but eventually resolves. Whereas complete recovery is the rule in children, adults may occasionally be left with residual renal impairment.

Antiglomerular Basement Membrane Disease   Anti-GBM disease is an autoimmune disease in which autoantibodies directed against type IV collagen induce RPGN and crescentic glomerulonephritis. Acute nephritic syndrome is rare. Between 50 and 70 percent of patients have lung hemorrhage; the clinical complex of anti-GBM nephritis and lung hemorrhage is referred to as *Goodpasture's syndrome*. Anti-GBM disease is a rare disorder of unknown etiology with an annual incidence of 0.5 per million. There is a bimodal peak in incidence. Patients with Goodpasture's syndrome are typically young males (5 to 40 years; male-female ratio of 6:1). In contrast, patients presenting during the second peak in the sixth decade rarely suffer lung hemorrhage and have an almost equal sex distribution. The target antigen is a component of the noncollagenous domain (NCI) of the α3 chain of type IV collagen, the α3 chain being preferentially expressed in glomerular and pulmonary alveolar basement membrane. The trigger(s) for loss of self-tolerance to this Goodpasture antigen has not been well defined. A genetic predisposition is suggested by an association with HLA-DRw2 and occasional occurrence in identical twins. Patients with lung hemorrhage are more likely to be cigarette smokers and to have suffered a recent upper respiratory tract infection or exposure to volatile hydrocarbon solvents. These observations suggest that diverse insults to the alveolar basement membrane may render previously sequestered Goodpasture antigens available for interaction with circulating autoantibodies. It is not clear whether environmental factors also trigger the onset of nephritis. Binding of anti-GBM antibodies to the GBM induces activation of complement, leukocyte recruitment, necrotizing proliferative glomerulonephritis, disruption of the glomerular capillary wall, leakage of fibrin into Bowman's space, and crescent formation (see Chap. 273). A similar sequence of events in the lung leads to disruption of the alveolar capillary wall and pulmonary hemorrhage.

Anti-GBM disease commonly presents with hematuria, nephritic urinary sediment, subnephrotic proteinuria, and rapidly progressive renal failure over weeks, with or without pulmonary hemorrhage. When pulmonary hemorrhage occurs, it usually predates nephritis by weeks or months. Hemoptysis can vary from fluffy pulmonary infiltrates on chest x-ray and mild dyspnea on exertion to life-threatening pulmonary hemorrhage. Hypertension is unusual and occurs in fewer than 20 percent of cases.

The diagnostic serologic marker is circulating anti-GBM antibodies with a specificity for the NCI domain of the α3 chain of type IV collagen (Fig. 274-1). Anti-GBM antibodies are detected in the serum of >90 percent of patients with anti-GBM nephritis by specific radioimmunoassay. If radioimmunoassay is not available, circulating anti-GBM antibodies can be detected in 60 to 80 percent of patients by indirect immunofluorescence, i.e., by incubating the patient's serum with stored sections of normal human kidneys. Complement levels are normal. About 20 percent of patients have low titers of ANCA, usually a perinuclear ANCA (see Chap. 275), the pathophysiologic significance of which is unclear. Occasional patients have a positive cytoplasmic ANCA, which may signal the presence of coexistent extraglomerular renal vasculitis. Patients with lung involvement frequently have microcytic, hypochromic, iron-deficiency anemia from alveolar hemorrhage, and abnormal bilateral hilar and basilar intersti-

tial shadowing on chest x-ray that may be difficult to distinguish from pulmonary edema or infection. The diffusion capacity for carbon dioxide is a useful tool for distinguishing among the latter diagnoses, being increased in patients with lung hemorrhage due to uptake of carbon monoxide by alveolar blood, and reduced in patients with infection or pulmonary edema.

Renal biopsy is the gold standard for diagnosis of anti-GBM nephritis. The typical morphologic pattern on light microscopy is diffuse proliferative glomerulonephritis, with focal necrotizing lesions and crescents in >50 percent of glomeruli (crescentic glomerulonephritis). Immunofluorescence microscopy reveals linear ribbon-like deposition of IgG along the GBM (Fig. 274-2). C3 is present in the same distribution in 70 percent of patients. Prominent IgG deposition along the tubule basement membrane and tubulointerstitial inflammation is found occasionally. Electron microscopy reveals nonspecific inflammatory changes without immune deposits. Typical features on lung biopsy include alveolar hemorrhage, disruption of alveolar septa, hemosiderin-laden macrophages, and linear staining of IgG along the alveolar capillary basement membrane.

It should be noted that Goodpasture's syndrome is not the only cause of the pulmonary-renal syndrome (i.e., renal failure and lung hemorrhage). Other important causes of this clinical complex include severe cardiac failure complicated by pulmonary edema (often blood-tinged) and prerenal azotemia; renal failure from any cause complicated by hypervolemia and pulmonary edema; immune-complex–mediated vasculitides such as systemic lupus erythematosus (SLE), Henoch-Schönlein purpura, and cryoglobulinemia; pauci-immune vasculitides such as Wegener's granulomatosis and polyarteritis nodosa; infections such as Legionnaire's disease; and renal vein thrombosis with pulmonary embolism. In general, these disorders can be differentiated by astute analysis of the clinical, serologic, and histopathologic findings.

TREATMENT

Prior to the introduction of immunosuppressive therapy, greater than 80 percent of patients with anti-GBM nephritis developed ESRD within 1 year, and many patients died from pulmonary hemorrhage or complications of uremia. With early and aggressive use of plasmapheresis, glucocorticoids, cyclophosphamide, and azathioprine, renal and patient survival have improved dramatically. In general, emergency plasmapheresis is performed daily or on alternate days until anti-GBM antibodies are not detected in the circulation (usually 1 to 2 weeks). Prednisone (1 mg/kg per day) is started simultaneously, in combination with either cyclophosphamide (2 to 3 mg/kg per day) or azathioprine (1 to 2 mg/kg per day) to suppress new synthesis of anti-GBM antibodies. The speed of initiation of therapy is a critical determinant of outcome. One-year renal survival approaches 90 percent if treatment is started before serum creatinine exceeds 442 μmol/L (5 mg/dL) and falls to about 10 percent if renal failure is more advanced. Patients who require dialysis at presentation rarely recover renal function. Serial anti-GBM titers are monitored to gauge response to therapy. Relapses are not unusual and are often heralded by rising antibody titers. In patients with ESRD, renal transplantation is a viable treatment option. Recurrence of anti-GBM nephritis in the allograft is extremely unusual provided that anti-GBM antibody titers have been consistently negative for 2 to 3 months prior to transplantation.

Pauci-Immune Glomerulonephritis   The major pauci-immune glomerulonephritides are *idiopathic renal-limited crescentic glomerulonephritis*, *microscopic polyarteritis nodosa*, and *Wegener's granulomatosis* (Fig. 274-1). RPGN is a more common clinical presentation than acute nephritic syndrome, and the usual pathology is necrotizing glomerulonephritis with crescents affecting >50 percent of glomeruli (crescentic glomerulonephritis). The marked overlap of clinical features and glomerular histopathology, and the presence of circulating

ANCA in most patients, suggest that these entities are a spectrum of a single disease. Here, we focus on idiopathic renal-limited crescentic glomerulonephritis. The ANCA-associated glomerulopathies with extrarenal features, namely Wegener's granulomatosis and microscopic polyarteritis nodosa, are discussed in Chap. 275.

Idiopathic Renal-Limited Crescentic Glomerulonephritis This is more common in middle-aged and older patients and shows a slight male preponderance. Patients typically present with RPGN, nephritic syndrome being rare. ANCA, usually a perinuclear ANCA IgG with specificity for myeloperoxidase (see Chap. 275), are detected in 70 to 90 percent of patients (Fig. 274-1). The erythrocyte sedimentation rate and C-reactive protein levels may be elevated; however, C3 levels are typically normal, and circulating immune complexes, cryoglobulins, and anti-GBM antibodies are not detected. Most patients have crescents on light microscopy, often associated with necrotizing glomerulonephritis. Immune deposits are scanty or absent. Immunofluorescence microscopy reveals abundant fibrin deposits within crescents (Fig. 274-2). Most cases are treated aggressively with glucocorticoids, with or without cyclophosphamide or azathioprine (see Chap. 275).

NEPHROTIC SYNDROME

GENERAL FEATURES AND COMPLICATIONS The *nephrotic syndrome* is a clinical complex characterized by a number of renal and extrarenal features, the most prominent of which are proteinuria of >3.5 g per 1.73 m^2 per 24 h (in practice, >3.0 to 3.5 g per 24 h), hypoalbuminemia, edema, hyperlipidemia, lipiduria, and hypercoagulability. It should be stressed that the key component is *proteinuria*, which results from altered permeability of the glomerular filtration barrier for protein, namely the GBM and the podocytes and their slit diaphragms. The other components of the nephrotic syndrome and the ensuing metabolic complications are all secondary to urine protein loss and can occur with lesser degrees of proteinuria or may be absent even in patients with massive proteinuria.

In general, the greater the proteinuria, the lower the serum albumin level. *Hypoalbuminemia* is compounded further by increased renal catabolism and inadequate, albeit usually increased, hepatic synthesis of albumin. The pathophysiology of *edema* formation in nephrotic syndrome is poorly understood. The *underfilling hypothesis* postulates that hypoalbuminemia results in decreased intravascular oncotic pressure, leading to leakage of extracellular fluid from blood to the interstitium. Intravascular volume falls, thereby stimulating activation of the renin-angiotensin-aldosterone axis and the sympathetic nervous system and release of vasopressin (antidiuretic hormone), and suppressing atrial natriuretic peptide release. These neural and hormonal responses promote renal salt and water retention, thereby restoring intravascular volume and triggering further leakage of fluid to the interstitium. This hypothesis does not, however, explain the occurrence of edema in many patients in whom plasma volume is expanded and the renin-angiotensin-aldosterone axis is suppressed. The latter finding suggests that *primary renal salt and water retention* may also contribute to edema formation in some cases.

Hyperlipidemia is believed to be a consequence of increased hepatic lipoprotein synthesis that is triggered by reduced oncotic pressure and may be compounded by increased urine loss of proteins that regulate lipid homeostasis. Low-density lipoproteins and cholesterol are increased in the majority of patients, whereas very low density lipoproteins and triglycerides tend to rise in patients with severe disease. Although not proven conclusively, hyperlipidemia may accelerate atherosclerosis and progression of renal disease.

Hypercoagulability is probably multifactorial in origin and is caused, at least in part, by increased urinary loss of antithrombin III, altered levels and/or activity of proteins C and S, hyperfibrinogenemia due to increased hepatic synthesis, impaired fibrinolysis, and increased platelet aggregability. As a consequence of these perturbations, patients can develop spontaneous *peripheral arterial or venous thrombosis*,

renal vein thrombosis, and *pulmonary embolism*. Clinical features that suggest acute renal vein thrombosis include sudden onset of flank or abdominal pain, gross hematuria, a left-sided varicocele (the left testicular vein drains into the renal vein), increased proteinuria, and an acute decline in GFR. Chronic renal vein thrombosis is usually asymptomatic. Renal vein thrombosis is particularly common (up to 40 percent) in patients with nephrotic syndrome due to membranous glomerulopathy, membranoproliferative glomerulonephritis, and amyloidosis.

Other metabolic complications of nephrotic syndrome include *protein malnutrition* and iron-resistant *microcytic hypochromic anemia* due to transferrin loss. *Hypocalcemia* and secondary hyperparathyroidism can occur as a consequence of vitamin D deficiency due to enhanced urinary excretion of cholecalciferol-binding protein, whereas loss of thyroxine-binding globulin can result in *depressed thyroxine levels*. An increased susceptibility to *infection* may reflect low levels of IgG that result from urinary loss and increased catabolism. In addition, patients are prone to unpredictable changes in the *pharmacokinetics* of therapeutic agents that are normally bound to plasma proteins.

ETIOLOGY AND DIFFERENTIAL DIAGNOSIS Proteinuria of greater than 150 mg per 24 h is abnormal and can result from a number of mechanisms. *Glomerular proteinuria* results from leakage of plasma proteins through a perturbed glomerular filtration barrier; *tubular proteinuria* results from failure of tubular reabsorption of low-molecular-weight plasma proteins that are normally filtered and then reabsorbed and metabolized by tubular epithelium; *overflow proteinuria* results from filtration of proteins, usually immunoglobulin light chains, that are present in excess in the circulation. Tubular proteinuria virtually never exceeds 2 g per 24 h and thus, by definition, never causes nephrotic syndrome. Overflow proteinuria should be suspected in patients with clinical or laboratory evidence of multiple myeloma or other lymphoproliferative malignancy. Suspicion is heightened when there is a discrepancy between proteinuria detected by dipsticks, which are sensitive to albumin but not light chains, and the sulfosalicylic acid precipitation method, which detects both.

Nephrotic syndrome can complicate any disease that perturbs the negative electrostatic charge or architecture of the GBM and the podocytes and their slit diaphragms. Six entities account for greater than 90 percent of cases of nephrotic syndrome in adults: minimal change disease (MCD), focal and segmental glomerulosclerosis (FSGS), membranous glomerulopathy, MPGN, diabetic nephropathy, and amyloidosis. Diabetic nephropathy and amyloidosis, being manifestations of systemic diseases, are discussed in Chap. 275. *Renal biopsy* is a valuable tool in adults with nephrotic syndrome for establishing a definitive diagnosis, guiding therapy, and estimating prognosis. Renal biopsy is not required in the majority of children with nephrotic syndrome as most cases are due to MCD and respond to empiric treatment with glucocorticoids.

MINIMAL CHANGE DISEASE This glomerulopathy accounts for about 80 percent of nephrotic syndrome in children of younger than 16 years and 20 percent in adults (Table 274-1). The peak incidence is between 6 and 8 years. Patients typically present

Table 274-1

Causes of Minimal Change Disease (Nil Disease, Lipoid Nephrosis)

Idiopathic (majority)
In association with systemic diseases or drugs
    Drug-induced interstitial nephritis induced by NSAIDs, rifampin, interferon α
    Hodgkin's disease and other lymphoproliferative malignancy
    Human immunodeficiency virus infection
    IgA nephropathy
    Diabetes mellitus
    Fabry's disease
    Sialidosis
    Heroin use
    Iron dextran administration

with nephrotic syndrome and benign urinary sediment. Microscopic hematuria is present in 20 to 30 percent. Hypertension and renal insufficiency are very rare.

MCD (also called nil disease, lipoid nephrosis, or foot process disease) is so named because glomerular size and architecture are normal by light microscopy. Immunofluorescence studies are typically negative for immunoglobulin and C3. Mild mesangial hypercellularity and sparse deposits of C3 and IgM may be detected. Occasionally, mesangial proliferation is associated with scanty IgA deposits, similar to those found in IgA nephropathy. However, the natural history of this variant and response to therapy resemble classic MCD. Electron microscopy reveals characteristic *diffuse effacement of the foot processes of visceral epithelial cells* (Fig. 274-3). This morphologic finding is referred to as foot process fusion in the older literature.

The etiology of MCD is unknown and the vast majority of cases are idiopathic (Table 274-1). MCD occasionally develops after upper respiratory tract infection, immunizations, and atopic attacks. Patients with atopy and MCD have an increased incidence of HLA-B12, suggesting a genetic predisposition. MCD, often in association with interstitial nephritis, is a rare side effect of nonsteroidal anti-inflammatory drugs (NSAIDs), rifampin, and interferon α. Rare cases occur in association with inherited and acquired metabolic diseases such as Fabry's disease, sialidosis, and diabetes mellitus (see Chap. 275). The occasional association with lymphoproliferative malignancies (such as Hodgkin's lymphoma), the tendency for idiopathic MCD to remit during intercurrent viral infection such as measles, and the good response of idiopathic forms to immunosuppressive agents (see below) suggest an immune etiology. In children, the urine contains albumin principally and minimal amounts of higher molecular weight proteins such as IgG and α_2-macroglobulin. This *selective proteinuria* in conjunction with foot process effacement suggests injury to podocytes and loss of the fixed *negative charge* in the glomerular filtration barrier for protein. Proteinuria is typically nonselective in adults, suggesting more extensive perturbation of membrane permeability.

℞ TREATMENT

MCD is highly steroid-responsive and carries an excellent prognosis. Spontaneous remission occurs in 30 to 40 percent of childhood cases, but is less common in adults. Approximately 90 percent of children and 50 percent of adults enter remission following 8 weeks of high-dose oral glucocorticoids. In a typical regimen, children receive 60 mg of prednisone per m^2 of body surface area daily for 4 weeks, followed by 40 mg/m^2 on alternate days for an additional 4 weeks. Adults receive 1 to 1.5 mg/kg body weight per day for 4 weeks, followed by 1 mg/kg per day on alternate days for 4 weeks. Up to 90 percent of adults enter remission if therapy is extended for 20 to 24 weeks. Nephrotic syndrome relapses in over 50 percent of cases following withdrawal of glucocorticoids. Alkylating agents are reserved for the small number of patients who fail to achieve lasting remission. These include patients who relapse during or shortly after withdrawal of steroids (steroid-dependent) and those who relapse more than three times per year (frequently relapsing). In these settings, cyclophosphamide (2 to 3 mg/kg per day) or chlorambucil (0.1 to 0.2 mg/kg per day) is started after steroid-induced remission and continued for 8 to 12 weeks. Cytotoxic agents may also induce remission in occasional steroid-resistant cases. These benefits must be balanced against the risk of infertility, cystitis, alopecia, infection, and secondary malignancies, particularly in children and young adults. Azathioprine has not been proven to be a useful adjunct to steroid therapy. Cyclosporine induces remission in 60 to 80 percent of patients; it is an alternative to cytotoxic agents and an option in patients who are resistant to cytotoxic agents. Unfortunately, relapse is usual when cyclosporine is withdrawn, and long-term therapy carries the risk of nephrotoxicity and other side effects. Long-term renal and patient survival is excellent in MCD.

FOCAL AND SEGMENTAL GLOMERULOSCLEROSIS WITH HYALINOSIS The pathognomonic morphologic lesion in FSGS is sclerosis with hyalinosis involving portions (segmental) of

FIGURE 274-3 Typical findings on electron microscopy of renal biopsy specimens from patients with minimal change glomerulopathy, membranous glomerulopathy, and membranoproliferative glomerulonephritis. The pathognomonic feature of minimal change glomerulopathy (*upper*) is effacement of foot processes of visceral epithelial cells (podocytes), giving the impression of foot process fusion. Foot process effacement is also evident in focal and segmental glomerulosclerosis (not shown here); in addition, there is typically detachment of podocytes from basement membrane, areas of glomerular capillary collapse, deposits of hyaline material, and sclerosis. Membranous nephropathy (*middle*) is characterized by immune complexes in the subepithelial space. These electron-dense immune deposits stimulate production of new GBM, which eventually surrounds and incorporates the immune deposits into the GBM. The hallmarks of type I membranoproliferative glomerulonephritis (*lower panel*) are increased mesangial cellularity and matrix and thickening and reduplication of the GBM. The latter is initiated by formation of electron-dense immune complexes on the subendothelial aspect of the GBM, which are subsequently covered by a new layer of GBM, probably produced by regenerating endothelial cells. (*Micrographs courtesy of Dr. Helmut Rennke.*)

fewer than 50 percent (focal) of glomeruli on a tissue section. Idiopathic (primary) FSGS accounts for 10 to 15 percent of nephrotic syndrome in children and 15 to 25 percent in adults. FSGS can complicate a number of systemic diseases and sustained glomerular capillary hypertension following nephron loss from any cause (Table 274-2 and Chap. 273).

Idiopathic FSGS typically presents as nephrotic syndrome (~66 percent) or subnephrotic proteinuria (~33 percent) in association with hypertension, mild renal insufficiency, and an abnormal urine sediment that contains red blood cells and leukocytes. Proteinuria is nonselective in most cases.

Light microscopy of renal biopsy tissue reveals FSGS with entrapment of amorphous hyaline material, a process that shows a predilection for juxtamedullary glomeruli. The sclerotic scars contain areas of glomerular capillary collapse and hyaline material composed of collagen types I, III, and IV. Adhesions occur between areas of capillary collapse and Bowman's capsule. Immunofluorescence studies are usually negative. Electron microscopy reveals evidence of damage to visceral epithelial cells, including swelling and detachment of podocytes from the GBM, effacement of foot processes, transition to foam cells, and overt cell degeneration and necrosis.

The etiology of primary FSGS is unclear (Table 274-2). The overlap of clinical and morphologic features between MCD and FSGS has prompted some authorities to speculate that they are a spectrum of morphologic manifestations of a single pathogenetic process. FSGS is a potential long-term consequence of nephron loss from any cause. It can complicate congenital renal diseases such as congenital oligomeganephronia, in which both kidneys have a reduced complement of nephrons, and congenital unilateral agenesis. In addition, FSGS may develop following acquired loss of nephrons from extensive surgical ablation of renal mass, reflux nephropathy, glomerulonephritis, interstitial nephritis, sickle cell disease, and the combined effects of ischemia, cyclosporine nephrotoxicity and rejection on renal allograft function (Table 274-2). It appears that >50 percent of nephrons must be lost for development of secondary FSGS.

℞ **TREATMENT**

In contrast to MCD, spontaneous remission of primary FSGS is rare and renal prognosis is relatively poor. Proteinuria remits in only 20 to 40 percent of patients treated with glucocorticoids for 8 weeks. Uncontrolled studies suggest that up to 70 percent respond when steroid therapy is prolonged for 16 to 24 weeks. Cyclophosphamide and cyclosporine, when used at doses described above for MCD,

induce partial or complete remission in 50 to 60 percent of steroid-responsive patients, but are generally ineffective in steroid-resistant cases. Poor prognostic factors at presentation include hypertension, abnormal renal function, black race, and persistent heavy proteinuria. Renal transplantation is complicated by recurrence of FSGS in the allograft in about 50 percent of cases and graft loss in about 10 percent. Factors associated with an increased risk of recurrence include a short time interval between the onset of the FSGS and ESRD, young age at onset, and possibly the presence of mesangial hypercellularity on renal biopsy.

MEMBRANOUS GLOMERULOPATHY This lesion is the most common cause of idiopathic nephrotic syndrome in adults (30 to 40 percent) and a rare cause in children (<5 percent). It has a peak incidence between the ages of 30 to 50 years and a male-female ratio of 2:1 (Table 274-3). Membranous glomerulopathy derives its name from the characteristic light-microscopic appearance on renal biopsy, namely diffuse thickening of the GBM, which is most apparent upon staining with periodic acid Schiff (PAS). Most patients (>80 percent) present with nephrotic syndrome, proteinuria usually being nonselective. Microscopic hematuria is present in up to 50 percent of cases, but red blood cells casts, macroscopic hematuria, and leukocytes are extremely rare. Hypertension is documented in only 10 to 30 percent of patients at the outset but is common later in patients with progressive renal failure. Serologic tests such as antinuclear antibody, ANCA, anti-GBM antibody, cryoglobulin titers, and complement levels are normal in the idiopathic form.

Light microscopy of renal biopsy sections reveals diffuse thickening of the GBM without evidence of inflammation or cellular proliferation. Silver staining demonstrates characteristic *spikes* along the GBM, which represent projections of new basement membrane engulfing subepithelial immune deposits. Immunofluorescence reveals granular deposition of IgG, C3, and the terminal components of complement (C_{5b-9}) along the glomerular capillary wall. Electron-microscopic appearances vary depending on the stage of disease. The earliest finding is the presence of subepithelial immune deposits (Fig. 274-3). As these deposits enlarge, spikes of new basement membrane extend out between the immune deposits and begin to engulf them. With time, the deposits are completely surrounded and incorporated into the basement membrane.

The pathogenesis of idiopathic human membranous glomerulopathy is incompletely understood. The presence of electron-dense immune deposits that contain IgG and C3 suggest an immune process. About one-third of adult membranous nephropathy occurs in association with systemic diseases such as SLE, infections such as hepatitis

Table 274-2

Etiology of Focal and Segmental Glomerulosclerosis

Idiopathic (majority)
In association with systemic diseases or drugs
  HIV infection
  Diabetes mellitus
  Fabry's disease
  Sialidosis
  Charcot-Marie-Tooth disease
As consequence of sustained glomerular capillary hypertension
  Congenital oligonephropathies
    Unilateral renal agenesis
    Oligomeganephronia
  Acquired nephron loss
    Surgical resection
    Reflux nephropathy
    Glomerulonephritis or tubulointerstitial nephritis
  Other adaptive responses
    Sickle cell nephropathy
    Obesity with sleep apnea syndrome
    Familial dysautonomia
Miscellaneous
  Heroin use

Table 274-3

Conditions Associated with Membranous Glomerulopathy

Idiopathic (majority)
In association with systemic diseases or drugs
  Infection
    Hepatitis B and C, secondary and congenital syphilis, malaria, schistosomiasis, leprosy, hydatid disease, filariasis, enterococcal endocarditis
  Systemic autoimmune diseases
    SLE, rheumatoid disease, Sjögren's syndrome, Hashimoto's disease, Graves' disease, mixed connective tissue disease, primary biliary cirrhosis, ankylosing spondylitis, dermatitis herpetiformis, bullous pemphigoid, myasthenia gravis
  Neoplasia
    Carcinoma of the breast, lung, colon, stomach, and esophagus; melanoma; renal cell carcinoma; neuroblastoma; carotid body tumor
  Drugs
    Gold, penicillamine, captopril, NSAIDs, probenecid, trimethadione, chlormethiazole, mercury
  Miscellaneous
    Sarcoidosis, diabetes mellitus, sickle cell disease, Crohn's disease, Guillain-Barré syndrome, Weber-Christian disease, Fanconi's syndrome, α_1 antitrypsin deficiency, angiofollicular lymph node hyperplasia

B, malignancy, and drug therapy with gold and penicillamine (Table 274-3).

CHAPTER 274
The Major Glomerulopathies

1543

Nephrotic syndrome remits spontaneously and completely in up to 40 percent of patients with membranous glomerulopathy. The natural history of another 30 to 40 percent is characterized by repeated relapses and remissions. The final 10 to 20 percent suffer a slow progressive decline in GFR that typically culminates in ESRD after 10 to 15 years. Presenting features that predict a poor prognosis include male gender, older age, hypertension, severe proteinuria and hyperlipidemia, and impaired renal function. Controlled trials of glucocorticoids have failed to show consistent improvement in proteinuria or renal protection. Cyclophosphamide, chlorambucil, and cyclosporine have each been shown to reduce proteinuria and/or slow the decline in GFR in patients with progressive disease in small or uncontrolled studies. These observations need to be confirmed in controlled prospective studies. Transplantation is a successful treatment option for patients who reach ESRD.

MEMBRANOPROLIFERATIVE GLOMERULONEPHRITIS This morphologic entity, also known as mesangiocapillary glomerulonephritis, is characterized by thickening of the GBM and proliferative changes on light microscopy (Table 274-4). It is equally common in males and females and more common in whites. Two major types are identified. Both are characterized by a diffuse increase in mesangial cellularity and matrix and thickening and reduplication of the GBM such that the lobular pattern of the glomerular tuft is exaggerated. The hallmark of type I MPGN is the presence of subendothelial and mesangial deposits on electron microscopy that contain C3 and IgG or IgM; rarely, IgA deposits are demonstrated by immunofluorescence microscopy (Fig. 274-3). The hallmark of type II MPGN (dense deposit disease) is the presence of electron-dense deposits within the GBM and other renal basement membranes (shown by electron microscopy) that stain for C3 but little or no immunoglobulin.

Most patients with type I MPGN present with heavy proteinuria or nephrotic syndrome, active urinary sediment, and normal or mildly impaired GFR. C3 levels are usually depressed, and C1q and C4 levels are borderline or low. Type I MPGN is an immune-complex glomerulonephritis and can be associated with a variety of chronic infections (e.g., bacterial endocarditis, human immunodeficiency virus, hepatitis B and C), systemic immune-complex diseases (e.g., SLE, cryoglobulinemia) and malignancies (e.g., leukemias, lymphomas). Type I MPGN is a relatively benign disease, and 70 to 85 percent of patients survive without clinically significant impairment of GFR.

Table 274-4

Causes of Membranoproliferative (Mesangiocapillary) Glomerulonephritis

Idiopathic	
Type I	With subendothelial and mesangial immune deposits
Type II	With intramembranous dense deposits containing sparse or no Ig; associated with C3 nephritic factor
Type III	Features of type I MPGN and membranous nephropathy
In association with systemic diseases or drugs*	
Systemic immune-complex disease	SLE, mixed cryoglobulinemia, Sjögren's syndrome
Chronic infections	Hepatitis B and C, human immunodeficiency virus, bacterial endocarditis, ventriculoatrial shunts, visceral abscess
Malignancy	Leukemias, lymphomas
Liver disease	Chronic active hepatitis and cirrhosis (usually associated with hepatitis B or C)
Miscellaneous	Partial lipodystrophy, heroin use, sarcoidosis, inherited C2 deficiency, thrombotic microangiopathies

* Usual with morphologic features of idiopathic type 1 MPGN (see above).

There is no proven therapy for patients with progressive disease beyond eradicating the underlying infection, malignancy, or systemic disease, when possible.

Type II MPGN can also present with proteinuria and nephrotic syndrome; however, some patients present with nephritic syndrome, RPGN, or recurrent macroscopic hematuria. Type II MPGN is an autoimmune disease in which patients have an IgG autoantibody, termed *C3 nephritic factor*, that binds to C3 convertase, the enzyme that metabolizes C3, and renders it resistant to inactivation (see Chap. 273). Type II MPGN runs a variable course; the GFR remains stable in some patients and declines gradually to ESRD over 5 to 10 years in others. There is no effective therapy for this disease.

FIBRILLARY-IMMUNOTACTOID GLOMERULOPATHY This emerging clinicopathologic entity accounts for 1 percent of diagnoses in most large renal biopsy series. Virtually all patients present with proteinuria, and >50 percent have nephrotic syndrome. The majority of patients also have hematuria, hypertension, and renal insufficiency. The light-microscopic appearances vary from mesangial expansion and basement membrane thickening with PAS-positive material to proliferative and crescentic glomerulonephritis. On electron microscopy, this PAS-positive material is observed to be composed of randomly arranged (fibrillary glomerulopathy) or organized bundles (immunotactoid glomerulopathy) of microfibrils and microtubules, the composition of which has yet to be defined. The etiology of fibrillary-immunotactoid glomerulopathy remains to be determined. Patients with the immunotactoid variant have an increased incidence of lymphoproliferative malignancy. There is no proven therapy for fibrillary-immunotactoid glomerulopathy, and many patients progress to ESRD over 1 to 10 years. Transplantation appears to be a viable option in the latter setting.

MESANGIAL PROLIFERATIVE GLOMERULONEPHRITIS In 5 to 10 percent of patients with idiopathic nephrotic syndrome, renal biopsy reveals a diffuse increase in glomerular cellularity, predominantly due to proliferation of mesangial and endothelial cells, and infiltration by monocytes. Findings on immunofluorescence microscopy vary and include deposits of IgA, IgG, IgM, and/or complement, or absence of immune reactants. It is likely that this morphologic entity is, in fact, a heterogeneous group of diseases that includes atypical forms of MCD and FSGS, and milder or resolving forms of the immune-complex and pauci-immune glomerulopathies described above under nephritic syndrome and RPGN. In keeping with the heterogeneity of this diagnosis, the prognosis is variable. In general, persistent nephrotic range proteinuria signals a poor prognosis, with many patients progressing to ESRD over 10 to 20 years despite immunosuppressive therapy.

℞ TREATMENT

Nephrotic Syndrome and Complications The treatment of nephrotic syndrome involves (1) specific treatment of the underlying morphologic entity and, when possible, causative disease (see above); (2) general measures to control proteinuria if remission is not achieved through immunosuppressive therapy and other specific measures; and (3) general measures to control nephrotic complications.

General measures may be warranted to control proteinuria in nephrotic syndrome if patients do not respond to immunosuppressive therapy and other specific measures and suffer progressive renal failure or severe nephrotic complications. Nonspecific measures that may reduce proteinuria include *dietary protein restriction, angiotensin-converting enzyme (ACE) inhibitors*, and *NSAIDs*. The first two of these measures aim to reduce proteinuria and slow the rate of progression of renal failure by lowering intraglomerular pressure and preventing the development of hemodynamically mediated focal segmental glomerulosclerosis. There is conclusive evidence that ACE inhibitors are renoprotective in human diabetic nephropathy (see Chap. 275) and that both ACE inhibitors and dietary protein restriction slow the development of secondary FSGS in experimental animals. Their role in the treatment of nephrotic syndrome in other settings is unproven. NSAIDs also reduce proteinuria in some patients with nephrotic syndrome, probably by altering glomerular hemodynamics or GBM permeability characteristics. This potential benefit must be balanced against the risk of inducing acute renal failure, hyperkalemia, salt and water retention, and other side effects.

Complications of nephrotic syndrome that may require treatment include edema, hyperlipidemia, thromboembolism, malnutrition, and vitamin D deficiency. Edema should be managed cautiously by moderate *salt restriction* usually 1 to 2 g/day, and the judicious use of *loop diuretics*. It is unwise to remove >1.0 kg of edema per day as more aggressive diuresis may precipitate intravascular volume depletion and prerenal azotemia. Administration of salt-poor albumin is not recommended as most is excreted within 24 to 48 h. Whereas many nephrologists advocate lowering low-density lipoproteins and cholesterol levels with *lipid-lowering drugs* to prevent accelerated atherosclerosis and slow the rate of decline of GFR, the value of such interventions in this setting has not been conclusively shown. *Anticoagulation* is indicated for patients with deep venous thrombosis, arterial thrombosis, and pulmonary embolism. Patients may be relatively resistant to heparin as a consequence of antithrombin III deficiency. Renal vein and vena caval angiography are probably indicated only when embolization occurs on anticoagulation and insertion of a caval filter is contemplated. There is no consensus regarding the optimal *diet* for patients with nephrotic syndrome. High-protein diets to prevent protein malnutrition are now in disfavor, since protein supplements have little, if any, effect on serum albumin levels and may hasten the progression of renal disease by increasing urinary protein excretion. The potential value of dietary protein restriction for reducing proteinuria and slowing the decline in GFR is discussed above. *Vitamin D* supplementation is advisable in patients with clinical or biochemical evidence of vitamin D deficiency.

ASYMPTOMATIC ABNORMALITIES OF THE URINARY SEDIMENT

HEMATURIA   Most asymptomatic glomerular hematuria is due to *IgA nephropathy* (Berger's disease) or *thin basement membrane (TBM) disease* (benign hematuria). A rarer but more ominous cause of isolated hematuria is *Alport's syndrome*. The latter is the most common form of hereditary nephritis, is usually transmitted as an X-linked dominant trait, and is associated with sensorineural deafness, ophthalmologic abnormalities, and progressive renal insufficiency (see Chap. 275). TBM disease is sometimes familial but, in contrast to Alport's syndrome, is a benign disorder. Asymptomatic hematuria may also be the presenting feature of indolent forms of most other primary and secondary proliferative glomerulopathies (see Fig. 274-1). Glomerular hematuria must be distinguished from a variety of renal parenchymal and extrarenal causes of hematuria. It is particularly important to exclude malignancy of the kidney or urinary tract, particularly in older male patients (see Chap. 96). Other potential diagnoses include vascular, cystic, and tubulointerstitial diseases; papillary necrosis; hypercalciuria and hyperuricosuria; benign prostatic hypertrophy; and renal calculi. Important clues to the presence of glomerular hematuria are the presence of urinary red blood cell casts, dysmorphic urinary red blood cells, proteinuria of greater than 2.0 g per 24 h, and clinical or serologic evidence of nephritic syndrome, RPGN, or a compatible systemic disease.

IgA Nephropathy (Berger's Disease)   IgA nephropathy is the most common glomerulopathy worldwide and accounts for 10 to 40 percent of glomerulonephritis in most series (Table 274-5). The disease is particularly common in southern Europe and Asia and appears to be more common in blacks than whites. Familial clustering has been reported but is rare. No consistent HLA association has emerged,

although HLA-B35 appears to be more common in French patients. Most cases are idiopathic. The renal and serologic abnormalities in IgA nephropathy and Henoch-Schönlein purpura (see Chap. 275) are indistinguishable, and most authorities consider these to be a spectrum of a single disease. Less commonly, IgA nephropathy is found in association with systemic diseases, including chronic liver disease, Crohn's disease, gastrointestinal adenocarcinoma, chronic obstructive bronchiolitis, idiopathic interstitial pneumonia, dermatitis herpetiformis, mycosis fungoides, leprosy, ankylosing spondylitis, relapsing polychondritis, and Sjögren's syndrome. In many of these conditions, IgA is deposited in the glomerulus without inducing inflammation, and this may be a clinically insignificant consequence of perturbed IgA homeostasis.

Patients with IgA nephropathy typically present with gross hematuria, often 24 to 48 h after a pharyngeal or gastrointestinal infection, vaccination, or strenuous exercise. Other cases are diagnosed upon detection of microscopic hematuria during routine physical examinations. Hypertension (20 to 30 percent) and nephrotic syndrome (~10 percent) are unusual at presentation. Light microscopy of renal biopsy specimens typically shows mesangial expansion by increased matrix and cells. Diffuse proliferation, cellular crescents, interstitial inflammation, and areas of glomerulosclerosis may be evident in severe cases. The diagnostic finding, for which the disease is named, is mesangial deposition of IgA, detected by immunofluorescence microscopy. C3 is usually detected in the area of immune deposits, and IgG is observed in 50 percent of cases. Electron microscopy reveals electron-dense deposits in the mesangium and, in severe cases, these extend into the paramesangial subendothelial space. The pathogenesis of IgA nephropathy is incompletely understood.

℞ TREATMENT

There is no proven therapy for IgA nephropathy. A recent, relatively large randomized controlled trial suggested a benefit of fish oils in patients with progressive disease and heavy proteinuria; however, this experience has not been universal. Some authorities advocate a trial of high-dose immunosuppressive therapy in patients with severe nephrotic syndrome and those with nephritic syndrome or RPGN and evidence of active inflammation on renal biopsy.

IgA nephropathy typically smolders for decades, with patients often suffering exacerbations of hematuria and renal impairment during intercurrent infections. As many as 20 to 50 percent of patients develop ESRD within 20 years. Clinical predictors of a poor prognosis include older age, male sex, hypertension, nephrotic-range proteinuria, and renal insufficiency at presentation. Histologic features that predict an aggressive course include diffuse severe disease, extracapillary proliferation (crescents), extension of immune attack into the paramesangial subendothelial space, glomerulosclerosis, interstitial fibrosis, and arteriolar hyalinosis.

Thin Basement Membrane Disease (Benign Hematuria)   This disorder can be heredofamilial or sporadic and is as common as IgA nephropathy in some series of asymptomatic hematuria. When familial,

Table 274-5

Diseases Associated with IgA Nephropathy

Idiopathic (majority)	
Renal-limited or as component of Henoch-Schönlein Purpura	
In association with systemic diseases or drugs*	
Liver	Chronic liver disease with involvement of biliary tree
Gastrointestinal	Celiac disease, Crohn's disease, adenocarcinoma
Respiratory	Idiopathic interstitial pneumonitis, obstructive bronchiolitis, adenocarcinoma
Skin	Dermatitis herpetiformis, mycosis fungoides, leprosy
Eyes	Episcleritis, anterior uveitis
Miscellaneous	Ankylosing spondylitis, relapsing polychondritis, Sjögren's syndrome, monoclonal IgA gammopathy, schistosomiasis

* Although prominent deposition of IgA has been reported with each of these conditions, significant glomerular inflammation and dysfunction is rare.

it is usually inherited as an autosomal dominant trait. TBM disease typically manifests in childhood as persistent hematuria. Intermittent hematuria and exacerbation of hematuria during upper respiratory tract infections have also been reported. The kidney is normal on light and immunofluorescence microscopy. The GBM is thin (usually <275 nm in children and <300 nm in adults) by comparison with normal subjects. TBM disease is almost always benign, and progressive renal impairment or proteinuria should prompt a search for an alternative diagnosis. The molecular basis for this disease has not been determined.

PROTEINURIA Between 0.5 and 10 percent of the population have isolated proteinuria, defined as proteinuria in the presence of an otherwise normal urinary sediment, a radiologically normal urinary tract, and the absence of known renal disease. The majority of these patients excrete <2 g of protein per day, and more than 80 percent have an excellent prognosis (*benign isolated proteinuria*). A minority (10 to 25 percent) are found to have persistent proteinuria (*persistent isolated proteinuria*), some of whom develop progressive renal insufficiency over 10 to 20 years.

Benign Isolated Proteinuria The major categories of benign isolated proteinuria are idiopathic transient proteinuria, functional proteinuria, intermittent proteinuria, and postural proteinuria. *Idiopathic transient proteinuria* is usually observed in young adults and refers to dipstick-positive proteinuria in an otherwise healthy individual that disappears spontaneously by the next clinic visit. *Functional proteinuria* refers to transient proteinuria during fever, exposure to cold, emotional stress, congestive cardiac failure, or obstructive sleep apnea. This phenomenon is presumed to be mediated through changes in glomerular ultrafiltration pressure and/or membrane permeability. Patients with *intermittent proteinuria* have proteinuria in approximately half of their urine samples in the absence of other renal or systemic abnormalities. *Postural proteinuria* is proteinuria (usually <2.0 g per 24 h) that is evident only in the upright position. This disorder affects 2 to 5 percent of adolescents and may be transient (~80 percent) or fixed (~20 percent). Fixed postural proteinuria resolves within 10 to 20 years in most cases. In each of these conditions, renal biopsy reveals either normal renal parenchyma or mild and nonspecific changes involving podocytes or the mesangium. All carry an excellent prognosis.

Persistent Isolated Proteinuria Isolated proteinuria detected on multiple ambulatory clinic visits in both the recumbent and upright position usually signals a structural renal lesion. Virtually all glomerulopathies that induce nephrotic syndrome (see above) can cause persistent isolated proteinuria. The most common lesion on renal biopsy is mild mesangial proliferative glomerulonephritis with or without focal and segmental glomerulosclerosis (30 to 70 percent), followed by focal or diffuse proliferative glomerulonephritis (~15 percent) and interstitial nephritis (~5 percent). Although this clinical entity carries a worse prognosis than benign isolated proteinuria, the prognosis is still relatively good, with only 20 to 40 percent of patients developing renal insufficiency after 20 years. Furthermore, progression to ESRD is extremely rare. It is wise to exclude monoclonal gammopathy by urinary electrophoresis in older patients.

CHRONIC GLOMERULONEPHRITIS

This syndrome is characterized by persistent proteinuria and/or hematuria and renal insufficiency that progresses slowly over years. Chronic glomerulonephritis usually comes to light (1) upon routine urinalysis, (2) when routine blood tests reveal unexplained anemia or elevated blood urea nitrogen and creatinine, (3) following discovery of bilateral small kidneys on abdominal imaging, (4) during evaluation for secondary causes of hypertension, or (5) during a clinical exacerbation of glomerulonephritis triggered by pharyngitis (synpharyngitic) or other infections. Chronic glomerulonephritis can be a manifestation of virtually all of the major glomerulopathies. Renal biopsy typically reveals a variable combination of proliferative, membranous, and sclerotic changes, depending on the causative glomerulopathy. Arteriosclerosis, induced by secondary hypertension, is a common finding in the renal vasculature. Tubulointerstitial inflammation and scarring are frequent

additional findings and portend a poor prognosis. Glomerular hypertension and hyperfiltration through remnant functioning nephrons can hasten progression to ESRD (see Chap. 273). Treatment is directed at lowering systemic and glomerular hypertension, usually with an ACE inhibitor, and controlling extracellular fluid volume, anemia, metabolic abnormalities, and the uremic syndrome through judicious use of diuretics, erythropoietin, and dietary modification (see "Chronic Renal Failure," Chap. 271). Some patients develop ESRD and require renal replacement therapy with dialysis or transplantation.

BIBLIOGRAPHY

BERNARD DB, SALANT DJ: Clinical approach to the patient with proteinuria and the nephrotic syndrome, in *The Principles and Practice of Nephrology*, 2d ed, HR Jacobsen, GE Striker, S Klahr (eds). St. Louis, Mosby, 1995, pp 110–121

COTRAN R, RENNKE HG: Sites and the mechanisms of proteinuria. N Engl J Med 309:1050, 1983

D'AMICO G: Immunoglobulin A nephropathy, in *The Principles and Practice of Nephrology*, 2d ed, HR Jacobsen, GE Striker, S Klahr (eds). St. Louis, Mosby, 1995, pp 133–138

FALK RJ: ANCA-associated renal disease. Kidney Int 38:998, 1990

GLASSOCK RJ et al: Primary glomerular diseases, in *The Kidney*, 5th ed, BM Brenner (ed). Philadelphia, Saunders, 1996, pp 1392–1497

KELLY PT, HAPONIK EF: Goodpasture's syndrome: Molecular and clinical advances. Medicine (Baltimore) 73:171, 1994

MEYER TW et al: Nephron adaptation to renal injury, in *The Kidney*, 5th ed, BM Brenner (ed). Philadelphia, Saunders, 1996, pp 2011–2048

---

275 | *Yvonne M. O'Meara, Hugh R. Brady, Barry M. Brenner*

GLOMERULOPATHIES ASSOCIATED WITH MULTISYSTEM DISEASES

An array of multisystem diseases can cause glomerular injury, with glomerulopathy being either the dominant presenting feature or a relatively benign and clinically insignificant manifestation that is overshadowed by involvement of other organs. Glomerulopathies associated with multisystem diseases are often classified as *secondary* glomerulopathies to distinguish them from the *primary* glomerulopathies (Chap. 274) in which the pathology is limited to the kidneys. It should be emphasized, however, that most morphologic patterns of glomerular injury (Table 273-1) can manifest as a renal-limited process (i.e., primary) or as part of a systemic disease (i.e., secondary). It is best to approach glomerular disease by first identifying the presenting clinical syndrome (e.g., nephritic, nephrotic), then defining the pathologic features (e.g., proliferative, crescentic, membranous), and finally attempting to establish the specific disease that provoked glomerular injury [e.g., systemic lupus erythematosus (SLE), Henoch-Schönlein purpura].

In this chapter, we focus on the epidemiology, clinicopathologic features, and management of the major glomerulopathies associated with systemic diseases. The pathogenesis of glomerular injury is discussed in Chap. 273, and the overall place of the major glomerulopathies in the differential diagnosis of the major renal syndromes is described in Chap. 274.

DIABETIC NEPHROPATHY (See also Chaps. 273 and 334)

Diabetic nephropathy is the leading cause of end-stage renal disease (ESRD) in western societies and accounts for 30 to 35 percent of patients on renal replacement therapy in North America. Insulin-dependent diabetes mellitus (IDDM) and non-insulin-dependent diabetes mellitus (NIDDM) affect 0.5 and 4 percent of the population, respectively. Nephropathy complicates 30 percent of cases of IDDM and approximately 20 percent of cases of NIDDM. However, the majority of diabetic patients with ESRD have NIDDM because of the greater prevalence of NIDDM worldwide (90 percent of all diabetics). For reasons that are unclear, ESRD from diabetic nephropathy is more common in blacks with NIDDM than in whites (4:1 ratio), whereas the reverse is true for IDDM.

The clinical and morphologic features of diabetic nephropathy are similar in IDDM and NIDDM. Glomerular hypertension and hyperfiltration are the earliest renal abnormalities in experimental and human diabetes and are observed within days to weeks of diagnosis. Microalbuminuria, so named because the abnormal albumin excretion of 30 to 300 mg per 24 h is below the limits of detection of standard dipsticks, develops after approximately 5 years of sustained glomerular hypertension and hyperfiltration. Microalbuminuria is the first manifestation of injury to the glomerular filtration barrier and predicts the development of overt nephropathy. Dipstick-positive proteinuria, ultimately reaching nephrotic levels, typically develops 5 to 10 years after the onset of microalbuminuria (i.e., 10 to 15 years after the onset of diabetes) and is associated with hypertension and progressive loss of renal function. In addition, patients can display features of tubulointerstitial disease such as hyperkalemia and type IV renal tubular acidosis. ESRD typically develops 5 to 10 years after the development of overt nephropathy. Diabetic nephropathy is usually diagnosed on clinical grounds without a renal biopsy. Supportive clues are the presence of normal sized or enlarged kidneys, evidence of proliferative diabetic retinopathy, and a bland urinary sediment. Retinopathy is found in 90 and 60 percent of patients with IDDM and NIDDM, respectively, who develop nephropathy.

The earliest morphologic abnormalities in diabetic nephropathy are thickening of the glomerular basement membrane (GBM) and expansion of the mesangium due to accumulation of extracellular matrix. With time, matrix accumulation becomes diffuse and is evident as eosinophilic, periodic acid Schiff–positive glomerulosclerosis on renal biopsy. Prominent areas of nodular matrix expansion (nodular glomerulosclerosis, the classic Kimmelstiel-Wilson lesion) are often superimposed on this background. The glomeruli and kidneys are typically normal or increased in size, distinguishing diabetic nephropathy from most other forms of chronic renal insufficiency (renal amyloidosis and polycystic kidney disease being other important exceptions). Immunofluorescence microscopy may reveal deposition of IgG along the GBM in a linear pattern, but this does not appear to be immunopathogenetic as in anti-GBM disease. Immune deposits are not seen. The renal vasculature typically displays evidence of atherosclerosis, as a consequence of hyperlipidemia, and hypertensive arteriosclerosis.

℞ TREATMENT

Therapy is aimed at retarding the progression of nephropathy through control of blood sugar, systemic blood pressure, and glomerular capillary pressure. Glycemic control is achieved through regulation of diet and administration of oral hypoglycemic agents and insulin (see Chap. 334). Angiotensin-converting enzyme (ACE) inhibitors are the drugs of choice as they control both systemic hypertension and intraglomerular hypertension by inhibiting the actions of angiotensin II on the systemic vasculature and renal efferent arterioles. ACE inhibitors also attenuate the stimulatory effect of angiotensin II on glomerular cell growth and matrix production. Because ACE inhibitors have been shown conclusively to delay the time to ESRD by 50 percent in patients with IDDM in a large randomized controlled trial and to delay progression significantly in NIDDM, it is felt that all diabetic patients should receive an ACE inhibitor upon the development of microalbuminuria, even in the absence of systemic hypertension (Fig. 275-1).

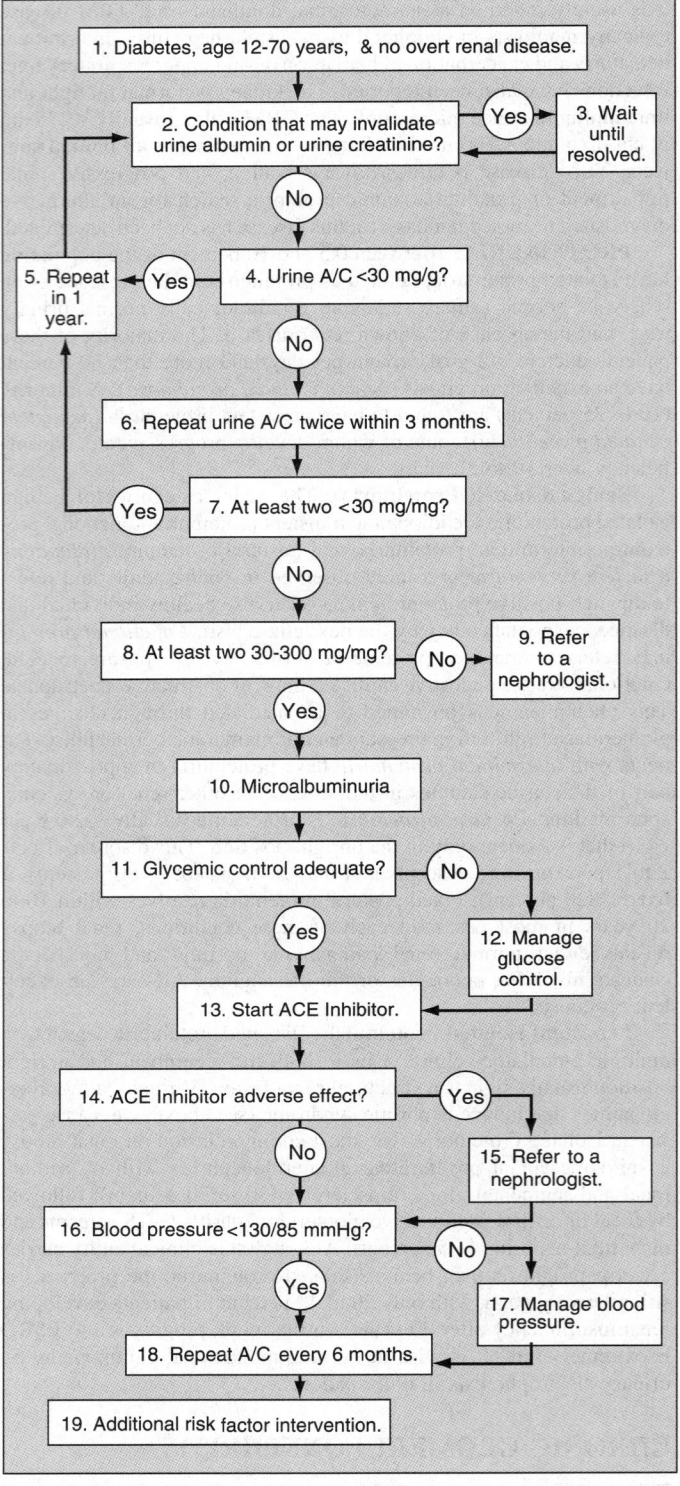

FIGURE 275-1 Algorithm for screening and management of microalbuminuria in patients with diabetes mellitus. A/C, albumin (in mg)/creatinine (in mg) in a spot urine sample. (*Reproduced with permission from Bennett et al.*)

Diabetic nephropathy is the most common cause of ESRD requiring renal replacement therapy, and diabetic patients have the highest annual mortality (20 to 30 percent) of any group on dialysis, in large part as a result of accelerated atherosclerosis. Survival of younger patients is comparable with either peritoneal dialysis or hemodialysis; however, older diabetics appear to have higher mortality on peritoneal dialysis. Transplantation is the preferred mode of renal replacement therapy in patients who are otherwise medically suitable.

The glomerulus is a frequent target of injury in a variety of immunologically mediated multisystem diseases, particularly systemic vasculitis and SLE. Systemic vasculitis is usually classified according to the size of the inflamed vessel (see Chap. 319). The major *large vessel* vasculitides are Takayasu's disease and giant cell arteritis. Glomerular injury is exceedingly rare in these diseases.

CLASSIC POLYARTERITIS NODOSA (See also Chap. 319) The typical glomerular lesion in classic polyarteritis nodosa (PAN) is ischemic collapse and obsolescence. Characteristic clinical and serologic features are hypertension, a bland urine sediment with subnephrotic proteinuria, slowly progressive renal insufficiency, normal serum complement levels, and absence of antineutrophil cytoplasmic antibodies (ANCA). Treatment with glucocorticoids and immunosupressive agents, such as cyclophosphamide, affords a 5-year patient survival of approximately 80 percent, as compared with 10 percent in untreated cases.

ANCA-ASSOCIATED SMALL-VESSEL VASCULITIS The ANCA-associated small-vessel vasculitides are Wegener's granulomatosis, the microscopic and Churg-Strauss variants of polyarteritis nodosa, and pauci-immune renal-limited glomerulonephritis. These diseases share a number of clinocopathologic and serologic features and may represent a spectrum of manifestations of a single disease. They are more common in whites and older patients (mean age 57 years) and show a slight male preponderance. Their incidence peaks in the winter months, and many patients have a viral-like prodrome, suggesting a pathogenetic role for an infective agent. Patients typically present with nonspecific constitutional symptoms and signs such as lethargy, malaise, anorexia, weight loss, fever, arthralgias, and myalgias. Nonspecific laboratory abnormalities include a rapid sedimentation rate, elevated C-reactive protein, leukocytosis, thrombocytosis, and normochromic, normocytic anemia. Serum complement levels are typically normal.

The majority of patients with these conditions have circulating ANCA. It is not clear whether ANCA are involved in the pathogenesis of vasculitis or merely represent an epiphenomenon of the vasculitic process, and there is debate whether serial ANCA titers are useful for monitoring disease activity and predicting relapse. Some ANCA activate cytokine-primed neutrophils in vitro and provoke them to injure endothelial cells, suggesting a pathogenetic role (see Chap. 273). It should be noted that ANCA are not entirely specific for vasculitis and are also found, albeit at low titers, in some cases (~20 percent) of anti-GBM disease and in patients with inflammatory bowel disease, primary biliary cirrhosis, and other autoimmune disorders.

Patients with ANCA-associated renal disease usually present with a nephritic urine sediment and moderate proteinuria. Renal dysfunction can vary from a mild decrement in glomerular filtration rate (GFR) to rapidly progressive glomerulonephritis (RPGN). Renal biopsy typically reveals focal, segmental, necrotizing glomerulonephritis with crescent formation. Immunofluorescence and electron microscopy are remarkable for the paucity or absence of immunoglobulin, complement, and immune deposits: so-called pauci-immune glomerulonephritis. These findings are in stark contrast to the prominent granular deposition of IgG and C3 in immune-complex glomerulonephritides such as Henoch-Schönlein purpura and lupus nephritis. ANCA-associated vasculitis is usually responsive to combined therapy with glucocorticoids and cyclophosphamide, and the 5-year patient survival usually exceeds 75 percent. The distinguishing features of individual ANCA-associated renal diseases are summarized below.

Wegener's Granulomatosis (See Chap. 319) Renal injury occurs in 80% of patients with Wegener's granulomatosis and varies from indolent smoldering inflammation to rapidly progressive renal failure. Cytoplasmic ANCA are detected at presentation in 80 percent of patients with renal disease and in a further 10 percent on follow-up. Renal biopsy typically reveals focal, segmental, necrotizing pauci-immune glomerulonephritis with crescent formation. In contrast to the lung, granulomas are rarely seen in the kidney.

℞ TREATMENT

Glucocorticoids and cyclophosphamide are the mainstay of treatment and dramatically ameliorate glomerular injury. Steroids are usually administered initially by pulse intravenous therapy on three consecutive days, followed by daily oral dosing of about 1 mg/kg body weight tapered to zero over 3 to 6 months. Cyclophosphamide is typically administered orally at a daily dose of 1 to 2 mg/kg or as monthly intravenous pulses of 1 g/m^2 of body surface area. Plasmapheresis may be a useful adjunct in patients with severe nephritis requiring dialysis. As many as 30% of patients relapse following treatment-induced remission. A persistently elevated or rising ANCA titer may predict relapse in individual patients; however, this relationship is not strong enough to justify treatment based on titers alone. Dialysis and renal transplantation afford excellent survival in patients with ESRD. Recurrence of Wegener's granulomatosis in the allograft is rare. ACE inhibitors may help to slow the progression to end–stage renal failure.

Microscopic Polyarteritis Nodosa (See Chap. 319) Microscopic PAN is a systemic disease characterized by leukocytoclastic vasculitis involving multiple organ systems including the lungs, skin, joints, and kidneys. Clinical renal disease ranges from a nephritic urinary sediment with mild impairment of GFR to RPGN. The usual histopathologic lesion is pauci-immune focal segmental necrotizing and crescentic glomerulonephritis. Circulating ANCA are detected in 70 to 80 percent of patients at presentation, cytoplasmic and perinuclear ANCA being equally prevalent. The treatment of microscopic PAN involves glucocorticoids and cyclophosphamide, as for Wegener's granulomatosis. Plasmapheresis may benefit patients with severe acute renal failure or massive pulmonary hemorrhage.

Churg-Strauss Syndrome (See Chap. 319) Clinical renal involvement in Churg-Strauss syndrome is relatively infrequent and usually limited to mild proteinuria and hematuria. Evolution to chronic renal failure is rare. Renal biopsy most frequently reveals extraglomerular pathology, with involvement of the renal vasculature and tubulointerstitium by granulomatous vasculitis. A minority of patients have focal segmental necrotizing glomerulonephritis.

Henoch-Schönlein Purpura (See Chap. 319) Nephritis is present in 80 percent of cases of Henoch-Schönlein purpura and manifests as a nephritic urine sediment and moderate proteinuria. Macroscopic hematuria and nephrotic-range proteinuria are uncommon. Light-microscopic appearances can vary from mild mesangial proliferation and expansion to diffuse proliferation with glomerular crescents. The glomerular lesion is identical to that found in IgA nephropathy (Berger's disease; see Chap. 274), suggesting that Henoch-Schönlein nephritis and IgA nephropathy are a spectrum of manifestations of a single disease. The *sine qua non* for diagnosis is the presence of mesangial IgA deposition on immunofluorescence microscopy. IgG and C3 are also detected. Electron microscopy reveals mesangial immune deposits. Immune complexes may also be seen in the peripheral glomerular capillary wall and paramesangial areas. Biopsy of involved skin reveals dermal IgA deposition and leukocytoclastic vasculitis. IgA deposition is also seen in areas of uninvolved skin.

℞ TREATMENT

Since there is no proven therapy for Henoch-Schönlein nephritis, treatment is supportive. Steroids and/or cytotoxic agents are often tried in patients with severe disease, but without compelling scientific evidence to support their use. The disease typically undergoes clinical exacerbations and remissions in the first year and then enters long-term remission. The prognosis is generally excellent; chronic renal failure and persistent hypertension occur in fewer than 10 percent of patients.

ESSENTIAL MIXED CRYOGLOBULINEMIA (See Chap. 319) Renal involvement is most common with the mixed cryoglobulinemias (types II and III), which are more common in females and usually begin in the sixth decade. Most patients present with a variable combination of leukocytoclastic vasculitis, skin ulcerations, arthralgias, fatigue, and Raynaud's phenomenon. Renal disease complicates 50 percent of cases and usually develops after 12 to 24 months. The typical clinical renal manifestations are nephrotic-range proteinuria, microscopic hematuria, and hypertension. Acute nephritic syndrome occurs in 20 to 30 percent, and oliguric acute renal failure in about 5 percent of patients with renal disease. The characteristic morphologic lesions are diffuse mesangial proliferative or membranoproliferative glomerulonephritis. The glomerular capillaries frequently contain eosinophilic hyaline "pseudothrombi" composed of precipitated immunoglobulins. Granular deposition of IgG, IgM, and C3 is usually prominent on immunofluorescence microscopy. Electron microscopy typically reveals subendothelial deposits containing microfibrils and microtubules that display a characteristic "thumbprint" appearance.

Circulating levels of C3, C4, and CH50 are depressed in about 80 percent of patients with renal involvement, and a transient antinuclear antibody (ANA) (speckled pattern) is sometimes detected. Abnormal liver function tests are found in about 15 percent of patients at presentation and in up to 50 percent subsequently. Many patients with "essential" mixed cryoglobulinemia (EMC) (i.e., idiopathic) are chronically infected with hepatitis C virus (HCV). In keeping with a pathogenetic role for this virus, HCV RNA has been isolated from the serum of patients with EMC, indicating active infection, and anti-HCV antibodies have been detected in both the serum and cryoprecipitates in association with viral antigens.

℞ TREATMENT

Traditionally, glucocorticoids, with or without cyclophosphamide, and plasmapheresis were the standard treatment for EMC. Recent reports indicate that interferon α controls viral replication and stabilizes renal function in most patients with EMC and HCV infection. Unfortunately, most patients relapse when interferon α is discontinued, a major problem given the prohibitive cost of the drug. In general, patient and renal survival are good in EMC, with 75 percent of patients being alive at 10 years.

SYSTEMIC LUPUS ERYTHEMATOSUS (See Chap. 312) Renal involvement is clinically evident in 40 to 85 percent of patients with SLE; it varies from isolated abnormalities of the urinary sediment to full-blown nephritic or nephrotic syndrome or chronic renal failure. Most glomerular injury is triggered by the formation of immune complexes within the glomerular capillary wall; however, thrombotic microangiopathy may be the dominant reason for renal dysfunction in a small subset of patients with the antiphospholipid antibody syndrome.

Immune Complex Mediated Lupus Nephritis The renal biopsy has proven very useful for identifying the different patterns of immune-complex glomerulonephritis in SLE, which are diverse, portend different prognoses, and do not necessarily correlate with the clinical findings. Indeed, clinically silent lupus nephritis is well described in which the urinalysis is virtually normal but renal biopsy demonstrates varying degrees of injury.

The World Health Organization categorizes lupus nephritis into six histologic classes. *Class I* consists of a normal biopsy on light microscopy with occasional mesangial deposits on immunofluorescence microscopy. Patients in this category usually do not have clinical renal disease. Patients with *class II* or mesangial lupus nephritis have prominent mesangial deposits of IgG, IgM, and C3 on immunofluorescence and electron microscopy. Mesangial lupus nephritis is designated as class IIA when the glomeruli are normal by light microscopy and class IIB when there is mesangial hypercellularity. Microscopic hematuria is common with this lesion, and 25 to 50 percent of patients

have moderate proteinuria. Nephrotic syndrome is not seen, and renal survival is excellent (>90 percent at 5 years). *Class III* describes focal segmental proliferative lupus nephritis with necrosis or sclerosis affecting fewer than 50 percent of glomeruli. Up to one-third of patients have nephrotic syndrome, and glomerular filtration is impaired in 15 to 25 percent. In *class IV* or diffuse proliferative lupus nephritis, most glomeruli show cell proliferation, often with crescent formation. Other features on light microscopy include fibrinoid necrosis and "wire loops," which are caused by basement membrane thickening and mesangial interposition between basement membrane and endothelial cells. Deposits of IgG, IgM, IgA, and C3 are evident by immunofluorescence, and crescents stain positive for fibrin. Electron microscopy reveals numerous immune deposits in mesangial, subepithelial, and subendothelial locations. Tubuloreticular structures are frequently seen in endothelial cells. These are not specific for lupus nephritis and are also seen in human immunodeficiency virus (HIV)-associated nephropathy. Electron microscopy may also reveal curvilinear parallel arrays of microfibrils, measuring approximately 10 to 15 nm in diameter, with "thumbprinting," similar to those seen in cryoglobulinemia. Nephrotic syndrome and renal insufficiency are present in at least 50 percent of patients with class IV disease. Diffuse proliferative lupus nephritis is the most aggressive renal lesion in SLE, and as many as 30 percent of these patients progress to terminal renal failure. *Class V* is termed membranous lupus nephritis because of its similarity to idiopathic membranous glomerulopathy. Thickening of the GBM is evident by light microscopy. Electron microscopy reveals predominant subepithelial deposits in addition to subendothelial and mesangial deposits. Proliferative changes may also be evident, but the predominant pattern is that of membranous glomerulopathy. Most patients present with nephrotic syndrome (90 percent), but significant impairment of GFR is relatively unusual (10 percent). Tubulointerstitial changes such as active infiltration by inflammatory cells, tubular atrophy, and interstitial fibrosis are seen to varying degrees in lupus nephritis and are most severe in classes III and IV, especially in patients with long-standing disease. *Class VI* probably represents the end stages of proliferative lupus nephritis and is characterized by diffuse glomerulosclerosis and advanced tubulointerstitial disease. These patients are often hypertensive, may have nephrotic syndrome, and usually have impaired GFR.

Transformation from one class to another is relatively frequent. For example, class III often progresses to class IV spontaneously, and class IV can transform to class II or class V following treatment. Class II and class V lupus nephritis may predate other manifestations of lupus, whereas class III or IV usually occurs in patients who have systemic features of SLE. A semiquantitative analysis can be performed using a variety of features on renal biopsy, scored 0 to 3+, to derive indices of disease activity and chronicity. Features that suggest active inflammation include endocapillary proliferation, glomerular leukocyte infiltration, wire loop deposits, cellular crescents, and interstitial inflammation. In contrast, features that suggest chronicity include glomerulosclerosis, fibrous crescents, tubular atrophy, and interstitial fibrosis. In some, but not all, studies, these indices have been useful in predicting response to therapy and renal prognosis.

Patients with active lupus nephritis have a range of serologic abnormalities. Hypocomplementemia is present in 75 to 90 percent of patients and is most striking with diffuse proliferative glomerulonephritis. ANA are usually detected (95 to 99 percent), although not specific for SLE. ANA titers tend to fall with treatment, and ANA may not be detected during remissions. Anti-double-stranded DNA (dsDNA) antibodies are highly specific for SLE, and changes in their titers correlate with the activity of lupus nephritis. It should be noted that almost 100 percent of patients taking procainamide and 65 percent of patients taking hydralazine develop ANA; however, overt lupus, including nephritis, occurs in fewer than 10 percent of these patients, and anti-DNA antibodies are not usually detected. Other antibodies found in patients with SLE include anti-Sm (17 to 30 percent; highly specific, but not sensitive); anti-RNP, which frequently accompanies anti-Sm in low titer; anti-Ro (35 percent); anti-La (15 percent); and anti-histone antibodies (70 percent of SLE and 95 percent of drug-induced lupus).

The treatment of lupus nephritis is controversial and based largely on the class of injury and disease activity. Because there is relatively poor correlation between clinical features (urinalysis findings, serum creatinine) and histologic class, the renal biopsy findings are an important guide to therapy. Treatment is not indicated for class I and most cases of class II lupus nephritis, as these histologic patterns portend an excellent prognosis (100 percent and >90 percent 5-year survival, respectively). Extrarenal manifestations may warrant treatment with glucocorticoids, salicylates, or antimalarials. Glucocorticoids and cyclophosphamide are the mainstays of therapy for patients with proliferative nephritis (classes III and IV). High-dose steroids given as intravenous boluses (pulse therapy) are usually effective at rapidly controlling acute glomerular inflammation. Cyclophosphamide and azathioprine are important adjuncts to steroid therapy and appear to afford better long-term preservation of renal function than steroids alone. Intravenous pulse cyclophosphamide is as efficacious as oral therapy and appears to be less toxic. Most authorities advocate an initial regimen of monthly intravenous boluses of cyclophosphamide for 6 months. Subsequent therapy is tailored to disease activity and typically involves dosing every 3 to 6 months for a total treatment period of 18 to 24 months. The initial dose of cyclophosphamide is 0.5 g/m^2, and the dose is increased gradually to a maximum of 1 g/m^2 unless patients develop leukopenia or other side effects. Steroids are usually started simultaneously at 1 mg/kg per day and are tapered over the first 6 months to a maintenance dose of 5 to 10 mg/day for the duration of cyclophosphamide therapy. Five-year renal survivals of 60 to 90 percent have been obtained with this and similar regimens. A large randomized, prospective trial indicated that plasmapheresis does not offer additional benefit in patients with severe proliferative lupus nephritis. Plasmapheresis may have a role, albeit unproven, in patients with antiphospholipid syndrome and thrombotic microangiopathy (see below).

The management of membranous lupus nephritis is less well defined. As with idiopathic membranous glomerulopathy, the incidence of spontaneous remission approaches 50 percent in membranous lupus nephritis, and the course of the disease is generally indolent, with 70 to 90 percent renal survival at 5 years. Some authorities advocate steroids and ACE inhibitors at the time of diagnosis, whereas others reserve them for patients with progressive renal insufficiency or severe nephrotic syndrome. Useful parameters for monitoring the response to therapy and predicting relapse include the activity of the urine sediment, proteinuria, GFR, serum complement levels, and anti-dsDNA titers. Despite maximal immunosuppressive therapy, about 20 percent of patients with aggressive lupus nephritis develop ESRD requiring dialysis. SLE tends to become quiescent with advanced uremia, and patients rarely develop systemic flares once they commence dialysis. Recurrence of nephritis and systemic flares are also very uncommon following renal transplantation, and allograft survival rates are comparable to those in patients with other causes of ESRD.

Antiphospholipid Antibody Syndrome and Thrombotic Microangiopathy Patients with this syndrome can develop a variable degree of renal impairment due to thrombotic microangiopathy. The latter typically affects the interlobular arteries, arterioles, and glomerular capillaries and is characterized by intravascular microthrombi and swelling of endothelial cells. Decreased levels of tissue plasminogen activator and increased level of α_2-antiplasmin, both of which would tend to promote thrombosis, have been described in this syndrome.

RHEUMATOID ARTHRITIS (See Chap. 313)   Although extra-articular manifestations are present in 35 percent of patients with rheumatoid arthritis, direct involvement of the kidney by rheumatoid disease is rare, and glomerular injury is usually secondary to AA amyloidosis or a side effect of drug therapy. AA amyloidosis complicates 10 to 20 percent of cases of rheumatoid arthritis, and renal involvement is evident clinically in 3 to 10 percent of these patients

(nephrotic syndrome, renal insufficiency). Amyloidosis is more frequent in patients with rheumatoid arthritis of long duration (>10 years), with circulating rheumatoid factor, and with destructive arthropathy. Less frequent glomerular lesions include mesangial proliferative glomerulonephritis and basement membrane thickening by subepithelial immune deposits. Gold and penicillamine may cause nephrotic syndrome by inducing membranous glomerulopathy, whereas nonsteroidal anti-inflammatory drugs (NSAIDs) can trigger the nephrotic syndrome by inducing minimal change nephropathy, usually in association with acute interstitial nephritis (see below).

SJÖGREN'S SYNDROME (See Chap. 316)   Tubulointerstitial injury is the most common form of renal involvement in Sjögren's syndrome and usually presents as either Fanconi's syndrome, distal renal tubular acidosis, or impairment of renal concentrating ability. Glomerulonephritis is relatively rare and should prompt a search for evidence of secondary causes. Membranous glomerulopathy and membranoproliferative glomerulonephritis (MPGN) are the most common lesions. Anecdotal reports describe successful therapy with glucocorticoids and cytotoxic agents.

POLYMYOSITIS AND DERMATOMYOSITIS (See Chap. 315)   Occasional cases of focal mesangial proliferative glomerulonephritis with mesangial deposition of IgG and complement have been described in polymyositis/dermatomyositis. Membranous glomerulopathy has also been reported, particularly when polymyositis/dermatomyositis is associated with malignancy.

MIXED CONNECTIVE TISSUE DISEASE (See Chap. 314)   Mixed connective tissue disease is a syndrome that includes features of SLE, scleroderma, and polymyositis and is associated with high titers of antiribonucleoprotein antibodies and negative antismooth muscle antibodies. Renal involvement occurs in fewer than 15 percent of patients and manifests as hematuria and subnephrotic proteinuria. The usual pathologic lesion is membranous or MPGN. The prognosis is usually excellent, and steroid therapy may be useful in rare patients with progressive renal disease.

GLOMERULAR DEPOSITION DISEASES

The glomerular deposition diseases are characterized by deposition of abnormal proteins, usually immunoglobulins or fragments thereof, within the glomerulus. They include amyloidosis, light and heavy chain deposition disease, cryoglobulinemia, and fibrillary/immunotactoid glomerulonephritis. Here, we focus on amyloidosis and light chain deposition disease (LCDD). Cryoglobulinemic nephropathy is described above in the discussion on systemic vasculitis. → *Fibrillary and immunotactoid glomerulopathy are discussed in Chap. 274.*

AMYLOIDOSIS (See Chap. 309)   Amyloidosis is classified according to the major component of its fibrils: for example, immunoglobulin light chains in AL amyloidosis, serum amyloid A in AA amyloidosis, β_2-microglobulin in dialysis-associated amyloidosis, and amyloid β protein in Alzheimer's disease and Down's syndrome. Amyloid deposits also contain a nonfibrillar component called the P component, a serum α_1 glycoprotein with a high affinity for the fibrillar components of all forms of amyloid. AL and AA amyloidosis frequently involve the kidneys, whereas involvement by other forms of amyloidosis is very rare.

There is substantial overlap in the renal clinicopathologic presentations of AL and AA amyloidosis. Glomeruli are involved in 75 to 90 percent of patients, usually in association with involvement of other organs. The clinical correlate of glomerular amyloid deposition is nephrotic-range proteinuria. In addition, over 50 percent of patients have impaired glomerular filtration at diagnosis. Hypertension is present in about 20 to 25 percent. Renal size is usually normal or slightly enlarged. A minority of patients present with renal failure due to amyloid deposition in the renal vasculature or with Fanconi's syndrome, nephrogenic diabetes insipidus, or renal tubular acidosis due to involvement of the tubulointerstitium. Rectal biopsy and abdominal fat pad biopsy reveal amyloid deposits in about 70 percent of patients and may obviate the need for renal biopsy.

Renal biopsy gives a very high yield if there is clinical evidence of renal involvement. The earliest pathologic changes are mesangial expansion by amorphous hyaline material and thickening of the GBM. Further amyloid deposition results in the development of large nodular eosinophilic masses. When stained with Congo red, these deposits show apple-green birefringence under polarized light. Immunofluorescence microscopy is usually only weakly positive for immunoglobulin light chains because amyloid fibrils are usually derived from the variable region of light chains. Electron microscopy reveals the characteristic nonbranching extracellular amyloid fibrils of 7.5 to 10 nm in diameter. Tubulointerstitial and vascular deposits of amyloid are also seen and may occasionally be more prominent than glomerular deposits.

℞ TREATMENT

Most patients with renal involvement by AL amyloidosis develop ESRD within 2 to 5 years. No treatment has been shown consistently to improve this prognosis; however, some success has been reported with a combination of melphalan and prednisone. Colchicine delays the onset of nephropathy in patients with familial Mediterranean fever but has not proved useful in patients with established disease or with other forms of amyloid. Remissions may be achieved in AA amyloidosis by eradication of the underlying cause. Renal replacement therapy is offered to patients who reach ESRD; however, 1-year survival on dialysis is low (~66 percent) by comparison with other causes of ESRD. Most patients die from extrarenal complications, particularly cardiovascular disease. Renal transplantation is a viable option in patients with AA amyloidosis whose primary disease has been eradicated. Transplantation is also an option for patients with AL amyloidosis, though a poor prognosis because of extrarenal organ involvement may preclude them as candidates. Here again, survival is lower by comparison with other causes of ESRD, most of the excess mortality being due to infectious and cardiovascular complications. Recurrence of amyloidosis in the allograft is common but rarely leads to graft loss.

LIGHT CHAIN DEPOSITION DISEASE (See Chap. 114) Renal involvement complicates 90 percent of cases of LCDD and is often the dominant feature. Nephrotic syndrome and renal impairment are the usual presenting features. Microscopic hematuria occurs in about 20 percent of cases. Defective hydrogen ion and potassium excretion and urinary concentration may be evident if light chains are deposited predominantly in the tubules. The most common pathologic lesion on renal biopsy is ribbon-like thickening of the tubular basement membrane due to light chain deposition. Mesangial expansion and nodular glomerulosclerosis are found in about 33 percent of patients. This light-microscopic appearance resembles that of idiopathic MPGN and diabetic nephropathy. Superimposed crescentic change is occasionally seen. Immunofluorescence studies are strongly positive for monoclonal light chains, in contrast to AL amyloid, because the constant region of the immunoglobulin is typically deposited. The tissue deposits in LCDD are granular rather than fibrillar on electron microscopy, appear more amorphous in character, do not stain with Congo red, and seem to have a greater affinity for basement membranes.

The prognosis of LCDD is poor when associated with multiple myeloma, and most patients progess rapidly to ESRD. Treatment with melphalan and prednisone has been reported to reduce proteinuria and stabilize renal function in uncontrolled studies. In the absence of myeloma, the prognosis is somewhat more variable, as several patients have undergone successful renal transplantation.

WALDENSTRÖM'S MACROGLOBULINEMIA (See Chap. 114) This disorder is characterized by monoclonal proliferation of an IgM-secreting clone of plasma cells. The circulating IgM paraprotein

frequently gives rise to the hyperviscosity syndrome, which may compromise renal blood flow and GFR. Direct renal involvement is rare and, when present, involves deposition of large amorphous deposits of eosinophilic material in the glomerular capillaries. Renal amyloidosis can also occur.

DRUG-INDUCED GLOMERULAR DISEASE

A variety of drugs damage the glomerular filtration barrier and induce proteinuria and nephrotic syndrome. In contrast, drug-induced proliferative glomerulonephritis is rare. The more common drug-induced glomerulopathies are discussed here. Additional associations are included in Table 275-1 and Table 69-1.

NSAIDs have a variety of renal side effects, including hemodynamically mediated acute renal failure, salt and water retention, hyponatremia, hyperkalemia, papillary necrosis, acute interstitial nephritis, nephrotic syndrome, and ESRD. Nephrotic syndrome and acute renal failure frequently coexist due to a combination of acute interstitial nephritis and a glomerular lesion that is identical to that of minimal change disease. This entity occurs most commonly in patients on propionic acid derivatives such as fenoprofen, ibuprofen, and naproxen but can occur with other NSAIDS, ampicillin, rifampin, and interferon α. Withdrawal of the drug usually results in resolution of renal disease.

Gold therapy, administered by injection or orally, induces proteinuria in 5 to 25 percent of patients with rheumatoid arthritis. Proteinuria develops after 4 to 6 months of therapy, and up to 33 percent of patients develop full-blown nephrotic syndrome. Renal biopsy typically reveals membranous glomerulopathy, though minimal change disease or mesangial proliferative lesions have also been described. Progressive renal impairment is rare. Nephrotic syndrome is more common in patients who are HLA-B8/DR3 positive, suggesting a genetic susceptibility. Withdrawal of the drug leads to gradual resolution of the proteinuria.

Penicillamine also induces proteinuria in 5 to 30 percent of patients. As with gold, the underlying glomerular lesion is usually membranous glomerulopathy, and proteinuria gradually resolves following withdrawal of the drug.

Intravenous heroin use is associated with an increased incidence of focal and segmental glomerulosclerosis (heroin-associated nephropathy). It is not clear whether the nephrotoxin in this setting is heroin itself or a contaminant. Heroin-associated nepropathy occurs predominantly in blacks and is characterized by nephrotic syndrome, hyperten-

Table 275-1

Drug-Induced Glomerular Disease

Morphologic Lesion	Causative Agent
Minimal change diseases (usually with interstitial nephritis)	Nonsteroidal anti-inflammatory agents
	Recombinant interferon α
	Rifampin
	Ampicillin
Membranous nephropathy	Penicillamine
	Gold
	Mercury
	Trimethadione
	Captopril
	Chlormethiazole
Focal segmental glomerulosclerosis	Heroin
Pauci-immune necrotizing GN	Ciprofloxacin
	Hydralazine
Proliferative GN with vasculitis	Allopurinol
	Penicillin
	Sulfonamides
	Thiazides
	Intravenous amphetamines
RPGN	Rifampin
	Warfarin
	Carbimazole
	Amoxicillin
	Penicillamine

NOTE: GN, glomerulonephritis; RPGN, rapidly progressive glomerulonephritis.

sion, and a gradual progression to ESRD over a period of 3 to 5 years. The pathologic features are similar to those of idiopathic focal segmental glomerulosclerosis, though mesangial deposition of IgM and C3 may be more prominent. The incidence of this disease appears to be declining steadily. Potential reasons for the decline include increased purity of street heroin and a bias to attribute focal segmental glomerulosclerosis to HIV infection when both risk factors coexist. Intravenous *amphetamine* abuse is a rare cause of systemic necrotizing vasculitis.

HEREDITARY DISEASES WITH GLOMERULAR INVOLVEMENT

ALPORT'S SYNDROME (See Chap. 348) Alport's syndrome is the most common hereditary nephritis and is usually transmitted as an X-linked dominant trait. The genetic defect resides in the gene for the α5 chain of type IV collagen located on the long arm of the X chromosome, type IV collagen being a major structural component of the GBM. Numerous genetic mutations have been detected, ranging from major deletions to point mutations, and this genetic heterogeneity is reflected in the phenotypic variations of the disease. In the X-linked forms, males usually present with microscopic hematuria, proteinuria (nephrotic-range in 30 percent), and progressive renal insufficiency. Common extrarenal manifestations include sensorineural hearing loss (~60 percent) and bilateral anterior lenticonus (~15 to 30 percent). Platelet defects are described but are rare. Female carriers usually have mild disease and do not develop renal insufficiency. An autosomal recessive form also exists in which there are mutations in the gene for the α3 chain of type IV collagen, and males and females are equally affected.

Typical light-microscopic features on renal biopsy include mesangial hypercellularity, focal and segmental glomerulosclerosis, chronic tubulointerstitial fibrosis, atrophy, and accumulation of foam cells. Electron microscopy reveals thickening, fragmentation, and lamellation of the lamina densa of the GBM. Patchy thinning of the GBM may also be seen, especially early in the course of the disease and in female carriers.

Males with the disease tend to progress to ESRD and are suitable candidates for dialysis and transplantation. About 5 percent of transplant recipients develop anti-GMB disease in the renal allograft; their immune system recognizes normal GBM of the transplanted kidney as a foreign antigen. These patients can have antibodies against the α3 (Goodpasture antigen) or α5 chains of type IV collagen, probably because defective synthesis of the α5 chain results in defective incorporation or orientation of the α3 chain in the GBM.

SICKLE CELL DISEASE (See Chap. 107) Glomerular disease is common (15 to 30 percent) in homozygotes for sickle cell disease. Glomerular hyperfiltration and hypertrophy occur within the first 5 years of life. Approximately 15 to 30 percent of patients develop proteinuria in the first three decades, and 5 percent develop ESRD. The glomerular pathology is usually focal segmental glomerulosclerosis, probably due to sustained glomerular capillary hypertension, or MPGN. Predictors of chronic renal failure are worsening anemia, proteinuria, nephrotic syndrome, and hypertension. ACE inhibitors may slow the progression of renal disease by lowering systemic and glomerular capillary hypertension.

FABRY'S DISEASE (See Chap. 346) In patients with Fabry's disease, renal biopsy reveals accumulation of neutral glycosphingo-lipids with terminal α-galactosyl moieties in lysosomes of glomerular, tubular, vascular, and interstitial cells. Focal and global glomerulosclerosis are later features. Electron microscopy reveals stacked, concentric lamellar profiles known as "myeloid" bodies, which are characteristic. Renal disease manifests in the late teens to early twenties with lipiduria, proteinuria with minimal hematuria, nephrotic syndrome, hypertension, and progressive renal insufficiency. The most striking systemic manifestations are skin lesions (angiokeratomas), corneal and lens opacities, painful dysesthesias of the extremities, and arthropathy of the terminal interphalangeal joints. The diagnosis of Fabry's disease can often be made by careful physical examination, especially

if many of the typical clinical features are present. Measurement of urinary glycosphingolipids and estimation of peripheral leukocyte α-galactosidase levels help confirm the diagnosis. The renal lesion is progressive, and these patients often tolerate hemodynamic changes during dialysis poorly because of progressive vascular disease. Successful renal transplantation has been reported despite recurrence in the allograft.

NAIL-PATELLA SYNDROME The nail-patella syndrome is a rare hereditary disorder transmitted as an autosomal dominant trait. It is characterized by multiple osseous abnormalities, primarily affecting the elbows and knees, and nail dysplasia. About 50 percent of cases have clinically evident nephropathy. The light-microscopic features on renal biopsy include local GBM thickening, tubular atrophy, interstitial fibrosis, and varying degrees of glomerular sclerosis. Electron microscopy reveals irregular thickening of the GBM, with electrolucent areas giving it a "moth-eaten" appearance. Cross-striated fibrils with the periodicity of collagen can be identified in the mesangium and basement membrane. The disease usually manifests clinically as asymptomatic hematuria and proteinuria, occasionally in the nephrotic range, but may be silent. The renal lesion is usually benign, and progression to ESRD is rare (<10 percent).

LIPODYSTROPHY (See Chap. 352) MPGN type II (dense deposit disease) is the most frequent glomerular lesion (80 percent) in this condition, whereas MPGN type I affects the remainder (20 percent). The disease occurs mostly in females between the ages of 5 to 15 years, and the clinical presentation and course is similar to that of idiopathic MPGN, namely nephrotic-range proteinuria and progressive renal insufficiency. Low C3 levels are common in association with C3 nephritic factor (see Chap. 274).

LECITHIN-CHOLESTEROL ACYLTRANSFERASE DEFICIENCY (See Chap. 341) Renal manifestations of this disease include proteinuria, microscopic hematuria, and progressive renal insufficiency. Renal biopsy typically reveals focal and segmental glomerulosclerosis. Electron-microscopic findings include irregular rounded, lucent lacunae that contain solid or laminated dense structures in the GBM, mesangial matrix, and Bowman's capsular and renal tubular basement membranes. Endothelial cell detachment is also evident, and capillary lumens may be occluded by vacuolated foam cells. Recurrence of the disease has been documented in the renal allograft but without marked impairment of graft function.

GLOMERULAR LESIONS ASSOCIATED WITH INFECTIOUS DISEASES

VIRAL INFECTIONS Hepatitis B, hepatitis C, and HIV are strongly associated with glomerular disease (Table 275-2). Glomerular lesions associated with *hepatitis B virus* (HBV) infection include membranous glomerulopathy, MPGN, IgA nephropathy, essential mixed cryoglobulinemia, and polyarteritis nodosa. Membranous glomerulopathy is most common. In endemic areas, such as Asia and Africa, 80 to 100 percent of children and 30 to 45 percent of adults with membranous glomerulopathy have HBV surface antigenemia. HBV antigens have been identified in renal immune deposits, suggesting in situ immune complex formation following planting of HBV antigens or trapping of circulating immune complexes containing HBV antigens. Patients typically present with nephrotic syndrome and microscopic hematuria. Hypertension and renal impairment are rare. The most common associated hepatic lesion is chronic persistent or chronic active hepatitis. There is a male preponderance, and many patients are intravenous drug users or have other risk factor for acquisition of HBV. The asymptomatic carrier state of HBV is frequently associated with MPGN in endemic areas. Hypertension and azotemia are more common with this morphologic pattern than with membranous glomerulopathy. Children with HBV-associated membranous glomerulonephritis have a good prognosis, and almost two-thirds enter spontaneous remission within 3 years. ESRD is rare. In contrast, 30 percent of

Table 275-2

Glomerular Lesions Associated with Infectious Diseases

Morphologic Lesion	Common Disease or Inciting Organism
Diffuse proliferative glomerulonephritis (classic postinfectious glomerulonephritis)	Streptococcal pharyngitis Acute/subacute bacterial endocarditis Visceral sepsis Typhoid fever Syphilis Leptospirosis (*Mycobacterium leprae*) Toxoplasmosis Falciparum malaria *Plasmodium falciparum* Varicella, mumps, echovirus, coxsackievirus, measles Infectious mononucleosis Hepatitis B and C
Membranoproliferative glomerulonephritis	Subacute bacterial endocarditis Ventriculoatrial shunt infection Visceral sepsis Hepatitis C infection Hepatitis B infection *P. falciparum* Schistosomiasis
Mesangial proliferative glomerulonephritis	Recovery phase of postinfectious glomerulonephritis
Membranous nephropathy	Hepatitis C infection Hepatitis B infection Syphilis Filiariasis Hydatid disease Schistosomiasis *Plasmodium malariae* Leprosy Enterococcal endocarditis
Focal segmental glomerulosclerosis	HIV infection Schistosomiasis
Renal amyloidosis	Any chronic infection

adults develop progressive renal failure within 5 years, with 10 percent reaching ESRD. Steroids and cytotoxic agents are contraindicated as they may lead to increased viral replication and worsening of liver disease. Interferon α may reduce proteinuria and stabilize renal function in patients with progressive disease.

Hepatitis C infection (Chap. 295) should be considered in all patients with cryoglobulinemic proliferative glomerulonephritis, MPGN, and membranous glomerulopathy. These three clinocopathologic entities may represent a spectrum of morphologic manifestations of the same pathogenetic process, namely HCV-induced immune-complex disease. Up to 30 percent of patients with chronic HCV infection have an abnormal urinary sediment. HCV infection accounts for 10 to 20 percent of type I MPGN and is a major cause of essential mixed cryoglobulinemia. Renal biopsy reveals typical features of type I MPGN and IgG, IgM, C3, and/or cryoglobulin deposits. Most patients present with nephrotic syndrome and microscopic hematuria and may have red blood cell casts. Liver function tests are usually abnormal, and C3 levels are typically depressed. Anti-HCV antibodies are detected in most patients, and viral RNA has been documented in blood and cryoglobulins. A variety of treatments have been reported to be useful in HCV-induced renal disease including steroids, cytotoxic agents, and plasmapheresis; however, controlled trials to support their use are lacking. More recently, interferon α has been demonstrated to clear antigenemia, lower cryoglobulin levels, and stabilize renal disease. Unfortunately, relapse is usual once the drug is discontinued.

HIV infection (Chap. 308) has been associated with focal segmental glomerulosclerosis, acute diffuse proliferative glomerulonephritis, and mesangioproliferative glomerulonephritis, including IgA nephropathy, MPGN, and membranous glomerulopathy. The classic and most com-

mon HIV-associated glomerulopathy is focal segmental glomerulosclerosis, an entity that is termed *human immunodeficiency virus–associated nephropathy (HIVAN)*. The latter may be the first manifestation of infection in otherwise asymptomatic patients. HIVAN is more common in blacks than in other ethnic groups and is more frequent in intravenous drug abusers with HIV infection than in homosexuals. The disease has been described in all high-risk groups, however, including infants of HIV-positive mothers. Renal biopsy typically reveals glomerular collapse, severe tubulointerstitial inflammation, and microcystic dilatation of renal tubules. A number of characteristic abnormalities are noted on electron microscopy, including tubuloreticular inclusions in glomerular endothelial cells, tubular cells and infiltrating leukocytes, fibrillogranular degeneration of tubular nuclei, and the presence of complex nuclear bodies. The morphologic features distinguish HIVAN from idiopathic focal segmental glomerulosclerosis. The mechanisms of renal cell injury are still being defined. Viral DNA has been demonstrated in the renal epithelia of HIV-infected patients with and without nephropathy, suggesting that pathogenetic factors, other than infection of cells, are required for induction of disease. The typical clinical correlates of HIVAN are severe nephrotic syndrome and rapid progression to ESRD, occurring in weeks to months. Survival on dialysis is particularly poor for patients with clinical AIDS, though asymptomatic carriers have a better prognosis. There is no proven therapy for HIVAN. Anecdotal reports suggest a benefit of steroids, ACE inhibitors, and zidovudine (AZT) in reducing proteinuria, but there are no controlled trials to support their use.

BACTERIAL INFECTIONS (See Table 275-2)   Immune-complex glomerulonephritis is a relatively frequent complication of inefective *endocarditis* (Chap. 126). Other mechanisms of renal injury in bacterial endocarditis include embolic renal infarction, septic abscesses, acute tubular necrosis secondary to septicemia and drug therapy, disseminated intravascular coagulation, and antibiotic-induced acute interstitial nephritis. Patients typically present with microscopic hematuria, urinary red blood cell casts, pyuria and modest proteinuria (nephrotic range in 25 percent of patients), and mild, if any, renal failure. Rheumatoid factor is present in 10 to 70 percent, and circulating immune complexes in 90 percent. Serum complement levels are usually depressed. Renal biopsy reveals mild focal proliferative glomerulonephritis with mesangial and capillary wall deposition of IgG and C3 by immunofluorescence microscopy and subendothelial, mesangial, and subepithelial electron-dense deposits by electron microscopy. Occasional patients develop diffuse necrotizing glomerulonephritis with crescent formation and present with nephritic syndrome or RPGN. Endocarditis-associated glomerulonephritis typically has a good prognosis and resolves with eradication of the underlying infection.

Immune-complex glomerulonephritis complicates 1 to 4 percent of cases of *infected ventriculoatrial shunts*. Nephritis can manifest weeks to years after shunt insertion and usually presents with microscopic hematuria. Nephrotic syndrome occurs in 50 to 60 percent. The usual renal pathology is a membranoproliferative pattern, though diffuse proliferation can also occur. Immunofluorescence reveals IgM and C3 in the capillary wall and mesangial area, while subendothelial deposits and mesangial interposition are seen by electron microscopy. Up to one-third of patients may have residual renal impairment despite removal of the infected shunt and resolution of the infection.

Suppurative infections such as intrathoracic and intraabdominal abscesses, osteomyelitis, and dental abscesses have been associated with glomerulonephritis. The usual presentation is hematuria, urinary red blood cell casts, proteinuria, and acute renal failure. Oliguria and hypertension are common. Pathologic renal lesions include mesangial proliferative, membranoproliferative and diffuse proliferative glomerulonephritis with crescents. Immunofluorescence reveals mesangial and capillary wall deposition predominantly of C3, though IgG and IgM may also be seen.

Nephrotic syndrome complicates 0.3 percent of cases of secondary *syphilis* and 8 percent of congenital syphilis. The usual pathology is membranous glomerulopathy; however, mild mesangial and endocapillary proliferation can occur. IgG and IgM are evident in affected regions by immunofluorescence microscopy, and treponemal antigens have been identified in diseased glomeruli. C3 and C4 are typically depressed in congenital syphilis. The treatment consists of penicillin to eradicate the infection.

Leprosy most commonly causes AA amyloidosis; however, a syndrome resembling acute poststreptococcal glomerulonephritis has also been described.

PROTOZOAN AND PARASITIC INFECTIONS Transient proteinuria (50 percent of cases) and nephrotic syndrome (<1 percent of cases) are complications of infection with *Plasmodium falciparum*. Membranoproliferative glomerulonephritis is the usual pathologic lesion and may respond to eradication of infection. *Plasmodium malariae* has been associated with diffuse or focal proliferative glomerulonephritis, membranous glomerulopathy, and minimal change disease. Eradication of the malarial infection does not consistently induce remission of the nephrotic syndrome. *Schistosoma mansoni* causes nephrotic syndrome in 5 to 10 percent of cases. The usual pathology is MPGN or mesangial proliferative glomerulonephritis, though membranous glomerulonephritis and amyloidosis are occasionally seen. *Filariasis* can trigger membranous glomerulonephritis (*Loa loa*) and occasionally induces proliferative glomerulonephritis (*Onchocerca volvulus*). *Congenital toxoplasmosis* infection occasionally induces immune-complex glomerulonephritis characterized by mesangial and subendothelial immune deposits that contain *Toxoplasma* antigens. Membranous glomerulopathy and proliferative glomerulonephritis occasionally complicate *hydatid disease* and *trichinosis*, respectively.

GLOMERULAR LESIONS ASSOCIATED WITH NEOPLASIA

Glomerulopathies associated with neoplasia include membranous glomerulopathy, minimal change disease, focal segmental glomerulosclerosis, immune-complex glomerulonephritis, fibrillary/immunotactoid glomerulonephritis, LCDD, and amyloidosis. Mild proteinuria is common in patients with *solid tumors*, but overt glomerulonephritis is rare. Patients with solid tumors of the lung, gastrointestinal tract, breast, kidney, and ovary have an increased incidence of nephrotic syndrome, frequently due to a membranous glomerulopathy. Estimates of the incidence of occult malignancy in patients presenting with membranous glomerulopathy range from 0.1 to 10 percent. Most authorities agree that an extensive search for malignancy is not indicated, unless there are other suggestive clinical features. As many as 35 percent of patients with renal cell carcinoma have mesangial deposition of IgG and C3 visible on immunofluorescence; however, morphologic abnormalities are detected in only 50 percent of these patients, and clinically significant glomerulopathy is rare. Glomerular amyloidosis has also been described in association with this tumor.

An array of glomerular disease has been reported in patients with lymphoproliferative malignancy. Nephrotic syndrome is a recognized complication of *Hodgkin's lymphoma*, 70 percent of cases being due to minimal change disease. The latter may occur concurrently with (40 to 45 percent), precede (10 to 15 percent), or follow (40 to 50 percent) diagnosis of the malignancy. It is postulated that a lymphokine or other mediator released by malignant T lymphocytes perturbs podocyte function and alters glomerular permeability in this setting. Nephrotic syndrome typically resolves with successful treatment and relapses with recurrence of disease. Less frequent associations with Hodgkin's lymphoma include focal segmental glomerulosclerosis, membranous glomerulopathy, MPGN, proliferative glomerulonephritis, and crescentic glomerulonephritis. Minimal change disease, membranous glomerulopathy, MPGN, and crescentic glomerulonephritis have also been reported in patients with *non-Hodgkin's lymphoma*. Glomerulopathy in the context of leukemia is rare. MPGN can complicate *chronic lymphatic leukemia* and related *B cell lymphomas*, particularly when associated with cryoglobulinemia. Other glomerular lesions associated with *paraproteinemia* include primary amyloid, LCDD, proliferative glomerulonephritis induced by cryoglobulinemia, and fibrillary/immunotactoid glomerulopathy. Here again, the renal lesion frequently improves or resolves with successful treatment of the underlying malignancy.

BIBLIOGRAPHY

ADLER SG et al: Secondary glomerular diseases, in *The Kidney*, 5th ed, BM Brenner (ed). Philadelphia, Saunders, 1996, pp. 1498–1596
BALOW J: Lupus nephritis. Ann Intern Med 79:106, 1987
BENNETT PH et al: Screening and management of microalbuminuria in patients with diabetes mellitus: Recommendations to the Scientific Advisory Board of the National Kidney Foundation from an ad hoc committee of the Council on Diabetes Mellitus of the National Kidney Foundation. Am J Kidney Dis 25:107, 1995
FALK RJ: ANCA-associated renal disease. Kidney Int 38:998, 1990
GREGORY MC, ATKIN CL: Alport syndrome, in *Diseases of the Kidney*, 5th ed, RW Schrier, CW Gottschalk (eds). Boston, Little, Brown, 1992, pp 571–592
HUMPHREYS MH: Human immunodeficiency virus–associated glomerulosclerosis. Kidney Int 48:311, 1995
JOHNSON R et al: Renal manifestations of hepatitis C virus infection. Kidney Int 46:1265, 1994
PARVING HH et al: Diabetic nephropathy, in *The Kidney*, 5th ed, BM Brenner (ed). Philadelphia, Saunders, 1996, pp 1864–1892
SEALY FD et al: Acquired immunodeficiency syndrome and the kidney. Am J Kidney Dis 16:1, 1990

276 *Barry M. Brenner, Elliott Levy, Thomas H. Hostetter*

TUBULOINTERSTITIAL DISEASES OF THE KIDNEY

An etiologically diverse group of renal diseases can be distinguished from those considered in Chaps. 274 and 275 because the histologic and functional abnormalities involve the tubules and interstitium to a greater degree than the glomeruli and renal vasculature (see Table 276-1). Both clinically and histologically, these disorders can be divided into acute and chronic forms. The chronic group may be due to sustained insults by a factor or factors that initially cause acute disease or to a slower, progressive, cumulative insult without an identifiable acute episode. Morphologically, acute forms of these disorders are characterized by interstitial edema, often associated with cortical and medullary infiltration by polymorphonuclear leukocytes and patchy areas of tubule cell necrosis. In more chronic forms, interstitial fibrosis predominates, inflammatory cells are typically mononuclear, and abnormalities of the tubules tend to be more widespread, as evidenced by atrophy, luminal dilatation, and thickening of tubule basement membranes. Because of the nonspecific nature of the histology, particularly in chronic tubulointerstitial diseases, biopsy specimens rarely provide a specific diagnosis. The urine sediment is also unlikely to be diagnostic, except in allergic forms of acute tubulointerstitial disease, in which eosinophils may predominate in the urinary sediment.

Defects in renal function often accompany these alterations of tubule and interstitial structure (see Table 276-2). Proximal tubule dysfunction may be manifested as selective reabsorptive defects leading to hypokalemia, aminoaciduria, glycosuria, phosphaturia, uricosuria, or bicarbonaturia (proximal or type II renal tubular acidosis; see Chap. 278). In combination, these defects constitute the *Fanconi syndrome*. Protein excretion is usually modest, rarely exceeding 2 g/d.

Defects in urinary acidification and concentrating ability often represent the most troublesome of the tubule dysfunctions encountered in patients with tubulointerstitial disease. Hyperchloremic metabolic acidosis often develops at a relatively early stage in the course. Patients with this finding generally elaborate urine of maximal acidity (pH of 5.3 or less). In such patients the defect in acid excretion is usually caused by a reduced capacity to generate and excrete ammonia due to the reduction in renal mass. Preferential damage to the collecting ducts, as in amyloidosis or chronic obstructive uropathy, also may predispose to distal or type I renal tubular acidosis, characterized by high urine pH (>5.5) during spontaneous or NH_4Cl-induced metabolic

Table 276-1

Principal Causes of Tubulointerstitial Disease of the Kidney

TOXINS

Exogenous toxins
  Analgesic nephropathy*
  Lead nephropathy (see Chap. 397)
  Miscellaneous nephrotoxins (e.g., antibiotics, cyclosporine, radiographic
    contrast media, heavy metals)*†
Metabolic toxins
  Acute uric acid nephropathy (see Chap. 344)
  Gouty nephropathy (see Chap. 344)*
  Hypercalcemic nephropathy (see Chap. 354)
  Hypokalemic nephropathy (see Chap. 49)
  Miscellaneous metabolic toxins (e.g., hyperoxaluria, cystinosis,
    Fabry's disease, see Chap. 346)

NEOPLASIA

Lymphoma (see Chap. 113)
Leukemia (see Chap. 112)
Multiple myeloma (see Chap. 114)*

IMMUNE DISORDERS

Hypersensitivity nephropathy*†
Sjögren's syndrome (see Chap. 316)
Amyloidosis (see Chap. 309)
Transplant rejection (see Chap. 272)†
Tubulointerstitial abnormalities associated with glomerulonephritis
  (see Chaps. 274 and 275)
HIV–associated nephropathy (see Chap. 308)

VASCULAR DISORDERS (see Chaps. 270 and 277)

Arteriolar nephrosclerosis*
Atheroembolic disease
Sickle cell nephropathy
Acute tubular necrosis*†

HEREDITARY RENAL DISEASES

Hereditary nephritis (Alport's syndrome) (see Chaps. 275 and 348)
Medullary cystic disease (see Chap. 278)
Medullary sponge kidney (see Chap. 278)
Polycystic kidney disease (see Chap. 278)

INFECTIOUS INJURY (see Chap. 131)

Acute pyelonephritis*†
Chronic pyelonephritis

MISCELLANEOUS DISORDERS

Chronic urinary tract obstruction (see Chap. 280)*
Vesicoureteral reflux*
Radiation nephritis

* Common.
† Typically acute.

Table 276-2

Transport Dysfunctions of Tubulointerstitial Disease

Defect	Cause(s)
Reduced GFR*	Obliteration of microvasculature and obstruction of tubules
Fanconi syndrome	Damage to proximal tubular reabsorption of glucose, amino acids, phosphate, and bicarbonate
Hyperchloremic acidosis*	1. Reduced ammonia production 2. Inability to acidify the collecting duct fluid (distal renal tubular acidosis) 3. Proximal bicarbonate wasting
Tubular or small-molecular-weight proteinuria*	Failure of proximal tubule protein reabsorption
Polyuria, isothenuria*	Damage to medullary tubules and vasculature
Hyperkalemia*	Potassium secretory defects including aldosterone resistance
Salt wasting	Distal tubular damage with impaired sodium reabsorption

* Common

pH of the fluid within most nephron segments may affect the ionization characteristics of potentially toxic compounds and thereby influence local concentration and solubility. Although these processes render the kidney vulnerable to toxic injury, the role of nephrotoxins in renal damage often goes unrecognized because the manifestations of such injury are usually nonspecific in nature and insidious in onset. Diagnosis largely depends on a history of exposure to a certain toxin. Particular attention should be paid to the occupational history, as well as to an assessment of exposure—current and remote—to drugs, especially antibiotics and analgesics. The recognition of a potential association between a patient's renal disease and exposure to a nephrotoxin is crucial, because, unlike many other forms of renal disease, progression of the functional and morphologic abnormalities associated with toxin-induced nephropathies may be prevented, and even reversed, by eliminating additional exposure.

EXOGENOUS TOXINS   Analgesic nephropathy   A distinct clinicopathologic syndrome has been described in heavy users of analgesic mixtures containing phenacetin in combination with aspirin, acetaminophen, or caffeine. These individuals have an approximately 20-fold increased risk of end-stage renal disease (ESRD). Analgesic nephropathy has been an important cause of chronic renal failure in Australia, Switzerland, Sweden, Belgium, and the southeastern United States.

Morphologically, analgesic nephropathy is characterized by papillary necrosis and tubulointerstitial inflammation. At an early stage, damage to the vascular supply of the inner medulla (vasa recta) leads to a local interstitial inflammatory reaction and, eventually, to papillary ischemia, necrosis, fibrosis, and calcification. The susceptibility of the renal papillae to damage by phenacetin is believed to be related to the establishment of a renal gradient for its acetaminophen metabolite, resulting in papillary tip concentrations tenfold higher than those in renal cortex. Hydration dissipates this gradient and may explain the protective effect of this maneuver in preventing phenacetin-induced papillary necrosis in animals. Aspirin in these analgesic compounds contributes to renal injury by uncoupling oxidative phosphorylation in renal mitochondria and by inhibiting the synthesis of renal prostaglandins, which are potent endogenous renal vasodilator hormones.

Analgesic nephropathy occurs some three to five times more commonly in women than in men. A direct relationship exists between the total amount of analgesic compounds ingested and the degree of renal impairment. The intake of 1.0 g phenacetin per day for 1 to 3 years or the total ingestion of 2 kg phenacetin in combination with other analgesics appears to represent minimum requirements for the development of analgesic nephropathy. In such patients, renal function usually declines gradually, in association with chronic necrosis of papillae and diffuse tubulointerstitial damage to the renal cortex. Occasionally, papillary necrosis may be associated with hematuria and even

acidosis. Patients with tubulointerstitial diseases affecting medullary and papillary structures predominantly also may evidence concentrating defects, with resultant nocturia and polyuria. Analgesic nephropathy and sickle cell disease are prototypes of this form of injury.

TOXINS

Although the kidneys constitute less than 1 percent of total body mass, they receive approximately 20 percent of the cardiac output, and 90 percent or more of renal blood flow is distributed to the renal cortex. Exposure of tubules and interstitium of the renal cortex to circulating toxins is therefore greater than is that of most other tissues. Transport processes in renal tubules contribute further to the intrarenal accumulation of toxins, enhancing local concentrations of noxious agents. The urinary concentrating mechanism also can establish high levels of toxins within medullary and papillary portions of the kidney, predisposing these regions to chemical injury. Finally, the relatively acid renal colic owing to obstruction of a ureter by necrotic tissue. More than half of patients with analgesic nephropathy have pyuria, which, if persistently associated with sterile urine, provides an important clue to the diagnosis. Nonetheless, active pyelonephritis may coexist in patients with analgesic nephropathy. Proteinuria, if present, is typically mild (less than 1 g/d). Patients with analgesic nephropathy are usually unable to generate maximally concentrated urine, reflecting the underlying medullary and papillary damage. An acquired form of distal renal tubular acidosis may contribute to the development of *nephrocalcinosis*. The occurrence of anemia out of proportion to the degree of azotemia also may provide a clue to the diagnosis of analgesic nephropathy. When analgesic nephropathy has progressed to renal insufficiency, the kidneys usually appear bilaterally shrunken on intravenous pyelography, and the calyces are deformed. A "ring sign" on the pyelogram is pathognomonic of papillary necrosis and represents the radiolucent sloughed papilla surrounded by the radiodense contrast material in the calyx. Renal sonography may reveal papillary calcifications surrounding the central sinus complex in a "garland" pattern. Transitional cell carcinoma may develop in the urinary pelvis or ureters as a late complication of analgesic abuse.

 TREATMENT
Every effort must be made to convince the patient who ingests excessive amounts of analgesic combinations to discontinue this hazardous practice. When renal damage is at an early stage, cessation of abuse usually arrests the progression of the nephrotoxic process; not infrequently, overall renal function improves with time. With continued abuse, however, progressive renal damage leads invariably to chronic renal failure.

Whether single-ingredient analgesics, used alone, cause renal disease is controversial. Recent reports have suggested a two- to threefold increase in the risk of ESRD among regular users of acetaminophen, and perhaps nonsteroidal antiinflammatory drugs (NSAIDs), but not among regular users of aspirin. Until conclusive evidence is available, physicians should consider screening regular users of acetaminophen and NSAIDs for evidence of renal disease. In patients with preexisting renal disease, the use of aspirin should be considered.

Lead Nephropathy (See also Chap. 397)   Lead intoxication may produce a chronic tubulointerstitial renal disease. Children who repeatedly ingest lead-based paints may develop kidney disease as adults. Significant occupational exposure may occur in a diverse variety of workplaces where lead-containing metals or paints are heated to high temperatures, such as battery factories, smelters, salvage yards, and firing ranges. Alcohol, illegally distilled in an apparatus constructed from automobile radiators (so-called moonshine), is another cause of lead poisoning. Environmental lead exposure, particularly in industrial regions, may be great enough to produce changes in renal function.

Tubule transport processes enhance the accumulation of lead within renal cells, particularly in the proximal convoluted tubule, leading to cell degeneration, mitochondrial swelling, and eosinophilic intranuclear inclusion bodies rich in lead. In addition to tubule degeneration and atrophy, lead nephropathy is associated with ischemic changes in the glomeruli, fibrosis of the adventitia of small renal arterioles, and focal areas of cortical scarring. Eventually, the kidneys become atrophic. Urinary excretion of lead, porphyrin precursors such as δ-aminolevulinic acid and coproporphyrin, and urobilinogen, may be increased. Patients with chronic lead nephropathy are characteristically *hyperuricemic*, a consequence of enhanced reabsorption of filtered urate. Acute gouty arthritis (so-called saturnine gout) develops in about 50 percent of patients with lead nephropathy, in striking contrast to other forms of chronic renal failure in which de novo gout is rare (also see Chap. 344). Hypertension is also a complication. Therefore, in any patient with slowly progressive renal failure, atrophic kidneys, gout, and hypertension, the diagnosis of lead intoxication should be considered. Features of acute lead intoxication (abdominal colic, anemia, peripheral neuropathy, and encephalopathy) are usually absent.

The diagnosis may be suspected by finding elevated serum levels of lead. However, because blood levels may not be elevated even in the presence of a toxic total-body burden of lead, the quantitation of lead excretion following infusion of the chelating agent calcium disodium edetate is a more reliable indicator of serious lead exposure. Urinary excretion of more than 0.6 mg/d of lead is indicative of overt or potential toxicity.

TREATMENT
Treatment includes removing the patient from the source of exposure and augmenting lead excretion with a chelating agent such as calcium disodium edetate.

Miscellaneous Nephrotoxins   Use of *lithium salts* for manic-depressive illness has been associated with polyuria and polydipsia caused by tubulointerstitial disease. There are only rare reports of chronic renal insufficiency attributable to this agent. Renal function should be followed in patients taking this drug, and caution should be exercised if lithium is employed in patients with underlying renal disease.

The immunosuppressant *cyclosporine* causes both acute and chronic renal injury. The acute injury and the use of cyclosporine in transplantation are discussed in Chap. 272. The chronic injury results in an irreversible reduction in glomerular filtration rate (GFR), with mild proteinuria and arterial hypertension. Hyperkalemia is a relatively common complication and results in part from tubule resistance to aldosterone. Hypomagnesemia due to urinary magnesium wasting is less common but can cause hypocalcemia. The histologic changes in renal tissue include patchy interstitial fibrosis and tubular atrophy. In addition, the intrarenal vasculature often demonstrates hyalinosis, and focal segmental glomerular sclerosis can be present as well. Fibrosis may be the result of a cyclosporine-induced increase in renal collagen production. Vasoconstrictive mediators, such as angiotensin II, or vasoconstriction itself may also play a role in chronic cyclosporine toxicity. In patients receiving this drug for renal transplantation (see Chap. 272), chronic rejection and recurrence of the primary disease may coincide with chronic cyclosporine injury, and on clinical grounds, distinction among these may be difficult. Although most patients experience stable, albeit reduced, renal function, progressive renal injury can occur without a progressive reduction in GFR. Dose reduction appears to mitigate cyclosporine-associated renal fibrosis, but may increase the risk of rejection and graft loss. The optimal dosage of cyclosporine in renal transplantation remains controversial. Treatment of any associated arterial hypertension may lessen renal injury.

Many agents that commonly lead to acute renal failure are also capable of producing tubulointerstitial injury (see Chap. 270). These include antibiotics (e.g., aminoglycosides, amphotericin B), radiographic contrast agents, various hydrocarbons (e.g., carbon tetrachloride), and heavy metals (e.g., mercury, cadmium, and bismuth).

METABOLIC TOXINS   Acute Uric Acid Nephropathy (See also Chap. 344)   Acute overproduction of uric acid and extreme hyperuricemia often lead to a rapidly progressive renal insufficiency, so-called acute uric acid nephropathy. This tubulointerstitial disease is usually seen in patients given cytotoxic drugs for the treatment of lymphoproliferative or myeloproliferative disorders but also may occur in these patients before such treatment is begun. The pathologic changes are largely the result of deposition of uric acid crystals in the kidneys and their collecting systems, leading to partial or complete obstruction of collecting ducts, renal pelvis, or ureter. Since obstruction is often bilateral, patients typically show the clinical course of acute renal failure, characterized by oliguria and rapidly rising serum creatinine concentration. In the early phase uric acid crystals can be found in urine, usually in association with microscopic or gross hematuria. Peak serum uric acid levels vary but are almost always above 1200 μmol/L (20 mg/dL) and may even exceed 3500 μmol/L (60 mg/dL).

Prevention of hyperuricemia in patients at risk by treatment with allopurinol in doses of 200 to 800 mg/d prior to cytotoxic therapy reduces the danger of acute uric acid nephropathy. Once hyperuricemia develops, however, efforts should be directed to preventing deposition of uric acid within the urinary tract. Increasing urine volume with potent diuretics (furosemide or mannitol) effectively lowers intratubular uric acid concentrations, and alkalinization of the urine to pH 7 or greater with sodium bicarbonate and/or a carbonic anhydrase inhibitor (acetazolamide) enhances uric acid solubility. If these efforts, together with allopurinol therapy, are ineffective in preventing acute renal failure, dialysis should be instituted to lower the serum uric acid concentration as well as to treat the acute manifestations of uremia.

Gouty Nephropathy (See also Chap. 344) Patients with less severe but prolonged forms of hyperuricemia are predisposed to a more chronic tubulointerstitial disorder, often referred to as *gouty nephropathy*. The severity of renal involvement correlates with the duration and magnitude of the elevation of the serum uric acid concentration. Histologically, the distinctive feature of gouty nephropathy is the presence of crystalline deposits of uric acid and monosodium urate salts in kidney parenchyma. These deposits not only cause intrarenal obstruction but also incite an inflammatory response, leading to lymphocytic infiltration, foreign-body giant cell reaction, and eventual fibrosis, especially of medullary and papillary regions of the kidney. Bacteriuria and pyelonephritis occur in about one-fourth of cases, presumably as complications of intrarenal urinary stasis. Since patients with gout frequently suffer from hypertension and hyperlipidemia, degenerative changes of the renal arterioles may constitute a striking feature of the histologic abnormality, often out of proportion to other morphologic defects. Clinically, gouty nephropathy is an insidious cause of renal insufficiency. Early in its course, GFR may be near normal, often despite focal morphologic changes in medullary and cortical interstitium, proteinuria, and diminished urinary concentrating ability. Whether reducing serum uric acid levels with allopurinol exerts a beneficial effect on the kidney remains to be demonstrated. Although such undesirable consequences of hyperuricemia as gout and uric acid stones respond well to allopurinol, use of this drug in asymptomatic hyperuricemia has not been shown to improve renal function consistently. On the other hand, uricosuric agents such as probenecid, which may increase uric acid stone production, clearly have no role in the treatment of renal disease associated with hyperuricemia.

Hypercalcemic Nephropathy (See also Chap. 354) Chronic hypercalcemia, as occurs in primary hyperparathyroidism, sarcoidosis, multiple myeloma, vitamin D intoxication, or metastatic bone disease, can cause tubulointerstitial damage and progressive renal insufficiency. The earliest lesion is a focal degenerative change in renal epithelia, primarily in collecting ducts, distal convoluted tubules, and loops of Henle. Tubule cell necrosis leads to nephron obstruction and stasis of intrarenal urine, favoring local precipitation of calcium salts and infection. Dilatation and atrophy of tubules eventually occur, as do interstitial fibrosis, mononuclear leukocyte infiltration, and interstitial calcium deposition (nephrocalcinosis). Calcium deposition also may occur in glomeruli and the walls of renal arterioles.

Clinically, the most striking defect is an inability to concentrate the urine maximally, resulting in polyuria and nocturia. Defective transport of NaCl in the ascending limb of Henle's loop is responsible, at least in part, for this concentrating defect. Additionally, reduced collecting duct responsiveness to vasopressin may contribute. Reductions in GFR and renal blood flow also occur, both in acute severe hypercalcemia and with prolonged hypercalcemia of lesser severity. Distal renal tubular acidosis and sodium and potassium wasting also have been described in these chronic states. Eventually, uncontrolled hypercalcemia leads to severe tubulointerstitial damage and overt renal failure. Abdominal x-rays may demonstrate nephrocalcinosis as well as nephrolithiasis, the latter due to the hypercalciuria that often accompanies hypercalcemia.

℞ **TREATMENT**

This consists of reducing the serum calcium concentration toward normal and correcting the primary abnormality of calcium metabolism. The management of hypercalcemia is discussed in Chap. 354. Prognosis for recovery of renal function depends on the severity of the renal lesion at the time hypercalcemia is corrected. Renal dysfunction of acute hypercalcemia may be completely reversible. Gradual, progressive renal insufficiency related to chronic hypercalcemia, however, may not improve with correction of the calcium disorder. Nonetheless, every effort should be made to return serum calcium concentration to normal to minimize further loss of renal function.

Hypokalemic Nephropathy (See also Chap. 49) Disturbances of renal structure and function occur commonly in patients with moderate to severe potassium depletion of at least several weeks' duration. Histologically, renal epithelial cells are often seen to contain numerous vacuoles, most marked in proximal tubules. Glomeruli are reduced in size and may become sclerotic. Whether prolonged or recurrent potassium deficiency results in irreversible tubulointerstitial fibrosis, scarring, and atrophy is unresolved. Loss of urinary concentrating ability is the most commonly encountered functional defect and is due, at least in part, to defective operation of the countercurrent multiplier system. Elevated rates of intrarenal prostaglandin synthesis also may contribute to this concentrating defect. Nocturia, polyuria, and polydipsia are frequently encountered in patients with chronic potassium depletion. The polydipsia is probably due to both the impaired renal concentrating ability and a primary disorder of the thirst mechanism, which is believed to be a common feature of chronic potassium depletion. Patients with hypokalemic nephropathy may have an enhanced susceptibility to pyelonephritis. Urinalysis often reveals no abnormalities except for mild proteinuria. Serum creatinine and urea nitrogen concentrations usually remain within normal limits.

℞ **TREATMENT**

This should be directed at repleting body potassium stores and correcting the primary process responsible for potassium loss. With correction of body potassium, functional and histologic abnormalities of the kidneys usually disappear, although maximal urinary concentrating ability may not return to normal for several months.

Miscellaneous Metabolic Toxins Urinary oxalate, derived from the metabolism of glycine and, to a variable extent, from ingested oxalate, may deposit as insoluble intratubular calcium oxalate crystals and result in chronic tubulointerstitial damage in patients with hereditary or acquired forms of *hyperoxaluria*. *Cystinosis* and *Fabry's disease* are other hereditary depositional disorders affecting the renal tubules and interstitium (see Chaps. 275, 278, and 279).

RENAL PARENCHYMAL DISEASE ASSOCIATED WITH EXTRARENAL NEOPLASM

Except for the glomerulopathies associated with lymphomas and several solid tumors (see Chap. 275), the renal manifestations of primary extrarenal neoplastic processes are confined mainly to the interstitium and tubules. Although metastatic renal involvement by solid tumors is unusual, the kidneys are often invaded by neoplastic cells in various lymphomas and leukemias and in multiple myeloma. In postmortem studies of patients with *lymphoma*, renal involvement is found in approximately half. The involvement may be focal, in the form of multiple discrete nodules, or diffuse, with lymphomatous infiltration throughout the renal parenchyma. Diffuse infiltration is seen most commonly in lymphomas other than Hodgkin's disease. There may be flank pain related to massive renal infiltration, and x-rays may show enlargement of one or both kidneys. Renal insufficiency occurs in a minority of cases, and overt uremia is rare. Treatment of the primary disease may improve renal function in these cases.

The kidneys are also commonly involved in various forms of *leukemia*. At postmortem examination, bilateral renal involvement is present in approximately 50 percent of cases. As with lymphoma, uremia is rarely, if ever, a consequence of leukemic infiltration of the kidneys. The kidneys also can be involved in leukemias because of the associated high incidence of hyperuricemia, hypercalcemia, and lysozymuria. The myelogenous leukemias, particularly of the monocytic type, may be complicated by tubule defects involving potassium and magnesium wasting.

In contrast, infiltration of the kidneys with *myeloma* cells is infrequent (see also Chap. 114). When it occurs, the process is usually focal, so renal insufficiency from this cause is also uncommon. The more usual lesion is *myeloma kidney*, characterized histologically by atrophic tubules, many with eosinophilic intraluminal casts, and numerous multinucleated giant cells within tubule walls and in the interstitium. The frequent occurrence of myeloma kidney in patients with Bence Jones proteinuria has suggested a causal relation. Bence Jones proteins are thought to cause myeloma kidney through direct toxicity to renal tubule cells. In addition, Bence Jones proteins may precipitate within the distal nephron where the high concentrations of these proteins and the acid composition of the tubule fluid favor intraluminal cast formation and intrarenal obstruction. Occasionally, acute renal failure occurs after intravenous pyelography in patients with multiple myeloma and is believed to result from the further precipitation of Bence Jones proteins induced by dehydration prior to radiographic study. Dehydration of the patient with myeloma in preparation for intravenous pyelography should therefore be avoided. Multiple myeloma also may affect the kidneys indirectly. Hypercalcemia or hyperuricemia may lead to the nephropathies described above. Proximal tubule disorders are also seen occasionally, including type II proximal renal tubular acidosis and the Fanconi syndrome. Additionally, intrarenal deposits of *amyloid* (see below) may contribute to impaired excretory function.

IMMUNE DISORDERS

HYPERSENSITIVITY NEPHROPATHY An acute diffuse tubulointerstitial reaction may result from hypersensitivity to a number of drugs, including sulfonamides, many penicillins and cephalosporins, the fluoroquinolone antibiotics ciprofloxacin and norfloxacin, and the antituberculous drugs isoniazid and rifampin. Acute tubulointerstitial damage has also occurred after use of thiazide and loop diuretics, antiulcer medications (cimetidine, ranitidine, and omeprazole), and NSAIDs. Of note, the tubulointerstitial nephropathy that develops in some patients taking NSAIDs may be associated with nephrotic-range proteinuria and histologic evidence of minimal change glomerulopathy. Grossly, the kidneys are usually enlarged. Histologically, the glomeruli appear normal. The principal pathologic abnormalities are in the interstitium of the kidney, which reveals pronounced edema and infiltration with polymorphonuclear leukocytes, lymphocytes, plasma cells, and, in some cases, large numbers of eosinophils. If the process is severe, tubule cell necrosis and regeneration also may be apparent. Immunofluorescence studies either have been unrevealing or have demonstrated a linear pattern of immunoglobulin and complement deposition along tubule basement membranes. In a few cases of methicillin-induced acute tubulointerstitial disease, circulating anti-tubule basement membrane antibodies also have been found, suggesting that autoantibody formation may have been induced by the penicilloyl hapten of methicillin (by conjugation of hapten with tubule basement membrane proteins, thereby altering the native antigenicity of the basement membrane).

Most patients require several weeks of drug exposure before developing evidence of renal injury. Rare cases have occurred after only a few doses or after a year of more of use. Azotemia is usually present; a diagnostic triad of fever, skin rash, and peripheral blood eosinophilia is highly suggestive of acute tubulointerstitial nephritis but is often absent. Examination of the urine sediment reveals hematuria and often pyuria; occasionally, eosinophils may be present. Proteinuria is usually mild to moderate, except in cases of NSAID-induced tubulointerstitial nephritis with minimal change glomerulopathy. The clinical picture may be confused with acute glomerulonephritis, but when acute azotemia

and hematuria are accompanied by eosinophilia, skin rash, and a history of drug exposure, a hypersensitivity reaction leading to acute tubulointerstitial nephritis should be regarded as the leading diagnostic possibility. Discontinuation of the drug usually results in complete reversal of the renal injury; rarely, renal damage may be irreversible. Glucocorticoids have been used, but their value has not been established.

SJÖGREN'S SYNDROME (See also Chap. 316) When the kidneys are involved in this disorder, the predominant histologic findings are those of chronic tubulointerstitial disease. Interstitial infiltrates are composed primarily of lymphocytes, causing the histology of the renal parenchyma in these patients to resemble that of the salivary and lacrimal glands. Renal functional defects include diminished urinary concentrating ability and distal (type I) renal tubular acidosis. Urinalysis may show pyuria (predominantly lymphocyturia) and mild proteinuria.

AMYLOIDOSIS (See also Chaps. 275 and 309) Glomerular pathology usually predominates and leads to heavy proteinuria and azotemia. However, tubule function also may be deranged, giving rise to a nephrogenic diabetes insipidus and to distal (type I) renal tubular acidosis. In several cases these functional abnormalities correlated with peritubular deposition of amyloid, particularly in areas surrounding vasa rectae, loops of Henle, and collecting ducts. Bilateral enlargement of the kidneys, especially in a patient with massive proteinuria and tubule dysfunction, should raise the possibility of amyloid renal disease.

HUMAN IMMUNODEFICIENCY VIRUS (HIV) INFECTION (See also Chap. 308) Chronic renal disease occurs in a small fraction of patients infected with HIV. This complication usually presents with nephrotic proteinuria and a rapid decline in renal function and may precede overt AIDS. Most patients have a characteristic renal lesion, HIV-associated nephropathy, comprising focal and segmental glomerulosclerosis with collapse of the glomerular tuft, tubular dilatation with cystic change, epithelial cell vacuolization, and a dense mononuclear cell infiltrate of the interstitium. A minority of patients have an immune-complex glomerulonephritis, with HIV-antigen-specific immune complexes. Uncertainty exists whether direct infection of renal cells by the virus or some indirect immune reaction is responsible for the renal disease. In addition to these HIV-specific renal diseases, a diverse array of mycobacterial, fungal, and viral diseases can affect the kidneys in HIV-infected individuals. Additional renal abnormalities may result from repeated exposure to nephrotoxic antibiotics. A thrombotic microangiopathy has also been reported. Black patients with HIV appear to be at particularly high risk for HIV-associated nephropathy. Once ESRD develops, survival depends primarily on the immunologic and functional status of the individual. The value of antiretroviral or steroid therapy in slowing the progression to ESRD has not been proved, whereas angiotensin-converting enzyme inhibitors appear to offer some benefit.

TUBULOINTERSTITIAL ABNORMALITIES ASSOCIATED WITH GLOMERULONEPHRITIS A number of primary glomerulopathies also may be associated with damage to tubules and interstitium. For example, in more than half of patients with the nephropathy of systemic lupus erythematosus, deposits of immune complexes can be identified in tubule basement membranes, usually accompanied by an interstitial mononuclear inflammatory reaction. Similarly, in many patients with glomerulonephritis associated with anti-glomerular basement membrane antibody, the same antibody is reactive against tubule basement membranes as well.

MISCELLANEOUS DISORDERS

VESICOURETERAL REFLUX (See also Chaps. 131 and 280) When the function of the ureterovesical junction is impaired, urine may reflux into the ureters due to the high intravesical pressure that develops during voiding. Clinically, reflux is often detected on the voiding and postvoiding films obtained during intravenous pyelography, although voiding cystourethrography may be required for definitive diagnosis. Bladder infection may ascend the urinary tract to the kidneys through incompetent ureterovesical sphincters. Not surprisingly, therefore, reflux is often discovered in patients with acute and/or chronic urinary tract infections. With more severe degrees of reflux, characterized by dilatation of ureters and renal pelves, progressive renal damage often appears, and although active infection also may be present, uncertainty exists as to the necessity of infection in producing the scarred kidney of reflux nephropathy. Substantial proteinuria is often present, and glomerular lesions similar to those of idiopathic focal glomerulosclerosis (Chap. 274) are often found in addition to the changes of chronic tubulointerstitial disease. Surgical correction of reflux is usually necessary only with the more severe degrees of reflux since renal damage correlates with the extent of reflux. Obviously, if extensive glomerulosclerosis already exists, urologic repair may no longer be warranted.

RADIATION NEPHRITIS Renal dysfunction can be expected to occur if 23 Gy (2300 rad) or more of x-ray irradiation is administered to both kidneys during a period of 5 weeks or less. Histologic examination of the kidneys reveals hyalinized glomeruli, atrophic tubules, extensive interstitial fibrosis, and hyalinization of the media of renal arterioles. Radiation-induced renal ischemia is believed to be the main pathogenic factor responsible for the tubulointerstitial damage, which may not become evident clinically for months after completion of radiation. The presentation of acute radiation nephritis includes rapidly progressive azotemia, moderate to malignant hypertension, anemia, and proteinuria that may reach the nephrotic range. More than 50 percent progress to chronic renal failure. A more insidious form is characterized by slower development of azotemia, anemia, and nephrotic syndrome. Malignant hypertension may follow unilateral renal irradiation and resolve with ipsilateral nephrectomy. Radiation nephritis has all but vanished because of heightened awareness of its pathogenesis by radiotherapists.

BIBLIOGRAPHY

ADLER SG et al: Hypersensitivity phenomena and the kidney: Role of drugs and environmental agents. Am J Kidney Dis 5:75, 1985

ARANT BS: Reflux nephropathy. Kidney 21:19, 1989

BENNET WM: Lead nephropathy. Kidney Int 28:218, 1985

———, DEBROE ME: Analgesic nephropathy. A preventable renal disease. N Engl J Med 320, 1269, 1989

KELLY CJ, NEILSON EG: Tubulointerstitial diseases, in The Kidney, 5th ed, BM Brenner (ed). Philadelphia, Saunders, 1996 pp 1655–1679

BOTON R et al: Prevalence, pathogenesis, and treatment of renal dysfunction associated with chronic lithium therapy. Am J Kidney Dis 10:329, 1987

CAMERON JS: Immunologically mediated interstitial nephritis: Primary and secondary. Adv Nephrol 18:207, 1989

LUKE RG: New issues in therapy after renal transplantation. N Engl J Med 331:393, 1994

MYERS BD et al: The long-term course of cyclosporine-associated chronic nephropathy. Kidney Int 33:590, 1988

PERNEGER TV et al: Risk of renal failure associated with the use of acetaminophen, aspirin, and nonsteroidal antiinflammatory drugs. N Engl J Med 331:1675, 1994

RAO TKS: Clinical features of human immunodeficiency virus associated nephropathy. Kidney Int 40(Suppl 35):S-13, 1991

277

Kamal F. Badr, Barry M. Brenner

VASCULAR INJURY TO THE KIDNEY

Adequate delivery of blood to the glomerular capillary network is crucial for glomerular filtration and overall salt and water balance. Thus, in addition to the threat to the viability of renal tissue, vascular injury to the kidney may compromise the maintenance of body fluid volume and composition. Involvement of the renal vessels by atherosclerotic, hypertensive, embolic, inflammatory, and hematologic disorders is usually a manifestation of generalized vascular pathology. The morphologic and clinical responses to these insults and the unique renal vasculopathy associated with the toxemias of pregnancy are considered in this chapter.

THROMBOEMBOLIC DISEASES OF THE RENAL ARTERIES Thrombosis of the major renal arteries or their branches is an important cause of deterioration of renal function, especially in the elderly. It is often difficult to diagnose and therefore requires a high index of suspicion. Thrombosis may occur as a result of intrinsic pathology in the renal vessels (posttraumatic, atherosclerotic, or inflammatory) or as a result of emboli originating in distant vessels, most commonly fat emboli, emboli originating in the left heart (mural thrombi following myocardial infarction, bacterial endocarditis, or aseptic vegetations), or "paradoxical" emboli passing from the right side of the circulation via a patent foramen ovale or atrial septal defect. Renal emboli are bilateral in 15 to 30 percent of cases.

The clinical presentation is variable, depending on the time course and the extent of the occlusive event. Acute thrombosis and infarction, such as follows embolization, may result in sudden onset of flank pain and tenderness, fever, hematuria, leukocytosis, nausea, and vomiting. If infarction occurs, renal enzymes may be elevated, namely aspartate aminotransferase (AST), lactic dehydrogenase (LDH; most reliable), and alkaline phosphatase, which rise and fall in the order listed. Urinary lactic dehydrogenase and alkaline phosphatase also may increase after infarction. Renal function deteriorates acutely, leading in bilateral thrombosis to acute oliguric renal failure. More gradual (i.e., atherosclerotic) occlusion of a single renal artery may go undetected. A spectrum of clinical presentations lies between these two extremes (Table 277-1). Hypertension usually follows renal infarction and results from renin release in the peri-infarction zone. Hypertension is usually transient but may be persistent. Diagnosis is established by renal arteriography.

℞ TREATMENT

Management of *acute* renal arterial thrombosis includes surgical intervention, anticoagulant therapy, conservative and supportive therapy, and control of hypertension. The choice of treatment depends mainly on (1) the condition of the patient, in particular the patient's ability to withstand major surgery, and (2) the extent of renovascular occlusion and amount of renal mass at risk of infarction. In general, supportive care and anticoagulant therapy are indicated in unilateral disease. In bilateral thrombosis, medical and surgical therapies yield comparable results. Twenty-five percent of patients die during the acute episode, usually from extrarenal complications. In *chronic* ischemic renal disease, surgical revascularization is more likely to preserve and improve renal function and to control the hypertension (see below).

ATHEROEMBOLIC DISEASE OF THE RENAL ARTERIES Atheroembolic disease typically results from multiple showers of cholesterol-containing microemboli dislodged from atheromatous plaques in large arteries. Such emboli occlude small (150- to 200-μm diameter) vessels in the kidneys and in other organs (retina, brain, pancreas, muscles, skin, and extremities). It usually occurs in an elderly individual with atherosclerotic disease elsewhere and usually follows aortic surgery or renal or coronary arteriography. Spontaneous atheroembolic disease has also been reported. Manifestations include deterioration of renal function (sudden or gradual), mild proteinuria, microscopic hematuria, and leukocyturia. Urine volume may remain normal or fall to oliguric levels depending on severity. Renal ischemia can induce or exacerbate preexisting hypertension.

Table 277-1

Clinical Presentations of Ischemic Renal Disease

Acute renal failure

Progressive azotemia in a patient with known renovascular hypertension (usually on medical therapy)

Unexplained progressive azotemia in an elderly patient with or without refractory hypertension

Hypertension and azotemia in a renal transplant patient

Antemortem diagnosis of atherosclerotic renal emboli is difficult. The demonstration of cholesterol emboli in the retina is helpful, but a firm diagnosis is established only by demonstration of cholesterol crystals in the smaller arteries and arterioles in renal biopsy or autopsy specimens. These also may be seen in asymptomatic skeletal muscle or skin. No specific treatment is available.

RENAL VEIN THROMBOSIS (RVT) Thrombosis of one or both main renal veins occurs in a variety of settings (Table 277-2). The pathogenesis is not always clear, particularly when it occurs in so-called hypercoagulable states such as may develop in pregnant women, users of oral contraceptives, subjects with nephrotic syndrome, or dehydrated infants. Nephrotic syndrome accompanying membranous glomerulopathy and certain carcinomas seems to predispose to the development of RVT, which occurs in 10 to 50 percent of patients with these disorders. RVT may exacerbate preexisting proteinuria but is infrequently the cause of the nephrotic syndrome.

The clinical manifestations depend on the severity and abruptness of its occurrence. Acute cases occur typically in children and are characterized by sudden loss of renal function, often accompanied by fever, chills, lumbar tenderness (with kidney enlargement), leukocytosis, and hematuria. Hemorrhagic infarction and renal rupture may lead to hypovolemic shock. In young adults RVT is usually suspected from an unexpected and relatively acute or subacute deterioration of renal function and/or exacerbation of proteinuria and hematuria in the appropriate clinical setting (underlying nephrotic syndrome, trauma, pregnancy, oral contraceptive use). In cases of gradual thrombosis, usually occurring in the elderly, the only manifestation may be recurrent pulmonary emboli or development of hypertension. A Fanconi-like syndrome and proximal renal tubular acidosis have been described.

The definitive diagnosis can only be established through selective renal venography with visualization of the occluding thrombus.

℞ TREATMENT

Treatment consists of anticoagulation, the main purpose of which is prevention of pulmonary embolization, although some authors have also claimed improvement in renal function and proteinuria. Encouraging reports have appeared concerning the use of streptokinase. Spontaneous recanalization with clinical improvement also has been observed. Anticoagulant therapy is more rewarding in the acute thrombosis seen in younger individuals. Nephrectomy is advocated in infants with life-threatening renal infarction. Thrombectomy is effective in some cases.

RENAL ARTERY STENOSIS/ISCHEMIC RENAL DISEASE Stenosis of the main renal artery and/or its major branches accounts for 2 to 5 percent of hypertension. The common cause in the middle-aged and elderly is an atheromatous plaque at the origin of the renal artery. In a large unselected autopsy series, stenosis producing > 50 percent renal artery diameter reduction was found in 18 percent of those between 65 and 74 years of age and in 42 percent of those older than 75 years. Bilateral involvement was found in half of the affected cases in both age groups. In younger women, stenosis is due to intrinsic structural abnormalities of the arterial wall caused by a heterogeneous group of lesions termed *fibromuscular dysplasia*.

Renal artery stenosis should be suspected when hypertension develops in a previously normotensive individual over 50 years of age or in the young (under 30 years) with suggestive features: symptoms of vascular insufficiency to other organs, high-pitched epigastric bruit on physical examination, symptoms of hypokalemia secondary to hyperal-

dosteronism (muscle weakness, tetany, polyuria), and metabolic alkalosis. If renovascular hypertension is suspected, a positive captopril test, which has a sensitivity and specificity of greater than 95 percent, constitutes an excellent screening procedure to assess the need for more invasive radiographic evaluation. The test relies on the exaggerated increase in plasma renin activity (PRA) following administration of captopril to patients with renovascular hypertension as compared with those with essential hypertension. It is considered positive when all the following criteria are satisfied: stimulated PRA of 12 (μg/L)/h, absolute increase in PRA of 10 (μg/L)/h or more, and increase in PRA of greater than 150 percent [or 400 percent if baseline PRA is less than 3 (μg/L)/h]. In the appropriate clinical setting, particularly in the presence of a positive captopril test, digital subtraction renal arteriography should be performed. This procedure obviates the need for cannulation of the arterial system and has a low incidence of false-positive (5 percent) and false-negative (10 percent) results. Since angiotensin I–converting enzyme (ACE) inhibitors magnify the impairment in renal blood flow and glomerular filtration rate (GFR) caused by functionally significant renal artery stenosis, use of these drugs in association with ^{99m}Tc-DTPA or ^{99m}MAG$_3$ renography greatly enhances the predictive value of radionuclide renography (>90 percent sensitivity and specificity). The most definitive diagnostic procedure is bilateral arteriography with repeated bilateral renal vein and systemic renin determinations. If renal vein renin measurements from the two kidneys differ by a factor of 1.5:1 or more (higher value from the affected kidney) in a patient with radiographic unilateral renal artery stenosis, the chance of cure of hypertension by surgical reconstruction is almost 90 percent, particularly if renal vein renin level from the unaffected kidney is equal to or less than systemic levels (suppressible). A ratio of less than 1.5:1, however, does not exclude the diagnosis of renovascular hypertension, particularly in the presence of bilateral disease. Two diagnostic modalities for the noninvasive evaluation of significant renal artery stenosis are duplex scanning (sensitivity 95 percent, specificity 90 percent) and magnetic resonance angiography (sensitivity 100 percent for lesions with ≥50 percent stenosis, specificity 92 percent).

℞ TREATMENT

The aims of treatment are control of the blood pressure and restoration of perfusion to the ischemic kidney. In general, it is now firmly established that interventional therapy (i.e., surgery or angioplasty) is superior to medical therapy, which, while controlling blood pressure, does little to salvage renal mass lost to ischemic injury. Success rates with percutaneous transluminal angioplasty in young patients with fibromuscular dysplasia are 50 percent cure and improvement in blood pressure control in another 30 percent. Angioplasty is best suited for noncalcified, segmental short lesions and is also useful in some elderly patients who are poor surgical risks. About half of elderly individuals with reduced renal function as a result of renal arterial stenosis improve following angioplasty or surgery, even when preintervention arteriography shows little evidence of cortical perfusion. Despite the risks associated with surgery, long-term follow-up studies demonstrate an advantage of surgery over angioplasty both with regard to the incidence of restenosis and to the preservation or improvement in GFR.

Renal artery stenosis, particularly if atherosclerotic, is a progressive disease that may lead to gradual and silent loss of renal functional tissue (ischemic renal disease). Progression of ipsilateral atherosclerotic narrowing can be expected in nearly 50 percent of individuals, resulting in complete occlusion in about 10 percent. Thus, these patients need careful follow-up of initially nonclinically significant narrowing (<70 percent) for the possibility of further occlusion or the development of contralateral disease (30 percent). Compensatory contralateral hypertrophy may maintain renal function until affected by superimposed pathologic processes, at which time azotemia supervenes. Ischemic renal disease is now recognized as a significant cause of end-stage renal dis-

Table 277-2

Conditions Associated with Renal Vein Thrombosis

Trauma
Extrinsic compression (lymph nodes, aortic aneurysm, tumor)
Invasion by renal cell carcinoma
Dehydration (infants)
Nephrotic syndrome
Pregnancy or oral contraceptives

ease in patients over 50 years of age (approximately 15 percent). Even if angioplasty or surgery fail to return blood pressure to normal, these procedures usually render medical therapy easier.

HEMOLYTIC UREMIC SYNDROME (HUS) AND THROMBOTIC THROMBOCYTOPENIC PURPURA (TTP) (See also Chap. 117)

HUS and TTP, consumptive coagulopathies characterized by microangiopathic hemolytic anemia and thrombocytopenia, have a particular predilection for the kidney and the central nervous system, the latter especially in TTP. The kidneys of patients with HUS or TTP often exhibit a "flea-bitten" appearance, the result of multiple cortical hemorrhagic infarcts. The major sites of pathology are the small renal arteries and afferent arterioles, which are nearly occluded as a result of marked intimal hyperplasia (particularly in TTP) and fibrin deposits in the subintimal regions. When the vasoocclusive process is extensive, bilateral cortical necrosis may occur. In addition, arteriolar microaneurysms, glomerular infarction, or nonspecific focal changes may be seen. In keeping with the focal nature of the vascular lesions, patchy areas of interstitial edema, tubular necrosis, and, eventually, fibrosis occur. By immunofluorescence staining, complement components and immunoglobulins may be demonstrated in the arterioles, and fibrinogen deposits are present in arteries, arterioles, and glomerular capillary loops.

Several mechanisms have been implicated in the etiology of the intravascular coagulopathy seen in HUS and TTP, including induction of a generalized Shwartzman phenomenon by microorganisms or endotoxin, genetic predisposition, and deficiency of platelet antiaggregatory substance(s) (e.g., prostacyclin). Some patients improve following exchange transfusion or plasmapheresis, suggesting accumulation of an as yet unidentified toxin.

Renal failure is common in both HUS and TTP, usually manifested by azotemia, mild proteinuria, microscopic and/or gross hematuria, and cylindruria. Patients with HUS have more severe renal failure, often marked by oligoanuria and hypertension and commonly progressing to chronic renal failure. The prognosis in HUS is better in children than in adults. In TTP, the course of which may span days to months, renal failure is usually less severe.

℞ TREATMENT

In the management of TTP, high-dose glucocorticoids and plasma exchange often provide complete remission or cure. Plasma exchange should be initiated as early as possible, and the treatment cycles can be repeated if thrombocytopenia recurs. Splenectomy and antiplatelet therapy also have been used with varying degrees of success in TTP patients. The success of plasma exchange in adult HUS is less well established than in TTP.

ARTERIOLAR NEPHROSCLEROSIS (See also Chap. 242)

Whether hypertension is "essential" or of known etiology, persistent exposure of the renal circulation to elevated intraluminal pressures results in development of intrinsic lesions of the renal arterioles (hyaline arteriolosclerosis) that eventually lead to loss of function (nephrosclerosis). Nephrosclerosis is divided into two distinct entities: "benign" and "malignant" (or accelerated).

Benign Arteriolar Nephrosclerosis Benign arteriolar nephrosclerosis is seen in patients who are hypertensive for an extended period of time (blood pressure more than 150/90 mmHg) but whose hypertension has not progressed to a malignant form (described below). Such patients, usually in the older age group, are often discovered to be hypertensive on routine physical examination or as a result of nonspecific symptomatology (e.g., headaches, weakness, palpitations).

Kidney size is normal to reduced, with loss of cortical mass leading to a fine granularity. Although the larger arteries may show atherosclerotic changes, the characteristic pathology is in the afferent arterioles, which have thickened walls due to deposition of homogeneous eosinophilic material (hyaline arteriolosclerosis). This material is composed of plasma proteins and fats that have been deposited in the arteriolar

wall due to injury to the endothelium, probably secondary to the elevated intraluminal hydraulic pressure. Narrowing of vascular lumina results, with consequent ischemic injury to glomeruli and tubules.

Nephrosclerosis accompanying long-standing systemic arterial hypertension is only one manifestation of a generalized process affecting the cardiovascular system. Physical examination, therefore, may reveal changes in retinal vessels (arteriolar narrowing and/or flame-shaped hemorrhages), cardiac hypertrophy, and possibly signs of congestive heart failure. Renal disease may manifest as a mild to moderate elevation of serum creatinine concentration, microscopic hematuria, and/or mild proteinuria. In general, clinical evaluation does not reveal significant renal abnormalities. More specialized examination may disclose elevated urinary albumin excretion, tapering and loss of caliber of intrarenal vessels on arteriography, and an exaggerated natriuresis in response to a fluid challenge. Patients with benign nephrosclerosis maintain a near-normal GFR despite a reduction in renal blood flow.

Malignant Arteriolar Nephrosclerosis Patients with long-standing benign hypertension or patients not known to be hypertensive previously may develop malignant hypertension characterized by a sudden (accelerated) elevation of blood pressure (diastolic often above 130 mmHg) accompanied by papilledema, central nervous system manifestations, cardiac decompensation, and acute progressive deterioration of renal function. The absence of papilledema does not rule out the diagnosis in a patient with markedly elevated blood pressure and rapidly declining renal function. The kidneys are characterized by a flea-bitten appearance resulting from hemorrhages in surface capillaries. Histologically, two distinct vascular lesions can be seen. The first, affecting arterioles, is fibrinoid necrosis, i.e., infiltration of arteriolar walls with eosinophilic material including fibrin. There is thickening of vessel walls and, occasionally, an inflammatory infiltrate (necrotizing arteriolitis). The second lesion, involving the interlobular arteries, is a concentric hyperplastic proliferation of the cellular elements of the vascular wall with deposition of collagen to form a hyperplastic arteriolitis (onion-skin lesion). Fibrinoid necrosis occasionally extends into the glomeruli, which also may undergo proliferative changes or total necrosis. Most glomerular and tubular changes are secondary to ischemia and infarction. The sequence of events leading to the development of malignant hypertension is poorly defined. Two pathophysiologic alterations appear central in its initiation and/or perpetuation: (1) increased permeability of vessel walls to invasion by plasma components, particularly fibrin, which activates clotting mechanisms leading to a microangiopathic hemolytic anemia, thus perpetuating the vascular pathology; and (2) activation of the renin-angiotensin-aldosterone system at some point in the disease process, which contributes to the acceleration and maintenance of blood pressure elevation and, in turn, to vascular injury.

Malignant hypertension is most likely to develop in a previously hypertensive individual, usually in the third or fourth decade of life. There is a higher incidence among men, particularly black men. The presenting symptoms are usually neurologic (dizziness, headache, blurring of vision, altered states of consciousness, and focal or generalized seizures). Cardiac decompensation and renal failure appear thereafter. Renal abnormalities include a rapid rise in serum creatinine, hematuria (at times macroscopic), proteinuria, and red and white blood cell casts in the sediment. Nephrotic syndrome may be present. Elevated plasma aldosterone levels cause hypokalemic metabolic alkalosis in the early phase. Uremic acidosis and hyperkalemia eventually obscure these early findings. Hematologic indices of microangiopathic hemolytic anemia (i.e., schistocytes) are often seen.

℞ TREATMENT

Control of hypertension is the principal goal of therapy for both benign and malignant forms. The time of initiation of therapy, its effectiveness, and patient compliance are crucial factors in arresting the progression of benign nephrosclerosis. Untreated, most of these patients succumb to the extrarenal complications of hypertension. In contrast, malignant hypertension is a medical emergency; its natural course includes a death rate of 80 to 90 percent within 1 year of onset, almost always due to uremia. Supportive measures should be instituted to control the neurologic, cardiac, and other complications of acute renal failure, but the mainstay of therapy is prompt and aggressive reduction of blood pressure, which, if successful, can reverse all complications in the majority of patients. Presently, 5-year survival is 50 percent, and some patients have evidence of partial reversal of the vascular lesions and a return of renal function to near-normal levels.

SCLERODERMA (PROGRESSIVE SYSTEMIC SCLEROSIS) (See also Chap. 314)

Renal vascular involvement in scleroderma is characterized by a distinctive lesion of the small arteries (diameters of 150 to 500 µm) consisting of intimal proliferation, medial thinning, and increased collagen deposition in the adventitial layer. Fibrinoid changes in the walls of afferent arterioles and microinfarcts may occur. Glomerular changes are generally nonspecific and secondary to ischemic damage. Tubules are often atrophic. As part of a generalized increase in vasomotor tone, a vasospastic (Raynaud-like) phenomenon at the level of the renal vasculature contributes to the renal insufficiency. Reduction in renal blood flow is the major mechanism underlying the deterioration in kidney function, being present in 80 percent of patients, even in the absence of other clinical abnormalities. As vascular narrowing progresses, hypertension, azotemia, and proteinuria eventually develop. Plasma renin rises in response to sustained renal ischemia. The resulting hypertension causes further renal injury and may play a role in the ultimate destruction of nephrons. As more and more nephrons are lost to the combined insults of ischemia and hypertension, development of azotemia heralds a particularly grim prognosis. Proteinuria, usually mild, is a consequence of ischemic and hypertensive glomerular injury.

Although the majority of patients with scleroderma present with extrarenal manifestations, renal involvement is eventually manifested in half of patients followed for up to 20 years. Renal involvement can present in one of two ways, depending on whether malignant hypertension is superimposed on the renal pathology: (1) *Persistent urinary abnormalities* with or without hypertension tend to follow an indolent course with mild proteinuria, occasional casts, cellular elements in the urinary sediment, and a propensity for development of hypertension. Azotemia is absent initially, but when it develops, dialysis is required within 1 year. (2) *Scleroderma renal crisis* is a rapid deterioration in renal function, usually accompanied by malignant hypertension, oliguria, fluid retention, microangiopathic hemolytic anemia, and central nervous system involvement. It may occur in patients with previously undemonstrable or slowly progressive renal disease. Untreated, it leads to chronic renal failure within days to months.

The prognosis of scleroderma renal disease is generally poor, particularly following the onset of azotemia. Aggressive antihypertensive therapy may be effective in delaying the progression of renal failure. In scleroderma renal crisis, prompt treatment with beta blockers, minoxidil, and particularly ACE inhibitors may reverse acute renal failure. The effect of these interventions on renal function over the long term is uncertain.

SICKLE CELL NEPHROPATHY (See also Chaps. 107 and 275)

Sickle cell disease causes renal complications that arise mainly as a result of sickling of red blood cells in the microvasculature. The hypertonic and relatively hypoxic environment of the renal medulla, coupled with the slow blood flow in the vasa recta, favors the sickling of red blood cells, with resultant local infarction (papillary necrosis). Functional tubule defects in patients with sickle cell disease are likely the result of partial ischemic injury to the renal tubules.

In addition to the intrarenal microvascular pathology described above, young patients with sickle cell disease are characterized by renal hyperperfusion, glomerular hypertrophy, and hyperfiltration. Many of these individuals eventually develop a glomerulopathy leading to glomerular proteinuria (present in as many as 30 percent) and, in some, the nephrotic syndrome. Mild azotemia and hyperuricemia also can develop, but advanced renal failure and uremia are rare. Pathologic examination reveals the typical lesion of "hyperfiltration nephropathy," namely, focal segmental glomerular sclerosis. This has led to the

suggestion that anemia-induced hyperfiltration in childhood is the principal cause of the adult glomerulopathy. Nephron loss secondary to ischemic injury also contributes to the development of azotemia in these patients.

In addition to the glomerulopathy described above, renal complications of sickle cell disease include the following: *Cortical infarcts* can cause loss of function, persistent hematuria, and perinephric hematomas. *Papillary infarcts*, demonstrated radiographically in 50 percent of patients with sickle trait, lead to an increased risk of bacterial infection in the scarred renal tissues and functional tubule abnormalities. Painless gross hematuria occurs with a higher frequency in sickle trait than in sickle cell disease and likely results from infarctive episodes in the renal medulla. *Functional tubule abnormalities* such as nephrogenic diabetes insipidus result from marked reduction in vasa recta blood flow, combined with ischemic tubule injury. This concentrating defect places these patients at increased risk of dehydration and, hence, sickling crises. The concentrating defect also occurs in individuals with sickle trait. Other tubule defects involve potassium and hydrogen ion excretion, occasionally leading to hyperkalemic metabolic acidosis and a defect in uric acid excretion which, combined with increased purine synthesis in the bone marrow, results in hyperuricemia.

Management of sickle nephropathy is not separate from that of overall patient management (see Chap. 107). In addition, however, the use of ACE inhibitors has been associated with improvement of the hyperfiltration glomerulopathy.

TOXEMIAS OF PREGNANCY (See also Chap. 7)

Renal function is "reset" at a higher level during normal pregnancy. Renal plasma flow and GFR both increase by 30 to 50 percent. Therefore, serum creatinine levels above 70 µmol/L (0.8 mg/dL) or blood urea nitrogen (BUN) levels above 4.6 mmol/L (13 mg/dL) are abnormal in pregnant women and should be investigated. Systolic and diastolic blood pressures decrease by an average of 10 to 15 mmHg below pregravid values. A diastolic pressure above 75 mmHg during the second trimester or above 85 mmHg during the third trimester is therefore abnormal. Vasodilation in the uterine, renal, and cutaneous beds, vasodilator prostaglandin release from the uteroplacental unit, and a decrease in arteriolar sensitivity to angiotensin II all play a role in the decline of blood pressure during pregnancy.

Preeclampsia-Eclampsia The toxemia syndrome, usually occurring in the third trimester of primigravidas, includes hypertension, proteinuria, edema, consumptive coagulopathy, sodium retention, hyperreflexia (preeclampsia), and, if uncontrolled, convulsions (eclampsia). In pure preeclampsia (i.e., not superimposed on previously existing hypertensive or renal disease), the primary sites of pathology are the glomerular endothelial cells. These cells show marked swelling due to an increase in cytoplasmic volume with vacuolization (endotheliosis) and encroach on the vascular lumen, rendering the enlarged glomeruli ischemic. The glomerular basement membrane and the extraglomerular blood vessels are intact. The pathogenesis is unknown. Coagulation abnormalities, hormonal factors, uteroplacental ischemia, and immune mechanisms have all been implicated. Recent evidence suggests that increased microvascular reactivity is a result of endothelial cell change, which, in turn, alters the balance of endothelium-derived vasodilator/vasoconstrictor autacoids. These include reduced synthesis of nitric oxide and altered eicosanoid (thromboxane/prostacyclin) balance. Despite sodium retention, intravascular volume is contracted as compared with pregravid values. An increased sensitivity to angiotensin II is the basis for the "roll-over test" (an increase in diastolic blood pressure of 20 mmHg or more upon changing the patient's position from lateral recumbent to supine, presumably due to alterations in circulating angiotensin levels). In the supine position, the reduction in venous return due to compression by the gravid uterus increases circulating levels of angiotensin II. This results in a hypertensive response in preeclamptic patients, who are hyperresponsive to angiotensin II, but not in normal women, in whom pregnancy leads to a relative resistance to the pressor effects of this hormone.

A diagnosis of preeclampsia-related hypertension can be made when repeated measurements over a 4- to 6-h period show a blood pressure of 140/85 mmHg or more. The rise in blood pressure tends to be more severe at night. When preeclampsia occurs in a previously hypertensive patient, a rapid acceleration of the blood pressure elevation is accompanied by an increase in proteinuria, oliguria, edema, and coagulopathy. This is a life-threatening syndrome and tends to recur with future pregnancies. In addition to proteinuria, which correlates with the severity of the renal lesion, GFR and renal plasma flow are depressed. In view of the preexisting high levels, however, GFR in preeclamptic women often remains above nonpregnant levels. Uric acid clearance also falls, resulting in hyperuricemia. In the postpartum period, these patients are particularly susceptible to the development of "postpartum renal failure," which is thought to be a form of adult HUS.

℞ TREATMENT

This consists of bed rest in a quiet environment and control of neurologic manifestations and blood pressure, the former with magnesium sulfate and the latter usually with vasodilators such as hydralazine and methyldopa. Diuretics are avoided. The ultimate "treatment" is delivery, which should be induced if fetal maturity is adequate or if life-threatening coagulopathy or renal failure occur. The long-term prognosis is generally favorable.

Development of acute renal failure/preeclampsia in a pregnant woman should alert the physician to potential preexisting renal disease and/or hypertension. The latter is particularly likely if systolic blood pressure is greater than 200 mmHg. Hypertension and preexisting proteinuria tend to worsen in 50 percent of women during pregnancy. In addition, these abnormalities may be unmasked during pregnancy as the first manifestations of an underlying glomerulopathy. Conversely, patients with established underlying renal disease should be followed closely during pregnancy, with monthly measurements of 24-h urinary protein excretion and GFR. Sudden deterioration should raise suspicion of superimposed preeclampsia. There is no convincing evidence that pregnancy has an adverse effect on the long-term outcome of immunologic glomerular diseases or diabetic nephropathy. In all situations, control of blood pressure should be the primary therapeutic goal in view of its established beneficial effects on the progression of renal injury.

Bilateral Cortical Necrosis Acute bilateral cortical necrosis is associated with septic abortions, abruptio placentae, and preeclampsia. Coagulation in cortical vessels and arterioles leads to renal tissue necrosis. Anuria and renal failure ensue and may be irreversible. In other cases, renal function returns partially, but on long-term follow-up most patients slowly progress to uremia.

BIBLIOGRAPHY

BARRÉ P et al: Successful treatment with streptokinase of renal vein thrombosis associated with oral contraceptive use. Am J Nephrol 6:316, 1986

BAYLIS C: Nitric oxide and preeclampsia, in *Nitric Oxide and the Kidney: Physiology and Pathophysiology*, MS Goligorsky (ed). London, Chapman Hall, in press

BREYER JA, JACOBSON HR: Ischemic nephropathy. Curr Opin Nephrol Hypertens 2:216, 1993

EKNOYAN G, RIGGS SA: Renal involvement in patients with thrombotic thrombocytopenic purpura. Am J Nephrol 6:117, 1986

GUASCH A et al: Early detection and the course of glomerular injury in patients with sickle cell anemia. Kidney Int 49:786–791, 1996

HARDING MB et al: Renal artery stenosis: Prevalence and associated risk factors in patients undergoing routine cardiac catheterization. J Am Soc Nephrol 2:1608, 1992

KASHGARIAN M: Pathology of small blood vessels in hypertension. Am J Kidney Dis 5:A104, 1985

LLACH F: *Renal Vein Thrombosis*. New York, Futura, 1983

MANN SJ, PICKERING TG: Screening for renovascular hypertension. Ann Intern Med 118:906, 1993

MCLEAN AG et al: Screening for renovascular disease with captopril-enhanced renography. Nephrol Dial Transplant 7:211, 1992

REDMAN CWG: Hypertension in pregnancy, in *Medical Disorders in Obstetric Practice*, M DeSwiet (ed). Oxford, Blackwell Scientific, 1995

RIMMER JM, GENNARI FJ: Atherosclerotic renovascular disease and progressive renal failure. Ann Intern Med 118:712, 1993

SYMPOSIUM ON ISCHEMIC RENAL DISEASE: Am J Kidney Dis 24:614, 1994

WILCOX CS: Use of angiotensin-converting enzyme inhibitors for diagnosing renovascular hypertension. Kidney Int 44:1379, 1993

WORKING GROUP ON RENOVASCULAR HYPERTENSION: Final Report: Detection, evaluation, and treatment of renovascular hypertension. Arch Intern Med 147:820, 1987

278

John R. Asplin, Fredric L. Coe

HEREDITARY TUBULAR DISORDERS

The hereditary renal tubular disorders and their morphologic and functional abnormalities, mode of inheritance, and associated abnormalities are summarized in Table 278-1. The individual disorders are discussed in detail below.

AUTOSOMAL DOMINANT POLYCYSTIC KIDNEY DISEASE

ETIOLOGY AND PATHOLOGY Autosomal dominant polycystic kidney disease (ADPKD) has a prevalence of 1:300 to 1:1000 and accounts for approximately 10 percent of end-stage renal disease (ESRD) in the United States. Ninety percent of cases are inherited as an autosomal dominant trait, and approximately 10 percent are spontaneous mutations. Three forms of ADPKD have been identified. ADPKD-1 accounts for 90 percent of cases, and the gene has been localized to the short arm of chromosome 16. The gene has recently been sequenced and found to encode a 4300-amino-acid protein; the function of the protein is unknown at this time. The gene for ADPKD-2 has been mapped to the short arm of chromosome 4. ADPKD-2 appears to have a later age of onset of symptoms and renal failure than ADPKD-1. A third form has been documented but has not been mapped to a gene at this point.

The kidneys are grossly enlarged, with multiple cysts studding the surface of the kidney. The cysts contain straw-colored fluid that may become hemorrhagic. The cysts are spherical, vary in size from a few millimeters to centimeters, and are distributed evenly throughout the cortex and medulla. Only 1 to 5 percent of nephrons will develop cysts. Hyperplastic polyps and renal adenomas are frequently found. The remaining renal parenchyma reveals varying degrees of tubular atrophy, interstitial fibrosis, and nephrosclerosis.

CLINICAL FEATURES The disease may present at any age but most frequently causes symptoms in the third or fourth decade. Patients may develop chronic flank pain from the mass effect of the enlarged kidneys. Acute pain indicates infection, urinary tract obstruction by clot or stone, or sudden hemorrhage into a cyst. Gross and microscopic hematuria are common, and impaired renal concentrating ability frequently leads to nocturia. Nephrolithiasis occurs in 15 to 20 percent of patients, calcium oxalate and uric acid stones being most common. Low urine pH, low urine citrate, and urinary stasis from distortion of the collecting system by cysts all play a role in stone formation. Hypertension is found in 20 to 30 percent of children and up to 75 percent of adults. It is secondary to intrarenal ischemia from distortion of the renal architecture, leading to activation of the renin-angiotensin system. Urinary tract infection is common and may involve the bladder or renal interstitium (pyelonephritis) or infect a cyst (pyocyst). Pyocysts can be difficult to diagnose but are more likely to be present if the patient has positive blood cultures, new renal pain, or failed to improve clinically after a standard course of antibiotic therapy.

Progressive decline in renal function is common, with approximately 50 percent of patients developing ESRD by age 60. However, there is considerable variation in age of onset of renal failure, even within the same family. Hypertension, recurrent infections, male sex, and early age of diagnosis are related to early onset renal failure. Renal failure usually progresses slowly; if a sudden decrement in kidney function occurs, ureteral obstruction from stone, clot, or compression by a cyst are likely causes. Patients usually have high hematocrits for their level of renal function, as erythropoietin production is high. Fluid overload is uncommon because of a tendency for renal salt wasting.

Extrarenal manifestations of this disease are frequent and underscore the systemic nature of the defect. Hepatic cysts occur in 50 to 70 percent of patients. Cysts are generally asymptomatic, and liver function is normal, though women may develop massive hepatic cystic disease on occasion. Cyst formation has also been observed in the spleen, pancreas, and ovaries. Intracranial aneurysms are present in 5 to 10 percent of asymptomatic patients, with potential for permanent neurologic injury or death from subarachnoid hemorrhage. Screening of all ADPKD patients for aneurysms is not recommended, but patients with a family history of subarachnoid hemorrhage should be studied noninvasively with magnetic resonance imaging angiography. Colonic diverticular disease is the most common extrarenal abnormality, and patients are more likely to develop perforation than the general population with colonic diverticula. Mitral valve prolapse is found in 25 percent of patients, and the prevalence of aortic and tricuspid valve insufficiency is increased.

Table 278-1

Renal Tubule Defects

Disease	Renal Morphologic Abnormalities	Renal Functional Abnormalities	Mode of Inheritance*	Associated Abnormalities
Autosomal dominant polycystic disease	Cortical and medullary cysts	Chronic renal failure, >20 yr	AD	Hepatic cysts, intracranial aneurysms, colonic diverticula
Autosomal recessive polycystic disease	Distal tubule and collecting duct cysts	Chronic renal failure, <20 yr	AR	Congenital hepatic fibrosis
Tuberous sclerosis	Renal cysts and angiomyolipomas	None	AD	Skin lesions, hamartomas of the central nervous system
Von Hippel–Lindau disease	Renal cysts, increased risk of renal cell cancer	None	AD	Hemangioblastoma of the retina and central nervous system
Medullary sponge kidney	Dilated collecting ducts	Nephrocalcinosis, hematuria	AD, S	None
Juvenile nephronophthisis	Medullary cysts, small kidneys	Chronic renal failure, <20 yr polyuria, salt wasting	AR	Hepatic fibrosis, retinal abnormalities
Medullary cystic disease	Medullary cysts, small kidneys	Chronic renal failure, >20 yr polyuria, salt wasting	AD	None
Liddle's syndrome	None	Hypokalemia, alkalosis, low aldosterone levels	AR	Hypertension
Bartter's syndrome	Juxtaglomerular apparatus hyperplasia	Hypokalemia, alkalosis, high aldosterone levels	AR, S	None
Congenital nephrogenic diabetes insipidus	None	Vasopressin renal concentrating defect	XL, AR	None
Renal tubular acidosis, type 1	Nephrocalcinosis	Impaired proton secretion in distal tubule, non-anion-gap metabolic acidosis	AD, AR, XL, S, ACQ	Rickets, osteomalacia, nephrolithiasis
Renal tubular acidosis, type 2	None	Reduced bicarbonate reabsorption, non-anion-gap metabolic acidosis	AR, AD, XL, ACQ	Fanconi syndrome, rickets
Renal tubular acidosis, type 4	Chronic renal insufficiency	Reduced proton and potassium secretion	ACQ	Renal insufficiency
X-linked hypophosphatemia	None	Reduced phosphate reabsorption	XL	Rickets, osteomalacia, normal serum 1,25(OH)$_2$D$_3$
Vitamin D–dependent rickets, type 1	None	Defective renal 1,25(OH)$_2$D$_3$ production	AR	Rickets, osteomalacia, low serum 1,25(OH)$_2$D$_3$
Vitamin D–dependent rickets, type 2	None	Renal resistance to 1,25(OH)$_2$D$_3$	AR, S	Rickets, osteomalacia, high serum 1,25(OH)$_2$D$_3$
Oncogenic osteomalacia	None	Reduced phosphate reabsorption	ACQ	Osteomalacia, mesenchymal tumors
X-linked recessive nephrolithiasis	Interstitial fibrosis, medullary calcifications	Hypercalciuria, low-molecular-weight proteinuria	XL	Renal failure
Isolated hyperuricemia	None	Reduced urate reabsorption	AR	Variable hypercalciuria
Hartnup disorder	None	Reduced reabsorption of neutral amino acids	AR	Dermatitis, diarrhea, dementia
Cystinuria	Cystine stones	Reduced reabsorption of dibasic amino acids	AR	Short stature
Iminoglycinuria	None	Reduced reabsorption of proline, hydroxyproline, and glycine	AR	None
Fanconi syndrome	Swan neck deformity of proximal tubule	Reduced reabsorption of bicarbonate, glucose, phosphate, uric acid, and amino acids	AR	Rickets, osteomalacia, hypokalemia, metabolic acidosis

* AD, autosomal dominant; AR, autosomal recessive; XL, X-linked; ACQ, acquired; S, sporadic

DIAGNOSIS Ultrasound is the preferred technique for diagnosis of symptomatic patients and for screening asymptomatic family members. The ability to detect cysts increases with the subject's age: 80 to 90 percent of ADPKD patients over the age of 20 will have detectable cysts, and almost 100 percent over the age of 30 will have cysts. At least three to five cysts in each kidney is the standard diagnostic criteria for ADPKD. Computed tomography scan may be more sensitive than ultrasound in detection of small cysts. Genetic linkage analysis is now available for diagnosis of ADPKD-1 but is reserved for cases where radiographic imaging is negative and the need for definitive diagnosis critical, such as screening family members for potential kidney donation.

TREATMENT

The goals of treatment are to slow the rate of progression of renal disease and minimize symptoms. Hypertension and renal infection should be treated aggressively to maintain renal function. Converting enzyme inhibitors are effective antihypertensive agents, though patients should be closely monitored as some develop renal insufficiency and hyperkalemia. Urinary infection is treated in a standard manner unless a pyocyst is suspected, in which case antibiotics that penetrate cysts should be used, such as trimethoprim-sulfamethoxazole, ciprofloxacin, and chloramphenicol. Chronic pain from cysts can be managed by cyst puncture and sclerosis with ethanol.

AUTOSOMAL RECESSIVE POLYCYSTIC KIDNEY DISEASE

ETIOLOGY AND PATHOLOGY Autosomal recessive polycystic kidney disease (ARPKD) is a rare genetic disease that has an incidence between 1:10,000 and 1:40,000. The gene for ARPKD has been localized to chromosome 6. In the past, ARPKD was considered to be a family of disorders, categorized as neonatal, infantile, and childhood forms depending on the age of onset and the relative degree of involvement of the kidneys and liver. However, variable clinical presentations within siblings in the same family, as well as the localization of the disease to chromosome 6 in multiple families, support the premise that this is a single genetic disease with variable phenotypic presentation.

At birth the kidneys are enlarged with a smooth external surface. The distal tubules and collecting ducts are dilated into elongated cysts that are arranged in a radial fashion. As the patient ages, the cysts may become more spherical and can be confused with ADPKD. Interstitial fibrosis is also seen as renal function deteriorates. Liver involvement includes proliferation and dilation of small intrahepatic bile ducts as well as periportal fibrosis.

CLINICAL FEATURES The majority of cases are diagnosed in the first year of life, presenting as bilateral abdominal masses. Death in the neonatal period is most commonly due to pulmonary hypoplasia. Hypertension and impaired urinary concentrating ability are common. The time course to ESRD is variable, though many children maintain adequate kidney function for years. Older children present with complications secondary to congenital hepatic fibrosis and generally have less severe kidney disease. Hepatosplenomegaly, portal hypertension, and esophageal varices are frequent complications of ARPKD.

DIAGNOSIS Ultrasound is the most common technique used to diagnose ARPKD, prenatally and in childhood. Ultrasound examination reveals enlarged kidneys with increased echogenicity. At times spherical cysts may be seen, potentially leading to an incorrect diagnosis of ADPKD. A thorough family history and imaging the kidneys of the parents aids in differentiation from other cystic diseases. The recent mapping of the gene should allow linkage studies to be used in diagnosis.

TREATMENT

Aggressive treatment of hypertension and urinary tract infection are the major goals of therapy in order to maintain native renal function as long as possible. Dialysis and transplant are appropriate when kidney failure occurs. Hepatic fibrosis may lead to life-threatening variceal hemorrhage, requiring sclerotherapy or portocaval shunting.

TUBEROUS SCLEROSIS

Patients with this multisystem disease most commonly present with skin lesions and benign tumors of the central nervous system (Chap. 375). Renal involvement is common; angiomyolipomas are the most frequent abnormality and are usually bilateral. Renal cysts may be present as well and can give an appearance similar to that of ADPKD. Histologically, the cysts are unique—the cyst lining cells are large with an eosinophilic staining cytoplasm and they may form hyperplastic nodules that can fill the cyst space. The disease is inherited as an autosomal dominant trait, though spontaneous mutations do occur. Gene mutations have been identified on chromosomes 9 and 16. Tuberous sclerosis may be confused with ADPKD if the extrarenal manifestations are minimal.

VON HIPPEL–LINDAU DISEASE

This autosomal dominant disease is characterized by hemangioblastomas of the retina and the central nervous system (Chap. 375). Renal cysts occur in the majority of cases and are usually bilateral. Linkage studies have localized the gene to the short arm of chromosome 3 and it has been identified as a tumor-suppressor gene. Renal cell carcinoma may be found in up to 25 percent of patients and is frequently multifocal. Yearly screening of adults using computed tomography scans has been recommended in an attempt to diagnose renal cell cancers at an early stage.

MEDULLARY SPONGE KIDNEY (MSK)

ETIOLOGY AND PATHOLOGY MSK is a congenital disorder. Although some cases have apparent autosomal dominant inheritance, most are sporadic. It is found in 0.5 to 1 percent of all intravenous pyelograms. Males and females are affected equally. The pathologic lesion is cystic dilation of the inner medullary and papillary collecting ducts, with collecting diameters ranging from 1 to 5 mm. Bilateral renal involvement is present in 70 percent of cases, but not all papillae are equally affected. The dilated ducts are lined by cuboidal epithelium with areas of pseudostratified and stratified squamous epithelium. Calculi are frequently found in the dilated collecting ducts.

CLINICAL FEATURES Patients generally present in the third or fourth decade with kidney stones, infection, or recurrent hematuria. The disease is most commonly diagnosed by intravenous pyelogram, which shows linear striations radiating into the renal papillae or small cystic collections of contrast in the dilated ducts (Fig. 278-1). Approximately 60 percent of patients with MSK have stones, and 12 percent of all stone formers will have MSK. Hypercalciuria occurs with the same frequency in MSK as it does in random stone formers. Papillary nephrocalcinosis occurs more frequently in patients with MSK than in the random stone former. Proteinuria is minimal, if present at all, and renal function is normally preserved unless there is renal damage from recurrent infection or severe stone disease.

TREATMENT

Asymptomatic patients require no specific therapy except to maintain high fluid intake to reduce the risk of nephrolithiasis. If stones are present, standard laboratory evaluation should be done and metabolic abnormalities treated as in any stone former (see Chap. 279). Infection should be treated aggressively, and instrumentation of the urinary tract should be minimized to avoid introducing infection.

JUVENILE NEPHRONOPHTHISIS/MEDULLARY CYSTIC DISEASE

ETIOLOGY AND PATHOLOGY Juvenile nephronophthisis (JN) and medullary cystic disease (MCD) have similar pathologic findings but differ in inheritance pattern and age of onset. JN is inherited as an autosomal recessive disease; linkage studies have shown 90 percent of the cases to map to a gene on the short arm of chromosome 2. MCD appears to be an autosomal dominant disease. In both conditions, the kidneys tend to be small, with cysts throughout the medulla; the cortex and papilla rarely have cysts. The cysts originate in the collecting ducts, distal convoluted tubules, and loops of Henle and range in size from 1 to 10 mm. Sclerotic glomeruli, tubule atrophy, and interstitial fibrosis are frequent findings on biopsy.

CLINICAL FEATURES Patients with JN present during childhood with symptoms of polyuria, growth retardation, anemia, and progressive renal insufficiency. Most patients develop ESRD prior to the age of 20; JN accounts for 2 to 10 percent of renal failure in children. Hepatic fibrosis, retinal abnormalities, and mental retardation have been reported in association with JN. MCD presents in the third or fourth decade, though some cases may be diagnosed in the elderly population. Presenting symptoms in MCD are the same as in JN except for growth retardation. In addition, MCD does not have extrarenal abnormalities. Severe salt wasting can be seen, though this is usually a transient phase that resolves as the disease progresses to ESRD. Other features of tubule damage are often found, including hyperkalemia and hyperchloremic metabolic acidosis. Proteinuria is mild, and hematuria is rare.

DIAGNOSIS The diagnosis is suggested by a family history of renal disease. The pattern of inheritance and age of onset aid in distinguishing JN/MCD from other inherited diseases. Radiographic studies show small kidneys, loss of the corticomedullary junction, and multiple cysts in the medulla. Computed tomography scan is more sensitive than ultrasound in making the diagnosis. Open renal biopsy, including medullary tissue, may be required for diagnosis in some cases.

℞ **TREATMENT**

Treatment is mainly supportive, as there is no specific therapy to prevent loss of renal function. Patients with salt wasting require a large oral intake of salt and water to maintain adequate extracellular volume. Alkali replacement and erythropoietin are required for acidosis and anemia, respectively. Renal transplantation has been performed in numerous patients, and the disease does not recur.

LIDDLE'S SYNDROME

Liddle's syndrome is a rare familial disease with a clinical presentation of hyperaldosteronism, consisting of hypertension, hypokalemia, and metabolic alkalosis. However, aldosterone levels are undetectable in these patients, and a nonaldosterone mineralocorticoid has not been isolated. Increased distal tubule sodium reabsorption, due to mutations in the β subunit of the amiloride-sensitive sodium channel, has been described in multiple families. Pharmacologic agents that block distal tubule sodium uptake, such as amiloride and triamterene, are effective in treating the hypertension and electrolyte abnormalities. As expected, spironolactone is ineffective, since the disease is not mediated via the aldosterone receptor.

BARTTER'S SYNDROME

CLINICAL FEATURES Hypokalemia secondary to renal potassium wasting, metabolic alkalosis, and normal to low blood pressure are the clinical features of Bartter's syndrome. Renin and aldosterone production are increased, and there is hyporesponsiveness to the pressor effects of angiotensin II infusion. Prostaglandin E_2, prostacyclin, kallikrein, and bradykinin production are frequently elevated. Hypomagnesemia with hypermagnesuria may be present. Most cases are diagnosed during childhood, with the presenting symptoms, such as polyuria and weakness, being attributable to hypokalemia. Inheritance is autosomal recessive, though sporadic cases do occur. Growth and developmental retardation may be associated with Bartter's syndrome. Although renal biopsy is rarely required for diagnosis, it reveals hyperplasia of the juxtaglomerular apparatus and prominence of medullary interstitial cells, with variable degrees of interstitial fibrosis.

PATHOGENESIS The pathogenesis of Bartter's syndrome is a matter of debate as the distinction between primary and secondary phenomena is difficult. Juxtaglomerular hyperplasia is most likely an epiphenomenon, as any form of chronic hyperreninemia will cause it. Resistance to the pressor effects of angiotensin II may be secondary to the high levels of vasodilatory prostaglandins. Inhibition of prostaglandin synthesis can reverse the vascular hyporesponsiveness. Prostaglandin overproduction has been implicated as the primary event, but variable clinical response to prostaglandin inhibitors suggests this is not the common etiology. Prostaglandin overproduction could be secondary to hypokalemia or volume depletion. Impaired chloride reabsorption in the thick ascending limb of the loop of Henle appears to be the most likely etiology. Inadequate chloride reabsorption would cause volume depletion and activate the renin-angiotensin system. Distal delivery of salt and water would be high in the presence of high aldosterone, promoting secretion of potassium and hydrogen ions. Hypokalemia and alkalosis would result. Prostaglandin synthesis would be increased by the volume contraction and hypokalemia. High aldosterone levels would increase production of kallikrein and bradykinin.

FIGURE 278-1 *A*. Radiographic appearance of medullary sponge kidney. Abdominal flat plate reveals multiple bilateral calcifications. *B*. Radiographic contrast material accumulates in the dilated and cystic terminal collecting ducts and obscures the calcifications.

However, Bartter's syndrome may be a disorder with a single phenotype caused by many physiologic abnormalities, further complicating investigation of its pathogenesis. Angiotensin II–receptor antagonists can produce some of the features of Bartter's syndrome in experimental studies. The gene for the angiotensin II receptor has been found to be abnormal in one of five Bartter's patients studied. Whether this will be a common finding in Bartter's syndrome remains to be seen.

DIAGNOSIS Most cases of Bartter's syndrome present during childhood. Symptoms such as weakness and cramps are secondary to the hypokalemia. Polyuria and nocturia are common due to the hypokalemia-induced nephrogenic diabetes insipidus (NDI). The disease is inherited as an autosomal recessive trait, though sporadic cases do occur. Differential diagnosis includes vomiting, surreptitious diuretic abuse, and magnesium deficiency. Chronic vomiting can be diagnosed by a low urine chloride concentration. Magnesium deficiency causes kaliuresis and alkalosis, simulating Bartter's syndrome. Serum and urine magnesium will be low in such cases. Diuretic abuse produces metabolic abnormalities indistinguishable from those of Bartter's syndrome. Urine should be screened for diuretics multiple times before the diagnosis of Bartter's syndrome is made in a patient without a family history of the disorder.

℞ TREATMENT
Dietary intake of sodium and potassium should be liberal. Potassium supplements are usually required. Magnesium supplements are needed in those patients with magnesuria. Spironolactone will reduce potassium wasting. Prostaglandin synthetase inhibitors are useful in some patients. Angiotensin-converting enzyme inhibitors have also been shown to be of use.

CONGENITAL NEPHROGENIC DIABETES INSIPIDUS

This rare genetic disorder is most commonly inherited as an X-linked disease, with full expression in males and variable penetrance in females. Vasopressin acts through two receptors; type 1 receptors are located in the vasculature, while type 2 receptors are found in the collecting ducts of the kidney. In NDI, only the actions requiring type 2 receptors are abnormal. Linkage analysis has localized the NDI gene to the long arm of the X chromosome in region 28 (Xq28), the same locus as the type 2 vasopressin receptor. Mutations in the gene that encodes the type 2 vasopressin receptor segregate with NDI, confirming it as the putative gene. Less frequently, NDI may be inherited as an autosomal recessive trait, in which mutations in the gene for the water channels in collecting duct cells (aquaporin 2) lead to abnormal cell routing of aquaporin 2.

Clinical presentation is that of persistent polyuria, dehydration, and hypotonic urine in the presence of hypernatremia. Vasopressin

levels are appropriately elevated in the hypertonic state, but renal response is lacking. The onset of the disorder is in infancy. The recurrent hypernatremia may lead to seizures or mental retardation. Once old enough to satisfy their thirst, children will be clinically stable though in a chronic state of polyuria and polydypsia. Renal function is normal, and radiographic studies of the urinary system reveal dilated ureters and bladder secondary to the chronically high urine flow. Since the most common form of the disease is X-linked, most patients are male. Heterozygous females generally have mild concentrating defects, though a few have phenotypic expression similar to males due to skewed X-chromosome inactivation. In the autosomal recessive form, males and females are affected equally.

℞ TREATMENT
Treatment is aimed at maintaining adequate hydration. In the infant, low-solute feedings and high water intake are generally adequate. Addition of a thiazide diuretic reduces urine flow by inhibiting sodium reabsorption in the distal convoluted tubule. This lowers free water production and, by causing extracellular volume contraction, increases proximal salt and water reabsorption, reducing delivery to the distal nephron. Administration of vasopressin and its analogues has no role in the management of this disorder.

RENAL TUBULAR ACIDOSIS (RTA)

RTA is a disorder of renal acidification out of proportion to the reduction in glomerular filtration rate. RTA is characterized by hyperchloremic metabolic acidosis with a normal serum anion gap [$Na^+ - (Cl^- + HCO_3^-)$]. There are multiple forms of RTA, depending on which aspects of renal acid handling have been affected. Defective bicarbonate reabsorption in the proximal tubule, suppressed renal ammoniagenesis, and inadequate distal tublule proton secretion are the abnormalities that produce RTA. Three types of RTA exist (Table 278-2). Types 1 and 2 may be inherited or acquired. Type 4 is acquired and is associated with either hypoaldosteronism or tubular hyporesponsiveness to mineralocorticoids. Type 3 was formerly used to define distal RTA with bicarbonate wasting in children; however, the bicarbonaturia resolves with age and is not truly part of a pathologic process. The term *type 3 RTA* is no longer used.

TYPE 1 (DISTAL) RTA In this disorder the distal nephron does not lower urine pH normally, either because the collecting ducts permit excessive back-diffusion of hydrogen ions from lumen to blood or because there is inadequate transport of hydrogen ions. Excretion of titratable acid is low, as inadequate proton secretion prevents titration of urinary buffers such as phosphate. Urine ammonium excretion is inappropriately low for the level of acidosis, as the defect in acidification reduces the ion trapping required for ammonium excretion. Urinary concentration and potassium conservation also tend to be impaired.

Chronic acidosis lowers tubule reabsorption of calcium, causing renal hypercalciuria and mild secondary hyperparathyroidism. Buffering of bone by the daily metabolic acid load contributes to hypercalciuria. Urine citrate excretion is low, as acidosis and hypokalemia stimulate proximal tubule reabsorption of citrate. The hypercalciuria, alkaline urine, and low levels of urine citrate, which normally complexes about 40 percent of urine calcium, cause calcium phosphate stones and nephrocalcinosis. Growth in children is stunted because of rickets; this growth defect responds to amelioration of the acidosis with alkali. In the adult, osteomalacia occurs. In both children and adults, bone diseases may result, in part, from acidosis-induced loss of bone material and inadequate production of 1,25-dihydroxyvitamin D_3 [$1,25(OH)_2D_3$]. Since

Table 278-2

Comparison of Normal Anion-Gap Acidoses

Finding	Type 1 RTA	Type 2 RTA	Type 4 RTA	GI Bicarbonate Loss
Normal anion-gap acidosis	Yes	Yes	Yes	Yes
Minimum urine pH	>5.5	<5.5	<5.5	5 to 6
% filtered bicarbonate excreted	<10	>15	<10	<10
Serum potassium	Low	Low	High	Low
Fanconi syndrome	No	Yes	No	No
Stones/nephrocalcinosis	Yes	No	No	No
Daily acid excretion	Low	Normal	Low	High
Urine anion gap	Positive	Positive	Positive	Negative
Daily bicarbonate replacement needs	<4 mmol/kg	>4 mmol/kg	<4 mmol/kg	Variable

the kidney does not conserve potassium or concentrate the urine normally, polyuria and hypokalemia occur. With the stress of an intercurrent illness, acidosis and hypokalemia can be life-threatening.

Type 1 RTA can be familial, with autosomal dominant as the most common form of inheritance. X-linked, autosomal recessive, and sporadic cases have been reported. Other hereditary diseases that cause type 1 RTA include galactosemia, Ehler-Danlos syndrome, Fabry's disease, medullary sponge kidney, Wilson's disease, and hereditary elliptocytosis. The majority of cases of type 1 RTA are secondary to a systemic disorder such as Sjögren's syndrome, hypergammaglobulinemia, chronic active hepatitis, or lupus.

The diagnosis of type 1 RTA is suggested by a normal anion gap metabolic acidosis with a simultaneous urine pH greater than 5.5. Osteomalacia or rickets and calcium phosphate stones or nephrocalcinosis support the diagnosis, though they are not present in all cases. Bicarbonaturia is not present, which distinguishes this disorder from type 2 RTA. If acidosis is not severe and urine pH is equivocal, the oral ammonium chloride (NH_4Cl) loading test should be carried out: 0.1 g (1.9 mmol) NH_4Cl per kilogram of body weight is administered, and blood and urine pH are measured repeatedly over the next 6 h. Although systemic acidosis worsens, urine pH does not fall below 5.5. Urinary tract infection must not be present during this test because bacteria may possess urease, which hydrolyzes urea to ammonia and produces an alkaline urine.

Chronic diarrheal states cause normal anion gap acidosis and hypokalemia; urine pH may be above 5.5 if ammonium production is very high. The urine anion gap ($Na^+ + K^+ - Cl^-$) can be used to estimate renal ammonium production and distinguish RTA from gastrointestinal bicarbonate loss. Normally the urine anion gap is positive, as unmeasured anions exceeds unmeasured cations. If urine ammonium levels are high, urine chloride concentration increases to balance the charge. Unmeasured cation (predominantly ammonium) now exceeds unmeasured anion, and the urine anion gap is negative. During metabolic acidosis, a negative urine anion gap suggests an extrarenal cause of acidosis, whereas a positive urine anion gap suggests RTA. The urine anion gap cannot be used if there are large amounts of unmeasured anions, such as bicarbonate or ketones, in the urine.

℞ TREATMENT

Alkali supplements are the standard therapy. Enough alkali is prescribed to titrate the daily metabolic acid production, usually in the range of 0.5 to 2.0 mmol/kg body weight in four to six divided doses per day. Sodium bicarbonate and Shohl's solution (1 mmol sodium citrate and 1 mmol citric acid per mL) are common treatments. Potassium alkali salts can be used if hypokalemia is a persistent problem. Citrate requires less frequent dosing than bicarbonate salts as it is metabolized to bicarbonate after absorption. The dose of alkali should be raised until acidosis and hypercalciuria are both eliminated, and the patients should be followed by measurements of serum potassium, chloride, and CO_2 content approximately twice yearly. Requirements for alkali usually rise during intercurrent illnesses but are usually below 4 mmol/kg body weight per day. The relatives of patients with idiopathic type 1 RTA should be screened for this disorder, as timely treatment can prevent growth retardation in children. Incomplete RTA secondary to idiopathic hypercalciuria is best treated using thiazide diuretics in conjunction with potassium citrate (Chap. 279).

TYPE 2 (PROXIMAL) RTA Type 2 RTA usually occurs as part of a generalized disorder of proximal tubule function, presenting as hyperchloremic acidosis with other features of Fanconi syndrome. Bicarbonate reabsorption in the proximal tubule is defective. At normal concentrations of plasma bicarbonate, large amounts of bicarbonate are delivered to the distal tubule, overwhelming the absorptive capacity of the distal tubule and resulting in bicarbonaturia. As plasma bicarbonate levels fall, the lower filtered load of bicarbonate can be reabsorbed by the proximal tubule, resulting in normal distal delivery of bicarbonate. At this point the distal nephron can acidify the urine normally, resulting in normal excretion of daily metabolic acid production, albeit

at a low serum bicarbonate level. Hypophosphatemia and low calcitriol levels are common and may lead to rickets or osteomalacia. Hypercalciuria occurs, but stone formation is unusual since urine citrate levels are normal or high because of reduced proximal tubule citrate reabsorption. Type 2 RTA may be inherited as autosomal dominant, autosomal recessive, or X-linked disorder. It may be acquired in association with other diseases (see "Fanconi Syndrome") or be secondary to drugs that inhibit carbonic anhydrase activity, such as acetazolamide.

Type 2 RTA may be distinguished from type 1 RTA by the ability to normally acidify urine during spontaneous or ammonium chloride–induced acidosis. Correction of acidosis with bicarbonate will result in bicarbonaturia in type 2 RTA but not type 1 RTA. Fractional excretion of bicarbonate is greater than 15 percent at normal or near-normal serum bicarbonate levels. In distal RTA it is less than 10 percent. It is unusual for serum bicarbonate levels to fall below 15 mmol/L in proximal RTA. The urine anion gap will be positive, as ammonium excretion is normal to handle daily acid production, but is not elevated as in nonrenal causes of acidosis.

℞ TREATMENT

Children should be treated to prevent growth retardation. Alkali must be given in large amounts daily, 5 to 15 mmol/kg body weight per day, because bicarbonate is rapidly excreted in the urine. A thiazide diuretic can be used in conjunction with a low-salt diet to reduce the amount of bicarbonate required. Potassium supplementation is often required.

TYPE 4 RTA In type 4 RTA, also called hyperkalemic distal RTA, distal tubule secretion of both potassium and hydrogen ions is abnormal, resulting in hyperchloremic acidosis with hyperkalemia. Type 4 RTA is an acquired disorder; a moderate degree of renal insufficiency is present in the majority of patients. Patients with type 4 RTA can be differentiated from patients with type 1 since they have an acid urine (pH < 5.5) during periods of acidosis (see Table 278-2) and hyperkalemia. They differ from type 2 patients by having a fractional excretion of bicarbonate less than 10 percent and a daily bicarbonate requirement of 1 to 3 mmol/kg body weight per day. Because potassium and hydrogen ion excretion are abnormal, such patients are considered to have generalized distal nephron dysfunction due to either insufficient aldosterone production or intrinsic renal disease causing aldosterone resistance. The resulting hyperkalemia reduces proximal tubule ammonia production, in addition to the inadequate proton secretion, leading to inadequate excretion of the daily metabolic proton load. These patients have an acid urine despite reduced proton secretion because there is inadequate ammonia to buffer protons in the distal tubule. If buffer delivery to the distal nephron is increased, urine pH will rise despite persistent acidosis.

Type 4 RTA due to inadequate aldosterone production has multiple etiologies. Hyporeninemic hypoaldosteronism is the most common cause of type 4 RTA. Plasma levels of renin and aldosterone are subnormal, even during extracellular volume depletion, and the most common causes of this are diabetic nephropathy and chronic tubulointerstitial nephropathies. Nonsteroidal anti-inflammatory drugs, angiotensin-converting enzyme inhibitors, and heparin can reduce aldosterone production and produce a type 4 RTA. Drug-induced type 4 RTA is usually seen in patients with preexisting renal insufficiency. Reduced aldosterone production may be due to adrenal disease, either occurring as an isolated defect or as part of a more generalized adrenal disorder (Chap. 332). Renin levels are normal to high in adrenal disorders.

Patients with tubular resistance to aldosterone present with the same clinical features as those with hyporeninemic hypoaldosteronism. A tubulointerstitial process damages the distal tubule, restricting potassium and hydrogen ion excretion, despite adequate aldosterone levels. Obstructive uropathy and sickle cell disease are the most common causes of acquired tubular resistance to aldosterone. Hyporeninemic hypoaldosteronism can be found in addition to tubular aldosterone resistance in many patients. Spironolactone, a competitive inhibitor of the aldosterone receptor, produces an aldosterone-resistant state. Amiloride and triamterene are diuretics that block sodium transport in the distal nephron, blunting the effect of aldosterone on the distal tubule.

 TREATMENT

This is aimed mainly at reducing serum potassium, as acidosis will usually improve once the hyperkalemic block of ammonium production is removed. All patients should be placed on a low-potassium diet. Any drug that suppresses aldosterone production or blocks aldosterone effect should be discontinued. Mineralocorticoid supplementation with fludrocortisone, 0.1 to 0.2 mg/d, will improve hyperkalemia and acidosis; however, the patients who also have a partial tubule resistance to mineralocorticoid will require a higher dose. Mineralocorticoid replacement may not be appropriate for patients with hypertension or a history of heart failure. In such situations, a loop diuretic with a liberal sodium intake can usually promote adequate potassium excretion. Exchange resins will reduce potassium levels but are usually not tolerated well enough to be used for long-term treatment.

IDIOPATHIC PSEUDOHYPOALDOSTERONISM This rare inherited disorder is transmitted as either an autosomal dominant or recessive trait. It is due to a defect in the high-affinity aldosterone receptor, resulting in hyperkalemia and metabolic acidosis unresponsive to mineralocorticoid supplementation. The disease presents during childhood and is usually complicated by salt wasting and volume depletion. Plasma renin and aldosterone levels are elevated. Treatment includes salt supplements, alkali, and potassium restriction.

VITAMIN D DISORDERS

X-LINKED HYPOPHOSPHATEMIC RICKETS (See also Chap. 355) This disorder, also called vitamin D–resistant rickets, is an X-linked dominant disorder characterized by hypophosphatemia with renal phosphate wasting, rickets, and short stature. Hypophosphatemia is present soon after birth; rachitic bowing of the legs develops when the child begins to walk. Children have growth retardation which is limited almost entirely to the lower extremities. Dentition is delayed, and skull abnormalities are common. Females generally have less severe disease than males. Presentation in adults ranges from disabling bone pain to no active symptoms, but generally some physical sign of childhood disease, such as short stature or bowed legs, is present. Overgrowth of bone at joints or sites of muscle attachment may reduce the mobility of the joint or cause nerve entrapment.

Hypophosphatemia secondary to reduced renal phosphate reabsorption is the hallmark of the disease. Intestinal phosphate absorption is low, worsening hypophosphatemia. Serum calcium levels are usually normal, with low intestinal absorption and renal excretion of calcium. Serum alkaline phosphatase and osteocalcin levels are elevated. Parathyroid hormone levels are normal, as would be expected with normal serum calcium. $1,25(OH)_2D_3$ levels are usually normal, though in the setting of hypophosphatemia $1,25(OH)_2D_3$ levels should be elevated. Inadequate 1α-hydroxylase activity appears to play some role in the disease. Linkage analysis has localized the gene to the Xp22.1 region of the X chromosome. A candidate gene has been identified and appears to be related to a family of endopeptidase genes.

 TREATMENT

The goal of therapy is to raise serum phosphorous to normal or near-normal levels to improve bone mineralization. Oral neutral phosphate, 1 to 4 g/d in four to six doses, combined with calcitriol is an effective therapy that improves growth rate, reduces bone pain, and leads to radiographically evident improvement of the bone disease. Patients should be closely monitored during therapy as they may develop nephrocalcinosis and renal insufficiency.

VITAMIN D–DEPENDENT RICKETS TYPE 1 This is an autosomal recessive disorder in which $1,25(OH)_2D_3$ levels are very low but 25-hydroxyvitamin D levels are normal. There appears to be a defect in renal 1α-hydroxylase activity, leading to a clinical syndrome of vitamin D deficiency. Symptoms usually appear before the age of 2, including rickets and growth retardation. Levels of serum calcium and phosphorous are low but that of alkaline phosphatase is elevated. Intestinal calcium absorption and urinary calcium excretion are low. Parathyroid hormone is elevated in response to the hypocalcemia, resulting in increased urinary phosphate losses.

 TREATMENT

Calcitriol (0.5 to 1 μg/d) leads to rapid correction of the biochemical abnormalities and resolution of the bone disease. Calcium and phosphorous supplementation are usually not required.

VITAMIN D–DEPENDENT RICKETS TYPE II (See also Chap. 355) End-organ resistance to $1,25(OH)_2D_3$ is the pathogenesis of this disorder. Serum calcium and phosphate levels are low, secondary hyperparathyroidism is present, and $1,25(OH)_2D_3$ levels are elevated. Inheritance is usually autosomal recessive, though sporadic cases have been reported. Most patients present during childhood with rickets, though some have a milder form of disease not recognized until adulthood. Alopecia is common and tends to be associated with the more severe childhood form of the disease. Multiple defects have been detected in $1,25(OH)_2D_3$ receptor interaction, including absent hormone binding to the receptor, decreased receptor affinity, deficient hormone-receptor localization, and abnormalities of the DNA-binding domain of the receptor. Pharmacologic doses of calcitriol (5 to 30 μg/d) along with mineral supplementation will improve the biochemical disorders and bone disease, though some patients have no response to massive doses of calcitriol.

ONCOGENIC OSTEOMALACIA This syndrome generally occurs in adults with highly vascular mesenchymal tumors. Patients present with bone pain and muscle weakness. Symptoms may be present for years before the correct diagnosis is made. Over 90 percent of the tumors are benign, and most are found in the extremities or maxillofacial region. Hypophosphatemia secondary to renal phosphate wasting and low levels of $1,25(OH)_2D_3$ are the major biochemical abnormalities. Serum calcium and parathyroid hormone levels are normal. It appears the tumor produces a humoral agent that reduces proximal tubule phosphate reabsorption and 1α-hydroxylase activity. Removal of the tumor leads to rapid resolution of the disease.

X-LINKED RECESSIVE NEPHROLITHIASIS

This disorder presents as calcium nephrolithiasis in male children and progresses to nephrocalcinosis and renal failure. Low-molecular-weight proteinuria and hypercalciuria are also prominent features of the disease. Kidney biopsy reveals tubular atrophy, interstitial fibrosis, and medullary calcifications. The gene has been mapped to the short arm of the X chromosome and encodes a voltage-gated chloride channel. Dent's disease has been mapped to the same gene and has a similar presentation, except for an increased incidence of rickets.

ISOLATED HYPOURICEMIA (See also Chap. 350)

This disorder is generally inherited as an autosomal recessive trait. Most commonly there is deficient urate reabsorption in the proximal tubule, though some patients have been demonstrated to oversecrete urate. Serum uric acid is usually below 120 μmol/L (2 mg/dL) and hyperuricosuria is common, possibly due to decreased intestinal urate excretion. Hypouricemia is usually an incidental finding, as patients with this disorder are asymptomatic except for an increased risk of nephrolithiasis. Other disorders associated with hypouricemia include Fanconi syndrome, Wilson's disease, Hodgkin's disease, and Hartnup disease. No treatment is required except for high fluid intake to prevent kidney stones. Alkali and allopurinol may be used to prevent stones if fluids alone are not sufficient. Hypercalciuria has been associated with isolated hypouricemia in some families.

SELECTED DISORDERS OF AMINO ACID TRANSPORT

HARTNUP DISEASE   This disorder is characterized by reduced intestinal absorption and renal reabsorption of neutral amino acids. The defect involves an amino acid transporter on the brush border of the jejunum and the proximal tubule. Intestinal absorption of free amino acids is reduced, though the neutral amino acids can be absorbed when present in di- and tripeptides. Degradation of unabsorbed tryptophan by intestinal bacteria produces indolic acids that are absorbed and subsequently excreted at high levels in the urine of these patients. The disorder is inherited as an autosomal recessive trait, affecting males and females equally. Widespread screening of newborns has estimated an incidence of 1 in 24,000 live births.

The majority of subjects with this disorder are asymptomatic. Approximately 10 to 20 percent present with clinical symptoms similar to those seen in pellagra, including a photosensitive erythematous scaly rash, intermittent cerebral ataxia, delirium, and diarrhea. Short stature is noted in some patients. The symptoms are thought to be due to deficiency in the essential amino acid tryptophan and resultant inadequate synthesis of nicotinamide. Though the inheritance of the disorder is Mendelian autosomal recessive, the development of symptomatic disease appears to be multifactorial. Diet, environment, and polygenic traits controlling plasma amino acid levels all contribute to development of symptoms.

Clinically affected patients can be differentiated from patients with pellagra by dietary history and the presence of aminoaciduria. Diagnosis is made by the characteristic finding of large amounts of neutral amino acids in the urine. It can easily be distinguished from generalized aminoaciduria by the normal excretion of proline. There are no other renal tubule defects as in Fanconi syndrome. Heterozygotes have normal urinary amino acid excretion.

 TREATMENT
Symptomatic individuals should receive oral nicotinamide, 40 to 200 mg/d, and a high-protein diet to compensate for the poor amino acid absorption. Some patients who do not respond to nicotinamide may improve with tryptophan ethyl ester, which is lipid soluble and can be absorbed without an active transport system.

FANCONI SYNDROME   Fanconi syndrome is a generalized defect in proximal tubule transport involving amino acids, glucose, phosphate, uric acid, sodium, potassium, bicarbonate, and proteins. Idiopathic Fanconi syndrome may be inherited as an autosomal dominant, autosomal recessive, or X-linked trait. Sporadic cases are also seen. A variety of inherited systemic disorders are also associated with Fanconi syndrome including Wilson's disease, galactosemia, tyrosinemia, cystinosis, fructose intolerance, and Lowe's oculocerebral syndrome. The syndrome may be acquired in multiple myeloma, amyloid, and heavy metal toxicity.

The patients may present with a wide array of laboratory abnormalities including proximal renal tubular acidosis, glucosuria with a normal serum glucose, hypophosphatemia, hypouricemia, hypokalemia, generalized aminoaciduria, and low-molecular-weight proteinuria. Some patients do not have abnormalities in all proximal tubule transporters and may present with only a few of the laboratory findings. Rickets and osteomalacia are common findings secondary to the hypophosphatemia; production of calcitriol may also be abnormal. Metabolic acidosis also contributes to the bone disease. Polyuria, salt wasting, and hypokalemia may be quite severe.

 TREATMENT
Treatment includes phosphate supplements and calcitriol to heal the bone lesions, alkali for the acidosis, and liberal intake of salt and water. Alkali in the form of potassium salts may be particularly useful in the patient with RTA and hypokalemia. Aminoaciduria, glucosuria, hypouricemia, and low-molecular-weight proteinuria do not require treatment.

BIBLIOGRAPHY

BUCKALEW VM JR: Calcium nephrolithiasis and renal tubular acidosis, in *Disorders of Bone and Mineral Metabolism*, FL Coe, MJ Favus (eds). New York, Raven Press, 1992, p 729

CANTANI A et al: Familial juvenile nephronophthisis: A review and differential diagnosis. Clin Pediatr 25:90, 1986

CLIVE DM: Bartter's syndrome: The unsolved puzzle. Am J Kidney Dis 25:813, 1995

ECONS MJ, DREZNER MK: Bone disease resulting from inherited disorders of renal tubule transport and vitamin D metabolism, in *Disorders of Bone and Mineral Metabolism*, FL Coe, MJ Favus (eds). New York, Raven Press, 1992, p 935

GABOW PA: Autosomal dominant polycystic kidney disease. N Engl J Med 329:332, 1993

GINALSKI JM et al: Does medullary sponge kidney cause nephrolithiasis. AJR 155:299, 1990

HALPERIN ML et al: Urine ammonium: The key to the diagnosis of distal renal tubular acidosis. Nephron 50:1, 1988

INTERNATIONAL POLYCYSTIC KIDNEY DISEASES CONSORTIUM: Polycystic kidney disease: The complete structure of the PKD1 gene and its protein. Cell 81:289, 1995

LLOYD SE et al: A common molecular basis for three inherited kidney stone diseases. Nature 379:445, 1996

MORRIS RC, IVES HE: Inherited disorders of the renal tubule, in *The Kidney*, 5th ed, BM Brenner (ed). Philadelphia, Saunders, 1996, p 1764

SCHILD L: A mutation in the epithelial sodium channel causing Liddle disease increases channel activity in the *Xenopus laevis* oocyte expression system. Proc Natl Acad Sci 92:5699, 1995

SCRIVER CR et al: The Hartnup phenotype: Mendelian transport disorder, multifactorial disease. Am J Hum Genet 40:401, 1987

SIRIS ES et al: Tumor-induced osteomalacia. Am J Med 82:307, 1987

VERGE CF et al: Effects of therapy in X-linked hypophosphatemic rickets. N Engl J Med 325:1843, 1991

WELLING LW, GRANTHAM JJ: Cystic and developmental diseases of the kidney, in *The Kidney*, 5th ed, BM Brenner (ed). Philadelphia, Saunders, 1996, p 1828

YOSHIDA H et al: Angiotensin II type 1 receptor gene abnormality in a patient with Bartter's syndrome. Kidney Int 46:1505, 1994

John R. Asplin, Fredric L. Coe, Murray J. Favus

NEPHROLITHIASIS

TYPES OF STONES

Calcium salts, uric acid, cystine, and struvite ($MgNH_4PO_4$) are the basic constituents of most kidney stones in the western hemisphere. Calcium oxalate and calcium phosphate stones make up 75 to 85 percent of the total (Table 279-1) and may be admixed in the same stone. Calcium phosphate in stones is usually hydroxyapatite [$Ca_5(PO_4)_3OH$] or, less commonly, brushite ($CaHPO_4 \cdot H_2O$).

Calcium stones are more common in men; the average age of onset is the third decade. Approximately 60 percent of people who form a single calcium stone eventually form another within the next 10 years, and the intervals between successive stones shorten or remain constant. The average rate of new stone formation in patients who have had a previous stone is about one stone every 2 or 3 years. Calcium stone disease is frequently familial.

In the urine, calcium oxalate monohydrate crystals (whewellite) usually grow as biconcave ovals that resemble red blood cells in shape and size but may occur in a larger, "dumbbell" form. In polarized light the crystals appear bright against a dark background, with an intensity that is dependent on orientation, a property known as *birefringence*. Calcium oxalate dihydrate crystals (weddellite) are bipyramidal and only weakly birefringent. Apatite crystals do not exhibit birefringence and appear amorphous because the actual crystals are too small to be resolved by light microscopy. Brushite produces elongated lathlike (narrow, long, rectangular) crystals.

Uric acid stones (see Table 279-1) are radiolucent and are also more common in men. Half of patients with uric acid stones have gout; uric acid lithiasis is usually familial whether or not gout is present. In urine, uric acid crystals are red-orange in color because they absorb the pigment uricine. Anhydrous uric acid produces small crystals that appear amorphous by light microscopy. They are indistinguishable from apatite crystals, except for their birefringence. Uric acid dihydrate tends to form teardrop-shaped crystals as well as flat, square plates; both are strongly birefringent. Uric acid gravel appears like red dust, and the stones are also orange or red on some occasions. *Cystine stones* are uncommon (see Table 279-1), are lemon yellow, and sparkle; radiopacity is due to the sulfur content. Cystine crystals appear in the urine as flat, hexagonal plates.

Struvite stones are common (see Table 279-1) and potentially dangerous. These stones occur mainly in women or patients who require chronic bladder catheterization and result from urinary tract infection with urease-producing bacteria, usually *Proteus* species. The stones can grow to a large size and fill the renal pelvis and calyces to produce a "staghorn" appearance. They are radiopaque and have a variable internal density. In urine, struvite crystals are rectangular prisms said to resemble coffin lids.

MANIFESTATIONS OF STONES

As stones grow on the surfaces of the renal papillae or within the collecting system, they need not produce symptoms. Asymptomatic stones may be discovered during the course of radiographic studies undertaken for unrelated reasons. Stones rank, along with benign and malignant neoplasms, renal cysts, and genitourinary tuberculosis, among the common causes of isolated hematuria. Much of the time, however, stones break loose and enter the ureter or occlude the ureteropelvic junction, causing pain and obstruction.

STONE PASSAGE A stone can traverse the ureter without symptoms, but passage usually produces pain and bleeding. The pain begins gradually, usually in the flank, but increases over the next 20 to 60 min to become so severe that narcotic drugs may be needed for its control. The pain may remain in the flank or spread downward and anteriorly toward the ipsilateral loin, testis, or vulva. Pain that migrates downward indicates that the stone has passed to the lower third of the ureter, but if the pain does not migrate, the position of the stone cannot be predicted. A stone in the portion of the ureter within the bladder wall causes frequency, urgency, and dysuria that may be confused with urinary tract infection. Hematuria is usual with passage of a stone.

OTHER SYNDROMES *Staghorn Calculi* Struvite, cystine, and uric acid stones often grow too large to enter the ureter. They

Table 279-1

Major Causes of Renal Stones

Stone Type and Causes	Percent of all Stones*	Percent Occurrence of Specific Causes*	Ratio of Males to Females	Etiology	Diagnosis	Treatment
Calcium stones	75–85		2:1 to 3:1			
Idiopathic hypercalciuria		50–55	2:1	Hereditary (?)	Normocalcemia, unexplained hypercalciuria†	Thiazide diuretic agents
Hyperuricosuria		20	4:1	Diet	Urine uric acid >750 mg per 24 h (women), >800 mg per 24 h (men)	Allopurinol or diet
Primary hyperparathyroidism		5	3:10	Neoplasia	Unexplained hypercalcemia	Surgery
Distal renal tubular acidosis		Rare	1:1	Hereditary	Hyperchloremic acidosis, minimum urine pH >5.5	Alkali replacement
Intestinal hyperoxaluria		~1–2	1:1	Bowel surgery	Urine oxalate >50 mg per 24 h	Cholestyramine or oral calcium loading
Hereditary hyperoxaluria		Rare	1:1	Hereditary	Urine oxalate and glycolic or l-glyceric acid increased	Fluids and pyridoxine
Hypocitraturia		15–60	2:1 to 5:1	Hereditary (?), diet	Urine citrate <320 mg per 24 h	Alkali supplements
Idiopathic stone disease		20	2:1	Unknown	None of the above present	Oral phosphate, fluids
Uric acid stones	5–8					
Gout		~50	3:1 to 4:1	Hereditary	Clinical diagnosis	Alkali to raise urine pH
Idiopathic		~50	1:1	Hereditary (?)	Uric acid stones, no gout	Allopurinol if daily urine uric acid above 1000 mg
Dehydration		?	1:1	Intestinal, habit	History, intestinal fluid loss	Alkali, fluids, reversal of cause
Lesch-Nyhan syndrome		Rare	Males only	Hereditary	Reduced hypoxanthine-guanine phosphoribosyltransferase level	Allopurinol
Malignant tumors		Rare	1:1	Neoplasia	Clinical diagnosis	Allopurinol
Cystine stones	1		1:1	Hereditary	Stone type; elevated cystine excretion	Massive fluids, alkali, D-penicillamine if needed
Struvite stones	10–15		2:10	Infection	Stone type	Antimicrobial agents and judicious surgery

* Values are percent of patients who form a particular type of stone and who display each specific cause of stones.
† Urine calcium above 300 mg per 24 h (men), 250 mg per 24 h (women), or 4 mg/kg per 24 h either sex. Hyperthyroidism, Cushing syndrome, sarcoidosis, malignant tumors, immobilization, vitamin D intoxication, rapidly progressive bone disease, and Paget's disease all cause hypercalciuria and must be excluded in diagnosis of idiopathic hypercalciuria.

gradually fill the renal pelvis and may extend outward through the infundibula to the calyces themselves.

Nephrocalcinosis Calcium stones grow on the papillae. Most break loose and cause colic, but they may remain in place so that multiple papillary calcifications are found by x-ray, a condition termed *nephrocalcinosis*. Papillary nephrocalcinosis is common in hereditary distal renal tubular acidosis (RTA) and in other types of severe hypercalciuria. In medullary sponge kidney disease (see Chap. 278) calcification may occur in dilated distal collecting ducts.

Sludge Sufficient uric acid or cystine in the urine may plug both ureters with precipitate. Calcium oxalate crystals do not do this because less than 100 mg oxalate usually is excreted daily in the urine even in severe hyperoxaluric states, compared with 1000 mg uric acid in patients with hyperuricosuria and 400 to 800 mg cystine in patients with cystinuria. Calcium phosphate crystals can render the urine milky but do not plug the urinary tract.

INFECTION Although urinary tract infection is not a direct consequence of stone disease, it can occur after instrumentation and surgery of the urinary tract, which are frequent in the treatment of stone disease. Stone disease and urinary tract infection can enhance the seriousness of one another and interfere with treatment. Obstruction of an infected kidney by a stone may lead to sepsis and extensive damage of renal tissue, since it converts the urinary tract proximal to the obstruction into a closed, or partially closed, space that can become an abscess. Stones may harbor bacteria in the stone matrix, leading to recurrent urinary tract infection. On the other hand, infection due to bacteria that possess the enzyme urease can cause stones composed of struvite.

ACTIVITY OF STONE DISEASE *Active disease* means that new stones are forming or that preformed stones are growing. Sequential radiographs of the renal areas are needed to document the growth or appearance of new stones and to ensure that passed stones are actually newly formed, not preexistent ones.

PATHOGENESIS OF STONES

Urinary stones usually arise because of the breakdown of a delicate balance. The kidneys must conserve water, but they must excrete materials that have a low solubility. These two opposing requirements must be balanced during adaptation to diet, climate, and activity. The problem is mitigated to some extent by the fact that urine contains substances that inhibit crystallization of calcium salts and others that bind calcium in soluble complexes. These protective mechanisms are less than perfect. When the urine becomes supersaturated with insoluble materials, because excretion rates are excessive and/or because water conservation is extreme, crystals form and may grow and aggregate to form a stone.

SUPERSATURATION In a solution in equilibrium with crystals of calcium oxalate, the product of the chemical activities of the calcium and oxalate ions in the solution is termed the *equilibrium solubility product*. If crystals are removed, and if either calcium or oxalate ions are added to the solution, the activity product increases, but the solution may remain clear; no new crystals form. Such a solution is *metastably supersaturated*. If new calcium oxalate seed crystals are now added, they will grow in size. Ultimately, the activity product reaches a critical value at which a solid phase begins to develop spontaneously. This value is called the *upper limit of metastability*, or the *formation product*. Stone growth in the urinary tract requires a urine that, on average, is above the equilibrium solubility product. Persistence of a stone requires an average activity product at least equal to the solubility product. Excessive supersaturation is common in stone formation.

Calcium, oxalate, and phosphate form many stable soluble complexes among themselves and with other substances in urine, such as citrate. As a result, their free ion activities are below their chemical concentrations and can be measured only by indirect techniques. Reduction in ligands such as citrate can increase ion activity without changing total urinary calcium. Urine supersaturation can be increased by dehydration or by overexcretion of calcium, oxalate, phosphate,

cystine, or uric acid. Urine pH is also important; phosphate and uric acid are weak acids that dissociate readily over the physiologic range of urine pH. Alkaline urine contains more urate and dibasic phosphate, favoring deposits of sodium hydrogen urate, brushite, and apatite. Below a urine pH of 5.5, uric acid crystals (pK 5.47) predominate, whereas phosphate crystals are rare. The solubility of calcium oxalate, on the other hand, is not influenced by changes in urine pH. Measurements of supersaturation in a pooled 24-h urine sample probably underestimate the risk of precipitation. Transient dehydration, variation of urine pH, and postprandial bursts of overexcretion may cause values considerably above average.

NUCLEATION **Homogeneous Nucleation** In urine that is supersaturated with respect to calcium oxalate, these two ions form clusters. Most small clusters eventually disperse because the internal forces that hold them together are too weak to overcome the random tendency of ions to move away. Clusters of over 100 ions can remain stable because attractive forces balance surface losses. Once they are stable, nuclei can grow at levels of supersaturation below that needed for their creation. The formation product marks the point at which stable nuclei become frequent enough to create a permanent solid phase.

Heterogeneous Nucleation If a supersaturated urine is seeded with preformed nuclei of a crystal that is similar in structure to calcium oxalate, calcium and oxalate ions in solution will bind to the crystal's surface as they would on a seed crystal of calcium oxalate itself. The organized growth of one crystal on the surface of another is called *epitaxial growth*, and the seeding of a supersaturated solution by foreign nuclei is called *heterogeneous nucleation*. Sodium hydrogen urate, uric acid, and hydroxyapatite crystals can serve as heterogeneous nuclei that permit calcium oxalate stones to form, even though urine calcium oxalate supersaturation never exceeds the metastable limit for homogeneous nucleation.

INHIBITORS OF CRYSTAL FORMATION Stable nuclei must grow and aggregate to produce a stone of clinical significance. Urine contains potent inhibitors of nucleation, growth, and aggregation for calcium oxalate and calcium phosphate but not for uric acid, cystine, or struvite. Inorganic pyrophosphate is a potent inhibitor that appears to affect calcium phosphate more than calcium oxalate crystals. Other urine components that appear to be glycoproteins inhibit all three processes of calcium oxalate stone formation. Slowing of crystal growth increases the apparent upper limit of metastability because the critical growth of ion clusters into stable nuclei is hindered. As a consequence of the presence of these inhibitors, crystal growth in urine is slow compared with growth in simple salt solutions, and the upper limit of metastability is higher. Citrate inhibits crystal growth and nucleation, though most of the stone inhibitory activity of citrate is due to lowering urine supersaturation via complexation of calcium.

EVALUATION AND TREATMENT OF PATIENTS WITH NEPHROLITHIASIS

Most patients with nephrolithiasis have remediable metabolic disorders that cause stones and can be detected by chemical analyses of serum and urine. A practical outpatient evaluation consists of two or three 24-h urine collections, each with a corresponding blood sample; measurements of serum and urine calcium, uric acid, electrolytes and creatinine and of urine pH, volume, oxalate, and citrate should be made. Since stone risks vary with diet, activity, and environment, at least one urine collection should be made on a weekend when the patient is at home and another on a work day. When possible, the composition of kidney stones should be determined because treatment depends on stone type (see Table 279-1). No matter what disorders are found, every patient should be counseled to avoid dehydration and to drink sufficient water so that they excrete at least 2 L of urine every day. Since treatment is prolonged, the use of medications must be justified by the activity and severity of stone disease and the importance of protection against new stones.

℞ TREATMENT

The management of stones already present in the kidneys or urinary tract requires a combined medical and surgical approach. The specific treatment depends on the location of the stone, the extent of obstruction, the function of the affected and unaffected kidney, the presence or absence of urinary tract infection, the progress of stone passage, and the risks of operation or anesthesia given the clinical state of the patient. In general, severe obstruction, infection, intractable pain, and serious bleeding are indications for removal of a stone.

In the past, stones were removed by operation or by passing a flexible basket retrograde up the ureter from the bladder during cystoscopy. There are now three alternatives. *Extracorporeal lithotripsy* causes the in situ fragmentation of stones in the kidney, renal pelvis, or proximal ureter by exposing them to shock waves. The kidney with the stone is centered at a focal point of parabolic reflectors, and high-intensity shock waves are created by high-voltage discharge. The waves are transmitted to the patient using water as a conduction medium, either by placing the patient in a water tank or by placing water-filled cushions between the patient and the shock-wave generators. The shock waves are focused by the reflectors so that they pass through the patient and fracture the stone as they pass. After multiple discharges, most stones are reduced to powder that moves through the ureter into the bladder. *Percutaneous ultrasonic lithotripsy* requires the passage of a rigid cystoscope-like instrument into the renal pelvis through a small incision in the flank. Stones can be disrupted by a small ultrasound transducer, and fragments can be removed directly. The last method is *laser lithotripsy via a ureteroscope* for removal of ureteral stones. These various forms of lithotripsy have largely replaced pyelolithotomy and ureterolithotomy.

CALCIUM STONES Idiopathic Hypercalciuria (See also Chap. 354)   This condition appears to be hereditary, and its diagnosis is straightforward (see Table 279-1). In some patients, primary intestinal hyperabsorption of calcium causes transient postprandial hypercalcemia that suppresses secretion of parathyroid hormone. The renal tubules are deprived of the normal stimulus to reabsorb calcium at the same time that the filtered load of calcium is increased. In other patients, reabsorption of calcium by the renal tubules appears to be defective, and secondary hyperparathyroidism is evoked by urinary losses of calcium. Renal synthesis of 1,25-dihydroxyvitamin D is increased, enhancing intestinal absorption of calcium. In the past, the separation of "absorptive" and "renal" forms of hypercalciuria was used to guide treatment. However, these may not be distinct entities but the extremes of a continuum of behavior. Vitamin D overactivity, either through high vitamin D levels or excess vitamin D receptor, is a likely explanation for the hypercalciuria in many of these patients. Hypercalciuria contributes to stone formation by raising urine saturation with respect to calcium oxalate and calcium phosphate.

℞ TREATMENT

Thiazide diuretics lower urine calcium in idiopathic hypercalciuria and are effective in preventing the formation of stones. Two 3-year randomized trials have shown a 50 percent decrease in stone formation in the thiazide-treated group as compared to the placebo-treated controls. The drug effect requires slight contraction of the extracellular fluid volume, and massive use of NaCl reduces its therapeutic effect. Thiazide-induced hypokalemia should be aggressively treated since hypokalemia will reduce urine citrate, increasing urine calcium ion levels.

Hyperuricosuria   About 20 percent of calcium oxalate stone formers are hyperuricosuric, primarily because of an excessive intake of purine from meat, fish, and poultry. The mechanism of stone formation probably is heterogeneous nucleation of calcium oxalate by crystals of sodium hydrogen urate or uric acid. A low-purine diet is desirable but difficult for many patients to achieve. The alternative is allopurinol, usually 100 mg bid.

Primary Hyperparathyroidism (See also Chap. 354)   The diagnosis of this condition is established by documenting that hypercalcemia that cannot be otherwise explained is accompanied by inappropriately elevated serum concentrations of parathyroid hormone. Hypercalciuria, usually present, raises the urine supersaturation of calcium phosphate and/or calcium oxalate (see Table 279-1). Prompt diagnosis is important because parathyroidectomy should be carried out before renal damage or bone disease occurs.

Distal Renal Tubular Acidosis (See also Chap. 278)   The defect in this condition seems to reside in the distal nephron, which cannot establish a normal pH gradient between urine and blood, leading to hyperchloremic acidosis. The diagnosis is suggested by a minimum urine pH in the presence of systemic acidosis above 5.5. If the diagnosis is in doubt because metabolic abnormalities are mild, oral challenge with NH$_4$Cl, 1.9 mmol/kg of body weight, will not lower urine pH below 5.5 in patients with distal RTA. Hypercalciuria, an alkaline urine, and a low urine citrate level cause supersaturation with respect to calcium phosphate. Calcium phosphate stones form, nephrocalcinosis is common, and osteomalacia or rickets may occur. Renal damage is frequent, and glomerular filtration rate falls gradually. Treatment with supplemental alkali reverses hypercalciuria and limits the production of new stones. The usual dose of sodium bicarbonate is 0.5 to 2.0 mmol/kg of body weight per day in four to six divided doses. An alternative is potassium citrate supplementation, given at the same dose per day but needing to be given only three to four times per day. In incomplete distal RTA, systemic acidosis is absent, but urine pH cannot be lowered below 5.5 after an exogenous acid load such as ammonium chloride. Incomplete RTA may develop in some patients who form calcium oxalate stones because of idiopathic hypercalciuria; the importance of the RTA in producing stones in this situation is uncertain, and thiazide treatment is a reasonable alternative. Some patients with incomplete RTA form calcium phosphate stones because of low urine citrate and an alkaline urine and are best treated with alkali as if RTA were complete.

Hyperoxaluria   Overabsorption of dietary oxalate and consequent oxaluria, i.e., so-called intestinal oxaluria, is one consequence of fat malabsorption (Chap. 285). The latter can be caused by a variety of conditions, including bacterial overgrowth syndromes, chronic disease of the pancreas and biliary tract, jejunoileal bypass in treatment of obesity, or ileal resection for inflammatory bowel disease. With fat malabsorption, calcium in the bowel lumen is bound by fatty acids instead of oxalate, which is left free for absorption in the colon. Delivery of unabsorbed fatty acids and bile salts to the colon may injure the colonic mucosa and enhance oxalate absorption. Dietary excess of oxalate in patients with normal intestinal function is a common cause of mild elevation of urine oxalate, but seldom to the level of urine oxalate seen in patients with enteric hyperoxaluria. Hereditary hyperoxaluria states are rare causes of severe hyperoxaluria; patients usually present with recurrent calcium oxalate stones during childhood. Type I hereditary hyperoxaluria is inherited as an autosomal recessive trait and is due to a deficiency in the peroxisomal enzyme alanine:glyoxylate aminotransferase. Type II is due to a deficiency of D-glyceric dehydrogenase. Ethylene glycol intoxication and methoxyflurane also can cause oxalate overproduction and hyperoxaluria. Hyperoxaluria from any cause can produce tubulointerstitial nephropathy (Chap. 276) and lead to stone formation.

℞ TREATMENT

The oxalate-binding resin cholestyramine at a dose of 8 to 16 g/d, correction of fat malabsorption, and a low-fat diet are effective treatments for oxaluria secondary to intestinal overabsorption. Calcium lactate, 8 to 14 g/d, which precipitates oxalate in the gut lumen, is an alternative form of therapy. Treatment for hereditary hyperoxaluria includes a high fluid intake, neutral phosphate, and pyridoxine (25 to 200 mg/d). Citrate supplementation may also have some benefit. Even with aggressive therapy, irreversible renal failure secondary to recurrent stone formation often occurs. Segmental liver transplant, to correct the enzyme defect, combined with a kidney transplant have been successfully utilized in patients with hereditary hyperoxaluria.

Hypocitraturia Urine citrate prevents calcium stone formation by creating a soluble complex with calcium, effectively reducing free urine calcium. Hypocitraturia is found in 15 to 60 percent of stone formers, either as a single disorder or in combination with other metabolic abnormalities. It can be secondary to systemic disorders, such as RTA, chronic diarrheal illness, or hypokalemia, or it may be a primary disorder, in which case it is called *idiopathic hypocitraturia*.

 TREATMENT

Treatment is with alkali, which increases urine citrate excretion; generally bicarbonate or citrate salts are used. Potassium salts are preferred as sodium loading increases urinary excretion of calcium, reducing the effectiveness of treatment. A recent randomized, placebo-controlled trial has demonstrated the effectiveness of potassium citrate in idiopathic hypocitraturia.

Idiopathic Calcium Lithiasis Some patients have no metabolic cause for stones despite a thorough metabolic evaluation (see Table 279-1). The best treatment appears to be high fluid intake so that the urine specific gravity remains at 1.005 or below throughout the day and night. Oral phosphate at a dose of 2 g phosphorus daily may lower urine calcium and increase urine pyrophosphate and thereby reduce the rate of recurrence. Orthophosphate causes mild nausea and diarrhea initially, but tolerance may improve with continued intake. Thiazide treatment to reduce calcium excretion and allopurinol to diminish uric acid output also may be helpful.

URIC ACID STONES These stones form because the urine becomes supersaturated with undissociated uric acid, uric acid that is protonated at its N-9 position. In gout, idiopathic uric acid lithiasis, and dehydration, the average pH is usually below 5.4 and often below 5.0. Undissociated uric acid therefore predominates and is soluble in urine only in concentrations of 100 mg/L. Concentrations above this level represent supersaturation that causes crystals and stones to form. Hyperuricosuria, when present, increases supersaturation, but urine of low pH can be supersaturated with undissociated uric acid even though the daily excretion rate is normal. Myeloproliferative syndromes, chemotherapy of malignant tumors, and the Lesch-Nyhan syndrome cause such massive production of uric acid and consequent hyperuricosuria that stones and uric acid sludge form even at a normal urine pH. Plugging of the renal collecting tubules by uric acid crystals can cause acute renal failure.

 TREATMENT

The two goals of treatment are to raise urine pH and to lower excessive urine uric acid excretion to less than 1 g/d. Supplemental alkali, 1 to 3 mmol/kg of body weight per day, should be given in three or four evenly spaced, divided doses, one of which should be given at bedtime. The form of the alkali may be important. Potassium citrate may reduce the risk of calcium salts crystallizing when urine pH is increased, whereas sodium citrate or sodium bicarbonate may increase the risk. If the overnight urine pH is below 5.5, the evening dose of alkali may be raised or 250 mg acetazolamide added at bedtime. A low-purine diet should be instituted in those uric acid stone formers with hyperuricosuria. Patients who continue to form uric acid stones despite treatment with fluids, alkali, and a low-purine diet should have allopurinol added to their regimen. If hypercalciuria is also present, it should be specifically treated as alkali alone could lead to calcium phosphate stone formation.

CYSTINURIA AND CYSTINE STONES (See also Chap. 349) In this disorder, proximal tubular and jejunal transport of the dibasic amino acids cystine, lysine, arginine, and ornithine are defective, and excessive amounts are lost in the urine. Clinical disease is due solely to the insolubility of cystine, which forms stones.

Pathogenesis Cystinuria probably occurs because of defective transport of amino acids by the brush borders of renal tubule and intestinal epithelial cells. Cystine, lysine, arginine, and ornithine appear to share a common renal transport pathway, since infusion of lysine decreases tubular reabsorption of the other three. However, cystine is also transported by a separate transport mechanism, because cystinuria and dibasic aminoaciduria can occur independently. The intestinal defects are not similar in all patients who are homozygous for cystinuria, and the extent of aminoaciduria in individuals who are heterozygous carriers of the defect varies from family to family. Three types of inheritance have been described (see Chap. 349).

Diagnosis Cystine stones are formed only by patients with cystinuria, but 10 percent of stones in cystinuric patients do not contain cystine; therefore, every stone former should be screened for the disease. The sediment from a first morning urine specimen in many patients with homozygous cystinuria reveals typical flat, hexagonal platelike cystine crystals. Cystinuria also can be detected using the urine sodium nitroprusside test. The test is positive with 75 to 125 mg cystine per gram of creatinine, a concentration lower than that in the urine of patients with cystinuria but above the levels in normal urine. Because the test is sensitive, it is positive in many asymptomatic heterozygotes for cystinuria. A positive nitroprusside test or the finding of cystine crystals in the urine sediment should be evaluated by measurement of daily cystine excretion. Normal adults excrete 40 to 60 mg cystine per gram of creatinine, heterozygotes usually excrete less than 300 mg/g, and homozygotes almost always excrete above 250 mg/g.

 TREATMENT

This consists of a high fluid intake, even at night. Daily urine volume should exceed 3 L. Raising urine pH with alkali is helpful, provided the urine pH exceeds 7.5. A low-salt diet (100 mmol/d) can reduce cystine excretion up to 40 percent. Because side effects are frequent, drugs such as penicillamine and tiopronin, which form the soluble disulfide cysteine-drug complexes, should be used only when fluid loading, salt reduction, and alkali therapy are ineffective. Captopril, which has a free sulfhydryl group to bind cysteine, has been used in a limited number of patients with some success. Low-methionine diets have not proved to be practical for clinical use, but patients should avoid protein gluttony.

STRUVITE STONES These stones are a result of urinary infection with bacteria, usually *Proteus* species, which possess urease, an enzyme that degrades urea to NH_3 and CO_2. The NH_3 hydrolyzes to NH_4^+ and raises urine pH to 8 or 9. The CO_2 hydrates to H_2CO_3 and then dissociates to CO_3^{2-} which precipitates with calcium as $CaCO_3$. The NH_4^+ precipitates PO_4^{3-} and Mg^{2+} to form $MgNH_4PO_4$ (struvite). The result is a stone of calcium carbonate admixed with struvite. Struvite does not form in urine in the absence of infection, because NH_4^+ concentration is low in urine that is alkaline in response to physiologic stimuli. Chronic *Proteus* infection can occur because of impaired urinary drainage, urologic instrumentation or surgery, and especially with chronic antibiotic treatment, which can favor the dominance of *Proteus* in the urinary tract.

 TREATMENT

Complete removal of the stone with subsequent sterilization of the urinary tract is the treatment of choice for patients who can tolerate the procedures. Open surgery is successful in debulking the stone and improving renal function if obstruction is present; however, there is recurrence of stone in 25 percent of the patients. Irrigation of the renal pelvis and calyces with hemiacidrin, a solution that dissolves struvite, can reduce recurrence after surgery. Newer procedures such as lithotripsy and percutaneous nephrolithotomy, alone or in combination, have largely replaced open surgery. Stone-free rates of 50 to 90 percent have been reported after these procedures.

Antimicrobial treatment is best reserved for dealing with acute infection and for maintenance of a sterile urine after surgery, in the hope of preventing recurrence or minimizing stone growth. Urine cultures and culture of stone fragments removed at surgery should guide the choice of antibiotic. Methenamine mandelate, which lowers urine pH and liberates formaldehyde, can be used for chronic suppression of infection when a stone is present. For patients who are not candidates for surgical removal of stone, acetohydroxamic acid, an inhibitor of urease, can be used. Though effective in treating the stones, acetohydroxamic acid has many side effects, such as headache, tremor, and thrombophlebitis, which limits its use. Lowering urine pH with chronic administration of NH_4Cl may retard stone growth but also may raise urine calcium level and promote the formation of calcium oxalate stones.

BIBLIOGRAPHY

BATAILLE P et al: Diet, vitamin D and vertebral mineral density in hypercalciuric calcium stone formers. Kidney Int 39:1193, 1991.

BARCELO P et al: Randomized double-blind study of potassium citrate in idiopathic hypocitraturic calcium nephrolithiasis. J Urol 150:1761, 1993

COE FL et al: The pathogenesis and treatment of kidney stones. N Engl J Med 327:1141, 1992

CONSENSUS CONFERENCE: Prevention and treatment of kidney stones. JAMA 260:977, 1988

GLEESON MJ, GRIFFITH DP: Struvite calculi. Br J Urol 71:503, 1993

LEMANN J JR: Pathogenesis or idiopathic hypercalciuria and nephrolithiasis, in *Disorders of Bone and Mineral Metabolism*, FL Coe, MJ Favus (eds). New York, Raven Press, 1992, p 685

LINGEMAN JE: Mechanisms of stone disruption and dissolution, in *Disorders of Bone and Mineral Metabolism*, FL Coe, MJ Favus (eds). New York, Raven Press, 1992, p 625

NEWMAN DM et al: Long-term follow-up of 1,900 ESWL treatments, in *Shock Wave Lithotripsy*, JE Lingeman, DM Newman (eds). New York, Plenum, 1988

RESNICK MI, PAK CYC: *Urolithiasis*. Philadelphia, Saunders, 1991

280

Julian L. Seifter, Barry M. Brenner

URINARY TRACT OBSTRUCTION

Obstruction to the flow of urine, with attendant stasis and elevation in urinary tract pressure, impairs renal and urinary conduit functions and is a common cause of acute and chronic renal failure. With early relief of obstruction, the defects in function usually disappear completely. However, chronic obstruction may produce permanent loss of renal mass (renal atrophy) and excretory capability, as well as enhanced susceptibility to local infection and stone formation. Early diagnosis and prompt therapy are therefore essential to minimize the otherwise devastating effects of obstruction on kidney structure and function.

ETIOLOGY Obstruction to urine flow can result from *intrinsic* or *extrinsic mechanical blockade* as well as from *functional defects* not associated with fixed occlusion of the urinary drainage system. Mechanical obstruction can occur at any level of the urinary tract, from the renal calyces to the external urethral meatus. Normal points of narrowing, such as the ureteropelvic and ureterovesical junctions, bladder neck, and urethral meatus, are common sites of obstruction. When blockage is above the level of the bladder, unilateral dilatation of the ureter (*hydroureter*) and renal pyelocalyceal system (*hydronephrosis*) occur; lesions at or below the level of the bladder cause bilateral involvement.

Common forms of obstruction are listed in Table 280-1. In childhood, *congenital malformations*, including marked narrowing of the ureteropelvic junction, anomalous (retrocaval) location of the ureter, and posterior urethral valves, predominate. The latter defect is the

most common cause of bilateral hydronephrosis in boys. Children also may have bladder dysfunction secondary to congenital urethral stricture, urethral meatal stenosis, or bladder neck obstruction. In adults, urinary tract obstruction is due mainly to *acquired defects*. Pelvic tumors, calculi, and urethral stricture predominate. Ligation of, or injury to, the ureter during pelvic or colonic surgery can lead to hydronephrosis which, if unilateral, may remain relatively silent and undetected. *Schistosoma haematobium* and genitourinary tuberculosis are infectious causes of ureteral obstruction. Obstructive uropathy also may result from extrinsic neoplastic (carcinoma of cervix or colon, retroperitoneal lymphoma) or inflammatory disorders. One such inflammatory disorder is retroperitoneal fibrosis, a process of unknown cause seen most commonly in middle-aged men, which occasionally leads to bilateral ureteral obstruction. Retroperitoneal fibrosis must be distinguished from other retroperitoneal causes of ureteral obstruction, particularly lymphomas and pelvic neoplasms.

Functional impairment of urine flow usually results from disorders that involve both the ureter and bladder. Common functional lesions include neurogenic bladder, often with adynamic ureter, and vesicoureteral reflux. Reflux of urine from bladder to ureter(s) is more common in children than in adults and may result in severe unilateral or bilateral hydroureter and hydronephrosis. Abnormal insertion of the ureter into the bladder is the most common cause of vesicoureteral reflux in children. Reflux in the absence of urinary tract infection or bladder neck obstruction usually does not lead to renal parenchymal damage and often resolves spontaneously as the child matures. Surgical reinsertion of the ureter into the bladder is indicated if reflux is severe and unlikely to improve spontaneously, if renal function deteriorates, or if urinary tract infections recur despite chronic antimicrobial therapy. Hydronephrosis, usually more marked on the right than on the left, is common in pregnancy, due both to ureteral compression by the enlarged uterus and to functional effects of progesterone.

Table 280-1

Common Mechanical Causes of Urinary Tract Obstruction

Ureter	Bladder Outlet	Urethra
CONGENITAL		
Ureteropelvic junction narrowing or obstruction	Bladder neck obstruction	Posterior urethral valves
Ureterovesical junction narrowing or obstruction	Ureterocele	Anterior urethral valves
Ureterocele		Stricture
Retrocaval ureter		Meatal stenosis
		Phimosis
ACQUIRED INTRINSIC DEFECTS		
Calculi	Benign prostatic hyperplasia	Stricture
Inflammation	Cancer of prostate	Tumor
Trauma	Cancer of bladder	Calculi
Sloughed papillae	Calculi	Trauma
Tumor	Diabetic neuropathy	Phimosis
Blood clots	Spinal cord disease	
Uric acid crystals	Anticholinergic drugs and alpha-adrenergic antagonists	
ACQUIRED EXTRINSIC DEFECTS		
Pregnant uterus	Carcinoma of cervix, colon	Trauma
Retroperitoneal fibrosis	Trauma	
Aortic aneurysm		
Uterine leiomyomata		
Carcinoma of uterus, prostate, bladder, colon, rectum		
Lymphoma, pelvic inflammatory disease		
Accidental surgical ligation		

CLINICAL FEATURES The pathophysiology and clinical features of urinary tract obstruction are summarized in Table 280-2. *Pain* is the symptom that most commonly provokes the need for medical attention. The pain of urinary tract obstruction is due to distention of the collecting system or renal capsule. The severity of the pain is influenced more by the rate at which distention develops than by the degree of distention. Acute supravesical obstruction, as from a stone lodged in a ureter (Chap. 279), is associated with excruciatingly severe pain, usually called *renal colic*. This pain is relatively steady and continuous, with little fluctuation in intensity, and often radiates to the lower abdomen, testes, or labia. By contrast, more insidious causes of obstruction, such as chronic narrowing of the ureteropelvic junction, may produce little or no pain yet result in total destruction of the affected kidney. Flank pain that occurs only with micturition is pathognomonic of vesicoureteral reflux.

Azotemia develops in urinary tract obstruction when overall excretory function is impaired. This may occur in the setting of bladder outlet obstruction, bilateral renal pelvic or ureteric obstruction, or unilateral disease in a patient with a solitary functioning kidney. Complete bilateral obstruction should be suspected when acute renal failure is accompanied by anuria. Any patient with renal failure otherwise unexplained or with a history of nephrolithiasis, hematuria, diabetes mellitus, prostatic enlargement, pelvic surgery, trauma, or tumor should be evaluated for urinary tract obstruction.

In the acute setting, bilateral obstruction may result in sodium and water retention that may mimic prerenal azotemia. However, with more prolonged obstruction, symptoms of *polyuria* and *nocturia* commonly accompany partial urinary tract obstruction and result from impaired renal concentrating ability. This defect usually does not improve with administration of vasopressin and is therefore a form of acquired nephrogenic diabetes insipidus. Disturbances in sodium chloride transport in the ascending limb of Henle and, in azotemic patients, the osmotic (urea) diuresis per nephron lead to decreased medullary hypertonicity and hence a concentrating defect. Partial obstruction, therefore, may be associated with increased rather than decreased urine output. Indeed, wide fluctuations in urine output in a patient with azotemia should always raise the possibility of intermittent or partial urinary tract obstruction. If fluid intake is inadequate, severe dehydration and

hypernatremia may develop. Hesitancy and straining to initiate the urinary stream, postvoid dribbling, urinary frequency, and (overflow) incontinence are common with obstruction at or below the level of the bladder (see Chap. 47).

In addition to loss of urinary concentrating ability and azotemia, partial bilateral urinary tract obstruction often results in other derangements of renal function, including *acquired distal renal tubular acidosis*, *hyperkalemia*, and *renal salt wasting*. These defects in tubule function are often accompanied by renal tubulointerstitial damage. Morphologic abnormalities appear early in the course of obstruction; initially the interstitium becomes edematous and infiltrated with mononuclear inflammatory cells. With continued obstruction, the interstitium becomes fibrotic; scarring and atrophy of the papillae and medulla occur and precede these processes in the cortex.

The possibility of urinary tract obstruction must always be considered in patients with urinary tract infections or urolithiasis. Urinary stasis encourages the growth of organisms as well as the formation of crystals, especially magnesium ammonium phosphate (struvite). *Hypertension* is frequent in acute and subacute unilateral obstruction and is usually a consequence of increased release of renin by the involved kidney. Chronic unilateral or bilateral hydronephrosis, in the presence of extracellular volume expansion or other renal disease, may result in significant hypertension. *Polycythemia*, an infrequent complication of obstructive uropathy, is probably secondary to increased erythropoietin production by the obstructed kidney.

DIAGNOSIS A history of difficulty in voiding, pain, infection, or changes in urinary volume is common. Evidence for distention of the kidney or urinary bladder often can be obtained by palpation and percussion of the abdomen. A careful rectal examination may reveal enlargement or nodularity of the prostate, abnormal rectal sphincter tone, or a rectal or pelvic mass. The penis should be inspected for evidence of meatal stenosis or phimosis. In the female, vaginal, uterine, and rectal lesions responsible for urinary tract obstruction are usually revealed by inspection and palpation.

Urinalysis and examination of the urine sediment may reveal hematuria, pyuria, and bacteriuria. Often, however, the urine sediment is normal, even when obstruction leads to marked azotemia and extensive structural damage. An abdominal scout film should be obtained to evaluate the possibility of nephrocalcinosis or a radiopaque stone at any level of the urinary collecting system. As indicated in Fig. 280-1, if urinary tract obstruction is suspected, a bladder catheter should be inserted. If diuresis does not follow, then abdominal ultrasonography should be performed to evaluate renal and bladder size, as well as pyelocalyceal contour. Ultrasonography is approximately 90 percent specific and sensitive for detection of hydronephrosis. False-positive results are associated with diuresis, renal cysts, or presence of an extrarenal pelvis, a normal congenital variant. Hydronephrosis may be absent on ultrasound when obstruction is associated with volume contraction, staghorn calculi, or retroperitoneal fibrosis.

In some cases, the intravenous urogram may define the site of obstruction. In the presence of obstruction, the appearance time of the nephrogram is often delayed. Eventually, however, the renal image becomes more dense than normal because of slow tubular fluid flow rate, which results in enhanced water reabsorption by the nephrons and greater concentration of contrast medium within tubules. The kidney involved by an acute obstructive process is usually slightly enlarged, and there is dilatation of the calyces, renal pelvis, and ureter above the obstruction. The ureter, however, is not tortuous, as is the case when the obstruction is chronic. In comparison with the nephrogram, the urogram may be extremely faint, especially if the dilated renal pelvis is voluminous, causing dilution of the contrast medium. The radiographic study should be continued until the site of obstruction is determined or the contrast medium is excreted. Radionuclide scans define less anatomic detail than intravenous urography and, like the urogram, are of limited value when renal function is poor. Nonetheless, such scans are sensitive for the detection of obstruc-

Table 280-2

Pathophysiology of Bilateral Ureteral Obstruction

Hemodynamic Effects	Tubule Effects	Clinical Features
ACUTE		
↑Renal blood flow	↑Ureteral and tubule pressures	Pain (capsule distention)
↓GFR	↑Reabsorption of Na⁺, urea, water	Azotemia
↓Medullary blood flow		Oliguria or anuria
↑Vasodilator prostaglandins		
CHRONIC		
↓Renal blood flow	↓Medullary osmolarity	Azotemia
↓↓GFR	↓Concentrating ability	Hypertension
↑Vasoconstrictor prostaglandins	Structural damage; parenchymal atrophy	ADH-insensitive polyuria
↑Renin-angiotensin production	↓Transport functions for Na⁺, K⁺, H⁺	Natriuresis
		Hyperkalemic, hyperchloremic acidosis
RELEASE OF OBSTRUCTION		
Slow ↑ in GFR (variable)	↓Tubule pressure	Postobstructive diuresis
	↑Solute load per nephron (urea, NaCl)	Potential for volume depletion and electrolyte imbalance due to losses of Na⁺, K⁺, PO₄²⁻, Mg²⁺, and water
	Natriuretic factors present	

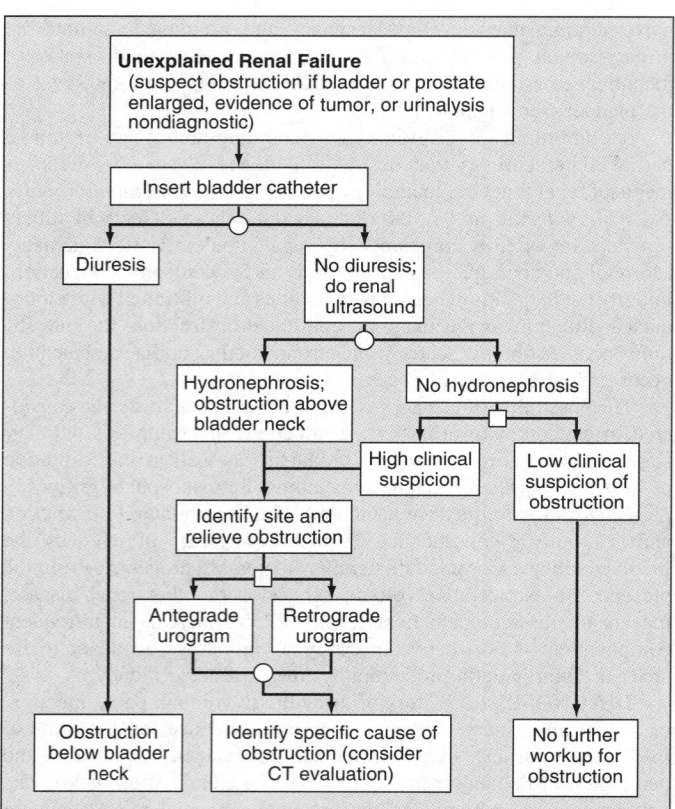

FIGURE 280-1 Diagnostic approach for urinary tract obstruction in unexplained renal failure. Circles represent diagnostic procedures, and squares indicate clinical decisions based on available data. CT, computed tomography.

tion and provide a substitute test in some patients at high risk for reaction to intravenous contrast.

To facilitate visualization of a suspected lesion in a ureter or renal pelvis, *retrograde* or *antegrade urography* should be attempted. These diagnostic studies may be preferable to the intravenous pyelogram in the azotemic patient, in whom poor excretory function precludes adequate visualization of the collecting system. Furthermore, intravenous urography carries the risk of contrast-induced renal failure in patients with renal insufficiency, diabetes mellitus, and multiple myeloma, particularly when performed under conditions of dehydration. The retrograde approach involves catheterization of the involved ureter under cystoscopic control, while the antegrade technique necessitates placement of a catheter into the renal pelvis via a needle inserted percutaneously under ultrasonic or fluoroscopic guidance. While the antegrade approach carries the added advantage of providing immediate decompression of a unilateral obstructing lesion, many urologists initially attempt the retrograde approach and resort to the antegrade method only when attempts at retrograde catheterization are unsuccessful or when cystoscopy or general anesthesia is contraindicated. Patients suspected of having intermittent ureteropelvic obstruction (whether functional or mechanical) should have radiologic evaluation while they are in pain, since a normal urogram is commonly seen during asymptomatic periods. Hydration often helps to provoke a symptomatic attack. Voiding cystourethrography is of great value in the diagnosis of vesicoureteral reflux and bladder neck and urethral obstructions. Patients with obstruction at or below the level of the bladder exhibit thickening, trabeculation, and diverticula of the bladder wall. Postvoiding films reveal residual urine. If these radiographic studies fail to provide adequate information for diagnosis, endoscopic visualization by the urologist often permits precise

identification of lesions involving the urethra, prostate, bladder, and ureteral orifices.

Computed tomography is useful in the diagnosis of specific intraabdominal and retroperitoneal causes of obstruction but is less practical as an initial test to establish the presence of obstruction. Magnetic resonance imaging also may be useful in the identification of specific obstructive causes.

℞ TREATMENT

An individual with any form of urinary tract obstruction complicated by infection requires relief of obstruction as soon as possible to prevent development of generalized sepsis and progressive renal damage. On a temporary basis, depending on the site of obstruction, drainage is often satisfactorily achieved by nephrostomy, ureterostomy, or ureteral, urethral, or suprapubic catheterization. The patient with acute urinary tract infection and obstruction should be given appropriate antibiotics based on in vitro bacterial sensitivity and ability of the drug to concentrate in the kidney and urine. Treatment may be required for 3 to 4 weeks. Chronic or recurrent infections in an obstructed kidney with poor intrinsic function may necessitate nephrectomy. When infection is not present, immediate surgery often is not required, even in the presence of complete obstruction and anuria (because of the availability of dialysis), at least until acid-base, fluid and electrolyte, and cardiovascular status are restored to normal. Nevertheless, the site of obstruction should be ascertained as soon as feasible, in part because of the possibility that sepsis may occur and necessitate prompt urologic intervention. Elective relief of obstruction is usually recommended in patients with urinary retention, recurrent urinary tract infections, persistent pain, or progressive loss of renal function. Infrequently, mechanical obstruction can be alleviated by nonsurgical means, as with radiation therapy for retroperitoneal lymphoma. Likewise, functional obstruction secondary to neurogenic bladder may be decreased with the combination of frequent voiding and cholinergic drugs. → *The approach to obstruction secondary to renal stones is discussed in Chap. 279.*

PROGNOSIS With relief of obstruction, the prognosis regarding return of renal function depends largely on whether irreversible renal damage has occurred. When obstruction is not relieved, the course will depend mainly on whether the obstruction is complete or incomplete, bilateral or unilateral, and whether urinary tract infection is also present. Complete obstruction with infection can lead to total destruction of the kidney within days. In dogs, relief of complete obstruction of 1 and 2 weeks' duration restores glomerular filtration rate to 60 and 30 percent of normal, respectively; after 8 weeks of obstruction, recovery does not occur. Nevertheless, in the absence of definitive evidence of irreversibility, every effort should be made to decompress in the hope of restoring renal function at least partially. A renal radionuclide scan, performed after a prolonged period of decompression, may be used to predict reversible renal function.

POSTOBSTRUCTIVE DIURESIS Relief of bilateral, but not unilateral, complete urinary tract obstruction commonly leads to a postobstructive diuresis, characterized by polyuria, which may be massive. The urine is usually hypotonic and may contain a large amount of sodium chloride. The natriuresis is due, at least in part, to the excretion of retained urea, which acts as a poorly reabsorbable solute and diminishes salt and water reabsorption in the tubules (osmotic diuresis). The increase in intratubular pressure very likely also contributes to the impairment in net sodium chloride reabsorption, especially in the terminal nephron segments. Natriuretic factors (other than urea) also may accumulate during uremia induced by obstruction and depress salt and water reabsorption when urine flow is reestablished. In the majority of patients this diuresis is physiologic, resulting in the *appropriate* excretion of the excesses of salt and water retained during the period of obstruction. When extracellular volume and composition return to normal, the diuresis usually abates spontaneously. Therefore, replacement of urinary losses should serve only to prevent hypovolemia, hypotension, or disturbances in serum electrolyte concentrations. Occasionally, iatrogenic expansion of extracellular volume, secondary to administration of excessive quantities of intravenous fluids, is responsible for, or sustains, the diuresis observed in the postobstructive period. Replacement of no more than two-thirds of urinary volume losses per day is usually effective in avoiding this complication. The loss of electrolyte-free water with urea may result in hypernatremia. Serum and urine sodium and osmolal concentrations should guide the use of appropriate intravenous replacement. Often replacement with 0.45% saline is required. In a rare patient, relief of obstruction may be followed by urinary salt and water losses severe enough to provoke profound dehydration and vascular collapse. In these patients, an intrinsic defect in tubule reabsorptive function is probably responsible for the marked diuresis. Appropriate therapy in such patients includes intravenous administration of large quantities of salt-containing solutions to replace sodium and volume deficits.

BIBLIOGRAPHY

Curhan GC, Zeidel ML: Urinary tract obstruction, in *The Kidney*, 5th ed, BM Brenner (ed). Philadelphia, Saunders, 1996, p 1936

Gillenwater JY: The pathophysiology of urinary obstruction, in *Campbell's Urology*, 6th ed, PC Walsh et al (eds). Philadelphia, Saunders, 1992, pp 499–532

Kaye AD, Pollack HM: Diagnostic imaging approach to the patient with obstructive uropathy. Semin Nephrol 2:55, 1982

Klahr S, Harris KPG: Obstructive uropathy, in *The Kidney: Physiology and Pathophysiology*, 2d ed, DW Seldin, G Giebisch (eds). New York, Raven Press, 1992, p 3327

Wilson DR: Renal function during and following obstruction. Annu Rev Med 28:329, 1977

Section 1

DISORDERS OF THE ALIMENTARY TRACT

281 Kurt J. Isselbacher, Daniel K. Podolsky

APPROACH TO THE PATIENT WITH GASTROINTESTINAL DISEASE

BIOLOGIC CONSIDERATIONS   The mucosal surface of the gastrointestinal (GI) tract is composed of a remarkably dynamic population of epithelial cells that are highly developed in their capacity for transmembrane absorption and secretion. These secretory and absorptive abilities facilitate the essential function of the digestive tract in digestion and nutrient uptake, which must be accomplished while maintaining the barrier between the host and potentially harmful pathogens and mutagens in the lumen. The latter is accomplished through both the physical integrity of the intact mucosal surface and the extensive population of resident immune cells.

The intestinal surface itself also contains the distinctive M cells that serve to sample the antigenic milieu of the lumen. They overlie lymphoid aggregates (Peyer's patches). The predominance of suppressor lymphocytes in the surface epithelial layer (intraepithelial lymphocytes) suggests that damping of the body's response to the enormous number of potentially antigenic substances in the lumen is necessary to prevent the constant and unrestrained activation of immune and inflammatory processes. Conversely, the presence of large numbers of helper lymphocytes as well as other cellular effectors of immune response in the lamina propria and submucosa attests to a large armamentarium ready to respond when surface defenses have been breached. No doubt the concentration of so many immune cells capable of attracting and activating inflammatory cells predisposes to the numerous inflammatory conditions to which the GI tract is subject.

The mucosal surface of the GI tract is also remarkable for the very rapid turnover of the epithelial cell population. It is likely that the epithelium turns over in its entirety every 24 to 72 h. This capacity may permit rapid restitution of a functional cell population following an acute insult and may reduce the risk of malignancy through the shedding of cells affected by the many mutagens in the luminal contents. Nevertheless, this proliferative potential creates the setting for neoplastic disorders, which are so common in the GI tract. Another fundamental feature of the GI mucosa is the spatial segregation of the proliferative compartment from the terminally differentiated cells. This is true throughout the GI tract but is most apparent in the small intestine, where a gradient of differentiation exists from the depths of the crypts of Lieberkühn to the villus tip. This organization has a strong effect on the histology and pathophysiology of many mucosal disorders, such as celiac sprue.

In view of the important secretory and absorptive activities of mucosal surface, diseases of the GI tract may result in clinical consequences owing to physical disruption of the mucosal layer (e.g., blood loss, fluid loss, pathogenic invasion) or to nutritional derangements caused by impaired digestion and nutrient absorption. In focal or localized disease processes the former effects predominate, whereas the latter may be especially prominent in disorders that affect extensive areas of the GI tract in a diffuse manner.

While the essential roles of the GI tract—the absorption of nutrients and the excretion of the products—are accomplished in large part at the luminal surface, these processes also depend on the deeper muscular layers for the coordinated propulsion of food through the lumen. The complexity of the local and distant neural and endocrine factors that contribute to the regulation of intestinal motility is only now becoming fully appreciated. Disruption of normal motility is quite common, with functional bowel complaints affecting as many as 15 percent of adults. Alterations in frequency of bowel movements, abdominal distention, abdominal pain, and nausea, individually or in varying combinations, may result from dysmotility. In addition, structural lesions may also indirectly lead to symptoms through their impact on motility involving some or all regions of the GI tract. These range from the *direct* effects of an obstructing lesion to the *indirect* actions of substances released by a primary mucosal disorder (e.g., inflammatory mediators such as arachidonic acid metabolites that also affect smooth-muscle activity).

Although valid unifying generalizations can be made about the GI tract in its entirety, the spectrum of diseases affecting this system and their clinical manifestations are significantly related to the constituent organ(s) involved (Table 281-1). Thus, esophageal disorders manifest themselves mainly through their relationship to swallowing; gastric disorders are dominated by features relating to acid secretion; and disease of the small and large intestine is evidenced mainly by disruption of nutrition and alterations of bowel movements. Similarly, diseases of the related ancillary organs, the exocrine pancreas and the hepatobiliary system, present characteristic clinical challenges. Finally, the GI tract may be affected by systemic disorders. These include vascular, inflammatory, infectious, and neoplastic conditions leading to focal or diffuse structural lesions. Metabolic and endocrine abnormalities as well as some drugs can disrupt normal bowel motility. Table 281-2 summarizes criteria that may be used to distinguish functional from organic or structural diseases of the GI tract.

CLINICAL CONSIDERATIONS   History   A thorough clinical history is essential in directing the clinician's attention to appropriate diagnostic considerations in the patient with GI symptoms. The most common complaints resulting from disorders involving the GI tract include pain and alterations in bowel habit, especially diarrhea or constipation. Of these complaints, *abdominal pain* is the most frequent and variable and may reflect a broad spectrum of problems, from the least threatening to the most urgent (see Chap. 14). In conjunction with an estimation of its intensity, an initial distinction should be made between pain of acute onset and more chronic discomfort. Pain of abrupt onset is often encountered in serious illness requiring urgent intervention, while a history of chronic discomfort is most often related to an indolent disorder. Dyspepsia, an ill-defined upper abdominal discomfort, is especially common. It is often accompanied in varying degrees by feelings of nausea, bloating, and distention. While it may be associated with peptic ulceration, non-ulcer dyspepsia (NUD) is common. A change in the pattern or character of pain may be equally important, possibly signifying the progression to a more critical stage of a problem (either recent or chronic) that was mild in onset. Ascertaining the location of the pain (upper or lower, localized or diffuse), its character (sharp, burning, cramping), and its relationship to meals will often provide significant insight into the most important diagnostic considerations. If eating produces the symptom, the clinician should determine whether the discomfort occurs while the patient is eating (as in esophageal disorders), shortly after the meal (as often occurs in biliary tract disease and abdominal angina), or 30 to 90 min later (as is typical of peptic disease). Pain that is not affected by eating suggests a process outside of the bowel lumen, such as abscess, peritonitis, pancreatitis, and some malignancies. Conversely, identification of factors that relieve the symptom is also helpful. For example, eating or antacid use typically gives relief in peptic ulcer disease or gastritis. A relationship of the discomfort to bowel movement, especially in association with an altered bowel habit, should focus attention on a disorder of the small or large bowel, such as inflammatory bowel disease.

Alterations in bowel habit can result from either disruption of normal intestinal motility or significant structural pathology. A thorough determination of the temporal evolution of the change and the nature of the alteration, in conjunction with other constitutional symptoms such as weight loss, fever, or anorexia, is important. A temporary variation in bowel habit in association with some life stress and in the absence of signs of systemic illness suggests the common "irritable bowel syndrome," especially when the alteration varies between diarrhea and constipation. Small, pellet-like stools are often described by the patient. Associated symptoms of dyspepsia (bloating, nausea, and "gas") are also common. This diagnosis can essentially be made on the basis of a thorough history and physical examination and very limited laboratory testing, to exclude structural disease. In contrast, the onset of worsening constipation in an adult with previously regular habits, especially when accompanied by systemic symptoms such as weight loss, suggests the possible presence of an underlying obstructing process, particularly malignancy. If diarrhea is present, one should determine the average number of stools, their consistency, their pattern, and the presence or absence of blood. Although *diarrhea* refers to an increased frequency of movements, patients will often use the term to describe loose or watery stools. The occurrence of nocturnal or true bloody diarrhea almost always reflects structural rather than functional bowel disease. A pungent stool odor or the presence of undigested meat in the movement are suggestive of pancreatic insufficiency. An alteration in color can be seen in cholestasis or steatorrhea (light-colored) or hemorrhage (melenic to maroon or bright red). Mucus in the movement is usually a sign of a functional bowel syndrome, while pus is more strongly suggestive of infectious or inflammatory disease. Less common but more dramatic are the symptoms of acute GI bleeding, including hematemesis, melena, and hematochezia, which usually lead to prompt efforts to find medical attention but should always be enquired after by the clinician.

In the evaluation of male patients, especially those with diarrhea, a tactful inquiry into sexual activity is essential. Homosexual males are at increased risk for a large variety of GI disorders, as well as AIDS, which may first manifest itself with GI symptoms. Such symptoms, especially diarrhea, are common in patients with AIDS. These patients are susceptible to a wide range of infections and neoplastic disorders of the GI tract, liver and biliary tract (see Chap. 308). Finally, careful attention must be given to a general medical history with an emphasis on present or past use of medications or nonprescription drugs. Thyroid and other metabolic disorders, especially those affecting calcium metabolism, can cause a variety of GI symptoms. Unless asked, patients may forget to mention that they take aspirin almost daily for headache, and this may account for occult blood found in the stool. The use of daily laxatives may explain chronic diarrhea.

Physical Examination, Endoscopy, and Radiology All of the cardinal methods of examination are helpful in evaluating the patient with GI symptoms. *Inspection* may disclose signs of cholestasis or nutritional deficiencies. Examination of the abdomen for an abnormal contour or inspection of the perianal region may reveal signs of a mass or a draining fistula. *Auscultation* is also important. A succussion splash may be elicited in the patients with symptoms of gastric outlet obstruction. The absence of bowel sounds or an alteration in pitch can lead to recognition of an evolving ileus or an obstructing process. A bruit may also be appreciated where there are symptoms of ischemic bowel disease. Careful *palpation* of the abdomen is especially important in detecting tenderness and masses, which in the appropriate clinical setting will lead to the recognition of cholecystitis, Crohn's disease, periappendiceal abscess, and many other disorders. Findings on abdominal palpation will often be complemented by *percussion*, which is essential to assessing liver and spleen size.

Elicitation of *rebound tenderness*, either direct or referred, after removal of the examining hand provides an important clue to localized or more generalized peritonitis, which is characteristic of many abdominal emergencies, including a perforated viscus, intraabdominal abscess, or tissue infarction. The clinician should be particularly alert to these signs in patients with severe pain of abrupt onset. Typically, the patient will remain immobile to avoid the accentuation of pain that may follow even slight movement and jarring of the abdomen. This contrasts with the sometimes frantic efforts to find a position of comfort in patients with severe pain deriving from visceral disease, e.g., pancreatitis or intestinal ischemia. In these disorders, the absence of findings on palpation of the abdomen may be in striking contrast to the evident distress of the patient. Only when the process progresses to tissue destruction (e.g., necrotizing pancreatitis or intestinal infarction) and secondary peritonitis will the abdominal examination prove remarkable, often in concert with striking signs of systemic illness, including hemodynamic instability. In addition to the examination of the abdomen, a carefully performed digital rectal examination is also essential. In the patient with complaints of incontinence, the integrity of the sphincter can be assessed. Most important, masses intrinsic to the rectum as well as abnormalities in the pelvis or the pouch of Douglas may only be detected by this examination, and the presence or absence of frank or occult blood in the stool is always important diagnostic information. Sigmoidoscopy should be viewed as a routine part of the physical examination in the patient with diarrhea or another alteration in bowel habit as well as when there is known or suspected blood loss from the lower bowel. Sigmoidoscopy, which can be performed with either a rigid or a flexible fiberoptic instrument, allows for direct inspection of the rectosigmoid mucosa, permitting the detection of cancers and polyps in this lower bowel segment that might well be missed by barium x-rays. Inflammatory changes of the mucosa can help identify patients with infectious dysentery or other forms of colitis, most notably ulcerative colitis. The findings of edema, granularity, and diffuse friability (easily induced mucosal bleeding) as well as superficial ulcerations are characteristic of the latter disorder. Fresh stool samples for microbiologic studies and superficial mucosal biopsies obtained at the time of sigmoidoscopy can also yield crucial diagnostic information.

Table 281-1

Distinguishing between Functional and Organic/Structural Disease of Gastrointestinal Tract

	Functional	Organic	
		Neoplastic	Inflammatory
Symptoms			
Weight loss	None	Common	Sometimes
Diarrhea	Daytime only	Nocturnal	Day and night
Blood loss	None	Frequent	Frequent
Fever	None	Rare	Frequent
Pain	Cramping, relieved by defecation	Minor to severe	May be localized; may be severe
Bowel habit (diarrhea or constipation)	Alternating diarrhea/constipation Pellet-like stools	Constipation (rarely diarrhea) Change in caliber	Diarrhea or normal
Laboratory tests			
Hematocrit	Normal	Often decreased	May be decreased
White blood cell count	Normal	Usually normal	Often elevated
Erythrocyte sedimentation rate	Normal	Usually increased	Usually increased

Definitive demonstration or exclusion of structural lesions of the GI tract, particularly the great majority of disorders that affect primarily the mucosal surface, often cannot be accomplished by physical examination alone. Many upper and lower GI tract disorders are accessible to inspection via fiberoptic instruments. As a result, endoscopy has supplanted conventional contrast x-ray studies for many clinical problems, both because of its heightened precision for diagnosis and the opportunity in many instances to accomplish meaningful therapeutic intervention. However, it should be emphasized that *no procedure should be considered routine* and used indiscriminately; there must be a rational basis for its use in the individual patient. These techniques are discussed in detail in Chap. 282. Upper GI endoscopy permits evaluation of the esophagus, stomach, duodenum, and, with specially designed instruments, proximal jejunum. When the clinical history warrants a diagnostic examination of the upper GI tract for a structural lesion, endoscopic examination is preferable to radiologic study in most patients when the choice is available. Side-viewing scopes permit inspection and cannulation of the ampulla of Vater, facilitating retrograde cholangiopancreatography. Evaluation of some patients will be further benefited by endoscopic ultrasound, which can delineate submucosal mass lesions and abnormalities in the pancreas. The colonoscope can be used to visualize the entire colon and often the terminal ileum, resulting in more accurate diagnosis of inflammatory bowel disease and mass lesions. Frequently, colonic polyps can be removed at the time of their initial identification.

Endoscopic techniques are relatively precise in defining many problems, but the limitations of these tools, as well as the continued advantages of x-ray studies in some situations, should be recognized. Endoscopic tools are not useful in assessing GI motility, which may be assessed more accurately by barium studies. In addition, some areas, notably the small intestine, remain relatively inaccessible to fiberoptic instruments. In hospitals where endoscopy is not feasible, the upper GI series and barium enema remain good diagnostic modalities to evaluate the upper and lower GI tract, especially when air-contrast techniques are employed. However, they should generally be avoided in patients with GI bleeding or suspected bowel obstruction. In addition the physician must exercise judgment in preparing the patient for these studies, recognizing that cathartics may markedly worsen the condition of a patient with obstructing lesions or colitis.

Although endoscopy has obviated the need for many conventional GI x-rays, other radiologic imaging modalities have assumed a crucial role in the approach to the patient with GI symptoms. These techniques include ultrasound (US), computed tomography (CT), and magnetic resonance imaging (MRI). Both US and CT are useful in the delineation of abdominal masses. CT, though more expensive, is often more effective in the evaluation of the lower abdomen, where inflammatory masses in patients with Crohn's disease or complications of diverticular disease may be accurately imaged. However, US is an effective and less expensive tool for the evaluation of the right upper quadrant, including the gall bladder and biliary tract. Imaging techniques are often complementary in the evaluation of pancreatic disease. In combination with Doppler analysis, US can be used to assess the patency and direction of blood flow in the portal vein in the patient with advanced liver disease. MRI may give exquisitely accurate information on the anatomic extent of invasive rectal cancers and blood flow in patients with vascular disorders, but the full range of its uses in GI disorders remains to be delineated. More sophisticated CT and MRI equipment can actually permit the performance of digital angiography without the invasive catheterization necessary in conventional visceral angiography.

DIAGNOSTIC APPROACHES **Abdominal Pain** Determination of the cause of abdominal pain remains an imposing clinical challenge. As noted above, disorders ranging from the acute and catastrophic to the chronic and indolent can cause abdominal pain. Further-

Table 281-2

Overview of Approach to Patients with Common Gastrointestinal Disorders

Site of Disorder	Common Symptoms	Possible Physical Signs	Potential Procedures or Laboratory Studies
Esophagus	Dysphagia Odynophagia Heartburn, chest pain Hematemesis/melena		Esophagoscopy Barium swallow Manometry Bernstein test
Stomach	Nausea and vomiting Epigastric pain Hematemesis/melena Early satiety	Distention Tenderness Succussion splash Mass	Gastroscopy Upper GI x-ray series Nasogastric aspiration Gastric emptying
Pancreas	Pain Weight loss Diarrhea Steatorrhea	Mass Jaundice	Kidney-ureter-bladder x-ray series Qualitative stool fat and muscle fiber US, CT, MRI, endoscopic retrograde cholangiopancreatography Pancreatic function tests
Small Intestine Duodenum	Pain Nausea/vomiting Hematemesis	Tenderness Altered bowel sounds Distention Mass	Duodenoscopy Small bowel follow-through, enteroclysis Kidney-ureter-bladder x-ray series D-Xylose absorption tests
Jejunum	Pain Diarrhea	Altered bowel sounds Distention Mass	CT Stool cultures, stool examination for ova and parasites Small bowel biopsy
Ileum	Pain Diarrhea	Altered bowel sounds Distention Mass	
Colon	Diarrhea Pain Blood	Tenderness Mass Distention	Sigmoidoscopy Colonoscopy Barium enema Stool culture, stool examination for ova and parasites *Clostridium difficile* toxin assay
Rectum	Pain Urgency Hematochezia Pruritus	Tenderness	Sigmoidoscopy Anoscopy
Nonspecific	Weight loss Fever Anorexia Nausea and vomiting		Complete blood count Erythrocyte sedimentation rate Fecal occult blood test

more, differential diagnostic considerations may encompass diseases extrinsic to the GI tract, such as disorders of the genitourinary tract (e.g., pelvic inflammatory disease) and the peritoneum. The history and physical examination are essential guides to a sensible diagnostic approach. The initial goal is to distinguish between an urgent problem requiring expeditious delineation and a nonacute disorder. In the former situation, initial clinical impressions based on the history and physical examination can be further refined through routine laboratory tests such as a complete blood count and differential as well as plain films of the abdomen. Particular features will dictate the appropriateness of urgent US or CT examination or the need to proceed promptly with surgery. In the patient with a long-standing and relatively stable problem, diagnostic evaluation can be more deliberate. The clinician may be able to reasonably establish a functional basis for the complaint on the strength of the history and physical examination alone. Radiologic contrast studies, other imaging modalities (e.g., US, CT), or endoscopic examination may be appropriate to exclude or identify certain of the gamut of disorders discussed above. If all these approaches do not determine the cause of the patient's symptoms, more unusual causes of abdominal pain may have to be excluded through specific urine or blood tests (e.g., porphyrins).

Problems of Swallowing   The approach should be as follows:

1. *Thorough determination of the nature of dysphagia.* Is the difficulty primarily in swallowing liquids, solids, or both? The location of the difficulty from the patient's perspective and presence or absence of accompanying *odynophagia* are important to ascertain. These historical clues are complemented by careful visual and neurologic examination of the oropharynx when appropriate.
2. *Routine esophageal x-rays* in the upright and lateral or Trendelenburg position. The horizontal views are essential for demonstration of the swallowing mechanism, unaided by gravity, and of the esophagogastric junction. For details of the pharyngoesophageal area, cineradiography is necessary because of the rapidity with which the contrast medium passes through. Hiatus hernia is extremely common (in 15 to 35 percent of persons over 50) and often is asymptomatic unless spontaneous reflux of gastric contents can be demonstrated to occur repeatedly. Careful attention is usually needed to detect lower esophageal rings or webs, which may be visible as indentations in the barium column only from a limited angle.
3. *Esophagoscopy.* This procedure is desirable for lesions suggested by x-ray or, if the lesion is unsuspected, to biopsy masses or abnormal mucosa and to obtain washings for exfoliative cytologic study. The diagnoses of peptic esophagitis and Barrett's esophagus are made endoscopically. Endoscopy is the most sensitive technique for identifying esophageal or gastric varices, although they are seldom important in the absence of hemorrhage. Fiberoptic instruments with a US probe at the tip (endoscopic ultrasound) are increasingly useful diagnostic tools for particular problems of the esophagus (and other sites of the GI tract).
4. *Manometric studies* of the upper esophagus, particularly in conjunction with cineradiography. At present, this procedure offers the best means of differentiating among disorders originating in the central nervous system, primary pharyngeal muscular disease, and cricopharyngeal dystonia. Manometry of the lower esophagus is useful in the diagnosis of diffuse esophageal spasm, achalasia, and infiltrative diseases that can alter esophageal motility.

Peptic or Digestive Disorders   The approaches to these disorders include the following.

1. *Insertion of a nasogastric tube.* This approach is used to establish whether significant gastric retention (more than 75 mL of gastric contents in the fasting state) exists and whether acid, bile, blood, or other materials are present. If pyloric obstruction or gastric atony is present, the tube is used to maintain suction while the

patient's electrolyte and fluid balance is restored to normal; the stomach is kept as clean as possible so that reliable diagnostic investigation may be carried out.

2. *Upper gastrointestinal endoscopy.* This procedure is most helpful in assessing the mucosa in gastritis or, together with biopsy and brushings for cytology, in differentiating between peptic and neoplastic ulcerating lesions. It may identify a specific bleeding site in clinical situations where several potential bleeding sites could exist, as in the patient with portal hypertension. In addition, it may be possible to cauterize or otherwise intervene to control hemorrhage via the endoscope (e.g., by injections of vasoconstricting agents such as epinephrine). The frequent association of gastritis with *Helicobacter pylori* in patients with actual peptic ulceration, as well as in those with nonulcer dyspepsia, has been well documented. Although, at this time, *H. pylori* infection can be most reliably confirmed in the individual patient by endoscopy and biopsy, this approach may be superseded by other, less invasive modalities including breath and serologic tests. Endoscopy can detect a number of potential sources of upper GI bleeding that are often missed by x-ray studies (e.g., erosive gastritis, Mallory-Weiss tear). Gastroscopy is particularly helpful in inspecting the postoperative stomach, especially in detecting stomal ulceration or so-called alkaline reflux gastritis. The first and second portions of the duodenum can also be routinely examined, and important information about ulcers and other lesions can be obtained. Radiologic studies may be useful when endoscopy is not readily available or in the assessment of suspected motility disorders (e.g., gastroparesis). In addition, radiologic examination may be preferred when there are contraindications to safe endoscopy.
3. *Gastric acid secretory studies.* Although not routinely necessary, these studies are useful in the diagnosis of the Zollinger-Ellison syndrome or atrophic gastritis and for determination of completeness of vagotomy. They should not be performed for the routine diagnosis of uncomplicated duodenal ulcer; also, there is no convincing evidence that they are useful in determining the choice of surgery for peptic ulcer.

Obstructive and Vascular Disorders of the Small Intestine
When intestinal problems present as obstructive syndromes, the plain x-ray film of the abdomen is the most important diagnostic adjunct to careful physical examination. Patterns of dilation of individual loops of intestine may be characteristic, as in volvulus or acute pancreatitis; erect and decubitus views will often show fluid levels in the affected segments. Motility disorders of the small intestine (temporary ileus or chronic intestinal pseudoobstruction) may also present with obstructive symptoms and similar x-ray findings but must be managed medically without surgical intervention. Air under the diaphragm is diagnostic of a perforated viscus; air in the portal vein usually results from intestinal necrosis secondary to mesenteric vascular occlusion. The diagnostic accuracy of the plain x-ray film in all types of intestinal obstruction is about 75 percent. In patients with symptoms of incomplete obstruction, the radiographic small-bowel series will often be diagnostic in defining the site and degree of obstruction. Infrequently, in this setting, all conventional x-ray studies are unremarkable. In such cases, the radiologist may perform a small bowel enteroclysis study by passing a special tube into the proximal jejunum; the rapid instillation of barium through the tube will distend the intestine and often reveal subtle lesions missed by other tests.

Vascular diseases of the small intestine are among the most difficult diseases to diagnose. In chronic mesenteric ischemia, radiographic, endoscopic, and laboratory tests are usually normal. Early in the course of acute mesenteric ischemia, the plain film of the abdomen may be unremarkable despite complaints of severe abdominal pain. In these settings, prompt mesenteric angiography is essential to confirm the diagnosis of vascular disease.

Inflammatory and Neoplastic Diseases of Small and Large Intestine   Patients with these conditions are usually identified by history, physical examination, and careful examination of the stools for exudate and blood. Examination of fresh stool samples for common bacterial pathogens and parasites by laboratories skilled in these techniques is important in identifying or excluding infectious causes of diarrhea, particularly in the patient with colitis. Sigmoidoscopy is valuable in identifying mucosal and neoplastic lesions of the rectum and distal colon. The mucosal surface of the entire colon and terminal ileum can be examined directly and biopsied through the fiberoptic sigmoidoscope or colonoscope. The radiologic examination of the small intestine is highly reliable in identifying the prestenotic and stenotic lesions of Crohn's disease. In the colon, a single barium enema examination in a well-prepared patient has a diagnostic accuracy of 80 to 85 percent; the addition of air-contrast technique brings the accuracy up over 90 percent. None of these figures is meaningful if the patient is poorly prepared for the examination, however. Colonoscopy may be preferable because of its greater accuracy and the fact that it enables the operator to remove the vast majority of polyps that are encountered as well as to obtain preoperative tissue confirmation in the patient who probably has cancer.

Peroral biopsy of the small intestine (now most often accomplished during endoscopy) and forceps biopsy of the rectosigmoid are of considerable importance in revealing mucosal disease. Rectal biopsy is an excellent means of demonstrating amyloidosis, schistosomiasis, and amebiasis. Submucosal disease is not seen in these superficial biopsies. Hirschsprung's disease is diagnosed histologically by a deep surgical biopsy of the lower part of the rectum.

Malabsorption Syndromes Malabsorption may be suspected on the basis of history and physical examination and confirmed by examination of the stool. Radiologic examination is helpful to rule out local lesions and to suggest motor and secretory dysfunction, but it is rarely diagnostic unless an abnormal small bowel mucosa or fistulas between the intestine and stomach are demonstrated.

The tests useful in the diagnosis of malabsorption are discussed in Chap. 285. A simple screening test for excessive fat in the stools can be accomplished by the microscopic examination of a stool specimen stained with Sudan. Chemical analysis of 3-day stool collection for fat, with the patient on a standard diet, is used to establish the diagnosis of steatorrhea. The D-xylose absorption test is about 90 percent accurate in distinguishing mucosal disease from pancreatic insufficiency. Peroral biopsy of the small intestine via the endoscope or a specialized biopsy device is of value in the diagnosis of celiac disease, and it may show the less common infiltrations of the mucosa by amyloid or bacterial mucoproteins (Whipple's disease). Leakage of protein into the intestinal lumen may cause hypoproteinemia and can be demonstrated by the recovery in stools of the serum protein α_1-antitrypsin or intravenously administrated markers such as albumin labeled with iodine or chromium isotopes.

Pancreas The pancreas is difficult to study because of its anatomic location and relative inaccessibility. Calcification of the pancreas on a plain abdominal film is highly suggestive of chronic pancreatitis and may be associated with fat malabsorption. Pancreatic exocrine insufficiency can be demonstrated by intubation of the duodenum and collection of pancreatic juice after stimulation with secretin or a test meal, but a stool collection for qualitative determination of fat and muscle fiber content is usually sufficient as an initial diagnostic approach. Abdominal US and CT are the best radiographic means of searching for pancreatic enlargement (see Chaps. 303 and 304). Both techniques may also be used to guide needle biopsies of the pancreas and may provide sufficient diagnostic information to obviate the need for exploratory surgery. The pancreatic duct can be cannulated via the fiberoptic duodenoscope and visualized by the injection of radiographic dye. Visualization of the duct may be helpful in the diagnosis of pancreatic pseudocysts, carcinoma, or chronic pancreatitis.

BIBLIOGRAPHY

JOHNSON LR et al: *Physiology of the Gastrointestinal Tract*, 3d ed. New York, Raven, 1995

SLEISENGER MH, FORDTRAN JS: *Gastrointestinal Disease*, 5th ed. Philadelphia, Saunders, 1993

YAMADA T et al: *Textbook of Gastroenterology*, 2d ed. Philadelphia, Lippincott, 1995

282 *Fred E. Silverstein*

GASTROINTESTINAL ENDOSCOPY*

Endoscopes have revolutionized the examination of the gastrointestinal (GI) tract. Because of the flexibility of the instrument and the controllability of the instrument tip, the operator can steer the endoscope around multiple bends under visual control. A channel permits the passage of a variety of endoscopic tools, such as biopsy forceps, cytology brushes, wash tubes, injecting devices, and electrocautery probes and snares. The viewing window and the light at the instrument's distal end can be washed free of obscuring material. Fluid can be aspirated from hollow organs, and air can be insufflated as needed to improve visualization. The videoendoscope is a modification of the original fiberendoscope in which a charge-coupled device on the tip of the instrument transmits the image to a TV screen. This system is being used increasingly because it permits storage, analysis, and transmission of the endoscopic images. → *The Color Atlas has plates of typical endoscopically visualized lesions.*

The usefulness of fiberendoscopy in diagnosing gastrointestinal disease is well established. Shallow lesions, such as erosions or healing ulcers, are missed by single-contrast x-ray examinations but not by endoscopy. The success of polypectomy via the colonoscope and of sphincterotomy via the duodenoscope have led to the development of other endoscopic therapeutic techniques, such as esophageal band ligation and endoscopic ultrasonography with fine needle aspiration; endoscopic approaches are now preferred to surgery in many situations.

Although esophagogastroduodenoscopy (EGD) is not a procedure for the occasional operator, it is widely available in both inpatient and outpatient settings. It is relatively easy to perform, but training and continued experience are necessary for optimal diagnostic accuracy and mastery of therapeutic techniques. The more complex procedures, such as colonoscopy and endoscopic retrograde cholangiopancreatography (ERCP), require special dexterity, a substantial investment of time for learning, and constant practice to maintain adequate skill; they are probably best performed by subspecialists. Complications are most frequent when the operator is inexperienced.

A history and physical examination should be done before any endoscopic procedure is undertaken. Special care is taken in patients with significant cardiac or pulmonary disease; blood clotting parameters should be checked in those with a history of excessive bleeding. Patients with prosthetic heart valves and those with a history of bacterial endocarditis or a significant right-to-left shunt should receive antibiotic prophylaxis. Contraindications to endoscopy in most situations include the inability of the patient to cooperate or give informed consent, an unstable cardiac or pulmonary condition, and an unstable neck prior to EGD. Intestinal perforation or full-thickness wall necrosis is also a contraindication to any endoscopic procedure.

Most endoscopists prefer to administer conscious sedation for endoscopic procedures other than flexible sigmoidoscopy and some screening upper endoscopies. After insertion of an intravenous catheter, a benzodiazepine such as diazepam or midazolam is titrated to light sedation. Supplementation with a narcotic such as meperidine also may be useful. Adequate monitoring of vital signs and oxygen saturation is important, as is the availability of oropharyngeal suction, resuscitation equipment, and antagonists to the sedative agents. Topical pharyngeal anesthesia with a gargle or spray of lidocaine or similar anesthetic is useful prior to upper endoscopic procedures.

Because of the risk of infection transmission, it is essential that every endoscope undergo meticulous cleaning and high-level disinfection or that the contaminated surfaces and tubing be replaced after each procedure.

---

* Dr. Michael Kimney contributed to this chapter in the 13th edition.

UPPER GASTROINTESTINAL ENDOSCOPY The tip of a forward-viewing endoscope is placed at the cricopharyngeal sphincter of the esophagus, and the patient is encouraged to swallow while gentle pressure is exerted. Small amounts of air are passed through the endoscope to visualize the esophageal lumen. The endoscope is then passed under direct vision into the stomach. The gastric body and antrum are carefully examined. The instrument tip is retroflexed in the stomach to view the gastric cardia, the fundus, and the whole lesser curvature. The pylorus is traversed, and the first and second portions of the duodenum are visualized. Visualized lesions can be recorded on photographs or videotape. Biopsies and brush cytologic examinations can be performed on suspicious areas.

EGD is a relatively safe procedure in experienced hands. Several large surveys suggest a risk of serious complications during diagnostic EGD of approximately 1 in 500 and a risk of death of approximately 1 in 10,000. The risks are higher in emergency procedures and in the elderly or seriously ill. In a survey of patients examined by endoscopy while experiencing upper GI bleeding, 1 in 200 had serious complications and 1 in 700 died from the procedure. The main causes of mortality were cardiopulmonary complications and perforations by the instrument. Endoscopy is preferred over x-ray examination in the urgent diagnosis of gastrointestinal illness in women who might be pregnant.

Gastroesophageal Reflux Disease (See Chap. 283) Esophageal pain may be confused with cardiac disease, or esophagitis may present as painless blood loss. Because esophagitis usually involves only the superficial mucosa, it cannot be diagnosed by routine single-contrast radiography. By endoscopy, friable mucosa, linear erosions, and ulcerations are clearly visible. Not every patient with heartburn requires esophagoscopy, but the procedure is indicated if the patient complains of dysphagia; if an x-ray shows a stricture, mass, or ulcer; if symptoms persist despite therapy; or if antireflux surgery is contemplated. Patients over age 40 with significant complaints of heartburn for over 10 years should be considered for endoscopy to detect Barrett's esophagus.

Barrett's esophagus is the progressive replacement of distal eroded squamous mucosa with metaplastic epithelium, which is more resistant to peptic digestion. This finding can be detected by visual inspection at endoscopy and confirmed by biopsy. Such epithelium is more prone to malignant transformation and, therefore, merits regular surveillance by esophagoscopy and biopsy every 12 to 24 months. Flow cytometry also may prove useful in the early detection of abnormal cell DNA populations (e.g., aneuploidy). If dysplasia is present, more frequent surveillance may be indicated to detect invasive carcinoma, or esophagectomy may be recommended, particularly if dysplasia is high-grade.

Esophagitis may progress to scarring and stricture formation. The endoscopic appearance of a benign stricture is characteristic but not diagnostic; a malignancy should be ruled out by biopsy and cytologic brushing; the whole length of the stricture should be sampled. Endoscopy may also facilitate dilatation of strictures (see below). Endoscopy is also indicated to biopsy the rim of an esophageal ulcer to rule out cancer.

The dilatation of a difficult stricture is best initiated by passing a flexible spring-tipped guidewire via the biopsy channel of the endoscope through the stricture under direct vision. The endoscope can then be withdrawn over the wire, which serves as a guide for passage of progressively larger polyvinyl dilators through the stricture under fluoroscopic control. An alternative technique uses balloon catheters passed via the endoscope channel or over a guidewire through the stricture. The balloon is inflated under endoscopic and/or fluoroscopic guidance to dilate the stricture.

Peptic Ulcer EDG is more accurate than upper GI x-ray examination for the detection of ulcers. It has been suggested that x-rays be abandoned entirely in favor of endoscopy for this purpose. Doing so makes sense when the source of acute upper GI bleeding is sought and urgent surgical intervention is being considered. However, in the workup of the patient with less pressing ulcer complaints, a double-contrast upper GI x-ray may still be used as the initial diagnostic test. Endoscopy may be indicated if the x-ray is equivocal or suggests that the ulcer may be malignant, if it is negative but the clinical picture suggests peptic ulceration, or if the patient is about to undergo surgery for ulcer. Patients with duodenal ulcers shown by x-ray or with classic ulcer deformities of the duodenal bulb do not require endoscopy for diagnosis if the presenting symptoms are characteristic and if the patient responds to antiulcer treatment. However, endoscopy also allows diagnosis of *Helicobacter pylori*, which is thought to cause most gastric and duodenal ulcers in patients not taking nonsteroidal antiinflammatory drugs. Screening endoscopy using small-diameter endoscopes without sedation is a reasonable alternative to contrast x-rays as the initial diagnostic test in a symptomatic patient.

Endoscopy is especially useful in visualizing postbulbar ulcers, giant duodenal ulcers, and stomal ulceration after partial gastrectomy, all of which can be missed by x-ray. Endoscopy is also of use in determining the cause of gastric outlet obstruction.

Cancer The endoscopic appearance of upper gastrointestinal cancer may seem obvious, especially if there is a mass growing into the lumen. On the other hand, malignant ulcers, infiltrative carcinomas, or small early carcinomas are frequently impossible to diagnose by their gross endoscopic appearance. Six to eight biopsy samples should be taken from the rim of a gastric ulcer to exclude malignancy. Experience and skill in choosing the biopsy sites improves the accuracy. A cytologic examination of lavage or brush specimens adds to the diagnostic accuracy in all areas of the upper gastrointestinal tract (see Chap. 92).

In patients with gastric ulcers, it has been standard practice to assess ulcer healing by endoscopy after 12 weeks of antiulcer therapy. Persistent ulcers should be biopsied if they were not biopsied at the time of the initial diagnosis or should be rebiopsied if they have not healed. Duodenal ulcers are rarely malignant and therefore do not need to be assessed for healing after therapy in most circumstances.

Primary gastric lymphoma can mimic benign gastric ulcer or adenocarcinoma on gastroscopy or x-ray. It can be diagnosed by biopsy or cytology, although the accuracy is not as high as in gastric adenocarcinoma. The diagnosis of lymphoma is aided by immunochemical staining of biopsy specimens.

If a polypoid lesion of the stomach is covered by mucosa that appears normal by gastroscopy, the likelihood of malignancy is small. Such lesions are often intramural subepithelial benign tumors such as leiomyomas or pancreatic rests. Biopsies are usually not diagnostic. These lesions can be evaluated by endoscopic ultrasonography, a technique that combines diagnostic ultrasound with endoscopy. Polyps covered by abnormal-appearing mucosa can be benign or malignant. Random biopsy can miss carcinoma within a polyp. If technically feasible, polyps should therefore be removed in their entirety by snare cautery for histologic examination. Polyps larger than 2 cm in diameter, are more likely to contain cancer (see Chap. 92). Large polyps may require surgical excision.

Ampullary carcinoma may be diagnosed by biopsy during duodenoscopy; a prior endoscopic sphincterotomy increases the diagnostic yield. Other primary duodenal malignancies are rare. Extensions from pancreatic or biliary tract cancer are difficult to diagnose because the tumor may not have extended into the mucosa and therefore may not be accessible for endoscopic biopsy or cytologic examination. In these secondary tumors, diagnosis must depend on some combination of ultrasonography (endoscopic and transabdominal), computed tomography, angiography, and ERCP with cytologic examination and/or biopsy of ductal strictures.

Upper GI Bleeding (See also Chap. 44) Endoscopy within the first 12 to 24 h of an upper GI hemorrhage is helpful in planning rational therapy by visualizing the bleeding source. Superficial lesions not visible by x-ray may be seen (esophagitis, a Mallory-Weiss tear, erosive gastritis, a stress ulcer, or telangiectasia). Moreover, lesions that are visible by x-ray may not be the source of bleeding. Endoscopy can determine the actual bleeding site and the degree of bleeding. For example, visualization of a spurting artery that is flooding the stomach indicates massive ongoing bleeding requiring prompt therapeutic intervention. Several studies have shown that the demonstration at endoscopy of any active bleeding whatsoever or of a nonbleeding 'visible' vessel (or "sentinel clot") in the ulcer base increases the likelihood of rebleeding. The diagnostic accuracy of emergency endoscopy in upper GI bleeding approaches 90 percent.

Every patient who is undergoing endoscopy for upper GI bleeding merits a complete endoscopic examination of the esophagus, stomach, and duodenum. Occasionally it is not possible to diagnose the exact lesion that is bleeding, but localizing the area of bleeding can be helpful; for example, bright red arterial blood may be seen pouring into the stomach from the duodenum when the esophagus and stomach show no signs of active bleeding.

There are three controversial areas relative to endoscopy and GI bleeding. First, *do all bleeders need endoscopy?* Endoscopy is indicated in all patients who may require surgery for continual bleeding or rebleeding, because the type of operation selected depends on the site and nature of the bleeding. Moreover, endoscopy provides critical information regarding the likelihood the bleeding will continue or recur. Finally, endoscopy permits therapeutic intervention. Second, *how early should endoscopy be performed in the acutely bleeding patient?* Most studies suggest that the diagnostic accuracy of EGD remains high for the first 12 to 24 h after the bleeding episode. All would agree that it is desirable to delay endoscopy if possible until vital signs have been stabilized after adequate blood replacement. Emergency endoscopy is critical in patients with continued massive bleeding or rebleeding requiring an immediate decision regarding surgery or other treatment. If the patient is exsanguinating, endoscopy can be performed after the induction of anesthesia and just before surgery. Thus, the patient's airway is protected by an endotracheal tube. Finally, *does endoscopy affect the clinical outcome?* Studies of the endoscopic treatment of bleeding lesions with heater probes, bipolar probes, and injection methods suggest that these methods are safe and reduce blood requirements, the need for surgery, and the risk of mortality in some patients.

Injection of various sclerosing solutions into or next to esophageal varices is an effective treatment for stopping active variceal bleeding. Rubber band ligation of varices at endoscopy has also been shown to stop bleeding and to obliterate varices with fewer sessions and less severe complications than occur with the use of sclerosing agents. Repeated injection sclerotherapy or band ligation may be performed to eradicate varices.

Percutaneous Endoscopic Gastrostomy (PEG)   The placement of feeding or decompression gastrostomy tubes can be facilitated with the use of an endoscope. Under sedation, a suitable location for a gastrostomy is identified, a needle is introduced into the stomach percutaneously, and a snare is passed through the endoscope to capture a wire or suture placed through the needle. Using this wire, a feeding tube is advanced into the stomach. Feedings are generally begun the same or following day. Hospitalization time and morbidity and mortality rates are reduced compared to those for operative gastrostomy.

Patients with transfer dysphagia secondary to strokes and degenerative neurologic disorders benefit the most from percutaneous endoscopic gastrostomy. Other indications include dysphagia produced by head and neck neoplasms and the inability to eat secondary to diffuse cerebral injury. Patients with severe gastroparesis can be fed through a jejunal feeding tube placed through the gastrostomy and then directed through the pylorus. Simultaneous gastric decompression is possible through a separate lumen in the gastrostomy.

Palliation of Esophageal Carcinoma   Patients with dysphagia caused by malignant esophageal strictures usually cannot be cured by esophagectomy. Surgical resection and radiation therapy are often chosen for palliation of dysphagia in this situation. The endoscopist also can help provide palliation in these patients when radiation therapy has failed or when surgical risks are too great.

Dilatation of malignant strictures is usually possible with polyvinyl dilators passed over an endoscopically placed guidewire. This procedure may improve the patient's swallowing initially, but more definitive therapy is usually needed. That can take the form of laser ablation or the placement of a prosthesis or stent. Tumor within the esophageal lumen can be destroyed by application of Nd:YAG laser energy using a laser waveguide placed through the biopsy channel of the endoscope. New approaches using photodynamic therapy are being evaluated. Alternatively, after stricture dilatation, large-caliber stents can be placed over a dilator. When the dilator is removed, the stent lumen is available for the passage of food. Stenting is especially useful in the palliation of malignant tracheoesophageal fistulas.

Other Indications   Upper GI endoscopy is usually substituted for x-ray examination in the urgent diagnosis of GI illness in *pregnancy*. Patients with *dysphagia* merit esophagoscopy because the cause is frequently structural, the lesion can be missed by x-ray, and biopsy confirmation is possible during endoscopy. Dysphagia caused by esophageal dysmotility is best diagnosed by manometry or cineradiography. *Painful swallowing* (odynophagia), especially in immunosuppressed or diabetic patients, may merit esophagoscopy because biopsy and brushings of the involved esophageal wall may reveal monilial, herpetic, or cytomegalovirus infections. Soon after ingestion of a corrosive agent, if there is no indication of wall necrosis, limited and gentle upper endoscopy is useful in evaluating the severity of injury. Many impacted foreign bodies can be removed from the esophagus or stomach with a snare or forceps; sharp foreign bodies are usually best removed by pulling them into a rigid open-lumen tubular esophagoscope or into a protective overtube around a fiberoptic endoscope. Careful esophagoscopy after removal of an esophageal foreign body is important to determine whether there is an underlying lesion that caused the impaction (e.g., cancer, benign stricture, peptic esophagitis).

In the postoperative stomach, gastroscopy is especially useful in detecting carcinoma, recurrent ulceration, retrograde intussusception, and stomal stricture. Several studies have suggested that there is an increased risk of carcinoma developing in the gastric stump more than 20 years after a Billroth II gastrectomy, although the magnitude of the risk, if there is one, is controversial. The diagnosis of such postoperative carcinomas may require many biopsies of seemingly normal mucosa near the anastomosis.

A new endoscopic application is the combination of ultrasound with endoscopy. This can be achieved by attaching an ultrasound system to the endoscope or passing an ultrasound probe down the biopsy channel of the endoscope. High-resolution ultrasound applied endoscopically is an accurate tool in the staging of esophageal and gastric malignancies, the detection of pancreatic neoplasia, and the determination of vascular extension in pancreatic cancers. Endoscopic ultrasound can be used to evaluate masses and to guide endoscopic needle aspiration.

ENDOSCOPIC RETROGRADE CHOLANGIOPANCREATOGRAPHY   ERCP involves placing a side-viewing instrument (duodenoscope) in the descending duodenum. The papilla of Vater is cannulated, x-ray contrast medium is injected, and the pancreatic ducts and hepatobiliary tree are visualized radiographically. Skilled operators can visualize 90 to 95 percent of pancreatic ducts and 90 percent of biliary ducts.

ERCP is performed on an x-ray table after sedation of the patient and induction of duodenal hypotonia with atropine or glucagon. The pancreatic duct is gently filled throughout its length with contrast material under constant fluoroscopic monitoring (Fig. 282-1*A*). Injection is continued until the first side branches are seen, and overfilling is avoided. Insertion of the cannula at a more acute cephalad angle makes it possible to visualize the common bile duct and the whole biliary tract including the gallbladder (Fig. 282-1*B*).

ERCP is a safe procedure when performed by an experienced operator. Asymptomatic amylase elevations occur in 40 to 75 percent of patients after pancreatography but are rarely of clinical significance. Pancreatitis occurs in approximately 1 to 7 percent of patients but is usually benign and self-limited. In a nationwide survey of complications, the morbidity rate was 3 percent and the mortality rate 0.2 percent. The main serious complication is retention of nonsterile con-

A

B

C

D

FIGURE 282-1 *A.* A tapering pancreatic duct of normal caliber is seen and may be compared to the endoscope (E) 1 cm in diameter. *B.* Normal cholangiogram. The diameter of the common bile duct (CBD) is normal. The intrahepatic ducts branch normally, and the gallbladder (GB) can be seen. The endoscope (E) is seen in the duodenum. *C.* Several stones *(arrows)* can be seen in an obstructed, dilated common duct. The gallbladder also contains several stones. Regurgitated contrast material is seen in the duodenum (D). *D.* The sharp cutoff *(arrow)* of the pancreatic duct is caused by a carcinoma of the body of the pancreas. *(Courtesy of Dr. Charles Rohrmann.)*

Remediable causes of obstructive jaundice that can be diagnosed by retrograde cholangiography include common duct stones (Fig. 282-1C) and benign and malignant strictures. In jaundiced patients with suspected primary liver disease, such as primary biliary cirrhosis, ERCP can assure that no operable obstruction is being missed.

Most physicians first use ultrasound or computed tomography to see whether the biliary ducts are dilated and to seek the cause of the patient's jaundice (stones, a pancreatic mass, etc.). A radionuclide biliary scintigraphy scan can help to determine if the cystic duct and bile ducts are patent. Direct visualization is undertaken if the diagnosis is not established. Percutaneous transhepatic cholangiography (PTC) is often attempted first if an intrahepatic or proximal bile duct obstruction is suggested by imaging. ERCP is used first if distal obstruction is suspected. Advantages of the endoscopic approach are that the papilla and the pancreatic duct are seen (in addition to the biliary ducts) and that therapy can be performed with endoscopic sphincterotomy or drainage when appropriate. In the event of a technical failure or if the information provided by either ERCP or PTC is incomplete, the other technique is tried. This approach detects most lesions requiring surgical intervention.

ERCP or PTC also can be useful in patients with biliary pain, cholangitis, or impaired liver function after previous biliary surgery. Remediable postoperative lesions such as strictures can be discovered and sometimes treated endoscopically. Should endoscopic therapy fail,

trast material proximal to an obstructed duct, causing cholangitis or pancreatic sepsis. If bile duct or pancreatic duct obstruction is first revealed by ERCP, the obstructed duct should be drained, if possible, either immediately by means of endoscopic techniques (papillotomy, stents, nasobiliary drains, etc.) or surgically within 36 h. Systemic antibiotics should be used immediately after filling an obstructed ductal system, especially if immediate endoscopic drainage cannot be accomplished.

Retrograde Cholangiography This procedure is especially useful in patients with persistent jaundice when the cause cannot be established by conventional diagnostic methods. The important differential diagnosis is between obstructive and nonobstructive jaundice. When the cause of jaundice is unclear, approximately 15 percent of patients thought to have nonobstructive jaundice prove to have extrahepatic biliary obstruction requiring endoscopic therapy or surgery; conversely, the same percentage of patients thought to have obstructive jaundice prove to have an open ductal system by ERCP.

the precise anatomy of the lesion still has been outlined, so that reoperation is less difficult. Biliary manometry also can be performed in this setting to diagnose dysfunction of the sphincter of Oddi. A perfused catheter is placed into the sphincter via the endoscope, and pressures are recorded. A high basal sphincter pressure may predict a beneficial effect of sphincterotomy.

Retrograde Pancreatography Patients with recurrent or chronic pancreatitis may be candidates for retrograde pancreatography to seek a lesion that can be approached endoscopically or surgically, such as localized pancreatitis in the tail of the gland or ductal pathology amenable to endoscopic stenting or surgical drainage.

In patients with symptoms, signs, or laboratory findings suggesting pancreatic carcinoma, the pancreatogram may suggest malignancy by showing a narrowed, encased, or sharply "cut-off" pancreatic duct (Fig. 282-1D). Differentiation of pancreatic carcinoma from benign inflammatory disease on the basis of such ductal findings can be difficult. Cytologic examination of pancreatic duct brushings obtained during ERCP may prove helpful. Unfortunately, most patients with symptomatic pancreatic cancer diagnosed by ERCP are inoperable.

Patients presenting with painless steatorrhea of pancreatic origin may have a ductal pattern suggesting chronic pancreatitis or pancreatic carcinoma. Pancreatography has not been useful in the study of obscure upper abdominal pain. Pancreatic cysts can be better diagnosed by noninvasive techniques such as ultrasound, and pancreatography should be reserved for cases in which it is desirable to outline the anatomy immediately before surgery. Pancreatography alone is not a reliable method of screening for early pancreatic carcinoma.

Therapeutic ERCP Access to the pancreatic and biliary tree for the removal of stones and the placement of stents is made possible by endoscopic retrograde sphincterotomy (ERS). The pancreatic or biliary sphincter mechanism is cut using electrosurgical current passed through a wire attached to the ERCP catheter. Complications in the form of bleeding, perforation, pancreatitis, or cholangitis occur in 5 to 8 percent of patients, with a resulting mortality rate of 0.5 to 1 percent. The role of pancreatic sphincterotomy in the management of pancreatic stones and strictures is evolving; however, biliary sphincterotomy is an established therapy for several conditions.

Common bile duct stones in patients with prior cholecystectomy can be successfully removed from the bile duct after ERS 90 percent of the time. Small stones pass spontaneously or are pulled into the duodenum with a balloon catheter or after being captured by a basket. Stones larger than 1.5 cm in diameter may be difficult to extract without prior fragmentation by mechanical or other techniques. With the increasing use of laparoscopic cholecystectomy, endoscopic removal of common bile duct stones is being performed in this setting. Older patients with increased surgical risks can sometimes be managed with ERS and stone extraction alone; cholecystectomy can be delayed or avoided entirely. Urgent ERS is also indicated for acute cholangitis and has assumed an increasing role in the initial treatment of severe biliary pancreatitis, in which early endoscopic stone removal has been shown to improve outcome.

Patients with benign and malignant bile duct strictures may benefit from the endoscopic placement of biliary stents after ERS. Benign strictures frequently remain dilated following removal of stents that have been left in place for several months. In patients with either pancreatic carcinoma or cholangiocarcinoma and obstructive jaundice, palliation can be achieved by placement of a plastic or metal biliary stent. Plastic stents usually occlude after 3 to 6 months and must be exchanged if recurrent jaundice or cholangitis develops; wire-mesh metal stents are preferred in patients likely to survive at least 6 months. Strictures involving the hilum of the liver (see Chap. 302) are difficult to palliate endoscopically; stents sometimes must be placed into both sides of the liver. These patients may require additional percutaneous radiologic procedures to achieve adequate biliary drainage.

COLONOSCOPY The interior of the entire length of the colon from anus to cecum can be visualized by the experienced colonoscopist. This is one of the most significant diagnostic and therapeutic applications of endoscopy, because it can diagnose potentially curable colonic cancers that would be missed by other techniques, and it

can be used for the removal of potentially precancerous adenomatous polyps.

Most initial colonoscopies are performed to investigate findings on an abnormal barium enema or to elucidate the cause of gastrointestinal bleeding. The ability to examine the whole colon is also useful in the management of some patients with inflammatory bowel disease and in patients with a strong family history of colonic polyps or cancer.

Patients are prepared for colonoscopy with laxatives and tap water enemas or by a total-gut lavage with a nonabsorbable electrolyte solution.

The main complications of colonoscopy are hemorrhage and perforation (morbidity rate, 0.5 to 1.3 percent; mortality rate, 0.02 percent). The complication rate for polypectomy is 1 to 2 percent. Diverticular or ischemic disease and prior irradiation make the procedure more difficult and hazardous. The risk of perforation is also increased in the patient with very active colitis; in most circumstances, colonoscopy should be avoided during the acute phase.

Polyps (See also Chap. 92) A polyp seen on barium enema merits colonoscopy for two reasons: It may be an artifact or a cancer, and a second polyp or cancer may have been missed. During colonoscopy, the polyp can usually be excised, with lower morbidity and mortality rates than with surgery. The best way to rule out cancer in a polyp is to remove the polyp completely for histologic examination. Hyperplastic polyps do not become malignant; colonic polyps that show benign neoplasia histologically may become malignant (tubular and villous adenomas). The risk that a neoplastic polyp is cancerous increases with its size. The risk is also higher in villous adenomas. Pedunculated polyps with moderately or well differentiated cancer confined to the mucosa and with an uninvolved stalk can be cured by removal with an electrocautery snare during colonoscopy. Thus, most colonoscopists will remove all polyps greater than 0.5 cm in diameter. Polyps smaller than 0.5 cm in diameter should be biopsied or removed, because more than 50 percent may be adenomatous, and the gross appearance of a polyp does not predict its histology. The wisdom of this course of action is suggested by several studies, including a sigmoidoscopic study in which the removal of all polyps reduced the expected incidence and invasiveness of subsequent cancers. Patients with adenomatous polyps are at increased risk of developing another polyp or cancer and therefore merit a regular screening program. The optimal frequency of follow-up examinations after polypectomy is not yet established. When a polyp is discovered, the entire colon should be examined for synchronous polyps or cancer. This examination should probably be repeated at 3- to 5-year intervals, and more frequently in patients with a history of colon cancer or multiple polyps. If stools are positive for occult blood or symptoms develop, immediate evaluation is indicated. In the average-risk patient without a known polyp, yearly digital examination and a stool test for occult blood are performed. Beginning at age 50, flexible sigmoidoscopy should be performed every 3 to 5 years.

Abnormal Findings on Barium Enema All filling defects on barium enema merit evaluation by colonoscopy. If the lesion is a pedunculated polyp, it can be removed for histologic examination; if its appearance suggests a cancer, it can be biopsied for histologic confirmation. When a polyp or a carcinoma is found, the remainder of the colon should be examined for additional polyps and synchronous carcinoma. A finding that is diagnosed as a mass by x-ray may be found on colonoscopy either not to exist or to represent a lesion such as a polyp rather than a cancer.

Narrowing Visualized by X-Ray Determining the cause of segmental narrowing may be difficult by x-ray but possible by colonoscopy, which can help in the differentiation of adenocarcinoma from inflammation secondary to ischemia, irradiation, diverticular disease, or Crohn's colitis. Even the most classic "apple-core" lesion seen on x-ray may be found on colonoscopy to be covered by normal mucosa, which suggests an extrinsic inflammatory lesion. In 10 to 30 percent of patients, narrowed segments seen on x-ray are not visualized during colonoscopy, probably because they were areas of temporary spasm.

Chronic Bleeding (X-Ray and Sigmoidoscopy Negative) Chronic bleeding is a common indication for colonoscopy. The x-ray is more likely to miss a lesion when a single-contrast technique is used rather than air contrast. The source of bleeding is found in approximately 40 percent of such patients and consists of such entities as an adenomatous polyp, an adenocarcinoma, and inflammatory bowel disease. If no bleeding site is found, it may be appropriate to search for an upper GI source with an upper GI x-ray or upper endoscopy, as well as to consider the possibiity of small intestinal bleeding.

Inflammatory Bowel Disease Colonoscopy may help in the initial diagnosis of this condition, especially in differentiating Crohn's colitis from ulcerative colitis. It also can aid the surgeon in assessing the activity and extent of the disease before surgery. Colonoscopy can help in the evaluation of radiographic abnormalities suggesting cancer, such as strictures, polyps, or masses. Colonoscopy is generally indicated in patients with ulcerative colitis of more than 10 years duration because of the increased risk of carcinoma; colonoscopy repeated at regular intervals helps to detect colonic dysplasia while the lesions are still curable. However, the benefit of such colonoscopic surveillance in terms of mortality and the optimal frequency of colonoscopy in such patients are still controversial. Nevertheless, if an expert gastrointestinal pathologist finds high-grade dysplasia in colonic biopsy samples from a patient with long-standing ulcerative colitis, most would consider it to be an indication for colectomy. Colonoscopy is contraindicated in patients with toxic megacolon, very active disease, or a possible intestinal perforation.

Other Indications The flexible sigmoidoscope has generally replaced the rigid 25-cm sigmoidoscope for routine screening because it can be passed to 40 to 60 cm with minimal preparation, less discomfort, and a higher diagnostic yield. After segmental colonic resection for carcinoma, colonoscopy may detect early mucosal recurrence and differentiate it from benign anastomotic strictures or bleeding suture granulomas. Colonoscopy is occasionally used during laparotomy to assist the surgeon in ruling out the presence of other lesions. The colonoscope can be advanced to the cecum rapidly with the surgeon's assistance, and additional polyps removed without colotomy. Colonoscopy is useful in the management of patients with lower GI bleeding (see Chap. 44). Bleeding polyps may be removed by snare electrocautery. Endoscopic hemostatic therapy may be useful in other bleeding lesions, such as colonic angiodysplasia.

Colonoscopy is usually not necessary for the diagnosis of familial polyposis because affected family members can be diagnosed by periodic flexible sigmoidoscopy. Carcinoma is a great threat in the familial polyposis syndromes that produce many adenomatous polyps (familial polyposis and Gardner's syndrome); in these conditions, polypectomy is useful for diagnosis, but colectomy is the only treatment that prevents development of carcinoma. These patients are also at risk of developing duodenal and periampullary adenomas and cancer and should probably undergo periodic surveillance with a side-viewing duodenoscope.

BIBLIOGRAPHY

HAGGITT RC et al: Prognostic factors in colorectal carcinomas arising in adenomas: Implications for lesions removed by endoscopic polypectomy. Gastroenterology 89:328, 1985
JENSEN DM, MACHICADO GA: Diagnosis and treatment of severe hematochezia: The role of urgent colonoscopy after purge. Gastroenterology 95:1569, 1988
LAI ECS et al: Endoscopic biliary drainage for severe acute cholangitis. N Engl J Med 326:1582, 1992
LAINE L: Multipolar electrocoagulation in the treatment of active upper gastrointestinal tract hemorrhage. N Engl J Med 316:1613, 1987
LIGHTDALE CJ et al: Localization of endocrine tumors of the pancreas with endoscopic ultrasonography. Cancer 68:1815, 1991
NIH CONSENSUS DEVELOPMENT CONFERENCE: Therapeutic endoscopy and bleeding ulcers. JAMA 262:1369, 1989
REID BJ et al: Flow cytometric and histologic progression to malignancy in Barrett's esophagus: Prospective endoscopic surveillance of a cohort. Gastroenterology 102:1212, 1992
SILVERSTEIN FE, TYTGAT GNJ: *Atlas of Gastrointestinal Endoscopy*, 3rd ed. London, Mosby-Wolfe, 1996
SPACH DH et al: Transmission of infection by gastrointestinal endoscopy and bronchoscopy. Ann Intern Med 118:117, 1993
STIEGMANN GV et al: Endoscopic sclerotherapy as compared with endoscopic ligation for bleeding esophageal varices. N Engl J Med 326:1527, 1992
TIO TL et al: Endosonography and computer tomography of esophageal carcinoma. Preoperative classification compared to the new TNM system. Gastroenterology 96:1478, 1989

283 *Raj K. Goyal*

DISEASES OF THE ESOPHAGUS

The two major functions of the esophagus are the transport of the food bolus from the mouth to the stomach and the prevention of retrograde flow of gastrointestinal contents. The transport function is achieved by peristaltic contractions (see Chap. 40). Retrograde flow is prevented by the two esophageal sphincters, which remain closed between swallows. The upper esophageal sphincter consists of the cricopharyngeus and inferior pharyngeal constrictor muscles, which are striated muscles and are innervated by excitatory somatic lower motor neurons. These muscles exhibit no myogenic tone and receive no inhibitory innervation. The upper sphincter remains closed owing to the elastic properties of its wall and to neurogenic tonic contraction of the sphincter muscles and is opened by inhibition of the sphincter muscles in concert with forward displacement of the larynx by the suprahyoid muscles. In contrast, the lower esophageal sphincter (LES) is composed of smooth muscle and is innervated by parallel sets of parasympathetic excitatory and inhibitory pathways. It remains closed because of its intrinsic myogenic tone, which is modulated by the excitatory and inhibitory nerves. It opens in response to the activity of the inhibitory nerves. The neuromuscular neurotransmitter of the excitatory nerves is acetylcholine, and those of the inhibitory nerves are vasoactive intestinal peptide (VIP) and nitric oxide. The function of the LES is supplemented by the striated muscle of diaphragmatic crura, which surrounds the sphincter and acts as external lower esophageal sphincter. A reflex decrease in the lower sphincter pressure occurs during belching and gastric distention. Fatty meals, smoking, and beverages with a high xanthine content (tea, coffee, cola) also cause a reduction in sphincter pressure. Many hormones and neurotransmitters can modify lower sphincter pressure. Muscarinic M_2 receptor agonists, alpha-adrenergic agonists, gastrin, substance P, and prostaglandin $F_{2\alpha}$ cause contraction; in contrast, nicotine, beta-adrenergic agonists, dopamine, cholecystokinin, secretin, VIP, calcitonin gene–related peptide (CGRP), adenosine, and nitric oxide donors such as nitrates cause relaxation of the sphincter.

SYMPTOMS

DYSPHAGIA → *See Chap. 40.*

ESOPHAGEAL PAIN *Heartburn*, or pyrosis, is characterized by burning retrosternal discomfort that may move up and down the chest like a wave. When severe, it may radiate to the sides of the chest, the neck, and the angles of the jaw. Heartburn is a characteristic symptom of reflux esophagitis and may be associated with regurgitation or a feeling of warm fluid climbing up the throat. It is aggravated by bending forward, straining, or lying recumbent and is worse after meals. It is relieved by an upright posture, by the swallowing of saliva or water, and, more reliably, by antacids. Heartburn appears to be produced by heightened mucosal sensitivity and can be reproduced by infusion of dilute (0.1 *N*) hydrochloric acid (Bernstein test) or neutral hyperosmolar solutions into the esophagus.

Odynophagia, or painful swallowing, is characteristic of nonreflux esophagitis, particularly monilial and herpes esophagitis. Odynophagia also may occur with peptic ulcer of the esophagus (Barrett's ulcer), carcinoma with periesophageal involvement, caustic damage of the esophagus, and esophageal perforation. Odynophagia is unusual in uncomplicated reflux esophagitis. Crampy chest pain associated with impaction of a food bolus should be distinguished from odynophagia.

Atypical chest pain other than heartburn and odynophagia occurs in reflux esophagitis or esophageal motility disorders such as diffuse esophageal spasm. The latter may occur spontaneously or during a meal. Chest pain due to periesophageal involvement caused by carcinoma or peptic ulcer may be constant and agonizing. Sometimes different types of esophageal pains exist together in the same patient, and frequently patients are not able to describe the pain accurately enough to allow its classification. Coronary artery disease should always be carefully excluded before the esophagus is considered as the cause of atypical chest pain. The most frequent esophageal cause of chest pain is reflux esophagitis. Some patients with atypical chest pain have nonspecific esophageal motor abnormalities of uncertain significance. Many of these patients have behavioral abnormalities, psychosomatic disorders, depression, anxiety, panic reactions, and other somatization disorders.

REGURGITATION *Regurgitation* is the effortless appearance of gastric or esophageal contents in the mouth. In distal esophageal obstruction and stasis, as in achalasia or the presence of a large diverticulum, the regurgitated material consists of tasteless mucoid fluid or undigested food. Regurgitation of sour or bitter-tasting material occurs in severe gastroesophageal reflux and is associated with incompetence of both the upper and lower esophageal sphincters. Regurgitation may result in laryngeal aspiration, with spells of coughing and choking that awaken the patient from sleep, and in aspiration pneumonia. Water brash is reflex salivary hypersecretion which occurs in response to peptic esophagitis; it should not be confused with regurgitation.

DIAGNOSTIC TESTS

RADIOLOGIC STUDIES Barium swallow with fluoroscopy and an esophagogram is the most widely used test for the diagnosis of esophageal disease and can be used to evaluate both structural and motor disorders. Since the oropharyngeal phase of swallowing lasts no more than a second, videofluoroscopy is necessary to permit detec-

tion and analysis of abnormalities of oral and pharyngeal function. The pharynx is examined to detect stasis of barium in the valleculae and piriform sinuses and regurgitation of barium into the nose and tracheobronchial tree. Spontaneous reflux of barium from the stomach into the esophagus should be sought in patients with suspected reflux esophagitis. Esophageal peristalsis is best studied in the recumbent position, because in the upright position the passage of most of the barium occurs by gravity alone. A double-contrast esophagogram, obtained by coating the esophageal mucosa with barium and distending the esophageal lumen with air using effervescent granules, is particularly useful in demonstrating mucosal ulcers and early cancers. A barium-soaked piece of bread or a 13-mm barium tablet is sometimes used to demonstrate an obstructive lesion. Figures 283-1 and 283-2 illustrate the radiographic appearance of some esophageal disorders.

ESOPHAGOSCOPY Fiberoptic esophagogastroduodenoscopy is described in Chap. 282. Esophagoscopy is the direct method of establishing the cause of mechanical dysphagia and of identifying mucosal lesions, such as superficial ulcers and esophagitis, which may not be identified by the usual barium swallow. If the lumen is markedly narrowed, it may be necessary to use a smaller-caliber endoscope, although on occasion a stricture must be dilated before the examination can be completed. Transendoscopic biopsies are useful in diagnosing carcinoma, reflux esophagitis, and other mucosal diseases. Obtaining cells by scraping the mucosa with a Teflon brush during endoscopy may enable the cytologist to detect carcinoma.

ESOPHAGEAL MOTILITY The study of esophageal motility entails simultaneous recording of pressures from different sites in the esophageal lumen using an assembly of pressure sensors that are positioned 5 cm apart. The upper and lower esophageal sphincters appear as zones of high pressure that relax on swallowing. The pharynx and esophageal body normally show peristaltic waves with each swallow.

Esophageal motility studies are very helpful in the diagnosis of achalasia, diffuse esophageal spasm and its variants, scleroderma, and other motor disorders of the esophagus (Fig. 283-3) but are of no value in the diagnosis of mechanical dysphagia. In patients with reflux

FIGURE 283-1 Radiographic appearance of some motor disorders of the pharynx and esophagus. *(1)* Pharyngeal paralysis with tracheal aspiration *(arrow)*. *(2)* Cricopharyngeal achalasia. Note the prominent cricopharyngeus, which is recognized by its smoothness and location in the posterior wall. *(3)* Diffuse esophageal spasm. Note typical corkscrew appearance of the lower part of the esophagus. *(4)* Achalasia, showing a dilated esophageal body with an air-fluid level and a closed lower esophageal sphincter. *(5)* Muscular (contractile) lower esophageal ring. Note that the asymmetric contraction visible in *5A* has disappeared in *5B*, obtained during the same examination. *(6)* Scleroderma esophagus showing dilated esophagus with a stricture *(6A)* and reflux of barium from the stomach into the esophagus *(6B)*. *(Courtesy of Dr. Harvey Goldstein.)*

FIGURE 283-2 Selected structural lesions of the esophagus. *(1)* Carcinoma of the esophagus, with typical annular narrowing with overhanging margins and destruction of the mucosa. *(2)* Leiomyoma of the esophagus, with a smooth filling defect and right angles of origin from the esophageal wall. *(3)* Esophageal ulcer in columnar-cell-lined esophagus (Barrett's esophagus). *(4)* Monilial esophagitis, with irregular plaquelike filling defects. *(5)* Long stricture secondary to lye ingestion. *(6)* Peptic stricture, short and tubular, with associated hiatus hernia. *(7)* Lower esophageal mucosal (Schatzki) ring. A thin, weblike annular constriction at the esophagogastric junction is associated with a small hiatal hernia. *(Courtesy of Dr. Harvey Goldstein.)*

esophagitis, esophageal manometry is useful in quantitating lower esophageal competence and providing information on the status of the esophageal body motor activity. The information obtained by manometry is quantitative and cannot be obtained by barium swallow or endoscopy.

Special tests for the evaluation of reflux esophagitis are described later.

MOTOR DISORDERS

STRIATED MUSCLE Oropharyngeal Paralysis Paralysis of oral muscle leads to difficulty in initiating swallowing and to drooling of food out of mouth. Pharyngeal paralysis is characterized by dysphagia, nasal regurgitation, and tracheobronchial aspiration during swallowing. It occurs in a variety of neuromuscular disorders (see Table 40-1). Some of these disorders also may involve laryngeal muscles, causing hoarseness. When the suprahyoid muscles are paralyzed, the upper sphincter does not open with swallowing, leading to paralytic achalasia of the upper esophageal sphincter and severe dysphagia.

Videofluoroscopy using barium of various consistencies may reveal difficulties in the oral phase of swallowing. There may be stasis of barium in the valleculae and piriform sinuses, nasal and tracheobronchial aspiration, failure of the upper sphincter to open, and/or abnormal movement of the hyoid bone and the larynx with a swallow (Fig. 283-1). Motility studies demonstrate a reduced amplitude of pharyngeal and upper esophageal contractions and reduced basal upper esophageal sphincter pressure without further relaxation on swallowing (Fig. 283-3). Patients with myasthenia gravis and polymyositis respond to treatment for these diseases (see Chap. 381). Dysphagia resulting from a cerebrovascular accident improves with time, although often not completely. Treatment consists of maneuvers to reduce pharyngeal stasis and enhance airway protection under the direction of a trained swallow therapist. Feeding by a nasogastric tube or an endoscopically placed gastrostomy tube may be necessary for nutritional support; however, these maneuvers do not provide protection against aspiration of salivary secretions. Cricopharyngeal myotomy is sometimes performed, but its usefulness is unproven. Extensive operative procedures to prevent aspiration are rarely needed. Death is often due to pulmonary complications.

Cricopharyngeal Bar Failure of the cricopharyngeus to relax on swallowing leads to a contracted cricopharyngeus, which appears as a prominent bar on the posterior wall of the pharynx on barium swallow (Fig. 283-1). A transient cricopharyngeal bar is seen in up to 5 percent of subjects without dysphagia undergoing upper gastrointestinal studies; it can be produced in normal subjects during a Valsalva maneuver. A persistent cricopharyngeal bar may be caused by fibrosis in the cricopharyngeus. Some of these patients complain of food sticking in their throats. Cricopharyngeal myotomy may be helpful, but it is contraindicated in the presence of gastroesophageal reflux because, in such patients, it may lead to pharyngeal and pulmonary aspiration.

Globus Pharyngeus A sensation of a constant lump in the throat, but with no difficulty in swallowing, occurs especially in subjects with emotional disorders, particularly women. Results of barium studies and manometry are normal. Treatment consists primarily of reassurance. Some patients with globus pharyngeus have associated reflux esophagitis, and they may respond to treatment of the esophagitis.

SMOOTH MUSCLE Achalasia Achalasia is a motor disorder of the esophageal smooth muscle in which the LES does not relax properly with swallowing, and the normal peristalsis of the esophageal body is replaced by abnormal contractions. Achalasia can be divided into two types on the basis of the changes in the esophageal body. In *classic achalasia*, simultaneous small-amplitude contractions occur, while in *vigorous achalasia*, contractions are simultaneous in onset, large in amplitude, and repetitive, resembling those seen in diffuse esophageal spasm.

Pathophysiology The underlying abnormality is the loss of intramural neurons, particularly the inhibitory neurons containing VIP and nitric oxide synthase, in the smooth-muscle portion of the esophageal body and the LES. Primary idiopathic achalasia accounts for most of the patients seen in the United States. Secondary achalasia may be caused by gastric carcinoma that infiltrates the esophagus, by lymphoma, by Chagas' disease, and by neuropathic chronic intestinal pseudoobstruction syndrome. A hypertensive or hypercontracting LES may be considered to represent a variant of achalasia.

Clinical features Achalasia affects patients of all ages and both sexes. Dysphagia, chest pain, and regurgitation are the main symptoms. Dysphagia appears early, occurs with both liquids and solids, and is worsened by emotional stress and hurried eating. Various maneuvers designed to increase intraesophageal pressure, including the Valsalva maneuver, may aid the passage of the bolus into the stomach. Chest pain is more pronounced in vigorous achalasia than in classic achalasia. Regurgitation and pulmonary aspiration occur because of retention of large volumes of saliva and ingested food in the esophagus. The presence of gastroesophageal reflux argues against achalasia, and in patients with long-standing heartburn, cessation of heartburn and appearance of dysphagia suggest development of achalasia in a patient with reflux esophagitis. The overall course is usually chronic, with progressive dysphagia and weight loss over months to years. Achalasia associated with carcinoma is characterized by severe weight loss and a rapid downhill course if untreated.

Diagnosis   A chest x-ray shows absence of the gastric air bubble and sometimes a tubular mediastinal mass beside the aorta. An air-fluid level in the mediastinum in the upright position represents retained food in the esophagus. Barium swallow shows esophageal dilation, and in advanced cases the esophagus may become sigmoid. On fluoroscopy, normal peristalsis is lost in the lower two-thirds of the esophagus. The terminal part of the esophagus shows a persistent beaklike narrowing representing the nonrelaxing LES (see Fig. 283-1). In patients with vigorous achalasia, there may be pronounced nonperistaltic contractions.

Manometry shows the basal lower esophageal sphincter pressure to be normal or elevated, and swallow-induced relaxation either does not occur or is reduced in degree, duration, and consistency. The esophageal body shows an elevated resting pressure. In response to swallows, primary peristaltic waves are replaced by simultaneous-onset contractions (Fig. 283-3). These contractions may be of poor amplitude (classic achalasia) or of large amplitude and long duration (vigorous achalasia). Administration of the cholinergic muscarinic agonist mecholyl causes a marked increase in baseline esophageal pressure, chest pain, and regurgitation of retained esophageal contents (Mecholyl test). Cholecystokinin (CCK), which normally causes a fall in the sphincter pressure, paradoxically causes contraction of the LES (the CCK test). This paradoxical response occurs because, in achalasia, the neurally transmitted inhibitory effect of CCK is absent owing to the loss of inhibitory neurons. Endoscopy is helpful in excluding the secondary causes of achalasia, particularly gastric carcinoma.

℞ TREATMENT

Medical treatment using soft foods, sedatives, and anticholinergic drugs is usually unsatisfactory. Nitroglycerin, 0.3 to 0.6 mg sublingually before meals and as needed for chest pain, is usually helpful. Isosorbide dinitrate, 2.5 to 5 mg sublingually or 10 to 20 mg orally before meals, can be used for longer-lasting relief of symptoms. Nitrates are associated with headache and postural hypotension. The calcium channel blocker nifedipine, 10 to 20 mg orally or sublingually before meals, is also effective. Injection of botulinum toxin in the LES during endoscopy has been reported to be effective. Botulinum toxin acts by blocking cholinergic excitatory nerves in the sphincter. A time-tested therapy involves balloon dilatation to reduce the basal LES pressure by tearing muscle fibers. In experienced hands, this technique is effective in about 85 percent of patients. Perforation and bleeding are potential complications. Heller's extramucosal myotomy of the lower sphincter, in which the circular muscle layer is incised, is equally effective. Reflux esophagitis and peptic stricture may follow successful treatment (more often with myotomy than with balloon dilatation). Laparoscopic myotomy of the sphincter also is successful.

Diffuse Esophageal Spasm and Related Motor Disorders   Diffuse esophageal spasm is a motor disorder of the esophageal smooth muscle characterized by multiple spontaneous contractions and by swallow-induced contractions that are of simultaneous onset. The contractions may be of large amplitude, long duration, and repetitive occurrence. Variants show some but not all of these motor abnormalities.

Pathophysiology   The pathogenesis of the various abnormalities of peristalsis in diffuse esophageal spasm is not known. Histopathologic studies show patchy neural degeneration localized to nerve processes, rather than the prominent degeneration of nerve cell bodies seen in achalasia.

Esophageal contractions that are peristaltic but of large amplitude constitute a condition (sometimes called "nutcracker" esophagus) that is diagnosed by manometry and is due to heightened excitatory activity. Cholinergic drugs cause large-amplitude contractions. Simultaneous contractions indicate loss of inhibitory nerve function; they frequently occur as a primary disease or in association with a variety of diseases as well as with emotional stress and aging. Collagen vascular disease, diabetic neuropathy, reflux esophagitis, irradiation esophagitis, esophageal obstruction, and anticholinergic drugs can cause simultaneous contractions. The relationship between reflux esophagitis and motor abnormalities is controversial. Overlapping features of diffuse esophageal spasm and achalasia occur in vigorous achalasia. The variant syndromes are more frequent in clinical practice than is classic diffuse esophageal spasm.

Clinical features   The symptomatic patient with diffuse spasm or one of its variants presents with chest pain, dysphagia, or both. Chest pain is particularly marked in patients with esophageal contractions of large amplitude and long duration. Chest pain usually occurs at rest but may be brought on by swallowing or by emotional stress. The pain is retrosternal; it may radiate to the back, the sides of the chest,

FIGURE 283-3   Motility patterns in selected esophageal and pharyngeal disorders. In normal subjects, the upper and lower esophageal sphincters (UES and LES) appear as zones of high pressure. With a swallow (indicated by ↑), pressure in the sphincters falls and a contraction wave starts in the pharynx and progresses down the esophagus. In scleroderma, the lower part of the esophagus (smooth muscle) shows a reduced amplitude of contractions, which may be peristaltic or simultaneous in onset, and hypotension of the lower sphincter. In achalasia, the lower part of the esophagus shows contractions that are reduced in amplitude and simultaneous in onset. In contrast to scleroderma, the lower esophageal sphincter in achalasia is hypertensive and fails to relax in response to a swallow. In diffuse esophageal spasm, the lower part of the esophagus shows simultaneous-onset, large-amplitude, prolonged, repetitive contractions. In pharyngeal paralysis, the smooth-muscle part of the esophagus is normal. The skeletal muscle part shows a reduced amplitude of contractions. The upper esophageal sphincter is hypotensive and may not relax normally on swallowing owing to associated weakness of the suprahyoid muscles.

both arms, or the sides of the jaw and may last from a few seconds to several minutes. It may be acute and severe, mimicking the pain of myocardial ischemia. Dysphagia for solids and liquids may occur with or without chest pain and is correlated particularly with simultaneous-onset contractions.

Diffuse esophageal spasm must be differentiated from other causes of chest pain, particularly ischemic heart disease with atypical angina. A complete cardiac workup should be done before an esophageal etiology is considered seriously. The presence of dysphagia in association with pain should point to the esophagus as the site of disease. Symptoms of esophageal spasm should be carefully distinguished from those of reflux esophagitis; the two conditions may coexist.

Diagnosis Barium swallow shows that normal sequential peristalsis below the aortic arch is replaced by uncoordinated simultaneous contractions that produce the appearance of curling or multiple ripples in the wall, sacculations, and pseudodiverticula—the "corkscrew" esophagus (Fig. 283-1). Sometimes an esophageal contraction obliterates the lumen, and barium is pushed away in both directions. The lower esophageal sphincter opens normally.

Manometry reveals the characteristic presence of prolonged, large-amplitude, repetitive contractions of simultaneous onset in the lower part of the esophagus (Fig. 283-3). Only one or two of these abnormalities may be present in variants of diffuse spasm. Because the disorder may be episodic, the results of manometry may be normal at the time of the study; therefore, several techniques are used in attempts to provoke esophageal spasm. Cold swallows produce chest pain but do not produce spasm on manometric studies. Solid boluses and pharmacologic agents, particularly edrophonium, induce both chest pain and motor abnormalities. However, there is a poor correlation between induction of pain and motility changes. Ergonovine can induce motor abnormalities but also may cause coronary artery spasm and therefore should not be used. Overall, the usefulness of pharmacologic provocative tests is limited.

℞ TREATMENT

Anticholinergics are usually of limited value. Agents that relax smooth muscle, such as sublingual nitroglycerin (0.3 to 0.6 mg) or longer-acting agents such as isosorbide dinitrate (10 to 30 mg orally before meals) and nifedipine (10 to 20 mg orally before meals) are helpful. Sublingual forms of these agents can also be used. Reassurance and tranquilizers are helpful in allaying patients' apprehension.

Scleroderma Involving the Esophagus The esophageal lesions in systemic sclerosis consist of atrophy of smooth muscle contraction, manifested by weakness in the lower two-thirds of the esophageal body and incompetence of the LES. The esophageal wall is thin and atrophic and may exhibit areas of patchy fibrosis. Patients usually present with dysphagia to solids. Liquids may cause dysphagia when the patient is in the recumbent position. Some patients present with heartburn and regurgitation due to gastroesophageal reflux and esophagitis, which in turn may lead to stricture formation and more pronounced dysphagia. Barium swallow shows dilation and loss of peristaltic contractions in the middle and distal portions of the esophagus. The LES is patulous, and gastroesophageal reflux may occur freely (Fig. 283-1). Mucosal changes due to esophageal ulceration may be detected, and esophageal stricture may be present. Motility studies show a marked reduction in the amplitude of smooth-muscle contractions, which may be peristaltic or nonperistaltic. The resting pressure of the LES is subnormal, but sphincter relaxation is normal (Fig. 283-3). Esophageal motor abnormalities are frequently found in patients with Raynaud's syndrome alone. Currently, there is no effective treatment for the motor difficulty. Reflux esophagitis and its complications should be treated aggressively, as described in the following section.

GASTROESOPHAGEAL REFLUX AND ESOPHAGITIS

Reflux esophagitis consists of esophageal mucosal damage caused by reflux of gastric or intestinal contents into the esophagus. Depending on the causative agent, it is referred to as *peptic*, *bile*, or *alkaline esophagitis*.

Pathophysiology Three considerations involved in the pathophysiology of reflux esophagitis are (1) the reflux episode, (2) the cumulative esophageal reflux, and (3) the pathogenesis of esophagitis.

Two conditions must be met for a *reflux episode* to occur: The gastrointestinal contents must be "ready" to reflux, and the antireflux mechanism at the lower end of the esophagus must be compromised. Gastrointestinal contents are most likely to reflux (1) when gastric volume is increased (after meals, in the presence of pyloric obstruction or gastric stasis syndrome, and in acid hypersecretory states), (2) when the gastric contents are located near the gastroesophageal junction (owing to recumbency, bending down, or the presence of a hiatus hernia), and (3) when gastric pressure is increased (owing to obesity, pregnancy, ascites, or tight binders or girdles).

The normal antireflux mechanisms consist of the LES and the anatomic configuration of the gastroesophageal junction. Reflux occurs only when the gradient of pressure between the LES and the stomach is lost. It can be caused by increased intragastric pressure or by a transient or sustained decrease in LES tone. The decrease in sphincter tone may be due to muscle weakness or to inappropriate sphincter relaxation mediated by inhibitory nerves. The secondary causes of LES incompetence include scleroderma-like diseases; a myopathic type of chronic intestinal pseudoobstruction syndrome; pregnancy; smoking; smooth-muscle relaxants (such as beta-adrenergic agents, aminophylline, nitrates, and calcium channel blockers); destruction of the sphincter by surgical resection, myotomy, or balloon dilatation; and esophagitis. Abnormal activity of the diaphragmatic crural muscle, which surrounds the esophageal hiatus in the diaphragm and changes the anatomic configuration of the esophagogastric junction—as occurs in hiatal hernia—also predisposes to gastroesophageal reflux.

The *cumulative esophageal reflux*—the amount and duration of refluxed noxious material remaining in the esophagus—depends on (1) the amount of refluxed material per episode, (2) the frequency of reflux episodes, (3) the rate of clearing of the esophagus by gravity and peristaltic contraction, and (4) the rate of neutralization of gastric acid by salivary secretion.

Esophagitis is a complication of reflux, and it develops when the mucosal defenses that normally counteract the effect of injurious agents on the esophageal mucosa succumb to the onslaught of the refluxed acid pepsin or bile. *Mild esophagitis* is manifested by microscopic changes of mucosal infiltration with granulocytes or eosinophils, hyperplasia of basal cells, and elongation of dermal pegs. It can occur with or without endoscopic abnormalities. *Erosive esophagitis* involves endoscopically visible damage to the mucosa in the form of marked redness, friability, bleeding, superficial linear ulcers, and exudates. *Peptic stricture* results from fibrosis that causes constriction of the esophageal lumen. Peptic strictures occur in about 10 percent of patients with reflux esophagitis. Short peptic strictures caused by spontaneous reflux are usually 1 to 3 cm long and are present in the distal esophagus near the squamocolumnar junction (see Fig. 283-2). Long, tubular peptic strictures can result from persistent vomiting or prolonged nasogastric intubation. Replacement of the squamous epithelium of the esophagus by columnar epithelium (*Barrett's esophagus*) also may result from reflux esophagitis. The columnar epithelium usually represents a specialized type of intestinal metaplasia, and the condition may be complicated further by a peptic ulcer or peptic stricture located in the upper part of the lower esophagus or in the midesophagus. Adenocarcinoma occurs in 2 to 5 percent of cases and is usually preceded by dysplasia of the columnar mucosa. Recently, a high prevalence of intestinal metaplasia localized to the gastroesophageal junction has been reported during upper endoscopic examination. This finding may explain the increased incidence of adenocarcinoma at the gastroesophageal junction.

Clinical Features Heartburn is the characteristic symptom and is produced by the contact of refluxed material with the inflamed esophageal mucosa. Angina-like or atypical chest pain occurs in some patients, while others experience no heartburn or chest pain. Dysphagia suggests development of a peptic stricture. Most patients with peptic stricture have a history of several years of heartburn preceding dysphagia. However, in one-third of patients, dysphagia is the presenting symptom. Rapidly progressive dysphagia and weight loss may indicate the development of adenocarcinoma in Barrett's esophagus. Bleeding occurs due to mucosal erosions or Barrett's ulcer. Reflux in the absence of esophagitis is usually asymptomatic. Severe reflux may reach the pharynx and mouth and result in laryngitis, morning hoarseness, and pulmonary aspiration. Recurrent pulmonary aspiration can cause aspiration pneumonia, pulmonary fibrosis, or chronic asthma.

Diagnosis The evaluation of reflux esophagitis is designed to assess the presence and severity of reflux, the nature of the refluxant, the presence and severity of esophagitis, and the pathophysiology of the reflux. A history is taken, and barium swallow, esophagoscopy, mucosal biopsy, esophageal motility testing, and a variety of special tests are performed.

The *presence of reflux* is suggested by the history. Spontaneous reflux from the stomach into the esophagus on barium examination suggests advanced reflux. Reflux of barium induced by stressful maneuvers is not very helpful, however, because of the high incidence of false-positive and false-negative results. A scintiscan using ^{99m}Tc-sulfur colloid has been used to quantitate gastroesophageal reflux. Several tests that involve the recording of the luminal pH of the esophagus with a small pH electrode have been proposed to detect and quantitate the reflux of gastric acid. In these tests, the pH electrode is swallowed, positioned in the stomach, gradually withdrawn across the LES, and then fixed at 5 cm above the sphincter. In the standard acid reflux test, a diagnosis of reflux can be made by failure of the pH to rise as the electrode enters the esophagus and by a decrease in esophageal pH with straining maneuvers. Quantitative information on acid reflux is obtained by ambulatory long-term (24-h) esophageal pH recording. The pH recordings are helpful only in the evaluation of acid reflux. The presence of bile or alkaline reflux is suggested by the occurrence of reflux symptoms in the absence of gastric acid and by the demonstration of bile in an aspirate of esophageal reflux fluid.

The *presence and complications of reflux esophagitis* are assessed by barium swallow, esophagoscopy, mucosal biopsy, and the Bernstein test. The results of barium swallow are usually normal in uncomplicated esophagitis but may reveal the complication of stricture or ulcer formation. A high esophageal peptic stricture, a deep ulcer, or adenocarcinoma suggest Barrett's esophagus. Uncomplicated Barrett's esophagus is not diagnosed reliably by barium studies. Esophagoscopy may reveal the presence of erosive esophagitis, distal peptic stricture, or a columnar-cell-lined lower esophagus with or without a proximally located peptic stricture, ulcer, or adenocarcinoma. Results of esophagoscopy may be normal in many patients with esophagitis; in such patients, mucosal biopsies and the Bernstein test are helpful. The mucosal biopsies should be performed at least 5 cm above the LES, because esophageal mucosal changes of chronic esophagitis are quite frequent in the most distal esophagus in otherwise normal subjects. Approximately 10 percent of biopsies yield a false-positive or false-negative result. Patients with Barrett's esophagus will show columnar mucosa lining the esophagus; the mucosa may be of a gastric fundic, cardiac, or specialized type. The Bernstein test consists of infusions of solutions of 0.1 N HCl and normal saline into the esophagus. It is useful in diagnosing reflux esophagitis that is not endoscopically obvious. In patients with reflux esophagitis, infusion of acid, but not of saline, reproduces the symptoms of heartburn. Infusion of acid in normal subjects usually produces no symptoms. Reflux esophagitis should be included in the differential diagnosis of chest pain, esophagitis, upper gastrointestinal bleeding, and dysphagia.

The *causative and predisposing factors* are assessed by the history and by studies of esophageal motility and esophageal clearance. Esophageal motility studies may provide useful quantitative information on the competence of the LES and on esophageal motor function. Barium swallow and scintiscans can be used to study esophageal clearance. An esophageal acid clearance test using a pH electrode quantifies the number of swallows necessary to clear the esophagus of 10 mL of instilled dilute 0.1 N HCl.

Full diagnostic evaluation is not necessary in every patient with reflux esophagitis. In transient and mild cases with a clear-cut history of reflux esophagitis, a therapeutic trial may be sufficient. In persistent cases and when the diagnosis is not clear, barium swallow, esophagoscopy, and esophageal motility with pH monitoring are indicated.

Patients with angina-like chest pain in whom coronary artery disease has been excluded may be investigated by the Bernstein test, 24-h ambulatory esophageal pH recording, and motility recording. Most of these patients are found to have reflux esophagitis, while a few have specific esophageal motor disorders. It also should be remembered that reflux esophagitis and nonspecific esophageal motility disorders frequently coexist with coronary artery disease.

℞ TREATMENT

The goals of treatment are to decrease gastroesophageal reflux, render the refluxate harmless, improve esophageal clearance, and protect the esophageal mucosa. These goals can be achieved by certain general measures and specific drug treatments. The management of uncomplicated cases generally includes weight reduction, sleeping with the head of the bed elevated by about 4 to 6 in with blocks, and elimination of factors that increase abdominal pressure. Patients should not smoke and should avoid consuming fatty foods, coffee, chocolate, alcohol, mint, orange juice, and certain medications (such as anticholinergic drugs, calcium channel blockers, and other smooth-muscle relaxants). They should also avoid ingesting of large quantities of fluids with meals. In mild cases, the use of H_2 receptor blocking agents (cimetidine, 300 mg; ranitidine, 150 mg; or famotidine, 20 mg) as needed may suffice.

In moderate to severe cases, the preceding measures are more strictly enforced. H_2 receptor blockers are used in higher doses (cimetidine, 300 mg qid; ranitidine, 150 mg bid; famotidine, 20 mg bid). If the patient does not respond fully, a prokinetic agent such as metoclopramide (10 mg) or cisapride (10 to 20 mg), taken 30 min before meals and at bedtime, is prescribed to raise sphincter pressure, hasten gastric emptying, and improve esophageal clearance. Metoclopramide may cause extrapyramidal central nervous system side effects. Inhibition of H^+,K^+-ATPase, the parietal cell pump that is responsible for acid secretion, with omeprazole (20 to 40 mg daily) is a most effective form of therapy that has been shown to heal erosive esophagitis. Reflux esophagitis requires prolonged therapy, for 3 to 6 months or longer if the disease recurs quickly. Patients with reflux esophagitis who have complications such as Barrett's esophagus (with or without a deep ulcer) should be treated vigorously. Patients who have an associated peptic stricture are treated with dilators to relieve dysphagia as well as with vigorous treatment for reflux. Patients who have specialized intestinal metaplasia must be monitored for the development of high-grade dysplasia and early adenocarcinoma, which must be treated if they occur. Monitoring consists of close follow-up with periodic endoscopic biopsies. Endoscopic surveillance is indicated every 1 to 2 years in patients without evidence of dysplasia; patients with dysplasia require more frequent surveillance. Suitable surgical candidates with high-grade dysplasia and early carcinoma are treated by esophagectomy and esophagogastric anastomosis.

Antireflux surgery, in which the gastric fundus is wrapped around the esophagus (fundoplication), increases the lower sphincter pressure and should be considered in patients with resistant and complicated reflux esophagitis that does not respond fully to medical therapy or in patients for whom long-term medical therapy is not desirable. Laproscopic fundoplication is used increasingly. In the ideal candidate for fundoplication, motility studies show persistently inadequate lower sphincter pressure but normal peristaltic contractions in the esophageal body.

Patients with alkaline esophagitis are treated with general antireflux measures and neutralization of bile salts with cholestyramine, aluminum hydroxide, or sucralfate. Sucralfate is particularly useful in these cases, as it also serves as a surface protector.

INFECTIOUS ESOPHAGITIS   With the recent increase in the frequency of immunodeficiency states, infectious esophagitis has become increasingly important. Infectious esophagitis can be due to viral, bacterial, fungal, or parasitic organisms. In severely immunocompromised patients, multiple organisms may coexist.

Viral Esophagitis (See also Chap. 184)   *Herpes simplex virus* (HSV) type 1 occasionally causes esophagitis in immunocompetent individuals, but either HSV type 1 or HSV type 2 may afflict patients who are immunosuppressed. These patients complain of an acute onset of chest pain, odynophagia, and dysphagia. Bleeding may occur in severe cases, and systemic manifestations such as nausea, vomiting, fever, chills, and mild leukocytosis may be present. Herpetic vesicles on the nose and lips sometimes provide a clue to the diagnosis. Barium swallow is inadequate to detect early lesions and cannot reliably distinguish HSV infection from other types of infections. Endoscopy shows vesicles and small, discrete, punched-out superficial ulcerations with or without a fibrinous exudate. In later stages, there is a diffuse erosive esophagitis caused by enlargement and coalescence of the ulcers. Mucosal cells from a biopsy sample taken at the edge of an ulcer or from a cytologic smear show ballooning degeneration, ground-glass changes in the nuclei with eosinophilic intranuclear inclusions (Cowdry type A), and giant cell formation on routine stains. Culture for HSV becomes positive within days and is helpful in diagnosis. For prophylaxis in a severely immunocompromised host, acyclovir, 800 mg orally twice daily or 250 mg per square meter of body surface every 12 h intravenously, is recommended. For treatment of esophagitis, intravenous therapy, 250 mg/m^2 every 8 h, is usually initiated. As swallowing improves, the therapy is changed to 200 to 400 mg orally five times daily. Symptoms usually resolve in 1 week, but large ulcerations may take longer to heal. Foscarnet (60 mg/kg intravenously every 8 h) may be useful if acyclovir resistance occurs. These patients also may have reflux esophagitis, which may worsen the symptoms and add to complications.

Varicella-zoster virus (VZV) (see also Chap. 185) sometimes produces esophagitis in children with chickenpox and adults with herpes zoster. Esophageal VZV also can be the source of disseminated VZV infection in the absence of skin involvement. In an immunocompromised host, VZV esophagitis causes vesicles and confluent ulcers and usually resolves spontaneously, but it may cause necrotizing esophagitis in a severely compromised host. On routine histologic examination of mucosal biopsy samples or cytology specimens, VZV is difficult to distinguish from HSV, but the distinction can be made immunohistologically or by culture. Acyclovir is effective in prevention and treatment of VZV esophagitis, but much higher doses are needed than for HSV.

Cytomegalovirus (CMV) infections occur only in immunocompromised patients. CMV is usually activated from a latent stage or may be acquired from blood product transfusions. CMV lesions initially appear as serpiginous ulcers in an otherwise normal mucosa. These may coalesce to form giant ulcers, particularly in the distal esophagus.

Patients present with painful swallowing, chest pain, hematemesis, nausea, and vomiting. Diagnosis requires endoscopy and biopsies of the center of the ulcer. Mucosal brushings are not useful. Routine histologic examination shows intranuclear and small intracytoplasmic inclusions in large fibroblasts and endothelial cells of blood vessels. Immunohistology with monoclonal antibodies to CMV and in situ hybridization of CMV DNA can be performed on centrifugation culture and are useful for early diagnosis. Ganciclovir (DHPG), 5 mg/kg every 12 h intravenously, is the treatment of choice. Foscarnet (60 mg/kg

every 8 h intravenously) is used in resistant cases. Therapy is continued until healing, which may take weeks to months.

Human immunodeficiency virus (HIV) may be associated with a self-limited syndrome of acute esophageal ulceration associated with oral ulcers and a maculopapular skin rash, which occurs at the time of HIV seroconversion. Some patients with advanced disease have deep, persistent esophageal ulcers. They require treatment with oral steroids or thalidomide. Some ulcers respond to local steroid injection.

Bacterial Esophagitis   *Bacterial esophagitis* is unusual, but esophagitis caused by *Lactobacillus* and beta-hemolytic streptococci has been described in the immunocompromised host. In profoundly granulocytopenic patients and in patients with cancer, bacterial esophagitis is often missed because it is commonly present with other organisms, including viruses and fungi, and because bacteria are difficult to identify on routine histologic examination. In patients with AIDS, infection with *Cryptosporidium* or *Pneumocystis carinii* may cause nonspecific inflammation, and *Mycobacterium tuberculosis* infection may cause deep ulcerations of the distal esophagus.

Candida **Esophagitis**   Many *Candida* species are normal commensals in the throat but become pathogenic and produce esophagitis in immunodeficiency states. Occasionally, monilial *Candida* esophagitis occurs in the absence of any predisposing factors. Patients may be asymptomatic or complain of odynophagia and dysphagia. Oral thrush or other evidence of mucocutaneous candidiasis may be absent. Rarely, *Candida* esophagitis is complicated by esophageal bleeding, perforation, and stricture or by systemic invasion. Results of barium swallow may be normal or may show multiple nodular filling defects of various sizes (Fig. 283-2). Large nodular defects may resemble clusters of grapes. Endoscopy shows small, yellow-white raised plaques with surrounding erythema in mild disease. In extensive disease, confluent linear and nodular plaques are seen. Diagnosis is made by demonstration of yeast or hyphal forms in plaque smears and exudate stained with Gram's, periodic acid–Schiff, or silver stains. Biopsy results usually are not positive. Culture is not useful in diagnosis but may be helpful in confirming the species and, if needed, the drug sensitivities of the yeast (see Chap. 209). In normal or minimally immunocompromised patients, nystatin or clotrimazole treatment is often successful. Nystatin is used as an oral suspension (100,000 units per milliliter) in doses of 10 to 20 mL every 6 h; clotrimazole is administered in the form of 10-mg tablets to be sucked five times a day. Ketoconazole (200 to 400 mg in a single daily oral dose) is an effective treatment; the higher dose is used in severely immunocompromised hosts. The bioavailability of ketoconazole is severely reduced at increased gastric pH; therefore, it should not be used concurrently with gastric acid suppression therapy or in achlorhydric subjects. Fluconazole (200 mg on the first day, followed by 100 mg daily) is the preferred treatment because its absorption is not affected by high gastric pH. Poorly responsive patients are treated with amphotericin, 10 to 15 mg as an intravenous infusion for 6 h daily to a total dose of 300 to 500 mg. Miconazole and amphotericin lozenges are currently not available in the United States. The treatment is for 7 to 10 days followed by nystatin, clotrimazole, ketoconazole, or fluconazole for as long as the host resistance remains low. In patients with AIDS and suspected *Candida* esophagitis, empirical treatment with fluconazole is often initiated.

OTHER TYPES OF ESOPHAGITIS   *Radiation esophagitis* is a common occurrence during radiation treatment for lung, mediastinal, or esophageal carcinoma. The frequency and severity of esophagitis increase with the amount of radiation delivered to the area and with the subsequent use of certain chemotherapeutic agents, such as doxorubicin, bleomycin, cyclophosphamide, and cisplatin. Dysphagia and odynophagia may last several weeks to several months after the conclusion of therapy. The esophageal mucosa becomes erythematous, edematous, and friable. Superficial erosions coalesce to form larger superficial ulcers. Submucosal fibrosis and degenerative changes in the blood vessels, muscles, and myenteric neurons may be present. The treatment is relief of pain with viscous lidocaine during the acute phase; indomethacin treatment may lessen the radiation damage. Esophageal stricture may develop and require dilatation.

Corrosive esophagitis is caused by the ingestion of caustic agents, such as strong alkalies or acids. When severe, corrosive injury may lead to esophageal perforation, bleeding, and death. Steroids have not been shown to be useful in acute corrosive esophagitis. Healing is usually associated with stricture formation. Caustic strictures are usually long and rigid (Fig. 283-2) and generally require dilatation with dilators passed over a guidewire through the stricture. *Pill-induced esophagitis* is associated with the ingestion of certain pills and accounts for many cases of erosive esophagitis. Antibiotics such as doxycycline, tetracycline, and clindamycin account for over half the cases. Other commonly prescribed pills that cause esophageal injury include aspirin, potassium chloride, ferrous sulfate, quinidine, alprenolol, and various steroidal and nonsteroidal anti-inflammatory agents. Pill esophagitis can be prevented by having patients take pills in the upright position and wash them down with copious amounts of fluids.

Sclerotherapy for bleeding esophageal varices usually produces transient retrosternal chest pain and dysphagia; esophageal ulcer, stricture, hematoma, or perforation may occur. *Esophagitis associated with mucocutaneous and systemic diseases* is usually associated with blister and bulla formation, epithelial desquamation, and thin, weblike or dense esophageal strictures. Pemphigus vulgaris and bullous pemphigoid form intraepithelial and subepithelial bullae, respectively, and can be distinguished by specific immunohistology; they are both characterized by sloughing of epithelium or the presence of esophageal casts. Glucocorticoid treatment is usually effective. Dystrophic epidermolysis bullosa is an inherited disease that presents in childhood in which local trauma is associated with bulla formation and scarring. Cicatricial pemphigoid, Stevens-Johnson syndrome, and toxic epidermolysis bullosa can produce esophageal bullous lesions and strictures requiring gentle dilatation. Graft-versus-host disease occurs in patients who have received allogeneic bone marrow transplants and is associated with generalized desquamation and esophageal strictures. Behçet's disease and eosinophilic gastroenteritis may involve the esophagus and may respond to steroid therapy. Crohn's disease and an erosive lichen planus also can involve the esophagus, and Crohn's disease may cause inflammatory strictures, sinus tract, filiform polyps, and fistulas in the esophagus.

OTHER ESOPHAGEAL DISORDERS

DIVERTICULA Diverticula are outpouchings of the wall of the esophagus. A *Zenker's diverticulum* appears in the natural zone of weakness in the posterior hypopharyngeal wall and causes halitosis and regurgitation of saliva and food particles consumed several days previously. When it becomes large and filled with food, such a diverticulum can compress the esophagus and cause dysphagia or complete obstruction. Nasogastric intubation and endoscopy should be performed with utmost care in these patients, since they may cause perforation of the diverticulum. A *midesophageal diverticulum* may be caused by traction from old adhesions or by propulsion associated with esophageal motor abnormalities. An *epiphrenic diverticulum* may be associated with achalasia. Small or medium-sized diverticula and midesophageal and epiphrenic diverticula are usually asymptomatic. *Diffuse intramural diverticulosis* of the esophagus is due to dilation of the deep esophageal glands. This condition may lead to chronic candidiasis or to the development of a stricture high up in the esophagus. These patients may present with dysphagia. Symptomatic Zenker's diverticula are treated by cricopharyngeal myotomy with or without diverticulectomy. Very large symptomatic esophageal diverticula are removed surgically. When they are associated with motor abnormalities, distal myotomy is performed. Strictures associated with diffuse intramural diverticulosis are treated with rubber dilators.

WEBS AND RINGS Weblike constrictions of the esophagus are usually congenital or inflammatory in origin. Asymptomatic hypopharyngeal webs are demonstrated in up to 10 percent of normal individuals. When concentric, they cause intermittent dysphagia to solids. The combination of symptomatic hypopharyngeal webs and iron-deficiency anemia in middle-aged women constitutes *Plummer-Vinson syndrome*. The clinical importance of this syndrome is uncer-

tain. Midesophageal webs are rare. A *lower esophageal mucosal ring* (Schatzki ring) is a thin, weblike constriction located at the squamocolumnar mucosal junction at or near the border of the LES (Fig. 283-2). It invariably produces dysphagia when the lumen diameter is less than 1.3 cm. Dysphagia to solids is the only symptom, and it is usually episodic. Asymptomatic rings may be present in about 10 percent of normal individuals. A lower esophageal ring is one of the common causes of dysphagia. Symptomatic webs and mucosal lower esophageal rings are easily treated by dilatation. A *lower esophageal muscular ring* (contractile ring) is located proximal to the site of mucosal rings and may represent an abnormal uppermost segment of the lower esophageal sphincter. These rings can be recognized by the fact that they are not constant in size and shape. They also may cause dysphagia and should be differentiated from peptic strictures, achalasia, and lower esophageal mucosal ring. They are treated by dilatation.

HIATAL HERNIA A *hiatal hernia* is a herniation of part of the stomach into the thoracic cavity through the esophageal hiatus in the diaphragm. A *sliding hiatal hernia* is one in which the gastroesophageal junction and fundus of the stomach slide upward. A sliding hernia may result from weakening of the anchors of the gastroesophageal junction to the diaphragm, from longitudinal contraction of the esophagus, or from increased intraabdominal pressure. Small sliding hernias can be demonstrated commonly during barium studies if intraabdominal pressure is increased. Their incidence increases with age; in the sixth decade of life, the prevalence of such hernias is around 60 percent. It is unlikely that a small sliding hiatal hernia by itself produces any clinical symptoms, but it plays a role in the pathogenesis of reflux esophagitis. A *paraesophageal hernia* is one in which the esophagogastric junction remains fixed in its normal location and a pouch of stomach is herniated beside the gastroesophageal junction through the esophageal hiatus. A paraesophageal or mixed paraesophageal and sliding hernia may become incarcerated and strangulate. This situation leads to acute chest pain, dysphagia, and a mediastinal mass and requires prompt operative treatment. A herniated gastric pouch may cause dysphagia and may be the site of gastritis and ulceration causing chronic blood loss. A large paraesophageal hernia should be surgically repaired.

MECHANICAL TRAUMA *Esophageal rupture* may be caused by (1) iatrogenic damage from instrumentation of the esophagus or external trauma, (2) increased intraesophageal pressure associated with forceful vomiting or retching (*spontaneous rupture* or *Boerhaave's syndrome*), or (3) diseases of the esophagus such as corrosive esophagitis, esophageal ulcer, and neoplasm. The site of perforation depends on the cause. Instrumental perforation usually occurs in the pharynx or lower esophagus, often just above the diaphragm in the posterolateral wall. Esophageal perforation causes severe retrosternal chest pain, which may be worsened by swallowing and breathing. Free air enters the mediastinum and spreads to neighboring structures and causes palpable subcutaneous emphysema in the neck, mediastinal crackling sounds on auscultation, and pneumothorax. With time, secondary infection supervenes, and mediastinal abscess and pleuropulmonary suppurative complications may develop. Esophageal perforation associated with vomiting usually deposits gastric contents in the mediastinum and causes severe mediastinal complications. On the other hand, instrumental perforation may be clinically mild and free of severe complications. Spontaneous rupture of the esophagus may mimic myocardial infarction, pancreatitis, or rupture of an abdominal viscus. Symptoms of chest pain may be mild, particularly in the elderly. Mediastinal emphysema may develop late. An x-ray of the chest shows abnormalities in most patients, but computed tomography of the chest is more sensitive in detecting mediastinal air. Fluid from pleural effusions may have a high content of (salivary) amylase. The diagnosis is confirmed by swallow of radiopaque contrast material. Treatment includes esophageal and gastric suction and parenteral administration of broad-spectrum antibiotics. Surgical drainage and repair of the laceration should be performed as soon as possible. In patients with terminal carcinoma, surgical repair may not be feasible, and patients with minor instrumental perforation can be treated conservatively. Extensive corrosive damage may require esophageal diversion and subsequent excision of the damaged portion of the esophagus.

Mucosal Tear (Mallory-Weiss Syndrome) This tear is usually caused by vomiting, retching, or vigorous coughing. The tear usually involves the gastric mucosa near the squamocolumnar mucosal junction. Patients present with upper gastrointestinal bleeding, which may be severe. In most patients bleeding ceases spontaneously; continued bleeding may respond to vasopressin therapy or angiographic embolization. Surgery is rarely needed.

Intramural Hematoma Emetogenic injury, particularly in patients with bleeding abnormalities, can cause bleeding between the mucosal and muscle layers of the esophagus. The patients develop sudden dysphagia. The diagnosis is made by barium swallow and computed tomography. Resolution is usually spontaneous.

FOREIGN BODIES Foreign bodies may lodge in the cervical esophagus just beyond the upper esophageal sphincter, near the aortic arch, or above the lower esophageal sphincter. Impaction of a bolus of food, particularly a piece of meat or bread, may occur when the esophageal lumen is narrowed due to stricture, carcinoma, or a lower esophageal ring. Acute impaction causes a complete inability to swallow and severe chest pain. Both foreign bodies and food boluses may be removed endoscopically. Use of a meat tenderizer to facilitate passage of an obstructed meat bolus is to be discouraged because of potential esophageal perforation and aspiration pneumonia.

For further discussion of cholinergic and anti-cholinergic agents and vasoconstrictors and vasodilators see Chaps. 7 and 32, in Goodman and Gilman's The Pharmacological Basis of Therapeutics, 9th ed, McGraw-Hill, New York, 1996.

BIBLIOGRAPHY

ALLEN ML, DIMARINO AJ JR: Manometric diagnosis of diffuse esophageal spasm. Dig Dis Sci 41:1346, 1996

BOTT S et al: Medication-induced esophageal injury: Survey of the literature. Am J Gastroenterol 82:758, 1987

CONKLIN JL, CHRISTENSEN J: Neuromuscular control of the oropharynx and esophagus in health and disease. Annu Rev Med 45:13, 1994

DODDS WJ: The pathogenesis of gastroesophageal reflux disease. Am J Roentgenol 151:49, 1988

KLINKENBERG-KNOL EC et al: Long-term treatment with omeprazole for refractory reflux esophagitis: Efficacy and safety. Ann Intern Med 121:161, 1994

MITTAL RK et al: Transient lower esophageal sphincter relaxation. Gastroenterology 109:601, 1995

PASRICHA PH et al: Intrasphincteric botulinum toxin for treatment of achalasia. N Engl J Med 322:774, 1995

RICHTER JE et al: Esophageal chest pain: Current controversies in pathogenesis, diagnosis, and therapy. Ann Intern Med 110:66, 1989

RUBESIN SE: Oral and pharyngeal dysphagia. Gastroenterol Clin North Am 24:331, 1995

SINGARAM C et al: Nitrinergic and peptidergic innervation of the human esophagus. Gut 35:1690, 1994

SPECHLER SJ, GOYAL RK: Barrett's esophagus. N Engl J Med 315:362, 1986
—— et al: Prevalence of metaplasia at the gastroesophageal junction. Lancet 344:1533, 1994

SUTTON FM et al: Infectious esophagitis. Gastrointest Endosc Clin North Am 4:713, 1994

VAEZI MF et al: Role of acid and duodenogastric reflux in esophageal mucosal injury: A review of animal and human studies. Gastroenterology 108:1897, 1995

WEBB WA: Management of foreign bodies of the upper gastrointestinal tract: Update. Gastrointest Endosc 41:39, 1995

WILCOX CM et al: Esophageal ulceration in human immunodeficiency virus infection. Causes, response to therapy, and long-term outcome. Ann Intern Med 123:143, 1995

PEPTIC ULCER AND RELATED DISORDERS*

A peptic ulcer is a mucosal lesion of the stomach or duodenum in which acid and pepsin play major pathogenic roles. The major forms of peptic ulcer are duodenal ulcer (DU) and gastric ulcer (GU), both of which are chronic diseases often caused by the bacterium *Helicobacter pylori*. *H. pylori* is also an important risk factor for gastric cancer and certain types of gastric lymphoma. The term *peptic ulcer* also encompasses GUs and DUs associated with stress or the ingestion of drugs, most commonly aspirin and other nonsteroidal anti-inflammatory drugs (NSAIDs). Ulcer associated with the Zollinger-Ellison syndrome (ZES), caused by gastrin-secreting islet cell tumors (gastrinomas), is also considered a form of peptic ulcer.

Although our knowledge of the cause of peptic ulcer is incomplete, available information supports a central role for *H. pylori* and a necessary role for acid and pepsin. Whether an ulcer develops depends on the balance between aggressive factors (principally gastric acid and pepsin) and factors that participate in mucosal defense or resistance to ulceration. Peptic ulcer results when gastroduodenal mucosal defenses are unable to protect the epithelium from the corrosive effects of acid and pepsin.

In the past, ideas concerning the pathogenesis of peptic ulcer focused on the role of acid and pepsin, but recent observations suggest that many of the reported abnormalities of gastric acid secretion in patients with peptic ulcer may be a direct consequence of infection with *H. pylori*. Nevertheless, an understanding of basic gastric physiology remains central to a consideration of ulcer pathogenesis.

GASTRIC PHYSIOLOGY RELATED TO PEPTIC ULCER

Aggressive Factors: Acid and Pepsin The gastric mucosa has an extraordinary capacity to secrete acid. The parietal cells scattered along the course of the mucosal glands (oxyntic mucosa) of the body and fundus of the stomach secrete hydrochloric acid by a process involving oxidative phosphorylation (Fig. 284-1). The estimated concentration of HCl secreted by parietal cells is approximately 160 mM. Each secreted hydrogen ion (H$^+$) is accompanied by a chloride ion (Cl$^-$). For each hydrogen ion secreted into the gastric lumen, one bicarbonate ion (HCO$_3^-$) is released into the gastric venous circulation, accounting for the so-called alkaline tide; bicarbonate is released from carbonic acid generated from carbon dioxide by parietal cell carbonic anhydrase. The final step in hydrogen ion secretion is accomplished by an H$^+$,K$^+$-ATPase "proton pump" located in the apical microvillus membrane and tubovesicular apparatus of the parietal cell. This H$^+$,K$^+$-ATPase exchanges hydrogen for potassium across the microvillus membrane.

Multiple chemical, neural, and hormonal factors participate in the regulation of gastric acid secretion. Acid secretion is stimulated by gastrin and by postganglionic vagal fibers via muscarinic cholinergic receptors on parietal cells. Gastrin, the most potent known stimulant of gastric acid secretion, is contained in and released into the circulation from cytoplasmic secretory granules of gastrin cells (G cells), which are scattered singly or in small clusters among the epithelial lining cells of the middle and deeper portions of the pyloric glands of the antrum. Gastrin release is stimulated by the neuropeptide gastrin-releasing peptide and inhibited by somatostatin produced by D cells in the antrum. Gastrin in tissues and in the circulation exists in several molecular forms. The principal form of gastrin in gastric antral mucosa is heptadecapeptide gastrin (G-17), which contains 17 amino acid residues; the active site region is the C-terminal tetrapeptide amide (Trp-Met-Asp-Phe-NH$_2$). Gastrin II is the form in which the tyrosyl residue at position 12 is sulfated, while gastrin I is the nonsulfated form. Although G-17 accounts for more than 90 percent of the gastrin in antral mucosa, approximately two-thirds of the gastrin in serum is a larger species containing 34 amino acids (G-34). Although G-17 has a shorter half-life than G-34, circulating G-17 is approximately as potent as G-34 in stimulating gastric acid

---

* James McGuigan, M.D., was the author of this chapter in the 13th edition.

FIGURE 284-1 Biology of the parietal cell. G_i and G_s, inhibitory and stimulatory G protein subunits; ECL, enterochromaffin-like.

secretion. Gastrin is also present in duodenal mucosa, particularly in the most proximal duodenum (at approximately 10 percent of the antral concentration). The mucosal concentration of gastrin and the proportion of G-17 decrease progressively down the duodenum.

The effects of gastrin and vagal stimulation on gastric acid secretion are intimately interrelated. Vagal stimulation increases gastric acid secretion by cholinergic stimulation of parietal cell secretion, by enhancing release of gastrin from antral G cells (by both inhibition of the release of somatostatin by antral D cells and by direct stimulation of G cells), and by lowering the parietal cell threshold for response to circulating gastrin concentrations.

The gastric mucosa contains large amounts of histamine contained in cytoplasmic granules of mast cells and enterochromaffin-like (ECL) cells; the latter are epithelial endocrine cells distributed singly in the oxyntic glands, often in direct contact with parietal cells. Recognition of the role of histamine in acid secretion was fostered by discovery of H_2 receptor antagonists that competitively inhibit the action of histamine on H_2 receptors, which are located on gastric parietal, cardiac atrial, and uterine smooth-muscle cells. These drugs exert negligible effects on H_1 receptors, which are inhibited readily by conventional antihistamines (H_1 receptor antagonists). H_2 receptor antagonists (e.g., cimetidine, ranitidine, famotidine, and nizatidine) inhibit basal acid secretion as well as secretion in response to feeding, gastrin, histamine, hypoglycemia, or vagal stimulation. Histamine is the most important stimulant of gastric acid secretion and is released from ECL cells by the action of both gastrin and cholinergic activity.

The basolateral membranes of parietal cells contain receptors for histamine, gastrin, and acetylcholine that stimulate acid secretion and for prostaglandins and somatostatin that inhibit acid secretion (Fig. 284-1). The parietal cell histamine receptor is a membrane-spanning G protein-coupled receptor. Histamine stimulates gastric acid secretion by increasing parietal cell cyclic adenosine monophosphate (AMP), thereby activating cyclic AMP–dependent protein kinase(s). Gastrin stimulates gastric acid secretion by direct stimulation of parietal cells and by stimulation of histamine release from ECL cells. Gastrin and acetylcholine do not stimulate cyclic AMP production but, instead, stimulate acid secretion by increasing parietal cell cytosolic calcium. Prostaglandins and somatostatin act through inhibitory G proteins that decrease the generation of cyclic AMP; somatostatin also inhibits histamine release from ECL cells.

The major physiologic stimulus for gastric acid secretion is ingestion of food. Traditionally, regulation of gastric acid secretion has been classified into three phases: cephalic, gastric, and intestinal. This classification is of some value in analyzing factors that participate in regulation of gastric acid secretion. The cephalic phase encompasses the gastric acid secretory response to the sight, smell, taste, and anticipation of food; the gastric phase is induced by food in the stomach; and the intestinal phase occurs after entry of food into the lumen of the small intestine. The cephalic phase, which includes cortical and hypothalamic components, is mediated primarily by vagal activation, which increases gastric acid secretion principally by direct stimulation of ECL and parietal cells and to a lesser extent by promoting gastrin release. The gastric phase results from stimulation of chemical and mechanical receptors in the gastric wall by luminal contents. Mechanical distention of the stomach stimulates gastric acid secretion but results in little gastrin release; this mechanical effect is inhibited by atropine and appears to be mediated by vagal reflexes. Food (principally protein and the products of protein digestion) in the stomach promotes gastric acid secretion by increasing gastrin release. Food in the proximal small intestine stimulates the intestinal phase of gastric acid secretion by inducing the release of small amounts of gastrin and other peptides that stimulate gastric acid secretion and by a direct effect of absorbed amino acids on parietal cells. Basal or interdigestive gastric acid secretion can be considered to be a fourth phase of acid secretion. This phase is unrelated to feeding and reaches its peak around midnight and its lowest point about 7 A.M.; neural pathways are probably most important in its regulation.

Ingestion of both caffeine-containing and caffeine-free coffee stimulates gastric acid secretion by stimulating gastrin release. Ingestion of beer and wine also stimulate gastric acid secretion, presumably owing to the effects of amines and other congeners, because pure ethanol is a weak stimulant of acid secretion. Intravenous calcium stimulates gastric acid secretion and produces minimal increases in serum gastrin levels. Oral calcium has been reported to stimulate gastric acid secretion directly, i.e., without an increase in serum calcium or gastrin concentrations. Except in patients who harbor a gastrinoma, hypercalcemia is not usually associated with gastric acid hypersecretion or with an increase in serum gastrin.

Gastric acid secretion can be inhibited by acid in the stomach or duodenum, by hyperglycemia, or by hypertonic fluids or fat in the duodenum. Reduction of the intragastric pH to 3.0 produces partial inhibition of gastrin release; further reduction to pH 1.5 or below completely blocks release of gastrin in response to almost all stimuli. Somatostatin appears to play an important role in this acid-induced feedback inhibition of gastrin release. Somatostatin-containing antral mucosal endocrine cells (D cells) have cytoplasmic processes that extend to neighboring gastrin cells and to parietal cells. Somatostatin reduces gastric acid secretion by inhibiting gastrin release, by directly inhibiting parietal cell secretion, and by inhibiting the release of histamine by ECL cells. Acid in the duodenum decreases gastric acid secretion by the stomach, most likely by stimulating release into the circulation of intestinal peptides such as secretin that inhibit gastric acid secretion. Fat in the duodenum also inhibits gastric acid secretion; gastric inhibitory peptide (GIP) has been proposed as a candidate for this action. The mechanisms by which hyperglycemia or intraduodenal hyperosmolality inhibit gastric acid secretion are not known. Additional small intestinal mucosal peptides possessing the capacity to inhibit gastric acid secretion include vasoactive intestinal peptide (VIP), enteroglucagon, neurotensin, peptide YY, and urogastrone, but the extent to which these peptides contribute to the physiologic regulation of gastric acid secretion has not been defined.

The proteolytic effects of pepsins in concert with the corrosive properties of secreted gastric acid contribute to the tissue injury that produces peptic ulcer. Gastric acid catalyzes the cleavage of inactive pepsinogen molecules, converting them to proteolytically active pepsins, and also provides the low pH required for pepsin activity. Pepsins are maximally active at a pH of approximately 2.0, have substantially reduced activity above a pH of 4.0, and are irreversibly inactivated and denatured at neutral or alkaline pH. A variety of pepsinogens and their respective active pepsins are present in gastric juice. Pepsinogens (and their corresponding pepsins) have been classified by immunochemical techniques as either pepsinogen I or A (comprising pepsinogens 1 through 5) or pepsinogen II or C (comprising pepsinogens 6 and 7). Pepsinogen I is found in chief and mucous cells in the body and fundus of the stomach. Pepsinogen II is located in mucous cells in the body and fundus as well as in cells of the pyloric glands, cells of Brunner's glands of the duodenum, and mucous cells of the gastric cardiac glands. Both pepsinogen I and pepsinogen II are present in plasma, whereas only pepsinogen I is detected in urine. In general, there is a direct correlation between pepsinogen I serum concentrations and maximal gastric acid secretion. Most agents that stimulate gastric acid secretion also stimulate pepsinogen secretion; cholinergic action is particularly potent in promoting pepsinogen secretion. However, secretin inhibits gastric acid secretion but stimulates pepsinogen secretion.

In addition to secretion of hydrochloric acid, parietal cells also secrete intrinsic factor. Agents that stimulate gastric acid secretion also lead to secretion of intrinsic factor.

Measurement of Gastric Acid Secretion Gastric acid output is measured by collecting four consecutive 15-min samples to determine the 1-h basal acid output (BAO). Secretion volume and acid concentration (titrated with sodium hydroxide to pH 7.0 or calculated by formula from the pH of the aspirated gastric juice) are measured. Pentagastrin (which contains the biologically active C-terminal tetrapeptide amide portion of gastrin) is the preferred agent to stimulate maximal acid output (MAO) by the stomach. Following collection of basal acid secretion, gastric juice is collected for four additional consecutive 15-min periods after the subcutaneous injection of pentagastrin (6 μg/kg). The MAO is the amount of acid aspirated during the 1 h after pentagastrin administration. Peak acid output (PAO) is calculated by combining the two highest consecutive 15-min acid outputs following pentagastrin injection and multiplying by 2.

Measurement of basal and stimulated gastric acid secretion was used in the past in the clinical assessment of some patients with peptic ulcer and is still used as a research tool. The range of values for normal subjects is extremely broad and overlaps substantially with those for patients with DU, GU, and even ZES. Mean BAO in normal males without known ulcer disease is about 0.8 μmol/s (2 to 3 mEq/h). Mean MAO in normal males is about 6.4 μmol/s (23 mEq/h). In general, basal and stimulated acid outputs in females are approximately two-thirds to three-fourths those found in males. In patients with DU, the mean BAO averages 1 to 1.7 μmol/s (4 to 6 mEq/h) and the mean MAO is 8 to 11 μmol/s (30 to 40 mEq/h), again with wide variation. Patients with GU tend to have acid secretory rates that are normal or often slightly less than those for normal subjects. Whether variations in acid output from normal in patients with peptic ulcer reflect the effects of *H. pylori* infection is controversial, but the preponderance of evidence suggests that slight gastric acid hypersecretion persists in many patients with DU after eradication of *H. pylori* (see below).

Measurement of gastric acid output may be of value in selected clinical situations, particularly when ZES is suspected. Specifically, when hypergastrinemia is identified, measurement of gastric acid output will distinguish between clinical conditions characterized by gastric acid hypersecretion (e.g., ZES) and those that involve achlorhydria (e.g., atrophic gastritis associated with pernicious anemia).

Mucosal Defense The mechanisms by which the normal stomach and duodenum resist the corrosive effects of acid and pepsin (i.e., the mechanisms of mucosal resistance to injury or mucosal defense) have not been defined completely. However, a variety of factors have been identified that contribute to or compromise mucosal defense (Fig. 284-2).

Gastric mucus secreted by mucous cells of the gastric mucosal epithelium and gastric glands is important in mucosal defense and in preventing peptic ulceration. Mucus secretion is stimulated by mechanical or chemical irritation and by cholinergic stimulation. Gastric mucus is present in two phases: in a soluble phase in gastric juice and as an insoluble mucus gel layer, approximately 0.2 mm thick, which coats the mucosal surface of the stomach. Normally, the mucus gel is secreted constantly by gastric mucous epithelial cells and is continuously solubilized by pepsins secreted into the gastric lumen. When intact, the mucus gel serves as an unstirred water layer which slows ionic diffusion and is impermeable to macromolecules such as pepsins (molecular weight, 34,000). Pepsin molecules secreted into the gastric lumen are denied return by the intact mucus gel, which thereby protects mucosal cells from proteolytic injury. Gel thickness is increased by the E prostaglandins and reduced by aspirin and other NSAIDs. Gastric mucus glycoproteins also contain antigenic determinants used to classify AB(O) blood group substances. Approximately three-fourths of the population secrete gastric juice containing these AB(O) substances, and such individuals are referred to as secretors.

Nonparietal gastric epithelial cells secrete bicarbonate ions into the mucus gel, which help to create a microenvironment with a substantial hydrogen ion gradient, ranging from pH 1 to 2 in the luminal side of the gel layer to pH 6 to 7 in the zone in contact with the gastric mucosal cells. As an unstirred water layer, the mucus gel slows the diffusion of hydrogen ion toward the gastric mucosal surface, allowing buffering by bicarbonate within the gel. Gastric bicarbonate secretion is stimulated by calcium, certain prostaglandins of the E and F series, cholinergic agents, and dibutyryl cyclic guanosine monophosphate. It is inhibited by aspirin and NSAIDs, acetazolamide, alpha-adrenergic agents, and ethanol.

Normally, the luminal surfaces and intercellular tight junctions of the gastric epithelial cells create a gastric mucosal barrier that is almost completely impermeable to diffusion of hydrogen ions from the lumen. This barrier can be interrupted by bile acids, salicylates, ethanol, and weak organic acids, permitting hydrogen ions to diffuse into gastric tissue. The result may be cell injury, release of histamine from mast cells, further stimulation of acid secretion, damage to small blood vessels, mucosal hemorrhage, and erosion or ulceration. Interruption of the gastric mucosal barrier appears to contribute to the hemorrhagic erosive gastropathy associated with salicylate or ethanol ingestion and with other forms of gastric mucosal injury. Because of the high metabolic activity and substantial oxygen requirements of the gastric mucosa, maintenance of normal blood flow to the gastric mucosa is an essential component of mucosal resistance to injury. Decreased mucosal blood flow, accompanied by diffusion of luminal hydrogen

FIGURE 284-2 Gastric mucosal defense mechanisms. These include stimulation of secretion of mucus by gastric glands and of biocarbonate by gastric epithelial cells, epithelial cell renewal, and the gastric microcirculation, which provides nutrients to cells. Administration of prostaglandins enhances all of these mechanisms.

ions, is thought to be important in producing gastric mucosal damage.

Prostaglandins are abundant in the gastric mucosa. Administration to animals of various prostaglandins, particularly those of the E series, has been shown to prevent gastric mucosal injury caused by a wide variety of agents. Endogenous prostaglandins stimulate secretion of gastric mucus and gastric and duodenal mucosal bicarbonate. They participate in the maintenance of gastric mucosal blood flow and of the integrity of the gastric mucosal barrier and promote epithelial cell renewal in response to mucosal injury.

DUODENAL ULCER

DU is characteristically a chronic and recurrent disease. In contrast to erosions, which are superficial and limited to the mucosa, DUs are usually deep and sharply demarcated. They penetrate through the mucosa and submucosa, often into the muscularis propria. The ulcer floor contains no intact epithelium and usually consists of a zone of eosinophilic necrosis resting on a base of granulation tissue surrounded by variable amounts of fibrosis. The ulcer bed may be clear or may contain blood or a proteinaceous exudate with entrapped erythrocytes and acute and chronic inflammatory cells.

More than 95 percent of DUs occur in the first portion of the duodenum, and approximately 90 percent of those are located within 3 cm of the junction of the pyloric and duodenal mucosa. DUs are usually less than 1 cm in diameter; rarely, they are extremely large, 3 to 6 cm in diameter ("giant DUs"), and may be mistaken radiographically for the entire duodenal bulb.

The prevalence of DU is estimated to range from 6 to 15 percent of Western populations. During the past 40 years, the frequency of DU has been decreasing in the United States and England, especially in males. The reasons for this reduction are not known but are likely to relate to the changing epidemiology of *H. pylori* (see below). DUs now appear to be approximately as common in males as in females. Current estimates suggest that approximately 10 percent of the population has clinical evidence of DU at some time in their lives. The natural history of untreated DU consists of spontaneous healing and recurrence; at least 60 percent of healed DUs recur within 1 year, and 80 to 90 percent recur within 2 years.

ETIOLOGY AND PATHOGENESIS Peptic ulcer disease is thought to result from an imbalance between aggressive factors, especially gastric acid and pepsin, and protective factors, including gastric mucus, bicarbonate, and prostaglandins. Evidence that *H. pylori* plays a principal role in the pathogenesis of peptic ulcer disease is compelling. Indeed, infection with *H. pylori* is associated with a greatly increased risk of duodenal and gastric ulceration: from 95 to 100 percent of patients with DU and 75 to 85 percent of patients with GU (including virtually all cases not associated with NSAIDs) harbor the organism. Nested case-controlled studies in which IgG antibodies to *H. pylori* were measured in stored serum samples have demonstrated that preexisting *H. pylori* infection increases the risk of the subsequent development of either DU or GU; the level of antibody in serum correlates positively with the risk of DU and GU. On the other hand, only 15 to 20 percent of persons infected with *H. pylori* will develop an ulcer in their lifetimes, implying that additional pathogenic factors must be involved.

HELICOBACTER PYLORI *H. pylori* is a short (0.2 to 0.5 μm long), spiral-shaped, microaerophilic gram-negative bacillus which invariably causes chronic active gastritis. With gastric colonization, *H. pylori* is found primarily in the deep portions of the mucus gel layer that coats the gastric mucosa and between the mucus gel layer and the apical surfaces of the gastric mucosal epithelial cells. *H. pylori* may adhere to the luminal surfaces of gastric epithelial cells but does not invade the gastric mucosa.

Pathophysiology *H. pylori* produces a variety of proteins that appear to mediate or facilitate its damaging effects on the gastric mucosa. Urease produced by *H. pylori* catalyzes the hydrolysis of urea to ammonia and carbon dioxide. Production of urease is required for gastric colonization by *H. pylori* and may protect *H. pylori* from

the effects of gastric acid, which normally prevents gastric colonization by other bacteria. Hydroxide ions generated by the equilibration of water with ammonia may contribute to gastric mucosal epithelial damage. *H. pylori* produces surface proteins that are chemotactic for human neutrophils and monocytes and secretes platelet-activating factor, which is also proinflammatory. *H. pylori* activates monocytes which express HLA-DR and interleukin 2 receptors on their cell surface and produce superoxides, interleukin 1, and tumor necrosis factor. The organism also produces proteases and phospholipases, which degrade the glycoprotein-lipid complex of the mucus gel layer. This activity reduces the thickness and viscosity of the mucus gel overlying the gastric mucosal epithelial cells, in spite of increased mucus synthesis and secretion. *H. pylori* produces an adhesin that facilitates its attachment to gastric epithelial cells. Different strains of *H. pylori* are thought to exist, and it has been proposed that only strains that have the cytotoxin-associated gene *cagA* and/or a 120-kDa vacuolating cytotoxin are associated with DU formation. In addition, there is some evidence that the likelihood of DU formation increases with increasing density of *H. pylori* (and hence urease activity) in the antrum.

Epidemiology In the United States, healthy persons under age 30 have prevalence rates of gastric colonization with *H. pylori* of approximately 10 percent. The prevalence of gastric colonization increases with age, with persons over age 60 having colonization rates that are approximately equal to their age. In contrast, in developing countries, *H. pylori* is generally acquired in childhood. Rates of *H. pylori* infection increase with deprived socioeconomic circumstances and also are increased in custodial institutions; they have been reported to be higher in black and Hispanic Americans. Transmission of *H. pylori* appears to be direct, from person to person; fecal-oral, oral-oral, and gastric-oral routes of transmission have been postulated. The risk of *H. pylori* infection is declining in developed countries, as is the risk of peptic ulcer. Most patients with gastric colonization by *H. pylori* never develop ulceration and remain asymptomatic.

Diagnosis *H. pylori* can be identified in gastric mucosal samples by histologic examination, culture, and detection of urease activity (Table 284-1). On stained tissue sections, *H. pylori* is positive for Giemsa and Warthin-Starry stains and faintly positive for hematoxylin. The organisms can be cultured successfully from biopsy samples but usually not from gastric secretions. *H. pylori* produces large amounts of urease. The rapid urease test of gastric biopsy material is a relatively simple and reliable method for presumptive identification of *H. pylori*. A positive test results from an increase in pH, with the phenol red indicator turning from light orange to red. The test is inexpensive, with a sensitivity of at least 90 percent and a specificity approaching 100 percent.

A urea breath test using ^{13}C or ^{14}C also has been developed for identifying *H. pylori* on the basis of urease production with release of labeled CO_2 (Fig. 284-3). This test has a sensitivity of 90 to 95 percent and a specificity of 98 to 99 percent.

Table 284-1

Diagnostic Tests for *Helicobacter pylori*

Test	Sensitivity (%)	Comments
Urease assay		
Breath	90–95	Simple; may be used to monitor therapy
Biopsy	90–98	Requires endoscopy
Histology	70–99	Requires endoscopy; may require special stains
Culture	70–95	Requires endoscopy; may be essential if antibiotic resistance emerges
Serology	95	Does not differentiate between active and remote infection; epidemiologic tool; titer decreases slowly after eradication

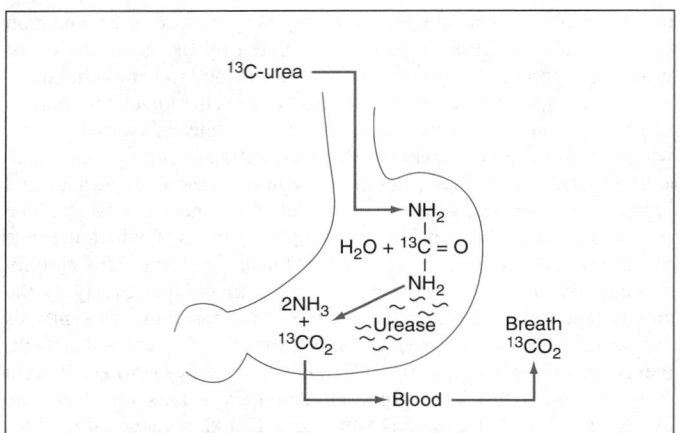

FIGURE 284-3 The urea breath test. Radiolabeled carbon dioxide is detectable in expired air after oral ingestion of radiolabeled urea in the presence of gastric urease produced by *H. pylori*.

Antibodies (IgG and IgA) to *H. pylori* have been identified in sera of individuals with *H. pylori* colonization. Serology is now used widely for routine detection of *H. pylori*. An enzyme-linked immunosorbent assay (ELISA) is the most commonly used serologic method, and a variety of diagnostic kits are available commercially. Compared with endoscopic detection of *H. pylori* infection, the ELISA has proved to be sensitive and specific and is particularly suited for epidemiologic studies. There is a high degree of correlation between the presence of serum antibodies and histologic evidence of gastritis.

Implications of Treatment The most compelling evidence for the role of *H. pylori* in the pathogenesis of peptic ulcer is that the 1-year relapse rate for DUs is less than 15 percent following therapy that successfully eradicates *H. pylori* but 70 to 80 percent after treatment only with H_2 receptor antagonists (see below) (Fig. 284-4). However, it should be emphasized that most persons with *H. pylori* infection never develop symptomatic DU or GU, suggesting that other factors have a role in the pathogenesis of peptic ulceration.

OTHER PATHOGENIC FACTORS It has long been observed that DU patients as a group secrete more acid than normal; however, most individual DU patients have acid secretory rates (BAO and MAO) within the normal range. In response to stimulation of gastric acid secretion, DU patients as a group also have comparable increases in gastric secretion of pepsin and in serum PGI levels. The variations in both groups are so large that most DU patients are in the normal range.

At initiation of infection by *H. pylori*, there may be a transient increase in gastric acid secretion. This phase is often followed by hypochlorhydria lasting for several months, after which rates of acid secretion return within a year to approximately their preinfection levels. Subsequently, *H. pylori* infection may be associated with an increase in basal and meal-stimulated serum gastrin levels, presumably owing to chronic antral inflammation. Somatostatin deficiency has been proposed as the mechanism responsible for enhanced gastrin release in patients with *H. pylori* infection, in whom gastric mucosal somatostatin levels are reduced and are correlated inversely with gastric luminal ammonia. An associated increase in gastric acid secretion (BAO and MAO in response to gastrin) in patients with DU has been attributed to an increase in parietal cell mass caused by the increased gastrin release, but a similar increase in gastric acid secretion is generally not observed in patients infected with *H. pylori* but without a DU, even though gastrin levels may be elevated. Therefore, increased gastric acid secretion in DU patients may be dependent on factors other than *H. pylori* infection. With eradication of *H. pylori*, the serum gastrin level and BAO slowly return to normal, but MAO in response to gastrin may remain mildly elevated.

The stomach tends to empty more rapidly in DU patients than in non-DU patients. This phenomenon, when coupled with relative gastric acid hypersecretion, may contribute to a greater rate of acid delivery to the first part of the duodenum in DU patients. In patients with DU and *H. pylori* infection, acidification of the proximal duodenum results in a smaller secretion of bicarbonate into the lumen by duodenal mucosal cells than in subjects not infected with *H. pylori*. Moreover, acidification of the proximal duodenum may lead to gastric metaplasia of the duodenal mucosa and subsequent colonization by *H. pylori*, which may in turn lead to ulcer formation.

A role for genetic factors in DU is suspected. DUs are approximately three times as common in first-degree relatives of DU patients than in the general population, although this finding may reflect a higher rate of *H. pylori* infection rather than genetic susceptibility. Patients with DUs have an increased frequency of blood group O and of the nonsecretor status [absence of secretion of AB(O) blood group antigens into the gastric juice], but these associations are weak. Moreover, the association with blood group O may relate to preferential binding of group O antigens to *H. pylori*. An increased incidence of HLA-B5 antigen has been reported in white male subjects with DU. Because the MAO in response to gastrin generally does not return to normal after eradication of *H. pylori* in patients with DU, despite return of serum gastrin elevations to normal, it is possible that at least some DU patients have an unusually large parietal cell mass (and hence MAO) on a genetic basis.

Cigarette smoking has been associated with an increased incidence of DU, a decreased response to DU therapy, and an increased mortality rate from DU. Although cigarette smoking does not increase gastric acid secretion, the increased incidence of DU among cigarette smokers may be due to inhibition of pancreatic bicarbonate secretion by nicotine or cigarette smoke, to accelerated emptying of gastric acid into the

FIGURE 284-4 Lifetime recurrence of duodenal ulcers for the year after successful healing with an H-2 receptor antagonist alone or triple therapy plus an H-2 receptor antagonist. No maintenance therapy was given; the recurrence rate of ulcers in patients healed with an H-2 receptor antagonist alone was significantly greater ($p < 0.01$) than in those who received triple therapy plus a histamine-2 receptor antagonist. *(From DY Graham et al., 1992, with permission.)*

duodenum, or to a predisposition to (or association with) *H. pylori* infection.

The incidence of DU appears to be increased in patients with chronic renal failure, alcoholic cirrhosis, renal transplantation, hyperparathyroidism, systemic mastocytosis, and chronic obstructive pulmonary disease. Antibodies to herpes simplex have been reported to be present more often and in higher titers in sera of patients with DU than in normal subjects.

The importance of psychological factors in the pathogenesis of DU remains controversial. Contrary to earlier views, there is no typical DU personality. Chronic anxiety and psychological stress may, however, be factors in exacerbation of ulcer activity.

DU is uncommon before age 15, but GU may develop in children as young as age 5. It has been proposed that DU develops only in persons who acquire *H. pylori* infection at the end of childhood or later, because parietal cell mass is conserved after that point (see below).

CLINICAL FEATURES Epigastric pain is the most frequent DU symptom. The pain is often described as sharp, burning, or gnawing. However, it may be ill-defined, boring, or aching or may be perceived as abdominal pressure or fullness or as a hunger sensation. In approximately 10 percent of patients, the pain is located to the right of the epigastrium. The pain of DU characteristically occurs 90 min to 3 h after eating and frequently awakens the patient at night. It is usually relieved within a few minutes by food or antacids, presumably as a result of partial neutralization of gastric acid. However, ingestion of food leading to transient partial neutralization of gastric acid is followed by a rebound of gastrin release, resulting again in stimulation of acid secretion. With subsequent gastric emptying and increasing gastric acid secretion, the pH in the stomach and first portion of the duodenum becomes low enough to cause recurrent pain. Acid-induced pain in DU patients is believed to be due to acid stimulation of chemical receptors and/or alterations in gastric motility.

Episodes of pain may persist for periods of several days to weeks or months. Although symptoms tend to be recurrent and episodic, DUs often recur in the absence of pain. Periods of remission usually last from weeks to years and are almost always longer than the episodes of pain. However, in some patients the disease is more aggressive, with frequent and persistent symptoms or development of complications.

Changes in the character of ulcer pain may signal the development of complications. For example, ulcer pain that becomes constant, is no longer relieved by food or antacids, or radiates to the back or to either upper quadrant may herald penetration of the ulcer (often posteriorly into the pancreas). Pain associated with DU that is accentuated rather than relieved by food and/or is accompanied by vomiting often indicates gastric outlet obstruction. Abrupt, severe, or generalized abdominal pain is characteristic of free ulcer perforation into the peritoneal cavity. DU may cause acute gastrointestinal (GI) hemorrhage, with vomiting of blood or "coffee grounds" material or with the passage of black, tarry stools or even frankly red blood, if the bleeding is massive. Uncommonly, blood loss with DU is more subtle, with occult blood loss detected by stool examination or by variable degrees of anemia which may be accompanied by iron deficiency. Weight loss, in the absence of some degree of gastric outlet obstruction, is unusual in patients with DU.

It is important to emphasize that many patients with active DU have no ulcer symptoms. This situation leads to a significant underestimation of DU frequency in the population. Prospective studies using upper GI endoscopy suggest that approximately half of DU recurrences are without symptoms. Endoscopic studies also show a lack of good correlation among ulcer activity, symptom resolution, and ulcer healing. The absence of ulcer pain does not exclude DU as a potential cause for acute or chronic GI hemorrhage, gastric outlet obstruction, or ulcer perforation.

On physical examination, epigastric tenderness is the most frequent finding. The area of tenderness is usually in the midline, often midway between the umbilicus and the xiphoid process. In approximately 20 percent of patients, the tender area is to the right of the midline. Acute DU perforation into the peritoneal cavity often produces a rigid, board-like abdomen, usually with generalized rebound tenderness. Ausculta-

tion of the abdomen initially may reveal hyperactive bowel sounds which, with clinical progression, may diminish or disappear. Patients with gastric outlet obstruction caused by a DU or a pyloric channel ulcer may have a succussion splash produced by retained fluid and air in the distended stomach.

The pyloric channel, which is 1 to 2 cm in length, is the narrowest portion of the gastric outlet. Because of their gastric acid secretory characteristics and clinical features, pyloric channel ulcers are classified with DU rather than with GU (Fig. 284-5). Ulcers in this location often produce symptoms similar to those of a DU; however, symptoms tend to be less responsive to food and antacids; food may accentuate rather than relieve ulcer pain and may produce vomiting due to partial gastric outlet obstruction. Surgery has been required more frequently for pyloric channel ulcers than for those in the duodenal bulb.

Nonulcer dyspepsia, also referred to as *essential* or *functional* dyspepsia, is a term used to describe a heterogeneous group of disorders characterized by persistent or recurrent upper abdominal pain or discomfort for which no underlying cause is detected. Although *H. pylori* is the primary cause of gastritis and an essential factor in the pathogenesis of peptic ulcer disease, it has not been proved to have a role in the pathogenesis of nonulcer dyspepsia. The prevalence of *H. pylori* infection in patients with nonulcer dyspepsia (50 percent) is no higher than that of the general population, and there is no convincing evidence that *H. pylori* accounts for the symptoms in these patients. Eradication of *H. pylori* infection with the subsequent resolution of histologic gastritis does not reliably lead to resolution of dyspepsia. Until and unless a clear association between *H. pylori* and nonulcer dyspepsia can be shown, there is no indication to treat such patients for *H. pylori*.

DIAGNOSIS Barium examination of the upper GI tract is of value in identifying DU and is still the most common initial method used to establish the diagnosis. Using conventional single-contrast barium techniques, 70 to 80 percent of DUs found at endoscopy can be identified by x-ray. With double-contrast barium examinations, the detection rate is about 90 percent. On x-ray, the typical DU appears as a discrete crater in the proximal portion of the duodenal bulb (Fig. 284-6). Marked deformity of the duodenal bulb, common in patients with chronic recurrent DU, may make radiographic identification of the ulcer difficult or impossible.

FIGURE 284-5 Barium radiograph of pyloric channel ulcer. *(Courtesy of Gary J. Whitman, M.D., Houston, TX)*

FIGURE 284-6 Barium radiograph of a DU. Note discrete ulcer in duodenal bulb (*arrow*). (*Courtesy of Gary J. Whitman, M.D., Houston, TX*)

Endoscopic examination of the upper GI tract is the most accurate means of diagnosing DU. Endoscopy is not required for this purpose when DU has been identified by barium radiographic examination. However, endoscopy may be of greatest value in (1) detecting DU suspected in the absence of a radiographically demonstrable ulcer, (2) evaluating patients with a radiographic deformity and uncertainty regarding ulcer activity, (3) identifying ulcers too small or too superficial to be recognized by x-ray, and (4) identifying (or excluding) an ulcer as the source of active GI hemorrhage. Endoscopy permits direct visualization and photographic documentation of the ulcer, including its size, shape, and location; permits mucosal biopsy of the antrum for detection of *H. pylori*; and may provide a reference base for assessment of ulcer healing.

In most patients with typical DUs, specific diagnostic testing for *H. pylori* may be unnecessary because the organism can be assumed to be present, as long as there is no recent history of NSAID use, symptoms or signs of a gastric hypersecretory state, or history of recent antibiotic therapy that might have eradicated *H. pylori*. Determination of the serum gastrin level is recommended only in patients for whom surgery is planned or in whom an underlying gastrinoma is suspected (see below). Patients with ulcer-like symptoms but no evidence of ulcer may be considered to have nonulcer dyspepsia.

Controversy exists as to the optimal approach to the patient presenting with chronic dyspepsia (see Chap. 41). Options include an initial trial of symptomatic treatment with an H_2 receptor antagonist, sucralfate, or omeprazole (see below), serologic testing for *H. pylori* and a course of therapy to eradicate the organism if it is present (see below), or immediate endoscopy followed by specific treatment based on the findings. Limited data suggest that early endoscopy gives precise guidance for diagnosis and treatment and reduces the number of patients treated inappropriately. While early endoscopy may be the most costly initial approach, its use may not lead to higher overall costs. In an individual case the approach to diagnosis and management may be influenced by other factors, such as the age and preference of the patient. Moreover, current practice is to limit treatment to eradicate *H. pylori* to patients with confirmed ulcers (see below).

℞ TREATMENT

Traditionally, the major objectives of DU therapy have been relief of pain, acceleration of ulcer healing, and prevention of ulcer recurrence and complications. Conclusions regarding the effectiveness

of therapy were confused by the spontaneous healing of DU (a component of the natural history of the disease), and by imprecise methods used to assess ulcer activity. With the recognition that *H. pylori* plays a central role in the pathogenesis of DU, the objective of therapy now is eradication of *H. pylori* and cure of the disease.

There is general agreement that the only uniformly accepted indication for treating *H. pylori* infection is to prevent recurrent ulcer disease. Although eradication of *H. pylori* was originally reserved for recurrent or complicated ulcers that were unrelated to NSAIDs, a National Institutes of Health Consensus Development Conference Report has advocated routine eradication of *H. pylori* on first presentation of a peptic ulcer. Thus, patients with documented evidence of DU (by upper GI contrast radiography or endoscopy) should be treated for *H. pylori*, regardless of the severity of symptoms or the presence of other risk factors for ulcer disease, such as NSAID use. Treatment may be extended to patients who have a *history* of documented DU and evidence of *H. pylori* infection by serologic or breath test methods. While patients with complicated (e.g., bleeding) ulcers have generally been placed on long-term maintenance therapy with H_2 receptor antagonists to prevent recurrent complications (see below), data are emerging to suggest that maintenance therapy may not be necessary after eradication of *H. pylori*. Recent studies have suggested that rebleeding from recurrent DU is prevented by eradication of *H. pylori*. However, maintenance antisecretory therapy may be continued in patients for whom recurrent bleeding could be especially life-threatening.

Numerous drugs have been evaluated in the treatment of *H. pylori* infection, including bismuth compounds, amoxicillin, tetracycline, clarithromycin, metronidazole, omeprazole, and H_2 receptor antagonists, singly or in various combinations. *No single agent is optimally effective against the organism.* Although *H. pylori* is susceptible in vitro to most antibiotics, in vivo susceptibility cannot be assumed, because of the possibility of poor drug bioavailability, drug resistance, or patient noncompliance. Currently, therapy should consist of the most efficacious combination of agents, designed to maximize the eradication rate but minimize side effects and ensure patient compliance. The therapy of *H. pylori* infection is still evolving, and new drug regimens continue to be evaluated in an attempt to determine the best drug combinations, dosing regimens, and duration of treatment (Table 284-2).

Bismuth compounds have been used for the treatment of peptic ulcer disease for several centuries. The mechanism of action of bismuth is uncertain but may involve cytoprotective effects, including binding of the agent to the ulcer base and the stimulation of mucus and prostaglandin production. In addition, bismuth is thought to exert an antibacterial effect through inhibition of proteolytic, lipolytic, and urease enzyme activities. When used as monotherapy, bismuth compounds result in eradication of *H. pylori* in only 20 percent of patients, but when used in combination with antibiotics, they are associated with eradication in up to 95 percent of patients with documented *H. pylori* infection.

Currently, the most successful therapy for *H. pylori* infection is so-called triple therapy, which consists of a bismuth compound, metronidazole, and either amoxicillin or tetracycline. The most widely used and most effective regimen is a 2-week course of bismuth [usually a preparation such as bismuth subsalicylate (PeptoBismol)] at a dosage of two tablets qid together with metronidazole (250, 400, or 500 mg tid or qid) and tetracycline (500 mg qid); this regimen leads to eradication of *H. pylori* in about 90 percent of cases. Although tetracycline may be replaced with oral amoxicillin (500 mg qid), this change slightly increases the cost and slightly decreases the efficacy. Some studies suggest that a 1-week course of triple therapy may be as effective as a 2-week course.

Triple therapy for 2 weeks in combination with administration of an H_2 receptor antagonist for 6 weeks improves the ulcer healing rate slightly compared with use of an H_2 receptor antagonist alone and reduces the rate of ulcer recurrence to less than 15 percent at 1 year (compared to 60 to 100 percent after conventional antisecretory therapy). Although the requirement for gastric acid suppression in addition to therapy aimed at eradicating *H. pylori* has been questioned, the addition of omeprazole to a triple drug regimen appears to increase the rate of *H. pylori* eradication to about 98 percent. The precise role of gastric acid suppression as an essential component of the therapeutic regimen for *H. pylori* remains to be defined, but such therapy does contribute to the relief of symptoms in patients with DU.

Although triple therapy is the most effective and least expensive regimen, it has some drawbacks. Patient compliance is one of the important factors. A typical 2-week treatment requires that a patient ingest a total of approximately 200 tablets and take medication four times daily. Troublesome side effects occur in 20 to 30 percent of patients. Bismuth may cause darkening of the tongue and stool and lead to constipation. Amoxicillin may cause antibiotic-associated diarrhea, including pseudomembranous colitis, and may be associated with nausea, vomiting, skin rash, and allergic reactions. Tetracycline has been associated with skin rash and, rarely, anaphylaxis and hepatotoxicity. Potential adverse effects of long-term metronidazole use include paresthesias and, rarely, seizures, and those of short-term use include nausea, vomiting, diarrhea, and an altered taste sensation. In addition, patients must be cautioned to abstain from alcohol while taking metronidazole to avoid a disulfiram-like reaction.

Resistance to metronidazole is also a potentially significant problem in the treatment of *H. pylori* and has been found in about 30 percent of isolates from North America. The treatment of metronidazole-resistant strains of *H. pylori* with triple therapy does not necessarily result in failure of eradication. In fact, triple therapy has been reported to result in eradication of *H. pylori* in 91 percent of patients infected with a metronidazole-susceptible strain and 63 percent of those infected with a metronidazole-resistant strain.

Owing to the limitations of triple therapy, alternative regimens may be used. Dual therapy with amoxicillin (500 mg qid) and omeprazole (20 mg bid) for 2 weeks is associated with fewer side effects and improved compliance. However, this regimen may yield an eradication rate for *H. pylori* of only 36 to 60 percent, and the use of higher doses of omeprazole (40 mg bid or tid) and amoxicillin (750 mg tid) does not reliably increase the eradication rate.

Clarithromycin, a newer macrolide antimicrobial, may be used in place of metronidazole in a dose of 250 mg four times daily and, as part of a triple regimen, has resulted in a 90 percent eradication rate. Similar eradication rates have been achieved when clarithromycin is used in a dose of 500 mg three times daily in combination with omeprazole, 40 mg a day or 20 mg twice daily. Eradication rates of about 85 percent have been reported for a regimen of clarithromycin and the combination drug ranitidine bismuth citrate (RBC). There is much interest in simpler triple regimens of omeprazole (or lansoprazole), clarithromycin, and either metronidazole or amoxicillin given twice daily for 1 week (see Table 284-2). Combination therapy using clarithromycin is well-tolerated and may be especially useful

in patients who are infected with metronidazole-resistant *H. pylori*, are allergic to penicillin, or have difficulty with compliance. However, resistance to clarithromycin may develop, and regimens that include omeprazole or clarithromycin are substantially more expensive than standard triple therapy.

Until now, confirmation that *H. pylori* has been eradicated has required repeat endoscopy with gastric mucosal biopsy and has generally been reserved for patients with complicated ulcer disease (e.g., bleeding). Serologic testing is unreliable for this purpose, because antibody levels generally decline slowly after successful therapy and often do not decline to zero. When eradication of *H. pylori* is demonstrated at least 1 month after the completion of treatment, subsequent reinfection is uncommon, with a frequency as low as 1 percent per year in Western countries. The availability of urea breath tests should make confirmation of *H. pylori* eradication simpler and less expensive.

Regardless of the treatment regimen used, it is becoming clear that eradication of *H. pylori* is the most cost-effective method of managing DU. In the past, drugs that neutralized or reduced secretion of gastric acid were the mainstays of DU therapy. With the advent

Table 284-2

Drugs Used in the Treatment of Peptic Ulcer

Drug and Mechanism	Dose	Side Effects
"Triple therapy": eradication of *H. pylori*	Bismuth subsalicylate 2 tabs qid, amoxicillin 500 mg qid or tetracycline 500 mg tid, plus metronidazole 250 mg tid. Treat for 2 weeks (combine with H_2 receptor antagonist or proton pump inhibitor)	Cumbersome; diarrhea, pseudomembranous colitis
"Dual therapy": eradication of *H. pylori* (plus proton pump inhibition)	Omeprazole 40 mg/d in the morning plus clarithromycin 500 mg tid. Treat for 2 weeks.	As for omeprazole and triple therapy, but frequency of side effects lower and cost greater
"New triple therapy": eradication of *H. pylori* (plus proton pump inhibition)	Omeprazole 20 mg bid plus either clarithromycin 250 mg bid and metronidazole 500 mg bid *or* clarithromycin 500 mg bid and amoxicillin 1 g bid. Treat for one week	Frequency of side effects lower than for standard triple therapy but cost greater
Ranitidine bismuth citrate plus antibiotic: eradication of *H. pylori*	Ranitidine bismuth citrate 400 mg bid for 4 weeks plus clarithromycin 500 mg tid for first 2 weeks	Taste disturbance and diarrhea most common
Cimetidine: H_2 receptor blockade	300 mg qid or 400 mg bid or 800 mg at bedtime	Uncommon: antiandrogen (high doses), ↑ creatinine, ↓ hepatic drug metabolism, ↑ serum aminotransferase levels, rare blood dyscrasias
Ranitidine: H_2 receptor blockade	150 mg bid or 300 mg at bedtime	As for cimetidine but antiandrogen and drug metabolism effects are less frequent; rare cases of hepatitis
Famotidine: H_2 receptor blockade	40 mg at bedtime	As for ranitidine
Nizatidine: H_2 receptor blockade	300 mg at bedtime	Probably as for ranitidine
Misoprostol: raises prostaglandin levels (enhances mucosal defense, reduces gastric acid secretion)	200 mg qid for prevention of NSAID-induced ulcers	Diarrhea, uterine contraction (do not use in women of childbearing age)
Sucralfate: coats ulcers, binds pepsin	1 g 1 h before meals and at bedtime or 2 g bid	Constipation, binding to coadministered drugs
Omeprazole: inhibits H^+, K^+-ATPase (proton pump) on gastric parietal cell	20 mg/d in the morning	↓ Hepatic drug metabolism; prolonged use in high doses in rats causes gastric carcinoids
Lansoprazole: proton pump inhibitor	30 mg/d in the morning	As for omeprazole
Antacids: acid neutralization	140 mmol 1 h and 3 h after eating and at bedtime (e.g., 30 mL Maalox); lower doses (15 mL after eating and at bedtime) appear to be as effective	Diarrhea (Mg), constipation (Al), osteomalacia, milk-alkali syndrome (elevated serum Ca, P, BUN, creatinine, HCO_3; due to $CaCO_3$)

of therapy aimed at eradicating *H. pylori*, these drugs are now used in an adjunctive role or for symptomatic relief of DUs. In addition, they still form the mainstay of therapy for gastroesophageal reflux disease (see Chap. 283).

Antacids Although antacids have been used for decades to treat DU, only in the past 20 years has their effectiveness in accelerating DU healing been verified. They are now generally used on an as-needed basis for symptomatic relief in ulcer patients. The most widely used antacid preparations are mixtures of aluminum hydroxide and magnesium hydroxide that neutralize HCl. Complications of aluminum hydroxide treatment include constipation and systemic phosphate depletion, which can result in weakness, malaise, and anorexia in patients with phosphate-poor diets (e.g., dietary deficiency accompanying chronic alcoholism or other states of reduced dietary protein intake). Magnesium hydroxide may produce loose stools. This laxative effect and the constipating effects of aluminum hydroxide can be overcome by using antacids that contain these agents in combination. Ionic magnesium stimulates gastrin release, leading to increased gastric acid secretion ("acid rebound"). Magnesium trisilicate, which is included in various antacid mixtures, is a slow-acting weak antacid.

Calcium carbonate is a potent and inexpensive antacid that is converted to calcium chloride in the stomach. Approximately 10 percent of the ingested calcium is absorbed. Like magnesium hydroxide, calcium carbonate ingestion is associated with acid rebound. Chronic excessive calcium carbonate administration may be associated with the milk-alkali syndrome, producing elevations of serum calcium, phosphate, urea nitrogen, creatinine, and bicarbonate levels and resulting in renal calcinosis and possibly progressive renal insufficiency. Sodium bicarbonate is a potent and rapidly acting antacid, but it has a tendency to induce systemic alkalosis.

H_2 Receptor Antagonists H_2 receptor antagonists are potent inhibitors of basal (unstimulated) and stimulated gastric acid secretion. H_2 receptor antagonists exhibit some structural similarities to histamine and to each other, with variations in ring structures and side chains (Fig. 284-7). Until recently, H_2 receptor antagonists were

the preferred drugs in the treatment of peptic ulcer because of their safety and effectiveness in accelerating healing. Healing rates for treatment with H_2 receptor antagonists are similar to those for antacid treatment, but compliance appears to be better. Until recently, a daily maintenance dose of H_2 receptor antagonists (one-half the standard dose) was often used to reduce DU recurrence, with a reduction of 1-year recurrence rates by 50 to 70 percent after initial ulcer healing. H_2 receptor antagonists are now often used for 4 to 6 weeks in combination with triple therapy against *H. pylori*, as discussed above.

Cimetidine was the first H_2 receptor antagonist developed. At 300 mg, it inhibits basal acid secretion by more than 80 percent and meal-stimulated acid secretion by approximately 70 percent. It strikingly reduces acid secretory responses to histamine, caffeine, hypoglycemia, and gastrin. Initially, the oral dose of cimetidine recommended and used in treatment of DU was 300 mg four times daily, with meals and at bedtime. A dose of 400 mg twice daily (morning and bedtime) or 800 mg once daily (at bedtime) is also effective in the treatment of DU.

Few serious adverse effects have been experienced with cimetidine. Slight and reversible increases in serum aminotransferase and creatinine levels and brief increases in serum prolactin may occur after intravenous and oral use. Cimetidine has been shown to inhibit some cytochrome P450 hepatic microsomal enzyme systems and therefore may increase the blood level, duration of action, and pharmacologic effects of drugs metabolized by those systems. Tender gynecomastia due to the weak antiandrogenic effect of cimetidine has been reported in patients with ZES who required and were treated with extremely large doses for months to years. Although reversible confusional states have been attributed to cimetidine in a small number of severely ill patients with preexisting hepatic and/or renal functional impairment, a causative effect has not been proven.

Ranitidine is about six times as potent as cimetidine in inhibiting gastric acid secretion. Both drugs have similar half-lives, approximately 1.5 to 2 h. In the past, the recommended dose of ranitidine for treatment of DU was 150 mg twice a day, but 300 mg at bedtime is equally effective. Ranitidine may increase levels of serum asparate aminotransferase and alanine aminotransferase. There have been occasional reports of reversible hepatitis with ranitidine administration. This drug appears to have no antiandrogen properties and has a smaller inhibitory effect on cytochrome P450 mixed oxygenase enzyme systems than does cimetidine.

Famotidine and *nizatidine* are two other potent H_2 receptor antagonists. The recommended daily dose of famotidine in the treatment of DU is 40 mg once daily at bedtime, while that for nizatidine is 300 mg at bedtime. Associated blood dyscrasias have been noted rarely, and hepatotoxicity, similar to that with ranitidine and cimetidine, also has been reported.

Anticholinergic Agents Anticholinergic agents, such as atropine, were used in the past to block parietal cell muscarinic acetylcholine receptors and thereby decrease gastric acid secretion. However, they were not as effective as H_2 receptor antagonists and were associated with a variety of side effects, including dryness of the mouth, blurring of vision, cardiac arrhythmias, and urinary retention. *Pirenzepine*, a relatively selective anticholinergic agent, is more specific in inhibiting gastric acid secretion and has fewer side effects than other anticholinergic agents but is not available in the United States and is unlikely to find a role in ulcer treatment.

Coating Agents Several drugs that act neither by neutralization of gastric acid nor by inhibition of its secretion have been used in the treatment of DU. Among these is *sucralfate*, a complex polyaluminum hydroxide salt of sucrose sulfate (Fig. 284-8). Sucralfate becomes highly polar at acid pH and binds to the ulcer bed for up to 12 h, whereas relatively little of it binds to intact gastric or duodenal mucosa. It is believed that the adherence of sucralfate to granulation tissue impedes diffusion of H^+ to the base of the ulcer. In addition, sucralfate binds bile acids and pepsins and may therefore reduce their injurious effects. Sucralfate may increase the level of endogenous tissue prostaglandins and may bind epidermal growth factors

FIGURE 284-7 Chemical structures of H_2 receptor antagonists.

and other growth factors and present them to the ulcer, thereby increasing mucosal defense. It is only minimally absorbed, with less than 5 percent appearing in the urine. Sucralfate is similar to antacids and H₂ receptor antagonists in its effectiveness in the treatment of DU and in prevention of DU recurrence. The recommended dose of sucralfate is 1 g 1 h before each meal and at bedtime.

Colloidal bismuth compounds also aid ulcer healing by forming (in an acid medium) a bismuth-protein coagulant which is believed to protect the ulcer from acid and pepsin digestion. Colloidal bismuth compounds have little acid-neutralizing effect and do not reduce gastric acid secretion. These compounds inhibit pepsin activity, bind to the gastric mucus gel layer, and may prevent diffusion of hydrogen ions. They stimulate gastric mucosal secretion of prostaglandins, bicarbonate, and glycoprotein mucus. As discussed above, the principal role of bismuth-containing compounds in the treatment of DU relates to their effects on *H. pylori*. Colloidal bismuth compounds are the only class of antiulcer drugs that eradicate *H. pylori* and cure the gastritis associated with its colonization (see below).

Prostaglandins A variety of prostaglandins, particularly those of the E series (PGE₁ and PGE₂), have been shown to be effective in clinical trials in the treatment of DU. They reduce basal and stimulated gastric acid secretion and appear to enhance mucosal resistance to tissue injury. In low doses, exogenous PGEs exert the following actions important in enhancing mucosal defense: they (1) stimulate gastric mucus secretion, (2) stimulate gastric and duodenal bicarbonate secretion, (3) maintain or increase gastric mucosal blood flow, (4) maintain the gastric mucosal barrier to diffusion of H⁺, and (5) stimulate mucosal cell replacement. Because of side effects (diarrhea, uterine contraction) and the availability of other therapies, prostaglandins generally have not been used to treat DU. In the United States, misoprostol, a PGE₁ analogue, has been approved for use only for preventing ulcers caused by NSAIDs (see below).

Proton Pump Inhibitors The final step of hydrogen ion secretion by parietal cells is accomplished by H⁺,K⁺-ATPase, a proton pump that exchanges hydrogen for potassium. The H⁺,K⁺-ATPase is located in the apical membrane and tubulovesicular apparatus of parietal cells. The luminal surface of the transmembrane enzyme is exposed to the gastric luminal acid. Omeprazole and lansoprazole, specific inhibitors of this H⁺,K⁺-ATPase, are extraordinarily potent in decreasing gastric acid secretion (Fig. 284-9). These are substituted benzimidazoles that bind to the proton pump and irreversibly inactivate it. Both omeprazole and lansoprazole produce prolonged inhibition of all phases of gastric acid secretion, with acid secretory recovery requiring synthesis of new enzyme. The maximum effect of omeprazole occurs within 2 h; 50 percent of the maximum inhibition remains at 24 h; and inhibition persists for up to 72 h. With once-daily dosing, a plateau is reached after 4 days, and after discontinuation, gastric acid secretory activity returns gradually to normal over 3 to 5 days.

Omeprazole and lansoprazole are approved for treatment of DU, erosive esophagitis, and gastric acid hypersecretory states, including ZES. For DU, these drugs are used in conjunction with triple therapy or with antibiotics such as amoxicillin and/or clarithromycin, as discussed above. The standard dose of omeprazole is 20 mg daily and that for lansoprazole is 30 mg daily in the morning before

FIGURE 284-9 Chemical structures of omeprazole and lansoprazole.

breakfast for periods of 4 to 8 weeks. These drugs cause a small to moderate increase in serum gastrin because of their effect on gastric acidity. Serum gastrin levels return to normal within 2 weeks after drug discontinuance. Hypergastrinemia-induced hyperplasia of gastric mucosal ECL cells and carcinoid tumors, which were noted in rats receiving omeprazole, have not been documented in humans.

DIET In the past, many different diet programs were used for treatment of patients with DU. There is no evidence that bland diets reduce gastric acid secretion or promote healing, although they may relieve symptoms of DU. Similarly, soft diets or diets free of spices or fruit juices have not been proved beneficial. Although traditionally milk and cream were prescribed for ulcer patients, there is no evidence that they promote ulcer healing. They actually stimulate gastric acid secretion, contribute to the development of the milk-alkali syndrome, and probably accelerate atherogenesis. Many physicians recommend that patients with DU avoid coffee, with or without caffeine, and other caffeine-containing beverages because of their effects on gastric secretion. It also may be desirable to restrict alcohol intake in these patients. It is reasonable to suggest that patients avoid foods that exacerbate their symptoms.

GASTRIC ULCER

The incidence of GU peaks in the sixth decade, approximately 10 years later than for DU. Slightly more than half of GUs occur in males. The precise incidence of GU is not known, since many GUs are asymptomatic. Although DU is identified clinically more frequently than GU, most autopsy studies show an equal or greater proportion of GUs.

GUs are deep, penetrating beyond the mucosa of the stomach, and are similar histologically to DUs, but usually with more extensive gastritis surrounding the ulcer. Almost all benign GUs are found immediately distal to the junction of the antral mucosa and the acid-secreting mucosa of the body of the stomach. The location of this junction is variable. In general, antral mucosa extends approximately two-thirds of the way up the lesser curvature and one-third of the way up the greater curvature of the stomach.

Benign GUs are rare in the fundus of the stomach. Benign GUs are virtually always accompanied by antral gastritis as a result of *H. pylori* infection, with variable amounts of mucosal atrophy. When GU is associated with aspirin and other NSAIDs, gastritis is often absent.

ETIOLOGY AND PATHOGENESIS As for DU, acid and pepsin are important in the pathogenesis of GU. In contrast to DU patients, GU patients as a group have acid secretion rates that are normal or reduced compared with nonulcer subjects, although true achlorhydria (in response to pentagastrin stimulation) almost never occurs with benign GU. About 10 percent of patients with GUs also

FIGURE 284-8 Chemical structure of sucralfate.

have a DU. Patients with both a DU and a GU tend to have acid secretory patterns that parallel those of DU.

Compelling evidence supports the primary importance of *H. pylori* in the pathogenesis of GU. Why some persons infected with *H. pylori* develop DU and others develop GU (in the absence of NSAID use) is not clear. It has been proposed that persons with GU, which can occur in children as young as age 5, acquire *H. pylori* infection earlier in life than do those with DU. Infection at a young age is more likely to result in chronic or atrophic gastritis (see below), with a subsequent decrease in gastric acid secretion and therefore a lower risk of DU but a higher risk of GU and gastric cancer. Serum gastrin levels are slightly higher than normal in a significant proportion of GU patients, reflecting gastric acid hyposecretion.

Gastric emptying is delayed in GU. Regurgitation of duodenal contents may contribute to gastric mucosal injury and subsequent GU by causing interruption of the gastric mucosal barrier with resulting diffusion of secreted hydrogen ions to the mucosa. NSAIDs are responsible for 15 to 25 percent of GUs, as is discussed below.

CLINICAL FEATURES As with DU, epigastric pain is the most common symptom, but the pattern is less characteristic. The pain may be precipitated or accentuated by food, and symptom relief with food or antacids is less consistent than with DU. Whereas in DU patients, nausea and vomiting almost always indicate gastric outlet obstruction, in patients with GU they may occur in the absence of mechanical obstruction. Weight loss may occur, due to anorexia or aversion to food developing from the discomfort produced by eating. GUs tend to heal but then recur, often in the same location.

Hemorrhage is a common complication of GU, occurring in approximately 25 percent of patients; gastric perforation is less common. The mortality rate with GU perforation is approximately three times that with DU perforation, owing partly to the greater average age of GU patients, the usually longer delay in diagnosis, and the greater soilage of the peritoneum with GU perforation. Gastric outlet obstruction may complicate GU in the distal antrum.

DIAGNOSIS While the history is of value in suggesting GU, it is not as characteristic as in DU. The two methods used for diagnosis are barium examination and endoscopy. GU usually can be identified by barium examination, although NSAID-associated GUs are frequently more superficial and are less often identified radiographically. Both benign GUs and malignant ulcers are more common on the lesser than on the greater curvature (Fig. 284-10). Radiation of gastric mucosal folds from the margin of the ulcer crater suggests a benign lesion. Large ulcers—i.e., those greater than 3 cm in diameter—are more often malignant than smaller ones. An ulcer within a mass, as defined radiographically, also suggests malignancy. From 1 to 8 percent of GUs that appear benign radiographically prove to be malignant (by endoscopic biopsy or at surgery). Because of false-positive and false-negative errors, radiographic appearance cannot be used as the sole criterion for judging the benign or malignant nature of an ulcer in the stomach.

Endoscopic visualization of the ulcer allows definition of its size, location, and, by biopsy, its histologic characteristics. To exclude malignancy at gastroscopy, a total of at least six biopsy samples are obtained from the inner margin of the ulcer. Brushings of the ulcer for cytology should be obtained prior to biopsy. The combination of radiographic, endoscopic, and histologic techniques makes it possible to distinguish malignant from benign ulcers with more than 97 percent confidence.

Gastric ulcer with pentagastrin-fast achlorhydria is rare. When it occurs, it almost always indicates gastric carcinoma. However, most patients with gastric carcinoma are capable of secreting gastric acid, although usually less than normal.

It is important in patients with GU to determine whether *H. pylori* is present, because the organism should be eradicated. Identification of *H. pylori* can be done by a rapid urease test on an antral mucosal biopsy specimen or histology preparation when endoscopy is the

method used to diagnose the ulcer or by serology or urea breath testing (where available) when radiography is the method used. When GU is associated with *H. pylori* infection, treatment aimed at eradicating *H. pylori* is indicated, even if the GU occurs in the setting of NSAID use (see below).

℞ TREATMENT

On the basis of preliminary studies, it appears that GUs associated with *H. pylori* infection should be treated with triple therapy combined with an acid-suppressive agent, as for DU. In general, whatever the medical treatment modality selected, GUs tend to heal more slowly than DUs, and larger GUs take longer to heal than smaller ones. Although GU patients have normal or reduced gastric acid secretion, acid-inhibiting agents have been effective in promoting the acute healing of GUs, and GUs heal more rapidly with omeprazole than with H_2 receptor antagonists.

Since salicylates and other NSAIDs are associated with the development of GU, these agents should be discontinued if in use. Milk and cream, as well as bland or homogenized diets, have not been shown to be of value in treatment. In general, it is probably sufficient to recommend that patients consume a diet of their own choice. As in the case of DU, patients should be advised to avoid coffee (caffeine-containing or caffeine-free), other caffeine-containing beverages, and alcohol.

Carbenoxolone has been used in many countries (although it is not available in the United States) in GU treatment. This drug, a hydrolytic product of glycyrrhizic acid (derived from licorice), has been shown to decrease symptoms and increase the rate of GU healing. It does not decrease gastric acid secretion, but rather increases the life span of gastric mucosal epithelial cells as well as the secretion and viscosity of gastric mucus. Carbenoxolone possesses aldosterone-like effects, producing sodium and water retention. Its side effects and the availability of effective alternatives have led to its decreased use.

Benign GUs should heal completely within 2 to 3 months of the start of therapy. The failure of a GU to decrease satisfactorily in size and to heal with medical treatment has been taken as a sign of malignancy. Therefore, it may be reasonable, at least in selected cases, to monitor GU healing by a repeat gastroscopy after treatment, to check for healing of apparently benign GUs. If the ulcer is not healed, malignancy must be suspected, and exfoliative cytology samples and biopsy specimens of the ulcer should be obtained. Apparently complete healing with potent acid-suppressive therapy

FIGURE 284-10 Barium radiograph of a benign GU. (*Courtesy of Gary J. Whitman, M.D., Houston, TX*)

does not guarantee the benign nature of a GU, since approximately 70 percent of ulcers that are eventually found to be malignant undergo significant (albeit usually incomplete) healing with such treatment.

COMPLICATIONS AND SURGERY FOR PEPTIC ULCER

Complications of ulcers include hemorrhage, obstruction, and perforation. Hemorrhage occurs in approximately 15 to 25 percent of patients with DUs; a recurrence of bleeding is estimated to occur in about 40 percent of patients with an initial hemorrhage if *H. pylori* eradication is not part of the treatment regimen or if maintenance therapy with an H₂ receptor antagonist is not prescribed. Hemorrhage related to an NSAID-associated ulcer occurs particularly frequently in the absence of prior peptic ulcer symptoms (approximately 50 percent of cases). In most patients, hemorrhage from a peptic ulcer is self-limited (see Chap. 44). In some cases, endoscopic intervention (use of a heater probe or bipolar electrocautery, laser photocoagulation, or injection of a vasoconstrictor or sclerosing agent) is needed to stop active bleeding or prevent recurrent bleeding in patients with ulcer characteristics, such as a *visible vessel*, that connote a high risk of rebleeding.

Free perforation into the peritoneal cavity occurs in approximately 2 to 3 percent of patients with DU. Of these patients, 5 to 10 percent will have had no recognizable prior ulcer symptoms. Simultaneous hemorrhage occurs in approximately 10 percent of patients with DU perforation; mortality is greatly increased in this group. DUs, especially those located posteriorly, may penetrate into adjacent structures, most often the pancreas, frequently resulting in modestly increased serum amylase levels. Less commonly, DUs penetrate into the liver, biliary tract, or colon.

Gastric outlet obstruction occurs in 2 to 4 percent of patients admitted to the hospital with duodenal or pyloric channel ulcers. Symptoms include abdominal bloating, nausea, vomiting, and weight loss. These patients usually have had ulcer symptoms for many years and, often, obstructive symptoms for several months.

℞ **TREATMENT**

For Duodenal Ulcer With the advent of curative therapy for ulcers associated with *H. pylori* infection as well as nonsurgical methods to arrest ulcer bleeding, the need for ulcer surgery has declined considerably. However, some patients will continue to need surgery for complicated ulcer disease, and there are many patients who have had ulcer surgery in the past. Therefore, there is a need for familiarity with the techniques and complications of ulcer surgery.

No single surgical procedure has been accepted universally as the most satisfactory DU operation. The most commonly performed surgical procedures are vagotomy with antrectomy, vagotomy with pyloroplasty, and proximal gastric vagotomy (also referred to as parietal cell or highly selective vagotomy) without a gastric drainage procedure (Table 284-3).

With truncal vagotomy and antrectomy, the vagal trunks are transected, the antrum is removed, and GI continuity is reestablished by anastomosis of the remaining stomach with the proximal duodenum (Billroth I anastomosis) or with a loop of jejunum (Billroth II anastomosis) (Fig. 284-11). Vagotomy with antrectomy has been an effective procedure with a low recurrence rate (approximately 1

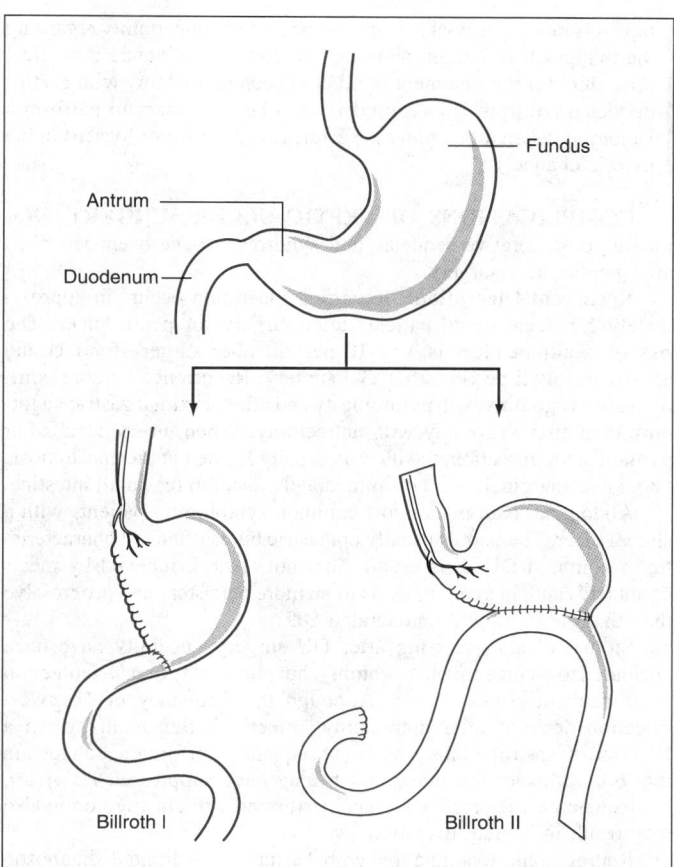

FIGURE 284-11 Diagram of Billroth I and II procedures.

percent), but morbidity and mortality rates have been slightly greater than with vagotomy with pyloroplasty and vary with patient selection and the skill of the surgeon.

With vagotomy and pyloroplasty, vagotomy is performed to inhibit vagal stimulation of gastric acid secretion, and a pyloroplasty is performed to facilitate gastric drainage after truncal or selective vagotomy. Three types of vagotomy have been used in the surgical treatment of duodenal or pyloric channel ulcer: truncal vagotomy, selective vagotomy, and proximal gastric vagotomy. Pyloroplasty with truncal vagotomy has been associated with a mortality rate of approximately 1 percent. Ulcer recurrence during the 5 years after surgery has been about 5 to 8 percent. With selective vagotomy, only the branches of the vagus that supply the stomach are transected, leaving intact the vagal innervation of other abdominal viscera. Selective vagotomy has been found by some surgeons to result in a more complete vagotomy, less ulcer recurrence, and fewer postvagotomy complications than truncal vagotomy. Proximal gastric vagotomy denervates only the acid-secreting portion of the stomach, sparing the branches of the vagus that innervate the antrum, which makes a gastric drainage procedure (e.g., pyloroplasty) unnecessary. Both immediate and late postoperative complications have been less common with proximal gastric vagotomy than with truncal vagotomy, and reductions in acid secretion are similar to those achieved with truncal or selective vagotomy. Mortality with proximal gastric vagotomy is less than 1 percent. With experience, recurrence has been comparable to that with vagotomy and pyloroplasty.

For Gastric Ulcer In the past, surgical treatment was required for GU patients who did not respond satisfactorily to medical therapy or who developed complications similar to those described for DU. With the current diagnostic accuracy of careful radiographic examination, endoscopy, biopsy of the ulcer margins, and exfoliative cytol-

Table 284-3

Principal Operations for Peptic Ulcer

Operation	Recurrence Rate, %	Complication Rate
Vagotomy + antrectomy (Billroth I or II)*	1	Highest
Vagotomy and pyloroplasty	10	Intermediate
Proximal gastric vagotomy	≥10	Lowest

* Billroth I, gastroduodenostomy; Billroth II, gastrojejunostomy.

ogy, it is rarely necessary to operate because of uncertainty regarding the malignant or benign nature of the ulcer. The standard surgical procedure for the treatment of GU has been antrectomy with gastroduodenal (Billroth I) anastomosis. It is not necessary to perform a vagotomy when antrectomy is performed for GU (not located in the pyloric channel).

COMPLICATIONS OF PEPTIC ULCER SURGERY Numerous postoperative sequelae and syndromes have been described after peptic ulcer surgery.

Recurrent Ulceration Recurrent ulceration occurs in approximately 5 percent of all patients after surgery for peptic ulcer. The risk of recurrent ulcer is 3 to 10 percent after surgery for DU and approximately 2 percent after GU surgery. Recurrence is more common after vagotomy with pyloroplasty and after proximal gastric vagotomy than after vagotomy with antrectomy. When ulcers occur after partial gastric resection, the ulcer is usually located at the anastomosis (stomal or marginal ulcer) or immediately distal in the small intestine.

Abdominal pain is the most common symptom in patients with a stomal ulcer. The pain is usually epigastric but is often not characteristic of common DU. It is usually, but not always, relieved by meals or antacids and, in general, tends to be more persistent and progressive than that observed with unoperated DU.

Stomal ulcers occurring after DU surgery generally have been attributed to an incomplete vagotomy, but persistent *H. pylori* infection is probably a critical factor. Although the frequency of *H. pylori* infection declines after antrectomy, infection often recurs when a Roux-en-Y gastrojejunostomy is subsequently performed, suggesting that bile refluxed into the stomach may have suppressed *H. pylori*. Inadequate gastric resection, when performed without vagotomy, also may result in stomal ulceration.

Radiographic examination with barium is of limited diagnostic value and identifies only 50 to 60 percent of stomal ulcerations. Surgical deformity at the anastomotic site often may either mimic or conceal a stomal ulcer. When stomal ulceration is suspected, endoscopic examination is required to identify it. H_2 receptor antagonists and proton pump inhibitors have been reported to induce healing of stomal ulcers, although the long-term effectiveness of these agents in promoting healing of stomal ulcers and preventing their recurrence is uncertain. Transthoracic vagotomy may be effective when recurrent ulcer results from an incomplete vagotomy. Whether eradication of *H. pylori* should play a role in the treatment of stomal ulcers is uncertain.

Recurrent Ulcer due to Retained Antrum In a small number of patients who undergo antrectomy with gastrojejunostomy (Billroth II anastomosis), the antral resection is not complete, and residual distal antrum remains in continuity with the duodenum. These patients usually develop or continue to have gastric acid hypersecretion due to gastrin release by the residual antral mucosa, which is no longer in contact with gastric acid, the normal inhibitor of gastrin release. Fasting serum gastrin levels in these patients may be normal to moderately increased. Patients with retained antrum can be distinguished from those with gastrinoma by intravenous injection of secretin and measurements of serum gastrin levels. Gastrinoma patients exhibit substantial increases in serum gastrin (an increase of >200 ng/L), whereas those with retained antrum exhibit decreased, unchanged, or only slightly increased serum gastrin levels. The diagnosis of retained antrum may be suggested by a careful review of the original operative report or surgical pathology slides. In addition, endoscopy with biopsy of the anastomosis may disclose antral mucosa. These patients improve with removal of the remaining antrum.

Afferent Loop Syndromes Patients who have undergone partial gastric resection and gastrojejunostomy (Billroth II anastomosis) may experience abdominal bloating and pain 20 min to 1 h after eating, frequently followed by nausea and vomiting. The vomitus often contains large amounts of bile. Characteristically, the bloating and abdominal discomfort are relieved by vomiting. This type of afferent loop

syndrome, which is uncommon, is believed to be caused by distention of an incompletely draining afferent intestinal loop by pancreatic and biliary secretions, which are stimulated by eating. Serum amylase levels may be mildly or moderately increased. Because of partial obstruction, it is often difficult to demonstrate the afferent loop by barium meal examination. Treatment is surgical correction of the incomplete afferent loop obstruction and, in some instances, revision to a gastroduodenal anastomosis.

A second form of afferent loop dysfunction is that due to stasis with bacterial overgrowth in the afferent loop. These patients may exhibit the same characteristics as those found with other forms of small intestinal bacterial overgrowth or blind loop syndromes (see Chap. 285), such as malabsorption, especially of fat and vitamin B_{12}. The syndrome can be corrected by surgical revision of the afferent loop.

Bile Reflux Gastropathy After peptic ulcer surgery, a small proportion of patients experience early satiety, abdominal discomfort, and vomiting, which is believed to be due to reflux of duodenal contents into the stomach. Endoscopic examination usually reveals regurgitated bile in the stomach and mucosal hyperemia, often involving the entire gastric remnant. Histologically, there is epithelial cell and foveolar injury with minimal inflammation. This entity has been referred to as alkaline reflux gastropathy, bile reflux gastropathy, duodenogastric reflux, and bilious vomiting. The substances in the refluxed intestinal contents that account for these symptoms have not been defined. Despite the term *bile reflux gastropathy*, there is no certainty that regurgitated bile is responsible for the syndrome. Administration of cholestyramine, intended to bind bile acids and facilitate their excretion, has not been proved of benefit in this disorder. In some cases, symptoms improve with administration of a gastric prokinetic agent such as cisapride, 10 to 20 mg before meals and at bedtime. Surgical diversion of duodenal contents from proximity to the stomach with a roux-en-Y anastomosis often alleviates bilious vomiting, particularly in patients in whom bile reflux is demonstrated by nuclear scanning after administration of ^{99m}Tc-HIDA; however, early satiety often does not improve with surgery.

Dumping Syndrome Following peptic ulcer surgery, some patients experience a spectrum of vasomotor symptoms after eating. These include palpitations, tachycardia, lightheadedness, diaphoresis, and, less frequently, postural hypotension. Abdominal discomfort and vomiting also may occur. This constellation of symptoms, called the *early dumping syndrome*, is usually experienced within 30 min after eating and is believed to result from rapid emptying of hyperosmolar gastric contents into the proximal small intestine, which leads to a shift of fluid into the gut lumen, intestinal distention, and contraction of plasma volume. Additional proposed mechanisms for these symptoms include stimulation of autonomic reflexes secondary to small intestinal distention and/or release of hormones from the gut and vasoactive substances into the circulation in response to the rapid entry of gastric contents into the duodenum or jejunum.

The *late dumping syndrome* is a symptom complex of dizziness, lightheadedness, palpitations, diaphoresis, confusion, and, in rare instances, syncope occurring 90 min to 3 h after eating. The symptoms can often be precipitated by meals rich in simple carbohydrates, especially sucrose, and appear to result from hypoglycemia due to excessive insulin release, which is stimulated by an abrupt increase in blood glucose secondary to rapid emptying of sugar-containing meals into the proximal small intestine.

Both forms of the dumping syndrome are treated by dietary measures, including limitation of simple sugar-continuing liquids and solids (sweets), elimination of liquids at mealtime, and the eating of frequent small meals. In severe cases, symptoms may improve with the somatostatin analogue octreotide (50 μg subcutaneously tid).

Postvagotomy Diarrhea Some patients experience diarrhea after peptic ulcer surgery, especially after truncal vagotomy. Diarrhea usually occurs within 2 h of eating. The mechanism of diarrhea is not clear but is thought to involve interruption of vagal fibers to the abdominal viscera. Loss of the pyloric regulatory emptying mechanism and rapid emptying of gastric contents into the small intestine, resulting in increased fluid volume within the intestinal lumen due to the osmotic action of the meal, also may contribute to the diarrhea.

Hematologic Complications   Intrinsic factor secreted by gastric parietal cells is necessary for active absorption of vitamin B_{12} by the distal ileum (see Chap. 108). Although total gastrectomy invariably results in malabsorption of vitamin B_{12}, megaloblastic anemia due to vitamin B_{12} deficiency is rare after partial gastric resection; however, reduced serum vitamin B_{12} levels have been observed in about 14 percent of these patients. Gastritis in the remaining stomach is present in more than 60 percent of DU patients after vagotomy with antrectomy or vagotomy with pyloroplasty; it may progress to gastric atrophy and also may contribute to decreased vitamin B_{12} absorption. Because the stomach secretes approximately 100 times more intrinsic factor than is needed, peptic ulcer patients treated with partial gastric resection do not develop vitamin B_{12} deficiency as a result of the amount of stomach resected. Moreover, the resected portion of the stomach is almost always mainly antrum, which contains few parietal cells. Nevertheless, after peptic ulcer surgery, patients may develop decreased serum vitamin B_{12} levels as a result of reduced absorption of vitamin B_{12}. The precise mechanism of the malabsorption of vitamin B_{12} is not known but may in part involve hypochlorhydria and bacterial overgrowth.

Anemia may result from iron deficiency due to impaired absorption of dietary iron in patients with a Billroth II gastrojejunostomy. These patients have normal absorption of iron salts and respond favorably to oral iron preparations. Folate deficiency may result from either reduced dietary intake or impaired folate absorption. Except for anemia from blood loss caused by early recurrent ulcer, development of anemia after peptic ulcer surgery is gradual, usually occurring over several years.

Osteomalacia and Osteoporosis   Osteoporosis and osteomalacia are common after partial or complete gastrectomy but are rare after vagotomy with pyloroplasty. Osteomalacia is extremely common after gastrojejunostomy or Billroth II anastomosis owing to malabsorption of calcium and vitamin D. The incidence of bone fractures in men following gastric resection has been estimated to be almost twice that of control subjects of similar age. Reduced bone density perceptible by x-ray requires years to develop. Patients may develop bone pain and pathologic fractures. Patients with osteomalacia usually have increased levels of serum alkaline phosphatase and may have reduced serum calcium concentrations. These patients should be treated with supplemental oral vitamin D and calcium. The frequency of osteoporosis and osteomalacia after partial or complete gastrectomy is sufficiently great to justify prophylactic treatment with vitamin D and calcium indefinitely after gastric resection, especially in females.

General Malabsorption   (See also Chap. 285)   Mild, chemically demonstrable steatorrhea is common after ulcer surgery. Weight loss is more common after partial gastric resection (approximately 60 percent of patients) than after vagotomy alone. The major cause of weight loss is reduced food intake. On a diet providing 100 g of fat per day, loss of stool fat seldom exceeds 15 g/d (normal, less than 7 g/d). The causes of maldigestion and malabsorption include rapid gastric emptying, a reduced dispersion of food in the stomach, reduced bile concentrations in the gut lumen, an increased rate of transit of the meal through the small intestine, and reduced or delayed pancreatic secretory responses to feeding. Steatorrhea and weight loss, sometimes accompanied by vitamin B_{12} malabsorption, also may develop as a result of bacterial overgrowth. Malabsorption after peptic ulcer surgery also may be due to preexisting conditions, including latent celiac sprue or chronic pancreatitis.

Carcinoma after Partial Gastrectomy   Several studies have reported an increased incidence of adenocarcinoma of the stomach in DU patients 15 or more years after partial gastric resection for DU. This complication should be considered when abdominal symptoms (which may be similar to or distinct from those due to the original ulcer) appear many years after apparently successful ulcer surgery.

NONGASTRITIS EPITHELIAL CELL INJURY

STRESS-RELATED MUCOSAL INJURY   Acute upper GI erosions and ulcers distinct from chronic peptic ulcer may occur in patients with shock, massive burns, sepsis, and severe trauma (Table 284-4). These lesions, called *stress erosions* and *ulcers*, are frequently multiple and are most common in the acid-secreting portion of the stomach. They occur in about 80 to 90 percent of patients with massive injuries and burns (in the latter case, they are called *Curling's ulcers*). The most common clinical finding is painless GI hemorrhage. In critically ill patients in medical intensive care units, the principal risk factors for bleeding are the need for mechanical ventilation and the presence of coagulopathy. Blood loss is usually minimal but may be substantial and life-threatening. Usually, erosions develop about 24 h after trauma or shock. When massive hemorrhage occurs, it typically happens more than 2 or 3 days after the acute insult. The diagnosis is best established by upper GI endoscopy. Erosions are usually too superficial to be recognized by barium examination.

Many theories have been proposed to explain stress-associated acute mucosal ulceration, but mucosal ischemia and tissue injury from gastric acid appear to be the most important factors. Although there is usually no evidence of acid hypersecretion, the lesions cannot be produced in experimental animals in the absence of acid. It is believed that ischemia of the gastric mucosa, which has enormous oxygen requirements, is the most important element in producing stress erosions and ulceration.

Cushing's ulcers are acute ulcers of the upper GI tract associated with intracranial injury or an increase in intracranial pressure (e.g., due to a brain tumor or subdural hematoma). These ulcers may involve the stomach, proximal duodenum, or esophagus and frequently lead to hemorrhage or perforation. They do not differ histologically from acute stress ulceration; however, they are frequently associated with gastric acid hypersecretion. Treatment includes correction of increased intracranial pressure, when possible, and the usual measures for treatment of acute erosions and ulcerations, including vigorous therapy with antacids or H_2 receptor antagonists.

Management of acute stress ulcerations and erosions is principally preventive. With improvements in the hemodynamic management of critically ill patients in the past 20 years, the frequency of bleeding from stress ulcers in intensive care units has fallen from 20 to 30 percent to 1.5 to 14 percent. In fact, the need for routine therapy to prevent stress ulcer bleeding has been questioned. However, it is still standard practice to administer prophylactic therapy to high-risk patients, including patients in an intensive care unit who are being mechanically ventilated, who have coagulopathy or multiorgan failure, or who are severely burned. Standard preventive therapy consists of liquid antacids administered via a nasogastric tube hourly or as needed to maintain a gastric pH of at least 3.5 and/or intravenous administration of an H_2 receptor antagonist, either as bolus injections or by continuous infusion. Alternatively, sucralfate administered by nasogastric tube as a 1-g slurry every 6 h is equally effective in preventing stress ulcer bleeding, and, because it does not raise gastric pH, it may be associated with a lower risk of late-onset (4 or more days after initiation) pneumonia than antacids and H_2 receptor antagonists. When bleeding occurs and does not subside with medical therapy, endoscopic intervention and, in some cases, surgery, including pyloroplasty with vagotomy or total gastrectomy, may be necessary.

MUCOSAL INJURY INDUCED BY ASPIRIN AND OTHER NSAIDS   Aspirin is associated with an increased incidence of GU and, to a lesser extent, DU and may cause hemorrhagic erosive gastro-

Table 284-4

Risk Factors for Stress-Related Mucosal Injury (Stress Erosions and Ulcers)

Mechanical ventilation
Coagulopathy
Sepsis and multiorgan failure
Burns (Curling's ulcers)
Central nervous system trauma (Cushing's ulcers)

pathy. Similar gastric mucosal injury is observed in patients ingesting other NSAIDs (e.g., indomethacin, ibuprofen, naproxen, tolmetin, sulindac, piroxicam, diflunisal, fenoprofen, and others). Several mechanisms by which salicylates and other NSAIDs induce ulcers and erosions have been proposed. NSAIDs are directly toxic to the gastric mucosa, and they deplete protective endogenous mucosal prostaglandins by inhibiting prostaglandin synthesis. They also may contribute to ulcer formation by interrupting the gastric mucosal barrier, permitting back-diffusion of hydrogen ions that may injure the gastric mucosa. They reduce gastric mucus secretion and gastric and duodenal bicarbonate secretion and may increase gastric acid secretion. Depletion of mucosal prostaglandins also impairs epithelial cell replacement after injury.

Gastric ulcers develop in 10 to 30 percent of patients receiving chronic NSAID treatment, while the prevalence of DU is 2 to 20 percent. Factors contributing to a high risk for ulcer are shown in Table 284-5. There is no convincing evidence that *H. pylori* infection, smoking, or caffeine or alcohol ingestion increase the risk of NSAID-induced ulcers. As yet, there is no conclusive evidence that any particular NSAID is associated with a lower or greater risk of gastroduodenal ulceration, but some observations suggest that newer NSAIDs, such as nabumetone, which selectively inhibit mucosal cyclooxygenase type 2, may be associated with a lower risk of ulceration than other NSAIDs. Glucocorticoids administered alone have not been proven to be ulcerogenic.

Most persons taking aspirin or NSAIDs experience some GI distress, but there is a poor correlation between symptoms and the development of chronic ulcers. In addition to causing GUs and DUs, NSAIDs have been implicated in occasional cases of small intestinal and colonic ulceration and strictures (which may be either broad or thin and diaphragm-like), as well as in exacerbations of Crohn's disease and ulcerative colitis.

Misoprostol, a PGE₁ analogue, in doses of 100 and 200 µg four times a day, reduces the risk of NSAID-associated GU by approximately 75 and 95 percent, respectively. Abdominal cramping and/or diarrhea may occur with abrupt initiation of the full dose. The drug causes uterine contraction and should not be used in women of childbearing age. NSAID-induced DUs can be prevented by H₂ receptor antagonists, and preliminary studies suggest that higher than standard doses (e.g., famotidine 40 mg orally bid) are also effective in preventing NSAID-induced GUs. These drugs and omeprazole are also effective in healing NSAID-induced ulcers, and omeprazole appears to accelerate the healing of such ulcers even if NSAID use is continued.

OTHER AGENTS THAT INDUCE MUCOSAL INJURY
Ethanol damage to the gastric mucosa is associated with subepithelial hemorrhages with surrounding edema and only slight to moderate increases in mucosal inflammatory cells. Possible mechanisms for cell injury include the inherent lipophilic and lipolytic properties of ethanol, interruption of the gastric mucosal barrier, and direct damage to small mucosal blood vessels.

Ingestion of corrosive chemicals can cause severe damage to the gastric mucosa. Causative agents include strong acids (e.g., hydrochloric acid, sulfuric acid) and strong alkalis (e.g., sodium hydroxide). The esophagus is particularly susceptible to severe injury by alkalies (particularly lye), with a risk of necrosis and subsequent stricture

Table 284-5

Risk Factors for NSAID-Induced Mucosal Injury

Older age
Female sex
High NSAID doses
Protracted NSAID use
Combined use of NSAID and glucocorticoids
Severe intercurrent illness
Unproven: *H. pylori*, smoking, caffeine, alcohol

formation. The stomach, especially the antrum, is more susceptible to acute injury from strong acid. Depending on the dose and concentration, these agents can cause injury ranging from mild inflammation to extensive tissue necrosis. Patients may describe burning of the mouth, throat, and retrosternal area. Epigastric pain and vomiting often signal gastric injury. Hemorrhage and/or perforation may occur. Treatment of strong acid ingestion includes dilution with water, followed by antacids and supportive therapy as required.

GASTRITIS

Gastritis, or inflammation of the gastric mucosa, is not a single disease but rather a group of disorders that all induce inflammatory changes in the gastric mucosa but that differ in their clinical features, histologic characteristics, and causative mechanisms. Several classifications of gastritis exist (Table 284-6). In general, these classifications have been based on (1) the acuteness or chronicity of the clinical manifestations, (2) histologic features, (3) anatomic distribution, or (4) proposed mechanism of pathogenesis. On the basis of clinical features, the two principal forms of gastritis are acute gastritis and chronic gastritis. Different types of chronic gastritis may be classified according to their presumed cause, their histologic features, and the anatomic distribution of the gastritis or associated mucosal atrophy.

ACUTE GASTRITIS ASSOCIATED WITH *H. PYLORI*
The onset of *H. pylori* infection may result in acute gastritis associated with a transient increase in gastric acid secretion followed by hypochlorhydria for up to 1 year. Patients may have mild epigastric discomfort, although most remain asymptomatic. Several epidemics of acute gastritis have been attributed to *H. pylori*, but the endoscopic and histologic features have not been well characterized. Acute *H. pylori* gastritis is a precursor to chronic active gastritis (see below).

OTHER CAUSES OF INFECTIOUS GASTRITIS Infectious causes of gastritis, other than gastric *H. pylori* colonization, are unusual. *Phlegmonous gastritis*, a rare form of bacterial gastritis, is a life-threatening disease with extensive infiltration of the gastric wall, tissue necrosis, and manifestations of generalized sepsis. Responsible organisms include streptococci, staphylococci, *Proteus* species, and *Escherichia coli*. Treatment includes appropriate intravenous antibiotics and necessary supportive care with fluid and electrolyte replacement as required. Lack of response to therapy may necessitate gastrectomy.

Infectious gastritis may be found in immunocompromised patients, including patients with AIDS. Gastric erosions may be produced by herpes simplex virus. Typical intranuclear inclusions of cytomegalovirus, with positive cultures, may occur in disseminated cytomegalovirus infection.

Table 284-6

Classification of Gastritis

Acute gastritis
  Acute *H. pylori* gastritis
  Other acute infectious gastritides
    Bacterial (other than *H. pylori*)
      Helicobacter helmmanii
      Phlegmonous
      Mycobacterial
      Syphilitic
    Viral
    Parasitic
    Fungal
Chronic atrophic gastritis
  Type A: Body-predominant, autoimmune
  Type B: Antral-predominant, *H. pylori*–related, environmental
  Type AB
  Indeterminant type
Uncommon forms of gastritis
  Lymphocytic gastritis
  Eosinophilic gastritis
  Crohn's disease
  Sarcoidosis
  Isolated granulomatous gastritis

CHRONIC GASTRITIS The inflammatory cell infiltrate in chronic gastritis consists mainly of lymphocytes and plasma cells. Polymorphonuclear leukocytes and eosinophils may be present in small numbers. Chronic gastritis is often patchy and irregular in distribution. It involves the superficial and glandular areas of the gastric mucosa initially and progresses to glandular destruction, which may be followed by gland metaplasia and a profound reduction in gland number (atrophy). Chronic gastritis has been classified descriptively on the basis of several characteristic histologic abnormalities.

Superficial gastritis appears to represent the initial stage in the development of chronic gastritis. Inflammatory changes are limited to the lamina propria of the superficial mucosa, with cellular infiltration and edema separating the gastric glands; the glands are preserved. There may be a decrease in the amount of mucus in glandular mucous cells and in the frequency of mitotic figures in cells of the glands.

Atrophic gastritis is the next stage in the development of chronic gastritis. The inflammatory infiltrate extends to the deep portions of the mucosa. There is progressive distortion and destruction of the glands, which become separated by the inflammatory process. In the more common form of chronic gastritis, the process begins in the antrum and extends proximally into the body and fundus of the stomach.

Gastric atrophy is the final stage of chronic gastritis. There is a profound loss of glandular structures, which are now separated widely by connective tissue, with a greatly reduced or absent inflammatory infiltrate. The mucosa becomes thin, and the underlying blood vessels may be evident on endoscopic examination.

There may be changes in the morphology of the gastric glandular elements as chronic gastritis progresses. *Intestinal metaplasia* is the conversion of gastric glands to a form resembling that of small intestinal mucosal glands containing goblet cells. Intestinal metaplasia may be patchy or extensive and is an important predisposing factor for gastric cancer (see Chap. 92); however, the magnitude of the risk is not sufficient to justify endoscopic surveillance for gastric cancer.

The two major forms of chronic gastritis traditionally have been called types A (body-predominant, autoimmune) and B (antral-predominant, related to *H. pylori* infection) on the basis of their distribution in the gastric mucosa coupled with implications regarding their pathogenesis, although the distinction is not always clear. In some cases, the designation *type AB gastritis* is used to reflect involvement of both body and antrum.

Type A Gastritis (Body-Predominant Gastritis, Autoimmune Chronic Atrophic Gastritis)   Type A gastritis is the less common form of chronic gastritis. It characteristically involves the fundus and body of the stomach, with relative sparing of the antrum. This is the form of gastritis that may be associated with pernicious anemia (see Chap. 108). The frequent presence of antibodies to parietal cells and to intrinsic factor in sera of patients with type A gastritis and pernicious anemia has suggested an immune or autoimmune pathogenesis for this form of gastritis, although autoimmune features are often not present and it appears that a substantial number of cases may result from *H. pylori* infection (see below). Antibodies to parietal cells have been shown to be cytotoxic for gastric mucosal cells. Cell-mediated immune mechanisms also have been proposed to participate in gastric mucosal cell injury in pernicious anemia and related forms of type A gastritis. Antibodies to parietal cells have been found in sera of approximately 90 percent of patients with pernicious anemia and in more than half of other patients with type A gastritis. Relatives of patients with pernicious anemia have a higher than normal frequency of serum antibodies to parietal cells, atrophic gastritis, and reduced gastric acid secretion. In control populations, parietal cell antibodies may be found in up to 20 percent of individuals over age 60 and in approximately 20 percent of all patients with hypoparathyroidism, Addison's disease, and vitiligo. About 50 percent of patients with pernicious anemia have antibodies to thyroid antigens, and approximately 30 percent of patients with thyroid disease have circulating antibodies to parietal cells. Serum antibodies to intrinsic factor are more specific for type A gastritis than parietal cell antibodies and are present in about 40 percent of patients with pernicious anemia.

In patients with pernicious anemia, the gastric glands that contain parietal cells are invariably destroyed, accounting for their inability to secrete hydrochloric acid. Since, in humans, parietal cells also secrete intrinsic factor, type A atrophic gastritis also results in malabsorption of vitamin B_{12}, with resulting hematologic and/or neurologic consequences characteristic of pernicious anemia.

In general, the reduction in gastric acid secretion, which is complete in patients with pernicious anemia, is proportionate to the severity of parietal cell destruction and mucosal atrophy in the body and fundus of the stomach. Serum gastrin levels are usually elevated substantially in patients with pernicious anemia and are in approximately the same range as those of patients with ZES (gastrinoma). Since the antral mucosa is relatively spared, the antral gastrin-containing cells, deprived of the feedback control normally exerted by acid in the stomach, release gastrin continuously. As a result of pronounced hypergastrinemia, ECL-cell hyperplasia and carcinoid tumors of the stomach may develop in these patients. Carcinoids may regress following antrectomy to remove gastrin-producing cells. Serum gastrin levels are also often similarly elevated in patients with type A gastritis with achlorhydria or profound hypochlorhydria who do not have pernicious anemia.

Type B Gastritis (Antral-Predominant Gastritis, *H. pylori* Gastritis, Environmental Gastritis)   Type B gastritis is the more common form of chronic gastritis. In younger patients, type B gastritis principally involves the antrum, whereas in older patients the entire stomach is affected. This transition is estimated to require about 15 to 20 years. The incidence of chronic gastritis, most of it type B gastritis, increases with age, reaching 78 percent in individuals over age 50 and virtually 100 percent after age 70.

Studies from various parts of the world have established that *H. pylori* is the agent responsible for type B gastritis and that eradication of *H. pylori* leads to resolution of the histologic findings. Gastric colonization with *H. pylori* is found in virtually all patients with chronic superficial gastritis, but fewer bacteria are demonstrable with progression to atrophic gastritis. In general, the degree of histologic abnormality correlates with the number of organisms identified histologically. Findings include a dense chronic inflammatory infiltrate of the lamina propria and invasion of the epithelial cell layer by polymorphonuclear leukocytes (Fig. 284-12). *H. pylori* are few in number or not demonstrated with severe gastric atrophy.

Patients with type B gastritis have fasting serum gastrin levels that are highly variable, not consistently elevated, and often in the normal range. A few patients with type B gastritis have serum antibodies to gastrin, leading some to propose an autoimmune mechanism for this form of gastritis. Alternatively, and probably more likely, these antibodies may represent responses to the inflammatory process rather than contributing factors.

Chronic *H. pylori* gastritis may lead to multifocal atrophic gastritis, gastric atrophy, and gastric metaplasia (Fig. 284-13). Moreover, treatment with acid-suppressive therapy (e.g., H_2 receptor antagonists or proton pump inhibitors) increases the rate of development of gastric atrophy, thereby possibly increasing the risk of gastric cancer. In addition, such therapy in patients infected with *H. pylori* may increase the activity of gastritis in the gastric body; this too may lead to atrophic gastritis and a predisposition to gastric cancer.

H. pylori appears to be an independent risk factor for the development of gastric cancer, although its effect may be indirect. The epidemiologic features of gastric carcinoma and *H. pylori* infection are similar, and socioeconomic conditions known to influence the risk of gastric cancer are also important determinants of *H. pylori* infection. Worldwide epidemiologic studies have shown a higher prevalence of *H. pylori* infection in patients with gastric cancer than in control subjects. Seropositivity for *H. pylori* is associated with a three- to sixfold increase in the risk of gastric cancer (as high as ninefold after adjustment for the inaccuracy of serological testing in the elderly), although no such association exists in patients with cancer located at the gastric cardia.

As for peptic ulcer, not all patients with gastric cancer are infected with *H. pylori*, and not all persons with *H. pylori* infection develop gastric cancer. In addition, gastric atrophy only sometimes progresses to gastric cancer. Therefore, the etiology of gastric cancer is most likely multifactorial, with *H. pylori* infection as one of several factors contributing to its development.

The mechanism by which *H. pylori* infection may initiate gastric carcinogenesis is not known. The organism alters the physical and chemical milieu of the gastric mucus, which may render the gastric mucosa less resistant to environmental or dietary carcinogens. *H. pylori* infection also causes a decrease in the gastric secretion of ascorbic acid, reduced levels of which may allow formation of carcinogenic *N*-nitroso compounds. In addition, the chronic inflammation produced by *H. pylori* infection may stimulate mucosal hyperproliferation in a manner similar to that observed in chronic ulcerative colitis. It remains to be determined if eradication of *H. pylori* will substantially reduce the risk of gastric cancer. Currently, eradication of *H. pylori* in asymptomatic persons to reduce gastric cancer risk is not recommended.

H. pylori may also be associated with gastric lymphoma. Whereas lymphoid tissue is not found in the normal stomach, gastric lymphoid tissue develops in response to local infection with *H. pylori*. Most primary gastric lymphomas are, in fact, derived from mucosa-associ-

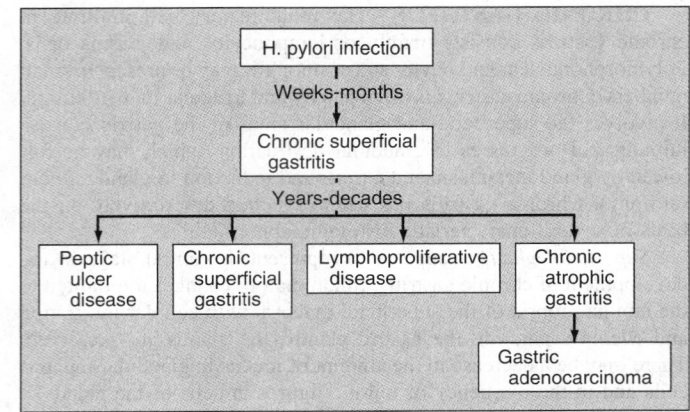

FIGURE 284-13 Possible long-term consequences of *H. pylori* infection.

ated lymphoid tissue (MALT). Epidemiologic studies in Europe have shown that regions with a high incidence of gastric lymphoma have higher rates of *H. pylori* infection than regions with a low incidence of gastric lymphoma. Moreover, patients with gastric lymphoma are more likely to have serologic evidence of *H. pylori* infection than matched controls. No association has been found between nongastric, non-Hodgkin's lymphoma and *H. pylori* infection.

The mechanism by which *H. pylori* infection leads to gastric lymphoma is unclear. Features of primary gastric B-cell lymphoma of MALT suggest that the tumor may be antigen-responsive; that is, the lymphoid follicles may result from chronic antigenic stimulation of the gastric mucosa by *H. pylori*. Given its close association with MALT lymphoma, *H. pylori* may initiate a malignant transformation by stimulating an immune response.

It has also been suggested that eradication of *H. pylori* from the gastric mucosa may result in the eventual loss of MALT, thereby removing the lymphoid precursor from which gastric lymphoma arises. Indeed, some studies have demonstrated that antibiotic treatment of *H. pylori* in patients with biopsy-proven low-grade B-cell MALT lymphoma results in eradication of the infection and regression of the lymphoma. It remains to be determined if prophylactic eradication of the infection will result in a substantially reduced risk of gastric lymphoma. Currently, the treatment of *H. pylori* in asymptomatic persons for the purpose of reducing the risk of gastric lymphoma is not recommended.

DIAGNOSIS Biopsy is the most reliable means of identifying and classifying gastritis as well as detecting *H. pylori*. However, caution must be exercised in the interpretation of a single gastric mucosal biopsy, because the patchy and irregular distribution of the gastritis may lead to substantial sampling error. Therefore, biopsy of several suspected areas is recommended when it is safe and possible.

℞ TREATMENT

In general, no specific treatment is required for type A or type B chronic gastritis with or without mucosal atrophy. However, pernicious anemia, a consequence of type A gastritis, requires lifelong regular parenteral vitamin B_{12} administration (see Chap. 108). In the absence of documented peptic ulcer or MALT lymphoma, eradication of *H. pylori* in patients with type B gastritis is generally not recommended.

OTHER TYPES OF GASTRITIS *Lymphocytic gastritis* is characterized histologically by intense lymphocytic infiltration of the gastric surface epithelium and the presence of superficial pits with a lymphocytosis of small mature T cells and plasmacytosis of the lamina propria. The cause is unknown, but some cases occur in patients with celiac sprue, and shared pathogenic mechanisms are suspected. Patients are usually asymptomatic, but endoscopy shows thickened gastric folds, often capped by small nodules with central depressions, an appearance often referred to as "varioliform gastritis." Lymphocytic gastritis has been treated with corticosteroids or sodium cromoglycate,

FIGURE 284-12 Chronic gastritis and *Helicobacter pylori* organisms. *A.* H&E stain of gastric mucosa showing surface foveolar cells, adherent mucus, and scattered bacillary forms within the mucus. *B.* Steiner silver stain of superficial gastric mucosa, showing abundant darkly staining microorganisms layered over the apical portion of the surface epithelium. Note that there is no tissue invasion. *[Courtesy of James M. Crawford, M.D., Ph.D. Reprinted with permission from JM Crawford, The oral cavity and gastrointestinal tract, in Basic Pathology, V Kumar, RS Cotran, and SL Robbins (eds.). Philadelphia, Saunders, 1997.]*

with variable response. There is controversy as to whether lymphocytic gastritis may be caused by *H. pylori.*

CHAPTER 284
Peptic Ulcer and Related Disorders

1613

Eosinophilic gastritis is characterized by extensive eosinophilic infiltration of the stomach wall, usually with circulating eosinophilia. It may occur as isolated involvement of the stomach or as a component of eosinophilic gastroenteritis. Biopsy reveals extensive eosinophilic infiltration, which may involve all layers of the stomach wall or may be limited to the mucosa, submucosa, or muscularis. The antrum is involved more often than the body or fundus. There may be prominent antral mucosal folds with edema and mucosal thickening, which uncommonly lead to gastric outlet obstruction. Epigastric pain, which may be accompanied by nausea and vomiting, is the most frequent symptom. Patients usually respond favorably to treatment with glucocorticoids.

A number of generalized diseases can involve the stomach, producing *granulomatous gastritis.* Crohn's disease may produce gastric ulceration, granulomatous infiltration, and/or scarring with stricture formation; associated small intestinal Crohn's disease is usually present. Infectious causes of granulomatous gastritis include histoplasmosis, candidiasis, syphilis, and tuberculosis. Multiple mucosal biopsies and cytology are usually required to establish the diagnosis of granulomatous gastritis and to exclude malignancy. If the diagnosis is not established by biopsy at endoscopy, surgical exploration may be required. Rarely, sarcoidosis, idiopathic granulomatous gastritis, and eosinophilic granulomas involve the stomach.

MÉNÉTRIER'S DISEASE

Ménétrier's disease is a clinical entity characterized by large, tortuous gastric mucosal folds, which may be localized or may involve the whole stomach. These mucosal folds are often most conspicuous in the gastric body and fundus. The mucosal thickening is due to massive foveolar hyperplasia (hyperplasia of surface and glandular mucous cells), which replaces most of the chief and parietal cells. The pits of the gastric glands elongate and may become extremely tortuous. The lamina propria may contain a mild chronic inflammatory infiltrate; however, technically Ménétrier's disease is not a form of gastritis.

The most common symptom is epigastric pain. Anorexia, nausea, vomiting, and weight loss are less frequent. Occult GI bleeding may occur, but overt bleeding is unusual and, when present, is due to superficial mucosal erosions. Uncommonly, GU or gastric carcinoma may develop. Patients often develop a protein-losing gastropathy resulting in hypoalbuminemia and edema. Gastric acid secretion is usually reduced or absent. Barium examination of the upper GI tract reveals the large gastric folds, which are readily confirmed by endoscopy. Deep mucosal biopsy (and cytology) is needed for diagnosis. The depth of these lesions and the disconcerting prominence of the folds may require a surgical full-thickness biopsy to exclude lymphoma or infiltrating carcinoma.

Anticholinergic agents and H_2 receptor antagonists have been reported to decrease protein loss in patients with Ménétrier's disease. Treatment includes a high-protein diet, when required, to replace protein losses. If ulcers are present, the treatment should be as for common GU. Severe disease with persistent and substantial protein loss may require total gastrectomy.

ZOLLINGER-ELLISON SYNDROME (GASTRINOMA)

Zollinger-Ellison syndrome (ZES) consists of ulcer disease of the upper GI tract, marked increases in gastric acid secretion, and non-beta islet cell tumors of the pancreas. These tumors are called gastrinomas because they contain gastrin, which circulates in large amounts, producing the pathophysiologic characteristics of ZES.

ETIOLOGY AND PATHOGENESIS In initial studies, gastrinomas were reported most often in the pancreas. They are most common in the head of the pancreas and may vary in size from 1 mm to more than 20 cm in diameter. One-half to two-thirds of patients have multiple gastrinomas. Recent studies suggest that, with careful searching, gastrinomas are found as frequently (or perhaps more frequently) in the wall of the duodenum as in the pancreas. Duodenal gastrinomas, approximately half of which are solitary, are usually found in the submucosa of the first or second part of the duodenum and are just as likely as pancreatic gastrinomas to be malignant. Rarely, gastrinomas are found in the stomach or in lymph nodes near to the pancreas, proximal duodenum, or spleen in the absence of demonstrated primary tumors. Approximately 90 percent of gastrinomas are found within an anatomic triangle ("the gastrinoma triangle") that is defined by the junction of the cystic and common bile ducts superiorly, the junction of the second and third portions of the duodenum inferiorly, and the junction of the pancreatic body and neck medially. In unusual instances, ZES has resulted from gastrinomas originating in remote organs, such as the parathyroids or ovaries.

About two-thirds of gastrinomas are histologically or biologically malignant; about one-third of all patients have metastatic disease on presentation. Malignant gastrinomas usually grow slowly; however, a small portion are rapidly invasive and may metastasize early and widely. Metastasis is most often to regional lymph nodes and the liver; other sites are peritoneal surfaces, spleen, bone, skin, and mediastinum. Gastrinomas have similarities by light microscopy to carcinoid tumors and may be mistaken for these tumors, especially when arising from the mucosa of the small intestine or stomach.

Pancreatic islet cell hyperplasia occurs in approximately 10 percent of patients with ZES. Islet hyperplasia accompanying recognized or unidentified gastrinoma appears to be a result, rather than a cause, of excess gastrin release, since gastrin is not present in the hyperplastic tissue.

In an estimated 20 to 60 percent of patients with ZES, the gastrinoma is a component of the multiple endocrine neoplasia type 1 (MEN 1) syndrome, an autosomal dominant disorder with a high degree of penetrance and great variability in expressivity (see Chap. 340). The MEN 1 locus is on chromosome 11 (11q11-q13). Patients with MEN 1 may have clinically recognized hyperplasia, adenomas, or carcinoma involving, in order of frequency, the parathyroid glands, pancreatic islets, and pituitary. Hyperparathyroidism has been reported in close to 90 percent of patients with MEN 1 syndrome, and gastrinoma has been reported in approximately half of them (see Chap. 340). However, a careful search would probably find involvement of all three organs in all patients with MEN 1, although frequently without overt clinical expression. Patients with MEN 1 usually present with multiple gastrinomas, which generally are smaller than sporadic gastrinomas. Gastrinomas with MEN 1 are located more frequently in the wall of the duodenum than in the pancreas. In fact, MEN 1 patients, including those with duodenal gastrinomas, usually have multiple pancreatic islet cell tumors, but most of these are not gastrinomas.

Most of the gastrin in gastrinomas is heptadecapeptide gastrin (G-17), with the remainder being mostly G-34. In contrast, approximately two-thirds of circulating gastrin in gastrinoma patients is G-34; most of the remainder is G-17. When examined carefully, almost all gastrin-secreting islet cell tumors contain multiple hormones, which are usually clinically silent. These may include adrenocorticotropic hormone (ACTH), glucagon, melanocyte-stimulating hormone, parathyroid hormone, growth hormone releasing factor (GRF), insulin, pancreatic polypeptide, and vasoactive intestinal peptide. Of these, ACTH is the most common; it is found in approximately one-third of gastrinomas. Cushing's syndrome with increased serum ACTH levels has been reported in 8 percent of patients with ZES. ACTH-releasing gastrinomas are often aggressively malignant. In contrast, ACTH may be released by pituitary tumors in patients with MEN 1, in whom symptoms of Cushing's syndrome are generally mild and gastrinomas are usually not metastatic. Approximately one-third of patients with gastrinomas have increases in serum concentrations of pancreatic polypeptide.

In patients with ZES, the parietal cell mass is substantially expanded (three to six times normal), owing to the trophic effects of circulating gastrin. Small, multicentric, noninvasive carcinoid tumors have been identified in the gastric mucosa of ZES patients. These tumors and associated focal areas of enterochromaffin-like (ECL) cell hyperplasia are believed to result from substantial and sustained hypergastrinemia and are more likely in patients with MEN 1 than in those with sporadic gastrinomas. Carcinoids and ECL hyperplasia also have been found in the gastric mucosa of patients with pernicious anemia and achlorhydria, who have increases in serum gastrin in the range of those found with gastrinoma.

CLINICAL FEATURES While the true incidence of ZES is not known, estimates are that it accounts for 0.1 to 1 percent of peptic ulcers. ZES may occur at any age, but initial manifestations occur most commonly between ages 30 and 60.

Most, if not all, patients with gastrinomas develop ulceration of the GI tract at some point in the course of their disease. Profound gastric acid hypersecretion is usually present. Especially early in the course of the disease, symptoms are usually similar to those of patients with typical peptic ulcer. However, ulcer symptoms may be more fulminant, progressive, and persistent and, in general, respond poorly to usual medical and surgical peptic ulcer treatments. The anatomic site of the ulcers in ZES is similar but not identical to that of common types of peptic ulcer. About 75 percent of ZES patients have ulcers in the first portion of the duodenum or in the stomach; these are usually single but may be multiple. When multiple ulcers occur, they are frequently located not only in the first portion of the duodenum, but also in the remainder of the duodenum and even the jejunum.

Diarrhea occurs in about 40 percent of patients owing to the outpouring of large amounts of hydrochloric acid into the proximal duodenum; it can be reduced or eliminated by aspiration of gastric juice. The excessive acid has been shown to reduce the pH of the contents of the proximal and distal jejunum to as low as 1 and 3.6, respectively. The large amounts of acid and pepsin may cause corrosive changes in the mucosa of the small intestine. Steatorrhea, which is less common than diarrhea, results from inactivation of pancreatic lipase by large concentrations of acid in the proximal small intestine and from decreases in luminal bile acids. The decrease in intraluminal bile acid concentration is caused by precipitation of the major bile acids at low pH, leading to impaired micelle formation, which, in turn, reduces intestinal absorption of fatty acids and monoglycerides (see Chap. 285). Vitamin B_{12} malabsorption not correctable by addition of intrinsic factor has been detected in some patients with ZES. Although gastric secretion of intrinsic factor appears normal, the reduced luminal pH prevents the activation of the pancreatic enzymes that are needed to split R proteins from vitamin B_{12} so that the vitamin can bind with intrinsic factor and undergo intestinal absorption (see Chap. 108).

DIAGNOSIS Gastrinoma should be suspected in patients with a compatible clinical history, especially in those with marked acid hypersecretion (Table 284-7). More than 90 percent of patients with ZES have a basal gastric acid output (BAO) that exceeds 4 μmol/s (15 mEq/h). In rare instances, the BAO may be greater than 40 μmol/s (150 mEq/h). However, there is substantial overlap in rates of gastric acid secretion among ZES patients, those with DU, and normal subjects. Patients with ZES often have a BAO that is greater than 60 percent of the output induced by maximal stimulation (the MAO). In most normal subjects and DU patients, the BAO is less than 60 percent of maximal secretion. However, exceptions are common, so the BAO/MAO ratio alone cannot be relied on to identify patients with gastrinoma.

Some radiographic and endoscopic features may suggest the diagnosis of ZES. Large mucosal folds may be demonstrated most prominently in the stomach but also in the duodenum and, in some instances, the jejunum. The lumen of the stomach and small intestine often contains large amounts of fluid. Radiographic and endoscopic features of most ulcers in these patients, except when they are distal in location, are similar to those of common peptic ulcer. *H. pylori* is usually absent.

The diagnosis of gastrinoma in a patient with clinical features consistent with ZES depends on the demonstration of increased serum gastrin levels by radioimmunoassay. Fasting serum gastrin levels in normal subjects and patients with typical DU average approximately 20 to 50 ng/L and usually do not exceed 150 ng/L. Patients with ZES almost always have fasting serum gastrin levels that are greater than 200 ng/L; levels may be as high as 450,000 ng/L. However, approximately half these patients have fasting serum gastrin levels less than 1000 ng/L (the approximate mean value for serum gastrin for patients with gastrinoma). Rarely, serum gastrin levels as measured by standard assays are normal in patients with ZES.

Several provocative tests have been used to evaluate patients with possible ZES, especially those who do not exhibit pronounced hypergastrinemia (i.e., serum gastrin of at least 1000 ng/L). These tests involve measurements of serum gastrin levels after intravenous secretin injection, calcium infusion, or ingestion of a standard test meal.

In the *secretin injection* test, secretin (Kabi secretin, 2 U/kg) is given intravenously over 30 to 60 s. Serum gastrin is measured in samples obtained immediately before injection of secretin, at 2 and 5 min after injection, and at 5-min intervals thereafter for a total of 30 min. In normal individuals and patients with common DU, secretin produces either no change or small reductions or increases in serum gastrin levels. However, in ZES patients, intravenous secretin induces substantial increases in serum gastrin; these levels increase promptly by at least 200 ng/L, usually at 5 min (and virtually always by 10 min), and then gradually decrease toward preinjection levels by 30 min.

In the *calcium infusion* test, serum gastrin measurements are obtained before and at 30-min intervals for 4 h after a 3-h constant-rate intravenous infusion of calcium gluconate (5 mg/kg per hour). In patients with ZES, serum gastrin concentrations usually increase above the basal serum gastrin level by more than 400 ng/L.

The third provocative test involves the *feeding of a standard meal*: gastrin is measured in serum samples obtained before the meal and at 15-min intervals thereafter for 90 min. This test has been used to attempt to distinguish between ZES patients and those with hypergastrinemia and gastric acid hypersecretion due to antral gastrin cell hypertrophy or hyperplasia (see below).

The secretin injection test is the most valuable provocative test in identifying patients with ZES. Positive serum gastrin response to intravenous secretin is found in more than 95 percent of ZES patients. Using the criteria suggested, substantial increases in serum gastrin following secretin injection occur only rarely in nongastrinoma patients. Because reduced gastric acid secretion (achlorhydria or profound hypochlorhydria) is the most common cause of hypergastrinemia, gastric acid secretion should be measured before using the secretin injection test (Table 284-8). Exaggerated release of gastrin in response to calcium infusion is found in more than 80 percent of ZES patients; however, this exaggerated response also occurs in some nongastrinoma patients with hypergastrinemia (e.g., with achlorhydria). Enhanced gastrin release with calcium infusion is rarely observed in ZES patients in the absence of the abnormally large gastrin release in response to secretin. Since the calcium infusion test does not add significantly to the sensitivity or specificity of the secretin injection

---

Table 284-7

Indications for Measuring Serum Gastrin Levels in Patients with Peptic Ulcer

Multiple ulcers or ulcers in unusual locations
Ulcers resistant to therapy or with frequent recurrences
Ulcers requiring surgery
Extensive family history of peptic ulcer disease
Postoperative ulcer recurrence
Severe esophagitis
Basal hyperchlorhydria
Unexplained diarrhea or steatorrhea
Hypercalcemia
Family history of pancreatic islet, pituitary, or parathyroid tumor
Prominent gastric or duodenal folds

Table 284-8

Causes of Hypergastrinemia

Hypochlorhydria or achlorhydria with or without pernicious anemia
Retained gastric antrum
Antral G-cell hyperplasia
Renal insufficiency
Massive small bowel resection
Gastric outlet obstruction
Pheochromocytoma

test, and since calcium infusion is potentially more hazardous, it is usually not necessary or recommended.

In a minority of DU patients (much less than 1 percent), gastric acid hypersecretion may be accompanied by increased serum gastrin levels due to hyperfunctioning and/or hyperplasia of antral gastrin cells (G cells). It is quite possible that this response is an effect, at least in part, of *H. pylori* infection. These patients can be distinguished from those with ZES by the secretin and meal stimulation tests. In patients with this antral gastrin cell abnormality, intravenous secretin does not produce the large increases in serum gastrin characteristic of ZES. On the other hand, serum gastrin concentrations may increase by greater than 200 percent after test meals in patients with gastrin cell hypertrophy or hyperplasia, suggesting that this response may be of value in distinguishing these patients from those with gastrinoma. More recently, however, other investigators have found similarly large amounts of gastrin released into the sera of patients with gastrinomas, suggesting that the meal-stimulated test is of limited value in distinguishing between patients with antral gastrin cell hyperplasia and those with ZES.

Gastrinomas are difficult to localize. In almost half of patients with clinical and laboratory evidence of ZES, the tumors cannot be identified at surgery. Selective arteriography identifies gastrinomas in about half of patients with clinical and biochemical evidence of ZES. Computed tomography (CT) localizes gastrinomas in 30 percent, and ultrasound in 20 percent, of ZES patients. Hepatic venous gastrin sampling after intra-arterial injection of secretin during arteriography appears to be useful in localizing duodenal gastrinomas. Magnetic resonance imaging is no better than CT in localizing primary tumors but is the most sensitive method of detecting hepatic metastases. Endoscopic retrograde pancreatography has not been helpful in the diagnosis or exclusion of pancreatic gastrinomas. A small number of duodenal wall gastrinomas have been identified and confirmed histologically by duodenoscopy and, more recently, by endoscopic ultrasonography, which shows great promise. Because gastrinomas express cell-surface receptors for somatostatin, nuclear scanning after intravenous injection of radiolabeled octreotide has proved useful for localizing small primary tumors and metastases.

℞ TREATMENT

In general, patients with ZES are resistant to the medical and surgical therapies that are effective in treating common peptic ulcer. In fact, partial gastric resection (with or without vagotomy) or pyloroplasty with vagotomy is frequently followed by prompt and often fulminant ulcer recurrence. In the past, many patients with gastrinoma underwent multiple surgical procedures, particularly in cases where the diagnosis was not established initially. The mortality rate was reported to be lowest in patients with ZES in whom gastrectomy was the initial gastric surgery. This report led to the conclusion that, when surgery was required in gastrinoma patients, total gastrectomy was the procedure of choice.

Development of effective drugs to reduce acid secretion and of more precise diagnostic techniques to locate gastrinomas have increased therapeutic options substantially. Management in these patients must be individualized, because patients with ZES are heterogeneous with respect to clinical manifestations and extent of disease. As with many other predominantly malignant tumors, the ideal treatment is removal of the gastrinoma.

H_2 receptor antagonists are effective in reducing gastric acid secretion, relieving symptoms, and inducing ulcer healing in patients with ZES. Improvement in clinical symptoms, a decrease in gastric acid output, and ulcer healing occur in 80 to 85 percent of patients. Daily doses four to eight times those used in the treatment of common DU may be required. H_2 receptor antagonist therapy must be continued indefinitely, since even temporary discontinuation is usually followed by ulcer recurrence. In approximately 25 percent of patients with ZES, ulcers fail to respond to treatment with H_2 receptor antagonists or recur during treatment. The dose of H_2 receptor antagonist required to maintain a satisfactory reduction in gastric acid secretion can be assessed by measuring the BAO during the hour immediately prior to the next anticipated dose of the drug; the goal is to reduce BAO to less than 2.8 μmol/s (10 mEq/h) at that time.

The parietal cell H^+,K^+-ATPase inhibitors omeprazole and lansoprazole are the most effective drugs and the agents of choice in reducing gastric acid secretion and healing ulcers in patients with ZES, including those with ulcers resistant to treatment with H_2 receptor antagonists. The usual initial daily recommended dose of omeprazole or lansoprazole is 60 mg in a single dose administered in the morning before breakfast. The dose is adjusted to maintain the BAO at less than 2.8 μmol/s (10 mEq/h) [or at less than 1.4 μmol/s (5 mEq/h) in patients who have had prior ulcer surgery] during the hour immediately before the next dose. Patients with esophagitis may require doses sufficient to reduce gastric hypersecretion to less than 0.25 μmol/s (1 mEq/h) to control symptoms. Twice-daily dosing is required in about one-third of patients. It may be possible to reduce the drug dose once symptoms are controlled.

Some patients with ZES in whom gastrinomas could not be identified or removed surgically have been treated with parietal cell vagotomy. In a few instances, this treatment has reduced the amount of H_2 receptor antagonist required or rendered the drug unnecessary.

In selecting the best therapy, the biologic behavior of the tumor and the clinical manifestations in each patient must be taken into consideration. Early studies indicated that morbidity and mortality in patients with ZES were due principally to complications of severe ulcer disease. However, with earlier diagnosis, more effective antiulcer treatment, and longer follow-up, more frequent consequences of the malignant properties of gastrinomas are being recognized. Approximately half of ZES patients in whom the gastrinoma has not been removed will die from malignant invasion by the tumor. Complete surgical resection of the tumors, when possible, is the optimal treatment. Exploratory surgery should include endoscopic transillumination of the duodenum and lateral duodenotomy with examination of the duodenum. The possible benefit of intraoperative ultrasonography remains to be determined. Complete surgical removal of gastrinoma, with cure, has been achieved in approximately 30 percent of patients with ZES.

Treatment with omeprazole or lansoprazole is indicated while the diagnosis is being established, while the location and extent of the tumor are being determined, and prior to anticipated surgery. At present, long-term treatment with omeprazole or lansoprazole is indicated for patients who are not suitable candidates for surgery, who refuse surgery, or in whom surgical removal of the tumor is not possible.

Patients with aggressively invasive gastrinoma have been treated with combinations of streptozotocin, 5-fluorouracil, and doxorubicin in attempts to reduce tumor bulk and associated symptoms. Response to chemotherapy is limited, with initial response rates of up to 65 percent and no complete responses. The efficacy of interferon and octreotide also appears limited. When metastatic or nonresectable gastrinoma is present, control of the ulcer disease may be achieved in most instances by treatment with omeprazole or lansoprazole or, rarely, when required, by total gastric resection. There is no convincing evidence that tumor progression is influenced by gastrectomy.

BIBLIOGRAPHY

PEPTIC ULCER AND *HELICOBACTER PYLORI*

EL-OMAR EM et al: *Helicobacter pylori* infection and abnormalities of acid secretion in patients with duodenal ulcer disease. Gastroenterology 109:681, 1995

FENDRICK AM et al: Alternative management strategies for patients with suspected peptic ulcer disease. Ann Intern Med 123:260, 1995

GRAHAM DY et al: Effect of treatment of *Helicobacter pylori* infection on the long-term recurrence of gastric or duodenal ulcer: a randomized, controlled study. Ann Intern Med 116:705, 1992

HENTSCHEL E et al: Effect of ranitidine and amoxicillin plus metronidazole on the eradication of *Helicobacter pylori* and the recurrence of duodenal ulcer. N Engl J Med 328:308, 1993

McGOWAN CC et al: *Helicobacter pylori* and gastric acid: Biological and therapeutic implications. Gastroenterology 110:926, 1996

MODLIN IM, TANG LH: The gastric enterochromaffin-like cell: An enigmatic cellular link. Gastroenterology 111:926, 1996

SOLL AH: Medical treatment of peptic ulcer disease: Practice guidelines. JAMA 275:622, 1996

TALLEY TJ: A critique of therapeutic trials in *Helicobacter pylori*-positive functional dyspepsia. Gastroenterology 106:1174, 1994

TAYLOR JL et al: Pharmacoeconomic comparison of treatments for the eradication of *Helicobacter pylori*. Arch Intern Med 157:87, 1997

WALSH JH, PETERSON WL: The treatment of *Helicobacter pylori* infection in the management of peptic ulcer disease. N Engl J Med 338:984, 1995

WOLFE MM, SOLL AH: The physiology of gastric acid secretion. N Engl J Med 319:1707, 1988

STRESS ULCERS AND EROSIONS

BEN-MENACHEM T et al: Prophylaxis for stress-related gastric hemorrhage in the medical intensive care unit: A randomized, controlled single-blind study. Ann Intern Med 121:568, 1994

PEURA DA, JOHNSON LF: Cimetidine for prevention and treatment of gastroduodenal lesions in patients in an intensive care unit. Ann Intern Med 103:173, 1985

PROD'HOM G et al: Nosocomial pneumonia in mechanically ventilated patients receiving antacid, ranitidine, or sucralfate as prophylaxis for stress ulcer: A randomized controlled trial. Ann Intern Med 10:653, 1994

ASPIRIN AND NSAID-INDUCED MUCOSAL INJURY

CRYER B, FELDMAN M: Effects of nonsteroidal anti-inflammatory drugs on endogenous GI prostaglandins and therapeutic strategies for prevention and treatment of nonsteroidal anti-inflammatory drug-induced damage. Arch Intern Med 152:1145, 1992

HOLLANDER G: GI complications of nonsteroidal anti-inflammatory drugs: Prophylactic and therapeutic strategies. Am J Med 96:274, 1994

SILVERSTEIN FE et al: Misoprostol reduces serious GI complications in patients with rheumatoid arthritis receiving nonsteroidal anti-inflammatory drugs: A randomized double-blind, placebo-controlled trial. Ann Intern Med 123:241, 1995

GASTRIC MUCOSAL DISEASE

APPLEMAN HD: Gastritis: Terminology, etiology, and clinical correlations: Another biased view. Hum Pathol 25:1006, 1994

KUIPERS EJ et al: Review article: The development of atrophic gastritis— *Helicobacter pylori* and the effects of acid suppressive therapy. Aliment Pharmacol 9:331, 1995

PARSONNET J et al: *Helicobacter pylori* infection and the risk of gastric carcinoma. N Engl J Med 325:1127, 1991

———— et al: *Helicobacter pylori* infection and gastric lymphoma. N Engl J Med 330:1267, 1994

WOLFSEN HC et al: Ménétrier's disease: A form of hypertrophic gastropathy or gastritis? Gastroenterology 104:1310, 1993

ZOLLINGER-ELLISON SYNDROME

GIBRIL F et al: Somatostatin receptor scintigraphy: Its sensitivity compared with that of other imaging methods in detecting primary and metastatic gastrinomas. Ann Intern Med 125:26, 1996

JENSEN RT et al: Zollinger-Ellison syndrome: Advances in the treatment of gastric hypersecretion and the gastrinoma. JAMA 271:1429, 1994

MATON PN: Review article: The management of Zollinger-Ellison syndrome. Aliment Pharmacol Ther 7:467, 1993

METZ DC et al: Use of omeprazole in Zollinger-Ellison syndrome: A prospective nine-year study of efficacy and safety. Aliment Pharmacol Ther 7:597, 1993

PIPELEERS-MARICHAL M et al: Gastrinomas in the duodenums of patients with multiple endocrine neoplasia type 1 and the Zollinger-Ellison syndrome. N Engl J Med 322:723, 1990

PISEGNA JR et al: Effects of curative gastrinoma resection on gastric secretory function and antisecretory drug requirement in the Zollinger-Ellison syndrome. Gastroenterology 102:767, 1992

TERMANINI B et al: Value of somatostatin receptor scintigraphy: A prospective study in gastrinoma of its effects in clinical management. Gastroenterology 112:335, 1997

---

285   *Norton J. Greenberger, Kurt J. Isselbacher*

DISORDERS OF ABSORPTION

MECHANISMS OF ABSORPTION

Diseases of the small intestine are frequently accompanied by alterations in intestinal function, and clinically, this impaired function is seen as the malabsorption syndrome. To obtain a better appreciation of the derangements that occur in the many disorders of intestinal function, the processes of normal absorption will first be reviewed.

It is important to distinguish between digestion and absorption, since an increased loss of nutrients in the stool may reflect a derangement of either process. Digestion involves the breakdown or hydrolysis of nutrients to smaller molecules to prepare the ingested substances for absorption, or transport across the intestinal cell. It will be recalled that most of the digestive process is initiated in the stomach by acid and pepsin and is continued in the upper small intestine primarily by the action of pancreatic enzymes such as lipase, amylase, and trypsin. As a result of these digestive actions, carbohydrates are broken down to monosaccharides and disaccharides, proteins to peptides and amino acids, and fats to monoglycerides and fatty acids. In the adult, it is in this form that nutrients are largely transported across the epithelial surface of the intestinal cell.

ANATOMIC AND PHYSIOLOGIC FACTORS The intestine has an enormous surface area. This fact can be attributed in large part to the length of the intestine, which in the adult is more than 4 m, and to the foldings of the surface plicae. At the light-microscopic level, the villi of the small intestine provide additional surface area, which is further augmented by the presence of microvilli (approximately $2 \times 10^8/cm^2$) on the brush border region of epithelial cells.

Bowel motility is an important process which permits nutrients to remain in intimate contact with the intestinal cells and influences the continued movement of the nutrients into and along the absorbing channels, such as the lymphatics. Two types of motility aid in this process: the gross motility of the intestine itself and the motility of individual villi. The entrance of the nutrients into the general circulation is achieved via the capillaries into the portal system or via the lacteals into the intestinal lymphatics.

TYPES OF ABSORPTION (See also Chap. 42) Four mechanisms have been considered to be important in the transport of substances across the intestinal cell membrane, namely, active transport, passive diffusion, facilitated diffusion, and endocytosis.

Active transport involves the transport of a substance across the cell against an electric or chemical gradient; this process requires energy, is carrier-mediated, and is subject to competitive inhibition. *Passive diffusion* is the opposite of this process; energy is not required, transport is with (rather than against) the electric or chemical gradient, the process is not carrier-mediated, and it does not show properties of competitive inhibition. Thus, active transport may be viewed as "uphill" transport, whereas passive diffusion is equivalent to "downhill" transport. *Facilitated diffusion* is similar to passive diffusion except that it shows evidence of being carrier-mediated and frequently is subject to competitive inhibition.

Endocytosis is a process akin to phagocytosis. By this mechanism, nutrients (dissolved or particulate) are surrounded by the components of the outer plasma cell membrane as they enter the cell. In the intestinal tract, endocytosis occurs in the neonatal period and also to a limited extent in the adult. While quantitatively limited, it appears to account, at least in part, for uptake of antigens.

SITES OF ABSORPTION While many substances are absorbed throughout the length of the small intestine, certain nutrients tend to be absorbed more in one region than in others. The proximal intestine is a major area for the absorption of iron, calcium, water-soluble vitamins, and fat (monoglycerides and fatty acids). Sugars are absorbed in the proximal intestine as well as the midintestine. While amino acids are absorbed primarily in the middle of the small intestine, or jejunum, some absorption also occurs in the upper and lower areas. The distal small intestine is the *major* absorptive area for bile salts and vitamin B_{12}. As is emphasized below, this fact is of clinical significance in circumstances where there has been removal or disease of the ileum.

The colon is important for the absorption of water and electrolytes, a process that occurs predominantly in the cecum. Although the rectum is not a usual site for absorption of ingested nutrients, drugs introduced by rectum may be absorbed there. Thus, drugs introduced by this route, such as salicylates or steroids, may have systemic as well as local effects.

ABSORPTION OF SPECIFIC NUTRIENTS **Carbohydrate Absorption** Much of the carbohydrate we ingest is in the form of starch, a complex polysaccharide consisting of many hexose units. By the action of salivary and pancreatic amylase, starch is hydrolyzed to oligosaccharides and then to disaccharides (mostly maltose). While monosaccharides such as glucose are readily absorbed, disaccharides are not. Disaccharides are split enzymatically into their component sugars by brush border disaccharidases (or oligosaccharidases). The two types of disaccharidases are β-galactosidases (lactase) and α-glucosidases (sucrase, maltase). By the action of these enzymes, lactose is split into glucose and galactose, sucrose into glucose and fructose, and maltose into two molecules of glucose. The resulting monosaccharides are then transported through the cell into the portal circulation. Most disaccharides are hydrolyzed so rapidly by brush border enzymes that the capacity of the transport mechanism is exceeded, and some monosaccharides diffuse back into the intestinal lumen. Lactose, however, is hydrolyzed at a slower rate, and thus lactose hydrolysis is the rate-limiting step in lactose absorption.

Sugars such as glucose and galactose are absorbed by an active transport mechanism. Glucose (and galactose) enter the cell via the Na^+-dependent glucose transporter. Energy is required for the movement of glucose into the cell, and it comes largely from the Na^+,K^+-ATPase of the basolateral membrane (see below).

Protein and Amino Acid Absorption Dietary proteins undergo initial degradation in the stomach by pepsin. However, complete hydrolysis is largely achieved by the action of pancreatic trypsin and chymotrypsin, as well as by other endopeptidases and exopeptidases such as carboxypeptidase. These enzymatic processes yield oligopeptides, dipeptides, and amino acids. Just as there are disaccharidases on the surface of mucosal cells to digest disaccharides, so there are oligopeptidases to split small peptides. However, dipeptidases are located in the cytoplasm as well as on the microvilli. Dipeptides are absorbed more rapidly than amino acids, and presumably their uptake involves a separate mechanism. Thus, digestion of proteins to amino acids occurs in three locations: the intestinal lumen, the brush border, and the cytoplasm of mucosal cells. As indicated above, proteins also can be absorbed by the adult intestine. Although quantitatively limited, protein absorption can be immunologically significant.

Most naturally occurring amino acids are L-amino acids, and these are subject to a number of different transport processes. *Neutral* amino acids share a common carrier mechanism; thus, amino acids such as tryptophan and alanine show competitive inhibition. Among the *dibasic* amino acids that appear to have a distinct transport mechanism are arginine, ornithine, and lysine. The neutral amino acid cystine shares this mechanism. There is a separate transport system for *glycine* and the *imino acids* proline and hydroxyproline. There is also a transport system for *dicarboxylic* acids, such as glutamic and aspartic acids. Therefore, in genetic disorders such as cystinuria, there is impaired absorption not only of cystine but also of arginine, ornithine, and lysine. Similarly, in Hartnup disease, a defect in the transport of neutral amino acids (especially of tryptophan, phenylalanine, and histidine) is found. In these genetic disorders, uptake and absorption of dipeptides is normal (see Chap. 350).

Absorption of amino acids is rapid in the duodenum and jejunum but slow in the ileum. Sodium ions are necessary for the entry of these acids, and energy is needed for their concentration within the cell. Some amino acids have affinity for more than one mechanism. For example, glycine can be transported by both the neutral and the imino acid transport systems.

Fat Absorption (Fig. 285-1) Most of the ingested dietary fats are in the form of long-chain triglycerides. These contain both saturated fatty acids (such as palmitic and stearic) and unsaturated fatty acids (such as oleic and linoleic). The particle size of the fat is decreased largely by the churning action of the stomach. The entry of fat into the duodenum, plus the presence of acid, causes release of secretin and cholecystokinin, which in turn stimulate the flow of bile and pancreatic juice.

Role of pancreatic lipase The hydrolysis of triglycerides by pancreatic lipase is a complex process involving lipase, colipase, and bile salts. Pancreatic lipase binds to the oil-water interface of an emulsified triglyceride substrate. The detergent properties of bile salts permit pancreatic lipase to gain access to water-insoluble lipids. One of the important functions of bile salts is to clear the oil-water interface of dietary fat from proteins of exogenous and endogenous origin, thus making it available for pancreatic lipolysis. Colipase, a protein present in pancreatic juice, is also essential for the action of lipase; its function is to anchor the lipase close to the surface of the triglyceride droplet. All three components—i.e., pancreatic lipase, colipase, and bile salts—form a *ternary complex*, which generates lipolytic products that diffuse away from the complex and are absorbed. With colipase present, lipase remains at the interface and forms 2-monoglycerides and fatty acids, which are the major end products of triglyceride hydrolysis. Less than 5 percent of ingested fat remains in the form of diglycerides and triglycerides. Without colipase, bile acids would actually wash pancreatic lipase away from the interface, and the rate of hydrolysis of triglycerides would be reduced.

Role of bile salts (Fig. 285-2) Bile salts play an important role in the digestion and absorption of fat. They are synthesized from

FIGURE 285-1 Scheme of intestinal digestion, absorption, esterification, and transport of dietary triglycerides. TG, triglycerides; FA, fatty acids; MG, monoglycerides; BS, bile salts.

cholesterol in the liver (in an amount of approximately 200 to 600 mg daily) and are excreted in the bile in the form of their glycine or taurine conjugates. In humans, the principal bile acids excreted are conjugates of cholic and chenodeoxycholic acid. Bile salts are good detergents, because they have both polar (hydrophilic) and nonpolar (hydrophobic) groups. During digestion, the concentration of conjugated bile salts in the lumen is in the range of 5 to 15 μmol/mL, and at these concentrations the bile salts aggregate to form *micelles*. Fatty acids and monoglycerides enter these micelles, forming mixed micelles. An emulsion of triglyceride is turbid; mixed micelles containing bile salts, fatty acids, and monoglycerides form clear solutions. The formation of *mixed micelles*, and hence the solubilization of fatty acids and monoglycerides, is much more effectively achieved with *conjugated bile salts* at the pH normally present in the intestinal lumen (see Fig. 285-2).

Most conjugated bile salts are absorbed in the ileum and, after entering the portal vein, are subject to an enterohepatic circulation. By this process, about 90 percent of the amount of conjugated bile salts reaching the ileum is reabsorbed. As a consequence, only about 200 to 600 mg of bile salts is excreted in the feces per day, even though the 3- to 4-g bile salt pool passes through the enterohepatic circulation many times each day, and, thus, 20 to 30 g of bile salts may enter the duodenum daily. When the enterohepatic circulation is intact, the size of the bile salt pool is determined largely by the rate of the enterohepatic circulation, i.e., the number of cycles occurring per day (see also Chap. 302). If the ileum is diseased or removed, absorption of bile salts is impaired, and a significant fecal loss of bile salts will occur. As a consequence of this bile salt depletion, the concentration of bile salts in the intestinal lumen also will decrease, leading to further impairment of fat absorption. A similar result will occur if bile salt reabsorption is prevented by chelating agents, such as cholestyramine (see "Regional Enteritis," below). Diarrhea per se may result in increased fecal excretion of bile salts. This effect has been demonstrated both in normal subjects in whom diarrhea has been induced and in patients with chronic idiopathic diarrhea.

Intramucosal aspects of fat absorption (Fig. 285-1) After triglycerides have been hydrolysed to fatty acids and monoglycerides and these products have interacted with bile salts to form mixed micelles, the lipids pass through an "unstirred" water layer covering the cell surface. The mixed micelles do not enter the cell; rather, the component fatty acids and monoglycerides are released from the micellar phase and then enter the cell by diffusion. In aqueous duodenal contents, large bile-salt mixed micelles saturated with products of lipolysis coexist with larger liquid crystal liposomes of the same lipids saturated with free fatty acids and mixed bile salts. These phases are interconvertible, and both may be important in fat digestion and absorption. Upon entry into the mucosal cell, fatty acids interact with specific fatty acid binding proteins. The subsequent fate of the intracellular lipid is strongly influenced by the fatty acid chain length. Fatty acids and monoglycerides derived from long-chain triglycerides (i.e., containing C_{16} to C_{18} fatty acids) are promptly *reesterified to triglycerides* by enzymes of the endoplasmic reticulum. These triglycerides then interact with specific apolipoproteins plus cholesterol and phospholipid to form chylomicrons and very low density lipoproteins. These initially accumulate in the Golgi region of the cell and then are secreted into the lacteals and the intestinal lymph. There are thus four major steps in the absorption of long-chain fatty acids and monoglycerides: (1) mucosal uptake and interaction with binding proteins, (2) reesterification to triglycerides, (3) lipoprotein formation, and (4) secretion into lymph.

By contrast, fatty acids derived from medium-chain triglycerides (i.e., those containing C_8 and C_{12} fatty acids) are *not reesterified* to any significant extent within the cell and are not incorporated into lipoproteins. Instead, they rapidly enter the portal venous system, where they are transported as fatty acids bound to albumin. The major aspects of fat absorption are summarized in Fig. 285-1.

Absorption of Cholesterol and Fat-Soluble Vitamins (A, D, E, K) In addition to contributing significantly to the total-body synthesis of cholesterol, the intestine also plays an active role in the absorption of cholesterol and its esters. Within the lumen, cholesterol esters from the bile and diet are hydrolyzed by a pancreatic esterase. There is also a separate cholesterol esterase in the intestinal microvilli which completes this hydrolysis. As a result, only free cholesterol enters the intestinal cell. However, just as in the case of long-chain fatty acids, much of the cholesterol is reesterified and is then secreted primarily into lymph.

The absorption mechanisms of the fat-soluble vitamins A, D, E, and K are not well understood. The intestine is able to convert β-carotene into vitamin A. The vitamin A thus formed or absorbed from the lumen is esterified in the mucosa primarily with palmitic acid, transported in the chylomicrons of the lymph, and stored as retinol palmitate in the liver. The other lipid-soluble vitamins also appear in lymph chylomicrons, but esterification with fatty acids does not appear to be necessary for their transport.

Water and Sodium Absorption (See also Chap. 42) The mechanisms responsible for fluid absorption differ in the jejunum, ileum, and colon. There are two pathways by which water and ions cross the intestinal mucosa: the paracellular and transcellular pathways. Individual intestinal mucosa cells are joined near their apex by a tight junction, and ions and water traverse this *paracellular* pathway during absorption and secretion. The tight-junction pathway contains water-filled channels or pores. Such intercellular spaces are closed in the resting state and dilated during absorption. Considerable evidence has accumulated indicating that pumps and carriers are involved in intestinal water and solute transport. For example, in the ileum, Na^+ enters in exchange for H^+, and Cl^- enters in exchange for HCO_3^-. Sodium entry into the cell also occurs coupled with glucose via the glucose-sodium carrier in the microvillus mem-

FIGURE 285-2 Scheme of hepatic and intestinal metabolism of bile salts and the enterohepatic circulation (from ileum to liver). Note that bacteria lead to the formation of secondary bile acids; of the latter, only deoxycholic acid is absorbed to any appreciable extent.

brane. Inside the cell, the Na^+ pump located in the basolateral membrane actively transports Na^+ out of the mucosal cell and into the intercellular space. *Transcellular* transport requires passage of ions through two membrane barriers, i.e., the apical brush border plasma membrane and the basolateral membrane. After Na^+ and Cl^- are transported across the brush border membrane into the cell, Na^+ is pumped across the basolateral membrane and Cl^- either follows passively or is also pumped into the intercellular space. The Na^+, K^+-ATPase is present in the basolateral but not in the brush border membrane and is the biochemical mediator of this pump. Bulk water movement obviously influences the movement of Na^+, K^+, and Cl^-. This "solvent drag" effect is explained by two mechanisms: (1) solutes may be caught in a moving stream of water and transported across a membrane, and (2) water movement results in increased concentration of solute on the side of the membrane from which water was transported, which causes solute to diffuse through the direction of flow. Diarrhea can be simply defined as impaired net absorption of water and electrolytes by the small intestine or colon. Some mechanisms producing diarrhea are listed in Table 285-1. The response to fasting is a practical way to distinguish secretory from osmotic diarrhea; stool volumes do not decrease with fasting in secretory diarrhea, whereas a reduction in stool volumes to under 300 g/d is characteristic of osmotic diarrhea. Steatorrheic stools are usually less than 700 g/d.

Calcium Absorption Calcium is actively transported by the small intestine, and this process is intimately linked to the active form of vitamin D_3, namely, 1,25-dihydroxycholecalciferol. The role of two other intestinal cell proteins, calcium-binding protein and calmodulin, in the absorption of calcium remains unclear. Recent studies indicate that calcium is absorbed to the same extent from various calcium salts (carbonate, citrate, gluconate, lactate, and acetate) and from milk in healthy subjects; an average of 32 percent of the ingested calcium was absorbed from the various sources.

Iron Absorption The formation of soluble iron complexes is important for maintaining intraluminal iron in an absorbable form. Gastric acid facilitates the chelation of inorganic iron with substances such as ascorbic acid, sugars, amino acids, and bile; these macromolecular complexes then remain soluble in the more alkaline duodenum and jejunum. In the average western diet, the iron intake averages 15 to 25 mg/d; iron absorption averages 0.5 to 1.0 mg/d in men and 1.0 to 2.0 mg/d in women during their reproductive years. Iron is actively transported by the small intestine, with the duodenum being the principal site of iron absorption. The transferrin receptor and also duodenal ferritin in small intestinal mucosal cells appear to have a regulatory/inhibitory role in iron absorption. The absorption of elemental iron in humans and animals involves at least two distinct steps: (1) mucosal uptake of iron from the lumen and (2) mucosal transfer of iron to the plasma. Much of the iron entering the mucosal cell is not transferred to the plasma but remains trapped in the cell and is excreted into the lumen when the cell is shed. The amount of iron lost by this mechanism seems to vary inversely with body iron stores. However, this mucosal regulatory mechanism can be overcome when pharmacologic doses of iron are ingested. Hemoglobin iron is also absorbed by human subjects in amounts that depend on body requirements for iron; the heme is split from globin in the lumen and absorbed as an intact metalloporphyrin. Organic iron in the form of hemoglobin is absorbed more effectively than iron from cereals and vegetables. The absorption of inorganic iron is increased by ascorbic acid. Similarly, the presence of anemia, liver injury, pregnancy, idiopathic hemochromatosis, or a portacaval shunt may result in increased iron absorption. Conversely, the prior ingestion of large doses of iron and the presence in the lumen of phosphates, carbonates, and phytates may lead to decreased absorption of inorganic iron. Impaired absorption of iron is frequent in disorders (such as celiac sprue) which involve the duodenal mucosa.

Water-Soluble Vitamins *Vitamin B_{12} absorption* is discussed in Chap. 108. In the case of *folic acid absorption*, it should be emphasized that folates exist in food conjugated with glutamyl peptides. These *polyglutamates* must be deconjugated (by folic deconjugase) to monoglutamates for absorption to occur. Certain drugs (such as oral

contraceptives, sulfasalazine, diphenylhydantoin, trimethoprim, and pyrimethamine) inhibit the absorption of dietary folate and hence can cause folate deficiency. Sulfasalazine, for example, competitively inhibits three enzymes important in the intestinal metabolism of folate: dihydrofolate reductase, methylene tetrahydrofolate reductase, and serine transhydroxymethylase. Thiamine and riboflavin appear to be absorbed by passive diffusion.

TESTS USEFUL IN THE DIAGNOSIS OF MALABSORPTION Most of the tests useful in the diagnosis of malabsorption indicate the presence of abnormal absorptive or digestive function, and only a few tests may suggest a specific diagnosis. Accordingly, it is frequently necessary to employ a combination of tests to establish a diagnosis. To illustrate the use of various tests, the characteristic

Table 285-1

Some Mechanisms in the Production of Diarrhea

SECRETORY DIARRHEA

Secretory agents associated with adenylate cyclase system
  Enterotoxin-producing bacteria (*Vibrio cholerae, Escherichia coli*)
  Methylxanthines (caffeine, theophylline)
  Prostaglandins
  Vasoactive intestinal peptide (VIP)
  Dihydroxy bile acids (affect colon primarily; effects seen after ileal resection)
Secretory agents *not associated* with adenylate cyclase system
  Glucagon, secretin, cholecystokinin-pancreozymin, serotonin, calcitonin, gastric inhibitory polypeptide (GIP)
  Some laxatives* (ricinoleic acid, bisacodyl, phenolphthalein, dioctyl sodium sulfosuccinate)
  Bacterial enterotoxins (*Shigella, Staphylococcus aureus, Clostridium perfringens*)
Mucosal injury, altered cell permeability
  Salmonella, Shigella, invasive *E. coli*, gastroenteritis viruses
  Celiac sprue
  Inflammatory bowel disease (ulcerative colitis, regional enteritis)
Neoplasms with or without hormone production
  Gastrinoma (gastrin)
  Carcinoid syndrome (serotonin, prostaglandins)
  Medullary carcinoma of thyroid (calcitonin, prostaglandins)
  Pancreatic cholera syndrome (VIP)
  Villous adenoma
Medications
  Diuretics
  Theophylline
  Colchicine
  Prostaglandins (misoprostol)
  Azodisalicylate
Congenital
  Microvillus inclusion disease
  Congenital chloridorrhea

OSMOTIC DIARRHEA

Impaired carbohydrate absorption
  Disaccharidase deficiency (lactose or sucrose-isomaltose intolerance)
  Glucose-galactose malabsorption
Nonabsorbable osmotically active agents (lactulose, sorbitol, mannitol, dietetic foods)
Laxative ingestion or abuse
  Saline purgatives (magnesium phosphate, magnesium hydroxide–containing antacids)
Postoperative disorders
  Vagotomy and pyloroplasty*
  Gastrojejunostomy* (Billroth I and II)

MOTILITY DISORDERS

Laxative abuse*
Irritable bowel syndrome
Diverticular disease of the colon
Diabetic diarrhea with visceral neuropathy
Hyperthyroidism

* Multiple mechanisms involved in production of diarrhea.

findings in celiac sprue, an example of a primary malabsorptive disorder, and pancreatic insufficiency, an example of impaired digestion, are compared in Table 285-2.

Stool Fat The qualitative examination of the stool for undigested muscle fibers, neutral fat, and split fat is a simple and reliable screening test for steatorrhea. The finding of an increased number of muscle fibers indicates impaired intraluminal digestion. Properly performed, the qualitative microscopic examination of a stool specimen with the Sudan III stain is of value and correlates well with the quantitative determination of fecal fat. The latter remains the most reliable measurement of steatorrhea. Normal fecal fat excretion is less than 6 g for 24 h, representing a coefficient of fat absorption of >94 percent. It has been demonstrated that diarrhea itself can induce mild secondary steatorrhea. When the quantitative fecal fat test is used in patients with diarrhea, mild abnormalities (up to 14 g/d) are not specific for a primary defect in fat digestion or absorption, i.e., they may represent false-positive results.

Although not used frequently, oral [^{14}C]triolein can be used as an effective test for fat absorption. During the digestive process, the triolein is hydrolyzed, and the labeled glycerol is absorbed and metabolized by the liver. The $^{14}CO_2$ produced is exhaled and can then be measured hourly (for 6 h) in the expired air. Normally, more than 3.5 percent of the administered label [0.185 MBq (5 μCi)] appears in the breath per hour.

Xylose Absorption In the most commonly employed test of carbohydrate absorption, the patient ingests 25 g D-xylose. A 5-h urine xylose excretion of 26 mmol (4.0 g) or greater is considered normal. Low values may be obtained in patients with ascites, intestinal bacterial overgrowth, or renal insufficiency; after the administration of certain drugs (e.g., aspirin, indomethacin); and, most commonly, if the urine collection is incomplete. To prevent difficulties in interpreting the test, it is advisable to determine the blood xylose level 2 h after ingestion of xylose. A blood xylose level of 2 mmol/L (30 mg/dL) or greater indicates normal absorption of D-xylose. Abnormal D-xylose absorption is found most frequently in disorders affecting the mucosa of the proximal small intestine, such as celiac sprue and tropical sprue.

Gastrointestinal X-Ray Studies All patients with malabsorption should have radiographic examinations of the small intestine and, in many cases, of the esophagus, stomach, and colon as well. Occasionally, the latter two examinations may provide important clues to the presence of such disorders as celiac sprue, scleroderma, Zollinger-Ellison syndrome, regional enteritis, ulcerative colitis, and intestinal fistulas. Traditional radiographic findings suggesting a diagnosis of malabsorption include flocculation of barium in fluid-filled loops, which causes fragmentation and segmentation of the barium column. However, these patterns are no longer demonstrated reliably in small-bowel series because of the widespread use of barium products that contain a nonflocculating suspension of micropulverized barium sulfate. In celiac sprue, the most consistent abnormalities are thickened and nodular duodenal folds and dilation of the small bowel. However, these findings are nonspecific and may be found in several of the disorders listed in Table 285-3. Some representative examples of abnormal small-bowel radiographs are shown in Fig. 285-3.

Small-Intestinal Biopsy The most commonly used instrument for obtaining peroral biopsy specimens from the small intestine is the upper gastrointestinal endoscope, which has largely superseded the use of the Crosby, Carey, and Ross-Moore biopsy capsules. Examination of small bowel biopsy specimens is of considerable value in the differential diagnosis of malabsorptive disorders. Table 285-3 lists disorders associated with abnormalities in intestinal biopsies, and Fig. 285-4 depicts some illustrative lesions.

Schilling Test for Vitamin B_{12} Absorption The Schilling test is valuable in the differential diagnosis of malabsorption and is frequently carried out in three stages: (1) without intrinsic factor, (2) with intrinsic factor, and (3) after a course of treatment with antibiotics or anti-inflammatory drugs. Since vitamin B_{12} is absorbed primarily in the

distal ileum, an abnormal response to a Schilling test may indicate a pathologic condition of the distal small bowel. In disorders affecting the terminal ileum, such as regional enteritis and lymphomas, the first- and second-stage Schilling tests are frequently abnormal. The ileal receptor site appears to be damaged in these disorders, and the impaired absorption of B_{12} is not corrected by the addition of intrinsic factor or the use of antibiotics. However, the Schilling test response may normalize after treatment with prednisone or sulfasalazine. The Schilling test also may be useful in establishing a diagnosis of intestinal bacterial overgrowth of the small bowel, as in disorders such as blind loop syndrome, scleroderma, and multiple small-bowel diverticula (see below). In the blind loop syndrome, for example, the bacteria can actually take up vitamin B_{12}, with resultant impaired absorption of B_{12}. Under these conditions, the first-stage Schilling test frequently gives an abnormal result, as does the second-stage test. After appropriate antibiotic treatment, the Schilling test response usually returns to normal. Vitamin B_{12} absorption is frequently abnormal in patients with exocrine pancreatic insufficiency (see Chap. 304).

Secretin and Other Pancreatic Tests The secretin test, secretin cholecystokinin test, intraduodenal perfusion with essential amino acids, and bentiromide test, which may be useful in establishing a diagnosis of pancreatic insufficiency, are discussed in detail in Chap. 303.

Serum Calcium, Albumin, Cholesterol, Magnesium, and Iron Abnormal serum calcium, albumin, cholesterol, magnesium, and iron values may be found in several malabsorptive disorders. The primary value of such findings is to suggest abnormal absorption. These tests are usually of limited value in the *differential diagnosis* of malabsorption, but an abnormal result may be helpful in supporting this diagnosis.

Serum Carotenes, Vitamin A, and Prothrombin Time Absorption of the fat-soluble vitamins A, D, K, and E is frequently impaired in patients with steatorrhea. Measurements of serum carotene and vitamin A levels are useful as screening tests for malabsorption. However, other tests not only are more sensitive but often give more specific information than the serum carotene and vitamin A levels. The blood prothrombin time is an important test, since patients with malabsorption may present with abnormal bleeding due to vitamin K deficiency. If the decreased prothrombin activity is due to malabsorption, it should be readily correctable with parenteral vitamin K.

Breath Tests The bile acid breath test utilizing [^{14}C]cholylglycine is a reasonably reliable screening test for bacterial overgrowth syndromes. Approximately two-thirds of patients with a positive small-bowel culture will have an abnormal bile acid breath test. However, in patients with suspected malabsorption of bile acids, the test is rather insensitive without the additional determination of fecal bile acid excretion. The excretion of breath hydrogen after ingestion of lactose is a sensitive, specific, and noninvasive test for detecting lactase deficiency. Lactulose and [^{14}C]xylose breath tests for bacterial overgrowth also have been found helpful.

PATHOPHYSIOLOGIC BASIS FOR SYMPTOMS AND SIGNS IN MALABSORPTIVE DISORDERS The common symptoms and signs found in malabsorptive disorders are listed in Table 285-4. The most frequent symptoms are those of malnutrition, weight loss, and diarrhea. However, in each of the clinical settings listed in Table 285-4, it is important to consider the cause of the malabsorption.

DISORDERS OF MALABSORPTION
See Table 285-5

INADEQUATE DIGESTION   Liver and Biliary Tract Disease It is not generally appreciated that patients with acute or chronic liver disease may develop malabsorption owing to impaired intraluminal digestion. Steatorrhea has been described in acute viral hepatitis, chronic extrahepatic biliary tract obstruction, primary biliary cirrhosis, and postnecrotic and nutritional cirrhosis. Absorption of D-xylose and vitamin B_{12} is usually normal, and small-intestinal mucosal biopsy specimens are generally unremarkable. The steatorrhea associated with

Table 285-2

Tests Useful in the Diagnosis of Malabsorptive Disorders

Test	Normal Values	Typical Findings Malabsorption (Celiac Sprue)	Typical Findings Maldigestion (Pancreatic Insufficiency)	Comment
Quantitative determination of stool fat	<6 g per 24 h: >95% coefficient of fat absorption	>6 g per 24 h	>6 g per 24 h	Best test for establishing presence of steatorrhea
Carbohydrate absorption				
D-Xylose absorption (25-g oral dose)	5-h urinary excretion >26 mmol (>4.5 g); peak blood level >2.0 mmol/L (>30 mg/dL)	↓	Normal	A good screening test for carbohydrate malabsorption
Small-intestine x-rays		Malabsorption pattern	Normal or minimal malabsorption pattern; occasionally pancreatic calcification	
Blood tests				
Serum calcium	2.2–2.7 mmol/L (9–11 mg/dL)	Frequently ↓	Usually normal	
Serum albumin	35–55 g/L (3.5–5.5 g/dL)	Frequently ↓	Usually normal	Decreased levels of both serum albumin and globulins should raise the question of protein-losing enteropathy
Serum cholesterol	3.90–6.45 mmol/L (150–250 mg/dL)	↓	Frequently ↓	Usually decreased in disorders associated with significant steatorrhea
Serum iron	14–24 μmol/L (80–150 μg/dL)	Frequently ↓	Normal	Low values may reflect decreased body iron stores
Serum magnesium	0.6–1.0 mmol/L (1.2–2.0 mEq/L)	Frequently ↓	Usually normal	
Serum zinc	12–20 μmol/L	Frequently ↓	Usually normal	Decreased levels common in malnutrition, cirrhosis, and malabsorption
Serum carotenes	>100 IU/dL	↓	Usually ↓	Fairly satisfactory screening tests for malabsorption
Serum vitamin A	>100 IU/dL	↓		
Prothrombin time	70–100%; 12–15 s	Frequently ↑	Frequently ↑ (prolonged)	
Small intestinal mucosal biopsy		Abnormal	Normal	A specific diagnosis can be established in a small number of disorders (see text)
Urine tests				
Vitamin B_{12} absorption	>8% urinary excretion in 48 h	Frequently ↓	Frequently ↓	Useful in determining whether vitamin B_{12} malabsorption is due to gastric or small-intestinal disorders or to pancreatic insufficiency
Urine 5-hydroxyindoleacetic acid (5-HIAA)	10–47 μmol per 24 h (2–9 mg per 24 h)	↑	Normal	Slightly increased level (12–16 mg per 24 h) characteristically found in celiac sprue
Breath tests				
Breath H_2 (after 50 g lactose)	Minimal breath H_2	May be ↑	Normal	Secondary to lactase deficiency (see text)
Breath H_2 (after 10 g lactulose)	Minimal breath H_2	May be normal or ↓	Normal	Early peak in bacterial overgrowth; can be used to determine intestinal transit time
Breath $^{14}CO_2$ (after [^{14}C]xylose)	Minute amounts $^{14}CO_2$	May be ↓	Usually normal	Increased in bacterial overgrowth
Glycocholic acid metabolism (oral glycine-1-[^{14}C]glycocholate)	<1% of dose excreted $^{14}CO_2$ in 4 h	Normal	Normal	Increased $^{14}CO_2$ excretion with bacterial overgrowth or bile acid malabsorption (due to ileal resection or inflammatory disease)
	<4% of dose excreted in stools	Normal	Normal	Increased fecal excretion of ^{14}C in bile acid malabsorption
[^{14}C]triolein absorption (breath test)	>3.5% of dose as breath $^{14}CO_2$ per hour	↓	↓	Correlates well with chemical stool fat; recently introduced test
Miscellaneous				
Bacteria (culture)	<10^3 organisms per milliliter	Normal	Normal	>10^5 organisms per milliliter indicates bacterial overgrowth
Secretin test	Volume >1.8 (mL/kg)/h Bicarbonate concentration >80 mmol/L	Normal	Abnormal	See discussion of pancreatic insufficiency in Chaps. 303 and 304
Bentiromide test	Urine excretion arylamines ≥50%	May be abnormal	Abnormal	See discussion of pancreatic disease in Chaps. 303 and 304

Table 285-3

Disorders Associated with Abnormalities in Small-Bowel Biopsy Specimens

BIOPSY HAS DIAGNOSTIC VALUE (DIFFUSE LESIONS)

Whipple's disease: Lamina propria infiltrated with macrophages containing PAS-positive glycoproteins
Abetalipoproteinemia: Villus structure normal; epithelial cells vacuolated due to excess fat
Agammaglobuinemia: Flattened or absent villi; increased lymphocyte infiltration; absence of plasma cells
Mycobacterium avium complex

BIOPSY MAY HAVE DIAGNOSTIC VALUE (PATCHY LESIONS)

Intestinal lymphoma: Infiltration of lamina propria and submucosa with malignant cells
Intestinal lymphangiectasia: Dilated lacteals and lymphatics in lamina propria; clubbed villi
Eosinophilic enteritis: Diffuse or patchy eosinophilic infiltration in lamina propria and mucosa
Amyloidosis: Presence of amyloid confirmed by special stains
Regional enteritis: Noncaseating granulomas
Parasitic infestations: Parasitic invasion of mucosa; adherence of trophozoites to mucosal surface, as in giardiasis
Systemic mastocytosis: Mast cell infiltration of lamina propria

BIOPSY IS ABNORMAL BUT NOT DIAGNOSTIC

Celiac sprue: Shortened or absent villi; hypertrophied crypts; damaged surface epithelium; mononuclear infiltrate
"Collagenous" sprue: Indistinguishable from celiac sprue; extensive subepithelial collagen deposition
Tropical sprue: Lesion similar to celiac sprue with shortened or absent villi; lymphocyte infiltration
Folate deficiency: Shortened villi; megalocytosis; decreased mitoses in crypts
Vitamin B_{12} deficiency: Similar to folate deficiency
Acute radiation enteritis: Similar to folate deficiency
Systemic scleroderma: Fibrosis around Brunner's glands
Bacterial overgrowth syndromes: Patchy damage to villi and increased lymphocyte infiltration

liver and biliary tract disease is thought to be due to impaired hepatic synthesis or excretion of conjugated bile salts, resulting in impaired formation of micellar lipid. In addition to steatorrhea, patients with liver disease may have impaired absorption of vitamin D and calcium, resulting in severe metabolic bone disease. This is particularly common in patients with primary biliary cirrhosis. Skeletal roentgenograms may show increased porosity of bone, cortical thinning, vertebral compression, and spontaneous pathologic fractures. Patients with alcohol-induced liver disease also may have exocrine pancreatic insufficiency. Accordingly, pancreatic function should be evaluated in patients with liver disease and malabsorption.

Postgastrectomy Malabsorption The presence of a malabsorption syndrome has been documented frequently in patients after subto-

B

A

C

FIGURE 285-3 *A*. Radiograph of a normal small intestine showing good mucosal pattern. *B*. Intestinal radiograph of a patient with celiac sprue. Note dilation of small bowel, lack of mucosal markings, and segmentation and clumping of barium. *C*. Intestinal radiograph of patient with obstructed lymphatics due to Köhlmeier-Degos disease, with "accordion-pleated" pattern (lower edge).

FIGURE 285-4 Typical peroral intestinal biopsy specimens. *A.* Jejunal mucosa of patient with celiac sprue. Note virtual absence of villi, elongated crypts (some cut in cross section), mononuclear infiltrate, and cuboidal instead of columnar epithelium on top of villi (300×). *B.* Biopsy specimen from the same patient as in *A*, after 9 months on a gluten-free diet. Note reappearance of villi with normal-appearing columnar cells and reduction in infiltrate and crypt height (300×). *C.* Biopsy specimen from patient with agammaglobulinemia. The features bear a striking resemblance to those of celiac sprue. There is a marked mononuclear infiltration, some of it in aggregates (200×). *D.* Close-up of villi of patient with protein-losing enteropathy. Note broadened and dilated tips, and lymphatic spaces (*arrows*). (450×). *E.* Intestinal biopsy specimen from patient with abetalipoproteinemia. The villus tips have a "lacy" appearance (*arrow*) due to retained fat (300×). *F.* High-power micrograph of villus in *E*. Vacuoles are filled with lipid (750×). Insert shows dark-staining (osmium) lipid droplets in mucosal cells (osmium counterstained with Giemsa; 800×).

Table 285-4

Pathophysiologic Basis for Symptoms and Signs in Malabsorptive Disorders

Symptom or Sign	Pathophysiology
GASTROINTESTINAL	
Generalized malnutrition and weight loss	Malabsorption of fat, carbohydrate, and protein → loss of calories, anorexia
Diarrhea	Impaired absorption or increased secretion of water and electrolytes; unabsorbed dihydroxy bile acids and fatty acids → decreased absorption of water and electrolytes; excess load of fluid and electrolytes presented to the colon may exceed its absorptive capacity
Flatus	Bacterial fermentation of unabsorbed carbohydrate
Glossitis, cheilosis, stomatitis	Deficiency of iron, vitamin B_{12}, folate, and other vitamins
Abdominal pain	Distention or inflammation of bowel, chronic pancreatitis
GENITOURINARY	
Nocturia	Delayed absorption of water, hypokalemia
Azotemia, hypotension	Fluid and electrolyte depletion
Amenorrhea, ↓ libido	Protein depletion and "caloric starvation" → secondary hypopituitarism
HEMATOPOIETIC	
Anemia	Impaired absorption of iron, vitamin B_{12}, folic acid, and pyridoxine
Hemorrhagic phenomena	Vitamin K malabsorption → hypoprothrombinemia
MUSCULOSKELETAL	
Bone pain	Protein depletion → impaired bone formation → osteoporosis; Calcium malabsorption → demineralization of bone → osteomalacia; Vitamin D malabsorption
Osteoarthropathy	Cause uncertain
Tetany, paresthesias	Calcium malabsorption → hypocalcemia; magnesium malabsorption → hypomagnesemia
Weakness	Anemia: electrolyte depletion (hypokalemia)
NERVOUS SYSTEM	
Night blindness	Impaired absorption vitamin A → vitamin A deficiency
Xerophthalmia	Vitamin A deficiency
Peripheral neuropathy	Vitamin B_{12}, thiamine deficiency
SKIN	
Eczema	Cause uncertain
Purpura	Vitamin K deficiency
Follicular hyperkeratosis and dermatitis	Deficiency of vitamin A, zinc, essential fatty acids, and other vitamins

tal gastrectomy. Steatorrhea is more common with a Billroth II than a Billroth I type of anastomosis. Usually the fat loss is minimal, ranging from 7 to 10 g per 24 h. Patients with gross steatorrhea usually have impaired intraluminal fat digestion due to several factors, as follows. (1) With a Billroth II anastomosis the duodenum is bypassed, and there is a decreased entry of stomach contents into the proximal duodenum (i.e., the afferent loop). This leads to a decreased stimulus for the release of *secretin* and *cholecystokinin* (CCK) from the duodenum and may result in a depressed pancreatic enzyme response. (2) There may be *inadequate mixing* of the pancreatic enzymes and bile

Table 285-5

Classification of the Malabsorption Syndromes

Inadequate digestion
 Postgastrectomy steatorrhea*
 Deficiency or inactivation of pancreatic lipase
  Exocrine pancreatic insufficiency
   Chronic pancreatitis
   Pancreatic carcinoma
   Cystic fibrosis
   Pancreatic resection
  Gastrinoma (Zollinger-Ellison syndrome)*
Reduced intestinal bile salt concentration (with impaired micelle formation)
 Liver disease
  Parenchymal liver disease
  Cholestasis (intrahepatic or extrahepatic)
 Abnormal bacterial proliferation in the small bowel
  Afferent loop stasis
  Strictures
  Fistulas
  Blind loops
  Multiple diverticula of the small bowel
  Hypomotility states (diabetes, scleroderma, intestinal pseudoobstruction)
 Interrupted enterohepatic circulation of bile sales
  Ileal resection
  Ileal inflammatory disease (Crohn's disease)
 Drugs (by sequestration or precipitation of bile salts)
  Neomycin
  Calcium carbonate
  Cholestyramine
Inadequate absorptive surface
 Intestinal resection or bypass
  Mesenteric vascular disease with massive intestinal resection
  Regional enteritis with multiple bowel resections
  Jejunoileal bypass
  Gastroileostomy (inadvertent)
Lymphatic obstruction
 Intestinal lymphangiectasia
 Lymphoma
Cardiovascular disorders
 Constrictive pericarditis
 Congestive heart failure
 Mesenteric vascular insufficiency
 Vasculitis
Primary mucosal absorptive defects
 Inflammatory, infiltrative disorders or infection
  Crohn's disease*
  Amyloidosis
  Scleroderma*
  Lymphoma*
  Radiation enteritis
  Eosinophilic enteritis
  Tropical sprue
  Infective enteritis (e.g., salmonellosis)
  Collagenous sprue
  Whipple's disease
  Nonspecific ulcerative jejunitis
  Mastocytosis
  Dermatologic disorders (e.g., dermatitis herpetiformis)
 Biochemical or genetic abnormalities
  Celiac sprue (gluten-induced enteropathy)
  Disaccharidase deficiency
  Hypogammaglobulinemia
  Abetalipoproteinemia
  Hartnup disease
  Cystinuria
  Monosaccharide malabsorption
Endocrine and metabolic disorders
 Diabetes mellitus*
 Hypoparathyrodism
 Adrenal insufficiency
 Hyperthyroidism
 Gastrinoma (Zollinger-Ellison syndrome)*
 Carcinoid syndrome

* Malabsorption caused by multiple defects.

salts secreted into the proximal duodenum with the gastric contents entering the jejunum. (3) There may be *stasis* of intestinal contents in the afferent loop, resulting in abnormal bacterial proliferation in the proximal small bowel. This in turn may lead to abnormalities in bile salt metabolism (see "Pathophysiology" under "Malabsorption Due to Bacterial Overgrowth of the Small Bowel," below). (4) The presence of maldigestion may lead to *protein depletion*, which in turn may produce further impairment in pancreatic function. (5) The *loss of the reservoir function of the stomach* may result in decreased intestinal transit time. Perhaps the most important factor is rapid gastric emptying, which results in low luminal concentrations of digestive secretions for the first 60 to 80 min after a meal. Such a disorder has been described in patients with subtotal gastrectomy and duodenostomy (Billroth I), gastrojejunostomy (Billroth II), and truncal vagotomy and pyloroplasty (V&P). That gastric emptying rates are somewhat slower in patients with V&P may account for the overall less severe nutritional deficiencies in such patients. In some patients, treatment with pancreatic enzymes leads to significant improvement. Specimens of duodenal or jejunal fluid should be obtained for culture of both aerobic and anaerobic organisms, and appropriate antibiotic therapy should be instituted if there is evidence of abnormal bacterial overgrowth (a colony count of $>10^5$/mL in jejunal fluid). Because the duodenum is the principal site of absorption of iron and calcium, in patients with a Billroth II anastomosis, impaired absorption of calcium and iron also may develop. Occult metabolic bone disease occurs frequently in this setting.

INADEQUATE ABSORPTIVE SURFACE (SHORT-BOWEL SYNDROME) Extensive intestinal resection often results in the short-bowel syndrome. The most common disorders resulting in this syndrome are (1) massive intestinal resection following a vascular insult to the small intestine, (2) regional enteritis with multiple bowel resections, and (3) a jejunoileal bypass for morbid obesity. In general, the absorption of nutrients will be influenced by the extent and site of small bowel resected, the presence of the ileocecal valve, and adaptation of the remaining small bowel. Resection of 40 to 50 percent of the small bowel is usually well tolerated, provided the proximal duodenum, the distal half of the ileum, and the ileocecal valve are spared. By contrast, resection of the ileum and the ileocecal valve alone may induce severe diarrhea and malabsorption, even though less than 30 percent of the small intestine is resected.

Several measures are important in the management of short-bowel syndrome: (1) The diet should contain at least 2500 kcal and consist primarily of carbohydrate and protein, with fat restricted to less than 40 g/d. A fat-restricted diet is effective in reducing diarrhea, presumably because there is decreased production of hydroxy fatty acids from long-chain fats. Such hydroxy fatty acids, in essence, are cathartics and increase net secretion of water and electrolytes by the colon as well as the small bowel. (2) It is often necessary to provide vitamin and mineral supplements, which usually include K^+, Cl^-, Mg^{2+}, Ca^{2+}, trace metals (Zn, Cd, Mn), iron, folate, vitamin B_{12}, other vitamins (A, D, E, K, B_1, B_2, B_6, biotin), and essential fatty acids. (3) Specific drugs (e.g., belladonna alkaloids, diphenoxylate, loperamide, and codeine) that decrease intestinal motility and prolong mucosal contact time are helpful in controlling diarrhea. These agents also decrease ileostomy outputs. (4) A bile salt–sequestering agent such as cholestyramine blunts the effects of bile salts, which stimulate net secretion of water and electrolytes by the colon. (5) Patients with short-bowel syndrome may have gastric acid hypersecretion, which is often transient and which results in dilution of pancreatic secretions as well as inactivation of pancreatic enzymes. Under these conditions, a histamine H_2 receptor antagonist or proton pump inhibitor is useful because it will suppress gastric acid secretion and decrease the volume of fluid entering the proximal small bowel, thus leading to an increased concentration of pancreatic enzymes. In addition, supplemental pancreatic enzyme therapy may be required. (6) A bypassed colon can be used to receive infusions of fluid and electrolytes, since a portion of the colon can still absorb 1000 to 1500 mL fluid per day. (7) Octreotide, a long-acting somatostatin analogue, reduces digestive secretions (biliary and pancreatic secretions and succus entericus) and thus

may ameliorate diarrhea. Finally, (8) total parenteral nutrition is frequently required during the first 6 months after massive intestinal resection, until some degree of adaptation has occurred. Such patients also may require long-term parenteral hyperalimentation with a silicone rubber catheter in the superior vena cava; this can be done at home.

→ *For a discussion of regional enteritis see Chap. 286.*

MALABSORPTION DUE TO BACTERIAL OVERGROWTH OF THE SMALL BOWEL The proximal small intestine is usually bacteriologically sterile because of three factors: (1) the acid milieu of the stomach, (2) intestinal peristalsis, which sweeps bacteria to the distal small bowel, and (3) secretion into the lumen of the intestine of immunoglobulins, which may serve as coproantibodies. When bacteria are isolated from the upper small bowel, they are frequently contaminants transported from the mouth and upper respiratory tract, and the colony count rarely exceeds 10^4 per milliliter of jejunal fluid. The major mechanism limiting the growth of bacteria in the small intestine is normal peristalsis. Any disorder leading to impaired intestinal motility may result in abnormal stasis of intestinal contents with ineffective mechanical cleansing of bacteria. This, in turn, may lead to abnormal bacterial proliferation and malabsorption. An intact ileocecal valve prevents reflux of colonic bacteria; loss of the ileocecal valve, as in the case of ileocecal resection, facilitates bacterial proliferation in the small bowel. Several malabsorptive disorders have been associated with bacterial overgrowth of the small bowel, and these are listed in Table 285-6.

Pathophysiology Bacterial overgrowth may result in changes in bile salt metabolism, leading directly and indirectly to steatorrhea. First, bacteria (especially anaerobic gram-positive bacteria) may lead to the intraluminal deconjugation of bile salts, with a consequent production of free bile acids. In contrast to conjugated bile salts, unconjugated bile salts may be absorbed in the proximal small bowel by nonionic diffusion, resulting in decreased intraluminal concentrations of bile salts in the jejunum. Second, the decreased bile salt concentrations, the increase of unconjugated bile salts, and the decrease of the conjugated salts all serve to contribute to impaired intraluminal micelle formation and hence fat malabsorption. In addition to these abnormalities, intestinal mucosal lesions have been demonstrated in patients with intestinal stasis. Such lesions are often patchy in distribu-

Table 285-6

Causes of Intestinal Bacterial Overgrowth (Intestinal Colonization)

Structural abnormalities producing stasis of intestinal contents
 Multiple small-bowel diverticula
 Strictures
  Crohn's disease*
  Radiation enteritis*
  Occlusive vascular disease: vasculitis
 Billroth II subtotal gastrectomy with afferent loop stasis*
 Multiple laparotomies resulting in adhesions and partial small-bowel
  obstruction
Fistulas: Gastrocolic, gastroileal, jejunoileal, jejunocolic
Motor abnormalities resulting in intestinal hypomotility
 Scleroderma*
 Amyloidosis*
 Diabetes mellitus*
 Hypothyroidism
 Vagotomy
 Intestinal pseudoobstruction (see Table 285-7)
Miscellaneous
 Hypogammaglobulinemia*
 Nodular lymphoid hyperplasia
 Pancreatic insufficiency
 Gastric hypochlorhydria/achlorhydria
  Subtotal gastrectomy
  Pernicious anemia
  Prolonged use of H_2 receptor antagonists, proton pump inhibitors

* No underlying disorder detected.

tion, and the histologic appearance ranges in severity from minimal changes in villous architecture to severe lesions with virtual absence of villi. The cause of these lesions is unclear; possible causes include damage caused by bacterial invasion, bacterial toxins, or metabolic products such as unconjugated bile salts. In this regard, certain bacteria such as *Bacteroides* elaborate proteases that solubilize brush border proteins and destroy disaccharidases such as sucrase and maltase. The impaired absorption of vitamin B_{12} is not related to the disturbed bile salt metabolism but appears to be due to uptake of vitamin B_{12} by microorganisms.

Many of the preceding abnormalities in bile salt metabolism may be reversed by appropriate antibiotic therapy. When such treatment is instituted, the level of unconjugated bile salts in the jejunal fluid decreases, the amount of micellar lipid phase increases, and steatorrhea diminishes or disappears. In addition, significant improvement in the absorption of vitamin B_{12} occurs with the use of broad-spectrum antibiotics such as tetracycline.

Clinical Manifestations Breath tests—i.e., tests with ^{14}C-labeled bile acid, [^{14}C]xylose, or lactulose—are useful screening tests for malabsorption syndromes due to abnormal bacterial overgrowth of the small intestine. The 2-h 50-g glucose breath hydrogen test reliably predicts the presence of bacterial overgrowth; a positive test is characterized by a rise in breath hydrogen of at least 12 parts per million (ppm) within 2 h of a 50-g glucose challenge *and* a high fasting breath hydrogen level of at least 15 ppm. A definitive diagnosis is established by demonstrating larger numbers of microorganisms (greater than 10^5/mL) and a polymicrobial flora in cultures of duodenal or jejunal fluid or in cultures of an unwashed mucosal biopsy specimen, especially when luminal secretions are scanty. Other clinical features include the following: (1) a moderate steatorrhea, usually in the range of 15 to 30 g fecal fat per 24 h, (2) macrocytic anemia with a megaloblastic bone marrow, (3) impaired absorption of vitamin B_{12} that is not corrected by intrinsic factor, and (4) correction of steatorrhea and impaired vitamin B_{12} absorption by antibiotic therapy. Absorption of D-xylose, peroral small-intestinal biopsy specimens, and results of other tests of absorptive function (see Table 285-2) may be normal in these patients. A single course or a series of intermittent courses (2 to 3 weeks per month) of therapy with antibiotics such as tetracycline, ciprofloxacin, clarithromycin, ampicillin, metronidazole, or trimethoprim-sulfamethoxazole is usually given. Finally, it should be noted that duodenal bacterial overgrowth occurs frequently after long-term treatment with omeprazole, and while it clearly causes impaired absorption of vitamin B_{12}, it is typically not associated with clinically significant fat or carbohydrate malabsorption.

Chronic Intestinal Pseudoobstruction (See also Chap. 288) Chronic intestinal pseudoobstruction is a heterogeneous syndrome with a variety of causes (Table 285-7). Primary or idiopathic intestinal pseudoobstruction is a chronic illness characterized by recurrent episodes of intestinal obstruction in which all known causes of mechanical obstruction and other illnesses known to produce intestinal pseudoobstruction have been excluded. In addition to abnormalities in small-bowel motility, derangements in esophageal, gastric, and colonic motility also have been described. The primary clinical manifestations are nausea and vomiting, abdominal pain, distention, constipation, diarrhea, and urinary tract symptoms. Patients typically exhibit a prolonged transit time for chyme along the gastrointestinal tract, especially the small bowel, where pressure-activity patterns are markedly disordered. Oral cisapride accelerates gastric emptying, normalizes intestinal transit, and improves propulsive small-bowel activity in patients with pseudoobstruction. Octreotide is also sometimes useful. Malabsorption secondary to stasis of intestinal contents with resultant abnormal bacterial proliferation in the small bowel is frequently a contributing factor.

Tropical Sprue Tropical sprue is a malabsorptive disorder of unknown cause affecting residents of or visitors to tropical regions. Both epidemic and endemic forms of the disease have been recognized.

Tropical sprue may have its onset months or even years after a patient has returned from the tropics. The etiology of the disorder has not been elucidated, but it might well result from one or more of the following: (1) a nutritional deficiency, (2) a transmissible infectious microorganism, and (3) a toxin elaborated by a microorganism or contained in the diet. It is of interest that coliform organisms, shown to produce an enterotoxin causing fluid secretion, have been isolated from the jejunum of tropical sprue patients but not from other patients with bacterial overgrowth of the proximal small bowel. Anorexia, diarrhea, weight loss, symptoms of anemia, sequelae of nutritional deficiency (see Table 285-4), and abdominal distention are common findings. Patients are frequently deficient in iron as well as vitamin B_{12} and folate. Laboratory studies usually reveal anemia (megaloblastic in 60 percent of cases) and impaired absorption of fat, xylose, and vitamin B_{12}. Malabsorption of at least two nutrients is considered essential for the diagnosis. Jejunal biopsy classically reveals shortened and thickened villi, increased crypt depth, and increased infiltration of mononuclear cells in the lamina propria and epithelium. Endoscopy may reveal scalloping of the valvulae conniventes and a mosaic-appearing mucosa (see Table 285-3). However, these biopsy findings are not specific, and the lesion may be patchy; in addition, interpretation is difficult because "control" biopsies from asymptomatic residents in the same tropical region are often considered abnormal when compared with normal biopsies from patients in temperate zones. Such histologic findings have been termed *tropical jejunitis*. Treatment with vitamin B_{12}, folate, and antibiotics have all been effective in inducing a remission. A short course (2 to 4 weeks) of combined therapy with a sulfonamide or tetracycline and folic acid is usually given. Occasional patients require more prolonged antibiotic therapy.

Scleroderma Although there are numerous reports of small-intestinal involvement in scleroderma, frank malabsorption has been reported in only one-third of patients. Malabsorption is due to three key factors: (1) impaired intestinal motility and jejunal pseudodiverticulosis leading to relative stasis of intestinal contents and hence bacterial overgrowth; (2) involvement of the intestinal wall by the disease; and (3) vascular ischemia. In some cases, abnormal bacterial proliferation in the upper small bowel can be documented, and in these patients antibiotic therapy with drugs such as ciprofloxacin, trimethoprim-sulfamethoxazole, and metronidazole may result in decreased steatorrhea, gain in weight, and increased absorption of vitamin B_{12}. In the intestinal wall there also may be extensive deposition of collagen, especially in the muscular mucosa, submucosa, and muscularis externa, with significant muscle atrophy. Studies of duodenal myoelectric activity in scleroderma revealed absence of migrating motor complexes in

Table 285-7

Causes of Chronic Intestinal Pseudoobstruction

Primary: Idiopathic
 Visceral myopathy
 Visceral neuropathy
Secondary
 Collagen vascular disease
  Scleroderma
  Dermatomyositis/polymyositis
  Systemic lupus erythematosus
 Amyloidosis
 Endocrine disorders
  Hypothyroidism
  Diabetes mellitus
 Neurologic diseases
  Chagas' disease
 Paraneoplastic visceral neuropathy
  Small cell lung carcinoma
 Drugs
  Chronic narcotic use (narcotic bowel syndrome)
  Tricyclic antidepressants
 Miscellaneous
  Jejunal diverticulosis
  Jejunoileal bypass

* See Chap. 288.

the basal state and decreased excitability of the bowel to mechanical stimuli, such as distention, and humoral stimuli, such as pentagastrin and secretin. This motor dysfunction is an important factor in the dilatation, atony, and stasis of intestinal contents in scleroderma. Therapy with prokinetic drugs such as octreotide, cisapride, and erythromycin may be beneficial.

Malabsorption in AIDS Diarrhea and weight loss occur frequently in patients with AIDS. These symptoms are often due to enteric infections or small-intestinal Kaposi's sarcoma. The jejunal mucosa is often abnormal in patients infected with human immunodeficiency virus (HIV), and such abnormalities can be masked by an opportunistic infection. However, such symptoms can be due to malabsorption, which has been well documented in patients with AIDS in whom identifiable enteric infections and intestinal involvement with Kaposi's sarcoma have been excluded. The presence of malabsorption in these patients has been documented by steatorrhea and abnormal D-xylose absorption tests. Serum zinc levels may be decreased. In addition, small-bowel biopsy specimens have revealed dense infiltration of mononuclear cells and histiocytes. Microorganisms also have been identified in the mucosa (see also Chap. 308).

DISORDERS ASSOCIATED WITH LYMPHATIC OBSTRUCTION Whipple's Disease This is a rare disorder characterized clinically by arthralgia, abdominal pain, diarrhea, progressive weight loss, dilated lacteals in the bowel wall, and impaired intestinal absorption. Wasting, low-grade fever, increased skin pigmentation, and peripheral lymphadenopathy are frequently present. In addition, heart failure, endocarditis, uveitis, and central nervous system manifestations, including confusion, memory loss, focal cranial nerve signs, nystagmus, and ophthalmoplegia, may be present. Laboratory examination usually reveals the presence of steatorrhea, impaired xylose absorption, abnormal small-bowel x-rays, hypoalbuminemia, and anemia. Hypoalbuminemia is due to excessive loss of serum albumin into the gastrointestinal tract as well as impaired synthesis of albumin.

The diagnosis is established by demonstrating the presence in the mucosa of macrophages containing large cytoplasmic granules that stain brilliant magenta with the periodic acid Schiff (PAS) reagent. Such macrophages also may be seen in other tissues, such as lymph nodes, spleen, or liver. The finding of PAS-positive macrophages in the lamina propria is not specific for Whipple's disease, but virtual replacement of most cellular elements in the lamina propria by these macrophages has been seen only in this disorder. In addition to the PAS-positive macrophages, jejunal biopsy specimens frequently show dilated lymphatics and some degree of blunting of the intestinal mucosal villi. Since many patients with Whipple's disease have bacteremia, testing of peripheral blood using the polymerase chain reaction is potentially useful in diagnosis.

Electron-microscopic studies have revealed the presence of rod-shaped structures (or bacilliform bodies) 0.3 by 1.5 to 2.5 μm in and adjacent to the macrophages in the lamina propria as well as in epithelial cells and polymorphonuclear leukocytes. The bacterium has not been cultured but has been identified as a gram-negative actinomycete with distinct morphologic characteristics and thus named *Tropheryma whippelii*. After treatment of the patient with antibiotics, the bacilliform bodies decrease or disappear together with a decrease in the number of PAS-positive macrophages. In addition, the reappearance of the bacteria often heralds the onset of a clinical relapse after antibiotics have been withdrawn. Positive blood tests for *T. whippelii* DNA have been reported in patients with AIDS.

Whipple's disease at one time was thought to be invariably fatal. However, it is now clear that therapy with antibiotics will usually induce a clinical remission. In a few cases there has been complete reversal of the histologic abnormalities in the jejunal mucosa, and some of these cases have been followed for more than 10 years. Patients with Whipple's disease should be treated with antibiotics such as trimethoprim-sulfamethoxazole for at least 1 year. Treatment with tetracycline alone or penicillin alone is not adequate initial therapy; relapse rates with these drugs are approximately 40 percent. The most important parameter for following the disease and predicting its course is the presence or absence of bacilli in sections of small-bowel biopsy specimens.

Intestinal Lymphoma Steatorrhea is a manifestation of *primary* intestinal lymphoma. The disease occurs predominantly in men, and the mean age of onset of symptoms is about 50 years. The diagnosis should be suspected in patients with malabsorption with the following findings: (1) a malabsorption syndrome in which clinical and biopsy features resemble those of celiac sprue but in which there is an incomplete response to a gluten-free diet, (2) the presence of *abdominal pain* and *fever*, and (3) signs and symptoms of intestinal obstruction. The usual stigmata of generalized lymphoma are frequently absent. Hepatomegaly, splenomegaly, palpable abdominal masses, and peripheral adenopathy are usually not found. Lymphangiography and computed tomography (CT) may reveal abnormal intraabdominal nodes. The diagnosis can be established by laparotomy and often may be made by thorough examination of multiple mucosal biopsy specimens obtained perorally. There may be a total absence of villi or lesser degrees of blunting and shortening of the villi. In contrast to celiac sprue, the lamina propria is usually massively infiltrated with lymphoid cells. Malignancy may be diagnosed by demonstrating lymphoid cells with the cytologic features of malignancy, the presence of reticulum cells outside germinal centers, and infiltration and destruction of crypts by pleomorphic lymphoid cells. Some patients elaborate or secrete a fragment of the heavy chain of IgA immunoglobulins (α-*chain disease*). The latter is probably a variant of intestinal lymphoma.

The mechanism of malabsorption in intestinal lymphoma may be related to several factors: (1) diffuse involvement of the small-intestinal mucosa, (2) involvement of the bowel wall with lymphatic obstruction, and (3) localized stenosis with stasis of intestinal contents and bacterial overgrowth. It should be emphasized that it is often difficult, by clinical and morphologic features alone, to distinguish Crohn's disease and celiac sprue from intestinal lymphoma. Indeed, there is evidence to suggest that lymphoma may develop as a late complication of celiac sprue.

The course of intestinal lymphoma has ranged from 4 months to 4 years from the onset of symptoms. Perforation, bleeding, and intestinal obstruction are common terminal complications. Multimodality treatment appears to be superior to therapy with either surgery or chemotherapy alone.

CARDIOVASCULAR DISORDERS Steatorrhea has been described in patients with chronic congestive heart failure, superior mesenteric artery insufficiency, and constrictive pericarditis. Abnormal dilated mucosal lymphatics and excessive enteric loss of protein have been demonstrated in patients with constrictive pericarditis. The mechanism of steatorrhea in patients with chronic heart failure remains uncertain. It might be due to congestion and edema of the mucosa, mucosal hypoxia, or abnormalities in pancreatic function. Although pronounced steatorrhea is uncommon in congestive heart failure, these patients are frequently anorectic, and a low fat intake could mask a latent steatorrhea. Steatorrhea is quite infrequent in patients with vasculitis and is thought to be due to segmental infarction of the small bowel in addition to intestinal ischemia.

DEFECTS IN MUCOSAL FUNCTION

INFLAMMATORY OR INFILTRATIVE DISORDERS Regional Enteritis The clinical features of regional enteritis are described in Chap. 286. Malabsorption in regional enteritis may result from several factors: (1) interruption of the enterohepatic circulation of bile salts by ileal disease or resection, (2) deconjugation of bile salts due to bacterial overgrowth, in turn related to strictures and/or fistulas, (3) active inflammatory bowel disease causing impaired mucosal cell function, (4) inadequate absorptive surface resulting from intestinal resection or fistulas, and (5) severe protein depletion producing impaired exocrine pancreatic function. Active ileal disease and/or ileal resection resulting in an interrupted enterohepatic circulation of and deficiency of conjugated bile salts appears to be the major factor responsible for steatorrhea as well as impaired absorption of vitamin B_{12}. Small-bowel absorptive function has been correlated with the extent of ileal disease or resection. When the length of dysfunctional ileum exceeds 90 to 100 cm, virtually all patients will have steatorrhea and vitamin B_{12} malabsorption. After intestinal resection, the functional capacity of the remaining small bowel will depend on the site and extent of resection as well as the presence of residual inflammatory disease. Massive intestinal resection usually results in impaired absorption of all food constituents. When the malabsorption is due to strictures and blind loops as a result of previous surgery, antibiotic therapy may be helpful, but surgical removal of these areas is usually necessary for long-term improvement. With diffuse inflammatory disease, a florid malabsorption syndrome may occur with steatorrhea, hypocalcemia, impaired vitamin B_{12} absorption, and hypoalbuminemia due to increased enteric protein loss. Treatment with sulfasalazine, glucocorticoids, and other immunosuppressive drugs may be beneficial (see Chap. 286).

After *ileal resection*, patients frequently have bothersome diarrhea. This appears to be due to *interruption of the enterohepatic circulation*, whereby increased amounts of bile salts reach the colon, where they interfere with water and electrolyte absorption and thus have a cathartic effect. The *bile salt–induced diarrhea* after ileal resection may respond to treatment with cholestyramine, an exchange resin that binds bile salts and causes them to lose their biochemical effect on the bowel. Patients with ileal resection of less than 100 cm and fecal fat excretion less than 20 g/d show the best symptomatic response to cholestyramine, usually at a dose of 4 g tid.

Chronic Nongranulomatous Ulcerative Jejunoileitis This disorder is characterized by abdominal pain, weight loss, fever, diarrhea, steatorrhea, hypoalbuminemia, and protein-losing enteropathy. Clinical features mimic those found in both regional enteritis and celiac sprue. Indeed, the intestinal lesion may be indistinguishable from celiac sprue. However, exclusion of gluten from the diet does not result in any benefit. Glucocorticoid treatment has resulted in transient improvement, but long-term effects are unpredictable.

Amyloidosis See Chap. 309

Radiation Injury to the Small Bowel Extensive morphologic damage of the small-intestinal mucosa often follows normal or excessive abdominal irradiation. These changes include a decrease in crypt mitoses, marked shortening of the villi, megalocytosis of epithelial cells, and inflammatory cell infiltration of the lamina propria. These may be associated with transient diarrhea and impaired intestinal absorption. However, restoration of normal intestinal architecture is usually complete within 2 weeks after cessation of therapy. Persistent diarrhea and malabsorption may develop shortly after x-ray therapy, or there may be a latent period of several years before the onset of diarrhea. Steatorrhea, ranging from 10 to 40 g/d, has been observed frequently, but impaired absorption of calcium, iron, D-xylose, or vitamin B_{12} is less common. In some patients, intestinal strictures due to vasculopathy and ischemia may develop following irradiation, and thus stasis of intestinal contents and abnormal bacterial proliferation may occur. In others, intestinal lymphangiectasia, presumably due to lymphatic obstruction, has been documented. Diarrhea and malabsorption may be refractory to all methods of management. Treatment with antibiotics, pancreatic enzymes, gluten-free diet, adrenal glucocorticoids, and opiates has met with but limited success.

Eosinophilic Enteritis Eosinophilic gastroenteritis is a disorder of the stomach, small bowel, and colon that is of unknown etiology and is characterized by peripheral blood eosinophilia and eosinophilic infiltration of the gut wall without evidence of vasculitis. The clinical manifestations, usually recurrent, are protean and relate to the site of gastrointestinal tract involvement. Three main patterns have been identified: (1) Predominant mucosal disease manifested by iron-deficiency anemia, hypoalbuminemia due to protein-losing enteropathy, and mild steatorrhea. Patients in this group often present with a malabsorption syndrome and a history of intolerance to specific foods. (2) Predominant muscle layer disease characterized by marked thick-

ening and rigidity of the stomach and proximal small bowel with obstructive symptoms and radiologic features of pyloric narrowing and obstruction. (Because of this pattern, eosinophilic enteritis should be considered in the differential diagnosis of gastric outlet obstruction, diffuse small-bowel disease, and ileocolitis. Indeed, eosinophilic enteritis often mimics regional enteritis.) (3) Predominant subserosal disease in which the cardinal manifestation is ascites with marked eosinophilia in the ascitic fluid. Although this classification based on the tissue layer of major involvement is useful in understanding the principal manifestations, it should be emphasized that mixed clinical forms— e.g., ascites (serosal involvement) plus obstruction (muscular involvement)—also occur. Diarrhea occurs in 30 to 60 percent of patients regardless of whether eosinophils infiltrate the gut mucosal, muscular, or serosal layers. *Ancylostoma caninum*, the canine hookworm present in domestic pets throughout Northeastern Australia and possibly worldwide, has been identified as a cause of obscure abdominal pain with biopsy-proven eosinophilic enteritis. The diagnosis can be confirmed by serologic tests.

Previous reports have emphasized food allergy and mucosal features of this disease. However, food allergy is related to symptoms in less than 20 percent of patients. In such patients, fasting serum IgE levels are often elevated, and challenge with offending foods frequently evokes symptoms of abdominal pain and diarrhea in addition to a marked increase in serum IgE levels. In most patients with eosinophilic enteritis, however, immunologic studies, including measurement of serum immunoglobulins, serum complement, lymphocytes, and lymphocyte response to nonspecific mitogens, reveal no abnormalities. Thus both IgE-mediated and IgE-independent mechanisms may be operative in different patients with eosinophilic gastroenteritis. It seems clear that evidence of allergy or food sensitivity is often absent and is not required for the diagnosis of eosinophilic enteritis. In addition, even in patients with food allergies, elimination diets are frequently ineffective, and such patients may require prolonged glucocorticoid therapy to remain well. Ketotifen and cromolyn are also useful therapeutic adjuncts. However, surgical treatment for relief of obstructive symptoms and use of glucocorticoids are the mainstays of therapy.

Dermatitis and Malabsorption A malabsorption syndrome, usually mild, has been reported in patients with a variety of dermatologic disorders, including psoriasis, eczematoid dermatitis, and dermatitis herpetiformis. Proximal intestinal mucosal abnormalities are almost invariably found in patients with dermatitis herpetiformis. In one study, 21 of 22 patients had lesions ranging in severity from a completely "flat" to an almost normal intestinal mucosa. The mucosal lesions were often patchy in distribution. Clinical and laboratory evidence of significant malabsorption was infrequent, possibly owing to the limited length of small intestine involved in this skin disorder. While the skin lesions of dermatitis herpetiformis respond to sulfone, the gut lesions do not. By contrast, in some patients with blunted and flattened intestinal mucosal lesions and steatorrhea, there may be a striking improvement in villous architecture and regression of steatorrhea after withdrawal of gluten from the diet without improvement in the skin lesions. Further, in patients with dermatitis herpetiformis and a morphologically normal small-intestinal mucosa, administration of a high-gluten diet may result in blunted and flattened mucosal lesions indistinguishable from those of celiac sprue. As in the latter disease, an increased frequency of HLA-A1 and HLA-B8 is also seen. These observations raise the interesting question as to whether certain patients with dermatitis herpetiformis and a malabsorption syndrome have latent celiac sprue.

BIOCHEMICAL OR GENETIC ABNORMALITIES Celiac Sprue Celiac sprue is a disorder characterized by malabsorption, abnormal small-bowel structure, and intolerance to gluten, a protein found in wheat and wheat products. It has been appropriately referred to as *gluten-induced enteropathy*. Celiac disease in children and celiac sprue in adults are probably the same disorder with the same pathogenesis.

There are insufficient data to provide an accurate estimation of the incidence of celiac sprue in any population. This is largely because the severity of the disease varies greatly, and individuals may have typical mucosal change and yet have no overt symptoms. In most reported series, 70 percent of the cases are in women. The incidence in siblings appears to be many times higher than that in the general population, and it has been suggested that sprue may be inherited through a dominant gene with incomplete penetrance. Celiac sprue patients have an increased frequency of some serum histocompatibility antigens, particularly of the HLA-DR3 and HLA-DQw2 types. The HLA-DR3 phenotype has been found in 70 to 90 percent of sprue patients, as compared with 20 to 25 percent in normal subjects. The HLA antigens may be linked to immune response genes which may determine the immunologic recognition of certain substances (see Chap. 306). It has been suggested that such genetic factors may predispose to immunologic tolerance of dietary proteins such as the peptides in gluten or to the production of pathogenic antigluten antibodies, which could result in the binding of gluten to epithelial cells with subsequent tissue damage. The discordance for celiac sprue among HLA-identical siblings and some identical twins raises the question of whether an additional susceptibility gene (or genes) not yet identified is required for the development of celiac sprue.

Pathophysiology Gluten and the related substance gliadin are high-molecular-weight proteins found especially in wheat. The alcohol-soluble fraction of gluten consists of glutamine-rich gliadin polypeptides, which can be fractionated into γ, β, δ, and α subgroups; peptides from all four gliadin subgroups are toxic to celiac sprue patients and induce the intestinal lesion when administered to patients with sprue in remission. The exact mechanism for this effect is not clear, but two theories have been proposed, namely, a "toxic" and an immunologic theory. One possible mechanism is that patients with celiac sprue lack a specific mucosal peptidase, so that gluten or its larger glutamine-containing peptides are not effectively hydrolyzed to smaller peptides (i.e., dipeptides or amino acids). As a consequence, "toxic" peptides might accumulate in the mucosa. It has been demonstrated that patients with celiac sprue in remission will develop steatorrhea and typical mucosal changes when they are given gluten. Similar results will occur with the administration of peptide hydrolysates containing at least eight amino acids with a terminal glutamine residue. It has been shown that when gluten is instilled into the *ileum* of celiac sprue patients, histologic changes begin to occur within hours. This does not occur in the *upper jejunum*, suggesting that the effect is immediate and is local rather than systemic. After surface absorptive cells are damaged by noxious gluten fractions, they are sloughed rapidly from the mucosal surface into the gut lumen. To compensate for this loss, cell proliferation increases, crypts undergo hypertrophy, and cell migration accelerates to replace the damaged and sloughed epithelial cells. This accelerated epithelial cell renewal can be reversed by a gluten-free diet.

The intestinal mucosa of patients with celiac sprue shows many enzyme alterations, including decreased levels of disaccharidases, alkaline phosphatase, and peptide hydrolases, as well as impaired ability to digest gluten peptides. However, these abnormalities usually revert toward normal after successful treatment with a gluten-free diet. There is additional evidence supporting the concept of toxicity of gluten and gluten breakdown products in celiac sprue. First, gliadin, especially the A-gliadin moiety, is toxic to sprue mucosa maintained in organ culture, causing ultrastructural changes and depression of disaccharidase activity. Second, sprue mucosa hydrolyzes a specific fraction of a gliadin digest (fraction 9) in a defective manner, and fraction 9 is selectively toxic to sprue mucosa. Third, specific fractions of gluten fed to celiac sprue patients cause transient alterations in mucosal histology and depression of disaccharidase activity, but full recovery is observed in 72 h. The rapid onset of these changes and the prompt recovery are consistent with a direct toxic effect. Two key tetrapeptide sequences present in cereals are toxic to patients with celiac disease— namely, Pro-Ser-Gly-Gly and Gly-Gly-Gly-Pro. Despite intensive study, however, no persistent, specific, or selective peptidase or other enzyme deficiency has been demonstrated.

It also has been suggested that gluten or gluten metabolites may initiate an *immune reaction* in the intestinal mucosa. Alternatively, the interaction of T lymphocytes with crypt epithelium may be a primary event in the pathogenesis of the intestinal lesion. The presence of a mononuclear inflammatory cell infiltrate in the lamina propria of the mucosa, the beneficial effect of glucocorticoid drugs, the finding of abnormal antibodies to gliadin in the serum of celiac sprue patients, the synthesis of increased amounts of antigliadin antibody by sprue mucosa maintained in organ culture, and the elaboration of lymphokines such as migration inhibitory factor (MIF) by sprue mucosa incubated with gliadin have all been cited as evidence in support of this hypothesis.

A possible role for adenovirus serotype 12 (Ad12) in the pathogenesis of celiac sprue has been proposed on the basis of two observations: (1) There is amino acid sequence homology between a portion of A-gliadin and a viral-encoded protein (E16) produced by Ad12, and (2) patients with untreated celiac sprue have a much higher frequency of antibodies to Ad12 than treated celiac sprue patients and controls. Although other studies have not confirmed these results, these findings are in accord with the hypothesis that there must be *environmental* factors as well as a *genetic predisposition* to explain why only certain people develop celiac sprue. Despite intensive studies, there is not yet enough information to integrate the distinctive dietary, immunologic, and genetic features of celiac sprue into a clear understanding of the pathogenesis of the disease.

Jejunal biopsy specimens from patients with celiac sprue show a characteristic lesion. There is blunting and flattening of the mucosal surface, with villi either absent or broad and short. The crypts are elongated, and there is generally a dense infiltration of inflammatory cells in the lamina propria. The surface epithelium is altered with a sparse brush border, cuboidal rather than the normal columnar cells, and infiltration of inflammatory cells in the epithelial layer. These changes are usually most severe in the proximal small bowel, presumably because this area of the bowel is exposed to the highest gluten concentration. The typical morphologic changes illustrated in Fig. 285-4 are characteristic of celiac sprue but are not specific. Similar changes have been described in other conditions, including lymphoma, tropical sprue, and hypogammaglobulinemia associated with malabsorption. Many biochemical abnormalities have been demonstrated in mucosal biopsy specimens from celiac sprue patients. Impaired esterification of fatty acids to triglycerides, decreased uptake of amino acids, and decreased activity of intestinal disaccharidases (especially lactase) have been well documented. The latter observation may account for the high incidence of milk intolerance in untreated celiac sprue patients or those in relapse. However, the greater abundance of undifferentiated crypt cells may be important, since crypt cells normally have a lower capacity for nutrient uptake than do villus cells.

Since the mucosa is damaged and altered in patients with celiac sprue, there may be *decreased release of pancreatotropic hormones* (secretin and CCK). This effect results in decreased stimulation of the pancreas and abnormally low intraluminal levels of pancreatic enzymes in response to a meal. In addition, the gallbladder appears to be resistant to the action of CCK, resulting in absent or minimal contractions of the gallbladder, in turn leading to sequestration of bile salts in an inert gallbladder. These two defects may result in impaired intraluminal digestion of fat and protein, which will be superimposed on the defect in intestinal transport caused by a damaged mucosa.

Diarrhea is common in celiac sprue patients and is due to a number of factors, including impaired *absorption* of salt and water by duodenum and jejunum, net *secretion* of water and electrolytes by an abnormally permeable jejunal mucosa, and net colonic secretion of water and electrolytes induced by unabsorbed fatty acids and hydroxy fatty acids. However, the distal small intestine in celiac sprue has the ability to adapt to the damage and loss of absorptive capacity in the proximal small intestine. Indeed, increased ileal absorption of sodium, chloride, and water has been demonstrated in celiac sprue patients.

Clinical features Most patients with celiac sprue will have a typical malabsorption syndrome characterized by weight loss, abdominal distention and bloating, diarrhea, steatorrhea, and abnormal results on tests of absorptive function. The characteristic alterations in responses to these tests are outlined in Table 285-2. It should be emphasized, however, that some patients present with isolated abnormalities that initially do not suggest the diagnosis of celiac sprue. Thus a patient may be admitted for investigation of iron-deficiency anemia without apparent blood loss or of abnormal bleeding due to hypoprothrombinemia but may not have diarrhea or overt steatorrhea. Likewise, celiac sprue patients may present with puzzling metabolic bone disease without diarrhea or steatorrhea. Such patients usually complain of bone pain and tenderness and frequently are found to have extensive demineralization of bone, compression deformities, kyphoscoliosis, and Milkman's fractures. Emotional disturbances are common in these patients, and many individuals with a diagnosis of weight loss initially considered related to severe anxiety and depression are subsequently found to have celiac sprue. Neurologic manifestations of celiac sprue include cerebellar ataxia, sensory neuropathy, myopathy hyporeflexia, and seizures. In each of the preceding clinical settings, celiac sprue should be considered in the differential diagnosis. In addition to dermatitis herpetiformis, there are established associations between celiac sprue and diabetes mellitus, selective IgA deficiency, primary sclerosing cholangitis, primary biliary cirrhosis, ulcerative colitis, and lymphocytic or microscopic colitis (see Chaps. 286 and 298).

Three criteria should be met for a definite diagnosis of celiac sprue to be made: (1) evidence of malabsorption, (2) the finding of an abnormal small-bowel (jejunal) biopsy specimen showing blunting and flattening of the villi along with changes in the surface epithelium, and (3) clinical, biochemical, and histologic improvement after institution of a gluten-free diet.

In recent studies, distinctive endoscopic changes were found in 22 of 28 patients with microscopic changes characteristic of sprue on biopsy (6 of 9 with sprue in relapse and 16 of 19 with initial symptoms). The mucosa was atrophic and had a mottled appearance, with patchy areas of pale mucosa alternating with more edematous mucosa; the pale areas had a pronounced mosaic appearance. Importantly, the valvulae conniventes exhibited a lesion now recognized to be characteristic of sprue—a distinctive scalloped appearance. The duodenal folds should always be examined at upper gastrointestinal endoscopy. If they are absent or reduced, duodenal biopsy is indicated. Abnormality of Kerkring's folds is a helpful sign of celiac disease, especially in patients with minimal or transient symptoms.

In equivocal cases, the patient can be challenged with 30 to 50 g gluten orally; if this challenge results promptly in increased diarrhea and steatorrhea, the diagnosis of gluten-induced enteropathy is established. It should be emphasized that tests of intestinal absorption may reveal abnormalities ranging from very minimal to severe. Abnormalities in absorption tests have been shown to correlate reasonably well with the length of small-bowel involvement and to a lesser extent with the severity of the proximal lesion. Antigliadin, antiendomysial, and antireticulin antibodies have been widely used in the diagnosis of celiac disease. Approximately 90 percent of patients with untreated clinically symptomatic celiac disease, and many patients with asymptomatic latent disease, have IgA and/or IgG antigliadin antibodies; titers frequently decrease after institution of a gluten-free diet. Elevated titers of antiendomysial antibodies are found in over 90 percent of patients with active celiac disease and also decrease with improvement following intitiation of a gluten-free diet. Antireticulin antibodies are less sensitive but more specific than antigliadin antibodies, which can be found in other disorders affecting the small-bowel mucosa, such as Crohn's disease. Combined determination of antigliadin, antiendomysial, and antireticulin antibodies offers optimal sensitivity and specificity for the detection of celiac disease. These antibodies are also useful in following the response to therapy and adherence to a gluten-free diet, and in screening for celiac disease among family members.

A possible variant of celiac sprue is *collagenous* sprue, in which small-bowel biopsy specimens characteristically reveal a blunted and flattened mucosa and large masses of eosinophilic hyaline material in the lamina propria. In one study of biopsy specimens from 145 patients with celiac sprue, 31 percent showed basement membrane thickening, which often was associated with collagen deposition, but dense collagen deposition was found in only 8 percent. Fatal, unremitting malabsorption developed in a third of the latter patients. These observations suggest that collagenous membrane thickening is a fairly frequent finding in jejunal biopsies of patients with sprue but that dense collagen deposits are unusual and may indicate a poor prognosis.

℞ TREATMENT

Despite the uncertainties concerned with the diagnosis of celiac sprue, approximately 80 percent improve after institution of a *gluten-free diet*. Symptomatic improvement usually occurs within a few weeks, but improvement in the response to tests of absorptive function and in small-bowel histologic characteristics may not occur for months. It has been demonstrated repeatedly that strict adherence to a gluten-free diet more consistently results in improvement than does suboptimal gluten restriction. Recent studies indicate that oats, when ingested in quantities of about 50 g/d, are safe for celiac sprue patients for a period of at least 6 to 12 months. Nevertheless, even with strict diet adherence, some patients show little improvement in intestinal histologic features. Patients with celiac sprue who are treated with glucocorticoids but continue to eat a normal gluten-containing diet have shown symptomatic improvement as well as improvement in intestinal histology and tests of intestinal absorptive function. The mechanism by which glucocorticoids protect the mucosa from the effects of gluten is not clear.

If a patient with celiac sprue does not respond to a gluten-free diet, other possibilities or complicating factors must be considered: (1) The diagnosis is incorrect; (2) the patient is not adhering strictly to the diet; (3) there may be another concurrent disease, such as pancreatic insufficiency; (4) the patient may have ulceration of the jejunum or ileum; (5) lactase deficiency may be present with resulting milk intolerance; (6) the patient may have collagenous sprue; (7) the patient may have developed intestinal lymphoma, a disease which appears to occur more frequently in patients with sprue than in the general population; and (8) the patient may have developed lymphocytic or microscopic colitis. Finally, it should be emphasized that a small number of patients show a markedly delayed response to a gluten-free diet, with significant improvement occurring only after 24 to 36 months of therapy. Approximately 50 percent of patients with refractory sprue respond to glucocorticoids; such patients also may require parenteral hyperalimentation or treatment with other immunosuppressive drugs such as 6-mercaptopurine.

Systemic Mastocytosis   Some evidence of malabsorption occurs in 30 percent of patients with systemic mastocytosis. Malabsorption is usually not severe and is manifested primarily as minimal or moderate steatorrhea and impaired absorption of D-xylose and vitamin B_{12}. Small-bowel biopsy specimens typically show moderate blunting of villi and mast cell infiltration. Treatment with histamine H_1 and H_2 receptor antagonists and cromolyn provides relief of diarrhea in some patients.

Disaccharidase Deficiency Syndromes   As indicated above, the hydrolysis of disaccharides occurs on or within the brush border (microvilli) of intestinal epithelial cells by specific disaccharidases. There are both primary (genetic or familial) and secondary (acquired) disaccharidase deficiencies.

Lactase deficiency in the adult   Instances of isolated deficiency of mucosal lactase occur; they are associated with symptoms of lactose intolerance. Since lactose is the principal carbohydrate of milk, such individuals show milk intolerance, with symptoms of abdominal cramps, bloating or distention, and diarrhea. Similar symptoms will occur following the ingestion of lactose. When lactose is not hydrolyzed, it is not absorbed, and its osmotic effect in the lumen leads to shifts of fluid into the intestinal tract. The pH of the stool also will decrease because of the production of lactic acid and short-chain fatty acids from the fermentation of lactose by colonic bacteria. Although primary intestinal lactase deficiency seems to be hereditary, lactose or milk intolerance may not become clinically evident until puberty or late adolescence. There are significant racial differences in the incidence of this entity. It would appear that about 5 to 15 percent of the adult white population shows intestinal lactase deficiency, but in African Americans, Bantus, and Asians, the incidence is as high as 80 to 90 percent.

The diagnosis may be suspected when one obtains a history of gastrointestinal symptoms following milk ingestion. Bloating, cramps, and flatulence, but not diarrhea, are usually produced with ingestion of moderate amounts of lactose. The vast majority of lactose-intolerant persons are aware that they are milk-intolerant and avoid milk. These symptoms are not due to allergic reactions to the proteins in milk (i.e., milk allergy or hypersensitivity) and can be demonstrated by measurement of breath hydrogen after ingestion of 50 g lactose, which is a sensitive and specific test. The rationale for this test is that hydrogen is released from unabsorbed lactose by colonic bacteria, and breath hydrogen excretion subsequently rises. The test is noninvasive and is not influenced by gastric emptying or metabolic factors. Approximately 70 percent of patients with primary lactose intolerance will respond to a lactose-restricted diet, while the remaining 30 percent will not because of an underlying irritable bowel syndrome. When lactose intake is limited to less than 240 mL of milk per day, gastrointestinal symptoms are likely to be negligible in many patients who identify themselves as severely lactose intolerant. These findings suggest that a variety of abdominal complaints are frequently misattributed to lactose intolerance. The use of lactase-containing digestive aids may be unnecessary for milk intakes of <8 oz/d.

Acquired lactase deficiency is often seen in association with a variety of gastrointestinal diseases, in many of which there is histologic evidence of mucosal damage. These include celiac and tropical sprue, regional enteritis, viral and bacterial infections of the intestinal tract, giardiasis, abetalipoproteinemia, cystic fibrosis, and ulcerative colitis.

Deficiency of other disaccharidases Damage to the intestinal mucosa may produce decreased levels of other disaccharidases, such as sucrase-isomaltase, but usually these enzymes are not as depressed as lactase, and symptoms of specific intolerance, such as sucrose intolerance, are uncommon. There are instances of primary and apparently hereditary sucrose intolerance, but these always occur in association with sucrase-isomaltase deficiency. Sucrase-isomaltase deficiency, while not as common as lactase deficiency, is nonetheless an important cause of diarrhea, bloating, and cramping abdominal pain in children. Such patients are often unable to adhere to a low-sucrose diet. Thus, the observation that the symptoms of sucrose malabsorption can be ameliorated by the simple expedient of ingesting viable yeast cells is of considerable practical importance.

Hypogammaglobulinemia See Chap. 307

Abetalipoproteinemia See Chap. 341

Hartnup Disease, Cystinuria See Chap. 350

ENDOCRINE AND METABOLIC DISORDERS Diabetes Mellitus The occurrence of diarrhea and steatorrhea in patients with diabetes mellitus has been well documented. When steatorrhea accompanies diabetes, it may be due to the presence of (1) exocrine pancreatic insufficiency, (2) coexisting celiac sprue (6 percent of insulin-requiring diabetics have shown histologic evidence of celiac sprue), (3) abnormal bacterial proliferation in the proximal small bowel, or (4) severe and uncontrolled diabetes per se (e.g., so-called diabetic diarrhea). Patients falling into the first three categories will usually respond satisfactorily to treatment with pancreatic extracts, a gluten-free diet, and antibiotics, respectively. The pathogenesis of diarrhea and steatorrhea in patients in the fourth category remains poorly understood. They may have involvement of the autonomic nervous system with degenerative changes in the sympathetic and parasympathetic nerves and ganglia; in some, bacterial overgrowth may occur and contribute to the malabsorption.

The clinical features in patients with diarrhea and steatorrhea due to diabetes seem to be fairly uniform. Diabetes usually developed at a young age and is often severe and difficult to control. There is a distinct male predominance. Several signs of autonomic neuropathy are usually present, including postural hypotension, anhydrosis, impotence, and bladder irregularities. Peripheral vascular disease and peripheral neuropathy are also common. Gastrointestinal x-rays may show delayed gastric emptying and disordered transit through the small bowel. Small-bowel biopsy specimens appear normal. Tests of intestinal absorptive function give normal results except for showing the presence of steatorrhea and azotorrhea. There has been no consistent response to therapy with pancreatic extracts, a gluten-free diet, or glucocorticoids. When bacterial overgrowth is present, broad-spectrum antibiotics may be helpful. Persistent diarrhea may also result from ingestion of dietetic food containing large amounts of sorbitol, which often are erroneously labeled "sugarless." Clonidine has proved useful in patients with large-volume diarrhea not responding to dietary measures and anticholinergics.

Hypoparathyroidism Steatorrhea has been documented in several patients with idiopathic hypoparathyroidism. In addition to hypocalcemia, impaired absorption of D-xylose and vitamin B_{12}, decreased serum iron values, and abnormal small-intestinal roentgenograms have been demonstrated in some cases. In such patients the serum phosphorus level is elevated (owing to the hypoparathyroidism) rather than low (as in primary malabsorption). The cause of malabsorption in this disorder is unclear.

Adrenal Insufficiency Although there are few studies on fat excretion in adrenal insufficiency in human beings, malabsorption, especially of fat, appears to occur more frequently than has been generally appreciated. Patients with adrenal insufficiency have been found to have steatorrhea that is corrected by therapy with adrenal glucocorticoids.

Hyperthyroidism There are few detailed studies on intestinal absorptive function in patients with hyperthyroidism. Mild to moderate steatorrhea and hypoalbuminemia have been reported, but absorption of D-xylose and vitamin B_{12} is frequently normal. Steatorrhea usually remits after successful treatment of hyperthyroidism. Clinical studies suggest that steatorrhea in hyperthyroidism is not due to any defect of pancreatic, biliary, or small-intestinal mucosal function but is a result of hyperphagia with ingestion of unusually large amounts of fat occurring in association with rapid gastric emptying and intestinal transit.

Gastrinoma (Zollinger-Ellison Syndrome) The clinical features of gastrinomas are described in Chaps. 95 and 284. Malabsorption is frequently found in this disease. The acidification and dilution of intestinal contents caused by gastric acid hypersecretion leads to major disturbances in fat digestion and absorption. Impaired formation of micellar lipid due to inactivation of pancreatic lipase is probably the major factor in the production of steatorrhea. Other factors contributing to fat malabsorption include (1) precipitation of glycine-conjugated bile salts due to low intraluminal pH, (2) alteration of the intestinal mucosa with ulceration and metaplasia, and (3) impaired fatty acid esterification and chylomicron formation.

Carcinoid Syndrome (See also Chap. 95) Although diarrhea is common in the carcinoid syndrome, malabsorption with significant steatorrhea is unusual. In many cases of carcinoid syndrome with steatorrhea, there has been a prior intestinal resection (usually ileal), and in these cases the resection is the major cause of steatorrhea. However, direct involvement of the bowel wall and mesentery by the carcinoid tumor has been well documented. That abnormalities in serotonin metabolism also may be important is suggested from the decrease in the steatorrhea observed in some of these patients when treated with the antiserotonin drug methysergide. Although side effects may occur, for control of diarrhea and steatorrhea, patients may be given a trial of 8 to 12 mg methysergide per day.

PROTEIN-LOSING ENTEROPATHY The gastrointestinal tract plays a significant role in the metabolism and physiologic degradation of plasma proteins. While the exact magnitude of the normal gastrointestinal protein loss is unclear, studies with labeled albumin suggest that between 10 and 20 percent of the normal turnover of albumin may be accounted for by enteric protein loss. However, under certain pathologic conditions, excessive gastrointestinal protein loss may develop. Many disorders have been found to be associated with intestinal protein loss. Some of these are listed in Table 285-8.

Pathophysiology Several mechanisms have been proposed for the passage of plasma proteins across the gastrointestinal mucosa, both normally and in certain disease states. First, plasma proteins may pass into the gastrointestinal tract through an inflamed or ulcerated mucosa and account for the protein loss occasionally seen in Crohn's disease and ulcerative colitis. Second, plasma protein loss may occur as a result of disordered mucosal cell structure. For example, patients with celiac sprue have abnormal villous structure and surface epithelium, and these changes facilitate the diffusion of plasma protein between the cells. Third, in the presence of increased lymphatic pressure, there may be increased passage of plasma proteins into the lumen via the intercellular spaces of the mucosal epithelium. This might be expected to occur in disorders in which there is granulomatous or neoplastic involvement of lymphatics. Fourth, dilated lymph vessels in the mucosa may rupture through the surface epithelium, discharging their contents into the intestinal lumen. This is thought to be important in the pathogenesis of steatorrhea and hypoproteinemia in patients with idiopathic intestinal lymphangiectasia (see "Intestinal Lymphangiectasia," below).

In the past, the detection and quantitation of gastrointestinal protein loss primarily involved the use of intravenously administered radiolabeled macromolecules such as ^{125}I-labeled serum albumin, ^{51}CrCl$_3$, ^{51}Cr-labeled albumin, and indium 111. Patients with excessive enteric protein loss may excrete from 2 to 40 percent of the injected radioactive label, versus 0.1 to 0.7 percent in normal subjects. False-positive results may be obtained if the stool specimen is contaminated with urine. However, tests with radiolabeled compounds have been superceded by a reliable and sensitive *nonisotopic* method to measure intestinal protein loss which involves the measurement of α_1-antitrypsin (AT). This serum enzyme, which has the same molecular weight as albumin (50,000), is resistant to proteolysis and, when leaked into the intestinal lumen, is not degraded. One can easily measure AT in serum and stool by radial immunodiffusion in order to measure the AT loss in stool (the normal loss is less than 2.6 mg per gram of stool) or intestinal clearance of AT (the normal value is less than 13 mL/d). Random fecal AT assays also can be used as a simple screening method for enteric protein loss.

Intestinal Lymphangiectasia *Pathophysiology* This disorder is characterized by increased enteric loss of protein, hypoproteinemia, edema, lymphocytopenia, malabsorption, and abnormal dilated lymphatic channels in the small intestine. The high incidence of chylous effusions and abnormal peripheral, retroperitoneal, and thoracic lymphatics indicates that intestinal lymphangiectasia is part of a generalized congenital disorder of the lymphatic system. It has been suggested that the hypoplastic visceral lymphatic channels result in obstruction to lymph flow, with the subsequent development of increased intestinal lymphatic pressure. This, in turn, may lead to dilated lymphatic vessels throughout the small-bowel wall and mesentery. Hypoproteinemia and steatorrhea are thought to be due to rupture of the dilated lymphatic vessels with discharge of lymph into the bowel lumen. In adults, approximately 1500 mL of lymph, containing 70 g fat and 50 g albumin, passes through the thoracic duct each day. The leakage of a small amount of this lymph might be expected to result in considerable loss of protein and fat into the intestinal lumen. In addition, absorption of dietary long-chain triglycerides stimulates lymph flow, and this may increase further the retrograde leakage of intestinal lymph into the lumen. Three lines of evidence support the concept of intestinal leakage of lymph in intestinal lymphangiectasia: (1) Chylous fluid has been recovered from the duodenum in these patients; (2) retrograde passage of contrast material from retroperitoneal lymphatics into the duodenum and jejunum has been documented; and (3) significant steatorrhea may persist in patients after institution of a completely fat-free diet, suggesting an increased enteric loss of endogenous fat present in lymph.

Clinical features The disease affects primarily children and young adults. All patients have edema, which may be asymmetric because of hypoplastic peripheral lymphatics. Chylous effusions and diarrhea are common symptoms. The primary laboratory finding is hypoproteinemia with decreased serum levels of albumin, immunoglobulins IgG, IgA, and IgM, transferrin, and ceruloplasmin. Despite moderate to severe hypogammaglobulinemia, there does not appear to be an increased incidence of pyogenic bacterial infections. In addition, the circulating antibody response to challenge with *Brucella* and typhoid antigens is normal. Steatorrhea is usually mild, although in some instances fat loss may be as much as 40 g/d. Some patients have hypocalcemia and impaired absorption of vitamin B$_{12}$. Lymphocytopenia (due to the loss of lymphocytes in lymph) is common, with lymphocyte counts ranging from 400 to 1000/mL (normal: 1500 to 4000/mL). This deficiency is associated with abnormal delayed hypersensitivity, as evidenced by prolonged homograft survival and impaired cutaneous responsiveness to antigens such as mumps and monilia.

Small-bowel roentgenograms are frequently abnormal, showing changes of mucosal edema and a malabsorption pattern. Lymphangiograms may demonstrate hypoplastic peripheral and visceral lymphatics, with the absence of groups of retroperitoneal lymph nodes. Specimens of jejunal mucosa characteristically reveal dilated and telangiectatic lymphatic vessels in the lamina propria and submucosa. The villi may be club-shaped because of distortion from grossly dilated lymphatics (see Fig. 285-4). Such changes in the intestinal mucosa may be reversed after appropriate therapy. The diagnosis of intestinal lymphangiectasia is therefore established by (1) small-intestinal biopsy and (2) demonstration of increased enteric protein loss using radiolabeled macromolecules.

℞ TREATMENT

A low-fat diet, by decreasing lymph flow, usually results in significant improvement with decreased fecal fat excretion, decreased enteric protein loss, increased serum calcium and albumin levels, and an increased half-life of injected ^{125}I-labeled albumin. Similar results may be obtained by the substitution of medium-chain triglycerides for dietary long-chain triglycerides, since the former are transported as medium-chain fatty acids by the portal vein rather than via the lymph.

For further discussion of drugs affecting gastrointestinal function, see Chaps. 37 and 38, in Goodman and Gilman's The Pharmacological Basis of Therapeutics, *9th ed., McGraw-Hill, New York, 1996.*

Table 285-8

Disorders Associated with Protein-Losing Enteropathy

Stomach	Colon
Gastric carcinoma	Colonic neoplasm
Ménétrier's disease	Ulcerative colitis
Atrophic gastritis	Granulomatous colitis
Postgastrectomy syndrome	Megacolon
Small intestine	**Heart**
Intestinal lymphangiectassia	Congestive heart failure
Celiac sprue	Constrictive pericarditis
Tropical sprue	Interatrial septal defect
Regional enteritis	Primary cardiomyopathy
Whipple's disease	**Miscellaneous**
Lymphoma	Esophageal carcinoma
Intestinal tuberculosis	Gastrocolic fistula
Acute infectious enteritis	Agammaglobulinemia
Scleroderma	Nephrosis
Jejunal diverticulosis	
Allergic gastroenteropathy	
Eosinophilic gastroenteritis	
Bacterial overgrowth	

AMER MH, EL-AKKAD S: Gastrointestinal lymphoma in adults: Clinical features and management of 300 cases. Gastroenterology 106:840, 1994

ARRANZ E, FERGUSON A: Intestinal antibody pattern in celiac disease: Occurrence in patients with normal jejunal biopsy histology. Gastroenterology 104:1263, 1993

CHIN JS et al: Paraneoplastic visceral neuropathy as a cause of severe gastrointestinal motor dysfunction. Gastroenterology 95:1279, 1988

CORAZZA G et al: Gliadin immune reactivity is associated with overt and latent enteropathy in relatives of celiac patients. Gastroenterology 102:1517, 1992

FERGUSON A et al: Clinical and pathological spectrum of coeliac disease—active, silent, latent, potential. Gut 34:150, 1993

FINE KD, FORDTRAN JS: The effect of diarrhea on fecal fat excretion. Gastroenterology 102:1936, 1992

FINE KD: The prevalence of occult gastrointestinal bleeding in celiac sprue. N Engl J Med 334:1163, 1996

FRIED M et al: Duodenal bacterial overgrowth during treatment in outpatients with omeprazole. Gut 35:23, 1994

HAMMER HF et al: Carbohydrate malabsorption: Its measurement and its contribution to diarrhea. J Clin Invest 86:1936, 1990

JANATUINEN ER et al: A comparison of diets with and without oats in adults with celiac disease. N Engl J Med 333:1033, 1995

KAGNOFF M et al: Evidence for the role of human intestinal adenovirus in the pathogenesis of coeliac disease. Gut 28:5, 1987

KERLIN P, WONG L: Breath hydrogen testing in bacterial overgrowth of the small intestine. Gastroenterology 95:982, 1988

LADINSER B et al: Endomysium antibodies in coeliac disease. Gut 35:776, 1994

LOUGHRAN TP et al: T-cell intestinal lymphoma associated with celiac sprue. Ann Intern Med 104:44, 1986

MARCUARD SP et al: Omeprazole therapy causes malabsorption of cyanocobalamin (vitamin B-12). Ann Intern Med 120:211, 1994

RELMAN DA et al: Identification of the uncultured bacillus of Whipple's disease. N Engl J Med 327:293, 1992

SALTZMAN JR et al: Bacterial overgrowth without clinical malabsorption in elderly hypochlorhydric subjects. Gastroenterology 106:615, 1994

SUAREZ FL et al: A comparison of symptoms after the consumption of milk or lactose-hydrolyzed milk by people with self reported lactose intolerance. N Engl J Med 333:1, 1995

SCHILLER LR et al: Studies on the prevalence and significance of radiolabeled bile acid malabsorption in a group of patients with idiopathic chronic diarrhea. Gastroenterology 92:151, 1987

TRIER JS: Medical progress: Celiac sprue. N Engl J Med 325:1709, 1991

TRONCONE R et al: Gluten-sensitive enteropathy. Pediatr Clin North Am 43:355, 1996

VAN ELBURG RM et al: Intestinal permeability in patients with coeliac disease and relatives of patients with coeliac disease. Gut 34:354, 1993

286   *Robert M. Glickman*

INFLAMMATORY BOWEL DISEASE: Ulcerative Colitis and Crohn's Disease

DEFINITION   *Inflammatory bowel disease* (IBD) is a general term for a group of chronic inflammatory disorders of unknown cause involving the gastrointestinal tract. Since these disorders have no pathognomonic features or specific diagnostic tests, in a strict sense they remain diagnoses of exclusion. Their features are sufficiently characteristic, however, to permit accurate diagnosis in most cases. Chronic IBD may be divided into two major groups, chronic nonspecific *ulcerative colitis* (UC) and *Crohn's disease* (CD). The original description of the latter disease by Crohn, Ginzberg, and Oppenheimer in 1932 localized it to segments of ileum. However, the same process may involve the buccal mucosa, esophagus, stomach, and duodenum, as well as the jejunum and ileum. Crohn's disease of the small bowel is also known as *regional enteritis*. A similar inflammatory picture may occur in the colon, either alone or with accompanying small intestinal involvement. In most instances, this form of colitis can be distinguished clinically and pathologically from ulcerative colitis and may be referred to as *Crohn's disease of the colon*. *Granulomatous colitis* is a less accurate term because only some cases exhibit granu-

lomas. Clinically these disorders are characterized by recurrent inflammatory involvement of intestinal segments with diverse clinical manifestations, often resulting in a chronic, unpredictable course.

EPIDEMIOLOGY   The epidemiology and etiology of UC and CD share many features and will be discussed together. These diseases are more common in whites than in blacks or Asians, and Jews have an incidence three to six times greater than that of non-Jews. The sexes are affected equally.

The incidence and prevalence of the two diseases differ slightly, UC being the more common. When analyzed in western Europe and the United States, UC (including ulcerative proctitis) has an incidence of approximately 6 to 8 cases per 100,000 population and an estimated prevalence of approximately 70 to 150 cases per 100,000 population. Estimates of the incidence of CD (colonic plus small bowel) are approximately 2 cases per 100,000 population; the prevalence is estimated at 20 to 40 per 100,000 population. Many believe the incidence of CD (especially colonic) to be increasing. In western Europe and North America, the incidence and prevalence of CD have been increasing five times faster than those of ulcerative colitis.

While the occurrence of both diseases peaks between the ages of 15 and 35, they have been reported from every decade of life. A familial incidence of IBD has been recorded, with estimates that 2 to 5 percent of persons with CD or UC will have one or more relatives affected. There is no specificity, however, for a given form of IBD within a given family. Such epidemiologic clustering of cases could be due to an effect of either genetic factors or common environmental influences on the development of these diseases (see below). It has been suggested that the pathogenesis of these disorders has both a probable hereditary basis and a strong environmental component.

ETIOLOGY AND PATHOGENESIS   While the causes of UC and CD remain unknown, certain features of these diseases have suggested several areas of possible importance. These include familial or genetic, infectious, immunologic, and psychological factors.

As mentioned, the increased incidence of inflammatory bowel disease in whites and in Jews and the occurrence of familial clustering suggest a *genetic* predisposition to the development of the disease. An increased incidence of CD in monozygotic twins also is strong evidence for a genetic component. A search for genetic markers that might be of value in identifying susceptible individuals has not identified any single marker (i.e., a histocompatibility antigen) in patients with IBD.

The chronic inflammatory nature of these diseases has prompted a continuing search for an *infectious* cause. Despite numerous attempts, no bacterial, fungal, or viral agents has thus far been isolated. Preliminary reports of isolates of cell wall variants of *Pseudomonas* or of transmissible agents producing cytopathic effects in tissue culture have yet to be confirmed. As discussed below, many infectious agents can produce *acute* colitis or ileitis; however, there is no evidence that these agents are involved in *chronic* IBD.

The idea that an *immune* mechanism is involved is based on the reasoning that the extraintestinal manifestations that may accompany these disorders (e.g., arthritis and pericholangitis) may represent autoimmune phenomena and that therapeutic agents such as glucocorticoids, azathioprine, and cyclosporine may act via immunosuppressive mechanisms. Patients with IBD may have *humoral antibodies* to colon cells, to bacterial antigens such as *Escherichia coli*, to lipopolysaccharide, and to foreign proteins such as cow's milk protein. In general, the presence and titer of these antibodies do not correlate with disease activity. It is likely that these antigens gain access to immunocompetent cells as a consequence of epithelial damage. In addition, IBD has been described in association with agammaglobulinemia as well as IgA deficiency, casting further doubt on the pathogenetic role of humoral antibodies. *Immune complexes* also have been invoked to explain extraintestinal manifestations of IBD. While there are well-defined examples of tissue injury resulting from immune complexes, studies using specific detection techniques have failed to demonstrate an increased frequency of immune complexes in patients with IBD.

Abnormalities of *cell-mediated immunity* that have been reported in association with IBD include cutaneous anergy, diminished responsiveness to various mitogenic stimuli, and a decreased number of peripheral T cells. Since many of these changes may revert to normal when the disease is quiescent, they are probably secondary phenomena. Many abnormalities of cell-mediated immunity in the mucosa of patients with IBD also have been described. They include an increased concentration of mucosal IgG cells and changes in subsets of T cells, suggesting antigenic stimulation. Activation of mucosal immune cells results in a complex expression of cytokines, which may contribute to the mucosal inflammatory response. In addition, noncytokine inflammatory mediators, such as prostaglandin and thromboxane products, are present in elevated levels in the mucosa of patients with IBD and would further stimulate the inflammatory response. Animal models of IBD, including a transgenic rat model that expresses human HLA-B27, a mouse deficient in interleukin 2, and the spontaneous chronic colitis of the cotton-top tamarin, also may yield important insights into the pathogenesis of IBD. No immunologic alterations specific for either UC or CD have yet been found, however.

The *psychological* features of patients with IBD also have been stressed. It is not uncommon for these diseases to present initially or to flare up in association with major psychological stresses such as the loss of a family member. It has been suggested that patients with IBD have a characteristic personality that renders them susceptible to emotional stresses. While there is little evidence directly relating emotional factors to the etiology of IBD, there is little doubt that a chronic disease of unknown cause, affecting individuals in the prime of life, often results in anger, anxiety, and some degree of depression. These reactions are undoubtedly important factors in modifying the course of these diseases and the response to therapy.

PATHOLOGY   In UC, there is an inflammatory reaction primarily involving the colonic mucosa. Grossly, the colon appears ulcerated, hyperemic, and usually hemorrhagic (Fig. 286-1). A striking feature of the inflammation is that it is *uniform* and *continuous*, with no intervening areas of normal mucosa. The rectum is usually involved (95 percent of cases), and the inflammation extends proximally in a continuous fashion for a variable distance. When the entire colon is involved, there may also be minimal involvement of a few centimeters of the terminal ileum, called "backwash ileitis." This involvement never leads to the thickening and narrowing characteristic of Crohn's disease. The surface mucosal cells as well as the crypt epithelium and submucosa are involved in an inflammatory reaction with neutrophilic infiltration (Fig. 286-2A). This reaction progresses to epithelial damage with loss of surface epithelial cells, resulting in multiple ulcerations. Infiltration of the crypts by neutrophils results in characteristic (but not specific) small crypt abscesses and eventual crypt destruction. There also may be loss of crypt epithelium, with a loss of goblet cells and submucosal edema. Repetitive cycles of inflammation lead to mild submucosal fibrosis. Regenerative activity is evidenced by crypts with irregular epithelium and often with a basal bifurcation. It is important to stress that, unlike Crohn's disease, deeper layers of the bowel, beneath the submucosa, usually are not involved. In severe UC, as seen with toxic megacolon, the bowel wall may become extremely thin and denuded of mucosa, with inflammation extending to the serosa, leading to dilation and subsequent perforation.

Recurrent inflammation may lead to characteristic features of chronicity. Fibrosis and longitudinal retraction result in shortening of the colon. Loss of the normal haustral pattern leads radiologically to a smooth, "lead-pipe" appearance of the colon. Regenerating islands of mucosa surrounded by areas of ulceration and denuded mucosa appear as "polyps" protruding into the lumen. However, these protrusions are inflammatory rather than neoplastic and are therefore called *pseudopolyps* (Fig. 286-2B).

With long-standing UC, the surface epithelium may show features of *dysplasia*. Nuclear and cellular atypia are thought to represent premalignant changes occurring in the setting of long-standing UC. Marked dysplasia in colonic biopsy samples in the setting of long-standing colitis is associated with a significant risk of a carcinoma elsewhere in the colon and may influence the decision to advise colectomy.

Crohn's disease, in contrast to ulcerative colitis, is characterized by chronic inflammation extending through *all layers of the intestinal wall* and involving the mesentery as well as regional lymph nodes. Whether or not the small bowel or colon is involved, the basic pathologic process is the same for small bowel and colonic involvement.

The earliest pathologic changes in CD are poorly defined, since surgery is usually not undertaken electively early in the course of the disease. At laparotomy, the terminal ileum appears hyperemic and boggy, with mesentery and mesenteric lymph nodes swollen and reddened. At this stage, the bowel wall, although edematous, is usually pliable. While some patients with this initial presentation subsequently develop typical regional enteritis, a significant number recover completely. This acute form of ileitis will undoubtedly be shown to have diverse causes. Indeed, a significant number of patients with this presentation have been shown to be infected with *Yersinia enterocolitica*, an organism capable of producing a self-limited, acute inflammatory ileitis.

As the disease progresses, the gross appearance becomes characteristic. The bowel appears greatly thickened and leathery with a narrowed lumen (Fig. 286-3). This characteristic stenosis can occur in any portion of the intestine and may be associated with some degree of intestinal obstruction. The mesentery appears greatly thickened and fatty and often extends over the serosal surface of the bowel in characteristic finger-like projections. The appearance of the mucosa depends on the severity and stage of the disease, but it may be relatively normal, in sharp contrast to the mucosa in UC. In more advanced cases, the mucosa has a nodular, "cobblestone" look. This appearance is the result of submucosal thickening and mucosal ulceration, often linear in the long axis of the bowel at the base of mucosal folds. These ulcerations may penetrate into the submucosa and muscularis and coalesce to form intramural channels that become manifest as fistulas and fissures.

Other morphologic features also distinguish CD from UC. In CD, the disease is often *discontinuous*; severely involved segments of bowel are separated by "skip areas" of apparently normal bowel. In approximately 50 percent of cases of CD of the colon, the rectum is spared. In sharp contrast, in UC, the involvement is contiguous and the rectum almost always is involved. In addition, in CD, the transmural inflammatory process, involving serosa and mesentery, accounts for the characteristic fistula and abscess formation. As a result of serosal inflammation, adjacent loops of small intestine may become adherent

FIGURE 286-1   Ulcerative colitis. Resected colon with portion of terminal ileum. The specimen showed uniform inflammation, erythema, and hemorrhage and a normal terminal ileum.

FIGURE 286-2 Colonic biopsy samples in inflammatory bowel disease. *A.* Ulcerative colitis. The surface mucosa is destroyed and the submucosa is diffusely infiltrated with polymorphonuclear leukocytes. Crypt abscesses are also present. *B.* Pseudopolyp. Regenerating island of mucosa with adjacent area of ulceration. *C.* Ulcerative colitis. Severe dysplasia occurring in long-standing chronic ulcerative colitis. Note atypical changes in the nuclei and marked palisading of nuclei of the crypt epithelium. *D.* Crohn's disease of the colon. Note the relatively intact mucosa with a solitary granuloma in the lamina propria.

FIGURE 286-3 Regional enteritis. Resected specimen of terminal ileum demonstrates thickened bowel wall and chronically inflamed mucosa. Note the relatively sharp demarcation of the diseased segment, with grossly normal mucosa on either side.

Pathologic and Clinical Features of IBD

Features	Ulcerative Colitis	Crohn's Disease
PATHOLOGIC FEATURES		
Segmental	0	+ +
Transmural involvement	+/−	+ +
Granulomas	0	+/+ + (50%)
Fibrosis	+	+ +
Fissuring, fistulas	+/−	+ +
Mesenteric fat, lymph node involvement	0	+ +
CLINICAL FEATURES		
Diarrhea	+ +	+ +
Rectal bleeding	+ +	+
Abdominal pain	+	+ +
Palpable mass	0	+ +
Fistulas	+/−	+ +
Strictures	+	+ +
Small bowel involvement	+/− ("backwash ileitis")	+ +
Rectal involvement	+ + (95%)	+/+ + (50%)
Extraintestinal disease	+ +	+ +
Toxic megacolon	+	+/−
Recurrence after colectomy	0	+
Malignancy (with long-standing disease)	+	+/−

NOTE: 0, never; +/−, rare; +, occasional; + +, frequent, common.

and matted together by a fibrinous peritoneal reaction, leading to a palpable mass, most often in the right lower quadrant. Fistulas may form between adherent structures, including loops of intestine or colon as well as adjacent organs such as the bladder or vagina. Fistulous tracts also may lead to the skin or end blindly in the peritoneum or retroperitoneum, surrounded by adherent loops of bowel and inflammatory tissue. Fistula formation is not seen in UC.

Microscopically, granulomas are most helpful in distinguishing CD from other forms of IBD; they do not occur in UC. They may be seen in rectal or colonoscopic biopsy samples (Fig. 286-2*D*). While granulomas are a helpful finding when present, it is the chronic inflammation involving all layers of the intestinal wall which is most characteristic of CD.

In most series reporting the distribution of CD, approximately 30 percent of cases involve only the small intestine (usually the terminal ileum), 30 percent have only colonic involvement, and 40 percent have ileocolic involvement, usually of the ileum and right colon. In a small number of patients (mostly children and adolescents) there is diffuse and extensive ulceration of the jejunum and ileum.

While there often are sufficient features to permit distinction between UC and CD of the colon (Table 286-1), in 10 to 20 percent of cases this distinction is not possible.

CLINICAL FEATURES

ULCERATIVE COLITIS The major symptoms of UC are bloody diarrhea and abdominal pain, often with fever and weight loss in more severe cases. With mild disease, there may be one or two semiformed stools per day, containing little blood, and there may be no systemic manifestations. In contrast, the patient with severe disease may have frequent liquid stools containing blood and pus, complain of severe cramps, and demonstrate symptoms and signs of dehydration, anemia, fever, and weight loss. With predominantly rectal involvement, constipation rather than diarrhea may be present, and tenesmus may be a major complaint. On occasion, intestinal symptoms may be overshadowed by fever, weight loss, or one of the extracolonic manifestations of the disease (see below).

The physical findings in UC are usually nonspecific; there may be some abdominal distention or tenderness along the course of the colon. In mild cases, the general physical examination will be normal. Extracolonic manifestations include arthritis, skin changes, or evidence of liver disease. Fever, tachycardia, and postural hypotension are usually associated with more severe disease. The laboratory findings are often nonspecific and usually reflect the degree and severity of bleeding and inflammation. There may be anemia, which reflects chronic disease as well as iron deficiency from chronic blood loss. Leukocytosis with

a left shift and an elevated erythrocyte sedimentation rate are often seen in the severely ill, febrile patient. Electrolyte abnormalities, especially hypokalemia, reflect the degree of diarrhea. Hypoalbuminemia is common with extensive disease and usually represents luminal protein loss through an ulcerated mucosa. An elevated alkaline phosphatase level may indicate associated hepatobiliary disease (see below).

The clinical course of UC is variable. Most patients will suffer a relapse within 1 year of the first attack, reflecting the recurrent nature of the disease. There may, however, be prolonged periods of remission with only minimal symptoms. In general, the severity of symptoms reflects the extent of colonic involvement and the intensity of the inflammation. At one end of the spectrum are patients who present with limited involvement of the rectum (ulcerative proctitis) or rectum and sigmoid (ulcerative proctosigmoiditis). Their disease usually is mild, with minimal systemic or extracolonic manifestations, although ulcerative proctitis is sometimes difficult to treat, exhibiting protracted bleeding and tenesmus. The major symptoms are rectal bleeding and tenesmus. Most of these patients, especially those with only rectal involvement, do not develop more extensive disease. In the remainder, the disease may extend proximally with variable involvement. Perhaps 85 percent of patients with UC have mild to moderate disease of an intermittent nature and can be managed without hospitalization. In approximately 15 percent of patients, the disease becomes more fulminant, involves the entire colon, and presents with severe bloody diarrhea and systemic signs and symptoms. These patients are at risk of developing toxic dilation and perforation of the colon (described below) and represent a medical emergency.

CROHN'S DISEASE As discussed above, the basic pathologic features of CD are the same whether the disease involves the small bowel or the colon. The clinical presentation, however, largely reflects the anatomic location of the disease and to some degree predicts which complications may develop. The clinical features are compared in Table 286-1.

The major clinical features of CD are fever, abdominal pain, diarrhea (often without blood), and generalized fatigability. There may be associated weight loss. With *colonic involvement*, diarrhea and pain are the most frequent symptoms. Rectal bleeding is distinctly less common than with UC and reflects (1) sparing of the rectum in many patients and (2) the transmural nature of the disease, with only irregular mucosal involvement. There may be associated severe anorectal complications such as fistulas, fissures, and perirectal abscess. Such features may antedate the clinical onset of colitis and should always raise the suspicion of associated Crohn's disease. Recurrent perirectal inflammation may result in a thickened anal canal, and perianal fistulas or scarring may be present. Extensive colonic involvement may lead to dilation of the colon. However, since CD often results in a thickened colonic wall, this feature is less common with CD than with UC. Extracolonic manifestations (discussed below), particularly arthritis, are seen more commonly with colonic than with small-bowel CD.

Involvement of the *small bowel* may be accompanied by additional presenting signs and symptoms. Typically, the disease presents in a young adult with a history of fatigue, variable weight loss, right lower quadrant discomfort or pain, and diarrhea. Low-grade fever, anorexia, nausea, and vomiting also may be present. The abdominal pain may be steady and localized to the right lower quadrant or may assume a colicky or crampy pattern, reflecting various degrees of intestinal stenosis. The diarrhea is often moderate, usually without gross blood; if there is no rectal involvement, tenesmus is absent. Physical examination at this time often reveals right lower quadrant tenderness with an associated fullness or mass reflecting adherent loops of bowel. At this time the patient may have mild anemia, mild to moderate leukocytosis, and an elevated erythrocyte sedimentation rate.

Since acute ileitis may have an abrupt onset with fever, leukocytosis, and right lower quadrant pain, the clinical picture may be indistinguishable from that of acute appendicitis. Often the diagnosis can be made only at laparotomy, when the characteristic beefy red terminal ileum, boggy mesenteric fat, and succulent mesenteric lymph nodes indicate that appendicitis alone cannot be the culprit.

While the symptoms of diarrhea and abdominal pain will usually alert the clinician to the possibility of regional enteritis, other symptoms may dominate the clinical presentation. In children and the aged, fever of undetermined origin and unexplained weight loss may be prominent and initially may suggest an underlying malignancy. In some patients, the first manifestation of the disease is intestinal obstruction; in others, the disease presents with perianal sepsis or urinary tract infection resulting from an enterovesical fistula. Similarly, right ureteral obstruction and hydronephrosis may occur as a result of external compression of the ureter by a right lower quadrant inflammatory mass. On occasion, often in the setting of extensive small-bowel involvement, features of malabsorption may be prominent. These features, along with anorexia and the catabolic effects of the chronic inflammatory process, may combine to produce striking weight loss. The complications of the disease are often local, resulting from intestinal inflammation and involvement of adjacent structures.

Intestinal obstruction is a frequent complication, occurring in 20 to 30 percent of patients during the course of the disease. In the initial stages, the obstruction usually is due to acute inflammation and edema of the involved intestinal segment, which is usually the terminal ileum. However, as the disease progresses and fibrosis develops, obstruction may be due to a fixed narrowing of the bowel.

Fistula formation is a frequent complication of chronic regional enteritis as well as of CD of the colon. Fistulas may occur between contiguous segments of intestine; they also may burrow into the retroperitoneal spaces and present as cutaneous fistulas or indolent abscesses. In a significant number of patients, the first indication of the disease may be the presence of persistent rectal fissures, a perirectal abscess, or a rectal fistula. Although uncommon, pneumaturia should raise the suspicion of enterovesical fistula and is often associated with a persistent urinary tract infection.

Since CD is a transmural disease in which the bowel wall is greatly thickened, free *intestinal perforation* is uncommon. Rarely, however, it is the presenting feature, and the disease is first discovered at the time of laparotomy for a perforated viscus. The passage per rectum of bright red blood should alert one to the possible coexistence of rectal involvement (i.e., ileocolitis). CD can involve any portion of the gastrointestinal tract. Aphthous ulcers are the most common *oral* manifestation of CD. CD also may involve the *stomach* and *duodenum*, most often the antrum and/or the first and second portions of the

duodenum. Symptoms may include pain mimicking peptic ulcer disease. Later in the course of the disease, chronic scarring may produce gastric outlet or duodenal obstruction.

There are increasing reports of *small-bowel* and *colonic malignancy* developing in the setting of long-standing CD. The frequency of malignancy in this setting is low compared with the frequency of malignancy in UC, however (see below). The presence of extensive ileal disease, resulting in *bile salt malabsorption*, is associated with a decreased bile salt pool and increased bile lithogenicity (see Chap. 285). Up to 30 percent of patients with extensive ileal disease develop gallstones. Also, in the setting of ileal disease and an intact colon, there is increased colonic absorption of dietary oxalate, with resulting hyperoxaluria and the development of *urinary oxalate stones*. Dehydration due to diarrhea is an additional predisposing factor in renal stone formation.

DIAGNOSIS

The diagnosis of IBD should be entertained in all patients presenting with diarrhea or bloody diarrhea, persistent perianal sepsis, and abdominal pain. Atypical presentations also occur, such as fever of unexplained origin either in the absence of bowel symptoms or with extracolonic manifestations such as arthritis or liver disease that antedate or overshadow the bowel involvement. Since CD also may involve the small intestine, it should be considered in the differential diagnosis of all types of malabsorption syndromes, intermittent intestinal obstruction, and abdominal fistulas.

The results of laboratory tests usually are nonspecific and reflect the extent and severity of the inflammatory reaction. When CD involves the small bowel, laboratory features of malabsorption also may be present. There may be a variable degree of anemia, caused by occult blood loss or the effect of chronic inflammation on the bone marrow. Folate or vitamin B_{12} malabsorption also may contribute to the anemia. While the Schilling test may give abnormal results in patients with extensive ileal disease, frank macrocytic anemia due to vitamin B_{12} malabsorption alone is unusual, attesting to the efficiency of ileal absorption of the vitamin. When there is significant diarrhea, electrolyte abnormalities (hypokalemia, hypomagnesemia) may be prominent. Hypocalcemia may reflect extensive mucosal involvement and malabsorption of vitamin D. Hypoalbuminemia may result from amino acid malabsorption as well as from protein-losing enteropathy. A variable degree of steatorrhea may result from bile salt depletion and mucosal damage. Mild abnormalities of liver function markers (especially an increased level of serum alkaline phosphatase) may reflect the development of hepatosteatosis in a malnourished patient or a coexisting early sclerosing cholangitis. Significant jaundice is unusual.

Sigmoidoscopy and *radiologic studies* of the bowel are most important in establishing the diagnosis of IBD. Sigmoidoscopy must be performed in all patients presenting with chronic diarrhea and in all instances of rectal bleeding. While meticulous air-contrast barium enema examination of a perfectly prepared colon may disclose the earliest mucosal changes in either UC or CD (see below), a conventional barium enema examination is often "normal" in early disease. Direct visualization of the colonic mucosa combined with biopsy is the most sensitive way of determining whether rectal inflammation is present. This procedure can often be performed without prior enema preparation in a patient having active diarrhea. The goal of this initial sigmoidoscopy is to establish *whether* mucosal inflammation is present, not necessarily to determine its full *extent*. Thus, if changes are encountered within the first 8 to 10 cm, it is not necessary to pass the instrument to its full length, which may cause discomfort when the bowel is acutely inflamed. In UC, findings include a loss of mucosal vascularity, diffuse erythema, friability of the mucosa, and often an exudate consisting of mucus, blood, and pus. Mucosal friability and uniform involvement are characteristic. Once diseased mucosa is encountered (usually in the rectum), there are no areas of intervening normal mucosa before the proximal limit of the disease is reached. Ulcers are shallow and may be small or confluent, but ulceration invariably occurs in segments of active colitis. Full colonoscopic examination of the colon in UC is not indicated in the acutely ill patient. Rectal biopsy may corroborate mucosal inflammation. With more chronic disease, the mucosa may appear granular and pseudopolyps may be present.

Endoscopic examination of the colon is also of value in the diagnosis of colonic CD. The salient finding is ulcerations, which may be tiny, aphthous erosions or deep, longitudinal fissures. They usually occur in segments of otherwise normal mucosa. Since the mucosa is not uniformly involved, friability and diffuse granularity—hallmarks of UC—are not characteristic. Rather, a cobblestone appearance—that is, coarse irregularity of the mucosal surface, reflecting submucosal inflammation—is characteristic of CD. Pseudopolyps, edema, and strictures may be seen in CD as well as in UC. Colonic mucosal biopsy reveals granulomas in 30 to 50 percent of specimens taken from involved areas. Features such as crypt abscesses, infiltration with inflammatory cells, or ulcerations are nonspecific but compatible. Since skip areas and rectal sparing are characteristic of CD, colonoscopy may be better than sigmoidoscopy for the evaluation of CD. Colonoscopic examination is also indicated when CD appears only to involve the small bowel. Ileal biopsy may be feasible, and coexisting colonic involvement occurs in a significant number of cases. Perianal inflammatory lesions as well as areas of rectal disease seen at endoscopy often show granulomatous inflammation. In 5 to 15 percent of patients, rectal biopsy samples of seemingly uninvolved areas show microscopic evidence of granulomatous inflammation.

The *radiologic evaluation* of the bowel provides essential information in the diagnosis of IBD. In UC, barium enema may reveal the extent of the disease and help to define associated features such as stricture, pseudopolyposis, or carcinoma. The earliest features seen in UC are irritability and incomplete filling due to associated inflammation. Fine ulcerations may be seen at this time as serrations along the contour of the bowel, producing a hazy margin (Fig. 286-4). The ulcerations may become deeper and, with more fulminant disease, produce a grossly ragged and irregular contour. Polypoid defects appear as a result of edematous mucosa between ulcerations. The diffuse pattern of ulceration is best seen on the evacuation film or on air-contrast barium enema. In the chronic stage of the disease (Fig. 286-5), the characteristic features are shortening of the bowel, depression of the flexures, narrowing of the bowel lumen, and rigidity. The bowel has a symmetric, ahaustral, tubular appearance with a decreased mucosal pattern. Although strictures are uncommon, when they occur, they have a concentric lumen with fusiform tapering margins. Eccentricity should raise the suspicion of an associated carcinoma.

On barium enema examination, CD of the colon usually has features that distinguish it from UC. These features include rectal sparing, the presence of skip lesions, and small ulcerations occurring on small irregular nodules. Small ulcerations often extend to produce longitudinal ulcers (Fig. 286-6) and transverse fissures, which in reality are limited sinus tracts. These may extend into adjacent tissues to produce fistulas. Irregular thickening and fibrosis may lead to stricture formation, which may be multiple. In 10 to 15 percent of cases, the disease involves the entire colon uniformly, making differentiation from UC more difficult. Reflux of barium into the terminal ileum during barium enema may reveal characteristic ileal changes of regional enteritis.

The terminal ileum is the portion of the small intestine most often involved by CD, with features similar to those of colonic involvement. Careful x-ray examination of the small bowel may demonstrate loss of mucosal detail and rigidity of involved segments resulting from submucosal edema or stenosis. The submucosal inflammation may lead to the characteristic radiologic cobblestone appearance of the mucosa (Fig. 286-7), and fistulous tracts may be seen, especially in the ileocecal area (Fig. 286-8). Involvement of the stomach and duodenum usually appears radiologically as stiffening and infiltration of the mucosa and can mimic an infiltrative tumor. If such an appearance is due to regional enteritis, there is almost always coexisting involvement of the jejunum or ileum. In CD, computed tomography (CT) of the abdomen may be of value in the evaluation of thickened, separated bowel loops and may help distinguish thickened, matted loops (phlegmon) from intraabdominal abscess.

While barium studies often provide information on the pattern and extent of IBD, caution must be exercised in performing these studies

FIGURE 286-4 Acute ulcerative colitis, air-contrast study. Note the diffuse fine ulceration of the entire colon, producing serration along the contour of the bowel. *(Courtesy of R. Gold, Columbia Presbyterian Medical Center.)*

FIGURE 286-5 Chronic ulcerative colitis. Note the loss of haustrations and the fusiform stricture in the transverse colon. *(Courtesy of R. Gold, Columbia Presbyterian Medical Center.)*

FIGURE 286-8   Regional enteritis. X-ray showing fistulas between loops of bowel. Insert is a compression film of this area; note fistulas between adjacent loops of bowel.

FIGURE 286-6   Crohn's colitis. Air-contrast study.

FIGURE 286-7   Crohn's ileocolitis. Note the nodularity and ulceration of the terminal ileum and the deformity of the cecum.

in acutely ill patients with severe colitis, as the procedure and the bowel cleansing that precedes it may cause a worsening of the disease and can precipitate toxic dilation of the colon.

Fiberoptic colonoscopy is a powerful tool in the diagnosis of colonic IBD. Areas beyond the reach of the sigmoidoscope can now be directly visualized and biopsied. Early in the course of colonic inflammation, endoscopic examination and biopsy are the most sensitive techniques for demonstrating mucosal involvement. Polypoid lesions, strictures, and unclear x-ray features can usually be defined fully. Periodic colonoscopic examination and biopsy are being used increasingly in cancer surveillance in patients with long-standing IBD (see below).

DIFFERENTIAL DIAGNOSIS

Many entities must be considered in the differential diagnosis of IBD. The focus of the differential diagnosis is determined largely by the presenting features of the disease. When *rectal bleeding* is the presenting complaint, a colonic source should be considered. While *hemorrhoids* are commonly found, they must be considered a tentative source of bleeding until sigmoidoscopy, colonoscopy, and/or barium enema examination have ruled out other colonic lesions. Colonic *neoplasms* (carcinoma, adenomatous polyps) also may present with rectal bleeding and can usually be diagnosed by barium enema with subsequent sigmoidoscopic or colonoscopic biopsy. It should be remembered that carcinoma may complicate long-standing colitis. Rectal bleeding from *colonic diverticula* or *arteriovenous malformations* usually presents no problem in differential diagnosis, since radiologic and endoscopic features of IBD are absent. *Radiation proctitis*, which may present as a localized area of colitis, is usually found in the setting of pelvic irradiation. The onset may be months to years after irradiation. Characteristic features on sigmoidoscopy include mucosal atrophy and telangiectasia along with friability and small ulcerations. A colitis sometimes indistinguishable from ulcerative colitis may occur in Behçet's syndrome and is associated with aphthous oral ulceration, uveitis, and urethritis.

Acute colitis may be caused by a variety of *infectious* agents (Chap. 128). Often presenting with bloody diarrhea, infectious colitis may be difficult to distinguish from IBD at initial presentation, and severe cases may present with colonic dilation mimicking toxic megacolon.

Rectal biopsy in infectious colitis shows marked polymorphonuclear infiltration with pronounced edema and relative sparing of the crypts, features that may distinguish this entity from idiopathic inflammatory bowel disease. A listing of these agents is given in Table 286-2. It should also be noted that an unexplained exacerbation of IBD symptoms may be due to a superimposed infectious colitis. Thus, in all cases of IBD exacerbation, appropriate cultures should be performed to rule out an associated infection.

Amebiasis may present with bloody diarrhea and may be indistinguishable by sigmoidoscopy from idiopathic ulcerative colitis. A history of recent foreign travel or homosexual exposure would be important. Serologic testing may be of value, although initial positive titers may indicate prior amebic infection at an indeterminate time in the past. Since specific amebicidal therapy is necessary to eradicate this infection and corticosteroids may be detrimental, every effort should be made to exclude this diagnosis in appropriate individuals via serologic titers and careful examination of colonic secretions and biopsy samples. Acute *bacillary dysentery* may be caused by *Shigella* and *Salmonella* or *Campylobacter*, all easily diagnosed by stool culture. *Yersinia enterocolitis* infection, which may present as acute ileitis, also can produce a self-limited colitis, sometimes with granulomatous reaction. Infectious agents may cause acute proctitis indistinguishable from idiopathic ulcerative proctitis. Such infections, often seen in homosexuals, may represent herpes simplex virus infection, *gonorrhea*, *lymphogranuloma venereum* (LGV), cytomegalovirus infection, *Isospora* infection, or *Treponema pallidum* infection, as well as *amebiasis*. In homosexual men, non-LGV strains of *Chlamydia* have been shown to produce a granulomatous proctitis closely resembling Crohn's disease of the rectum.

Pseudomembranous colitis (antibiotic-associated colitis) is caused by a necrolytic toxin elaborated by *Clostridium difficile*, which proliferates the bowel under certain circumstances (see Chap. 148). Most often the disease is a result of antibiotic therapy, which presumably upsets the normal ecologic balance of the bowel flora and permits *C. difficile* to proliferate. Almost every antibiotic has been implicated, although cases related to the use of vancomycin or aminoglycosides are rare. Most often diarrhea is profuse and watery, although bloody diarrhea occurs in 5 percent of cases. Characteristic multiple, discrete yellowish plaques are seen on sigmoidoscopy, which on biopsy show features of acute inflammation and ulceration with a pseudomembrane of fibrin and necrotic material. On occasion, lesions may be beyond the reach of the sigmoidoscope and require colonoscopy. Diagnosis is best made by detecting *C. difficile* toxin in the stool. Treatment is initially directed at eradicating *C. difficile* from the stool. Vancomycin (250 mg orally qid for 7 to 14 days) is the treatment of choice for more severely ill patients and should produce clinical improvement within 5 days. Since vancomycin therapy is expensive, alternative therapies have been proposed. The use of metronidazole (500 mg orally qid for 7 to 14 days) has been shown to be as effective as vancomycin. Bacitracin (20,000 units qid for 7 to 14 days) is also

Table 286-2

Microbiologic Causes of Colitis

Shigella infection
Salmonella infection
Amebiasis (infection with *Entamoeba histolytica*)
Yersinia enterocolitica infection
Campylobacter jejuni infection
Lymphogranuloma venereum (LGV)
"Non-LGV" *Chlamydia* infection
Neisseria gonorrhoeae infection
Pseudomembranous colitis (caused by *Clostridium difficile* toxin)
Tuberculosis (*Mycobacterium tuberculosis* infection)
Infection with enteropathogenic *Escherichia coli* O157:H7
Aeromonas hydrophila infection
Plesiomonas shigelloides infection

quite effective. With all forms of therapy, relapse rates of 15 to 30 percent have been observed, and a second course of therapy may be required to eradicate the organism.

Occasionally, infectious colitis is superimposed on an unsuspected case of UC or CD. In this situation, once the acute infection has subsided, symptoms and inflammatory mucosal changes may persist, raising the possibility of associated idiopathic IBD. Similar considerations apply to the rare patient with IBD who develops associated *pseudomembranous colitis*. The finding of *C. difficile* toxin in the stool and subsequent treatment will serve to clarify this presentation.

Abdominal pain in association with rectal bleeding, especially in older patients, may be due to *ischemic colitis*; this condition may be most difficult to distinguish from IBD, especially CD. Because of an excellent collateral circulation, the rectum is usually spared. Radiologic features are often characteristic, showing submucosal edema or hemorrhage (thumb-printing) which typically resolves spontaneously over several weeks.

IBD may be difficult to distinguish from functional diarrhea early in the course of disease. The presence of constitutional symptoms such as fatigue, fever, weight loss, and nocturnal diarrhea, coupled with laboratory findings of anemia, an elevated erythrocyte sedimentation rate, or occult blood in the stool, should alert the clinician to the possibility of IBD. Similarly, the presence of leukocytes in a stained stool specimen points to an inflammatory basis for the diarrhea. In all cases, stool cultures and parasitologic examination of the stool are required to rule out enteric bacterial pathogens or amebiasis. In the *irritable bowel syndrome*, sigmoidoscopy, rectal biopsy, and barium enema examination all give normal results (see Chap. 287).

Once the diagnosis of idiopathic IBD has been established, it is usually possible to distinguish between UC and CD of the colon (see Table 286-1).

With small-intestinal involvement (regional enteritis), the differential diagnosis should include disorders presenting with intraabdominal abscesses, fistulas, intestinal obstruction, and malabsorption. The finding of associated colonic involvement in patients with ileal disease will often serve to distinguish CD from other ileal disorders. With diffuse involvement of the jejunum and ileum, regional enteritis must be distinguished from *nongranulomatous ulcerative jejunoileitis*. Abdominal pain and diarrhea are prominent features of the latter disorder, and weight loss, malabsorption, and hypoproteinemia tend to be more prominent than in regional enteritis. Small-bowel biopsy shows a more diffuse lesion with flattened villi (similar to celiac sprue), infiltration of the lamina propria, and mucosal ulceration. *Abdominal lymphoma* likewise may present with clinical and radiologic features difficult to distinguish from those of regional enteritis. Hepatosplenomegaly and peripheral adenopathy, when present, are helpful clues, but often disease is confined to the intestine. In such cases, laparotomy is usually required to make the definitive histologic diagnosis.

The advanced presentation of regional enteritis with areas of stenosis and draining fistulas also may be confused with *chronic fungal infection of the bowel*, including actinomycosis, aspergillosis, and blastomycosis. These infections often are seen in debilitated patients with impaired host defenses. Fungal skin tests and examination of fistula drainage and biopsy material for characteristic granules and fungi are helpful in making the diagnosis.

Intestinal tuberculosis characteristically produces stenotic lesions, usually in the terminal ileum and often also involving the contiguous cecum and ascending colon. Unlike regional enteritis, skip areas are unusual. Histologically, the granulomatous inflammation seen with *Mycobacterium tuberculosis* infection may be indistinguishable from regional enteritis; acid-fast stains and cultures are required for diagnosis. Fortunately, in western countries, primary intestinal tuberculosis is now rare.

COMPLICATIONS OF INFLAMMATORY BOWEL DISEASE

The complications of IBD may be classified as local or systemic, the former being direct consequences of inflammation or its extension

(Table 286-3). Local complications of IBD including fistulas, abscesses, and strictures are described above. In addition, perforation, toxic dilation, and the development of carcinoma may complicate both UC and CD.

CHAPTER 286
Inflammatory Bowel Disease: Ulcerative Colitis and Crohn's Disease 1641

PERFORATION Intestinal perforation can occur in severe UC because extensive ulceration may greatly thin the bowel wall. The clinical features are those of acute peritonitis, with signs of peritoneal inflammation and the demonstration of free air under the diaphragm on upright film of the abdomen. These signs are an indication for immediate colectomy.

Toxic dilation of the colon may occur in CD but is more common in UC. This complication can best be considered as a severe form of ulcerative colitis with the additional feature of colonic dilation. The dilation is thought to result from an effect of the severe inflammation on the neuromuscular tone of the bowel. Injudicious use of hypomotility agents (codeine, diphenoxylate, loperamide, paregoric, anticholinergic agents) to treat diarrhea in the setting of acute colitis can precipitate this complication. Similarly, cathartic preparation for a barium enema examination, as well as the examination and superimposed hypokalemia, may be contributing factors. Clinically, features of severe colitis are present, with high fever, tachycardia, volume depletion, electrolyte imbalance, and abdominal pain. On examination, the patient appears toxic, and colonic dilation may be evident. There is abdominal tenderness, and, if perforation has already occurred, peritoneal signs. Diarrhea may actually decrease markedly owing to colonic atony, creating the false impression that the colitis is clinically improved. Plain film of the abdomen will show colonic dilation with a colon diameter of more than 6 cm. There may be air in the wall of the colon, and irregular, ulcerated islands of mucosa may be silhouetted against the air shadow. While the transverse colon is the most common site of dilation, this effect is probably largely positional, since with the patient supine this is the highest portion of the colon. This presentation of colitis represents a true medical emergency and is associated with a mortality of greater than 30 percent if perforation has occurred. Appropriate therapy is discussed below.

CARCINOMA AND INFLAMMATORY BOWEL DISEASE Patients with chronic IBD have a higher incidence of carcinoma than the general population, especially patients who have extensive mucosal involvement (i.e., pancolitis) and those whose disease is of long duration. The cumulative risk of cancer begins to rise 10 years after the disease is diagnosed. While the incidence of cancer varies among patient populations, the overall incidence of cancer is estimated to be 0.5 to 1 percent per year after 10 years. For patients with pancolitis, the risk of cancer has been estimated to be 12 percent at 15 years, 23 percent at 20 years, and 42 percent at 24 years, although estimates in community-based practices have been lower (a 10 percent risk of colon cancer at 26 years). In children, the risk of cancer appears to rise more sharply after the first 10 years of disease, perhaps because of the higher incidence of pancolitis in children. Patients with ulcerative proctitis (disease limited to the rectum) have no increased risk of cancer. Rates of malignancy in patients with CD of the colon or small bowel are less well documented, but the incidence of both small- and large-bowel malignancy is higher than in the general population. However, it is lower than in patients with UC, perhaps because less mucosa usually is chronically involved with CD than with UC.

The development of colon carcinoma in the setting of IBD differs in important ways from that of carcinoma arising in a noncolitic population. Many of the earlier warning signs of a colonic neoplasm (rectal bleeding, a change in bowel habits) are difficult to interpret in the setting of colitis. In colitic patients, carcinomas are distributed more uniformly throughout the colon than in noncolitic patients; in the latter, most carcinomas are in the rectosigmoid region, within reach of the sigmoidoscope. In colitis patients, the tumors are more often multiple, flat, and infiltrating and appear to have a higher grade of malignancy. There is some evidence that these features may reflect the younger age at which they occur rather than the associated colitis. Further adding to the difficulty of diagnosis is the frequent occurrence of mucosal irregularities, ulcerations, and pseudopolyps, which make a small carcinoma difficult to diagnose radiologically or endoscopically.

Efforts have been made to devise effective screening procedures to detect carcinoma developing in the setting of IBD. Plasma levels of carcinoembryonic antigen may be elevated in UC, but this finding is nonspecific and therefore of limited value. Periodic barium enema examination and/or sigmoidoscopy or colonoscopy has been suggested, but interpretation of these studies is sometimes hampered by abnormalities related to the colitis itself. The addition of colonic mucosal biopsy may add a significant dimension. It was originally suggested that a generalized precancerous lesion may be present in high-risk patients with colitis who either harbor an occult malignancy or will develop cancer. Subsequent studies in patients who had long-standing colitis and subsequently underwent colectomy showed that if severe dysplasia was present, there was approximately a 50 percent chance that an associated malignancy also was present. Complicating these findings was the fact that dysplastic changes were found by rectal biopsies only 60 percent of the time, making colonoscopy with multiple biopsies desirable. In addition, in some patients who did not undergo colectomy, dysplasia was not a consistent finding on subsequent biopsies. In any event, it seems prudent to examine patients with colonic IBD of greater than 8 to 10 years' duration with colonoscopy and multiple mucosal biopsies at regular intervals. The optimal frequency for such examinations has not been established; recommendations vary from every 6 months to every 2 years. If severe dysplasia is found, confirmation at less than 6-month intervals seems prudent. While most authorities would not advise "prophylactic" colectomy in patients with long-standing colitis and mild or moderate dysplasia, the finding of severe dysplasia may well identify a subgroup who already harbor an occult carcinoma or are at high risk for carcinoma. There can be no uniform recommendation for this small group of patients, but many physicians will advise colectomy in this setting.

EXTRAINTESTINAL MANIFESTATIONS OF INFLAMMATORY BOWEL DISEASE

A variety of nonintestinal symptoms and signs may be associated with IBD and occur in both UC and CD (see Table 286-3). Because some of these manifestations may not coincide with or may overshadow

Table 286-3

Some Systemic Complications of Inflammatory Bowel Disease

Nutritional and metabolic complications
  Weight loss, reduced muscle mass, growth retardation (children)
  Electrolyte deficiency (K^+, Ca^{2+}, Mg^{2+})
  Hypoalbuminemia (inadequate nutrition, protein-losing enteropathy)
  Anemia (chronic disease, iron deficiency; rarely folate or vitamin B_{12} deficiency in Crohn's disease)
  Bile salt deficiency with ileal disease (steatorrhea and fat-soluble vitamin deficiency; increased colonic oxalate absorption leading to renal stones; increased lithogenicity of bile leading to gallstones)
Musculoskeletal complications
  Peripheral arthralgia, arthritis
  Ankylosing spondylitis, sacroileitis
  Granulomatous myositis (rare)
Hepatobiliary disease
  Hepatosteatosis
  Cholelithiasis
  Pericholangitis, biliary cirrhosis (rare)
  Sclerosing cholangitis
  Bile duct carcinoma
  Chronic active hepatitis and cirrhosis
Skin and mucous membrane complications
  Erythema nodosum
  Pyoderma gangrenosum
  Aphthous stomatitis
  Crohn's disease of buccal mucosa, gingiva, vagina
Ocular complications: iritis, uveitis, episcleritis
Venous thrombosis and thromboembolism (hypercoagulability, dehydration, stasis)

the underlying bowel disease, they sometimes pose difficult diagnostic problems. Their cause is currently unknown.

Joint manifestations occur in 25 percent of patients with IBD. They range from arthralgia to an acute arthritis with painful, swollen joints. The nondeforming arthritis is mono- or polyarticular and often migratory. Knees, ankles, and wrists are most commonly involved, but any joint may be affected. Joint fluid, if aspirated, reveals findings of an acute arthritis without crystals or evidence of infection. Tests for markers of specific forms of arthritis (rheumatoid factor, antinuclear antibody, and lupus erythematosus factor) are negative. Typically, the severity of arthritis varies with the activity of the underlying bowel disease. Rarely, peripheral arthritis truly predates clinical bowel symptoms. Arthritis is more common in patients with colonic than with only small-bowel involvement (regional enteritis).

In contrast, the central arthritis or ankylosing spondylitis associated with IBD is unrelated to the activity of the underlying bowel disease. It may antedate the bowel disease by years and persist after surgical or medical remission of the disease has been achieved. Symptoms consist of low backache and stiffness with eventual limitation of motion. Sacroileitis may be present as well. X-rays usually reveal characteristic changes. In contrast to the peripheral arthritis, there is a strong association of HLA-B27 with ankylosing spondylitis, whether or not IBD is present.

Like the peripheral arthritis, *skin manifestations* are more common with colonic disease. They occur in about 15 percent of patients, and their severity correlates with activity of the bowel disease. *Erythema nodosum* may be seen and heals without scarring. *Pyoderma gangrenosum*, an ulcerating lesion often occurring on the trunk, is relatively painless and may heal with scarring. In rare patients, the lesion persists even after colectomy for UC. *Aphthous ulcers* resemble "canker sores" of the mouth, and in approximately 5 to 10 percent of patients they are present during periods of active disease and then resolve. Their cause is unknown, and they are treated symptomatically. *Ocular manifestations* such as episcleritis, recurrent iritis, and uveitis occur in approximately 5 percent of patients and may represent a severe manifestation of the disease. In general, their activity parallels the course of the bowel disease, and they may respond dramatically when colectomy is done for other indications.

Abnormalities of *liver function* are common in IBD. In the severely ill, malnourished patient, mild abnormalities of serum levels of aminotransferases and alkaline phosphatase are often seen and represent nonspecific focal hepatitis or fatty infiltration. Factors favoring hepatosteatosis in the severely ill patient are poor nutrition and, often, concomitant steroid therapy. The lesion is not progressive and resolves with disease remission. *Pericholangitis* is characterized histologically by portal tract inflammation, some bile ductular proliferation, and concentric fibrosis around bile ductules. Some workers think that this lesion represents the intrahepatic form of sclerosing cholangitis. Most often, the lesion is clinically insignificant, and its sole manifestation is an elevated serum alkaline phosphatase level. It is usually nonprogressive and requires no therapy. Rarely, there is apparent progression to cirrhosis of either the postnecrotic or biliary type. Uncommonly, patients with IBD develop *sclerosing cholangitis* (Chap. 302), a chronic inflammation of unknown cause involving the extrahepatic and intrahepatic bile ducts, which may produce various degrees of extrahepatic biliary obstruction. Corticosteroids and immunosuppressive therapy are not beneficial. The disease only sometimes reverses after colectomy and should not be the sole indication for colectomy. Cholangiocarcinoma, arising in the extrahepatic biliary tree, has an increased incidence in patients with chronic UC, especially patients with sclerosing cholangitis. Such patients will present with extrahepatic biliary obstruction, which must be distinguished from sclerosing cholangitis. Finally, *autoimmune chronic active hepatitis*, which may progress to *cirrhosis*, may be seen in IBD, although the exact relationship between these disorders is unknown. There is no clear evidence that colectomy influences the course of this form of liver disease.

℞ TREATMENT

Certain common principles govern the treatment of UC and CD. Initial treatment of all forms of uncomplicated IBD is primarily medical, and the principles of medical therapy are similar for the two types of disease. Surgery is reserved for (1) specific complications and (2) intractable disease. There are important differences between the treatment of UC and CD however: the response to drug therapy may differ, complications often differ, and the prognosis after surgical therapy is not the same.

Ulcerative Colitis **MEDICAL THERAPY** Once the diagnosis is established, the severity of the disease must be assessed. Mild UC, including ulcerative proctitis, can usually be treated on an ambulatory basis. It should be noted that the disease is occasionally severe, even though it is limited to the rectum. The disease can worsen rapidly, and the course of a given attack cannot be predicted at the outset. The aims of therapy are to control the inflammatory process and to replace nutritional losses. A degree of improvement usually follows intravenous correction of fluid and electrolyte disturbances. Blood transfusions may be required, especially when there is continued active bleeding. Agents to control diarrhea (diphenoxylate, loperamide, codeine, anticholinergics) should be used with extreme caution for fear of precipitating colonic dilation and toxic megacolon. The decision to institute specific nutritional replacement therapy is determined by the patient's nutritional status and by whether the clinical course is expected to be protracted. In the severely ill patient, even clear liquids taken orally may stimulate colonic activity, and it is often wise to give the patients nothing by mouth. In this setting, intravenous alimentation, either peripheral or central, has been used as interim nutritional replacement therapy (see Chap. 78). While there is no evidence that intravenous alimentation is effective as primary therapy, it is an important component of a treatment program. In less severely ill patients able to tolerate fluids by mouth, the use of elemental oral diets may be beneficial, providing supplemental nutrition with low fecal volume.

The principal drugs used in the therapy of ulcerative colitis are the anti-inflammatory agents *sulfasalazine* (Azulfidine) and *glucocorticoids*. Sulfasalazine consists of a sulfonamide (sulfapyridine) moiety chemically bound to a salicylate (5-aminosalicylate); it undergoes bacterial cleavage in the colon. The liberated sulfapyridine is efficiently absorbed and largely excreted in the urine; the liberated 5-aminosalicylate, believed to be the active component, remains largely in the colon and is excreted in the stool. The salicylate moiety is thought to exert its action through inhibition of prostaglandin synthesis. While most physicians are familiar with the use of sulfasalazine to prevent recurrences of UC, it is less well appreciated that this agent is effective in the therapy of acute UC of mild to moderate severity. Therapeutic doses of 4 to 6 g/d are required. The drug is usually started at a dose of 500 mg bid and then increased daily or every other day by 1 g until the therapeutic dose is achieved. Topical preparations of 5-aminosalicylate (mesalamine) given as an enema are effective in the control of distal proctocolitis. Some of the oral and rectal 5-aminosalicylic acid products and their uses are listed in Table 286-4.

In the severely ill patient who may not tolerate oral medication, and for whom more rapid therapy is often desired, initial therapy is begun with glucocorticoids. While adrenocorticotropic hormone is as effective as glucocorticoids when given in equivalent dosages and by comparable routes of administration, most physicians seldom use it. The choice is one of individual preference; oral prednisone (45 to 60 mg/d) is usually employed initially. In the severely ill patient, parenteral administration of corticosteroids (i.e., intravenous prednisolone, 45 to 60 mg/d) is preferable to avoid the uncertainty of oral absorption. Improvement is usually noted after 7 to 10 days of such therapy by a reduction in fever, a decrease in bloody diarrhea, and improvement in appetite.

After initial improvement, low-roughage oral feedings can be resumed. At this point, the dose of steroids can be tapered. While there is no specific tapering schedule, the guiding principle is that, once clinical remission is achieved, there is no evidence that chronic glucocorticoid administration improves the long-term outlook or helps to prevent recurrences. In practice, steroid therapy can be tapered and discontinued over a 2- to 3-month period after discharge. In some patients (10 to 15 percent), efforts to completely eliminate steroids may be associated with a flare-up of the disease, and low to moderate steroid doses (10 to 15 mg prednisone daily) may be required to suppress disease activity. This regimen should not be confused with prophylactic administration of steroids to patients in remission but rather represents treatment of incompletely responsive disease. Once the acutely ill patient is taking oral feedings, sulfasalazine should be added as described above in a daily dose of 2 g. Controlled trials have shown that this dose of sulfasalazine, when administered chronically to patients with UC, is effective in decreasing the frequency of relapses and should be continued chronically after glucocorticoids have been discontinued. Patients with glucose phosphate dehydrogenase deficiency and those exhibiting severe allergic reactions to the sulfa moiety of the drug unfortunately cannot be maintained on it. Patients who exhibit intolerance for the drug (headache, nausea) or allergic reactions can be treated with one of the oral preparations of 5-aminosalicylate listed in Table 286-4. Mesalamine enemas are effective topical therapy for distal UC and are necessary to maintain remission.

The use of immunosuppressive therapy with drugs such as azathioprine is less well established in UC. As a single agent in the therapy of acute UC, the drug is ineffective. However, it may be added to the regimen at a dose of 1.5 to 2.0 mg/kg when glucocorticoids fail or when the steroid dose needed to reduce inflammation is too high. It is desirable to monitor the blood count and observe the patient carefully for infection. Azathioprine also may have a limited role as a "steroid-sparing agent" in the patient with chronic UC who must be maintained on glucocorticoids to control disease activity. Cyclosporine (4 mg/kg per day), a potent immunosuppressive agent, is also beneficial in severely ill patients, producing marked improvement in patients who otherwise would require colectomy.

Toxic megacolon is a major complication of severe UC that requires rapid, intensive management, best carried out jointly by the internist or gastroenterologist and the surgeon. Once the diagnosis is established, prompt and vigorous use of intravenous fluids, electrolyte replacement therapy, and blood transfusions are indicated. Because of the fear of perforation and high likelihood that bacteremia and occult perforation have occurred, many physicians institute broad-spectrum antibiotic coverage after appropriate cultures have been obtained. The patient is given nothing by mouth and nasogastric suction is instituted. Full intravenous glucocorticoid therapy is also begun. Most workers favor an initial period of medical stabilization for the first 24 to 48 h. If significant objective improvement has not occurred, and if perforation seems imminent, emergency colectomy should be carried out. While some patients slowly improve under maximal medical therapy and thus avoid colectomy, this approach is risky, because mortality rates rise sharply if perforation occurs,

approaching 50 percent in patients who subsequently undergo colectomy.

At the other end of the spectrum is the patient with mild UC limited to the rectum or rectosigmoid. Therapy is started with sulfasalazine, 0.5 to 1.0 g four times a day with meals. Alternatively, in the sulfa-allergic patient, 5-aminosalicylate enemas or oral 5-aminosalicylate preparations can be given. If rectal symptoms such as tenesmus are prominent, topical steroid enemas may produce marked improvement. The equivalent of 100 mg of hydrocortisone (20 mg of prednisone) in 60 to 100 mL of saline is used as a bedtime enema. On occasion, steroid foam preparations may be better tolerated in patients with severe tenesmus. Retention enemas have been shown to deliver medication as far as the descending colon, and absorption of steroid is slight (10 to 20 percent). If large doses of rectal steroids are required for control, it is preferable to use oral prednisone at a moderate dosage (20 mg/d).

PSYCHOTHERAPY The elements of trust and mutual understanding combined with the compassion and expertise of the physician are essential in the therapy of any chronic disease and are particularly important in the long-term management of patients with IBD. Often these patients are intelligent young adults, who frequently are resentful of a disease that affects them during their most productive years. However, through the vigorous participation of the physician, many patients are able to lead reasonably stable and productive lives. More formal psychiatric assistance may be required in chronically ill patients, in particular children or adolescents, and in the elderly, in whom severe depressive reactions are common. This is particularly true when colectomy is being advised and for the emotional adjustment that must be made after colectomy.

PREGNANCY AND ULCERATIVE COLITIS While many physicians are apprehensive about the management and prognosis of UC in the pregnant patient, the outcome for the patient and fetus is excellent. In general, the pregnancy is not threatened by coexisting colitis, with no increase in stillbirths or premature deliveries when compared with the general population. When patients with inactive colitis become pregnant, approximately 50 percent have an exacerbation of their disease, with some clustering of these flare-ups during the first trimester and in the postpartum period. The therapy of UC during pregnancy is largely the same as in the nonpregnant patient. Sulfasalazine is used to treat mild to moderate disease, since there is no evidence that the drug is harmful to the fetus or leads to fetal malformations. Women with inactive colitis who enter a pregnancy on maintenance sulfasalazine should be continued on the drug to protect the mother during the postpartum period from a relapse of disease. Both sulfasalazine and 5-aminosalicylate preparations may be taken during breast feeding. Corticosteroids should be used in the same dosage and for the same indications as in the nonpregnant patient. However, other immunosuppressive agents should not be

Table 286-4

5-Aminosalicylic Acid Products and Their Uses

Drug	Delivery Method	Dose	Use in Ulcerative Colitis	Use in Crohn's Disease
Sulfasalazine (Azulfidine)	Colonic bacterial azo reductases	2–4 g	Active colitis Maintenance	Active colonic disease
Olsalazine (Dipentum)	Colonic bacterial azo reductases	1 g	Active colitis Maintenance	Active colonic disease
Mesalamine (Asacol)	Eudragit-S Release at pH > 7	800–2400 mg	Active colitis Maintenance	Active colonic disease
Mesalamine (Pentasa)	Ethylcellulose microgranules Time-release	1500–4000 mg	Active colitis Maintenance	Active disease Maintenance
Mesalamine enemas (Rowasa)	Directly available	4 g	Active left-sided disease Maintenance	Distal colonic disease
Mesalamine suppositories (Rowasa)	Directly available	500 mg	Active proctitis Maintenance	Crohn's proctitis

SOURCE: Modified from Griffin and Miner.

used during pregnancy. Similar therapeutic approaches apply to the management of CD during pregnancy.

SURGICAL THERAPY Approximately 20 to 25 percent of patients with UC require colectomy during the course of their disease. A major indication for colectomy is failure to respond to intensive medical management. This group includes patients who do not improve after 7 to 10 days of optimal medical therapy, even if they do not show signs of colonic dilation. Fever, persistent bloody diarrhea, and severe fatigue may persist, and consideration should be given to semielective colectomy. Elective colectomy may be performed in patients whose disease remains chronically active and who require continuous glucocorticoid administration. Such patients are at risk of developing the complications of chronic steroid therapy. After colectomy, these patients often feel more energetic and usually gain weight to their preillness level. As discussed above, the patient with long-standing colitis is at high risk for colonic cancer. While most authorities do not advise "prophylactic" colectomy in patients with quiescent disease, the finding of marked dysplasia on colonoscopic biopsies performed as a part of a surveillance program should make the physician think seriously about advising colectomy.

The decision to advise colectomy in other than emergency circumstances is difficult for both patient and physician. Many patients have an understandable reluctance to undergo colectomy and have difficulty in viewing life with an ileostomy. In most metropolitan centers there are ileostomy groups who visit patients preoperatively and can provide answers to many practical questions. It is also desirable for the patient to be visited by a nurse familiar with stoma care to instruct the patient on the practical aspects of handling the ileostomy.

While total proctocolectomy with permanent ileostomy has been the standard surgical procedure for almost all patients undergoing colectomy, several alternative approaches are available. The *continent ileostomy* is an ileal loop reservoir fashioned under the skin with a nipple valve to prevent spilling of ileal contents. Ileal effluent collects in this reservoir, which must be emptied with a soft rubber catheter. Only a small stoma is externally visible, thus eliminating an external ileostomy appliance. Problems with leakage and frequent revisions have made this procedure less attractive. There is great enthusiasm for *ileal-rectal anastomosis* with an internal ileal pouch created to act as a reservoir. This often produces a highly satisfactory result, with continence and five to seven stools per day. Complications such as pouchitis or the need for surgical revision seem less frequent than with the continent ileostomy. Refinement in technique has permitted an *ileoanal anastomosis* with an internal pouch fashioned from small intestine anastomosed to the anal canal. When the procedure is performed by experienced surgeons, continence is excellent; however, nocturnal leakage occurs in about 20 percent of patients. Since some residual rectal mucosa may remain after these anastomotic procedures, surveillance proctoscopy for dysplasia should be performed.

Crohn's Disease The medical management of colonic CD is similar in most respects to that of UC. In a multicenter study (National Cooperative Crohn's Disease Study), sulfasalazine was shown to be effective in the therapy of active colonic disease. Glucocorticoids also were efficacious, but less so than with small-bowel involvement. The indications and dosages for these medications are similar to those for UC. Since, in CD, intraabdominal sepsis can result from fistula or abscess formation, glucocorticoids must be used with caution, and constant attention is required to detect sepsis, which can be masked by these agents. In general, the disease is less explosive in onset, and toxic dilation and perforation are less common than in UC. The principles of management are the same. Because of the indolent nature of the disease, the response to therapy is often less complete than in UC, and the disease tends to progress despite apparent clinical inactivity. It may be more difficult to achieve a clinical remission and to withdraw steroids completely.

As in UC, controlled studies have shown no benefit to continuing steroids after remission, since the frequency of recurrence is not altered by prophylactic steroid therapy. Disappointingly, sulfasalazine has not decreased recurrence rates in CD.

While response to treatment of the initial attack of Crohn's colitis may be satisfactory, many patients continue to have persistently active disease. This may express itself as progressive weight loss, diarrhea, and deterioration of general health. Perianal disease with predominantly left-sided colonic involvement (fistula formation and perirectal abscesses) may be a recurrent problem. In one controlled study, *metronidazole* (20 mg/kg per day in divided doses) resulted in marked improvement in some patients with chronic perineal fistulas associated with CD. It is not clear whether the drug is active because of its antibacterial properties or through anothermechanism. It is possible that metronidazole may be of value in treating the perineal complications of CD before surgical therapy is attempted. In patients taking these doses of metronidazole on a chronic basis, peripheral sensory neuropathy is a significant side effect and may necessitate reducing the dose or discontinuing the drug if symptoms persist. The role of immunosuppressive therapy in the treatment of CD has become better established in recent years. The use of 6-mercaptopurine or azathioprine (1.5 to 2.0 mg/kg) has been shown to decrease disease activity, cause fistulas to close or become less active, and exert a steroid-sparing effect; it may decrease the relapse rate if used as maintenance therapy. Often, adding these drugs to a maximal program in a nonresponding patient produces beneficial results. However, a positive response may take 3 to 4 months to appear.

The management of CD of the small intestine (regional enteritis) is similar to that for colonic CD, and, as noted, many patients have both small- and large-bowel disease. Several additional considerations are pertinent, however. *Intestinal obstruction* is not uncommonly a presenting feature with ileal involvement. Initially, this problem may be secondary to acute inflammation and will respond to glucocorticoids. With recurrent involvement and the development of fibrosis, steroid therapy is less effective, and surgical decompression is required. *Nutritional problems* often are more severe with involvement of the small intestine than with colonic involvement alone. Added to the general catabolic nature of the disease may be loss of absorptive surface, either from progressive involvement or because of surgical resection. Refinements in the technique of parenteral alimentation have made it possible to provide a patient's total daily caloric intake intravenously for a period of weeks or even months (see Chap. 78). Parenteral alimentation has been employed with increasing frequency in severely ill patients as a means of "resting" the gastrointestinal tract and in preparing the malnourished patient for surgery. However, disease activity frequently recurs when oral feedings are resumed. On occasion, prolonged intravenous alimentation, administered at home, may be required when oral feedings are not effective or in children exhibiting severe growth failure associated with CD. Most often it is possible to design a dietary program of oral supplementation to nourish the patient adequately.

In patients with extensive small-bowel involvement and in those with a short bowel resulting from extensive intestinal resection, supplementation of electrolytes, minerals, and vitamins will be necessary. Extensive ileal disease or resection often results in diarrhea induced by impaired bile salt absorption; cholestyramine may be needed to control the diarrhea, and medium-chain triglycerides may need to be added to reduce fat malabsorption (see Chap. 285). In patients with stenotic segments of intestine, a low-residue (low-fiber) diet should be recommended. A lactose-free diet should be instituted if there is an associated lactase deficiency. Other dietary modifications have not been shown to have any beneficial effect on the primary disease process. Patients should be encouraged to eat a nutritious, appealing diet of their own choosing.

Surgical therapy in general should be reserved for the complications of CD rather than used as a primary form of therapy. More patients with CD than with UC require surgery in the chronic management of the disease. Approximately 70 percent of patients require at least one operation during the course of their disease. Although each case must be assessed individually, surgery may be required (1) for persistent or fixed bowel narrowing or obstruction, (2) for symptomatic fistula formation to the bladder, vagina, or skin, (3) for persistent anal fistulas or abscesses, and (4) for intraabdominal abscesses, toxic dilation of the colon, or perforation. In contrast to UC, where colectomy is curative, in CD surgical resection of the small or large intestine is followed by a high rate of recurrence. With resection of segments of small bowel or ileum and reanastomosis, a recurrence rate of 50 to 75 percent over a 5-year period is not unusual. The site of recurrence invariably is proximal to the created anastomosis. When total colectomy and ileostomy are performed for CD of the colon without significant small-intestinal involvement, recurrence rates are lower, varying from 10 to 30 percent. Despite these recurrences, most patients do not develop a short bowel syndrome, and most can expect significant improvement. Faced with the possibility of recurrent disease, many physicians are reluctant to advise surgery in CD, except for the clear-cut complications described above. Alternatively, surgery may be indicated for patients with persistently active disease that requires chronic maintenance therapy with unacceptably high levels of corticosteroids. While patients with Crohn's colitis without major small-bowel involvement also have a definite rate of recurrence, such recurrences often are not disabling. When extensive small-bowel disease is present, surgical therapy often is not feasible and should only be reserved for specific disease complications.

The therapy of CD in children presents special problems, since active disease may retard normal growth and development. In addition to conventional drug therapy, intensive nutritional therapy or the judicious use of surgery may be required.

PROGNOSIS

The overall prognosis of IBD has been improved by the use of glucocorticoids and sulfasalazine, as well as supportive measures such as intravenous alimentation. In *acute* UC, these therapeutic modalities can produce a remission in almost 90 percent of patients. The mortality rate from an initial acute attack is less than 5 percent. The prognosis is poorer and the mortality rate higher when there is total colonic involvement, when disease onset is after age 60, and when toxic megacolon develops.

The long-term prognosis of *chronic* UC is more difficult to assess owing to the variable and intermittent nature of the disease and improvements in therapy. Left-sided colitis and ulcerative proctitis have a very favorable prognosis and probably cause no increase in mortality rate; similarly, the long-term prognosis for extensive colitis has improved greatly. Previous studies suggested a poor prognosis for extensive colitis, with less than 50 percent of patients surviving 15 years after onset. However, more recent observations (longest follow-up, 11 years) show 10-year mortality rates of 5 and 10 percent for severe first attacks (excluding toxic megacolon). Approximately 75 percent of patients will experience relapses, and 20 to 25 percent will require colectomy. The problem of carcinoma developing in the setting of long-standing chronic UC is important in determining the long-term prognosis of UC. As discussed above, periodic colonoscopic surveillance with multiple biopsies to detect dysplastic changes is indicated to detect a high-risk group in whom to advise colectomy.

The prognosis for CD is not as favorable as for UC. An exception is *acute regional enteritis*, often discovered during laparotomy for suspected appendicitis; this condition has an excellent prognosis. More than two-thirds of such patients may show no subsequent evidence of regional enteritis, and this form of acute ileitis may well be due to *Yersinia* infection (see above). Surgical opinion favors a conservative approach in this situation, and in general operative resection is not advised.

In most patients with CD, the course is chronic and intermittent regardless of the site of involvement. The disease responds less well to medical therapy with time, and over two-thirds of patients develop complications requiring surgery at some point in their disease. In contrast to UC, where mortality appears greatest early in the disease, in CD the mortality rate increases with the duration of the disease and probably ranges from 5 to 10 percent. Most deaths are caused by peritonitis and sepsis. As indicated above, patients with CD often have recurrence and relapses after surgery. Nevertheless, therapy results in reasonably stable and productive lives for most CD patients.

BIBLIOGRAPHY

GENERAL

KIRSNER JB, SHORTER RG (eds): *Inflammatory Bowel Disease*, 4th ed. Philadelphia, Lea & Febiger, 1995

PODOLSKY DK: Inflammatory bowel disease. N Engl J Med 325:928, 1991

SLEISENGER MH, FORDTRAN JS (eds): *Gastrointestinal Diseases*, 5th ed. Philadelphia, Saunders, 1993

STENSON WF, MACDERMOTT RP: Inflammatory bowel disease, in *Textbook of Gastroenterology*, 2d ed, T Yamada et al (eds). Philadelphia, Lippincott, 1995

ETIOLOGY AND DIAGNOSTIC ASPECTS

BLASER MJ, RELLER LB: *Campylobacter* enteritis. N Engl J Med 305:1444, 1981

COLOMBEL JF et al: Clinical characteristics of Crohn's disease. Gastroenterology 111:604, 1996

GOLDBERG HI et al: Computed tomography in the evaluation of Crohn's disease. Am J Roentgenol 140:277, 1983

MACDERMOTT RP, STENSON WF: Alterations of the immune system in ulcerative colitis and Crohn's disease. Adv Immunol 42:285, 1988

SURAWICZ CM, BELIC L: Rectal biopsy helps to distinguish acute self limited colitis from idiopathic inflammatory bowel disease. Gastroenterology 86:104, 1984

THERAPY OF INFLAMMATORY BOWEL DISEASE

BOHR J et al: Collagenous colitis: A retrospective study of clinical presentation and treatment in 163 patients. Gut 39:846, 1996

COLLINS RH et al: Colon cancer in ulcerative colitis. Gastroenterology 94:1089, 1988

EKBOM A et al: Ulcerative colitis and colorectal cancer. N Engl J Med 323:1228, 1990

FARMER RG et al: Long-term follow-up of patients with Crohn's disease. Relationship between clinical pattern and prognosis. Gastroenterology 88:1818, 1985

GAGINELLA TS, WALSH RE: Sulfasalazine: Multiplicity of action. Dig Dis Sci 37:801, 1992

GIONCHETTI P, CAMPIERI M: Medical treatment of ulcerative colitis. Curr Opin Gastroenterol 12:352, 1996

GRIFFIN MG, MINER PB JR: Conventional drug therapy in inflammatory bowel disease. Gastroenterol Clin North Am 24:509, 1995

HANAUER SB: Drug therapy: Inflammatory bowel disease. N Engl J Med 334:841, 1996

LICHTIGER S et al: Cyclosporine in severe ulcerative colitis refractory to steroid therapy. N Engl J Med 330:1841, 1994

PEMBERTON JH et al: Ileal ulcerative colitis—anal anastomosis for chronic ulcerative colitis. Long-term results. Ann Surg 206:504, 1987

PEPPERCORN MA: Advances in drug therapy for inflammatory bowel disease. Ann Intern Med 112:50, 1990

PRESENT DH et al: 6-Mercaptopurine in the management of inflammatory bowel disease: short- and long-term toxicity. Ann Intern Med 111:641, 1989

PROVENCALE D et al: Prophylactic colectomy or surveillance for chronic ulcerative colitis. Gastroenterology 109:1188, 1995

RANSOHOFF DF et al: Ulcerative colitis and colon cancer: Problems in analyzing the diagnostic usefulness of mucosal dysplasia. Dis Colon Rectum 28:383, 1985

RIDDELL RH et al: Dysplasia in inflammatory bowel disease. Hum Pathol 14:931, 1983

SANDBORN WJ et al: Ulcerative colitis disease activity following treatment of associated primary sclerosing cholangitis with cyclosporine. Gut 34:242, 1993

SCHROEDER KW et al: Coated oral 5-aminosalicylate acid therapy for mild to moderately active ulcerative colitis. A randomized study. N Engl J Med 317:1625, 1987

SUGITA A et al: Colorectal cancer in ulcerative colitis: Influence of anatomical extent and age at onset in colitis-cancer interval. Gut 32:169, 1991

287

Richard B. Lynn, Lawrence S. Friedman

IRRITABLE BOWEL SYNDROME

The irritable bowel syndrome (IBS) is the most common gastrointestinal disease in clinical practice. Although not a life-threatening illness, it can cause great distress to patients and a feeling of frustration for physicians. IBS is characterized by abdominal pain and altered bowel habits, including diarrhea, constipation, or alternating diarrhea and constipation. Symptoms are typically intermittent but may be continuous and should be present for at least 3 months before a diagnosis of IBS is considered.

DEFINITION AND CLINICAL PRESENTATION   Abdominal pain and altered bowel habits are nonspecific symptoms found in patients with a wide variety of illnesses (see Table 287-1). However, several characteristic symptoms, known as the *Manning criteria*, have been identified that, when present, increase the likelihood of IBS. The Manning criteria include abdominal pain or discomfort that is relieved by defecation or associated with a change in stool frequency or consistency, abdominal distention, the sensation of incomplete evacuation, and the passage of mucus. Diagnostic criteria for IBS that incorporate the Manning criteria have been established to standardize research and may be useful in clinical practice (Table 287-2). Patients presenting with abdominal pain in the absence of altered bowel habits or with altered bowel habits in the absence of abdominal pain may be considered to have IBS if no alternative explanation for the symptoms is found. However, patients with otherwise unexplained chronic constipation in the absence of abdominal pain are generally considered to have a distinct disorder (see Chap. 42).

In addition to altered bowel habits and abdominal pain, patients with IBS may have symptoms referable to the upper gastrointestinal (GI) tract, including noncardiac chest pain, heartburn, dysphagia, and globus sensation. Patients with IBS also may have a broad range of nongastrointestinal symptoms, such as fatigue, urologic dysfunction, and gynecologic complaints.

EPIDEMIOLOGY   Estimates of the prevalence of IBS vary depending on the definition used and the population studied. Symptoms compatible with IBS are reported by 10 to 22 percent of the U.S. adult population, with a female predominance > 2:1 among patients presenting to a physician. However, fewer than half of adults with symptoms seek medical attention (see below). Symptoms typically begin in young adulthood, and the prevalence of IBS is similar in elderly and younger adults. IBS is a worldwide disorder with similar prevalence rates reported in a variety of industrialized and nonindustrialized countries. Until now, patients with symptoms of IBS have constituted fully 25 to 50 percent of outpatients referred to gastroenterologists, a reflection of the high prevalence and chronicity of IBS as well as the difficulty in treating the disorder.

ETIOLOGY AND PATHOGENESIS   IBS is often considered a "functional" disorder because no structural, biochemical, or infectious etiology has been found. The fundamental disturbance is thought to relate to disordered motor or sensory function of the GI tract. Other functional disorders of the GI tract include noncardiac chest pain, nonulcer dyspepsia, and biliary dyskinesia. Similarities among these disorders and IBS suggest that they share underlying pathophysiologic mechanisms. Functional bowel disorders are often attributed erroneously to stress. Despite extensive investigation, however, there is no proof that emotional stress is the cause of IBS, but for many patients stress can lead to exacerbations of IBS.

IBS is probably a heterogeneous group of disorders. Numerous studies have reported motility or sensory abnormalities of the GI tract in some patients with IBS, but none of the findings is present in all patients nor accounts for the entire symptom complex. Some of these findings may characterize subgroups of patients with IBS. Studies describing motility and sensory abnormalities in IBS have generally been performed on patients either at rest or subjected to acute stimulation but not while experiencing the spontaneous painful episodes characteristic of IBS. Therefore, the relevance of the observed abnormalities to the pathophysiology of IBS remains uncertain.

IBS is often assumed to be caused by altered colonic motility because the characteristic symptoms are consistent with colonic dysfunction and the abdominal pain is frequently located in areas referable to the colon. Abnormal colonic motility has been reported in some patients, but these findings have not been convincingly linked with the pathogenesis of IBS. Similarly, continuous recording techniques have identified abnormalities of small intestinal motility, but their relevance to IBS is unclear. The most reproducible finding in IBS patients is altered visceral sensation. Balloon distention of the rectum, sigmoid colon, or small intestine causes abdominal pain in IBS patients at volumes usually not painful in control subjects. Little is understood, however, about either the mechanism of this abnormality in pain sensation or whether the fundamental defect resides in sensory recep-

Table 287-1

Some Conditions That May Present with Symptoms Similar to IBS

Intestinal malabsorption: Lactose intolerance
Infections: Giardiasis
Inflammatory bowel diseases: Crohn's disease, ulcerative colitis, collagenous colitis, lymphocytic colitis
Neoplasms: Colon cancer, villous adenoma, small-bowel tumors
Obstructing disorders: Fecal impaction, intermittent sigmoid volvulus, megacolon
Vascular insufficiency: Abdominal angina, ischemic colitis
Gynecologic disorders: Endometriosis
Psychiatric disorders: Depression, panic disorders, somatization, anxiety
Chronic idiopathic intestinal pseudoobstruction

Table 287-2

Evaluation of Patients with Symptoms of IBS

I. Diagnositc criteria for IBS
  A. At least 3 months of continuous or recurrent symptoms of
    1. Abdominal pain or discomfort that is
      a. Relieved with defecation
      b. Associated with a change in frequency of stool, or
      c. Associated with a change in consistency of stool, and
    2. Two or more of the following, at least on one-fourth of occasions or days:
      a. Altered stool frequency (>3 bowel movements daily or <3 bowel movements weekly)
      b. Altered stool consistency (lumpy/hard or loose/watery stool)
      c. Altered stool passage (straining, urgency, or feeling of incomplete evacuation),
      d. Passage of mucus,
      e. Bloating or feeling of abdominal distention
II. Essential history to exclude other causes
  A. Exclude symptoms not compatible with IBS only:
    1. Visible or occult blood in the stool
    2. Weight loss
    3. Fever
    4. Pain or diarrhea awakening the patient from sleep
  B. Obtain dietary history to exclude lactose intolerance or excessive use of sorbitol, fructose, or caffeine
  C. Review medications with possible GI side effects
  D. Consider depression or panic disorders
III. Physical examination: Should be unremarkable; if positive, further evaluation required
IV. Laboratory examination
  A. Complete blood count; erythrocyte sedimentation rate; chemistry panel
  B. Flexible sigmoidoscopy (patients >40 years old; all patients with diarrhea)
  C. If diarrhea is predominant symptom:
    1. Examine stool for ova and parasites, fecal leukocytes, excessive fat
    2. Thyroid function tests
    3. Mucosal biopsy of rectosigmoid for microscopic colitis

SOURCE: Adapted from Thompson et al, with permission.

tors and neurons in the bowel wall or in the central nervous system where pain sensation is processed and reaches awareness. Lower pain thresholds have been found at multiple locations in the gut in patients with IBS, suggesting that the disease involves a generalized disorder of visceral pain sensation.

PSYCHOSOCIAL FACTORS Psychosocial factors play an important role in IBS. Only 15 to 50 percent of adults with IBS symptoms seek medical attention. Compared to non-IBS controls and persons with symptoms of IBS who do not seek medical attention, patients with symptoms of IBS presenting to a physician have an increased frequency of psychiatric diagnoses, including personality disorders, anxiety, depression, hysteria, and somatization. Symptomatic patients not seeking medical attention are not psychologically different from healthy subjects. Therefore, while psychosocial factors do not cause the IBS symptoms, they can influence how symptomatic patients respond. While presenters report more severe GI distress, it is unclear whether they actually have more severe symptoms because their psychiatric disturbances affect pain sensation or whether they experience similar symptoms but report them as more severe.

The origin of psychosocial dysfunction in IBS patients probably varies. One hypothesis is that symptomatic IBS patients who seek medical attention have a learned illness behavior originating in childhood. In some cases, there may be a history of childhood sexual or physical abuse.

DIAGNOSTIC EVALUATION A diagnosis of IBS is based on a careful history to identify characteristic symptoms (e.g., Manning criteria), physical examination, selected laboratory tests, and, if necessary, further testing to exclude other disorders (see Table 287-2). In most cases, postponing designation of IBS as the likely diagnosis until all other possible etiologies of abdominal pain and altered bowel habits have been excluded by additional radiologic or endoscopic studies is unnecessary. Such an approach can lead to expensive, often invasive testing that increases the patient's anxiety and reinforces the unrealistic expectation that a demonstrable abnormality needs to be found. On the other hand, in persons with the recent onset of symptoms, particularly those over age 40, and those with previously stable IBS who have a change in symptoms, a thorough investigation of the GI tract may be indicated.

The history should include a detailed description of the abdominal pain, but it should be recognized that wide variations may be found in patients with IBS. Careful description of bowel frequency, consistency, and volume should be elicited. A complete list of medications should be reviewed, as many medications cause diarrhea or constipation (see Chap. 42). A careful dietary history is essential, including excessive use of caffeinated beverages or foods and beverages sweetened with fructose or sorbitol, which may cause diarrhea, bloating, or cramps. Consideration should be given to a 3-week trial of a lactose-free diet to exclude lactose intolerance. It is especially important to explore the psychosocial factors that may have influenced the patient to seek medical attention, including the specific events prompting the patient's initial visit. Panic disorders and depression often present with GI symptoms.

The physical examination in IBS patients is generally unremarkable. Abdominal tenderness, often in the left lower quadrant, may be elicited but is typically mild. A mass, an enlarged liver or spleen, or a positive fecal occult-blood test are not compatible with IBS alone and require further evaluation. In women, a pelvic examination should be performed to look for endometriosis.

Certain procedures may be needed to exclude other disorders. Flexible sigmoidoscopy is generally included in the evaluation of all patients over age 40 to exclude colonic neoplasms. In younger patients with IBS in whom diarrhea is the predominant symptom, flexible sigmoidoscopy is also indicated to exclude inflammatory bowel disease. If there is persistent diarrhea, sigmoidoscopic biopsies should be performed to exclude disorders such as collagenous or lymphocytic colitis. In many patients with suspected IBS, barium enema or colonoscopy may not be needed but should be considered if the patient is over age 40 or if there is a strong family history of colorectal neoplasms. Symptoms suggestive of upper GI or biliary tract disease may require additional evaluation.

℞ TREATMENT

The most important aspect of treatment is to establish a therapeutic physician-patient relationship. A beneficial outcome is most likely when the physician is nonjudgmental, establishes realistic expectations and consistent limits, encourages the patient's understanding of the illness, and involves the patient in treatment decisions. Discussion of the circumstances leading to the decision to seek medical attention may be particularly beneficial. The patient needs to be reassured of the benign nature of the illness and of the excellent long-term prognosis. It may be helpful to emphasize that although there is no cure for IBS, there are steps that both the physician and patient can take to improve the symptoms.

Initial recommendations generally focus on dietary modifications. These include avoidance of dairy products; foods, beverages, or medications containing fructose or sorbitol; excessive caffeine; or gas-forming foods such as legumes. Fiber supplements can often be recommended regardless of the presenting complaint but are particularly useful when constipation is the predominant symptom (see Table 287-3). Natural fiber, such as wheat bran, is inexpensive, but fiber supplements such as psyllium, polycarbophil, and methylcellulose may cause less bloating and discomfort. In fact, all fiber supplements can cause bloating and discomfort, but these symptoms often resolve within a few weeks. Although the efficacy of fiber supplements in IBS has never been proven, in part because of the high placebo response rate in controlled trials, a trial of fiber is generally safe and reasonable.

While most patients will improve with the simple measures outlined above, some with persistent symptoms may benefit from additional medications as shown in Table 287-3. While no medication has been proven effective in controlled trials, some patients may benefit from one or more of them. On the other hand, a trial-and-error approach using a series of medications should be avoided, as it may mislead the patient that a cure can be found.

Treatment should be directed to the predominant symptom. With diarrhea-predominant IBS, an antidiarrheal agent such as loperamide or diphenoxylate with atropine may be used. For symptoms of abdominal pain and bloating, an anticholinergic agent (e.g., belladonna)

Table 287-3

Drugs of Potential Benefit in IBS

Drug Type and Examples	Typical Starting Dose	Indications
Fiber supplements		Constipation-predominant IBS
Wheat bran	1/2 cup; 10–30 g/d	May be tried for any IBS symptom complex
Psyllium	1/2 to 1 tbsp qd to bid	
Antispasmodics (anticholinergics)		Pain-predominant IBS
Tincture of belladonna	5–10 drops PO tid	Prevention of postcibal abdominal pain
Dicyclomine	10–20 mg tid–qid	
Cimetropium bromide	50 mg tid	
Antidiarrheals		Diarrhea-predominant IBS
Diphenoxylate	2.5–5 mg qid	
Loperamide	2 mg bid	
Cholestyramine	1/2–1 pck qd to bid	
Tricyclic antidepressants		Pain-predominant IBS
Amitriptyline	10–25 mg qhs	
Desipramine	50 mg qhs	
Prokinetic agents		Constipation-predominant IBS
Cisapride	5–10 mg tid	
Domperidone	10–20 mg qid	
Benzodiazepine-type anxiolytics		Anxiety, use for brief periods

may be used as an antispasmodic. Newer anticholinergic agents (e.g., dicyclomine and cimetropium) appear to act more selectively on GI smooth muscle than older anticholinergic agents and therefore may have fewer side effects. Tricyclic antidepressants, which have proven effective in some chronic pain syndromes, may also benefit some patients with pain-predominant IBS; however, it is unclear whether a response to tricyclic antidepressants is due to their antidepressant or anticholinergic effects or to a direct effect on sensory pathways mediating pain perception. Anxiolytic agents may be used for brief periods when there are stress-related exacerbations of symptoms but should not be used on a long-term basis because of the risk of habituation, rebound effect on withdrawal, and drug interactions.

Other medications may be useful in selected cases. For example, cholestyramine may be helpful in some patients with apparent diarrhea-predominant IBS, in whom diarrhea is the result of bile salt malabsorption by the terminal ileum (see Chap. 42). Cisapride may improve constipation and abdominal pain in patients with constipation-predominant IBS. Other drugs being tried in the treatment of IBS include calcium channel blockers, gonadotropin-releasing hormone, serotonin-receptor antagonists, somatostatin agonists, and kappa opioid agonists. In refractory or severe cases, psychotherapy, hypnotherapy, and biofeedback may be helpful. In all cases, efforts should be directed toward firm and empathetic psychosocial support in the context of a sustained physician-patient relationship.

BIBLIOGRAPHY

CAMILLERI M, PRATHER CM: The irritable bowel syndrome: Mechanisms and a practical approach to management. Ann Intern Med 116:1001, 1992

DROSSMAN DA et al: Psychosocial factors in the irritable bowel syndrome: A multivariate study of patients and nonpatients with irritable bowel syndrome. Gastroenterology 95:701, 1988

———: Sexual and physical abuse and gastrointestinal illness. Ann Intern Med 123:782, 1995

———, THOMPSON WG: The irritable bowel syndrome: Review and a graduated multicomponent treatment approach. Ann Intern Med 116:1009, 1992

KLEIN KB: Controlled treatment trials in the irritable bowel syndrome: A critique. Gastroenterology 95:232, 1988

LYNN RB, FRIEDMAN LS: Irritable bowel syndrome. N Engl J Med 329:1940, 1993

———, ———: Irritable bowel syndrome: managing the patient with abdominal pain and altered bowel habits. Med Clin North Am 79:373, 1995

MANNING AP et al: Towards positive diagnosis of the irritable bowel. BMJ 2:653, 1978

TALLEY NJ et al: Psychological treatments for irritable bowel syndrome: A critique of controlled treatment trials. Am J Gastroenterol 91:277, 1996

THOMPSON WG et al: Functional bowel disorders and functional abdominal pain, in *The Functional Gastrointestinal Disorders*, DA Drossman et al (eds). Boston, Little, Brown, 1994

WHITEHEAD WE et al: Symptoms of psychologic distress associated with irritable bowel syndrome: Comparison of community and medical clinic samples. Gastroenterology 95:709, 1988

288   *Kurt J. Isselbacher, Alan Epstein*

DIVERTICULAR, VASCULAR, AND OTHER DISORDERS OF THE INTESTINE AND PERITONEUM

DIVERTICULAR DISEASE

Diverticula may be either congenital or acquired and may affect either the small or large intestine. Congenital diverticula are herniations of the entire thickness of intestinal wall, while the more common acquired diverticula consist of herniations of the mucosa through the muscularis, generally at the site of a nutrient artery.

SMALL-INTESTINAL DIVERTICULA   Diverticula may occur in any portion of the small intestine; however, with the exception of Meckel's diverticulum, the most common locations are in the duodenum and jejunum. Most often diverticula are asymptomatic and discovered incidentally on upper gastrointestinal x-rays. On occasion, however, they may cause symptoms either because of their anatomic proximity to other structures or rarely from inflammation or bleeding.

Duodenal diverticula arise singly from the medial surface of the second portion of the duodenum. In most patients, they cause no symptoms. Rarely, they may present as acute diverticulitis with abdominal pain, fever, gastrointestinal bleeding, or, most rarely, perforation. Periampullary diverticula are occasionally associated with cholangitis or pancreatitis. Jejunal diverticula, while less common, also may be the site of acute inflammation, bleeding, or perforation with resulting abscess or peritonitis.

Multiple jejunal diverticula may be associated with malabsorption related to bacterial overgrowth within the diverticula, similar to other situations where intestinal stasis (e.g., blind loops) permits bacterial proliferation. The consequences of bacterial proliferation with resultant mucosal damage, deconjugation of bile salts, and vitamin B$_{12}$ malabsorption are discussed in Chap. 285.

Meckel's diverticulum, a persistent omphalomesenteric duct, is the most frequent congenital anomaly of the digestive tract, occurring in approximately 2 percent of autopsied adults. The diverticulum is widemouthed, about 5 cm long, and arises from the antimesenteric border of the ileum, usually within 100 cm of the ileocecal valve. The sac may be lined with normal ileal mucosa (approximately 50 percent) or contain gastric, duodenal, pancreatic, or colonic mucosa. While rarely symptomatic after age 5, Meckel's diverticulum may produce hemorrhage, inflammation, and obstruction in children and teenagers.

Hemorrhage occurs almost exclusively before age 10 and invariably results from peptic ulceration of ileal mucosa adjacent to a Meckel's diverticulum lined with gastric mucosa. The diagnosis may be established by isotope scanning of the abdomen after injection of technetium, which is taken up by the ectopic gastric mucosa in the diverticulum. False-negative and false-positive Meckel's scans are not uncommon; thus, other clinical and laboratory features must be assessed carefully before recommending surgery. In older children and young adults, inflammation of the diverticulum may mimic acute appendicitis. Mechanical obstruction also may occur if the diverticulum intussuscepts into the lumen of the bowel or twists on a fibrous remnant of the omphalomesenteric duct which extends from the diverticulum to the abdominal wall. The treatment of any of these complications of Meckel's diverticulum is surgical excision.

COLONIC DIVERTICULA   Diverticula of the colon are herniations or saclike protrusions of the mucosa through the muscularis, at the point where a nutrient artery penetrates the muscularis. Diverticula occur most commonly in the sigmoid colon and decrease in frequency in the proximal colon. They increase with age, and the incidence ranges between 20 and 50 percent in western populations over age 50. The exact mechanism for their formation is unknown but may be related to an increase in intraluminal pressure. Thickening of the muscle coat of the colon in most patients with diverticula suggests that herniations of mucosa are caused by increased pressure produced by colonic muscle contractions. The rarity of colonic diverticula in underdeveloped nations has led to the speculation that diverticula result from the highly refined western diet, which is deficient in dietary fiber or roughage. It is proposed that such diets result in decreased fecal bulk, narrowing of the colon, and an increase in intraluminal pressure in order to move the smaller fecal mass. However, the role of dietary fiber in the etiology and treatment of diverticular disease remains to be determined.

Colonic diverticula are usually asymptomatic and are an incidental finding on barium enema or colonoscopy. The major complications of inflammation, both acute and chronic, and hemorrhage occur in only a small percentage of individuals with diverticulosis. Since diverticulosis is quite common in older patients, one must avoid the temptation of attributing pain or bleeding to the diverticula unless other conditions, especially colonic neoplasm, have been excluded.

DIVERTICULITIS Inflammation can occur in or around the diverticular sac. The cause of diverticulitis is probably mechanical, related to retention in the diverticula of undigested food residues and bacteria, which may form a hard mass called a *fecalith*. This compromises the blood supply to the thin-walled sac (made up solely of mucosa and serosa) and renders it susceptible to invasion by colonic bacteria. The inflammatory process may vary from a small intramural or pericolic abscess to generalized peritonitis. Some attacks are accompanied by minimal symptoms and seem to heal spontaneously. Studies of resected specimens indicate that most perforations of the diverticular sac are small and result in inflammation of the sac itself and the adjacent serosal surface. Diverticulitis occurs more often in men than in women and three times as often in the left as in the right colon. This suggests that diverticulitis may be related to the higher intraluminal pressures and the more solid fecal material in the sigmoid and descending colon.

Acute colonic diverticulitis is a disease of variable severity characterized by fever, left lower quadrant abdominal pain, and signs of peritoneal irritation—muscle spasm, guarding, rebound tenderness. Rectal examination may reveal a tender mass if the area of inflammation is close to the rectum. Although constipation may not have been noted prior to onset of the illness, the inflammation around the colon often results in some degree of acute constipation or obstipation. Rectal bleeding, usually microscopic, is noted in 25 percent of cases; it is rarely massive. Polymorphonuclear leukocytosis is common. Complications include free perforation, which results in acute peritonitis, sepsis, and shock, particularly in the elderly. The perforation may be walled off by adherent omentum or neighboring structures such as the bladder or small bowel. Abscess formation or fistulas then occur as the inflammatory mass burrows into other organs. Severe pericolitis may cause a fibrous stricture around the bowel, which can be associated with colonic obstruction and may mimic a neoplasm.

Diagnosis During the acute phase of diverticulitis, barium enema and sigmoidoscopy may be hazardous, since contrast material or air under pressure may lead to rupture of an inflamed diverticulum and convert a walled-off inflammatory lesion to a free perforation. These examinations are usually safe after adequate treatment and healing of the diverticulitis. The radiologic findings on barium enema suggestive of diverticulitis are leakage of barium from a diverticular sac, stricture formation, and the presence of a pericolic inflammatory mass. In many patients, the distortion caused by inflammation prevents a clear distinction between cancer and diverticulitis. In these cases, colonoscopy or surgical excision may be required for accurate diagnosis. Abdominal computed tomography scan may be useful in demonstrating the presence of a pericolic abscess.

 TREATMENT
Most patients with acute diverticulitis require bowel rest, intravenous fluids, and broad-spectrum antibiotics. Repeated attacks of diverticulitis in the same area generally require surgical resection. Severe attacks with acute peritoneal signs, suspected abscess, or perforation require intravenous antibiotics directed against gram-negative anaerobic bacteria, followed by surgical drainage or resection. The usual procedure is a diverting colostomy with resection of the involved colon; reanastomosis is then performed at a second operation.

PAINFUL DIVERTICULAR DISEASE WITHOUT DIVERTICULITIS Some patients with diverticulosis develop recurrent left lower quadrant colicky pain without clinical or pathologic evidence of acute diverticulitis. They often have bouts of alternating constipation and diarrhea, and the pain may be relieved by defecation or passage of flatus. These features suggest the coexistence of the irritable bowel syndrome (see below). Examination during a bout of pain reveals tenderness of the sigmoid colon, but signs of peritoneal inflammation such as rebound tenderness, muscle guarding, fever, and leukocytosis are absent. Barium enema shows typical diverticula without evidence of inflammation and stricture, plus a "sawtooth" irregularity of the lumen reflecting muscle hypertrophy and spasm. In some patients the pain is severe enough to warrant observation in a hospital and restriction of food, since feeding aggravates the pain by causing colonic contraction. Anticholinergics, which reduce sigmoid contractions, and mild sedation are usually all that is required. After recovery, the patient should be started on a high-residue diet or given a bulk laxative such as hemicellulose, unprocessed bran, or psyllium extract. Surgical excision is usually not indicated unless acute diverticulitis or its complications occur.

HEMORRHAGE FROM DIVERTICULA Massive hemorrhage from colonic diverticula is one of the most common causes of hematochezia in patients over age 60. This complication of diverticulosis is caused by erosion of a vessel by a fecalith within the diverticular sac. The bleeding is painless and not accompanied by signs or symptoms of diverticulitis. Most cases of mild or moderate hemorrhage stop spontaneously with bed rest and blood transfusion. Localization of bleeding can be obtained by bleeding scan or angiography. In patients with severe hemorrhage, mesenteric angiography can be both diagnostic in localizing the bleeding site and therapeutic, since vasoconstrictive drugs or artificial blood clot infused intraarterially can sometimes effectively control hemorrhage. Colonoscopy is also useful in evaluating acute hematochezia and the endoscopist may be able to cauterize angiodysplasias (see Chap. 44). The location of bleeding diverticula demonstrated at angiography on several series has been more commonly in the right colon, particularly the ascending colon, in contrast to the sigmoid colon, where diverticula are more numerous.

MOTILITY DISORDERS

Normal intestinal motility involves the delicate interplay of the gut motor system, neural influences of the autonomic and central nervous system, as well as hormonal factors, specifically gut neuropeptides. In addition, many drugs used in the treatment of disease (e.g., opioids, antibiotics) affect and influence intestinal motility directly or indirectly. The reader is referred to several excellent reviews cited in the bibliography, dealing with the complex mechanism involved in the regulation of intestinal motility.

Table 288-1 lists some of the common and unusual disorders of the enteric motor and neural system. Only some of the more clinically relevant and important ones are discussed below.

MEGACOLON Megacolon, or giant colon, is characterized by massive distention of the colon, usually accompanied by severe constipation or obstipation. This condition can be either congenital or acquired and is seen in all age groups. Acute toxic megacolon is a severe complication of ulcerative colitis (see Chap. 286).

Aganglionic Megacolon (Hirschsprung's Disease) This is a congenital disorder due to absence of enteric neurons (ganglions) in the distal colon and rectum. This aganglionic segment loses its neural inhibition and remains contracted. Hirschsprung's disease is a heterogeneous genetic disorder—some patients have an autosomal dominant form of the disease with mutations in the *RET* gene; many have an autosomal recessive form with a mutation in the endothelin-B receptor gene. These defects result in the gestational failure of neural crest cells to migrate to the distal colon. The disease becomes manifest in early infancy, occurring more frequently in males, and is often familial. These infants have massive abdominal distention, absent bowel movements, and impaired nutrition due to chronic obstruction of the colon. In some individuals with less severe symptoms, the disease may not be diagnosed until adolescence or early adulthood. The aganglionic and contracted segment of bowel is unable to relax to permit passage of stool, causing the normal proximal colon to become greatly dilated. On rectal examination, the ampulla is empty of feces and the anal sphincter is normal. Barium enema reveals a narrowed segment in the rectosigmoid, with massive dilatation above. Diagnosis is made by full-thickness surgical biopsy under anesthesia and demonstration of absent ganglion cells in the diseased segment. In most patients the aganglionic segment is in the rectosigmoid colon. The treatment of choice is a pull-through procedure in which normally innervated colon is anastomosed to the distal rectum just above the internal sphincter, thus bypassing the contracted aganglionic segment and restoring normal defecation.

Acquired Megacolon In Central and South America, infection with *Trypanosoma cruzi* (Chagas' disease) can result in destruction of the ganglion cells of the colon, producing a clinical picture similar to congenital megacolon, except that the onset is in adult life rather than childhood. A number of other diseases are associated with megacolon in adults. Patients with schizophrenia or depression, particularly institutionalized patients, may have obstipation and massive colonic dilatation. Severe neurologic disorders, including cerebral atrophy, spinal cord injury, and parkinsonism, also may cause megacolon. Myxedema, infiltrative diseases such as amyloidosis, and primary systemic sclerosis also can reduce colonic motility and produce marked colonic distention. Narcotic drugs, particularly morphine and codeine, can cause severe constipation, especially when administered to bedridden patients. Digital rectal examination of adults with acquired megacolon reveals a rectum distended with feces, as opposed to the empty rectum in aganglionic megacolon. Treatment is aimed at the underlying disease, as well as the careful use of enemas and cathartics.

INTESTINAL PSEUDOOBSTRUCTION Intestinal pseudoobstruction is an acute or chronic motility disorder characterized by distention or dilatation of the small and large intestine. Abdominal pain, nausea, and vomiting may lead to diagnostic confusion with mechanical obstruction, but as the name of this condition implies, the underlying cause is not obstruction but rather a severe dysmotility resulting in distention. Pseudoobstruction may be primary or secondary and acute or chronic. In primary or idiopathic pseudoobstruction, no other contributing condition can be identified, and the motility disorder is attributed to abnormalities of sympathetic innervation or of the muscle layers of the intestine. Secondary pseudoobstruction may result from primary systemic sclerosis, diabetes, amyloidosis, neurologic diseases, drugs, or sepsis.

Chronic or Intermittent Secondary Pseudoobstruction Numerous medical conditions can cause chronic dilatation of the large and small bowel. Some of these may involve the intestinal smooth muscle, such as primary systemic sclerosis, amyloidosis, or muscular dystrophy. Endocrine disorders, including myxedema and diabetes mellitus, may result in chronic distention, which in the diabetic patient results from autonomic visceral neuropathy. Chronic neurologic diseases, including Parkinson's disease and stroke, may be complicated by chronic pseudoobstruction; in these patients, drugs and relative immobility are contributing features. Finally, psychotic patients (especially those who are institutionalized) may suffer from prolonged megacolon.

The symptoms of chronic secondary pseudoobstruction are chronic or intermittent constipation, crampy abdominal pain, anorexia, and bloating. Gastric distention and disordered swallowing may be present. Abdominal x-rays reveal gaseous distention of the large and small

Table 288-1

Some Motility Disorders of the Enteric Nervous System

Disorder	Comment
Intestinal pseudo-obstruction	
Visceral neuropathy	Autosomal dominant disorder characterized by dilatation of jejunum and ileum and degeneration and loss of neurons.
Visceral neuropathy with basal ganglia calcifications	Autosomal recessive disorder with dilatation of duodenum and small bowel and mental retardation. Calcification of basal ganglia and degeneration of myenteric plexus.
Megacolon	
Hirschsprung's disease	Congenital disorder characterized by colonic dilatation proximal to an aganglionic, contracted distal colon and rectum. Caused by gestational failure of neural crest cells to migrate to distal colon. An autosomal dominant form is associated with mutations of the *RET* gene, and an autosomal recessive form with mutation of the endothelin, B–receptor gene.
Multiple endocrine neoplasia type 2A (MEN-2A)	Features similar to those of Hirschsprung's disease. Medullary thyroid cancer, parathyroid hyperplasia, and pheochromocytoma are characteristic. ? Mutation of *RET* gene.
Generalized, with hyperganglionosis	
MEN-2B (Sipple's syndrome)	Achalasia and pseudoobstruction reported with ganglioneuromatosis of myenteric and submucosal plexuses. Medullary thyroid cancer, pheochromocytoma, and mucosal neuromas are characteristic. Mutation of *RET* gene reported.
Neurofibromatosis(von Recklinghausen's disease)	Achalasia and megacolon reported, with neuronal dysplasia of the myenteric plexus. Central nervous system tumors, neurofibromas, pigmented iris, hamartomas, café au lait spots, and mental retardation are characteristic.
Generalized, with hypoganglionosis	
Chagas' disease	Achalasia, intestinal, and colonic pseudoobstruction; megaloureter; and myocarditis due to infection with *Trypanosoma cruzi*. Possible autoimmune response to parasitic antigen.
Paraneoplastic syndrome	Achalasia, gastroparesis, and intestinal pseudoobstruction reported in some patients with small-cell lung cancer and carcinoid tumors. Serum antibodies reactive to enteric neurons.
Cytomegalovirus infection	Esophageal dysmotility, delayed gastric emptying, achalasia, and pseudoobstruction reported, with intranuclear neuronal viral inclusions and loss of myenteric neurons.
Myotonic dystrophy	Autosomal dominant disorder with impaired esophageal and gastric transit and intestinal pseudoobstruction, selective loss of substance P– and enkephalin-containing enteric neurons and preservation of neurons containing neuropeptide Y or vasoactive intestinal polypeptide. Myotonia, weakness, cataracts, cardiac abnormalities, gonadal atrophy, and mental retardation are characteristic.
Generalized, other	
Parkinson's disease	Achalasia, pseudoobstruction, and megacolon reported in some patients, with Lewy bodies in the myenteric plexus of the esophagus and colon.
Diabetes mellitus	Gastroparesis and intestinal and colonic dysmotility, with generalized autonomic neuropathy. Myenteric plexus morphologically intact.
Amyloidosis	Achalasia, gastroparesis, and pseudoobstruction, with amyloid deposits in both smooth muscle and the myenteric plexus.
Fabry's disease	Impaired gastric emptying, jejunal and colonic diverticulosis, and malabsorption, with glycolipid deposition in neurons of the myenteric plexus and decreased numbers of enlarged ganglion cells. Cutaneous angiokeratoma, renal insufficiency, and cardiovascular and central nervous system damage are also seen.
Disorders caused by exogenous neural toxins	Intestinal and colonic pseudoobstruction, with increased argyrophilia of the myenteric plexus.

SOURCE: Modified from Goyal and Hirano, with permission.

bowel and occasionally of the stomach. Air-fluid levels are unusual and should raise the possibility of mechanical obstruction. Upper gastrointestinal series and barium enema do not reveal specific abnormalities of the intestine such as tumor, stricture, or volvulus. The presence of an autoimmune disorder or endocrinopathy may require confirmation by serologic or blood tests; biopsy may be needed as in amyloidosis or muscular dystrophy.

The treatment of chronic intestinal pseudoobstruction is made difficult by the complexity and chronicity of the underlying systemic disease. Patients with primary systemic sclerosis may respond to broad-spectrum antibiotics if intestinal bacterial overgrowth is suspected. Metoclopramide may benefit gastric dysmotility in the diabetic patient. Discontinuation of psychotropic or anti-Parkinson drugs occasionally may result in improvement. Cathartics and enemas may be required to relieve fecal impaction, and the regular use of stool softeners and a high-fiber diet may help prevent recurrences.

Idiopathic Intestinal Pseudoobstruction This term is used to describe the condition of patients with signs and symptoms of pseudoobstruction in whom no systemic disease can be identified. The typical patient has recurrent attacks of abdominal pain and distention with nausea and vomiting. The small intestine is primarily involved, and chronic constipation is much less frequent than in secondary pseudoobstruction. Steatorrhea secondary to bacterial overgrowth of the small intestine is common and may lead to chronic diarrhea and malnutrition. Many patients exhibit abnormalities of motility in the esophagus and urinary bladder, in addition to the small and large intestine. Neuromuscular defects have been described in patients with this syndrome, including abnormalities of the mesenteric plexus and myopathy of the intestinal and urinary bladder smooth muscle (so-called hollow visceral myopathy). Elevated prostaglandin E levels have been reported in some patients.

Management of idiopathic pseudoobstruction is unsatisfactory. Surgery to relieve "obstruction" is to be avoided, since the condition is often worsened by abdominal surgery. Medical therapy with metoclopramide and cholinergic agents has been unsuccessful. Nutritional support in the form of low-residue elemental diets or parenteral hyperalimentation may be helpful. Unfortunately, the lack of effective therapy and the progressive nature of the illness make the prognosis of idiopathic pseudoobstruction rather unfavorable. Death from malnutrition and steatorrhea are common. The long-term impact of total parenteral nutrition on this disease is not yet clear.

Acute Intestinal Pseudoobstruction This entity, sometimes referred to as *Ogilvie's syndrome*, is characterized by acute intestinal dilatation involving primarily the colon but occasionally also the small intestine. As in other forms of pseudoobstruction, the clinical features are difficult to distinguish from mechanical obstruction. The patient may complain of colicky lower abdominal pain and acute constipation. Examination reveals a distended, tympanitic abdomen, with reduced or absent bowel sounds. Localized tenderness over the distended colon is common, but diffuse abdominal tenderness, rigidity, or rebound tenderness are unusual. Abdominal films reveal massive dilatation of the colon and small intestine, occasionally with the presence of air-fluid levels. The cecum, being the most capacious part of the colon, is often massively dilated and tender. The onset of these symptoms usually occurs in patients who have recently undergone severe surgical or medical stress such as major surgery, myocardial infarction, sepsis, or respiratory failure. Patients with acute pseudoobstruction are frequently on respirators, have received narcotics or sedatives, and have metabolic and electrolyte disturbances. Ogilvie's syndrome may also be due to paraneoplastic obstruction.

Management of acute pseudoobstruction requires careful correction of fluid and electrolyte abnormalities, intubation of the stomach or small intestine for decompression, and avoidance of drugs that depress intestinal motility. Barium enema may be hazardous because of the risk of perforating the already dilated bowel. Decompressive colonoscopy is beneficial in some patients, and cecostomy may be required in some patients with massive cecal dilatation. The outcome depends in large part on the prognosis of the associated medical or surgical conditions. Patients who recover from the underlying medical or surgical conditions usually have a return of normal colonic function.

IRRITABLE BOWEL SYNDROME See Chap. 287

CHRONIC CONSTIPATION The mechanism of defecation is discussed in Chap. 42. Chronic constipation is widespread in western society, with approximately 10 percent of the population taking laxatives on a regular basis. Most cases of chronic constipation arise from habitual neglect of afferent impulses, failure to initiate defecation, and accumulation of large, dry fecal masses in the rectum. This voluntary suppression of the call to stool may arise during the period of toilet training in childhood or later in life because of a sense of social impropriety, unaccustomed surroundings, uncomfortable toilet facilities, or illnesses that require confinement to bed. Chronic constipation is much more common in women, with onset typically in late adolescence or early adulthood. As constant distention of the rectum with feces becomes chronic, the patient grows less aware of rectal fullness. Bowel movements become progressively more difficult, and painful hemorrhoids or anal fissures reinforce suppression of the urge to defecate. To avoid these problems, the patient begins the chronic use of laxatives or enemas, without which defecation becomes impossible.

℞ TREATMENT

The physician should make every attempt to educate the patient about the chain of events that has led to chronic constipation. Attempts should be made to alter patterns of many years' duration, and the patient must recognize the importance of responding to, rather than suppressing, the urge to defecate. It is helpful to initiate a routine whereby defecation is attempted at a given time each day. In most individuals the call to stool occurs in the morning after breakfast. Physical exercise such as a brisk walk just before attempts at defecation may be helpful. Patients are instructed to increase dietary bulk with foods rich in fiber, such as green vegetables and unprocessed cereal grains, or by the regular use of bulk laxatives, such as hemicellulose, psyllium extract, and powdered unprocessed bran. The success of such a regimen depends to some extent on the duration of symptoms. Elderly patients with long-standing constipation and reliance on enemas or laxatives are more resistant to these measures than younger patients whose bowel patterns are less established. Moreover, poor muscle tone, reduced physical activity, and increased incidence of other medical conditions make the problem more difficult in the older age group. Bedridden elderly patients often develop severe constipation and even fecal impaction unless preventive measures are taken. This applies not only to patients with previous constipation but also to those with regular bowel movements prior to their confining illness. Regular administration of stool softeners, bulk laxatives, or mild cathartics is necessary until full ambulation and a normal diet are resumed. The onset of fecal impaction in bedridden patients is heralded by a feeling of rectal distention, urgency of defecation, or tenesmus. Occasionally, the fecal impaction will result in low-grade chronic obstruction with dilatation and increased fluid content proximal to the impaction; "paradoxical diarrhea" may thus occur as fluid moves past the obstructing fecal mass. This situation will be aggravated if antidiarrheal drugs are given because the underlying constipation will be worsened. The appropriate maneuver is to disimpact the rectum manually or to administer gentle enemas if the impaction is beyond the reach of the finger.

DISORDERS OF THE MESENTERIC CIRCULATION

Ischemia of the intestine is the end result of interruption or reduction of its blood supply. However, the clinical manifestations of intestinal ischemia range from mild chronic symptoms to a catastrophic acute episode, depending on the vascular supply involved, the extent of the occlusion or ischemia, and the rapidity of the process. The clinician should be aware of the spectrum of clinical manifestations (Table 288-2). The gut derives its arterial blood supply from the celiac axis and the superior and inferior mesenteric arteries. The small intestine is supplied by the celiac and superior mesenteric arteries; the colon by branches of the superior and inferior mesenteric arteries. A rich network of anastomotic vessels and the possible development of collateral circulation determine the clinical picture of acute or chronic intestinal arterial insufficiency.

MESENTERIC ISCHEMIA AND INFARCTION Acute intestinal ischemia may be classified as occlusive or nonocclusive. *Occlusion* may result from an arterial thrombus or embolus of the celiac or superior mesenteric arteries or from venous occlusion in the same distribution. Arterial embolus occurs most commonly in patients with chronic or recurrent atrial fibrillation, artificial heart valves, or valvular heart disease; arterial thrombosis is usually associated with extensive atherosclerosis or low cardiac output. Venous occlusion is rare; it is occasionally seen in women taking oral contraceptives. Approximately one-half of patients with mesenteric ischemia have no definite occlusion of a major vessel, a condition referred to as *nonocclusive ischemia*. The exact cause of nonocclusive disease is obscure; systemic arterial hypotension, cardiac arrhythmias, prolonged heart failure, digitalis therapy, dehydration, and endotoxemia can be contributing factors.

The major clinical feature of acute mesenteric ischemia is severe abdominal pain, often colicky and periumbilical at the onset, later becoming diffuse and constant. Vomiting, anorexia, diarrhea, and constipation are also frequent but of little diagnostic help. Examination of the abdomen may reveal tenderness and distention. Bowel sounds are often normal even in the face of severe infarction. Some patients have a surprisingly normal abdominal examination in spite of severe pain. Mild gastrointestinal bleeding is often detected by examination of stool for occult blood; gross hemorrhage is unusual except in ischemic colitis (see below). A typical laboratory finding is a pronounced polymorphonuclear leukocytosis. Late in the course of the disease (24 to 72 h), gangrene of the bowel occurs with diffuse peritonitis, sepsis, and shock. Abdominal plain films in patients with mesenteric ischemia may reveal air-fluid levels and distention. Barium study of the small intestine reveals nonspecific dilatation, poor motility, and evidence of thick mucosal folds ("thumbprinting") (Fig. 288-1).

Acute mesenteric ischemia is a grave condition with a high morbidity and mortality. Patients suspected of having acute arterial embolus should undergo immediate celiac and mesenteric angiography to localize the embolus, followed by embolectomy. Restoration of normal circulation may allow complete recovery if performed before irreversible necrosis or gangrene has occurred. Unfortunately, infarction and transmural necrosis are frequently found at surgery, necessitating resection. Arterial or venous thrombosis is not generally amenable to surgical removal of the thrombus, and resection of the affected bowel is required. Similarly, patients with nonocclusive ischemia are not candidates for corrective vascular surgery (as major vessels are patent).

FIGURE 288-1 Barium enema showing "thumbprinting" or submucosal edema of the inferior margin of the transverse colon in a patient with acute ischemic colitis.

These individuals often have extensive necrosis of the small or large intestine because of the widespread nature of the ischemic event. The decision to operate when mesenteric ischemia is suspected is often difficult, because the typical patient is a poor surgical risk owing to advanced age, dehydration, sepsis, and other serious medical conditions.

Chronic arterial insufficiency may precede acute vascular insufficiency, producing so-called abdominal angina. As in angina pectoris, the pain of chronic mesenteric insufficiency occurs under conditions of increased demand for splanchnic blood flow. The patient complains of intermittent dull or cramping midabdominal pain 15 to 30 min after a meal, lasting for several hours postprandially. There may be significant weight loss due to decreased food intake; however, Chronic intestinal ischemia also may produce mucosal damage and malabsorption, which in turn aggravates the weight loss. Since abdominal angina may progress to bowel infarction, serious consideration should be given to performing arteriographic studies to confirm the diagnosis in those patients who are candidates for abdominal vascular surgery. The only definitive treatment is vascular surgery or balloon angioplasty to remove the thrombus or the construction of bypass arterial grafts to the ischemic bowel.

A number of systemic conditions are associated with *vasculitis* of the large and small arteries supplying the intestine. Most often these disorders can be recognized by the associated extraintestinal manifestations, as in polyarteritis nodosa, lupus erythematosus, dermatomyositis, Henoch-Schönlein purpura (allergic vasculitis), and rheumatoid vasculitis. When larger arteries are involved, as in polyarteritis nodosa, the picture of acute intestinal infarction is similar to that of embolic or atherosclerotic vascular occlusion. Often the involvement of smaller vessels leads to areas of intramural hemorrhage and edema resulting in abdominal pain, variable degrees of intestinal obstruction, and bleeding. Barium enema may show "thumbprinting" and "spiculation" due to localized edema, hemorrhage, and ulceration (see Fig. 288-1). In many instances, treatment of the underlying disorder may lead to regression of symptoms. If signs of an acute abdomen develop, surgical exploration is usually indicated.

Intramural small-intestinal hemorrhage may occur with vasculitis, trauma, or impaired coagulation, especially in patients receiving anticoagulants. The clinical and radiologic features resemble those seen with vasculitis and local mucosal hemorrhage.

ISCHEMIC COLITIS Ischemia of the colon most often affects the elderly because of the greater frequency of vascular disease in that group. Ischemic colitis is almost always a nonocclusive disease. Shunting of blood away from the mucosa may contribute to this condition, but the mechanism of ischemia is not known.

Table 288-2

Patterns of Intestinal Ischemia

Condition	Etiology	Clinical Features	Management
Mesenteric artery embolus	Arterial embolus associated with atrial fibrillation or rheumatic heart disease	Acute central abdominal pain, shock, peritonitis	Immediate angiography and embolectomy if possible
Abdominal angina	Atherosclerosis of celiac and superior mesenteric arteries	Chronic postprandial pain, weight loss	Angiography and surgery in selected cases
Ischemic colitis	Low-flow state	Acute lower abdominal pain, rectal bleeding	Sigmoidoscopy; surgery only for peritonitis

The clinical picture depends on the degree of ischemia and its rate of development. In *acute fulminant ischemic colitis*, the major manifestations are severe lower abdominal pain, rectal bleeding, and hypotension. Dilatation of the colon and physical signs of peritonitis are seen in severe cases. Abdominal films may reveal thumbprinting from submucosal hemorrhage and edema (Fig. 288-1). Barium enema is hazardous in the acute situation because of the risk of perforation. Sigmoidoscopy or colonoscopy may detect ulcerations, friability, and bulging folds from submucosal hemorrhage. Angiography is not helpful in the management of patients with presumed ischemic colitis because a remediable occlusive lesion is very rarely found. Surgical resection may be required in some patients with fulminant ischemic colitis to remove gangrenous bowel; others with lesser degrees of ischemia may respond to conservative medical management.

Subacute ischemic colitis is the most common clinical variant of ischemic colonic disease. It produces lesser degrees of pain and bleeding, often occurring over several days or weeks. The left colon may be involved, but the rectum is usually spared because of the collateral blood supply, a feature distinguishing it from acute ulcerative colitis. Barium enema reveals edema, cobblestoning, thumbprinting, and occasionally superficial ulceration. Angiography is not indicated because almost all cases are nonocclusive. Occasionally, *stricture formation* may follow a bout of ischemic colitis or may present de novo without a history of antecedent pain or bloody diarrhea. Most cases of nonocclusive ischemic colitis resolve in 2 to 4 weeks and do not recur. Surgery is not required except for obstruction secondary to postischemic stricture.

ANGIODYSPLASIA OF THE COLON These are vascular ectasias or arteriovenous malformations (AVMs) that occur in the right colon of many older individuals and may cause bleeding (see Chap. 44). Angiodysplasia is a degenerative lesion consisting of dilated, distorted, thin-walled vessels lined by vascular endothelium. It may result from partial obstruction of the submucosal venous plexus by the tension generated in the cecal wall during muscular contraction. Grossly, angiodysplasias look similar to spider angiomas of the skin and on colonoscopy appear as star-shaped branching vessels in the submucosa measuring from 2 mm to 1 cm in diameter. The lesions are usually multiple and are found primarily in the cecum and ascending colon, but in some patients they may be distributed from the stomach to rectum.

Cecal angiodysplasia is important because of the likelihood of bleeding, either massively or chronically. In patients over age 60, approximately one-quarter of colonic bleeding episodes are secondary to angiodysplasia. The diagnosis is easiest to establish by colonoscopy, which allows treatment by laser photocoagulation, electrocautery, or injection with sclerosant. Some patients with massive uncontrolled bleeding or multiple sites of angiodysplasia may require right hemicolectomy. Angiodysplasias also may respond to chronic estrogen-progesterone therapy.

ANORECTAL PROBLEMS

HEMORRHOIDS The internal hemorrhoidal plexus of veins is located in the submucosal space above the valves of Morgagni. The anal canal separates it from the external hemorrhoidal venous plexus, but the two spaces communicate under the anal canal, the submucosa of which is attached to underlying tissue to form the interhemorrhoidal depression. Whenever the internal hemorrhoidal plexus is enlarged, there is associated increase in supporting tissue mass, and the resultant venous swelling is called an *internal hemorrhoid*. When veins in the external hemorrhoidal plexus become enlarged or thrombosed, the resultant bluish mass is called an *external hemorrhoid*.

Both types of hemorrhoids are very common and are associated with increased hydrostatic pressure in the portal venous system, such as during pregnancy, straining at stool, or with cirrhosis. When internal hemorrhoids enlarge, pain is not a usual feature until the situation is complicated by thrombosis, infection, or erosion of the overlying mucosal surface. Most persons complain of bright red blood on the toilet tissue or coating the stool, with a feeling of vague anal discomfort.

The discomfort is increased when the hemorrhoid enlarges or prolapses through the anus: prolapse is often accompanied by edema and sphincteric spasm. Prolapse, if not treated, usually becomes chronic as the muscularis stays stretched, and the patient complains of constant soiling of underclothing with very little pain. Prolapsed hemorrhoids may be detected or thrombosed; the overlying mucous membrane may bleed profusely from the trauma of defecation.

External hemorrhoids, because they lie under the skin, are quite often painful, particularly if there is a sudden increase in their mass. These episodes result in a tender blue swelling at the anal verge due to thrombosis of a vein in the external plexus and need not be associated with enlargement of the internal veins. Since the thrombus usually lies at the level of the sphincteric muscles, anal spasm often occurs.

The diagnosis of internal and external hemorrhoids is made by inspection, digital examination, and direct vision through the anoscope and proctoscope. Since such lesions are very common, they must not be regarded as the cause of rectal bleeding or chronic hypochromic anemia until a thorough investigation has been made of the more proximal gastrointestinal tract. Acute blood loss can occasionally be attributed to internal hemorrhoids. Chronic anemia or occult blood in the stool in the presence of large but not definitely bleeding hemorrhoids requires a search for a polyp, cancer, or ulcer.

℞ TREATMENT

Most hemorrhoids respond to conservative therapy such as sitz baths or other forms of moist heat, suppositories, stool softeners, and bed rest. Internal hemorrhoids that remain permanently prolapsed are best treated surgically; milder degrees of prolapse or enlargement with pruritus ani or intermittent bleeding can be handled successfully by banding or injection of sclerosing solutions. External hemorrhoids that become acutely thrombosed are treated by incision, extraction of the clot, and compression of the incised area following clot removal. No surgical procedure should be carried out in the presence of acute inflammation of the anus, ulcerative proctitis, or ulcerative colitis. Proctoscopy or colonoscopy should always be performed before a patient is subjected to hemorrhoidectomy.

ANAL INFLAMMATION Perianal inflammatory lesions may be primary or may be associated with inflammatory bowel disease or diverticular disease, as mentioned above. *Anal fissures* are superficial erosions of the anal canal which usually heal rapidly with conservative therapy. *Anal ulcers* are more chronic and deep and give symptoms largely as the result of painful spasm of the external anal sphincter during and after defecation. Bleeding may occur with either fissure or ulcer; healing of the ulcer often is associated with a hypertrophied anal papilla and some degrees of anal contracture. *Fistula in ano*, a tract leading from the rectal lumen to the perianal skin, usually results from local crypt abscesses. The fistula is a chronically inflamed canal made up of fibrous tissue surrounding granulation tissue, the lumen of which may be difficult to demonstrate. *Perirectal abscesses* often represent the tracking down into the anal area of purulent material escaping from the rectosigmoid; diverticulitis, Crohn's disease, ulcerative colitis, or previous surgery may be the underlying cause. Fistulas between the rectum and vagina or the rectum and bladder represent serious complications of granulomatous, septic, or malignant disorders and require the patient to be hospitalized for definitive diagnostic and therapeutic procedures.

PERITONEAL AND MESENTERIC DISEASES

ACUTE PERITONITIS Peritonitis is a localized or generalized inflammatory process of the peritoneum that may appear in both acute and chronic forms. In the acute form, the motor activity of the intestine is decreased, and the intestinal lumen becomes distended with gas and fluid. Fluid accumulates as a result of failure to reabsorb the 7 or 8 L normally secreted daily into the lumen and absorbed from the distal small bowel and colon. Because of accumulation of fluid in the peritoneal cavity as well as decreased oral intake, rapid depletion of the plasma volume with impaired cardiac and renal function may occur.

Etiology *Bacterial peritonitis* may be due to entry of bacteria into the peritoneal cavity from a perforation in the gastrointestinal tract or from an external penetrating wound. *Chemical peritonitis* results from spillage of pancreatic enzymes, gastric acid, or bile as a result of injury or perforation of the intestine or biliary tract. *Sterile peritonitis* occurs in patients with systemic lupus erythematosus, porphyria, and familial Mediterranean fever (FMF) during attacks of their disease (see below).

The most common causes of bacterial peritonitis are appendicitis, perforations associated with diverticulitis, peptic ulcer, gangrenous gallbladder, and gangrenous obstruction of the small bowel from adhesive bands, incarcerated hernia, or volvulus. Any lesion leading to the escape of intestinal bacteria may be a source, including a perforating carcinoma, foreign body, and ulcerative colitis. The peritoneal cavity is remarkably resistant to contamination, and unless continuing contamination occurs, the peritonitis remains localized. Patients with alcoholic cirrhosis and ascites have an increased susceptibility to *spontaneous bacterial peritonitis*, usually from enteric pathogens. This complication occurs in the absence of recognizable perforation of a viscus and may be due to leakage of bacteria through the intestinal wall (see Chap. 299).

Clinical Features The cardinal manifestations of peritonitis are acute abdominal pain and tenderness. The location of the pain and tenderness depends on the underlying cause and whether the inflammation is localized or generalized. In *localized peritonitis*, as seen in uncomplicated appendicitis or diverticulitis, the physical findings are limited to the area of inflammation. With widespread peritoneal inflammation there is *generalized peritonitis* with diffuse abdominal tenderness and rebound. Rigidity of the abdominal wall is a common finding in peritonitis and may be localized or generalized.

Peristalsis may be present initially but usually disappears as the illness progresses and bowel sounds disappear. Hypotension, tachycardia, oliguria, and leukocytosis, with cell counts greater than 20,000 cells per microliter, are common, especially in generalized peritonitis. Plain abdominal films may reveal dilatation of the large and small bowel with edema of the small-bowel wall, as evidenced by the distance between adjacent loops of gas-filled small intestine. Diagnostic paracentesis is sometimes valuable in determining the nature of the exudate as well as whether bacteria can be demonstrated or cultured.

GONOCOCCAL PERITONITIS This usually involves an extension of gonococcal infection from a primary focus in the female reproductive tract. The signs of inflammation usually are limited to the pelvis, but there may be findings of a mild generalized peritonitis. Occasionally, the patient has right upper quadrant pain and tenderness caused by gonococcal perihepatitis involving the liver capsule and adjacent peritoneum (Fitz-Hugh–Curtis syndrome; see also Chap. 150).

STARCH PERITONITIS An acute granulomatous peritonitis can develop in some patients as a foreign-body reaction to cornstarch used to powder surgical gloves. The clinical picture is that of acute abdominal pain and fever 10 to 30 days after an abdominal operation. The diagnosis can be made by paracentesis and demonstration of starch granules in monocytes. However, most patients are reexplored because of the fear of abscess or bacterial peritonitis, with the finding of foreign-body granuloma studding the peritoneum.

PSEUDOMYXOMA PERITONEI This is a rare condition resulting from rupture of a mucocele of the appendix, a mucinous ovarian cyst, or mucin-secreting intestinal or ovarian adenocarcinoma. The abdomen becomes filled with masses of jelly-like mucus. Occasionally, with removal of the mucocele or the ovarian cyst and most of the myxomatous material, a cure may ensue. In other cases, however, the mucoid material recurs, leading to progressive wasting and eventual death. Colloid carcinoma arising from the stomach or colon with peritoneal implants may resemble pseudomyxoma at laparotomy. The course of this type of highly malignant tumor is one of rapid cachexia and early death. The diagnosis usually can be made by the appearance of many highly malignant cells in the peritoneal implants.

PNEUMATOSIS CYSTOIDES INTESTINALIS This is a condition in which multiple gas-filled blebs or cysts accumulate in the intestinal wall beneath the serosal surface of the bowel. The exact source of the gas has not been explained satisfactorily. In some instances, this disease is associated with specific ulceration of the intestinal mucosa, in particular peptic ulcer with outlet obstruction. Cysts in the wall of the small bowel are seen as an occasional complication of mesenteric vascular occlusion. In the large bowel, these cysts are usually benign, may be seen with a variety of other disorders, and usually disappear over time.

There are no specific physical findings secondary to the pneumatosis, and the diagnosis is made either by x-ray or at laparotomy. Occasionally, the subserosal cysts may rupture, resulting in pneumoperitoneum.

CHYLOUS ASCITES See Chap. 46

MESENTERIC LIPODYSTROPHY This is a rare disorder usually affecting middle-aged women and characterized pathologically by infiltration of the mesentery with lipid-laden macrophages and fibrous tissue. These patients present with ill-defined abdominal pain and occasionally an abdominal mass. The diagnosis is made at laparotomy by demonstration of thick fibrofatty masses at the root of the mesentery with retraction and distortion of the bowel loops.

FAMILIAL MEDITERRANEAN FEVER*

Familial Mediterranean fever (FMF, familial paroxysmal polyserositis) is an inherited disorder of unknown etiology, characterized by recurrent episodes of fever, peritonitis, and/or pleuritis. Arthritis, skin lesions, and amyloidosis are seen in some patients.

FMF occurs predominantly in patients of non-Ashkenazi (Sephardic) Jewish, Armenian, and Arabic ancestry. However, the disease has been seen in patients of Italian, Ashkenazi Jewish, and Anglo-Saxon descent as well as others.

The earliest studies of the genetics of FMF were done in Israel, where the disease appears to be inherited in an autosomal recessive manner. Consanguinity among the parents of FMF patients is as high as 20 percent, a figure that may be an underestimate. Approximately 60 percent of patients are male. The gene believed to cause FMF is located in the short arm of chromosome 16.

ETIOLOGY The cause of FMF is unknown. Fever and inflammation are such prominent signs that frequent attempts have been made to implicate infectious agents and/or their products. However, extensive studies have failed to implicate these or any other specific infectious agents. Others have suggested a deficiency in an inhibitor of C5a, thus implicating alterations in the immune system. The demonstration that FMF is inherited as an autosomal recessive disorder has led to the thesis that it is an inborn error of metabolism. However, no such error has been found.

PATHOLOGY Despite the striking clinical manifestations during an acute attack of FMF, no specific pathologic alterations have been found. At laparotomy, there is acute peritoneal inflammation with an exudate that contains a predominance of polymorphonuclear leukocytes. A disproportionately large number of male patients develop gallbladder disease with and without cholelithiasis. Pleural and joint inflammation are also nonspecific.

In the amyloidosis that accompanies FMF, amyloid is deposited in the intima and media of the arterioles, the subendothelial region of venules, the glomeruli, and the spleen. Aside from their vessels, the heart and liver are uninvolved.

MANIFESTATIONS The symptoms of FMF often begin between the ages of 5 and 15, although attacks sometimes commence during infancy and onset has occurred as late as age 50. The duration

---

* The late Sheldon M. Wolff was the previous author of this topic.

and frequency of attacks vary greatly in the same patient, and there is no set pattern to their occurrence. The usual acute episode lasts 24 to 48 h, but some may be prolonged for 7 to 10 days. The attacks range in frequency from twice weekly to once a year, but 2 to 4 weeks is the commonest interval. Spontaneous remissions lasting years have been seen. There may be a decrease in the severity and frequency of the attacks with age or with development of amyloidosis.

Fever Fever is a cardinal manifestation and is present during most attacks. Rarely, fever may be present without serositis. The temperature may be preceded by a chill and will peak in 12 to 24 h. Defervescence is often accompanied by diaphoresis. The fever ranges from 38.5 to 40°C but is quite variable.

Abdominal Pain Abdominal pain occurs in more than 95 percent of patients and may vary in severity in the same patient. Minor premonitory discomfort may precede an acute episode by 24 to 48 h. The pain usually starts in one quadrant and then spreads to involve the whole abdomen. The initial site is usually very tender. Tenderness may remain localized with referred pain in other areas, and there may be radiation to the back. There may be splinting of the chest and pain in one or both shoulders, typical of diaphragmatic irritation. Nausea and vomiting sometimes occur. The abdomen is usually distended and may become rigid, with decreased or absent bowel sounds. On x-ray, the wall of the small intestine may appear edematous, transit of barium is slowed, and fluid levels may be seen. An abdominal operation may precipitate an acute attack of FMF, which may be confused with other postoperative complications.

Chest Pain Most patients with abdominal attacks have referred chest pain at one time or another, and 75 percent also develop acute pleuritic pain with or without abdominal symptoms. In 30 percent, the attacks of pleuritis precede the onset of abdominal attacks by varying periods of time, and a small number of patients never develop abdominal attacks. Chest pain is usually unilateral and is associated with diminished breath sounds, a friction rub, or a transient pleural effusion.

Joint Pain In Israel, 75 percent of patients report at least one episode of acute arthritis. Arthritis can be distinct from abdominal or pleural attacks, can be acute or, rarely, chronic, and may involve one or several joints. Effusions are common, with large joints most frequently involved. Radiologic findings are nonspecific. Despite careful search, frank arthritis rarely has been seen in the United States. Some patients have a history of rheumatic fever–like illness in childhood, but in a large series of patients, including 30 from the Middle East, acute arthritis was not observed. Mild arthralgia is common during acute attacks but is nonspecific.

Skin Manifestations Skin involvement occurs in a third of patients. These lesions consist of painful, erythematous areas of swelling from 5 to 20 cm in diameter, usually located on the lower legs, the medial malleolus, or the dorsum of the foot. They may occur without abdominal or pleural pain and subside within 24 to 48 h.

Other Signs and Symptoms Involvement of other serosal membranes has been reported, but pericarditis and meningitis are rare. Hematuria, splenomegaly, and small white dots called *colloid bodies* in the ocular fundus are findings of questionable significance. Rarely migraine-like headaches accompany acute abdominal attacks, and some patients have become somewhat irrational or show extreme emotional lability during attacks. Whether these are primary manifestations of FMF or secondary effects of pain and fever is unclear.

Complications Depression and lack of motivation are common, and patients with FMF require considerable support. A striking number of patients have developed gallbladder disease.

Amyloidosis has been reported in Israel, North Africa, and elsewhere in the Middle East, but its occurrence is rare in the United States. These findings are even more striking because there are probably as many known FMF patients in the United States as in Israel. Thus, environmental or nutritional, as well as genetic, factors may play a role in the development of amyloidosis in FMF.

LABORATORY FINDINGS Polymorphonuclear leukocytosis ranging from 10,000 to 30,000 cells/μL is almost invariable during acute attacks. The erythrocyte sedimentation rate is elevated during

attacks but returns to normal between attacks. Plasma fibrinogen, serum haptoglobin, ceruloplasmin, and C-reactive protein increase during the episodes. Plasma lipids are normal, and there are no consistent abnormalities of hepatic or renal function. When amyloidosis is present, laboratory findings are typical of a nephrotic syndrome followed by renal insufficiency.

DIAGNOSIS When the typical acute attacks of FMF occur in an individual of appropriate ethnic background with a family history of FMF, the diagnosis is easy. When a patient is seen for the first time, a variety of other febrile illnesses must be excluded, such as acute appendicitis, pancreatitis, porphyria, cholecystitis, intestinal obstruction, and other major abdominal catastrophes.

Some inherited hyperlipidemias may mimic the clinical picture of FMF, but lipid analysis will eliminate them from consideration. The FMF patient is not immune to other diseases, and when an attack differs from the usual pattern or is more prolonged, consideration should be given to other diagnostic possibilities. The pleural form of the disease is sometimes difficult to differentiate from acute pulmonary infection or infarction, but the rapid disappearance of signs and symptoms resolves the problem. The erythema is sometimes difficult to differentiate from superficial thrombophlebitis or cellulitis.

The most difficult diagnostic problem in FMF is the patient who presents with fever alone. In this situation, an extensive diagnostic workup for fever of unknown origin may be required. Fortunately, such patients are rare, and all eventually develop serosal involvement. Until specific diagnostic tests for FMF are available, patients with recurrent fever but without signs of inflammation of one of the serosal membranes should not be categorized as having FMF.

PROGNOSIS Despite the severity of the symptoms during some acute attacks, most patients are remarkably free of debilitation between attacks and are able to lead fairly normal lives. The greatest hazard to patients is prolonged periods of hospitalization due to erroneous diagnoses or failure to understand the disease. In the United States, the prognosis of patients with FMF does not seem to be different from that of patients with other chronic nonfatal illnesses. Death usually results from causes unrelated to the underlying disease.

In the past, approximately 25 percent of FMF patients in Israel developed amyloidosis, and this complication usually led to death. However, the widespread use of colchicine has resulted in dramatically decreasing the incidence of amyloidosis.

℞ **TREATMENT**

Among the therapies tried have been antibiotics, hormones (including estrogens and glucocorticoids), antipyretic drugs, immunotherapy, psychotherapy, elimination and low-fat diets, chloroquine, and phenylbutazone. When carefully studied and followed up, none of these therapies proved effective.

During the past 25 years, the outlook of patients with FMF has been altered dramatically. In 1972, Goldfinger showed that the prophylactic use of colchicine dramatically reduced the number of attacks. Subsequently, controlled trials in the United States and Israel have shown that chronic administration of colchicine greatly reduces the number of acute attacks of FMF. It is recommended that 0.6 mg colchicine be taken by mouth three times a day. Patients often develop gastrointestinal side effects with this dose, however, in which case the dose should be reduced to 0.6 mg taken twice a day. Although an occasional patient will respond to 0.6 mg taken only once a day, this amount is less likely to be beneficial. Most FMF patients will respond favorably to colchicine prophylaxis.

BIBLIOGRAPHY

DISORDERS OF MOTILITY

COLEMONT LJ, CAMILLERI M: Chronic intestinal pseudo-obstruction: Diagnosis and treatment. Mayo Clin Proc 64:60, 1989

DROSSMAN DA, THOMPSON WG: The irritable bowel syndrome: Review and a graduated multicomponent treatment approach. Ann Intern Med 116:1009, 1992

GOYAL RK, HIRANO I: Mechanisms of disease: The enteric nervous system. N Engl J Med 334:1106, 1996

JOHNSON LR (ed): *Physiology of the Gastrointestinal Tract*, 2d ed. New York, Raven Press, 1987

KELLOW JE, MALCOLM A: Motility. Curr Opin Gastroenterol 12:134, 1996

LYNN RB, FRIEDMAN LS: Irritable bowel syndrome. Managing the patient with abdominal pain and altered bowel habits. Med Clin North Am 79:373, 1995

PRESTON DM, LENNARD-JONES JE: Severe chronic constipation of young women: Idiopathic slow transit constipation. Gut 27:41, 1986

DIVERTICULAR DISEASES

BRIAN JE, STAIR JM: Non-colonic diverticular disease. Surg Gynecol Obstet 161:189, 1985

STEFANSSON T et al: Increased risk of left sided colon cancer in patients with diverticular disease. Gut 34:499, 1993

THOMPSON WG, PATEL DG: Clinical picture of diverticular disease of the colon. Clin Gastroenterol 15:903, 1986

INTESTINAL ISCHEMIA AND ANGIODYSPLASIA

CLAVIN PA: Diagnosis and management of mesenteric infarction. Br J Surg 77:601, 1990

KITCHENS CS: Evolution of our understanding of the pathophysiology of primary mesenteric venous thrombosis. Am J Surg 163:346, 1992

NAVEAU S et al: Long-term results of treatment of vascular malformation of the gastrointestinal tract by neodynium YAG laser photocoagulation. Dig Dis Sci 35:821, 1990

SARGEANT IR et al: Laser ablation of upper gastrointestinal vascular ectasias: Long term results. Gut 34:470, 1993

VAN CUTSEM et al: Treatment of bleeding gastrointestinal vascular malformations with oestrogen-progesterone. Lancet I:953, 1990

PERITONEAL AND MESENTERIC DISEASES

GORTINE SR: Treatment of benign anal disease with topical nitroglycerine. Dis Colon Rectum 38:453, 1995

PRESS OW et al: Evaluation and management of chylous ascites. Ann Intern Med 96:358, 1982

SCHWARTZ SI et al: *Principles of Surgery*, 6th ed. New York, McGraw-Hill, 1994

TITO L et al: Spontaneous bacterial peritonitis. Hepatology 8:27, 1988

YAMADA T et al (eds): *Textbook of Gastroenterology*, 2d ed. Philadelphia, Lippincott, 1995

FAMILIAL MEDITERRANEAN FEVER

DANIELS M et al: Familial Mediterranean fever: High gene frequency among the Jewish populations in Israel. Am J Med Genet 55:311, 1995

DINARELLO CA et al: Colchicine therapy for familial Mediterranean fever. A double-blind trial. N Engl J Med 291:934, 1974

MEYERHOFF J: Familial Mediterranean fever: Report of a large family, review of the literature, and discussion of the frequency of amyloidosis. Medicine 59:66, 1980

PRAS E et al: Mapping of a gene causing familial Mediterranean fever to the short arm of chromosome 16. N Engl J Med 326:1509, 1992

ZEMER D et al: Colchicine in the prevention and treatment of the amyloidosis of familial Mediterranean fever. N Engl J Med 314:1001, 1986

289	*William Silen*

ACUTE INTESTINAL OBSTRUCTION

ETIOLOGY AND CLASSIFICATION Intestinal obstruction may be *mechanical* or *nonmechanical* (resulting from neuromuscular disturbances that produce either *adynamic* or *dynamic ileus*). The causes of mechanical obstruction of the lumen are conveniently divided into (1) lesions *extrinsic* to the intestine, e.g., adhesive bands, internal and external hernias; (2) lesions *intrinsic* to the wall of the intestine, e.g., diverticulitis, carcinoma, regional enteritis; and (3) obturation of the lumen, e.g., gallstone obstruction, intussusception. Clinically, however, it is most useful to consider whether the obstructive mechanism involves the small or large intestine, because the causes, symptoms, and treatments are different (see below). Adhesions and external hernias are the most common causes of obstruction of the small intestine, constituting 70 to 75 percent of cases of this type. Adhesions, however, almost never produce obstruction of the colon, whereas carcinoma, sigmoid diverticulitis, and volvulus, in that order, are the most common causes and together account for about 90 percent of the cases. Primary intestinal pseudoobstruction (see Chap. 288) is a chronic motility disorder that frequently mimics mechanical obstruction. Unnecessary operations in such patients should be avoided.

Adynamic ileus is probably the most common overall cause of obstruction. The development of this condition is mediated via the hormonal component of the sympathoadrenal system. Adynamic ileus may occur after any peritoneal insult, and its severity and duration will be dependent to some degree on the type of peritoneal injury. Hydrochloric acid, colonic contents, and pancreatic enzymes are among the most irritating substances, whereas blood and urine are less so. Adynamic ileus occurs to some degree after any abdominal operation. Retroperitoneal hematomas, particularly associated with vertebral fracture, commonly cause severe adynamic ileus, and the latter may occur with other retroperitoneal conditions, such as ureteral calculus or severe pyelonephritis. Thoracic diseases, including lower-lobe pneumonia, fractured ribs, and myocardial infarction, frequently produce adynamic ileus, as do electrolyte disturbances, particularly potassium depletion. Finally, intestinal ischemia, whether the result of vascular occlusion or intestinal distention itself, may perpetuate an adynamic ileus.

Spastic ileus or *dynamic ileus* is very uncommon and results from extreme and prolonged contraction of the intestine. It has been observed in heavy metal poisoning, uremia, porphyria, and extensive intestinal ulcerations.

PATHOPHYSIOLOGY Distention of the intestine is caused by the accumulation of gas and fluid proximal to and within the obstructed segment. Between 70 and 80 percent of intestinal gas consists of swallowed air, and because this is composed mainly of nitrogen, which is poorly absorbed from the intestinal lumen, removal of air by continuous gastric suction is a useful adjunct in the treatment of intestinal distention. The accumulation of fluid proximal to the obstructing mechanism results not only from ingested fluid, swallowed saliva, gastric juice, and biliary and pancreatic secretions but also from interference with normal sodium and water transport. During the first 12 to 24 h of obstruction, there is a marked depression of flux from lumen to blood of sodium and consequently water in the distended proximal intestine. After 24 h, there is movement of sodium and water into the lumen, contributing further to the distention and fluid losses. Intraluminal pressure rises from a normal of 2 to 4 cmH$_2$O to 8 to 10 cmH$_2$O. During peristalsis, when simple obstruction or a "closed loop" is present, pressures reach 30 to 60 cmH$_2$O. Closed-loop obstruction of the small intestine results when the lumen is occluded at two points by a single mechanism such as a hernial ring or adhesive band, thus producing a closed loop whose blood supply is often obstructed at the same time. Strangulation of the loop itself is thus common in association with marked distention proximal to the involved loop. A form of closed-loop obstruction is encountered when complete obstruction of the colon exists in the presence of a competent ileocecal valve (85 percent of individuals). Although the blood supply of the colon is not entrapped within the obstructing mechanism, distention of the cecum is extreme because of its greater diameter (Laplace's law), and impairment of the intramural blood supply is considerable with consequent gangrene of the cecal wall, usually anteriorly. Necrosis of the small intestine may occur by the same mechanism of interference with intramural blood flow when distention is extreme, but this sequence is uncommon in the small intestine. Once impairment of blood supply occurs, bacterial invasion supervenes, and peritonitis develops. The systemic effects of extreme distention include elevation of the diaphragm with restricted ventilation and subsequent atelectasis. Venous return via the inferior vena cava also may be impaired.

The loss of fluids and electrolytes may be extreme and, unless replacement is prompt, leads to hemoconcentration, hypovolemia, renal insufficiency, shock, and death. Vomiting, accumulation of fluids within the lumen by the mechanisms described above, and the sequestration of fluid into the edematous intestinal wall and peritoneal cavity as a result of impairment of venous return from the intestine all contribute to massive loss of fluid and electrolytes, especially potassium. As soon as significant impedance to venous return is present, the intestine becomes severely congested, and blood begins to seep into the intestinal lumen. Blood loss may reach significant levels when long segments of intestine are involved.

SYMPTOMS *Mechanical small-intestinal obstruction* is characterized by cramping midabdominal pain, which tends to be more severe the higher the obstruction. The pain occurs in paroxysms, and the patient is relatively comfortable in the intervals between the pains. Audible borborygmi are often noted by the patient simultaneously with the paroxysms of pain. The pain may become less severe as distention progresses, probably because motility is impaired in the edematous intestine. When strangulation is present, the pain is usually more localized and may be steady and severe without a colicky component, a fact that often causes delay in diagnosis of obstruction. Vomiting is almost invariable, and it is earlier and more profuse the higher the obstruction. The vomitus initially contains bile and mucus and remains as such if the obstruction is high in the intestine. With low ileal obstruction, the vomitus becomes feculent, i.e., orange-brown in color with a foul odor, which results from the overgrowth of bacteria proximal to the obstruction. Hiccups (singultus) are common. Obstipation and failure to pass gas by rectum are invariably present when the obstruction is complete, although some stool and gas may be passed spontaneously or after an enema shortly after onset of the complete obstruction. Diarrhea is occasionally observed in partial obstruction. Blood in the stool is rare but does occur in cases of intussusception. Other than some minor but inconsistent differences in pain patterns noted above, the symptoms of strangulating obstructions cannot be distinguished from those of nonstrangulating obstructions.

Mechanical colonic obstruction produces colicky abdominal pain similar in quality to that of small-intestinal obstruction but of much lower intensity. Complaints of pain are occasionally absent in stoic elderly patients. Vomiting occurs late, if at all, particularly if the ileocecal valve is competent. Paradoxically, feculent vomitus is very rare. A history of recent alterations in bowel habits and blood in the stool is common because carcinoma and diverticulitis are the most frequent causes. Constipation becomes progressive, and obstipation with failure to pass gas ensues. Acute symptoms may develop over a period of a week. Cecal volvulus more closely resembles obstruction of the small intestine clinically, whereas patients with sigmoid volvulus more typically have the picture of colonic obstruction in which marked distention predominates, with relatively less pain.

In *adynamic ileus*, colicky pain is absent, and only discomfort from distention is evident. Vomiting may be frequent but is rarely profuse. It usually consists of gastric contents and bile and is almost never feculent. Complete obstipation may or may not occur. Singultus (hiccups) is common.

PHYSICAL FINDINGS *Abdominal distention* is the hallmark of all forms of intestinal obstruction. It is least marked in cases of obstruction high in the small intestine and most marked in colonic obstruction. Early, especially in closed-loop strangulating small-bowel obstruction, distention may be barely perceptible or absent. Tenderness and rigidity are usually minimal; the temperature is rarely above 37.8°C (100°F) in nonstrangulating obstruction of the small and large intestine. Contrary to popular belief, the same is true of strangulating obstruction until very late, a fact that has often resulted in unfortunate delay in treatment. Signs and symptoms of shock also occur *very late* in strangulating obstruction. The appearance of shock, tenderness, rigidity, and fever often means that there has been contamination of the peritoneum with infected intestinal content. Hernial orifices should always be carefully examined for the presence of a mass.

The presence of a palpable abdominal mass usually signifies a closed-loop strangulating small-bowel obstruction because the tense fluid-filled loop is the palpable lesion. Auscultation may reveal loud, high-pitched borborygmi coincident with the colicky pain, but this finding is often absent late in strangulating or nonstrangulating obstruction. A quiet abdomen does not eliminate the possibility of obstruction, nor does it necessarily establish the diagnosis of adynamic ileus.

LABORATORY AND X-RAY FINDINGS Leukocytosis, with shift to the left, usually occurs when strangulation is present, but a normal white blood cell count does not exclude strangulation. Elevation of the serum amylase level is encountered occasionally in all forms of intestinal obstruction, especially the strangulating variety.

The x-ray is extremely valuable but under certain circumstances also may be misleading. In nonstrangulating complete small-bowel obstruction, x-rays are almost completely reliable. Distention of fluid- and gas-filled loops of small intestine usually arranged in a "stepladder" pattern with air-fluid levels and an absence or paucity of colonic gas are pathognomonic (Fig. 289-1). These findings, however, are absent in slightly over half the cases of strangulating small-bowel obstruction, especially early in the disease. A general haze due to peritoneal fluid and sometimes a "coffee bean"–shaped mass are seen in strangulating obstruction. Occasionally, the films are normal, but when symptoms are consistent with obstruction of the small intestine, a normal film should suggest strangulation. Roentgenographic differentiation of partial mechanical small-bowel obstruction from adynamic ileus may be impossible because gas is present in both the small and large intestines; however, colonic distention is usually more prominent in adynamic ileus. A radiopaque dye given by mouth is useful in making this distinction.

Colonic obstruction with a competent ileocecal valve is easily recognized because distention with gas is mainly confined to the colon. Barium enema, sigmoidoscopy, or colonoscopy, depending on the suspected site of obstruction, is usually advisable to determine the nature of the lesion, except when concomitant perforation is suspected,

FIGURE 289-1 Acute mechanical obstruction of small intestine (upright film). Note air-fluid levels, marked distention of bowel loops, and absence of colonic gas.

a rare occurrence. Sigmoidoscopy may be therapeutic in cases of sigmoid volvulus. When the ileocecal valve is incompetent, the films resemble those of partial small-bowel obstruction or adynamic ileus, and barium enema or colonoscopy is necessary to establish the correct diagnosis. Barium given by mouth is perfectly safe when obstruction is in the small intestine, since the barium sulfate does not become inspissated in this location. *Barium should never be given by mouth to a patient with possible colonic obstruction* until that possibility has been excluded by barium enema.

℞ **TREATMENT**

 Small-Intestinal Obstruction The overall mortality rate for obstruction of the small intestine is about 10 percent, even under the most optimal conditions. While the mortality rate for nonstrangulating obstruction is as low as 5 to 8 percent, that for strangulating obstruction has been reported to be between 20 and 75 percent. Well over half the deaths from small-bowel obstruction occur in those with strangulation; however, the latter constitute only one-fourth to one-third of the cases. Careful studies indicate that the clinical, laboratory, and x-ray findings are not reliable in distinguishing strangulating from nonstrangulating obstruction when obstruction is complete. Complete obstruction is suggested when there has been a total cessation in the passage of gas or stool per rectum and when gas is absent in the distal intestine by x-ray. Since strangulating small-bowel obstruction is always complete, operation should always be undertaken in such patients after suitable preparation. Prior to operation, fluid and electrolyte balance should be restored and decompression instituted by means of a nasogastric tube. Replacement of potassium is especially important because intake is nil and losses in vomitus are large. Six to eight hours of preparation may be necessary. During this period, broad-spectrum antibiotics are indicated if strangulation is felt to be likely, but operation should not be delayed unless there is unequivocal clinical and roentgenographic evidence of resolution of the obstruction during the period of preparation. Attempts to pass a long tube into the small intestine usually fail while putting the patient through uncomfortable, unproductive manipulations that delay appropriate fluid replacement and decompression. *There are probably few, if any, indications for the use of a long intestinal tube.* Procrastination of operation because of improvement in well-being of the patient during resuscitation and gastric decompression usually leads to unnecessary and hazardous delay in proper treatment. Purely nonoperative therapy is safe only in the presence of incomplete obstruction and is best utilized in patients with (1) repeated episodes of partial obstruction, (2) recent postoperative partial obstruction, and (3) partial obstruction following a recent episode of diffuse peritonitis.

 Colonic Obstruction The mortality rate for colonic obstruction is about 20 percent. As in small-bowel obstruction, nonoperative treatment is contraindicated unless the obstruction is incomplete. Occasionally, but not always, when the obstruction is incomplete, nonoperative therapy may result in sufficient decompression that a definitive operative procedure can be undertaken at a later date. This usually can be accomplished by discontinuation of all oral intake and perhaps by nasogastric suction, although attempts to decompress a *completely* obstructed colon by intubation are almost invariably futile. A long intestinal tube will not decompress an obstructed colon with a competent ileocecal valve. When obstruction is complete, early operation is mandatory, especially when the ileocecal valve is competent; cecal gangrene is likely if the cecal diameter exceeds 10 cm on plain abdominal film. For obstruction on the left side of the colon, the most common site, preliminary operative decompression by cecostomy or transverse colostomy followed by definitive resection of the primary lesion has been the treatment of choice. Recently, primary resection of obstructing left-sided lesions with on-table washout of the colon has been accomplished safely. For a lesion of the right or transverse colon, primary resection and

anastomosis can be performed safely because distention of the ileum with consequent discrepancy in size and hazard in suture are not present.

 Adynamic Ileus This type of ileus usually responds to nonoperative continuous decompression and adequate treatment of the primary disease. The prognosis is usually good. Successful decompression of severe colonic ileus has been accomplished by colonoscopy, but this should be avoided if tenderness in the right lower quadrant suggests possible cecal gangrene. Rarely, adynamic colonic distention may become so great that cecostomy is required if cecal gangrene is feared. Spastic ileus usually responds to treatment of the primary disease.

BIBLIOGRAPHY

BULKLEY GB et al: Intraoperative determination of small intestinal viability following ischemic injury: Prospective controlled trial of two adjuvant methods (Doppler and fluorescein) compared with standard clinical judgement. Ann Surg 193:628, 1981

DUBOIS A et al: Postoperative ileus: Physiopathology, etiology and treatment. Ann Surg 178:781, 1973

ESKELINEN M et al: Contributions of history-taking, physical examination, and computer assistance to diagnosis of acute small-bowel obstruction. A prospective study of 1333 patients with acute abdominal pain. Scand J Gastroenterol 29:715, 1994

HOFSETTER SR: Acute adhesive obstruction of the small intestine. Surg Gynecol Obstet 152:141, 1981

JACKSON BR: The diagnosis of colonic obstruction. Dis Colon Rectum 25:603, 1982

PESCHIERA JL, BEERMAN SP: Intestinal dysfunction associated with acute thoracolumbar fractures. Orthop Rev 19:284, 1990

SILEN W: *Cope's Early Diagnosis of the Acute Abdomen*, 18th ed. London, Oxford, 1991

290 *William Silen*

ACUTE APPENDICITIS

 INCIDENCE AND EPIDEMIOLOGY The maximum incidence of acute appendicitis occurs in the second and third decades of life. While the disease may be encountered at any time of life, it is relatively rare at the extremes of age. Males and females are equally affected, except between puberty and age 25, when males predominate in a 3:2 ratio. Perforation is relatively much more common in infancy and in the aged, during which periods mortality rates are highest. The mortality rate has decreased steadily in Europe and the United States from 8.1 per 100,000 of the population in 1941 to less than 1 per 100,000 in 1970 and subsequently. The absolute incidence of the disease also decreased by about 40 percent between 1940 and 1960 but since then has remained unchanged. Although various factors such as changing dietary habits, altered intestinal flora, and better nutrition and intake of vitamins have been suggested to explain the reduced incidence, the exact reasons have not been elucidated. The overall incidence of appendicitis is much lower in underdeveloped countries, especially parts of Africa, and in lower socioeconomic groups.

 PATHOGENESIS The primary pathogenetic hallmark has always been thought to be luminal obstruction. While obstruction can be identified in 30 to 40 percent of cases, recent studies have shown that ulceration of the mucosa is the initial event in the majority. The causation of the ulceration is unknown, although a viral etiology has been postulated. It has been suggested that infection with *Yersinia* organisms may cause the disease, since high complement fixation titers have been found in as many as 30 percent of cases of proven appendicitis 1 week after operation. Whether the inflammatory reaction attendant with ulceration is sufficient to obstruct the tiny appendiceal lumen even transiently is not clear. Obstruction, when present, is most commonly caused by a fecalith, which results from accumulation and inspissation of fecal matter around vegetable fibers. Enlarged lymphoid follicles associated with viral infections (e.g., measles), inspissated barium, worms (e.g., pinworms, *Ascaris*, and *Taenia*), and tumors (e.g., carcinoid or carcinoma) also may obstruct the lumen. Secretion of mucus distends the organ, which has a capacity of only 0.1 to 0.2 mL, and luminal pressures rise as high as 60 cmH2O. Luminal bacteria multiply and invade the appendiceal wall as venous engorgement and subsequent arterial compromise result from the high intraluminal pressures. Finally, gangrene and perforation occur. If the process evolves slowly, adjacent organs such as the terminal ileum, cecum, and omentum may wall off the appendiceal area so that a localized abscess will develop, whereas rapid progression of vascular impairment may cause perforation with free access to the peritoneal cavity. Subsequent rupture of primary appendiceal abscesses may produce fistulas between the appendix and bladder, small intestine, sigmoid, or cecum. Occasionally, acute appendicitis may be the first manifestation of Crohn's disease. While chronic infection of the appendix with tuberculosis, amebiasis, and actinomycosis may occur, a useful clinical aphorism states that *chronic appendiceal inflammation is not usually the cause of prolonged abdominal pain of weeks' or months' duration.* In contrast, it is clear that recurrent acute appendicitis does occur, often with complete resolution of inflammation and symptoms between attacks. Recurrent acute appendicitis may become more frequent as antibiotics are dispensed more freely and if a long appendiceal stump becomes more prevalent as laparoscopic appendectomy is used more often.

CLINICAL MANIFESTATIONS The history and sequence of symptoms are among the most important diagnostic features of appendicitis. The initial symptom is almost invariably *abdominal pain* of the visceral type, resulting from appendiceal contractions or distention of the lumen. It is usually poorly localized in the periumbilical or epigastric region. There is often an accompanying urge to defecate or pass flatus, neither of which relieves the distress. This visceral pain is mild, often cramping, and rarely catastrophic in nature, usually lasting 4 to 6 h, but it may not be noted by stoic individuals or by some patients during sleep. As inflammation spreads to the parietal peritoneal surfaces, the pain becomes somatic, steady, and more severe, aggravated by motion or cough, and usually located in the *right lower quadrant*. *Anorexia* is so frequent that the presence of hunger should arouse suspicion of the diagnosis of acute appendicitis. *Nausea* and *vomiting* occur in 50 to 60 percent of cases, but vomiting is rarely profuse and protracted. The development of nausea and vomiting before the onset of pain is extremely rare. Change in bowel habit is of little diagnostic value, since any or no alteration may be observed, although the presence of diarrhea caused by an inflamed appendix in juxtaposition to the sigmoid may cause serious diagnostic difficulties. Urinary frequency and dysuria occur if the appendix lies adjacent to the bladder. The typical sequence of symptoms (poorly localized periumbilical pain followed by nausea and vomiting with subsequent shift of pain to the right lower quadrant) occurs in only 50 to 60 percent of patients, and some variations are considered below.

Physical findings vary with time after onset of the illness and according to the location of the appendix, which may be situated deep in the pelvic cul-de-sac; in the right lower quadrant in any relation to the peritoneum, cecum, and small intestine; in the right upper quadrant (especially during pregnancy); or even in the left lower quadrant. *The diagnosis cannot be established unless tenderness can be elicited.* While tenderness is sometimes absent in the early visceral stage of the disease, it ultimately always develops and is found in any location corresponding to the position of the appendix. Abdominal tenderness may be completely absent if a retrocecal or pelvic appendix is present, in which case the sole physical finding may be tenderness in the flank or on rectal or pelvic examination. Percussion, rebound tenderness, and referred rebound tenderness are often, but not invariably, present; they are most likely to be absent early in the illness. Flexion of the right hip and guarded movement by the patient are due to parietal peritoneal involvement. Hyperesthesia of the skin of the right lower quadrant and a positive psoas or obturator sign are often late findings and are rarely of diagnostic value. When the inflamed appendix is in close proximity to the anterior parietal peritoneum, muscular rigidity is present yet is often minimal early. The temperature is usually normal

or slightly elevated [37.2 to 38°C (99 to 100.5°F)], but a temperature above 38.3°C (101°F) should always suggest the presence of perforation. Tachycardia is commensurate with the elevation of the temperature. Rigidity and tenderness become more marked as the disease progresses to perforation and localized or diffuse peritonitis. Distention is rare unless severe diffuse peritonitis has developed. The alleged disappearance of pain and tenderness just prior to perforation is extremely unusual. A mass may develop if localized perforation has occurred but usually will not be detectable before 3 days after onset of the disease. Earlier presence of a mass suggests carcinoma of the cecum or Crohn's disease. Perforation is rare before 24 h after onset of symptoms, but the rate may be as high as 80 percent after 48 h.

Laboratory examination does not establish the diagnosis because the latter is based primarily on clinical grounds. Although moderate leukocytosis of 10,000 to 18,000 cells/μL is frequent (with a concomitant shift to immature cells), the absence of leukocytosis does not eliminate the possibility of acute appendicitis. Leukocytosis of greater than 20,000 cells/μL should alert the clinician to the probability of perforation. Anemia and blood in the stool suggest a primary diagnosis of carcinoma of the cecum, especially in elderly individuals. The urine may contain a few white or red blood cells without bacteria if the appendix lies close to the right ureter or bladder.

Urinalysis is most useful, however, in excluding genitourinary conditions that may mimic acute appendicitis. X-rays are rarely of value except when an opaque fecalith (5 percent of patients) is observed in the right lower quadrant (especially in children) together with other clinical findings consistent with appendicitis. Consequently, there is no routine need to obtain films of the abdomen unless there is a possibility of other conditions such as intestinal obstruction or ureteral calculus. In some patients in whom symptoms are either recurrent or more prolonged, a careful barium enema or computed tomography scan may disclose an extrinsic defect on the medial wall of the cecum or a calcified fecalith. The diagnosis also may be established by the ultrasonic demonstration of an enlarged and thick-walled appendix, but if the appendix cannot be seen, the diagnosis cannot be excluded. Ultrasound is most useful to exclude ovarian cysts, ectopic pregnancy, or tuboovarian abscess.

While the typical historical sequence and physical findings are present in 50 to 60 percent of cases, it is obvious that a wide variety of atypical patterns of disease are encountered, especially at the age extremes and during pregnancy. The 70 to 80 percent incidence of perforation and generalized peritonitis in infants under 2 years of age is dramatic testimony to the importance of the history in the early detection of the disease. Any infant or child with diarrhea, vomiting, and abdominal pain is highly suspect. Fever is much more common in this age group, and abdominal distention is often the only physical finding. In the elderly, pain and tenderness are often obtunded, and thus the diagnosis is frequently delayed. A 30 percent incidence of perforation in patients over 70 attests to the importance of this delay. Elderly patients often present themselves initially with a slightly painful mass (a primary appendiceal abscess) or sometimes appear with adhesive intestinal obstruction 5 or 6 days after a previously undetected perforated appendix. Appendicitis occurs about once in every 1000 pregnancies and is the most common extrauterine condition requiring abdominal operation. The diagnosis may be missed or delayed because of the frequent occurrence of mild abdominal discomfort and nausea and vomiting during pregnancy. During the last trimester, when the mortality rate from appendicitis is highest, uterine displacement of the appendix to the right upper quadrant and laterally leads to confusion in diagnosis because pain and tenderness are similarly displaced.

DIFFERENTIAL DIAGNOSIS A listing of the differential diagnoses of acute appendicitis would produce an encyclopedic compendium of all conditions that cause abdominal pain, since appendicitis may simulate any of these diseases. Diagnostic accuracy is about 75 to 80 percent for experienced clinicians and must be based solely on the clinical criteria outlined above. It is probably better to err slightly in the direction of overdiagnosis, since delay is associated with perforation and increased morbidity and mortality. In unperforated appendicitis, the mortality rate is 0.1 percent, little more than that associated with general anesthesia; for perforated appendicitis, there is an overall mortality of 3 percent, a figure that increases to 15 percent in the elderly. In doubtful cases, 4 to 6 h of observation is always more beneficial than harmful, however. The most common conditions discovered at operation when acute appendicitis is erroneously diagnosed are, in rough order of frequency, mesenteric lymphadenitis, no organic disease, acute pelvic inflammatory disease, ruptured graafian follicle or corpus luteum cyst, and acute gastroenteritis. In addition, acute cholecystitis, perforated ulcer, acute pancreatitis, acute diverticulitis, strangulating intestinal obstruction, ureteral calculus, and pyelonephritis frequently present diagnostic difficulties.

It is useful to consider separately some of the more common and difficult diagnostic possibilities, especially in the female. Differentiation of *pelvic inflammatory disease* from acute appendicitis may be virtually impossible. Gram-negative intracellular diplococci on cervical smear are not pathognomonic unless *Neisseria gonorrhoeae* can be cultured. Pain on movement of the cervix is not specific and may occur in appendicitis if perforation has occurred or if the appendix lies adjacent to the uterus or adnexa. *Rupture of a graafian follicle* (mittelschmerz) occurs at midcycle with spill of blood and fluid to produce pain and tenderness more diffuse and usually of a less severe degree than in appendicitis. Fever and leukocytosis are usually absent. *Rupture of a corpus luteum cyst* is identical clinically to rupture of a graafian follicle but develops about the time of menstruation. The presence of an adnexal mass, evidence of blood loss, and a positive pregnancy test help differentiate *ruptured tubal pregnancy*, but a negative pregnancy test is present when tubal abortion has occurred. *Twisted ovarian cyst* and *endometriosis* occasionally are difficult to distinguish from appendicitis. In all these female conditions, ultrasonic examination of the pelvis and laparoscopy may be of great value.

Acute mesenteric lymphadenitis is the appellation usually given when enlarged, slightly reddened lymph nodes at the root of the mesentery and a normal appendix are encountered at operation in a patient who usually has right lower quadrant tenderness and a somewhat higher temperature than most patients with acute appendicitis. Whether this is a single, discrete entity is unclear, since the causative factor is not known. It has been recognized that some of these patients have infection with *Y. pseudotuberculosis* or *Y. enterocolitica*, in which case the diagnosis can be established by culture of the mesenteric nodes or by serologic titers (see Chap. 164). The diagnosis is essentially impossible clinically, although retrospectively there often appears to have been more diffuse pain and tenderness. Children seem to be affected more frequently than adults. Operation should be undertaken unless there is rapid resolution of all symptoms and findings. *Acute gastroenteritis* usually causes profuse watery diarrhea, often with nausea and vomiting, but without localized findings. Between cramps, the abdomen is completely relaxed. In *Salmonella* gastroenteritis, the abdominal findings are similar, although the pain may be more severe and more localized, and fever and chills are common. The occurrence of similar symptoms among other members of the family may be helpful. When the diagnosis of acute pelvic appendicitis with perforation has been missed, gastroenteritis is the most common previous working diagnosis. Persistent abdominal or rectal tenderness should eliminate the diagnosis of gastroenteritis. *Regional enteritis* (Crohn's disease) is usually associated with a more prolonged history, often with previous exacerbations regarded by the patient or physician as episodes of gastroenteritis unless the diagnosis has been established previously. *Meckel's diverticulitis* usually cannot be distinguished from acute appendicitis but is very rare.

℞ TREATMENT

Cathartics and enemas should be avoided if appendicitis is under consideration, and antibiotics should not be administered when the diagnosis is in question, since they will only mask the presence or development of perforation. The treatment is early operation and appendectomy as soon as the patient can be prepared. Appendectomy is increasingly accomplished laparoscopically, but there is no demonstrable value of this technique over open operation except where a diagnostic dilemma exists. Preparation rarely takes more than 1 to 2 h in early appendicitis but may require 6 to 8 h in cases of severe sepsis and dehydration associated with late perforation. The *only* circumstance in which operation is *not* indicated is the presence of a palpable mass 3 to 5 days after the onset of symptoms. Should operation be undertaken at that time, a phlegmon rather than a definitive abscess will be found, and complications from dissection of such a phlegmon are frequent. Such patients treated with broad-spectrum antibiotics, parenteral fluids, and rest usually show resolution of the mass and symptoms within 1 week. *Interval appendectomy* can and should be done safely 3 months later. Should the mass enlarge or the patient become more toxic, drainage of the abscess is necessary. The complications of subphrenic, pelvic, or other intra-abdominal abscesses usually follow perforation with generalized peritonitis and can be avoided by early diagnosis of the disease.

BIBLIOGRAPHY

BUTLER C: Surgical pathology of acute appendicitis. Hum Pathol 12:870, 1981

SARFATI MR et al: Impact of adjunctive testing on the diagnosis and clinical course of patients with acute appendicitis. Am J Surg 166:660, 1993

TATE JJ et al: Conventional versus laparoscopic surgery for acute appendicitis. Br J Surg 80:761, 1993

WADE DS et al: Accuracy of ultrasound in the diagnosis of acute appendicitis compared with the surgeon's clinical impression. Arch Surg 128:1039, 1993

SECTION 2

LIVER AND BILIARY TRACT DISEASE

291

Kurt J. Isselbacher, Daniel K. Podolsky

APPROACH TO THE PATIENT WITH LIVER DISEASE

BIOLOGIC CONSIDERATIONS An understanding of diseases of the liver and their clinical manifestations can be derived from a knowledge of fundamental normal hepatic structure and function. An appreciation of anatomic aspects of the liver and biliary tree from the gross level to that of the individual hepatocyte and other cellular constituents is needed to understand the spectrum of clinical manifestations of liver disease. The dual blood supply, unique to the liver and including the portal venous system, makes the liver an intermediate filter for most of the venous drainage of the abdominal viscera. This often leads to secondary hepatic involvement in a number of extrahepatic diseases and makes the liver a relatively common site of solid tumor metastases. Furthermore, an appreciation of the relevant anatomy, especially that of the portal venous system, is important in understanding clinically important manifestations of portal hypertension, a common complication of chronic liver disease when scarring and regeneration lead to distortion of the intrahepatic microvasculature. These anatomic considerations lead the clinician to look for evidence of splenic enlargement and hypersplenism, gastrointestinal bleeding, accumulation of ascites, and signs of portal-systemic encephalopathy. An understanding of the anatomy of the biliary tract from canaliculus to common bile duct is integral to understanding the basis and sequelae of obstructive jaundice. While inflammation of the gallbladder may lead to fever and pain, choledocholithiasis will cause biliary colic as well as jaundice. Diffuse processes affecting the intrahepatic ducts, such as primary sclerosing cholangitis, will lead to cholestasis and its attendant symptoms, while a focal process affecting a single branch of the biliary tree, such as a neoplasm, usually will not.

The structural organization at a level intermediate between the gross anatomic and the cellular also contributes to the clinical patterns seen with disorders of the liver. While various concepts have been offered, the most useful is that of the traditional liver lobule. Blood emanates from the portal venules at the periphery and passes through the hepatic sinusoids to the central vein. The portal venules, terminal bile ductules, and hepatic arterioles are arranged in a *triad*. Appreciation of this organization and the presence of concentric zones of function within the lobule explain distinct patterns of injury such as the centrilobular injury resulting from ischemia. These structural features no doubt also provide the basis for the relative preservation of hepatocellular function in many disorders that can lead to significant portal hypertension, such as schistosomiasis and biliary cirrhosis.

As important as the anatomic features are in understanding liver disease, many liver disorders and their manifestations can only be appreciated in the context of the functional complexity of the liver at the cellular level. As detailed in Chap. 293, the hepatocyte plays an important role in diverse general metabolic processes that may be deranged as a consequence of liver disease. In addition, this metabolic diversity leads to hepatic involvement in many inborn errors of metabolism, including a wide variety of storage diseases, and less well-understood disorders of iron metabolism (hemosiderosis and hemochromatosis) and copper homeostasis (Wilson's disease).

Some other functional aspects also should be emphasized. The hepatocyte modifies numerous endogenous (e.g., bilirubin) and exogenous (e.g., alcohol, acetaminophen) potentially toxic compounds through oxidation, reduction, and conjugation carried out by several enzymes of the endoplasmic reticulum. Conjugation of substrates generally facilitates their hepatic excretion, converting water-insoluble substances to water-soluble derivatives. It is therefore not surprising that parenchymal liver disease may lead to either conjugated or unconjugated hyperbilirubinemia and jaundice. Metabolic modifications may significantly alter the pharmacologic activity of drugs through formation of derivatives with either decreased or enhanced activity. These metabolic processes may create intermediates that are toxic to the liver itself. This explains the selective susceptibility of the liver to the toxicity of carbon tetrachloride, acetaminophen, and, most important, alcohol, which is converted initially to acetaldehyde.

Additional functions of the hepatocyte that may have significant clinical ramifications include the production of a variety of soluble proteins for secretion into the circulation and the presence of receptors specific for various circulating ligands. The latter is a property shared with the Kupffer cell, which fulfills much of its function as a constituent of the reticuloendothelial system by clearing a number of serum glycoproteins through asialoglycoprotein receptor–mediated endocytosis. There is evidence to suggest that some of the substances taken up by this endocytotic mechanism may subsequently pass to and through the hepatocyte to complete an enterohepatic circulation. Carcinoembryonic antigen (CEA) is a glycoprotein and tumor-associated marker that is handled in this manner, leading to artifactual elevations in hepatobiliary disease. In contrast to the Kupffer cell, the spectrum of ligands taken up by hepatocytes via specific receptors is much broader. In addition to ligands targeted for lysosomal degradation, the hepatocyte possesses receptors for ligands that are metabolically active after

their uptake and dissociation from their receptors. These include transferrin-bound iron and, most important, low-density lipoprotein, which contributes to regulation of overall body cholesterol metabolism. Disruption of lysosomal degradation of specific ligands in hereditary storage disease leads to hepatomegaly and a variety of infiltrative disorders. Disruption of the nonlysosomal endocytotic pathway ligands can lead to systemic disorders. It is not clear whether specific receptors or other hepatocyte membrane components play a role in the relative or absolute tropism of infectious agents (particularly the hepatitis viruses) that account for a large proportion of both acute and chronic liver disease. However, the relative selectivity of the hepatitis viruses (A, B, C, E, and indirectly D) for the hepatocyte is essential in understanding the clinical features of the illnesses caused by these agents, which derive from the extent of hepatocyte destruction, largely due to immune destruction rather than direct cytopathic effects of the virus. At the same time, the hepatocyte may be infected by less strictly organotropic agents including other viruses (e.g., Epstein-Barr virus) and a wide variety of bacterial and parasitic organisms. The vascular supply of the liver leads to its frequent involvement in disseminated infections.

A final feature of hepatocyte cell biology that contributes to the expression of liver disease is the potential for proliferation and regeneration. Although few mitotic figures are seen in normal hepatic parenchyma, rapid regeneration involving both proliferation and cellular hypertrophy occurs following hepatic resection in experimental animals and humans. The capacity for hepatocellular regeneration is evident in the complete recovery that usually occurs following fulminant hepatitis (due either to viral or toxic agents) if the patient can be sustained through the period of acute injury. Architecturally disordered regeneration in concert with fibrosis is an essential factor in the development of cirrhosis and leads both to disruption of blood flow through the hepatic parenchyma and to uneven hepatocellular function due to distortion of normal lobular structure.

CLINICAL CONSIDERATIONS In approaching the patient with known or suspected liver disease, consideration of the patient's problem in the context of a few salient questions permits the clinician to focus on the most important diagnostic possibilities and the severity of the illness. Is the problem primarily hepatocellular or cholestatic? Was the onset of the illness abrupt or gradual? Has the problem led to clinically significant impairment of normal hepatocellular function, such as signs of altered mentation or coagulopathy? Are there signs or symptoms of portal hypertension? Important and reliable clues that address these questions often may be obtained from a careful history and physical examination.

Clinical History   A number of historic features may distinguish cholestatic and hepatocellular disease processes. A history of marked right upper quadrant pain or previous indigestion suggests cholelithiasis, cholecystitis, or choledocholithiasis, whereas vague, nagging discomfort suggests hepatocellular or infiltrative disease with hepatomegaly causing pain due to acute distention of Glisson's capsule. Additional important symptoms that should be elicited include pruritus, jaundice, anorexia, weight loss, and fever. Complaints of easy bruising or mental confusion by the patient (or family) should be regarded as ominous signs of either fulminant acute or advanced chronic liver disease.

Family history is important with respect to jaundice, anemia, splenectomy, or cholecystectomy; a positive history may be helpful in diagnosing hemolytic anemia, congenital or familial hyperbilirubinemia, or gallstones. *Occupation* should be reviewed in detail, and *environmental factors* need to be examined. Note should be made of the use of any medications or exposure to known or putative toxins such as carbon tetrachloride, beryllium, or vinyl chloride. The patient should be asked about travel to other countries, especially to areas where hepatitis may be endemic. Careful questioning regarding alcohol intake is important in most cases. Since the alcoholic often denies or understates the amounts consumed, it may be desirable to check the validity of the history with relatives or close friends. History of concomitant use of acetaminophen and alcohol may be particularly important.

Contact with jaundiced patients (especially intimate or sexual relations) should be noted. If the patient has had any *injections*, hepatitis B or C infection may be the underlying disease. Injections include blood or plasma transfusions, tattooing, and dental treatment. Postoperative jaundice may be due to the anesthetic, especially after multiple uses of halothane, or to impaired hepatic excretory function resulting from relative hypoxemia of liver cells during the operative or postoperative period.

As suggested, the manner of the *onset of the illness* should be ascertained. The relatively abrupt onset of nausea, anorexia, and aversion to smoking followed by progressive jaundice suggests viral hepatitis. A gradual development of jaundice associated with pruritus suggests cholestasis. Intermittent right upper quadrant abdominal pain followed by cholestatic jaundice points to gallstone disease, while the gradual onset of painless jaundice with weight loss is suggestive of tumor, such as carcinoma of the head of the pancreas. Jaundice associated with fever and chills makes cholangitis and extrahepatic biliary obstruction likely possibilities. The awareness of progressive abdominal swelling, perhaps first noticed because of tightness of clothing, suggests ascites, which may be due to malignancy or an insidious first manifestation of cirrhosis. The patient with hepatitis generally feels ill, and dark urine and light stools occur before the appearance of scleral or skin icterus. In cholestatic hepatitis, the patient may feel relatively well and complain only of symptoms due to the obstruction, such as pruritus.

Physical Examination   Jaundice is looked for in the sclera as well as the skin. Pallor indicative of anemia may be a reflection of hemolysis, cirrhosis, or neoplasm. Significant cachexia, especially of the extremities, may be associated with cancer or cirrhosis. In the cirrhotic patient, one should look for stigmata of alcohol abuse such as parotid and lacrimal gland enlargement and Dupuytren's contracture, as well as other features of cirrhosis, such as gynecomastia, testicular atrophy, and diminished axillary or pubic hair.

The *skin examination* may reveal ecchymoses due to prothrombin deficiency or purpura due to thrombocytopenia. *Palmar erythema* or *spider angiomas* may reflect acute or chronic liver disease. Spider angiomas are usually found above the umbilicus and especially on the face, neck, shoulders, forearms, and dorsum of the hands. The presence of a few spider angiomas is not abnormal in women, especially during pregnancy. However, their appearance in men is always abnormal and should be carefully searched for. In chronic cholestasis, *scratch marks, finger clubbing*, and *xanthoma* of the eyelids and extensor surfaces of the tendons of the wrists and ankles may be found. A *slate color* to the skin due to increased iron or bronze discoloration resulting from melanin deposition should suggest the presence of hemochromatosis.

Evaluation of the *mental state* and *neurologic function* is important. Slight deterioration of the intellect and minimal personality changes may suggest hepatocellular disease or the presence of portal-systemic venous shunts, but care must be taken to exclude other causes such as neurologic disease. The presence of flapping tremor of the hands (asterixis) may be found in association with portal-systemic encephalopathy or impending hepatic coma.

Abdominal examination may reveal ascites, which, together with dilated periumbilical veins, suggests cirrhosis and extensive portal collateral circulation. If additional features of liver disease are lacking, malignancy must be considered more seriously. A very large, nodular, and rock-hard liver suggests the presence of hepatoma or hepatic metastases. Careful percussion is necessary to evaluate the size of a nonpalpable liver. A small liver may indicate cirrhosis (especially postnecrotic); a small liver that diminishes in size suggests severe hepatitis or massive hepatic necrosis. In the alcoholic, fatty infiltration and cirrhosis often produce a uniform enlargement of the liver. The liver edge is tender in hepatitis, in congestive heart failure, and occasionally in malignant disease and with alcoholism (especially "alcoholic hepatitis").

A palpable, enlarged gallbladder (Courvoisier's sign) suggests extrahepatic biliary obstruction, often due to pancreatic cancer. A tender gallbladder and positive Murphy's sign suggest cholelithiasis or choledocholithiasis. A palpable spleen may indicate hepatitis or cirrhosis; significant splenomegaly may be a reflection of portal hypertension.

Table 291-1

Suggested Guidelines for Ordering Hepatobiliary Imaging Studies in Various Clinical Situations

Clinical Problem	Initial Imaging Study	Supplemental Imaging Studies (if Necessary)
Suspected gallbladder disease	US to detect stones or evidence of acute or chronic cholecystitis Nuclear medicine biliary scan for suspicion of acute cholecystitis	OCG to assess gallbladder function and number of stones CT if abscess suspected
Suspected bile duct abnormalities	US to detect dilatation, stones, or mass ERCP or THC to define ductal anatomy	CT to detect stones or cause of extrinsic compression
Jaundice	US to detect biliary obstruction, liver masses, or obvious hepatic parenchymal disease	CT if dilated ducts to detect obstructing lesion or if suspicion of a mass in the pancreas or porta hepatis ERCP or THC to determine site and exact cause of dilated ducts
Hepatic parenchymal disease	US ^{99m}TC-labeled sulfur colloid scan MRI	Doppler, color Doppler, or MRI with flow sequences if a vascular abnormality is suspected and in some instances of portal hypertension
Screening for liver mass	US ^{99m}Tc-labeled sulfur colloid scan	MRI
Characterizing known liver mass		
Suspicion of malignancy	US- or CT-directed biopsy	CT portogram MRI Intraoperative US
Suspicion of benign lesion (hemangioma, regenerative nodule, focal nodular hyperplasia, adenoma)	MRI (after detection on US or CT) Nuclear medicine scan (e.g., ^{99m}TC-labeled red blood cell scan for suspected hemangioma)	Angiography US- or CT-directed biopsy
Suspicion of abscess	US or CT US- or CT-directed aspiration	Nuclear medicine abscess scan (gallium or ^{111}In-labeled white blood cell scan)

NOTE: US, ultrasound; OCG, oral cholecystogram; CT, computed tomography; THC, transhepatic cholangiography; ERCP, endoscopic retrograde cholangiopancreatography; MRI, magnetic resonance imaging; Tc, technetium; In, indium.

Table 291-2
Classification of Liver Disease

PARENCHYMAL

1. Hepatitis (viral, drug-induced, toxic, ischemic)
   a. Acute
   b. Chronic (persistent or active)
2. Cirrhosis
   a. Alcoholic (portal, nutritional, Lacnnec's cirrhosis)
   b. Postnecrotic
   c. Biliary
   d. Hemochromatosis
   e. Rare types (e.g., Wilson's disease, galactosemia, cystic fibrosis of pancreas, alpha$_1$-antitrypsin deficiency)
3. Infiltrations
   a. Glycogen
   b. Fat (neutral fat, cholesterol, gangliosides, cerebrosides)
   c. Amyloid
   d. Lymphoma, leukemia
   e. Granuloma (e.g., sarcoidosis, tuberculosis, idiopathic)
4. Space-occupying lesions
   a. Hepatocellular carcinoma, metastatic tumor
   b. Abscess (pyogenic, amoebic)
   c. Cysts (polycystic disease, *Echinococcus*)
   d. Gummas
5. Functional disorders associated with jaundice (hereditary or acquired)
   a. Gilbert's syndrome
   b. Crigler-Najjar syndrome
   c. Dubin-Johnson and Rotor syndromes
   d. Cholestasis of pregnancy and benign recurrent cholestasis

HEPATOBILIARY

1. Extrahepatic biliary obstruction (by stone, stricture, or tumor)
2. Cholangitis (septic, primary biliary cirrhosis, primary sclerosing cholangitis, drug, toxic)

VASCULAR

1. Chronic passive congestion and cardiac cirrhosis
2. Hepatic vein thrombosis (Budd-Chiari syndrome)
3. Portal vein thrombosis
4. Pylophlebitis
5. Arteriovenous malformations
6. Venocclusive disease

Abdominal auscultation may reveal the presence of a venous hum over dilated collateral veins radiating from the umbilicus, the so-called caput medusae. In advanced cirrhosis this venous hum is virtually diagnostic of significant portal hypertension. A bruit may sometimes be heard over large regenerating nodules in cirrhosis and occasionally over hepatomas and metastatic nodules in the liver. A friction rub occasionally may be heard over hepatomas and metastatic liver nodules.

Laboratory Evaluation   Serum assays for biochemical markers of liver disease are an integral part of the proper evaluation of liver and biliary tract disease. In general, the serum bilirubin level is measured to confirm the presence and severity of jaundice and determine the extent of bilirubin conjugation. Aminotransferase (transaminase) elevations reflect the severity of active hepatocellular damage, though not necessarily the aggregate severity of liver injury (e.g., aminotransferase levels may actually decline with near-complete hepatic parenchymal destruction), while alkaline phosphatase elevations are found with cholestasis and hepatic infiltrates. Serum albumin level and the prothrombin time are used as indexes of hepatic synthetic function. → *These and other tests are reviewed in Chaps. 45 and 292.*

The further evaluation of patients with hepatobiliary disease should be individualized depending on the history, physical findings, and initial screening laboratory tests. Hepatocellular disease such as hepatitis is often sufficiently clear that only serologic tests are needed. Nonetheless, in many patients, computed tomography (CT), ultrasound, scintiscans, magnetic resonance imaging (MRI), or liver biopsy may be needed to determine the nature of the liver disease. When hepatic tumors are suspected, CT, ultrasound, MRI, or scintiscan may be performed followed by liver biopsy or laparoscopy for a more specific diagnosis. When biliary obstruction is suspected, the first examination is usually an ultrasound study to determine the size of

the bile ducts, whether gallstones are present, or whether there is the suggestion of a mass in the head of the pancreas. Frequently, more information is needed, and thus a cholangiogram, performed through the endoscope (endoscopic retrograde cholangiopancreatography) or through percutaneous puncture under ultrasound or CT guidance, should be obtained. An overview of the utilization of imaging studies in the evaluation of patients with suspected hepatic and biliary disorders is provided in Table 291-1. More detailed consideration of imaging modalities is presented in the context of the discussion of specific conditions (Chaps. 302 and 304).

CLASSIFICATION OF LIVER DISEASE   No single classification of the various types of liver disease is entirely satisfactory because in many instances the etiology and pathogenetic mechanism are obscure. As a consequence, one finds an abundance of labels and names applied to hepatic disorders. Some individuals use the term *hepatitis* to imply viral infection; others, simply to connote evidence of hepatic inflammation. The often used words *acute*, *subacute*, and *chronic* are ambiguous. *Chronicity* should refer to continuing or recurrent disease (i.e., duration). *Activity* should refer to evidence of the presence of perpetuation of liver cell injury; this is most readily identified by serum transaminase elevations and by the degree of hepatocellular necrosis on biopsy.

Because of the difficulties involved in defining the etiology of many types of liver disease, in most instances the process is best defined and described by an examination of the morphologic character of the lesion. Therefore, a *morphologic classification* of liver disease, as outlined in Table 291-2, appears at present more practical than one based on etiology.

BIBLIOGRAPHY

M illward-S adler GH et al: *Wright's Liver and Biliary Disease*, 3d ed. London, Saunders, 1992
S herlock S, D ooley J: *Diseases of the Liver and Biliary System*, 9th ed., Oxford, Blackwell, 1993
Z akim D, B oyer TD: *Hepatology: A Textbook of Liver Disease*, 3d ed. Philadelphia, Saunders, 1996

292   *Daniel K. Podolsky, Kurt J. Isselbacher*

EVALUATION OF LIVER FUNCTION

The diversity of normal liver functions and the disruption of these functions by the spectrum of disorders that may affect the liver preclude the use of any single test as a reliable measure of overall liver function. Many disease processes may lead to severe impairment of some liver functions, while others remain entirely unaffected. Since no battery of tests is universally applicable, those most appropriate to a given clinical problem must be selected, their potential value and risks considered, and the results interpreted in relation to the clinical findings.

In assessing the severity and course of liver disease, the physician should be guided by several practical principles. The tests selected should (1) assess different parameters of liver function, (2) be used *serially* in order to evaluate the evolution or course of the disease, and (3) be interpreted within the total clinical context, with recognition that any single laboratory test may be fallible.

BLOOD TESTS OF LIVER FUNCTION
See Table 292-1

BILIRUBIN   Bilirubin metabolism and its assessment are discussed in detail in Chaps. 45 and 294. Spectrophotometric determinations of serum bilirubin in the clinical laboratory measure two pigment

Table 292-1

Abnormalities Shown by Tests of Liver Function

Test	Type of Liver Disease	
	Obstructive	Parenchymal
AST and ALT (SGOT and SGPT)	↑	↑–↑↑↑
Alkaline phosphatase	↑↑↑	↑
Albumin	N	↓–↓↓↓
Prothrombin time	N–↑*	↑–↑↑↑
Bilirubin	N–↑↑↑	N–↑↑↑
γ-Glutamyl transpeptidase (GGT)	↑↑↑	N–↑↑↑
5'-Nucleotidase	↑–↑↑↑	N–↑

* Correctable with parenteral vitamin K if elevated.
NOTE: N, normal; ↑, elevated; ↓, decreased.

fractions: (1) the water-soluble conjugated fraction that gives a *direct reaction* with the diazo reagent and consists largely of conjugated bilirubin (as the mono- and diglucuronide) and (2) the lipid-soluble *indirect-reaction* fraction (total minus direct) that represents primarily unconjugated bilirubin. The serum of normal adults (when measured by the van den Bergh reaction) contains less than 4.2 μmol/L (0.25 mg/dL) direct-reacting bilirubin and 17 μmol/L (1 mg/dL) or less of total bilirubin. Studies with high-performance liquid chromatography suggest that even these levels may be artifactually high in normal persons (see Chap. 45).

Conjugated hyperbilirubinemia with elevated direct- and indirect-reacting material indicates impairment of secretion into the bile, while unconjugated hyperbilirubinemia reflects impaired conjugation. The latter is found in a limited number of processes, including such nonhepatic conditions as hemolytic anemia and ineffective erythropoiesis (increased pigment load) and a few hepatic disorders, principally Gilbert's syndrome or the relatively rare Crigler-Najjar syndrome. Although measurement of both the direct and total serum bilirubin will determine whether the patient has predominantly unconjugated or conjugated hyperbilirubinemia, this distinction is of limited usefulness, since the majority of hepatobiliary disorders lead to conjugated hyperbilirubinemia. In most instances, fractionation of serum bilirubin does not distinguish cholestasis due to parenchymal disease from that arising from biliary tract disease.

Bilirubin appears in the urine only after it is converted to a water-soluble form; generally this involves conjugation with polar glucuronide groups that enhance water solubility. Rapid assessment of bilirubinuria is possible using commercially available dipsticks and may be helpful as an initial screening measure. Bilirubinuria occurs with even minimal degrees of jaundice and may be detected before jaundice is clinically evident. Its usefulness is otherwise quite limited. Urobilinogen, a product of luminal bacterial metabolism of bilirubin, is reabsorbed from the bowel and secreted in the urine. Complete bile duct obstruction blocks excretion of bilirubin into the gut and results in disappearance of urobilinogen from the urine. Assessment of urobilinogen in a freshly collected 2-h urine specimen by the Watson method (normal values 0.2 to 1.2 units) may distinguish biliary tract obstruction from parenchymal dysfunction, but this test has been largely superseded by other methods.

SERUM ENZYME ASSAYS A number of serum enzymes have been used to distinguish and assess hepatocellular injury and biliary tract dysfunction or obstruction. All have inherent limitations in sensitivity and specificity, and none truly distinguishes these processes definitively. Elevations in enzyme activities also may be seen in association with nonhepatic disorders. Nevertheless, with proper and careful interpretation, a number of serum enzymes provide important clinical tools.

Aminotransferases (Transaminases) Assays of many serum enzymes have been proposed as indicators of hepatocellular damage. Of these, aspartate aminotransferase (AST, SGOT) and alanine aminotransferase (ALT, SGPT) activities have proven most useful. These enzymes catalyze the transfer of the γ-amino groups of aspartate and alanine, respectively, to the γ-keto group of ketoglutarate, leading to the formation of oxaloacetic acid and pyruvic acid. In contrast to ALT, which is found primarily in the liver, AST is present in many tissues, including heart, skeletal muscle, kidney, and brain, and is thus somewhat less specific as an indicator of liver function. The source of serum AST and ALT in the normal person [less than 0.58 μkat/L (35 U/L)] is unclear, and the mechanism responsible for clearance of these enzymes is uncertain. In the hepatocyte, ALT is found exclusively in the cytosol, while different isoenzymes of AST exist in the mitochondria and the cytosol. Although elevated serum levels of AST or ALT may be observed in a variety of nonhepatic diseases, notably in myocardial infarction and skeletal muscle disorders, these disorders can usually be distinguished clinically from liver disease. Conversely, uremia may lead to spuriously low aminotransferase values.

Serum AST and ALT are elevated to some extent in nearly all liver disorders. Highest levels are found in association with conditions causing extensive hepatic necrosis, such as severe viral hepatitis, toxin-induced liver injury, or prolonged circulatory collapse. Lesser elevations are encountered in mild acute viral hepatitis as well as in both diffuse and focal chronic liver diseases (e.g., chronic active hepatitis, cirrhosis, and hepatic metastases). However, the absolute levels of aminotransferases correlate poorly with severity of liver injury or prognosis, and serial determinations are usually most helpful. Thus, in the patient with massive hepatic necrosis, there may be marked elevations in the early phase (i.e., 24 to 48 h), but by the time the patient is tested 3 to 5 days later, the levels may be in the range of 3.34 to 5.8 μkat/L (200 to 350 U/L). It is noteworthy that in severe alcoholic hepatitis one commonly finds only modest increases in these enzymes (generally less than 5.0 μkat/L). Minimal elevations of AST and ALT (less than 1.67 μkat/L) also may be found in association with biliary tract obstruction; higher levels suggest the development of cholangitis with resultant hepatic cell necrosis.

In general AST and ALT levels parallel each other, with a couple of exceptions. In alcoholic hepatitis the AST/ALT ratio may be greater than 2; this appears to result from a reduction in hepatic ALT content due to a deficiency in the cofactor pyridoxine-5-phosphate. An increase in the ratio of AST/ALT (>1) also can be seen occasionally in patients with the fatty liver associated with pregnancy, but is typically <1 in other causes of steatohepatitis.

Alkaline Phosphatase Human serum contains several forms of alkaline phosphatase, a plasma membrane–derived enzyme of uncertain physiologic function that hydrolyzes synthetic phosphate esters at pH 9. These activities arise from bone, intestine, liver, and placenta. A number of different assays have been developed that utilize different substrates.

In the absence of bone disease or pregnancy, elevated levels of alkaline phosphatase activity usually reflect impaired biliary tract function. The increased levels reflect increased synthesis of the enzyme by hepatocytes and biliary tract epithelium rather than regurgitation of enzyme due to obstruction. Bile acids may play a role both by inducing synthesis and by promoting solubilization of the membrane-associated enzyme activity.

Slight to moderate increases in alkaline phosphatase (one to two times normal) occur in many patients with parenchymal liver disorders such as hepatitis and cirrhosis; transient increases may occur in all types of liver disease. Occasionally very high levels of alkaline phosphatase may be found in association with some infiltrative disorders, e.g., mycobacterial infection. However, striking increases in alkaline phosphatase (10 times normal or more) occur more consistently with extrahepatic biliary tract (mechanical) obstruction or with intrahepatic (functional) cholestasis, as in drug-induced cholestasis or primary biliary cirrhosis. Conversely, it is unusual for the serum alkaline phosphatase to remain normal when there is obstructive jaundice, and a normal enzyme level argues strongly against the presence of cholestasis. The alkaline phosphatase is usually mildly elevated in metastatic or infiltrative liver disease (e.g., leukemia, lymphoma, and sarcoid). The enzyme may be elevated in the presence of incomplete biliary obstruction or when there is obstruction of only one hepatic duct, conditions in which the serum bilirubin is often normal or only slightly elevated. Serum alkaline phosphatase is also elevated in nonhepatic disorders, most notably in some bone disorders (e.g., Paget's disease, osteomalacia, and metastases to bone) and sometimes with malignancy. Occasionally, tumors produce an alkaline phosphatase that is identical or similar to the placental form (Regan isoenzyme).

Although one can usually make a reasonable assessment as to whether an elevation of the alkaline phosphatase is of hepatic or nonhepatic origin, several methods can distinguish the different isoenzymes, facilitating resolution of any uncertainty. In contrast to that derived from bone, the hepatic isozyme is stable to treatment with heat (56°C for 15 min) or urea. These enzymes also can be separated by electrophoresis, but this is usually impractical. Parallel determination of serum 5'-nucleotidase activity is also helpful; an increase of both 5'-nucleotidase and alkaline phosphatase is consistent with an hepatobiliary source of the enzyme elevation. Even after correction for age and sex (higher levels being found in the young and in older women), isolated elevations in alkaline phosphatase may occasionally be encountered in adults with no apparent disease.

5'-Nucleotidase This enzyme catalyzes the hydrolysis of phosphate from the 5' position of the pentose component of the nucleotide. Although tissue distribution is widespread, elevations are generally associated with hepatobiliary disease. The principal value of the 5'-nucleotidase measurement is to confirm the hepatic origin of an elevated alkaline phosphatase level in children or pregnant women or in those settings where coincident bone disease may be present. However, 5'-nucleotidase levels do not always parallel alkaline phosphatase in liver disease, and lack of elevation does not exclude an hepatic source of elevated serum alkaline phosphatase.

γ-Glutamyltranspeptidase (GGT) GGT catalyzes the transfer of the γ-glutamyl group from peptides such as glutathione to other amino acids and may play a role in amino acid transport. It is found throughout the hepatobiliary system as well as in other tissues. In liver disease, GGT correlates with alkaline phosphatase levels and is the most sensitive indicator of biliary tract disease. However, elevations of GGT are nonspecific and may be associated with pancreatic, cardiac, renal, and pulmonary disorders as well as with diabetes and alcoholism. The overall lack of specificity of GGT has limited its clinical usefulness.

Other Enzymes Measurement of total serum lactic dehydrogenase (LDH) or its isoenzymes is usually not helpful in diagnosis of liver disease because of this enzyme's nearly ubiquitous body distribution. Moderate LDH elevations are common in acute viral hepatitis, cirrhosis, and metastatic carcinoma to the liver. Biliary tract disease also may produce slight elevations. Marked elevations of LDH in association with abnormal results of other tests of liver function may reflect a hematologic malignancy such as lymphoma. Elevation of serum ornithine carbamyl transferase, a urea cycle enzyme present only in liver and intestine, occurs primarily in liver disease, but its lack of association with any specific type of liver disease has limited its diagnostic usefulness.

SERUM PROTEINS Extensive liver injury may lead to *decreased* blood levels of albumin, prothrombin, fibrinogen, and other proteins synthesized exclusively by hepatocytes. In contrast to measurements of serum enzymes, serum protein levels reflect liver synthetic function rather than just cell injury. There are three important caveats in the interpretation of serum protein levels: (1) they are neither early nor sensitive indicators of liver disease (because of the extent of hepatic reserve and their half-life, see below), (2) they are of little value in the differential diagnosis of liver disease, and (3) decreases in their serum levels are not specific for liver disease.

Albumin and Globulin Albumin is quantitatively the most important serum protein synthesized by the liver; the normal serum value ranges from 35 to 55 g/L (see Chap. 293). Albumin has a fairly long half-life (14 to 20 days), with less than 5 percent turnover daily; it is therefore not a good indicator of acute or mild liver injury. Further-

more, there is a substantial reserve of hepatic albumin synthesis; thus adequate synthesis may continue until there is extensive hepatocellular injury. Serum levels are influenced by a variety of nonhepatic factors, most notably nutritional status, hormonal factors, and plasma oncotic pressure. Routes of degradation in health remain undefined, but nonhepatic conditions may lead to depressed serum albumin levels mainly due to excessive loss (e.g., nephrotic syndrome or protein-losing enteropathy) despite adequate synthetic function. Nonetheless, reduction in the serum albumin levels provides an excellent indication of the severity of chronic liver disease. In the patient with ascites, an increased volume of distribution as well as an absolute reduction in protein synthesis may contribute to hypoalbuminemia.

Serum globulins are a heterogeneous group of proteins whose production in a variety of tissues is influenced by a number of factors. Serum globulins (normal value ranges from 20 to 35 g/L) include alpha and beta globulins as well as serum immunoglobulins, the latter largely accounting for the gamma fraction. Serum globulins are often diffusely elevated in association with chronic liver disease and in other nonhepatic disorders. In cirrhosis, varying degrees of hyperglobulinemia may occur; this may reflect increased stimulation of the peripheral reticuloendothelial compartment due to shunting of antigens past the liver and impaired clearance by hepatic Kupffer cells. Although some have suggested that elevations in different globulin fractions as assessed by electrophoretic or other means may have a differential diagnostic value, this remains a largely unfulfilled promise. Similarly, the albumin/globulin ratio has no physiologic significance.

Clotting Factors The liver is the major site of synthesis of virtually all coagulation proteins (factors I, II, V, VII, IX, X, XII, and XIII). With the exception of factors V, XII, and XIII, production of functional proteins requires the presence of the cofactor vitamin K. Because most of these factors are normally present in excess concentrations, impaired coagulation is usually seen only in severe liver disease. Abnormalities of these factors can be most efficiently determined by the one-stage *prothrombin time*, which measures the rate of prothrombin conversion to thrombin in the presence of thromboplastin and calcium and requires the integrity of most of the vitamin K–dependent clotting factors (see Chap. 60). Factor VII is the rate-limiting factor in this pathway and thus has the greatest influence on the prothrombin levels. The prothrombin time is dependent on normal hepatic synthesis of clotting factors and sufficient intestinal uptake of vitamin K. Absorption of this fat-soluble vitamin itself requires adequate dietary intake and normal function of intestinal mucosa and biliary secretion. Severe acute or chronic parenchymal liver injury may lead to prolongation of the prothrombin time due to impaired synthesis of the clotting proteins. Because these proteins have a shorter half-life than that of albumin, the prothrombin time may be an earlier indicator than serum albumin level of severe liver injury. In both acute and chronic hepatocellular injury, an increase in the prothrombin time serves as an ominous prognostic sign. Because vitamin K is a fat-soluble vitamin, prolongation of the prothrombin time can result from vitamin K malabsorption, which may occur with cholestasis due to biliary tract disease or due to fat malabsorption (steatorrhea) of any cause (e.g., pancreatic insufficiency). Poor dietary intake, antibiotic therapy, and use of warfarin-type anticoagulants are additional causes of a prolonged prothrombin time, owing to deficiencies of active vitamin K. These processes can be distinguished from hepatic synthetic failure by demonstrating normalization of the prothrombin time (within 24 to 48 h) after parenteral injections of vitamin K. The *partial thromboplastin time*, which reflects the activities of fibrinogen, prothrombin, and factors V, VIII, IX, X, XI, and XII, also may be prolonged in severe liver disease. Clotting functions should be assessed in all patients with liver disease prior to any surgical procedure, including liver biopsy (see Chaps. 60 and 118). Of interest, hepatocellular carcinomas have been found to produce an abnormal form of prothrombin that has not been fully carboxylated by vitamin K–dependent mechanisms (des-γ-prothrombin).

BLOOD AMMONIA   Ammonia is elevated in the blood of some patients with either acute or chronic liver disease. Although influenced by a number of factors (summarized in Chap. 293), elevations in blood ammonia reflect disruption of the pathways of urea synthesis by which the liver detoxifies amine groups. A markedly elevated blood ammonia usually reflects severe hepatocellular injury. Cirrhotic patients, especially those with endogenous or surgically created portal-systemic shunting, often have varying degrees of hyperammonemia and hepatic encephalopathy. However, there is only a rough correlation between blood ammonia levels and the degree of hepatic encephalopathy; some patients will function normally with a twofold elevation, while others will be stuporous at the same concentration. Ammonia levels may increase before the onset of coma; similarly, they may return to normal some 48 to 72 h before improvement of the neurologic status.

SERUM LIPIDS AND LIPOPROTEINS AND BILE ACIDS-

Abnormalities in serum lipids and lipoproteins are sensitive but nonspecific indicators of liver diseases. Acute parenchymal liver disease is commonly associated with increased plasma triglycerides, decreased cholesterol esters, and abnormal lipoproteins. The absence of alpha and prebeta bands with a concomitant increase in the beta fraction is typical of acute viral hepatitis. Less marked but more persistent abnormalities are found in patients with chronic parenchymal disease, reflecting deficiencies in lecithin:cholesterol acyltransferase (LCAT) and hepatic triglyceride lipase. Either intra- or extrahepatic cholestasis may lead to an increase in unesterified cholesterol and in serum phospholipids.

Removal of bile acids from portal blood is impaired in liver disease because of parenchymal damage and portal-systemic shunts; there also may be reentry of bile acids into blood from injured hepatocytes or an obstructed biliary tract. Although there are a variety of techniques for measuring serum bile acids, these determinations are not yet of proven value for routine clinical use.

IMMUNOLOGIC AND OTHER TESTS

A number of immunologic derangements may be seen in liver disease. These are summarized in Table 292-2. Antimitochondrial antibodies (AMA) are found in 85 to 90 percent of patients with primary biliary cirrhosis. These antibodies appear to be directed against components of the pyruvate dehydrogenase complex and other related mitochondrial enzyme complexes. In this test, serum is incubated with rabbit hepatocytes. The presence of AMA can then be assessed after subsequent staining with a fluorescein-tagged second antibody. However, this marker is not entirely specific and is occasionally found in patients

Table 292-2

Immunologic Tests in Diagnosis of Hepatic Disorders

Test	Disease Association	Comment
Antimitochondrial antibody (AMA)	Primary biliary cirrhosis (90%); chronic active hepatitis (occasional)	Antibodies against component of pyruvate dehydrogenase and other 2-oxo-acid complexes
Antinuclear antibody (ANA)	Autoimmune hepatitis (10%)	
Anti-smooth-muscle antibody (ASM)	Autoimmune hepatitis	
Antineutrophil cytoplasmic antibody (ANCA)	Primary sclerosing cholangitis	Perinuclear pattern; antigen unknown but distinct from myeloperoxidase
Anti-liver/kidney microsomal antibody (anti-LKM)	Autoimmune hepatitis, type II	

with autoimmune hepatitis and drug-induced hepatitis. Its primary value is in helping to distinguish primary biliary cirrhosis from extrahepatic biliary obstruction. In autoimmune hepatitis, the *lupus erythematosus–cell test* may be positive, and *antinuclear antibodies* (ANA) as well as *anti-smooth-muscle antibodies* (ASM) may be present (see Chap. 312). Patients with autoimmune hepatitis have clinical and histologic features similar to those of primary biliary cirrhosis but serologic tests resembling those of autoimmune hepatitis (negative AMA and positive ANA or ASM). Alpha fetoprotein is of value in the diagnosis of hepatocellular carcinoma (see Chap. 93). Measurements of serum α_1-antitrypsin and ceruloplasmin should be performed in infants with cirrhosis or hepatitis since they may reflect α_1-antitrypsin deficiency or Wilson's disease, respectively (see Chaps. 300 and 345).

Studies assessing iron stores are essential in the evaluation of those patients suspected of hemochromatosis on clinical grounds, those exhibiting compatible nonspecific abnormal liver function tests results (e.g., unexplained mild to moderate elevation of aminotransferase), or those with evidence of liver disease, early or advanced, of uncertain cause. Routine tests include iron, total serum iron-binding capacity (TIBC), and ferritin. Hemochromatosis is associated with elevated levels of both iron and TIBC and an increased ratio of iron/TIBC, consistent with a high degree of saturation of iron-binding capacity. While iron-binding saturations of >90% are typical, hemochromatosis should be suspected at levels about 50%, especially in women. Although high iron saturation may be seen in many chronic systemic illnesses, the overall levels of iron and TIBC will be diminished. Serum levels of ferritin, the intrahepatic ion storage protein, are typically markedly elevated in hemochromatosis. Somewhat less pronounced increases may be seen in other forms of liver injury, including alcoholic liver disease and other diseases (e.g., lymphoma). Particular confusion may arise in distinguishing secondary hemosiderosis, most commonly seen in alcoholics but also encountered in patients receiving numerous transfusions (e.g., sickle cell anemia), from primary hemochromatosis by these initial serum determinations. Diagnosis often ultimately requires percutaneous liver biopsy or other more specific tests. → *For further discussion, see Chap. 342.*

OTHER DIAGNOSTIC PROCEDURES   **Percutaneous Needle Biopsy of the Liver**   Percutaneous needle biopsy is a safe, simple, and valuable method for the diagnostic evaluation of liver disease. *Diffuse parenchymal disorders* such as cirrhosis, hepatitis, and drug reactions may be diagnosed with remarkable accuracy. In *disseminated focal diseases* (such as granulomas or tumor infiltrates), serial sections may demonstrate characteristic lesions.

Biopsy is usually performed "blindly," under local anesthesia, by either a transpleural or subcostal approach. If the operator is skillful and patients are carefully selected, morbidity should be quite low and limited to occasional postbiopsy pain or vasovagal reactions.

Some of the most frequent indications for needle biopsy are (1) unexplained hepatomegaly or hepatosplenomegaly; (2) cholestasis of uncertain cause; (3) persistently abnormal liver function tests; (4) suspected systemic or infiltrative diseases such as sarcoidosis, miliary tuberculosis, or fever of unknown origin; and (5) suspected primary or metastatic liver tumor. Percutaneous liver biopsy may be performed either for diagnostic purposes or to evaluate the extent and severity of a known disease process. However, other new and improved noninvasive diagnostic methods have obviated the need for biopsy in many circumstances, and thus biopsy should be performed only when information from these other techniques is inadequate.

Needle biopsy should not be performed if (1) the patient is unable to cooperate; (2) clinical or laboratory evidence indicates impaired hemostasis (prothrombin time prolonged by 3 s or more over control, thrombocytopenia less than 80 × 10^9 platelets per liter, or partial thromboplastin time or bleeding time prolonged); (3) there is infection of the right pleural space or septic cholangitis; (4) tense ascites is present, with risk of continued leakage of ascitic fluid; (5) compatible blood is not available for transfusion in case of hemorrhage; (6) high-grade biliary obstruction is suspected and there is an increased risk of bile peritonitis; (7) there is a possible echinococchal cyst; or (8) a vascular lesion is suspected. In patients in whom a percutaneous biopsy cannot be performed safely due to impaired hemostasis or ascites, biopsy can sometimes be carried out by a transjugular approach, in which the tissue is obtained via the hepatic vein and any bleeding occurs directly into the vascular space. With the increasing use of computed tomography scanning and ultrasonography, it is possible to perform "directed" aspiration biopsies of isolated focal lesions with very thin needles. Aspirated material can be used for cytology (tumors) and culture (abscesses) but is often inadequate for assessment of liver architecture.

BIBLIOGRAPHY

SCHIFF L, SCHIFF ER: *Diseases of the Liver*, 7th ed. Philadelphia, Lippincott, 1993

ZAKIM D, BOYER TD: *Hepatology: A Textbook of Liver Disease*, 3d ed. Philadelphia, Saunders, 1996

293 *Daniel K. Podolsky, Kurt J. Isselbacher*

DERANGEMENTS OF HEPATIC METABOLISM

The liver plays a central role in the maintenance of metabolic homeostasis. It is therefore not surprising that the development of clinically important liver disease is accompanied by diverse manifestations of disordered metabolism. Although some functions are more sensitive than others, the liver has considerable reserve capacity, so minimal or even moderate cell injury may not be reflected by measurable metabolic changes. However, a variety of defects may be seen, depending on the nature and extent of the initial insult.

The biochemical functions in which the liver plays a major role include (1) the intermediate metabolism of amino acids and carbohydrates, (2) synthesis and degradation of proteins and glycoproteins, (3) metabolism and degradation of drugs and hormones, and (4) regulation of lipid and cholesterol metabolism. The derangements of these functions are discussed in connection with their occurrence in various forms of parenchymal liver disease. Alterations of bilirubin, bile salt, and porphyrin metabolism are discussed elsewhere (Chaps. 45, 285, and 343).

Metabolic derangements are most evident in the patient with advanced liver disease, and the manifestations are similar regardless of the initial etiologic insult. To a varying degree, similar abnormalities are observed in patients with severe chronic hepatitis, micronodular cirrhosis, and postnecrotic cirrhosis. Since the many functions of the liver may be affected to varying degrees in individual patients, no single test effectively measures the overall state of liver function. The proper evaluation of tests of liver function is discussed in Chap. 292.

CARBOHYDRATE METABOLISM The liver functions to maintain normal levels of blood sugar by a combination of glycogenesis, glycogenolysis, glycolysis, and gluconeogenesis. These pathways are regulated by a number of hormones, including insulin, glucagon, growth hormone, and certain catecholamines. Although it has been presumed that exquisite sensitivity of the hepatocytes to insulin is responsible for the uptake of an oral glucose load by the liver, there are also data that have challenged the importance of insulin-mediated glucose uptake by the hepatocyte. In the fasting state, the liver contributes to glucose homeostasis by glycogenolysis and gluconeogenesis in response to hypoinsulinemia and hyperglucagonemia. Maintenance of normal blood glucose levels through gluconeogenesis is ultimately related to catabolism of muscle protein, which provides the necessary amino acid precursors, especially alanine. In a complementary fashion, in the postprandial state, the liver directs alanine and branched-chain amino acids to the peripheral tissues, where they are then incorporated into muscle protein. These reciprocal pathways form a glucose-alanine shuttle, which is modulated by ambient changes in the hormones mentioned above. While it has been presumed that synthesis of glyco-

gen and fatty acid in the postprandial state arises from direct conversion of glucose, there are data to suggest that, in fact, these pathways are *indirect*, with products deriving from three-carbon metabolites of glucose or other gluconeogenic compounds such as lactate, fructose, and alanine.

Abnormalities of glucose homeostasis are common in cirrhosis (Table 293-1). Most frequently, hyperglycemia and glucose intolerance are observed. Glucose intolerance is associated with normal or increased levels of plasma insulin (except in patients with hemochromatosis), suggesting that insulin resistance rather than insulin deficiency may be responsible. One of the factors that may play a role in the apparent insulin resistance is an absolute decrease in the liver's ability to metabolize a glucose load because of a decrease in functioning hepatocellular mass. There is also evidence that response to insulin is diminished due to both receptor and postreceptor defects in hepatocytes of patients with cirrhosis. In addition, both hyperinsulinemia and hyperglucagonemia may be present due to decreased hepatic clearance of this hormone resulting from portal-systemic shunting. In patients with hemochromatosis, however, insulin levels, may indeed be low due to pancreatic iron deposition and sometimes concomitant diabetes mellitus. Patients with cirrhosis also may have elevated serum lactate levels, reflecting the decreased capacity of the liver to utilize lactate for gluconeogenesis.

Hypoglycemia, although more common in acute fulminant hepatitis, also may be seen with end-stage cirrhosis. Because the capacity of the liver to store glycogen is limited (approximately 70 g) and glucose consumption continues at a constant rate (approximately 150 g/d), hepatic glycogen stores are depleted after 1 day of fasting. Hypoglycemia in end-stage cirrhosis may be due to decreased hepatic glycogen stores, diminished glucagon responsiveness, or decreased capacity to synthesize glycogen due to extensive parenchymal destruction.

AMINO ACID AND AMMONIA METABOLISM Through a variety of anabolic and catabolic processes, the liver is the major site of amino acid interconversion. Amino acids utilized for hepatic protein synthesis are derived from dietary protein, metabolic turnover of endogenous protein (primarily from muscle), and direct synthesis in the liver. Most of the amino acids entering the liver via the portal vein are catabolized to urea (except for the branched-chain amino acids leucine, isoleucine, and valine). Some of these amino acids are released into the general circulation as free amino acids and may play an important role in the glucose-alanine cycle mentioned above. In addition, amino acids are utilized for the synthesis of liver intracellular proteins, plasma proteins, and special compounds such as glutathione, glutamine, taurine, carnosine, and creatine. Disruption of normal amino acid metabolism may be reflected in altered plasma amino acid concentrations. In general, levels of aromatic amino acids normally metabolized by the liver (as well as methionine) are elevated, while those of

Table 293-1

Alteration of Glucose Metabolism in Cirrhosis

Factors Leading to Hyperglycemia
  Decreased hepatic glucose uptake
  Decreased hepatic glycogen synthesis
  Hepatic resistance to insulin
  Portal-systemic glucose shunting
  Peripheral insulin resistance
  Hormonal abnormalities (serum)
    ↑ Glucagon
    ↓ Cortisol
    ↑ Insulin (↓ in hemochromatosis)
Factors Leading to Hypoglycemia
  Decreased gluconeogenesis
  Decreased hepatic glycogen content
  Hepatic resistance to glucagon
  Poor oral intake
  Hyperinsulinemia secondary to portal-systemic shunting

the branched-chain amino acids, largely utilized by skeletal muscle, tend to be normal or depressed. It was previously suggested that an alteration in the ratio of these two types of amino acids plays a role in the development of hepatic encephalopathy (see below), but there is not agreement on this concept.

Hepatic catabolism or degradation of amino acids involves two major reactions: transamination and oxidative deamination. In transamination, an amino group of an amino acid is transferred to a keto acid. This process is catalyzed by aminotransferases, which are found in very high amounts in liver but are also present in other tissues, such as kidney, muscle, heart, lung, and brain. Glutamic-oxaloacetic acid transaminase (aspartate aminotransferase, AST) has been studied most extensively, and increased levels are found in the serum secondary to various types of liver injury (e.g., acute viral and drug-induced hepatitis). As a result of transamination, amino acids can enter the citric acid cycle and then function in the intermediary metabolism of carbohydrates and lipids. Most of the nonessential amino acids are also synthesized in the liver by transamination. Oxidative deamination, which results in conversion of amino acids to keto acids (and ammonia), is catalyzed by L-amino acid oxidase with two exceptions: glycine oxidation is catalyzed by glycine oxidase, and glutamic oxidation is catalyzed by glutamic dehydrogenase. With severe liver damage (e.g., massive hepatic necrosis), utilization of amino acids is impaired, free amino acids in the bloodstream increase, and an "overflow" type of aminoaciduria may occur (unless renal function is also impaired).

Urea production is intimately related to the metabolic pathways outlined above, providing a means for disposal of ammonia, the toxic product of nitrogen metabolism. Disruption of this process is of particular clinical importance in the patient with severe acute and chronic liver disease. The fixation of amino acid–derived NH_3 in the form of urea is carried out via the Krebs-Henseleit cycle. The final step of this cycle, the formation of urea by arginase, is irreversible. In advanced liver disease, urea synthesis is often depressed, leading to an accumulation of NH_3, usually with a significant reduction in blood urea nitrogen, an ominous sign of liver failure. This finding may be obscured by superimposed renal impairment, which often develops in patients with severe hepatic failure. Urea is mostly excreted by the kidney, but approximately 25 percent will diffuse into the intestine, where it is converted to NH_3 by bacterial urease. The intestinal production of ammonia also occurs from the bacterial deamination of unabsorbed amino acids and of protein derived from the diet, exfoliated cells, or blood in the gastrointestinal tract.

Gut NH_3 is absorbed and transported to the liver via the portal vein, where it is again converted to urea. The kidney also produces varying amounts of NH_3, largely by the deamination of glutamine. The contributions of the gut and kidney to ammonia synthesis have important implications for the management of the hyperammonemic state frequently seen in patients with advanced liver disease, usually in association with portal-systemic shunting of blood.

While the exact chemical mediators of hepatic encephalopathy remain unknown and may include endogenous benzodiazepine compounds, elevated levels of blood NH_3 are generally associated with the development of encephalopathy, although approximately 10 percent of such patients have normal levels of blood ammonia (see Chap. 299). In addition, therapeutic measures that reduce serum NH_3 levels also usually lead to clinical improvement. The several mechanisms known to lead to increased blood NH_3 levels in patients with cirrhosis are illustrated in Fig. 293-1 and include the following:

1. If there is excessive nitrogenous material in the intestine (from bleeding or dietary protein), excessive amounts of NH_3 will be formed by bacterial deamination of amino acids. If intestinal motility is diminished, as manifest by constipation, bacterial production of ammonia will increase due to prolonged time for degradation of luminal protein and amino acids.

2. If renal function declines (as in the hepatorenal syndrome), blood urea nitrogen rises, leading to increased diffusion of urea into the intestinal lumen, where bacterial urease converts it to NH_3.

3. If hepatic function is significantly depressed, diminished urea synthesis may occur with a resultant decrease in the removal of NH_3.

4. If alkalosis (often due to central hyperventilation) and hypokalemia accompany hepatic decompensation, there may be a decrease in the renal availability of H^+ ions; as a result, the NH_3 produced from glutamine by the action of renal glutaminase is permitted to enter the renal vein (rather than being excreted as NH_4^+), leading to increased peripheral blood NH_3 levels. In addition, hypokalemia itself leads to increased renal NH_3 production.

5. If portal hypertension is present and anastomoses exist between the portal vein and systemic venous channels, these portal-systemic shunts will allow NH_3 from the gut to bypass hepatic detoxification, leading to elevated blood NH_3 levels. Thus, with portal-systemic shunting of blood, elevated NH_3 levels may develop with relatively modest hepatocellular dysfunction.

It is unclear what effects these same factors may have on other compounds that may play a role in the development of hepatic encephalopathy.

An additional factor important in determining whether a given NH_3 level in the blood will be detrimental to the central nervous system is the blood pH. The more alkaline the pH, the more toxic a given level of NH_3 is likely to be. At 37°C, the pK of NH_3 is 8.9; this is close enough to the pH of blood that minor changes in pH can affect the NH_4^+/NH_3 ratio. Because un-ionized NH_3 crosses membranes more readily than NH_4^+ ions, alkalosis favors the entry of ammonia into the brain (with subsequent changes in cell metabolism) by shifting the equilibrium of the following reaction to the right

$$NH_4^+ + OH^- \rightleftharpoons NH_3 + HOH$$

As a result, alkalosis not only increases peripheral blood NH_3 levels by renal mechanisms but also increases tissue levels by influencing the diffusion of NH_3 across membranes. Similarly, alterations in the pH of intestinal luminal contents also will affect the equilibrium between NH_4^+ and NH_3; a more alkaline lumen will shift the balance in favor of NH_3, permitting increased absorption. In theory, laxatives that cause relative acidification of luminal contents (e.g., lactulose) may be more effective than others as agents for the treatment of hepatic encephalopathy. However, this theoretical effect on the equilibrium

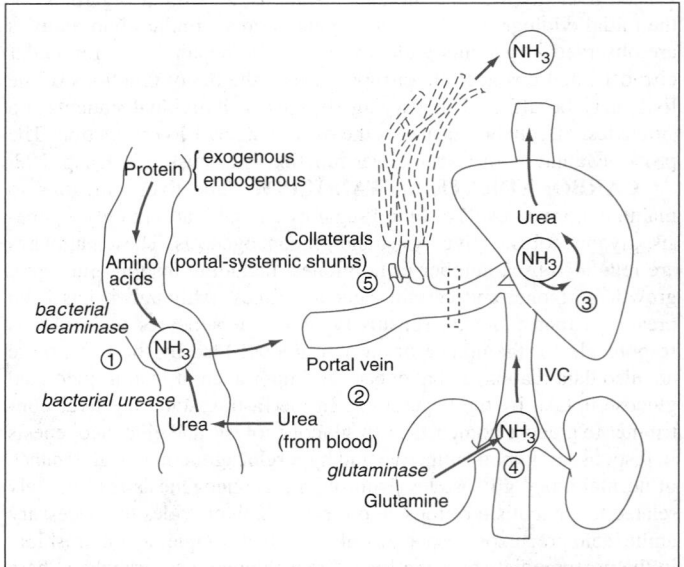

FIGURE 293-1 Major factors (steps 1 to 4) influencing the level of blood ammonia. In cirrhosis with portal hypertension, venous collaterals allow ammonia to bypass the liver (step 5), permitting the entry of ammonia into the systemic circulation (portal-systemic shunting).

between NH_4^+ and NH_3 has never been convincingly demonstrated for available laxatives.

PROTEIN SYNTHESIS AND DEGRADATION The liver is an important site of protein synthesis and degradation. Although the body muscle mass produces the greatest total amount of protein, the liver has the highest rate of synthesis per gram of tissue. The liver synthesizes not only the proteins it needs, but also produces numerous export proteins. Among the latter, albumin is the most important; *it is produced at a rate of approximately 12 g/d*, representing 25 percent of total hepatic protein synthesis and half of all exported protein. The average normal half-life of serum albumin is 17 to 20 days. The proportion of hepatocytes carrying out active albumin synthesis varies from 10 to 60 percent, depending on the body's requirements. Approximately 60 percent of albumin is found in the extravascular spaces, but plasma albumin is still the most abundant circulating protein.

Albumin contributes significantly to the plasma oncotic pressure. In addition, it is the principal binding and transport protein for numerous substances, including some hormones, fatty acids, trace metals, tryptophan, bilirubin, and other organic anions of both endogenous and exogenous origin. Despite the many important functions of albumin, rare individuals with congenital analbuminemia appear to have no major physiologic derangements other than the excessive accumulation of extravascular fluid. While many of the less hydrophobic ligands may be transported in the unbound form, this suggests that other serum proteins also may play a role in binding and transport.

Much has been learned about the mechanisms involved in the synthesis of secretory proteins, especially albumin. Polyribosomes bound to the rough endoplasmic reticulum (RER) of the hepatocyte are the principal site of translation of messenger RNA coding for export proteins; in contrast, proteins destined for intracellular use, such as ferritin, are synthesized on free rather than bound polyribosomes in the cytoplasm. Albumin, like secretory proteins produced by other organs, appears to be synthesized initially as a larger precursor, preproalbumin. This precursor molecule contains an additional 24 extra amino acid residues on the *N* terminus, referred to as a *signal peptide*, which undergoes two sequential cleavages (or "processing"). The "pre" portion of preproalbumin is cleaved within the RER even before protein synthesis is completed; the "pro" segment is removed within the lumen of the RER. The molecule is then transported to the Golgi apparatus prior to secretion. Once synthesis and processing are completed, albumin is transported from the Golgi vesicles to the hepatocyte surface by mechanisms that are unclear but almost certainly involve the microfilaments and microtubule apparatus of the cell. Although the hepatic lymph space of Disse provides a potential avenue for the newly released albumin, most secreted proteins such as albumin enter the plasma.

Albumin synthesis is subject to a number of regulatory influences. These include the rate of transcription of specific messenger RNAs and the availability of the substrate transfer RNA. At the translational level, the integrity of polyribosomes and their synthetic abilities are modified by factors affecting initiation, elongation, and release of peptides and proteins as well as by the availability of ATP, GTP, and magnesium ions. The rate of albumin synthesis is also influenced by the availability of amino acid precursors, especially tryptophan, the scarcest of the essential amino acids. Indeed, in patients with large carcinoid tumors, albumin synthesis may decrease precipitously when tryptophan is consumed by carcinoid cells in the production of 5-hydroxytryptophan (serotonin) (see Chap. 95). The rate of albumin synthesis is also affected by colloid oncotic pressure, with increased production occurring in response to falling oncotic pressure. Finally, influences of hormones such as insulin and glucagon on hepatic protein metabolism are closely integrated with the nutritional factors discussed above.

The liver also produces a wide variety of other secretory proteins, most of which have a synthetic pathway and processing procedure similar to that of albumin. The presence of a signal peptide such as the "prepro" segment of albumin, which is subsequently removed during protein maturation, appears to be a general mechanism for orienting proteins in the membranes of the endoplasmic reticulum and directing them for export rather than for intracellular use or degrada-

tion. Most proteins undergo even further modification in the form of sequential *glycosylation* in the RER and Golgi apparatus. The carbohydrate moieties of these glycoproteins appear to be important in determining their site of action and their rate of tissue uptake after secretion. Some of the clinically important secretory glycoproteins include ceruloplasmin, α_1-antitrypsin, and most other alpha and beta globulins. While the site of albumin catabolism is uncertain, the removal of terminal sialic acid residues after secretion and the resultant exposure of penultimate galactose or *N*-acetylglucosamine residues appears to result in receptor-mediated uptake of "aged" proteins by hepatocytes and Kupffer cells, followed by their subsequent degradation. Reduced amounts of the hepatic receptor for asialoglycoproteins appear to result in elevated serum concentrations of these glycoproteins in patients with severe and chronic liver disease.

One of the clinically most important derangements in protein metabolism is the development of *hypoalbuminemia*, which results largely from reduced synthetic activity. Decreased synthesis may be caused by a decrease in the number as well as the function of hepatocytes. A decrease in the dietary supply of amino acids also can contribute to deficient synthesis. To some extent the body attempts to compensate for decreased albumin synthesis by reducing the rate of degradation. Attempts to raise the serum albumin level by intravenous infusions are often futile because this compensatory mechanism can be blunted and the decrease in albumin degradation may not occur. The reduced degradation of albumin is not a general phenomenon in chronic liver disease because other proteins such as fibrinogen are degraded more rapidly than normal. In the patient with ascites, the degree of hypoalbuminemia is worsened by the loss of large amounts of the body's albumin into the ascitic fluid. When there is increased hepatic venous pressure (as in postsinusoidal or hepatic vein outflow block), there may be increased hepatic lymph production with extravasation into the peritoneal cavity. In contrast to intestinal lymph, the protein content of hepatic lymph appears to be relatively uninfluenced by ascitic oncotic pressure, most likely reflecting the lack of tight junctions between sinusoidal endothelial cells.

Other proteins produced by the liver include many of the blood-clotting factors: fibrinogen (factor I), prothrombin (factor II), and factors V, VII, IX, X, XII, and XIII, as well as inhibitors of both coagulation and fibrinolysis. Factors II, VII, IX, and X are vitamin K–responsive and are dependent on normal intestinal fat absorption. Vitamin K activates an enzyme system in liver endoplasmic reticulum which catalyzes the γ carboxylation of selected glutamyl residues in clotting factor precursors. The γ carboxylation enhances the Ca^{2+}- and phospholipid-binding capacity of prothrombin and permits its rapid conversion to thrombin in the presence of factors V and X (Chap. 118).

The liver is involved in the process of hemostasis by virtue of both anabolic and catabolic functions. As expected, severe liver disease leads to reduced synthesis of prothrombin, a vitamin K–dependent clotting factor. The presence of malnutrition, the use of broad-spectrum antibiotics, or concomitant impairment of fat absorption due to reduction in intestinal bile salt concentration (e.g., cholestasis) may accentuate hypoprothrombinemia by decreasing the amount of vitamin K that can be absorbed from the intestine. In these situations, prothrombin levels may be at least partially corrected by parenteral vitamin K administration. However, when the coagulopathy results from impaired hepatocellular function and not cholestasis or intestinal factors, exogenous vitamin K is unlikely to correct or improve prothrombin synthesis. The vitamin K–dependent clotting proteins have a substantially shorter serum half-life than albumin; therefore, hypoprothrombinemia usually precedes the development of hypoalbuminemia, especially in the patient with acute hepatocellular disease. In cirrhosis, coagulopathy may be further aggravated by the thrombocytopenia resulting from hypersplenism.

Since the liver is also the site of production of non-vitamin K–dependent clotting factors, severe liver disease injury may lead to decreased plasma concentrations of factor V. It is unusual for fibrinogen to be reduced significantly, unless there is an associated disseminated intravascular coagulation. For unclear reasons, the damaged liver may actually produce increased amounts of fibrinogen as well as other proteins, collectively designated *acute-phase reactants* (C-reactive proteins, haptoglobin, ceruloplasmin, and transferrin). The latter are produced both in response to liver injury and in association with systemic illnesses such as cancer, rheumatoid arthritis, bacterial infections, burns, and myocardial infarctions. Cytokines, including interleukins 1 and 6, appear to be major stimuli of hepatic synthesis of acute-phase reactants. However, while the diseased liver may produce normal or increased amounts of fibrinogen, the molecules themselves may be qualitatively abnormal (i.e., structurally and functionally), reflecting more subtle derangements in protein synthesis. These functionally abnormal fibrinogen molecules may contribute to the altered hemostasis frequently found in patients with chronic liver disease.

DETOXIFICATION MECHANISMS Water-soluble drugs and endogenous substances usually are excreted unchanged in the urine or bile. However, lipid-soluble compounds tend to accumulate in the body and affect cellular processes, unless they are converted to less active compounds or to more water-soluble metabolites that are more easily excreted. Hepatic blood flow, protein binding, and the intrinsic capacity of the liver to eliminate a drug are all primary determinants of hepatic drug clearance. The liver has an important role in the metabolism of many exogenous drugs and endogenous hormones by virtue of several enzyme systems involved in biochemical transformation, as well as the "first-pass effect" of blood flow from virtually the entire gastrointestinal tract through the liver via the portal circulation. The relative importance of these various factors differs depending on how well a drug is extracted by the liver. There are two major types of reactions. The first, *phase I reactions*, results in chemical modification of reactive groups by oxidation, reduction, hydroxylation, sulfoxidation, deamination, dealkylation, or methylation. Such modifications usually involve one of several enzymatic systems, including the mixed-function oxidases, cytochromes b_5 and P450 (microsomal), and the glutathione *S*-acyltransferases (cytoplasmic). These biochemical reactions usually lead to *inactivation* of drugs such as benzodiazepines. However, *activation* also may occur. For example, cortisone is activated to cortisol and prednisone to prednisolone (both products being more potent than the parent compounds); imipramine, a depressant, is converted to desmethylimipramine, an antidepressant. In the same manner, phase I reactions may even convert a nontoxic compound to a toxic one, as in the metabolism of isoniazid and acetaminophen. Similarly, some carcinogens may be activated by formation of highly reactive epoxide intermediates in the liver, while other carcinogens may be detoxified.

The enzymes responsible for phase I reactions, especially those involving the cytochrome P450 system, can be induced by drugs such as ethanol, barbiturates, haloperidol, and glutethimide. Conversely, hepatic microsomal enzymes may be inhibited by agents such as chloramphenicol, cimetidine, disulfiram, dextropropoxyphene, allopurinol, and, paradoxically, ethanol. The concomitant administration of two drugs metabolized by the same microsomal enzyme may result in modification, potentiation, or diminution of the pharmacologic efficacy of either or both drugs. Activity of phase I reactions also may change with aging.

Phase II reactions involve the conversion of substances to their glucuronide, sulfate, acetyl, taurine, or glycine derivatives, thereby converting lipophilic substances to water-soluble derivatives and permitting their excretion in bile or urine. Conjugation catalyzed by microsomal UDP (uridine diphosphate)-glucuronosyltransferases to form glucuronide derivatives is one of the most common phase II reactions. In general, the conjugates are more soluble than the parent compound and are pharmacologically inactive.

An awareness that there may be varying degrees of impairment in the hepatic uptake, detoxification, and excretion of certain drugs is important in the clinical management of patients with chronic liver disease. Portal-systemic shunting of blood may decrease the first-pass effect of drugs absorbed from the gut. In cirrhosis, altered intrahepatic hemodynamics due to a disordered liver architecture also may reduce the rates of hepatic drug clearance. Hypoalbuminemia will permit drugs usually bound to albumin to be present in increased concentrations of their unbound form in the circulation and extracellular spaces; this may result in their increased activity. Most important, a decrease in the amount of functional microsomal enzymes responsible for phase I and phase II reactions will result in slower rates of drug inactivation and elimination. Drugs for which there may be a decreased hepatic clearance include anticonvulsants (e.g., phenytoin, phenobarbital), anti-inflammatory agents (e.g., acetaminophen, phenylbutazone, glucocorticoids), minor tranquilizers, cardioactive drugs (e.g., lidocaine, quinidine, propranolol), and antibiotics (e.g., nafcillin, chloramphenicol, tetracyclines, clindamycin, trimethoprim, rifampin, pyrazinamide). This will lead to decreased dosage requirements and a narrowing of the range between therapeutic and toxic drug levels. Finally, the patient with chronic liver disease may demonstrate alterations in the pharmacologic effects of drugs in addition to or independent of changes in their pharmacokinetics, such as an increased central nervous system sensitivity to opiates and other sedatives.

The difficulties in safely administering pharmacologic agents to patients with both acute and chronic liver disease are underscored by the frequency with which administration of benzodiazepines precipitates hepatic coma. It may be very difficult clinically to determine whether agitation, confusion, and irrational behavior are due to early hepatic encephalopathy or are related to the concurrent use of benzodiazepines, opiates, barbiturates, and other depressants. It should be recognized that there is great variation of drug clearance in patients with liver disease; although data on average clearances may provide a reasonable estimate for initial dosages, subsequent adjustments in dose need to be individualized in order to attain the desired plasma drug concentration.

The mechanism by which some agents exert a hepatotoxic effect may involve the same metabolic pathways responsible for normal drug detoxification. The mechanism of acetaminophen toxicity is particularly illustrative. Acetaminophen is metabolized and detoxified by the hepatic mixed-function oxygenase system, but one of the intermediate products is a potent free radical (postulated metabolite *N*-acetylimidoquinone) that can inactivate many enzymes and proteins by binding irreversibly to their sulfhydryl groups. Normally, this interaction can be prevented by reduced glutathione. In the presence of excessive amounts of the acetaminophen free radical (e.g., from overdosage or underlying liver disease), the glutathione levels of the hepatocytes are readily exhausted, and the excess free radicals can lead to inactivation of cellular proteins and produce widespread hepatocellular necrosis. In the case of acetaminophen overdosage, the very early administration of sulfhydryl groups in the form of *N*-acetylcysteine can often prevent this drug-induced liver injury.

HORMONE METABOLISM In addition to its role in the metabolism of diverse pharmacologic agents, the liver is also responsible for inactivation or modification of several endogenous hormones; therefore, chronic liver disease may be accompanied by signs of apparent hormonal imbalance. Some hormones (e.g., insulin and glucagon) are inactivated in the liver by proteolysis or deamination. Thyroxine and triiodothyronine are metabolized in the liver by reactions involving deiodination. Steroid hormones, such as glucocorticoids and aldosterone, are first inactivated to their tetrahydro derivative (by reduction of the Δ^4 double bond and the 3-keto group), followed by conjugation, mostly with glucuronic acid. Testosterone is metabolized to the isomeric 17-ketosteroids androsterone and etiocholanolone and excreted in the urine mostly as sulfate conjugates. Estrogens, such as estradiol, may be converted to estriol and estrone and then conjugated with glucuronic acid or sulfate. Abnormalities in estrogen (and testosterone) metabolism are believed to be involved in the development of the spider angiomas, loss of axillary or pubic hair, and testicular atrophy frequently seen in patients with chronic liver disease. In addition, increased portal-systemic shunting of testosterone and androstenedione secondary to portal hypertension may lead to the development of gynecomastia in cirrhotic males due to increased peripheral conversion to estradiol and estrone, especially in patients with alcoholic cirrhosis. In patients with alcoholic liver disease, feminization also may be related to the direct toxic effects of alcohol on the gonadal-pituitary-hypothalamic axis, which lead to an overall reduction in serum testosterone. Similar effects are also seen in patients with hemochromatosis due to deposition of iron in these sites. However, gynecomastia is often lacking in the latter, apparently due to a coincident reduction in plasma concentration of androstenedione, a major precursor for estrogen synthesis.

Estrogens also act directly on the liver to impair hepatic secretory activity. Estradiol and related estrogens, such as those present in contraceptive pills, interfere with bile salt excretion and worsen the preexisting defect in secretion of conjugated bilirubin in patients with Dubin-Johnson syndrome; they also may elevate plasma alkaline phosphatase levels (see Chap. 292). Related steroids such as etiocholanolone and pregnanediol have been shown to stimulate δ-aminolevulinic acid (ALA) synthetase activity, leading to increased porphobilinogen excretion. Since these steroids exert their effects only in their unconjugated form, the increased hepatic levels of δ-aminolevulinic acid synthetase in patients with alcoholic cirrhosis may be secondary to the action of gonadal steroids. The liver also serves to remove some important circulating vasoactive substances, including epinephrine and bradykinin. Elevated levels of epinephrine, perhaps reflecting in part diminished hepatic uptake, may promote the hyperdynamic state that contributes to the development of ascites and the hepatorenal syndrome.

LIPID METABOLISM: FATTY ACIDS AND TRIGLYCER-IDES Under normal conditions, most of the fatty acids taken up by the liver and esterified to triglyceride are derived from adipose tissue or the diet. Some fatty acids (especially saturated ones) are synthesized in the liver from acetate. The fatty acids may then be converted enzymatically to triglyceride, esterified with cholesterol, incorporated into phospholipids, or oxidized to CO_2 or ketone bodies. Most of the triglyceride is produced for export, but in order to be secreted it must be converted to lipoproteins by combining with relatively specific apoprotein moieties. This emphasizes the importance of protein synthesis for the release and secretion of triglyceride from the liver. The liver plays a major role in regulating lipoprotein levels by virtue of both its degradative and synthetic functions. Thus the liver is quantitatively the major site of low-density lipoprotein (LDL) catabolism, with dual high- and low-affinity receptor-mediated pathways playing a role. In addition, chylomicron remnants are removed and degraded by the liver, where their constituents have a number of metabolic effects. The liver is not only the primary site of very low density lipoprotein (VLDL) secretion but also accounts for a major portion of its subsequent degradation by mechanisms similar to that of chylomicron remnant degradation and the conversion to LDL. The liver also may play a role in high-density lipoprotein (HDL) catabolism. It is noteworthy that with the exception of cholestatic disease (see below), clinically significant alterations in lipoprotein and cholesterol metabolism are usually not found in patients with chronic liver disease.

Studies on the production of fatty liver have shown that, singly or in combination, one or more of the steps depicted in Fig. 293-2 may be involved. An increased influx of fatty acids mobilized from adipose tissue due to drugs (e.g., ethanol or glucocorticoids) or secondary to diabetic ketosis may lead to a fatty liver. Similarly, increased levels of fatty acids in the liver, either from enhanced fatty acid synthesis or from decreased fatty acid oxidation, may lead to increased triglyceride formation. In some instances (e.g., ethanol excess) there also may be increases in the carbohydrate backbone, α-glycerophosphate, involved in fatty acid esterification to triglyceride. Since release of triglyceride involves the formation of lipoproteins, lipid accumulation may occur because of decreased apoprotein synthesis. This appears to be the case in fatty livers seen in patients with protein-calorie malnutrition (kwashiorkor) and due to toxins such as carbon tetrachloride, phosphorus, or ethionine, as well as following excessive doses of antibiotics such as tetracycline that can inhibit protein synthesis. Finally, there may be impaired lipoprotein secretion from the liver.

Different alterations disrupting hepatic fat metabolism may lead to different patterns of fat accumulation designated *macrovesicular* (most common) and *microvesicular*; these are reviewed in Chap. 300. Alcohol is perhaps the most common agent leading to hepatic steatosis, but the mechanism(s) whereby alcohol leads to increased liver triglyceride is not clear. Depending on factors such as dose or duration, alcohol ingestion may affect any of the seven steps shown in Fig. 293-2; however, the primary factor for the production of the alcohol-induced fatty liver remains to be determined. The alterations in the redox state due to excessive accumulation of NADH resulting from oxidation of alcohol also may contribute.

CHOLESTEROL Cholesterol and bile acid synthesis is carried out primarily by the liver. Cholesterol synthesis is subject to a number of metabolic controls, most of them mediated via the rate-limiting biosynthetic enzyme 3-hydroxy-3-methylglutaryl coenzyme A reductase (HMG-CoA reductase). Cholesterol exists either free or combined with fatty acids in the form of cholesterol esters; in the plasma, both are found primarily in association with β-lipoproteins. The plasma and liver also contain lecithin–cholesterol acyltransferase (LCAT), an enzyme involved in the conversion of free cholesterol to its esterified form. Since there is exchange of free cholesterol between tissues, changes in plasma cholesterol levels reflect changes in total body cholesterol. However, decreases in plasma cholesterol esters may reflect hepatic damage and impaired hepatic cholesterol esterification.

Severe liver injury often leads to a decrease in *total* serum cholesterol levels, including both free and esterified fractions. This may be due to decreased synthesis of cholesterol and cholesterol esters, decreased apoprotein synthesis, or both. In cholestasis (either intra- or extrahepatic), total serum cholesterol often increases strikingly. Disorders of cholestasis are associated with marked abnormalities of lipoprotein metabolism. In primary biliary cirrhosis there are pronounced elevations in serum free cholesterol and LDL; conversely, serum HDL is reduced and may disappear from the serum in patients with long-standing disease. Similar but less marked changes are seen in other cholestatic conditions.

The increase in serum free cholesterol (and phospholipid) and the concomitant decrease in esterified cholesterol in cholestasis may be related to a decrease in the hepatic production of LCAT. Reduced levels of LCAT are also correlated with the appearance of an abnormal

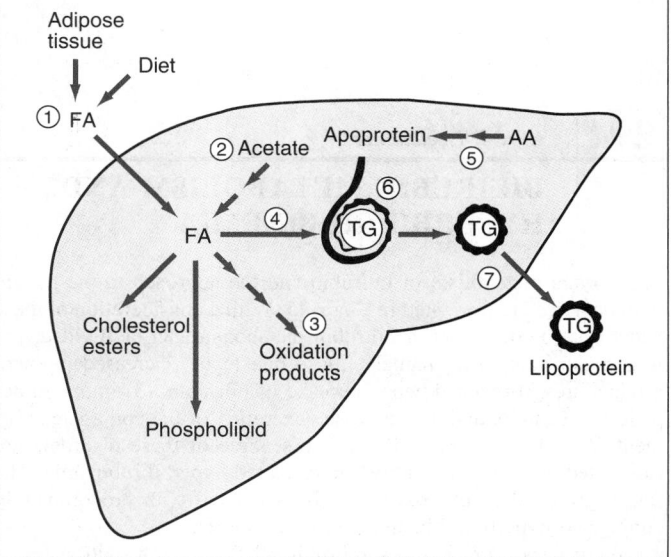

FIGURE 293-2 Factors in the uptake and esterification of fatty acids to triglyceride by the liver, including the formation and release of triglyceride as lipoprotein. The numbers refer to steps, which, if altered, may result in increased liver triglyceride (i.e., fatty liver).

LDL, referred to as *lipoprotein X* (LP-X). Although LP-X, which has a high content of free cholesterol and triglyceride, was originally thought to be a specific indicator of biliary tract obstruction, it is evident that it appears in any cholestatic condition. While the depressed hepatic production of LCAT may be responsible for altered lipid content and composition of lipoproteins, the factors leading to the overall increase in total serum cholesterol are not clear. In experimental animals, bile duct ligation results in a net increase in hepatic cholesterol synthesis and in "regurgitation" of bile salts, cholesterol, and LP-X into venous radicals. However, it is difficult to translate these experimental findings to the patient with primary biliary cirrhosis unless any insult to cells lining the biliary canaliculi and ductules can impair the delicate balance of lipid synthesis and removal.

The alterations in cholesterol and related substances resulting from liver disease may lead to significant changes in the composition of erythrocyte membranes. Such changes in composition lead to altered morphology with the development of spur and burr cell forms. The presence of these altered erythrocytes is usually an ominous sign of advanced liver disease.

BIBLIOGRAPHY

ARIAS IM et al: *The Liver: Biology and Pathophysiology*, 3d ed. New York, Raven, 1994

COOPER AD: Role of the liver in the degradation of lipoproteins. Gastroenterology 88:192, 1984

FLANNERY DB et al: Current status of hyperammonemic syndromes. Hepatology 2:495, 1982

HOYUMPA AM et al: Hepatic encephalopathy. Gastroenterology 77:803, 1979

KLEG HK et al: Conversion of androgens to estrogens in idiopathic hemochromatosis: Comparison with alcoholic liver disease. J Clin Endocrinol Metab 61:1, 1985

OWEN OE et al: Hepatic, gut and renal substrate flux rates in patients with hepatic cirrhosis. J Clin Invest 68:240, 1981

PETRIDES A et al: Pathogenesis of glucose intolerance and diabetes mellitus in cirrhosis. Hepatology 19:616, 1994

ROTHSCHILD MA et al: Serum albumin. Hepatology 8:355, 1988

SCHIFF L, SCHIFF ER: *Diseases of the Liver*, 7th ed. Philadelphia, JB Lippincott, 1993

SMITH AR et al: Alteration in plasma and CSF amino acids, amines and metabolites in hepatic coma. Ann Surg 187:343, 1978

WILLIAMS RC: Drug administration in hepatic disease. N Engl J Med 309:1616, 1983

ZAKIM D, BOYER TD: *Hepatology: A Textbook of Liver Disease*, 3d ed. Philadelphia, Saunders, 1996

294 *Kurt J. Isselbacher*

BILIRUBIN METABOLISM AND HYPERBILIRUBINEMIA

The normal metabolism of bilirubin and the approach to the patient with jaundice are presented in Chap. 45. With a consideration of these pathways, the disorders of bilirubin metabolism can be divided into four major categories, namely, those due to (1) increased pigment production, (2) reduced hepatic uptake of bilirubin, (3) impaired hepatic conjugation, and (4) decreased excretion of the conjugated pigment from the liver into bile. The first three of these disorders are associated with predominantly unconjugated hyperbilirubinemia. The fourth group, defective excretion, is associated with predominantly conjugated hyperbilirubinemia and bilirubinuria.

As discussed in Chap. 45, bilirubin UDP-glucuronosyltransferase (UGT) is essential for the normal excretion of bilirubin mono- or diglucuronide from liver to bile. There are two isoforms of UGT that are encoded by the UGT1 gene by the process of alternative splicing. Mutation in either the variable or common exons of this gene accounts

for the hereditary unconjugated hyperbilirubinemic syndromes described below.

DISORDERS CAUSING PREDOMINANTLY UNCONJUGATED HYPERBILIRUBINEMIA

The plasma concentration of unconjugated bilirubin is determined by (1) the rate at which newly synthesized bilirubin enters the plasma (bilirubin turnover) and (2) the rate of removal of bilirubin by the liver (hepatic bilirubin clearance). Disturbances of the latter can result from derangements of hepatic bilirubin uptake, conjugation, or both. Measurements of these variables, although not routinely available, permit a classification of patients into those with *increased bilirubin turnover* (e.g., hemolysis), those with *decreased bilirubin clearance* (e.g., Gilbert's syndrome), and those in whom both mechanisms operate.

OVERPRODUCTION OF BILIRUBIN (INCREASED TURNOVER) Increased Destruction of Circulating Erythrocytes (Intravascular and Extravascular Hemolysis) In disorders associated with hemolysis, most commonly the hemolytic anemias, the rate of bilirubin production is increased and may even exceed the amount that can be removed by a normal liver. The resulting jaundice is primarily an unconjugated hyperbilirubinemia. There is often also a small increase in the serum conjugated bilirubin. If significant anemia or other adverse factors are present (e.g., fever, sepsis, hypoxemia, or vascular collapse), the ability of the liver to handle the pigment load will be compromised, and the degree of jaundice will be greater.

The clinical and diagnostic features of the various hemolytic anemias are described in Chap. 109. The presence of reticulocytosis, shortened red blood cell survival, and increased fecal urobilinogen, in the absence of clinical and laboratory evidence of liver disease, strongly suggest hemolysis and overproduction of bilirubin as the cause of the jaundice. It is obvious, however, that in some cases (e.g., cirrhosis, tumors, and sepsis), hemolysis *plus* deranged liver function may be present. In most cases of uncomplicated hemolytic states, the mean serum bilirubin level will be in the range of 51 to 68 μmol/L (3 to 4 mg/dL); rarely, higher levels may be seen.

Jaundice due to increased pigment production also may be seen as a consequence of *tissue infarction* (e.g., pulmonary infarcts) and large *collections of blood in tissues* (e.g., leakage from blood vessels after catheterization studies, rupture of an aortic aneurysm). If hypotension and hypoxemia also supervene, jaundice is usually more pronounced, and the resulting impairment of liver function also may lead to a significant increase in the serum conjugated bilirubin level (see "Postoperative Jaundice," below).

Except in early infancy, elevations of serum unconjugated bilirubin levels are not harmful per se, and the prognosis is that of the hemolytic process itself. However, in the neonatal state and infancy, unconjugated bilirubin levels above 340 μmol/L (20 mg/dL) may lead to *kernicterus* due to bilirubin deposition in the lipid-rich basal ganglia. Chronic overproduction of bilirubin may result in the formation of gallstones composed predominantly of bilirubin ("pigment stones"). In this situation, all the potential complications of calculus disease of the biliary tract (Chap. 302) may be superimposed on the chronic hemolytic state that produced it.

Increased Production of Bilirubin from Sources Other Than Circulating Erythrocytes About 15 to 20 percent of the circulating bilirubin is normally derived from sources other than the destruction of circulating red blood cells. This represents the so-called early-labeled fraction; it includes the synthesis of bilirubin from nonhemoglobin heme in the liver and from hemoglobin heme in the marrow.

In some conditions, jaundice results from an increased destruction of red blood cells or their precursors in the marrow—a process referred to as *ineffective erythropoiesis* (see Chap. 59). In patients with thalassemia, pernicious anemia, and congenital erythropoietic porphyria, such an increased rate of formation of the early-labeled bilirubin fraction has been demonstrated. It is possible that some cases of unexplained unconjugated hyperbilirubinemia may be caused by an increased hepatic production of bilirubin from nonhemoglobin heme, but this phenomenon has not been demonstrated clinically.

IMPAIRED HEPATIC UPTAKE OF BILIRUBIN Drugs Only a few drugs have been definitely shown to influence the uptake of bilirubin by the liver. Flavaspidic acid, used in the treatment of tapeworm infestation, may cause unconjugated hyperbilirubinemia during its administration. The jaundice readily subsides with cessation of the drug. Flavaspidic acid competes with bilirubin for binding to ligandin, leading thereby to unconjugated hyperbilirubinemia. The jaundice that may occur with novobiocin and some cholecystogrphic dyes is also apparently due to an interference in bilirubin uptake.

Gilbert's Syndrome Some cases of this syndrome of chronic unconjugated hyperbilirubinemia may be due to a defect in hepatic uptake. In most cases, however, a mild deficiency of bilirubin glucuronosyltransferase can be demonstrated. Hence this syndrome is best considered as a defect in bilirubin conjugation (see below).

IMPAIRED BILIRUBIN CONJUGATION (DECREASED ACTIVITY OF BILIRUBIN GLUCURONOSYLTRANSFER-ASE) Neonatal Jaundice (Physiologic Jaundice of the Newborn) Almost every infant exhibits some transient unconjugated hyperbilirubinemia between the second and fifth days of life. While during gestation the placenta serves to clear bilirubin from the fetus, after birth infants must detoxify the pigments themselves. However, at this stage the hepatic enzyme glucuronosyltransferase is still "immature." In addition, lack of intestinal bacteria prevents bilirubin conversion to urobilinogen, permitting unconjugated bilirubin to be absorbed. As a result, unconjugated bilirubinemia develops, usually not exceeding 86 µmol/L (5 mg/dL). The activity of glucuronosyltransferase increases within several days to 2 weeks after birth, and concomitantly, the serum bilirubin level returns to normal. In infants with a superimposed hemolytic process (e.g., erythroblastosis), the excessive pigment load leads to more pronounced jaundice, and bilirubin levels may exceed 340 µmol/L (20 mg/dL). It should be emphasized that neonatal jaundice is not present at the time of delivery; if jaundice is present at birth, other causes must be considered.

The cytoplasmic liver cell protein ligandin (glutathione-S-transferase B) binds bilirubin in the hepatocyte and may assist in the transfer of bilirubin to the endoplasmic reticulum for conjugation (Chap. 45).

An additional facet of the "immature" liver is a concomitant defect in the excretion of *conjugated* bilirubin. Rarely this defect persists beyond the time needed for the development of adequate glucuronide conjugation and may explain the occasional presence of conjugated hyperbilirubinemia in infants with erythroblastosis (*inspissated bile syndrome*).

When in the neonatal state unconjugated bilirubin levels approach or exceed 340 µmol/L (20 mg/dL), the infants may develop and die of kernicterus (bilirubin encephalopathy). This condition results from unconjugated bilirubin deposition in the lipid-rich basal ganglia. The current therapeutic approach involves *phototherapy*; intense illumination of these patients with strong white or blue light leads to the *photoisomerization* of bilirubin to water-soluble isomers that are rapidly excreted in the bile without the prior need for conjugation. Another novel approach involves decreasing bilirubin production from heme by inhibitors of heme oxygenase. Synthetic protoporphyrins, such as tin protoporphyrin, have been administered successfully to patients with neonatal hyperbilirubinemia with marked reduction in the serum bilirubin and with no major side effects.

Hereditary Glucuronosyltransferase Deficiency There are currently three syndromes that fall into this category. As indicated in Table 294-1, they reflect progressive decreases in the activity of glucuronosyltransferase and thus may be part of a spectrum, i.e., from minimal deficiency to complete absence of bilirubin glucuronosyltransferase.

Gilbert's syndrome Since the original report by Gilbert in 1907, there has been an increased recognition of this benign but chronic disorder characterized by mild, persistent, unconjugated hyperbilirubinemia. The patient usually does not manifest this disorder until after the second decade and is often unaware of the jaundice until it is detected by physical examination or routine laboratory testing. The total serum bilirubin level usually ranges and fluctuates from 21 to 51 µmol/L (1.2 to 3 mg/dL) and rarely exceeds 86 µmol/L (5 mg/

dL). With the van den Bergh diazo reaction, less than 20 percent of bilirubin gives a direct reaction; however, studies using more accurate methods (such as high-pressure liquid chromatography) show that *the serum bilirubin in patients with Gilbert's syndrome is almost all unconjugated*. Typically, the jaundice fluctuates and is exacerbated following prolonged fasting (see below), surgery, fever or infection, and excessive exertion or alcohol ingestion. Liver function tests are normal, and the liver cells usually appear normal by light microscopy.

With the exception of hemolytic anemias, Gilbert's syndrome is probably the most common cause of mild unconjugated hyperbilirubinemia. On the basis of serum bilirubin levels, 3 to 10 percent of the general population are estimated to have Gilbert's syndrome. These patients have a partial deficiency of bilirubin glucuronosyltransferase; their hepatic glucuronidating activity is approximately 30 percent of normal.

Genetic data indicate that patients with Gilbert's syndrome have reduced expression of the UGT1 gene due to the presence of two extra nucleotides (TA) in the promotor region (the TATAA element) of the gene. This expanded nucleotide repeat interferes with the binding for the transcription factor IID resulting in reduced expresion of UGT1. Some patients also manifest decreased bilirubin uptake and increased hemolysis. Decreased glucuronosyltransferase alone or together with a decrease in bilirubin uptake appears to account for the observed *decrease in hepatic bilirubin clearance*. A decreased clearance and hepatic uptake of bile salts also have been shown.

Previously, Gilbert's syndrome was traditionally defined as mild, chronic, unconjugated hyperbilirubinemia occurring in the absence of hemolysis. However, with the use of radiobilirubin kinetics and erythrocyte half-life studies, at least two forms of Gilbert's syndrome have been described. One group includes patients with decreased bilirubin clearance and *no hemolysis*. A second group includes those who also have *evidence of hemolysis* (often occult) and hence increased bilirubin turnover. The simultaneous presence of both derangements appears to be a chance occurrence of two not uncommon disorders in the same patient and does not imply a causal relationship. There is additional evidence of the heterogeneity of patients with Gilbert's syndrome. Thus, some patients have an increase in hepatocyte lipofuscin and an increase in the smooth endoplasmic reticulum (SER); others show an increase in hepatic lysosomal enzymes.

A feature of Gilbert's syndrome that can be useful diagnostically is the increase in serum bilirubin following prolonged fasting or calorie deprivation. Patients with this disorder, when placed on 1260 kJ (300 kcal) per day for 2 days, will increase their serum bilirubin by 25 µmol/

Table 294-1

Hereditary Unconjugated Hyperbilirubinemias with Deficiency of Glucuronosyltransferase

Features	Mild (Gilbert's Syndrome)	Moderate (Crigler-Najjar Syndrome Type II)	Severe (Crigler-Najjar Syndrome Type I)
Inheritance	Unclear*	Dominant†	Recessive
Serum bilirubin, µmol/L (mg/dL)	17–102 (1–6)	102–340 (6–20)	340–770 (20–45)
Kernicterus	No	Rare	Yes
Conjugated bilirubin in bile	Yes (↑ monoconjugates)	Yes (↑↑ monoconjugates)	No
Response to phenobarbital	Yes	Yes	No
Bilirubin conjugation	↓‡	↓↓	Absent

* Many cases have no familial incidence.
† Variable expressivity.
‡ Other defects such as occult hemolysis and decreased bilirubin uptake may coexist.

L (1.5 mg/dL) or more, the major increase being in the unconjugated fraction. A decrease in glucuronosyltransferase activity is needed to obtain this effect. Patients with hemolysis do not show an increase in serum bilirubin with fasting. As a reflection of the mild decrease in glucuronosyltransferase in Gilbert's syndrome, (1) serum bilirubin levels will diminish when the enzyme activity is enhanced following phenobarbital administration, and (2) the bile shows a modest increase in monoconjugates of bilirubin (see Table 294-1).

In general, the diagnosis of this benign but not uncommon disorder is made by exclusion. The syndrome is suspected in a patient with low-grade unconjugated hyperbilirubinemia with (1) no systemic symptoms, (2) *no overt* or clinically recognizable hemolysis, (3) normal tests of routine liver function, and (4) a liver biopsy (although usually not necessary) that is normal by light microscopy.

Crigler-Najjar syndrome (types I and II) This disorder exists in two forms. Type I is the clinically *severe* form (originally described by Crigler and Najjar) and is due to *absence of glucuronosyltransferase activity* as a result of a mutation in one of the common 3′ regions of the UGT1 gene (or lack of function of one or more isoenzymes of the transferase). Type II has more *moderate* clinical findings due to *partial deficiency of glucuronosyltransferase* resulting from a mutation in the variable region (exon 1) of the UGT1 gene. The major differences of types I and II are summarized in Table 294-1.

Type I (Crigler-Najjar) is a rare disorder. Infants develop high unconjugated bilirubin levels in the serum [340 to 770 μmol/L (20 to 45 mg/dL)]. Absence of the enzyme can be demonstrated in the liver by enzymatic or molecular genetic techniques. Routine liver function tests are normal, as is liver histology. Because of the lack of glucuronosyltransferase activity, no conjugated bilirubin is formed by the liver; hence no bilirubin is secreted into the bile and liver, and the bile is colorless.

Phototherapy may temporarily and transiently reduce the unconjugated bilirubin level. Phenobarbital has no effect, since the enzyme defect is complete and no drug "induction" is therefore possible. Other options include plasmapheresis, orthotopic liver transplantation, and, perhaps in the future, gene therapy with insertion of the normal UGT gene. Affected infants usually die within the first year of life, although some patients have survived to the second or third decade of life. Death is usually from kernicterus. A strain of rats (Gunn rat) with the type I defect exists and is widely used as an animal model of the Crigler-Najjar syndrome (type I).

Type II patients with only a *partial deficiency* of glucuronosyltransferase have a less severe disorder. Serum unconjugated bilirubin levels are lower [103 to 340 μmol/L (6 to 20 mg/dL)], jaundice may not appear until adolescence, and neurologic complications are uncommon. The bile contains variable amounts of conjugated bilirubin with a significant increase in monoconjugates. Phenobarbital is effective in lowering the serum bilirubin level in type II patients. However, the disorder is relatively benign in those patients with bilirubin levels less than 308 to 340 μmol/L (18 to 20 mg/dL).

Acquired Deficiency of Glucuronosyltransferase (UGT) As with any enzyme, glucuronosyltransferase is susceptible to inhibition by a variety of agents, and because of the decreased activity of the enzyme in the neonatal state, such inhibition may be more evident at that time. Neonatal jaundice may be aggravated or prolonged in infants treated with *drugs* such as chloramphenicol or novobiocin or with *vitamin K*. In some breast-fed infants, jaundice has been ascribed to glucuronosyltransferase inhibitors in *breast milk*, including pregnane-3β,20α-diol and free fatty acids. When the infant is removed from the breast, the "breast-milk jaundice" subsides.

Hypothyroidism delays the normal "maturation" of glucuronosyltransferase. In cretins, neonatal jaundice may be prolonged for weeks or months. In fact, the presence of prolonged unconjugated hyperbilirubinemia after birth may be a clue to an underlying hypothyroidism.

In the infant, as well as in the adult, *liver cell damage* leads to impairment in glucuronide conjugation as a result of decreased transferase activity. However, since excretion is probably the rate-limiting step in bilirubin metabolism, and since this step appears to be interfered with to a greater extent than conjugation in parenchymal liver disease, the pigment that accumulates in the blood is predominantly conjugated bilirubin.

DISORDERS CAUSING COMBINED CONJUGATED AND UNCONJUGATED HYPERBILIRUBINEMIA

In jaundice due to primary liver disease, the plasma usually exhibits elevated levels of both conjugated and unconjugated bilirubin, and the *urine contains bilirubin*. The relative proportions of the two pigments are highly variable. In many familial hepatic abnormalities (described below) and in some forms of liver injury, the jaundice is largely due to increases in conjugated bilirubin. Such a serum pigment pattern is also seen with extrahepatic biliary obstruction. One *cannot differentiate* intrahepatic and extrahepatic causes of jaundice from either the levels or proportions of unconjugated and conjugated bilirubin in serum. Thus the main purpose of the initial fractionation of the serum bilirubin is to distinguish hepatic parenchymal and biliary obstructive disease from the disorders associated with predominantly unconjugated hyperbilirubinemia.

FAMILIAL DEFECTS IN HEPATIC EXCRETORY FUNCTION Dubin-Johnson Syndrome This relatively rare disorder, also called *chronic idiopathic jaundice*, is a benign, autosomally inherited hyperbilirubinemia characterized by the presence of a dark pigment in the centrilobular region of the liver cells. On direct visual inspection, the liver is black. Functionally, there exists a *defect in biliary excretion* of bilirubin, cholephilic dyes, and porphyrins. Using the diazo method for measuring bilirubin, the serum pigment in these patients typically is in the range of 51 to 257 μmol/L (3 to 15 mg/dL) and predominantly of the conjugated type. However, with the newer and more accurate method (alkaline methanolysis and high-pressure liquid chromatography), homozygous patients with the Dubin-Johnson syndrome have been shown to also have significant levels of serum *unconjugated bilirubin*. The latter finding may in part reflect pigment that, after conjugation by the liver, is deconjugated in the hepatobiliary system and refluxed back into the plasma. Moreover, the serum contains more diconjugated than monoconjugated bilirubin, just the reverse of what is seen in acquired hepatobiliary disease and Rotor syndrome. This reversed ratio is believed to be characteristic and diagnostic for homozygous patients.

Patients with Dubin-Johnson syndrome may be asymptomatic or have vague constitutional or gastrointestinal symptoms. Pruritus is absent, and serum bile acid levels are normal. The degree of jaundice is increased by intercurrent illness, oral contraceptives, and pregnancy. Not infrequently the liver is slightly enlarged; in about one-fourth of cases there is mild hepatic tenderness. Oral and intravenous cholangiography fail to visualize the biliary tract. There is typically and characteristically a late rise in the plasma sodium sulfobromophthalein (BSP) elimination curve at *90 min*. This is caused by the reflux from the liver of the conjugated dye and reflects the defect in the hepatic excretory transport maximum. It is noteworthy that there is no such secondary rise in plasma when dyes that are not conjugated by the liver are given, such as indocyanine green. When bile salts such as ursodeoxycholic acid are given, these patients show a decreased hepatic uptake and clearance. In the liver the striking feature is the presence of a *brown or black pigment in the hepatocytes*. Some findings suggest that this unique pigment is "melanin-like"; others indicate it to be a polymer of epinephrine metabolites.

These patients also show an abnormality in coproporphyrin excretion. Normal urine contains mostly coproporphyrin III and small amounts of coproporphyrin I; Dubin-Johnson patients show the opposite, i.e., they excrete predominantly coproporphyrin I. Heterozygotes show an intermediate excretory pattern.

There is impaired excretion of many metabolites, including conjugated bilirubin, BSP, and iodinated dyes. Excretion of bile acids, however, is normal. Oral contraceptive agents may accentuate hyperbilirubinemia or may produce jaundice for the first time. Features of cholestasis such as pruritus or steatorrhea are usually lacking, and specifically, serum alkaline phosphatase levels are *not* elevated. The overall prognosis of the disorder is excellent.

Rotor Syndrome This is similar in many respects to the Dubin-Johnson syndrome. However, *there is no pigment in the liver cells*, and the serum conjugated bilirubin has more monoconjugates than diglucuronide conjugates. The liver looks grossly normal. The gallbladder is usually visualized on cholecystography, and there is an increase in the *total* urinary coproporphyrins but *not* an increased percentage in excretion of coproporphyrin I. The BSP excretion pattern does *not* show a secondary rise at 90 min. The impairment in excretion that is typical of Dubin-Johnson syndrome is not present; instead, in most cases with Rotor syndrome there is impairment of *hepatic storage capacity*. This rare syndrome is inherited as an autosomal recessive trait and is genetically distinct from Dubin-Johnson syndrome.

Benign Recurrent Intrahepatic Cholestasis This is a relatively rare syndrome characterized by recurrent attacks of pruritus and jaundice. During an attack, the serum alkaline phosphatase and bile acid levels are markedly elevated, and liver biopsy shows the morphologic features of cholestasis. However, there is no mechanical biliary obstruction, with cholangiography revealing a patent biliary tree. Remissions are the rule, and at such times hepatic function tests and liver morphologic features are normal. The cause of the disorder is unknown; cirrhosis does not develop, and the disorder is benign. A congenital origin has been postulated on the basis of the early age of onset and familial incidence.

Recurrent Jaundice of Pregnancy This form of jaundice is also known as *intrahepatic cholestasis of pregnancy*. During a normal pregnancy, some derangements in liver function occur, especially during the last trimester. Usually these consist of slight increases in BSP retention and in serum alkaline phosphatase. This mild increase in alkaline phosphatase during pregnancy is normally of placental rather than of hepatic origin. With a normal pregnancy, elevations of serum bilirubin level either do not occur or are less than 34 μmol/L (2 mg/dL).

In a small number of pregnant women, intrahepatic cholestasis may appear. This usually occurs in the third trimester but may develop any time after the seventh week of gestation. The clinical features consist primarily of pruritus and jaundice. Serum bilirubin levels are usually less than 103 μmol/L (6 mg/dL). The serum alkaline phosphatase and cholesterol levels are elevated significantly, while other liver function tests are only mildly deranged. Histologically, the liver shows varying degrees of cholestasis but only a few parenchymal cell changes. The clinical and laboratory abnormalities subside promptly after delivery and are usually normal within 7 to 14 days.

This condition has been seen more frequently in Scandinavia and Europe than in the United States. Since steroid hormones and specifically estrogens can induce changes in hepatic excretory function in normal individuals (see Chap. 293), these patients probably have an increased susceptibility or sensitivity to the hepatic effects of estrogenic and progestational hormones. The intrahepatic cholestasis is usually termed *recurrent*, since the syndrome often (but not always) reappears in subsequent pregnancies. The process is benign and self-limited, and treatment is usually not needed, but cholestyramine administration will diminish the pruritus. This disorder must be distinguished from the many other causes of jaundice not unique to pregnancy, such as viral hepatitis. It also must be distinguished from the idiopathic *acute fatty liver of pregnancy* and the *tetracycline-induced fatty liver*. The latter two conditions are rare, occur in the last trimester, and have a high fatality rate; however, in these disorders there is evidence of diffuse parenchymal damage and not only cholestasis.

ACQUIRED DEFECTS OF HEPATIC EXCRETORY FUNCTION Drug-Induced Cholestasis A condition entirely analogous to the intrahepatic cholestasis of pregnancy may occur in some women following the use of oral contraceptive agents. In some, mild cholestatic jaundice may occur, liver function returns to normal when the drugs are withdrawn, and chronic liver disease does not result. It is relevant that one-third of the reported patients with jaundice due to oral contra-

ceptives also have a history of recurrent intrahepatic cholestasis of pregnancy.

The nature of these changes produced by the natural and synthetic female sex hormones is very similar to those resulting from the administration of certain testosterone analogues, especially those with α substitutions at the 17 position of the steroid nucleus. These agents (such as methyltestosterone and norethandrolone), unlike the female hormones, have been implicated as a cause of chronic liver disease, especially biliary cirrhosis.

Because of these phenomena, synthetic steroid sex hormones should not be used in patients with liver disease. Conversely, in individuals using these agents, the appearance of jaundice or elevations in serum aminotransferase or alkaline phosphatase levels contraindicates their further use.

There are many drugs that may produce not only cholestasis but liver injury resembling acute hepatitis or cholestatic hepatitis. In contrast to the jaundice produced by the steroid hormones, the clinical features are those of fever, rash, arthralgia, and sometimes eosinophilia, with the liver showing a pronounced inflammatory reaction. These features suggest that such reactions are *allergic* or *toxic* in nature and therefore differ from the effects caused by the steroid hormones, which probably represent an exaggerated response by the liver to the normal action of these hormones. → *For further discussion, see Chap. 296.*

Postoperative Jaundice The occurrence of postoperative jaundice is a problem of increasing importance. It is perhaps seen more frequently now than in earlier years because patients are able to undergo more major surgical procedures (i.e., cardiac surgery, repair of ruptured aneurysms) and survive. In approaching this problem, the possible pathogenic mechanisms listed in Table 294-2 need to be considered. The patient may have *pigment overload*, especially from blood transfusions (with hemolysis of stored blood), from resorption of blood in extravascular spaces, and, less commonly, from hemolytic anemia. *Hepatocellular damage* and decreased liver cell function may occur due to concurrent use of hepatotoxic drugs (Chap. 296) or anesthetics such as halothane. Hepatocellular necrosis may follow profound shock; with lesser degrees of hypotension or hypoxemia, morphologic damage may be slight, but significant impairment of function may occur. Hence prior shock or hypotension plus pigment overload may produce significant jaundice. Extensive sepsis also can produce jaundice, often of a cholestatic type. Concurrent renal impairment due to hypotension and hypoxemia may enhance the degree of jaundice because the renal excretion of conjugated bilirubin is decreased. *Extrahepatic obstruction* due to surgical damage or stones needs to be considered and may be excluded by sonography.

A form of jaundice referred to as *benign postoperative intrahepatic cholestasis* may be seen. In the typical case, the patient has had major

Table 294-2

Conditions Causing or Contributing to Postoperative Jaundice

I. Increased pigment load
  A. Hemolytic anemia
  B. Transfusions (especially of stored blood)
  C. Resorption of hematomas, blood in extravascular spaces
II. Impaired hepatocellular function
  A. Hepatitis-like picture
    1. Anesthetic agents (e.g., halothane)
    2. Drugs
    3. Shock
    4. Infection with hepatitis viruses
  B. Cholestatic picture
    1. Hypotension, hypoxemia
    2. Drugs
    3. Sepsis
III. Extrahepatic obstruction
  A. Bile duct injury
  B. Choledocholithiasis

and prolonged surgery for a catastrophic event such as a ruptured aortic aneurysm complicated by hypotension and hypoxemia, extensive blood loss into tissues, and massive blood replacement. Jaundice may be noted on the second or third postoperative day, and the serum bilirubin, predominantly conjugated, may reach 340 to 680 μmol/L (20 to 40 mg/dL) by the eighth to tenth day. Serum alkaline phosphatase levels may be elevated three- to tenfold. Typically, the serum aspartate aminotransferase (AST, SGOT) is only mildly elevated. The liver morphology is striking in that necrosis is not seen, only cholestasis and erythrophagocytosis.

The cause of this type of postoperative cholestatic jaundice is uncertain. However, it probably reflects (1) increased pigment load, (2) decreased liver function due to hypoxemia and hypotension, and (3) decreased renal bilirubin excretion due to varying degrees of tubular necrosis as a result of shock. This diagnostic possibility must be considered in the postoperative patient with marked cholestatic jaundice. The course of the jaundice is self-limited and will subside if the other systemic complications do not predominate and lead to death.

Hepatitis and Cirrhosis These disorders constitute the *most common disorders associated with jaundice*. As has been stated previously, when the liver cell is damaged, as in viral hepatitis, there is often impairment in all three major hepatic phases of bilirubin metabolism, namely, uptake, conjugation, and excretion. Since the excretory step is the one which is rate-limiting and most readily affected by injury, significant amounts of conjugated bilirubin reenter the systemic circulation. There are also lesser increases in the serum unconjugated bilirubin. This phenomenon is probably a reflection of the impaired uptake and conjugation and is due in part to the shortened life span of red blood cells often found in liver disease. In most patients with hepatitis and cirrhosis, the total serum bilirubin levels tend not to exceed 860 μmol/L (50 mg/dL). (For a summary of laboratory features in icteric states, see Table 294-3.) → *For detailed discussion, see Chaps. 295 to 298.*

EXTRAHEPATIC BILIARY OBSTRUCTION Anatomic or mechanical obstruction of the bile ducts is most commonly due to stones, tumors, or strictures. The clinical picture is quite similar to that of intrahepatic cholestasis, with pronounced elevations of the serum conjugated bilirubin and alkaline phosphatase levels. Usually, but not always, fever, pain, and chills may be present. In contrast to hepatitis and cirrhosis, the serum bilirubin level often tends to plateau and rarely exceeds levels of 600 μmol/L (35 mg/dL). The reason for this plateau is not clear but may be related to renal excretion of conjugated bilirubin or alternative pathways of bilirubin catabolism in obstructive jaundice.

Table 294-3

Laboratory Features in Icteric States

Bilirubin Disorder	Serum Bilirubin		Urine Bilirubin	Comments
	Unconjugated	Conjugated		
OVERPRODUCTION				
I. Hemolysis (intra- and extravascular)	↑	N	0	↑ Bilirubin turnover; serum bilirubin rarely exceeds 68 μmol/L (4 mg/dL)
II. Ineffective erythropoiesis	↑	N	0	Splenomegaly; normal RBC survival; normoblasts in marrow
DEFECTIVE HEPATIC UPTAKE				
I. Some drugs (e.g., flavaspidic acid, novobiocin)				
II. Gilbert's syndrome (some cases)	↑	N	0	Normal liver biopsy
DEFECTIVE CONJUGATION				
I. Neonatal jaundice	↑	Low	0	↓ Glucuronosyltransferase; ↓ conversion of bilirubin to urobilinogen
II. Gilbert's syndrome	↑	Low	0	↓ Glucuronosyltransferase and ↓ bilirubin uptake; some may have ↑ hemolysis; bile contains ↑ monoconjugates
III. Crigler, Najjar syndrome (types I and II)	↑	Low	0	Type I = absence of transferase Type II = deficiency of transferase; bile contains ↑↑ monoconjugates
DEFECTIVE EXCRETION				
I. Intrahepatic obstruction				
A. Familial syndromes				
1. Dubin-Johnson	↑	↑	+	Abnormal BSP curve, hepatic lipochrome pigment; ↑ urinary coproporphyrin type I
2. Rotor	↑	↑		No liver pigment; ↑ total urinary coproporphyrin
B. Drugs (e.g., chloramphenicol, methyltestosterone)	↑	↑	+	↑ Alkaline phosphatase but other function tests usually normal
C. Benign recurrent intrahepatic cholestasis	↑	↑	+	↑ Alkaline phosphatase
D. Recurrent jaundice of pregnancy (third trimester)	↑	↑	+	↑ Alkaline phosphatase; may be reproduced in afflicted subjects by estrogens or progesterone
II. Extrahepatic obstruction (tumors, stone, stricture of bile duct)				↑↑ Alkaline phosphatase (often > fourfold)
A. Partial	↑	↑	+	
B. Complete	↑	↑	+	
HEPATOCELLULAR DISEASE*				
I. Hepatitis	↑	↑	+	Conjugated/total serum bilirubin >50–70%; liver biopsy important for diagnosis
II. Cirrhosis: Same as hepatitis	↑	↑		

* Note that in hepatocellular disease there is generally an interference in all pathways of bilirubin metabolism (i.e., impaired uptake, conjugation, and excretion).

BENIGN RECURRENT INTRAHEPATIC CHOLESTASIS

DePAGTER AGF et al: Familial benign intrahepatic cholestasis. Gastroenterology 71:202, 1976

ENDO T et al: Bile acid metabolism in benign recurrent intrahepatic cholestasis. Gastroenterology 76:1002, 1979

DUBIN-JOHNSON AND ROTOR SYNDROMES

PAULUSMA CC et al: Congenital jaundice in rats with a mutation in a multidrug resistance-associated protein gene. Science 271:1126,1996

ROSENTHAL P et al: Homozygous Dubin-Johnson syndrome exhibits a characteristic serum bilirubin pattern. Hepatology 1:540, 1981

SWARTZ HM et al: On the nature and excretion of the hepatic pigment in the Dubin-Johnson syndrome. Gastroenterology 76:958, 1979

WOLPERT E et al: Abnormal sulfobromophthalein metabolism in Rotor's syndrome and obligate heterozygotes. N Engl J Med 206:1099, 1977

BILIRUBIN GLUCURONOSYL TRANSFERASE (UGT) DEFICIENCY STATES

AONO S et al: Analysis of genes for bilirubin UDP-glucuronosyltransferase in Gilbert's syndrome. Lancet 345:958, 1995

BOSMA PJ et al: The genetic basis of the reduced expression of UDP-glucuronosyltransferase 1 in Gilbert's syndrome. N Engl J Med 333:1171, 1995

BURCHELL B et al: Function and regulation of UDP-glucuronosyltransferase genes in health and liver disease. Hepatology 20:1622, 1994

CHOWDURY JR et al: Hereditary jaundice and disorders of bilirubin metabolism, in *The Metabolic and Molecular Bases of Inherited Disease*, 7th ed. CR Scriver et al (eds). New York, McGraw-Hill, 1995, pp 2161–2208

————, CHOWDURY NR: Unveiling the mysteries of inherited disorders of bilirubin glucuronidation. Gastroenterology 105:288, 1993

MONAGHAN G et al: Genetic variation in bilirubin UDP-glucuronosyltransferase gene promotor and Gilbert's syndrome. Lancet 347:578, 1996

RITTER JK et al: Identification of a genetic alteration in the code for bilirubin UDP-glucuronosyltransferase in the UGT1 gene complex of a Crigler-Najjar type I patient. J Clin Invest 90:150, 1992

SEPPEN J et al: Discrimination between Crigler-Najjar type I and II by expression of mutant bilirubin uridine diphosphate-glucuronosyltransferase. J Clin Invest 94:2385, 1994

SOEDA Y et al: Predicted homozygous missense mutation in Gilbert's syndrome. Lancet 346:1494, 1995

POSTOPERATIVE JAUNDICE

HOOTEGEM PV et al: Serum bilirubins in hepatobiliary disease: Comparison with other liver function tests and changes in the postobstructive period. Hepatology 5:112, 1985

LAMONT JT, ISSELBACHER KJ: Postoperative jaundice, in *Wright's Liver and Biliary Disease*, 3d ed, GH Millward-Sadler et al (eds). Philadelphia, Saunders, 1992, pp 1372–1380

295 *Jules L. Dienstag, Kurt J. Isselbacher*

ACUTE VIRAL HEPATITIS

Acute viral hepatitis is a systemic infection affecting the liver predominantly. Almost all cases of acute viral hepatitis are caused by one of five viral agents: hepatitis A virus (HAV), hepatitis B virus (HBV), hepatitis C virus (HCV), the HBV-associated delta agent or hepatitis D virus (HDV), and hepatitis E virus (HEV). A sixth agent, hepatitis G virus (HGV), has been discovered, but its role in acute viral hepatitis remains to be established. All these human hepatitis viruses are RNA viruses, except for hepatitis B, which is a DNA virus. Although these agents can be distinguished by their molecular and antigenic properties, all types of viral hepatitis produce clinically similar illnesses. These range from asymptomatic and inapparent to fulminant and fatal acute infections common to all types, on the one hand, and from subclinical persistent infections to rapidly progressive chronic liver disease with cirrhosis and even hepatocellular carcinoma, common to the blood-borne types (HBV, HCV, and HDV), on the other.

VIROLOGY AND ETIOLOGY   Hepatitis A   Hepatitis A virus is a nonenveloped 27-nm, heat-, acid-, and ether-resistant RNA virus in the hepatovirus genus of the picornavirus family (Fig. 295-1). Its virion contains four capsid polypeptides, designated VP1 to VP4, which are cleaved posttranslationally from the polyprotein product of a 7500-nucleotide genome. Inactivation of viral activity can be achieved by boiling for 1 min, by contact with formaldehyde and chlorine, or by ultraviolet irradiation. Despite nucleotide sequence variation of up to 20 percent among isolates of HAV, all strains of this virus are immunologically indistinguishable and belong to one serotype. Hepatitis A has an incubation period of approximately 4 weeks. Its replication is limited to the liver, but the virus is present in the liver, bile, stools, and blood during the late incubation period and acute preicteric phase of illness. Despite persistence of virus in the liver, viral shedding in feces, viremia, and infectivity diminish rapidly once jaundice becomes apparent. HAV is the only one of the human hepatitis viruses that can be cultivated in vitro.

Antibodies to HAV (anti-HAV) can be detected during acute illness when serum aminotransferase activity is elevated and fecal HAV shedding is still occurring. This early antibody response is predominantly of the IgM class and persists for several months, rarely for 6 to 12 months. During convalescence, however, anti-HAV of the IgG class becomes the predominant antibody (Fig. 295-2). Therefore, the diagnosis of hepatitis A is made during acute illness by demonstrating anti-HAV of the IgM class. Following acute illness, anti-HAV of the IgG class remains detectable indefinitely, and patients with serum anti-HAV are immune to reinfection. Indeed, neutralizing antibody activity parallels the appearance of anti-HAV, and the IgG anti-HAV present in immune globulin accounts for the protection it affords against HAV infection.

Hepatitis B   Hepatitis B virus is a DNA virus with a remarkably compact genomic structure; despite its small, circular, 3200-base-pair size, HBV DNA codes for four sets of viral products and has a complex, multiparticle structure. HBV achieves its genomic economy by relying on an efficient strategy of encoding proteins from four overlapping genes: S, C, P, and X (Fig. 295-3), as detailed below. Once thought to be unique among viruses, HBV is now recognized as one of a family of animal viruses, hepadnaviruses (hepatotropic DNA viruses), and is classified as hepadnavirus type 1. Similar viruses infect certain species of woodchucks, ground and tree squirrels, and Pekin ducks, to mention the most carefully characterized. Like HBV, all have the same distinctive three morphologic forms, have counterparts to the envelope and nucleocapsid virus antigens of HBV, replicate within the liver but exist in extrahepatic sites, contain their own endogenous DNA polymerase, have partially double-stranded and partially single-stranded genomes, are associated with acute and chronic hepatitis and hepatocellular carcinoma, and rely on a replicative strategy unique among DNA viruses but typical of retroviruses. Instead of DNA replication directly from a DNA template, hepadnaviruses rely on reverse transcription (effected by the DNA polymerase) of minus-strand DNA from a "pregenomic" RNA intermediate. Then plus-strand DNA is transcribed from the minus-strand DNA template by the DNA-dependent DNA polymerase. Viral proteins are translated by the pregenomic RNA, and the proteins and genome are packaged into virions and secreted from the hepatocyte. Although HBV is difficult to cultivate in vitro in the conventional sense from clinical material, several cell lines have been transfected with HBV DNA. Such transfected cells support in vitro replication of the intact virus and its component proteins.

Three particulate forms of HBV (Table 295-1) can be demonstrated by electron microscopy (see Fig. 295-1). The most numerous are the 22-nm particles, which appear as spherical or long filamentous forms; these are antigenically indistinguishable from the outer surface or envelope protein of HBV and are thought to represent excess viral envelope protein. Outnumbered in serum by a factor of 100 or 1000 to 1 compared with the spheres and tubules are large, 42-nm, double-shelled spherical particles, which represent the intact hepatitis B virion. The envelope protein expressed on the outer surface of the virion and on the smaller spherical and tubular structures is referred to as *hepatitis B surface antigen* (HBsAg). The concentration of HBsAg and virus

FIGURE 295-1 *A.* Electron micrograph of 27-nm hepatitis A virus particles purified from stool of a patient with acute hepatitis A virus infection and aggregated by hepatitis A antibody. *B.* Electron micrograph of concentrated serum from a patient with acute hepatitis B infection, demonstrating the 42-nm virions, tubular forms, and spherical 22-nm particles of hepatitis B surface antigen. 132,000×. (Hepatitis D resembles 42-nm virions of hepatitis B but is smaller, 35 to 37 nm; hepatitis E resembles hepatitis A virus but is slightly larger, 32 to 34 nm; hepatitis C has not been visualized definitively.)

particles in the blood may reach 500 µg/mL and 10 trillion particles per milliliter, respectively. The envelope protein, HBsAg, is the product of the S gene of HBV.

HBsAg consists primarily of two major polypeptides, one of 24,000 mol wt and its glycosylated counterpart of 28,000 mol wt. A number of different HBsAg subdeterminants have been identified. There is a common group-reactive antigen, *a*, shared by all HBsAg isolates. In addition, HBsAg may contain one of several subtype-specific antigens, namely, *d* or *y*, *w* or *r*, as well as other more recently characterized specificities. These HBsAg subtypes provide additional epidemiologic markers in evaluating the transmission of hepatitis B infection in that subtypes "breed true." For example, studies of hepatitis outbreaks have shown that index cases and their contacts have identical HBsAg subtypes. Clinical course and outcome, however, are independent of subtype.

Upstream of the S gene are the pre-S genes (Fig. 295-3), which code for pre-S gene products, including receptors on the HBV surface of polymerized human serum albumin and for hepatocyte membrane proteins. The pre-S region actually consists of both pre-S1 and pre-S2. Depending on where translation is initiated, three potential HBsAg gene products are synthesized. The protein product of the S gene is HBsAg (*major protein*), the product of the S region plus the adjacent pre-S2 region is the *middle protein*, and the product of the pre-S1 plus pre-S2 plus S regions is the *large protein*. Compared with the smaller spherical and tubular particles of HBV, complete 42-nm virions are enriched in the large protein. Both pre-S proteins and their respective antibodies can be detected during HBV infection, and the period of pre-S antigenemia appears to coincide with other markers of virus replication, as detailed below.

The intact 42-nm virion can be disrupted by mild detergents, and the 27-nm nucleocapsid core particle isolated. Nucleocapsid proteins

are coded for by the C gene. The antigen expressed on the surface of the nucleocapsid core is referred to as *hepatitis B core antigen* (HBcAg), and its corresponding antibody is anti-HBc. A third HBV antigen is *hepatitis B e antigen* (HBeAg), a soluble, nonparticulate, nucleocapsid protein that is immunologically distinct from intact HBcAg but is a product of the same C gene. The C gene has two initiation codons, a precore and a core region (Fig. 295-3). If translation is initiated at the precore region, the protein product is HBeAg, which has a signal peptide that binds it to the smooth endoplasmic reticulum and leads to its secretion into the circulation. If translation begins with the core region, HBcAg is the protein product; it has no signal peptide, it is not secreted, but it assembles into nucleocapsid particles, which bind to and incorporate RNA and which, ultimately, contain HBV DNA. Also packaged within the nucleocapsid core is a DNA polymerase, which directs replication and repair of HBV DNA. In vitro, the polymerase can repair the single-stranded gap and render it double-stranded; it directs the synthesis of plus-strand DNA from a minus-strand template. When packaging within viral proteins is complete, synthesis of the incomplete plus strand stops; this accounts for the single-stranded gap and for differences in the size of the gap. HBcAg particles remain in the hepatocyte, where they are readily detectable by immunohistochemical staining, and are exported after encapsidation by an envelope of HBsAg. Therefore, naked core parti-

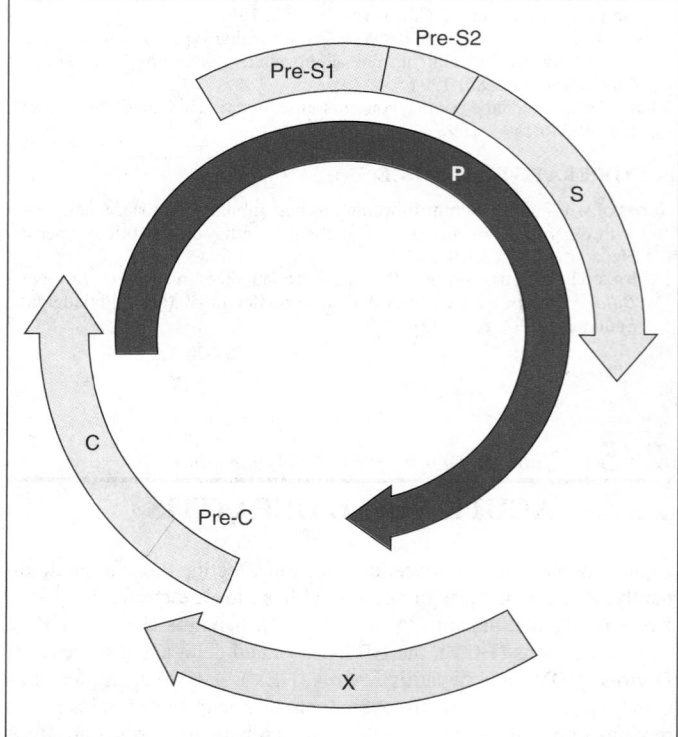

FIGURE 295-3 Its compact genomic structure, with overlapping genes, permits HBV to code for multiple proteins. The S gene codes for the "major" envelope protein, HBsAg. Pre-S1 and pre-S2, upstream of S, combine with S to code for two larger proteins, "middle" protein, the product of pre-S2 + S, and "large" protein, the product of pre-S1 + pre-S2 + S. The largest gene, P, codes for DNA polymerase. The C gene codes for two nucleocapsid proteins, HBeAg, a soluble, secreted protein (initiation from the pre-C region of the gene) and HBcAg, the intracellular core protein (initiation after pre-C). The X gene codes for HBxAg, which can transactivate the transcription of cellular and viral genes; its clinical relevance is not known.

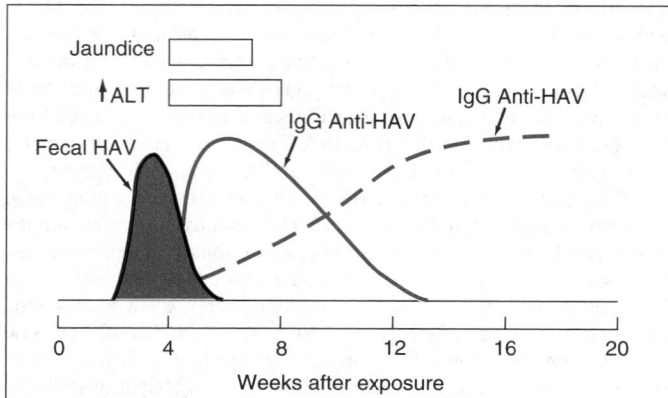

FIGURE 295-2 Scheme of typical clinical and laboratory features of viral hepatitis type A.

Table 295-1

Nomenclature and features of hepatitis viruses

Hepatitis Type	Virus Particle	Morphology	Genome*	Classification	Antigen(s)	Antibodies	Remarks
HAV	27 nm	Icosahedral nonenveloped	7.5-kb RNA, linear, ss, +	Hepatovirus	HAV	anti-HAV	Early fecal shedding Diagnosis: IgM anti-HAV Previous infection: IgG anti-HAV
HBV	42 nm	Double-shelled virion (surface and core) spherical	3.2-kb DNA, circular, ss/ds	Hepadnavirus	HBsAg HBcAg HBeAg	anti-HBs anti-HBc anti-HBe	Bloodborne virus; carrier state Acute diagnosis: HBsAg, IgM anti-HBc Chronic diagnosis: IgG anti-HBc, HBsAg Markers of replication: HBeAg, HBV DNA Liver, lymphocytes, other organs.
	27 nm	Nucleocapsid core			HBcAg HBeAg	anti-HBc anti-HBe	Nucleocapsid contains DNA and DNA polymerase; present in hepatocyte nucleus; HBcAg does not circulate; HBeAg (soluble, nonparticulate) and HBV DNA circulate—correlate with infectivity and complete virions.
	22 nm	Spherical and filamentous; represents excess virus coat material			HBsAg	anti-HBs	HBsAg detectable in >95% of patients with acute hepatitis B; found in serum, body fluids, hepatocyte cytoplasm; anti-HBs appears following infection—protective antibody.
HCV	Approx. 30–60 nm	Enveloped	9.4-kb RNA, linear, ss, +	Flavivirus-like	HCV C100-3 C33c C22-3 NS5	anti-HCV	Bloodborne agent, formerly labeled non-A, non-B hepatitis Acute diagnosis: anti-HCV (C33c, C22-3, NS5), HCV RNA Chronic diagnosis: anti-HCV (C100-3, C33c, C22-3, NS5) and HCV RNA; cytoplasmic location in hepatocytes
HDV	35–37 nm	Enveloped hybrid particle with HBsAg coat and HDV core	1.7-kb RNA, circular, ss, −	Resembles viroids and plant satellite viruses	HBsAg HDV antigen	anti-HBs anti-HDV	Defective RNA virus, requires helper function of HBV (hepadnaviruses); HDV antigen present in hepatocyte nucleus Diagnosis: anti-HDV, HDV RNA; HBV/HDV coinfection—IgM anti-HBc and anti-HDV; HDV superinfection—IgG anti-HBc and anti-HDV.
HEV	32–34 nm	Nonenveloped icosahedral	7.6-kb RNA, linear, ss, +	Alphavirus-like	HEV antigen	anti-HEV	Agent of enterically transmitted hepatitis; rare in USA; occurs in Asia, Mediterranean countries, Central America Diagnosis: IgM/IgG anti-HEV (assays being developed); virus in stool, bile, hepatocyte cytoplasm
HGV	?	?	9.4-kb RNA, linear, ss, +	Flavivirus-like	?	?	Bloodborne agent, definitive role as pathogen inconclusive Diagnosis: HGV RNA, serologic assays being developed

* ss, single-stranded; ss/ds, partially single-stranded, partially double-stranded; −, minus-stranded; +, plus-stranded.

cles do not circulate in the serum. The secreted nucleocapsid protein, HBeAg, provides a convenient, readily detectable, qualitative marker of HBV replication and relative infectivity.

HBsAg-positive serum containing HBeAg is more likely to be highly infectious and to be associated with the presence of hepatitis B virions (and DNA polymerase and HBV DNA, see below) than HBeAg-negative or anti-HBe-positive serum. For example, HBsAg carrier mothers who are HBeAg-positive almost invariably (>90 percent) transmit hepatitis B infection to their offspring, while HBsAg carrier mothers with anti-HBe rarely (10 to 15 percent) infect their offspring.

Early during the course of acute hepatitis B, HBeAg appears transiently; its disappearance may be a harbinger of clinical improvement and resolution of infection. Persistence of HBeAg in serum beyond the first 3 months of acute infection may be predictive of the development of chronic infection, and the presence of HBeAg during chronic hepatitis B is associated with ongoing viral replication, infectivity, and inflammatory liver injury.

The third of the HBV genes is the largest, the P gene (Fig. 295-3), which codes for the DNA polymerase; as noted above, this enzyme has both DNA-dependent DNA polymerase and RNA-dependent reverse transcriptase activities. The fourth gene, X, codes for a small, nonparticulate protein that has been shown to be capable of transactivating the transcription of both viral and cellular genes (Fig. 295-3). Such transactivation may enhance the replication of HBV, leading to the clinical association observed between the expression of the product of the X gene, hepatitis B x antigen (HBxAg), and antibodies to it in patients with severe chronic hepatitis and hepatocellular carcinoma. The transactivating activity can enhance the transcription of other viruses besides HBV, such as human immunodeficiency virus (HIV). Therefore, HBV may be responsible for enhanced replication of other viruses. Cellular processes transactivated by X include the human interferon γ gene and class I major histocompatibility genes; potentially, these effects could contribute to enhanced susceptibility of HBV-infected hepatocytes to cytolytic T cells. The X gene and its protein product, however, are absent in nonmammalian hepadnaviruses; therefore, X is not essential for hepadnavirus replication.

After infection with HBV, the first virologic marker detectable in serum is HBsAg (Fig. 295-4). Circulating HBsAg precedes elevations of serum aminotransferase activity and clinical symptoms and remains

FIGURE 295-4 Scheme of typical clinical and laboratory features of acute viral hepatitis type B.

detectable during the entire icteric or symptomatic phase of acute hepatitis B and beyond. In typical cases, HBsAg becomes undetectable 1 to 2 months following the onset of jaundice and rarely persists beyond 6 months. After HBsAg disappears, antibody to HBsAg (anti-HBs) becomes detectable in serum and remains detectable indefinitely thereafter. Because HBcAg is sequestered within an HBsAg coat, HBcAg is not detectable routinely in the serum of patients with HBV infection. On the other hand, anti-HBc is readily demonstrable in serum, beginning within the first 1 to 2 weeks after the appearance of HBsAg and preceding detectable levels of anti-HBs by weeks to months. Because variability exists in the time of appearance of anti-HBs following HBV infection, occasionally a gap of several weeks or longer may separate the disappearance of HBsAg and the appearance of anti-HBs. During this "gap" or "window" period, anti-HBc may represent serologic evidence of current or recent HBV infection, and blood containing anti-HBc in the absence of HBsAg and anti-HBs has been implicated in the development of transfusion-associated hepatitis B. In part because the sensitivity of immunoassays for HBsAg and anti-HBs has increased, however, this window period is rarely encountered. In some persons, years after HBV infection, anti-HBc may persist in the circulation longer than anti-HBs. Therefore, isolated anti-HBc does not necessarily indicate active virus replication; most instances of isolated anti-HBc represent hepatitis B infection in the remote past. Rarely, however, isolated anti-HBc represents low-level hepatitis B viremia, with HBsAg below the detection threshold; occasionally, isolated anti-HBc represents a cross-reacting or false-positive immunologic specificity. Distinction between recent and remote HBV infection can be accomplished by determination of the immunoglobulin class of anti-HBc. Anti-HBc of the IgM class (IgM anti-HBc) predominates during the first 6 months approximately after acute infection, whereas IgG anti-HBc is the predominant class of anti-HBc beyond 6 months. Therefore, patients with current or recent acute hepatitis B, including those in the anti-HBc window, have IgM anti-HBc in their serum. In patients who have recovered from hepatitis B in the remote past as well as those with chronic HBV infection, anti-HBc is predominantly of the IgG class. Infrequently, in no more than 1 to 5 percent of patients with acute HBV infection, levels of HBsAg are too low to be detected; in such cases, the presence of IgM anti-HBc establishes the diagnosis of acute hepatitis B. When isolated anti-HBc occurs in the rare patient with chronic hepatitis B whose HBsAg level is below the sensitivity threshold of contemporary immunoassays (a low-level carrier), the anti-HBc is of the IgG class. Generally, in persons who have recovered from hepatitis B, anti-HBs and anti-HBc persist indefinitely.

The temporal association between the appearance of anti-HBs and resolution of HBV infection as well as the observation that persons

with anti-HBs in serum are protected against reinfection with HBV suggest that *anti-HBs is the protective antibody*. Therefore, strategies for prevention of HBV infection are based on providing susceptible persons with circulating anti-HBs (see below). Occasionally, in 10 to 20 percent of patients with chronic hepatitis B, low-level, low-affinity anti-HBs can be detected. This antibody is directed against a subtype determinant different from that represented by the patient's HBsAg; its presence is thought to reflect the stimulation of a related clone of antibody-forming cells, but it has no clinical relevance and does not signal imminent clearance of hepatitis B.

The other readily detectable serologic marker of HBV infection, HBeAg, appears concurrently with or shortly after HBsAg. Its appearance coincides temporally with high levels of virus replication and reflects the presence of circulating intact virions, DNA polymerase, and HBV DNA. Pre-S1 and pre-S2 proteins are also expressed during periods of peak replication, but assays for these gene products are not routinely available. In self-limited HBV infections, HBeAg becomes undetectable shortly after peak elevations in aminotransferase activity, before the disappearance of HBsAg, and anti-HBe then becomes detectable, coinciding with a period of relatively lower infectivity (see Fig. 295-4). Because markers of HBV replication appear transiently during acute infection, testing for such markers is of little clinical utility in typical cases of acute HBV infection. In contrast, markers of HBV replication provide valuable information in patients with protracted infections. Departing from the pattern typical of acute HBV infections, in chronic HBV infection, HBsAg remains detectable beyond 6 months, anti-HBc is primarily of the IgG class, and anti-HBs is either undetectable or detectable at low levels (see "Laboratory Features," below) (Fig. 295-5). During early chronic HBV infection, HBV DNA can be detected both in serum and in hepatocyte nuclei, where it is present in free or episomal form. This *replicative stage* of HBV infection is the time of maximal infectivity and liver injury; HBeAg is a qualitative marker and HBV DNA a quantitative marker of this replicative phase, during which all three forms of HBV circulate, including intact virions. Over time, the replicative phase of chronic HBV infection gives way to a relatively *nonreplicative phase*. This occurs at a rate of approximately 10 percent per year and is accompanied by seroconversion from HBeAg-positive to anti-HBe-positive. In most cases, this seroconversion coincides with a transient, acute hepatitis–like elevation in aminotransferase activity, believed to reflect cell-mediated clearance of virus-infected hepatocytes. In the nonreplicative phase of chronic infection, when HBV DNA is demonstrable in hepatocyte nuclei, it tends to be integrated into the host genome. In this phase, only spherical and tubular forms of HBV, *not intact*

FIGURE 295-5 Scheme of typical laboratory features of chronic viral hepatitis type B. HBeAg and HBV DNA can be detected in serum during the *replicative phase* of chronic infection, which is associated with infectivity and liver injury. Seroconversion from the replicative phase to the *nonreplicative phase* occurs at a rate of approximately 10 to 15 percent per year and is heralded by an acute hepatitis–like elevation of ALT activity; during the nonreplicative phase, infectivity and liver injury are limited.

virions, circulate, and liver injury tends to subside. Most such patients would be characterized as asymptomatic HBV *carriers*. In reality, the designations *replicative* and *nonreplicative* are only relative; even in the so-called nonreplicative phase, HBV replication can be detected with highly sensitive amplification probes such as the polymerase chain reaction. Still, the distinctions are pathophysiologically and clinically meaningful. Occasionally, nonreplicative HBV infection converts back to replicative infection. Such spontaneous reactivations are accompanied by reexpression of HBeAg and HBV DNA as well as by exacerbations of liver injury.

Molecular variants of HBV have been recognized. Variation occurs throughout the HBV genome, and clinical isolates of HBV that do not express typical viral proteins have been attributed to mutations in individual or even multiple gene locations. For example, variants have been described that lack nucleocapsid proteins, envelope proteins, or both. Two categories of HBV have attracted the most attention. One of these was identified initially in Mediterranean countries among patients with an unusual serologic-clinical profile. They have severe chronic HBV infection and detectable HBV DNA but with anti-HBe instead of HBeAg. These patients were found to be infected with an HBV mutant that contained an alteration in the precore region rendering the virus incapable of encoding HBeAg. Although several potential mutation sites exist in the pre-C region, the region of the C gene necessary for the expression of HBeAg (see "Virology and Etiology," above), the most commonly encountered in such patients is a single base substitution, from G to A, which occurs in the second to last codon of the pre-C gene at nucleotide 1896. This substitution results in the replacement of the TGG tryptophan codon by a stop codon (TAG), which prevents the translation of HBeAg. Another mutation in the core promoter region prevents transcription of the coding region for HBeAg and yields an HBeAg-negative phenotype. Patients with such precore mutants that are unable to secrete HBeAg tend to have severe liver disease that progresses rapidly to cirrhosis and that does not respond readily to antiviral therapy. Both "wild-type" HBV and precore mutant HBV can coexist in the same patient, or mutant HBV may arise during wild-type HBV infection. In addition, clusters of fulminant hepatitis B in Israel and Japan have been attributed to common-source infection with a precore mutant. Fulminant hepatitis B in North America and western Europe, however, occurs in patients infected with wild-type HBV, in the absence of precore mutants, and both precore mutants and other mutations throughout the HBV genome occur commonly even in patients with typical, self-limited, milder forms of HBV infection. Therefore, additional investigation will be necessary to define the effect of precore mutants on the pathogenicity and natural history of HBV infection.

The second important category of HBV mutants consists of *escape mutants*, in which a single amino acid substitution, from glycine to arginine, occurs at position 145 of the immunodominant *a* determinant common to all subtypes of HBsAg. This change in HBsAg leads to a critical conformational change that results in a loss of neutralizing activity by anti-HBs. This specific HBV/*a* mutant has been observed in two situations, active and passive immunization, in which humoral immunologic pressure may favor evolutionary change ("escape") in the virus—in a small number of hepatitis B vaccine recipients who acquired HBV infection despite the prior appearance of neutralizing anti-HBs and in liver transplant recipients who underwent the procedure for hepatitis B and who were treated with a high-potency human monoclonal anti-HBs preparation. Although such mutants have not been appreciated frequently, their existence raises a concern that may complicate vaccination strategies and serologic diagnosis.

Hepatitis B antigens and HBV DNA have been identified in extrahepatic sites, including lymph nodes, bone marrow, circulating lymphocytes, spleen, and pancreas. Although the virus does not appear to be associated with tissue injury in any of these extrahepatic sites, its presence in these "remote" reservoirs has been invoked to explain the recurrence of HBV infection after orthotopic liver transplantation. A more complete understanding of the clinical relevance of extrahepatic HBV remains to be defined.

Hepatitis D The delta hepatitis agent, or HDV, is a defective RNA virus that coinfects with and requires the helper function of HBV (or other hepadnaviruses) for its replication and expression. Slightly smaller than HBV, delta is a formalin-sensitive, 35- to 37-nm virus with a hybrid structure. Its nucleocapsid expresses delta antigen, which bears no antigenic homology with any of the HBV antigens, and contains the virus genome. The delta core is "encapsidated" by an outer envelope of HBsAg, indistinguishable from that of HBV except in its relative compositions of major, middle, and large HBsAg component proteins. The genome is a small, 1700-nucleotide, circular, single-stranded RNA (minus strand) that is nonhomologous with HBV DNA (except for a small area of the polymerase gene) but that has features and the rolling circle model of replication common to genomes of plant satellite viruses or viroids. HDV RNA contains many areas of internal complementarity; therefore, it can fold on itself by internal base pairing to form an unusual, very stable, rodlike structure. HDV RNA replicates via RNA-directed RNA synthesis by transcription of genomic RNA to a complementary antigenomic (plus strand) RNA; the antigenomic RNA, in turn, serves as a template for subsequent genomic RNA synthesis. Between the genomic and antigenomic RNAs of HDV, there are coding regions for nine proteins. Delta antigen, which is a product of the antigenomic strand, exists in two forms, a small, 195-amino-acid species, which plays a role in facilitating HDV RNA replication, and a large, 214-amino-acid species, which appears to suppress replication but is required for assembly of the antigen into virions. Although complete hepatitis D virions and liver injury require the cooperative helper function of HBV, intracellular replication of HDV RNA can occur without HBV. Genomic heterogeneity among HDV isolates has been described; however, pathophysiologic and clinical consequences of this genetic diversity have not been recognized.

HDV can either infect a person simultaneously with HBV (*coinfection*) or superinfect a person already infected with HBV (*superinfection*); when HDV infection is transmitted from a donor with one HBsAg subtype to an HBsAg-positive recipient with a different subtype, the HDV agent assumes the HBsAg subtype of the recipient, rather than the donor. Because HDV relies absolutely on HBV, the duration of HDV infection is determined by the duration of (and cannot outlast) HBV infection. HDV antigen is expressed primarily in hepatocyte nuclei and is occasionally detectable in serum. During acute HDV infection, anti-HDV of the IgM class predominates, and 30 to 40 days may elapse after symptoms appear before anti-HDV can be detected. In self-limited infection, anti-HDV is low titer and transient, rarely remaining detectable beyond the clearance of HBsAg and HDV antigen. In chronic HDV infection, anti-HDV circulates in high titer, and both IgM and IgG anti-HDV can be detected. HDV antigen in the liver and HDV RNA in serum and liver can be detected during HDV replication.

Hepatitis C Hepatitis C virus, which, before its identification was labeled "non-A, non-B hepatitis," is a linear, single-stranded, positive-sense, 9500-nucleotide RNA virus, the genome of which is similar in organization to that of flaviviruses and pestiviruses; HCV constitutes its own genus in the family Flaviviridae. The HCV genome contains a single large open reading frame (gene) that codes for a virus polyprotein of approximately 3000 amino acids. The 5' end of the genome consists of an untranslated region adjacent to the genes for structural proteins, the nucleocapsid core protein and two envelope glycoproteins, E1 and E2/NS1. The 5' untranslated region and core gene are highly conserved among genotypes, but the envelope proteins are coded for by the hypervariable region, which varies from isolate to isolate and may allow the virus to evade host immunologic containment directed at accessible virus-envelop proteins. The 3' end of the genome contains the genes for nonstructural (NS) proteins. The first reported HCV clone, 5-1-1, and the nucleotide sequence coding for C100-3, the recombinant virus protein used in the first immunoassay for antibodies to HCV, reside within the NS4 gene, and the RNA-dependent RNA polymerase, through which HCV replicates, is encoded by the NS5 region (Fig. 295-6). Because HCV does not replicate via a DNA

FIGURE 295-6 Organization of the hepatitis C virus genome and its associated proteins. Structural genes at the 5′ end include the nucleocapsid region, C, and the envelope regions, E1 and E2. The 5′ untranslated region and the C region are highly conserved among isolates, while the envelope domain E2/NS1 contains the hypervariable region. At the 3′ end are five nonstructural (NS) regions. Viral proteins included in the first-generation (C100-3), second-generation (C200, a fusion protein of C100-3 and C33c, and C22-3), and third-generation (C22-3, C200, or C33c and C100-3, and NS5) immunoassays and in the recombinant immunoblot assay (5-1-1, C100-3, C33c, C22-3, NS5) are presented below their corresponding genes (AA = amino acid).

intermediate, it does not integrate into the host genome. Because HCV tends to circulate in very low titer, visualization of virus particles has been difficult. Although in vitro HCV replication remains difficult to accomplish convincingly, the chimpanzee has proven to be an invaluable experimental animal model.

At least six distinct genotypes, as well as subtypes within genotypes, of HCV have been identified by nucleotide sequencing. Because divergence of HCV isolates within a genotype or subtype, and within the same host, may vary insufficiently to define a distinct genotype, these intragenotypic differences are referred to as *quasispecies*. The genotypic and quasispecies diversity of HCV, resulting from its high mutation rate, interferes with effective humoral immunity. Neutralizing antibodies to HCV have been demonstrated, but they tend to be short-lived, and HCV infection has not been shown to induce lasting immunity against reinfection with different virus isolates or even the same virus isolate. Thus, neither *heterologous* nor *homologous* immunity appears to develop after acute HCV infection. Some HCV genotypes are distributed worldwide, while others are more geographically confined. In addition, differences in pathogenicity and responsiveness to antiviral therapy have been reported among genotypes; however, the biological impact of genotype and quasispecies differences remains incompletely defined.

As noted above, the first assay detected antibodies to C100-3, a recombinant polypeptide derived from the NS4 region of the genome. In most patients with acute hepatitis C, antibody detected with this assay appears between 1 to 3 months after the onset of acute hepatitis but sometimes not for a year or longer. Second-generation assays incorporate recombinant proteins from the nucleocapsid core region, C22-3, and the NS3 region, C33c (expressed in combination with C100-3 as C200); these assays are more sensitive (by approximately 20 percent) and detect anti-HCV 30 to 90 days earlier, during the period of acute hepatitis. A third-generation immunoassay, which incorporates proteins from the NS5 region and replaces some recombinant proteins with synthetic peptides, may detect anti-HCV even earlier. Because nonspecificity has been encountered in clinical samples tested for anti-HCV, a supplementary recombinant immunoblot assay was introduced. Reactivity in an immunoassay is "confirmed" by incubation with a nitrocellulose strip that contains individual bands of recombinant or synthetic HCV proteins. This approach allows the demonstration of individual antibodies to nonstructural and structural viral proteins and identifies false-positive reactivity associated with nonviral specificities. It is useful to support the validity of anti-HCV-

reactive samples, especially in patients with a low prior probability of true infection (e.g., blood donors) or in patients with confounding activity in serum (such as a rheumatoid factor) that may yield false-positive antibody reactivity. Still, detection of anti-HCV is insufficient to identify all persons infected with HCV. The most sensitive indicator is the presence of HCV RNA, which requires molecular amplification by polymerase chain reaction (PCR) (Fig. 295-7). An alternative method for detection of HCV RNA, more easily automated but one or two orders of magnitude less sensitive, is branched-chain complementary DNA hybridization. HCV RNA can be detected within a few days of exposure to HCV, well before the appearance of anti-HCV, and tends to persist for the duration of HCV infection; however, in patients with chronic HCV infection, occasionally, HCV RNA may be detectable only intermittently. Application of sensitive molecular probes for HCV RNA has revealed the presence of replicative HCV in peripheral blood lymphocytes of infected persons; however, as is the case for HBV in lymphocytes, the clinical relevance of HCV lymphocyte infection is not known.

Hepatitis E Previously labeled *epidemic* or *enterically transmitted non-A, non-B hepatitis*, HEV is an enterically transmitted virus that occurs primarily in India, Asia, Africa, and Central America. This agent, with epidemiologic features resembling those of hepatitis A, is a 32- to 34-nm, nonenveloped, HAV-like virus with a 7600-nucleotide, single-stranded, positive-sense RNA genome. HEV has three open reading frames (genes), the largest of which encodes nonstructural proteins involved in virus replication. A middle-sized gene encodes the nucleocapsid protein, and the smallest, whose function is not known, encodes protein specificities to which antibodies appear in human serum. All HEV isolates appear to belong to a single serotype, despite genomic heterogeneity of up to 25 percent. There is no genomic or antigenic homology, however, between HEV and HAV or other picornaviruses, and HEV, although resembling caliciviruses, appears to be sufficiently distinct from any known agent to merit a new classification of its own within the alphavirus group. The virus has been detected in stool, bile, and liver from infected patients as well as from experimentally infected nonhuman primates. Studies in humans and experimental animals have shown that HEV is excreted in the stool during the late incubation period and that immune responses to viral antigens occur very early during the course of acute infection. Both IgM anti-HEV and IgG anti-HEV can be detected, but both fall rapidly after acute infection, reaching low levels within 9 to 12 months. Currently, serologic testing for HEV infection is not available routinely.

Hepatitis G A sixth hepatitis virus was discovered independently by two different groups, one calling it hepatitis G (HGV), the other calling it GB virus C (GBV-C; a viral agent isolated in the 1960s from a surgeon with viral hepatitis and transmitted in tamarins). This

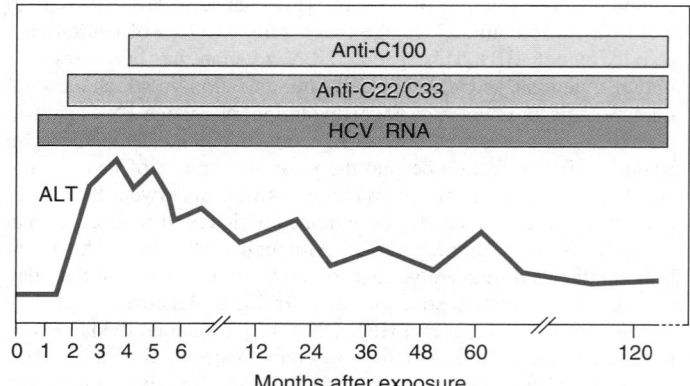

FIGURE 295-7 Scheme of typical laboratory features during acute hepatitis type C progressing to chronicity. HCV RNA is the first detectable event, preceding ALT elevation and the appearance of anti-HCV. The appearance of antibody to C100, detectable with first-generation assays, is delayed from 1 to 3 months after the appearance of antibody to C22 and C33, antibodies that are included in second-generation immunoassays. Anti-HCV detectable with second-generation assays appears during acute hepatitis C.

agent may contribute to cases of acute and chronic viral hepatitis unaccounted for by the other five hepatitis viruses. Like HCV, HGV is a bloodborne RNA virus with a flavivirus-like genomic structure. Its 2900-amino-acid polyprotein is encoded by a 9400 nucleotide genome, the 5′ end of which codes for structural (nucleocapsid and envelope) proteins and the 3′ end of which codes for nonstructural proteins with replicative function (helicase, protease, and RNA polymerase). HGV and GBV-C share almost complete nucleotide and amino acid sequence homology, and they are distantly related to HCV (approximate nucleotide homology of 25 percent), from which they diverged evolutionarily in the remote past. Infection with this agent, identified reliably by PCR amplification of RNA (much less reliably by antibody testing), occurs in approximately 1.5 percent of blood donors, is transmitted by blood transfusion, and can be detected in some patients with acute, chronic, and fulminant hepatitis. Data available to date, however, indicate that a sizable proportion of clinically apparent HGV infections occur in patients coinfected with hepatitis C, that HGV does not alter the severity of hepatitis C, and that most isolated instances of HGV infection are not associated with acute or chronic liver injury. Thus, although HGV may play a small role in viral hepatitis and may be transmitted by transfusion, its contribution to acute and chronic liver disease requires better definition.

PATHOGENESIS Under ordinary circumstances, none of the hepatitis viruses is known to be directly cytopathic to hepatocytes. Evidence suggests that the clinical manifestations and outcomes following acute liver injury associated with viral hepatitis are determined by the immunologic responses of the host. Among the viral hepatitides, the immunopathogenesis of hepatitis B has been studied most extensively. Certainly for this agent, the existence of asymptomatic hepatitis B carriers with normal liver histology and function suggests that the virus is not directly cytopathic. The facts that lymphoid cells are juxtaposed with necrotic hepatocytes in the livers of patients with liver injury and that patients with defects in cellular immune competence are more likely to remain chronically infected rather than to clear the virus are cited to support the role of cellular immune responses in the pathogenesis of hepatitis B–related liver injury. The model that has the most experimental support involves cytolytic T cells sensitized specifically to recognize host and hepatitis B viral antigens on the liver cell surface. Although HBsAg was initially thought to be the most likely viral target antigen on the hepatocyte surface, recent laboratory observations suggest that nucleocapsid proteins (HBcAg and possibly HBeAg), present on the cell membrane in minute quantities, are the viral target antigens that, with host antigens, invite cytolytic T cells to destroy HBV-infected hepatocytes. Still, this hypothesis is insufficient to explain differences in outcomes between those who recover after acute hepatitis and those who progress to chronic hepatitis or between those with mild and severe (fulminant) acute HBV infection. As convincing as are the cumulative data supporting nucleocapsid proteins as the target of cell-mediated immunologic injury, attention has been refocused on the envelope protein, HBsAg, by the demonstration that in transgenic mice with the gene for HBsAg inserted into their genomes, cytolytic T cells directed against HBsAg can be shown to destroy hepatocytes. Therefore, HBsAg cannot be dismissed as a potential immunologic target.

Moreover, debate continues over the relative importance of viral and host factors in the pathogenesis of HBV-associated liver injury and its outcome. As noted above, precore genetic mutants of HBV have been associated with the more severe outcomes of HBV infection (severe chronic and fulminant hepatitis), suggesting that, under certain circumstances, relative pathogenicity is a property of the virus, not the host. The fact that concomitant HDV and HBV infections are associated with more severe liver injury than HBV infection alone and the fact that cells transfected in vitro with the gene for HDV (delta) antigen express HDV antigen and then become necrotic in the absence of any immunologic influences are also consistent with a viral effect on pathogenicity. Similarly, in patients who undergo liver transplantation for end-stage chronic HBV infection, occasionally, rapidly progressive liver injury appears in the new liver. This clinical pattern is associated with an unusual histologic pattern in the new

liver, *fibrosing cholestatic hepatitis*, which, ultrastructurally, appears to represent a choking of the cell with overwhelming quantities of HBsAg. This observation suggests that under the influence of the potent immunosuppressive agents required to prevent allograft rejection, HBV may have a direct cytopathic effect on liver cells, independent of the immune system.

Although the precise mechanism of liver injury in HBV infection remains elusive, studies of nucleocapsid proteins have shed light on the profound immunologic tolerance to HBV of babies born to mothers with highly replicative (HBeAg-positive), chronic HBV infection. In HBeAg-expressing transgenic mice, in utero exposure to HBeAg, which is sufficiently small to traverse the placenta, induces T cell tolerance to both nucleocapsid proteins. This, in turn, may explain why, when infection occurs so early in life, immunologic clearance does not occur, and protracted, lifelong infection ensues.

Immune complex–mediated tissue damage appears to play a pathogenetic role in the extrahepatic manifestations of acute hepatitis B. The occasional prodromal serum sickness–like syndrome observed in acute hepatitis B appears to be related to the deposition in tissue blood vessel walls of circulating immune complexes leading to activation of the complement system. The clinical consequences are urticarial rash, angioedema, fever, and arthritis. During the early prodrome of HBV infection in these patients, HBsAg in high titer in association with small amounts of anti-HBs leads to the formation of soluble, circulating immune complexes (in antigen excess). Complement components in the serum are depressed during the arthritic phase of the illness and are also detectable in the circulating immune complexes. In addition to complement components, these complexes contain HBsAg, anti-HBs, IgG, IgM, IgA, and fibrin. After the patient recovers from the serum sickness–like syndrome, these immune complexes disappear.

In patients with chronic hepatitis B, other types of immune-complex disease may be seen. Glomerulonephritis with the nephrotic syndrome is occasionally observed; HBsAg, immunoglobulin, and C3 deposition has been found in the glomerular basement membrane. While polyarteritis nodosa develops in considerably fewer than 1 percent of patients with HBV infection, 20 to 30 percent of patients with polyarteritis nodosa have HBsAg in serum. In these patients, the affected small and medium-sized arterioles have been shown to contain HBsAg, immunoglobulins, and complement components. Another extrahepatic manifestation of viral hepatitis, essential mixed cryoglobulinemia (EMC), was reported initially to be associated with hepatitis B. The disorder is characterized clinically by arthritis and cutaneous vasculitis (palpable purpura) and serologically by the presence of circulating cryoprecipitable immune complexes of more than one immunoglobulin class. Many patients with this syndrome have chronic liver disease, but the association with HBV infection has always been controversial. Recent reevaluation of patients with EMC suggests instead that a substantial proportion have chronic HCV infection. Their circulating immune complexes contain HCV RNA at a concentration that exceeds its serum concentration; this observation argues against secondary trapping of HCV in the immune complexes and favors a primary role for the virus in the pathogenesis of EMC.

PATHOLOGY The typical morphologic lesions of all types of viral hepatitis are similar and consist of panlobular infiltration with mononuclear cells, hepatic cell necrosis, hyperplasia of Kupffer cells, and variable degrees of cholestasis. Hepatic cell regeneration is present, as evidenced by numerous mitotic figures, multinucleated cells, and "rosette" or "pseudoacinar" formation. The mononuclear infiltration consists primarily of small lymphocytes, although plasma cells and eosinophils are occasionally seen. Liver cell damage consists of hepatic cell degeneration and necrosis, cell dropout, ballooning of cells, and acidophilic degeneration of hepatocytes (forming so-called Councilman-like bodies). Large hepatocytes with a ground glass appearance of the cytoplasm may be seen in chronic but not in acute HBV infection; these cells have been shown to contain HBsAg and can be identified histochemically with orcein or aldehyde fuchsin. In uncomplicated viral hepatitis, the reticulin framework is preserved.

In hepatitis C, the histologic lesion is often remarkable for a relative paucity of inflammation, a marked increase in activation of sinusoidal lining cells, lymphoid aggregates, the presence of fat, and, occasionally, bile duct lesions in which biliary epithelial cells appear to be piled up without interruption of the basement membrane. Occasionally, microvesicular steatosis occurs in hepatitis D. In hepatitis E, a common histologic feature is marked cholestasis. A cholestatic variant of slowly resolving acute hepatitis A also has been described.

A more severe histologic lesion, *bridging hepatic necrosis*, also termed *subacute* or *confluent necrosis*, is occasionally observed in some patients with acute hepatitis. "Bridging" between lobules results from large areas of hepatic cell dropout, with collapse of the reticulin framework. Characteristically, the bridge consists of condensed reticulum, inflammatory debris, and degenerating liver cells that span adjacent portal areas, portal to central veins, or central vein to central vein. This lesion had been thought to have prognostic significance; in many of the originally described patients with this lesion, a subacute course terminated in death within several weeks to months, or severe chronic hepatitis and postnecrotic cirrhosis developed. More recent investigations have failed to uphold the association between bridging necrosis and such a poor prognosis in patients with acute hepatitis. Although the frequency of bridging may be higher among hospitalized patients with severe acute hepatitis, and although cirrhosis, chronic hepatitis, and even death have been observed in this group, the frequency of bridging necrosis in uncomplicated acute viral hepatitis is probably on the order of 1 to 5 percent. Prospective studies have failed to demonstrate a difference in prognosis between patients with acute hepatitis who have bridging necrosis and those who do not. Therefore,

although demonstration of this lesion in patients with chronic hepatitis has prognostic significance (see Chap. 297), its demonstration during acute hepatitis is less meaningful, and liver biopsies to identify this lesion are no longer undertaken routinely in patients with acute hepatitis. In *massive hepatic necrosis* (fulminant hepatitis, acute yellow atrophy), the striking feature at postmortem examination is the finding of a small, shrunken, and soft liver. Histologic examination reveals massive necrosis and dropout of liver cells of most lobules with extensive collapse and condensation of the reticulin framework.

Immunofluorescence and immunoperoxidase antibody studies have localized HBsAg to the cytoplasm and plasma membrane of infected liver cells. In contrast, HBcAg predominates in the nucleus, but occasionally, scant amounts are also seen in the cytoplasm and on the cell membrane. Electron-microscopic studies of liver biopsy material have demonstrated the presence of HBsAg particles in the cytoplasm and HBcAg particles in the nucleus of liver cells during hepatitis B infection. These morphologic observations suggest that DNA is synthesized and packaged within core particles in the nucleus, while the envelope is assembled in the cytoplasm, resulting in the formation of intact hepatitis B virus. HDV antigen is localized to the hepatocyte nucleus, while HAV, HCV, and HEV antigens are localized to the cytoplasm.

EPIDEMIOLOGY Prior to the availability of serologic tests for hepatitis viruses, all viral hepatitis cases were labeled either as "infectious" or "serum" hepatitis. Modes of transmission overlap, however, and *a clear distinction among the different types of viral hepatitis cannot be made solely on the basis of clinical or epidemiologic features* (Table 295-2). The most accurate means to distinguish the various types of viral hepatitis involves specific serologic testing.

Hepatitis A *This agent is transmitted almost exclusively by the fecal-oral route.* Person-to-person spread of HAV is enhanced by poor personal hygiene and overcrowding, and large outbreaks as well as sporadic cases have been traced to contaminated food, water, milk, and shellfish. Intrafamily and intrainstitutional spread are also com-

Table 295-2

Clinical and Epidemiologic Features of Viral Hepatitis

Feature	HAV	HBV	HCV	HDV	HEV
Incubation (days)	15–45, mean 30	30–180, mean 60–90	15–160, mean 50	30–180, mean 60–90	14–60, mean 40
Onset	Acute	Insidious or acute	Insidious	Insidious or acute	Acute
Age preference	Children, young adults	Young adults (sexual and percutaneous), babies, toddlers	Any age, but more common in adults	Any age (similar to HBV)	Young adults (20–40 years)
Transmission:					
Fecal-oral	+++	−	−	−	+++
Percutaneous	Unusual	+++	+++	+++	−
Perinatal	−	+++	±[a]	+	−
Sexual	±	++	±[a]	++	−
Clinical:					
Severity	Mild	Occasionally severe	Moderate	Occasionally severe	Mild
Fulminant	0.1%	0.1–1%	0.1%	5–20%[b]	1–2%[e]
Progression to chronicity	None	Occasional (1–10%) (90% of neonates)	Common (50–70% chronic hepatitis; 80–90% chronic infection)	Common[d]	None
Carrier	None	0.1–30%[c]	0.5–1.0%	Variable[f]	None
Cancer	None	+ (neonatal infection)	+	±	None
Prognosis	Excellent	Worse with age, debility	Moderate	Acute, good Chronic, poor	Good
Prophylaxis	IG Inactivated vaccine	HBIG Recombinant vaccine	None	HBV vaccine (none for HBV carriers)	Unknown
Therapy	None	Interferon 40% effective	Interferon 50% response; sustained response <15%	Unknown	None

[a] Primarily with HIV coinfection and high-level viremia in index case; risk approximately 5 percent.
[b] Up to 5% in acute HBV/HDV coinfection; up to 20% in HDV superinfection of chronic HBV infection.
[c] Varies considerably throughout the world and in subpopulations within countries; see text.
[d] In acute HBV/HDV coinfection, the frequency of chronicity is the same as that for HBV; in HDV superinfection, chronicity is invariable.
[e] 10–20% in pregnant women.
[f] Common in Mediterranean countries, rare in North America and western Europe.

mon. Early epidemiologic observations suggested that there is a predilection for hepatitis A to occur in late fall and early winter. In temperate zones, epidemic waves have been recorded every 5 to 20 years as new segments of nonimmune population appeared; however, in developed countries, the incidence of type A hepatitis has been declining, presumably as a function of improved sanitation, and these cyclic patterns are no longer being observed. No HAV carrier state has been identified after acute type A hepatitis; perpetuation of the virus in nature depends presumably on nonepidemic, inapparent subclinical infection.

In the general population, anti-HAV, an excellent marker for previous HAV infection, increases in prevalence as a function of increasing age and of decreasing socioeconomic status. In the 1970s, serologic evidence of prior hepatitis A infection occurred in about 40 percent of urban populations in the United States, most of whom never recalled having had a symptomatic case of hepatitis. In subsequent decades, however, the prevalence of anti-HAV has been declining in the United States. In developing countries, exposure, infection, and subsequent immunity are almost universal in childhood. As the frequency of subclinical childhood infections declines in developed countries, a susceptible cohort of adults emerges. Hepatitis A tends to be more symptomatic in adults; therefore, paradoxically, as the frequency of HAV infection declines, the likelihood of clinically apparent, even severe, HAV illnesses increases in the susceptible adult population. Travel to endemic areas is a common source of infection for adults from nonendemic areas. More recently recognized epidemiologic foci of HAV infection include child-care centers, neonatal intensive care units, promiscuous homosexual men, and intravenous drug users. Although hepatitis A is rarely bloodborne, several outbreaks have been recognized in recipients of clotting factor concentrates.

Hepatitis B It has long been recognized that a major route of hepatitis B transmission is percutaneous, but the outmoded designation "serum hepatitis" is an inaccurate label for the epidemiologic spectrum of HBV infection recognized today. As detailed below, most of the hepatitis transmitted by blood transfusion is not caused by HBV; moreover, in approximately half of patients with acute type B hepatitis, there is no history of an identifiable percutaneous exposure. We now recognize that many cases of type B hepatitis result from less obvious modes of nonpercutaneous or covert percutaneous transmission. HBsAg has been identified in almost every body fluid from infected persons—saliva, tears, seminal fluid, cerebrospinal fluid, ascites, breast milk, synovial fluid, gastric juice, pleural fluid, and urine, and even rarely in feces. Although there is abundant evidence to suggest that feces are not infectious, at least some of these body fluids—most notably semen and saliva—have been shown to be infectious, albeit less so than serum, when administered percutaneously or nonpercutaneously to experimental animals. Among the nonpercutaneous modes of HBV transmission, oral ingestion has been documented as a potential route of exposure but one whose efficiency is quite low. On the other hand, the two nonpercutaneous routes considered to have the greatest impact are intimate (especially sexual) contact and perinatal transmission.

In sub-Saharan Africa, intimate contact among toddlers is considered instrumental in contributing to the maintenance of the high frequency of HBsAg in the population. Perinatal transmission occurs primarily in infants born to HBsAg carrier mothers or mothers with acute hepatitis B during the third trimester of pregnancy or during the early postpartum period. Perinatal transmission is uncommon in North America and western Europe but occurs with great frequency and is the most important mode of HBV perpetuation in the Far East and developing countries. Although the precise mode of perinatal transmission is unknown, and although approximately 10 percent of infections may be acquired in utero, epidemiologic evidence suggests that most infections occur approximately at the time of delivery and are not related to breast feeding. The likelihood of perinatal transmission of HBV correlates with the presence of HBeAg; 90 percent of HBeAg-positive mothers but only 10 to 15 percent of anti-HBe-positive mothers transmit HBV infection to their offspring. In most cases, acute infection in the neonate is clinically asymptomatic, but the child is very likely to become an HBsAg carrier.

The more than 200 million HBsAg carriers in the world constitute the main reservoir of hepatitis B in human beings. Serum HBsAg is infrequent (0.1 to 0.5 percent) in normal populations in the United States and western Europe; however, a prevalence of up to 5 to 20 percent has been found in the Far East and in some tropical countries and in persons with Down's syndrome, lepromatous leprosy, leukemia, Hodgkin's disease, polyarteritis nodosa, patients with chronic renal disease on hemodialysis, and needle-using drug addicts.

Other groups with high rates of HBV infection include spouses of acutely infected persons, sexually promiscuous persons (especially promiscuous homosexual men), health care workers exposed to blood, persons who require repeated transfusions especially with pooled blood product concentrates (e.g., hemophiliacs), residents and staff of custodial institutions for the mentally retarded, prisoners, and, to a lesser extent, family members of chronically infected patients. In volunteer blood donors, the prevalence of anti-HBs, a reflection of previous HBV infection, ranges from 5 to 10 percent, but the prevalence is higher in lower socioeconomic strata, older age groups, and persons—including those mentioned above—exposed to blood products.

Prevalence of infection, modes of transmission, and human behavior conspire to mold geographically different epidemiologic patterns of HBV infection. In the Far East and Africa, hepatitis B, a disease of the newborn and young children, is perpetuated by a cycle of maternal-neonatal spread. In North America and western Europe, hepatitis B is primarily a disease of adolescence and early adulthood, the time of life when intimate sexual contact as well as recreational and occupational percutaneous exposures tend to occur.

Hepatitis D Infection with HDV has a worldwide distribution, but two epidemiologic patterns exist. In Mediterranean countries (northern Africa, southern Europe, the Middle East), HDV infection is endemic among those with hepatitis B, and the disease is transmitted predominantly by nonpercutaneous means, especially close personal contact. In nonendemic areas, such as the United States and northern Europe, HDV infection is confined to persons exposed frequently to blood and blood products, primarily drug addicts and hemophiliacs. HDV infection can be introduced into a population through drug addicts or by migration of persons from endemic to nonendemic areas. Thus, patterns of population migration and human behavior facilitating percutaneous contact play important roles in the introduction and amplification of HDV infection. Occasionally, the migrating epidemiology of hepatitis D is expressed in explosive outbreaks of severe hepatitis, such as those which have occurred in remote South American villages as well as in urban centers in the United States. Ultimately, such outbreaks of hepatitis D—either of coinfections with acute hepatitis B or of superinfections in those already infected with HBV—may blur the distinctions between endemic and nonendemic areas.

Hepatitis C Routine screening of blood donors for HBsAg and the elimination of commercial blood sources in the early 1970s reduced the frequency of, but did not eliminate, transfusion-associated hepatitis. During the 1970s, the likelihood of acquiring hepatitis after transfusion of voluntarily donated, HBsAg-screened blood was approximately 10 percent per patient (up to 0.9 percent per unit transfused). Although hepatitis B accounted for up to 5 to 10 percent of these cases, the remaining 90 to 95 percent were classified, based on serologic exclusion, as "non-A, non-B" hepatitis. For patients requiring transfusion of pooled products, such as clotting factor concentrates, the risk was even higher, up to 20 to 30 percent, while for those receiving such products as albumin and immune globulin, because of prior treatment of these materials by heating to 60°C or cold ethanol fractionation, there was no risk of hepatitis.

During the 1980s, voluntary self-exclusion of blood d⁻ risk factors for AIDS and then the introduction of ⁻ for anti-HIV reduced further the likelihood of tra⁻ hepatitis to under 5 percent. During the late 1980s⁻ the introduction first of "surrogate" screening tests fc⁻ hepatitis [alanine aminotransferase (ALT) and anti-HE⁻

to identify blood donors with a higher likelihood of transmitting non-A, non-B hepatitis to recipients] and, subsequently, after the discovery of HCV, first-generation immunoassays for anti-HCV reduced the frequency of transfusion-associated hepatitis even further. A prospective analysis of transfusion-associated hepatitis conducted between 1986 and 1990 showed that the incidence of transfusion-associated hepatitis at one urban university hospital fell from a baseline of 3.8 percent per patient (0.45 percent per unit transfused) to 1.5 percent per patient (0.19 percent per unit) after the introduction of surrogate testing and to 0.6 percent per patient (0.03 percent per unit) after the introduction of first-generation anti-HCV assays. The introduction of second-generation anti-HCV assays has reduced the frequency of transfusion-associated hepatitis C to almost imperceptible levels.

In addition to being transmitted by transfusion, hepatitis C can be transmitted by other percutaneous routes, such as self-injection with intravenous drugs. In addition, this virus can be transmitted by occupational exposure to blood, and the likelihood of infection is increased in hemodialysis units. Although the frequency of transfusion-associated hepatitis C fell as a result of blood donor screening, the overall frequency of hepatitis C remained the same until the early 1990s, when the overall frequency fell in parallel with a reduction in the number of new cases in intravenous drug users. After the exclusion of anti-HCV-positive plasma units from the donor pool, rare, sporadic instances have occurred of hepatitis C among recipients of immune globulin preparations for intravenous (but not intramuscular) use.

Serologic evidence for HCV infection occurs in >90 percent of patients with transfusion-associated hepatitis, hemophiliacs, and intravenous drug users; 60 to 70 percent of patients with sporadic non-A, non-B hepatitis (in the absence of a known risk factor); 0.5 percent of volunteer blood donors; and 1.5 percent of the general population. The vast majority of asymptomatic blood donors found to have circulating, reproducible anti-HCV do not belong to high-risk groups. How they become infected remains a mystery. The potential exists that such infections of undefined source represent sexually transmitted infection or infection acquired by perinatal transmission. Although these routes of infection can occur (in some studies especially when the source of infection is also infected with HIV, in other studies primarily when the level of viremia in the source is very high), their efficiency is low; the risk of sexual (primarily in those with multiple sexual partners, rarely for monogamous couples) and perinatal transmission is only approximately 5 percent, insufficient to account for the large reservoir of epidemiologically unexplained cases. In all likelihood, the inefficiency of these less than direct routes of transmission is a reflection of the relatively low infectivity titer of HCV. Infections of household contacts are rare as well. Among patients with reported cases of acute hepatitis C, 40 percent have no readily identifiable risk factor, but they do have in common the fact that they tend to belong to lower socioeconomic groups.

The risk of HCV infection is increased in organ transplant recipients and in patients with AIDS; in all immunosuppressed groups, levels of anti-HCV may be undetectable, and a diagnosis may require testing for HCV RNA. Chronic hepatitis C occurs in as many as 20 percent of renal transplant recipients. In the early years after transplantation, the death rate in these patients with hepatitis is increased not as a result of liver failure but of severe infections outside the hepatobiliary tree. This effect has been attributed to the immunosuppressive impact of HCV infection on the host. Five to 10 years after transplantation, however, complications of chronic liver disease account for increased morbidity and mortality. The impact of HCV infection on liver transplant recipients is controversial, associated with severe liver disease in some series but with trivial morbidity in others.

Hepatitis E   The enteric form of non-A, non-B hepatitis identified in India, Asia, Africa, and Central America resembles hepatitis in its primarily enteric mode of spread. The commonly recognized ~s occur after contamination of water supplies such as after mon~ flooding, but sporadic, isolated cases occur. An epidemiologic feature that distinguishes HEV from other enteric agents is the rarity of secondary person-to-person spread from infected persons to their close contacts. Infections arise in populations that are immune to HAV and favor young adults. It is not known if hepatitis E occurs outside of recognized endemic areas, for example, in the United States, but preliminary studies suggest that HEV does not account for any of the sporadic "non-A, non-B" cases in nonendemic areas. Cases imported from endemic areas have been found in the United States.

Hepatitis G   Hepatitis G is a bloodborne agent whose modes of transmission have not been defined adequately but tend to parallel those of HCV infection. Evidence for infection occurs in approximately 1.5 percent of blood donors, but the frequency of infection is the same in blood donors with normal and with elevated ALT levels. Among sporadic, community-acquired cases of acute viral hepatitis unexplained by hepatitis viruses A through E, HGV accounts for only 10 to 15 percent, which represents less than 0.5 percent of all community-acquired cases.

CLINICAL AND LABORATORY FEATURES   Symptoms and Signs   Acute viral hepatitis occurs after an incubation period that varies according to the responsible agent. Generally, incubation periods for hepatitis A range from 15 to 45 days (mean 4 weeks), for hepatitis B and D from 30 to 180 days (mean 4 to 12 weeks), for hepatitis C from 15 to 160 days (mean 7 weeks), and for hepatitis E from 14 to 60 days (mean 5 to 6 weeks). The *prodromal symptoms* of acute viral hepatitis are systemic and quite variable. Constitutional symptoms of anorexia, nausea and vomiting, fatigue, malaise, arthralgias, myalgias, headache, photophobia, pharyngitis, cough, and coryza may precede the onset of jaundice by 1 to 2 weeks. The nausea, vomiting, and anorexia are frequently associated with alterations in olfaction and taste. A low-grade fever between 38 and 39°C (100 to 102°F) is more often present in hepatitis A and E than in hepatitis B or C, except when hepatitis B is heralded by a serum sickness–like syndrome; rarely, a fever of 39.5 to 40°C (103 to 104°F) may accompany the constitutional symptoms. Dark urine and clay-colored stools may be noticed by the patient from 1 to 5 days prior to the onset of clinical jaundice.

With the onset of *clinical jaundice*, the constitutional prodromal symptoms usually diminish, but in some patients mild weight loss (2.5 to 5 kg) is common and may continue during the entire icteric phase. The liver becomes enlarged and tender and may be associated with right upper quadrant pain and discomfort. Infrequently, patients present with a cholestatic picture, suggesting extrahepatic biliary obstruction. Splenomegaly and cervical adenopathy are present in 10 to 20 percent of patients with acute hepatitis. Rarely, a few spider angiomas appear during the icteric phase and disappear during convalescence. During the *recovery phase*, constitutional symptoms disappear, but usually some liver enlargement and abnormalities in liver biochemical tests are still evident. The duration of the posticteric phase is variable, ranging from 2 to 12 weeks, and usually is more prolonged in acute hepatitis B and C. Complete clinical and biochemical recovery is to be expected 1 to 2 months after all cases of hepatitis A and E and 3 to 4 months after the onset of jaundice in three-quarters of uncomplicated cases of hepatitis B and C. In the remainder, biochemical recovery may be delayed. A substantial proportion of patients with viral hepatitis never become icteric.

Infection with HDV can occur in the presence of acute or chronic HBV infection; the duration of HBV infection determines the duration of HDV infection. When acute HDV and HBV infection occur simultaneously, clinical and biochemical features may be indistinguishable from those of HBV infection alone, although occasionally they are more severe. As opposed to patients with *acute* HBV infection, patients with *chronic* HBV infection can support HDV replication indefinitely. This can happen when acute HDV infection occurs in the presence of a nonresolving acute HBV infection. More commonly, acute HDV infection becomes chronic when it is superimposed on an underlying chronic HBV infection. In such cases, the HDV superinfection appears as a clinical exacerbation or an episode resembling acute viral hepatitis in someone already chronically infected with HBV. Superinfection with HDV in a patient with chronic hepatitis B often leads to clinical deterioration (see below).

In addition to superinfections with other hepatitis agents, acute hepatitis-like clinical events in persons with chronic hepatitis B may accompany spontaneous HBeAg-to–anti-HBe seroconversion or spontaneous reactivation, i.e., reversion from nonreplicative to replicative infection. Such reactivations can occur as well in therapeutically immunosuppressed patients with chronic HBV infection when cytotoxic-immunosuppressive drugs are withdrawn; in these cases, restoration of immune competence is thought to allow resumption of previously checked cell-mediated cytolysis of HBV-infected hepatocytes. Occasionally, acute clinical exacerbations of chronic hepatitis B may represent the emergence of a precore mutant (see "Virology and Etiology," above).

Laboratory Features The serum aminotransferases AST and ALT (previously designated SGOT and SGPT) show a variable increase during the prodromal phase of acute viral hepatitis and precede the rise in bilirubin level (see Figs. 295-2 and 295-4). The acute level of these enzymes, however, does not correlate well with the degree of liver cell damage. Peak levels vary from 400 to 4000 IU or more; these levels are usually reached at the time the patient is clinically icteric and diminish progressively during the recovery phase of acute hepatitis. The diagnosis of anicteric hepatitis is difficult and requires a high index of suspicion; it is based on clinical features and on aminotransferase elevations, although mild increases in conjugated bilirubin also may be found.

Jaundice is usually visible in the sclera or skin when the serum bilirubin value exceeds 43 μmol/L (2.5 mg/dL). When jaundice appears, the serum bilirubin typically rises to levels ranging from 85 to 340 μmol/L (5 to 20 mg/dL). The serum bilirubin may continue to rise despite falling serum aminotransferase levels. In most instances, the total bilirubin is equally divided between the conjugated and unconjugated fractions. Bilirubin levels above 340 μmol/L (20 mg/dL) extending and persisting late into the course of viral hepatitis are more likely to be associated with severe disease. In certain patients with underlying hemolytic anemia, however, such as glucose-6-phosphate dehydrogenase deficiency and sickle cell anemia, a high serum bilirubin level is common, resulting from superimposed hemolysis. In such patients, bilirubin levels greater than 513 μmol/L (30 mg/dL) have been observed and are not necessarily associated with a poor prognosis.

Neutropenia and lymphopenia are transient and are followed by a relative lymphocytosis. Atypical lymphocytes (varying between 2 and 20 percent) are common during the acute phase. These atypical lymphocytes are indistinguishable from those seen in infectious mononucleosis. Measurement of the prothrombin time (PT) is important in patients with acute viral hepatitis, for a prolonged value may reflect a severe synthetic defect, signify extensive hepatocellular necrosis, and indicate a worse prognosis. Occasionally, a prolonged PT may occur with only mild increases in the serum bilirubin and aminotransferase levels. Prolonged nausea and vomiting, inadequate carbohydrate intake, and poor hepatic glycogen reserves may contribute to hypoglycemia noted occasionally in patients with severe viral hepatitis. Serum alkaline phosphatase may be normal or only mildly elevated, while a fall in serum albumin is uncommon in uncomplicated acute viral hepatitis. In some patients, mild and transient steatorrhea has been noted as well as slight microscopic hematuria and minimal proteinuria.

A diffuse but mild elevation of the gamma globulin fraction is common during acute viral hepatitis. Serum IgG and IgM are elevated in about one-third of patients during the acute phase of viral hepatitis, but serum IgM elevation is seen more characteristically during acute hepatitis A. During the acute phase of viral hepatitis, antibodies to smooth muscle and other cell constituents may be present, and low titers of rheumatoid factor, antinuclear antibody, and heterophil antibody also can be found occasionally. In hepatitis C and D, antibodies to liver-kidney microsomes (LKM) may occur; however, the species of LKM antibodies in the two types of hepatitis are different from each other as well as from the LKM antibody species characteristic of autoimmune chronic hepatitis type 2 (see Chap. 297). The autoantibodies in viral hepatitis are nonspecific and also can be associated with other viral and systemic diseases. In contrast, virus-specific antibodies, which appear during and after hepatitis virus infection, are serologic markers of diagnostic importance.

As described above, serologic tests are available with which to establish a diagnosis of hepatitis A, B, D, and C. Tests for fecal or serum HAV are not routinely available. Therefore, a diagnosis of type A hepatitis is based on detection of IgM anti-HAV during acute illness (see Fig. 295-2). Rheumatoid factor can give rise to false-positive results in this test.

A diagnosis of HBV infection can usually be made by detection of HBsAg in serum. Infrequently, levels of HBsAg are too low to be detected during acute HBV infection, even with the current generation of highly sensitive immunoassays. In such cases, the diagnosis can be established by the presence of IgM anti-HBc.

The titer of HBsAg bears little relation to the severity of clinical disease. Indeed, there may be an inverse correlation between the serum concentration of HBsAg and the degree of liver cell damage. For example, titers are highest in immunosuppressed patients, lower in chronic liver disease (but higher in mild chronic than in severe chronic hepatitis), and very low in acute fulminant hepatitis. These observations suggest that in hepatitis B the degree of liver cell damage and the clinical course are probably related to variations in the patient's immune response to HBV rather than to the amount of circulating HBsAg. In immunocompetent persons, however, there is a correlation between markers of HBV *replication* and liver injury (see below).

Another serologic marker that may be of value in patients with hepatitis B is HBeAg. Its principal clinical usefulness is as an indicator of relative infectivity. Because HBeAg is invariably present during early acute hepatitis B, HBeAg testing is indicated primarily during follow-up of chronic infection.

In patients with hepatitis B surface antigenemia of unknown duration, e.g., blood donors found to be HBsAg-positive and referred to a physician for evaluation, testing for IgM anti-HBc may be useful to distinguish between acute or recent infection (IgM anti-HBc-positive) and chronic HBV infection (IgM anti-HBc-negative, IgG anti-HBc-positive). A false-positive test for IgM anti-HBc may be encountered in patients with high-titer rheumatoid factor.

Anti-HBs is rarely detectable in the presence of HBsAg in patients with *acute* hepatitis B, but 10 to 20 percent of persons with *chronic* HBV infection may harbor low-level anti-HBs. This antibody is directed not against the common group determinant, *a*, but against the heterotypic subtype determinant (e.g., HBsAg of subtype *ad* with anti-HBs of subtype *y*). In most cases, this serologic pattern cannot be attributed to infection with two different HBV subtypes, and the presence of this antibody is not a harbinger of imminent HBsAg clearance. When such antibody is detected, its presence is of no recognized clinical significance (see "Virology and Etiology," above).

After immunization with hepatitis B vaccine, which consists of HBsAg alone, anti-HBs is the only serologic marker to appear. A summary of the commonly encountered serologic patterns of hepatitis B and their interpretations appears in Table 295-3. Tests for the detection of HBV DNA in liver and serum are now available. Like HBeAg, serum HBV DNA is an indicator of HBV replication, but tests for HBV DNA are more sensitive and quantitative. These markers are useful in following the course of HBV replication in patients with chronic hepatitis B receiving antiviral chemotherapy, e.g., with interferon (see Chap. 297). In immunocompetent persons, a general correlation does appear to exist between the level of HBV replication, as reflected by the level of HBV DNA in serum, and the degree of liver injury. High serum HBV DNA levels, increased expression of viral antigens, and necroinflammatory activity in the liver go hand in hand unless immunosuppression interferes with cytolytic T cell responses to virus-infected cells; reduction of HBV replication with antiviral drugs, such as interferon, tends to be accompanied by an improvement in liver histology.

In patients with hepatitis C, an episodic pattern of aminotransferase elevation is common. A specific serologic diagnosis of hepatitis C can be made by demonstrating the presence in serum of anti-HCV. When a second- or later-generation immunoassay (that detects antibodies to nonstructural and nucleocapsid proteins) is used, anti-HCV can be detected in acute hepatitis C during the initial phase of elevated aminotransferase activity. This antibody may never become detectable in 5 to 10 percent of patients with acute hepatitis C, and levels of anti-HCV may become undetectable after recovery from acute hepatitis C. In patients with chronic hepatitis C, anti-HCV is detectable in >90 percent of cases. Because nonspecificity can confound immunoassays for anti-HCV, a supplementary recombinant immunoblot assay should be done, especially in persons with a low prior probability of infection, to establish the specific viral proteins to which anti-HCV is directed (see "Virology and Etiology," above). Assays for HCV RNA are the most sensitive tests for HCV infection. HCV RNA can be detected even before acute elevation of aminotransferase activity and before the appearance of anti-HCV in patients with acute hepatitis C. In addition, HCV RNA remains detectable indefinitely, continuously in most but intermittently in some, in patients with chronic hepatitis C (even detectable in some persons with normal liver tests, i.e., asymptomatic carriers). Thus a diagnosis of hepatitis C can be supported by detection of anti-HCV and by exclusion of false-positive reactivity. In the small minority of patients with hepatitis C who lack anti-HCV, a diagnosis can be supported by detection of HCV RNA. If all these tests are negative and the patient has a well-characterized case of hepatitis following percutaneous exposure to blood or blood products, a diagnosis of hepatitis G or, perhaps, hepatitis caused by another agent as yet unidentified can be entertained. A proportion of patients with hepatitis C have isolated anti-HBc in their blood, a reflection of a common risk in certain populations to multiple bloodborne hepatitis agents. The anti-HBc in such cases is almost invariably of the IgG class and usually represents HBV infection in the remote past, rarely current HBV infection with low-level virus carriage.

The presence of HDV infection can be identified by demonstrating intrahepatic HDV antigen or, more practically, an anti-HDV seroconversion (a rise in titer of anti-HDV or de novo appearance of anti-HDV). Circulating HDV antigen, also diagnostic of acute infection, is detectable only briefly, if at all. Because anti-HDV is often undetectable once HBsAg disappears, retrospective serodiagnosis of acute self-limited, simultaneous HBV and HDV infection is difficult. Early diagnosis of acute infection may be hampered by a delay of up to 30 to 40 days in the appearance of anti-HDV.

When a patient presents with acute hepatitis and has HBsAg and anti-HDV in the serum, determination of the class of anti-HBc is helpful in establishing the relationship between infection with HBV and HDV. Although IgM anti-HBc does not distinguish *absolutely* between acute and chronic HBV infection, its presence is a reliable indicator of recent infection and its absence a reliable indicator of infection in the remote past. In simultaneous acute HBV and HDV infections, IgM anti-HBc will be detectable, while in acute HDV infection superimposed on chronic HBV infection, anti-HBc will be of the IgG class.

Tests for the presence of HDV RNA are useful for determining the presence of ongoing HDV replication and relative infectivity. Currently, probes for this marker are restricted to a limited number of research laboratories. Similarly, diagnostic tests for hepatitis E and G are confined to a small number of research laboratories.

Liver biopsy is rarely necessary or indicated in acute viral hepatitis, except when there is a question about the diagnosis or when there is clinical evidence suggesting a diagnosis of chronic hepatitis.

A diagnostic algorithm can be applied in the evaluation of cases of acute viral hepatitis. A patient with acute hepatitis should undergo four serologic tests, HBsAg, IgM anti-HAV, IgM anti-HBc, and anti-HCV (Table 295-4). The presence of HBsAg, with or without IgM anti-HBc, represents HBV infection. If IgM anti-HBc is present, the HBV infection is considered acute; if IgM anti-HBc is absent, the HBV infection is considered chronic. A diagnosis of acute hepatitis B can be made in the absence of HBsAg when IgM anti-HBc is detectable. A diagnosis of acute hepatitis A is based on the presence of IgM anti-HAV. If IgM anti-HAV coexists with HBsAg, a diagnosis of simultaneous HAV and HBV infections can be made; if IgM anti-HBc (with or without HBsAg) is detectable, the patient has simultaneous acute hepatitis A and B, and if IgM anti-HBc is undetectable, the patient has acute hepatitis A superimposed on chronic HBV infection. The presence of anti-HCV, if confirmable, supports a diagnosis of acute hepatitis C. Occasionally, repeat anti-HCV testing later during the illness is necessary to establish the diagnosis. Absence of all serologic markers is consistent with a diagnosis of "non-A, non-B, non-C" hepatitis, if the epidemiologic setting is appropriate.

In patients with chronic hepatitis, initial testing should consist of HBsAg and anti-HCV. Anti-HCV supports the diagnosis of chronic hepatitis C. If a

Table 295-4

Simplified Diagnostic Approach in Patients Presenting with Acute Hepatitis

Serologic Tests of Patient's Serum				
HBsAg	IgM Anti-HAV	IgM Anti-HBc	Anti-HCV	Diagnostic Interpretation
+	−	+	−	Acute hepatitis B
+	−	−	−	Chronic hepatitis B
+	+	−	−	Acute hepatitis A superimposed on chronic hepatitis B
+	+	+	−	Acute hepatitis A and B
−	+	−	−	Acute hepatitis A
−	+	+	−	Acute hepatitis A and B (HBsAg below detection threshold)
−	−	+	−	Acute hepatitis B (HBsAg below detection threshold)
−	−	−	+	Acute hepatitis C

Table 295-3

Commonly Encountered Serologic Patterns of Hepatitis B Infection

HBsAg	Anti-HBs	Anti-HBc	HBeAg	Anti-HBe	Interpretation
+	−	IgM	+	−	Acute HBV infection, high infectivity
+	−	IgG	+	−	Chronic HBV infection, high infectivity
+	−	IgG	−	+	Late-acute or chronic HBV infection, low infectivity
+	+	+	+/−	+/−	1. HBsAg of one subtype and heterotypic anti-HBs (common) 2. Process of seroconversion from HBsAg to anti-HBs (rare)
−	−	IgM	+/−	+/−	1. Acute HBV infection 2. Anti-HBc window
−	−	IgG	−	+/−	1. Low-level HBsAg carrier 2. Remote past infection
−	+	IgG	−	+/−	Recovery from HBV infection
−	+	−	−	−	1. Immunization with HBsAg (after vaccination) 2. Remote past infection (?) 3. False-positive

serologic diagnosis of chronic hepatitis B is made, testing for HBeAg and anti-HBe is indicated to evaluate relative infectivity. Testing for HBV DNA in such patients provides a more quantitative and sensitive test for the level of virus replication and, therefore, is very helpful during antiviral therapy (see Chap. 297). In patients with hepatitis B, testing for anti-HDV is useful under the following circumstances: severe and fulminant cases, severe chronic cases, cases of acute hepatitis-like exacerbations in patients with chronic hepatitis B, persons with frequent percutaneous exposures, and persons from areas where HDV infection is endemic.

PROGNOSIS Virtually all previously healthy patients with hepatitis A recover completely from their illness with no clinical sequelae. Similarly, in acute hepatitis B, 95 percent of patients have a favorable course and recover completely. There are, however, certain clinical and laboratory features that suggest a more complicated and protracted course. Patients of advanced age and with serious underlying medical disorders may have a prolonged course and are more likely to experience severe hepatitis. Initial presenting features such as ascites, peripheral edema, and symptoms of hepatic encephalopathy suggest a poorer prognosis. In addition, a prolonged PT, low serum albumin level, hypoglycemia, and very high serum bilirubin values suggest severe hepatocellular disease. Patients with these clinical and laboratory features deserve prompt hospital admission. The case-fatality rate in hepatitis A and B is very low (approximately 0.1 percent) but is increased by advanced age and underlying debilitating disorders. Among patients ill enough to be hospitalized for acute hepatitis B, the fatality rate is 1 percent. Hepatitis C occurring after transfusion is less severe during the acute phase than type B hepatitis and is more likely to be anicteric; fatalities are rare, but the precise case-fatality rate is not known. In outbreaks of waterborne hepatitis E in India and Asia, the case-fatality rate is 1 to 2 percent and up to 10 to 20 percent in pregnant women. Patients with simultaneous acute hepatitis B and hepatitis D do not necessarily experience a higher mortality rate than do patients with acute hepatitis B alone; however, in several recent outbreaks of acute simultaneous HBV and HDV infection among drug addicts, the case fatality rate has been approximately 5 percent. In the case of HDV superinfection of a person with chronic hepatitis B, the likelihood of fulminant hepatitis and death is increased substantially. Although the case-fatality rate for hepatitis D has not been defined adequately, in outbreaks of severe HDV superinfection in isolated populations with a high hepatitis B carrier rate, the mortality rate has been recorded in excess of 20 percent.

COMPLICATIONS AND SEQUELAE A small proportion of patients with hepatitis A experience *relapsing hepatitis* weeks to months after apparent recovery from acute hepatitis. Relapses are characterized by recurrence of symptoms, aminotransferase elevations, occasionally jaundice, and fecal excretion of HAV. Another unusual variant of acute hepatitis A is *cholestatic hepatitis*, characterized by protracted cholestatic jaundice and pruritus. Rarely, liver test abnormalities persist for many months, even up to a year. Even when these complications occur, hepatitis A remains self-limited and does not progress to chronic liver disease. During the prodromal phase of acute hepatitis B, a serum sickness–like syndrome characterized by arthralgia or arthritis, rash, angioedema, and rarely hematuria and proteinuria may develop in 5 to 10 percent of patients. This syndrome occurs prior to the onset of clinical jaundice, and these patients are often erroneously diagnosed as having rheumatoid arthritis or other rheumatologic diseases such as systemic lupus erythematosus. The diagnosis can be established by measuring serum aminotransferase levels, which are almost invariably elevated, and serum HBsAg. As noted above, EMC is an immune-complex disease that can complicate hepatitis C. Attention has been drawn as well to associations between hepatitis C and such cutaneous disorders as porphyria cutanea tarda and lichen planus. A mechanism for these associations is unknown.

The most feared complication of viral hepatitis is *fulminant hepatitis* (massive hepatic necrosis); fortunately, this is a rare event. This is primarily seen in hepatitis B and D, as well as hepatitis E, but rare fulminant cases of hepatitis A occur primarily in older adults and in persons with underlying chronic liver disease. Hepatitis B accounts for more than 50 percent of fulminant hepatitis cases, a sizable proportion of which are associated with HDV infection. Participation of HDV can be documented in approximately one-third of patients with acute fulminant hepatitis B and two-thirds of patients with fulminant hepatitis superimposed on chronic hepatitis B. Fulminant hepatitis is seen rarely in hepatitis C, but hepatitis E, as noted above, can be complicated by fatal fulminant hepatitis in 1 to 2 percent of all cases and in up to 20 percent of cases occurring in pregnant women. Patients usually present with signs and symptoms of encephalopathy that may evolve to deep coma. The liver is usually small and the PT excessively prolonged. The combination of rapidly shrinking liver size, rapidly rising bilirubin level, and marked prolongation of the PT, together with clinical signs of confusion, disorientation, somnolence, ascites, and edema, indicates that the patient has hepatic failure with encephalopathy. Cerebral edema is common; brainstem compression, gastrointestinal bleeding, sepsis, respiratory failure, cardiovascular collapse, and renal failure are terminal events. The mortality is exceedingly high (greater than 80 percent in patients with deep coma), but patients who survive may have a complete biochemical and histologic recovery. If a donor liver can be located on time, liver transplantation may be life-saving in patients with fulminant hepatitis.

It is particularly important to document the disappearance of HBsAg following apparent clinical recovery from acute hepatitis B. Before laboratory methods were available to distinguish between acute and acute hepatitis–like exacerbations (*spontaneous reactivations*) of chronic hepatitis B, observations suggested that approximately 10 percent of patients remained HBsAg-positive for longer than 6 months after the onset of clinically apparent acute hepatitis B. Half these persons were found to clear the antigen from their circulations during the next several years, but the other 5 percent remained chronically HBsAg-positive. More recent observations suggest that the true rate of chronic infection after clinically apparent acute hepatitis B is as low as 1 percent in normal, immunocompetent, young adults. Earlier, higher estimates may have been biased by inadvertent inclusion of acute exacerbations in chronically infected patients; these patients, chronically HBsAg-positive before exacerbation, were unlikely to seroconvert to HBsAg-negative thereafter. Whether the rate of chronicity is 10 or 1 percent, such patients have anti-HBc in serum; anti-HBs is either undetected or detected at low titer against the opposite subtype specificity of the antigen (see "Laboratory Features," above). These patients may (1) be asymptomatic carriers, (2) have low-grade, mild chronic hepatitis, or (3) have moderate to severe chronic hepatitis with or without cirrhosis. The likelihood of becoming an HBsAg carrier after acute HBV infection is especially high among neonates, persons with Down's syndrome, chronically hemodialyzed patients, and immunosuppressed patients, including persons with HIV infection.

Chronic hepatitis is an important late complication of acute hepatitis B occurring in a small proportion of acute cases but more common in those who present with chronic infection without having experienced an acute illness (see Chap. 297). Certain clinical and laboratory features suggest progression of acute hepatitis to chronic hepatitis: (1) lack of complete resolution of clinical symptoms of anorexia, weight loss, and fatigue and the persistence of hepatomegaly; (2) the presence of bridging or multilobular hepatic necrosis on liver biopsy during protracted, severe acute viral hepatitis; (3) failure of the serum aminotransferase, bilirubin, and globulin levels to return to normal within 6 to 12 months following the acute illness; and (4) the continued presence of HBsAg and HBeAg 6 months or more after acute hepatitis, suggesting chronic, replicative viral infection of the liver.

Although acute hepatitis D infection does not increase the likelihood of chronicity of simultaneous acute hepatitis B, hepatitis D has the potential for contributing to the severity of chronic hepatitis B. Hepatitis D superinfection can transform asymptomatic or mild chronic hepatitis B into severe, progressive chronic hepatitis and cirrhosis; it also can accelerate the course of chronic hepatitis B. Some HDV superinfections in patients with chronic hepatitis B lead to fulminant hepatitis. Although HDV and HBV infections are associated with severe liver disease, mild hepatitis and even asymptomatic carriage have been identified in some patients. After transfusion-associated acute hepatitis C, at least 50 percent of patients have abnormal biochemical liver tests for more than a year. In some experiences, the frequency of progression to chronicity after acute hepatitis C is as high as 70 percent. In most of these patients, liver histology is consistent with moderate to severe chronic hepatitis. Even among those who recover biochemically, the likelihood of retaining circulating HCV RNA is high. Thus, after acute HCV infection, the likelihood of remaining chronically *infected* approaches 85 to 90 percent. Although many patients with chronic hepatitis C have no symptoms, cirrhosis may develop in as many as 20 percent within 10 years of acute illness; in some series of cases, cirrhosis has been reported in as many as 50 percent of patients with chronic hepatitis C. Although chronic hepatitis C accounts for a quarter of cases of chronic liver disease and a quarter of patients undergoing liver transplantation for end-stage liver disease in the United States and Europe, in the majority of patients with chronic hepatitis C, morbidity and mortality are limited during the initial 20 years after the onset of infection. Progression of chronic hepatitis C may be influenced by hepatitis C genotype, level of hepatitis C viremia, age of acquisition, duration of infection, immunosuppression, as well as coexisting excessive alcohol use or other hepatitis virus infection. In contrast, neither HAV nor HEV causes chronic liver disease.

Rare complications of viral hepatitis include pancreatitis, myocarditis, atypical pneumonia, aplastic anemia, transverse myelitis, and peripheral neuropathy. *Carriers* of HBsAg, particularly those infected in infancy or early childhood, have an enhanced risk of hepatocellular carcinoma. The risk of hepatocellular carcinoma is increased as well in patients with chronic hepatitis C, almost exclusively in patients with cirrhosis, and almost always after at least a decade, usually after three decades of disease (see Chap. 93). In children, hepatitis B may present rarely with anicteric hepatitis, a nonpruritic papular rash of the face, buttocks, and limbs, and lymphadenopathy (papular acrodermatitis of childhood or Gianotti-Crosti syndrome).

DIFFERENTIAL DIAGNOSIS Viral diseases such as infectious mononucleosis; those due to cytomegalovirus, herpes simplex, and coxsackieviruses; and toxoplasmosis may share certain clinical features with viral hepatitis and cause elevation in serum aminotransferase and less commonly in serum bilirubin levels. Tests such as the differential heterophile and serologic tests for these agents may be helpful in the differential diagnosis if HBsAg, anti-HBc, IgM anti-HAV, and anti-HCV determinations are negative. Aminotransferase elevations can accompany almost any systemic viral infection; other rare causes of liver injury confused with viral hepatitis are infections with *Leptospira, Candida, Brucella, Mycobacteria,* and *Pneumocystis.* A complete drug history is particularly important, for many drugs and certain anesthetic agents can produce a picture of either acute hepatitis or cholestasis (see Chap. 296). Equally important is a past history of unexplained "repeated episodes" of acute hepatitis. This should alert the physician to the possibility that the underlying disorder is chronic hepatitis. Alcoholic hepatitis also must be considered, but usually the serum aminotransferase levels are not as markedly elevated and other stigmata of alcoholism may be present. The finding on liver biopsy of fatty infiltration, a neutrophilic inflammatory reaction, and "alcoholic hyaline" would be consistent with alcohol-induced rather than viral liver injury. Because acute hepatitis may present with right upper quadrant abdominal pain, nausea and vomiting, fever, and icterus, it is often confused with acute cholecystitis, common duct stone, or ascending cholangitis. Patients with acute viral hepatitis may tolerate surgery poorly; therefore, it is important to exclude this diagnosis, and in confusing cases, a percutaneous liver biopsy may be necessary prior to laparotomy. Viral hepatitis in the elderly is often misdiagnosed as obstructive jaundice resulting from a common duct stone or carcinoma of the pancreas. Because acute hepatitis in the elderly may be quite severe and the operative mortality high, a thorough evaluation including biochemical tests, radiographic studies of the biliary tree,

and even liver biopsy may be necessary to exclude primary parenchymal liver disease. Another clinical constellation that may mimic acute hepatitis is right ventricular failure with passive hepatic congestion or hypoperfusion syndromes, such as those associated with shock, severe hypotension, and severe left ventricular failure. Also included in this general category is any disorder that interferes with venous return to the heart, such as right atrial myxoma, constrictive pericarditis, hepatic vein occlusion (Budd-Chiari syndrome), or venoocclusive disease. Clinical features are usually sufficient to distinguish between these vascular disorders and viral hepatitis. Acute fatty liver of pregnancy, cholestasis of pregnancy, eclampsia, and the HELLP syndrome (hemolysis, elevated liver tests, and low platelets) can be confused with viral hepatitis during pregnancy. Very rarely, malignancies metastatic to the liver can mimic acute or even fulminant viral hepatitis. Occasionally, genetic or metabolic liver disorders (e.g., Wilson's disease, α_1-antitrypsin deficiency) are confused with viral hepatitis.

℞ TREATMENT

Treatment of Acute Attack There is no specific treatment for *typical acute viral hepatitis.* Although hospitalization may be required for clinically severe illness, most patients do not require hospital care. Forced and prolonged bed rest is not essential for full recovery, but many patients will feel better with restricted physical activity. A high-calorie diet is desirable, and because many patients may experience nausea late in the day, the major caloric intake is best tolerated in the morning. Intravenous feeding is necessary in the acute stage if the patient has persistent vomiting and cannot maintain oral intake. Drugs capable of producing adverse reactions such as cholestasis and drugs metabolized by the liver should be avoided. If severe pruritus is present, the use of the bile salt–sequestering resin cholestyramine will usually alleviate this symptom. Glucocorticoid therapy has no value in acute viral hepatitis. Even in severe cases associated with *bridging necrosis,* controlled trials have failed to demonstrate the efficacy of steroids. In fact, such therapy may be hazardous.

Physical isolation of patients with hepatitis to a single room and bathroom is rarely necessary except in the case of fecal incontinence for hepatitis A and E or uncontrolled, voluminous bleeding for hepatitis types B (with or without concomitant hepatitis D) and hepatitis C. Because most patients hospitalized with hepatitis A excrete little if any HAV, the likelihood of HAV transmission from these patients during their hospitalization is low. Therefore, burdensome *enteric precautions are no longer recommended.* Although gloves should be worn when the bedpans or fecal material of patients with hepatitis A are handled, these precautions do not represent a departure from sensible procedure for all hospitalized patients. For patients with hepatitis types B and C, emphasis should be placed on blood precautions, i.e., avoiding direct, ungloved hand contact with blood and other body fluids. Enteric precautions are unnecessary. The importance of simple hygienic precautions, such as hand washing, cannot be overemphasized. Universal precautions that have been adopted for all patients apply to patients with viral hepatitis.

Hospitalized patients may be discharged when there is substantial symptomatic improvement, a significant downward trend in the serum aminotransferase and bilirubin values, and a return to normal of the PT. Mild aminotransferase elevations should not be considered contraindications to the gradual resumption of normal activity.

In *fulminant hepatitis,* the goal of therapy is to support the patient by maintenance of fluid balance, support of circulation and respiration, control of bleeding, correction of hypoglycemia, and treatment of other complications of the comatose state in anticipation of liver regeneration and repair. Protein intake should be restricted, and oral lactulose or neomycin administered. Glucocorticoid therapy has been shown in controlled trials to be ineffective. Likewise, exchange transfusion, plasmapheresis, human cross-circulation, porcine liver cross-perfusion, and hemoperfusion have not been proven to enhance survival. Meticulous intensive care is the one factor that does appear to improve survival. Orthotopic liver transplantation is resorted to with increasing frequency, with excellent results, in patients with fulminant hepatitis (see Chap. 301).

PROPHYLAXIS Because there is no therapy for acute viral hepatitis, and because antiviral therapy for chronic viral hepatitis is effective in only a proportion of patients (see Chap. 297), emphasis is placed on prevention through immunization. The prophylactic approach differs for each of the types of viral hepatitis. In the past, immunoprophylaxis relied exclusively on passive immunization with antibody-containing globulin preparations purified by cold ethanol fractionation from the plasma of hundreds of normal donors. Currently, for hepatitis A and B, active immunization with vaccines is available as well.

Hepatitis A Both passive immunization with immune globulin (IG) and active immunization with a killed vaccine are available. All preparations of IG contain anti-HAV. Although the titers may vary, all IG preparations have an antibody concentration sufficient to be protective. When administered before exposure or during the early incubation period, IG is effective in preventing clinically apparent type A hepatitis. In some cases, IG does not abort infection but, by attenuating it, renders it inapparent. As a result, long-lasting "passive-active" immunity occurs; however, this is now considered to be the exception rather than the rule. For postexposure prophylaxis of intimate contacts (household, institutional) of persons with hepatitis A, administration of 0.02 mL/kg is recommended as early after exposure as possible; it may be effective even when administered as late as 2 weeks after exposure. Prophylaxis is not necessary for casual contacts (office, factory, school, or hospital), for most elderly persons, who are very likely to be immune, or for those known to have anti-HAV in their serum. In day-care centers, recognition of hepatitis A cases in children or staff should provide a stimulus for immunoprophylaxis in the center and in the children's family members. By the time most common-source outbreaks of type A hepatitis are recognized, it is usually too late in the incubation period for IG to be effective; however, prophylaxis may limit the frequency of secondary cases. For travelers to tropical countries, developing countries, and other areas outside standard tourist routes, IG prophylaxis had been recommended, before a vaccine became available. When such travel lasted less than 3 months, 0.02 mL/kg was given; for longer travel or residence in these areas, a dose of 0.06 mL/kg every 4 to 6 months was recommended. The high-dose, repeated approach was recommended as well for certain primate handlers and laboratory personnel who work with HAV or fecal specimens. Administration of plasma-derived globulin is safe; it has not been associated with transmission of AIDS to recipients, and the AIDS virus (HIV) is inactivated by 25% alcohol, to which plasma is subjected during the cold ethanol fractionation process.

A formalin-inactivated vaccine made from a strain of HAV attenuated in tissue culture has been shown to be safe, immunogenic, and effective in preventing hepatitis A. It is approved for use in persons who are at least 2 years old and appears to provide adequate protection 4 weeks after a primary inoculation. If it can be given within 4 weeks of an expected exposure, such as by travel to an endemic area, hepatitis A vaccine is the preferred approach to *preexposure* immunoprophylaxis. If travel is more imminent, IG (0.02 mL/kg) should be administered at a different injection site, along with the first dose of vaccine. Because vaccination provides long-lasting protection (protective levels of anti-HAV should last 20 years after vaccination), persons whose risk will be sustained (e.g., frequent travelers or those remaining in endemic areas for prolonged periods) should be vaccinated, and vaccine should supplant the need for repeated IG injections. Other groups who are candidates for hepatitis A vaccination include military personnel, populations with cyclic outbreaks of hepatitis A (e.g., Alaskan natives), employees of day-care centers, primate handlers, laboratory workers exposed to hepatitis A or fecal specimens, and other populations whose recognized risk of hepatitis A is increased. For adults, a complete course of hepatitis A vaccine consists of two intramuscular injections (a 1-mL dose contains 1440 enzyme immunoassay units of viral antigen) given 6 to 12 months apart. For children, aged 2 to 18, three transmuscular injections (a 0.5-mL dose contains 360 enzyme immunoassay units) are recommended, the first two a month apart and the third 6 to 12 months after the first. The role of hepatitis A vaccine in *postexposure* prophylaxis remains to be demonstrated.

Hepatitis B Until 1982, prevention of hepatitis B was based on *passive* immunoprophylaxis either with standard IG, containing modest levels of anti-HBs, or hepatitis B immune globulin (HBIG), containing high-titer anti-HBs. The efficacy of standard IG has never been established and remains questionable; even the efficacy of HBIG, demonstrated in several clinical trials, has been challenged, and its contribution appears to be in reducing the frequency of clinical *illness*, not in preventing *infection*. The first vaccine for *active* immunization, introduced in 1982, was prepared from purified, noninfectious 22-nm spherical forms of HBsAg derived from the plasma of healthy HBsAg carriers. In 1987, the plasma-derived vaccine was supplanted by a genetically engineered vaccine derived from recombinant yeast. The latter vaccine consists of HBsAg particles that are nonglycosylated but are otherwise indistinguishable from natural HBsAg. Current recommendations can be divided into those for preexposure and postexposure prophylaxis.

For *preexposure* prophylaxis against hepatitis B in settings of frequent exposure (health workers exposed to blood, hemodialysis patients and staff, residents and staff of custodial institutions for the developmentally handicapped, intravenous drug abusers, inmates of long-term correctional facilities, promiscuous homosexual men as well as promiscuous heterosexuals, persons such as hemophiliacs who require long-term, high-volume therapy with blood derivatives, household and sexual contacts of HBsAg carriers, persons living in or traveling extensively in endemic areas, and unvaccinated children under the age of 11 who are Alaskan natives, Pacific Islanders, or residents in households of first-generation immigrants from endemic countries), three intramuscular (deltoid, not gluteal) injections of hepatitis B vaccine are recommended at 0, 1, and 6 months. Pregnancy is *not* a contraindication to vaccination. In areas of low HBV endemicity such as the United States, despite the availability of safe and effective hepatitis B vaccines, a strategy of vaccinating persons in high-risk groups has not been effective. The incidence of new hepatitis B cases continued to increase in the United States after introduction of vaccines; fewer than 10 percent of all targeted persons in high-risk groups have actually been vaccinated, and approximately 30 percent of persons with sporadic acute hepatitis B do not fall into any high-risk-group category. Therefore, to have an impact on the frequency of HBV infection in an area of low endemicity such as the United States, universal hepatitis B vaccination in childhood has been recommended. For unvaccinated children born after the implementation of universal infant vaccination, vaccination during early adolescence, at age 11 to 12 years, has been recommended.

There are two comparable recombinant hepatitis B vaccines available, one containing 10 μg of HBsAg (Recombivax-HB) and the other containing 20 μg of HBsAg (Engerix-B), and recommended doses for each injection vary between the two preparations. For Recombivax-HB, 2.5 μg is recommended for children <11 years of age of HBsAg-negative mothers, 5 μg for infants of HBsAg-positive mothers (see below) and for children and adolescents 11 to 19 years of age; 10 μg for immunocompetent adults; and 40 μg for dialysis patients and other immunosuppressed persons. For Engerix-B, 10 μg is recommended for children aged 10 and under, 20 μg for immunocompetent children older than 10 years of age and adults, and 40 μg for dialysis patients and other immunocompromised persons.

For unvaccinated persons sustaining an exposure to HBV, *postexposure* prophylaxis with a combination of HBIG (for rapid achievement of high-titer circulating anti-HBs) and hepatitis B vaccine (for achievement of long-lasting immunity as well as its apparent efficacy in attenuating clinical illness after exposure) is recommended. For *perinatal* exposure of infants born to HBsAg-positive mothers, a single dose of HBIG, 0.5 mL, should be administered intramuscularly in the thigh *immediately after birth*, followed by a complete course of three injections of recombinant hepatitis B vaccine (see doses above) to be started within the first 12 h of life. For those experiencing a direct percutaneous inoculation or transmucosal exposure to HBsAg-positive blood or body fluids (e.g., accidental *needle stick*, other mucosal penetration, or ingestion), a single intramuscular dose of HBIG, 0.06 mL/ kg, administered as soon after exposure as possible, is followed by a complete course of hepatitis B vaccine to begin within the first week. For those exposed by *sexual* contact to a patient with acute hepatitis B, a single intramuscular dose of HBIG, 0.06 mL/kg, should be given within 14 days of exposure, to be followed by a complete course of hepatitis B vaccine. When both HBIG and hepatitis B vaccine are recommended, they may be given at the same time but at separate sites.

The precise duration of protection afforded by hepatitis B vaccine is unknown; however, approximately 80 to 90 percent of immunocompetent vaccinees retain protective levels of anti-HBs for at least 5 years. Thereafter and even after anti-HBs becomes undetectable, protection persists against clinical hepatitis B, hepatitis B surface antigenemia, and chronic HBV infection. Currently, *booster* immunizations are not recommended routinely, except in immunosuppressed persons who have lost detectable anti-HBs or immunocompetent persons who sustain percutaneous HBsAg-positive inoculations after losing detectable antibody. Specifically, for hemodialysis patients, annual anti-HBs testing is recommended after vaccination; booster doses are recommended when anti-HBs levels fall below 10 mIU/mL.

Hepatitis D Infection with hepatitis D can be prevented by vaccinating susceptible persons with hepatitis B vaccine. No product is available for immunoprophylaxis to prevent HDV superinfection in HBsAg carriers; for them, avoidance of percutaneous exposures and limitation of intimate contact with persons who have HDV infection are recommended.

Hepatitis C IG has been shown to be ineffective in preventing hepatitis C and is no longer recommended for postexposure prophylaxis in cases of perinatal, needle stick, or sexual exposure. Although a prototype vaccine that induces antibodies to HCV envelope protein has been developed, currently, hepatitis C vaccination is not feasible practically. Genotype and quasispecies viral heterogeneity, as well as rapid evasion of neutralizing antibodies by this rapidly mutating virus, conspire to render HCV a difficult target for immunoprophylaxis with a vaccine. Prevention of transfusion-associated hepatitis C has been accomplished by the following successively introduced measures: Exclusion of commercial blood donors and reliance on a volunteer blood supply; screening donor blood with surrogate markers such as ALT (no longer recommended) and anti-HBc, markers that identify segments of the blood donor population with an increased risk of bloodborne infections; exclusion of blood donors in high-risk groups for AIDS and the introduction of anti-HIV screening tests; and progressively sensitive serologic screening tests for anti-HCV. Chemical and heat treatment of blood products used for large-pool and concentrated blood derivates are being pursued.

Hepatitis E Whether IG prevents hepatitis E remains undetermined. Development of a vaccine is in progress.

BIBLIOGRAPHY

ADVISORY COMMITTEE ON IMMUNIZATION PRACTICES: Licensure of inactivated hepatitis A vaccine and recommendations for use among international travelers. Morb Mort Week Rep 44:559, 1995

ALTER HJ: To C or not to C: These are the questions. Blood 85:1681, 1995

ALTER MJ et al: The epidemiology of viral hepatitis in the United States. Gastroenterol Clin North Am 23:437, 1994

———: Acute non-A-E hepatitis in the United States and the role of hepatitis G virus infection. N Engl J Med 336:741, 1997

BARRERA JM et al: Persistent hepatitis C viremia after acute self-limiting posttransfusion hepatitis C. Hepatology 21:639, 1995

CENTERS FOR DISEASE CONTROL: Update: Recommendations to prevent hepatitis B virus transmission—United States. Morb Mort Week Rep 44:574, 1995

CHOO Q-L et al: Isolation of a cDNA clone derived from a blood-borne non-A, non-B viral hepatitis genome. Science 244:359, 1989

COHEN JI: Hepatitis A virus: Insights from molecular biology. Hepatology 9:889, 1989

DI BISCEGLIE AM et al: Long-term clinical and histologic follow-up of chronic posttransfusion hepatitis. Hepatology 14:969, 1991

DIENSTAG JL: Non-A, non-B hepatitis: I. Recognition, epidemiology, and clinical features. II. Experimental transmission, putative virus agents and markers, and prevention. Gastroenterology 85:439, 743, 1983

——— (ed): Viral hepatitis. Semin Liver Dis 11:73, 1991

DOBSON S et al: Assessment of a universal, school-based hepatitis B vaccination program. JAMA 274:1209, 1995

DONAHUE JG et al: The declining risk of post-transfusion hepatitis C virus infection. N Engl J Med 327:369, 1992

FARCI P et al: Lack of protective immunity against reinfection with hepatitis C virus. Science 258:135, 1992

HOOFNAGLE JH: Type D (delta) hepatitis. JAMA 261:1321, 1989

HOUGHTON M et al: Molecular biology of the hepatitis C viruses: Implications for diagnosis, development and control of viral disease. Hepatology 14:381, 1991

INNIS BL et al: Protection against hepatitis A by an inactivated vaccine. JAMA 271:1328, 1994

KRAWCZYNSKI K: Hepatitis E. Hepatology 17:932, 1993

LEMON SM, THOMAS DL: Vaccines to prevent viral hepatitis. N Engl J Med 336:196, 1997

LINNEN J et al: Molecular cloning and disease association of hepatitis G virus: A transfusion-transmissible agent. Science 271:505, 1996

MARGOLIS HS et al: Prevention of hepatitis B virus transmission by immunization: An economic analysis of current recommendations. JAMA 274:1201, 1995

MILLER RH et al: Compact organization of the hepatitis B virus genome. Hepatology 9:322, 1989

NISHIOKA K et al (eds): *Viral Hepatitis and Liver Disease*. New York, Springer-Verlag, 1994

NOUSBAUM J-B et al: Hepatitis C virus type 1b (II) infection in France and Italy. Ann Intern Med 122:161, 1995

OKAMOTO H et al: Superinfection of chimpanzees carrying hepatitis C virus of genotype II/1b with that of genotype III/2a or I/1a. Hepatology 20:1131, 1994

PURCELL RH: Hepatitis viruses: Changing patterns of human disease. Proc Natl Acad Sci USA 91:2401, 1994

REYES GR et al: Isolation of a cDNA from the virus responsible for enterically transmitted non-A, non-B hepatitis. Science 247:1335, 1990

SATO S et al: Hepatitis B virus strains with mutations in the core promoter in patients with fulminant hepatitis. Ann Intern Med 122:241, 1995

SEEFF LB: Natural history of viral hepatitis, type C. Semin Gastrointest Dis 6:20, 1995

———: Hepatitis C. Semin Liver Dis 15:1, 1995

SHAKIL AO et al: Volunteer blood donors with antibody to hepatitis C virus: Clinical, biochemical, virologic, and histologic features. Ann Intern Med 123:330, 1995

SHETH SG et al: Nonalcoholic steatohepatitis. Ann Intern Med 126:137, 1997

SIMMONDS P: Variability of hepatitis C virus. Hepatology 21:570, 1995

SIMONS JN et al: Isolation of novel virus-like sequences associated with human hepatitis. Nature 1:564, 1995

——— et al: Identification of two flavivirus-like genomes in the GB hepatitis agent. Proc Natl Acad Sci USA 92:3401, 1995

TAKAHASHI M et al: Natural history of chronic hepatitis C. Am J Gastroenterol 88:240, 1993

THOMAS DL et al: Sexual transmission of hepatitis C virus among patients attending sexually transmitted disease clinics in Baltimore—an analysis of 309 sex partnerships. J Infect Dis 171:768, 1994

TONG MJ et al: Clinical outcomes after transfusion-associated hepatitis C. N Engl J Med 332:1463, 1995

296 *Jules L. Dienstag, Kurt J. Isselbacher*

TOXIC AND DRUG-INDUCED HEPATITIS

Liver injury may follow the inhalation, ingestion, or parenteral administration of a number of pharmacologic and chemical agents. These include industrial toxins (e.g., carbon tetrachloride, trichloroethylene, and yellow phosphorus), the heat-stable toxic bicyclic octapeptides of certain species of *Amanita* and *Galerina* (hepatotoxic mushroom poisoning), and more commonly, pharmacologic agents used in medical therapy. It is essential that any patient presenting with jaundice or altered biochemical liver tests be questioned carefully about exposure to chemicals used in work or at home and drugs taken by prescription or bought "over the counter." In general, two major types of chemical hepatotoxicity have been recognized: (1) direct toxic type and (2) idiosyncratic type.

As shown in Table 296-1, direct toxic hepatitis occurs with predictable regularity in individuals exposed to the offending agent and is dose-dependent. The latent period between exposure and liver injury is usually short (often several hours), although clinical manifestations may be delayed for 24 to 48 h. Agents producing toxic hepatitis are generally systemic poisons or are converted in the liver to toxic metabolites. The direct hepatotoxins result in morphologic abnormalities that are reasonably characteristic and reproducible for each toxin. For example, carbon tetrachloride and trichloroethylene characteristically produce a centrilobular zonal necrosis, whereas yellow phosphorus poisoning typically results in periportal injury. The hepatotoxic octapeptides of *Amanita phalloides* usually produce massive hepatic necrosis. The lethal dose of the toxin is about 10 mg, the amount found in a single deathcap mushroom. Tetracycline, when administered in intravenous doses greater than 1.5 g daily, leads to microvesicular fat deposits in the liver. Liver injury, which is often only one facet of the toxicity produced by the direct hepatotoxins, may go unrecognized until jaundice appears.

In idiosyncratic drug reactions the occurrence of hepatitis is usually infrequent and unpredictable, the response is not dose-dependent, and it may occur at any time during or shortly after exposure to the drug. Extrahepatic manifestations of hypersensitivity, such as rash, arthralgias, fever, leukocytosis, and eosinophilia, occur in about one-quarter of patients with idiosyncratic hepatotoxic drug reactions; this observation and the unpredictability of idiosyncratic drug hepatotoxicity contributed to the hypothesis that this category of drug reactions is immunologically mediated. More recent evidence, however, suggests that, in most cases, even idiosyncratic reactions represent direct hepatotoxity but are caused by drug metabolites rather than by the intact compound. Even the prototype of idiosyncratic hepatoxicity reactions, halothane hepatitis, and isoniazid hepatotoxicity, associated frequently with hypersensitivity manifestations, are now recognized to be mediated by toxic metabolites that damage liver cells directly. Currently, most idiosyncratic reactions are thought to result from differences in metabolic reactivity to specific agents; host susceptibility is mediated by the kinetics of toxic metabolite generation, which differs among individuals. Occasionally, however, the clinical features of an allergic reaction (prominent tissue eosinophilia, autoantibodies, etc.) are difficult to ignore. In vitro models have been described in which lymphocyte cytotoxicity can be demonstrated against rabbit hepatocytes altered by incubation with the potential offending drug. Similarly, in selected cases, a drug or its metabolite has been shown to bind to a host cellular component forming a hapten; the immune response to this "neoantigen" is postulated to play a role in the pathogenesis of liver injury. Therefore, some authorities subdivide idiosyncratic drug hepatotoxicity into hypersensitivity (allergic) and "metabolic" categories. Several unusual exceptions notwithstanding, true drug allergy is difficult to support in most cases of idiosyncratic drug-induced liver injury.

Idiosyncratic reactions lead to a morphologic pattern that is more variable than those produced by direct toxins; a single agent is often capable of causing a variety of lesions, although certain patterns tend to predominate. Depending on the agent involved, idiosyncratic hepatitis may result in a clinical and morphologic picture indistinguishable from that of viral hepatitis (e.g., halothane) or may simulate extrahepatic bile duct obstruction clinically with morphologic evidence of cholestasis and minimal hepatocellular damage (e.g., chlorpromazine). Morphologic alterations also may include bridging hepatic necrosis (e.g., methyldopa), or, infrequently, hepatic granulomas (e.g., sulfonamides).

Not all adverse hepatic drug reactions can be classified as either toxic or idiosyncratic in type. For example, oral contraceptives, which combine estrogenic and progestational compounds, may result in impairment of hepatic tests and occasionally in jaundice. However, they do not produce necrosis or fatty change, manifestations of hypersensitivity are generally absent, and susceptibility to the development of oral contraceptive–induced cholestasis appears to be genetically determined.

Because drug-induced hepatitis is often a presumptive diagnosis and many other disorders produce a similar clinicopathologic picture, evidence of a causal relationship between the use of a drug and subsequent liver injury may be difficult to establish. The relationship is most convincing for the direct hepatotoxins, which lead to a high frequency of hepatic impairment after a short latent period. Idiosyncratic reactions may be reproduced, in some instances, when rechallenge, after an asymptomatic period, results in a recurrence of signs, symptoms, and morphologic and biochemical abnormalities. Rechallenge, however, is often ethically unfeasible, because severe reactions may occur.

℞ **TREATMENT**

Treatment of toxic and drug-induced hepatic disease is largely supportive, as in acute viral hepatitis, except in acetaminophen hepatotoxicity (see below). Withdrawal of the suspected agent is indicated at the first sign of an adverse reaction. In the case of the direct toxins, liver involvement should not divert attention from renal or other organ involvement, which also may threaten survival.

In Table 296-2, several classes of chemical agents are listed, together with examples of the pattern of liver injury produced by them. Certain drugs appear to be responsible for the development of chronic as well as acute hepatic injury. For example, oxyphenisatin, alpha methyldopa, and isoniazid have been associated with moderate to severe chronic hepatitis, and halothane and methotrexate have been implicated in the development of cirrhosis. A syndrome resembling primary biliary cirrhosis has been described following treatment with chlorpromazine, methyl testosterone, tolbutamide, and other drugs. Portal hypertension in the absence of cirrhosis may result from alterations in hepatic architecture produced by vitamin A or arsenic intoxication, industrial exposure to vinyl chloride, or administration of thorium dioxide. The latter three agents also have been associated with

Table 296-1

Some Features of Toxic and Drug-Induced Hepatic Injury

Features	Direct Toxic Effect		Idiosyncratic			Other
	(Carbon Tetrachloride, e.g.)	(Acetaminophen, e.g.)	(Halothane, e.g.)	(Isoniazid, e.g.)	(Chlorpromazine, e.g.)	(Oral Contraceptive Agents, e.g.)
Predictable and dose-related toxicity	+	+	0	0	0	+
Latent period	Short	Short	Variable	Variable	Variable	Variable
Arthralgia, fever, rash, eosinophilia	0	0	+	0	+	0
Liver morphology	Necrosis, fatty infiltration	Centrilobular necrosis	Similar to viral hepatitis	Similar to viral hepatitis	Cholestasis *with* portal inflammation	Cholestasis *without* portal inflammation, vascular lesions

Table 296-2

Principal Alterations of Hepatic Morphology Produced by Some Commonly Used Drugs and Chemicals*

Principal Morphologic Change	Class of Agent	Example
Cholestasis	Anabolic steroid	Methyl testosterone.
	Anti-inflammatory	Sulindac
	Antithyroid	Methimazole
	Antibiotic	Erythromycin estolate, nitrofurantoin, rifampin
	Oral contraceptive	Norethynodrel with mestranol
	Oral hypoglycemic	Chlorpropamide
	Tranquilizer	Chlorpromazine†
	Oncotherapeutic	Anabolic steroids, busulfan, tamoxifen
	Immunosuppressive	Cyclosporine
	Anticonvulsant	Carbamazine
	Calcium channel blocker	Nifedipine, verapamil
Fatty liver	Antibiotic	Tetracycline
	Anticonvulsant	Sodium valproate
	Antiarrhythmic	Amiodarone
	Antiviral	Dideoxynucleosides (e.g., zidovudine)
	Oncotherapeutic	Asparaginase, methotrexate
Hepatitis	Anesthetic	Halothane‡
	Anticonvulsant	Phenytoin, carbamazine
	Antihypertensive	Methyldopa,‡ captopril, enalapril
	Antibiotic	Isoniazid,‡ rifampin, nitrofurantoin
	Diuretic	Chlorothiazide
	Laxative	Oxyphenisatin‡
	Antidepressant	Iproniazid, amitriptyline, imipramine
	Anti-inflammatory	Ibuprofen, indomethacin, diclofenac, sulindac
	Antifungal	Ketoconazole, fluconazole, itraconazole
	Antiviral	Zidovudine, dideoxy inosine
	Calcium channel blocker	Nifedipine, verapamil, diltiazem
	Antiandrogen	Flutamide
Mixed hepatitis/ cholestatic	Immunosuppressive	Azathioprine
	Lipid-lowering	Nicotinic acid, lovastatin
Toxic (necrosis)	Hydrocarbon	Carbon tetrachloride
	Metal	Yellow phosphorus
	Mushroom	*Amanita phalloides*
	Analgesic	Acetaminophen
	Solvent	Dimethylformamide
Granulomas	Anti-inflammatory	Phenylbutazone
	Antibiotic	Sulfanomides
	Xanthine oxidase inhibitor	Allopurinol
	Antiarrhythmic	Quinidine
	Anticonvulsant	Carbamazine

* Several agents cause more than one type of liver lesion and appear under more than one category.
† Rarely associated with primary biliary cirrhosis–like lesion.
‡ Occasionally associated with chronic hepatitis or bridging hepatic necrosis or cirrhosis.

angiosarcoma of the liver. Oral contraceptives have been implicated in the development of hepatic adenoma and, rarely, hepatocellular carcinoma and occlusion of the hepatic vein (Budd-Chiari syndrome). Another unusual lesion, peliosis hepatis (blood cysts of the liver), has been observed in some patients treated with anabolic steroids. The existence of these hepatic disorders expands the spectrum of liver injury induced by chemical agents and emphasizes the need for a thorough drug history in all patients with liver dysfunction.

The following are the patterns of adverse hepatic reactions for some prototypic agents.

ACETAMINOPHEN HEPATOTOXICITY (DIRECT TOXIN) Acetaminophen has caused severe centrolobular hepatic necrosis when ingested in large amounts in suicide attempts or accidentally by children. A single dose of 10 to 15 g, occasionally less, may produce clinical evidence of liver injury. Fatal fulminant disease is usually (although not invariably) associated with ingestion of 25 g or more. Blood levels of acetaminophen correlate with the severity of hepatic injury (levels above 300 μg/mL 4 h after ingestion are predictive of the development of severe damage, while levels below 150 μg/mL suggest that hepatic injury is highly unlikely). Nausea, vomiting, diarrhea, abdominal pain, and shock are early manifestations occurring 4 to 12 h after ingestion. Then 24 to 48 h later, when these features are abating, hepatic injury becomes apparent. Maximal abnormalities and hepatic failure may not be evident until 4 to 6 days after ingestion, and aminotransferase levels approaching 10,000 units are not uncommon. Renal failure and myocardial injury may be present.

Acetaminophen hepatotoxicity is mediated by a toxic reactive metabolite formed from the parent compound by the cytochrome P450 mixed-function oxidase system of the hepatocyte. This metabolite is detoxified by binding to glutathione. When excessive amounts of the metabolite are formed, glutathione levels in the liver fall, and the metabolite is covalently bound to nucleophilic hepatocyte macromolecules. This process is believed to lead to hepatocyte necrosis; the precise sequence and mechanism are unknown. Hepatic injury may be potentiated by prior administration of alcohol or other drugs, by conditions that stimulate the mixed-function oxidase system, or by conditions such as starvation that reduce hepatic glutathione levels. Cimetidine, which inhibits P450 enzymes, has the potential to reduce generation of the toxic metabolite. In chronic alcoholics, the toxic dose of acetaminophen may be as low as 2 g.

℞ **TREATMENT**

Treatment of acetaminophen overdosage includes gastric lavage, supportive measures, and oral administration of activated charcoal or cholestyramine to prevent absorption of residual drug. Neither of these agents appears to be effective if given more than 30 min after acetaminophen ingestion; if they are used, the stomach lavage should be done before other agents are administered orally. In patients with high acetaminophen blood levels (>200 μg/mL measured at 4 h or >100 μg/mL at 8 h after ingestion), the administration of sulfhydryl compounds (e.g., cysteamine, cysteine, or N-acetylcysteine) appears to reduce the severity of hepatic necrosis. These agents appear to act by providing a reservoir of sulfhydryl groups to bind the toxic metabolites or by stimulating synthesis and repletion of hepatic glutathione. Therapy should be begun within 8 h of ingestion but may be effective even if given as late as 24 to 36 h after overdose. Later administration of sulfhydryl compounds is of uncertain value. Routine use of N-acetylcysteine has reduced substantially the occurrence of fatal acetaminophen hepatotoxicity. When given orally, N-acetylcysteine is diluted to yield a 5% solution. A loading dose of 140 mg/kg is given, followed by 70 mg/kg every 4 h for 15 to 20 doses. Treatment can be stopped when plasma acetominophen levels indicate that the risk of liver damage is low.

Survivors of acute acetaminophen overdose usually have no evidence of hepatic sequelae. In a few patients, prolonged or repeated administration of acetaminophen in therapeutic doses appears to have led to the development of chronic hepatitis and cirrhosis.

HALOTHANE HEPATOTOXICITY (IDIOSYNCRATIC REACTION) Administration of halothane, a nonexplosive fluorinated hydrocarbon anesthetic agent that is structurally similar to chloroform, results in severe hepatic necrosis in a small number of individuals, many of whom have previously been exposed to this agent. The failure to produce similar hepatic lesions reliably in animals, the rarity of hepatic impairment in human beings, and the delayed appearance of hepatic injury suggest that halothane is not a direct hepatotoxin but rather a sensitizing agent. However, manifestations of hypersensitivity are seen in fewer than 25 percent of cases. A genetic predisposition leading to an idiosyncratic metabolic reactivity has been postulated and appears to be the most likely mechanism of halothane hepatotoxicity. Adults (rather than children), obese people, and women appear to be particularly susceptible. Fever, moderate leukocytosis, and eosinophilia may occur in the first week following halothane administration. Jaundice usually is noted 7 to 10 days after exposure but may occur earlier in previously exposed patients. Nausea and vomiting may precede the onset of jaundice. Hepatomegaly is often mild, but liver tenderness is common. The serum aminotransferase levels are elevated. The pathologic changes at autopsy are indistinguishable from massive hepatic necrosis resulting from viral hepatitis. The case-fatality rate of halothane hepatitis is not known but may vary from 20 to 40 percent in cases with severe liver involvement. It is strongly suggested that patients in whom unexplained spiking fever, especially delayed fever, or jaundice develops after halothane anesthesia not receive this agent again. Because cross-reactions between halothane and methoxyfluorane have been reported, the latter agent should not be used after halothane reactions. Later-generation halogenated hydrocarbon anesthetics, which have supplanted halothane except in rare instances, are felt to be associated with a lower risk of hepatotoxicity.

METHYLDOPA HEPATOTOXICITY (TOXIC AND IDIO-SYNCRATIC REACTION) Minor alterations in liver tests are reported in about 5 percent of patients treated with this antihypertensive agent. These trivial abnormalities typically resolve despite continued drug administration. In fewer than 1 percent of patients, acute liver injury resembling viral or chronic hepatitis or, rarely, a cholestatic reaction is seen 1 to 20 weeks after methyldopa is started. In 50 percent of cases the interval is shorter than 4 weeks. A prodrome of fever, anorexia, and malaise may be noted for a few days before the onset of jaundice. Rash, lymphadenopathy, arthralgia, and eosinophilia are rare. Serologic markers of autoimmunity are detected infrequently, and fewer than 5 percent of patients have a Coombs-positive hemolytic anemia. In about 15 percent of patients with methyldopa hepatotoxicity, the clinical, biochemical, and histologic features are those of moderate to severe chronic hepatitis, with or without bridging necrosis and macronodular cirrhosis. With discontinuation of the drug, the disorder usually resolves.

ISONIAZID HEPATOTOXICITY (TOXIC AND IDIOSYN-CRATIC REACTION) In approximately 10 percent of adults treated with the antituberculosis agent isoniazid, elevated serum aminotransferase levels develop during the first few weeks of therapy; this appears to represent an adaptive response to a toxic metabolite of the drug. Whether or not isoniazid is continued, these values (usually below 200 units) return to normal in a few weeks. In about 1 percent of treated patients, an illness develops that is indistinguishable from viral hepatitis; approximately half of these cases occur within the first 2 months of treatment, while in the remainder, clinical disease may be delayed for many months. Liver biopsy reveals morphologic changes similar to those of viral hepatitis or bridging hepatic necrosis. The disease may be severe, with a case-fatality rate of 10 percent. Important liver injury appears to be age-related, increasing substantially after age 35; the highest frequency is in patients over age 50, the lowest under the age of 20. Isoniazid hepatotoxicity is enhanced by alcohol and rifampicin. Fever, rash, eosinophilia, and other manifestations of drug allergy are distinctly unusual. A reactive metabolite of acetylhydrazine, a metabolite of isoniazid, may be responsible for liver injury, and patients who are rapid acetylators would be more prone to such injury. A picture resembling chronic hepatitis has been observed in a few patients.

SODIUM VALPROATE HEPATOTOXICITY (TOXIC AND IDIOSYNCRATIC REACTION) Sodium valproate, an anticonvulsant useful in the treatment of petit mal and other seizure disorders, has been associated with the development of severe hepatic toxicity and, rarely, fatalities in both children and adults. Asymptomatic elevations of serum aminotransferase levels have been recognized in as many as 45 percent of treated patients. These "adaptive" changes,

however, appear to have no clinical importance, for major hepatotoxicity is not seen in the majority of patients despite continuation of drug therapy. In those rare patients in whom jaundice, encephalopathy, and evidence of hepatic failure are found, examination of liver tissue reveals microvesicular fat and bridging hepatic necrosis, predominantly in the centrolobular zone. Bile duct injury also may be apparent. It seems likely that sodium valproate is not directly hepatotoxic but that its metabolite, 4-pentenoic acid, may be responsible for hepatic injury.

PHENYTOIN HEPATOTOXICITY (IDIOSYNCRATIC RE-ACTION) Phenytoin, formerly diphenylhydantoin, a mainstay in the treatment of seizure disorders, has been associated in rare instances with the development of severe hepatitis-like liver injury leading to fulminant hepatic failure. In many patients the hepatitis is associated with striking fever, lymphadenopathy, rash (Stevens-Johnson syndrome or exfoliative dermatitis), leukocytosis, and eosinophilia, suggesting an immunologically mediated hypersensitivity mechanism. Despite these observations, there is also evidence that metabolic idiosyncrasy may be responsible for hepatic injury. In the liver, phenytoin is converted by the cytochrome P450 system to metabolites, which include the highly reactive electrophilic arene oxides. These metabolites are normally metabolized further by epoxide hydrolases. A defect (genetic or acquired) in epoxide hydrolase activity could permit covalent binding of arene oxides to hepatic macromolecules, thereby leading to hepatic injury. Regardless of the mechanism, hepatic injury is usually manifest within the first 2 months after beginning phenytoin therapy. With the exception of an abundance of eosinophils in the liver, the clinical, biochemical, and histologic picture resembles that of viral hepatitis. In rare instances, bile duct injury may be the salient feature of phenytoin hepatotoxicity, with striking features of intrahepatic cholestasis. Asymptomatic elevations of aminotransferase and alkaline phosphatase levels have been observed in a sizable proportion of patients receiving long-term phenytoin therapy. These liver changes are believed by some authorities to represent the potent hepatic enzyme–inducing properties of phenytoin and are accompanied histologically by swelling of hepatocytes in the absence of necroinflammatory activity or evidence of chronic liver disease.

CHLORPROMAZINE HEPATOTOXICITY (CHOLE-STATIC IDIOSYNCRATIC REACTION) In about 1 percent of patients receiving chlorpromazine, intrahepatic cholestasis with jaundice develops after 1 to 4 weeks of treatment. In rare instances, jaundice has been reported after a single exposure. Anicteric reactions are frequent. The onset may be abrupt, with fever, rash, arthralgias, lymphadenopathy, nausea, vomiting, and epigastric or right upper quadrant pain. Pruritus may precede the appearance of jaundice, dark urine, and light stools. Eosinophilia with or without mild leukocytosis may be present, and conjugated hyperbilirubinemia, moderately elevated serum alkaline phosphatase, and mildly elevated serum aminotransferase levels (100 to 200 units) are noted. Liver biopsy reveals cholestasis, bile plugs in dilated bile canaliculi, and a dense portal infiltrate of polymorphonuclear, eosinophilic, and mononuclear leukocytes. Occasionally, scattered foci of hepatic parenchymal necrosis may be evident. Jaundice and pruritus usually subside within 4 to 8 weeks following cessation of therapy, without sequelae, and fatalities are rare. Cholestyramine may be of value in relieving severe pruritus. In a small number of patients, jaundice is prolonged for several months to years; rarely, a disorder resembling but distinct from primary biliary cirrhosis may develop.

AMIODARONE HEPATOTOXICITY (TOXIC AND IDIO-SYNCRATIC REACTION) Therapy with this potent antiarrhythmic drug is accompanied in 15 to 50 percent of patients by modest elevation of serum aminotransferase levels that may remain stable or diminish despite continuation of the drug. Such abnormalities may appear days to many months after beginning therapy. A proportion of those with elevated aminotransferase levels have detectable hepatomegaly, and clinically important liver disease develops in fewer than 5 percent of patients. Features that represent a direct effect of the drug on the liver and that are common to the majority of long-term recipients are ultrastructural phospholipidosis, unaccompanied by clinical liver disease, and interference with hepatic mixed-function oxidase metabolism of other drugs. The relatively common elevations in aminotransferase levels are also considered a predictable, dose-dependent, direct hepatotoxic effect. On the other hand, in the rare patient with clinically apparent, symptomatic liver disease, liver injury resembling that seen in alcoholic liver disease is observed. The so-called pseudoalcoholic liver injury can range from steatosis, to alcoholic hepatitis–like neutrophilic infiltration and Mallory's hyaline, to cirrhosis. Electron-microscopic demonstration of phospholipid-laden lysosomal lamellar bodies can help to distinguish amiodarone hepatotoxicity from typical alcoholic hepatitis. This category of liver injury appears to be a metabolic idiosyncracy that allows hepatotoxic metabolites to be generated. Rarely, an acute idiosyncratic hepatocellular injury resembling viral hepatitis or cholestatic hepatitis occurs. Hepatic granulomas have occasionally been observed. Because amiodarone has a long half-life, liver injury may persist for months after the drug is stopped.

ERYTHROMYCIN HEPATOTOXICITY (CHOLESTATIC IDIOSYNCRATIC REACTION)   The most important adverse effect associated with erythromycin is the infrequent occurrence of a cholestatic reaction. Although most of these reactions have been associated with erythromycin estolate, other erythromycins also may be responsible. The reaction usually begins during the first 2 or 3 weeks of therapy and includes nausea, vomiting, fever, right upper quadrant abdominal pain, jaundice, leukocytosis, and moderately elevated aminotransferase levels. The clinical picture can resemble acute cholecystitis or bacterial cholangitis. Liver biopsy reveals variable cholestasis; portal inflammation comprising lymphocytes, polymorphonuclear leukocytes, and eosinophils; and scattered foci of hepatocyte necrosis. Symptoms and laboratory findings usually subside within a few days of drug withdrawal, and evidence of chronic liver disease has not been found on follow-up. The precise mechanism remains ill-defined.

ORAL CONTRACEPTIVE HEPATOTOXICITY (CHOLESTATIC REACTION)   The administration of oral contraceptive combinations of estrogenic and progestational steroids leads to intrahepatic cholestasis with pruritus and jaundice in a small number of patients weeks to months after taking these agents. Especially susceptible seem to be patients with recurrent idiopathic jaundice of pregnancy, severe pruritus of pregnancy, or a family history of these disorders. With the exception of liver biochemical tests, laboratory studies are normal, and extrahepatic manifestations of hypersensitivity are absent. Liver biopsy reveals cholestasis with bile plugs in dilated canaliculi and striking bilirubin staining of liver cells. In contrast to chlorpromazine-induced cholestasis, portal inflammation is absent. The lesion is reversible on withdrawal of the agent. The two steroid components appear to act synergistically on hepatic function, although the estrogen may be primarily responsible. Oral contraceptives are contraindicated in patients with a history of recurrent jaundice of pregnancy. Primarily benign, but rarely malignant, neoplasms of the liver, hepatic vein occlusion, and peripheral sinusoidal dilatation have also been associated with oral contraceptive therapy.

17,α-ALKYL-SUBSTITUTED ANABOLIC STEROIDS (CHOLESTATIC REACTION)   In the majority of patients receiving these agents, used therapeutically mainly in the treatment of bone marrow failure but used surreptitiously and without medical indication by athletes to improve their performance, mild hepatic dysfunction develops. Impaired excretory function is the predominant defect, but the precise mechanism is uncertain. Jaundice, which appears to be dose-related, develops in only a minority of patients and may be the sole clinical manifestation of hepatotoxicity, although anorexia, nausea, and malaise may occur. Pruritus is not a prominent feature. Serum aminotransferase levels are usually under 100 units, and serum alkaline phosphatase levels are normal, mildly elevated, or, in fewer than 5 percent of patients, three or more times the upper limit of normal. Examination of liver tissue reveals cholestasis without inflammation or

necrosis. Hepatic sinusoidal dilatation and peliosis hepatis have been found in a few patients. The cholestatic disorder is usually reversible on cessation of treatment, although fatalities have been linked to peliosis. An association with hepatic adenoma and hepatocellular carcinoma has been reported.

TRIMETHOPRIM-SULFAMETHOXAZOLE   HEPATO-TOXICITY (IDIOSYNCRATIC REACTION)   This antibiotic combination is used routinely for urinary tract infections in immunocompetent persons and for prophylaxis against and therapy of *Pneumocystis carinii* pneumonia in immunosuppressed persons (transplant recipients, patients with AIDS). With its increasing use, its occasional hepatotoxicity is being recognized with growing frequency. Its likelihood is unpredictable, but when it occurs, trimethoprim-sulfamethoxazole hepatotoxicity follows a relatively uniform latency period of several weeks and is often accompanied by eosinophilia, rash, and other features of a hypersensitivity reaction. Biochemically and histologically, acute hepatocellular necrosis predominates, but cholestatic features are quite frequent. Occasionally, cholestasis without necrosis occurs, and very rarely, a severe cholangiolytic pattern of liver injury is observed. In most cases, liver injury is self-limited, but rare fatalities have been recorded. The hepatotoxicity is attributable to the sulfamethoxazole component of the drug and is similar in features to that seen with other sulfonamides; tissue eosinophilia and granulomas may be seen.

BIBLIOGRAPHY

BLACK M et al: Isoniazid-associated hepatitis in 114 patients. Gastroenterology 69:389, 1975

———: Acetaminophen hepatotoxicity. Ann Rev Med 35:577, 1984

HARRISON PM et al: Improved outcome of paracetamol-induced fulminant hepatic failure by late administration of acetylcysteine. Lancet 335:1572, 1990

KAPLOWITZ N et al: Drug-induced hepatotoxicity. Ann Intern Med 104:826, 1986

——— (ed): Recent advances in drug metabolism and hepatotoxicity. Semin Liver Dis 10:233, 1990

LEE WM: Drug-induced hepatotoxicity. N Engl J Med 333:1118, 1995

LEWIS JH et al: Amiodarone hepatotoxicity: Prevalence and clinicopathologic correlations among 104 patients. Hepatology 9:679, 1989

LUDWIG J, AXELSEN R: Drug effects on the liver: An updated tabular compilation of drugs and drug-related hepatic diseases. Dig Dis Sci 28:651, 1983

MORGAN DJ, SMALLWOOD RA: Drug-induced liver disease. Curr Opinion Gastroenterol 12:246, 1996

RABINOVITZ M et al: Hepatotoxicity of nonsteroidal anti-inflammatory drugs. Am J Gastroenterol 87:1696, 1992

SEEFF LB et al: Acetaminophen hepatotoxicity in alcoholics: A therapeutic misadventure. Ann Intern Med 104:399, 1986

SMILKSTEIN MJ et al: Efficacy of N-acetylcysteine in the treatment of acetaminophen overdose. N Engl J Med 319:1557, 1988

TARAZI EM et al: Sulindac-associated hepatic injury: Analysis of 91 cases reported to the Food and Drug Administration. Gastroenterology 104:569, 1993

WHITCOMB DC et al: Association of acetaminophen hepatotoxicity with fasting and ethanol use. JAMA 272:1845, 1994

ZIMMERMAN HJ, ISHAK KG: Valproate-induced hepatic injury: Analysis of 23 fatal cases. Hepatology 2:591, 1982

297   *Jules L. Dienstag, Kurt J. Isselbacher*

CHRONIC HEPATITIS

Chronic hepatitis represents a series of liver disorders of varying causes and severity in which hepatic inflammation and necrosis continue for at least 6 months. Milder forms are nonprogressive or only slowly progressive, while more severe forms may be associated with scarring and architectural organization, which, when advanced, lead ultimately to cirrhosis. Several categories of chronic hepatitis have been recognized. These include chronic viral hepatitis (see Chap. 295), drug-induced chronic hepatitis (see Chap. 296), and autoimmune chronic hepatitis. In many cases, clinical and laboratory features are insufficient to allow assignment into one of these three categories; these "idiopathic" cases are also believed to represent autoimmune chronic hepatitis. Finally, clinical and laboratory features of chronic hepatitis are observed occasionally in patients with such hereditary/metabolic disorders as Wilson's disease (copper overload) and even occasionally in patients with alcoholic liver injury (see Chap. 298). Although all types of chronic hepatitis share certain clinical, laboratory, and histopathologic features, chronic viral and chronic autoimmune hepatitis are sufficiently distinct to merit separate discussions.

CLASSIFICATION OF CHRONIC HEPATITIS Common to all forms of chronic hepatitis are histopathologic distinctions based on localization and extent of liver injury. These vary from the milder forms, previously labeled chronic persistent hepatitis and chronic lobular hepatitis, to the more severe form, formerly called chronic active hepatitis. When first defined, these designations were felt to have prognostic implications, which have been challenged by more recent observations. Compared to the time more than two decades ago when the histologic designations chronic persistent, chronic lobular, and chronic active hepatitis were adopted, much more information is currently available about the causes, natural history, pathogenesis, serologic features, and therapy of chronic hepatitis. Therefore, categorization of chronic hepatitis based primarily upon histopathologic features has been replaced by a more informative classification based upon a combination of clinical, serologic, and histologic variables. Classification of chronic hepatitis is based upon (1) its *cause*, (2) its histologic activity, or *grade*, and (3) its degree of progression, or *stage*. Thus, neither clinical features alone nor histologic features—requiring liver biopsy—alone are sufficient to characterize and distinguish among the several categories of chronic hepatitis.

Classification by Cause Clinical and serologic features allow the establishment of a diagnosis of *chronic viral hepatitis*, caused by hepatitis B, hepatitis B plus D, hepatitis C, or other viruses; *autoimmune hepatitis*, including several subcategories, types 1, 2, and 3, based on serologic distinctions; *drug-associated chronic hepatitis*; and a category of unknown cause, or *cryptogenic* chronic hepatitis (Table 297-1). These are addressed in more detail below.

Classification by Grade Grade, a histologic assessment of necroinflammatory activity, is based upon examination of the liver biopsy. An assessment of important histologic features includes the degree of *periportal necrosis* and the disruption of the limiting plate of periportal hepatocytes by inflammatory cells (so-called *piecemeal necrosis*); the

Table 297-2

Histologic Activity Index (Knodell-Ishak Score) in Chronic Hepatitis

Histologic Feature	Severity	Score
1. Periportal necrosis, including piecemeal necrosis (PN), and/or bridging necrosis (BN)	None	0
	Mild PN	1
	Moderate PN	3
	Marked PN	4
	Moderate PN + BN	5
	Marked PN + BN	6
	Multilobular necrosis	10
2. Intralobular necrosis	None	0
	Mild	1
	Moderate	3
	Marked	4
3. Portal inflammation	None	0
	Mild	1
	Moderate	3
	Marked	4
4. Fibrosis	None	0
	Expanding portal tract	1
	Bridging fibrosis	3
	Cirrhosis	4
Maximum score		22

degree of confluent necrosis that links, or forms bridges between vascular structures—between portal tract and portal tract or even more important bridges between portal tract and central vein—referred to as *bridging necrosis*; the degree of hepatocyte degeneration and focal necrosis within the lobule; and the degree of *portal inflammation*. Several scoring systems that take these histologic features into account have been devised, and the most popular is the numerical histologic activity index (HAI), based on the work of Knodell and Ishak (Table 297-2). Technically, the HAI, which is primarily a measure of *grade*, also includes an assessment of fibrosis, which is currently used to categorize *stage* of the disease, as described below. Such precise HAI scoring tends to be used more in measuring disease activity before and after therapy in clinical studies. In clinical practice, more qualitative grading suffices. Based on the presence and degree of these features of histologic activity, chronic hepatitis can be graded as mild, moderate, or severe.

Classification by Stage The stage of chronic hepatitis, which reflects the level of progression of the disease, is based on the degree of fibrosis. When fibrosis is so extensive that fibrous septa surround parenchymal nodules and alter the normal architecture of the liver lobule, the histologic lesion is defined as cirrhosis. Staging is based on the degree of fibrosis as follows:

0 = no fibrosis
1 = mild fibrosis
2 = moderate fibrosis
3 = severe fibrosis, including bridging fibrosis
4 = cirrhosis

Reconciliation Between Histologic Classification and New Classification For historical purposes, and to provide the basis for navigating several decades worth of literature on chronic hepatitis, the histologic categories chronic persistent hepatitis, chronic lobular hepatitis, and chronic active hepatitis are worth reviewing and linking with their new-classification counterparts (Table 297-3).

In *chronic persistent hepatitis*, a mononuclear inflammatory infiltrate expands, but is localized to and contained within, portal tracts. The "limiting plate" of periportal hepatocytes is intact, and there is no extension of the necroinflammatory process into the liver lobule. A "cobblestone" arrangement of liver cells, indicative of hepatic regenerative activity, is a common feature, and although minimal periportal fibrosis may be present, *cirrhosis is absent*. As a general rule, patients with chronic persistent hepatitis are asymptomatic or have relatively

Table 297-1

Clinical and Laboratory Features of Chronic Hepatitis

Type of Hepatitis	Diagnostic Test(s)	Autoantibodies	Therapy
Chronic hepatitis B	HBsAg, IgG anti-HBc, HBeAg, HBV DNA	Uncommon	Interferon α
Chronic hepatitis C	Anti-HCV (EIA and RIBA), HCV RNA	Anti-LKM1*	Interferon α
Chronic hepatitis D	Anti-HDV, HDV RNA, HBsAg, IgG anti-HBc	Anti-LKM3	Interferon α (?)
Other viral	?Anti-HGV, ?HGV RNA	?	?
Autoimmune hepatitis	ANA† (homogeneous), anti-LKM1(±), hyperglobulinemia	ANA, anti-LKM1, anti-SLA‡	Prednisone, azathioprine
Drug-associated	—	Uncommon	Withdraw drug
Cryptogenic	All negative	None	Prednisone (?), azathioprine (?)

* Antibodies to liver-kidney microsomes type 1 (autoimmune hepatitis type II and some cases of hepatitis C).
† Antinuclear antibody (autoimmune hepatitis type I).
‡ Antibodies to soluble liver antigen (autoimmune hepatitis type III).

NOTE: HBsAg, hepatitis B surface antigen; EIA, enzyme immunoassay; RIBA, recombinant immunoblot assay; HGV, hepatitis G virus.

Table 297-3

Correlation Between Earlier and Contemporary Nomenclature of Chronic Hepatitis

Old Classification	Contemporary Classification	
	Grade (Activity)	Stage (Fibrosis)
Chronic persistent hepatitis	Minimal or mild	None or mild
Chronic lobular hepatitis	Mild or moderate	Mild
Chronic active hepatitis	Mild, moderate, or severe	Mild, moderate, or severe

mild constitutional symptoms (e.g., fatigue, anorexia, nausea); have normal physical findings, except perhaps for liver enlargement, without the usual stigmata of chronic liver disease (see below); and have modest elevations of aminotransferase activities. Progression to more severe lesions (chronic active hepatitis and cirrhosis) was felt to be very unlikely, especially in patients with autoimmune or idiopathic chronic persistent hepatitis; however, progressive disease occurs in patients with chronic persistent *viral* hepatitis and in those with chronic persistent hepatitis following spontaneous or therapeutic remission of autoimmune hepatitis. In the new nomenclature, chronic persistent hepatitis would be classified by *grade* as minimal or mild chronic hepatitis and by *stage* as absent or mild fibrosis.

In patients with *chronic lobular hepatitis*, in addition to portal inflammation, histologic examination of the liver reveals foci of necrosis and inflammation in the liver lobule. Morphologically, chronic lobular hepatitis resembles slowly resolving acute hepatitis. The limiting plate remains intact, periportal fibrosis is absent or limited, lobular architecture is preserved, and progression to chronic active hepatitis and cirrhosis was felt to be rare. Thus chronic lobular hepatitis can be considered a variant of chronic persistent hepatitis with a lobular component, and clinical/laboratory features are comparable. Occasionally, the clinical activity of chronic lobular hepatitis may increase spontaneously; elevation of aminotransferase activity may resemble that seen in acute hepatitis, and transient histologic deterioration can be documented. The same qualifications in prognostic import mentioned above for chronic persistent hepatitis apply to chronic lobular hepatitis. Chronic lobular hepatitis corresponds in the new nomenclature to a mild or moderate *grade* and a *stage* of absent or minimal fibrosis.

Chronic active hepatitis is characterized clinically by continuing hepatic necrosis, portal/periportal and, to a lesser extent, lobular inflammation, and fibrosis. Varying in severity from mild to severe, chronic active hepatitis was recognized to be a progressive disorder that can lead to cirrhosis, liver failure, and death. Morphologic characteristics of chronic active hepatitis include (1) a dense mononuclear infiltrate of the portal tracts, which are substantially expanded into the liver lobule (in the autoimmune type, plasma cells represent a component of the infiltrate); (2) destruction of the hepatocytes at the periphery of the lobule, with erosion of the limiting plate of hepatocytes surrounding the portal triads (piecemeal necrosis); (3) connective tissue septa surrounding portal tracts and extending from the portal zones into the lobule, isolating parenchymal cells into clusters and enveloping bile ducts; and (4) evidence of hepatocellular regeneration—"rosette" formation, thickened liver cell plates, and regenerative "pseudolobules." This process may be patchy, with individual liver lobules spared, or it may be diffuse. Histologic evidence of single-cell coagulative necrosis, Councilman or acidophilic bodies, appear in the periportal areas. Piecemeal necrosis is the minimal histologic requirement to establish a diagnosis of chronic active hepatitis, but this change is seen even in mild, relatively nonprogressive forms of chronic active hepatitis. A more severe lesion, *bridging hepatic necrosis* (originally termed *subacute hepatic necrosis*), characterizes a more severe and progressive form of chronic active hepatitis. Although bridging necrosis can be seen occasionally in patients with acute hepatitis, in whom it carries no prognostic importance, in chronic active hepatitis this

lesion is associated with progression to cirrhosis. Bridging necrosis is characterized by hepatocellular dropout that spans lobules (i.e., between portal tracts—the periphery of the lobule—or between portal tracts and central veins—the centrizonal part of the lobule). Collapse of the reticulin network is a hallmark of bridging necrosis, and bridging fibrosis follows, leading ultimately to architectural reorganization by nodular regeneration, i.e., cirrhosis. A more extensive and ominous variant of bridging necrosis is multilobular collapse, in which bridging necrosis is widespread throughout the liver and which is associated clinically with rapid deterioration and even acute liver failure.

Although progression to cirrhosis is difficult to demonstrate in patients with chronic active hepatitis who have isolated piecemeal necrosis, in more severe forms of chronic active hepatitis, progression to cirrhosis is common. Among patients with chronic active hepatitis on liver biopsy, 20 to 50 percent also have cirrhosis, even early during the course of the disease. Generally, chronic active hepatitis is more severe clinically than chronic persistent and lobular hepatitis. Although a sizable proportion of patients with chronic active hepatitis are asymptomatic, the majority tend to have mild to severe constitutional symptoms, especially fatigue. Generally, physical findings associated with chronic liver disease and portal hypertension are more common, aminotransferase levels tend to be higher, and jaundice and hyperbilirubinemia are more frequent in this form of chronic hepatitis.

In the new nomenclature for chronic hepatitis, what used to be called chronic active hepatitis spans the entire spectrum of activity *grade* from minimal, to mild, to severe chronic hepatitis, based on the degree of periportal and piecemeal necrosis, on the degree of lobular inflammation and injury, and on the degree of portal inflammation. Similarly, *stage* in chronic active hepatitis can translate to mild, moderate, or severe fibrosis as well as to cirrhosis.

CHRONIC VIRAL HEPATITIS   Both the enterically transmitted forms of viral hepatitis, hepatitis A and E, are self-limited and do not cause chronic hepatitis (rare reports notwithstanding in which acute hepatitis A serves as a trigger for the onset of autoimmune hepatitis in genetically susceptible patients). In contrast, the entire clinicopathologic spectrum of chronic hepatitis occurs in patients with chronic viral hepatitis B and C as well as in patients with chronic hepatitis D superimposed on chronic hepatitis B.

Chronic Hepatitis B   The likelihood of chronicity after acute hepatitis B varies as a function of age. Infection at birth is associated with a clinically silent acute infection but a 90 percent chance of chronic infection, while infection in young adulthood in immunocompetent persons is associated typically with clinically apparent acute hepatitis but a risk of chronicity of only approximately 1 percent. Most cases of chronic hepatitis B among adults, however, occur in patients who never had a recognized episode of clinically apparent acute viral hepatitis. The degree of liver injury (grade) in patients with chronic hepatitis B is variable, ranging from none in asymptomatic carriers, to mild, to severe. Among adults with chronic hepatitis B, histologic features are of prognostic importance. In one long-term study of patients with chronic hepatitis B, investigators found a 5-year survival of 97 percent for patients with chronic persistent hepatitis (mild chronic hepatitis), of 86 percent for patients with chronic active hepatitis (moderate to severe chronic hepatitis), and of only 55 percent for patients with chronic active hepatitis and postnecrotic cirrhosis. On the other hand, more recent observations do not allow us to be so sanguine about the prognosis in patients with mild chronic hepatitis; among patients with what used to be labeled chronic persistent hepatitis followed for 1 to 13 years, progression to more severe chronic hepatitis and cirrhosis has been observed in more than a quarter of cases.

Probably more important to consider than histology alone in patients with chronic hepatitis B is the degree of hepatitis B virus (HBV) replication. As reviewed in Chap. 295, chronic hepatitis B can be divided into two phases based on the relative level of HBV replication. The relatively *replicative phase* is characterized by the presence in the serum of markers of HBV replication [hepatitis B e antigen (HBeAg) HBV DNA], by the presence in the liver of detectable intrahepatocyte nucleocapsid antigens [primarily hepatitis B core antigen (HBcAg)], by high infectivity, and by accompanying liver injury;

HBV DNA can be detected in the liver but is extrachromosomal. In contrast, the relatively *nonreplicative phase* is characterized by the absence of conventional markers of HBV replication (HBeAg and HBV DNA detectable by hybridization) but associated with anti-HBe, the absence of intrahepatocytic HBcAg, limited infectivity, and minimal liver injury; HBV DNA can be detected in the liver but is integrated into the host genome. Those in the replicative phase tend to have more severe chronic hepatitis, while those in the nonreplicative phase tend to have minimal or mild chronic hepatitis or to be asymptomatic hepatitis B carriers; however, distinctions in HBV replication and in histologic category do not always coincide. The likelihood of converting spontaneously from relatively replicative to nonreplicative chronic HBV infection is approximately 10 to 15 percent per year. As noted in Chap. 295, the conversion from replicative to nonreplicative chronic hepatitis B is associated with a transient elevation in aminotransferase activity resembling acute hepatitis; occasionally, spontaneous resumptions of replicative activity occur in nonreplicative infection; and occasionally, HBV variants occur in which serologic markers of replication (HBeAg) are absent, despite the presence of replicative infection. As reviewed in Chap. 93, chronic HBV infection, especially when acquired at birth or in early childhood, is associated with an increased risk of hepatocellular carcinoma. A discussion of the pathogenesis of liver injury in patients with chronic hepatitis B appears in Chap. 295.

The spectrum of *clinical features* of chronic hepatitis B is broad, ranging from asymptomatic infection to debilitating disease or even end-stage, fatal hepatic failure. As noted above, the onset of the disease tends to be insidious in most patients, with the exception of the very few in whom chronic disease follows failure of resolution of clinically apparent acute hepatitis B. The clinical and laboratory features associated with progression from acute to chronic hepatitis B are discussed in Chap. 295. *Fatigue* is a common symptom, and persistent or intermittent *jaundice* is a common feature in severe or advanced cases. Intermittent deepening of jaundice and recurrence of malaise and anorexia, as well as worsening fatigue, are reminiscent of acute hepatitis; such exacerbations may occur spontaneously, often coinciding with evidence of virologic reactivation, may lead to progressive liver injury, and, when superimposed on well-established cirrhosis, may cause hepatic decompensation. Complications of cirrhosis occur in end-stage chronic hepatitis and include ascites, edema, bleeding gastroesophageal varices, hepatic encephalopathy, coagulopathy, or hypersplenism. Occasionally, these complications bring the patient to initial clinical attention. Extrahepatic complications of chronic hepatitis B, similar to those seen during the prodromal phase of acute hepatitis B, are associated with deposition of circulating hepatitis B antigen–antibody immune complexes. As reviewed in Chap. 295, these include arthralgias and arthritis, which are common, and the more rare purpuric cutaneous lesions (leukocytoclastic vasculitis), immune-complex glomerulonephritis, and generalized vasculitis (polyarteritis nodosa).

Laboratory features of chronic hepatitis B do not distinguish adequately between histologically mild and severe hepatitis. Aminotransferase elevations tend to be modest for chronic hepatitis B but may fluctuate in the range of 100 to 1000 units. As is true for acute viral hepatitis B, alanine aminotransferase (ALT, or SGPT) tends to be more elevated than aspartate aminotransferase (AST, or SGOT); however, once cirrhosis is established, AST tends to exceed ALT. Levels of alkaline phosphatase activity tend to be normal or only marginally elevated. In severe cases, moderate elevations in serum bilirubin [51.3 to 171 μmol/L (3 to 10 mg/dL)] occur. Hypoalbuminemia and prolongation of the prothrombin time occur in severe or end-stage cases. Hyperglobulinemia and detectable circulating autoantibodies are distinctly absent in chronic hepatitis B (in contrast to autoimmune hepatitis). → *Viral markers of chronic HBV infection are discussed in Chap. 295.*

℞ **TREATMENT**
Management of chronic hepatitis B depends on the level of virus replication. Although progression to cirrhosis is more likely in severe chronic than in mild or moderate chronic hepatitis B, all forms of chronic viral hepatitis can be progressive. Randomized, prospective, controlled trials have established that patients with well-compensated

chronic replicative hepatitis B, selected to have chronic hepatitis on liver biopsy and aminotransferase elevations, regardless of histologic features, respond to antiviral therapy with interferon α. A 4-month (16-week) course of subcutaneous injections, daily at a dose of 5 million units or three times a week at a dose of 10 million units, is associated with an approximately 40 percent seroconversion from replicative (HBeAg and HBV DNA detectable in serum) to nonreplicative (anti-HBe detectable) HBV infection, with a concomitant improvement in liver histologic features and an approximately 10 percent chance of losing detectable HBsAg. In most cases, successful interferon therapy and seroconversion is accompanied by an acute hepatitis–like elevation in aminotransferase activity, which is believed to represent an immunostimulatory effect of interferon on the interaction between the cellular immune system and virus-infected hepatocytes. Relapse after successful therapy is rare indeed (1 to 2 percent). The likelihood of responding to interferon is greater in patients with moderate to low levels of HBV DNA (<200 pg/mL) and in patients with substantial elevations of aminotransferase activities (e.g., >100 to 200 units). The likelihood of losing HBsAg *during therapy* is increased in patients with brief-duration disease (mean duration 1½ years); if patients are followed sufficiently long after successful interferon-induced loss of replicative markers, approximately 60 to 70 percent have been estimated to lose HBsAg, i.e., all serologic markers of infection, over a 5-year period. Immunosuppressed patients with chronic hepatitis B and children infected at birth do not appear to be responsive to interferon therapy. Indications for interferon therapy in patients with chronic hepatitis B are summarized in Table 297-4.

Complications of interferon therapy include systemic "flulike" symptoms, marrow suppression, emotional lability (irritability commonly, depression rarely), autoimmune reactions (especially autoimmune thyroiditis), and miscellaneous side effects such as alopecia, rashes, diarrhea, and numbness and tingling of the extremities. With the possible exception of autoimmune thyroiditis, all these side effects are reversible upon dose lowering or cessation of therapy.

In patients with chronic hepatitis B, long-term therapy with glucocorticoids is not only ineffective but also detrimental. Under certain circumstances, however, the predicted impact of glucocorticoids on HBV and the immune system can be exploited for the patient's benefit. Glucocorticoids increase HBV replication and expression in hepatocytes and depress the activity of cytolytic T cells. Theoretically, if steroids are administered for a brief time and then withdrawn, cytolytic T cells, suppressed while HBV replication was being steroid-induced, could resume their presteroid function and be capable of attacking and destroying the new crop of HBV antigen–expressing hepatocytes. Such appears to be the case; an acute hepatitis–like elevation of aminotransferase activity follows and may be accompanied by a dramatic drop in, or even a loss of, HBV replication. A preliminary 6-week period of glucocorticoid therapy (prednisone at doses of 60 mg for 2 weeks, 40 mg for 2 weeks, and 20 mg for 2 weeks), followed by its abrupt withdrawal, has been shown to be of benefit in conjunction with interferon therapy (5 million units subcutaneously daily for 4 months) in patients with chronic hepatitis B, primarily those with near-normal or only modest eleva-

Table 297-4

Characteristics of Patients with Chronic Hepatitis B Who Are Candidates for Interferon Therapy

Detectable markers of chronic, replicative hepatitis B (HBeAg and HBV DNA)
Elevated ALT activity
Immunocompetence
Acquisition of HBV infection in adulthood
Compensated liver disease
"Wild-type" chronic hepatitis B (not "pre-core" mutants)

tions in aminotransferase levels. This approach, however, has not attracted broad acceptance by clinicians and is used rarely.

No treatment is indicated or available for asymptomatic, nonreplicative hepatitis B carriers, and antiviral therapy should be withheld from patients with decompensated hepatitis B, in whom treatment may be associated with hepatic decompensation. Such patients should be referred to research centers involved in clinical trials. Several nucleoside analogues active against HBV are being evaluated in experimental trials. Famciclovir and ganciclovir have activity against hepatitis B, but the dideoxynucleoside lamivudine (3 thiacytidine), active against reverse transcriptase activity of human immunodeficiency virus and HBV, is a more potent inhibitor of HBV replication than these other antivirals and has shown promise in initial trials among patients with chronic replicative hepatitis B.

For patients with end-stage chronic hepatitis B, liver transplantation is the only potential lifesaving intervention. Reinfection of the new liver is almost universal; however, the likelihood of liver injury associated with hepatitis B in the new liver is variable. The majority of patients become high-level viremic carriers with minimal liver injury. Unfortunately, an unpredictable proportion experience severe hepatitis B–related liver injury, sometimes a fulminant-like hepatitis, sometimes a rapid recapitulation of the original severe chronic hepatitis B (see Chap. 301). Prevention of recurrent hepatitis B after liver transplantation has been achieved by *prophylaxis* with hepatitis B immune globulin and with nucleoside analogues; in addition, nucleoside analogues have been used successfully to *reverse* posttransplantation liver injury associated with recurrent hepatitis B (see Chap. 301).

Chronic Hepatitis D (Delta Hepatitis) The clinical and laboratory features of chronic hepatitis D virus (HDV) infection are summarized in Chap. 295. Chronic hepatitis D may follow acute coinfection with HBV but at a rate no higher than the rate of chronicity of hepatitis B. That is, although HDV coinfection can increase the severity of acute hepatitis B, HDV does not increase the likelihood of progression to chronic hepatitis B. However, when HDV superinfection occurs in a person who is already chronically infected with HBV, long-term HDV infection is the rule and a worsening of the liver disease the expected consequence. Except for severity, chronic hepatitis B plus D has similar clinical and laboratory features to those seen in chronic hepatitis B alone. Relatively severe chronic hepatitis, with or without cirrhosis, is the rule, and mild chronic hepatitis the exception. A distinguishing serologic feature of chronic hepatitis D is the presence in the circulation of antibodies to liver-kidney microsomes (anti-LKM); however, the anti-LKM seen in hepatitis D are designated anti-LKM3 and are distinct from anti-LKM1 seen in patients with autoimmune hepatitis and in a subset of patients with chronic hepatitis C (see below).

℞ **TREATMENT**

Management is not well defined. Glucocorticoids are ineffective and are not used. Preliminary experimental trials of interferon α suggested that conventional doses and durations of therapy lower levels of HDV RNA and aminotransferase activity only transiently during treatment but have no impact on the natural history of the disease. Although high-dose interferon α (9 million units) three times a week for 12 months may be associated with a sustained loss of HDV replication and clinical improvement in up to 50 percent of patients, ultimately recurrent HDV replication becomes universal after cessation of therapy. Antiviral therapy for chronic hepatitis D remains the subject of experimental trials. In patients with end-stage liver disease secondary to chronic hepatitis D, liver transplantation has been effective. If hepatitis D recurs in the new liver without the expression of hepatitis B (an unusual serologic profile in immunocompetent persons, but common in transplant patients), liver injury is limited. In fact, the outcome of transplantation for chronic hepatitis D is superior to that for chronic hepatitis B (see Chap. 301).

Chronic Hepatitis C Regardless of the epidemiologic mode of acquisition of hepatitis C virus (HCV) infection, chronic hepatitis follows acute hepatitis C in 50 to 70 percent of cases. Furthermore, in patients with chronic transfusion-associated hepatitis followed for 10 years, progression to cirrhosis occurs in about 20 percent. Such is the case even for patients with relatively clinically mild chronic hepatitis, including those without symptoms, with only modest elevations of aminotransferase activity, and with mild chronic hepatitis on liver biopsy. Even in cohorts of well-compensated patients with chronic hepatitis C (no complications of chronic liver disease and with normal hepatic synthetic function), the prevalence of cirrhosis may be as high as 50 percent. Many cases of hepatitis C are identified in asymptomatic patients who have no history of acute hepatitis C, e.g., those discovered while attempting to donate blood or as a result of routine laboratory screening tests. The source of HCV infection in most of these cases is not defined, although a long-forgotten percutaneous exposure in the remote past can be elicited in a substantial proportion. The natural history of chronic hepatitis C identified under these circumstances remains to be determined. Among asymptomatic persons with anti-HCV, even when aminotransferase levels are normal, between a third and a half have been reported to have chronic hepatitis on liver biopsy, although mild in most cases. In these asymptomatic persons with normal aminotransferase levels, the presence of detectable circulating HCV RNA appears to distinguish those with chronic hepatitis on biopsy from those with normal liver histology.

Despite this substantial rate of progression of chronic hepatitis C, and despite the fact that liver failure can result from end-stage chronic hepatitis C, the long-term prognosis for chronic hepatitis C in a majority of patients is relatively benign. Mortality over 10 to 20 years among patients with transfusion-associated chronic hepatitis C has been shown not to differ from mortality in a matched population of transfused patients in whom hepatitis C did not develop. Although death in the hepatitis group is more likely to result from liver failure, and although hepatic decompensation may occur in approximately 15 percent of such patients over the course of a decade, the majority (almost 60 percent) of patients remain asymptomatic and well compensated, with no clinical sequelae of chronic liver disease. Overall, then, chronic hepatitis C tends to be very slowly and insidiously progressive, if at all, in the vast majority of patients, while in approximately a quarter of cases, chronic hepatitis C will progress eventually to end-stage cirrhosis. The degree of progression of liver disease in chronic hepatitis C has been shown to be greater in patients with higher levels of HCV RNA and longer durations of infection; HCV-associated liver disease also tends to be worse in patients with certain genotypes (e.g., 1b). Among these variables, however, duration of infection appears to be the most important. In addition, severity of chronic hepatitis is greater and progression of chronic liver disease is more accelerated in patients who have chronic hepatitis C as well as other liver processes, including alcoholic liver disease, chronic hepatitis B, hemochromatosis, and α_1-antitrypsin deficiency. No other epidemiologic or clinical features of chronic hepatitis C (e.g., severity of acute hepatitis, level of aminotransferase activity, presence or absence of jaundice) are predictive of eventual outcome. Despite the relative benignity of chronic hepatitis C over time, cirrhosis following chronic hepatitis C has been associated with the late development, after several decades, of hepatocellular carcinoma (see Chap. 93).

Clinical features of chronic hepatitis C are similar to those described above for chronic hepatitis B. Generally, *fatigue* is the most common symptom; jaundice is rare. Immune-complex–mediated extrahepatic complications of chronic hepatitis C are less common than in chronic hepatitis B, with the exception of essential mixed cryoglobulinemia (see Chap. 295). This is the case, despite the fact that assays for immune-complex–like activity are often positive in patients with chronic hepatitis C. In addition, chronic hepatitis C has been associated with extrahepatic complications unrelated to immune-complex injury. These include Sjögren's syndrome, lichen planus, and porphyria cutanea tarda. *Laboratory features* of chronic hepatitis C are similar to those in patients with chronic hepatitis B, but aminotransferase levels tend to fluctuate more (the characteristic episodic pattern of aminotransferase activity) and to be lower, especially in patients with long-standing disease. An interesting and occasionally confusing finding in patients with chronic hepatitis C is the presence of autoantibodies. Rarely, patients with autoimmune hepatitis (see below) and hyperglobulinemia have false-positive enzyme immunoassays for anti-HCV. On the other hand, some patients with serologically confirmable chronic hepatitis C have circulating anti-LKM. These antibodies are anti-LKM1, as seen in patients with autoimmune hepatitis *type 2* (see below), and are directed against a 33-amino-acid sequence of P450 IID6. The occurrence of anti-LKM1 in some patients with chronic hepatitis C may result from the partial sequence homology between the epitope recognized by anti-LKM1 and two segments of the HCV polyprotein. In addition, the presence of this autoantibody in some patients with chronic hepatitis C suggests that autoimmunity may be playing a role in the pathogenesis of chronic hepatitis C. Histopathologic features of chronic hepatitis C, especially those that distinguish hepatitis C from hepatitis B, are described in Chap. 295.

℞ TREATMENT

In the management of chronic hepatitis C, glucocorticoids are ineffective. Based on the outcome of prospective, randomized, controlled clinical trials, interferon α has been approved for the treatment of chronic hepatitis C. Doses ranging from 2 to 5 million units three times a week have been shown to be effective in these trials, but the initial dose recommendation was 3 million units by subcutaneous injection three times a week for 6 months (24 weeks). This regimen is associated with a likelihood of biochemical response (return of ALT to normal or a 50 percent reduction of ALT to within 1.5 times the upper limit of normal) in approximately 50 percent of patients. Other regimens are being evaluated (see below). Unlike in hepatitis B, in chronic hepatitis C a successful response to interferon is not accompanied by an acute hepatitis–like elevation in aminotransferase activity; instead, ALT levels fall precipitously. Between 85 and 90 percent of responses occur within the first 3 months of therapy; responses thereafter are rare. In addition, histologic improvement in periportal and lobular inflammation has been demonstrated, primarily in biochemically responding patients but also in biochemical nonresponders. Clinical trials have demonstrated that, after 6 months of therapy, at least 50 percent of responding patients experience a biochemical relapse; based on this relapse rate, the likelihood of a sustained response would be 25 percent. In practice, however, the relapse rate can approach 90 percent, and the likelihood of a sustained response is probably no greater than 10 to 15 percent. Still, in a proportion of cases, all markers of HCV infection can be eradicated by interferon therapy, and durable responses have been documented many years after successful therapy. In those who relapse after responding, retreatment with interferon invariably leads to a subsequent response. A small proportion of patients, approximately 10 percent, experience biochemical "breakthrough" *during* interferon therapy. In general, they remain refractory to retreatment thereafter; some such breakthroughs are associated with interferon antibodies, while others may reflect mutations in the HCV genome that render HCV nonresponsive to interferon.

Levels of HCV RNA fall in tandem with ALT levels during interferon therapy, but loss of detectable HCV RNA does not preclude relapse. When a patient experiences an apparently sustained biochemical response after discontinuing interferon but continues to remain viremic, as reflected by the persistence of detectable HCV RNA, future biochemical relapse is likely. Patient variables that tend to correlate with *sustained* responsiveness to interferon include a low baseline level of HCV RNA and histologically mild hepatitis. Patients with cirrhosis can respond, but they are less likely to do so and especially unlikely to have a *sustained* response. In certain countries, patients with HCV genotype 1b are less likely to respond than patients with other genotypes, but in the United States, where most patients are infected with either genotypes 1a or 1b, genotype appears to have less of an impact on interferon responsiveness. Other variables reported to correlate with increased responsiveness include brief duration of infection, low HCV quasispecies diversity, a high

baseline ALT, immunocompetence, and low liver iron levels. High levels of HCV RNA, more histologically advanced liver disease, and high quasispecies diversity all go hand in hand with advanced duration of infection, which may be the single most important variable determining interferon responsiveness. The ironic fact, then, is that patients whose disease is *least* likely to progress are the ones *most* likely to respond to interferon and vice versa. Finally, among patients with genotype 1b, responsiveness to interferon is enhanced in those with amino-acid-substitution mutations in the nonstructural protein 5A gene.

Among the approaches to increasing the response rate and decreasing the relapse rate associated with interferon therapy are longer-duration, higher-dose, and/or higher-frequency therapy. In several European studies, durations of therapy of 12 to 18 months increased the frequency of sustained responses, but this effect has not been observed as conclusively in studies conducted in the United States. Other approaches that have been suggested but not yet supported by adequate clinical trials include the initiation of therapy with a higher dose followed by maintenance with a standard dose; reliance on alternative types of interferons; tapering therapy slowly rather than discontinuing therapy abruptly; and, because of the observation that a high liver iron level is associated with nonresponsiveness, the addition of phlebotomy to interferon therapy. Pending clinical trials to the contrary, none of these approaches can be recommended. Several small clinical trials have suggested that the nucleoside analogue ribavirin, which is ineffective when used alone, may increase the efficacy of interferon when given as combination therapy; large-scale, multicenter trials are underway to pursue this potential approach. Whether sustained, long-term (even indefinite) therapy will be necessary or effective in those who relapse remains to be determined. Similarly, the impact of short-term therapy on the long-term natural history of chronic hepatitis C continues to be studied.

Although a consensus exists that patients with symptomatic chronic hepatitis C should be treated with interferon, treatment of asymptomatic patients and those with mild chronic hepatitis remains controversial. Because progression to cirrhosis can occur in an unpredictable proportion of such cases, the potential benefit of therapy should not be dismissed out of hand in these patients. Additional study is needed. Currently, the treatment of asymptomatic hepatitis C "carriers" with normal aminotransferase levels or patients with decompensated cirrhosis secondary to chronic hepatitis C is not recommended. Interferon therapy has been advocated for patients with symptomatic essential mixed cryoglobulinemia, but results are mixed (Table 297-5). For those with decompensated, end-stage disease, liver transplantation is an option. Although the likelihood of reexpressing detectable anti-HCV after transplantation is low, the likelihood of reinfection of the new liver is almost universal. Nevertheless, and the occasional exception notwithstanding, most patients who undergo liver transplantation for chronic hepatitis C experience little, if any, morbidity, allograft loss, or mortality associated with recurrent hepatitis C infection during the early postoperative years (see Chap. 301).

AUTOIMMUNE HEPATITIS Definition Autoimmune hepatitis (formerly called autoimmune chronic active hepatitis) is a chronic disorder characterized by continuing hepatocellular necrosis and inflammation, usually with fibrosis, which tends to progress to cirrhosis and liver failure. When fulfilling criteria of severity, this type of chronic hepatitis may have a 6-month mortality of as high as 40 percent. The prominence of extrahepatic features of autoimmunity as well as seroimmunologic abnormalities in this disorder supports an autoimmune process in its pathogenesis, and this concept is reflected in the labels "lupoid," plasma cell, or autoimmune hepatitis. Because autoantibodies and other typical features of autoimmunity do not occur in all cases, however, a broader, more appropriate designation for this type of chronic hepatitis is "idiopathic" or cryptogenic. Cases in which

Table 297-5

Indications for Interferon Therapy in Patients with Chronic Hepatitis C

ACCEPTED INDICATIONS

Elevated ALT activity ($\geq$1.5 times the upper limit of normal)
Chronic hepatitis of moderate severity on liver biopsy
Detectable HCV RNA

CONTROVERSIAL INDICATIONS

Histologically mild hepatitis
Near-normal ALT activity (<1.5 times the upper limit of normal)
History of relapse after an initial course of interferon
Hepatitis C–associated essential mixed cryoglobulinemia

FEATURES ASSOCIATED WITH REDUCED RESPONSIVENESS

Advanced histologic lesion (e.g., advanced cirrhosis)
Long-duration disease
High-level HCV RNA
Genotype 1b (especially so in Europe and Japan, less so in the United
  States)
High HCV RNA quasispecies diversity

ABSENCE OF BENEFIT

Decompensated liver disease
Normal aminotransferase activity
Failure to respond to a previous course of interferon

hepatotropic viruses, metabolic/genetic derangements, and hepatotoxic drugs have been excluded merit this designation and probably include a spectrum of heterogeneous liver disorders of unknown cause, a proportion of which have characteristic autoimmune features.

Immunopathogenesis The weight of evidence suggests that the progressive liver injury in patients with idiopathic/autoimmune hepatitis is the result of a cell-mediated immunologic attack directed against liver cells; in all likelihood, predisposition to autoimmunity is inherited, while the liver specificity of this injury is triggered by environmental (e.g., chemical or viral) factors. For example, patients have been described in whom apparently self-limited cases of acute hepatitis A or B led to autoimmune hepatitis, presumably because of genetic susceptibility or predisposition. Evidence to support an autoimmune pathogenesis in this type of hepatitis includes the following: (1) In the liver, the histopathologic lesions are composed predominantly of cytotoxic T cells and plasma cells; (2) circulating autoantibodies (nuclear, smooth muscle, thyroid, etc.; see below), rheumatoid factor, and hyperglobulinemia are common; (3) other autoimmune disorders—such as thyroiditis, rheumatoid arthritis, autoimmune hemolytic anemia, ulcerative colitis, proliferative glomerulonephritis, juvenile diabetes mellitus, and Sjögren's syndrome—occur with increased frequency in patients who have autoimmune hepatitis and in their relatives; (4) histocompatibility haplotypes associated with autoimmune diseases, such as HLA-B1, -B8, -DRw3, and -DRw4, are common in patients with autoimmune hepatitis; and (5) this type of chronic hepatitis is responsive to glucocorticoid/immunosuppressive therapy, effective in a variety of autoimmune disorders.

Cellular immune mechanisms appear to be important in the pathogenesis of autoimmune hepatitis. In vitro studies have suggested that in patients with this disorder, lymphocytes are capable of becoming sensitized to hepatocyte membrane proteins and of destroying liver cells. Abnormalities of immunoregulatory control over cytotoxic lymphocytes (impaired suppressor cell influences) may play a role as well. Studies of genetic predisposition to autoimmune hepatitis demonstrate that certain haplotypes are associated with the disorder, as enumerated above. The precise triggering factors, genetic influences, and cytotoxic and immunoregulatory mechanisms involved in this type of liver injury remain poorly defined.

Intriguing clues into the pathogenesis of autoimmune hepatitis come from the observation that circulating autoantibodies are prevalent in patients with this disorder. Among the autoantibodies described in these patients are antibodies to nuclei [so-called antinuclear antibodies (ANA), primarily in a homogeneous pattern] and smooth muscle (so-called anti-smooth-muscle antibodies, directed at actin), anti-LKM (see below), antibodies to "soluble liver antigen" (directed at cytokeratins), as well as antibodies to the liver-specific asialoglycoprotein receptor (or "hepatic lectin") and other hepatocyte membrane proteins. Although some of these provide helpful diagnostic markers, their involvement in the pathogenesis of autoimmune hepatitis has not been established.

Humoral immune mechanisms have been shown to play a role in the extrahepatic manifestations of autoimmune/idiopathic hepatitis. Arthralgias, arthritis, cutaneous vasculitis, and glomerulonephritis occurring in patients with autoimmune hepatitis appear to be mediated by the deposition in affected tissue vessels of circulating immune complexes, followed by complement activation, inflammation, and tissue injury. While specific viral antigen-antibody complexes can be identified in acute and chronic viral hepatitis, the nature of the immune complexes in autoimmune hepatitis has not been defined.

Many of the *clinical features* of autoimmune hepatitis are similar to those described for chronic viral hepatitis. The onset of disease may be insidious or abrupt; the disease may present initially like, and be confused with, acute viral hepatitis; and a history of recurrent bouts of what had been labeled acute hepatitis is not uncommon. A subset of patients with autoimmune hepatitis has distinct features. Such patients are predominantly young to middle-aged women with marked hyperglobulinemia and high-titer circulating ANA. This is the group with positive LE preparations (initially labeled "lupoid" hepatitis) in whom other autoimmune features are common. Fatigue, malaise, anorexia, amenorrhea, acne, arthralgias, and jaundice are common. Occasionally, arthritis, maculopapular eruptions (including cutaneous vasculitis), erythema nodosum, colitis, pleurisy, pericarditis, anemia, azotemia, and sicca syndrome (keratoconjunctivitis, xerostomia) occur. In some patients, complications of cirrhosis, such as ascites and edema (associated with hypoalbuminemia), encephalopathy, hypersplenism, coagulopathy, or variceal bleeding, may bring the patient to initial medical attention.

The course of autoimmune hepatitis may be variable. In those with mild disease or limited histologic lesions (e.g., piecemeal necrosis without bridging), progression to cirrhosis is limited. In those with severe symptomatic autoimmune hepatitis (aminotransferase levels >10 times normal, marked hyperglobulinemia, "aggressive" histologic lesions—bridging necrosis or multilobular collapse, cirrhosis), then 6-month mortality without therapy may be as high as 40 percent. Such severe disease accounts for only 20 percent of cases; the natural history of milder disease is variable, often accentuated by spontaneous remissions and exacerbations. Especially poor prognostic signs include multilobular collapse at the time of initial presentation and failure of the bilirubin to improve after 2 weeks of therapy. Death may result from hepatic failure, hepatic coma, other complications of cirrhosis (e.g., variceal hemorrhage), and intercurrent infection. In patients with established cirrhosis, hepatocellular carcinoma may be a late complication (see Chap. 93).

Laboratory features of autoimmune hepatitis are similar to those seen in chronic viral hepatitis. Liver biochemical tests are invariably abnormal but may not correlate with the clinical severity or histopathologic features in individual cases. Many patients with autoimmune hepatitis have normal serum bilirubin, alkaline phosphatase, and globulin levels with only minimal aminotransferase elevations. Serum AST and ALT levels are increased and fluctuate in the range of 100 to 1000 units. In severe cases, the serum bilirubin level is moderately elevated [51 to 171 μmol/L (3 to 10 mg/dL)]. Hypoalbuminemia occurs in patients with very active or advanced disease. Serum alkaline phosphatase levels may be moderately elevated or near normal. In a small proportion of patients, marked elevations of alkaline phosphatase activity occur; in such patients, clinical and laboratory features overlap with those of primary biliary cirrhosis (see Chap. 298). The prothrombin time is often prolonged, particularly late in the disease or during active phases.

Hypergammaglobulinemia (>2.5 g/dL) is common in autoimmune hepatitis. Rheumatoid factor is common as well. As noted above, circulating autoantibodies are also common. The most characteristic are ANA in a homogeneous staining pattern. Smooth-muscle antibodies are less specific, seen just as frequently in chronic viral hepatitis. Because of the high levels of globulins achieved in the circulation of some patients with autoimmune hepatitis, occasionally the globulins may bind nonspecifically in solid-phase binding immunoassays for viral antibodies. This has been recognized most commonly in tests for antibodies to hepatitis C virus, as noted above. In fact, studies of autoantibodies in autoimmune hepatitis have led to the recognition of new categories of autoimmune hepatitis. *Type I autoimmune hepatitis* is the classic syndrome occurring in young women, associated with marked hyperglobulinemia, lupoid features, and circulating ANA. *Type II autoimmune hepatitis*, often seen in children and more common in Mediterranean populations, is associated not with ANA but with anti-LKM. Actually, anti-LKM represent a heterogeneous group of antibodies. In type II autoimmune hepatitis, the antibody is anti-LKM1, directed against P450 IID6. This is the same anti-LKM seen in some patients with chronic hepatitis C. Anti-LKM2 is seen in drug-induced hepatitis, and anti-LKM3 is seen in patients with chronic hepatitis D. Type II autoimmune hepatitis has been subdivided by some authorities into two categories, one more typically autoimmune and the other associated with viral hepatitis type C. Autoimmune hepatitis type IIa is felt to be autoimmune, is more likely to occur in young women, is associated with hyperglobulinemia, is associated with high-titer anti-LKM1, responds to glucocorticoid therapy, and is seen commonly in western Europe and the United Kingdom. Type IIb autoimmune hepatitis is associated with hepatitis C virus infection, tends to occur in older men, is associated with normal globulin levels and low-titer anti-LKM1, responds to interferon, and occurs most commonly in Mediterranean countries. In addition, another type of autoimmune hepatitis has been recognized, *autoimmune hepatitis type III*. These patients, who lack ANA and anti-LKM1, have circulating antibodies to soluble liver antigen, which are directed at hepatocyte cytoplasmic cytokeratins 8 and 18. Most of these patients are women and have clinical features similar to those of patients with type I autoimmune hepatitis.

℞ TREATMENT

The mainstay of management in autoimmune or idiopathic (nonviral) hepatitis is glucocorticoid therapy. Several controlled clinical trials have documented that such therapy leads to symptomatic, clinical, biochemical, and histologic improvement as well as increased survival. A therapeutic response can be expected in up to 80 percent of patients. Unfortunately, therapy has not been shown to prevent ultimate progression to cirrhosis. Although some advocate the use of prednisolone, the hepatic metabolite of prednisone, prednisone is just as effective and is favored by most authorities. Therapy may be initiated at 20 mg/d, but a popular regimen in the United States relies on an initiation dose of 60 mg/d. This high dose is tapered successively over the course of a month down to a maintenance level of 20 mg/d. An alternative, but equally effective, approach is to begin with half the prednisone dose (30 mg/d) along with azathioprine (50 mg/d). With azathioprine maintained at 50 mg/d, the prednisone dose is tapered over the course of a month down to a maintenance level of 10 mg/d. The advantage of the combination approach is a reduction, over the span of an 18-month course of therapy, in serious, life-threatening complications of steroid therapy from 66 percent down to under 20 percent. Azathioprine alone, however, is not effective in achieving remission, nor is alternate-day glucocorticoid therapy. Although therapy has been shown to be effective for severe autoimmune hepatitis, therapy is not indicated for mild forms of chronic hepatitis (which used to be labeled chronic persistent hepatitis or chronic lobular hepatitis), and the efficacy of therapy in mild or asymptomatic autoimmune hepatitis (which used to be labeled mild chronic active hepatitis) has not been established.

Improvement of fatigue, anorexia, malaise, and jaundice tends to occur within days to several weeks; biochemical improvement occurs over the course of several weeks to months, with a fall in serum bilirubin and globulin levels and an increase in serum albumin. Serum aminotransferase levels usually drop promptly, but improvements in AST and ALT alone do not appear to be a reliable marker of recovery in individual patients; histologic improvement, characterized by a decrease in mononuclear infiltration and in hepatocellular necrosis may be delayed for 6 to 24 months. Still, if interpreted cautiously, aminotransferase levels are valuable indicators of relative disease activity, and many authorities do *not* advocate serial liver biopsies to assess therapeutic success or to guide decisions to alter or stop therapy. Therapy should continue for at least 12 to 18 months. After tapering and cessation of therapy, the likelihood of relapse is at least 50 percent, even if posttreatment histology has improved to show mild chronic hepatitis, and the majority of patients require therapy at maintenance doses indefinitely. Continuing azathioprine alone after cessation of prednisone therapy may reduce the frequency of relapse.

If medical therapy fails, or when chronic hepatitis progresses to cirrhosis and is associated with life-threatening complications of liver decompensation, liver transplantation is the only recourse (see Chap. 301). Recurrence of autoimmune hepatitis in the new liver has not been documented to occur.

DIFFERENTIAL DIAGNOSIS Early during the course of chronic hepatitis, the disease may resemble typical *acute viral hepatitis*. Without histologic assessment, severe chronic hepatitis cannot be readily distinguished based on clinical or biochemical criteria from mild chronic hepatitis. In adolescence, *Wilson's disease* may present with features of chronic hepatitis long before neurologic manifestations become apparent and before the formation of Kayser-Fleischer rings; in this age group, serum ceruloplasmin and serum and urinary copper determinations and measurement of liver copper levels will establish the correct diagnosis. *Postnecrotic* or *cryptogenic cirrhosis* and *primary biliary cirrhosis* share clinical features with autoimmune hepatitis; biochemical, serologic, and histologic assessments are usually sufficient to allow these entities to be distinguished from autoimmune hepatitis. Of course, the distinction between autoimmune ("idiopathic") and viral chronic hepatitis is not always straightforward, especially when viral antibodies occur in patients with autoimmune disease or when autoantibodies occur in patients with viral disease. Finally, the presence of extrahepatic features such as arthritis, cutaneous vasculitis, or pleuritis—not to mention the presence of circulating autoantibodies—may cause confusion with *rheumatologic disorders* such as rheumatoid arthritis and systemic lupus erythematosus. The existence of clinical and biochemical features of progressive necroinflammatory liver disease distinguishes chronic hepatitis from these other disorders, which are not associated with severe liver disease.

For further discussion of interferon and other antiviral agents, see Chap. 50, in Goodman and Gilman's The Pharmacological Basis of Therapeutics, 9th ed., McGraw-Hill, New York, 1996.

BIBLIOGRAPHY

ALTER HJ: The cloning and clinical implications of HGV and HGBV-C. N Engl J Med 334:1536, 1996

BRILLANTI S et al: A pilot study of combination therapy with ribavirin plus interferon alfa for interferon alfa-resistant chronic hepatitis C. Gastroenterology 107:812, 1994

CHEMELLO L et al: Randomized trial comparing three different regimens of alpha-2a-interferon in chronic hepatitis C. Hepatology 22:700, 1995

CZAJA AJ et al: Frequency and significance of antibodies to liver/kidney microsome type 1 in adults with chronic active hepatitis. Gastroenterology 103:1290, 1992

———: Autoimmune hepatitis: Evolving concepts and treatment strategies. Dig Dis Sci 40:435, 1995

———: The variant forms of antoimmune hepatitis. Ann Intern Med 125:588, 1996

DAVIS GL et al: Treatment of chronic hepatitis C with recombinant interferon alfa: A multicenter randomized, controlled trial. N Engl J Med 321:1501, 1989

DESMET VJ et al: Classification of chronic hepatitis: Diagnosis, grading, and staging. Hepatology 19:1513, 1994

DIENSTAG JL et al: A preliminary trial of lamivudine for chronic hepatitis B infection. N Engl J Med 333:1657, 1995

ENOMOTO N et al: Mutations in the nonstructural protein 5A gene and response to interferon in patients with chronic hepatitis C virus 1b infection. N Engl J Med 334:77, 1996

FARCI P et al: Treatment of chronic hepatitis D with interferon alfa-2a. N Engl J Med 330:88, 1994

GARSON JA et al: Analysis of clinical and virological factors associated with response to alpha interferon therapy in chronic hepatitis C. J Med Virol 45:348, 1995

HOOFNAGLE JH, DiBISCEGLIE AM: The treatment of chronic viral hepatitis. N Engl J Med 336:347, 1997

————, JONES EA (GUEST EDS.): Interferon therapy of chronic viral hepatitis. Semin Liver Dis 9:231, 1989

————: Therapy of acute and chronic viral hepatitis. Adv Intern Med 39:241, 1994

ISHAK K et al: Histologic grading and staging of chronic hepatitis. J Hepatol 22:696, 1995

JOHNSON PJ et al: Azathioprine for long-term maintenance of remission in autoimmune hepatitis. N Engl J Med 333:958, 1995

KASAHARA A et al: Ability of prolonged interferon treatment to suppress relapse after cessation of therapy in patients with chronic hepatitis C: A multicenter randomized controlled trial. Hepatology 21:291, 1995

KATKOV WN, DIENSTAG JL: Prevention and therapy of viral hepatitis. Semin Liver Dis 11:165, 1991

KORENMAN J et al: Long-term remission of chronic hepatitis B after alpha-interferon therapy. Ann Intern Med 114:629, 1991

KRAWITT EL: Autoimmune hepatitis. N Engl J Med 334:897, 1996

MADDREY WC: Chronic hepatitis. Dis Mon 39:53, 1993

MASUKO K et al: Infection with hepatitis GB virus C in patients on maintenance dialysis. N Engl J Med 334:1485, 1996

NIEDERAU C et al: Long-term follow-up of HBeAg-positive patients treated with interferon alfa for chronic hepatitis B. N Engl J Med 334:1422, 1996

PERRILLO RP et al: A randomized, controlled trial of interferon alpha-2b alone and after prednisone withdrawal for the treatment of chronic hepatitis B. N Engl J Med 323:295, 1990

POYNARD T et al: A comparison of three interferon alfa-2b regimens for the long-term treatment of chronic non-A, non-B hepatitis. N Engl J Med 332:1457, 1995

REICHARD O et al: High sustained response rate and clearance of viremia in chronic hepatitis C after treatment with interferon-α2b for 60 weeks. Hepatology 19:280, 1994

———— et al: Two-year biochemical, virological, and histological follow-up in patients with chronic hepatitis C responding in a sustained fashion to interferon alfa-2b treatment. Hepatology 21:918, 1995

ROMEO R et al: Eradication of hepatitis C virus RNA after alpha-interferon therapy. Ann Intern Med 121:276, 1994

SHINDO M et al: Hepatic hepatitis C virus RNA as a predictor of a long-term response to interferon-α therapy. Ann Intern Med 122:586, 1995

TONG MJ et al: Clinical outcomes after transfusion-associated hepatitis C. N Engl J Med 332:1463, 1995

298

Daniel K. Podolsky, Kurt J. Isselbacher

CIRRHOSIS AND ALCOHOLIC LIVER DISEASE

Cirrhosis is a pathologically defined entity that is associated with a spectrum of characteristic clinical manifestations. The cardinal pathologic features reflect irreversible chronic injury of the hepatic parenchyma and include extensive fibrosis in association with the formation of regenerative nodules. These features result from hepatocyte necrosis, collapse of the supporting reticulin network with subsequent connective tissue deposition, distortion of the vascular bed, and nodular regeneration of remaining liver parenchyma. The pathologic process should be viewed as a final common pathway of many types of chronic liver injury. Clinical features of cirrhosis derive from the morphologic alterations and often reflect the severity of hepatic damage rather than the etiology of the underlying liver disease. Loss of functioning hepatocellular mass may lead to jaundice, edema, coagulopathy, and a variety of metabolic abnormalities; fibrosis and distorted vasculature lead to portal hypertension and its sequelae, including gastroesophageal varices and splenomegaly. Ascites and hepatic encephalopathy result from both hepatocellular insufficiency and portal hypertension.

Classification of the various types of cirrhosis based on either etiology or morphology alone is unsatisfactory. A single pathologic pattern may result from a variety of insults, while the same insult may produce several morphologic patterns. Nevertheless, most types of cirrhosis may be usefully classified by a mixture of etiologically and morphologically defined entities as follows: (1) alcoholic; (2) cryptogenic and postviral or postnecrotic; (3) biliary; (4) cardiac; (5) metabolic, inherited, and drug-related; and (6) miscellaneous. This chapter considers the various types of cirrhosis. → *The major complications of cirrhosis are discussed in Chap. 299.*

ALCOHOLIC LIVER DISEASE AND CIRRHOSIS

Definition *Alcoholic cirrhosis*, historically referred to as *Laennec's cirrhosis*, is the most common type of cirrhosis encountered in North America and many parts of western Europe and South America. It is characterized by diffuse fine scarring, fairly uniform loss of liver cells, and small regenerative nodules, and therefore it is sometimes referred to as *micronodular cirrhosis*. However, micronodular cirrhosis also may result from other types of liver injury (e.g., following jejunoileal bypass), and thus alcoholic cirrhosis and micronodular cirrhosis are not necessarily synonymous. Conversely, alcoholic cirrhosis may progress to macronodular cirrhosis with time.

Alcoholic cirrhosis is only one of many consequences resulting from chronic alcohol ingestion, and it often accompanies other forms of alcohol-induced liver injury. The three principal alcohol-induced hepatic lesions are designated (1) *alcoholic fatty liver (steatosis)*, (2) *alcoholic hepatitis*, and (3) *alcoholic cirrhosis*. These morphologic categories are rarely found in a pure form, and features of each may be present to varying degrees in an individual patient.

Etiology Although chronic alcoholism is the most common cause of cirrhosis, the quantity and duration of drinking necessary to cause cirrhosis remain unclear. The typical alcoholic patient with cirrhosis has had a daily consumption of a pint or more of whiskey, several quarts of wine, or an equivalent amount of beer for at least 10 years. The amount and duration of ethanol ingestion, rather than the type of alcoholic beverage or the pattern of ingestion, appear to be the important determinants of liver injury. In general, the latent period preceding the development of cirrhosis is inversely related to the level of daily alcohol intake. Rates of ethanol metabolism are under genetic control, but no metabolic defect has been identified in cirrhotic patients or their families to suggest a unique "susceptibility" to ethanol or its toxic effects. Although malnutrition per se does not appear to lead to cirrhosis, it is possible that nutritional factors may augment the detrimental effects of chronic alcohol ingestion on the liver. The finding that only 10 to 15 percent of alcoholics develop cirrhosis suggests that other factors may affect the impact of alcohol on the liver. Women, on average, appear to develop alcohol-induced liver injury at lesser levels of consumption than men, suggesting that hormonal factors may play a role in susceptibility. Lower levels of alcohol dehydrogenase in gastric mucosa and resultant diminished rates of alcohol metabolism may also contribute to a greater predisposition to alcohol-related liver injury in women. The finding of increased concordance of alcoholic liver disease among monozygotic twins compared to dizygotic twins ingesting excessive amounts of alcohol suggests that genetic factors contribute, though no genetic alterations have yet been consistently identified. Other observations suggest that immune mechanisms may also play a significant role.

Alcoholic fatty liver occurs in most heavy drinkers but is reversible on cessation of alcohol consumption and is not thought to be an inevitable precursor of alcoholic hepatitis or cirrhosis. In contrast, alcoholic hepatitis, an inflammatory lesion characterized by infiltration of the liver with leukocytes, liver cell necrosis, and alcoholic hyaline, is thought to be the major precursor of cirrhosis. Subsequent healing accompanied by fibrosis distorts the normal lobular architecture. Indeed, *deposition of collagen in perivenular spaces* may be the earliest manifestation of the process that ultimately leads to cirrhosis.

Pathology and Pathogenesis *Alcoholic fatty liver* The liver is enlarged, yellow, greasy, and firm. Hepatocytes are distended by large macrovesicular cytoplasmic fat vacuoles that push the hepatocyte nucleus against the cell membrane. Accumulation of fat in the liver of the alcoholic results from the combination of impaired fatty acid oxidation, increased uptake and esterification of fatty acids to form triglycerides, and diminished lipoprotein biosynthesis and secretion (see Fig. 293-3).

Alcoholic hepatitis Morphologic features include hepatocyte degeneration and necrosis, often with ballooned cells, and an infiltrate of polymorphonuclear leukocytes and lymphocytes. The polymorphonuclear cells may encircle damaged hepatocytes that contain *Mallory bodies*, or *alcoholic hyaline*. These are clumps of perinuclear, deeply eosinophilic material believed to represent aggregated intermediate filaments. Mallory bodies are highly suggestive of, but *not specific* for, alcoholic hepatitis, since morphologically similar material is seen in association with morbid obesity, jejunoileal bypass surgery, poorly controlled diabetes mellitus, and a variety of other disorders, including Wilson's disease and Indian childhood cirrhosis. Deposition of collagen around the central vein and in perisinusoidal areas, often termed *central hyaline sclerosis*, is associated with an increased likelihood of progression to cirrhosis.

Alcoholic cirrhosis With continued alcohol intake and destruction of hepatocytes, fibroblasts (including myofibroblasts with contractile properties) appear at the site of injury and stimulate collagen formation. Weblike septa of connective tissue appear in periportal and pericentral zones and eventually connect portal triads and central veins. This fine connective tissue network surrounds small masses of remaining liver cells, which regenerate and form nodules. Although regeneration occurs within the small remnants of parenchyma, cell loss generally exceeds replacement. With continuing hepatocyte destruction and collagen deposition, the liver shrinks in size, acquires a nodular appearance, and becomes hard as "end-stage" cirrhosis develops. Although alcoholic cirrhosis is usually a progressive disease, appropriate therapy and strict avoidance of alcohol may arrest the disease at most stages and permit functional improvement.

Clinical Features *Signs and symptoms* Clinical manifestations of *alcoholic fatty liver* are often minimal or entirely absent, and the disorder may not be recognized unless another illness (frequently alcohol-related) brings the patient to medical attention. Hepatomegaly, at times accompanied by tenderness, may be the only finding. Jaundice, ascites, and edema are seen only with more serious liver injury.

The clinical severity of *alcoholic hepatitis* varies enormously, ranging from asymptomatic or mild illness to fatal hepatic insufficiency. Typically, the clinical features of alcoholic hepatitis resemble those of viral or toxic liver injury. Patients often experience anorexia, nausea and vomiting, malaise, weight loss, abdominal distress, and jaundice. Fever sometimes as high as 39.4°C (103°F) is seen in about half of cases. On physical examination, tender hepatomegaly is common, and splenomegaly is found in about one-third of patients. The patient may have cutaneous arterial "spider" angiomas and jaundice. More severe cases may be complicated by ascites, edema, bleeding, and encephalopathy. At the time of initial presentation, the central nervous system findings may be difficult to distinguish from manifestations of concurrent alcohol intoxication or withdrawal (see below).

Although jaundice, ascites, and encephalopathy may subside with abstinence, continued alcohol excess and poor dietary habits usually lead to repeated acute episodes of hepatic decompensation. Some patients die during these acute exacerbations, but most recover after several weeks or months. Even after complete abstinence, clinical recovery may be protracted, and histologic abnormalities can persist up to 6 months or longer. Cholestatic jaundice mimicking biliary tract obstruction also may develop in some cases of acute alcoholic hepatitis.

Alcoholic cirrhosis also may be clinically silent and many (10 to 40 percent) cases are discovered incidentally at laparotomy or autopsy.

In many cases symptoms are insidious in onset, occurring usually after 10 or more years of excessive alcohol use and progressing slowly over subsequent weeks and months. Anorexia and malnutrition lead to weight loss and a reduction in skeletal muscle mass. The patient may experience easy bruising, increasing weakness, and fatigue. Eventually the clinical manifestations of hepatocellular dysfunction and portal hypertension ensue, including progressive jaundice, bleeding from gastroesophageal varices, ascites, and encephalopathy. The abrupt onset of one of these complications may be the first event prompting the patient to seek medical attention. In other cases, cirrhosis first becomes evident when the patient requires treatment of symptoms related to alcoholic hepatitis.

A firm, nodular liver may be an early sign of disease; the liver may be either enlarged, normal, or decreased in size. Other frequent findings include jaundice, palmar erythema, spider angiomas, parotid and lacrimal gland enlargement, clubbing of fingers, splenomegaly, muscle wasting, and ascites with or without peripheral edema. Men may have decreased body hair and/or gynecomastia and testicular atrophy, which, like the cutaneous findings, result from disturbances in hormonal metabolism, including increased peripheral formation of estrogren due to diminished hepatic clearance of the precursor androstenedione. Testicular atrophy may reflect hormonal abnormalities or the toxic effect of alcohol on the testes. In women, signs of virilization or menstrual irregularities may occasionally be encountered. Dupuytren's contractures resulting from fibrosis of the palmar fascia with resulting flexion contracture of the digits are associated with alcoholism but are not specifically related to cirrhosis.

Although the cirrhotic patient may stabilize if drinking is discontinued, over a period of years, the patient may become emaciated, weak, and chronically jaundiced. Ascites and other signs of portal hypertension may become increasingly prominent. Ultimately, most patients with advanced cirrhosis die in hepatic coma, commonly precipitated by hemorrhage from esophageal varices or intercurrent infection. Progressive renal dysfunction often complicates the terminal phase of the illness.

Laboratory findings Routine hematologic and biochemical blood tests are usually normal in patients with alcoholic fatty liver, except for minimal elevations of the serum AST (aspartate aminotransferase); occasionally alkaline phosphatase and bilirubin levels are also elevated. In more advanced alcoholic liver disease, abnormalities of laboratory tests are more common. Anemia may result from acute and chronic gastrointestinal blood loss, coexistent nutritional deficiency (notably of folic acid and vitamin B_{12}), hypersplenism, and a direct suppressive effect of alcohol on the bone marrow. Hemolytic anemia, presumably due to effects of hypercholesterolemia on erythrocyte membranes resulting in unusual spurlike projections (acanthocytosis), has been described in some alcoholics with cirrhosis. Leukocytosis is often present in severe alcoholic hepatitis; however, some patients with this disorder may have leukopenia and thrombocytopenia due to hypersplenism or an inhibitory effect of alcohol on the bone marrow. Mild or pronounced hyperbilirubinemia may be found, usually in association with varying elevations of serum alkaline phosphatase levels. Levels of serum AST are frequently elevated, but levels greater than 5 μkat (300 units) are unusual and should prompt one to look for other coincident or complicating factors. In contrast to viral hepatitis, the serum AST is usually disproportionately elevated relative to ALT (alanine aminotransferase), i.e., AST/ALT ratio >2. In nonalcoholic steatohepatitis, the ALT level is also typically greater than the AST level. This discrepancy in alcoholic hepatitis may result from the proportionally greater inhibition of ALT synthesis by ethanol, which may be partially reversed by pyridoxal phosphate.

The serum prothrombin time is frequently prolonged, reflecting reduced synthesis of clotting proteins, most notably the vitamin K–dependent factors (see "Coagulopathy" in Chap. 299). The serum albumin level is usually depressed, while serum globulins are increased. Hypoalbuminemia reflects in part overall impairment in hepatic protein synthesis, while hyperglobulinemia is thought to result from nonspecific stimulation of the reticuloendothelial system. Elevated blood ammonia levels in patients with hepatic encephalopathy reflect diminished hepatic clearance because of impaired liver function and shunting of portal venous blood around the cirrhotic liver into the systemic circulation (see Chaps. 293 and 299).

A variety of metabolic disturbances may be detected. Glucose intolerance due to endogenous insulin resistance may be present; however, clinical diabetes is uncommon. Central hyperventilation may lead to respiratory alkalosis in patients with cirrhosis. *Dietary deficiency* and *increased urinary losses* lead to hypomagnesemia and *hypophosphatemia*. In patients with ascites and dilutional hyponatremia, hypokalemia may occur from increased urinary potassium losses due in part to hyperaldosteronism. Prerenal azotemia is also observed in such patients.

Diagnosis   *Alcoholic fatty liver* should be suspected in alcoholic patients with hepatomegaly and normal or minimally deranged liver function tests. Alcoholic fatty liver may be seen in combination with alcoholic hepatitis or established cirrhosis. *Alcoholic hepatitis* should be considered in an alcoholic who has been drinking heavily and demonstrates jaundice, fever, an enlarged, tender liver, or ascites. The clinical impression is often supported by the deranged results of tests of liver function and other laboratory abnormalities described above. Alcoholic hepatitis or fatty liver may be present in association with alcoholic cirrhosis.

Alcoholic cirrhosis should be strongly suspected in patients with a history of prolonged or excessive alcohol intake and physical signs of chronic liver disease. However, since only 10 to 15 percent of individuals with excessive alcohol intake develop cirrhosis, other causes and types of liver disease may have to be excluded. The clinical features and laboratory findings are usually sufficient to provide reasonable indication of the presence and extent of hepatic injury. Although a percutaneous needle biopsy of the liver is not usually necessary to confirm the typical findings of alcoholic hepatitis or cirrhosis, it may be helpful in distinguishing patients with less advanced liver disease from those with cirrhosis and in excluding other forms of liver injury such as viral hepatitis. Biopsy also may be helpful as a diagnostic tool in evaluating patients with clinical findings suggestive of alcoholic liver disease who deny alcohol intake. In patients with features of cholestasis, ultrasonography may be appropriate to exclude the presence of extrahepatic biliary obstruction. When the clinical status of an otherwise stable cirrhotic patient deteriorates without an obvious explanation, complicating conditions, such as infection, portal vein thrombosis, and hepatocellular carcinoma, should be sought.

Prognosis   The patient with an alcoholic fatty liver and no complications has a good prognosis; rapid and complete resolution usually follows cessation of alcohol intake. In patients with alcoholic hepatitis, the presence of marked hyperbilirubinemia, rising serum creatinine, marked prolongation of the prothrombin time (>1.5 times control), ascites, and encephalopathy are associated with a poor short-term prognosis; the in-hospital mortality in these patients may exceed 50 percent. A discriminant function calculated as $4.6 \times$ [prothrombin time − control time (seconds)] + serum bilirubin $(\mu m/L)/17$ can be used to distinguish between those with especially poor prognosis (value > 32). In milder cases, clinical recovery may be complete, but repeated bouts of alcoholic hepatitis usually lead to irreversible and progressive chronic liver injury. Abstinence from alcohol as well as early and appropriate medical care can decrease long-term morbidity and mortality and delay or prevent the appearance of further complications. Patients who have had a major complication of cirrhosis and who continue to drink have a 5-year survival of less than 50 percent. However, those patients who remain abstinent have a substantially better prognosis. In general, overall outlook in patients with advanced liver disease remains poor; most of these patients eventually die as a result of massive variceal hemorrhage and/or profound hepatic encephalopathy (see Chap. 299).

℞ TREATMENT

Alcoholic hepatitis and cirrhosis are serious illnesses that require long-term medical supervision and careful management. Therapy of the underlying liver disease is largely supportive. Specific treatment is directed at particular complications such as variceal bleeding and ascites (see Chap. 299). Some studies suggest that administration of prednisone or prednisolone in moderately large doses may be helpful in patients with severe alcoholic hepatitis and encephalopathy. However, the use of glucocorticoids in acute alcoholic hepatitis remains controversial and should probably be reserved for those with a discriminant function greater than 32, as described above. Maintenance therapy with colchicine (0.6 mg PO bid) has been shown to slow disease progression and increase longevity of the patient with alcoholic liver disease in one long-term study.

In the absence of signs of impending hepatic coma, the patient should be placed on a diet containing at least 1 g protein per kilogram of body weight and 8500 to 12,500 kJ (2000 to 3000 kcal) per day. Use of diets enriched in branched-chain amino acids has been advocated in patients predisposed to hepatic encephalopathy, but the value of these diets in patients with compensated cirrhosis is unproven. Daily multivitamin supplements should be prescribed, with the addition of large parenteral doses of thiamine in patients with Wernicke-Korsakoff disease (see Chap. 380). The patient should be made to realize that there is no medication that will protect the liver against the effects of further alcohol ingestion. Therefore, alcohol should be absolutely forbidden. An important component of the complete care of such patients is encouragement to become involved in an appropriate alcohol counseling program.

All medicines must be administered with caution in the patient with cirrhosis, especially those eliminated or modified through hepatic metabolism or biliary pathways. In particular, care must be taken to avoid overzealous use of drugs that may directly or indirectly precipitate complications of cirrhosis. For example, vigorous treatment of ascites with diuretics may result in electrolyte abnormalities or hypovolemia, which can lead to coma. Similarly, even modest doses of sedative can lead to deepening encephalopathy. Furthermore, patients may be sensitive to the toxic effects of acetaminophen, particularly in conjunction with alcohol, which can lead to excess concentrations of a toxic metabolite even at doses that are not generally toxic.

POSTNECROTIC CIRRHOSIS, POSTVIRAL CIRRHOSIS

Definition   Postnecrotic cirrhosis represents the final common pathway of many types of advanced liver injury. *Coarsely nodular*, *posthepatitic*, and *multilobular cirrhosis* are terms synonymous with *postnecrotic cirrhosis*. The term *cryptogenic cirrhosis* has been used interchangeably with *postnecrotic cirrhosis*, but this designation should be reserved for those cases in which the etiology of cirrhosis is unknown (approximately 10 percent of all patients with cirrhosis).

Postnecrotic cirrhosis is characterized morphologically by (1) extensive confluent loss of liver cells, (2) stromal collapse and fibrosis resulting in broad bands of connective tissue containing the remains of many portal triads, and (3) irregular nodules of regenerating hepatocytes, varying in size from microscopic to several centimeters in diameter.

Etiology   *Postnecrotic cirrhosis* is a morphologic term referring to a defined stage of advanced chronic liver injury of both specific and unknown (cryptogenic) causes. Epidemiologic and serologic evidence suggests that viral hepatitis (hepatitis B or hepatitis C) may be an antecedent factor in from one-fourth to three-fourths of cases of apparently cryptogenic postnecrotic cirrhosis. In areas where hepatitis B virus infection is endemic (e.g., Southeast Asia, sub-Saharan Africa), up to 15 percent of the population may acquire the infection in early childhood, and cirrhosis may ultimately develop in one-fourth of these chronic carriers. Although hepatitis B infection is much less prevalent in the United States, it is relatively common among certain high-risk groups (e.g., promiscuous homosexual men, intravenous drug abusers) and contributes to an increased incidence of cirrhosis. In the United States, hepatitis C accounts for many cases of cirrhosis following blood transfusions. Before hepatitis C screening of blood donors was introduced, hepatitis C occurred in 5 to 10 percent of blood recipients. In over 20 percent of those surviving 20 years or more, cirrhosis may ultimately develop. More than half of patients who would previously have been designated as having cryptogenic chronic liver disease have evidence of hepatitis C infection. Postnecrotic cirrhosis also may develop in patients with autoimmune hepatitis (see Chap. 297).

Other probable causes of postnecrotic cirrhosis, including drugs and toxins, are listed in Table 298-1. In some instances, advanced alcoholic liver disease and primary biliary cirrhosis may lead to postnecrotic cirrhosis.

Pathology   The postnecrotic liver is typically shrunken in size, distorted in shape, and composed of nodules of liver cells separated by dense and broad bands of fibrosis. The microscopic picture is consistent with the gross impression: Nodules are highly variable in size, with large amounts of connective tissue separating the disorganized islands of regenerating parenchyma.

Clinical Features   In patients with cirrhosis of known etiology in whom there is progression to a postnecrotic stage, the clinical manifestations are an extension of those resulting from the initial disease process. Usually clinical symptoms are related to portal hypertension and its sequelae, such as ascites, splenomegaly, hypersplenism, encephalopathy, and bleeding esophageal varices. The hematologic and liver function abnormalities resemble those seen with other types of cirrhosis. In a few patients with postnecrotic cirrhosis the diagnosis may be made incidentally at operation, at postmortem, or by a needle biopsy of the liver performed to investigate asymptomatic hepatosplenomegaly.

Table 298-1

Cirrhosis and/or Liver Disease Associated with Various Disorders

INFECTIOUS DISEASES

Brucellosis (Chap. 162)
Echinococcus (Chap. 225)
Schistosomiasis (Chap. 224)
Toxoplasmosis (Chap. 219)
Viral hepatitis [hepatitis B, C, D, E, G; cytomegalovirus (Chaps. 187, 295, and 297)]

INHERITED AND METABOLIC DISORDERS (see also Chap. 300)

Alpha$_1$-antitrypsin deficiency (Chap. 300)
Fanconi's syndrome (Chap. 346)
Galactosemia (Chap. 351)
Gaucher's disease (Chap. 346)
Glycogen storage disease (Chap. 347)
Hemochromatosis (Chap. 342)
Hereditary fructose intolerance (Chap. 351)
Hereditary tyrosinemia (Chap. 349)
Wilson's disease (Chap. 345)

DRUGS AND TOXINS (Chap. 296)

Arsenicals
Isoniazid
Methotrexate
Methyldopa
Oral contraceptives (Budd-Chiari)
Oxyphenisatin
Perhexilene maleate
Pyrrolidizine alkaloids (venooclusive disease)

OTHER OR UNPROVEN CAUSES

Chronic inflammatory bowel disease (Chap. 286)
Cystic fibrosis (Chap. 257)
Diabetes mellitus (Chap. 334)
Graft-versus-host disease (Chap. 116)
Jejunoileal bypass (Chap. 43)
Sarcoidosis (Chap. 320)

Diagnosis and Prognosis   Postnecrotic cirrhosis should be suspected in patients with signs and symptoms of cirrhosis or portal hypertension. Needle or operative liver biopsies confirm the diagnosis, although nonuniformity of the pathologic process may result in sampling errors. The diagnosis of cryptogenic cirrhosis is reserved for those patients in whom no known etiology can be demonstrated. About 75 percent of patients have progressive disease despite supportive therapy and die within 1 to 5 years from complications, including exsanguinating variceal hemorrhage, hepatic encephalopathy, or superimposed hepatocellular carcinoma.

℞ **TREATMENT**

Management is usually limited to treatment of the complications of portal hypertension, including control of ascites, avoidance of drugs or excessive protein intake that may induce hepatic coma, and prompt treatment of infections (see Chap. 299). In patients with asymptomatic cirrhosis, expectant management alone is appropriate. In those patients in whom postnecrotic cirrhosis has developed as a result of a treatable condition, therapy directed at the primary disorder may limit further progression (e.g., Wilson's disease, hemochromatosis).

BILIARY CIRRHOSIS

Biliary cirrhosis results from injury to or prolonged obstruction of either the intrahepatic or extrahepatic biliary system. It is associated with impaired biliary excretion, destruction of hepatic parenchyma, and progressive fibrosis. Primary biliary cirrhosis is characterized by chronic inflammation and fibrous obliteration of intrahepatic bile ductules. Secondary biliary cirrhosis is the result of long-standing obstruction of the larger extrahepatic ducts. Although primary and secondary biliary cirrhosis are separate pathophysiologic entities with respect to the initial insult, many clinical features are similar.

PRIMARY BILIARY CIRRHOSIS   Etiology and Pathogenesis   The cause of primary biliary cirrhosis (PBC) remains unknown. Several observations suggest that a disordered immune response may be involved. PBC is frequently associated with a variety of disorders presumed to be autoimmune in nature, such as the syndrome of calcinosis, Raynaud's phenomenon, esophageal dysmotility, sclerodactyly, telangiectasia (CREST); the sicca syndrome (dry eyes and dry mouth); autoimmune thyroiditis; and renal tubular acidosis.

Most important, a circulating IgG antimitochondrial antibody (AMA) is detected in more than 90 percent of patients with primary biliary cirrhosis and only rarely in other forms of liver disease. It has been demonstrated that these autoantibodies recognize three to five inner mitochondrial membrane proteins identified as enzymes of the pyruvate dehydrogenase complex (PDC), the branched chain α-keto-acid dehydrogenase complex (BCKDC), and the α-ketoglutarate dehydrogenase complex (KGDC). The major autoantigen in PBC (found in 90 percent of patients) has been identified as the 74-kDa E2 component of the PDC, dihydrolipoamide acetyltransferase. The antibodies are directed to a region essential for binding of a lipoic acid cofactor and inhibit the overall enzymatic activity of the PDC. Other AMA autoantibodies in PBC patients are directed to similar constituents of BCKDC and KGDC and also inhibit their enzymatic function. It remains unclear whether these properties have a direct pathogenetic role in the development of PBC. In addition to AMA, elevated serum levels of IgM and cryoproteins consisting of immune complexes capable of activating the alternative complement pathway are found in 80 to 90 percent of patients. Aberrant expression of major histocompatibility complex class II molecules has been found on biliary epithelium in association with PBC, suggesting that these cells may serve as antigen-presenting cells in this setting. Lymphocytes are prominent in the portal regions and surround damaged bile ducts. These histologic findings resemble those noted in graft-versus-host disease following liver and bone marrow transplantation and suggest that damage to bile ducts may be immunologically mediated, perhaps reflecting a defect in a suppressor cell population.

Pathology PBC is often divided into four stages based on morphologic findings. The earliest recognizable lesion (stage I), termed *chronic nonsuppurative destructive cholangitis*, is a necrotizing inflammatory process of the portal triads. It is characterized by destruction of medium and small bile ducts, a dense infiltrate of acute and chronic inflammatory cells, mild fibrosis, and occasionally, bile stasis. At times, periductal granulomas and lymph follicles are found adjacent to affected bile ducts. Subsequently, the inflammatory infiltrate becomes less prominent, the number of bile ducts is reduced, and smaller bile ductules proliferate (stage II). Progression over a period of months to years leads to a decrease in interlobular ducts, loss of liver cells, and expansion of periportal fibrosis into a network of connective tissue scars (stage III). Ultimately, cirrhosis, which may be micronodular or macronodular, develops (stage IV).

Clinical Features *Signs and symptoms* Many patients with PBC are asymptomatic, and the disease is initially detected on the basis of elevated serum alkaline phosphatase levels during routine screening. The majority of such patients remain asymptomatic for prolonged periods, although many may ultimately develop progressive liver injury.

Among patients with symptomatic disease, 90 percent are women aged 35 to 60. Often the earliest symptom is pruritus, which may be either generalized or limited initially to the palms and soles. In addition, fatigue is commonly a prominent early symptom. After several months or years, jaundice and gradual darkening of the exposed areas of the skin (melanosis) may ensue. Other early clinical manifestations of PBC reflect impaired bile excretion. These include steatorrhea and the malabsorption of lipid-soluble vitamins, often resulting in easy bruising (vitamin K deficiency); bone pain due to osteomalacia (vitamin D deficiency), which is typically present in conjunction with osteoporosis; occasionally night blindness (vitamin A deficiency); and dermatitis (possibly vitamin E and/or essential fatty acid deficiency). Protracted elevation of serum lipids, especially cholesterol, leads to subcutaneous lipid deposition around the eyes (xanthelasmas) and over joints and tendons (xanthomas). Over a period of months to years, the itching, jaundice, and hyperpigmentation slowly worsen. Eventually signs of hepatocellular failure and portal hypertension develop and ascites appears. Progression may be quite variable. Whereas a proportion of asymptomatic patients may show no signs of progression for a decade or longer, in others, death due to hepatic insufficiency may occur within 5 to 10 years after the first signs of the illness. Such decompensation is often precipitated by uncontrolled variceal hemorrhage or infection.

Physical examination may be entirely normal in the early phase of the disease, when patients are asymptomatic or pruritus is the sole complaint. Later, there may be jaundice of varying intensity, hyperpigmentation of the exposed skin areas, xanthelasmas and tendinous and planar xanthomas, moderate to striking hepatomegaly, splenomegaly, and clubbing of the fingers. Bone tenderness, signs of vertebral compression, ecchymoses, glossitis, and dermatitis may all be noted. Clinical evidence of the sicca syndrome can be found in as many as 75 percent of patients, and serologic evidence of autoimmune thyroid disease in 25 percent. Other conditions encountered with increased frequency include rheumatoid arthritis, CREST syndrome, scleroderma, pernicious anemia, and renal tubular acidosis. Bone disease is often a significant problem encountered over the course of the disease. While osteomalacia occurs due to diminished vitamin D absorption, accelerated osteoporosis in this patient population (the majority of whom are postmenopausal women) is even more common.

Laboratory findings PBC is increasingly diagnosed at a presymptomatic stage, prompted by the finding of a two- to fivefold elevation of the serum alkaline phosphatase during routine screening. Serum 5'-nucleotidase activity is also elevated. In this setting, serum bilirubin and aminotransferase levels are usually normal, but the diagnosis is supported by a positive antimitochondrial antibody test (titer > 1:40). The latter is both *relatively* specific and sensitive; a positive test is found in over 90 percent of symptomatic patients. As the disease evolves, the serum bilirubin level rises progressively and may reach

510 μmol/L (30 mg/dL) or more in the final stages. Serum aminotransferase values rarely exceed 2.5 to 3.3 μkat (150 to 200 units). Hyperlipidemia is common, and a striking increase of the serum unesterified cholesterol is often noted. An abnormal serum lipoprotein (lipoprotein X) may be present in PBC but is not specific and appears in other cholestatic conditions. A deficiency of bile salts in the intestine leads to moderate steatorrhea and impaired absorption of the fat-soluble vitamins and hypoprothrombinemia. Patients with PBC have elevated liver copper levels, but this finding is not specific and is found in all disorders in which there is prolonged cholestasis.

Diagnosis PBC should be considered in middle-aged women with unexplained pruritus or an elevated serum alkaline phosphatase level and in whom there may be other clinical or laboratory features of protracted impairment of biliary excretion. Although a positive serum AMA determination provides important diagnostic evidence, false-positive results do occur, and therefore, liver biopsy should be performed to confirm the diagnosis. Rarely, the AMA test may be negative in patients with histologic features of PBC. Frequently, patients have antibodies to the E2 protein in tests using these specific antigens. In some cases with histologic features of PBC and a negative AMA, antinuclear or smooth muscle antibodies are present (as in autoimmune hepatitis), and the designation *autoimmune cholangitis* is applied. In most cases the biliary tract should be evaluated to exclude remediable extrahepatic biliary tract obstruction, especially in view of the frequent presence of coexisting cholelithiasis.

℞ TREATMENT

There is no specific therapy for PBC. Glucocorticoids are ineffective and may actually worsen the bone disease. D-Penicillamine has been tried because of its ability to chelate copper and because of its possible antifibrotic and immunomodulating activities. However, the drug appears to be ineffective and has a high incidence of unacceptable side effects. While some have suggested that azathioprine may be helpful in slowing the progression of disease, this has not been established. Colchicine has been shown to have some limited effectiveness in slowing the progression of disease in symptomatic patients and should be tried (0.6 mg PO bid) unless gastrointestinal intolerance is limiting. Treatment with either low-dose methotrexate or cyclosporine has been reported to halt or reverse progression of PBC, but definitive trials have not been reported and these drugs are not appropriate for routine use. Only ursodiol treatment (13 to 15 mg/kg per day) has been consistently observed to achieve both symptomatic improvement and "improvement" in serum biochemical markers in patients with clinically overt PBC. The mechanism of action of ursodeoxycholic acid in achieving this benefit remains obscure. This agent is generally well tolerated and safe and should be considered for use in PBC patients. However, it may have limited ability to prevent ultimate progression to advanced cirrhosis.

Treatment is generally directed toward the relief of symptoms. As noted, ursodiol may be helpful in controlling symptoms and improving the patient's sense of well-being. Although the mechanism of the protracted pruritus is not entirely clear, cholestyramine, an oral bile salt–sequestering resin, may be helpful in doses of 8 to 12 g/d to decrease both the pruritus and the hypercholesterolemia. Occasionally orthotopic liver transplantation has been performed for intractable pruritus. Rifampin, opiate antagonists, plasmapheresis, and ultraviolet light have all been tried for control of pruritus with varying results. Steatorrhea can be reduced by a low-fat diet and substituting medium-chain triglycerides for dietary long-chain triglycerides. Fat-soluble vitamins A and K should be given by parenteral injection at regular intervals to prevent or correct night blindness and hypoprothrombinemia, respectively. Zinc supplementation may be necessary if night blindness is refractory to vitamin A therapy. Osteomalacia and osteoporosis may be ameliorated by dietary calcium supplements in conjunction with oral vitamin D. In advanced disease, $25(OH)D_3$ or $1,25(OH_2)D_3$ may be preferred to vitamin D, since poor hepatic function may limit conversion of vitamin D to the active metabolites. Progression of PBC leads to the typical complications of advanced liver disease.

The management of ascites, variceal hemorrhage, and encephalopathy are described in Chap. 299. In recent years, it has become evident that orthotopic liver transplantation is a highly effective treatment for patients with advanced PBC. Stratified analysis of patients with a wide variety of risk levels utilizing a validated prognostic model has demonstrated enhanced survival for all. Thus, hepatic transplantation is the treatment of choice for advanced PBC.

SECONDARY BILIARY CIRRHOSIS Etiology Secondary biliary cirrhosis (SBC) results from prolonged partial or total obstruction of the common bile duct or its major branches. In adults, obstruction is most frequently caused by postoperative strictures or gallstones, usually with superimposed infectious cholangitis. Chronic pancreatitis may lead to biliary stricture and secondary cirrhosis. SBC also may develop in patients with pericholangitis or primary sclerosing cholangitis. Patients with malignant tumors of the common bile duct or pancreas rarely survive long enough to develop SBC. In children, congenital biliary atresia and cystic fibrosis are common causes of SBC. Choledochal cysts, if unrecognized, also may be a rare cause of SBC.

Pathology and Pathogenesis Unrelieved obstruction of the extrahepatic bile ducts leads to (1) bile stasis and focal areas of centrilobular necrosis followed by periportal necrosis, (2) proliferation and dilatation of the portal bile ducts and ductules, (3) sterile or infected cholangitis with accumulation of polymorphonuclear infiltrates around bile ducts, and (4) progressive expansion of portal tracts by edema and fibrosis. Extravasation of bile from ruptured interlobular bile ducts into areas of periportal necrosis leads to the formation of "bile lakes" surrounded by cholesterol-rich pseudoxanthomatous cells. As in other forms of cirrhosis, injury is accompanied by regeneration in residual parenchyma. These changes gradually lead to a finely nodular cirrhosis. In general, at least 3 to 12 months is required for biliary obstruction to result in cirrhosis. Relief of the obstruction is frequently accompanied by biochemical and morphologic improvement.

Clinical Features *Signs and symptoms* The signs and symptoms of SBC are similar to those of PBC. Jaundice and pruritus are usually the most prominent features. In addition, fever and/or right upper quadrant pain, reflecting bouts of cholangitis or biliary colic, are typical. The manifestations of portal hypertension are found only in advanced cases.

Laboratory tests Elevations in serum alkaline phosphatase and 5′-nucleotidase as well as conjugated hyperbilirubinemia are almost always present. There is a moderate increase in serum aminotransferases. When the disease is complicated by cholangitis, elevations in aminotransferase levels and leukocytosis are more pronounced. As in PBC, there are abnormalities in serum lipids (including the presence of lipoprotein X) and laboratory findings consistent with steatorrhea. However, the antimitochondrial antibody test is usually negative.

Diagnosis SBC should be considered in any patient with clinical and laboratory evidence of prolonged obstruction to bile flow, especially when there is a history of previous biliary tract surgery or gallstones, bouts of ascending cholangitis, or right upper quadrant pain. Cholangiography (either percutaneous or endoscopic) usually demonstrates the underlying pathologic process. Liver biopsy, although not always necessary from a clinical standpoint, can document the development of cirrhosis.

℞ TREATMENT

Relief of obstruction to bile flow, by either endoscopic or surgical means, is the most important step in the prevention and therapy of SBC. Effective decompression of the biliary tract results in a significant improvement in both symptoms and survival, even in patients with established cirrhosis. When obstruction cannot be relieved, as in sclerosing cholangitis, antibiotics may be helpful acutely in controlling superimposed infection or, when administered on a chronic basis, as prophylactic therapy in suppressing recurring episodes of ascending cholangitis. Without relief of obstruction, there is a steady progression to end-stage cirrhosis and its terminal manifestations.

CARDIAC CIRRHOSIS

Definition Prolonged, severe right-sided congestive heart failure may lead to chronic liver injury and cardiac cirrhosis. The characteristic pathologic features of fibrosis and regenerative nodules distinguish cardiac cirrhosis from both reversible passive congestion of the liver due to acute heart failure and acute hepatocellular necrosis ("ischemic hepatitis" or "shock liver") resulting from systemic hypotension and hypoperfusion of the liver.

Etiology and Pathology In right-sided heart failure, retrograde transmission of elevated venous pressure via the inferior vena cava and hepatic veins leads to congestion of the liver. Hepatic sinusoids become dilated and engorged with blood, and the liver becomes tensely swollen. With prolonged passive congestion and ischemia from poor perfusion secondary to reduced cardiac output, necrosis of centrilobular hepatocytes ensues and leads to fibrosis in these central areas. Ultimately, centrilobular fibrosis develops, with collagen extending outward in a characteristic stellate pattern from the central vein. Gross examination of the liver shows alternating red (congested) and pale (fibrotic) areas, a pattern often referred to as "nutmeg liver." Improvement in management of cardiac disorders, particularly advances in surgical treatment, has reduced the frequency of cardiac cirrhosis.

Clinical Features In acute passive congestion, the liver becomes enlarged and tender, and the patient may complain of severe right upper quadrant pain due to stretching of Glisson's capsule. A range of abnormalities of liver function tests may be found, though none is uniformly present. The serum bilirubin is usually only mildly increased and may be predominantly either conjugated or unconjugated. Mild to moderate elevation in alkaline phosphatase and prothrombin time prolongation are sometimes present. The AST level is also typically mildly elevated but may be transiently very high following a period of marked systemic hypotension (shock liver), when the clinical picture can mimic acute viral or drug-induced hepatitis. In cases of tricuspid insufficiency the liver may be pulsatile, but this finding disappears as cirrhosis develops. With prolonged right-sided heart failure the liver becomes enlarged, firm, and usually nontender. The signs and symptoms of heart failure usually overshadow the liver disease. Bleeding from esophageal varices is rare, but chronic encephalopathy may be prominent, with a waxing and waning course reflecting variations in the severity of right-sided heart failure. Ascites and peripheral edema, often primarily related to the underlying cardiac dysfunction, may be worsened by the superimposed liver disease.

Diagnosis The presence of a firm, enlarged liver with signs of chronic liver disease in a patient with valvular heart disease, constrictive pericarditis, or cor pulmonale of long duration (>10 years) should suggest cardiac cirrhosis. Liver biopsy can confirm the diagnosis but is usually contraindicated because of coagulopathy or ascites. Coexistent chronic heart and liver disease should also raise the possibility of hemochromatosis, amyloidosis, or other infiltrative diseases.

Budd-Chiari syndrome resulting from the occlusion of the hepatic veins or inferior vena cava may be confused with acute congestive hepatomegaly. In this condition the liver is grossly enlarged and tender, and severe intractable ascites is present. However, signs and symptoms of heart failure are notably absent. The most common cause is thrombosis of the hepatic veins, often in the setting of polycythemia rubra vera, myeloproliferative syndromes, paroxysmal nocturnal hemoglobinuria, oral contraceptive use, or other hypercoagulable states; it also may result from invasion of the inferior vena cava by tumor, such as renal cell or primary hepatocellular carcinoma. Idiopathic membranous obstruction of the inferior vena cava is the most common cause of this syndrome in Japan. Hepatic venography or liver biopsy showing centrilobular congestion and sinusoidal dilatation in the absence of right-sided heart failure establishes the diagnosis of Budd-Chiari syndrome. Venoocclusive disease affecting the sublobular branches of the hepatic veins and the hepatic venules may result from hepatic irradiation, treatment with certain antineoplastic agents, or ingestion

Table 298-2

Some Causes of Noncirrhotic Hepatic Fibrosis

Idiopathic portal hypertension (noncirrhotic portal fibrosis, Banti's syndrome); three variants:
    Intrahepatic phlebosclerosis and fibrosis
    Portal and splenic vein sclerosis
    Portal and splenic vein thrombosis
Schistosomiasis ("pipe-stem" fibrosis with presinusoidal portal hypertension)
Congenital hepatic fibrosis (may be associated with polycystic disease of liver and kidneys)

of pyrrolidizine alkaloids present in some herbal teas ("bush tea disease") and can mimic congestive hepatomegaly.

  TREATMENT
Prevention or treatment of cardiac cirrhosis depends on the diagnosis and therapy of the underlying cardiovascular disorder. Improvement in cardiac function frequently results in improvement of liver function and stabilization of the liver disease.

METABOLIC, HEREDITARY, DRUG-RELATED, AND OTHER TYPES OF CIRRHOSIS (See Table 298-1)

Cirrhosis or hepatitis may result from a wide variety of other processes encompassing the spectrum of etiologic factors listed in Table 298-2. Although some of these disorders have distinctive clinical or morphologic features, the manifestations of cirrhosis are largely independent of the underlying pathogenic mechanism.

NONCIRRHOTIC FIBROSIS OF THE LIVER

Several diseases, either congenital or acquired, may be associated with localized or generalized hepatic fibrosis. They are distinguished from cirrhosis by the absence of hepatocellular damage and the lack of nodular regenerative activity. The clinical manifestations in such cases are largely secondary to portal hypertension. The different types of these disorders are indicated in Table 298-2; with the exception of schistosomiasis, all these conditions are relatively rare.

BIBLIOGRAPHY

ALCOHOLIC AND POSTNECROTIC CIRRHOSIS

ARROYO V, GINÉS P: Arteriolar vasodilation and the pathogenesis of the hyperdynamic circulation and renal sodium and water retention in cirrhosis. Gastroenterology 102:1077, 1992

BACON BR et al: Nonalcoholic steatohepatitis: An expanded clinical entity. Gastroenterology 107:1103, 1994

BROWN J et al: Seroprevalence of hepatitis C virus nucleocapsid antibodies in patients with cryptogenic chronic liver disease. Hepatology 15:175, 1992

CARITHERS RL et al: Methylprednisolone therapy in patients with severe alcoholic hepatitis: A randomized multicenter trial. Ann Intern Med 110:685, 1989

JEFFERS LJ et al: Prevalence of antibodies to hepatitis C virus among patients with cryptogenic chronic hepatitis and cirrhosis. Hepatology 15:187, 1992

LIEBER CS: Alcohol and the liver: 1994 update. Gastroenterology 106:1085, 1994

RAMOND M-J et al: A randomized trial of prednisolone in patients with severe alcoholic hepatitis. N Engl J Med 326:507, 1992

SHETH SG et al: Nonalcoholic steatohepatitis. Ann Intern Med 126:137, 1997

BILIARY CIRRHOSIS

CHRISTENSEN E et al: Updating prognosis in primary biliary cirrhosis using a time-dependent cox regression model. Gastroenterology 105:1865, 1993

COMBES B et al: A randomized, double-blind, placebo-controlled trial of ursodeoxycholic acid in primary biliary cirrhosis. Hepatology 22:759, 1995

FREGEAU DR et al: Antimitochondrial antibodies of primary biliary cirrhosis recognize dihydrolipoamide acyltransferase and inhibit enzyme function of the branched chain α-ketoacid dehydrogenase complex. J Immunol 142:3815, 1989

KAPLAN MM: Medical progress: Primary biliary cirrhosis. N Engl J Med 335:1570, 1996

LOCKE III GR et al: Time course of histological progression in primary biliary cirrhosis. Hepatology 23:52, 1996

MARKUS BH et al: Efficacy of liver transplantation in patients with primary biliary cirrhosis. N Engl J Med 320:1709, 1989

METCALF JV et al: Natural history of early primary biliary cirrhosis. Lancet 348:1399, 1996

POUPON RE et al: Ursodial for the long-term treatment of primary biliary cirrhosis. N Engl J Med 330:1342, 1994

TSUNEYAMA K et al: Abnormal expression of the E2 component of the pyruvate dehydrogenase complex on the luminal surface of biliary epithelium before major histocompatibility complex class II and BB1/BB7 expression. Hepatology 21:103, 1995

299 *Daniel K. Podolsky, Kurt J. Isselbacher*

MAJOR COMPLICATIONS OF CIRRHOSIS

The clinical course of patients with advanced cirrhosis is often complicated by a number of important sequelae that are independent of the etiology of the underlying liver disease. These include portal hypertension and its consequences (e.g., gastroesophageal varices and splenomegaly), ascites, hepatic encephalopathy, spontaneous bacterial peritonitis, hepatorenal syndrome, and hepatocellular carcinoma.

PORTAL HYPERTENSION Definition and Pathogenesis
Normal pressure in the portal vein is low (10 to 15 cm saline) because vascular resistance in the hepatic sinusoids is minimal. Portal hypertension (>30 cm saline) most commonly results from increased resistance to portal blood flow. Because the portal venous system lacks valves, resistance at any level between the right side of the heart and splanchnic vessels results in retrograde transmission of an elevated pressure. Increased resistance can occur at three levels relative to the hepatic sinusoids: (1) presinusoidal, (2) sinusoidal, and (3) postsinusoidal. Obstruction in the *presinusoidal* venous compartment may be anatomically outside the liver (e.g., portal vein thrombosis) or within the liver itself but at a functional level proximal to the hepatic sinusoids so that the liver parenchyma is not exposed to the elevated venous pressure (e.g., schistosomiasis).

Postsinusoidal obstruction also may occur outside the liver at the level of the hepatic veins (e.g., Budd-Chiari syndrome), the inferior vena cava, or, less commonly, within the liver (e.g., venoocclusive disease in which the central hepatic venules are the primary site of injury). When cirrhosis is complicated by portal hypertension, the increased resistance is usually *sinusoidal*. While distinctions between pre-, post-, and sinusoidal processes are conceptually appealing, functional resistance to portal flow in a given patient may occur at more than one level. Portal hypertension also may arise from increased blood flow (e.g., massive splenomegaly or arteriovenous fistulas), but the low outflow resistance of the normal liver makes this a rare clinical problem.

Cirrhosis is the most common cause of portal hypertension in the United States. Clinically significant portal hypertension is present in greater than 60 percent of patients with cirrhosis. *Portal vein obstruction* is the second most common cause; it may be idiopathic or occur in association with cirrhosis, infection, pancreatitis, or abdominal trauma. Portal vein thrombosis may develop in a variety of hypercoagulable states including polycythemia vera, essential thrombocythemia, and deficiencies of protein C, protein S, or antithrombin III. Portal vein thrombosis may be idiopathic, though some of these patients may have a subtle myeloproliferative disorder. *Hepatic vein thrombosis* (Budd-Chiari syndrome) and hepatic venoocclusive disease are relatively infrequent causes of portal hypertension (see above). Portal vein occlusion may result in massive hematemesis from gastroesophageal varices, but ascites is usually found only when cirrhosis is present. Noncirrhotic portal fibrosis accounts for only a few cases of portal hypertension.

Clinical Features The major clinical manifestations of portal hypertension include hemorrhage from gastroesophageal varices, splenomegaly with hypersplenism, ascites, and acute and chronic hepatic encephalopathy. These are related, at least in part, to the development of portal-systemic collateral channels. The absence of valves in the portal venous system facilitates retrograde (hepatofugal) blood flow from the high-pressure portal venous system to the lower-pressure systemic venous circulation. Major sites of collateral flow involve the veins around the rectum (hemorrhoids), cardioesophageal junction (esophagogastric varices), retroperitoneal space, and the falciform ligament of the liver (periumbilical or abdominal wall collaterals). Abdominal wall collaterals appear as tortuous epigastric vessels that radiate from the umbilicus toward the xiphoid and rib margins (caput medusae).

Diagnosis In patients with known liver disease, the development of portal hypertension usually becomes evident by the appearance of splenomegaly, ascites, encephalopathy, and/or esophageal varices. Conversely, the finding of any of these features should lead one to evaluate the patient for the presence of underlying portal hypertension and liver disease. Varices are most reliably documented by fiberoptic esophagoscopy; their presence lends indirect support to the diagnosis of portal hypertension. Although rarely necessary, portal venous pressure may be measured directly by percutaneous transhepatic "skinny needle" catheterization or indirectly through transjugular cannulation of the hepatic veins. Both free and wedged hepatic vein pressure (WHVP) should be measured. While WHVP is elevated in sinusoidal and postsinusoidal portal hypertension, including cirrhosis, this measurement is usually normal in presinusoidal portal hypertension. In patients in whom additional information is necessary (e.g., preoperative evaluation before portal-systemic shunt surgery) or when percutaneous catheterization is not feasible, mesenteric and hepatic angiography may be helpful. Particular attention should be directed to the venous phase to assess the patency of the portal vein and the direction of portal blood flow.

R̲x̲ **TREATMENT**

Although treatment is usually directed toward a specific complication of portal hypertension, attempts are sometimes made to reduce the pressure in the portal venous system. Surgical decompression procedures have been used for many years to lower portal pressure in patients with bleeding esophageal varices (see below). However, portal-systemic shunt surgery does not result in improved survival rates in patients with cirrhosis. Decompression can now be accomplished without surgery through the percutaneous placement of a portal-systemic shunt, termed a transjugular intrahepatic portosystemic shunt (TIPS). Beta-adrenergic blockade with propranolol or nadolol reduces portal pressure through vasodilatory effects on both the splanchnic arterial bed and the portal venous system in combination with reduced cardiac output. Such therapy has been shown to be effective in preventing both a first variceal bleed and subsequent episodes after an initial bleed. Treatment of patients with clinically significant sequelae of portal hypertension, especially variceal bleeding, with doses of propranolol titrated to reduce the resting pulse by 25 percent is reasonable if no contraindications exist.

Vigorous treatment of patients with alcoholic hepatitis and cirrhosis, chronic active hepatitis, and other liver diseases may lead to a fall in portal pressure and to a reduction in variceal size. In general, however, portal hypertension due to cirrhosis is not reversible. In appropriately selected patients hepatic transplantation will be beneficial.

VARICEAL BLEEDING Pathogenesis While vigorous hemorrhage may arise from any portal-systemic venous collaterals, bleeding is most common from varices in the region of the gastroesophageal junction. The factors contributing to bleeding from gastroesophageal varices are not entirely understood but include the degree of portal hypertension and the size of the varices.

Clinical Features and Diagnosis Variceal bleeding often occurs without obvious precipitating factors and usually presents with painless but massive hematemesis with or without melena. Associated signs range from mild postural tachycardia to profound shock, depending on the extent of blood loss and degree of hypovolemia. Because patients with varices may bleed from other gastrointestinal lesions (e.g., peptic ulcer, gastritis), exclusion of other bleeding sources is important even in patients with prior variceal hemorrhage. Fiberoptic endoscopy is the best approach to evaluate upper gastrointestinal hemorrhage in patients with known or suspected portal hypertension.

R̲x̲ **TREATMENT**

(See Fig. 299-1) Variceal bleeding is a life-threatening emergency. Prompt estimation and vigorous replacement of blood loss to maintain intravascular volume are essential and take precedence over diagnostic studies and more specific intervention to stop the bleeding. However, excessive fluid administration can increase portal pressure with resultant further bleeding and should therefore be avoided. Replacement of clotting factors with fresh frozen plasma is important in patients with coagulopathy. Patients are best managed in an intensive care unit and require close monitoring of central venous or pulmonary capillary wedge pressures, urine output, and mental status. Only when the patient is hemodynamically stable should attention be directed toward specific diagnostic studies (especially endoscopy) and other therapeutic modalities to prevent further or recurrent bleeding.

About half of all episodes of variceal hemorrhage cease without intervention, although the risk of rebleeding is very high. The medical management of acute variceal hemorrhage includes the use of vasoconstrictors (vasopressin or somatostatin), balloon tamponade, and endoscopic sclerosis of varices (sclerotherapy) or endoscopic ligation of varices and beta-adrenergic blockade (see Chap. 44). Intravenous infusion of *vasopressin* at a rate of 0.1 to 0.4 U/min results in generalized vasoconstriction leading to diminished blood flow in the portal venous system. Intravenous infusion of vasopressin is as effective as selective intraarterial administration. Control of bleeding can be achieved in up to 80 percent of cases, but bleeding recurs

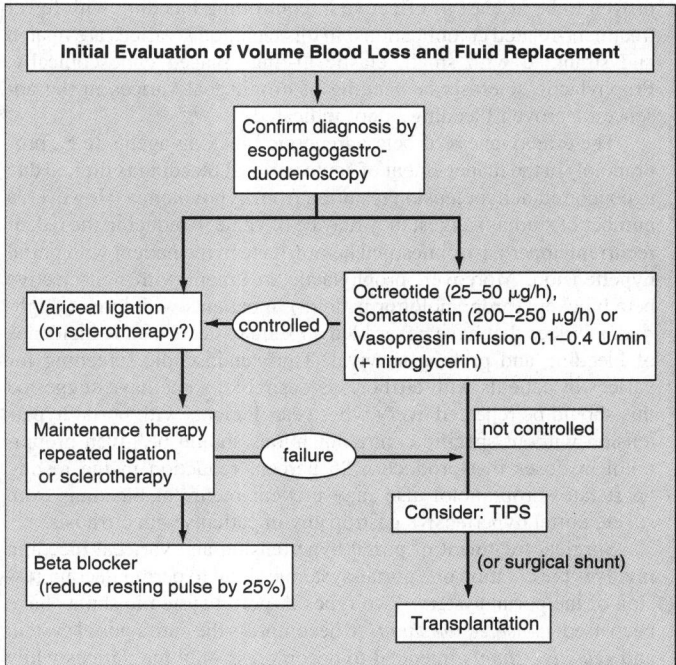

FIGURE 299-1 Approach to the patient with variceal bleeding. Use of a beta blocker is the only intervention demonstrated to offer prophylactic benefit in a patient who has never bled.

in more than half after the vasopressin is tapered and discontinued. Furthermore, a number of serious side effects, including cardiac and gastrointestinal tract ischemia, acute renal failure, and hyponatremia, may be associated with vasopressin therapy. Concurrent use of veno-dilators such as nitroglycerin as an intravenous infusion or isosorbide dinitrate sublingually may enhance the effectiveness of vasopressin and reduce complications. Somatostatin and its analogue, octreotide, are direct splanchnic vasoconstrictors. In some studies somatostatin, given as an initial 250-μg bolus followed by constant infusion (250 μg/h), has been found to be as effective as vasopressin. Octreotide at doses of 25 to 50 μg/h is also effective. These agents may be preferable to vasopressin, offering equivalent efficacy with fewer complications. If bleeding is too vigorous or endoscopy is not available, *balloon tamponade* of the bleeding varices may be accomplished with a triple-lumen (Sengstaken-Blakemore) or four-lumen (Minnesota) tube with esophageal and gastric balloons. Because of the high risk of aspiration, endotracheal intubation should be performed prior to placing one of these tubes. After the tube is introduced into the stomach, the gastric balloon is inflated and pulled back into the cardia of the stomach. If bleeding does not stop, the esophageal balloon is inflated for additional tamponade. Complications occur in 15 percent or more of patients and include aspiration pneumonitis as well as esophageal rupture.

Where available, *endoscopic intervention* should be employed as the first line of treatment to control bleeding acutely (see Chap. 44). Over the past 15 years, endoscopic sclerosis of varices has been extensively employed. In this procedure, the varices are injected with one of several sclerosing agents via a needle-tipped catheter passed through the endoscope. After endoscopic identification of varices as the presumed source of bleeding, sclerotherapy controls acute bleeding in up to 90 percent of cases. In addition, repeated sclerotherapy can be performed until obliteration of all varices is accomplished in an effort to prevent recurrent bleeding. While available data support the efficacy of sclerotherapy in controlling bleeding acutely, repeated sclerotherapy has not been documented to prolong survival. Mucosal ulceration resulting from injection of the caustic sclerosant may occur and result in further hemorrhage or stenosis. More recently, endoscopic ligation (rubber banding) of varices has proven to be at least as effective in controlling bleeding with fewer treatment-related complications. In this technique, varices are ligated and strangled with small, elastic O-rings placed endoscopically. Prophylactic sclerosis or banding of esophageal varices in the absence of proven bleeding is not indicated.

The effectiveness of beta-adrenergic blocking agents (e.g., propranolol) in the management of acute variceal bleeding is limited due to concomitant hypotension resulting from hypovolemia. However, a number of studies suggest they may be of value in reducing the risk of recurrent upper gastrointestinal hemorrhage in the patient with portal hypertension. Moreover, prophylactic treatment with nonselective beta blockers (propranolol or nadolol) in patients with large ("high-risk") varices that have never bled appears to decrease the incidence of bleeding and prolong survival. Thus, endoscopic screening for varices in patients with cirrhosis is desirable; some have suggested this should be repeated every other year. Patients with portal hypertension without specific contraindications should be given propranolol in doses that produce a 25 percent reduction in the resting heart rate. Propranolol also may prevent recurrent bleeding from severe portal hypertensive gastropathy in patients with cirrhosis.

Surgical treatment of portal hypertension and variceal bleeding involves the creation of a portal-systemic shunt to permit decompression of the portal system. Two types of portal systemic shunts have been used: *nonselective shunts* to decompress the entire portal system and *selective shunts* intended to decompress only the varices while maintaining blood flow to the liver itself. Nonselective shunts include end-to-side or side-to-side portacaval and proximal splenorenal anastomoses; selective shunts include the distal splenorenal shunt. Nonse

lective shunts are more likely to be complicated by encephalopathy than selective shunts. Emergency portal-systemic nonselective shunts may control acute hemorrhage, but such surgery is usually used only as a last resort because early operative mortality is greater than 30 percent. The role of portal-systemic shunt surgery after initial control of bleeding by nonoperative means is also uncertain. Surgically created shunts effectively reduce the risk of recurrent hemorrhage, but the overall mortality of patients undergoing such surgery is comparable to that of unoperated patients. Although patients who have undergone portal-system surgery succumb to recurrent bleeding less commonly than unoperated patients, this improvement is counterbalanced by increased morbidity from encephalopathy and death from progressive liver failure. Increasingly, therapeutic portal-systemic shunts have been reserved for patients who experience further bleeding despite serial endoscopic sclerotherapy or band ligation. Using TIPS, a technique developed to create a portal-systemic shunt by a percutaneous approach, an expandable metal stent is advanced to the hepatic veins under angiographic guidance and then through the substance of the liver to create a direct portacaval channel. This technique offers an alternative to surgery for refractory bleeding due to portal hypertension, but stents frequently undergo stenosis or occlude over a period of months, prompting the need for a second TIPS or an alternative approach. Encephalopathy may be encountered after TIPS just as in the surgical shunts. Procedures such as esophageal transection also have been advocated for the management of acute variceal bleeding, but their efficacy remains unproven. Even though recent trials found that esophageal transection was as effective as endoscopic sclerotherapy, transection is usually considered a last resort.

Portal Hypertensive Gastropathy   Although variceal hemorrhage is the most commonly encountered bleeding complication of portal hypertension, many patients will develop a congestive gastropathy due to the venous hypertension. In this condition, identified by endoscopic examination, the mucosa appears engorged and friable. Indolent mucosal bleeding occurs rather than the brisk hemorrhage typical of a variceal source. Beta-adrenergic blockade with propranolol (reducing splanchnic arterial pressure as well as portal pressure) is sometimes effective in ameliorating this condition. H_2 receptor antagonists or other agents useful in the treatment of peptic disease are usually not helpful.

SPLENOMEGALY   Definition and Pathogenesis   Congestive splenomegaly is common in patients with severe portal hypertension. Rarely, massive splenomegaly from nonhepatic disease leads to portal hypertension due to increased blood flow in the splenic vein.

Clinical Features   Although usually asymptomatic, splenomegaly may be massive and contribute to the thrombocytopenia or pancytopenia of cirrhosis. In the absence of cirrhosis, splenomegaly in association with variceal hemorrhage should suggest the possibility of splenic vein thrombosis.

 TREATMENT

Splenomegaly usually requires no specific treatment, although massive enlargement of the spleen may occasionally necessitate splenectomy at the time of shunt surgery. However, it should be noted that splenectomy without an accompanying shunt may actually increase portal pressure. Splenectomy also may be indicated if splenomegaly is the cause rather than the result of portal hypertension. Thrombocytopenia alone is rarely severe enough to necessitate removal of the spleen.

ASCITES   Definition   Ascites is the accumulation of excess fluid within the peritoneal cavity. It is most frequently encountered in patients with cirrhosis and other forms of severe liver disease, but a number of other disorders may lead to either transudative or exudative ascites (see Chap. 46).

Pathogenesis   The accumulation of ascitic fluid represents a state of total-body sodium and water excess, but the event that initiates this imbalance is unclear. Three theories have been proposed (see Fig.

The "underfilling" theory suggests that the primary abnormality is inappropriate sequestration of fluid within the splanchnic vascular bed due to portal hypertension and a consequent decrease in effective circulating blood volume. According to this theory, an apparent decrease in intravascular volume (underfilling) is sensed by the kidney, which responds by retaining salt and water. The "overflow" theory suggests that the primary abnormality is inappropriate renal retention of salt and water in the absence of volume depletion. A third theory, the peripheral arterial vasodilation hypothesis, has been proposed to account for the constellation of arterial hypotension and increased cardiac output in association with high levels of vasoconstrictor substances that are routinely found in patients with cirrhosis and ascites. Again, sodium retention is considered secondary to arterial vascular underfilling and the result of a disproportionate increase of the vascular compartment due to arteriolar vasodilation rather than from decreased intravascular volume. According to this theory, portal hypertension results in splanchnic arteriolar vasodilation, possibly mediated by nitric oxide, and leading to underfilling of the arterial vascular space and baroreceptor-mediated stimulation of renin-angiotensin, sympathetic output, and antidiuretic hormone release.

Regardless of the initiating event, a number of factors contribute to accumulation of fluid in the abdominal cavity (see Fig. 299-2). Elevated levels of serum epinephrine and norepinephrine have been well documented. *Increased central sympathetic outflow* is found in patients with cirrhosis and ascites but not in those with cirrhosis alone. Increased sympathetic output results in diminished natriuresis by activation of the renin-angiotensin system and diminished sensitivity to atrial natriuretic peptide. *Portal hypertension* plays an important role in the formation of ascites by raising hydrostatic pressure within the splanchnic capillary bed. *Hypoalbuminemia* and *reduced plasma oncotic pressure* also favor the extravasation of fluid from plasma to the peritoneal cavity, and thus ascites is infrequent in patients with cirrhosis unless both portal hypertension and hypoalbuminemia are present. *Hepatic lymph* may weep freely from the surface of the cirrhotic liver due to distortion and obstruction of hepatic sinusoids and lymphatics and contribute to ascites formation. In contrast to the contribution of transudative fluid from the portal vascular bed, hepatic lymph may weep into the peritoneal cavity even in the absence of marked hypoproteinemia because the endothelial lining of the hepatic sinusoids is discontinuous. This mechanism may account for the high protein con-

centration present in the ascitic fluid of some patients with the Budd-Chiari syndrome.

Renal factors also play an important role in perpetuating ascites. Patients with ascites fail to excrete a water load in a normal fashion. They have increased renal sodium reabsorption by both proximal and distal tubules, the latter due largely to increased plasma renin activity and secondary hyperaldosteronism. Insensitivity to circulating atrial natriuretic peptide, often present in elevated concentrations in patients with cirrhosis and ascites, may be an important contributory factor in many patients. This insensitivity has been documented in those patients with the most severely impaired sodium excretion, who typically also exhibit low arterial pressure and marked overactivity of the renin-aldosterone axis. Renal vasoconstriction, perhaps resulting from increased serum prostaglandin or catecholamine levels, also may contribute to sodium retention. Recently a role for endothelin, a potent vasoconstrictor peptide, has been proposed. While elevated levels have been reported by some, this has not been observed by others.

As discussed in Chap. 46, ascites may arise in a number of clinical settings in addition to cirrhosis and portal hypertension. Although historically ascites was classified as either transudative or exudative, similar to the characterization of pleural fluids, this schema has limitations. Instead, the serum-ascites albumin gradient (SAAG) provides a better classification than total protein content or other parameters. Ascites resulting from cirrhosis typically has a high SAAG (>1.1 g/dL), reflecting indirectly the abnormally high hydrostatic pressure gradient between the portal bed and the ascitic compartment.

Clinical Features and Diagnosis Usually ascites is first noticed by the patient because of increasing abdominal girth. More pronounced accumulation of fluid may cause shortness of breath because of elevation of the diaphragm. When peritoneal fluid accumulation exceeds 500 mL, ascites may be demonstrated on physical examination by the presence of shifting dullness, a fluid wave, or bulging flanks. Ultrasound examination, preferably with a Doppler study, can detect smaller quantities of ascites and should be performed when physical examination is equivocal or when the cause of the recent onset of ascites is not clear (e.g., exclude Budd-Chiari syndrome or portal vein thrombosis).

℞ **TREATMENT**
(See Fig. 299-3) A thorough search should be made for precipitating factors in the patient with recent onset of or worsening ascites, e.g., excessive salt intake, medication noncompliance, superimposed infection, worsening liver disease, portal vein thrombosis, or development of hepatocellular carcinoma. When ascites develops in the setting of severe, acute liver disease, resolution of ascites is likely to follow improvement in liver function. More commonly, ascites develops in patients with stable or steadily worsening liver function. Paracentesis usually should be performed with a small-gauge needle at the time of initial evaluation or at the time of any clinical deterioration of a cirrhotic patient with ascites. A small amount of fluid (<200 mL) should be obtained and examined for evidence of infection, tumor, or other possible causes and complications of ascites. Therapeutic intervention is indicated both to prevent potential complications and to control progressive increase in ascites, which may become pronounced enough to cause physical discomfort. For the patient with a modest accumulation, therapy can be undertaken as an outpatient and should be gentle and incremental (see below). The goal is the loss of no more than 1.0 kg/d if both ascites and peripheral edema are present and no more than 0.5 kg/d in patients with ascites alone. In some patients, particularly those with a large accumulation of fluid, it may be desirable to hospitalize the patient so that daily weights and frequent serum electrolyte levels can be monitored and compliance ensured. Although abdominal girth measurements are frequently used as an index of fluid loss, they tend to be unreliable.

Strict bed rest is often recommended because of improved renal clearance in the supine position. However, salt restriction is the most important cornerstone of therapy. A diet containing 800 mg sodium

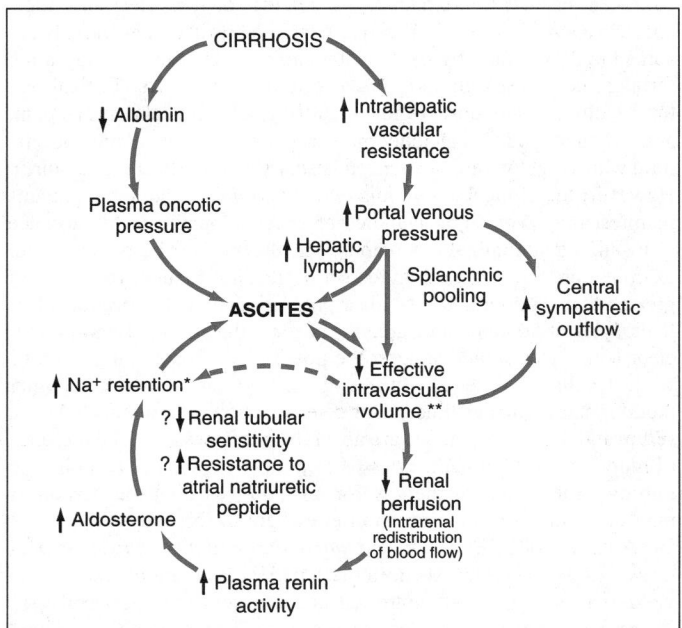

FIGURE 299-2 Multiple factors involved in development of ascites. Current concepts suggest that initiating factor may be primary sodium retention (*"overflow"), diminished effective intravascular volume (**"underfilling"), or arteriolar vasodilation.

FIGURE 299-3 Approach to the patient with ascites [and spontaneous bacterial peritonitis (SBP)]. PMN, polymorphonuclear leukocytes; TIPS, transjugular intrahepatic portosystemic shunt. *Calculate SAAG [serum ascites albumin gradient = serum albumin − ascites albumin (g/dL)] to confirm low gradient (<1.1 g/dL) in portal hypertension. †If PMN > 250/μL but culture is negative = culture negative neutrocytic ascites; begin empiric antibiotic and retap at 48 h; if culture is positive but PMN < 250/μL normal = monomicrobial non-neutrocytic bacterascites; retap; treat if PMN > 250/μL; if polymicrobial infection, exclude secondary peritonitis.

(2 g NaCl) is often adequate to induce a negative sodium balance and permit diuresis. Response to salt restriction and bed rest alone is more likely to occur if the ascites is of recent onset, the underlying liver disease is reversible, a precipitating factor can be corrected, or the patient has a high urinary sodium excretion (~25 mmol/d) and normal renal function. Fluid restriction of approximately 1000 mL/d does little to enhance diuresis but may be necessary to correct hyponatremia. If sodium restriction alone fails to result in diuresis and weight loss, diuretics should be prescribed. Because of the role of hyperaldosteronism in sustaining salt retention, spironolactone or other distal tubule–acting diuretics (triamterene, amiloride) are the drugs of choice. These agents are also preferred because of their gentle action and specific potassium-sparing properties. Spironolactone is initially given in a dose of 25 mg four times a day and is increased as needed by 100 mg/d every several days to a maximum dose that should rarely exceed 400 mg/d. An indication of the minimum effective dose of spironolactone may be obtained by monitoring urinary electrolyte concentrations for a rise in sodium and fall in potassium levels, reflecting effective competitive inhibition of aldosterone. Conversely, the development of azotemia or hyperkalemia may be dose-limiting or even warrant a reduction in the amount of this medication. In some patients, diuresis cannot be initiated despite maximal doses of distal tubule–acting agents (e.g., 400 mg spironolactone) because of avid proximal tubular sodium absorp-

tion. More potent and proximally acting diuretics (furosemide, thiazide, or ethacrynic acid) may then be added cautiously to the regimen. Spironolactone plus furosemide, 20 or 80 mg/d, is usually sufficient to initiate a diuresis in most patients. However, such aggressive therapy must be used with great caution to avoid plasma volume depletion, azotemia, and hypokalemia, which may lead to encephalopathy.

In patients with pronounced ascites, particularly those requiring hospitalization, large-volume paracentesis has proven to be an effective and less costly approach to initial management than prolonged bed rest and conventional diuretic treatment. In this approach, ascitic fluid is removed by peritoneal cannula using strict aseptic techniques and monitoring hemodynamic and renal function. This can be safely accomplished in a single session. The need for concomitant albumin replacement by intravenous infusion remains controversial but may be prudent in the patient without peripheral edema, to avoid depleting the intravascular space and precipitating hypotension. Maintenance diuretic therapy in conjunction with sodium restriction may then be instituted to avoid recurrent ascites.

A minority of patients with advanced cirrhosis have "refractory ascites" or rapidly reaccumulate fluid after control by paracentesis. In some patients, a side-to-side *portacaval shunt* may result in improvement in ascites, although generally these patients are extremely poor surgical risks. In the past, intractable ascites has also been treated with the surgical implantation of a plastic *peritoneovenous shunt*, which has a pressure-sensitive, one-way valve allowing ascitic fluid to flow from the abdominal cavity to the superior vena cava. However, the usefulness of this technique is limited by a high rate of complications such as infection, disseminated intravascular coagulation, and thrombosis of the shunt. More recently, TIPS has been used effectively to control refractory ascites, although portal decompression, while mobilizing ascitic fluid, has precipitated severe hepatic encephalopathy in some patients.

SPONTANEOUS BACTERIAL PERITONITIS (SBP) Patients with ascites and cirrhosis may develop acute bacterial peritonitis without an obvious primary source of infection. Patients with very advanced liver disease are particularly susceptible to SBP. The ascitic fluid in these patients typically has especially low concentrations of albumin and other so-called opsonic proteins, which normally may provide some protection against bacteria. Although key steps in the pathogenesis of SBP remain to be elucidated, it is clear that most bacteria contributing to SBP derive from the bowel and eventually are spread to ascitic fluid by the hematogenous route after transmigration through the bowel wall and transversing the lymphatics. Typical features include abrupt onset of fever, chills, generalized abdominal pain, and rebound abdominal tenderness accompanied by cloudy ascitic fluid with a high white cell count and usually positive bacterial cultures. However, the clinical symptoms *may be minimal*, and some patients manifest only worsening jaundice or encephalopathy in the absence of localizing abdominal complaints. The diagnosis is based on careful examination of the ascitic fluid. An ascitic fluid leukocyte count of greater than 500 cells/μL (with a proportion of polymorphonuclear leukocytes of 50 percent or greater) or more than 250 polymorphonuclear leukocytes should suggest the possibility of bacterial peritonitis while results of bacterial cultures of ascitic fluid are pending. Other measurements such as fluid pH or determination of gradients between serum and fluid pH or lactate are generally not necessary. The presence of more than 10,000 leukocytes/μL, multiple organisms, or failure to improve after standard therapy for 48 h suggest that the peritonitis may be secondary to an infection elsewhere in the body.

A variant of SBP, designated *monomicrobial nonneutrocytic bacterascites*, is sometimes seen. In these patients, culture of ascitic fluid yields bacteria, but the neutrophil count is less than 250 cells/μL. These patients often have less severe liver disease than those found initially to have typical SBP. While many patients with this variant have cleared the bacterascites at the time of a subsequent paracentesis, nearly 40 percent will develop typical SBP; thus follow-up paracentesis is usually warranted in this setting.

TREATMENT

Empirical therapy with cefotaxime or ampicillin and an aminoglycoside should be initiated when the diagnosis is first suspected because enteric gram-negative bacilli are found in the majority of cases; less frequently, the infection is caused by pneumococci and other gram-positive bacteria. Cefotaxime may be preferable due to the lower rate of renal toxicity. Specific antibiotic therapy can be selected once the specific organism is identified. Therapy is usually administered for 10 to 14 days, although one controlled study has suggested that a 5-day course of intravenous antibiotics may be as effective when repeat paracentesis at 48 h demonstrates a decline in the ascitic polymorphonuclear leukocytes count by more than 50 percent and negative cultures.

While appropriate antibiotic therapy is usually effective in the treatment of an episode of SBP, recurrent episodes are relatively common; as many as 70 percent of patients will experience at least one recurrence within a year of the first episode. The risk of recurrence likely reflects the predisposing role of the underlying advanced liver disease that contributed to the development of the first episode of SBP. Recent trials have demonstrated that prophylactic maintenance therapy with norfloxacin (400 mg/d) can reduce the frequency of recurrent SBP. This agent presumably causes elective decontamination of the intestine, eliminating many aerobic gram-negative bacilli. Trimethoprim-sulfamethoxazole given for 5 days a week has also proven effective. Antibiotics may be administered as infrequently as once a week (e.g., ciprofloxacin, 750 mg once weekly). While maintenance therapy reduces the frequency of SBP and need for hospitalization, it is unclear whether this is associated with prolonged survival.

HEPATORENAL SYNDROME **Definition and Pathogenesis** Hepatorenal syndrome is a serious complication in the patient with cirrhosis and ascites and is characterized by worsening azotemia with avid sodium retention and oliguria in the absence of identifiable specific causes of renal dysfunction. The exact basis for this syndrome is not clear, but altered renal hemodynamics appear to be involved. The kidneys are structurally intact; urinalysis and pyelography are usually normal. Renal biopsy, although rarely needed, is also normal, and in fact, kidneys from such patients have been used successfully for renal transplantation. There are indications that an imbalance in certain metabolites of arachidonic acid (prostaglandins and thromboxane) may play a pathogenetic role.

Clinical Features and Diagnosis Worsening azotemia, hyponatremia, progressive oliguria, and hypotension are the hallmarks of the hepatorenal syndrome. This syndrome, which is distinct from prerenal azotemia, may be precipitated by severe gastrointestinal bleeding, sepsis, or overly vigorous attempts at diuresis or paracentesis; it also may occur without an obvious cause. It is essential to exclude other causes of renal impairment often seen in these patients. These include prerenal azotemia or acute tubular necrosis due to hypovolemia (e.g., secondary to gastrointestinal bleeding or diuretic therapy) or an increased nitrogen load such as that seen as a result of bleeding. Drug nephrotoxicity is also often a consideration, particularly in the patient who has received agents such as aminoglycosides or contrast dye. The diagnosis is supported by the demonstration of avid urinary sodium retention. Typically, the urine sodium concentration is less than 5 mmol/L, a concentration lower than that generally found in uncomplicated prerenal azotemia. The urinary sediment is unremarkable.

 TREATMENT

Treatment is usually unsuccessful. Although some patients with hypotension and decreased plasma volume may respond to infusions of salt-poor albumin, volume expansion must be undertaken with caution to avoid precipitating variceal bleeding. Vasodilator therapy, including intravenous infusion of dopamine, is not effective.

HEPATIC ENCEPHALOPATHY **Definition** Hepatic (portal-systemic) encephalopathy is a complex neuropsychiatric syndrome

characterized by disturbances in consciousness and behavior, personality changes, fluctuating neurologic signs, asterixis or "flapping tremor," and distinctive electroencephalographic changes. Encephalopathy may be *acute* and reversible or *chronic* and progressive. In severe cases, irreversible coma and death may occur. Acute episodes may recur with variable frequency.

Pathogenesis The specific cause of hepatic encephalopathy is unknown. The most important factors in the pathogenesis are severe hepatocellular dysfunction and/or intrahepatic and extrahepatic shunting of portal venous blood into the systemic circulation so that the liver is largely bypassed. As a result of these processes, various toxic substances absorbed from the intestine are not detoxified by the liver and lead to metabolic abnormalities in the central nervous system (CNS). Ammonia is the substance most often incriminated in the pathogenesis of encephalopathy. Many, but not all, patients with hepatic encephalopathy have elevated blood ammonia levels, and recovery from encephalopathy is often accompanied by declining blood ammonia levels. Other compounds and metabolites that may contribute to the development of encephalopathy include mercaptans (derived from intestinal metabolism of methionine), short-chain fatty acids, and phenol. Several observations suggest that excessive concentrations of gamma-aminobutyric acid (GABA), an inhibitory neurotransmitter, in the CNS are important in the reduced levels of consciousness seen in hepatic encephalopathy. Increased CNS GABA may reflect failure of the liver to extract precursor amino acids efficiently or to remove GABA produced in the intestine. False neurochemical transmitters (e.g., octopamine), resulting in part from alterations in plasma levels of aromatic and branched-chain amino acids, also may play a role. An increase in the permeability of the blood-brain barrier to some of these substances may be an additional factor involved in the pathogenesis of hepatic encephalopathy. There is also evidence to suggest that endogenous benzodiazepines may contribute to the development of hepatic encephalopathy. This evidence includes isolation of 1,4-benzodiazepines from brain tissue of patients with fulminant hepatic failure as well as the partial response observed in some patients and experimental animals after administration of flumazenil, a benzodiazepine antagonist. The benzodiazepine receptor is closely associated with the GABA receptor and may facilitate GABA neurotransmission. However, the inconsistent effect of flumazenil in patients with encephalopathy, as well as potential methodologic pitfalls in the measurement of endogenous benzodiazepines, precludes definitive attribution of a role to these substances in the pathogenesis of hepatic encephalopathy.

In the patient with otherwise stable cirrhosis, hepatic encephalopathy often follows a clearly identifiable precipitating event (see Table 299-1). Perhaps the most common predisposing factor is *gastrointestinal bleeding*, which leads to an increase in the production of ammonia

Table 299-1

Common Precipitants of Hepatic Encephalopathy

Increased Nitrogen Load
  Gastrointestinal bleeding
  Excess dietary protein
  Azotemia
  Constipation
Electrolyte and Metabolic Imbalance
  Hypokalemia
  Alkalosis
  Hypoxia
  Hyponatremia
Drugs
  Narcotics, tranquilizers, sedatives
  Diuretics (see "Electrolyte imbalance")
Miscellaneous
  Infection
  Surgery
  Superimposed acute liver disease
  Progressive liver disease

and other nitrogenous substances which are then absorbed. Similarly, *increased dietary protein* may precipitate encephalopathy as a result of increased production of nitrogenous substances by colonic bacteria. *Electrolyte disturbances*, particularly hypokalemic alkalosis secondary to overzealous use of diuretics, vigorous paracentesis, or vomiting, may precipitate hepatic encephalopathy. Systemic alkalosis causes an increase in the amount of nonionic ammonia (NH_3) relative to ammonium ions (NH_4^+). Only nonionic (uncharged) ammonia readily crosses the blood-brain barrier and accumulates in the central nervous system. Hypokalemia also directly stimulates renal ammonia production. Hypoxia, injudicious use of CNS-depressing drugs (e.g., barbiturates, benzodiazepines), and acute infection may trigger or aggravate hepatic encephalopathy, although the mechanisms involved are not clear. Other potential precipitating factors include superimposed acute viral hepatitis, alcoholic hepatitis, extrahepatic bile duct obstruction, surgery, and other coincidental medical complications.

Clinical Features and Diagnosis   Hepatic encephalopathy has protean manifestations, and any neurologic abnormality, including focal deficits, may be encountered. In patients with acute encephalopathy, neurologic deficits are completely reversible upon correction of underlying precipitating factors and/or improvement in liver function, but in patients with chronic encephalopathy, the deficits may be irreversible and progressive. Cerebral edema is frequently present and contributes to the clinical picture and overall mortality in patients with both acute and chronic encephalopathy.

The diagnosis of hepatic encephalopathy should be considered when four major factors are present: (1) acute or chronic hepatocellular disease and/or extensive portal-systemic collateral shunts (the latter may be either spontaneous, e.g., secondary to portal hypertension, or surgically created, e.g., portacaval anastomosis); (2) disturbances of awareness and mentation, which may progress from forgetfulness and confusion to stupor and finally coma; (3) shifting combinations of neurologic signs, including asterixis, rigidity, hyperreflexia, extensor plantar signs, and rarely, seizures; and (4) a characteristic (but nonspecific) symmetric, high-voltage, slow-wave (2 to 5 per second) pattern on the electroencephalogram. Asterixis ("liver flap," "flapping tremor") is a nonrhythmic asymmetric lapse in voluntary sustained position of the extremities, head, and trunk. It is best demonstrated by having the patient extend the arms and dorsiflex the hands. Because elicitation of asterixis depends on sustained voluntary muscle contraction, it is not present in the comatose patient. Asterixis is nonspecific and also occurs in patients with other forms of metabolic brain disease. Disturbances of sleep with reversal of sleep/wake cycles are among the earliest signs of encephalopathy. Alterations in personality, mood disturbances, confusion, deterioration in self-care and handwriting, and daytime somnolence are additional clinical features of encephalopathy. *Fetor hepaticus*, a unique musty odor of the breath and urine believed to be due to mercaptans, may be noted in patients with varying stages of hepatic encephalopathy. Some patients may develop spastic paraparesis or *chronic progressive hepatocerebral degeneration*, the latter a clinical variant of hepatic encephalopathy characterized by a slow decline in intellectual function, tremor, cerebellar ataxia, choreoathetosis, and psychiatric symptoms.

Grading or classifying the stages of hepatic encephalopathy is often helpful in following the course of the illness and assessing response to therapy. One useful classification is shown in Table 299-2.

The diagnosis of hepatic encephalopathy is usually one of exclusion. There are no diagnostic liver function test abnormalities, although an elevated serum ammonia level in the appropriate clinical setting is highly suggestive of the diagnosis. Examination of the cerebrospinal fluid is unremarkable, and computed tomography of the brain shows no characteristic abnormalities. A number of conditions, particularly disorders related to acute and chronic alcoholism, can mimic the clinical features of hepatic encephalopathy. These include acute alcohol intoxication, sedative overdose, delirium tremens, Wernicke's encephalopathy, and Korsakoff's psychosis (see Chap. 379). Subdural

Table 299-2

Clinical Stages of Hepatic Encephalopathy

Stage	Mental Status	Asterixis	EEG
I	Euphoria or depression, mild confusion, slurred speech, disordered sleep	$+/-$	Usually normal
II	Lethargy, moderate confusion	+	Abnormal
III	Marked confusion, incoherent speech, sleeping but arousable	+	Abnormal
IV	Coma; initially responsive to noxious stimuli, later unresponsive	−	Abnormal

hematoma, meningitis, and hypoglycemia or other metabolic encephalopathies also must be considered, especially in patients with alcoholic cirrhosis. In young patients with liver disease and neurologic abnormalities, Wilson's disease should be excluded.

℞ TREATMENT

(See Fig. 299-4) Early recognition and prompt treatment of hepatic encephalopathy are essential. Patients with acute, severe hepatic encephalopathy (stage IV) require the usual supportive measures for the comatose patient. Specific treatment of hepatic encephalopathy is aimed at (1) elimination or treatment of precipitating factors and (2) lowering of blood ammonia (and other toxin) levels by decreasing the absorption of protein and nitrogenous products from the intestine. In the setting of acute gastrointestinal bleeding, blood in the bowel should be promptly evacuated with laxatives (and enemas if necessary) in order to reduce the nitrogen load. Protein should be excluded from the diet, and constipation should be avoided. Ammonia absorption can be decreased by the administration of lactulose, a nonabsorbable disaccharide that acts as an osmotic laxative. Metabolism of lactulose by colonic bacteria also may result in an acid pH that favors conversion of ammonia to the poorly absorbed ammonium ion. In addition, lactulose may actually diminish ammonia production through its direct effects on bacterial metabolism. Acutely, lactulose syrup can be administered in a dose of 30 to 50 mL every hour until diarrhea occurs; thereafter the dose is adjusted (usually 15 to 30 mL three times daily) so that the patient has two to four soft stools daily.

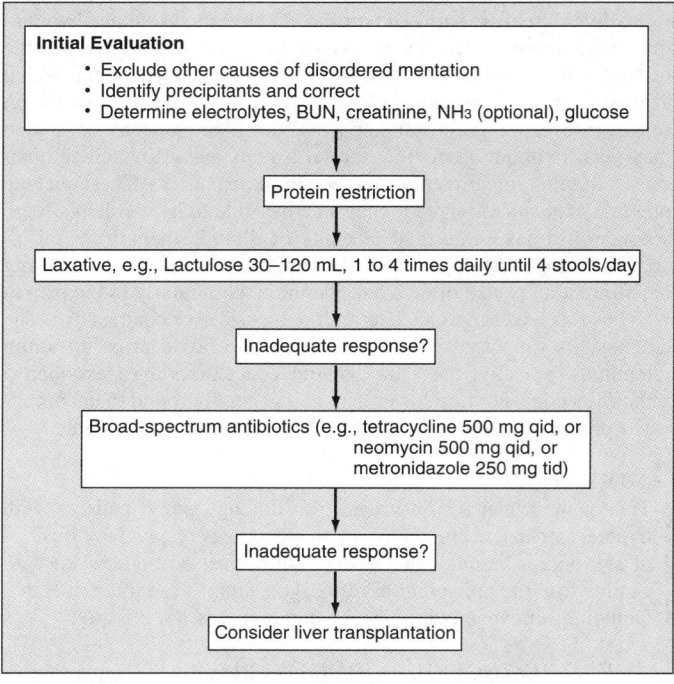

FIGURE 299-4   Approach to the patient with hepatic encephalopathy.

Intestinal ammonia production by bacteria also can be decreased by oral administration of a "nonabsorbable" antibiotic such as neomycin (0.5 to 1.0 g every 6 h). However, despite poor absorption, neomycin may reach sufficient concentrations in the bloodstream to cause real toxicity. Equal benefits may be achieved with broad-spectrum antibiotics such as tetracycline, ampicillin, or metronidazole. The use of agents such as levodopa, bromocriptine, keto analogues of essential amino acids, and intravenous amino acid formulations rich in branched-chain amino acids in the treatment of acute hepatic encephalopathy remains of unproven benefit. Flumazenil, a short-acting benzodiazepine antagonist, may have a role in management of hepatic encephalopathy precipitated by use of benzodiazepines, if there is a need for urgent therapy. Hemoperfusion to remove toxic substances and therapy directed primarily toward coincident cerebral edema in acute encephalopathy are also of unproven value.

Chronic encephalopathy may be effectively controlled by administration of lactulose. Management of patients with chronic encephalopathy should include dietary protein restriction (usually to 60 g/d) in combination with low doses of lactulose or neomycin. Nephrotoxicity or ototoxicity may be limiting in prolonged usage of neomycin. There are suggestions that vegetable protein may be preferable to animal protein.

OTHER SEQUELAE OF CIRRHOSIS Coagulopathy Patients with cirrhosis often demonstrate a variety of abnormalities in both cellular and humoral clotting function. Thrombocytopenia may result from hypersplenism. In the alcoholic patient, there may be direct bone marrow suppression by ethanol. Diminished protein synthesis may lead to reduced production of fibrinogen (factor I), prothrombin (factor II), and factors V, VII, IX, and X. Reduction in levels of all factors except factor V may be worsened by the coincident malabsorption of the fat-soluble cofactor vitamin K due to cholestasis (see Chap. 285). Recent reports have documented the appearance of normal factor VIII levels following liver transplantation in patients with classical hemophilia, probably as a result of production by nonhepatocellular components of the donor organ.

Hepatocellular Carcinoma See Chap. 93.

**HYPOXEMIA AND HEPATOPULMONARY SYNDROME
Definition and Pathogenesis** Mild hypoxemia occurs in approximately one-third of patients with chronic liver disease. The hepatopulmonary syndrome is manifest by dyspnea, platypnea, and orthopnea. Hypoxemia results from right-to-left intrapulmonary shunts through dilatations in intrapulmonary vessels that can be detected by contrast-enhanced echocardiography.

℞ TREATMENT

No specific treatment is consistently effective, though large arteriovenous shunts may be embolized.

BIBLIOGRAPHY

HEPATIC ENCEPHALOPATHY

BASILE AS et al: Elevated brain concentrations of 1,4-benzodiazepines in fulminant hepatic failure. N Engl J Med 325:473, 1991
FRASER CL, ARIEFF AI: Hepatic encephalopathy. N Engl J Med 313:865, 1985
JALAN R et al: Review article: Pathogenesis and treatment of chronic hepatic encephalopathy. Aliment Pharmacol Ther 10:681, 1996
JONES EA et al: The neurobiology of hepatic encephalopathy. Hepatology 4:1235, 1984
MORGAN MY, HAWLEY KE: Lactitol vs. lactulose in the treatment of acute hepatic encephalopathy in cirrhotic patients: A double-blind randomized study. Hepatology 7:1278, 1987
SKOLNICK P: The γ-aminobutyric acid A (GABA_A)-benzodiazepine receptor complex, pp 534–536, in, Jones EA, moderator: The γ-aminobutyric A (GABA_A) receptor complex and hepatic encephalopathy: Some recent advances. Ann Intern Med 110:532, 1989

VARICEAL HEMORRHAGE

LAINE L et al: Endoscopic ligation compared with sclerotherapy for treatment of esophageal variceal bleeding: A meta-analysis. Ann Intern Med 123:280, 1995

———— et al: Endoscopic ligation compared with sclerotherapy for the treatment of bleeding esophageal varices. Ann Intern Med 119:1, 1993
LO G-H et al: A prospective, randomized trial of sclerotherapy versus ligation in the management of bleeding esophageal varices. Hepatology 22:466, 1995
PAGLIARO L et al: Prevention of first bleeding in cirrhosis: A meta-analysis of randomized trials of nonsurgical treatment. Ann Intern Med 117:59, 1992
PLANAS R et al: A prospective randomized trial comparing somatostatin and sclerotherapy in the treatment of acute variceal bleeding. Hepatology 20:370, 1994
STIEGMANN GV et al: Endoscopic sclerotherapy as compared with endoscopic ligation for bleeding esophageal varices. N Engl J Med 326:1527, 1992
SUNG JJY et al: Octreotide infusion or emergency sclerotherapy for variceal haemorrhage. Lancet 342:637, 1993

PORTAL HYPERTENSION AND ASCITES

D'AMICO G et al: The treatment of portal hypertension: A meta-analytic review. Hepatology 22:332, 1995
FLORAS JS et al: Increased sympathetic outflow in cirrhosis and ascites: Direct evidence from intraneural recordings. Ann Intern Med 114:373, 1991
GINÉS P et al: Comparison of paracentesis and diuretics in the treatment of cirrhotics with tense ascites: Results of a randomized study. Gastroenterology 93:234, 1987
———— et al: Paracentesis with intravenous infusion of albumin as compared with peritoneovenous shunting in cirrhosis with refractory ascites. N Engl J Med 325:829, 1991
———— et al: Incidence, predictive factors, and prognosis of the hepatorenal syndrome in cirrhosis with ascites. Gastroenterology 105:229, 1993
JAFFE D et al: Management of portal hypertension and its complications. Med Clin North Am 80:1021, 1996
OCHES A et al: The transjugular intrahepatic portosystemic stent-shunt procedure for refractory ascites. N Engl J Med 332:1192, 1995
PINTO PC et al: Large-volume paracentesis in nonedematous patients with tense ascites: Its effect on intravascular volume. Hepatology 8:207, 1988
PYNARD T et al: Beta-adrenergic-antagonist drugs in the prevention of gastrointestinal bleeding in patients with cirrhosis and esophageal varices. N Engl J Med 324:1532, 1991
RING EJ et al: Using transjugular intrahepatic portosystemic shunts to control variceal bleeding before liver transplantation. Ann Intern Med 116:304, 1992
STANLEY AJ et al: Long-term follow up of transjugular mitrahepatic portosystemic stent shunt (TIPSS) for the treatment of portal hypertension: Results in 130 patients. Gut 39:479, 1996
STIEGMANN GV et al: Endoscopic sclerotherapy as compared with endoscopic ligation for bleeding esophageal varices. N Engl J Med 326:1527, 1992

SPONTANEOUS BACTERIAL PERITONITIS

NAVASA M et al: Randomized, comparative study of oral ofloxacin versus intravenous cefotaxime in spontaneous bacterial peritonitis. Gastroenterology 111:1011, 1996
ROLACHON A et al: Ciprofloxacin and long-term prevention of spontaneous bacterial peritonitis: Results of a prospective controlled trial. Hepatology 22:1171, 1995
RUNYON BA et al: Short-course versus long-course antibiotic treatment of spontaneous bacterial peritonitis: A randomized controlled study of 100 patients. Gastroenterology 100:1737, 1991

300   *Kurt J. Isselbacher, Daniel K. Podolsky*

INFILTRATIVE AND METABOLIC DISEASES AFFECTING THE LIVER

Many disseminated, systemic, or metabolic diseases involve the liver in a diffuse manner by the infiltration of abnormal cells or the accumulation of chemical substances or metabolites. Chemical accumulation may be extracellular or intracellular and may involve hepatocytes, Kupffer cells, or other elements of the reticuloendothelial system. Although infiltrative diseases may vary widely in cause and extrahepatic manifestations, the findings in the liver may be quite similar.

Generalized enlargement and firmness of the liver, gradual and nonspecific deterioration of liver function, and, less often, signs of portal hypertension or ascites are typical features of this group of diseases. Differential diagnosis by clinical means may be difficult on occasion, but in patients in whom ancillary clinical findings do not establish the diagnosis, the diffusely infiltrated liver provides an excellent source of tissue for diagnostic purposes.

HEPATIC STEATOSIS (FATTY LIVER) AND STEATOHEPATITIS (See also Chap. 293)

Slight to moderate enlargement of the liver due to a diffuse accumulation of neutral fat (triglycerides) in hepatocytes is an important clinical and pathologic finding. Imaging techniques such as computed tomography (CT), ultrasound, and magnetic resonance imaging (MRI) may each yield alterations suggesting increased fat in the liver. As discussed in Chap. 293, several mechanisms can contribute to lipid accumulation in the liver. Fatty liver can be separated into two categories based on whether the fat droplets in the hepatocytes are macrovesicular or microvesicular (Table 300-1). In addition, fatty infiltration may be accompanied by necroinflammatory activity, a condition designated *steatohepatitis.*

MACROVESICULAR FATTY LIVER This is the most common type of fatty liver and is seen most frequently in alcoholism or alcoholic liver disease, diabetes mellitus, obesity, and prolonged parenteral nutrition. Hematoxylin and eosin–stained liver sections show hepatocytes with large, empty vacuoles with the nucleus "pushed" to the periphery of the cell. In general, fat in the liver is not damaging per se, and the fat will disappear with improvement or elimination of the predisposing condition.

Etiology The major causes of fatty liver with macrovesicular fat depend on the age, geographic location, and metabolic-nutritional status of the patient population. *Chronic alcoholism* is the most common cause of hepatic steatosis in this country and in other countries with a high alcohol intake. The severity of fatty involvement is roughly proportional to the duration and degree of alcoholic excess. *Protein malnutrition*, especially in infancy and early childhood, accounts for most cases of severe fatty liver in the tropical zones of Africa, South America, and Asia. The hepatic changes may be associated with other clinical and pathologic features of kwashiorkor. Patients with adult-onset *diabetes mellitus*, especially those who are overweight and are poorly controlled, often have fatty livers. *Obesity* is commonly associated with fatty infiltration of the liver; this recedes as weight reduction occurs. *Jejunoileal bypass* for surgical treatment of morbid obesity was sometimes associated with severe fatty liver and hepatic failure that could be fatal. In patients with Cushing's syndrome and in those receiving large doses of glucocorticoids, fatty infiltration of the liver may occur. In many *chronic illnesses*, especially those complicated

Table 300-1

Causes of Hepatic Steatosis

MACROVESICULAR (LARGE FAT DROPLETS IN HEPATOCYTES)

Alcohol, alcoholic liver disease*
Diabetes mellitus*
Obesity*
Protein-calorie malnutrition
Total parenteral nutrition*, jejunoileal bypass
Drugs*, e.g., methotrexate, aspirin, vitamin A, glucocorticoids, amiodarone, and synthetic estrogen

MICROVESICULAR (SMALL FAT DROPLETS IN HEPATOCYTES)

Reye's syndrome
Acute fatty liver of pregnancy
Jamaican vomiting sickness
Drugs, e.g., valproic acid, tetracycline

---

* May also be associated with necroinflmmatory activity

by impaired nutrition or malabsorption, increased fat is found in liver cells. For example, patients with severe ulcerative colitis, chronic pancreatitis, or protracted heart failure frequently have moderate hepatic steatosis at the time of death. Patients maintained on prolonged *total parenteral nutrition* also may develop a fatty liver. In some cases, fatty infiltration and steatohepatitis may occur in the absence of an identifiable cause.

Acute fatty liver is caused by a number of hepatotoxins and is frequently accompanied by signs and symptoms of liver failure. Carbon tetrachloride intoxication, DDT poisoning, and ingestion of substances containing yellow phosphorus result in severe hepatic steatosis. Acute and prolonged alcohol ingestion also may be considered in this category and may be associated with a rapidly enlarging and fat-laden liver.

Clinical Features The signs and symptoms of hepatic steatosis are related to the degree of fat infiltration, the time course of its accumulation, and the underlying cause. The obese or diabetic patient with a chronic fatty liver is usually asymptomatic and has only mild tenderness over the enlarged liver. The liver function tests are normal or show mild elevations of alkaline phosphatase or aminotransferases. In contrast, the rapid accumulation of fat seen in the setting of hyperalimentation may lead to marked tenderness, presumably resulting from stretching of Glisson's capsule. Similarly, alcoholic patients with acute fatty liver following a bout of heavy drinking may have right upper quadrant pain and tenderness often with laboratory evidence of cholestasis. The clinical presentation of fatty liver from hepatotoxins is similar to that of fulminant hepatic failure arising from any cause, with evidence of hepatic encephalopathy, marked elevations of prothrombin time and aminotransferases, and variable degrees of jaundice. Although steatohepatitis is generally thought to have a benign clinical course with improvement following elimination of the associated precipitant, in some individuals it may result in significant fibrosis and even cirrhosis.

Diagnosis The findings of a firm, nontender, and generally enlarged liver with minimal hepatic dysfunction in a patient with chronic alcoholism, malnutrition, poorly controlled diabetes mellitus, or obesity should suggest hepatic steatosis. This can usually be detected by CT, MRI, or ultrasound. Modest elevations of aminotransferases are often found in association with hepatic steatohepatitis. A disproportional elevation in AST leading to an AST/ALT ratio greater than 2 is generally associated with alcoholic hepatitis; ratios below one are usually found in non-alcoholic steatohepatitis. When diagnostic uncertainty exists, needle biopsy of the liver will demonstrate the increased fat content and possibly the underlying primary disorder.

℞ TREATMENT

Adequate nutritional intake, removal of alcohol or offending toxins, and correction of any associated metabolic disorders usually result in recovery. There is no clinical rationale for the use of lipotropic agents such as choline. When indicated, attention should be directed to abstinence from alcohol, careful control of diabetes, weight loss, or correction of intestinal absorptive defects. In the alcoholic fatty liver there is gradual disappearance of fat from the liver after 4 to 8 weeks of adequate diet and abstinence from alcohol. Similarly, fatty infiltration usually resolves within 2 weeks after discontinuation of parenteral hyperalimentation.

MICROVESICULAR FATTY LIVER This is the less common form of fatty liver. On microscopic examination, the fat is present in many small vacuoles. Although the droplets consist of triglycerides in both the macrovesicular and microvesicular forms, the reason for this difference in morphologic appearance is not clear.

Acute fatty liver of pregnancy is a syndrome that occurs late in pregnancy and is often associated with jaundice and hepatic failure. In half the cases it is associated with preeclampsia. If diagnosed in time, the disease usually resolves with termination of the pregnancy.

Microvesicular fat accumulation also may be seen as a toxic reaction to *valproic acid* and with excessive doses of *tetracycline*. It is a typical finding in *Jamaican vomiting sickness*, which is caused by hypoglycin A present in unripened ackee fruit.

REYE'S SYNDROME (FATTY LIVER WITH ENCEPHA-LOPATHY) This acute illness is encountered exclusively in children below 15 years of age. It is characterized clinically by vomiting and signs of progressive central nervous system damage, signs of hepatic injury, and hypoglycemia. Morphologically, there is extensive fatty vacuolization of the liver and renal tubules. There is mitochondrial dysfunction with decreased activity of hepatic mitochondrial enzymes. The cause is unknown, although viral agents and drugs, especially salicylates, have been implicated. Increased aspirin use and much higher serum salicylate levels in children with this illness than in the general population have been described during outbreaks of Reye's syndrome. Recognition of this relationship and reduced aspirin use in this setting may account for the decreasing incidence of Reye's syndrome. However, this illness may occur in the absence of exposure to salicylates. In fatal cases, the liver is enlarged and yellow with striking diffuse fatty microvacuolization of cells. Peripheral zonal hepatic necrosis also has been present in some cases. Fatty changes of the renal tubular cells, cerebral edema, and neuronal degeneration of the brain are the major extrahepatic changes. Electron-microscopic studies show structural alterations of mitochondria in liver, brain, and muscle.

The onset usually follows an upper respiratory tract infection, especially influenza or chickenpox. Within 1 to 3 days, persistent vomiting occurs, together with stupor, which usually progresses rapidly to generalized convulsions and coma. The liver is enlarged, but *jaundice is characteristically absent or minimal.* Elevations in serum aminotransferases and prothrombin time, hypoglycemia, metabolic acidosis, and elevated serum ammonia levels are the major laboratory findings. The mortality rate in Reye's syndrome is approximately 50 percent. Therapy consists of infusions of glucose and fresh frozen plasma, as well as intravenous mannitol to reduce the cerebral edema. Chronic liver disease has not been reported in survivors.

STORAGE DISEASES

Lipid storage diseases include the hereditary disorders of Gaucher's and Niemann-Pick disease. Other rare diseases associated with increased fat in the liver include abetalipoproteinemia, Tangier disease, Fabry's disease, and types I and V hyperlipoproteinemia (see Chap. 341 for details). Hepatic enlargement caused by distention of liver cells with glycogen is present in some poorly controlled diabetics and frequently in juvenile diabetes. More often, however, hepatomegaly is due to fatty infiltration (see above). Ketoacidosis and vigorous insulin therapy may further enhance hepatic enlargement.

HEPATIC MINERAL ACCUMULATION

WILSON'S DISEASE This is a rare disorder, predominantly of young people, in which excess copper accumulates in the liver and other tissues. Deficiency of the plasma copper protein ceruloplasmin is a characteristic feature. The accumulation appears to result from impaired copper excretion due to a mutation in a gene that encodes a P-type ATPase copper transporter. Clinically, patients may present in teenage or early adult years with chronic hepatitis, cirrhosis or their complications. A small number of patients will present with fulminant hepatitis. Liver disease is often accompanied by softening and degeneration of the basal ganglia (hepatolenticular degeneration) due to copper deposition, which results in extrapyramidal neurologic and psychiatric symptoms. Pigmentation of the cornea (Kayser-Fleischer rings) is frequently present. Hemolytic anemia is also common, especially with fulminant disease. Liver biopsy may reveal findings ranging from fulminant hepatitis to macronodular cirrhosis in addition to excess copper levels. Typically, liver cells are ballooned and show increased glycogen with glycogen vacuolization in the nuclei. All patients under age 40 with unexplained chronic hepatitis or cirrhosis should be evaluated for possible Wilson's disease. Prompt diagnosis is important; treatment, which must be continued throughout life, can prevent progression of end-organ damage. → *For further discussion, see Chap. 345.*

HEMOCHROMATOSIS Hemochromatosis may be the most common genetic disorder of humans; it involves accumulation of abnormal amounts of iron due to inappropriate absorption from the intestine. The liver, as a primary site of iron storage, is affected most directly. There is diffuse deposition of excess iron in hepatocytes, in contrast to the characteristic accumulation of iron in the reticuloendothelial compartment typical of secondary iron overload and hemosiderosis. Excess hepatic iron commonly results in hepatomegaly. Although liver function is initially well preserved, if the disease is untreated, progressive impairment is followed by the development of cirrhosis. Prompt diagnosis can permit the institution of effective lifelong therapy to reduce the iron load and halt progression of the disease. → *For further discussion, see Chap. 342.*

OTHER INFILTRATIVE DISEASES

HURLER'S SYNDROME This is an uncommon hereditary disease that is characterized by the widespread tissue deposition of mucopolysaccharide (chondroitin sulfate B and heparan sulfate) in many tissues. The liver is frequently enlarged and firm. Microscopically, Kupffer cells and other macrophages are enlarged and filled with metachromatic granular material. Cirrhosis may be a late complication. → *For further discussion, see Chap. 346.*

α_1**-ANTITRYPSIN DEFICIENCY** Patients with homozygous deficiency of serum α_1-antitrypsin (α_1AT) are prone to develop emphysema in adult life. The disease is suggested by the absence of alpha$_1$ globulin on serum electrophoresis (α_1AT makes up 90 percent of this fraction normally) and confirmed by direct measurement of α_1AT. The exact phenotype can then be determined by starch electrophoresis. Although there are approximately 75 recognized alleles, only PiZ and PiS are associated with clinical disease. The molecular bases of these altered products have been related to single nucleic acid substitutions, e.g., PiZ is caused by a G (guanine) to A (adenine) transposition, which results in a substitution of a glutamic acid for lysine at residue 292 in the α_1AT protein. Hepatocytes of some patients with this deficiency contain globules positive to the periodic acid Schiff reaction. Approximately 10 percent of children with homozygous deficiency (PiZZ phenotype) of α_1AT will develop significant liver disease, including neonatal hepatitis and progressive cirrhosis. It has been suggested that 15 to 20 percent of all chronic liver disease in infancy may be attributed to α_1AT deficiency. In adults, the most common manifestation of α_1AT deficiency is asymptomatic cirrhosis, which may progress from a micronodular to a macronodular state and may be complicated by the development of hepatocellular carcinoma. The occurrence of liver disease in these patients is not dependent on the development of lung disease. → *For further discussion, see Chap. 258).*

RETICULOENDOTHELIAL DISORDERS (See also Chaps. 61 and 113)

Moderate to massive hepatomegaly and splenomegaly occur frequently in the various types of *leukemia* and *lymphoma.* Jaundice, when present, is usually slight and results from hemolysis, although cholestasis may occasionally be associated with lymphoma as a paraneoplastic syndrome. Deep and protracted jaundice is distinctly rare and is caused by obstruction of the intrahepatic or extrahepatic bile ducts by tumor. Liver biopsy specimens reveal portal and sinusoidal infiltrates in most cases of leukemia, but the cellular pattern may be mixed and nonspecific. Liver biopsy is diagnostic in only 5 percent of patients with *Hodgkin's disease.* This percentage is increased in those with advanced disease or splenomegaly. Directed biopsy at laparoscopy or laparotomy is more likely to be positive than "blind" needle biopsy. Nonspecific histologic changes in the liver have been described in patients with lymphoma and may contribute to the abnormal liver function tests.

Myeloid metaplasia and other myeloproliferative disorders associated with extramedullary hematopoiesis produce hepatomegaly which may reach huge proportions, especially following splenectomy. Serum alkaline phosphatase elevations are often found. Ascites and portal hypertension, resulting from diffuse involvement of portal venules and lymphatics, are rare complications.

GRANULOMATOUS INFILTRATIONS

Perhaps as a result of the large population of mononuclear phagocytes, a number of systemic granulomatous diseases involve the liver, including sarcoidosis, miliary tuberculosis, histoplasmosis, brucellosis, schistosomiasis, berylliosis, and drug reactions (Table 300-2). In addition, isolated granulomas of no diagnostic importance may be found occasionally in patients with various forms of cirrhosis and hepatitis. The liver infiltrated by granulomas may be slightly enlarged and firm, but hepatic dysfunction is usually limited. Increases in serum alkaline phosphatase are common and may range from mild to marked. Occasionally mild serum elevations in aminotransferases are also present. In a few patients with sarcoidosis or brucellosis, portal hypertension may develop, and extensive postnecrotic scarring or postnecrotic cirrhosis may follow healing of the granulomatous lesions, as in schistosomiasis.

In AIDS, evidence of liver disease is quite common but is usually mild with minimal morbidity. In these patients, hepatic granulomatous disease is often present and may be caused by opportunistic infections, with *Mycobacterium avium-intracellulare* being the most frequent pathogen. Cytomegalovirus hepatitis and hepatic mycoses are less common. These patients are frequently being treated for *Pneumocystis carinii* infections with sulfonamides, which also may cause hepatic granulomatous disease. AIDS cholangiopathy has become a well recognized entity. It exhibits features similar to those found in primary sclerosing cholangitis and is typically associated with cryptosporidia, microsporidia, and/or cytomegalovirus infection in the biliary tract. Papillary stenosis is frequently present.

Needle biopsy of the liver often provides the first definite evidence of a systemic or disseminated granulomatous disease. In patients with sarcoidosis who have neither clinical nor laboratory evidence of hepatic involvement, needle biopsy is positive in about 80 percent of cases. In cases of suspected miliary tuberculosis, a portion of the biopsy should be cultured and stained for mycobacteria. The organism can be detected in the majority of cases, particularly when caseating granulomas are present. Serial sections of the biopsy specimen should be examined if granulomas are not apparent. Individual granulomas are rarely specific in their microscopic appearance, and final diagnosis usually requires other clinical, laboratory, or histologic data.

In approximately 20 percent of patients it is not possible to identify a cause for the granulomatous infiltration. When these infiltrates are accompanied by fever of unknown origin, the diagnosis of granulomatous hepatitis should be considered. This is an uncommon disorder of unknown cause and is diagnosed by exclusion. While granulomatous hepatitis invariably responds to moderate doses of glucocorticoids, relapses are frequent, and such therapy should never be undertaken unless tuberculous disease or other causes of granulomatous infiltration have been excluded. This may include an initial empiric trial of antituberculous therapy.

AMYLOIDOSIS (See also Chap. 309)

Systemic amyloidosis, whether primary and idiopathic, familial, or secondary to chronic inflammatory or neoplastic diseases, often involves the liver. Grossly, the liver infiltrated with amyloid is enlarged and pale and rubbery in consistency. Microscopically, the birefringent amyloid deposits appear as homogeneous waxy material within the space of Disse, often being concentrated in the periportal areas and associated with atrophy of adjacent liver cell plates. Selective involvement of the walls of blood vessels, especially of the hepatic arterioles, may be a striking feature of primary amyloidosis. With this possible exception, however, the hepatic lesions are the same in all forms of amyloidosis and are present in 60 to 90 percent of cases.

An enlarged and firm liver is found in about 60 percent of patients, and ascites occurs in advanced stages of the disease in about 20 percent. Jaundice, portal hypertension, and other signs of chronic liver disease are usually absent. Liver function changes, although frequent, correlate poorly with the extent of liver infiltration. Hypoalbuminemia and elevated serum alkaline phosphatase are common. Hypoalbuminemia, however, may be related to the presence of nephrosis; the prothrombin time is usually normal. The diagnosis is established by biopsy of rectum, skin, liver, or other involved organs and demonstration of the characteristic Congo red–staining deposits by polarizing microscopy.

BIBLIOGRAPHY

ARIAS IM et al: *The Liver: Biology and Pathobiology*, 3d ed. New York, Raven Press, 1994

CRYSTAL RG: Alpha 1-antitrypsin deficiency, emphysema and liver disease: Genetic basis and strategy for therapy. J Clin Invest 85:1343, 1990

HURWITZ ES et al: Public Health Service Study on Reye's syndrome and medications. N Engl J Med 313:842, 1985

HUTCHISON DC: Natural history of alpha 1-protease inhibitor deficiency. Am J Med 84:3, 1988

LEE WM: Drug-induced hepatotoxicity. N Engl J Med 333:1118, 1995

MINAKAMI H et al: Pre-eclampsia: A microvesicular fat disease of the liver. Am J Obstet Gynecol 159:1043, 1988

PERLMUTTER DH: The cellular basis for liver injury in alpha 1-antitrypsin deficiency. Hepatology 13:172, 1991

RILEY C et al: Acute fatty liver of pregnancy: A reassessment based on observations in nine patients. Ann Intern Med 106:703, 1987

RUSTGI VK: Liver disease in pregnancy. Med Clin North Am 73:1041, 1989

SCHIFF L, SCHIFF ER: *Diseases of the Liver*, 7th ed. Philadelphia, Lippincott, 1993

SCRIVER CR et al (eds): *The Metabolic and Molecular Bases of Inherited Disease*, 7th ed. New York, McGraw-Hill, 1995

SHERLOCK S, DOOLEY J: *Diseases of the Liver and Biliary System*, 9th ed. Oxford, Blackwell, 1993

STERNLIEB I: Perspectives on Wilson's disease. Hepatology 12:1234, 1990

VAN COSTA RN et al: Adult Reye's syndrome: A review with new evidence for a generalized defect in intramitochondrial enzyme processing. Neurology 41:1815, 1991

ZAKIM D, BOYER TD: *Hepatology: A Textbook of Liver Disease*, 3d ed. Philadelphia, Saunders, 1996

Table 300-2

Some Causes of Hepatic Granulomas

SYSTEMIC DISEASE	
Sarcoidosis	Crohn's disease
Hodgkin's and non-Hodgkin's lymphoma	Wegener's granulomatosis
	Granulomatous hepatitis, idiopathic
Primary biliary cirrhosis	
Berylliosis	

INFECTIONS	
Bacterial	Parasitic
Tuberculosis	Schistosomiasis
Mycobacterium avium intracellulare	Rickettsial
	Q fever
Brucellosis	Spirochetes
Leprosy	Syphilis
Viral	Drugs
Epstein-Barr virus	Sulfonamides
Cytomegalovirus	Isoniazid
Chicken pox	Allopurinol

LIVER TRANSPLANTATION

Liver transplantation, the replacement of the native, diseased liver by a normal organ (allograft) recovered from a brain-dead donor, has matured from an experimental procedure reserved for desperately ill patients to an accepted, lifesaving operation applied much earlier in the natural history of end-stage liver disease. The preferred and technically most advanced approach is *orthotopic transplantation*, in which the native organ is removed and the donor organ is inserted in the same anatomic location. Pioneered in the 1960s by Starzl at the University of Colorado and, later, at the University of Pittsburgh and by Calne in Cambridge, England, liver transplantation is now performed routinely by dozens of centers throughout North America and western Europe. Success and survival have improved from approximately 30 percent in the 1970s to >80 percent today. These improved prospects for prolonged survival, dating back to the early 1980s, resulted from refinements in operative technique (including the introduction of venovenous bypass to allow venous return from the extremities and visceral circulation during clamping of the inferior vena cava), improvements in organ procurement and preservation, advances in immunosuppressive therapy, and, perhaps most influentially, more enlightened patient selection and timing. Despite the perioperative morbidity and mortality, the technical and management challenges of the procedure, and its costs, liver transplantation has become the approach of choice for selected patients whose chronic or acute liver disease is progressive, life-threatening, and unresponsive to medical therapy. Based on the current level of success, the number of liver transplants has continued to grow each year; in 1995, 3700 patients received liver allografts in the United States. Still, the demand for new livers continues to outpace availability; in 1995, as many as 6000 patients in the United States were on a waiting list for a donor liver.

INDICATIONS Potential candidates for liver transplantation are children and adults who, in the absence of contraindications (see below), suffer from severe, irreversible liver disease for which alternative medical or surgical treatments have been exhausted or are unavailable. *Timing of the operation is of critical importance.* Indeed, improved timing and better patient selection are felt to have contributed more to the increased success of liver transplantation in the 1980s and beyond than all the impressive technical and immunologic advances combined. Although the disease should be advanced, and although opportunities for spontaneous or medically induced stabilization or recovery should be allowed, the procedure should be done sufficiently early to give the surgical procedure a fair chance for success. Ideally, transplantation should be considered in patients with end-stage liver disease who are experiencing or have experienced a life-threatening complication of hepatic decompensation, whose quality of life has deteriorated to unacceptable levels, or whose liver disease will result predictably in irreversible damage to the central nervous system (CNS). If this is done sufficiently early, the patient will not have developed any contraindications or extrahepatic systemic deterioration. Although patients with well-compensated cirrhosis can survive for many years, many patients with quasi-stable chronic liver disease have much more advanced disease than may be apparent. As discussed below, the better the status of the patient prior to transplantation, the higher will be the anticipated success rate of transplantation. The decision about *when* to transplant is complex and requires the combined judgment of an experienced team of hepatologists, transplant surgeons, anesthesiologists, and specialists in support services, not to mention the well-informed consent of the patient and the patient's family.

Transplantation in Children Indications for transplantation in children are listed in Table 301-1. The most common is *biliary atresia*. *Inherited or genetic disorders of metabolism* associated with liver failure constitute another major indication for transplantation in children and adolescents. In Crigler-Najjar disease type I and in certain hereditary disorders of the urea cycle and of amino acid or lactate-pyruvate metabolism, transplantation may be the only way to prevent

impending deterioration of CNS function, despite the fact that the native liver is structurally normal. Combined heart and liver transplantation has yielded dramatic improvement in cardiac function and in cholesterol levels in children with homozygous familial hypercholesterolemia; combined liver and kidney transplantation has been successful in patients with hereditary oxalosis. In hemophiliacs with transfusion-associated hepatitis and liver failure, liver transplantation has been associated with recovery of normal factor VIII synthesis.

Transplantation in Adults Liver transplantation is indicated for end-stage *cirrhosis* of all causes (see Table 301-1). In sclerosing cholangitis and *Caroli's disease* (multiple cystic dilatations of the intrahepatic biliary tree), recurrent infections and sepsis associated with inflammatory and fibrotic obstruction of the biliary tree may be an indication for transplantation. Because prior biliary surgery complicates, and is a relative contraindication for, liver transplantation, surgical diversion of the biliary tree has been all but abandoned for patients with sclerosing cholangitis. In patients who undergo transplantation for *hepatic vein thrombosis (Budd-Chiari syndrome)*, postoperative anticoagulation is essential; underlying myeloproliferative disorders may have to be treated but are not a contraindication to liver transplantation. If a donor organ can be located quickly, before life-threatening complications—including cerebral edema—set in, patients with *fulminant hepatitis* are candidates for liver transplantation. More controversial as candidates for liver transplantation are patients with *alcoholic cirrhosis*, *chronic viral hepatitis*, and *primary hepatocellular malignancies*. Although all three of these categories are considered to be high risk, liver transplantation can be offered to carefully selected patients. Patients with alcoholic cirrhosis can be considered as candidates for transplantation if they meet strict criteria for abstinence and reform. Patients with chronic hepatitis C have done as well as any other subset of patients after transplantation, despite the fact that recurrent infection in the donor organ is the rule. In patients with chronic hepatitis B, in the absence of measures to prevent recurrent hepatitis B, survival after transplantation is reduced by approximately 10 to 20 percent; however, prophylactic use of hepatitis B immune globulin (HBIG) during and after transplantation increases the success of transplantation compared to that seen in patients with nonviral causes of liver decompensation. Issues of disease recurrence are discussed in more detail below. Patients with nonmetastatic primary hepatobiliary tumors—primary hepatocellular carcinoma, cholangiocarcinoma, hepatoblastoma, angiosarcoma, epithelioid hemangioendothelioma, and multiple or massive hepatic adenomata—have undergone liver transplantation; however, for hepatobiliary malignancies,

Table 301-1

Indications for Liver Transplantation

Children	Adults
Biliary atresia	Primary biliary cirrhosis
Neonatal hepatitis	Secondary biliary cirrhosis
Congenital hepatic fibrosis	Primary sclerosing cholangitis
Alagille's disease*	Caroli's disease‡
Byler's disease†	Cryptogenic cirrhosis
α₁-Antitrypsin deficiency	Chronic hepatitis with cirrhosis
Inherited disorders of metabolism	Hepatic vein thrombosis
Wilson's disease	Fulminant hepatitis
Tyrosinemia	Alcoholic cirrhosis
Glycogen storage diseases	Chronic viral hepatitis
Lysosomal storage diseases	Primary hepatocellular malignancies
Protoporphyria	Hepatic adenomas
Crigler-Najjar disease type I	
Familial hypercholesterolemia	
Hereditary oxalosis	
Hemophilia	

* Arteriohepatic dysplasia, with paucity of bile ducts, and congenital malformations, including pulmonary stenosis.
† Intrahepatic cholestasis, progressive liver failure, mental and growth retardation.
‡ Multiple cystic dilatations of the intrahepatic biliary tree.

overall survival is significantly lower than that for other categories of liver disease. To minimize the very high likelihood of recurrent tumor after transplantation, some centers are evaluating experimental adjuvant chemotherapy protocols. Some transplantation centers have reported excellent long-term, recurrence-free survival in patients with unresectable hepatocellular carcinoma for single tumors <5 cm in diameter or for three or fewer lesions all <3 cm. Because the likelihood of recurrent cholangiocarcinoma is almost universal, this tumor is no longer considered an indication for transplantation.

CONTRAINDICATIONS *Absolute contraindications* for transplantation include life-threatening systemic diseases, uncontrolled extrahepatic bacterial or fungal infections, preexisting advanced cardiovascular or pulmonary disease, multiple uncorrectable life-threatening congenital anomalies, metastatic malignancy, active drug or alcohol abuse, and human immunodeficiency virus (HIV) infection. Because carefully selected patients in their sixties and even seventies have undergone transplantation successfully, advanced age per se is no longer considered an absolute contraindication; however, in older patients, a more thorough preoperative evaluation should be undertaken to exclude ischemic cardiac disease. Advanced age (>60 years), however, may be considered a *relative contraindication*, that is, a factor to be taken into account with other relative contraindications. Other relative contraindications include highly replicative hepatitis B, portal vein thrombosis, preexisting renal disease not associated with liver disease, intrahepatic or biliary sepsis, severe hypoxemia resulting from right-to-left intrapulmonary shunts, previous extensive hepatobiliary surgery, and any uncontrolled serious psychiatric disorder. Any one of these relative contraindications is insufficient in and of itself to preclude transplantation. For example, the problem of portal vein thrombosis can be overcome by constructing a graft from the donor liver portal vein to the recipient's superior mesenteric vein.

TECHNICAL CONSIDERATIONS **Donor Selection** Donor livers for transplantation are procured primarily from victims of head trauma. Organs from brain-dead donors up to age 60 are acceptable if the following criteria are met: hemodynamic stability, adequate oxygenation, absence of bacterial or fungal infection, serologic exclusion of hepatitis B and C viruses and HIV, absence of abdominal trauma, and absence of hepatic dysfunction. Cardiovascular and respiratory functions are maintained artificially until the liver can be removed. Compatibility in ABO blood group and organ size between donor and recipient are important considerations in donor selection; however, ABO-incompatible or reduced-donor-organ transplants can be performed in emergency or marked donor-scarcity situations. Tissue typing for HLA matching is not required, and preformed cytotoxic HLA antibodies do not preclude liver transplantation. Following perfusion with cold electrolyte solution, the donor liver is removed and packed in ice. The use of University of Wisconsin (UW) solution, rich in lactobionate and raffinose, has permitted the extension of cold ischemic time up to 20 h; however, 12 h may be a more reasonable limit. Improved techniques for harvesting multiple organs from the same donor have increased the availability of donor livers, but the availability of donor livers is far outstripped by the demand. Currently, in the United States, all donor livers are distributed through a nationwide organ-sharing network (United Network of Organ Sharing) designed to allocate available organs based on regional considerations and recipient acuity. Recipients who require the highest level of care (intensive care) have the highest priority.

Surgical Technique Removal of the recipient's native liver is technically difficult, particularly in the presence of portal hypertension with its associated collateral circulation and extensive varices, and even more so in the presence of scarring from previous abdominal operations. The combination of portal hypertension and coagulopathy (elevated prothrombin time and thrombocytopenia) translates into large blood product transfusion requirements. After the portal vein and infrahepatic and suprahepatic inferior vena cavae are dissected, a pump-driven venovenous bypass system is applied to reroute blood

from the portal vein and inferior vena cava, preventing congestion of visceral organs. After the hepatic artery and common bile duct are dissected, the native liver is removed and the donor organ inserted. During the anhepatic phase, coagulopathy, hypoglycemia, hypocalcemia, and hypothermia are encountered and must be managed by the anesthesiology team. Caval, portal vein, hepatic artery, and bile duct anastomoses are performed in succession, the last by end-to-end suturing of the donor and recipient common bile ducts or by choledochojejunostomy to a Roux en Y loop if the recipient common bile duct cannot be used for reconstruction (e.g., in sclerosing cholangitis). A typical transplant operation lasts 8 h, with a range of 6 to 18 h. Because of excessive bleeding, large volumes of blood, blood products, and volume expanders may be required during surgery.

POSTOPERATIVE COURSE AND MANAGEMENT **Immunosuppressive Therapy** The introduction in 1980 of cyclosporine as an immunosuppressive agent contributed substantially to the improvement in survival after liver transplantation. Cyclosporine inhibits early activation of T cells and is specific for T cell functions that result from the interaction of the T cell with its receptor and that involve the calcium-dependent signal transduction pathway; as a result, the activity of cyclosporine leads to inhibition of lymphokine gene activation, blocking interleukins 2, 3, and 4, tumor necrosis factor α, as well as other lymphokines. Cyclosporine also inhibits B cell functions. This process occurs without affecting rapidly dividing cells in the bone marrow, which may account for the reduced frequency of posttransplantation systemic infections. The most common and important side effect of cyclosporine therapy is nephrotoxicity. Cyclosporine causes dose-dependent renal tubular injury and direct renal artery vasospasm. Following renal function, therefore, is important in monitoring cyclosporine therapy, perhaps even a more reliable indicator than blood levels of the drug. Nephrotoxicity is reversible and can be managed by dose reduction. Other adverse effects of cyclosporine therapy include hypertension, hyperkalemia, tremor, hirsutism, glucose intolerance, and gum hyperplasia.

Tacrolimus (originally labeled FK 506) is a macrolide lactone antibiotic isolated from a Japanese soil fungus, *Streptomyces tsukubaensis*. It has the same mechanism of action as cyclosporine but is 10 to 100 times more potent. Initially applied as "rescue" therapy for patients in whom rejection occurred despite the use of cyclosporine, tacrolimus has been shown in two large, multicenter, randomized trials to be associated with a reduced frequency of acute rejection, refractory rejection, and chronic rejection. Although patient and graft survival are the same with these two drugs, the advantage of tacrolimus in minimizing episodes of rejection, reducing the need for additional glucocorticoid doses, and reducing the likelihood of bacterial and cytomegalovirus infection has simplified the management of patients undergoing liver transplantation. In addition, the oral absorption of tacrolimus is more predictable than that of cyclosporine, especially during the early postoperative period when T-tube drainage interferes with the enterohepatic circulation of cyclosporine. As a result, in most transplantation centers, tacrolimus has now supplanted cyclosporine for primary immunosuppression, and many centers rely on oral, rather than intravenous, administration from the outset. For transplantation centers that prefer cyclosporine, a new, better-absorbed, microemulsion preparation is now available.

Although tacrolimus is more potent than cyclosporine, it is also more toxic and more likely to be discontinued for adverse events. The toxicity of tacrolimus is similar to that of cyclosporine; nephrotoxicity and neurotoxicity are the most commonly encountered adverse effects, and neurotoxicity (tremor, seizures, hallucinations, psychoses, coma) is more likely and more severe in tacrolimus-treated patients. Both drugs can cause diabetes mellitus, but tacrolimus does not cause hirsutism or gingival hyperplasia. Because of overlapping toxicity between cyclosporine and tacrolimus, especially nephrotoxicity, and because tacrolimus reduces cyclosporine clearance, these two drugs should not be used together. Because 99 percent of tacrolimus is metabolized by the liver, hepatic dysfunction reduces its clearance; in primary graft nonfunction (when, for technical reasons or because of ischemic damage prior to its insertion, the allograft is defective and does not function normally from the outset) tacrolimus doses have to be reduced substantially, especially in children. Both cyclosporine and tacrolimus are metabolized by the cytochrome P450 IIIA system, and so drugs that induce cytochrome P450 (e.g., phenytoin, phenobarbital, carbamazepine, rifampin) reduce available levels of cyclosporine and tacrolimus; drugs that inhibit cytochrome P450 (e.g., erythromycin, fluconazole, ketoconazole, clotrimazole, itraconazole, verapamil, diltiazem, nicardipine, cimetidine, danazol, metoclopramide, bromocriptine) increase cyclosporine and tacrolimus blood levels. Like azathioprine, cyclosporine and tacrolimus appear to be associated with a risk of lymphoproliferative malignancies (see below), which may occur earlier after cyclosporine or tacrolimus than after azathioprine therapy. Because of these side effects, combinations of cyclosporine or tacrolimus with prednisone and azathioprine—all at reduced doses—are preferable regimens for immunosuppressive therapy.

In patients with pretransplant renal dysfunction or renal deterioration that occurs intraoperatively or immediately postoperatively, tacrolimus or cyclosporine therapy may not be practical; under these circumstances, induction or maintenance of immunosuppression with monoclonal antibodies to T cells, OKT3, may be appropriate. Therapy with OKT3 has been especially effective in reversing acute rejection in the posttransplant period and is the standard treatment for acute rejection that fails to respond to methylprednisolone boluses. Intravenous infusions of OKT3 may be complicated by transient fever, chills, and diarrhea. When this drug is used to induce immunosuppression initially or to provide "rescue" in those who reject despite "conventional" therapy, the incidence of bacterial, fungal, and especially cytomegalovirus infections is increased during and after such therapy. In some centers, ganciclovir antiviral therapy is initiated prophylactically as a routine along with OKT3. Another immunosuppressive drug that is likely to be used in the future for patients undergoing liver transplantation is mycophenolic acid, a nonnucleoside purine metabolism inhibitor derived as a fermentation product from several *Penicillium* species. Mycophenolate has been shown to be better than azathioprine, when used with other standard immunosuppressive drugs, in preventing rejection after renal transplantation and has been approved for use in renal transplantation. Rapamycin, an inhibitor of later events in T cell activation, is yet another drug undergoing experimental evaluation as an immunosuppressive agent.

The most important principle of immunosuppression is that the ideal approach strikes a balance between immunosuppression and immunologic competence. Given sufficient immunosuppression, acute liver allograft rejection is always reversible; however, if the cumulative dose of immunosuppressive therapy is too large, the patient will succumb to opportunistic infection. Therefore, immunosuppressive drugs must be used judiciously, with strict attention to the infectious consequences of such therapy.

Postoperative Complications Complications of liver transplantation can be divided into hepatic and nonhepatic categories. In addition, both immediately postoperative and late complications are encountered. Patients who undergo liver transplantation as a rule have been chronically ill for protracted periods and may be malnourished and wasted. The impact of such chronic illness and the multisystem failure that accompanies liver failure continues to require attention in the postoperative period. Because of the massive fluid losses and fluid shifts that occur during the operation, patients may remain fluid overloaded during the immediate postoperative period, straining cardiovascular reserve; this effect can be amplified in the face of transient renal dysfunction and pulmonary capillary vascular permeability. Continuous monitoring of cardiovascular and pulmonary function, measures to maintain the integrity of the intravascular compartment and to treat extravascular volume overload, and scrupulous attention to potential sources of and sites of infection are of paramount importance. Cardiovascular instability may result as well from the electrolyte imbalance that may accompany reperfusion of the donor liver. Pulmonary function may be compromised further by paralysis of the right hemidiaphragm associated with phrenic nerve injury. The hyperdynamic state with increased cardiac output that is characteristic of patients with liver failure reverses rapidly after successful liver transplantation.

Other immediate management issues include renal dysfunction; prerenal azotemia, acute kidney injury associated with hypoperfusion (acute tubular necrosis), and renal toxicity caused by antibiotics, tacrolimus, or cyclosporine are frequently encountered in the postoperative period, sometimes necessitating dialysis. Occasionally, postoperative intraperitoneal bleeding may be sufficient to increase intraabdominal pressure, which, in turn, may reduce renal blood flow—this effect is rapidly reversible when abdominal distention is relieved by exploratory laparotomy to identify and ligate the bleeding site and to remove intraperitoneal clot. Anemia also may result from acute upper gastrointestinal bleeding or from transient hemolytic anemia, which may be autoimmune, especially when blood group O livers are transplanted into blood group A or B recipients. This autoimmune hemolytic anemia is mediated by donor intrahepatic lymphocytes that recognize red blood cell A or B antigens on recipient erythrocytes. Transient in nature, this process resolves once the donor liver is repopulated by recipient bone marrow–derived lymphocytes; the hemolysis can be treated by transfusing blood group O red blood cells and/or by administering higher doses of glucocorticoids. Transient thrombocytopenia is encountered commonly as well. Aplastic anemia, a late occurrence, is rare but has been reported in almost 30 percent of patients who underwent liver transplantation for acute, severe hepatitis of unknown cause.

Bacterial, fungal, or viral infections are common and may be life-threatening postoperatively. Early after transplant surgery, common postoperative infections predominate—pneumonia, wound infections, infected intraabdominal collections, urinary tract infections, and intravenous line infections—rather than opportunistic infections; these infections may involve the biliary tree and liver as well. Beyond the first postoperative month, the toll of immunosuppression becomes evident, and opportunistic infections—cytomegalovirus, herpes viruses, fungal infections (*Aspergillus*, *Candida*, cryptococcal disease), mycobacterial infections, parasitic infections (*Pneumocystis*, *Toxoplasma*), bacterial infections (*Nocardia*, *Legionella*, and *Listeria*)—predominate. Rarely, early infections represent those transmitted with the donor liver, either infections present in the donor or infections acquired during procurement processing. De novo viral hepatitis infections acquired from the donor organ or from transfused blood products occur after typical incubation periods for these agents (well beyond the first month). Obviously, infections in an immunosuppressed host demand early recognition and prompt management; prophylactic antibiotic therapy is administered routinely in the immediate postoperative period. Use of sulfamethoxazole with trimethoprim reduces the incidence of postoperative *Pneumocystis carinii* pneumonia.

Neuropsychiatric complications include seizures (commonly associated with cyclosporine and tacrolimus toxicity), encephalopathy, depression, and difficult psychosocial adjustment. Rarely, diseases are transmitted by the allograft from the donor to the recipient. In addition to viral and bacterial infections, malignancies of donor origin have occurred. Lymphoproliferative malignancies, especially B cell lymphoma, are a recognized complication associated with immunosuppressive drugs such as azathioprine, tacrolimus, and cyclosporine (see above). Epstein-Barr virus has been shown to play a contributory role in some of these tumors, which may regress when immunosuppressive therapy is reduced.

Hepatic Complications Hepatic dysfunction after liver transplantation is similar to the hepatic complications encountered after major abdominal and cardiothoracic surgery; however, in addition, there may be complications such as primary graft failure, vascular compromise, failure or obstruction of the biliary anastomoses, and rejection. As in nontransplant surgery, postoperative jaundice may result from prehepatic, intrahepatic, and posthepatic sources. *Prehepatic* sources represent the massive hemoglobin pigment load from transfusions, hemolysis, hematomas, ecchymoses, and other collections of blood. *Early intrahepatic* liver injury includes effects of hepatotoxic drugs and anesthesia; hypoperfusion injury associated with hypotension, sepsis, and shock; and benign postoperative cholestasis. *Late intrahepatic* sources of liver injury include posttransfusion hepatitis and recurrent primary disease (see below). *Posthepatic* sources of hepatic dysfunction include biliary obstruction and reduced renal clearance of conjugated bilirubin. Hepatic complications unique to liver transplantation include primary graft failure associated with ischemic injury to the organ during harvesting; vascular compromise associated with thrombosis or stenosis of the portal vein or hepatic artery anastomoses; stenosis, obstruction, or leakage of the anastomosed common bile duct; and rejection.

Transplant Rejection Despite the use of immunosuppressive drugs, rejection of the transplanted liver still occurs in a majority of patients, beginning 1 to 2 weeks after surgery. Clinical signs suggesting rejection are fever, right upper quadrant pain, and reduced bile pigment and volume. Leukocytosis may occur, but the most reliable indicators are increases in serum bilirubin and aminotransferase levels. Because these tests lack specificity, distinguishing among rejection and biliary obstruction, primary graft nonfunction, vascular compromise, viral hepatitis, cytomegalovirus infection, drug hepatotoxicity, and recurrent primary disease may be difficult. Radiographic visualization of the biliary tree and/or percutaneous liver biopsy often help to establish the correct diagnosis. Morphologic features of acute rejection include portal infiltration, bile duct injury, and/or endothelial inflammation ("endothelialitis"); some of these findings are reminiscent of graft-versus-host disease and primary biliary cirrhosis. As soon as transplant rejection is suspected, treatment consists of intravenous methylprednisolone in repeated boluses; if this fails to abort rejection, many centers use antibodies to lymphocytes, such as OKT3, or polyclonal antilymphocyte globulin.

Chronic rejection is a relatively rare outcome that may follow repeated bouts of acute rejection or that occurs unrelated to preceding rejection episodes. Morphologically, chronic rejection is characterized by progressive cholestasis, focal parenchymal necrosis, mononuclear infiltration, vascular lesions (intimal fibrosis, subintimal foam cells, fibrinoid necrosis), and fibrosis. This process may be reflected as ductopenia—the vanishing bile duct syndrome. Some of the histologic hallmarks of chronic rejection may be so similar to those of chronic viral hepatitis that differentiation between the two may be difficult. Reversibility of chronic rejection is limited; in patients with therapy-resistant chronic rejection, retransplantation has yielded encouraging results.

OUTCOME **Survival** The survival rate for patients undergoing liver transplantation has improved steadily since 1983. One-year survival rates have increased from approximately 70 percent in the early 1980s to 80 to 90 percent in the mid-1990s. Currently, the 5-year survival rate approaches 60 percent. An important observation is the relation between clinical status before transplantation and outcome. For patients who undergo liver transplantation when their level of compensation is high (e.g., still working or only partially disabled), a 1-year survival rate of 85 percent is common. For those whose level of decompensation mandates continuous in-hospital care prior to transplantation, the 1-year survival rate is about 70 percent, while for those who are so decompensated that they require life support in an intensive care unit, the 1-year survival rate is approximately 50 percent. Indeed, the trend toward transplantation earlier in the natural history of end-stage liver disease is a major factor in the increased success of liver transplantation during the 1980s and 1990s. Another important distinction in survival has been drawn between high-risk and low-risk patient categories. For patients who do not fit any "high-risk" designations, 1-year and 5-year survival rates of 85 and 80 percent, respectively, have been recorded. In contrast, among patients in high-risk categories—cancer, fulminant hepatitis, hepatitis B, age >65, concurrent renal failure, respirator dependence, portal vein thrombosis, and history of a portacaval shunt or multiple right upper quadrant operations—survival statistics fall into the range of 60 percent at 1 year and 35 percent at 5 years. Survival after retransplantation for primary graft nonfunction is approximately 50 percent. Causes of failure of liver transplantation vary with time. Failures within the first 3 months result primarily from technical complications, postoperative infections, and hemorrhage. Transplant failures after the first 3 months are more likely to result from infection, rejection, or recurrent disease (such as malignancy or viral hepatitis).

Recurrence of Primary Disease The recurrence of autoimmune hepatitis or primary sclerosing cholangitis has not been reported. There have been reports of recurrent primary biliary cirrhosis after liver transplantation; however, the histologic features of primary biliary cirrhosis and acute rejection are virtually indistinguishable and occur as frequently in patients with primary biliary cirrhosis as in patients undergoing transplantation for other reasons. Hereditary disorders such as Wilson's disease and α_1-antitrypsin deficiency have not recurred after liver transplantation; however, recurrence of disordered iron metabolism has been observed in some patients with hemochromatosis. Hepatic vein thrombosis (Budd-Chiari syndrome) may recur; this can be minimized by treating underlying lymphoproliferative disorders and by anticoagulation. Cholangiocarcinoma recurs almost invariably; therefore, few centers now transplant such patients. In patients with hepatocellular carcinoma, tumor recurrence in the liver is common after approximately 1 year, although better success has been reported in patients with an unresectable isolated lesion <5 cm or with three or fewer lesions all <3 cm. Trials are underway to assess the benefit of adjuvant chemotherapy.

Hepatitis A can recur after transplantation for fulminant hepatitis A, but such acute reinfection has no serious clinical sequelae. In fulminant hepatitis B, recurrence is not the rule; however, in the absence of any prophylactic measures, hepatitis B usually recurs after transplantation for end-stage chronic hepatitis B. With sufficient immunosuppressive therapy to prevent allograft rejection, levels of hepatitis B viremia increase markedly, regardless of pretransplantation values. A majority of patients undergoing transplantation for chronic hepatitis B become carriers of hepatitis B virus (HBV) with high levels of virus replication but without liver injury; however, some patients experience a rapid recapitulation of severe injury—severe chronic hepatitis or even fulminant hepatitis—after transplantation. *Fibrosing cholestatic hepatitis* is a histologic feature linked to rapidly progressive liver injury in approximately 10 percent of patients who undergo liver transplantation for hepatitis B. These patients experience marked hyperbilirubinemia, substantial prolongation of the prothrombin time (both out of proportion to relatively modest elevations of aminotransferase activity), and rapidly progressive liver failure. This lesion has been suggested to represent a "choking off" of the hepatocyte by an overwhelming density of HBV proteins. Complications such as sepsis and pancreatitis also have been observed more frequently in patients undergoing liver transplantation for hepatitis B. Although the risk of recurrent hepatitis B is approximately 20 percent higher in patients with pretransplantation markers of HBV replication (hepatitis B e antigen and HBV DNA), recurrent hepatitis B occurs in at least 60 percent of patients whose replicative markers were undetectable prior to transplantation, probably because of the enhancing impact of immunosuppressive drugs on HBV replication. Most transplantation centers will not undertake liver transplantation in patients with hepatitis B unless immunoprophylaxis with HBIG is used. Neither preoperative hepatitis B vaccination, preoperative or postoperative interferon therapy, nor short-term (≤2 months) HBIG prophylaxis has been shown to be effective, but a retrospective analysis of data from several hundred patients followed for 3 years after transplantation has shown that long-term (≥6 months) prophylaxis with HBIG is associated with a lowering of the risk of HBV reinfection from approximately 75 percent to 35 percent and a reduction in mortality from approximately 50 percent to 20 percent. Passive immunoprophylaxis with HBIG is begun during the anhepatic stage of surgery, repeated daily for the first 6 postoperative days, then continued with infusions that are given either at regular intervals of 4 to 6 weeks or, alternatively, when anti-HBs levels fall below a threshold of 100 mIU/mL. In all likelihood, indefinite HBIG infusions will be required, and, occasionally "breakthrough" HBV infection occurs. This approach is very expensive, approximately $20,000 per year, and involves the intravenous administration of a globulin preparation designed for intramuscular injection. Although this approach is now practiced universally, it has not been approved officially by the U.S. Food and Drug Administration; clinical trials of HBIG preparations produced specifically for intravenous administration are in progress.

An alternative, promising but still experimental approach to the prophylaxis of patients with chronic hepatitis B undergoing liver transplantation is the use of nucleoside analogues such as famciclovir and lamivudine (see Ch. 297). Limited evidence available to date suggests that they have the potential to prevent recurrence of HBV infection when administered *prior* to transplantation, to treat hepatitis B that recurs *after* transplantation, including in patients who break through HBIG prophylaxis, and to reverse the course of otherwise fatal fibrosing cholestatic hepatitis. Clinical trials are underway to define the role of these antiviral agents in the management of patients undergoing liver transplantation for chronic hepatitis B.

Patients who undergo liver transplantation for chronic hepatitis B plus D have a better survival rate than patients undergoing transplantation for hepatitis B alone. Recurrence of hepatitis C virus (HCV) after liver transplantation can be documented in almost every patient, if sufficiently sensitive virus markers are used. Although acute and chronic liver injury occur after transplantation in patients with chronic hepatitis C, and although histologic analyses reveal moderate to severe HCV-associated hepatic injury in approximately half of all patients, HCV-induced liver injury is mild or absent in the other half of patients, and clinical consequences of recurrent hepatitis C are limited during the first 5 years after transplantation. About 5 to 10 percent of patients have sufficiently severe recurrent hepatitis C to merit antiviral therapy with interferon (which can *suppress* HCV-associated liver injury in approximately half of patients but rarely leads to *sustained* benefit), a small number succumb to HCV-associated liver injury, and a syndrome reminiscent of fibrosing cholestatic hepatitis (see above) has been observed rarely. Because patients with more episodes of rejection receive more immunosuppressive therapy, and because immunosuppressive therapy enhances HCV replication, patients with severe or multiple episodes of rejection are more likely to experience early recurrence of hepatitis C after transplantation. In addition, patients with HCV genotype 1b are more likely to have recurrent HCV-induced liver disease and to experience disease recurrence earlier after transplantation than patients with other genotypes. On the other hand, in the vast majority of patients, the impact of recurrent hepatitis C on graft and patient survival appears to be negligible, at least for the first 5 years after transplantation.

Patients who undergo liver transplantation for end-stage alcoholic cirrhosis are at risk of resorting to drinking again after transplantation, a potential source of recurrent alcoholic liver injury. Currently, alcoholic liver disease is one of the most common indications for liver transplantation, and most transplantation centers screen candidates carefully for predictors of continued abstinence. Recidivism is more likely in patients whose sobriety prior to transplantation was shorter than 6 months.

Posttransplantation Quality of Life   Full rehabilitation is achieved in the majority of patients who survive the early postoperative months and escape chronic rejection or unmanageable infection. Psychosocial maladjustment interferes with medical compliance in a small number of patients, but most manage to adhere to immunosuppressive regimens, which must be continued indefinitely. In one study, 85 percent of patients who survived their transplants returned to gainful activities. In fact, some women have conceived and carried pregnancies to term after transplantation without demonstrable injury to their infants.

BIBLIOGRAPHY

BISMUTH H (ed): Consensus conference on indications of liver transplantation. Hepatology 20(Suppl):1, 1994

DAVIES SE et al: Hepatic histological findings after transplantation for chronic hepatitis B virus infection, including a unique pattern of fibrosing cholestatic hepatitis. Hepatology 13:150, 1991

EUROPEAN FK506 MULTICENTRE LIVER STUDY GROUP: Randomised trial comparing tacrolimus (FK506) and cyclosporin in prevention of liver allograft rejection. Lancet 344:423, 1994

FÉRAY C et al: Reinfection of liver graft by hepatitis C virus after liver transplantation. J Clin Invest 89:1361, 1992

————: Influence of the genotype of hepatitis C virus on the severity of recurrent liver disease after liver transplantation. Gastroenterology 108:1088, 1995

GANE EJ et al: Long-term outcome of hepatitis C infection after liver transplantation. N Engl J Med 334:815, 1996

KEEFE EB, ESQUIVEL CO: Liver transplantation. Current Opinion in Gastroenterology 12:290, 1996

LAU JYN et al: High-level expression of hepatitis B viral antigens in fibrosing cholestatic hepatitis. Gastroenterology 102:956, 1992

LUCEY MR et al: Selection for and outcome of liver transplantation in alcoholic liver disease. Gastroenterology 102:1736, 1992

MAZZAFERRO V et al: Liver transplantation for the treatment of small hepatocellular carcinoma in patients with cirrhosis. N Engl J Med 334:693, 1996

OSORIO RW et al: Predicting recidivism after orthotopic liver transplantation for alcoholic liver disease. Hepatology 20:105, 1994

SAMUEL D et al: Liver transplantation in European patients with the hepatitis B surface antigen. N Engl J Med 329:1842, 1993

STARZL TE et al: Liver transplantation. N Engl J Med 321:1014, 1092, 1989

TODO S et al: Orthotopic liver transplantation for patients with hepatitis B virus–related liver disease. Hepatology 13:619, 1991

U.S. MULTICENTER FK506 LIVER STUDY GROUP: A comparison of tacrolimus (FK506) and cyclosporine for immunosuppression in liver transplantation. N Engl J Med 331:1110, 1994

WADE JJ et al: Bacterial and fungal infections after liver transplantation: An analysis of 284 patients. Hepatology 21:1328, 1995

WRIGHT TL: Liver transplantation for chronic hepatitis C viral infection. Gastroenterol Clin North Am 22:231, 1993

———— et al: Interferon-α therapy for hepatitis C infection after liver transplantation. Hepatology 20:773, 1994

ZETTERMAN RK (guest ed): Long-term management of the liver transplant patient. Semin Liver Dis 15:123, 1995

---

302   *Norton J. Greenberger, Kurt J. Isselbacher*

DISEASES OF THE GALLBLADDER AND BILE DUCTS

PHYSIOLOGY OF BILE PRODUCTION AND FLOW   **Bile Secretion and Composition**   Bile formed in the hepatic lobules is secreted into a complex network of canaliculi, small bile ductules, and larger bile ducts that run with lymphatics and branches of the portal vein and hepatic artery in portal tracts situated between hepatic lobules. These interlobular bile ducts coalesce to form larger septal bile ducts that join to form the right and left hepatic ducts, which in turn unite to form the common hepatic duct. The common hepatic duct is joined by the cystic duct of the gallbladder to form the common bile duct (CBD), which enters the duodenum (often after joining the main pancreatic duct) through the ampulla of Vater.

Hepatic bile is a pigmented isotonic fluid with an electrolyte composition resembling blood plasma. The electrolyte composition of gallbladder bile differs from that of hepatic bile because most of the inorganic anions, chloride and bicarbonate, have been removed by reabsorption across the basement membrane.

Major components of bile by weight include water (82 percent), bile acids (12 percent), lecithin and other phospholipids (4 percent), and unesterified cholesterol (0.7 percent). Other constituents include conjugated bilirubin, proteins (IgA, by-products of hormones, and other proteins metabolized in the liver), electrolytes, mucus, and, often, drugs and their metabolic by-products.

The total daily basal secretion of hepatic bile is approximately 500 to 600 mL. The metabolic products of hepatocyte uptake and synthesis are secreted into the bile canaliculi, which are lined by microvillus membrane components associated with microfilaments of actin, microtubules, and other contractile elements. Within the hepato-cyte, conjugation of many of the bile constituents may occur, while other components of bile, such as primary bile acids, lecithin, and some cholesterol, are synthesized de novo. Three mechanisms are important in regulating bile flow: (1) active transport of bile acids from hepatocytes into the canaliculi, (2) bile acid–independent ATPase-mediated transport of sodium, and (3) ductular secretion. The last is a secretin-mediated and cyclic AMP–dependent phenomenon that appears to result from the active transport of sodium and bicarbonate into the ductule, with resulting passive movement of water across the cell membrane.

The Bile Acids The primary bile acids, cholic and chenodeoxy-cholic acids, are synthesized from cholesterol in the liver, conjugated with glycine or taurine, and excreted into the bile. Secondary bile acids, including deoxycholate and lithocholate, are formed in the colon as bacterial metabolites of the primary bile acids. However, lithocholic acid is much less efficiently absorbed from the colon than deoxycholic acid. Other secondary bile acids, found in trace amounts, which include ursodeoxycholic acid [(UDCA) a stereoisomer of chenodeoxycholate (CDCA)] and a variety of other unusual or "aberrant" bile acids, may be produced in increased amounts in patients with chronic cholestatic syndromes. In normal bile, the ratio of glycine to taurine conjugates is about 3:1, while in patients with cholestasis, increased concentrations of sulfate and glucuronide conjugates of bile acids are often found.

Bile acids are detergents that in aqueous solutions and above a critical concentration of about 2 mM form molecular aggregates called *micelles*. Cholesterol alone is poorly soluble in aqueous environments, and its solubility in bile depends on both the lipid concentration and the relative molar percentages of bile acids and lecithin. Normal ratios of these constituents favor the formation of solubilizing *mixed micelles*, while abnormal ratios promote the precipitation of cholesterol crystals in bile.

In addition to facilitating the biliary excretion of cholesterol, bile acids are necessary for the normal intestinal absorption of dietary fats via a micellar transport mechanism (see Chap. 285). Bile acids also serve as a major physiologic driving force for hepatic bile flow and aid in water and electrolyte transport in the small bowel and colon.

Enterohepatic Circulation Bile acids are efficiently conserved under normal conditions. Conjugated and unconjugated bile acids are absorbed by *passive diffusion* along the entire gut. Quantitatively much more important for bile salt recirculation, however, is the *active transport* mechanism for conjugated bile acids in the distal ileum (see Chap. 285). The reabsorbed bile acids enter the portal bloodstream and are taken up rapidly by hepatocytes, reconjugated, and resecreted into bile (enterohepatic circulation).

The normal bile acid pool size is approximately 2 to 4 g. During digestion of a meal, the bile acid pool undergoes at least one or more enterohepatic cycles, depending on the size and composition of the meal. Normally, the bile acid pool circulates approximately 5 to 10 times daily. Intestinal absorption of the pool is about 95 percent efficient, so fecal loss of bile acids is in the range of 0.3 to 0.6 g/d. This fecal loss is compensated by an equal daily synthesis of bile acids by the liver, and thus the size of the bile salt pool is maintained. Bile acids returning to the liver suppress de novo hepatic synthesis of primary bile acids from cholesterol by inhibiting the rate-limiting enzyme 7α-hydroxylase. While the loss of bile salts in stool is usually matched by increased hepatic synthesis, the maximum rate of synthesis is approximately 5 g/d, which may be insufficient to replete the bile acid pool size when there is pronounced impairment of intestinal bile salt reabsorption.

Gallbladder and Sphincteric Functions In the fasting state, the sphincter of Oddi offers a high-pressure zone of resistance to bile flow from the common bile duct into the duodenum. This tonic contraction serves to (1) prevent reflux of duodenal contents into the pancreatic and bile ducts and (2) promote bile filling of the gallbladder. The major factor controlling the evacuation of the gallbladder is the

peptide hormone cholecystokinin (CCK), which is released from the duodenal mucosa in response to the ingestion of fats and amino acids. CCK produces (1) powerful contraction of the gallbladder, (2) decreased resistance of the sphincter of Oddi, (3) increased hepatic secretion of bile, and thus (4) enhanced flow of biliary contents into the duodenum.

Hepatic bile is "concentrated" within the gallbladder by energy-dependent transmucosal absorption of water and electrolytes. Almost the entire bile acid pool may be sequestered in the gallbladder following an overnight fast for delivery into the duodenum with the first meal of the day. The normal capacity of the gallbladder is 30 to 75 mL of bile.

DISEASES OF THE GALLBLADDER

CONGENITAL ANOMALIES Anomalies of the biliary tract may be found in 10 to 20 percent of the population, including abnormalities in number, size, and shape (e.g., agenesis of the gallbladder, duplications, rudimentary or oversized "giant" gallbladders, and diverticula). Phrygian cap is a clinically innocuous entity in which a partial or complete septum (or fold) separates the fundus from the body. Anomalies of position or suspension are not uncommon and include left-sided gallbladder, intrahepatic gallbladder, retrodisplacement of the gallbladder, and "floating" gallbladder. The latter condition predisposes to acute torsion, volvulus, or herniation of the gallbladder.

GALLSTONES Pathogenesis Gallstones are quite prevalent in most western countries. In the United States, autopsy series have shown gallstones in at least 20 percent of women and in 8 percent of men over the age of 40. It is estimated that 16 to 20 million persons in the United States have gallstones and that approximately 1 million new cases of cholelithiasis develop each year.

Gallstones are crystalline structures formed by concretion or accretion of normal or abnormal bile constituents. These stones are divided into three major types; cholesterol and mixed stones account for 80 percent of the total, with pigment stones comprising the remaining 20 percent. Mixed and cholesterol gallstones usually contain more than 70 percent cholesterol monohydrate plus an admixture of calcium salts, bile acids and bile pigments, proteins, fatty acids, and phospholipids. Pigment stones are composed primarily of calcium bilirubinate; they contain less than 10 percent cholesterol.

Cholesterol and mixed stones and biliary sludge Cholesterol is relatively water insoluble and requires aqueous dispersion into either micelles or vesicles, both of which require the presence of a second lipid to "liquefy" the cholesterol. When the cholesterol content of bile exceeds the amount that can be solubilized by bile salt and bile salt–lecithin micelles, the excess is dispersed in larger lipid vesicles (Fig. 302-1). Vesicles are spherical particles composed of lecithin and cholesterol and contain only traces of bile salts. Vesicles and micelles are important cholesterol-solubilizing and -transport agents in bile supersaturated with cholesterol.

There are several important mechanisms in the formation of lithogenic (stone-forming) bile. The most important is increased biliary secretion of cholesterol. This may occur in association with obesity, high-caloric diets, or drugs (e.g., clofibrate) and may result from increased activity of hydroxymethylglutaryl–coenzyme A (HMG-CoA) reductase, the rate-limiting enzyme of hepatic cholesterol synthesis. In some patients, impaired hepatic conversion of cholesterol to bile acids also may occur, resulting in an increase of the lithogenic cholesterol/bile acid ratio. Lithogenic bile also results from decreased hepatic secretion of bile salts and phospholipids, which may follow impaired hepatic synthesis (e.g., rare inborn errors of metabolism such as cerebrotendinous xanthomatosis), or conditions affecting the enterohepatic circulation of these constituents (e.g., prolonged parenteral alimentation or ileal disease or resection). In addition, most patients with gallstones appear to have reduced activity of hepatic cholesterol 7α-hydroxylase, the rate-limiting enzyme for primary bile acid synthesis.

Thus an excess of biliary cholesterol in relation to bile acids and phospholipids may be due to hypersecretion of cholesterol, hyposecretion of bile acids, or both. While cholesterol saturation of bile is an important prerequisite for gallstone formation, it is not sufficient by itself to produce cholesterol precipitation in vivo. Most people with supersaturated bile do not develop stones because the time required for cholesterol crystals to nucleate and grow is longer than the time bile spends in the gallbladder. Two additional disturbances of bile acid metabolism that are likely to contribute to supersaturation of bile with cholesterol are (1) reduction of the bile acid pool and (2) enhanced conversion of cholic acid to deoxycholic acid, with replacement of the cholic acid pool by an expanded deoxycholic acid pool. The first disorder may be caused by more rapid loss of primary bile acid from the small intestine into the colon. The second disturbance may result from enhanced dehydroxylation of cholic acid and increased absorption of newly formed deoxycholic acid.

A second important abnormality is defective vesicle formation. Ordinarily, cholesterol and phospholipid are secreted into bile as unilamellar bilayered vesicles, which are unstable and are converted, along with bile acids, into other lipid aggregates such as micelles. During micellation of vesicles, more phospholipid than cholesterol is transferred to mixed micelles, leading to unstable cholesterol-rich vesicles

that aggregate into larger multilamellar vesicles from which cholesterol crystals aggregate.

A third important mechanism is *nucleation* of cholesterol monohydrate crystals, which is greatly accelerated in human lithogenic bile; it is this feature rather than the degree of cholesterol supersaturation that distinguishes lithogenic from normal gallbladder bile. Accelerated nucleation of cholesterol monohydrate in bile may be due to either an *excess of pronucleating factors* or a *deficiency of antinucleating factors*. Nonmucin and mucin glycoproteins and lysine phosphatidylcholine appear to be pronucleating factors, while apolipoproteins AI and AII and other glycoproteins appear to be antinucleating factors. However, the characterization of additional pronucleating and antinucleating factors remains incomplete. Cholesterol monohydrate crystal nucleation and crystal growth probably occur within the mucin gel layer. Vesicle fusion leads to liquid crystals, which, in turn, nucleate into solid cholesterol monohydrate crystals. Continued growth of the crystals occurs by direct nucleation of cholesterol molecules from supersaturated unilamellar or multilamellar biliary vesicles.

A fourth important mechanism in cholesterol gallstone formation concerns *biliary sludge*. Biliary sludge is a thick mucous material that upon microscopic examination reveals lecithin-cholesterol crystals, cholesterol monohydrate crystals, calcium bilirubinate, and mucin thread or mucous gels. Biliary sludge typically forms a crescent-like layer in the most dependent portion of the gallbladder and is recognized by characteristic echoes on ultrasonography (see below). In vitro, cholesterol monohydrate crystals (>50 μm) mixed with mucus produce echoes that are indistinguishable from gallbladder sludge observed in patients. The presence of biliary sludge implies two abnormalities: (1) the normal balance between gallbladder mucin secretion and elimination has become deranged; and (2) nucleation from biliary solutes has occurred. That biliary sludge is a precursor form of gallstone disease is evident from several observations. In one study, 96 patients with gallbladder sludge were followed prospectively by serial ultrasound studies. In 17 patients (18 percent), biliary sludge disappeared and did not recur for at least 2 years. In 58 patients (60 percent), biliary sludge disappeared and reappeared. Importantly, gallstones developed in 14 patients, in 8 of whom the gallstones were "silent." In 12 patients, cholecystectomies were performed, 6 for gallstone-associated biliary pain and 3 in symptomatic patients with sludge but without gallstones who had prior attacks of pancreatitis; the latter did not recur after cholecystectomy. It should be emphasized that biliary sludge can develop with disorders that cause gallbladder hypomotility, i.e., surgery, burns, total parenteral nutrition, pregnancy, and oral contraceptives—all of which are associated with gallstone formation. Finally, biliary sludge can account for the observation that most cholesterol gallstones have a pigmented center.

Two other conditions are associated with cholesterol stone or biliary sludge formation: pregnancy and very low calorie diet. There appear to be two key changes during pregnancy that contribute to a "cholelithogenic state." First, the composition of the bile acid pool and the cholesterol-carrying capacity of bile change, with a resultant marked increase in cholesterol saturation during the third trimester. Second, ultrasonographic studies have demonstrated that gallbladder contraction in response to a standard meal is sluggish, resulting in impaired gallbladder emptying. That these changes are related to pregnancy per se is supported by several studies that show reversal of these abnormalities after delivery. During pregnancy, gallbladder sludge develops in 20 to 30 percent of women and gallstones in 5 to 12 percent. While biliary sludge is a common finding during pregnancy, it is usually asymptomatic and often resolves spontaneously after delivery. Gallstones that are less common and frequently associated with biliary colic may also disappear after delivery because of spontaneous dissolution related to bile becoming unsaturated with cholesterol post partum.

Ten to 20 percent of people having rapid weight reduction through very low calorie dieting develop gallstones. In a study involving close

FIGURE 302-1 Scheme showing pathogenesis of gallstone formation. Conditions or factors that increase the ratio of cholesterol to bile acids and lecithin favor gallstone formation (HMG-CoAR, hydroxymethylglutaryl–coenzyme A reductase; 7-α-OHase, 7α-hydroxylase).

to 800 patients who completed a 16-week, 520-kcal/d diet, UDCA in a dosage of 600 mg/d proved highly effective in preventing gallstone formation; gallstones developed in only 2 percent of UDCA recipients compared to 28 percent of placebo-treated patients.

There is increasing evidence for the association between dietary cholesterol and gallstone formation. In patients with gallstones, an increase in dietary cholesterol further *increases* biliary cholesterol secretion and *decreases* bile acid synthesis and pool size, changes known to predispose to cholesterol gallstone formation. These changes do not occur in control (non-gallstone) patients on high-cholesterol diets. These findings help explain the presence of supersaturated bile in individuals predisposed to form gallstones.

To summarize, cholesterol gallstone disease occurs because of several defects, which include (1) bile supersaturation with cholesterol, (2) nucleation of cholesterol monohydrate with subsequent crystal retention and stone growth, and (3) abnormal gallbladder motor function with delayed emptying and stasis. Other important factors known to predispose to cholesterol stone formation are summarized in Table 302-1.

Pigment stones Gallstones composed largely of calcium bilirubinate are much more common in the orient than in western countries.

Table 302-1

Predisposing Factors for Cholesterol and Pigment Gallstone Formation

CHOLESTEROL AND MIXED STONES

1. Demography
   a. Northern Europe and North and South America greater than Asia, native Americans, probable familial, hereditary aspects
2. Obesity
   a. Normal bile acid pool and secretion but increased biliary secretion of cholesterol
3. Weight loss
   a. Mobilization of tissue cholesterol leads to increased biliary cholesterol secretion while enterohepatic secretion of bile salt is decreased
4. Female sex hormones
   a. Estrogens stimulate hepatic lipoprotein receptors, increase uptake of dietary cholesterol, increase biliary cholesterol secretion, and inhibit synthesis of chenodeoxycholic acid
   b. Natural estrogens, other estrogens, and oral contraceptives lead to decreased bile salt secretion and decreased conversion of cholesterol to cholesteryl esters
5. Ileal disease or resection
   a. Malabsorption of bile acids leads to decreased bile acid pool, decreased biliary secretion of bile salts, and decreased 7α-hydroxylase activity
6. Increasing age
   a. Increased biliary secretion of cholesterol, decreased size of bile acid pool, decreased biliary secretion of bile salts
7. Gallbladder hypomotility leading to stasis and formation of sludge/stools
   a. Prolonged parenteral nutrition
   b. Fasting
   c. Pregnancy
   d. Drugs such as octreotide
8. Clofibrate therapy
   a. Increased biliary secretion of cholesterol
9. Decreased bile acid secretion
   a. Primary biliary cirrhosis
   b. Chronic intrahepatic cholestasis
10. Miscellaneous
    a. High-calorie, high-fat diet
    b. Spinal cord injury

PIGMENT STONES

1. Demographic/genetic factors: Asia, rural setting
2. Chronic hemolysis
3. Alcoholic cirrhosis
4. Chronic biliary tract infection, parasite infestation
5. Increasing age

The presence of increased amounts of unconjugated, insoluble bilirubin in bile results in the precipitation of bilirubin, which may aggregate to form pigment stones or may fuse to form the nidus for growth of mixed cholesterol gallstones. In western countries, chronic hemolytic states (with increased conjugated bilirubin in bile) or alcoholic liver disease are associated with an increased incidence of pigment stones. Deconjugation of soluble bilirubin mono- and diglucuronide may be mediated by the enzyme β-glucuronidase, which is sometimes produced when bile is chronically infected by bacteria. Pigment stone formation is especially prominent in Asians and is often associated with infections in the biliary tree (see Table 302-1).

Diagnosis Procedures of potential use in the diagnosis of cholelithiasis and other diseases of the gallbladder are detailed in Table 302-2. The plain abdominal film may detect gallstones containing sufficient calcium to be radiopaque (10 to 15 percent of cholesterol and mixed stones and approximately 50 percent of pigment stones). Plain radiography also may be of use in the diagnosis of emphysematous cholecystitis, porcelain gallbladder, limey bile, and gallstone ileus.

Ultrasonography of the gallbladder is very accurate in the identification of cholelithiasis and has several advantages over oral cholecystography (see Fig. 302-2A). The gallbladder is easily visualized with the technique, and in fact, failure to image the gallbladder successfully in a fasting patient correlates well with the presence of underlying gallbladder disease. Stones as small as 2 mm in diameter may be confidently identified provided that firm criteria are used [e.g., acoustic "shadowing" of opacities that are within the gallbladder lumen and that change with the patient's position (by gravity)]. In major medical centers, the false-negative and false-positive rates for ultrasound in gallstone patients are about 2 to 4 percent. Biliary sludge is material of low echogenic activity that typically forms a layer in the most dependent position of the gallbladder. This layer shifts with postural changes but fails to produce acoustic shadowing; these two characteristics distinguish sludges from gallstones.

Oral cholecystography (OCG) is a useful procedure for the diagnosis of gallstones but has been largely replaced by ultrasound. However, OCG is still useful for the selection of patients for nonsurgical therapy of gallstone disease such as lithotripsy or bile acid dissolution therapy. In both these settings, OCG is used to assess the patency of the cystic duct and gallbladder emptying function. Further, OCG can also delineate the size and number of gallstones and determine whether they are calcified. Factors that may produce nonvisualization of the OCG are summarized in Table 302-2.

Radiopharmaceuticals such as ^{99m}Tc-labeled *N*-substituted iminodiacetic acids (HIDA, DIDA, DISIDA, etc.) are rapidly extracted from the blood and are excreted into the biliary tree in high concentration even in the presence of mild to moderate serum bilirubin elevations. Failure to image the gallbladder in the presence of biliary ductal visualization may indicate cystic duct obstruction, acute or chronic cholecystitis, or surgical absence of the organ. Such scans have their greatest application in the diagnosis of acute cholecystitis.

Symptoms of Gallstone Disease Gallstones usually produce symptoms by causing inflammation or obstruction following their migration into the cystic duct or CBD. The most specific and characteristic symptom of gallstone disease is biliary colic. Obstruction of the cystic duct or CBD by a stone produces increased intraluminal pressure and distention of the viscus that cannot be relieved by repetitive biliary contractions. The resultant visceral pain is characteristically a severe, steady ache or pressure in the epigastrium or right upper quadrant (RUQ) of the abdomen with frequent radiation to the interscapular area, right scapula, or shoulder.

Biliary colic begins quite suddenly and may persist with severe intensity for 1 to 4 h, subsiding gradually or rapidly. An episode of biliary pain is sometimes followed by a residual mild ache or soreness in the RUQ, which may persist for 24 h or so. Nausea and vomiting frequently accompany episodes of biliary colic, and mild elevations of serum bilirubin [not exceeding 85.5 μmol/L (5 mg/dL)] occur in 25 percent of patients. Persistence of a high serum bilirubin level suggests common duct stones. Fever or chills (rigors) with biliary colic usually imply an underlying complication, i.e., cholecystitis, pancreatitis, or cholangitis. Complaints of vague epigastric fullness, dyspepsia, eructation, or flatulence, especially following a fatty meal, should not be confused with biliary colic. Such symptoms are frequently elicited from patients with gallstone disease but are not specific for biliary calculi. Biliary colic may be precipitated by eating a fatty meal, by consumption of a large meal following a period of prolonged fasting, or by eating a normal meal.

Natural History   Gallstone disease discovered in an asymptomatic patient or in a patient whose symptoms are not referable to cholelithiasis is a common clinical problem. The natural history of "silent" or asymptomatic gallstones has occasioned much debate. In contrast to previous reports, a study of predominantly male silent gallstone patients suggests that the cumulative risk for the development of symptoms or complications requiring surgery is relatively low— 10 percent at 5 years, 15 percent at 10 years, and 18 percent at 15 years. Patients remaining asymptomatic for 15 years were found to be unlikely to develop symptoms during further follow-up, and most patients who did develop complications from their gallstones experienced *prior* warning symptoms. Similar conclusions apply to diabetics with silent gallstones. Decision analysis has suggested that (1) the cumulative risk of death due to gallstone disease while on expectant management is small, and (2) prophylactic cholecystectomy is not warranted.

Complications requiring cholecystectomy appear to be much more common in gallstone patients who have developed symptoms of biliary colic. Patients found to have gallstones at a young age are more likely to develop symptoms from cholelithiasis than are patients older than 60 years at the time of initial diagnosis. Patients with diabetes mellitus and gallstones may be somewhat more susceptible to septic complications, but the magnitude of risk of septic biliary complications in diabetic patients is incompletely defined. In addition, asymptomatic gallstone patients with nonvisualization of the gallbladder on OCG appear to have an increased tendency to develop symptoms and complications.

 TREATMENT

Surgical Therapy   Although the management of silent gallstones remains controversial, the risk of developing symptoms or complications requiring surgery is quite small (in the range of 1 to 2 percent per year) in most asymptomatic gallstone patients. Thus a recommendation for prophylactic cholecystectomy in a patient with gallstones should probably be based on assessment of three factors: (1) the presence of symptoms that are frequent enough or severe enough to interfere with the patient's general routine; (2) the presence of a prior complication of gallstone disease, i.e., history of acute cholecystitis, pancreatitis, gallstone fistula, etc.; or (3) the presence of an underlying condition predisposing the patient to increased risk of gallstone complications (e.g., calcified or porcelain gallbladder, cholesterolosis, adenomyomatosis, and/or a previous attack of acute cholecystitis regardless of current symptomatic status). Patients with very large gallstones (over 2 cm in diameter) and patients having gallstones in a congenitally anomalous gallbladder also might be considered for prophylactic cholecystectomy. Although age under 50 years is a worrisome factor in asymptomatic gallstone patients, few authorities would now recommend routine cholecystectomy in all young patients with silent stones. Laparoscopic cholecystectomy is a minimal-access approach for the removal

Table 302-2

Diagnostic Evaluation of the Gallbladder

Diagnostic Advantages	Diagnostic Limitations	Comment
PLAIN ABDOMINAL X-RAY		

Low cost
Readily available
	Relatively low yield
	?Contraindicated in pregnancy
		Pathognomonic findings in:
		  Calcified gallstones
		  Limey bile, porcelain GB
		  Emphysematous cholecystitis
		  Gallstone ileus

ORAL CHOLECYSTOGRAM		

Low cost
Readily available
Accurate identification of gallstones (90–95%)
Identification of GB anomalies, hyperplastic cholecystoses
Identification of chronic GB disease after nonvisualization on double dose
	?Contraindicated in pregnancy
	?Contraindicated with history of reaction to iodinated contrast
	Nonvisualization with:
	  Serum bilirubin >34–68 μmol/L (2–4 mg/dL)
	  Failure to ingest or absorb tablets
	  Impaired hepatic excretion
	Very small stones may be undetected
	More time-consuming than GBUS
		Largely replaced by GBUS
		A useful procedure in identification of gallstones if diagnostic limitations prevent GBUS

GALLBLADDER ULTRASOUND		
Rapid Accurate identification of gallstones (>95%) Simultaneous scanning of GB, liver, bile ducts, pancreas "Real-time" scanning allows assessment of GB volume, contractility Not limited by jaundice, pregnancy May detect very small stones	Bowel gas Massive obesity Ascites Recent barium study	Procedure of choice for detection of stones
RADIOISOTOPE SCANS (HIDA, DIDA, ETC.)		
Accurate identification of cystic duct obstruction Simultaneous assessment of bile ducts	?Contraindicated in pregnancy Serum bilirubin >103–205 μmol/L (6–12 mg/dL) Cholecystogram of low resolution	Indicated for confirmation of suspected acute cholecystitis; less sensitive and less specific in chronic cholecystitis; useful in diagnosis of acalculous cholecystopathy, especially if given with CCK to assess gallbladder emptying

NOTE: GB, gallbladder; GBUS, gallbladder ultrasound.

of the gallbladder together with its stones. Because of a markedly shortened hospital stay as well as decreased cost and a mortality rate of less than 1 percent, it is the procedure of choice for most patients referred for elective cholecystectomy; in only 4 to 5 percent of patients are surgeons compelled to convert to open cholecystectomy.

From several studies involving over 4000 patients undergoing laparoscopic cholecystectomy, the following key points emerge: (1) complications develop in about 4 percent of patients; (2) conversion to laparotomy occurs in 5 percent; (3) the death rate is remarkably low (i.e., <0.1 percent); and (4) bile duct injuries are unusual (i.e., 4 percent). Preoperative endoscopic retrograde cholangiopancreatography (ERCP) was carried out in about 5 percent, intraoperative cholangiography in about 30 percent, and postoperative ERCP in approximately 1.5 percent of patients. These data indicate why laparoscopic cholecystectomy has become the "gold standard" for treating symptomatic cholelithiasis.

Medical Therapy—Gallstone Dissolution UDCA and CDCA decrease HMG-CoA reductase activity, which in turn results in decreased hepatic cholesterol synthesis. UDCA administration also appears to produce a lamellar liquid crystalline phase in bile that allows a dispersion of cholesterol from stones by physiochemical means. UDCA also may retard cholesterol crystal nucleation. In carefully selected patients with a functioning gallbladder and with radiolucent stones <15 mm in diameter, complete dissolution can be achieved in 50 to 60 percent of patients within 2 years with UDCA at a dose of 10 to 13 mg/kg per day. The highest success rate (i.e., >70 percent) occurs in patients with small (<5 mm) floating radiolucent gallstones. Probably no more than 10 percent of patients with *symptomatic* cholelithiasis are candidates for such treatment. However, in addition to the vexing problem of recurrent stones (30 to 50 percent over 3 to 12 years of follow-up), there is also the factor of taking an expensive drug for an indefinite period of time. The advantages and success of laparoscopic cholecystectomy have largely reduced the role of gallstone dissolution to patients who either refuse or are not candidates for elective cholecystectomy. One role for UDCA is in the treatment of patients with recurrent calculous disease after cholecystectomy.

Gallbladder stones may be fragmented by extracorporeal shock waves generated by the use of electrohydraulic, piezoceramic, or electromagnetic devices. While such shock wave lithotripsy combined with medical litholytic therapy is safe and effective in carefully selected patients with gallbladder calculi, the procedure is employed infrequently for several reasons: (1) the rapid emergence of laparoscopic cholystectomy as the procedure of choice for symptomatic cholelithiasis and/or chronic cholecystitis, (2) recurrence of gallstones in 10 to 15 percent of patients within 2 years after lithotripsy combined with medical litholytic therapy, and (3) the considerable cost of taking UDCA or UDCA plus CDCA for an indefinite period.

ACUTE AND CHRONIC CHOLECYSTITIS **Acute Cholecystitis** Acute inflammation of the gallbladder wall usually follows obstruction of the cystic duct by a stone. Inflammatory response can be evoked by three factors: (1) *mechanical inflammation* produced by increased intraluminal pressure and distention with resulting ischemia of the gallbladder mucosa and wall, (2) *chemical inflammation* caused by the release of lysolecithin (due to the action of phospholipase on lecithin in bile) and other local tissue factors, and (3) *bacterial inflammation*, which may play a role in 50 to 85 percent of patients with acute cholecystitis. The organisms most frequently isolated by culture of gallbladder bile in these patients include *Escherichia coli*, *Klebsiella* species, group D *Streptococcus*, *Staphylococcus* species, and *Clostridium* species.

Acute cholecystitis often begins as an attack of biliary colic that progressively worsens. Approximately 60 to 70 percent of patients report having experienced prior attacks that resolved spontaneously. As the episode progresses, however, the pain of acute cholecystitis becomes more generalized in the right upper abdomen. As with biliary colic, the pain of cholecystitis may radiate to the interscapular area, right scapula, or shoulder. Peritoneal signs of inflammation such as increased pain with jarring or on deep respiration may be apparent. The patient is anorectic and often nauseated. Vomiting is relatively common and may produce symptoms and signs of vascular and extracellular volume depletion. Jaundice is unusual early in the course of acute cholecystitis but may occur when edematous inflammatory changes involve the bile ducts and surrounding lymph nodes.

A low-grade fever is characteristically present, but shaking chills or rigors are not uncommon. The RUQ of the abdomen is almost invariably tender to palpation. An enlarged, tense gallbladder is palpa-

FIGURE 302-2 Examples of ultrasound and radiologic studies of the biliary tract. *A.* An ultrasound study showing a distended gallbladder containing a single large stone (*arrow*) which casts an acoustic shadow. *B.* Endoscopic retrograde cholangiopancreatogram (ERCP) showing normal biliary tract anatomy. In addition to the endoscope and large vertical gallbladder filled with contrast dye, the common hepatic duct (chd), common bile duct (cbd), and pancreatic duct (pd) are shown. The arrow points to the ampulla of Vater. *C.* Percutaneous transhepatic cholangiogram (PTHC) showing choledocholithiasis. The biliary tract is dilatated and contains multiple radiolucent calculi (*small arrows*). The dilatation is due to obstruction by a large stone in the distal portion of the duct (*large arrow*). *D.* ERCP showing sclerosing cholangitis. The common bile duct is to the right of the endoscope. Following retrograde cholangiography, the common bile duct shows thickening of the wall with a narrow, beaded lumen typical of sclerosing cholangitis.

ble in one-quarter to one-half of patients. Deep inspiration or cough during subcostal palpation of the RUQ usually produces increased pain and inspiratory arrest (Murphy's sign). A light blow delivered to the right subcostal area may elicit a marked increase in pain. Localized rebound tenderness in the RUQ is common, as are abdominal distention and hypoactive bowel sounds from paralytic ileus, but generalized peritoneal signs and abdominal rigidity are usually lacking, absent perforation.

The diagnosis of acute cholecystitis is usually made on the basis of a characteristic history and physical examination. The triad of sudden onset of RUQ tenderness, fever, and leukocytosis is highly suggestive. Typically, leukocytosis in the range of 10,000 to 15,000 cells per microliter with a left shift on differential count is found. The serum bilirubin is mildly elevated [<85.5 μmol/L (5 mg/dL)] in 45 percent of patients, while 25 percent have modest elevations in serum aminotransferases (usually less than a fivefold elevation). The radionuclide (e.g., HIDA) biliary scan may be confirmatory if bile duct imaging is seen without visualization of the gallbladder. Ultrasound will demonstrate calculi in 90 to 95 percent of cases.

Approximately 75 percent of patients treated medically have remission of acute symptoms within 2 to 7 days following hospitalization. In 25 percent, however, a complication of acute cholecystitis will occur despite conservative treatment (see below). In this setting, prompt surgical intervention is required. Of the 75 percent of patients with acute cholecystitis who undergo remission of symptoms, approximately one-quarter will experience a recurrence of cholecystitis within 1 year, and 60 percent will have at least one recurrent bout within 6 years. In view of the natural history of the disease, acute cholecystitis is best treated by early surgery whenever possible.

Acalculous cholecystitis In 5 to 10 percent of patients with acute cholecystitis, calculi obstructing the cystic duct are not found at surgery. In over 50 percent of such cases an underlying explanation for acalculous inflammation is not found. An increased risk for the development of acalculous cholecystitis is especially associated with serious trauma or burns, with the postpartum period following prolonged labor, and with orthopedic and other nonbiliary major surgical operations in the postoperative period. Other precipitating factors include vasculitis, obstructing adenocarcinoma of the gallbladder, diabetes mellitus, torsion of the gallbladder, "unusual" bacterial infections of the gallbladder (e.g., *Leptospira, Streptococcus, Salmonella,* or *Vibrio cholerae*), and parasitic infestation of the gallbladder. Acalculous cholecystitis also may be seen with a variety of other systemic disease processes (sarcoidosis, cardiovascular disease, tuberculosis, syphilis, actinomycosis, etc.) and may possibly complicate periods of prolonged parenteral hyperalimentation.

Although the clinical manifestations of acalculous cholecystitis are indistinguishable from those of calculous cholecystitis, the setting of acute gallbladder inflammation complicating severe underlying illness is characteristic of acalculous disease. Ultrasound, computed tomography (CT) scanning, or radionuclide examinations demonstrating a large, tense, static gallbladder without stones and with evidence of poor emptying over a prolonged period may be diagnostically useful in some cases. The complication rate for acalculous cholecystitis exceeds that for calculous cholecystitis. Successful management of acute acalculous cholecystitis appears to depend primarily on early diagnosis and surgical intervention, with meticulous attention to postoperative care.

Acalculous cholecystopathy Disordered motility of the gallbladder can produce recurrent biliary pain in patients without gallstones. Infusion of an octapeptide of CCK can be used to measure the gallbladder ejection fraction during cholescintigraphy. In a representative study, CCK cholescintigraphy using ^{99m}Tc-diisopropyl iminodiacetic acid (DIDA) identified 21 patients with an abnormal gallbladder ejection fraction (<40 percent at 45 min); 10 of 11 patients who underwent surgery became asymptomatic, whereas all 10 who did not undergo surgery showed abnormalities, i.e., chronic cholecystitis, gallbladder muscle hypertrophy, and/or a markedly narrowed cystic duct. From this and other similar studies, the following criteria can be used to identify patients with acalculous cholecystopathy: (1) recurrent epi-

sodes of typical RUQ pain characteristic of biliary tract pain, (2) abnormal CCK cholescintigraphy demonstrating a gallbladder ejection fraction of less than 40 percent, (3) infusion of CCK reproduces the patient's pain, and (4) prior history of transient abnormalities in liver tests that accompanied episodes of RUQ pain. An additional clue would be the identification of a large gallbladder on ultrasound examination. Finally, it should be noted that sphincter of Oddi dysfunction also can give rise to recurrent RUQ pain and CCK-scintigraphic abnormalities.

Emphysematous cholecystitis So-called emphysematous cholecystitis is thought to begin with acute cholecystitis (calculous or acalculous) followed by ischemia or gangrene of the gallbladder wall and infection by gas-producing organisms. Bacteria most frequently cultured in this setting include anaerobes, such as *Clostridium welchii* or *Clostridium perfringens*, and aerobes, such as *E. coli*. This condition occurs most frequently in elderly men and in patients with diabetes mellitus. The clinical manifestations are essentially indistinguishable from those of nongaseous cholecystitis. The diagnosis is usually made on plain abdominal film by the finding of gas within the gallbladder lumen, dissecting within the gallbladder wall to form a gaseous ring, or in the pericholecystic tissues. The morbidity and mortality rates with emphysematous cholecystitis are considerable. Prompt surgical intervention coupled with appropriate antibiotics is mandatory.

Chronic Cholecystitis Chronic inflammation of the gallbladder wall is almost always associated with the presence of gallstones and is thought to result from repeated bouts of subacute or acute cholecystitis or from persistent mechanical irritation of the gallbladder wall. The presence of bacteria in the bile occurs in more than one-quarter of patients with chronic cholecystitis. Although the presence of infected bile in a patient with *chronic* cholecystitis undergoing elective cholecystectomy probably adds little to the operative risk, intraoperative Gram's staining and routine culturing of bile have been advocated to identify those patients whose gallbladder is colonized with *Clostridium* species. Appropriate antibiotics intra- and postoperatively are recommended in such patients because colonization with these organisms may be associated with devastating septic complications following surgery. Chronic cholecystitis may be asymptomatic for years, may progress to symptomatic gallbladder disease or to acute cholecystitis, or may present with complications (see below).

Complications of Cholecystitis *Empyema and hydrops* Empyema of the gallbladder usually results from progression of acute cholecystitis with persistent cystic duct obstruction to superinfection of the stagnant bile with a pus-forming bacterial organism. The clinical picture resembles that of cholangitis with high fever, severe RUQ pain, marked leukocytosis, and often, prostration. Empyema of the gallbladder carries a high risk of gram-negative sepsis and/or perforation. Emergency surgical intervention with proper antibiotic coverage is required as soon as the diagnosis is suspected.

Hydrops or mucocele of the gallbladder also may result from prolonged obstruction of the cystic duct, usually by a large solitary calculus. In this instance, the obstructed gallbladder lumen is progressively distended, over a period of time, by mucus (mucocele) or by a clear transudate (hydrops) produced by mucosal epithelial cells. A visible, easily palpable, nontender mass often extending from the RUQ into the right iliac fossa may be found on physical examination. The patient with hydrops of the gallbladder frequently remains asymptomatic, although chronic RUQ pain also may occur. Cholecystectomy is indicated, since empyema, perforation, or gangrene may complicate the condition.

Gangrene and perforation Gangrene of the gallbladder results from ischemia of the wall and patchy or complete tissue necrosis. Underlying conditions often include marked distention of the gallbladder, vasculitis, diabetes mellitus, empyema, or torsion resulting in arterial occlusion. Gangrene usually predisposes to perforation of the gallbladder, but perforation also may occur in chronic cholecystitis without premonitory warning symptoms. *Localized perforations* are usually contained by the omentum or by adhesions produced by recurrent inflammation of the gallbladder. Bacterial superinfection of the walled-off gallbladder contents results in abscess formation. Most patients are best treated with cholecystectomy, but some seriously ill patients may be managed with cholecystostomy and drainage of the abscess. *Free perforation* is less common but is associated with a mortality rate of approximately 30 percent. Such patients may experience a sudden transient relief of RUQ pain as the distended gallbladder decompresses; this is followed by signs of generalized peritonitis.

Fistula formation and gallstone ileus   *Fistulization* into an adjacent organ adherent to the gallbladder wall may result from inflammation and adhesion formation. Fistulas into the duodenum are most common, followed in frequency by those involving the hepatic flexure of the colon, stomach or jejunum, abdominal wall, and renal pelvis. Clinically "silent" biliary-enteric fistulas occurring as a complication of chronic cholecystitis have been found in up to 5 percent of patients undergoing cholecystectomy. Asymptomatic cholecystoenteric fistulas may sometimes be diagnosed by finding gas in the biliary tree on plain abdominal films. Barium contrast studies or endoscopy of the upper gastrointestinal tract or colon may demonstrate the fistula, but oral cholecystography will almost never result in opacification of either the gallbladder or the fistulous tract. Treatment in the symptomatic patient usually consists of cholecystectomy, CBD exploration, and closure of the fistulous tract.

Gallstone ileus refers to mechanical intestinal obstruction resulting from the passage of a large gallstone into the bowel lumen. The stone customarily enters the duodenum through a cholecystoenteric fistula at that level. The site of obstruction by the impacted gallstone is usually at the ileocecal valve, provided that the more proximal small bowel is of normal caliber. The majority of patients do not give a history of either prior biliary tract symptoms or complaints suggestive of acute cholecystitis or fistulization. Large stones over 2.5 cm in diameter are thought to predispose to fistula formation by gradual erosion through the gallbladder fundus. Diagnostic confirmation may occasionally be found on the plain abdominal film (e.g., small-intestinal obstruction with gas in the biliary tree and a calcified, ectopic gallstone) or following an upper gastrointestinal series (cholecystoduodenal fistula with small bowel obstruction at the ileocecal valve). Laparotomy with stone extraction (or propulsion into the colon) remains the procedure of choice to relieve obstruction. Evacuation of large stones within the gallbladder should also be performed. In general, the gallbladder and its attachment to the intestines should be left alone.

Limey (milk of calcium) bile and porcelain gallbladder   Calcium salts may be secreted into the lumen of the gallbladder in sufficient concentration to produce calcium precipitation and diffuse, hazy opacification of bile or a layering effect on plain abdominal roentgenography. This so-called limey bile or milk of calcium bile is usually clinically innocuous, but cholecystectomy is recommended because limey bile most often occurs in a hydropic gallbladder. In the entity called *porcelain gallbladder*, calcium salt deposition within the wall of a chronically inflamed gallbladder may be detected on the plain abdominal film. Cholecystectomy is advised in all patients with porcelain gallbladder because in a high percentage of cases this finding appears to be associated with the development of carcinoma of the gallbladder.

℞ TREATMENT

Medical Therapy   Although surgical intervention remains the mainstay of therapy for acute cholecystitis and its complications, a period of in-hospital stabilization may be required before cholecystectomy. Oral intake is eliminated, nasogastric suction is initiated, and extracellular volume depletion and electrolyte abnormalities are repaired. Meperidine or pentazocine are usually employed for analgesia because they may produce less spasm of the sphincter of Oddi than drugs such as morphine. Intravenous antibiotic therapy

is usually indicated in patients with severe acute cholecystitis even though bacterial superinfection of bile may not have occurred in the early stages of the inflammatory process. Postoperative complications of wound infection, abscess formation, or sepsis are reduced in antibiotic-treated patients. Effective single-agent antibiotics include ampicillin, cephalosporins, ureidopenicillins, or aminoglycosides, but in diabetic or debilitated patients and in those with signs of gram-negative sepsis, combination antibiotic treatment may be preferable (see also Chap. 138).

Surgical Therapy   The optimal timing of surgical intervention in patients with acute cholecystitis depends on stabilization of the patient. The clear trend is toward earlier surgery, and this is due in part to requirements for shorter hospital stays. Urgent (emergency) cholecystectomy or cholecystostomy is probably appropriate in most patients in whom a complication of acute cholecystitis such as empyema, emphysematous cholecystitis, or perforation is suspected or confirmed. In uncomplicated cases of acute cholecystitis, up to 30 percent of patients fail to resolve their symptoms on appropriate medical therapy, and progression of the attack or a supervening complication leads to the performance of early operation (within 24 to 72 h). The technical complications of surgery are not increased in patients undergoing early as opposed to delayed cholecystectomy. Delayed surgical intervention is probably best reserved for (1) patients in whom the overall medical condition imposes an unacceptable risk for early surgery and (2) patients in whom the diagnosis of acute cholecystitis is in doubt. Early cholecystectomy is the treatment of choice for most patients with acute cholecystitis. Mortality figures for emergency cholecystectomy in most centers approach 3 percent, while the mortality risk for elective or early cholecystectomy approximates 0.5 percent in patients under age 60. Of course, the operative risks increase with age-related diseases of other organ systems and with the presence of long- or short-term complications of gallbladder disease. Seriously ill or debilitated patients with cholecystitis may be managed with cholecystostomy and tube drainage of the gallbladder. Elective cholecystectomy may then be done at a later date.

Postcholecystectomy Complications   Early complications following cholecystectomy include atelectasis and other pulmonary disorders, abscess formation (often subphrenic), external or internal hemorrhage, biliary-enteric fistula, and bile leaks. Jaundice may indicate absorption of bile from an intraabdominal collection following a biliary leak or mechanical obstruction of the CBD by retained calculi, intraductal blood clots, or extrinsic compression. Routine performance of intraoperative cholangiography during cholecystectomy has helped to reduce the incidence of these early complications.

Overall, cholecystectomy is a very successful operation that provides total or near-total relief of preoperative symptoms in 75 to 90 percent of patients. The most common cause of persistent postcholecystectomy symptoms is an overlooked extrabiliary disorder (e.g., reflux esophagitis, peptic ulceration, postgastrectomy syndrome, pancreatitis, or irritable bowel syndrome). In a small percentage of patients, however, a disorder of the extrahepatic bile ducts may result in persistent symptomatology. These so-called postcholecystectomy syndromes may be due to (1) biliary strictures, (2) retained biliary calculi, (3) cystic duct stump syndrome, (4) stenosis or dyskinesia of the sphincter of Oddi, or (5) bile salt–induced diarrhea or gastritis.

Cystic duct stump syndrome   In the absence of cholangiographically demonstrable retained stones, symptoms resembling biliary colic or cholecystitis in the postcholecystectomy patient have frequently been attributed to disease in a long (>1 cm) cystic duct remnant (cystic duct stump syndrome). Careful analysis, however, reveals that postcholecystectomy complaints are attributable to other causes in almost all patients in whom the symptom complex was originally thought to result from the existence of a long cystic duct stump. Accordingly, considerable care should be taken to investigate the possible role of other factors in the production of postcholecystectomy symptoms before attributing them to cystic duct stump syndrome.

Papillary dysfunction, papillary stenosis, spasm of the sphincter of Oddi, and biliary dyskinesia Symptoms of biliary colic accompanied by signs of recurrent, intermittent biliary obstruction may be produced by papillary stenosis, papillary dysfunction, spasm of the sphincter of Oddi, and biliary dyskinesia. Papillary stenosis is thought to result from acute or chronic inflammation of the papilla of Vater or from glandular hyperplasia of the papillary segment. Five criteria have been used to define papillary stenosis: (1) upper abdominal pain, usually RUQ or epigastric, (2) abnormal liver tests, (3) dilatation of the common bile duct upon ERCP examination, (4) delayed (>45 min) drainage of contrast material from the duct, and (5) increased basal pressure of the sphincter of Oddi, a finding that may be of only minor significance. A useful alternative to ERCP is hepatobiliary scintigraphy using ^{99m}Tc-DIDA, especially if ERCP and/or biliary manometry are either unavailable or not feasible. In patients with papillary stenosis, quantitative hepatobiliary scintigraphy has revealed delayed transit from the common bile duct to the bowel, ductal dilatation, and abnormal time-activity dynamics. This technique also can be used before and after sphincterotomy to document improvement in biliary emptying. Treatment consists of endoscopic or surgical sphincteroplasty to ensure wide patency of the distal portions of both the bile and pancreatic ducts. The greater the number of the preceding criteria present, the greater the likelihood that a patient does have a degree of papillary stenosis sufficient to justify correction. The factors usually considered as indications for sphincterotomy include (1) prolonged duration of symptoms, (2) lack of response to symptomatic treatment, (3) presence of severe disability, and (4) the patient's choice of sphincterotomy over surgery (given a clear understanding on his or her part of the risks involved in both procedures).

Criteria for diagnosing dyskinesia of the sphincter of Oddi are even more controversial than those for papillary stenosis. Proposed mechanisms include spasm of the sphincter, denervation sensitivity resulting in hypertonicity, and abnormalities of the sequencing or frequency rates of sphincteric contraction waves. When thorough evaluation has failed to demonstrate another cause for the pain, and when cholangiographic and manometric criteria suggest a diagnosis of biliary dyskinesia, medical treatment with nitrites or anticholinergics to attempt pharmacologic relaxation of the sphincter has been proposed. Endoscopic sphincterotomy or surgical sphincteroplasty may be indicated in patients who fail to respond to a 2- to 3-month trial of medical therapy, especially if basal sphincter of Oddi pressures are elevated.

Bile salt–induced catharsis and gastritis Postcholecystectomy patients may develop symptoms and signs of gastritis, which has been attributed to duodenogastric reflux of bile. However, firm data linking an increased incidence of bile gastritis with surgical removal of the gallbladder are lacking. Similarly, the occurrence of cholestyramine-responsive diarrhea in a small number of patients following cholecystectomy has been attributed to an alteration of the enterohepatic circulation of bile acids induced or unmasked by removal of the gallbladder.

THE HYPERPLASTIC CHOLECYSTOSES The term *hyperplastic cholecystoses* is used to denote a group of disorders of the gallbladder characterized by excessive proliferation of normal tissue components.

Adenomyomatosis is characterized by a benign proliferation of gallbladder surface epithelium with glandlike formations, extramural sinuses, transverse strictures, and/or fundal nodule ("adenoma" or "adenomyoma") formation. Outpouchings of mucosa termed *Rokitansky-Aschoff sinuses* may be seen on oral cholecystography in conjunction with hyperconcentration of contrast medium. Characteristic dimpled filling defects also may be seen.

Cholesterolosis is characterized by abnormal deposition of lipid, especially cholesterol esters, in the lamina propria of the gallbladder wall. In its diffuse form ("strawberry gallbladder"), the gallbladder mucosa is brick red and speckled with bright yellow flecks of lipid. The localized form shows solitary or multiple "cholesterol polyps" studding the gallbladder wall. Cholesterol stones of the gallbladder are found in nearly half the cases. Cholecystectomy is indicated in both adenomyomatosis and cholesterolosis when symptomatic or when cholelithiasis is present.

DISEASES OF THE BILE DUCTS

CONGENITAL ANOMALIES **Biliary Atresia and Hypoplasia** Atretic and hypoplastic lesions of the extrahepatic and major intrahepatic bile ducts are the most common biliary anomalies of clinical relevance encountered in infancy. The clinical picture is one of severe obstructive jaundice during the first month of life, with pale stools. The diagnosis is confirmed by surgical exploration with operative cholangiography. Approximately 10 percent of cases of biliary atresia are treatable with roux-en-Y choledochojejunostomy, with the Kasai procedure (hepatic portoenterostomy) being attempted in the remainder in an effort to restore some bile flow. Most patients, even those having successful biliary-enteric anastomoses, eventually develop chronic cholangitis, extensive hepatic fibrosis, and portal hypertension.

Choledochal Cysts Cystic dilatation may involve the free portion of the CBD, i.e., choledochal cyst, or may present as diverticulum formation in the intraduodenal segment. In the latter situation, chronic reflux of pancreatic juice into the biliary tree can produce inflammation and stenosis of the extrahepatic bile ducts leading to cholangitis or biliary obstruction. Because the process may be gradual, approximately 50 percent of patients present with onset of symptoms after age 10. The diagnosis may be made by ultrasound, abdominal CT, or cholangiography. Only one-third of patients show the classic triad of abdominal pain, jaundice, and an abdominal mass. Ultrasonographic detection of a cyst separate from the gallbladder should suggest the diagnosis of choledochal cyst, which can be confirmed by demonstrating the entrance of extrahepatic bile ducts into the cyst. Surgical treatment involves excision of the "cyst" and biliary-enteric anastomosis. Patients with choledochal cysts are at increased risk for the subsequent development of cholangiocarcinoma.

Congenital Biliary Ectasia Cystic dilatation of the intrahepatic bile ducts may involve either the major intrahepatic radicles (Caroli's disease), the inter- and intralobular ducts (congenital hepatic fibrosis), or both. In Caroli's disease, clinical manifestations include recurrent cholangitis, abscess formation in and around the affected ducts, and, sometimes, gallstone formation within portions of ectatic intrahepatic biliary radicles. The CT scan and cholangiographic patterns are usually diagnostic, and treatment with ongoing antibiotic therapy is usually undertaken in an effort to limit the frequency and severity of recurrent bouts of cholangitis. Progression to secondary biliary cirrhosis with portal hypertension, amyloidosis, extrahepatic biliary obstruction, cholangiocarcinoma, or recurrent episodes of sepsis with hepatic abscess formation is common.

CHOLEDOCHOLITHIASIS **Pathophysiology and Clinical Manifestations** Passage of gallstones into the CBD occurs in approximately 10 to 15 percent of patients with cholelithiasis. The incidence of common duct stones increases with increasing age of the patient so that up to 25 percent of elderly patients may have calculi in the common duct at the time of cholecystectomy. Undetected duct stones are left behind in approximately 1 to 5 percent of cholecystectomy patients. The overwhelming majority of bile duct stones are cholesterol or mixed stones formed in the gallbladder, which then migrate into the extrahepatic biliary tree through the cystic duct. Primary calculi arising de novo in the ducts are usually pigment stones developing in patients with (1) chronic hemolytic diseases, (2) hepatobiliary parasitism or chronic, recurrent cholangitis, (3) congenital anomalies of the bile ducts (especially Caroli's disease), or (4) dilated, sclerosed, or strictured ducts. Common duct stones may remain asymptomatic for years, may pass spontaneously into the duodenum, or (most often) may present with biliary colic or a complication.

Complications *Cholangitis* Cholangitis may be acute or chronic, and symptoms result from inflammation, which usually requires at least partial obstruction to the flow of bile. Bacteria are present on bile culture in approximately 75 percent of patients with acute cholangitis early in the symptomatic course. The characteristic presentation of acute cholangitis involves biliary colic, jaundice, and spiking fevers with chills (Charcot's triad). Blood cultures are frequently positive, and leukocytosis is typical. *Nonsuppurative* acute cholangitis is most common and may respond relatively rapidly to supportive measures and to treatment with antibiotics. In *suppurative* acute cholangitis, however, the presence of pus under pressure in a completely obstructed ductal system leads to symptoms of severe toxicity—mental confusion, bacteremia, and septic shock. Response to antibiotics alone in this setting is relatively poor, multiple hepatic abscesses are often present, and the mortality rate approaches 100 percent unless prompt surgical correction of the obstructing lesion and drainage of infected bile is carried out. Endoscopic management of bacterial cholangitis is as effective as surgical intervention. ERCP with endoscopic sphincterotomy is safe and the preferred initial procedure for both establishing a definitive diagnosis and providing effective therapy.

Obstructive jaundice Gradual obstruction of the CBD over a period of weeks or months usually leads to initial manifestations of jaundice or pruritus without associated symptoms of biliary colic or cholangitis. Painless jaundice may occur in patients with choledocholithiasis, but this manifestation is much more characteristic of biliary obstruction secondary to malignancy of the head of pancreas, bile ducts, or ampulla of Vater.

In patients whose obstruction is secondary to choledocholithiasis, associated chronic calculous cholecystitis is very common, and the gallbladder in this setting may be relatively indistensible. The absence of a palpable gallbladder in most patients with biliary obstruction from duct stones is the basis for *Courvoisier's law*, i.e., that the presence of a palpably enlarged gallbladder suggests that the biliary obstruction is secondary to an underlying malignancy rather than to calculous disease. Biliary obstruction causes progressive dilatation of the intrahepatic bile ducts as intrabiliary pressures rise. Hepatic bile flow is suppressed, and regurgitation of conjugated bilirubin into the bloodstream leads to jaundice accompanied by dark urine (bilirubinuria) and light-colored (acholic) stools.

CBD stones should be suspected in any patient with cholecystitis whose serum bilirubin level exceeds 85.5 μmol/L (5 mg/dL). The maximum bilirubin level is seldom over 256.5 μmol/L (15.0 mg/dL) in patients with choledocholithiasis unless concomitant hepatic disease or another factor leading to marked hyperbilirubinemia exists. Serum bilirubin levels of 342.0 μmol/L (20 mg/dL) or more should suggest the possibility of neoplastic obstruction. The serum alkaline phosphatase level is almost always elevated in biliary obstruction. A rise in alkaline phosphatase often precedes clinical jaundice and may be the only abnormality in routine liver function tests. There may be a two- to tenfold elevation of serum aminotransferases, especially in association with acute obstruction. Following relief of the obstructing process, serum aminotransferase elevations usually return rapidly to normal, while the serum bilirubin level may take 1 to 2 weeks to return to normal. The alkaline phosphatase level usually falls slowly, lagging behind the decrease in serum bilirubin.

Pancreatitis The most common associated entity discovered in patients with nonalcoholic acute pancreatitis is biliary tract disease. Biochemical evidence of pancreatic inflammation complicates acute cholecystitis in 15 percent of cases and choledocholithiasis in over 30 percent, and the common factor appears to be the passage of gallstones through the common duct. Coexisting pancreatitis should be suspected in patients with symptoms of cholecystitis who develop (1) back pain or pain to the left of the abdominal midline, (2) prolonged vomiting with paralytic ileus, or (3) a pleural effusion, especially on the left side. Surgical treatment of gallstone disease is usually associated with resolution of the pancreatitis.

Secondary biliary cirrhosis Secondary biliary cirrhosis may complicate prolonged or intermittent duct obstruction with or without recurrent cholangitis. Although this complication may be seen in patients with choledocholithiasis, it is more common in cases of prolonged obstruction from stricture or neoplasm. Once established, secondary biliary cirrhosis may be progressive even after correction of the obstructing process, and increasingly severe hepatic cirrhosis may lead to portal hypertension or to hepatic failure and death. Prolonged biliary obstruction also may be associated with clinically relevant deficiencies of the fat-soluble vitamins A, D, and K.

Diagnosis and Treatment The diagnosis of choledocholithiasis is usually made by cholangiography (Table 302-3), either preoperatively by ERCP or intraoperatively at the time of cholecystectomy. As many as 20 percent of patients undergoing cholecystectomy will prove to have CBD stones. With the advent of laparoscopic cholecystectomy, the management of CBD stones in the presence of gallstones is gradually being clarified. Preoperative ERCP with endoscopic papillotomy and stone extraction is the preferred approach. It not only provides stone clearance but also defines the anatomy of the biliary tree in relationship to the cystic duct. ERCP is indicated in gallstone patients who have any of the following risk factors: (1) a history of jaundice or pancreatitis, (2) abnormal tests of liver function, and (3) ultrasonographic evidence of a dilated CBD or stones in the duct. Alternatively, if routine cholangiography of the cystic duct reveals retained stones, postoperative ERCP can be carried out. The need for preoperative ERCP is expected to decrease further as laparoscopic techniques improve.

The widespread use of laparoscopic cholecystectomy and ERCP has decreased the incidence of complicated biliary tract disease and the need for choledocholithotomy and T-tube drainage of the bile ducts. Endoscopic sphincterotomy followed by spontaneous passage or stone extraction is a nonoperative alternative in the management of patients with common duct stones, especially in elderly or poor-risk patients.

TRAUMA, STRICTURES, AND HEMOBILIA Benign strictures of the extrahepatic bile ducts result from surgical trauma in approximately 95 percent of cases and occur in about 1 in 500 cholecystectomies. Strictures may present with bile leak or abscess formation in the immediate postoperative period or with biliary obstruction or cholangitis as long as 2 years or more following the inciting trauma. The diagnosis is established by percutaneous or endoscopic cholangiography. Endoscopic brushing of biliary strictures is an effective way to establish the nature of the lesion and is more accurate than bile cytology alone. When positive exfoliative cytology is obtained, the diagnosis of a neoplastic stricture is established. This procedure is especially important in patients with primary sclerosing cholangitis who are predisposed to the development of cholangiocarcinomas. Successful operative correction by a skilful surgeon with duct-to-bowel anastomosis is usually possible, although mortality rates from surgical complications, recurrent cholangitis, or secondary biliary cirrhosis are high.

Hemobilia may follow traumatic or operative injury to the liver or bile ducts, intraductal rupture of a hepatic abscess or aneurysm of the hepatic artery, biliary or hepatic tumor hemorrhage, or mechanical complications of choledocholithiasis or hepatobiliary parasitism. Diagnostic procedures such as liver biopsy, percutaneous transhepatic cholangiography (PTHC), and transhepatic biliary drainage catheter placement also may be complicated by hemobilia. Patients often present with a classic triad of biliary colic, obstructive jaundice, and melena or occult blood in the stools. The diagnosis is sometimes made by cholangiographic evidence of blood clot in the biliary tree, but selective angiographic verification may be required. Although minor episodes of hemobilia may resolve without operative intervention, surgical ligation of the bleeding vessel is frequently required.

EXTRINSIC COMPRESSION OF THE BILE DUCTS Partial or complete biliary obstruction may sometimes be produced by extrinsic compression of the ducts. The most common cause of this form of obstructive jaundice is carcinoma of the head of the pancreas. Biliary obstruction also may occur as a complication of either acute or chronic pancreatitis or involvement of lymph nodes in the porta hepatis by lymphoma or metastatic carcinoma. The latter should be distinguished from cholestasis resulting from massive replacement of the liver by tumor.

Table 302-3

Diagnostic Evaluation of the Bile Ducts

Diagnostic Advantages	Diagnostic Limitations	Contraindications	Complications	Comment
HEPATOBILIARY ULTRASOUND				
Rapid Simultaneous scanning of GB, liver, bile ducts, pancreas Accurate identification of dilated bile ducts Not limited by jaundice, pregnancy Guidance for fine-needle biopsy	Bowel gas Massive obesity Ascites Barium Partial bile duct obstruction Poor visualization of distal CBD	None	None	Initial procedure of choice in investigating possible biliary tract obstruction
COMPUTED TOMOGRAPHY				
Simultaneous scanning of GB, liver, bile ducts, pancreas Accurate identification of dilated bile ducts, masses Not limited by jaundice, gas, obesity, ascites High-resolution image Guidance for fine-needle biopsy	Extreme cachexia Movement artifact Ileus Partial bile duct obstruction High cost May not be readily available	Pregnancy	Reaction to iodinated contrast, if used	Indicated for evaluation of hepatic or pancreatic masses Procedure of choice in investigating possible biliary obstruction if diagnostic limitations prevent HBUS
MAGNETIC RESONANCE CHOLANGIOPANCREATOGRAPHY				
Useful modality for visualizing pancreatic and biliary ducts Can identify pancreatic duct dilatation or stricture, pancreatic duct stenosis, and pancreas divisum Has excellent sensitivity for bile duct dilatation, biliary stricture, and intraductal abnormalities	Cannot offer therapeutic intervention			
PERCUTANEOUS TRANSHEPATIC CHOLANGIOGRAM				
Extremely successful when bile ducts dilated Best visualization of proximal biliary tract Possible separate visualization of obstructed left ductal system Bile cytology/culture Percutaneous transhepatic drainage	Nondilated or sclerosed ducts	Pregnancy Uncorrectable coagulopathy Massive ascites ? Hepatic abscess	Bleeding Hemobilia Bile peritonitis Bacteremia, sepsis	Usually, initial cholangiogram of choice when bile ducts are dilated
ENDOSCOPIC RETROGRADE CHOLANGIOPANCREATOGRAM				

Simultaneous pancreatography
Visualization/biopsy of ampulla and duodenum
Best visualization of distal biliary tract
Bile or pancreatic cytology
Endoscopic sphincterotomy and stone removal
Biliary manometry
Not limited by ascites, coagulopathy, abscess
	Gastroduodenal obstruction
	? Roux en Y biliary-enteric anastomosis
		Pregnancy
		? Acute pancreatitis
		? Severe cardiopulmonary disease
			Pancreatitis
			Cholangitis, sepsis
			Infected pancreatic pseudocyst
			Perforation (rare)
			Hypoxemia, aspiration
				Cholangiogram of choice in:
				  Absence of dilated ducts
				  ? Pancreatic, ampullary or gastroduodenal disease
				  Prior biliary surgery
				  PTHC contraindicated or failed
				Endoscopic sphincterotomy a treatment possibility

NOTE: GB, gallbladder; HBUS, hepatobiliary ultrasound. Intravenous cholangiography is an obsolete technique because 40 percent of common duct stones are missed and there is poor resolution even with tomography. There are few indications for its use, especially since other cholangiographic techniques are usually available.

HEPATOBILIARY PARASITISM Infestation of the biliary tract by adult helminths or their ova may produce a chronic, recurrent pyogenic cholangitis with or without multiple hepatic abscesses, ductal stones, or biliary obstruction. This condition is relatively rare but does occur in inhabitants of southern China and elsewhere in Southeast Asia. The organisms most commonly involved are trematodes or flukes, including *Clonorchis sinensis*, *Opisthorchis viverrini* or *Opisthorchis felineus*, and *Fasciola hepatica*. The biliary tract also may be involved by intraductal migration of adult *Ascaris lumbricoides* from the duodenum or by intrabiliary rupture of hydatid cysts of the liver produced by *Echinococcus* species. The diagnosis is made by cholangiography and the presence of characteristic ova on stool examination. When obstruction is present, the treatment of choice is laparotomy under antibiotic coverage, with common duct exploration and a biliary drainage procedure. It should be emphasized that in the Orient, one also sees cholangiohepatitis associated with pigment lithiasis, which may, in fact, be more common than cholangitis due to parasites.

SCLEROSING CHOLANGITIS Primary or idiopathic sclerosing cholangitis is a disorder characterized by a progressive, inflammatory, sclerosing, and obliterative process affecting the extrahepatic and, often, the intrahepatic bile ducts. The lesion may appear as an isolated entity or may occur in association with inflammatory bowel disease, especially ulcerative colitis, or with multifocal fibrosclerosis syndromes such as retroperitoneal, mediastinal, and/or periureteral fibrosis; Riedel's struma; or pseudotumor of the orbit. In patients with AIDS, cholangiopancreatography may demonstrate a broad range of biliary tract changes as well as pancreatic duct obstruction and occasionally pancreatitis (see Chap. 308). Further, biliary tract lesions in AIDS include infection and cholangiopancreatographic changes similar to primary sclerosing cholangitis. Changes noted include: (1) diffuse involvement of intrahepatic bile ducts alone, (2) involvement of both intra- and extrahepatic bile ducts, (3) ampullary stenosis, (4) stricture of the intrapancreatic portion of the common bile duct, and (5) pancreatic duct involvement. Associated infectious organisms include *Cryptosporidium*, *Mycobacterium avium-intracellulare*, cytomegalovirus, *Microsporidia*, and *Isospora*. In addition, acalculous cholecystitis occurs in up to 10 percent of patients. ERCP sphincterotomy, while not without risk, provides significant pain reduction in patients with AIDS-associated papillary stenosis. Secondary sclerosing cholangitis may occur as a long-term complication of choledocholithiasis, cholangiocarcinoma, operative or traumatic biliary injury, or contiguous inflammatory processes.

Patients with primary sclerosing cholangitis often present with signs and symptoms of chronic or intermittent biliary obstruction: jaundice, pruritus, RUQ abdominal pain, or acute cholangitis. Late in the course, complete biliary obstruction, secondary biliary cirrhosis, hepatic failure, or portal hypertension with bleeding varices may occur. The diagnosis is usually established by finding thickened ducts with narrow, beaded lumina on cholangiography (see Fig. 302-2*D*). The cholangiographic technique of choice in suspected cases is probably ERCP, since intrahepatic ductal involvement may make PTHC difficult. When a diagnosis of sclerosing cholangitis has been established, a search for associated diseases, especially for chronic inflammatory bowel disease, should be carried out.

 TREATMENT
Therapy with cholestyramine may help control symptoms of pruritus, and antibiotics are useful when cholangitis complicates the clinical picture. Vitamin D and calcium supplementation may help prevent the loss of bone mass frequently seen in patients with chronic cholestasis. Glucocorticoids, UDCA, methotrexate, and cyclosporine have not been shown to be efficacious. In cases where complete or high-grade biliary obstruction has occurred, balloon dilatation or surgical intervention may be appropriate. Efforts at biliary-enteric anastomosis or stent placement may, however, be complicated by recurrent cholangitis and further progression of the stenosing process. The role of colectomy in patients with sclerosing cholangitis complicating chronic ulcerative colitis is uncertain. The prognosis is unfavorable, with a mean survival of 4 to 10 years following the diagnosis, regardless of therapy. Four variables (age, serum bilirubin level, histologic stage, and splenomegaly) predict survival in patients with primary sclerosing cholangitis and serve as the basis for a risk score. Primary sclerosing cholangitis is one of the most common indications for liver transplantation. In one study, the mean follow-up time from the diagnosis of primary sclerosing cholangitis to the time of liver transplantation was 5.8 years.

BIBLIOGRAPHY

ABEI M et al: Isolation and characterization of a cholesterol crystallization promoter from human bile. Gastroenterology 104:539, 1993

BARKUN JS et al: Randomised controlled trial of laparoscopic versus mini cholecystomy. Lancet 340:1116, 1992

CAREY MC et al: Whither biliary sludge? Gastroenterology 95:508, 1988

DICKSON ER: Primary sclerosing cholangitis: Refinement and validation of survival models. Gastroenterology 103:1893, 1992

EVERSON GT: Pregnancy and gallstones. Hepatology 17:160, 1993

GEENEN JE et al: The efficacy of endoscopic sphincterotomy after cholecystectomy in patients with sphincter-of-Oddi dysfunction. N Engl J Med 320:82, 1989

GRACIE WA, RANSOHOFF DF: The natural history of silent gallstones. The innocent gallstone is not a myth. N Engl J Med 307:798, 1982

JOHNSTON DE, KAPLAN MM: Medical progress: Pathogenesis and treatment of gallstones. N Engl J Med 328:412, 1993

LEE SP et al: Origin and fate of biliary sludge. Gastroenterology 94:170, 1988

MARINGHINI A et al: Gallstones, gallbladder cancer, and other gastrointestinal malignancies: An epidemiologic study in Rochester, Minnesota. Ann Intern Med 107:30, 1987

MEYERS WC: A prospective analysis of 1518 laparoscopic cholecystectomies. N Engl J Med 324:1073, 1991

PAUMGARTNER G et al: Gallstones: Pathogenesis. Lancet 338:1117, 1991

PODDA M et al: Efficacy and safety of a combination of dienodeoxycholic acid and ursodeoxycholic acid for gallstone dissolution. Gastroenterology 96:222, 1989

PORAYKO MK et al: Patients with asymptomatic primary sclerosing cholangitis frequently have progressive disease. Gastroenterology 98:1594, 1990

SHAFFER EA et al: Cholescintigraphic detection of functional obstruction of the sphincter of Oddi: Effect of papillotomy. Gastroenterology 90:728, 1986

SHIFFMAN M et al: Prophylaxis against gallstone formation with ursodeoxycholic acid in patients. Ann Intern Med 122:999, 1995

SOTO JA et al: Magnetic resonance cholangiography: Comparison with endoscopic retrograde cholangiopancreatography. Gastroenterology 110:598, 1996

WIESNER RH et al: Comparison of clinicopathologic features of primary sclerosing cholangitis and primary biliary cirrhosis. Gastroenterology 88:108, 1985

YAP L et al: Acalculous biliary pain: Cholecystectomy alleviates symptoms in patients with abnormal cholescintigraphy. Gastroenterology 101:786, 1991

303

Phillip P. Toskes, Norton J. Greenberger

APPROACH TO THE PATIENT WITH PANCREATIC DISEASE

GENERAL CONSIDERATIONS

Inflammatory disease of the pancreas may be acute or chronic. Although good data exist concerning the frequency of acute pancreatitis (about 5000 new cases per year in the United States, with a mortality rate of about 10 percent), the number of patients who suffer with recurrent acute pancreatitis or chronic pancreatitis is largely undefined. Only one prospective study on the incidence of chronic pancreatitis is available; it showed an incidence of 8.2 new cases per 100,000 per year and a prevalence of 26.4 cases per 100,000. These numbers probably underestimate considerably the true incidence and prevalence, since non-alcohol-induced pancreatitis was largely ignored. At autopsy, the prevalence of chronic pancreatitis ranges from 0.04 to 5 percent. The relative inaccessibility of the pancreas to direct examination and the nonspecificity of the abdominal pain associated with pancreatitis make the diagnosis of pancreatitis difficult and usually dependent on elevation of blood amylase levels. Many patients with chronic pancreatitis do not have elevated blood amylase levels. Some patients with chronic pancreatitis develop signs and symptoms of pancreatic exocrine insufficiency, and thus objective evidence for pancreatic disease can be demonstrated. However, there is a very large reservoir of pancreatic exocrine function. More than 90 percent of the pancreas must be damaged before maldigestion of fat and protein is manifested. Even the secretin stimulation test, which is the most sensitive method of assessing pancreatic exocrine function, is probably abnormal only when more than 60 percent of exocrine function has been lost. Noninvasive, indirect tests of pancreatic exocrine function (bentiromide, serum trypsinogen) are much more likely to give abnormal results in patients with obvious pancreatic disease, i.e., pancreatic calcification, steatorrhea, or diabetes mellitus, than in patients with occult disease. Thus, the number of patients who have subclinical exocrine dysfunction (less than 90 percent loss of function) is unknown.

The clinical manifestations of acute and chronic pancreatitis and pancreatic insufficiency are protean. Thus, patients may present with hypertriglyceridemia, vitamin B_{12} malabsorption, hypercalcemia, hypocalcemia, hyperglycemia, ascites, pleural effusions, and chronic abdominal pain with normal blood amylase levels. Indeed, if the clinician considers pancreatitis as a possible diagnosis only when presented with a patient having classic symptoms (i.e., severe, constant epigastric pain that radiates through to the back, along with an elevated blood amylase level), only a minority of patients with pancreatitis will be diagnosed correctly.

As emphasized in Chap. 304, the etiologies as well as the clinical manifestations of pancreatitis are quite varied. Although it is well appreciated that pancreatitis is frequently secondary to alcohol abuse and biliary tract disease, it can also be caused by drugs, trauma, and viral infections and is associated with metabolic and connective tissue disorders. In approximately 30 percent of patients with acute pancreatitis and 25 to 40 percent of patients with chronic pancreatitis, the etiology is obscure.

TESTS USEFUL IN THE DIAGNOSIS OF PANCREATIC DISEASE

Several tests have proved of value in the evaluation of pancreatic exocrine function. Examples of specific tests and their usefulness in the diagnosis of acute and chronic pancreatitis are summarized in Table 303-1. At most institutions, pancreatic function tests are performed if the diagnosis of pancreatic disease remains a possibility after noninvasive tests [ultrasound, computed tomography (CT)] and invasive tests [endoscopic retrograde cholangiopancreatography (ERCP)] have given normal or inconclusive results. In this regard, tests employing *direct* stimulation of the pancreas are the most sensitive.

PANCREATIC ENZYMES IN BODY FLUIDS The serum amylase level is widely used as a screening test for acute pancreatitis in the patient with acute abdominal pain or back pain. A value greater than 65 U/L should raise the question of acute pancreatitis. Levels greater than 130 U/L make the diagnosis more likely, and values greater than three times normal virtually clinch the diagnosis if gut perforation or infarction is excluded. In acute pancreatitis, the serum amylase is usually elevated within 24 h of onset and remains so for 1 to 3 days. Levels return to normal within 3 to 5 days unless there is extensive pancreatic necrosis, incomplete ductal obstruction, or pseudocyst formation. Approximately 85 percent of patients with acute pancreatitis will have an elevated serum amylase level. This index may be normal, however, if (1) there is a delay (of 2 to 5 days) before blood samples are obtained, (2) the underlying disorder is chronic pancreatitis rather than acute pancreatitis, or (3) hypertriglyceridemia is present. Patients with hypertriglyceridemia and proven pancreatitis have been found to have spuriously low levels of amylase and lipase activity.

The serum amylase is often elevated in other conditions (Table 303-2), in part because the enzyme is found in many organs in addition to the pancreas (salivary glands, liver, small intestine, kidney, fallopian tube) and can be produced by various tumors (carcinomas of the lung, esophagus, breast, and ovary). Isoenzymes of amylase fall into two general categories: those arising from the pancreas (P isoamylases) and those arising from nonpancreatic sources (S isoamylases). The measurement of serum isoamylases is of clinical importance. In normal serum, about 35 to 45 percent of the amylase is of pancreatic origin. For example, in patients with acute pancreatitis, the total serum amylase level returns to normal more rapidly than the level of pancreatic isoamylase. Thus, in patients seen after the first day, the pancreatic isoamylase level is a more sensitive indicator of pancreatitis than the total serum amylase level. In the past, elevations in serum amylase seen in certain conditions, such as the postoperative state, acute alcohol intoxication, and diabetic ketoacidosis, were assumed to indicate acute pancreatitis. However, the elevation of serum amylase in such conditions has been shown to be due to an elevation of the S isoamylase. Simple tests to distinguish pancreatic from nonpancreatic amylase are no longer readily available, and such tests are often not reliable when the total amylase is minimally to moderately elevated. An assay of serum trypsinogen (performed by several commercial laboratories) is quite helpful in this regard. Since this enzyme is secreted specifically by the pancreas, a normal serum trypsinogen level in a patient with minimal elevation of serum amylase essentially rules out acute pancreatitis. Urinary amylase measurements, including the amylase/creatinine clearance ratio, are no more sensitive or specific than blood amylase levels.

Elevation of ascitic fluid amylase occurs in acute pancreatitis as well as in (1) pancreatogenous ascites due to disruption of the main pancreatic duct of a leaking pseudocyst and (2) other abdominal disorders that simulate pancreatitis (e.g., intestinal obstruction, intestinal infarction, and perforated peptic ulcer). Elevation of pleural fluid amylase occurs in acute pancreatitis, chronic pancreatitis, carcinoma of the lung, and esophageal perforation.

Lipase may now be the single best enzyme to measure for the diagnosis of acute pancreatitis. Improvements in substrates and technology offer clinicians improved options, especially when a turbidometric assay is used. The newer lipase assays have colipase as a cofactor and are fully automated.

An assay for trypsinogen (or for trypsin-like immunoreactivity) has a theoretical advantage over amylase and lipase determinations

Table 303-1

Tests Useful in the Diagnosis of Acute and Chronic Pancreatitis and Pancreatic Tumors

Test	Principle	Comment
PANCREATIC ENZYMES IN BODY FLUIDS		
Amylase		
1. Serum	Pancreatic inflammation leads to increased enzyme levels	Simple; 20–40% false negatives and positives; reliable if test results are three times the upper limit of normal
2. Urine	Renal clearance of amylase is increased in acute pancreatitis	May be abnormal when serum levels normal; false negatives and positives
3. Amylase/creatinine clearance ratio (C_{am}/C_{cr})	Renal clearance of amylase greater than clearance of creatinine	No more sensitive than serum amylase; many false positives
4. Ascitic fluid	Disruption of gland or main pancreatic duct leads to increased amylase concentration	Can establish diagnosis of pancreatitis; false positives occur with intestinal obstruction and perforated ulcer
5. Pleural fluid	Exudative pleural effusion with pancreatitis	False positives occur with carcinoma of the lung and esophageal perforation
6. Isoenzymes	P isoamylases arise from the pancreas; S isoamylases are from other sources	More sensitive than total serum amylase in diagnosis of acute pancreatitis; useful in identifying non-pancreatic causes of hyperamylasemia
Serum lipase	Pancreatic inflammation leads to increased enzyme levels	New methods have greatly simplified determination; positive in 70–85% of cases.
Serum trypsin-like immunoreactivity (TLI)	Pancreatic inflammation leads to increased levels	*Elevated* in acute pancreatitis; *decreased* in chronic pancreatitis *with* steatorrhea; normal in chronic pancreatitis *without* steatorrhea and in steatorrhea with normal pancreatic function
Pancreatic polypeptide (PP)	PP confined almost totally to the pancreas; release stimulated by nutrients and hormones; such release parallels pancreatic enzyme secretion	Basal, meal-simulated, and hormone-stimulated (by secretin or CCK) PP levels *decreased* in chronic pancreatitis; a fasting PP level >125 pg/mL argues against chronic pancreatitis and pancreatic cancer
STUDIES PERTAINING TO PANCREATIC STRUCTURE		
Radiologic and radionuclide tests		
1. Plain film of the abdomen	Abnormal in acute and chronic pancreatitis	Simple; normal in >50% of cases of both acute and chronic pancreatitis
2. Upper gastrointestinal x-rays	Abnormally thickened duodenal folds; displacement of stomach or widening of duodenal loop suggests a pancreatic mass (inflammatory, neoplastic, cystic)	Simple; frequently normal; largely superseded by US and CT scanning
3. Ultrasonography (US)	Can provide information on edema, inflammation, calcification, pseudocysts, and mass lesions	Simple, noninvasive; sequential studies quite feasible; useful in diagnosis of pseudocyst
4. CT scan	Permits detailed visualization of pancreas and surrounding structures	Useful in the diagnosis of pancreatic calcification, dilated pancreatic ducts, and pancreatic tumors; may not be able to distinguish between inflammatory and neoplastic mass lesions
5. Selective angiography	Can identify pancreatic neoplasms (1) by sheathing of celiac or superior mesenteric branches by tumor or (2) by tumor staining; displacement of vessels by tumor	Indicated (1) in suspected islet cell tumors and (2) prior to pancreatic or duodenal resection; most reliable features reflect nonresectable pancreatic cancer
6. Endoscopic retrograde cholangiopancreatography (ERCP)	Cannulation of pancreatic and common bile duct permits visualization of pancreatic-biliary ductal system	Provides diagnostic data in 60–85% of cases; differentiation of chronic pancreatitis from pancreatic carcinoma may be difficult
Pancreatic biopsy with US or CT guidance	Percutaneous biopsy with skinny needle and localization of lesion by US	High diagnostic yield; laparotomy avoided; requires special technical skills
TESTS OF EXOCRINE PANCREATIC FUNCTION		
Direct stimulation of the pancreas with analysis of duodenal contents		
1. Secretin-pancreozymin (CCK) test	Secretin leads to increased output of pancreatic juice and HCO_3^-; CCK leads to increased output of pancreatic enzymes; pancreatic secretory response is related to the functional mass of pancreatic tissue	Sensitive enough to detect occult disease; involves duodenal intubation and fluoroscopy; poorly defined normal enzyme response; overlap in chronic pancreatitis; large secretory reserve capacity of the pancreas
Indirect stimulation of pancreas with measurement of pancreatic enzymes		
1. Lundh test meal	Test meal (fat, carbohydrate, and protein) causes increased release of CCK, which causes increased enzyme output; trypsin concentration measured	Useful in pancreatic exocrine insufficiency; false negatives with delayed gastric emptying; false positives in primary mucosal disease of the gut and choledocholithiasis; does not measure secretory capacity
2. Benzoyl-tyrosyl-*p*-aminobenzoic acid (Bz-Ty-PABA, bentiromide) test	Synthetic peptide (Bz-Ty-PABA) is specifically cleaved by chymotrypsin, liberating PABA, which is absorbed; PABA metabolite is excreted in the urine	Simple and reliable test of pancreatic exocrine function. Measurement of blood PABA level increases sensitivity.

(continued)

Table 303-1—(Continued)

Tests Useful in the Diagnosis of Acute and Chronic Pancreatitis and Pancreatic Tumors

Test	Principle	Comment
3. Pancreolauryl test	Fluorescein dilaurate is hydrolyzed by pancreatic elastase and absorbed; fluorescein is measured in urine	Sensitivity and specificity similar to those of Bentiromide test
Measurement of intraluminal digestion products		
1. Microscopic examination of stool for undigested meat fibers and fat	Lack of proteolytic and lipolytic enzymes causes decreased digestion of meat fibers and triglycerides	Simple, reliable; not sensitive enough to detect milder cases of pancreatic insufficiency
2. Quantitative stool fat determination	Lack of lipolytic enzymes brings about impaired fat digestion	Reliable, reference standard for defining severity of malabsorption; does not distinguish between maldigestion and malabsorption
3. Fecal nitrogen	Lack of proteolytic enzymes leads to impaired protein digestion, resulting in an increase in stool nitrogen	Does not distinguish between maldigestion and malabsorption; low sensitivity
Measurement of pancreatic enzymes in feces		
1. Chymotrypsin	Pancreatic secretion of proteolytic enzymes	May be useful in cystic fibrosis; tedious; 10% false-positive and false-negative results
Miscellaneous tests		
1. Dual-labeled Schilling test	Intrinsic factor [^{57}Co]cobalamin and Hog R protein [^{58}Co]cobalamin are given together. Since proteases are necessary to cleave R protein, the ratio of labeled cobalamin excreted in urine is an index of exocrine dysfunction.	Time-consuming and expensive

in that the pancreas is the only organ that contains this enzyme. The test appears to be useful in the diagnosis of both acute and chronic pancreatitis. Sensitivity and specificity are comparable to those of amylase and lipase determinations. Since trypsinogen is also excreted by the kidney, elevated serum values are found in renal failure, as is the case with serum amylase and lipase levels. *No single blood test is reliable for the diagnosis of acute pancreatitis in patients with renal failure.* Determinating whether a patient with renal failure and abdominal pain has pancreatitis remains a difficult clinical problem. A recent study found that serum amylase levels were elevated in patients with renal dysfunction only when creatinine clearance was less than 50 mL/min. In such patients, the serum amylase level was invariably less than 500 IU/L in the absence of objective evidence of acute pancreatitis. In that study, serum lipase and trypsin levels paralleled serum amylase values.

A recent study evaluated the sensitivity and specificity of five assays used to diagnose acute pancreatitis: two for amylase, one for lipase, one for trypsin-like immunoreactivity (TLI), and one for pancreatic isoamylase. The data obtained (1) show that, if the best cutoff level is used, all these assays have similar specificities and (2) suggest that total serum amylase is as good an indicator of acute pancreatitis as any of the alternatives. However, inherent in many such studies is the problem that the recognition and diagnosis of acute pancreatitis hinge on the finding of an elevated serum amylase level. The question arises as to whether any diagnostic test result can be proved superior to the total serum amylase level if hyperamylasemia is required for the diagnosis. In other studies, when "objective" confirmation of the clinical diagnosis of pancreatitis was required (ultrasonography, CT, laparotomy), the sensitivity of the serum amylase has been found to be as low as 68 percent. With these limitations in mind, the recommended screening tests for acute pancreatitis are *total serum amylase* and *serum lipase activities.* Serum amylase values greater than three times normal are highly specific.

STUDIES PERTAINING TO PANCREATIC STRUCTURE **Radiologic Tests** Plain films of the abdomen provide useful information in 30 to 50 percent of patients with acute pancreatitis. The most frequent abnormalities include (1) a localized ileus, usually involving the jejunum ("sentinel loop"), (2) a generalized ileus with air-fluid levels, (3) the "colon cutoff sign," which results from isolated distention of the transverse colon, (4) duodenal distention with air-fluid levels, and (5) a mass, which is frequently a pseudocyst. In chronic pancreatitis, an important radiographic finding is pancreatic calcification, which characteristically is localized adjacent to and superimposed on the second lumbar vertebra (see Fig. 304-3*A*).

Upper gastrointestinal x-rays may reveal displacement of the stomach by the retroperitoneal mass (see Fig. 304-2*A*) or widening and effacement of the duodenal C loop, which also suggest the presence of a pancreatic mass, which could be inflammatory, cystic, or neoplastic. However, the use of x-ray films has been largely superseded by ultrasound.

Ultrasonography can provide important information in patients with acute pancreatitis, chronic pancreatitis, pancreatic calcification, pseudocyst, and pancreatic carcinoma. Echographic appearances can indicate the presence of edema, inflammation, and calcification (not

Table 303-2

Causes of Hyperamylasemia and Hyperamylasuria

PANCREATIC DISEASE

I. Pancreatitis
  A. Acute
  B. Chronic: ductal obstruction
  C. Complications of pancreatitis
    1. Pancreatic pseudocyst
    2. Pancreatogenous ascites
    3. Pancreatic abscess
II. Pancreatic trauma
III. Pancreatic carcinoma

NONPANCREATIC DISORDERS

I. Renal insufficiency
II. Salivary gland lesions
  A. Mumps
  B. Calculus
  C. Irradiation sialadenitis
  D. Maxillofacial surgery
III. "Tumor" hyperamylasemia
  A. Carcinoma of the lung
  B. Carcinoma of the esophagus
  C. Breast carcinoma, ovarian carcinoma
IV. Macroamylasemia
V. Burns
VI. Diabetic ketoacidosis
VII. Pregnancy
VIII. Renal transplantation
IX. Cerebral trauma
X. Drugs: morphine

OTHER ABDOMINAL DISORDERS

I. Biliary tract disease: cholecystitis, choledocholithiasis
II. Intraabdominal disease
  A. Perforated or penetrating peptic ulcer
  B. Intestinal obstruction or infarction
  C. Ruptured ectopic pregnancy
  D. Peritonitis
  E. Aortic aneurysm
  F. Chronic liver disease
  G. Postoperative hyperamylasemia

obvious on plain films of the abdomen), as well as pseudocysts, mass lesions, and gallstones (see Figs. 304-2*B* and 304-3*B*). In acute pancreatitis, the pancreas is characteristically enlarged. In pancreatic pseudocyst, the usual appearance is that of an echo-free, smooth, round fluid collection. Pancreatic carcinoma distorts the usual landmarks, and mass lesions greater than 3.0 cm are usually detected as localized, echo-free solid lesions. Ultrasound is often the initial investigation for most patients with suspected pancreatic disease. However, obesity, excess small- and large-bowel gas, and recently performed barium contrast examinations can interfere with ultrasound studies.

CT is the best imaging study for initial evaluation of a suspected chronic pancreatic disorder and for the complications of acute and chronic pancreatitis. It is especially useful in the detection of pancreatic tumors, fluid-containing lesions such as pseudocysts and abscesses, and calcium deposits (see Figs. 304-3*C* and 304-4*A*). Most lesions are characterized by (1) enlargement of the pancreatic outline, (2) distortion of the pancreatic contour, and/or (3) a fluid filling that has a different attenuation coefficient than normal pancreas. However, it is occasionally difficult to distinguish between inflammatory and neoplastic lesions. Oral water-soluble contrast agents may be used to opacify the stomach and duodenum during CT scans; this strategy permits more precise delineation of various organs as well as mass lesions. Dynamic CT (using rapid intravenous administration of contrast)is useful in estimating the degree of pancreatic necrosis and in predicting morbidity and mortality. Spiral (helical) CT provides clear images much more rapidly and essentially negates artifact caused by patient movement (Fig. 304-2*D*).

Selective catheterization of the celiac and superior mesenteric arteries combined with superselective catheterization of others arteries, such as the hepatic, splenic, and gastroduodenal arteries permits visualization of the pancreas and detection of pancreatic neoplasms and pseudocysts. Pancreatic neoplasms can be identified by the sheathing of blood vessels by a mass lesion (see Fig. 304-1*D*). Hormone-producing pancreatic tumors are especially likely to exhibit increased vascularity and tumor staining. Angiographic abnormalities are noted in many patients with pancreatic carcinoma but are uncommon in patients without pancreatic disease. Angiography complements ultrasonography and ERCP in the study of patients with a suspected pancreatic lesion and may be carried out if ERCP is either unsuccessful or nondiagnostic. The recently introduced technique of *magnetic resonance cholangiopancreatography* (MRCP) appears to be of value under these conditions.

ERCP may provide useful information on the status of the pancreatic ductal system and thus aid in the differential diagnosis of pancreatic disease (see Figs. 304-1*C*, 304-3*D*, and 304-4*B*). Pancreatic carcinoma is characterized by stenosis or obstruction of either the pancreatic duct or the common bile duct; both ductal systems are often abnormal. In chronic pancreatitis, ERCP abnormalities include (1) luminal narrowing, (2) irregularities in the ductal system with stenosis, dilation, sacculation, and ectasia, and (3) blockage of the pancreatic duct by calcium deposits. The presence of ductal stenosis and irregularity can make it difficult to distinguish chronic pancreatitis from carcinoma. It is important to be aware that ERCP changes interpreted as indicating chronic pancreatitis actually may be due to the effects of aging on the pancreatic duct or to the fact that the procedure was performed within several weeks of an attack of acute pancreatitis. Although aging may cause impressive ductal alterations, it does not affect the results of pancreatic function tests (i.e., the secretin test). Elevated serum and/or urine amylase levels following ERCP have been reported in 25 to 75 percent of patients, but clinical pancreatitis is uncommon. In a series of 300 patients, pancreatitis occurred in only 5 patients following ERCP. If no lesion is found in the biliary and/or pancreatic ducts in a patient with repeated attacks of acute pancreatitis, manometric studies of the sphincter of Oddi may be indicated. Such studies, however, do increase the risk of post-ERCP/manometry acute pancreatitis. Such pancreatitis appears to be more common in patients with a nondilated pancreatic duct.

Pancreatic Biopsy with Radiologic Guidance Percutaneous aspiration biopsy of a pancreatic mass often distinguishes a pancreatic inflammatory mass from a pancreatic neoplasm.

TESTS OF EXOCRINE PANCREATIC FUNCTION

Pancreatic function tests (Table 303-1) can be divided into the following:

1. *Direct stimulation of the pancreas* by intravenous infusion of secretin or secretin plus cholecystokinin (CCK) followed by collection and measurement of duodenal contents
2. *Indirect stimulation of the pancreas* using nutrients or amino acids, fatty acids, and synthetic peptides followed by assays of proteolytic, lipolytic, and amylolytic enzymes
3. Study of *intraluminal digestion products,* such as undigested meat fibers, stool fat, and fecal nitrogen
4. *Measurement of fecal pancreatic enzymes* such as chymotrypsin

The secretin test, used to detect diffuse pancreatic disease, is based on the physiologic principle that the pancreatic secretory response is directly related to the functional mass of pancreatic tissue. In the standard assay, secretin is given intravenously in a dose of 1 clinical unit (CU) per kilogram, as either a bolus or a continuous infusion. Obviously, the results will vary with the secretin preparation used, the dose, the mode of administration, and the completeness with which the duodenal contents are collected. Normal values for the standard secretin test are (1) volume output >2.0 mL/kg per hour, (2) bicarbonate (HCO_3^-) concentration >80 mmol/L, and (3) HCO_3^- output >10 mmol in 1 h. The most reproducible measurement, giving the highest level of discrimination between normal subjects and patients with chronic pancreatitis, appears to be the maximal bicarbonate concentration.

The *combined secretin-CCK test* permits measurement of pancreatic amylase, lipase, trypsin, and chymotrypsin. Although there is overlap in the distributions of enzyme output in normal subjects and patients with pancreatitis in response to this test, markedly low enzyme outputs suggest advanced damage and destruction of acinar cells. With frank exocrine pancreatic insufficiency, there is usually an overall reduction in both HCO_3^- concentration and output of several enzymes. However, with lesser degrees of pancreatic damage there may be a dissociation between HCO_3^- concentration and enzyme output. There also may be a dissociation between the results of the secretin test and those of tests of absorptive function. For example, patients with chronic pancreatitis often have abnormally low outputs of HCO_3^- after secretin but have normal fecal fat excretion. Thus the secretin test measures the secretory capacity of ductular epithelium, while fecal fat excretion indirectly reflects intraluminal lipolytic activity. Steatorrhea does not occur until intraluminal levels of lipase are markedly reduced, underscoring the fact that only small amounts of enzymes are necessary for intraluminal digestive activities. An abnormal secretin test result suggests only that chronic pancreatic damage is present; it will not consistently distinguish between chronic pancreatitis and pancreatic carcinoma.

Another test of exocrine pancreatic function, which indirectly reflects intraluminal chymotrypsin activity, has been evaluated in patients with pancreatic disease. This test (the *tripeptide hydrolysis* or *bentiromide test*) uses a synthetic peptide, *N*-benzoyl-L-tyrosyl-*p*-aminobenzoic acid (Bz-Ty-PABA), that is specifically cleaved by chymotrypsin to Bz-Ty and PABA. Normally, after oral administration, the peptide is hydrolyzed in the small intestine by chymotrypsin with the liberation of PABA, which is rapidly absorbed and excreted in the urine. Results in several hundred patients with chronic pancreatitis and other disorders indicate that PABA excretion is significantly lower in patients with chronic pancreatitis than in control subjects. Depending on the severity of pancreatic exocrine impairment, the overall sensitivity is 60 percent (range, 46 to 74 percent), and the specificity if coupled with a D-xylose test approximates 90 percent. Measurement of blood PABA levels increases sensitivity.

Measurement of *intraluminal digestion products*, i.e., undigested muscle fibers, stool fat, and fecal nitrogen, is discussed in Chap. 285. The amount of chymotrypsin in stool reflects the pancreatic output of this proteolytic enzyme. Decreased chymotrypsin activity in stool has been reported in patients with chronic pancreatitis and cystic fibrosis. However, normal values may occur in patients with pancreatic insufficiency, and false-positive results have been reported in up to 10 percent of normal individuals. → *Tests useful in the diagnosis of exocrine pancreatic insufficiency and the differential diagnosis of malabsorption are also discussed in Chaps. 285 and 304*

304

Norton J. Greenberger, Phillip P. Toskes, Kurt J. Isselbacher

ACUTE AND CHRONIC PANCREATITIS

BIOCHEMISTRY AND PHYSIOLOGY OF PANCREATIC EXOCRINE SECRETION

GENERAL CONSIDERATIONS The pancreas secretes 1500 to 3000 mL of isosmotic alkaline (pH >8.0) fluid per day containing about 20 enzymes and zymogens. The pancreatic secretions provide the enzymes needed to effect the major digestive activity of the gastrointestinal tract and provide an optimal pH for the function of these enzymes.

REGULATION OF PANCREATIC SECRETION The exocrine pancreas is influenced by intimately interacting hormonal and neural systems. *Gastric acid* is the stimulus for the release of secretin, a peptide with 27 amino acids. Sensitive radioimmunoassay studies for secretin suggest that the pH threshold for its release from the duodenum and jejunum is 4.5. Secretin stimulates the secretion of pancreatic juice rich in *water and electrolytes*. Release of cholecystokinin (CCK) from the duodenum and jejunum is largely triggered by long-chain fatty acids, certain essential amino acids (tryptophan, phenylalanine, valine, methionine), and gastric acid itself. CCK evokes an *enzyme-rich secretion from the pancreas*. Gastrin, although it has the same terminal tetrapeptide as CCK, is a weak stimulus for pancreatic enzyme output. The *parasympathetic nervous system* (via the vagus nerve) exerts significant control over pancreatic secretion. Secretion evoked by secretin and CCK depends on permissive roles of vagal afferent and efferent pathways. This is particularly true for enzyme secretion, whereas water and bicarbonate secretion is heavily dependent on the hormonal effects of secretin and CCK. Also, vagal stimulation effects the release of vasoactive intestinal peptide (VIP), a secretin agonist. Bile salts also stimulate pancreatic secretion, thereby integrating the functions of the biliary tract, pancreas, and small intestine.

Somatostatin acts on multiple sites to induce inhibition of pancreatic secretion. The appropriate roles of other peptides, such as peptide YY, pancreastatin, gastrin-releasing peptide, pituitary adenylate cyclase–activating polypeptide, calcitonin gene–related peptide, and galanin are still being defined. Nitric oxide is an important neurotransmitter in the regulation of pancreatic exocrine secretion, although its mechanism of action has not been fully elucidated.

WATER AND ELECTROLYTE SECRETION Although sodium, potassium, chloride, calcium, zinc, phosphate, and sulfate are found in pancreatic secretions, *bicarbonate is the ion of primary physiologic importance*. In the acini and in the ducts, secretin causes the cells to add water and bicarbonate to the fluid. In the ducts, an exchange occurs between bicarbonate and chloride. There is a good correlation between the maximal bicarbonate output after stimulation with secretin and the pancreatic mass. The bicarbonate output of 120 to 300 mmol/d helps neutralize gastric acid and creates the appropriate pH for the activity of the pancreatic enzymes.

ENZYME SECRETION The pancreas secretes amylolytic, lipolytic, and proteolytic enzymes. *Amylolytic enzymes*, such as amy-

lase, hydrolyze starch to oligosaccharides and to the disaccharide maltose. The *lipolytic enzymes* include lipase, phospholipase A, and cholesterol esterase. Bile salts *inhibit* lipase in isolation, but colipase, another constituent of pancreatic secretion, binds to lipase and prevents this inhibition. Bile salts *activate* phospholipase A and cholesterol esterase. *Proteolytic enzymes* include *endopeptidases* (trypsin, chymotrypsin), which act on internal peptide bonds of proteins and polypeptides; *exopeptidases* (carboxypeptidases, aminopeptidases), which act on the free carboxyl- and amino-terminal ends of peptides, respectively; and elastase. The proteolytic enzymes are secreted as inactive precursors (zymogens). Ribonucleases (deoxyribonucleases, ribonuclease) are also secreted. While parallel secretion of pancreatic enzymes usually occurs, nonparallel secretion can occur as a result of exocytosis from heterogeneous sources in the pancreas. *Enterokinase*, an enzyme found in the duodenal mucosa, cleaves the lysine-isoleucine bond of trypsinogen to form trypsin. Trypsin then activates the other proteolytic zymogens in a cascade phenomenon. All pancreatic enzymes have pH optima in the alkaline range.

AUTOPROTECTION OF THE PANCREAS Autodigestion of the pancreas is prevented by the packaging of proteases in precursor form and by the synthesis of protease inhibitors. These protease inhibitors are found in the acinar cell, the pancreatic secretions, and the alpha₁- and alpha₂-globulin fractions of plasma.

EXOCRINE-ENDOCRINE RELATIONSHIPS Insulin appears to be needed locally for secretin and CCK to promote exocrine secretion; thus, it acts in a permissive role for these two hormones.

ENTEROPANCREATIC AXIS AND FEEDBACK INHIBITION Pancreatic enzyme secretion is controlled, at least in part, by a negative feedback mechanism induced by the presence of active serine proteases in the duodenum. To illustrate, perfusion of the duodenal lumen with phenylalanine causes a prompt increase in plasma CCK levels as well as increased secretion of chymotrypsin. However, simultaneous perfusion with trypsin blunts both responses. Conversely, perfusion of the duodenal lumen with protease inhibitors actually leads to enzyme hypersecretion. It appears that serine proteases inhibit pancreatic secretion by acting on a CCK-releasing peptide in the lumen of the small intestine.

ACUTE PANCREATITIS

GENERAL CONSIDERATIONS Pancreatic inflammatory disease may be classified as (1) acute pancreatitis and (2) chronic pancreatitis. The pathologic spectrum of acute pancreatitis varies from *edematous pancreatitis*, which is usually a mild and self-limited disorder, to *necrotizing pancreatitis*, in which the degree of pancreatic necrosis correlates with the severity of the attack and its systemic manifestations. The term *hemorrhagic pancreatitis* is less meaningful in a clinical sense because variable amounts of interstitial hemorrhage can be found in pancreatitis as well as in other disorders such as pancreatic trauma, pancreatic carcinoma, and severe congestive heart failure.

The incidence of pancreatitis varies in different countries and depends on cause, e.g., alcohol, gallstones, metabolic factors, and drugs (Table 304-1). In the United States, for example, acute pancreatitis is related to alcohol ingestion more commonly than to gallstones; in England, the opposite obtains.

ETIOLOGY AND PATHOGENESIS There are many causes of acute pancreatitis (Table 304-1), but the mechanisms by which these conditions trigger pancreatic inflammation have not been identified. Alcoholic patients with pancreatitis may represent a special subset, since most alcoholics do not develop pancreatitis. The list of identifiable causes is growing, and it is likely that pancreatitis related to viral infections, drugs, and as yet undefined factors is more common than heretofore recognized.

Approximately 5 percent of cases of acute pancreatitis are drug-related (Table 304-1). Drugs cause pancreatitis either by a hypersensi-

Table 304-1

Causes of Acute Pancreatitis

Alcohol ingestion (acute and chronic alcoholism)
Biliary tract disease (gallstones)
Postoperative state (after abdominal or nonabdominal operation)
Endoscopic retrograde cholangiopancreatography (ERCP), especially
    manometric studies of sphincter of Oddi
Trauma (especially blunt abdominal type)
Metabolic causes
    Hypertriglyceridemia
    Apolipoprotein CII deficiency syndrome
    Hypercalcemia (e.g., hyperparathyroidism), drug-induced
    Renal failure
    After renal transplantation*
    Acute fatty liver of pregnancy†
Hereditary pancreatitis
Infections
    Mumps
    Viral hepatitis
    Other viral infections (coxsackievirus, echovirus, cytomegalovirus)
    Ascariasis
    Infections with *Mycoplasma, Campylobacter, Mycobacterium avium*
        complex, other bacteria
Drugs
    Drugs for which association is definite
        Azathioprine, 6-mercaptopurine
        Sulfonamides
        Thiazide diuretics
        Furosemide
        Estrogens (oral contraceptives)
        Tetracycline
        Valproic acid
        Pentamidine
        Dideoxyinosine (ddI)
    Drugs for which association is probable
        Acetaminophen
        Nitrofurantoin
        Methyldopa
        Erythromycin
        Salicylates
        Metronidazole
        Nonsteroidal anti-inflammatory drugs
        Angiotensin-converting enzyme (ACE) inhibitors
Vascular causes and vasculitis
    Vascular
        Ischemic-hypoperfusion state (after cardiac surgery)
        Atherosclerotic emboli
    Connective tissue disorders with vasculitis
        Systemic lupus erythematosus
        Necrotizing angiitis
        Thrombotic thrombocytopenic purpura
Penetrating peptic ulcer
Obstruction of the ampulla of Vater
    Regional enteritis
    Duodenal diverticulum
Pancreas divisum
Causes to be considered in patients having recurrent bouts of acute
    pancreatitis without an obvious cause
        Occult disease of the biliary tree or pancreatic ducts, especially occult
            gallstones (microlithiasis, sludge)
        Drugs
        Hypertriglyceridemia
        Pancreas divisum
        Pancreatic cancer
        Sphincter of Oddi dysfunction
        Cystic fibrosis
        Truly idiopathic

---

* Pancreatitis occurs in 3 percent of renal transplant patients and is due to many factors,
    including surgery, hypercalcemia, drugs (glucocorticoids, azathioprine, L-asparaginase,
    diuretics), and viral infections.
† Pancreatitis also occurs in otherwise uncomplicated pregnancy and is most often associ-
    ated with cholelithiasis.

tivity reaction or by the generation of a toxic metabolite, although in some cases it is not clear which of these mechanisms is operative.

Autodigestion is one pathogenetic theory, according to which pancreatitis results when proteolytic enzymes (e.g., trypsinogen, chymotrypsinogen, proelastase, and phospholipase A) are activated in the pancreas rather than in the intestinal lumen. A number of factors (e.g., endotoxins, exotoxins, viral infections, ischemia, anoxia, and direct trauma) are believed to activate these proenzymes. Activated proteolytic enzymes, especially trypsin, not only digest pancreatic and peripancreatic tissues but also can activate other enzymes, such as elastase and phospholipase. The active enzymes then digest cellular membranes and cause proteolysis, edema, interstitial hemorrhage, vascular damage, coagulation necrosis, fat necrosis, and parenchymal cell necrosis. Cellular injury and death result in the liberation of activated enzymes. In addition, activation and release of bradykinin peptides and vasoactive substances (e.g., histamine) are believed to produce vasodilation, increased vascular permeability, and edema. Thus, a cascade of events culminates in the development of acute necrotizing pancreatitis.

The autodigestion theory has largely eclipsed two older theories. First, according to the "common channel" theory, the existence of a common anatomic channel for pancreatic secretions and bile permits reflux of bile into the pancreatic duct, which results in activation of pancreatic enzymes. (Actually, a common channel with free communication between the common bile duct and the main pancreatic duct is infrequently encountered.) The second theory is that obstruction and hypersecretion are pivotal in the development of pancreatitis. Obstruction of the main pancreatic duct, however, produces pancreatic edema but generally not pancreatitis.

A recent hypothesis to explain the intrapancreatic activation of zymogens is that they become activated by *lysosomal hydrolases* in the pancreatic acinar cell itself. In two different types of experimental pancreatitis, it has been demonstrated that digestive enzymes and lysosomal hydrolases become admixed; as a result, the latter can activate the former in the acinar cell. In vitro, lysosomal enzymes such as cathepsin B can activate trypsinogen, and trypsin can activate the other protease precursors. It is still not clear, however, whether the human acinar cell can provide the pH (about 3.0) necessary for activation of trypsinogen by lysosomal hydrolases. It is now believed that ischemia/hypoperfusion can alone result in activation of trypsinogen and pancreatic injury.

CLINICAL FEATURES *Abdominal pain* is the major symptom of acute pancreatitis. Pain may vary from a mild and tolerable discomfort to severe, constant, and incapacitating distress. Characteristically, the pain, which is steady and boring in character, is located in the epigastrium and periumbilical region and often radiates to the back as well as to the chest, flanks, and lower abdomen. The pain is frequently more intense when the patient is supine, and patients often obtain relief by sitting with the trunk flexed and knees drawn up. Nausea, vomiting, and abdominal distention due to gastric and intestinal hypomotility and chemical peritonitis are also frequent complaints.

Physical examination frequently reveals a distressed and anxious patient. Low-grade fever, tachycardia, and hypotension are fairly common. Shock is not unusual and may result from (1) hypovolemia secondary to exudation of blood and plasma proteins into the retroperitoneal space (a "retroperitoneal burn"); (2) increased formation and release of kinin peptides, which cause vasodilation and increased vascular permeability; and (3) systemic effects of proteolytic and lipolytic enzymes released into the circulation. Jaundice occurs infrequently; when present, it usually is due to edema of the head of the pancreas with compression of the intrapancreatic portion of the common bile duct. Erythematous skin nodules due to subcutaneous fat necrosis may occur. In 10 to 20 percent of patients, there are pulmonary findings, including basilar rales, atelectasis, and pleural effusion, the latter most frequently left-sided. Abdominal tenderness and muscle rigidity are present to a variable degree, but, compared with the intense pain, these signs may be unimpressive. Bowel sounds are usually diminished or absent. A pancreatic pseudocyst may be palpable in the upper abdomen. A faint blue discoloration around the umbilicus

(Cullen's sign) may occur as the result of hemoperitoneum, and a blue-red-purple or green-brown discoloration of the flanks (Turner's sign) reflects tissue catabolism of hemoglobin. The latter two findings, which are uncommon, indicate the presence of a severe necrotizing pancreatitis.

LABORATORY DATA The diagnosis of acute pancreatitis is usually established by the detection of an increased level of serum amylase. Values threefold or more above normal virtually clinch the diagnosis if overt salivary gland disease and gut perforation or infarction are excluded. However, there appears to be no definite correlation between the severity of pancreatitis and the degree of serum amylase elevation. After 48 to 72 h, even with continuing evidence of pancreatitis, total serum amylase values tend to return to normal. However, pancreatic isoamylase and lipase levels may remain elevated for 7 to 14 days. It will be recalled that amylase elevations in serum and urine occur in many conditions other than pancreatitis (see Table 303-2). Importantly, patients with *acidemia* (arterial pH $\leq$7.32) may have spurious elevations in serum amylase. In one study, 12 of 33 acidemic patients had elevated serum amylase, but only 1 had an elevated lipase value; in 9, salivary-type amylase was the predominant serum isoamylase. This finding explains why patients with diabetic ketoacidosis may have marked elevations in serum amylase without any other evidence of acute pancreatitis. The urine amylase:creatinine clearance ratio (C_{am}/C_{cr}) is usually elevated in patients with severe pancreatitis; this ratio usually is not increased in patients with a normal level of serum amylase. Serum lipase activity increases in parallel with amylase activity, and measurement of both enzymes increases the diagnostic yield. An elevated serum lipase or trypsin value is usually diagnostic of acute pancreatitis; these tests are especially helpful in patients with nonpancreatic causes of hyperamylasemia (see Table 303-2). Markedly increased levels of peritoneal or pleural fluid amylase [>1500 nmol/L (>5000 U/dL)] are also helpful, if present, in establishing the diagnosis.

Leukocytosis (15,000 to 20,000 leukocytes per microliter) occurs frequently. More severe cases may show hemoconcentration with hematocrit values exceeding 50 percent because of loss of plasma into the retroperitoneal space and peritoneal cavity. *Hyperglycemia* is common and is due to multiple factors, including decreased insulin release, increased glucagon release, and an increased output of adrenal glucocorticoids and catecholamines. *Hypocalcemia* occurs in approximately 25 percent of cases, and its pathogenesis is incompletely understood. While earlier studies suggested that the response of the parathyroid gland to a decrease in serum calcium is impaired, subsequent observations have failed to confirm this idea. Intraperitoneal saponification of calcium by fatty acids in areas of fat necrosis occurs occasionally, with large amounts (up to 6.0 g) dissolved or suspended in ascitic fluid. Such "soap formation" also may be significant in patients with pancreatitis, mild hypocalcemia, and little or no obvious ascites. *Hyperbilirubinemia* [serum bilirubin >68 μmol/L (>4.0 mg/dL)] occurs in approximately 10 percent of patients. However, jaundice is transient, and serum bilirubin levels return to normal in 4 to 7 days. Serum alkaline phosphatase and aspartate aminotransferase (AST) levels are also transiently elevated and parallel serum bilirubin values. Markedly elevated serum lactic dehydrogenase (LDH) levels [>8.5 μmol/L (>500 U/dL)] suggest a poor prognosis. Serum albumin is decreased to $\leq$30 g/L ($\leq$3.0 g/dL) in about 10 percent of cases; this sign is associated with more severe pancreatitis and a higher mortality rate (Table 304-2). *Hypertriglyceridemia* occurs in 15 to 20 percent of cases, and serum amylase levels in these patients are often spuriously normal (see Chap. 303). Most patients with hypertriglyceridemia and pancreatitis, when subsequently examined, show evidence of an underlying derangement in lipid metabolism which probably antedated the pancreatitis (see below). Approximately 25 percent of patients have *hypoxemia* (arterial P_{O_2} $\leq$ 60 mmHg), which may herald the onset of adult respiratory distress syndrome. Finally, the electrocardiogram is occasionally abnormal in acute pancreatitis with ST-segment and T-wave abnormalities simulating myocardial ischemia.

Radiologic studies useful in the diagnosis of acute pancreatitis are discussed in Chap. 303 and listed in Table 303-1. Although one or more radiologic abnormalities are found in over 50 percent of patients, the findings are inconstant and nonspecific. The chief value of conventional x-rays [chest films; kidney, ureter, and bladder (KUB) studies] in acute pancreatitis is to help exclude other diagnoses, especially a perforated viscus. Upper gastrointestinal tract x-rays have been superseded by ultrasonography and computed tomography (CT). A CT scan may confirm the clinical impression of acute pancreatitis even in the face of normal serum amylase levels. Importantly, CT is quite helpful in indicating the severity of acute pancreatitis and the risk of morbidity and mortality (see below). Sonography and radionuclide scanning [*N-p*-isopropylacetanilide-iminodiacetic acid (PIPIDA) scan; hepatic 2,6-dimethyliminodiacetic acid (HIDA) scan] are useful in acute pancreatitis to evaluate the gallbladder and biliary tree.

DIAGNOSIS Any severe acute pain in the abdomen or back should suggest acute pancreatitis. The diagnosis is usually entertained when a patient with a possible predisposition to pancreatitis presents with severe and constant abdominal pain, nausea, emesis, fever, tachycardia, and abnormal findings on abdominal examination. Laboratory studies frequently reveal leukocytosis, an abnormal appearance on x-rays of the abdomen and chest, hypocalcemia, and hyperglycemia. The diagnosis is usually confirmed by the finding of an elevated level of serum amylase and/or lipase. Obviously, not all the above features have to be present for the diagnosis to be established.

The *differential diagnosis* should include the following disorders: (1) perforated viscus, especially peptic ulcer, (2) acute cholecystitis and biliary colic, (3) acute intestinal obstruction, (4) mesenteric vascular occlusion, (5) renal colic, (6) myocardial infarction, (7) dissecting aortic aneurysm, (8) connective tissue disorders with vasculitis, (9) pneumonia, and (10) diabetic ketoacidosis. A penetrating duodenal ulcer usually can be identified by upper gastrointestinal x-rays and/or endoscopy. A perforated duodenal ulcer is readily diagnosed by the presence of free intraperitoneal air. It may be difficult to differentiate acute cholecystitis from acute pancreatitis, since an elevated serum amylase may be found in both disorders. Pain of biliary tract origin is more right-sided and gradual in onset, and ileus is usually absent; sonography and radionuclide scanning are helpful in establishing the diagnosis of cholelithiasis and cholecystitis. Intestinal obstruction due to mechanical factors can be differentiated from pancreatitis by the history of colicky pain, findings on abdominal examination, and x-rays of the abdomen showing changes characteristic of mechanical

Table 304-2

Factors That Adversely Affect Survival in Acute Pancreatitis

Ranson/Imrie criteria
  At admission or diagnosis
    Age >55 years
    Leukocytosis >16,000/μL
    Hyperglycemia >11 mmol/L (>200 mg/dL)
    Serum LDH >400 IU/L
    Serum AST >250 IU/L
  During initial 48 h
    Fall in hematocrit by >10 percent
    Fluid deficit of >4000 mL
    Hypocalcemia [calcium concentration <1.9 mmol/L (<8.0 mg/dL)]
    Hypoxemia (P_{O_2} <60 mmHg)
    Increase in BUN to >1.8 mmol/L (>5 mg/dL) after IV fluid
      administration
    Hypoalbuminemia [albumin level <32 g/L (<3.2 g/dL)]
Acute physiology and chronic health evaluation (APACHE II) score > 12
Hemorrhagic peritoneal fluid
Obesity
Key indicators of organ failure
  Hypotension (blood pressure <90 mmHg) or tachycardia >130 beats per
    minute
  P_{O_2} <60 mmHg
  Oliguria (<50 mL/h) or increasing blood urea nitrogen (BUN), creatinine
  Metabolic indicators: serum calcium <1.9 mmol/L (<8.0 mg/dL) or
    serum albumin <32 g/L (<3.2 g/dL)

obstruction. Acute mesenteric vascular occlusion is usually evident in elderly debilitated patients with brisk leukocytosis, abdominal distention, and bloody diarrhea, in whom paracentesis shows sanguineous fluid and arteriography shows vascular occlusion. Serum as well as peritoneal fluid amylase levels are increased, however, in patients with intestinal infarction. Systemic lupus erythematosus and polyarteritis nodosa may be confused with pancreatitis, especially since pancreatitis may develop as a complication of these diseases. Diabetic ketoacidosis is often accompanied by abdominal pain and elevated total serum amylase levels, thus closely mimicking acute pancreatitis. However, the serum lipase and pancreatic isoamylase levels are not elevated in diabetic ketoacidosis.

COURSE OF THE DISEASE AND COMPLICATIONS It is important to identify patients with acute pancreatitis who have an increased risk of dying. Ranson and Imrie have used multiple prognostic criteria and have demonstrated that there is an increased mortality rate when three or more risk factors are identifiable either at the time of admission to the hospital or during the initial 48 h of hospitalization (see Table 304-2). Recent studies indicate that obesity is a major risk factor for severe pancreatitis, presumably because the increased deposits of peripancreatic fat in such patients may predispose them to more extensive pancreatic and peripancreatic necrosis. The acute physiology and chronic health evaluation scoring system (APACHE II) uses the worst values of 12 physiologic measurements plus age and previous health status and provides a good description of illness severity for a wide range of common diseases; this score also correlates with outcome. Prospective studies have compared APACHE II with multiple prognostic criteria, i.e., Ranson and Imrie scores, in predicting the severity of acute pancreatitis. On admission, APACHE II identified approximately two-thirds of severe attacks, and after 48 h, the prognostic accuracy of APACHE II is comparable with that of Ranson and Imrie's scoring system. The drawbacks of APACHE II are (1) its complexity, (2) the requirement of a computer for scoring, and (3) standardization regarding peak values and cutoff scores. McMahon and colleagues have shown that the presence of a "toxic broth" or dark (hemorrhagic) fluid in abdominal pancreatitis is also an important prognostic indicator in acute pancreatitis. These multiple-factor scoring systems are difficult to use and have not been embraced consistently by clinicians. There is a great need for a reliable, simple biochemical test that consistently predicts outcome in patients with acute pancreatitis. Three candidate markers that show great promise are C-reactive protein, serum granulocyte elastase, and urinary trypsinogen activation peptide (TAP). The key indicators of a severe attack of acute pancreatitis are also listed in Table 304-2. Importantly, the presence of any one of these factors is associated with an increased risk of complications, and the presence of any two, with a 20 to 30 percent mortality rate. The high mortality rate of such severely ill patients is due in large part to infection and warrants intensive radiologic intervention and monitoring and/or a combination of radiologic and surgical means, as discussed in detail below.

The local and systemic complications of acute pancreatitis are listed in Table 304-3. Patients frequently develop an inflammatory mass in the first 2 to 3 weeks after pancreatitis. This may be due to pancreatic necrosis (with or without infection) or may represent an abscess or pseudocyst (see below). Systemic complications include pulmonary, cardiovascular, hematologic, renal, metabolic, and central nervous system abnormalities. Pancreatitis and hypertriglyceridemia constitute an association in which cause and effect remain incompletely understood. However, several reasonable conclusions can be drawn. First, hypertriglyceridemia can precede and apparently cause pancreatitis. Second, the vast majority (>80 percent) of patients with acute pancreatitis do not have hypertriglyceridemia. Third, almost all patients with pancreatitis and hypertriglyceridemia have preexisting abnormalities in lipoprotein metabolism. Fourth, many of the patients with this association have persistent hypertriglyceridemia after recovery from pancreatitis and are prone to recurrent episodes of pancreatitis. Fifth,

Table 304-3

Complications of Acute Pancreatitis

LOCAL

Necrosis
  Sterile
  Infected
Pancreatic fluid collections
  Pancreatic abscess
  Pancreatic pseudocyst
    Pain
    Rupture
    Hemorrhage
    Infection
    Obstruction of gastrointestinal tract (stomach, duodenum, colon)
Pancreatic ascites
  Disruption of main pancreatic duct
  Leaking pseudocyst
Involvement of contiguous organs by necrotizing pancreatitis
  Massive intraperitoneal hemorrhage
  Thrombosis of blood vessels (splenic vein, portal vein)
  Bowel infarction
Obstructive jaundice

SYSTEMIC

Pulmonary
  Pleural effusion
  Atelectasis
  Mediastinal abscess
  Pneumonitis
  Adult respiratory distress syndrome
Cardiovascular
  Hypotension
    Hypovolemia
    Hypoalbuminemia
  Sudden death
  Nonspecific ST-T changes in electrocardiogram simulating myocardial infarction
  Pericardial effusion
Hematologic
  Disseminated intravascular coagulation
Gastrointestinal hemorrhage*
  Peptic ulcer disease
  Erosive gastritis
  Hemorrhagic pancreatic necrosis with erosion into major blood vessels
  Portal vein thrombosis, variceal hemorrhage
Renal
  Oliguria
  Azotemia
  Renal artery and/or renal vein thrombosis
  Acute tubular necrosis
Metabolic
  Hyperglycemia
  Hypertriglyceridemia
  Hypocalcemia
  Encephalopathy
  Sudden blindness (Purtscher's retinopathy)
Central nervous system
  Psychosis
  Fat emboli
Fat necrosis
  Subcutaneous tissues (erythematous nodules)
  Bone
  Miscellaneous (mediastinum, pleura, nervous system)

* Aggravated by coagulation abnormalities (disseminated intravascular coagulation).

any factor (e.g., drugs or alcohol) that causes an abrupt increase in serum triglycerides to levels greater than 11 mmol/L (1000 mg/dL) can precipitate a bout of pancreatitis that can be associated with significant complications and even become fulminant. To avert the risk of triggering pancreatitis, a fasting serum triglyceride measurement should be obtained before estrogen replacement therapy is begun in postmenopausal women. Fasting levels less than 300 mg/dL pose no risk, whereas levels greater than 750 mg/dL are associated with a high probability of developing pancreatitis. Finally, patients with a deficiency of apolipoprotein CII have an increased incidence of pancreatitis; apolipoprotein CII activates lipoprotein lipase, which is important in clearing chylomicrons from the bloodstream.

Purtscher's retinopathy, a relatively unusual complication, is manifested by a sudden and severe loss of vision in a patient with acute pancreatitis. It is characterized by a peculiar funduscopic appearance with cotton-wool spots and hemorrhages confined to an area limited by the optic disk and macula; it is believed to be due to occlusion of the posterior retinal artery with aggregated granulocytes.

The two most common causes of acute pancreatitis are alcoholism and biliary tract disease; other causes are listed in Table 304-1. However, after a conventional workup, a specific cause will not be identified in about 30 percent of patients. It is important to note that ultrasound examinations will fail to detect gallstones, especially microlithiasis and/or sludge, in 4 to 7 percent of patients. In one series of 31 patients diagnosed initially as having idiopathic acute pancreatitis, 23 were found to have occult gallstone disease. Thus, approximately two-thirds of patients with recurrent acute pancreatitis without an obvious cause actually have occult gallstone disease due to microlithiasis. Examination of duodenal aspirates in such cases often reveals cholesterol crystals, which confirm the diagnosis. Other diseases of the biliary tree and pancreatic ducts that can cause acute pancreatitis include choledochocele, ampullary tumors, pancreas divisum, and pancreatic duct stones, stricture, and tumor. Approximately 2 percent of patients with pancreatic carcinoma present with acute pancreatitis.

Pancreatitis in AIDS Patients   The incidence of acute pancreatitis is increased in patients with AIDS for two reasons: (1) the high incidence of infections involving the pancreas, such as infections with cytomegalovirus, *Cryptosporidium*, and the *Mycobacterium avium* complex; and (2) the frequent use by AIDS patients of medications such as didanosine, pentamidine, and trimethoprim-sulfamethoxazole (see also Chap. 308).

℞ TREATMENT

In most patients (approximately 85 to 90 percent) with acute pancreatitis, the disease is self-limited and subsides spontaneously, usually within 3 to 7 days after treatment is instituted. Conventional measures include (1) analgesics for pain, (2) intravenous fluids and colloids to maintain normal intravascular volume, (3) no oral alimentation, and (4) nasogastric suction to decrease gastrin release from the stomach and prevent gastric contents from entering the duodenum.

Recent controlled trials, however, have shown that nasogastric suction offers no clear-cut advantages in the treatment of mild to moderately severe acute pancreatitis. Its use, therefore, must be considered elective rather than mandatory.

It has been demonstrated that CCK-stimulated pancreatic secretion is almost abolished in four different experimental models of acute pancreatitis. This probably explains why drugs to block pancreatic secretion in acute pancreatitis have failed to have any therapeutic benefit. For this and other reasons, anticholinergic drugs are not indicated in acute pancreatitis. In addition to nasogastric suction and anticholinergic drugs, other therapies designed to "rest the pancreas" by inhibiting pancreatic secretion have not changed the course of the disease. Although antibiotics have been used in the treatment of acute pancreatitis, randomized, prospective trials have shown no benefit from their use in acute pancreatitis of mild to moderate severity. However, recent studies of antibiotic use in patients with extensive pancreatic necrosis have demonstrated a reduced mortality rate. Furthermore, because secondary infection of necrotic pancreatic tissue (abscess, pseudocyst) or obstructed biliary passages (ascending cholangitis, complicating choledocholithiasis) contributes to much of the late mortality from pancreatitis, appropriate *antibiotic therapy of established infection* is obviously quite important. Several other drugs have been evaluated by prospective, controlled trials and found *ineffective* in the treatment of acute pancreatitis. The list, by no means complete, includes glucagon, H₂ blockers, protease inhibitors such as aprotinin, glucocorticoids, calcitonin, somatostatin analogues such as octreotide, and nonsteroidal anti-inflammatory drugs (NSAIDs). However, prophylactic treatment with gabexate, a protease inhibitor, has reduced pancreatic damage related to endoscopic retrograde cholangiopancreatography (ERCP).

A CT scan, especially a contrast-enhanced dynamic CT (CECT) scan, provides valuable information on the severity and prognosis of acute pancreatitis (Fig. 304-1 and Table 304-4). In particular, CECT allows estimation of the presence and extent of pancreatic necrosis. Recent studies suggest that the likelihood of prolonged pancreatitis or a serious complication is negligible when the CT severity index is 1 or 2 and low with scores of 3 to 6. However, patients with scores of 7 to 10 had a 92 percent morbidity and 17

A

B

FIGURE 304-1   Acute pancreatitis: CT evolution. *A*. Contrast-enhanced CT scan of the abdomen performed on admission of a patient with clinical evidence of acute pancreatitis. Note the mildly decreased density of the body of the pancreas to the left of the midline (*arrow*). There are a few linear strands in the peripancreatic fat, suggesting inflammation (*open arrows*). A small amount of fluid is seen in the anterior pararenal space (*arrowhead*). *B*. Nine days after admission, there is a marked worsening with severe inflammation of the pancreas evidenced by anterior displacement of the posterior gastric wall (*arrows*), increased inflammation of the peripancreatic fat, and increased pancreatic effusion in the anterior perirenal space and around the splenic vein (*open arrows*). (*Courtesy of Dr. PR Ros, University of Florida College of Medicine.*)

Table 304-4

Severity Index in Acute Pancreatitis

	Points
Grade of Acute Pancreatitis	
A. Normal pancreas	0
B. Pancreatic enlargement alone	1
C. Inflammation compared with pancreas and peripancreatic fat	2
D. One peripancreatic fluid collection	3
E. Two or more fluid collections	4
Degree of Pancreatic Necrosis	
A. No necrosis	0
B. Necrosis of one-third of pancreas	2
C. Necrosis of one-half of pancreas	4
D. Necrosis of more than one-half of pancreas	6

percent mortality. A CECT scan is indicated in patients with three or more of Ranson's signs, in all seriously ill patients, and in patients who show evidence of clinical deterioration. The patient with mild to moderate pancreatitis usually requires treatment with intravenous fluids, fasting, and possibly nasogastric suction for 2 to 4 days. A clear liquid diet is frequently started on the third to sixth day, and a regular diet by the fifth to seventh day. The patient with unremitting *fulminant pancreatitis* usually requires inordinate amounts of fluid and close attention to complications such as cardiovascular collapse, respiratory insufficiency, and pancreatic infection. The latter should be managed by a combination of radiologic and surgical means (see below). While earlier uncontrolled studies suggested that *peritoneal lavage* via a percutaneous dialysis catheter was helpful in severe pancreatitis, subsequent studies indicate that this treatment does not influence the outcome of such attacks. Laparotomy with adequate drainage and removal of necrotic tissue should be considered if conventional therapy does not halt the patient's deterioration. The use of parenteral nutrition makes it possible to give nutritional support to patients with severe, acute, or protracted pancreatitis who are unable to eat normally. Patients with severe gallstone-induced pancreatitis may improve dramatically if papillotomy is carried out within the first 36 to 72 h of the attack. Recent studies indicate that only those patients with gallstone pancreatitis who are in the very severe group should be considered for urgent ERCP. Finally, the treatment for patients with hypertriglyceridemia-associated pancreatitis include (1) weight loss to ideal weight, (2) a lipid-restricted diet, (3) exercise, (4) avoidance of alcohol and of drugs that can elevate serum triglycerides (i.e., estrogens, vitamin A, thiazides, and beta-blockers), and (5) control of diabetes.

INFECTED PANCREATIC NECROSIS, ABSCESS, AND PSEUDOCYST Infected pancreatic necrosis should be differentiated from pancreatic abscess. The former is a diffuse infection of an acutely inflamed, necrotic pancreas occurring in the first 1 to 2 weeks after the onset of pancreatitis. In contrast, a pancreatic abscess is an ill-defined, liquid collection of pus that evolves over a longer period, often 4 to 6 weeks. It tends to be less life-threatening and is associated with a lower rate of surgical mortality. Infected pancreatic necrosis should be treated by surgical debridement because the solid component of the infected pancreas is not amenable to effective radiologically guided percutaneous evacuation. Pancreatic abscess can be treated surgically or, in selected cases, by percutaneous drainage. The necrotic pancreas becomes secondarily infected in 40 to 60 percent of patients, most frequently with gram-negative bacteria of alimentary origin. Whether infection occurs depends on several factors, including the extent of pancreatic and peripancreatic necrosis, the degree of pancreatic ischemia and hypoperfusion, and the presence of organ or multi-organ failure.

The early diagnosis of pancreatic infection can be accomplished by CT-guided needle aspiration. In one study, 60 patients, representing 5 percent of all admissions for acute pancreatitis, were suspected of harboring a pancreatic infection on the basis of fever, leukocytosis, and an abnormal CT scan (phlegmon, pseudocyst, or extrapancreatic fluid collection). Importantly, 60 percent of these patients had a pancreatic infection, and 55 percent of these infections developed in the first 2 weeks. These findings suggest that only guided aspiration can reliably distinguish sterile from infected pancreatic necrosis. The following are guidelines for patients meeting the above selection criteria: (1) Pseudocysts and phlegmons should be aspirated promptly, because more than half may be infected; (2) extrapancreatic fluid collections need not be aspirated promptly, because most are sterile; (3) if a phlegmon is found initially to be sterile but fever and leukocytosis persist, several days of observation should be allowed to pass before reaspiration is considered, as clinical improvement frequently occurs; and (4) if fever and leukocytosis recur after an interval of well-being, reaspiration should be considered.

Severe pancreatitis with the presence of three or more risk factors, postoperative pancreatitis, early oral feeding, early laparotomy, and perhaps injudicious use of antibiotics predispose to the development of pancreatic abscess, which occurs in 3 to 4 percent of patients with acute pancreatitis. Pancreatic abscess also may develop because of a communication between a pseudocyst and the colon, inadequate surgical drainage of a pseudocyst, or needling of a pseudocyst. The characteristic signs of abscess are fever, leukocytosis, ileus, and rapid deterioration in a patient previously recovering from pancreatitis. Sometimes, however, the only manifestations are persistent fever and signs of continuing pancreatic inflammation. Drainage of pancreatic abscesses by percutaneous catheter techniques, using CT guidance, has been only moderately successful (resolution in 50 to 60 percent of patients). Accordingly, laparotomy with radical sump drainage and possibly resection of necrotic tissue is usually required, because the mortality rate for undrained pancreatic abscess approaches 100 percent. Multiple abscesses are common, and reoperation is frequently necessary.

Pseudocysts of the pancreas are collections of tissue, fluid, debris, pancreatic enzymes, and blood which develop over a period of 1 to 4 weeks after the onset of acute pancreatitis; they form in approximately 15 percent of patients with acute pancreatitis. In contrast to true cysts, pseudocysts do not have an epithelial lining, the walls consisting of necrotic tissue, granulation tissue, and fibrous tissue. Disruption of the pancreatic ductal system is common. However, the subsequent course of this disruption varies widely, ranging from spontaneous healing to continuous leakage of pancreatic juice, which results in tense ascites. Pseudocysts are preceded by pancreatitis in 90 percent of cases and by trauma in 10 percent. Approximately 85 percent are located in the body or tail of the pancreas and 15 percent in the head. Some patients have two or more pseudocysts. Abdominal pain, with or without radiation to the back, is the usual presenting complaint. A palpable, tender mass may be found in the middle or left upper abdomen. The serum amylase level is elevated in 75 percent of patients at some point during their illness and may fluctuate markedly.

On x-ray examination, 75 percent of pseudocysts can be seen to displace some portion of the gastrointestinal tract (Fig. 304-2). Sonography, however, is reliable in detecting pseudocysts. Sonography also permits differentiation between an edematous, inflamed pancreas (pancreatic phlegmon), which can give rise to a palpable mass, and an actual pseudocyst. Furthermore, serial ultrasound studies will indicate whether a pseudocyst has resolved. CT complements ultrasonography in the diagnosis of pancreatic pseudocyst (Fig. 304-2), especially when the pseudocyst is infected.

In studies using sonography, pseudocysts were seen to resolve in 25 to 40 percent of patients. Pseudocysts that are greater than 5 cm in diameter and that persist for longer than 6 weeks should be considered for drainage. Recent natural history studies have suggested that noninterventional, expectant management is the best course in selected patients with minimal symptoms and no evidence of active alcohol use in whom the pseudocyst appears mature by radiography and does not resemble a cystic neoplasm. A significant number of these pseudocysts will resolve spontaneously more than 6 weeks after their formation. Also, these studies demonstrate that large pseudocyst size is not an absolute indication for interventional therapy and that many peripancreatic fluid collections detected on CT in cases of acute pancreatitis resolve spontaneously. A pseudocyst that does not resolve spontaneously may lead to serious complications, such as (1) pain caused by expansion of the lesion and pressure on other viscera, (2) rupture, (3) hemorrhage, and (4) abscess. Rupture of a pancreatic pseudocyst is a particularly serious complication. Shock almost always supervenes, and mortality rates range from 14 percent if the rupture is not associated with hemorrhage to over 60 percent if hemorrhage has occurred. Rupture and hemorrhage are the prime causes of death from pancreatic pseudocyst. A triad of findings—an increase in the size of the mass, a localized bruit over the mass, and a sudden decrease in hemoglobin level and hematocrit without obvious external blood loss—should alert one to the possibility of hemorrhage from a pseudocyst. Thus, in patients who are stable and free of complications and in whom serial ultrasound studies show that the pseudocyst is shrinking, conservative

therapy is indicated. Conversely, if the pseudocyst is expanding and is complicated by rupture, hemorrhage, or abscess, the patient should be operated on. Using ultrasound or CT guidance, sterile chronic pseudocysts can be treated safely with single or repeated needle aspiration or more prolonged catheter drainage with a success rate of 45 to 75 percent. The success rate of these techniques for infected pseudocysts is considerably less (40 to 50 percent). Patients who do not respond to drainage require surgical therapy for internal or external drainage of the cyst.

Pseudoaneurysms develop in up to 10 percent of patients with acute pancreatitis at sites reflecting the distribution of pseudocysts and fluid collections (Fig. 304-2D). The splenic artery is most frequently involved, followed by the inferior and superior pancreatic duodenal

A

B

C

D

FIGURE 304-2 Pseudocyst of pancreas. *A.* Upper gastrointestinal x-ray showing displacement of stomach by pseudocyst. *B.* Sonogram showing pseudocyst (*cyst*). GB, gallbladder; MVP, portal vein. Behind the large pseudocyst is seen the calcified head of the pancreas. A dilated common bile duct (*asterisk*) is noted. *C.* CT scan showing pseudocyst. Note the large, lobulated fluid collection (*arrows*) surrounding the tail of the pancreas (*arrowheads*). Note also the dense, thin rim in the periphery representing the fibrous capsule of

the pseudocyst. *D.* Spiral CT showing a pseudocyst (*small arrow*) with a pseudoaneurysm (light area in pseudocyst). Note the demonstration of the main pancreatic duct (*big arrow*), even though this duct is minimally dilated by ERCP. (*A, B courtesy of Dr. CE Forsmark, University of Florida College of Medicine; C, D courtesy of Dr. PR Ros, University of Florida College of Medicine.*)

arteries. This diagnosis should be suspected in patients with pancreatitis who develop upper gastrointestinal bleeding without an obvious cause or in whom thin-cut CT scanning reveals a contrast-enhanced lesion within or adjacent to a suspected pseudocyst. Arteriography is necessary to confirm the diagnosis.

PANCREATIC ASCITES AND PANCREATIC PLEURAL EFFUSIONS Pancreatic ascites is usually due to disruption of the main pancreatic duct, often by an internal fistula between the duct and the peritoneal cavity or a leaking pseudocyst (see also Chap. 43). This diagnosis is suggested in a patient with an elevated serum amylase level in whom the ascites fluid has both increased levels of albumin [>30 g/L (>3.0 g/dL)] and a markedly elevated level of amylase. The fluid in true pancreatic ascites usually has an amylase concentration of >20,000 U/L as a result of the ruptured duct or leaking pseudocyst. Lower amylase elevations may be found in the peritoneal fluid of patients with acute pancreatitis. In addition, ERCP will often demonstrate passage of contrast material from a major pancreatic duct or a pseudocyst into the peritoneal cavity. As many as 15 percent of patients with pseudocysts have concurrent pancreatic ascites. The differential diagnosis should include intraperitoneal carcinomatosis, tuberculous peritonitis, constrictive pericarditis, and Budd-Chiari syndrome.

If the pancreatic duct disruption is posterior, an internal fistula may develop between the pancreatic duct and the pleural space, producing a pleural effusion, which is usually left-sided and often massive. This complication often requires thoracentesis or chest tube drainage.

Treatment usually involves using nasogastric suction and parenteral alimentation to decrease pancreatic secretion. In addition, paracentesis is performed to keep the peritoneal cavity free of fluid and, it is hoped, to effect sealing of the leak. The long-acting somatostatin analogue octreotide, which inhibits pancreatic secretion, is useful in cases of pancreatic ascites and pleural effusion. If ascites continues to recur after 2 to 3 weeks of medical management, the patient should be operated on following pancreatography to define the anatomy of the abnormal duct. A disrupted main pancreatic duct can also be treated effectively by stenting. Patients in whom ERCP identifies two or more sites of extravasation are unlikely to respond to conservative management and/or stenting.

CHRONIC PANCREATITIS AND PANCREATIC EXOCRINE INSUFFICIENCY

GENERAL AND ETIOLOGIC CONSIDERATIONS Chronic inflammatory disease of the pancreas may present as episodes of acute inflammation in a previously injured pancreas or as chronic damage with persistent pain or malabsorption. The causes of relapsing chronic pancreatitis are similar to those of acute pancreatitis (Table 304-1), except that there is an appreciable incidence of cases of undetermined origin. In addition, the pancreatitis associated with gallstones is predominantly acute or relapsing-acute in nature. A cholecystectomy is almost always performed in patients after the first or second attack of gallstone-associated pancreatitis. Patients with chronic pancreatitis may present with persistent abdominal pain, with or without steatorrhea; some present with steatorrhea and no pain.

Patients with chronic pancreatitis in whom there is extensive destruction of the pancreas (less than 10 percent of exocrine function remaining) will have steatorrhea and azotorrhea. Among American adults, alcoholism is the most common cause of clinically apparent pancreatic exocrine insufficiency, while cystic fibrosis is the most frequent cause in children. In up to 25 percent of American adults with chronic pancreatitis, the cause is not known; that is, they have idiopathic chronic pancreatitis. In other parts of the world, severe protein-calorie malnutrition is a common cause. Table 304-5 lists other causes of pancreatic exocrine insufficiency, but they are relatively uncommon.

PATHOPHYSIOLOGY Unfortunately, the events that initiate an inflammatory process in the pancreas are still not well understood.

Table 304-5

Causes of Pancreatic Exocrine Insufficiency

Alcohol, chronic alcoholism
Idiopathic pancreatitis
Cystic fibrosis
Hypertriglyceridemia
Severe protein-calorie malnutrition with hypoalbuminemia
   Tropical pancreatitis (Africa, Asia)
Pancreatic and duodenal neoplasms
Pancreatic resection
Gastric surgery
   Subtotal gastrectomy with Billroth I anastomosis
   Subtotal gastrectomy with Billroth II anastomosis
   Truncal vagotomy and pyloroplasty
Gastrinoma (Zollinger-Ellison syndrome)
Hereditary pancreatitis
Traumatic pancreatitis
Abdominal radiotherapy
Hemochromatosis
Shwachman's syndrome (pancreatic insufficiency and bone marrow
   dysfunction)
Trypsinogen deficiency
Enterokinase deficiency
Isolated deficiencies of amylase, lipase, or proteases
α_1-Antitrypsin deficiency

The many hypotheses will not be reviewed here. In the case of alcohol-induced pancreatitis, however, it has been suggested that the primary defect may be the precipitation of protein (inspissated enzymes) in the ducts. The resulting ductal obstruction could lead to duct dilation, diffuse atrophy of the acinar cells, fibrosis, and eventual calcification of some of the protein plugs. However, the fact that some alcoholic patients with recurrent acute pancreatitis show no evidence of chronic pancreatitis does not support this hypothesis. In fact, experimental and clinical observations have shown that alcohol has direct toxic effects on the pancreas. While patients with alcohol-induced pancreatitis generally consume large amounts of alcohol, some consume very little (50 g/d or less). Thus prolonged consumption of "socially acceptable" amounts of alcohol is compatible with the development of pancreatitis. In addition, the finding of extensive pancreatic fibrosis in patients who died during their first attack of clinical acute alcohol-induced pancreatitis supports the concept that such patients already have chronic pancreatitis.

CLINICAL FEATURES Patients with relapsing chronic pancreatitis may present with symptoms identical to those of acute pancreatitis, but pain may be continuous, intermittent, or absent. The pathogenesis of this pain is poorly understood. Although the classic description is of epigastric pain radiating through the back, the pain pattern is often atypical; the pain may be worst in the right or left upper quadrant of the back or may be diffuse throughout the upper abdomen; it may even be referred to the anterior chest or flank. Characteristically it is persistent, deep-seated, and unresponsive to antacids. It often is worsened by ingestion of alcohol or a heavy meal (especially one rich in fat). Often the pain is severe enough to necessitate the frequent use of narcotics.

Weight loss, abnormal stools, and other signs or symptoms suggestive of malabsorption (see Table 285-5) are common in chronic pancreatitis. However, clinically apparent deficiencies of fat-soluble vitamins are surprisingly rare. The physical findings in these patients are usually not impressive, so that there is a disparity between the severity of the abdominal pain and the physical signs (other than some abdominal tenderness and mild temperature elevation).

DIAGNOSTIC EVALUATION (See Chap. 303) In contrast to relapsing acute pancreatitis, the serum amylase and lipase levels are usually not elevated in chronic pancreatitis. Elevations of serum bilirubin and alkaline phosphatase levels may indicate cholestasis secondary to chronic inflammation around the common bile duct (Fig. 304-3). Many patients demonstrate impaired glucose tolerance, and some have an elevated fasting blood glucose level.

The classic triad of pancreatic calcification, steatorrhea, and diabetes mellitus usually establishes the diagnosis of chronic pancreatitis and exocrine pancreatic insufficiency but is found in less than one-third of chronic pancreatitis patients. Accordingly, it is often necessary to perform an intubation test such as the *secretin stimulation test*, which usually gives abnormal results when 60 percent or more of pancreatic exocrine function has been lost. Approximately 40 percent of patients with chronic pancreatitis have *cobalamin (vitamin B₁₂) malabsorption*, which can be corrected by the administration of oral pancreatic enzymes. There is usually a marked excretion of fecal fat (see Chap. 285), which can be reduced by the administration of oral pancreatic enzymes. The bentiromide test (Chap. 303) and the D-xylose urinary excretion test are useful in patients with "pancreatic steatorrhea," since the bentiromide test will be abnormal, and D-xylose excretion usually is normal. A decreased serum trypsinogen level strongly suggests pancreatic exocrine insufficiency.

The radiographic hallmark of chronic pancreatitis is the presence of scattered calcification throughout the pancreas (Fig. 304-3). Diffuse pancreatic calcification indicates that significant damage has occurred and obviates the need for a secretin test. While alcohol is by far the most common cause, pancreatic calcification also may be seen in cases of severe protein-calorie malnutrition, hereditary pancreatitis, posttraumatic pancreatitis, hyperparathyroidism, islet cell tumors, and idiopathic chronic pancreatitis. A large prospective study has shown convincingly that pancreatic calcification decreases or even disappears spontaneously in one-third of patients with severe chronic pancreatitis; this outcome may also follow ductal decompression. Pancreatic calcification is a dynamic process that is incompletely understood.

Sonography, CT, and ERCP greatly aid the diagnosis of pancreatic disease. In addition to excluding pseudocysts and pancreatic cancer, sonography and CT may show calcification or dilated ducts associated with chronic pancreatitis (Fig. 304-4). ERCP is the only major technique that provides a direct view of the pancreatic duct. In patients with alcohol-induced pancreatitis, ERCP may reveal a pseudocyst missed by sonography or CT.

COMPLICATIONS OF CHRONIC PANCREATITIS The complications of chronic pancreatitis are protean. *Cobalamin (vitamin B₁₂) malabsorption* occurs in 40 percent of patients with alcohol-induced chronic pancreatitis and in virtually all with cystic fibrosis. It is consistently corrected by the administration of pancreatic enzymes (containing proteases). It may be due to excessive binding of cobalamin by cobalamin-binding proteins other than intrinsic factor, which ordinarily are destroyed by pancreatic proteases and therefore do not

A

C

B

D

FIGURE 304-3 Radiologic abnormalities in chronic pancreatitis. *A*. Pancreatic calcification (*arrows*) and stenosis (tapering) of the intrahepatic portion of the common bile duct demonstrated by percutaneous transhepatic cholangiography. *B*. Pancreatic calcification (*large white arrow*) demonstrated by sonography. Note dilated pancreatic duct (*thin white arrow*) and splenic vein (*open arrow*). *C*. Pancreatic calcification (*vertical arrows*) and dilated pancreatic duct (*horizontal arrow*) demonstrated by CT scan. *D*. Endoscopic retrograde cholangiogram shows grossly dilated pancreatic ducts (*arrows*) in a patient with long-standing pancreatitis.

patients with chronic pancreatitis who have been followed for 2 or more years. Perhaps the most common and troublesome complication is addiction to narcotics.

FIGURE 304-4 Chronic pancreatitis and pancreatic calculi: CT scan and ERCP appearance. *A.* In this contrast-enhanced CT scan of the abdomen, there is evidence of an atrophic pancreas with multiple calcifications (*arrows*). Note the markedly dilated pancreatic duct seen in this section through the body and tail (*open arrows*). *B.* ERCP in the same patient demonstrates the dilated pancreatic duct as well as an intrapancreatic duct calculus (*arrows*). These findings correlate nicely with the CT scan appearance.

compete with intrinsic factor for cobalamin binding. Although most patients show *impaired glucose tolerance*, diabetic ketoacidosis and coma are uncommon. Similarly, end-organ damage (retinopathy, neuropathy, nephropathy) is also uncommon, and the appearance of these complications should raise the question of concomitant genetic diabetes mellitus. A nondiabetic retinopathy, peripheral in location and secondary to vitamin A and/or zinc deficiency, is common in these patients. *Effusions* containing high concentrations of amylase may occur into the pleural, pericardial, or peritoneal space. *Gastrointestinal bleeding* may occur from peptic ulceration, gastritis, a pseudocyst eroding into the duodenum, or ruptured varices secondary to splenic vein thrombosis due to inflammation of the tail of the pancreas. *Icterus* may occur, caused either by edema of the head of the pancreas, which compresses the common bile duct, or by chronic cholestasis secondary to a chronic inflammatory reaction around the intrapancreatic portion of the common bile duct (Fig. 304-3). The chronic obstruction may lead to cholangitis and ultimately to biliary cirrhosis. *Subcutaneous fat necrosis* may appear as tender red nodules on the lower extremities. *Bone pain* may be secondary to intramedullary fat necrosis. Inflammation of the large and small joints of the upper and lower extremities may occur. The incidence of pancreatic carcinoma is increased in

TREATMENT

Therapy for patients with chronic pancreatitis is directed toward two major problems—pain and malabsorption. Patients with intermittent attacks of pain are treated essentially like those with acute pancreatitis (see above). Patients with severe and persistent pain should avoid alcohol completely and avoid large meals rich in fat. Since the pain is often severe enough to require frequent use of narcotics (and hence addiction), a number of surgical procedures have been developed for pain relief. ERCP allows the surgeon to plan the operative approach. If there is a stricture of the pancreatic duct, a *local resection* may ameliorate the pain. Unfortunately, isolated localized strictures are not common. In most patients with alcohol-induced disease, the pancreas is diffusely involved, and surgically correctible localized ductal disease is rare. When there is primary ductal obstruction and dilation, ductal decompression may provide effective pain palliation. Short-term pain relief may be achieved in up to 80 percent of patients, while long-term pain relief occurs in approximately 50 percent. In some of these patients, however, pain relief can be achieved only by resecting 50 to 95 percent of the gland. Although pain relief is achieved in three-quarters of these patients, they tend to develop pancreatic endocrine and exocrine insufficiency and must be treated with pancreatic enzyme replacement therapy. It is important to screen patients carefully, for such radical surgery is contraindicated in those who are severely depressed or suicidal or who continue to drink. Procedures such as splanchnicectomy, celiac ganglionectomy, and nerve blocks usually bring only temporary relief and are not recommended. Endoscopic treatment of chronic pancreatitis may involve sphincterotomy of the minor or major pancreatic sphincter, dilatation of strictures, removal of calculi, or stenting of the ventral or dorsal pancreatic duct. While many of these techniques are technically impressive, none has been subjected to a randomized trial in patients with chronic pancreatitis. In addition, significant complications—acute pancreatitis, pancreatic abscess, damage to the pancreatic duct, and death—have occurred in up to 36 percent of patients following stent placement.

Three double-blind trials have demonstrated that administration of pancreatic enzymes decreases abdominal pain in selected patients with chronic pancreatitis. In these trials, approximately 75 percent of the patients evaluated experienced pain relief. The patients most likely to respond are those with mild to moderate exocrine pancreatic dysfunction, as evidenced by an abnormal secretin test, normal fat absorption, and minimal abnormalities on ERCP examination. These clinical observations seem to fit with data from human beings and experimental animals demonstrating a negative feedback regulation for pancreatic exocrine secretion controlled by the amount of proteases within the lumen of the proximal small intestine. It seems reasonable to use the following approach for patients with severe, persistent or continuous abdominal pain thought to be caused by chronic pancreatitis. After other causes of abdominal pain (peptic ulcer, gallstones, etc.) have been excluded, a pancreatic *sonogram* should be done. If no mass is found, a *secretin test* may be performed, because its results usually are abnormal in cases of chronic pancreatitis with pain. If the results are abnormal (i.e., decreased bicarbonate concentration or volume output), a 3- to 4-week *trial of pancreatic enzyme administration* is appropriate. Eight conventional tablets or capsules are taken at meals and at bedtime. There are a number of studies suggesting that patients may have small-duct chronic pancreatitis and chronic abdominal pain with a normal appearance on radiographic evaluations (ultrasound, CT, ERCP) but abnormal results on hormone stimulation tests (secretin test) and/or abnormal pancreatic histology. Such minimal-change chronic pancreatitis may respond well to pancreatic enzyme therapy (non-enteric-coated) for relief of abdominal pain. If no relief is obtained, and especially if the volume secreted during the secretin test is very low, ERCP should be performed. If a pseudocyst or a localized ductal obstruction is found, surgery should be considered. A patient who has dilated ducts may be a candidate for a surgical ductal decompression procedure. This procedure provides short-term relief in up to 80 percent of patients, although long-term results are closer to 50 percent. Some studies have shown octreotide to be effective in decreasing abdominal pain in patients with severe large-duct disease. If no surgically remediable lesion is found and severe pain continues despite abstinence from alcohol, subtotal pancreatic resection may be necessary.

The treatment of malabsorption rests on the use of pancreatic enzyme replacement therapy. Diarrhea and steatorrhea are usually improved by this treatment, although the steatorrhea may not be completely corrected. The major problem is delivering enough active enzyme into the duodenum. Steatorrhea could be abolished if 10 percent of the normal amount of lipase could be delivered to the duodenum at the proper time. This concentration of lipase cannot be achieved with the current preparations of pancreatic enzymes, even if the latter are given in large doses. The reason for these poor results may be that lipase is inactivated by gastric acid, that food empties from the stomach faster than do the pancreatic enzymes, and that batches of commercially available pancreatic extracts vary in enzyme activity.

For the usual patient, two or three enteric-coated capsules or eight conventional (non-enteric-coated) tablets of a potent enzyme preparation should be administered with meals. Some patients using conventional tablets require adjuvant therapy to improve enzyme replacement treatment. H_2 receptor antagonists, sodium bicarbonate, and proton pump inhibitors are effective adjuvants. Antacids containing calcium carbonate or magnesium hydroxide are not effective and may actually result in increased steatorrhea. Adjuvant therapy should not be given with enteric-coated microsphere preparations, because the resulting increase in gastric pH might cause these preparations to release their enzymes into the stomach rather than the small intestine. Several publications have reported colonic strictures in patients with cystic fibrosis receiving extraordinarily high doses of high-potency pancreatic enzyme preparations. Such lesions have not been reported in adults with chronic pancreatitis.

Supportive measures include diet restriction and pain medications. The diet should be moderate in fat (30 percent), high in protein (24 percent), and low in carbohydrate (40 percent). Restriction of long-chain triglyceride intake can help patients who do not respond satisfactorily to pancreatic enzyme therapy. Use of foods containing mainly medium-chain fatty acids, which do not require lipase for digestion, may be beneficial. Nonnarcotic analgesics should be emphasized. Patients taking narcotic drugs for pain relief often become addicted and continue to have pain.

Patients with severe exocrine pancreatic insufficiency secondary to alcohol who continue to drink have a high mortality rate (in one series, 50 percent of patients who were followed for 5 to 12 years died during this period) and significant morbidity (weight loss, lassitude, vitamin deficiency, and narcotic addiction). Chronic pancreatitis carries significant medical and social costs. A recent study found that pancreatitis led to retirement in 11 percent of patients with the disease, accounting for 45 percent of all retirements. In 87 percent of patients with chronic pancreatitis unable to maintain gainful employment, alcoholism was a contributing factor. Patients with chronic pancreatitis also use substantial medical resources. In 1987 in the United States, this diagnosis accounted for 122,000 recorded outpatient visits and 56,000 hospital admissions. Pain may abate if progressive severe exocrine insufficiency continues. Patients who abstain from alcohol and use vigorous replacement therapy for maldigestion-malabsorption do reasonably well.

HEREDITARY PANCREATITIS Hereditary pancreatitis is a rare disease that is similar to chronic pancreatitis except for an early age of onset and evidence of hereditary factors (involving an autosomal dominant gene with incomplete penetrance). These patients have recurring attacks of severe abdominal pain which may last from a few days to a few weeks. The serum amylase and lipase levels may be elevated during acute attacks but usually are normal. Patients frequently develop pancreatic calcification, diabetes mellitus, and steatorrhea, and, in addition, they have an increased incidence of pancreatic carcinoma. Such patients often require ductal decompression for pain relief. Abdominal complaints in relatives of patients with hereditary pancreatitis should raise the question of pancreatic disease.

PANCREATIC ENDOCRINE TUMORS

→ *Pancreatic endocrine tumors are summarized in Table 304-6 and are discussed in Chap. 95.*

OTHER CONDITIONS

ANNULAR PANCREAS When the ventral pancreatic anlage fails to migrate correctly to make contact with the dorsal anlage, the result may be a ring of pancreatic tissue encircling the duodenum. Such an annular pancreas may cause intestinal obstruction in the neonate or the adult. Symptoms of postprandial fullness, epigastric pain, nausea, and vomiting may be present for years before the diagnosis is entertained. The radiographic findings are symmetric dilation of the proximal duodenum with bulging of the recesses on either side of the annular band, effacement but not destruction of the duodenal mucosa, accentuation of the findings in the right anterior oblique position, and lack of change on repeated examinations. The differential diagnosis should include duodenal webs, tumors of the pancreas or duodenum, postbulbar peptic ulcer, regional enteritis, and adhesions. Patients with annular pancreas have an increased incidence of pancreatitis and peptic ulcer. Because of these and other potential complications, the treatment is surgical even if the condition has been present for years. Retrocolic duodenojejunostomy is the procedure of choice, although some surgeons advocate Billroth II gastrectomy, gastroenterostomy, and vagotomy.

PANCREAS DIVISUM Pancreas divisum occurs when the embryologic ventral and dorsal pancreatic anlagen fail to fuse, so that pancreatic drainage is accomplished mainly through the accessory papilla. Pancreas divisum is the most common congenital anatomic variant of the human pancreas. Current evidence indicates that this anomaly does not predispose to the development of pancreatitis in the great majority of patients who harbor it. However, the combination of pancreas divisum and a small accessory orifice could result in dorsal duct obstruction. The challenge is to identify this subset of patients with dorsal duct pathology. Cannulation of the dorsal duct by ERCP is not as easily done as is cannulation of the ventral duct. Patients with pancreatitis and pancreas divisum demonstrated by ERCP should be treated with conservative measures, including pancreatic enzyme therapy. In many of these patients, the pancreatitis is idiopathic and unrelated to the pancreas divisum and will respond well to pancreatic enzyme therapy. Endoscopic or surgical intervention is indicated only when the above methods fail. If marked dilation of the dorsal duct can be demonstrated, surgical ductal decompression should be performed. The appropriate therapy for patients without dilation of the dorsal duct is not yet defined. It should be stressed that the ERCP appearance of pancreas divisum—i.e., a small-caliber ventral duct with an arborizing pattern—may be mistaken as representing an obstructed main pancreatic duct secondary to a mass lesion.

MACROAMYLASEMIA In macroamylasemia, amylase circulates in the blood in a polymer form too large to be easily excreted by the kidney. Patients with this condition demonstrate an elevated serum amylase value, a low urinary amylase value, and a C_{am}/C_{cr} ratio of less than 1 percent. The presence of macroamylase can be documented by chromatography of the serum. The prevalence of macroamylasemia is 1.5 percent of the nonalcoholic general adult hospital population. Usually macroamylasemia is an incidental finding and is not related to disease of the pancreas or other organs. It is important

Table 304-6

Pancreatic Endocrine Tumors

Syndrome	Hormone(s) Produced	Primary Hormone Effects	Pathologic Features	Clinical Features
Zollinger-Ellison	Gastrin	Gastric acid hypersecretion with basal acid outputs usually >15 mmol/h (>15 mEq/h)	Delta cell islet tumors; 10% aberrant (duodenal); 60% malignant	Severe peptic ulcer disease often refractory to therapy; ectopic ulcers; diarrhea; multiple endocrine adenomas (parathyroid, pituitary, adrenal, thyroid)
Insulinoma	Insulin	Hypoglycemia with inappropriately increased serum insulin levels	Beta cell islet tumors; 80–90% benign	Hypoglycemic symptoms
Glucagonoma	Glucagon; pancreatic polypeptide	Hyperglucagonemia → glucose intolerance	Alpha cell islet tumors; 60% malignant	Slow-growing pancreatic tumor; hyperglycemia; bullous and eczematoid dermatitis; weight loss; anemia; gastric and intestinal motor abnormalities
Somatostatinoma	Somatostatin; pancreatic polypeptide	Somatostatin inhibits insulin, gastrin, and pancreatic enzyme secretion; decreased bile flow	Delta cell islet tumor	Pancreatic tumor; diarrhea; steatorrhea; gallstones; diabetes mellitus; anemia
Pancreatic cholera	Vasoactive intestinal peptide ? Gastric inhibitory polypeptide ? Prostaglandin E ? Pancreatic peptide	Net secretion of salt and water by gut	? Delta cell tumor; >50% malignant	Pancreatic tumor with severe watery diarrhea; flushing; weight loss; hypokalemia; hypercalcemia; hypochlorhydria; hyperglycemia; inordinate fecal water and electrolyte losses
Carcinoid	Serotonin; prostaglandins	Altered gut motility; diarrhea	Enterochromaffin cells; non-beta-cell islet tumors	Carcinoid syndrome with flushing; wheezing; diarrhea; alcohol intolerance; hepatomegaly

to be aware of this fact, so that patients with macroamylasemia will not be needlessly evaluated and treated for pancreatic disease.

Macrolipasemia has now been documented in a few patients with cirrhosis or non-Hodgkin's lymphoma. In these patients, the pancreas appeared normal on ultrasound and CT examination. Lipase was shown to be complexed with immunoglobulin A. Thus, the possibility of *both* macroamylasemia and macrolipasemia should be considered in patients with elevated blood levels of these enzymes.

BIBLIOGRAPHY

BALTHAZAR EJ et al: Acute pancreatitis: Value of CT in establishing prognosis. Radiology 174:331, 1990

BOZKURT T et al: Comparison of pancreatic morphology and exocrine functional impairment in patients with chronic pancreatitis. Gut 35:1132, 1994

CAVALLINI G et al: Gabexate for the prevention of pancreatic damage related to endoscopic retrograde cholangiopancreatography. N Engl J Med 335:919, 1996

FAN ST et al: Early treatment of acute biliary pancreatitis by endoscopic papillotomy. N Engl J Med 328:228, 1993

FERNANDEZ DEL CASTILLO C et al: Acute pancreatitis. Lancet 342:475, 1993

KARIMGANI I et al: Prognostic factors in sterile pancreatic necrosis. Gastroenterology 103:1636, 1992

LEE SP et al: Biliary sludge as a cause of acute pancreatitis. N Engl J Med 326:589, 1992

NEOPTOLEMOS JP et al: Control trial of urgent endoscopic retrograde cholangiopancreatography and endoscopic sphincterotomy versus conservative treatment for acute pancreatitis due to gallstones. Lancet 2:979, 1988

SAINIO V et al: Early antibiotic treatment in acute necrotizing pancreatitis. Lancet 346:663, 1995

STEER ML et al: Chronic pancreatitis. N Engl J Med 332:1482, 1995

STEINBERG WM et al: Diagnostic assays in acute pancreatitis: A study of sensitivity and specificity. Ann Intern Med 102:576, 1985

———, TENNER S: Medical progress. Acute pancreatitis. N Engl J Med 330:1198, 1994

WHITCOMB DC et al: Hereditary pancreatitis is caused by a mutation in the cationic trypsinogen gene. Nature Genetics 13:141, 1996

WILSON C et al: Prediction of outcome in acute pancreatitis: A comparative study of APACHE II, clinical assessment, and multiple screening systems. Br J Surg 77:1260, 1990

305

Barton F. Haynes, Anthony S. Fauci

INTRODUCTION TO THE IMMUNE SYSTEM

Basic research in immunology has resulted in advances in a wide range of clinical disciplines, from allergy and rheumatology to neurology and cardiology. Monoclonal antibody technology has revolutionized the study of cell surface molecules of effector and regulatory immune cells and has provided specific reagents for essentially any target molecule. Advances in cell biology have resulted in the ability to expand and characterize isolated immune cell populations with specific functions in vitro. The ability to manipulate ("overexpress" or "knock-out") genes in the living animal has created the opportunity to study the immune function of virtually any protein in vivo. The cloning and sequencing of genes for antigen receptors and their associated molecules on B cells and T cells, the delineation of the structures of major histocompatibility complex (MHC) class I and class II molecules (see Chap. 306), the identification of soluble mediators (cytokines) as cell-to-cell messengers in the immune system, and the elucidation of the molecular and biochemical mechanisms of signal transduction in immune competent cells have provided the information necessary to understand immune cell recognition and effector function. Thus, in recent years, breakthroughs in new technology have provided molecular explanations for specificity and diversity of the immune system, induction and maintenance of self-tolerance (self-antigen nonreactivity), and regulation of immune cell growth and differentiation.

The normal function of the immune system is essential for health, and dysfunction of the immune system leads to a wide diversity of diseases (Table 305-1). Deficiency of immune cell production or defective immune cell function can lead to a spectrum of immunodeficiency diseases (see Chap. 307). Overactivity of various components of the immune system leads to the development of allergic or autoimmune diseases. Leukemias and lymphomas are the result of malignant transformation in cells of the immune system (see Chaps. 112 and 113). With these new insights into immune system function have come new and specific modes of therapy for autoimmune, immunodeficiency, and malignant immune system diseases. The aim of this chapter is to provide the essentials of the cellular and molecular basis of immunity, with emphasis on those principles relevant to understanding at a basic level the protean clinical and laboratory manifestations of disordered immunity.

THE CD CLASSIFICATION OF HUMAN LYMPHOCYTE DIFFERENTIATION ANTIGENS The development of monoclonal antibody technology led to the discovery of a large number of new leukocyte surface molecules. In 1982, the First International Workshop on Leukocyte Differentiation Antigens was held to establish a nomenclature for cell surface molecules of human leukocytes. From this and subsequent leukocyte differentiation workshops has come the cluster of differentiation (CD) classification of leukocyte antigens (Table 305-2). The data presented in Table 305-2 establish a context to facilitate study of the extraordinarily complex series of events that transpire during normal and aberrant human immune system function.

CYTOKINES Cytokines are soluble proteins produced by a wide variety of hematopoietic and nonhematopoietic cell types. They are critical for normal immune system function, and their expression may be perturbed in disease states. They are involved in the regulation of the growth, development, and activation of immune system cells

and the mediation of the inflammatory response. In general, cytokines are characterized by considerable redundancy in that different cytokines have similar functions. In addition, many cytokines are pleotropic in that they are capable of acting on many different cell types. This pleotropism results from the expression on multiple cell types of receptors for the same cytokine (see below), leading to the formation of "cytokine networks." The action of cytokines may be: (1) autocrine when the target cell is the same cell that secretes the cytokine, (2) paracrine when the target cell is nearby, and (3) endocrine when the cytokine is secreted into the circulation and acts distal to the source. A number of categorizations have been proposed for the grouping of cytokines according to functions. However, these are all imperfect because of the fact that a number of cytokines overlap these groupings. One empiric categorization divides the cytokines into the following three groups: (1) Immunoregulatory cytokines that are involved in the activation, growth, and differentiation of lymphocytes and monocytes, e.g., interleukin (IL)-2, IL-4, and transforming growth factor beta (TGFβ); (2) proinflammatory cytokines that are produced predominantly by mononuclear phagocytes in response to infectious agents, e.g., IL-1, tumor necrosis factor (TNF) alpha, and IL-6, and the chemokine family of inflammatory cytokines, within which are included IL-8, monocyte chemotactic protein (MCP)-1, MCP-2, MCP-3, macrophage inflammatory protein (MIP)-1α, MIP-1β, and regulation-upon-activation, normal T expressed and secreted (RANTES) (see also Chap. 62); and (3) cytokines that regulate immature leukocyte growth and differentiation, e.g., IL-3, IL-7, and granulocyte-macrophage colony stimulating factor (GM-CSF). In general, cytokines exert their effects by influencing gene activation that results in cellular activation, growth, differentiation, functional cell surface molecule expression, and cellular effector function. In this regard, cytokines can have dramatic effects on the regulation of immune responses and the pathogenesis of a variety of diseases. Indeed, T cells have been categorized on the basis of the pattern of cytokines that they secrete that results in either an allergic humoral immune response or a cell-mediated immune response (see below).

Cytokine receptors can be grouped into five general families based on similarities in their extracellular amino acid sequences and conserved structural domains (Fig. 305-1). The immunoglobulin (Ig) superfamily represents a large number of cell surface and secreted proteins. All members of the Ig superfamily must have at least one domain in their protein structure. The IL-1 receptors (type 1, type 2) are examples of cytokine receptors with extracellular Ig domains. The hallmark of the hematopoietic growth factor (type 1) receptor family is that the extracellular regions of each receptor contain two conserved motifs. One motif located at the N terminus is rich in cysteine residues. The other motif is located at the C terminus proximal to the transmembrane region and comprises five amino acid residues, tryptophan-serine-X-tryptophan-serine (WSXWS). Cytokine receptors expressing the WSXWS motif are also referred to as "type I family of cytokine receptors." This family can be further grouped on the basis of the number of receptor subunits they have and utilization of shared subunits. The shared common receptors often have a critical role in signal transduction. A number of cytokine receptors, i.e., IL-6, IL-11, IL-12, and leukemia inhibitory factor, are paired with gp130. There is also a common 150-kDa subunit shared by IL-3, IL-5, and GM-CSF receptors. The gamma chain (γ$_c$) of the IL-2 receptor is common to the IL-2, IL-4, IL-7, IL-9, and IL-15 receptors. Thus, the specific cytokine receptor is responsible for ligand-specific binding, while the subunits such as gp130, the 150-kDa subunit, and γ$_c$ are important in

Table 305-1

Disorders of the Immune System

IMMUNODEFICIENCIES

Primary immunodeficiencies
Combined immunodeficiencies
  Severe combined immunodeficiency
    X-linked
    Autosomal recessive
  Adenosine deaminase (ADA) deficiency
  Purine nucleoside phosphorylase (PNP)
    deficiency
  MHC class II deficiency
  MHC class I deficiency (bare leukocyte
    syndrome)
  Reticular dysgenesis
  CD3γ or CD3ε deficiency
  CD8 deficiency
Predominantly antibody deficiencies
  X-linked agammaglobulinemia (Bruton)
  Hyper-IgM syndrome
    X-linked
    Other
  Ig heavy chain gene deletions
  κ chain deficiency
  IgA deficiency
  Selective deficiency of IgG subclasses
  Common variable immunodeficiency (CVID)
  Antibody deficiency with normal Igs
  Transient hypogammaglobulinemia of infancy
  Secretory component deficiency
Other well-defined immunodeficiency
  syndromes
  Wiskott-Aldrich syndrome

Ataxia-telangiectasia
DiGeorge anomaly
Syndromes associated with immunodeficiency
  Chromosomal instability or defective repair
    Bloom syndrome
    Fanconi anaemia
    ICF syndrome
    Nijmegen breakage syndrome
    Seckel syndrome
    Xeroderma pigmentosa
  Chromosomal defects
    Down syndrome
    Turner syndrome
    Chromosome 18 rings and deletions
  Skeletal abnormalities
    Short-limbed skeletal dysplasia
    Cartilage-hair hypoplasia
  Immunodeficiency with generalized growth
    retardation
    Schimke immunoosseous dysplasia
    Immunodeficiency with absent thumbs
    Dubowitz syndrome
    Growth retardation, facial anomalies, and
      immunodeficiency
    Progeria (Hutchinson-Gilford syndrome)
  Immunodeficiency with dermatologic defects
    Partial albinism
    Dyskeratosis congenita

Netherton syndrome
Acrodermatitis enteropathica
Anhidrotic ectodermal dysplasia
Papillon-Lefèvre syndrome
  Hereditary metabolic defects
    Transcobalamin 2 deficiency
    Methylmalonic acidaemia
    Type I hereditary orotic aciduria
    Biotin-dependent carboxylase deficiency
    Mannosidosis
    Glycogen storage disease, type 1b
    Chédiak-Higashi syndrome
  Hypercatabolism of immunoglobulin
    Familial hypercatabolism
    Intestinal lymphangiectasia
  Other
    Hyper-IgE syndrome
    Chronic mucocutaneous candidiasis
    Hereditary or congenital hypo- or
      asplenia
    Ivermark syndrome
    X-linked lymphoproliferative syndrome
Acquired immunodeficiencies
Acquired immunodeficiency syndrome (AIDS)
Iatrogenic
Idiopathic CD4+ T lymphocytopenia

ALLERGIC DISEASES

Generalized
  Anaphylaxis
  Serum sickness
  Generalized drug reactions
  Food allergy
  Insect venom allergy
  Mastocytosis
Airways
  Allergic rhinitis

Asthma
Hypersensitivity pneumonitis
Skin
  Urticaria
  Angioedema
  Eczema
  Atopic dermatitis
  Allergic contact dermatitis

Erythema multiforme and Stevens-Johnson
  syndrome
Ocular allergy
  Allergic conjunctivitis
  Atopic keratoconjunctivitis
  Venereal keratoconjunctivitis
  Giant papillary conjunctivitis
  Contact allergy

AUTOIMMUNITY

Organ specific
Endocrine system
  Thyroid gland
    Hashimoto's thyroiditis
    Graves' disease
    Thyroiditis with hyperthyroidism
  Type I autoimmune polyglandular syndrome
  Type II autoimmune polyglandular syndrome
  Insulin-dependent diabetes mellitus
  Immune-mediated infertility
  Autoimmune Addison's disease
Skin
  Pemphigus vulgaris
  Pemphigus foliaceus
  Paraneoplastic pemphigus
  Bullus pemphigoid
  Dermatitis herpetiformis
  Linear IgA disease
  Epidermolysis bullosa acquisita
  Autoimmune alopecia
  Erythema nodosum
  Pemphigoid gestationis
  Cicatricial pemphigoid
  Chronic bullous disease of childhood
Hematologic system
  Autoimmune hemolytic anemia
  Autoimmune thrombocytopenic purpura
    Idiopathic
    Drug-related
  Autoimmune neutropenia

Neuromuscular system
  Myasthenia gravis
  Eaton-Lambert myasthenic syndrome
  Stiff-man syndrome
  Acute disseminated encephalomyelitis
  Multiple sclerosis
  Guillain-Barré syndrome
  Chronic inflammatory demyelinating
    polyradiculoneuropathy
  Multifocal motor neuropathy with
    conduction block
  Chronic neuropathy with monoclonal
    gammopathy
  Paraneoplastic neurologic disorders
    Opsoclonus-myoclonus syndrome
    Cerebellar degeneration
    Encephalomyelitis
    Retinopathy
Hepatobiliary system
  Autoimmune chronic active hepatitis
  Primary biliary sclerosis
  Sclerosing cholangitis
Gastrointestinal tract
  Gluten-sensitive enteropathy
  Pernicious anemia
  Inflammatory bowel disease
Organ nonspecific
Connective tissue diseases
  Systemic lupus erythematosus

Rheumatoid arthritis
Systemic sclerosis (scleroderma)
Ankylosing spondylitis
Reactive arthritides
Polymyositis/dermatomyositis
Sjögren's syndrome
Mixed connective tissue disease
Behçet's syndrome
Psoriasis
Vasculitic syndromes
  Systemic necrotizing vasculitides
    Classic polyarteritis nodosa
    Allergic angiitis and granulomatosis
      (Churg-Strauss disease)
    Polyangiitis overlap syndrome
  Hypersensitivity vasculitis
  Wegener's granulomatosis
  Temporal arteritis
  Takayasu's arteritis
  Kawasaki's disease
  Isolated vasculitis of the central nervous
    system
  Thromboangiitis obliterans
  Miscellaneous vasculitides
Sarcoidosis
Graft-versus-host disease
Cryopathies

(continued)

Table 305-1 (*continued*)

Disorders of the Immune System

NEOPLASMS

T cell neoplasms
  Adult T cell leukemia/lymphoma
  Cutaneous T cell lymphoma
  Non-Hodgkin's lymphoma
  Acute lymphoblastic leukemia
  Chronic lymphocytic leukemia (rare)
B cell neoplasms
  Chronic lymphocytic leukemia
  Multiple myeloma
  Burkitt's lymphoma
  Hairy cell leukemia

Acute lymphoblastic leukemia
Non-Hodgkin's lymphoma
Waldenström's macroglobulinemia
Primary amyloidosis
Heavy chain diseases
  Gamma (Franklin's disease)
  Alpha (Seligmann's disease)
  Mu
Monocyte neoplasms
  Acute monocytic leukemia
  Hodgkin's disease

True histiocytic lymphoma
Histiocytosis X
  Eosinophilic granuloma
  Letterer-Siwe disease
  Hand-Schüller-Christian disease
Malignant histiocytosis (histiocytic medullary
  reticulosis)
Other
  Large granular lymphocyte (LGL) leukemia

Table 305-2

CD Classification of Human Lymphocyte Surface Molecule

CD	Other Names	Molecular Mass, kDa	Chromosome Location	Molecular Structure	Tissue/Lineage	Function
CD1	T6	49	1q22-23	Ig superfamily associated with β2M	Cortical thymocytes, Langerhans cells, interdigitating cells	Antigen presentation to TCRγδ cells
CD2	T11, LFA-3 receptor, E-rosette receptor	50	1p13	Ig superfamily	T lymphocytes	Binds LFA-3 (CD58) on RBC, monocytes, thymic epithelial cells; alternative pathway of T cell activation
CD3	T3, CD3 complex, Leu4	CD3γ—26 CD3δ—20 CD3ε—20 CD3ζ—16 CD3η—28	11q23 11q23 11q23 1q22 1q22	CD3γ,δ,ε Ig superfamily; CD3η, ζ; homologous to each other and with FcRε ζ chain comprise α family of signal transducers	CD3γ,δ,ε,ζ,η, T lymphocytes, cytoplasmic CD3ε, NK cells	T cell–associated molecules; transduce signals from T cell receptors
CD4	T4, Leu3a	59	12pter-p12	Ig superfamily	T lymphocytes, monocytes, tissue macrophages, microglial cells, EBV-transformed B lymphocytes	Receptor for HIV env gp120; binds to MHC class II; associated with p56-lck tyrosine kinase
CD5	T1	67	11q13	Ig superfamily	T lymphocytes, B lymphocyte subset	Comitogenic for T lymphocytes; ligand for CD72
CD6	T12	100	?	Scavenger receptor type I superfamily	Subset of T and B lymphocytes	?
CD7	3A1, Leu9	40	17	Ig superfamily	T lymphocytes, NK cells; on subsets of T, B, and myeloid precursors	Comitogenic for T lymphocytes; Ca²⁺ inducible gene; signals T and NK cells through phosphoinositide-3-phosphate kinase
CD8	T8, Leu2a	CD8α—38 CD8β—38	2p12 2	CD8 α, β, Ig superfamily	T cell subset	Receptor for MHC class I; associated with p56-lck tyrosine kinase
CD9	p24	24	12p13	Type III transmembrane protein	Platelets, megakaryocytes, monocytes, pre B cells, activated T cells	Plays a signal transduction role in platelet activation and aggregation
CD10	J5, CALLA, neutral endopeptidase	100	3q21-27	Endopeptidase enzyme	B lymphoid progenitor cells	Peptide cleavage
CD11a	LFA-1α chain	180	16p13.1-11	αL integrin	T, B, NK lymphocytes, monocytes	With β2 integrin, ligand for ICAM-1 (CD54), ICAM-2, and ICAM-3; mediates leukocyte adhesion and leukocyte-endothelial adherence

(continued)

Table 305-2 (*continued*)

CD Classification of Human Lymphocyte Surface Molecule

CD	Other Names	Molecular Mass, kDa	Chromosome Location	Molecular Structure	Tissue/Lineage	Function
CD11b	MAC-1, MO-1α chain, CR3	165	16p13.1-11	α^M integrin	NK cells, PMNs, monocytes	With β2 integrin, receptor for C3bi, fibrinogen, factor X
CD11c	gp150/95 α chain, CR4	150	16p13.1-11	α^X integrin	NK cells, PMNs, monocytes	With β2 integrin, mediates cell binding to C3bi
CD14	LeuM3, MO-2	55	5q31	Phosphoinositol-linked transmembrane glycoprotein	Monocytes	Endotoxin-binding protein
CD15	Sialyl Lewis X (sLe^x)	Carbohydrate	11q	Neu Acα 2–3 Gal β1–4 (Fucα1–3) GlcNac	Granulocytes; cryptic form of CD15 is on T cells [Cutaneous lymphocyte antigen (CLA)]	Ligand for ELAM-1 on endothelial cells; CLA mediates T cell homing to skin
CD16	Fc receptor for IgG (low affinity) FcRγIII	50–65	1q23	Ig superfamily, PI and TM forms	NK cells, PMN, macrophages	FcR for IgG
CD18	LFA-1β chain	95	21q22.3	β2 integrin	T, B, NK lymphocytes, monocytes	Ligand for ICAM-1, (CD54), ICAM-2, and ICAM-3; mediates leukocyte-endothelial interactions
CD19	B4	90	?	Ig superfamily	B lymphocytes	Regulates B cell activation
CD20	B1, Bp35	35–37	11q12-13.1	Calcium channel	B lymphocytes	Mediates B cell activation
CD21	B2	140	1q32	Complement regulatory protein family	B lymphocytes	C3d/EBV receptor, complement receptor 2 (CR2), ligand for CD23
CD22	Bgp135	135	19p13.1	Ig superfamily, homology with N-CAM, myelin-associated glycoprotein (MAG)	B lymphocytes	Comitogenic for B cell activation, interacts with CD45RO on T cells and CD75 on B cells
CD23	Low-affinity receptor for IgE FcεRII	45–50	19	Homology with asialoglycoprotein receptor (lectin)	Activated B lymphocytes, subset of activated T lymphocytes, thymic epithelial cells, macrophages, eosinophils, platelets	FcεRII, soluble CD23 activates immature T cells, ligand for CD21
CD25	TAC, IL-2 receptor α chain	55	10p15-14	Type I transmembrane protein	Activated T and B lymphocytes, monocytes	Low-affinity receptor for IL-2
CD26	Dipeptidylpeptidase IV, gp120	120	11pter-p11.2	Dipeptidylpeptidase IV enzyme	Activated T and B lymphocytes, monocytes	Serine exopeptidase; binds collagen
CD27		55	12p13	TNF receptor family	T cells	Involved in T cell activation; CD70 ligand
CD28	Tp44	44	2q33-34	Ig superfamily	T lymphocytes and activated B cells	Comitogenic for T lymphocytes, regulates T cell cytokine stability, Ligand for B7/BB1 (CD80) molecules
CD29	Integrin β1 chain; common β subset of VLA-1-6, GPIIa	130	10p11.2	β1 integrin	Panhematopoietic, many other cell types	Ligand for many extracellular matrix molecules; conserved cytoplasmic domain binds to cytoskeleton
CD30	Ki-1	105–120	1p36	TNF receptor family	Activated T and B cells	Involved in T cell activation
CD30 ligand		40	9q33	TNF receptor family	Activated T cells and monocytes	Activates or kills CD30+ cells
CD32	FcδRII, gp40	39, 48	1q23	Polymorphic transmembrane glycoproteins, two chains	Macrophages, PMNs, B cells, eosinophils	Fc receptor for aggregated IgG, ligation leads to cell activation

(*continued*)

Table 305-2 (continued)

CD Classification of Human Lymphocyte Surface Molecule

CD	Other Names	Molecular Mass, kDa	Chromosome Location	Molecular Structure	Tissue/Lineage	Function
CD34	MY10	105–120	1q32	Sialomucin with unique protein sequence	Pluripotent stem cells, other hematopoietic precursors, endothelial cells	Phosphorylated upon cell activation
CD35	CR1, C3b receptor	160–250	1q32	Type I transmembrane receptor	B cells, subset NK cells, PMNs, monocytes, RBC	Binds immune complexes; ? Binds complement-opsonized HIV
CD38	OKT10, T10	45	4	Single-chain glycoprotein	T and B cells, NK cells, and macrophages	Ligand for hyaluronate; modulates immune cell function via ADP-ribosylation of intracellular signal-transducing mediators
CD39	gp80	70–100	?	—	Activated B lymphocytes, T lymphocytes, and NK cells	Mediates homotypic adhesion of B cells
CD40	gp50	44–48	20	Homology with nerve growth factor receptor, fas(APO-1), and TNF receptor	B cells, follicular dendritic cells, macrophages	B cell activation, homotypic adhesion; binds to a TNF-like molecule, gp39, that is defective in X-linked hyper-IgM syndrome
CD40 ligand	gp39	39	Xq26	TNF receptor family	Activated CD4+ cells	Induces activation of CD40-expressing cells
CD43	Leukosialin, sialophorin, leukocyte sialoglycoprotein	95	16p11.2	Cell surface sialomucin	T, B, NK cells, monocytes	Involved in leukocyte activation, deficient in Wiskott-Aldrich syndrome, ligand for ICAM-1 (CD54)
CD44	Pgp-1, In(Lu)-related p80, Hermes, extracellular matrix receptor III	80–120	11p13	Cartilage link protein, core proteoglycan homology; multiple isoforms generated by alternative splicing	T, B, NK cells, monocytes, RBC	Transmembrane hyaluronate receptor, promotes leukocyte adhesion; comitogenic for T cells, mediates leukocyte-endothelial binding; promotes carcinoma metastasis
CD45	Leukocyte common antigen, T200	CD45RO—180 CD45RA—220 CD45RB—220, 205, 190	1q31-32 1q31-31 1q31-32	Multiple isoforms generated by alternative splicing	Leukocytes	Cytoplasmic domain is a tyrosine phosphatase, regulates lymphocyte activation, CD45RO in T cells is a ligand for CD22 on B cells
CD49a	VLA-1	210	5	α1 integrin, assembles with CD29 to form α1β1 integrin	Activated T cells, monocytes	Laminin and collagen receptor
CD49b	VLA-2α chain	170	5q23-31	α2 integrin, assembles with CD29, β1 integrin	Activated T cells, platelets	With β1 integrin (CD29), binds collagen types I, II, III, and IV
CD49c	VLA-3	125	17	α3 integrin, assembles with CD29, β1 integrin	B cells	Laminin, collagen, fibronectin receptor
CD49d	VLA-4α chain	150	2q31-32	α4 integrin, assembles with CD29, β1 integrin	T and B lymphocytes, monocytes	With β integrin (CD29), is the receptor for endothelial VCAM-1; mediates leukocyte-endothelial cell binding in Peyer's patches

(continued)

Table 305-2 (continued)

CD Classification of Human Lymphocyte Surface Molecule

CD	Other Names	Molecular Mass, kDa	Chromosome Location	Molecular Structure	Tissue/Lineage	Function
CD54	ICAM-1	40	19	Ig superfamily	Endothelial cells, activated lymphocytes	Ligand for LFA-1, rhinoviruses, falciparum malaria, CD43
CD55	Decay accelerating factor	70	1q32	Complement control protein superfamily	Hematopoietic and nonhematopoietic cells	Binds C3b, C3/C5 convertase
CD56	N-CAM, NKH-1	140	11q23-24	Ig superfamily, homology with N-CAM	NK cells, neuroectodermal cells	Mediates NK cell homotypic adhesion
CD57	HNK1, Leu7	110	?		NK cells, subset of T cells	?
CD58	LFA-3	40–65	1p13	Ig superfamily	Widespread, activated lymphocytes	Ligand for CD2
CD62E	ELAM; E-selectin; LECAM-2	140	1q12-qter	Selectin family; C-type lectin	Endothelium	Binds sialyl Lewis X; mediates neutrophil-endothelial interactions
CD62L	LAM-1, L-selectin, LECAM-1, Leu-8, MEL-14	75–80	1q23-25	Selectin family; C-type lectin	B, T, NK cells, monocytes	Binds CD34, GlyCAM, mediates leukocyte-endothelial interactions; leukocyte rolling
CD62P	P-selectin, PADGEM; LECAM-3	140	1q21-24	Selectin family; C-type lectin	Platelets, endothelium	Binds sialyl Lewis X; mediates platelet interaction with leukocytes and neutrophil-endothelial cell interactions
CD64	FcγRI, high-affinity receptor for IgG	72	1q	Ig superfamily	Monocytes, tissue macrophages	Binds monomeric IgG with high affinity, leads to cell activation
CD69	Activation inducer molecule, EA-1, gp34/28; Leu-23	28, 34	12p12.3-13.2	Homodimer; type II membrane protein related to NK cell activation protein family	Activated B, T, NK cells, monocytes	Ligand binding to CD69 triggers cytolytic activity of NK and TCR γδ T cells
CD70	Ki-24	75, 95, 170	19p13	Type II membrane protein	Activated T cells	CD27 ligand; involved in T cell activation
CD71	T9, transferrin receptor	95	3q26.2-qter	Heterodimer	Activated T and B lymphocytes, monocytes, proliferating cells of many types	Binds transferrin
CD72	Mouse Lyb2	39, 43	9p	Heterodimer	B cells	Ligand for CD5 molecule
CD73	Ecto-5′ nucleotidase L-VAP-2	69	6q14-21	Nucleotidase enzyme	Subsets of B and T lymphocytes	Regulates uptake of nucleotides; mediates binding of lymphocytes to endothelial cells
CD74	Invariant chain of MHC class II	33–43	5q31-33	Glycoprotein	MHC class II–positive cells	MHC class II–associated invariant chains prevents binding of endogenous peptide to class II; associates with CD44
CD79α, β	B cell receptor–associated molecules	α:32–33 β:37–39	?	Ig superfamily	B cells	Component of B cell antigen receptor involved in signal transduction
CD80	B7, BB1	60	3q13.3-21	Ig superfamily	Antigen-presenting cells, B cells, NK cells	Ligand for CTLA-4 and CD28; involved in co-stimulation of T cells

(continued)

Table 305-2 (*continued*)

CD Classification of Human Lymphocyte Surface Molecule

CD	Other Names	Molecular Mass, kDa	Chromosome Location	Molecular Structure	Tissue/Lineage	Function
CD81	TAPA-1	26	11p	Tetraspanning membrane protein	Lymphocytes	Associates with CD19 and CD21 to form B cell signal–transduction complex
CD83	HB15	43	6p23-21.3	Type I transmembrane protein	Activated B, T cells, bone marrow dendritic cells	Unknown
CD86	B7-2, FUN-1	80	3q13.3-21	Ig superfamily	Monocytes, activated B cells	Ligand for CD28 and CTLA-4
CD87	UPA-R	50–65	19q13.1-13.2	Glycoprotein	Granulocytes, monocytes-macrophages, activated T cells	Urokinase plasminogen activator receptor
CD89	FcαR	50–70	19q13.4	Ig superfamily	Leukocytes	Receptor for IgA
CD95	fas/APO-1	43	10q24.1	TNF receptor family	Wide variety of leukocytes, thymic epithelial cells	Binds fas ligand, induces programmed cell death (apoptosis)
CD98	4F2	80, 40	11q12-22	Glycoprotein heterodimer	Monocytes, activated T cells	Involved in T cell activation
CD99	E2, MIC2	32	Xp22.32-pter or Yp11.2-pter (pseudoautosomal)	Glycoprotein	T, B, NK cells, erythrocytes	Involved in T cell activation and adhesion
CD102	ICAM-2	55–65	17q23	Ig superfamily	Lymphocytes, monocytes, endothelial cells	Ligand for CD11a/ CD18 (LFA-1)
CD115	M-CSF, c-fms	150	5q33.2-33.3	Ig superfamily, transmembrane tyrosine kinase receptor	Monocytes-macrophages	Receptor for M-CSF
CDw116	GM-CSFRα	70–85	Xp22.32; Yp11.3; pseudoautosomal	Hematopoietin receptor family	Granulocytes, endothelium	GM-CSF receptor α chain
CD117	SCFR, c-kit	145	4cen-q21	Ig superfamily	Hematopoietic progenitors	Tyrosine kinase that is receptor for stem cell factor (kit ligand)
CD119	IFN γR	90–100	6q23-24	Glycoprotein	Monocytes, B cells, endothelium	IFN γ receptor
CD120a,b	TNFRI(a) TNFRII(b)	55 75–85	12p13.2 1p36.3-36.2	TNF receptor family	Hematopoietic and nonhematopoietic cells	Binds both TNFα and TNFβ
CD121a	IL-1R type I	80	2q12	Ig superfamily	Thymocytes, T cells	Binds IL-1α and IL-1β
CD121b	IL-1R type II	60–70	2q12	Ig superfamily	Monocytes, B cells	Binds IL-1α and IL-1β
CD122	IL-2Rβ	75	2q12-22	Hematopoietin receptor family	NK cells, T and B cells	Binds IL-2
CD123	IL-3Rα	70	?	Hematopoietin receptor family	Stem cells, granulocytes, monocytes	Binds IL-3
CD124	Il-4R	130–150	16p12.1-11.2	Hematopoietin receptor family	T and B cells, hematopoietic precursors	Binds IL-4
CD125	IL-5R	55–60	?	Hematopoietin receptor family	Eosinophils, basophils	Binds IL-5
CD126	IL-6Rα	80	1	Hematopoietin receptor and Ig superfamilies	Activated B cells, granulocytes, monocytes	Binds IL-6
CD127	IL-7R	75	?	Hematopoietin receptor family	Lymphoid precursors, T cells, monocytes	Binds IL-7
CD128	IL-8R	58–67	2	Chemokine (rhodopsin) family	Neutrophils, basophils, T cell subset	Binds IL-8
CD130	IL-6Rβ, IL-11Rβ, OSMRβ, L1FRβ	130	?	Hematopoietin and Ig superfamilies	Activated B cells, monocytes, T cells, NK cells	Common β subunit of IL-6, IL-11, oncostatin M, and leukemia inhibitory factor receptors

NOTE: LFA, lymphocyte function-associated (glycoprotein); RBC, red blood cell; EBV, Epstein-Barr virus; ICAM, intercellular adhesion molecule; PMNs, polymorphonuclear leukocytes; ELAM, endothelial-leukocyte adhesion molecule; VCAM, vascular cell adhesion molecule; VLA, very late activation (antigen).

SOURCE: After Haynes and Denning; Janeway and Travers; and SF Schlossman et al (eds), *Leucocyte Typing V. White Cell Differentiation Antigens,* vols 1 and 2, Oxford, Oxford Univ Press, 1995, with permission.

signal transduction. The members of the interferon (IFN) (type II) receptor family include the receptors for IFN γ, and IFN α/β, which share a similar 210-amino-acid binding domain with conserved cysteine pairs at both the amino and carboxy termini. The receptors for the interferons consist of at least two distinct subunits. The members of the TNF (type III) receptor family share a common binding domain composed of repeated cysteine-rich regions. Members of this family include the p55 and p75 receptors for TNF (TNFR1 and TNFR2, respectively); CD40 antigen, which is an important B cell surface marker involved in isotype switching; fas/Apo-1, whose triggering induces apoptosis; CD27 and CD30, which are found on activated T cells and B cells; and nerve growth factor receptor. The common motif for the seven transmembrane helix family was originally found in receptors that are linked to GTP-binding proteins. This family includes receptors for chemokines, beta-adrenergic receptors, and retinal rhodopsin. It is important to note that two members of the chemokine receptor family, CXC chemokine receptor type 4 (CXCR4) and beta chemokine receptor type 5 (CCR5), have recently been found to serve as coreceptors during infection of CD4-expressing host cells for syncytium-inducing and non-syncytium-inducing HIV, respectively. Both cytokines and their receptors share similar structures and functions. For example, ligands for the TNF receptor family of receptors regulate and determine cell death (apoptosis) program activation and all ligate molecules of the same structural family. Similarly IL-3, IL-5, and GM-CSF are all produced by T helper (TH) 2 cells, and the receptors of these cytokines share common β chains. Thus, cytokines and their receptors may have diversified together during evolution.

Significant advances have been made in defining the signaling pathways through which cytokines exert their effects intracellularly. This is particularly true with regard to the diverse family of hematopoietin receptors. The Janus family of protein tyrosine kinases (JAK) is a critical element involved in signaling via the hematopoietin receptors. There are four known JAK kinases, JAK1, JAK2, JAK3, and Tyk2, which preferentially bind different receptor subunits. Cytokine binding to its receptor brings the subunits into apposition and allows a pair of JAKs to transphosphorylate and activate one another. The JAKs then phosphorylate the receptor on the tyrosine residues and allow signaling molecules to bind to the receptor, where these molecules in turn can become phosphorylated. These signaling molecules can bind the receptor because they have domains (SH2, or src homology 2 domains) that can bind phosphorylated tyrosine residues. There are a number of these important signaling molecules that bind the receptor, such as the adapter molecule SHC, which can couple the receptor to

the activation of the mitogen-activated protein kinase pathway. In addition, a very important class of substrate of the JAKs is the signal transducers and activators of transcription (STAT) family of transcription factors. STATs have SH2 domains that enable them to bind to phosphorylated receptors, where they are then phosphorylated by the JAKs. It appears that different STATs have specificity for different receptor subunits. The STATs then dissociate from the receptor and translocate to the nucleus, bind to DNA motifs that they recognize, and regulate gene expression. The STATs preferentially bind DNA motifs that are slightly different from one another and thereby presumably control transcription of specific genes. The importance of this pathway is particularly relevant to lymphoid development. The receptors for IL-2, IL-4, IL-7, IL-9, and IL-15 all contain a common receptor subunit termed the *common γ subunit*, or γc. The gene for γc is on the X chromosome, and mutations of γc result in the disease X-linked severe combined immunodeficiency (SCID). Mutations of JAK3 itself also result in a disorder identical to X-SCID; however, since JAK3 is found on chromosome 19 and not on the X chromosome, JAK3 deficiency occurs in boys and girls (see Chap. 307). In this chapter the cytokines that affect various cell types are discussed in the context of each type of immune cell.

PHENOTYPE AND FUNCTION OF IMMUNE CELLS

The host defense system is divided into two major categories: immune and nonimmune. Immunity is characterized by an antigen-specific response to a foreign antigen or pathogen and generally takes several days or longer to materialize. A key feature of immunity is memory for the antigen such that subsequent exposure leads to more rapid and often a more vigorous response. Nonimmune host defense is not antigen-specific and is an immediate response system (beginning within minutes of an insult) without memory for the eliciting stimulus. This process is called inflammation. Neutrophils, eosinophils, basophils, natural killer (NK) cells, monocytes, and macrophages are the mediators of this immediate response system. They also play a role in the subsequent development of an immune response.

The dual limbs of the immune system consist of cellular and humoral immunity. The principal effector of cellular immunity is the thymus-derived (T) lymphocyte, and of humoral immunity is the bone marrow–derived or bursa-equivalent (B) lymphocyte. Both B and T lymphocytes derive from a common stem cell. Other key effector and regulator cells of the immune system are large granular lymphocytes (LGL), monocytes-macrophages, and dendritic/Langerhans cells (Fig. 305-2).

FIGURE 305-1 Cytokine family receptor members. Cytokine receptors have been segregated into several large families based on similarities in their extracellular amino acid sequences and conserved structural domains. There are five cytokine receptor family members. See text for details. (*After Abbas et al, with permission.*)

The proportion and distribution of immunocompetent cells in various tissues reflect cell traffic, homing patterns, and functional capabilities. Bone marrow is the major site of maturation of B cells, monocytes-macrophages, and granulocytes and contains pluripotent stem cells which, under the influence of various colony stimulating factors, are capable of giving rise to all hematopoietic cell types (Table 305-3). Granulocyte colony stimulating factor (G-CSF) stimulates the production of neutrophils and stem cell division; GM-CSF stimulates neutrophil, monocyte, eosinophil, and erythroid and megakaryocytoid cell growth and synergizes with IL-3, IL-11, and stem cell factor (SCF) for stem cell activation. Macrophage colony stimulating factor (M-CSF) drives monocyte differentiation; GM-CSF, IL-4, and TNFα drive dendritic/Langerhans cell differentiation; IL-3 drives neutrophil, monocyte, eosinophil, basophil, and erythroid and megakaryocytoid cell differentiation and promotes hematopoietic stem cell survival (see Chap. 105). T cell precursors also arise from hematopoietic stem cells but leave the yolk sac, fetal liver, or bone marrow while they are immature and home to the thymus for completion of maturation. Mature T lymphocytes, B lymphocytes, monocytes, and dendritic/Langerhans cells enter the circulation and home to peripheral lymphoid organs (lymph nodes, spleen) and the gut-associated lymphoid tissue (tonsil, Peyer's patches, and appendix) as well as the skin and mucous membranes and await activation by foreign antigen.

T CELLS   T lymphocytes differ from other immune effector cell types in that the pool of effector T cells is established in the thymus early in life and is maintained throughout life by antigen-driven expansion of virgin peripheral T cells into "memory" T cells that reside primarily in peripheral lymphoid organs. Mature T lymphocytes constitute 70 to 80 percent of normal peripheral blood lymphocytes (only 2 percent of the total body lymphocytes are contained in peripheral blood), 90 percent of thoracic duct lymphocytes, 30 to 40 percent of lymph node cells, and 20 to 30 percent of spleen lymphoid cells. In lymph nodes, T cells occupy deep paracortical areas around B cell germinal centers, and in the spleen, they are located in periarteriolar areas of white pulp (see Chap. 61). T cells are the primary effectors of cell-mediated immunity, with subsets of T cells maturing into cytotoxic cells capable of lysis of virus-infected or foreign cells. T cells are also the primary regulatory cells of T and B lymphocyte and monocyte function by the production of cytokines and by direct cell contact. In addition, T cells regulate erythroid cell maturation in bone marrow.

Human T cells express cell surface proteins that mark stages of intrathymic T cell maturation or identify specific functional subpopulations of mature T cells. Many of these molecules mediate or participate in important T cell function (Table 305-2; Fig. 305-3).

A number of cytokines regulate the process of T cell proliferation and differentiation (Table 305-4). The earliest identifiable cells of T lineage are CD34+ pro-T cells (i.e., cells in which T cell receptor genes are neither rearranged nor expressed); they are found in fetal liver, yolk sac, and postnatal bone marrow. In the thymus, CD7lo+, CD34+ T cell precursors begin cytoplasmic (c) synthesis of components of the CD3 complex of T cell receptor–associated molecules (see Fig. 305-3). Within CD7+, CD2+, and cCD3+ T cell precursors, T cell receptor (TCR) gene rearrangement begins under the influence of IL-7 and eventuates in two T cell lineages, expressing either TCRαβ chains or TCRγδ chains (see Chap. 307). T cells expressing the TCRαβ

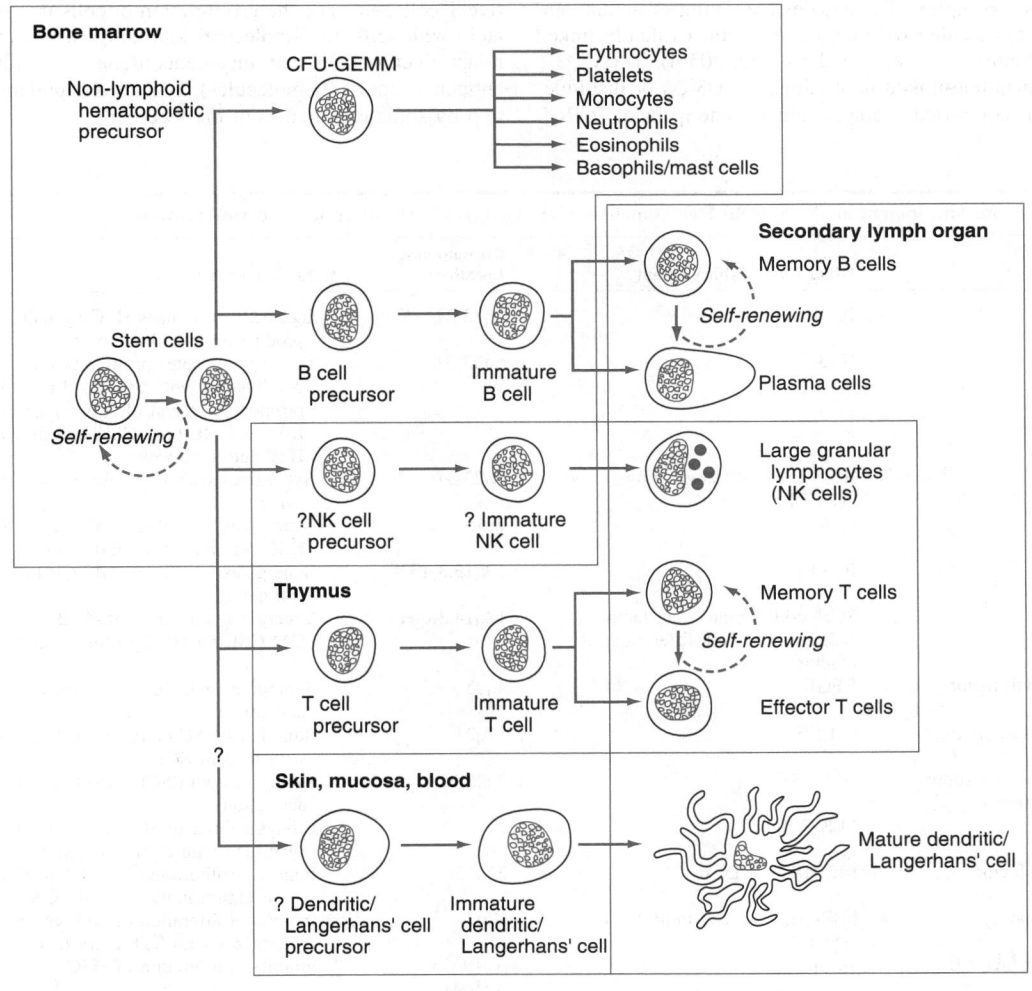

FIGURE 305-2 Hematopoietic stem cell differentiation in bone marrow, thymus, and secondary lymphoid organs. *(After Haynes and Denning, with permission.)*

chains comprise the majority of peripheral T cells in blood, lymph node, and spleen and terminally differentiate into either CD4 + or CD8 + cells. Cells expressing TCRγδ chains circulate as a minor population in blood; their functions, although not fully known, have been postulated as immune surveillance at epithelial surfaces and as cellular defenses against mycobacterial organisms and other intracellular bacteria. Immature cortical thymocytes express, in addition to CD1, both CD4 and CD8 (i.e., they are double positive); however, upon reaching functional maturity, T cell expression of CD1 ceases, and CD4 and CD8 are reciprocally expressed. Mature CD4 + TCRαβ + cells induce B cell differentiation, induce CD8 + cytotoxic T cell proliferation, produce various cytokines, and regulate certain stages of erythropoiesis. A subset of CD4 + cells also functions as cytotoxic effector cells, recognizing foreign peptide antigen fragments that are physically associated with MHC class II molecules on antigen-presenting cells (APC). CD8 + TCRαβ + cells function as cytotoxic effector T cells or as immunoregulatory cells that modulate B and T cell function; CD8 + T cells recognize foreign peptide antigen fragments associated with MHC class I molecules (see Chap. 306).

Elucidation of the stages of T cell development has found clinical relevance in the understanding of T cell malignancies. T cell acute lymphoblastic leukemia and lymphomas are malignancies of pro-T, pre-T, or immature T cells, while forms of cutaneous T cell lymphoma (mycosis fungoides, Sézary syndrome), peripheral T cell lymphomas, and the syndrome of adult T cell leukemia (associated with HTLV-I infection) share the phenotype of mature (usually CD4 +) T cells.

Molecular Basis of T Cell Recognition of Antigen The T cell antigen receptor is a complex of molecules consisting of an antigen-binding heterodimer of either αβ or γδ chains noncovalently linked with five CD3 subunits (γ, δ, ε, ζ, and η) (Fig. 305-4). The CD3 ζ chains are either disulfide-linked homodimers (CD3-ζ₂) or disulfide-linked heterodimers composed of one ζ chain and one η chain. TCRαβ

or TCRγδ molecules must be associated with CD3 molecules to be inserted into the T cell surface membrane, TCRα being paired with TCRβ and TCRγ being paired with TCRδ. Molecules of the CD3 complex mediate transduction of T cell activation signals via T cell receptors, while TCRα and β or γ and δ molecules combine to form the TCR antigen-binding site.

The α, β, γ, and δ T cell antigen receptor molecules have amino acid sequence homology and structural similarities to immunoglobulin heavy and light chains and are thus members, along with other important molecules of immune cells (e.g., MHC class I or II, CD2, CD4, CD8), of the *immunoglobulin gene superfamily* of molecules. The genes encoding the TCR molecules are encoded as clusters of gene segments that rearrange during the course of T cell maturation. This creates an efficient and compact mechanism for housing the diversity requirements of antigen receptor molecules. The TCRβ and δ chains contain four separate regions, namely, the V (variable), D (diversity), J (joining), and C (constant) regions, each encoded by a different gene segment; the TCRα and γ chains consist of V, J, and C regions. Thus, molecules of the T cell antigen receptor have constant (framework) and variable regions, and the gene segments encoding the α, β, γ, and δ chains of these molecules are selected in an antigen-independent fashion during T cell maturation in the thymus, culminating in synthesis of the completed molecule.

TCR diversity is created by the different V, (D), and J segments that are possible for each receptor chain, extensive junctional diversity due to large numbers of possible segments, "N-region diversification" due to the addition of nucleotides at the junction of rearranged gene segments, and the pairing of individual chains to form a TCR dimer. As T cells mature in the thymus, the repertoire of antigen-reactive T cells is modified by selection processes that eliminate many autoreactive T cells, enhance the proliferation of cells that function appropriately with self-MHC molecules and antigen, and allow T cells with nonproductive TCR rearrangements to die (see below). Unlike B cell antigen receptors (Ig molecules), TCRs do not undergo affinity maturation by somatic mutation of the receptor.

Table 305-3

Cytokines That Regulate Multipotent or Pluripotent Hematopoietic Stem Cell (HSC) Proliferation and Differentiation

Cytokine	Other Names/Abbreviation	Chromosome Location	Effect on Stem Cells
Interleukin 1α,β	IL-1αβ	2q13-21	Indirectly stimulates HSC by inducing IL-6 production from bone marrow stromal cells
Interleukin 3	IL-3	5q23-31	Directly promotes proliferation of progenitors in combination with SCF, GM-CSF, or M-CSF; promotes survival of HSC; synergizes with IL-11, LIF, SCF, IL-6, G-CSF, and flt-3 ligand for entry of HSC into cell cycle
Interleukin 4	IL-4, B cell differentiating factor (BCDF)	5q23-31	Synergizes with IL-11 for entry of HSC into cell cycle
Interleukin 6	IL-6	7p15	Synergizes with IL-3, GM-CSF, G-CSF, or SCF for HSC differentiation into myeloid lineages
Interleukin 11	IL-11	19q13.3-13.4	Synergizes with IL-3 and SCF for entry of HSC into cell cycle
Stem cell factor	SCF, c-kit ligand, steel factor (SLF), mast cell differentiating factor	12q14.3-qter	Synergizes with IL-3, IL-6, IL-11, G-CSF, and GM-CSF for HSC proliferation
Basic fibroblast growth factor	BFGF	4q25	Synergizes with IL-3 and GM-CSF for HSC activation
Granulocyte colony stimulating factor	G-CSF	17q21	Stimulates HSC entry into cell cycle and synergizes with IL-3 or SCF
Granulocyte/monocyte-macrophage colony stimulating factor	GM-CSF	5q23-31	Synergizes with SCF, IL-11, and IL-3 for HSC activation
Flt-3 ligand	FLK-2 ligand	?	Effects similar to SCF but, in contrast, does not synergize with erythropoietin (EPO)
Leukemia inhibitory factor	LIf, HILDA, DIA	22q12	Inhibits proliferation of HSC alone but enhances proliferation induced by IL-3, M-CSF, and SCF
Macrophage inflammatory protein 1α	MIP-1α, stem cell inhibitor 1 (SCI-1)	17q	Inhibits proliferation of embryonic stem cells but synergizes with SCF entry of HSC into cell cycle
Transforming growth factor β	TGFβ	β₁:19q13 β₂:1q41	Inhibits proliferation of HSC

SOURCE: After Haynes and Denning, with permission.

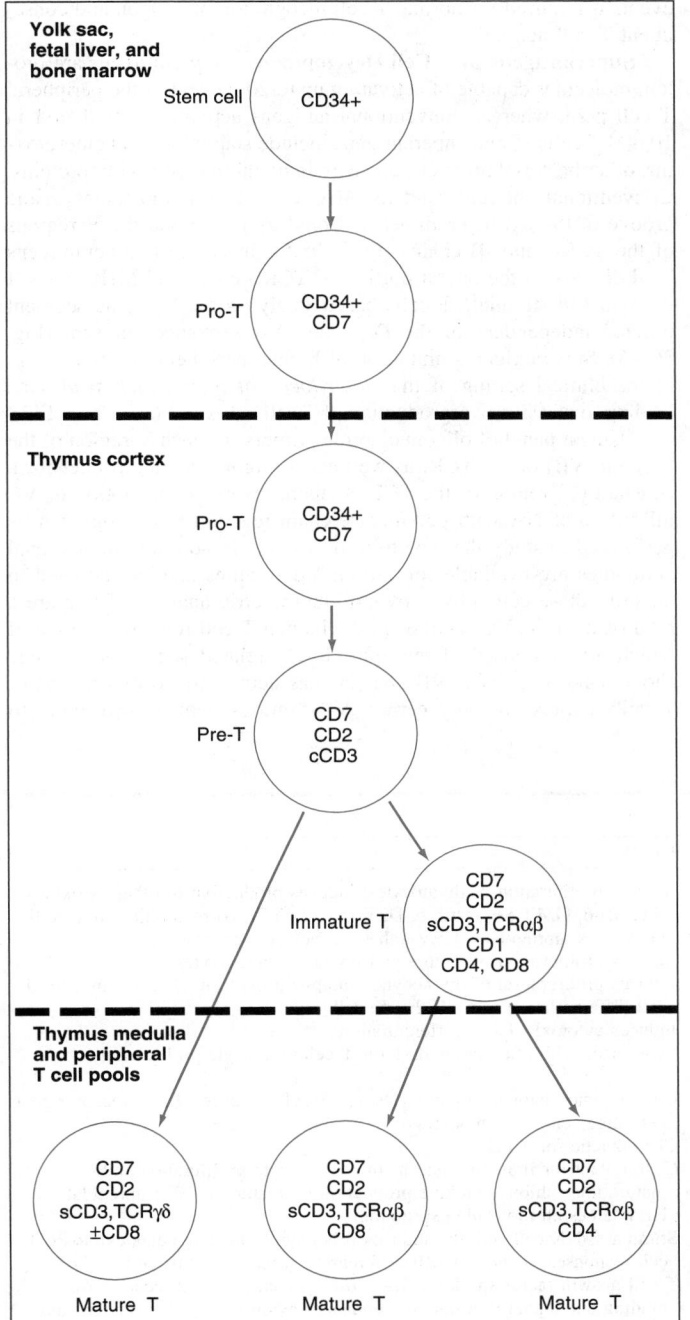

FIGURE 305-3 Human T cell maturation. sCD3, surface CD3 expression; cCD3, cytoplasmic CD3 expression.

T cells do not recognize native protein or carbohydrate antigens. Instead, T cells recognize only short (approximately 9 to 13 amino acids) peptide fragments derived from protein antigens taken up or produced in APC. Foreign antigens (such as mycobacteria pathogens) may be taken up by endocytosis into acidified intracellar vesicles and degraded into small peptides that associate with MHC class II molecules (exogenous antigen-presentation pathway). Other foreign antigens arise endogenously in the cytosol (such as from replicating viruses) and are broken down into small peptides that associate with MHC class I molecules (endogenous antigen-presenting pathway). Thus, APC proteolytically degrade foreign proteins and display peptide fragments embedded in the MHC class I or II antigen-recognition site on the MHC molecule surface (Fig. 305-5), where foreign peptide fragments are available to bind to TCRαβ or TCRγδ chains of reactive T cells. CD4 molecules act as an adhesive and, by direct binding to MHC class II (DR, DQ, or DP) molecules, stabilize the interac-

tion of TCR with peptide antigen (see Fig. 305-4). Similarly, CD8 molecules also act as adhesives to stabilize the TCR-antigen interaction by direct CD8 molecule binding to MHC class I (A, B, or C) molecules.

Antigens that arise in the cytosol and are processed via the endogenous antigen-presentation pathway are cleaved into small peptides by a 28-subunit complex of proteases called the *proteasome*. From the proteasome, antigen peptide fragments are transported from the cytosol into the lumen of the endoplasmic reticulum by a heterodimeric complex termed *transporters associated with antigen processing*, or TAP proteins. There, MHC class I molecules in the endoplasmic reticulum membrane physically associate with processed cytosolic peptides. Following peptide association with class I molecules, peptide–class I complexes are exported to the Golgi apparatus, and then to the cell surface, for recognition by CD8+ T cells.

Antigens that are taken up from the extracellular space via endocytosis into intracellular acidified vesicles are degraded by vesicle proteases into peptide fragments. Intracellular vesicles containing MHC class II molecules fuse with peptide-containing vesicles, thus allowing peptide fragments to physically bind to MHC class II molecules. Peptide–MHC class II complexes are then transported to the cell surface for recognition by CD4+ T cells.

Whereas it is generally agreed that the TCRαβ receptor recognizes peptide antigens in MHC class I or class II molecules, recent data suggest that lipids in the cell wall of intracellular bacteria such as mycobacteria can be presented to TCRγδ T cells in the context of MHC-related CD1 molecules.

Just as foreign antigens are degraded and their peptide fragments presented in the context of MHC class I or class II molecules on APC, endogenous self-proteins are also degraded and self-peptide fragments are presented to T cells in the context of MHC class I or class II molecules on APC. In peripheral lymphoid organs, T cells are present that are capable of recognizing self-protein fragments but normally are *anergic*, i.e., nonresponsive to self-antigenic stimulation.

The immune repertoire of mature T cells is largely determined within the thymus during fetal and early postnatal development. In the thymus, the recognition of self-peptides on thymic epithelial cells and thymic macrophages and dendritic cells is thought to play an important role in shaping the T cell repertoire to recognize foreign antigen (*positive selection*) and in eliminating highly autoreactive T cells (*negative selection*). As immature cortical thymocytes begin to express surface TCR, autoreactive thymocytes are destroyed (negative selection), thymocytes with TCR capable of interacting with foreign antigen peptides in the context of self–MHC antigens are activated and develop to maturity (positive selection), and thymocytes with TCR that are incapable of binding to self–MHC antigens die of attrition (*no selection*). Mature thymocytes that are positively selected are either CD4+ helper T cells or MHC class II–restricted cytotoxic (killer) T cells, or they are CD8+ T cells destined to become MHC class I–restricted cytotoxic T cells. For T cells to be *MHC class I–* or *class II–restricted* means that T cells recognize antigen peptide fragments as immunogenic only when they are presented in the antigen-recognition site of a class I or class II MHC molecule, respectively.

Once engagement of mature T cell TCR by foreign peptide occurs in the context of self–MHC class I or class II molecules (see Fig. 305-4), binding of non-antigen-specific adhesion ligand pairs such as CD54-CD11/CD18 and -CD58/CD2 stabilizes MHC peptide–TCR binding and the expression of these adhesion molecules is upregulated (see Fig. 305-4).

Once TCR-MHC binding is stabilized, activation signals are transmitted through the cell to the nucleus that lead to the expression of gene products that are important in mediating the wide diversity of T cell functions. The TCR does not have intrinsic signaling activity but is linked to a variety of signaling pathways via tyrosine-based activation motifs expressed on the various CD3 chains that bind to enzymes that mediate signal transduction. Each of the pathways results in the activation of particular transcription factors that control the expression of cytokine and cytokine receptor genes. Thus, antigen-MHC binding to the TCR induces the activation of the src family kinases, fyn and lck (lck is associated with CD4 or CD8 co-stimulatory molecules); phosphorylation of CD3ζ chain; activation of the related tyrosine kinases ZAP-70 and syk; and downstream activation of the calcium-dependent calcineurin pathway, the ras pathway, and the protein kinase pathway. Each of these pathways leads to activation of specific families of transcription factors (including NF-AT, fos and jun, and rel/NF-κB) that form heteromultimers capable of inducing expression of IL-2, IL-2 receptor, IL-4, TNF, and other T cell mediators. The src family kinases require dephosphorylation of an inactivation site by CD45 phosphatase before they can be phosphorylated on an activation site. Furthermore, the activity through the receptor is downregulated by the csk kinase, which inactivates the src family kinases.

In addition to the signals delivered to the T cell from the TCR and CD4 and CD8 molecules, other co-stimulatory receptors [including CD2 activated by CD58, and CD28 activated by CD80 (B7/BB1)] also deliver important signals that affect the function of the T cell. The CD28 signal transduction pathway appears particularly important. CD28 signals through phosphoinositide-3-phosphate kinase; its downstream effects are not completely clear. However, if signal transduction through CD28 is blocked, the T cell becomes inactivated or anergic rather than activated. Thus, a concert of molecular and biochemical

events is required for normal T cell recognition of antigen and consequent T cell activation.

Superantigens in T Cell Development   *Superantigens* are protein molecules capable of activating up to 20 percent of the peripheral T cell pool, whereas conventional antigens activate fewer than 1 in 10,000 T cells. T cell superantigens include staphylococcal enterotoxins, other bacterial products, and certain nonhuman retroviral proteins. Conventional antigens bind to MHC class I or II molecules in the groove of the $\alpha\beta$ heterodimer and bind to T cells via the V regions of the TCRα and -β chains (Fig. 305-5). In contrast, superantigens bind directly to the lateral portion of TCRβ chain and MHC class II β chain and stimulate T cells based solely on the Vβ gene segment utilized independent of the D, J, and Vα sequences present (Fig. 305-6). Superantigen stimulation of human peripheral T cells occurs in the clinical setting of the *staphylococcal toxic shock syndrome*, leading to massive overproduction of T cell cytokines (see Chap. 142).

Using a panel of oligonucleotide primers for each V region of the β chain (Vβ) of the TCR, as well as an oligonucleotide primer for a constant (C) region of the TCR β chain, reverse transcription of Vβ mRNA to cDNA with polymerase chain reaction technology can be performed to study the repertoire of T cells. In addition, monoclonal antibodies are available for certain Vβ families and can be used to quantify these cell subsets by cytofluorometric analysis. There are a total of 24 TCR Vβ families in the human T cell repertoire, some of which are composed of multiple closely related segments. In toxic shock syndrome, TCR Vβ analysis has demonstrated expansions of T cells expressing only certain Vβ families, which correspond to

Table 305-4

Roles of Cytokines in T Cell Proliferation and Differentiation

Cytokine	Source	Function
IL-1α,β	Macrophages, E cells, fibroblasts, endothelial cells, dendritic cells	Induces proliferation of thymocytes; induces production of other cytokines (i.e., IL-6, GM-CSF); with sCD23, induces TCR$\alpha\beta$ maturation in T cell precursors; upregulates HEV adhesion molecule expression
IL-2	Activated T cells	Induces proliferation of mature and immature thymocytes
IL-4	T cells	Induces proliferation of thymocytes; inhibits growth of TE cells; induces T cell differentiation to a TH-2 type cell
IL-5	Activated T cells	Induces cytotoxic T cell differentiation
IL-6	Activated T and B cells, macrophages, fibroblasts, TE cells, endothelial cells	Synergizes with mitogen or IL-1 for T cell/thymocyte proliferation
IL-7	Fibroblasts, BM stromal cell line	Comitogenic factor for thymocytes and T cells; induces T cell receptor gene rearrangement in thymocytes
IL-8	Monocytes-macrophages	Chemotactic for T cells
IL-10	Fetal and postnatal thymocytes, B cells	Costimulant for immature and mature thymocyte proliferation and maturation; inhibits cytokine production by mature T cells; upregulates HEV adhesion molecule expression
IL-12	B cells, macrophages	Stimulates NK cell activity; induces IFNγ synthesis; augments cytotoxic T cell responses; induces T cell differentiation to TH-1 type cell
IL-15	Activated monocytes-macrophages; wide variety of tissues; not T cells	T cell growth factor similar to IL-2; uses β chain of IL-2 receptor for binding and signal transduction; enhances cytotoxic function of NK and CD8+ T cells
Soluble CD23 (FcϵRII)	TE cells, B cells	With IL-1, induces TCR$\alpha\beta$ maturation in T cell precursors
GM-CSF	Activated T cells, fibroblasts, endothelial cells, T cells	Promotes growth of early T cell leukemias; promotes proliferation of immature thymocytes
G-CSF	TE cells, macrophages, fibroblasts	?Mitogenic for immature thymocytes
M-CSF	TE cells, monocytes, fibroblasts, endothelial cells	Supports differentiation of progenitors committed to the monocyte-macrophage lineages; ?mitogenic for immature thymocytes
LIF	TE cells, activated cells	?Prevents multilineage differentiation of intrathymic stem cells prior to signal to become T cell precursors
IFNγ	Activated T cells, thymocytes	Upregulates expression of TE, fibroblast, and macrophage CD54 (ICAM-1) and MHC class II; antiproliferative effect on thymocytes via adenylate cyclase pathway; induced HEV adhesion molecule expression
TNFα	Macrophages, activated T and B cells, thymocytes	IL-1–like effects
TGFα	Activated macrophages, TE cells	Regulates production of other cytokines (IL-1 and IL-6) by TE cells; drives TE cell proliferation and/or differentiation via EGF receptor
TGFβ	?TE cells, T cells	Regulates expression of several oncogenes; suppresses lymphocyte responses to other cytokines; ?inhibits TE cell proliferation
EGF	?Monocytes-macrophages, ?fibroblasts, ?TE cells	Drives TE and other epithelial cell proliferation

NOTE: Unless otherwise stated, effect reported or postulated is in humans, TE; thymic epithelial; BM, bone marrow; EGF, epidermal growth factor; LIF, leukemia inhibitory factor; IFNγ, interferon γ; TNF, tumor necrosis factor; TGF, transforming growth factor; HEV, high endothelial venule; FcϵRII, Fc receptor for IgE type II; IL, interleukin.
SOURCE: After BF Haynes et al, Semin Immunol 2:67, 1990.

Antigen presenting cell

CD58 (LFA-3)   CD54 (ICAM-1)
HLA Class II   B7
? Ligand   α β
CD2   CD45   CD4   TCR   CD28
    CD3
    α β
    γ σ ε ς η
    G
PKC   ? p56-lck   ZAP-70
Activated
    ? pp59-fyn
    ? PLCγ1
Tyrosine   CD11, CD18
Phosphatase   (LFA-1)
Vav
    Stabilize
    Cytokine
    mRNA
Ras   PiP₂ → IP₃, DG
Raf-1   Increase in intracellular
    calcium
Mek   Calcineurin
MAP-Kinase   NF-AT_c → NF-AT_c*
Fos/Jun
NF-AT_n   NF-AT_c
    IL-2 Gene

FIGURE 305-4 Molecules involved in human T cell recognition of antigen and in human T cell activation. The black circle at the tip of the αβ chains of MHC class II molecules represents a peptide fragment of "processed" protein antigen. See text for details of the activation and signal transduction process. The asterisk on NF-AT_c represents the activated form of the molecule. *(After Robey and Allison; and Weiss and Littman, with permission.)*

those Vβ families capable of binding to (and being activated by) the staphylococcal enterotoxin superantigen of *Staphylococcus aureus*. The demonstration of selective expansions of certain Vβ subsets in diseases such as rheumatoid arthritis (see Chap. 313) and Kawasaki disease (see Chap. 319) has led to suggestions that various microbes might be the inducing stimuli of these diseases; however, the role of superantigens in such diseases remains speculative.

B CELLS Mature B cells comprise 10 to 15 percent of human peripheral blood lymphocytes, 50 percent of splenic lymphocytes, and approximately 10 percent of bone marrow lymphocytes. B cells express on their surface intramembrane immunoglobulin (Ig) molecules that function as B cell antigen receptors in a complex of Ig-associated α and β signaling molecules with intracellular signaling events similar to those in T cells (Fig. 305-7). Unlike T cells, which recognize only processed peptide fragments of conventional antigens embedded in the notches of MHC class I and class II antigens of APC, B cells are capable of recognizing and proliferating to whole and unprocessed native antigens via antigen binding to B cell surface Ig (sIg) receptors.

B cells also express surface receptors for the Fc region of IgG molecules (CD32) as well as receptors for activated complement components (C3d or CD21, C3b or CD35). The primary function of B cells is to produce antibodies. B cells also serve as APC and are highly efficient at antigen processing. Their antigen-presenting function is enhanced by a variety of cytokines. Mature B cells are derived from bone marrow precursor cells that arise continuously throughout life (see Fig. 305-2).

B lymphocyte development can be separated into antigen-independent and antigen-dependent phases (see Chap. 307). Antigen-independent B cell development occurs in primary lymphoid organs, including fetal liver and bone marrow, and includes all stages of B cell maturation up to the sIg+ mature B cell. Antigen-dependent B cell maturation is driven by the interaction of antigen with B cell sIg, leading to memory B cell induction, Ig class switching, and plasma cell formation. Antigen-dependent stages of B cell maturation occur in secondary lymphoid organs, including lymph node, spleen, and gut Peyer's patches. In contrast to the T cell repertoire that is for the most part generated intrathymically before contact with foreign antigen, the repertoire of B cells expressing diverse antigen-reactive sites is modified by further alteration of Ig genes after stimulation by antigen—a process called *somatic mutation*—which occurs in lymph node germinal centers.

During B cell development, diversity of the antigen-binding variable region of Ig is generated by an ordered set of Ig gene rearrangements. Heavy chain rearrangements precede those for light chains. For the heavy chain, there is first a rearrangement of D segments to J segments, followed by a second rearrangement between a V gene segment and the newly formed D-J sequence; the C segment is aligned to the V-D-J complex to yield a functional Ig heavy chain gene (V-D-J-C). During later stages, a functional κ or λ light chain gene is generated by rearrangement of a V segment to a J segment, ultimately yielding an intact Ig molecule composed of heavy and light chains (see Chaps. 114 and 307).

The process of Ig gene rearrangement is regulated to result in a single antibody specificity produced by each B cell with each Ig molecule comprising one type of heavy chain and one type of light chain. Although each B cell contains two copies of Ig light and heavy chain genes, only one gene of each type in each B cell is productively rearranged and expressed, a process termed *allelic exclusion*.

There are approximately 300 V_κ genes and 5 J_κ genes, resulting in the pairing of V_κ and J_κ genes to create 1500 different light chain combinations. The number of distinct κ light chains that can be generated is increased by somatic mutations within the V_κ and J_κ genes, thus creating large numbers of possible specificities from a limited amount of germ-line genetic information. As noted above, in heavy chain Ig gene rearrangement, the VH domain is created by the joining of three types of germ-line genes called V_H, D_H, and J_H, thus allowing for even greater diversity in the variable region of heavy chains than for light chains (see Chap. 307).

The most immature B cell precursors (pro-B cells) express surface CD10 and CD34, lack B lineage–specific antigens CD19 and CD22, and also lack cytoplasmic Ig (cIg) and surface sIg (Fig. 305-8). The next stage in B cell development, the pre-B cell I, is marked by the acquisition of CD19 and CD22 B cell antigens. Ig genes undergo rearrangement in pre-pre-B cells, but Ig heavy chain protein is not expressed. The hallmark of the next maturation stage, the pre-B cell II, is expression of cμ heavy chain in association with expression of CD73 and CD21 surface proteins. Immature B cells have rearranged Ig light chain genes and express sIgM. As immature B cells develop into mature B cells, sIgD is expressed as well as sIgM and CD23. At this point, B lineage development in bone marrow is complete, and B cells exit into the peripheral circulation and migrate to secondary lymphoid organs.

A number of cytokines synergize to drive sequential stages of B cell maturation (Table 305-5). Bone marrow stromal cell– and T cell–

derived IL-3 and IL-7 drive the earliest stages of B cell differentiation. Low-molecular-weight B cell growth factor binds to high-affinity receptors expressed on all B cell precursors except pro-B cells and also triggers B cell differentiation. IL-1, -2, -4, -5, and -6 synergize to drive mature B cells to proliferate and differentiate into Ig-secreting cells. TGFβ can be an antagonistic cytokine for B cells in that it can block the synthesis of κ light chains.

Evidence exists that the murine B cell compartment contains three B cell subsets, each derived from a distinct cell lineage. B-1a B cells are produced early in fetal development, express the pan–T cell marker CD5, and produce high levels of autoantibodies. B-1b B cells have similar properties to B-1a cells except that B-1b cells are CD5 negative. Both B-1a and B-1b B cells are capable of self-replenishment in the adult and are found in the peritoneum of adult animals. In contrast, B-2 B cells are conventional B cells that are continuously generated in adult bone marrow, produce low levels of autoantibodies, and are the predominant B cell type in lymph nodes, Peyer's patches, and peripheral blood. B-1a, B-1b, and B-2 B cells each display unique $V_H D J_H$ repertoires that are formed at distinct stages of fetal or adult development, confirming their separate lineages. Some evidence suggests that similar B cells are present in humans, with elevated levels of CD5+ B cells found in autoimmune diseases such as rheumatoid arthritis (see Chap. 313).

LARGE GRANULAR LYMPHOCYTES   LGL constitute approximately 5 to 10 percent of peripheral blood lymphocytes. LGL are nonadherent, nonphagocytic cells with large azurophilic cytoplasmic granules. LGL express surface receptors for the Fc portion of IgG

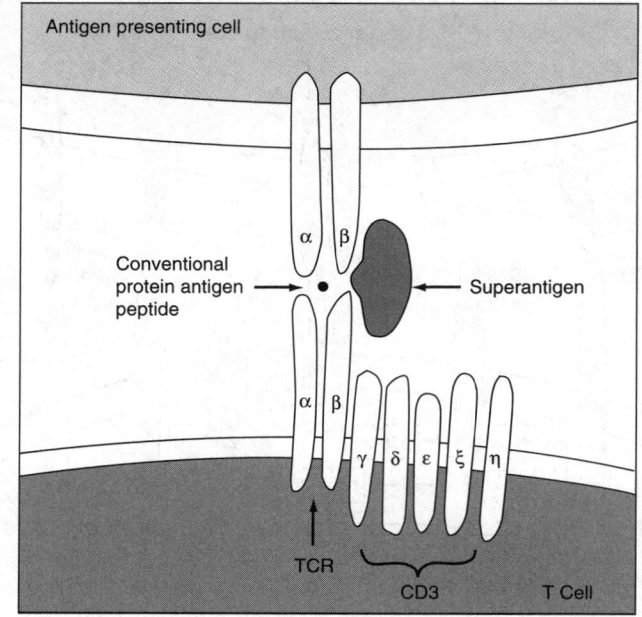

FIGURE 305-6   Comparison of site of superantigen binding to T cell receptor with the site of binding to T cell receptor of processed conventional antigen.

(CD16) and for NCAM-1 (CD56), and many LGL express some T lineage markers, particularly CD8, and proliferate in response to IL-2. LGL arise in both bone marrow and thymic microenvironments (see Fig. 305-2).

Functionally, LGL share features with both monocytes-macrophages and neutrophils in that subsets of LGL mediate antibody-dependent cellular cytotoxicity (ADCC) and NK activity. ADCC is the binding of an opsonized (antibody-coated) target cell to an Fc receptor–bearing effector cell via the Fc region of antibody, resulting in lysis of the target by the effector cell. NK cell activity is the nonimmune (i.e., effector cell never having had previous contact with the target), MHC-unrestricted, non-antibody-mediated killing of target cells, which are usually malignant cell types, transplanted foreign cells, or virus-infected cells. Thus, LGL that mediate NK activity may play an important role in immune surveillance and destruction of cells that spontaneously undergo malignant transformation in vivo. Subsets of NK cells may play a role in hematopoietic cell engraftment; some subsets stimulate bone marrow stem cells, and others stimulate engraftment. Lymphokine-activated killer (LAK) cells are NK lymphocytes that proliferate in vitro to high levels of IL-2 and develop the ability to kill tumor cells more efficiently than unstimulated NK cells. Rare patients with complete absence of NK cells have been described who lack both NK activity and CD56+, CD16+ lymphocytes but have normal T and B cell function. NK cell hyporesponsiveness is also observed in patients with the *Chédiak-Higashi syndrome*, an autosomal recessive disease associated with fusion of

FIGURE 305-5   Structure of MHC class I and MHC class II molecules. *A* and *B*. Top and schematic side views of an MHC class I molecule. *C* and *D*. Top and schematic side views of an MHC class II molecule. Peptide-binding cleft is location of short peptide fragments derived from proteolytic cleavage of either foreign or self-proteins. Whereas the peptide-binding cleft comprises the α1, α2, and α3 domains of the class I α chain, the peptide-binding cleft of class II comprises the β1 and α1 domains of the class IIβ and α chains, respectively. (*From Janeway and Travers, with permission.*)

Membrane IgM

Antigen

L — L

β — β
μH — μH
α — α

CD45

FIGURE 305-7 B cell antigen receptor for antigen-associated molecules. Immunoglobulin (Ig) associated α (CD79α) and β (CD79β) chains are disulfide-linked molecules that mediate the delivery of intracellular activation signals to B cells following interaction of membrane Ig with antigen. CD45 modulates the activation state of B cells by the tyrosine phosphatase activity of the cytoplasmic domain of CD45 molecules.

cytoplasmic granules and defective degranulation of neutrophil lysosomes. Recently, a series of studies has suggested that subsets of NK cells can specifically recognize normal allogeneic cells in a clonal fashion. Studies of allogeneic target cells suggest that the genetic locus controlling NK alloantigen lysis is different from conventional MHC products, is inherited as an autosomal recessive trait, and is located on chromosome 6 in the same region as MHC class I genes.

The ability of NK cells to kill target cells is inversely related to target cell expression of MHC class I molecules. Thus, NK cells kill target cells with low or negative levels of MHC class I expression and are prevented from killing target cells with high levels of class I expression. Some viruses and cancers downregulate host cell MHC class I molecule expression, thereby making infected or transformed cells unable to be targeted by CD8 + MHC class I–restricted cytotoxic T cells. One hypothesis is that NK cells evolved to fill a niche in the host immune response to viruses and tumors by providing a surveillance component of the immune system that could kill MHC class I–negative infected or malignant cells. Recently, the NK surface receptors that bind to MHC class I molecules and prevent NK cell killing of class I–expressing target cells have been cloned in humans and shown to be a group of molecules in the Ig gene superfamily.

MONOCYTES-MACROPHAGES

Monocytes arise from precursor cells within bone marrow (see Fig. 305-2) and circulate with a half-life ranging from 1 to 3 days. Monocytes leave the peripheral circulation by marginating in capillaries and then migrating into a vast extravascular pool. Tissue macrophages arise by migration of monocytes from the circulation and by proliferation of macrophage precursors in tissue. Common locations of tissue macrophages (and some of their specialized names) are lymph node, spleen, bone marrow, perivascular connective tissue, serous cavities such as the peritoneum, pleura, skin connective tissue, lung (alveolar macrophage), liver (Kupffer cell), bone (osteoclast), central nervous system (microglia), and synovium (type A lining cell).

The monocyte-macrophage system plays a major role in the expression of

immune reactivity by mediation of functions such as the presentation of antigen to T lymphocytes and the secretion of factors such as IL-1 and IL-6 that are central to antigen-specific activation of T and B lymphocytes. Although monocytes-macrophages were first thought to be the major APC of the immune system, it is now clear that dendritic/ Langerhans cells are the most potent and effective APC in the body (see below). Monocytes-macrophages mediate effector functions such as destruction of antibody-coated bacteria, tumor cells, or even normal hematopoietic cells in certain types of autoimmune cytopenias. Activated macrophages also can mediate antigen-nonspecific lytic activity and eliminate cell types such as tumor cells in the absence of antibody. This activity is largely mediated by cytokines (i.e., TNF and IL-1). Monocytes-macrophages express lineage-specific molecules (e.g., CD14) as well as surface receptors for a number of molecules, including the Fc region of IgG (CD16, CD32, CD64), activated complement components (CD35) (see Table 305-2), and various cytokines (see Tables 305-3 to 305-5). Finally, macrophage secretory products are more diverse than those known for any other cell of the immune system. These secretory products allow the macrophage to exert both pro- and anti-inflammatory effects and to regulate other cell types. Among monocyte-macrophage–secreted products are hydrolytic enzymes, products of oxidative metabolism, TNFα, IL-1, -6, -12, -15, and a number of chemoattractant cytokines (chemokines) involved in the orchestration of an immune response in tissues.

DENDRITIC/LANGERHANS CELLS Dendritic/Langerhans cells are bone marrow–derived APC that are distinct from monocytes-macrophages. They lack the standard T, B, NK, and monocyte cell markers and have very little expression of C3 and Fc receptors; they express CD83 and other molecules that aid in their identification. They can be expanded in culture and their function enhanced by the cytokines GM-CSF, IL-1, IL-4, and TNFα. They are distinguished by an exceptional ability to present antigen, by expression of high levels of MHC class II and adhesion molecules, and dendritic morphology with multiple thin membrane projections (veils). Their antigen-processing capability has not been well studied. When present in the skin and beneath the mucosal surfaces, they are referred to as *Langerhans cells*. They are the dendritic cells of the blood and the spleen, the veiled cells of afferent lymphatics, and form part of the interdigitating cell network of the lymphoid organs. Dendritic cells are present in the blood in very small numbers, fewer than 0.1 percent of total blood leukocytes;

	Stem Cell	Pro-B	Pre-B I	Pre-B II (Large)	Pre-B II (Small)	Immature B	Mature B
	CD34	CD34	CD34	CD34	-	-	-
		CD10	CD10	CD10	CD10	-	-
			CD19	CD19	CD19	CD19	CD19
			CD40	CD40	CD40	CD40	CD40
				CD73	CD73	CD73	CD73
				CD22	CD22	CD22	CD22
				CD38	CD38	-	-
					CD21	CD21	CD21
							CD23
IL-7 Receptor	-	+	+	-	-	-	-
IL-3 Receptor	-	+	+	+	+	-	-
IL-4 Receptor	-	-	-	-	+	+	+
Immunoglobulin gene rearrangement	-	-	+	+	+	+	+
IgM Expression	-	-	-	-	cytoplasm	surface	surface
IgD Expression	-	-	-	-	-	-	surface

FIGURE 305-8 Antigen-independent human B lymphocyte maturation. (*After Haynes and Denning, with permission.*)

Table 305-5

Cytokines That Regulate Human B Cell Development

Cytokine	Source	Function
IL-7	T cells, bone marrow stromal cells	Drives pro-B and pre-pre-B cells to proliferate and differentiate
BCG-F (low-molecular-weight B cell growth factor)	Activated T cells	B cell precursor proliferation
IL-3	T cells, stromal cells	Induces B cell precursor proliferation
IL-1, IL-2, IL-4, IL-5, IL-6	T cells (IL-2, IL-4, IL-5), monocytes (IL-1, IL-6)	Drives mature B cells to proliferate and differentiate into Ig-secreting cells
TGFβ	T cells, ?thymic epithelial cells	Blocks synthesis of κ light chains

their presence in the blood suggests that these cells traffic among different organs.

FOLLICULAR DENDRITIC CELLS Follicular dendritic cells (FDC) are APC for B cells and are distinct from the dendritic/ Langerhans cells, which are APC for T cells. They are located in the germinal centers or follicles of secondary lymphoid organs. The origin of FDC is unclear. Their main function is to trap and retain antigen in the germinal centers of lymphoid organs and present the antigen to B cells. Antigen is retained on their membranes in the form of antigen-antibody complexes that bind to the cell via the cellular receptor for C3. The FDC have extensive, thin, finger-like projections that surround the B cells in the germinal centers, allowing for maximal exposure of trapped antigen. FDC show very little evidence of endocytosis. The retention of antigen on the surface of the FDC membranes is felt to be critical for the selection and growth of high-affinity clones of B cells and for the maintenance of B cell memory. CD4 + T cells migrate into the germinal centers to provide immunologic help to the B cells. Of note, the human immunodeficiency virus (HIV) is trapped in large quantities on the processes of FDC in lymphoid organs, allowing the lymphoid tissue to serve as a reservoir of virus and a source of infection for CD4 + T cells migrating into the area to provide help to B cells in the initiation and propagation of an HIV-specific humoral response (see Chap. 308).

NEUTROPHILS, EOSINOPHILS, AND BASOPHILS Granulocytes are present in nearly all forms of inflammation and are nonspecific amplifiers and effectors of specific immune responses. Unchecked accumulation and activation of granulocytes can lead to host tissue damage, as seen in neutrophil- and eosinophil-mediated *systemic necrotizing vasculitis*. Granulocytes are derived from stem cells in bone marrow (see Fig. 305-2). Each type of granulocyte (neutrophil, eosinophil, or basophil) is derived from a different subclass of progenitor cell, which is stimulated to proliferate by colony stimulating factors. During terminal maturation of granulocytes, class-specific nuclear morphology and cytoplasmic granules appear that allow for histologic identification of granulocyte type.

Neutrophils express Fc receptors for IgG (CD16) and receptors for activated complement components (C3b or CD35) (see Table 305-2). Upon interaction of neutrophils with immune complexes, azurophilic granules (containing myeloperoxidase, lysozyme, elastase, and other enzymes) and specific granules (containing lactoferrin, lysozyme, collagenase, and other enzymes) are released, and microbicidal superoxide radicals (O_2) are generated at the neutrophil surface. The generation of superoxide leads to inflammation by direct injury to tissue and by alteration of macromolecules such as collagen and DNA.

Eosinophils express Fc receptors for IgG (CD32) and are potent cytotoxic effector cells for various parasitic organisms. Intracytoplasmic contents of eosinophils, such as major basic protein, eosinophil

cationic protein, and eosinophil-derived neurotoxin, are capable of directly damaging tissues and may be responsible in part for the organ system dysfunction in the *hypereosinophilic syndromes* (see Chap. 62). Since the eosinophil granule contains anti-inflammatory types of enzymes (histaminase, arylsulfatase, phospholipase D), eosinophils may downregulate or terminate ongoing inflammatory responses in normal inflammation homeostasis.

The normal functions of basophils and tissue mast cells are not completely understood; the capacity of basophil mediators to increase local delivery of antibodies and complement by increasing vascular permeability is hypothetical. Thus, the basophil is identified principally with allergic reactions and some delayed cutaneous hypersensitivity states. Certainly the promotion of increased vascular permeability by basophils is important in the genesis of inflammatory lesions in some vasculitis syndromes (see Chap. 319). Basophils express high-affinity surface receptors for IgE (Fc RI) and, upon cross-linking of basophil-bound IgE by antigen, release histamine, eosinophil chemotactic factor of anaphylaxis, and neutral protease—all mediators of immediate (anaphylaxis) hypersensitivity responses (Table 305-6). In addition, basophils express surface receptors for activated complement components (C3a, C5a), through which mediator release can be directly effected. → *For further discussion of tissue mast cells, see Chap. 310.*

HUMORAL MEDIATORS OF SPECIFIC IMMUNITY: IMMUNOGLOBULINS

Immunoglobulins are the products of differentiated B cells and mediate the humoral arm of the immune response. The primary functions of antibodies are to bind specifically to antigen and bring about the inactivation or removal of the offending toxin, microbe, parasite, or other foreign substance from the body. The structural basis of Ig molecule function and Ig gene organization has provided insight into the role of antibodies in normal protective immunity, pathologic immune-mediated damage by immune complexes, and autoantibody formation against host determinants.

All immunoglobulins have the basic structure of two heavy and two light chains (Fig. 305-9). Immunoglobulin isotype (i.e., G, M, A, D, E) is determined by the type of Ig heavy chain present. IgG and IgA isotypes can be divided further into subclasses (G1, G2, G3, G4, and A1, A2) based on specific antigenic determinants on Ig heavy chains. The characteristics of human immunoglobulins are outlined in Table 305-7. The four chains are covalently linked by disulfide bonds. Each chain is made up of a V region and C regions (also called *domains*), themselves made up of units of approximately 110 amino acids. Light chains have one variable (VL) and one constant (CL) unit; heavy chains have one variable unit (VH) and three or four constant (CH) units, depending on isotype. As the name suggests, the

Table 305-6

Mediators Released from Human Mast Cells and Basophils

Mediator	Actions
Histamine	Smooth-muscle contraction, increased vascular permeability
Slow reacting substance of anaphylaxis (SRSA) (leukotriene C_4, D_4, E_4)	Smooth-muscle contraction
Eosinophil chemotactic factor of anaphylaxis (ECF-A)	Chemotactic attraction of eosinophils
Platelet-activating factor	Activates platelets to secrete serotonin and other mediators; smooth-muscle contraction; induces vascular permeability
Neutrophil chemotactic factor (NCF)	Chemotactic attraction of neutrophils
Leukotactic activity (leukotriene B_4)	Chemotactic attraction of neutrophils
Heparin	Anticoagulant
Basophil kallikrein of anaphylaxis (BK-A)	Cleaves kininogen to form bradykinin

FIGURE 305-9 Schematic structure of the immunoglobulin G (IgG) molecule.

C regions of Ig molecules are made up of homologous sequences and share the same primary structure as all other Ig chains of the same isotype and subclass. Constant regions are involved in biologic functions of Ig molecules. The CH2 domain of IgG and the CH4 units of IgM are involved with the binding of the C1q portion of C1. The CH region at the carboxy-terminal end of the IgG molecule, the Fc region (see Fig. 305-9), binds to surface Fc receptors (CD16, CD32, CD64) of macrophages, LGL, B cells, neutrophils, and eosinophils.

Variable regions (VL and VH) constitute the antibody-binding (Fab) region of the molecule. Within the VL and VH regions are hypervariable regions (extreme sequence variability) that constitute the antigen-binding site unique to each Ig molecule. The idiotype is defined as the specific region of the Fab portion of the Ig molecule to which antigen binds. Antibodies against the idiotype portion of an antibody molecule are called *anti-idiotype antibodies*. The formation of such antibodies in vivo during a normal B cell antibody response

may generate a negative (or "off") signal to B cells to terminate antibody production.

IgG comprises approximately 75 to 85 percent of total serum immunoglobulin. The four IgG subclasses are numbered in order of their level in serum, IgG1 being found in greatest amounts and IgG4 the least. IgG subclasses have clinical relevance in their varying ability to bind macrophage and neutrophil Fc receptors and to activate complement (see Table 305-7). Moreover, selective deficiencies of certain IgG subclasses give rise to clinical syndromes in which the patient is inordinately susceptible to bacterial infections. IgG antibodies are frequently the predominant antibody made after rechallenge of the host with antigen (secondary antibody response).

IgM antibodies normally circulate as a 950-kDa pentamer with 160-kDa bivalent monomers joined by a molecule called the *J chain*, a 15-kDa nonimmunoglobulin molecule that also effects polymerization of IgA molecules. IgM is the first immunoglobulin to appear in the immune response (primary antibody response) and is the initial type of antibody made by neonates. Membrane IgM in the monomeric form also functions as a major antigen receptor on the surface of mature B cells (see Fig. 305-7). IgM is an important component of immune complexes in autoimmune diseases. For instance, IgM antibodies against IgG molecules (rheumatoid factors) are present in high titers in *rheumatoid arthritis*, other collagen diseases, and some infectious diseases (*subacute bacterial endocarditis*). IgM antibody binds the C1 component of complement via the CH4 domain and thus is a potent activator of complement.

IgA comprises only 7 to 15 percent of total serum immunoglobulin but is the predominant class of immunoglobulin in secretions. IgA in secretions (tears, saliva, nasal secretions, gastrointestinal tract fluid, and human milk) is in the form of secretory IgA (sIgA), a polymer consisting of two IgA monomers, a joining molecule, again called the J chain, and a glycoprotein called the *secretory protein*. Of the two IgA subclasses, IgA1 is primarily found in serum, whereas IgA2 is more prevalent in secretions. IgA fixes complement via the alternative complement pathway and has potent antiviral activity in humans by

Table 305-7

Physical, Chemical, and Biologic Properties of Human Immunoglobulins

Property	IgG	IgA	IgM	IgD	IgE
Usual molecular form	Monomer	Monomer, dimer	Pentamer, hexamer	Monomer	Monomer
Other chains	None	J chain, SC	J chain	None	None
Subclasses	G1, G2, G3, G4	A1, A2	None	None	None
Heavy chain allotypes	Gm (≈30)	No A1, A2m (2)	None	None	None
Molecular mass, kDa	150	160, 400	950, 1150	175	190
Sedimentation constant, Sw20	6.6S	7S, 11S	19S	7S	8S
Carbohydrate content, %	3	7	10	9	13
Serum level in average adult, mg/mL	9.5–12.5	1.5–2.6	0.7–1.7	0.04	0.0003
Percentage of total serum Ig	75–85	7–15	5–10	0.3	0.019
Serum half-life, days	23	6	5	3	2.5
Synthesis rate, mg/kg per day	33	65	7	0.4	0.016
Antibody valence	2	2, 4	10, 12	2	2
Classical complement activation	+(G1, 2?, 3)	−	+ +	−	−
Alternate complement activation	+(G4)	+	−	+	−
Binding cells via Fc	Macrophages, neutrophils, large granular lymphocytes	Lymphocytes	Lymphocytes	None	Mast cells, basophils, B cells
Biologic properties	Placental transfer, secondary Ab for most antipathogen responses	Secretory immunoglobulin	Primary Ab responses	Marker for mature B cells	Allergy, antiparasite responses

SOURCE: After L Carayannopoulos and JD Capra, in Paul, with permission.

prevention of virus binding to respiratory and gastrointestinal epithelial cells.

IgD is found in minute quantities in serum (see Table 305-7) and along with IgM is a major receptor for antigen on the B cell surface. Present in serum in very low concentrations (see Table 305-7), IgE is the major class of immunoglobulin involved in arming mast cells and basophils by binding to these cells via the Fc region. Antigen cross-linking of IgE molecules on basophil and mast cell surfaces results in release of mediators of the immediate hypersensitivity response (see Table 305-6).

CELLULAR INTERACTIONS IN REGULATION OF THE NORMAL IMMUNE RESPONSE

The net result of activation of the humoral (B cell) and cellular (T cell) arms of the immune system by foreign antigen is the elimination of antigen directly by immune effector cells or in concert with specific antibody. In addition, a series of regulatory cells is activated that modulate T effector cell activation and B cell antibody production. Figure 305-10 is a simplified schematic diagram of the immune system outlining some of these cellular interactions.

T CELL–T CELL AND T CELL–B CELL INTERACTIONS The expression of immune cell function is the result of a complex series of immunoregulatory events that occur in phases. Both T and B lymphocytes mediate immune functions, and each of these cell types, when given appropriate signals, passes through stages, from activation and induction through proliferation, differentiation, and ultimately effector functions. The effector function expressed may be at the end point of a response, such as secretion of antibody by a differentiated plasma cell, or it might serve a regulatory function that modulates other functions, such as is seen with CD4 + inducer or CD8 + regulatory T lymphocytes, which modulate both differentiation of B cells and activation of CD8 + or CD4 + cytotoxic T cells.

CD4 inducer (or helper) T cells can be subdivided on the basis of cytokines produced (Fig. 305-11). Activated TH1-type inducer T cells secrete IL-2, IFNγ, and TNFβ, while activated TH2-type inducer T cells secrete IL-4, -5, -6, and -10. TH1 CD4 + T cells provide T cell help for generation of cytotoxic T cells and generally respond to

FIGURE 305-11 CD4 + T helper 1 (TH1) cells and TH2 T cells and their precursors (TH0 cells) secrete distinct but overlapping sets of cytokines. TH1 cells are frequently activated in immune and inflammatory reactions that involve CD8 + cytotoxic T cell induction and/or granuloma formation, while TH2 cells are frequently activated for certain types of antibody production and are activated in allergic diseases. *(From Janeway and Travers, with permission.)*

antigens that lead to delayed hypersensitivity types of immune responses (such as *Mycobacterium tuberculosis*). In contrast, TH2 cells regulate the intensity of immune responses by the secretion of a cytokine, IL-10, that inhibits the production of other cytokines (see Table 305-4). In addition, TH2 CD4 + T cells provide help to B cells for specific Ig production and respond to antigens that require high antibody levels for foreign antigen elimination (such as in certain parasite infections). Different cytokines can drive the immune response preferentially towards a TH1 or a TH2 response. For example, IL-12 induces T cell differentiation towards a TH1 type cell, whereas IL-4 drives differentiation towards a TH2 type cell.

As shown in Fig. 305-10, upon activation by APC, regulatory T cell subsets that produce IL-2, IL-3, IFNγ, and/or IL-4, -5, -6, and -10 are generated that exert positive and negative influences on effector T and B cells. For B cells, trophic effects are mediated by a variety of cytokines, particularly T cell–derived IL-3, -4, and -5, which act at sequential stages of B cell maturation, resulting in B cell proliferation, differentiation, and ultimately antibody secretion (see Table 305-5). For cytotoxic T cells, trophic factors include inducer T cell secretion of IL-2, IFNγ, IL-12, and IL-15 (see Table 305-4). In addition, B cells themselves are capable of serving as APC, processing and presenting antigens to T cells, and secreting TNFα and IL-6.

Although B cells recognize native antigen via B cell surface Ig receptors, B cells require T cell help to produce high-affinity antibody of multiple isotypes that will be the most effective antibody response in eliminating foreign antigen. This T cell dependence likely functions in the regulation of B cell responses and in protection against excessive autoantibody production. T cell–B cell interactions that lead to high-affinity antibody production require: (1) processing of native antigen by B cells and expressing peptide fragments on the B cell surface for presentation to TH cells, (2) the ligation of B cells both by the T

FIGURE 305-10 Schematic model of intercellular interactions of immune competent cells during the ontogeny and activation stages of immune responses.

cell receptor complex and the CD40 ligand, (3) induction of the process termed *antibody isotype switching* in antigen-specific B cell clones, and (4) induction of the process of *affinity maturation* of antibody in the germinal centers of B cell follicles of lymph node and spleen.

Naive B cells express cell-surface IgD and IgM, and initial contact of naive B cells with antigen is via B cell surface IgM binding to native antigen. T cell cytokines, released following TH cell contact with B cells or by a "bystander" effect, induce changes in Ig gene conformation that promote recombination of Ig genes. These events then result in the "switching" of expression of heavy chain exons in a triggered B cell, leading to IgG, IgA, or, in some cases, IgE antibody types secreted with the same V region antigen specificity as the original IgM antibody produced. Class switching may also occur by a posttranscriptional mechanism acting at the RNA level. The T cell cytokines that induce antibody isotype switching are IL-4, TGFβ, IL-5, and IFNγ. CD40 ligand expression by TH cells is critical for induction of antibody isotype switching, and patients with mutations in T cell CD40 ligand have B cells that are unable to undergo isotype switching, resulting in the immunodeficiency syndrome of *X-linked hyper-IgM syndrome* (see Chap. 307).

The gradual increase in the affinity of antibodies for antigen over time occurs in the germinal centers of lymph node and spleen and results from continued alteration of Ig V region genes, through a process of *somatic hypermutation*. Somatic hypermutation is a process whereby many mutations in V region genes occur, leading to a wide range of possibilities for changes in antibody specificity. Those changes that result in higher affinity antibodies are selected for continued usage by germinal center B cells by the firm binding of B cells to antigen on the surface of antigen-presenting FDC (see above), leading to B cell proliferation and clonal expansion.

ANTIGEN-PRESENTING CELL–T CELL INTERACTIONS

The three cell types that are the primary presenters of antigen peptide fragments to T cells are dendritic/Langerhans cells, monocytes-macrophages, and B lymphocytes. Many of the activation and regulatory effects of these cell types occur via cytokines that regulate T and B cell maturation following direct APC–T cell contact (see Tables 305-3 to 305-5). APC are required for optimal activation of T cells by antigens or by mitogens (nonspecific activators of lymphocytes). Two signals are required to activate T cells by APC: signal 1, delivered to the T cell receptor/CD3 complex by antigen peptides embedded in MHC class I or class II clefts or grooves; and signal 2, delivered by an antigen-nonspecific co-stimulatory signal, mediated on APC by molecules, termed B7-1 (CD80) and B7-2 (CD86), that bind to the T cell molecule, CD28 (Fig. 305-4). Ligation of the T cell receptor/CD3 complex by MHC molecule/peptide complexes in the presence of co-stimulatory molecule ligation leads to T cell activation and clonal expansion of antigen-specific T cells; whereas, ligation of the T cell receptor in the absence of T cell CD28 ligation leads to T cell nonresponsiveness, termed *anergy*. Ingestion of foreign antigens such as bacteria by macrophage APC leads to induction of macrophage B7 molecule expression and the ability to activate bacteria-specific T cells, whereas presentation of host (self) peptides in APC MHC molecules does not lead to APC expression of B7, thus promoting the normal state of host T cell anergy to self-antigens. Upon contact with antigens or mitogens, APC secrete IL-1, IL-6, and TNFα, the effects of which are (1) the induction of receptors for IL-2 on T cells, and (2) the induction of T cell secretion of IL-2, IL-4, and other cytokines. These cytokines, in turn, activate other T cells in an antigen-nonspecific fashion, resulting in recruitment of effector and regulatory T cells that also have been induced to express IL-2, -4, and -7 receptors (see Fig. 305-10). Effector T cells mediate a variety of functions, including the killing of virus-infected cells, graft rejection, graft-versus-host reaction, delayed-type hypersensitivity, and the release of a wide spectrum of immunoregulatory cytokines (see Tables 305-3 to 305-5).

THE COMPLEMENT SYSTEM

The complement system is a cascading series of plasma enzymes, regulatory proteins, and proteins capable of cell lysis whose principal site of synthesis is the liver. There are two arms of the complement system (Fig. 305-12). Activation of the classic complement pathway via C1, C4, and C2 and activation of the alternative complement pathway via factor D, C3, and factor B both lead to cleavage and activation of C3. C3 is a protein whose activation fragments, when bound to target surfaces such as bacteria and other foreign antigens, are critical for opsonization (coating by antibody and complement) in preparation for phagocytosis.

The protein fragment C3b, split from C3, is necessary for activation of the terminal complement components C5–9. These form the membrane attack complex which, when inserted into cell membranes, brings about osmotic lysis of the cell.

C3b also joins with a cleavage product of factor B (called Bb) to form C3bBb, also known as the *alternative pathway C3 convertase*. Activation of the classic complement pathway results in cleavage of C4 and C2 with a resulting complex of fragments, C4b2a, also called the *classic pathway C3 convertase*. Both the classic pathway C3 convertase (C4b2a) and the alternative pathway C3 convertase (C3bBb) function to cleave C3 to form active C3b, thus driving activation of the C5–9 membrane attack complex. The fact that C3b can combine with Bb to form the alternative pathway C3 convertase gives rise to a potent positive feedback loop for production of C3b and thus continued activation of terminal complement components.

The classic complement pathway is activated by interaction of antigen and antibody to form immune complexes that bind C1q, a subunit of C1. Immunoglobulin isotypes that bind C1q and activate the classic pathway are IgM, IgG1, IgG2, and IgG3. In contrast, IgA1, IgA2, and IgD activate complement via the alternative pathway. Activation of the complement cascade via the classic pathway by IgG- or IgM-containing immune complexes is a rapid and efficient pathway to activation of terminal complement components. In contrast, activation of the alternative complement pathway via IgA-containing immune complexes or by bacterial endotoxin is a slower and less efficient pathway to terminal component activation. Thus the immunoglobulin isotype composition of immune complexes is a critical factor in determining complement activation and the efficiency of clearance of immune complexes by C3 receptor–bearing cells.

FIGURE 305-12 Components of the complement system. (*After Paul, with permission.*)

In addition to the role of complement in opsonization of bacteria and cell lysis, several complement fragments are potent mediators of immune cell activation. C3a and C5a bind to receptors on mast cells and basophils, resulting in release of histamine and other mediators of anaphylaxis. C5a is also a potent chemoattractant for neutrophils and monocytes-macrophages (Table 305-8).

MECHANISMS OF IMMUNE DAMAGE

Several responses by the host to foreign antigen culminate in the rapid and efficient elimination of nonself substances. In these scenarios, the classic weapons of the immune system (T cells, B cells, macrophages) interface with cells and soluble products that are mediators of inflammatory responses (neutrophils, eosinophils, basophils, kinin and coagulation systems, and complement cascade) (see Chaps. 62 and 310).

There are four general phases of host defenses: (1) migration of leukocytes to sites of antigen localization; (2) specific and nonspecific recognition of foreign antigens mediated by T and B lymphocytes, macrophages, and the alternative complement pathway; (3) amplification of the inflammatory response with recruitment of specific and nonspecific effector cells by complement components, lymphokines and monokines, kinins, arachidonic acid metabolites, and mast cell–basophil products; and (4) macrophage, neutrophil, and lymphocyte participation in antigen destruction with ultimate removal of antigen particles by phagocytosis (by macrophages or neutrophils) or by direct cytotoxic mechanisms (involving macrophages, neutrophils, and lymphocytes). Under normal circumstances, orderly progression of host defenses through these phases results in a well-controlled immune and inflammatory response that protects the host from the offending antigen. However, dysfunction of any of the host defense systems can damage host tissue and produce clinically apparent disease. Furthermore, for certain pathogens or antigens, the normal immune response itself might contribute substantially to the tissue damage. For example, the immune and inflammatory response in the brain to certain pathogens such as *M. tuberculosis* may be responsible for much of the morbidity of this disease in that organ system (see Chap. 171). In addition, the morbidity associated with certain pneumonias such as that caused by *Pneumocystis carinii* may be associated more with inflammatory infiltrates than with the tissue destructive effects of the microorganism itself (see Chap. 211).

THE MOLECULAR BASIS OF LYMPHOCYTE–ENDO-THELIAL CELL INTERACTIONS The control of lymphocyte

circulatory patterns between the bloodstream and peripheral lymphoid organs operates at the level of lymphocyte–endothelial cell interactions to control the specificity of lymphocyte subset entry into organs. Similarly, lymphocyte–endothelial cell interactions regulate the entry of lymphocytes into inflamed tissue. Adhesion molecule expression on lymphocytes and endothelial cells regulates the retention and subsequent egress of lymphocytes within tissue sites of antigenic stimulation, delaying cell exit from tissue and preventing reentry into the circulating lymphocyte pool. All types of lymphocyte migration begin with lymphocyte attachment to specialized regions of vessels, termed *high endothelial venules* (HEV). An important concept for many of the adhesion molecules listed in Table 305-9 is that the molecules do not generally bind their ligand until a conformational change (ligand activation) occurs in the adhesion molecule that allows ligand binding. Induction of a conformation-dependent determinant on an adhesion molecule can be accomplished by cytokines or via ligation of other adhesion molecules on the cell.

The first stage of lymphocyte–endothelial cell interactions, *attachment and rolling*, occurs when lymphocytes leave the stream of flowing blood cells in a postcapillary venule and roll along venule endothelial cells (Fig. 305-13). Lymphocyte rolling is mediated by the L-selectin molecule (LECAM-1, LAM-1) (see Table 305-9). Lymphocyte L-selectin ligands on HEV are sulfated oligosaccharides present on three different molecules: glycosylation-dependent cell adhesion molecule 1 (GlyCAM-1), CD34, and mucosal addressin cell adhesion molecule 1 (MAdCAM-1), leading to adhesion of lymphocytes to HEV. Lymphocyte rolling slows cell transit time through venules, allowing time for activation of adherent cells.

The second stage of lymphocyte–endothelial cell interactions, *adhesion triggering*, requires stimulation of lymphocytes by chemoattractants or by endothelial cell–derived cytokines. Cytokines thought to participate in adherent cell triggering include members of the IL-8–intercrine family, platelet-activation factor, leukotriene B$_4$, and C5a. Following activation by chemoattractants, lymphocytes shed L-selectin from the cell surface and upregulate cell CD11b/18 (MAC-1) or CD11a/18 (LFA-1) molecules (see Tables 305-2 and 305-9), resulting in firm attachment of lymphocytes to HEV.

Lymphocyte homing to peripheral lymph nodes involves adhesion of L-selectin to carbohydrate of peripheral node HEV, whereas homing of lymphocytes to intestine Peyer's patches primarily involves adhesion of the α4,β7 integrin to MAdCAM-1 oligosaccharides on Peyer's patch HEV. However, for migration to mucosal Peyer's patch lymphoid aggregates, naive lymphocytes primarily use L-selectin, whereas memory lymphocytes use α4,β7 integrin. α4, β1 (CD49d/CD29, VLA-4)–VCAM-1 interactions are important in the initial interaction of memory lymphocytes with HEV of multiple organs in sites of inflammation.

The third stage of leukocyte emigration in HEV, *sticking and arrest*, is sticking, of the lymphocyte and arrest at the site of sticking, mediated predominantly by ligation of αL,β2 integrin LFA-1 to the integrin ligands, ICAM-1 and ICAM-2 on HEV. While the first three stages of lymphocyte attachment to HEV takes only a few seconds, the fourth stage of lymphocyte emigration, *transendothelial migration*, takes approximately 10 min. Although the molecular mechanisms that control lymphocyte transendothelial migration are not fully characterized, the HEV CD44 molecule and molecules of the HEV glycocalyx (extracellular matrix) are thought to play important regulatory roles in this process (Fig. 305-13). Finally, expression of matrix metalloproteases capable of digesting the subendothelial basement membrane, rich in nonfibrillar collagen, appears to be required for the penetration of lymphoid cells into the extravascular sites.

Abnormal induction of HEV formation and use of the molecules discussed above have been implicated in the induction and maintenance of inflammation in a number of chronic inflammatory diseases. In animal models of insulin-dependent diabetes mellitus (IDDM), MAdCAM–1 and GlyCAM-1 have been shown to be highly expressed on HEV in inflamed pancreatic islets, and treatment of these animals with inhibitors of L-selectin and α4 integrin function blocked the development of IDDM (see Chap. 334). A similar role in human chronic inflammatory disease for abnormal induction of the adhesion

Table 305-8

Biologic Activities of Some Complement Components

Component	Activity
C4a weak anaphylatoxin	Evokes histamine release from basophils and mast cells
C3a	Anaphylatoxin; evokes histamine release from basophils and mast cells
C5a	Anaphylatoxin; evokes histamine release from basophils and mast cells; potent chemoattractant for monocytes and neutrophils
C3b, C3bi	Enhancement of phagocytosis by neutrophils and monocytes; promotes immune-complex binding to cells within monocyte-macrophage system, as well as neutrophils; C3b with Bb forms alternative pathway C3 convertase and amplifies alternative pathway; promotes solubilization of immune complexes
C5–9	Membrane attack complex; forms transmembrane channels leading to cell destruction

SOURCE: After S Ruddy, in Kelley et al, with permission.

Table 305-9

Leukocyte–Endothelial Cell Adhesion Molecules

Molecule	Distribution	Ligand	Functions
SELECTIN FAMILY			
L-selectin (LECAM-1, LAM-1)	Leukocyte	Sulfated oligosaccharides on GlyCAM-1, MAdCAM-1, and CD34	Regulates leukocyte binding to inflamed endothelium; lymph node homing receptor
P-selectin (GMP-140)	Endothelial cells, alpha granules of platelets	Sialylated derivatives of Lewis X oligosaccharides	Involved in some initial PMN leukocyte–endothelial cell interactions
E-selectin (ELAM-1)	Endothelial cells	Sialylated derivatives of Lewis X oligosaccharides	Involved in some initial PMN leukocyte–endothelial cell interactions
INTEGRIN FAMILY			
α1β1 (VLA-1, CD49a)	Activated T cells, monocytes, endothelial cells	Laminin, collagen	Activation-dependent adhesion receptor; marker for memory T cells
α2β1 (VLA-2, CD49b)	Lymphocytes, endothelial cells, widespread	Collagen, laminin	Activation-dependent adhesion receptor
α3β1 (VLA-3, CD49c)	Lymphocytes, endothelial cells, widespread	Fibronectin, collagen, laminin	Activation-dependent adhesion receptor
α4β1 (VLA-4, CD49d)	Lymphocytes	VCAM-1, fibronectin fragment, vascular addressin	Involved in organ-specific homing in inflammation; activation upregulates adhesion
α4β7	Lymphocytes	MAdCAM-1	Involved in organ-specific homing to Peyer's patches and to a variety of tissues in chronic diseases
α5β1 (VLA-5, CD49c)	Lymphocytes, endothelial cells, widespread	Fibronectin	Activation-dependent adhesion receptor; marker for memory T cells
α6β1 (VLA-6, CD49f)	Widespread	Laminin	Adhesion to endothelial cells
αLβ2 (LFA-1, CD11a)	Leukocytes	ICAM-1, ICAM-2, ICAM-3	Activation-dependent adhesion receptor
αMβ2 (MAC-1, CD11b)	Myeloid, NK cells	ICAM-1, C3bi, factor X	Activation-dependent adhesion receptor; mediates adhesion of myeloid cells to endothelial cells
αXβ1 (p150, 95, CD11c)	Myeloid cells, subset of lymphocyte	?	Activation-dependent adhesion receptor; mediates binding of myeloid cells to ligands derived from complement cascade
CD2	T cells, NK cells	CD58 (LFA-3)	Activation-dependent adhesion receptor; can transmit proliferation signal
CD54 (ICAM-1)	Activated lymphocytes, thymic epithelium, cytokine (IL-1, TNFα, IFNγ)–stimulated endothelial cells	LFA-1, rhinoviruses, *P. falciparum*	Upregulated expression on many tissues; mediates endothelial-leukocyte adherence
ICAM-2	Endothelial cells	LFA-1	Mediates leukocyte-endothelial adherence
ICAM-3	All resting leukocytes	LFA-1	Leukocyte-leukocyte interactions prior to leukocyte activation
CD58 (LFA-3)	Most tissue cell types	CD2	Upregulated expression in lymphoid tissues; involved in CTL–target cell interactions
VCAM-1 (InCAM-110)	TNFα– and IL-1–stimulated endothelial cells, follicular dendritic cells	VLA-4 (α4β1)	Mediates homing of VLA-4 + leukocytes to Peyer's patches; mediates binding of B cells to germinal centers
CARTILAGE LINK PROTEIN FAMILY			
CD44 (Hermes, Pgpl, EcMRIII)	Leukocytes, widespread	Hyaluronan (hyaluronic acid)	Mediates leukocyte adhesion to extracellular matrix, probably by activation-dependent adhesion; binds to various cytokines; possibly involved in memory lymphocyte transendothelial migration

NOTE: ELAM, endothelial-leukocyte adhesion molecule; PMN, polymorphonuclear leukocytes; VLA, very late activation (antigen); VCAM, vascular cell adhesion molecule; LFA, lymphocyte function-associated (glycoprotein); ICAM, intercellular adhesion molecule; MAC, membrane attack complex.

SOURCE: From Haynes and Denning, with permission.

FIGURE 305-13 Lymphocyte emigration in high endothelial venules (HEV). *A.* Lymphocytes circulating in blood initiate contact with high endothelial cells via microvilli. This initial adhesion is transient and is often manifested in rolling of the interacting cells along the HEV endothelium (step 1: attachment and rolling). Activation of lymphocyte adhesiveness (step 2: adhesion triggering) results in firm attachment, which becomes stable to physiologic shear force (step 3: sticking and arrest). Lymphocytes then migrate through endothelial cell junctions and enter lymphoid tissue after crossing the HEV basal lamina (stage 4: transendothelial migration). The luminal surface of HEV is coated by a prominent glycocalyx, and this may play an important role in lymphocyte emigration (see text for details). *B.* The initial interaction of lymphocytes with HEV in peripheral lymph nodes (PLNs) is mediated by L-selectin, which recognizes the following HEV mucin-like counter-receptors: CD34 and glycosylation-dependent cell adhesion molecule 1 (GlyCAM-1). Activation of lymphocyte adhesiveness occurs via G protein–coupled receptors, but the local factors involved in physiologic activation of lymphocytes in HEV are not yet characterized. The integrin leukocyte function–associated molecule 1 (LFA-1) (αβ; CD11a/CD18) and its HEV counterreceptors intercellular adhesion molecule 1 (ICAM-1) and ICAM-2 play a major role in lymphocyte arrest in PLN HEV. The molecular mechanisms involved in lymphocyte transendothelial migration remain poorly characterized. *(After JP Girard, TA Springer. Immunology Today 16:449, 1995, with permission.)*

molecules of lymphocyte emigration has been suggested in rheumatoid arthritis (see Chap. 313), Hashimoto's thyroiditis (see Chap. 331), Graves' disease (see Chap. 331), multiple sclerosis (see Chap. 376), Crohn's disease (see Chap. 286), and ulcerative colitis (see Chap. 286). Cytokines that induce HEV expression of MAdCAM-1 and GlyCAM-1 are IFNγ, TNFα, IL-1, and IL-10.

IMMUNE-COMPLEX FORMATION Clearance of antigen by immune-complex formation between antigen and antibody is a highly effective mechanism of host defense. However, depending on the level of immune complexes formed and their physicochemical properties, immune complexes may or may not result in host and foreign cell damage. After antigen exposure, certain types of soluble antigen-antibody complexes freely circulate and, if not cleared by the reticuloendothelial system, can be deposited in blood vessel walls and in other tissues such as renal glomeruli. The precise mechanisms whereby immune complexes damage tissues, particularly blood vessels, are discussed in Chap. 319.

IgE-MEDIATED ALLERGIC REACTIONS—ANAPHYLAXIS T helper cells that drive antiallergen IgE responses are usually TH2-type inducer T cells that secrete IL-4, IL-5, IL-6, and IL-10. Mast cells and basophils have high-affinity receptors for the Fc portion of IgE (Fc RI), and cell-bound antiallergen IgE effectively "arms" basophils and mast cells. Mediator release is triggered by antigen (allergen) interaction with Fc receptor–bound IgE; the mediators released are responsible for the pathophysiologic changes of allergic diseases (see Table 305-6). Mediators released from mast cells and basophils can be divided into three broad functional types: (1) those that increase vascular permeability and contract smooth muscle (histamine, platelet-activating factor, SRS-A, BK-A); (2) those that are chemotactic for or activate other inflammatory cells (ECF-A, NCF, leukotriene B₄); and (3) those that modulate the release of other mediators (BK-A, platelet-activating factor) (see Chap. 310).

CYTOTOXIC REACTIONS OF ANTIBODY In this type of immunologic injury, complement-fixing (C1-binding) antibodies against normal or foreign cells or tissues (IgM, IgG1, IgG2, IgG3) bind complement via the classic pathway and initiate a sequence of events similar to that initiated by immune-complex deposition, resulting in cell lysis or tissue injury. Examples of antibody-mediated cytotoxic reactions include red cell lysis in *transfusion reactions*, *Goodpasture's syndrome* with anti-glomerular basement membrane antibody formation, and *pemphigus vulgaris* with antiepidermal antibodies inducing blistering skin disease.

CLASSIC DELAYED-TYPE HYPERSENSITIVITY REACTIONS Inflammatory reactions initiated by mononuclear leukocytes and not by antibody alone have been termed *delayed-type hypersensitivity reactions*. The term *delayed* has been used to contrast a secondary cellular response that appears 48 to 72 h after antigen exposure with an *immediate* hypersensitivity response generally seen within 12 h of antigen challenge and initiated by basophil mediator release or preformed antibody. For example, in an individual previously infected with *M. tuberculosis* organisms, intradermal placement of tuberculin purified-protein derivative as a skin test challenge results in an indurated area of skin at 48 to 72 h, indicating previous exposure to tuberculosis.

The cellular events that result in classic delayed-type hypersensitivity responses are centered around T cells (predominantly IFNγ, IL-2, and TNFβ-secreting TH1-type helper T cells) and macrophages. First, local immune and inflammatory responses at the site of foreign antigen upregulate endothelial cell adhesion molecule expression, promoting the accumulation of lymphocytes at the tissue site. In the general scheme outlined in Fig. 305-10, antigen is processed by dendritic/Langerhans cells or monocytes-macrophages and presented to small numbers of TH1 cells expressing a TCR specific for the antigen. IL-1 and IL-6 secreted by APC amplify the clonal expansion of antigen-specific T cells, and lymphokines (primarily IL-2, IFNγ, and TNFβ) are secreted that promote recruitment of diverse populations of T cells and macrophages to the site of the cellular inflammatory response. In particular, CD8+ cytotoxic T cells are induced to become active killer cells by IL-2. Once recruited, macrophages frequently undergo epithelioid cell transformation and form giant cells in response to IL-4 and IFNγ. This type of mononuclear cell infiltrate is termed *granulomatous inflammation*. Examples of diseases in which delayed-type hypersensitivity plays a major role are fungal infections (*histoplasmosis*) (see Chap. 203), mycobacterial infections (*tuberculosis*, *leprosy*) (see Chaps. 171 and 172), chlamydial infections (*lymphogranuloma venereum*) (see Chap. 181), helminth infections (*schistosomiasis*) (see Chap. 224), reactions to toxins (*berylliosis*) (see Chap. 254), and hypersensitivity reactions to organic dusts (*hypersensitivity pneu-*

responses play important roles in tissue damage in autoimmune diseases such as *rheumatoid arthritis*, *temporal arteritis*, and *Wegener's granulomatosis* (see Chaps. 313 and 319).

AUTOIMMUNE DISEASE Autoimmune disease is characterized by production of either antibodies that react with host tissue or immune effector T cells that are autoreactive to endogenous self-peptides. Because most B cell responses in humans require helper T cells, a B cell autoantibody response generally implies disordered T cell immunoregulatory control. Exceptions to this rule are seen with T cell–independent and anti-idiotypic B cell responses. In some instances, autoantibodies may arise from normal T and B cell responses to foreign organisms or substances that contain antigens, particularly polysaccharides, that cross-react with similar self-antigens in body tissues. This phenomenon is called *molecular mimicry*. Examples of clinically relevant autoantibodies are antibodies against the acetylcholine receptor in *myasthenia gravis* (see Chap. 382) and anti-DNA, antierythrocyte, and antiplatelet antibodies in *systemic lupus erythematosus* (see Chap. 312).

As mentioned above in the description of immunoglobulins, the unique portion of the variable region of the immunoglobulin molecule where antigen binds is called the *idiotype*, and an antibody that reacts specifically with that region is called an *anti-idiotype antibody*. Anti-idiotype antibodies may arise during the course of the normal immune response. For example, anti-idiotypes against antitetanus antibodies develop during normal immunization of humans to tetanus toxoid and serve to deliver "off" signals to B cells secreting antitetanus antibodies. Antibodies may be an important component of the normal immunoregulatory network. Anti-idiotype antibodies also may be relevant to two types of autoimmunity: (1) dysfunction of the idiotype–anti-idiotype antibody system could lead to B cell hyperreactivity by failure to generate "off" signals for B cell differentiation, and (2) some antireceptor antibodies produced in autoimmune diseases (anti-insulin receptor antibodies in forms of type 1 diabetes mellitus and antithyrotropin receptor antibodies in autoimmune thyroid disease) may be anti-idiotype antibodies made against the antibody-combining site (idiotype) of an autoantibody. Despite these mechanistic considerations, the precise role, if any, of anti-idiotype antibodies in human disease remains speculative.

Genetic factors play a role in the genesis of many autoimmune diseases, as shown in studies of familial aggregation and high concordance for disease in monozygotic, but not dizygotic, twins. Based upon analogy to murine autoimmune disorders and on limited human data, polygenic inheritance (e.g., multiple independent genes) of autoimmune susceptibility is likely. It is possible that genetic factors operate via an influence on inherent B or T cell hyperreactivity via presentation of self- or foreign peptides that stimulate an inappropriate antiself response, or via abnormal downregulatory mechanisms. In this regard, many autoimmune disorders are associated with specific haplotypes (e.g., combinations of allelic genes) of the MHC, strongly suggesting that inherited differences in APC molecules or in APC–T cell interactions might influence susceptibility to autoimmunity. The strongest known association between an MHC molecule and an autoimmune disease is the class I molecule HLA-B27 and inflammatory spondyloarthropathy (ankylosing spondylitis) (see Chap. 317). In type 1 diabetes mellitus, a genome-wide search for disease genes has demonstrated that several genes contribute to diabetes, but that MHC-linked genes are the most important. Other genetic association studies have implicated the Ig heavy chain locus in some forms of autoimmunity.

Whereas organ-specific autoimmune diseases are likely the result of the combined effects of several factors that lead to inappropriate targeting of a particular organ or system to immune damage by induction of HEV adhesion molecules for memory and effector lymphocytes, generalized autoimmune diseases such as systemic lupus erythematosus (see Chap. 312) can be thought of as diseases in which there is episodic breakdown of immunologic tolerance to self-molecules. Recent studies have demonstrated that in a mouse model of autoimmunity (the MRL mouse), the cause of autoimmune disease is a defect in a cell surface molecule (fas/APO-1) on T cells that is required for the intrathymic death of autoreactive T lymphocytes. The defective fas/

APO-1 molecule prevents negative selection of autoreactive T cells, leading to seeding of peripheral lymphoid organs with excessive numbers of autoreactive T cells. It is thought that rare serious multisystem lupus erythematosus–like syndromes in children may be the human homologues of murine MRL autoimmune disease. Instead of a defect in central (thymic) tolerance, adult acquired systemic lupus erythematosus is more likely to result from a generalized defect in maintenance of peripheral tolerance in which the peripheral immune system lacks the ability to maintain anergy to self-antigens. While the molecules involved in maintenance of peripheral tolerance/anergy to self-antigens are not fully known, recent data suggest that T cell CD28 and B cell B7/BB1 molecules are involved in regulating this process.

THE CELLULAR AND MOLECULAR CONTROL OF PROGRAMMED CELL DEATH (APOPTOSIS) The process of programmed cell death, or apoptosis, plays a crucial role in the tissue organization and modeling that occur during normal embryogenesis and development of many tissues. Induction of apoptosis leads to the removal of superfluous and damaged cells in many cell systems and is particularly critical to regulating normal responses to antigen in the immune system. In general, a wide variety of stimuli trigger cell surface receptors (e.g., TNF receptor family members or related proteins) or cytoplasmic receptors (e.g., ceramide, glucocorticosteroids) that activate groups of proteases such as IL-1β converting enzyme. These proteases either cleave molecules that lead to cell death themselves or activate other enzymes to cleave molecules that eventuate in cell death (Fig. 305-14). The end stages of this sequence of events lead to cell death characterized by degradation of cytoplasmic (actin) and nuclear cytoskeletal proteins as well as cleavage of DNA at regular intervals (nucleosomes), leading to nuclear disintegration seen on electron microscopy and "laddering" of DNA when analysed by agarose

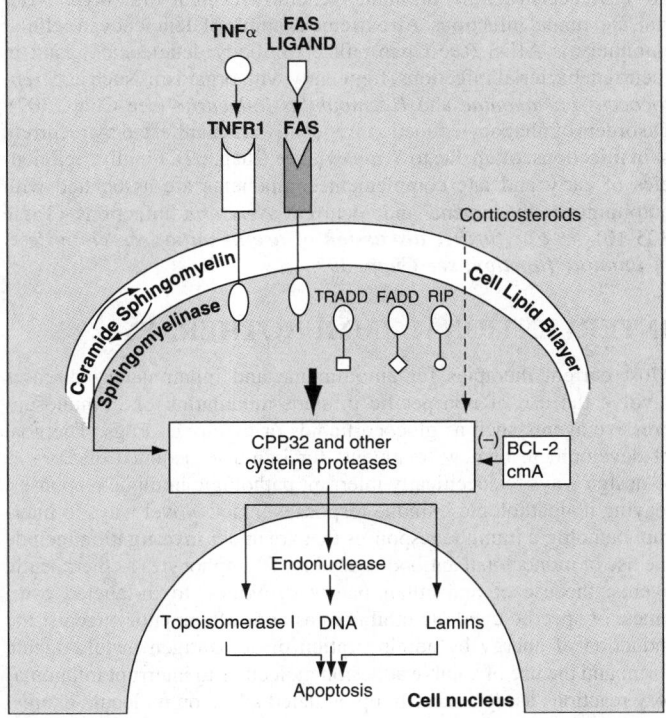

FIGURE 305-14 Pathways that regulate programmed cell death. Ceramide production via fas/APO-1 ligation or other stimuli, ligation of fas or TNFR1, and, for some cell types, stimulation with corticosteroids, can lead to triggering of cytosolic and nuclear proteases that degrade cytoskeletal proteins and DNA, leading to cell death. BCL-2 and crmA are two proteins that inhibit programmed cell death. TRADD, FADD, and RIP are cytoplasmic proteins thought to associate with either TNFR1 or fas via their cytoplasmic domains in the mediation of programmed cell death.

gel electrophoresis. The level of expression of certain cytosolic proteins, such as CrmA and Bcl-2, negatively regulates the process of apoptosis by inhibiting activation of cytosolic proteases that induce cell death. For example, T cells that are negatively selected in the thymus are induced to undergo apoptosis and have low levels of proteins such as Bcl-2, whereas medullary thymocytes that have been triggered to proliferate and survive thymocyte selection (positive selection) have high levels of Bcl-2.

Thus, in the immune system, apoptosis is a mechanism induced to remove autoreactive T cells from the thymus during negative selection, to remove autoreactive B and T cells from peripheral lymphoid organs upon immune cell contact with antigen or antigen-reactive T helper cells in spleen and lymph node, and to remove virus-infected or malignant cells after contact with antigen-specific CD8 + cytotoxic T lymphocytes. Induction of apoptosis is one of two principal mechanisms of target cell lysis by cytotoxic T lymphocytes, the other consisting of the release of cytotoxic perforin molecules.

CLINICAL EVALUATION OF IMMUNE FUNCTION

Clinical assessment of immunity requires investigation of the four major components of the immune system that participate in host defense and in pathogenesis of autoimmune diseases: (1) humoral immunity (B cells); (2) cell-mediated immunity (T cells, monocytes); (3) phagocytic cells of the reticuloendothelial system (macrophages), as well as polymorphonuclear leukocytes; and (4) complement. Clinical problems that require an evaluation of immunity include chronic infections, recurrent infection, unusual infecting agents, and certain autoimmune syndromes. The type of clinical syndrome under evaluation can provide information regarding possible immune defects (see Chap. 307). Defects in cellular immunity generally result in viral, mycobacterial, and fungal infections. An extreme example of deficiency in cellular immunity is AIDS (see Chap. 308). Antibody deficiencies result in recurrent bacterial infections, frequently with organisms such as *Streptococcus pneumoniae* and *Haemophilus influenzae* (see Chap. 307). Disorders of phagocyte function frequently are manifested by recurrent skin infections, often due to *S. aureus* (see Chap. 62). Finally, deficiencies of early and late complement components are associated with autoimmune phenomena and recurrent *Neisseria* infections (Table 305-10). → *For further discussion of useful initial screening tests of immune function, see Chap. 307.*

INTERVENTIONAL IMMUNOTHERAPY

Most current therapies for autoimmune and inflammatory diseases involve the use of nonspecific immune-modulating or immunosuppressive agents such as glucocorticoids or cytotoxic drugs. The goal of development of new treatments for immune-mediated diseases is to design ways to specifically interrupt pathologic immune responses, leaving nonpathologic immune responses intact. Novel ways to interrupt pathologic immune responses that are under investigation include the use of monoclonal antibodies against T lymphocytes as therapeutic agents; the use of anti-inflammatory cytokines, toxin-labeled cytokines, or specific cytokine inhibitors as anti-inflammatory agents; the induction of anergy by administration of autoantigen in tolerogenic form; and the use of soluble adhesion molecules to interrupt inflammatory reactions associated with upregulated adhesion molecule expression. For some animal models of organ-specific autoimmune disease, the TCR types of pathogenic T cells have been found to be oligoclonal or monoclonal, raising hope that anti-TCR therapy (TCR peptides, inducing anti-TCR antibodies or anti-TCR regulatory T cells) may be feasible. However, to date, pathologic T cells in human autoimmune disease have remained difficult to define, and specific TCR-directed therapy of T cell–mediated autoimmune diseases remains only a theoretical possibility.

Table 305-10

Complement Deficiencies and Associated Diseases

Component	Associated Diseases
CLASSIC PATHWAY	
C1q, C1r, C1s, C4	Immune-complex syndromes,* pyogenic infections
C2	Immune-complex syndromes,* few with pyogenic infections
C1 inhibitor	Rare immune-complex disease, few with pyogenic infections
C3 AND ALTERNATIVE PATHWAY C3	
C3	Immune-complex syndromes,* pyogenic infections
D	Pyogenic infections
Properdin	*Neisseria* infections
I	Pyogenic infections
H	Hemolytic uremic syndrome
MEMBRANE ATTACK COMPLEX	
C5, C6, C7, C8	Recurrent *Neisseria* infections, immune-complex disease
C9	Rare *Neisseria* infections

* Immune-complex syndromes include systemic lupus erythematosus (SLE) and SLE-like syndromes, glomerulonephritis, and vasculitis syndromes.
SOURCE: After JA Schifferli and DK Peters, Lancet 88:957, 1983, with permission.

Immune-based therapy has been used with varying success to enhance host defense mechanisms as well as specific and nonspecific immune responses in a variety of host defense defects and immune deficiency diseases (see Chaps. 62, 307, 308). Of particular note has been the successful use of IFNγ in the treatment of the phagocytic cell defect in chronic granulomatous disease (see Chap. 62). Intermittent infusions of IL-2 in HIV-infected individuals in the early or intermediate stages of disease has resulted in substantial and sustained increases in CD4 + T cells. However, the long-term benefit of this therapeutic modality remains to be determined.

BIBLIOGRAPHY

ABBAS AK et al (eds): *Cellular and Molecular Immunology*, 2d ed. Philadelphia, Saunders, 1994

FINKEL TH et al: T-cell development and transmembrane signaling: Changing biological responses through an unchanging receptor. Immunol Today 12:79, 1991

GIRARD JP, SPRINGER TA: High endothelial venules (HEVs): Specialized endothelium for lymphocyte migration. Immunol Today 16:449, 1995

GLEICH GJ: Eosinophils, basophils and mast cells. J Allergy Clin Immunol 84:1024, 1989

HAYNES BF, DENNING SM: Lymphopoiesis, in *The Molecular Basis of Blood Diseases*, 2d ed, G Stamatoyannopoulos et al (eds). Philadelphia, Saunders, 1993, pp 425–462

HERMAN A et al: Superantigens: Mechanism of T-cell stimulation and the role in immune responses. Annu Rev Immunol 9:745, 1991

JANEWAY CA, TRAVERS P (eds): *Immunobiology. The Immune System in Health and Disease*. New York, Garland, 1994

KAYE PM: Costimulation and the regulation of anti-microbial immunity. Immunol Today 16:423, 1995

KELLEY WN et al (eds): *Textbook of Rheumatology*, 4th ed. Philadelphia, Saunders, 1993, chaps. 6, 7, 10, 13, 15, 16

MARTIN SJ, GREEN DR: Protease activation during apoptosis: Death by a thousand cuts. Cell 82:349, 1995

PAUL WE (ed): *Fundamental Immunology*, 2d ed. New York, Raven, 1989

RETH M et al: The B-cell antigen receptor complex. Immunol Today 12:196, 1991

ROBEY E, ALLISON JP: T-cell activation: Integration of signals from the antigen receptor and costimulatory molecules. Immunol Today 16:306, 1995

ROLINK A et al: B-cell development in mouse and man. The Immunologist 3:125, 1995

SPRINGER TA: Traffic signals for lymphocyte recirculation and leukocyte emigration: The multistep paradigm. Cell 76:301, 1994

WEISS A, LITTMAN DR: Signal transduction by lymphocyte antigen receptors. Cell 76:263, 1995

THE MAJOR HISTOCOMPATIBILITY GENE COMPLEX

Antigenic differences between members of a species are called *alloantigens*, and when these play a determining role in the rejection of allogeneic tissue grafts, they are called *histocompatibility antigens*. Evolution has conserved a single closely linked region of histocompatibility genes, the products of which are prominently displayed on cell surfaces and provide a strong barrier to allotransplantation. The terms *major histocompatibility antigens* and *major histocompatibility gene complex* (MHC) refer to the gene products and genes of this chromosomal region. Their principal function is to bind peptide fragments of potentially pathogenic microbes and present them to T lymphocytes for recognition. Cell-surface antigen receptors on T lymphocytes [T cell receptors (TCR)] are virtually identical for each member of a clone, and they engage antigenic peptide fragments that have been previously bound to MHC molecules. Direct TCR binding to peptides in solution, or to antigenic determinants present on the surface of an intact protein molecule, does not occur. Much of the early evidence for MHC genetic control of the immune response came from work in animal models in which immune response genes were mapped within the mouse (H-2), rat (RT1), and guinea pig (GPLA) MHC. The response to a given antigenic determinant is now known to require the binding of the appropriate peptide fragment to an MHC molecule. In humans, the MHC is called HLA and is located on the short arm of chromosome 6. The individual letters of HLA have various unofficial meanings, and by international agreement HLA is the logo for the human MHC.

Several generalizations can be made about the MHC. *First*, three classes of gene products are encoded within the 4000-kilobase region of HLA. Class I molecules, expressed on virtually all cell surfaces, consist of one heavy and one light polypeptide chain and are the products of three reduplicated loci: HLA-A, HLA-B, and HLA-C. Class II molecules, restricted in expression to B lymphocytes, dendritic cells, monocytes, antigen-activated T lymphocytes, and to epithelial and endothelial cells that have been activated by interferon, consist of two noncovalently linked polypeptide chains (α and β) of unequal length. They are the products of several closely linked genes, collectively termed the *HLA-D region*. The class II heterodimers form a structure similar to that of class I. Class III molecules are the C4, C2,

and Bf components of complement and share little structural similarity to classes I and II. *Second*, the expressed MHC genes in the thymus play a crucial role in the selection of the T cell receptor repertoire during maturation. Various self-peptide + MHC combinations promote survival or elimination of newly formed T cells. Clones with too high or too low an affinity to MHC are eliminated. Self versus nonself discrimination, based upon moderate affinity to self-peptide + MHC, is thereby imprinted on the T cell repertoire, providing the means for selective, also called restricted, recognition of peptides bound to self-peptide + MHC molecules. *Third*, genes for enzyme systems having no apparent relationship to immunity are located in the region of the MHC, as are genes of importance in skeletal growth and development. *Fourth*, genes for tumor necrosis factor (TNF) α and TNFβ, heat shock protein (Hsp$_{70}$), and peptide processing (LMP) and transport (TAP) lie also within the MHC (Fig. 306-1).

In contrast to the single linkage group for the MHC, many *minor* histocompatibility antigen genes are encoded throughout the genome. They represent weaker allotypic differences on molecules that serve functions apparently unrelated to the immune system, except that they can be a target for rejection of transplants. Whereas the MHC is a powerful stimulus to the immune system during a primary response, minor histocompatibility differences can be of clinical significance only after priming has occurred. Antibody responses to minor histocompatibility antigens are generally weak or absent, whereas cytotoxic CD8 + T cell responses, restricted to presentation of peptides derived from minor antigens by self-peptide + MHC molecules, are common.

LOCI OF THE HLA SYSTEM   Class I Antigens   HLA antigens of the class I type are defined serologically by human immune sera, principally from multiparous females, and to a limited extent by monoclonal antibodies. They are present in varying densities in most body tissues, including B cells, T cells, and platelets, but not in mature red blood cells. CD8 + T cells preferentially bind to MHC class I molecules via a CD8 binding site on class I. The number of serologically defined specificities is large, and the HLA system is the most polymorphic genetic system known in humans. Three clearly defined loci are recognized within the HLA complex for class I HLA antigens. Each class I antigen consists of an 11.5-kDa β_2-microglobulin subunit and a 44-kDa heavy chain that carries the antigenic specificities (Fig. 306-2). There are over 80 serologically defined A and B specificities, and 8 C-locus specificities are known. Antigens of the major complex are prefixed by HLA, but this may be omitted when the context is

FIGURE 306-1   Schematic representation of human chromosome 6 showing the location of the HLA region in the 21 region of the short arm. The HLA-A, -B, and -C loci encode class I heavy chains (44 kDa), while the β_2-microglobulin light chain (11.5 kDa) of the class I molecule is encoded by genes of chromosome 15. HLA-D region (class II) is centromeric to the A, B, and C loci, with genes for closely linked complement components C4A, C4B, Bf, and C2 in the B–D region. Two genes for tumor necrosis factor (TNFα,β) also lie between HLA-B and the complement genes. The order of the complement genes is uncertain. Additional loci shown are P for the proteosome (LMP) and T for the peptide transporter (TAP) genes and the Hsp$_{70}$ heat-shock protein gene. Each D region class II molecule is made up of an α and β chain (their

genes are written as A and B). They appear on the cell surface in distinct heterodimers, DP, DQ, and DR. The numbers following A or B indicate that there are different genes for the chains of a given set; e.g., for DR, there are 9 β-chain genes (three are shown). The expressed molecule may be $\beta1\alpha$(B1A) or $\beta3\alpha$(B3A), for example. The $\beta2$ gene is not expressed (pseudogene). The antigens DR51, DR52, and DR53 are on the expressed B5, B3, and B4 chains, respectively, while the other DR antigens are on B1. DRA is not polymorphic, while the molecules bearing the DQ antigens have polymorphism in both A1 and B1 chains. DQA2 and DQB2 are pseudogenes. Polymorphism in DP is greater for B1 than for A1. The overall length of the HLA region is about 3 cM (3400 kilobases).

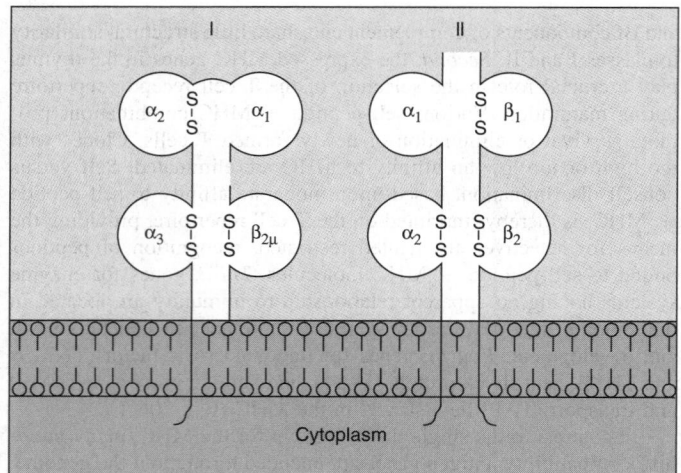

FIGURE 306-2 Schematic representation of class I and class II molecules on the cell surface. Class I molecules are composed of two polypeptide chains. The 44-kDa heavy chain passes through the plasma membrane. Its external portion consists of three domains (α_1, α_2, α_3) formed by disulfide bonding. The β_2-microglobulin ($\beta_{2\mu}$) light chain (11.5 kDa) encoded by chromosome 15 is noncovalently bound to the heavy chain. Amino acid sequence homology among class I molecules is 80 to 85 percent, falling to 50 percent or less in portions of α_1 and α_2 that represent the sites of alloantigenic polymorphism. Class II molecules consist of two noncovalently associated polypeptide chains, a 34-kDa α and a 29-kDa β. Each chain has two domains formed by disulfide bridging (the α_1 domains lack a sulfide bridge). (*From Carpenter and Strom.*)

clear. The number following the locus designation is the name of the antigen (e.g., HLA-A2). HLA antigens of African, Asian, and Oceanic peoples include many of the antigens commonly found in people of western European ancestry. However, the distribution of HLA antigens is distinctive for certain racial groups and can serve as anthropologic markers in the study of migration patterns and diseases.

Class II Antigens The HLA-D region is separated from the class I loci on the short arm of chromosome 6 by 1000 kilobases (see Fig. 306-1). This region encodes a series of class II molecules, each consisting of a 29-kDa β chain and a 34-kDa α chain (see Fig. 306-2). Incompatibility for this region, particularly concerning the DR antigens, determines the in vitro proliferative response of lymphocytes to mismatched haplotypes. CD4 + T cells preferentially bind to MHC class II molecules via a CD4 binding site on class II. Since chromosomes are paired, each individual has 12 HLA-A, HLA-B, HLA-C, HLA-DR, HLA-DQ, and HLA-DP antigens, 6 from each parent. Each of these chromosomal sets is termed a *haplotype*, and by simple Mendelian inheritance, one-fourth of siblings have identical haplotypes, one-half share a haplotype, and the remaining one-fourth are completely incompatible (Fig. 306-3). Evidence that this gene complex plays the major role in the transplantation response comes from the fact that haplotype-matched sibling donor-recipient combinations show excellent results in kidney transplantation, in the vicinity of 85 to 90 percent long-term survival (see Chap. 272).

The mixed lymphocyte response (MLR) is assessed by the degree of proliferation of a *mixed lymphocyte culture* (MLC) and is positive even when HLA-A, HLA-B, and HLA-C antigens are identical (see Fig. 306-3). When parental recombination has occurred between HLA-B and -DR, for example, a new haplotype appears in the child, who will be identical for class I but different for class II (a versus a_r in Fig. 306-3). HLA-D antigens are defined by stimulation with reference lymphocytes that are homozygous for HLA-D and are inactivated by x-irradiation or mitomycin C to make the reaction unidirectional. There are over 35 such antigens recognized by homozygous typing cells.

Attempts to define HLA-D by serology first established a series of D-related (DR) antigens expressed on class II molecules of B lympho-

Haplotypes:
a = A1,Cw3,B8,Dw3
b = A29,Cw4,B35,Dw1
a_r = A1,Cw3,B8,Dw1
b_r = A29,Cw4,B35,Dw3

Inheritance:
ab x cd
ac ad bc bd

FIGURE 306-3 HLA region, chromosome 6: inheritance of HLA haplotypes. Each chromosomal segment of linked genes is termed a *haplotype*, and each individual inherits one haplotype from each parent. The A, B, C, and D antigens of haplotypes a and b are shown for this hypothetical individual in chromosomal order on the diagram and also below as they would be written in text. If individual ab were to marry cd, their offspring would be of four types only, as far as HLA is concerned. Occasionally (*dashed cross*) recombination occurs in the germ line (meiosis) of a parent, resulting in an altered haplotype. The frequency of recombinant children is a measure of the map distance (1 percent recombination frequency = 1 cM; see Fig. 306-1). (*From CB Carpenter, Kidney Int 14:283, 1978.*)

cytes, monocytes, and activated T lymphocytes. Macrophages, dendritic cells, and skin Langerhans cells are also class II–positive. There are 22 DR, 8 DQ, and 8 DP antigens recognized by serology. The class II gene map shown in Fig. 306-1 describes a minimal number of genes and molecular sets. Although a class II molecule may be composed of a DQα (DQA1 gene) from one parental haplotype and a DQβ (DQB1 gene) from the other parent (transcomplementation), α and β combinations among DP, DQ, and DR sets rarely, if ever, occur. DR, and to some extent DQ, molecules provide the stimuli for the primary MLR. A second round of MLR stimulation in culture (secondary MLR) is called the *primed lymphocyte test* (PLT) and occurs rapidly over 24 to 36 h instead of 6 to 7 days. DP alloantigens were discovered from their ability to provide PLT stimulation, although they do not contribute much to a primary MLR. DQ and DP molecules also can be identified serologically. While B lymphocytes and activated T lymphocytes express all three sets of class II molecules, DQ antigens are not expressed on 60 to 90 percent of monocytes, which are virtually all DP- and DR-positive.

Three-Dimensional Structure of HLA X-ray diffraction studies of crystallized HLA class I molecules show a groove or cleft on the surface facing away from the cell membrane with dimensions sufficient to bind a linearly extended peptide fragment 8 to 15 amino acids long. In fact, class I molecules usually bind sequences of 9 amino acids. The margins of the binding site are formed by α helices, and the base is floored by eight antiparallel β strands, with the α1 and α2 domains contributing equally to each side of the structure (Fig. 306-4). The HLA variable regions that are recognized by alloantibodies or cytotoxic T cells lie along the surfaces of the α helices and β strands that form the margins of the groove. When the bound materials released by acidification of affinity purified, or redissolved, HLA class I crystals were analyzed by high-performance liquid chromatography (HPLC), hundreds of different peptides were found. Of those analyzed further, a 9-amino-acid length and a binding consensus motif at positions 2 and 9 were characteristic. The class II heterodimeric molecule is remarkably similar to class I in core structure. The amino acid carbon backbone for α helices and β strands of class II is superimposable upon that of class I. Therefore, the overall size and shape of the binding grooves are the same, and the class II polymorphic regions are also arrayed along the margins of the α helices and β strands. The main difference is that the ends of the class II groove are more open, allowing peptides as long as 26 amino acids to bind.

Antigen Processing T lymphocyte receptors bind efficiently only to peptide fragments of proteins presented in the groove of a self-MHC molecule. Virtually all MHC molecules come to the surface of the cell with a peptide in place. These peptides may have originated from an intracellular or extracellular source. In the case of class I, the pathway is primarily one of selection of peptides generated from endogenous proteins within the cytosolic compartment (e.g., from intracellular viral infection); for class II, the pathway is primarily an exogenous one that processes endocytosed or pinocytosed proteins. Any cell that expresses MHC class II can serve as an antigen-presenting cell (APC) to CD4 + lymphocytes; in addition, the macrophage can also process exogenous proteins into the class I pathway for presentation to CD8 + lymphocytes, thereby providing a means for activating both CD4 + and CD8 + subsets to fragments of the same antigen.

Cytosolic proteins subject to proteolysis include normal cellular constituents, including self-peptide + MHC molecules, and foreign invaders such as viruses. Proteosome genes mapped to the class II region of the MHC (Fig. 306-1) encode cytosolic structures that cleave proteins into short peptides (8 to 9 amino acids); however, these particular genes (LMP2 and LMP7) do not account for all the immunogenic peptides formed in the cytosol. A heterodimeric channel encoded by TAP1 and TAP2 genes then transports peptides to the endoplasmic reticulum (ER) where binding to class I heavy chains and association with β_2-microglobulin complete the class I assembly before transport to the cell surface. The class II pathway utilizes proteases in acidic endocytic vesicles to produce random proteolysis of ingested proteins. The peptide-rich endosome then fuses with the ER where class II assembly occurs. The 13- to 26-amino-acid length of peptides eluted from class II molecules frequently consists of a nested set of sequences of various lengths, having a consensus binding region of 9 or so amino acids, and variably sized tails at either end of the groove. Eluted class II bound peptides also contain a high proportion of self-MHC fragments.

Understanding the precise topography of TCR binding to MHC + peptide awaits the full crystal structure of the α and β chains of the TCR; however, sequence analysis of TCR genes indicates three hypervariable regions (CDR) for each chain. A likely model is that the CDR-1 and CDR-2 regions of the TCR α chain bind to one of the MHC α helices, while the analogous CDRs of the TCR β chain bind to the other MHC α helix. Both CDR-3 regions would, by this model, contact the peptide. Alternatively, it may be possible that all contact points are to portions of the MHC α helices, the shape of which is modified by the peptide.

Molecular Genetics Each polypeptide chain of class I and class II molecules bears several polymorphic sites. The "private" antigen (e.g., B27 or B35) defined by alloantisera frequently depends upon more than one site on the face of the molecule. In the *cell-mediated lympholysis* (CML) test, the specificity of killer T cells (T_c), which arise during the proliferative events in MLR, is determined by testing on target cells from donors other than those providing the MLR stimulus. Antigen systems defined by this method show a close but imperfect correlation with class I private antigens. Cloning of cytotoxic cells has revealed the presence of a variety of polymorphic target determinants on HLA molecules, some of which are identifiable by alloantisera or monoclonal antibodies derived from immunization of mice with human cells. Some of these reagents can be used to identify private determinants of HLA, while others are directed to more "public" (sometimes called *supertypic*) determinants. The latter are epitopes found to be identical on molecules that have different private specificities. One such system of public HLA-B antigens has two alleles, Bw4 and Bw6. Most HLA-B private antigens are associated with either Bw4 or Bw6. HLA-B–bearing heavy chains carry additional sites that are common to B7, B27, B22, and B40, and others to B5, B15, B18, and B35. Other types of shared antigenic determinants exist, as exemplified by a monoclonal antibody that reacts with a site shared between HLA-A and HLA-B heavy chains. Increasingly, these complexities are more easily resolved by analysis of DNA sequences than by serology.

When genomic DNA for HLA is examined, typical exon-intron sequences of DNA have been found for class I and class II, exons having been identified for signal peptides (5'), each of the domains, a transmembrane hydrophobic segment, and a cytoplasmic segment (3'). cDNA probes are available for most of the HLA chains, and enzymatic digests have been used to study patterns of *restriction fragment length polymorphisms* (RFLP), many of which correlate with class II serologic and MLR patterns. There are 20 to 30 class I genes, however, making assessment of polymorphism by RFLP difficult. Many of these genes are not expressed (pseudogenes), while some could represent additional class I loci that are expressed only on activated T cells and are of uncertain function. Tissue typing by the detection of variable nucleotide sequences begins with the polymerase

FIGURE 306-4 Structure of the HLA class I molecule as determined by x-ray crystallography. *A.* Shown is the face of the HLA-A2 molecule that points away from the cell surface. This ribbon diagram shows the groove that is formed by two α helices and is supported by a floor of eight β strands. N is the amino terminal of the α_1 domain; the two small circles represent a disulfide bond. *B.* Composite display of polymorphic sites from several human and mouse class I alleles using the HLA-A2 structure as the model. The symbols show a composite of the polymorphisms along the groove. Localization of variable amino acids and/or sites for alloantibody and/or cytotoxic T cell recognition is shown to be along the α helices (*circles*). Polymorphic sites exist also in the β strands (*squares*). The numbers indicate the amino acid sequence. (*After PJ Bjorkman et al.*)

chain reaction (PCR) technique to amplify specific segments of DNA, as defined by oligonucleotide primers, from genomic DNA obtained from a small sample of blood or tissue. The primers are usually locus-specific (e.g., the β1 chain of HLA-DR) or may be allele-specific (e.g., amplifying only genes having a particular polymorphic sequence). The products are then analyzed by hybridization with sequence-specific labeled probes or by RFLP analysis of the amplified DNA. The technique has already demonstrated ability to identify sequences in the human population in a more accurate fashion than with the established serologic technique. The official HLA nomenclature has been changed to reflect the definition of distinct sequences and to document the presence of polymorphisms not previously appreciated from the definitions of classical serology. To illustrate, HLA-DR1 is written as DRB1*0101. DRB1 indicates the β1 chain of the DR locus, and *0101 indicates that it is antigen 1, first variant. In similar fashion, DQA1*0302 indicates the α1 chain of the DQ locus, antigen 3, variant 2. Many recent observations of disease associations with HLA antigens use this more precise nomenclature in order to define the molecular basis for peptide binding, as well as to provide better genetic markers for ethnic and population diversity. Molecular typing for HLA-DR is proving to be of value in clinical typing for organ and bone marrow transplantation.

Complement (Class III)   Structural genes for three complement components, C4, C2, and Bf (factor B), are present in the HLA-BD region (see Fig. 306-1). There are two loci for C4, coding for C4A and C4B, formerly recognized as the Rodgers and Chido red blood cell antigens, respectively. These antigens are, in fact, adsorbed plasma C4 molecules. Other complement components are not closely linked to HLA. No crossovers have been found between the C2, Bf, and C4 loci. They are all encoded within a 100-kilobase segment between HLA-B and HLA-DR. There are two alleles of C2, four of Bf, seven of C4A, and three of C4B, plus blanks (null genes) for each locus (QO). The extensive polymorphism of complement types (complotypes) makes them useful for genetic studies. The four most common extended haplotypes found in people of western European ancestry are shown in Table 306-1. Such identical extended haplotypes may be conserved from a common ancestor. MLRs between unrelated individuals who are matched for these extended haplotypes are nonreactive, whereas some reactivity is common if unrelated individuals are serologically matched for only HLA-DR antigens.

Other Linked Sixth-Chromosome Genes   Deficiency of steroid 21-hydroxylase, an autosomal recessive trait, results in the syndrome of congenital adrenal hyperplasia (see Chaps. 332 and 339). The genes for the enzyme are also localized in the HLA-B-D region. The 21-hydroxylase gene adjacent to C4A is deleted in affected individuals along with C4A (C4AQO), and the HLA-B locus gene may have been altered to convert B13 to the rare B47 found only in affected haplotypes. A late-onset variant of 21-hydroxylase deficiency is also linked to HLA. Congenital adrenal hyperplasia due to 11β-hydroxylase deficiency is not HLA-linked. Idiopathic hemochromatosis, an autosomal recessive disorder, is linked to HLA, as has been shown in several family studies (see Chap. 342). Although the pathogenesis of this disease is unknown, the gene that modulates gastrointestinal iron absorption is near HLA-A (Table 306-2).

Immune-Response Genes   As originally defined in the guinea pig and the mouse, high and low immune responsiveness to haptens

or synthetic peptide motifs was shown to be determined by genes in the region of the MHC. It is now clear that these genes encode the class II molecules and that the ability to bind the relevant antigen is the major determinant of a strong T cell–dependent response initiated by CD4+ T cells. Class I genes are also important in the effector phases of a response, especially with regard to recognition by CD8+ T cells of foreign peptide bound to class I molecules. For example, human cell lines infected with the influenza virus are lysed by immune cytotoxic T cells (T_c) only if a class I (HLA-A or HLA-B) antigen is shared between the attacking and target cells. Class I and II molecules are said to be the *restriction elements* in immune responsiveness because they must be able to bind and present peptide fragments properly to T cells. In the allogeneic response, there is evidence that recognition may be of either the amino acid differences on the external face of the intact MHC molecule or of an MHC peptide fragment presented by a responder strain MHC molecule. In this special case, instead of restricting the response, the MHC antigenic differences become the stimulus. In transplantation, the induction and effector phases of a rejection response follow the general rules of CD4+ T_H (T helper cell) and CD8+ T_c interacting with MHC class II and I, respectively (Fig. 306-5). Although B lymphocytes can be directly activated via their surface immunoglobulin receptors, they also express high concen-

Table 306-2

Linkage of Genetic Defects to HLA

	Gene Location	Common Haplotype Found
C2 deficiency	HLA-B-D	A25, B18, BfS, DR2
21-OH deficiency	HLA-B-D	A3, B47, BfF, DR7
21-OH deficiency (late onset)	HLA-B-D	B14, BfS, DR1
Idiopathic hemochromatosis	HLA-A	A3, B14
Paget's disease	HLA-A-D	
Spinocerebellar ataxia	HLA-A-D	
Hodgkin's disease	HLA-A-D	

FIGURE 306-5   Schema of the relative roles of HLA-A, -B, -C, and -D antigens in initiation of the alloimmune response and in the development of effector cells and antibodies. Two main classes of T lymphocytes recognize antigens: T_c, the precursors to the cytotoxic "killer" cells, and T_H, the helper cells for amplification of the cytotoxic response. T_H also provide help to B lymphocytes for production of a fully mature IgG response. Note that T_c generally recognize class I antigens, while the T_H signal is provided by antigens of the HLA-D region (class II). (*From CB Carpenter, Kidney Int 14:283, 1978.*)

Table 306-1

Common Extended HLA Haplotypes

HLA-B	HLA-DR	Bf	C2	C4A	C4B
8	3	S	C	QO	1
7	2	S	C	3	1
57	7	S	C	6	1
44	7	F	C	3	1

trations of class I and II molecules and can process antigens for presentation on the cell surface. It is the response of the T cell to such antigen presentation that provides the "help" required for a mature IgG secretory response by the B cells.

DISEASE ASSOCIATIONS   Not all genes involved in regulating the immune response are in the MHC region. It is nevertheless a fact that most human inflammatory diseases thought to have some autoimmune basis are in some way promoted by genes of the HLA region. In most cases, these are *associations* of particular HLA antigens in populations of individuals with certain diseases. Since it is becoming apparent that the extensive polymorphism of the MHC is directly related to the ability of a given molecule to bind a particular peptide sequence, the critical biologic function of MHC polymorphism may be to ensure survival of the species in relation to the large numbers of microbiologic agents present in the environment. Self-tolerance that happens to crossreact with microbiologic agents would produce a high degree of susceptibility, resulting in lethal infection, whereas the polymorphism of the HLA system ensures that some individuals in segments of the human population will recognize offending agents as foreign and initiate the appropriate response. The value of the MHC for species survival is of such importance that there is need for local

mechanisms, not entirely understood, to prevent allorecognition in the special case of pregnancy. The extent to which the MHC plays a role in immune surveillance against neoplasia and whether such a role contributes to survival in an evolutionary sense are not established.

Table 306-3 summarizes the most significant HLA and disease associations. Overall, the mechanisms in the induction of these diseases are not yet explained. It should be noted that such associations do not in themselves prove that variations in antigen presentation to T cells is necessarily at the root of autoimmunity. It also can be that HLA genes are markers for haplotypes in which mutations have occurred in other linked genes. A possible example of effects of linked genes is the recent observation that insulin-dependent diabetes is associated with a low density of MHC class I molecules on the patient's cells, explained by a defect in TAP peptide transporters. Since the genes for the latter map to the HLA class II region (Fig. 306-1), associations of diabetes with class II antigens could in part be on this basis.

Most striking is the increased frequency of HLA-B27 in certain rheumatic diseases, particularly ankylosing spondylitis, a condition

Table 306-3

HLA Antigens and Disease, Showing the Most Highly Associated Antigens

Disease	Antigen	Relative Risk*	Disease	Antigen	Relative Risk*
RHEUMATIC			**ENDOCRINE**		
Ankylosing spondylitis	B27	69.1	Type 1 diabetes mellitus	DR4	3.6
Reiter's syndrome	B27	37.0		DR3	4.8
Acute anterior uveitis	B27	8.2		DR2	0.2
Reactive arthritis (*Yersinia*,	B27	18.0		BfF1	15.0
Salmonella, gonococcus)			Hyperthyroidism (Graves')	B8	2.5
Psoriatic arthritis, central	B27	10.7		DR3	3.7
	B38	9.1	Hyperthyroidism (Japanese)	B35	4.4
Psoriatic arthritis, peripheral	B27	2.0		A2	2.2
	B38	6.5		DP5	4.4
Juvenile rheumatoid arthritis	B27	3.9		A2 + DP5	10.5
	DR8	3.6	Adrenal insufficiency	Dw3	10.5
Juvenile arthritis, pauciarticular	DR5	3.3	Subacute thyroiditis (de Quervain)	B35	13.7
Rheumatoid arthritis	Dw4/DR4	3.8	Hashimoto's thyroiditis	DR5	3.2
Sjögren's syndrome	Dw3	5.7	Congenital adrenal hyperplasia	B47	15.4
Systemic lupus erythematosus			**NEUROLOGIC**		
Caucasian	DR3	2.6			
Japanese	DR2	5.3	Myasthenia gravis	B8	2.7
Chinese	DQ3	11.5		DR3	2.5
Systemic lupus erythematosus	DR4	5.6	Multiple sclerosis	DR2	6.0
(hydralazine)			Manic-depressive disorder	B16	2.3
			Narcolepsy	DR2	130.0
GASTROINTESTINAL			Schizophrenia	A28	2.3
Gluten-sensitive enteropathy	DR3	11.6	**RENAL**		
Chronic active hepatitis	DR3	6.8			
Ulcerative colitis	B5	3.8	Idiopathic membranous	DR3	5.7
			glomerulonephritis		
HEMATOLOGIC			Goodpasture's syndrome (anti-	DR2	15.9
Idiopathic hemochromatosis	A3	6.7	GBM)		
	B14	2.7	Minimal change disease (steroid	B12	4.2
	A3, B14	90.0	response)		
Pernicious anemia	DR5	5.4	Polycystic kidney disease	B5	2.6
Hodgkin's disease			IgA nephropathy		
Caucasian	DP3	2.0	Caucasian	DR2	0.6
Japanese	DP4	0.2	French, Japanese	DR4	3.1
			Gold nephropathy	DR3	14.0
SKIN				DR4	0.3
Dermatitis herpetiformis	Dw3	17.3	**INFECTIOUS**		
Psoriasis vulgaris	Cw6	7.5			
Psoriasis vulgaris (Japanese)	Cw6	8.5	Tuberculoid leprosy (Asians)	B8	6.8
Pemphigus vulgaris (Jews)	DR4	14.6	Paralytic polio	B16	4.3
	A26	4.8	Low vs. high response to vaccinia	Cw3	12.7
Behçet's disease			virus		
Caucasian	B5	3.8	**IMMUNODEFICIENCY**		
Japanese	B51	12.4			
Chinese	B51	5.5	IgA deficiency (blood donors)	DR3	13.0

* Relative risk $= \dfrac{(\% \text{ antigen-positive patients})(\% \text{ antigen-negative controls})}{(\% \text{ antigen-negative patients})(\% \text{ antigen-positive controls})}$.

with a strong familial tendency. B27 is present in about 7 percent of people of western European ancestry, while it appears in 80 to 90 percent of patients with ankylosing spondylitis. Expressed as a relative risk, the antigen B27 confers a susceptibility to the development of ankylosing spondylitis that is 69 times that in the general population. Similarly, acute anterior uveitis, Reiter's syndrome, and reactive arthritis to at least three bacterial infections (*Yersinia*, *Salmonella*, and gonococcus) show a high degree of association with B27. Although the ordinary form of juvenile rheumatoid arthritis (JRA) also shows a similar association with B27, the pauciarticular form of JRA with iritis is DR5-associated. The increased incidence of B27 in psoriatic arthritis is also significant for the central type (axial skeleton) of the disorder, while B38 is associated with both the central and peripheral types. Psoriasis is associated with Cw6. Patients with degenerative arthritis or gout show no alteration in antigen frequencies.

Most other disease associations are with HLA-D region antigens. The rheumatoid arthritis associations with DR4 involve 3 of the 22 DR4 variants (DRB1*0401, *0404, and *0405), as well as DRB1*0101 and DRB1*1402 in some ethnic groups. Such specificity adds weight to the argument for disease being the result of binding and presentation of particular peptides. Narcolepsy is virtually 100 percent associated with DR2 in both Japanese and Caucasians. Affected individuals need inherit only a single gene dose of DR2. Although there is no apparent autoimmune component to this condition, there is speculation that an abnormality in a neurotransmitter or its receptor may be influenced by the DR2 gene or another closely linked gene. Gluten-sensitive enteropathy (celiac disease, nontropical sprue) in children and adults is associated with DR3 (relative risk = 12). Recent DNA typing shows a higher relative risk of 52 with DQA1*0501 and DQB1*0201. The actual percentage of such patients having DR3 ranges from 63 to 96 percent compared with 22 to 27 percent of controls. The same antigen is also present in increased frequency in patients with chronic active hepatitis and in patients with dermatitis herpetiformis who also have gluten-sensitive enteropathy. Juvenile-onset insulin-dependent diabetes mellitus (type 1) is associated with DR4 and DR3 and is negatively associated with DR2. Resistance to type 1 diabetes is strongly associated with the inheritance of aspartate at position 57 of the β chain of HLA-DQ, in linkage disequilibrium with HLA-DR2. Other amino acids at position 57, especially when HLA-DR3 or -DR4 are on the same haplotype, are associated with an increased risk of disease. Recent studies show that not having aspartate at position 57 of DQB1 of both haplotypes confers a relative risk for type 1 diabetes of 7.4, whereas a single or double dose of aspartate at position 57, as with DQB1*0601 or *0602, provides protection (relative risk of 0.2). A rare allele of Bf (F1) is also found in 17 to 25 percent of patients with type 1 diabetes. Maturity-onset diabetes is not HLA-associated. Hyperthyroidism is an example of a disease in which racial differences display different HLA associations, in contrast with rheumatoid arthritis and type 1 diabetes, in which the DR4 associations are more universal. The common DR2 and DQ haplotype found in normal individuals (DRB1*1501, DQA1*0102, DQB1*0602) is also most commonly increased in multiple sclerosis. Renal diseases strongly HLA-DR–associated are Goodpasture's syndrome due to an autoantibody to glomerular basement membrane (DR2); idiopathic membranous glomerulonephritis (DR3 in Caucasians, DR2 in Japanese), which involves antibodies to an antigen of the glomerulus; and gold-induced nephritis (DR3). Studies of HLA associations with AIDS suggest that HLA-B35 is a risk factor for more rapid progression of the disease (see Chap. 308).

LINKAGE DISEQUILIBRIUM The most salient feature of population genetics of HLA antigens is the random distribution of HLA antigens within a given racial or ethnic group. The term *linkage disequilibrium* means that antigens of closely linked loci appear together more frequently than predicted by random association. In other words, nonrandom distribution of HLA antigens occasionally is found. The classic example is the frequency of the A-locus antigen HLA-

A1 and the B-locus antigen HLA-B8 in people of western European ancestry. The coincidence of A1 and B8 should be the product of their individual gene frequencies ($0.17 \times 0.11 \cong 0.02$). The observed frequency of A1 and B8 is 0.08, four times that expected, an increase of 0.06. The latter value is termed Δ (delta) and is a measure of the disequilibrium. Other A- and B-locus haplotype disequilibria have been recognized and include (A3, B7), (A2, B12), (A29, B12), and (A11, B35). Furthermore, some D-region determinants are in linkage disequilibrium with B-locus antigens (e.g., DR3 and B8), as are some B- and C-locus antigens. Serologically defined HLA antigens can serve as markers for the genes of an entire haplotype within a family, but cannot predict other alleles within a population unless a linkage disequilibrium exists. Selective pressures during the course of evolution may have been the major factor in the survival of certain gene combinations in a haplotype. The conservation of certain extended haplotypes, mentioned above, supports this view.

On the other hand, the selection hypothesis is not necessary to explain linkage disequilibrium. When a population lacking certain antigens migrates into an area in which HLA antigens are in equilibrium, a Δ can develop within a few generations. For example, the increasing Δ value for A1, B8 found in populations from east to west, from India to western Europe, can be explained on the basis of migration and fusion. In smaller groups, consanguinity, founder effects, and gene drift may account for disequilibria. Finally, certain linkage disequilibria could occur as a result of nonrandom crossing over during gametic meiosis because of chromosomal segments that are either more or less likely to break. Unless there are selective pressures or restrictions in crossing over, linkage disequilibria disappear over a period of several generations.

LINKAGE VERSUS ASSOCIATION The diseases listed in Table 306-2 are examples of HLA linkage wherein the inherited conditions are marked within families by the relevant HLA haplotypes. For C2 deficiency, 21-hydroxylase deficiency, and idiopathic hemochromatosis, the mode of inheritance is recessive, with heterozygotes showing partial deficiencies. These genetic defects are also HLA-associated, with an excess of certain HLA alleles in affected unrelated individuals. Also, C2 deficiency is commonly linked to the HLA-A25, -B18, -BfS, Dw/DR2 haplotype, and idiopathic hemochromatosis exhibits both linkage and strong association with HLA-A3 and -B14. The high degree of linkage disequilibria in these HLA-linked diseases may result from mutations in a single founder, and a sufficient period of time may not have passed to bring the gene pool back into equilibrium. In this view, the HLA antigens are simple markers for the linked gene. Alternatively, expression of the defect may require interaction with specific HLA alleles. This latter hypothesis would require a higher mutation rate, with defective gene expression occurring only when linked with certain HLA genes.

HLA linkage can be demonstrated in the absence of association with a particular allele. Paget's disease and spinocerebellar ataxia are HLA-linked autosomal dominant traits, and Hodgkin's disease shows an HLA-linked recessive pattern of inheritance. As no HLA associations have been discerned for these disorders, it is suggested that there were multiple founders with mutations of as yet undefined genes in linkage with different HLA alleles.

CLINICAL APPLICATIONS The clinical value of HLA typing for diagnosis of disease is limited to B27 and ankylosing spondylitis, where nevertheless there are 10 percent false-positive and false-negative rates. HLA studies are also of value in genetic counseling and early recognition of disease in families with idiopathic hemochromatosis or congenital adrenal hyperplasia due to steroid 21-hydroxylase deficiency, particularly since HLA typing can be performed on cells obtained by amniocentesis. The high degree of polymorphism of the HLA system also makes it a powerful tool for paternity testing and other medicolegal applications. The implications for diseases such as type 1 diabetes mellitus and the other diseases showing HLA associations require further study of the components of the HLA system and their role in the pathogenesis of disease. Matching for HLA antigens in allogeneic transplantation shows the superiority of HLA identical sibs as donors and the immunodominance of HLA-A, -B, and -DR loci. Compatibility for these loci yields superior results in unrelated renal transplantation from cadaveric donors (see Chap. 272).

BIBLIOGRAPHY

BJORKMAN PJ et al: The foreign antigen binding site and T cell recognition regions of class I histocompatibility antigen. Nature 329:512, 1987

BODMER LG et al: Nomenclature for factors of the HLA system, 1995. Hum Immunol 43:149, 1995

BROWN JH et al: Three-dimensional structure of the human class II histocompatibility antigen HLA-DR1. Nature 364:33, 1993

CARPENTER CB, STROM TB: Immunobiology of renal transplantation, in *Contemporary Issues in Nephrology*, vol 19: *Renal Transplantation*, EL Milford et al (eds). New York, Churchill Livingstone, 1989

CHICZ RM et al: Specificity and promiscuity among naturally processed peptides bound to HLA-DR alleles. J Exp Med 178:27, 1993

GERMAIN RN: MHC-dependent antigen processing and peptide presentation: Providing ligands for T lymphocyte activation. Cell 76:287, 1994

ITESCU S et al: HLA-B35 is associated with accelerated progression to AIDS. J Acquir Immune Defic Syndr 5:37, 1992

POWIS SH et al: Alleles and haplotypes of the MHC-encoded ABC transporters TAP1 and TAP2. Immunogenetics 37:373, 1993

ROOPENIAN DC: What are minor histocompatibility loci? A new look at an old question. Immunol Today 13:7, 1992

SAYEGH MH et al: Mechanisms of T cell recognition of alloantigen: The role of peptides. Transplantation 57:1295, 1994

THOMSON G: HLA disease associations: Models for the study of complex human genetic disorders. Crit Rev Clin Lab Sci 32:183, 1995

WUCHERPFENNIG KW, STROMINGER JL: Selective binding of self peptides to disease-associated major histocompatibility complex (MHC) molecules: A mechanism for MHC-linked susceptibility to human autoimmune diseases. J Exp Med 181:1597, 1995

---

307 Max D. Cooper, Alexander R. Lawton III

PRIMARY IMMUNE DEFICIENCY DISEASES

Immunologic functions are mediated by developmentally independent, but functionally interacting, families of lymphocytes. The activities of B and T lymphocytes and their products in host defense are closely integrated with the functions of other cells of the reticuloendothelial system. Macrophages, dendritic cells, and the Langerhans' cells in the skin play an important role in the trapping and presentation of antigens to T and B cells to initiate the immune response. Macrophages also become effector cells, especially when activated by cytokine products of lymphocytes. The scavenger activity of polymorphonuclear leukocytes is directed and made specific by antibodies in concert with cytokines and the complement system. Natural killer (NK) cells, a population of granular lymphocytes, may spontaneously kill tumor and virus-infected cells, activities that are enhanced by the cytokine products of immune and inflammatory cells. Killing by NK cells also can be targeted by IgG antibodies for which NK cells have cell-surface receptors. The interaction of basophils and tissue mast cells with IgE antibodies in causation of immediate-type hypersensitivity is discussed in Chap. 310. Consideration of these interrelationships is an important part of the analysis of patients with suspected immune deficiency.

CLINICAL DISEASE FEATURES COMMON TO IMMUNE DEFICIENCY Immunodeficiency syndromes, whether congenital, spontaneously acquired, or iatrogenic, are characterized by unusual susceptibility to infection and not infrequently to autoimmune disease and lymphoreticular malignancies. The types of infection often provide the first clue to the nature of the immunologic defect.

Patients with *defects in humoral immunity* have recurrent or chronic sinopulmonary infection, meningitis, and bacteremia, most commonly caused by pyogenic bacteria such as *Haemophilus influenzae*, *Streptococcus pneumoniae*, and staphylococci. These and other pyogenic organisms also cause frequent infections in individuals who have either neutropenia or a deficiency of the pivotal third component of complement (C3). The tripartite collaboration of antibody, comple-

ment, and phagocytes in host defense against pyogenic organisms makes it important to assess all three systems in individuals with unusual susceptibility to bacterial infections.

Antibody-deficient patients in whom cell-mediated immunity is intact have an interesting response to viral infections. The clinical course of primary infection with viruses such as varicella zoster or rubeola, unless complicated by bacterial infection, does not differ significantly from that of the normal host. However, long-lasting immunity may not develop, and as a result, multiple bouts of chickenpox and measles may occur. Such observations suggest that intact T cells may be sufficient for control of established viral infections, while antibodies play an important role in limiting the initial dissemination of virus and in providing long-lasting protection. Exceptions to this generalization are becoming more widely recognized. Agammaglobulinemic patients fail to clear hepatitis B virus from their circulation and have a progressive, and often fatal, course. Poliomyelitis has occurred following live-virus vaccination in some patients. Chronic encephalitis, which may progress over a period of months to years, is a particular threat in congenitally agammaglobulinemic boys. Echoviruses and adenoviruses have been isolated from brain, spinal fluid, or other sites in such patients.

The occurrence of an unusually serious infection, for example, *H. influenzae* meningitis in an older child or adult, warrants consideration of humoral immune deficiency. Recurrent bacterial pneumonias also suggest this possibility. Chronic otitis media occurs frequently in patients with hypogammaglobulinemia and is significant because of its relative rarity in normal adults. Pansinusitis, although almost invariably present in immunoglobulin deficiency, is a less helpful finding because it is not rare in apparently normal people. Bacterial infections of the skin or urinary tract are less frequent problems in hypogammaglobulinemic patients.

Infestation with the intestinal parasite *Giardia lamblia* is a frequent cause of diarrhea in antibody-deficient patients.

Abnormalities of cell-mediated immunity predispose to disseminated virus infections, particularly with latent viruses such as herpes simplex (see Chap. 184), varicella zoster (see Chap. 185), and cytomegalovirus (see Chap. 187). In addition, patients so affected almost invariably develop mucocutaneous candidiasis and frequently acquire systemic fungal infections. Pneumonia caused by *Pneumocystis carinii* is also common (see Chap. 211).

T cell deficiency is always accompanied by some abnormality of antibody responses (see Fig. 307-1), although this may not be reflected by hypogammaglobulinemia. This explains in part why patients with primary T cell defects are also subject to overwhelming bacterial infection.

The most severe form of immune deficiency occurs in individuals, often infants, who lack both cell-mediated and humoral immune functions. Individuals with severe combined immunodeficiency (SCID) are susceptible to the whole range of infectious agents including organisms not ordinarily considered pathogenic. Multiple infections with viruses, bacteria, and fungi occur, often simultaneously. Because donor lymphocytes cannot be rejected by these recipients, blood transfusions can produce fatal graft-versus-host disease.

DIFFERENTIATION OF T AND B CELLS The functional deficits that occur in both congenital and acquired immunodeficiencies are usefully viewed as being caused by defects at various points along the differentiation pathways of immunocompetent cells. For this reason, certain features of the development and differentiation of T and B cells that are especially relevant to the analysis of immunodeficiency are briefly presented here; Chap. 305 provides a general account of their roles in cellular and humoral immunity.

A subpopulation of hematopoietic stem cells may become restricted to lymphoid differentiation prior to migration to the thymus, where T cells are generated, or to the fetal liver and adult bone marrow, where B cell development begins (see Fig. 307-1). A major function of these central lymphoid tissues is to generate the clonal diversity characteristic of the immune system. Each T or B lymphocyte expresses surface receptor molecules of a unique specificity for antigen. The receptors of B lymphocytes are immunoglobulin molecules that are formed by paired heavy and light chains of either κ or λ type. The heavy chain gene loci are on the long arm of chromosome 14; the 5′-3′ order of these is V_H (variable), D_H (diversity), and J_H (joining) minigene families followed by the C_H (constant region) genes, C_μ, C_δ, $C_{\gamma3}$, $C_{\gamma1}$, $C_{\alpha1}$, $C_{\gamma2}$, $C_{\gamma4}$, C_ϵ, and $C_{\alpha2}$. The κ gene family, consisting of V_κ, J_κ, and C_κ genes, is located on chromosome 2 and the homologous λ gene loci on chromosome 22.

The T cell receptors are related cell-surface molecules with antigen-binding specificity. The receptor on most T cells is composed of two polypeptide chains, called α and β. The β-chain family is located on chromosome 7 and consists of V_β, D_β, J_β, and C_β minigene loci. The α-chain family on chromosome 14 similarly consists of a series of V_α, D_α, J_α, and C_α genes. A smaller subpopulation of T cells express a T cell receptor composed of γ and δ polypeptide chains. The γ-chain gene family is located on chromosome 7, and the δ-chain family is located in the midst of the α gene locus on chromosome 14.

The genetic strategy for creating functional gene complexes encoding antigen receptors is similar for T and B cells. For example, a functional V region gene of the immunoglobulin heavy chain is formed by productive rearrangement of one each of the V_H, D_H, and J_H genes and deletion of the intervening DNA to generate a contiguous coding structure that is then transcribed together with the nearest C_H gene. Functional light chain genes are formed by a V-J rearrangement in either the κ or λ gene loci. The V_β gene is similarly composed of a rearranged set of V_β, D_β, and J_β genes forming a contiguous coding structure, which the T cell then transcribes along with the nearest C_β gene. Conserved flanking sequences serve as recombination signals for the V, D, and J gene segments in the T cell receptor (TCR) and immunoglobulin gene assembly processes. In both T and B cell precursors this DNA cutting and splicing operation involves the same recombinase proteins: the recombinase-activating gene (RAG) 1 and RAG-2, a DNA-dependent protein kinase, and at least two other proteins essential for DNA repair. Because there are many different V, D, and J genes, they can be put together in various combinations to encode a large number of receptor molecules having different antigen-binding specificities. Antibody and TCR variability are amplified further by nuclease nibbling around the DNA cuts needed to join the V, D, and J region segments and by addition of nonencoded nucleotides in the joins, a task that is performed by the nuclear enzyme, terminal deoxynucleotidyl transferase (TdT).

Generation of clonal diversity requires cellular proliferation, such that each of the different receptor specificities encoded in the genome

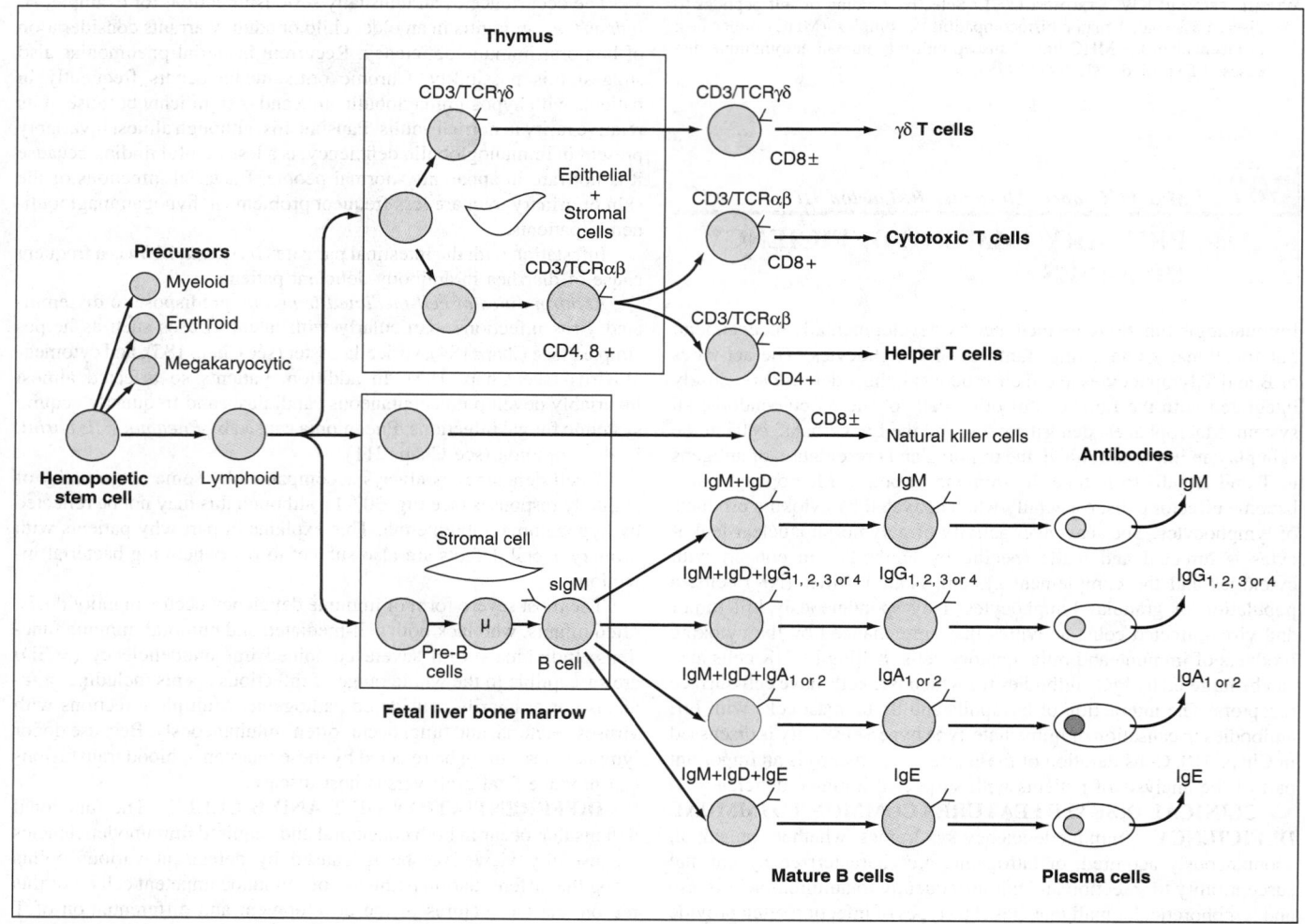

FIGURE 307-1 Hypothetical model outlining the differentiation of hemopoietic stem cells along T, B, and NK cell lineages. Failure to develop T and B cells may result from defective stem cells or from inborn metabolic errors affecting both cell types. Rarely, other hematopoietic cell lines are also absent. Absence of either T or B cells suggests malfunction of central lymphoid tissues, including the thymus and the fetal liver–bone marrow complex. B cell deficiency may result from failure to generate pre-B cells from their stem cell precursors or from failure of pre-B cells to give rise to their B lymphocyte progeny.

Similarly, differentiation may be arrested at several levels within the T cell lineage; arrests at the thymocyte level and failure to develop the helper subset have been observed in immunodeficient patients. Agammaglobulinemia and deficiencies of some T cell functions may occur despite the presence of normal numbers of B or T cells in the circulation. Failure of B lymphocytes to differentiate to plasma cells can be due to intrinsic cellular abnormalities or to faulty T cell regulation.

comes to be uniquely expressed by individual cells. A clone consists of cells that express the identical antigen-binding receptors. Estimates for the total number of B cell clones usually vary between 10 and 100 million. T cell clonal diversity may be equally extensive. The initial step in clonal development is independent of antigen and reflects a genetically programmed sequence of differentiation analogous to that of primary erythropoiesis or myelopoiesis. This phase, termed *primary differentiation*, begins early in human fetal development and continues in adult life, albeit at reduced levels.

The most primitive morphologically identifiable cell in the B lineage is called a *pro-B cell*. These cells are marked by the cell surface CD19 antigen and nuclear TdT expression. Pro-B cells undergo productive $V_H D_H J_H$ rearrangement to express cytoplasmic μ chains (the heavy chain of IgM) and become pre-B cells. Since light chain gene rearrangement usually occurs later, pre-B cells lack the characteristic membrane-bound immunoglobulin receptors that characterize B lymphocytes but they may express μ chain/surrogate light chain receptors encoded by the nonrearranged V pre-B and 14.1 genes in the λ light chain gene locus. Pre-B cells are generated in the fetal liver and in bone marrow throughout life, dividing in response to interleukin (IL)7 and other growth factors made by neighboring stromal cells. After undergoing a productive rearrangement of light chain VJ genes, pre-B cells become immature B lymphocytes that express surface IgM receptors. These B lymphocytes differ from their more mature counterparts in an important physiologic characteristic; they are highly susceptible to inactivation when their receptors bind antigen. Consequently, immature B cells encountering self-antigens may be eliminated or rendered anergic. The antigen receptors on B cells are multichain units. In order for membrane-bound immunoglobulins to reach the B cell surface, they require association with Ig-α and Ig-β chains, which serve as signal transduction elements for the antigen receptor complex. Antigen-mediated crosslinkage of the B cell receptors triggers the phosphorylation of tyrosines located in short conserved stretches of amino acids, called *immunomodulatory tyrosine activation motifs* in the cytoplasmic domains of the Ig-α and Ig-β chains. A cascade of enzymatic interactions is thus initiated that culminates in the binding of nuclear transcriptional factors to promoter regions of genes that determine the B cell's fate: death, survival, growth, or differentiation. A pivotal enzyme in this B cell activation cascade is the *Syk* tyrosine kinase.

The developmental sequence for expression of diverse immunoglobulin classes by B lymphocytes begins with expression of IgM. The expression of IgD on immature IgM-bearing cells occurs after they leave the bone marrow. Lymphocytes committed to synthesis of IgG, IgA, and IgE are derived from the IgM- and IgD-bearing precursors via a genetic switch mechanism. Each of the heavy chain constant region genes except C_δ is preceded by a switch region composed of repetitive nucleotide sequences. The heavy chain class switch is accomplished by splicing of the switch region of μ with the switch region in front of the downstream heavy chain gene to be expressed next and deletion of the C_μ, C_δ, and other C_H genes in the intervening DNA. The switch process involves antigenic stimulation and the help of T cells. Class switching occurs within the germinal centers of peripheral lymphoid tissues, where pairs of B and T cells cooperate in an antigen response. Essential to this process is the signal-inducing interaction of the CD40 molecule on the B cell with the CD40 ligand that is transiently expressed on the antigen-activated T cell partner. The helper T cell also produces soluble factors that can direct the class switch. IL-4 and transforming growth factor β can promote IgE and IgA responses, for example. The germinal center B cells also undergo somatic mutations in the variable regions of their immunoglobulin genes, and those with the highest antigen affinity are selected for survival as memory B cells or for terminal differentiation into antibody-secreting plasma cells.

During their development T lineage cells also undergo sequential rearrangements of the minigene families encoding their antigen receptors. On entering the epithelial thymus, the precursor cells may follow one of two major pathways. The first involves rearrangement of V_γ and J_γ genes to express γ chains and rearrangement of V_δ, D_δ, and J_δ genes to express δ chains. These associate with the CD3 proteins to

form the CD3/$\gamma\delta$ TCR complex of $\gamma\delta$ T cells. Pre-T cells beginning development along the second differentiation pathway in the thymus rearrange one each of the V_β, D_β, and J_β genes prior to the expression of a complete β chain together with a newly discovered pre-T chain. At a later differentiation stage, rearrangements of V_α and J_α genes occur in the α-chain family, and then the completed antigen receptor molecule of one α chain and one β chain is expressed together with the CD3 protein complex on the cell surface of an immature $\alpha\beta$ T cell. Initially, the $\alpha\beta$ T cells express both the CD4 and CD8 accessory molecules on their surface. As these cells mature under the influence of a selfantigen selection process, they either downregulate the CD8 molecule to become CD4+ T cells with helper cell potential or they cease to express the CD4 molecule to become CD8+ T cells with cytotoxic potential. The CD4+ $\alpha\beta$ T cells leaving the thymus have been selected to recognize peptide fragments presented in the groove of class II major histocompatibility complex (MHC) molecules of antigen presenting cells. The CD8+ $\alpha\beta$ T cells migrating from the thymus have been selected to recognize peptide fragments in the cleft of class I MHC molecules expressed by virtually all types of nucleated cells. The CD4 and CD8 molecules are called *accessory receptors* because they have binding affinity for class II or class I MHC molecules, respectively, and are coupled to tyrosine kinase molecules that are active in signal transduction. While the $\gamma\delta$ T cells express neither CD4 nor CD8 molecules during their intrathymic development, they may express CD8 molecules as mature T cells in the periphery. Expression of these and other cell surface molecules can be defined by specific monoclonal antibodies, thus providing a powerful tool for elucidating the developmental status of both T and B lymphocytes (see Fig. 307-1).

The $\alpha\beta$ T cells bearing the CD4 markers constitute approximately 70 percent of circulating T cells and function as helper cells that facilitate the effector functions of B cells, other T cells, NK cells, and macrophages. The $\alpha\beta$ T cells expressing CD8 molecules constitute 20 to 30 percent of circulating T cells, mediate cytotoxic reactions, and may suppress immune responses. The $\gamma\delta$ T cells constitute a minor population of T cells. They may serve a protective role along epithelial surfaces, where they predominate, and may modulate immune-based tissue damage. Developmental arrests or failure of function of one or more of these T cell subsets may result in immunodeficiency or autoimmune diseases.

The events designated *secondary differentiation* follow stimulation of specific clones of lymphocytes by antigen. These processes are synonymous with the immune response (see Chap. 305). Particularly important in consideration of immunodeficiencies are the collaborative interactions among macrophages, T cells, and B cells. While B lymphocytes may differentiate to become IgM-secreting plasma cells when stimulated by thymus-independent antigens, such as lipopolysaccharides, most antibody responses, particularly those of the IgG, IgA, and IgE classes, require intimate collaboration between T and B cells. Antigens bound to the antibody receptors on B cells are internalized, partially digested, and recycled to the cell surface, where they are presented on class II molecules to the T cell. The activated T cell in turn produces soluble factors that promote growth and differentiation of the B cell or inflammatory responses. These factors, which include interleukins IL-2, IL-4, IL-5, IL-6, IL-10, IL-12 and interferon γ (IFNγ), may be differentially produced by individual T cells. Depending on their initial activation stimulus, helper CD4 T cells may differentiate into different types of effector cells. The subset of helper T cells, designated TH1 cells, produces IL-2, IFNγ, tumor necrosis factor α, and other cytokines that regulate cell-mediated immunity, while the TH2 subset of cells typically produces IL-4, IL-5, IL-10, and other cytokines that regulate humoral immune responses. Antigenpresenting monocytes may produce IL-12 to bias the immune response toward TH1 effector cells, while IL-4 produced by a special subset of T cells or mast cells favors a TH2 effector cell response.

Differentiation of T or B cells may be arrested at either the primary or secondary stages. Reflecting the complex cellular interactions involved in immune responses and the pivotal role played by T lymphocytes, immune deficiencies primarily involving T cells are usually also associated with abnormal B cell function. Conversely, immunodeficiencies manifested primarily by inability to produce antibodies may be caused by T cell defects not associated with abnormal cell-mediated immunity.

EVALUATION OF IMMUNODEFICIENT PATIENTS A careful history and physical examination will usually indicate whether the major problem involves the antibody-complement-phagocyte system or cell-mediated immunity. A history of a normal response to smallpox vaccination or of contact dermatitis due to poison ivy suggests intact cellular immunity. Persistent mucocutaneous candidiasis suggests deficient cell-mediated immunity. Lymphopenia and the absence of palpable lymph nodes may be important findings. However, patients with profound immunodeficiency may have diffuse lymphoid hyperplasia. Most immunodeficiencies may be diagnosed by thoughtful use of tests available in local or regional clinical laboratories. More precise evaluation of immunologic functions and treatment may require referral to specialized centers. Table 307-1 presents a résumé of widely available laboratory investigations.

Humoral Immunity With rare exceptions, deficiency of humoral immunity is accompanied by diminished serum concentration of one or more classes of immunoglobulin. Normal values vary with age, and adult concentrations of IgM (1.0 g/L) are reached at about 1 year, of IgG (8.0 g/L) at 5 to 6 years, and of IgA (2.0 g/L) by puberty (see Chap. 305). Also, the wide range of values among normal adults creates difficulty in defining the lower limits of normal. Reasonable estimates for low normal values are 0.4 g/L for IgM, 5 g/L for IgG, and 0.5 g/L for IgA. In the presence of borderline hypogammaglo-

Table 307-1

Laboratory Evaluation of Host Defense Status

INITIAL SCREENING ASSAYS*

Complete blood count with differential smear
Serum immunoglobulin levels: IgM, IgG, IgA, IgD, IgE

OTHER READILY AVAILABLE ASSAYS

Quantification of blood mononuclear cell populations by immunofluorescence assays employing monoclonal antibody markers[†]
  T cells: CD3, CD4, CD8, TCRαβ, TCRγδ
  B cells: CD19, CD20, CD21, Ig(μ, δ, γ, α, κ, λ), Ig-associated molecules
     (α, β)
  NK cells: CD16
  Monocytes: CD15
  Activation markers: HLA-DR, CD25, CD80 (B cells)
T cell functional evaluation
  1. Delayed hypersensitivity skin tests (PPD, *Candida* histoplasmin, tetanus toxoid)
  2. Proliferative response to mitogens (anti-CD3 antibody, phytohemagglutinin, concanavalin A) and allogeneic cells (mixed lymphocyte response)
  3. Cytokine production
B cell functional evaluation
  1. Natural or commonly acquired antibodies: isohemagglutinins; antibodies to common viruses (influenza, rubella, rubeola) and bacterial toxins (diphtheria, tetanus)
  2. Response to immunization with protein (tetanus toxoid) and carbohydrate (pneumococcal vaccine, *H. influenzae* B vaccine) antigens
  3. Quantitative IgG subclass determinations
Complement
  1. CH$_{50}$ assays (classic and alternative pathways)
  2. C3, C4, and other components
Phagocyte function
  1. Reduction of nitroblue tetrazolium
  2. Chemotaxis assays
  3. Bactericidal activity

---

* Together with a history and physical examination, these tests will identify more than 95 percent of patients with primary immunodeficiencies.
[†] The menu of monoclonal antibody markers may be expanded or contracted to focus on particular clinical questions.

bulinemia, assessing the patient's capacity to produce specific antibodies becomes particularly important. Isohemagglutinins, anti-streptolysin O, and "febrile agglutinins" are valuable standard assays, and measurements of pre- and postimmunization titers to tetanus toxoid, diphtheria toxoid, *H. influenzae* capsular polysaccharide, and *S. pneumoniae* serotypes provide a comprehensive assessment of humoral responsiveness.

Estimation of numbers of circulating B and T lymphocytes is of value in determining the pathogenesis of certain types of immune deficiency. B lymphocytes are identified by the presence of membrane-bound immunoglobulins, their associated α- and β-chain units, and other lineage-specific molecules on the B cell surface (Table 307-1), which can be identified and enumerated by specific monoclonal antibodies.

Since antibody deficiency may be mimicked clinically by deficiency of complement components, measurement of total hemolytic complement (CH$_{50}$) should be a part of the evaluation of host defense. Measurement of C3 alone is inadequate for screening, since deficiencies of both early and late complement components may predispose to bacterial infection (see Chap. 305).

Cellular Immunity T lymphocytes may be enumerated by their expression of the TCR/CD3 complex of surface molecules. The CD2 antigenic molecule is also expressed by almost all of the T cells and a few non-T lineage lymphocytes. The CD4 molecule serves as a marker for helper T cells, although macrophages also express this molecule in relatively low levels. Conversely, CD8αβ heterodimers are expressed by cytotoxic T cells. These cell-surface molecules are also expressed by some γδ T cells and by NK cells, although usually as CD8αα homodimeric molecules.

Normal levels of serum immunoglobulins and antibody responsiveness are reliable indices of intact helper T cell function. T lymphocyte function can be measured directly by delayed hypersensitivity skin testing using a variety of antigens to which the majority of older children and adults have been sensitized. A generally useful skin test antigen is a 1:5 dilution of tetanus toxoid injected intradermally, since almost all individuals will have been sensitized. Purified protein derivative (PPD), histoplasmin, mumps antigen, and extracts of *Candida* or *Trichophyton* also may be used.

T lymphocyte function may be estimated in vitro by the capacity of cells to proliferate in response to antigens to which the patient has been sensitized, to lymphocytes from an unrelated donor, to antibodies that cross-link the CD3/TCR complex, or to the T cell mitogens, which include phytohemagglutinin, concanavalin A, and pokeweed mitogen. The response is usually quantified by measurement of incorporation of radioactive thymidine into newly synthesized DNA. It is also possible to measure the production of cytokines (or interleukins) by activated T cells. The ability of T cells activated in mixed lymphocyte culture to lyse target cells can be measured. Finally, assays exist for detection of defects in T cell surface receptors and specific elements of the signal transduction pathways that they activate in T cell responses.

CLASSIFICATION *Primary immunodeficiencies* may be either congenital or acquired and are currently classified according to mode of inheritance and whether the defect involves T cells, B cells, or both (Table 307-2). The following discussion emphasizes three related concepts: (1) that immunodeficiencies are most logically viewed as defects of cellular differentiation, (2) that these defects may involve either primary development of T or B cells or the antigen-dependent phase of their differentiation, and (3) that defects of B cell differentiation may in some instances reflect faulty T-B collaboration.

Secondary immunodeficiencies are those not caused by intrinsic abnormalities in development or function of T and B cells. The best known of these is AIDS, which may follow infection with the human immunodeficiency virus (see Chap. 308). Other examples are immune deficiency associated with malnutrition, protein-losing enteropathy, and intestinal lymphangiectasia. Also considered secondary are immunodeficiencies resulting from hypercatabolic states such as occur in myotonic dystrophy, immunodeficiency associated with lymphoreticu-

Table 307-2

WHO Classification of Primary Immunodeficiencies

COMBINED IMMUNODEFICIENCIES

Severe combined immunodeficiency (SCID):
  X-linked
  Autosomal recessive ("Swiss-type agammaglobulinemia")
Adenosine deaminase (ADA) deficiency
Purine nucleoside phosphorylase (PNP) deficiency
MHC class II deficiency
Reticular dysgenesis
CD3γ or CD3ε deficiency
CD8 deficiency

PREDOMINANTLY ANTIBODY DEFICIENCIES

X-linked agammaglobulinemia
Hyper-IgM syndrome:
  X-linked
  Other
Ig heavy chain–gene deletions
κ-Chain deficiency
IgA deficiency
Selective deficiency of IgG subclasses (with or without IgA deficiency)
Common variable immunodeficiency (CVID)
Antibody deficiency with normal immunoglobulins
Transient hypogammaglobulinemia of infancy

OTHER WELL-DEFINED IMMUNODEFICIENCY SYNDROMES

Wiskott-Aldrich syndrome
Ataxia telangiectasia
DiGeorge anomaly

IMMUNODEFICIENCY ASSOCIATED WITH OR SECONDARY TO OTHER DISEASES

Chromosomal instability or defective repair
  Bloom syndrome
  Fanconi anaemia
  ICF syndrome
  Nijmegen breakage syndrome
  Seckel syndrome
  Xeroderma pigmentosa
Chromosomal defects
  Down syndrome
  Turner syndrome
  Chromosome 18 rings and deletions
Skeletal abnormalities
  Short-limbed skeletal dysplasia
  Cartilage-hair hypoplasia
Immunodeficiency with generalized growth retardation
  Schimke immunoosseous dysplasia
  Immunodeficiency with absent thumbs
  Dubowitz syndrome
  Growth retardation, facial anomalies and immunodeficiency
  Progeria (Hutchinson-Gilford syndrome)
Immunodeficiency with dermatologic defects
  Partial albinism
  Dyskeratosis congenita
  Netherton syndrome
  Acrodermatitis enteropathica
  Anhidrotic ectodermal dysplasia
  Papillon-Lefevre syndrome
Hereditary metabolic defects
  Transcobalamin 2 deficiency
  Methylmalonic acidaemia
  Type 1 hereditary orotic aciduria
  Biotin-dependent carboxylase deficiency
  Mannosidosis
  Glycogen storage disease, type 1b
  Chédiak–Higashi syndrome
Hypercatabolism of immunoglobulin
  Familial hypercatabolism
  Intestinal lymphangiectasia
Other
  Hyper-IgE syndrome
  Chronic mucocutaneous candidiasis
  Hereditary or congenital hypo- or asplenia
  Ivermark syndrome

lar malignancy, and immunodeficiency resulting from treatment with x-rays, antilymphocyte serum, or cytotoxic drugs.

Incidence As a group, the primary immunodeficiencies are relatively common. The most frequent, isolated IgA deficiency, occurs in approximately 1 in 600 individuals in North America.

The more severe forms of primary immunodeficiency have their onset early in life and all too frequently result in death during childhood. Immunodeficiencies may become apparent at any age, however, and patients with congenital hypogammaglobulinemia may survive to middle age or beyond. In a referral center for patients with immunodeficiency diseases, approximately two-thirds of the immunodeficient patients will be adults.

Severe Combined Immunodeficiency The SCID syndrome is characterized by gross functional impairment of both humoral and cell-mediated immunity and by susceptibility to devastating fungal, bacterial, and viral infections. It is usually congenital, may be inherited either as an X-linked or autosomal recessive defect, or may occur sporadically. Affected infants rarely survive beyond 1 year without treatment.

The syndrome has been associated with a diversity of defects in development of immunocompetent cells, some of which are related to specific enzymatic abnormalities.

One form of SCID is characterized by severe lymphopenia and is inherited as an autosomal recessive disorder. The failure in both T and B cell development in some patients is due to *mutations in the RAG-1 or RAG-2 genes*, the combined activities of which are needed for V(D)J recombination. A function-loss *mutation in the DNA-dependent tyrosine kinase gene* is present in SCID mice and also may prove to be a cause for SCID in humans. Rarely, other hematopoietic cell lines fail to develop in a variant form of SCID called *reticular dysgenesia*. About half of patients with autosomal recessive SCID are deficient in an enzyme involved in purine metabolism, adenosine deaminase (ADA), due to deletions or point *mutations in the ADA gene*. Studies of the pathophysiologic relationship of ADA deficiency to abortive lymphoid differentiation suggest that intracellular accumulation of adenosine and deoxyadenosine nucleotides interferes with critical metabolic functions, including DNA synthesis. Improvement of both clinical status and immunologic function occurs in some patients treated with exogenous ADA conjugated to polyethylene glycol to prolong its half-life. The cellular defect in the lymphopenic forms of SCID logically rests with the precursor cells for both T and B lineages. The immunologic defects in all these types of SCID patients have been repaired following transplantation of bone marrow or fetal liver as a source of stem cells, indicating that the stromal microenvironments of the thymus and bone marrow of these patients are intact and capable of supporting T and B cell differentiation of normal stem cells.

SCID also may occur with an X-linked inheritance pattern. Aborted thymocyte differentiation and an absence of peripheral T cells and NK cells is seen in *X-linked SCID*. B lymphocytes are present in normal numbers but are functionally defective. The defective gene encodes a common γ chain of the receptors for IL-2, -4, -7, -9, and -15, thus disrupting the action of an important set of lymphokines. This developmental disorder can be repaired by transplantation of bone marrow stem cells from a histocompatible sibling. Transplants of haploidentical bone marrow, depleted of donor T cells to prevent graft-versus-host disease, also may correct the T cell deficit. However, antibody deficiency requiring immunoglobulin replacement therapy may persist for years unless the defective B cells are replaced by normal B cells of donor origin.

JAK3 protein kinase deficiency The same T⁻NK⁻B⁺ SCID phenotype seen in X-linked SCID can be inherited as an autosomal recessive disease due to mutations in the gene for JAK3 protein kinase. This enzyme associates with the common γ chain of the receptors for IL-2, -4, -7, -9, and -15 as a key element in their signal transduction pathways.

TREATMENT

Treatment of SCID patients should be performed in centers with a strong research interest in this problem. It is crucial that these patients be recognized early and not be given live viral vaccines or blood transfusions, which may cause fatal graft-versus-host disease.

T Cell Immunodeficiency Reflecting the diversity of T cell functions, abnormalities of T cell development may be responsible for a wide spectrum of immune deficiencies, including SCID, selective defects in cell-mediated immunity, and syndromes presenting as antibody deficiency. These defects may be acquired (see Chap. 308) as well as congenital.

DiGeorge's syndrome This classic example of isolated T cell deficiency results from maldevelopment of thymic epithelial elements derived from the third and fourth pharyngeal pouches. The gene defect has been mapped to chromosome 22q11. Defective development of organs dependent on cells of embryonic neural crest origin includes congenital cardiac defects, particularly those involving the great vessels; hypocalcemic tetany, due to failure of parathyroid development; and absence of a normal thymus. Facial abnormalities may include abnormal ears, shortened philtrum, micrognathia, and hypertelorism. Serum immunoglobulin concentrations are frequently normal, but antibody responses, particularly of IgG and IgA isotypes, are usually impaired. T cell levels are reduced, whereas B cell levels are normal. Affected individuals usually have a small, histologically normal thymus located near the base of the tongue or in the neck, allowing most patients to develop functional T cells in numbers that may or may not be adequate for host defense. Therapeutic intervention in the form of an epithelial thymic transplant is recommended only for the most severe cases of DiGeorge's syndrome.

T cell receptor deficiency Since the expression and function of antigenspecific TCR is dependent on their companion CD3γ, δ, ϵ, and ζ-η chains, defective genes for any of these receptor components can impair T cell development and function. Immunodeficiencies due to inherited CD3γ and CD3ϵ mutations have been identified. CD3γ mutations result in a selective deficit in CD8 T cells, whereas CD3ϵ mutations lead to a preferential reduction in CD4 T cells, thus implying differences in the signal transduction roles for each CD3 component.

MHC class II deficiency Because T cells are required for B cell responses to most antigens, any gene defect (or acquired disorder) that interferes with T cell development and cell-mediated immunity will also compromise antibody production and humoral immunity. MHC class II deficiency results in one such immunodeficiency in that the TCR must see protein antigens as peptide fragments held within the α helical grooves of class II and class I molecules encoded by the MHC. Antigen-presenting cells in individuals with this relatively rare disorder fail to express the class II molecules DP, DQ, and DR on their surface. Limited numbers of helper CD4 T cells are therefore generated in the thymus, and they fail to see antigen in the periphery. Affected individuals experience recurrent bronchopulmonary infections, chronic diarrhea, and severe viral infections that usually prove fatal before 4 years of age. The defect is caused by mutations in genes that encode essential transcription factors that bind to promoter elements for the MHC class II genes. In one subgroup of such patients the class II transactivator gene is mutated, whereas in other families mutations in genes encoding additional transcriptional factors for MHC class II genes are responsible for the defective development and function of CD4 T cells.

ZAP70 tyrosine kinase deficiency Recurrent and opportunistic infections begin within the first year of life in individuals with a deficiency in ZAP70 tyrosine kinase, a pivotal component in the TCR/CD3 signal transduction cascade. The rare inheritance of mutations in both alleles of the ZAP70 gene results in a selective deficiency of CD8 T cells and dysfunction of CD4 T cells, which are present in

normal numbers. Severe immunodeficiency is the inevitable consequence.

Purine nucleoside phosphorylation deficiency Function-loss mutations of the purine nucleoside phosphorylase (PNP) gene are associated with an often severe and selective deficiency of T lymphocyte function. This enzyme functions in the same purine salvage pathway as ADA; toxic effects of the PNP deficiency may be related to intracellular accumulation of deoxyguanosine triphosphate.

Ataxia-telangiectasia Ataxia-telangiectasia (AT) is an autosomal recessive genetic disorder characterized by cerebellar ataxia, oculocutaneous telangiectasia, and immunodeficiency. The gene responsible is located in the q22–23 region on chromosome 11. The mutant AT gene has sequence similarity to the phosphatidyl-inositol-3 kinases that are involved in signal transduction. The AT gene belongs to a conserved family of genes that monitor DNA repair and coordinate DNA synthesis with cell division. The deleterious effects of the AT gene are widespread. Onset of truncal ataxia usually occurs in infancy and is progressive. Immunodeficiency may be clinically manifest by recurrent and chronic sinopulmonary infection leading to bronchiectasis, although not all patients have overt immunodeficiency. Ovarian agenesis is a frequent occurrence. Persistence of very high serum levels of oncofetal proteins, including alpha fetoprotein and carcinoembryonic antigen, may be of diagnostic value. Frequent causes of death are chronic pulmonary disease and malignancy. Lymphomas are most common, although carcinomas also have occurred.

The immunologic abnormalities seem to be related to maldevelopment of the thymus. The thymus is markedly hypoplastic and similar in appearance to an embryonic thymus. The peripheral T cell pool is frequently reduced in size, especially in lymphoid tissue compartments. Cutaneous anergy and delayed rejection of skin grafts are common. Although B lymphocyte development is normal, most patients are deficient in serum IgE and IgA, and a smaller number have reduced serum levels of IgG, particularly of the IgG2, IgG4 subclasses. IgM and IgD are usually normal.

The defect in DNA repair mechanisms in these patients renders their cells highly susceptible to radiation-induced chromosomal damage and results in a high incidence of malignancies.

Only symptomatic treatment is available. Unless a severe IgG deficiency is present, therapy with immunoglobulin is not indicated. Exposure to x-irradiation should be avoided in AT patients. AT is a rare disorder, one in 10,000 to 100,000 incidence, but 1 percent of the population is heterozygous for an AT mutation. The heterozygous state predisposes to enhanced cellular radiosensitivity and cancer, especially breast cancer in females.

Immunoglobulin deficiency syndromes *X-linked agammaglobulinemia* Males with this syndrome often begin to have recurrent bacterial infections late in the first year of life, when maternally derived immunoglobulins have disappeared. Affected individuals have very few immunoglobulin-bearing B lymphocytes in their circulation and lack primary and secondary lymphoid follicles. However, B cell progenitors are found in normal frequency in the bone marrow. This developmental block at the pre-B cell level contrasts with earlier and later arrests in B cell differentiation characterizing other immunodeficiencies (see below and Fig. 307-1). The defective Bruton's tyrosine kinase (Btk) gene responsible for X-linked agammaglobulinemia is located in the Xq 22 region. B cells from heterozygous female carriers utilize the X chromosome with the normal Btk gene exclusively, while T cells and myeloid cells express either X chromosome. *X-linked agammaglobulinemia with growth hormone deficiency* is a rare variant disorder caused by another gene defect that maps to the same region of the X chromosome.

Agammaglobulinemia is a misnomer, since most patients with this and other forms of severe panhypogammaglobulinemia synthesize some immunoglobulins. Within the same family, some affected males have had substantial levels of IgM, IgG, and IgA, while others have been nearly agammaglobulinemic. All of the Btk-deficient patients are very deficient in circulating B lymphocytes. This observation indicates that the few B lymphocytes that escape the block in differentiation are capable of plasma cell maturation and immunoglobulin synthesis.

However, antibody replacement therapy is needed in all these patients because of the limited number of B cell clones that are generated.

Sinopulmonary infections constitute the most frequent clinical problem. A form of arthritis with some of the features of rheumatoid disease occurs in some of these patients. *Mycoplasma* organisms are sometimes the cause of the arthritis. Chronic encephalitis of viral etiology can be a fatal complication. Some of these patients have an associated dermatomyositis. The frequency with which these complications occur is reduced by adequate treatment with intravenous immunoglobulin.

Transient hypogammaglobulinemia of infancy This diagnosis is reserved for those rare instances in which normal physiologic hypogammaglobulinemia of infancy is unusually prolonged and severe. IgG levels normally drop to 3.0 to 4.0 g/L between 3 and 6 months of age as maternally derived IgG is catabolized. The IgG levels subsequently rise, reflecting the infants' increased synthetic capacity. Periodic immunologic assessment is needed to differentiate transient hypogammaglobulinemia from other forms of antibody deficiency. Antibody replacement therapy is recommended only in the face of severe or recurrent infections.

Isolated deficiency of IgA This immunodeficiency occurs with a frequency of approximately 1 in 600 individuals of European origin. IgA deficiency is much less common in people of Asian and African origin. In Japan, for example, the incidence is approximately 1 in 18,500. While the precise genetic basis for this difference in incidence is unknown, IgA deficiency is frequently associated with certain MHC haplotypes in Caucasians.

With rare exceptions, IgA1 and IgA2 subclasses are both deficient in serum and in mucous secretions. While most individuals with isolated IgA deficiency appear healthy, others have an increased number of respiratory infections of varying severity, and a few have severe pulmonary disease such as bronchiectasis. Chronic diarrheal disease also occurs. The incidence of asthma and other atopic diseases among IgA-deficient patients is high, and conversely, the incidence of IgA deficiency among atopic children has been found to be 20 to 40 times that in the normal population. IgA deficiency is also significantly associated with autoimmune diseases such as rheumatoid arthritis (see Chap. 313) and systemic lupus erythematosus (see Chap. 312). Selective reductions in the IgG2 and IgG4 subclasses have been associated with the increased infections seen in some IgA-deficient individuals. Finally, IgA-deficient patients may develop significant levels of antibodies to IgA. These patients may have severe anaphylactic reactions when transfused with normal blood or blood products.

IgA deficiency is often familial. It also can occur in association with congenital intrauterine infections, such as toxoplasmosis, rubella, and cytomegalovirus infection, or following treatment with phenytoin, penicillamine, or other medications in genetically susceptible individuals.

The pathogenesis of IgA deficiency, whether genetic or induced by environmental insult, involves a block in terminal differentiation of B lymphocytes. The IgA-bearing lymphocytes in these patients also bear surface IgM. This immature phenotype, also prevalent in normal neonates, may reflect a primary defect in essential regulatory interactions between T and B cells.

Treatment of IgA deficiency is essentially symptomatic. IgA cannot be effectively replaced by exogenous immunoglobulin or plasma, and use of either can increase the risk of development of antibodies to IgA. IgA-deficient patients in need of transfusion should be screened for the presence of antibodies to IgA and ideally should be given blood only from IgA-deficient donors. Treatment with immunoglobulin may benefit the exceptional IgA-deficient person in whom IgG2 and IgG4 subclass deficiencies are associated with severe infections. The risk of anaphylactic reactions to contaminating IgA must always be considered in treating IgA-deficient patients.

IgG subclass deficiencies Selective deficiencies in one or more of the four IgG subclasses are seen in some patients with repeated infections. The IgG subclass deficiency may easily go undetected when the total serum IgG level is measured, because IgG2, IgG3, and IgG4 together account for only 30 to 40 percent of the IgG antibodies. Even

a deficiency in IgG1 may be masked by increases in the remaining IgG isotypes. However, the availability of subclass-specific monoclonal antibodies allows precise measurement of IgG subclass levels.

Homozygous deletions of genes encoding the constant region of the different γ chains is the basis for the IgG subclass deficiency in some individuals. For example, deletion of the $C_{\alpha 1}$, $C_{\gamma 2}$, $C_{\gamma 4}$, and C_{ϵ} genes on both chromosomes 14 was responsible for one individual's inability to make IgA1, IgG2, IgG4, and IgE. Interestingly, individuals with this and other patterns of C_H-gene deletions may not have unusual infections.

Most of the IgG subclass–deficient individuals with repeated infections appear to have regulatory defects that prevent normal B cell differentiation. The defect may extend to other isotypes. IgA deficiency may accompany IgG2 and IgG4 subclass deficiencies (see "Isolated Deficiency of IgA," above), and an inability to produce IgM antibodies to polysaccharide antigens often reflects a broader defect in antibody responsiveness. While patients with IgG subclass deficiency may benefit from administration of immunoglobulin, a thorough immunologic assessment is needed to identify the relatively few who need this therapy.

Common variable immunodeficiency This diagnostic category includes a heterogeneous group of males and females, mostly adults, who have in common the clinical manifestations of deficient production of all major immunoglobulin classes. The majority of these panhypogammaglobulinemic patients have normal numbers of B lymphocytes that are clonally diverse but phenotypically immature. B lymphocytes in these patients are able to recognize antigens and can proliferate in response but fail to differentiate to become plasma cells. This abortive differentiation pattern leads to the frequent occurrence of nodular lymphoid hyperplasia, including splenomegaly and intestinal lymphoid hyperplasia. Several types of defects in B lymphocyte differentiation have been suggested. An intrinsic abnormality of B lymphocytes may prevent their differentiation into immunoglobulin-secreting plasma cells even when provided with differentiation factors from normal T cells. Alternatively, the defective B cell response may reflect a deficiency of helper T cell function which may be associated with reduced numbers of CD4 + T cells. Other possible causes include a deficiency in complement components, such as C4A, which facilitate antigen-mediated triggering of B cells.

Common variable immunodeficiency and IgA deficiency may represent polar ends of a clinical spectrum due to the same underlying gene defect in a large subset of these patients. The two disorders feature similar B cell differentiation arrests, differing only in the numbers of immunoglobulin classes involved. Both disorders occur frequently within the same family, and the same MHC haplotypes are associated with both immunodeficiency patterns. The data suggest an underlying susceptibility gene in both disorders.

It is important to consider the diagnosis of common variable immunodeficiency in adults with chronic pulmonary infections, some of whom will present with unexplained bronchiectasis. Intestinal diseases, including chronic giardiasis, intestinal malabsorption, and atrophic gastritis with pernicious anemia, are common in this group of patients. Patients with common variable immunodeficiency also may present with signs and symptoms highly suggestive of lymphoid malignancy, including fever, weight loss, splenomegaly, generalized lymphadenopathy, and lymphocytosis. Routine histologic examination of lymphoid tissues usually reveals germinal center hyperplasia which may be difficult to distinguish from nodular lymphoma (see Chap. 113). Demonstration of a normal distribution of immunoglobulin isotypes and light chain classes on circulating and tissue B lymphocytes can serve to distinguish these patients from those having a monoclonal B cell malignancy with secondary hypogammaglobulinemia. The monthly administration of intravenous immunoglobulin in adequate doses (see below) is an essential part of the prevention and treatment of all these complications.

X-linked immunodeficiency with increased levels of IgM In this syndrome, IgG and IgA levels are very low, while IgD levels may be high. The normal development of B lymphocytes bearing IgM and IgD and the absence of IgG and IgA B lymphocytes indicate a defect in isotype switching. The defective gene in most of these patients encodes a transmembrane molecule on activated T cells that is the ligand for the CD40 molecule on B cells. Gene mutations that preclude normal expression of this CD40 ligand prevent normal T and B cell cooperation, germinal center formation, and isotype switching. The clinical patterns of infection are similar to but more severe than those occurring with other hypogammaglobulinemic states. Probably because of a subtle defect in T cell responsiveness, pneumonia caused by *P. carinii*, severe enteritis due to cryptosporidial infection, and fungal infections sometimes occur. Neutropenia in affected males also can increase their vulnerability to infections. Adequate antibody replacement by immunoglobulin administration may reverse the neutropenia and reduce the frequency of infections requiring antibiotic therapy. Bone marrow transplantation can be curative, but this treatment presently is reserved for exceptional circumstances.

Isolated deficiency of IgM This syndrome has been reported rarely in the United States but was detected frequently in a British population. Approximately 60 percent of these patients had severe recurrent infections, often with bacteremia. Pneumococcal pneumonia and meningococcal meningitis have been noted in IgM-deficient patients. Other associated conditions included gastrointestinal disease, atopy, splenomegaly, and development of malignancy. The condition was frequently familial and was four times more common in males than in females. The number of circulating B lymphocytes has varied from very low to normal.

Miscellaneous Immunodeficiency Syndromes Infection with *Candida albicans* is the almost universal accompaniment of severe deficiencies in cell-mediated immunity. *Chronic mucocutaneous candidiasis* is different because superficial candidiasis is usually the only major manifestation of immunodeficiency in this syndrome. These patients rarely develop systemic infection with *Candida* or other fungal agents and are not unusually susceptible to virus or bacterial disease. The syndrome is often congenital and may be associated with single or multiple endocrinopathies as well as iron deficiency. Treatment of associated conditions may lead to improvement or even cure of *Candida* infection.

No uniformity of immunologic defects has been identified in these patients, although defects of antibody formation have been detected occasionally. Humoral immunity, including ability to make specific anti-*Candida* antibodies, is usually normal. Many patients are anergic, some to a variety of antigens and some only to *Candida*; anergy in some patients has been related to inability of their lymphocytes to produce the cytokine called *migration inhibition factor*.

Results of treatment with antifungal agents, such as amphotericin B, have been variable. In some patients, intensive treatment with amphotericin B coupled with surgical removal of infected nails has led to sustained improvement. Oral antifungal agents, such as fluconazole and itraconazole, also may be effective.

Immunodeficiency with thymoma The association of hypogammaglobulinemia with spindle cell thymoma usually occurs relatively late in adult life. Bacterial infections and severe diarrhea often reflect the antibody deficiency, whereas fungal and viral infections are infrequent complications. T cell numbers and cell-mediated immunity are usually intact, but these patients are very deficient in circulating B lymphocytes and pre-B cells in the bone marrow. They also frequently have eosinopenia and may develop erythroid aplasia. Complete bone marrow failure has occurred in a few immunodeficient patients with thymoma. The relationship between the thymoma and apparent abnormalities of hematopoietic stem cells remains conjectural.

Wiskott-Aldrich syndrome This is an X-linked genetic disease characterized by eczema, thrombocytopenia, and repeated infections. The platelets are small and have a shortened half-life. Affected male infants often present with bleeding, and most do not survive childhood,

dying of complications of bleeding, infection, or lymphoreticular malignancy. The immunologic defects are well characterized phenotypically but are poorly understood. Serum concentrations of IgM are usually decreased, while IgA and IgG are normal and IgE is frequently increased. Synthetic rates for all three classes may be elevated, indicating a significant element of hypercatabolism. The number and class distribution of B lymphocytes are usually normal. Functionally, these boys are consistently unable to make antibodies to polysaccharide antigens normally; responses to protein antigens are often impaired late in the course of the disease. While most patients acquire T cell deficiencies, serial appraisal suggests that the T cell defects are secondary. Affected boys frequently become anergic, and their T cells do not respond normally to challenge with ubiquitous antigens. Mutations in the WASP gene on the short arm of the X chromosome are responsible for this disease. The WASP protein may serve an important role in transduction of cellular signals.

Transplantation of histocompatible bone marrow from a sibling donor has corrected both hematologic and immunologic abnormalities in several patients. In patients lacking a suitable donor, intravenous immunoglobulin infusions or splenectomy may improve platelet counts and reduce the risk of serious hemorrhage. Because of the increased risk of pneumococcal bacteremia, splenectomized patients should probably receive prophylactic penicillin.

X-linked lymphoproliferative syndrome This is an X-linked recessive disease in which there appears to be a selective impairment in immune elimination of Epstein-Barr virus (EBV). Infectious mononucleosis in affected males may have a fulminant and fatal outcome, may be associated with development of B cell malignancies, or may result in acquired hypogammaglobulinemia, aplastic anemia, or agranulocytosis. Antibodies to EBV can be detected in some patients but are often absent in the face of infection. Generation of cytotoxic T cells appears to be the primary mechanism of control of EBV infection in normal persons, and NK cells also may play a role in eliminating EBV-infected B cells. The gene defect has been mapped to the Xq 25 region, and the mutant gene responsible for the X-linked lymphoproliferative syndrome should be identified soon. Bone marrow transplantation from an HLA-matched donor may be curative, especially in younger children with this syndrome. Intravenous immunoglobulins should be administered to affected males who develop hypogammaglobulinemia.

Hyper-IgE syndrome The hyper IgE syndrome (see Chap. 62) is characterized by recurrent abscesses involving skin, lungs, and other organs and very high IgE levels. Staphylococcal infection is common to all patients, but most have infections with other pyogenic organisms as well. Males and females of all races are affected in an inheritance pattern suggesting an autosomal dominant defect with variable penetrance. A specific immunologic defect has not been identified. Abnormal neutrophil chemotaxis is an inconsistent finding, and diminished antibody responses to secondary immunization have been noted in some patients. Prophylaxis with penicillinase-resistant penicillins or cephalosporins is highly recommended to prevent staphylococcal infections. Pneumatocoeles, a frequent complication of penumonias, may require surgical excision.

Metabolic Abnormalities Associated with Immunodeficiency The relation of deficiencies of the purine salvage enzymes adenosine deaminase and purine nucleoside phosphorylase to immunodeficiency was discussed earlier. The syndrome of *acrodermatitis enteropathica* includes severe desquamating skin lesions, intractable diarrhea, bizarre neurologic symptoms, variable combined immunodeficiency, and an often fatal outcome. This disease is apparently caused by an inborn error of metabolism resulting in malabsorption of dietary zinc and can be treated effectively by parenteral or large oral doses of zinc. Zinc deficiency might in part account for the immunodeficiency that accompanies severe malnutrition. Inherited *deficiency of transcobalamin II*, the serum carrier molecule responsible for transport of vitamin B_{12} to tissues, is associated with failure of immunoglobulin production as well as megaloblastic anemia, leukopenia, thrombocytopenia, and severe malabsorption. All abnormalities of this rare disorder are reversed by administration of vitamin B_{12}.

℞ **TREATMENT**

Immunodeficiency diseases involving severe abnormalities of T cell function, with or without hypogammaglobulinemia, are often treatable with bone marrow transplants (see Fig. 307-1). Histocompatible marrow from a sibling donor is preferred, but haploidentical marrow may be used after removal of T cells. This therapy is complex and is best done by experienced research teams.

Replacement therapy with human immunoglobulin currently should be used in patients who have recurrent bacterial infections and are deficient in IgG. Maintenance of serum IgG levels above 5.0 g/L is sufficient to prevent most systemic infections and, together with antibiotic therapy, enhances reversal of chronic sinopulmonary infection. These serum levels usually can be achieved by intravenous administration of IgG, 400 mg/kg, at monthly intervals. In patients with mild to moderate IgG deficiency (3.0 to 4.0 g/L), the decision to treat should be based on clinical symptoms and response to antigenic challenge.

Immunoglobulin treatment is of no value in patients with deficiencies of immunoglobulins other than IgG, and this treatment is not benign. Some patients develop symptoms of diaphoresis, tachycardia, flank pain, and hypotension during or immediately following immunoglobulin administration. This reaction may be mediated by aggregates of IgG or other biologically active substances, but it also may occur as a consequence of antibodies produced by the patient against donor immunoglobulins, particularly IgA (see Chap. 115).

Therapy with exogenous IgG may not suffice to eliminate the chronic sinopulmonary inflammation and its progression to pulmonary fibrosis and bronchiectasis. Therefore, maintenance of good pulmonary toilet with regular postural drainage can be an especially important part of immunodeficient patient management. The principles of antibiotic therapy are not different in these than in other patients, except that the index of suspicion of bacterial infection should remain very high.

The availability of purified INFγ and other biologically active cytokines may prove to be valuable in the therapy of certain immunologic disorders. Gene replacement has been partially successful so far only in SCID patients with ADA deficiency. However, gene therapy holds great promise for treatment of a variety of genetic defects of the immune system, provided that the difficult problem of gene replacement in hemopoietic stem cells can be solved.

BIBLIOGRAPHY

ALARCON R et al: Familial defect in the surface expression of the T cell receptor-CD3 complex. N Engl J Med 319:1203, 1988

BLAESE MR et al: T lymphocyte-directed gene therapy for ADA⁻ SCID: Initial trial results after 4 years. Science 270:475, 1995

BUCKLEY RH, SHIFF RI: The use of intravenous immune globulin in immunodeficiency diseases. N Engl J Med 325:110, 1991

ELDER ME et al: Human SCID due to a defect in ZAP70, a T cell tyrosine kinase. Science 264:4596, 1994

FISCHER A, ARNAIZ-VILLENA A: Immunodeficiencies of genetic origin. Immunol Today 16:510, 1995

HOLLENBAUH D et al: The role of CD40 and its ligand in the regulation of the immune response. Immunol Rev 138:23, 1994

MACH B: MHC class II regulation: Lessons from a disease. N Engl J Med 332:120, 1995

PAUL WE: *Fundamental Immunology*, 3d ed. New York, Raven Press, 1993

ROSEN FS et al: Primary immunodeficiency diseases. N Engl J Med 333:341, 1995

——— et al: Primary immunodeficiency diseases. Report of a WHO Scientific Group. Clin Exp Immunol 99(Suppl 1):1, 1995

SAVITSKY K et al: A single ataxia telangiectasia gene with a product similar to PI-3 kinase. Science 268:1749, 1995

SIDERAS P, SMITH CIE: Molecular and cellular aspects of X-linked agammaglobulinemia. Adv Immunol 59:135, 1995

308 Anthony S. Fauci, H. Clifford Lane

HUMAN IMMUNODEFICIENCY VIRUS (HIV) DISEASE: AIDS AND RELATED DISORDERS

The acquired immune deficiency syndrome (AIDS) was first recognized in the United States in the summer of 1981, when the Centers for Disease Control and Prevention (CDC) reported the unexplained occurrence of *Pneumocystis carinii* pneumonia in five previously healthy homosexual men in Los Angeles and of Kaposi's sarcoma in 26 previously healthy homosexual men in New York and Los Angeles. Within months, the disease became recognized in male and female injection drug users (IDUs) and soon thereafter, in recipients of blood transfusions and in hemophiliacs. Because of the disproportionate number of cases of AIDS among Haitians in the United States early in the epidemic, this group was incorrectly designated as a "risk" group. Studies among Haitians in the United States and in Haiti soon revealed that the disease among Haitians was following a pattern of homosexual as well as heterosexual transmission; the latter was virtually identical to the predominant mode of transmissibility that was being recognized in developing countries in sub-Saharan Africa and elsewhere in the world (see below). As the epidemiologic pattern of the disease unfolded, it became clear that a microbe transmissible by sexual contact and blood or blood products was the most likely etiologic agent of the epidemic.

In 1983, human immunodeficiency virus (HIV) was isolated from a patient with lymphadenopathy, and by 1984 it was demonstrated clearly to be the causative agent of AIDS. The virus, which belongs to the lentivirus subfamily of the large family of retroviruses (Retroviridae) (see Chap. 192) was formerly called *lymphadenopathy associated virus* (LAV), *human T lymphotropic virus* (HTLV) *type III*, and *AIDS-associated retrovirus* (ARV). In 1985, a sensitive enzyme-linked immunosorbent assay (ELISA) was developed, which has led to an appreciation of the scope of HIV infection among cohorts of individuals in the United States who admit to practicing high-risk behavior (see below) as well as among selected populations that had been screened, such as blood donors, military recruits and active-duty military personnel, Job Corps applicants, and patients in selected sentinel hospitals. In addition, seroprevalance studies revealed the enormity of the global pandemic, particularly in developing countries (see below). Such surveillance approaches, when combined with monitoring of CD4+ T cell counts as a parameter of immunosuppression, led to the realization that there is a broad spectrum of HIV disease, ranging from asymptomatic infection and clinical latency to advanced clinical disease, the latter constituting AIDS.

During the early years of the AIDS epidemic in the 1980s, the care of HIV-infected individuals in the United States was, with few exceptions, confined to relatively restricted groups of physicians and hospitals, located predominantly in urban areas, particularly on the northeastern and western seaboards. Today, it is clear that virtually every practicing physician in the country and worldwide will be required to have some degree of familiarity with the workup, diagnosis, management, and specific treatment of HIV-infected individuals. HIV-infected patients are presenting in increasing numbers to family practice physicians, internists, obstetricians/gynecologists, pediatricians, and surgeons, with clinical problems that may be directly or indirectly related, or totally unrelated, to their HIV infection.

The staggering worldwide growth of the HIV pandemic is matched by an explosion of information in the areas of HIV virology, the pathogenesis (both immunologic and virologic) and treatment of HIV disease, the treatment and prophylaxis of the opportunistic diseases associated with HIV infection, and vaccine development. The information flow related to HIV disease is much greater than that for any other infectious or immunologic disease, or in fact for any other single disease in any subspecialty. It becomes almost impossible for the health care generalist to stay abreast of the literature. The purpose of this chapter is to present the most current information available on the scope of the epidemic; on its pathogenesis, treatment, and prevention; and on prospects for vaccine development. Above all, the aim is to provide a solid scientific basis and practical guidelines for a state-of-the-art approach to the HIV-infected patient.

DEFINITION AIDS was originally defined for surveillance purposes by the CDC (prior to the identification of HIV as the etiologic agent) as the presence of a reliably diagnosed "opportunistic" disease that is at least moderately predictive of an underlying defect in cell-mediated immunity in the absence of known causes of underlying immune defects, such as iatrogenic immunosuppression or malignant neoplasms. With the identification of HIV as the etiologic agent of AIDS and with the availability of sensitive and specific diagnostic tests for HIV infection, the case definition of AIDS has undergone several revisions. The latest revision took place in 1993; this revised CDC classification system for HIV-infected adolescents and adults categorizes persons on the basis of clinical conditions associated with HIV infection and CD4+ T lymphocyte counts. The system is based on three ranges of CD4+ T lymphocyte counts and three clinical categories and is represented by a matrix of nine mutually exclusive categories (Tables 308-1 and 308-2). Using this system, any HIV-infected individual with a CD4+ T cell count of <200/μL has AIDS by definition, regardless of the presence of symptoms or opportunistic diseases (Table 308-1). The clinical conditions in clinical category C now include pulmonary tuberculosis, recurrent pneumonia, and invasive cervical cancer (Table 308-2). Once individuals have had a clinical condition in category B, their disease cannot again be classified as category A, even if the condition resolves; the same holds true for category C in relation to category B.

While the definition of AIDS is complex and comprehensive, the clinician should not focus on whether AIDS is present but should view HIV disease as a spectrum ranging from primary infection, with or without the acute syndrome, to the asymptomatic stage, to advanced disease (see below). The definition of AIDS was established not for the practical care of patients but for surveillance purposes.

ETIOLOGIC AGENT

The etiologic agent of AIDS is HIV, which belongs to the family of human retroviruses and the subfamily of lentiviruses. Nononcocgenic lentiviruses cause disease in other animal species, including sheep, horses, goats, cattle, cats, and monkeys. The four recognized human retroviruses belong to two distinct groups: the human T lymphotropic viruses, HTLV-I and HTLV-II, which are transforming retroviruses; and the human immunodeficiency viruses, HIV-1 and HIV-2, which are cytopathic viruses. The reader is referred to Chap. 192 for a detailed description of the biology of the human retroviruses. The most common cause of HIV disease throughout the world, and certainly in the United

Table 308-1

1993 Revised Classification System for HIV Infection and Expanded AIDS Surveillance Case Definition for Adolescents and Adults*

CD4+ T Cell Categories	Clinical Categories		
	A Asymptomatic, Acute (Primary) HIV or PGL†	**B** Symptomatic, Not A or C Conditions	**C** AIDS-Indicator Conditions
>500/μL	A1	B1	C1
200–499/μL	A2	B2	C2
<200/μL	A3	B3	C3

* The shaded areas indicate the expanded AIDS surveillance case definition.
† PGL, progressive generalized lymphadenopathy.
SOURCE: Morb Mort Week Rep 42(No. RR-17), December 18, 1992.

Table 308-2

Clinical Categories of HIV Infection

Category A: Consists of one or more of the conditions listed below in an adolescent or adult (>13 years) with documented HIV infection. Conditions listed in categories B and C must not have occurred.
  Asymptomatic HIV infection
  Persistent generalized lymphadenopathy
  Acute (primary) HIV infection with accompanying illness or history of acute HIV infection
Category B: Consists of symptomatic conditions in an HIV-infected adolescent or adult that are not included among conditions listed in clinical category C and that meet at least one of the following criteria: (1) The conditions are attributed to HIV infection or are indicative of a defect in cell-mediated immunity; or (2) the conditions are considered by physicians to have a clinical course or to require management that is complicated by HIV infection. Examples include, but are not limited to, the following:
  Bacillary angiomatosis
  Candidiasis, oropharyngeal (thrush)
  Candidiasis, vulvovaginal; persistent, frequent, or poorly responsive to therapy
  Cervical dysplasia (moderate or severe)/cervical carcinoma in situ
  Constitutional symptoms, such as fever (38.5°C) or diarrhea lasting >1 month
  Hairy leukoplakia, oral
  Herpes zoster (shingles), involving at least two distinct episodes or more than one dermatome
  Idiopathic thrombocytopenic purpura
  Listeriosis
  Pelvic inflammatory disease, particularly if complicated by tuboovarian abscess
  Peripheral neuropathy
Category C: Conditions listed in the AIDS surveillance case definition.
  Candidiasis of bronchi, trachea, or lungs
  Candidiasis, esophageal
  Cervical cancer, invasive*
  Coccidioidomycosis, disseminated or extrapulmonary
  Cryptococcosis, extrapulmonary
  Cryptosporidiosis, chronic intestinal (>1 month's duration)
  Cytomegalovirus disease (other than liver, spleen, or nodes)
  Cytomegalovirus retinitis (with loss of vision)
  Encephalopathy, HIV-related
  Herpes simplex: chronic ulcer(s) (>1 month's duration); or bronchitis, pneumonia, or esophagitis
  Histoplasmosis, disseminated or extrapulmonary
  Isosporiasis, chronic intestinal (>1 month's duration)
  Kaposi's sarcoma
  Lymphoma, Burkitt's (or equivalent term)
  Lymphoma, primary, of brain
  Mycobacterium avium complex or *M. kansasii*, disseminated or extrapulmonary
  Mycobacterium tuberculosis, any site (pulmonary* or extrapulmonary)
  Mycobacterium, other species or unidentified species, disseminated or extrapulmonary
  Pneumocystis carinii pneumonia
  Pneumonia, recurrent*
  Progressive multifocal leukoencephalopathy
  Salmonella septicemia, recurrent
  Toxoplasmosis of brain
  Wasting syndrome due to HIV

* Added in the 1993 expansion of the AIDS surveillance case definition.
SOURCE: Morb Mort Week Rep 42(No. RR-17), December 18, 1992.

States, is HIV-1. HIV-1 comprises several subtypes with different geographic distributions (see below). HIV-2 was first identified in 1986 in West African patients and was originally confined to West Africa. However, a number of cases have been identified in Europe, South America, Canada, and the United States. HIV-2 is more closely related phylogenetically to the simian immunodeficiency virus (SIV) found in sooty mangabeys than it is to HIV-1. HIV-1 is more closely related to an SIV isolated from chimpanzees in 1990. The taxonomic relationship among primate lentiviruses is shown in Fig. 308-1.

MORPHOLOGY OF HIV Electron microscopy shows that the HIV virion is an icosahedral structure (Fig. 308-2A) containing numerous external spikes formed by the two major envelope proteins, the external gp120 and the transmembrane gp41. The virion buds from

FIGURE 308-1 Five groups of primate lentiviruses. Five discrete groups of primate lentiviruses have been identified thus far on the basis of genetic sequence analysis. Members of each group share the same genomic organization and are more closely related to each other than to members of different groups. The percentages refer to the approximate amino acid identities in the relatively conserved *pol* gene. *(Adapted from RC Desrosiers, Nature 345:288, 1990; also from Desrosiers and Fauci.)*

the surface of the infected cell and incorporates a variety of host proteins, including major histocompatibility complex (MHC) class I and II antigens (see Chap. 306), into its lipid bilayer. The structure of HIV-1 is schematically diagrammed in Fig. 308-2*B* (see also Chap. 192).

LIFE CYCLE OF HIV   HIV is an RNA virus whose hallmark is the reverse transcription of its genomic RNA to DNA by the enzyme *reverse transcriptase*. The life cycle of HIV begins with the high-affinity binding of the gp120 protein via a portion of its V1 region near the N terminus to its receptor on the host cell surface, the CD4 molecule (Fig. 308-3). The CD4 molecule is a 55-kDa protein found predominantly on a subset of T lymphocytes that are responsible for helper or inducer function in the immune system (see Chap. 305). It is also expressed on the surface of monocytes/macrophages and dendritic/Langerhans cells. It has recently been demonstrated that the coreceptor that must be present together with the CD4 molecule for fusion and entry of T cell–tropic strains of HIV-1 is a molecule termed CXCR4, while the coreceptor for macrophage-tropic strains of HIV-1 is the β-chemokine receptor CCR5. Both receptors belong to the family of seven-transmembrane-domain G protein–coupled cellular receptors (see below for details). Following binding, fusion with the host cell membrane occurs via the gp41 molecule, and the HIV genomic RNA is uncoated and internalized into the target cell. The reverse transcriptase enzyme, which is contained in the infecting virion, then catalyzes the reverse transcription of the genomic RNA into double-stranded DNA. The DNA translocates to the nucleus, where it is integrated randomly into the host cell chromosomes through the action of another virally encoded enzyme, *integrase*. This provirus may remain transcriptionally inactive (latent), or it may manifest varying levels of gene expression, up to active production of virus.

Cellular activation plays an important role in the life cycle of HIV and is critical to the pathogenesis of HIV

disease (see below). Following initial binding and internalization of virions into the target cell, incompletely reverse-transcribed DNA intermediates are labile in quiescent cells and will not integrate efficiently into the host cell genome unless cellular activation occurs shortly after infection. Furthermore, activation of the host cell is required for the initiation of transcription of the integrated proviral DNA into either genomic RNA or mRNA. In this regard, activation of HIV expression from the latent state depends on the interaction of a number of cellular and viral factors. Following transcription, HIV mRNA is translated into proteins that undergo modification through glycosylation, myristylation, phosphorylation, and cleavage. The viral core is formed by the assembly of HIV proteins, enzymes, and genomic RNA at the plasma membrane of the cells. Budding of the progeny virion occurs through the host cell membrane, where the core acquires its external envelope (see Chap. 192). Each point in the life cycle of HIV is a real or potential target for therapeutic intervention (see below). Thus far, the reverse transcriptase and protease enzymes have proven to be susceptible to pharmacologic disruption (see below).

HIV GENOME   Figure 308-4 schematically illustrates the arrangement of the HIV genome. Like other retroviruses, HIV-1 has genes that encode the structural proteins of the virus: *gag* encodes the proteins that form the core of the virion (including p24 antigen); *pol* encodes the enzymes responsible for reverse transcription and integration; and *env* encodes the envelope glycoproteins. However, HIV-1 is more complex than other retroviruses, particularly those of the nonprimate group, in that it also contains at least six other genes (*tat, rev, nef, vif, vpr,* and *vpu*), which code for proteins involved in the regulation of gene expression (see Chap. 192). Flanking these genes are the long terminal repeats (LTRs), which contain regulatory elements involved in gene expression (see below), such as the poly-adenylation signal sequence, the TATA promotor sequence, the NF-κB and SP1 enhancer binding sites, the transactivating response (TAR) sequences, where the *tat* protein binds, and the negative regulatory element (NRE), whose deletion increases the level of gene expression (Fig. 308-4). The major difference between the genomes of HIV-1 and HIV-2 is the fact that HIV-2 lacks the *vpu* gene and has a *vpx* gene not contained in HIV-1.

MOLECULAR HETEROGENEITY OF HIV-1   Molecular analysis of various HIV isolates reveals sequence variation over many parts of the viral genome. For example, in different isolates, the degree of difference in the coding sequences of the viral envelope protein ranges from a few percent (very close) to 50 percent. These changes

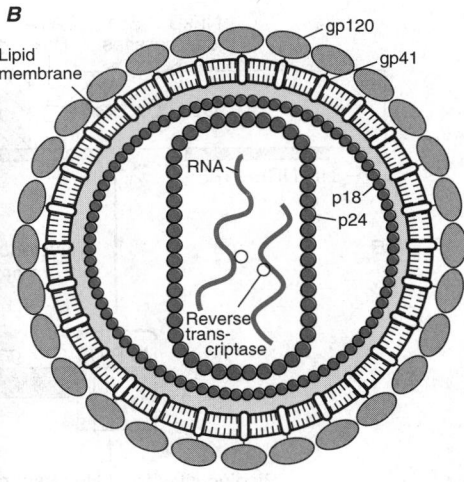

FIGURE 308-2   *A.* Electron micrograph of HIV. Figure illustrates a typical virion following budding from the surface of a CD4+ T lymphocyte, together with two additional incomplete virions in the process of budding from the cell membrane. *B.* Structure of HIV-1, including the gp120 outer membrane, gp41 transmembrane components of the envelope, genomic RNA, enzyme reverse transcriptase, p18(17) inner membrane, and p24 core protein. *[Adapted from RC Gallo. The human immunodeficiency virus (HIV), Sci Am, January 1987.]*

FIGURE 308-3   The life cycle of HIV. See text for description. *(From AS Fauci, Science 239:617, 1988.)*

tend to cluster in hypervariable regions. One such region, called V3, is a target for neutralizing antibodies and contains recognition sites for T cell responses (see below). Variability in this region is likely due to selective pressure from the host immune system. The extraordinary variability of HIV-1 is in marked contrast to the relative genetic stability of HTLV-I and -II.

There are two groups of HIV-1: group M (major), which is responsible for most of the infections in the world, and group O (outlier), a relatively rare viral form found at this time in Cameroon, Gabon, and France (see Chap. 192). The M group comprises at least eight sequence subtypes, or clades, designated A through H, which are distinguished by the fact that, at this time, they differ from each other by 30 percent in their *env* coding sequences and by 14 percent in their *gag* coding sequences. Curiously, the O-group viral sequences display subtype distances among each other of the same magnitude. As a result of the evolutionary process underlying these sequence differences, phylogenetic tree analyses produce starlike configurations suggestive of radiation from single ancestral viruses, one for the M group and one for the O group (Fig. 308-5).

0.10

FIGURE 308-5   A phylogenetic tree constructed from HIV-1 M (major) and O (outlier) viral envelope sequences. Within the M group, subtypes A through G are represented (H is not shown); subtype B viruses predominate in the United States at this time. HIV-1 viruses are related to immunodeficiency viruses found in chimpanzees in the wild (CPZGAB). The M- and recently discovered O-group viruses each display a star-like configuration suggestive of two separate introductions of viruses into the human population. The scale-bar at the bottom indicates a 10 percent difference at the nucleotide level. *(Courtesy of Bette Korber and Gerald Myers, Los Alamos National Laboratory, Los Alamos, NM.)*

The global patterns of HIV-1 variation likely result from accidents of viral trafficking. Subtype B viruses, which now differ by up to 17 percent in their *env* coding sequences, are uniformly seen in the United States. It is thought that, purely by chance, this viral subtype was seeded into the United States in the late 1970s, thereby establishing

FIGURE 308-4   *A.* The genome of HIV. *B.* The long terminal repeat of HIV. *(A adapted from WC Greene, N Engl J Med 324:308, 1991; B from ZF Rosenberg, AS Fauci, Immunol Today 11:176, 1990.)*

an overwhelming founder effect. Subtype A viruses (of the M group) appear to be the most common form worldwide; many countries have cocirculating viral subtypes that are giving rise to recombinant forms. Figure 308-6 schematically diagrams the worldwide distribution of HIV-1 subtypes by region. The predominant subtype in Europe and the Americas is subtype B. In Africa, more than 75 percent of strains recovered to date have been of subtypes A, C, and D. In Asia, HIV-1 isolates of subtypes E, C, and B are found. Subtype E accounts for most infections in Southeast Asia, while subtype C is prevalent in India (see "HIV Infections and AIDS Worldwide," below). Sequence analyses of HIV-1 isolates from infected individuals indicate that recombination among viruses of different clades likely occurs as a result of infection of an individual with viruses of more than one clade, particularly in geographic areas where clades overlap.

TRANSMISSION

HIV is transmitted by both homosexual and heterosexual contact; by blood and blood products; and by infected mothers to infants either intrapartum, perinatally, or via breast milk. After more than 15 years of scrutiny, there is no evidence that HIV is transmitted by casual contact or that the virus can be spread by insects, such as by a mosquito bite.

SEXUAL TRANSMISSION HIV infection is predominantly a sexually transmitted disease worldwide. Although approximately one-half of reported cases of AIDS in the United States are still among homosexual men, heterosexual transmission is clearly the most common mode of infection worldwide, particularly in developing countries. Furthermore, the yearly incidence of new cases of AIDS contracted through heterosexual transmission is steadily increasing in the United States, mainly among minorities, particularly women minorities (see below).

HIV has been demonstrated in seminal fluid both within infected mononuclear cells and in the cell-free state. The virus appears to concentrate in the seminal fluid, particularly in situations where there are increased numbers of lymphocytes and monocytes in the fluid, as in genital inflammatory states such as urethritis and epididymitis, conditions closely associated with other sexually transmitted diseases (see below). The virus has also been demonstrated in cervical smears and vaginal fluid. There is a strong association of transmission of HIV with receptive anal intercourse, likely owing to the fact that only a thin and fragile rectal mucosal membrane separates the deposited semen from potentially susceptible cells in and beneath the mucosa, as well as the fact that trauma may be associated with anal intercourse. Anal douching and sexual practices such as insertion of hard objects or a clenched fist into the rectum ("fisting") traumatizes the rectal mucosa, thereby increasing the likelihood of infection during receptive anal intercourse. It is likely that anal intercourse provides at least two modalities of infection: direct inoculation into blood in cases of traumatic tears in the mucosa, and infection of susceptible target cells, such as Langerhans cells, in the mucosal layer in the absence of trauma (see below). Although the vaginal mucosa is several layers thicker than the rectal mucosa and less likely to be traumatized during intercourse, it is clear that the virus can be transmitted to either partner through vaginal intercourse. In the United States, there is approximately a 20-fold greater chance of transmission of HIV from a man to a

woman than from a woman to a man through vaginal intercourse. This difference may be due in part to the prolonged exposure to infected seminal fluid of the vaginal and cervical mucosa, as well as the endometrium (when semen enters through the cervical os). By comparison, the penis and urethral orifice are exposed relatively briefly to infected vaginal fluid. Bidirectional heterosexual transmission appears to occur much more readily in Thailand than in the United States. The predominant strain of HIV-1 in Thailand is clade E, and the predominant strain in the United States is clade B (see above and below). Clade E has been observed to infect Langerhans cells, which reside in and beneath the mucosal surfaces of the vagina and other genital tract organs, more readily than does HIV clade B. It has been hypothesized that these differences account at least in part for the observed differences in transmission rates, but this hypothesis requires further investigation.

There is a close association between genital ulcerations and transmission, from the standpoints of both susceptibility to infection and infectivity. Infections with microorganisms such as *Treponema pallidum* (see Chap. 174), *Haemophilus ducreyi* (see Chap. 152), and herpes simplex virus (see Chap. 184) are important causes of genital ulcerations linked to transmission of HIV. Furthermore, there have been reports of associations of cervical ectopy as well as cervical erosions resulting from infection due to *Chlamydia trachomatis* (see Chap. 181) and *Neisseria gonorrhoeae* (see Chap. 150) with transmission of HIV infection. In a randomized trial, empirical treatment of genital ulcer disease was associated with a decrease in the risk of HIV infection. Finally, lack of circumcision has been reported to be associated with a higher risk of HIV infection in certain cohorts. This difference may be due to the higher risk of genital ulcerative disease in uncircumcised men as well as to other factors, such as microtrauma and a hospitable environment for the virus in the folds of the prepuce. Thus, in certain cases, all of these phenomena can be considered as *cofactors* for HIV transmission.

Oral sex appears to be a much less efficient mode of transmission of HIV than receptive anal intercourse. In this regard, there is a misperception by some people that oral sex, particularly among homosexual men, can be proposed as a form of "safe sex" and a substitute

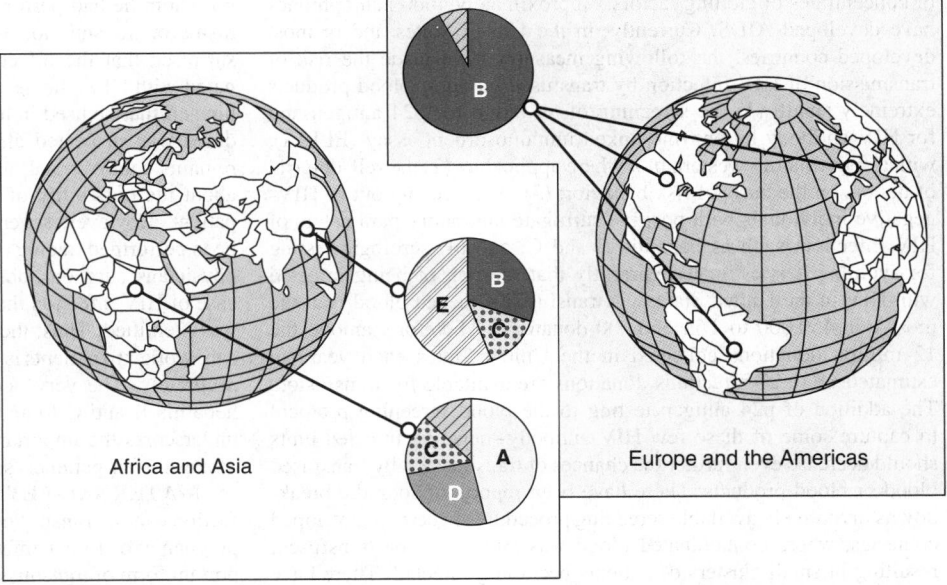

FIGURE 308-6 Geographic distribution of HIV-1 subtypes. The prevalence of HIV-1 genetic subtypes varies by geographic region. The proportions of subtypes in a particular region are indicated by the pie chart. The cross-hatched portion of the charts indicates the proportion of all other subtypes combined. Systematic evaluations of HIV-1 subtypes are needed to confirm and extend these initial observations. *(Courtesy of Dr. Francine E. McCutchan and Dr. Mika O. Salminen of The Henry Jackson Foundation for the Advancement of Military Medicine and of Col. Donald S. Burke of the Walter Reed Army Institute of Research.)*

for receptive anal intercourse. This is a dangerous approach, as there have been reports of documented HIV transmission resulting solely from receptive fellatio and insertive cunnilingus. There are probably many more cases that go unreported because of the frequent practice of both oral sex and receptive anal intercourse by the same person. In this regard, studies in the SIV model have clearly demonstrated the ease with which SIV infection can be transmitted by deposition of virus in the oral cavity. The association of alcohol consumption and crack cocaine use with unsafe sexual behavior, both homosexual and heterosexual, leads to an increased risk of sexual transmission of HIV.

TRANSMISSION BY BLOOD AND BLOOD PRODUCTS
HIV can be transmitted by blood and blood products, both among individuals who share contaminated paraphernalia (needles and syringes) for injection drug use and in those who receive transfusions of blood and blood products. Among IDUs, HIV infection occurs through parenteral exposure to infected blood via contaminated drug paraphernalia. The risk of infection increases with the duration of injection drug use, the frequency of needle sharing, participation in the "shooting gallery" drug culture, where several individuals share the same paraphernalia, and the use of injection drugs in a geographic location with a high prevalence of HIV infection, such as inner city areas.

From the late 1970s until the spring of 1985, when mandatory testing of donated blood for HIV-1 was initiated, it has been estimated that over 10,000 individuals in the United States were infected through transfusions of blood or blood products (see Chap. 115). Approximately 7250 individuals who survived the illness for which the transfusion was administered have developed AIDS. It is estimated that 90 to 100 percent of individuals who were transfused with HIV-infected blood became infected. Transfusions of whole blood, packed red blood cells, platelets, leukocytes, and plasma are all capable of transmitting HIV infection. In contrast, hyperimmune gamma globulin, hepatitis B immune globulin, plasma-derived hepatitis B vaccine, and Rh_o immune globulin have not been associated with transmission of HIV infection. The procedures involved in processing these products either inactivate or remove the virus.

In addition to the above, several thousand hemophiliacs were infected with HIV by receipt of HIV-contaminated fresh frozen plasma or concentrates of clotting factors. Approximately 4000 hemophiliacs have developed AIDS. Currently, in the United States and in most developed countries, the following measures have made the risk of transmission of HIV infection by transfused blood or blood products extremely small: (1) the screening of all blood for p24 antigen and for HIV antibody by enzyme-linked immunosorbent assay (ELISA), with a confirmatory western blot where applicable; (2) the self-deferral of donors on the basis of risk behavior; (3) the screening out of HIV-negative individuals with positive surrogate laboratory parameters of HIV infection, such as hepatitis B and C; and (4) serologic testing for syphilis. It is estimated currently that the risk of being infected with HIV in the United States via transfused screened blood is at the most 1 in 450,000 to 1 in 660,000 donations. Therefore, among the 12 million donations collected in the United States each year, an estimated 18 to 27 infectious donations are available for transfusion. The addition of p24 antigen testing to the blood screening protocol to capture some of these few HIV antibody–negative infected units should decrease even further the chances of transmission by transfused blood or blood products. There have been reports of sporadic breakdowns in routinely available screening procedures in certain developed countries, where contaminated blood was allowed to be transfused, resulting in small clusters of patients becoming infected. There have been no reported cases of transmission of HIV-2 in the United States via donated blood, and, currently, donated blood is screened for both HIV-1 and HIV-2 antibodies. The chance of infection of a hemophiliac via clotting factor concentrates has essentially been eliminated because of the added layer of safety resulting from heat treatment of the concentrates.

Prior to the screening of donors, a small number of cases of transmission of HIV via semen used in artificial insemination and tissues used in organ transplantation were well documented. At present, donors of such tissues are screened for HIV infection prior to transplantation.

OCCUPATIONAL TRANSMISSION OF HIV: HEALTH CARE AND LABORATORY WORKERS There is a small, but definite, occupational risk of HIV transmission among health care workers, laboratory personnel, and potentially others who work with HIV-infected specimens, particularly when sharp objects are used. It is estimated that 250,000 to 1 million health care workers are stuck with needles or other sharp medical instruments in the United States each year. Large, multiinstitutional studies have indicated that the risk of HIV transmission following skin puncture from a needle or a sharp object that was contaminated with blood from a person with documented HIV infection is approximately 0.3 percent (see "HIV and the Health Care Worker" below). The risk of hepatitis B infection following a similar type of exposure is 20 to 30 percent (see Chap. 295). An increased risk for HIV infection following percutaneous exposures to HIV-infected blood is associated with exposures involving a relatively large quantity of blood, as in the case of a device visibly contaminated with the patient's blood, a procedure that involves a needle placed directly in a vein or artery, or a deep injury. In addition, the risk increases for exposures to blood from patients with advanced-stage disease, probably owing to the higher titer of HIV in the blood as well as to other factors, such as the presence of more virulent strains of virus.

There have been reports of health care workers who became infected through the exposure of mucous membranes or abraded skin to HIV-infected material; however, the risk associated with mucocutaneous exposure has been difficult to quantify, because transmission by this route is rare. The risk that has been estimated by pooling data from several studies is 0.1 percent (95 percent confidence interval, 0.01 to 0.5 percent). Factors that might be associated with mucocutaneous transmission of HIV include exposure to an unusually large volume of blood, prolonged contact, and a potential portal of entry. The use of antiretroviral drugs after the exposure may be protective for occupationally exposed health care workers. Transmission of HIV through intact skin has not been documented (see "HIV and the Health Care Worker" below).

In 1990, the CDC reported that an HIV-infected dentist in Florida, by then deceased, had transmitted HIV infection to five of his patients on whom he had performed invasive dental procedures. The mechanisms of transmission were never fully delineated, although it was surmised that the infections occurred through instruments contaminated with HIV; the dentist supposedly used the same instruments on himself that he used in his practice, and a breakdown in sterile procedures was suspected although never proven. To this day, this case remains controversial, and for a time it caused considerable concern about the possibility of spread of HIV from health care provider to patient. However, several epidemiologic studies have subsequently been performed tracing thousands of patients of HIV-infected dentists, physicians, surgeons, obstetricians, and gynecologists, and not a single case of HIV infection that could be linked to the health care providers was identified. Thus, the risk of transmission from an infected health care worker to patients is extremely low; in fact, too low to be measured accurately. The very occurrence of transmission of HIV as well as hepatitis B and C to and from health care workers in the workplace underscores the importance of the use of universal precautions when caring for all patients (see below and Chap. 138).

MATERNAL-FETAL/INFANT TRANSMISSION HIV infection can be transmitted from an infected mother to her fetus during pregnancy or to her infant during delivery. This is an extremely important form of transmission of HIV infection in developing countries, where the proportion of infected women to infected men is approximately 1:1. In the United States, approximately 1600 newborns per year are infected with HIV from their mother. Virologic analysis of aborted fetuses indicate that HIV can be transmitted to the fetus during pregnancy, as early as the first and second trimester. However, maternal transmissions to the fetus occur most commonly in the perinatal period.

This conclusion is based on a number of considerations, including the time frame of identification of infection by the sequential appearance of classes of antibodies to HIV (i.e., the appearance of HIV-specific IgA antibody within 3 to 6 months after birth); a positive viral culture; the appearance of p24 antigenemia weeks to months after delivery, but not at the time of delivery; a polymerase chain reaction (PCR) assay of infant blood following delivery that is negative at birth and positive several months later; the demonstration that the firstborn twin of an infected mother is more commonly infected than is the second twin; and the evidence that cesarean section results in decreased transmission to the infant.

The rate of transmission of HIV from untreated mother to infant/fetus in the United States is approximately 25 percent. Studies in a variety of countries indicate a wide range of transmission rates, with a low of 12.9 percent in a European collaborative study to a high of approximately 45 to 48 percent in Nairobi, Kenya, and other cities in developing countries. These differences may relate to the adequacy of prenatal care as well as to the stage of HIV disease and the general health of the mother during pregnancy. Higher rates of transmission have been associated with advanced-stage disease, a low CD4+ T cell count, high levels of viremia, and vitamin A deficiency in the mother, as well as with chorioamniitis and funisitis. In addition, prolonged labor, a long interval between membrane rupture and delivery, and factors that increase the exposure of the infant to the mother's blood, including fetal-scalp electrodes, episiotomy, and severe cervical and vaginal lacerations, may contribute to transmission to the infant. With regard to levels of viremia, one report indicated that when the level of plasma viral RNA in the mother is less than 100,000 copies per milliliter, there is only a 3 percent likelihood that the infection will be passed to the infant. Finally, it has been speculated that if the mother experiences acute primary HIV infection during pregnancy, there is a higher rate of transmission to the fetus, owing to the high levels of viremia that follow primary infection (see below). Zidovudine treatment of HIV-infected pregnant women from the beginning of the second trimester through delivery and of the infant for 6 weeks following birth has dramatically decreased the rate of intrapartum and perinatal transmission of HIV infection from 22.6 percent in the untreated group to 7.6 percent in the zidovudine-treated group. It is expected that the rate of transmission will decrease even further as more potent combinations of drugs are used in HIV-infected pregnant women (see below and Table 308-26).

Postnatal transmission of HIV from mother to infant has been clearly documented, strongly implicating colostrum and breast milk as the vehicles of infection; virus can be isolated from both fluids. In rare cases, mothers have been infected by transfusions following delivery and have transmitted the infection to their infants, with the only risk factor being breast feeding. This is an important modality of transmission of HIV infection in developing countries, particularly where mothers continue to breast-feed for longer than is usual in developed countries. A meta-analysis of several prospective studies indicated that the risk attributable to breast feeding was 7 to 22 percent. Women with low CD4+ T cell counts, especially those with vitamin A deficiency, may be at increased risk of transmitting HIV to their infants through breast milk. Certainly, in developed countries breast feeding by an infected mother should be avoided. However, there is disagreement regarding recommendations for breast feeding in certain developing countries, where breast milk is the only source of adequate nutrition as well as immunity against potentially serious infections for the infant.

TRANSMISSION BY OTHER BODY FLUIDS There is no convincing evidence that saliva can transmit HIV infection, either through kissing or through other exposures, such as occupationally to health care workers. Although HIV can be isolated from saliva, this has been achieved in only a small percentage of infected individuals. Furthermore, a protein contained in saliva, called secretory leukocyte protease inhibitor, has been demonstrated to possess anti-HIV-1 activity in vitro. There have been outlier cases of suspected transmission by saliva, but these have probably been blood-to-blood transmissions. One case was reported of a 91-year-old man who was bitten during a robbery attempt by an HIV-infected person. He seroconverted, and

there was no question that the source of the infection was the human bite. However, the individual who bit him had bleeding gums, and it was thought that the infection was actually transmitted via blood. In addition, a most unusual form of HIV transmission from infected children to mothers in the former Soviet Union has been identified. In those cases, the children (infected through transfusion) were said to have bleeding sores in the mouth, and the mothers were said to have lacerations and abrasions on and around the nipples of the breast resulting from trauma from the children's teeth. Breast feeding had been continued until the children were older than is usual in other developed countries.

Although virus can be identified, if not isolated, from virtually any body fluid, there is no evidence that HIV transmission can occur as a result of exposure to tears, sweat, and urine. However, there have been isolated cases of transmission of HIV infection by body fluids that may or may not have been contaminated with blood. For example, there is a documented case of a mother who very likely contracted HIV infection from her child who had a colostomy. The mother regularly rendered colostomy care, often without wearing gloves, and was exposed to potentially infected material from the colostomy as well as from blood and nasal secretions. Without question, bodily wastes of patients should be handled according to universal precautions (see below).

EPIDEMIOLOGY

HIV INFECTION AND AIDS WORLDWIDE HIV infection/AIDS is a global pandemic, with cases reported from virtually every country. The current estimate of the number of cases of HIV infection among adults worldwide is approximately 22 million, and among children it is approximately 1 million; the global distribution of these cases is illustrated in Fig. 308-7. The World Health Organization (WHO) estimates that approximately 2.6 million HIV-infected children have been born since the start of the HIV pandemic, and approximately one-half of these have developed AIDS and have died. The global projections for the total number of HIV-infected individuals by the year 2000 range from 40 to 100 million. The HIV epidemic has occurred in "waves" in different regions of the world, each wave having somewhat different characteristics depending on the demographics of the country and region in question and the timing of the introduction of HIV into the population. Of note is the fact that different subtypes or clades of HIV-1 are prevalent in different regions of the world (see above and Fig. 308-6). The potential relevance of these differences relate in part to the development of vaccines. It is unlikely that a single vaccine will be applicable to all regions of the world, because of the substantial variations among viral subtypes throughout the world. In addition, it is likely that there will be gradual introduction of diverse HIV-1 genetic subtypes into the western hemisphere. In this regard, HIV-1 subtypes A, D, and E have been detected in United States and South American servicemen who had been deployed in southeast Asia and sub-Saharan Africa.

Figure 308-8 illustrates the beginnings, real and projected peaks, plateaus, and declines of the epidemic in different regions of the world. Although the epidemic was first recognized in the United States and shortly thereafter in western Europe, it very likely began in sub-Saharan Africa (see above and Chap. 192). The number of new cases of AIDS per year has already peaked and is plateauing in North America and western Europe (Fig. 308-8). The incidence in these areas is projected to decline toward the year 2000. Despite this plateau, the demographics of the epidemic in the United States and western Europe is shifting with regard to the target populations (see below). Sub-Saharan Africa has been particularly devastated by the epidemic, with the prevalance of infection in many cities in the double digits. Indeed, in certain sub-Saharan African countries such as Uganda, available seroprevalence data indicate that more than 10 percent of the entire population may be infected, with much higher prevalences in large trading centers. The epidemic is projected to peak in sub-

Saharan Africa by the year 2000; however, it is possible that the epidemic will continue to accelerate there beyond the year 2000. Although the epidemic in Asian countries, particularly India and Thailand, has lagged somewhat behind that in Africa, the number of new cases in this region is accelerating rapidly, and the magnitude of the epidemic is projected to exceed that of sub-Saharan Africa as we enter the twenty-first century.

The actual reported cases of AIDS worldwide are a gross underestimate of the true prevalence, mainly because of the incomplete reporting mechanisms in certain developing countries. The reported cumulative cases of AIDS as of November 1996 are shown in Table 308-3.

The major mode of transmission of HIV worldwide is unquestionably heterosexual sex; this is particularly true in developing countries, where the numbers of infected men and women are approximately equal. Countries such as those in sub-Saharan Africa with a predominantly heterosexual mode of transmission have been termed by WHO as *pattern II* countries. In contrast, pattern I countries are those in which the vast majority of cases are among men who have sex with men or among IDUs. Originally, the United States and Canada, most countries in South America, western Europe, Scandinavia, Australia, and New Zealand were clearly pattern I countries. However, in most of these countries, including the United States, the pattern is gradually shifting, with a growing proportion of new cases among heterosexuals (see below). Pattern III countries are those in which there are relatively few cases of HIV infection/AIDS, and most of the infected individuals have had contact with individuals from pattern I or II countries. A striking index of the spread of the epidemic is the fact that, just a few years ago, India and Thailand, along with other Asian countries, countries in eastern Europe, North Africa, and the Middle East, and certain countries in the Pacific were considered pattern III countries. Both India and Thailand have rapidly evolved into pattern II countries. If educational and behavior-modification programs fail in other pattern III countries, there is no doubt that many of them will evolve to patterns I or II.

Apart from the tragic situation in certain countries in sub-Saharan Africa (see above), the potential for explosive spread of the epidemic can be illustrated dramatically by the situation in Thailand. A single HIV-positive person was identified in Thailand among 101 male prostitutes in Bangkok in 1985, and it was expected that gay men would experience the first wave of rapid transmission. From 1985 through 1987, serosurveys among IDUs in Thailand revealed a prevalence of 0 to 1 percent, and similar surveys conducted among female prostitutes from 1985 through 1989 reported prevalance rates of less than 1 percent. There was very little appreciation of the potential of the epidemic to emerge into the general population, and it was anticipated that it would remain confined largely to men who have sex with men and possibly to IDUs. However, a remarkable pattern began to emerge in 1988. There was an extraordinary explosion of HIV prevalence among IDUs, from 1 percent at the beginning of 1988 to 32 to 43 percent by August–September of 1988. Thus, unexpectedly, the first wave of HIV infection spread rapidly among IDUs. This was followed by successive waves of transmission, first to female commercial sex workers, then to their non-IDU male clients, and ultimately into the low-risk wives and girlfriends of these men in the general population. At present in Thailand, more than 70 percent of reported cases of AIDS are attributable to heterosexual transmission, and the major risk factor for infection is a history of sexual intercourse with commercial sex workers. The prevalence of HIV infection among military recruits bears witness to the growing rate of HIV infection among young men in Thailand, which is boosted by the frequent use of female commercial sex workers by young men in that country. Young men aged 19 to 23 are conscripted by lottery into the Royal Thai Army and Air Force and undergo mandatory HIV testing. Serosurveys of conscripts indicate that in the northern provinces of Thailand, including Chiang Mai, the overall prevalence of HIV infection has reached as high as 18 percent. Fortunately, an aggressive public health campaign to promote the use of condoms is showing signs of decreasing this accelerated spread of HIV in Thailand (see "Prevention" below). Such explosive patterns are being seen in other Asian countries, particularly developing countries such as India. It is projected that this region will equal and surpass sub-Saharan Africa as the most severely afflicted region in the remainder of the twentieth century and into the twenty-first century.

AIDS IN THE UNITED STATES AIDS has had and will continue to have an extraordinary public health impact in the United States. It is the leading cause of death among Americans aged 25 to 44 years (Fig. 308-9). As of January 1, 1997, more than 570,000 cumulative cases of AIDS had been reported in adults and adolescents in the United States (Table 308-4); approximately 60 percent of these patients have died so far. When one looks at the totality of data collected from the beginning of the epidemic, approximately one-half of cases are among men who have had sex with men. Given the large numbers of such individuals who are HIV-infected but do not yet have advanced HIV disease, it is clear that large numbers of new cases of AIDS will continue to emerge in this group. Although there have been progressively smaller annual increases in cases of AIDS among men who have sex with men, male-to-male sexual contact continues to represent the most frequently reported mode of HIV transmission among persons with AIDS. However, over the past few years, the numbers of newly reported cases of AIDS among other groups, including IDUs and heterosexuals (particularly women) from certain large cities such as New York City, have surpassed the numbers of newly reported cases among men who have had sex with men. The proportion of new cases of AIDS per year attributed to heterosexual contact has increased dramatically over the past 10 years in the United States. In the mid-1980s, this proportion was less than 2 percent; in 1995 it was approximately 15 percent (Fig. 308-10). The relationship between geographic areas of the country and the demography of HIV infection and AIDS compellingly links geography, injection

Male:Female Proportions

750,000
270,000
1.3 million
200,000
14 million
510,000
50,000
100,000
5.2 Million
13,000

Global Total: 22.6 million

FIGURE 308-7 Estimated cases of adult HIV infection and AIDS as of January 1, 1997 (*From WHO.*)

drug use, and heterosexual transmission, particularly among women, with consequent spread to children intrapartum or perinatally (see above). The rates of reported AIDS cases per 100,000 population in the United States by state from January 1996 through December 1996 are shown in Fig. 308-11. Most cases of transmission by injection drug use and heterosexual contact are reported from the northeast and southeast regions of the country, particularly among minorities. HIV infection and AIDS have disproportionately affected minority populations in the United States. African-Americans and Hispanics constitute only 12 and 9 percent of the population, respectively, yet they account for 35 and 18 percent, respectively, of adult/adolescent AIDS cases and for 58 and 23 percent, respectively, of AIDS cases in children.

As of January 1, 1997, 7629 cases of AIDS in children less than 13 years old had been reported, and more than

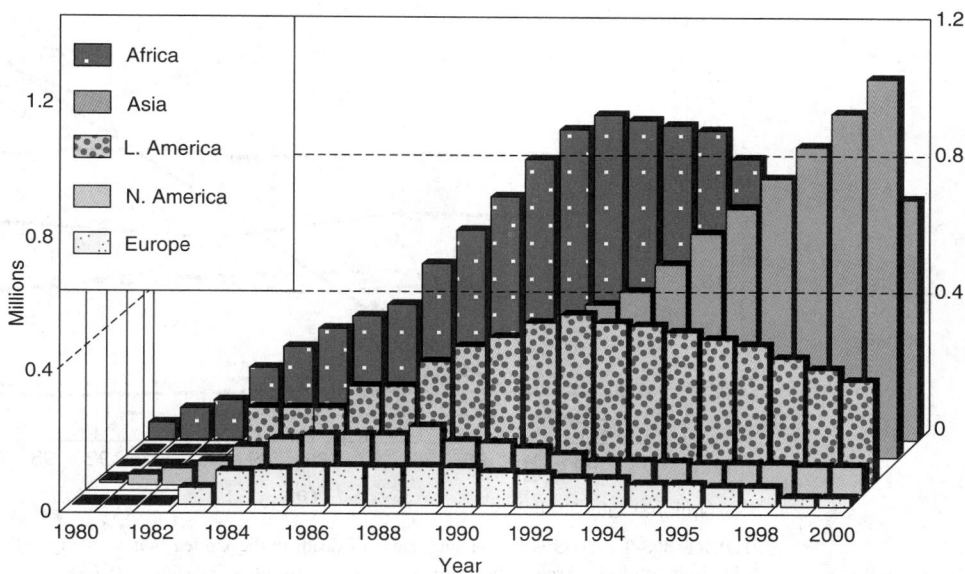

FIGURE 308-8 Estimated/projected annual adult HIV infections *(From WHO.)*

50 percent of these children have died (Table 308-5). Approximately 90 percent of these children were born to HIV-infected mothers, and, in approximately 60 percent of those cases, the mother was either an IDU or the heterosexual partner of an IDU. Forty-five percent of women with AIDS have become infected through injection drug use, compared to 22 percent of men with AIDS; 38 percent of women have become infected by heterosexual contact, compared to 3 percent of men with AIDS (Table 308-4). Only 1 percent of AIDS cases are among hemophiliacs, and 1 percent are among recipients of blood transfusions, blood products, or transplanted tissue. The relative contribution of the latter groups will gradually decrease, even though individuals infected previously through this mode of transmission will continue to develop AIDS. The risk of additional infections via this mode of transmission in the United States is extremely small (see above).

In recent years, the incidence of AIDS has reached a plateau with approximately 40,000 new cases per year. This trend likely reflects both reduced infection rates since the mid-1980s and more widespread use of prophylactic therapies, which delay the onset of AIDS (see below). Also, the demography of newly infected individuals has changed considerably since the mid-1980s (see below).

HIV PREVALENCE IN THE UNITED STATES Using "back-calculation" mathematical modeling based on the national AIDS database compiled by the CDC and the distribution of the incubation period from initial infection with HIV to diagnosis with AIDS, it is estimated that between 630,000 and 897,000 adults and adolescents in the United States were living with HIV infection as of January, 1993, including 107,000 to 150,000 women. This estimate results in an overall nationwide prevalence of HIV infection of approximately 0.3 to 0.4 percent. The estimated incidence of HIV infection has declined among white males, especially those older than 30 years. In contrast, HIV incidence appears to have remained relatively constant among women and minorities (Fig. 308-12). As of January 1993, prevalence was highest among young adults in their late twenties and thirties and among minorities. An estimated 3 percent of black men and 1 percent of black women in their thirties were living with HIV infection as of that date. The estimated prevalence of HIV infection in the United States among different groups is shown in Table 308-6. The number of new infections per year is estimated to be approximately 40,000.

The seroprevalence rates differ greatly among groups practicing high-risk behaviors, and seroprevalence studies have given insight into the variability of HIV prevalence among diverse cohorts and the risk factors associated with seroconversion. There is a great deal of variability in seroprevalence and seroconversion rates related to geography, race, economic status, age, sex and, of course, behavior.

Rates of seroconversion and seroprevalence have remained stable among certain groups and have increased or decreased among others over the past few years.

The routine and periodic nature of HIV-1 testing in the United States Army has allowed the direct measurement of the incidence of new infections among soldiers. Between November 1985 and October 1993, 978 HIV-1 seroconversions were noted among 1,061,768 soldiers with over 3.6 million person-years of follow-up. The seroconversion rate was 0.27 per 1000 person-years. A significant decreasing trend in seroconversion rates was seen over the period of analysis. The rate of new infections declined significantly from the first interval, 1985–1987 (0.43 per 1000 person-years), to the second interval, 1987–1988 (0.28 per 1000 person-years), but stabilized at approximately 0.22 per 1000 person-years after 1988. The latter figure represents approximately 100 to 150 new infections among soldiers annually. Subgroup analysis revealed that being young, male, of a minority race/ethnicity, and unmarried were strongly associated with HIV-1 seroconversion.

An important source of information regarding seroprevalence in various communities is the screening of patients who visit hospital emergency departments. A typical example of trends in inner-city HIV prevalence that is similar to results from a number of comparable studies is seen with data from the Johns Hopkins Hospital Department of Emergency Medicine. Of 1606 patients screened in 1992, 183 (11.4 percent) were HIV-positive, compared with 6.0 percent from an identical study conducted in 1988. The seroprevalence rose over this interval from 10.0 to 17.0 percent in black males, from 3.8 to 8.5 percent in black females, from 5.5 to 9.8 percent in white males, and from 1.6 to 1.9

Table 308-3

Cumulative Worldwide Cases of AIDS Reported to the World Health Organization as of November 1996

Country/Region	Cases
Africa	553,291
Americas	749,800
Canada	13,810
Caribbean/Bahamas	17,444
Central America	9997
Mexico	29,954
South America	113,498
United States of America	565,097
Asia	53,974
Europe	179,339
Oceania	7596
TOTAL	1,544,000

FIGURE 308-9 AIDS is the leading cause of death in the United States among individuals 25 to 44 years old. *, Preliminary data. *(From Centers for Disease Control and Prevention, 1997.)*

FIGURE 308-10 Percentage of AIDS cases attributed to heterosexual HIV transmission in the United States from 1981 through 1995. *(From CDC.)*

percent in white females. Seroprevalence rates among patients whose only risk was heterosexual contact increased more than fourfold.

Other studies indicate high rates of seroprevalence among homeless people, inmates of prisons, and teenagers. In a cross-sectional study of inner-city shelters and free-meal programs in San Francisco, HIV seroprevalence was 8.5 percent. Of note, the prevalence of *Myco-*

bacterium tuberculosis infection was 32 percent, and 19 percent of the HIV-seropositive subjects had positive tuberculin skin tests (see below). Voluntary testing programs for HIV infection among prison inmates reveal a range of results depending on geographic location, from less than 1.0 percent in Oregon to 8.5 percent in Maryland. In anonymous, cross-sectional serosurveys of HIV infection among teenagers conducted in 130 clinics in 24 cities, the median clinic-specific prevalence was 0.2 percent in 22 adolescent medicine clinics, 0.3 percent in 33 correctional facilities, 0.5 percent in 70 sexually transmitted disease (STD) clinics, and 1.1 percent in 5 homeless youth centers. Rates were highest among young men who have sex with men; however, most teenagers practicing risk behaviors reported heterosexual activity as their only potential risk of exposure to HIV.

The seroprevalence and incidence rates among men who have sex with men has evolved dramatically since the beginning of the AIDS epidemic. The rate of new infection among homosexual men attending STD clinics in San Francisco in 1982 and 1983 was approximately 19 percent per year, and the prevalence of infection among this cohort was estimated at greater than 50 percent. By the mid and late 1980s, the seroconversion rate had dropped to less than 1 percent per year, likely owing to a combination of a saturation effect and significant behavioral modification. However, in the early 1990s, a disturbing upward trend in the annual rate of new infection was noted among young homosexual men who were "coming out." As a group, young homosexual men have not witnessed firsthand the devastation of the epidemic to the degree that their older counterparts have and are

Table 308-4

AIDS Cases in Adults/Adolescents in the United States as of January 1, 1997

Exposure Category	White, not Hispanic, No. (%)	Black, not Hispanic, No. (%)	Hispanic, No. (%)	Asian/Pacific Islander, No. (%)	Native American/ Alaskan Native, No. (%)	Total,* No. (%)
Men who have sex with men	188,022 (70)	58,795 (30)	36,928 (36)	2768 (68)	778 (50)	287,576 (51)
Injection drug user (female and heterosexual male)	30,494 (11)	76,527 (38)	38,621 (38)	264 (6)	306 (20)	146,359 (25)
Men who have sex with men and inject drugs	19,590 (7)	11,568 (6)	5635 (6)	120 (3)	219 (14)	37,152 (6)
Hemophilia/coagulation disorder	3456 (1)	505 (0)	389 (0)	61 (1)	26 (2)	4443 (1)
Heterosexual contact	11,315 (4)	26,221 (13)	11,774 (12)	296 (7)	118 (8)	49,764 (9)
Receipt of transfusion of blood, blood components, or tissue	4702 (2)	1970 (1)	1002 (1)	185 (5)	17 (1)	7888 (1)
Other/undetermined	9908 (4)	23,194 (12)	6904 (7)	396 (10)	80 (5)	40,618 (7)
Subtotal	267,487 (47)	198,780 (35)	101,253 (18)	4090 (<1)	1544 (<1)	573,800 (100)

* Includes 646 persons of unknown race/ethnicity. Also includes 1648 women who reported sexual contact with other women in addition to the exposure categories listed above.

SOURCE: Centers for Disease Control and Prevention, USPHS.

engaging in a greater degree of high-risk behavior. A survey was conducted among 425 young (17 to 22 years) homosexual and bisexual men in public venues in San Francisco and Berkeley, California, including street corners, sidewalks, dance clubs, bars, and parks. HIV seroprevalence was 9.4 percent and was significantly higher among African-Americans (21.2 percent) than among other racial/ethnic groups. Approximately one-third of the participants reported unprotected anal intercourse, and 11.8 percent reported injection drug use in the previous 6 months. Of the HIV-infected men, 70 percent did not know that they were HIV seropositive.

During the earlier years of the epidemic, the HIV seroprevalence among IDUs in treatment programs in several metropolitan areas ranged from 0 to greater than 50 percent. The rates varied considerably with geographic location, with the highest rates observed on the eastern seaboard and much lower rates in the West and Southwest. To determine the

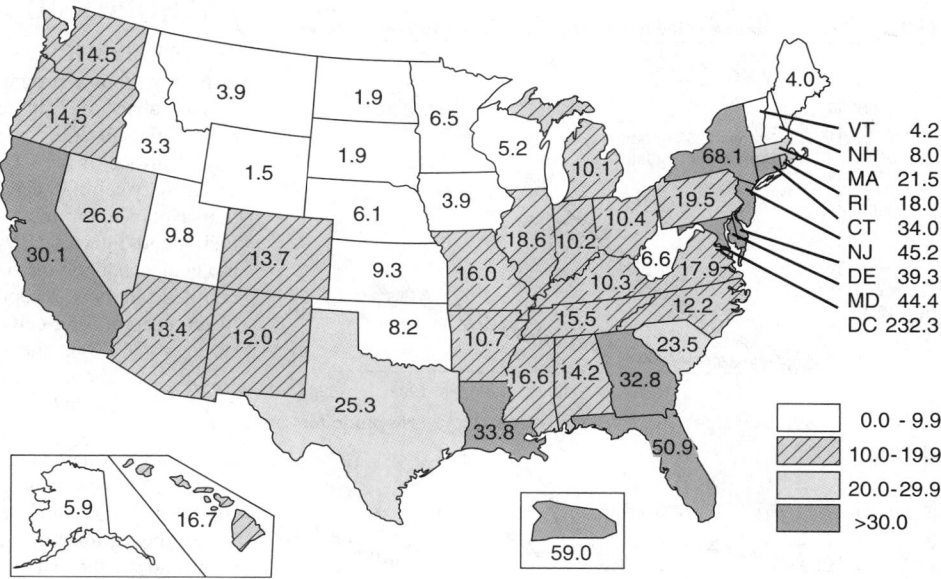

FIGURE 308-11 Annual rates of AIDS cases in the United States per 100,000 population by state (January through December 1996). *(From CDC HIV/AIDS Surveillance Report, 1996.)*

trends in HIV seroprevalence and risk behavior among IDUs in New York City, comparisons were made between two surveys of IDUs at the same hospital-based drug abuse detoxification program. One survey was conducted among 141 IDUs in 1984, and the other among 974 IDUs from 1990 through 1992. The HIV seroprevalence remained stable over this period at slightly more than 50 percent. The estimated seroconversion rate among the new IDUs in the study was 6.6 per 100 person-years at risk. While still high, this rate was approximately half that of the rate of 13 per 100 person-years at risk estimated for IDUs seen at the same detoxification program from 1978 through 1983 and for whom historically collected serum samples were available for HIV testing. Large-scale decreases in risk behaviors were observed; for example, the use of potentially contaminated syringes declined from 51 percent to 7 percent of injections. Additional risk reduction was associated with the use of the underground syringe exchanges. In other studies, HIV prevalence rates among female prostitutes also varied greatly, from 0 to approximately 50 percent, with the rates directly reflecting the degree of injection drug use among the groups surveyed as well as the prevalence of HIV in the IDUs in that geographic location at the time of the survey.

Further information regarding changes in trends of HIV seroprevalence was obtained by annual studies of patients attending sentinel clinics for STDs in 40 metropolitan areas throughout the United States

from 1988 through 1992. From 1988 to 1992, 552,665 specimens were tested in 80 STD clinics. The overall HIV prevalence was 33 percent (range among metropolitan areas, 5 to 52 percent) among homosexual and bisexual men; 3 percent (range, 0.3 to 11 percent) among heterosexual men; 2 percent (range, 0.1 to 11 percent) among women, and 10 percent (range, 0.5 to 45 percent) among heterosexual IDUs. HIV seroprevalence decreased among all homosexual and bisexual men, but especially among white homosexual and bisexual men, for whom it fell from 32 percent in 1989 to 22 percent in 1992. Among heterosexual men and women, HIV seroprevalence decreased among whites and, to a lesser degree, Hispanics, but it remained essentially stable among African-Americans over time. Among heterosexual IDUs, seroprevalence was also unchanged. This study clearly demonstrates a shift in the HIV epidemic in the United States, with an increasing burden of infection among heterosexuals and IDUs, particularly in minority populations (see above).

Thus, HIV infection and AIDS is widespread in the United States, and, although the epidemic on the whole is plateauing, it is spreading rapidly among certain populations, stabilizing in others, and decreasing in others. Similar to other STDs, HIV infection will not spread homogeneously throughout the population of the United States. However, it is clear that anyone who practices high-risk behavior is at risk for HIV infection. In addition, the alarming increase in infections and

Table 308-5

Pediatric (<13 Years) AIDS Cases in the United States as of January 1, 1997

Exposure Category	White, not Hispanic, No. (%)	Black, not Hispanic, No. (%)	Hispanic, No. (%)	Asian/Pacific Islander, No. (%)	Native American/ Alaskan Native, No. (%)	Total,* No. (%)
Hemophilia/coagulation disorder	157 (11)	34 (1)	36 (2)	3 (7)	1 (4)	231 (3)
Mother with/at risk for AIDS/HIV infection	1006 (73)	4201 (95)	1619 (91)	27 (66)	24 (96)	6891 (90)
IV drug–related	614	2306	1109	8	18	4061
Sex with bisexual male	56	52	36	2	—	146
Sex with person with hemophilia	16	5	5	—	—	26
Receipt of blood transfusion, blood components, or tissue	43	74	31	1	—	149
Other	277	1764	438	16	6	2509
Receipt of transfusion of blood, blood components, or tissue	183 (13)	89 (2)	91 (5)	10 (24)	—	373 (5)
Undetermined	23 (2)	85 (2)	24 (1)	1 (2)	—	134 (2)
Subtotal	1369 (18)	4409 (58)	1770 (23)	41 (<1)	25 (<1)	7629 (100)

* Includes 15 children of unknown race/ethnicity.

SOURCE: Centers for Disease Control and Prevention, USPHS.

PATHOPHYSIOLOGY AND PATHOGENESIS

The hallmark of HIV disease is a profound immunodeficiency resulting primarily from a progressive quantitative and qualitative deficiency of the subset of T lymphocytes referred to as *helper* or *inducer T cells*. This subset of T cells is defined phenotypically by the presence on its surface of the CD4 molecule (see Chap. 305), which serves as the primary cellular receptor for HIV. It has recently been demonstrated that a coreceptor must be present together with CD4 for efficient fusion and entry of HIV-1 into its target cells. These coreceptors are molecules that belong to the seven-transmembrane-domain G protein–coupled family of receptors. The molecule termed *fusin* or CXCR4 is the coreceptor for T cell–tropic strains of HIV-1, and the β-chemokine receptor CCR5 is the coreceptor for macrophage-tropic strains of HIV-1 (see above and below). Although a number of mechanisms responsible for cytopathicity and immune dysfunction of CD4+ T cells have been demonstrated in vitro, particularly direct infection and destruction of these cells by HIV (see below), it remains unclear which mechanisms or combination of mechanisms is primarily responsible for their progressive depletion and functional impairment in vivo. When the number of CD4+ T cells declines below a certain level (see below), the patient is at high risk of developing a variety of opportunistic diseases, particularly the infections and neoplasms that are AIDS-defining illnesses. Some features of AIDS, such as Kaposi's sarcoma and neurologic abnormalities, cannot be explained completely by the immunosuppressive effects of HIV, since these complications may occur prior to the development of severe immunologic impairment.

The combination of viral pathogenic and immunopathogenic events that occur during the course of HIV disease from the moment of initial (primary) infection through the development of advanced-stage disease is complex and varied. It is important to appreciate that the pathogenic mechanisms of HIV disease are multifactorial and multiphasic and are different at different stages of the disease. Therefore, it is essential to consider the typical clinical course of an HIV-infected individual in order to more fully appreciate these pathogenic events (Fig. 308-13).

PRIMARY HIV INFECTION, INITIAL VIREMIA, AND DISSEMINATION OF VIRUS The events associated with primary HIV infection are likely critical to the determination of the subsequent course of HIV disease. In particular, the phenomenon of dissemination of virus to lymphoid organs is a major factor in the establishment of a chronic and persistent infection (see below). The initial infection of susceptible cells may vary somewhat with the route of infection. Virus that enters directly into the bloodstream via infected blood or blood products (i.e., transfusions, use of contaminated needles for injecting drugs, sharp-object injuries, maternal-to-fetal transmission either intrapartum or perinatally, or, in certain cases, sexual intercourse where there is enough trauma to cause bleeding) is likely cleared from the circulation to the spleen and other lymphoid organs, where it replicates

FIGURE 308-12 Monthly incidence of AIDS in the United States from 1982 through January, 1993. *A.* Monthly AIDS incidence for the total U.S. population (squares) and for individuals born in 1959 or earlier (diamonds) and in 1960 or later (triangles). *B.* Monthly AIDS incidence for white, black, and Hispanic men and women. Locally weighted regression smoothing with a bandwidth of 40 percent of the time axis was used to highlight trends in incidence (solid curves). The date axes mark 1 January of the years indicated. *(From Rosenberg.)*

AIDS cases among heterosexuals, particularly sexual partners of IDUs, women, infants born of infected women, and adolescents, as well as spread in certain inner city areas, particularly among underserved minority populations with inadequate access to health care, testifies to the fact that the epidemic of HIV infection in the United States is a public health problem of major proportions.

Table 308-6

Prevalence of HIV-1 Infection in the United States as of January 1, 1993, Estimated by Back-Calculation from AIDS Incidence Data*

Group	Alive with HIV-1 Infection†	HIV-1 Positive, Ages 18 to 59 y‡
MALES		
White	255 (248–370)	0.49 (0.48–0.70)
Black	184 (176–236)	2.29 (2.20–2.91)
Hispanic	97 (91–131)	1.44 (1.37–1.87)
Total	536 (523–747)	0.78 (0.77–1.04)
FEMALES		
White	25 (23–34)	0.05 (0.04–0.06)
Black	67 (63–82)	0.74 (0.69–0.90)
Hispanic	24 (21–32)	0.34 (0.31–0.45)
Total	116 (107–150)	0.16 (0.15–0.20)
Grand Total	652 (630–897)	0.47 (0.46–0.62)

* Plausible ranges, given in parentheses, reflect some uncertainty about the incubation distribution.
† Data given in thousands.
‡ Prevalence (%)

SOURCE: From Rosenberg.

FIGURE 308-13 Typical course of an HIV-infected individual. See text for detailed description. *(From Fauci et al.)*

to a critical level and then leads to a burst of viremia that disseminates virus throughout the body. It is uncertain which cell in the blood or lymphoid tissue is the first actually to become infected. Certainly, CD4 + T cells and cells of monocyte lineage are the major ultimate targets of infection. Recent data indicate that dendritic cells are efficient transporters or presenters of HIV to CD4 + T cells, which is consistent with their role as extremely efficient antigen-presenting cells in the course of the normal immune response to antigen (see Chap. 305). The likely scenario in infection contracted via blood exposure is that free virus or virus-infected cells are cleared by the reticuloendothelial system and come into contact with susceptible target cells in these tissues, or that blood dendritic cells carry virus to tissues, particularly lymph nodes, where they put the virus in contact with susceptible CD4 + T cells. This is somewhat different from the role of follicular dendritic cells that reside in the germinal centers of lymphoid tissue and serve as traps or filters for the virus (see below). Dendritic cells have been reported to express low levels of CD4. However, there are conflicting reports as to whether blood dendritic cells themselves can actually become infected with HIV. Certain studies have shown that dendritic cells form conjugates with several CD4 + T cells and that active virus replication takes place within the conjugates. Data from the SIV-macaque model indicate that mucosal dendritic cells, known as Langerhans cells, become infected following mucosal exposure to the virus, as might occur when infected seminal fluid comes into contact with mucosal surfaces of the urogenital tract, the upper gastro-intestinal tract, or the rectum. This mechanism likely operates when the virus enters "locally" (as opposed to directly into the blood), as via the vagina, rectum, or urethra during intercourse, or via the upper gastrointestinal tract from swallowed infected semen, vaginal fluid, or breast milk. The common denominator of local infection is the drainage of Langerhans cells to the regional lymph nodes; these cells either are themselves infected or carry virus to the lymphoid tissue. CD4 + T cells in the regional lymph nodes become infected after contact with the Langerhans cells, and virus replication intensifies prior to the initiation of an HIV-specific immune response (see below), leading to a burst of viremia (Fig. 308-13), which then leads to rapid dissemination of virus to other lymphoid organs, the brain, and other tissues. It is well documented that individuals who experience the "acute HIV syndrome" following primary infection have high levels of viremia which last for several weeks (see below). The acute mononu-cleosis-like symptoms are well correlated with the presence of viremia. It is highly likely that most patients develop some degree of viremia, which contributes to virus dissemination, even though they remain asymptomatic or do not recall experiencing symptoms. Many patients who have progressed to AIDS and who clearly have had wide dissemi-nation of virus do not report having experienced such an acute viral syndrome. Careful examination of lymph nodes from more than one site in patients with established HIV infection who did not report symptoms that could have been related to primary infection strongly indicate that wide dissemination to lymphoid tissue occurs in most patients. A more detailed description of the role of lymphoid tissue in the immunopathogenesis of HIV disease is given below. It is unclear whether a high level of initial plasma viremia is associated with a poor prognosis. However, the set point of the level of steady state plasma viremia after approximately 1 year does seem to correlate with the rapidity of disease progression (see below).

ESTABLISHMENT OF CHRONIC AND PERSISTENT IN-FECTION   HIV infection is relatively unique among human viral in-fections in that, despite the robust cellular and humoral immune re-sponses that are mounted following primary infection (see below), the virus is, with very few exceptions, not cleared completely from the body. Rather, a chronic infection develops that persists with varying degrees of virus replication for a median of approximately 10 years before the patient becomes clinically ill (see below). It is this establishment of a chronic infection that is the hallmark of HIV disease. Throughout the often protracted course of chronic infection, virus replication can almost invariably be detected, if not by measurable plasma viremia, then by demonstration of virus replication in lymphoid tissue. In the vast major-ity of human viral infections, if the host survives, the virus is completely cleared from the body and a state of immunity against subsequent infec-tion develops. HIV infection very rarely kills the host during primary infection. Certain viruses, such as herpes simplex virus (see Chap. 184), are not completely cleared from the body after infection but instead enter a latent state; in these cases, clinical latency is accompanied by microbiologic latency. This is not the case with HIV infection, in which some degree of virus replication invariably occurs during the period of clinical latency (see below). Chronicity associated with persistent virus replication can be seen in certain cases of hepatitis B and C infections (see Chap. 297); however, in these infections the immune system is not a target. As mentioned above, HIV usually does not abruptly kill the host; rather it generally succeeds in escaping from a rather vigorous immune response and establishing a state of chronic infection with per-sistently active virus replication.

HIV uses a number of mechanisms to evade elimination by the immune system. HIV has an extraordinary ability to mutate, but this mechanism probably acts mainly after the establishment of chronic infection and contributes to the maintenance of chronicity. Since the transmitted virus and the virus that initially becomes established as a chronic infection are relatively homogeneous, the initial escape from immune system control likely involves other mechanisms. Molecular analysis of clonotypes has demonstrated that clones of CD8 + cytolytic T lymphocytes (CTLs) that expand greatly during primary HIV infec-tion and likely represent the high-affinity clones that would be expected to be most efficient in eliminating virus-infected cells disappear after their initial burst of expansion. The disappearance of these HIV-specific cells cannot be explained by mutations in the viral epitope to which they are directed, since virus sequencing studies indicate that the initial viral epitope is still present when the clones are no longer detected. Furthermore, other, less expanded clones of CD8 + T cells that recognize the same viral epitope persist and likely account for the partial control of virus replication. It is thought that the initially expanded clones are deleted owing to the overwhelming exposure to viral antigens during the initial burst of viremia, similar to the exhaus-tion of CD8 + CTLs that has been reported in the murine model of lymphocytic choriomeningitis virus (LCMV) infection. To compound this phenomenon, virus replication and thus saturation of antigen-presenting cells with viral antigen take place in the lymphoid tissue (see below), which is also the site of generation of HIV-specific CTLs.

Another important mechanism of HIV escape is related to the fact that, during primary HIV infection and the transition to established chronic infection, both activated HIV-specific CTLs and CTL precur-sors are preferentially and paradoxically segregated in the peripheral blood, where very little active virus replication takes place, rather than in the lymphoid tissue, which is the main site of virus replication and spreading and the major source of plasma viremia. Finally, the escape of HIV from elimination during primary infection allows the formation of a large pool of latently infected cells that cannot be eliminated by virus-specific CTLs. Thus, despite a potent immune response and the marked downregulation of virus replication following primary HIV in-fection, HIV succeeds in establishing a state of chronic infection with a variable degree of persistent virus replication. In most cases, during this period the patient makes the clinical transition from acute primary infection to a relatively prolonged state of clinical latency (see below).

Viral Dynamics   It was originally thought that very little virus replication occurred during clinical latency. However, studies of lymphoid tissue using PCR analysis for HIV RNA and in situ hybridi-zation for individual virus-expressing cells clearly demonstrated that HIV replication occurs throughout the course of HIV infection, even during clinical latency, when it is very difficult to culture virus from unfractionated peripheral blood mononuclear cells. The availability of sensitive PCR techniques led to the demonstration that plasma viremia is present at all stages of HIV disease. Subsequently, the dynamics of viral production and turnover were quantified using mathematical modeling in the setting of the administration of reverse transcriptase and protease inhibitors to HIV-infected individuals in clinical studies.

Treatment with these drugs resulted in a precipitous decline in the level of plasma viremia, which typically fell by 99 percent within 2 weeks. The number of CD4+ T cells in the blood increased concurrently, which implies that the killing of CD4+ T cells is linked directly to the levels of replicating virus. However, a contribution by redistribution of cells into the peripheral blood from other body compartments following the decrease in viremia has not been completely ruled out. It was determined on the basis of the emergence of resistant mutants during therapy that 99 percent of the circulating virus originated from recently infected cells. It was also determined that the half-life of a circulating virion was approximately 6 h and that of productively infected cells was 1.6 days. Given the relatively steady level of plasma viremia and of infected cells, it appears that extremely large amounts of virus (approximately 10^{10} virions) are produced and cleared from the circulation each day. In addition, data suggest that the minimum duration of the HIV-1 life cycle in vivo averages 1.2 days; the average generation time (the time from release of a virion until it infects another cell and causes the release of a new generation of viral particles) is estimated to be 2.6 days. Other studies have demonstrated that the decrease in plasma viremia that results from antiretroviral therapy correlates closely with a decrease in virus replication in lymph nodes, further confirming that lymphoid tissue is the main site of HIV replication and the main source of plasma viremia.

The level of steady-state viremia, called the viral *set point*, at approximately 1 year has important prognostic implications for the progression of HIV disease. It has been demonstrated that HIV-infected individuals who have a low set point at 6 months to 1 year progress to AIDS much more slowly than individuals whose set point is very high at that time. Levels of viremia generally increase as disease progresses. Measurement of the level of viremia is playing an increasingly important role in the guiding of therapeutic decisions in HIV-infected individuals (see below).

Immunopathogenic Events during Clinical Latency   With few exceptions, the level of CD4+ T cells in blood decreases gradually and progressively in HIV-infected individuals. The slope of this decline, together with the level of plasma viremia (see above), predicts well the pattern of the clinical course and the development of advanced disease. Most patients are entirely asymptomatic while this progressive decline is taking place (see below), which led to the term *clinical latency*. However, clinical latency does not mean disease latency, since progression is generally relentless during this period. Furthermore, clinical latency should not be confused with microbiologic latency since, as mentioned above, although there are cells that are latently infected with virus, there is virtually always some degree of virus replication, even during the early stages of HIV disease.

ADVANCED HIV DISEASE   After a variable period, usually measured in years, the CD4+ T cell count falls below a critical level (less than 200 cells per microliter), and the patient becomes highly susceptible to opportunistic disease. For this reason, the CDC case definition of AIDS was modified to include all HIV-infected individuals with CD4+ T cell counts below this level (see Table 308-1). Patients may experience constitutional signs and symptoms, or they may develop an opportunistic disease abruptly without any prior symptoms, although the latter scenario is unusual. The depletion of CD4+ T cells continues to be progressive and unrelenting in this phase. It is not uncommon for CD4+ T cell counts to drop as low as 10/μL or even to zero, yet the patients may survive for months or even for more than 1 year. This situation has become increasingly common as patients are treated more aggressively and are given prophylaxis against the common life-threatening opportunistic infections (see below). Ultimately, patients who progress to this severest form of immunosuppression usually succumb to opportunistic infections or neoplasms (see below).

LONG-TERM SURVIVORS AND LONG-TERM NONPROGRESSORS   The median time from primary HIV infection to the development of AIDS is approximately 10 years. The definitions of *long-term survivor* and *long-term nonprogressor* continue to evolve as more data are collected from prospective cohort studies. Predictions from one study estimate that approximately 13 percent of homosexual/bisexual men who were infected at an early age may remain free of clinical AIDS for longer than 20 years. Currently, individuals are considered to be long-term survivors if they remain alive for 10 to 15 years after initial infection. In most such individuals the disease has progressed, in that they have significant immunodeficiency and many have experienced opportunistic diseases. Some of these individuals have CD4+ T cell counts that have decreased to 200/μL or lower but have remained stable at that level for years. The mechanisms of this stabilization are not entirely clear but may relate to the beneficial effects of antiretroviral therapy and prophylaxis against opportunistic infections. In addition, a number of viral and/or host determinants likely contribute to the long-term survival of these individuals. In some individuals, the virus may either have been less virulent initially or have mutated to a less virulent form. Quantitative and qualitative aspects of the HIV-specific immune response, as well as unrecognized genetic factors, may also contribute to the long-term survival of these individuals.

Less than 5 percent of HIV-infected individuals are characterized as *long-term nonprogressors*. While all long-term nonprogressors are long-term survivors the reverse is not true. Although different sets of empirical criteria have been proposed for the definition of long-term nonprogression, there is a common denominator. Individuals who have been infected with HIV for a long period (approximately 10 or more years), whose CD4+ T cell counts are in the normal range and have remained stable over years, and who have not received antiretroviral therapy are considered to be long-term nonprogressors. These patients are characterized by a low viral burden (low number of HIV-infected cells), low levels of plasma viremia, generally normal immune function according to commonly measured parameters (skin tests, in vitro lymphocyte responses to various mitogens and antigens), and normal-appearing lymphoid tissue architecture as determined on lymph node biopsy. In general, long-term nonprogressors manifest robust HIV-specific immune responses, both humoral (neutralizing antibodies) and cell-mediated (HIV-specific CTLs). Although viremia is consistently low in these patients, many have persistent viremia by the most sensitive PCR assays. No qualitative abnormalities in the virus could be detected in most of these patients. However, a small subset of patients do have defective virus; in particular, in one of five long-term nonprogressors, the virus had a defect in the *nef* gene. In another report, a blood donor in Australia who was HIV-infected and a group of six individuals who were infected by blood or blood products from that donor remain free of HIV-related disease and have normal and stable CD4+ T cell counts 10 to 14 years after infection. Sequence analysis of viruses isolated from the donor and recipients revealed similar deletions in the *nef* gene and the region of overlap of *nef* and the U3 region of the HIV LTR (see Fig. 308-4). The precise role of host factors in long-term nonprogression remains unclear. There is no obvious and consistent genetic determinant for nonprogression. However, recent studies indicate that the frequency of individuals heterozygous for a defect in the gene for CCR-5 (see below), which is the receptor for macrophage-tropic strains of HIV-1 (see above), may be increased among long-term nonprogressors, suggesting that heterozygosity for the genetic defect may provide some degree of protection. Although long-term nonprogressors have robust HIV-specific immune responses as well as competent CD8+ T cell suppressors of HIV replication, it is unclear whether these factors are directly responsible for the state of nonprogression. A substantial proportion of HIV-infected individuals manifest comparable immune responses early in the course of their disease and still experience disease progression. Long-term nonprogressors likely represent a heterogeneous group. The lack of disease progression may be explained in some by a defect in the virus, in others by any of a variety of host factors, including recognized and as yet unrecognized genetic factors, and in others by a combination of both.

ROLE OF LYMPHOID ORGANS IN HIV PATHOGENESIS   The lymph nodes are the major anatomic sites for the establishment and propagation of HIV infection (see above). For practical reasons, most studies on the pathogenesis of HIV infection have focused on peripheral-blood mononuclear cells. However, lymphocytes in the peripheral blood represent only approximately 2 percent of the total body lymphocyte pool and so may not always accurately reflect the status of the entire immune system; most of the body's lymphocytes reside in lymphoid organs, such as the lymph nodes, spleen, and gut-associated lymphoid tissue. Furthermore, virus replication occurs mainly in lymphoid tissue and not in blood; the level of plasma viremia reflects virus production in lymphoid tissue. Finally, since HIV disease is an infectious disease of the immune system, it is critical to appreciate the pathogenic events that occur in the lymphoid tissue in HIV infection.

Certain patients experience progressive generalized lymphadenopathy (see below) early in the course of the infection; others experience varying degrees of transient lymphadenopathy. Lymphadenopathy reflects the cellular activation and immune response to the virus in the lymphoid tissue, which is generally characterized by follicular or germinal-center hyperplasia. Lymph node involvement is a common denominator of virtually all patients with HIV infection, even those without easily detectable lymphadenopathy. It has been suggested that progressive generalized lymphadenopathy represents an exaggerated immune response to HIV and carries a more favorable prognosis; however, long-term follow-up of such patients has not borne out this hope.

Simultaneous examination of lymph node and peripheral blood in the same patients during various stages of HIV disease, including the early asymptomatic stage (when CD4+ T cell counts generally are greater than 500/μL), the intermediate stage (when counts are usually 200 to 500/μL) and the advanced stage (when counts are <200/μL) has led to substantial insight into the pathogenesis of HIV disease. Using a combination of PCR techniques for HIV DNA and RNA in tissue and RNA in plasma, in situ hybridization for HIV RNA, and light and electron microscopy, the following picture has emerged. In most patients, early in the course of infection prior to significant immunodeficiency (CD4+ T cell counts >500/μL), plasma viremia generally is low, the viral burden (number of infected cells) in the peripheral blood is extremely low, and expression of HIV in these cells is minimal or undetectable. Remarkably, at this time copious amounts of extracellular virions are trapped on the processes of the follicular dendritic cells (FDCs) in the germinal centers of the lymph nodes (Fig. 308-14A). In situ hybridization reveals expression of virus in individual cells of the paracortical area and, to a lesser extent, the germinal center (Fig. 308-14B). The number of cells expressing virus is very low early in the course of disease and increases as disease progresses. Examination of lymph nodes during primary HIV infection in humans (see above) and SIV infection in macaques indicates that during the transition from primary infection to established chronic infection, germinal centers form and virus is trapped. This trapping, together with the generation of a vigorous HIV-specific immune response, likely contributes to the rapid decrease in plasma viremia seen in most patients following the initial burst of viremia associated with primary infection. A considerable amount of virus can be trapped during the period of high viremia associated with primary infection. The persistence of trapped virus after chronic infection has been established likely reflects a steady state whereby trapped virus turns over and is replaced by fresh virions, which are produced persistently, albeit usually at low levels during the early, clinically latent stage of disease.

During early-stage HIV disease, the architecture of the germinal centers is generally preserved and may even be hyperplastic owing to in situ proliferation of cells (mostly B lymphocytes) and recruitment to the lymph nodes of a number of cell types (B cells, CD4+ and CD8+ T cells). Electron microscopy demonstrates a fine network of FDCs with many long, finger-like processes that envelop virtually every lymphocyte in the germinal center (Fig. 308-14C). Extracellular virions can be seen attached to the processes, yet the FDCs appear to be relatively healthy. The trapping of antigen is a physiologically normal function for the FDCs, which present antigen to B cells and contribute to the generation of B cell memory. However, in the case of HIV, the trapped virions serve as a persistent source of cellular activation, resulting in the secretion of proinflammatory cytokines such as interleukin (IL) 1β, tumor necrosis factor (TNF)-α, and IL-6, which can upregulate virus replication in infected cells (see below). Furthermore, although trapped virus is coated by neutralizing antibodies, it has been demonstrated that these virions remain infectious for CD4+ T cells while attached to the processes of the FDCs. CD4+ T cells that migrate into the germinal center to provide help to B cells in the generation of an HIV-specific immune response thus are susceptible to infection by these trapped virions. Thus, in HIV infection, a normal physiologic function of the immune system, which contributes to the clearance of virus as well as to the generation of a specific immune response, can also have deleterious consequences. It is difficult to demonstrate infection of the FDCs at this point, or even in advanced disease; however, rare examples of virus budding off FDCs have been reported.

As the disease progresses, the architecture of the germinal centers begins to show disruption, and the trapping efficiency of the lymph node diminishes. Electron microscopy reveals swollen organelles, and the FDCs begin to undergo cell death. The mechanisms of FDC death remain unclear; there is no indication by electron microscopy of copious virus replication or budding of virions off the cell in great quantities. At this stage, the level of plasma viremia generally increases. In addition, both the relative number of infected cells in the blood and the expression of virus from these cells increases, approaching the levels in the lymph nodes. As the disease progresses to an advanced stage, there is complete disruption of the architecture of the germinal centers, accompanied by dissolution of the FDC network and massive dropout of FDCs (Fig. 308-14D). The trapping function of the lymph nodes is completely lost, and virus freely spills out into the circulation. Simultaneous PCR analysis of lymph node and peripheral blood mononuclear cells indicates that the relative number of infected cells in the blood and their expression of virus begins to equal the levels in the lymph nodes at this stage. Advanced disease is accompanied by high levels of plasma viremia, which represent a true increase in virus replication, due in part to a further diminution of immune control of virus replication (see below) as well as to the loss of the mechanical trapping function of the lymph nodes. At this point, the lymph nodes are "burnt out." This destruction of lymphoid tissue compounds the immunodeficiency of HIV disease and contributes to the inability to mount adequate immune responses against opportunistic pathogens. The events from primary infection to the ultimate destruction of the immune system are illustrated in Fig. 308-15.

ROLE OF CELLULAR ACTIVATION IN HIV PATHOGENESIS The immune system is normally in a state of homeostasis, awaiting perturbation by foreign antigenic stimuli. Activation of the immune system is an essential component of an appropriate immune response to a foreign antigen. Once the immune response deals with and clears the antigen, the system returns to relative quiescence (see Chap. 305). In HIV infection, however, the immune system is chronically activated owing to the chronicity of infection and the persistence of virus replication (see above). This activated state is reflected by hyperactivation of B cells leading to hypergammaglobulinemia; spontaneous lymphocyte proliferation; activation of monocytes; expression of activation markers on CD4+ and CD8+ T cells; lymph node hyperplasia, particularly early in the course of disease (see above); increased secretion of proinflammatory cytokines (see below); elevated levels of neopterin, β2-microglobulin, acid-labile interferon, and soluble IL-2 receptors; and autoimmune phenomena (see below).

Persistent immune activation may have several deleterious consequences. From a virologic standpoint, although quiescent CD4+ T cells can be infected with HIV, reverse transcription, integration, and virus spread are much more efficient in activated cells. Furthermore, cellular activation induces expression of virus in cells latently infected with HIV. From an immunologic standpoint, chronic exposure of the immune system to a particular antigen over an extended period may ultimately lead to an inability to sustain an adequate immune response to the antigen. Furthermore, the ability of the immune system to respond to a broad spectrum of antigens may be compromised if immune-competent cells are maintained in a state of chronic activation. In addition, activation of the immune system may favor the elimination of cells via programmed cell death (apoptosis) (see below) as well as the secretion of certain cytokines that can induce HIV expression (see below).

Role of Apoptosis *Apoptosis* is a form of programmed cell death that is a normal mechanism for the elimination of effete cells in organogenesis as well as in the cellular proliferation that occurs during a normal immune response (see Chap. 305). Apoptosis is strictly dependent on cellular activation. It has been hypothesized that, in HIV infection, sequential activation signals delivered to CD4+ T cells induce apoptosis. Cross-linking of the CD4 molecule by gp120 or gp120/anti-gp120 complexes delivers the first of two signals required for apoptosis. The second signal supposedly leading to cell death is delivered via the T cell receptor by a conventional antigen or a superantigen (see below and Chap. 305). By this hypothesis, direct infection of CD4+ T cells is not required for apoptosis to occur, although it has been demonstrated that alterations in tyrosine kinase

activity of HIV-infected cells may induce the cell to undergo apoptosis. A number of studies, including those examining lymphoid tissue, have demonstrated that the rate of apoptosis is elevated in HIV infection and that apoptosis is seen in CD8+ T cells and B cells as well as in CD4+ T cells. Furthermore, the intensity of apoptosis correlates with the general state of activation of the immune system and not with the stage of disease or with viral burden. It is likely that apoptosis of immune-competent cells contributes to the immune abnormalities in HIV disease; however, this is probably a nonspecific mechanism that merely reflects the aberrant state of immune activation.

Superantigens and HIV Pathogenesis It has been hypothesized that *superantigens*, either retrovirally coded or related to other microorganisms, may contribute to the pathogenesis of HIV disease. Conventional antigens bind in the groove of the MHC molecule of the antigen-presenting cell (see Chap. 305) and interact with the variable (V) components of the T cell receptor α and β chains to activate the T cell. Thus, any conventional antigenic peptide can stimulate only a very small fraction (<1/100,000) of total T cells. In contrast, certain microbial antigens are capable of binding to and activating entire subsets of T cells, not through true antigen-receptor binding, but by binding to another site on the V region of the β chain of the T cell receptor. There are 24 families or subsets of T cells that can be

A

B

C

D

FIGURE 308-14 HIV in the lymph nodes of HIV-infected individuals. *A.* Cervical lymph node from an asymptomatic individual with very low levels of plasma viremia. In situ hybridization using a molecular probe for HIV RNA reveals copious virus demarcating the numerous germinal centers (bright areas) of the node. The virus was extracellular and bound to the processes of the follicular dendritic cells which form a matrix within the confines of the germinal centers. Original ×25. *B.* Individual cells infected with HIV. Two cells in the paracortical area of the lymph node are shown expressing HIV RNA by in situ hybridization using a radiolabeled molecular probe. Original ×250. *C.* Follicular dendritic cells in cervical node of an asymptomatic HIV-infected

individual. Electron microscopy reveals a follicular dendritic cell with a prominant nucleolus surrounded by several lymphocytes within the germinal center of the node. Higher magnification of several fields indicates that multiple processes of the follicular dendritic cells are in contact with several lymphocytes. Original ×1920. *D.* Dissolution of follicular dendritic cells in the germinal center of a cervical lymph node from a patient with advanced HIV disease. Widespread death of follicular dendritic cells is associated with a loss of ability of the lymph node to trap virus late in the course of HIV disease. Original ×3744. *(A and B courtesy of Dr. Cecil Fox; C and D courtesy of Dr. Jan Orenstein. Adapted from G Pantaleo et al, N Engl J Med 328:327, 1993.)*

identified on the basis of their Vβ usage. Binding of a superantigen to all members of a particular Vβ subset of T cells (1 to 10 percent of all T cells) can induce massive stimulation of T cells and/or, depending on the original state of activation of the T cell, can result in deletion or anergy of T cells bearing the specific Vβs. There is no convincing evidence that HIV codes for a superantigen, nor is there any convincing evidence supporting the concept of true deletion of Vβ subsets by a superantigen mechanism in HIV disease. However, if superantigens associated with other microorganisms play any role in HIV disease, this role probably is related to the fact that superantigens can activate large numbers of CD4+ T cells and render them more susceptible to efficient virus infection (see above).

Autoimmune Phenomena   The autoimmune phenomena that are common in HIV-infected individuals reflect, at least in part, chronic immune system activation. Although these phenomena usually occur in the absence of autoimmune disease, a wide spectrum of clinical manifestations that may be associated with autoimmunity have been described (see below). Autoimmune phenomena include antibodies to lymphocytes and, less commonly, to platelets and neutrophils. Antiplatelet antibodies have some clinical relevance, in that they may contribute to the thrombocytopenia of HIV disease (see below). Antibodies to nuclear and cytoplasmic components of cells have been reported, as have antibodies to cardiolipin, CD4 molecules, CD43 molecules, and IL-2. In addition, autoantibodies to a range of serum proteins, including albumin, immunoglobulin, and thyroglobulin, have been reported. There is antigenic cross-reactivity between HIV viral proteins (gp120 and gp41) and MHC class II determinants, and anti-MHC class II antibodies have been reported in HIV infection. These antibodies could potentially lead to the elimination of MHC class II-bearing cells via antibody-dependent cellular cytotoxicity (ADCC) (see Chap. 305). In addition, regions of homology exist between HIV envelope glycoproteins and IL-2 as well as MHC class I molecules.

Cofactors Contributing to HIV Pathogenesis   Both endogenous and exogenous factors can contribute to HIV pathogenesis by a number of mechanisms; paramount among these is the upregulation of virus expression, a process intimately connected with cellular activation. The main endogenous factors that regulate HIV expression are cytokines (see below). Among exogenous factors, other microbes likely have important effects on HIV replication and HIV pathogenesis. They can thus be considered real or potential *cofactors* in the pathogenesis of HIV disease. Coinfection or simultaneous cotransfection of cells with HIV and other heterologous viruses or viral genes has demonstrated that certain viruses, such as herpes simplex virus type 1, cytomegalovirus, human herpesvirus 6, Epstein-Barr virus, hepatitis B virus, adenovirus, pseudorabies virus, and HTLV-I can upregulate HIV expression. Other microbes, such as *Mycoplasma* have been reported to contribute to the induction of HIV expression. *Mycobacterium tuberculosis* is a common opportunistic infection in HIV-infected individuals (see below and Chap. 171). In addition to the fact that HIV-infected individuals are more likely to develop active tuberculosis after exposure, it has been demonstrated that active tuberculosis can accelerate the course of HIV infection. It has also been shown that levels of plasma viremia are greatly elevated in HIV-infected individuals with active tuberculosis, compared to pretuberculosis levels and levels of viremia after successful treatment of the active tuberculosis. In vitro studies demonstrated that virus replication was markedly enhanced in lymphocytes of HIV-infected individuals who were skin test–positive for purified protein derivative (PPD) when PPD antigen was added to culture, resulting in cellular activation. Confirmatory evidence that antigen-induced activation was a major contributor to the accelerated viremia in HIV-infected individuals with active tuberculosis was provided by studies in which HIV-infected individuals were immunized with common recall antigens such as tetanus toxoid, influenza, or pneumococcal polysaccharide. Under these circumstances, a transient elevation of plasma viremia accompanied the cellular activation induced by the immunization.

THE CYTOKINE NETWORK IN HIV PATHOGENESIS   The immune system is homeostatically regulated by a complex network of immunoregulatory cytokines, which are pleiotropic and

FIGURE 308-15   Events that transpire from primary HIV infection through the establishment of chronic persistent infection to the ultimate destruction of the immune system. See text for details.

redundant and operate in an autocrine and paracrine manner. They are expressed continuously, even during periods of apparent quiescence of the immune system. On perturbation of the immune system by antigenic challenge, the expression of cytokines increases to varying degrees (see Chap. 305). Cytokines that are important components of this immunoregulatory network have been demonstrated to play a major role in the regulation of HIV expression in vitro. A number of in vitro model systems of chronically infected monocyte or T cell lines, primary cultures of peripheral blood or lymph node mononuclear cells from HIV-infected individuals, and acutely infected primary cell cultures have been used to demonstrate the role of cytokines in the regulation of HIV expression. Potent modulation of HIV expression has been demonstrated either by manipulating endogenous cytokines or by adding exogenous cytokines to culture. Cytokines that induce HIV expression in one or more of these systems include IL-1, IL-2, IL-3, IL-6, IL-12, TNFα, and TNFβ, macrophage colony stimulating factor (M-CSF), and granulocyte-macrophage colony stimulating factor (GM-CSF). Among these cytokines, the most consistent and potent inducers of HIV expression are the *proinflammatory cytokines* TNFα, IL-1β, and IL-6. Interferon (INF) α and INFβ suppress HIV replication, whereas transforming growth factor (TGF)-β, IL-4, IL-10, and IFNγ can either induce or suppress HIV expression, depending on the system involved. The β-*chemokines* RANTES, macrophage inflammatory protein (MIP) 1α, and MIP-1β (see Chap. 305) inhibit infection by and spread of macrophage-tropic HIV-1 strains, while *stromal cell–derived factor* (SDF) 1 inhibits infection by and spread of T cell–tropic strains (see below). Several of these cytokines act synergistically in regulating HIV infection and replication, and others function in an autocrine and paracrine manner, similar to their physiologic function in the regulation of the immune system. Blocking of endogenous HIV-inducing cytokines or addition of inhibitors of HIV suppressor cytokines in cultures of peripheral blood and lymph node mononuclear cells from HIV-infected individuals has demonstrated that HIV replication is controlled tightly by endogenous cytokines acting in an autocrine and paracrine manner. Indeed, the net level of virus replication in an HIV-infected individual at least in part reflects a balance between inductive and suppressive host factors, mediated mainly by cytokines. An example of this endogenous regulation is the case of IL-10, which inhibits HIV replication in acutely infected monocyte/macrophages by blocking the secretion of the HIV-inducing cytokines TNFα and IL-6. In addition, IL-4, IL-13, and TGFβ inhibit HIV expression in chronically infected monocytic cell lines stimulated by lipopolysaccharide and GM-CSF by increasing the ratio of expression of endogenous IL-1 receptor antagonist to IL-1β.

The molecular mechanisms of HIV regulation are best understood for TNFα, which activates NF-κB proteins that function as transcriptional activators of HIV expression. The HIV-inducing effect of IL-1β is thought to occur at the level of viral transcription in an NF-κB-independent manner. IL-6, GM-CSF, and IFNγ regulate HIV expression mainly by posttranscriptional mechanisms. Elevated levels of TNFα and IL-6 have been demonstrated in plasma and cerebrospinal fluid, and increased expression of TNFα, IL-1β, IFNγ, and IL-6 have been demonstrated in the lymph nodes of HIV-infected individuals. The mechanisms whereby the β-chemokines RANTES, MIP-1α, and MIP-1β inhibit infection of macrophage-tropic strains of HIV very likely involve blocking of the binding of the virus to its coreceptor, the β-chemokine receptor CCR5 (see above and below).

HIV-infected individuals show an imbalance in the T cell limbs of the immune response, which are defined by the patterns of cytokine secretion. T helper (TH)-1 cells are characterized by secretion of IL-2 and IFNγ and favor cell-mediated immune responses, whereas TH-2 cells are characterized by secretion of IL-4, IL-5, and IL-10 and favor humoral immune responses (see Chap. 305). Since several cell types in addition to CD4+ T cells secrete these cytokines, it is more accurate to refer to immune responses that reflect one or the other cytokine pattern as *TH-1* or *TH-2 type responses*. HIV-infected individ-

uals show a decrease in TH-1 type responses relative to TH-2 type cytokine patterns. It has also been demonstrated that in vitro apoptosis can be inhibited in T cells from HIV-infected donors by antibodies to IL-4 and IL-10 and enhanced by antibodies to IL-12. Although it has been proposed that a clear-cut switch from a TH-1 type to a TH-2 type of cytokine pattern is a critical step in the pathogenesis of HIV disease, no sharp dichotomy between these two types of cytokine patterns that is directly related to progression of disease has been corroborated.

CELLULAR TARGETS OF HIV Although the CD4+ T lymphocytes and CD4+ cells of monocyte lineage are the principal targets of HIV, virtually any cell that expresses the CD4 molecule together with coreceptor molecules (see above and below) can potentially be infected with HIV. Circulating dendritic cells have been reported to express low levels of CD4, and there have been conflicting reports on whether these cells can be infected with HIV. Epidermal Langerhans cells express CD4 and have been infected by HIV in vivo. In vitro, HIV has been reported also to infect a wide range of cells and cell lines that express low levels of CD4, no detectable CD4, or only CD4 mRNA; among these are follicular dendritic cells; megakaryocytes; eosinophils; astrocytes; oligodendrocytes; microglial cells; CD8+ T cells; B cells; natural killer cells; renal epithelial cells; cervical cells; rectal and bowel mucosal cells such as enterochromaffin, goblet, and columnar epithelial cells; trophoblastic cells; and cells from a variety of organs, such as liver, lung, heart, salivary gland, eye, prostate, testis, and adrenal gland. Since the only cells that have been shown unequivocally to be infected with HIV and to support replication of the virus are CD4+ T lymphocytes and cells of monocyte/macrophage lineage, the relevance of the in vitro infection of these other cell types is unclear and is questionable at present.

Of potentially important clinical relevance is the demonstration that thymic precursor cells, which were assumed to be negative for CD3, CD4, and CD8 molecules, actually do express low levels of CD4 and can be infected with HIV in vitro. In addition, human thymic epithelial cells transplanted into an immunodeficient mouse can be infected with HIV by direct inoculation of virus into the thymus. Since these cells may play a role in the normal replenishment of CD4+ T cells, it is possible that their infection and depletion contributes, at least in part, to the inability of the CD4+ T cell pool to replenish itself in infected individuals, including those in whom antiretroviral therapy has at least temporarily suppressed viral replication (see below). In addition, CD34+ monocyte precursor cells have been shown to be infected in vivo in patients with advanced HIV disease. It is likely that these cells express low levels of CD4, and therefore it is not essential to invoke CD4-independent mechanisms to explain the infection.

DETERMINANTS OF CELL TROPISM OF HIV The ability of HIV to infect different cell types varies from isolate to isolate. Many primary isolates of HIV replicate well in both primary T lymphocytes and monocytes, but not in transformed T cell lines. These isolates are often called *monocyte-tropic* or *macrophage-tropic* viruses, despite the fact that they actually can infect both primary T cells and monocytes. Isolates that replicate well only in primary macrophages, and not in lymphocytes, have been only rarely identified. Other isolates, particularly those that have been passaged in vitro in lymphoid cells (T cell line–adapted strains), infect primary T lymphocytes but not monocyte/macrophages; these isolates are referred to as *T cell–tropic* viruses. The viral determinant of cellular tropism maps to the gp120 subunit of the HIV-1 envelope protein, particularly the third variable region (V3 loop) of gp120 (see below). Early in the course of disease, macrophage-tropic viruses predominate in blood, whereas over time and as disease progresses, T cell–tropic viruses predominate. Similarly, viruses isolated from patients early in disease have been characterized as non-syncytia-inducing (NSI) in in vitro assays, while viruses isolated late in the course of disease are typically syncytia-inducing (SI) (see below). Thus, the term *macrophage-tropic* is often used synonymously with *NSI*, and the term *T cell–tropic* with *SI*. The transition from macrophage-tropic/NSI to T cell–tropic/SI virus in an infected individual (which may involve the transient appearance of dual-tropic viruses) is associated with the onset of a more rapid decline in CD4+ T cells. Transmitting viruses are usually macrophage-tropic. However, since most of these studies were done in homosexual men who were infected via receptive anal intercourse, this bias may be influenced somewhat by the route of transmission. Macrophage-tropic viruses are more efficient in infecting monocyte/macrophages and microglial cells of the brain. The *galactosyl ceramide* molecule can serve as an alternative receptor for HIV in CD4-negative neuronal and epithelial cells (see "Neuropathogenesis" below). The *env* gene is primarily responsible for the differences in the ability of different isolates to infect particular cell types, i.e., lymphocytes versus monocytes and primary mononuclear cells versus propagated cell lines. The V3 region of the viral envelope protein is a major determinant of cell tropism, and V3 appears to play a role in envelope protein–mediated fusion of viral and target cell membranes. Sequences within the envelope protein but outside of V3 can also influence the tropism of virus for different cells; however, the mechanisms involved have not been elucidated.

In mid-1996, it was demonstrated that cellular tropism actually reflects the presence of coreceptors specific for macrophage-tropic versus T cell-tropic strains of HIV-1. These coreceptors belong to the seven-transmembrane-domain G protein–coupled family of receptors. The coreceptor for T cell–tropic viruses is *fusin* or CXCR4, which is required for entry and fusion of these strains of virus. Its natural ligand is *stromal cell–derived factor* (SDF)-1. This ligand, as well as antibodies to fusin, can effectively block entry and infection of target cells by T cell–tropic viruses. The main coreceptor for macrophage-tropic viruses is the β chemokine receptor *CCR5*. This receptor binds all three of the β-chemokines (RANTES, MIP-1α, and MIP-1β) that have been shown to inhibit infection with macrophage-tropic strains of HIV-1. However, there is a great deal of redundancy among the β-chemokine receptors, and other members of this family, particularly CCR2b and CCR3, can support infection of dual-tropic strains of HIV-1. The mechanisms of inhibition of entry of macrophage-tropic and T cell–tropic strains of HIV-1 into their target cells by the β-chemokines and SDF-1, respectively, are not entirely clear. However, certain experiments indicate that at least for the β-chemokines, the mechanism involves a receptor blockade and not inhibition of signal transduction (Fig. 308-16). Given the already determined complexity in the interaction between HIV and its human host, it is highly likely that other coreceptors for HIV-1 entry will be identified.

T CELL ABNORMALITIES The range of T cell abnormalities in advanced HIV infection is broad. The defects are both quantitative and qualitative and involve virtually every limb of the immune system (see below), indicating the critical dependence of the integrity of the immune system on the inducer/helper function of CD4+ T cells. Virtually all of the immune defects in advanced HIV disease can ultimately be explained by the quantitative depletion of CD4+ T cells. However, T cell dysfunction (see below) can be demonstrated in patients early in the course of infection, even when the CD4+ T cell count is in the low-normal range. The degree and spectrum of dysfunctions increase as the disease progresses. One of the first abnormalities to be detected is a defect in response to remote recall antigens, such as tetanus toxoid and influenza, at a time when mononuclear cells can still respond normally to mitogenic stimulation. Defects in responses to soluble antigens are followed in time by the loss of T cell proliferative responses to alloantigens, and subsequently to mitogens. Essentially every T cell function has been reported to be abnormal at some stage of

HIV infection. These abnormalities include defective T cell cloning and colony-forming efficiencies, impaired expression of IL-2 receptors, defective IL-2 production, decreased IFNγ production in response to antigens, and decreased help to B cells to produce immunoglobulins.

The level of CD8+ T cells varies throughout the course of disease. Following the resolution of acute primary infection, CD8+ T cells generally rebound to higher than normal levels, and they may remain that way throughout the clinically latent stage of disease. This CD8+ T lymphocytosis may in part reflect the expansion of clones of HIV-specific CD8+ CTLs. In addition, homeostatic mechanisms responsible for maintaining the total T cell count in the normal range in the face of CD4+ T cell destruction would replace lost CD4+ T cells with CD4+ T cells as well as with CD8+ T cells, thus leading to a CD8+ T lymphocytosis, at least prior to the advanced stage of disease (see below). However, during the late stages of HIV infection, there is a significant reduction in the numbers of CD8+ T cells. HIV-specific CD8+ CTLs have been demonstrated in HIV-infected individuals early in the course of disease (see below). As the disease progresses, this functional capability decreases and may be lost entirely. The cause of this loss of cytolytic activity is unclear. However, it has been demonstrated that, as disease progresses, CD8+ T cells assume an abnormal phenotype characterized by expression of activation markers such as HLA-DR with an absence of expression of the IL-2 receptor (CD25) and a loss of clonogenic potential. It has been reported that the phenotype of CD8+ T cells in HIV-infected individuals may be of prognostic significance. Those individuals whose CD8+ T cells developed a phenotype of HLA-DR+/CD38− following seroconversion had stabilization of their CD4+ T cell counts, whereas those whose CD8+ T cells developed a phenotype of HLA-DR+/CD38+ had a more aggressive course and a poorer prognosis. In addition to the defects in HIV-specific CTLs, functional defects in other MHC-restricted CTLs, such as those directed against influenza and cytomegalovirus, have been demonstrated. Since the integrity of CD8+ T cell function depends in part on adequate inductive signals from CD4+ T cells, the defect in CD8+ CTLs is likely compounded by the quantitative loss of CD4+ T cells.

Mechanisms of CD4+ T Lymphocyte Depletion and Dysfunction It is difficult to explain completely the profound immunodeficiency noted in HIV-infected individuals solely on the basis of direct infection and quantitative depletion of CD4+ T cells. This is particu-

T Cell Line-Tropic Strain of HIV-1

Macrophage-Tropic Strain of HIV-1

FIGURE 308-16 Model for the role of coreceptors fusin and CCR5 in the efficient binding and entry of T cell–tropic and macrophage-tropic strains of HIV-1, respectively, into CD4+ target cells. Blocking of this initial event in the virus life cycle can be accomplished by inhibition of binding to the coreceptor by the ligand for the receptor in question. The ligand for fusin is stromal cell–derived factor (SDF-1); the ligands for the β chemokine receptor CCR5 are RANTES, MIP-1α, and MIP-1β.

larly apparent during the early stages of HIV disease, when CD4+ T cell numbers may be only marginally decreased. Certainly, at the stage of advanced disease when the CD4+ T cell count is in the range of 0 to 50/μL, quantitative depletion alone can explain the immune defects. However, it is likely that CD4+ T cell dysfunction results from a combination of depletion of cells due to direct infection and a number of virus-related but indirect effects on the cell (Table 308-7).

Single-cell killing and the formation of syncytia between infected and uninfected cells have been demonstrated clearly in vitro, although the precise mechanisms of cell death in vivo have not been determined. Cytopathicity in an infected cell in vitro may result from a number of mechanisms, including copious budding of virions from the cell surface with resulting disruption of the integrity of the cell membrane; interference with cellular RNA processing or the accumulation of high levels of heterodisperse RNA molecules; disruption of cellular protein synthesis owing to high levels of viral RNA; accumulation of high levels of unintegrated viral DNA in the cell cytoplasm; induction of aberrant patterns of protein tyrosine phosphorylation; and the interaction between HIV gp120 and CD4 intracellularly. Strain differences in single-cell killing are determined largely by gp120 sequences, which supports the importance of the viral envelope in this process. *Syncytia formation* involves fusion of the cell membrane of an infected cell with the cell membranes of variable numbers of uninfected CD4+ cells. Although cell fusion has not been shown to be an important pathogenic process in vivo, a direct relationship between the presence of syncytia and the degree of cytopathic effect has been demonstrated in vitro, and a correlation has been reported between the presence of virus isolates that readily induce syncytia in vitro and a more aggressive clinical course in the patient. Efficient syncytia formation depends on the leukocyte adhesion molecule LFA-1 (see Chap. 305) on human CD4+ T cells acutely infected with HIV in vitro.

Humoral and cellular immune responses to HIV may contribute to protective immunity by eliminating virus and virus-infected cells (see below). However, since the main targets of HIV infection are immune-competent cells, these responses may contribute to immune-cell depletion and immunologic dysfunction by eliminating both infected cells and "innocent bystander" cells. Soluble viral proteins, particularly gp120, can bind with high affinity to the CD4 molecules on uninfected T cells and monocytes; in addition, virus and/or viral protein can bind to dendritic cells or follicular dendritic cells. HIV-specific antibody can recognize these bound molecules and potentially collaborate in the elimination of the cells by ADCC.

Nonpolymorphic determinants of MHC class I products share a degree of homology with gp120 and gp41 proteins of HIV. Such similarities may lead to the generation of autoantibodies to self-MHC determinants. In fact, anti-HLA-DR antibodies have been demonstrated in the sera of HIV-infected individuals (see "Autoimmune Phenomena," above). These antibodies could contribute to the elimination of HLA-DR–expressing cells by ADCC; in addition, it has been

Table 308-7

Potential Mechanisms of CD4+ T Lymphocyte Dysfunction/Depletion in HIV Infection

HIV-mediated direct cytopathicity (single-cell killing)
HIV-mediated syncytia formation
Virus-specific immune responses
   HIV-specific cytolytic T lymphocytes
   Antibody-dependent cellular cytotoxicity (ADCC)
   Natural killer cells
Autoimmune mechanisms
Anergy caused by inappropriate cell signaling via gp120/CD4 interaction
Superantigen-mediated perturbation of T cell subsets
Programmed cell death (apoptosis)
Defect in CD4+ T cell regeneration

SOURCE: Adapted from G Pantaleo et al., N Engl J Med 328:327, 1993.

suggested that these antibodies may inhibit certain T cell functions that involve HLA-DR molecules.

It has been proposed that attempts by the immune system to maintain T cell homeostasis contribute to the progressive decline in numbers of CD4+ T cells. The theory of "blind" T cell homeostasis states that when CD4+ or CD8+ T cells are depleted selectively, the immune system is programmed to restore the total number of T cells blindly, without regard for which subset is depleted (see below). In HIV-infected individuals who experience a selective decrease in CD4+ T cells, both CD4+ and CD8+ T cells are produced to restore homeostasis. Thus, CD4+ T cells are further decreased relative to CD8+ T cells as the total number of T cells is maintained. This theory, if correct, can only apply to the early stages of HIV disease, since both CD4+ and CD8+ T cells decline as disease progresses to the advanced stages.

After gp120/anti-gp120 complexes bind to cell-surface CD4 molecules and cause cross-linking of these molecules, CD4+ T cells may become refractory to further stimulation in vitro via the CD3 molecule. Cross-linking of CD4 by gp120 and/or gp120/anti-gp120 complexes may result in cellular signal-transduction abnormalities, inhibition of IL-2 production and IL-2 receptor expression, steric interference with the MHC class II-CD4–mediated cell adhesion that is necessary for the induction of antigen-specific responses, and even inappropriate activation of the cell (see above). Inappropriate and sustained cellular activation play critical roles in the phenomenon of apoptosis, which may be an important mechanism of death of uninfected cells in HIV infection. In addition, putative superantigens associated with other microbes may contribute to this heightened state of cellular activation, and hence may contribute to immune dysfunction (see "Role of Cellular Activation in HIV Pathogenesis," above).

Finally, the inexorable decline in CD4+ T cell counts that occurs in most HIV-infected individuals may result in part from the inability of the immune system to regenerate the CD4+ T cell pool rapidly enough to compensate for both HIV-mediated destruction of cells and natural attrition of cells. At least two major mechanisms may contribute to the failure of the CD4+ T cell pool to adequately reconstitute itself over the course of HIV infection. The first is the destruction of lymphoid precursor cells, including thymic and bone marrow progenitor cells (see above); the other is the gradual disruption of the lymphoid tissue microenvironment, which is essential for efficient regeneration of immune-competent cells (see above).

B CELL ABNORMALITIES B cells from HIV-infected individuals manifest abnormal activation, which is reflected by spontaneous proliferation and immunoglobulin secretion and by increased spontaneous secretion of TNFα and IL-6. The enhanced spontaneous in vitro transformation of B cells with Epstein-Barr virus (EBV) is probably due to defective T cell immune surveillance and has as its in vivo counterpart an increase in the incidence of EBV-related B cell lymphomas. Untransformed B cells cannot be infected with HIV. However, HIV or its products can activate B cells directly; portions of the HIV gp41 envelope protein have been reported to induce polyclonal B cell activation. In addition, it has been reported that products of the VH$_3$ genes on the surface of B cells can serve as a receptor for HIV. It is likely that in vivo activation of B cells by virus products accounts at least in part for the spontaneous activation of these cells noted ex vivo. In vivo, this activated state manifests itself by hypergammaglobulinemia and by the presence of circulating immune complexes and autoantibodies (see above). The B cells are also defective in that they respond poorly to in vitro stimulation with antigens and mitogens. HIV-infected individuals respond poorly to primary and secondary immunizations with protein and polysaccharide antigens. These B cell defects are likely responsible in part for the increase in certain bacterial infections seen in advanced HIV disease in adults, as well as for the important role of bacterial infections in the morbidity and mortality of HIV-infected children, who cannot mount an adequate humoral response to common bacterial pathogens. The absolute number of circulating B cells may be depressed in primary HIV infection; however, this phenomenon is usually transient and likely reflects in part a redistribution of cells out of the circulation and into the lymphoid tissue. In certain patients, the number of circulating B cells decreases in advanced-stage disease.

CHAPTER 308
HIV Disease: AIDS and Related Disorders

1811

MONOCYTE/MACROPHAGE ABNORMALITIES Circulating monocytes are generally normal in number in HIV-infected individuals. Monocytes express the CD4 molecule and coreceptor for HIV on their surface and thus are targets of HIV infection. Of note is the fact that the degree of cytopathicity of HIV for cells of the monocyte lineage is low, and HIV can replicate extensively in cells of the monocyte lineage with little cytopathic effect. Hence, monocyte-lineage cells can serve as reservoirs of HIV infection and may play a role in the dissemination of HIV in the body. In vivo infection of circulating monocytes is difficult to demonstrate; however, infection of tissue macrophages and macrophage-lineage cells in the brain (infiltrating macrophages or resident microglial cells) and lung (pulmonary alveolar macrophages) can be demonstrated easily. Infection of monocyte precursors in the bone marrow may directly or indirectly be responsible for certain of the hematologic abnormalities in HIV-infected individuals. A number of abnormalities of circulating monocytes have been reported in HIV-infected individuals, including defects in chemotaxis, secretion of IL-1, antigen presentation and induction of T cell responses, Fc receptor function, C3 receptor–mediated clearance, oxidative burst responses, and certain cytotoxic functions. The mechanisms of the monocyte defects are uncertain, but almost certainly they cannot be explained by direct infection with HIV. Exposure of monocytes to gp120 as well as to certain cytokines can cause abnormal activation, and this may play a role in cellular dysfunction (see above).

ABNORMALITIES OF DENDRITIC AND LANGERHANS CELLS There has been considerable disagreement regarding the HIV infectibility and hence the depletion as well as the dysfunction of circulating dendritic cells. Certain groups have reported infection and cellular dysfunction, particularly a decreased ability to present antigen to T cells, and other groups have found little if any HIV infection or functional abnormalities. There is more agreement regarding the ability of skin and mucous membrane Langerhans cells to be infected (see above). These latter cells likely play an important role in the initiation and propagation of HIV infection. The discrepancies in reported depletions and functional abnormalities in these cell types likely reflect the existence of different subsets of cells as well as the differences in isolation techniques and culture systems employed by various groups.

ABNORMALITIES OF NATURAL KILLER CELLS The presumed role of natural killer (NK) cells is to provide immunosurveillance against virus-infected cells, certain tumor cells, and allogeneic cells (see Chap. 305). Functional abnormalities in NK cells have been observed throughout the course of HIV disease, and the severity of these abnormalities increases as disease progresses. Most studies report that NK cells are normal in number and phenotype in HIV-infected individuals; however, a numerical decrease in the CD16+/CD56+ subpopulation of NK cells has been reported. The abnormality in NK cell function is thought to result from a defect in post-binding lysis. However, the lytic machinery does not appear to be impaired, since NK cells from HIV-infected individuals mediate ADCC normally. The addition of either IL-2 or IL-12 to cultures improves the defective in vitro NK cell function of HIV-infected individuals. The in vivo mechanisms for defective NK cell activity is unknown; however, it may be related to the lack of normal inductive signals from CD4+ T cells.

GENETIC FACTORS IN HIV PATHOGENESIS Several reports have described MHC alleles and other host factors that may influence the pathogenesis and course of HIV disease. These include associations with certain HIV-related manifestations, such as Kaposi's sarcoma and diffuse lymphadenopathy, or with the type of clinical course, such as long-term survival or rapid progression (Table 308-8). A number of mechanisms have been proposed whereby MHC-encoded molecules might predispose an individual either to rapid progression or to nonprogression to AIDS. These proposed mechanisms include the ability to present certain immunodominant HIV T helper or CTL epitopes, leading to a relatively protective immune response against HIV and hence to slow progression of disease. In

contrast, certain MHC class I or class II alleles might predispose an individual to an immunopathogenic response against viral epitopes in certain tissues, such as the central nervous system or lungs, or against certain HIV-infected cell types, such as macrophages or dendritic cells/Langerhans cells. In addition, certain rare MHC class I and class II alleles might facilitate rapid recognition of HIV-infected cells from the infecting partner in primary HIV infection and promote rejection of these cells by alloreactive responses. Similarly, common MHC alleles could lead to less effective removal of HIV-infected allogeneic cells. Other data have indicated that transporter associated with antigen-presenting (TAP) genes play a role in determining the outcome of HIV infection. HLA profiles that reflect certain combinations of MHC-encoded TAP and class I and class II genes are strongly associated with different rates of progression to AIDS.

The most compelling data regarding the role of host genetic factors in the pathogenesis of HIV infection were reported in 1996. Rare individuals had been reported who had had repetitive sexual exposure to HIV in high-risk situations but who had remained uninfected. The peripheral blood mononuclear cells of two such individuals were found to be highly resistant to infection in vitro with macrophage-tropic strains of HIV-1, but they were readily infected with T cell–tropic strains. Genetic analysis revealed that these two individuals inherited a homozygous defect in the gene that codes for CCR5, the cellular coreceptor for macrophage-tropic strains of HIV-1. The defective

Table 308-8

Genetic Factors Implicated in the Pathogenesis of HIV Disease

Factor	Association
MAJOR HISTOCOMPATIBILITY LOCI-ENCODED GENES	
B35, C4, DR1, DQ1	Kaposi's sarcoma
DR1	Kaposi's sarcoma
DR2, DR5	Kaposi's sarcoma
DR5	Kaposi's sarcoma
Aw23, Bw49	Kaposi's sarcoma
B62	Fever, skin rash in primary HIV infection
Aw19	HIV seropositivity in individuals multiply exposed to HIV
A1, A24, C7, B8, DR3	Rapid progression to AIDS
DR4, DQB1*0302	Rapid progression to AIDS
DR3, DQ1	Rapid progression to AIDS
B35	Rapid progression to AIDS
TAP2.1	Promotes HIV progression to AIDS
DR5	Thrombocytopenia and lymphadenopathy in HIV infection
DR5, DR6	Diffuse infiltrative CD8+ lymphocytosis with Sjögren-like syndrome in HIV infection
Bw4	Slow decline in CD4+ T cell count
B13, B27, B51, B57, DQB1*0302,0303	Protects from progression to AIDS
A26, B38, TAP1.4, TAP2.3	Ability to clear HIV infection in transiently infected seronegative individuals
A28, Bw70, Aw69, B18	Protection from HIV infection
A32, B4, C2	Long-term survival in HIV infection
A11, A32, B13, C2, DQA1*0301, DQB1*0302, DRB1*0400, DRB4*0101	Long-term survival in HIV infection
OTHER GENES	
p53 tumor suppressor gene	Controls HIV replicative patterns and determinant of viral latency
CCR-5 gene	Homozygous defect results in resistance to infection; heterozygous defect appears to result in partial protection against disease progression

SOURCES: Haynes et al; Liu et al; Samson et al.

CCR5 allele contained a 32-base-pair deletion corresponding to the second extracellular loop of the receptor. The encoded protein was severely truncated, and the receptor was nonfunctional, explaining the refractoriness to infection with macrophage-tropic strains of HIV-1. Population studies revealed that approximately 1 percent of the Caucasian population of western European ancestry possessed the homozygous defect. Twenty percent of this group had the heterozygous defect. Of note, cohort studies of hundreds of DNA samples originating from western and central Africa and Japan did not reveal a single mutant allele, suggesting that the allele is either absent or extremely rare in Africa and Japan. In a cohort of 1400 HIV-1–infected Caucasian individuals, no subject homozygous for the mutation was found, strongly supporting the concept that the homozygous defect confers protection against infection. This finding is particularly compelling in light of the fact that transmitting viruses are strongly biased towards macrophage-tropic strains of HIV-1 (see above). Furthermore, there was a higher frequency of individuals heterozygous for the genetic defect among HIV-infected patients who were long-term nonprogressors compared to HIV-infected individuals who progressed more rapidly.

NEUROPATHOGENESIS HIV-infected individuals can experience a variety of neurologic abnormalities due either to opportunistic infections and neoplasms (see below) or to direct effects of HIV or its products. With regard to the latter, HIV has been demonstrated in the brain and cerebrospinal fluid of infected individuals with and without neuropsychiatric abnormalities. The main cell types that are infected in the brain in vivo are those of the monocyte/macrophage lineage, including monocytes that have migrated to the brain from the peripheral blood as well as resident microglial cells. HIV entry into brain is felt to be due, at least in part, to the ability of virus-infected and immune-activated macrophages to induce adhesion molecules such as E-selectin and vascular cell adhesion molecule-1 (VCAM-1) on brain endothelium. Other studies have demonstrated that HIV gp120 enhances the expression of intercellular adhesion molecule-1 (ICAM-1) in glial cells, and this effect may facilitate entry of HIV-infected cells into the central nervous system and may promote syncytia formation. Virus isolates from the brain are preferentially monocytotropic as opposed to T cell–tropic (see above); in addition, distinct HIV envelope sequences are associated with the clinical expression of the AIDS dementia complex (see below). Although there have been reports of infrequent HIV infection of neuronal cells and astrocytes, there is no convincing evidence that brain cells other than those of monocyte/macrophage lineage can be infected in vivo. Nonetheless, it has been demonstrated that galactosyl ceramide may be an essential component of the HIV gp120 receptor on neural cells, and antibodies to galactosyl ceramide inhibit entry of HIV into neural cell lines in vitro.

HIV-infected individuals may manifest white matter lesions as well as neuronal loss. Given the relative absence of evidence of HIV infection of neurons either in vivo or in vitro, it is unlikely that direct infection of these cells accounts for their loss. Rather, the HIV-mediated effects on brain tissue are thought to be due to a combination of direct effects, either toxic or function-inhibitory, of gp120 on neuronal cells and effects of a variety of neurotoxins released from infiltrating monocytes, resident microglial cells, and astrocytes. Neurotoxins can be released from monocytes as a consequence of infection and/or immune activation. Monocyte-derived neurotoxic factors have been reported to kill neurons via the N–methyl-D-aspartate (NMDA) receptor. In addition, HIV gp120 shed by virus-infected monocytes could cause neurotoxicity by antagonizing the function of vasoactive intestinal peptide (VIP), by elevating intracellular calcium levels, and by decreasing nerve growth factor levels in the cerebral cortex. A variety of monocyte-derived cytokines can contribute directly or indirectly to the neurotoxic effects in HIV infection; these include TNFα, IL-1, IL-6, TGFβ, INFγ, platelet-activating factor, and endothelin. In addition, infection and/or activation of monocyte-lineage cells can result in increased production of eicosanoids, nitric oxide, and quinolinic acid, which may contribute to neurotoxicity. Astrocytes may play

diverse roles in HIV neuropathogenesis. Reactive gliosis or astrocytosis has been demonstrated in the brains of HIV-infected individuals, and TNFα and IL-6 have been shown to induce astrocyte proliferation. In addition, astrocyte-derived IL-6 can induce HIV expression in infected cells in vitro. Furthermore, it has been suggested that astrocytes may downregulate macrophage-produced neurotoxins. The likelihood that HIV or its products are involved in neuropathogenesis is supported by the observation that neuropsychiatric abnormalities may undergo remarkable and rapid improvement upon the initiation of antiretroviral therapy, particularly in HIV-infected children.

PATHOGENESIS OF KAPOSI'S SARCOMA Kaposi's sarcoma is an opportunistic disease in HIV-infected individuals. Unlike opportunistic infections, its occurrence is not strictly related to the level of depression of CD4+ T cell counts (see below). Kaposi's sarcoma does not result from a neoplastic transformation of cells in the classic sense, and so is not truly a sarcoma. It is a manifestation of excessive proliferation of spindle cells that are believed to be of vascular origin and have features in common with endothelial and smooth muscle cells. The initiation and/or propagation of Kaposi's sarcoma is mediated, at least in part, by cytokines. A number of factors, including TNFα, IL-1β, IL-6, GM-CSF, basic fibroblast growth factor, and oncostatin M, function in an autocrine and paracrine manner to sustain the growth and chemotaxis of the Kaposi's sarcoma spindle cells. In addition, the HIV-1 Tat protein has been shown to act synergistically with basic fibroblast growth factor in the induction of lesions resembling Kaposi's sarcoma lesions in mice. Glucocorticoids have been shown to have a stimulatory effect, and human chorionic gonadotrophin an inhibitory effect, on Kaposi's sarcoma spindle cells, suggesting that modulation of the balance of autocrine factors may have therapeutic potential in Kaposi's sarcoma.

The identification of Kaposi's sarcoma in HIV-seronegative homosexual men at high risk for HIV infection, as well as the disproportionate occurrence of Kaposi's sarcoma among HIV-infected homosexual men compared to other HIV-infected groups, has led to the suggestion that Kaposi's sarcoma is caused by a sexually transmitted agent other than HIV. In 1994, a molecular procedure called representational difference analysis succeeded in identifying unique herpesvirus sequences in more than 90 percent of Kaposi's sarcoma tissues obtained from HIV-infected individuals. The sequences showed similarities to herpesvirus saimiri of squirrel monkeys and to EBV. The virus is referred to as *Kaposi's sarcoma–associated herpesvirus* or *human herpesvirus* (HHV)-8. PCR analysis indicated that these same sequences were present not only in HIV-associated Kaposi's sarcoma, but also in classic Kaposi's sarcoma and the Kaposi's sarcoma that occurs in HIV-negative homosexual men (see above). In addition, the sequences were identified in AIDS-related, body cavity–based B cell lymphomas. HHV-8 has been detected in the blood of more than 50 percent of individuals with Kaposi's sarcoma of the skin. In addition, detection of HHV-8 in the blood is felt to be strongly predictive of later development of Kaposi's sarcoma. In 1996, the successful propagation of HHV-8 in culture made possible the performance of seroepidemiologic studies that strongly indicated that HHV-8 has a specific etiologic role in Kaposi's sarcoma. It is likely that the combination of immune activation, cytokine secretion, and HHV-8 act synergistically in the ultimate expression of this disease.

IMMUNE RESPONSE TO HIV

As detailed above and below, following the initial burst of viremia during primary infection, HIV-infected individuals generally mount a robust immune response that usually substantially curtails the levels of plasma viremia and almost certainly contributes to slowing the progression of infection and to delaying the ultimate development of clinically apparent disease for a median of 10 years. This immune response contains elements of both humoral and cell-mediated immunity (Table 308-9) and is directed against multiple antigenic determinants of the HIV virion, as well as against viral proteins produced in infected cells. Paradoxically, those CD4+ cellular elements of the immune system with T cell receptors specific for HIV are theoretically

Table 308-9

CHAPTER 308
HIV Disease: AIDS and Related Disorders **1813**

Elements of the Immune Response to HIV

Humoral immunity
  Binding antibodies
  Neutralizing antibodies
    Type specific
    Group specific
  Antibodies participating in ADCC
    Protective
    Pathogenic (bystander killing)
  Enhancing antibodies
Cell-mediated immunity
  Helper CD4 + T lymphocytes
  Class I MHC–restricted cytotoxic CD8 + T lymphocytes
  CD8 + T cell–mediated inhibition (noncytolytic)
  Antibody-dependent cellular cytotoxicity
  Natural killer cells

those CD4 + T cells most likely to bind to infected cells and themselves be infected and destroyed. Thus, relatively early in the course of HIV infection, it is likely that the cellular components of host defense that are most important for the control of HIV infection are preferentially infected and destroyed.

Although a great deal of investigation has been directed toward attempting to delineate and understand the individual elements of this immune response, it remains unclear which of these phenomena are most important in delaying progression of infection and which, if any, may actually be playing a role in the pathogenesis of HIV disease.

HUMORAL IMMUNE RESPONSE Antibodies to HIV usually appear within 2 weeks and almost invariably within 8 weeks of the onset of primary infection (Fig. 308-17). Detection of these antibodies forms the basis of most diagnostic screening tests for HIV infection. It should be noted that the appearance of HIV-binding antibodies detected by ELISA and western blot assays (see below) occurs prior to the appearance of neutralizing antibodies. The latter generally appear following the downregulation of plasma viremia, which is more closely associated with the appearance of HIV-specific CD8 + CTLs (see below). Despite earlier claims to the contrary, there is currently no evidence to suggest that, apart from extremely rare exceptions, the period between initial infection and development of an antibody response is any longer than 3 months. The first antibodies detected are those directed against the structural or *gag* proteins of HIV, p24 and p17, and the *gag* precursor p55. The development of antibodies to p24 is associated with a decrease in the serum levels of free p24 antigen. Antibodies to the *gag* proteins are followed by the appearance of antibodies to the envelope proteins (gp160, gp120, p88, and gp41) and to the products of the *pol* gene (p31, p51, and p66). In addition, one may see antibodies to low-molecular-weight proteins from HIV-infected cells corresponding to antibodies to the regulatory proteins produced by the HIV genes *vpr*, *vpu*, *vif*, *rev*, *tat*, and *nef*.

While antibodies are produced to multiple antigens of HIV, their precise functional significance is unclear. The best studied have been the antibodies directed toward the envelope proteins of the virus. As noted above, the envelope of HIV consists of an outer envelope glycoprotein, with a molecular weight of 120 kDa, and a transmembrane glycoprotein, with a molecular weight of 41 kDa. These are initially synthesized as a 160-kDa precursor. Most of the antienvelope antibodies are directed toward either an epitope in the gp41 region comprising amino acids 579 through 613, or towards a hypervariable region of the gp120 molecule known as the V3 loop region, comprising amino acids 303 through 338. This V3 region is a major site for the development of mutations that lead to variants of HIV that are not as well recognized by the immune system.

Antibodies directed toward the envelope proteins of HIV have been characterized both as being protective and as possibly contributing to the pathogenesis of HIV disease. Among the protective antibodies are those that function to neutralize HIV directly and prevent the infection of additional cells, as well as those that participate in ADCC. Neutralizing antibodies appear to be of two forms, type-specific and group-specific. Type-specific neutralizing antibodies are generally directed to the V3 loop region. These antibodies only neutralize viruses of a given strain and are present in low titer in most infected individuals. Group-specific antibodies, on the other hand, are capable of neutralizing a wide variety of HIV isolates. At least two forms of group-specific antibodies have been identified, those binding to amino acids 423 to 437 of gp120 and those binding to amino acids 728 to 745 of gp41. The other major class of protective antibodies are those that participate in ADCC. ADCC is actually a form of cell-mediated immunity (see Chap. 305) in which NK cells that bear Fc receptors and are armed with specific anti-HIV antibodies (which bind via their Fc portion to the cellular Fc receptors) bind to and destroy cells expressing HIV antigens (Fig. 308-18). Antibodies to both gp120 and gp41 have been shown to participate in ADCC-mediated killing of HIV-infected cells. The levels of antienvelope antibodies capable of mediating ADCC are highest in the earlier stages of HIV infection. ADCC-mediated killing can be augmented in vitro by IL-2.

In addition to playing a role in host defense, HIV-specific antibodies also have been implicated in the pathogenesis of the disease. In vitro, antibodies directed to gp41, when present in low titer, have been shown to be capable of facilitating infection of cells through an Fc receptor–mediated mechanism known as antibody enhancement. The same regions of the envelope protein of HIV that give rise to antibodies capable of mediating ADCC also elicit the production of antibodies that can facilitate infection of uninfected cells in vitro. In addition, it has been postulated that anti-gp120 antibodies that participate in the ADCC killing of HIV-infected cells might also kill uninfected CD4 + T cells if the uninfected cells had bound free gp120 from the circulation, a phenomenon referred to as *bystander killing* (Fig. 308-18).

CELLULAR IMMUNE RESPONSE Given the fact that T cell–mediated immunity is known to play a major role in host defense against most viral infections (see Chap. 305), it is generally thought to be an important component of the host immune response to HIV. T cell immunity can be divided into two major categories, mediated respectively by the helper/inducer or CD4 + T cells and the cytotoxic/immunoregulatory or CD8 + T cells.

It has been very difficult to demonstrate directly the presence of HIV-specific CD4 + T cells in HIV-infected patients. This difficulty may be related to the fact that these cells, with their high affinity for binding to HIV-infected cells, may be among the first to be infected and destroyed during HIV infection. Nonetheless, through the use of computer modeling, several regions of the HIV-1 envelope molecule have been identified that are structurally analogous to other known T cell epitopes by virtue of having structures known as *amphipathic helices*. Peptides from these envelope regions have been used to dem-

FIGURE 308-17 Relationship between antigenemia and the development of antibodies to HIV. Antibodies to HIV proteins are generally seen 6 to 12 weeks following infection and 3 to 6 weeks after the development of plasma viremia. Late in the course of illness, antibody levels to p24 decline, generally in association with a rising titer of p24 antigen.

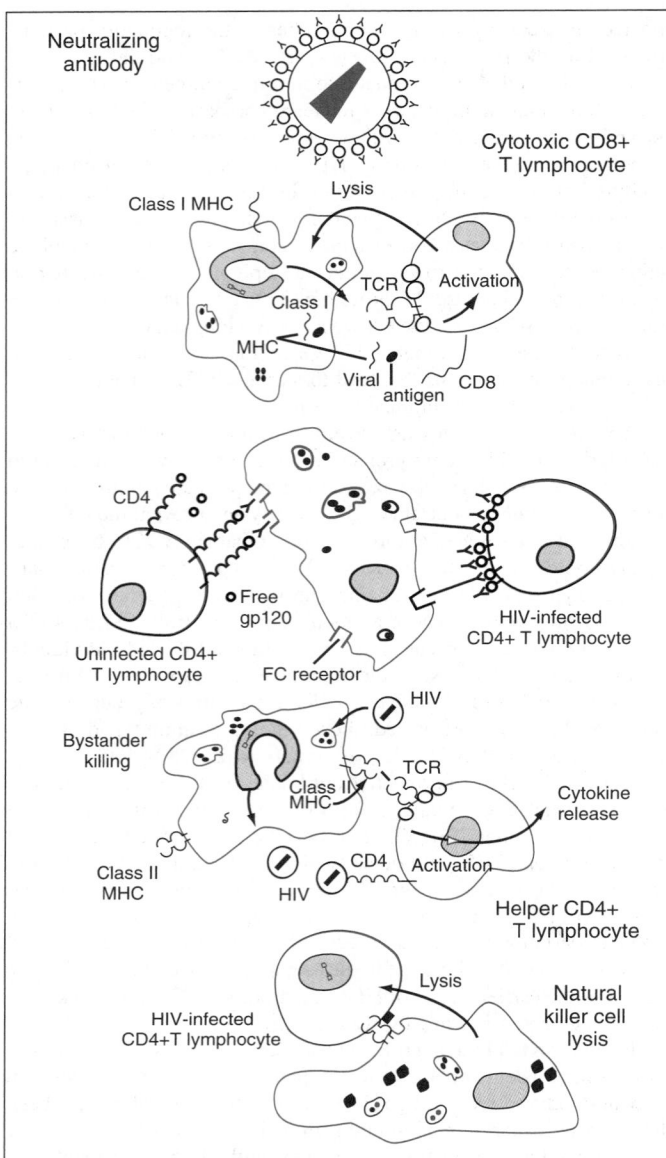

FIGURE 308-18 Schematic representation of the different immunologic effector mechanisms felt to be active in the setting of HIV infection. Detailed descriptions are given in the text.

onstrate the presence of CD4+ T cells specific for these regions in the peripheral blood of HIV-infected individuals. Other studies have demonstrated that peripheral blood T cells of some healthy, HIV-negative individuals also react to the envelope proteins of HIV.

Classic, MHC class I–restricted, HIV-specific CD8+ CTLs have been identified in the peripheral blood of patients within weeks of HIV infection. These CD8+ T lymphocytes, through their HIV-specific antigen receptors, bind to and cause the lytic destruction of target cells bearing identical MHC class I molecules associated with HIV antigens (Fig. 308-18). Two types of CD8+ CTL activity can be demonstrated in the peripheral blood and lymph node mononuclear cells of HIV-infected individuals. The first type directly lyses appropriate target cells in culture without in vitro stimulation (spontaneous CTL activity). The other type of CTL activity reflects the precursor frequency of CTLs (CTL$_p$); this type of CTL activity can be demonstrated by stimulation of CD8+ T cells in vitro with a mitogen such as phytohemagglutinin or anti-CD3 antibody. Following primary HIV infection, the qualitative nature of the HIV-specific CTL responses is an important predictor of

eventual outcome. Patients who mount a broad CD8+ CTL response, involving several CD8+ T cell clonotypes none of which exhibits more than minor expansion, generally have a more favorable clinical course than patients who mount a more restricted CTL response, characterized by major expansions of a very restricted repertoire of CD8+ T cell clonotypes (see above). Longitudinal studies have demonstrated that the gradual loss of CD4+ T lymphocytes is paralleled by a loss of HIV-specific CD8+ CTL activity, which reinforces the concept that the CD4+ T lymphocyte is an important element in maintaining antigen-specific CTL responses. Multiple HIV antigens can elicit HIV-specific CTL responses. Class I–restricted CTLs directed against products of at least six HIV genes—*gag, env, pol, tat, rev,* and *nef*—have been identified. CD4+ CTLs, which are class II MHC–restricted, have also been identified in HIV-infected individuals and in uninfected individuals following vaccination with HIV proteins. The pathophysiologic significance of these CD4+ CTLs is unclear at present.

At least three other forms of cell-mediated immunity to HIV have been described. These are CD8+ T cell–mediated suppression of HIV replication, ADCC, and NK cell activity. *CD8+ T cell–mediated suppression of HIV replication* refers to the ability of CD8+ T cells from an HIV-infected patient to inhibit the replication of HIV in tissue culture in a noncytolytic manner. There is no requirement for HLA compatibility between the CD8+ T cells and the infected CD4+ T cells. In most culture systems that have been employed, the CD8+ T cells must be derived from an HIV-infected individual to suppress HIV replication. However, in certain systems, CD8+ T cells from uninfected individuals can also have this effect. It has been demonstrated that this effector mechanism is mediated by a soluble factor(s). CD8+ T cells, as well as monocytes, CD4+ T cells, and B cells, secrete the β-chemokines RANTES, MIP-1α, and MIP-1β (see above). These chemokines are potent suppressors of HIV replication and operate at least in part via blockade of the coreceptor (CCR5) for macrophage-tropic strains of HIV on peripheral blood mononuclear cells (see above). It is clear that other CD8+ T cell–derived soluble factors besides the β-chemokines suppress HIV replication; one of the mechanisms of suppression of HIV replication by these factors has been reported to be the inhibition of HIV transcription. The identity of these factors remain unknown.

ADCC, as described above in relation to humoral immunity, involves the killing of HIV-expressing cells by NK cells armed with specific antibody directed against HIV antigens. Finally, NK cells alone have been shown to be capable of killing HIV-infected target cells in tissue culture. This primitive cytotoxic mechanism of host defense is geared toward nonspecific surveillance for neoplastic transformation and viral infection through recognition of altered class I MHC molecules. Both NK and ADCC activity can be enhanced by IL-2.

DIAGNOSIS AND LABORATORY MONITORING OF HIV INFECTION

Before HIV-1 was identified as the causative agent of AIDS, a diagnosis of AIDS was made solely on clinical grounds. The establishment of HIV as the causative agent of AIDS and related syndromes early in 1984 was followed by the rapid development of sensitive screening tests for HIV infection, and by March 1985, blood donors in the United States were screened routinely for antibodies to HIV. In June 1996, blood banks in the United States added the p24 antigen capture assay to help identify the rare infected individuals who donate blood in the window of time before they develop antibodies, who would not have been identified by the standard screening assays (see below). At present, a wide array of laboratory tests are available for diagnosing and monitoring patients with HIV infection.

DIAGNOSIS OF HIV INFECTION The diagnosis of HIV infection depends on the demonstration of antibodies to HIV and/or the direct detection of HIV or one of its components. As noted above, antibodies to HIV generally appear in the circulation 4 to 8 weeks after infection.

The standard screening test for HIV is the *enzyme-linked immunosorbent assay* (ELISA). This solid-phase assay is an extremely good screening test, with a sensitivity of over 99.5 percent. Most diagnostic laboratories use a commercial ELISA kit that contains antigens from both HIV-1 and HIV-2 and that will detect either. These kits use both natural and recombinant antigens and are continuously updated to increase their sensitivity to newly discovered species, such as group O viruses (see Fig. 308-5). ELISA tests are generally scored as positive (highly reactive), negative (nonreactive), or indeterminate (partially reactive). While the ELISA is extremely sensitive, it is not optimal with regard to specificity. In fact, in studies of low-risk individuals, such as volunteer blood donors, only 13 percent of ELISA-positive individuals actually had HIV infection. Among the factors associated with false-positive ELISA tests are antibodies to class II antigens, autoantibodies, hepatic disease, and recent influenza vaccination. For these reasons, anyone suspected of having HIV infection on the basis of an inconclusive or positive ELISA result must have the result confirmed with a more specific assay.

The most commonly used confirmatory test is the *western blot* (Fig. 308-19). It takes advantage of the fact that multiple HIV antigens having different, well-characterized molecular weights elicit the production of specific antibodies. These antigens can be separated on the basis of molecular weight, and antibodies to each component can be detected as discrete bands on the western blot. A negative western blot is one in which no bands are present at molecular weights corresponding to HIV gene products. In a patient with a positive or indeterminate ELISA and a negative western blot, one can conclude with certainty that the ELISA reactivity was a false positive. On the other hand, a western blot demonstrating antibodies to products of all three of the major genes of HIV (*gag*, *pol*, and *env*) is conclusive evidence of infection with HIV. In fact, according to most experts, as well as the criteria established by the Association of State and Territorial Public Health Laboratory Directors and adopted by the CDC, a western blot can be considered positive for HIV-1 if it contains bands to at least two of the following gene products: p24, gp41, and gp120/160. By definition, western blot patterns of reactivity that do not fall into the positive or negative categories are considered "indeterminate." There are two possible explanations for an indeterminate western blot result. The most likely explanation is that the patient being tested has antibodies that cross-react with one of the proteins of HIV. The most common patterns of cross reactivity are antibodies that react with p24 and/or p55. The least likely explanation for an indeterminate western blot is that the individual is infected with HIV and is in the process of mounting a classic antibody response. In either instance, the western blot should be repeated in 1 month to confirm whether or not the indeterminate pattern is a pattern in evolution. In addition, one may attempt to confirm a diagnosis of HIV infection with the p24 antigen capture assay or one of the tests for HIV RNA (discussed below). While the western blot is an excellent confirmatory test for HIV infection in patients with a positive or indeterminate ELISA, it is a poor screening test. Among individuals with a negative ELISA and PCR for HIV, 20 to 30 percent may show one or more bands on western blot. While these bands are usually faint and represent cross reactivity, their presence creates a situation in which other diagnostic modalities (such as DNA PCR, RNA PCR, the bDNA assay, or p24 antigen capture) must

be employed to ensure that the bands do not indicate early HIV infection.

A guideline for the use of these serologic tests in attempting to make a diagnosis of HIV infection is depicted in Fig. 308-20. In a patient in whom HIV infection is suspected, the appropriate initial test is the ELISA. If the result is negative, unless there is strong reason to suspect early HIV infection (as in a patient exposed within the previous 3 months), the diagnosis is ruled out and retesting should be performed only as clinically indicated. If the ELISA is indeterminate or positive, the test should be repeated. If the repeat is negative on two occasions, one can assume that the initial positive reading was due to a technical error in the performance of the assay and that the patient is negative. If the repeat is indeterminate or positive, one should proceed to the western blot. If the western blot is positive, the diagnosis is HIV infection. If the western blot is negative, the ELISA can be assumed to have been false positive, and the diagnosis of HIV infection is ruled out. If the western blot is indeterminate, it should be repeated in 1 month; in addition, one may proceed to a p24 antigen capture assay, HIV RNA assay, or HIV DNA PCR. If the p24 and HIV RNA assays are negative and there is no progression in the western blot, a diagnosis of HIV is ruled out. If either the p24 or HIV RNA assay is positive and/or the western blot shows progression, a tentative diagnosis of HIV infection can be made and later confirmed with a follow-up western blot demonstrating a positive pattern.

As mentioned earlier a variety of laboratory tests are available for the direct detection of HIV or its components (Table 308-10). These tests may be of considerable help in making a diagnosis of HIV infection when the western blot results are indeterminate. In addition, several of these can be used to assess the antiviral activity of therapies for HIV. The easiest to perform of these is the *p24 antigen capture assay*. This is an ELISA-type assay in which the solid phase consists of antibodies to the p24 antigen of HIV. It detects the viral protein p24 in the blood of HIV-infected individuals, where it exists either as free antigen or complexed to anti-p24 antibodies. Overall, approxi-

A
1. Virus digested: digest separated into components by molecular weight
2. Proteins transferred to filter paper: reaction with test serum
3. Enzyme-conjugated antihuman antibody added
4. Substrate added and color noted

B
1. Positive HIV-1 infection
2. gp 160 immunization
3. Indeterminate (HIV-2 infection)
4. Indeterminate (cross-reacting antibody to p24)
5. Negative

FIGURE 308-19 *A.* Schematic representation of how a western blot is performed. *B.* Examples of patterns of western blot reactivity. In each instance the western blot strip contains antigens to HIV-1. The sera from the patient immunized to the HIV-1 envelope only contains antibodies to the HIV-1 envelope proteins. The sera from the patient with HIV-2 infection cross-reacts with both reverse transcriptase and *gag* gene products of HIV-1.

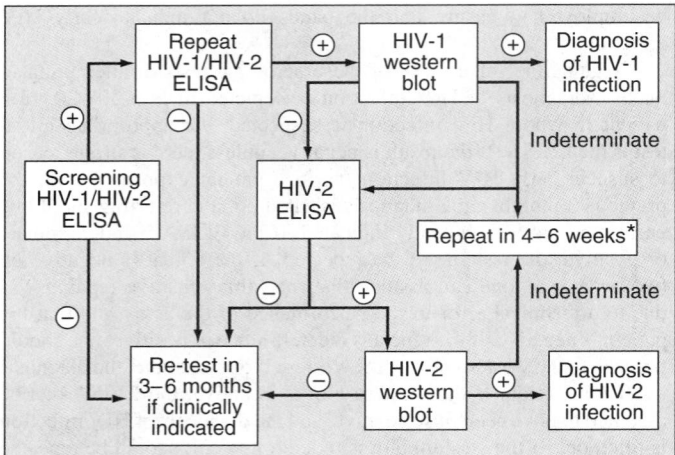

FIGURE 308-20 Algorithm for the use of serologic tests in the diagnosis of HIV-1 or HIV-2 infection. * Stable indeterminate western blot 4–6 weeks makes HIV infection unlikely. However, it should be repeated twice at 3-month intervals to rule out HIV infection. Alternatively, one may test for HIV-1 p24 antigen on HIV RNA.

mately 30 percent of individuals with HIV infection have detectable levels of free p24 antigen. This percentage increases to about 50 percent when samples are treated with a weak acid to dissociate antigen-antibody complexes prior to assay. Throughout the course of HIV infection, an equilibrium appears to exist between p24 antigen and anti-p24 antibodies. During the first few weeks of infection, before an immune response develops, there is a brisk rise in p24 antigen levels. After the development of anti-p24 antibodies, these levels decline. Late in the course of infection, when circulating levels of free virus are high, p24 antigen levels also increase, particularly when detected by techniques involving dissociation of antigen-antibody complexes. While the precise pathophysiologic significance of p24 antigenemia is unclear, it has been shown that, for a group of asymptomatic HIV-infected patients having similar CD4+ T cell counts, those with detectable levels of p24 antigen are three times more likely on average to show progression to AIDS over a period of 3 years than those in whom p24 antigen levels cannot be detected. In addition, multiple clinical trials have demonstrated that patients receiving antiretroviral therapy show a decline in their circulating levels of p24 antigen. Some workers have advocated the use of this assay for monitoring the effectiveness of such treatment, but the validity of this recommendation has yet to be established. Moreover, the second- and third-generation PCR-based and bDNA assays are assuming a much greater

role in the decisions to initiate and/or modify antiretroviral therapy (see below). At present, the p24 antigen capture assay seems to be most useful as a screening test for HIV infection in patients suspected of having the acute HIV syndrome, as high levels of p24 antigen are present prior to the development of antibodies. It is currently used along with the HIV ELISA to screen blood donors in the United States for evidence of HIV infection.

The *polymerase chain reaction* is a diagnostic technique that has gained acceptance in many areas of clinical microbiology. Although the extreme sensitivity of this technique leads in many cases to false-positive results, in a well-controlled setting PCR has been of extraordinary value in furthering our understanding of the pathogenesis of HIV disease and has provided a gold standard for the diagnosis of HIV infection. This is particularly true for the diagnosis of HIV infection in at-risk neonates. Two forms of PCR are used in the study of HIV infection, DNA PCR and RNA PCR. The DNA PCR can be used for making a diagnosis of HIV infection by amplifying proviral DNA. In performing a DNA PCR test for HIV, peripheral blood mononuclear cells are lysed, and the DNA region of interest is amplified using primer pairs from relatively constant regions of the HIV genome. Primer pairs from both the *gag* and LTR regions are usually employed. The amplified DNA is then characterized using nucleic acid hybridization techniques. With the proper controls to check for contamination and success of amplification, it is possible to determine whether or not HIV proviral DNA is present at a frequency of one copy per 10,000 to 100,000 cells. Studies of this type have clearly documented that the interval between HIV infection and antibody positivity is on the order of 1 to 3 months. In addition to being a diagnostic tool, DNA PCR is also useful for amplifying defined areas of proviral DNA for sequence analysis and has become an important technique for studies of sequence diversity and microbial resistance to antiretroviral agents. While RNA PCR has been used most frequently for monitoring changes in the level of the HIV genome present in plasma, it can also be used for making an early diagnosis of HIV infection. In this technique, following DNAase treatment, a cDNA copy is made of all RNA species present in plasma. Insofar as HIV is an RNA virus (see above and Chap. 192), this will result in the production of DNA copies of the HIV genome in amounts proportional to the amount of HIV present in plasma. This proviral cDNA is then amplified and characterized using the PCR technique, employing primer pairs that can distinguish genomic cDNA from messenger cDNA. In patients with a positive or indeterminate ELISA test and an indeterminate western blot, and in patients in whom serologic testing may be unreliable (such as patients with hypogammaglobulinemia), PCR is a valuable diagnostic tool for making a diagnosis of HIV infection. Given its cost and the problem of artifacts resulting from contamination, however, it should be used as a diagnostic tool only when standard serologic testing has failed to provide a definitive result.

LABORATORY MONITORING OF PATIENTS WITH HIV INFECTION The epidemic of HIV infection and AIDS has provided the clinician with new challenges in the integration of clinical and laboratory data. The close relationship between clinical manifestations of HIV infection and CD4+ T cell count has made measurement of the latter quantity a routine part of the evaluation of HIV-infected individuals. Coupled with knowledge of the levels of HIV RNA in serum or plasma (see below), CD4+ T cell counts make a powerful set of tools for determining prognosis and monitoring response to therapy. While the CD4+ T cell count provides information on the current immunologic status of the patient, the HIV RNA level predicts what will happen to that CD4+ T cell count in the near future and hence predicts the clinical prognosis for the

Table 308-10

Characteristics of Tests for Direct Detection of HIV

Test	Technique	Sensitivity	Cost/Test
Immune complex–dissociated p24 antigen capture assay	Measurement of levels of HIV-1 core protein in an ELISA-based format following dissociation of antigen-antibody complexes by weak acid treatment	Positive in 50% of patients. Detects down to 15 pg/mL of p24 protein	$1–2
HIV RNA by PCR	PCR amplification of cDNA generated from viral RNA (target amplification)	Positive in >98% of patients. Detects down to 40 copies/mL of HIV RNA	$150
HIV RNA by bDNA	Measurement of levels of particle-associated HIV RNA in a nucleic acid capture assay employing signal amplification	Positive in 90% of patients. Detects down to 500 copies/mL of HIV RNA	$150

patient. Other tests, such as the p24 antigen capture assay (described above) and measurement of serum levels of neopterin and β_2-microglobulin, may also provide information of value to the clinician (see below).

The direct cultivation of HIV from plasma or peripheral blood mononuclear cells is a technique employed in many research laboratories and has proven very useful for generating HIV isolates for studies of antiviral resistance and analysis of genomic drift. Most of the techniques employed involve cocultivation of patient material with an indicator cell line capable of supporting HIV replication, most commonly peripheral blood mononuclear cells that have been activated with phytohemagglutinin. Cultures generally need to be maintained for up to 28 days, during which time they are periodically observed for the formation of syncytia or giant cells, and supernatants are sampled for the presence of either HIV p24 (using the antigen capture assays mentioned above) or reverse transcriptase. There is no role at present for HIV culture in the diagnosis or routine management of patients with HIV infection; however, such tests may be used more commonly as attempts are made to tailor antiretroviral therapy to the sensitivities of patient-derived viral isolates.

The CD4+ T cell count is the laboratory test generally accepted as an indicator of the immunologic competence of the patient with HIV infection. This measurement, which is the product of the percent of CD4+ T cells (determined by flow cytometry) and the total lymphocyte count [determined by the white blood cell count (WBC) and the differential count] has been shown to correlate very well with clinical progression. Patients with CD4+ T cell counts below 200/µL are at high risk of infection with *Pneumocystis carinii*, while patients with CD4+ T cell counts below 100/µL are at high risk of infection with cytomegalovirus and the *Mycobacterium avium-intracellulare* complex (Fig. 308-21). Patients with an initial diagnosis of HIV infection should have CD4+ T cell measurements performed approximately every 6 months, and more frequently if a declining trend is noted. At a minimum, antiretroviral therapy is generally indicated when the CD4+ T cell count falls below 500/µL, and a declining CD4+ T cell count may provide an indication for changing therapy (see below). Once the CD4+ T cell count is below 200/µL, patients should be placed on a regimen for *P. carinii* pneumonia (PCP) prophylaxis. All effective forms of antiretroviral therapy to date have been associated with at least a transient increase in either CD4+ T cell count or CD4 percent (see below).

Direct Measurements of HIV RNA
Facilitated by techniques for the precise quantitation of small amounts of nucleic acids, the measurement of serum or plasma levels of HIV RNA has become the most commonly used approach for the direct detection of HIV. Two basic techniques are used: the reverse transcriptase PCR (RT-PCR) assay and the branched DNA (bDNA) assay. The RT-PCR assay involves the PCR amplification of cDNA generated from viral RNA. The bDNA assay involves the use of a solid-phase nucleic acid capture system and signal amplification through successive nucleic acid hybridizations to detect small quantities of HIV RNA. Both assays generate data in the form of number of copies of HIV RNA per milliliter of serum or plasma. The RT-PCR assay can detect as few as 40 copies of HIV RNA per milliliter and is positive in >98 percent of patients. The bDNA assay can detect as few as 500 copies of HIV RNA per milliliter and is positive in >90 percent of patients. Measurements of levels of HIV RNA over time have been of great value in delineating the relationship between levels of virus and

rates of disease progression (Fig. 308-22), the rates of viral turnover, the relationship between immune system activation and viral replication, and the time to development of antiviral drug resistance. While the p24 antigen capture assays reflect changes in total viral burden over an extended period, the HIV RNA assays allow an evaluation of the changes in viral burden that occur over a matter of hours. Measurements of HIV RNA levels should be made approximately every 6 months and more frequently in the setting of changes in antiretroviral therapy. While precise guidelines have yet to be established, a level of HIV RNA of >20,000 copies per milliliter is felt by many experts to be an indication for antiretroviral therapy, regardless of the CD4+ T cell count. All effective forms of antiretroviral therapy to date have been associated with a drop in levels of HIV RNA.

β_2-Microglobulin Levels β_2-Microglobulin is an 11-kDa protein that is expressed on the surface of most nucleated cells. It forms a heterodimer with class I MHC molecules and exhibits amino acid homology with the constant region of immunoglobulin. Free β_2-microglobulin can be measured in both serum and urine. Levels of β_2-microglobulin are elevated in a variety of conditions characterized by lymphocyte activation and/or lymphocyte destruction; among these are lymphoproliferative syndromes, autoimmune diseases, and viral infections, including HIV infection. In addition, β_2-microglobulin is excreted by the renal tubules, and levels may be elevated in patients with renal disease. Levels of β_2-microglobulin correlate with the degree of progression of HIV disease. The highest levels are seen in patients with AIDS; the lowest levels in patients with asymptomatic HIV infection. The β_2-microglobulin level has a predictive value for progression to AIDS that is independent of its inverse relationship to CD4+ T cell counts. In one large study, the level of serum β_2-microglobulin was the single most important predictor of development of AIDS. In another study, 34 percent of patients with a β_2-microglobulin level of >3.8 µg/mL went on to develop AIDS over a 3-year period, compared to only 7 percent of patients with a β_2-microglobulin level of <2.9 µg/mL. Levels of β_2-microglobulin have been shown to decrease in a dose-dependent fashion in patients treated with zidovudine (AZT).

FIGURE 308-21   Relationship between CD4+ T cell counts and the development of opportunistic diseases. Boxplot of the median (line inside the box), first quartile (bottom of the box), third quartile (top of the box), and mean (asterisk) CD4+ lymphocyte count at the time of the development of opportunistic disease. Can, candidal esophagitis; CMV, cytomegalovirus infection; Crp, cryptosporidiosis; Cry, cryptococcal meningitis; DEM, AIDS dementia complex; HSV, herpes simplex virus infection; HZos, herpes zoster; KS, Kaposi's sarcoma; MAC, *Mycobacterium avium* complex bacteremia; NHL, non-Hodgkin's lymphoma; PCP, primary *Pneumocystis carinii* pneumonia; PCP2, secondary *Pneumocystis carinii* pneumonia; PML, progressive multifocal leukoencephalopathy; Tox, *Toxoplasma gondii* encephalitis; WS, wasting syndrome. (*From Moore & Chaisson.*)

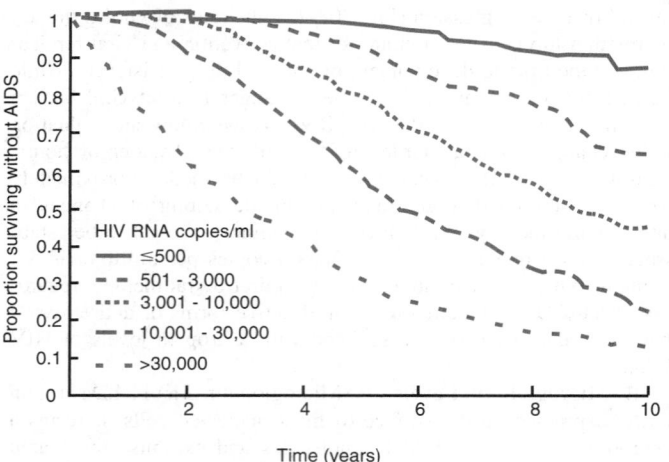

FIGURE 308-22 Relationship between levels of virus and rates of disease progression. Kaplan-Meier curves for AIDS-free survival stratified by baseline HIV-1 RNA categories (molecules per milliliter). *(From Mellors.)*

Neopterin Levels *Neopterin* (6-D-erythrotrihydroxypropylpterin) is a low-molecular-weight compound derived from an intermediate product of the de novo biosynthesis of tetrahydrobiopterin from guanosine triphosphate (GTP). It is produced by activated monocytes, and increased levels have been observed in patients with HIV infection. Elevated levels have also been reported in patients with other viral infections, autoimmune diseases, and atypical phenylketonuria, and in patients receiving immunostimulant therapy. As in the case of β_2-microglobulin, serum or urine levels of neopterin are highest in patients with advanced HIV disease and, in asymptomatic patients, higher levels are associated with an increased risk of progression to AIDS that is independent of CD4 + T cell count. Neopterin levels appear to measure a parameter linked to the same factor(s) that result in elevations in the level of β_2-microglobulin. The predictive value of these two parameters together does not exceed that provided by either one alone.

A variety of other nonviral laboratory tests have been studied as potential markers of HIV disease activity. Among these are circulating levels of soluble IL-2 receptor, IgA, acid-labile endogenous interferon, and TNFα. While each of these quantities may have some value as a marker of disease activity, they have not been evaluated as carefully as the parameters discussed above and at present do not play a major role in the laboratory monitoring of patients with HIV-1 infection.

CLINICAL MANIFESTATIONS

The clinical consequences of HIV infection encompass a spectrum ranging from an acute syndrome associated with primary infection to a prolonged asymptomatic state to advanced disease. It is best to regard HIV disease as beginning at the time of primary infection and progressing through various stages. As mentioned above, active virus replication and progressive immunologic impairment occur throughout the course of HIV infection in most patients. With the exception of long-term nonprogressors (see above), HIV disease inexorably progresses even during the clinically latent stage. HIV disease can be divided empirically on the basis of the degree of immunodeficiency into an early stage (CD4 + T cell count >500/µL), an intermediate stage (CD4 + T cell count 200 to 500/µL), and an advanced stage (CD4 + T cell count <200/µL). Most AIDS-defining opportunistic infections and true malignancies occur in the advanced stage of disease, while neurologic disease and Kaposi's sarcoma (see above) are not as strictly related to the degree of immunodeficiency. The two major classification systems for staging HIV disease are the CDC system (Table 308-11) and the Walter Reed Medical Center System (Table 308-12); these are to be distinguished from the case definition for

AIDS, which is used for surveillance purposes (Table 308-1). Each classification system has advantages and disadvantages; the CDC system relies more on clinical condition, and the Walter Reed system more on markers of immunologic status, such as the CD4 + T cell count and the presence or absence of delayed cutaneous hypersensitivity. For the purposes of describing the clinical syndromes seen in patients with HIV disease, this chapter devotes sections to the acute syndrome, the asymptomatic stage, early symptomatic disease, neurologic disease, secondary infections, neoplasms, and organ-specific syndromes.

THE ACUTE HIV SYNDROME It is estimated that 50 to 70 percent of individuals with HIV infection experience an acute clinical syndrome approximately 3 to 6 weeks after primary infection (Fig. 308-23). Varying degrees of clinical severity have been reported, and it has been suggested that symptomatic seroconversion leading to the seeking of medical attention indicates an increased risk for an accelerated course of disease. The typical clinical findings are listed in Table 308-13; they occur along with a burst of plasma viremia and p24 antigenemia. The syndrome is typical of an acute viral syndrome and has been likened to acute infectious mononucleosis. Symptoms usually persist for 1 to several weeks and gradually subside as an immune response to HIV develops and the levels of plasma viremia decrease. Opportunistic infections have been reported during this stage of infection, reflecting the immunodeficiency that results from reduced numbers of CD4 + T cells and likely also from functional suppression of CD4 + T cells owing to cross-linking of the CD4 molecule on the cell surface (see "Mechanisms of CD4 + T Lymphocyte Depletion and Dysfunction," above) as a result of the extremely high levels of plasma viremia. A number of immunologic abnormalities accompany the acute HIV syndrome, including multiphasic perturbations of the numbers of circulating lymphocyte subsets. Total lymphocyte and T cell subsets (CD4 + and CD8 +) are initially reduced. An inversion of the CD4 +/CD8 + T cell ratio occurs later because of a rise in the number of CD8 + T cells. In fact, there may be a selective and transient expansion of CD8 + T cell subsets, as determined by T cell receptor analysis (see above). The total circulating CD8 + T cell count may remain elevated or return to normal; however, CD4 + T cell levels usually remain somewhat depressed, although there may be a slight rebound towards normal. Lymphadenopathy occurs in approximately 70 percent of individuals with primary HIV infection. Most patients recover spontaneously from this syndrome and have a mildly depressed CD4 + T cell count that remains stable for a variable period before beginning its progressive decline (see below); in some individuals, the CD4 + T cell count returns to the normal range. Approximately 10 percent of patients manifest a fulminant course of immunologic and clinical deterioration after primary infection, even after the disappearance of symptoms. In most patients, primary infection with or without the acute syndrome is followed by a prolonged period of clinical latency.

THE ASYMPTOMATIC STAGE—CLINICAL LATENCY Although the length of time from initial infection to the development of clinical disease varies greatly, the median time is approximately 10 years. As emphasized above, HIV disease with active virus replication usually progresses during this asymptomatic period. The rate of disease progression is directly correlated with HIV RNA levels. Patients with

Table 308-11

Centers for Disease Control Classification System for HIV Disease

Group I	Acute HIV syndrome
Group II	Asymptomatic infection
Group III	Persistent generalized lymphadenopathy
Group IV	Other diseases
Subgroup A	Constitutional disease
Subgroup B	Neurologic disease
Subgroup C	Secondary infectious diseases
Subgroup D	Secondary neoplasms
Subgroup E	Other conditions

SOURCE: Modified from the Centers for Disease Control and Prevention, USPHS, 1986 and 1987.

Table 308-12

Walter Reed Staging Classification of HIV Infection

Stage	HIV Antibody	Chronic Lymphadenopathy	CD4+ Cell Count, Cells/μL	DTH Skin Testing	Thrush	Opportunistic Infections
WR0	−	−	>400	Normal (reactive to ≥2 skin test antigens)	−	−
WR1	+	−	>400	Normal	−	−
WR2	+	+	>400	Normal	−	−
WR3	+	+/−	<400	Normal	−	−
WR4	+	+/−	<400	Partial defect (reactive to 1 skin test antigen)	−	−
WR5	+	+/−	<400	Anergy and/or thrush (reactive to 0 skin test antigens)		−
WR6	+	+/−	<400	Normal, partial defect or anergy	+/−	+

NOTE: [   ], absolute criteria to be fulfilled for stage assignment; +, present; −, absent; DTH, delayed-type hypersensitivity.

SOURCE: Modified from Redfield et al.

high levels of HIV RNA progress to symptomatic disease faster than do patients with low levels of HIV RNA (Fig. 308-22). Some patients, called long-term nonprogressors (see above), show little if any decline in CD4+ T cell counts over an extended period. These patients generally have extremely low levels of HIV RNA. Certain other patients remain entirely asymptomatic despite the fact that their CD4+ T cell counts fall extremely low. In these patients, the appearance of an opportunistic disease may be the first manifestation of HIV infection. Some patients, otherwise asymptomatic, develop persistent generalized lymphadenopathy during this time (Table 308-11) (see below). With few exceptions, CD4+ T cell counts fall progressively during this asymptomatic period at an average rate of approximately 50 cells/μL per year. When the CD4+ cell count falls below about 200/μL, the resulting state of immunodeficiency is severe enough to place the patient at high risk for opportunistic infections and neoplasms, and hence for clinically apparent disease.

EARLY SYMPTOMATIC DISEASE As noted above, viral replication continues during the period of clinical latency, and the immunologic function of the HIV-infected individual usually declines progressively. At some point, usually after the CD4+ T cell count has fallen below 500/μL, patients begin to develop signs and symptoms of clinical illness (Table 308-14). Many of these problems can be traced to minor opportunistic infections, not sufficiently indicative of a defect in cell-mediated immunity to be considered AIDS-defining illnesses, while some of them appear to be direct effects of long-standing HIV infection. This stage of HIV infection has been given a variety of names in the past, among them *pre-AIDS* and *AIDS-related complex* (ARC); however, these terms are rarely used today. The clinical findings at this stage of disease (described below), while indicative of a decline in immune function, are generally less predictive

of the patient's overall status than are the data obtained from serial measurements of CD4+ T cell counts.

Generalized Lymphadenopathy This condition, defined as the presence of enlarged lymph nodes (>1 cm) in two or more extrainguinal sites for more than 3 months without an obvious cause, is often the earliest symptom of HIV infection after primary infection. It is due to marked follicular hyperplasia in response to HIV infection, and the nodes are generally discrete and freely movable. This feature of HIV disease, which may be seen at any point in the spectrum of immune dysfunction, is not associated with an increased likelihood of developing AIDS. Paradoxically, a loss in lymphadenopathy or a decrease in lymph node size may be a prognostic marker of disease progression. In the early and intermediate stages of HIV infection (CD4+ T cell counts >200/μL), the main differential diagnosis is an adenopathic form of Kaposi's sarcoma. Late in the course of disease, differential diagnosis expands to include lymphoma, mycobacterial infection, toxoplasmosis, systemic fungal infection, and bacillary angiomatosis. Lymph node biopsy is not indicated in patients with early-stage disease unless there are signs and symptoms of systemic illness, such as fever and weight loss, or unless the nodes begin to enlarge, become fixed, or coalesce.

Oral Lesions Oral lesions, including thrush, hairy leukoplakia, and aphthous ulcers, are particularly common during this phase of HIV infection. Thrush, due to *Candida* infection, and oral hairy leukoplakia, presumed due to Epstein-Barr virus, are usually indicative of fairly advanced immunologic decline, generally occurring in patients with fewer than 300 CD4+ T cells per microliter. In one study, 59 percent of patients with oral candidiasis went on to develop AIDS in the next year. Thrush appears as a white, cheesy exudate, often on an erythematous mucosa **(see Plate ID-42)**. While most commonly seen on the soft palate, early lesions are often found along the gingival border. The diagnosis is made by direct examination of a scraping for pseudohyphal elements. Culturing is of no value, as most patients with HIV infection have a positive throat culture for *Candida* even in the absence of thrush. Oral hairy leukoplakia presents as a filamentous white lesion, generally along the lateral borders of the tongue **(see**

Table 308-13

Clinical Findings in the Acute HIV Syndrome

General	Neurologic
Fever	Meningitis
Pharyngitis	Encephalitis
Lymphadenopathy	Peripheral neuropathy
Headache/retroorbital pain	Myelopathy
Arthralgias/myalgias	Dermatologic
Lethargy/malaise	Erythematous maculopapular rash
Anorexia/weight loss	Mucocutaneous ulceration
Nausea/vomiting/diarrhea	

SOURCE: From Tyndal and Cooper.

FIGURE 308-23 The acute HIV syndrome. See text for detailed description. (*From G Pantaleo et al, N Engl J Med 328:327, 1993.*)

Table 308-14

Clinical Characteristics of Early Symptomatic Disease

Generalized lymphadenopathy
Thrush
Oral hairy leukoplakia
Shingles
Thrombocytopenia
Molluscum contagiosum
Recurrent herpes simplex
Condyloma acuminata
Aphthous ulcers

Plate ID-41). While usually more a sign of HIV-induced immunodeficiency than a clinical problem, severe cases have responded to therapy with acyclovir. Aphthous ulcers of the posterior oropharynx are also seen with regularity in patients with HIV infection. These lesions are of unknown etiology and can be quite painful and interfere with swallowing. Topical anesthetics provide immediate symptomatic relief of short duration. The fact that thalidomide is an effective treatment for this condition suggests that the pathogenesis may involve the action of tissue-destructive cytokines.

Reactivation Herpes Zoster (Shingles) This condition (**see Plate ID-37**) is seen in 10 to 20 percent of patients with HIV infection. This reactivation syndrome of varicella-zoster virus indicates a modest decline in immune function and is often the first clinical indication of immunodeficiency. In one series, patients who developed shingles did so an average of 5 years after HIV infection. In a cohort of patients with HIV infection, AIDS developed in 1 percent per month of the cohort after a diagnosis of localized zoster. In that study, AIDS was more likely to develop in patients with severe pain, extensive disease, or disease involving cranial or cervical dermatomes. In patients who developed shingles and oral hairy leukoplakia or thrush, shingles preceded the oral lesions by approximately 1 year. The clinical manifestations of reactivation zoster in HIV-infected patients, although indicative of immunologic compromise, are not as severe as those seen in other immunodeficient conditions. Thus, while lesions may extend over several dermatomes and frank cutaneous dissemination may be seen, visceral involvement has not been reported. In contrast to patients without a known underlying immunodeficiency state, patients with HIV infection tend to have recurrences of zoster, with a relapse rate of approximately 20 percent.

Thrombocytopenia Thrombocytopenia also may be an early consequence of HIV infection. Approximately 3 percent of patients with HIV infection and CD4+ T cell counts above $400/\mu L$ have platelet counts under $150,000/\mu L$. For patients with CD4+ T cell counts below $400/\mu L$, this incidence increases to 10 percent. Thrombocytopenia is rarely a serious clinical problem in these patients. Most such patients retain platelet counts above $50,000/\mu L$, and the condition can be managed conservatively. As in other forms of thrombocytopenia, bleeding is rare unless the count falls below $10,000/\mu L$, and bleeding of the gums, extremity petechiae, and easy bruisability are common presenting features. Bone marrow examination, which should be done to rule out other causes of thrombocytopenia, including drug toxicity, lymphoma, fungal infection, and mycobacterial infection, generally reveals a normal or increased number of megakaryocytes. In this regard, the idiopathic thrombocytopenia seen in patients with HIV infection is very similar to the thrombocytopenia seen in patients with idiopathic thrombocytopenic purpura (see Chap. 117). Immune complexes containing anti-gp120 antibodies and anti-anti-gp120 antibodies have been noted in the circulation and on the surface of platelets in patients with HIV infection. Patients with HIV infection also have been noted to have a platelet-specific antibody directed toward a 25-kDa component of the surface of the platelet. Because these data point to an immunologic basis for the thrombocytopenia seen in patients with AIDS, most of the therapeutic interventions that have been em-

ployed have been immune-based. Both high-dose intravenous immunoglobulin (IVIG) and glucocorticoids can induce a transient increase in platelet count, but they do not generally provide a long-term solution. It has been suggested that the thrombocytopenia in patients with HIV infection may be due to a direct effect of HIV on megakaryocytes, as evidenced by a decrease in platelet production. Consistent with this idea is the fact that the most effective medical approach to this problem has been the use of antiretroviral agents. Even in patients without thrombocytopenia, therapy with zidovudine has been associated with a significant increase in platelet count. Approximately 70 percent of patients with HIV-associated thrombocytopenia show a satisfactory response to zidovudine. Before combination antiretroviral therapy became the preferred treatment for HIV infection (see below), zidovudine alone was considered the treatment of choice for HIV-associated thrombocytopenia. Now, a combination of antiretroviral drugs that includes zidovudine is the treatment of choice. For patients with platelet counts below $20,000/\mu L$, the approach should be initial treatment with IVIG or glucocorticoids for an immediate response, coupled with combination antiretroviral therapy for a more lasting response. Splenectomy is an option in patients refractory to medical management. Most patients with HIV-associated thrombocytopenia will respond to this surgical treatment. Because of the risk of serious infections with encapsulated organisms, physicians should ensure that all patients with HIV infection, especially those about to undergo splenectomy, are immunized with pneumococcal polysaccharide. It should be noted that, in addition to causing an increase in the platelet count, removal of the spleen will result in an increase in the peripheral blood lymphocyte count, making CD4+ T cell counts unreliable. In this situation, one should rely on the CD4 percent for making diagnostic decisions with respect to the likelihood of opportunistic infections. In patients with early HIV infection, thrombocytopenia has also been reported as a consequence of classic thrombotic thrombocytopenic purpura (see Chap. 117). This clinical syndrome, consisting of fever, thrombocytopenia, hemolytic anemia, and neurologic and renal dysfunction, is a rare complication of early HIV infection. As in other settings, the appropriate management is the use of salicylates and plasma exchange.

Miscellaneous Clinical Conditions Other conditions frequently seen in patients with early-stage HIV infection include molluscum contagiosum, basal cell carcinomas of the skin, headache, condyloma acuminata, and recurrent bouts of oral or genital herpes simplex. In the past, unexplained fever, weight loss, and diarrhea were included under the general heading of ARC. Many of these cases are now being diagnosed as specific opportunistic infections. In addition, this syndrome has been classified as an AIDS-defining illness in patients in whom no other diagnosis can be found; it is discussed below in the section "Generalized Wasting."

NEUROLOGIC DISEASE Clinical disease of the nervous system accounts for a significant degree of morbidity in a high percentage of patients with HIV infection (Table 308-15). The neurologic problems that occur in HIV-infected individuals may be either primary to the pathogenic processes of HIV infection or secondary to opportunistic infections or neoplasms. Among the opportunistic infections and neoplasms that involve the central nervous system (CNS) are toxoplasmosis, cryptococcosis, progressive multifocal leukoencephalopathy, infection with cytomegalovirus, HTLV-I, or *Mycobacterium tuberculosis*, syphilis, and primary CNS lymphoma. As a group, these diseases occur in about one-third of patients with AIDS; they are discussed in more detail below. Primary processes related to HIV infection of the nervous system are somewhat similar to those seen with other lentiviruses, such as the Visna-Maedi virus of sheep. Neurologic problems occur throughout the course of disease and may be inflammatory, demyelinating, or degenerative in nature. While only one of these, the AIDS dementia complex, or HIV encephalopathy, is considered an AIDS-defining illness, most HIV-infected patients have some neurologic problem during the course of their disease. As noted in the section on pathogenesis, damage to the CNS may be a direct result of viral infection of CNS macrophages or glial cells or may be secondary to the release of neurotoxins and potentially toxic cytokines such

Table 308-15

Table 308-15

Neurologic Diseases in Patients with HIV Infection

Opportunistic infections
  Toxoplasmosis
  Cryptococcosis
  Progressive multifocal leukoencephalopathy
  Cytomegalovirus
  Syphilis
  Mycobacterium tuberculosis
  HTLV-I infection
Neoplasms
  Primary CNS lymphoma
  Kaposi's sarcoma
Result of HIV-1 infection
  Aseptic meningitis
  AIDS dementia complex (HIV encephalopathy)
  Myelopathy
    Vacuolar myelopathy
    Pure sensory ataxia
    Paresthesia/dysesthesia
  Peripheral neuropathy
    Acute demyelinating polyneuropathy
    Mononeuritis multiplex
    Distal symmetric polyneuropathy
  Myopathy

as IL-1β, TNFα, IL-6, and TGFβ. Virtually all patients with HIV infection have some degree of involvement of the nervous system with HIV. This is evidenced by the fact that cerebrospinal fluid (CSF) findings are abnormal in approximately 90 percent of patients, even during the asymptomatic stage of HIV infection. Included among these abnormalities are pleocytosis (50 to 65 percent of patients), isolation of virus (approximately 50 percent), elevated CSF protein level (35 percent), and evidence of intrathecal synthesis of anti-HIV antibodies (89 percent). It should be pointed out, however, that evidence of infection of the CNS with HIV does not imply impairment of cognitive function, and, while neurologic problems related to HIV infection can be seen at all stages of disease, the mere presence of HIV infection in the CNS does not mean that the patient has a clinically relevant neurologic problem. The neurologic function of an HIV-infected individual should be considered normal unless clinical signs and symptoms suggest otherwise.

Aseptic Meningitis Aseptic meningitis may be seen in any but the very late stages of HIV infection. In the setting of acute primary infection (see above) patients may experience a syndrome of headache, photophobia, and, in some instances, frank encephalitis. CSF findings include a lymphocytic pleocytosis, elevated protein level, and normal glucose level. Cranial nerve involvement may be seen, predominantly cranial nerve VII, occasionally V, and/or VIII. This syndrome usually resolves spontaneously within 2 to 4 weeks; however, in some patients, signs and symptoms persist chronically. Such episodes may occur any time in the course of HIV infection; however, they become increasingly rare following the development of AIDS. This fact suggests that aseptic meningitis in the context of HIV infection is an immune-mediated disease.

HIV Encephalopathy HIV encephalopathy, also called *HIV-associated dementia* or *AIDS dementia complex*, consists of a constellation of signs and symptoms of CNS disease that generally occurs late in the course of HIV infection (Table 308-16). A major feature of this entity is the development of dementia, which is defined as a decline in cognitive ability from a previous level. It may present as impaired ability to concentrate, increased forgetfulness, difficulty reading, or increased difficulty performing complex tasks. Initially these symptoms may be indistinguishable from findings of situational depression or fatigue. In addition to dementia, patients with HIV encephalopathy also may have motor and behavioral abnormalities. Among the motor problems are unsteady gait, poor balance, tremor, and difficulty with rapid alternating movements. Increased tone and deep tendon reflexes may be found in patients with spinal cord involvement (see below). Late stages may be complicated by bowel and/or bladder incontinence.

Behavioral problems include apathy and lack of initiative, with progression to a vegetative state in some instances. Some patients develop a state of agitation or mild mania. These changes usually occur without significant changes in level of alertness, in contrast to the findings in patients with dementia due to toxic/metabolic encephalopathies.

HIV encephalopathy is the initial AIDS-defining illness in approximately 3 percent of patients with HIV infection and thus only rarely precedes clinical evidence of immunodeficiency. Clinically significant HIV encephalopathy eventually develops in approximately one-fourth of patients with HIV infection. As immunologic function declines, the risk and severity of HIV encephalopathy increase. Autopsy series suggest that 80 to 90 percent of patients with HIV infection have histologic evidence of CNS involvement. Several classification schemes have been developed for grading HIV encephalopathy. The most commonly used clinical staging system is outlined in Table 308-16.

The precise cause of HIV encephalopathy remains unclear, although the condition is thought to be a result of direct effects of HIV on the CNS. HIV has been found in the brains of patients with HIV encephalopathy by Southern blot, in situ hybridization, PCR, and electron microscopy. Multinucleated giant cells, macrophages, and microglial cells appear to be the main cell types harboring virus in the CNS. Histologically, the major changes are seen in the subcortical areas of the brain and thus fall in the general category of subcortical dementia. In this regard, HIV encephalopathy is similar to the dementia seen in patients with Parkinson's disease (see Chap. 368) and Huntington's chorea (see Chap. 367) and distinct from that seen in patients with Alzheimer's disease (see Chap. 367). Among the histopathologic changes are pallor and gliosis, multinucleated giant cell encephalitis, and vacuolar myelopathy. Less commonly, diffuse or focal spongiform changes in the white matter occur.

There are no specific criteria for a diagnosis of HIV encephalopathy, and this syndrome thus must be distinguished from a number of other diseases that affect the CNS of HIV-infected patients (Table 308-17). The diagnosis of dementia depends on demonstrating a de-

Table 308-16

Clinical Staging of HIV Encephalopathy (AIDS Dementia Complex)

Stage	Definition
Stage 0 (normal)	Normal mental and motor function
Stage 0.5 (equivocal/ subclinical)	Absent, minimal, or equivocal symptoms without impairment of work or capacity to perform activities of daily living. Mild signs (snout response, slowed ocular or extremity movements) may be present. Gait and strength are normal.
Stage 1 (mild)	Able to perform all but the more demanding aspects of work or activities of daily living but with unequivocal evidence (signs or symptoms that may include performance on neuropsychological testing) of functional, intellectual, or motor impairment. Can walk without assistance.
Stage 2 (moderate)	Able to perform basic activities of self-care but cannot work or maintain the more demanding aspects of daily life. Ambulatory, but may require a single prop.
Stage 3 (severe)	Major intellectual incapacity (cannot follow news or personal events, cannot sustain complex conversation, considerable slowing of all output) or motor disability (cannot walk unassisted, usually with slowing and clumsiness of arms as well).
Stage 4 (end-stage)	Nearly vegetative. Intellectual and social comprehension and output are at a rudimentary level. Nearly or absolutely mute. Paraparetic or paraplegic with urinary and fecal incontinence.

SOURCE: Adapted from JJ Sidtis, RW Price, Neurology 40:197, 1990.

Table 308-17

Characterization of the Most Common Central Nervous System Diseases in Patients with HIV Infection

Disease	Approximate Incidence, %	Clinical Features	Characteristic CSF Findings	Characteristic Radiologic Findings
HIV encephalopathy (AIDS dementia complex)	25	Personality changes, dementia, unsteady gait, seizures	Nonspecific increases in cells and protein	Cortical atrophy, ventricular dilation, bright spots on T2-weighted MRI
Toxoplasmosis	15	Fever, headache, focal neurologic deficits, seizures, + antibodies in 95%	Nonspecific	Single or multiple ring-enhancing lesions in multiple locations
Cryptococcal meningitis	6–12	Fever, nausea, vomiting, confusion, headache	Elevated protein, low glucose, positive cryptococcal antigen or culture	Nonspecific
Progressive multifocal leukoencephalopathy	4	Multiple focal deficits without changes in level of consciousness	Nonspecific	Multiple white matter lesions on T2-weighted MRI images
Neurosyphilis	1	Meningitis, neuroretinitis, deafness, focal neurologic deficits	Positive VDRL, elevated protein, increase in cells	Nonspecific
Lymphoma	1	Seizure, focal neurologic deficits, headache	Nonspecific in primary CNS lymphoma; malignant cells in systemic lymphoma	Single or few ring-enhancing lesions
Tuberculous meningitis	1	Fever, headache, confusion, meningitis, cough	Elevated protein, low glucose, pleocytosis, positive smear/culture for acid-fast bacilli (AFB)	Mass lesions in approximately 50%, abnormal chest x-ray

cline in cognitive function. This can be accomplished objectively with the use of the Mini-Mental Status Examination (Table 308-18) in patients for whom prior scores are available. For this reason, it is advisable for all patients with a diagnosis of HIV infection to have a baseline Mini-Mental Status Examination. Imaging studies of the CNS, by either computed tomography (CT) or magnetic resonance imaging (MRI), often demonstrate evidence of cerebral atrophy (Fig. 308-24). MRI may also reveal small areas of increased density on T2-weighted images.

Table 308-18

The Folstein Mini-Mental Status Examination

Question	Scoring	Maximum Score
1. Where are you (state, county, city, hospital, clinic)?	1 point for each	5
2. What are the (day, date, month, season, year, time)?	1 point for each	5
3. "Say these three words after me: (yellow, apple, Ohio)."	1 point for each	3
4. Ask patient to begin with 100 and count backwards by 7's. Or, if patient refuses, ask to spell "world" backwards.	Stop after 5, score no. correct Or 1 point for each correct letter	5
5. Recall the three words given in question no. 3.	1 point for each	3
6. Ask the patient to name "watch" then "pencil".	1 point for each	2
7. Ask the patient to repeat "No ifs, ands, or buts."	1 point if correct	1
8. Three-stage command: Take this paper in your right hand, fold it in half, and put it on the door.	1 point for each correct	3
9. Ask the patient to read silently and obey the command (print in block letters): CLOSE YOUR EYES.	1 point if correct	1
10. Ask the patient to write a sentence.	1 point if contains a subject and verb and makes sense (ignore spelling and grammar)	1
11. Draw a clock with numbers and hands showing the time to be 8:20	2 points if correct	2
12. Have the patient copy this design:	1 point if all sides and angles are preserved and if intersecting sides form a quadrangle	1

While a lumbar puncture is an important element of the evaluation of patients with HIV infection and neurologic abnormalities, it is generally most helpful in the diagnosis of opportunistic infections. In HIV encephalopathy, patients may have an increase in CSF cells and protein level; however, these findings are nonspecific, and the diagnosis is truly one that can be made only after opportunistic pathogens and neoplasms have been ruled out. While HIV can often be isolated from the CSF of these patients, this finding is not specific for HIV encephalopathy and, in fact, there appears to be no correlation between the presence of HIV in the CSF and the presence of HIV encephalopathy. Elevated levels of β_2-microglobulin, neopterin, and quinolinic acid (a metabolite of tryptophan reported to cause CNS injury) have been noted in the CSF of patients with AIDS dementia complex. These findings suggest that these factors as well as inflammatory cytokines may be involved in the pathogenesis of this syndrome; however, at this time definitive evidence is still lacking.

While there is no specific treatment for HIV encephalopathy, multiple reports suggest that treatment with antiretroviral agents may be of benefit. Improvement in neuropsychiatric test scores have been noted for both adult and pediatric patients treated with either zidovudine or didanosine. In fact, the rapid symptomatic improvement in cognitive function noted with the initiation of antiretroviral therapy suggests that at least some component of this problem is quickly reversible, again supporting at least a partial role of soluble mediators in the pathogenesis. It should also be noted that these patients have an increased sensitivity to the side effects of neuroleptic drugs. The use of these drugs for symptomatic treatment is associated with an increased risk of extrapyramidal

FIGURE 308-24 Computed tomogram of the central nervous system of a patient with AIDS dementia complex. CT demonstrates cortical thinning and dilation of the ventricles.

side effects, so patients with HIV encephalopathy who receive these agents must be monitored carefully.

Seizures Seizures are a relatively frequent complication of HIV infection and may be a consequence of opportunistic infections, neoplasms, or HIV encephalopathy (Table 308-19). The seizure threshold is often lower than normal in these patients owing to the frequent presence of electrolyte abnormalities. Seizures are seen in 15 to 40 percent of patients with cerebral toxoplasmosis, 15 to 35 percent of patients with primary CNS lymphoma, 8 percent of patients with cryptococcal meningitis, and 7 to 50 percent of patients with HIV encephalopathy. Seizures may also be seen in patients with CNS tuberculosis, aseptic meningitis, and progressive multifocal leukoencephalopathy. Seizures may be the presenting clinical symptom of HIV disease. In one study of 100 patients with HIV infection presenting with a first seizure, cerebral mass lesions were the most common cause, responsible for 32 of the 100 new-onset seizures. Of these 32 cases, 28 were due to toxoplasmosis and 4 to lymphoma. HIV encephalopathy accounted for an additional 24 new-onset seizures. Cryptococcal meningitis was the third most common diagnosis, responsible for 13 of the 100 seizures. In 23 cases, no cause could be found; it is possible that these cases represent a subcategory of HIV encephalopathy. Of these 23 cases, 16 (70 percent) had two or more seizures, suggesting that anticonvulsant therapy is indicated in all patients with HIV infection and seizures unless a rapidly correctable cause is found. While phenytoin remains the initial treatment of choice, hypersensitivity reactions to this drug have been reported in over 10 percent of patients with AIDS, and therefore the use of phenobarbital or valproic acid must be considered as alternatives.

Table 308-19

Causes of Seizures in Patients with HIV Infection

Disease	Overall Contribution to First Seizure, %	Fraction of Patients Who Have Seizures, %
AIDS dementia complex	24–47	7–50
Cerebral toxoplasmosis	28	15–40
Cryptococcal meningitis	13	8
Primary central nervous system lymphoma	4	15–30
Progressive multifocal leukoencephalopathy	1	

SOURCE: From Holtzman et al.

Spinal Cord Disease Spinal cord disease, or myelopathy, is present in approximately 20 percent of patients with AIDS, often as part of HIV encephalopathy. In fact, 90 percent of the patients with HIV-associated myelopathy have some evidence of dementia, suggesting that similar pathologic processes may be responsible for both conditions. Three main types of spinal cord disease are seen in patients with AIDS. The first of these is a vacuolar myelopathy, as discussed above under HIV encephalopathy. This condition is pathologically similar to subacute combined degeneration of the cord such as occurs with pernicious anemia. Although vitamin B_{12} deficiency is common in patients with AIDS, it does not appear to be responsible for the cord disease seen in these patients, given that there is no response to treatment with parenteral vitamin B_{12}. Vacuolar myelopathy is characterized by a subacute onset and often presents with gait disturbances, predominantly ataxia and spasticity; it may progress to include bladder and bowel dysfunction. Physical findings include evidence of increased deep tendon reflexes and extensor plantar responses. The second form of spinal cord disease involves the dorsal columns and presents as a pure sensory ataxia. The third form is also sensory in nature and presents with paresthesias and dysesthesias of the lower extremities. In contrast to the cognitive problems seen in patients with HIV encephalopathy, these spinal cord syndromes do not generally respond to therapy with antiretroviral drugs, and therapy is mainly supportive. One exception is a polyradiculopathy associated with cytomegalovirus (CMV). This entity is generally seen late in the course of HIV infection and is fulminant in onset, with lower extremity and sacral paresthesias, difficulty in walking, areflexia, ascending sensory loss, and urinary retention. CSF examination reveals a predominantly neutrophilic pleocytosis. Therapy with ganciclovir or foscarnet can lead to rapid improvement. Other diseases involving the spinal cord in patients with HIV infection include HTLV-I-associated myelopathy (HAM) (see Chap. 192), neurosyphilis (see Chap. 174), herpesvirus infections (varicella-zoster, simplex, and CMV) (see Chaps. 184 and 185), tuberculosis (see Chap. 171), and lymphoma (see Chap. 113).

Peripheral Neuropathies Peripheral neuropathies are common in patients with HIV infection; they occur at all stages of illness and take a variety of forms. Early in the course of HIV infection, an acute inflammatory demyelinating polyneuropathy resembling Guillain-Barré syndrome may occur (see Chap. 376). Patients commonly present with progressive weakness, areflexia, and minimal sensory changes. CSF examination reveals a pleocytosis, and peripheral nerve biopsy demonstrates a perivascular infiltrate suggesting an autoimmune etiology. Although generally a self-limited disease, in severe cases plasma exchange, intravenous immunoglobulin, or systemic glucocorticoids have been tried with variable degrees of success. Because of the immunosuppressive effects of glucocorticoids, they should be reserved for severe cases refractory to other measures. Another autoimmune peripheral neuropathy seen in patients with AIDS is mononeuritis multiplex (see Chap. 319). This necrotizing arteritis of peripheral nerves generally occurs in patients with a moderate degree of immunodeficiency and may be managed as outlined above. The most common peripheral neuropathy in patients with HIV infection is a distal sensory polyneuropathy, generally seen in patients with advanced HIV infection. Although it is present clinically in 30 to 40 percent of patients, two-thirds of patients with AIDS may be shown by electrophysiologic studies to have some evidence of peripheral nerve disease. This polyneuropathy, which is felt to be due to HIV-mediated axonal degeneration, most often presents as symmetric bilateral painful burning sensations in the feet and lower extremities. Antiretroviral agents have been of little benefit in the management of this problem and in fact may be the causative agent in some instances. Dideoxynucleoside-associated peripheral neuropathy may be a painful complication of didanosine, zalcitabine, or stavudine therapy, is most commonly seen at higher doses, and usually resolves following discontinuation of therapy. It is discussed in more detail below in relation to antiretroviral agents. Other entities in the differential diagnosis include diabetes mellitus, vitamin B_{12} deficiency, and side effects from flagyl or dapsone. For distal sensory polyneuropathy of unknown cause that fails to resolve following the discontinuation of dideoxynucleosides, therapy is symptomatic, involving the use of tricyclics and analgesics. Nerve growth factor is being investigated as a possible agent in this setting.

Myopathy Myopathy may also complicate the course of HIV infection. Among the causes of myopathy in the setting of HIV infection are HIV itself, zidovudine, and the generalized wasting syndrome. HIV-associated myopathy may range in severity from an asymptomatic elevation in creatine kinase to a subacute syndrome characterized by proximal muscle weakness and myalgias. Quite pronounced elevations in creatine kinase may occur in asymptomatic patients, particularly after exercise. The clinical significance of this finding is unclear. A variety of both inflammatory and noninflammatory pathologic processes have been noted in patients with more severe myopathy, including myofiber necrosis with inflammatory cells, nemaline rod bodies, cytoplasmic bodies, and mitochondrial abnormalities. Profound muscle wasting may be seen after prolonged zidovudine therapy. This toxic side effect of the drug appears to be related to its ability to interfere with the function of mitochondrial polymerases and is reversible following discontinuation of treatment. Histologically, red ragged fibers are a characteristic feature.

OPPORTUNISTIC INFECTIONS

Opportunistic infections are late complications of HIV infection, for the most part occurring in patients with less than 200 CD4+ T cells per microliter. While the causative agents characteristically are opportunistic organisms, such as *Pneumocystis carinii*, *Mycobacterium avium* complex, CMV, and other organisms that do not ordinarily cause disease in the absence of a compromised immune system, they also include common bacterial and mycobacterial pathogens. Opportunistic infections are the leading cause of morbidity and mortality in patients with HIV infection. Approximately 80 percent of AIDS patients die as a direct result of an infection other than HIV, with bacterial infections heading the list. The clinical spectrum of diseases caused by opportunistic infections is constantly changing as patients live longer and as new and better approaches to treatment and prophylaxis are developed.

PROTOZOAL INFECTIONS Pneumocystis carinii Infection (See Chap. 211) *P. carinii* is one of the most common causes of infection in patients with HIV infection; however, with the development of effective prophylactic regimens, the incidence of *P. carinii* infection and its relative contribution to morbidity and mortality have been decreasing. *P. carinii* pneumonia (PCP) is the initial AIDS-defining illness in close to 20 percent of patients, and approximately 50 percent of patients with HIV infection experience at least one bout of PCP during the course of their disease. As a result of increased awareness, improved diagnosis, and better treatment, the probability of death from a single episode of PCP has decreased from as high as 50 percent to 2 percent. Because of the AIDS epidemic, PCP has become a growing cause of community-acquired pneumonia. While the mode of transmission is unclear, infections with PCP probably represent reactivation of latent infection or failure of host defense mechanisms to suppress a ubiquitous microorganism. In the hospital setting, person-to-person spread of infection has been suggested anecdotally, and some feel it is prudent not to place a patient at risk for PCP (for example, an HIV-infected patient with fewer than 200 CD4+ T cells/μL) in the same room with someone suffering from an acute episode of PCP. Data are insufficient to make this a recommendation as standard practice. The risk of infection with *P. carinii* increases as the CD4+ T cell count declines. Among HIV-infected patients, PCP is most commonly seen among those who have experienced a previous bout of PCP and those who have fewer than 200 CD4+ T cells per microliter. In the absence of PCP prophylaxis, following a primary bout of PCP, 31 percent of HIV-infected individuals experience a second bout within 6 months, and 66 percent within 12 months. For

patients with more than 200 CD4+ T cells per microliter, the attack rate for PCP is approximately 0.5 percent over a 6-month period. In contrast, for patients with less than 200 CD4+ T cells per microliter, the attack rate is 8 percent over 6 months and 18 percent over 12 months. For this reason, it is recommended that all patients with HIV infection who have either experienced a previous bout of PCP or have a CD4+ T cell count of <200/μL (or a CD4 percentage of less than 15), receive some form of PCP prophylaxis (discussed below). Owing to the implementation of these guidelines, the incidence of primary PCP for patients with HIV infection and CD4+ T cell counts of <300/μL has dropped to 8.9 cases per 100 person-years, and the incidence of secondary PCP has dropped to 5.1 cases per 100 person-years. Primary PCP is now occurring at a median CD4+ T cell count of 36/μL, while secondary PCP is occurring at a median CD4+ T cell count of 10/μL.

As suggested by its name, the most common manifestation of infection with *P. carinii* is pneumonia. Patients generally present with fever and a cough that is usually nonproductive or productive of only scant amounts of white sputum. They may complain of a characteristic retrosternal chest pain, which is usually worse on inspiration and described as either sharp or burning. In more severe cases, patients usually note dyspnea on exertion, fatigue, and weight loss. In stark contrast to PCP in the non-HIV setting, which is often a fulminant disease with patients usually presenting within 5 days of the onset of symptoms, HIV-associated PCP may have an indolent course characterized by weeks of vague symptoms prior to presentation or diagnosis. PCP should be included in the differential diagnosis of fever, pulmonary symptoms, or unexplained weight loss in any patient with HIV infection and fewer than 200 CD4+ T cells per microliter. Findings on physical examination are minimal, and the usual findings for pneumonia may not be present. Breath sounds are usually clear but may be slightly diminished. While occasional rhonchi or wheezes may be heard, especially in patients with some other underlying pulmonary disease, findings of consolidation are usually absent. While chest x-ray may reveal a variety of patterns, the most common finding is either a normal film, if the disease is suspected early, or a faint bilateral interstitial infiltrate. The classic finding of a dense, perihilar infiltrate described in patients with non-HIV-associated PCP is rarely seen in patients with AIDS. In patients with PCP who have been receiving aerosolized pentamidine for prophylaxis, one may see a chest x-ray pattern with upper lobe cavitary disease, reminiscent of tuberculosis. Other less common findings on chest film include lobar infiltrates and pleural effusions.

PCP is complicated by pneumothorax in approximately 2 percent of cases. Pneumothorax is more common in patients with prior episodes of PCP and in patients who have received aerosolized pentamidine for prophylaxis, presumably owing to the tendency of these patients to have apical cavitary disease. The mortality for patients with PCP-associated pneumothorax is approximately 10 percent, and aggressive medical (sclerotherapy) and/or surgical intervention may be required.

The laboratory evaluation is usually of little help in the differential diagnosis of PCP. A mild leukocytosis is common; however, given the fact that HIV-infected patients generally have leukopenia with baseline WBC values in the range of 1500 to 3000 cells/μL, a WBC on the order of 4000 to 6000/μL may represent an elevation. The serum lactate dehydrogenase (LDH) level is often elevated, and arterial blood gases may indicate hypoxemia, with a decline in Pa_{O_2} and an increase in the arterial-alveolar (a-A) gradient. Arterial blood gas measurements not only aid in making the diagnosis of PCP but also provide important information for staging the severity of the disease and directing treatment (see below and Chap. 211).

A definitive diagnosis of PCP requires demonstration of the trophozoite or cyst form of the organisms in samples obtained from induced sputum, bronchoalveolar lavage, transbronchial biopsy, or open lung biopsy (see Chap. 211). The diagnosis may be somewhat more difficult to make in patients who have been receiving aerosolized pentamidine for PCP prophylaxis, as the burden of organisms may be reduced. In this setting, the diagnostic yield from induced sputum decreases from 92 percent to 64 percent, while the yield from bronchoalveolar lavage

Table 308-20

CHAPTER 308
HIV Disease: AIDS and Related Disorders **1825**

Extrapulmonary Manifestations of *Pneumocystis carinii* Infection in Patients with HIV Infection

Acute otitis
Retinitis
Visceral cystic calcifications
Necrotizing vasculitis
Intestinal obstruction
Lymphadenopathy
Bone marrow involvement
Ascites
Thyroiditis

drops from 95 percent to 80 percent. More recently, PCR has been used in an attempt to identify specific DNA sequences for *P. carinii* in clinical specimens. This technique may provide somewhat better sensitivity than that obtained through histologic staining. The differential diagnosis of PCP in patients with HIV infection includes CMV pneumonia, fungal pneumonia, nonspecific interstitial pneumonitis, tuberculosis, and Kaposi's sarcoma (see below).

In addition to pneumonia, a number of other clinical problems have been reported in the HIV-infected patients as a result of infection with *P. carinii*. Many of these reports involve patients receiving aerosolized pentamidine as prophylaxis for PCP. This form of prophylaxis, while quite effective in preventing PCP, is ineffective in preventing disease outside the lung and has largely been replaced by oral systemic prophylaxis. *P. carinii* appears to be capable of hematogenous spread and of seeding a variety of organ systems as well as causing a primary infection of the ear (Table 308-20). "Extrapulmonary" manifestations of *P. carinii* infection occur in approximately 2.5 to 5.0 percent of patients with HIV infection.

Otic involvement with *P. carinii* is most commonly seen as a primary infection, i.e., in patients with no evidence of pulmonary disease. It usually presents as a unilateral polypoid mass that involves the external auditory canal. It may also involve the middle ear and may extend to the mastoid, resulting in radiographic abnormalities on plain films of the skull. Patients often complain of ear pain and decreased hearing. Perforation of the tympanic membrane has been reported in over half of the cases. In contrast, most of the other extrapulmonary forms of pneumocystosis are seen in patients with a history of PCP. Most common in this group are ophthalmic lesions of the choroid, which are usually noted on routine examination or in the context of evaluation for CMV retinitis. Multiple, bilateral lesions 0.5 to 2 disc diameters in size that appear as slightly elevated yellow-white plaques are generally seen. They are usually asymptomatic and are often confused with the cotton-wool spots of the retina associated with HIV infection. *P. carinii* has also been reported to cause a necrotizing vasculitis that resembles Buerger's disease, bone marrow hypoplasia, and intestinal obstruction. Other organs that have been involved include lymph nodes, spleen, liver, kidney, pancreas, pericardium, heart, thyroid, and adrenals. The presence of infection in either liver, kidney, or spleen may be asymptomatic and may be associated with cystic lesions that appear calcified on CT or ultrasound.

℞ TREATMENT

A variety of therapeutic options are available for the patient with PCP or disseminated pneumocystis (Table 308-21) (see Chap. 211). The gold standard for therapy at present is trimethoprim/sulfamethoxazole, which is available in both intravenous and oral forms and is effective in approximately 90 percent of patients. The major disadvantage of this therapy is the relatively high incidence of side effects. In contrast to the non-HIV population, in which there is a 10 percent incidence of side effects, the HIV-infected population has a 50 to 65 percent incidence of side effects, including rash, fever, leukopenia, thrombocytopenia, and hepatitis. Although therapy need not be discontinued when these occur, it is important to remain vigilant for more serious hypersensitivity reactions, such as Stevens-Johnson syndrome. In addition, it may be advisable to withhold

other myelotoxic drugs, such as zidovudine and ganciclovir, during therapy with trimethoprim/sulfamethoxazole. In patients with mild disease, side effects may be minimized by slightly reducing dosage. Ideally, treatment with trimethoprim/sulfamethoxazole or the other agents mentioned below should be continued for 21 days. In contrast to many other infections, in which one expects to see stabilization, if not improvement, within 24 to 48 h of the initiation of appropriate antimicrobial therapy, AIDS patients with PCP often do not begin to improve until the end of the first week. In fact, during the first 5 days of treatment, particularly in moderate to severe cases, the patient's condition often worsens, presumably owing to the inflammatory response resulting from the death of large numbers of organisms in the lung. This inflammatory response and its adverse clinical consequences can be markedly reduced by the adjunct use of glucocorticoids. Glucocorticoids are indicated for use in the treatment of any patient with HIV infection and PCP in whom the Pa_{O_2} is under 70 mmHg or in whom the a-A gradient is over 35 mmHg. In this setting, several clinical trials have shown clear benefit from glucocorticoids, with approximately a 50 percent decrease in mortality (from 40 to 20 percent) and a 50 percent decrease in the number of patients requiring mechanical ventilatory support. The only significant side effect has been an increased incidence of thrush. Adjunct glucocorticoid therapy should be started as soon as possible after the diagnosis is made, preferably no later than 36 to 72 h. In fact, glucocorticoids added later in the course of disease have not been shown to confer any clinical benefit and have been associated with an increased risk of other opportunistic infections. The recommended length of glucocorticoid therapy is 21 days (Table 308-21), although some prefer to stop the drug 48 to 72 h prior to stopping antimicrobial therapy, to make it possible to assess the baseline status when the patient is still receiving antimicrobials but no longer receiving glucocorticoids.

Several options are available in patients unable to tolerate trimethoprim/sulfamethoxazole. Pentamidine isethionate is also licensed for treatment of PCP; this drug must be administered parenterally. The development of sterile abscesses following intramuscular administration makes intravenous administration the route of choice. In addition, it has been proposed that, for mild cases, the drug may be administered as an aerosol. Although some therapeutic successes have been noted with this route of administration, it is ineffective for extrapulmonary disease, and aerosolized pentamidine should be reserved for prophylaxis of PCP in the rare patient unable to tolerate systemic prophylaxis (see below). When given by the intravenous route, pentamidine must be administered slowly to prevent cardiovascular effects. Although comparable in efficacy to trimethoprim/sulfamethoxazole therapy, pentamidine therapy is associated with a greater number of serious side effects, including nephrotoxicity (which often necessitates reducing the dose by 20 to 50 percent), pancreatitis (necessitating discontinuation), thrombocytopenia, and dysregulation of glucose metabolism resulting in either hyper- or hypoglycemia. The latter side effect is seen in 14 percent of patients receiving pentamidine and is probably secondary to pancreatic injury during therapy. Fatal hypoglycemia as well as the development of insulin-requiring diabetes mellitus have occurred. These disorders of glucose metabolism are more common in patients who develop renal damage during therapy, generally occur late in the course of therapy, and are more common in patients receiving total doses above 4 g and in patients who have received pentamidine in the past. Pentamidine-associated hypoglycemia has been reported as late as 2 weeks following the discontinuation of drug; thus, patients must be alerted to watch for this side effect.

Among the alternatives to trimethoprim/sulfamethoxazole and intravenous pentamidine are trimethoprim/dapsone (oral only), clindamycin/primaquine (oral and parenteral), atovaquone (oral only), trimetrexate/leucovorin (oral and parenteral), and eflornithine (DFMO, oral and parenteral). The combination of trimethoprim and

Table 308-21

Manifestations and Treatment of Secondary Infections in Patients with HIV Disease

Infecting Agent	Manifestations	Treatment	Prophylaxis	Drug Toxicities	Comment
Pneumocystis carinii			TMP/SMX 1 DS tablet daily, or 3×/wk, or	Rash, fever, neutropenia	Begin once CD4+ T cell count <200/μL or CD4% <15
			Aerosolized pentamidine 300 mg/month, or	Bronchospasm	
			Dapsone 50 mg/d PO + Pyrimethamine 50 mg/wk PO + Folinic acid 25 mg/wk PO	Methemoglobinemia, neutropenia	Contraindicated in patients with G6PD deficiency
	Mild to moderate pneumonia [Pa$_{O_2}$ ≥ 70 mmHg and (A-a)dO$_2$ ≤ 35 mmHg]	TMP/SMX 15–20 mg/kg/d PO		Rash, fever, neutropenia	Treat for 21 d if possible; no less than 14 d
		TMP 20 mg/kg/d PO qd + Dapsone 100 mg PO qd		Methemoglobinemia, *C. difficile* colitis	Contraindicated in patients with G6PD deficiency
		Clindamycin 600 mg PO q6h + Primaquine 15 mg PO qd		Rash, neutropenia, nephritis, pancreatitis, hypoglycemia, diabetes	Contraindicated in patients with G6PD deficiency
		IV Pentamidine 3–4 mg/kg/d Atovaquone, 750 mg, PO, tid for 21 d			
		Aerosolized pentamidine 300 mg/d		Bronchospasm	Provides no systemic effects. Not recommended but an option for multidrug-allergic patient with mild pneumonia
	Severe pneumonia [Pa$_{O_2}$ < 70 mmHg or (A-a)dO$_2$ > 35 mmHg]	TMP/SMX 15–20 mg/kg/d IV initially (total course 14–21 d) Pentamidine 3–4 mg/kg/d IV for 14–21 d Clindamycin 900 mg IV q8h then 450 mg PO q6h +		Rash, fever, leukopenia, thrombocytopenia, hepatitis, nephritis, pancreatitis, hypoglycemia, diabetes, *C. difficile* colitis	Prednisone, 40 mg bid for 2 d, then 40 mg/d for 5 d, then 20 mg/d to the end of therapy (21 d total) added to specific antimicrobial ASAP and no later than 36 h after diagnosis
		Primaquine 30 mg PO qd for total of 14–21 d		Rash, neutropenia	Contraindicated in patients with G6PD deficiency
		Trimetrexate 45 mg/m^2 IV (over 60–90 min) qd × 21 d + Leucovorin, 20 mg/m^2 IV q6h × 24 d		Rash, neutropenia	For patients intolerant of other regimens. Less effective than standard therapy. Bone marrow–suppressive effects blunted by use of leucovorin
		Eflornithine (DFMO) 100 mg/kg IV q6h for 14 d followed by 75 mg/kg PO q6h for 4–6 wk		Thrombocytopenia	Call 1-800-TRIALSA for information
	Disseminated disease	Any of the systemic therapies outlined above			
Toxoplasma gondii			TMP/SMX 1 DS tablet qd	Rash, fever, neutropenia	Alternative is dapsone, 50 mg, PO qd + pyrimethamine, 50 mg, PO weekly + folinic acid, 25 mg, PO weekly
	Encephalitis, brain abscess, chorioretinitis, myocarditis	Sulfadiazine 1–2 g PO q6h + Pyrimethamine 25–100 mg qd + Folinic acid 10–20 mg PO qd		Crystalluria, rash	Treatment is generally for life. Leucovorin to minimize bone marrow suppression
		Clindamycin initially 200–400 mg IV q6h +		Rash, fever, neutropenia *C. difficile* colitis	

(continued)

Table 308-21—*(continued)*

Manifestations and Treatment of Secondary Infections in Patients with HIV Disease

Infecting Agent	Manifestations	Treatment	Prophylaxis	Drug Toxicities	Comment
Toxoplasma gondii—*(continued)*		Pyrimethamine 25–100 mg qd + Folinic acid 10–20 mg qd followed by Clindamycin 300–900 mg PO q8h + Pyrimethamine 25–100 mg qd		Rash, fever, neutropenia	Leucovorin to minimize bone marrow suppression
		Atovaquone 250 mg PO tid + Pyrimethamine 25–100 mg qd + Folinic acid 10–20 mg qd		Rash, fever, neutropenia	Leucovorin to minimize bone marrow suppression
		Macrolides (clarithromycin or azithromycin) + Pyrimethamine			Early results disappointing
Isospora belli	Diarrhea	TMP/SMX 1 DS tablet PO qid for 10 d then bid for 3 weeks		Rash, fever, neutropenia	TMP/SMX 1 DS tablet PO 3×/week for maintenance
Cryptosporidia Microsporidia	Diarrhea	No known specific therapy; supportive measures include parenteral nutrition			NTZ; bovine colostrum in trials
Mycobacterium avium complex			Clarithromycin 500 mg PO bid or Azithromycin 1200 mg weekly or Rifabutin 300 mg PO qd		Begin prophylaxis once CD4+ T cell count <100/μL or <50/μL. Treatment is generally for life. Macrolides + rifabutin may be more effective; however, more toxic and costly
	Disseminated disease that may involve lung, bone marrow, liver	Ethambutol 15 mg/kg qd + Rifabutin 600 mg/qd + Clarithromycin 100 mg PO bid		Hepatitis, neuropathy (peripheral/optic)	
Mycobacterium tuberculosis	Asymptomatic, PPD test positive	Isoniazid 15 mg/kg up to 900 mg PO twice a wk or 300 mg PO daily for 1 y + Pyridoxine 50 mg/d		Hepatitis	
	Active disease	Isoniazid, 300 mg PO qd × 1 y + Rifampin 600 mg PO qd × 1 y + Pyrazinamide 30 mg/kg/d in 2 doses		Hepatitis Hepatitis Hepatitis	Treat with 3 drugs for 2 mo. If isolate is sensitive to isoniazid and rifampin, then switch to those 2 drugs. Treat a minimum of 9 mo and at least 6 mo after third negative culture. Quinolones may also be considered as a fifth drug
	Active disease in a setting where there is a possibility of multidrug resistance	Add ethambutol 15–25 mg/kg/d and Streptomycin or Amikacin		Neuropathy (peripheral/optic) Nephrotoxicity, hearing loss	
Candida albicans	Thrush, vaginitis	Clotrimazole troches, Nystatin prn Fluconazole 200 mg PO qd for 7–14 d Amphotericin B 0.25 mg/kg/d IV for 7–10 d	Fluconazole 200 mg PO qd (optional)	Hepatotoxicity Hepatotoxicity Nephrotoxicity, fever/chills	Primary prophylaxis generally not indicated. Treatment is generally prn
Cryptococcus neoformans	Meningitis, brain abscess, pneumonia, disseminated disease	Amphotericin B 0.3 mg/kg/d IV + Flucytosine 150 mg/kg/d PO for 6 wk followed by Fluconazole 100–200 mg PO qd indefinitely	Fluconazole 200 mg PO qd (optional)	Hepatotoxicity Nephrotoxicity, fever/chills, bone marrow suppression Hepatotoxicity	Begin prophylaxis if CD4+ T cell count <50/μL (optional; depending on risk). Approximately 50% will need to have flucytosine held during therapy due to neutropenia. An alternative is amphotericin B alone at a dose of 0.8 mg/kg/d

(continued)

Table 308-21—*(continued)*

Manifestations and Treatment of Secondary Infections in Patients with HIV Disease

Infecting Agent	Manifestations	Treatment	Prophylaxis	Drug Toxicities	Comment
Histoplasma capsulatum	Disseminated disease, pneumonia	Amphotericin B 0.6–1 mg/kg/d to a total 1 g then Itraconazole 200 mg qd indefinitely		Nephrotoxicity, fever/chills	
Bartonella henselae, (quintana)	Nodular skin lesions, peliosis hepatitis, trench fever	Erythromycin 500 g PO or IV qd for 2 months			
Penicillium marneffei	Disseminated disease, umbilicated skin lesions	Amphotericin B, 0.6–1 mg/kg/d to a total of 1 g then Itraconazole 200 mg qd indefinitely		Nephrotoxicity, fever, chills, hepatitis	
Cytomegalovirus	Retinitis, esophagitis, colitis, and pneumonia		Ganciclovir 1.0 g PO tid with food (optional)	Neutropenia	Expensive, marginal efficacy. Neutropenia may be ameliorated by colony-stimulating factors
		Ganciclovir 5 mg/kg q12h for 14 d followed by 5 mg/kg qd IV indefinitely			Retinitis may also be treated with ocular implant Oral ganciclovir, 1 g PO tid with food may be used for maintenance
		Foscarnet 90 mg/kg q12h for 14 d followed by 90–120 mg/kg qd IV indefinitely		Interstitial nephritis, seizure, hypocalcemia	Should be preceded by saline infusion to minimize nephrotoxicity
Herpes simplex virus	Recurrent perioral, perirectal, or genital ulcers	Acyclovir 200–400 mg PO 5id as needed			Foscarnet 60 mg/kg q8h × 14 d for patients with acyclovir-resistant herpes simplex or zoster
	Esophagitis; acute retinal necrosis	Acyclovir 5 mg/kg IV q8h for 10–14 d			
Varicella-zoster virus	Cutaneous (local or disseminated); retinal necrosis	Acyclovir 800 mg PO 5id or 10 mg/kg IV q8h for 10–14 d or longer			Famciclovir 500 mg PO q8h × 7 d is an alternative
Treponema pallidum	Early syphilis	Benzathine penicillin G 2.4 million units IM weekly for 3 wk			Approximately 20% relapse, need retreatment. Immunologic abnormalities may cause inaccurate serology
	Late or neurosyphilis	Aqueous penicillin G 12–24 million units IV daily for 10–14 d Procaine penicillin G 2.4 million units IM daily for 10–14 d + Probenicid 500 mg PO qid Ceftriaxone 1–2 g IM or IV qd 10–14 d			

ABBREVIATIONS: DS, double-strength; NTZ, nitazoxanide; TMP/SMX, trimethoprim/sulfamethoxazole.

dapsone has been shown to be similar in efficacy to trimethoprim/sulfamethoxazole and to be associated with fewer toxicities. Some clinicians choose this combination as first-line treatment in patients with mild disease. One side effect of dapsone therapy is the development of methemoglobinemia, and its use is contraindicated in patients with glucose-6-phosphate dehydrogenase (G6PD) deficiency. Dapsone as a single agent is not effective. Similarly, while neither clindamycin alone nor primaquine alone is effective for the treatment of pneumocystosis, when they are used in combination, response rates are as high as 86 percent. The main side effects are rash and methemoglobinemia. Atovaquone is a hydroxynapthoquinone that interferes with electron transport in mitochondria and, as such, interferes with pyrimidine synthesis in protozoa. In a series of clinical trials, this drug has been shown to have activity against *P. carinii*. The incidence of side effects is lower than for trimethroprim/sulfamethoxazole, but overall response rates also are somewhat lower, and relapses are more common, so this agent must be considered second-line therapy. Trimetrexate, an inhibitor of dihydrofolate reductase, is another agent shown to be effective in the treatment of patients with PCP. This drug, whose side effect of bone marrow suppression can be greatly minimized by the concomitant use of folinic acid (leucovorin), is associated with response rates of approximately 70 percent. While not appropriate as initial therapy, trimetrexate may be of use in patients unable to tolerate or failing other forms of treatment. Eflornithine is an irreversible inhibitor of decarboxylase and thus interferes with the synthesis of polyamines. Its main side effect is thrombocytopenia. As in the case of trimetrexate, this drug has been shown to have some efficacy as a salvage treatment; however, the overall response rates to this agent are lower than for trimethoprim/sulfamethoxazole, which suggests that it not be used for initial therapy.

Once infection with *P. carinii* is diagnosed or suspected, appropriate systemic therapy is initiated with one of the agents or combinations discussed above. For patients with moderate to severe disease, glucocorticoids are included as part of the treatment regimen, and specific antimicrobial therapy should be administered parenterally (see above). After 7 to 14 days of therapy, clear-cut clinical improvement should be seen. If it is not, a change in therapy must be considered, with the general practice being to switch treatment regimens rather than add new drugs. If the situation is worsening, one should consider a repeat bronchoscopy to confirm the diagnosis and to rule out the possibility of a second infection. For patients who develop respiratory failure, intubation and mechanical ventilation remain an option; given the current range of therapeutic options available for treatment, such patients have been successfully treated and extubated.

Prophylaxis *Pneumocystis* prophylaxis is one of the cornerstones in the management of the HIV-infected patient. Prophylaxis is indicated for any HIV-infected individual who has experienced a previous bout of PCP, any patient who has fewer than 200 CD4+ T cells per microliter or a CD4 percentage of 15 or lower, any patient with unexplained fever (>100°F) for ≥2 weeks, and any patient with a history of oropharyngeal candidiasis. As in treatment, the preferred medication for prophylaxis is trimethoprim/sulfamethoxazole, which is given as a single double-strength tablet from three times a week to twice a day. The most common regimen is a single double-strength tablet daily. In studies of the twice-a-day regimen, no cases of PCP occurred in the treatment group, whereas 16 cases occurred in the untreated control group. In addition, in this study, which had a minimum follow-up of 24 months, the median survival in the treatment group was 22.9 months, compared to 12.6 months for the control group. In trials comparing a once-a-day regimen of trimethoprim/sulfamethoxazole to aerosolized pentamidine at a dose of 300 mg every 4 weeks, 1-year and 18-month recurrence rates of 4.5 percent and 11.4 percent, respectively, were found for the trimethoprim/sulfamethoxazole group, compared to 18.5 percent and 27.6 percent, respectively, for the aerosolized pentamidine group. These data, coupled with the increased incidence of pneumothorax and disseminated pneumocystosis seen with aerosolized pentamidine, point to systemic therapy with trimethoprim/sulfamethoxazole as the preferred regimen of prophylaxis. Unfortunately, however, some patients are unable to tolerate trimethoprim/sulfamethoxazole, and there is a great need for alternative regimens. Many such regimens, most of them variations on the treatment themes outlined above, have been proposed. A study of dapsone was stopped when it was observed that there was a higher incidence of death due to bacterial infections in the dapsone group than in the trimethoprim/sulfamethoxazole group. This result may have been due to the broad-spectrum antibacterial activity of the combination regimen or to some adverse effect of dapsone on neutrophil function. The combination of dapsone, pyrimethamine, and leucovorin has been recommended by some as a systemic alternative for those unable to tolerate trimethoprim/sulfamethoxazole. This regimen also provides protection against toxoplasmosis but not against most bacterial infections. Aerosolized pentamidine, 300 mg every 4 weeks delivered by a Respirgard II or equivalent nebulizer, remains an option for patients unable to tolerate systemic therapy.

Toxoplasmosis (See Chap. 219) *Toxoplasma gondii*, the etiologic agent of toxoplasmosis, is the most common cause of secondary CNS infection in patients with AIDS, accounting for 38 percent of all such infections. It accounts for 50 to 60 percent of all mass lesions in the CNS of patients with HIV infection and is responsible for 28 percent of first seizures. Overall, toxoplasmosis is seen in approximately 15 percent of patients with AIDS and is most common in patients from the Caribbean and from France. Toxoplasmosis is generally a late complication of HIV infection and usually occurs in patients with less than 100 CD4+ T cells per microliter. It is the initial AIDS-defining condition in 2 percent of AIDS patients in the United States. It is thought to represent a reactivation syndrome and is 10 times more common in patients with antibodies to the organisms, an indicator of prior infection, than in patients who are seronegative. However, owing to the abnormalities of B cell function seen in patients with HIV infection, serologic testing cannot be used to rule out a diagnosis of toxoplasmosis, and approximately 5 percent of cases occur in HIV-infected patients who are seronegative for *T. gondii*. Approximately 30 percent of AIDS patients with antibodies to *T. gondii* go on to develop CNS infection at some time during the course of their disease. Patients diagnosed with HIV infection should be screened for IgG antibody to *Toxoplasma* as part of their initial workup. Those who are seronegative should be counseled about ways to avoid infection, including avoiding the consumption of undercooked meat and careful hand washing after contact with soil or changing the cat litter box.

Primary infection with *T. gondii* is usually asymptomatic and occurs early in life, although some experience a chorioretinitis such as is seen following congenital infection. While primary infection in an immunocompromised host may result in a disseminated lethal infection involving lung, myocardium, and brain, this syndrome is rarely seen in patients with HIV infection. The most common clinical presentation in patients with HIV infection is one of fever, headache, and focal neurologic deficits, with the latter occurring in approximately 90 percent of patients. Patients may present with seizure, hemiparesis, or aphasia as a manifestation of focal neurologic defects or with a picture more related to accompanying cerebral edema and consisting of confusion, dementia, lethargy, and progression to coma. The latter manifestations are obviously similar to problems encountered in patients with HIV encephalopathy. In this clinical setting, the diagnosis is suspected on the basis of radiologic findings. MRI or double-dose contrast CT are the preferred techniques; MRI is clearly the most sensitive. Findings generally include multiple lesions in multiple locations, although in some cases only a single lesion is seen. Pathologically, these lesions generally exhibit inflammation and central necrosis and, as a result, show ring enhancement on contrast CT or MRI (Fig. 308-25). There is usually evidence of surrounding edema. The definitive diagnostic procedure is a brain biopsy. However, given the morbidity frequently associated with this procedure, it is usually more appropriate in the patient in whom one suspects toxoplasmosis (multiple ring-enhancing lesions on CT, seropositivity) to initiate specific therapy (see below) and proceed to biopsy only if there is no therapeutic response by 2 to 4 weeks. In a seronegative patient, the likelihood that a mass lesion of the CNS is due to *Toxoplasma* is less than 10 percent. In this setting, one may choose to be more aggressive and perform a biopsy sooner.

In addition to the classic presentation as a CNS mass lesion, *T. gondii* has been reported to cause a variety of other clinical problems in HIV-infected patients, including a CNS presentation more characteristic of herpes simplex, with a negative CT scan, chorioretinitis, pneumonia, peritonitis with ascites, gastrointestinal tract involvement, cystitis, and orchitis.

℞ TREATMENT

The standard treatment is combination therapy with pyrimethamine and sulfadiazine (Table 308-21). This regimen has a response rate of approximately 90 percent; however, since the relapse rate is over 50 percent at 6 months, the requirement for therapy is generally lifelong. Leukopenia, the main side effect of this combination, may be ameliorated by the concomitant use of folinic acid (leucovorin). If the patient is receiving other myelosuppressive agents, such as

FIGURE 308-25 Contrast-enhanced MRI scan of the brain of a patient with CNS toxoplasmosis. Several ring-enhancing lesions can be seen in the temporo-parietal area.

zidovudine or ganciclovir, the dosages of these medications may have to be modified. Other complications of therapy include fever, rash, thrombocytopenia, and renal failure due to sulfadiazine crystalluria. Crystalluria can be managed by administering fluids and alkalinizing the urine without discontinuing the medications. Overall, 45 to 70 percent of patients will develop side effects of treatment, and approximately 33 percent of patients will require a change in therapy. Treatment with clindamycin in combination with pyrimethamine is almost as good as treatment with sulfadiazine in combination with pyrimethamine and is an alternative for sulfa-allergic patients. Other treatment options include atovaquone plus pyrimethamine and azithromycin plus rifabutin plus pyrimethamine. Atovaquone has activity against a wide range of protozoa. Both as a single agent and in combination with pyrimethamine, it has been shown to be a viable alternative for treatment of toxoplasmosis in patients who have failed or developed adverse reactions to standard therapy. In patients for whom the sulfa component of treatment appears to cause side effects, the use of pyrimethamine alone as a maintenance regimen has been advocated. Although not as effective as the combination, it does appear to provide some protection from relapse. While animal model data suggest that the macrolide antibiotics clarithromycin and azithromycin might be of benefit for treatment of toxoplasmosis, clinical trial results thus far have been disappointing. Anecdotal reports suggest that the combination of a macrolide with rifabutin and pyrimethamine may have some activity. Glucocorticoids are recommended for the management of patients with cerebral edema.

Prophylaxis Given the frequency of toxoplasmosis in the HIV-infected population (overall incidence approximately 15 percent), there is a great need to develop effective prophylaxis. Unfortunately, aside from atovaquone, most of the agents and combinations of agents with therapeutic activity have severe enough side effects to make them dubious choices for primary prophylaxis. Fortunately, patients receiving trimethoprim/sulfamethoxazole or dapsone and pyrimethamine for prophylaxis of PCP have a decreased incidence of toxoplasmosis, which again underscores the potential importance of these particular regimens for antimicrobial prophylaxis.

Protozoal Diarrhea Cryptosporidia, microsporidia, and *Isospora belli* (see Chap. 220) are the most common opportunistic protozoa that infect the gastrointestinal tract and cause diarrhea in HIV-infected patients. *Cryptosporidium* is a well-known cause of diarrhea in animals and may cause a self-limited diarrheal infection in the immunocompetent host. It is spread through fecal-oral contact, and nosocomial outbreaks have been reported. In HIV-infected individuals, cryptosporidial infection may present in a variety of ways, ranging from a self-limited or intermittent diarrheal illness in patients in the early stages of HIV disease to a severe, life-threatening diarrhea in severely immunodeficient individuals. In patients with CD4+ T cell counts of <300/μL, the incidence of cryptosporidiosis is approximately 1 percent per year. Patients generally give a history of several months of intermittent diarrhea evolving to a several-month history of persistent diarrhea with copious watery stools, often up to several liters per day. In 75 percent of cases, diarrhea is accompanied by crampy abdominal pain; approximately 25 percent of patients have nausea and/or vomiting. This intestinal infection may be complicated by lactose intolerance and malabsorption. In addition to involving the intestinal tract, cryptosporidia may cause biliary tract disease in the HIV-infected population, which may present as cholecystitis with or without accompanying cholangitis. Radiographic studies of the biliary tree reveal thickening of the gallbladder wall with luminal abnormalities accompanying bile duct dilation and stricture. Cryptosporidia have also been noted in pulmonary specimens; however, the clinical significance of this finding is unclear. The diagnosis of cryptosporidial diarrhea is made by stool examination. The diarrhea is noninflammatory, and the characteristic finding is the presence of oocysts that stain with acid-fast dyes. Use of a sucrose flotation technique followed by procedures to concentrate the cysts and to separate them from other particles in the specimen may enhance detection. Organisms may be seen adhering to the brush border of intestinal epithelium on electron microscopy of small bowel biopsy specimens. Therapy is purely symptomatic at present. Patients can minimize their risk of developing cryptosporidiosis by avoiding contact with human and animal feces and by not drinking water from lakes or rivers.

Microsporidia are small, unicellular, obligate intracellular parasites that reside in the cytoplasm of enteric cells (see Chap. 220). The main species causing disease in humans is *Enterocytozoon bieneusi*. The clinical manifestations are similar to those described for *Cryptosporidium* and include abdominal pain and diarrhea. The small size of the organism may make it difficult to detect; however, with the use of chromotrope-based stains, organisms can be identified in stool samples by light microscopy. Definitive diagnosis generally depends on electron microscopic examination of a stool specimen, intestinal aspirate, or intestinal biopsy specimen. In contrast to cryptosporidia, microsporidia have been noted in a variety of extraintestinal locations, including the eye, muscle, and liver, and have been associated with conjunctivitis and hepatitis. As in the case of cryptosporidia, no effective therapy is known, and treatment is purely symptomatic.

Isospora belli is a coccidian parasite (see Chap. 220) most commonly found as a cause of diarrhea in patients from the Caribbean and Africa. Its cysts appear in the stool as large, acid-fast structures that can be differentiated from those of cryptosporidia on the basis of size, shape, and number of sporocysts. The clinical syndromes caused by these organisms appear to be identical to those caused by cryptosporidia; however, one important difference is that this infection can be treated with trimethoprim/sulfamethoxazole. While relapses are common, a three-times-a-week regimen, similar to that used to provide prophylaxis against PCP, appears adequate to prevent recurrence.

Entamoeba histolytica (see Chap. 215) and *Giardia lamblia* (see Chap. 220), although not strictly opportunistic pathogens in that they can also cause disease in immunocompetent individuals, are more common in patients with HIV infection. These treatable protozoal infections should be carefully looked for in any patient with HIV infection and persistent diarrhea. Other strains of Entamoeba and *Blastocystis hominis* are also seen with increased frequency in homosexual men with HIV infection; however, they are felt to be of little if any clinical significance.

Miscellaneous Protozoal Infections Miscellaneous protozoal infections are being reported with increased frequency as the AIDS epidemic spreads through the world. Visceral leishmaniasis (see Chap. 217) is recognized with increasing frequency in patients who live in or travel to endemic areas. The clinical presentation is one of hepatosplenomegaly, fever, and hematologic abnormalities. Lymphadenopathy and other constitutional symptoms may be present. Organisms can be isolated from cultures of bone marrow aspirates, while histologic stains are often negative and antibody titers are of little help in diagnosis. Patients usually respond well initially to standard therapy, although, as with most infections in HIV-infected individuals, eradication of the organisms is difficult and relapses are common. Among other protozoal infections that have been reported are severe and recurrent babesiosis (Chap. 179), Chagas' disease (Chap. 218) presenting as a CNS mass lesion, and meningoencephalitis due to *Acanthamoeba* or *Naegleria* (Chap. 215). No significant changes have been noted in the clinical manifestations of malaria in HIV-infected patients. Infections with *Cyclospora* species have been reported in HIV-infected individuals. Although infections in the general population have been linked to contaminated water, in 1996 outbreaks of infection with *Cyclospora cayetanensis* have been reported in association with the consumption of contaminated fruit, particularly strawberries and raspberries. Signs and symptoms include prolonged watery diarrhea, nausea, vomiting, crampy abdominal pain, and fever; these may be particularly severe and prolonged in HIV-infected individuals.

BACTERIAL INFECTIONS Bacterial infections are the leading cause of death in patients with HIV infection. While bacterial infections are often the terminal event in AIDS patients with multiple other problems, they also account for a substantial proportion of opportunistic infections earlier in the course of HIV disease. In the United States, disseminated mycobacterial infection, particularly due to the *Mycobacterium avium* complex (MAC), is the most common opportunistic bacterial infection. It is diagnosed antemortem in approximately 40 percent of HIV-infected patients and is seen at autopsy in 80 percent of patients. MAC accounts for 95 percent of the atypical mycobacterial infections seen in patients with AIDS in the United States; however, infections with at least 12 different mycobacteria, including *Mycobacterium bovis* and representatives of all four Runyon groups, have been reported. Infections with MAC, which consists of *M. avium* and *Mycobacterium intracellulare*, are seen mainly in patients in the United States and are rare in Africa. It has been suggested that prior infection with *M. tuberculosis* decreases the risk of MAC infection.

Infections with Atypical Mycobacteria MAC infection probably represents an acute infection with organisms that are ubiquitous in the environment in both soil and water. The presumed portals of entry are the gastrointestinal and respiratory tract. MAC infection is a late complication of HIV infection, occurring in patients with CD4 + T cell counts of <100/μL. Prior to the introduction of prophylactic regimens for MAC infections, the median CD4 + T cell count for patients with MAC was approximately 50/μL. Now, with more widespread MAC prophylaxis, the CD4 + T cell count at the time of diagnosis is approximately 10/μL. HIV-infected patients presenting with MAC infection have been reported to have a median survival of approximately 6 to 10 months. This fact likely reflects the late stage of their HIV infection. While a variety of clinical syndromes have been attributed to MAC infections, the most common presentation is fever, weight loss, and night sweats, presumably due to disseminated disease. At least 85 percent of HIV-infected patients with MAC infection are mycobacteremic, and enormous numbers of organisms can often be demonstrated on bone marrow biopsy. Liver involvement is common, and MAC infection should be suspected in any HIV-infected individual with a low CD4 + T cell count, unexplained fever, and an elevated alkaline phosphatase level. The chest x-ray is abnormal in approximately 25 percent of patients; the most common radiographic pattern is a bilateral lower lobe interstitial infiltrate, suggestive of miliary spread. In addition, alveolar or nodular infiltrates and hilar and/or mediastinal adenopathy occur. Endobronchial lesions have also been reported. Other clinical findings include lymphadenopathy, abdominal pain, and diarrhea. The diagnosis is suggested by the demonstration of long, slender acid-fast bacilli in biopsy specimens of bone marrow, lymph node, or liver or in stool specimens and is confirmed by culture of blood or involved tissue. The finding of two consecutive sputum samples positive for MAC is highly suggestive of pulmonary infection. Cultures generally turn positive within 2 weeks. In earlier studies, treatment with various combination regimens, which usually included ethambutol, clofazimine, and rifabutin, with or without an aminoglycoside, were shown to have little effect on mycobacteremia and to increase only marginally the median survival of patients with MAC infection (from 6 months to 8 months). The availability of the newer macrolide antibiotics (clarithromycin and azithromycin) changed this scenario considerably. Treatment with clarithromycin and ethambutol is thought by many to be the treatment of choice of MAC infection in patients with HIV infection. Some elect to add a third agent, either rifabutin, rifampin, clofazimine, ciprofloxacin, or amikacin, to the combination of ethambutol and a macrolide. At present, the data supporting the value of the third agent, particularly given the increased cost and complexity of such regimens, are weak. As with all of the potentially life-threatening infections seen in patients with AIDS, prophylactic regimens should be employed when available. In this regard, the use of rifabutin in patients with advanced HIV infection has been shown to delay the onset of bacteremia and death. Rifabutin has commonly been used as a prophylactic agent for patients with less than 75 to 100 CD4 + T cells per microliter. More recently, better results have been obtained with clarithromycin or azithromycin prophylaxis in patients with CD4 + T cell counts of less than 75/μL, and many experts now recommend single-agent macrolide prophylaxis in preference to rifabutin.

A number of other atypical mycobacteria cause infections in patients with HIV infection. Infection with *Mycobacterium kansasii* generally presents as a pulmonary infection, with 20 to 30 percent of patients showing evidence of disseminated disease. Patients usually present with fever, cough, and night sweats. Chest x-ray reveals upper lobe cavitation in approximately half of these patients, while a lower lobe interstitial pattern consistent with hematogenous spread may be seen in other patients. Organisms are usually identified easily in pulmonary secretions; evidence of disease is found in over 75 percent of patients with a positive culture. It is particularly important to diagnose correctly *M. kansasii* infection, since it is relatively easy to treat with a combination regimen of isoniazid, rifampin, and ethambutol. *Mycobacterium fortuitum*, *Mycobacterium chelonae*, *Mycobacterium marinum*, *Mycobacterium scrofulaceum*, and *Mycobacterium haemophilum* all cause cutaneous lesions in patients with HIV infection; *M. haemophilum* also causes disseminated disease and septic arthritis. *Mycobacterium gordonae*, generally a nonpathogen in humans, and *Mycobacterium xenopi*, a colonizer of water storage tanks, may cause disseminated disease. Therapy of the latter organisms is extremely difficult.

Tuberculosis *M. tuberculosis*, once thought to be on its way to extinction in the United States, experienced a resurgence associated with the HIV epidemic (see Chap. 171). A 20-year decline in the number of new cases of tuberculosis in the United States ended in 1986, and the number of new cases per year increased for several years before reaching a new plateau. Approximately 5 percent of AIDS patients have active tuberculosis. While the prevalence and incidence of infection with *M. tuberculosis* in a given risk group, as determined by purified protein derivative (PPD) skin testing, appear not to be affected strongly by HIV status, HIV infection increases the risk of developing active tuberculosis by a factor of 15 to 30. For the patient with HIV infection and a positive PPD skin test, the rate of reactivation is 7 to 10 percent per year. Tuberculosis is a particularly important problem in patients with HIV infection. HIV disease progresses more rapidly in patients with tuberculosis; the level of plasma viremia increases during active tuberculosis; and successful treatment of tuberculosis causes plasma viremia to fall back to baseline levels. Although most cases of tuberculosis in the HIV-infected population are thought to represent reactivation, acute infection and reinfection are being seen increasingly often, especially in the context of outbreaks of multidrug resistant (MDR) tuberculosis. Active tuberculosis appears to be most common in patients 25 to 44 years of age, in African-Americans and Hispanics, in patients in New York City and Miami, and in patients in developing countries; in these demographic groups, 20 to 70 percent of the new cases of active tuberculosis are in patients with HIV infection. Given the fact that, in contrast to HIV infection, infection with *M. tuberculosis* can be spread via respiratory droplets and close, nonsexual contact, this epidemic of tuberculosis probably represents the greatest health risk to the general public and the health care profession associated with the HIV epidemic. In contrast to infection with MAC, active tuberculosis often develops relatively early in the course of HIV infection and may be among the earliest clinical signs of HIV infection. In one study, the median CD4+ T cell count at presentation of tuberculosis was 326/μL. The clinical manifestations of tuberculosis in HIV-infected patients are quite varied and generally show different patterns as a function of the CD4+ T cell count. In patients with relatively high CD4+ T cell counts, a typical pattern of pulmonary reactivation occurs in which patients present with fever, cough, dyspnea on exertion, weight loss, night sweats, and a chest x-ray revealing cavitary apical disease of the upper lobes. Disseminated disease is more common in patients with low CD4+ T cell counts. The chest x-ray in patients with disseminated disease may reveal diffuse or lower lobe bilateral reticulonodular infiltrates consistent with miliary spread, pleural effusions, and hilar and/or mediastinal adenopathy. Infection may be present in bone, brain, meninges, gastrointestinal tract, lymph nodes (particularly cervical nodes), and viscera. Abscesses of the liver and prostate have been reported. Approximately 60 to 80 percent of patients have pulmonary disease, and 30 to 40 percent have extrapulmonary disease.

Respiratory isolation and a negative-pressure room should be used for patients in whom a diagnosis of pulmonary tuberculosis is being considered. This approach is critical to limit nosocomial and community spread of infection. A definitive diagnosis is made by culture of the organisms from an involved site. Blood cultures are positive in 15 percent of cases. However, given the importance of making an early diagnosis and initiating treatment, especially with the emergence of MDR tuberculosis (see below), a presumptive diagnosis should be made based on a positive acid-fast stain or positive PCR and consistent clinical presentation while culture results are awaited. In such patients, treatment as indicated below should be initiated. PPD skin testing in HIV-infected individuals poses a particular problem. A positive PPD test in an HIV-infected person is defined as an area of induration ≥5 mm in diameter. While this test can be used to support the diagnosis and identify candidates for isoniazid prophylaxis, up to 50 percent of patients with HIV infection and active tuberculosis are anergic, and thus a negative skin test does not rule out a diagnosis. This fact underscores the importance of the anergy panel in evaluating a patient for tuberculosis. Some experts recommend that any anergic patient with HIV infection who is at high risk for tuberculosis should be given a 1-year course of isoniazid.

℞ **TREATMENT**

Standard therapy for tuberculosis is generally as successful in the HIV-infected patient as in the HIV-negative patient. Tuberculosis is one of the totally curable conditions seen in patients with HIV infection. Given the potential for the occurrence of MDR tuberculosis, a standard course of action for the HIV-infected patient with active tuberculosis is to initiate therapy with four drugs for 4 months followed by two drugs (four drugs if the isolate turns out to be resistant) for an additional 4 months and for no less than 6 months after a third negative culture. Given the plethora of gastrointestinal problems in patients with HIV infection, malabsorption should be considered in any patient in whom a tuberculosis infection fails to clear despite appropriate therapy. To ensure the best possible treat-

ment outcome, daily therapy should be observed directly by a health care professional.

A major emerging problem is the increasing identification of strains of *M. tuberculosis* resistant to two or more first-line drugs, usually isoniazid and rifampin, so-called MDR tuberculosis (see Chap. 171). Of the first 87 reported cases of MDR tuberculosis, 83 occurred in HIV-infected patients. Owing to delays in obtaining results of antimicrobial sensitivity testing, patients often received inadequate treatment regimens, and the initial mortality from MDR tuberculosis was as high as 72 to 89 percent. Up to 20 percent of cases of tuberculosis in some series were due to resistant strains. Owing to more aggressive treatment strategies, particularly ones employing directly observed therapy, the incidence of MDR tuberculosis is decreasing.

Prevention Effective prevention of active tuberculosis can be a reality if the health care profession is aggressive in looking for evidence of latent tuberculosis by making sure that all patients at risk for tuberculosis and all patients with HIV infection receive a PPD skin test. The therapeutic approach to an HIV-infected patient with a positive PPD result or to an anergic HIV-infected patient at risk for tuberculosis is discussed above.

Infections with Bacteria Other than Mycobacteria Nonmycobacterial bacteria account for a high number of infections in patients with AIDS and are the leading cause of death in this patient population. Bacterial infections most frequently present clinically as respiratory tract infections, sepsis, and/or gastroenteritis. In addition, syphilis and bacillary angiomatosis may present with atypical features. Patients with HIV infection appear to be particularly prone to infections with encapsulated organisms, perhaps as a consequence of altered B cell activation and/or defects in neutrophil function that may be secondary to disease or drugs. *Streptococcus pneumoniae* (see Chap. 141) and *Haemophilus influenzae* (see Chap. 152) are among the most common bacterial causes of infection seen in patients with HIV infection. These two organisms are responsible for most cases of bacterial pneumonia in patients with AIDS and contribute to the increased incidence of sinusitis that has been reported in this patient population. Patients with HIV infection have a sixfold increase in the incidence of pneumococcal pneumonia and a 100-fold increase in the incidence of pneumococcal bacteremia. For these reasons, all patients with HIV infections should receive immunization with pneumococcal polysaccharide. *Staphylococcus aureus* infections (see Chap. 142) are seen with increased frequency in the setting of HIV infection and account for approximately one-third of all episodes of bacteremia in HIV-infected individuals. HIV-infected individuals also have about twice the rate of carriage of staphylococcal organisms as the general population. Staphylococcal infections are usually responsible for catheter-related sepsis, with the risk increasing as the CD4+ T cell count declines. Pyomyositis is another complication of staphylococcal infection and is seen with increased frequency in HIV-infected patients. This disease, which was formerly rare in the United States, is generally seen in association with muscle injury; it has been postulated that the myopathy of HIV infection may be a predisposing factor.

Infections with enteric pathogens such as *Salmonella*, *Shigella*, and *Campylobacter* are more common in homosexual men and are often more severe and more apt to relapse in patients with HIV infection. These patients have approximately a 20-fold increased risk of infection with *Salmonella typhimurium* (see Chap. 158). They may present with a variety of nonspecific symptoms, including fever, anorexia, fatigue, and malaise of several weeks' duration. Diarrhea is common but may be absent. Diagnosis is made by culture of blood and stool. Although treatment generally is not indicated for *Salmonella* gastroenteritis in the general population, among HIV-infected patients this disease often follows a protracted course and has a high rate of recurrence, and long-term therapy is usually prescribed for *Salmonella* infection in this setting. The greatest success has been reported with oral ciprofloxacin. HIV-infected patients also have an increased incidence of infection with *Salmonella typhi* in areas of the world where typhoid is a problem (see Chap. 158).

Shigella infections (see Chap. 159) cause particularly severe gastrointestinal disease in HIV-infected individuals, characterized by diarrhea and fever. *Shigella flexneri* is the most common species isolated, and up to 50 percent of patients with HIV infection and shigellosis are bacteremic, in contrast to otherwise healthy hosts, in whom bacteremia is rare.

Campylobacter infections (see Chap. 160) occur at an increased frequency in HIV-infected patients. While *Campylobacter fetus* and *Campylobacter jejuni* are the strains most frequently isolated, infections with many other strains have been reported. Patients usually present with crampy abdominal pain, fever, and bloody diarrhea; infection may also present as proctitis. Stool examination reveals the presence of fecal leukocytes. Systemic infection can occur, with up to 10 percent of infected patients exhibiting bacteremia. As in the case of the other enteric pathogens, infections with *Campylobacter* species are often persistent or recurrent, and prolonged therapy is usually required. Most strains are sensitive to erythromycin; however, resistant strains have been reported.

Infections with *Treponema pallidum*, the etiologic agent of syphilis, play an important role in the HIV epidemic (see Chap. 174). In HIV-negative individuals, genital syphilitic ulcers rank with the ulcers of chancroid as major predisposing factors for heterosexual transmission of HIV (see above). While most HIV-infected individuals with syphilis have a typical presentation, a variety of formerly rare clinical problems may be encountered. Among them are lues maligna, an ulcerating lesion of the skin due to a necrotizing vasculitis; unexplained fever; nephrotic syndrome; and neurosyphilis. The most common presentation is that of condyloma lata, a form of secondary syphilis. Neurosyphilis may be asymptomatic or may present as acute meningitis, neuroretinitis, deafness, or stroke. In one series, 44 percent of all cases of neurosyphilis occurred in patients with HIV infection; the rate of neurosyphilis in this population may be as high as 1.5 percent. The incidence is particularly high in users of crack cocaine. Given the immunologic abnormalities seen in patients with HIV infection, diagnosis of syphilis through standard serologic testing may be challenging. On the one hand, a significant number of patients have a false positive Venereal Disease Research Laboratories (VDRL) test due to polyclonal B cell activation. On the other hand, the development of a positive VDRL result may be delayed in patients with new infections, and the anti-fluorescent treponema antibody (anti-FTA) test may be negative owing to immunodeficiency. Dark-field examination of appropriate specimens should be performed in any patient in whom syphilis is suspected, even if the patient has a negative VDRL test. Similarly, given that the diagnosis of neurosyphilis may be difficult to make, any patient with a positive serum VDRL test, neurologic findings, and abnormal findings on spinal fluid examination, whether or not the CSF VDRL test is positive, should be considered to have possible neurosyphilis. In the HIV-infected patient with syphilis, standard treatment may be inadequate; treatment may need to be repeated in patients who fail to respond or show evidence of relapse. In these patients, it is necessary to have a high index of suspicion for neurosyphilis and to treat accordingly with high-dose intravenous penicillin if this diagnosis is suspected.

Infections with species of the small, gram-negative rickettsia-like organism *Bartonella* (see Chap. 165) are seen with increased frequency among HIV-infected patients. Among the clinical manifestations of *Bartonella* infection are bacillary angiomatosis, cat-scratch disease, and trench fever. Bacillary angiomatosis is usually due to infection with *Bartonella henselae*. It is characterized by a vascular proliferation that leads to a variety of skin lesions, which have been confused with Kaposi's sarcoma. In contrast to the lesions of Kaposi's sarcoma, the lesions of bacillary angiomatosis generally blanch and are painful, and they are often associated with systemic symptoms. Infection can also extend to the lymph nodes, liver (peliosis hepatis), spleen, bone, heart, nervous system, respiratory tract, and gastrointestinal tract. This infection is usually seen in relatively advanced HIV infection, with an average CD4+ T cell count of 60/μL. Cat-scratch disease generally begins with a papule at the site of inoculation. This is followed several weeks later by the development of regional adenopathy and malaise.

Infection with *Bartonella quintana* is transmitted by lice and has been associated with case reports of trench fever, endocarditis, adenopathy, and bacillary angiomatosis.

FUNGAL INFECTIONS   Candidiasis   *Candida* infections are the most common fungal infections in patients with HIV infection; virtually all patients experience some type of *Candida* infection over the course of their illness (see Chap. 207). *Candida* infections often occur early in the course of HIV disease and may mark the onset of clinically apparent immunodeficiency. Although they are a significant cause of morbidity, *Candida* infections are generally easy to control and usually involve only the mucosal surfaces. Invasive disease is extremely rare and occurs predominantly as a consequence of iatrogenic measures, such as use of indwelling catheters or broad-spectrum antibiotics and/or drug-induced neutropenia.

Superficial infection of the oral cavity with *Candida* (thrush) generally presents as a white, cheesy exudate on the posterior oropharynx **(see Plate ID-42)**. Early lesions also may be detected along the gingival-labial margins. The exudate is easy to scrape, and branching pseudohyphae are readily detectable on wet-mount KOH preparations. In women with HIV infection, vaginal yeast infections are an early sign of immunodeficiency.

Later in the course of HIV infection, generally in association with CD4+ T cell counts below 100/μL, *Candida* infections of the esophagus, trachea, bronchi, or lungs may occur. These infections are thought to indicate a serious defect in cell-mediated immunity and are among the AIDS-defining conditions (Table 308-2). The most common of these is esophagitis. While generally a late manifestation of HIV infection, *Candida* esophagitis has also been reported during the acute syndrome associated with primary HIV infection. Esophagitis generally presents as odynophagia and retrosternal pain or burning. Oral thrush is often present as well, although it may be absent in patients who have been receiving topical oral medications. A definitive diagnosis is made through upper gastrointestinal endoscopy and observation of characteristic white plaques shown by wet mount to contain pseudohyphae. However, a high index of suspicion based on history and/or a barium swallow demonstrating a grossly irregular mucosa (Fig. 308-26) is sufficient to justify an empirical trial of antifungal therapy. If improvement does not occur after 4 to 6 days of therapy, upper gastrointestinal endoscopy should be performed to eliminate the other possible causes of esophagitis, namely CMV infection, herpes simplex, Kaposi's sarcoma, and lymphoma.

℞ TREATMENT

Oral and vaginal *Candida* infections can be treated with topical nystatin or clotrimazole troches; the frequency of administration should match the severity of disease. In severe cases, many clinicians find it more convenient to use systemic therapy with either ketoconazole or fluconazole, both of which are effective in most cases. Although fluconazole is more expensive, somewhat better results have been achieved with it, which may, at least in part, reflect the poor absorption of ketoconazole in patients with high gastric pH. A short course of intravenous therapy with amphotericin B followed by oral therapy with fluconazole may be indicated in particularly severe cases of *Candida* infection.

Cryptococcosis   *Cryptococcus neoformans* is the leading cause of meningitis in patients with AIDS (see Chap. 206). This ubiquitous yeast-like fungus, which has a polysaccharide capsule, causes serious, life-threatening infection in 6 to 12 percent of patients with AIDS. It is the initial AIDS-defining condition in 2 percent of patients, generally occurring in patients with fairly advanced disease in whom CD4+ T cell counts are below 100/μL. The median survival of a patient with HIV infection following a diagnosis of cryptococcal infection is 9 months. Cryptococcal meningitis is particularly common in patients with AIDS in Africa, occurring in approximately 20 percent of individuals; it was the illness that first suggested that a new epidemic of

FIGURE 308-26 Barium swallow of a patient with *Candida* esophagitis. The flow of barium along the mucosal surface is grossly irregular.

immunodeficiency was occurring in Africa. Although the organism is thought to invade via the respiratory route, the most common sites of infection are the brain and meninges. CNS infection is seen in 67 to 85 percent of AIDS patients with cryptococcal disease; most patients present with a picture of subacute meningoencephalitis. In addition to meningitis, patients may develop cryptococcomas, which appear on MRI as multiple ring-enhancing lesions. Patients with CNS cryptococcal disease often experience symptoms for weeks to months prior to diagnosis; as with many AIDS-associated opportunistic infections, a high index of suspicion is essential to making an early diagnosis. Among the common symptoms are fever (in virtually 100 percent of patients), nausea and vomiting (40 percent), and altered mental status, headache, and meningeal signs (25 percent). The incidence of seizures and focal neurologic defects is low. Pulmonary disease occurs in 40 percent of patients, 90 percent of whom also have CNS infection. Patients with pulmonary disease present with fever, cough, dyspnea, and, in some cases, hemoptysis. A focal or diffuse interstitial infiltrate is seen on chest x-ray in over 90 percent of patients with pulmonary disease. Chest x-ray may also reveal lobar disease, cavitary disease, pleural effusions, and hilar or mediastinal adenopathy. Over half of patients are fungemic. In patients with fungemia, fever, malaise, and fatigue are common. While most patients with cryptococcal disease present with CNS infection, 4 to 10 percent present with pulmonary disease in the absence of other manifestations, and 4 to 8 percent present with fungemia as the only manifestation of infection. Uncommon manifestations of cryptococcal infection in patients with HIV infection include skin lesions resembling molluscum contagiosum, lymphadenopathy, palatal and glossal ulcers, arthritis, gastroenteritis, myocarditis, and prostatitis. The prostate gland may serve as a reservoir for smoldering infection.

A presumptive diagnosis of cryptococcal infection can be made by the identification of organisms in spinal fluid with India ink exami-

nation, by the detection of cryptococcal antigen in blood or spinal fluid, or by histologic evidence of cryptococcal infection in a biopsy specimen. A definitive diagnosis is made by culturing organisms from spinal fluid, blood, bone marrow, sputum, or tissue. A positive culture for *Cryptococcus neoformans*, regardless of site, should be considered significant and an indication for treatment. Cryptococcal antigen is present in the CSF of virtually all patients with cryptococcal meningitis, although in 15 percent of these patients, all other findings are normal. In cryptococcal meningitis, the CSF WBC exceeds $20/\mu L$ in less than 50 percent of patients, the protein level is elevated in 35 to 70 percent, and the glucose level is low in about 50 percent. In patients with CNS cryptococcomas, both CSF antigen and culture may be negative, and biopsy may be required to make the diagnosis.

℞ TREATMENT

Therapy should be initiated immediately in any patient with evidence of cryptococcal infection, either by antigen or culture. Standard therapy in the HIV-infected patient consists of 6 weeks of amphotericin B at a daily dose of 0.3 to 0.5 mg/kg in combination with 150 mg/kg of flucytosine. In approximately 50 percent of patients the flucytosine will have to be omitted for at least part of the course of therapy owing to neutropenia. Given that over 50 percent of patients will relapse with this therapy alone, it is recommended that at the termination of amphotericin therapy, patients be placed on fluconazole, 100 to 200 mg daily, indefinitely. Many physicians choose to treat all patients with HIV infection with fluconazole, 100 to 200 mg daily, once the CD4+ T cell count falls below $100/\mu L$ as prophylaxis against both candidal and cryptococcal infections.

Histoplasmosis Histoplasmosis is an opportunistic infection that is seen most frequently in patients in the Mississippi and Ohio River valleys, Puerto Rico, the Dominican Republic, and South America; all of these are areas in which infection with *Histoplasma encapsulatum* is endemic (see Chap. 203). Because of this limited geographic distribution, the percentage of AIDS cases in the United States with histoplasmosis is only approximately 0.5 percent. In endemic areas, however, the incidence is much higher. The organism exists in the mycelial phase in soil, and large numbers of organisms are found in soil that contains droppings from birds or bats. The organism exists in the yeast phase at body temperature. Histoplasmosis is generally a late manifestation of HIV infection; however, it may be the initial AIDS-defining condition. The median CD4+ T cell count for patients with histoplasmosis was $33/\mu L$ in one study. While disease due to *H. encapsulatum* may present as a primary infection of the lung, disseminated disease, presumably due to reactivation, is the most common presentation in HIV-infected patients. These patients usually present with a 4- to 8-week history of fever and weight loss. Hepatosplenomegaly and lymphadenopathy are each seen in about 25 percent of patients. CNS disease, either meningitis or a mass lesion, is seen in 15 percent of patients. Bone marrow involvement is common, with thrombocytopenia, neutropenia, and anemia occurring in 33 percent of patients. Approximately 7 percent of patients have mucocutaneous lesions, consisting of a maculopapular rash and skin or oral ulcers. Although respiratory symptoms are usually minimal, with cough and dyspnea seen in 10 to 30 percent of patients, the chest x-ray is abnormal in about 50 percent of patients, revealing either a diffuse interstitial infiltrate or diffuse small nodules. The diagnosis is made by culturing the organisms from blood, bone marrow, or tissue. Fungal polysaccharide antigen may be detectable and quantifiable in the blood and can be used to follow the course of therapy; however, this test is not readily available commercially. Treatment consists of an initial course of amphotericin B, 0.6 mg/kg daily to a total dose of 1 g, followed by an indefinite maintenance regimen of either amphotericin, 1 mg/kg biweekly, or oral itraconazole.

***Penicillium marneffei* Infection** Following the spread of HIV infection to southeast Asia, disseminated infection with *Penicillium marneffei* was recognized as a complication of HIV infection. Clinical features include fever, generalized lymphadenopathy, hepatosplenomegaly, anemia, thrombocytopenia, and papular skin lesions with central umbilication. Treatment is with amphotericin B followed by itraconazole.

CHAPTER 308
HIV Disease: AIDS and Related Disorders
1835

Coccidioidomycosis *Coccidioides immitis* is a mold that resides in the soil and causes a mainly pulmonary infection in both immunologically intact hosts and patients with HIV infection (see Chap. 204). As in the case of histoplasmosis, infection with *C. immitis* is limited to certain geographic areas; it is endemic in the southwest United States. In these endemic areas, the annual rate of infection is approximately 3 percent, and most of the disease seen in patients with HIV infection is thought to be a result of reactivation. Although coccidioidal infection may develop relatively early in the course of HIV infection, most patients with this condition have CD4+ T cell counts below 250/μL. Patients generally present with fever, weight loss, cough, and fairly extensive abnormalities on chest x-ray. Diffuse reticulonodular infiltrates are the most common finding on chest x-ray, although nodules, cavities, pleural effusions, and hilar adenopathy also occur. While pulmonary disease is the most common manifestation of infection, seen in almost 70 percent of patients, 12 percent develop meningitis; 9 percent, lymphadenopathy; 9 percent, hepatic involvement; and 5 percent, cutaneous disease. Abdominal infection and peritonitis have also been reported. Diagnosis is made by culture. While serologic testing is usually helpful in the immunocompetent host, serologies are negative in 25 percent of HIV-infected individuals with coccidioidal infection. Treatment is with amphotericin B, 1 mg/kg daily to a total dose of 1 g, followed by indefinite maintenance with either fluconazole or itraconazole.

Aspergillosis Invasive aspergillosis (see Chap. 208) is not an AIDS-defining illness and is generally not seen in patients with AIDS in the absence of neutropenia or administration of glucocorticoids. It does have an unusual presentation in the respiratory tract of patients with AIDS, where it gives the appearance of a pseudomembranous tracheobronchitis. As in other settings, treatment is with amphotericin B.

VIRAL INFECTIONS Herpesvirus Infections Human herpesvirus infections present substantial problems throughout the course of HIV infection. In addition to causing clinical disease in their own right, mainly in the form of reactivation syndromes, these DNA viruses are also thought to act as cofactors, enhancing the replication of HIV. Among the members of this group that are particularly disabling of patients with HIV infection are CMV (see Chap. 187), herpes simplex viruses (see Chap. 184), varicella-zoster viruses (see Chap. 185), Epstein-Barr virus (see Chap. 186) and HHV-8 (see above).

Cytomegalovirus infections CMV causes an acute infection, generally early in life, after which it exists in a latent state (see Chap. 187). Over 95 percent of patients with HIV infection are seropositive for CMV, and at autopsy 90 percent of patients have some evidence of reactivated CMV disease. Clinical manifestations of CMV generally occur late in the course of HIV infection, for the most part in patients with less than 50 CD4+ T cells per microliter; however, evidence of active CMV replication, such as excretion of CMV in throat washings or urine, can be detected quite early in the course of HIV disease. Retinitis, esophagitis, and colitis are the most common manifestations of CMV infection in patients with AIDS.

Among the most devastating manifestations of CMV is retinitis, occurring in 25 to 30 percent of patients. CMV retinitis usually presents as a painless, progressive loss of vision; patients may complain of "floaters." The disease is usually bilateral, affecting one eye more than the other, and the diagnosis is made purely on clinical grounds by an experienced ophthalmologist. The characteristic retinal appearance is that of perivascular hemorrhage and exudate (**see Plate III-1**). CMV infection of the retina results in a necrotic inflammatory process, and the visual loss that develops is irreversible. As a consequence of retinal atrophy in areas of prior inflammation, CMV retinitis may be complicated by rhegmatogenous retinal detachment.

CMV esophagitis presents with substernal chest pain and odynophagia. Diagnosis usually requires endoscopy, which characteristically reveals a single large, shallow ulcer in the distal esophagus. Biopsy reveals characteristic intranuclear and intracytoplasmic inclusion bodies. While CMV may also involve the stomach and small intestine, the most frequent gastrointestinal manifestation of CMV infection is

colitis, which is seen in 5 to 10 percent of all patients with AIDS and presents as diarrhea, abdominal pain, weight loss, and anorexia. The diarrhea is usually nonbloody and, as in the case of esophagitis, diagnosis is usually achieved through endoscopy and biopsy; characteristically, multiple mucosal ulcerations are seen. Barium enema examination is of little value and, in fact, may appear normal. Patients with CMV colitis may experience abdominal perforation and become bacteremic as a result. One consequence of CMV involvement of the gastrointestinal tract may be diffuse, generalized wasting.

Other manifestations of CMV disease are much less common in the HIV-infected patient. While histologic evidence of hepatitis is seen in 33 to 50 percent of patients who have CMV disease elsewhere in the body, clinical hepatitis is rare outside the setting of primary infection, which is almost exclusively seen in children. Approximately 33 percent of patients show some biochemical evidence of biliary tract disease, and CMV may cause a syndrome of papillary stenosis and sclerosing cholangitis. In patients with CMV-associated papillary stenosis, dilation of the extrahepatic common bile duct is usually demonstrated on ultrasound.

While the rate of pulmonary infection with CMV, as evidenced by positive cultures of pulmonary secretions, is quite high, the incidence of actual pulmonary disease due to CMV is quite low. In contrast to other manifestations of CMV infection in AIDS patients, CMV pneumonia responds quite poorly to therapy, as is the case in individuals without HIV infection.

CMV can cause an ascending myelitis and subacute polyneuropathy, which may respond to treatment. Other manifestations of CMV infection include adrenalitis, epididymitis, cervicitis, and pancreatitis.

The diagnosis of clinically significant CMV infection can be difficult. Given the fact that most patients with advanced HIV infection excrete CMV, positive throat, urine, blood, and/or tissue cultures are quite common and of little diagnostic significance. Aside from CMV retinitis, where the diagnosis is made on clinical grounds, a diagnosis of CMV infection requires the histologic demonstration of large intranuclear bodies and cytoplasmic inclusions in the suspect tissue, in the absence of other possible pathologic processes.

℞ TREATMENT

Three drugs—ganciclovir, foscarnet, and cidofovir—are currently licensed for systemic treatment of CMV infection, and formulations of ganciclovir and cidofovir are available for use as ocular implants. Initial response rates of retinitis to treatment with ganciclovir or foscarnet are approximately 80 to 90 percent; however, relapse rates are extremely high, and patients must receive long-term maintenance therapy. Of the two drugs, ganciclovir is somewhat easier to administer for initial therapy; it is given as a short infusion twice a day for 14 days. However, it is associated with a high incidence of bone marrow suppression and usually cannot be given in combination with zidovudine or trimethoprim/sulfamethoxazole. Foscarnet therapy is associated with a high incidence of renal and electrolyte disorders and, for initial therapy, foscarnet must be given as three 2-h infusions daily for 14 days. Maintenance therapy for both drugs consists of a single daily infusion. While both drugs were shown to have similar efficacy in a randomized controlled trial, patients without renal insufficiency treated with foscarnet had a slightly longer survival than patients treated with ganciclovir. The reason for this finding is unclear; however, it may be related to the fact that, in addition to being a potent anti-CMV agent, foscarnet also has activity against HIV. Hence, some clinicians recommend that patients with CMV retinitis be treated with an initial course of the more convenient drug, ganciclovir, followed by maintenance with foscarnet. Strains of CMV that are resistant to ganciclovir have been identified; foscarnet or cidofovir are clearly the agents of choice in this situation. Cidofovir was licensed for treating AIDS-related CMV retinitis based on two studies involving a total of 148 patients. One study showed that cidofovir was capable of delaying the progression of CMV retinitis.

The other demonstrated that cidofovir was effective in patients with relapsing CMV retinitis who had received other CMV therapy previously. While cidofovir may not be as potent as ganciclovir or foscarnet, it is clearly easier to administer. It is given once weekly for the first 2 weeks of treatment and once every 2 weeks thereafter. The major side effects include leukopenia, weakness, nausea, diarrhea, and decreased intraocular pressure. Another convenient way to treat CMV retinitis is to use intraocular implants that slowly release ganciclovir into the intraocular fluid. Although this approach is associated with an increased incidence of retinal detachments, it avoids the need for intravenous infusions. For the small percentage of HIV-infected individuals who are antibody-negative for CMV and who require blood products, such products should be obtained from CMV-negative donors if at all possible. The use of oral ganciclovir in the context of a medical center–based controlled clinical trial as a form of CMV prophylaxis has been associated with a delay in the development of CMV disease, and oral ganciclovir is licensed for this indication. A similar study taking place in a community-based setting failed to show any value for this form of prophylaxis.

Herpes simplex virus infections   Infection with herpes simplex virus (HSV) in HIV-infected individuals is associated with recurrent orolabial, genital, and perianal lesions (see Chap. 184). As HIV disease progresses and the CD4+ T cell count declines, these infections become more frequent and severe. Lesions often appear beefy red, are exquisitely painful, and have a tendency to occur high in the gluteal cleft (Fig. 308-27). Perirectal HSV may be associated with proctitis and anal fissures. HSV should be high on the differential diagnosis in any HIV-infected patient with a poorly healing, painful perirectal lesion. As in the case of CMV, HSV may cause esophagitis. HSV esophagitis often occurs together with active orolabial lesions. In contrast to CMV, where esophagitis is usually associated with a single, large ulcer, HSV esophagitis generally occurs as multiple small ulcers.

FIGURE 308-27   Severe, erosive perirectal herpes simplex in a patient with AIDS.

Recurrent *herpetic whitlow* is another problem in patients with HIV infection. It may present with painful vesicles or extensive cutaneous erosion and is a more severe version of the form seen in the immunologically intact host. Both HSV and varicella-zoster virus (see below) rarely cause a widespread, bilateral necrotizing retinitis referred to as the *acute retinal necrosis syndrome*. This syndrome, in contrast to CMV retinitis, is associated with pain, keratitis, and iritis. It is often associated with orolabial HSV or trigeminal zoster. Ophthalmologic examination reveals widespread pale gray peripheral lesions; this condition is often complicated by retinal detachment. Herpetic encephalitis is extremely rare in HIV-infected patients, despite its association with other immunocompromised conditions.

℞ TREATMENT

The treatment for severe or recurrent HSV infection is acyclovir. For most cases, 200 mg is given orally five times per day for 10 to 14 days; for more severe cases, the drug is given intravenously at higher doses. A more convenient alternative is famciclovir, 500 mg orally every 8 h for 7 days. Valacyclovir is licensed as a treatment for recurrent herpes simplex in the immunocompetent host; however, it has been associated with fatal cases of thrombotic thrombocytopenic purpura and should be avoided in immunocompromised patients, including patients with HIV infection. The development of microbial resistance to acyclovir due to alterations in the viral thymidine kinase enzyme is becoming an increasing problem in the HIV-infected population. These resistant strains are also resistant to ganciclovir; however, they are usually sensitive to foscarnet. The possibility of acyclovir resistance should be considered in patients with herpetic lesions refractory to acyclovir therapy.

Varicella-zoster virus infections   Varicella-zoster virus (VZV), the etiologic agent of chickenpox, assumes a latent form in dorsal root ganglia following primary infection (see Chap. 185). Later in life, reactivation is associated with shingles; the appearance of shingles in any patient under 50 years of age should be an indication for workup of an underlying immunodeficiency, particularly HIV. Shingles is an early manifestation of HIV-induced immunodeficiency and, in one African study, 91 percent of patients developing shingles had underlying HIV infection. VZV infection in a patient with HIV infection is almost exclusively confined to the skin, although the skin eruptions may be extensive, over several dermatomes, and extremely painful **(see Plate ID-37)**. A recurrence rate of 23 percent was noted in one report. A disseminated cutaneous form of zoster that very much resembles a mild form of chickenpox may be seen in patients with advanced HIV disease. As noted above, a small number of patients may develop the acute retinal necrosis syndrome, often in association with trigeminal shingles. Progression to visceral involvement is extremely rare as a reactivation syndrome in an HIV-infected patient, in contrast to many other severe immunodeficiency states. Hence, patients need not be hospitalized nor placed in strict isolation. Primary infection, on the other hand, can be lethal and should be treated aggressively with acyclovir and hyperimmune globulin. While treatment of shingles is not required, it can often result in a reduction in the time to resolution of lesions, and most physicians choose to treat it with high-dose oral or intravenous acyclovir or oral famciclovir. Acyclovir-resistant strains exist and characteristically produce hyperkeratotic lesions; under these circumstances, foscarnet is a useful alternative.

Epstein-Barr virus infections   EBV, one of the causative agents of infectious mononucleosis, is also a very common infection in patients with HIV infection (see Chap. 186). Many patients with HIV actively shed EBV throughout the course of their illness. Aside from the association with lymphoma (discussed below), EBV is thought to play a causative role in *oral hairy leukoplakia*. This condition presents as white, frondlike lesions on the lateral aspect of the tongue and sometimes on the adjacent buccal mucosa **(see Plate ID-41)**. These lesions are sometimes confused with candidiasis; however, they are quite distinct and, in contrast to *Candida* lesions, cannot be removed by scraping. The EBV genome has been demonstrated in these lesions by in situ hybridization. This observation, coupled with the fact that these lesions have been reported to regress following therapy with high-dose oral acyclovir, support the concept that EBV plays a causative role in this condition. Despite this therapeutic option, these lesions are rarely of sufficient clinical consequence to require therapy; they have a relatively high spontaneous remission rate (25 to 50 percent) and are more important for what they represent, namely, the presence of immunodeficiency.

Other human herpesvirus infections Human herpesvirus-8 (HHV-8) has been recognized in association with the lesions of Kaposi's sarcoma. It has also been associated with body cavity lymphoma in HIV-infected individuals. There is no specific therapy for HHV-8 infection at present (see "Pathogenesis of Kaposi's Sarcoma," above, for further details).

Human herpesvirus-6 is the first known human T-lymphotropic herpesvirus. It is the causative agent of exanthem subitum in infants. HHV-6 has been shown in some in vitro studies to act as a cofactor leading to an enhancement of HIV replication, and it is felt by some to accelerate the course of HIV disease. While antibodies to HHV-6 are present in 80 to 100 percent of individuals regardless of HIV status, HHV-6 replication is increased in patients with HIV infection, as evidenced by an increase in the fraction of patients harboring HHV-6 proviral DNA in peripheral blood (21 percent, versus 3 percent in HIV-negative individuals). HHV-6 is found in the retinal tissues of approximately 50 percent of HIV-infected individuals in whom it was sought, and it has been suggested that it may play a role in the subsequent development of CMV retinitis.

JC Virus Infection JC virus, a human papovavirus that is the etiologic agent of *progressive multifocal leukoencephalopathy* (PML), is an important opportunistic pathogen in patients with AIDS (see Chap. 379). While approximately 70 percent of the general adult population have antibodies to JC virus, indicative of prior infection, fewer than 10 percent of healthy adults show any evidence of ongoing viral replication. In contrast, close to 33 percent of HIV-infected individuals have evidence of active replication of JC virus. PML, the only known clinical manifestation of JC virus infection, is seen in 4 percent of HIV-infected individuals and is a late manifestation of AIDS. PML is a demyelinating disease; it begins as small foci in subcortical white matter, and the lesions eventually coalesce. The cerebral hemispheres, cerebellum, and brainstem may all be involved. Histologically, swollen oligodendritic nuclei with inclusions due to the nucleocapsid proteins of JC are seen. Death of the oligodendrocyte leads to demyelination without inflammation. Patients have a protracted clinical course, often developing multifocal neurologic deficits without changes in mental status. Patients with PML may exhibit ataxia, hemiparesis, visual field defects, aphasia, and sensory defects. The diagnosis is usually made by MRI, which reveals multiple white matter lesions on T2-weighted images. The clinical picture is generally much more impressive than the findings on MRI. Death usually occurs within 3 to 6 months of the onset of symptoms. Intrathecal administration of cytosine arabinoside has been reported to lead to improvement in some cases; however, no consistently effective therapy is currently available.

Human Papillomavirus Infection Evidence of infection with human papillomavirus is approximately twice as common in HIV-infected individuals (81 percent of patients in one series) as in the general population. The association of this virus with epidermal dysplasia suggests that both anal and cervical carcinomas will be seen in the HIV-infected population with increased frequency as survival is prolonged through the use of better antiretroviral regimens (see below).

Infection with Hepatitis Viruses Over 95 percent of HIV-infected individuals have evidence of infection with hepatitis B virus; coinfection with hepatitis C and/or D viruses is also quite common. HIV infection has several effects on hepatitis virus infection. It is associated with approximately a threefold increase in the development of persistent hepatitis B surface antigenemia. However, patients infected with both hepatitis B virus and HIV have decreased evidence of inflammatory liver disease, presumably owing to the effects of HIV on the immune system. Hepatitis D is a defective RNA virus that requires concomitant infection with hepatitis B in order to replicate,

and thus infection is only seen together with hepatitis B infection. Hepatitis D infection is more common in patients with HIV infection, is associated with higher levels of hepatitis B virus replication, and seems to be associated with slightly worse hepatic disease, as evidenced by slightly higher levels of hepatic transaminases. Patients with HIV infection respond more poorly to treatment of hepatitis B with interferon-α than do HIV-negative individuals.

NEOPLASTIC DISEASES

A variety of neoplastic and premalignant diseases occur with increased frequency in HIV-infected individuals. Among them are Kaposi's sarcoma, lymphoma, and intraepithelial dysplasia of the cervix and anus. These diseases are significant contributors to the morbidity and mortality of patients with HIV infection. The clinical manifestations of these complications, as well as their epidemiologic profiles, have undergone considerable change as new approaches to treatment develop and as the epidemic involves different demographic groups.

KAPOSI'S SARCOMA Kaposi's sarcoma is a multicentric neoplasm consisting of multiple vascular nodules appearing in the skin, mucous membranes, and viscera. The course ranges from indolent, with only minor skin or lymph node involvement, to fulminant, with extensive cutaneous and visceral involvement. In the initial period of the AIDS epidemic, Kaposi's sarcoma was a prominent clinical feature of the first cases of AIDS, occurring in 79 percent of the patients diagnosed in 1981. By 1989 it was seen in only 25 percent of cases, and by 1992 this number had decreased to 9 percent. Part of this decrease is a reflection of the fact that AIDS-related Kaposi's sarcoma, in contrast to classic or endemic forms, occurs predominantly in homosexual men, with 96 percent of all cases occurring in that risk group. As the percentage of AIDS cases in other risk groups increases, the percentage of cases complicated by Kaposi's sarcoma decreases. This, however, is only a partial explanation for the observed decreased incidence of Kaposi's sarcoma in patients with AIDS. A growing body of epidemiologic and virologic data points to the high likelihood that a sexually transmitted cofactor plays an important role in the development of Kaposi's sarcoma. HHV-8 has been strongly implicated as this viral cofactor (see above). In this regard, Kaposi's sarcoma is four times more common in women who have had sexual contact with bisexual men than in other women, has been seen in homosexual men without evidence of HIV infection, and is more common among homosexual men in New York and Los Angeles than among homosexual men in the central states. As safer sex practices are employed, especially in the homosexual community, the risk of transmission of this cofactor and thus the risk of Kaposi's sarcoma has decreased. Kaposi's sarcoma can be an early manifestation of HIV infection, at times occurring in patients with normal CD4 + T cell counts. Thus, the rate of new cases of Kaposi's sarcoma may be influenced as much by the rate of new HIV infections as by the total number of HIV infections. As the rate of new HIV infections among homosexual men decreased, so did the incidence of new cases of Kaposi's sarcoma. However, as secondary opportunistic infections are better controlled, Kaposi's sarcoma is now appearing as a late complication of HIV infection. In these more advanced patients, Kaposi's sarcoma may be either quite indolent or aggressive. Overall, patients with Kaposi's sarcoma are more likely to die from causes other than those directly related to their tumor.

From a pathophysiologic perspective, Kaposi's sarcoma seems to be more a consequence of disordered cytokine regulation of cell growth than a true cancer (see above). Generally speaking, the tumor respects tissue planes and is rarely invasive.

Clinically, Kaposi's sarcoma may present in a variety of ways and may be seen at any stage of HIV infection, even in the presence of a normal CD4 + T cell count. The initial lesion may be a small, raised reddish-purple nodule on the skin, a discoloration on the oral mucosa, or a swollen lymph node (**see Plate IB-22**). Lesions often appear in sun-exposed areas, particularly the tip of the nose, and have a propensity to occur in areas of trauma (Koebner phenomenon). Because of the vascular nature of the tumors and the presence of extravasated red blood cells in the lesions, their color ranges from reddish to purple to brown and often take the appearance of a bruise, with yellowish discoloration and tattooing. Lesions range in size from a few millimeters to several centimeters in diameter and may be either discrete or confluent. Kaposi's sarcoma lesions most commonly appear as raised macules; however, they also can be papular, particularly in patients with higher CD4+ T cell counts. Confluent lesions may give rise to surrounding lymphedema and may be quite disfiguring when they involve the face and disabling when they involve the lower extremities or the surfaces of joints. Apart from the skin, the lymph nodes, gastrointestinal tract, and lung are the organ systems most commonly affected by Kaposi's sarcoma; however, lesions have been reported in virtually every organ, including the heart and the CNS. In contrast to most malignancies, in which lymph node involvement implies metastatic spread and a poor prognosis, lymph node involvement may be seen very early in Kaposi's sarcoma and is of no special clinical significance. In fact, some patients may present with disease limited to the lymph nodes. These are generally patients with relatively intact immune function and thus with the best prognosis. Pulmonary involvement generally presents as shortness of breath. Eighty percent of patients with pulmonary Kaposi's sarcoma have cutaneous lesions. The chest x-ray characteristically shows bilateral lower lobe infiltrates that obscure the margins of the mediastinum and diaphragm (Fig. 308-28). Pleural effusions are seen in 70 percent of cases of pulmonary Kaposi's sarcoma, a fact that is often helpful in the differential diagnosis. Gastrointestinal involvement is seen in 50 percent of patients and usually takes one of two forms. The first is mucosal involvement, which may lead to bleeding that can be severe. These patients sometimes also develop symptoms of gastrointestinal obstruction if lesions become large. The second gastrointestinal manifestation is biliary tract involvement. Kaposi's sarcoma lesions may infiltrate the gallbladder and biliary tree, leading to a clinical picture of obstructive jaundice similar to that seen with sclerosing cholangitis.

Several systems have been proposed for staging the extent of Kaposi's sarcoma. Given the unique nature of this disorder, standard oncologic staging systems have not been useful. An excellent staging system has been developed by the National Institute of Allergy and Infectious Diseases AIDS Clinical Trials Group; it distinguishes patients on the basis of tumor extent, immunologic function, and presence or absence of systemic disease (Table 308-22).

A diagnosis of Kaposi's sarcoma is based on biopsy of a suspicious lesion. Histologically one sees a proliferation of spindle cells and

FIGURE 308-28 Chest x-ray of a patient with AIDS and pulmonary Kaposi's sarcoma. The characteristic findings include dense bilateral lower lobe infiltrates obscuring the heart borders and a pleural effusion.

endothelial cells, extravasation of red blood cells, hemosiderin-laden macrophages, and, in early cases, an inflammatory cell infiltrate. Included in the differential diagnoses are lymphoma (oral lesions), bacillary angiomatosis, and cutaneous mycobacterial infections.

℞ TREATMENT

Management of Kaposi's sarcoma (Table 308-23) should be carried out in consultation with an expert, since definitive therapeutic guidelines do not exist. In some cases, lesions remain quite indolent, and many of these patients can be managed with no specific treatment. Given the fact that less than 10 percent of AIDS patients with Kaposi's sarcoma die as a consequence of their malignancy and that death from opportunistic infections is much more common, whenever possible one should avoid treatment regimens that may further suppress the immune system and render the patients more susceptible to opportunistic infections. Furthermore, treatment is palliative and is not associated with improved survival.

Treatment is indicated under two main circumstances. The first is when a single lesion or a limited number of lesions are causing significant discomfort or cosmetic problems, such as with prominent facial lesions, lesions overlying a joint, or lesions in the posterior oropharynx that interfere with swallowing. Under these circumstances, treatment with localized irradiation, intralesional vinblastine, or cryotherapy may be indicated. It should be noted that patients with HIV infection are particularly sensitive to the side effects of radiation therapy. This is especially true with respect to the development of radiation-induced mucositis; doses of radiation directed at mucosal surfaces, particularly in the head and neck region, should be adjusted accordingly. The use of single-agent systemic chemotherapy should be considered in patients with a large number of lesions. Response rates varying from 26 to 80 percent have been seen with etoposide, vinblastine, doxorubicin, bleomycin, or IFNα. The single most important determinant of response appears to be the CD4+ T cell count. It is ironic that the patients most likely to respond to therapy are those who need it the least and who generally should not be treated aggressively for fear of further compromising immune function. This relationship between response rate and baseline CD4+ T cell count is particularly true for IFNα, where the response rate for patients with CD4+ T cell counts of >600/μL is approximately 80 percent, while the response rate for patients with counts of <150/μL is less than 10 percent. In contrast to the other single therapy agents, IFNα provides an added advantage of having antiretroviral activity; thus, it may be an appropriate first choice for single-agent systemic therapy for the early patient with disseminated disease. Combination chemotherapy offers the best overall response rate for patients with life-threatening disease, with close to 90 percent of all patients responding to a low-dose combination regimen of doxorubicin, bleomycin, and vinblastine. Liposome-encapsulated doxorubicin offers the potential for enhanced tumor uptake of this agent and thus lesser systemic side effects. As noted above, Kaposi's sarcoma is a radiation-sensitive tumor, and for patients with severe pulmonary involvement, one may also consider radiation therapy.

LYMPHOMAS Lymphomas occur with an increased frequency in patients with congenital or acquired T cell immunodeficiencies (see Chap. 307). AIDS is no exception; at least 6 percent of all patients develop lymphoma at some time during the course of their illness, which represents a 120-fold increase in incidence compared to the general population. Lymphoma occurs in all risk groups, with the highest incidence in patients with hemophilia and the lowest in patients from the Caribbean or Africa with heterosexually acquired infection. Lymphoma is a late manifestation of HIV infection, generally occurring in patients with less than 200 CD4+ T cells per microliter. As HIV disease progresses, the risk of lymphoma increases. In contrast to Kaposi's sarcoma, which occurs at a relatively constant rate (2.4 percent per year) throughout the course of illness, the attack rate for lymphoma rises exponentially with increasing duration of HIV infection and decreasing level of immunologic function. At 3 years after infection, the risk of lymphoma is 0.8 percent per year; by 8 years after infection, it is 2.6 percent per year. As people with HIV infection live longer because of improved antiretroviral therapy and more aggressive treatment and prophylaxis of opportunistic infections, the incidence of lymphomas may increase.

Three main categories of lymphoma are seen in patients with HIV infection: grade III or IV immunoblastic lymphoma, Burkitt's lymphoma, and primary CNS lymphoma (see Chap. 113). Approximately 90 percent of these lymphomas are B cell in phenotype, and half contain Epstein-Barr virus DNA. These tumors may be either monoclonal or oligoclonal in origin and are probably in some way related to the pronounced polyclonal B cell activation seen in patients with AIDS (see "Pathophysiology and Pathogenesis," above). Body cavity lymphomas have been associated with HHV-8.

Immunoblastic lymphomas account for approximately 60 percent of the cases of lymphoma in patients with AIDS. These are generally high-grade and would have been classified as diffuse histiocytic lymphomas in earlier classification schemes. This tumor is more common in older patients, increasing in incidence from 0 percent in HIV-infected individuals less than 1 year old to over 3 percent in those over 50 years old.

Small noncleaved cell lymphoma (Burkitt's lymphoma) accounts for approximately 20 percent of the cases of lymphoma in patients with AIDS. They are most frequent in patients 10 to 19 years old and usually demonstrate characteristic *c-myc* translocations from chromosome 8 to chromosomes 14 or 22. Burkitt's lymphoma is not commonly seen in the setting of immunodeficiency other than that due to HIV, and the incidence of this tumor in the setting of HIV infection is over 1000-fold higher than that in the general population. In contrast to African Burkitt's lymphoma, where 97 percent of cases contain an Epstein-Barr virus genome, only 50 percent of HIV-associated Burkitt's lymphomas are Epstein-Barr positive.

Primary CNS lymphoma accounts for approximately 20 percent of the cases of lymphoma in patients with HIV infection. In contrast to HIV-associated Burkitt's lymphoma, primary CNS lymphomas are usually positive for Epstein-Barr virus; in one study, the incidence of positivity was 100 percent, and the lymphomas did not appear to have a predilection for any particular age group. The median CD4+ T cell count at time of diagnosis of primary CNS lymphoma in AIDS patients is approximately 40/μL. CNS lymphoma generally presents at a later stage of HIV infection than does systemic lymphoma, and this fact may explain at least in part the poorer prognosis for this subset of patients (see below).

Table 308-22

National Institute of Allergy and Infectious Diseases AIDS Clinical Trials Group TIS Staging System for Kaposi's Sarcoma

Parameter	Good Risk (stage 0): All of the Following	Poor Risk (stage 1): Any of the Following
Tumor (T)	Confined to skin and/or lymph nodes and/or minimal oral disease	Tumor-associated edema or ulceration Extensive oral lesions Gastrointestinal lesions Nonnodal visceral lesions
Immune system (I)	CD4+ T cell count ≥200/μL	CD4+ T cell count <200/μL
Systemic illness (S)	No B symptoms*	B symptoms* present
	Karnofsky performance status >70	Karnofsky performance status <70
	No history of opportunistic infection, neurologic disease, lymphoma, or thrush	History of opportunistic infection, neurologic disease, lymphoma, or thrush

* Defined as unexplained fever, night sweats. >10% involuntary weight loss, or diarrhea persisting for more than 2 weeks.

The clinical presentation of lymphoma in patients with HIV infection is quite varied, ranging from focal seizures to rapidly growing mass lesions in the oral mucosa (Fig. 308-29) to persistent unexplained fever. At least 80 percent of patients present with extranodal disease, and a similar percentage have B-type symptoms of fever, night sweats, or weight loss. Virtually any site in the body may be involved. The most common extranodal site is the CNS, which is involved in approximately one-third of all patients with lymphoma; approximately 60 percent of these cases are primary CNS lymphoma. Primary CNS lymphoma generally presents with focal neurologic deficits, including cranial nerve findings, headaches, and/or seizures. MRI or CT generally reveals a limited number (one to three) of 3- to 5-cm lesions. The lesions often show ring-enhancement on contrast administration and may occur in any location. The main disease to be considered in the differential diagnosis is cerebral toxoplasmosis, although cerebral Chagas' disease may manifest a similar clinical picture. The prognosis is poor; the median survival following diagnosis is 2 to 3 months.

In addition to the 20 percent of all lymphomas in HIV-infected individuals that are primary CNS lymphomas, CNS disease is also seen in HIV-infected patients with systemic lymphoma; approximately 20 percent of patients with systemic lymphoma have CNS disease in the form of leptomeningeal involvement. This fact underscores the importance of a lumbar puncture in the staging evaluation of patients with systemic lymphoma.

Another common extranodal site of lymphoma in HIV-infected patients is the gastrointestinal tract, with involvement noted in 25 percent of patients. Any site in the gastrointestinal tract may be involved, and patients may complain of difficulty swallowing or abdominal pain. The diagnosis is usually suspected on the basis of CT or MRI of the abdomen. Bone marrow involvement occurs in approximately 20 percent of patients and may be associated with pancytopenia. Liver and lung involvement are each seen in approximately 10 percent of patients. Pulmonary disease may present as either a mass lesion, multiple nodules, or an interstitial infiltrate.

Table 308-23

Management of AIDS-Associated Kaposi's Sarcoma

Observation
Single or limited number of lesions
  Radiation
  Intralesional vinblastine
  Cryotherapy
Extensive, non-life-threatening disease
  Single-agent chemotherapy (etoposide, vinblastine, adriamycin, or bleomycin)
  Interferon-α (if CD4+ T cell >150/μL)
Life-threatening disease
  Combination chemotherapy with low-dose doxorubicin, bleomycin, and vinblastine (ABV)
  Radiation treatment

FIGURE 308-29 Diffuse histiocytic lymphoma involving the hard palate of a patient with AIDS.

℞ **TREATMENT**

Both conventional and unconventional approaches have been employed in an effort to treat HIV-related lymphomas. Initial attempts using standard intensive therapeutic regimens have largely been abandoned due to low response rates (20 to 30 percent) and a high incidence of fatal opportunistic infections. The median survival for patients treated with intensive regimens is approximately 4 to 6 months. These figures mainly reflect results in patients with fairly advanced HIV infection and low CD4+ T cell counts. Patients with higher CD4+ T cell counts do better with intensive chemotherapy, and in these earlier-stage patients, response rates as high as 72 percent and disease-free intervals exceeding 15 months have been reported. Clinical trials are under way comparing standard chemotherapeutic approaches with low-dose modified regimens. The median survival for patients with HIV-related systemic lymphoma is 10 months. Treatment of primary CNS lymphoma is almost uniformly unsuccessful. Palliative measures, such as radiation therapy and/or glucocorticoids, aimed at reducing the size of the lesion(s) and the accompanying edema may provide some symptomatic relief. The prognosis is poor for patients with primary CNS lymphoma; median survival is 2 to 4 months.

INTRAEPITHELIAL DYSPLASIA OF THE CERVIX OR ANUS This condition has been recognized increasingly as a complication of long-standing HIV infection. This human papillomavirus–associated condition correlates with the subsequent development of intraepithelial neoplasia and eventually invasive cancer. In two separate studies, HIV-infected men without anorectal symptoms were studied for evidence of dysplasia, and Papanicolaou smears were found to be abnormal in about 40 percent. These changes were persistent at 1 year follow-up, raising the possibility of a subsequent transition to a more malignant condition. While the incidence of an abnormal Papanicolaou smear of the cervix is approximately 5 percent in otherwise healthy women, the incidence of abnormal cervical smears in women with HIV infection is 60 percent. Based on this finding, invasive cervical carcinoma was added to the list of AIDS-defining conditions. Thus far, however, only small increases in the incidence of cervical or anal cancer have been seen as a consequence of HIV infection. However, given these findings, as patients with HIV infection live longer through the use of improved treatment strategies, it is likely that such conditions will begin to appear more frequently. For these reasons, all patients with HIV infection should have periodic pelvic examinations and/or rectal examinations with Papanicolaou smears to look for evidence of cellular dysplasia.

OTHER NEOPLASTIC CONDITIONS A variety of other neoplastic conditions have been described in patients with HIV infection. While none of these other conditions have been reported

to occur at a higher rate than that seen in the general population, these cancers may be more fulminant and difficult to treat in HIV-infected patients. In this regard, Hodgkin's disease in the setting of HIV infection often presents as extensive disease, with mixed cellular or lymphocyte depletion pathologic types. In contrast to the excellent results and high cure rates for Hodgkin's disease in the general population, patients with advanced HIV infection and Hodgkin's disease have a median survival of only 12 to 15 months. As the epidemic of HIV infection continues, additional neoplastic complications are to be expected.

ORGAN-SPECIFIC SYNDROMES

Virtually every organ in the body is vulnerable to disease either as a direct consequence of HIV infection or secondary to other infectious or neoplastic conditions. While most of these diseases are due to opportunistic infections or neoplasms (see above), there are also a variety of clinical problems for which no specific pathogens are clearly identified.

PULMONARY DISEASE Pulmonary disease is seen in virtually every patient with HIV infection. Its evaluation is one of the most critical components in management, given the importance of early diagnosis and initiation of specific therapy. The most common manifestation of pulmonary disease is pneumonia. The two most common causes of pneumonia are bacterial infections and *P. carinii* infection. Other major causes of pneumonia include nonspecific interstitial pneumonitis, Kaposi's sarcoma, mycobacterial infections, and fungal infections. Although there are some distinguishing clinical and radiographic characteristics (Table 308-24), in most cases an accurate diagnosis is based on histologic or microbiologic identification of the causative organisms. Specimens for examination are derived from induced sputum, bronchoalveolar lavage, transbronchial biopsy, percutaneous aspiration, or open lung biopsy. In most of the conditions seen in HIV-infected patients, the chest x-ray reveals bilateral diffuse interstitial infiltrates. In patients with mycobacterial or fungal infections, hilar or mediastinal adenopathy may also be seen. *Aspergillus* may cause a pseudomembranous tracheobronchitis. In Kaposi's sarcoma, the infiltrates are dense and often obliterate the borders of the heart and diaphragm; there is usually an accompanying pleural effusion. Upper lobe cavitary disease is suggestive of reactivation tuberculosis or PCP in a patient receiving aerosolized pentamidine. The presence of a pneumothorax is most consistent with the latter condition. With the exception of bacterial pneumonias, sputum production is usually scant. Hemoptysis may be seen in the setting of cryptococcal pneumonia, tuberculosis, or Kaposi's sarcoma.

Two forms of *idiopathic interstitial pneumonia* have been described in patients with HIV infection: *lymphoid interstitial pneumonitis* (LIP) and *nonspecific interstitial pneumonitis* (NIP). LIP, a common finding in HIV-infected children, is rare in adults, occurring in approximately 1 percent of patients. This disorder is characterized by a benign lymphocytic infiltrate of the lung and is felt to be part of the systemic polyclonal activation of lymphocytes seen in the context of HIV and EBV infections. Transbronchial biopsy is diagnostic in 50 percent of cases; an open lung biopsy is required for diagnosis in the remainder. This condition is generally self-limited, and no specific treatment is necessary. Severe cases have been managed with a brief course of glucocorticoids. NIP is seen in up to half of all patients with AIDS and in some series is responsible for up to one-third of all pulmonary disease. Interstitial infiltrates with lymphocytes and plasma cells in a perivascular and peribronchial distribution are seen on histologic examination. Symptoms include fever and nonproductive cough, occasionally accompanied by mild chest discomfort. Chest x-ray, which is normal in 50 percent of cases, may reveal a faint

Table 308-24

Characteristics of Pneumonia in Patients with HIV Infection

Etiology	Sputum	Chest X-Ray
Pneumocystis carinii	Scant	Normal/interstitial infiltrate
Pneumocystis carinii in setting of aerosolized pentamidine	Scant	Upper lobe cavitary lesions; pneumothorax
Bacterial	Neutrophils, organisms	Consolidation
Atypical mycobacteria	Scant	Interstitial infiltrate; hilar adenopathy
Reactivation *Mycobacterium tuberculosis*	White blood cells, organisms, occasional hemoptysis	Cavitary or miliary infiltrates; hilar adenopathy
Nonspecific interstitial pneumonitis (NIP)	Scant	Normal/interstitial infiltrate
Kaposi's sarcoma	Scant, occasional hemoptysis	Dense, bilateral lower lobe infiltrates; pleural effusions

interstitial pattern. Like LIP, this is a self-limited process for which no therapy is indicated.

In addition to pneumonia, *sinusitis* is a common respiratory tract complication of HIV infection and is seen at all stages of disease. More severe cases are seen in patients with lower CD4+ T cell counts. Sinusitis presents as fever, nasal congestion, and headache; the diagnosis is best made by CT or MRI. The maxillary sinuses are most commonly involved; however, disease is also frequently seen in the ethmoid, sphenoid, and frontal sinuses. Although over 80 percent of patients show clinical improvement regardless of whether or not antibiotics are given, radiographic improvement is quicker and more pronounced in patients who have received antimicrobial therapy. It is postulated that this high incidence of sinusitis results from the increased frequency of infections with encapsulated organisms such as *Haemophilus influenzae* and *Streptococcus pneumoniae*, although this relationship has not been formally proven.

GASTROINTESTINAL DISEASE Gastrointestinal disease is a common feature of HIV infection and is most frequently due to a secondary infection. The oral mucosa, in addition to being involved with thrush, oral hairy leukoplakia, and Kaposi's sarcoma, may also be affected by large, shallow, painful aphthous ulcers. These lesions, which may be painful enough to result in a decrease in oral intake, are of unknown cause; however, they have been associated with dideoxynucleoside therapy in some instances. Brief courses of thalidomide have resulted in clearance of persistent aphthous ulcers. Esophagitis (Fig. 308-26) generally presents with odynophagia and retrosternal pain and may be due to *Candida*, CMV, or HSV. In addition, the esophagus may be involved with Kaposi's sarcoma and lymphoma. The esophageal mucosa, like the oral mucosa, may have large, painful ulcers of unclear etiology. These lesions are somewhat similar in appearance to the ulcers of CMV esophagitis but do not respond to antiviral therapy and can pose a significant problem with regard to nutrition. They may respond to therapy with thalidomide. Achlorhydria is a common problem in patients with HIV infection; however, gastric problems are otherwise rare. Kaposi's sarcoma as well as lymphoma may involve the stomach. Infections of the small and large intestine are among the most significant gastrointestinal problems in the HIV-infected patients. They usually present with diarrhea, abdominal pain, occasionally fever, and, in severe cases, weight loss. In addition to specific secondary infections, patients with HIV infection may also experience a chronic diarrheal syndrome for which no etiologic agent other than HIV can be identified and which is generally referred to as *AIDS* or *HIV enteropathy*. This is a clinical condition resembling chronic gastroenteritis with diarrhea of more than 1 month's duration for which no cause can be found. This condition is most likely a direct result of HIV infection in the gastrointestinal tract. Histologic examination of the small bowel in these patients reveals low-grade mucosal atrophy with a decrease in mitotic figures suggesting a hyporegenerative state. Patients often have decreased or absent small bowel lactase and malabsorption with accompanying weight loss.

In working up a patient with HIV infection and gastrointestinal problems, a set of stool examinations, including culture, examination for ova and parasites, and examination for *Clostridium difficile* toxin should form the initial part of the evaluation. Approximately 50 percent of the time, this workup will demonstrate infection with pathogenic bacteria, such as *Salmonella*, *Shigella*, or *Campylobacter*; mycobacteria (both atypical mycobacteria and *M. tuberculosis*); protozoa such as *Giardia*, *Entamoeba histolytica*, cryptosporidia, or *Isospora*; or *Clostridium difficile*. If these stool examinations are negative, additional evaluation, including upper and/or lower endoscopy with biopsy, establishes a diagnosis of microsporidial or mycobacterial infection of the small intestine or of CMV colitis in over half of patients. In patients for whom this diagnostic evaluation is nonrevealing, and if diarrhea has persisted for over 1 month, a presumptive diagnosis of HIV enteropathy can be made. An algorithm for the evaluation of diarrhea in patients with HIV infection is given in Fig. 308-30.

Rectal lesions are common in HIV-infected patients, particularly the perirectal ulcers and erosions due to the reactivation of HSV (Fig. 308-27). These may appear quite atypical, without vesicles, and

respond well to treatment with acyclovir. Other rectal lesions more commonly seen in HIV-infected patients include condyloma acuminatum, Kaposi's sarcoma, and intraepithelial neoplasia.

Several different forms of hepatobiliary disease occur in patients with HIV infection. Biliary tract disease in the form of papillary stenosis or sclerosing cholangitis has been reported in the context of cryptosporidiosis, CMV infection, and Kaposi's sarcoma. Hepatic disease may take the form of hepatocellular injury due to hepatitis viruses, granulomatous hepatitis due to mycobacterial or fungal infections, or hepatic masses secondary to tuberculous abscess or peliosis hepatis. Fatty infiltration has also been reported; in some patients it may be related to nucleoside therapy. Asymptomatic hyperbilirubinemia may be seen as a consequence of indinavir therapy.

Pancreatic injury is most commonly due to drug toxicity, notably that secondary to pentamidine or dideoxynucleosides. While up to 50 percent of patients with HIV infection have biochemical evidence of pancreatic injury, and there is often evidence of pancreatic infection with CMV and/or MAC at autopsy, fewer than 5 percent of patients show any clinical evidence of pancreatitis that is not linked to a drug toxicity.

HEMATOLOGIC PROBLEMS Hematologic problems are common throughout the course of HIV infection and may be direct results of HIV, manifestations of secondary infections and neoplasms, or side effects of therapy (Table 308-25). Bone marrow suppression may be associated with disseminated mycobacterial infections, fungal infections, and lymphoma. Direct histologic examination and culture of bone marrow in patients with HIV infection and unexplained hematologic abnormalities are often diagnostic. A significant percentage of bone marrow aspirates have been reported to contain lymphoid aggregates, the precise significance of which is unknown.

Anemia is the most common hematologic abnormality in HIV-infected individuals, being present in 18 percent of asymptomatic seropositive individuals, 50 percent of patients with early symptoms, and 75 percent of patients with AIDS. While generally mild, anemia can be quite severe and may require chronic blood transfusions. Among the specific reversible causes of anemia in HIV-infected individuals are drug toxicity, systemic fungal and mycobacterial infections, nutritional deficiencies, and parvovirus B19 infections.

Zidovudine is a major contributor to the anemia seen in patients with advanced HIV infection. This nucleoside analogue (discussed

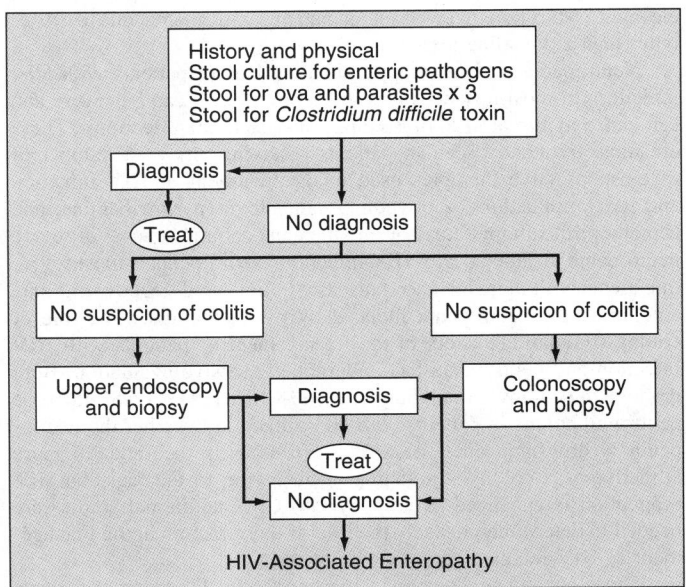

FIGURE 308-30 Algorithm for the evaluation of diarrhea in a patient with HIV infection. HIV-associated enteropathy is a diagnosis of exclusion and can be made only after other, generally treatable, forms of diarrheal illness have been ruled out.

Table 308-25

Causes of Bone Marrow Suppression in Patients with HIV Infection

HIV infection	Medications:
Mycobacterial infections	Zidovudine
Fungal infections	Dapsone
B19 parvovirus infection	Trimethoprim/sulfamethoxazole
Lymphoma	Pyrimethamine
	5-Flucytosine
	Ganciclovir
	Interferon-α
	Trimetrexate
	Foscarnet

below) has a somewhat selective ability to block erythroid maturation, an effect that precedes effects on other marrow elements. A characteristic feature of zidovudine therapy is an elevated mean corpuscular volume (MCV). Another drug with selective effects on the erythroid series is dapsone. This agent can cause a serious hemolytic anemia in patients who are G6PD-deficient and can create a functional anemia in others through induction of methemoglobinemia.

Folate levels are usually normal in HIV-infected individuals; however, vitamin B_{12} levels may be depressed in patients with AIDS, presumably as a consequence of long-standing achlorhydria and malabsorption. Replacement therapy with vitamin B_{12} seems to have a minimal effect on HIV-associated anemia. True autoimmune hemolytic anemia is rare, although approximately 20 percent of patients with HIV infection have a positive direct antiglobulin test, presumably as a consequence of polyclonal B cell activation.

In addition to the more common secondary infections described above, patients with HIV infection have been reported to develop anemia secondary to infection with parvovirus B19. It is important to be aware of this cause of anemia, as it responds to treatment with intravenous immunoglobulin.

Baseline erythropoietin levels in patients with HIV infection and anemia are generally less than expected, given the degree of anemia. The exception is zidovudine-associated anemia, in which levels may be quite high. In patients with zidovudine-associated anemia and low erythropoietin levels, treatment with erythropoietin at a dose of 100 μg/kg three times a week may result in an increase in hemoglobin levels. Erythropoietin seems to be of less benefit in patients with elevated erythropoietin levels and in patients with anemia due to causes other than zidovudine toxicity.

Neutropenia is seen in approximately half of patients with HIV infection. In most instances it is mild; however, it can be severe and can put patients at risk of spontaneous bacterial infections. These are most frequently seen in patients receiving any of a number of myelosuppressive therapies used in the treatment of HIV infection and its complications. Zidovudine, ganciclovir, pyrimethamine, and trimethoprim/sulfamethoxazole are the most common causes of severe neutropenia in patients with HIV infection. Neutropenia is most severe in patients with more advanced disease. Folinic acid (leucovorin) may ameliorate the neutropenia induced by pyrimethamine. The role of colony-stimulating factors in the management of patients with HIV infection and neutropenia has undergone extensive evaluation. Both granulocyte colony-stimulating factor (G-CSF) and GM-CSF increase neutrophil counts in patients with HIV infection, whether the neutropenia is drug-induced or not. While G-CSF is theoretically more attractive as a colony-stimulating agent owing to the fact that HIV replication is enhanced in vitro by GM-CSF, additional studies are needed to determine precisely the role of these factors in the management of HIV-infected patients with neutropenia.

Thrombocytopenia occurs in approximately 40 percent of patients with HIV infection and, in contrast to neutropenia and anemia, is often an early, primary manifestation of HIV infection. The thrombocytopenia seen as a direct result of HIV infection resembles that of idiopathic thrombocytopenic purpura (see Chap. 117) and responds not only to conventional strategies but, in a large number of cases, to therapy with antiretroviral agents. Thrombocytopenia may also be seen as a side effect of medications; however, it is rarely dose limiting. Other causes of thrombocytopenia in patients with HIV infection include bone marrow involvement by lymphoma, mycobacterial infection, and fungal infections.

LYMPHADENOPATHY Lymphadenopathy is also a common finding in patients with HIV infection, ranging from the generalized follicular hyperplasia seen early in disease (see above) to involvement secondary to opportunistic infections and neoplasms. Lymph node biopsy is not indicated in the lymphadenopathy seen early in disease unless it is associated with rapid enlargement, unusual consistency, or coalescence of nodes. While Kaposi's sarcoma may present in a lymphadenopathic form early in disease, there are no data to suggest that early treatment is indicated. In contrast, new-onset lymphadenopathy in the setting of more advanced HIV infection (CD4+ T cell counts under 200/μL) may be the first sign of a secondary infection or neoplasm and should be examined both histologically and microbiologically. Among the secondary infections commonly associated with lymphadenopathy are mycobacterial infections, fungal infections, and bacillary angiomatosis. In addition to Kaposi's sarcoma, lymphoma may also present as lymphadenopathy.

RENAL DISEASE Renal disease may be associated with HIV infection (see Chaps. 275 and 276). Although renal disease is often drug-induced, a significant portion of patients with AIDS (up to 10 percent in some series) develop renal disease as a direct consequence of HIV infection; this is designated *AIDS- or HIV-associated nephropathy*. Secondary infections rarely result in significant renal impairment; however, one may see nephrocalcinosis as a result of infection with mycobacteria or *P. carinii*.

Among the drugs commonly associated with renal damage in patients with AIDS are pentamidine, amphotericin, and foscarnet. In addition, trimethoprim/sulfamethoxazole may compete for tubular secretion with creatinine and cause an increase in the serum creatinine level. Sulfadiazine may crystallize in the kidney and result in an easily reversible form of renal shutdown, while the protease inhibitor indinavir can lead to renal calculi.

HIV-associated nephropathy closely resembles the heroin-associated nephropathy seen in IDUs and initially was thought to be that condition in patients with HIV infection; however, it is now recognized as a true direct complication of HIV infection. HIV-associated nephropathy can be an early manifestation of HIV infection and is also seen in children. The severity of renal disease and the propensity to develop end-stage renal failure appear to be a function of race and are much more of a problem among African Americans than whites, perhaps more so than any other manifestation of HIV infection. Given that in most series over 50 percent of patients with HIV-associated nephropathy were IDUs, it was originally thought that this racial predilection merely reflected the disproportionate number of African Americans in the IDU group rather than being a true race-related phenomenon. However, the incidence by race of HIV-associated end-stage renal failure in non-IDU homosexual men suggests that race does play a major role and that end-stage renal failure occurs disproportionately among African Americans.

The prototypic lesion of HIV-associated nephropathy is a focal segmental glomerulosclerosis, which is seen in approximately 80 percent of patients with this complication. Patients present with heavy proteinuria without edema or hypertension. Ultrasound examination usually reveals enlarged, hyperechogenic kidneys; a definitive diagnosis is obtained through renal biopsy. Progression to end-stage renal failure usually occurs within 1 year. The remainder of patients (approximately 20 percent) with HIV-associated nephropathy present with a mesangial hyperplasia with minimal glomerulosclerosis. It is believed that this may be the precursor lesion to focal segmental glomerulosclerosis.

There is no successful treatment for HIV-associated nephropathy. Antiretroviral therapy seems to have little overall beneficial effect on it, although temporary improvement following initiation of zidovudine therapy has been noted by some investigators. In patients in whom renal disease is detected relatively early, at the stage of mesangial hyperplasia with minimal glomerulosclerosis, it has been proposed that a short course of glucocorticoids may be of value. While this seems a reasonable therapeutic option, it must be carried out with awareness of the potential negative effects of long-term glucocorticoid use in patients with HIV infection.

DERMATOLOGIC PROBLEMS Dermatologic problems are common in patients with HIV infection (see Chap. 57). From the macular, roseola-like rash seen with the acute seroconversion syndrome to extensive end-stage Kaposi's sarcoma, cutaneous manifestations can be seen throughout the entire course of HIV infection. While many of these manifestations are covered elsewhere in this chapter under their respective causes and in the section "Early Symptomatic Disease," some additional ones occur (see Chaps. 55, 56, and 58). Among these are seborrheic dermatitis, eosinophilic pustular folliculitis, and several minor cutaneous infections.

Seborrheic dermatitis occurs in 3 percent of the general population, but it is seen in up to 50 percent of patients with HIV infection and is among the most common noninfectious manifestations of HIV infection. Seborrheic dermatitis increases in prevalence and severity as the CD4+ T cell count declines. In HIV-infected patients, seborrheic dermatitis may be aggravated by concomitant infection with *Pityrosporon*, a yeast-like fungus; use of topical antifungal agents has been recommended in cases refractory to standard topical treatment.

Eosinophilic pustular folliculitis is a rare dermatologic condition that is seen with increased frequency in patients with HIV infection. It presents as multiple urticarial perifollicular papules that may coalesce into plaque-like lesions. Skin biopsy reveals an eosinophilic infiltrate of the hair follicle, which in certain cases has been associated with the presence of a mite. Patients typically have an elevated IgE level and may respond to treatment with topical anthelmintics. There is at least one report of a patient with AIDS developing a severe form of Norwegian scabies with hyperkeratotic, psoriaform skin lesions.

Both psoriasis and ichthyosis, although they are not reported to be increased in frequency, may be particularly severe when they occur in patients with HIV infection. Preexisting psoriasis may become guttate in appearance and more refractory to treatment.

As mentioned above, a variety of secondary infections in HIV-infected patients can present with cutaneous manifestations. Among them are HSV infection, which can cause severe erosive orolabial, genital, and perirectal ulcers (Fig. 308-27) or whitlow lesions, and VZV infection, which can cause either shingles or a forme fruste of chickenpox secondary to cutaneous dissemination. Similarly, molluscum contagiosum and condyloma acuminatum may be significantly more serious in HIV-infected individuals. Atypical mycobacterial infections may present as erythematous cutaneous nodules, as may certain fungal infections and *Bartonella* infections. Extrapulmonary pneumocystosis may result in necrotizing vasculitis.

The skin of patients with HIV infection is often a target organ for drug reactions (see Chap. 56). Although most skin reactions are mild and not necessarily an indication to discontinue treatment, patients may have particularly severe cutaneous eruptions, including erythroderma and Stevens-Johnson syndrome, as a reaction to drugs, particularly sulfa drugs. Similarly, patients with HIV infection are often very photosensitive and burn easily following exposure to sunlight or as a side effect of radiation therapy (see Chap. 58).

HIV infection and treatment may be accompanied by cosmetic changes of the skin that are not of great clinical importance but nonetheless are troubling to patients. Both yellowing of the nails and straightening of the hair, particularly in African-American patients, have been reported as a consequence of HIV infection. Zidovudine therapy has been associated with elongation of the eyelashes and the development of a bluish discoloration to the nails, again more commonly among African Americans. Therapy with clofazimine may cause a yellow-orange discoloration of the skin.

HEART DISEASE While heart disease is a relatively common postmortem finding in HIV-infected patients (25 to 75 percent in autopsy series), it is rarely a clinical problem. The most common clinically significant finding is a dilated cardiomyopathy associated with congestive heart failure (see Chap. 239); this generally occurs as a late complication of HIV infection and, histologically, most closely resembles a myocarditis. HIV has been detected in cardiac tissue, and there is debate over whether it plays a direct role in this condition. Patients present with the classic findings of congestive heart failure, i.e., edema and shortness of breath. Treatment is no different than for any other patient with congestive heart failure, although one must be certain that drug toxicity is not the cause. Both IFNα and nucleoside analogues have been reported to cause a cardiomyopathy in patients with HIV infection that reverses once therapy is discontinued. Similarly, Kaposi's sarcoma, cryptococcosis, and toxoplasmosis can involve the myocardium, resulting in cardiomyopathy. In one series, most patients with a treatable myocarditis were found to have myocarditis associated with toxoplasmosis. Most of these patients also had evidence of CNS toxoplasmosis. Thus, an MRI or double-dose contrast CT scan of the brain should be included in the workup of any patient with advanced HIV infection and an unexplained cardiomyopathy.

A variety of other cardiovascular problems have been found in the setting of HIV infection. Pericardial disease may be due to Kaposi's sarcoma, mycobacterial infections, cryptococcal disease, or lymphoma. Tamponade and death have occurred in association with pericardial Kaposi's sarcoma, presumably owing to acute hemorrhage. Clinically significant ischemic heart disease is not seen to an increased degree in HIV-infected individuals, even though a high percentage of patients have hypertriglyceridemia, and coronary artery disease has been a relatively frequent finding at autopsy. Nonbacterial thrombotic endocarditis has been reported and should be considered in patients with unexplained embolic phenomena. Intravenous pentamidine, when given rapidly, can result in hypotension as a consequence of cardiovascular collapse.

IMMUNOLOGIC AND RHEUMATOLOGIC DISORDERS Disorders of these types are common in patients with HIV infection and range from excessive immediate hypersensitivity-type reactions (see Chap. 310) to an increase in the incidence of reactive arthritis (see Chap. 317) to conditions characterized by a diffuse infiltrative lymphocytosis. These phenomena occur in an apparent paradox to the profound immunodeficiency that characterizes this infection. Drug allergies are the most significant allergic reactions occurring in HIV-infected patients and seem to become more common as the disease progresses; they occur in 65 percent of patients who receive therapy with trimethoprim/sulfamethoxazole for PCP. In general, these drug reactions are characterized by an erythematous, morbilliform eruption that is pruritic, tends to coalesce, and is often associated with fever. Nonetheless, approximately 33 percent of patients can be maintained successfully on the offending therapy, and thus these reactions are not an immediate indication to stop the drug. Anaphylaxis is extremely rare in patients with HIV infection, and patients who have a cutaneous eruption during a single course of therapy can still be considered candidates for future treatment or prophylaxis with the same agent. In addition, desensitization regimens are moderately successful in HIV-infected patients. While the mechanisms underlying these allergic-type phenomena remain unknown, patients with HIV infection have been noted to have elevated IgE levels that increase as the CD4+ T cell count declines, and there are numerous examples of patients with multiple drug reactions, suggesting some common pathway. It is anticipated that allergic drug reactions will become an increasingly difficult aspect of managing patients with HIV infection, especially with the expanding need for multidrug regimens for the treatment of HIV infection itself and the treatment of tuberculosis, as well as for prophylaxis for opportunistic infections.

HIV infection shares many similarities with a variety of autoimmune diseases, including a substantial polyclonal B cell activation that is associated with a high incidence of antiphospholipid antibodies, such as anticardiolipin antibodies, VDRL antibodies, and lupus-like anticoagulants. In addition, HIV-infected individuals have an increased incidence of positive antinuclear antibodies. However, there is no evidence that HIV-infected individuals have an increase in two of the more common autoimmune diseases, namely systemic lupus erythematosus and rheumatoid arthritis. In fact, it has been observed that these diseases may be somewhat ameliorated by the concomitant presence of HIV infection, suggesting that an intact CD4 + T cell limb of the immune response plays an integral part in their pathogenesis. Similarly, there are anecdotal reports of patients with common variable immunodeficiency (see Chap. 307), characterized by hypogammaglobulinemia, who have had a normalization of Ig levels following the development of HIV infection, suggesting a possible role for overactive CD4 + T cell immunity in certain forms of that disease. The one autoimmune disease that may occur with an increased frequency in patients with HIV infection is a variant of primary Sjögren's syndrome (see Chap. 316). Patients with HIV infection may develop a syndrome consisting of parotid gland enlargement, dry eyes, and dry mouth that is characterized by lymphocytic infiltrates of the salivary gland and lung. In contrast to Sjögren's syndrome, in which these infiltrates are composed predominantly of CD4 + T cells, in patients with HIV infection the infiltrates are composed predominantly of CD8 + T cells. In addition, while patients with Sjögren's syndrome are mainly women who have autoantibodies to Ro and La and who frequently have HLA-DR3 or -B8, HIV-infected individuals with this syndrome are usually African-American men who do not have anti-Ro or anti-La and who most often have HLA-DR5. In at least one case, the syndrome improved following zidovudine therapy. The term *diffuse infiltrative lymphocytosis syndrome* (DILS) has been proposed to describe this entity and to distinguish it from Sjögren's syndrome.

Approximately 33 percent of HIV-infected individuals experience arthralgias; furthermore, 5 to 10 percent are diagnosed as having some form of reactive arthritis, such as Reiter's syndrome or psoriatic arthritis. These syndromes occur with increasing frequency as the competency of the immune system declines; this effect may be related to an increase in the number of infections with organisms that may trigger a reactive arthritis. These arthritides generally respond adequately to standard treatment (see Chap. 317); however, therapy with methotrexate has been associated with an increase in the incidence of opportunistic infections and should be used with caution and only in severe cases.

HIV-infected individuals also experience a variety of joint problems with no obvious cause, which are referred to generically as *HIV- or AIDS-associated arthropathy*. This syndrome is characterized by subacute obligoarticular arthritis developing over a period of 1 to 6 weeks and lasting 6 weeks to 6 months. It generally involves the large joints, predominantly knees and ankles, and is nonerosive with only a mild inflammatory response. X-rays of the joint are nonrevealing. Nonsteroidal anti-inflammatory drugs are marginally helpful; however, relief has been noted with the use of intraarticular steroids. A second form of arthritis also thought to be secondary to HIV infection is called "painful articular syndrome." This condition, described in as many as 10 percent of a cohort of AIDS patients, presents as acute, severe, sharp pain in the joint. It affects mainly the knees, elbows, and shoulders, lasts 2 to 24 h, and may be severe enough to require narcotic analgesics. The cause of this arthropathy is unclear; however, it is thought to result from a direct effect of HIV on the joint. This is a reasonable assumption, given the fact that other lentiviruses, in particular the caprine arthritis-encephalitis virus, are capable of causing arthritis.

A variety of other immunologic or rheumatologic diseases have been reported in HIV-infected individuals, either de novo or in association with opportunistic infections or drugs. Using the criteria of widespread musculoskeletal pain of at least 3 months' duration and the presence of at least 11 of 18 possible tender points by digital palpation, 11 percent of an HIV-infected cohort consisting of 55 percent IDUs could be diagnosed as having fibromyalgia (see Chap. 326). While the incidence of frank arthritis was less in this population than in other studied populations that consisted predominantly of homosexual men, these data support the concept that there are musculoskeletal problems that occur as a direct result of HIV infection. In addition, there have been reports of leukocytoclastic vasculitis in the setting of zidovudine therapy (see Chap. 319). CNS angiitis (see Chap. 319) and polymyo-

sitis (see Chap. 315) have also been reported in HIV-infected individuals. Septic arthritis is surprisingly rare, especially given the increased incidence of staphylococcal bacteremias seen in this population. When septic arthritis has been reported, it has usually been due to systemic fungal infections with *Sporothrix schenckii*, *Cryptococcus neoformans*, or *Histoplasma capsulatum*, or systemic mycobacterial infection with *Mycobacterium haemophilum*.

OPHTHALMIC PROBLEMS Ophthalmic problems are seen in over 50 percent of HIV-infected individuals, generally as a late manifestation of disease. The most common abnormal findings on funduscopic examination are cotton-wool spots—hard white spots that appear on the surface of the retina and often have an irregular edge. They represent areas of retinal ischemia secondary to microvascular disease. At times they are associated with small areas of hemorrhage and thus are difficult to distinguish from CMV retinitis. In contrast to CMV retinitis, however, these spots are not associated with visual loss and tend to remain stable or improve over time.

Apart from cotton-wool spots, the most common disease of the eye in HIV-infected individuals is CMV retinitis. This is almost invariably a late manifestation of HIV disease, occurring in patients with less than 50 CD4 + T cells per microliter. CMV causes a progressive necrotizing retinitis that results in permanent visual loss. Funduscopically one sees perivascular hemorrhage and exudate that is usually bilateral and progressive over time **(see Plate III-1)**. Retinal detachment may occur in areas of retinal scarring secondary to burned-out infection. Treatment is detailed above and at present is limited to either ganciclovir, foscarnet, or cidofovir.

Several other secondary infections may cause ocular problems in HIV-infected patients. Among them are *Pneumocystis carinii* infection, toxoplasmosis, and herpesvirus infections. *P. carinii* causes a severe choroiditis that is most commonly seen in the absence of pulmonary disease. Lesions appear as slightly raised yellow-white plaques and may be confused with cotton-wool spots. Toxoplasma retinitis is usually an accompaniment of CNS toxoplasmosis. It may be very difficult to distinguish from CMV retinitis and should be considered in anyone with a diagnosis of CMV retinitis who is not responding well to initial therapy. In contrast, infections of the retina caused by HSV and VZV, referred to as *acute retinal necrosis syndrome*, are quite distinct, causing a painful inflammation of the eye that may be associated with keratitis or iritis. Funduscopic examination reveals multiple, usually bilateral pale gray lesions. This entity is often seen in association with trigeminal zoster or orolabial herpes simplex and is associated with an increased risk of retinal detachment.

ENDOCRINE AND METABOLIC ABNORMALITIES Disorders of these types are frequently seen in HIV-infected individuals. The most common abnormality is hyponatremia, seen in up to 30 percent of patients. This is usually related to the syndrome of inappropriate antidiuretic hormone (vasopressin) secretion (SIADH) as a consequence of increased free water intake and decreased free water excretion (see Chap. 49). SIADH is generally seen in the context of pulmonary or CNS disease. A second cause of hyponatremia is adrenal insufficiency; the presence of a low serum sodium level combined with a high serum potassium level should alert one to this possibility. Although most HIV-infected individuals studied at autopsy had involvement of the adrenal gland, less than 10 percent had prior evidence of adrenal insufficiency. CMV is the most common cause of adrenal gland disease in HIV infection. Other causes include mycobacterial infections, Kaposi's sarcoma, cryptococcal disease, histoplasmosis, and ketoconazole toxicity.

Hypogonadism Hypogonadism is seen in approximately 50 percent of HIV-infected individuals and is generally a complication of the underlying illness. Testicular dysfunction may also be induced by ganciclovir therapy. In several surveys, 67 percent of patients with HIV infection reported decreased libido and 33 percent complained of impotence. Twenty-five percent of women with HIV infection in African studies were amenorrheic. Thyroid function is generally normal, despite histologic evidence of thyroid gland involvement with several pathologic processes, including Kaposi's sarcoma and infection with CMV, *Cryptococcus neoformans*, or *Pneumocystis carinii*.

PANCREATITIS As noted above, pancreatitis leading to abnormalities of glucose metabolism may be seen in HIV-infected individuals; however, this is most often due to complications of therapy with either pentamidine or dideoxynucleosides.

GENERALIZED WASTING Generalized wasting, defined as involuntary weight loss of greater than 10 percent associated with intermittent or constant fever and chronic diarrhea or fatigue lasting more than 30 days in the absence of a defined cause other than HIV infection, is an AIDS-defining condition (Table 308-11). It is the initial AIDS-defining illness in 9 percent of patients with AIDS in the United States and, thus, is currently the leading initial clinical indication of AIDS. A constant feature of this syndrome is major muscle wasting with scattered myofiber degeneration and occasional evidence of myositis. Glucocorticoids may be of some benefit; however, this approach must be carefully weighed against the risk of compounding the immunodeficiency of HIV infection. While similar findings may be seen with CMV disease or MAC bacteremia in the setting of advanced HIV infection, the generalized wasting syndrome appears to be a true direct effect of HIV. Androgenic steroids, growth hormone, and total parental nutrition have been used as therapeutic interventions with variable success.

IDIOPATHIC CD4+ T LYMPHOCYTOPENIA

A syndrome was recognized in 1992 that was characterized by an absolute CD4+ T cell count of less than 300/μL or less than 20 percent of total T cells on more than one occasion, no evidence of HIV-1, HIV-2, HTLV-I, or HTLV-II on testing, and the absence of any defined immunodeficiency or therapy associated with decreased levels of CD4+ T cells. By mid-1993, approximately 100 patients had been described. After extensive multicenter investigations, a series of reports were published in early 1993 which together allowed a number of conclusions. Idiopathic CD4+ lymphocytopenia (ICL) is a very rare syndrome, as determined by studies of blood donors and cohorts of HIV-seronegative homosexual men. Cases were clearly identified as early as 1983, and cases remarkably similar to ICL had been identified decades ago. The definition of ICL based on CD4+ T cell counts coincided with the ready availability of testing for CD4+ T cells in patients suspected of being immunosuppressed. Although, as a result of immunosuppression, certain patients with ICL develop some of the opportunistic diseases, particularly cryptococcosis, seen in HIV-infected patients, the syndrome is demographically, clinically, and immunologically unlike HIV infection and AIDS. Less than half of the ICL patients had risk factors for HIV infection, and there were wide geographic and age distributions. The fact that a significant proportion of patients did have risk factors probably reflects a selection bias, in that physicians who take care of HIV-infected patients are more likely to monitor CD4+ T cells. Approximately one-third of the patients are women, compared to 14 percent of women among HIV-infected individuals in the United States. Many patients with ICL remained clinically stable, and their condition did not progressively deteriorate as is common with seriously immunodeficient HIV-infected patients. Certain patients with ICL even experienced spontaneous reversal of the CD4+ T lymphocytopenia. Immunologic abnormalities in ICL are somewhat different from those of HIV infection. ICL patients often also have decreases in CD8+ T cells and in B cells. Furthermore, immunoglobulin levels were either normal or, more commonly, decreased in patients with ICL, compared to the usual hypergammaglobulinemia of HIV-infected individuals. Finally, virologic studies revealed no evidence of HIV-1, HIV-2, HTLV-I, or HTLV-II or of any other mononuclear cell–tropic virus. Furthermore, there was no epidemiologic evidence to suggest that a transmissible microbe was involved. The cases of ICL were widely dispersed, with no clustering. Close contacts and sexual partners who were studied were clinically well and were serologically, immunologically, and virologically negative for HIV. ICL is a heterogeneous syndrome, and it is highly likely that there is no common cause; however, there may be common causes among subgroups of patients that are currently unrecognized.

Patients who present with laboratory data consistent with ICL should be worked up for underlying diseases that could be responsible for the immunosuppression. If no underlying cause is detected, no specific therapy should be initiated. However, if opportunistic diseases occur, they should be treated appropriately (see above). Depending on the level of the CD4+ T cell count, patients should receive prophylaxis for the commonly encountered opportunistic infections.

TREATMENT OF HIV INFECTION AND ITS COMPLICATIONS

GENERAL PRINCIPLES OF PATIENT MANAGEMENT The treatment of patients with HIV infection requires not only a comprehensive knowledge of the possible disease processes but also the ability to deal with the problems of a chronic, life-threatening illness. Specific antiretroviral therapy and antimicrobial treatment and prophylaxis are critical measures in prolonging an acceptable quality of life; however, counseling and education are also of paramount importance in providing patients with optimal overall care. Patients must be educated about the potential transmission of their infection, including frank discussions concerning sexual practices and sharing of intravenous needles. The treating physician must not only be aware of the latest medications available for HIV infection and its complications but must also educate patients concerning the natural history of their illness and listen to and be sensitive to their fears and concerns. As with other diseases, therapeutic decisions should be made in consultation with the patient when possible and with the patient's proxy if the patient is incapable of making decisions. In this regard, it is recommended that all patients with HIV infection, and in particular those with less than 200 CD4+ T cells per microliter, designate a trusted individual with durable power of attorney to make medical decisions on their behalf, if necessary.

No matter how well prepared a person feels for adversity, the discovery of a diagnosis of HIV infection is a devastating event. For this reason it is recommended that anyone about to undergo testing have "pretest counseling" to prepare them at least partially should the results be positive. Following a diagnosis of HIV infection, the physician should be prepared to activate support systems immediately for the newly diagnosed patient; these should include an experienced social worker or nurse who can spend time talking to the person and ensuring that he or she is emotionally stable. Most communities have HIV crisis centers that can be of great help in these difficult situations.

Following a diagnosis of HIV infection, there are several examinations and laboratory studies that should be performed to help determine the extent of disease and provide baseline standards for future reference. In addition to routine chemistry, hematology screening panels, and chest x-ray, one should also obtain a CD4+ T cell count, two separate plasma HIV RNA levels, a VDRL test, and an anti-*Toxoplasma* antibody titer. A PPD skin test should be done and a Mini-Mental Status Examination performed and recorded (Table 308-18). In addition, patients should be counseled with regard to sexual practices and needle sharing, and counseling should be offered to those whom the patient knows or suspects may also be infected. Once these baseline activities are performed, short-term and long-term medical management strategies should be based on the most recent information and modified as new information becomes available.

ANTIRETROVIRAL THERAPY The cornerstone of medical management of HIV infection is antiretroviral therapy. Suppression of HIV replication is an important component in prolonging life as well as in improving the quality of life of patients with HIV infection. Many questions currently lack definitive answers, including when antiretroviral therapy should be started, what is the best regimen to start with, when therapy should be changed, and what it should be changed to. Nonetheless, the physician and patient must come to a mutually agreeable plan based on the best available data. At present an extensive clinical trials network, involving both clinical investigators and patient advocates, is in place, attempting to develop improved approaches to therapy. Consortia comprising representatives of academia, industry, and the governments of the United States and other nations are involved in the process of drug development and clinical trials. As a result, new therapies and new therapeutic strategies are continually emerging; in addition, new drugs are often available through expanded access programs prior to official licensure. For these reasons, management of patients with HIV infection is best accomplished primarily by or with significant input from someone who is an expert in the field.

Nucleoside Analogues *Zidovudine* Zidovudine (AZT; 3'-az-ido-2',3'-dideoxythymidine) was the first drug approved for the treatment of HIV infection and is the prototype drug for the class of compounds referred to as nucleoside analogues (Table 308-26). These compounds, in which the hydroxyl group in the 3' position of the ribose moiety is substituted with a hydrogen or other chemical group, act as DNA chain terminators owing to their inability to form a 3'-5' phosphodiester linkage with another nucleoside. They bind much more avidly to the active site of the RNA-dependent DNA polymerase of HIV (reverse transcriptase) than to the active site of mammalian cell DNA polymerases. This fact may, at least in part, explain their selective effect on HIV replication. Zidovudine also has a relatively high avidity for the DNA polymerase γ of human mitochondria, which may contribute to the development of the myopathy sometimes observed in patients receiving zidovudine. The active form of zidovudine is the triphosphate, and the rate of phosphorylation, a thymidine kinase–dependent pathway, may be different in different cells. This may explain why zidovudine is more effective at inhibiting HIV replication in some cells than others. Zidovudine is well absorbed orally, with a serum half-life of approximately 1 h. Hence, the earliest dosing regimens employed an every-4-h (five times daily) schedule. Given that the intracellular half-life may be much longer than the plasma half-life (as is also true for didanosine; see below), the rationale for this dosing schedule is unsubstantiated, and a variety of more convenient schedules involving twice- or thrice-daily dosing are often employed, particularly when zidovudine is given as part of a combination regimen.

The clinical efficacy of zidovudine was clearly established in a phase II, placebo-controlled trial in which 282 patients who had either experienced a single bout of PCP or had a variety of AIDS-associated symptoms were randomized to receive either placebo or zidovudine at a dose of 200 mg every 4 h. The trial was stopped prematurely when it became clear that there were far fewer deaths and far fewer new opportunistic infections among the patients receiving zidovudine. In addition to this clinical benefit, patients treated with zidovudine had increases in lymphocyte counts, including CD4 + T cell counts, declines in circulating levels of p24 antigen, and weight gain. In subsequent trials, a beneficial effect was also noted in patients with neurologic disease. Considerable controversy arose regarding the use of zidovudine as monotherapy in asymptomatic HIV-infected individuals with CD4 + T cell counts greater than 200/μL. Initial studies indicated that elevations of CD4 + T cell counts resulted from this approach. At that time, the CD4 + T cell count was thought to be an adequate surrogate marker for monitoring antiretroviral therapy. However, subsequent studies demonstrated that this approach offered no clinical benefit over waiting until there was clear evidence of disease progression. Thus, these studies called into question the relevancy of CD4 + T cell counts as surrogate markers for monitoring therapy. In addition, it became clear that zidovudine monotherapy was not associated with a clear-cut clinical benefit in asymptomatic HIV-infected individuals with CD4 + T cell counts greater than 200/μL. More recent data have demonstrated that combination regimens of nucleosides are more effective than zidovudine monotherapy, and, at present, zidovudine is most appropriately used as part of combination antiretroviral therapy for patients with HIV infection and less than 500 CD4 + T cells per microliter and as monotherapy for the prevention of maternal-fetal transmission of HIV infection. These recommendations are based on the U.S. Food and Drug Administration (FDA) approval and licensure process, which in turn is based solely on the results of controlled clinical trials. Only such trials can indicate whether antiretroviral therapy should be started earlier than the point at which CD4 + T

cell counts reach 500/μL. It should be pointed out that plasma levels of HIV RNA are assuming increasing importance in the decision as to when to initiate and/or modify antiretroviral therapy (see below).

A great deal of effort has been directed toward defining the optimal dose of zidovudine. While the earliest clinical trials employing doses of 1200 mg/d showed benefit, there was also substantial toxicity. Subsequent trials have demonstrated that doses as low as 400 to 600 mg/d are as effective as higher-dose regimens and significantly less toxic. At present, the dose usually employed is 200 mg three times a day in combination with other antiretroviral agents. The use of zidovudine monotherapy is currently restricted to the prevention of maternal-fetal transmission of HIV. Given the considerable advantage of combination regimens over monotherapy in other clinical settings, it is highly likely that combination regimens will also prove more effective in the prevention of maternal-fetal transmission and that recommendations for therapy in this setting will change accordingly.

While many patients experience fatigue, malaise, nausea, and headache on initiation of zidovudine therapy, these side effects often subside over time. The major toxicities of zidovudine involve the bone marrow. Patients often develop a macrocytic anemia which, when associated with low serum erythropoietin levels, may be ameliorated somewhat by injections of recombinant erythropoietin beginning at a dose of 100 μg/kg three times a week. Although zidovudine-induced anemia is macrocytic, there is no evidence that deficiencies in vitamin B_{12} or folate play a role; exogenous administration of these vitamins is of no benefit. In addition to anemia, patients receiving zidovudine, especially patients with advanced disease, may experience neutropenia and in some cases thrombocytopenia. Other common toxicities of zidovudine include a proximal myopathy characterized by weakness, muscle wasting, and in some patients an elevation in creatine kinase, which is felt to be secondary to mitochondrial dysfunction. This mechanism of action has also been postulated to play a role in some forms of zidovudine-associated cardiomyopathy, as well as in some cases of lactic acidosis associated with fatty infiltration of the liver. A bluish discoloration of the nails, which is particularly noticeable in black patients, has been observed. An increased incidence of tumors of the vaginal epithelium has been found in rodents treated with extremely high doses of zidovudine. In addition, in transplacental carcinogenicity studies, an increase in solid tumors occurred in adult mice whose mothers were treated with high doses of zidovudine during pregnancy. However, no increases in cancers in HIV-infected patients have thus far been attributed to zidovudine therapy. Given these potential side effects, it is recommended that patients starting therapy with zidovudine be monitored for toxicity at least every other week for the first month and then monthly.

Considerable concern has been raised over the existence of strains of HIV that are resistant to zidovudine. These have usually been identified in patients receiving zidovudine for periods of 6 months or longer; however, they have also been reported in isolates obtained at the time of seroconversion. Resistance emerges more rapidly in late-stage patients, in whom there is presumably a greater degree of viral replication and thus more chance for mutation. This resistance is secondary to mutations in the HIV reverse transcriptase; at least five different mutations have been identified that are associated with zidovudine resistance (codons Met41→Leu; Asp67→Asn; Lys70→Arg; Thr215→Tyr; and Phe/Lys219→Gln). While zidovudine resistance is not associated with resistance to either didanosine or zalcitabine, patients treated with zidovudine monotherapy are often less responsive to subsequent therapy with nucleoside analogues. The emergence of zidovudine-resistant strains of HIV certainly contributes to the limited long-term usefulness of this drug as monotherapy and provides a strong rationale for the use of combination regimens.

Didanosine Didanosine (ddI; 2',3'-dideoxyinosine) was the second drug licensed for the treatment of HIV infection. In a series of open trials, didanosine therapy resulted in increases in CD4 + T cell counts and declines in p24 antigen levels. Licensure was based on the demonstration in a controlled, randomized trial that patients who had received zidovudine for a minimum of 16 weeks and were switched to didanosine experienced increases in CD4 + T cell counts and fewer

Table 308-26

Antiretroviral Drugs Used in the Treatment of HIV Infection

Drug	Status	Indication	Dose as Monotherapy	Dose in Combination	Supporting Data	Toxicity
REVERSE TRANSCRIPTASE INHIBITORS						
Zidovudine (AZT, azidothymidine, Retrovir, 3′azido-3′-deoxythymidine)	Licensed	Patients with AIDS or ARC	100 mg q4h	200 mg q8h	19 vs 1 death in original placebo-controlled trial in 281 patients with AIDS or ARC	Anemia, granulocytopenia, myopathy, lactic acidosis, hepatomegaly with steatosis, headache, nausea
		Patients with HIV infection and CD4+ T cell count <500/μL	100 mg q4h	200 mg q8h	Decreased progression to AIDS in patients with CD4+ T cell counts <500/μL, n = 2051	
		Prevention of maternal-fetal HIV transmission	*Mother:* 100 mg 5id until the start of labor, then 2 mg/kg over 1 h IV, followed by 1 mg/kg/h IV until clamping of umbilical cord; *Infant:* 2 mg/kg PO q6h beginning within 12 h birth, or 1.5 mg/kg IV over 30 min q6h		In pregnant women with CD4+ T cell count ≥200/μL, AZT PO beginning at weeks 14–34 of gestation plus IV drug during labor and delivery plus PO AZT to infant for 6 wk decreased transmission of HIV by 67.5% (from 25.5% to 8.3%), n = 363	
Didanosine (Videx, ddI, dideoxyinosine, 2′,3′-dideoxyinosine)	Licensed	Alone or in combination with AZT for treatment of HIV infection in patients with CD4+ T cell count <500/μL	Requires 2 tablets to achieve adequate buffering of stomach acid; should be administered on an empty stomach		Clinically superior to AZT as monotherapy in 913 patients with prior AZT therapy. Clinically superior to AZT and comparable to AZT + ddI and AZT + ddC in 1067 AZT-naive patients with CD4+ T cell counts of 200–500/μL	Pancreatitis, peripheral neuropathy, abnormalities on liver function tests
			≥60 kg: 200 mg bid <60 kg: 125 mg bid	200 mg bid 125 mg bid		
Zalcitabine (ddC, HIVID, 2′3′-dideoxycytidine)	Licensed	In combination with AZT for treatment of patients with CD4+ T cell counts <500/μL As monotherapy for patients with advanced disease that is progressing despite AZT or who are intolerant to AZT	0.75 mg tid	0.75 mg tid in combination with AZT	Clinically inferior to AZT monotherapy as initial treatment. Clinically as good as ddI in advanced patients intolerant to AZT. In combination with AZT, was clinically superior to AZT alone in patient with AIDS or CD4+ T cell count <350/μL	Peripheral neuropathy, pancreatitis, lactic acidosis, hepatomegaly with steatosis, oral ulcers
Stavudine (d4T, Zerit, 2′3′-didehydro-3′-dideoxythymidine)	Licensed	Treatment of adults with advanced disease who are intolerant of approved therapies or whose disease is progressing despite other therapies	≥60 kg: 40 mg bid <60 kg: 30 mg bid	40 mg bid 30 mg bid	Superior to AZT with respect to changes in CD4+ T cell counts in 359 patients who had received ≥24 wk of AZT. Following 12 wk of randomization, the CD4+ T cell count had decreased in AZT-treated controls by a mean of 22/μL, while in stavudine-treated patients, it had increased by a mean of 22/μL	Peripheral neuropathy, pancreatitis

(continued)

Table 308-26—*(continued)*

Antiretroviral Drugs Used in the Treatment of HIV Infection

Drug	Status	Indication	Dose as Monotherapy	Dose in Combination	Supporting Data	Toxicity
Lamivudine (Epivir, 2'3'-dideoxy-3'-thiacytidine, 3TC)	Licensed	In combination with AZT for the treatment of HIV infection when treatment is indicated	Not licensed as monotherapy	150 mg bid	Superior to AZT alone with respect to changes in CD4 counts in 495 patients who were zidovudine-naive and 477 patients who were zidovudine-experienced. Overall CD4+ T cell counts for the zidovudine group were at baseline by 24 wk, while in the group treated with zidovudine plus lamivudine, they were 10–50 cells/μL above baseline. 54% decrease in progression to AIDS/death compared to AZT alone	
Delavirdine (Rescriptor)	Expanded access: 1-800-779-0070	Not to be used as monotherapy		400 mg tid		Skin rash, abnormalities in liver function tests
Nevirapine (Viramune)	Licensed	In combination with nucleoside analogues for treatment of progressive HIV infection	200 mg qd x 1 wk then 200 mg bid	200 mg bid	Increases in CD4+ T cell count, decrease in HIV RNA when used in combination with nucleosides	Skin rash, abnormalities in liver function tests

PROTEASE INHIBITORS

Drug	Status	Indication	Dose as Monotherapy	Dose in Combination	Supporting Data	Toxicity
Saquinavir mesylate (Invirase)	Licensed	In combination with nucleoside analogues for treatment of advanced HIV infection	600 mg q8h	600 mg q8h	Increases in CD4+ T cell counts, reduction in HIV RNA most pronounced in combination therapy with ddC. 50% reduction in first AIDS-defining event or death in combination with ddC compared to either agent alone.	Nausea
Ritonavir (Norvir)	Licensed	In combination with nucleoside analogues for treatment of HIV infection when treatment is warranted	600 mg bid	600 mg bid	Reduction in the cumulative incidence of clinical progression or death from 34% to 17% in patients with CD4+ T cell count <100/μL treated for a median of 6 months	Nausea, abdominal pain, may alter levels of many other drugs, including saquinavir
Indinavir sulfate (Crixivan)	Licensed	For treatment of HIV infection when antiretroviral treatment is warranted	800 mg q8h	800 mg q8h 1000 mg q8h with nevirapine 400–600 mg q8h with delavirdine	Increase in CD4+ T cell count by 100/μL and 2-log decrease in HIV RNA levels when given in combination with zidovudine and lamivudine	Nephrolithiasis, indirect hyperbilirubinemia
Nelfinavir mesylate (Viracept)	Licensed	Patients with <200 CD4+ T cells/μL unable to tolerate other protease inhibitors	750 mg tib	750 mg tid	2.0-log decline in HIV RNA when given in combination with stavudine	Diarrhea, loose stools

new opportunistic infections compared to patients remaining on zidovudine. Two randomized trials comparing zidovudine to didanosine as initial therapy yielded different results. In the first study, zidovudine was found to be superior to didanosine as initial therapy. In the second study, involving a larger number of patients, didanosine was found to be superior to zidovudine with respect to survival and to development of AIDS-defining illnesses (Table 308-26). At present, didanosine is an FDA-approved agent for any patient with HIV infection who has received prolonged zidovudine therapy or as initial therapy in patients with less than 500 CD4 + T cells/μL. While this is the licensed indication, the more common practice is to initiate therapy with didanosine as part of a combination regimen. As is the case with most antiretroviral drugs, strains of HIV that are resistant to didanosine emerge in patients receiving the drug. At least some of these isolates, occurring in patients who had originally developed zidovudine-resistant isolates as a consequence of prior zidovudine therapy, have regained some degree of sensitivity to zidovudine. Strains of HIV that are resistant to didanosine are generally also resistant to zalcitabine.

The standard dose of didanosine is 200 mg twice a day for patients over 60 kg and 125 mg twice a day for patients under 60 kg. Didanosine is best absorbed on an empty stomach at a neutral pH. For this reason, the current formulations of didanosine contain a buffer, and each dose must be administered in no less than two tablets. Thus, a patient who requires 100 mg twice a day should take two 50 mg tablets twice a day rather than one 100 mg tablet twice a day.

The toxicity profile of didanosine is quite different from that of zidovudine. The most frequent toxicity is a painful sensory peripheral neuropathy, which occurs in approximately 30 percent of patients receiving more than 200 mg twice a day; it generally resolves with discontinuation of drug and may not recur when the drug is resumed at a reduced dose. The other major toxicity is pancreatitis; it was reported to occur in 9 percent of patients in early clinical trials, although the frequency was somewhat less in later studies using lower doses. Pancreatitis can be fatal, and for this reason all patients receiving didanosine should be monitored carefully. Didanosine should be discontinued if a patient experiences abdominal pain consistent with pancreatitis or if an elevated serum level of amylase and/or lipase is found and ultrasound examination shows an edematous pancreas. Such patients should not be treated again with didanosine, and, in general, didanosine is contraindicated for patients with a prior history of pancreatitis, regardless of etiology. Didanosine has minimal effects on the bone marrow and can be given in combination with bone marrow–toxic drugs such as zidovudine, ganciclovir, and trimethoprim/sulfamethoxazole.

Zalcitabine Zalcitabine (ddC; 2′,3′-dideoxycytidine) was the third drug licensed for the treatment of HIV infection. It is officially licensed as monotherapy for patients who are intolerant of zidovudine or whose disease progresses while they are receiving zidovudine, and as part of a combination regimen with zidovudine as initial therapy for patients with CD4 + T cell counts of less than 500/μL (Table 308-26). The latter indication reflects the results of the first clinical trials designed to assess the efficacy of zalcitabine in the initial therapy of HIV infection. A direct comparison of zalcitabine to zidovudine was stopped prematurely when it was noted that significantly more deaths were occurring in the zalcitabine-treated group (59 vs. 33). In a separate trial, however, the combination of zalcitabine and zidovudine was shown to cause greater and more sustained elevations in CD4 + T cell counts than zidovudine alone. Based on these results, zalcitabine (0.75 mg/kg three times a day) was licensed as part of a combination regimen with zidovudine (200 mg three times a day) for patients with advanced HIV infection. Subsequent trials in the United States and Europe (Table 308-26) have demonstrated the clinical superiority of this combination over zidovudine alone. As for didanosine, the major toxicity of zalcitabine is a reversible peripheral neuropathy. While cases of pancreatitis have been reported in patients receiving zalcitabine, it has not been observed to the same degree as with didanosine. Nonetheless, zalcitabine is also contraindicated in patients with a prior history of pancreatitis. The zidovudine/zalcitabine combination regimen is an option for the initial treatment of HIV infection. As in the case of other nucleoside analogues, the development of

resistant strains of HIV is a common problem. Among the mutations in reverse transcriptase associated with resistance to zalcitabine are Lys65→Arg or Asn; Leu74→Val; Thr69→Asp; Val75→Thr; Met184→Val; and Tyr215→Cys. These mutations may also result in resistance to other nucleosides, including zidovudine, didanosine, stavudine, and lamivudine.

Stavudine Stavudine (d4T; 2′,3′-didehydro-3′-deoxythymidine) was the fourth nucleoside analogue licensed for the treatment of HIV infection. This agent is currently indicated for treatment of adults with advanced HIV disease who are intolerant of approved therapies with known clinical benefit or whose disease has progressed while they were receiving other therapies (Table 308-26). In preclinical studies, stavudine had an activity profile comparable to that of zidovudine. It demonstrates cross-resistance to ddI by mechanisms that have not yet been elucidated in vitro. Its activity is additive to that of ddI and in some situations antagonistic to that of zidovudine. For this reason, one should avoid the use of this agent in combination with zidovudine until definitive clinical data are available. Thus far, clinical trials have demonstrated that stavudine therapy is associated with increases in CD4 + T cell counts, declines in p24 antigen levels, and an improved sense of well-being. In a study of 359 zidovudine-experienced patients randomized to remain on zidovudine or switch to stavudine, the CD4 + T cell count in the patients who switched to stavudine increased by 22/μL, while in those remaining on zidovudine, it decreased by 22/μL. In contrast to zidovudine, stavudine appears to have minimal myelosuppressive toxicity. Peripheral neuropathy and elevations in the serum level of glutamic pyruvic transaminase have been the primary toxicities observed to date.

Lamivudine Lamivudine (3TC; 2′,3′-dideoxy-3′-thiacytidine) is the fifth of the nucleoside analogues to be licensed in the United States. This cytidine analogue is licensed for use only in combination with zidovudine in situations where zidovudine is indicated. However, it is often used as part of other combinations (Table 308-26). The broad language incorporated into the licensure of lamivudine reflects the increasing complexity of the field of antiretroviral therapy and acknowledges the fact that it will be impossible to test formally every monotherapy and combination regimen in every potential therapeutic setting. The combination of zidovudine and lamivudine in vitro is the most potent combination of nucleosides studied to date and is felt by many experts to be the preferred nucleoside combination. This potency may be due in part to the fact that strains of HIV that are resistant to lamivudine (Met184→Val) have an increased sensitivity to zidovudine, so that the development of dual resistance is more difficult. Another potential advantage of the combination regimen is the fact that some lamivudine-resistant mutants of the HIV reverse transcriptase are less able to generate errors in reverse transcription, thus potentially slowing the mutation rate of the virus. Licensure of this agent was based on laboratory data. Patients receiving the combination of zidovudine and lamivudine had increases in CD4 + T cell counts that were in the range of 40 to 70/μL greater than that seen with monotherapy. It is the opinion of many experts in the field that this is the most potent combination of nucleosides and should be considered first-line therapy either alone or together with a protease inhibitor (see below) as initial antiretroviral therapy. However, clinical data are not yet available to support this approach. Although the main toxicities of lamivudine are peripheral neuropathy and pancreatitis, it is among the best tolerated of the nucleoside analogues.

Nonnucleoside Reverse Transcriptase Inhibitors The nonnucleoside reverse transcriptase inhibitors interfere with the function of the viral enzyme reverse transcriptase by binding to regions outside the active site and causing conformational changes in the enzyme that render it inactive. Although these agents are potent in the nanomolar range, they are also very selective for the reverse transcriptase of HIV-1, have no activity against HIV-2, and, when used as monotherapy, are associated with the rapid emergence of drug-resistant mutants (Table 308-26). Two members of this class, *nevirapine* and *delavirdine*, are currently available for use. Nevirapine is licensed for use in combination with nucleoside analogues for the treatment of HIV-infected adults who have experienced clinical and/or immunologic deterioration. Delavirdine is licensed for use in combination with appropriate anti-HIV medications to treat patients with HIV infection when treatment is warranted. The main toxicities of these drugs are a maculopapular rash that generally resolves without the need for discontinuation of therapy and elevations in hepatic enzyme levels. In order to decrease the incidence of rash associated with nevirapine, it is recommended that it be given at a starting dose of 200 mg once a day for 2 weeks, followed by the full dose of 200 mg twice daily. When administered as part of combination regimens with nucleoside analogues, these agents lead to increases in CD4 + T cell counts and decreases in viral burden that are slightly greater and longer-lasting than those observed with nucleosides alone. These agents may play a valuable role in future multidrug combinations involving nucleosides and protease inhibitors.

Protease Inhibitors The licensure of four separate HIV-1 protease inhibitors (saquinavir, ritonavir, indinavir, and nelfinavir) heralded a major change in the options available for antiretroviral therapy of HIV infection. Unlike reverse transcriptase inhibitors, which interfere with cellular DNA polymerases as well as inhibiting the reverse transcriptase of HIV-1, the HIV protease inhibitors are exquisitely selective for the protease enzyme of HIV-1. These compounds are active in the nanomolar range and, thus far, are considerably less toxic than the reverse transcriptase inhibitors. Unfortunately, as in the case of the nonnucleoside reverse transcriptase inhibitors, this potency is accompanied by the rapid emergence of resistant isolates when these drugs are used alone. Thus, these compounds should be used in combination with other antiretroviral drugs.

Saquinavir Saquinavir was the first of the protease inhibitor compounds to be licensed (Table 308-26). In patients who had discontinued or were unable to take zidovudine, treatment with the combination of saquinavir and zalcitabine resulted in greater increases in CD4 + T cell counts and more pronounced decreases in plasma levels of HIV RNA than were seen with either agent alone. Subsequent clinical data revealed that at approximately 500 days of follow-up, there was a 50 percent decrease in the risk of either a first AIDS-defining event or death (rates of 15 percent, 27 percent, and 24 percent for saquinavir plus zalcitabine, zalcitabine alone, and saquinavir alone, respectively). Saquinavir is licensed to be given in combination with nucleoside analogues for the treatment of advanced HIV disease. Genotypic and/or phenotypic resistance to saquinavir has been observed in approximately 45 percent of patients. Viral resistance to the protease inhibitors is quite complex. Among the mutations in the HIV-1 protease codons associated with resistance to saquinavir are Leu90→Met and Gly48→Val. Of note is the fact that strains of HIV that are resistant to saquinavir are generally not resistant to either indinavir or ritonavir, suggesting that combination therapy with different protease inhibitors may be of considerable value. This possibility must be approached with caution, however, since saquinavir is metabolized by the cytochrome P450 system, and ritonavir therapy results in an inhibition of cytochrome P450 action. Thus, when both drugs are administered together, there is the potential for unpredictable increases in saquinavir levels. Of the first three protease inhibitors licensed for use in patients with HIV infection, saquinavir is among the better tolerated; however, it appears to be the least potent (Fig. 308-31).

Ritonavir Ritonavir is licensed for the treatment of HIV infection when treatment is warranted, either as monotherapy or in combination with nucleoside analogues. It was the first protease inhibitor for which clinical efficacy was demonstrated (Table 308-26). In a study of 1090 patients with CD4 + T cell counts less than 100/μL who were randomized to receive either placebo or ritonavir in addition to any other licensed medications, patients receiving ritonavir had a reduction in the cumulative incidence of clinical progression or death from 34 percent to 17 percent. Mortality decreased from 10.1 percent to 5.8 percent. Resistance to ritonavir has been associated with a variety of amino acid substitutions. Among them, a Val82→Phe substitution appears to be

necessary but not sufficient for the development of phenotypic resistance. Other common mutations that have been described are Ile84→Val, Ala71→Val, and Met46→Ile. Strains of HIV-1 that are resistant to ritonavir are resistant to indinavir. The main side effects of ritonavir are nausea, diarrhea, abdominal pain, and circumoral paresthesias; these can be reduced somewhat by initiating therapy at 300 mg bid and then rapidly escalating the dose over 5 days to the full dose of 600 mg bid. Ritonavir has a high affinity for several isoforms of cytochrome P450, and thus it can produce large increases in the plasma concentrations of drugs metabolized by this pathway. Among the agents affected in this manner are saquinavir, macrolide antibiotics, R-warfarin, ondansetron, rifampin, most calcium channel blockers, glucocorticoids, and some of the chemotherapeutic agents used to treat Kaposi's sarcoma. In addition, ritonavir may increase the activity of glucuronyltransferases, thus decreasing the levels of drugs metabolized by this pathway. Overall, great care must be taken when prescribing additional drugs to patients taking ritonavir. Ritonavir is more potent than saquinavir, but it is generally the most poorly tolerated of these drugs because of the gastrointestinal side effects.

Indinavir Indinavir was the third protease inhibitor licensed for the treatment of HIV-1 infection. It is indicated for the treatment of HIV infection in adults in whom antiretroviral therapy is warranted (Table 308-26). As in the case of saquinavir, this indication is based on laboratory data demonstrating substantial increases in CD4 + T cell counts and reductions in plasma levels of HIV RNA during therapy. The strongest results were observed in treatment regimens that included zidovudine and lamivudine. Resistance to indinavir has been associated with over 10 different amino acid substitutions. Isolates of HIV-1 that are resistant to indinavir show cross-resistance to ritonavir and variable degrees of cross-resistance to saquinavir. The main side effects of indinavir are nephrolithiasis (seen in 4 percent of patients) and asymptomatic indirect hyperbilirubinemia (seen in 10 percent of patients). Indinavir is metabolized mainly by the liver, and the dose should be lowered in patients with cirrhosis. It shares metabolic pathways with terfenadine, astemizole, cisapride, triazolam, and midazolam. For this reason, these drugs should not be administered to patients taking indinavir, to avoid the potential for cardiac arrhythmias or prolonged sedation. Similarly, levels of indinavir are decreased during concurrent therapy with rifabutin and increased during concurrent therapy with ketoconazole. Dosages should be modified when these circumstances arise. Acidic conditions in the stomach favor the absorption of indinavir but decrease the availability of didanosine. Both are best absorbed on an empty stomach. Thus, when these drugs are prescribed together, they should be administered at different times. Compared to saquinavir and ritonavir, indinavir is both well tolerated and quite potent.

Nelfinavir Nelfinavir (Viracept) was approved early in March 1997 for the treatment of adult or pediatric HIV infection when antiretroviral therapy is warranted. This approval was based upon analysis of surrogate markers. In approximately 300 patients who had not previously received antiretroviral therapy, the combination of zidovudine, lamivudine, and nelfinavir (750 mg three times a day) resulted in an average decrease of at least 98 percent in viral load and a CD4 cell increase of 150 cells/μL. At present, no clinical data are available. Mild diarrhea, seen in approximately 20 percent of patients, is the main side effect.

℞ TREATMENT

Choice of Antiretroviral Treatment Strategy The large number of available antiretroviral agents coupled with a relative paucity of clinical end point studies make the subject of antiretroviral therapy one of the more controversial in the management of HIV-infected individuals. The relative merits of different therapeutic strategies should be discussed with the patient throughout the course of the illness, and new findings should be incorporated as they are reported. It is clear from our knowledge of the pathogenesis of HIV infection that there is a sufficient rationale for attempting to suppress viral replication from the time of initial infection. Indeed, the limited data on the treatment of patients with the acute seroconversion syndrome suggest that immediate intervention is of value in delaying the progression of disease. Unfortunately, at present, it is unclear whether currently available drugs are either potent enough or safe enough to be used over an indefinite period in multidrug combinations. The obvious hope is that virus replication will be suppressed to a low enough level and for long enough that the residual or regenerated immune system would be able to protect the patient from opportunistic diseases indefinitely. The best approach for this goal is unclear at present. For this reason, a variety of antiretroviral treatment strategies are currently employed. In an attempt to provide a range of potential approaches to therapy of the HIV-infected individual, we present a conservative approach, an aggressive approach, and our current approach (Table 308-27). The reader should bear in mind that the field of HIV therapeutics is evolving so rapidly that new drugs and new information on the use of currently available drugs may call for substantial modifications of the recommendations given. Nonetheless, the principles delineated will likely remain constant.

A *conservative approach*, which uses only strategies that have been shown to be of clinical benefit, would generally involve withholding antiretroviral therapy until the CD4+ T cell count falls below 500/μL. A choice would then be made among the proven options of didanosine monotherapy, zidovudine plus didanosine, zidovudine plus zalcitabine, and zidovudine plus lamivudine. The chosen regimen would be used until the disease demonstrated progression, as defined by a fall in the CD4+ T cell count below 200/μL. Therapy would then be changed. While a wide array of choices for the new regimen are available, the most prudent would seem to be one containing one or two new nucleosides and a protease inhibitor.

An *aggressive approach* would involve using combination therapy from the time of diagnosis of HIV infection. If the therapeutic decision were based on surrogate marker data, one option would be to use a combination of zidovudine, lamivudine, and indinavir. The patient would be monitored carefully for changes in CD4+ T cell count and plasma levels of HIV RNA. Evidence of increased disease activity, defined as a 0.5 log increase in plasma levels of HIV RNA or a 25 percent decrease in the CD4+ T cell count, would indicate that it was time for a change in therapy. Options would include the use of other nucleosides in combination with saquinavir; a combination of nucleosides, saquinavir, and ritonavir; and possibly the addition of a nonnucleoside reverse transcriptase inhibitor.

The *current approach of the authors* falls between these two options and is influenced by the fact that the median time from infection to clinical disease is 10 years and that some patients, particularly those with low levels of plasma viremia (Fig. 308-22), may do extremely well without therapy for extended periods of time. For the asymptomatic patient with a stable CD4+ T cell count of more than 500/μL and plasma viremia less than 20,000 copies of HIV RNA per milliliter, we would not treat but would perform repeat evaluations every 6 months. If the plasma levels of HIV RNA are greater than 20,000 copies per milliliter or the CD4+ T cell count is less than 500/μL, or if the patient is symptomatic, or if there is indication of progressive disease, therapy with two nucleosides and a protease inhibitor would be initiated. The goal of therapy, once begun, is to decrease plasma viremia as low as possible for as long as possible. We would then monitor the patient every 3 to 4 months. Therapy would be modified to replace the current regimen with two new nucleosides or one new nucleoside and a nonnucleoside in combination with one or two different protease inhibitors if the plasma HIV level rose above the baseline by 0.5 log or the

CD4+ T cell count fell by more than 25 percent. The same holds true for a new patient whose care we assume and who is already receiving antiretroviral therapy. In the rare setting of diagnosing a patient with the acute retroviral syndrome, we would treat with two nucleosides and a protease inhibitor. This regimen should be continued for at least 1 year; many experts would continue treatment indefinitely. Definitive recommendations await the results of clinical trials. In any event, the patient should be evaluated every 3 to 4 months following initiation of therapy, and changes in therapy instituted where appropriate as indicated above.

Experimental Antiretroviral Agents In addition to the licensed drugs discussed above, a large number of experimental agents are being evaluated as possible therapies for HIV infection. Therapeutic strategies are being directed at virtually every step of the viral life cycle (Fig. 308-3). In addition, as more is learned about the role of the immune system in controlling viral replication, additional strategies, generically called *immune-based therapies*, are being developed as a complement to antiviral therapy. Among the antiviral agents in early clinical trials are additional nucleoside analogues, nucleotide analogues, additional protease inhibitors, integrase inhibitors, and antisense nucleic acids. Among the immune-based therapies being tested are IFNα, bone marrow transplantation with adoptive

Nucleoside Analogues

Zidovudine   Didanosine   Zalcitabine

Stavudine   Lamivudine

Non-nucleoside Reverse Transcriptase Inhibitors

Delavirdine   Nevirapine

Protease Inhibitors

Ritonavir   Nelfinavir mesylate

Saquinavir mesylate   Indinavir sulfate

FIGURE 308-31 Molecular structures of antiretroviral agents.

Table 308-27

Different Antiviral Treatment Strategies*

	Aggressive	Conservative
When to start	Time of diagnosis	CD4 + T cell count <500/μL
What to start with	AZT plus lamivudine plus protease inhibitor	Didanosine AZT plus zalcitabine AZT plus didanosine AZT plus lamivudine
When to change	0.5-log increase in HIV RNA or 10% decrease in CD4 + T cell count	CD4 + T cell count <200/μL
What to change to	Two new nucleosides (or a new nucleoside and a nonnucleoside) plus a new protease inhibitor	Two new nucleosides plus a protease inhibitor

* See text for current approach of the authors.

transfer of lymphocytes, thymic implants, active immunotherapy with subunit envelope vaccines or autologous cells genetically engineered to express viral proteins, passive immunotherapy with inactivated anti-HIV antisera or HIV-specific monoclonal antibodies, and intermittent administration of IL-2. In addition, clinical trials are under way that use the techniques of molecular biology to inhibit HIV replication and spread through the infusion of CD4 + T cells genetically modified to resist infection with HIV or the infusion of CD8 + T cells genetically modified to enhance their ability to eliminate HIV-infected cells.

Secondary Infections, Kaposi's Sarcoma, and Lymphomas
Treatment guidelines are outlined in Tables 308-21 and 308-23 and discussed in detail in the sections dealing with the secondary infections and neoplastic complications of HIV infection.

PROPHYLAXIS AGAINST SECONDARY INFECTIONS
The improvements in survival and quality of life that have been achieved in patients with HIV infection are due not only to the introduction of antiretroviral compounds but also to improved regimens for preventing secondary infections. As a result, the clinical profile of HIV-infected patients is continually evolving as immunodeficient patients live longer and are at less risk of formerly inevitable problems such as PCP. Some secondary infections occur predictably only when the competence of the immune system, as measured by the CD4 + T cell count, has fallen below a certain level, and this knowledge can be used to help devise effective strategies to minimize these risks.

PCP rarely occurs before the CD4 + T cell count drops below 200/μL or the CD4 percentage declines below 15 percent. At that point, patients should be started on a regimen of PCP prophylaxis. The preferred regimen, for patients who can tolerate it, is trimethoprim/sulfamethoxazole at a dose of one double-strength tablet daily. A benefit of this regimen is that it also provides protection against toxoplasmosis as well as certain bacterial infections. Alternative strategies for PCP prophylaxis include dapsone/pyrimethamine and clindamycin/primaquine. These are currently being evaluated for patients who are sulfa intolerant. Aerosolized pentamidine remains an option for individuals unable to tolerate any systemic therapy.

Another opportunistic infection for which primary prophylaxis is clearly indicated is MAC. This infection is extremely common among patients in the United States; it is rarely seen with CD4 + T cell counts above 100/μL. Rifabutin, 100 mg/d, was effective in a clinical trial in delaying the onset of MAC bacteremia by an average of 6 months. Based on these data, rifabutin has been licensed for use as primary prophylaxis for MAC infection in patients with HIV infection and less than 100 CD4 + T cells per microliter. Even better results have been seen with the macrolides clarithyomycin and azithromycin. The median survival for patients receiving clarithromycin prophylaxis was

>700 days, compared to 573 days for those receiving rifabutin. In a separate study, patients receiving azithromycin prophylaxis had an overall mortality of 10.5 percent, compared to 31 percent for those taking rifabutin. Of interest is the recent observation that patients with prior tuberculosis seem to have a decreased incidence of MAC. This finding raises the idea that it may be possible to develop a prophylactic vaccine for this complication.

Given the resurgence of tuberculosis in the HIV-infected population, any patient with HIV infection and at least 5 mm of induration upon PPD skin testing should receive a 1-year course of isoniazid. In addition, any patient with HIV infection who is anergic and at high risk of tuberculosis should be given 1 year of isoniazid therapy. These measures could be quite effective not only in helping the patient but also in curtailing the spread of tuberculosis in the community. All patients with tuberculosis should be treated with directly observed therapy to increase the chance of eradicating the infection and minimizing the risk of spread.

Patients with HIV infection are at increased risk for infection with encapsulated bacteria, particularly *H. influenzae* and *S. pneumoniae*. For this reason, these patients, and especially those in whom splenectomy is being considered, should be given the pneumococcal polysaccharide vaccine and possibly also the *H. influenzae* type b vaccine.

While no generally accepted guidelines exist, many physicians recommend primary prophylaxis against cryptococcal and candidal infections with fluconazole; clinical trials of a candidate cryptococcal vaccine are under way. In addition, clinical trials are being conducted to evaluate the role of intermittent clindamycin/pyrimethamine as primary prophylaxis for toxoplasmosis in patients unable to tolerate trimethoprim/sulfamethoxazole. Patients who are seronegative for *Toxoplasma gondii* should be encouraged to avoid ingestion of partially cooked meat and to use care when handling cat litter.

Secondary prophylaxis—the prevention of second or subsequent episodes of a given infection—is indicated for virtually every opportunistic infection experienced by patients with AIDS. These infections are usually impossible to eradicate and, with the exception of tuberculosis, life-long therapy or secondary prophylaxis is the rule (see Table 308-21). It is obvious that as the number of medications given to a patient increases, so do the chances of untoward drug reactions and interactions. Thus, patients must be monitored carefully for such reactions. However, the judicious use of prophylactic regimens clearly can yield a significant improvement in the quality and duration of life for the HIV-infected patient with advanced immunodeficiency.

HIV AND THE HEALTH CARE WORKER

Health care workers, especially those who deal with large numbers of HIV-infected patients, have a small but definite risk of becoming infected with HIV as a result of professional activities. By 1997, there were a total of 52 well-documented seroconversions in health care workers that occurred as a direct result of exposure to contaminated blood or bloody body fluids. Forty-five of these infections were due to percutaneous exposures, five were associated with mucous membrane exposures, one involved both percutaneous and mucous membrane exposures, and in one the route of exposure was unknown. Forty-seven of these accidents involved blood, one involved bloody pleural fluid, one involved an unspecified fluid, and three involved concentrated virus stocks. In addition, another 111 HIV-infected heath care workers have been identified with no identifiable risk for HIV infection other than possible occupational exposure. Taken together, the data from several large studies suggest that the risk of HIV infection following a percutaneous injury with an HIV-contaminated hollow-bore needle (in contrast to a solid-bore needle, i.e., a suture needle) is approximately 0.3 percent. A seroprevalence survey of 3420 orthopedic surgeons, 75 percent of whom practiced in an area with a relatively high prevalence of HIV infection and 39 percent of whom reported percutaneous exposure to patient blood, usually through an accident involving a suture needle, failed to reveal any cases of possible occupational infection, suggesting that the risk of infection with a suture needle may be considerably less than that with a blood-drawing needle.

Most cases of health care worker seroconversion occur as a result of needle-stick injuries. When one considers the circumstances that result in needle-stick injuries, it is immediately obvious that adhering to the standard guidelines for dealing with sharp objects would result in a significant decrease in this type of accident. In one study, 27 percent of needle-stick injuries resulted from improper disposal of the needle (over half of these were due to recapping the needle), 23 percent occurred during attempts to start an intravenous line, 22 percent occurred during blood drawing, 16 percent were associated with an intramuscular or subcutaneous injection, and 12 percent were associated with giving an intravenous infusion.

There is debate concerning the best management for a percutaneous injury with a needle contaminated with blood from an HIV-infected patient. The wound should be cleansed immediately and antiseptic applied. While there are multiple anecdotes of heath care workers who have seroconverted despite immediately beginning zidovudine prophylaxis, a case-control study among health care workers revealed that zidovudine postexposure prophylaxis was associated with a 79 percent decrease in the risk for HIV seroconversion after percutaneous exposure to HIV-infected blood. Based on this finding, a United States Public Health Service working group recommended that chemoprophylaxis be given after occupational exposure. While the precise regimen remains a topic of debate and will undoubtedly evolve, the authors currently recommend a combination of zidovudine, lamivudine, and indinavir. The side effects in this setting are considerable. In one study, 70 percent of health care workers taking zidovudine for postexposure prophylaxis reported one or more side effects, particularly nausea, malaise, and headache. The ultimate decision must be individualized and reached after careful discussion between the injured health care worker and the physician. Since antiretroviral prophylaxis, if it is going to be given, should probably be started as soon as possible after the injury, health care workers at potential risk should think beforehand about what they want to do. Given the prevalence of zidovudine resistance in the community, many experts advocate the use of combination therapy under such circumstances. Even if postexposure treatment fails to prevent primary infection, it almost certainly will decrease the initial burst of viremia (see above), which may have a significant long-term benefit.

Health care workers can minimize their risk of occupational HIV infection by following the CDC guidelines of July 1991, which include adherence to universal precautions; refraining from direct patient care if one has exudative lesions or weeping dermatitis; and disinfecting and sterilizing reusable devices employed in invasive procedures. The premise of universal precautions is that every specimen should be handled as if it came from someone infected with a bloodborne pathogen. All samples should be double-bagged, gloves should be worn when drawing blood, and spills should be immediately disinfected with bleach.

In attempting to put this small but definite risk to the health care worker in perspective, it is important to point out that approximately 200 health care workers die each year as a result of occupationally acquired hepatitis B infection. The tragedy in this instance is that these infections and deaths due to hepatitis B could be greatly decreased by more extended use of the hepatitis B vaccine. The risk of hepatitis B infection following a needle-stick injury from a hepatitis antigen–positive patient is much higher than the risk of HIV infection (see "Transmission," above). There are multiple examples of needle-stick injuries where the patient was positive for both hepatitis B and HIV and the health care worker became infected only with hepatitis B. For these reasons, it is advisable, given the high prevalence of hepatitis B infection in HIV-infected individuals, that all health care workers dealing with HIV-infected patients be immunized with the hepatitis B vaccine.

Tuberculosis is another infection common to HIV-infected patients that can be transmitted to the health care worker. For this reason, all health care workers should know their PPD status, have it checked yearly, and receive one year of isoniazid treatment if their skin test converts to positive. In addition, all patients in whom a diagnosis of tuberculosis is being entertained should be placed immediately in respiratory isolation, pending results of the diagnostic evaluation. The emergence of drug-resistant organisms has made tuberculosis an increasing problem for health care workers. This is particularly true for the health care worker with preexisting HIV infection.

One of the most charged issues ever to come between health care workers and patients is that of transmission of infection from HIV-infected health care workers to their patients. By the end of 1992, the well-publicized case of the Florida dentist (see above) was the only known or suspected case of such transmission, despite extensive investigation, including the testing of over 8000 patients who had received care from HIV-infected dentists or surgeons. This puts the risk of acquiring HIV infection from a doctor or dentist during an exposure-prone procedure at less than 1/1,000,000. That is one-half the risk that a given unit of screened blood is HIV-positive and 1/100th the risk of dying from general anesthesia. Thus, this level of risk seems acceptable and is within the scope of other risks taken by patients in the context of receiving health care. Theoretically, the same universal precautions that are used to protect the health care worker from the HIV-infected patient will also protect the patient from the HIV-infected health care worker.

VACCINES

Given the fact that human behavior, especially human sexual behavior, is extremely difficult to change, the best hope for preventing the spread of HIV infection rests with the development of a safe and effective vaccine. This task is extremely problematic for a number of reasons, including the high mutability of the virus, the fact that the infection can be transmitted by cell-free or cell-associated virus, and the likely need for the development of effective mucosal immunity. The fact that some HIV-infected individuals are long-term nonprogressors (see above), as well as the fact that a number of individuals have been exposed to HIV multiple times but remain uninfected, suggest that there are protective elements of an HIV-specific immune response. In addition, studies using animal models have been encouraging and suggest that an HIV vaccine is possible. It should be pointed out that while the ideal goal of an HIV vaccine is to prevent infection, a vaccine given to an uninfected individual that significantly alters the course of disease or the infectivity of the individual, should that person become infected, could have an impact not only on the individual in question, but on the spread of infection in the community.

Preclinical work in the area of vaccine development has been greatly facilitated by the use of animal models of lentivirus infections. Perhaps the most useful model to date has been the simian immunodeficiency virus (SIV) infection of rhesus monkeys. SIV, a lentivirus that is closely related to HIV-2 and differs from HIV-1 in lacking a *vpu* gene and having a *vpx* gene, causes an acute infection that leads to immunodeficiency, secondary infections, and death when administered to susceptible animals. Studies by several groups have clearly demonstrated that infection can be prevented by prior immunization of animals with either inactivated virus, recombinant vaccinia virus expressing the SIV envelope protein followed by a booster immunization with recombinant protein, or attenuated virus lacking an intact *nef* gene. Even in studies using antigens that did not confer protection from infection, the progression of disease following infection appeared to be decreased. Of note is the fact that in those studies that demonstrated protection it was not always obvious what components of the immune response conferred the protection. In fact, in certain studies of inactivated virus vaccines it was shown that the protective elements of the immune response were not directed toward genetic components of the virus at all but toward components of the cells used in growing up the viral stocks, which were incorporated into the viral envelope as the particles budded from the infected cells. These data suggest that antibodies to certain cell-surface proteins that participate in SIV binding may provide excellent protection against infection, a hypothesis that has been supported in studies of CD4-immunized monkeys. While the protection studies carried out with envelope-expressing recombinant vaccinia virus and recombinant envelope boosting point to an immune response to the envelope as potentially protective, there is still much to be learned about the correlates of immunity involved in protection against infection and/or disease.

The most suitable animal model for HIV infection is the chimpanzee. However, chimpanzees are expensive, they are an endangered species, and although they can be infected with HIV, they rarely develop disease over 10 years of observation. Thus, unless a candidate vaccine prevents infection in this model, its impact on disease progression is difficult to assess. Most recently, however, immunization of chimps either with whole inactivated virus followed by protein or peptide boosting or with recombinant envelope proteins has been shown to confer protection against infection with HIV-1. These data from animal models suggest the feasibility of inducing at least partial protection against HIV infection in humans by vaccination.

While clear signals from the preclinical animal studies are awaited, clinical trials of candidate vaccines have begun in humans. Both recombinant envelope proteins and recombinant viruses expressing a number of HIV proteins have been demonstrated to be safe and immunogenic in healthy uninfected volunteers. Certain of these vaccines are also being tested as forms of active immunotherapy in patients who are already infected. Different vaccine strategies lead to different immune responses. Live-virus vaccines and DNA vaccines are strategies in which the viral antigens are synthesized within the human cell. These types of vaccines tend to promote cytotoxic T cell responses. Recombinant proteins or killed-virus vaccines tend to promote antibody responses. A combination of these strategies tends to promote both. At present, one can state with a fair degree of certainty that humans can safely be immunized to several of the antigens of HIV. One or more of these vaccines candidates will be tested in vaccine efficacy trials. It is clear, however, that it will take several years of clinical trials to establish the efficacy or lack thereof of a candidate vaccine for HIV.

PREVENTION

Education, counseling, and behavior modification are the cornerstones of an HIV prevention strategy. Widespread voluntary testing of individuals who have practiced or are practicing high-risk behavior, together with counseling of infected individuals, is recommended. Information gathered from such an approach should serve as the basis for behavior-modification programs, both for infected individuals who may be unaware of their HIV status and who could infect others and for uninfected individuals practicing high-risk behavior. The practice of safe sex is the most effective way for sexually active uninfected individuals to avoid contracting HIV infection and for infected individuals to avoid spreading infection. Abstinence from sexual relations is the only absolute way to prevent sexual transmission of HIV infection. However, this may not be feasible, and there are a number of relatively safe practices that can markedly decrease the chances of transmission of HIV infection. Partners engaged in monogamous sexual relationships who wish to be assured of safety should both be tested for HIV antibody. If both are negative, it must be understood that any divergence from monogamy puts both partners at risk; open discussion of the importance of honesty in such relationships should be encouraged. When the HIV status of either partner is not known, or when one partner is positive, there are a number of options. Use of condoms, preferably together with the HIV-inhibiting spermicide nonoxynol-9, can markedly decrease the chance of HIV transmission. It should be remembered that condoms are not 100 percent effective in preventing transmission of HIV infection, and there is an approximately 10 percent failure rate of condoms used for contraceptive purposes. Most condom failures result from breakage or improper usage, such as not wearing the condom for the entire period of intercourse. Latex condoms are preferable, since virus has been shown to leak through natural skin condoms. Petroleum-based gels should never be used for lubrication of the condom, since they increase the likelihood of condom rupture. Mutual masturbation is considered safe provided there is no oral or open-cut exposure to or ingestion of semen, vaginal secretions, or other potentially infected body fluids. There has been a tendency among homosexual men to practice fellatio as a "minimal risk" activity compared to receptive anal intercourse. It should be emphasized that receptive oral fellatio is definitely not safe sex, and there has been clear-cut documentation of transmission of HIV where receptive fellatio was the only sexual act performed (see "Transmission," above). Topical microbicides for vaginal use are being pursued actively as a means by which women could avoid infection when the male partner cannot be relied on to use a condom. Kissing is considered safe, although there is a theoretical possibility of transmission via virus in saliva. The low concentration of virus in saliva of infected individuals, as well as the presence in saliva of HIV-inhibitory proteins (see above), lessens any risk of transmission by kissing.

The most effective way to prevent transmission of HIV infection among IDUs is to stop the use of injecting drugs. Unfortunately, that is extremely difficult to accomplish unless the addict enters a treatment program. For those who will not or cannot participate in a drug treatment program and who will continue to inject drugs, the avoidance of sharing of needles and other paraphernalia ("works") is the next best way to avoid transmission of infection. The cultural and social factors that contribute to the sharing of paraphernalia are complex and difficult to overcome. In addition, needles and syringes may be in short supply. Under these circumstances, paraphernalia should be cleaned after each usage with a virucidal solution, such as undiluted sodium hypochlorite (household bleach). Data from a number of studies have indicated that programs that provide sterile needles to addicts in exchange for used needles have resulted in a decrease in HIV transmission without increasing the use of injection drugs. It is important for IDUs to be tested for HIV infection and counseled, to avoid transmission to their sexual partners. Secondary and tertiary spread of HIV infection by the heterosexual route within settings of a high level of injection drug use has increased greatly in the United States (see above).

Transmission of HIV via transfused blood or blood products has been decreased dramatically by a combination of screening of all blood donors for HIV infection by assays for both HIV antibody and p24 antigen and self-deferral of individuals at risk for HIV infection. In addition, clotting factor concentrates are heat-treated, essentially eliminating the risk to hemophiliacs who require these products. Autologous transfusions are preferable to transfusions from another individual. However, logistic constraints as well as the unpredictability of the need for most transfusions limit the feasibility of this approach. At present the risk of becoming HIV-infected from a contaminated blood transfusion is approximately 2 in 1 million.

HIV can be transmitted via breast milk and colostrum. The avoidance of breast feeding may not be practical in developing countries, where nutritional concerns override the risk of HIV transmission. However, it is becoming appreciated that transmission by breast milk accounts for a considerable proportion of infections in infants in developing countries who were born of HIV-infected mothers and who were fortunate enough not to have been infected intrapartum or peripartum. Therefore, even in developing countries, breast feeding from an infected mother should be avoided if at all possible. In developed countries such as the United States, where bottled formula and milk are readily accessible, breast feeding is absolutely contraindicated when a mother is HIV positive.

BIBLIOGRAPHY

ALKHATIB G et al: CC CKR5: A RANTES, MIP-1α, MIP-1β receptor as a fusion cofactor for macrophage-tropic HIV-1. Science 272:1955, 1996

BLEUL CC et al: The lymphocyte chemoattractant SDF-1 is a ligand for LESTR/fusin and blocks HIV-1 entry. Nature 382:829, 1996

BRODINE SK et al: Detection of diverse HIV-1 genetic subtypes in the USA. Lancet 346:1198, 1995

CAO Y et al: Virologic and immunologic characterization of long-term survivors of human immunodeficiency virus type-1 infection. N Engl J Med 332:201, 1995

CARPENTER CJ et al: Antiretroviral therapy for HIV infection in 1996. Recommendations of an international panel. JAMA 276:146, 1996

CENTERS FOR DISEASE CONTROL AND PREVENTION: Update: Trends in AIDS diagnosis and reporting under the expanded surveillance definition for adolescents and adults—United States, 1993. Morb Mort Week Rep 43:826, 1994

———: Update: Trends in AIDS among men who have sex with men—United States, 1989–1994. Morb Mort Week Rep 44:401, 1995

———: Update: Mortality attributable to HIV infection among persons aged 25–44 years. Morb Mort Week Rep 45:121, 1996

———: Provisional recommendations for chemoprophylaxis after occupational exposure to human immunodeficiency virus. Morb Mort Week Rep 45:468, 1996

CESARMAN E et al: Kaposi's sarcoma-associated herpesvirus-like DNA sequences in AIDS-related body-cavity-based lymphomas. N Engl J Med 332:1186, 1995

CHANG Y et al: Identification of herpes-like DNA sequences in AIDS-associated Kaposi's sarcoma. Science 266:1865, 1994

CHOE H et al: The β-chemokine receptors CCR3 and CCR5 facilitate infection by primary HIV-1 isolates. Cell 85:1135, 1996

CLARK SJ, SHAW GM: The acute retroviral syndrome and the pathogenesis of HIV-1 infection. Semin Immunol 5:149, 1993

CLERICI M, SHEARER GM: The Th-1-Th-2 hypothesis of HIV infection: New insights. Immunol Today 15:575, 1994

COCCHI F et al: Identification of RANTES, MIP-1α, and MIP-1β as the major HIV-suppressive factors produced by CD8+ T cells. Science 270:1811, 1995

COLLIER AC et al: Treatment for human immunodeficiency virus infection with saquinavir, zidovudine, and zalcitabine. N Engl J Med 334:1011, 1996

CONNOR EM et al: Reduction of maternal-infant transmission of human immunodeficiency virus type 1 with zidovudine treatment. N Engl J Med 331:1173, 1994

D'AQUILA RT et al: Nevirapine, zidovudine and didanosine compared with zidovudine and didanosine in patients with HIV-1 infection. A randomized, double-blind, placebo controlled trial. Ann Intern Med 124:1019, 1996

DEACON NJ et al: Genomic structure of an attenuated quasi species of HIV-1 from a blood transfusion donor and recipients. Science 270:988, 1995

DEEKS SG et al: HIV-1 protease inhibitors. A review for clinicians. JAMA 277:145, 1997

DENG HK et al: Identification of a major co-receptor for primary isolates of HIV-1. Nature 381:661, 1996

DESROSIERS RC, FAUCI AS: Retroviral pathogenesis, Part II, in Retroviruses, H Varmus et al (eds). Cold Spring Harbor, NY, Cold Spring Harbor Laboratory Press, 1996

DICKOVER RE et al: Identification of levels of maternal HIV-1 RNA associated with risk of perinatal transmission. Effect of maternal zidovudine treatment on viral load. JAMA 275:599, 1996

DORANZ BJ et al: A dual-tropic primary HIV-1 isolate that uses fusin and the β-chemokine receptors CKR5, CKR3, and CKR-2b as fusion cofactors. Cell 85:1149, 1996

DRAGIC T et al: HIV-1 entry into CD4+ cells is mediated by the chemokine receptor CC-CKR-5. Nature 381:667, 1996

EMERY S, LANE HC: Immune-based therapies in HIV infection: Recent developments. AIDS 10(Suppl A):S159, 1996

ENSOLI B et al: Synergy between basic fibroblast growth factor and HIV-1 Tat protein in induction of Kaposi's sarcoma. Nature 371:674, 1994

ERON JJ et al: Treatment with lamivudine, zidovudine, or both in HIV-positive patients with 200 to 500 CD4+ cells per cubic millimeter. N Engl J Med 333:1662, 1995

EUROPEAN COLLABORATIVE STUDY: Caesarean section and risk of vertical transmission of HIV-1 infection. Lancet 343:1464, 1994

FANG G et al: Maternal plasma human immunodeficiency virus type 1 RNA level: A determinant and project threshold for mother-to-child transmission. Proc Natl Acad Sci USA 92:12100, 1995

FAUCI AS: CD4+ T lymphocytopenia without HIV infection—no lights, no camera, just facts. N Engl J Med 328:429, 1993

———: Multifactorial nature of human immunodeficiency virus disease: Implications for therapy. Science 262:1011, 1993

———: An HIV vaccine: Breaking the paradigms. Proc Assoc Am Physicians 108:6, 1996

———: Host factors and the pathogenesis of HIV-induced disease. Nature 384:529, 1996

——— et al: Immunopathogenic mechanisms of HIV infection. Ann Intern Med 124:654, 1996

FONG IW et al: The natural history of progressive multifocal leukoencephalopathy in patients with AIDS. Clin Infect Dis 20:1305, 1995

GALLANT JE et al: Prophylaxis for opportunistic infections in patients with HIV infection. Ann Intern Med 120:932, 1994

GERBERDING JL: Management of occupational exposures to blood-borne viruses. N Engl J Med 332:444, 1995

HAYNES BF et al: Toward an understanding of the correlates of protective immunity to HIV infection. Science 271:324, 1996

HO DD et al: Rapid turnover of plasma virions and CD4 lymphocytes in HIV infection. Nature 373:123, 1995

HOLTZMAN DM et al: New-onset seizures associated with human immunodeficiency virus infection: Causation and clinical features in 100 cases. Am J Med 87:173, 1989

JACOBSEN H et al: In vivo resistance to human immunodeficiency virus type 1 proteinase inhibitor: Mutations, kinetics and frequencies. J Infect Dis 173:1379, 1996

KAPLAN JE et al: USPHS/IDSA guidelines for the prevention of opportunistic infections in persons infected with human immunodeficiency virus. Clin Infect Dis 21(Suppl 1):1, 1995

——— et al: 14-year followup of HIV-infected homosexual men with lymphadenopathy syndrome. J Acquired Immune Defic Syndr Hum Retrovirol 11:206, 1996

KASLOW RA et al: Influence of combinations of human major histocompatibility complex genes on the course of HIV-1 infection. Nature Med 2:405, 1996

KELEN GD et al: Trends in human immunodeficiency virus (HIV) infection among a patient population of an inner-city emergency department: Implications for emergency department-based screening programs for HIV infection. Clin Infect Dis 21:867, 1995

KINLOCH-DE LOES S et al: A controlled trial of zidovudine in primary human immunodeficiency virus infection. N Engl J Med 333:408, 1995

KIRCHHOFF F et al: Brief report: Absence of intact nef sequences in a long-term survivor with nonprogressive HIV-1 infection. N Engl J Med 332:228, 1995

KORBER BTM et al: Mutational trends in V3 loop protein sequences observed in different genetic lineages of human immunodeficiency virus type 1. J Virol 68:6730, 1994

KOVACS JA et al: Controlled trial of interleukin-2 infusions in patients infected with the human immunodeficiency virus. N Engl J Med 335:1350, 1996

KROWN SE et al: Kaposi's sarcoma in the acquired immunodeficiency syndrome: A proposal for a uniform evaluation, response and staging criteria. J Clin Oncol 7:1201, 1989

KUHN L et al: Cesarean deliveries and maternal-infant HIV transmission: Results from a prospective study in South Africa. J Acquired Immune Defic Syndr Hum Retrovirol 11:478, 1996

LACKRITZ EM et al: Estimated risk of HIV transmission by screened blood in the United States. N Engl J Med 333:1721, 1995

LANE HC: Recent advances in the management of AIDS-related opportunistic infections. Ann Intern Med 120:945, 1994

LEVY JA: Pathogenesis of human immunodeficiency virus infection. Microbiol Rev 57:183, 1993

LIU R et al: Homozygous defect in HIV-1 coreceptor accounts for resistance of some multiply-exposed individuals to HIV-1 infection. Cell 86:367, 1996

LUSSO P, GALLO RC: Human herpesvirus 6 in AIDS. Immunol Today 2:67, 1995

MANNHEIMER SB, SOAVE R: Protozoal infections in patients with AIDS. Cryptosporidiosis, isosporiasis, cyclosporiasis, and microsporidiosis. Infect Dis Clin North Am 8:483, 1994

MELLORS JW et al: Prognosis in HIV-1 infection predicted by the quantity of virus in plasma. Science 272:1167, 1996

MOORE PS, CHANG Y: Detection of herpesvirus-like DNA sequences in Kaposi's sarcoma in patients with and those without HIV infection. N Engl J Med 332:1181, 1995

MOORE RD, CHAISSON RE: Natural history of opportunistic diseases in an HIV-infected urban clinical cohort. Ann Intern Med 124:633, 1996

NDUATI RW et al: Human immunodeficiency virus type 1-infected cells in breast milk: Association with immunosuppression and vitamin A deficiency. J Infect Dis 172:1461, 1995

OBERLIN E et al: The CXC chemokine receptor SDF-1 is the ligand for LESTR/fusin and prevents infection by T-cell-line-adapted HIV-1. Nature 382:833, 1996

O'BRIEN WA et al: Changes in plasma HIV-1 RNA and CD4+ lymphocyte count and the risk of progression to AIDS. N Engl J Med 334:426, 1996

PANTALEO G et al: Studies in subjects with long-term nonprogressive human immunodeficiency virus infection. N Engl J Med 332:209, 1995

———, FAUCI AS: New concepts in the pathogenesis of HIV infection. Annu Rev Immunol 13:487, 1995

——— et al: HIV infection is active and progressive in lymphoid tissue during the clinically latent stage of disease. Nature 362:355, 1993

PECKHAM C, GIBB D: Mother-to-child transmission of the human immunodeficiency virus. N Engl J Med 333:298, 1995

PERELSON AS et al: HIV-1 dynamics in vivo: Virion clearance rate, infected cell life-span, and viral generation time. Science 271:1582, 1996

PIATAK M et al: High levels of HIV-1 in plasma during all stages of infection determined by competitive PCR. Science 259:1749, 1993

PRICE RW: Neurological complications of HIV infection. Lancet 348:445, 1996

REDFIELD RR et al: The Walter Reed staging classification for HTLV-III/LAV infection. N Engl J Med 314:131, 1986

ROBERTSON DL et al: Recombination in HIV-1. Nature 374:124, 1995

ROSENBERG PS: Scope of the AIDS epidemic in the United States. Science 270:1372, 1995

SAMSON M et al: Resistance to HIV-1 infection in Caucasian individuals bearing mutant alleles of the CCR-5 chemokine receptor gene. Nature 382:722, 1996

SCHACKER T et al: Clinical and epidemiologic features of primary HIV infection. Ann Intern Med 125:257, 1996

SMITH KJ et al: Cutaneous findings in HIV-1 positive patients: a 42-month prospective study. J Am Acad Dermatol 31:746, 1994

SPARANO JA: Treatment of AIDS-related lymphomas. Curr Opin Oncol 7:442, 1995

SPECTOR SA et al: Oral ganciclovir for the prevention of cytomegalovirus disease in persons with AIDS. N Engl J Med 334:1491, 1996

SOCA ACTG: Mortality in patients with the acquired immunodeficiency syndrome treated with either foscarnet or ganciclovir for cytomegalovirus retinitis. N Engl J Med 326:213, 1992

SOTO-RAMIREZ LE et al: HIV-1 Langerhans' cell tropism associated with heterosexual transmission of HIV. Science 271:1291, 1996

SPIRA AI et al: Cellular targets of infection and route of viral dissemination after an intravaginal inoculation of simian immunodeficiency virus into rhesus macaques. J Exp Med 183:215, 1996

STANLEY SK, FAUCI AS: T cell homeostasis in HIV infection: Part of the solution or part of the problem? J Acquired Immune Defic Syndr Hum Retrovirol 6:142, 1993

TINDALL B, COOPER DA: Primary HIV infection. Host responses and intervention strategies. AIDS 5:1, 1991

WALKER CM et al: CD8 + lymphocytes can control HIV infection in vitro by suppressing virus replication. Science 234:1563, 1986

WEI X et al: Viral dynamics in human immunodeficiency virus type 1 infection. Nature 373:117, 1995

WHALEN C et al: Accelerated course of human immunodeficiency virus infection after tuberculosis. Am J Respir Crit Care Med 151:129, 1995

ZINKERNAGEL RM et al: Immunology taught by viruses. Science 271:173, 1996

309 *Jean D. Sipe, Alan S. Cohen*

AMYLOIDOSIS

DEFINITION AND CLASSIFICATION *Amyloidosis* results from the deposition of insoluble, fibrous amyloid proteins, nearly always in the extracellular spaces of organs and tissues. Named by Virchow in 1854 on the basis of color after staining with iodine and sulfuric acid, all amyloid proteins share a unique fibrillar ultrastructure. Depending upon the biochemical nature of the amyloid precursor protein, amyloid fibrils can be deposited locally or may involve virtually every organ system of the body. Amyloid fibril deposition may have no apparent clinical consequences or may lead to severe pathophysiologic changes. Often the disease falls between these two extremes. Regardless of etiology, the clinical diagnosis of amyloidosis is usually not made until the disease is far advanced.

There are multiple clinically and biochemically distinct forms of amyloid that share a unique morphology and secondary structure; some are systemic and others are localized or organ-limited (Table 309-1). Although the fibril precursors differ in their amino acid sequences, the polypeptide backbones of these protein precursors assume an identical secondary structure, the β-pleated sheet conformation, and similar fibrillar morphologies that render them resistant to proteolysis. All amyloid deposits contain an identical nonfibrillar component, the pentraxin or serum amyloid P (SAP). The amyloidoses are classified according to the biochemical nature of the fibril-forming protein. *Systemic amyloidoses* include biochemically distinct forms that are neoplastic, inflammatory, genetic, or iatrogenic in origin, while *localized* or *organ-limited amyloidoses* are associated with aging and diabetes and occur in isolated organs, often endocrine, without evidence of systemic involvement.

Despite their biochemical and clinical differences, the various amyloidoses share common features. These include the presence of an amyloidogenic precursor in appropriate concentration; the appropriate genetic background of the host; abnormalities in proteolysis of fibril precursors and nascent amyloid fibrils; and alterations in extracellular matrix constituents such as glycosaminoglycans, together with the presence of amyloid-enhancing factor (AEF). The most recent guidelines for nomenclature and classification of amyloid and amyloidosis were recommended in 1990 by the Nomenclature Committee of the International Society for Amyloidosis. Amyloid deposits should be classified using the capital letter A as the first letter of designation followed by the protein designation without any open space; for example, AL for amyloidosis involving immunoglobulin light chains (Table 309-1).

ETIOLOGY AND PATHOGENESIS **Light Chain Amyloidosis (AL)** The most common form of systemic amyloidosis seen in current clinical practice is AL (primary idiopathic amyloidosis, or that associated with multiple myeloma) resulting from fibril formation by monoclonal antibody light chains in primary amyloidosis and in some cases of multiple myeloma (see Chap. 114). Less than 20 percent of patients with AL have myeloma. The rest have other monoclonal gammopathies, light chain disease, or even agammablobulinemia (producing light chains, but not intact immunoglobulin). About 15 to 20 percent of patients with myeloma have amyloidosis. A monoclonal population of bone marrow plasma cells is present and consistently produces either small lambda or kappa fragments or immunoglobulins that are processed (cleaved) in an abnormal fashion by macrophage enzymes to produce the partially degraded light chains responsible for AL amyloidosis. Lambda chain class predominates over kappa in AL by a 2:1 ratio, whereas in multiple myeloma and normal immunoglobulin synthesis, the reverse is true. Indeed, almost all lambda VI family chains have been associated with amyloid. The primary structure of each amyloid-forming light chain is unique, reflecting the features of the B cell clone that produced it. In patients with multiple myeloma, light chains can be deposited as casts in kidney tubules or as punctate deposits on basement membranes. Also, nonfibrillar amyloid deposition diseases have been described; thus there are three forms of human light chain–associated renal and systemic diseases: AL amyloidosis, cast nephropathy, and light chain deposition disease. Rarely, heavy chain amyloid deposition has been reported.

Amyloid A Amyloidosis (AA) AA amyloidosis (secondary, reactive, or acquired amyloidosis) occurs most frequently as a complication of chronic inflammatory disease. Effective treatment of the underlying inflammatory condition has reduced incidence in developed countries. In the past in the United States, tuberculosis (see Chap. 171), osteomyelitis (see Chap. 132), and leprosy (see Chap. 172) were the most common precipitating diseases, and they remain so in developing countries. Familial deposition of the AA protein occurs in some groups of patients with familial Mediterranean fever (FMF) (see Chap. 288). However colchicine treatment has been very effective in reducing the incidence of AA amyloidosis in association with FMF. During inflammation, proinflammatory cytokines such as interleukin (IL) 1, IL-6, and tumor necrosis factor stimulate the synthesis in liver of serum amyloid A (apoSAA), a transient, injury-specific component of high-density lipoprotein (HDL). Thus, effective treatment of the underlying inflammatory disorder blocks the stimulus for precursor synthesis. SAA, the final protein product, is a chemokine, a chemoattractant cytokine that amplifies an inflammatory response.

Heredofamilial Amyloidoses Until the advent of biochemical studies, there was no generally accepted nosology for the heredofamilial amyloid syndromes. Some researchers emphasized the site of predominant organ involvement, classifying the disease as neuropathic, nephropathic, or cardiopathic amyloidosis, while others stressed the genetic aspects. With one exception, the amyloidosis of FMF, which is inherited as an autosomal recessive disorder and is an AA type of amyloid, the mode of inheritance of the heredofamilial amyloidoses is autosomal dominant. FMF is a disorder subdivided into phenotype I, with irregularly occurring fever and abdominal, chest, or joint pain, preceding or accompanying renal amyloid; and phenotype II, in which renal amyloidosis is the first or only manifestation of the disease (see

Chap. 288). Colchicine treatment prevents attacks of FMF and appears to prevent subsequent deposition of amyloid either by blocking precursor apoSAA production or by blocking AEF formation.

CHAPTER 309
Amyloidosis   1857

The heredofamilial amyloidoses primarily involve the nervous system. Familial amyloid polyneuropathies (FAP) are dominant hereditary diseases affecting kinships originating in Portugal, Japan, Sweden, Finland, Greece, Italy, and elsewhere. FAP can be subclassified based on clinical symptoms and the biochemical nature of the fibrils; in nearly all cases the fibrils are variants of transthyretin (TTR), apolipoprotein AI, gelsolin, cystatin C, and rarely the α chain of fibrinogen A or lysozyme. FAP are autosomal dominant conditions in which the mutant proteins, although present from birth, result in a delayed onset of disease symptoms, usually after three to seven decades of life. The FAP prototype is the lower limb neuropathy first described in Portugal, which has a poor prognosis and is characterized by progressively severe neuropathy, including marked autonomic nervous system involvement. In some of these individuals, bilateral "scalloped" pupils are pathognomonic of the disease.

ATTR   The most frequently occurring form of FAP involves TTR, a 14-kDa protein originally described as prealbumin, that transports thyroxine and retinol-binding protein in the blood. The first mutation to be identified in Portuguese families and in families of Swedish origin was a single amino acid substitution, methionine for valine at position 30. To date, more than 50 TTR variants have been defined. Variant TTR gene carriers exhibit clinically heterogeneous amyloidoses according to the position and nature of the amino acid substitution. Substitution of proline for leucine at position 55 results in an early onset and rapidly progressing disease, whereas substitution of methionine for threonine at position 119 appears to protect against amyloid fibril formation. In Denmark, patients with a methionine substitution for leucine at position 111 have a severe cardiopathy. Nonpathogenic TTR mutants such as the substitution of serine for glycine at position 6 also exist, and several are associated with changes in association with retinol-binding protein.

AApoAI   An autosomal dominant form of hereditary amyloidosis results from deposition of an apolipoprotein AI variant in which arginine is substituted for glycine at position 26 or for tryptophan at position 50 or for leucine at position 60. Gene carriers exhibit low levels of HDL and exhibit peripheral neuropathy that is clinically similar to the type of familial amyloidosis that is caused by variants of TTR. Another kindred carrying the same mutation presents clinically with renal failure but without neurologic symptoms.

AGel   Two mutations at position 187, within the actin-binding domain of gelsolin, are associated with a unique form of hereditary systemic amyloidosis. Gelsolin is a calcium-binding protein that binds to and fragments actin filaments. The disease has been reported primarily in Finland but also in patients of Japanese and Dutch backgrounds. Fibrils of gelsolin fragments are deposited in blood vessels and basement membranes, leading to clinical manifestations of lattice corneal dystrophy and cranial neuropathy, followed by peripheral neuropathy, dystrophic skin changes, and involvement of other organs.

ALys   Hereditary nonneuropathic systemic amyloidosis has been described in English families in which lysozyme is the major fibril protein. Two mutations have been described: one in

which threonine is substituted for isoleucine at position 56, and the second in which histidine is substituted for aspartic acid at position 67.

AFib   Hereditary nonneuropathic renal amyloidosis has been described in families with mutations in the fibrinogen A α chains.

Aβ₂M   Deposition of β₂-microglobulin as amyloid fibrils in the musculoskeletal system can occur in the presence of renal problems that require long-term hemodialysis usually with cuprophane membranes. β₂-microglobulin contains a significant amount of β-pleated sheet structure and is thought to form amyloid fibrils because of high local concentrations of the precursor protein.

Localized or Organ-Limited Amyloidoses   Depending upon the biochemical nature of the amyloid fibril protein, instead of systemic deposition involving the cardiovascular and gastrointestinal systems along with lymph nodes, spleen, liver, kidneys, and adrenals, amyloid deposition may be limited to a single organ such as the pancreas, brain, or heart.

Polypeptide hormone–derived amyloidosis   Polypeptide hormone–derived amyloid deposits are common in polypeptide hormone–producing tissues and tumors. Calcitonin is deposited in the hereditary amyloid syndrome, medullary carcinoma of the thyroid (ACal) (see Chap. 331). Also AANF (atrial natriuretic factor–derived) amyloid deposits are found in the sarcolemma of ~80 percent of persons over 80 years of age. AIAPP (islet amyloid polypeptide–derived, or amylin) is deposited as amyloid fibrils in >90 percent of individuals with type 2 diabetes (see Chap. 334), in endocrine tumors (see Chap. 95), and in insulinoma (see Chap. 95). It is produced in β cells of the pancreas and stored and released together with insulin. Human insulin does not naturally form amyloid fibrils, although fibrils of porcine insulin, AIns, are sometimes found as subcutaneous nodules at sites of insulin injection in diabetic individuals.

Amyloidosis associated with Alzheimer's disease   Alzheimer's disease (AD) is characterized by three lesions in the brain, i.e., senile or neuritic plaques, neurofibrillary tangles, and vascular lesions (see

Table 309-1

Abbreviated Classification of Amyloid

Amyloid Protein	Protein Precursor	Clinical Syndrome
AA	apoSAA	Reactive (secondary) Familial Mediterranean fever Muckle-Wells syndrome
AL	Igλ, Igκ	Idiopathic (primary) Multiple myeloma Local nodular
AH	γ1 heavy chain	Macroglobulinemia
Aβ₂M	β₂ microglobulin	Chronic hemodialysis arthropathy
Aβ	β-protein precursor	Alzheimer's disease Down's syndrome Hereditary cerebral angiopathy with bleeding (Dutch)
APrPˢᶜ	Prion protein	Creutzfeldt-Jakob disease Gerstmann-Straussler syndrome Kuru
AIAPP	Amyloid insulin polypeptide	Diabetes mellitus type 2 Insulinoma
AANF	Atrial natriuretic factor	Senile cardiac amyloid
ATTR	Transthyretin	FAP; multiple point mutations Senile systemic cardiac
AGel	Gelsolin	FAP-Finnish
AApoA1	Apolipoprotein A1	FAP-Iowa (Irish)
ACys	Cystatin C	Hereditary cerebral angiopathy with bleeding (Iceland)
AFibA	Fibrinogen A α	Nonneuropathic hereditary amyloid with renal disease
ALys	Lysozyme	Nonneuropathic hereditary amyloid with renal disease

Chap. 367). A novel protein, β-amyloid protein (Aβ), is the major fibril protein in the amyloid deposits of the cerebrovascular walls and the cores of neuritic plaques of AD patients and also in individuals with Down's syndrome (see Chap. 66). The intracellular neurofibrillary tangles are composed of paired helical filaments arranged in a twisted conformation and have as their major component an abnormally phosphorylated τ-protein, a microtubule-associated protein that, in spite of its intracellular localization, is sometimes considered to be amyloid in nature, i.e., APHF. Aβ varies in length from 39 to 43 amino acids and is derived from a large transmembrane glycoprotein called amyloid β-precursor protein (AβPP). Mutations in AβPP are associated with familial AD and also with a different type of amyloidosis, hereditary cerebral hemorrhage with amyloidosis (Dutch type).

Scrapie-associated prion proteins Prions are a unique class of infectious proteins associated with a group of neurodegenerative diseases, the transmissible spongiform encephalopathies. In humans, these diseases include kuru, Creutzfeldt-Jakob disease, Gerstmann-Straussler-Scheinker syndrome, and fatal familial insomnia (see Chap. 379); in animals, scrapie and bovine spongiform encephalopathy (mad cow disease). PrP^{Sc} is a pathogenic, transmissible spongiform encephalopathy-specific form of the host-encoded prion protein (PrP); PrP^{Sc} differs from PrP in that it contains a high amount of β-pleated sheet structure and is insoluble and resistant to proteolytic enzymes. PrP^{Sc} deposits either consist of or can be readily converted to amyloid fibrils. APrP is similar to Aβ and ATTR in that both familial and sporadic forms occur. It has been suggested that the earlier onset familial forms of amyloidosis are due to accelerated fibril formation from mutant precursors, whereas in sporadic cases, amyloid fibrils are formed more slowly from normal precursor molecules. The mutant PrP molecules are nearer the threshold for transition to the amyloidogenic PrP^{Sc} than are the normal. The transition from normal to amyloidogenic PrP^{Sc} is irreversible but very slow. The disease progresses because, once formed, amyloidogenic PrP^{Sc} can seed the conversion of normal molecules into an amyloidogenic form.

CLINICAL MANIFESTATIONS The clinical manifestations of amyloidosis are varied and depend entirely on the biochemical nature of the fibril protein and thus the area of the body that is involved (Table 309-2). The diagnosis of amyloidosis is usually not made until

Table 309-2

Clinical Presentation of Systemic Amyloidosis

Disease	Symptoms
AL (primary)	Monoclonal immunoglobulin in urine or serum plus any of the following: Unexplained nephrotic syndrome, Hepatomegaly, Carpal tunnel syndrome, Macroglossia, Malabsorption or unexplained diarrhea or constipation, Peripheral neuropathy, Cardiomyopathy
AA (secondary)	Chronic infection (osteomyelitis, tuberculosis) or chronic inflammation (rheumatoid arthritis, granulomatous ileitis) plus development of any of the following: Proteinuria, Hepatomegaly, Unexplained gastrointestinal disease
Hereditary amyloidosis	Family history of neuropathy plus any of the following: Early sensorimotor disassociation, Vitreous opacities, Renal disease, Autonomic nervous system symptoms, Cardiovascular disease, Gastrointestinal disease

after the point of irreversible organ damage. Proteinuria is often the first symptom associated with systemic amyloidosis, particularly of the AA and AL type; peripheral neuropathies are associated with FAP, and dementia and cognitive dysfunction with amyloid deposits in brain. Organ enlargement, especially of the liver, kidney, spleen, and heart, may be prominent; however, this does not occur in FAP, AD, or PrP.

Kidney Renal involvement may consist of mild proteinuria or frank nephrosis. In some cases, the urinary sediment may show a few red blood cells. The renal lesion is usually not reversible and in time leads to progressive azotemia and death. The prognosis does not appear to be related to the degree of the proteinuria; when azotemia finally develops, the prognosis is grave. Treatment by peritoneal or hemodialysis or kidney transplantation improves the prognosis considerably. Hypertension is rare, except in long-standing amyloidosis. Renal tubular acidosis or renal vein thrombosis may occur. Localized accumulation of amyloid may be noted in the ureter, bladder, or other parts of the genitourinary tract.

Heart With respect to systemic amyloidoses, cardiac amyloidosis is common in primary (AL) and heredofamilial amyloidosis and very rare in the secondary (AA) form. With respect to localized amyloidosis, cardiac amyloidosis of the TTR type is common after 80 years of age; also atrial natriuretic factor may be present in the atria. In systemic amyloidosis, cardiac manifestations consist primarily of congestive failure and cardiomegaly (with or without murmurs) and a variety of arrhythmias and are comparable in AL and FAP, the predominant forms with cardiomyopathy (see Chap. 239). Although these manifestations predominantly reflect diffuse myocardial amyloid, the endocardium, valves, and pericardium may also be involved. Pericarditis with effusion is rare, although the differential diagnosis of constrictive pericarditis versus restrictive cardiomyopathy frequently arises. Echocardiography has demonstrated symmetric thickening of the left ventricular wall; hypokinesia and decreased systolic contraction and thickening of the interventricular septum and left ventricular posterior wall; and left ventricular cavities of small to normal size. Two-dimensional echocardiography produces the characteristic findings of thickened right and left ventricles, a normal left ventricular cavity, and, especially, a diffuse hyperrefractile "granular sparkling" appearance. Hearts that are heavily infiltrated with amyloid may or may not show an enlarged silhouette. Fluoroscopy usually shows decreased mobility of the ventricular wall; angiographic studies usually demonstrate thickened ventricular wall, decreased ventricular mobility, and absence of rapid ventricular filling in early diastole. Cardiac amyloidosis can present as intractable heart failure. Electrocardiographic abnormalities include a low-voltage QRS complex and abnormalities in atrioventricular and intraventricular conduction, often resulting in varying degrees of heart block. Owing to their propensity to develop conduction defects and arrhythmias, patients with cardiac amyloidosis appear to be especially sensitive to digitalis, and this drug should be used with caution.

Liver While hepatic involvement is common except in heredofamilial amyloidosis of the TTR type, liver function abnormalities are minimal and occur late in the disease. Portal hypertension occurs but is uncommon. Intrahepatic cholestasis has been noted in about 5 percent of patients with AL (primary) amyloidosis. Hepatomegaly is common, and AL hepatic amyloid is usually accompanied by the nephrotic syndrome and congestive heart failure. Prognosis is poor, and one group of 80 patients with proven severe AL hepatic amyloid had a median survival of 9 months. Amyloidosis of the spleen characteristically is not associated with leukopenia and anemia.

Skin Involvement of the skin is one of the most characteristic manifestations of primary (AL) amyloidosis (see Chap. 57). Other forms of amyloidosis such as lichen amyloidosis are thought to involve forms of keratin. In AL amyloidosis, the lesions may consist of slightly raised, waxy papules or plaques that usually are clustered in the folds of the axillae, anal, or inguinal regions, the face and neck, or mucosal areas such as ear or tongue. Periorbital ecchymoses ("black eye" or "raccoon syndrome") have been reported. The lesions are seldom pruritic. Involvement of the skin or mucosa may not be apparent clinically but may induce bleeding into the skin, leading to purpura.

Cutaneous involvement can also be seen on biopsy in secondary amyloidosis; in one series it was found in 42 percent of such patients, in 55 percent of a group of patients with primary disease, and in all 11 patients with hereditary amyloid neuropathy.

Gastrointestinal Tract Gastrointestinal symptoms are common in all systemic types of amyloidosis. They may result from direct involvement of the gastrointestinal tract at any level or from infiltration of the autonomic nervous system with amyloid. The symptoms include those of obstruction, ulceration, malabsorption, hemorrhage, protein loss, and diarrhea (see Chap. 285). Infiltration of the tongue occasionally leads to macroglossia. When not enlarged, the tongue may become stiffened and firm to palpation. Infiltration of the tongue is characteristic of primary amyloidosis (AL) or amyloidosis accompanying multiple myeloma. Gastrointestinal bleeding may occur from any of a number of sites, notably the esophagus, stomach, or large intestine, and may be severe. Amyloid infiltration of the esophagus may lead to an incompetent or nonrelaxing lower esophageal sphincter, nonspecific motility disorders of the esophageal body, or rarely achalasia. Small-bowel lesions may lead to clinical and x-ray changes of obstruction. A malabsorption syndrome is common. Amyloidosis (AA or secondary) may also develop in association with other entities involving the gastrointestinal tract, especially tuberculosis (see Chap. 171), granulomatous enteritis (see Chap. 286), lymphoma (see Chap. 113), and Whipple's disease (see Chap. 285); differentiation of these conditions, which give rise to secondary amyloidosis, from diffuse primary amyloidosis of the small bowel may be difficult. Similarly, amyloidosis of the stomach may closely mimic gastric carcinoma, with obstruction, achlorhydria, and the radiologic appearance of tumor masses.

Nervous System Neurologic manifestations may include peripheral neuropathy, postural hypotension, inability to sweat, Adies's pupil, hoarseness, and sphincter incompetence. These manifestations are especially prominent in the heredofamilial amyloidoses. The cranial nerves are generally spared, except in the Finnish hereditary amyloidosis. Carpal tunnel syndrome may be caused by several amyloidoses, especially primary (AL) and chronic hemodialysis ($A\beta_2M$) amyloid. Peripheral neuropathy is frequent in the former type. $A\beta$ amyloid occurs in the central nervous system as a component of senile plaques and in blood vessels ("congophilic angiopathy"). The protein concentration in the cerebrospinal fluid may be increased. Infiltrates of the cornea or vitreous body may be present in hereditary amyloid syndromes. Certain of these syndromes (advanced FAP) are characterized by a bilateral scalloping appearance of the pupil.

Endocrine Amyloid may infiltrate the thyroid or other endocrine glands but rarely causes endocrine dysfunction. Local amyloid deposits almost invariably accompany medullary carcinoma of the thyroid. Amyloid is often found in the adrenal gland, pituitary gland, and pancreas. Little if any clinical dysfunction is present unless there is massive replacement of the gland by amyloid.

Joints and Muscles Amyloid can directly, although rarely, involve articular structures by its presence in the synovial membrane and synovial fluid or in the articular cartilage. In these cases it is almost always of the AL type and associated with multiple myeloma. Amyloid arthritis can mimic a number of the rheumatic diseases because it can present as a symmetric arthritis of small joints with nodules, morning stiffness, and fatigue (see Chap. 321). The synovial fluid usually has a low white blood cell count, a good to fair mucin clot, a predominance of mononuclear cells, and no crystals. Studies of surgical specimens suggest a significant incidence of amyloid in cartilage, capsule, and synovium in osteoarthritis (see Chap. 322). Amyloid infiltration of muscle may lead to a pseudomyopathy. Shoulder muscle infiltration can produce the "shoulder pad" sign. Amyloid is found in muscle inclusion body disease, where $A\beta$ and/or PrP have been identified.

Respiratory System The nasal sinuses, larynx, and trachea may be involved by accumulation of AL amyloid, which blocks the ducts, in the case of the sinuses, or the air passages. Amyloidosis of the lung involves the bronchi and alveolar septa diffusely. The lower respiratory tract is affected most frequently in primary (AL) amyloidosis and in the disease associated with dysproteinemia. Pulmonary symptoms

attributable to amyloid are present in about 30 percent of cases. In secondary (AA) amyloidosis, pulmonary disease is a frequent histopathologic accompaniment but seldom gives rise to clinically significant symptoms. Amyloid also may be localized in the bronchi or pulmonary parenchyma and may resemble a neoplasm. In these cases, local excision should be attempted and, when successful, may be followed by prolonged remissions.

Hematopoietic System Hematologic changes may include fibrinogenopenia, increased fibrinolysis, and selective deficiency of clotting factors. Deficient factor X seems to be due to nonspecific calcium-dependent binding to the polyanionic amyloid fibrils. Splenectomy in the patient with such a factor X deficiency can relieve the deficiency and the associated bleeding disorder, since factor X has been shown to bind to the large masses of splenic amyloid. Endothelial damage together with the clotting abnormalities lead to a propensity toward abnormal bleeding.

DIAGNOSIS Amyloid fibrils are identified in biopsy or necropsy tissue sections (Table 309-3). The systemic amyloidoses offer a choice of biopsy sites; abdominal fat aspirates or renal or rectal biopsies are often performed. Microscopically, amyloid deposits stain pink with the hematoxylin-eosin stain and show metachromasia with crystal violet. The Congo red stain imparts a unique green birefringence when stained tissue sections are viewed using the polarizing microscope. This is the single most widely used and useful procedure for establishing the presence of systemic amyloid. Fluorescent dyes such as thioflavin are sensitive screening stains for amyloid deposits in brain and other tissues; however, specificity should be confirmed. After amyloid has been identified by staining, it can be chemically classified by protein studies and by immunohistochemistry. In the case of FAP, the presence of mutant TTR (or gelsolin, apoAI, etc.) establishes the specific diagnosis of the disease. In order to establish the relationship of immunoglobulin-related amyloid to multiple myeloma, electrophoretic and immunoelectrophoretic studies on serum and urine should be performed when the biopsy reveals amyloid deposition. Most of these patients will have only relatively small paraprotein components, and only a few will have frank multiple myeloma.

PROGNOSIS Generalized amyloidosis is usually a slowly progressive disease that leads to death in several years, but in some instances, prognosis is improving. The average survival in most large series of AL amyloid is ~12 months and in FAP is ~7 to 15 years. A number of individuals with amyloid have been followed 5 to 10 years and longer. The course of amyloidosis is difficult to document, because dating the time of origin of the disease is rarely possible. When amyloidosis develops in patients with rheumatoid arthritis, it seldom becomes evident when the arthritis is less than 2 years in

Table 309-3

Diagnosis of Amyloidosis

BIOPSY	APPROPRIATE STAIN
Common sites	Congo red, viewed by polarization
Subcutaneous abdominal fat	microscopy
aspirate	Thioflavin (less specific)
Rectum	Potassium permanganate pretreatment,
Skin	then Congo red stain
Gingiva	Other:
Occasional sites	Cotton dyes (comparable with Congo
Small intestine	red)
Muscle	Crystal violet (less sensitive)
Nerve	
Rare sites	**PROTEIN OR DNA STUDIES**
Kidney	
Liver	Mutant protein identification
Bone marrow	Immunocytochemistry: immuno-
Synovium	fluorescent or immunoperoxidase
Spleen	stains with specific antisera

duration. When amyloidosis develops in patients with multiple myeloma, manifestations leading to initial hospitalization are more apt to be related to amyloid disease than to myeloma. In these cases, prognosis is very poor, and life expectancy is usually less than 6 months.

℞ TREATMENT

Rational therapy should be directed at (1) reducing precursor production, (2) inhibiting the synthesis and extracellular deposition of amyloid fibrils, and (3) promoting lysis or mobilization of existing amyloid deposits. There are new specific therapies for the various amyloidoses. In certain of the heredofamilial amyloidoses, genetic counseling is an important aspect of treatment, and the removal of the site of synthesis of the mutant protein by liver transplantation has proven remarkably successful. Liver transplantation has been carried out since 1990 for FAP patients in Sweden, the United States, Portugal, Spain, and other countries. It appears that disease progression is halted and that there is some improvement in autonomic nervous system function.

While instances have been reported of remission of amyloidosis accompanying treatable infections or inflammation, often these reports are not substantiated by biopsy proof of resorption. In one series, the mean survival of patients with renal amyloid from the time of biopsy was 29 months, but in a few cases, there was presumptive evidence of regression of the renal amyloid. The utilization of chronic hemodialysis and of kidney transplantation has clearly improved the prognosis of renal amyloid.

In the case of AL amyloid, the fact that immunoglobulin light chain is made by plasma cells has lead to the use of alkylating agents. However, these agents are toxic and not very effective. Recent trials have indicated that a prednisone/melphalan/colchicine program prolongs life. Hematopoietic stem cell transplantation appears promising. A novel anthracycline, iododoxorubicin, has been shown to bind to AL amyloid (similar to Congo red) in vivo and promote amyloid resorption. Only a small number of patients have received this experimental agent, but the majority have had objective improvement. Cardiac transplantation in selected cases of AL or FAP amyloidosis has its advocates.

Patients with severe renal amyloidosis and azotemia have been treated by dialysis or kidney transplantation with very good outcomes. This has significantly improved the prognosis in patients whose major manifestations are renal.

Colchicine has been shown to be effective in preventing acute attacks in patients with FMF (see Chap. 288). It has been determined from inhibition of AA amyloid deposition in the mouse model that colchicine inhibits formation of AEF. One large study has shown colchicine to be effective in prolonging life in primary (AL) amyloidosis using a life-table survivorship analysis, and it putatively reverses AA renal amyloid lesions.

The major causes of death are heart disease and renal failure. Sudden death, presumably due to arrhythmias, is common. Occasionally, gastrointestinal hemorrhage, respiratory failure, intractable heart failure, and superimposed infections are the terminal events.

BIBLIOGRAPHY

BENSON MD: Inherited amyloidosis. J Med Genet 28:73, 1991
COHEN AS: Amyloidosis. Bull Rheum Dis 40:1, 1991
———, JONES LA: Advances in amyloidosis. Curr Opin Rheumatol 5:62, 1993
———, SIPE JD: Amyloidosis; in *Clinical Immunology*, RR Rich et al (eds). St. Louis, Mosby Year Book, 1995, pp 1264–1272
GLENNER GG, MURPHY MA: Amyloidosis of the nervous system. J Neurol Soc 94:1, 1989
HUSBY G et al: The 1990 guidelines for nomenclature and classification of amyloid and amyloidosis, in *Amyloid and Amyloidosis*, JB Natvig et al (eds). Dordrecht, Netherlands, Kluwer, 1990, pp 813–816
——— et al: Serum amyloid A (SAA): Biochemistry, genetics and the pathogenesis of AA amyloidosis. Amyloid Int J Exp Clin Invest 1:119, 1994
LEWIS WD, SKINNER M: Liver transplantation for familial amyloidotic polyneuropathy: A potentially curative treatment. Amyloid Int J Exp Clin Invest 1:143, 1994
PRUSINER SB, DEARMOND SJ: Prion protein amyloid and neurodegeneration. Amyloid Int J Exp Clin Invest 2:39, 1995
SIPE JD: Amyloidosis. Crit Rev Clin Lab Sci 31:325, 1994
ZEMER D et al: Colchicine in the prevention and treatment of the amyloidosis of familial Mediterranean fever. N Engl J Med 314:1001, 1986

SECTION 2
DISORDERS OF IMMUNE-MEDIATED INJURY

---

310 *K. Frank Austen*

DISEASES OF IMMEDIATE TYPE HYPERSENSITIVITY

The term *atopic allergy* implies a familial tendency to manifest such conditions as asthma, rhinitis, urticaria, and eczematous dermatitis (atopic dermatitis) alone or in combination. However, individuals without an atopic background also may develop hypersensitivity reactions, particularly urticaria and anaphylaxis, associated with the same class of antibody, IgE, found in atopic individuals. The designation *diseases of immediate type hypersensitivity* presents a more suitable framework than the broad term *allergy* or the restrictive definition of atopy.

The fixation of IgE to human mast cells and basophils, a process termed *sensitization*, prepares these cells for subsequent antigen-specific activation. The high-affinity receptor for IgE, designated FcεRI, is composed of one α, one β, and two disulfide-linked γ chains, which together cross the plasma membrane seven times. The α chain is solely responsible for IgE binding, and the β and γ chains are responsible for signal transduction that results from the aggregation of the tetrameric receptors by polymeric antigen.

Aggregation causes activation of an Src family–related tyrosine kinase, termed *Lyn*, which is constitutively associated with the β chain and which phosphorylates a particular motif [antigen recognition activation motif (ARAM)] in the γ chain. The phosphorylation of this motif in the γ chain induces an interaction with certain SH2 domains of a ZAP70/Syk family tyrosine kinase. The subsequent activation of Syk leads to phorphorylation and activation of phospholipase Cγ-1. This polyphosphatidyl inositol–selective phospholipase C elaborates 1,2-diacylglycerols (1,2-DAG) and inositol-1,4,5-*tris*-phosphate (IP$_3$), which in turn activate protein kinase C and mobilize intracellular calcium ions, respectively. These events may be augmented by the formation of calcium ion channels and attenuated by the activation of adenylate cyclase with formation of cyclic 3′,5′-adenosine monophosphate (cyclic AMP) and activation of cyclic AMP–dependent protein kinase. The calcium ion–dependent activation of phospholipases cleaves membrane phospholipids to generate lysophospholipids, which, like 1,2-DAG, are fusogenic and may facilitate the fusion of the secretory granule perigranular membrane with the cell membrane, a step that releases the membrane-free granule containing the preformed or primary mediators of mast cell effects.

The secretory granule of the human mast cell has a crystalline structure, unlike mast cells of lower species, and IgE-dependent cell activation can be characterized morphologically by solubilization and swelling of the granule contents within the first minute of receptor perturbation; this reaction is followed by the ordering of intermediate filaments about the swollen granule, movement toward the cell surface, and fusion of the perigranular membrane with that of other granules and with the plasmalemma to form extracellular channels for mediator release while maintaining cell viability.

In addition to exocytosis, aggregation of FcεRI initiates two other pathways for generation of bioactive products, namely, lipid mediators and cytokines. The biochemical steps involved in expression of such cytokines as tumor necrosis factor α (TNFα), interleukin (IL)-6, IL-4, IL-5, granulocyte-macrophage colony-stimulating factor (GM-CSF), and others have not been defined for mast cells in a manner comparable to T cells. Nonetheless, inhibition studies of cytokine production (IL-1β, TNFα, and IL-6) in mouse mast cells with cyclosporine or FK506 reveal binding to the ligand-specific immunophilin and attenuation of the calcium ion- and calmodulin-dependent serine/threonine phosphatase, calcineurin.

Lipid mediator generation (Fig. 310-1) involves translocation of calcium ion–dependent cytosolic phospholipase A_2 to the perinuclear membrane, with subsequent release of arachidonic acid for metabolic processing by the distinct prostanoid and leukotriene pathways. The constitutive prostaglandin endoperoxide synthase (PGHS-1/cyclooxygenase-1) or the de novo inducible PGHS-2 convert released arachidonic acid to the sequential intermediates prostaglandin (PG) G_2 and PGH_2. The glutathione-dependent hematopoietic PGD_2 synthase then converts PGH_2 to PGD_2, the predominant mast cell prostanoid.

For processing by the leukotriene pathway, the released arachidonic acid is translocated to an integral perinuclear membrane protein, the 5-lipoxygenase activating protein (FLAP). The calcium ion–dependent activation of 5-lipoxygenase involves translocation to the perinuclear membrane, which allows conversion of the arachidonic acid to the sequential intermediates, 5-hydroperoxyeicosatetraenoic acid and leukotriene (LT) A_4. LTA_4 is conjugated with reduced glutathione by LTC_4 synthase, an integral membrane protein with significant homology to FLAP. Intracellular LTC_4 is released by a carrier-specific export step for extracellular conversion to the receptor-active cysteinyl leukotrienes LTD_4 and LTE_4 by sequential removal of glumatic acid and glycine. A cytosolic LTA_4 hydrolase converts some LTA_4 to the dihydroxy leukotriene LTB_4, which then undergoes specific export for extracellular receptor–mediated actions. The lysophospholipid formed during release of arachidonic acid from 1-O-alkyl-2-acyl-sn-glyceryl-3-phosphorylcholine can be acetylated in the second position to form platelet-activating factor (PAF).

Unlike other cells of bone marrow origin, mast cells do not mature in the marrow and do not circulate in a recognized mature form. In tissue they appear as mature populations with tissue-related phenotypes. It is thus assumed that unrecognized mast cell progenitors enter the tissue and undergo regulated proliferation, differentiation, and maturation. Based on the immunodetection of secretory granule neutral proteases, mast cells in the lung parenchyma and intestinal mucosa selectively express tryptase; those in the intestinal and airway submucosa, skin, lymph nodes, and breast parenchyma express tryptase, chymase, and carboxypeptidase A (CPA); and occasional mast cells in intestinal submucosa express chymase and CPA but not tryptase. The secretory granules of mast cells selectively positive for tryptase in lung and intestinal mucosa exhibit closed scrolls with a periodicity suggestive of a crystalline structure by electron microscopy; whereas the secretory granules of mast cells with mutiple proteases residing in skin, lymph nodes, breast parenchyma, and submucosa of airways and intestine are scroll-poor with an amorphous or latticelike appearance. These phenotypic distinctions are accompanied by differences in their T cell dependence; for example, intestinal mucosal but not submucosal mast cells are absent in patients with inborn or acquired cellular immunodeficiency.

Mast cells are distributed at cutaneous and mucosal surfaces and in deeper tissues about venules, are an expansile population during T cell stimulation, and could regulate the entry of foreign substances by their rapid response capability (Fig. 310-2). Upon stimulus-specific activation in vitro, histamine and selected secretory granule–associated acid hydrolases are solubilized, whereas the neutral proteases, which are cationic, remain largely complexed to the anionic proteoglycans, heparin and chrondroitin sulfate E. It is speculated that the macromolecular complex serves to deliver the neutral proteases so that the endo- and exoproteases can function in concert at the substrate site to clear damaged tissue and facilitate repair. Histamine and the various lipid mediators (PGD_2, LTD_4/E_4, PAF) alter venular permeability, thereby allowing influx of plasma proteins such as complement and immunoglobulins, whereas LTB_4 mediates leukocyte–endothelial cell adhesion with subsequent directed migration (chemotaxis). The accumulation of leukocytes and opsonins would facilitate defense of the microenvironment. The cysteinyl leukotrienes constrict both vascular and nonvascular smooth muscle and are much more potent than histamine in constricting human airway smooth muscle when administered by aerosol.

The cellular component of the inflammatory response elicited by preformed secretory granule–associated and membrane-derived lipid mediators would be augmented and sustained by the addition of cytokines of mast cell or T cell origin to the microenvironment. Activation of human skin mast cells in situ elicits TNFα production and augmented venular permeability and would provide endothelial cell responses favoring leukocyte adhesion. Activation of purified human lung mast cells in vitro results in substantial production of IL-5 and lesser quantities of IL-4. Biopsies of patients with bronchial asthma reveal that mast cells are immunohistochemically positive for IL-4 and IL-5, but that the predominant localization of IL-4, IL-5, and GM-CSF is to T cells, defined as TH2 by this profile. It is speculated that IL-4 modulates the T cell phenotype to the TH2 subtype, and that IL-5 or GM-CSF converts infiltrating eosinophils to an activated, autoaggressive phenotype with augmented capacity for cytotoxicity and generation of O_2^- and the cysteinyl leukotrienes.

FIGURE 310-1 Pathways for biosynthesis and release of membrane-derived lipid mediators from mast cells. In the 5-lipoxygenase pathway leukotriene A_4 (LTA_4) is the intermediate from which the terminal-pathway enzymes generate the distinct final products, leukotriene C_4 (LTC_4) and leukotriene B_4 (LTB_4), which leave the cell by separate saturable transport systems. Gamma glutamyl transpeptidase and a dipeptidase then cleave glutamic acid and glycine from LTC_4 to form LTD_4 and LTE_4, respectively, for which there appears to be a common receptor. The only mast cell product of the cyclooxygenase system is PGD_2.

The view of immediate and late, or cellular, phases of allergic inflammation is supported by the response of the skin, nose, or lung of allergic humans to local allergen challenge; greater quantities of allergen are needed to elicit the cellular phase. In the immediate phase of a local challenge, there is pruritus and watery discharge from the nose, bronchospasm and mucous secretion in the lungs, and a wheal-and-flare response with pruritus in the skin. The reduced nasal patency, pulmonary function, or evident erythema with swelling at the skin site in a late-phase response at 6 to 8 h are associated with biopsy findings of infiltrating and activated TH2 type T cells, eosinophils, and even some basophils and neutrophils. This allergic inflammation proceeding from early mast cell activation to late cellular infiltration is believed to promote end-organ hyperresponsivity, as would be characteristic of perennial rhinitis or bronchial asthma; for attenuation, it requires introduction of an anti-inflammatory agent such as a glucocorticoid. The particular cytokines responsible for eosinophil and T cell adhesion with subsequent directed migration are not yet defined, although numerous candidates are identified.

Consideration of the mechanism of immediate type hypersensitivity diseases in the human has focused largely on the IgE-dependent recognition of otherwise nontoxic substances. Support for this thesis has come from the finding that clinical atopic allergy is sometimes associated with elevated total levels of IgE and in some instances with an immune response that is specifically linked to the histocompatibility locus. IgE distribution in normal families is consistent with the dominant inheritance of the low-IgE phenotype. As a result of the action of a single IgE regulator gene, the majority of family members would have elevated IgE levels as a possible basis for their atopic state. The association between HLA histocompatibility type and the immediate hypersensitivity response has been noted in persons of the low-IgE phenotype who were studied with highly purified allergens, generally of small size. Such presumptive evidence of immune-response (Ir) genes by linkage disequilibrium, i.e., the association of the hypersensitivity response with a particular histocompatibility haplotype, represents an additional element in the polygenic atopic allergic state. It is also likely that diseases of immediate type hypersensitivity may occur because of deficient intracellular controls of mediator generation or release, or both, or that the extracellular controls directed against mediator inactivation may be impaired.

The induction of allergic disease requires sensitization of a predisposed individual to specific allergen. This sensitization can occur anytime in life, although the greatest propensity for the development of allergic disease appears to occur in childhood and early adolescence. Exposure of a susceptible individual to an allergen results in processing of the allergen by antigen-presenting cells, including macrophage-like cells located throughout the body at surfaces that contact the outside environment, such as the nose, lungs, eyes, skin, and intestine. These antigen-presenting cells process the allergen protein and present it in the context of select cell surface proteins to CD4+ T cells, which, in turn, become activated specifically by the peptide epitope resulting from processing of the allergen. T cells can potentially induce several responses to an allergen, including those typical of contact dermatitis, known as the TH1 type response; responses consistent with immediate hypersensitivity responses, known as TH2; or anergic, or nonresponses, known as TH0. These varying forms of T cell responsivity are associated with discrete cytokine products; interferon γ production is associated with TH1 responses, and IL-4, -5, and -6 and GM-CSF generation with TH2 responses. The TH2 response is associated with activation of specific B cells that transform into plasma cells that produce allergen-specific IgE. Release into the serum of allergen-specific IgE by plasma cells results in sensitization of IgE Fc receptor–bearing cells including mast cells and basophils, which subsequently are capable of becoming activated upon exposure to the specific allergen. In certain diseases, including those associated with atopy, the monocyte and eosinophil populations can express the high-affinity receptor, FcεRI, and respond to its aggregation.

ANAPHYLAXIS **Definition** The life-threatening anaphylactic response of a sensitized human appears within minutes after administration of specific antigen and is manifested by respiratory distress often followed by vascular collapse or by shock without antecedent respiratory difficulty. Cutaneous manifestations exemplified by pruritus and urticaria with or without angioedema are characteristic of such systemic anaphylactic reactions. Gastrointestinal manifestations include nausea, vomiting, crampy abdominal pain, and diarrhea.

Predisposing Factors and Etiology There is no convincing evidence that age, sex, race, occupation, or geographic location predisposes a human to anaphylaxis except through exposure to some immunogen. According to most studies, atopy does not predispose individuals to anaphylaxis from penicillin therapy or venom of a stinging insect.

The materials capable of eliciting the systemic anaphylactic reaction in humans include the following: heterologous proteins in the form of hormones (insulin, vasopressin, parathormone), enzymes (trypsin, chymotrypsin, penicillinase), pollen extracts (ragweed, grass, trees), nonpollen extracts (dust mites, cat dander), food (eggs, seafoods, nuts, grains, beans), antiserum (antilymphocyte gamma globulin), occupation-related proteins (rubber products), and Hymenoptera venom (yellow jacket, yellow and baldfaced hornets, paper wasp, honey bee, imported fire ants); polysaccharides such as dextran; and most commonly drugs such as antibiotics (penicillins, cephalosporins, amphotericin B, nitrofurantoin), local anesthetics (procaine, lidocaine), vitamins (thiamine, folic acid), diagnostic agents (sodium dehydrocholate, sulfobromophthalein), and occupation-related chemicals (ethylene oxide), which are considered to function as haptens that form immunogenic conjugates with host proteins. The conjugating hapten may be the parent compound, a nonenzymatically derived storage product, or a metabolite formed in the host.

Pathophysiology and Manifestations Individuals differ in the time of appearance of symptoms and signs, but the hallmark of the anaphylactic reaction is the onset of some manifestation within seconds to minutes after introduction of the antigen, generally by injection or less commonly by ingestion. There may be upper or lower airway obstruction or both. Laryngeal edema may be experienced as a "lump" in the throat, hoarseness, or stridor, while bronchial obstruction is associ-

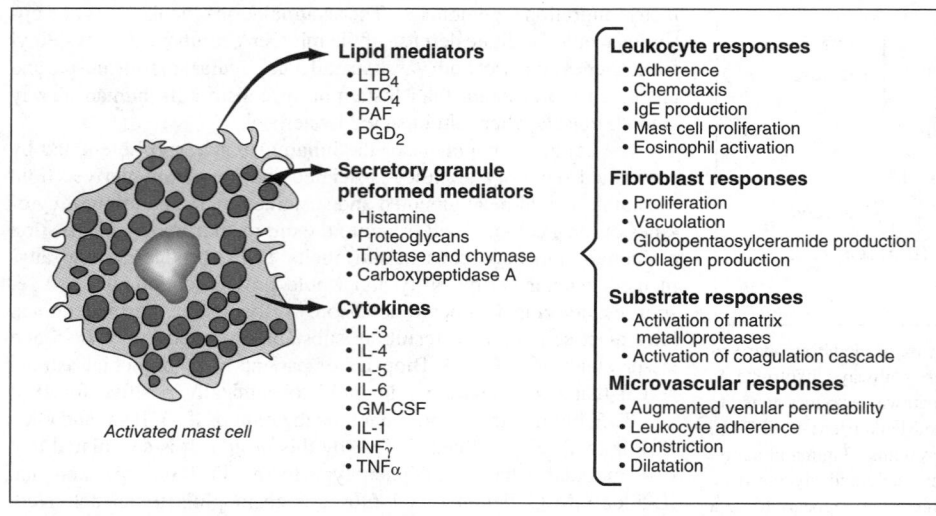

FIGURE 310-2 Bioactive mediators of three categories generated by IgE-dependent activation of murine mast cells can elicit common but sequential target cell effects leading to acute and sustained inflammatory responses.

ated with a feeling of tightness in the chest and/or audible wheezing. A characteristic feature is the eruption of well-circumscribed, discrete cutaneous wheals with erythematous, raised, serpiginous borders and blanched centers. These urticarial eruptions are intensely pruritic and may be localized or disseminated. They may coalesce to form giant hives, and they seldom persist beyond 48 h. A localized, nonpitting, deeper edematous cutaneous process, angioedema, also may be present. It may be asymptomatic or cause a burning or stinging sensation.

In fatal cases with clinical bronchial obstruction, the lungs show marked hyperinflation on gross and microscopic examination. The microscopic findings in the bronchi, however, are limited to luminal secretions, peribronchial congestion, submucosal edema, and eosinophilic infiltration, and the acute emphysema is attributed to intractable bronchospasm that subsides with death. The angioedema resulting in death by mechanical obstruction occurs in the epiglottis and larynx, but the process is also evident in the hypopharynx and to some extent in the trachea; on microscopic examination there is wide separation of the collagen fibers and the glandular elements; vascular congestion and eosinophilic infiltration are also present. Patients dying of vascular collapse without antecedent hypoxia from respiratory insufficiency have visceral congestion with a presumptive loss of intravascular blood volume. The associated electrocardiographic abnormalities, with or without infarction, noted in some patients may reflect a primary cardiac event or be secondary to a critical reduction in blood volume.

The angioedematous and urticarial manifestations of the anaphylactic syndrome have been attributed to release of endogenous histamine. A role for the cysteinyl leukotrienes in altering pulmonary mechanics by causing marked bronchiolar constriction seems likely. Vascular collapse without respiratory distress in response to experimental challenge with the sting of a hymenopteran was associated not only with marked and prolonged elevations in blood histamine but also with evidence of intravascular coagulation and kinin generation. Based on the findings that patients with systemic mastocytosis and episodic hypotension proceeding to vascular collapse excrete large amounts of PGD_2 in addition to histamine and are controlled by administration of a nonsteroidal agent but not by antihistamines alone, it may be that PGD_2 is also of importance in the hypotensive anaphylactic reactions. The cysteinyl leukotrienes may be involved in the pathobiologic process in patients with myocardial ischemia without or with infarction.

Diagnosis The diagnosis of an anaphylactic reaction depends largely on an accurate history revealing the onset of the appropriate symptoms and signs within minutes after the responsible material is encountered. When only a portion of the full syndrome is present, such as isolated urticaria, sudden bronchospasm in a patient with asthma, or vascular collapse after intravenous administration of an agent, it is difficult to exclude a nonimmunologic, toxicologic, or idiosyncratic response. Intravenous administration of a chemical mast cell–degranulating agent, including opiate derivatives and radiographic contrast media, may elicit generalized urticaria, angioedema, and a sensation of retrosternal oppression with or without clinically detectable bronchoconstriction or hypotension. Furthermore, nonsteroidal anti-inflammatory agents such as indomethacin, aminopyrine, mefenamic acid, and aspirin may precipitate a life-threatening episode of obstruction of upper or lower airways in patients with asthma that is clinically reminiscent of anaphylaxis but is not associated with a detectable IgE response. This syndrome, which is commonly associated with nasal polyposis, may reflect a unique reactivity to an imbalance in the ratio of prostaglandin to leukotriene biosynthesis when cyclooxygenase is inhibited.

The presence of specific IgE in the heart blood of patients dying of systemic anaphylaxis has been demonstrated at postmortem by passive transfer of the serum intradermally into a normal recipient, followed in 24 h by antigen challenge into the same site, with subsequent development of a wheal and flare, the Prausnitz-Küstner reaction. In order to avoid the hazards of transferring hepatitis or other infections to a recipient, it is preferable to employ a less sensitive monkey recipient or a human leukocyte suspension enriched with basophils for subsequent antigen challenge. Furthermore, radioimmunoassays

have demonstrated specific IgE antibodies in patients with anaphylactic reactions, but such approaches require purified antigens. Elevations of tryptase levels in serum implicate mast cell activation in an adverse systemic reaction and are particularly informative with episodes of hypotension during general anesthesia or when there has been a fatal outcome. In the transfusion anaphylactic reaction that occurs in patients with IgA deficiency, the responsible specificity resides in IgG or IgE anti-IgA; the mechanism of the reaction mediated by IgG anti-IgA is presumed to be complement activation with secondary mast cell participation.

℞ TREATMENT

Early recognition of an anaphylactic reaction is mandatory, since death occurs within minutes to hours after the first symptoms. Mild symptoms such as pruritus and urticaria can be controlled by administration of 0.2 to 0.5 mL of 1:1000 epinephrine subcutaneously, with repeated doses as required at 20-min intervals for a severe reaction. If the antigenic material was injected into an extremity, the rate of absorption may be reduced by prompt application of a tourniquet proximal to the reaction site, administration of 0.2 mL of 1:1000 epinephrine into the site, and removal without compression of an insect stinger, if present. An intravenous infusion should be initiated to provide a route for administration of 2.5 mL epinephrine, diluted 1:10,000, at 5- to 10-min intervals, volume expanders such as normal saline, and vasopressor agents such as dopamine if intractable hypotension occurs. Replacement of intravascular volume due to postcapillary venular leakage may require several liters of saline. Epinephrine provides both alpha- and beta-adrenergic effects, resulting in vasoconstriction, bronchial smooth-muscle relaxation, and attenuation of enhanced venular permeability. Beta blockers are relatively contraindicated in persons at risk for anaphylactic reactions, especially those sensitive to Hymenoptera venom or those undergoing immunotherapy for respiratory system allergy. When epinephrine fails to control the anaphylactic reaction, hypoxia due to airway obstruction or related to a cardiac arrhythmia, or both, must be considered. Oxygen via a nasal catheter or intermittent positive-pressure breathing of oxygen with 0.5 mL isoproterenol diluted 1:200 in saline may be helpful, but either endotracheal intubation or a tracheostomy is mandatory for oxygen delivery if progressive hypoxia develops. Ancillary agents such as the antihistamine diphenhydramine, 50 to 100 mg intramuscularly or intravenously, and aminophylline, 0.25 to 0.5 g intravenously, are appropriate for urticaria-angioedema and bronchospasm, respectively. Intravenous glucocorticoids are not effective for the acute event but may alleviate later recurrence of bronchospasm, hypotension, or urticaria.

Prevention Prevention of anaphylaxis must take into account the sensitivity of the recipient, the dose and character of the diagnostic or therapeutic agent, and the effect of the route of administration on the rate of absorption. If there is a definite history of a past anaphylactic reaction, even though mild, it is advisable to select another agent or procedure. A knowledge of cross-reactivity among agents is critical since, for example, cephalosporins share a common β-lactam ring with the penicillins. A skin test should be performed before the administration of certain materials that are likely to elicit anaphylactic reactions, such as allergenic extracts, or when the nature of the past adverse reaction is unknown. A scratch test should precede an intradermal test in very sensitive patients. With regard to penicillin, two-thirds of patients with a positive reaction history and positive skin tests to benzylpenicilloyl-polylysine (BPL) and/or the minor determinant mixture (MDM) of benzylpenicillin products experience allergic reactions with treatment, and these are almost uniformly of the anaphylactic type in those patients with minor determinant reactivity. Even patients without a history of previous clinical reactions have a 2 to 6 percent incidence of positive skin tests to the two test materials, and about 3 per 1000 with a negative history experience anaphylaxis with therapy, with a mortality of about 1 per 100,000. Skin testing for antibiotics should be performed only on patients with a positive clinical history consistent with an immediate hypersensitivity reaction and in imminent need of the antibiotic in question; skin testing is of no value for non-IgE-mediated eruptions. Desensitization with most antibiotics can proceed by the intravenous, subcutaneous, or oral route. Typically, graded quantities of the antibiotic are given by the selected route using double doses until a therapeutic dosage is achieved. Due to the risk of systemic anaphylaxis during the course of desensitization, such a procedure should be performed only in a setting in which resuscitation equipment is at hand and an intravenous line is in place. It is critical to give the therapeutic agent at regular intervals to prevent the reestablishment of a sensitized cell pool of large size.

A different form of protection involves the development of blocking antibody of the IgG class, which is protective against Hymenoptera venom–induced anaphylaxis by interacting with antigen so that less reaches the sensitized tissue mast cells; to be effective, this immunotherapy requires the use of specific or cross-reacting Hymenoptera venom.

Because sensitization can be transient, the maximal risk for systemic anaphylactic reactions in persons with Hymenoptera sensitivity occurs in association with a currently positive skin test. Although there is only low-grade cross-reactivity between honey bee and yellow jacket venoms, there is a high degree of cross-reactivity between yellow jacket venom and the rest of the vespid venoms (yellow or baldfaced hornets and wasps). Prevention involves modification of outdoor activities to exclude bare feet, wearing perfumed toiletries, eating in certain areas, clipping hedges or grass, and hauling away trash or fallen fruit. As with each anaphylactic sensitivity, the individual should wear an informational bracelet and have immediate access to an unexpired epinephrine kit. The limitations of lifestyle and the psychological duress can be addressed by venom immunotherapy to achieve a venom-specific IgG titer above 3.0 μg/mL of serum. Although it has been recommended that venom therapy be continued indefinitely or until the skin and specific serum IgE tests are unremarkable, there is evidence that 5 years of treatment induces a state of resistance to sting reactions that is independent of serum levels of specific IgG or IgE. This contrasts with the definite relation of sting immunity to specific IgG earlier in the treatment regime. For children with a systemic reaction limited to skin, the likelihood of progression to more serious respiratory or vascular manifestations is low, and thus immunotherapy is not recommended.

URTICARIA AND ANGIOEDEMA **Definition** Urticaria and angioedema may appear separately or together as cutaneous manifestations of localized nonpitting edema; a similar process may occur at mucosal surfaces of the upper respiratory or gastrointestinal tract. *Urticaria* involves only the superficial portion of the dermis, presenting as well-circumscribed wheals with erythematous raised serpiginous borders with blanched centers that may coalesce to become giant wheals. *Angioedema* is a well-demarcated localized edema involving the deeper layers of the skin, including the subcutaneous tissue. Recurrent episodes of urticaria and/or angioedema of less than 6 weeks' duration are considered acute, whereas attacks persisting beyond this period are designated chronic.

Predisposing Factors and Etiology The occurrence of urticaria and angioedema is probably more frequent than usually described because of the evanescent, self-limited nature of such eruptions, which seldom require medical attention when limited to the skin. Although persons in any age group may experience acute or chronic urticaria and/or angioedema, these lesions increase in frequency after adolescence, with the highest incidence occurring in persons in the third decade of life; indeed, one survey of college students indicated that 15 to 20 percent had experienced a pruritic wheal reaction.

The classification of urticaria-angioedema presented in Table 310-1 focuses on the different mechanisms for eliciting clinical disease. Only the IgE-dependent and the IgG-mediated reactions in IgA-

deficient persons should be considered immediate hypersensitivity. However, the other mechanisms are important for differential diagnosis, and most cases of chronic urticaria are idiopathic. The appearance of urticaria and angioedema in atopic persons in the absence of a specific exposure is attributed to the atopic diathesis and implies an IgE-dependent mechanism. Urticaria and/or angioedema occurring during the appropriate season in patients with seasonal respiratory allergy or as a result of exposure to animals or molds is attributed to inhalation or physical contact with pollens, animal dander, and mold spores, respectively. However, urticaria and angioedema secondary to inhalation are relatively uncommon compared to urticaria and angioedema elicited by ingestion of fresh fruits, shellfish, fish, milk products, chocolate, legumes including peanuts, and various drugs that may elicit not only the anaphylactic syndrome with prominent gastrointestinal complaints but also chronic urticaria.

Additional etiologies include physical stimuli such as cold, heat, solar rays, exercise, and mechanical irritation. The physical urticarias can be distinguished by the precipitating event and other aspects of the clinical presentation. *Dermographism*, which occurs in 1 to 4 percent of the population, is defined by the appearance of a linear wheal at the site of a brisk stroke with a firm object or by any configuration appropriate to the eliciting event. Dermographism has a prevalence that peaks in the second to third decades. It is not influenced by an atopic diathesis and has a duration generally of less than 5 years. *Pressure urticaria*, which often accompanies dermographism or chronic idiopathic urticaria, presents in response to a sustained stimulus such as a shoulder strap or belt, running (feet), or manual labor (hands). *Cholinergic urticaria* is distinctive in that the pruritic wheals are of small size (1 to 2 mm) and are surrounded by a large area of erythema; attacks are precipitated by fever, a hot bath or shower, or exercise and are presumptively attributed to a rise in core body temperature. *Exercise-related anaphylaxis* begins with erythema and pruritic urticaria but progresses to angioedema of the face, oropharynx, larynx, or intestine or to vascular collapse; it is distinguished from cholinergic urticaria by presenting with wheals of conventional size and by not occurring with fever or a hot bath. *Cold urticaria*, either acquired or hereditary, is local at the exposed site (ice cube) or exposed body areas (ambient temperature) but can progress to vascular collapse with immersion in cold water (swimming). *Solar urticaria* is subdivided into three groups by the response to specific portions of the light spectrum. *Vibratory angioedema* may occur after years of occupational exposure or can be idiopathic; it may be accompanied by cholinergic urticaria. Other rare forms of physical allergy, always defined by stimulus-specific elicitation, include *local heat urticaria, aquagenic urticaria* from contact with water of any temperature, and *contact urticaria* from direct interaction with some chemical substance.

Angioedema without urticaria occurs with C$\overline{1}$ inhibitor (C$\overline{1}$INH) deficiency that may be inborn as an autosomal dominant characteristic or may be acquired. The urticaria and angioedema associated with

Table 310-1

Classification of Urticaria with Angioedema

1. IgE-dependent
   a. Specific antigen sensitivity (pollens, foods, drugs, fungi, molds, Hymenoptera venom, helminths)
   b. Physical: dermographism, cold, solar, cholinergic, vibratory, exercise-related
2. Complement-mediated
   a. Hereditary angioedema: type 1, type 2
   b. Acquired angioedema: type 1, type 2
   c. Necrotizing vasculitis
   d. Serum sickness
   e. Reactions to blood products
3. Nonimmunologic
   a. Direct mast cell–releasing agents: opiates, antibiotics, curare, D-tubocurarine, radiocontrast media
   b. Agents that presumably alter arachidonic acid metabolism: aspirin and nonsteroidal anti-inflammatory agents, azo dyes, and benzoates
4. Idiopathic

---

classical serum sickness or with idiopathic cutaneous necrotizing angiitis are believed to be an immune-complex disease when hypocomplementemia is a concomitant. The idiosyncratic drug reactions to mast cell granule–releasing agents and to nonsteroidal anti-inflammatory drugs may be systemic, resembling anaphylaxis, or limited to cutaneous sites.

Pathophysiology and Manifestations Urticarial eruptions are distinctly pruritic, involve any area of the body from the scalp to the soles of the feet, and appear in crops of 24- to 72-h duration, with old lesions fading as new ones appear. The most common sites are the extremities, external genitalia, and face, particularly the region of the eyes and lips. Although self-limited in duration, angioedema of the upper respiratory tract may be life-threatening due to laryngeal obstruction, while gastrointestinal involvement may present with abdominal colic, with or without nausea and vomiting, and may precipitate unnecessary surgical intervention. No residual discoloration occurs with either urticaria or angioedema unless there is an underlying process leading to superimposed extravasation of erythrocytes.

The pathology of urticaria and angioedema is usually characterized by massive edema of the dermis in urticaria and of the subcutaneous tissue as well as the dermis in angioedema. Collagen bundles in affected areas are widely separated, and the venules are sometimes dilated. The perivenular infiltrate may consist of lymphocytes, eosinophils, and neutrophils that are present in varying combination and number throughout the dermis.

Perhaps the best-studied example of IgE- and mast cell–mediated urticaria and angioedema is *cold urticaria.* Cryoglobulins may be recognized, but not in the majority of patients. Immersion of an extremity in an ice bath precipitates angioedema of the distal portion with urticaria at the air interface within minutes of the challenge. Histologic studies reveal marked mast cell degranulation with associated edema of the dermis and subcutaneous tissues. The venous effluent of the cold-challenged and angioedematous extremity reveals a marked rise in plasma content of histamine, whereas the venous effluent of the contralateral normal extremity contains none of this mediator. Elevated levels of histamine have been found in the plasma content of venous effluent and in the fluid of suction blisters at experimentally induced lesional sites in patients with dermographism, pressure urticaria, vibratory angioedema, light urticaria, and heat urticaria. By ultrastructural analysis, the pattern of mast cell degranulation in cold urticaria resembles an IgE-mediated response with solubilization of granule contents, fusion of the perigranular and cell membranes, and discharge of granule contents, whereas in a dermographic lesion there is an additional superimposed zonal (piecemeal) degranulation. Elevations of plasma histamine levels with biopsy-proven mast cell degranulation have also been demonstrated with systemic attacks of *cholinergic urticaria* and *exercise-related anaphylaxis* precipitated experimentally by exercise on a treadmill while wearing a wet suit; however, only in cholinergic urticaria is there a concomitant decrease in pulmonary function.

Diagnosis The rapid onset and self-limited nature of urticarial and angioedematous eruptions are distinguishing features. Additional characteristics are the occurrence of the urticarial crops in various stages of evolution and the asymmetric distribution of the angioedema. Urticaria and/or angioedema involving IgE-dependent mechanisms are often appreciated by historical considerations implicating specific allergens or physical stimuli, by seasonal incidence, and by exposure to certain environments. Direct reproduction of the lesion with physical stimuli is particularly valuable because it so often establishes the cause of the lesion. The diagnosis of an environmental allergen based on the clinical history can be confirmed by skin testing or assay for allergen-specific IgE in serum. IgE-mediated urticaria and/or angioedema may or may not be associated with an elevation of total IgE or with peripheral eosinophilia. Fever, leukocytosis, and an elevated sedimentation rate are absent.

The classification of urticarial and angioedematous states noted in Table 310-1 in terms of possible mechanisms necessarily includes some differential diagnostic points. Hypocomplementemia is not observed in IgE-mediated mast cell disease and may reflect either an acquired abnormality generally attributed to the formation of immune complexes or a genetic deficiency of $\overline{\text{C1}}$INH. Chronic recurrent urticaria, generally in females, associated with arthralgias, an elevated sedimentation rate, and normo- or hypocomplementemia suggests an underlying cutaneous necrotizing angiitis. Vasculitic urticaria typically persists longer than 72 h, whereas conventional urticaria often has a duration of less than 24 to 48 h. Confirmation depends on a biopsy that reveals cellular infiltration, nuclear debris, and fibrinoid necrosis of the venules. The same pathobiologic process accounts for the urticaria in association with such diseases as systemic lupus erythematosus or viral hepatitis with or without an associated arteritis. Serum sickness per se or a similar clinical entity due to drugs includes not only urticaria but also pyrexia, lymphadenopathy, myalgia, and arthralgia or arthritis. Urticarial reactions to blood products or intravenous administration of immunoglobulin are defined by the event and generally are not progressive unless the recipient is IgA-deficient in the former case or the reagent is aggregated in the latter.

Hereditary angioedema is an autosomal dominant disease due to a deficiency of antigenic and/or functional $\overline{\text{C1}}$INH. The diagnosis is suggested not only by family history but also by the lack of pruritus and of urticarial lesions, the prominence of recurrent gastrointestinal attacks of colic, and episodes of laryngeal edema. Laboratory diagnosis depends on demonstrating a deficiency of $\overline{\text{C1}}$INH antigen (type 1) in most kindreds, but some kindreds have an antigenically intact nonfunctional protein (type 2) and require a functional assay to establish the diagnosis. The natural substrates of uninhibited $\overline{\text{C1}}$, C4 and C2, are chronically depleted but fall further during attacks due to the activation of additional C1. Because the $\overline{\text{C1}}$INH protein also regulates the Hageman factor–initiated activation of kallikrein and of plasmin, the vasoactive peptides responsible for the angioedema are likely some combination of bradykinin and a plasmin-derived fragment of $\overline{\text{C1}}$-cleaved C2. An acquired form of $\overline{\text{C1}}$INH deficiency, associated with lymphoproliferative disorders, has the same clinical manifestations but differs in the lack of a familial element; in the reduction of C1/$\overline{\text{C1}}$ as well as $\overline{\text{C1}}$INH, C4, and C2; and in the presence of an anti-idiotypic antibody to the monoclonal immunoglobulin expressed on the B cells. In a second acquired form of $\overline{\text{C1}}$INH deficiency with angioedema due to the appearance of IgG anti-$\overline{\text{C1}}$INH, B cell malignancy has not been prominent.

Urticaria and angioedema must be differentiated from contact sensitivity, a vesicular eruption that progresses to chronic thickening of the skin with continued allergenic exposure. They must also be differentiated from atopic dermatitis, a condition that may present as erythema, edema, papules, vesiculation, and oozing proceeding to a subacute and chronic stage in which vesiculation is less marked or absent and scaling, fissuring, and lichenification predominate in a distribution that characteristically involves the flexor surfaces. In cutaneous mastocytosis, the reddish brown macules and papules, characteristic of urticaria pigmentosa, urticate with pruritus upon trauma; and in systemic mastocytosis, without or with urticaria pigmentosa, there is an episodic systemic flushing with or without urticaria but no angioedema.

℞ TREATMENT

Identification of the etiologic factor(s) and their elimination provide the most satisfactory therapeutic program; this approach is feasible to varying degrees with IgE-mediated reactions to allergens or physical stimuli. For most forms of urticaria, H_1 antihistamines such as chlorpheniramine or diphenhydramine, and including the nonsedating class represented by astemizole, are effective in attenuating both urtication and pruritus. Cyproheptadine and especially hydroxyzine have proven effective when H_1 antihistamines have been inadequate. Doxepin, a dibenzoxepin tricyclic compound with both H_1 and H_2 receptor antagonist activity, is yet another alternative. Topical glucocorticoids are of no value in the management of urticaria and/or angioedema. Systemic glucocorticoids are generally avoided in idiopathic, allergen-induced, or physical urticarias due to their long-term toxicity. However, systemic glucocorticoids are useful in the management of patients with pressure urticaria, with vasculitic urticaria (especially with eosinophil prominence), or with idiopathic angioedema with or without urticaria. With persistent vasculitic urticaria, hydroxychloroquine or colchicine may be added to the regimen after hydroxyzine and before or along with systemic glucocorticoids.

The therapy of inborn $\overline{C1}$INH deficiency has been simplified by the finding that attenuated androgens correct the biochemical defect and afford prophylactic protection. Since the affected individuals are heterozygous, with the depletion of $\overline{C1}$INH being due to deficient synthesis and consequent excessive utilization of the limited amount available, the efficacy of the attenuated androgens is attributed to production by the normal gene of an amount of functional $\overline{C1}$INH sufficient to control the spontaneous activation of C1 to $\overline{C1}$. Since the use of such agents for children and pregnant women is not yet accepted, the antifibrinolytic agent ϵ-aminocaproic acid may be used occasionally to control spontaneous attacks or for preoperative prophylaxis in some patients. Infusion of isolated $\overline{C1}$INH protein appears useful in prophylaxis but is not widely available.

SYSTEMIC MASTOCYTOSIS

Definition *Systemic mastocytosis* is defined by mast cell hyperplasia that in most instances is indolent and nonneoplastic. Since human mast cells originate from pluripotent bone marrow cells (CD34+), circulate as nonmetachromatically staining, c-*kit*-positive mononuclear cells, and undergo tissue-specific proliferation and maturation, the hyperplasia is generally recognized only in bone marrow and in the normal peripheral distribution sites of the cells, such as skin, gastrointestinal mucosa, liver, and spleen. Mastocytosis occurs at any age and has a slight preponderance in males. The prevalence of systemic mastocytosis is not known, and a familial occurrence has not been established.

Classification, Pathophysiology, and Clinical Manifestations A recent consensus classification for systemic mastocytosis recognizes four forms (Table 310-2). The form designated as *indolent* accounts for the majority of patients and is not known to alter life expectancy. When a patient is classified as having indolent systemic mastocytosis, the concomitant clinical findings must be carefully noted, since they define the complications and directions for management. In systemic mastocytosis *associated with hematologic disorders*, the prognosis is determined by the nature of that disorder, which can range from dysmyelopoiesis to leukemia. In *aggressive* systemic mastocytosis, mast cell proliferation in parenchymal organs such as liver, spleen, and lymph nodes is marked and in a subset of patients is associated with prominent eosinophilia; the prognosis is poor. *Mast cell leukemia* is the rarest form of the disease and is invariably fatal at present. In types II and IV systemic mastocytosis there is a point mutation of the c-*kit* tyrosine kinase in the leukocytes and mast cells, respectively. In types I and III there is excessive production of the c-*kit* ligand (stem cell factor) in the microenvironment of the mast cells, and this may be autocrine in type III. The clinical manifestations of systemic mastocytosis, distinct from a leukemic complication, are due to tissue occupancy by the mast cell mass, the tissue response to that mass, and the release of bioactive substances acting at both local and distal sites.

Table 310-2

Classification of Systemic Mastocytosis

Type	Description
I	*Indolent* with cutaneous manifestations, vascular collapse, ulcer disease, malabsorption, skeletal disease, hepatosplenomegaly, or lymphadenopathy
II	*Concomitant hematologic disorder*, either myelodysplastic or myeloproliferative
III	*Aggressive* per se or lymphadenopathic mastocytosis with eosinophilia
IV	*Mastocytic leukemia*

The pharmacologically induced manifestations are pruritus, flushing, palpitations and vascular collapse, gastric distress, lower abdominal crampy pain, and recurrent headache. The increase in cell burden is evidenced by the small, reddish brown macules or papules, termed *urticaria pigmentosa*, at skin sites, but it also contributes to bone pain and malabsorption. The mast cell–mediated fibrotic changes are limited to liver, spleen, and bone marrow and presumably relate to the functional characteristics of mast cells developing at those sites, as opposed to those at sites without fibrosis, such as the gastrointestinal tissue or skin. Immunofluorescent analysis of bone marrow and skin lesions in indolent mastocytosis and of spleen and skin in aggressive systemic mastocytosis has revealed only one mast cell phenotype, namely, scroll-poor cells expressing tryptase, chymase, and carboxypeptidase A.

The cutaneous lesions of urticaria pigmentosa respond to trauma with urtication and erythema (Darier's sign). The apparent incidence of these lesions is 90 percent or greater in patients with indolent systemic mastocytosis. Approximately 1 percent of patients with indolent mastocytosis have skin lesions that appear as tan-brown macules with striking patchy erythema and associated telangiectasia (telangiectasia macularis eruptive perstans). In the upper gastrointestinal tract, histamine-mediated hypersecretion is the most common problem, with resultant gastritis and peptic ulcer. In the lower intestinal tract, the occurrence of diarrhea and abdominal pain is attributed to increased motility due to mast cell mediators, and this can be aggravated by malabsorption with secondary nutritional insufficiency and osteomalacia. The periportal fibrosis associated with mast cell infiltration and a prominence of eosinophils may lead to portal hypertension and ascites. In some patients, flushing and recurrent vascular collapse are markedly aggravated by an idiosyncratic response to a minimal dosage of nonsteroidal anti-inflammatory agents. The neuropsychiatric disturbances are clinically most evident as impaired recent memory and "migraine-like" headaches. Patients in every category of systemic mastocytosis may experience exacerbation of a specific clinical sign or symptom with alcohol ingestion, use of mast cell–interactive narcotics, or ingestion of nonsteroidal anti-inflammatory agents.

Diagnosis Although the diagnosis is generally suspected on the basis of the clinical history and physical findings, the contention can be strengthened by certain laboratory procedures and established only by a tissue diagnosis. A 24-h urine collection for measurement of histamine, histamine metabolites, or metabolites of PGD_2 is currently the most common noninvasive approach. A convenient alternative, but with a lesser incidence of positivity, is to measure blood levels of histamine or the mast cell–derived neutral protease tryptase. Additional studies directed by the presentation include a bone scan or skeletal survey; contrast studies of the upper gastrointestinal tract with small-bowel follow-through, computed tomography (CT) scan, or endoscopy; and a neuropsychiatric evaluation, including an EEG. The tissue diagnosis is straightforward if there are lesions of urticaria pigmentosa, but the diagnosis of systemic mastocytosis requires involvement of other organs and is most frequently established by bone marrow biopsy and aspiration. The bone marrow lesions consist of focal and paratrabecular aggregates of mast cells, often mixed with eosinophils, lymphocytes, and, on occasion, plasma cells, histiocytes, and fibroblasts.

The differential diagnosis requires the exclusion of other flushing disorders. The 24-h urine assessment of 5-hydroxy-indoleacetic acid and metanephrines should exclude a carcinoid tumor or a pheochromocytoma. Most patients with recurrent anaphylaxis, including the idiopathic group, present with angioedema, which is not a manifestation of systemic mastocytosis.

℞ **TREATMENT**

The management of systemic mastocytosis uses a stepwise and symptom-sign–directed approach that includes an H_1 antihistamine for flushing and pruritus, an H_2 antihistamine or proton pump inhibitor for gastric acid hypersecretion, oral cromolyn sodium for diarrhea and abdominal pain, and a nonsteroidal anti-inflammatory agent for severe flushing associated with vascular collapse despite use of H_1 and H_2 antihistamines to block biosynthesis of PGD_2. Systemic glucocorticoids appear to alleviate the malabsorption. Headaches are generally managed with the medications customarily utilized for migraine disease. Ketotifen has been used to alleviate flushing in patients intolerant to nonsteroidal anti-inflammatory agents and in patients with bone pain or intractable headaches. The efficacy of α interferon in aggressive systemic mastocytosis is controversial, and this may relate to the difficulty in achieving the necessary dosage in some patients due to the attendant side effects. Chemotherapy is not appropriate for patients with indolent mastocytosis and apparently does not prolong survival in patients with mast cell leukemia. It is appropriate for leukemia of other cell types and for the aggressive form of systemic mastocytosis.

ALLERGIC RHINITIS **Definition** Allergic rhinitis is characterized by sneezing; rhinorrhea; obstruction of the nasal passages; conjunctival, nasal, and pharyngeal itching; and lacrimation, all occurring in a temporal relationship to allergen exposure. Although commonly seasonal due to elicitation by airborne pollens, it can be perennial in an environment of chronic exposure. The incidence of allergic rhinitis in North America is about 7 percent, with the peak occurring in childhood and adolescence.

Predisposing Factors and Etiology Allergic rhinitis generally presents in atopic individuals, i.e., in persons with a family history of a similar or related symptom complex and a personal history of collateral allergy expressed as eczematous dermatitis, urticaria, and/or asthma (see Chap. 252). Symptoms generally appear before the fourth decade of life and tend to diminish gradually with aging, although complete spontaneous remissions are uncommon. A relatively small number of weeds that depend on wind rather than insects for cross-pollination, as well as certain grasses and trees, produce sufficient quantities of pollen suitable for wide distribution by air currents to elicit seasonal allergic rhinitis. The dates of pollination of these species generally vary little from year to year in a particular locale but may be quite different in another climate. In the temperate areas of North America, trees typically pollinate from March through May, grasses in June and early July, and ragweed from mid-August to early October. Molds, which are widespread in nature because they occur in soil or decaying organic matter, may propagate spores in a pattern dependent on climatic conditions. Perennial allergic rhinitis occurs in response to allergens that are present throughout the year such as in desquamating epithelium in animal dander or cockroach dander, the processed materials or chemicals utilized in an industrial setting, or the dust accumulating at work or at home. Dust has a diverse allergen content including *Dermatophagoides farinae* and *D. pteronyssinus*, which may be present alone or together in house dust. Dust mites are scavengers of flecks of human skin and coat the digestate with mite-specific protein for subsequent excretion as part of a fecal ball. Dust mites are perennially present in warm, humid climates, but their presence diminishes in the winter in colder climates due to lack of indoor humidity. Some patients with perennial rhinitis are sensitive only to house dust. In up to two-thirds of patients with perennial rhinitis, no clear-cut allergen can be demonstrated. The ability of allergens to cause rhinitis rather than lower respiratory symptoms may be attributed to their size, 10 to 100 μm, and retention within the nose.

Pathophysiology and Manifestations Episodic rhinorrhea, sneezing, and obstruction of the nasal passages with lacrimation and pruritus of the conjunctiva, nasal mucosa, and oropharynx are the hallmarks of allergic rhinitis. The nasal mucosa is pale and boggy, but the nares are not reddened or excoriated. The conjunctiva may be congested and edematous; the pharynx is generally unremarkable but may appear injected. Swelling of the turbinates and mucous membranes with obstruction of the sinus ostia and eustachian tubes precipitates secondary infections of the sinuses and middle ear, respectively, commonly in perennial but rarely in seasonal disease. Nasal polyps often arise concurrently with edema and/or infection within the sinuses and increase obstructive symptoms.

The nose presents a large mucosal surface area through the folds of the turbinates and serves to adjust the temperature and moisture content of inhaled air and to filter out particulate materials. The convoluted nasal passages readily filter out particles above 10 μm in size by impingement in a mucous blanket at bends in their course; ciliary action then moves the entrapped particles toward the pharynx. Entrapment of pollen and digestion of the outer coat by mucosal enzymes such as lysozymes release protein allergens generally of 10,000 to 40,000 molecular weight. Although the initial interaction occurs between the allergen and intraepithelial mast cells sensitized with specific IgE, the bulk of the mast cells are located beneath the mucosal surface and are recruited secondarily. During the symptomatic season when the mucosa are already swollen and hyperemic, there is enhanced adverse reactivity to the seasonal pollen as well as to antigenically unrelated pollens for which there is underlying hypersensitivity. This priming effect is attributed to improved penetration of the allergens to the deeper perivenular mast cells. Biopsy specimens of nasal mucosa during an episodic allergic reaction show profound submucosal edema with infiltration predominantly by eosinophils, although some neutrophil polymorphonuclear leukocytes are present. Polyps, a feature in perennial rhinitis, are mucosal protrusions containing chiefly edema fluid with variable degrees of eosinophilic infiltration.

The mucosal surface fluid contains not only IgA that is present preferentially because of its secretory piece but also IgE, which apparently arrives by diffusion from plasma cells distributed in proximity to mucosal surfaces. IgE fixes to mucosal and submucosal mast cells, and the intensity of the clinical response to inhaled allergens is quantitatively related to the naturally occurring or experimentally defined pollen dose. Specific IgE is distributed not only to tissue mast cells but also to circulating basophilic leukocytes; patients with more severe clinical disease have basophils that release histamine in response to lesser concentrations of allergen in vitro than do cells from patients with milder disease. Human nasal polyps from ragweed-sensitive patients release histamine, eosinophilotactic factor(s), and leukotrienes upon challenge with ragweed allergen in vitro. In sensitive individuals, the introduction of allergen into the nose is associated with sneezing, "stuffiness," and discharge, and the fluid contains histamine, PGD₂, and leukotrienes. Thus the mast cells of nasal polyp tissue, and of the nasal mucosa and submucosa, generate and release mediators through IgE-dependent reactions that are capable of producing tissue edema and eosinophilic infiltration.

Diagnosis The diagnosis of seasonal allergic rhinitis depends largely on an accurate history of occurrence coincident with the pollination of the offending weeds, grasses, or trees. The continuous character of perennial allergic rhinitis due to contamination of the home or place of work makes historical analysis difficult, but there may be a variability in symptoms that can be related to exposure to animal dander, dust mite allergens, cockroach dander, or work-related allergens such as latex. Patients with perennial rhinitis commonly develop the problem in adult life, are more often women than men, and manifest nasal polyps and thickening of the sinus membranes demonstrated by radiography. The term *vasomotor rhinitis* designates a condition of enhanced reactivity of the nasopharynx in which a symptom complex resembling perennial allergic rhinitis occurs with nonspecific stimuli and in the absence of any established allergic basis. Other entities to be excluded are structural abnormalities of the nasopharynx; exposure to irritants; upper respiratory infection; pregnancy with prominent nasal mucosal edema; prolonged topical use of alpha-adrenergic agents in the form of nose drops (rhinitis medicamentosa); and the use of certain therapeutic agents such as rauwolfia, beta-adrenergic antagonists, or estrogens. Nasal polyps may be present independently of ostomeatal sinus obstruction on an allergic basis, especially in individuals with sensitivity to nonsteroidal anti-inflammatory agents, rhinosinusitis, and bronchial asthma.

The nasal secretions of allergic patients are rich in eosinophils, and peripheral eosinophilia with elevations in relation to clinical exacerbations is a common feature. Local or systemic neutrophilia implies infection. Total serum IgE is frequently elevated, but the demonstration of immunologic specificity for IgE is critical to an etiologic diagnosis.

A skin test by the epicutaneous route (scratch or prick) with the allergens of interest provides a rapid and reliable approach to identifying allergen-specific IgE that has sensitized cutaneous mast cells. An intradermal test may follow if indicated by history when the epicutaneous test is negative, but it is less reliable due to the reactivity by this route of some asymptomatic individuals at the test dose. Skin testing by scratch or prick for food allergens is controversial but does seem to have predictive value for the absence of specific IgE sensitivity; false-positive results may occur due to the histamine content of the allergen preparation, and false-negative results due to denaturation of the epitopes of importance. A double-blind, placebo-controlled challenge may document a food allergy, but such a procedure does bear the risk of an anaphylactic reaction. An elimination diet is safer but is tedious and less definitive. Food allergy is uncommon as a significant cause of allergic rhinitis.

Newer methodology for detecting total IgE, including the development of enzyme-linked immunosorbent assays (ELISA) employing anti-IgE bound to either a solid-phase or a liquid-phase paramagnetic particle, provides rapid and cost effective determinations. More important for patient management are the measurements of specific anti-IgE in serum by its binding to a solid-phase allergen and quantitation by subsequent uptake of radiolabeled anti-IgE. The radioallergosorbent technique (RAST) correlates with the bioassay of specific IgE by skin test, which is mast cell–dependent, and by histamine release from peripheral blood leukocytes, which is basophil-dependent. As compared to the skin test, the assay of specific IgE in serum is less sensitive, which is of concern for assessing patients with an equivocal clinical history. However, the serum assay has high specificity, with false-positive results being of much less concern than false-negative ones. Furthermore, ELISA utilizing reactions that generate visible light or fluorescence have replaced the radioimmunoassays, and newer chemiluminescent tracers provide additional sensitivity for detection of minute quantities of allergen-specific IgE.

Prevention Avoidance of exposure to the offending allergen is the most effective means of controlling allergic diseases; removal of pets from the home to avoid animal danders, utilization of air filtration devices to minimize the concentrations of airborne pollens, elimination of cockroach dander by chemical destruction of the pest and careful food storage, travel to nonpollinating areas during the critical periods, and even a change of domicile to eliminate a mold spore problem may be necessary. Control of dust mites by allergen avoidance includes use of plastic-lined and covers for mattresses, pillows, and comforters, elimination of carpets and drapes, and avoidance of humidification steps.

℞ TREATMENT

Management with pharmacologic agents represents the standard approach to seasonal or perennial allergic rhinitis. Antihistamines of the H_1 class are effective for nasopharyngeal itching, sneezing, and watery rhinorrhea and for such ocular manifestations as itching, tearing, and erythema, but they are not efficacious for the nasal congestion. The older antihistamines are sedating, and their anticholinergic (muscarinic) effects include visual disturbance, urinary retention, and even arrhythmias. Because the newer H_1 antihistaminics such as terfenadine or astemizole are less lipophilic, their ability to cross the blood-brain barrier is reduced, and thus their sedating and anticholinergic side effects are minimized. Because life-threatening ventricular arrhythmias with some fatalities have occurred due to inhibition of the metabolism of terfenadine or astemizole by the interactions of macrolide antibiotics such as erythromycin and clarithromycin or broad-spectrum antifungal agents of the ketoconazole class, these nonsedating H_1 antihistamines are contraindicated in combinations with such drugs or with concomitant medical illnesses impairing hepatic function or predisposing to an arrhythmia. Alpha-adrenergic agents such as phenylephrine or oximetazoline are generally used topically to alleviate nasal congestion and obstruction, but

the duration of efficacy is limited because of rebound rhinitis and such systemic responses as insomnia, irritability, and hypertension. The latter are more frequent with use of oral alpha-adrenergic agonists. Nonetheless, oral alpha-adrenergic agonists are useful in enhancing the efficacy of antihistamines in relieving nasal congestion and may diminish their sedating effects. Cromolyn sodium, a liquid nasal metered-dose spray, is essentially without side effects and is the only intervention of a prophylactic nature; thus it is used to attenuate episodic allergen activation of nasal mast cells. To be efficacious, cromolyn sodium must be administered on a continuous basis during seasonal allergen exposure, generally four times daily, or immediately prior to a discrete exposure such as animal dander. The clinical efficacy of cromolyn sodium and that of nonsedating antihistamines are roughly equivalent. Intranasal high-potency glucocorticoids are the most potent drugs available for the relief of established rhinitis, seasonal or perennial, and even vasomotor rhinitis; they provide efficacy with substantially reduced side effects as compared with this same class of agent administered orally. Their most frequent side effect is local irritation, with *Candida* overgrowth being a rare occurrence. The topical-to-systemic activity of flunisolide or budesonide is significantly greater than for beclomethasone or triamcinolone with much less systemic absorption. Topical high-potency glucocorticoids exhibit superior efficacy as compared to antihistamines throughout the pollen seasons, especially when there is high pollen exposure. Thus, for patients who do not benefit adequately from a full dosage of nonsedating H_1 antihistamine and a maintenance dosage of cromolyn sodium, an alpha-adrenergic agent for short-term relief should be replaced by high-potency topical glucocorticoids. For systemic symptoms not related to the nasopharynx, such as allergic conjunctivitis, treatment may be local or by addition of an oral antihistamine.

Immunotherapy, often termed *hyposensitization*, consists of repeated subcutaneous injections of gradually increasing concentrations of the allergen(s) considered to be specifically responsible for the symptom complex. Controlled studies of ragweed, grass, dust mite, and cat dander allergens administered for treatment of allergic rhinitis have demonstrated at least partial relief of symptoms and signs. The duration of such immunotherapy is 3 to 5 years, with discontinuation being based upon minimal symptoms over two consecutive seasons of exposure. Clinical benefit appears related to the administration of a high dose of allergen at weekly or biweekly intervals. Patients should remain at the treatment site for at least 20 min after allergen administration so that any anaphylactic consequence can be managed. Local reactions with erythema and induration are not uncommon and may persist for 1 to 3 days. Immunotherapy is contraindicated in patients with significant cardiovascular disease or unstable asthma and should be conducted with particular caution in any patient requiring beta-adrenergic blocking therapy because of the difficulty in managing an anaphylactic complication. The immunologic characteristics of a response include a rise in antibodies of the IgG class, a small increase in specific IgE early in the treatment course followed by a plateau or decline, and a decline in the percentage of histamine released from peripheral blood basophilic leukocytes challenged with a fixed concentration of the allergen. The antibodies of the IgG class might well reduce or neutralize the quantity of allergen available for interaction with the tissue mast cells but, more important, could modify the seasonal booster response in specific IgE synthesis. None of the individual parameters of the response to immunotherapy correlates well with the assessments of clinical efficacy, suggesting that benefit is derived from a complex of effects that likely includes a reduction in T cell cytokine production. Immunotherapy should be reserved for clearly documented seasonal or perennial rhinitis, clinically related to defined allergen exposure with confirmation by the presence of allergen-specific IgE, which has failed management by allergen avoidance and pharmacotherapy due to lack of efficacy or side effects. A sequence for the management of allergic or perennial rhinitis based upon an allergen-specific diagnosis and stepwise management as required for symptom control would include the following: (1)

identification of the offending allergen(s) by history with confirmation of the presence of allergen-specific IgE by skin test (epicutaneous) and/or serum assay; (2) avoidance of the offending allergen; (3) for mild symptoms, prophylactic management with topical cromolyn sodium or treatment with a single bedtime dose of chlorpheniramine (if the latter is associated with undue side effects, substitute astemizole or terfenadine providing that there is no contraindication due to a concomitant medication or disease; (4) for prominent symptoms, utilization of topical beclomethasone with replacement by budesonide or flunisolide as needed for a satisfactory clinical outcome; and (5) for management failures despite avoidance and pharmacotherapy, progression to immunotherapy.

BIBLIOGRAPHY

Austen KF, Metcalfe DD: Anaphylactic syndrome, in *Immunological Diseases*, 5th ed, M Frank et al (eds). Boston, Little, Brown, 1995

Craig SS et al: Ultrastructural analysis of human T and TC mast cells identified by immunoelectron microscopy. Lab Invest 58:682, 1988

Gordon JR et al: Mast cells as a source of multifunctional cytokines. Immunol Today 11:458, 1990

Lewis RA et al: Leukotrienes and other products of the 5-lipoxygenase pathway: Biochemistry and relation to pathobiology in human diseases. N Engl J Med 323:645, 1990

McNeil HP, Austen KF: Biology of the mast cell, in *Immunological Diseases*, 5th ed, M Frank et al (eds). Boston, Little, Brown, 1995

Metcalfe DD, Austen KF: Mastocytosis, in *Immunological Diseases*, 5th ed, M Frank et al (eds). Boston, Little, Brown, 1995

Naclerio RM: Allergic rhinitis. N Engl J Med 325:860, 1991

Ravetch JV, Kinet J-P: Fc receptors. Annu Rev Immunol 9:457, 1991

Soter NA: Urticaria and angioedema, in *Dermatology In General Medicine*, 4th ed, TB Fitzpatrick et al (eds). New York, McGraw-Hill, 1993

Valentine MD: Insect venom allergy, in *Immunological Diseases*, 5th ed, M Frank et al (eds). Boston, Little, Brown, 1995

311 *Kim B. Yancey, Thomas J. Lawley*

IMMUNOLOGICALLY MEDIATED SKIN DISEASES

A number of immunologically mediated skin diseases and the cutaneous manifestations of immunologically mediated systemic disorders are now recognized as distinct entities with relatively consistent clinical, histologic, and immunopathologic findings. Many of these disorders are due to autoimmune mechanisms. Clinically, they are characterized by morbidity (pain, pruritus, disfigurement) and in some instances by mortality (largely due to loss of epidermal barrier function and/or secondary infection). The major features of the more common immunologically mediated skin diseases are summarized in this chapter (see Table 311-1).

PEMPHIGUS VULGARIS Pemphigus vulgaris (PV) is a blistering skin disease seen predominantly in elderly patients. Patients with PV have an increased incidence of the HLA-DR4 and -DRw6 serologically defined haplotypes. This disorder is characterized by the loss of cohesion between epidermal cells (a process termed *acantholysis*) with the resultant formation of intraepidermal blisters. Clinical lesions of PV typically consist of flaccid blisters on either normal-appearing or erythematous skin. These blisters rupture easily, leaving denuded areas that may crust and enlarge peripherally. Substantial portions of the body surface may be denuded in severe cases. Manual pressure to the skin of these patients may elicit the separation of the epidermis (Nikolsky's sign). This finding, while characteristic of PV, is not specific to this disorder and is also seen in toxic epidermal necrolysis, Stevens-Johnson syndrome, and a few other skin diseases. Lesions in PV typically present on the scalp, face, neck, axilla, trunk, and oral cavity. In half or more of patients, lesions begin in the mouth; approximately 90 percent of patients have oromucosal involvement at some time during the course of their disease. Involvement of other mucosal surfaces (e.g., pharyngeal, laryngeal, esophageal, conjuncti-

val, vulval, or rectal) can occur in severe disease. Pruritus may be a feature of early pemphigus lesions; extensive denudation may be associated with severe pain. Lesions usually heal without scarring, except at sites complicated by secondary infection or mechanically induced dermal wounds. Nonetheless, postinflammatory hyperpigmentation is usually present at sites of healed lesions for some time.

Biopsies of early lesions demonstrate intraepidermal vesicle formation secondary to loss of cohesion between epidermal cells (i.e., acantholytic blisters). Blister cavities contain acantholytic epidermal cells, which appear as round homogeneous cells containing hyperchromatic nuclei. Basal keratinocytes remain attached to the epidermal basement membrane, hence blister formation is within the suprabasal portion of the epidermis. Lesional skin may contain focal collections of intraepidermal eosinophils within blister cavities; dermal alterations are slight, usually limited to an eosinophil-predominant leukocytic infiltrate. Direct immunofluorescence microscopy of lesional or normal skin shows deposits of IgG on the surface of keratinocytes; in contrast, deposits of complement are typically found in lesional but not normal skin. Keratinocyte IgG deposits are derived from a circulating autoantibody directed against cell surface antigens. Circulating autoantibodies can be demonstrated in 80 to 90 percent of PV patients by indirect immunofluorescence microscopy; monkey esophagus is the optimal substrate for demonstration of these autoantibodies. In PV, autoantibodies are directed against a 130-kDa desmosomal cadherin molecule (desmoglein 3) that forms a complex with plakoglobin, an 85-kDa protein found in both desmosomal and adherens junctions. Anti-desmoglein 3 autoantibodies in patients with PV are responsible for dysadhesion of epidermal cells. The titer of circulating autoantibody (determined by indirect immunofluorescence microscopy) correlates roughly with disease activity. These immunopathologic findings aid the diagnosis of PV and its differentiation from other blistering skin diseases.

PV can be life-threatening. Prior to the availability of glucocorticoids, the mortality ranged from 60 to 90 percent. The current mortality is approximately 5 to 15 percent. Common causes of morbidity and mortality are infection and complications of treatment with glucocorticoids. Bad prognostic factors include advanced age, widespread involvement, and the requirement for high doses of glucocorticoids (with or without other immunosuppressive agents) for control of disease. The course of PV in individual patients is variable and difficult to predict. Some patients achieve remission after variable periods (40 percent of patients in some series), but others may require long-term treatment or succumb to complications of their disease or its treatment. The mainstay of treatment is systemic glucocorticoids. Patients with moderate to severe disease are usually started on prednisone 60 to 80 mg/d. If new lesions continue to appear after 1 to 2 weeks of treatment, the dose should be increased. Many regimens have combined an immunosuppressive agent with systemic glucocorticoids for control of PV. The two most frequently used are either azathioprine (1 mg/kg per day) or cyclophosphamide (1 mg/kg per day). It is important to bring severe or progressive disease under control quickly to lessen the severity and/or duration of this disorder.

PEMPHIGUS FOLIACEUS Pemphigus foliaceus (PF) is distinguished from PV by several features. In PF, acantholytic blisters are located high within the epidermis, usually just beneath the stratum corneum. Hence PF is a more superficial blistering disease than PV. The distribution of lesions in the two disorders is much the same, except that in PF mucous membrane lesions are rare. Patients with PF rarely demonstrate intact blisters but rather exhibit shallow erosions associated with erythema, scale, and crust formation. Mild cases of PF resemble severe seborrheic dermatitis; severe PF may cause extensive exfoliation. Sun exposure (ultraviolet irradiation) may be an aggravating factor. A blistering skin disease endemic to south central Brazil known as fogo selvagem or Brazilian pemphigus is clinically, histologically, and immunopathologically indistinguishable from PF.

Patients with PF have immunopathologic features in common with PV. Specifically, direct immunofluorescence microscopy of normal, perilesional skin demonstrates IgG on the surface of keratinocytes. As in PV, patients with PF frequently have circulating IgG autoantibodies against keratinocyte cell surface antigens. Guinea pig esophagus is the optimal substrate for indirect immunofluorescence microscopy studies of sera from patients with PF. In PF, autoantibodies are directed against desmoglein 1, a 160-kDa desmosomal cadherin that (like PV antigen) is complexed to plakoglobin.

Although pemphigus has been associated with several autoimmune diseases, its association with thymoma and/or myasthenia gravis is particularly notable. To date, more than 30 cases of thymoma and/or myasthenia gravis have been reported in association with pemphigus, usually with PF. Patients also may develop pemphigus as a consequence of drug exposure. The most frequently implicated agent is penicillamine; other offenders include captopril, rifampin, piroxicam, penicillin, and phenobarbital. Drug-induced pemphigus usually resembles PF rather than PV; autoantibodies in these patients have the same antigenic specificity as they do in other pemphigus patients. In most patients, lesions resolve following discontinuation of the drug; however, some patients require treatment with systemic glucocorticoids and/or immunosuppressive agents.

PF is generally a far less severe disease than PV and carries a better prognosis. Localized disease can be treated conservatively with topical or intralesional glucocorticoids; more active cases can usually be controlled with systemic glucocorticoids.

PARANEOPLASTIC PEMPHIGUS Paraneoplastic pemphigus is a recently described autoimmune acantholytic mucocutaneous disease associated with an occult or confirmed neoplasm. Patients with paraneoplastic pemphigus typically show painful mucosal erosive lesions in association with pruritic papulosquamous eruptions that often progress to blisters. Palm and sole involvement is common in these patients and raises the possibility that prior reports of neoplasia-associated erythema multiforme actually may have represented unrecognized cases of paraneoplastic pemphigus. Biopsies of lesional skin from these patients show varying combinations of acantholysis, keratinocyte necrosis, and vacuolar-interface dermatitis. Direct immunofluorescence microscopy of patient skin shows deposits of IgG and complement on the surface of keratinocytes as well as similar immunoreactants in the epidermal basement membrane zone. Patients with paraneoplastic pemphigus have IgG autoantibodies that react with the surface of tissues containing desmosomes (i.e., complex and simple epithelia as well as myocardium). These autoantibodies immunoprecipitate a unique complex of four polypeptides (250, 230, 210, and 190 kDa) from keratinocyte cell extracts. In sodium dodecyl sulfate–polyacrylamide gel electrophoresis, the 250- and 210-kDa antigens comigrate with the desmosomal plaque–associated proteins desmoplakins I and II, respectively, whereas the 230-kDa antigen comigrates with bullous pemphigoid antigen (see below); the identity of the other antigen in this complex has not yet been conclusively determined. Interestingly, passive transfer of patient immunoglobulin to neonatal mice produces keratinocyte detachment, indicating that autoantibodies from patients with paraneoplastic pemphigus are pathogenic mediators of tissue damage. Paraneoplastic pemphigus is generally treatment-resistant, although patients may improve (or even remit) following resection of underlying benign neoplasms. The predominant neoplasms associated with this disorder are non-Hodgkin's lymphoma, chronic lymphocytic leukemia, Castleman's disease, thymoma, and spindle cell neoplasms.

BULLOUS PEMPHIGOID Bullous pemphigoid (BP) is a subepidermal blistering skin disease usually seen in the elderly. Lesions typically consist of tense blisters on either normal-appearing or erythematous skin. The lesions are usually distributed over the lower abdomen, groin, and flexor surface of the extremities; oral mucosal lesions are found in 10 to 40 percent of patients. Pruritus may be nonexistent or severe. As lesions evolve, tense blisters tend to rupture and be replaced by flaccid lesions or erosions with or without surmounting crust. Nontraumatized blisters heal without scarring. There is no ethnic or HLA association. Despite isolated reports, several studies have shown that patients with BP do not have an increased incidence of malignancy in comparison with appropriately age- and sex-matched controls.

While biopsies of early lesional skin demonstrate subepidermal blisters, the histologic features depend on the character of the particular lesion. Lesions on normal-appearing skin generally show a sparse perivascular leukocytic infiltrate with some eosinophils. Biopsies of inflammatory lesions typically show an eosinophil-rich, leukocytic infiltrate within the papillary dermis at sites of vesicle formation and in perivascular areas. In addition to eosinophils, these cell-rich lesions also contain mononuclear cells and neutrophils. It is not always possible to distinguish BP from other subepidermal blistering skin diseases by routine histologic techniques.

Immunopathologic studies have broadened our understanding of this disease and aided its diagnosis. Direct immunofluorescence microscopy of normal-appearing perilesional skin shows linear deposits of IgG and/or C3 in the epidermal basement membrane. The sera of approximately 70 percent of these patients contain circulating IgG autoantibodies that bind the epidermal basement membrane of normal human skin in indirect immunofluorescence microscopy. An even higher percentage of patients shows reactivity to the epidermal side of 1 M NaCl split skin

Table 311-1

Immunologically Mediated Blistering Skin Diseases

Disease	Clinical	Histology	Immunopathology
Pemphigus vulgaris	Flaccid blisters, denuded skin, oromucosal lesions	Blister formed in suprabasal layer of epidermis	Cell surface deposits of IgG on keratinocytes
Pemphigus foliaceus	Crusts and shallow erosions on scalp, central face, neck, upper chest, and back	Blister formed in superficial layers of epidermis	Cell surface deposits of IgG on keratinocytes
Bullous pemphigoid	Large tense blisters on flexor surfaces, oromucosal lesions	Blister formed in subepidermal region, usually eosinophil-rich	Linear band of IgG and/or C3 at BMZ*
Dermatitis herpetiformis	Extremely itchy small papules and vesicles on elbows, knees, buttocks, and posterior nuchal area	Subepidermal blister with neutrophils in dermal papillae	Granular deposits of IgA in dermal papillae
Linear IgA disease	Extremely itchy small papules and vesicles on extensor surfaces, occasionally larger arciform blisters	Subepidermal blister with neutrophils in dermal papillae	Linear band of IgA at BMZ
Epidermolysis bullosa acquisita	Blisters, scarring, and milia on dorsum of hands, elbows, knees; oromucosal lesions	Blister is subepidermal and can be inflammatory or not	Linear band of IgG and/or C3 at BMZ
Cicatricial pemphigoid	Erosive and/or blistering lesions of mucous membranes and possibly the skin; scarring at some sites	Blister is subepithelial and may or may not be associated with a mononuclear cell–rich infiltrate	Linear band of IgG, IgA, and/or C3 at BMZ

* BMZ, basement membrane zone of epidermis.

[an alternative immunofluorescence microscopy test substrate that is commonly used to distinguish circulating IgG anti-basement membrane autoantibodies in patients with BP from those in patients with similar, yet different, subepidermal blistering diseases (e.g., epidermolysis bullosa acquisita, see below)]. No correlation exists between the titer of these autoantibodies and disease activity. In BP, circulating autoantibodies recognize 230- and (in approximately 50 percent of BP patients) 180-kDa hemidesmosome-associated proteins in basal keratinocytes. Autoantibodies are thought to develop against these antigens, deposit in situ, and activate complement that subsequently produces dermal mast cell degranulation and granulocyte-rich leukocytic infiltrates that cause tissue damage and blister formation.

BP is generally benign, but it may persist for months to years, with exacerbations or remissions. Although extensive involvement may result in widespread erosions and compromise cutaneous integrity, the mortality rate is low even in the absence of treatment. Nonetheless, deaths may occur in elderly and/or debilitated patients. The mainstay of treatment is systemic glucocorticoids. Patients with local or minimal disease can sometimes be controlled with topical glucocorticoids alone; patients with more extensive lesions generally respond to systemic glucocorticoids either alone or in combination with immunosuppressive agents. Patients will usually respond to prednisone, 40 to 60 mg/d. In some instances, azathioprine (1 mg/kg per day) or cyclophosphamide (1 mg/kg per day) are necessary adjuncts.

PEMPHIGOID GESTATIONIS Pemphigoid gestationis (PG), also known as herpes gestationis, is a rare, nonviral, subepidermal blistering disease of pregnancy and the puerperium. PG may begin during any trimester of pregnancy or present shortly after delivery. Lesions are usually distributed over the abdomen, trunk, and extremities; mucous membrane lesions are rare. Skin lesions in these patients may be quite polymorphic and consist of erythematous urticarial papules and plaques, vesiculopapules, and/or frank bullae. Lesions are almost always very pruritic. Severe exacerbations of PG frequently occur after delivery, typically within 24 to 48 h. PG tends to recur in subsequent pregnancies, often beginning earlier during such gestations. Brief flare-ups of disease may occur with resumption of menses and may develop in patients later exposed to oral contraceptives. Occasionally, infants of affected mothers demonstrate transient skin lesions.

Biopsies of early lesional skin show teardrop-shaped subepidermal vesicles forming in dermal papillae in association with an eosinophil-rich leukocytic infiltrate. Differentiation of PG from other subepidermal bullous diseases by light microscopy is often difficult. However, direct immunofluorescence microscopy of normal perilesional skin from PG patients reveals the immunopathologic hallmark of this disorder—linear deposits of C3 in the epidermal basement membrane zone. These deposits develop as a consequence of complement activation produced by a low titer IgG anti-basement membrane zone autoantibody. Recent studies have shown that the majority of PG sera contain autoantibodies that recognize the same 180-kDa hemidesmosome-associated protein that is targeted by autoantibodies in roughly 50 percent of patients with BP—a subepidermal bullous disease that resembles PG morphologically, histologically, and immunopathologically.

The goals of therapy in patients with PG are to prevent the development of new lesions, relieve intense pruritus, and care for erosions at sites of blister formation. Most patients require treatment with moderate doses of daily glucocorticoids (i.e., 20 to 40 mg of prednisone) at some point in their course. Mild cases (or brief flare-ups) may be controlled by vigorous use of potent topical glucocorticoids. Although PG was once thought to be associated with an increased risk of fetal morbidity and mortality, the best evidence now suggests that these infants may only be at increased risk of being slightly premature or "small for dates." Current evidence suggests that there is no difference in the incidence of uncomplicated live births in PG patients treated with systemic glucocorticoids and in those managed more conservatively. If systemic glucocorticoids are administered, newborns are at risk for development of reversible adrenal insufficiency.

DERMATITIS HERPETIFORMIS Dermatitis herpetiformis (DH) is an intensely pruritic, chronic papulovesicular skin disease characterized by lesions symmetrically distributed over extensor surfaces (i.e., elbows, knees, buttocks, back, scalp, and posterior neck). The primary lesion in this disorder is a papule, papulovesicle, or urticarial plaque. Because pruritus is prominent, patients may present with excoriations and crusted papules but no observable primary lesions. Patients sometimes report that their pruritus has a distinctive burning or stinging component; the onset of such local symptoms reliably heralds the development of distinct clinical lesions 12 to 24 h later. Almost all DH patients have an associated, usually subclinical, gluten-sensitive enteropathy (see also Chap. 285), and more than 90 percent express the HLA-B8/DRw3 and HLA-DQw2 haplotypes. DH may present at any age, including childhood; onset in the second to fourth decades is most common. The disease is typically chronic.

Biopsy of early lesional skin reveals neutrophil-rich infiltrates within dermal papillae. Neutrophils, fibrin, edema, and microvesicle formation at these sites are characteristic of early disease. Older lesions may demonstrate nonspecific features of a subepidermal bulla or an excoriated papule. Because the clinical and histologic features of this disease can be variable and resemble other subepidermal blistering disorders, the diagnosis can be confirmed by direct immunofluorescence microscopy of normal-appearing perilesional skin. Such studies demonstrate granular deposits of IgA (with or without complement components) in the papillary dermis and along the epidermal basement membrane zone. IgA deposits in the skin are unaffected by control of disease with medication; however, these immunoreactants may diminish in intensity or disappear in patients maintained for long periods on a strict gluten-free diet (see below). Patients with granular deposits of IgA in their epidermal basement membrane zone typically do not have circulating IgA anti-basement membrane autoantibodies and should be distinguished from individuals with linear IgA deposits at this site (see below).

Although most DH patients do not report overt gastrointestinal symptoms or laboratory evidence of malabsorption, biopsies of small bowel usually reveal blunting of intestinal villi and a lymphocytic infiltrate in the lamina propria. As is true for patients with celiac disease, this gastrointestinal abnormality can be reversed by a gluten-free diet. Moreover, if maintained, this diet alone may control the skin disease and eventuate in clearance of IgA deposits from these patients' epidermal basement membrane zone. Subsequent gluten exposure in the latter patients alters the morphology of their small bowel, elicits a flare-up of their skin disease, and is associated with the reappearance of IgA in their epidermal basement membrane zone. Patients with DH also have an increased incidence of thyroid abnormalities, achlorhydria, atrophic gastritis, and antigastric parietal cell antibodies. These associations likely relate to the high frequency of the HLA-B8/DRw3 haplotype in these patients, since this marker is commonly linked to autoimmune disorders. The mainstay of treatment of DH is dapsone. Patients respond rapidly (24 to 48 h) to dapsone but require careful pretreatment evaluation and close follow-up to ensure that complications are avoided or controlled. All patients on more than 100 mg/d dapsone will have some hemolysis and methemoglobinemia. These are expected pharmacologic side effects of dapsone. It is important to employ the lowest possible maintenance dose of dapsone to control symptoms and lesions. Gluten restriction can control DH and lessen dapsone requirements; this diet must rigidly exclude gluten to be of maximal benefit. Moreover, many months of dietary restriction may be necessary before a beneficial result is achieved. Good dietary counselling by a trained dietitian is essential.

LINEAR IgA DISEASE Linear IgA disease, once considered a variant form of dermatitis herpetiformis, is actually a separate and distinct entity. Clinically, these patients may resemble typical cases of DH, bullous pemphigoid, or other subepidermal blistering diseases. Lesions typically consist of papulovesicles, bullae, and/or urticarial plaques, predominantly on extensor (as seen in "classic" DH), central, or flexural sites. Oral mucosal involvement does occur in some patients. Severe pruritus resembles that in patients with DH. Patients with linear IgA disease do not have an increased frequency of the HLA-B8/DRw3 haplotype or an associated enteropathy and hence are not candidates for a gluten-free diet.

The histologic alterations in early lesions may be virtually indistinguishable from those in DH. However, direct immunofluorescence microscopy of normal-appearing perilesional skin reveals linear deposits of IgA (and often C3) in the epidermal basement membrane zone. Many patients with linear IgA disease demonstrate circulating IgA autoantibodies against a 97-kDa protein in normal epidermal basement membrane. These patients generally respond to treatment with dapsone, 50 to 200 mg/d.

EPIDERMOLYSIS BULLOSA ACQUISITA (EBA) EBA is a rare, noninherited, polymorphic, subepidermal blistering disease. (The inherited form is discussed in Chap. 348.) Patients with classic or noninflammatory EBA have blisters on noninflamed skin, atrophic scars, milia, nail dystrophy, and oral lesions. Because lesions generally occur at sites exposed to minor trauma, classic EBA is considered to be a mechanobullous disease. Other patients with EBA have widespread inflammatory, scarring, bullous lesions and oromucosal involvement that resembles severe BP. Interestingly, some patients present with an inflammatory bullous skin disease that subsequently evolves into the classic noninflammatory form of this disorder. In general, EBA is chronic; associations with multiple myeloma, amyloidosis, inflammatory bowel disease, and diabetes mellitus have been reported. The HLA-DR2 haplotype is found with increased frequency in these patients.

The histology of lesional skin varies depending on the type or character of the lesion being studied. Noninflammatory bullae show subepidermal blisters with a sparse leukocytic infiltrate and resemble those in patients with porphyria cutanea tarda. Inflammatory vesiculobullous lesions consist of a subepidermal blister and neutrophil-rich leukocytic infiltrates in the superficial dermis. EBA patients have continuous deposits of IgG (and frequently C3 as well as other complement components) in a linear pattern within the epidermal basement membrane zone. Ultrastructurally, these immunoreactants are found in the sublamina densa region in association with anchoring fibrils, wheat stack–like structures that extend from the lamina densa into the underlying papillary dermis. Approximately 25 to 50 percent of EBA patients have circulating IgG autoantibodies directed against type VII collagen—the collagen species found in anchoring fibrils. Such IgG anti-basement membrane autoantibodies bind the dermal side of 1 M NaCl split skin (in contrast to IgG anti-basement membrane autoantibodies in patients with BP that bind either epidermal or both sides of this indirect immunofluorescence microscopy test substrate).

Treatment of EBA is generally unsatisfactory. Some patients with inflammatory EBA may respond to systemic glucocorticoids, either alone or in combination with immunosuppressive agents. Other patients (especially those with neutrophil-rich inflammatory lesions) may respond to dapsone. The chronic, noninflammatory form of this disease is largely resistant to treatment.

CICATRICIAL PEMPHIGOID Cicatricial pemphigoid (CP) is a rare, acquired, subepithelial blistering disease characterized by erosive lesions of mucous membranes and skin that result in scarring of at least some sites of involvement. Immunopathologically, perilesional mucosa and skin of patients with CP demonstrate in situ deposits of immunoreactants in epithelial basement membranes. Common sites of involvement include the oral mucosa (especially the gingiva) and conjunctiva; other sites that may be affected include the nasopharyngeal, laryngeal, esophageal, genital, and rectal mucosa. Skin lesions (present in about one-third of patients) tend to predominate on the scalp, face, and upper trunk and generally consist of a few scattered erosions or tense blisters on an erythematous or urticarial base. Less commonly, skin lesions present as a few blisters that occur repeatedly on the same sites on the head or neck; such lesions eventually scar and may not be associated with mucosal involvement. CP is typically a chronic and progressive disorder. Serious complications may arise as a consequence of ocular, laryngeal, or esophageal lesions. Erosive conjunctivitis may result in shortened fornices, symblephara, ankylo-

blepharon, entropion, corneal opacities, and (in severe cases) blindness. Similarly, erosive lesions of the larynx may cause hoarseness, pain, and tissue loss that if unrecognized and untreated may eventuate in complete destruction of the airway. Esophageal lesions may result in stenosis and/or strictures that may place patients at risk for aspiration.

Biopsies of lesional tissue generally demonstrate subepithelial vesiculobullae and a mononuclear leukocytic infiltrate. Neutrophils and eosinophils may be seen in biopsies of early lesions; older lesions may demonstrate a scant leukocytic infiltrate and fibrosis. Direct immunofluorescence microscopy of perilesional tissue typically demonstrates deposits of IgG, IgA, and/or C3 in these patients' epithelial basement membranes. Because many of these patients show no evidence of circulating anti-basement membrane autoantibodies, testing of perilesional skin is important diagnostically. Although CP was once thought to be a single nosologic entity, it is now largely regarded as a disease phenotype that may develop as a consequence of an autoimmune reaction against a variety of different molecules in epithelial basement membranes (e.g., bullous pemphigoid antigens, laminin 5, or other antigens yet to be completely defined). Treatment of CP is largely dependent upon sites of involvement. Due to potentially severe complications, ocular, laryngeal, and/or esophageal involvement require aggressive systemic treatment with dapsone, prednisone, or the latter in combination with another immunosuppressive agent (e.g., azathioprine or cyclophosphamide). Less threatening forms of the disease may be managed with topical or intralesional glucocorticoids.

AUTOIMMUNE SYSTEMIC DISEASES WITH PROMINENT CUTANEOUS FEATURES

DERMATOMYOSITIS The cutaneous manifestations of dermatomyositis (see Chap. 315) are often distinctive but at times may resemble those of systemic lupus erythematosus (SLE) (see Chap. 312), scleroderma (see Chap. 314), or other overlapping connective tissue diseases (see Chap. 314). The extent and severity of cutaneous disease may or may not correlate with the extent and severity of the myositis. Patients with severe muscle involvement may have relatively minor skin changes, whereas patients with marked skin involvement may have mild muscle disease. The cutaneous manifestations of dermatomyositis are similar whether the disease appears in childhood or old age, except that calcification of subcutaneous tissue is a common late sequela in childhood dermatomyositis.

The cutaneous signs of dermatomyositis may precede or follow the development of myositis by weeks to years. Cases lacking muscle involvement (i.e., dermatomyositis sine myositis) also have been reported. The most common manifestation is a purple-red discoloration of the upper eyelids, sometimes associated with scaling ("heliotrope" erythema) and periorbital edema. Erythema on the cheeks and nose in a "butterfly" distribution may resemble the eruption in SLE. Erythematous or violaceous scaling patches are common on the upper anterior chest, posterior neck, scalp, and the extensor surfaces of the arms, legs, and hands. Erythema and scaling may be particularly prominent over the elbows, knees, and the dorsal interphalangeal joints. Approximately one-third of patients have violaceous, flat-topped papules over the dorsal interphalangeal joints that are pathognomonic of dermatomyositis (Gottron's sign or Gottron's papules). These lesions can be contrasted with the erythema and scaling on the dorsum of the fingers in some patients with SLE which spares the skin over the interphalangeal joints. Periungual telangiectasia may be prominent, and a lacy or reticulated erythema may be associated with fine scaling on the extensor surfaces of the thighs and upper arms. Other patients, particularly those with long-standing disease, develop areas of hypopigmentation, hyperpigmentation, mild atrophy, and telangiectasia known as *poikiloderma vasculare atrophicans*. Poikiloderma is rare in both SLE and scleroderma and thus can serve as a clinical sign that distinguishes dermatomyositis from these two diseases. However, cutaneous changes may be similar in scleroderma and dermatomyositis and may include thickening and binding down of the skin of the hands (sclerodactyly) as well as Raynaud's phenomenon. However, the presence of severe muscle disease, Gottron's papules, heliotrope erythema, and poikiloderma serve to distinguish these patients as having dermatomyositis. Skin biopsy of erythematous, scaling lesions of dermatomyositis may reveal only mild nonspecific inflammation but sometimes may show changes indistinguishable from those found in SLE, including epidermal atrophy, hydropic degeneration of basal keratinocytes, edema of the upper dermis, and a mild mononuclear cell infiltrate. Direct immunofluorescence microscopy of lesional skin is usually negative. Treatment should be directed at the systemic disease. In the few instances where adjunctive cutaneous therapy is desirable, topical glucocorticoids are sometimes useful. These patients should avoid exposure to ultraviolet irradiation and use photoprotective measures such as sunscreens.

LUPUS ERYTHEMATOSUS The cutaneous manifestations of lupus erythematosus (LE) (see Chap. 312) can be divided into acute, subacute, and chronic (i.e., discoid LE) types. *Acute cutaneous LE* is characterized by erythema of the nose and malar eminences in a "butterfly" distribution. The erythema is often sudden in onset, accompanied by edema and fine scale, and correlated with systemic involvement. Patients may have widespread involvement of the face as well as erythema and scaling of the extensor surfaces of the extremities and upper chest. These acute lesions, while sometimes evanescent, usually last for days and are often associated with exacerbations of systemic disease. Skin biopsy of acute lesions may show only a sparse dermal infiltrate of mononuclear cells and dermal edema. In some instances, cellular infiltrates around blood vessels and hair follicles are notable, as is hydropic degeneration of basal cells of the epidermis. Direct immunofluorescence microscopy of lesional skin frequently reveals deposits of immunoglobulin(s) and complement in the epidermal basement membrane zone. Treatment is aimed at control of systemic disease; photoprotection in this, as well as in other forms of LE, is very important.

Subacute cutaneous lupus erythematosus (SCLE) is characterized by a widespread photosensitive, nonscarring eruption. About half of these patients have SLE in which severe renal and central nervous system involvement is uncommon. SCLE may present as a papulosquamous eruption that resembles psoriasis or annular lesions that resemble those seen in erythema multiforme. In the papulosquamous form, discrete erythematous papules arise on the back, chest, shoulders, extensor surfaces of the arms, and the dorsum of the hands but are uncommon on the face, flexor surfaces of the arms, and below the waist. The slightly scaling papules tend to merge into large plaques, some with a reticulate appearance. The annular form involves the same areas and also begins as an erythematous papule but tends to develop oval, circular, or polycyclic lesions. The lesions of SCLE are more widespread but have less tendency for scarring than do lesions of discoid LE. Skin biopsy reveals a dense mononuclear cell infiltrate around hair follicles and blood vessels in the superficial dermis, combined with hydropic degeneration of basal cells in the epidermis. Direct immunofluorescence microscopy of lesional skin reveals deposits of immunoglobulin(s) in the epidermal basement membrane zone in about half these cases. Most SCLE patients have anti-Ro antibodies. Local therapy is usually unsuccessful, and most patients require treatment with aminoquinoline antimalarials. Low-dose therapy with oral glucocorticoids is sometimes necessary; photoprotective measures against both ultraviolet B and A wavelengths are very important.

Discoid lupus erythematosus (DLE) is characterized by discrete lesions, most often on the face, scalp, or external ears. The lesions are erythematous papules or plaques with a thick, adherent scale that occludes hair follicles (follicular plugging). When the scale is removed, its underside will show small excrescences that correlate with the openings of hair follicles and is termed a "carpet tack" appearance. This finding is relatively specific for DLE. Long-standing lesions develop central atrophy, scarring, and hypopigmentation but frequently have erythematous, sometimes raised borders at the periphery. These lesions persist for years and tend to expand slowly. Only 5 to 10 percent of patients with DLE meet the American Rheumatism Association criteria for SLE. However, typical discoid lesions are frequently seen in patients with SLE. Biopsy of DLE lesions shows hyperkeratosis, follicular plugging, and atrophy of the epidermis. The dermal-epidermal junction reveals hydropic degeneration of basal keratinocytes, and a mononuclear cell infiltrate surrounds hair follicles and blood vessels. Direct immunofluorescence microscopy demonstrates immunoglobulin(s) and complement deposits at the basement membrane zone in about 90 percent of cases. Treatment is focused on control of local cutaneous disease and consists mainly of photoprotection and topical or intralesional glucocorticoids. If local therapy is ineffective, use of aminoquinoline antimalarials may be indicated.

SCLERODERMA AND MORPHEA The skin changes of scleroderma (see Chap. 314) usually begin on the hands, feet, and face, with episodes of recurrent nonpitting edema. Sclerosis of the skin begins distally on the fingers (sclerodactyly) and spreads proximally, usually accompanied by resorption of bone of the fingertips, which may have punched out ulcers, stellate scars, or areas of hemorrhage. The fingers may actually shrink in size and become sausage-shaped, and since the fingernails are usually unaffected, the nails may curve over the end of the fingertips. Periungual telangiectasias are usually present, but periungual erythema is rare. In advanced cases, the extremities show contractures and calcinosis cutis. Face involvement includes a smooth, unwrinkled brow, taut skin over the nose, shrinkage of tissue around the mouth, and perioral radial furrowing. Matlike telangiectasias are often present, particularly on the face and hands. Involved skin feels indurated, smooth, and bound to underlying structures; hyperpigmentation and hypopigmentation are also often present. Raynaud's phenomenon, i.e., cold-induced blanching, cyanosis, and reactive hyperemia, is present in almost all patients with scleroderma and can precede development of scleroderma by many years. The combination of calcinosis cutis, Raynaud's phenomenon, esophageal dysmotility, sclerodactyly, and telangiectasia has been termed the *CREST syndrome*. Anticentromere antibodies have been reported in a very high percentage of patients with the CREST syndrome but in only a small minority of patients with scleroderma. Skin biopsy reveals thickening of the dermis and homogenization of collagen bundles. Direct immunofluorescence microscopy of lesional skin is usually negative.

Morphea, which has been called *localized scleroderma*, is characterized by localized thickening and sclerosis of skin, usually affecting young adults or children. Morphea begins as erythematous or flesh-colored plaques that become sclerotic, develop central hypopigmentation, and demonstrate an erythematous border. In most cases, patients have one or a few lesions, and the disease is termed *localized morphea*. In some patients, widespread cutaneous lesions may occur, without systemic involvement. This form is called *generalized morphea*. Most patients with morphea do not have autoantibodies. Skin biopsy of morphea is indistinguishable from that of scleroderma. Linear scleroderma is a limited form of disease that presents in a linear, bandlike distribution and tends to involve deep as well as superficial layers of skin. Scleroderma and morphea are usually quite resistant to therapy with medications. For this reason, physical therapy to prevent joint contractures and to maintain function is employed and is often helpful.

Diffuse fasciitis with eosinophilia is a clinical entity that can sometimes be confused with scleroderma. There is usually the sudden onset of swelling, induration, and erythema of the extremities frequently following significant physical exertion. The proximal portions of extremities (arms, forearms, thighs, legs) are more often involved than are the hands and feet. While the skin is indurated, it is usually not bound down as in scleroderma. These skin findings are accompanied by peripheral blood eosinophilia, increased erythrocyte sedimentation rate, and sometimes hypergammaglobulinemia. Deep biopsy of affected areas of skin reveals inflammation and thickening of the deep fascia overlying muscle. An inflammatory infiltrate composed of eosinophils and mononuclear cells is usually found. Patients with eosinophilic fasciitis appear to be at increased risk to develop bone marrow failure or other hematologic abnormalities. While the ultimate course of eosinophilic fasciitis is uncertain, many patients respond favorably to treatment with prednisone in doses ranging from 40 to 60 mg/d.

The *eosinophilia-myalgia syndrome*, a disorder reported in epidemic numbers in 1989 and linked to ingestion of tryptophan manufactured by a single company in Japan, is a multisystem disorder characterized by debilitating myalgias and absolute eosinophilia in association with varying combinations of arthralgias, pulmonary symptoms, and peripheral edema. In a later phase (i.e., 3 to 6 months after initial symptoms), these patients often develop localized sclerodermatous skin changes, weight loss, and/or neuropathy (see Chap. 314). The precise cause of this syndrome, which may resemble other sclerotic skin conditions, is unknown. However, the clustering of cases suggests that an impurity or contaminant in a manufactured tryptophan preparation is likely.

BIBLIOGRAPHY

ANHALT GJ et al: Paraneoplastic pemphigus: An autoimmune mucocutaneous disease associated with neoplasia. N Engl J Med 323:1729, 1990

BRAVERMAN IM: Connective tissue diseases, in *Skin Signs of Systemic Disease.* Philadelphia, Saunders, 1981

FINE JD: Management of acquired bullous skin disease. N Engl J Med 333:1475, 1995

GAMMON WR et al: Epidermolysis bullosa acquisita—A pemphigoid-like disease. J Am Acad Dermatol 11:820, 1984

HALL RP: Dermatitis herpetiformis. J Invest Dermatol 99:873, 1992

KATZ SI et al: Dermatitis herpetiformis: The skin and the gut. Ann Intern Med 93:857, 1980

KORMAN N: Pemphigus. J Am Acad Dermatol 18:1219, 1988

SHORNICK JK: Herpes gestationis. J Am Acad Dermatol 17:539, 1987

SHULMAN LE: Diffuse fasciitis with eosinophilia: A new syndrome. Arthritis Rheum 20(Suppl):205, 1977

STANLEY JR: Cell adhesion molecules as targets of autoantibodies in pemphigus and pemphigoid, bullous diseases due to defective epidermal cell adhesion. Adv Immunol 53:291, 1992

YANCEY KB: Adhesion molecules. II: Interactions of keratinocytes with epidermal basement membrane. J Invest Dermatol 104:1008, 1995

| 312 | *Bevra Hannahs Hahn* |

SYSTEMIC LUPUS ERYTHEMATOSUS

DEFINITION AND PREVALENCE Systemic lupus erythematosus (SLE) is a disease of unknown etiology in which tissues and cells are damaged by pathogenic autoantibodies and immune complexes. Ninety percent of cases are in women, usually of childbearing age, but children, men, and the elderly can be affected. In the United States, the prevalence of SLE in urban areas varies from 15 to 50 per 100,000 population; it is more common in blacks than in whites. Hispanic and Asian populations are also susceptible.

PATHOGENESIS AND ETIOLOGY SLE results from tissue damage caused by pathogenic subsets of autoantibodies and immune complexes. The abnormal immune responses include (1) polyclonal and antigen-specific T and B lymphocyte hyperactivity, and (2) inadequate regulation of that hyperactivity. These abnormal immune responses probably depend upon interactions between susceptibility genes and environment. Evidence for genetic predisposition includes increased concordance for disease in monozygotic (24 to 58 percent) compared with dizygotic (0 to 6 percent) twins, a 10 to 15 percent frequency of patients with more than one affected family member, and correlations of certain genes [especially major histocompatibility complex (MHC) class II and class III] with disease and with selected autoantibodies. C4AQO, a defective class III allele that fails to encode a functional C4A protein, is the most common genetic marker associated with SLE in many ethnic groups (found in 40 to 50 percent of patients compared with 15 percent of healthy controls). Most individuals with homozygous deficiencies of early complement components

develop SLE or lupus-like diseases. Certain extended haplotypes, such as B8.DR3.DQw2.C4AQO, predispose to SLE in some populations. Single-gene associations occur between HLA class II (especially DQ$_{beta}$) and autoantibodies that define clinical subsets of lupus. For example, high titers of IgG anti-DNA are associated with lupus nephritis and with DQB1*0201, *0602, and *0302 inherited with either DR2 or DR3. Antibodies to Ro/La (SS-A/SS-B) are associated with the dermatitis of subacute cutaneous lupus and with certain DQA and DQB genes inherited with DR3 (occasionally DR2). The lupus anticoagulant, correlated clinically with clotting, is associated with DQB*0301, *0302, *0303, and *0602 inherited with DR4 or DR7. The DQA or DQB susceptibility genes in each group share amino acid sequences that may determine the ability to make a particular autoantibody. Family studies suggest that genes unlinked to HLA also confer susceptibility, and that females are more likely than males to express the autoimmune manifestations of their genotypes. The more susceptibility genes one has, the higher is the relative risk for SLE; for most individuals at least three or four different genes are probably required.

Environmental factors that cause flares of SLE are largely unknown, with the exception of ultraviolet (UV)-B (and sometimes UV-A) light. As many as 70 percent of patients are photosensitive. Other factors, such as ingested alfalfa sprouts, and chemicals, such as hydrazines, have been implicated. Searches for viral/retroviral disease inducers have been inconclusive. Although some drugs can induce lupus-like disease, there are notable clinical and autoantibody differences between drug-induced and spontaneous lupus. Femaleness is clearly a susceptibility factor, since the prevalence in women of child-bearing years is seven to nine times higher than in men, whereas the female:male ratio is 3:1 in pre- and postmenopausal years. Metabolism of estrogenic and androgenic hormones may be abnormal in lupus patients. Sex hormones also influence immune tolerance.

Abnormal immune responses permit sustained production of pathogenic subsets of autoantibodies and immune complexes. No immunoglobulin genes have been identified that exclusively encode harmful autoantibodies, although certain V-region genes (especially V_H) seem to be preferentially used, and there is probably clonal selection of B cells secreting high-avidity antibodies to autoantigens. In most murine lupus models, T cell help is critical to development of full-blown disease; cells of CD4 + CD8 −, CD4 − CD8 +, and CD4 − CD8 − phenotypes all help autoantibody production in murine and human SLE. The abnormalities that permit hyperactivated self-reactive B and T cells to dominate immune repertoires in murine and human SLE are multiple and include defects in tolerance, apoptosis, idiotypic networks, immune complex clearance, generation of regulatory cells, and production of autoantibodies that can affect quantities and functions of living cells. The structure of antigens that stimulate autoantibodies is under investigation. Some are clearly derived from self (nucleosomes, ribonucleoprotein, erythrocyte and lymphocyte surface antigens); others may be from the external environment and mimic self (e.g., components of vesicular stomatitis virus mimic peptides in Sm antigen). Some autoantibodies induce disease by direct reaction with their antigens, such as those directed against surface antigens on erythrocytes or platelets. Others may attach to cell membranes [such as glomerular basement membrane (GBM)] via cationic charge, or because they cross-react with tissue constituents (e.g., some anti-DNA antibodies react with laminin in GBM). If these antibodies when complexed with antigen can fix complement, tissue damage occurs. Alteration of cell function after antibodies bind to membranes also occurs independent of complement activation. Autoantibodies characteristic of SLE are listed in Table 312-1.

In summary, some individuals are genetically predisposed to SLE. Under the influence of multiple genes, often triggered by environmental challenges and highly influenced by sex, they may develop a number of different clinical syndromes that fulfill diagnostic criteria for SLE. The etiology of these syndromes is complex and probably differs between patients.

CLINICAL MANIFESTATIONS At onset, SLE may involve only one organ system (additional manifestations occur later) or may be multisystemic. Clinical manifestations are listed in Table 312-2;

those that fulfill American Rheumatism Association (currently the American College of Rheumatology) criteria for a diagnosis of SLE are listed in Table 312-3. Autoantibodies are detectable at disease onset. Severity varies from mild and intermittent to persistent and fulminant. Most patients experience exacerbations interspersed with periods of relative quiescence. True remissions with no symptoms and requiring no therapy occur in up to 20 percent. Systemic symptoms are usually prominent and include fatigue, malaise, fever, anorexia, and weight loss.

Musculoskeletal Manifestations Almost all patients experience arthralgias and myalgias; most develop intermittent arthritis. Pain is often out of proportion to physical findings of symmetric fusiform swelling in joints [most frequently proximal interphalangeal (PIP) and metacarpophalangeal (MCP) joints of the hands, wrists, and knees], diffuse puffiness of hands and feet, and tenosynovitis. Joint deformities are unusual, with 10 percent of patients developing swan-neck deformities of fingers and ulnar drift at MCP joints. Erosions are rare; subcutaneous nodules occur. Myopathy can be inflammatory (during periods of active disease), or secondary to treatment (hypokalemia, glucocorticoid myopathy, hydroxychloroquine myopathy). Ischemic necrosis of bone is a common cause of hip, knee, or shoulder pain in patients receiving glucocorticoids.

Cutaneous Manifestations The malar ("butterfly") rash is a fixed erythematous rash, flat or raised, over the cheeks and bridge of the nose, often involving the chin and ears. It is photosensitive. Scarring is absent; telangiectases may develop. A more diffuse maculopapular rash, predominant in sun-exposed areas, is also common and usually indicates disease flare. Loss of scalp hair is usually patchy but can be extensive; hair often regrows in SLE lesions but not in lesions of discoid lupus erythematosus (DLE). DLE occurs in about 20 percent of patients with SLE and can be disfiguring, since the lesions have central atrophy and scarring, with permanent loss of appendages. DLE lesions are circular and characterized by an erythematous raised rim, scaliness, follicular plugging, and telangiectasia. They occur over the scalp, ears, face, and sun-exposed areas of the arms, back, and chest.

Only 5 percent of patients with DLE subsequently develop SLE. Less frequent SLE skin lesions include urticaria, bullae, erythema multiforme, lichen planus–like lesions, and panniculitis ("lupus profundus").

Patients with subacute cutaneous lupus erythematosus (SCLE) are a distinct subset with recurring extensive dermatitis. Arthritis and fatigue are frequent; central nervous system and renal involvement are not. Some patients are antinuclear antibody (ANA)–negative. Most have antibodies to Ro (SS-A) or to single-stranded (ss) DNA and are HLA-DR3, -DQw1, or -DQw2. Skin lesions are photosensitive and may be annular or papulosquamous psoriasiform lesions over the arms, trunk, and face; they become hypopigmented but do not scar.

Patients with SLE, DLE, or SCLE can develop vasculitic skin lesions. These include purpura, subcutaneous nodules, nail fold infarcts, ulcers, vasculitic urticaria, panniculitis, and gangrene of digits. Shallow, slightly painful ulcers in the mouth and nose are frequent in patients with SLE.

Renal Manifestations Most patients with SLE have immunoglobulins deposited in glomeruli, but only one-half have clinical nephritis, defined by proteinuria. Early in the disease most are asymptomatic, although some develop the edema of nephrotic syndrome. Urinalysis shows hematuria, cylindruria, and proteinuria. Most patients with mesangial or mild focal proliferative nephritis (see discussion under "Pathology" below) maintain good renal function. Patients with diffuse proliferative nephritis develop renal failure if untreated. Because severe nephritis requires aggressive immunosuppression with high-dose glucocorticoids and cytotoxic drugs and mild lesions do not, renal biopsy may provide information that affects therapy. Patients with rapidly deteriorating renal function and active urine sediment require prompt, aggressive therapy; biopsy is not necessary unless they fail to respond. However, patients with a slow rise in serum creatinine to levels >265 μmol/L (>3 mg/dL) may show a high

Table 312-1

Autoantibodies in Patients with SLE

	Incidence, %	Antigen Detected	Clinical Importance
Antinuclear antibodies	98	Multiple nuclear	Human cell substrates are more sensitive than murine. Repeatedly negative tests make SLE unlikely.
Anti-DNA	70	DNA (ds)	Anti-dsDNA is relatively disease-specific; anti-ssDNA is not. High titers are associated with nephritis and clinical activity.
Anti-Sm	30	Protein complexed to 6 species of small nuclear RNA	Specific for SLE.
Anti-RNP	40	Protein complexed to U1RNA	High titer in syndromes with features of polymyositis, lupus, scleroderma, and mixed connective tissue disease. If present in SLE without anti-DNA, risk for nephritis is low.
Anti-Ro (SS-A)	30	Protein complexed to y_1–y_5 RNA	Associated with Sjögren's syndrome, subacute cutaneous lupus, inherited C′ deficiencies, ANA-negative lupus, lupus in the elderly, neonatal lupus, congenital heart block. Can cause nephritis.
Anti-La (SS-B)	10	Phosphoprotein	Always associated with anti-Ro. Risk for nephritis is low if present. Associated with Sjögren's syndrome.
Antihistone	70	Histones	More frequent in drug-induced LE (95%) than in spontaneous SLE.
Antiphospholipid	50	Phospholipids	Three types—lupus anticoagulant (LA), anticardiolipin (aCL), and false-positive test for syphilis (BFP). The LA and aCL (particular high-titer IgG) are associated with clotting, fetal loss, thrombocytopenia, and valvular heart disease.
Antierythrocyte	60	Erythrocyte	A small proportion of these patients develop overt hemolysis.
Antiplatelet		Platelet surface	Associated with thrombocytopenia.
Antilymphocyte	70	Lymphocyte surface	Probably associated with leukopenia and abnormal T cell function.
Antineuronal	60	Neuronal and lymphocyte surface	In some series, high titers of IgG correlate with diffuse CNS lupus.
Antiribosomal P	20	Ribosomal P protein	In some series, antibody in serum correlates with psychosis or depression due to CNS SLE.

Table 312-2

Clinical Manifestations of SLE

	Percent of Patients Positive during Course of Disease
Systemic	95
Fatigue, malaise, fever, anorexia, nausea, weight loss	
Musculoskeletal	95
Arthralgias/myalgias	95
Nonerosive polyarthritis	60
Hand deformities	10
Myopathy/myositis	40/5
Ischemic necrosis of bone	15
Cutaneous	80
Malar rash	50
Discoid rash	15
Photosensitivity	70
Oral ulcers	40
Other rashes—maculopapular, urticarial, bullous, subacute cutaneous lupus	40
Alopecia	40
Vasculitis	20
Panniculitis	5
Hematologic	85
Anemia (of chronic disease)	70
Hemolytic anemia	10
Leukopenia (<4000/mm³)	65
Lymphopenia (<1500/mm³)	50
Thrombocytopenia (<100,000/mm³)	15
Circulating anticoagulant	10–20
Splenomegaly	15
Lymphadenopathy	20
Neurologic	60
Cognitive dysfunction	50
Organic brain syndromes	35
Psychosis	10
Seizures	20
Headache	25
Other CNS (see text)	15
Peripheral neuropathy	15
Cardiopulmonary	60
Pleurisy	50
Pericarditis	30
Myocarditis	10
Endocarditis (Libman-Sachs)	10
Pleural effusions	30
Lupus pneumonitis	10
Interstitial fibrosis	5
Pulmonary hypertension	<5
ARDS/hemorrhage	<5
Renal	50
Proteinuria >500 mg/24 h	50
Cellular casts	50
Nephrotic syndrome	25
Renal failure	5–10
Gastrointestinal	45
Nonspecific (anorexia, nausea, mild pain, diarrhea)	30
Vasculitis with bleeding or perforation	5
Ascites	<5
Abnormal liver enzymes	40
Thrombosis	15
Venous	10
Arterial	5
Fetal loss	30 (of pregnancies)
Ocular	15
Retinal vasculitis	5
Conjunctivitis/episcleritis	10
Sicca syndrome	15

Table 312-3

The 1982 Criteria for Classification of Systemic Lupus Erythematosus

1. Malar rash	Fixed erythema, flat or raised, over the malar eminences
2. Discoid rash	Erythematous raised patches with adherent keratotic scaling and follicular plugging; atrophic scarring may occur
3. Photosensitivity	
4. Oral ulcers	Includes oral and nasopharyngeal, observed by physician
5. Arthritis	Nonerosive arthritis involving two or more peripheral joints, characterized by tenderness, swelling, or effusion
6. Serositis	Pleuritis or pericarditis documented by ECG or rub or evidence of pericardial effusion
7. Renal disorder	Proteinuria greater than 0.5 g/d or greater than 3 +, or cellular casts
8. Neurologic disorder	Seizures without other cause or psychosis without other cause
9. Hematologic disorder	Hemolytic anemia or leukopenia (less than 4000/μL) or lymphopenia (less than 1500/μL) or thrombocytopenia (less than 100,000/μL) in the absence of offending drugs
10. Immunologic disorder	Positive LE cell preparation or anti-dsDNA or anti-Sm antibodies or false-positive VDRL
11. Antinuclear antibodies	An abnormal titer of ANAs by immunofluorescence or an equivalent assay at any point in time in the absence of drugs known to induce ANAs

If four of these criteria are present at any time during the course of disease, a diagnosis of systemic lupus can be made with 98 percent specificity and 97 percent sensitivity.

SOURCE: Criteria published by EM Tan et al, Arthritis Rheum 25:1271, 1982

proportion of sclerotic glomeruli on biopsy; they are unlikely to respond to immunosuppressive therapies and are candidates for dialysis or transplantation. Patients with persistently abnormal urinalyses, high titers of anti-dsDNA, and/or hypocomplementemia are at risk for severe nephritis; kidney biopsy may guide therapy.

Nervous System Any region of the brain can be involved in SLE, as can the meninges, spinal cord, and cranial and peripheral nerves. Central nervous system (CNS) events may be single or multiple and often occur when SLE is active in other organ systems. Mild cognitive dysfunction is the most frequent manifestation. Headaches are common and may be migrainelike or nonspecific. Seizures of any type may occur. Less frequent manifestations include psychosis, organic brain syndromes, focal infarcts, extrapyramidal disorders, cerebellar dysfunction, hypothalamic dysfunction with inappropriate antidiuretic hormone (ADH) secretion, pseudotumor cerebri, subarachnoid hemorrhage, aseptic meningitis, transverse myelitis, optic neuritis, cranial nerve palsies, and peripheral sensorimotor neuropathy. Depression and anxiety, usually related to being chronically ill and not to active SLE, are frequent.

Laboratory diagnosis of CNS lupus can be difficult. Abnormal electroencephalograms occur in about 70 percent of patients and usually show diffuse slowing or focal abnormalities. Cerebrospinal fluid (CSF) shows elevated protein levels in 50 percent and increased mononuclear cells in 30 percent of patients; oligoclonal bands, increased Ig synthesis, and antineuronal antibodies may be found. Lumbar puncture should be performed whenever CNS symptoms could result from infection, especially in immunosuppressed patients. Computed tomography (CT) scans and angiograms are most likely to be positive when focal neurologic deficits are present and are less helpful in cases with diffuse manifestations. Magnetic resonance imaging is the most sensitive radiographic technique to detect changes of SLE; changes are often nonspecific. Laboratory measures of disease activity often do not correlate with neurologic manifestations. Neurologic problems (with the exception of deficits resulting from large infarcts) usually improve with immunosuppressive therapy and/or time; recurrences are seen in approximately one-third of patients.

Vascular System Thrombosis in vessels of any size can be a major problem. Although vasculitis may underly thrombosis, there is increasing evidence that antibodies against phospholipids (lupus anticoagulant, anticardiolipin) are associated with clotting without inflammation. In addition, degenerative vascular changes after years of exposure of blood vessels to circulating immune complexes and hyperlipidemia from glucocorticoid therapy predispose to degenerative coronary artery disease in lupus patients. Therefore, anticoagulation is more appropriate than immunosuppression in some patients.

Hematologic Manifestation Anemia of chronic disease occurs in most patients when lupus is active. Hemolysis occurs in a small proportion of those with positive Coombs' tests; it is usually responsive to high-dose glucocorticoids; resistant cases may respond to splenectomy. Leukopenia (usually lymphopenia) is common but is rarely associated with recurrent infections and does not require treatment. Mild thrombocytopenia is common; severe thrombocytopenia with bleeding and purpura occurs in 5 percent of patients and should be treated with high-dose glucocorticoids. Short-term improvement can be achieved by administration of intravenous gamma globulin. If the platelet count fails to reach acceptable levels in 2 weeks, addition of cytotoxic drugs and/or splenectomy should be considered.

The lupus anticoagulant (LA) belongs to a family of antiphospholipid antibodies. It is recognized by prolongation of the partial thromboplastin time and failure of added normal plasma to correct the prolongation. More sensitive tests include the Russell viper venom time and the rabbit brain neutral phospholipid test. Antibodies to cardiolipin (aCL) are detected in enzyme-linked immunosorbent assays (ELISA). Clinical manifestations of LA and aCL include thrombocytopenia, recurrent venous or arterial clotting, recurrent fetal loss, and valvular heart disease. If the LA is associated with hypoprothrombinemia or thrombocytopenia, bleeding may occur. Less commonly, antibodies to clotting factors (VIII, IX) arise; they cause bleeding. Bleeding syndromes usually respond to glucocorticoids; clotting syndromes do not.

Cardiopulmonary System Pericarditis is the most frequent manifestation of cardiac lupus; effusions can occur and occasionally lead to tamponade; constrictive pericarditis is rare. Myocarditis can cause arrhythmias, sudden death, and/or heart failure. Valvular insufficiency (usually aortic or mitral) is an uncommon sequel of Libman Sachs endocarditis and may be a source of cerebral emboli; this syndrome is probably associated with antiphospholipid antibodies. Myocardial infarcts usually result from degenerative disease, although they can result from vasculitis.

Pleurisy and pleural effusions are common manifestations of SLE. Lupus pneumonitis causes fever, dyspnea, and cough; x-rays show fleeting infiltrates and/or areas of platelike atelectasis; this syndrome responds to glucocorticoids. However, *the most common cause of pulmonary infiltrates in patients with SLE is infection.* Interstitial pneumonitis leading to fibrosis occurs occasionally; the inflammatory phase may respond to treatment; the fibrosis does not. Pulmonary hypertension is an uncommon, grave manifestation of SLE. Infrequent pulmonary manifestations with high mortality include adult respiratory distress syndrome and massive intraalveolar hemorrhage.

Gastrointestinal System Common gastrointestinal (GI) symptoms include nausea, diarrhea, and vague discomfort. Symptoms may result from lupus peritonitis and may herald a flare of SLE. Vasculitis of the intestine is the most dangerous manifestation, presenting with acute crampy abdominal pain, vomiting, and diarrhea. Intestinal perforation can occur and usually requires immediate surgery. Patients with pseudoobstruction have abdominal pain; x-rays show dilated loops of small bowel which may be edematous; surgery should be avoided unless frank obstruction is present. Glucocorticoid therapy is useful for all these GI syndromes. Some patients have GI motility disorders similar to those in scleroderma; they are not benefited by steroids. Acute pancreatitis occurs and can be severe, resulting from active SLE or from therapy with glucocorticoids or azathioprine. Elevated amylase levels may reflect pancreatitis, salivary gland inflammation, or macroamylasemia. Elevated serum transaminase levels are common

in patients with active SLE but are not associated with significant hepatic damage; they return to normal as the disease is treated.

Ocular Manifestation Retinal vasculitis is a serious manifestation; blindness can develop over a few days, and aggressive immunosuppression should be instituted. Examination shows areas of sheathed, narrow retinal arterioles and cytoid bodies (white exudates) adjacent to vessels. Other ocular abnormalities include conjunctivitis, episcleritis, optic neuritis, and the sicca syndrome.

PATHOLOGY **Cutaneous Lesions** Lesions of acute SLE, DLE, and SCLE show similar histopathology, with degeneration of the basal layer of the epidermis, disruption of the dermal-epidermal junction (DEJ), and mononuclear infiltrates around vessels and appendages in the upper dermis. In DLE, follicular plugging and hyperkeratosis are prominent. Deposits of Ig and C' are seen in the DEJ in 80 to 100 percent of lesional and 50 percent of nonlesional skin in active SLE; the proportions are lower during remissions. Only 50 percent of SCLE lesions are positive for Ig and C' deposits. Ig deposition in the DEJ is not specific for SLE. Vasculitic skin lesions usually show leukocytoclastic angiitis.

Renal Lesions Glomerulonephritis (GN) is caused by deposition of circulating immune complexes or in situ complex formation in mesangium and GBM. Renal biopsy should be considered when results would affect therapy. Information regarding location of immune deposits, histologic pattern of renal damage, and activity and chronicity of lesions are all useful in predicting prognosis and selecting appropriate treatment. In mild GN unlikely to lead to renal failure, Ig deposits are confined to the mesangium, and histology shows no changes or mesangial proliferation. If Ig and C' are deposited outside the mesangium in capillary GBM, prognosis worsens. Histologic changes that should be treated with aggressive immunosuppression include focal proliferative, membranoproliferative, and diffuse proliferative GN (see Chap. 275). Progression from focal to diffuse lesions can occur. Membranous changes without proliferation are uncommon but have a better prognosis than proliferative GN. Activity and chronicity scores indicate severity and reversibility of lesions. *Reversible "active" lesions* associated with high risk of progression to renal failure are glomerular necrosis, cellular epithelial crescents, hyaline thrombi, interstitial inflammatory infiltrates, and necrotizing vasculitis. *Irreversible changes unlikely to respond to immunosuppression* and highly associated with renal failure include glomerular sclerosis, fibrous crescents, interstitial fibrosis, and tubular atrophy. In patients with high chronicity scores, treatment of lupus should be determined by extrarenal disease.

LABORATORY MANIFESTATIONS The presence of characteristic antibodies (Table 312-1) confirms the diagnosis of SLE. ANAs are the best screening test. If the test substrate contains human nuclei (WIL-2 or HEP-2 cells), more than 95 percent of lupus patients will be positive. A positive ANA test is not specific for SLE; ANA occur in some normal individuals (usually in low titer); the frequency increases with aging. Other autoimmune diseases, viral infections, chronic inflammatory processes, and several drugs induce ANA. Therefore, a positive ANA test supports the diagnosis of SLE but is not specific; a negative ANA test makes the diagnosis unlikely but not impossible. Antibodies to double-stranded DNA (dsDNA) and to Sm are relatively specific for SLE; other autoantibodies listed in Table 312-1 are not. However, determining the complete autoantibody profile of each patient helps predict clinical subsets. High serum levels of ANA and anti-dsDNA and low levels of complement usually reflect disease activity, especially in patients with nephritis. Total functional hemolytic complement (CH_{50}) levels are the most sensitive measure of complement activation but are also most subject to laboratory error. Quantitative levels of C3 and C4 are widely available. Very low levels of CH_{50} with normal levels of C3 suggest inherited deficiency of a complement component, which is highly associated with SLE and with ANA negativity.

Hematologic abnormalities include anemia (usually normochromic normocytic but occasionally hemolytic), leukopenia, lymphopenia, and thrombocytopenia. The Westergren erythrocyte sedimentation rate correlates with disease activity in some patients.

Urinalysis should be performed and serum creatinine levels should be measured periodically in patients with SLE. With active nephritis, the urinalysis usually shows proteinuria, hematuria, and cellular or granular casts. Urinary protein excretion measured over 24 h increases during periods of activity. (See the discussion under "Pathology" for a description of renal biopsy.)

PREGNANCY   Fertility rates are normal in patients with SLE, but spontaneous abortion and stillbirths are frequent (10 to 30 percent), especially in women with LA and/or aCL. Treatment of women with prior fetal loss and antiphospholipid antibodies is controversial. Options are no intervention, daily low-dose aspirin until the last month, low-dose aspirin plus daily high-dose glucocorticoids, and twice daily subcutaneous heparin in full anticoagulating doses; there are data to support each approach.

Pregnancy has varied effects on SLE activity. Disease flares in a small proportion, especially during the 6 weeks postpartum. If severe renal or cardiac disease is absent and SLE activity is controlled, most patients complete pregnancy safely and deliver normal infants. Glucocorticoids (except dexamethasone and betamethasone) are inactivated by placental enzymes and do not cause fetal abnormalities in humans; they should be used to suppress disease activity. Neonatal lupus, caused by transmission of maternal anti-Ro across the placenta, consists of transient skin rash and (rarely) permanent heart block. Transient thrombocytopenia from maternal antiplatelet antibodies also occurs.

DIFFERENTIAL DIAGNOSIS   The American Rheumatism Association published diagnostic criteria for SLE (Table 312-3). Any four of the manifestations listed establish a diagnosis of SLE. Early disease confined to a few systems is more difficult to classify; it may take several years for a patient to fulfill criteria. Disorders with which SLE can be confused include rheumatoid arthritis; various forms of dermatitis; neurologic disorders such as epilepsy, multiple sclerosis, and psychiatric disorders; and hematologic diseases such as idiopathic thrombocytopenic purpura. Many autoimmune disorders have overlapping features so that exact classification may be difficult. Mixed connective tissue disease has features of SLE, rheumatoid arthritis, polymyositis, and scleroderma, accompanied by high titers of anti-RNP antibodies (Chap 314); patients have a low incidence of nephritis and CNS disease and a high incidence of pulmonary manifestations and evolution into scleroderma. The possibility of drug-induced lupus should always be considered. Figure 312-1 presents an algorithm for diagnosis of SLE.

DRUG-INDUCED LUPUS   Several drugs can cause a syndrome resembling SLE, including procainamide, hydralazine, isoniazid, chlorpromazine, D-penicillamine, practolol, methyldopa, quinidine, interferon α, and possibly hydantoin, ethosuximide, and oral contraceptives. The syndrome is rare with all but procainamide, the most frequent offender, and hydralazine. There is genetic predisposition to drug-induced lupus, partly determined by drug acetylation rates. Procainamide induces ANA in 50 to 75 percent of individuals within a few months; hydralazine induces ANA in 25 to 30 percent. Between 10 and 20 percent of ANA-positive individuals develop lupuslike symptoms. Most common are systemic complaints and arthralgias; polyarthritis and pleuropericarditis occur in 25 to 50 percent. Renal and CNS diseases are rare. All patients have ANA and most have antibodies to histones. Antibodies to dsDNA and hypocomplementemia are rare—a helpful point in distinguishing drug-induced from idiopathic lupus. Anemia, leukopenia, LA, aCL, thrombocytopenia, cryoglobulins, rheumatoid factors, and false-positive VDRL, and positive direct Coombs' tests can occur. The initial therapeutic approach is withdrawal of the offending drug; most patients improve in a few weeks. If symptoms are severe, a short course (2 to 10 weeks) of glucocorticoids is indicated. Symptoms rarely persist more than 6 months; ANA may persist for years. Most lupus-inducing drugs can be used safely in patients with idiopathic SLE.

FIGURE 312-1   Algorithm for the diagnosis of SLE. ANA, antinuclear antibody; ARA, American Rheumatism Association; CTD, connective tissue disease; CBC, complete blood count; *, ANA titer ≥ 1 : 80.

PROGNOSIS   Survival in patients with SLE is 90 to 95 percent at 2 years, 82 to 90 percent at 5 years, 71 to 80 percent at 10 years, and 63 to 75 percent at 20 years. The following factors have been associated with poor prognosis (approximately 50 percent mortality in 10 years) in multiple studies: high serum creatinine levels (>1.4 mg/dL), hypertension, nephrotic syndrome (24-h urine protein excretion >2.6 g), anemia, hypoalbuminemia and hypocomplementemia at the time of diagnosis, and low socioeconomic status. Other factors associated with a poor prognosis in some but not all studies include thrombocytopenia, serious CNS involvement, antibodies to phospholipids, and non-Caucasian race. Disability in SLE patients is common. However, aproximately 20 percent of patients experience disease remissions (with a mean duration of 5 years), regardless of the severity of disease at diagnosis. Some 50 percent in remission remain in remission for decades, and the likelihood of remission increases with each decade after diagnosis. Infections and renal failure are the leading causes of death in the first decade of disease. Thromboembolic events are frequent causes of death in the second decade.

℞ **TREATMENT**
There is no cure for SLE. Complete remissions are rare. Therefore, patient and physician should plan (1) to control acute, severe flares, and (2) to develop maintenance strategies in which symptoms are suppressed to an acceptable level, usually at the cost of some drug side effects. Approximately 25 percent of SLE patients have mild disease with no life-threatening manifestations, although pain and fatigue may be disabling. These patients should be managed without glucocorticoids. Arthralgias, arthritis, myalgias, fever, and mild sero-

sitis may improve on nonsteroidal anti-inflammatory drugs (NSAIDs) including salicylates. However, NSAID toxicities such as elevated serum transaminases, aseptic meningitis, and renal impairment are especially frequent in SLE. The dermatitides of SLE, fatigue, and lupus arthritis may respond to antimalarials. Doses of 400 mg hydroxychloroquine daily may improve skin lesions in a few weeks. Side effects are uncommon and include retinal toxicity, rash, myopathy, and neuropathy. Regular ophthalmologic examinations should be performed at least annually, since retinal toxicity is related to cumulative dose. Other therapies for rash include sunscreens (an SPF rating ≥ 15 is recommended), topical or intralesional glucocorticoids, quinacrine, retinoids, and dapsone. Recent studies suggest that daily oral doses of dihydroepiandrosterone (DHEA) may lower disease activity in patients with mild SLE. Systemic glucocorticoids should be reserved for patients with disabling disease unresponsive to these conservative measures.

Life-threatening, severely disabling manifestations of SLE that are responsive to immunosuppression should be treated with high doses of *glucocorticoids* (1 to 2 mg/kg per day). When disease is active, glucocorticoids should be given in divided doses every 8 to 12 h. After the disease is controlled, therapy should be consolidated to one morning dose; thereafter the daily dose should be tapered as rapidly as clinical disease permits. Ideally, patients should be slowly converted to alternate-day therapy with a single morning dose of short-acting glucocorticoid (prednisone, prednisolone, methylprednisolone) to minimize side effects. However, the disease may flare on the day off steroids, in which case the lowest single daily dose that suppresses disease should be used. Acutely ill lupus patients, including those with proliferative GN, can be treated with 3 to 5 days of 1000 mg intravenous "pulses" of methylprednisolone, followed by maintenance daily or alternate-day glucocorticoids. Disease flares are probably controlled more rapidly by this approach, but it is unclear whether long-term outcome is changed.

Undesirable effects of chronic glucocorticoid therapy include cushingoid habitus, weight gain, hypertension, infection, capillary fragility, acne, hirsutism, accelerated osteoporosis, ischemic necrosis of bone, cataracts, glaucoma, diabetes mellitus, myopathy, hypokalemia, irregular menses, irritability, insomnia, and psychosis. Prednisone doses of 15 mg daily (or less) given before noon usually do not suppress the hypothalamic-pituitary axis. Some side effects can be minimized; hyperglycemia, hypertension, edema, and hypokalemia should be treated; infections should be identified and treated early; immunizations with influenza and pneumococcal vaccines are safe and should be given if disease is stable. To minimize osteoporosis, supplemental calcium (1000 mg daily) should be added in most patients; in those with 24-h urinary calcium excretion <120 mg, vitamin D, 50,000 units one to three times weekly, can be added (monitor for hypercalcemia). Estrogen replacement therapy (ERT) should be considered at menopause. There is debate regarding the ability of oral contraceptives or ERT to cause flares of SLE in some patients; these therapies should be withheld from patients with a history of thrombosis. Calcitonin and bisphosphonates are also useful in preventing and treating osteoporosis.

The use of *cytotoxic agents* (azathioprine, chlorambucil, cyclophosphamide) in SLE is probably beneficial in controlling active disease, reducing the rate of disease flares, and reducing steroid requirements. Patients with lupus nephritis have significantly less renal failure if treated with combinations of glucocorticoids plus cyclophosphamide; azathioprine as the second drug is less beneficial but is also effective. However, overall survival is not different, probably because renal failure usually leads to dialysis or transplantation rather than to death. Undesirable side effects of cytotoxic drugs include bone marrow suppression, increased infection with opportunistic organisms such as herpes zoster, irreversible ovarian failure, hepatotoxicity (azathioprine), bladder toxicity (cyclophosphamide), alopecia, and increased risk for malignancy. Azathioprine is the least toxic; recommended doses are 2 to 3 mg/kg per day orally. Cyclophosphamide is the most effective and the most toxic. Intravenous pulse doses (10 to 15 mg/kg) once every 4 weeks have less

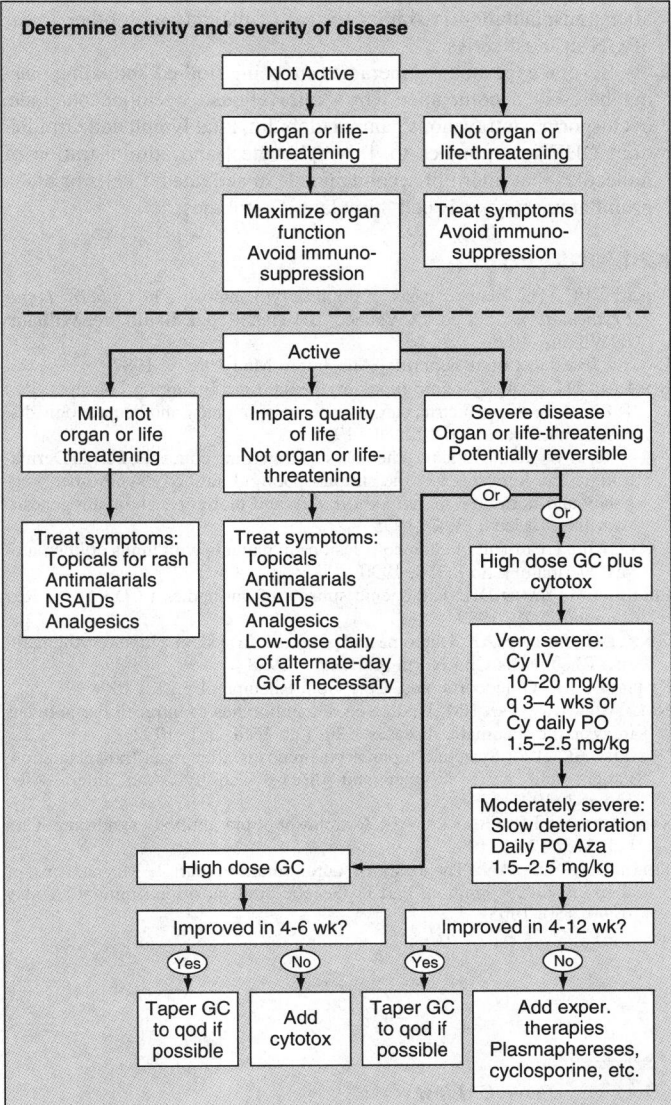

FIGURE 312-2 Algorithm for the treatment of SLE. GC, glucocorticoids; high-dose GC, methylprednisolone 1000 mg, IV, qd × 3, then 1 to 2 mg/kg prednisone per day orally, or 1 to 2 mg/kg prednisone per day orally; cytotox, cytotoxic drugs such as cyclophosphamide (Cy) and azathioprine (Aza); qod, alternate day therapy.

urinary bladder toxicity than daily oral doses, but bone marrow suppression can be severe. Cyclophosphamide can also be used in daily oral doses (1.5 to 2.5 mg/kg per day of each). After disease activity has been controlled for a few months, tapering of cytotoxic agents and attempts to discontinue them are appropriate. Figure 312-2 presents an algorithm for treatment of SLE.

Some manifestations of SLE do not respond to immunosuppression, including clotting disorders, some behavioral abnormalities, and end-stage GN. Anticoagulation is the therapy of choice for prevention of clotting; chronic warfarin therapy in relatively high doses (maintaining INR at 2.5 to 3.0) is effective in preventing venous and arterial clotting in patients with antiphospholipid syndromes; the effects of aspirin and heparin on arterial thrombosis are unclear. Psychoactive drugs should be used when appropriate. "Pure" membranous GN may not respond to immunosuppression; several weeks of therapy can be tried but should be abandoned if improvement is not obvious. The survival of lupus patients on dialysis or after transplantation is similar to that of patients with other forms of GN in most series.

Several experimental therapies are being studied, including plasmapheresis accompanied by intravenous cyclophosphamide, cyclosporine, intravenous gamma globulin, total lymph node irradiation, DHEA, antibodies to T lymphocytes, and administration of molecules that interrupt second signals in activated T cells or block proinflammatory or B cell stimulating cytokines.

BIBLIOGRAPHY

ARNETT FC: The genetic basis of lupus erythematosus, in *Dubois' Lupus Erythematosus*, 5th ed, D Wallace, BH Hahn (eds). Baltimore, Williams & Wilkins, 1996

BALOW JE et al: Lupus nephritis. Ann Intern Med 106:79, 1987

BOUMPAS DT et al: Systemic lupus erythematosus: Emerging concepts. Part 1: Renal, neuropychiatric, cardiovascular, pulmonary and hematologic disease. Ann Intern Med 122:940, 1995

———— et al: Systemic lupus erythematosus: Emerging concepts. Part 2: Dermatologic and joint disease, the antiphospholipid antibody syndrome, pregnancy and hormonal therapy, morbidity and mortality, and pathogenesis. Ann Intern Med 123:42, 1995

CALLEN JP: Treatment of cutaneous lesions in patients with lupus erythematosus. Dermatol Clin 8:355, 1990

EBLING FM, HAHN BH: Pathogenic subsets of antibodies to DNA. Int Rev Immunol 5:79, 1989

GINZLER E, SCHORN AK: Outcome and prognosis in systemic lupus erythematosus. Rheum Dis Clin North Am 14:67, 1988

KIMBERLY RP: Glucocorticoids. Curr Opin Rheumatol 6:273, 1994

NAKAMURA RM, TAN EM: Update on autoantibodies to intracellular antigens in systemic rheumatic diseases. Clin Lab Med 12:1, 1992

NOSSENT HC et al: Systemic lupus erythematosus after renal transplantation: Patient and graft survival and disease activity. Ann Intern Med 114:183, 1991

SAMMARITANO LR, GHARAVI AE: Antiphospholipid antibody syndrome. Clin Lab Med 12:41, 1992

THEOFILOPOULOS AN: The basis of autoimmunity: Part I. Mechanisms of aberrant self-recognition. Part II. Genetic predisposition. Immunol Today 16:90, 150, 1995

---

313 *Peter E. Lipsky*

RHEUMATOID ARTHRITIS

Rheumatoid arthritis (RA) is a chronic multisystem disease of unknown cause. Although there are a variety of systemic manifestations, the characteristic feature of RA is persistent inflammatory synovitis, usually involving peripheral joints in a symmetric distribution. The potential of the synovial inflammation to cause cartilage destruction and bone erosions and subsequent changes in joint integrity is the hallmark of the disease. Despite its destructive potential, the course of RA can be quite variable. Some patients may experience only a mild oligoarticular illness of brief duration with minimal joint damage, whereas others will have a relentless progressive polyarthritis with marked functional impairment.

EPIDEMIOLOGY AND GENETICS The prevalence of RA is approximately 0.8 percent of the population (range 0.3 to 2.1 percent); women are affected approximately three times more often than men. The prevalence increases with age, and sex differences diminish in the older age group. RA is seen throughout the world and affects all races. However, the incidence and severity seem to be less in rural sub-Saharan Africa and in Caribbean blacks. The onset is most frequent during the fourth and fifth decades of life, with 80 percent of all patients developing the disease between the ages of 35 and 50. The incidence of RA is more than six times as great in 60- to 64-year-old women compared to 18- to 29-year-old women.

Family studies indicate a genetic predisposition. For example, severe RA is found at approximately four times the expected rate in first-degree relatives of individuals with disease associated with the presence of the autoantibody, rheumatoid factor; approximately 10 percent of patients with RA will have an affected first-degree relative. Moreover, monozygotic twins are at least four times more likely to be concordant for RA than dizygotic twins, who have a similar risk of developing RA as nontwin siblings. Approximately only 15 to 20 percent of monozygotic twins are concordant for RA, however, implying that factors other than genetics play an important etiopathogenic role. One of the major genetic factors in the etiology of RA is the class II major histocompatibility complex (MHC) gene product HLA-DR4. As many as 70 percent of patients with classic or definite RA express HLA-DR4 compared with 28 percent of control individuals. An association with HLA-DR4 has been noted in many populations, including North American and European whites, Chippewa Indians, Japanese, and native populations in India, Mexico, South America, and southern China. In a number of groups, including Israeli Jews, Asian Indians, and Yakima Indians of North America, however, there is no association between the development of RA and HLA-DR4. In these individuals, there is an association between RA and HLA-DR1 in the former two groups and HLA-Dw16 in the latter. Molecular analysis of HLA-DR antigens has provided insight into these apparently disparate findings. The HLA-DR molecule is composed of two chains, a nonpolymorphic α chain and a highly polymorphic β chain. Allelic variations in the HLA-DR molecule reflect differences in the amino acids of the β chain, with the major amino acid changes occurring in the three hypervariable regions of the molecule. Each of the HLA-DR molecules that is associated with RA has the same or a very similar sequence of amino acids in the third hypervariable region of the β chain of the molecule (Table 313-1). Thus the β chains of the HLA-DR molecules associated with RA, including HLA-Dw4 (DRβ1*0401), HLA-Dw14 (DRβ1*0404), HLA-Dw15 (DRβ1*0405), HLA-DR1 (DRβ1*0101), and HLA-Dw16 (DRβ1*1402), contain the same amino acids at positions 67 through 74, with the exception of a single change of one basic amino acid for another (arginine → lysine) in position 71 of HLA-Dw4. All other HLA-DR β chains have amino acid changes in this region that alter either their charge or hydrophobicity. These results indicate that a particular amino acid sequence in the third hypervariable region of the HLA-DR molecule is a major genetic element conveying susceptibility to RA, regardless of whether it occurs in HLA-DR4, HLA-Dw16, or HLA-DR1. It has been estimated that the risk of developing RA in a person with HLA-Dw4 (DRβ1*0401) or HLA-Dw14 (DRβ1*0404) is 1 in 35 and 1 in 20, respectively, whereas the presence of both alleles puts persons at an even greater risk. The lack of association of HLA-DR4 and RA in certain populations is explained by the major member of the DR4 family found in that population. HLA-DR4 is a family of closely related, serologically defined molecules, including HLA-Dw4, -Dw10, -Dw13, and -Dw15. Different members of the HLA-DR family of molecules are found to predominate in different ethnic groups. Thus, in HLA-DR4–positive North American

---

Table 313-1

Amino Acid Sequence of the Third Hypervariable Region of the β Chains of HLA-DR Alleles Associated with Rheumatoid Arthritis

HLA-DR	β Chain	Amino Acid*								Associated with Rheumatoid Arthritis
		67	68	69	70	71	72	73	74	
DR4/Dw4	β1*0401	L	L	E	Q	K	R	A	A	+
DR4/Dw14	β1*0404	—	—	—	—	R	—	—	—	+
DR4/Dw15	β1*0405	—	—	—	—	R	—	—	—	+
DR1	β1*0101	—	—	—	—	R	—	—	—	+
Dw16	β1*1402	—	—	—	—	R	—	—	—	+
DR4/Dw10	β1*0402	I	—	—	D	E	—	—	—	—
DR4/Dw13	β1*0403	—	—	—	—	R	—	—	E	—

* Single-letter amino acid code.

whites, HLA-Dw4 and -Dw14 are the most frequent, whereas HLA-Dw15 is most frequent in Japanese and southern Chinese. Each of these is associated with RA. By contrast, HLA-Dw10, which is not associated with RA and contains nonconservative amino acid changes in positions 70 and 71 of the β chain, is most common in Israeli Jews. Therefore, HLA-DR4 is not associated with RA in this population. In certain groups of patients, there does not appear to be a clear association between HLA-DR4–related epitopes and RA. Thus, nearly 75 percent of African-American RA patients do not have this genetic element. Moreover, there is an association with HLA-DR10 (DRβ1*1001) in Spanish and Italian patients.

Additional genes in the HLA-D complex also may convey altered susceptibility to RA. Certain HLA-DR alleles, including HLA-DR5 (DRβ1*1101), HLA-DR2 (DRβ1*1501), HLA-DR3 (DRβ1*0301), and HLA-DR7 (DRβ1*0701) may protect against the development of RA in that they tend to be found at lower frequency in RA patients than in controls. Moreover, the HLA-DQ alleles, DQβ1*0301, DQβ1*0302, and DQβ1*0501, that are frequently linked to HLA-DR4 or -DR1 have also been associated with RA. Disease manifestations have also been associated with HLA phenotype. Thus, early aggressive disease and extraarticular manifestations are more frequent in patients with DRβ1*0401 or DRβ1*0404, and more slowly progressive disease with DRβ1*0101. The presence of both DRβ1*0401 and DRβ1*0404 appears to increase the risk for both aggressive articular and extraarticular disease. It has been estimated that HLA genes contribute only a portion of the genetic susceptibility to RA. Thus genes outside the HLA complex also contribute. These include genes controlling the expression of the antigen receptor on T cells and both immunoglobulin heavy and light chains.

Genetic risk factors do not fully account for the incidence of RA, suggesting that environmental factors also play a role in the etiology of the disease. This is emphasized by epidemiologic studies in Africa that have indicated that climate and urbanization have a major impact on the incidence and severity of RA in groups of similar genetic background.

Besides an association between the development of RA and genes of the MHC, there appears to be a genetic predisposition for the development of certain toxic reactions induced by drugs used to treat RA. For example, the presence of the HLA-DR3 (DRβ1*0301) allele is highly associated with the development of side effects to gold therapy, including proteinuria, thrombocytopenia, and perhaps skin rash. Similarly, the presence of this allele appears to predispose to the development of proteinuria following therapy with D-penicillamine. In general, no association has been noted between HLA type and the response to therapy.

ETIOLOGY The cause of RA remains unknown. It has been suggested that RA might be a manifestation of the response to an infectious agent in a genetically susceptible host. Because of the worldwide distribution of RA, it has been hypothesized that if an infectious agent is involved, the organism must be ubiquitous. A number of possible causative agents have been suggested, including *Mycoplasma*, Epstein-Barr virus, cytomegalovirus, parvovirus, and rubella virus, but convincing evidence that these or other infectious agents cause RA has not emerged. The process by which an infectious agent might cause chronic inflammatory arthritis with a characteristic distribution also remains a matter of controversy. One possibility is that there is persistent infection of articular structures or retention of microbial products in the synovial tissues which generates a chronic inflammatory response. Alternatively, the microorganism or response to the microorganism might induce an immune response to components of the joint by altering its integrity and revealing antigenic peptides. In this regard, reactivity to type II collagen and heat shock proteins has been demonstrated. Another possibility is that the infecting microorganism might prime the host to cross-reactive determinants expressed within the joint as a result of "molecular mimicry." Recent evidence of similarity between products of certain gram-negative bacteria and the HLA-DR molecule itself has supported this possibility. Finally, products of infecting microorganisms might induce the disease. Recent work has focused on the possible role of "superantigens" produced

by a number of microorganisms, including staphylococci, streptococci and *M. arthritidis*. Superantigens are proteins with the capacity to bind to HLA-DR molecules and particular V_β segments of the heterodimeric T cell receptor and stimulate specific T cells expressing the V_β gene products (see Chap. 305). The role of superantigens in the etiology of RA remains speculative.

PATHOLOGY AND PATHOGENESIS Microvascular injury and an increase in the number of synovial lining cells appear to be the earliest lesions in rheumatoid synovitis. The nature of the insult causing this response is not known. Subsequently, an increased number of synovial lining cells is seen along with perivascular infiltration with mononuclear cells. As the process continues, the synovium becomes edematous and protrudes into the joint cavity as villous projections.

Light-microscopic examination discloses a characteristic constellation of features which include hyperplasia and hypertrophy of the synovial lining cells; focal or segmental vascular changes, including microvascular injury, thrombosis, and neovascularization; edema; and infiltration with mononuclear cells, often collected into aggregates around small blood vessels. The endothelial cells of the rheumatoid synovium have the appearance of high endothelial venules (HEV) of lymphoid organs and have been altered by cytokine exposure to facilitate entry of cells into tissue. Rheumatoid synovial endothelial cells express increased amounts of various adhesion molecules involved in this process. Although this pathologic picture is typical of RA, it also can be seen in a variety of other chronic inflammatory arthritides. The mononuclear cell collections are variable in composition and size. The predominant infiltrating cell is the T lymphocyte. CD4+ T cells predominate over CD8+ T cells and are frequently found in close proximity to HLA-DR+ macrophages and dendritic cells. An increased number of a separate population of T cells expressing the γδ form of the T cell receptor also has been found in the synovium, although they remain a minor population there and their role in RA has not been delineated. The major population of T cells in the rheumatoid synovium is composed of CD4+ memory T cells that form the majority of cells aggregated around postcapillary venules. Scattered throughout the tissue are CD8+ T cells. Both populations express the early activation antigen, CD69. Besides the accumulation of T cells, rheumatoid synovitis is also characterized by the infiltration of large numbers of B cells that differentiate locally into antibody-producing plasma cells. These cells produce both polyclonal immunoglobulin and the autoantibody rheumatoid factor that results in the local formation of immune complexes. Finally, the synovial fibroblasts in RA manifest evidence of activation in that they produce a number of enzymes such as collagenase and cathepsins that can degrade components of the articular matrix. These activated fibroblasts are particularly prominent in the lining layer and at the interface with bone and cartilage. Osteoclasts are also prominent at sites of bone erosion.

The rheumatoid synovium is characterized by the presence of a number of secreted products of activated lymphocytes, macrophages, and fibroblasts. The local production of these cytokines and chemokines appears to account for many of the pathologic and clinical manifestations of RA. These effector molecules include those that are derived from T lymphocytes such as interleukin (IL) 2, interferon γ (IFNγ), IL-6, IL-10, granulocyte-macrophage colony stimulating factor (GM-CSF), tumor necrosis factor α (TNFα), and transforming growth factor β (TGFβ); those originating from activated macrophages, including IL-1, TNFα, IL-6, IL-8, IL-10, GM-CSF, macrophage CSF, platelet-derived growth factor, insulin-like growth factor, and TGFβ; as well as those secreted by other cell types in the synovium, such as fibroblasts and endothelial cells, including IL-1, IL-6, IL-8, GM-CSF, and macrophage CSF. The activity of these chemokines and cytokines appears to account for many of the features of rheumatoid synovitis, including the synovial tissue inflammation, synovial fluid inflammation, synovial proliferation, and cartilage and bone damage, as well as the systemic manifestations of RA. In addition to the production of effector molecules that propagate the inflammatory process, local factors are produced that tend to slow the inflammation, including specific inhibitors of cytokine action and additional cytokines, such as TGFβ, which inhibits many of the features of rheumatoid synovitis including T cell activation and proliferation, B cell differentiation, and migration of cells into the inflammatory site.

These findings have suggested that the propagation of RA is an immunologically mediated event, although the original initiating stimulus has not been characterized. One view is that the inflammatory process in the tissue is driven by the CD4 + T cells infiltrating the synovium. Evidence for this includes (1) the predominance of CD4 + T cells in the synovium; (2) the increase in soluble IL-2 receptors, a product of activated T cells, in blood and synovial fluid of patients with active RA; and (3) amelioration of the disease by removal of T cells by thoracic duct drainage or peripheral lymphapheresis or suppression of their function by drugs, such as cyclosporine. In addition, the association of RA with certain HLA-DR alleles, whose only known functions are to shape the repertoire of CD4 + T cells during ontogeny in the thymus and bind and present antigenic peptides to CD4 + T cells in the periphery, strongly implies a role for CD4 + T cells in the pathogenesis of the disease. Finally, patients with established RA who become infected with the human immunodeficiency virus (HIV) also have been noted to improve, although this has not been a uniform finding. T lymphocytes produce a number of cytokines, including IFNγ and GM-CSF, that can lead to activation of macrophages and also increased expression of HLA molecules. Moreover, T lymphocytes produce a variety of cytokines that promote B cell proliferation and differentiation into antibody-forming cells and therefore also may promote local B cell stimulation. The resultant production of immunoglobulin and rheumatoid factor can lead to immune-complex formation with consequent complement activation and exacerbation of the inflammatory process by the production of the anaphylatoxins, C3a and C5a, and the chemotactic factor C5a. The tissue inflammation is reminiscent of delayed type hypersensitivity reactions occurring in response to soluble antigens or microorganisms, although it has become clear that the number of T cells producing cytokines such as IFNγ is less than is found in typical delayed type hypersensitivity reactions. It remains unclear whether the persistent T cell activity represents a response to a persistent exogenous antigen or to altered autoantigens such as collagen, immunoglobulin, or one of the heat shock proteins. Alternatively, it could represent persistent responsiveness to activated autologous cells such as might occur as a result of Epstein-Barr virus infection or persistent response to a foreign antigen or superantigen in the synovial tissue. Finally, rheumatoid inflammation could reflect persistent stimulation of T cells by synovial-derived antigens that cross-react with determinants introduced during antecedent exposure to foreign antigens or infectious microorganisms.

Overriding the chronic inflammation in the synovial tissue is an acute inflammatory process in the synovial fluid. The exudative synovial fluid contains more polymorphonuclear leukocytes than mononuclear cells. A number of mechanisms play a role in stimulating the exudation of synovial fluid. Locally produced immune complexes can activate complement and generate anaphylatoxins and chemotactic factors. Local production by mononuclear phagocytes of factors such as IL-1, TNFα, and leukotriene B₄, as well as products of complement activation, can stimulate the endothelial cells of postcapillary venules to become more efficient at binding circulating cells, whereas TNFα, IL-8, C5a, and leukotriene B₄ stimulate the migration of polymorphonuclear leukocytes into the synovial site. In addition, vasoactive mediators such as histamine produced by the mast cells that infiltrate the rheumatoid synovium also may facilitate the exudation of inflammatory cells into the synovial fluid. Finally, the vasodilatory effects of locally produced prostaglandin E₂ also may facilitate entry of inflammatory cells into the inflammatory site. Once in the synovial fluid, the polymorphonuclear leukocytes can ingest immune complexes, with the resultant production of reactive oxygen metabolites and other inflammatory mediators, further adding to the inflammatory milieu.

Locally produced cytokines and chemokines such as TNFα, IL-8, and GM-CSF can additionally stimulate polymorphonuclear leukocytes. The production of large amounts of cyclooxygenase and lipoxygenase pathway products of arachidonic acid metabolism by cells in the synovial fluid and tissue further accentuates the signs and symptoms of inflammation.

The precise mechanism by which bone and cartilage destruction occurs has not been completely resolved. Although the synovial fluid contains a number of enzymes potentially able to degrade cartilage, the majority of destruction occurs in juxtaposition to the inflamed synovium, or pannus, that spreads to cover the articular cartilage. This vascular granulation tissue is composed of proliferating fibroblasts, small blood vessels, and a variable number of mononuclear cells and produces a large amount of degradative enzymes, including collagenase and stromelysin, that may facilitate tissue damage. The cytokines IL-1 and TNFα play an important role by stimulating the cells of the pannus to produce collagenase and other neutral proteases. These same two cytokines also activate chondrocytes in situ, stimulating them to produce proteolytic enzymes that can degrade cartilage locally. Finally, these two cytokines may contribute to the local demineralization of bone by activating osteoclasts. Prostaglandin E₂ produced by fibroblasts and macrophages also may contribute to bone demineralization. The common final pathway of bone erosion is likely to involve the activation of osteoclasts that are present in large numbers at these sites. Systemic manifestations of RA can be accounted for by release of inflammatory effector molecules from the synovium. These include IL-1, TNFα, and IL-6, which account for many of the manifestations of active RA, including malaise, fatigue, and elevated levels of serum acute phase reactants. The importance of TNFα in producing these manifestations is emphasized by the prompt amelioration of symptoms following administration of a monoclonal antibody to TNFα to patients with RA. In addition, immune complexes produced within the synovium and entering the circulation may account for other features of the disease, such as systemic vasculitis.

As shown in Fig. 313-1, the pathology of RA evolves over the duration of this chronic disease. The earliest event appears to be a nonspecific inflammatory response initiated by an unknown stimulus. Subsequently, an initial, and perhaps specific, response of CD4 + T cells is induced that amplifies and perpetuates the inflammation. The presence of activated T cells can induce polyclonal B cell stimulation and the local production of rheumatoid factor. As tissue damage occurs, additional autoantigens are revealed and the nature of the T cell response broadens as additional clones of CD4 + T cells are recruited to the inflammatory site. Finally, as a result of persistent exposure to the inflammatory milieu, the function of synovial fibroblasts is altered and they may acquire destructive potential that no longer requires stimulation from T cells or macrophages. Important features of this model include the following: (1) the pathologic events vary with time in this chronic disease; (2) the time required to progress from one

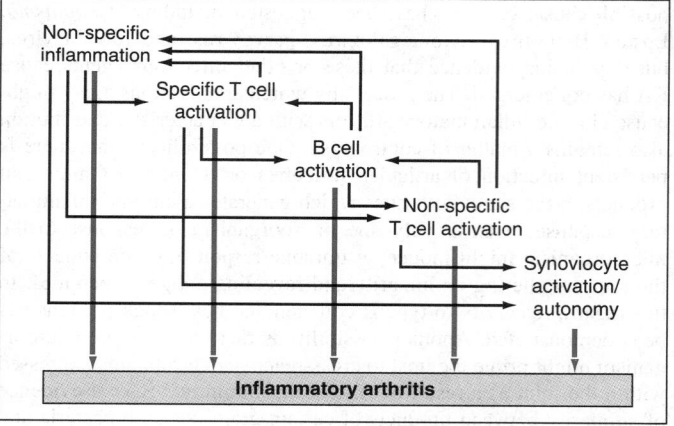

FIGURE 313-1 The progression of rheumatoid synovitis. This figure depicts the evolution of the pathogenic mechanisms and ultimate pathologic changes involved in the development of rheumatoid synovitis.

step to the next may vary in different patients; (3) once established, the major pathogenic events operative in an individual patient may vary at different times. These considerations have important implications with regard to appropriate treatment.

CLINICAL MANIFESTATIONS **Onset** Characteristically, RA is a chronic polyarthritis. In approximately two-thirds of patients, it begins insidiously with fatigue, anorexia, generalized weakness, and vague musculoskeletal symptoms until the appearance of synovitis becomes apparent. This prodrome may persist for weeks or months and defy diagnosis. Specific symptoms usually appear gradually as several joints, especially those of the hands, wrists, knees, and feet, become affected in a symmetric fashion. In approximately 10 percent of individuals, the onset is more acute, with a rapid development of polyarthritis, often accompanied by constitutional symptoms, including fever, lymphadenopathy, and splenomegaly. In approximately one-third of patients, symptoms may initially be confined to one or a few joints. Although the pattern of joint involvement may remain asymmetric in a few patients, a symmetric pattern is more typical.

Signs and Symptoms of Articular Disease Pain, swelling, and tenderness may initially be poorly localized to the joints. Pain in affected joints, aggravated by movement, is the most common manifestation of established RA. It corresponds in pattern to the joint involvement but does not always correlate with the degree of apparent inflammation. Generalized stiffness is frequent and is usually greatest after periods of inactivity. Morning stiffness of greater than 1-h duration is an almost invariable feature of inflammatory arthritis and may serve to distinguish it from various noninflammatory joint disorders. Recent evidence suggests, however, that the presence of morning stiffness may not reliably distinguish between chronic inflammatory and noninflammatory arthritides, as it is also found frequently in the latter. The majority of patients will experience constitutional symptoms such as weakness, easy fatigability, anorexia, and weight loss. Although fever to 40°C occurs on occasion, temperature elevation in excess of 38°C is unusual and suggests the presence of an intercurrent problem such as infection.

Clinically, synovial inflammation causes swelling, tenderness, and limitation of motion. Warmth is usually evident on examination, especially of large joints such as the knee, but erythema is infrequent. Pain originates predominantly from the joint capsule, which is abundantly supplied with pain fibers and is markedly sensitive to stretching or distention. Joint swelling results from accumulation of synovial fluid, hypertrophy of the synovium, and thickening of the joint capsule. Initially, motion is limited by pain. The inflamed joint is usually held in flexion to maximize joint volume and minimize distention of the capsule. Later, fibrous or bony ankylosis or soft tissue contractures lead to fixed deformities.

Although inflammation can affect any diarthrodial joint, RA most often causes symmetric arthritis with characteristic involvement of certain specific joints such as the proximal interphalangeal and metacarpophalangeal joints. The distal interphalangeal joints are rarely involved. Synovitis of the wrist joints is a nearly uniform feature of RA and may lead to limitation of motion, deformity, and median nerve entrapment (carpal tunnel syndrome). Synovitis of the elbow joint often leads to flexion contractures that may develop early in the disease. The knee joint is commonly involved with synovial hypertrophy, chronic effusion, and frequently ligamentous laxity. Pain and swelling behind the knee may be caused by extension of inflamed synovium into the popliteal space (Baker's cyst). Arthritis in the forefoot, ankles, and subtalar joints can produce severe pain with ambulation as well as a number of deformities. Axial involvement is usually limited to the upper cervical spine. Involvement of the lumbar spine is not seen, and lower back pain cannot be ascribed to rheumatoid inflammation. On occasion, inflammation from the synovial joints and bursae of the upper cervical spine leads to atlantoaxial subluxation. This usually presents as pain in the occiput but on rare occasions may lead to compression of the spinal cord.

With persistent inflammation, a variety of characteristic deformities develop. These can be attributed to a number of pathologic events, including laxity of supporting soft tissue structures; destruction or weakening of ligaments, tendons, and the joint capsule; cartilage destruction; muscle imbalance; and unopposed physical forces associated with the use of affected joints. Characteristic deformities of the hand include (1) radial deviation at the wrist with ulnar deviation of the digits often with palmar subluxation of the proximal phalanges ("Z" deformity), (2) hyperextension of the proximal interphalangeal joints, with compensatory flexion of the distal interphalangeal joints (swanneck deformity), (3) flexion deformity of the proximal interphalangeal joints and extension of the distal interphalangeal joints (boutonnière deformity), and (4) hyperextension of the first interphalangeal joint and flexion of the first metacarpophalangeal joint with a consequent loss of thumb mobility and pinch. Typical deformities also may develop in the feet, including eversion at the hindfoot (subtalar joint), plantar subluxation of the metatarsal heads, widening of the forefoot, hallux valgus, and lateral deviation and dorsal subluxation of the toes.

Extraarticular Manifestations RA is a systemic disease with a variety of extraarticular manifestations. Although these occur frequently, not all of them have clinical significance. However, on occasion, they may be the major evidence of disease activity and source of morbidity and require management per se. As a rule, these manifestations occur in individuals with high titers of autoantibodies to the Fc component of immunoglobulin G (rheumatoid factors).

Rheumatoid nodules develop in 20 to 30 percent of persons with RA. They are usually found on periarticular structures, extensor surfaces, or other areas subjected to mechanical pressure, but they can develop elsewhere, including the pleura and meninges. Common locations include the olecranon bursa, the proximal ulna, the Achilles tendon, and the occiput. Nodules vary in size and consistency and are rarely symptomatic, but on occasion they break down as a result of trauma or become infected. They are found almost invariably in individuals with circulating rheumatoid factor. Histologically, rheumatoid nodules consist of a central zone of necrotic material including collagen fibrils, noncollagenous filaments, and cellular debris; a midzone of palisading macrophages that express HLA-DR antigens; and an outer zone of granulation tissue. Examination of early nodules has suggested that the initial event may be a focal vasculitis.

Clinical weakness and atrophy of skeletal muscle are common. Muscle atrophy may be evident within weeks of the onset of RA and usually is most apparent in musculature approximating affected joints. Muscle biopsy may show type II fiber atrophy and muscle fiber necrosis with or without a mononuclear cell infiltrate.

Rheumatoid vasculitis (see Chap. 319), which can affect nearly any organ system, is seen in patients with severe RA and high titers of circulating rheumatoid factor. Rheumatoid vasculitis is very uncommon in African Americans. In its most aggressive form, rheumatoid vasculitis can cause polyneuropathy and mononeuritis multiplex, cutaneous ulceration and dermal necrosis, digital gangrene, and visceral infarction. While such widespread vasculitis is very rare, more limited forms are not uncommon, especially in white patients with high titers of rheumatoid factor. Neurovascular disease presenting either as a mild distal sensory neuropathy or as mononeuritis multiplex may be the only sign of vasculitis. Cutaneous vasculitis usually presents as crops of small brown spots in the nail beds, nail folds, and digital pulp. Larger ischemic ulcers, especially in the lower extremity, also may develop. Myocardial infarction secondary to rheumatoid vasculitis has been reported, as has vasculitic involvement of lungs, bowel, liver, spleen, pancreas, lymph nodes, and testes. Renal vasculitis is rare.

Pleuropulmonary manifestations, which are more commonly observed in men, include pleural disease, interstitial fibrosis, pleuropulmonary nodules, pneumonitis, and arteritis. Evidence of pleuritis is found commonly at autopsy, but symptomatic disease during life is infrequent. Typically, the pleural fluid contains very low levels of glucose in the absence of infection. Pleural fluid complement is also low compared with the serum level when these are related to the total protein concentration. Pulmonary fibrosis can produce impairment of the diffusing capacity of the lung. Pulmonary nodules may appear singly or in clusters. When they appear in individuals with pneumoconiosis, a diffuse nodular fibrotic process (Caplan's syndrome) may develop. On occasion, pulmonary nodules may cavitate and produce a pneumothorax or bronchopleural fistula. Rarely, pulmonary hypertension secondary to obliteration of the pulmonary vasculature occurs. In addition to pleuropulmonary disease, upper airway obstruction from cricoarytenoid arthritis or laryngeal nodules may develop.

Clinically apparent heart disease attributed to the rheumatoid process is rare, but evidence of asymptomatic pericarditis is found at autopsy in 50 percent of cases. Pericardial fluid has a low glucose level and is frequently associated with the occurrence of pleural effusion. Although pericarditis is usually asymptomatic, on rare occasions death has occurred from tamponade. Chronic constrictive pericarditis also may occur.

RA tends to spare the central nervous system directly, although vasculitis can cause peripheral neuropathy. *Neurologic manifestations* also may result from atlantoaxial or midcervical spine subluxations. Nerve entrapment secondary to proliferative synovitis or joint deformities may produce neuropathies of median, ulnar, radial (interosseous branch), or anterior tibial nerves.

The rheumatoid process involves the *eye* in fewer than 1 percent of patients. Affected individuals usually have long-standing disease and nodules. The two principal manifestations are episcleritis, which is usually mild and transient, and scleritis, which involves the deeper layers of the eye and is a more serious inflammatory condition. Histologically, the lesion is similar to a rheumatoid nodule and may result in thinning and perforation of the globe (scleromalacia perforans). Fifteen to twenty percent of persons with RA may develop Sjögren's syndrome with attendant keratoconjunctivitis sicca.

Felty's syndrome consists of chronic RA, splenomegaly, neutropenia, and on occasion anemia and thrombocytopenia. It is most common in individuals with long-standing disease. These patients frequently have high titers of rheumatoid factor, subcutaneous nodules, and other manifestations of systemic rheumatoid disease. Felty's syndrome is very uncommon in African Americans. It may develop after joint inflammation has regressed. Circulating immune complexes are often present, and evidence of complement consumption may be seen. The leukopenia is a selective neutropenia with polymorphonuclear leukocyte counts of less than 1500 cells per microliter and sometimes less than 1000 cells per microliter. Bone marrow examination usually reveals moderate hypercellularity with a paucity of mature neutrophils. However, the bone marrow may be normal, hyperactive, or hypoactive; maturation arrest may be seen. Hypersplenism has been proposed as one of the causes of leukopenia, but splenomegaly is not invariably found and splenectomy does not always correct the abnormality. Excessive margination of granulocytes caused by antibodies to these cells, complement activation, or binding of immune complexes may contribute to granulocytopenia. Patients with Felty's syndrome have increased frequency of infections usually associated with neutropenia. The cause of the increased susceptibility to infection is related to the defective function of polymorphonuclear leukocytes as well as the decreased number of cells.

Osteoporosis secondary to rheumatoid involvement is common and may be aggravated by glucocorticoid therapy. Glucocorticoid treatment may cause significant loss of bone mass, especially early in the course of therapy, even when low doses are employed. Osteopenia involves both juxtaarticular bone and long bones distant from involved joints. RA is associated with a modest decrease in mean bone mass and a moderate increase in the risk of fracture. Bone mass appears to be adversely affected by functional impairment and active inflammation, especially early in the course of the disease.

RA in the Elderly   The incidence of RA continues to increase past age 60. It has been suggested that elderly onset RA might have a poorer prognosis, as manifested by more persistent disease activity, more frequent radiographically evident deterioration, more frequent systemic involvement, and more rapid functional decline. Aggressive

disease is largely restricted to those patients with high titers of rheumatoid factor. By contrast, elderly patients who develop RA without elevated titers of rheumatoid factor (seronegative disease) generally have less severe, often self-limited disease.

LABORATORY FINDINGS   No tests are specific for diagnosing RA. However, rheumatoid factors, which are autoantibodies reactive with the Fc portion of IgG, are found in more than two-thirds of adults with the disease. Widely utilized tests largely detect IgM rheumatoid factors. The presence of rheumatoid factor is not specific for RA. Rheumatoid factor is found in 5 percent of healthy persons. The frequency of rheumatoid factor in the general population increases with age, and 10 to 20 percent of individuals over 65 years old have a positive test. In addition, a number of conditions besides RA are associated with the presence of rheumatoid factor. These include systemic lupus erythematosus, Sjögren's syndrome, chronic liver disease, sarcoidosis, interstitial pulmonary fibrosis, infectious mononucleosis, hepatitis B, tuberculosis, leprosy, syphilis, subacute bacterial endocarditis, visceral leishmaniasis, schistosomiasis, and malaria. In addition, rheumatoid factor may appear transiently in normal individuals after vaccination or transfusion and also may be found in relatives of individuals with RA.

The presence of rheumatoid factor does not establish the diagnosis of RA but can be of prognostic significance because patients with high titers tend to have more severe and progressive disease with extraarticular manifestations. Rheumatoid factor is uniformly found in patients with nodules or vasculitis. The predictive value of the presence of rheumatoid factor in determining a diagnosis of RA is poor. Thus fewer than one-third of unselected patients with a positive test for rheumatoid factor will be found to have RA. The test is not useful as a screening procedure but can be employed to confirm a diagnosis in individuals with a suggestive clinical presentation and, if present in high titer, to designate patients at risk for severe systemic disease.

Normochromic, normocytic anemia is frequently present in active RA. It is thought to reflect ineffective erythropoiesis; large stores of iron are found in the bone marrow. In general, anemia and thrombocytosis correlate with disease activity. The white blood cell count is usually normal, but a mild leukocytosis may be present. Leukopenia also may exist without the full-blown picture of Felty's syndrome. Eosinophilia, when present, usually reflects severe systemic disease.

The erythrocyte sedimentation rate is increased in nearly all patients with active RA. The levels of a variety of other acute phase reactants including ceruloplasmin and C-reactive protein are also elevated, and generally such elevations correlate with disease activity and the likelihood of progressive joint damage.

Synovial fluid analysis confirms the presence of inflammatory arthritis, although none of the findings is specific. The fluid is usually turbid, with reduced viscosity, increased protein content, and a slightly decreased or normal glucose concentration. The white cell count varies between 5 and 50,000 cells per microliter; polymorphonuclear leukocytes predominate. A synovial fluid white blood cell count of more than 2000 cells per microliter with more than 75 percent polymorphonuclear leukocytes is highly characteristic of inflammatory arthritis, although not diagnostic of RA. Total hemolytic complement, C3, and C4 are markedly diminished in synovial fluid relative to total protein concentration as a result of activation of the classic complement pathway by locally produced immune complexes.

RADIOGRAPHIC EVALUATION   Early in the disease, roentgenograms of the affected joints are usually not helpful in establishing a diagnosis. They reveal only that which is apparent from physical examination, namely, evidence of soft tissue swelling and joint effusion. As the disease progresses, abnormalities become more pronounced, but none of the radiographic findings is diagnostic of RA. The diagnosis, however, is supported by a characteristic pattern of abnormalities, including the tendency toward symmetric involvement. Juxtaarticular osteopenia may become apparent within weeks of onset. Loss of articular cartilage and bone erosions develop after months of sustained activity. The primary value of radiography is to determine the extent of cartilage destruction and bone erosion produced by the disease, particularly when one is monitoring the impact of therapy with disease-modifying drugs or surgical intervention. Other means of imaging bones and joints, including ^{99m}Tc bisphosphonate bone scanning and magnetic resonance imaging, may be capable of detecting early inflammatory changes that are not apparent from standard radiography but are rarely necessary in the routine evaluation of patients with RA.

CLINICAL COURSE AND PROGNOSIS The course of RA is quite variable and difficult to predict in an individual patient. Most patients experience persistent but fluctuating disease activity, accompanied by a variable degree of joint abnormalities and functional impairment. After 10 to 12 years, fewer than 20 percent of patients will have no evidence of disability or joint abnormalities. A number of features are correlated with a greater likelihood of developing joint abnormalities or disability. These include the presence of more than 20 inflamed joints, a markedly elevated erythrocyte sedimentation rate, radiographic evidence of bone erosions, the presence of rheumatoid nodules, high titers of serum rheumatoid factor, the presence of functional disability, persistent inflammation, advanced age at onset, the presence of comorbid conditions, low socioeconomic status or educational level, or the presence of HLA-DRβ1*0401 or -DRβ*0404. The presence of one or more of these implies the presence of more aggressive disease with a greater likelihood of developing progressive joint abnormalities and disability. Patients who lack these features have more indolent disease with a slower progression to joint abnormalities and disability. The pattern of disease onset does not appear to predict the development of disabilities. Approximately 15 percent of patients with RA will have a short-lived inflammatory process that remits without major disability. These individuals tend to lack the aforementioned features associated with more aggressive disease.

Several features of patients with RA appear to have prognostic significance. Remissions of disease activity are most likely to occur during the first year. White females tend to have more persistent synovitis and more progressively erosive disease than males. Persons who present with high titers of rheumatoid factor, C-reactive protein, and haptoglobin also have a worse prognosis, as do individuals with subcutaneous nodules or radiographic evidence of erosions at the time of initial evaluation. Although sustained disease activity of more than 1 year's duration portends a poor outcome, the rate of progression of joint abnormalities is not constant; the greatest progression takes place during the first 6 years of disease and at a much slower rate thereafter. Indeed, the rate of progression of joint damage is greater during the first year of observation compared with the second and third years. Within 3 years of disease, as many as 70 percent of patients will have some radiographic evidence of damage to joints; more than 50 percent of these persons will have had evidence of erosions in the first year of disease. Foot joints are affected more frequently than hand joints. Despite the decrease in the rate of progressive joint damage with time, functional disability, which develops early in the course of the disease, continues to worsen at the same rate, although the most rapid rate of functional loss occurs within the first 2 years of disease.

The median life expectancy of persons with RA is shortened by 3 to 7 years. Of the 2.5-fold increase in mortality rate, RA itself is a contributing feature in 15 to 30 percent. The increased mortality rate seems to be limited to patients with more severe articular disease and can be attributed largely to infection and gastrointestinal bleeding. Drug therapy also may play a role in the increased mortality rate seen in these individuals. Factors correlated with early death include disability, disease duration or severity, glucocorticoid use, age at onset, and low socioeconomic or educational status.

DIAGNOSIS The mean delay from disease onset to diagnosis is 9 months. This is often related to the nonspecific nature of initial symptoms. The diagnosis of RA is easily made in persons with typical established disease. In a majority of patients, the disease assumes its characteristic clinical features within 1 to 2 years of onset. The typical picture of bilateral symmetric inflammatory polyarthritis involving small and large joints in both the upper and lower extremities with sparing of the axial skeleton except the cervical spine suggests the diagnosis. Constitutional features indicative of the inflammatory nature of the disease, such as morning stiffness, support the diagnosis. Demonstration of subcutaneous nodules is a helpful diagnostic feature.

Table 313-2

The 1987 Revised Criteria for the Classification of Rheumatoid Arthritis

1. Guidelines for classification
   a. Four of seven criteria are required to classify a patient as having rheumatoid arthritis.
   b. Patients with two or more clinical diagnoses are not excluded.
2. Criteria*
   a. Morning stiffness: Stiffness in and around the joints lasting 1 h before maximal improvement.
   b. Arthritis of three or more joint areas: At least three joint areas, observed by a physician simultaneously, have soft tissue swelling or joint effusions, not just bony overgrowth. The 14 possible joint areas involved are right or left proximal interphalangeal, metacarpophalangeal, wrist, elbow, knee, ankle, and metatarsophalangeal joints.
   c. Arthritis of hand joints: Arthritis of wrist, metacarpophalangeal joint, or proximal interphalangeal joint.
   d. Symmetric arthritis: Simultaneous involvement of the same joint areas on both sides of the body.
   e. Rheumatoid nodules: Subcutaneous nodules over bony prominences, extensor surfaces, or juxtaarticular regions observed by a physician.
   f. Serum rheumatoid factor: Demonstration of abnormal amounts of serum rheumatoid factor by any method for which the result has been positive in less than 5 percent of normal control subjects.
   g. Radiographic changes: Typical changes of RA on posteroanterior hand and wrist radiographs which must include erosions or unequivocal bony decalcification localized in or most marked adjacent to the involved joints.

* Criteria a–d must be present for at least 6 weeks. Criteria b–e must be observed by a physician.
SOURCE: Arnett et al.

Additionally, the presence of rheumatoid factor, inflammatory synovial fluid with increased numbers of polymorphonuclear leukocytes, and radiographic findings of juxtaarticular bone demineralization and erosions of the affected joints substantiate the diagnosis.

The diagnosis is somewhat more difficult early in the course when only constitutional symptoms or intermittent arthralgias or arthritis in an asymmetric distribution may be present. A period of observation may be necessary before the diagnosis can be established. A definitive diagnosis of RA depends predominantly on characteristic clinical features and the exclusion of other inflammatory processes. The isolated finding of a positive test for rheumatoid factor or an elevated erythrocyte sedimentation rate, especially in an older person with joint pains, should not itself be used as evidence of RA.

In 1987, the American College of Rheumatology developed revised criteria for the classification of rheumatoid arthritis (Table 313-2). These criteria demonstrate a sensitivity of 91 to 94 percent and a specificity of 89 percent when used to classify patients with RA compared with control subjects with rheumatic diseases other than RA. Although these criteria were developed as a means of disease classification for epidemiologic purposes, they are useful as guidelines for establishing the diagnosis. Failure to meet these criteria, however, especially during the early stages of the disease, does not exclude the diagnosis.

 TREATMENT

General Principles The goals of therapy of RA are (1) relief of pain, (2) reduction of inflammation, (3) protection of articular structures, (4) maintenance of function, and (5) control of systemic involvement. Since the etiology of RA is unknown, the pathogenesis is speculative, and the mechanisms of action of many of the therapeutic agents employed are uncertain, therapy remain empirical. None of the therapeutic interventions is curative, and therefore all must be viewed as palliative, aimed at relieving the signs and symptoms of the disease. The various therapies employed are directed at nonspecific suppression of the inflammatory or immunologic process in the hope of ameliorating symptoms and preventing progressive damage to articular structures.

Management of patients with RA involves an interdisciplinary approach, which attempts to deal with the various problems that these individuals encounter with functional as well as psychosocial interactions. A variety of physical therapy modalities may be useful in decreasing the symptoms of RA. Rest ameliorates symptoms and can be an important component of the total therapeutic program. In addition, splinting to reduce unwanted motion of inflamed joints may be useful. Exercise directed at maintaining muscle strength and joint mobility without exacerbating joint inflammation is also an important aspect of the therapeutic regimen. A variety of orthotic and assistive devices can be helpful in supporting and aligning deformed joints to reduce pain and improve function. Patient and family education is an important component of the therapeutic plan to help those involved become aware of the potential impact of the disease and make appropriate accommodations in life-style to maximize satisfaction and minimize stress on joints.

Medical management of RA involves four general approaches. The first is the use of aspirin and other nonsteroidal anti-inflammatory drugs (NSAIDs) and simple analgesics to control the symptoms and signs of the local inflammatory process. These agents are rapidly effective at mitigating signs and symptoms, but they appear to exert minimal effect on the progression of the disease. The second line of therapy involves use of low-dose oral glucocorticoids. Although these agents have been widely used to suppress signs and symptoms of inflammation, recent evidence suggests that low-dose oral glucocorticoids may also retard the development and progression of bone erosions. The third line of agents includes a variety of agents that have been classified as the disease-modifying or slow-acting antirheumatic drugs. These agents appear to have the capacity to decrease elevated levels of acute phase reactants in treated patients and, therefore, are thought to modify the destructive capacity of the disease. Other agents are the immunosuppressive and cytotoxic drugs that have been shown to ameliorate the disease process in some patients. The fourth approach involves the use of intraarticular glucocorticoids that can provide transient relief when systemic medical therapy has failed to resolve inflammation. A final approach that can be entertained when standard therapy has failed to control disease activity involves the use of a variety of investigational therapies, including combinations of disease-modifying antirheumatic drugs (DMARDs) and other more experimental agents. Recently, substituting omega-3 fatty acids such as eicosapentaenoic acid found in certain fish oils for dietary omega-6 essential fatty acids found in meat also has been shown to provide symptomatic improvement in patients with RA. A variety of nontraditional approaches also have been claimed to be effective in treating RA, including diets, plant and animal extracts, vaccines, hormones, and topical preparations of various sorts. Many of these are costly, and none has been shown to be effective. However, belief in their efficacy ensures their continued use by some patients.

Nonsteroidal Anti-Inflammatory Drugs Besides aspirin, there are now several additional NSAIDs available to treat RA. As a result of the capacity of these agents to block the activity of the enzyme cyclooxygenase and therefore the production of prostaglandins, prostacyclin, and thromboxanes, they have analgesic, anti-inflammatory, and antipyretic properties. In addition, the agents may exert other anti-inflammatory effects. These agents are all associated with a wide spectrum of toxic side effects. Some, such as gastric irritation, azotemia, platelet dysfunction, and exacerbation of allergic rhinitis and asthma, are related to the inhibition of cyclooxygenase activity, while a variety of others, such as rash, liver function abnormalities, and bone marrow depression, may not be. Elderly patients on diuretics may be at higher risk for certain toxic effects. None of the NSAIDs has been shown to be more effective than aspirin in the

treatment of RA. However, these nonaspirin drugs are associated with a lower incidence of gastrointestinal intolerance. None of the newer NSAIDs appears to show significant therapeutic advantages over the other available agents. In addition, there is no consistent advantage of any of these newer agents over the others with respect to the incidence or severity of toxic manifestations. Recent evidence indicates that two separate enzymes, cyclooxygenase 1 and 2, are responsible for the initial metabolism of arachidonic acid into various inflammatory mediators. The former is constitutively present in many cells and tissues, including the stomach and the platelet, whereas the latter is specifically induced in response to inflammatory stimuli. Inhibition of cyclooxygenase 2 accounts for the anti-inflammatory effects of NSAIDs, and suppression of cyclooxygenase 1 induces much of the mechanism-based toxicity. As the currently available NSAIDs inhibit both enzymes, therapeutic benefit and toxicity are intertwined. Newer, specific cyclooxygenase 2 inhibitors are being developed that promise therapeutic benefit with less toxicity.

DISEASE-MODIFYING ANTIRHEUMATIC DRUGS Clinical experience has delineated a number of agents that appear to have the capacity to alter the course of RA. This group of agents includes gold compounds, D-penicillamine, the antimalarials, and sulfasalazine. Despite having no chemical or pharmacologic similarities, in practice these agents share a number of characteristics. They exert minimal direct nonspecific anti-inflammatory or analgesic effects, and therefore NSAIDs must be continued during their administration, except in a few cases when true remissions are induced with them. The appearance of benefit from DMARD therapy is usually delayed for weeks or months. As many as two-thirds of patients develop some clinical improvement as a result of therapy with any of these agents, although the induction of true remissions is unusual. In addition to clinical improvement, there is frequently an improvement in serologic evidence of disease activity, and titers of rheumatoid factor and C-reactive protein and the erythrocyte sedimentation rate frequently decline. Despite this, there is minimal evidence that DMARDs actually retard the development of bone erosions or facilitate their healing.

Each of these drugs is associated with considerable toxicity, and therefore careful patient monitoring is necessary. Which DMARD should be the drug of first choice remains controversial, and trials have failed to demonstrate a consistent advantage of one over the other. Toxicity of the various agents thus becomes important in determining the drug of first choice. Failure to respond or development of toxicity to one agent does not preclude responsiveness to another. For example, a similar percentage of RA patients who have failed to respond to gold will respond to D-penicillamine when it is given as the second disease-modifying drug.

No characteristic features of patients have emerged that predict responsiveness to a DMARD. Moreover, the indications for the initiation of therapy with one of these agents are not well defined, although recently the trend has been to begin DMARD therapy early in the course of the disease.

The folic acid antagonist methotrexate, given in an intermittent low dose (7.5 to 20 mg once weekly), is currently a frequently utilized DMARD. Most rheumatologists recommend use of methotrexate as the initial DMARD, especially in individuals with evidence of aggressive RA. Recent trials have documented the efficacy of methotrexate and have indicated that its onset of action is more rapid than other DMARDs, and patients tend to remain on therapy with methotrexate longer than they remain on other DMARDs because of better clinical responses and less toxicity. Long-term trials have indicated that methotrexate does not induce remission but rather suppresses symptoms while it is being administered. Maximal improvement is observed after 6 months of therapy, with little additional improvement thereafter. Major toxicity includes gastrointestinal upset, oral ulceration, and liver function abnormalities that appear to be dose-related and reversible and hepatic fibrosis that can be quite insidious, requiring liver biopsy for detection in its early stages. Drug-induced pneumonitis also has been reported. Liver biopsy is recommended for individuals with persistent or repetitive liver function abnormalities. Concurrent administration of folic acid or folinic acid may diminish the frequency of some side effects.

GLUCOCORTICOID THERAPY Systemic glucocorticoid therapy can provide effective symptomatic therapy in patients with RA. Low-dose (less than 7.5 mg/d) prednisone has been advocated as useful additive therapy to control symptoms. Moreover, recent evidence suggests that low-dose glucocorticoid therapy may retard the progression of bone erosions. Monthly pulses with high-dose glucocorticoids may be useful in some patients and may hasten the response when therapy with a DMARD is initiated.

IMMUNOSUPPRESSIVE THERAPY The immunosuppressive drugs azathioprine and cyclophosphamide have been shown to be effective in the treatment of RA and to exert therapeutic effects similar to those of the DMARDs. However, these agents appear to be no more effective than the DMARDs. Moreover, they cause a variety of toxic side effects, and cyclophosphamide appears to predispose the patient to the development of malignant neoplasms. Therefore, these drugs have been reserved for patients who have clearly failed therapy with DMARDs. On occasion, extraarticular disease such as rheumatoid vasculitis may require cytotoxic immunosuppressive therapy.

Recent trials have suggested that cyclosporine also may be effective in the treatment of RA. Although high-dose therapy may induce rapid improvement, it is associated with frequent renal and gastrointestinal toxicity. Lower doses of cyclosporine (<5 mg/kg per day), however, appear to cause slower but nonetheless significant improvement in disease activity with fewer toxic side effects that are reversed upon lowering the dose. In addition, concomitant use of methotrexate and cyclosporine may afford additional benefit. Currently, cyclosporine has not been approved for use in RA.

SURGERY Surgery plays a role in the management of patients with severely damaged joints. Although arthroplasties and total joint replacements can be done on a number of joints, the most successful procedures are carried out on hips, knees, and shoulders. Realistic goals of these procedures are relief of pain and reduction of disability. Reconstructive hand surgery may lead to cosmetic improvement and some functional benefit. Open or arthroscopic synovectomy may be useful in some patients with persistent monarthritis, especially of the knee. Although synovectomy may offer short-term relief of symptoms, it does not appear to retard bone destruction or alter the natural history of the disease. In addition, early tenosynovectomy of the wrist may prevent tendon rupture.

APPROACH TO THE PATIENT WITH RA An approach to the medical management of patients with rheumatoid arthritis is depicted in Fig. 313-2. The principles underlying care of these patients reflect the variability of the disease, the frequent persistent nature of the inflammation and its potential to cause disability, the relationship between sustained inflammation and bone erosions, and the need to reevaluate the patient frequently for symptomatic response to therapy, progression of disability and joint damage,

and side effects of treatment. At the onset of disease it is difficult to predict the natural history of an individual patient's illness. Therefore, the usual approach is to attempt to alleviate the patient's symptoms with NSAIDs. Some patients may have mild disease that requires no additional therapy.

At some time during most patients' course, the possibility of initiating DMARD therapy and/or low-dose oral glucocorticoids is entertained. With aggressive disease this might occur sooner, often within 1 to 3 months of diagnosis, whereas in patients with more indolent disease, smoldering activity may not require such therapy for many years. The development of bone erosions or radiographic evidence of cartilage loss is clear-cut evidence of the destructive potential of the inflammatory process and indicates the need for DMARD therapy. The other indications as outlined above, including persistent pain, joint swelling, or functional impairment, are much more subjective, however. The decision to begin use of a DMARD and/or low-dose oral glucocorticoids requires experience and clinical judgment as well as the ability to assess joint swelling and functional activity and the patient's pain tolerance and expectation of therapy accurately. In this setting, the fully informed patient must play an active role in the decision to begin DMARD and/or low-dose oral glucocorticoid therapy, after careful review of the therapeutic and toxic potential of the various drugs.

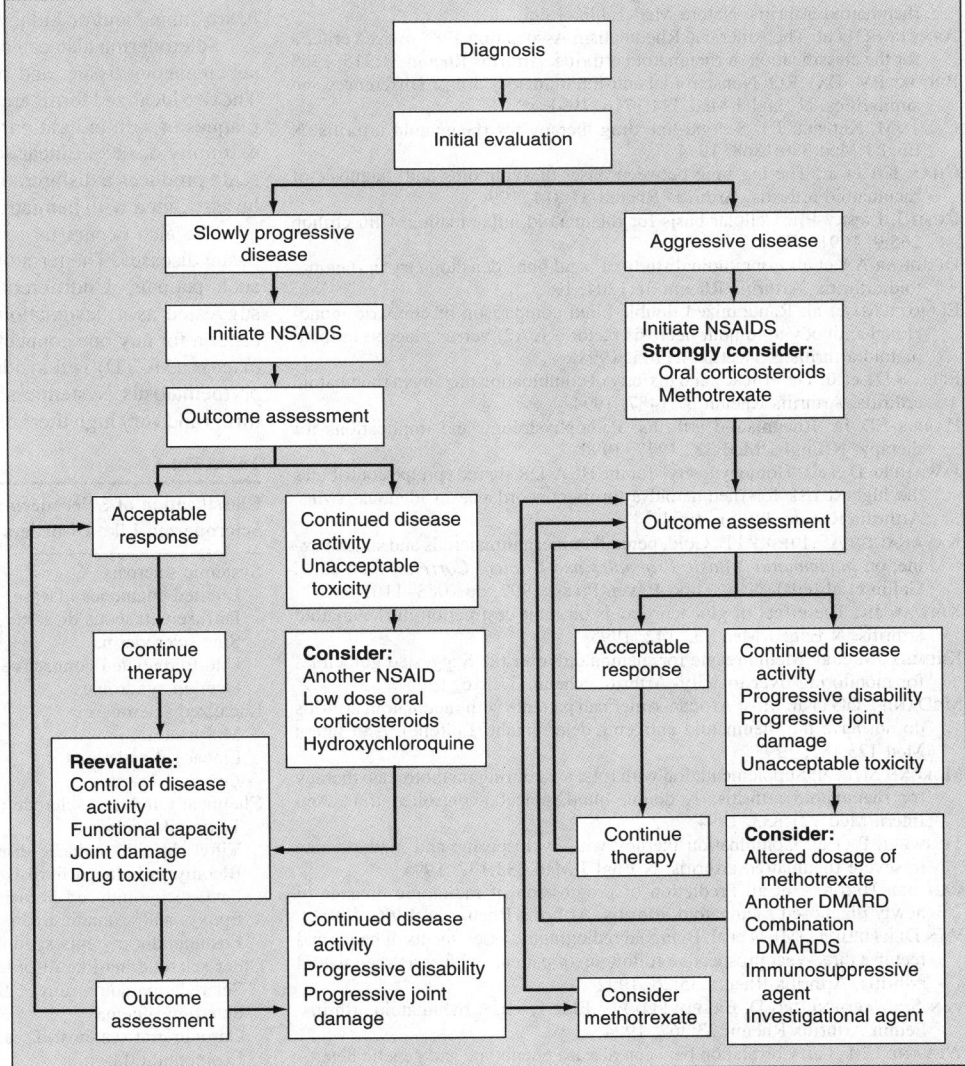

FIGURE 313-2 Algorithm for the medical management of rheumatoid arthritis. (*Courtesy of the University of Texas Southwestern Medical Center, Office of Continuing Education.*)

If a patient responds to a DMARD, therapy is continued with careful monitoring to avoid toxicity. All DMARDs provide a suppressive effect and therefore require prolonged administration. Even with successful therapy, local injection of glucocorticoids may be necessary to diminish inflammation that may persist in a limited number of joints. In addition, NSAIDs may be necessary to mitigate symptoms. Even after inflammation has totally resolved, symptoms from loss of cartilage and supervening degenerative joint disease or deformities may require additional treatment. Surgery also may be necessary to relieve pain or diminish the functional impairment secondary to deformity. Only when patients have persistent inflammatory disease or severe extraarticular manifestations is the use of cytotoxic immunosuppressive drugs or experimental procedures justified. Recently an alternative approach to treat patients with RA has been suggested. This involves the initiation of therapy with multiple agents early in the course of disease in an attempt to control inflammation, followed by maintenance on one or more agents as necessary to control disease activity. The effectiveness of this therapeutic alternative has not been proven.

BIBLIOGRAPHY

ALBANI S et al: Positive selection in autoimmunity: Abnormal immune responses to a bacterial dnaJ antigenic determinant in patients with early rheumatoid arthritis. Nature Med 1:448, 1995

ARNETT FC et al: The American Rheumatism Association 1987 revised criteria for the classification of rheumatoid arthritis. Arthritis Rheum 31:315, 1988

BROOKS PM, DAY RO: Nonsteroidal anti-inflammatory drugs: Differences and similarities. N Engl J Med 324:1716, 1991

CASH JM, KLIPPEL JH: Second-line drug therapy for rheumatoid arthritis. N Engl J Med 330:1368, 1994

CHAN KA et al: The lag time between onset of symptoms and diagnosis of rheumatoid arthritis. Arthritis Rheum 37:814, 1994

CUSH J, LIPSKY PE: Cellular basis for rheumatoid inflammation. Clin Orthop 265:9, 1991

DEODHAR AA et al: Longitudinal study of hand bone densitometry in rheumatoid arthritis. Arthritis Rheum 38:1204, 1995

ELLIOTT MJ et al: Randomized double-blind comparison of chimeric monoclonal antibody to tumour necrosis factor α (cA2) versus placebo in rheumatoid arthritis. Lancet 344:1105, 1994

FELSON DT et al: The efficacy and toxicity of combination therapy in rheumatoid arthritis. Arthritis Rheum 37:1487, 1994

HARRIS ED JR: Rheumatoid arthritis: Pathophysiology and implications for therapy. N Engl J Med 322:1277, 1990

JAWAHEER D et al: "Homozygosity" for the HLA-DR shared epitope contributes the highest risk for rheumatoid arthritis concordance in identical twins. Arthritis Rheum 37:681, 1994

KAVANAUGH AF, LIPSKY PE: Gold, penicillamine, antimalarials and sulfasalazine, on *Inflammation: Basic Principles and Clinical Correlates*, 2d ed, JI Gallin et al (eds). New York, Raven Press, 1992, pp 1083–1101

KIRWAN JR: The effect of glucocorticoids on joint destruction in rheumatoid arthritis. N Engl J Med 333:142, 1995

KREMER JM et al: Methotrexate for rheumatoid arthritis: Suggested guidelines for monitoring liver toxicity. Arthritis Rheum 37:316, 1994

MCDANIEL DO et al: Most African-American patients with rheumatoid arthritis do not have the rheumatoid antigenic determinant (Epitope). Ann Intern Med 123:181, 1995

MORGAN SL et al: Supplementation with folic acid during methotrexate therapy for rheumatoid arthritis: A double-blind, placebo-controlled trial. Ann Intern Med 121:833, 1994

TUGWELL P et al: Combination therapy with cyclosporine and methotrexate in severe rheumatoid arthritis. N Engl J Med 333:137, 1995

VAN DER HEIDE A et al: Prediction of progression of radiologic damage in newly diagnosed rheumatoid arthritis. Arthritis Rheum 38:1466, 1995

VAN DER HEIJDE DMFM et al: Biannual radiographic assessments of hands and feet in a three-year prospective follow-up of patients with early rheumatoid arthritis. Arthritis Rheum 35:26, 1992

VAN SCHAARDENBURG D, BREEDVELD FC: Elderly-onset rheumatoid arthritis. Semin Arthritis Rheum 23:367, 1994

WEYAND CM et al: Correlation between disease phenotype and genetic heterogeneity in rheumatoid arthritis. J Clin Invest 95:2120, 1995

ZVAIFLER NJ, FIRESTEIN GS: Pannus and pannocytes: Alternative models of joint destruction in rheumatoid arthritis. Arthritis Rheum 37:783, 1994

314   Bruce C. Gilliland

SYSTEMIC SCLEROSIS (SCLERODERMA)

DEFINITION Systemic sclerosis (SSc) is a multisystem disorder of unknown cause characterized by fibrosis of the skin, blood vessels, and visceral organs, including the gastrointestinal tract, lungs, heart, and kidneys (Table 314-1). The degree and rate of skin and internal organ involvement vary among patients. Two subsets, however, can be identified, even though there is some overlap (Table 314-2). One subset is referred to as *diffuse cutaneous scleroderma* and is characterized by the rapid development of symmetric skin thickening of proximal and distal extremity, face, and trunk. These patients are at greater risk for developing kidney and other visceral disease early in their course. The other subset is *limited cutaneous scleroderma*, which is defined by symmetric skin thickening limited to distal extremities and face. This subset frequently has features of the *CREST syndrome*, an acronym standing for calcinosis, Raynaud's phenomenon, esophageal dysmotility, sclerodactyly, and telangiectasia. The prognosis in limited cutaneous scleroderma is better except for the occasional patient who, after many years, develops pulmonary arterial hypertension or biliary cirrhosis. Systemic sclerosis of visceral organs also may occur in the absence of any skin involvement, which is referred to as *systemic sclerosis sine scleroderma*. Survival is determined by the severity of visceral disease, especially involving the heart, lungs, and/or kidneys.

Scleroderma also can occur in a localized form limited to the skin, subcutaneous tissue, and muscle and without systemic involvement. The two localized forms are morphea, which occurs as single or multiple plaques of skin induration, and linear scleroderma, which involves an extremity or face. Linear scleroderma of one side of the forehead and scalp produces a disfiguration referred to as *en coup de sabre* and may be associated with hemiatrophy of the same side of the face.

SSc also occurs in association with features of other connective tissue diseases. The term overlap syndrome has been used to describe such patients. Undifferentiated connective tissue disease has been suggested as a designation for patients who do not have diagnostic criteria for any one connective tissue disease. *Mixed connective tissue disease* (MCTD) is a syndrome involving features of systemic lupus erythematosus, systemic sclerosis, polymyositis, and rheumatoid arthritis and very high titers of circulating antibody to nuclear ribonucleo-

Table 314-1

Classification of Scleroderma/Systemic Sclerosis and Scleroderma-Like Disorders

Systemic sclerosis
   Limited cutaneous disease
   Diffuse cutaneous disease
   Sine scleroderma
   Undifferentiated connective tissue disease
   Overlap syndromes
Localized scleroderma
   Morphea
   Linear scleroderma
   En coup de sabre
Chemically induced scleroderma-like disorders
   Toxic-oil syndrome
   Vinyl chloride–induced disease
   Bleomycin-induced fibrosis
   Pentazocine-induced fibrosis
   Epoxy- and aromatic hydrocarbons–induced fibrosis
   Eosinophilia-myalgia syndrome
Other scleroderma-like disorders
   Sclerederma adultorum of Buschke
   Scleromyxedema
   Chronic graft-vs.-host disease
   Eosinophilic fasciitis
   Digital sclerosis in diabetes
   Primary amyloidosis and amyloidosis associated with multiple myeloma

protein antigen, will be discussed later in the chapter. *Eosinophilic fasciitis* and the *eosinophilia-myalgia syndrome* associated with L-tryptophan ingestion are scleroderma-like illnesses and will also be discussed in this chapter.

EPIDEMIOLOGY SSc has a worldwide distribution and affects all races. The onset of disease is unusual in childhood and young men. The incidence increases with age, peaking in the third to fifth decade. Women overall are affected approximately three times as often as men, and even more often during the childbearing years (as high as 15:1). SSc is more frequent and severe in young black women. The annual incidence has been estimated to be 14.1 cases per million population based on a 20-year study performed in Allegheny County, Pennsylvania. The prevalence of SSc has been reported between 19 and 75 per 100,000 persons. An exceptionally high prevalence of SSc was recently reported in the Choctaw Native Americans in Oklahoma. The prevalence was 472 per 100,000 persons, which is the highest found to date in any ethnic group. Both incidence and prevalence may be underestimated because patients with early and atypical disease may be overlooked in surveys. The role of heredity has not been clarified. Several examples of familial SSc have been reported, and the finding of other connective tissue diseases and autoantibodies in relatives of involved patients suggests a hereditary predisposition. However, an increased incidence of antinuclear antibodies in spouses of SSc patients suggests an environmental role. Immunogenetic studies have not shown strong associations between the major histocompatibility complex and susceptibility to SSc. Some studies have shown an association of SSc with HLA-DR1, -DR2, -DR3, and -DR5. C4A null alleles and HLA-DQA2 have been reported by some investigators to be markers for disease susceptibility. A more consistent relationship has been found between certain HLA types and the occurrence of specific autoantibodies in SSc patients. Anticentromere antibodies have been shown to be associated with HLA-DR1, -DR4, and -DR5, and antitopoisomerase antibodies with HLA-DR5. Both autoantibodies appear to be more closely associated with HLA-DQB1 alleles.

Several environmental factors have been associated with the development of SSc and scleroderma-like illnesses. SSc appears to be more common in coal and gold miners, especially in those with more extensive exposure, suggesting that silica dust may be a predisposing factor. Workers exposed to polyvinyl chloride may develop Raynaud's phenomenon, acroosteolysis, scleroderma-like skin lesions, and nail fold capillary abnormalities similar to those observed in SSc. These workers also may develop hepatic fibrosis and angiosarcoma. The development of scleroderma has been associated with exposure to vinyl chloride, epoxy resins, and aromatic hydrocarbons such as benzine and toluene. In 1981, in Spain, a multisystem disease resembling scleroderma occurred following the ingestion of adulterated cooking oil (rapeseed oil). Approximately 20,000 people were affected. The

patients initially develop interstitial pneumonitis, eosinophilia, arthralgias, arthritis, and myositis, followed subsequently by joint contractures, skin thickening, Raynaud's phenomenon, pulmonary hypertension, sicca syndrome, and resorption of the distal fingertips. Extensive sclerosis of the dermis and subcutaneous tissue has been noted in patients receiving pentazocine, a nonnarcotic analgesic agent. Bleomycin, an anticancer agent, produces fibrotic skin nodules, linear hyperpigmentation, alopecia, gangrene of fingers, and pulmonary fibrosis affecting mainly the lower lobes. Scleroderma and other connective tissue diseases have been reported in women who have had silicone breast implants. At present, the evidence is not conclusive that women with these implants carry an increased risk for developing scleroderma or other connective tissue diseases. Localized fibrosis, however, can occur around the implant. The development of a scleroderma-like illness has been associated with the ingestion of products containing L-tryptophan and is referred to as the *eosinophilia-myalgia syndrome* (see below and Chap. 315).

PATHOGENESIS The outstanding feature of SSc is overproduction and accumulation of collagen and other extracellular matrix proteins in skin and other organs. While the pathogenesis of SSc remains to be further elucidated, the disease process involves immunologic mechanisms, vascular damage, and activation of fibroblasts.

An early event in SSc that precedes fibrosis is vascular damage involving small arteries, arterioles, and capillaries in the skin, gastrointestinal tract, kidneys, heart, and lungs. Raynaud's phenomenon, the initial symptom of SSc in the majority of patients, is a clinical expression of the abnormal regulation of blood flow resulting from vascular injury. Injury to endothelial cells and basal lamina occurs early and is followed by thickening of the intima, narrowing of the lumen, and eventual obliteration of the vessel. As vascular damage progresses, the microvascular bed in the skin and other sites is diminished, producing a state of chronic ischemia. Vascular damage can be observed in the nail folds by wide-field microscopy, which shows drop-out of capillaries with dilatation and tortuosity of remaining ones. In the skin, remaining capillaries may proliferate and dilate to become visible telangiectasia.

Several mechanisms for endothelial injury in SSc patients have been proposed. In the sera of some patients an endothelial cytotoxic factor secreted by activated T cells has been found that degrades type IV collagen. This factor, termed granzyme A, is a serine proteinase and may be responsible for disruption of the basal lamina. The sera of some patients mediate antibody-dependent cellular cytotoxicity directed against human endothelial cells. Circulating antiendothelial antibodies, present in some patients, may be yet another mechanism for cell injury. Tumor necrosis factor also can induce endothelial injury as well as stimulate fibrosis. Vasoconstriction in SSc also contributes to endothelial damage through a mechanism of reperfusion injury resulting in fibrosis and vascular occlusion. Factors regulating vascular tone favor vasoconstriction. Endothelin 1, a vasoconstricting factor released from endothelial cells on cold exposure, is increased in SSc patients. Endothelin 1 has also been shown to stimulate fibroblasts and smooth-muscle cells. Its vasoconstriction action is normally opposed by endothelium-derived relaxation factor (EDRF, nitric oxide), also secreted by endothelial cells. The normal compensatory increase in EDRF was not seen in some patients with SSc, suggesting impairment of its synthesis. A deficiency of vasodilatory neuropeptides resulting from sensory system nerve damage may also contribute to a state favoring vasoconstriction.

Endothelial cell damage is reflected by elevated levels of factor VIII/von Willebrand factor in the sera of many but not all patients with SSc. The binding of von Willebrand factor to subendothelium mediates platelet activation with release of factors that alter vascular permeability, leading to edema. Activated platelets also release platelet-derived growth factor (PDGF), which is chemotactic and mitogenic for both smooth-muscle cells and fibroblasts, and transforming growth factor β (TGFβ), which stimulates fibroblast collagen synthesis. These

Table 314-2

Subsets of Systemic Sclerosis

	Diffuse	Limited*
Skin involvement	Distal and proximal extremities, face, trunk	Distal to elbows, face
Raynaud's phenomenon	Onset within 1 year or at time of skin changes	May precede skin disease by years
Organ involvement	Pulmonary (interstitial fibrosis); renal (renovascular hypertensive crisis); gastrointestinal; cardiac	Gastrointestinal; pulmonary arterial hypertension after 10–15 years of disease in fewer than 10% of patients; biliary cirrhosis
Nail fold capillaries	Dilatation and dropout	Dilatation without significant dropout
Antinuclear antibodies	Antitopoisomerase 1	Anticentromere

* Also referred to as CREST (calcinosis, Raynaud's, esophageal dysmotility, sclerodactyly, telangiectasia).

and other cytokines stimulate intimal fibrosis and with their passage through the injured endothelium also could account for adventitial and perivascular fibrosis. Endothelial damage along with a deficiency of tissue plasminogen activator factor enhances intravascular coagulation and, when extensive, can lead to microangiopathic hemolytic anemia observed in those patients at risk for developing acute renal failure.

Existing evidence indicates that cell-mediated immunity plays an important role in the development of fibrosis. Perivascular and diffuse mononuclear infiltrates consisting predominantly of T cells and monocytes are found in macroscopically normal appearing skin adjacent to areas of skin fibrosis. The T cells in these infiltrates are mostly helper T cells (CD4). Elevated levels of circulating interleukin (IL) 2, IL-2 receptors, CD4 antigens, and adenine deaminase are found in SSc patients, indicating activation of helper T cells. In early SSc, elevated levels of circulating IL-2 and IL-2 receptors have been shown to be associated with disease progression. IL-4 and IL-6 have also been detected in the sera of SSc patients. IL-4 is produced by activated T cells and mast cells and stimulates fibroblast proliferation and collagen synthesis (see Chap. 305). It also enhances T cell adhesion to endothelial cells. IL-6 is produced by several cells including fibroblasts, T and B cells, and endothelial cells. One of its roles is induction of IL-2 and IL-2R, which are involved in immune activation in SSc. The CD4+/CD8+ T cell ratio is increased in peripheral blood of SSc patients due usually to an increased number of CD4+ T cells and a decreased number of CD8+ T cells. Laminin and type IV collagen, components of the endothelial basement membrane, induce in vitro transformation of lymphocytes from SSc patients, suggesting that the target of cell-mediated immunity might be endothelium. T cell interaction with endothelial cells is mediated by a group of molecules known as selectins (E-selectin and P-selectin) and adhesion molecules including intercellular adhesion molecule 1 (ICAM-1), and vascular cell adhesion molecule 1 (VCAM-1) (see Chap. 305). Correlation has been shown between serum, skin, and endothelial expression of ICAM-1, VCAM-1, and P-selectin and disease activity in early SSc. Increased levels of circulating IL-1 and tumor necrosis factor in SSc patients indicate in vivo activation of monocytes. These two cytokines have been shown to stimulate fibroblasts. Additional support for involvement of cell-mediated immunity in the pathogenesis of SSc is the appearance of scleroderma-like lesions in patients with graft-versus-host disease (GVHD) after bone marrow transplantation and in a murine model of chronic GVHD, conditions known to be associated with activated T cells. Mast cells also may be involved in the development of fibrosis. Increased numbers of mast cells are found in the dermis in both involved and uninvolved skin. Mast cell degranulation has been noted in skin that subsequently became fibrosed. Interaction with T cells may be one mechanism for mast cell degranulation resulting in release of products that stimulate fibroblast collagen synthesis. Release of histamine from mast cells also may contribute to edema observed in early disease.

Humoral immune abnormalities are also present in patients with SSc. Antinuclear antibodies are found in approximately 95 percent of patients (see "Laboratory Findings," below), and antibodies to type IV collagen and laminin may be present. The role of these antibodies in the pathogenesis of SSc is not presently understood.

Regulatory mechanisms control fibroblast growth and synthesis of collagen, fibronectin, and glycosaminoglycans. Compared with fibroblasts from normal persons, the fibroblasts from SSc appear to have aberrant regulation of growth. When fibroblasts from affected SSc skin are removed and cultured in vitro, they continue to produce excessive quantities of collagen. The collagen is biochemically normal, and the proportion of type I to type III is the same as in normal skin. Fibroblasts from SSc patients appear to be in a state of permanent activation most likely as a result of stimulation by cytokines. These activated cells are thought to represent an expanded subpopulation of fibroblasts that inherently express increased matrix genes. Studies have revealed a subpopulation of SSc fibroblasts that produces two to three times more collagen than other cells from the same tissue. Fibroblasts expressing elevated levels of messenger RNA for types I and III collagen have been demonstrated by in situ hybridization, particularly around dermal blood vessels in affected SSc skin. A small number of fibroblasts expressed increased levels of mRNA for type VI and type VII collagen. Type VII collagen is normally found at the dermal-epidermal basement membrane zone and is the major component of anchoring fibrils that act to stabilize the attachment of the basement membrane to the underlying dermis. In SSc patients, type VII collagen is found throughout the dermis and may account for the indurated, tightly bound skin in this disease. PDGF receptors are expressed on SSc fibroblasts not only from affected areas but also from macroscopically normal appearing skin. Fibroblasts from normal persons lack expression of these receptors. TGFβ has been shown to upregulate the expression of these receptors in SSc fibroblasts but not in normal cells and, in conjunction with PDGF, stimulates SSc fibroblast proliferation. Macrophages and fibroblasts are capable of secreting PDGF and TGFβ, and activated T cells release TGFβ.

Fibroblasts may activate T cells to release cytokines that stimulate fibrosis. Fibroblasts in SSc patients have been shown to have increased expression of an adhesion molecule, ICAM-1, which binds to specific integrins on T cells. This binding allows interaction between T cell antigen receptor and class II molecules and antigen on fibroblasts resulting in T cell activation and cytokine release. T cells also may be activated by their interaction with extracellular matrix molecules including collagen, fibronectin, and laminin.

Chromosomal abnormalities have been noted in greater than 90 percent of SSc patients. These acquired abnormalities include chromatid breaks, acentric fragments, and ring chromosomes and are found in approximately 30 percent of mitotic cells. A chromosomal breakage factor has been found in the serum of SSc patients and their first-degree relatives. The significance of these chromosomal abnormalities is unknown.

PATHOLOGY **Skin** In the skin, a thin epidermis overlies compact bundles of collagen that lie parallel to the epidermis. Finger-like projections of collagen extend from the dermis into the subcutaneous tissue and bind the skin to the underlying tissue. Dermal appendages are atrophied, and rete pegs are lost. In early stages of disease, increased numbers of T cells, monocytes, plasma cells, and mast cells are found, particularly in the lower dermis of involved skin.

Gastrointestinal Tract In the lower two-thirds of the esophagus, the histologic findings consist of a thin mucosa and increased collagen in the lamina propria, submucosa, and serosa. The degree of fibrosis is less than in the skin. Atrophy of the muscularis in the esophagus and throughout the involved portions of the gastrointestinal tract is more prominent than the amount of fibrotic replacement of muscle. Ulceration of the mucosa is often present and may be due to either SSc or superimposed peptic esophagitis. Striated muscles in the upper third of the esophagus are relatively spared. Similar changes may be found throughout the gastrointestinal tract, especially in the second and third portions of the duodenum, in the jejunum, and in the large intestine. Atrophy of the muscularis of the large intestine may lead to the development of large-mouth diverticula. In the later stages of the disease, the involved portions of the gastrointestinal tract become dilated. Infiltration of lymphocytes and plasma cells in the lamina propria is also present.

Lung With pulmonary involvement, diffuse interstitial fibrosis, thickening of the alveolar membrane, and peribronchial fibrosis are observed. Bronchiolar epithelial proliferation accompanies the pulmonary fibrosis. Rupture of septa produces small cysts and areas of bullous emphysema. Small pulmonary arteries and arterioles show intimal thickening, fragmentation of the elastica, and muscular hypertrophy; this may occur without interstitial pulmonary fibrosis and produce pulmonary hypertension.

Musculoskeletal System The synovium in patients with arthritis is similar to that seen in early rheumatoid arthritis and shows edema with infiltration of lymphocytes and plasma cells. A characteristic finding is a thick layer of fibrin overlying and within the synovium. Later in the disease the synovium may become fibrotic. Fibrinous deposits appear on the surfaces of tendon sheaths and in the overlying fascia and may lead to audible creaking over moving tendons.

Histologic features of primary myopathy consist of interstitial and perivascular lymphocytic infiltrations, degeneration of muscle fibers, and interstitial fibrosis. Arterioles may be thickened, and capillaries may be decreased in number. Pathologic and electrophysiologic findings of polymyositis in proximal muscles are present in the few patients who are considered to have the overlap syndrome of SSc and polymyositis.

Heart   Cardiac involvement consists of degeneration of myocardial fibers and irregular areas of interstitial fibrosis that are most prominent around blood vessels. Fibrosis also involves the conduction system, leading to atrioventricular conduction defects and arrhythmias. The wall of smaller coronary arteries may be thickened. Fibrinous pericarditis and pericardial effusions are found in some patients.

Kidney   Renal involvement is found in over half the patients and consists of intimal hyperplasia of the interlobular arteries; fibrinoid necrosis of the afferent arterioles, including the glomerular tuft; and thickening of the glomerular basement membrane. Small cortical infarctions and glomerulosclerosis may be present. The renal pathologic change is often indistinguishable from that observed in malignant hypertension. Renal vascular lesions, however, may be present in the absence of hypertension. Immunofluorescence studies of kidney have shown IgM, complement components, and fibrinogen in the walls of affected vessels. Angiographic renal studies in patients with SSc may show constriction of the intralobular arteries, a finding that simulates the vasospasm of the digital arteries observed in Raynaud's phenomenon. Cold-induced Raynaud's phenomenon has been shown to decrease renal blood flow.

Other Organs   Primary liver involvement is not common. Primary biliary cirrhosis occurs in some patients, particularly in those with the limited cutaneous form of SSc. Fibrosis of the thyroid gland may develop in the presence or absence of autoimmune thyroiditis.

Thickening of the periodontal membrane with replacement of the lamina dura is demonstrated radiographically as widening of the periodontal space and rarely causes loosening of the teeth.

CLINICAL MANIFESTATIONS (See Table 314-3)   **Raynaud's phenomenon**   Systemic sclerosis usually begins insidiously; the first symptoms are frequently Raynaud's phenomenon and puffy fingers. Ninety-five percent of patients will experience Raynaud's phenomenon, which is defined as episodic vasoconstriction of small arteries and arterioles of fingers, toes, and sometimes the tip of the nose and earlobes. Episodes are brought on by cold exposure, vibration, or emotional stress. Patients experience pallor and/or cyanosis followed by rubor on rewarming. Pallor and/or cyanosis is usually associated with coldness and numbness of fingers and/or toes, and rubor with pain and tingling. Not all patients appreciate the three color phases. A history of digit pallor appears to be the most reliable symptom for the presence of Raynaud's phenomenon. Raynaud's phenome-

non may precede skin changes by several months or even years in those patients who subsequently develop the limited cutaneous form of SSc. In diffuse cutaneous SSc, skin changes are seen typically within a year of the onset of Raynaud's phenomenon. After 2 or more years of Raynaud's phenomenon, few patients who have this as their only symptom will subsequently develop SSc.

Skin Features   In early disease, fingers and hands are swollen. Swelling also may involve forearms, feet, lower legs, and face. However, lower extremities are relatively spared. This edematous phase may last for a few weeks, months, or even longer. The edema may be pitting or nonpitting and accompanied by erythema. The skin changes begin distally in the extremities and advance proximally. The skin gradually becomes firm, thickened, and eventually tightly bound to underlying subcutaneous tissue (indurative phase). In patients with diffuse cutaneous scleroderma, skin changes will become generalized, involving initially the extremities, followed by the face and trunk over a period of time, varying from months to a few years. In some patients, the skin changes may develop gradually over several years. Rapid progression of these changes over a 2- to 3-year period is associated with a greater risk of visceral disease, particularly of the lungs, heart, or kidneys. Also in diffuse cutaneous SSc, the skin changes usually peak in 3 to 5 years and then slowly improve. On the other hand, patients with limited cutaneous scleroderma will usually have a more gradual progression of skin changes, which are restricted to fingers or distal extremity and face and may continue to worsen. In both subsets of SSc, skin thickening is usually greater in the distal extremity. After many years of disease, the skin may soften and return to normal thickness or become thin and atrophic.

In the extremities, the taut skin over fingers gradually limits full extension, and flexion contractures develop. Ulcers may appear on the volar pads of the fingertips and over bony prominences such as elbows, malleoli, and the extensor surface of the proximal interphalangeal joints of the hands. These ulcers may become secondarily infected. The volar pads of the fingertips develop pitting scars and lose soft tissue. In some instances, resorption of the terminal phalanges occurs. Skin over the extremities, face, and trunk may become darkly pigmented, even without exposure to the sun. Pigmentation of the skin may occur over superficial blood vessels and tendons. Areas of hypopigmentation may also develop. The skin loses hair, oil, and sweat glands and so becomes dry and coarse. Vaginal dryness occurs and may cause dyspareunia.

In some patients, particularly those with the limited cutaneous form of disease, calcific deposits develop in intracutaneous and subcutaneous tissue. The sites commonly involved are periarticular tissue, digital pads, olecranon and prepatellar bursae, and skin along the extensor surface of the forearms. The overlying skin may break down, with drainage of calcific material. Involvement of the face results in loss of skin wrinkles and facial expression, as well as microstomia, which may make eating and dental hygiene difficult. The nose takes on a pinched or beaklike appearance. Wrinkles appear around the mouth perpendicular to the lips. Small telangiectatic mats may appear on the fingers, face, lips, tongue, and buccal mucosa after several years. They are seen more frequently in patients with limited cutaneous SSc but also are observed in patients with long-standing diffuse cutaneous SSc. The capillary beds of nail folds of the fingers may show enlargement of capillaries with little or no capillary loss, usually indicative of limited cutaneous scleroderma. In diffuse cutaneous scleroderma, there is disorganization of the capillary beds with dilated capillaries interspersed with areas where capillaries have disappeared. These capillary changes, which are observed by wide-angle microscopy or with an ophthalmoscope used as a magnifier, are not found in patients who have only Raynaud's phenomenon.

Musculoskeletal Features   More than half the patients with SSc complain of pain, swelling, and stiffness of the fingers and knees. A symmetric polyarthritis resembling rheumatoid arthritis may be seen. In more advanced stages of the disease, leathery crepitation can be

Table 314-3

Clinical Features of Systemic Sclerosis

Clinical Feature	Percent of Patients with Clinical Feature during Course of Disease	
	Limited*	Diffuse*
Raynaud's phenomenon	95–100	90–95
Skin thickening	98†	100
Subcutaneous calcinosis	50	10
Telangiectasia	85	40
Arthralgias/arthritis	40	70
Myopathy	5	50
Esophageal dysmotility	80	80
Pulmonary fibrosis	35	40
Isolated pulmonary arterial hypertension	<10	<1
Congestive heart failure	<1	30
Renal crisis	<1	15

*Limited cutaneous and diffuse cutaneous subsets of SSc
†2% or fewer of patients have SSc sine scleroderma

palpated over moving joints, especially the knee. Extensive fibrotic thickening of the tendon sheaths in the wrist can produce a carpal tunnel syndrome. Muscle weakness usually is present in patients with severe skin involvement and, in most cases, is due to disuse atrophy. There is a distinctive histologic myopathy that accompanies SSc that is not associated with muscle enzyme abnormalities. A few patients develop a myositis characterized by proximal muscle weakness and muscle enzyme elevations that are identical to polymyositis (overlap syndrome). In addition to terminal phalanges, resorption of bone may involve ribs, clavicle, and angle of mandible.

Gastrointestinal Features The majority of patients from both subsets of SSc have gastrointestinal involvement. Symptoms attributable to esophageal involvement are present in more than 50 percent of patients and include epigastric fullness, burning pain in the epigastric or retrosternal regions, and regurgitation of gastric contents. These symptoms, most noticeable when the patient is lying flat or bending over, are due to the reduced tone of the gastroesophageal sphincter and to dilatation of the distal esophagus. Peptic esophagitis frequently occurs and may lead to strictures and narrowing of the lower esophagus. However, it seldom results in bleeding. Barrett's metaplasia may develop, but transition to adenocarcinoma is uncommon. Dysphagia, particularly of solid foods, may occur independent of other esophageal symptoms and is caused by loss of esophageal motility due to neuromuscular dysfunction. Manometry or cineradiography reveals decreased amplitude or disappearance of peristaltic waves in the lower two-thirds of the esophagus. Raynaud's phenomenon in the absence of a connective tissue disease is also associated with esophageal dysmotility. Later in the course of the illness, dilatation and atony of the lower portion of the esophagus as well as reflux are seen. With gastric involvement, barium studies show dilatation, atony, and delayed gastric emptying.

Hypomotility of the small intestine produces symptoms of bloating and abdominal pain and may suggest an intestinal obstruction or paralytic ileus (pseudoobstruction). Malabsorption syndrome with weight loss, diarrhea, and anemia is due to bacterial overgrowth in the atonic intestine or possibly to obliteration of lymphatics by fibrosis. Roentgenographic features of the second and third portions of the duodenum and of the jejunum include dilatation, loss of the usual feathery pattern, and delayed disappearance of barium. Pneumatosis intestinalis occasionally occurs and appears as radiolucent cysts or linear streaks within the wall of the small intestine. Benign pneumoperitoneum may result from the rupture of these cysts. Involvement of the large intestine may cause chronic constipation and fecal impaction with episodes of bowel obstruction. A segment of atonic bowel may act as a fulcrum for intussuception to occur. Barium studies of the large intestine may show dilatation, atony, and large-mouth diverticula. Laxity of the anal sphincter may cause incontinence or rarely anal prolapse. Some patients may have gastrointestinal features of SSc with little or no cutaneous or other organ involvement, referred to as SSC sine scleroderma. Telangiectasia may develop in the stomach and intestine and can be the source of gastrointestinal bleeding.

Pulmonary Features Pulmonary involvement occurs in at least two-thirds of SSc patients and is now the leading cause of death in SSc, replacing renal disease, which usually can be treated effectively. The most common symptom is exertional dyspnea, often accompanied by a dry, nonproductive cough. Symptoms may occur in the absence of pulmonary fibrosis, and patients with pulmonary fibrosis can be relatively asymptomatic. Bilateral basilar rales may be present. Restriction of chest movement caused by extensive skin involvement of the thorax rarely occurs. Aspiration pneumonia may result from gastric reflux due to lower esophageal atony. Superimposed bacterial or viral pneumonia can be a serious complication in patients with pulmonary fibrosis. There is an increased frequency of alveolar cell and bronchogenic carcinoma in patients with pulmonary fibrosis. Pulmonary function tests are frequently abnormal and show a reduction in vital capacity and decreased lung compliance. Impairment of gas exchange is re-

flected by a low diffusing capacity and low P_{O_2} with exercise. These abnormalities may be present even when the chest radiograph is normal. Chest film may show a pattern of linear densities, mottling, and honeycombing involving most prominently the lower two-thirds of the lung. Early pulmonary disease can be detected by high-resolution computed tomography (HRCT) and bronchoalveolar lavage (BAL). The recovery by BAL of increased number of cells, mostly alveolar macrophages accompanied by neutrophils and eosinophils, is evidence for alveolitis. Treatment of alveolitis with drugs such as cyclophosphamide conceivably may be more effective when alveolitis is detected early, although this is not proven. A controlled study of the effect of cyclophosphamide in diffuse cutaneous SSc patients with early active alveolitis is under consideration. In the absence of significant interstitial fibrosis, a severe form of pulmonary arterial hypertension develops after many years of disease in patients with limited cutaneous scleroderma. Fewer than 10 percent of patients will develop this complication, which is caused by narrowing and obliteration of pulmonary arteries and arterioles by intimal fibrosis and medial hypertrophy. Pulmonary hypertension is manifested by progressive worsening of dyspnea and eventually by the appearance of right-sided heart failure. Electrocardiographic evidence of pulmonary hypertension is usually present. The prognosis is extremely poor with the development of pulmonary hypertension; the mean duration of survival is approximately 2 years.

Cardiac Features Primary cardiac involvement in SSc includes pericarditis with or without effusions, heart failure, and varying degrees of heart block or arrhythmias. The majority of patients with diffuse cutaneous SSc have cardiac abnormalities. Cardiomyopathy attributable to myocardial fibrosis appears in fewer than 10 percent of patients and involves primarily those patients with diffuse cutaneous scleroderma. Radionuclide studies have shown abnormalities of left ventricular function due to myocardial fibrosis. Cold-induced vasospasm of the hands produces defects in myocardial thallium perfusion. The characteristic pathologic feature of contraction band necrosis results from cardiac muscle damage caused by intermittent vasospasm of coronary vessels. Patients may experience angina pectoris even though coronary angiograms are normal. Patients also can develop left ventricular failure secondary to systemic hypertension or cor pulmonale secondary to pulmonary arterial hypertension.

Renal Features Renal failure was the leading cause of death in SSc until the advent of effective treatment. Significant renal disease occurs mostly in those patients with diffuse cutaneous scleroderma. A high risk of renal crisis is present in those patients who have rapidly progressive widespread skin thickening in their first 2 to 3 years of disease. Renal crisis is characterized by malignant hypertension, which can rapidly progress to renal failure. These patients manifest hypertensive encephalopathy, severe headache, retinopathy, seizures, and left ventricular failure. Hematuria and proteinuria are followed by oliguria and renal failure. The mechanism for the hypertensive crisis is activation of the renin-angiotensin system. Before the advent of effective antihypertensive drugs, the majority of these patients died within 6 months. A small number of patients may develop renal crises in the absence of hypertension. Renal failure also can develop insidiously later in the course of disease in the setting of mild to moderate hypertension and proteinuria. In these patients or those with clinically unrecognized renal disease, reduction of renal plasma flow secondary to heart failure or volume depletion resulting from overdiuresis may precipitate renal crisis. An indicator of impending renal failure is microangiopathic anemia, which may occur in a normotensive patient. The presence of a chronic pericardial effusion may also herald subsequent renal failure.

Other Features Symptoms of dry eyes and/or dry mouth are frequently present in patients with SSc. Lip biopsy may show lymphocytic infiltration of minor salivary glands characteristic of Sjögren's syndrome or intraglandular or periglandular fibrosis secondary to SSc. Antibodies to SS-A (Ro) and/or SS-B (La) are found in those patients with lip biopsies consistent with Sjögren's syndrome and not in those with salivary gland fibrosis.

Hypothyroidism occurs in a significant number of patients and may be associated with high levels of antithyroid antibodies. Fibrosis of the thyroid gland may be present but also occurs in the absence of autoimmune thyroiditis. Other manifestations of SSc include trigeminal neuralgia and male impotence secondary to decreased penile tumescence. These men have normal serum levels of testosterone and gonadotropins. Pathogenesis of this abnormality has been considered to be vascular and/or autonomic nervous system abnormalities. Biliary cirrhosis is occasionally observed in patients with limited cutaneous SSc.

LABORATORY FINDINGS The erythrocyte sedimentation rate may be elevated. Hypoproliferative anemia related to chronic inflammation is the most common cause of anemia in SSc. Anemia also may be caused by iron deficiency secondary to gastrointestinal bleeding. Bacterial overgrowth due to atony of the small bowel may lead to vitamin B_{12} and/or folic acid–deficiency anemia. Microangiopathic hemolytic anemia is most often associated with renal involvement and is caused by the presence of intravascular fibrin in renal arterioles. Hypergammaglobulinemia, consisting mostly of IgG, is found in approximately half the patients. Rheumatoid factor, in low titer, is present in 25 percent of patients. Antinuclear antibodies detected by using a cultured human laryngeal carcinoma cell line (HEp-2) substrate are present in 95 percent of patients (Table 314-4). Antinuclear antibodies that have a high specificity for SSc are antitopoisomerase 1 (Scl-70), antinucleolar, and anticentromere. Antitopoisomerase 1, originally called anti-Scl-70, recognizes the nuclear enzyme DNA topoisomerase 1. These antibodies are found in about 20 percent of all SSc patients and in approximately 40 percent of those with diffuse cutaneous SSc. They are associated with diffuse cutaneous involvement, interstitial pulmonary disease, and other visceral organ involvement. A very high frequency of these antibodies has been reported in Choctaw Native Americans in association with diffuse cutaneous SSc. They are seldom present in other disorders or in conjunction with anticentromere antibodies. Anticentromere antibodies react with protein antigens located in the kinetochore region of chromosomes and are present in 60 to 80 percent of patients with limited cutaneous scleroderma or CREST syndrome. Anticentromere antibodies are found in only about 10 percent of patients with diffuse cutaneous scleroderma and rarely in other connective tissue diseases. They are found occasionally in patients with only Raynaud's phenomenon and may indicate subsequent development of limited cutaneous disease. Antinucleolar antibodies are relatively specific for SSc and are present in approximately 20 to 30 percent of patients. Several antinucleolar antibodies have been associated with SSc: Anti-RNA polymerases I, II, and III are found in patients with diffuse cutaneous SSc who have a higher prevalence of renal and cardiac involvement. Anti-Th ribonucleoprotein (RNP) has been found in patients with limited cutaneous SSc, and anti-PM-Scl, formerly referred to as anti-PM1, may be found in a subset of patients with overlapping features of limited cutaneous SSc and polymyositis. *Anti-U₃ RNP (anti-fibrillarin) is also highly specific for SSc and may be associated with skeletal muscle disease, bowel involvement, and pulmonary arterial hypertension.* Anti-U₁ RNP is found in approximately 5 to 10 percent of SSc patients and 95 to 100 percent of those patients with the overlap syndrome of MCTD. The titers in MCTD are usually high (see below). Anti-SS-A and/or anti-SS-B are present in those patients with overlap syndrome of SSc and Sjögren's syndrome.

Table 314-4

Autoantibodies in Systemic Sclerosis

Autoantibody	Clinical Association	Percent*
Antitopoisomerase 1	Diffuse cutaneous SSc	40
Anticentromere	Limited cutaneous SSc	60–80
Anti-RNA polymerase I, II, III	Diffuse cutaneous SSc	5–40
Anti-Th RNP	Limited cutaneous SSc	14
Anti-U₁ RNP	Limited cutaneous SSc	5–10
	Mixed connective tissue disease	95–100
Anti-PM/Scl	Overlap (SSc, polymyositis)	25

* Approximate percentages for the predominant clinical association.

DIAGNOSIS The diagnosis of SSc presents no difficulty in the presence of Raynaud's phenomenon, with typical skin lesions and visceral involvement. Although Raynaud's phenomenon may be the first symptom of SSc, most patients with Raynaud's phenomenon alone do not develop a connective tissue disease. Other causes of Raynaud's phenomenon include thoracic outlet (scalenus anticus and cervical rib) syndromes, shoulder-hand syndrome, trauma (jackhammer or vibratory machine operators), previous cold injury, vinyl chloride exposure, and circulating cryoglobulins or cold agglutinins. Linear scleroderma and morphea are localized forms of scleroderma that can usually be distinguished clinically. In early disease, SSc may initially be confused with rheumatoid arthritis, systemic lupus erythematosus, or polymyositis when articular or muscle involvement is prominent. SSc without cutaneous involvement should be considered in patients with unexplained pulmonary fibrosis, pulmonary hypertension, cardiomyopathies, heart block, dysphagia, or malabsorption syndrome. Several conditions have scleroderma-like features but lack the visceral involvement. Scleredema (scleredema adultorum of Buschke) occurs predominantly in children and is characterized by painless edematous induration involving the face, scalp, neck, trunk, and proximal portions of the extremities. Involvement of the hands and feet usually does not occur. Scleredema may be associated with previous streptococcal infection and is usually self-limited, resolving in 6 to 12 months. Histology reveals accumulation of mucopolysaccharides in the dermis and skeletal muscle. A rare entity, scleromyxedema is manifested by yellowish or pale red papules in association with diffuse skin thickening that may involve the face and hands. Acid mucopolysaccharide deposits are found in the dermis. Monoclonal IgG may be detected in some of these patients. Patients with insulin-dependent diabetes mellitus may develop digital sclerosis and contractures. Primary amyloidosis and amyloidosis associated with multiple myeloma may involve the skin of the extremities and face diffusely to give the appearance of scleroderma. Biopsy will clearly differentiate these entities.

COURSE AND PROGNOSIS The course of SSc is quite variable. Until the disease differentiates into recognizable subsets, prognosis in early disease is difficult to predict. Patients with limited cutaneous scleroderma, especially those with anticentromere antibodies, have a good prognosis, with the notable exception of those few patients, fewer than 10 percent, who after 10 to 20 years or longer develop pulmonary arterial hypertension. Malabsorption syndrome and primary biliary cirrhosis are the causes of morbidity and mortality in some patients with limited cutaneous disease. On the other hand, the prognosis is generally worse in patients with diffuse cutaneous disease, particularly when the onset occurs at an older age. In addition, males have a worse prognosis. Renal and other visceral organ disease may develop early in the course of those patients with rapidly progressive generalized skin thickening. Death occurs most often from cardiac, renal, or pulmonary involvement. With the advent of effective therapy for renal crisis along with renal dialysis for those patients with renal failure, the 10-year cumulative survival rate has increased to approximately 65 percent. In patients with diffuse cutaneous disease, the 10-year cumulative survival rate is approximately 55 percent, and in limited cutaneous disease is 75 percent.

Skin may spontaneously soften after years of disease. Softening occurs in the reverse order of original skin involvement, beginning with the trunk and followed by the proximal and then the distal extremities. Sclerodactyly and flexion contractures may persist. Skin thickness may eventually approach normal; however, the skin may be atrophic.

℞ TREATMENT

Even though SSc cannot be cured, treatment of involved organ systems can relieve symptoms and improve function. The doctor-patient relationship is extremely important in caring for patients with this chronic debilitating illness. Once the diagnosis of SSc has been made, the patient and family should be instructed about this disorder. The patient will need repeated explanations and reassurances throughout his or her illness. Depending on the severity of illness, the patient will require monitoring of blood pressure, blood counts, urinalysis, and monitoring of renal and pulmonary function on a regular basis.

Effectiveness of drug therapy in SSc is difficult to evaluate because of the variable course and severity of the disease. Many drugs have been used in the treatment of SSc without any consistent or prolonged benefit. In uncontrolled studies, D-penicillamine has been reported to reduce skin thickening and prevent development of significant organ involvement. This drug interferes with inter- and intramolecular cross-linking of collagen and is also immunosuppressive. Its immunosuppressive activity also may lead to decreased collagen production. Penicillamine is better tolerated when started at a low dose, usually 250 mg/d, and then increased at 1- to 3-month intervals up to 1.5 g/d as tolerated. Although a few patients can tolerate higher doses, most patients are maintained on a dose between 0.5 and 1 g/d. For optimal absorption, it is important to give this drug 1 h before or 2 h after a meal. This drug can be quite toxic; its more serious complications include glomerulonephritis with nephrotic syndrome, aplastic anemia, leukopenia, thrombocytopenia, and myasthenia gravis. Other side effects are fever, rash, anorexia, nausea, and loss of taste. Patients should have monthly complete blood counts (including platelet count) and urinalyses. Azathioprine and other immunosuppressives also have been used in SSc and should be reserved for those patients with rapidly progressive and life-threatening disease. Control studies are lacking. Trials of treatment with recombinant interferon γ, 5-fluorouracil, and *extracorporeal photochemotherapy* have shown improvement in some disease parameters. No therapy, however, has been clearly demonstrated in a controlled, prospective study to suppress or reverse the disease process of SSc.

Antiplatelet therapy may play a role in the treatment of SSc, since the biologic products of platelets affect blood vessels. Low doses of aspirin block the formation of thromboxane A_2, a powerful vasoconstrictor and platelet aggregator. In addition, dipyridamole, 200 to 400 mg in divided daily doses, also decreases platelet adhesion to damaged vessel walls. While these drugs have a reasonable therapeutic rationale, a 2-year double-blind study did not show any benefit from their use. Reports of beneficial effects of colchicine or chlorambucil have not been documented in controlled studies.

Glucocorticoids are indicated in those patients with inflammatory myositis or pericarditis. The initial dose is 40 to 60 mg/d and is tapered based on clinical improvement. They should not be used for the indolent primary form of muscle disease of SSc. Prednisone in the range of 20 to 40 mg/d may decrease edema associated with the edematous phase of early skin involvement. Glucocorticoids are not otherwise indicated in the long-term treatment of SSc. High doses of glucocorticoids may play a role in precipitating acute renal failure. However, this association remains unclear.

The management of Raynaud's phenomenon is directed at control of vasospasm. Patients should be advised to dress warmly and wear mittens and socks, not to smoke, to remove causes of external stress, and to avoid drugs such as amphetamine and ergotamine. Beta blocking drugs may make Raynaud's phenomenon worse. Warmth of the central body induces peripheral vasodilatation. Drugs that block sympathetic vasoconstriction, such as reserpine, α-methyldopa, phenoxybenzamine, and prazosin, may be useful in the treatment of Raynaud's phenomenon, but their side effects often curtail extended use. The calcium channel blockers nifedipine and diltiazem can be effective in alleviating Raynaud's phenomenon, but side effects of light-headedness and palpitations may limit their use. The sustained-release form of nifedipine is better tolerated; the dose is 30 mg/d up to 60 or 90 mg/d as required to control symptoms. Ketanserin, an oral serotonin antagonist, also has been shown to be effective. Studies with iloprost, a prostacyclin analogue, have shown a decrease in frequency and severity of Raynaud's phenomenon and healing of digital ulcers in some patients. Iloprost is still not available in the United States for general use. Pentoxifylline may also improve perfusion by increasing the deformability of the red cell plasma membranes. Techniques of biofeedback also have been used with variable success for teaching patients to control the temperature of their hands. Stellate ganglion blockage may be useful in temporarily alleviating severe ischemic pain in the fingers. Surgical sympathectomy usually provides only temporary improvement, and it, along with other forms of therapy, does not prevent progression of the vascular lesion. The response to any therapy for Raynaud's phenomenon is limited by the degree of existing structural narrowing of digital arteries. Gangrene of distal digits may occur and require surgical amputation.

Numerous drugs have been claimed to soften the hidebound skin, but documentation in controlled studies is lacking. These drugs include D-penicillamine, colchicine, *p*-aminobenzoic acid, and vitamin E. Dryness of the skin may be reduced by avoiding frequent use of detergent soaps and by regularly applying hydrophilic ointments and bath oils. Regular exercise helps to maintain flexibility of extremities and pliability of skin. Massaging the skin several times a day also may be beneficial. Fingertip ulcerations can be protected by applying a guard or cage over the end of the finger. The use of an occlusive dressing, such as the hydrocolloid duoDERM or other membranes, over a noninfected ulcer may promote healing and protect the finger. Skin ulcers should be kept clean by soaking or by surgical or chemical debridement. Sympatholytic drugs or local nitroglycerine paste applied to or adjacent to the ulcer may be beneficial in promoting healing. Infected ulcers can usually be treated with topical antibiotics but may require systemic antibiotics, especially when there is a question of underlying osteomyelitis. The development of calcinosis cannot be prevented, nor can deposits be dissolved. Warfarin has been reported to reduce calcinosis in a few patients.

Patients with reflux esophagitis are treated with small, frequent meals, antacids between meals, and elevation of the head of the bed. Patients should be advised not to lie down for a few hours after a meal and to avoid coffee, tea, and chocolate, which reduce the pressure of the lower esophageal sphincter. Cimetidine, ranitidine or other newer H_2 blockers may be beneficial. Omeprazole, a gastric acid (proton) pump inhibitor, has been effective in treating erosive esophagitis in some patients. Metoclopramide and cisapride increase gastrointestinal motility but do not significantly improve esophageal motility. They both increase lower esophageal sphincter tone and can be of help in some patients. Nifedipine and, to a lesser extent, diltiazem reduce lower esophageal sphincter tone resulting in esophageal reflux. Patients with dysphagia should be instructed to chew their food thoroughly and wash it down with fluids. Malabsorption syndrome due to duodenal hypomotility and bacterial overgrowth may improve with intermittent use of appropriate antibiotics. Patients with severe debilitating malabsorption may benefit from parenteral hyperalimentation. Stool softeners and mild laxatives are usually adequate for treating constipation caused by hypomotility of the colon.

Articular symptoms are treated with nonsteroidal anti-inflammatory agents. Low-dose prednisone (10 mg/d or less) may improve symptoms in those not responding to these agents. Physical therapy may help to reduce the loss of joint mobility that occurs in SSc.

In patients with diffuse cutaneous SSc, the early recognition of alveolitis as previously described (see "Pulmonary Features") may allow treatment that might slow or prevent the development of pulmonary fibrosis. Cyclophosphamide has been reported in uncontrolled studies to be beneficial, and a controlled study is presently under consideration by the American College of Rheumatology. The role of glucocorticoids in preventing progression of interstitial lung disease is not clear but may be of benefit in early disease. Pulmonary fibrosis is not reversible, and therefore treatment is directed at symptoms or complications. Pulmonary infection requires prompt treatment with antibiotics. Hypoxia necessitates giving low concentrations of oxygen. Patients should receive polyvalent pneumoccal vaccine (Pneumovax) and yearly influenza immunizations.

For patients with limited cutaneous SSc who develop isolated pulmonary arterial hypertension, the treatment is inadequate. A calcium channel blocker such as nifedipine lowers pulmonary arterial resistance and improves cardiac function, but in most patients this is only for a short period of time. Few patients survive more than 5 years. Heart-lung or single-lung transplantation may be a therapeutic option in those patients without other significant systemic involvement. Recognition of early signs of renal hypertensive crisis is important in order to preserve renal function and prevent hypertensive encephalopathy. Renal involvement is often accompanied by hypertension and mild to moderate proteinuria. An occasional patient may be normotensive. Antihypertensive agents are often effective in lowering blood pressure and stabilizing or reversing renal failure. These drugs include propranolol, clonidine, and minoxidil. Particularly effective are the angiotensin-converting enzyme inhibitors, which include captopril, enalapril, and lisinopril. Dialysis may be required in patients with progressive renal failure. Some patients, however, have a slow return of renal function after several months and may no longer require dialysis. Patients are usually not candidates for kidney transplantation because of the other systemic manifestations of SSc.

Patients with cardiac failure require careful monitoring of digitalis and diuretic administration. Noninflammatory pericardial effusions also may improve with diuretics. Care should be taken to avoid overdiuresis, which may lead to decreased renal blood flow, decreased cardiac output, and renal failure.

MIXED CONNECTIVE TISSUE DISEASE MCTD is an overlap syndrome characterized by combinations of clinical features of systemic lupus erythematosus (SLE) (see Chap. 312), SSc, polymyositis (see Chap. 315), and rheumatoid arthrisis (see Chap. 313) and the presence of very high titers of circulating autoantibodies to nuclear RNP antigen. This antibody in high titer, now referred to as *anti-U₁ RNP*, has been a justification for considering MCTD as a distinct clinical entity. MCTD has been challenged as a distinct disorder by those who consider it as a subset of SLE or scleroderma. Others prefer to classify MCTD as an undifferentiated connective tissue disease. MCTD occurs worldwide and in all races. The peak onset of disease is in the second and third decades, but MCTD is seen in children and the elderly. Women are predominantly affected. The pathogenic mechanisms in MCTD reflect the disorders making up this syndrome.

Clinical Features The presenting symptoms of MCTD are most often Raynaud's phenomenon, puffy hands, arthralgias, myalgias, and fatigue. Occasionally, patients may present with the acute onset of high fever, polymyositis, arthritis, and neurologic features such as trigeminal neuralgia and aseptic meningitis. The various features of the connective tissue disorders making up MCTD develop over months and years.

The fingers as well as the entire hand may be puffy, followed later by sclerodactyly. Sclerodermal changes are usually limited to the distal extremities and sometimes the face but spare the trunk. Telangiectasia and calcinosis may develop. Some patients have mucocutaneous features of SLE including a classic malar rash, photosensitivity, discoid lesions, alopecia, and painful oral ulcerations. An erythematous rash over the knuckles, elbows, and knees and heliotropic eyelids, typical of dermatomyositis, are uncommon.

Joint pain, stiffness, and swelling involving the peripheral joints occur frequently. Deformities of the hands similar to those of rheumatoid arthritis may develop but usually without bony erosions. A destructive polyarthritis is occasionally observed. Myalgias are a frequent symptom. Some patients develop typical symptoms of polymyositis with proximal muscle weakness, abnormal electromyographic findings, elevated levels of muscle enzymes, and inflammatory changes on muscle biopsy.

Approximately 85 percent of patients have pulmonary involvement, which is often asymptomatic. Diffusing capacity for carbon monoxide may be the only abnormality. Pleurisy commonly occurs but is seldom associated with large pleural effusions. Some patients develop interstitial lung disease. Pulmonary arterial hypertension is the most common cause of death in MCTD.

Approximately 25 percent of patients develop renal disease. Membranous glomerulonephritis is most common and usually mild but can cause nephrotic syndrome. Diffuse proliferative glomerulonephritis is unusual in MCTD, perhaps because of the protective role played by the high titers of anti-U₁ RNP. Renal crisis secondary to malignant renovasculature hypertension, as occurs in scleroderma, is seen in a few patients.

Gastrointestinal involvement is seen in approximately 70 percent of patients. The most common manifestations are esophageal dysmotility, lower esophageal sphincter laxity, and gastroesophageal reflux. Bowel manifestations mimic those of scleroderma bowel disease.

Pericarditis occurs in 30 percent of patients. Other cardiac features include myocarditis, arrhythmia, conduction disturbances, and mitral valve prolapse. Other clinical features of MCTD include trigeminal neuropathy, peripheral neuropathy, aseptic meningitis, lymphadenopathy, and Sjögren's syndrome. The majority of patients have developed, or will develop within 5 years of presentation, diagnostic clinical criteria for one of the overlapping connective tissue diseases, most often SLE or SSc.

Laboratory Findings Anemia of chronic inflammation is seen in the majority of patients. A positive direct Coombs' test is found in about 60 percent of patients, but hemolytic anemia is unusual. Leukopenia, thrombocytopenia, or both are present in some patients. Hypergammaglobulinemia is common, and rheumatoid factor is present in 50 percent of patients.

All patients, by definition of MCTD, have antibodies to U₁ RNP. The specificity of this antibody is to the 70-kDa protein complexed to small nuclear RNA. The anti-U₁ RNP antibodies are associated with HLA-DR4 but not with -DR2 and -DR3 as found in SLE. Molecular mimicry has been demonstrated between U₁ RNP and retroviral antigens by some laboratories.

℞ TREATMENT
The treatment of MCTD is essentially the same as would be indicated for the respective connective tissue diseases defining this syndrome. More than half the patients have a favorable course. The 10-year survival rate overall is approximately 80 percent but varies depending on the connective tissue disease that may eventually develop.

EOSINOPHILIC FASCIITIS Eosinophilic fasciitis is a scleroderma-like syndrome of unknown cause characterized by inflammation followed later by sclerosis of the dermis, subcutis, and deep fascia. The disease affects adults and often occurs after strenuous physical activity. Patients do not have Raynaud's phenomenon or internal organ involvement. Several immunologic abnormalities have been associated with eosinophilic fasciitis and include aplastic anemia, myelodysplastic syndrome, and thrombocytopenia. Patients usually have the abrupt onset of symmetric tenderness and swelling of the extremities which is rapidly followed by induration of the skin and subcutaneous tissue. The skin takes on a cobblestone or puckered appearance. Carpal tunnel syndrome appears early in the course, and flexion contractures develop later. A low-grade myositis is often present, but creatinine kinase levels are usually normal. A marked eosinophilia is found in the early stage of disease and subsequently decreases. Increased levels of polyclonal IgG and immune complexes are often present in the serum. A full-thickness biopsy consisting of skin, fascia, and superficial muscle shows perivascular infiltration of histiocytes, eosinophils, lymphocytes, and plasma cells. Biopsies later in the course show sclerosis. Spontaneous improvement and occasionally complete remission may occur after 2 to 5 years of disease. Some patients have persistent disease, while others are left with flexion contractures. Administration of glucocorticoids may provide symptomatic improvement and will decrease the eosinophilia. Improvement has been reported with the use of the H₂ blocker cimetidine.

EOSINOPHILIA-MYALGIA SYNDROME In 1989, reports of patients with scleroderma-like skin changes, myalgias, and eosinophilia dramatically increased. Most, but not all, of these cases were associated with ingestion of L-tryptophan manufactured by a single Japanese company. Batches of L-tryptophan implicated in eosinophilia-myalgia syndrome (EMS) were found to contain trace amounts of a contaminant identified as a dimer of L-tryptophan that appeared in 1988 after changes were made in the method of manufacturing this drug. It is not clear whether this chemical contaminant is the etiologic agent or whether another unidentified substance is responsible. *L-Tryptophan products were taken off the market in 1990.* The onset of EMS can be either abrupt or insidious. In the early phases of the disease, clinical manifestations include low-grade fever, fatigue, dyspnea, cough, arthralgias/arthritis, evanescent erythematous rashes, muscle cramping, and severe myalgias. Pulmonary infiltrates may be present. Over the next 2 to 3 months, scleroderma-like skin changes appear. Some patients develop a peripheral neuropathy which may persist. An ascending polyneuropathy may lead to paralysis and respiratory failure requiring ventilatory assistance. Cognitive dysfunction with impairment of memory and concentration has been recognized in this syndrome. Myocarditis and cardiac arrhythmias occur in some patients, and a few patients develop pulmonary hypertension. Approximately a third of patients have features of eosinophilic fasciitis. EMS most closely resembles toxic oil syndrome; however, Raynaud's phenomenon does not occur, and there is a lower prevalence of pulmonary hypertension and thromboembolic disease. The peripheral eosinophil count is greater than 1000 cells per cubic millimeter in most patients. The histologic findings on biopsy of skin, fascia, and superficial muscle are similar to that found in eosinophilic fasciitis. The clinical features of EMS may persist after L-tryptophan has been discontinued. EMS may run a chronic course, and response to therapy has been variable. Treatment has included glucocorticoids, antimalarial drugs, immunosuppressive drugs, and plasmapheresis. Prednisone was beneficial during the acute inflammatory phase of the disease in the majority of patients and resulted in resolution of pulmonary infiltrates, peripheral edema, and eosinophilia. In the later phase of the illness, no treatment was found to be of particular value. The pathogenesis of this disease is not known. A follow-up of patients 2 years after their onset of illness showed that most symptoms and physical findings had resolved or improved except for cognitive dysfunction, which became worse in approximately one-third of the patients, and peripheral neuropathy, which remained unchanged (see also Chap. 315).

BIBLIOGRAPHY

ARNETT FC: HLA and autoimmunity in scleroderma (systemic sclerosis). Int Rev Immunol 12:107, 1995

BENNETT RM: Mixed connective tissue disease and other overlap syndromes, in *Textbook of Rheumatology*, 4th ed, WN Kelley et al (eds). Philadelphia, Saunders, 1993, p 1057

BLACK CM: The aetiopathogenesis of systemic sclerosis: Thick skin—thin hypotheses. J R Coll of Physicians Lond 29:119, 1995

CARPENTIER PH, MARICQ HR: Microvasculature in systemic sclerosis. Rheum Dis Clin North Am 16:75, 1990

HERTZMAN PA et al: The eosinophilia-myalgia syndrome: status of 205 patients and results of treatment 2 years after onset. Ann Intern Med 122:851, 1995

KAHALEH B, MATUCCI-CERINIC M: Raynaud's phenomenon and scleroderma. Dysregulated neuroendothelial control of vascular tone. Arthritis Rheum 38:1, 1995

LAKHANPAL S et al: Eosinophilic fasciitis: Clinical spectrum and therapeutic response in 52 cases. Semin Arthritis Rheum 17:221, 1988

LEGERTON CW III et al: Systemic sclerosis (scleroderma). Clinical management of its major complications. Rheum Dis Clin North Am 21:203, 1995

LEROY ED et al: Scleroderma (systemic sclerosis): Classification, subset and pathogenesis. J Rheumatol 15:202, 1988

MEDSGER TA JR: Systemic sclerosis (scleroderma), localized forms of scleroderma, and calcinosis, in *Arthritis and Allied Conditions*, 12th ed, DJ McCarty, WJ Koopman (eds). Philadelphia, Lea & Febiger, 1993, p 1253

POSTLETHWAITE AE: Role of T cells and cytokines in effecting fibrosis. Int Rev Immunol 12:247, 1995

SEIBOLD J: Scleroderma, in *Textbook of Rheumatology*, 4th ed, WN Kelley et al (eds). Philadelphia, Saunders, 1993, p 1113

SHARP GC, SINGSEN BH: Mixed connective tissue disease, in *Arthritis and Allied Conditions*, 12th ed, DJ McCarty, WJ Koopman (eds), Philadelphia, Lea & Febiger, 1993, p 1213

STEEN VD: Renal involvement in systemic sclerosis. Clin Dermatol 12:253, 1994

———— et al: Therapy for severe interstitial lung disease in systemic sclerosis. A retrospective study. Arthritis Rheum 37:1290, 1994

VARGA J, BASHEY RI: Regulation of connective tissue synthesis in systemic sclerosis. Int Rev Immunol 12:187, 1995

V'AZQUEZ AD, ROTHFIELD NF: Autoantibodies in systemic sclerosis. Int Rev Immunol 12:145, 1995

---

315   *Rup Tandan*

DERMATOMYOSITIS AND POLYMYOSITIS*

Dermatomyositis and polymyositis are conditions of presumed autoimmune etiology in which the skeletal muscle is damaged by a nonsuppurative inflammatory process dominated by lymphocytic infiltration. The term *polymyositis* is applied when the condition spares the skin, and the term *dermatomyositis* when polymyositis is associated with a characteristic skin rash. One-third of cases are associated with various connective tissue disorders, such as rheumatoid arthritis, lupus erythematosus, mixed connective tissue disorder, and progressive systemic sclerosis, and one-tenth with a malignancy. *Inclusion body myositis* is a distinct clinicopathologic entity characterized by the presence of vacuolated inclusions containing tubulofilaments in muscle.

ETIOLOGY   The precise cause of these diseases is unknown, but interplay between host genetic factors, viral infection of muscle, and autoimmune mechanisms is probably contributory. Familial occurrence of these diseases, and the increased frequency of HLA-DR3 and -DRw52 antigens in patients, suggest an underlying genetic and immunologic predisposition. Experimental viral myositis can be induced in animals by coxsackievirus. A mild inflammatory myopathy can occur with influenza and coxsackieviruses in humans. However, the several electron-microscopic observations of virus-like particles in muscle fibers in dermatomyositis or polymyositis have not been confirmed by virus isolation or demonstration of rising viral antibody titers, and the disease has not been passed into animals by injection of extracts of skeletal muscles. Nevertheless, the presence of serum antibodies to several cytoplasmic ribonucleoproteins involved in translation [especially histidyl tRNA synthetase or Jo-1 and signal recognition particle (SRP)] may result from an immune response to an altered virus that serves as an immunogen in polymyositis. These antibodies probably represent a cross-reactive phenomenon.

A lymphocyte-mediated disease resembling polymyositis has been reported in laboratory animals injected with muscle antigens together with Freund's adjuvant (experimental allergic myositis). Immunohistochemical and muscle co-culture studies indicate that muscle fiber necrosis in polymyositis and inclusion body myositis probably derive from activation of CD8 + T lymphocytes, accompanied by CD4 + T lymphocytes and macrophages present in the inflammatory infiltrates. In dermatomyositis, deposition of immunoglobulins and the C_{5b-9} complement membrane attack complex has been demonstrated on intramuscular blood vessels even in unaffected or minimally involved regions of muscle, suggesting that humorally mediated blood vessel damage initiates the angiopathy that precedes muscle destruction. The final pathway for muscle fiber damage in dermatomyositis may be T cell–dependent stimulation of B cells, with resultant antibody-mediated cytotoxicity. In inclusion body myositis, the accumulation of amyloid, paired helical filaments, and several other proteins typically seen at autopsy in brain specimens of patients with Alzheimer's disease suggest some overlap of pathogenic mechanisms in these disorders.

---

* The author acknowledges the contribution of Walter G. Bradley to this chapter in previous editions.

CLASSIFICATION A widely used classification of the dermatomyositis-polymyositis group is shown in Table 315-1. Other diseases uncommonly associated with polymyositis are sarcoidosis, giant cell myositis with thymoma, and myositis in systemic infections due to viruses, toxoplasma, or parasites. A focal infective myositis due to streptococcal or staphylococcal infection is mostly seen in the tropics. Focal nodular myositis is a variant of polymyositis in which focal areas of myositis cause hot, often painful, multifocal muscle masses.

INCIDENCE Current estimates of the annual incidence of the inflammatory myopathies are approximately five cases per million population. These estimates are probably low, however; the true incidence may be as high as two to three per hundred thousand.

CLINICAL MANIFESTATIONS **Group I: Primary Idiopathic Polymyositis** This group comprises about one-third of all cases of inflammatory myopathy. It is usually insidiously progressive over weeks, months, or even years. Rarely the disease is acute, producing severe muscle weakness in a matter of days or even rhabdomyolysis. The disease may develop at any age. Affected females outnumber males 2:1.

Patients first become aware of weakness of the proximal limb muscles, especially the hips and thighs, and find difficulty in arising from the squatting or kneeling position and in climbing or descending stairs. When shoulder girdle muscles are involved, placing an object on a high shelf or combing the hair becomes difficult. Occasionally the disease is more restricted, affecting only the neck, the shoulder, or the quadriceps muscles. Aching pain in the buttocks, thighs, and calves is experienced in about 10 percent of the cases, and tenderness on palpation in another 20 percent. In the majority of patients the disorder is painless. Early symptoms of dysphagia and weakness of flexor muscles of the neck in a patient with a chronic myopathy suggest the diagnosis of polymyositis.

When the patient is first seen, there may be weakness of the muscles of the trunk, the pectoral and pelvic girdles, the upper arms and thighs, the neck, and the pharynx. Ocular muscles are almost never affected except in a rare association with myasthenia gravis. The distal muscles are spared in about 75 percent of cases. Muscle atrophy, contractures, and diminished tendon reflexes are rare in early myositis and never as pronounced as in muscular dystrophies and denervating conditions. When the reflexes are disproportionately reduced, carcinoma with polymyositis and polyneuropathy or the Lambert-Eaton syndrome should be considered. Occasionally, the reflexes may be paradoxically brisk in dermatomyositis-polymyositis, perhaps due to irritation of muscle spindle receptors by the inflammation.

At presentation about 25 percent of patients have dysphagia, about 5 percent have significant respiratory impairment, and 5 percent are unable to walk. Dysphagia is due to involvement of striated muscles of the pharynx and upper esophagus. At some time in the course of the disease, cardiac abnormalities are observed in about 30 percent of cases; these include electrocardiogram (ECG) changes, arrhythmias, and heart failure secondary to myocarditis. About half of the fatal cases have pathologic evidence of cardiac disease with necrosis of myocardial fibers, usually with only modest inflammatory reaction. The frequency of myocardial infarction may be increased in those treated for long periods with glucocorticoids. In a few cases there is dyspnea due to lymphocytic pneumonitis, obliterating bronchiolitis, pulmonary edema, or pulmonary fibrosis. Arthralgia, Raynaud's phenomenon, and, rarely, low-grade fever may also be present.

Table 315-1

Classification of Polymyositis-Dermatomyositis

Group I	Primary idiopathic polymyositis
Group II	Primary idiopathic dermatomyositis
Group III	Dermatomyositis (or polymyositis) associated with neoplasia
Group IV	Childhood dermatomyositis (or polymyositis) associated with vasculitis
Group V	Polymyositis (or dermatomyositis) with associated collagen vascular disease

SOURCE: Classification suggested by Bohan et al.

Group II: Primary Idiopathic Dermatomyositis This group comprises just over one-third of all cases of myositis. The skin changes may precede or follow the muscle syndrome and include a localized or diffuse erythema, maculopapular eruption, scaling eczematoid dermatitis, or, rarely, an exfoliative dermatitis. The classic lilac-colored (heliotrope) rash is on the eyelids, bridge of the nose, cheeks (butterfly distribution), forehead, chest, elbows, knees and knuckles, and around the nail beds. Itching may be troublesome in some cases. The skin lesions may be subtle and easily overlooked. Periorbital edema is frequent, particularly in acute cases. The skin lesions may occasionally ulcerate. Subcutaneous calcification may occur, especially in children.

The typical rash and myositis allow a diagnosis of dermatomyositis, and such cases may be placed in this category (group II, Table 315-1) if idiopathic and into groups III, IV, and V if there are other features, namely malignancy, vasculitis in children, and an established collagen vascular disease. There should be concern about an underlying malignancy in patients over the age of 40 with dermatomyositis.

Group III: Polymyositis or Dermatomyositis with Neoplasia This syndrome, which comprises about 8 percent of all cases of myositis, is categorized separately, although muscle and skin changes are indistinguishable from those in the other groups. Malignancy, however, is uncommon in myositis seen in children and in association with a connective tissue disorder. The malignancy may antedate or postdate the onset of the myositis by up to 2 years. The incidence of neoplasia is higher in patients over the age of 40 and is particularly high in patients over age 60; therefore, in such patients a thorough history and clinical examination (including breast, gynecologic, and rectal) should be supplemented by complete blood count, biochemical profile, serum protein electrophoresis and immunofixation, screening for carcinoembryonic antigen, urine analysis for blood and cytology, stool samples for occult blood, chest x-ray, sputum for cytology, and bone scan seeking clues for an underlying malignancy. This relatively inexpensive search uncovers most malignancies; undirected radiologic screening procedures are costly and unhelpful in improving the yield. The most common malignancies are lung, ovary, breast, gastrointestinal tract, and lymphoproliferative disorders. The myositis is a paraneoplastic syndrome, the cause of which may lie in an altered immune status, cross-reactive antigens between tumor and muscle, or an occult viral infection of the muscle.

Group IV: Childhood Polymyositis and Dermatomyositis Associated with Vasculitis This group comprises about 8 to 20 percent of all cases of myositis in various series. Inflammatory myopathy in childhood is frequently associated with skin involvement and clinical or histologic evidence of vasculitis in skin, muscles, gastrointestinal tract, and other organs. Degeneration and loss of capillaries in a perifascicular distribution occur in the skeletal muscles; often necrotizing lesions of the skin, and ischemic infarction of kidneys, gastrointestinal tract, and rarely brain may be seen. Consequently, some authors have reported mortality rates of up to one-third in childhood dermatomyositis, though most have found that the prognosis is better than in adult dermatomyositis-polymyositis. Based upon current data, it is unclear whether or not all cases of childhood myositis should be included in group IV. Subcutaneous calcification is frequently present in childhood dermatomyositis.

Group V: Polymyositis or Dermatomyositis with an Associated Connective Tissue Disorder This "overlap group" of myositis comprises about one-fifth of all cases that occur in association with several connective tissue diseases. Progressive systemic sclerosis, rheumatoid arthritis, mixed connective tissue disease (the rheumatologic overlap disorder), and lupus erythematosus are the most common associated conditions; polyarteritis nodosa and rheumatic fever are more rarely associated. Criteria for placement in the "overlap group" combine the demonstration of the appropriate clinical and laboratory abnormalities required for the diagnosis of the connective tissue disorder together with clinical and laboratory evidence of myositis. The diagnosis of myositis is often difficult in patients with a connective tissue disorder producing arthritis with secondary (disuse) muscle weakness with type II fiber atrophy. Moreover, perivascular inflammatory foci are common in muscle in connective tissue disorders. Demonstration of increased serum creatine kinase (CK), electromyography (EMG), and muscle biopsy are often required to make this diagnosis. Though patients in this overlap group usually respond to glucocorticoid therapy, the prognosis for recovery of function is poorer than in pure dermatomyositis-polymyositis. Dysphagia in group V patients with progressive systemic sclerosis is often due to involvement of the smooth muscle of the distal third of the esophagus.

Other Disorders Associated with Myositis *Sarcoidosis and polymyositis* The skeletal muscle contains noncaseating granulomas with Langhans-type multinuclear giant cells in at least one-quarter of patients with sarcoidosis (Chap. 320). Symptomatic polymyositis is, however, uncommon. Regenerating multinuclear myoblasts resemble Langhans' giant cells, which has led to the misdiagnosis in many of the cases reported in the literature of "sarcoid myositis." Giant cell or granulomatous polymyositis and myocarditis, sometimes associated with myasthenia gravis, have been recorded in patients with thymomas.

Focal nodular myositis A syndrome of acutely developing and painful focal inflammatory nodules, sometimes occurring sequentially in different muscles, has been termed *focal nodular myositis*. The pathologic appearance and response to therapy are similar to those in generalized polymyositis. The differential diagnosis includes, when single, a muscle tumor (sarcoma or rhabdomyosarcoma) or proliferative fasciitis and myositis and, when multiple, muscle infarcts such as can occur in polyarteritis nodosa.

Infectious polymyositis Rare cases of polymyositis have been found to result from infection with known pathogens such as toxoplasma (Chap. 219), viruses (Chap. 195), and spirochetes (Lyme disease). Antibody screening will suggest the diagnosis in such cases. Trichinosis may be confused with idiopathic polymyositis, particularly if the history of raw or undercooked pork ingestion is not obtained (see Chap. 221). The symptoms of trichinosis are variable and depend upon the parasitic load. Low-grade fever, muscle pain of variable degree, conjunctival and periorbital edema, and fatigue are frequent. Weakness is generally mild. Heavy infestation is often associated with central nervous system symptoms of delirium, coma, or focal neurologic deficits. Myocardial involvement is common, manifested by tachycardia and ECG changes. The diagnosis is made by the history of ingestion of undercooked pork, marked eosinophilia, a positive skin test to *Trichina* antigen, and the appearance of serum antibodies to *Trichina* during the course of the disease. Occasionally the diagnosis is not recognized until a muscle is biopsied. Pyomyositis, a suppurative inflammation of muscle due to staphylococci or streptococci, is mainly seen in the tropics but has recently been reported in patients with AIDS. The presentation is that of a diffuse abscess of the muscle.

Myopathy in infection caused by human immunodeficiency virus (HIV) Polymyositis occurs in AIDS (see Chap. 308). It may be the presenting manifestation of the disorder or be due to therapy with zidovudine (AZT), which inhibits DNA polymerase gamma and presumably mitochondrial DNA replication. Weight loss greater than 10 percent of baseline body weight with associated chronic diarrhea or weakness characterizes the HIV wasting syndrome; a myopathy, among other causes, may underlie this entity. Raised serum CK, EMG evidence of myopathy, and muscle fiber necrosis with or without inflammatory infiltrates occur in AIDS myopathy. Rhabdomyolysis can occur in HIV-infected patients, possibly related to the use of drugs (such as didanosine or sulfonamides), or, in late cases, as part of opportunistic infection in muscle (such as *Staphylococcus aureus*), toxemia, or severe electrolyte disturbances. HIV antigens are present in macrophages associated with muscle inflammatory infiltrates but are absent in muscle fibers. The inflammatory myopathy associated with early HIV infection usually responds to glucocorticoids. AZT myopathy is dose related and usually improves after discontinuation

of the drug or reduction of the dose. Structural and functional mitochondrial abnormalities are usually associated with AZT myopathy.

Polymyositis also occurs in patients displaying the spectrum of diseases associated with human T lymphotropic virus type I infection, especially in the Caribbean islands and Japan. Almost all such patients show other neurologic features, such as a myelopathy or neuropathy. Response to glucocorticoids is usually poor.

Inclusion Body Myositis The clinical features of this typically sporadic, but rarely familial, disorder are similar to those of chronic idiopathic polymyositis, except that onset is at an older age, focal and distal muscle involvement are more frequent, and disease duration is longer. Early and prominent involvement of finger or forearm flexors and leg extensors is characteristic. Muscle biopsy shows interstitial and occasional perivascular inflammatory infiltrates, necrosis, and regeneration of muscle fibers, but in addition there are "rimmed vacuoles" in the fibers that stain positively with Congo-red, like amyloid. Inflammation is rarely seen in the familial disorder. Electron microscopy reveals paramyxovirus-like 15- to 18-nm filaments in the nuclei and sarcoplasm. Immunohistochemistry reveals abnormal accumulation of beta-amyloid protein, α_1-antichymotrypsin, phosphorylated tau, apolipoprotein E, and ubiquitin within vacuolated muscle fibers. The nature of the inflammatory infiltrate and the mechanism of muscle fiber damage are probably similar to that in polymyositis. Immunocytochemical and in situ hybridization studies suggest that a previously reported etiologic link with the mumps virus seems unlikely. This disorder usually responds poorly to glucocorticoids and immunosuppressive therapy; however, some patients may improve following treatment with intravenous immunoglobulin. Prognosis is for a chronically progressive disorder with loss of ambulation about 5 to 10 years after presentation.

Eosinophilic Myositis This rare disease probably represents one manifestation of the spectrum of hypereosinophilic syndrome. There are a number of subtypes. Subacute onset of muscle pain and proximal weakness, elevated serum CK, myopathic features on EMG, and histologic appearance of a myositis with an eosinophilic inflammatory infiltrate are characteristic. Some patients may respond to glucocorticoids, methotrexate, or leukapheresis.

Eosinophilia-myalgia syndrome A syndrome that is more common in women has been associated with ingestion of the essential amino acid L-tryptophan. Fever, rash, arthralgia, cough, dyspnea, and edema are commonly accompanied by eosinophilia (more than 1000 cells per microliter), peripheral neuropathy, and myositis with endomysial, perimysial, and fascial infiltration of lymphocytes and eosinophils. 1,1′-Ethylidenebis (tryptophan), a contaminating by-product of the manufacture of some batches of L-tryptophan, has been incriminated. Immune-mediated muscle damage by cytotoxic T cells alone or with accompanying macrophages has been reported.

Eosinophilic fasciitis This disorder is characterized by painful swelling and thickening of the skin in the extremities, limitation of movement due to contractures, and mild muscle weakness. Raised sedimentation rate, peripheral eosinophilia, hypergammaglobulinemia, and mildly elevated CK are seen. The EMG may show myopathic features. Histologically there is marked thickening and infiltration of the deep fascia with mononuclear cells and eosinophils, some involvement of the epimysium and perimysium, and variable muscle degeneration. Most patients respond to treatment with glucocorticoids.

Relapsing eosinophilic perimyositis This disease is characterized by recurrent painful and tender areas in the neck or lower extremities, but without muscle weakness. An elevated sedimentation rate and peripheral eosinophilia are frequent, serum CK is sometimes raised, and histologically there is eosinophilic infiltration of the perimysium. Response to glucocorticoids is usually good.

LABORATORY FINDINGS In all forms of polymyositis there may be elevated serum levels of the enzymes present in skeletal muscle, such as CK, aldolase, serum glutamic oxaloacetic transaminase, lactic acid dehydrogenase, and serum glutamic pyruvate transaminase. The degree of elevation decreases from the first to the last in this series of enzymes, and the pattern is the reverse of that seen in liver disease. The erythrocyte sedimentation rate is elevated in about two-thirds of cases. Tests for circulating rheumatoid factor are positive in less than one-half and for antinuclear antibodies in about three-quarters of the cases. Most other hematologic indexes are normal. Several autoantibodies seem to be associated with clinically distinct groups of patients. Anti-Jo-1 antibodies are more common in polymyositis, especially in patients with interstitial lung disease, and anti-nRNP antibodies are often associated with polymyositis seen in lupus erythematosus. Other antibodies seen in patients with dermatomyositis and polymyositis in association with connective tissue diseases include anti-Scl-70 (progressive systemic sclerosis), anti-Sm (lupus erythematosus), anti-Ro and anti-La (Sjögren's syndrome and lupus erythematosus), and anti-ENA (mixed connective tissue disease). Myoglobin can be found in the urine when muscle destruction is acute and extensive; rarely, acute polymyositis causes the full syndrome of rhabdomyolysis and myoglobinuria. In about 40 percent of cases EMG reveals a markedly increased insertional activity (muscle irritability), together with the typical myopathic triad of motor unit action potentials, which are of low amplitude, are polyphasic, and have an abnormally early recruitment. In a further 40 percent of the patients only myopathic changes are present. The ECG is abnormal in about 5 to 10 percent of the cases at presentation. Since the pathologic process in myositis is patchy, greater diagnostic yield is accomplished by obtaining a biopsy from two clinically affected muscles and by skip serial sectioning of all specimens. Magnetic resonance imaging may serve to identify sites of muscle involvement. Muscles recently used for EMG or intramuscular injection must be avoided as these procedures can produce inflammatory changes and muscle fiber damage, leading to false-positive results. In about two-thirds of cases, the biopsies will demonstrate the typical pathologic changes of myositis, but despite following the above recommendations, about 10 percent of cases have normal muscle biopsy.

Skeletal Muscle Pathology The principal changes in muscle consist of infiltrates of inflammatory cells (lymphocytes, macrophages, plasma cells, and rare eosinophils and neutrophils) and destruction of muscle fibers with a phagocytic reaction. Perivascular (usually perivenular) inflammatory cell infiltration is the hallmark of polymyositis. Interstitial inflammatory cell infiltration is also a prominent feature of the disease, but lesser degrees of it may be seen in other conditions as a secondary reaction (e.g., in facioscapulohumeral and Becker's muscular dystrophy). Evidence of muscle fiber degeneration and regeneration is almost invariably present. Many of the residual muscle fibers are small, with increased numbers of sarcolemmal nuclei. Either the degeneration of muscle fibers or the infiltration of inflammatory cells may predominate in any given biopsy specimen. Blood vessel changes and perifascicular atrophy are more prominent in childhood dermatomyositis than in adult dermatomyositis and polymyositis. Capillary loss due to endothelial cell necrosis occurs particularly in the periphery of fascicles and may explain the perifascicular atrophy. Other features include reduplication of capillary basement membrane and the presence of tubular inclusions within endothelial cells. Type II muscle fiber atrophy and muscle infarcts also may be found. Vasculitis is also seen in polymyositis or dermatomyositis associated with connective tissue disorders.

DIAGNOSIS Patients with dermatomyositis who have the characteristic skin rash, muscle weakness, EMG changes, and elevation of serum CK may not require a muscle biopsy to confirm the diagnosis. In the case of idiopathic polymyositis, however, a firm diagnosis must be based on the presence of a typical clinical picture, a typical EMG, elevation of serum CK, and a diagnostic muscle biopsy. All four of these criteria are required to be certain of the diagnosis, since inflammatory changes may occasionally occur in other myopathies (e.g., facioscapulohumeral muscular dystrophy) and in other connective tissue disorders without clear muscle weakness. However, in fewer than one-third of cases of polymyositis are *all* these criteria satisfied. It may be particularly difficult to obtain a diagnostic muscle biopsy because of the patchy nature of the disease. Thus, a therapeutic trial of glucocorticoids should be given when full investigation of a patient with significant disability leaves a diagnosis of "possible polymyositis," usually because of a nondiagnostic muscle biopsy.

DIFFERENTIAL DIAGNOSIS The clinical picture of skin rash and proximal or diffuse muscle weakness has few causes other than dermatomyositis. However, proximal muscle weakness without skin involvement can be due to many conditions other than polymyositis and necessitates detailed investigation to establish the correct diagnosis.

Subacute or Chronic Progressive Muscle Weakness This may be due to denervating conditions such as the spinal muscular atrophies or amyotrophic lateral sclerosis (Chap. 370). Upper motor neuron signs in the latter in addition to the muscle weakness aid in the diagnosis. The muscular dystrophies, such as those of Duchenne and Becker and the limb-girdle and facioscapulohumeral types, may appear similar to polymyositis (Chap. 383). However, the muscular dystrophies usually develop more slowly (over years rather than weeks or months); rarely present after the age of 30; usually spare the pharyngeal, posterior neck, and deltoid muscles until late in the course; and may selectively involve other muscles, such as the biceps and brachioradialis, early in the course. Nevertheless, in rare patients it may be difficult, even with a muscle biopsy, to distinguish chronic polymyositis from a rapidly advancing muscular dystrophy. This is particularly true of facioscapulohumeral muscular dystrophy, where interstitial inflammatory cell infiltration is commonly found early in the disease. Such doubtful cases should always be given an adequate trial of glucocorticoid therapy. Myotonic dystrophy produces a characteristic facies with ptosis, facial myopathy, temporalis muscle wasting, and grip myotonia (Chap. 383). Some metabolic myopathies, including glycogen storage disease due to carnitine and carnitine palmityltransferase deficiency, produce exertional cramps, rhabdomyolysis, and muscle weakness; diagnosis rests upon biochemical studies of the muscle biopsy (Chap. 383). Glycogen storage disease due to acid maltase deficiency also requires muscle biopsy for diagnosis. The endocrine myopathies such as those due to hypercorticosteroidism, hyper- and hypothyroidism, and hyper- and hypoparathyroidism require the appropriate laboratory investigations for diagnosis. Muscle wasting in patients with an underlying neoplasm may be true polymyositis, but it can be due to a protein-wasting state (cachexia), a paraneoplastic neuropathy, or type II fiber atrophy.

Muscle Weakness with Marked Exercise-Induced Fatigue Fatigue without much muscle wasting may be due to neuromuscular junction disorders including myasthenia gravis or the Lambert-Eaton syndrome. Repetitive nerve stimulation and single-fiber EMG studies aid in the diagnosis of these conditions (Chap. 382).

Acute Muscle Weakness This may be caused by an acute neuropathy such as that due to the Guillain-Barré syndrome or a neurotoxin. When combined with painful muscle cramps, rhabdomyolysis, and myoglobinuria, it may be due to metabolic disorders including some of the glycogen storage diseases such as myophosphorylase deficiency (McArdle's disease), carnitine palmityltransferase deficiency, and myoadenylate deaminase deficiency. Acute viral infections may cause a similar syndrome. Chronic alcoholics may develop a painful myopathy with myoglobinuria after a bout of heavy drinking or may present with a painless acute hypokalemic myopathy, which is completely reversible, or may show an asymptomatic elevation of serum CK and myoglobin. Acute muscle weakness with myoglobinuria may occur in prolonged severe hypokalemia due to potassium loss or with hypophosphatemia and hypomagnesemia, often seen in chronic alcoholics and in patients on nasogastric suction receiving parenteral hyperalimentation. An acute necrotizing myopathy with myoglobinuria can rarely accompany hyper- and hyponatremia.

Drug-Induced Myopathies Rhabdomyolysis and myoglobinuria have been associated with intake of amphotericin B, ε-aminocaproic acid, fenfluramine, heroin, and phencyclidine. A predominantly hypokalemic myopathy may result from prolonged use of diuretics, carbenoxolone, and azathioprine. Penicillamine has been reported to produce a myositis. The use of clofibrate, cimetidine, chloroquine, colchicine, carbimazole, cyclosporine, emetine, gemfibrozil, growth hormone, ketoconazole, leuprolide, lovastatin, phenytoin, provastatin, tretinoin, and, recently, AZT has been associated with a myopathy. Toxic myopathies usually have a different pathology from polymyositis and require a careful drug history for diagnosis. In other cases investigation reveals no etiology, and these may be due to a true acute autoimmune polymyositis or to an as yet undiscovered metabolic defect.

Pain on Movement and Muscle Tenderness Patients with muscle pain and little or no weakness may be thought to be neurotic or hysterical. A number of conditions including *polymyalgia rheumatica* (Chap. 319) and arthritic disorders of adjacent joints enter into the differential diagnosis of polymyositis. The muscle biopsy either is normal or discloses type II fiber atrophy, but in polymyalgia rheumatica the temporal artery biopsy may show giant cell arteritis (Chap. 319). *Fibrositis* and *fibromyalgia* are syndromes that frequently enter into the differential diagnosis of polymyositis. Patients complain of focal or diffuse muscle tenderness, aching, and weakness, which is sometimes poorly separated from joint pain. In other patients there may be minor signs of a collagen vascular disorder, such as an increased erythrocyte sedimentation rate, antinuclear antibody, or rheumatoid factor, and occasionally there is slight elevation of the serum CK. The muscle biopsy occasionally shows a few interstitial inflammatory cells. Where there is a focal "trigger point," biopsy may show inflammatory infiltration of the connective tissue. Rarely does this syndrome develop into frank polymyositis, and the prognosis is therefore more benign than that of polymyositis (see below). Many such patients show some response to nonsteroidal anti-inflammatory agents, though most continue to have indolent complaints. *Chronic fatigue syndrome*, which

may follow a viral infection, can present with debilitating fatigue, fever, sore throat, painful lymphadenopathy, myalgia, arthralgia, sleep disorder, and headache (Chap. 384). The presence of other cognitive and behavioral features, such as impaired memory and concentration, depression, and irritability, and a normal muscle biopsy usually help in the diagnosis.

℞ TREATMENT

(See Fig. 315-1) Glucocorticoids in high dosage is the accepted treatment for severe dermatomyositis-polymyositis, though there is no controlled trial to prove its effectiveness. Prednisone is generally started at a dose of 1 to 2 mg/kg body weight per day (60 to 100 mg/d for adults). Improvement may begin within 1 to 4 weeks, though in some patients treatment may need to be continued for 3 months before improvement occurs. When improvement is noted, the daily dose may be reduced by 5 mg every 4 weeks. Repeated manual muscle testing and serum CK determinations should be performed to ensure that the myositis does not relapse. At about 40 mg/d, the schedule is changed gradually to 80 mg every other day in order to reduce the incidence of glucocorticoid side effects. There is some evidence that the use of alternate-day glucocorticoids from the outset may be effective, particularly in patients with milder disease. Adults with acute to subacute dermatomyositis-polymyositis tend to improve more rapidly than those with chronic polymyositis; children also respond in most cases. If the dose is reduced too rapidly, or to too low a level, relapse will occur, necessitating return to high dosage. Prednisone therapy may have to be continued for several years, but an attempt should be made every year to withdraw the therapy from patients who are clinically stable in order to determine if the disease is still active.

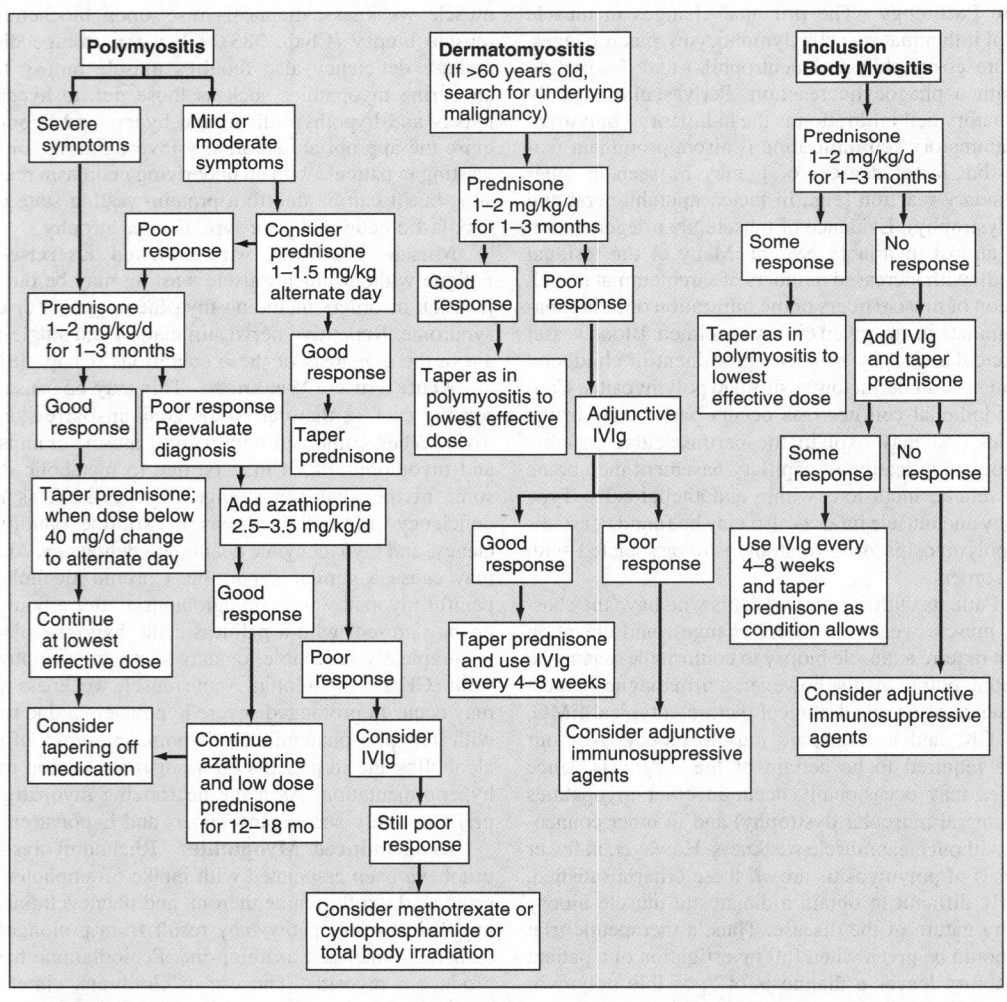

FIGURE 315-1 Algorithm for the treatment of polymyositis, dermatomyositis, and inclusion body myositis.

Cytotoxic drugs should be tried when the response to glucocorticoids is inadequate after 1 to 3 months or when relapses are frequent. The combined use of glucocorticoids and a cytotoxic drug usually allows a lower dose of glucocorticoids to be used. Azathioprine (2.5 to 3.5 mg/kg body weight per day in divided doses) is the most commonly used cytotoxic drug in this disease; preliminary studies have shown a benefit of azathioprine as adjunctive therapy in glucocorticoid-treated patients. The aim of therapy with azathioprine is to lower the total lymphocyte count to about 750/µL, while maintaining the hemoglobin level above 12 g/dL, the total white cell count above 3000/µL, and the platelet count about 125,000/µL. Periodic blood counts are required to monitor the cytotoxic drug therapy. Uncontrolled studies have shown some benefit with methotrexate, cyclophosphamide, and cyclosporine. Methotrexate is effective at doses that do not produce lymphopenia (usual dose about 0.5 mg/kg body weight per week achieved by slowly increasing from a starting dose of 10 mg). In a small controlled study, high-dose intravenous immunoglobulin (IVIg) therapy (0.4 g/kg daily for 5 consecutive days) produced improvement in patients with steroid-resistant dermatomyositis and probably should be used in severe or refractory cases. Anecdotal reports have suggested that IVIg may also be effective in polymyositis resistant to other forms of therapy. Total-body irradiation has been successfully used in some patients with disease refractory to glucocorticoids and immunosuppressants, but long-term follow-up and controlled studies are lacking for this potentially dangerous therapy. A controlled trial of plasma exchange and leukapheresis in a small number of patients with dermatomyositis-polymyositis resistant to glucocorticoids showed no benefit over sham pheresis. Bed rest has been recommended in the acute phase of the disease but is harmful in the long term. Physiotherapy and rehabilitative devices are important in the long-term treatment of patients with dermatomyositis-polymyositis.

Patients older than age 40, particularly those with dermatomyositis, should be followed closely for the possibility of malignant disease. If a malignant lesion is found, it should be treated, since the muscle weakness may disappear if the neoplasm is eradicated. However, a response to glucocorticoids can usually be obtained even in patients with dermatomyositis-polymyositis associated with a malignancy.

Monitoring serum CK levels during reduction of immunosuppressive therapy is useful, since a rise in level generally indicates an incipient clinical relapse. CK levels are not used to monitor initial response to prednisone, because prednisone reduces CK levels independent of any effects on the disease process.

Side effects of high-dose daily glucocorticoid therapy (see Chap. 332) are relatively common in patients treated for polymyositis and may limit therapy. However, these can be minimized by appropriate use of alternate-day therapy and judicious use of calcium supplements, vitamin D, and H_2-receptor blockers. When patients who have been stable on a static dose of prednisone develop increasing muscle weakness, this may be due to either a relapse of the myositis or to glucocorticoid myopathy. An EMG, serum CK measurement, and, rarely, muscle biopsy may help in differentiating these two conditions if the changes of myositis are present. Often, however, the only way to distinguish between these two conditions is to reduce the dose of prednisone slowly; if glucocorticoid myopathy is the cause of the weakness, it will improve as the dose is reduced; if a relapse of the myositis is responsible, the weakness will increase with reduction in the dose.

Side effects of cytotoxic drugs include marrow suppression, alopecia, gastrointestinal tract disorders, damage to the testes and ovaries, infections, and potential for malignancy.

PROGNOSIS The overall mortality rate of individuals with dermatomyositis-polymyositis is about four times that of the general population; death is usually due to pulmonary, renal, and cardiac complications. Females, blacks, and those severely affected at presentation or treated after long delays have a worse prognosis. Unfavorable outcome is also seen in patients with significant dysphagia, associated

cancer or connective tissue diseases, and serum antibodies to Jo-1 and SRP. Evidence from several series suggests that patients seen at tertiary referral centers may have less favorable outcome when compared with patients seen at smaller community hospitals, probably because they represent a population with more severe disease that is less responsive to therapy. Nevertheless, the 5-year survival rate is about 75 percent overall, and is higher yet in children. Most patients improve with therapy. Many make a full functional recovery, though some weakness of the shoulders and hips, usually not disabling, remains at the conclusion of treatment. Relapse may occur at any time. Glucocorticoids should not be discontinued too soon, for the relapse that may follow is often more difficult to treat than the original presentation. About one-half of the patients with this disease recover and can discontinue therapy within 5 years after the onset of the symptoms; about 20 percent still have active disease requiring continued therapy. The remaining 30 percent have inactive disease but residual muscle weakness.

BIBLIOGRAPHY

BOHAN A et al: A computer-assisted analysis of 153 patients with polymyositis and dermatomyositis. Medicine 56:255, 1977

CALLEN JP: Relationship of cancer to inflammatory muscle diseases. Dermatomyositis, polymyositis, and inclusion body myositis. Rheum Dis Clin North Am 20(4):943, 1994

CARPENTER S, KARPATI G: *Pathology of Skeletal Muscle*. New York, Churchill Livingstone, 1984, pp 515–592

CHARIOT P et al: Acute rhabdomyolysis in patients infected by human immunodeficiency virus. Neurology 44:1692, 1994

CHERIN P, HERSON S: Indications for intravenous gammaglobulin therapy in inflammatory myopathies. J Neurol Neurosurg Psychiatry 57:50, 1994

DALAKAS MC: How to diagnose and treat the inflammatory myopathies. Semin Neurol 14:137, 1994

——— et al: A controlled trial of high dose intravenous immune globulin infusions as treatment for dermatomyositis. N Engl J Med 329:1993

DEVERE R, BRADLEY WG: Polymyositis: Its presentation, mortality, and morbidity. Brain 98:637, 1975

ENGEL AG et al: The polymyositis and dermatomyositis syndromes, in *Myology*, 2d ed, AG Engel, C Franzini-Armstrong (eds). New York, McGraw-Hill, 1994, pp 1335–1383

GARLEPP MJ, MASTAGLIA FL: Inclusion body myositis. J Neurol Neurosurg Psychiatry 60:251, 1996

GRIGGS RC et al: Inclusion body myositis and myopathies. Ann Neurol 38:705, 1995

HOHLFELD R, ENGEL AG: The immunobiology of muscle. Immunol Today 15:269, 1994

JOFFE MM et al: Drug therapy of the idiopathic inflammatory myopathies: Predictors of response to prednisone, azathioprine, and methotrexate and a comparison of their efficacy. Am J Med 94:379, 1993

MARTIN RW et al: The clinical spectrum of the eosinophilia-myalgia syndrome associated with L-tryptophan ingestion. Ann Intern Med 113:124, 1990

MCKENZIE R, STRAUS SE: Chronic fatigue syndrome. Adv Intern Med 40:119, 1995

SIGURGEIRSSON B et al: Risk of cancer in patients with dermatomyositis or polymyositis: A population-based study. N Engl J Med 326:363, 1992

TARGOFF IN: Immune manifestations of inflammatory muscle disease. Rheum Dis Clin North Am 20(4):857, 1994

316 *Haralampos M. Moutsopoulos*

SJÖGREN'S SYNDROME

DEFINITION Sjögren's syndrome is a chronic, slowly progressive autoimmune disease characterized by lymphocytic infiltration of the exocrine glands resulting in xerostomia and dry eyes. Approximately one-third of patients present with systemic manifestations. A small but significant number of the patients may develop malignant lymphoma. The disease can be seen alone (primary Sjögren's syndrome) or in association with other autoimmune rheumatic diseases (secondary Sjögren's syndrome) (Table 316-1).

INCIDENCE AND PREVALENCE The disease affects predominantly middle-aged women (female-to-male ratio 9:1), although it can be seen in all ages, including childhood. The prevalence of primary Sjögren's syndrome is approximately 0.5 to 1.0 percent. In addition to the primary syndrome, 30 percent of patients with autoimmune rheumatic diseases suffer from secondary Sjögren's syndrome.

PATHOGENESIS Sjögren's syndrome is characterized by lymphocytic infiltration of the exocrine glands and B lymphocyte hyperreactivity, as illustrated by circulating autoantibodies. The latter is accompanied by an oligomonoclonal B cell process, which is characterized by serum and urine monoclonal light chains and cryoprecipitable monoclonal immunoglobulins.

Sera of patients with Sjögren's syndrome often contain a number of autoantibodies directed against non-organ-specific antigens such as immunoglobulins (rheumatoid factors) and extractable nuclear and cytoplasmic antigens (Ro/SS-A, La/SS-B). Ro/SS-A autoantigen consists of three polypeptide chains (52, 54, and 60 kDa) in conjunction with RNAs, whereas the 48-kDa La/SS-B protein is bound to RNA III polymerase transcripts. The presence of autoantibodies to Ro/SS-A and La/SS-B antigens in Sjögren's syndrome is associated with earlier disease onset, longer disease duration, salivary gland enlargement, severity of lymphocytic infiltration of minor salivary glands, and certain extraglandular manifestations such as lymphadenopathy, purpura, and vasculitis.

Phenotypic and functional studies have shown that the predominant cell infiltrating the affected exocrine glands is the helper/inducer T cell with characteristics of memory cells. Both B and T infiltrating lymphocytes are activated, as illustrated by production of immunoglobulins with autoantibody activity, spontaneous release of interleukin 2, as well as expression on the T cell surface of activation markers such as class II HLA molecules and lymphocyte function–associated antigen 1. Macrophages and natural killer cells are rarely detected in infiltrates, while epithelial cells of the affected glands inappropriately express class II molecules and possess messages for c-*myc* protooncogene and proinflammatory cytokines. All these phenomena suggest that the epithelial cell of the exocrine glands in Sjögren's syndrome may act as an antigen-presenting cell, and recent studies indicate that a retrovirus may be the initiator of the autoimmune process.

Immunogenetic studies have demonstrated that HLA-B8, -DR3, and -DRw52 are prevalent in primary Sjögren's syndrome patients as compared with the normal control population. Molecular analysis of HLA class II genes has revealed that Sjögren's syndrome patients, regardless of their ethnic origin, are highly associated with HLA DQA$_1$*0501 allele.

CLINICAL MANIFESTATIONS The majority of the patients with Sjögren's syndrome have symptoms related to diminished lacrimal and salivary gland function. In most patients, the primary syndrome runs a slow and benign course. The initial manifestations can be mucosal dryness or nonspecific, and 8 to 10 years elapse from the initial symptoms to full-blown development of the disease.

The principal oral symptom of Sjögren's syndrome is dryness (xerostomia). This is described as difficulty in swallowing dry food, inability to speak continuously, a burning sensation, increase in dental

caries, and problems in wearing complete dentures. Physical examination shows a dry, erythematous, sticky oral mucosa. There is atrophy of the filiform papillae on the dorsum of the tongue, and saliva from the major glands is either not expressible or is cloudy. Enlargement of the parotid or other major salivary glands occurs in two-thirds of patients with primary Sjögren's syndrome but is uncommon in those with the secondary syndrome. Diagnostic tests include sialometry, sialography, and scintigraphy. The labial minor salivary gland biopsy permits histopathologic confirmation of the focal lymphocytic infiltrates.

Ocular involvement is the other major manifestation of Sjögren's syndrome. Patients usually complain of dry eyes, with a sandy or gritty feeling under the eyelids. Other symptoms include burning, accumulation of thick strands at the inner canthi, decreased tearing, redness, itching, eye fatigue, and increased photosensitivity. These symptoms are attributed to the destruction of corneal and bulbar conjunctival epithelium, defined as keratoconjunctivitis sicca. Diagnostic evaluation of keratoconjunctivitis sicca includes measurement of tear flow by Schirmer's I test and tear composition as assessed by the tear breakup time or tear lysozyme content. Slit-lamp examination of the cornea and conjunctiva after rose Bengal staining reveals punctate corneal ulcerations and attached filaments of corneal epithelium.

Involvement of other exocrine glands occurs less frequently and includes a decrease in mucous gland secretions of the upper and lower respiratory tree, resulting in dry nose, throat, and trachea (xerotrachea), and diminished secretion of the exocrine glands of the gastrointestinal tract, leading to esophageal mucosal atrophy, atrophic gastritis, and subclinical pancreatitis. Dyspareunia due to dryness of the external genitalia and dry skin also may occur.

Extraglandular (systemic) manifestations are seen in one-third of patients with Sjögren's syndrome (Table 316-2), while they are very rare in patients with Sjögren's syndrome associated with rheumatoid arthritis. These patients complain more often of easy fatigability, low-grade fever, myalgias, and arthralgias. Most patients with primary Sjögren's syndrome experience at least one episode of nonerosive arthritis during the course of their disease. Manifestations of pulmonary involvement are frequent but rarely important clinically, with subclinical diffuse interstitial lung disease being the most common. Renal involvement includes interstitial nephritis, clinically manifested by hypostenuria and renal tubular dysfunction with or without acidosis and Fanconi's syndrome. Untreated acidosis may lead to nephrocalcinosis. Glomerulonephritis is a rare finding that occurs in patients with systemic vasculitis, cryoglobulinemia, or systemic lupus erythematosus overlapping with Sjögren's syndrome. Vasculitis affects small and medium-sized vessels. The most common clinical features are purpura, recurrent urticaria, skin ulcerations, glomerulonephritis, and mononeuritis multiplex.

It has been suggested that primary Sjögren's syndrome with vasculitis also may present with multifocal, recurrent, and progressive nervous system disease, such as hemiparesis, transverse myelopathy, hemisensory deficits, seizures, and movement disorders. Aseptic meningitis and multiple sclerosis also have been reported in these patients.

Table 316-1

Association of Sjögren's Syndrome with Other Autoimmune Diseases

Rheumatoid arthritis
Systemic lupus erythematosus
Scleroderma
Mixed connective tissue disease
Primary biliary cirrhosis
Vasculitis
Chronic active hepatitis

Table 316-2

Incidence of Extraglandular Manifestations in Primary Sjögren's Syndrome

Clinical Manifestation	Percent
Arthralgias/arthritis	60
Raynaud's phenomenon	37
Lymphadenopathy	14
Lung involvement	14
Vasculitis	11
Kidney involvement	9
Liver involvement	6
Lymphoma	6
Splenomegaly	3
Peripheral neuropathy	2
Myositis	1

Table 316-3

CHAPTER 316
Sjögren's Syndrome

1903

Diagnostic Criteria for Sjögren's Syndrome*

Criteria	Definitions
1. Ocular symptoms	Dry eyes every day for more than 3 months, recurrent sensation of sand or gravel in the eyes, or use of tear substitutes more than three times a day
2. Oral symptoms	Daily feeling of dry mouth for more than 3 months, recurrent or persistently swollen salivary glands, or use of liquids to aid in swallowing dry food
3. Ocular signs	Positive Schirmer's I test (<5 mm in 5 min), or a rose Bengal score of ≥4 according to van Bijsterveld's scoring system
4. Histopathology	Focus score 1 in a minor salivary gland biopsy
5. Salivary gland involvement	Positive result in one of the following tests: salivary scintigraphy, parotid sialography, salivary flow (≤1.5 mL in 15 min)
6. Autoantibodies	Antibodies to Ro(SS-A) or La(SS-B), antinuclear antibodies, or rheumatoid factor

* Probable Sjögren's syndrome: three items are present.
  Definite Sjögren's syndrome: four or more items are present.

Table 316-4

Differential Diagnosis of Sicca Symptoms

Xerostomia	Dry Eye	Bilateral Parotid Gland Enlargement
Viral infections	Inflammation	Viral infections
Drugs	Stevens-Johnson	Mumps
Psychotherapeutic	syndrome	Influenza
Parasympatholytic	Pemphigoid	Epstein-Barr
Antihypertensives	Chronic conjunctivitis	Coxsackievirus A
Psychogenic	Chronic blepharitis	Cytomegalovirus
Irradiation	Sjögren's syndrome	HIV
Diabetes mellitus	Toxicity	Sarcoidosis
Trauma	Burns	Amyloidosis
Sjögren's	Drugs	Sjögren's syndrome
syndrome	Neurologic conditions	Metabolic
	Impaired lacrimal gland	Diabetes mellitus
	function	Hyperlipoproteinemias
	Impaired eyelid function	Chronic pancreatitis
	Miscellaneous	Hepatic cirrhosis
	Trauma	Endocrine
	Hypovitaminosis A	Acromegaly
	Blink abnormality	Gonadal hypofunction
	Lid scarring	
	Anesthetic cornea	
	Epithelial irregularity	

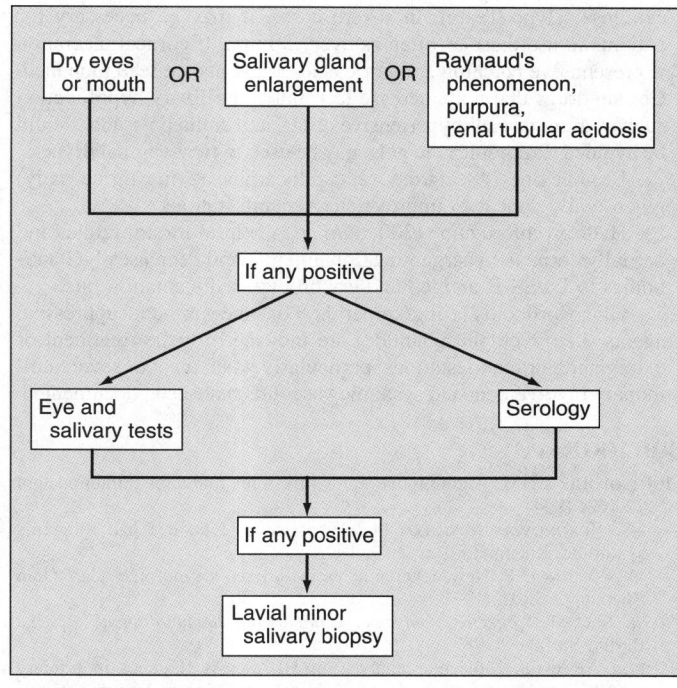

FIGURE 316-1   Algorithm for the diagnosis of Sjögren's syndrome.

tract, can be affected. Lymphomas may appear in Sjögren's syndrome patients after several years of an apparently benign course and are observed more often in patients with systemic disease.

Routine laboratory tests reveal mild normochromic, normocytic anemia. An elevated erythrocyte sedimentation rate is found in approximately 70 percent of patients.

DIAGNOSIS AND DIFFERENTIAL DIAGNOSIS   A European multicenter study has developed diagnostic criteria of Sjögren's syndrome (Table 316-3), which have been validated and present high specificity and sensitivity. A diagnostic algorithm is depicted in Fig. 316-1.

The differential diagnosis of Sjögren's syndrome includes other conditions that may cause dry mouth or eyes or parotid salivary gland enlargement (Table 316-4). Human immunodeficiency virus (HIV) infection (see Chap. 308) and sarcoidosis (see Chap. 320) appear to produce a clinical picture indistinguishable from Sjögren's syndrome (Table 316-5).

Rx   TREATMENT

Sjögren's syndrome remains fundamentally an incurable disease. Hence treatment of Sjögren's syndrome is aimed at symptomatic relief and limiting the damaging local effects of chronic xerostomia and keratoconjunctivitis sicca by substitution of the missing secretions.

The sicca complex is treated with fluid replacement supplied as often as necessary. To replace deficient tears, there are several readily available ophthalmic preparations (Tearisol; Liquifilm; 0.5% methyl-

Lymphoma and Waldenström's macroglobulinemia are well-known manifestations of Sjögren's syndrome. Most lymphomas are of B cell origin. Pseudolymphoma or frank lymphoma should always be suspected when persistent major salivary gland enlargement, lymphadenopathy, lung nodules, or hilar or mediastinal lymphadenopathy is observed. Parenchymal organs, such as lungs and gastrointestinal

Table 316-5

Differential Diagnosis of Sjögren's Syndrome with HIV Infection

HIV Infection and Sicca Syndrome	Sjögren's Syndrome	Sarcoidosis
Predominant in young males	Predominant in middle-aged women	Invariable
Lack of autoantibodies to Ro/SS-A and/or La/SS-B	Presence of autoantibodies	Lack of autoantibodies to Ro/SS-A and/or La/SS-B
Lymphoid infiltrates of salivary glands by CD8+ lymphocytes	Lymphoid infiltrates of salivary glands by CD4+ lymphocytes	Granulomas in salivary glands
Association with HLA-DR5	Association with HLA-DR3 and -DRw52	Unknown
Positive serologic tests for HIV	Negative serologic tests for HIV	Negative serologic tests for HIV

cellulose; Hypo Tears). In severe cases, it may be necessary for patients to use these as often as every 30 min. If corneal ulceration is present, eye patching and boric acid ointments are recommended. Certain drugs that may increase lacrimal and salivary hypofunction such as diuretics, antihypertensive drugs, and antidepressants should be avoided. Propionic acid gels may be used to treat vaginal dryness.

Bromhexine (48 mg/day) and pilocarpine (5 mg thrice daily) given orally appear to improve sicca manifestations.

Hydroxychloroquine (200 mg/day) is helpful for arthralgias and partially corrects hypergammaglobulinemia and decreases IgG antibodies to La/SS-B antigen and erythrocyte sedimentation rate.

Glucocorticoids (1 mg/kg per day) or other immunosuppressive agents (i.e., cyclophosphamide) are indicated for the treatment of extraglandular manifestations, particularly when renal or severe pulmonary involvement and systemic vasculitis have been documented.

BIBLIOGRAPHY

MOUTSOPOULOS HM: Autoimmune epithelitis. Clin Immunol Immunopathol 72:162, 1994

———, VLACHOYIANNOPOULOS PG: What would I do if I had Sjögren's syndrome. Rheumatol Rev 2:17, 1993

———, YOUINOU P: New developments in Sjögren's syndrome. Curr Opin Rheumatol 3:815, 1991

TALAL N et al: *Sjögren's syndrome. Clinical and Immunological Aspects.* Berlin, Springer, 1987

TAMBUR AR et al: Molecular analysis of HLA class II genes in primary Sjögren's syndrome: A study of Israeli and Greek non-Jewish patients. Hum Immunol 36:235, 1993

TZIOUFAS AG, MOUTSOPOULOS HM: Sjögren's syndrome, in *Connective Tissue Diseases*. JJF Belch, RB Zurier (eds). London, Chapman and Hall, 1995

VITALI C et al: Preliminary criteria for the classification of Sjögren's syndrome: Results of a prospective concerted action supported by the European Community. Arthritis Rheum 36:340, 1992

317 *Joel D. Taurog, Peter E. Lipsky*

ANKYLOSING SPONDYLITIS, REACTIVE ARTHRITIS, AND UNDIFFERENTIATED SPONDYLOARTHROPATHY

The spondyloarthropathies are a group of disorders that share certain clinical features and an association with the HLA-B27 allele. These disorders include ankylosing spondylitis, Reiter's syndrome, reactive arthritis, psoriatic arthritis and spondylitis, enteropathic arthritis and spondylitis, juvenile-onset spondyloarthropathy, and undifferentiated spondyloarthropathy. The similarity in clinical manifestations and in genetic predisposition suggests that these disorders share pathogenic mechanisms. Specific definitions and diagnostic criteria for the individual conditions will be provided in subsequent sections of this chapter.

ANKYLOSING SPONDYLITIS

Ankylosing spondylitis (AS) is an inflammatory disorder of unknown cause that primarily affects the axial skeleton; peripheral joints and extraarticular structures also may be involved. The disease usually begins in the second or third decade; the prevalence in men is approximately three times that in women. It is considered the prototype of the spondyloarthropathies. Older names include *Marie-Strümpell disease* or *Bechterew's disease*.

EPIDEMIOLOGY AS shows a striking correlation with the histocompatibility antigen HLA-B27 and occurs worldwide roughly in proportion to the prevalence of this antigen (see Chap. 306). In North American Caucasians, the general prevalence of B27 is 7 per-

cent, whereas over 90 percent of patients with AS have inherited this antigen. The association with B27 is independent of disease severity.

In population surveys, 1 to 2 percent of adults inheriting B27 have been found to have AS. In contrast, in families of patients with AS, the prevalence is 10 to 20 percent among adult first-degree relatives inheriting B27. The concordance rate in identical twins is estimated to be 50 percent. These findings indicate that both genetic and environmental factors play a role in the pathogenesis of the disease and that the genetic factors probably include allelic genes in addition to B27. AS is strongly associated with inflammatory bowel disease (IBD), including both ulcerative colitis and Chrohn's disease. IBD is a risk factor for AS independent of HLA–B27, although 50 to 75 percent of patients with both AS and IBD are B27 positive. → See also Chap. 286.

PATHOLOGY Sacroiliitis is usually one of the earliest manifestations of AS. The early lesion consists of subchondral granulation tissue containing lymphocytes, plasma cells, mast cells, macrophages, and chondrocytes. Usually, the thinner iliac cartilage is eroded before the thicker sacral cartilage. The irregularly eroded, sclerotic margins of the joint are gradually replaced by fibrocartilage regeneration and then by ossification. Ultimately, the joint may be totally obliterated. This progression is evident radiographically (see below).

In the spine, the initial lesion consists of inflammatory granulation tissue at the junction of the annulus fibrosus of the disk cartilage and the margin of vertebral bone. The outer annular fibers are eroded and eventually replaced by bone, forming the beginning of a bony excrescence called a *syndesmophyte*, which then grows by continued enchondral ossification, ultimately bridging the adjacent vertebral bodies. Ascending progression of this process leads to the "bamboo spine" observed radiographically. Other lesions in the spine include diffuse osteoporosis, erosion of vertebral bodies at the disk margin, "squaring" of vertebrae, and inflammation and destruction of the disk-bone border. Inflammatory arthritis of the apophyseal joints is common, with erosion of cartilage by pannus, often followed by bony ankylosis.

Peripheral arthritis in AS can show synovial hyperplasia, lymphoid infiltration, and pannus formation, but the process lacks the exuberant synovial villi, fibrin deposits, ulcers, and plaques of plasma cells seen in rheumatoid arthritis (see Chap. 313). Central cartilaginous erosions caused by proliferation of subchondral granulation tissue are common in AS but rare in rheumatoid arthritis.

The enthesis, the site of tendinous or ligamentous attachment to bone, is another common site of pathology in AS, especially at sites localized around the spine and pelvis. Enthesitis is characterized by erosive, inflammatory lesions that may eventually undergo ossification.

Acute anterior uveitis (iritis) occurs in approximately 20 percent of patients with AS. Few cases have been studied histologically, none at an early stage. After recurrent attacks, the iris shows nonspecific inflammatory changes, scarring, increased vascularity, and pigment-laden macrophages.

Aortic insufficiency develops in a small percentage of cases. There is thickening of the aortic valve cusps and the aorta near the sinuses of Valsalva, with dense adventitial scar tissue and intimal fibrous proliferation. The scar tissue can extend into the ventricular septum with resultant heart block.

Microscopic inflammatory lesions of the colon and ileocecal valve have been found in 25 to 50 percent of patients with AS, even in those lacking any clinical evidence of inflammatory bowel disease. IgA nephropathy has been reported with increased frequency.

PATHOGENESIS The pathogenesis of AS is incompletely understood. A number of features of the disease implicate immune-mediated mechanisms, including elevated serum levels of IgA and acute phase reactants, inflammatory histology, and close association with HLA-B27. No specific event or exogenous agent that triggers the onset of disease has been identified, although overlapping features with reactive arthritis and inflammatory bowel disease suggest that enteric bacteria may play a role. Elevated serum titers of antibodies to certain enteric bacteria, particularly *Klebsiella pneumoniae*, are common in AS patients. Furthermore, antigenic interrelatedness between B27 and certain enteric bacteria has been documented, but it is not yet known whether these factors contribute to the pathogenesis of AS. Evidence that B27 plays a direct role is provided by the finding that rats transgenic for B27 spontaneously develop spondylitis, along with colitis, peripheral arthritis, and other lesions characteristic of the spondyloarthropathies (see below).

CLINICAL MANIFESTATIONS The symptoms of the disease are usually first noticed in late adolescence or early adulthood; onset after age 40 is unusual. The initial symptom is usually dull pain, insidious in onset, felt deep in the lower lumbar or gluteal region, accompanied by low-back morning stiffness of up to a few hours' duration that improves with activity and returns following periods of inactivity. Within a few months of onset, the pain usually has become persistent and bilateral. Nocturnal exacerbation of pain that forces the patient to rise and move around may be frequent.

In some patients bony tenderness may accompany back pain or stiffness, while in others it may be the predominant complaint. Common sites include the costosternal junctions, spinous processes, iliac crests, greater trochanters, ischial tuberosities, tibial tubercles, and heels. Occasionally, bony chest pain is the presenting complaint. Arthritis in the hips and shoulders ("root" joints) occurs in 25 to 35 percent of patients, in many cases early in the disease course. Arthritis of peripheral joints other than the hips and shoulders, usually asymmetric, occurs in up to 30 percent of patients and can occur at any stage of the disease. Neck pain and stiffness from involvement of the cervical spine are usually relatively late manifestations. Occasional patients present with predominantly constitutional symptoms such as fatigue, anorexia, fever, weight loss, or night sweats.

AS often has a juvenile onset in developing countries. In these individuals, peripheral arthritis and enthesitis usually predominate, with axial symptoms supervening in late adolescence.

The most common extraarticular manifestation is acute anterior uveitis, which can antedate the spondylitis. Attacks are typically unilateral and tend to recur, causing pain, photophobia, and increased lacrimation. Aortic insufficiency, sometimes producing symptoms of congestive heart failure, occurs in a few percent of patients, occasionally early in the course of the spinal disease. Up to half the patients have inflammation in the colon or ileum. This is usually asymptomatic, but in 5 to 10 percent of patients with AS, frank IBD will develop.

Initially, physical findings mirror the inflammatory process. The most specific findings involve loss of spinal mobility, with limitation of anterior and lateral flexion and extension of the lumbar spine and of chest expansion. Limitation of motion is usually out of proportion to the degree of bony ankylosis, reflecting muscle spasm secondary to pain and inflammation. Pain in the sacroiliac joints may be elicited either with direct pressure or with maneuvers that stress the joints, but these techniques are unreliable in discriminating inflammatory sacroiliitis. In addition, there is commonly tenderness upon palpation at the sites of symptomatic bony tenderness and paraspinous muscle spasm.

The Schober test is a useful measure of flexion of the lumbar spine. The patient stands erect, with heels together, and marks are made directly over the spine 5 cm below and 10 cm above the lumbosacral junction (identified by a horizontal line between the posterosuperior iliac spines.) The patient then bends forward maximally, and the distance between the two marks is measured. The distance between the two marks increases 5 cm or more in the case of normal mobility and less than 4 cm in the case of decreased mobility. Chest expansion is measured as the difference between maximal inspiration and maximal forced expiration in the fourth intercostal space in males or just below the breasts in females. Normal chest expansion is 5 cm or greater.

Limitation or pain with motion of the hips or shoulders is usually present if either of these joints is involved. Careful examination is also necessary to detect inflammatory disease of peripheral joints. It should be emphasized that early in the course of mild cases, symptoms may be subtle and nonspecific, and the physical examination may be completely normal.

The course of the disease is extremely variable, ranging from the individual with mild stiffness and radiographically equivocal sacroiliitis to the patient with a totally fused spine and severe bilateral hip arthritis, possibly accompanied by severe peripheral arthritis and extra-

articular manifestations. Pain tends to be persistent early in the disease and then to become intermittent, with alternating exacerbations and quiescent periods. In a typical severe untreated case with progression of the spondylitis to syndesmophyte formation, the patient's posture undergoes characteristic changes. The lumbar lordosis is obliterated with accompanying atrophy of the buttocks. The thoracic kyphosis is accentuated. If the cervical spine is involved, there may be a forward stoop of the neck. Hip involvement with ankylosis may lead to flexion contractures, compensated by flexion at the knees. The progression of the disease may be followed by measuring the patient's height, chest expansion, Schober test, and occiput-to-wall distance when the patient stands erect with the heels and back flat against the wall. Occasional individuals are encountered with advanced physical findings suggestive of long-standing AS who report having never had significant symptoms.

Onset of the disease in adolescence correlates both with a worse prognosis and more frequent and severe hip involvement. The disease in women tends to progress less frequently to total spinal ankylosis, although there is some evidence for an increased prevalence of isolated cervical ankylosis and peripheral arthritis in women. In industrialized countries, peripheral arthritis (distal to hips and shoulders) occurs overall in about 25 percent of patients, usually as a late manifestation, whereas in developing countries, the prevalence is much higher, with onset typically early in the disease course.

The most serious complication of the spinal disease is spinal fracture, which can occur with even minor trauma to the rigid, osteoporotic spine. The cervical spine is most commonly involved, and this can lead to quadriplegia. Cauda equina syndrome and slowly progressive upper pulmonary lobe fibrosis are rare complications of long-standing AS. The prevalence of aortic insufficiency and of cardiac conduction disturbances, including third-degree heart block, increases with prolonged disease. Prostatitis has been reported to have an increased prevalence in men with AS. Amyloidosis is only rarely associated (see Chap. 309).

Despite the persistence of the disease, most patients with AS remain gainfully employed. Only in uncommon instances does the disease appear to shorten life, these being largely the result of spinal trauma, complications of therapy such as upper gastrointestinal hemorrhage, aortic insufficiency, respiratory failure, or amyloid nephropathy.

LABORATORY FINDINGS No laboratory test is diagnostic of AS. In most ethnic groups, the HLA-B27 gene is present in approximately 90 percent of patients with AS. Most patients with active disease have an elevated erythrocyte sedimentation rate and an elevated level of C-reactive protein. A mild normochromic, normocytic anemia may be present. Patients with severe disease may show an elevated alkaline phosphatase level. Elevated serum IgA levels are common. Rheumatoid factor and antinuclear antibodies are uniformly absent unless caused by a coexistent disease unrelated to AS. Synovial fluid from inflamed peripheral joints in AS is not distinctly different from that of other inflammatory joint diseases. In cases with restriction of chest wall motion, decreased vital capacity and increased functional residual capacity are common, but airflow measurements are normal and ventilatory function is usually well maintained.

RADIOGRAPHIC FINDINGS Radiographically demonstrable sacroiliitis is usually present in AS. The earliest changes in the sacroiliac joints demonstrable by standard radiography are blurring of the cortical margins of the subchondral bone, followed by erosions and sclerosis. Progression of the erosions leads to "pseudowidening" of the joint space; as fibrous and then bony ankylosis supervene, the joints may become obliterated radiographically. The changes and progression of the lesions are usually symmetric.

In mild cases, years may elapse before unequivocal sacroiliac abnormalities are evident on plain radiographs. Computed tomography (CT) and magnetic resonance imaging can detect abnormalities reliably at an earlier stage than plain radiography, but the role of these techniques in routine diagnosis is not yet settled.

Roentgenographic abnormalities generally appear in the sacroiliac joints before appearing elsewhere in the spine. In the lumbar spine, progression of the disease leads to straightening, caused by loss of lordosis, and reactive sclerosis, caused by osteitis of the anterior corners of the vertebral bodies with subsequent erosion, leading to "squaring" of the vertebral bodies. Progressive ossification of the superficial layers of the annulus fibrosus leads to eventual formation of marginal syndesmophytes, visible on plain films as bony bridges connecting successive vertebral bodies anteriorly and laterally.

DIAGNOSIS The diagnosis of early AS before the development of irreversible deformity can be difficult to establish. Currently, modified New York criteria (1984) are widely used for diagnosis. These consist of the following: (1) a history of inflammatory back pain (see below); (2) limitation of motion of the lumbar spine in both the sagittal and frontal planes; (3) limited chest expansion, relative to standard values for age and sex; and (4) definite radiographic sacroiliitis. Under these criteria, the presence of radiographic sacroiliitis plus any one of the other three criteria is sufficient for a diagnosis of definite AS.

Several studies have identified a sizable population of B27-positive individuals with symptoms suggestive of AS who lack definite radiographic sacroiliitis. Over time, most of these patients eventually develop radiographic changes. This indicates that diagnostic criteria based on plain radiographic findings may often be too insensitive for the diagnosis of early AS. The presence of B27 is neither necessary nor sufficient for the diagnosis, but the B27 test can be helpful in patients who have not yet developed radiographic sacroiliitis.

AS must be differentiated from numerous other causes of low-back pain, some of which are far more common than AS. The inflammatory back pain of AS is usually distinguished by the following five features: (1) age of onset below 40, (2) insidious onset, (3) duration greater than 3 months before medical attention is sought, (4) morning stiffness, and (5) improvement with exercise or activity. The most common causes of back pain other than AS are primarily mechanical or degenerative rather than inflammatory and do not show these features. Less common metabolic, infectious, and malignant causes of back pain also must be differentiated from AS.

Marked calcification and ossification of paraspinous ligaments occur in *diffuse idiopathic skeletal hyperostosis* (DISH). Although DISH is often categorized as a variant of osteoarthritis, diarthrodial joints are not involved. Ligamentous calcification and ossification are usually most prominent in the anterior spinal ligament and give the appearance of "flowing wax" on the anterior bodies of the vertebrae. However, a radiolucency may be seen between the newly deposited bone and the vertebral body, differentiating DISH from the marginal osteophytes in spondylosis. Intervertebral disk spaces are preserved, and sacroiliac and apophyseal joints appear normal, helping to differentiate DISH from spondylosis and from AS, respectively.

DISH occurs in the middle-aged and the elderly and is more common in men than in women. Patients are frequently asymptomatic but may have stiffness. Radiographic changes are generally much more severe than might be predicted from the mild symptoms caused by DISH.

℞ **TREATMENT**

There is no definitive treatment for AS. The principal goal of management is the conscientious participation by the patient in an exercise program designed to maintain functional posture and to preserve range of motion. There is evidence that exercise increases mobility and improves function. Most patients require anti-inflammatory agents to achieve sufficient symptomatic relief to be able to remain functional and carry out the exercise program. It is not known whether drug treatment alone can alter the progression of the disease.

Several nonsteroidal anti-inflammatory drugs (NSAIDs) have proved effective in reducing the pain and stiffness of AS and are commonly used. Indomethacin is particularly effective as a 75-mg slow-release preparation taken once or twice daily. Although phenyl-

butazone, at doses of 200 to 400 mg/d, has been considered by several authorities to be the most effective agent in AS, because of its greater potential for serious side effects such as aplastic anemia and agranulocytosis, its use in the United States is confined to patients with very severe disease whose symptoms do not respond at all to other agents. Recent controlled trials suggest that sulfasalazine,[1] in doses of 2 to 3 g/d, is useful in reducing peripheral joint symptoms as well as reversing laboratory evidence of inflammation. Some studies have not shown it to benefit axial arthritis, and its effect on natural progression of the disease is unproven. The peripheral arthritis also may respond to the folic acid antagonist methotrexate.[1] No therapeutic role for gold, penicillamine, immunosuppressive drugs, or systemic glucocorticoids has been documented in AS. Occasionally, intralesional or intraarticular glucocorticoid injections may be beneficial in patients with persistent enthesopathy or synovitis unresponsive to anti-inflammatory agents. Recent studies have suggested that symptomatic benefit can be achieved from CT-guided glucocorticoid injections into the sacroiliac joints.

The most common indication for surgery in patients with AS is severe hip joint arthritis, the pain and stiffness of which are often dramatically relieved by total hip arthroplasty. A small number of patients may benefit from surgical correction of extreme flexion deformities of the spine or of atlantoaxial subluxation.

Attacks of iritis are usually effectively managed with local glucocorticoid administration in conjunction with mydriatic agents. Coexistent cardiac disease may require pacemaker implantation or aortic valve replacement.

REACTIVE ARTHRITIS AND UNDIFFERENTIATED SPONDYLOARTHROPATHY

Reactive arthritis (ReA) refers to acute nonpurulent arthritis complicating an infection elsewhere in the body. In recent years, the term has been used primarily to refer to spondyloarthropathies following enteric or urogenital infections and occurring predominantly in individuals with the histocompatibility antigen HLA-B27. Included in this category is the constellation of clinical findings formerly commonly called *Reiter's syndrome*. Other forms of reactive arthritis not associated with B27 and showing a different spectrum of clinical features, such as rheumatic fever, are discussed elsewhere (see Chap. 236).

HISTORICAL BACKGROUND The association of acute arthritis with episodes of diarrhea or urethritis has been recognized for centuries. A large number of cases during World Wars I and II focused attention on the triad of arthritis, urethritis, and conjunctivitis, which became known as Reiter's syndrome, often occurring with additional mucocutaneous lesions.

The identification of bacterial species capable of triggering the clinical syndrome and the finding that up to three-fourths of the patients possess the B27 antigen have led to the unifying concept of ReA as a clinical syndrome triggered by specific etiologic agents in a genetically susceptible host. A similar spectrum of clinical manifestations can be triggered by enteric infection with any of several *Shigella*, *Salmonella*, *Yersinia*, and *Campylobacter* species, by genital infection with *Chlamydia trachomatis*, and possibly by other agents as well. Although Reiter's syndrome can be said to represent one part of the spectrum of the clinical manifestations of ReA, particularly that induced by *Shigella* or *Chlamydia*, the term is now largely of historical interest only. Since most patients with spondyloarthropathy do not have the classic features of Reiter's syndrome, it has become customary to employ the term *reactive arthritis*, regardless of whether or not there is evidence for a triggering infection. For the purposes of this chapter, the use of ReA will be restricted to those cases of spondyloarthropathy in which there is at least presumptive evidence for a related antecedent infection. Patients with clinical features of ReA who lack both evidence of an antecedent infection and the classic findings of Reiter's syndrome

---

[1] Azathioprine, methotrexate, and sulfasalazine have not been approved for this purpose by the Food and Drug Administration at the time of publication.

will be considered to have *undifferentiated spondyloarthropathy*, which is discussed at the end of this chapter.

CHAPTER 317
Ankylosing Spondylitis, Reactive Arthritis **1907**

EPIDEMIOLOGY   Like AS, ReA occurs predominantly in individuals who have inherited the B27 gene; in most series, 60 to 85 percent of patients are B27 positive. In epidemics of arthritogenic bacterial infection, e.g., *S. flexneri*, it has been estimated that ReA develops in ~20 percent of exposed B27-positive individuals. In families with multiple cases of AS or ReA, the two conditions have been said to "breed true," i.e., to be uncommonly found together within an individual family. Whether this is caused by genetic or environmental factors is not known. The disease is most common in individuals 18 to 40 years of age, but it can occur both in children over 5 years of age and in older adults.

The sex ratio in ReA following enteric infection is nearly 1:1, whereas venereally acquired ReA is predominantly a male disease. The overall prevalence and incidence of ReA are difficult to assess because of the variable prevalence of the triggering infections and genetic susceptibility factors in different populations. For example, in Olmsted County, MN, the incidence was estimated as 3.5 cases per 100,000 population per year. In contrast, in a population with a high rate of genitourinary and/or gastrointestinal infections such as urban homosexual and bisexual men, the prevalence may approach 1 per 1000.

A particularly severe form of peripheral spondyloarthropathy has been described in patients with AIDS (see Chap. 308). Most of these patients are HLA-B27 positive, but human immunodeficiency virus (HIV) infection per se is not an independent risk factor for spondyloarthropathy.

PATHOLOGY   Synovial histology is similar to that of other inflammatory arthropathies. Enthesitis is a common clinical finding in ReA; the histology of this lesion resembles that of AS. Microscopic histopathologic evidence of inflammation has occasionally been noted in the colon and ileum of patients with postvenereal ReA, but much less commonly than in postenteric ReA. The skin lesions of keratoderma blenorrhagica, which is associated mainly with venereally acquired ReA, are histologically indistinguishable from psoriatic lesions.

ETIOLOGY AND PATHOGENESIS   The first bacterial infection noted to be causally related to ReA was *S. flexneri*. An outbreak of shigellosis among Finnish troops in 1944 resulted in numerous cases of ReA. Of the four species *S. sonnei*, *S. boydii*, *S. flexneri*, and *S. dysenteriae*, *S. flexneri* has most often been implicated in cases of ReA, both sporadic and epidemic. *S. sonnei*, although responsible for the majority of cases of shigellosis in the United States, has only rarely been implicated in cases of ReA.

Other bacteria that have been definitively identified as triggers of ReA include several *Salmonella* species, *Y. enterocolitica*, *C. jejuni*, and *C. trachomatis*. There is suggestive evidence implicating several other microorganisms, including *Y. pseudotuberculosis*, *Clostridium difficile*, *Neisseria gonorrhoeae*, and *Ureaplasma urealyticum*. *Chlamydia pneumoniae*, a respiratory pathogen, has also recently been implicated in triggering ReA. There are also numerous isolated reports of acute arthritis preceded by other bacterial, viral, or parasitic infections, but whether the microorganisms involved are actual triggers of ReA remains to be determined.

It has not been determined whether ReA occurs by the same pathogenic mechanism following infection with each of these microorganisms, nor has the mechanism been fully elucidated in the case of any one of the known bacterial triggers. Most, if not all, of the triggering organisms share a capacity to attack mucosal surfaces, to invade host cells, and survive intracellularly. Antigens from *Chlamydia*, *Yersinia*, *Salmonella*, and *Shigella* have been shown to be present in the synovium of patients with ReA for long periods following the acute attack. In the case of *C. trachomatis*, synovial persistence of microbial DNA and RNA suggests the presence of viable organisms, despite uniform failure to culture the organism from these specimens. It is thus conceivable that the disorder may be a form of chronic infection, rather than solely "reactive." T cells that specifically respond to antigens of the inciting organism are typically found in inflamed synovium but not in peripheral blood of patients with ReA. These T cells are predominantly CD4+, but CD8+ B27-restricted bacteria-specific cytolitic T cells

have also been isolated in *Yersinia*- and *C. trachomatis*-induced ReA. The antibody response to *Yersinia*, *Salmonella*, and, in some studies, *C. trachomatis* tends to be more prolonged in patients developing ReA triggered by infection with these organisms than in individuals with uncomplicated infection. The role of these various immune responses in disease pathogenesis is not yet known.

The role of HLA-B27 in ReA remains to be determined. Transgenic rats with high expression of B27 spontaneously develop a multiple organ system inflammatory disease affecting the gut, peripheral and axial joints, male genital tract, and skin that resembles these human conditions clinically and histologically. When raised in a germ-free environment, the B27 rats do not develop gut or joint inflammation, but the skin and genital lesions are not prevented. These findings suggest that bacteria are necessary, and normal gut bacteria are sufficient, to induce B27-related joint inflammation. In both the rat and human diseases, it remains to be determined whether the primary process is an autoimmune response against host tissues or an immune response against antigens of the triggering organism that have disseminated to the target tissues, and the specific role of B27 itself remains to be determined.

CLINICAL FEATURES   The clinical manifestations of ReA constitute a spectrum that ranges from an isolated, transient monarthritis to severe multisystem disease. In the majority of cases, a careful history will elicit some evidence of an antecedent infection 1 to 4 weeks before the onset of symptoms of the reactive disease. However, in a sizable minority, no clinical or laboratory evidence of an antecedent infection can be found. In many cases of presumed venereally acquired reactive disease, there is a history of a recent new sexual partner, even in the absence of laboratory evidence of infection.

Constitutional symptoms are common, including fatigue, malaise, fever, and weight loss. The musculoskeletal symptoms are usually acute in onset. Arthritis is usually asymmetric and additive, with involvement of new joints occurring over a period of a few days to 1 to 2 weeks. The joints of the lower extremities, especially the knee, ankle, and subtalar, metatarsophalangeal, and toe interphalangeal joints, are the most common sites of involvement, but the wrist and fingers can be involved as well. The arthritis is usually quite painful, and tense joint effusions are not uncommon, especially in the knee. Dactylitis, or "sausage digit," a diffuse swelling of a solitary finger or toe, is a distinctive feature of both ReA and psoriatic arthritis (see Chap. 325). Tendinitis and fasciitis are particularly characteristic lesions, producing pain at multiple insertion sites, especially the Achilles insertion, the plantar fascia, and sites along the axial skeleton. Spinal and low-back pain are quite common and may be caused by insertional inflammation, muscle spasm, acute sacroiliitis, or, presumably, arthritis in intervertebral articulations.

Urogenital lesions may occur throughout the course of the disease. In males, urethritis may be marked or relatively asymptomatic and may be either an accompaniment of the triggering infection or a result of the reactive phase of the disease. Prostatitis is also common. Similarly, in females, cervicitis or salpingitis may be caused either by the infectious trigger or by the sterile reactive process.

Ocular disease is common, ranging from transient, asymptomatic conjunctivitis to an aggressive anterior uveitis that occasionally proves refractory to treatment and may result in blindness.

Mucocutaneous lesions are frequent. Oral ulcers tend to be superficial, transient, and often asymptomatic. The characteristic skin lesions, *keratoderma blenorrhagica*, consist of vesicles that become hyperkeratotic, ultimately forming a crust before disappearing. They are most common on the palms and soles but may occur elsewhere as well. In patients with HIV infection, these lesions are often extremely severe and extensive, to the point of dominating the clinical picture (see Chap. 308). Lesions on the glans penis, termed *circinate balanitis*, are common; these consist of vesicles that quickly rupture to form painless superficial erosions, which in circumcised individuals can form crusts similar to those of keratoderma blenorrhagica. Nail changes are common and consist of onycholysis, distal yellowish discoloration, and/or heaped-up hyperkeratosis.

Less frequent or rare manifestations of ReA include cardiac conduction defects, aortic insufficiency, central or peripheral nervous system lesions, and pleuropulmonary infiltrates.

Long-term follow-up studies suggest that some joint symptoms persist in 30 to 60 percent of patients with ReA. Recurrences of the acute syndrome are common, and as many as 25 percent of patients either become unable to work or are forced to change occupations because of persistent joint symptoms. Chronic heel pain is often a particularly distressing symptom. Some aspects of ankylosing spondylitis are also common sequelae (see below). In some but not all studies, HLA-B27-positive patients have shown a worse outcome than B27-negative patients. The extent to which the long-term prognosis varies with different inciting agents is not known. However, patients with *Yersinia*-induced arthritis appear to have less chronic disease than those whose initial episode follows epidemic shigellosis.

LABORATORY AND RADIOGRAPHIC FINDINGS The erythrocyte sedimentation rate is elevated during the acute phase of the disease. Mild anemia may be present, and acute phase reactants tend to be increased. Synovial fluid is nonspecifically inflammatory, showing an elevated white cell count with a predominance of neutrophils. In most ethnic groups, 50 to 75 percent of the patients are B27 positive, although some recent studies of ReA following *Salmonella* epidemics have shown a B27 prevalence of 30 percent or less. It is unusual for the triggering infection to persist at the site of primary mucosal infection through the time of onset of the reactive disease, but it may occasionally be possible to culture the organism, e.g., in the case of *Yersinia*- or *Chlamydia*-induced disease. Serologic evidence of a recent infection may be present, such as a marked elevation of antibodies to *Yersinia*, *Salmonella*, or *Chlamydia*.

In early or mild disease, radiographic changes may be absent or confined to juxtaarticular osteoporosis. With long-standing persistent disease, marginal erosions and loss of joint space can be seen in affected joints. Periostitis with reactive new bone formation is characteristic of the disease, as it is with all the spondyloarthropathies. Spurs at the insertion of the plantar fascia are common.

Sacroiliitis and spondylitis may be seen as late sequelae. The sacroiliitis is more commonly asymmetric than in AS, and the spondylitis, rather than ascending symmetrically from the lower lumbar segments, can begin anywhere along the lumbar spine. The syndesmophytes may be coarse and nonmarginal, arising from the middle of a vertebral body, a pattern rarely seen in primary AS. Progression to spinal fusion as a sequela of ReA is uncommon.

DIAGNOSIS ReA is a clinical diagnosis, there being no definitively diagnostic laboratory test or radiographic finding. The diagnosis should be entertained in any patient with an acute inflammatory, asymmetric, additive arthritis or tendinitis. The evaluation of such a patient should include careful questioning regarding possible antecedent triggering events such as an episode of diarrhea or dysuria. On physical examination, careful attention must be paid to the distribution of the joint and tendon involvement and to possible sites of extraarticular involvement, such as the eyes, mucous membranes, skin, nails, and genitalia. Synovial fluid aspiration and analysis may be helpful in excluding septic or crystal-induced arthritis.

Although typing for B27 is not needed to secure the diagnosis in clear-cut cases, it may have prognostic significance in terms of severity, chronicity, and the propensity for spondylitis and uveitis. Furthermore, it can be helpful diagnostically in atypical cases, a positive test increasing and a negative test decreasing the probability of ReA.

It is particularly important to differentiate ReA from disseminated gonococcal disease, both of which can be venereally acquired and associated with urethritis (see Chap. 150). Gonococcal arthritis and tenosynovitis tend to involve both upper and lower extremities equally, whereas in ReA lower extremity symptoms usually predominate. Back pain is common in ReA but is not a feature of gonococcal disease, whereas the vesicular skin lesions characteristic of disseminated gonococcal disease are not found in ReA. A positive gonococcal culture from the urethra or cervix does not exclude a diagnosis of ReA; however, culturing gonococci from blood, skin lesion, or synovium establishes the diagnosis of disseminated gonococcal disease. Occasionally, the only definitive way to distinguish the two is through a therapeutic trial of antibiotics.

ReA shares many features in common with psoriatic arthropathy, including the asymmetry of the arthritis, a propensity for "sausage digits" and nail involvement, an association with uveitis, and skin lesions of similar histology (see Chap. 325). However, psoriatic arthritis is usually gradual in onset, the arthritis tends to affect primarily the upper extremities, and there is less associated periarthritis. Psoriatic arthritis is not associated with mouth ulcers or urethritis, or, usually, with bowel symptoms. Although psoriatic arthropathy shows some distinctive radiographic features that are not found in ReA, these occur only late in the disease and are of little help diagnostically. Only psoriatic spondylitis, not the peripheral arthritis, is associated with B27, about 50 percent of patients being positive. Occasional patients, usually B27 positive, following what appears to be a typical episode of ReA, will develop typical psoriasis and persistent arthritis such that the two entities become indistinguishable.

Undifferentiated spondyloarthropathy, or simply "spondyloarthropathy," is diagnosed in patients who lack evidence of an antecedent infection that might trigger ReA and who do not meet criteria for AS but who show clinical features of these disorders.

℞ TREATMENT

Most patients with ReA are benefitted to some degree by NSAIDs, although rarely are symptoms of the acute arthritis completely ameliorated, and some patients fail to respond at all. Indomethacin, 75 to 150 mg/d in divided doses, is the initial treatment of choice. Other NSAIDs may be tried, with phenylbutazone, 100 mg tid or qid, being the NSAID of last resort, to be used only in severe, refractory cases because of its potentially serious side effects.

It is unclear whether antibiotics have a role in the therapy of ReA. One controlled study suggested that prolonged administration of a long-acting tetracycline may accelerate recovery from *Chlamydia*-induced ReA, but subsequent results have been less encouraging, and therapy for other bacterial triggers of ReA has shown little or no benefit. However, there is evidence that prompt, appropriate antibiotic treatment of acute chlamydial urethritis may prevent subsequent reactive arthritis.

Two recent multicenter trials have suggested that sulfasalazine, up to 3 g/d in divided doses, may be beneficial to patients with persistent ReA.[1] Patients with debilitating symptoms refractory to NSAID and sulfasalazine therapy may respond to immunosuppressive agents such as azathioprine, 1 to 2 mg/kg per day, or to methotrexate, 7.5 to 15 mg per week. Systemic glucocorticoids are not generally used but in rare instances may be helpful in mobilizing a severely affected bedridden patient. Antimalarials, gold, and penicillamine are not useful in the treatment of ReA.

Tendinitis and other enthesitic lesions occasionally may benefit from intralesional glucocorticoids. Uveitis may require aggressive treatment with glucocorticoids to prevent serious sequelae. Skin lesions ordinarily require only symptomatic treatment. In patients with HIV infection and ReA, many of whom have severe skin lesions, the skin lesions in particular appear to respond to systemic treatment with zidovudine (see Chap. 308). Cardiac complications are managed conventionally; management of neurologic complications is symptomatic.

Patients need to be educated about the nature of the disease and the factors that predispose to its recurrence. Comprehensive management includes counseling of patients in the avoidance of sexually transmitted disease and exposure to enteropathogens, as well as appropriate use of physical therapy, vocational counseling, and continued surveillance for long-term complications such as ankylosing spondylitis.

FIGURE 317-1 Algorithm for diagnosis of the spondyloarthropathies.

UNDIFFERENTIATED AND JUVENILE-ONSET SPONDYLOARTHROPATHY

It is not uncommon for clinicians to encounter patients, usually young adults, who do not have inflammatory bowel disease or psoriasis, lack evidence of an antecedent triggering infection, and do not have the classic triad of Reiter's syndrome or meet criteria for ankylosing spondylitis, who nonetheless present with some features of one or more of the spondyloarthropathies discussed above. For example, a patient may present with inflammatory synovitis of one knee, Achilles tendinitis, and dactylitis of one digit ("sausage digit"). It is now common to consider such patients as having *undifferentiated spondyloarthropathy*, or simply *spondyloarthropathy*. Other terms for this condition have included *seronegative oligoarthritis*, *undifferentiated oligoarthritis*, and the now-outmoded *incomplete Reiter's syndrome*. It is likely that some, perhaps most, of these patients have ReA in which the triggering infection remains undetected. In some other cases, the patient subsequently develops inflammatory bowel disease or psoriasis or the process eventually meets criteria for ankylosing spondylitis. Approximately half the patients with undifferentiated spondyloarthropathy are HLA-B27 positive, and thus the absence of B27 is not useful in establishing or excluding the diagnosis.

In *juvenile-onset spondyloarthropathy*, which begins most commonly in boys between ages 7 and 16, an asymmetric, predominantly lower extremity oligoarthritis and enthesitis without extraarticular features is the typical mode of presentation. The prevalence of B27 in this condition, which has been termed the *SEA syndrome* (seronegative,

enthesopathy, arthropathy), is approximately 80 percent. Many of these patients go on to develop typical ankylosing spondylitis in late adolescence or adulthood.

Management of undifferentiated spondyloarthropathy is similar to that of the other spondyloarthropathies, with NSAIDs and physical therapy forming the mainstays of treatment. Textbooks of pediatrics should be consulted for information on management of juvenile-onset spondyloarthropathy. An algorithm for the diagnosis of the spondyloarthropathies in adults is presented in Fig. 317-1.

BIBLIOGRAPHY

CALIN A AND TAUROG JD (eds): *The Spondyloarthritides*. Oxford, Oxford University Press, 1997

DOUGADOS M et al: Sulfasalazine in the treatment of spondylarthrapathy. A randomized, multicenter, double-blind, placebo-controlled study. Arthritis Rheum 38:618, 1995

GALL V: Exercise in the spondyloarthropathies. Arthritis Care Res 7:214, 1994

LEIRISALO-REPO M: Are antibiotics of any use in reactive arthritis? APMIS 101:575, 1993

MIELANTS H et al: The evolution of spondyloarthropathy in relation to gut histology. J Rheumatol 22:2266, 1995

NANAGARA R et al: Alteration of *Chlamydia trachomatis* biologic behavior in synovial membranes: Suppression of surface antigen production in reactive arthritis and Reiter's syndrome. Arthritis Rheum 38:1410, 1995

TAUROG JD et al: The germfree state prevents development of gut and joint inflammatory disease in HLA-B27 transgenic rats. J Exp Med 180:2359, 1994

318   *Haralampos M. Moutsopoulos*

BEHÇET'S SYNDROME

DEFINITION   Behçet's syndrome is a multisystem disorder presenting with recurrent oral and genital ulcerations as well as ocular involvement. Recently, internationally agreed diagnostic criteria have been proposed (Table 318-1).

PREVALENCE, PATHOGENESIS, AND PATHOLOGY
The disease has a worldwide distribution. The prevalence of Behçet's syndrome ranges from 1:10,000 in Japan to 1:500,000 in North America and Europe. It affects mainly young adults, with males having more severe disease than females.

The etiology and pathogenesis of this syndrome remain obscure; it is considered an autoimmune disease since vasculitis is the main pathologic lesion and circulating autoantibodies to human oral mucous membrane are found in approximately 50 percent of the cases. Familial occurrence has been reported, and in patients from eastern Mediterranean countries and Japan, the disease appears to be linked to HLA-B5 and -DR5 alloantigens.

CLINICAL FEATURES   The recurrent aphthous ulcerations are a *sine qua non* for the diagnosis. The ulcers are usually painful, shallow or deep with a central yellowish necrotic base, appear singly or in crops, and are located anywhere in the oral cavity. The ulcers persist for 1 to 2 weeks and subside without leaving scars. The genital ulcers resemble the oral ones.

Skin involvement includes folliculitis, erythema nodosum, an acne-like exanthem, and infrequently vasculitis. Nonspecific skin inflammatory reactivity to any scratches or intradermal saline injection (pathergy test) is a common and specific manifestation.

Eye involvement is the most dreaded complication, since it occasionally progresses rapidly to blindness. The eye disease is usually present at the onset but also may develop within the first few years. In addition to iritis, posterior uveitis, retinal vessel occlusions, and optic neuritis can be seen in some cases of the syndrome. Hypopyon uveitis, which is considered the hallmark of Behçet's syndrome, is in fact a rare manifestation.

The arthritis of Behçet's syndrome is not deforming and affects the knees and ankles.

Superficial or deep peripheral vein thrombosis is seen in one-fourth of the patients. Pulmonary emboli are a rare complication. The superior vena cava is obstructed occasionally, producing a dramatic clinical picture. Arterial involvement occurs infrequently and presents with aortitis or peripheral arterial aneurysm and arterial thrombosis. Pulmonary artery vasculitis presenting with dyspnea, cough, chest pain, hemoptysis, and infiltrates on chest roentgenograms has been reported recently in 5 percent of patients.

Central nervous system involvement is found more frequently in northern Europe and the United States. The most common lesions are benign intracranial hypertension, a multiple sclerosis–like picture, pyramidal involvement, and psychiatric disturbances.

Gastrointestinal involvement is reported in patients from Japan and includes mucosal ulcerations of the gut.

Laboratory findings are mainly nonspecific indices of inflammation such as leukocytosis and elevated erythrocyte sedimentation rate as well as C-reactive protein levels; antibodies to human oral mucosa are also found.

TREATMENT

The severity of the syndrome usually abates with time. Apart from the cases with neurologic complications, the life expectancy seems to be normal, and the only serious complication is blindness.

Treatment of Behçet's syndrome is symptomatic and empirical. Mucous membrane involvement may respond to topical glucocorticoids in the form of mouthwash or paste. Thrombophlebitis is treated with aspirin, 500 mg/d, and dipyridamole, 150 mg/d. Colchicine or interferon α can be beneficial for the arthritis of the syndrome. Uveitis and central nervous system involvement require systemic glucocorticoid therapy (prednisone, 1 mg/kg per day) and azathioprine, 2 to 3 mg/kg per day, or cyclosporine, 5 to 10 mg/kg per day.

BIBLIOGRAPHY

HAMURGUDAN V et al: Systemic interferon α2b treatment in Behçet's syndrome. J Rheumatol 21:1098, 1994

INTERNATIONAL STUDY GROUP FOR BEHÇET'S DISEASE: Criteria of diagnosis of Behçet's disease. Lancet 335:1078, 1990

MASUDA K et al: Double masked trial of cyclosporin in Behçet's disease. Lancet 1:1093, 1989

PAPIRIS SA, MOUTSOPOULOS HM: Rare rheumatic disorders: Behçet's disease. Baillieres Clin Rheumatol 7:173, 1993

RAZ I et al: Pulmonary manifestations in Behçet's syndrome. Chest 95:585, 1989

YAZICI H et al: A controlled trial of azathioprine in Behçet's syndrome. N Engl J Med 322:281, 1990

————: Behçet's syndrome, in *Rheumatology*. JH Klippel, PA Dieppe (eds). London, Mosby, 1995

319   *Anthony S. Fauci*

THE VASCULITIS SYNDROMES

DEFINITION   *Vasculitis* is a clinicopathologic process characterized by inflammation of and damage to blood vessels. The vessel lumen is usually compromised, and this is associated with ischemia of the tissues supplied by the involved vessel. A broad and heterogeneous group of syndromes may result from this process, since any type, size, and location of blood vessel may be involved. Vasculitis and its consequences may be the primary or sole manifestation of a disease; alternatively, vasculitis may be a secondary component of another primary disease. Vasculitis may be confined to a single organ such as the skin, or it may simultaneously involve several organ systems.

PATHOPHYSIOLOGY AND PATHOGENESIS   Generally, most of the vasculitic syndromes are assumed to be mediated at least in part by immunopathogenic mechanisms (see Table 319-1). However, evidence to this effect is for the most part indirect and may reflect epiphenomena as opposed to true causality. Vasculitis is generally considered within the broader category of *immune complex diseases* that include serum sickness and certain of the connective tissue diseases of which systemic lupus erythematosus (see Chap. 312) is the prototype. Although deposition of immune complexes in vessel walls is the most widely accepted pathogenic mechanism of vasculitis, the causal role of immune complexes has not been clearly established in most of the vasculitic syndromes. Circulating immune complexes need not result in deposition of the complexes in blood vessels with ensuing vasculitis, and many patients with active vasculitis do not have demonstrable circulating or deposited immune complexes. The actual antigen contained in the immune complex has only rarely been identified in vasculitic syndromes. In this regard, hepatitis B antigen has been identified in both the circulating and deposited immune complexes in a subset of patients with systemic vasculitis, most notably within the polyarteritis nodosa group (see below). Essential mixed cryoglobulinemia has been associated with hepatitis C virus infection; hepatitis

Table 318-1

Diagnostic Criteria of Behçet's Disease

Recurrent oral ulceration plus 2 of the following:
  Recurrent genital ulceration
  Eye lesions
  Skin lesions
  Pathergy test

C virions and hepatitis C virus antigen-antibody complexes have been identified in the cryoprecipitates of these patients. In addition, an association between persistent parvovirus B19 infection and certain vasculitides including Wegener's granulomatosis, polyarteritis nodosa, and Kawasaki's disease has been reported; however, the pathogenic mechanisms related to this association are unclear.

The mechanisms of tissue damage in immune-complex–mediated vasculitis resemble those described for serum sickness. In this model, antigen-antibody complexes are formed in antigen excess and are deposited in vessel walls whose permeability has been increased by vasoactive amines such as histamine, bradykinin, and leukotrienes released from platelets or from mast cells as a result of IgE-triggered mechanisms. The deposition of complexes results in activation of complement components, particularly C5a, which is strongly chemotactic for neutrophils. These cells then infiltrate the vessel wall, phagocytose the immune complexes, and release their intracytoplasmic enzymes, which damage the vessel wall. As the process becomes subacute or chronic, mononuclear cells infiltrate the vessel wall. The common denominator of the resulting syndrome is compromise of the vessel lumen with ischemic changes in the tissues supplied by the involved vessel.

In addition to the classic immune-complex–mediated mechanisms of vasculitis, other immunopathogenic mechanisms may be involved in damage to vessels. The most prominent of these are delayed hypersensitivity and cell-mediated immune injury as reflected in the histopathologic feature of granulomatous vasculitis. However, immune complexes themselves may induce granulomatous responses. Vascular endothelial cells can express HLA class II molecules following activation by cytokines such as interferon γ (IFNγ). This allows these cells to participate in immunologic reactions such as interaction with CD4 + T lymphocytes in a manner similar to antigen-presenting macrophages. Endothelial cells can secrete interleukin (IL)-1 which may activate T lymphocytes and initiate or propagate in situ immunologic processes within the blood vessel. In addition, IL-1 and tumor necrosis factor α (TNFα) are potent inducers of endothelial-leukocyte adhesion molecule 1 (ELAM-1) and vascular cell adhesion molecule 1 (VCAM-1), which may enhance the adhesion of leukocytes to endothelial cells in the blood vessel wall. Other mechanisms such as direct cellular cytotoxicity or antibody directed against vessel components or antibody-dependent cellular cytotoxicity have been suggested in certain types of vessel damage. However, there is no convincing evidence to support their causal contribution to the pathogenesis of any of the recognized vasculitic syndromes.

Antineutrophil Cytoplasmic Antibodies (ANCA) ANCA are antibodies directed against certain proteins in the cytoplasm of neutrophils. They are present in a high percentage of patients with systemic vasculitis, particularly Wegener's granulomatosis, as well as in patients with necrotizing and crescentic glomerulonephritis. They are important for the diagnosis and classification of Wegener's granulomatosis and other systemic vasculitides (see sections on individual diseases). There are two major categories of ANCA based on different targets for the antibodies. The terminology of cytoplasmic (c) ANCA refers to the diffuse, granular cytoplasmic staining pattern observed by immunofluorescence microscopy when serum antibodies bind to indicator neutrophils. Proteinase-3, the 29-kDa neutral serine proteinase present in neutrophil azurophilic granules is the major c-ANCA antigen. More than 90 percent of patients with typical Wegener's granulomatosis and active glomerulonephritis have a positive c-ANCA titer. The terminology of perinuclear (p) ANCA refers to the more localized perinuclear or nuclear staining pattern of the indicator neutrophils. The major target for p-ANCA is the enzyme myeloperoxidase; elastase is infrequently the target of p-ANCA. p-ANCA have been reported to occur in variable percentages of patients with polyarteritis nodosa, Churg-Strauss syndrome, polyangiitis overlap syndrome, crescentic glomerulonephritis, and Goodpasture's syndrome, as well as in some patients with characteristics of Wegener's granulomatosis.

It is unclear why patients with these vasculitis syndromes develop ANCA, whereas ANCA are rare in other inflammatory diseases. However, once ANCA are present, there are a number of in vitro observations that suggest feasible mechanisms whereby these antibodies can contribute to the pathogenesis of the vasculitis syndromes. When neutrophils are in the resting state, proteinase-3 exists in the azurophilic granules of the cytoplasm, apparently inaccessible to serum antibodies. However, when neutrophils are primed by TNFα or IL-1, proteinase-3 translocates to the cell membrane where it can interact with extracellular ANCA. The neutrophils then degranulate and produce reactive oxygen species that can cause tissue damage. Endothelial cells also translocate their cytoplasmic proteinase-3 to the cell membrane upon priming with TNFα, IL-1, or INFγ thus rendering them susceptible to interaction with ANCA and leading possibly to tissue damage due to complement-mediated cytotoxicity or antibody-dependent cellular cytotoxicity. Despite the attractiveness of these in vitro data, there is no conclusive evidence that ANCA are directly involved in the pathogenesis of the vasculitis syndromes, and they may represent merely an epiphenomenon; in fact, a number of clinical and laboratory observations argue against a primary pathogenic linkage. Patients may have vasculitis in the absence of ANCA; the absolute height of the antibody titers does not correlate well with disease activity; and patients with vasculitis, particularly Wegener's granulomatosis, in remission may continue to have high c-ANCA titers for years. Thus, their role in the pathogenesis of systemic vasculitis remains an open question.

It is unknown why certain individuals develop vasculitis in response to certain antigenic stimuli, whereas others do not. However, it is likely that a number of factors are involved in the ultimate expression of a vasculitic syndrome. These include the genetic predisposition and the regulatory mechanisms associated with immune response to certain antigens. When immune complexes are involved in the pathogenic process, the ability of the reticuloendothelial system to clear circulating complexes from the blood, the size and physicochemical properties of immune complexes, the relative degree of turbulence of blood flow, the intravascular hydrostatic pressure in different vessels, and the preexisting integrity of the vessel endothelium likely explain why only certain types of immune complexes cause vasculitis and why the vasculitic process is selective for only certain vessels in individual patients.

CLASSIFICATION OF VASCULITIC SYNDROMES A major feature of the vasculitic syndromes as a group is the fact that there is a great deal of heterogeneity at the same time as there is considerable overlap among them. This has led to both difficulty and confusion with regard to the categorization of these diseases. The classification scheme listed in Table 319-2 takes into account this heterogeneity and overlap and will serve as a matrix to emphasize the fact that certain syndromes are predominantly systemic in nature and

---

Table 319-1

Potential Pathogenic Mechanisms of Blood Vessel Damage in the Vasculitis Syndromes

IMMUNOPATHOGENIC MECHANISMS

In situ formation or deposition of immune complexes in blood vessel wall
Antineutrophil cytoplasmic antibody (ANCA)–mediated blood vessel damage
Direct antibody-mediated damage via antibodies directed at endothelial cells or other tissue components
Antibody-dependent cellular cytotoxicity directed against blood vessel tissue
Cytotoxic T lymphocytes directed at blood vessel components
Granuloma formation in blood vessel wall or adjacent to blood vessel
Cytokine (i.e., IL-1, TNFα)-induced mechanisms: expression of adhesion molecules for leukocytes on endothelial cells; induction of cytokine secretion by endothelial cells; procoagulant effects; prime neutrophils for ANCA-induced degranulation

NONIMMUNOPATHOGENIC MECHANISMS

Infiltration of blood vessel wall or surrounding tissue by microbial agents
Direct invasion of blood vessel wall by neoplastic cells
Unidentified mechanisms

almost invariably lead to irreversible organ system dysfunction and even death if untreated, while others are usually localized to the skin and rarely result in irreversible dysfunction of vital organs. The distinguishing and overlapping features of the diseases listed in Table 319-2, which justify this classification scheme, will be discussed below.

Approach to the Patient

Given the heterogeneous nature of the vasculitis syndromes, workup of a patient with suspected vasculitis should follow a series of progressive steps that establish the diagnosis of vasculitis, determine where possible the category of the vasculitis syndrome (Table 319-2), and determine the pattern and extent of disease activity. This information should then be utilized to determine the choice of therapeutic options (Fig. 319-1). This approach is of considerable importance since several of the vasculitis syndromes require aggressive therapy with glucocorticoids and immunosuppressive agents, while other syndromes usually resolve spontaneously and require symptomatic treatment only. Vasculitis is often suspected on clinical and laboratory grounds (see individual syndromes below). Depending on the individual category of vasculitis, measurement of ANCA titers may be helpful in this regard. However, a diagnosis of a vasculitis syndrome should not be made nor should treatment be initiated on the basis of a positive ANCA titer alone. The definitive diagnosis of vasculitis is made upon biopsy of involved tissue. The yield of "blind" biopsies of organs with no subjective or objective evidence of involvement is very low and should be avoided. When syndromes such as classic polyarteritis nodosa, Takayasu's arteritis, or the polyangiitis overlap syndrome are suspected, angiogram of organs with suspected involvement should be performed. However, angiograms should not be routinely performed when patients present with localized cutaneous vasculitis with no clinical indication of visceral involvement.

The constellation of clinical, laboratory, biopsy, and radiographic findings usually allows proper categorization to a specific syndrome, and therapy where appropriate should be initiated according to this information (see individual syndromes below). If an offending antigen that precipitates the vasculitis is recognized, the antigen should be

Table 319-2

Classification of the Vasculitis Syndromes

I. Systemic necrotizing vasculitis
  A. Polyarteritis nodosa (PAN)
    1. Classic PAN
    2. Microscopic polyangiitis
  B. Allergic angiitis and granulomatosis of Churg-Strauss
  C. Polyangiitis overlap syndrome
II. Wegener's granulomatosis
III. Temporal arteritis
IV. Takayasu's arteritis
V. Henoch-Schönlein purpura
VI. Predominantly cutaneous vasculitis (hypersensitivity vasculitis)
  A. Exogenous stimuli proven or suspected
    1. Drug-induced vasculitis
    2. Serum sickness and serum sickness–like reactions
    3. Vasculitis associated with infectious diseases
  B. Endogenous antigens likely involved
    1. Vasculitis associated with neoplasms (particularly lymphoid malignancies)
    2. Vasculitis associated with connective tissue diseases
    3. Vasculitis associated with other underlying diseases
    4. Vasculitis associated with congenital deficiencies of the complement system
VII. Other vasculitic syndromes
  A. Kawasaki disease
  B. Isolated central nervous system vasculitis
  C. Thromboangiitis obliterans (Buerger's disease)
  D. Behçet's syndrome
  E. Miscellaneous vasculitides

FIGURE 319-1 Algorithm for the approach to a patient with suspected diagnosis of vasculitis.

removed where possible. If the syndrome resolves, no further action should be taken. If disease activity continues, treatment should be initiated. If the vasculitis is associated with an underlying disease such as an infection, neoplasm, or connective tissue disease, the underlying disease should be treated. If the syndrome resolves, no further action should be taken. If the syndrome does not resolve or if there is no recognizable underlying disease and the vasculitis persists, treatment should be initiated according to the category of the vasculitis syndrome. Treatment options will be considered under the individual syndromes, and general principles of therapy will be considered at the end of the chapter.

SYSTEMIC NECROTIZING VASCULITIS

POLYARTERITIS NODOSA   **Definition**   *Classic polyarteritis nodosa* (PAN) was described in 1866 by Kussmaul and Maier. It is a multisystem, necrotizing vasculitis of small and medium-sized muscular arteries in which involvement of the renal and visceral arteries is characteristic. Classic PAN does not involve pulmonary arteries, although bronchial vessels may be involved; granulomas, significant eosinophilia, and an allergic diathesis are not part of the classic syndrome. The term *microscopic polyangiitis* (microscopic polyarteritis) was introduced into the literature by Davson in 1948. The Chapel Hill Consensus Conference on the Nomenclature of Systemic Vasculitis held in 1992 officially adopted the term to connote a necrotizing vasculitis with few or no immune complexes (pauci-immune) affecting small vessels (capillaries, venules, or arterioles). Since necrotizing arteritis involving small and medium-sized arteries may also be present, it shares features with classic PAN except that glomerulonephritis is very common in microscopic polyangiitis, and pulmonary capillaritis often occurs.

Incidence and Prevalence   It is difficult to establish an accurate incidence of this disease because of the fact that many reports of PAN actually have included both classic PAN and microscopic polyangiitis as well as other related vasculitides. Both diseases are uncommon, but classic PAN is felt to be more uncommon than microscopic polyangiitis. The mean age at onset in reports of PAN is 48 years, and the male-to-female ratio is 1.6:1.

Pathophysiology and Pathogenesis The vascular lesion in classic PAN is a necrotizing inflammation of small and medium-sized muscular arteries. The lesions are segmental and tend to involve bifurcations and branchings of arteries. They may spread circumferentially to involve adjacent veins. However, involvement of venules is not seen in classic PAN and, if present, suggests microscopic polyangiitis or the polyangiitis overlap syndrome (see below). In the acute stages of disease, polymorphonuclear neutrophils infiltrate all layers of the vessel wall and perivascular areas, which results in intimal proliferation and degeneration of the vessel wall. Mononuclear cells infiltrate the area as the lesions progress to the subacute and chronic stages. Fibrinoid necrosis of the vessels ensues with compromise of the lumen, thrombosis, infarction of the tissues supplied by the involved vessel, and, in some cases, hemorrhage. As the lesions heal, there is collagen deposition, which may lead to further occlusion of the vessel lumen. Aneurysmal dilatations up to 1 cm in size along the involved arteries are characteristic of classic PAN. Granulomas and substantial eosinophilia with eosinophilic tissue infiltrations are not characteristically found and suggest allergic angiitis and granulomatosis (see below).

Multiple organ systems are involved, and the clinicopathologic findings reflect the degree and location of vessel involvement and the resulting ischemic changes. As mentioned above, pulmonary arteries are not involved in classic PAN, and bronchial artery involvement is uncommon, whereas pulmonary capillaritis occurs frequently in microscopic polyangiitis. The pathology in the kidney in classic PAN is predominantly that of arteritis without glomerulonephritis. In contrast, glomerulonephritis is very common in microscopic polyangiitis. In patients with significant hypertension, typical pathologic features of glomerulosclerosis may be seen alone or superimposed on lesions of glomerulonephritis. In addition, pathologic sequelae of hypertension may be found elsewhere in the body.

The presence of hepatitis B antigenemia in approximately 20 to 30 percent of patients with systemic vasculitis, particularly of the classic PAN type, together with the isolation of circulating immune complexes composed of hepatitis B antigen and immunoglobulin, and the demonstration by immunofluorescence of hepatitis B antigen, IgM, and complement in the blood vessel walls, strongly suggest the role of immunologic phenomena in the pathogenesis of this disease. Hepatitis C infection has been reported in approximately 5 percent of patients with PAN; however, its pathogenic role in the vasculitis is unclear at present. Hairy cell leukemia can be associated with classic PAN; the pathogenic mechanisms of this association are unclear.

Clinical and Laboratory Manifestations Nonspecific signs and symptoms are the hallmarks of classic PAN. Fever, weight loss, and malaise are present in over one-half of cases. Patients usually present with vague symptoms such as weakness, malaise, headache, abdominal pain, and myalgias. Specific complaints related to the vascular involvement within a particular organ system also may dominate the presenting clinical picture as well as the entire course of the illness (Table 319-3). In classic PAN, renal involvement most commonly manifests as ischemic changes in the glomeruli, whereas in microscopic polyangiitis glomerulonephritis is the predominant renal lesion. Hypertension may be related to both the renal polyarteritis and the glomerulitis and may dominate the clinical picture. Classic PAN may involve any organ system; the clinical manifestations related to specific organ system involvement are listed in Table 319-3.

There are no diagnostic serologic tests for classic PAN. In over 75 percent of patients, the leukocyte count is elevated with a predominance of neutrophils. Eosinophilia is seen only rarely and, when present at high levels, suggests the diagnosis of allergic angiitis and granulomatosis. The anemia of chronic disease may be seen, and an elevated erythrocyte sedimentation rate (ESR) is almost always present. Other common laboratory findings reflect the particular organ involved. Hypergammaglobulinemia may be present, and up to 30 percent of patients have a positive test for hepatitis B surface antigen. Positive ANCA titers (usually of the p-ANCA type) are found in variable percentages of patients with classic PAN. Microscopic polyangiitis is strongly associated with ANCA that are usually of the p-ANCA type, but c-ANCA have also been reported. In contrast, the ANCA in Wegener's granulomatosis (see below) are almost always of the c-ANCA type, which can be helpful in distinguishing Wegener's granulomatosis from microscopic polyangiitis when both present with a pulmonary-renal syndrome. Arteriograms may demonstrate characteristic abnormalities such as aneurysms in the small and medium-sized muscular arteries of the kidneys and abdominal viscera.

Diagnosis The diagnosis of classic PAN is based on the demonstration of characteristic findings of vasculitis on biopsy material of involved organs. In the absence of easily accessible tissue for biopsy, the angiographic demonstration of involved vessels, particularly in the form of aneurysms of small and medium-sized arteries in the renal, hepatic, and visceral vasculature, is sufficient to make the diagnosis. Aneurysms of vessels are not pathognomonic of classic PAN; furthermore, aneurysms need not always be present, and angiographic findings may be limited to stenotic segments and obliteration of vessels. Biopsy of symptomatic organs such as nodular skin lesions, painful testes, and muscle groups provides the highest diagnostic yields, while blind biopsy of asymptomatic organs is frequently negative. The presence of small vessel vasculitis, particularly in the setting of glomerulonephritis and pulmonary capillaritis distinguishes microscopic polyangiitis from classic PAN.

Prognosis The prognosis of untreated classic PAN as well as that of microscopic polyangiitis is extremely poor. The usual clinical course is characterized either by fulminant deterioration or by relentless progression associated with intermittent acute flare-ups. Death usually results from renal failure; from gastrointestinal complications, particularly bowel infarcts and perforation; and from cardiovascular causes. Intractable hypertension often compounds dysfunction in other organ systems, such as the kidneys, heart, and central nervous system, leading to additional late morbidity and mortality. The 5-year survival rate of untreated patients has been reported to be 13 percent, while glucocorticoid treatment may increase this figure to over 40 percent.

℞ **TREATMENT**

Extremely favorable therapeutic results have been reported in classic PAN with the combination of prednisone, 1 mg/kg per day, and cyclophosphamide, 2 mg/kg per day (see "Wegener's Granulomatosis" for a detailed description of this therapeutic regimen). This regimen has been reported to result in up to a 90 percent long-term remission rate even following the discontinuation of therapy. In

Table 319-3

Clinical Manifestations Related to Organ System Involvement in Classic PAN

Organ System	Percent Incidence	Clinical Manifestations
Renal	60	Renal failure, hypertension
Musculoskeletal	64	Arthritis, arthralgia, myalgia
Peripheral nervous system	51	Peripheral neuropathy, mononeuritis multiplex
Gastrointestinal tract	44	Abdominal pain, nausea and vomiting, bleeding, bowel infarction and perforation, cholecystitis, hepatic infarction, pancreatic infarction
Skin	43	Rash, purpura, nodules, cutaneous infarcts, livedo reticularis, Raynaud's phenomenon
Cardiac	36	Congestive heart failure, myocardial infarction, pericarditis
Genitourinary	25	Testicular, ovarian, or epididymal pain
Central nervous system	23	Cerebral vascular accident, altered mental status, seizure

SOURCE: From Cupps and Fauci, p 29.

addition, long-term remissions have been reported in PAN associated with hepatitis B virus antigenemia using the antiviral agent vidarabine in combination with plasma exchange with and without glucocorticoids. Favorable results have also been reported in the treatment of PAN related to hepatitis B virus with IFNα and plasma exchange. Careful attention to the treatment of hypertension can lessen the acute and late morbidity and mortality associated with renal, cardiac, and central nervous system complications of PAN. The treatment regimen for microscopic polyangiitis is similar to that for classic PAN, particularly if glomerulonephritis is present.

ALLERGIC ANGIITIS AND GRANULOMATOSIS (CHURG-STRAUSS DISEASE)

Definition *Allergic angiitis and granulomatosis* was described in 1951 by Churg and Strauss and is a disease characterized by granulomatous vasculitis of multiple organ systems, particularly the lung. It is similar in many respects to classic PAN, except that the former has a high frequency of lung involvement, vasculitis of blood vessels of various types or sizes (including veins and venules), intra- and extravascular granuloma formation together with eosinophilic tissue infiltration, and a strong association with severe asthma and peripheral eosinophilia.

Incidence and Prevalence Allergic angiitis and granulomatosis is an uncommon disease whose exact incidence, similar to classic PAN, is difficult to determine due to the grouping of multiple types of vasculitic syndromes in many reported series. The disease can occur at any age with the possible exception of infants. The mean age of onset is 44 years, with a male-to-female ratio of 1.3:1.

Pathophysiology and Pathogenesis The vasculitis that is characteristic of allergic angiitis and granulomatosis is similar to that of classic PAN (see above) with certain notable exceptions. In addition to small and medium-sized muscular arteries, capillaries, veins, and venules can be involved in the former disease. The characteristic histopathologic features of allergic angiitis and granulomatosis are granulomatous reactions that may be present in the tissues or even within the walls of the vessels themselves. These are usually associated with infiltration of the tissues with eosinophils. This process can occur in any organ in the body; however, in sharp contrast to classic PAN, lung involvement is predominant, with skin, cardiovascular system, kidney, peripheral nervous system, and gastrointestinal tract also commonly involved. Although the precise pathogenesis of this disease is uncertain, its strong association with asthma, its clinicopathologic manifestations which strongly suggest hypersensitivity phenomena, and its close similarity to classic PAN point to aberrant immunologic phenomena.

Clinical and Laboratory Manifestations Patients with allergic angiitis and granulomatosis exhibit nonspecific manifestations such as fever, malaise, anorexia, and weight loss similar to patients with classic PAN. In contrast to the latter disease, the pulmonary findings in allergic angiitis and granulomatosis clearly dominate the clinical picture with severe asthmatic attacks and the presence of pulmonary infiltrates. Clinically recognizable heart disease occurs in approximately one-third of patients. Heart involvement is seen at autopsy in 62 percent of cases and is the cause of death in 23 percent of patients. Skin lesions occur in approximately 70 percent of patients and include purpura in addition to cutaneous and subcutaneous nodules. Apart from the characteristic pulmonary findings, the multisystem involvement in this disease is quite similar to that of classic PAN (see above); an important exception is the fact that the renal disease in allergic angiitis and granulomatosis is less common and generally less severe than that of classic PAN.

The characteristic laboratory finding in virtually all patients with allergic angiitis and granulomatosis is a striking eosinophilia which reaches levels greater than 1000 cells/μL in more than 80 percent of patients. The other laboratory findings are similar to those of classic PAN and reflect the organ systems involved. Allergic angiitis and granulomatosis is associated with p-ANCA.

Diagnosis Similar to classic PAN, the diagnosis of allergic angiitis and granulomatosis is made by biopsy, demonstrating vasculitis in a patient with the characteristic clinical manifestations. The biopsy findings are distinctive in the latter disease in that granulomatous vasculitis with eosinophilic tissue involvement together with peripheral eosinophilia are typical. Furthermore, pulmonary involvement is extremely common and is usually manifested by severe asthma associated with pulmonary infiltrates that may be fleeting in nature.

Prognosis The prognosis of untreated allergic angiitis and granulomatosis is poor, with a reported 5-year survival of 25 percent. Unlike classic PAN, the cause of death is more likely to be related to pulmonary and cardiac disease as opposed to renal or gastrointestinal involvement.

℞ TREATMENT

Glucocorticoid therapy has been reported to increase the 5-year survival to more than 50 percent. In certain patients, the disease may be quite mild and may remit spontaneously or with short courses of glucocorticoids. In glucocorticoid failures or in patients who present with fulminant multisystem disease, the treatment of choice is a combined regimen of cyclophosphamide and alternate-day prednisone, which has resulted in a high rate of complete remission similar to the experience with classic PAN (see above).

POLYANGIITIS OVERLAP SYNDROME Many patients with systemic vasculitis manifest clinicopathologic characteristics that do not fit precisely into any classification but that have overlapping features of classic PAN, allergic angiitis and granulomatosis, Wegener's granulomatosis, Takayasu's arteritis, and the hypersensitivity group of vasculitides. This subgroup has been referred to as the *polyangiitis overlap syndrome* and is part of the major grouping of systemic necrotizing vasculitis. This entity has been designated with a distinct classification in order to avoid confusion in attempting to fit such overlap syndromes into one or other of the more classic vasculitic syndromes. This subgroup is truly a systemic vasculitis with the same potential for resulting in irreversible organ system dysfunction as the other systemic necrotizing vasculitides. The diagnostic and therapeutic considerations as well as the prognosis for this subgroup are the same as those for classic PAN and allergic angiitis and granulomatosis.

WEGENER'S GRANULOMATOSIS

DEFINITION *Wegener's granulomatosis* is a distinct clinicopathologic entity characterized by granulomatous vasculitis of the upper and lower respiratory tracts together with glomerulonephritis. In addition, variable degrees of disseminated vasculitis involving both small arteries and veins may occur.

INCIDENCE AND PREVALENCE Wegener's granulomatosis is an uncommon disease whose true incidence is difficult to determine. It is extremely rare in blacks compared with whites; the male-to-female ratio is 1:1. The disease can be seen at any age; approximately 15 percent of patients are less than 19 years of age, and only rarely does the disease occur before adolescence; the mean age of onset is approximately 40 years.

PATHOPHYSIOLOGY AND PATHOGENESIS The histopathologic hallmarks of Wegener's granulomatosis are necrotizing vasculitis of small arteries and veins together with granuloma formation which may be either intravascular or extravascular (Fig. 319-2). Lung involvement typically appears as multiple, bilateral, nodular cavitary infiltrates (Fig. 319-3), which on biopsy almost invariably reveal the typical necrotizing granulomatous vasculitis. Endobronchial disease, either in its active form or as a result of fibrous scarring, may lead to obstruction with atelectasis. Upper airway lesions, particularly those in the sinuses and nasopharynx, typically reveal inflammation, necrosis, and granuloma formation with or without vasculitis.

In its earliest form, renal involvement is characterized by a focal and segmental glomerulitis that may evolve into a rapidly progressive crescentic glomerulonephritis. Granuloma formation is only rarely seen on renal biopsy. In addition to the classic triad of upper and

FIGURE 319-2 Lung biopsy in a patient with Wegener's granulomatosis. Biopsy revealed necrotizing vasculitis of medium-sized artery in the lung. Compromise of the vessel lumen, fibrinoid necrosis of the vessel wall, and mononuclear cell infiltration of vessel wall with early granuloma formation are seen.

lower respiratory tracts and kidney disease, virtually any organ can be involved with vasculitis, granuloma, or both.

The immunopathogenesis of this disease is unclear, although the involvement of upper airways and lungs suggests an aberrant hypersensitivity response to an exogenous or even endogenous antigen that enters through or resides in the upper airway. Chronic nasal carriage of *Staphylococcus aureus* has been reported to be associated with a higher relapse rate of Wegener's granulomatosis; however, there is no evidence for a role of this organism in the pathogenesis of the disease.

Although circulating and deposited immune complexes have been demonstrated in certain patients with Wegener's granulomatosis, there is no convincing evidence that immune complexes play a causal pathogenic role in this disease. The presence of granulomas with copious, well-defined multinucleated giant cells, particularly in involved pulmonary tissue, suggests delayed hypersensitivity and/or foreign-body reactions. However, direct evidence for either of these mechanisms is lacking.

A high percentage of patients with Wegener's granulomatosis develop ANCA; c-ANCA are the predominant ANCA in this disease. As with the other categories of vasculitis, there is no clear evidence that ANCA play a primary role in the pathogenesis of Wegener's granulomatosis.

The bronchoalveolar lavage fluid of patients with active Wegener's granulomatosis contains a high percentage of neutrophils compared

with that of other granulomatous lung diseases such as sarcoidosis, in which increased numbers of lymphocytes are noted (see Chap. 320). The pathogenic significance of this difference is unclear.

CLINICAL AND LABORATORY MANIFESTATIONS A typical patient presents with severe upper respiratory tract findings such as paranasal sinus pain and drainage and purulent or bloody nasal discharge with or without nasal mucosal ulceration (Table 319-4). Nasal septal perforation may follow, leading to saddle nose deformity. Serous otitis media may occur as a result of eustachian tube blockage.

Pulmonary involvement may be manifested as asymptomatic infiltrates or may be clinically expressed as cough, hemoptysis, dyspnea, and chest discomfort. It is present in 85 to 90 percent of patients. Subglottic stenosis resulting from active disease or scarring occurs in approximately 16 percent of patients and may result in severe airway obstruction.

Eye involvement (52 percent of patients) may range from a mild conjunctivitis to dacryocystitis, episcleritis, scleritis, granulomatous sclerouveitis, ciliary vessel vasculitis, and retroorbital mass lesions leading to proptosis.

Skin lesions (46 percent of patients) appear as papules, vesicles, palpable purpura, ulcers, or subcutaneous nodules; biopsy reveals vasculitis, granuloma, or both. Cardiac involvement (8 percent of patients) manifests as pericarditis, coronary vasculitis, or, rarely, cardiomyopathy. Nervous system manifestations (23 percent of patients) include

Table 319-4

Wegener's Granulomatosis: Frequency of Clinical Manifestations in 158 Patients Studied at the National Institutes of Health

Manifestation	Percent at Disease Onset	Percent Throughout Course of Disease
Kidney		
Glomerulonephritis	18	77
Ear/nose/throat	73	92
Sinusitis	51	85
Nasal disease	36	68
Otitis media	25	44
Hearing loss	14	42
Subglottic stenosis	1	16
Ear pain	9	14
Oral lesions	3	10
Lung	45	85
Pulmonary infiltrates	25	66
Pulmonary nodules	24	58
Hemoptysis	12	30
Pleuritis	10	28
Eyes		
Conjunctivitis	5	18
Dacryocystitis	1	18
Scleritis	6	16
Proptosis	2	15
Eye pain	3	11
Visual loss	0	8
Retinal lesions	0	4
Corneal lesions	0	1
Iritis	0	2
Other*		
Arthralgias/arthritis	32	67
Fever	23	50
Cough	19	46
Skin abnormalities	13	46
Weight loss (greater than 10 percent body weight)	15	35
Peripheral neuropathy	1	15
Central nervous system disease	1	8
Pericarditis	2	6
Hyperthyroidism	1	3

FIGURE 319-3 Computed tomography scan of a patient with Wegener's granulomatosis. The patient developed multiple, bilateral, and cavitary infiltrates.

* Fewer than 1 percent had parotid, pulmonary artery, breast, or lower genitourinary (urethra, cervix, vagina, testicular) involvement.

SOURCE: Hoffman et al., 1992.

cranial neuritis, mononeuritis multiplex, or, rarely, cerebral vasculitis and/or granuloma.

Renal disease (77 percent of patients) generally dominates the clinical picture and, if left untreated, accounts directly or indirectly for most of the mortality in this disease. Although it may smolder in some cases as a mild glomerulitis with proteinuria, hematuria, and red blood cell casts, it is clear that once clinically detectable renal functional impairment occurs, rapidly progressive renal failure usually ensues unless appropriate treatment is instituted.

While the disease is active, most patients have nonspecific symptoms and signs such as malaise, weakness, arthralgias, anorexia, and weight loss. Fever may indicate activity of the underlying disease but more often reflects secondary infection, usually of the upper airway.

Characteristic laboratory findings include a markedly elevated ESR, mild anemia and leukocytosis, mild hypergammaglobulinemia (particularly of the IgA class), and mildly elevated rheumatoid factor. Thrombocytosis may be seen as an acute-phase reactant; hypocomplementemia is not seen despite the presence of circulating immune complexes in some patients. In typical Wegener's granulomatosis with granulomatous vasculitis of the respiratory tract and glomerulonephritis, approximately 90 percent of patients have a positive c-ANCA. However, in the absence of renal disease, the sensitivity drops to approximately 70 percent.

DIAGNOSIS The diagnosis of Wegener's granulomatosis is a clinicopathologic one made by the demonstration of necrotizing granulomatous vasculitis on biopsy of appropriate tissue in a patient with the clinical findings of upper and lower respiratory tract disease together with evidence of glomerulonephritis. Pulmonary tissue, preferably obtained by open thoracotomy, offers the highest diagnostic yield, almost invariably revealing granulomatous vasculitis. Biopsy of upper airway tissue usually reveals granulomatous inflammation with necrosis but may not show vasculitis. Renal biopsy confirms the presence of glomerulonephritis.

The specificity of a positive c-ANCA titer for Wegener's granulomatosis is very high, especially if active glomerulonephritis is present. However, the presence of c-ANCA should be adjunctive and should not substitute for a tissue diagnosis. False-positive ANCA titers have been reported in certain infectious and neoplastic diseases. Furthermore, in evaluating patients for relapse, the ANCA titer can be misleading. Many patients who achieve remission continue to have elevated titers for years. In addition, over 40 percent of patients who were in remission and had a fourfold increase in c-ANCA titer did not have a relapse of disease.

In its typical presentation, the classic clinicopathologic complex of Wegener's granulomatosis usually provides ready differentiation from other disorders. However, if all the typical features are not present at once, it needs to be differentiated from the other vasculitides, particularly allergic angiitis and granulomatosis, Goodpasture's syndrome (see Chap. 275), tumors of the upper airway or lung, and infectious diseases such as mucocutaneous leishmaniasis (see Chap. 217) and rhinoscleroma (see Chap. 30) as well as noninfectious granulomatous diseases.

Of particular note is the differentiation from *midline granuloma* and *upper airway neoplasms*, which are part of the spectrum of *midline destructive diseases*. These diseases lead to extreme tissue destruction and mutilation localized to the midline upper airway structures including the sinuses; erosion through the skin of the face commonly occurs, a feature that is extremely rare in Wegener's granulomatosis. Although blood vessels may be involved in the intense inflammatory reaction and necrosis, primary vasculitis is seen rarely. When systemic involvement occurs, it usually declares itself as a neoplastic process. In this regard, it is likely that midline granuloma is part of the spectrum of *angiocentric immunoproliferative lesions* (AIL). The latter are considered to represent a spectrum of postthymic T cell proliferative lesions and should be treated as such (see Chap. 113). The term *idiopathic* has been applied to midline granuloma when extensive diagnostic workup including multiple biopsies has failed to reveal anything other than inflammation and necrosis. Under these circumstances, it is possible that the tumor cells were masked by the intensive inflammatory response. Such cases have responded to local irradiation with 50 Gy (5000 rad). Upper airway lesions should never be irradiated in Wegener's granulomatosis.

Wegener's granulomatosis must also be differentiated from *lymphomatoid granulomatosis*, the latter also being a part of the spectrum of AIL. Lymphomatoid granulomatosis is characterized by lung, skin, central nervous system, and kidney involvement in which atypical lymphocytoid and plasmacytoid cells infiltrate tissue in an angioinvasive manner. In this regard, it clearly differs from Wegener's granulomatosis in that it is not an inflammatory vasculitis in the classic sense but an infiltration of vessels with atypical mononuclear cells; granuloma may be present in involved tissues. Approximately 50 percent of patients develop a true malignant lymphoma. The presence of c-ANCA proves extremely helpful in the differentiation from all the preceding diseases.

℞ TREATMENT

Wegener's granulomatosis was formerly universally fatal, usually within a few months after the onset of clinically apparent renal disease. Glucocorticoids alone led to some symptomatic improvement, with little effect on the ultimate course of the disease. It has been well established that the treatment of choice in this disease is cyclophosphamide given in doses of 2 mg/kg per day orally. The leukocyte count should be monitored closely during therapy, and the dosage should be adjusted in order to maintain the count above $3000/\mu L$, which generally maintains the neutrophil count at approximately $1500/\mu L$. With this approach, clinical remission can usually be induced and maintained without causing severe leukopenia with its associated risk of infection. Cyclophosphamide should be continued for 1 year following the induction of complete remission and gradually tapered and discontinued thereafter.

At the initiation of therapy, glucocorticoids should be administered together with cyclophosphamide. This can be given as prednisone, 1 mg/kg per day initially (for the first month of therapy) as a daily regimen, with gradual conversion to an alternate-day schedule followed by tapering and discontinuation after approximately 6 months.

Using the above regimen, the prognosis of this disease is excellent; marked improvement is seen in more than 90 percent of patients, and complete remissions are achieved in 75 percent of patients. A number of patients who developed irreversible renal failure but who achieved subsequent remission on appropriate therapy have undergone successful renal transplantation.

Despite the dramatic remissions induced by the therapeutic regimen described above, long-term follow-up of patients has revealed that approximately 50 percent of remissions are later associated with one or more relapses. Reinduction of remission is almost always achieved; however, a high percentage of patients ultimately have some degree of morbidity from irreversible features of their disease, such as varying degrees of renal insufficiency, hearing loss, tracheal stenosis, saddle nose deformity, and chronically impaired sinus function.

Certain types of morbidity are related to toxic side effects of treatment. Since the preceding therapeutic regimen calls for conversion to alternate-day glucocorticoid therapy within 3 months and ultimate discontinuation within 6 to 12 months, glucocorticoid-related side effects such as diabetes mellitus, cataracts, life-threatening infectious disease complications, serious osteoporosis, and severe cushingoid features are infrequently encountered except in those patients requiring prolonged courses of daily glucocorticoids. However, cyclophosphamide-related toxicities are more frequent and severe. Cystitis to varying degrees occurs in 43 percent of patients, bladder cancer in 5 percent, and myelodysplasia in 2 percent.

Despite its life-saving effects in patients with Wegener's granulomatosis, cyclophosphamide cannot be tolerated by certain patients, such as those who develop severe neutropenia at low doses of drug or those who develop severe cystitis or bladder cancer. In these patients, alternative treatment regimens should be initiated. In one study, weekly methotrexate was shown to be an acceptable alternative therapy for selected patients with Wegener's granulomatosis who did not have immediately life-threatening disease or had developed serious cyclophosphamide-associated toxicity. Patients in this category were given oral prednisone as described above, and methotrexate was administered orally starting at a dosage of 0.3 mg/kg, with a maximum of 15 mg/week. If the treatment was well tolerated after 1 to 2 weeks, the dosage was increased by 2.5 mg weekly up to a dosage of 20 to 25 mg/week and maintained at that level. Remissions were achieved in 30 of 42 patients (71 percent). Eleven patients relapsed; eight of these were treated with a second course of methotrexate and prednisone and six of eight achieved a second remission. Toxicities of methotrexate included elevated transaminase levels (24 percent), leukopenia (7 percent), opportunistic infection (9.5 percent), methotrexate pneumonitis (7 percent), and stomatitis (2 percent). Azathioprine, in doses of 1 to 2 mg/kg per day, has proven effective in some patients, particularly in maintaining remission in those in whom remission was induced by cyclophosphamide. The drug should be administered together with the glucocorticoid regimen described above. Anecdotal reports have indicated therapeutic success with less frequent and severe toxic side effects using intermittent boluses of intravenous cyclophosphamide (1 g/m^2 per month) in place of daily drug administered orally. However, we have found that although 6 months of such a regimen induced improvement in approximately 90 percent of patients with remissions in 50 percent, 72 percent of patients were unable to maintain remission despite further treatment over 6 to 24 months. Although certain reports have indicated that trimethoprim-sulfamethoxazole may be of benefit in the treatment of Wegener's granulomatosis, there are no firm data to substantiate this, particularly in patients with serious renal and pulmonary disease.

TEMPORAL ARTERITIS

DEFINITION *Temporal arteritis,* also referred to as *cranial* or *giant cell arteritis,* is an inflammation of medium- and large-sized arteries. It characteristically involves one or more branches of the carotid artery, particularly the temporal artery, hence the name. However, it is a systemic disease that can involve arteries in multiple locations.

INCIDENCE AND PREVALENCE The incidence of temporal arteritis varies widely in different studies and in different geographic regions. A high incidence has been found in Scandanavia and in regions of the United States with large Scandanavian populations, compared to a lower incidence in southern Europe. The annual incidence rates in individuals 50 years of age and older range from 0.49 to 23.3 per 100,000 population. It occurs almost exclusively in individuals older than 55 years; however, well-documented cases have occurred in patients 40 years old or younger. It is more common in women than in men and is rare in blacks. Familial aggregation has been reported, as has an association with HLA-DR4. In addition, genetic linkage studies have demonstrated an association of temporal arteritis with alleles at the HLA-DRB1 locus, particularly HLA-DRB1*04 variants. The disease is closely associated with *polymyalgia rheumatica,* which is more common than temporal arteritis. In Olmsted County, Minnesota, the annual incidence of polymyalgia rheumatica in individuals 50 years of age and older is 52.5 per 100,000 population.

PATHOPHYSIOLOGY AND PATHOGENESIS Although the temporal artery is most frequently involved in this disease, patients often have a systemic vasculitis of multiple medium- and large-sized arteries, which may go undetected. Histopathologically, the disease is a panarteritis with inflammatory mononuclear cell infiltrates within the vessel wall with frequent giant cell formation. There is proliferation of the intima and fragmentation of the internal elastic lamina. Pathophysiologic findings in organs result from the ischemia related to the involved vessels. Distinct cytokine patterns as well as T lymphocytes expressing specific antigen receptors have been described suggesting the involvement of immunopathogenic mechanisms in temporal arteritis. IL-6 and IL-1β expression has been detected in a majority of circulating monocytes of patients with temporal arteritis and polymyal-

gia rheumatica. T cells recruited to vasculitic lesions in patients with temporal arteritis produce predominantly IL-2 and IFNγ, and the latter has been suggested to be involved in the progression to overt arteritis. Sequence analysis of the T cell receptor of tissue-infiltrating T cells in lesions of temporal arteritis indicates restricted clonal expansion, suggesting that an antigen residing in the arterial wall is recognized by a small fraction of T cells.

CLINICAL AND LABORATORY MANIFESTATIONS The disease is characterized clinically by the classic complex of fever, anemia, high ESR, and headaches in an elderly patient. Other manifestations include malaise, fatigue, anorexia, weight loss, sweats, and arthralgias. The polymyalgia rheumatica syndrome is characterized by stiffness, aching, and pain in the muscles of the neck, shoulders, lower back, hips, and thighs.

In patients with involvement of the temporal artery, headache is the predominant symptom and may be associated with a tender, thickened, or nodular artery, which may pulsate early in the disease but become occluded later. Scalp pain and claudication of the jaw and tongue may occur. A well-recognized and dreaded complication of temporal arteritis, particularly in untreated patients, is ocular involvement due primarily to ischemic optic neuritis, which may lead to serious visual symptoms, even sudden blindness in some patients. However, most patients have complaints relating to the head or eyes for months before objective eye involvement. Attention to such symptoms with institution of appropriate therapy (see below) will usually avoid this complication. Claudication of the extremities, strokes, myocardial infarctions, aortic aneurysms and dissections, and infarctions of visceral organs have been reported.

Characteristic laboratory findings in addition to the elevated ESR include a normochromic or slightly hypochromic anemia. Liver function abnormalities are common, particularly increased alkaline phosphatase levels. Increased levels of IgG and complement have been reported. Levels of enzymes indicative of muscle damage such as serum creatine kinase are not elevated.

DIAGNOSIS The diagnosis of temporal arteritis and its associated clinicopathologic syndrome often can be made clinically by the demonstration of the classic picture of fever, anemia, and high ESR with or without symptoms of polymyalgia rheumatica in an elderly patient. The diagnosis is confirmed by biopsy of the temporal artery. Since involvement of the vessel may be segmental, the diagnosis may be missed on routine biopsy; serial sectioning of biopsy specimens is recommended. When the temporal arteries appear clinically normal, but temporal arteritis is strongly suspected, a biopsy segment of a few centimeters may be required to establish the diagnosis. A temporal artery biopsy should be obtained as quickly as possible in the setting of ocular signs and symptoms, and under these circumstances therapy should not be delayed pending a biopsy. In this regard, it has been reported that temporal artery biopsies may show vasculitis even after more than 14 days of glucocorticoid therapy. A dramatic clinical response to a trial of glucocorticoid therapy can confirm the diagnosis.

℞ **TREATMENT**
Temporal arteritis and its associated symptoms are exquisitely sensitive to glucocorticoid therapy. Treatment should begin with prednisone, 40 to 60 mg per day for approximately 1 month, followed by a gradual tapering to a maintenance dose of 7.5 to 10 mg per day. In order to lessen glucocorticoid side effects in elderly individuals, conversion to alternate-day therapy may be attempted, but only after the disease has been put into remission with daily therapy. When ocular signs and symptoms occur, it is important that therapy be initiated or adjusted to control them. Because of the possibility of relapse, therapy should be continued for at least 1 to 2 years. The ESR can serve as a useful indicator of inflammatory disease activity in monitoring and tapering therapy and can be used to judge the pace of the tapering schedule. However, minor increases in the ESR can occur as glucocorticoids are being tapered and do not necessarily reflect an exacerbation

of arteritis, particularly if the patient remains symptom free. Under these circumstances, the tapering should continue with caution. If one attempts to maintain a normal ESR throughout the tapering period, glucocorticoid toxicity will almost surely occur. The prognosis is generally good, and most patients achieve complete remission that is often maintained after withdrawal of therapy.

TAKAYASU'S ARTERITIS

DEFINITION *Takayasu's arteritis* is an inflammatory and stenotic disease of medium- and large-sized arteries characterized by a strong predilection for the aortic arch and its branches. For this reason, it is often referred to as the *aortic arch syndrome*.

INCIDENCE AND PREVALENCE Takayasu's arteritis is an uncommon disease, much less common than temporal arteritis. It is most prevalent in adolescent girls and young women. Although it is more common in the Orient, it is neither racially nor geographically restricted. An association of the disease has been described with HLA-DR2, MB1 in Japan and HLA-DR4, MB3 in the United States.

PATHOPHYSIOLOGY AND PATHOGENESIS The disease involves medium- and large-sized arteries, with a strong predilection for the aortic arch and its branches; the pulmonary artery also may be involved. The most commonly affected arteries seen by angiography are listed in Table 319-5. The involvement of the major branches of the aorta is much more marked at their origin than distally. The disease is a panarteritis with inflammatory mononuclear cell infiltrates and occasionally giant cells. There is marked intimal proliferation and fibrosis, scarring and vascularization of the media, and disruption and degeneration of the elastic lamina. Narrowing of the lumen occurs with or without thrombosis. The vasa vasorum are frequently involved. Pathologic changes in various organs reflect the compromise of blood flow through the involved vessels.

Immunopathogenic mechanisms, the precise nature of which is uncertain, are suspected in this disease. As with several of the vasculitis syndromes, circulating immune complexes have been demonstrated, but their pathogenic significance is unclear.

CLINICAL AND LABORATORY MANIFESTATIONS Takayasu's arteritis is a systemic disease with generalized as well as local symptoms. The generalized symptoms include malaise, fever, night sweats, arthralgias, anorexia, and weight loss which may occur months before vessel involvement is apparent. These symptoms may merge into those related to pain over the involved vessels, followed by symptoms of ischemia in organs supplied by the compromised vessels. Pulses are commonly absent in the involved vessels, particularly the subclavian artery. The frequency of arteriographic abnormalities and the potentially associated clinical manifestations are listed in Table 319-5.

The clinical course may be fulminant, may progress gradually, or may stabilize. Complications are related to the distribution of the involved vessels. Death usually occurs from congestive heart failure or cerebrovascular accidents.

Characteristic laboratory findings include an elevated ESR, mild anemia, and elevated immunoglobulin levels.

DIAGNOSIS The diagnosis of Takayasu's arteritis should be suspected strongly in a young woman who develops a decrease or absence of peripheral pulses, discrepancies in blood pressure, and arterial bruits. The diagnosis is confirmed by the characteristic pattern on arteriography, which includes irregular vessel walls, stenosis, poststenotic dilatation, aneurysm formation, occlusion, and evidence of increased collateral circulation. Complete aortic arteriography should be obtained unless this is renally contraindicated in order to fully delineate the distribution and degree of arterial disease. Histopathologic demonstration of inflamed vessels adds confirmatory data; however, tissue is rarely readily available for examination.

℞ TREATMENT

The course of the disease is variable, and spontaneous remissions may occur. Reported mortality statistics range from less than 10 percent to 75 percent. Although glucocorticoid therapy in doses of 40 to 60 mg prednisone per day alleviates symptoms, there are no convincing studies that indicate that they alone increase survival. The combination of glucocorticoid therapy for acute signs and symptoms and an aggressive surgical and/or angioplastic approach to stenosed vessels has markedly improved survival and decreased morbidity by lessening the risk of stroke, correcting hypertension due to renal artery stenosis, and improving blood flow to ischemic viscera and limbs. Unless it is urgently required, surgical correction of stenosed arteries should be undertaken only when the vascular inflammatory process is well controlled with medical therapy. Most recent mortality figures using this therapeutic approach are less than 10 percent. In individuals who are refractory to glucocorticoids, methotrexate in doses up to 25 mg per week has yielded encouraging results; however, long-term studies will be needed to confirm this.

HENOCH-SCHÖNLEIN PURPURA

DEFINITION *Henoch-Schönlein purpura*, also referred to as *anaphylactoid purpura* is a distinct systemic vasculitis syndrome that is characterized by palpable purpura (most commonly distributed over the buttocks and lower extremities), arthralgias, gastrointestinal signs and symptoms, and glomerulonephritis. It is a small vessel vasculitis.

INCIDENCE AND PREVALENCE Henoch-Schönlein purpura is usually seen in children; most patients range in age from 4 to 7 years; however, the disease may also be seen in infants and adults. It is not a rare disease; in one series it accounted for between 5 and 24 admissions per year at a pediatric hospital. The male to female ratio is 1.5:1. A seasonal variation with a peak incidence in spring has been noted.

PATHOPHYSIOLOGY AND PATHOGENESIS The presumptive pathogenic mechanism for Henoch-Schönlein purpura is immune-complex deposition. A number of inciting antigens have been suggested including upper respiratory tract infections, various drugs, foods, insect bites, and immunizations. IgA is the antibody class most often seen in the immune complexes and has been demonstrated in the renal biopsies of these patients.

CLINICAL AND LABORATORY MANIFESTATIONS In pediatric patients, presenting symptoms related to the skin, gut, and joints are present in 50 percent of cases. In adults, presenting symptoms

Table 319-5

Frequency of Arteriographic Abnormalities and Potential Clinical Manifestations of Arterial Involvement in Takayasu's Arteritis

Artery	Percent of Arteriographic Abnormalities	Potential Clinical Manifestations
Subclavian	93	Arm claudication, Raynaud's phenomenon
Common carotid	58	Visual changes, syncope, transient ischemic attacks, stroke
Abdominal aorta*	47	Abdominal pain, nausea, vomiting
Renal	38	Hypertension, renal failure
Aortic arch or root	35	Aortic insufficiency, congestive heart failure
Vertebral	35	Visual changes, dizziness
Coeliac axis*	18	Abdominal pain, nausea, vomiting
Superior mesenteric*	18	Abdominal pain, nausea, vomiting
Iliac	17	Leg claudication
Pulmonary	10–40	Atypical chest pain, dyspnea
Coronary	<10	Chest pain, myocardial infarction

* Arteriographic lesions at these locations are usually asymptomatic but may potentially cause these symptoms.

SOURCE: G. Kerr et al., 1994.

related to the skin are seen in over 70 percent of patients, while initial complaints related to the gut or the joints are noted in fewer than 20 percent of cases. The typical palpable purpura is seen in virtually all patients; most patients develop polyarthralgias in the absence of frank arthritis. Gastrointestinal involvement, which is seen in almost 70 percent of pediatric patients, is characterized by colicky abdominal pain usually associated with nausea, vomiting, diarrhea, or constipation and is frequently accompanied by the passage of blood and mucus per rectum; bowel intussusception may occur rarely. The renal involvement is usually characterized by mild glomerulonephritis leading to proteinuria and microscopic hematuria, with red blood cells casts in the majority of patients (see also Chap. 275); it usually resolves spontaneously without therapy. Rarely, a progressive glomerulonephritis will develop. Renal failure is the most common cause of death in the rare patient who dies of Henoch-Schönlein purpura. Although certain studies have found that renal disease is more severe in adults, this has not been a consistent finding. However, the course of renal disease in adults may be more insidious and thus requires close follow-up. Myocardial involvement can occur in adults but is rare in children.

Routine laboratory studies generally show a mild leukocytosis, a normal platelet count, and occasionally eosinophilia. Serum complement components are normal, and IgA levels are elevated in about one-half of patients.

℞ TREATMENT

The prognosis of Henoch-Schönlein purpura is excellent. Most patients recover completely, and some do not require therapy. Treatment is similar for adults and children. When glucocorticoid therapy is required, prednisone in doses of 1 mg/kg per day and tapered according to clinical response has been shown to be useful in decreasing tissue edema, arthralgias, and abdominal discomfort; however, it has not proven beneficial in the treatment of skin or renal disease and does not appear to shorten the duration of active disease or lessen the chance of recurrence. Patients with rapidly progressive glomerulonephritis have been anecdotally reported to benefit from intensive plasma exchange combined with immunosuppressive drugs.

PREDOMINANTLY CUTANEOUS VASCULITIS

DEFINITION   The term *predominantly cutaneous vasculitis* has been used in the literature interchangeably with the terms *hypersensitivity vasculitis* and *cutaneous leukocytoclastic vasculitis*. Due to the heterogeneity of this group of disorders, none of these terms is totally adequate. The common denominator of this group of diseases is the involvement of small vessels of the skin. The syndrome is presumed to be associated with an aberrant hypersensitivity reaction to an antigen such as an infectious agent, a drug, or other foreign or endogenous substances. In most instances, however, an antigen is never identified and the disease remains idiopathic. The Chapel Hill Consensus Conference on Nomenclature of Systemic Vasculitis does not use the term *hypersensitivity vasculitis*. Indeed, this is easily a misleading term since most of the other groups of vasculitis syndromes are probably also associated with some form of hypersensitivity or aberrant immunologic reaction to as yet unidentified antigens. The term *cutaneous leukocytoclastic vasculitis* is a better term; however, not all of these vasculitides are truly leukocytoclastic in nature. We have elected to use the term *"predominantly" cutaneous vasculitis* since skin involvement generally dominates the clinical picture, but the skin is not always the exclusive organ involved. Indeed, any organ system can be involved with this type of vasculitis; however, the extracutaneous involvement is usually much less severe than that of the systemic necrotizing vasculitides.

INCIDENCE AND PREVALENCE   Although the exact incidence of this group of vasculitis syndromes is uncertain, it is clearly more common than the systemic necrotizing vasculitis group. The disease can occur at any age and in both sexes; however, different subgroups have a higher incidence in certain age groups, and some are more common in males than females, or vice versa.

PATHOPHYSIOLOGY AND PATHOGENESIS   The typical histopathologic feature of the predominantly cutaneous vasculitides

is the presence of vasculitis of small vessels. Postcapillary venules are the most commonly involved vessels; capillaries and arterioles may be involved less frequently. This vasculitis is characterized by a *leukocytoclasis*, a term that refers to the nuclear debris remaining from the neutrophils that have infiltrated in and around the vessels during the acute stages. In the subacute or chronic stages, mononuclear cells predominate; in certain subgroups, eosinophilic infiltration is seen. Erythrocytes often extravasate from the involved vessels, leading to palpable purpura.

Immune-complex deposition is generally considered to be the immunopathogenic mechanism of this type of vasculitis; however, formal proof that this is the case has not been established for all subgroups (see above). The predominantly cutaneous vasculitides can be broken down empirically into two major categories depending on the type of putative antigen involved in the hypersensitivity reaction. In the originally described group, the antigen was foreign to the host, i.e., a drug, microbe, or foreign protein. In this regard, essential mixed cryoglobulinemia has been associated with hepatitis C virus infection. In the second category, the antigen is felt to be endogenous to the host. Examples of these are the "self" proteins such as DNA or immunoglobulin, which form immune complexes with their respective antibodies and lead to vasculitic complications in systemic lupus erythematosus and rheumatoid arthritis, respectively; other examples are the recognized and putative tumor antigens that form immune complexes with antibody and lead to vasculitis associated with certain neoplasms. Certain lymphoid malignancies also may secrete cytokines that contribute to the pathogenic process (see Table 319-1).

CLINICAL   AND   LABORATORY   MANIFESTATIONS

The hallmark of this broad group of vasculitides is the predominance of skin involvement. Skin lesions may appear typically as palpable purpura; however, other cutaneous manifestations of the vasculitis may occur, including macules, papules, vesicles, bullae, subcutaneous nodules, ulcers, and recurrent or chronic urticaria. Despite the fact that skin lesions predominate, other organ systems may be involved to varying degrees, and the extent to which this occurs may define a relatively distinct subgroup. Even in patients with isolated cutaneous involvement, the disease may be characterized by systemic signs and symptoms such as fever, malaise, myalgia, and anorexia. The skin lesions may be pruritic or even quite painful, with a burning or stinging sensation. Lesions most commonly occur in the lower extremities in ambulatory patients or in the sacral area in bedridden patients due to the effects of hydrostatic forces on the postcapillary venules. Edema may accompany certain lesions, and hyperpigmentation often occurs in areas of recurrent or chronic lesions.

There are no specific laboratory tests diagnostic of this category of vasculitis. A mild leukocytosis with or without eosinophilia is characteristic, as is an elevated ESR. Cryoglobulins and rheumatoid factor may be seen in certain cases, and serum complement levels follow no definite pattern. Laboratory abnormalities related to specific organ dysfunction reflect the involvement of these organs in the particular syndrome in question.

Drug-Induced Vasculitis   Cutaneous drug reactions take a number of forms, and vasculitis is only one of these (see Chaps. 56 and 57). Vasculitis associated with drug reactions usually presents as palpable purpura that may be generalized or limited to the lower extremities or other dependent areas; however, urticarial lesions, ulcers, and hemorrhagic blisters may also occur (see Chap. 56). Signs and symptoms may be limited to the skin, although systemic manifestations such as fever, malaise, and polyarthralgias may occur. Although the skin is the predominant organ involved, systemic vasculitis may result from drug reactions. Drugs that have been implicated in vasculitis include allopurinol, thiazides, gold sulfonamides, phenytoin, and penicillin.

Serum Sickness and Serum Sickness–Like Reactions   These reactions are characterized by the occurrence of fever, urticaria, polyarthralgias, and lymphadenopathy 7 to 10 days after primary exposure and 2 to 4 days after secondary exposure to a heterologous protein (classic serum sickness) or a nonprotein drug such as penicillin or sulfa (serum sickness–like reaction). Most of the manifestations are not due to a vasculitis; however, occasional patients will have typical cutaneous venulitis that may progress rarely to a systemic vasculitis.

Vasculitis Associated with Other Underlying Primary Diseases   A number of diseases have vasculitis as a secondary manifestation of the underlying primary process. Foremost among these are the connective tissue diseases, particularly *systemic lupus erythematosus* (Chap. 312), *rheumatoid arthritis* (Chap. 313), and *Sjögren's syndrome* (Chap. 316). The most common form of vasculitis in these conditions is the small vessel venulitis isolated to the skin and clinically indistinguishable from the predominantly cutaneous vasculitides noted in response to an exogenous antigen. However, certain patients may develop a fulminant systemic necrotizing vasculitis indistinguishable from the PAN group.

Cryoglobulinemia may be seen in a number of the diverse vasculitic syndromes. *Essential mixed cryoglobulinemia* (see Chap. 275) may present as a typical predominantly cutaneous vasculitis. However, typically, it is associated with glomerulonephritis, arthralgias, hepatosplenomegaly, and lymphadenopathy in addition to skin involvement.

Vasculitis can be associated with certain *malignancies*, particularly lymphoid or reticuloendothelial neoplasms. Leukocytoclastic venulitis confined to the skin is the most common finding; however, widespread systemic vasculitis may occur. Of particular note is the association of *hairy cell leukemia* (Chap. 113) with classic PAN.

A leukocytoclastic vasculitis predominantly involving the skin with occasional involvement of other organ systems may be a minor component of many other diseases. These include *subacute bacterial endocarditis, Epstein-Barr virus infection, human immunodeficiency virus infection, chronic active hepatitis, ulcerative colitis, congenital deficiencies of various complement components, retroperitoneal fibrosis,* and *primary biliary cirrhosis*. Association of predominantly cutaneous vasculitis with α_1-*antitrypsin deficiency, intestinal bypass surgery,* and *relapsing polychondritis* has been reported.

DIAGNOSIS   The diagnosis of this category of vasculitis is made by the demonstration of vasculitis on biopsy. Given the predominance of cutaneous involvement, biopsy material is generally readily available. An important principle in the diagnostic approach to patients with presumed isolated cutaneous vasculitis is to search for an etiology of the vasculitis—be it an exogenous agent such as a drug or an infection or an endogenous condition such as an underlying disease (Fig. 319-1). In addition, a careful physical and laboratory examination should be performed to rule out the possibility of systemic disease. This should start with the least invasive diagnostic approach and proceed to the more invasive only if clinically indicated.

℞ TREATMENT

Most cases of predominantly cutaneous vasculitis resolve spontaneously, and others remit and relapse before finally remitting completely. In those patients in whom persistent cutaneous disease evolves or in whom extracutaneous organ system involvement occurs, a variety of therapeutic regimens have been tried with variable results. In general, the treatment of this type of vasculitis has not been satisfactory. This is in contrast to the systemic necrotizing vasculitis group and Wegener's granulomatosis (see above), which generally are much more serious diseases than predominantly cutaneous vasculitis but usually respond dramatically to the combination of prednisone and cyclophosphamide. Fortunately, since the disease is generally limited to the skin, this lack of consistent response to therapy usually does not lead to a life-threatening situation. When an antigenic stimulus is recognized as the precipitating factor in the vasculitis, it should be removed; if this is a microbe, appropriate antimicrobial therapy should be instituted. If the vasculitis is associated with another underlying disease, treatment of the latter often results in resolution of the former. In situations where disease is apparently self-limited,

no therapy, except possibly symptomatic therapy, is indicated. When disease persists or results in progressive organ system dysfunction, as may occur with the vasculitis that may be associated with certain connective tissue diseases, treatment according to the regimen for systemic necrotizing vasculitis should be initiated. Glucocorticoid therapy should be instituted, usually as prednisone, 1 mg/kg per day, in a regimen aimed at rapid tapering where possible, either directly to discontinuation or by conversion to an alternate-day regimen followed by ultimate discontinuation. In cases that prove refractory to glucocorticoids in which irreversible organ system dysfunction is likely, a trial of a cytotoxic agent such as cyclophosphamide in the regimen described above for systemic vasculitis is warranted. Patients with chronic vasculitis isolated to cutaneous venules rarely respond dramatically to any therapeutic regimen, and cytotoxic agents should be used only as a last resort in these patients. Plasmapheresis has been used with some success in fulminant cases. Dapsone has been tried in a number of patients with isolated cutaneous vasculitis with rare anecdotal reports of success. However, this drug has been consistently beneficial as therapy for cutaneous vasculitis only in patients with erythema elevatum diutinum (see below).

KAWASAKI DISEASE

Kawasaki disease (mucocutaneous lymph node syndrome) is an acute, febrile, multisystem disease of children. It is characterized by unresponsiveness to antibiotics, nonsuppurative cervical adenitis, and changes in the skin and mucous membranes such as edema, congested conjunctivae, erythema of the oral cavity, lips, and palms, and desquamation of the skin of the fingertips. Although the disease is generally benign and self-limited, it is associated with coronary artery aneurysms in approximately 25 percent of cases, with an overall case fatality rate of 0.5 to 2.8 percent. These complications usually occur between the third and fourth weeks of illness during the convalescent stage. Vasculitis of the coronary arteries is seen in almost all the fatal cases that have been autopsied. There is typical intimal proliferation and infiltration of the vessel wall with mononuclear cells. Beadlike aneurysms and thromboses may be seen along the artery. Most investigators agree that many of the cases of PAN formerly reported in children were actually arteritic complications of unrecognized Kawasaki disease. Other manifestations include pericarditis, myocarditis, myocardial ischemia and infarction, and cardiomegaly.

It is likely that immune-mediated injury to blood vessel endothelium is involved in the pathogenesis of this disease. Patients with Kawasaki disease have been demonstrated to have evidence of increased immune activation characterized by increased activated helper T cells and monocytes, elevated serum-soluble IL-2 receptor levels, elevated levels of spontaneous IL-1 production by peripheral blood mononuclear cells, anti-endothelial cell antibodies, and increased cytokine-inducible activation antigens on their vascular endothelium. A strong association has been reported between a novel form of *S. aureus* that releases toxic shock syndrome toxin 1 and Kawasaki disease, suggesting that this was the causative organism and was acting as a superantigen similar to the superantigen effect in toxic shock syndrome. However, analysis of the T cell receptor repertoire of patients with Kawasaki disease suggests that the T cell response is driven by a conventional antigen and not a superantigen.

Apart from the up to 2.8 percent of patients who develop fatal complications, the prognosis of this disease for uneventful recovery is excellent. High-dose intravenous gamma globulin (2 g/kg as a single infusion over 10 h) together with aspirin (100 mg/kg per day for 14 days followed by 3 to 5 mg/kg per day for several weeks) have been shown to be effective in reducing the prevalence of coronary artery abnormalities when administered early in the course of the disease.

ISOLATED VASCULITIS OF THE CENTRAL NERVOUS SYSTEM

Isolated vasculitis of the central nervous system is an uncommon clinicopathologic entity characterized by vasculitis restricted to the vessels of the central nervous system without other apparent systemic vasculitis. Although the arteriole is most commonly affected, vessels of any size can be involved. The inflammatory process is usually composed of mononuclear cell infiltrates with or without granuloma formation. Cases have been associated with cytomegalovirus, syphilis, pyogenic bacterial, and varicella-zoster infections, as well as with Hodgkin's disease and amphetamine abuse; however, in most cases no underlying disease process has been identified.

Patients may present with severe headaches, altered mental function, and focal neurologic defects. Systemic symptoms are generally absent. Devastating neurologic abnormalities may occur depending on the extent of vessel involvement. The diagnosis is generally made by demonstration of characteristic vessel abnormalities on arteriography and confirmed by biopsy of the brain parenchyma and leptomeninges. In the absence of a brain biopsy, care should be taken not to misinterpret angiographic abnormalities that might actually be vessel spasm related to another cause with true primary vasculitis. The prognosis of this disease is poor; however, in certain patients the disease may remit spontaneously, and some reports indicate that glucocorticoid therapy alone or together with cyclophosphamide in steroid-resistant patients administered as described above for the systemic vasculitides has induced sustained clinical remissions in a small number of patients.

THROMBOANGIITIS OBLITERANS (BUERGER'S DISEASE)

Thromboangiitis obliterans is an inflammatory occlusive peripheral vascular disease of unknown etiology that affects arteries and veins. Thrombosis of the vessels is likely the primary event, and so this disease is not a classic vasculitis. However, it is considered among the vasculitides because of the intense inflammatory response within the thrombus and the fact that there is often a vasculitis of the vasa vasorum in the arterial wall. → *The disease is discussed in detail in Chap. 248.*

BEHÇET'S SYNDROME

Behçet's syndrome is a clinicopathologic entity characterized by recurrent episodes of oral and genital ulcers, iritis, and cutaneous lesions. The underlying pathologic process is a leukocytoclastic venulitis, although vessels of any size and in any organ can be involved. → *This disorder is described in detail in Chap. 318.*

MISCELLANEOUS VASCULITIDES

A variety of disorders, many of which are uncommon, are characterized by varying degrees of inflammatory responses involving blood vessels. *Cogan's syndrome* is a disease characterized by nonsyphilitic interstitial keratitis together with vestibuloauditory symptoms. It may be associated with a systemic vasculitis involving vessels of different sizes as well as the aortic valve.

Erythema elevatum diutinum is a rare chronic skin disorder of unknown etiology characterized by persistent red, purple, and yellowish papules, plaques, and nodules usually distributed symmetrically over the extensor surface of the limbs; on biopsy, they demonstrate a leukocytoclastic venulitis together with a marked dermal inflammatory infiltrate. An association with streptococcal infections has been reported. The disease responds dramatically to dapsone therapy.

Certain *infections* may directly trigger an inflammatory vasculitic process. For example, rickettsias can invade and proliferate in the endothelial cells of small blood vessels causing a vasculitis (see Chap. 179). In addition, the inflammatory response around blood vessels associated with certain systemic fungal diseases such as histoplasmosis (see Chap. 203) may mimic a primary vasculitic process.

℞ TREATMENT

Once a diagnosis of vasculitis has been established, a decision regarding therapeutic strategy must be made (Fig. 319-1). The vasculitis syndromes represent a wide spectrum of diseases with varying degrees of severity. Some require immediate and aggressive therapy with glucocorticoids and immunosuppressive agents, while others should be treated conservatively and symptomatically, usually with nonsteroidal anti-inflammatory drugs. Since the potential toxic side effects of certain therapeutic regimens may be substantial, the risk-versus-benefit ratio of any therapeutic approach should be weighed carefully. Specific therapeutic regimens are discussed above for the individual vasculitis syndromes; however, certain general principles regarding therapy should be considered. On the one hand, glucocorticoids and/or immunosuppressive therapy should be instituted immediately in diseases where irreversible organ system dysfunction and high morbidity and mortality have been clearly established. Wegener's granulomatosis is the prototype of a severe systemic vasculitis requiring such a therapeutic approach (see above). On the other hand, when feasible, aggressive therapy should be avoided for vasculitic manifestations that rarely result in irreversible organ system dysfunction and that usually do not respond to such therapy. For example, isolated cutaneous vasculitis usually resolves with symptomatic treatment, and prolonged courses of glucocorticoids uncommonly result in clinical benefit. Immunosuppressive agents have not proven to be beneficial in isolated cutaneous vasculitis, and their toxic side effects generally outweigh any potential beneficial effects. Glucocorticoids should be initiated in those systemic vasculitides that cannot be specifically categorized or for which there is no established standard therapy; immunosuppressive therapy should be added in these diseases only if an adequate response does not result or if remission can only be achieved and maintained with an unacceptably toxic regimen of glucocorticoids. When remission is achieved, one should continually attempt to taper glucocorticoids to an alternate-day regimen and discontinue when possible. When using immunosuppressive regimens, one should taper and discontinue the drug as soon as is feasible upon induction of remission (see below).

When glucocorticoids are used, prednisone is generally the formulation of choice and is administered as 1 mg/kg per day orally, first in divided doses and then converted to a single daily dose. After clinical improvement is noted (usually within a month), the regimen is gradually converted to an alternate-day schedule, followed by tapering and discontinuation after approximately 6 months or as the clinical response dictates. When an immunosuppressive agent is required, cyclophosphamide is the drug of choice and its efficacy has been clearly established in Wegener's granulomatosis and the severe systemic vasculitides (see above). It should be given in doses of 2 mg/kg per day orally. It is recommended that the drug be taken as a single dose in the morning together with large amounts of fluid. Dose adjustments should be based on the leukocyte count, which should be maintained above 3000/μL. Leukocyte counts at any given time will reflect the dosage of cyclophosphamide taken the previous week. Of note, neutropenia may become more pronounced as glucocorticoids are tapered. The regimen that has proven successful in Wegener's granulomatosis (see above) and that should be followed for the other severe systemic vasculitides has called for continuation of cyclophosphamide for approximately 1 year following the induction of complete remission, with gradual tapering (by 25-mg decrements of the daily dose) over several months until discontinuation. No other drug has proven to be as effective as cyclophosphamide for severe life-threatening vasculitis. However, immediate and long-range toxic side effects may be severe. Alternative immunosuppressive regimens may be instituted where indicated in those patients who cannot tolerate cyclophosphamide due to unacceptable side effects or who do not wish to take cyclophosphamide because of the potential side effects, particularly infertility or sterility in individuals of child-bearing age. Methotrexate has been shown to be an acceptable alternative to cyclophosphamide when the latter drug cannot be used. Methotrexate is administered initially at a dosage of 0.3 mg/kg, not to exceed 15 mg per week. If the treatment is well tolerated after 1 to 2 weeks, the dosage should be increased by 2.5 mg weekly up to a dosage of 20 to 25 mg/week and maintained at that level. Azathioprine at a

Table 319-6

Major Toxic Side Effects of Drugs Commonly Used in the Treatment of Systemic Vasculitis

GLUCOCORTICOIDS

Osteoporosis	
Cataracts	Growth suppression in children
Glaucoma	Hypertension
Diabetes mellitus	Avascular necrosis of bone
Electrolyte abnormalities	Myopathy
Metabolic abnormalities	Alterations in mood
Suppression of inflammatory and immune responses leading to opportunistic infections	Psychosis Pseudotumor cerebri Peptic ulcer diathesis
Cushingoid features	Pancreatitis

CYCLOPHOSPHAMIDE

Bone marrow suppression	Hypogammaglobulinemia
Cystitis	Pulmonary fibrosis
Bladder carcinoma	Myelodysplasia
Gonadal suppression	Oncogenesis
Gastrointestinal intolerance	

METHOTREXATE

Gastrointestinal intolerance	Pneumonitis
Stomatitis	Teratogenicity
Neutropenia	Opportunistic infections
Hepatotoxicity (may lead to fibrosis or cirrhosis)	

dosage of 2 mg/kg per day orally has also been employed as an alternative to cyclophosphamide in severe systemic vasculitis with less favorable results. In unusual cases in which none of the above regimens have resulted in remission of the vasculitis, certain experimental approaches have been used, such as plasmapheresis together with immunosuppressive drugs, with anecdotal reports of limited success. In addition, other immunosuppressive agents such as cyclosporine have been employed with minimal success.

Physicians should be thoroughly aware of the toxic side effects of therapeutic agents employed (Table 319-6). Side effects of glucocorticoid therapy are markedly decreased in frequency and duration in patients on alternate-day regimens compared to daily regimens. When cyclophosphamide is administered chronically in doses of 2 mg/kg per day for substantial periods of time (one to several years), the incidence of cystitis as defined by nonglomerular hematuria is approximately 40 percent and the incidence of bladder cancer is 5 percent. Significant alopecia is unusual in the chronically administered, low-dose regimen. When patients are receiving low-dose cyclophosphamide, the white blood count (WBC) is maintained above 3000/μL, and the patient is not receiving daily glucocorticoids, the incidence of life-threatening opportunistic infections is very low. However, the WBC is not an accurate predictor of risk of opportunistic infections in patients receiving methotrexate; infections with *Pneumocystis carinii* and certain fungi can be seen in the face of WBC that are within normal limits.

Finally, it should be emphasized that each patient is unique and requires individual decision-making. The above outline should serve as a framework to guide therapeutic approaches; however, flexibility should be practiced in order to provide maximal therapeutic efficacy with minimal toxic side effects in each patient.

BIBLIOGRAPHY

CUPPS TR, FAUCI AS: *The Vasculitides*. Philadelphia, Saunders, 1981
———— et al: Isolated angiitis of the central nervous system. Prospective diagnostic and therapeutic experience. Am J Med 74:97, 1983
FAUCI AS et al: Wegener's granulomatosis: Prospective clinical and therapeutic experience with 85 patients for 21 years. Ann Intern Med 98:76, 1983

GIORDANO JM et al: Experience with surgical treatment of Takayasu's disease. Surgery 109:252, 1991
GUILLEVIN L et al: Treatment of polyarteritis nodosa related to hepatitis B virus with interferon-alpha and plasma exchanges. Ann Rheum Dis 53:334, 1994
HAYNES BF: Vasculitis: Pathogenic mechanisms of vessel damage, in *Inflammation: Basic Principles and Clinical Correlates*, JI Gallin et al (eds). New York, Raven Press, 1992, pp 921–941
HOFFMAN GS et al: Wegener's granulomatosis: An analysis of 158 patients. Ann Intern Med 116:488, 1992
HUNDER GG: Giant cell (temporal arteritis). Rheum Dis Clin North Am 16:399, 1990
JENNETTE JC et al: Nomenclature of systemic vasculitis. Proposal of an international consensus conference. Arthritis Rheum 37:187, 1994
KALLENBERG CGM et al: ANCA—pathophysiology revisited. Clin Exp Immunol 100:1, 1995
KERR G et al: Limited prognostic value of changes in antineutrophil cytoplasmic antibody titer in patients with Wegener's granulomatosis. Arthritis Rheum 36:365, 1993
———— et al: Takayasu arteritis. Ann Intern Med 120:919, 1994
NEWBURGER JW et al: A single intravenous infusion of gamma globulin as compared with four infusions in the treatment of acute Kawasaki disease. N Engl J Med 324:1633, 1991
NILES JL: Value of tests for antineutrophil cytoplasmic autoantibodies in the diagnosis and treatment of vasculitis. Curr Opin Rheumatol 5:18, 1993
PIETRA BA et al: TCR Vβ family repertoire and T cell activation markers in Kawasaki disease. J Immunol 153:1881, 1994
SNELLER MC et al: An analysis of forty-two Wegener's granulomatosis patients treated with methotrexate and prednisone. Arthritis Rheum 38:608, 1995
SOMER T, FINEGOLD SM: Vasculitis associated with infections, immunization, and antimicrobial drugs. Clin Infect Dis 20:1010, 1995
WEYLAND CM et al: Distinct vascular lesions in giant cell arteritis share identical T cell clonotypes. J Exp Med 179:951, 1994
———— et al: Tissue cytokine patterns in patients with polymyalgia rheumatica and giant cell arteritis. Ann Intern Med 121:484, 1994

320   *Ronald G. Crystal*

SARCOIDOSIS

DEFINITION   Sarcoidosis is a chronic, multisystem disorder of unknown cause characterized in affected organs by an accumulation of T lymphocytes and mononuclear phagocytes, noncaseating epithelioid granulomas, and derangements of the normal tissue architecture. Although there are usually skin anergy and depressed cellular immune processes in the blood, sarcoidosis is characterized at the sites of disease by exaggerated T helper lymphocyte immune processes. All parts of the body can be affected, but the organ most frequently affected is the lung. Involvement of the skin, eye, and lymph nodes is also common. The disease is often acute or subacute and self-limiting, but in many individuals it is chronic, waxing and waning over many years.

ETIOLOGY   The cause of sarcoidosis is unknown. A variety of infectious and noninfectious agents have been implicated, but there is no proof that any specific agent is responsible. However, all available evidence is consistent with the concept that the disease results from an exaggerated cellular immune response (acquired, inherited, or both) to a limited class of persistent antigens or self-antigens.

INCIDENCE AND PREVALENCE   Sarcoidosis is a relatively common disease affecting individuals of both sexes and almost all ages, races, and geographic locations. Females appear to be slightly more susceptible than males. Cases of sarcoid have been described in all of the major races, and the disease is found throughout the world. It has been suggested that sarcoid is more common in certain geographic areas such as the southeastern part of the United States, but when case-matched controls have been used, these geographic differences are less convincing. There is a remarkable diversity of the prevalence of sarcoidosis among certain ethnic and racial groups, with a range of <1 to 64 per 100,000 worldwide. The prevalence of sarcoidosis is from 10 to 40 per 100,000 in the United States and Europe. In the United States, the majority of patients are black, with a ratio of blacks to whites ranging from 10:1 to 17:1. In Europe, however, the disease affects mostly whites. Furthermore, while the prevalence per 100,000 in Sweden is 64, in France it is 10, in Poland 3, yet for Irish females living in London it is 200. In contrast, the disease is very rare among Inuit, Canadian Indians, New Zealand Maoris, and Southeast Asians.

Most patients present with sarcoidosis between the ages of 20 and 40, but it can occur in children and in the elderly. Several hundred kindred groups with familial sarcoidosis have been described, and the disease has been observed in twins, more commonly in monozygotic than in dizygotic pairs. There also have been several instances of husband-wife pairs identified, and geographic foci of sarcoid among unrelated individuals living closely within a community, arguing for some environmental factors in the pathogenesis of the disease. Although the disease is believed to result from exaggerated cellular immune responses to a limited class of antigens, no clear patterns in any HLA locus have emerged. Unlike many diseases in which the lung is involved, sarcoidosis favors nonsmokers.

PATHOPHYSIOLOGY AND IMMUNOPATHOGENESIS

The first manifestation of the disease is an accumulation of mononuclear inflammatory cells, mostly T helper lymphocytes and mononuclear phagocytes, in affected organs. This inflammatory process is followed by the formation of granulomas, aggregates of macrophages and their progeny, epithelioid cells, and multinucleated giant cells. The typical sarcoid granuloma is a compact structure composed of an aggregate of mononuclear phagocytes surrounded by a rim of T helper-inducer lymphocytes and, to a far lesser extent, B lymphocytes. The overall structure is relatively discrete and is interspersed with fine collagen fibrils, presumably remnants of the underlying connective tissue matrix. The giant cells within the granuloma can be of the Langhans' or foreign-body variety and often contain inclusions such as Schaumann bodies (conchlike structures), asteroid bodies (stellate-like structures), and residual bodies (refractile calcium-containing inclusions).

Together the accumulated T cells, mononuclear phagocytes, and granulomas represent the active disease. Other than the fact that they take up space and thus their bulk modifies the local architecture, there is no evidence that the mononuclear inflammatory cells dispersed in the tissue or in the granuloma injure the affected organ by releasing mediators that damage the normal parenchymal cells or the extracellular matrix. Rather, organ dysfunction in sarcoid results mostly from the accumulated inflammatory cells distorting the architecture of the affected tissue; if a sufficient number of structures vital to the function of the tissue are involved, the disease becomes clinically apparent in that organ. Thus, while autopsy series show that, to some extent, sarcoidosis involves most organs in the majority of patients, the disease manifests clinically only in organs where it affects function (such as the lung and eye) or in organs where it is readily observed (such as the skin or, by x-ray, the hilar nodes). For example, in the lung, the inflammatory cells and granulomas distort the walls of the alveoli, bronchi, and blood vessels (Fig. 320-1A), thus altering the intimate relationships between air and blood necessary for normal gas exchange. When a sufficient amount of pulmonary tissue is involved, it is sensed by the individual as dyspnea. In contrast, most individuals with sarcoidosis have granulomatous mononuclear cell inflammation in the liver but usually do not have symptoms or functional derangements referable to that organ, likely because the disease process does not modify the local structures sufficiently to affect function.

If the disease is suppressed, either spontaneously or with therapy, the mononuclear inflammation is reduced in intensity and the number of granulomas is reduced. The granulomas resolve either by dispersion of the cells or by centripetal proliferation of fibroblasts from the periphery of the granuloma inward, to form a small scar. In chronic cases, the mononuclear cell inflammation persists for years. If the intensity of the inflammation is sufficiently high for a sufficiently long period, the derangements to the affected tissues result in extensive damage, the development of fibrosis, and permanent loss of organ function.

All available evidence suggests that active sarcoidosis results from an exaggerated cellular immune response to a variety of antigens or self-antigens, in which the process of T lymphocyte triggering, proliferation, and activation is skewed in the direction of helper-

inducer T lymphocyte processes (Fig. 320-1B). The result is an exaggerated helper-inducer T cell response and thus the accumulation of large numbers of activated T cells in the affected organs. Since the activated helper-inducer T lymphocyte releases mediators that attract and activate mononuclear phagocytes, it is likely that the process of granuloma formation is a secondary phenomenon that is a consequence of the exaggerated helper-inducer T cell process. In this context, the current hypotheses of the cause of sarcoidosis, not mutually exclusive, include the following: (1) The disease is caused by a class of persistent antigens, nonself or self, that trigger only the helper-inducer T cell arm of the immune response; (2) the disease results from an inadequate suppressor arm of the immune response, such that helper-inducer T cell processes cannot be shut down in a normal fashion; or (3) the disease results from inherited (and/or acquired) differences in immune response genes, such that the response to a variety of antigens is an exaggerated, helper-inducer T cell process.

Independent of the inciting agent(s) or the reason why there is an exaggerated helper-inducer T cell response, there is a general understanding of the processes responsible for the maintenance of the inflammation and the development of the granuloma. The T helper-inducer lymphocytes accumulate at the sites of disease, at least in part, because they proliferate in these sites at an exaggerated rate. This T cell proliferation is maintained by the spontaneous release of interleukin (IL) 2, the T cell growth factor, by activated T helper-inducer cells in the local milieu. In this regard, sarcoidosis is a remarkable example of compartmentalization of the immune system and a dramatic illustration of why disease activity of sarcoidosis cannot be assessed by evaluating the immune system only in the blood. Whereas the T helper-inducer cells in the involved organs are releasing IL-2 and proliferating at an enhanced rate, the T cells in other sites, such as blood, are quiescent. Furthermore, while there is a marked enhancement of the number of T helper-inducer cells at the sites of disease, the numbers of T helper-inducer cells in the blood are normal or slightly reduced. In the involved organs, the ratio of helper-inducer to suppressor-cytotoxic T cells may be as high as 10:1 compared to the ratio of 2:1 found in normal tissues or in the blood of affected individuals.

In addition to driving other T helper-inducer cells in the affected organs to proliferate, the T helper-inducer cells at the sites of disease are activated and release mediators that both recruit and activate mononuclear phagocytes. The activated T helper-inducer cells accomplish this by releasing a variety of mediators (lymphokines) including proteins capable of recruiting blood monocytes to the local milieu of the activated T cells and interferon γ, a protein that, among its many actions, activates mononuclear phagocytes. Together with other cytokines released locally, these mediators recruit blood monocytes to the affected organs and activate them, providing the building blocks for the formation of the granuloma.

In addition to these exaggerated cellular immune processes, active sarcoid is also characterized by hyperglobulinemia. Included among the immunoglobulins are antibodies against a variety of infectious agents as well as IgM anti-T cell antibodies. However, there is no evidence that any of these antibodies plays a role in the pathogenesis of the disease, and they are thought to result from the nonspecific polyclonal stimulation of B cells by the activated T cells at the site of disease.

If the damage in the affected organs is sufficiently extensive that the remaining parenchymal cells cannot reestablish the normal tissue architecture, the usual result is fibrosis, the proliferation of mesenchymal cells, and deposition of their connective tissue products. There is convincing evidence that the fibroblast proliferation is directed by tissue macrophages spontaneously releasing growth signals for fibroblasts, including platelet-derived growth factor, fibronectin, and insulin-like growth factor 1. It is not known, however, why this fibrotic process occurs only in a relatively small proportion of individuals with sarcoidosis.

CLINICAL MANIFESTATIONS Sarcoidosis is a systemic disease, and thus the clinical manifestations may be generalized or focused on one or more organs. However, because the lung is almost always involved, most patients have symptoms referable to the respiratory system. Independent of the site, the clinical manifestations of the disease relate directly to the exaggerated helper-inducer T cell–mononuclear phagocyte granulomatous inflammatory process itself or to the sequelae resulting from the permanent damage caused by this process.

Sarcoidosis is occasionally discovered in a completely asymptomatic individual, but more commonly it presents abruptly over 1 to 2 weeks or the affected individual develops symptoms insidiously over several months. Independent of the mode of presentation, about 75 percent of all cases present when the individual is less than 40 years of age.

The asymptomatic form is usually detected by a routine examination, such as a chest film. In the United States, this represents about 10 to 20 percent of all cases, but in countries where chest films are mandatory in preemployment screening programs, the proportion of asymptomatic patients is higher.

So-called acute or subacute sarcoidosis develops abruptly over a period of a few weeks and represents 20 to 40 percent of all cases. These individuals usually have constitutional symptoms such as fever, fatigue, malaise, anorexia, or weight loss. These symptoms are usually mild, but in approximately 25 percent of the acute cases the constitutional complaints are extensive. Many patients have respiratory symptoms, including cough, dyspnea, a vague retrosternal chest discomfort and/or polyarthritis. Two syndromes have been identified in the acute group. Löfgren's syndrome, frequent in Scandinavian, Irish, and Puerto Rican females, includes the complex of erythema nodosum and x-ray findings of bilateral hilar adenopathy, often accompanied by joint symptoms, including arthritis at the ankles, knees, wrists, or elbows. The Heerfordt-Waldenström syndrome describes individuals with fever, parotid enlargement, anterior uveitis, and facial nerve palsy.

The insidious form of sarcoidosis develops over months and is associated usually with respiratory complaints without constitutional symptoms. In the United States, 40 to 70 percent of all sarcoid patients are in this category. About 10 percent of these individuals have symptoms referable to organs other than the lung. It is the individuals who present with the insidious form of sarcoidosis who most commonly go on to develop chronic sarcoidosis, with permanent damage to the lung and other organs.

Despite the fact that sarcoidosis is a systemic disease and some evidence of inflammation can be detected in most organs in the majority of patients, sarcoidosis is important clinically because of the pulmonary abnormalities and, to a lesser extent, lymph node, skin, and eye involvement. Far less commonly, other organs are involved significantly.

Lung Of individuals with sarcoidosis, 90 percent have an abnormal chest x-ray at some time during their course (Fig. 320-2A). Overall, approximately 50 percent develop permanent pulmonary abnormalities, and 5 to 15 percent have progressive fibrosis of the lung parenchyma. Sarcoidosis of the lung is primarily an interstitial lung disease (see Chap. 259) in which the inflammatory process involves the alveoli, small bronchi, and small blood vessels. These individuals typically have symptoms of dyspnea, particularly with exercise, and a dry cough. In acute and subacute cases, physical examination usually reveals dry rales. Hemoptysis is rare, as is production of sputum. Occasionally, the large airways are involved to a degree sufficient to cause dysfunc-

FIGURE 320-1 Pathogenesis of sarcoidosis. *A.* Histologic abnormalities. Normal alveoli (*left*) and alveoli in active sarcoidosis (*right*). The latter are distorted by the accumulated T helper-inducer lymphocytes, alveolar macrophages, and macrophages aggregated into granulomas. There is mild damage to alveolar epithelial and endothelial cells. *B.* The exaggerated processes of T helper-inducer lymphocytes in affected organs result in the accumulation of these cells along with macrophages and macrophages aggregated into granulomas. The trigger for the T helper-inducer cells is unknown. It may be a limited class of antigens or self-antigens presented in the context of class II HLA surface molecules by mononuclear phagocytes to the T helper-inducer lymphocyte. The antigen class II HLA complex is identified by the T cell antigen receptor, and the T cell is activated. Consequent to this process the immune response is exaggerated and skewed to produce activated T helper-inducer cells that release interleukin 2, which drives the accumulation of more T helper cells. The activated T helper-inducer cells also release interferon γ (INF-γ). Together with cytokines such as macrophage inflammatory protein 1α and granulocyte-macrophage colony stimulating factor released in the local milieu, there is recruitment and activation of blood monocytes and subsequent granuloma formation.

tion. Distal atelectasis can result from endobronchial sarcoidosis or from external compression from enlarged intrathoracic nodes. Rarely, wheezing is heard, incorrectly suggesting asthma. Large-vessel pulmonary granulomatous arteritis is common, but it rarely causes major problems. If it dominates the pulmonary lesions, it is sometimes called *necrotizing sarcoidal granulomatosis*. The pleura is involved in 1 to 5 percent of cases, almost always manifesting as a unilateral pleural effusion with characteristics of an exudate containing lymphocytes. The effusions usually clear within a few weeks, but chronic pleural thickening can result. Pneumothorax is very rare.

Lymph Nodes Lymphadenopathy is very common in sarcoidosis. Intrathoracic nodes are enlarged in 75 to 90 percent of all patients; usually this involves the hilar nodes, but the paratracheal nodes are commonly involved (Fig. 320-2A). Less frequently, there is enlargement of subcarinal, anterior mediastinal, or posterior mediastinal nodes. Peripheral lymphadenopathy is very common, particularly involving the cervical, axillary, epitrochlear, and inguinal nodes. The nodes in the retroperitoneal area and in the mesenteric chain also can enlarge. All these nodes are nonadherent, with a firm, rubbery texture. Palpation causes no pain. Unlike nodes in tuberculosis, the nodes do not ulcerate. The lymphadenopathy rarely causes a problem for the affected individual; however, if it is massive, it can be disfiguring and can impinge on other organs and lead to functional impairment.

Skin Sarcoidosis involves the skin in about 25 percent of cases. The most common lesions are erythema nodosum, plaques, maculopapular eruptions, subcutaneous nodules, and lupus pernio. Erythema nodosum, comprising bilateral, tender red nodules on the anterior surface of the legs, is not specific for sarcoidosis but is common, particularly in acute sarcoidosis, in combination with systemic symptoms and polyarthralgias. Treatment is not required, since the lesions resolve spontaneously in 2 to 4 weeks. Erythema nodosum is much more common among sarcoid patients in Europe than in the United States. Skin plaques associated with sarcoid are purple, indolent lesions, often raised, and usually occur on the face, buttocks, and extremities. The maculopapular eruptions occur on the face around the eyes and nose, on the back, and on the extremities. These are elevated lesions less than 1 cm in diameter with a flat, waxy top. Subcutaneous nodules are most common on the trunk and extremities. Lupus pernio is characterized by indurated blue-purple, swollen, shiny lesions on the nose, cheeks, lips, ears, fingers, and knees. The lesions on the tip of the nose cause a bulbous appearance, sometimes associated with varicosities. The nasal mucosa is usually involved, and underlying bone can be destroyed. Sarcoidosis also can involve old surgical scars and tattoos. Although it may be disfiguring, cutaneous sarcoidosis rarely causes major problems. Clubbing of the fingers is occasionally observed in sarcoidosis, usually in association with extensive pulmonary fibrosis.

Eye Eye involvement occurs in approximately 25 percent of patients with sarcoidosis, and it can cause blindness. The usual lesions involve the uveal tract, iris, ciliary body, and choroid. Of those cases with eye involvement, approximately 75 percent have anterior uveitis and 25 to 35 percent have posterior uveitis. There is blurred vision, tearing, and photophobia. The uveitis can develop rapidly and may clear spontaneously over a 6- to 12-month period. It also can develop insidiously and be chronic. Conjunctival involvement is also common, usually with small, yellow nodules. When the lacrimal gland is involved, a keratoconjunctivitis sicca syndrome, with dry, sore eyes, can result.

Upper Respiratory Tract The nasal mucosa is involved in up to 20 percent of patients, usually presenting with nasal stuffiness. Any of the structures of the mouth can be involved, particularly the tonsils. Sarcoidosis involves the larynx in about 5 percent of cases. The epiglot-

FIGURE 320-2 Common laboratory findings of sarcoidosis. *A*. Schematic view of the abnormal findings on the chest x-ray. Shown are changes observed with the average frequency of occurrence. *B*. Typical gallium 67 scan of an individual with active sarcoidosis. The isotope has accumulated in the lung parenchyma (LP), liver (L), spleen (S), parotid (P), hilar nodes (HN), and pelvic nodes (PN). *C*. Cells recovered by bronchoalveolar lavage of an individual with active pulmonary sarcoidosis. The lavage analysis reflects the inflammation in the tissue. Shown are alveolar macrophages (*large cells*) and lymphocytes (*small cells*). The cell population is dominated by lymphocytes, in contrast to normal individuals, in whom lymphocytes represent <20 percent of the cell population.

tis and areas around the true vocal cords are usually involved, but the cords themselves are not. These individuals are usually hoarse, and they have dyspnea, wheezing, and stridor; complete obstruction can occur.

Bone Marrow and Spleen Sarcoidosis of the marrow is reported in 15 to 40 percent of cases, but it rarely causes hematologic abnormalities other than a mild anemia, neutropenia, eosinophilia, and occasionally, thrombocytopenia. Although splenomegaly occurs in only 5 to 10 percent of patients, celiac angiography or splenic biopsy reveals involvement in 50 to 60 percent of cases. The presentation and complications of splenomegaly in sarcoidosis are similar to those of splenomegaly in general.

Liver Although liver biopsy reveals liver involvement in 60 to 90 percent of cases, liver dysfunction is usually not important clinically. Sarcoidosis involves generally the periportal areas. Approximately 20 to 30 percent have hepatomegaly and/or biochemical evidence of liver involvement. Usually these changes reflect a cholestatic pattern and include an elevated alkaline phosphatase level; the bilirubin and aminotransferase levels are only mildly elevated, and jaundice is rare. Rarely, portal hypertension can occur, as can intrahepatic cholestasis with cirrhosis.

Kidney Clinically apparent primary renal involvement in sarcoidosis is rare, although tubular, glomerular, and renal artery diseases have been reported. More commonly, but still in only 1 to 2 percent of all cases, there is a disorder of calcium metabolism with hypercalciuria, with or without hypercalcemia. If chronic, nephrocalcinosis and nephrolithiasis can result. It is believed that the calcium abnormalities are associated with enhanced calcium absorption in the gut, which is related to an abnormally high level of circulating 1,25-dihydroxyvitamin D produced by mononuclear phagocytes in the granulomas.

Nervous System All components of the nervous system can be involved in sarcoidosis. Neurologic findings are observed in about 5 percent of patients. Seventh nerve involvement with unilateral facial paralysis is most common. It occurs suddenly and is usually transient. Other common manifestations of neurosarcoid include optic nerve dysfunction, papilledema, palate dysfunction, hearing abnormalities, hypothalamic and pituitary abnormalities, chronic meningitis, and occasionally, space-occupying lesions. Psychiatric disturbances have been described, and seizures can occur. Rarely, multiple lesions occur that mimic multiple sclerosis, spinal cord abnormalities, and peripheral neuropathy.

Musculoskeletal System The bones, joints, and/or muscles can be involved in sarcoidosis. Bone lesions are observed in 5 percent of patients and include variable-sized cysts in areas of expanded bone; well-defined, round, punched-out lesions; or lattice-like changes. Hand and foot bones are the common sites, but most bones can be involved. Occasionally, the bone lesions are tender and painful. Joint involvement is more common, with an incidence of 25 to 50 percent in known cases of sarcoidosis. Arthralgias and frank arthritis occur mostly in large joints; they can be migratory and are usually transient, but they can be chronic and result in deformities. Although muscle biopsy frequently demonstrates granulomatous inflammation, muscle dysfunction is rare. However, nodules, polymyositis, and chronic myopathy have been described.

Heart Approximately 5 percent of patients have significant heart involvement, with clinical evidence of cardiac dysfunction. Left ventricular wall involvement is common. Arrhythmias are frequent, and serious conduction disturbances, including complete heart block, can occur. Papillary muscle dysfunction, pericarditis, and congestive heart failure are also observed. Cor pulmonale secondary to chronic pulmonary fibrosis may occur but is uncommon.

Endocrine and Reproductive System The hypothalamic-pituitary axis is the part of the endocrine system most commonly involved; this usually presents as diabetes insipidus. Anterior pituitary dysfunction is also seen, manifesting as a deficiency in one or more pituitary hormones. Complete hypopituitarism is rare. Much less frequently, sarcoidosis can cause primary dysfunction of other endocrine glands.

Adrenal cortical involvement resulting in Addison's syndrome has been described. Involvement of the reproductive organs occurs, but infertility is rare. Pregnancy is not affected by sarcoidosis, and patients with sarcoidosis who become pregnant usually improve during pregnancy. However, the disease may flare post partum; presumably this variation results from fluctuations in endogenous glucocorticoid production.

Exocrine Glands Parotid enlargement is a classic feature of sarcoidosis, but clinically apparent parotid involvement occurs in fewer than 10 percent of patients. Bilateral involvement is the rule. The gland is usually nontender, firm, and smooth. Xerostomia can occur; other exocrine glands are affected only rarely.

Gastrointestinal Tract Although sarcoidosis involvement of the gastrointestinal tract is found occasionally at autopsy, it rarely has clinical importance. Occasionally, patients have esophageal or gastric symptoms.

COMPLICATIONS The respiratory tract abnormalities cause most of the morbidity and mortality associated with sarcoidosis. The major problems are those characteristic of interstitial lung disease (see Chap. 259), particularly dyspnea and insufficient oxygen delivery to vital organs. Respiratory failure with carbon dioxide retention is rare. In some patients, lung destruction results in formation of bullae that may harbor mycetomas, which are usually aspergillomas; erosion into the parenchyma can result in massive bleeding. The most common complications apart from the lung are associated with the eye; however, with therapy, blindness is rare. Complications of other organs include a gamut of abnormalities. The most serious are CNS lesions or cardiac involvement leading to congestive heart failure or sudden death.

LABORATORY ABNORMALITIES Common abnormalities in the blood include lymphocytopenia, an occasional mild eosinophilia, an increased erythrocyte sedimentation rate, hyperglobulinemia, and an elevated level of angiotensin-converting enzyme. False-positive tests for rheumatoid factor or antinuclear antibodies can be observed. Hypercalcemia is rare. Other serum abnormalities relate to involvement of specific organs such as liver, kidney, or endocrine glands.

Because the lung is involved so commonly, the routine chest film is almost always abnormal (Fig. 320-2A). The three classic x-ray patterns of pulmonary sarcoidosis are type I—bilateral hilar adenopathy with no parenchymal abnormalities; type II—bilateral hilar adenopathy with diffuse parenchymal changes; and type III—diffuse parenchymal changes without hilar adenopathy. The type III pattern is sometimes split into two categories, with films that show fibrosis and upper lobe retraction classified separately. Although patients with type I x-rays tend to have the acute or subacute, reversible form of the disease while those with types II and III often have the chronic, progressive disease, these patterns do not represent consecutive "stages" of sarcoidosis. Thus, except for epidemiologic purposes, this x-ray categorization is mostly of historic interest. The hilar adenopathy is almost always bilateral, but unilateral node enlargement can be seen. Nodes are also common in the paratracheal region. The diffuse parenchymal changes are typically reticulonodular infiltrates, but an acinar pattern is observed occasionally. Large nodules, similar to those of metastatic disease, are unusual but can occur. When there is massive fibrosis, the hila are pulled upward and there are conglomerate masses in the midlung zones. Some of the unusual chest x-ray findings in sarcoidosis include "egg shell" calcification of hilar nodes, pleural effusions, cavitation, atelectasis, pulmonary hypertension, pneumothorax, and cardiomegaly. Computed tomography of the chest is rarely helpful but can identify early fibrosis, and a "ground-glass" appearance is thought to be consistent with an active alveolitis.

The lung function abnormalities of sarcoidosis are typical for interstitial lung disease (see Chap. 259) and include decreased lung volumes and diffusing capacity with a normal or supernormal ratio of the forced expiratory volume in 1 s to the forced vital capacity. Occasionally there is evidence of airflow limitation. There is usually mild hypoxemia and a mild, compensated hypocarbia.

The gallium 67 lung scan is usually abnormal, showing a pattern of diffuse uptake. If present, enlarged nodes are detected in these scans, as is inflammation in a variety of extrathoracic sites that usually have no clinical importance (Fig. 320-2*B*). Bronchoalveolar lavage typically demonstrates an increased proportion of lymphocytes, most of which are activated helper-inducer T lymphocytes (Fig. 320-2*C*). The remainder of the cells are mostly alveolar macrophages. In patients with significant fibrosis, a small number of neutrophils are also found. Eosinophils are rare.

The other laboratory features of sarcoidosis depend on the specific organ involved.

DIAGNOSIS For a typical case, the diagnosis of sarcoidosis is made by a combination of clinical, radiographic, and histologic findings (Fig. 320-3*A*). In a young adult with constitutional complaints, respiratory symptoms, erythema nodosum, blurred vision, and bilateral hilar adenopathy, the diagnosis is almost always sarcoidosis. Commonly, however, the findings are more subtle. Furthermore, because sarcoidosis can occur in almost any place in the body, like tuberculosis or syphilis, it can be confused with many other disorders. In this context, the differential diagnosis of sarcoidosis must cover a wide range. However, it is confused most commonly with neoplastic diseases such as lymphoma or with disorders characterized also by a mononuclear cell granulomatous inflammatory process, such as the mycobacterial and fungal disorders.

The presence of skin anergy is typical but not diagnostic of sarcoidosis. Individuals with sarcoidosis who develop active tuberculosis react strongly to skin tests with purified protein derivative. The Kveim-Siltzbach skin test, the intradermal injection of a heat-treated suspension of a sarcoidosis spleen extract which is biopsied 4 to 6 weeks later, yields sarcoidosis-like lesions in 70 to 80 percent of individuals with sarcoidosis, with fewer than 5 percent false-positive results. However, the material is not widely available, and with the use of the transbronchial biopsy to obtain lung parenchyma for diagnostic purposes, the Kveim-Siltzbach test is not in general use.

No blood findings are diagnostic of the disease. Angiotensin-converting enzyme is elevated in the serum in approximately two-thirds of patients with sarcoidosis. Approximately 5 percent of all positive tests are not sarcoidosis and are seen in a variety of disorders, including asbestosis, silicosis, berylliosis, fungal infection, granulomatous hepatitis, hypersensitivity pneumonitis, leprosy, lymphoma, and tuberculosis. An elevated 24-h urine calcium level is consistent with the diagnosis but is not specific.

The chest x-ray cannot be used as the sole criterion for the diagnosis of sarcoidosis. While the finding of bilateral hilar adenopathy is the hallmark of this disease, a similar pattern is occasionally observed in lymphoma, tuberculosis, coccidioidomycosis, brucellosis, and bronchogenic carcinoma.

The pattern of the gallium 67 scan is not diagnostic for sarcoidosis, nor is the finding of an increased proportion of lymphocytes among the cells recovered by bronchoalveolar lavage. However, the typical patterns of these tests (Fig. 320-2*B* and *C*) put the diagnosis in the general category of granulomatous lung disorders.

Whether or not the presentation is "classic," biopsy evidence of a mononuclear cell granulomatous inflammatory process is mandatory in order to make a definitive diagnosis of sarcoidosis. Because the lung is involved so frequently, it is the most common site to be biopsied, usually through a fiberoptic bronchoscope. Less common, but acceptable, sites for biopsy are the hilar nodes (by mediastinoscopy), the skin, conjunctiva, or lip. Rarely, the spleen, intraabdominal nodes, muscle, parotid or other salivary glands, upper respiratory tract, or the heart is biopsied for diagnostic purposes. At any of these sites, the findings must include the typical noncaseating granulomas. However, although histologic evidence is mandatory for a definitive diagnosis of sarcoidosis, the histologic findings are not sufficiently specific to make the diagnosis by themselves, since noncaseating granulomas are found in a number of other diseases, including

infections and malignancy. Furthermore, although the liver or scalene nodes often reveal "positive" biopsies in cases of sarcoidosis, noncaseating granulomas from other causes are so frequent in these sites that they are not considered acceptable sites for establishing the diagnosis. Thus the definitive diagnosis of sarcoidosis is based on the biopsy in the context of the history, physical examination, blood tests, x-ray, lung function, and, if available, gallium 67 scan and bronchoalveolar lavage. Patients with human immunodeficiency virus (HIV) infection commonly have lymphocytopenia, chest x-ray abnormalities, positive gallium 67 chest scans, and increased proportions of lavage lymphocytes (early in the course of the disease), and they can have lung granulomas; thus, serologic testing for HIV infection should always be done in individuals suspected of having sarcoidosis.

PROGNOSIS Overall, the prognosis in sarcoidosis is good. Most individuals who present with the acute disease are left with no significant sequelae. Approximately half of all patients have some permanent organ dysfunction, but for most this is mild, stable, and progresses rarely. In approximately 15 to 20 percent of cases, the disease remains active or recurs intermittently. Death is attributable directly to the disease in about 10 percent of all those affected.

FIGURE 320-3 Diagnostic and therapeutic algorithms relevant to sarcoidosis. *A.* Diagnosis of sarcoidosis. If the history and physical examination suggest sarcoidosis, the diagnosis is made by a combination of history, physical examination, and diagnostic test. No tests are definitive for sarcoidosis; the diagnosis is made by a combination of findings. The major diagnostic tests carry the most weight, with biopsy and histologic assessment of the relevant organ the most important. Assessment of function of the organ systems that appear to be affected help with diagnosis and decisions about therapy. *B.* Therapy of sarcoidosis. Once the definitive diagnosis is made, the decision to not treat or to institute treatment with glucocorticoids is based on the presence or absence of disabling symptoms, organ dysfunction, organ derangement, and results of various tests of disease activity. Any organ can be threatened by sarcoidosis, but lung, eye, heart, and central nervous system are at greatest risk. The disease can wax and wane, and periodic assessments at 3- to 6-month intervals are used to reevaluate decisions regarding therapy.

℞ **TREATMENT**

The therapy of choice for sarcoidosis is glucocorticoids (Fig. 320-3*B*), A variety of other drugs have been tried, including indomethacin, oxyphenbutazone, chloroquine, methotrexate, *p*-aminobenzoate, allopurinol, levamisole, and cyclophosphamide, but there is no evidence, apart from anecdotal, uncontrolled reports, to support their efficacy. Cyclosporine is ineffective for the pulmonary manifestations of the disease; anecdotal reports suggest that it may be useful in extrathoracic sarcoid not responding to glucocorticoids.

The major problem in treating sarcoidosis is in deciding when to treat. Because the disease clears spontaneously in about 50 percent of patients, and because the permanent organ derangements often do not improve with glucocorticoids, there is controversy among clinicians as to the criteria for treatment. However, there is no question that glucocorticoids suppress effectively the activated T helper-inducer cell processes occurring at the sites of disease. Thus the major problem in making decisions concerning therapy in sarcoidosis is to determine the extent and activity of the inflammatory process in the organs at greatest risk, such as the lung, eye, heart, and central nervous system.

For the lung, this is based on a combination of history, physical findings, chest x-ray, and pulmonary function tests. Centers that see large numbers of these individuals also use criteria based on gallium 67 lung scans and bronchoalveolar lavage findings. The serum level of the angiotensin-converting enzyme has been suggested as a criterion for disease activity, but it is not specific for the lung. Unless the respiratory impairment is devastating, active pulmonary sarcoidosis is observed usually without therapy for 2 to 3 months; if the inflammation does not subside spontaneously, therapy is instituted. For the eye, decisions concerning therapy are based on slit-lamp examination and tests for visual acuity. For the heart and central nervous system, decisions are based on an estimate of the severity of the involvement; patients with minor dysfunction are usually observed, while patients with significant cardiac or neurologic abnormalities are treated. Usually, it is not necessary to treat the systemic symptoms, but occasionally the extent of the fevers, fatigue, and/or weight loss will necessitate therapy.

The usual therapy for sarcoidosis is prednisone, 1 mg/kg, for 4 to 6 weeks, followed by a slow taper over 2 to 3 months. This is repeated if the disease again becomes active. Alternate-day therapy is used by some clinicians, but there is no evidence that it is as effective. High-dose bolus intravenous glucocorticoids are used occasionally but are probably not as effective as oral therapy. There is no evidence that inhaled glucocorticoids are efficacious. Mild ocular disease responds usually to local therapy, but suppression of the uveitis often requires systemic glucocorticoids.

BIBLIOGRAPHY

CONSENSUS CONFERENCE: Activity of sarcoidosis. Third WASOG Meeting. Eur Respir J 7:624, 1994

CRYSTAL RG: Interstitial lung disease of unknown etiology: Disorders characterized by chronic inflammation of the lower respiratory tract. N Engl J Med 310:154, 235, 1984

DU BOIS RM: Corticosteroids in sarcoidosis: Friend or foe? Eur Respir J 7:1203, 1994

—— et al: Granulomatous processes, in *The Lung: Scientific Foundations*, 2d ed, RG Crystal et al (eds). Philadelphia, Lippincott-Raven, 1996, pp 2395–2409

FANBURG BL, PITT EA: Sarcoidosis, in *Textbook of Respiratory Medicine*, JF Murray, JA Nadel (eds). Philadelphia, Saunders, 1988, pp 1486–1500

JAMES DG (ed): *Sarcoidosis and Other Granulomatous Disorders*. New York, Marcel Dekker, 1994

MOLLER DR et al: Bias toward use of a specific T-cell receptor β-chain variable region in a subgroup of individuals with sarcoidosis. J Clin Invest 82:1183, 1988

NAGAI S, IZUMI T: Pulmonary sarcoidosis: Population differences and pathophysiology. South Med J 88:1001, 1995

PINKSTON P et al: Spontaneous release of interleukin-2 by lung T-lymphocytes in active pulmonary sarcoidosis. N Engl J Med 208:793, 1983

ROBINSON BWS et al: Gamma interferon is spontaneously released by alveolar macrophages and lung T-lymphocytes in patients with pulmonary sarcoidosis. J Clin Invest 75:1488, 1985

ROBINSON DS et al: Granulomatous processes, in *The Lung: Scientific Foundations*, 2d ed, RG Crystal et al (eds). Philadelphia, Lippincott-Raven, 1996, pp 2395–2410

SALTINI C et al: Spontaneous release of interleukin-2 by lung T-lymphocytes in active pulmonary sarcoidosis is primarily from the Leu3 + DR + T-cell subset. J Clin Invest 77:1962, 1986

SHARMA OP: Pulmonary sarcoidosis and corticosteroids. Am Rev Resp Dis 147:1598, 1993

VENET A et al: Enhanced alveolar macrophage-mediated antigen-induced T-lymphocyte proliferation in sarcoidosis. J Clin Invest 75:293, 1985

SECTION 3

DISORDERS OF THE JOINTS

321 | *John J. Cush, Peter E. Lipsky*

APPROACH TO ARTICULAR AND MUSCULOSKELETAL DISORDERS

Musculoskeletal complaints account for more than 315,000,000 outpatient visits per year. Many of the musculoskeletal complaints that cause patients to seek medical attention are related to self-limited conditions requiring minimal evaluation and only symptomatic therapy and reassurance. However, some patients with similar symptoms have a more serious condition that requires further evaluation or additional laboratory testing to confirm the suspected diagnosis or determine the extent and nature of the pathologic process. The initial goal of the clinician is to formulate a differential diagnosis that leads to accurate diagnosis and timely therapy while avoiding excessive diagnostic testing and unnecessary treatment (Table 321-1).

Individuals with musculoskeletal complaints should be evaluated in a uniform, logical manner by means of a thorough history, a comprehensive physical examination, and if appropriate, laboratory testing. The goals of the initial encounter are to determine whether the musculoskeletal complaint is (1) *articular* or *nonarticular* in origin, (2) *inflammatory* or *noninflammatory* in nature, (3) *acute* or *chronic*, and (4) *localized*, *widespread*, or *systemic*.

With such an approach and an understanding of the pathophysiologic processes that underlie musculoskeletal complaints, an adequate diagnosis can be made in the vast majority of individuals. However, some patients will not fit immediately into an established diagnostic category. Many musculoskeletal disorders resemble each other at the outset, and some take months to evolve into a readily recognizable diagnostic entity. This consideration should temper the desire always to establish a definitive diagnosis at the first encounter.

ARTICULAR VERSUS NONARTICULAR SITE OF ORIGIN The musculoskeletal evaluation must discriminate the anatomic site(s) of origin of the patient's complaint. For example, ankle pain can result from a variety of pathologic conditions involving disparate anatomic structures, including gonococcal arthritis, calcaneal fracture, Achilles tendinitis, cellulitis, and peripheral neuropathy. Articular structures include the synovium, synovial fluid, articular cartilage, intraarticular ligaments, joint capsule, and juxtaarticular bone. Nonarticular (or periarticular) structures, such as supportive extraarticular ligaments, tendons, bursae, muscle, fascia, bone, nerve, and overlying skin, may be involved in the pathologic process. Pain from these structures may mimic true articular pain because of their proximity to the joint. Distinguishing between articular and nonarticular disease requires a careful and detailed examination. Articular disorders may be characterized by pain and limited range of motion on active and passive movement, swelling caused by synovial proliferation or effusion or bony enlargement, crepitation, instability, locking, or deformity. By contrast, nonarticular disorders tend to be painful on active but not passive range of motion, demonstrate point or focal tenderness in regions distinct from articular structures, and have physical findings remote from the joint capsule. Moreover, nonarticular disorders seldom demonstrate crepitus, instability, or deformity.

INFLAMMATORY VERSUS NONINFLAMMATORY DISORDERS In the course of a musculoskeletal evaluation, the examiner should elicit symptoms and signs that will narrow or establish the diagnosis. A primary objective is to identify the nature of the underlying pathologic process. Musculoskeletal disorders are generally classified as inflammatory or noninflammatory. Inflammatory disorders may be infectious (infection with *Neisseria gonorrhoea* or *Mycobacterium tuberculosis*), crystal-induced (gout, pseudogout), immune-related [rheumatoid arthritis (RA), systemic lupus erythematosus (SLE)], reactive (rheumatic fever, Reiter's syndrome), or idiopathic. Inflammatory disorders may be identified by the presence of some or all of the four cardinal signs of inflammation (erythema, warmth, pain, and swelling), by systemic symptoms (prolonged morning stiffness, fatigue, fever, weight loss), or by laboratory evidence of inflammation (elevated erythrocyte sedimentation rate or C-reactive protein level or thrombocytosis). Articular stiffness is common in chronic musculoskeletal disorders. However, the chronology and magnitude of stiffness may be diagnostically important. Morning stiffness related to inflammatory disorders (such as RA) is precipitated by prolonged rest, often lasts several hours, and may improve with activity and anti-inflammatory medications. By contrast, intermittent stiffness associated with noninflammatory conditions, such as osteoarthritis, is precipitated by brief periods of rest, usually lasts less than 60 min, and is exacerbated by activity. Noninflammatory disorders may be related to trauma (rotator cuff tear), ineffective repair (osteoarthritis), cellular overgrowth (pigmented villonodular synovitis), or pain amplification (fibromyalgia). They are often characterized by pain without swelling or warmth, the absence of inflammatory or systemic features, little or no morning stiffness, and normal laboratory findings.

Identification of the nature of the underlying process and the site of the complaint will enable the examiner to narrow the diagnostic considerations and to assess the need for immediate diagnostic or therapeutic intervention or for continued observation. Figure 321-1 presents a logical approach to the evaluation of patients with musculoskeletal complaints.

CLINICAL HISTORY Additional historic features may be helpful in establishing the nature and extent of the pathologic process and may provide important clues to the diagnosis. Aspects of the patient profile, including age, sex, race, and family history, can provide important information. Certain diagnoses are more frequent in specific age groups. SLE, rheumatic fever, and Reiter's syndrome are more common in the young, whereas fibromyalgia is most common in middle

age, and osteoarthritis and polymyalgia rheumatica in old age. Some diseases are more common in a particular gender or race. Gout and the spondyloarthropathies (e.g., ankylosing spondylitis, Reiter's syndrome) are more common in men, whereas rheumatoid arthritis and fibromyalgia are more common in women. Polymyalgia rheumatica, giant cell arteritis, and Wegener's granulomatosis preferentially affect whites, whereas sarcoidosis and systemic lupus erythematosus are more common in blacks. *Familial aggregation* occurs in some disorders, such as ankylosing spondylitis, gout, RA, and Heberden's nodes of osteoarthritis.

The chronology of the complaint (*onset, evolution,* and *duration*) is an important diagnostic feature. The onset of disorders such as septic arthritis and gout tends to be abrupt, whereas osteoarthritis, rheumatoid arthritis, and fibromyalgia may develop more indolently In terms of evolution, disorders are classified as chronic (e.g., osteoarthritis), intermittent (e.g., gout), migratory (e.g., rheumatic fever, gonococcal or viral arthritis), or additive (e.g., RA, Reiter's syndrome). Musculoskeletal disorders typically are called *acute* if they last less than 6 weeks and *chronic* if they last longer. Acute arthropathies tend to be infectious, crystal-induced, or reactive. Noninflammatory and immune-related arthritides, such as osteoarthritis and RA, respectively, are often chronic. The duration of the patient's complaints may alter the diagnostic considerations. For example, the musculoskeletal signs and symptoms of hepatitis B virus infection may be identical with those of early RA at the onset but rarely persist beyond 3 weeks.

The *number and distribution* of involved articulations should be noted. Articular disorders are classified as *monarticular* (one joint involved), *oligoarticular* or *pauciarticular* (two to three joints involved), or *polyarticular* (more than three joints involved). Nonarticular disorders can be classified as either *focal* or *widespread.* Complaints secondary to trauma and gout are typically focal or monarticular, whereas polymyositis, RA, and fibromyalgia are more diffuse or polyarticular. Joint involvement tends to be symmetric in RA but is often asymmetric in the spondyloarthropathies and in gout. The upper extremities are frequently involved in rheumatoid arthritis, whereas lower extremity arthritis is characteristic of Reiter's syndrome and gout at their onset. Involvement of the axial skeleton is common in osteoarthritis and ankylosing spondylitis but infrequent in RA, with the notable exception of the cervical spine.

The clinical history should also identify *precipitating events,* such as trauma, drug administration, or antecedent or intercurrent illnesses, that may have contributed to the patient's complaint. Last, a thorough *rheumatic review of systems* may disclose associated features outside the musculoskeletal system and provide useful diagnostic information. A variety of musculoskeletal disorders may be associated with systemic features such as fever (SLE, infection), rash (SLE, Reiter's syndrome, dermatomyositis), myalgias, weakness (polymyositis, polymyalgia rheumatica), and morning stiffness (inflammatory arthritis). In addition, some conditions are associated with involvement of other organ systems, including the eyes (Behçet's disease, sarcoidosis, Reiter's syndrome), gastrointestinal tract (scleroderma, inflammatory bowel disease), genitourinary tract (Reiter's syndrome, gonococcemia), and nervous system (Lyme disease, vasculitis).

PHYSICAL EXAMINATION The goal of the physical examination is to ascertain the structures involved, the nature of the underlying pathology, the extent and functional consequences of the process, and the presence of systemic or extraarticular manifestations (Table 321-2). A knowledge of topographic anatomy is necessary to identify the primary site(s) of involvement and differentiate articular from nonarticular disorders. The musculoskeletal examination depends largely on careful inspection, palpation, and a variety of specific physical maneuvers to elicit diagnostic signs. Although most articulations of the appendicular skeleton can be examined in this manner, adequate inspection and palpation are not possible for many axial (e.g., zygapophyseal) and inaccessible (e.g., sacroiliac or hip) joints. For such

Table 321-1

Evaluation of Patients with Musculoskeletal Complaints

Goals
  Accurate diagnosis
  Timely provision of therapy
  Avoidance of unnecessary diagnostic testing
Approach
  Anatomic localization of complaint (articular vs. nonarticular)
  Determination of the nature of the pathologic process (inflammatory vs. noninflammatory)
  Determination of the extent of involvement (monarticular, polyarticular, focal, widespread)
  Determination of chronology (acute vs. chronic)
  Formulation of a differential diagnosis

joints, there is a greater reliance on specific maneuvers and imaging for assessment.

Examination of involved and uninvolved joints will determine whether *warmth*, *erythema*, or *swelling* is present. The examination should distinguish true articular swelling caused by synovial effusion or synovial proliferation from nonarticular or periarticular involvement, which usually extends beyond the normal joint margins or the full extent of the synovial space. Synovial effusion can be distinguished from synovial hypertrophy or bony hypertrophy by palpation or specific maneuvers. For example, small to moderate knee effusions may be identified by the "bulge sign" or "ballottement of the patella." Bursal effusions (e.g., effusions of the olecranon or prepatellar bursa) overlie bony prominences and are fluctuant with sharply defined bor-

ders. Joint *stability* can be assessed by palpation and by the application of manual stress. Subluxation or dislocation, which may be secondary to traumatic, mechanical, or inflammatory causes, can be assessed by inspection and palpation. Joint *volume* can be assessed by palpation. Distention of the articular capsule usually causes pain. The patient will attempt to minimize the pain by keeping the joint in the position of least intraarticular pressure and greatest volume, usually partial flexion. Clinically, joint distention may be detected as obvious swelling, voluntary or fixed flexion deformities, or diminished range of motion—especially on extension, which decreases joint volume. Active and passive *range of motion* should be assessed in all planes, with contralateral comparison. Serial evaluations of joint motion may be made using a goniometer to quantify the arc of movement. Each joint should be passively manipulated through its full range of motion (including, as appropriate, flexion, extension, rotation, abduction, adduction, inversion, eversion, supination, pronation, and medial or lateral deviation or bending). Limitation of motion is frequently caused by effusion, pain, deformity, or contracture. *Contractures* may reflect antecedent synovial inflammation or trauma. Joint *crepitus* may be felt during palpation or maneuvers and may be prominent in osteoarthritis. Joint *deformity* usually indicates a long-standing or aggressive pathologic process. Deformities may result from ligamentous destruction, soft tissue contracture, bony enlargement, ankylosis, erosive disease, or subluxation. Examination of the musculature will permit assessment of strength and reveal atrophy, pain, or spasm. The examiner should look carefully for nonarticular or periarticular involvement, especially when articular complaints are not supported by objective findings referable to the joint capsule. The identification of musculoskeletal pain of soft tissue origin (nonarticular pain) will prevent unwarranted and often expensive additional evaluations. Specific maneuvers may reveal nonarticular abnormalities, such as a carpal tunnel syndrome (which can be identified by Tinel's or Phalen's sign). Other examples of soft tissue abnormalities include olecranon bursitis, epicondylitis (tennis elbow), enthesitis (e.g., Achilles tendinitis), and trigger points associated with fibromyalgia.

LABORATORY INVESTIGATIONS The vast majority of musculoskeletal disorders can be diagnosed easily by a complete history and physical examination. An additional objective of the initial encounter is to determine whether additional investigations or immediate therapy are required. A number of features indicate the need for additional evaluation. *Monarticular* conditions require additional evaluation, as do *traumatic* or *inflammatory* conditions and conditions accompanied by *neurologic changes* or *systemic manifestations* of serious disease. Finally, individuals with *chronic* symptoms (lasting more than 6 weeks), especially when there has been a lack of response to symptomatic measures, are candidates for additional evaluation. The extent and nature of the

FIGURE 321-1 Algorithm for the diagnosis of musculoskeletal complaints. An approach to formulating a differential diagnosis (shown in italics). (ESR, erythrocyte sedimentation rate; CRP, C-reactive protein; DIP, distal interphalangeal; CMC, carpometacarpal; PIP, proximal interphalangeal; MCP, metacarpophalangeal; MTP, metatarsophalangeal; PMR, polymyalgia rheumatica; SLE, systemic lupus erythematosus; JA, juvenile arthritis.)

Glossary of Musculoskeletal Terms

Subluxation Alteration of joint alignment such that articulating surfaces incompletely approximate each other

Dislocation Abnormal displacement of articulating surfaces such that the surfaces are not in contact

Range of motion For diarthrodial joints, the arc of measurable movement through which the joint moves in a single plane

Contracture Loss of full movement resulting from a fixed resistance due either to tonic spasm of muscle (reversible) or to fibrosis of periarticular structures (permanent)

Deformity Abnormal shape or size of a structure; may result from bony hypertrophy, malalignment of articulating structures, or damage to periarticular supportive structures

Enthesitis Inflammation of the entheses (tendinous or ligamentous insertions on bone)

Epicondylitis Infection or inflammation involving an epicondyle

additional investigation should be dictated by the clinical features and suspected pathologic process. Broad batteries of diagnostic tests and radiographic procedures are rarely useful or cost-effective.

Besides a complete blood count, including a white blood cell and differential count, the routine evaluation should include determination of an acute-phase indicator, such as the erythrocyte sedimentation rate (ESR) or C-reactive protein (CRP), which can be useful in discriminating inflammatory from noninflammatory musculoskeletal disorders. Both tests are inexpensive and easily performed; the resulting values may be elevated with infections, inflammatory arthritis, autoimmune disorders, neoplasia, pregnancy, and advanced age. Serum uric acid determinations are only useful when gout has been diagnosed and therapy contemplated.

Serologic tests for rheumatoid factor, antinuclear antibodies, complement levels, Lyme disease antibodies, or antistreptolysin O (ASO) titer should be carried out only when there is substantive clinical evidence suggesting a relevant diagnosis, as these tests have poor predictive value when used in a screening fashion. They should not be performed arbitrarily in patients with minimal or nonspecific musculoskeletal complaints. IgM rheumatoid factor (autoantibodies against the Fc portion of IgG) is found in 80 percent of patients with RA and may also be seen in low titers in patients with chronic infections (tuberculosis, leprosy), other autoimmune diseases (SLE, Sjögren's syndrome), or chronic pulmonary, hepatic, or renal diseases. Antinuclear antibodies (ANAs) are found in nearly all patients with SLE and may also be seen in patients with other autoimmune diseases (polymyositis, scleroderma), drug-induced lupus (resulting from hydralazine, procainamide, or quinidine administration), or chronic hepatitic or renal disorders. The interpretation of a positive ANA determination may depend on the titer and on the pattern observed by immunofluorescence microscopy. Diffuse and speckled patterns are the least specific, whereas a peripheral, or rim, pattern is highly specific and is suggestive of autoantibodies against double-stranded (native) DNA. This pattern is seen only in patients with SLE.

Aspiration and analysis of synovial fluid is always indicated in acute monarthritis or when an infectious or crystal-induced arthropathy is suspected. Synovial fluid analysis may be crucial in distinguishing between noninflammatory and inflammatory processes. This distinction can be made on the basis of the appearance, viscosity, and cell count of the synovial fluid. Tests for synovial fluid glucose, protein, lactate dehydrogenase, lactic acid, or autoantibodies are not recommended, as they are insensitive or have little discriminatory value. Noninflammatory synovial fluid is clear, viscous, and amber-colored, with a white blood cell count of <2000/μL and a predominance of mononuclear cells. The viscosity of synovial fluid is assessed by expressing fluid from the syringe one drop at a time. Normally there is a stringing effect, with a long tail behind each drop. Effusions due to osteoarthritis or trauma usually have this typical viscosity. Inflammatory fluid is turbid and yellow, with an increased white cell count (2000 to 50,000 cells per microliter) and a predominance of polymorphonuclear leukocytes. Inflammatory fluid has a reduced vis-

cosity, with little or no tail following each drop of synovial fluid. Such effusions are found in RA, gout, other inflammatory arthritides, and septic arthritis. Infectious fluid is turbid and opaque, with a white cell count usually >50,000/μL, a predominance of polymorphonuclear leukocytes (>75%), and low viscosity. Such effusions are typical of septic arthritis, but they occur rarely with sterile inflammatory arthritides such as RA or gout. In addition, hemorrhagic synovial fluid may be seen with hemarthrosis or trauma. An algorithm for synovial fluid aspiration and analysis is shown in Fig. 321-2. Synovial fluid should be analyzed immediately for appearance, viscosity, and cell count. Cellularity and the presence of crystals may be assessed by light or polarizing microscopy, respectively. Monosodium urate crystals, seen in gouty effusions, are long, needle-shaped, negatively birefringent, and usually intracellular, whereas calcium pyrophosphate dihydrate crystals, found in chondrocalcinosis and pseudogout, are usually short, rhomboid-shaped, and positively birefringent. Whenever infection is

FIGURE 321-2 Algorithmic approach to the use and interpretation of synovial fluid aspiration and analysis.

suspected, synovial fluid should be Gram stained and cultured appropriately. If gonococcal arthritis is suspected, immediate plating of the fluid on appropriate culture medium is indicated. Synovial fluid from chronic monarthritis patients should also be cultured for *M. tuberculosis* and fungi. Last, it should be noted that crystal-induced arthritis and infection occasionally occur together in the same joint.

DIAGNOSTIC IMAGING IN JOINT DISEASES Conventional radiography has been a valuable tool in the diagnosis and staging of articular disorders. Plain x-rays are most appropriate when there is a history of trauma, suspected chronic infection, progressive disability, or monarticular involvement; when therapeutic alterations are considered; or when a baseline assessment is desired for what appears to be a chronic process. However, in most inflammatory disorders, early radiography is rarely helpful in establishing a diagnosis and may only reveal soft tissue swelling or juxtaarticular demineralization. As the disease progresses, calcification (of soft tissues, cartilage, or bone), joint space narrowing, erosions, bony ankylosis, new bone formation (sclerosis, osteophyte formation, or periostitis), or subchondral cysts may develop and suggest specific clinical entities. Proper technique and positioning can prevent the need for further studies.

Newer imaging techniques enhance diagnostic sensitivity and facilitate early diagnosis in a limited number of articular disorders and are indicated in selected circumstances when conventional radiography is not adequate (Table 321-3). *Ultrasonography* is useful in the detection of soft tissue abnormalities that cannot be appreciated fully by clinical examination. Although ultrasonography is inexpensive and easily performed, only in a limited number of circumstances is it the preferred method of evaluation. The foremost application of ultrasound is in the diagnosis of synovial (Baker's) cysts, although rotator cuff tears and various tendon injuries may be evaluated with ultrasound by an experienced operator. *Radionuclide scintigraphy* provides useful information regarding the metabolic status of bone and, along with radiography, is well suited for total-body assessment of the extent and distribution of musculoskeletal involvement. It is a very sensitive but poorly specific means of detecting inflammatory or metabolic alterations in bone or periarticular soft tissue structures. The limited tissue resolution of scintigraphy may obscure the distinction between bony and periarticular processes and may necessitate the use of additional imaging modalities. Scintigraphy, using ^{99m}Tc, ^{67}Ga, or white blood cells (WBCs) labeled with ^{111}In, has been applied to a variety of articular disorders with variable success (Table 321-2). [^{99m}Tc]pertechnetate or [^{99m}Tc]diphosphonate scintigraphy may be useful in identifying infection, neoplasia, inflammation, increased blood flow, bone remodeling, heterotopic bone formation, or avascular necrosis (Fig. 321-3). However, the poor specificity of ^{99m}Tc scanning has limited its use to investigational and serial assessments of joint or bone involvement, assessment of inflammatory or infectious processes, and surveys for bone metastases. ^{67}Ga binds to serum and cellular transferrin and lactoferrin and is preferentially taken up by neutrophils, macrophages, bacteria, and tumor tissue (e.g., lymphoma tissue) and is useful in the identification of infection and malignancies. Scanning with ^{111}In-labeled WBCs has been used to detect both infectious and inflammatory arthritis. Although both have been used with success, ^{111}In-labeled WBC scanning is superior to ^{67}Ga in the early diagnosis of osteomyelitis and infected prosthetic joints. Prior treatment with antibiotics may reduce the diagnostic sensitivity of both ^{67}Ga and ^{111}In-labeled WBC scintigraphy.

Computed tomography (CT) provides rapid reconstruction of sagittal, coronal, and axial images and thus of the spatial relationships among anatomic structures. It has proved most useful in the assessment of the axial skeleton because of its ability to visualize in the axial plane. Articulations that are difficult to visualize by conventional radiography, such as the zygapophyseal, sacroiliac, sternoclavicular, and hip joints, can be evaluated effectively using CT. CT has been demonstrated to be useful in the diagnosis of low back pain syndromes, sacroiliitis, osteoid osteoma, tarsal coalition, osteomyelitis, intraarticular osteochondral fragments, and advanced osteonecrosis.

Magnetic resonance imaging (MRI) has significantly advanced the ability to image musculoskeletal structures. MRI can provide multiplanar images with fine anatomic detail and contrast resolution (Fig. 321-4). Other advantages are the absence of ionizing radiation and adverse effects and the superior ability to visualize bone marrow and soft tissue periarticular structures. However, the high cost and long procedural time of MRI limit its use in the evaluation of musculoskeletal disorders. MRI should be used only when it will provide necessary information that cannot be obtained by less expensive and noninvasive means.

MRI can image fascia, vessels, nerve, muscle, cartilage, ligaments, tendons, pannus, synovial effusions, cortical bone, and bone marrow. Visualization of particular structures can be enhanced by altering the pulse sequence to produce either T1-weighted or T2-weighted spin echo, gradient echo, or inversion recovery (including STIR) images (Fig. 321-5). Because of its sensitivity to changes in marrow fat, MRI is a sensitive although nonspecific means of detecting osteonecrosis and osteomyelitis. Because of its greater ability to resolve soft tissue contrasts, MRI is more sensitive than arthrography or CT for the diagnosis of soft tissue injuries (e.g., meniscal and rotator cuff tears), intraarticular derangements, and spinal cord damage following injury, subluxation, or synovitis of the vertebrae.

RHEUMATOLOGIC EVALUATION OF THE ELDERLY Muscu-

Table 321-3

Diagnostic Imaging Techniques for Musculoskeletal Disorders

Method	Imaging Time, h	Cost*	Current Indications
Ultrasound†	<1	+	Synovial cysts Rotator cuff tears Tendon injury
Radionuclide scintigraphy			
^{99m}Tc	1–4	+ +	Metastatic bone survey Evaluation of Paget's disease Quantitative joint assessment Acute infection Acute and chronic osteomyelitis
^{111}In-WBC	24	+ + +	Acute infection Prosthetic infection Acute osteomyelitis
^{67}Ga	24–48	+ + + +	Acute and chronic infection Acute osteomyelitis
Computed tomography	<1	+ + +	Herniated intervertebral disk Sacroiliitis Spinal stenosis Spinal trauma Osteoid osteoma Tarsal coalition
Magnetic resonance imaging	1/2–2	+ + + + +	Avascular necrosis Osteomyelitis Intraarticular derangement and soft tissue injury Derangements of axial skeleton and spinal cord Pigmented villonodular synovitis Inflammatory and metabolic muscle pathology

* Relative cost for imaging study.
† Results depend on operator.

L R

FIGURE 321-5 Coronal magnetic resonance images of the wrist in a 54-year-old woman with rheumatoid arthritis. *A.* T1-weighted image demonstrates an erosion of the triquetrum (*arrow*). *B.* Gadopentetate dimeglumine enhanced T1-weighted image demonstrates enhancement of the same erosion (*arrow*), indicating the presence of vascularized pannus. *C.* Inversion-recovery (STIR) image demonstrates a fluid-dense, high-intensity signal near the triquetrum (*arrow*) and in the intercarpal spaces, suggesting widespread intercarpal inflammation.

FIGURE 321-3 [^{99m}Tc]diphosphonate scintigraphy of the feet of a 33-year-old black male with Reiter's syndrome, manifested by sacroiliitis, urethritis, uveitis, asymmetric oligoarthritis, and enthesitis. This bone scan demonstrates increased uptake indicative of enthesitis involving the insertions of the left Achilles tendon, plantar aponeurosis, and right tibialis posterior tendon as well as arthritis of the right first interphalangeal joint.

loskeletal disorders in elderly patients are often not diagnosed because the signs and symptoms may be insidious or chronic in these patients. In addition, the nature of the problem is often obscured by the presence of multiple interacting factors, including other medical conditions and therapies. These difficulties are compounded by the diminished reliability of laboratory testing in the elderly, which is secondary to the wider range of nonpathologic variability. For example, erythrocyte sedimentation rates may be misleadingly high and titers of rheumatoid factor or antinuclear antibodies misleadingly low. Although nearly all rheumatic disorders can afflict the elderly, certain diseases and drug-induced disorders are more common in this age group. The elderly should be approached in the same manner as other patients with musculoskeletal complaints, but with additional inquiries to exclude common geriatric musculoskeletal disorders. An emphasis on identifying the rheumatic consequences of intercurrent medical conditions and therapies is extremely important. Drug-induced lupus erythemato-

sus, polymyalgia rheumatica, gout, and chronic salicylate toxicity are all more common in the elderly than in other individuals. The physical examination should put an emphasis on coexisting diseases that may influence the diagnosis and choice of treatment.

Approach to the Patient

With Regional Rheumatic Complaints Although all patients should be evaluated in a logical and thorough manner, many cases of focal musculoskeletal complaints are caused by commonly encountered disorders that exhibit a predictable pattern of onset, evolution, and localization and that often can be diagnosed immediately on the basis of limited historical information and selected maneuvers or tests. Although nearly every joint can be approached in this manner, the evaluation of four commonly involved anatomic regions—the hand, shoulder, hip, and knee—are reviewed here.

HAND PAIN Focal or unilateral hand pain may result from trauma, overuse, infection, or a reactive or crystal-induced arthritis. By contrast, bilateral hand complaints suggest osteoarthritis or a systemic or inflammatory/immune etiology. Patterns of joint involvement are highly suggestive of certain disorders. The distribution of affected joints in the hand may provide important diagnostic information. Thus, osteoarthritis (or degenerative arthritis) may manifest as distal interphalangeal (DIP) and proximal interphalangeal (PIP) joint pain with bony hypertrophy sufficient to produce Heberden's and Bouchard's nodes, respectively. Pain, with or without bony swelling, involving the base of the thumb (first carpometacarpal joint) is also highly suggestive of osteoarthritis. By contrast, RA tends to involve the proximal interphalangeal, metacarpophalangeal, intercarpal, and carpometacarpal joints (wrist) with pain, prolonged stiffness, and palpable synovial tissue hypertrophy. Psoriatic arthritis may also involve the DIP and PIP joints and the carpus with inflammatory pain, stiffness, and synovitis. Moreover, the diagnosis of psoriatic arthritis can be suggested by nail pitting or onycholysis. Soft tissue swelling may also be noted over the dorsum of the hand and wrist and may suggest an inflammatory extensor tendon tenosynovitis, possibly caused by gonococcal infection, gout, or inflammatory arthritis. The diagnosis of tenosynovitis may be suggested by local warmth and edema and is confirmed when pain is induced by maintaining the wrist in a fixed, neutral position and flexing the digits distal to the metacarpophalangeal joints to stretch the extensor tendon sheaths.

Focal wrist pain localized to the radial aspect may be caused by DeQuervain's tenosynovitis resulting from inflammation of the tendon sheath(s) involving the abductor pollicis longus or extensor pollicis brevis. This condition commonly results from overuse or develops after pregnancy and may be diagnosed with Finkelstein's test. A positive result in Finkelstein's test is present when local wrist pain is induced after the thumb is flexed across the palm and placed inside a clenched fist and the examiner passively deviates the hand towards the ulnar side. Carpal tunnel syndrome is another common disorder of the upper extremity and results from compression of the median

FIGURE 321-4 Superior sensitivity of magnetic resonance imaging in the diagnosis of osteonecrosis of the femoral head. A 25-year-old white man taking high-dose glucocorticoids for idiopathic thrombocytopenic purpura developed bilateral hip pain. Conventional x-ray films (*A*) demonstrated abnormalities only in the right hip consistent with stage II osteonecrosis (*arrow*). A bone scan (*B*) revealed increased uptake in the right hip only (*arrow*). MRI using spin-echo proton density images (*C* and *D*) demonstrated low-density signals from both femoral heads (*arrows*), indicative of bilateral osteonecrosis.

nerve within the carpal tunnel to produce paresthesias in the thumb and the second, third, and radial half of the fourth fingers as well as, sometimes, atrophy of thenar musculature. Carpal tunnel syndrome is commonly associated with pregnancy, edema, trauma, osteoarthritis, inflammatory arthritis, and infiltrative disorders (e.g., amyloidosis). The diagnosis is suggested by a positive Tinel's or Phalen's sign. With each test, paresthesia in a median nerve distribution is induced or increased by either "thumping" the volar aspect of the wrist (Tinel's sign) or pressing the extensor surfaces of the two flexed wrists against each another (Phalen's sign).

SHOULDER PAIN   During the evaluation of shoulder disorders, the examiner should carefully note any history of trauma, infection, inflammatory disease, occupational hazards, or previous cervical disease. In addition, the patient should be questioned as to the activities or movement(s) that elicit shoulder pain. Shoulder pain frequently is referred from the cervical spine, but it may also be referred from intrathoracic lesions (e.g., a Pancoast tumor) or from gallbladder, hepatic, or diaphragmatic disease. The shoulder should be put through its full range of motion both actively and passively (with examiner assistance): forward flexion, extension, abduction, adduction, and rotation. Manual inspection of the periarticular structures will often provide important diagnostic information. The examiner should apply direct manual pressure over the subacromial bursa, which lies lateral to and immediately beneath the acromion. Subacromial bursitis is a frequent cause of shoulder pain. Anterior to the subacromial bursa, the bicipital tendon traverses the bicipital groove. This tendon is best identified by palpating it in its groove as the patient rotates the humerus internally and externally. Direct pressure over the tendon may reveal pain indicative of bicipital tendinitis. Palpation of the acromioclavicular joint may disclose local pain, bony hypertrophy, or synovial swelling. Whereas osteoarthritis and RA commonly affect the acromioclavicular joint, osteoarthritis seldom involves the glenohumeral joint, unless there is a traumatic or occupational cause. The glenohumeral joint is best palpated anteriorly by placing the thumb over the humeral head (just medial and inferior to the coracoid process) and having the patient rotate the humerus internally and externally. Pain localized to this region is indicative of glenohumeral pathology. Synovial effusion or tissue is seldom palpable, but if present may suggest infection, RA, or an acute tear of the rotator cuff.

Rotator cuff tendinitis or tear is a very common cause of shoulder pain. The rotator cuff is formed by the tendons of the supraspinatus, infraspinatus, teres minor, and subscapularis muscles. Rotator cuff tendinitis is suggested by pain on active abduction (but not passive abduction), pain over the lateral deltoid muscle, night pain, and evidence of the impingement sign. This maneuver is performed by the examiner raising the patient's arm into forced flexion while stabilizing the scapula and preventing it from rotating. A positive sign is present if pain develops before 180° of forward flexion. A complete tear of the rotator cuff, which often results from trauma, may manifest in the same manner but is less common than tendinitis. The diagnosis is suggested by the drop arm test, in which the patient is asked to maintain the arm outstretched as it is passively abducted. If the patient is unable to hold the arm up once 90° of abduction is reached, the test is positive. Tendinitis or tear of the rotator cuff can be confirmed by MRI (tendinitis and tear) or arthrography (tear only).

KNEE PAIN   A careful history should delineate the chronology of the knee complaint and whether there are predisposing conditions, trauma, or medications that might underlie the complaint. Observation of the patient's gait is also important. The knee should be carefully inspected in the upright (weight-bearing) and prone positions for swelling, erythema, contusion, laceration, and malalignment. The most common form of malalignment in the knee is genu varum (bow-legs) and genu valgum (knock-knees). Bony swelling of the knee joint commonly results from hypertrophic osseous changes seen with disorders such as osteoarthritis and neuropathic arthropathy. Swelling caused by hypertrophy of intrasynovial structures (synovial enlarge-

ment or effusion) may manifest as a fluctuant, ballotable, or soft tissue enlargement in the suprapatellar pouch (superior reflection of the synovial cavity) or lateral and medial to the patella. Synovial effusions may also be detected by balloting the patella downward toward the femoral groove or by eliciting a bulge sign. To elicit this sign, the examiner positions the knee extended and manually compresses or milks synovial fluid down from the suprapatellar pouch and lateral to the patellae. Manual pressure lateral to the patella may cause an observable shift in synovial fluid (bulge) to the medial aspect. This maneuver is only effective for detecting small to moderate effusions (smaller than 100 mL). Inflammatory disorders such as RA, gout, and Reiter's syndrome may involve the knee joint and produce significant pain, stiffness, swelling, or warmth.

Anserine bursitis is an often missed cause of knee pain in adults. The pes anserine bursa underlies the semimembranosus tendon and may become inflamed and painful owing to trauma, overuse, or inflammation. Anserine bursitis manifests primarily as point tenderness inferior and medial to the patella and overlying the medial tibial plateau. Swelling and erythema may not be present. Other forms of bursitis may also present as knee pain. The prepatellar bursa is superficial and is located over the inferior portion of the patella. The infrapatellar bursa is deeper and lies beneath the patellar ligament before its insertion on the tibial tubercle.

Internal derangement of the knee may result from trauma or degenerative processes. Damage to the meniscal cartilage (medial or lateral) frequently presents as chronic or intermittent knee pain. Such an injury should be suspected when there is a history of trauma or athletic activity and when the patient relates symptoms of locking, clicking, or "giving way" of the joint. Pain may be detected during direct palpation over the medial or lateral joint line. The diagnosis may also be suggested by ipsilateral joint-line pain when the knee is stressed laterally or medially. A positive McMurray test may indicate a meniscal tear. To perform this test, the knee is first flexed at 90°, and the leg is then extended while simultaneously the lower extremity is torqued medially or laterally. A painful click during inward rotation may indicate a lateral meniscus tear, and pain during outward rotation may indicate a tear in the medical meniscus. Finally, damage to the cruciate ligaments should be suspected if there is pain of acute onset, possibly with swelling, a history of trauma, or a synovial fluid aspirate that is grossly bloody. Examination of the cruciate ligaments is best accomplished by eliciting a drawer sign. With the patient recumbent, the knee should be partially flexed and the foot stabilized on the examining surface. The examiner should manually attempt to displace the tibia anteriorly or posteriorly with respect to the femur. If anterior movement is detected, then anterior cruciate ligament damage is likely. Conversely, significant posterior movement may indicate posterior cruciate damage. Contralateral comparison will assist the examiner in detecting significant anterior or posterior movement.

HIP PAIN   The hip is best evaluated by observing the patient's gait and assessing range of motion. The vast majority of patients reporting "hip pain" localize their pain unilaterally to the posterior or gluteal musculature. Such pain may or may not be associated with low back pain and tends to radiate down the posterolateral aspect of the thigh. Range of movement may be limited by pain. This presentation frequently results from degenerative arthritis of the lumbosacral spine and commonly follows a dermatomal distribution with involvement of nerve roots between L2 and S1. Some individuals instead localize their "hip pain" laterally to the area overlying the trochanteric bursa. Because of the depth of this bursa, swelling and warmth are usually absent. Diagnosis of trochanteric bursitis can be confirmed by inducing point tenderness over the trochanteric bursa. Pain in the hip joint is less common and tends to be located anteriorly, over the inguinal ligament; it may radiate medially to the groin or along the anteromedial thigh. Uncommonly, iliopsoas bursitis may mimic true hip joint pain. Diagnosis of iliopsoas bursitis may be suggested by a history of trauma or inflammatory arthritis. Pain associated with an iliopsoas bursitis tends to worsen with hyperextension of the hip, and many patients prefer to flex and externally rotate the hip to reduce the pain from a distended bursa.

BROWER AC: Imaging techniques and modalities, in *Arthritis in Black and White*, AC Brower (ed). Philadelphia, Saunders, 1988, p 1

GALL EP: Evaluation of the patient. A: History and physical examination, in *Primer on the Rheumatic Diseases*, 10th ed, HR Schumacher et al (eds). Atlanta, Arthritis Foundation, 1993, pp 60–64

HASSELBACHER P: Arthrocentesis, synovial fluid analysis and synovial biopsy, in *Primer on the Rheumatic Diseases*, 10th ed, HR Schumacher et al (eds). Atlanta, Arthritis Foundation, 1993, pp 67–72

LICHTENSTEIN MJ, PINCUS T: How useful are combinations of blood tests in "rheumatic panels" in diagnosis of rheumatic disease? J Gen Intern Med 3:435, 1988

SCHUMACHER HR JR: Arthritis of recent onset. A guide to evaluation and initial therapy for primary care physicians. Postgrad Med 97:52, 1995

SHMERLING RH, LIANG MH: Laboratory evaluation of rheumatic diseases, in *Primer on the Rheumatic Diseases*, 10th ed, HR Schumacher et al (eds). Atlanta, Arthritis Foundation, 1993, pp 64–66

——— et al: Synovial fluid tests: What should be ordered? JAMA 264:1009, 1990

WERNICK R: Avoiding laboratory test misinterpretation. Geriatrics 44:61, 1989

322	*Kenneth D. Brandt*

OSTEOARTHRITIS

Osteoarthritis (OA), also erroneously called degenerative joint disease, represents failure of a diarthrodial (movable, synovial-lined) joint. In idiopathic (primary) OA, the most common form of the disease, no predisposing factor is apparent. Secondary OA is pathologically indistinguishable from idiopathic OA but is attributable to an underlying cause (Table 322-1).

EPIDEMIOLOGY AND RISK FACTORS   OA is the most common joint disease of humans. Among the elderly, knee OA is the leading cause of chronic disability in developed countries; some 100,000 people in the United States are unable to walk independently from bed to bathroom because of OA of the knee or hip.

Under the age of 55 years, the joint distribution of OA in men and women is similar; in older individuals, hip OA is more common in men, while OA of interphalangeal joints and the thumb base is more common in women. Similarly, radiographic evidence of knee OA and, especially *symptomatic* knee OA, is more common in women than in men (Table 322-2).

Racial differences exist in both the prevalence of OA and the pattern of joint involvement. The Chinese in Hong Kong have a lower incidence of hip OA than whites; OA is more frequent in native Americans than in whites. Interphalangeal joint OA and, especially, hip OA are much less common in South African blacks than in whites in the same population. Whether these differences are genetic or are due to differences in joint usage related to life-style or occupation is unknown.

In other cases, the relation of heredity to OA is less ambiguous. Thus, the mother and sister of a woman with distal interphalangeal joint OA (Heberden's nodes) are, respectively, twice and thrice as likely to exhibit OA in these joints as the mother and sister of an unaffected woman. Point mutations in the cDNA coding for articular cartilage collagen have been identified in families with chondrodysplasia and polyarticular secondary OA.

Age is the most powerful risk factor for OA. In a radiographic survey of women less than 45 years old, only 2 percent had OA; between the ages of 45 to 64 years, however, the prevalence was 30 percent, and for those older than 65 years it was 68 percent. In males, the figures were similar but somewhat lower in the older age groups.

Major trauma and repetitive joint use are also important risk factors for OA. In both humans and animal models, anterior cruciate ligament insufficiency and meniscus damage (and also meniscectomy) lead to

knee OA. Although damage to the articular cartilage may occur at the time of injury or subsequently, with use of the affected joint, even normal cartilage will degenerate if the joint is unstable. A person with a trimalleolar fracture will almost certainly develop ankle OA.

The pattern of joint involvement in OA is influenced by prior vocational or avocational overload. Thus, ankle OA is common in

Table 322-1

Classification of OA

I. **Idiopathic**
   A. Localized OA
      1. Hands: Heberden's and Bouchard's nodes (nodal), erosive interphalangeal arthritis (nonnodal), carpal–1st metacarpal
      2. Feet: hallux valgus, hallux rigidus, contracted toes (hammer/cock-up toes), talonavicular
      3. Knee:
         a. Medial compartment
         b. Lateral compartment
         c. Patellofemoral compartment
      4. Hip:
         a. Eccentric (superior)
         b. Concentric (axial, medial)
         c. Diffuse (coxae senilis)
      5. Spine:
         a. Apophyseal joints
         b. Intervertebral joints (disks)
         c. Spondylosis (osteophytes)
         d. Ligamentous (hyperostosis, Forestier's disease, diffuse idiopathic skeletal hyperostosis
      6. Other single sites, e.g., glenohumoral, acromioclavicular, tibiotalar, sacroiliac, temporomandibular
   B. Generalized OA includes 3 or more of the areas listed above (Kellgren-Moore)

II. **Secondary**
   A. Trauma
      1. Acute
      2. Chronic (occupational, sports)
   B. Congenital or developmental
      1. Localized diseases: Legg-Calvé-Perthes, congenital hip dislocation, slipped epiphysis
      2. Mechanical factors: unequal lower extremity length, valgus/varus deformity, hypermobility syndromes
      3. Bone dysplasias: epiphyseal dysplasia, spondyloapophyseal dysplasia, osteonychondystrophy
   C. Metabolic
      1. Ochronosis (alkaptonuria)
      2. Hemochromatosis
      3. Wilson's disease
      4. Gaucher's disease
   D. Endocrine
      1. Acromegaly
      2. Hyperparathyroidism
      3. Diabetes mellitus
      4. Obesity
      5. Hypothyroidism
   E. Calcium deposition diseases
      1. Calcium pyrophosphate dihydrate deposition
      2. Apatite arthropathy
   F. Other bone and joint diseases
      1. Localized: fracture, avascular necrosis, infection, gout
      2. Diffuse: rheumatoid (inflammatory) arthritis, Paget's disease, osteopetrosis, osteochondritis
   G. Neuropathic (Charcot joints)
   H. Endemic
      1. Kashin-Beck
      2. Mseleni
   I. Miscellaneous
      1. Frostbite
      2. Caisson disease
      3. Hemoglobinopathies

Supported in part by grant AR 20582 from the National Institute of Arthritis and Musculoskeletal and Skin Diseases.

SOURCE: HJ Mankin et al: Workshop on etiopathogenesis of osteoarthritis. *J Rheumatol* 13:1127, 1986.

ballet dancers, elbow OA in baseball pitchers, and metacarpophalangeal joint OA in prize fighters, although OA is not very common at any of these sites in the general population.

Given the growing participation of the population of this country in sports, it is important to note that there are no convincing data to support an association between specific athletic activities and arthritis if major trauma is excluded. Neither long distance running nor jogging has been shown to cause OA. This apparent lack of association may, however, be due to the lack of good long-term studies, the difficulty of retrospective assessment of activities, and selection bias, i.e., early discontinuation of the activity by those incurring joint damage. In contrast, vocational activities, such as those performed by jackhammer operators, cotton mill and shipyard workers, and coal miners may lead to OA in the joints exposed to repetitive occupational use. Men whose jobs required knee bending and at least medium physical demands had a higher rate of radiographic evidence of knee OA, and more severe radiographic changes, than men whose jobs required neither.

Obesity is a risk factor for knee OA and hand OA. For those in the highest quintile for body mass index at baseline examination, the relative risk for developing knee OA in the ensuing 36 years was 1.5 for men and 2.1 for women. For *severe* knee OA, the relative risk rose to 1.9 for men and 3.2 for women, suggesting that obesity plays an even larger role in the etiology of the most serious cases of knee OA. Furthermore, obese subjects who have not yet developed OA can reduce their risk: A weight loss of only 5 kg was found to be associated with a 50 percent reduction in the odds of developing symptomatic knee OA.

The correlation between the pathologic severity of OA and symptoms is poor. Many individuals with radiographic changes of advanced OA have no symptoms. The risk factors for *pain and disability* in affected individuals are poorly understood. Disability in subjects with knee OA is more strongly associated with quadriceps muscle weakness than with either joint pain or radiographic severity of the disease. For the same degree of pathologic severity, women are more likely to be symptomatic than men, those on welfare more likely than those who are working, and those who are divorced more likely than those who are married. For individuals with OA who had poor social support, periodic telephone calls from a trained lay interviewer were as effective as a nonsteroidal anti-inflammatory drug (NSAID) in reducing joint pain, emphasizing the importance of psychosocial factors as determinants of pain.

PATHOLOGY The most striking changes in OA are usually seen in load-bearing areas of the articular cartilage. In the early stages the cartilage is thicker than normal, but with progression of OA, the joint surface thins, the cartilage softens, the integrity of the surface is breached, and vertical clefts develop (fibrillation) (Fig. 322-1). Deep cartilage ulcers, extending to bone, may appear. Areas of fibrocartilaginous repair may develop, but the repair tissue is inferior to pristine hyaline articular cartilage in its ability to withstand mechanical stress. All of the cartilage is metabolically active, and the chondrocytes replicate, forming clusters (clones). Later, however, the cartilage becomes hypocellular.

Remodeling and hypertrophy of bone are also major features of OA. Appositional bone growth occurs in the subchondral region, leading to the bony "sclerosis" seen radiographically. The abraded bone under a cartilage ulcer may take on the appearance of ivory (eburna-

Table 322-2

Risk Factors for OA	
Age	Repetitive stress, e.g., vocational*
Female sex	Obesity*
Race	Congenital/developmental defects*
Genetic factors	Prior inflammatory joint disease
Major joint trauma*	Metabolic/endocrine disorders

* Potentially modifiable

SOURCE: Adapted from M Hochberg: J Rheum 18:1438, 1991.

tion). Growth of cartilage and bone at the joint margins leads to osteophytes (spurs), which alter the contour of the joint and may restrict movement. A patchy chronic synovitis and thickening of the joint capsule may further restrict movement. Periarticular muscle wasting is common and may play a major role in symptoms and, as indicated above, in disability.

PATHOGENESIS The main load on articular cartilage—the major target tissue in OA—is produced by contraction of the muscles that stabilize or move the joint. Although cartilage is an excellent shock absorber in terms of its bulk properties, at most sites it is only 1 to 2 mm thick—too thin to serve as the sole shock-absorbing structure in the joint. Additional protective mechanisms are provided by subchondral bone and periarticular muscles.

Articular cartilage serves two essential functions in the joint, both of which are mechanical. First, it provides a remarkably smooth bearing surface, so that, with joint movement, the bones glide effortlessly over each other. With synovial fluid as lubricant, the coefficient of friction for cartilage rubbed against cartilage, even under physiologic loading, is 15 times lower than that of two ice cubes passed across each other! Second, articular cartilage prevents concentration of stresses, so the bones do not shatter when the joint is loaded.

OA develops in either of two settings: (1) the biomaterial properties of the articular cartilage and subchondral bone are normal, but excessive loading of the joint causes the tissues to fail, or (2) the applied load is reasonable, but the material properties of the cartilage or bone are inferior.

Although articular cartilage is highly resistant to wear under conditions of repeated oscillation, repetitive impact loading soon leads to joint failure. This fact accounts for the high prevalence of OA at specific sites related to vocational or avocational overloading. In general, the earliest changes occur at the sites in the joint that are subject to the greatest compressive loads. More than 80 percent of all cases of "idiopathic" OA of the hip may be due to subtle congenital or developmental defects, such as congenital subluxation/dislocation, acetabular dysplasia, Legg-Calvé-Perthes disease, or slipped capital femoral epiphysis, which increase joint congruity and concentrate the dynamic load. Notably, institution in the 1940s of screening of newborns and infants for congenital hip disease has been accompanied by a marked decrease in the prevalence of hip OA in adults in Brittany.

Clinical conditions that reduce the ability of the cartilage or subchondral bone to deform are associated with development of OA. In ochronosis, for example, accumulation of homogentisic acid polymers leads to stiffening of the cartilage; in osteopetrosis, stiffness of the subchondral trabeculae occurs. In both conditions, severe generalized OA is usually apparent by the age of 40. If the subchondral bone is stiffened experimentally, repetitive impact loading soon leads to breakdown of the overlying cartilage. Conversely, osteoporosis, in which the bone is abnormally soft, may protect against OA.

The Extracellular Matrix of Normal Articular Cartilage Articular cartilage is composed of two major macromolecular species: proteoglycans (PGs), which are responsible for the compressive stiffness of the tissue and its ability to withstand load, and collagen, which provides tensile strength and resistance to shear. Although lysomal proteases (cathepsins) have been demonstrated within the cells and matrix of normal articular cartilage, their low pH optimum makes it likely that the proteoglycanase activity of these enzymes will be confined to an intracellular site or the immediate pericellular area. However, cartilage also contains a family of matrix metalloproteinases (MMPs), including stromelysin, collagenase, and gelatinase, which can degrade all the components of the extracellular matrix at neutral pH. Each is secreted by the chondrocyte as a latent proenzyme that must be activated by proteolytic cleavage of its N-terminal sequence. The level of MMP activity in the cartilage at any given time represents the balance between activation of the proenzyme and inhibition of the active enzyme by tissue inhibitors.

The turnover of normal cartilage is effected through a degradative cascade, for which many investigators consider the driving force to be interleukin (IL) 1, a cytokine produced by mononuclear cells (including synovial lining cells) and synthesized by chondrocytes. IL-1 stimulates the synthesis and secretion of the latent MMPs and of tissue plasminogen activator. Plasminogen, the substrate for the latter enzyme, may be synthesized by the chondrocyte or may enter the cartilage from the synovial fluid. Both plasminogen and stromelysin may play a role in activation of the latent MMPs. In addition to its catabolic effect on cartilage, at concentrations even lower than those needed to stimulate cartilage degradation, IL-1 suppresses PG synthesis by the chondrocyte, inhibiting matrix repair (see below).

The balance of the system lies with at least two inhibitors, tissue inhibitor of metalloproteinase (TIMP) and plasminogen activator inhibitor-1 (PAI-1), which are synthesized by the chondrocyte and limit the degradative activity of MMPs and plasminogen activator, respectively. If TIMP or PAI-1 is destroyed or is present in concentrations that are insufficient relative to those of active enzymes, stromelysin and plasmin are free to act on matrix substrates. Stromelysin can degrade the protein core of the PG and activate latent collagenase. Conversion of latent stromelysin to an active, highly destructive protease by plasmin provides a second mechanism for matrix degradation.

Polypeptide mediators, e.g., insulin-like growth factor-1 (IGF-1) and transforming growth factor β (TGF-β), stimulate biosynthesis of PGs. They regulate matrix metabolism in normal cartilage and may play a role in matrix repair in OA. Notably, these growth factors modulate catabolic as well as anabolic pathways of chondrocyte metabolism; by down-regulating chondrocyte receptors for IL-1, they may decrease PG degradation.

In addition to its responsiveness to cytokines and a variety of other biologic mediators, chondrocyte metabolism in normal cartilage can be modulated directly by mechanical loading. Whereas static loading and prolonged cyclic loading inhibit synthesis of PGs and protein, loads of relatively brief duration may stimulate matrix biosynthesis.

Pathophysiology of Cartilage Changes in OA   Most investigators feel that the primary changes in OA begin in the cartilage. A change in the arrangement and size of the collagen fibers is apparent. The biochemical data are consistent with the presence of a defect in the collagen network of the cartilage, perhaps due to disruption of the "glue" that binds adjacent fibers together in the matrix. This is among the earliest matrix changes observed and appears to be irreversible.

Although "wear" may be a factor in the loss of cartilage, strong evidence supports the concept that lysosomal enzymes and MMPs account for much of the loss of cartilage matrix in OA. Whether their synthesis and secretion are stimulated by IL-1 or by other factors (e.g., mechanical stimuli), MMPs, plasmin, and cathepsins all appear to be involved in the breakdown of articular cartilage in OA. TIMP and PAI-1 may work to stabilize the system, at least temporarily, while growth factors, such as IGF-1, TGF-β, and basic fibroblast growth factor (FGF), are implicated in repair processes that may heal the lesion or, at least, stabilize the process. A stoichiometric imbalance exists between the levels of active enzyme and the level of TIMP, which may be only modestly increased.

The chondrocytes in OA cartilage undergo active cell division and are very active metabolically, producing increased quantities of DNA, RNA, collagen, PG, and noncollagenous proteins. (For this reason, it is inaccurate to call OA a "degenerative" joint disease). Prior to cartilage loss and PG depletion, this marked biosynthetic activity may lead to an increase in PG concentration, which may be associated with thickening of the cartilage and a stage of homeostasis referred to as "compensated" OA. These mechanisms may maintain the joint in a reasonably functional state for years. The repair tissue, however,

Table 322-3

Causes of Joint Pain in Patients with OA

Source	Mechanism
Synovium	Inflammation
Subchondral bone	Medullary hypertension, microfractures
Osteophyte	Stretching of periosteal nerve endings
Ligaments	Stretch
Capsule	Inflammation, distention
Muscle	Spasm

often does not hold up as well under mechanical stresses as normal hyaline cartilage, and eventually, at least in some cases, the rate of PG synthesis falls off and "end-stage" OA develops, with full-thickness loss of cartilage.

CLINICAL FEATURES   The joint pain of OA is often described as a deep ache and is localized to the involved joint. Typically, the pain of OA is aggravated by joint use and relieved by rest, but, as the disease progresses, it may become persistent. Nocturnal pain, interfering with sleep, is seen particularly in advanced OA of the hip and may be enervating. Stiffness of the involved joint on arising in the morning or after a period of inactivity (e.g., an automobile ride) may be prominent but usually lasts less than 20 min. Systemic manifestations are not a feature of primary OA.

Because articular cartilage is aneural, the joint pain in OA must arise from other structures (Table 322-3). In some patients it may be due to stretching of nerve endings in the periosteum covering osteophytes. In others it may arise from microfractures in subchondral bone or from medullary hypertension caused by distortion of blood flow by thickened subchondral trabeculae. Joint instability, leading to stretching of the joint capsule, and muscle spasm also may be sources of pain.

In some patients with OA, joint pain may be due to synovitis. In advanced OA, histologic evidence of synovial inflammation may be as marked as that in the synovium of a patient with rheumatoid arthritis. Synovitis in OA may be due to phagocytosis of shards of cartilage and bone from the abraded joint surface (wear particles), to release from the cartilage of soluble matrix macromolecules, or to crystals of calcium pyrophosphate or hydroxyapatite. In other cases, immune complexes, containing antigens derived from cartilage matrix, may be sequestered in collagenous tissue of the joint, leading to low-grade

FIGURE 322-1   *A.* Normal articular cartilage. Note the intact surface and even distribution of chondrocytes. Mitotic figures are not present in normal adult articular cartilage. *B.* Osteoarthritic cartilage. Note the disruption of surface integrity, with vertical fissures (fibrillation) and irregular distribution of cells. Many of the chondrocytes have replicated and exist in clusters. Stained with safranin-O, which binds to the sulfated glycosaminoglycan chains of proteoglycans. Note patchy areas of diminished staining (pale extracellular matrix) due to proteoglycan depletion.

chronic synovitis. In contrast, in the earlier stages of OA, even in the patient with chronic joint pain, synovial inflammation may be absent, suggesting that the joint pain is due to one of the other factors mentioned above.

Physical examination of the OA joint may reveal localized tenderness and bony or soft tissue swelling. Bony crepitus (the sensation of bone rubbing against bone, evoked by joint movement) is characteristic. Synovial effusions, if present, are usually not large. Palpation may reveal some warmth over the joint. Periarticular muscle atrophy may be due to disuse or to reflex inhibition of muscle contraction. In the advanced stages of OA, there may be gross deformity, bony hypertrophy, subluxation, and marked loss of joint motion. The notion that OA is inexorably progressive, however, is incorrect. In many patients the disease stabilizes; in some, regression of joint pain and even of radiographic changes occurs.

Although the diagnosis of OA is often straightforward because of the high prevalence of radiographic changes of OA in asymptomatic individuals, it is important to ensure that joint pain in a patient with radiographic evidence of OA is not due to some other cause, such as soft tissue rheumatism (e.g., anserine bursitis at the knee, trochanteric bursitis at the hip), radiculopathy, referral of pain from another joint (e.g., 25 percent of patients with hip disease have pain referred to the knee, for example), entrapment neuropathy, vascular disease (claudication), or some other type of arthritis (e.g., crystal-induced synovitis, septic arthritis). These are all common pitfalls in the diagnosis of OA. It is usually not difficult to differentiate OA from a systemic rheumatic disease, such as rheumatoid arthritis, because, in the latter diseases, joint involvement is usually symmetric and polyarticular, with arthritis in wrists and metacarpophalangeal joints (which are generally not involved in OA), and there are also constitutional features such as prolonged morning stiffness, fatigue, and, occasionally, weight loss or fever (see Chap. 313).

LABORATORY AND RADIOGRAPHIC FINDINGS   The diagnosis of OA is usually based on clinical and radiographic features. In the early stages, the radiograph may be normal, but joint space narrowing becomes evident as articular cartilage is lost. Other characteristic radiographic findings include subchondral bone sclerosis, subchondral cysts, and osteophytosis. A change in the contour of the joint due to bony remodeling and subluxation may be seen. Although tibiofemoral joint space narrowing has been considered to be a radiographic surrogate for articular cartilage thinning, in patients with early OA who do not have radiographic evidence of bony changes (e.g., subchondral sclerosis or cysts, osteophytes), joint space narrowing alone does not accurately indicate the status of the articular cartilage. Similarly, osteophytosis alone, in the absence of other radiographic features of OA, may be due to aging rather than to OA.

As indicated above, there is often great disparity between the severity of radiographic findings, the severity of symptoms, and functional ability in OA. Thus, while more than 90 percent of persons over the age of 40 have some radiographic changes of OA in weight-bearing joints, only 30 percent of these persons are symptomatic.

No laboratory studies are diagnostic for OA, but specific laboratory testing may help in identifying one of the underlying causes of secondary OA (Table 322-1). Because primary OA is not systemic, the erythrocyte sedimentation rate, serum chemistry determinations, blood counts, and urinalysis are normal. Analysis of synovial fluid reveals mild leukocytosis (<2000 white blood cells per microliter), with a predominance of mononuclear cells. Synovial fluid analysis is of particular value in excluding other conditions, such as calcium pyrophosphate dihydrate (CPPD) deposition disease (see Chap. 323), gout (see Chap. 344), or septic arthritis (see Chap. 324).

Prior to the appearance of radiographic changes, the ability to clinically diagnose OA without an invasive procedure (e.g., arthroscopy) is limited. Approaches such as magnetic resonance imaging (MRI) and ultrasonography have not been sufficiently validated, and their limits of resolution and cost do not justify their routine clinical use for diagnosis of OA or monitoring of disease progression.

OA AT SPECIFIC JOINT SITES   **Interphalangeal Joints** Heberden's nodes, bony enlargements of the distal interphalangeal joints, are the most common form of idiopathic OA (Fig. 322-2). A similar process at the proximal interphalangeal joints leads to Bouchard's nodes. Often, Heberden's nodes develop gradually, with little or no discomfort. However, they may present acutely with pain, redness, and swelling, sometimes triggered by minor trauma. Gelatinous dorsal cysts filled with hyaluronic acid may develop at the insertion of the digital extensor tendon into the base of the distal phalanx.

Erosive OA   In erosive OA distal and/or proximal interphalangeal joints of the hands are most prominently affected. Erosive OA tends to be more destructive than typical nodal OA. Radiographic evidence of collapse of the subchondral plate is characteristic, and bony ankylosis may occur. Joint deformity and functional impairment may be severe. Pain and tenderness are commonly episodic. The synovium is much more extensively infiltrated with mononuclear cells than in other forms of OA.

Generalized OA   Generalized OA is characterized by involvement of three or more joints or groups of joints (distal interphalangeal and proximal interphalangeal joints are counted as one group each). Heberden's and Bouchard's nodes are prominent. Symptoms may be episodic, with "flare-ups" of inflammation marked by soft tissue swelling, redness, and warmth. The erythrocyte sedimentation rate may be elevated, but serum rheumatoid factor tests are negative.

Thumb Base   The second most frequent area of involvement in OA is the thumb base. Swelling, tenderness, and crepitus on movement of the joint are typical. Osteophytes may lead to a "squared" appearance of the thumb base (Fig. 322-3). In contrast to Heberden's nodes, which usually do not interfere significantly with function, thumb base OA frequently causes loss of motion and strength. Pain with pinch leads to adduction of the thumb and contracture of the first web space, often resulting in compensatory hyperextension of the first metacarpophalangeal joint and swan-neck deformity of the thumb.

The Hip   Congenital or developmental defects (e.g., acetabular dysplasia, Legg-Calvé-Perthes disease, slipped capital epiphysis) may be implicated in as many as 80 percent of cases of hip OA. Twenty percent of patients will develop bilateral involvement. Pain from hip OA is generally referred to the inguinal area but may be referred to the buttock or proximal thigh. Less commonly, hip OA presents as knee pain. Pain can be evoked by putting the involved hip through its range of motion. Flexion may be painless initially, but internal rotation will exacerbate pain. Loss of internal rotation occurs early, followed by loss of extension, adduction, and flexion due to capsular fibrosis and/or buttressing osteophytes.

FIGURE 322-2   Nodal osteoarthritis. Note bony enlargement of distal and proximal interphalangeal joints (Heberden's nodes and Bouchard's nodes, respectively). *(Reprinted from the Clinical Slide Collection on the Rheumatic Diseases, © 1991, 1995. Used by permission of the American College of Rheumatology.)*

FIGURE 322-3 Osteoarthritis of the first carpometacarpal joint. Note the squared appearance of the thumb base, due to bony enlargement and remodeling of the joint.

The Knee OA of the knee may involve the medial or lateral femorotibial compartment and/or the patellofemoral compartment. Palpation may reveal bony hypertrophy (osteophytes) and tenderness. Effusions, if present, are generally small. Joint movement commonly elicits bony crepitus. OA in the medial compartment may result in a varus (bow-leg) deformity; in the lateral compartment it may produce a valgus (knock-knee) deformity. A positive "shrug" sign (pain when the patella is compressed manually against the femur during quadriceps contraction) may be a sign of patellofemoral OA.

Chondromalacia patellae, which also is characterized by anterior knee pain and a positive shrug sign, is a syndrome of patellofemoral pain, often bilateral, in teenagers and young adults. It is more common in females than in males. It may be caused by a variety of factors (e.g., abnormal quadriceps angle, patella alta, trauma). Although exploration of the knee may reveal softening and fibrillation of cartilage on the posterior aspect of the patella, this change is usually not progressive; chondromalacia patellae is usually not a precursor of OA. In most cases, analgesics or NSAIDs and physical therapy are effective; in some, pain may be relieved by surgical correction of patellar malalignment.

The Spine Degenerative disease of the spine can involve the apophyseal joint, intervertebral disks, and/or paraspinous ligaments. *Spondylosis* refers to degenerative *disk* disease. The diagnosis of spinal OA should be reserved for cases showing involvement of the apophyseal joints (true diarthrodial joints). Symptoms of spinal OA include localized pain and stiffness. Nerve root compression by an osteophyte blocking a neural foramen, prolapse of a degenerated disk, or subluxation of an apophyseal joint may cause radicular pain and motor weakness.

Marked calcification and ossification of paraspinous ligaments occur in diffuse idiopathic skeletal hyperostosis (DISH). Although DISH is often categorized as a variant of OA, diarthrodial joints are not involved. Ligamentous calcification and ossification in the anterior spinal ligaments give the appearance of "flowing wax" on the anterior vertebral bodies. However, a radiolucency may be seen between the newly deposited bone and the vertebral body, differentiating DISH from the marginal osteophytes in spondylosis. Intervertebral disk spaces are preserved, and sacroiliac and apophyseal joints appear normal, helping to differentiate DISH from spondylosis and from ankylosing spondylitis, respectively. DISH occurs in the middle-aged and elderly and is more common in men than in women. Patients are frequently asymptomatic but may have musculoskeletal stiffness. The radiographic changes are generally much more severe than might be predicted from the mild symptoms.

℞ TREATMENT

Treatment of OA is aimed at reducing pain, maintaining mobility, and minimizing disability. The vigor of the therapeutic intervention should be dictated by the severity of the condition in the individual patient. For those with only mild disease, reassurance, instruction in joint protection, and an occasional analgesic may be all that is required; for those with more severe OA, especially of the knee or hip, a comprehensive program comprising a spectrum of nonpharmacologic measures supplemented by an analgesic and/or anti-inflammatory drug is appropriate.

Nonpharmacologic measures REDUCTION OF JOINT LOADING OA may be caused or aggravated by poor body mechanics. Correction of poor posture and a support for excessive lumbar lordosis can be helpful. Excessive loading of the involved joint should be avoided. Patients with OA of the knee or hip should avoid prolonged standing, kneeling, and squatting. Obese patients should be counseled to lose weight. In patients with medial-compartment knee OA, a wedged insole may decrease joint pain.

Rest periods during the day may be of benefit, but complete immobilization of the painful joint is rarely indicated. In patients with unilateral OA of the hip or knee, a cane, held in the contralateral hand, may reduce joint pain by reducing the joint contact force. Bilateral disease may necessitate use of crutches or a walker.

PHYSICAL THERAPY Application of heat to the OA joint may reduce pain and stiffness. A variety of modalities are available; often, the least expensive and most convenient is a hot shower or bath. Occasionally, better analgesia may be obtained with ice than with heat.

Disuse of the OA joint because of pain will lead to muscle atrophy. Reflex inhibition of muscle contraction may have a similar effect. Because periarticular muscles play a major role in protecting the articular cartilage from stress, strengthening them is important. Exercises should be designed to maintain range of motion as well as to strengthen muscles surrounding the joint. In subjects with knee OA, strengthening of the periarticular muscles may result, within weeks, in a decrease in joint pain as great as that seen with NSAIDs.

Drug therapy of OA Therapy for OA today is palliative; no pharmacologic agent has been shown to prevent, delay the progression of, or reverse the pathologic changes of OA in humans.

Although NSAIDs often decrease joint pain and improve mobility in OA, the magnitude of this improvement is generally modest—on average, about 30 percent reduction in pain and 15 percent improvement in function. Patients with OA may obtain symptomatic benefit from an NSAID even when evidence of synovitis is lacking, consistent with the fact that these drugs have analgesic effects independent of their anti-inflammatory actions. In a double-blinded, controlled trial in patients with symptomatic knee OA, an anti-inflammatory dose of ibuprofen was no more effective than a low (i.e., essentially analgesic) dose of ibuprofen or than acetaminophen, a drug with essentially no anti-inflammatory effect. Other studies confirm that an analgesic dose of ibuprofen may be as effective as anti-inflammatory doses of other NSAIDs, including the potent agent phenylbutazone, in symptomatic treatment of patients with knee OA. Furthermore, even in the presence of clinical signs of inflammation (synovial swelling, tenderness), relief of joint pain by acetaminophen may be superior to that achieved with an NSAID. Nonetheless, if simple analgesics are inadequate, it is reasonable to cautiously prescribe an NSAID for a patient with OA. Although some NSAIDs have been claimed to have a "chondroprotective" effect, adequately controlled clinical trials of these claims in humans with OA are lacking.

Furthermore, concern is growing with respect to the appropriateness of NSAID administration in OA because of the side effects of these agents, especially those related to the gastrointestinal tract. The segment of the population at greatest risk for OA, i.e., the elderly, appears also to be at greater risk than younger individuals for gastrointestinal symptoms, ulceration, hemorrhage, and death as a result of NSAID use. The annual rate of hospitalization for peptic ulcer disease among elderly current NSAID users was 16 per 1000—four times greater than that for subjects not taking an NSAID.

Among people aged 65 and older, as many as 30 percent of all hospitalizations and deaths related to peptic ulcer disease have been attributed to NSAID use.

Systemic glucocorticoids have no place in the treatment of OA. However, intra- or periarticular injection of a depot glucocorticoid preparation may provide marked symptomatic relief for weeks to months. Because studies in animal models have suggested that glucocorticoids may produce cartilage damage, and frequent injections of large amounts of steroids have been associated with joint breakdown in humans, the injection should be generally not be repeated in a given joint more often than every 4 to 6 months.

Capsaicin cream, which depletes local sensory nerve endings of substance P, a neuropeptide mediator of pain, may reduce joint pain and tenderness when applied topically by patients with hand or knee

OA, even when used as monotherapy, i.e., without NSAIDs or systemic analgesics.

A rational approach to the nonsurgical management of OA　It is being increasingly recognized that nonpharmacologic management is as important—and often more important—than drug treatment in the management of OA and that drugs should serve an *adjunctive* role in the management of this disease. Nonpharmacologic measures may comprise instruction of the patient in principles of joint protection; thermal modalities; exercises to strengthen periarticular muscles; weight reduction if the patient is obese; avoidance of excessive loading of the arthritic hip or knee joint by use of shoes with well-cushioned soles and a cane or walker, when appropriate; and prescription of orthotics for the patient with varus or valgus knee deformity. Medial taping of the patella may reduce knee pain in patients with patellofemoral OA. In patients with knee OA, if the above measures are ineffective, tidal irrigation of the painful joint warrants consideration. A health education program designed to assist the

FIGURE 322-4　Algorithm for management of a newly diagnosed patient with knee OA. *(Modified from Brandt, 1996.)*

Figure 322-4 provides an algorithm which might be applied to treatment of a newly diagnosed patient with knee OA. The progressive levels of treatment are associated with increasing cost, decreasing convenience for the patient, and increasing risk of side effects. The scheme should not be interpreted dogmatically as a fixed progression of steps; rather, treatment of OA must be individualized. The treatment program should be flexible. For example, in some patients it may be reasonable to institute patellar taping or prescribe a wedged insole on the initial visit, or an intraarticular steroid injection on a later visit.

Because the symptomatic relief afforded by NSAIDs is often no greater than that achieved by a simple analgesic, because the side effects of NSAIDs are more frequent and more severe than those of acetaminophen, and because prescription NSAIDs cost considerably more than acetaminophen, when an analgesic drug is required for treatment of OA pain it is reasonable to prescribe acetaminophen initially, up to 4000 mg/d, as an adjunct to the nonpharmacologic measures mentioned above. If this regimen does not control joint symptoms in a reasonable period of time, a *low dose* or an NSAID (e.g., ibuprofen, 1200 mg/d; naproxen, 500 mg/d) may be substituted for, or added to, the acetaminophen. Should this modification be insufficient, tramadol, a weak opioid for which the risk of tolerance and addiction appear to be minimal, may be prescribed. If the above approach is not satisfactory, an antiinflammatory dose of an NSAID should be used.

Because the risk of an NSAID-associated gastrointestinal catastrophe (e.g., perforation, hemorrhage) is dose-dependent, the lowest effective dose should be employed. Salsalate and other nonacetylated salicylates, which have only a minimal effect on prostaglandin synthase, are as effective as other NSAIDs as have a lower rate of serious gastrointestinal side effects. When NSAIDs are required, they may be prescribed on an "as needed" basis, rather than in a fixed daily dose; pain control has been shown to be comparable and the risk of toxicity will be reduced. Once treatment with an NSAID or simple analgesic is initiated, the need for continuation of that treatment requires ongoing assessment. For many patients with OA, it will be possible eventually to reduce the dose of drug or to use the agent only intermittently, during exacerbations of joint pain.

Orthopedic surgery Joint replacement surgery should be reserved for patients with advanced OA in whom aggressive medical management has failed. In such cases it may be remarkably effective in relieving pain and increasing mobility. Osteotomy, which is surgically more conservative, can eliminate concentrations of peak dynamic loading and may provide effective pain relief in patients with hip or knee OA. It is of greatest benefit when the disease is only moderately advanced. Arthroscopic removal of loose cartilage fragments can prevent locking and relieve pain. Lavage of the OA knee with large quantities of saline or Ringer's lactate to flush out fibrin, cartilage shards, and other debris may provide months of comfort for the patient whose joint pain has been refractory to analgesics, NSAIDs, and intraarticular steroid injections. However, invasive procedures such as this are accompanied by a large placebo effect, and studies that include a sham lavage control group have not yet been reported.

Chondroplasty (abrasion arthroplasty) also has gained some popularity as treatment for OA, but well-controlled studies of its efficacy are lacking, and the fibrocartilage that resurfaces the abraded bone is inferior to normal hyaline cartilage in its ability to withstand mechanical loads. Notably, in patients who had undergone tibial osteotomy for medial compartment knee OA, knee pain and function were not related to the degree of cartilage regeneration seen at arthroscopy two years later.

BIBLIOGRAPHY

ANDERSON JJ, FELSON DT: Factors associated with osteoarthritis of the knee in the first national health and nutrition examination survey (HANES I).

Evidence for an association with overweight, race, and physical demands of work. Am J Epidemiol 128:179, 1988
BRADLEY JD et al: Comparison of an anti-inflammatory dose of ibuprofen, an analgesic dose of ibuprofen, and acetaminophen in the treatment of patients with osteoarthritis of the knee. N Engl J Med 325:87, 1991
BRANDT KD: Management of osteoarthritis, in *Textbook of Rheumatology,* 5th ed, WN Kelley et al (eds). Philadelphia, Saunders, 1995
———: Nonsurgical management of osteoarthritis with an emphasis on non-pharmacologic measures. Arch Fam Med 4:1057, 1995
———: *Diagnosis and Nonsurgical Management of Osteoarthritis.* Caddo, OK, Professional Communications, Inc., 1996
———, FLUSSER D: Osteoarthritis, in *Prognosis in the Rheumatic Diseases,* N Bellamy (ed). Kluwer Academic Publishers, Lancaster, UK, 1991, pp 11–35
———, MANKIN HJ: Pathogenesis of osteoarthritis, in *Textbook of Rheumatology,* 4th ed, WN Kelley et al (eds). Philadelphia, Saunders, 1993
———, RADIN E: The physiology of articular stress: Osteoarthrosis. Hosp Pract 22: 103, 1987
GRIFFIN MR et al: Practical management of osteoarthritis: Integration of pharmacologic and nonpharmacologic measures. Arch Fam Med 4:1049, 1995
HOCHBERG MC et al: Guidelines for the medical management of osteoarthritis: Part I. Arthritis Rheum 38:1535, 1995
——— et al: Guidelines for the medical management of osteoarthritis: Part II. Arthritis Rheum 38:1541, 1995
MANKIN HJ: Clinical feature of osteoarthritis, in *Textbook of Rheumatology,* 3d ed, WN Kelley et al (eds). Philadelphia, Saunders, 1989, pp 1480–1500
——— et al: Workshop on etiopathogenesis of osteoarthritis. J Rheumatol 13:1127, 1986

323 | *Antonio J. Reginato, Gary S. Hoffman*

ARTHRITIS DUE TO DEPOSITION OF CALCIUM CRYSTALS

"GOUT" CRYSTALLOGRAPHY AND ARTHRITIS The use of polarizing microscopy during synovial fluid analysis, and the application of other research tools such as electron microscopy, energy-dispersive elemental analysis, and x-ray diffraction have established the role of different microcrystals, including monosodium urate (MSU), calcium pyrophosphate dihydrate (CPPD), calcium hydroxyapatite (HA), and calcium oxalate (CaOx), in inducing arthritis (See Chap. 344). Each of these crystals may cause acute or chronic arthritis or periarthritis. In spite of differences in crystal morphology, chemistry, and physical properties, the clinical events that result from deposition and release of MSU, CPPD, HA, and CaOx may be indistinguishable. Prior to the use of crystallographic techniques in rheumatology, much of what was considered to be MSU gouty arthritis in fact was not. Simkin has suggested that the generic term *gout* be used to describe the whole group of crystal-induced arthritides (MSU gout, CPPD gout, HA gout, and CaOx gout). This concept further emphasizes the identical clinical presentations of these entities and the need to perform synovial fluid analysis to distinguish the type of crystal involved. In the setting of acute articular or periarticular inflammation, aspiration and analysis of effusions are most important to assess the possibility of infection and to identify the type of crystals present. Polarization microscopy alone can identify most typical crystals and allow diagnosis. HA, however, is an exception. Because these crystals are not birefringent and are extremely small, alizarin red S stain may be used as screening test, and more sophisticated techniques are required to confirm the presence of these crystals. Apart from the identification of specific microcrystalline materials or organisms, synovial fluid characteristics are nonspecific, and synovial fluid can be inflammatory or noninflammatory. The presence of crystals does not exclude the existence of an associated acute or, more rarely, chronic infection.

CPPD DEPOSITION DISEASE Pathogenesis The deposition of CPPD crystals in articular cartilage, synovium, and periarticular ligaments and tendons is most common in the elderly, affecting 10 to

15 percent of persons 65 to 75 years old and 30 to 60 percent of those more than 85 years old. In most cases this process is asymptomatic, and the cause of CPPD deposition is uncertain. Because over 80 percent of patients are more than 60 years old and 70 percent have preexisting joint damage from other conditions, it is likely that physical and chemical changes in aging cartilage favor crystal nucleation. Examples of such chemical alterations include the following. (1) There is an increased production of inorganic pyrophosphate and decreased levels of pyrophosphatases in cartilage extracts from patients with CPPD arthritis. The increase in pyrophosphate production appears to be related to enhanced activity of ATP pyrophosphohydrolase and 5′-nucleotidase, which catalyze the reaction of ATP to adenosine and pyrophosphate. This pyrophosphate could combine with calcium to form CPPD crystals in matrix vesicles. (2) There is a diminution in the levels of cartilage glycoproteins that normally inhibit and regulate crystal nucleation. These deficiencies may lead to increased crystal deposition. (3) In vitro studies have demonstrated that transforming growth factor β1 and epidermal growth factor both stimulate the production of pyrophosphate by articular cartilage and thus may contribute to the deposition of CPPD crystals. The release of CPPD crystals into the joint space is followed by the phagocytosis of these crystals by neutrophils, which respond by releasing inflammatory substances. In addition, neutrophils release a glycopeptide that is chemotactic for other neutrophils, thus augmenting the inflammatory events. The same substance is present in MSU gout. The production of this glycopeptide can be suppressed by colchicine.

A minority of patients with CPPD arthropathy have metabolic abnormalities or hereditary CPPD disease (Table 323-1). These associations suggest that a variety of different metabolic products may enhance CPPD deposition. Included among these conditions are hyperparathyroidism, hemochromatosis, gout, hypophosphatasia, hypomagnesemia, and ochronosis. Hemochromatosis and hyperparathyroidism are good examples. Ferrous ions and hypercalcemia may either directly alter cartilage or inhibit inorganic pyrophosphatases, leading to enhanced susceptibility to CPPD deposition. The presence of CPPD arthritis in individuals less than 50 years old should lead to consideration of these metabolic disorders and inherited forms of disease, including those identified in a variety of ethnic groups (Table 323-1). Genomic DNA studies performed on three different kindreds have shown a possible location of the genetic defects on chromosomes 5p and 8q. Identification of these genes will help elucidate the pathogenesis of both the familial and the more common sporadic form of the disease. Investigation should include inquiry for evidence of familial aggregation and evaluation of serum calcium, phosphorus, alkaline phosphatase, magnesium, serum ferritin, and transferritin saturation.

Clinical Manifestations CPPD arthropathy may be asymptomatic, acute, subacute, or chronic or cause acute synovitis superimposed on chronically involved joints. Acute CPPD arthritis was originally termed *pseudogout* by McCarty and coworkers because of its striking similarity to MSU gout. He and others have since recognized that the clinical sequelae of CPPD deposition include (1) induction or

Table 323-1

Conditions Associated with CPPD Disease

Aging
Disease-associated:
  Primary hyperparathyroidism
  Hemochromatosis
  Hypophosphatasia
  Hypomagnesemia
  Chronic tophaceous gout
  Post-meniscectomy
Epiphyseal dysplasias
Hereditary: Slovakian-Hungarian, Chilean-Spanish, French, Swedish, Dutch, Canadian, Mexican-American, Italian-American, German-American, Japanese, Tunisian, Jewish, English

FIGURE 323-1 Intracellular and extracellular calcium pyrophosphate dihydrate crystals, as seen in a fresh preparation of synovial fluid, illustrate rectangular, rod-shaped, and rhomboid weakly birefringent crystals (compensated polarized light microscopy; 400×).

enhancement of peculiar forms of osteoarthritis, (2) induction of severe resorptive disease that may radiographically mimic neuropathic arthritis, (3) production of symmetric proliferative synovitis, clinically similar to rheumatoid arthritis and frequently seen in familial forms with early onset, (4) intervertebral disk and ligament calcification with restriction of spine mobility, mimicking ankylosing spondylitis (also seen in hereditary forms), and (5) rarely spinal stenosis (most commonly seen in the elderly).

The knee is the joint most frequently affected in CPPD arthropathy. Other sites include the wrist, shoulder, ankle, elbow, and hands. Rarely, the temporomandibular joint and ligamentum flavum of the spinal canal are involved. Clinical and radiographic evidence indicates that CPPD deposition is polyarticular in at least two-thirds of patients. When acute synovitis occurs, diagnosis is made by identification of rod-shaped or rhomboid crystals with weak positive birefringence (Fig. 323-1) in synovial fluid. When the clinical picture resembles that of slowly progressive osteoarthritis, diagnosis may be more difficult. Joint distribution may provide important clues suggesting CPPD disease. For example, primary osteoarthritis rarely involves a metacarpophalangeal, wrist, elbow, shoulder, or ankle joint. If radiographs reveal punctate and/or linear radiodense deposits in fibrocartilaginous joint menisci or articular hyaline cartilage (chondrocalcinosis), the diagnostic certainty of CPPD is further enhanced. *Definitive diagnosis* requires demonstration of typical crystals in synovial fluid or articular tissue. In the absence of joint effusion or indications to obtain a synovial biopsy, chondrocalcinosis is presumptive of CPPD deposition. One exception is chondrocalcinosis due to CaOx in some patients with chronic renal failure.

Acute attacks of CPPD arthritis may be precipitated by trauma, such as physical injury to an extremity, joint surgery, a sprain, or even a long walk. Rapid diminution of serum calcium concentration, as may occur in severe medical illness or after surgery (especially parathyroidectomy), also can lead to pseudogout. How transient calcium disequilibrium may facilitate CPPD release is unclear.

In as many as 50 percent of cases, CPPD gout is associated with low-grade fever and, on occasion, temperatures as high as 40°C. Whether or not radiographic proof of chondrocalcinosis is evident in the involved joint(s), synovial analysis with microbial stains and cultures is essential to rule out the possibility of infection. In fact, infection in a joint with any microcrystalline deposition process can lead to crystal shedding and subsequent synovitis from both crystals and microorganisms. Synovial fluid in acute CPPD gout has inflammatory qualities. The white blood cell (WBC) count can range from several thousand cells to 100,000 cells/µL, the mean being about 24,000 cells/µL and the predominant cell being the neutrophil. Polarization microscopy usually reveals crystals with weak positive birefringence in the extracellular fluid and in neutrophils.

℞ TREATMENT

Untreated acute attacks may last a few days to as long as a month. *Treatment* by joint aspiration (to decrease intraarticular pressure) and nonsteroidal anti-inflammatory agents or intraarticular glucocorticoid injection may result in return to prior status in 10 days or less. For patients with frequent recurrent attacks of CPPD gout, daily prophylactic treatment with low doses of colchicine may be helpful in decreasing the frequency of the attacks. Severe polyarticular attacks usually require short courses of corticosteroids. Unfortunately, there is no effective way to remove CPPD deposits from cartilage and synovium. Uncontrolled studies suggest that radioactive synovectomy (with yttrium 90) or the administration of antimalarial agents may be helpful in controlling persistent synovitis. Patients with progressive destructive large joint arthropathy usually require joint replacement. There is no subsequent increased risk of soft tissue heterotopic calcification around the prosthesis.

Table 323-2

Conditions Associated with HA Deposition Disease

Aging
Osteoarthritis
Hemorrhagic shoulder effusions in the elderly (Milwaukee shoulder)
Destructive arthropathy
Tendinitis, bursitis
Tumoral calcinosis (sporadic cases)
Disease-associated
    Hyperparathyroidism
    Milk alkali syndrome
    Renal failure/long-term dialysis
    Connective tissue diseases (e.g., progressive systemic sclerosis, CREST syndrome, idiopathic myositis)
    Heterotopic calcification following neurologic catastrophes (e.g., stroke, spinal cord injury)
Hereditary
    Bursitis, arthritis
    Tumoral calcinosis

CALCIUM HA DEPOSITION DISEASE Pathogenesis HA is the primary mineral of bone and teeth. Abnormal accumulation can occur in areas of tissue damage (dystrophic calcification), in hypercalcemic or hyperparathyroid states (metastatic calcification), and in certain conditions of unknown cause (Table 323-2). In chronic renal failure, hyperphosphatemia enhances HA deposition both in and around joints.

HA may be released from exposed bone and cause the acute synovitis occasionally seen in chronic stable osteoarthritis (e.g., "hot" Heberden's nodes). HA deposition is also an important factor in an extremely destructive chronic arthropathy of the elderly that occurs most often in knees and shoulders (Milwaukee shoulder). Joint destruction is associated with attenuation or rupture of supporting structures, leading to instability and deformity. Progression tends to be indolent, and synovial fluid WBC counts are usually less than 1000 cells/µL. Symptoms range from minimal to severe pain and disability that may lead to joint replacement surgery. Whether severely affected patients merely represent an extreme synovial tissue response to the HA crystals that are so common in osteoarthritis is uncertain. Observations that favor the idea that articular HA deposition and joint destruction constitute a unique entity rather than just a sequel of osteoarthritis include the following. (1) Primary osteoarthritis of the shoulders is infrequent. (2) High levels of activated collagenase and neutral protease, as well as fragments of collagen, have been found in the noninflammatory synovial fluids of patients with severe HA arthropathy; the concentration of these enzymes exceeded those found in rheumatoid arthritis and uncomplicated osteoarthritis. (3) Synovial membrane tissue cultures exposed to HA (or CPPD) crystals markedly increased release of these enzymes, underscoring the destructive potential of abnormally stimulated synovial lining cells.

Clinical Manifestations Periarticular and articular deposits may coexist and be associated with acute and/or chronic damage to the joint capsule, tendons, bursa, or articular surfaces. The most common sites of HA deposition include those in and/or around the knees, shoulders, hips, and fingers. Clinical manifestations include asymptomatic radiographic abnormalities, acute synovi-

tis or tendinitis, and chronic destructive arthropathy. Most patients with HA arthropathy are elderly. Although the true incidence of HA arthritis is not known, 30 to 50 percent of patients with osteoarthritis have HA microcrystals in their synovial fluid. Such crystals can frequently be identified in clinically stable osteoarthritic joints, but they are more likely to come to attention in persons experiencing acute or subacute worsening of joint pain and swelling. The synovial fluid WBC count in HA arthritis is usually low (<2000 cells/µL) but may at times have as many as 50,000 cells/µL. Most synovial fluid analyses reveal a predominance of mononuclear cells. Occasionally, neutrophils may dominate.

Diagnosis Radiographic findings in HA arthropathy are not diagnostic. Intra- and/or periarticular calcifications with or without erosive, destructive, or hypertrophic changes may be present. X-ray films also may be normal.

Definitive diagnosis of HA arthropathy depends on identification of crystals from synovial fluid or tissue (Fig. 323-2). Individual crystals are very small, nonbirefringent, and can only be seen by electron microscopy. Clumps of crystals may appear as 1- to 20-µm shiny intra- or extracellular globules that stain purplish with Wright's stain and bright red with alizarin red S. Absolute identification depends on electron microscopy with energy-dispersive elemental analysis, x-ray diffraction, or infrared spectroscopy.

FIGURE 323-2 *A.* Cytoplasmic round inclusions inside synovial fluid cells represent aggregates of apatite crystals (fresh preparation, ordinary light microscopy; 288×). *B.* An electron micrograph demonstrates a cluster of dark apatite crystals within a synovial fluid mononuclear cell (21,600×).

TREATMENT

Treatment of HA arthritis is nonspecific. Acute attacks of synovitis may be self-limiting, resolving in from days to several weeks. Aspiration of effusions and the use of either nonsteroidal anti-inflammatory agents or oral colchicine for 2 weeks or of intraarticular injection of glucocorticoid salts appear to shorten the duration and intensity of symptoms. In patients with underlying severe destructive articular changes, response to medical therapy is usually less rewarding.

CaOx DEPOSITION DISEASE   Pathogenesis   *Primary oxalosis* is a rare hereditary metabolic disorder (Chap. 349). Enhanced production of oxalic acid may result from at least two different enzyme defects, leading to hyperoxalemia and deposition of calcium oxalate crystals in tissues. Nephrocalcinosis, renal failure, and death usually occur before age 20. Acute and/or chronic CaOx arthritis and periarthritis may complicate primary oxalosis during later years of illness.

Secondary oxalosis is more common than the primary disorder. It is one of the many metabolic abnormalities that complicate end-stage renal disease (ESRD). In ESRD, calcium oxalate deposits have long been recognized in visceral organs, blood vessels, bones, and even cartilage. However, it was not until 1982 that such deposits were demonstrated to be one of the causes of arthritis in chronic renal failure. Thus far, reported patients have been dependent on long-term hemodialysis or peritoneal dialysis (see also Chap. 272), and many had received vitamin C (ascorbic acid) supplements. Ascorbic acid is metabolized to oxalate, which is inadequately cleared in uremia and by dialysis. Such supplements are now usually avoided in dialysis programs because of the risk of enhancing hyperoxalosis and its sequelae.

Clinical Manifestations and Diagnosis   As was noted for the other calcium salts, CaOx aggregates can be found in bone, articular cartilage, synovium, and periarticular tissues. From these sites, crystals may be shed, causing acute synovitis. Persistent aggregates of CaOx may, like HA and CPPD, stimulate synovial proliferation and enzyme release, resulting in progressive articular destruction. Deposits have been documented in fingers, wrists, elbows, knees, ankles, and feet. Any articular site could potentially be involved.

Each of the known microcrystalline arthropathies may be a complication of ESRD, and rare patients have more than one type of crystal present in a joint effusion. The advent of crystallographic techniques has made it clear that most arthritic problems in ESRD are not, as was once believed, due to MSU gout. Clinical features of acute CaOx arthritis may not be distinguishable from those due to sodium urate, CPPD, or HA. Radiographs may reveal chondrocalcinosis, a feature of either CPPD or CaOx deposition. CaOx-induced synovial effusions are usually noninflammatory, with less than 2000 leukocytes/μL. Neutrophils or mononuclear cells have predominated. In most instances, crystals are extracellular, although CaOx has been identified in neutrophils. Synovial membranes show modest signs of inflammation. CaOx crystals have a variable shape and variable birefringence to polarized light. The most easily recognized forms are bipyramidal and have strong positive birefringence (Fig. 323-3).

 TREATMENT

Treatment of CaOx arthropathy with nonsteroidal anti-inflammatory agents, colchicine, intraarticular glucocorticoids, and/or an increased frequency of dialysis has produced only slight improvement. In primary oxalosis, liver transplantation has induced a significant reduction in crystal deposits (see Chap. 349).

BIBLIOGRAPHY

ALVARELLOS A, SPILBERG I: Colchicine prophylaxis in pseudogout. J Rheumatol 13:804, 1986

BETH A et al: Articular cartilage vesicles generate calcium pyrophosphate dihydrate-like crystals in vitro. Arthritis Rheum 35:231, 1992

DIEPPE PA et al: Apatite deposition disease: A new arthropathy. Lancet 1:266, 1976

BALDWIN CT et al: Linkage of early onset osteoarthritis and chondrocalcinosis to human chromosome 8q. Am J Hum Genet 56:692, 1995

DOHERTY M et al: Inorganic pyrophosphate in metabolic diseases predisposing to calcium pyrophosphate dihydrate crystal deposition. Arthritis Rheum 34:1297, 1991

HOFFMAN GS et al: Calcium oxalate microcrystalline-associated arthritis in end-stage renal disease. Ann Intern Med 97:36, 1982

HUGHES A et al: Localisation of a gene for chondrocalcinosis to chromosome 5p. Hum Mol Genet 4:1225, 1995

McCARTHY DJ: Crystals and arthritis. Dis Month 40:255, 1994

REGINATO AJ et al: Familial calcium pyrophosphate crystal deposition disease or calcium pyrophosphate gout. Rev Rheum [Engl Ed] 62:376, 1995

REGINATO AJ, SCHUMACHER HR: Apatite crystals in joint fluid; clinical relevance and search for a simple and accurate diagnostic test. Rheumatol Rev 3, 1994

ROSENTHAL AK, RYAN LM: Treatment of refractory crystal-associated arthritis. Rheum Dis Clin North Am 21:151, 1995

SIMKIN PA: Oxalate crystals and the taxonomy of gout. JAMA 260:1285, 1988

FIGURE 323-3   Bipyramidal and small polymorphic calcium oxalate crystals (ordinary light microscopy; 400×).

324   *Scott J. Thaler, James H. Maguire*

INFECTIOUS ARTHRITIS

INTRODUCTION AND APPROACH TO THE PATIENT
While *Staphylococcus aureus*, *Neisseria gonorrhoeae*, and other bacteria are the most common causes of infectious arthritis, various mycobacteria, spirochetes, fungi, and viruses also infect joints. Since acute bacterial infection can rapidly destroy articular cartilage, all inflamed joints must be evaluated without delay to exclude noninfectious processes and to determine appropriate antimicrobial therapy and drainage procedures. For more detailed information on infectious arthritis due to specific organisms, the reader is referred to the chapters on those organisms.

Acute bacterial infection typically involves a single joint or a few joints. Subacute or chronic monarthritis or oligoarthritis suggests mycobacterial or fungal infection; episodic inflammation is seen in syphilis, Lyme disease, and the reactive arthritis that follows enteric infections and chlamydial urethritis (Table 324-1). Acute polyarticular inflammation occurs as an immunologic reaction during the course of endocarditis, rheumatic fever, disseminated neisserial infection, and acute hepatitis B. Bacteria and viruses occasionally infect multiple joints, the former most commonly in persons with rheumatoid arthritis.

Aspiration of synovial fluid, an essential element in the evaluation of potentially infected joints, can be performed without difficulty in most cases by the insertion of a large-bore needle into the site of maximal fluctuation or tenderness or by the route of easiest access. Ultrasonography or fluoroscopy may be used to guide aspiration of difficult-to-localize effusions of the hip and, occasionally, the shoulder and other joints. Normal synovial fluid contains fewer than 180 cells (predominantly mononuclear cells) per microliter. Synovial cell counts averaging 100,000/μL (range, 25,000 to 250,000/μL), with more than 90 percent neutrophils, are characteristic of acute bacterial infections. Crystal-induced, rheumatoid, and other noninfectious inflammatory arthritides are usually associated with fewer than 30,000 to 50,000 cells/μL; cell counts of 10,000 to 30,000/μL, with 50 to 70 percent neutrophils and the remainder lymphocytes, are common in mycobacterial and fungal infections. Definitive diagnosis of an infectious process relies on identification of the pathogen in stained smears of synovial fluid, isolation of the pathogen from cultures of synovial fluid and blood, or detection of microbial nucleic acids and proteins by polymerase chain reaction (PCR)–based assays and immunologic techniques.

ACUTE BACTERIAL ARTHRITIS **Pathogenesis** Bacteria enter the joint from the bloodstream, from a contiguous site of infection in bone or soft tissue, or by direct inoculation during surgery, injection, or trauma. In hematogenous infection, bacteria escape from synovial capillaries, which have no limiting basement membrane, and within hours provoke neutrophilic infiltration of the synovium. Neutrophils and bacteria enter the lumen of the joint; later, bacteria adhere to articular cartilage. Degradation of cartilage begins within 48 h as a result of increased intraarticular pressure, release of proteases and cytokines from chondrocytes, and invasion of the cartilage by bacteria and inflammatory cells. Histologic studies reveal bacteria lining the synovium and cartilage as well as abscesses extending into the synovium, cartilage, and—in severe cases—subchondral bone. Synovial proliferation results in the formation of a pannus over the cartilage, and thrombosis of inflamed synovial vessels develops. Bacterial factors that appear important in the pathogenesis of infective arthritis include collagen receptors in *S. aureus* that permit adherence to cartilage and endotoxins that promote chondrocyte-mediated breakdown of cartilage.

Microbiology The hematogenous route of infection is the most common route in all age groups. In infants, group B streptococci, gram-negative enteric bacilli, and *S. aureus* are the usual pathogens. Since the advent of the *Haemophilus influenzae* vaccine, *S. aureus* and *Streptococcus pyogenes* (group A *Streptococcus*) have predominated in children less than 5 years of age. Among young adults and adolescents, *N. gonorrhoeae* is the most commonly implicated organism. *S. aureus* accounts for most nongonococcal isolates in adults of all ages; gram-negative bacilli, pneumococci, and group B and other streptococci are involved in up to one-third of cases in older adults, especially those with underlying comorbid illnesses.

Infections following surgical procedures or penetrating injuries are due most often to *S. aureus* and occasionally to other gram-positive bacteria or gram-negative bacilli. Infections with coagulase-negative staphylococci are unusual except after the implantation of prosthetic joints or arthroscopy. Anaerobic organisms, often in association with aerobic or facultative bacteria, are found after human bites and when decubitus ulcers or intraabdominal abscesses spread into adjacent joints. Polymicrobial infections complicate traumatic injuries with extensive contamination. Cat bites or scratches may introduce *Pasteurella multocida* into joints.

Nongonococcal Bacterial Arthritis *Epidemiology* Although hematogenous infections with virulent organisms such as *S. aureus*, *H. influenzae*, and pyogenic streptococci occur in healthy persons, there is an underlying host predisposition in many cases of septic arthritis. Patients with rheumatoid arthritis have the highest incidence of infective arthritis, most often secondary to *S. aureus*, because of chronically inflamed joints, glucocorticoid therapy, and frequent breakdown of rheumatoid nodules, vasculitic ulcers, and skin overlying deformed joints. Diabetes mellitus, glucocorticoid therapy, hemodialysis, and malignancy all carry an increased risk of infection with *S. aureus* and gram-negative bacilli. Pneumococcal infections complicate alcoholism, deficiencies of humoral immunity, and hemoglobinopathies. Intravenous drug users acquire staphylococcal and streptococcal infections from their own flora and acquire pseudomonal and other gram-negative infections from drugs and injection paraphernalia.

Clinical manifestations Ninety percent of patients present with involvement of a single joint: most commonly the knee, less frequently the hip, and still less often the shoulder, wrist, or elbow. Small joints of the hands and feet are more likely to be affected after direct inoculation or a bite. Among intravenous drug users, infections of the spine, sacroiliac joints, or sternoclavicular joints are more common than infections of the appendicular skeleton. Polyarticular infection is most common among patients with rheumatoid arthritis and may resemble a flare of the underlying disease.

The usual presentation consists of moderate to severe pain that is uniform around the joint, effusion, muscle spasm, and decreased range of motion. Fever in the range of 38.3 to 38.9°C (101 to 102°F) and sometimes higher is common but may be lacking, especially in persons with rheumatoid arthritis, renal or hepatic insufficiency, or conditions requiring immunosuppressive therapy. The inflamed, swollen joint is usually evident on examination except in the case of a deeply situated joint, such as the hip or the sacroiliac joint. Cellulitis, bursitis, and acute osteomyelitis, which may produce a similar clinical picture, should be distinguished from septic arthritis by their greater range of motion and less-than-circumferential swelling. A focus of extraarticular infection, such as a boil or pneumonia, should be sought. Peripheral-blood leukocytosis and a left shift are common findings.

Plain radiographs show evidence of soft tissue swelling, joint-space widening, and displacement of tissue planes by the distended capsule. Narrowing of the joint space and bony erosions indicate

Table 324-1

Differential Diagnosis of Arthritis Syndromes

Acute Monarticular Arthritis	Chronic Monarticular Arthritis	Polyarticular Arthritis
Staphylococcus aureus	*Mycobacterium tuberculosis*	*Neisseria meningitidis*
Streptococcus pneumoniae	Nontuberculous mycobacteria	*Neisseria gonorrhoeae*
β-Hemolytic streptococci	*Borrelia burgdorferi*	Nongonococcal bacterial arthritis
Gram-negative bacilli	*Treponema pallidum*	Bacterial endocarditis
Neisseria gonorrhoeae	*Candida* species	*Candida* species
Candida species	*Sporothrix schenckii*	Poncet's disease (tuberculous
Crystal-induced arthritis	*Coccidioides immitis*	rheumatism)
Fracture	*Blastomyces dermatitidis*	Hepatitis B virus
Hemarthrosis	*Aspergillus* species	Parvovirus B19
Foreign body	*Cryptococcus neoformans*	Human immunodeficiency virus
Osteoarthritis	*Nocardia* species	Human T lymphotropic virus
Ischemic necrosis	*Brucella* species	type I
Monarticular rheumatoid	Legg-Calvé-Perthes disease	Rubella virus
arthritis	Osteoarthritis	Sickle cell disease flare
		Reactive arthritis
		Serum sickness
		Acute rheumatic fever
		Inflammatory bowel disease
		Systemic lupus erythematosus
		Rheumatoid arthritis/Still's
		disease
		Other vasculitides
		Sarcoidosis

advanced infection and a poor prognosis. Ultrasound is useful for detecting effusions in the hip, and computed tomography or magnetic resonance imaging can demonstrate infections of the sacroiliac joint and the spine very well.

Laboratory findings Specimens of peripheral blood and synovial fluid should be obtained before antibiotics are administered. Blood cultures are positive in up to 50 percent of *S. aureus* infections but are less frequently positive in infections due to other organisms. The synovial fluid is turbid, serosanguineous, or frankly purulent. Gram-stained smears confirm the presence of large numbers of neutrophils. Levels of total protein and lactate dehydrogenase in synovial fluid are elevated, and the glucose level is depressed; however, measurement of these levels is not necessary to make the diagnosis. The synovial fluid should be examined for crystals, because gout and pseudogout can resemble septic arthritis clinically, and infection and crystal-induced disease occasionally occur together. Organisms are seen on synovial fluid smears in nearly three-quarters of infections with *S. aureus* and streptococci and in 30 to 50 percent of infections due to gram-negative and other bacteria. Cultures of synovial fluid are positive in more than 90 percent of cases. Inoculation of synovial fluid into bottles containing liquid media for blood cultures increases the yield of culture.

℞ TREATMENT

Prompt administration of systemic antibiotics and drainage of the involved joint can prevent destruction of cartilage, postinfectious degenerative arthritis, joint instability, or deformity. Once cultures of blood and synovial fluid have been obtained, empirical antibiotics should be given that are directed against bacteria visualized on smears or against the pathogens that are likely, given the patient's age and risk factors. Initial therapy should consist of the intravenous administration of bactericidal agents; direct instillation of antibiotics into the joint is not necessary to achieve adequate levels in synovial fluid and tissue. An intravenous combination of a third-generation cephalosporin such as cefotaxime (1 g every 8 h) or ceftriaxone (1 to 2 g every 24 h) and either oxacillin or nafcillin (2 g every 4 h) will provide adequate coverage for most infections in adults. Intravenous vancomycin (1 g every 12 h) should be given if methicillin-resistant *S. aureus* is a possible pathogen in a hospitalized patient. In addition, an aminoglycoside should be given to intravenous drug users or other patients in whom *Pseudomonas aeruginosa* may be the responsible agent.

Definitive therapy is based on the identity and antibiotic susceptibility of the bacteria isolated in culture. Infections due to staphylococci are treated with oxacillin, nafcillin, or vancomycin for 4 weeks. Pneumococcal and streptococcal infections due to penicillin-susceptible organisms respond to 2 weeks of therapy with penicillin G (2 million units intravenously every 4 h); infections caused by *H. influenzae* and by strains of *S. pneumoniae* that are resistant to penicillin are treated with cefotaxime or ceftriaxone for 2 weeks. Most enteric gram-negative infections can be cured in 3 to 4 weeks by a second- or third-generation cephalosporin given intravenously. *P. aeruginosa* infection should be treated with at least 3 weeks of combination therapy with an aminoglycoside plus either an extended-spectrum penicillin such as mezlocillin (3 g intravenously every 4 h) or an antipseudomonal cephalosporin such as ceftazidime (1 g intravenously every 8 h). If tolerated, this regimen is continued for an additional 2 to 3 weeks; alternatively, a fluoroquinolone such as ciprofloxacin (750 mg orally twice daily) is substituted for the aminoglycoside.

Timely drainage of pus and necrotic debris from the infected joint is required for a favorable outcome. Needle aspiration of readily accessible joints such as the knee may be adequate if loculations or particulate matter in the joint does not prevent its thorough decompression. Arthroscopic drainage and lavage may be employed initially or within several days if repeated needle aspiration fails to relieve symptoms, decrease the volume of the effusion and the synovial white cell count, and clear bacteria from smears and cul-

tures. In some cases, arthrotomy is necessary to remove loculations and debride infected synovium, cartilage, or bone. Septic arthritis of the hip is best managed with arthrotomy, particularly in young children, in whom infection threatens the viability of the femoral head. Septic joints do not require immobilization except for pain control before symptoms are alleviated by treatment. Weight bearing should be avoided until signs of inflammation have subsided, but frequent passive motion of the joint is indicated to maintain full mobility.

Gonococcal Arthritis *Epidemiology* Gonococcal arthritis, accounting for 70 percent of episodes of infectious arthritis in persons under 40 years of age, results from bacteremia arising from gonococcal infection or, more frequently, from asymptomatic gonococcal mucosal colonization of the urethra, cervix, or pharynx. Women are at greatest risk during menses and overall are two to three times more likely than men to develop disseminated gonococcal infection and arthritis. Persons with complement deficiencies, especially of the terminal components, are prone to recurrent episodes of gonococcemia. Strains of gonococci that are most likely to cause disseminated infection include those that produce transparent colonies in culture, have the type IA outer-membrane protein, or are of the AUH-auxotroph type.

Clinical manifestations and laboratory findings The most common manifestation of disseminated gonococcal infection is a syndrome of fever, chills, rash, and articular symptoms. Small numbers of papules that progress to hemorrhagic pustules develop on the trunk and the extensor surfaces of the distal extremities. Migratory arthritis and tenosynovitis of the knees, hands, wrists, feet, and ankles are prominent. The cutaneous lesions and articular findings are believed to be the consequence of an immune reaction to circulating gonococci and immune-complex deposition in tissues. Thus, cultures of synovial fluid are consistently negative, and blood cultures are positive in fewer than 45 percent of patients. Synovial fluid may be difficult to obtain from inflamed joints and usually contains only 10,000 to 20,000 leukocytes/μL.

True gonococcal septic arthritis is less common than the disseminated gonococcal infection syndrome and always follows disseminated infection, which is unrecognized in one-third of patients. A single joint, such as the hip, knee, ankle, or wrist, is usually involved. Synovial fluid that contains more than 50,000 leukocytes/μL can be obtained with ease; the gonococcus is only occasionally evident in gram-stained smears, and cultures of synovial fluid are positive in fewer than 40 percent of cases. Blood cultures are almost always negative.

Because it is difficult to isolate gonococci from synovial fluid and blood, specimens for culture should be obtained from potentially infected mucosal sites. Cultures and gram-stained smears of skin lesions occasionally are positive. All specimens for culture should be plated onto Thayer-Martin agar directly or in special transport media at the bedside and transferred promptly to the microbiology laboratory in an atmosphere of 5% CO_2, as generated in a candle jar. PCR-based assays are extremely sensitive in detecting gonococcal DNA in synovial fluid. A dramatic alleviation of symptoms within 12 to 24 h after the initiation of appropriate antibiotic therapy supports a clinical diagnosis of the disseminated gonococcal infection syndrome if cultures are negative.

℞ TREATMENT

Initial treatment consists of ceftriaxone (1 g intravenously or intramuscularly every 24 h) to cover possible penicillin-resistant organisms. Once local and systemic signs are clearly resolving, the 7-day course of therapy can be completed with an oral agent such as cefixime (400 mg twice daily) or ciprofloxacin (500 mg twice daily) or, if penicillin-susceptible organisms are isolated, amoxicillin (500 mg three times daily). Suppurative arthritis usually responds to needle aspiration of involved joints and 7 to 10 days of antibiotic treatment. Arthroscopic lavage or arthrotomy is rarely required.

It is noteworthy that arthritis symptoms similar to those seen in disseminated gonococcal infections occur in meningococcemia. A dermatitis-arthritis syndrome, purulent monarthritis, and reactive polyarthritis have been described. All respond to treatment with intravenous penicillin.

SPIROCHETAL ARTHRITIS   Lyme Disease   Lyme disease due to infection with the spirochete *Borrelia burgdorferi* causes arthritis in up to 70 percent of persons who are not treated. Intermittent arthralgias and myalgias, but not arthritis, occur within days or weeks of inoculation of the spirochete by the *Ixodes* tick. Later, there are three patterns of joint disease: (1) Fifty percent of untreated persons experience intermittent episodes of monarthritis or oligoarthritis involving the knee and/or other large joints. The symptoms wax and wane without treatment over months, and each year 10 to 20 percent of patients report loss of joint symptoms. (2) Twenty percent of untreated persons develop a pattern of waxing and waning arthralgias. (3) Ten percent of patients develop chronic inflammatory synovitis resulting in erosive lesions and destruction of the joint.

℞ **TREATMENT**

Lyme arthritis generally responds well to therapy. A regimen of oral doxycycline, oral amoxicillin plus probenecid, or parenteral ceftriaxone for a period of 3 to 4 weeks is recommended. Patients who do not respond to such a regimen are unlikely to benefit from additional therapy. Failure of therapy is associated with host features such as the HLA-DR4 genotype or persistent reactivity to OspA (outer surface protein A). New techniques using PCR amplification of spirochetal DNA may be useful in the monitoring of patients in whom conventional therapy fails. Patients who have negative results of synovial-fluid PCR and who fail to respond to initial therapy are highly unlikely to benefit from additional antimicrobial therapy.

Syphilitic Arthritis   Articular manifestations occur in different stages of syphilis. In early congenital syphilis, periarticular swelling and immobilization of the involved limbs (Parrot's pseudoparalysis) complicate osteochondritis of long bones. Clutton's joint, a late manifestation of congenital syphilis that typically develops between the ages of 8 and 15, is caused by chronic painless synovitis with effusions of large joints, particularly the knees and elbows. Secondary syphilis may be associated with arthralgias; symmetric arthritis of the knees and ankles and occasionally of the shoulders and wrists; and sacroiliitis. The arthritis follows a subacute to chronic course with a mixed mononuclear and neutrophilic synovial-fluid pleocytosis (typical cell counts, 5,000 to 15,000/μL). Immunologic mechanisms may contribute to the arthritis, and symptoms usually improve rapidly with penicillin therapy. In tertiary syphilis, Charcot's joint is a result of sensory loss due to tabes dorsalis. Penicillin is not helpful in this setting.

MYCOBACTERIAL ARTHRITIS   Tuberculous arthritis accounts for about 1 percent of all cases of tuberculosis and for 10 percent of extrapulmonary cases. The most common presentation is chronic granulomatous monarthritis. An unusual syndrome, Poncet's disease, is a reactive symmetric form of polyarthritis that affects persons with visceral or disseminated tuberculosis. No mycobacteria are found in the joints, and symptoms resolve with antituberculous therapy.

Unlike tuberculous osteomyelitis, which typically involves the thoracic and lumbar spine (50 percent of cases), tuberculous arthritis primarily involves the large weight-bearing joints, in particular the hips, knees, and ankles, and only occasionally involves smaller non-weight-bearing joints. Progressive monarticular swelling and pain develop over months to years, and systemic symptoms are seen in only half of all cases. Coexistent active pulmonary tuberculosis is unusual.

Aspiration of the involved joint yields fluid with an average cell count of 20,000/μL, with approximately 50 percent neutrophils. Acid-fast staining of the fluid yields positive results in fewer than one-third of cases, and cultures are positive in 80 percent. Culture of synovial tissue taken at biopsy is positive in about 90 percent of cases and shows granulomatous inflammation in most. Radiographs reveal peripheral erosions at the points of synovial attachment, periarticular osteopenia, and eventually joint-space narrowing. Therapy for tuberculous arthritis is the same as that for tuberculous pulmonary disease, requiring the administration of multiple agents for 6 to 9 months. Therapy is more prolonged in immunosuppressed individuals, such as those infected with human immunodeficiency virus (HIV).

Various atypical mycobacteria found in water and soil may cause chronic indolent arthritis. Such disease results from trauma and direct inoculation associated with farming, gardening, or aquatic activities. Smaller joints, such as the digits, wrists, and knees, are usually involved. Involvement of tendon sheaths and bursae is typical. The mycobacterial species involved include *M. marinum*, *M. avium-intracellulare*, *M. terrae*, *M. kansasii*, *M. fortuitum*, and *M. chelonae*. In persons who have HIV infection or are receiving immunosuppressive therapy, hematogenous spread to the joints has been reported for *M. kansasii*, *M. avium-intracellulare*, and *M. haemophilum*. Diagnosis usually requires biopsy and culture, and therapy is based on antimicrobial susceptibility patterns.

FUNGAL ARTHRITIS   Fungi are an unusual cause of chronic monarticular arthritis. Granulomatous articular infection with the endemic dimorphic fungi *Coccidioides immitis*, *Blastomyces dermatitidis*, and (less commonly) *Histoplasma capsulatum* results from hematogenous seeding or direct extension from bony lesions in persons with disseminated disease. Joint involvement is an unusual complication of sporotrichosis (infection with *Sporothrix schenckii*) among gardeners and other persons who work with soil or sphagnum moss. Articular sporotrichosis is six times more common among men than among women, and alcoholics and other debilitated hosts are at risk for polyarticular infection.

Candida infection involving a single joint, usually the knee, hip, or shoulder, results from surgical procedures, intraarticular injections, or (among critically ill patients with debilitating illnesses such as diabetes mellitus or hepatic or renal insufficiency and patients receiving immunosuppressive therapy) hematogenous spread. *Candida* infections in intravenous drug users typically involve the spine, sacroiliac joints, or other fibrocartilaginous joints. Unusual cases of arthritis due to *Aspergillus* species, *Cryptococcus neoformans*, *Pseudallescheria boydii*, and the dematiaceous fungi have also resulted from direct inoculation or disseminated hematogenous infection in immunocompromised persons.

The synovial fluid in fungal arthritis usually contains 10,000 to 40,000 cells/μL, with about 70 percent neutrophils. Stained specimens and cultures of synovial tissue often confirm the diagnosis of fungal arthritis when studies of synovial fluid give negative results. Treatment consists of drainage and lavage of the joint and systemic administration of amphotericin B, fluconazole, or itraconazole (the exact drug depending on the species involved). The doses and duration of therapy are the same as for disseminated disease. Intraarticular instillation of amphotericin B has been used in addition to intravenous therapy.

VIRAL ARTHRITIS   Viruses produce arthritis by infecting synovial tissue during systemic infection or by provoking an immunologic reaction that involves joints. As many as 50 percent of women report persistent arthralgias and 10 percent frank arthritis within 3 days of the rash that follows natural infection with *rubella virus* and within 2 to 6 weeks after receipt of live virus vaccine. Episodes of symmetric inflammation of fingers, wrists, and knees uncommonly recur for longer than a year, but a syndrome of chronic fatigue, low-grade fever, headaches, and myalgias can persist for months or years. Intravenous immunoglobulin has been helpful in selected cases. Self-limited monarticular or migratory polyarthritis may develop within 2 weeks of the parotitis of *mumps*; this sequela is more common in men than in women. Approximately 10 percent of children and 60 percent of women develop arthritis after infection with *parvovirus B19*. In adults, arthropathy sometimes occurs without fever or rash. Pain and stiffness, with less prominent swelling (primarily of the hands but also of the knees, wrists, and ankles), usually resolve within weeks, although a small proportion of women develop chronic arthropathy.

About 2 weeks before the onset of jaundice, up to 10 percent of persons with acute *hepatitis B* develop an immune complex–mediated, serum sickness–like reaction with maculopapular rash, urticaria, fever, and arthralgias. Less common developments include symmetric arthritis involving the hands, wrists, elbows, or ankles and morning stiffness that resembles a flare of rheumatoid arthritis. Symptoms resolve at the time jaundice develops. Painful arthritis involving larger joints often accompanies the fever and rash of several arthropod-borne viral infections, including those caused by *chikungunya, O'nyong-nyong, Ross River, Mayaro,* and *Barmah Forest* viruses. Symmetric arthritis involving the hands and wrists may occur during the convalescent phase of infection with *lymphocytic choriomeningitis virus.* Patients infected with an *enterovirus* frequently report arthralgias, and *echovirus* has been isolated from patients with acute polyarthritis.

Several arthritis syndromes are associated with *HIV* infection. Reiter's syndrome with persistent, painful, lower-extremity oligoarthritis often follows an episode of urethritis in HIV-infected persons. HIV-associated Reiter's syndrome appears to be extremely common among persons with the HLA-B27 haplotype, but sacroiliac joint disease is unusual. Up to one-third of HIV-infected persons with psoriasis develop psoriatic arthritis. Painless monarthropathy and persistent symmetric polyarthropathy occasionally complicate HIV infection. Chronic persistent oligoarthritis of the shoulders, wrists, hands, and knees occurs in women infected with human T-lymphotropic virus type I. Synovial thickening, destruction of articular cartilage, and leukemic-appearing atypical lymphocytes in synovial fluid are characteristic, but progression to T cell leukemia is unusual.

PARASITIC ARTHRITIS Arthritis due to parasitic infection is rare. The guinea worm *Dracunculus medinensis* may cause destructive joint lesions in the lower extremities as migrating gravid female worms invade joints or cause ulcers in adjacent soft tissues that become secondarily infected. Hydatid cysts infect bones in 1 to 2 percent of cases of infection with *Echinococcus granulosus.* The expanding destructive cystic lesions may spread to and destroy adjacent joints, particularly the hip and pelvis. In rare cases, chronic synovitis has been associated with the presence of schistosomal eggs in synovial biopsies. Monarticular arthritis in children with lymphatic *filariasis* appears to respond to therapy with diethylcarbamazine despite the absence of microfilariae in synovial fluid. Reactive arthritis has been attributed to *hookworm, Strongyloides, Cryptosporidium,* and *Giardia* infection in case reports, but confirmation is required.

REACTIVE ARTHRITIS OR REITER'S SYNDROME A syndrome of reactive arthritis associated with rash, urethritis, conjunctivitis, uveitis, and oral ulcers develops several weeks after approximately 1 percent of cases of nongonococcal urethritis and 2 percent of enteric infections, particularly with those due to *Yersinia enterocolitica, Shigella flexneri, Campylobacter jejuni,* and *Salmonella* species. Studies have identified microbial DNA or antigen in synovial fluid or blood in some cases, but the pathogenesis of this condition is poorly understood.

Reactive arthritis is most common among young men (except after *Yersinia* infection) and has been linked to the HLA-B27 locus as a potential genetic predisposing factor. Patients report painful, asymmetric oligoarthritis affecting mainly the knees, ankles, and feet. Low-back pain is common, and radiographic evidence of sacroiliitis is found in patients with long-standing disease. Most patients recover within 6 months, but prolonged recurrent disease is more common in cases following nongonococcal urethritis. Anti-inflammatory agents help to relieve symptoms, but the role of prolonged antibiotic therapy in eliminating microbial antigen from the synovium is controversial.

INFECTIONS IN PROSTHETIC JOINTS Infection complicates 1 to 4 percent of total joint replacements. The majority of infections are acquired intraoperatively or immediately postoperatively as a result of wound breakdown or infection; less commonly, these joint infections develop later after joint replacement and are the result of hematogenous spread or direct inoculation. The presentation may be acute, with fever, pain, and local signs of inflammation, especially in infections due to *S. aureus,* pyogenic streptococci, and enteric bacilli. Alternatively, infection may persist for months or years without causing constitutional symptoms when less virulent organisms, such as coagulase-negative staphylococci or diphtheroids, are involved. Such indolent infections are usually acquired during joint implantation and are discovered during evaluation of chronic unexplained pain or after a radiograph shows loosening of the prosthesis; the erythrocyte sedimentation rate is usually elevated in such cases.

The diagnosis is best made by needle aspiration of the joint; accidental introduction of organisms during aspiration must be meticulously avoided. Synovial fluid pleocytosis with a predominance of polymorphonuclear leukocytes is highly suggestive of infection, since other inflammatory processes uncommonly affect prosthetic joints. Culture and Gram's stain usually yield the responsible pathogen. Use of special media for unusual pathogens such as fungi, atypical mycobacteria, and *Mycoplasma* may be necessary if routine and anaerobic cultures are negative.

℞ TREATMENT

Treatment includes surgery and high doses of parenteral antibiotics, which are given for 4 to 6 weeks because bone is usually involved. In most cases, the prosthesis must be replaced to cure the infection. Implantation of a new prosthesis is best delayed for several weeks or months because relapses of infection occur most commonly within this time frame. In some cases, reimplantation is not possible, and the patient must manage without a joint, with a fused joint, or even with amputation. Cure of infection without removal of the prosthesis is occasionally possible in cases that are due to streptococci or pneumococci and that lack radiologic evidence of loosening of the prosthesis. In these cases, antibiotic therapy must be initiated within several days of the onset of infection, and the joint should be drained vigorously either by open arthrotomy or arthroscopically.

Prevention To avoid the disastrous consequences of infection, candidates for joint replacement should be selected with care. Rates of infection are particularly high among patients with rheumatoid arthritis, persons who have undergone previous surgery on the joint, and persons with medical conditions requiring immunosuppressive therapy. Perioperative antibiotic prophylaxis, usually with cefazolin, and measures to decrease intraoperative contamination, such as laminar flow, have lowered the rates of perioperative infection to <1 percent in many centers. After implantation, measures should be taken to prevent and rapidly treat extraarticular infections that might give rise to hematogenous spread to the prosthesis. The effectiveness of prophylactic antibiotics for the prevention of hematogenous infection following dental procedures has not been demonstrated; in fact, viridans streptococci and other components of the oral flora are extremely unusual causes of prosthetic joint infection.

BIBLIOGRAPHY

Baker DG, Schumacher HR: Acute monoarthritis. N Engl J Med 329:1013, 1993

Brower AC: Septic arthritis. Radiol Clin North Am 34:293, 1996

Calabrese LH: Human immunodeficiency virus (HIV) infection and arthritis. Rheum Dis Clin North Am 19:477, 1993

Cuckler JM et al: Diagnosis and management of the infected total joint arthroplasty. Orthop Clin North Am 22:523, 1991

Cunningham R et al: Clinical and molecular aspects of the pathogenesis of *Staphylococcus aureus* bone and joint infections. J Med Microbiol 44:157, 1996

Eustace SJ et al: Lyme arthropathy. Radiol Clin North Am 34:454, 1996

Evans J: Lyme disease. Curr Opin Rheumatol 7:322, 1995

Gardner GC, Weisman MH: Pyarthrosis in patients with rheumatoid arthritis: A report of 13 cases and a review of the literature from the past 40 years. Am J Med 88:503, 1990

Goldenberg DL: Bacterial arthritis. Curr Opin Rheumatol 7:310, 1995

———, Reed JI: Bacterial arthritis. N Engl J Med 312:764, 1985

Hughes RA, Keat AC: Reiter's syndrome and reactive arthritis: A current view. Semin Arthritis Rheum 24:190, 1994

Keat A: Reiter's syndrome and reactive arthritis in perspective. N Engl J Med 309:1606, 1983

Liebling MR et al: Identification of *Neisseria gonorrhoeae* in synovial fluid using the polymerase chain reaction. Arthritis Rheum 37:702, 1994

Meier JL, Beekmann SE: Mycobacterial and fungal infections of bones and joints. Curr Opin Rheumatol 7:329, 1995

Mitchell LA et al: Chronic rubella vaccine-associated arthropathy. Arch Intern Med 153:2268, 1993

MURADALI D et al: Multifocal osteoarticular tuberculosis: Report of four cases and review of management. Clin Infect Dis 17:204, 1993

PINALS RS: Polyarthritis and fever. N Engl J Med 330:769, 1994

PURVIS RS et al: Sporotrichosis presenting as arthritis and subcutaneous nodules. J Am Acad Dermatol 28:879, 1993

REGINATO AJ: Syphilitic arthritis and osteitis. Rheum Dis Clin North Am 19:379, 1993

SHMERLING R et al: Synovial fluid tests: What should be ordered? JAMA 264:1009, 1990

SILVEIRA LH et al: *Candida* arthritis. Rheum Dis Clin North Am 19:427, 1993

TSUKAYAMA DT et al: Infection after total hip arthroplasty. A study of the treatment of one hundred and six infections. J Bone Joint Surg [Am] 78A:512, 1996

WISE CM et al: Gonococcal arthritis in an era of increasing penicillin resistance. Arch Intern Med 154:2690, 1994

325   *Peter H. Schur*

PSORIATIC ARTHRITIS AND ARTHRITIS ASSOCIATED WITH GASTROINTESTINAL DISEASE

PSORIATIC ARTHRITIS

Psoriatic arthritis (PsA) is a chronic inflammatory arthritis that affects 5 to 42 percent of people with psoriasis.

ETIOLOGY AND PATHOGENESIS   To date, the cause and pathogenesis of PsA are unknown. Indirect evidence has suggested that infections, trauma, increased cellular immunity (e.g., to streptococci), decreased suppressor cell activation, immune complexes, complement activation, adhesion molecules, dendritic cells, keratinocytes, and abnormal fibroblast and polymorphonuclear leukocyte (PMN) function may each play a role. Polyarthritis has developed in patients with psoriasis and hepatitis treated with interferon α. Most studies have observed an increased frequency of HLA-B17, CW6, DQ2, and/or B27 in patients with psoriatic spondylitis, while B27, BW62, B38, B39, and DR7a have been noted in association with peripheral arthritis in different studies. Fulminant disease should make one suspect human immunodeficiency virus (HIV) disease (see Chap. 308).

CLINICAL MANIFESTATIONS   Three major types of psoriatic arthritis are generally recognized: asymmetric inflammatory arthritis, symmetric arthritis, and psoriatic spondylitis. A mean of 47 percent of patients (range, 16 to 70 percent) have an asymmetric inflammatory arthritis. Disease appears equally in men and women. Psoriasis tends to precede the arthritis by years, although many patients complain of morning stiffness. The proximal interphalangeal (PIP) and distal interphalangeal (DIP) joints are commonly involved [with characteristic sausage-shaped digits (dactylitis)], while knees, hips, ankles, temporomandibular joints, and wrists are less frequently involved. Most patients have onychodystrophy (onycholysis, ridging and pitting of nails), the course of which does not parallel that of the synovitis. The prognosis is good, with only one-fourth of the patients developing progressive destructive disease; one-third develop inflammatory ocular complications (conjunctivitis, iritis, episcleritis).

A mean of 25 percent of patients (range, 15 to 39 percent) develop symmetric arthritis resembling rheumatoid arthritis (see Chap. 313). This disease occurs twice as frequently in women. Psoriasis and inflammatory arthritis usually develop simultaneously; most patients experience morning stiffness. The DIP, PIP, metacarpophalangeal (MCP), metatarsophalangeal (MTP), sternoclavicular, and, in particular, large peripheral joints are involved. Practically all patients have onychodystrophy, which helps distinguish them from patients with rheumatoid arthritis. Over half of the patients in this group go on to develop destructive arthritis, including arthritis mutilans. Eye complications are uncommon. Subcutaneous nodules are not present, but one-fourth of patients have rheumatoid factors. Unilateral upper limb edema has been described.

A mean of 23 percent of the patients (range 5 to 40 percent) have psoriatic "spondylitis," with or without peripheral joint involvement. Psoriasis tends to precede the arthritis by a few years, and low back pain with morning stiffness is common. Psoriatic spondylitis is more common in men. About half the patients in this group have spondylitis and the other half have sacroiliitis. The back disease is usually slowly progressive, with little clinical deterioration as compared with ankylosing spondylitis; the peripheral disease also tends not to be destructive except for the occasional patient with arthritis mutilans. Enthesopathy, i.e., inflammation of tendons and ligamentous attachments to bone, is characteristic, viz., of the tendo Achillis, or of the plantar fascia causing heel pain. Many patients have onychodystrophy, but few have inflammatory ocular complications. Gut inflammation occurs in 30 percent (no gut inflammation was noted in patients with only peripheral arthritis).

Some authors have described additional subsets of psoriatic arthritis: predominant DIP joint involvement, arthritis mutilans, juvenile psoriatic arthritis, and SAPHO (synovitis, acne, pustulosis, hyperostosis, osteomyelitis).

The pathology of PsA is similar to that seen in rheumatoid arthritis: synoviocytic hyperplasia, early PMN infiltration and later mononuclear cell infiltration, cartilage erosion, and pannus formation. However, in PsA, the synovium is more vascular and there are fewer macrophages and less expression of endothelial cell leukocyte adhesion molecule-1 (ELAM-1). Skin lesions have more CD45RO+ cells in psoriasis. Fibrosis of the joint capsule and marrow is prominent in many patients.

LABORATORY FINDINGS   There are a few laboratory abnormalities. Elevated erythrocyte sedimentation rates, C-reactive proteins, and complement levels reflect inflammation. Rheumatoid factors are uncommon and are more likely to be observed in those with symmetric arthritis. Immunoglobulin levels, especially IgA levels, may be elevated (IgA antibodies to cytokeratins and antienterobacteria antibodies are elevated). Uric acid levels may be elevated; sodium urate crystals in joint fluids suggest gout.

Radiologic investigation reveals findings similar to those of rheumatoid arthritis: soft tissue swelling, loss of the cartilage space, erosions, bony ankylosis of fingers, subluxations, and subchondral cysts; there is less demineralization, however. However, more unique and suggestive of psoriatic arthritis are erosions at DIP joints, expansion of the base of the terminal phalanx, tapering of the proximal phalanx and cuplike erosions of and bony proliferation of the distal terminal phalanx ("pencil-in-cup" appearance), proliferation of bone near osseous erosions, terminal phalangeal osteolysis, bone proliferation and periostitis (especially of phalanges), and telescoping of one bone into its neighbor, leading to the "opera-glass" deformity. The axial skeleton shows asymmetric or unilateral sacroiliitis, often asymptomatic paravertebral ossification, including cervical involvement, and large asymmetric nonmarginal syndesmophytes. Echocardiographic abnormalities resemble those of ankylosing spondilitis.

DIAGNOSIS   The diagnosis of psoriatic arthritis should be considered in individuals with arthritis and psoriasis. Psoriasis should be distinguished from seborrheic dermatitis and eczema. Psoriatic lesions may be quite small peripherally and often are hidden in the scalp, umbilicus, and gluteal folds. Fungal infection of nails can be distinguished from psoriasis, for the latter will demonstrate pitting and onycholysis. Furthermore, onychodystrophy is uncommon (20 percent of cases) in uncomplicated psoriasis. It is often difficult to distinguish Reiter's syndrome (see Chap. 317) from psoriatic arthritis, since both manifest dactylitis. Reiter's syndrome usually presents in younger individuals, especially males, is less frequently progressive or destructive and is more likely to be associated with characteristic skin lesions (keratoderma blenorrhagica), urethritis, and conjunctivitis. Gout can be distinguished by the presence of intraarticular sodium urate crystals (see Chap. 344). Psoriasis in association with Heberden's nodes or Bouchard's nodes of the DIP and PIP joints, respectively, rather suggests osteoarthritis (see Chap. 322). Psoriatic arthritis differs from rheumatoid arthritis by the relative lack of rheumatoid factors; the tendency to asymmetry, dactylitis, iritis, enthesopathy, and onychodystrophy; the high frequency of HLA-B27, especially in patients with axial skeletal involvement; and characteristic radiologic features.

℞ TREATMENT

The treatment of psoriatic arthritis begins with patient education and physical and occupational therapy to maintain muscle strength and joint and muscle function. Orthotics and occasional intraarticular glucocorticoids for isolated acutely and severely inflamed joints may be added as needed (Fig. 325-1). The mainstay, however, is the use of nonsteroidal anti-inflammatory drugs (NSAIDs), which reduce inflammation and alleviate pain for most patients. For patients with more severe involvement, a disease-modifying antirheumatic drug should be used. While hydroxychloroquine is often successful in producing either amelioration or remission, it carries a significant risk of exacerbation of psoriasis and exfoliation. For more severe cases, especially with extensive skin involvement, 5 to 25 mg methotrexate per week is recommended. Most patients respond well with respect to both skin lesions and arthritis. Patients who are resistant to oral therapy may respond to intravenous therapy. Folic acid (1 mg/d) is recommended to prevent hematologic complications. Renal and liver function tests and a complete blood count should be performed frequently, and any abnormalities should suggest modification of the dosage. Liver biopsies are recommended after a total of 1.5 g methotrexate have been given and then every 2 years to identify the rare patient with fibrosis and cirrhosis, which necessitate withdrawal of the drug. Increased serum levels of the N-terminal propeptide of type III procollagen may predict liver fibrogenesis. However, patients are advised to avoid nephrotoxic and hepatotoxic (e.g., ethanol) drugs. Patients with HIV infection may have worsening of their disease when treated with methotrexate. Sulfasalazine (3 to 4 g/d), intramuscular gold, cyclosporine (2 to 5 mg/kg per day), etretinate (0.5 mg/kg per day), 6-mercaptopurine, and azathioprine have also proved successful. The arthritis may also respond to heliotherapy.

ARTHRITIS ASSOCIATED WITH GASTROINTESTINAL DISEASE

INFLAMMATORY BOWEL DISEASE Peripheral arthritis occurs in 9 to 22 percent of patients with inflammatory bowel disease (IBD) (e.g., ulcerative colitis or Crohn's disease; see Chap. 286), and arthralgia is more common. Arthritis is somewhat more likely to occur in patients with large-bowel disease and in those patients with complications such as abscesses, pseudomembranous polyposis, perianal disease, massive hemorrhage, erythema nodosum, stomatitis, uveitis, and pyoderma gangrenosum. Males and females are affected equally. The arthritis tends to be acute, is associated with a flare-up of the bowel disease, occurs early in the course of the bowel disease, is self-limiting (90 percent of cases resolve within 6 months), and does not result in destruction. Most patients have a symmetric, migratory polyarthritis affecting primarily large joints of the lower extremity. Rheumatoid factors are not present. There is some association with HLA-BW62. Synovial fluids have 5000 to 12,000 white blood cells per microliter, mostly PMNs. Radiographs demonstrate soft tissue swelling and effusions without erosions or destruction. Pathologic examination of synovial biopsy specimens reveals only nonspecific inflammation. The peripheral arthritis responds to successful treatment of the bowel disease, such as colectomy (for ulcerative colitis), or administration of glucocorticoids, methotrexate, or sulfasalazine. NSAIDs relieve pain and inflammation but should be used with caution because of possible gastrointestinal side effects.

Spondylitis occurs in 1.1 to 43 percent of patients with IBD (while IBD develops in 5 percent of patients with ankylosing spondylitis). Spondylitis often precedes IBD; their clinical courses are unrelated.

FIGURE 325-1 Algorithm for the treatment of psoriatic arthritis. See text for detailed description. NSAID, non-steroidal anti-inflammatory drugs; CBC, complete blood count; UA, urinalysis; LFTs, liver function tests.

Males are affected more frequently. Patients typically complain of stiffness in the back and/or buttocks in the morning or after rest. The stiffness and associated pain are often relieved by exercise. Gastrointestinal infection/inflammation is thought to play a role in exacerbation of spondylitis. Physical examination reveals limitation of spinal flexion and reduced chest expansion. Some patients may have peripheral arthritis, especially of the hips and/or shoulders. Iritis is a frequent complication. Radiographs of the back show the typical findings of ankylosing spondylitis and bilateral sacroiliitis. HLA-B27 is found in 53 to 75 percent of these patients. Treatment includes physical therapy, NSAIDs, glucocorticoids for the bowel disease, and sulfasalazine. NSAIDs should be used with caution lest they exacerbate the IBD. The axial disease progresses slowly in a manner akin to that of ankylosing spondylitis.

Asymptomatic sacroiliitis detected by radiography occurs in 4 to 25 percent of patients with IBD. By contrast, 52 percent of patients with IBD have abnormalities on technetium pyrophosphate bone scans of the sacroiliac joint. There is no increased frequency of HLA-B27 in these patients. This "disease" does not necessarily progress to spondylitis.

Other complications of chronic IBD include (1) finger clubbing (observed in 4 to 13 percent of patients with Crohn's disease, especially those with small-bowel involvement), which may regress after surgery; (2) development of amyloid, especially in association with Crohn's disease; and (3) osteoporosis resulting from inactivity, malabsorption, and/or treatment with glucocorticoids. Osteomalacia can result from malabsorption. In this setting, with acutely increased back pain, one should suspect compression fracture.

INTESTINAL BYPASS ARTHRITIS Intestinal bypass surgery was developed for the treatment of obesity in 1952; 11 years later arthritis was recognized as a postoperative complication. Polyarthralgia and sometimes arthritis occur weeks, even years, after surgery in 8 to 36 percent of patients. Tenosynovitis is common, with episodes sometimes lasting for days and even months; it tends to affect the knee, wrist, ankle, shoulder, and finger joints and cause pain in the neck and back. This syndrome occurs more often after jejunocolic than after jejunoileal surgery and more often in females than in males. There is often an associated urticarial, vesicular, pustular, macular, or nodular eruption. Raynaud's symptoms appear in one-third of patients. X-rays generally show no joint damage, except marginal erosions in patients with persistent arthritis. Synovial fluids generally have white blood cell counts of 500 to 27,000 cells/μL, mostly PMNs. Synovial biopsy specimens show chronic synovitis with lymphocytes but without lymphoid follicles. Tests for rheumatoid factors, antinuclear antibodies, and HLA-B27 are usually negative, while immune complexes (and cryoglobulins) are often present. They contain bacterial antigens, the corresponding antibodies, IgA secretory component, and various complement components. These observations suggest that the syndrome has the following pathogenesis: Bacteria proliferate in intestinal blind loops; bacterial antigens are absorbed; and antibodies to these antigens develop and combine with them to form immune complexes, which deposit in synovial tissue to cause arthritis. NSAIDs and glucocorticoids can relieve the joint symptoms, but more lasting results can be achieved by tetracycline therapy to decrease the bacterial load; even better is reanastomosis of the bowel or resection of the blind loop.

WHIPPLE'S DISEASE (INTESTINAL LIPODYSTROPHY)

Whipple's disease is rare and occurs mostly in middle-aged Caucasian males, who develop arthritis, prolonged diarrhea, malabsorption, and weight loss. Up to 90 percent of patients with the disease develop arthritis, usually prior to other symptoms. Knees and ankles and, to a lesser extent, fingers, hips, shoulders, elbows, and wrists are involved. The arthritis is acute in onset, migratory, usually lasts just a few days, and is rarely chronic or a cause of permanent joint damage. Associated symptoms may include fever (54 percent), edema, serositis (pleurisy, pericarditis, endocarditis), pneumonia, hypotension, lymphadenopathy (54 percent), hyperpigmentation (54 percent), subcutaneous nodules, clubbing, and uveitis. Central nervous system involvement may develop (43 percent), with loss of memory, confusion, depression, headache, diplopia, and papilledema, and may be appreciated by abnormalities in magnetic resonance images of the brain. Laboratory abnormalities include anemia (75 percent), low serum levels of carotene (95 percent), and albumin (93 percent). The presence of HLA-B27 (8 to 30 percent) occurs in those patients with axial arthritis. Synovial fluids have been reported to contain 450 to 36,000 white blood cells per microliter (30 to 95 percent neutrophils) or a mild monocytosis. Joint x-rays rarely show erosions but may show a sacroiliitis in the occasional patients who have axial skeletal symptoms; abdominal computed tomographic scans may reveal lymphadenopathy. The lamina propria and/or foamy macrophages in small intestine contain PAS-staining bacterial remnants, presumably of *Tropheryma whippelii* or related bacteria. Diagnosis is often established by polymerase chain reaction (PCR) of the 165 ribosomal gene sequences of these bacteria. These inclusion-containing foamy macrophages also have been detected in the synovium, lymph nodes, and other tissues. The syndrome responds best to long-term therapy with trimethoprim-sulfamethoxazole. However, CNS relapse may develop, which has been treated with cefixime.

REACTIVE ARTHRITIS A Reiter's-like syndrome of arthritis can develop 2 to 3 weeks following diarrhea caused by *Shigella*, *Salmonella*, *Yersinia*, *Chlamydia trachomatis*, or *Campylobacter* organisms. → *This condition is described in Chap. 289.*

BIBLIOGRAPHY

BRUCKLE W et al: Treatment of psoriatic arthritis with auranofin and gold sodium thiomalate. Clin Rheumatol 13:209, 1994

DOUGADOS M et al: Sulfasalazine in the treatment of spondylarthropathy. A randomized multicenter, double-blind, placebo-controlled study. Arthritis Rheum 38:618, 1995

ESPINOZA LR et al: Psoriatic arthritis: Clinical response and side effects to methotrexate therapy. J Rheumatol 19:872, 1992

GLADMAN DD: Natural history of psoriatic arthritis. Baillieres Clin Rheumatol 8:379, 1994

———, FAREWELL VT: The role of HLA antigens as indicators of disease progression in psoriatic arthritis. Multivariate relative risk model. Arthritis Rheum 38:845, 1995

——— et al: Clinical and radiological progression in psoriatic arthritis. J Rheumatol 17:809, 1990

GOUPILLE P et al: Treatment of psoriatic arthritis. Semin Arthritis Rheum 21:355, 1992

HELLIWELL P et al: A re-evaluation of the osteoarticular manifestations of psoriasis. Br J Rheumatol 30:339, 1991

KAHN MF, CHAMOT AM: SAPHO syndrome. Rheum Dis Clin North Am 18:225, 1992

LEIRISALO-REPO M, REPO H: Gut and spondyloarthropathies. Rheum Dis Clin North Am 18:23, 1992

MAHRLE G et al: Low-dose short-term cyclosporine versus etretinate in psoriasis: Improvement of skin, nail, and joint involvement. J Am Acad Dermatol 32:78, 1995

PANAYI GS: Immunology of psoriasis and psoriatic arthritis. Baillieres Clin Rheumatol 8:419, 1994

PORTER GG: Psoriatic arthritis. Plain radiology and other imaging techniques. Baillieres Clin Rheumatol 8:465, 1994

SNELLMAN E et al: Effect of heliotherapy on skin and joint symptoms in psoriasis. A 6-month follow-up study. Br J Dermatol 128:172, 1993

TROUGHTON PR, MORGAN AW: Laboratory findings and pathology of psoriatic arthritis. Baillieres Clin Rheumatol 8:439, 1994

VEALE D et al: Classification of clinical subsets in psoriatic arthritis. Br J Rheumatol 33:133, 1994

WHITING-O'KEEFE QE et al: Methotrexate and histologic hepatic abnormalities: A meta-analysis. Am J Med 90:711, 1991

---

326 *Bruce C. Gilliland*

RELAPSING POLYCHONDRITIS AND OTHER ARTHRITIDES

RELAPSING POLYCHONDRITIS

Relapsing polychondritis is an episodic and often progressive inflammatory disorder of unknown cause affecting predominantly the cartilage of the ears, nose, and tracheobronchial tree, as well as internal structures of the eyes and ears. Other manifestations include polyarthritis, vasculitis, cardiac abnormalities, skin lesions, and glomerulonephritis. It is most common between the ages of 40 to 60 years but may affect children and the elderly. Relapsing polychondritis is an uncommon disorder which has been found in all races. Both sexes are equally affected, and no familial tendency is apparent. Approximately 30 percent of patients with relapsing polychondritis will have another rheumatologic disorder, the most frequent being systemic vasculitis, followed by rheumatoid arthritis, systemic lupus erythematosus, or Sjögren's syndrome. A significantly higher frequency of HLA-DR4 has been found in patients with relapsing polychondritis than in normal individuals. A predominant subtype of HLA-DR4 was not found, as has been the experience in patients with rheumatoid arthritis who are HLA-DR4 positive.

PATHOLOGY AND PATHOPHYSIOLOGY The earliest abnormality of cartilage noted histologically is a focal or diffuse loss of basophilic staining indicating depletion of proteoglycan from the cartilage matrix. Inflammatory infiltrates are found adjacent to involved cartilage and consist predominantly of mononuclear cells and occasional plasma cells. In acute disease, polymorphonuclear white cells also may be present. Destruction of cartilage begins at the outer edges and advances centrally. There is lacunar breakdown and loss of chondrocytes. Degenerating cartilage is replaced by granulation tissue and later by fibrosis and focal areas of calcification. Small loci of cartilage regeneration may be present. Immunofluorescence studies have shown immunoglobulins and complement at sites of involvement. Fine granular material observed in the degenerating cartilage matrix by electron microscopy has been interpreted to be enzymes or immunoglobulins.

Immunologic mechanisms play a role in the pathogenesis of relapsing polychondritis. Immunoglobulin and complement deposits are found at sites of inflammation. In addition, antibodies to type II collagen and immune complexes are detected in the sera of some patients. The possibility that an immune response to type II collagen may be important in the pathogenesis is supported experimentally by the occurrence of auricular chondritis in rats immunized with type II collagen. Antibodies to type II collagen are found in the sera of these animals, and immune deposits are detected at sites of ear inflammation. Cell-mediated immunity also may be operative in causing tissue injury, since lymphocyte transformation can be demonstrated when lymphocytes of patients are exposed to cartilage extracts. Humoral and cellular immune responses to type IX and type XI collagen have been demonstrated in some patients.

Dissolution of cartilage matrix can be induced by the intravenous injection of crude papain, a proteolytic enzyme, into young rabbits, which results in collapse of their normally rigid ears within 4 h. Reconstitution of the matrix occurs in about 7 days. In relapsing polychondritis, loss of cartilage matrix also most likely results from action of proteolytic enzymes released from chondrocytes, polymorphonuclear white cells, and monocytes that have been activated by inflammatory mediators.

CLINICAL MANIFESTATIONS Auricular chondritis is the most frequent presenting manifestation of relapsing polychondritis in 40 percent of patients and eventually affects about 85 percent of patients (Table 326-1). Usually both ears are involved. Patients experience the sudden onset of pain, tenderness, and swelling of the cartilaginous portion of the ear. Earlobes are spared because they do not contain cartilage. The overlying skin has a beefy red or violaceous color. Prolonged or recurrent episodes result in a flabby or droopy ear. Swelling may close off the eustachian tube (causing otitis media) or the external auditory meatus, either of which can impair hearing. Inflammation of the internal auditory artery or its cochlear branch produces hearing loss, vertigo, ataxia, nausea, and vomiting. The cartilage of the nose becomes inflamed during the first or subsequent attacks. Approximately 50 percent of patients will eventually have nose involvement. Patients may experience nasal stuffiness, rhinorrhea, and epistaxis. The bridge of the nose becomes red, swollen, and tender and may collapse, producing a saddle deformity. In some patients, the saddle deformity develops insidiously without overt inflammation. Saddle nose is observed more frequently in younger patients, especially in women.

Arthritis is the presenting manifestation in relapsing polychondritis in approximately one-third of patients and may be present for several months before other features appear. Eventually, more than half the patients will have arthritis. The arthritis usually is asymmetric and oligo- or polyarticular, and involves both large and small peripheral joints. An episode of arthritis lasts from a few days to several weeks and resolves spontaneously without residual joint deformity. Attacks of arthritis may not be temporally related to other manifestations of relapsing polychondritis. The joints are warm, tender, and swollen. Joint fluid has been reported to be noninflammatory. In addition to peripheral joints, inflammation may involve the costochondral, sternomanubrial, and sternoclavicular cartilages. Destruction of these cartilages may result in a pectus excavatum deformity or even a flail anterior chest wall. Relapsing polychondritis may occur in patients with preexisting rheumatoid arthritis, Reiter's syndrome, psoriatic arthritis, or ankylosing spondylitis. Myelodysplastic syndrome has been reported in several patients with relapsing polychondritis.

Eye manifestations occur in more than half of patients and include conjunctivitis, episcleritis, scleritis, iritis, and keratitis. Ulceration and perforation of the cornea may occur and cause blindness. Other manifestations include eyelid and periorbital edema, proptosis, cataracts, optic neuritis, extraocular muscle palsies, retinal vasculitis, and renal vein occlusion.

Laryngotracheal involvement occurs in approximately 50 percent of patients. Symptoms include hoarseness, a nonproductive cough, and tenderness over the larynx and proximal trachea. Mucosal edema, strictures, and/or collapse of laryngeal or tracheal cartilage may cause stridor and life-threatening airway obstruction necessitating tracheostomy. Collapse of cartilage in bronchi leads to pneumonia and, when extensive, to respiratory insufficiency.

Aortic regurgitation occurs in about 5 percent of patients and is due to progressive dilation of the aortic ring or to destruction of the valve cusps. Mitral and other heart valves are less often affected. Other cardiac manifestations include pericarditis, myocarditis, and conduction abnormalities. Aneurysms of the proximal, thoracic, or abdominal aorta may occur and occasionally rupture.

Systemic vasculitis may occur in association with relapsing polychondritis. Vasculitides include leukocytoclastic vasculitis, polyarteritis, temporal arteritis, and Takayasu's arteritis (see Chap. 319). Neurologic abnormalities usually occur as a result of underlying vasculitis, manifesting as seizures, strokes, ataxia, and peripheral and cranial nerve neuropathies. Cranial nerves VI and VII are most often involved. Approximately 25 percent of patients have skin lesions, none of which are characteristic for relapsing polychondritis. These include purpura, erythema nodosum, erythema multiforme, angioedema/urticaria, livedo reticularis, and panniculitis. Segmental necrotizing glomerulonephritis with crescent formation has been noted in some patients in the absence of systemic vasculitis.

The course of disease is highly variable, with episodes lasting from a few days to several weeks and then subsiding spontaneously. In other patients, the disease has a chronic, smoldering course. In one study, the 5-year estimated survival rate was 74 percent and the 10-year survival rate 55 percent. In contrast to earlier series, only about half the deaths could be attributed to relapsing polychondritis or complications of treatment. Pulmonary complications accounted for only 10 percent of all fatalities. In general, patients with more widespread disease have a worse prognosis.

LABORATORY FINDINGS Mild leukocytosis and normocytic, normochromic anemia are often present. The erythrocyte sedimentation rate is usually elevated. Rheumatoid factor and antinuclear antibody tests are occasionally positive in low titers. Antibodies to type II collagen are present in most patients, but they are not specific. Circulating immune complexes may be detected, especially in patients with early active disease. Elevated levels of gamma globulin may be present. Antineutrophil cytoplasmic antibodies (ANCA), either cytoplasmic (C-ANCA) or perinuclear (P-ANCA), are found in some patients with active disease. The upper and lower airways can be evaluated by imaging techniques such as linear tomography, laryngotracheography, and computed tomography, and by bronchoscopy. Bronchography is performed to demonstrate bronchial narrowing. Intrathoracic airway obstruction also can be evaluated by inspiratory-expiratory flow studies. The chest film may show narrowing of the main bronchi, widening of the ascending or descending aorta due to an aneurysm, and cardiomegaly when aortic insufficiency is present. Radiographs may show calcification at previous sites of cartilage damage involving ear, nose, larynx, or trachea.

DIAGNOSIS Diagnosis is based on recognition of the typical clinical features. Biopsies of the involved cartilage from the ear, nose, or respiratory tract will confirm the diagnosis but are only necessary when clinical features are not typical. Patients with Wegener's granulomatosis may have a saddle nose and pulmonary involvement but can be distinguished by the absence of auricular involvement and the presence of granulomatous lesions in the tracheobronchial tree. Patients with Cogan's syndrome have interstitial keratitis and vestibular and auditory abnormalities, but this syndrome does not involve the respiratory tract or ears. Reiter's syndrome may initially resemble relapsing polychondritis because of oligoarticular arthritis and eye involvement, but it is distinguished in time by the appearance of

Table 326-1

Clinical Manifestations of Relapsing Polychondritis

	Frequency, %	
Clinical Feature	Presenting	Cumulative
Auricular chondritis	40	85
Hearing loss	10	30
Nasal chondritis	25	55
Saddle nose deformity	20	30
Ocular deformities	20	50
Respiratory disease	25	50
Arthritis	35	50
Aortic regurgitation	—	5
Vasculitis	3	10

SOURCE: Modified from Isaak et al.

urethritis and typical mucocutaneous lesions and the absence of nose or ear cartilage involvement. Rheumatoid arthritis may initially suggest relapsing polychondritis because of arthritis and eye inflammation. The arthritis in rheumatoid arthritis, however, is erosive and symmetric. In addition, rheumatoid factor titers are usually high compared with those in relapsing polychondritis. Bacterial infection of the pinna may be mistaken for relapsing polychondritis but differs by usually involving only one ear, including the earlobe. Auricular cartilage also may be damaged by trauma or frostbite.

Relapsing polychondritis may develop in patients with a variety of autoimmune disorders, including systemic lupus erythematosus, rheumatoid arthritis, Sjögren's syndrome, and vasculitis. In most cases, these disorders antedate the appearance of polychondritis, usually by months or years. It is likely that these patients have an immunologic abnormality that predisposes them to development of this group of autoimmune disorders.

℞ TREATMENT

In patients with active chondritis or associated vasculitis, prednisone, 40 to 60 mg/d, is often effective in suppressing disease activity; it is tapered gradually once disease is controlled. In some patients, prednisone can be stopped, while in others low doses in the range of 10 to 15 mg/d are required for continued suppression of disease. Immunosuppressive drugs such as cyclophosphamide or azathioprine should be reserved for patients who fail to respond to prednisone or who require high doses for control of disease activity. Dapsone and cyclosporine have been reported to be beneficial in a few patients. Patients with significant ocular inflammation often require intraocular steroids as well as high doses of prednisone. Heart valve replacement or repair of an aortic aneurysm may be necessary. In patients with obstructive subglottic disease, tracheostomy is required. Stents may be necessary in patients with tracheobronchial collapse.

OTHER ARTHRITIDES

NEUROPATHIC JOINT DISEASE   Neuropathic joint disease (Charcot's joint) is a severe form of osteoarthritis associated with loss of pain sensation, proprioception, or both. In addition, normal muscular reflexes that modulate joint movement are decreased. Without these protective mechanisms, joints are subjected to repeated trauma, resulting in progressive cartilage damage. The distribution of joint involvement depends on the underlying neurologic disorder (Table 326-2). In tabes dorsalis, knees, hips, and ankles are most commonly affected; in syringomyelia, the glenohumeral joint, elbow, and wrist; and in diabetes mellitus, the tarsal and tarsometatarsal joints. Resorption of metatarsals and phalanges is also seen in diabetic patients. In children, neuropathic joint disease is caused by congenital indifference to pain or meningomyelocele. Neuropathic joint disease is also observed in patients with amyloidosis and leprosy or following frequent repeated intraarticular glucocorticoid injections. The mechanism of injury in the latter situation is thought to be an analgesic effect of steroids leading to overuse of a previously damaged joint, which results in accelerated cartilage deterioration.

Neuropathic joint disease usually begins in a single joint and then progresses to involve other joints, depending on the underlying neurologic disorder. The involved joint progressively becomes enlarged from bony overgrowth and synovial effusion. Loose bodies may be palpated in the joint cavity. Joint instability, subluxation, and crepitus occur as the disease progresses. Charcot's joints may develop rapidly, and a totally disorganized joint with multiple bony fragments may evolve in a patient within weeks or months. The amount of pain

Table 326-2

Disorders Associated with Neuropathic Joint Disease

Diabetes mellitus	Amyloidosis
Tabes dorsalis	Leprosy
Meningomyelocele	Congenital indifference to pain
Syringomyelia	

experienced by the patient is less than would be anticipated based on the degree of joint involvement. Patients may experience sudden joint pain from intraarticular fractures of osteophytes or condyles. Initially, radiographs show early features of osteoarthritis followed subsequently by marked destructive and hypertrophic changes. Large, bizarre-shaped osteophytes and intraarticular bone fragments are observed. The radiographic findings of the diabetic Charcot's foot may be difficult to distinguish from those of osteomyelitis. Osteomyelitis is often suspected when the diabetic patient has an infected cutaneous ulcer on the foot. The Charcot's joint radiographically shows osteopenia, sharp cortical margins, and severe disruption and disorganization of the midtarsal and tarsometatarsal joints. In osteomyelitis, the bone margins are indistinct. The synovial fluid from a neuropathic joint is usually noninflammatory, may be bloody or xanthochromic, and may contain fragments of synovium, cartilage, and/or bone.

℞ TREATMENT

The primary focus of treatment is to provide stabilization of the joint. Treatment of the underlying disorder, even if successful, usually does not alter the joint disease. Braces and splints are helpful. Their use requires close surveillance, since patients may be unable to appreciate pressure from a poorly adjusted brace. In the diabetic patient, early recognition and treatment of a Charcot's foot by prohibiting weight bearing of the foot for at least 8 weeks may possibly prevent severe disease from developing. Fusion of a very unstable joint may improve function, but nonunion is frequent, especially when immobilization of the joint is inadequate.

HYPERTROPHIC OSTEOARTHROPATHY AND CLUBBING   Hypertrophic osteoarthropathy (HOA) is characterized by clubbing of digits and, in more advanced stages, by periosteal new bone formation and synovial effusions. HOA occurs in primary and familial forms and begins usually in childhood. The secondary form of HOA is associated with intrathoracic malignancies, suppurative lung disease, congenital heart disease, and a variety of other disorders and is more common in adults. Clubbing is almost always a feature of HOA but can occur as an isolated manifestation (Fig. 326-1). The presence of clubbing in isolation is generally considered to represent either an early stage or an element in the spectrum of HOA. The presence of only clubbing in a patient usually has the same clinical significance as HOA.

Pathology and Pathophysiology   In HOA, the bone changes in the distal extremities begin as a low-grade inflammatory process in the periosteum followed by new bone formation. At this stage, a radiolucent area may be observed between the new periosteal bone and subjacent cortex. As the process progresses, multiple layers of new bone are deposited, which become contiguous with the cortex

FIGURE 326-1   Clubbing of fingers. (*Reprinted from the Clinical Slide Collection on the Rheumatic Diseases, Copyright 1991, 1995. Used by permission of the American College of Rheumatology.*)

and result in cortical thickening. The outer portion of bone is laminated in appearance, with an irregular surface. Initially, the process of periosteal new bone formation involves the proximal and distal diaphyses of the tibia, fibula, radius, and ulna and, less frequently, the femur, humerus, metacarpals, metatarsals, and phalanges. Occasionally, scapulae, clavicula, ribs, and pelvic bones are also affected. In long-standing disease, these changes extend to involve metaphyses and musculotendinous insertions. The adjacent interosseous membranes may become ossified. The distribution of the bone manifestations is usually bilateral and symmetric. The soft tissue overlying the distal third of the arms and legs may be thickened. Mononuclear cell infiltration may be present in the adjacent soft tissue. Proliferation of connective tissue occurs in the nail bed and volar pad of digits, giving the distal phalanges a clubbed appearance. Small blood vessels in the clubbed digits are dilated and have thickened walls. In addition, the number of arteriovenous anastomoses is increased. The synovium of involved joints shows edema, varying degrees of synovial cell proliferation, thickening of the subsynovium, vascular congestion, vascular obliteration with thrombi, and small numbers of lymphocyte infiltrates.

Several theories have been suggested for the pathogenesis of HOA. Most have either been disproved or have not explained the development in all clinical disorders associated with HOA. Previously proposed neurogenic and humoral theories are no longer considered likely explanations for HOA. The neurogenic theory was based on the observation that vagotomy resulted in symptomatic improvement in a small number of patients with lung tumors and HOA. It was postulated that vagal stimuli from the tumor site led via a neural reflex to efferent nerve impulses to the distal extremities, resulting in HOA. This theory, however, did not explain HOA in conditions where vagal stimulation did not occur, as in cyanotic congenital heart disease or arterial aneurysms. The humoral theory postulated that soluble substances that normally are inactivated or removed during passage through the lung reached the systemic circulation in an active form and stimulated the changes of HOA. Substances proposed included prostaglandins, ferritin, bradykinin, estrogen, and growth hormone. These substances seemed unlikely candidates, since their blood levels in HOA patients overlapped those in individuals without HOA. Furthermore, these substances did not explain the development of localized HOA associated with arterial aneurysms or infected arterial grafts.

Recent studies have suggested a role for platelets in the development of HOA. It has been observed that megakaryocytes and large platelet particles, present in venous circulation, were fragmented in their passage through normal lung. In patients with cyanotic congenital heart disease and in other disorders associated with right-to-left shunts, these large platelet particles may bypass the lung and reach the distal extremities, where they can interact with endothelial cells. Platelet clumps have been demonstrated to form on an infected heart valve in bacterial endocarditis, in the wall of arterial aneurysms, and on infected arterial grafts. These platelet particles may also reach the distal extremities and interact with endothelial cells. Platelet-endothelial activation in the distal portion of extremities would then result in the release of platelet-derived growth factor (PDGF) and other factors leading to the proliferation of connective tissue and periosteum. Stimulation of fibroblasts by PDGF and transforming growth factor β (TGFβ) results in cell growth and collagen synthesis. Elevated plasma levels of von Willebrand factor antigen have been found in patients with both primary and secondary forms of HOA indicating endothelial activation or damage. Abnormalities of collagen synthesis have been demonstrated in the involved skin of patients with primary HOA. Fibroblasts from affected skin were shown to have increased collagen synthesis, increased $\alpha1$ (I) procollagen mRNA, and evidence for upregulation of collagen transcription. Other factors are undoubtedly involved in the pathogenesis of HOA, and further studies are needed to better understand this disorder.

Clinical Manifestations Primary HOA, also referred to as *pachydermoperiostitis* or *Touraine-Solente-Golé syndrome*, usually begins insidiously at puberty. In a smaller number of patients, the onset is in the first year of life. The disorder is inherited as an autosomal dominant trait with variable expression and is nine times more common in boys than in girls. Approximately one-third of patients have a family history of primary HOA.

Primary HOA is characterized by clubbing, periostosis, and unusual skin features. A small number of patients with this syndrome do not express clubbing. The skin changes and periostitis are prominent features of this syndrome. The skin becomes thickened and coarse. Deep nasolabial folds develop, and the forehead may become furrowed. Patients may have heavy-appearing eyelids and ptosis. The skin is often greasy, and there may be excessive sweating of the hands and feet. Patients also may experience seborrhea and folliculitis. In a few patients, the skin over the scalp becomes very thick and corrugated, a feature that has been descriptively termed *cutis verticis gyrata*. The distal extremities, particularly the legs, become thickened owing to proliferation of new bone and soft tissue; when the process is extensive, the ankles resemble elephant feet. The periostosis is usually not painful, as it may be in secondary HOA. Clubbing of the fingers may be extensive, producing large, bulbous deformities and clumsiness. Clubbing also affects the toes. Patients may experience articular and periarticular pain, especially in the ankles and knees, and joint motion may be mildly restricted owing to periarticular bone overgrowth. Noninflammatory effusions occur in the wrists, knees, and ankles. Synovial hypertrophy is not found. Associated abnormalities observed in patients with primary HOA include hypertrophic gastropathy, bone marrow failure, female escutcheon, and cranial suture defects. In patients with primary HOA, the symptoms disappear when adulthood is reached.

HOA secondary to an underlying disease occurs more frequently than primary HOA. It accompanies a variety of disorders and may precede clinical features of the associated disorder by months. Clubbing is more frequent than the full syndrome of HOA in patients with associated illnesses. Because clubbing evolves over months and is usually asymptomatic, it is often recognized first by the physician and not the patient. Patients may experience a burning sensation in their fingertips. Clubbing is characterized by widening of the fingertips, enlargement of the distal volar pad, convexity of the nail contour, and the loss of the normal 15° angle between the proximal nail and cuticle. The thickness of the digit at the base of the nail is greater than the thickness at the distal interphalangeal joint. The base of the nail feels spongy when compressed, and the nail can be easily rocked on its bed. Marked periungual erythema is usually present. When clubbing is advanced, the finger may have a drumstick appearance. Periosteal involvement in the distal extremities may produce a burning or deepseated aching pain. The pain can be quite incapacitating and is aggravated by dependency and relieved by elevation of the affected limbs. The overlying soft tissue may be swollen, and the skin slightly erythematous. Pressure applied over the distal forearms and legs may be quite painful.

Patients may also experience joint pain, most often in the ankles, wrists, and knees. Joint effusions may be present; usually they are small and noninflammatory. The small joints of the hands are rarely affected. Severe joint or bone pain may be the presenting symptom of an underlying lung malignancy and may precede the appearance of clubbing. In addition, the progression of HOA tends to be more rapid when associated with malignancies, most notably bronchogenic carcinoma. Unlike primary HOA, excessive sweating and oiliness of the skin and thickening of the facial skin are uncommon in secondary HOA.

HOA occurs in 5 to 10 percent of patients with intrathoracic malignancies, the most common being bronchogenic carcinoma and pleural tumors (Table 326-3). Lung metastases infrequently cause HOA. HOA is also seen in patients with intrathoracic infections, including lung abscesses, empyema, bronchiectasis, chronic obstructive lung disease, and, uncommonly, pulmonary tuberculosis. HOA also may accompany chronic interstitial pneumonitis, sarcoidosis, and cystic fibrosis. In the latter, clubbing is more common than the full syndrome of HOA. Other causes of clubbing include congenital heart

Disorders Associated with Hypertrophic Osteoarthropathy

Pulmonary
  Bronchogenic carcinoma and other neoplasms
  Lung abscesses, empyema, bronchiectasis
  Chronic interstitial pneumonitis
  Cystic fibrosis
  Chronic obstructive lung disease
  Sarcoidosis
Gastrointestinal
  Inflammatory bowel disease
  Sprue
  Neoplasms: esophagus, liver, bowel
Cardiovascular
  Cyanotic congenital heart disease
  Subacute bacterial endocarditis
  Infected arterial grafts*
  Aortic aneurysm*
  Aneurysm of major extremity artery*
  Patent ductus arteriosus
  Arteriovenous fistula of major extremity vessel*
Thyroid (thyroid acropachy)
  Hyperthyroidism (Graves' disease)

* Unilateral involvement

disease with right-to-left shunts, bacterial endocarditis, Crohn's disease, ulcerative colitis, sprue, and neoplasms of the esophagus, liver, and small and large bowel. In patients with congenital heart disease with right-to-left shunts, clubbing alone occurs more often than the full syndrome of HOA.

Unilateral clubbing has been found in association with aneurysms of the aorta or the subclavian or innominate artery and with arteriovenous fistulas of brachial vessels. Clubbing of the toes but not fingers has been associated with an infected abdominal aortic aneurysm and patent ductus arteriosus. Clubbing of a single digit may follow trauma and has been reported in tophaceous gout and sarcoidosis. While clubbing occurs more commonly than the full syndrome in most diseases, periostosis in the absence of clubbing has been observed in the affected limb of patients with infected arterial grafts.

Hyperthyroidism (Graves' disease), treated or untreated, occasionally is associated with clubbing and periostitis of the bones of the hands and feet. This condition is referred to as *thyroid acropachy*. Periostitis is asymptomatic and occurs in the midshaft and diaphyseal portion of the metacarpal and phalangeal bones. The long bones of the extremities are seldom affected. Elevated levels of long-acting thyroid stimulator (LATS) are found in the serum of these patients.

Laboratory Findings The laboratory abnormalities reflect the underlying disorder. The synovial fluid of involved joints has fewer than 500 white cells per microliter, and the cells are predominantly mononuclear. Radiographs show a faint radiolucent line beneath the new periosteal bone along the shaft of long bones at their distal end. These changes are observed most frequently at the ankles, wrists, and knees. The ends of the distal phalanges may show osseous resorption. Radionuclide studies show pericortical linear uptake along the cortical margins of long bones that may be present before any radiographic changes.

℞ **TREATMENT**

The treatment of hypertrophic osteoarthropathy is to identify the associated disorder and treat it appropriately. The symptoms and signs of hypertrophic osteoarthropathy may disappear completely with removal or effective chemotherapy of a tumor or with antibiotic therapy and drainage of a chronic pulmonary infection. Vagotomy or percutaneous block of the vagus nerve leads to symptomatic relief in some patients. Aspirin, other nonsteroidal anti-inflammatory drugs, or analgesics may help control symptoms of hypertrophic osteoarthropathy.

FIBROMYALGIA Fibromyalgia is a commonly encountered disorder characterized by widespread musculoskeletal pain, stiffness, paresthesia, nonrestorative sleep, and easy fatigability along with mul-

tiple tender points which are widely and symmetrically distributed. Fibromyalgia affects predominantly women. This disorder is found in most countries, in most ethnic groups, and in all types of climates. The prevalence of fibromyalgia in the general population of a community in the United States using the 1990 American College of Rheumatology classification criteria was reported recently to be 3.4 percent in women and 0.5 percent in men. Contrary to some previous reports, fibromyalgia was not found to be present mainly in young women but, rather, to be most prevalent in women aged 50 and older. The prevalence increased with age, being 7.4 percent in women between the ages of 70 and 79 years. Although not common, fibromyalgia also occurs in children. The reported prevalence of fibromyalgia in some rheumatology clinics has been as high as 20 percent. Several causative mechanisms for fibromyalgia have been postulated. Disturbed sleep has been implicated as a factor in the pathogenesis. Nonrestorative sleep or awakening unrefreshed has been observed in most patients with fibromyalgia. Sleep electroencephalographic studies in patients with fibromyalgia have shown disruption of normal stage 4 sleep [non–rapid eye movement (NREM) sleep] by many repeated alpha-wave intrusions. The idea that stage 4 sleep deprivation has a role in causing this disorder was supported by the observation that symptoms of fibromyalgia developed in normal subjects whose stage 4 sleep was disrupted artificially by induced alpha-wave intrusions. This sleep disturbance, however, has been demonstrated in healthy individuals, in emotionally distressed individuals, and in patients with sleep apnea, fever, osteoarthritis, or rheumatoid arthritis. Low levels of serotonin metabolites have been reported in the cerebrospinal fluid of patients with fibromyalgia, suggesting that a deficiency of serotonin, a neurotransmitter that regulates pain and NREM sleep, might also be involved in the pathogenesis of fibromyalgia. Drugs that affect serotonin metabolism have not had a dramatic effect on fibromyalgia, however. Since patients experience pain from muscle and musculotendinous sites, many studies have been done to examine muscle, both structurally and physiologically. Inflammation or diagnostic muscle abnormalities have not been found. Evidence indicates deconditioning of muscles, and patients experience a greater degree of postexertional pain than do unaffected persons. Fibromyalgia patients as a group have been reported by some investigators to have lower levels of somatomedin C than normal individuals. Since somatomedin C is the major mediator of the anabolic function of growth hormone and is important for muscle repair and strength, low levels of somatomedin C therefore might retard the healing process in muscles of fibromyalgia patients and account for the extended periods of pain following exertion. The low levels of somatomedin C in these patients may result from lack of exercise or a disturbance in stage 4 sleep, both of which stimulate production of growth hormone. The observation of low somatomedin C levels therefore may indicate a mechanism connecting sleep abnormality and muscle pain. The level of the neurotransmitter substance P has been reported to be increased in the cerebrospinal fluid of fibromyalgia patients and may play a role in spreading muscle pain. Many patients with fibromyalgia have psychological abnormalities; there has been disagreement as to whether some of these abnormalities represent reactions to the chronic pain or whether the symptoms of fibromyalgia are a reflection of psychiatric disturbance. Many patients fit a psychiatric diagnosis, the most common being depression, anxiety, somatization, and hypochondriases. Studies have also shown a high prevalence of sexual and physical abuse and eating disorders. However, fibromyalgia also occurs in patients without significant psychiatric problems. Patients with fibromyalgia may have a lower pain threshold than usual, although not all investigators in the field agree on this point. A better understanding of fibromyalgia awaits further studies.

Symptoms are generalized aching and stiffness of the trunk, hip, and shoulder girdles. Other patients complain of generalized muscle aching and weakness. Patients may complain of low back pain, which may radiate into the buttocks and legs. Others complain of pain and tightness in the neck and across the upper posterior shoulders. Patients complain of muscle pain after even mild exertion. Some degree of pain is always present. The pain has been described as a burning or gnawing pain or as soreness, stiffness, or aching. While pain may begin in one region, such as the shoulders, neck, or lower back, it eventually becomes widespread. Patients may complain of joint pain and perceive that their joints are swollen; however, joint examination yields normal findings. Stiffness is usually present on arising in the morning; usually it improves during the day, but in some patients it lasts all day. Patients may complain of numbness of their hands and feet. They also may feel colder overall than others in the home, and some may experience Raynaud's-like phenomena or actual Raynaud's phenomenon. Patients complain of feeling fatigued and exhausted and wake up tired. They also awaken frequently at night and have trouble falling back to sleep. Symptoms are made worse by stress or anxiety, cold, damp weather, and overexertion. Patients often feel better during warmer weather and vacations.

The characteristic feature on physical examination is the demonstration of specific tender points, which are exclusively more tender or painful than adjacent areas. The American College of Rheumatology (ACR) Criteria for Fibromyalgia defines 18 tender points (Fig. 326-2). These points of tenderness are remarkably constant in location. Approximately 4 kg of force ($4 \text{ kg} \cdot \text{f/cm}^2$) should be used in digital palpation of these tender points. Some workers recommend that the tender site be palpated using a rolling motion, which may be more effective in eliciting the tenderness. The tender sites can also be examined using a dolorimeter, which is a spring-loaded pressure gauge. Digital palpation appears to be as effective and accurate for the diagnosis of fibromyalgia as dolorimetry. The amount of pressure applied by the examiner introduces variability in the interpretation, however. If too much pressure is applied, the pain will be produced even in normal subjects. Likewise, tenderness will not be appreciated if too little pressure is applied or the

site is missed on palpation. Some investigators have quantitated their response, but the number of tender points sites is more diagnostic. Some patients are tender all over and not just at the specific tender point sites. These patients are still more tender over the specific tender point sites, however. Sites where there usually is no tenderness and which can be used as controls are the dorsum of the third digit between the proximal interphalangeal and distal interphalangeal joints, the medial third of the clavicle, the medial malleolus, and the forehead. If tenderness at these sites is also present, the diagnosis of fibromyalgia should be questioned, and possible psychiatric disorders investigated. Whether such patients can be diagnosed as also having fibromyalgia is debatable.

Skinfold tenderness may be present, particularly over the upper scapular region. Subcutaneous nodules may be felt at sites of tenderness. Nodules in similar locations are present in normal persons but are not tender.

Fibromyalgia may be triggered by emotional stress, medical illness, surgery, hypothyroidism, and trauma. It has appeared in some patients with human immunodeficiency virus (HIV) infection, parvovirus B19 infection, or Lyme disease. In the latter situation, fibromyalgia persisted despite adequate antibiotic treatment for Lyme disease. Disorders commonly associated with fibromyalgia include irritable bowel syndrome, irritable bladder, headaches (including migraine headaches), dysmenorrhea, premenstrual syndrome, restless legs syndrome, temporomandibular joint pain, and sicca syndrome.

The course of fibromyalgia is variable. Symptoms wax and wane in some patients, while in others pain and fatigue are persistent regardless of therapy. Studies from tertiary medical centers indicate a poor prognosis for most patients. The prognosis may be better in community-treated patients. In a community-based study reported after 2 years of treatment, 24 percent of patients were in remission, and 47 percent no longer fulfilled the ACR criteria for fibromyalgia.

Fibromyalgia is diagnosed by a history of widespread pain and the demonstration of at least 11 of the 18 tender point sites on digital palpation (Fig. 326-2). The ACR criteria are useful for standardizing the diagnosis; however, not all patients with fibromyalgia meet these criteria (Table 326-4). Some patients have fewer tender sites and more regional pain and may be considered to have probable fibromyalgia.

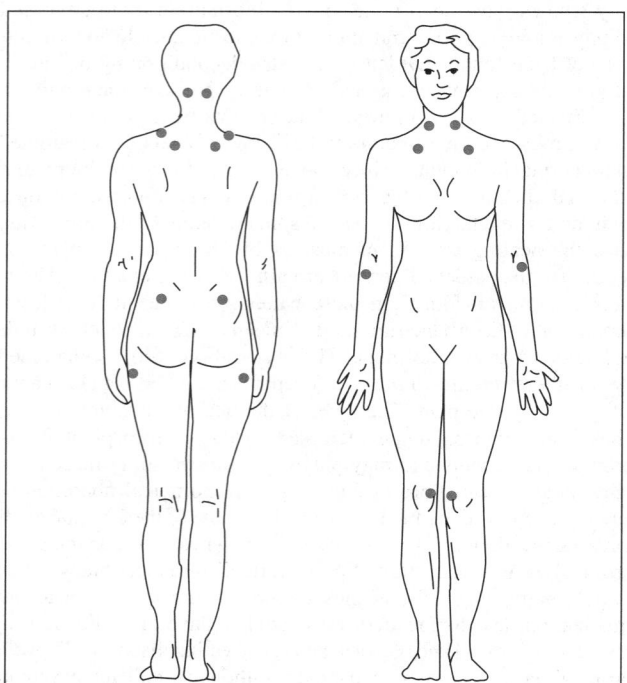

FIGURE 326-2 Tender points in fibromyalgia. Suboccipital muscle insertion at base of skull; anterior aspect of intertransverse process spaces at C5–7; midpoint of upper border of trapezius muscle; above scapular spine near medial border of scapula; second costochondral junction; lateral epicondyle; upper outer quadrant of buttocks; posterior aspect of trochanteric prominence; medial fat pad of knee (all bilateral). *(From the brochure "Fibromyalgia," Arthritis Information, Advise and Guidance, Disease Series. Used by permission of the Arthritis Foundation.)*

Table 326-4

The American College of Rheumatology 1990 Criteria for the Classification of Fibromyalgia*

A. History of widespread pain. Pain is considered widespread when all of the following are present:
1. Pain in the left side of the body
2. Pain in the right side of the body
3. Pain above the waist
4. Pain below the waist
5. Axial skeletal pain (cervical spine or anterior chest or thoracic spine or low back)

B. Pain on digital palpation in at least 11 of the following 18 tender point sites (see Fig. 326-2):
1. Occiput: bilateral, at the suboccipital muscle insertion
2. Low cervical: bilateral, at the anterior aspect of the intertransverse spaces at C5–7
3. Trapezius: bilateral, at the midpoint of the upper border
4. Supraspinatus: bilateral, at the origin, above the scapular spine near the medial border
5. Second rib: bilateral, at the second costochondral junction, just lateral to the junction on the upper surface
6. Lateral epicondyle: bilateral, 2 cm distal to the epicondyle
7. Gluteal: bilateral, in the upper outer quadrant of the buttock in the anterior fold of muscle
8. Greater trochanter: bilateral, posterior to the trochanteric prominence
9. Knee: bilateral, at the medial fat pad proximal to the joint line

Digital palpation should be performed with an approximate force of 4 kg. For a tender point to be considered positive, the subject must state that the palpation was painful. "Tender" is not to be considered painful.

---

* For purposes of classification, patients will be said to have fibromyalgia if both criteria are satisfied. Widespread pain must have been present for at least three months. The presence of a second clinical disorder does not exclude the diagnosis of fibromyalgia.

SOURCE: Modified from F Wolfe et al: Arthritis Rheum 33:171, 1990.

Results of joint and muscle examinations are normal in fibromyalgia patients, and there are no laboratory abnormalities. Fibromyalgia may occur in patients with rheumatoid arthritis, other connective tissue diseases, or other medical illness. A distinction is no longer made between primary and secondary fibromyalgia (concomitant with other disease), as the signs and symptoms are similar. Fibromyalgia and chronic fatigue syndrome have many similarities (see Chap. 384). Both are associated with fatigue, abnormal sleep, musculoskeletal pain, and psychiatric conditions such as less severe forms of depression and anxiety. Patients with chronic fatigue syndrome, however, are more likely to have symptoms suggesting a viral illness. These include mild fever, sore throat, and pain in the axillary and anterior and posterior cervical lymph nodes. The onset of chronic fatigue syndrome is usually sudden; patients are usually able to date the onset. Patients also have impaired memory and concentration. While many patients with chronic fatigue syndrome have tender points, the diagnosis does not require their presence. Polymyalgia rheumatica is distinguished from fibromyalgia in an elderly patient by the presence of more proximal muscle stiffness and pain and an elevated erythrocyte sedimentation rate. Patients should be evaluated for hypothyroidism, which may have symptoms similar to fibromyalgia or may accompany fibromyalgia.

The diagnosis of fibromyalgia has taken on a more complex significance in regard to labor and industry issues. This has become a significant issue since it has been reported that 10 to 25 percent of patients are not able to work in any capacity, while others require modification of their work. Disability evaluation in fibromyalgia is controversial. The diagnosis of fibromyalgia is not accepted by all. It is hard to evaluate patients' perceptions of their inability to function. The determination of tender points can also be subjective, on the part of both the physician and the patient, particularly when issues of compensation are pending. Patients also encounter difficulty in having their illness recognized as a disability. Physicians have been placed in the inappropriate role of assessing the patient's disability. Physicians are not in a position to quantitate disability at the workplace; that is better done by a work evaluation specialist. Better instruments are clearly needed for measuring disability, particularly in patients with fibromyalgia.

Patients should be informed that they have a condition that is not crippling, deforming, or degenerative, and that treatment is available. Salicylates or other nonsteroidal anti-inflammatory drugs only partially improve symptoms. Glucocorticoids have been of little benefit and should not be used in these patients. Opiate analgesics should be avoided. Local measures such as heat, massage, injection of tender sites with steroids or lidocaine, and acupuncture provide only temporary relief of symptoms. Other therapies that may help to varying degrees including biofeedback, hypnotherapy, and stress management and relaxation response training. The use of tricyclics such as amitriptyline (10 to 25 mg) and doxepin (10 to 25 mg) or a pharmacologically similar drug, cyclobenzaprine (10 to 20 mg), 1 to 2 h before bedtime will give the patient restorative sleep, resulting in clinical improvement. Higher doses of these medications may be necessary. Depression and anxiety should be treated with appropriate drugs and, when indicated, with psychiatric counseling. Alprazolam can be used for anxiety, while trazodone, sertraline, or fluoxetine can be used as antidepressants. Patients also may benefit by regular aerobic exercises. Exercise should be of a low-impact type and begun at a low level. Eventually, the patient should be exercising 20 to 30 min 3 to 4 days a week. Regular stretching exercises are also very important. Life stresses should be identified and discussed with the patient, and the patient should be provided with help on how to cope with these stresses. Patients may benefit from a multidisciplinary team approach involving a mental health professional, a physical therapist, and a physical medicine and rehabilitation specialist. Group therapy may be beneficial. Patients should be well educated about their disorder and taught the importance of self help. There are patient support groups in many communities. While treatment of fibromyalgia is effective in some patients, others continue to have chronic disease, which is relieved only partially if at all.

MYOFASCIAL PAIN SYNDROME   Myofascial pain syndrome is characterized by localized musculoskeletal pain and tenderness in association with trigger points. The pain is deep and aching and may be accompanied by a burning sensation. Myofascial pain may follow trauma, overuse, or prolonged static contraction of a muscle or muscle group, which may occur when reading or writing at a desk or working at a computer. In addition, this syndrome may be associated with underlying osteoarthritis of the neck or low back. Trigger points are a diagnostic feature of this syndrome. Pain is referred from trigger points to defined areas distant from the original tender points. Palpation of the trigger point reproduces or accentuates the pain. The trigger points are usually located in the center of a muscle belly, but they can occur at other sites, such as costosternal junctions, the xyphoid process, ligamentous and tendinous insertions, fascia, and fatty areas. Trigger point sites in muscle have been described as feeling indurated and taut, and palpation may cause the muscle to twitch. These findings, however, have been shown not to be unique for myofascial pain syndrome, since in a controlled study they were also present in fibromyalgia patients and normal subjects. Myofascial pain most often involves the posterior neck, low back, shoulders, and chest. Chronic pain in the muscles of the posterior neck may involve referral of pain from the trigger point in the erector neck muscle or upper trapezius to the head, leading to persistent headaches which may last for days. Trigger points in the paraspinal muscles of the low back may refer pain to the buttock. Pain may be referred down the leg from a trigger point in the gluteus medius and can mimic sciatica. A trigger point in the infraspinatus muscle may produce local and referred pain over the lateral deltoid and down the outside of the arm into the hand. Injection of a local anesthetic such as 1% lidocaine into the trigger point site often results in pain relief. Another useful technique is first to spray from the trigger point toward the area of referred pain with an agent such as ethyl chloride and then to stretch the muscle. This maneuver may need to be repeated several times. Massage and application of ultrasound to the affected area may also be beneficial. Patients should be instructed in methods to prevent muscle stresses related to work and recreation. Posture and resting positions are important in preventing muscle tension. The prognosis in most patients is good. In some patients, myofascial pain syndrome may evolve into fibromyalgia. Patients at risk for developing fibromyalgia are thought to be those with anxiety, depression, nonrestorative sleep, and fatigue.

PSYCHOGENIC RHEUMATISM   Patients may experience severe joint pain involving a few to several joints without physical findings of arthritis. These patients are often convinced that they have rheumatoid arthritis, systemic lupus erythematosus, or another connective tissue disease. This disorder is recognized by the inconsistencies, exaggerations, and emotional lability of the patient during the history and physical examination. Results of laboratory studies are normal. Organic disease needs to be excluded, which necessitates seeing the patient at regular intervals. This condition also needs to be distinguished from fibromyalgia. Anti-inflammatory or other drugs are not helpful.

REFLEX SYMPATHETIC DYSTROPHY SYNDROME
The reflex sympathetic dystrophy syndrome (RSDS) is characterized by pain and swelling, usually of a distal extremity, accompanied by vasomotor instability, trophic skin changes, and the rapid development of bony demineralization. RSDS occasionally involves an isolated site such as a knee, hip, or one or two digits of a foot or hand. The contralateral side is affected clinically in approximately 25 percent of patients and may be involved in virtually all patients with RSOS, as shown by scintigraphic studies. A precipitating event can be identified in at least two-thirds of cases. These events include trauma, such as fractures and crush injuries; myocardial infarction; strokes; peripheral nerve injury; and use of certain drugs, including barbiturates, antituberculous drugs, and, more recently, cyclosporine administered to patients undergoing renal transplantation. The pathogenesis of RSDS is poorly understood and is thought to involve abnormal activity of the sympathetic nervous system following a precipitating event.

RSDS evolves through three clinical phases. The first phase is characterized by an intense burning pain and swelling of a distal extremity. The involved extremity is warm, edematous, and very tender, especially around joints. Sweating and hair growth are increased. Light touch causes pain, which may continue after the stimulus is removed. Passive or active motion of joints is very painful, and the joints are stiff. In the first phase, especially when both sides are involved, the clinical findings may suggest early rheumatoid arthritis. Redness and swelling over a distal extremity such as an ankle or wrist may also mimic inflammatory arthritis, or even an infectious arthritis. In 3 to 6 months, the skin gradually becomes thin, shiny, and cool. This is the second phase of the disease. The clinical features of the first and second phases often overlap. In another 3 to 6 months (third phase), the skin becomes atrophic and dry, and irreversible flexion contractures, palmar fibromatosis, and Dupuytren's contractures develop, resulting in a claw-like hand deformity. Similar changes occur in the feet. When RSDS occurs in the upper extremity, motion of the shoulder on the affected side may be painful and restricted, a condition referred to as *shoulder-hand syndrome* (see "Adhesive Capsulitis," below). → *Reflex sympathetic dystrophy syndrome, including its treatment, is covered in greater detail in Chap. 371.*

TIETZE'S SYNDROME AND COSTOCHONDRITIS Tietze's syndrome is manifested by painful swelling of one or more costochondral articulations. The age of onset is usually before 40, and both sexes are affected equally. In most patients only one joint is involved, usually the second or third costochondral joint. The onset of anterior chest pain may be sudden or gradual. The pain may radiate to the arms or shoulder and is aggravated by sneezing, coughing, deep inspirations, or twisting motions of the chest. The term *costochondritis* is often used interchangeably with *Tietze's syndrome*, but some workers restrict the former term to pain of the costochondral articulations without swelling. Costochondritis is observed in patients over age 40, tends to affect the third, fourth, and fifth costochondral joints, and occurs more often in women. Both syndromes may mimic cardiac or upper abdominal causes of pain. Rheumatoid arthritis, ankylosing spondylitis, and Reiter's syndrome may involve costochondral joints but are distinguished easily by their other clinical features. Other skeletal causes of anterior chest wall pain are xiphoidalgia and the slipping rib syndrome, which usually involves the tenth rib. Malignancies such as breast cancer, prostate cancer, plasma cell cytoma, and sarcoma can invade the ribs, thoracic spine, or chest wall and produce symptoms suggesting Tietze's syndrome. They should be easily distinguishable by radiographs and biopsy. Analgesics, anti-inflammatory drugs, and local steroid injections usually relieve symptoms.

MUSCULOSKELETAL DISORDERS ASSOCIATED WITH HYPERLIPIDEMIA Musculoskeletal manifestations may be the first indication of a hereditary disorder of lipoprotein metabolism. Patients with type II hyperlipoproteinemia may have recurrent migratory polyarthritis involving knees and other large peripheral joints and, to a lesser degree, peripheral small joints. In a few patients, the arthritis is monarticular. Fever may accompany the arthritis. Pain ranges from moderate to very severe to incapacitating. The involved joints can be warm, erythematous, swollen, and tender. Arthritis usually has a sudden onset, lasts from a few days to 2 weeks, and does not cause joint damage. Several attacks occur a year. Synovial fluid from involved joints is not inflammatory and contains few white cells and no crystals. Joint involvement may actually represent inflammatory periarthritis or peritendinitis and not intraarticular disease. The recurrent, transient nature of the arthritis may suggest rheumatic fever, especially since patients with lipoproteinemia have an elevated erythrocyte sedimentation rate, a falsely elevated antistreptolysin O titer, and, in some cases, aortic valvular disease secondary to atherosclerosis. Patients heterozygous for type II hyperlipoproteinemia may also experience Achilles tendinitis, which can be very painful. Attacks of tendinitis come on gradually and last only a few days. Fever is not present. Patients may be asymptomatic between attacks. During an attack the Achilles tendon is warm, erythematous, swollen, and tender to palpation. Achilles tendinitis and other joint manifestations often precede

the appearance of xanthomas and may be the first clinical indication of hyperlipoproteinemia. Patients with type II hyperlipoproteinemia also have tendinous xanthomas in the Achilles, patellar, and extensor tendons of the hands and feet. Xanthomas have also been reported in the peroneal tendon, the plantar aponeurosis, and the periosteum overlying the distal tibia. These xanthomas are located within tendon fibers. They appear in childhood in homozygous patients and after the age of 30 in heterozygous patients. Tuberous xanthomas appear only in patients homozygous for type II hyperlipoproteinemia. They are soft subcutaneous masses located over the extensor surfaces of the elbows, knees, and hands, as well as on the buttocks. Patients with type IV hyperlipoproteinemia also may have a mild inflammatory arthritis affecting large and small peripheral joints, usually in an asymmetric pattern with only a few joints involved at a time. The onset of arthritis is usually in middle age. Arthritis may be persistent or recurrent with episodes lasting a few days to weeks. Joint pain is severe in some patients. Patients may experience morning stiffness. Joint tenderness and periarticular hyperesthesia may also be present. Joint fluid is noninflammatory and without crystals. Radiographs may show juxtaarticular osteopenia and cystic lesions. Large bone cysts have been noted in a few patients. The pathogenesis of arthritis in both types of hyperlipoproteinemia is not well understood. Salicylates, other nonsteroidal anti-inflammatory drugs (NSAIDs), or analgesics usually provide relief of symptoms. Xanthomas and bone cysts are also observed in other hyperlipoproteinemias. Tendinous and tuberous xanthomas are seen in type III disorder. Also in type III disorder, lipids are deposited in the palms to form plane xanthomas. Eruptive xanthomas are found over the knees, shoulders, back, and buttocks in types I, IV, and V disorders. Large cystic lesions in both proximal femurs were reported in a patient with type V disorder.

ARTHROPATHY OF ACROMEGALY Acromegaly is the result of excessive production of growth hormone by an adenoma in the anterior pituitary gland (see Chap. 328). Middle-aged persons are most often affected. The excessive secretion of growth hormone along with insulin-like growth factor I stimulates proliferation of cartilage, periarticular connective tissue, and bone, resulting in several musculoskeletal abnormalities, including osteoarthritis, back pain, muscle weakness, and carpal tunnel syndrome.

An arthropathy resembling osteoarthritis is a common feature, affecting most often the knees, shoulders, hips, and hands. Single or multiple joints may be affected. The overgrowth of cartilage initially produces widening of the joint space. The newly synthesized cartilage is not developed in an organized manner, making it susceptible to fissuring, ulceration, and destruction. Ligamental laxity of the joint resulting from the growth of connective tissue also contributes to the development of osteoarthritis. With breakdown and loss of cartilage, the joint space narrows, and subchondral sclerosis and osteophytes appear on radiographs. Joint examination reveals marked crepitus and hypermobility. Joint fluid is noninflammatory. Calcium pyrophosphate dehydrate crystals are found in the cartilage in some cases of acromegaly arthropathy and, when shed into the joint, can produce attacks of pseudogout. Chondrocalcinosis may also be observed radiographically. Approximately half of the patients with acromegaly experience back pain, which is predominantly lumbosacral. Hypermobility of the spine may be a contributing factor in back pain. Radiograph of the spine shows normal or increased intervertebral disk spaces, hypertrophic anterior osteophytes, and ligamental calcification. These changes are similar to those observed in patients with diffuse idiopathic skeletal hyperostosis. Dorsal kyphosis in conjunction with elongation of the ribs contributes to the development of the barrel chest seen in acromegalic patients. The hands and feet become enlarged owing to soft tissue proliferation. The fingers are thickened and have spade-like distal tufts. One-third of patients have a thickened heel pad. Approximately 25 percent of patients have Raynaud's phenomenon.

Carpal tunnel syndrome occurs in about half of patients. The median nerve is compressed by the excessive growth of connective tissue in the carpal tunnel. The median nerve also becomes enlarged. Patients with acromegaly also develop proximal muscle weakness, which is thought to be caused by the effect of growth hormone on muscle. Results of muscle enzyme assays and electromyography are normal. Muscle biopsy specimens show muscle fibers of varying size and no inflammatory changes.

ARTHROPATHY OF HEMOCHROMATOSIS Hemochromatosis is a disorder of iron storage. Excessive amounts of iron are absorbed from the intestine, leading to iron deposition in parenchymal cells, which results in tissue damage and impairment of organ function (see Chap. 342). Symptoms of hemochromatosis usually begin between the ages of 40 and 60 but can occur earlier. Arthritis, which occurs in 20 to 40 percent of patients, usually begins after the age of 50 years and may be the first clinical feature of hemochromatosis. The arthropathy is an inflammatory osteoarthritis-like disorder affecting the small joints of the hands, followed later by larger joints such as knees, ankles, shoulders, and hips. The second and third metacarpophalangeal joints of both hands are often the first joints affected; they can provide an important clue to the possibility of hemochromatosis. Patients experience stiffness and pain. Morning stiffness usually lasts less than half an hour. The affected joints are enlarged and mildly tender. Synovial tissue is not appreciatively increased. Radiographs show irregular narrowing of the joint space, subchondral sclerosis, and subchondral cysts. There is juxtaarticular proliferation of bone, with frequent hook-like osteophytes. The synovial fluid is noninflammatory. The synovium shows mild to moderate proliferation of lining cells, fibrosis, and a low number of inflammatory cells, which are mononuclear. In approximately half of patients, there is evidence of calcium pyrophosphate deposition disease. Iron can be demonstrated in the lining cells of the synovium and also in chondrocytes.

Iron may damage the articular cartilage in several ways. Promotion by iron of superoxide-dependent lipid peroxidation may play a role in joint damage. In animal models, ferric iron has been shown to interfere with collagen formation. Iron has also been shown to increase the release of lysosomal enzymes from cells in the synovial membrane. Iron may also play a role in the development of chondrocalcinosis. Iron inhibits synovial tissue pyrophosphatase in vitro and, therefore, may inhibit pyrophosphatase in vivo, resulting in chondrocalcinosis. Iron in synovial cells may also inhibit the clearance of calcium pyrophosphate from the joint.

℞ **TREATMENT**

The treatment of hemochromatosis is repeated phlebotomy. Unfortunately, this treatment has little effect on the arthritis, which, along with chondrocalcinosis, usually continues to progress. Treatment of the arthritis consists of administration of acetaminophen and NSAIDs. Placement of a hip or knee prosthesis has been successful in advanced disease.

HEMOPHILIC ARTHROPATHY Hemophilia is a sex-linked recessive genetic disorder characterized by the absence or deficiency of factor VIII (hemophilia A, or classic hemophilia) or factor IX (hemophilia B, or Christmas disease) (see Chap. 118). Hemophilia A is by far the more common type, constituting 85 percent of cases. Spontaneous hemarthrosis is a common problem with both types of hemophilia and can lead to a chronic deforming arthritis. The frequency and severity of hemarthrosis are related to the degree of clotting factor deficiency. Hemarthrosis is not common in other inherited disorders of coagulation, such as von Willebrand's disease or factor V deficiency.

Hemarthrosis becomes evident after 1 year of age, when the child begins to walk and run. In order of frequency, the joints most commonly affected are the knees, ankles, elbows, shoulders, and hips. Small joints of the hands and feet are occasionally involved.

In the initial stage of arthropathy, hemarthrosis produces a warm, tensely swollen, and painful joint. The patient holds the affected joint in flexion and guards against any movement. Blood in the joint remains liquid because of the absence of intrinsic clotting factor and the absence of tissue thromboplastin in the synovium. The blood in the joint space is resorbed over a period of a week or longer, depending on the size of the hemarthrosis. Joint function usually returns to normal or baseline in about 2 weeks.

Recurrent hemarthrosis leads to the development of a chronic arthritis. The involved joints remain swollen, and flexion deformities develop. In the later stages of arthropathy, joint motion is restricted and function is severely limited. Joint ankylosis, subluxation, or laxity are features of end-stage disease.

Bleeding into muscle and soft tissue also causes musculoskeletal disorders. When bleeding into the iliopsoas muscle occurs, the hip is held in flexion because of the pain, resulting in a hip flexion contracture. Rotation of the hip is preserved, which distinguishes this problem from intraarticular hemorrhage. Expansion of the hematoma may place pressure on the femoral nerve, resulting in a femoral neuropathy. Another problem is shortening of the heel cord secondary to bleeding into the gastrocnemius. Hemorrhage into a closed compartment space, such as the volar compartment in the forearm, can result in muscle necrosis and flexion deformities of the wrist and fingers. When bleeding involves periosteum or bone, a pseudotumor forms. These occur distal to the elbows or knees in children and improve with treatment of the hemophilia. Surgical removal is indicated if the pseudotumor continues to enlarge. In adults, they occur in the femur and pelvis and are usually refractory to treatment. When bleeding occurs in muscle, cysts may develop over the muscle. Needle aspiration of a cyst is contraindicated because it can induce bleeding.

Septic arthritis can occur in hemophilia and is difficult at times to distinguish from acute hemarthrosis. Whenever there is suspicion of an infected joint, the joint should be aspirated immediately, the fluid cultured, and the patient started on a broad-spectrum antibiotic. The patient should be infused with the deficient clotting factor before the joint is tapped.

Radiographs of joints reflect the stage of disease. In early stages there is only capsule distention; later, juxtaarticular osteopenia, marginal erosions, and subchondral cysts develop. In late disease, the joint space is narrowed and there is bony overgrowth. The changes are similar to those observed in osteoarthritis. Unique features of hemophilic arthropathy are widening of the femoral intercondylar notch, enlargement of the proximal radius, and squaring of the distal end of the patella.

Recurrent hemarthrosis produces synovial hyperplasia and hypertrophy. A pannus covers the cartilage. Cartilage is damaged by collagenase and other degradative enzymes released by mononuclear cells in the overlying synovium. Hemosiderin is found in synovial lining cells, the subsynovium, and chondrocytes and may also play a role in cartilage destruction.

℞ **TREATMENT**

The treatment of hemarthrosis consists in the immediate infusion of factor VIII or IX at the first sign of joint or muscle hemorrhage. The patient is placed at bed rest, with the involved joint in as much extension as the patient can tolerate. Analgesic NSAIDs and local icing may help with the pain. NSAIDs can be given safely for short periods even though they have a stabilizing effect on platelets. Studies have shown no significant abnormalities in platelet function or bleeding time in hemophiliacs receiving ibuprofen. Synovectomy, open or arthroscopic, may be indicated in patients with chronic synovial proliferation and recurrent hemarthrosis. Hypertrophied synovium is very vascular and subject to bleeding. Both types of synovectomy reduce the number of hemarthroses and slow the roentgenographic progression of hemophilic arthropathy. Open surgical synovectomy, however, is associated with some loss of range of motion. Radiosynovectomy with either yttrium 90 silicate or phosphorus 31 colloid has also been effective and may be a useful alternative when surgical synovectomy is not practical. Total joint replacement is indicated for severe joint destruction and incapacitating pain. Because of the young age of hemophilic patients, total-joint prostheses may need to be replaced more than once during their lives.

ARTHROPATHIES ASSOCIATED WITH HEMOGLOBINOPATHIES **Sickle Cell Disease** Sickle cell disease (see Chap.

Table 326-5

Musculoskeletal Abnormalities in Sickle Cell Disease

Sickle cell dactylitis
Joint effusions in sickle cell crises
Osteomyelitis
Infarction of bone
Infarction of bone marrow
Avascular necrosis
Bone changes secondary to marrow hyperplasia
Septic arthritis
Gouty arthritis

---

107) is associated with several musculoskeletal abnormalities (Table 326-5). Children under the age of 5 may develop diffuse swelling, tenderness, and warmth of the hands and feet lasting from 1 to 3 weeks. The condition referred to as *sickle cell dactylitis* or *hand-foot syndrome* has also been observed in sickle cell disease and sickle cell thalassemia. Dactylitis is believed to result from infarction of the bone marrow and cortical bone leading to periostitis and soft tissue swelling. Radiographs show periosteal elevation, subperiosteal new bone formation, and areas of radiolucency and increased density involving the metacarpals, metatarsals, and proximal phalanges. These bone changes disappear after several months. The syndrome leaves little or no residual damage. Because hematopoiesis ceases in the small bones of hands and feet with age, the syndrome is rarely seen after age 4 or 5 and does not occur in adults.

Sickle cell crisis is often associated with periarticular pain and joint effusions. The joint and periarticular area are warm and tender. Knees and elbows are most often affected, but other joints can be involved. Joint effusions are noninflammatory, with fewer than 1000 white cells/μL; mononuclear cells predominate. There have been a few reports of sterile inflammatory effusion with high cell counts consisting of mostly polymorphonuclear white cells. Synovial biopsies have shown mild lining cell proliferation and microvascular thrombosis. Scintigraphic studies have shown decreased marrow uptake adjacent to the involved joint. The joint effusion and periarticular pain are considered to be the result of ischemia and infarction of the synovium and adjacent bone and marrow. The treatment is that for sickle cell crisis (see Chap. 107).

Patients with sickle cell disease may also develop osteomyelitis, which commonly involves the long tubular bones (see Chap. 132). These patients are particularly susceptible to bacterial infections, especially *Salmonella* infections, which are found in more than half of cases (see Chap. 158). Radiographs of the involved site show periosteal elevation initially, followed by disruption of the cortex. Treatment of the infection results in healing of the bone lesion. Sickle cell disease is also associated with bone infarction resulting from thrombosis secondary to the sickling of red cells. Bone infarction also occurs in hemoglobin S-C disease and sickle cell thalassemia (see Chap. 107). The bone pain in sickle cell crisis is due to bone and bone marrow infarction. In children, infarction of the epiphyseal growth plate interferes with normal growth of the affected extremity. Radiographically, infarction of the bone cortex results in periosteal elevation and irregular thickening of the bone cortex. Infarction in the bone marrow leads to lysis, fibrosis, and new bone formation.

Avascular necrosis of the head of the femur is seen in about 5 percent of patients. It also occurs in the humeral head and less commonly in the distal femur, tibial condyles, distal radius, vertebral bodies, and other juxtaarticular sites. The mechanism for avascular necrosis is most likely the same as for bone infarction. Subchondral hemorrhage may play a role in the deterioration of articular cartilage. Irregularity of the femoral head or of other bone surfaces affected by avascular necrosis eventually results in degenerative joint disease. Radiograph of the affected joint may show patchy radiolucency and density followed by flattening of the bone. Magnetic resonance imag-

ing is a sensitive technique for detecting early avascular necrosis as well as bone infarction elsewhere. Total hip replacement and placement of prostheses in other joints may improve function and relieve pain in those patients with severe joint destruction.

Septic arthritis is occasionally encountered in sickle cell disease (see Chap. 324). Multiple joints may be infected. Joint infection may result from spread of contiguous osteomyelitis. Microorganisms identified include staphylococcus, *Streptococcus*, *Escherichia coli*, and *Salmonella*. The latter is not seen as frequently in septic arthritis as it is in osteomyelitis. Acute gouty arthritis is uncommon in sickle cell disease, even though 40 percent of patients are hyperuremic. Hyperuricemia is due to overproduction of uric acid secondary to increased red cell turnover. Attacks may be polyarticular.

The bone marrow hyperplasia in sickle cell disease results in widening of the medullary cavities, thinning of the cortices, coarse trabeculations and central cupping of the vertebral bodies. These changes are also seen to a lesser degree in hemoglobin S-C disease and sickle cell thalassemia. In normal individuals, red marrow is located mostly in the axial skeletal, but in sickle cell disease, red marrow is found in the bones of the extremities and even in the tarsal and carpal bones. Vertebral compression may lead to dorsal kyphosis, and softening of the bone in the acetabulum may result in protrusio acetabuli.

Thalassemia β-Thalassemia is a congenital disorder of hemoglobin synthesis characterized by impaired production of β chains (see Chap. 107). Bone and joint abnormalities occur in β-thalassemia, being most common in the major and intermedia groups. In one study, approximately 50 percent of patients with β-thalassemia had evidence of symmetric ankle arthropathy, characterized by a dull aching pain aggravated by weight bearing. The onset was most often in the second or third decade of life. The degree of ankle pain in these patients varied. Some patients experienced self-limited ankle pain, which occurred only after strenuous physical activity and lasted several days to weeks. Other patients had chronic ankle pain which became worse with walking. Symptoms eventually abated in a few patients. Compression of the ankle, calcaneus, or forefoot was painful in some patients. Synovial fluid from two patients was noninflammatory. Radiographs of ankle showed osteopenia, widened medullary spaces, thin cortices, and coarse trabeculations. These findings were largely the result of bone marrow expansion. The joint space was preserved. Specimens of bone from three patients revealed osteomalacia, osteopenia, and microfractures. Increased osteoblasts as well as increased foci of bone resorption were present on the bone surface. Iron staining was found in the bone trabeculae, in osteoid, and in the cement line. Synovium showed hyperplasia of lining cells which contained deposits of hemosiderin. This arthropathy was considered to be related to the underlying bone pathology. The role of iron overload or abnormal bone metabolism in the pathogenesis of this arthropathy is not known. This arthropathy was treated with analgesics and splints. Patients were also transfused to decrease hematopoiesis and marrow expansion.

Patients with β-thalassemia major and intermedia also have involvement of other joints, including the knees, hips, and shoulders. Acquired hemochromatosis with arthropathy has been described in a patient with thalassemia. Gouty arthritis and septic arthritis can occur. Avascular necrosis is not a feature of thalassemia because there is no sickling of red cells leading to thrombosis and infarction.

β-Thalassemia minor (trait) is also associated with joint manifestations. Chronic seronegative oligoarthritis affecting predominantly ankles, wrists, and elbows has been described. These patients had mild persistent synovitis without large effusions. Joint erosions were not seen. Recurrent episodes of an acute asymmetric arthritis also have been reported; episodes last less than a week and may affect knees, ankles, shoulders, elbows, wrists, and metacarpal phalangeal joints. The mechanism for this arthropathy is unknown. Treatment with nonsteroidal drugs was not particularly effective.

PERIARTICULAR DISORDERS Bursitis Bursitis is inflammation of a bursa, which is a thin-walled sac lined with synovial tissue. The function of the bursa is to facilitate movement of tendons and muscles over bony prominences. Excessive frictional forces, trauma, systemic disease (e.g., rheumatoid arthritis, gout), or infection may cause bursitis. Subacromial bursitis (subdeltoid bursitis) is the most common form of bursitis. Another form is trochanteric bursitis, which involves the bursa around the insertion of the gluteus medius onto the greater trochanter of the femur. Patients experience pain over the lateral aspect of the hip and upper thigh and have tenderness over the posterior aspect of the greater trochanter. External rotation and resisted abduction of the hip elicit pain. Olecranon bursitis occurs over the posterior elbow, and when the area is acutely inflamed, infection should be excluded by aspirating and culturing fluid from the bursa. Achilles bursitis involves the bursa located above the insertion of the tendon to the calcaneus and results from overuse and wearing tight shoes. Retrocalcaneal bursitis involves the bursa that is located between the calcaneus and posterior surface of the Achilles tendon. The pain is experienced at the back of the heel, and swelling appears on the medial and/or lateral side of the tendon. It occurs in association with spondyloarthropathies, rheumatoid arthritis, gout, and trauma. Ischial bursitis (weaver's bottom) affects the bursa separating the gluteus medius from the ischial tuberosity and develops from prolonged sitting on hard surfaces. Iliopsoas bursitis affects the bursa that lies between the iliopsoas muscle and hip joint and is lateral to the femoral vessels. Pain is experienced over this area and is made worse by hip extension and flexion. Bursitis results from trauma or overuse but can also be seen in patients with rheumatoid arthritis. Anserine bursitis is an inflammation of the sartorius bursa located over the medial side of the tibia just below the knee and is manifested by pain on climbing stairs. Tenderness is present over the insertion of the conjoint tendon of the sartorius, gracilis, and semitendinosus. Prepatellar bursitis (housemaid's knee) occurs in the bursa situated between the patella and overlying skin and is caused by kneeling on hard surfaces. Treatment of bursitis consists of prevention of the aggravating situation, rest of the involved part, administration of a NSAID, and local steroid injection.

Rotator Cuff Tendinitis and Impingement Syndrome Tendinitis of the rotator cuff is the major cause of a painful shoulder and is currently thought to be caused by impingement on the tendon(s). Of the tendons forming the rotator cuff, the supraspinatus tendon is the most often affected, probably because of its repeated confinement between the humeral head and the undersurface of the anterior third of the acromion and coracoacromial ligament above as well as the reduction in its blood supply that occurs with abduction of the arm (Fig. 326-3). The tendon of the infraspinatus or the long head of the biceps is less commonly involved. The process begins with edema

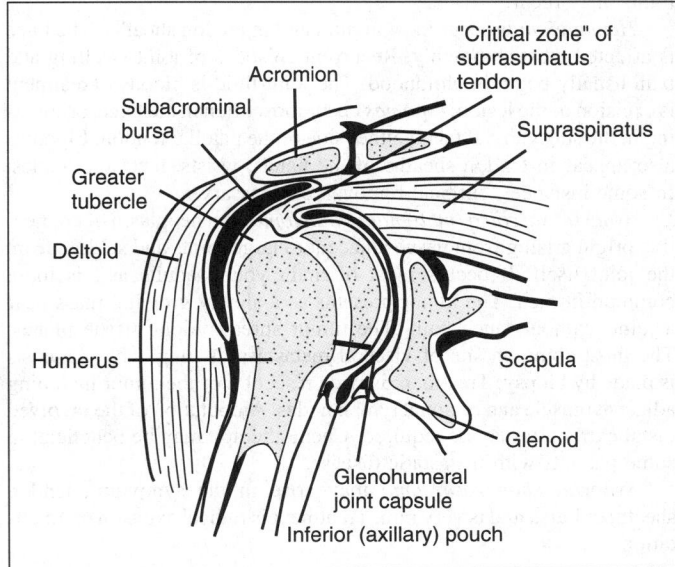

FIGURE 326-3 Coronal section of the shoulder illustrating the relationships of the glenohumeral joint, the joint capsule, the subacromial bursa, and the rotator cuff (supraspinatus tendon). *(From Kozin.)*

and hemorrhage of the rotator cuff, which evolves to fibrotic thickening and eventually to rotator cuff degeneration with tendon tears and bone spurs. Subacromial bursitis also accompanies this syndrome. Symptoms usually appear after injury or overuse, especially with activities involving elevation of the arm with some degree of forward flexion. Impingement syndrome occurs in persons participating in baseball, tennis, swimming, or occupations that require repeated elevation of the arm. Those over age 40 are particularly susceptible. Patients complain of a dull aching in the shoulder, which may interfere with sleep. Severe pain is experienced when the arm is actively abducted into an overhead position. The arc between 60 and 120° is especially painful. Tenderness is present over the lateral aspect of the humeral head just below the acromion. Nonsteroidal anti-inflammatory drugs, local steroid injection, and physical therapy may relieve symptoms.

Patients may tear the supraspinatus tendon acutely by falling on an outstretched arm or lifting a heavy object. Symptoms are pain, along with weakness of abduction and external rotation of the shoulder. Atrophy of the supraspinatus muscles develops. The diagnosis is established by arthrogram or ultrasound. Surgical repair may be necessary in patients who fail to respond to conservative measures. In patients with moderate to severe tears and functional loss, surgery is indicated.

Calcific Tendinitis This condition is characterized by deposition of calcium salts, primarily hydroxyapatite, within a tendon. The exact mechanism of calcification is not known but may be initiated by ischemia or degeneration of the tendon. The supraspinatus tendon is most often affected because it is frequently impinged on and has a reduced blood supply when the arm is abducted. The condition usually develops after age 40. Calcification within the tendon may evoke acute inflammation, producing sudden and severe pain in the shoulder. However, it may be asymptomatic or not related to the patient's symptoms.

Bicipital Tendinitis and Rupture Bicipital tendinitis, or tenosynovitis, is produced by friction on the tendon of the long head of the biceps as it passes through the bicipital groove. When the inflammation is acute, patients experience anterior shoulder pain which radiates down the biceps into the forearm. Abduction and external rotation of the arm are painful and limited. The bicipital groove is very tender to palpation. Pain may be elicited along the course of the tendon by resisting supination of the forearm with the elbow at 90° (Yergason's supination sign). Acute rupture of the tendon may occur with vigorous exercise of the arm and is often painful. In a young patient, it should be repaired surgically. Rupture of the tendon in an older person may be associated with little or no pain and is recognized by the presence of persistent swelling of the biceps ("Popeye" muscle) produced by the retraction of the long head of the biceps. Surgery is usually not necessary in this setting.

Adhesive Capsulitis Often referred to as "frozen shoulder," adhesive capsulitis is characterized by pain and restricted movement of the shoulder, usually in the absence of intrinsic shoulder disease. Adhesive capsulitis, however, may follow bursitis or tendinitis of the shoulder or be associated with systemic disorders such as chronic pulmonary disease, myocardial infarction, and diabetes mellitus. Prolonged immobility of the arm contributes to the development of adhesive capsulitis, and reflex sympathetic dystrophy is thought to be a pathogenic factor. The capsule of the shoulder is thickened, and a mild chronic inflammatory infiltrate and fibrosis may be present.

Adhesive capsulitis occurs more commonly in women after age 50. Pain and stiffness usually develop gradually over several months to a year but progress rapidly in some patients. Pain may interfere with sleep. The shoulder is tender to palpation, and both active and passive movement are restricted. Radiographs of the shoulder show osteopenia. The diagnosis is confirmed by arthrography, in that only a limited amount of contrast material, usually less than 15 mL, can be injected under pressure into the shoulder joint.

In most patients, the condition improves spontaneously 12 to 18 months after onset, but some have permanent restriction of movement.

Early mobilization of the arm following an injury to the shoulder may prevent the development of this disease. Slow but forceful injection of contrast material into the joint may lyse adhesions and stretch the capsule, resulting in improvement of shoulder motion. Manipulation under anesthesia may be helpful in some patients. Once the disease is established, therapy may have little effect on its natural course. Local injections of glucocorticoids, nonsteroidal anti-inflammatory drugs and physical therapy may provide relief of symptoms.

Lateral Epicondylitis (Tennis Elbow)   Lateral epicondylitis, or tennis elbow, is a painful condition involving the soft tissue over the lateral aspect of the elbow. The pain originates at or near the site of attachment of the common extensors to the lateral epicondyle and may radiate into the forearm and dorsum of the wrist. This painful condition is thought to be caused by small tears of the extensor aponeurosis resulting from repeated resisted contractions of the extensor muscles. The pain usually appears after work or recreational activities involving repeated motions of wrist extension and supination against resistance. Most patients with this disorder injure themselves in activities other than tennis, such as pulling weeds, carrying suitcases or briefcases, or using a screwdriver. The injury in tennis usually occurs when hitting a backhand with the elbow flexed. Shaking hands and opening doors can reproduce the pain. Striking the lateral elbow against a solid object may also induce pain.

The treatment is usually rest along with administration of a nonsteroidal anti-inflammatory drug. Ultrasound, icing, and friction massage may also help relieve pain. When pain is severe, the elbow is placed in a sling or splinted at 90° of flexion. When the pain is acute and well localized, injection of a steroid using a small-gauge needle may be effective. Following injection, the patient should be advised to rest the arm for at least 1 month and avoid activities that would aggravate the elbow. Once symptoms have subsided, the patient should begin rehabilitation to strengthen and increase flexibility of the extensor muscles before resuming physical activity involving the arm. A forearm band placed 2.5 to 5.0 cm (1 to 2 in) below the elbow may help to reduce tension on the extensor muscles at their attachment to the lateral epicondyle. The patient should be advised to restrict activities requiring forcible extension and supination of the wrist. Improvement may take several months. The patient may continue to experience mild pain but, with care, usually can avoid the return of debilitating pain. In an occasional patient, surgical release of the extensor aponeurosis may be necessary.

Medial Epicondylitis   Medial epicondylitis is an overuse syndrome resulting in pain over the medial side of the elbow with radiation into the forearm. The cause of this syndrome is considered to be repetitive resisted motions of wrist flexion and pronation, which lead to microtears and granulation tissue at the origin of the pronator teres and forearm flexors, particularly the flexor carpi radialis. This overuse syndrome is usually seen in patients older than 35 years and is much less common than lateral epicondylitis. It occurs most often in work-related repetitive activities but also occurs with recreational activities such as swinging a golf club (golfer's elbow) or throwing a baseball. On physical examination, there is tenderness just distal to the medial epicondyle over the origin of the forearm flexors. Pain can be reproduced by resisting wrist flexion and pronation with the elbow extended. Radiographs are usually normal. The differential diagnosis of patients with medial elbow symptoms include tears of the pronator teres, acute medial collateral ligament tear, and medial collateral ligament instability. Ulnar neuritis has been found in 25 to 50 percent of patients with medial epicondylitis and is associated with tenderness over the ulnar nerve at the elbow as well as hypesthesia and paresthesias on the ulnar side of the hand.

The initial treatment of medial epicondylitis is conservative, involving rest, nonsteroidal anti-inflammatory drugs, friction massage, ultrasound, and icing. Some patients may require splinting. Injections of glucocorticoids at the painful site may also be effective. Patients should be instructed to rest at least 1 month. Also, patients should be started on physical therapy once the pain has subsided. In patients with chronic debilitating medial epicondylitis that remains unresponsive after at least a year of treatment, surgical release of the flexor muscle at its origin may be necessary and is often successful.

TUMORS OF JOINTS   Primary tumors and tumor-like disorders of synovium are uncommon but should be considered in the differential diagnosis of monarticular joint disease. In addition, metastases to bone and primary bone tumors adjacent to a joint may produce joint symptoms.

Pigmented villonodular synovitis is characterized by exuberant proliferation of synovial cells, usually involving a single joint. It occurs most often in young adults and affects both sexes equally. The cause of this disorder is unknown.

The synovium has a brownish color and numerous large, fingerlike villi which fuse to form pedunculated nodules. There is marked hyperplasia of synovial cells in the stroma of the villi. Hemosiderin granules and lipids are found in the cytoplasm of macrophages and in the interstitial tissue. Multinucleated giant cells may be present. The proliferative synovium grows into the subsynovial tissue and invades adjacent cartilage and bone.

The clinical picture of pigmented villonodular synovitis is characterized by the insidious onset of swelling and pain in one joint, most commonly the knee. Other joints affected include the hips, ankles, calcaneocuboid joints, elbows, and small joints of the fingers or toes. The disease also may involve the common flexor sheath of the hand. Symptoms may be mild and intermittent and may be present for years before the patient seeks medical attention. Radiographs may show joint space narrowing, erosions, and subchondral cysts. The joint fluid contains blood and is dark red or almost black in color. Lipid-containing macrophages may be present in the fluid. The joint fluid may be clear if hemorrhages have not occurred.

The treatment of pigmented villonodular synovitis is complete synovectomy. With incomplete synovectomy, the villonodular synovitis recurs, and the rate of tissue growth may be faster than originally. Irradiation of the involved joint has been successful in some patients.

Synovial chondromatosis is a disorder characterized by multiple focal metaplastic growths of normal-appearing cartilage in the synovium or tendon sheath. Segments of cartilage break loose and continue to grow as loose bodies. When calcification and ossification of loose bodies occur, the disorder is referred to as *synovial osteochondromatosis*. The disorder is usually monarticular and affects young to middle-aged individuals. The knee is most often involved, followed by hip, elbow, and shoulder. Symptoms are pain, swelling, and decreased motion of the joint. Radiographs may show several rounded calcifications within the joint cavity. Treatment is synovectomy; however, the tumor may recur.

Hemangiomas occur in synovium and in tendon sheaths. The knee is affected most commonly. Recurrent episodes of joint swelling and pain usually begin in childhood. The joint fluid is bloody. Treatment is excision of the lesion. *Lipomas* occur most often in the knee, originating in the subsynovial fat on either side of the patellar tendon. Lipomas also appear in tendon sheaths of the hands, wrists, feet, and ankles. In some instances, surgical removal is necessary.

Synovial sarcoma (malignant synovioma) is a neoplasm of connective origin arising from tissue adjacent to large joints and seldom from the joint itself. It occurs most often in young adults and is more common in men. The tumor presents as a slowly growing mass near a joint, without much pain. The tumor spreads along tissue planes. The most common site of visceral metastasis is lung. The diagnosis is made by biopsy. Treatment is wide resection of the tumor including adjacent muscle and regional lymph nodes. Amputation of the involved distal extremity may be required. Chemotherapy may be beneficial in some patients with metastatic disease.

Synovial chondrosarcoma may arise in the synovium, tendon sheath, or bursa and is very rare. Treatment is radical excision or amputation.

BIBLIOGRAPHY

ALTMAN RD, TENENBAUM J: Hypertrophic osteoarthropathy, in *Textbook of Rheumatology*, 5th ed, WN Kelley et al (eds). Philadelphia, Saunders, 1997

ARMAN MI et al: Brief report. Frequency and features of rheumatic findings in thalassaemia minor: A blind controlled study. Br J Rheumatol 31:197, 1992

BENNETT RM: The fibromyalgia syndrome, in *Textbook of Rheumatology*, 5th ed, WN Kelley et al (eds). Philadelphia, Saunders, 1997

BERKOVITCH M et al: Arthropathy in thalassaemia patients receiving deferiprone. Lancet 343:1471, 1994

CARELESS DJ, COHEN MG: Rheumatic manifestations of hyperlipidemia and antihyperlipidemia drug therapy. Semin Arthritis Rheum 23:90, 1993

CRONIN ME: Rheumatic aspects of endocrinopathies, in *Arthritis and Allied Conditions,* 13th ed, WJ Koopman (ed). Baltimore, Williams & Wilkins, 1997

ELLMAN MH: Neuropathic joint disease (Charcot joints), in *Arthritis and Allied Conditions,* 13th ed, WJ Koopman (ed). Baltimore, Williams & Wilkins, 1997

GOLDENBERG DL: Fibromyalgia: Why such controversy? Ann Rheum Dis 54:3, 1995

HECK LW JR: Arthritis associated with hematologic disorders, storage diseases, disorders of lipid metabolism, and dysproteinemias, in *Arthritis and Allied Conditions,* 13th ed, WJ Koopman (ed). Baltimore, Williams & Wilkins, 1997

HOCHBERG ME: Relapsing Polychondritis, in *Textbook of Rheumatology*, 5th ed, WN Kelley et al (eds). Philadelphia, Saunders, 1997

ISAAK BL et al: Ocular and systemic findings in relapsing polychondritis. Ophthalmology 93:681, 1986

KOZIN F: Painful shoulder and the reflex sympathetic dystrophy syndrome, in *Arthritis and Allied Conditions*, 13th ed, WJ Koopman (ed). Baltimore, Williams & Wilkins, 1997

LAMBERT RE, McGUIRE JL: Iron storage disease, in *Textbook of Rheumatology*, 5th ed, WN Kelley et al (eds). Philadelphia, Saunders, 1997

LANG B et al: Susceptibility to relapsing polychondritis is associated with HLA-DR4. Arthritis Rheum 36:660, 1993

LINTNER SA et al: Sports medicine, in *Textbook of Rheumatology*, 5th ed, WN Kelley et al (eds). Philadelphia, Saunders, 1997

MARTINEZ-LAVIN M: Hypertrophic osteoarthropathy, in *Rheumatology*, JF Klippel, PA Dieppe (eds). St. Louis, Mosby, 1993, pp 40.1–40.4

MATSEN FA III, ARNTZ CT: Subacromial impingement, in *The Shoulder*, L Reines (ed). Philadelphia, Saunders, 1990

MICHET CJ: Relapsing polychondritis, in *Arthritis and Allied Conditions,* 13th ed, WJ Koopman (ed). Baltimore, Williams & Wilkins, 1997

NEER CS II: Impingement lesions. Clin Orthop 173:70, 1983

ROSENBERG EA, SCHILLER AC: Tumors and tumor-like lesions of joints and related structures, in *Textbook of Rheumatology*, 5th ed, WN Kelley et al (eds). Philadelphia, Saunders, 1997

SCHUMACHER RH JR: Hemoglobinopathies and arthritis, in *Textbook of Rheumatology*, 5th ed, WN Kelley et al (eds). Philadelphia, Saunders, 1997

UPCHURCH KS, BRETTLER DB: Hemophilic arthropathy, in *Textbook of Rheumatology*, 5th ed, WN Kelley et al (eds). Philadelphia, Saunders, 1997

WILKE WS: Treatment of "resistant" fibromyalgia. Rheum Dis Clin North Am 21:247, 1995

WOLFE F: When to diagnose fibromyalgia. Rheum Dis Clin North Am 20:485, 1994

——— et al: The prevalence and characteristics of fibromyalgia in the general population. Arthritis Rheum 38:19, 1995

327 | Jean D. Wilson

APPROACH TO THE PATIENT WITH ENDOCRINE AND METABOLIC DISORDERS

Communication between cells is mediated by the endocrine, nervous, and immune systems, which constitute an interlocking network. Not only do neurotransmitters such as norepinephrine circulate in blood as hormones, but neural impulses have major effects on the release of chemical mediators such as testosterone and insulin. Likewise, the immune system is subject to neural and hormonal modulation, and cytokine formation by lymphocytes can influence endocrine function. The interlocking nature of this relationship is most apparent in the hypothalamus, where a neuroendocrine-immunologic system evolved to integrate and coordinate the metabolic activities of higher organisms. Endocrinology deals largely with the chemical mediators that are secreted into the bloodstream, but in fact the functions of the three systems interlap at every level.

The term *hormone* originally referred to substances that are synthesized in a limited number of tissues and secreted into the circulation to act as chemical effectors in other tissues. However, the capacity to form such chemical mediators is not limited to so-called endocrine organs. Some hormones, such as angiotensins II and III, are formed in the bloodstream itself. Others, such as testosterone in women and dihydrotestosterone and estradiol in men, are both secreted from the gonads and formed in extraglandular tissues from circulating precursors (prohormones). Still other hormones circulate only in restricted compartments, such as the hypothalamic-pituitary portal system, and do not reach the systemic circulation in appreciable quantities. Finally, hormones such as insulin and dihydrotestosterone have *autocrine* actions in the cells of origin, *paracrine* actions in cells in the same tissues in which they are formed, *juxtacrine* actions on adjacent cells, and *endocrine* actions at distal sites. Other chemical mediators, such as müllerian-inhibiting hormone, appear to exert paracrine actions exclusively.

BIOCHEMISTRY

SYNTHESIS The approximately 150 known chemical mediators fall into three major categories—peptides or peptide derivatives, steroids, and amines. In the case of peptide hormones, genes code for messenger RNA, which is then translated into protein precursors. These proteins undergo posttranslational cleavage (preproparathyroid hormone → proparathyroid hormone → parathyroid hormone) and/or processing (thyroglobulin → thyroxine → triiodothyronine) to form the active hormone recognized by the target tissues. The distinct feature of peptide hormones is that one or a few structural genes code for the amino acid sequence of the peptide, and other genes are responsible for the alteration of the peptide to its final form. In the case of peptide hormones with subunits, the different subunits may be derived either from a single precursor (insulin) or from separate precursors [luteinizing hormone (LH)]. Furthermore, the same peptide hormone (somatostatin) can be formed from different prohormones encoded by distinct genes; individual prohormones such as proopiomelanocortin can be metabolized to different hormones in different cells, depending on the complement of processing enzymes in the cell in question; and the initial RNA transcripts of the calcitonin gene can be alternatively spliced in different tissues to form messenger RNA for either calcitonin or calcitonin gene–related peptide. Peptide hormones may also be formed ectopically in malignancies of nonendocrine origin, such as carcinoma of the lung, and in small amounts in normal nonendocrine tissues (see Chap. 102).

In the case of steroid hormones, the precursor—cholesterol (for most steroid hormones) or 7-dehydrocholesterol (for vitamin D metabolites)—undergoes a series of enzymatic transformations to form the final products. At least six enzymes, and consequently a minimum of six genes, are required to transform cholesterol to estradiol. Because of the number of enzymes required, the formation of steroid hormones is unusual in nonendocrine malignancies. However, many tissues—malignant and nonmalignant—that cannot synthesize steroid hormones from cholesterol contain enzymes that convert circulating steroids to other hormones; examples are the conversion of androgens to estrogens by trophoblastic tumors and by normal adipocytes and the conversion of progesterone to deoxycorticosterone by the kidney.

Amine hormones are formed by a process similar to that involved in steroid hormone synthesis except that the precursors are amino acids. For example, tyrosine is the precursor for epinephrine and norepinephrine (see Chap. 70).

STORAGE Most endocrine organs have a limited capacity to store the hormones they synthesize. For example, the normal adult testes contain only about one-fifteenth the quantity of testosterone secreted each day, and the testicular pool turns over several times to provide the normal daily output of hormone. Even when tissues have special storage organelles for hormones, the amount of hormone stored is usually limited: The insulin granules in the pancreatic beta cell ordinarily contain amounts of insulin sufficient only for short-term, reserve needs. (In contrast, nerve endings may contain a several-day supply of norepinephrine.) The limited storage capacity for hormones in tissues is due to the unsuitability of these compounds for incorporation into any of the three main storage compartments of the body (lipids, glycogen, or protein). For example, most steroid hormones are too polar to be stored in large quantities in lipid compartments, and peptide and amine hormones are unsuitable for incorporation into proteins. As a consequence, the body pools of most hormones tend to be small. The major exceptions to this rule occur when hormone precursors can be stored either as protein or in neutral lipid compartments; the normal thyroid gland contains the equivalent of a 2-week supply of thyroid hormones in the form of the protein thyroglobulin, and the precursor and intermediate forms of vitamin D can be stored in considerable quantity in hepatic lipid.

RELEASE Release of hormones into the blood stream can involve conversion of insoluble to soluble derivatives (proteolysis of thyroglobulin to thyroid hormones), exocytosis of storage granules (insulin, glucagon, prolactin, growth hormone), or passive diffusion of newly synthesized molecules such as steroid hormones down activity gradients into plasma.

Because of the limited capacity for storage, most hormones are released into plasma at a pace reflecting their rates of formation, and most trophic hormones enhance both the synthesis and release of their target hormones. Even when peptide hormones are stored in granules, release of the stored material is followed by an enhanced rate of synthesis (as, for instance, the two-phase release of insulin induced by glucose infusion). For some hormones, diurnal, sleep-related, developmental, and neural factors influence hormone release, and in most of these instances, synthesis and release are also tightly linked.

Hormone release may be periodic or rhythmic, the cycle varying in frequency from minutes to hours (*ultradian*) to daily (*circadian*) to months or years (*infradian*). The release of hormones such as LH and follicle-stimulating hormone (FSH) is *pulsatile*, with bursts of secretion occurring in a repetitive pattern; the release of adrenocorticotropic hormone (ACTH) (and of cortisol) varies over a 24-h cycle; and thyroid hormone release can vary on longer cycles. Whether this intermittent release is a function of alterations in synthetic rates, changes in blood flow, or other mechanisms is uncertain, but most such cycles are under neurogenic control. In some instances the physiologic significance of pulsatile release is not fully understood, but changes in frequency or amplitude of the release pattern on occasion have profound effects on hormone function; i.e., the pulsatile administration of luteinizing hormone–releasing hormone (LHRH) stimulates the release of LH by the pituitary, whereas the constant infusion of the same amount of hormone per unit time has the opposite effect. Furthermore, changes in frequency or amplitude of hormone release are characteristic of some disease states; the diurnal rhythm of cortisol release is lost in the early phase of Cushing's disease, and pulsatile release of LHRH is blunted in anorexia nervosa. Understanding the rhythms by which hormones are released is essential for interpreting plasma hormone levels.

TRANSPORT   Hormones are transported via lymph, blood, and extracellular fluids to sites of cellular action and ultimately of metabolic inactivation and degradation. The plasma is probably a passive diluent for most peptide and amine hormones, and this feature explains the short half-lives (3 to 7 min) of most nonglycosylated peptide hormones. [Glycoprotein hormones such as human chorionic gonadotropin (hCG) have longer half-lives.] The more insoluble a hormone in water, the more important the role of transport proteins; for example, thyroid and steroid hormones are transported largely in protein-bound form. However, no transport protein is the sole carrier of its hormone; for example, testosterone can be transported both by a specific binding protein [testosterone-binding globulin (TeBG); also called sex hormone–binding globulin (SHBG)] and by albumin; thyroxine can be transported both by prealbumin and by thyroxine-binding globulin (TBG). Protein-bound hormone (HP) cannot enter most cellular compartments and serves as a reservoir from which free hormone (H) is liberated for diffusion into intracellular compartments:

$$H + P \rightleftharpoons HP$$

Distribution of bound and free hormone in plasma is determined by the amount of hormone, the amount of binding protein(s), and the binding affinity of hormone for the proteins. The relation between free and bound hormone is complex. First, the free (dialyzable) fraction in vitro is usually an underestimate of the actual free fraction in vivo, because hormone bound to weakly binding proteins, such as albumin (in contrast to that bound to high-affinity binding proteins), dissociates rapidly as the free fraction diffuses from the capillary; consequently, the albumin-bound hormone approximates the free fraction in some capillary beds. In tissues, such as liver, that clear hormone-transport protein complexes, free hormone levels have less impact on hormone uptake by the tissue.

Second, the distribution of hormones between plasma and tissue is a function of the balance between tissue binding proteins and plasma binding proteins. Therefore, free hormone levels may not reflect the amounts of hormone within cells.

Third, only the free hormone interacts with receptors in target cells and participates in the regulatory feedback control of hormone synthesis. As a consequence, changes in the amount of transport protein cannot cause endocrine pathology in the steady state, provided the remainder of the endocrine feedback loop is intact. For example, profound elevations or decreases in TBG (because of either genetic or other factors) are both compatible with a euthyroid state. To illustrate, an increase in TBG would lower the level of free (dialyzable)

hormone and lower the amount bound to albumin; as a consequence, secretion of thyroid-stimulating hormone (TSH) would increase, and the output of thyroxine by the thyroid would increase *until* TBG again became saturated and the level of free hormone returned to the normal range, at which time TSH levels and the rate of thyroid hormone secretion also would return to normal. Likewise, a decrease in TBG would temporarily increase the level of free hormone, and TSH secretion and thyroxine output would fall until the free level returns to normal.

To summarize, a change in the level of a transport protein can cause profound alterations in total hormone levels but does not cause either hormone excess or deficiency of the hormone, provided the regulatory feedback mechanisms that control hormone synthesis are intact. However, alterations in the level of transport protein can cause endocrine pathology when hormone formation is not regulated by feedback control mechanisms or when feedback control mechanisms are deranged. For example, testosterone production in women is not regulated by testosterone levels, and alterations in TeBG levels in women can change the steady-state levels of free testosterone. Likewise, changes in TBG levels in a hypothyroid patient receiving a fixed dose of levothyroxine can cause alterations in free thyroxine levels.

DEGRADATION AND TURNOVER   The plasma level (PL) of any hormone is dependent on the secretion rate (SR) of the hormone and the rates of metabolism and excretion, the so-called metabolic clearance rate (MCR):

$$PL = SR/MCR \qquad or \qquad SR = MCR \times PL$$

Metabolic clearance of hormones is accomplished by several mechanisms. Small amounts of hormones are excreted intact in urine or bile. The largest fraction is degraded and/or inactivated in target tissues and in the liver and kidneys. Peptide hormones are inactivated by proteases, largely in target tissues. Catabolism of steroid and thyroid hormone facilitates their excretion by rendering them soluble in urine or bile. Thyroid hormones are deiodinated, deaminated, and deconjugated largely by the liver. Steroid hormones are reduced, hydroxylated, and converted into water-soluble glucuronide and sulfate conjugates. Biliary conjugates may be hydrolyzed in the gastrointestinal tract and reabsorbed into the circulation. The degradative mechanisms for different hormones have one common feature, namely, that alternative pathways exist for the catabolism of all hormones described to date.

Because of the nature of feedback control of hormone secretion, changes in rates of hormone degradation alone, like changes in plasma protein binding, do not cause endocrine pathology, provided the feedback control mechanisms that regulate synthesis are intact. For example, in severe liver disease and in hypothyroidism, the degradation of glucocorticoids by the liver is impaired; as a consequence, the turnover of cortisol slows, but the plasma level does not rise above the normal range because secretion of ACTH is inhibited. Thus, a normal level of free hormone is maintained by a decrease in the rate of cortisol secretion. The opposite is the case when glucocorticoid degradation is enhanced (as in thyrotoxicosis); in this situation, cortisol secretion increases to keep the level of the hormone normal.

Although changes in hormone degradation rates alone do not cause hormone deficit or excess, they can alter endocrine pharmacology. For example, ordinary doses of glucocorticoids can cause Cushing's syndrome when glucocorticoid metabolism is impaired by hypothyroidism or liver disease, and consequently glucocorticoid dosage must be reduced appropriately in both states. Likewise, doses of glucocorticoids may have to be increased in patients with hyperthyroidism. In addition, the development of hyperthyroidism in a patient with inadequate adrenal reserve can precipitate an adrenal crisis by accelerating glucocorticoid metabolism. Thus, when the normal control mechanisms that regulate hormone synthesis are circumvented or inoperative, changes in rates of hormone degradation can cause or aggravate pathology.

REGULATION OF HORMONE PRODUCTION

As stated above, hormone levels are determined primarily by the rates of formation. A unifying feature of all endocrine systems is the fact that the production of most hormones is regulated directly or indirectly by the metabolic activity of the hormone itself. This regulation is accomplished through a series of negative (and positive) feedback loops (Fig. 327-1). For example, hormones produced under the control of pituitary trophic hormones (cortisol, thyroxine, gonadal steroids) feed back on the hypothalamic-pituitary system to regulate their own rates of secretion. Similarly, the secretion of parathyroid hormone and insulin is controlled by feedback signals from serum calcium and glucose levels, respectively. When the hormone itself acts as the direct regulator of feedback (testosterone on the hypothalamic-pituitary axis), the effect is mediated by the same receptor system by which the hormone acts in other target tissues. An example of positive feedback is the stimulation of LH release by estradiol prior to ovulation. Nonhormonal and environmental factors can alter both positive and negative feedback control mechanisms or the response to such control.

Most feedback control systems operate within minutes or hours in response to varying metabolic demands to maintain homeostatic control within a narrow range. The main exceptions relate to spermatogenesis (see Chap. 336). Spermatogenesis and sperm export require approximately 2.5 months from initiation of differentiation to ejaculation of mature sperm, so that changes in FSH levels may not alter the numbers of sperm in the ejaculate for long periods.

The fact that the secretion of hormones is under regulatory control has important clinical implications. First, the plasma levels of hormones may be interpretable only if the appropriate regulatory factors are taken into account (Fig. 327-2). The meaning of a borderline-low plasma thyroxine level may be clear only when TSH is measured simultaneously; likewise, plasma insulin and parathyroid hormone levels may be interpretable only in conjunction with simultaneous measurements of plasma glucose and calcium, respectively. Second, the finding of simultaneous elevation of a hormone pair (or of a hormone and its regulatory factor) in the absence of evidence of hormone excess suggests the presence of a hormone-resistance state. For example, simultaneous elevation of plasma glucose and insulin is characteristic of insulin resistance, and simultaneous elevation of LH and testosterone suggests androgen resistance. In contrast, simultaneous elevation of hormone pairs with signs of hormone excess suggests a hormone-secreting tumor. Third, the fact that hormone secretion is under regulatory control is the basis for the various dynamic tests of hormone reserve and hormone secretion for the evaluation of subtle derangements of endocrine pathology (see below).

MECHANISMS OF HORMONE ACTION

In some instances, the first step in hormone action is the metabolism of the circulating hormone into its active form, either in plasma (as in the formation of angiotensin II from angiotensin), in target tissues

FIGURE 327-1 Feedback control of target endocrine organs such as the adrenal, thyroid, or gonads by the pituitary.

FIGURE 327-2 Relation between target hormone level and trophic hormone level in normal and disease states (e.g., TSH and thyroid hormones, ACTH and cortisol, LH and testosterone).

(as in the conversion of testosterone to dihydrotestosterone), or in secondary tissues for retransport back into plasma (as in the conversion of thyroxine to triiodothyronine and of testosterone to estradiol). All hormones then act by binding to receptors that are located either intracellularly or in the cell membrane.

INTRACELLULAR RECEPTORS Most intracellular hormones gain access to cell cytoplasm by what is believed to be a passive diffusion mechanism down an activity gradient and then bind to a specific receptor protein to form a hormone-receptor complex (Fig. 327-3). The hormone-receptor complex, which can either form in the cytoplasm and move into the nucleus or form within the nucleus itself, has the capacity to attach to specific regulatory sequences in DNA (so-called hormone regulatory elements) and acts to control the rate of RNA transcription from genes under the control of these regulatory elements. As the result, the synthesis of messenger RNA (mRNA) is either increased or decreased, and the synthesis of cytoplasmic proteins that mediate the effects of the hormone increases or decreases.

The receptors of this class bear a striking sequence homology to each other, suggesting that they evolved from a common ancestral transcription regulatory factor. Each contains a hormone-binding domain, a DNA-binding domain, and an *N*-terminal variable or immunodominant domain (Fig. 327-4). More than one receptor exists for certain hormones (thyroid hormones, retinoic acid). The hormone-receptor complexes are believed to act as dimers, and additional transcription regulatory factors are involved in their control of RNA transcription. Elucidation of the structures of these receptors made it possible to analyze the mutations that impair hormone action and cause hormone-resistance syndromes (see below).

MEMBRANE-BOUND RECEPTORS Membrane-bound hormone receptors can be divided into several classes, each of which

FIGURE 327-3 Mechanism of action of hormones with intracellular receptors. H, hormone; P, plasma transport protein; R, receptor; R*, activated receptor; mRNA, messenger RNA.

FIGURE 327-4 Intracellular receptors of the thyroid-steroid-retinoic acid class. The areas of greatest homology (DNA-binding domain) are shown by the light blue bars; the areas of intermediate homology (hormone-binding domain) are shown by the dark blue bars; and the areas with the least homology are shown by the open regions.

works by different mechanisms: seven-transmembrane-domain receptors, protein tyrosine kinase receptors, guanylyl cyclase receptors, and growth hormone/prolactin (cytokine family) receptors (Table 327-1 and Fig. 327-5).

Seven-Transmembrane-Domain Receptors This receptor family includes the α- and β-adrenergic receptors and receptors for parathyroid hormone, vasopressin, angiotensin II, glucagon, serotonin, dopamine, LH, FSH, TSH, and prostaglandins. Each of these receptors interacts within the plasma membrane with a member of another family of proteins, the guanine nucleotide–binding proteins (G proteins). The G protein family includes: G_s, which mediates adenyl cyclase stimulation; G_i, which mediates adenylyl cyclase inhibition; and G_q, which mediates phospholipase C activation. The G proteins are heterotrimers, composed of α, β, and γ subunits. The α subunits are unique to each G protein (some 15 different α subunits having been characterized), whereas the β and γ subunits of different G proteins are similar. The interaction of hormone-receptor complexes of this class with G proteins initiates reactions that cause the release of a variety of intracellular second messenger molecules that influence cellular metabolism. The classic second messenger is cyclic adenosine monophosphate (cyclic AMP), and many hormone actions are mediated by effects on adenylyl cyclase to increase or decrease cellular cyclic AMP, including actions of epinephrine and norepinephrine (the β-adrenergic receptor), vasopressin (V_2 receptors), glucagon, ACTH, LH, FSH, and TSH. Other hormone-receptor interactions activate phospholipase C to increase free cytosolic calcium and enhance protein kinase C, including epinephrine and norepinephrine (α-adrenergic receptors), vasopressin (V_1 receptors), and angiotensin II.

Protein Tyrosine Kinases Receptors of this class include the insulin receptor and receptors for epidermal growth factor (EGF), insulin-like growth factor I, fibroblast growth factor, and platelet-derived growth factor. The insulin receptor is a tetramer composed of two α and two β subunits, which are linked by sulfhydryl bonds (Fig. 327-5). The α subunits are extracellular and contain the insulin binding site, and the β subunits have one transmembrane domain and exhibit insulin-dependent tyrosine kinase activity; autophosphorylation of tyrosine residues on the receptor enhances the tyrosine kinase activity and enables the enzyme to phosphorylate other proteins that are components of downstream signaling pathways. The tyrosine kinase activity is essential for insulin action, as evidenced by the fact that point mutations in the coding sequence of the receptor gene that impair kinase activity cause profound resistance to insulin action (see below).

Receptors for Growth Hormone and Prolactin (the Cytokine Receptor Family) Receptors of this type do not have kinase domains, but ligand binding results in the rapid phosphorylation of tyrosine residues on the receptors themselves and on cellular proteins. This tyrosine phosphorylation is mediated by a family of cytoplasmic tyrosine kinases, the Janus kinases (JAK) (Fig. 327-5), which associate physically with intracellular domains of the receptors and are themselves activated to phosphorylate *s*ignal *t*ransducers and *a*ctivators of *t*ranscription (STATs), which mediate the actions of the hormones. The high-affinity growth hormone–binding protein in plasma corresponds to the extracellular hormone-binding domain of the growth hormone receptor and is believed to be cleaved from the receptor, but the role of the plasma protein in the regulation of growth is undefined. The growth hormone receptor has approximately 25 percent homology with the prolactin receptor, which suggests that the two receptors have evolved from a common ancestral gene. Mutations that impair the function of the growth hormone receptor are responsible for Laron dwarfism (see below).

Guanylyl Cyclase Receptors The receptor for atrial natriuretic peptide (ANP) is a guanylyl cyclase that spans the plasma membrane; the extracellular domain of the receptor binds the hormone, and the intracellular domain synthesizes guanosine-3′,5′-monophosphate (cyclic GMP) which serves as the second messenger for the hormone. The mechanism(s) by which cyclic GMP mediates the actions of ANP are not known, but in some cells cyclic GMP acts to maintain cation channels in an open configuration.

Table 327-1

Classification of Hormone Receptors

Type	Characteristic Hormones	Disease States due to Impairment of Receptor Function
INTRACELLULAR RECEPTORS		
Transcription regulatory proteins	Glucocorticoids, mineralocorticoids, estradiol, androgens, progesterone, triiodothyronine, 1,25-dihydroxyvitamin D, retinoic acid	Testicular feminization and other androgen resistance syndromes; cortisol resistance; vitamin D–dependent rickets, type II; thyroid hormone resistance; estrogen resistance
MEMBRANE RECEPTORS		
Seven-transmembrane-domain receptors	LH, TSH, parathyroid hormone, epinephrine, somatostatin, vasopressin, glucagon, angiotensin II, FSH, prostaglandins, serotonin	Pseudohypoparathyroidism, nephrogenic diabetes insipidus, male pseudohermaphroditism due to mutations of the LH receptor, Jansen's metaphyseal chondrodysplasia
Protein tyrosine kinases	Insulin, insulin-like growth factor I, platelet-derived growth factor, epidermal growth factor, fibroblast growth factor	Diabetes mellitus with profound insulin resistance
Growth hormone–prolactin family	Growth hormone, prolactin, cytokines, nerve growth factor	Laron dwarfism
Guanylate cyclase	Atrial natriuretic peptide	—

Endocrinopathy can result from hormone deficiency, hormone excess, resistance to hormone action, or constitutive mutations that activate hormone response systems in the absence of ligand; abnormalities in more than one endocrine system may coexist in the same individual.

DEFICIENCY STATES With few exceptions (calcitonin), hormone deficiency results in pathologic manifestations. The investigation of clinical deficiency states played an important role in the evolution of the discipline of endocrinology. Recognition of the effects of hormone deficiency was followed by extraction of the responsible hormone from normal endocrine tissues, characterization of the chemical nature of the molecule (and, ultimately, organic synthesis of it), and administration of the hormone to replace the deficit. The treatment of hypothyroidism by the administration of thyroid hormone is probably as successful as any therapeutic measure in medicine. Because clinical deficiency states can be induced in experimental animals by destruction or removal of the endocrine organ, an enormous amount is known about the pathophysiology of deficiency states, such as diabetes mellitus, pituitary and adrenal insufficiency, hypothyroidism, and hypogonadism.

The destructive processes that cause failure of the endocrine organs are also understood in many instances and include infections (as in adrenal insufficiency due to tuberculosis), tissue death due to infarction (as in postpartum pituitary failure) or inflammation (as in diabetes mellitus secondary to pancreatitis), tumors (as in null cell tumors of the pituitary), autoimmune processes that either destroy endocrine organs (as in Hashimoto's thyroiditis) or block the binding of trophic hormones (as in idiopathic hypothyroidism), dietary inadequacy (as in hypothyroidism due to iodine deficiency), and hereditary defects in hormone synthesis (as in pituitary dwarfism). In type I diabetes mellitus, the cause may be a hereditary predisposition that renders the pancreas subject to destruction by several mechanisms (see Chap. 334). In some instances (congenital anorchia) the etiology of the defect is unknown.

HORMONE EXCESS With few exceptions (testosterone in men, progesterone in men and women) hormone excess causes pathologic effects. Four general types of hormone excess are recognized. In one, the hormone is overproduced by the gland that is the usual site of its production (hyperthyroidism, acromegaly, Cushing's disease). In this situation, excess hormone production is due to failure or circumvention of the feedback mechanisms that control normal production

and can arise by several mechanisms, including autoantibodies that mimic the action of natural hormones (as in the case of thyroid-stimulating immunoglobulins in hyperthyroidism), mutations in receptor-effector mechanisms that impair feedback (as in mutation of G proteins in growth-hormone secreting pituitary adenomas), and development of tumors of uncertain provenance (such as Leydig cell tumors). A second type of hormone excess results when a hormone is produced by a tissue (usually malignant) that does not synthesize it ordinarily (for example, ACTH production by oat cell carcinoma of the lung, thyroid hormone secretion by struma ovarii). A third type of hormone excess involves the overproduction of hormones in peripheral tissues from circulating precursors, for example, overproduction of estrogen in liver disease because of diversion of the precursor androstenedione from its usual sites of catabolism in the liver to sites of extraglandular estrogen formation. Finally, hormone excess all too commonly results from iatrogenic causes (as in the complications resulting from glucocorticoid therapy; see Chap. 332) or from self-administration of hormones such as levothyroxine or insulin.

An excess of a given hormone may result from more than one cause. Thyrotoxicosis can result from overproduction of hormone by the thyroid as a result of overproduction of TSH (rare), from the action of thyroid-stimulating immunoglobulins on the thyroid, from autonomous thyroid hyperfunction, from leakage of preformed hormone due to an inflammatory injury of the thyroid, or from excess hormone arising from sources other than the thyroid itself, as in thyroid hormone overdosage, accidental ingestion of meats contaminated with thyroid tissue, or secretion by struma ovarii (see Chap. 331). The unraveling of the cause of specific hormone-excess states can be one of the most challenging problems of clinical endocrinology.

PRODUCTION OF ABNORMAL HORMONES In some instances abnormal hormones cause endocrine disease. One form of diabetes mellitus is the result of a single-gene mutation that results in the production of an abnormal insulin molecule that is ineffective because of defective binding to the insulin receptor. In other cases, hormone precursors, hormone subunits, or incompletely processed peptide hormones may be released into the circulation, as is common in so-called ectopic hormone production of neoplasia. Alternatively, immunoglobulins may bind to hormone receptors and thus exert hormonal actions, as is the case with the thyroid-stimulating immunoglobulins that exert TSH-like actions in hyperthyroidism (see Chap. 331) or the antibodies to the insulin receptor that have insulin-like actions (see Chap. 334).

HORMONE RESISTANCE The concept that an endocrinopathy can result because the tissues cannot respond to normal (or increased) levels of a hormone evolved from the deduction that pseudohypoparathyroidism is due to peripheral resistance to the action of parathyroid hormone (see Chap. 354). Diseases are now known to result from resistance to most hormones. Such hormone-resistance states frequently are due to mutations that impair hormone action, but they can be due to acquired defects in receptors and postreceptor effector mechanisms for hormones, to development of antibodies that block hormones or hormone receptors, or to the absence of target cells. Abnormalities of receptors also cause disease outside the endocrine domain, including familial hypercholesterolemia. Hormone resistance is not always the same in all tissues; selective resistance to thyroid hormone

FIGURE 327-5 Schematic representation of different classes of hormone receptors on the cell surface. Seven-transmembrane-domain receptor (β-adrenergic receptor); protein tyrosine kinases (insulin receptor); guanylate cyclase receptor [atrial natriuretic peptide (ANP) receptor]; growth hormone-prolactin receptor family [growth hormone (GH) receptor].

can be restricted to the pituitary itself, and androgen resistance may be more severe in the testis than in other target tissues.

A common feature of hormone-resistance states is the presence of a normal or *elevated* level of the hormone in the circulation despite deficient hormone action. This feature is a consequence of the fact that hormones are normally under regulatory feedback control and that failure of hormone action leads to increased hormone production.

The elucidation of the structures of hormone receptors and the cloning of the cDNAs for these proteins has made it possible to define the molecular defects in many hormone-resistance states (Table 327-1). Several clinical implications of these studies are apparent. First, in the past it was only possible to identify receptor defects that caused profound hormone resistance, but now that subtle defects in receptor function can be identified, it is clear that hormone resistance is more common than previously recognized. Second, at the molecular level, disorders are genetically heterogeneous. Unrelated families with mutations of the insulin receptor, the growth hormone receptor, or the androgen receptor rarely have identical mutations. Furthermore, in regard to individual receptors such as the androgen receptor, mutations may be due to gross deletions or gene rearrangements that completely disrupt the coding sequence, but more commonly they are due to point mutations that cause single amino acid substitutions in the protein or create premature termination codons. It is thus necessary to analyze each family separately. Third, the analysis of these mutations has provided major insight into hormone action—for example, establishing the critical importance of the tyrosine kinase function of the insulin receptor and making it possible to define the various domains of the intracellular receptors.

GAIN-OF-FUNCTION MUTATIONS Mutations that cause constitutive activity of hormone receptors or cause hormone receptors to lose ligand-binding specificity can cause the manifestations of hormone excess even when the hormone itself is undetectable. For example, mutations that cause constitutive activation of the LH receptor cause testitoxicosis, the most common cause of premature puberty in boys, and mutations of the androgen receptor in advanced prostatic cancer may allow activation of the receptor by ligands that would normally be ineffective.

DISEASES AFFECTING MULTIPLE ENDOCRINE SYSTEMS The fact that disorders can affect more than one endocrine system has been known since the description of panhypopituitarism in the nineteenth century. Such disorders have diverse causes, including autoimmunity [as in polyglandular autoimmune syndromes (PGAs)], receptor abnormalities (as in resistance to parathyroid hormone, gonadotropins, and thyrotropin in pseudohypoparathyroidism), tumors [multiple endocrine neoplasia (MEN)], and hereditary disorders of unknown etiology (such as the lipodystrophies) (see Chap. 340). They include both hypo- and hyperfunctioning states, and some clinical syndromes may occur in the context of more than one polyendocrine state (e.g., pheochromocytoma in MEN 2A, MEN 2B, and von Hippel-Lindau disease; diabetes mellitus in PGA II and lipodystrophy).

Because each endocrinopathy in such a constellation can also occur alone, all endocrine patients must be approached with a high index of suspicion for abnormalities of multiple systems. This is of particular importance because treatment of one condition may cause worsening of another (for example, surgical procedures such as thyroidectomy can cause worsening of unrecognized pheochromocytoma) and because in certain of the familial syndromes it is mandatory to make systematic searches for the disease in potentially affected family members.

ASSESSMENT OF ENDOCRINE FUNCTION

Endocrine status is assessed by measuring plasma hormone levels or the urinary excretion of hormones or hormone metabolites, measuring hormone reserve and regulation by dynamic tests, measuring the levels of hormone receptors, assessing hormone actions in target tissues, or performing appropriate combinations of these tests.

MEASUREMENT OF PLASMA HORMONE LEVELS The plasma levels of steroid and thyroid hormones range between 1 nmol/L and 1 μmol/L, while those of peptide hormones are generally in the range of 1 pmol/L to 0.1 nmol/L. The application of chemical, chromatographic, bioassay, radioreceptor, radioimmunoassay, and immunometric techniques for the assessment of plasma levels has made clinical endocrinology one of the most quantitative of clinical disciplines. In the case of hormones whose plasma levels are relatively constant from moment to moment and day to day (such as thyroxine and triiodothyronine), single hormone level measurements provide a reliable assessment of the hormone status in most clinical situations.

In the case of hormones that undergo pulsatile secretion (such as LH or testosterone), a single value may not be representative of mean plasma levels. In such instances it is necessary either to measure levels in several samples drawn at random or to pool aliquots of three or more samples of plasma drawn at 20- to 30-min intervals for a single determination.

When plasma levels undergo a characteristic, predictable fluctuation, such as the diurnal variation of plasma cortisol, the timing of plasma sampling must be designed to provide a useful index of the hormone status. In women, appropriate interpretation of plasma levels of gonadotropins, progesterone, and estradiol during the reproductive years requires knowledge of the phase of the ovulatory and menstrual cycles in which the measurement was made, and it may be necessary to obtain sequential samples over many days to provide interpretable data. Seasonal variations also occur in the levels of certain hormones (such as thyroxine and testosterone), but these changes are generally so small that they do not affect the interpretation of individual values. In some situations, variation in hormone levels is not the result of any obvious rhythmicity but rather the consequence of waxing and waning of a disease process; repeated measurements of cortisol or of calcium and parathyroid hormone levels over many months may be necessary to establish the diagnosis of Cushing's syndrome or of hyperparathyroidism.

In the case of steroids, thyroid hormones, and some peptide hormones, such as growth hormone, that are transported in plasma largely bound to proteins, measurement of total hormone concentration provides an index of endocrine status *only* to the extent that it allows the level of the free or unbound hormone to be deduced. Methods for directly measuring the level of free hormone (usually 1 percent or less of the total level) are available for some of these hormones. Since the amount of free hormone is a function of the amount and binding affinity of the transport proteins and the amount of hormone, the total hormone level reflects the amount of free hormone only as long as the level of binding protein(s) remains constant or fluctuates only within narrow limits. In those instances in which the level of binding protein is increased (as are the levels of TBG and TeBG in pregnancy) or decreased [as in the case of hereditary low levels of TBG or cortisol-binding globulin (CBG)], it is essential to assess the amount of binding protein to allow estimation of the free hormone level (for example, by T_3 resin uptake for TBG or by direct measurement for TBG, TeBG, or CBG).

Finally, most hormones show a broad range of plasma levels within a normal population. As a consequence, the level of a hormone in an individual may be halved or doubled (and thus be abnormal for that person) but still be within the so-called normal range. For this reason, it is useful to assess appropriate hormone pairs simultaneously (e.g., LH and testosterone, thyroxine and thyroid-stimulating hormone); indeed, measurement of TSH by itself is a useful index of thyroid hormone status in people with normal pituitary glands. Likewise, a borderline low testosterone level in the presence of elevated plasma LH is indicative of testicular failure, whereas the same level of testosterone in the presence of a normal LH level implies that the endocrine status is normal (see Fig. 327-2).

URINARY EXCRETION Measurement of the urinary excretion rate of a hormone or a hormone metabolite that reflects plasma levels or secretory rates offers certain advantages over the measurement of isolated plasma levels; for example, urinary excretion reflects the average of the plasma levels over the time of collection. Thus, a 24-h urine free cortisol value may provide a better estimate of the function of the adrenal cortex than isolated measurements of plasma cortisol. Such measurements do have the following limitations, however.

CHAPTER 327
Approach to the Patient with Endocrine and Metabolic Disorders   **1971**

1. Urinary creatinine should be measured routinely to document the adequacy of the urine collection. Women excrete on average about 1 g/d of creatinine, and men, about 1.8 g/d. The day-to-day variation in this quantity should not exceed 20 percent.
2. The amounts of individual metabolites in urine may not reflect changes in hormone secretion under all conditions. For example, the formation of the 18-oxo derivative of aldosterone may be influenced by drugs that do not alter secretion or plasma levels of the hormone.
3. Urine values are obviously meaningless for those hormones (thyroxine, triiodothyronine) that are excreted into bile. Peptide hormones such as gonadotropins may be metabolized differently in different individuals before being excreted in the urine, so that establishment of the range of normal is difficult.
4. Hormones from more than one source may be excreted as a given metabolite; urinary 17-ketosteroids are derived from both adrenal and gonadal androgens, and consequently their measurement is of little value in assessing testicular androgen production in men.
5. Changes in renal function may influence rates of hormone excretion into urine. Such changes can in part be corrected for by measurement of urine creatinine, but in the case of metabolites or conjugates formed in the kidney itself excretion patterns may be distorted out of proportion to the decrease in creatinine clearance.

DYNAMIC TESTS OF HORMONE RESERVE AND REGULATION   When hypo- or hyperfunction is severe, measurement of the level of hormone in blood or urine may be satisfactory for making a diagnosis, particularly when the tests demonstrate appropriate feedback relationships; for example, low plasma testosterone coupled with high plasma LH indicates primary testicular failure. In less clear-cut instances, however, stimulation tests are useful in establishing the significance of borderline-low values. Likewise, suppression tests are used to demonstrate the presence of hyperfunction of endocrine systems. All such dynamic tests are designed to take advantage of the known feedback control mechanisms for various hormones (Fig. 327-1).

Two types of *stimulation tests* are in common use. In one, endogenous hormone production or action is blocked (e.g., cortisol production by metyrapone, estradiol action by clomiphene), and the capacity of the pituitary to respond by increasing endogenous production of the trophic hormone, and/or the capacity of the target tissue to respond, are then assessed; ideally, such tests measure the integrity of the hypothalamic-pituitary-target tissue loop. In the other type of stimulation test, the trophic hormone itself is administered under some standardized regimen, and the capacity of the target tissue to respond is determined (as in measurement of cortisol levels before and after ACTH administration). Stimulation tests are particularly useful in four situations: (1) in assessing hormone status when precise quantification of plasma levels is difficult or imperfect (as for ACTH), (2) in assessing endocrine status when static tests give borderline-low values, (3) in distinguishing primary from secondary (pituitary) causes of endocrine failure, and (4) in assessing gonadal reserve in prepubertal subjects in whom plasma levels of gonadotropins and gonadal steroids are difficult to interpret.

Suppression tests are useful for the diagnosis of endocrine hyperfunction, because, by definition, hyperfunctioning glands do not operate under normal control mechanisms. The suppression of endocrine function can be either quantitatively or qualitatively abnormal. For example, the feedback control of the pituitary may be reset to respond to high levels of the suppressing hormone (pituitary ACTH secretion in Cushing's disease), or secretion can be completely autonomous (ACTH secretion by carcinoma of the lung). In principle, the feedback regulator is administered, and the degree of inhibition of hormone secretion is assessed (e.g., by the change in radioactive iodine uptake after administration of thyroid hormones, the change in cortisol secretion after the administration of potent exogenous glucocorticoids, or the suppressibility of plasma growth hormone by glucose).

The clinical usefulness of all dynamic tests is limited by the fact that endocrine control systems are subject to influence by a multitude of secondary factors. Age, coexisting disease states, and concurrent drug regimens all interact to influence responsiveness and hence to limit the diagnostic specificity of such tests. For example, psychiatric disorders such as endogenous depression can impair responses to endocrine dynamic tests in the absence of specific endocrine pathology.

HORMONE RECEPTORS AND ANTIBODIES   The measurement of hormone receptors in biopsy material from target tissues or in fibroblasts propagated from biopsy material is useful—for example, in the diagnosis of partial hormone-resistance states such as rickets due to vitamin D resistance, hyperglycemia and hyperinsulinemia associated with insulin resistance, and male pseudohermaphroditism due to androgen resistance. Certain laboratories can apply the techniques of molecular biology to provide specific information about the structure of mutant receptors. Likewise, measurement of antibodies to hormones (such as antibodies to thyroid hormones that can cause hypothyroidism) or antibodies to target tissues (adrenal gland, gonads, thyroid) may be essential for the assessment of endocrine status. With certain exceptions (e.g., assays for antibodies to thyroid tissue), these tests are not widely available.

TISSUE EFFECTS   At the theoretical level, the ideal means of assessing endocrine function is to measure the result of hormone action in target tissues for the hormone. Such an assay would provide insight into hormone levels, hormone receptors, second messengers, and tissue responses. For example, demonstration of the capacity to concentrate urine maximally following water restriction indicates that the hypothalamic mechanisms that control the function of the posterior pituitary are intact, that the posterior pituitary has a normal capacity to secrete vasopressin, that the vasopressin receptor is intact, and that the postreceptor effector mechanisms for the hormone are operative. Ideally, such a test assesses the function of the entire pathway of hormone secretion and action. In practice, many such tests are imperfect. For example, even if vasopressin secretion is normal, intrinsic renal disease can cause a fixed low urine osmolality and thus distort the interpretation of the functional test of vasopressin action. In other instances, such tests are difficult to perform and subject both to artifacts and to influences from diverse parameters (for example, the metabolic rate is increased by fever even when thyroid function is normal). For these reasons, the identification of additional specific tissue markers for hormone action would be very useful.

IMAGING PROCEDURES   Developments in imaging have made possible the noninvasive identification of abnormalities in almost every endocrine organ, including visualization of small lesions of the pituitary and hypothalamus, bone density assessments for metabolic bone disease, and localization of functioning parathyroid tissue in patients with persistent or recurrent hyperparathyroidism.

A major problem in imaging stems from the fact that small nodules of no functional significance are known from autopsy studies to occur in the pituitary, the adrenal, and, less commonly, the testes. The natural history of these nonfunctioning adenomas is not well understood; most appear to remain limited in size and nonfunctional for life, but in rare instances they evolve into autonomous and/or hyperfunctioning tumors. In addition, malignancies—both metastatic and primary—can occur in these tissues. As a consequence, adrenal and pituitary masses are common incidental findings in computed tomography (CT) and magnetic resonance imaging (MRI) scans performed for other reasons. Several types of criteria have been proposed for deciding whether a mass of the pituitary or adrenal is likely to be benign or should be removed. By one guideline, solid, endocrinologically silent lesions of the adrenal smaller than 3.5 cm may be followed safely with serial CT scans, whereas larger lesions deserve sonographically guided percutaneous needle biopsy or exploratory surgery. Additional experience will be required to establish the validity of these and other criteria for the assessment of such masses.

Another unresolved issue stems from the fact that it is not always clear which imaging procedure is best in a given clinical situation. In many instances, evidence has accumulated for the superiority of one or the other imaging procedure in a given situation. In other instances, definitive guidelines may be harder to develop, as in the choice between MRI and CT for delineation of the anatomy of the hypothalamic-pituitary system. In some patients, small lesions are best seen with MRI, whereas in others, lesions in the same areas—equally small and with similar histologic features—are better delineated with CT. In consequence, there is a tendency in the workup of suspected pituitary tumors to order both procedures routinely. Although this practice is justified in some cases, it inflates the cost of diagnostic workups.

An unexpected dividend of the developments in imaging is that it is now possible to chart the natural history of endocrine disease in a different way, as in the occasional documentation of hemorrhage into a pituitary tumor that eventuates in development of the empty sella syndrome or the uncovering of a functioning adrenal adenoma when biochemical or clinical evidence of Cushing's disease is minimal.

BIBLIOGRAPHY

BERRIDGE MJ: Inositol triphosphate and calcium signalling. Nature 361:315, 1993

BELLDEGRUN A et al: Incidentally discovered mass of the adrenal gland. Surg Gynecol Obstet 163:203, 1986

DOHLMAN HG et al: Model systems for the study of seven transmembrane segment receptors. Annu Rev Biochem 60:653, 1991

EXTON JH: Signalling through phosphatidyl choline breakdown. J Biol Chem 265:l, 1990

GODOWSKI PG et al: Characterization of the human growth hormone receptor gene and demonstration of a partial gene deletion in two patients with Laron-type dwarfism. Proc Natl Acad Sci USA 86:8083, 1989

GORDEN P, WEINTRAUB BD: Radioreceptor and other functional hormone assays, in *Williams Textbook of Endocrinology*, 8th ed, JD Wilson, DW Foster (eds). Philadelphia, Saunders, 1992, pp 1647–1661

GRIFFIN JE: Dynamic tests of endocrine function, in *Williams Textbook of Endocrinology*, 8th ed, JD Wilson, DW Foster (eds). Philadelphia, Saunders, 1992, pp 1663–1670

HAMPER UM et al: Primary adrenocortical carcinoma: Sonographic evaluation with clinical and pathologic correlation in 26 patients. Am J Roentgenol 148:915, 1987

KAHN CR, GOLDSTEIN BJ: Molecular defects in insulin action. Science 245:13, 1989

MENDELSON CR: Mechanisms of hormone action, in *Textbook of Endocrine Physiology*, 3d ed, JE Griffin, SR Ojeda (eds). New York, Oxford, 1996, pp 29–66

PARDRIDGE WM: Serum bioavailability of sex steroid hormones. Clin Endocrinol Metab 15:259, 1986

PEKARY AE, HERSHMAN JM: Hormone assays, in *Endocrinology and Metabolism*, 3d ed, P Felig et al (eds). New York, McGraw-Hill, 1995, p 201

QUIGLEY CA et al: Androgen receptor defects: Historical, clinical and molecular perspectives. Endocr Rev 16:271, 1991

REFETOFF S et al: The syndromes of resistance to thyroid hormone. Endocr Rev 14:348, 1993

TAYLOR SL et al: Mutations in the insulin receptor gene. Endocr Rev 13:566, 1992

TSAI MJ et al: Molecular mechanisms of action of steroid/thyroid receptor superfamily members. Annu Rev Biochem 63:451, 1994

328

Beverly M.K. Biller, Gilbert H. Daniels

NEUROENDOCRINE REGULATION AND DISEASES OF THE ANTERIOR PITUITARY AND HYPOTHALAMUS

The pituitary, appropriately titled the *master gland*, produces six major hormones and stores an additional two hormones (Fig. 328-1). Growth hormone (GH) regulates growth and has important influences on intermediary metabolism (see Chap. 329). Prolactin (PRL) is necessary

for lactation (see Chap. 338). Luteinizing hormone (LH) and follicle-stimulating hormone (FSH) control the gonads in men and women. Thyroid-stimulating hormone (TSH, thyrotropin) regulates thyroid function. Adrenocorticotropin (ACTH) controls glucocorticoid function of the adrenal cortex. These hormones are all synthesized in the anterior pituitary. Vasopressin (AVP; also called antidiuretic hormone, ADH) and oxytocin are produced in neurons of the hypothalamus and stored in the posterior lobe of the pituitary (see Chap. 330). AVP controls water conservation by the kidneys; oxytocin is necessary for milk let-down during lactation and may aid in parturition.

A feedback relationship exists between the anterior pituitary and its three target endocrine glands—the gonads, the adrenal cortex, and the thyroid. When the gonads fail or are removed, the concentrations of LH and FSH rise, a condition known as *primary hypogonadism*. When the adrenal cortex is removed or destroyed, *primary adrenal insufficiency* (Addison's disease) results, and the serum ACTH concentration increases. Thyroid failure results in the characteristic rise in TSH of *primary hypothyroidism*.

When the pituitary gland is removed or destroyed, loss of the trophic hormones results in *secondary* hypogonadism, adrenal insufficiency, or hypothyroidism. Growth hormone and prolactin function are also lost. The functions of AVP and oxytocin are not affected by destruction of the pituitary, provided their site of origin in the hypothalamus is intact.

The pituitary is, in turn, under the control of the hypothalamus, which produces a number of chemical mediators. These hormones are synthesized in the hypothalamus and enter the portal vascular system, which carries them through the pituitary stalk to the anterior lobe (Fig. 328-1). Interruption of the pituitary stalk is followed by reduction in the release of GH, LH, FSH, TSH, and ACTH from the anterior pituitary. This fact implies that stimulatory influences from the hypothalamus are necessary for release of these hormones. In contrast, the level of prolactin rises after interruption of the stalk, implying that the normal hypothalamic influence on prolactin secretion is inhibitory. The rise in prolactin secretion also indicates that stalk section does not lead to pituitary destruction. If the stalk section is not at too high a level, AVP and oxytocin release continue, principally from axons that terminate in the median eminence of the hypothalamus. With

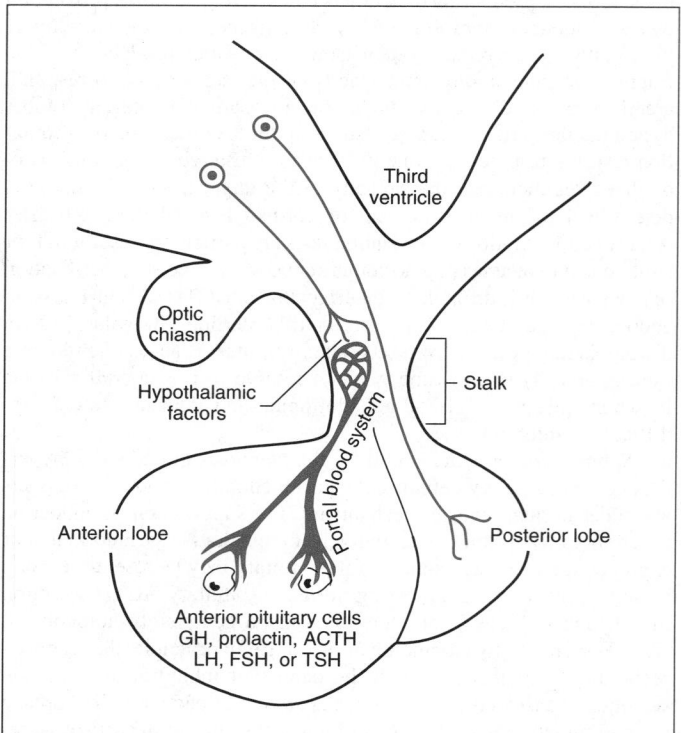

FIGURE 328-1 The relationship between the hypothalamus and the pituitary. See text for details.

Table 328-1

CHAPTER 328
Neuroendocrine Regulation **1973**

Anterior Pituitary and Hypophysiotropic Hormones

Pituitary Hormone	Hypophysiotropic Hormones	
	Name	Structure
Thyrotropin (TSH)	Thyrotropin-releasing hormone (TRH)	Tripeptide
Adrenocorticotropin (ACTH)	Corticotropin-releasing hormone (CRH)	41 amino acids
	Vasopressin (AVP)*	Peptide
Luteinizing hormone (LH)	Luteinizing hormone–releasing hormone (LHRH)	Decapeptide
Follicle-stimulating hormone (FSH)	LHRH	Decapeptide
Growth hormone (GH)	Growth hormone–releasing hormone (GHRH)	44 amino acids
	Growth hormone release–inhibiting hormone† (somatostatin, GIH)	14 amino acids
Prolactin	Prolactin release–inhibiting factor (PIF)	Dopamine
	Prolactin-releasing factor (PRF)‡	Peptide

* Other peptides are also important in ACTH release.
† Somatostatin also inhibits TRH-stimulated TSH release.
‡ TRH stimulates prolactin release.

hypothalamic ablation, the levels of GH, LH, FSH, TSH, ACTH, AVP, and oxytocin fall, whereas prolactin levels increase (Fig. 328-1).

Most hypothalamic factors that control secretion of the pituitary hormones are peptides (Table 328-1). Growth hormone–releasing hormone (GHRH) is the dominant influence on GH release, and somatostatin acts as an inhibitory hormone for GH release. Although LH and FSH levels vary independently in physiologic states, one releasing hormone [luteinizing hormone–releasing hormone (LHRH), also called gonadotropin-releasing hormone (GnRH)] plays a major role in controlling their release. Thyrotropin-releasing hormone (TRH) controls TSH release and also may influence prolactin release. Corticotropin-releasing hormone (CRH) and other factors control ACTH release. Dopamine acts as the major prolactin inhibitory factor (PIF).

Pituitary tumors may lead to hormonal over- or underproduction or may cause mechanical problems by impinging on neighboring structures. The most common syndromes produced by pituitary tumors are due to prolactin and GH excess. Prolactin excess leads to galactorrhea and/or hypogonadism; GH excess leads to gigantism and acromegaly. ACTH-secreting tumors produce Cushing's disease, and TSH-secreting tumors are a rare cause of hyperthyroidism. Paradoxically, gonadotropin-secreting tumors are most often associated with hypogonadism. Large pituitary tumors may cause partial or complete hypopituitarism by compression of the adjacent normal gland or pituitary stalk and are associated with visual field disturbances due to compression of the optic chiasm.

Other neurologic disturbances occur if the tumor invades the cavernous sinuses or cranial fossae.

Hypothalamic disease may cause hypopituitarism, with the exception that secretion of prolactin may be increased. Diabetes insipidus due to AVP deficiency is virtually diagnostic of hypothalamic disease or of high interruption of the pituitary stalk. Disturbances of thirst, temperature regulation, appetite, and blood pressure may occur with hypothalamic disorders as well. Large hypothalamic masses may lead to visual field disturbances, obstruction of the third ventricle, and invasion of surrounding brain tissue.

ANATOMY AND EMBRYOLOGY

The pituitary gland (hypophysis) sits within the sella turcica ("Turkish saddle") of the sphenoid bone at the base of the skull and is composed principally of the anterior lobe (adenohypophysis) and posterior lobe (neurohypophysis). The intermediate lobe is rudimentary in humans. The normal adult pituitary gland weighs between 0.4 and 0.8 g.

The pituitary is separated from the brain by the diaphragma sella, an extension of the dura mater, and from the sphenoid sinus anteriorly and inferiorly by a thin layer of bone. The lateral walls of the sella abut on the cavernous sinuses, which contain the internal carotid arteries and cranial nerves III, IV, V, and VI. The optic chiasm is located slightly anterior to the pituitary stalk, just above the diaphragma sella. Thus, tumors of the pituitary may lead to visual field defects, to cranial nerve palsies, or to invasion of the sphenoid sinus (Fig. 328-2).

The hypothalamus extends anteriorly to the margin of the optic chiasm and posteriorly to include the mammillary bodies. Superiorly, the hypothalamic sulcus of the third ventricle separates the thalamus

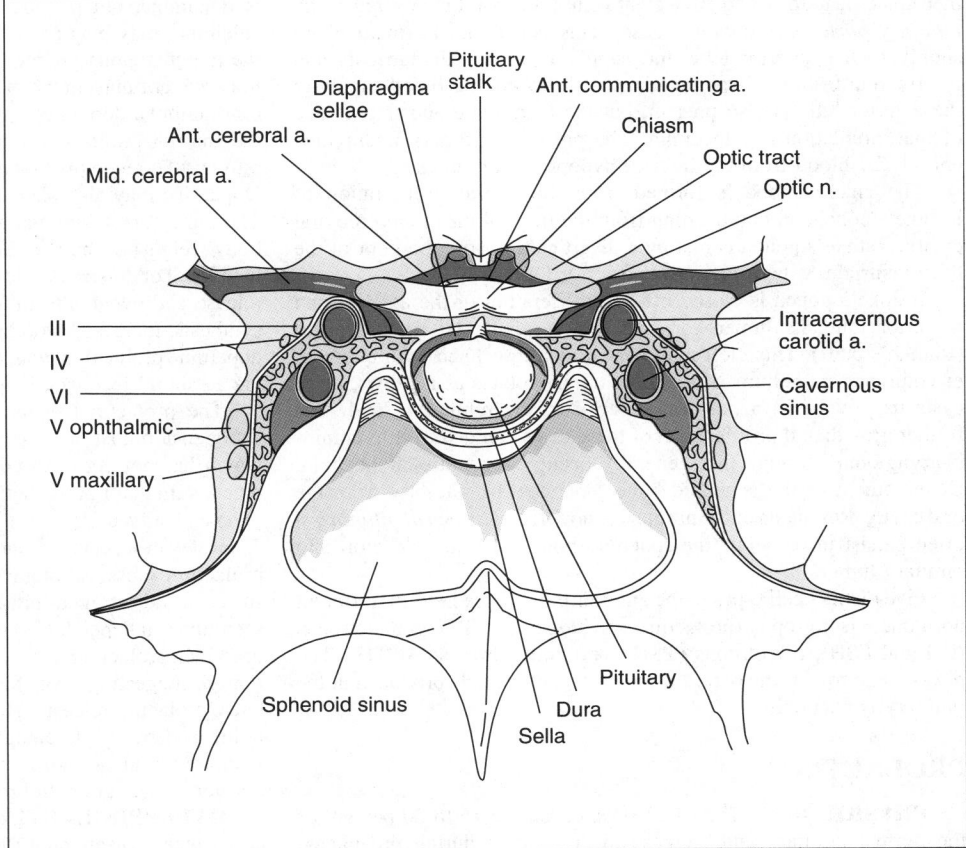

FIGURE 328-2 The relationship between the pituitary, the cranial nerves, and the cavernous sinus as viewed in a coronal section through the sella. *[From JA Taren, in Correlative Neurosurgery, 3d ed, RC Schneider et al (eds). Springfield, IL, Charles C Thomas, 1982.]*

from the hypothalamus. The rounded inferior base of the hypothalamus forms the tuber cinereum. The central portion of the base (termed the *infundibulum* or *median eminence*) is formed by the floor of the third ventricle and continues inferiorly to form the pituitary stalk. The releasing factors are synthesized in neurons situated along the margins of the third ventricle. They project fibers that terminate in the median eminence adjacent to the portal capillaries. The same releasing factors are produced by hypothalamic neurons that project to other parts of the brain.

The cell bodies of the supraoptic and paraventricular nuclei of the hypothalamus produce vasopressin and oxytocin, which travel down nerve axons in the supraopticohypophyseal and paraventriculohypophyseal tracts to reach the posterior lobe.

The communication between the hypothalamus and the anterior pituitary is chemical rather than physical. Releasing factors produced by hypothalamic neurons reach the anterior pituitary via the portal system to stimulate or inhibit hormone production. Some of the vasopressin-containing neurons also terminate in the median eminence, and vasopressin can stimulate release of ACTH and GH.

The anterior pituitary has the highest blood flow of any tissue in the body [0.8 (mL/g)/min]. The blood supply reaches the anterior pituitary by a circuitous route through the hypothalamus. Two derivatives of the internal carotid arteries, the superior hypophyseal arteries (SHA), branch in the subarachnoid space around the pituitary stalk and terminate in the capillary network of the median eminence. These capillaries have a fenestrated endothelium that allows easy access to the hypothalamic releasing hormones. Neurons containing vasoactive intestinal peptide (VIP) terminate on precapillary arterioles and may play a role in regulating blood flow. Transport of substances from the capillaries to the median eminence is also facilitated because the median eminence lies outside the blood-brain barrier. The capillaries then coalesce to form 6 to 10 straight veins known as the *hypothalamic-pituitary portal circulation*. These veins constitute the main blood supply to the anterior lobe and supply it with both nutrients and information from the hypothalamus. A direct arterial blood supply to the anterior lobe is also present, but the magnitude and importance of that circulation are uncertain. The posterior pituitary is supplied entirely by blood from the inferior hypophyseal arteries.

The anterior lobe is formed from the lateral proliferation of Rathke's pouch, an outpouching from the floor of the embryonic oral cavity. Rathke's pouch is met by a diverticulum from the floor of the third ventricle, which forms the posterior lobe.

Rathke's pouch is closed off by proliferation of the anterior and posterior lobe; its lumen forms a thin residual cleft in the gland (Rathke's cleft). This cleft may persist as a cyst lined with cuboidal or columnar epithelium. Since the pituitary rotates as it grows, these cysts usually lie in a position superior to the pituitary gland. The further growth and proliferation of these cysts can give rise to craniopharyngiomas, tumors that generally occupy a suprasellar position. Development of the sphenoid bone separates the pituitary from the oral cavity. Remnants of the pituitary, known as *pharyngeal pituitaries*, often persist in or below the sphenoid bone but rarely develop into pituitary tumors.

Five distinct cell types in the anterior pituitary secrete six different hormones: lactotrophs (prolactin), somatotrophs (GH), gonadotrophs (LH and FSH), thyrotrophs (TSH), and corticotrophs (ACTH). The physiologic role of the other hormones and chemicals produced in the pituitary is uncertain.

PROLACTIN

PHYSIOLOGY   The lactotrophs constitute 15 to 20 percent of the normal pituitary and increase to 70 percent during pregnancy. These cells share many electrical characteristics with neurons. The prolactin gene on chromosome 6 codes for a precursor molecule that is larger than the circulating hormone. The predominant form of the processed hormone contains 198 amino acids (23,000 mol wt) in a single polypeptide chain containing three intrachain disulfide bonds. Higher-molecular-weight forms of prolactin represent dimers, polymers, aggregates, and protein-bound species. They may be present in small amounts in the circulation of normal persons and in larger amounts in patients with pituitary adenomas. These molecules have variable but generally decreased immunologic and biologic activity. The role of prolactin fragments and glycosylated forms is under investigation.

Prolactin is essential for lactation. Prolactin receptors are members of the cytokine receptor family and are found in breast, gonads, liver, kidney, and adrenal (see Chap. 327). Prolactin promotes breast cancer in rodents; a similar connection has not been established in human breast cancer (see Chap. 91). A possible role for prolactin in immune modulation has been suggested.

During pregnancy, increasing estrogen production stimulates the growth and replication of the pituitary lactotrophs and causes increased prolactin secretion. The pituitary doubles in size during pregnancy and returns to normal after delivery. Prolactin during pregnancy prepares the breast for postpartum lactation. High estrogen levels inhibit prolactin action at the breast, so that lactation does not commence until estrogen levels decline post partum. Prolactin levels rise in the fetus beginning at about 25 weeks, probably owing to maternal estrogen transfer and stimulation of the fetal pituitary. The level falls rapidly after delivery, reaching a nadir by 2 to 4 weeks post partum. High concentrations of prolactin are present in amniotic fluid, probably of both uterine and placental origin. The functional significance of this prolactin is unknown.

Under normal circumstances, prolactin secretion by the anterior pituitary is restrained by the hypothalamus. With hypothalamic destruction or pituitary stalk section, prolactin secretion increases, and serum concentrations rise. The release of prolactin from pituitary cells after stalk section in animals requires the autocrine release of VIP by pituitary cells. The major hypothalamic inhibitory factor for prolactin is dopamine, but peptide inhibitory factors such as endothelin and calcitonin may play a role. The arcuate and paraventricular nuclei of the hypothalamus produce dopamine; dopamine travels down axons to nerve terminals in the median eminence, where it is released (tuberoinfundibular dopamine system) into the portal circulation and reaches the anterior pituitary to inhibit prolactin release via interactions with pituitary D_2 receptors (adenylate cyclase–linked dopamine receptors). Dopamine may also play an important role in the posterior pituitary. The intravenous administration of dopamine (2 μg/min per kilogram body weight) or the oral administration of dopamine precursors (e.g., levodopa) or dopamine agonists (e.g., bromocriptine) inhibits prolactin release and eventually inhibits lactotrope proliferation and prolactin synthesis. Increased blood prolactin appears to increase hypothalamic dopamine production, which, in turn, partially inhibits prolactin release via a "short" feedback loop.

The prolactin rise during suckling, sleep, and stress and after estrogen administration appears to require a prolactin-releasing factor, which has not yet been conclusively identified. Although TRH is a potent stimulator of prolactin release, TSH and prolactin are controlled independently under most circumstances; lactation does not lead to TSH elevation, and primary hypothyroidism may or may not cause prolactin excess. Serotonin antagonists such as methysergide inhibit suckling and estrogen-induced prolactin increase, but resting prolactin secretion is independent of serotonin. Opiate antagonists such as naloxone block prolactin release after stress, suckling, and estrogen administration, suggesting a role for endogenous opioids, and morphine stimulates prolactin release. However, basal prolactin secretion is not influenced by opiate antagonists. An abrupt rise in prolactin occurs within an hour of eating in normal individuals and pregnant women but not in patients with prolactinomas. The mechanism is unknown.

HYPERPROLACTINEMIA Clinical Features   Prolactin excess (hyperprolactinemia) has many causes, is often associated with hypogonadism and/or galactorrhea, and may indicate the presence of a pituitary adenoma or hypothalamic disease. Of women with amenorrhea, 10 to 40 percent have hyperprolactinemia, and about 30 percent of women with amenorrhea and galactorrhea have prolactin-secreting pituitary tumors.

The hypogonadism associated with hyperprolactinemia appears to be due to inhibition of hypothalamic release of LHRH, resulting in defective LH and FSH secretion. This functional hypogonadism can be regarded, in part, as a desirable physiologic mechanism whereby breast feeding causes decreased fertility and delayed resumption of menses. In general, the higher the plasma prolactin, the greater the likelihood of estrogen deficiency and amenorrhea. The wide variability in the clinical manifestations, despite similar degrees of hyperprolactinemia, is likely due to differing bioactivity of abnormal forms of prolactin produced by the tumors. Hyperprolactinemia in women can also cause either irregular menses or infertility despite regular menses, due at least in part to a shortened luteal phase. Prolactin excess in men can cause decreased libido, impotence, and infertility. In some series, 8 percent of men with impotence and 5 percent of men with infertility had hyperprolactinemia. With prolactin elevation, FSH and LH levels in men decline, and serum testosterone is often low.

Galactorrhea, defined as milk production in a patient who is not postpartum, is present in 30 to 90 percent of hyperprolactinemic women (see Chap. 338). The variation in incidence reflects, in part, variation in the intensity with which clinicians search for this finding. Galactorrhea may occur without hyperprolactinemia, particularly in parous women. However, galactorrhea is often a clue to prolactin excess; when galactorrhea is coupled with amenorrhea, hyperprolactinemia is present in 75 percent of patients. Hyperprolactinemia in men is a rare cause of gynecomastia or galactorrhea (see Chap. 338).

Differential Diagnosis Prolactin excess has many causes (Table 328-2) and several mechanisms: (1) autonomous production (pituitary adenomas), (2) decreased dopamine or dopamine inhibitory action (due, for example, to hypothalamic disease or to drugs that block the synthesis, release, or action of dopamine), (3) stimuli that overcome

Table 328-2

Causes of Hyperprolactinemia

PHYSIOLOGIC STATES

Pregnancy	Sleep
Nursing (early)	Nipple stimulation
"Stress"	Food ingestion

DRUGS

Dopamine receptor antagonists	Dopamine-depleting agents
Phenothiazines	Methyldopa
Butyrophenones	Reserpine
Thioxanthenes	Hormones
Metoclopramide	Estrogens
Sulpiride	Antiandrogens
Respiradone	Opiates
	Verapamil

DISEASE STATES

Pituitary tumors
  Prolactinomas
  Adenomas secreting GH and prolactin
  Adenomas secreting ACTH and prolactin (Nelson's syndrome and Cushing's disease)
  Nonfunctioning chromophobe adenomas with pituitary stalk compression
Hypothalamic and pituitary stalk disease
  Granulomatous diseases, especially sarcoidosis
  Craniopharyngiomas and other tumors
  Cranial irradiation
  Stalk section
  Empty sella
  Vascular abnormalities, including aneurysm
  Lymphocytic hypophysitis
  Metastatic carcinoma
Primary hypothyroidism
Chronic renal failure
Cirrhosis
Chest wall trauma (including surgery, herpes zoster)
Seizures

the normal dopaminergic inhibition (e.g., estrogens, possibly hypothyroidism), and (4) decreased clearance of prolactin (renal failure). No test can distinguish between physiologic and pharmacologic or pathologic causes of hyperprolactinemia.

Prolactin concentrations are slightly higher in women (<20 μg/L) than in men (<15 μg/L). During pregnancy, prolactin concentrations begin to increase during the second trimester and peak at term; maximal values are 100 to 300 μg/L, usually less than 200 μg/L. A pregnancy test is mandatory in all patients with hyperprolactinemic amenorrhea, as it is with amenorrhea alone. The mean prolactin level declines post partum but rises with each suckling episode. Over several months, basal and suckling-stimulated prolactin concentrations diminish; by 4 to 6 months post partum, basal prolactin levels are normal, and the suckling-induced rise is diminished or absent despite continued nursing. Prolactin levels rise within 1 h of eating and after seizures.

A careful drug history should be obtained in hyperprolactinemic patients. Dopamine-blocking drugs (e.g., phenothiazines, butyrophenones, metoclopramide, respiridone) and dopamine-depleting drugs (e.g., methyldopa and reserpine) are important causes of hyperprolactinemia. Chronic cocaine use causes modest hyperprolactinemia. In the absence of renal failure, prolactin levels are usually less than 100 μg/L with these agents (respiridone being a notable exception). However, concentrations as high as 275 μg/L have been reported. Although high-dose estrogens cause hyperprolactinemia, oral contraceptives containing low doses of estrogen do not.

End-stage renal failure is associated with elevated serum prolactin in 70 to 90 percent of women and 25 to 60 percent of men. This effect contributes to hypogonadism in some patients with renal failure. Both decreased prolactin clearance and increased prolactin secretion may contribute to this elevation. The increased serum prolactin level in cirrhosis of the liver has not been adequately explained.

Severe primary hypothyroidism may cause a mild elevation in serum prolactin level, due either to an elevation in the TRH level or to a decrease in dopaminergic tone. Since primary hypothyroidism also may cause enlargement of the sella turcica, mimicking a pituitary adenoma, thyroid function tests are essential in all patients with elevated serum prolactin. Rarely, primary adrenal insufficiency causes reversible serum prolactin elevation.

In 10,000 "normal" adults working at a single plant in Japan, the prevalence of hyperprolactinemia greater than 75 μg/L was 0.4 percent. Many different etiologies were found.

If a fasting hyperprolactinemic subject is not pregnant or in the postpartum period and is not cirrhotic, postictal, taking medications, hypothyroid, or in renal failure, disease of the pituitary or hypothalamus is likely. Ectopic production of prolactin by nonpituitary tumors occurs rarely if at all. Diseases of the hypothalamus or pituitary stalk cause moderate prolactin elevation (usually less than 150 μg/L). Hyperprolactinemia occurs in 20 to 50 percent of patients with hypothalamic tumors.

Prolactin-secreting pituitary adenomas (prolactinomas) are arbitrarily divided into microadenomas (<10 mm) and macroadenomas (≥10 mm). Large, nonfunctioning pituitary adenomas also may cause modest prolactin elevation, thought to be due to stalk compression and impairment of dopamine delivery to the gland. Some acromegalic persons (25 to 45 percent), some patients with Nelson's syndrome, and rare Cushing's patients have elevated serum prolactin levels due either to cosecretion of prolactin by the tumor or to stalk compression.

Laboratory Evaluation Serum prolactin levels should be measured in all people with unexplained hypogonadism, galactorrhea, or infertility. If a random prolactin concentration is elevated, further evaluation is warranted after it is established that the observed elevations are not simply normal minimal elevations (e.g., less than 30 μg/L) due to stress or food intake. Levels should be assessed after fasting or more than 1 h after eating. Although there is no simple test to distinguish the various causes of hyperprolactinemia, a serum prolactin level of over 300 μg/L is nearly always diagnostic of a prolactinoma; a serum prolactin of over 150 μg/L in a nonpregnant patient is usually caused by a pituitary adenoma. Administration of a dopamine agonist, such as bromocriptine, lowers the prolactin level regardless of the etiology and, therefore, is not useful as a differential test (Fig. 328-3). Most patients with prolactinomas show little or no rise in prolactin in response to TRH, as compared with the rise of 200 percent or more in normal individuals and the intermediate response (usually a doubling of serum prolactin) in patients with hypothalamic disease and in those taking dopamine-blocking agents. Unfortunately, the response to TRH is too variable to be of diagnostic value in individual patients. Antiprolactin antibodies may cause spuriously high (or low) prolactin levels in radioimmunoassays but not in immunoradiometric assays; the presence of normal menses in a woman with a serum prolactin level of >100 ng/dL suggests this phenomenon.

Patients with unexplained hyperprolactinemia require magnetic resonance imaging (MRI) of the hypothalamus and pituitary. Pituitary macroadenomas and most microadenomas are easily visualized on these scans, particularly with gadolinium enhancement. Any mass that impairs the flow of dopamine from the hypothalamus to the pituitary can cause hyperprolactinemia, a phenomenon termed "stalk hyperprolactinemia." MRI is essential to distinguish intrasellar lesions such as microprolactinomas and large "nonfunctioning" adenomas from suprasellar lesions such as craniopharyngiomas, germinomas, and meningiomas. When no radiologic abnormalities are found, the disorder is called *idiopathic hyperprolactinemia*, although a microadenoma may still be present.

Microprolactinomas do not cause hypopituitarism (except for hypogonadism). If a small pituitary lesion is seen in a patient with hypopituitarism and hyperprolactinemia, sarcoidosis or other lesions involving the pituitary stalk should be suspected, rather than a microprolactinoma. In patients with macroprolactinomas or hypothalamic lesions, evaluation of pituitary function and formal visual field examinations are essential.

Prolactinomas *Pathology* Prolactinomas are the most common functional pituitary adenomas. Small, unsuspected microadenomas are found in 6 to 24 percent of unselected autopsies; 40 percent of these small tumors contain prolactin by immunologic staining tech-

niques, but the fraction that actually secrete prolactin is unknown. About 70 percent of macroadenomas previously thought to be nonfunctioning are, in fact, prolactinomas. Prolactin-secreting pituitary carcinomas are rare.

The size of a prolactinoma correlates with its hormone output; in general, the larger the tumor, the higher the prolactin levels. Large pituitary tumors accompanied by a modest prolactin elevation (50 to 100 μg/L) are not true prolactinomas and differ in their biologic behavior. Microprolactinomas cause only hyperprolactinemia and hypogonadotropism, whereas macroprolactinomas may influence other pituitary hormones and cause headaches, visual field disturbances, and other mass effects.

The pathophysiology of prolactinoma development is not understood. Known oncogenes do not play a role in most prolactinomas. However, a *ras* mutation may be important in rare, highly invasive prolactinomas and metastatic pituitary carcinomas.

Clinical presentation Microprolactinomas are more common than macroprolactinomas, and 90 percent of patients with microprolactinomas are women. In contrast, 60 percent of patients with macroprolactinomas are men. Irregular menses, amenorrhea, and galactorrhea are likely to result in early diagnosis, and this fact may partially explain the preponderance of microadenomas in women. Sexual dysfunction occurs in most men with prolactinomas, but this is the presenting complaint in 15 percent or less. Although a delay in seeking medical help probably explains the larger size of tumors in men, the possibility of more aggressive tumor behavior in men has not been excluded.

Estrogens promote the growth of lactotrophs, but an etiologic role has not been established for oral contraceptives in the pathogenesis of prolactinomas. Many women with prolactinomas first develop galactorrhea while on oral contraceptives or develop amenorrhea when the drug is discontinued. Some of these women may have been started on oral contraceptives for irregular menses that were the consequence of a prolactinoma. Although amenorrhea after discontinuance of oral contraceptives is rare (about 2 percent), about a third of patients with post-pill amenorrhea have a prolactinoma. Development of galactorrhea in a woman using oral contraceptives mandates a prolactin determination. About 5 to 7 percent of prolactinoma patients have never menstruated (primary amenorrhea), making prolactinoma an important treatable cause of primary amenorrhea. Prolactinomas may grow during pregnancy, and 15 percent of prolactinoma patients are first diagnosed in the postpartum period.

Women with prolactinomas who desire pregnancy need special consideration. Medical treatment of patients with microprolactinomas results in an uneventful pregnancy 95 to 98 percent of the time; the remaining patients may develop headaches or visual field disturbances due to tumor enlargement that rarely requires therapy. Asymptomatic enlargement of microprolactinomas, as ascertained by radiologic studies, occurs in about 5 percent of patients. With macroprolactinomas, the complications of tumor growth during pregnancy are more common. Symptomatic tumor enlargement occurs in about 15 percent of these patients, although prior therapy with bromocriptine may decrease this risk.

In prolactinoma patients, the effect of pregnancy on prolactin secretion is variable. A further rise in prolactin during pregnancy may not occur even in patients in whom tumor growth occurs. Rarely, macroprolactinomas in men grow during replacement testosterone therapy, presumably as a result of extraglandular conversion of testosterone to estrogen. The safety of oral contraceptives in women with microprolactinomas is uncertain, but some data suggest that such therapy is unlikely to cause a rise in prolactin levels or significant tumor growth.

℞ **TREATMENT**

The natural history of untreated hyperprolactinemia is incompletely understood. Although large pituitary adenomas must begin as small tumors, most microadenomas do not progress to macroadenomas. In general, 90 to 95 percent of untreated microprolactinomas remain stable or exhibit decreased serum prolactin concentrations over 7 years of follow-up. Serum prolactin returns to normal in a third

FIGURE 328-3 Changes in serum prolactin concentration in a woman with "idiopathic" hyperprolactinemia after an initial 5-mg dose of bromocriptine and when maintained on 7.5 mg daily. (*From GH Besser, MO Thorner, Postgrad Med J 52:66, 1976.*)

of patients with idiopathic hyperprolactinemia (who may harbor microprolactinomas) who are followed for 5 years without therapy; this number increases to two-thirds if the basal prolactin is less than 40 μg/L. In 30 patients with varying degrees of hyperprolactinemia (30 to 260 μg/L) followed for a mean of 5.2 years, the prolactin level increased by more than 50 percent in one-fifth, and another fifth had signs of enlargement on computed tomography (CT) scans. The prolactin level decreased by more than 50 percent in one-third of the patients and returned to normal in one-fifth. The abnormal x-ray findings returned to normal in one-sixth of the patients.

Thus, not all patients with microprolactinomas need therapy. Women with microprolactinomas require therapy when they desire pregnancy or have amenorrhea (because of the risk of osteoporosis), acne or hirsutism, decreased libido, or troublesome galactorrhea. Men with microadenomas should be treated when they have hypogonadism (because of the risk of osteoporosis), decreased potency or libido, or infertility. Patients with macroprolactinomas require therapy to prevent or reverse the mass effects of the tumor.

The treatment of choice is medical therapy. Dopamine agonist drugs lower prolactin concentrations in virtually all hyperprolactinemic patients (Fig. 328-3). Bromocriptine, an ergot derivative with dopamine agonist actions, is the only effective prolactin-lowering agent licensed for this purpose in the United States. Bromocriptine should be given twice daily with food or a snack to prevent gastrointestinal irritation; in some patients, prolactin levels return to normal with once-daily dosing. Therapy should begin with a low dose of 0.625 to 1.25 mg with a snack at bedtime to minimize the side effects of nausea, vomiting, fatigue, nasal stuffiness, and postural hypotension. The dosage is gradually increased to an average of 2.5 mg twice daily. In some patients with microadenomas, control is achieved with 2.5 mg at bedtime, whereas up to 15 mg/d may be required with macroprolactinomas. Treatment success should be monitored by assessing clinical manifestations, prolactin levels in serum, and tumor size by MRI. Although the drug is expensive, it is effective in all forms of hyperprolactinemia and often abolishes nonhyperprolactinemic galactorrhea as well. Long-lasting parenteral and oral dopamine agonists and newer non-ergot-derived oral dopamine agonists are effective and in some cases better tolerated than bromocriptine; gastrointestinal intolerance to oral bromocriptine can be circumvented by vaginal administration. Neither the new agents nor vaginal administration is licensed in the United States.

Bromocriptine is the therapy of choice for patients with microprolactinomas who have one of the indications for treatment discussed above. Prolactin concentrations return to normal in almost all patients who tolerate the medication, usually within days of achieving the full therapeutic dosage (see Fig. 328-3). Menses usually resume within 2 months but may be delayed by up to a year. Since pregnancy may occur without resumption of menses, a barrier contraceptive is recommended until menses become regular. With this approach, bromocriptine can be stopped with the first missed period when pregnancy has occurred. Bromocriptine is not approved for use during pregnancy in the United States, but its use during pregnancy is not associated with an increased risk of congenital anomalies or fetal wastage. The effects of bromocriptine are usually not permanent, but one-sixth of microprolactinoma patients maintain normal prolactin concentrations after discontinuation of the drug.

In patients with macroprolactinomas, bromocriptine usually lowers the serum prolactin level and decreases tumor size (Fig. 328-4), but both effects may be incomplete. In men, testosterone concentrations usually begin to increase after 3 months of therapy, but they may remain subnormal. In some men sperm counts return to normal. Almost 90 percent of premenopausal women regain cyclic menses.

Tumor shrinkage is most rapid in the first 3 months of therapy. By 3 months 40 percent of tumors have shrunk by more than 50 percent. Of patients treated for a year 90 percent show tumor shrinkage of more than 50 percent. Most tumors shrink to some degree; more important, abnormal visual fields improve with medical therapy in 90 percent of patients. If the visual field defect does not resolve within a short period (1 to 3 months), surgery should be performed.

FIGURE 328-4 Frontal CT scan of a man with a large prolactin-secreting macroadenoma. *Top:* pretreatment scan. *Bottom:* scan after 1 year of treatment with bromocriptine. The upper border of the tumor is shown by arrows. *(From ME Molitch, 1987.)*

Prolactin levels fall to 20 percent of the baseline level in more than 90 percent of patients and return to normal in about a third. The dosage of bromocriptine can often be reduced after 2 years or more of therapy, but the drug rarely can be discontinued. In patients who have persistent symptomatic hyperprolactinemia despite a partial response to bromocriptine, surgical debulking or radiation therapy may be appropriate.

Although prolactin concentrations usually return rapidly to pretreatment levels when long-term bromocriptine treatment is stopped, tumor regrowth may be delayed for months or years. When pregnancy is considered by a patient with a macroprolactinoma, this slow regrowth should be kept in mind. Patients who conceive after prolonged bromocriptine therapy may be at less risk of tumor growth during pregnancy. In the United States, bromocriptine is generally stopped when pregnancy is confirmed; however, if tumor-related symptoms develop during pregnancy, bromocriptine should be reinstituted. Many physicians outside the United States use bromocriptine throughout pregnancy in patients with macroprolactinomas. There is no evidence that bromocriptine has an adverse effect on the fetus. Pregnant women with macroprolactinomas should have frequent testing of visual fields to monitor for tumor growth.

Patients who have large nonprolactinoma masses in the sella that cause stalk-compression hyperprolactinemia are sometimes treated mistakenly with bromocripitine. Although prolactin levels return to normal in such cases, the size of the mass is not affected. These patients should be treated surgically if debulking the mass or obtaining a tissue diagnosis is important.

While medical treatment is appropriate for most prolactinomas, surgery, usually by the transsphenoidal approach, is indicated in some situations, as in women with microprolactinomas who desire pregnancy and cannot tolerate bromocriptine. Following resection of microprolactinomas, serum prolactin levels return to normal in 80 to 90 percent of patients, usually within 24 h. However, recurrence rates may be as high as 40 percent within 6 years. Surgery may be more difficult and have a higher complication rate in microprolactinoma patients who are treated for more than 3 months with bromocriptine.

Surgery may also be necessary for macroprolactinoma patients in whom visual field defects persist despite bromocriptine treatment, who have tumor growth despite bromocriptine treatment, or who are intolerant of dopamine agonists. Tumors with a large cystic or hemorrhagic component may require surgical decompression for relief of visual symptoms or headaches. Surgery may also be appropriate for prolactinoma patients who need neuroleptic agents for psychiatric illness, because dopamine agonists counteract these medications and may precipitate psychotic episodes.

Surgery is rarely curative for macroprolactinomas. Prolactin concentrations return to normal in about 30 percent of patients treated surgically, but recurrence rates may be as high as 80 percent in this subgroup. Long-term bromocriptine therapy is therefore usually required after surgical therapy.

Radiation therapy plays a limited role in the treatment of prolactinomas. Conventional radiation therapy [4500 cGy (4500 rad) over 25 days] causes a slow decline in serum prolactin concentration. Although prolactin concentrations return to normal in about 30 percent of patients with microprolactinomas by 2 to 10 years after radiation therapy, we rarely treat microprolactinomas with radiation. The risks of hypopituitarism make this a poor fourth choice after medical therapy, surgery, or no therapy. Radiation therapy may be necessary for macroprolactinomas that grow rapidly or persistently despite dopamine agonist therapy and surgery or after surgery alone in patients intolerant of dopamine agonists. The respective roles of conventional radiation, focused gamma radiation ("gamma knife"), and heavy-particle (proton beam) radiation are not established.

PROLACTIN DEFICIENCY Prolactin deficiency is manifested as an inability to lactate. Failure of lactation is often the earliest clue to panhypopituitarism resulting from pituitary infarction during the peripartum period. The lateral wings of the pituitary, where most lactotrophs reside, have a precarious blood supply. During pregnancy, the hypertrophied and hyperplastic lactotrophs are at risk for necrosis. If systemic hypotension develops, as with postpartum hemorrhage, the pituitary may undergo infarction (Sheehan's syndrome). Patients with diabetes mellitus are susceptible to peripartum pituitary infarction even in the absence of significant hemorrhage. Autoimmune pituitary destruction (lymphocytic hypophysitis) also may occur during late pregnancy but often is associated with elevated prolactin levels.

Many prolactin radioimmunoassays cannot distinguish normal from low prolactin concentrations; hence, prolactin stimulation tests may be necessary to diagnose prolactin insufficiency. After administration of TRH or chlorpromazine, a rise in serum prolactin of less than 200 percent suggests prolactin deficiency. If prolactin deficiency is present, evaluation of other pituitary hormones is necessary to determine whether other manifestations of hypopituitarism are present.

GROWTH HORMONE

PHYSIOLOGY Growth hormone (GH, somatotropin) is secreted by somatotrophs, which make up about 50 percent of the anterior pituitary cells. The normal pituitary contains 3 to 5 mg of GH and secretes 500 to 875 μg of GH per day. GH shares an 85 percent structural identity with human placental lactogen (hPL, chorionic somatomammotropin). The GH and hPL genes are on chromosome 17 and appear to have originated by gene duplication. Human growth hormone consists of a single polypeptide chain of 191 amino acids (22,000 mol wt) with two intrachain disulfide bonds; it is cleaved from a larger precursor molecule (28,000 mol wt). Alternative splicing of this precursor yields a 20-kDa GH molecule with a lower biologic and immunologic activity. GH is stored in cytoplasmic granules in a high-molecular-weight polymeric form. A variant form of GH (GH-V) is found in the placenta, is the dominant form of GH circulating in the third trimester of pregnancy, and is a potent somatogen.

Multiple forms of GH exist in the circulation. The dominant form is monomeric GH (22 kDa), but larger, oligomeric forms (e.g., "big" GH, 44,000 mol wt) and smaller forms (e.g., the 20-kDa form) are present as well. All these variants contribute to the total circulating GH concentration. Several binding proteins for GH contribute to the heterogeneity of circulating GH. The high-affinity GH-binding protein, which is specific for the 22-kDa form of GH, appears to be a cleavage product of the extracellular domain of the GH receptor. A lower-affinity binding protein binds both the 22-kDa active and 20-kDa inactive forms of GH.

Pulsatile release of GH is characteristic. Circulating levels are immeasurably low for much of the day, and this base line level is punctuated by four to eight bursts, which occur after meals or exercise, during slow-wave sleep, or without an obvious cause. The half-life of the hormone in plasma is 20 to 30 min. GH secretion is low in infancy, slightly higher during early childhood, and dramatically increased during puberty. GH secretion is lower in adulthood than during puberty. After the third decade, a progressive (but individually variable) decline in GH secretion occurs.

GH is necessary for normal linear growth. GH deficiency causes short stature; GH excess (prior to epiphyseal closure) leads to gigantism. GH does not appear to be the principal direct stimulator of growth but rather acts indirectly by stimulating the formation of other hormones. These factors, known as *somatomedins* (SMs, somatotropin-mediating hormones) or *insulin-like growth factors* (IGFs), are GH-dependent and are responsible for growth stimulation (see also Chap. 329). IGF-I (formerly termed *somatomedin C*), the most important somatomedin for postnatal growth, is produced in the liver, chondrocytes, kidney, muscle, pituitary, and gastrointestinal tract. The liver is the main source of circulating IGF-I. IGF-I is a basic protein (7600 mol wt) that circulates bound to six distinct IGF binding proteins (IGF-BPs). IGF-BP3 is the major binding protein and is itself growth hormone–dependent. The net effect of the binding proteins is to increase the half-life of circulating IGF-I to 3 to 18 h, as compared with the half-life of 20 to 30 min for unbound hormone. The role of specific IGF-BPs in regulating IGF action is under investigation. Local tissue generation of IGF-I/SM-C, particularly in bone, may play an important role in growth mediation through its paracrine effects.

IGF-I is structurally similar to proinsulin and exerts some insulin-like actions. Furthermore, GH is a trophic factor for insulin release, facilitating release in response to various secretagogues, and GH-deficient individuals have impaired insulin release to glucose challenge. Technically, one might consider insulin a somatomedin.

During the prenatal and neonatal period, growth is independent of GH, as shown by the normal birth length of GH-deficient children born to GH-deficient mothers. Nevertheless, IGF-I levels are elevated during pregnancy; the concentration correlates with that of hPL, which may regulate IGF-I production. IGF-I levels at birth are lower than those of adults and rise gradually during childhood to reach the adult range by age 8 to 10 years. The levels also depend on nutritional status, declining in states of malnourishment. Serum IGF-I levels are elevated during the pubertal growth spurt, presumably accounting for pubertal growth acceleration.

Although IGF-I levels correlate with linear growth, the correlation is inexact, and, therefore, GH may have some direct influence on growth or cause somatomedin generation in target cells.

GH exerts additional metabolic effects, including stimulation of the incorporation of amino acids into protein. Although most of this action is IGF-mediated, GH can directly stimulate amino acid uptake in certain systems. Some amino acids, such as arginine, are potent stimuli for GH release.

GH may act as an insulin antagonist to inhibit glucose uptake by tissues. Patients with GH deficiency are prone to insulin-induced hypoglycemia; patients with GH excess develop insulin resistance. GH is one of the counterregulatory hormones that help restore a low blood sugar to normal (see Chap. 335). Hypoglycemia is a potent stimulus for GH release, and an acute rise in blood sugar inhibits GH release. Paradoxically, patients with type I diabetes mellitus have increased GH concentrations. GH increases the release of free fatty acids from adipocytes. The absence of this effect may be responsible for the pudgy appearance of children with GH deficiency and the high percentage of body fat in adults with GH deficiency. Increased serum free fatty acid concentrations tend to blunt GH release. GH opposes the action of insulin on sugar uptake and fatty acid release and complements the anabolic action of insulin on amino acid uptake.

GH is controlled by a dual hypothalamic regulation (Table 328-3). Secretion is stimulated by growth hormone–releasing hormone (GHRH, somatocrinin) and inhibited by somatostatin (growth hormone release–inhibiting hormone, somatotropin release–inhibiting factor, SRIF). GHRH appears to play the more important role, since pituitary stalk section leads to failure of GH release. Although GHRH and somatostatin are synthesized in separate neurons, these neurons have reciprocal interconnections.

Growth Hormone–Releasing Hormone GHRH has 44 amino acids, 29 of which are necessary for full potency. GHRH belongs to a family of molecules that includes secretin, glucagon, VIP, and gastric inhibitory peptide (GIP). The arcuate nucleus of the hypothalamus is the major site of GHRH production, although a few GHRH-producing neurons are found in the ventromedial nucleus. Axons containing the peptide project to the median eminence and terminate on the portal vessels. GHRH is also present in the mucosa of the small intestine.

The GHRH receptor is a G protein–coupled transmembrane receptor, and GHRH stimulates both the transcription of the GH gene and the synthesis and release of GH, an effect mediated by cyclic adenosine monophosphate (AMP). Intravenous injection of GHRH (0.1 to 3.3 μg/kg body weight) produces a peak GH response at 30 to 60 min with a return to baseline by 2 to 3 h after injection (Fig. 328-5).

Somatostatin Somatostatin, a cyclic tetradecapeptide, is the most widely distributed of the hypothalamic releasing hormones. The primary hypothalamic sources are the periventricular and medial preoptic areas of the anterior hypothalamus. Somatostatin is found in neurosecretory granules of axons that terminate in the median eminence. In addition to its function as a hormone, somatostatin is synthesized and distributed throughout the brain and serves as a neurotransmitter in many areas, including the spinal cord, brainstem, and cerebral cortex. Somatostatin is also present in the gastrointestinal tract and other organs. Somatostatin-secreting cells (D cells) of the pancreatic islets participate in the regulation of insulin and glucagon secretion, an example of paracrine regulation by this hormone (see Chap. 334). Somatostatin acts via a family of at least five G protein–coupled membrane receptors that utilize a number of different second messenger pathways.

Somatostatin is produced by processing of a larger precursor molecule and exists in both 28- and 14-amino-acid forms. The 28-amino-acid somatostatin has a longer half-life and is a more potent inhibitor of GH, TSH, and insulin secretion. Somatostatin 14 is the most abundant form but is less bioactive in inhibiting GH. It has a greater affinity for

Table 328-3

Growth Hormone Regulation

Class of Agent	Stimulation	Inhibition
Hypothalamic factors	GHRH	Somatostatin
Amines	Alpha-2-adrenergic stimuli (norepineph-rine, clonidine)	Beta-adrenergic stimuli
	Beta-adrenergic blockers (propranolol)	Alpha-2-adrenergic blockers (yohimbine)
	Dopaminergic stimuli (levodopa, bromocriptine, apomorphine)	Dopamine blockers (chlorpromazine)
	Serotonergic stimuli (L-tryptophan)	Serotonin blockers (methysergide, cyproheptadine)
Hormones	Decreased IGF-I/SM-C	Increased IGF-I/SM-C (obesity)
	Estrogen	Progestogens
	Vasopressin	Glucocorticoids*
	Glucagon†	
Fuels	Hypoglycemia‡	Increased blood sugar
	Decreased free fatty acids	Increased free fatty acids
	Amino acid (arginine)†	
Others	Exercise‡	Muscarinic cholinergic antagonists (atropine)
	Stress‡	
	Sleep†	
	Cholinergic (muscarinic stimuli) (pyridostigmine)	

* Acutely, glucocorticoids stimulate GH release.
† Probably mediated through cholinergic stimulation.
‡ Probably mediated through alpha-adrenergic stimulation.

hypothalamic and cortical receptors and is more potent in inhibition of glucagon release, splanchnic blood flow, intestinal motility, and gastric exocrine secretion. Somatostatin analogues are effective in the therapy of acromegaly, TSH-secreting pituitary adenomas, secretory pancreatic tumors, carcinoid syndrome, and other conditions.

Somatostatin inhibits GH secretion and decreases the GH response to secretagogues without altering GH mRNA levels. Somatostatin also lowers serum TSH levels in normal and hypothyroid individuals and blunts TSH release in response to TRH. Somatostatin probably mediates the secondary hypothyroidism that may develop in GH-deficient children treated with GH. Somatostatin has no significant effect on the release of prolactin, gonadotropins, or ACTH in normal subjects but may lower ACTH concentrations in patients with Nelson's syndrome.

FIGURE 328-5 Response to GHRH-44 (1 μg/kg) in eight men and eight women. The shaded area shows the full range of responses at each time point, and the error bars indicate the mean ± 1 SD. (*From MC Gelato et al, J Clin Endocrinol Metab 59:200, 1984.*)

Somatostatinomas are rare pancreatic islet cell or duodenal tumors that secrete somatostatin (see Chap. 95).

Growth hormone release is under complex physiologic control (see Table 328-3). The various mediators appear to act through GHRH and somatostatin. IGF-I has an important feedback effect on GH secretion. An increased IGF-I concentration inhibits GH release both through increased somatostatin production and by a direct action on the pituitary. A decrease in IGF-I, as induced by starvation, leads to a compensatory increase in GH release.

A number of neurotransmitters influence GH release, as follows.

1. Alpha-adrenergic agonists such as clonidine stimulate GHRH and GH release, an effect probably mediated through decreased hypothalamic somatostatin secretion. Several stimuli for GH release, including insulin hypoglycemia, exercise, and galanin, act through alpha-adrenergic mechanisms. Beta-adrenergic blockers potentiate the GH stimulatory effect of clonidine and some other agents. Alpha$_2$-adrenergic blocking agents, such as yohimbine, decrease GH release.
2. Stimulation of muscarinic cholinergic receptors, for example with acetylcholinesterase inhibitors, facilitates GH release, and this effect also is thought to be due to inhibition of somatostatin release. The induction of GH release by arginine, glucagon, or sleep is inhibited by muscarinic receptor antagonists. Atropine is the most effective blocker of opioid peptide–mediated GH release.
3. Oral administration of dopamine precursors or agonists that cross the blood-brain barrier, such as levodopa, apomorphine, or bromocriptine, causes an increase in serum GH levels. Although these stimuli can be used to test the adequacy of GH secretion (the so-called GH reserve), the mechanism of dopamine stimulation remains controversial; it is probably mediated by GHRH. Dopamine agonists may inhibit GH release from growth hormone–secreting adenomas.
4. Although serotonin agonists stimulate GH release, the role of serotonin in the physiologic control of GH is uncertain.

Obesity blunts GH release in response to many stimuli, including GHRH itself. Weight reduction restores normal GH dynamics. In contrast, malnourished individuals, including women with anorexia nervosa, often have an increase in the secretion and plasma concentration of GH. This effect results partly from a decreased serum IGF-I level, which is possibly the result of resistance to GH at the cellular level. Oral glucose administration decreases serum GH and the GH response to GHRH. Arginine also stimulates GH release by inhibiting somatostatin release. Both basal and stimulated GH release are reduced in patients with major depression.

A number of hormones influence GH release. Most factors that stimulate GH release are more potent in women than in men, an effect mediated by estrogen. However, androgen administration enhances GH release in prepubertal boys. In testing the GH reserve in children, estrogen priming may be necessary before adequate GH release can be demonstrated. Although estrogen increases the concentration of GH, it decreases the biologic effect of the hormone by blocking IGF-I production. This is similar to the estrogen effect on prolactin, in which secretion is stimulated but its action in promoting lactation is inhibited. Chronic glucocorticoid administration inhibits GH release and may blunt somatomedin action as well, resulting in the inhibition of growth in children. Acute administration of glucocorticoids stimulates GH release, although this response is reduced or absent in obese individuals. Deficiencies of ACTH and TSH may be associated with reversible GH deficiency. GH-releasing peptide (GHRP) is a synthetic hexapeptide that stimulates pituitary GH release but does not interact with GHRH or opiate receptors. The therapeutic potential of this and similar compounds is being explored.

GROWTH HORMONE EXCESS: ACROMEGALY AND GIGANTISM Clinical Features GH excess results in acromegaly, an insidious, chronic, debilitating disease associated with bony and soft tissue overgrowth (Table 328-4). Acromegaly is equally prevalent in men and women and occurs most frequently in middle age. It is uncommon, with an estimated prevalence of 50 to 70 cases per million and an incidence of 3 to 4 cases per million per year. These figures may be an underestimation due to underdiagnosis of the disorder. When GH excess develops prior to epiphyseal closure in children, increased linear growth can cause gigantism. Tumors may be more aggressive and cause more rapid onset of acromegaly in younger patients.

Most patients have soft tissue and bone enlargement, which results in increased hand, foot, and hat size, prognathism, enlargement of the tongue, wide spacing of the teeth, and coarsening of facial features; these are rarely the presenting complaints. Acromegalics are said to look more like each other than like their own family members (Fig. 328-6). Laryngeal hypertrophy and sinus enlargement with hyperpneumatization of the skull lead to a hollow-sounding voice. A moist, doughy handshake, increased skin tags, acanthosis nigricans, and oily skin are common.

Acromegaly is more than a cosmetically disfiguring disease. Patients feel weak and tired. The basal metabolic rate increases, which, in turn, causes increased sweating. Obstructive sleep apnea may be an important cause of hypersomnolence. Most patients have neurologic and musculoskeletal symptoms, including headaches, nerve entrapments and paresthesias (often due to carpal tunnel syndrome), muscle weakness, and arthralgias (particularly involving the shoulders, back, and knees). The cartilage hypertrophy and osseous overgrowth often lead to degenerative arthritis, kyphoscoliosis, and on occasion spinal stenosis. Hypertension occurs in about one-third of patients and is characterized by suppressed renin and aldosterone secretion associated with expansion of plasma volume and an increase in total body sodium.

Table 328-4

Manifestations of Acromegaly

Location	Symptoms	Signs
General	Fatigue	
	Increased sweating	
	Heat intolerance	
	Weight gain	
Skin and subcutaneous tissue	Enlarging hands, feet	Moist, warm, fleshy, doughy handshake
	Coarsening facial features	Skin tags
	Oily skin	Acanthosis nigricans
	Hypertrichosis	Increased heel pad
Head	Headaches	Parotid enlargement, frontal bossing
Eyes	Decreased vision	Visual field defects
Ears		Otoscope speculum cannot be inserted
Nose, throat, paranasal sinuses	Sinus congestion	Enlarged, furrowed tongue
	Increased tongue size	Tooth marks on tongue
	Malocclusion	Widely spaced teeth
	Voice change	Prognathism
Neck		Goiter
		Obstructive sleep apnea
		Enlarged sinuses
Cardiorespiratory system	Congestive heart failure	Hypertension
		Cardiomegaly
		Left ventricular hypertrophy
Genitourinary system	Decreased libido	
	Impotence	
	Oligomenorrhea	
	Infertility	
	Kidney stones	
Neurologic system	Paresthesias	Carpal tunnel syndrome
	Hypersomnolence	
Muscles	Weakness	Proximal myopathy
Skeletal system	Joint pains (shoulders, back, knees)	Osteoarthritis

FIGURE 328-6 Serial photographs of a patient with acromegaly taken at ages 28, 49, 55, and 65 years, 6 months after removal of a GH-secreting adenoma. Note the gradual increase in the size of the nose, lips, and skin folds, particularly the nasolabial skin fold and forehead. *(From S Reichlin, Med Grand Rounds 1:9, 1982.)*

Almost all hypertensive acromegalics and about half of nonhypertensive acromegalics have increased left ventricular mass or left ventricular wall thickness. Although it is not established whether a specific cardiomyopathy occurs, acromegalics may develop congestive heart failure in the absence of another known underlying heart disease. Amenorrhea may occur with or without hyperprolactinemia, and hirsutism is often noted. Many organs, including the liver and kidneys, increase in size with no evidence of functional impairment. Goiter, which probably results from IGF-I stimulation of thyroid cell growth, occurs in about 40 percent of patients, and 3 to 7 percent of patients have hyperthyroidism. Some series report abdominal pain and inguinal hernias, each occurring in about one-third of patients, and nasal polyps in as many as 15 percent. Intracranial aneurysms coexist in 10 percent or fewer of patients.

Patients with untreated acromegaly have a shortened life expectancy with increased rates of death from cardiovascular, cerebrovascular, and respiratory disease and, in some studies, from malignancies. In studies in which modern therapy was available, deleterious effects on life expectancy were less striking. Patients with coexisting diabetes mellitus have increased mortality. Skin tags appear to correlate with increased prevalence of colonic polyps and possibly with an increased risk for carcinoma of the colon. Bowel surveillance by colonoscopy has been suggested.

Laboratory Investigations Insulin resistance occurs in 80 percent of patients, although abnormal glucose tolerance (20 to 40 percent) and clinical diabetes mellitus (13 to 20 percent) are less common. Hypercalciuria is frequent, apparently due to increased levels of circulating 1,25-dihydroxyvitamin D; renal stones occur in about one-fifth of patients. Hypercalcemia, when it occurs, is not due to acromegaly

per se but suggests primary hyperparathyroidism as part of the multiple endocrine neoplasia 1 (MEN 1) syndrome (see Chap. 340). GH causes increased renal tubular reabsorption of phosphate by an undefined mechanism. Elevation of serum phosphate occurs in about one-half of patients. Hyperprolactinemia occurs in up to one-half of patients and is responsible for much of the associated galactorrhea, amenorrhea, and decreased libido.

Pathophysiology Well-defined pituitary adenomas are found in almost all patients with acromegaly and gigantism. The tumors tend to occur in the lateral wings of the sella, where somatotrophs normally are found in abundance. Occasionally, tumors are found in ectopic locations along the lines of migration of Rathke's pouch, such as the sphenoid sinus or parapharyngeal regions.

GH levels correlate, on average, with tumor size. Tumors tend to be larger and may be more aggressive in younger patients. At the time of diagnosis, 75 percent of somatotroph adenomas are macroadenomas; however, 70 percent are less than 20 mm in diameter at diagnosis. This feature is different than in prolactinomas, two-thirds of which are microadenomas at the time of diagnosis. Aggressive screening for acromegaly on the basis of subtle clinical clues might lead to early diagnosis while tumors are small and more easily curable.

Immunohistochemical staining and electron microscopy of somatotroph tumors help to predict their behavior. Densely granulated tumors have slower growth. GH-secreting carcinomas are rare and should be diagnosed only in the presence of distant metastases. Tumors that cause local invasion are called *invasive adenomas*.

Current evidence suggests a primary pituitary etiology for acromegaly. Most GH-secreting (and other pituitary) tumors are monoclonal in origin. A cellular mutation may lead to GH hypersecretion (and presumably tumor growth as well) in some patients. About 40 percent of somatotroph tumors have a mutation in the α subunit of a stimulatory G (G_s) protein. These G proteins normally couple surface signals to cyclic AMP production within the cells. Activation of G_s proteins is associated with binding of guanosine triphosphate (GTP) to the α subunit, which allows the α subunit to stimulate cyclic AMP production. The normal free subunit has intrinsic GTPase activity, which inactivates GTP, preventing continued cyclic AMP stimulation. The mutant α subunit in acromegalic patients does not possess GTPase activity; hence, continued cyclic AMP stimulation leads to autonomous GH production.

Another mechanism for tumor growth in somatotroph adenomas is deletion of the 11q13 region of chromosome 11, a loss believed to involve a normal suppressor gene. This loss occurs both as a part of the MEN 1 syndrome (see Chap. 340) and in sporadic tumors. Further evidence for a primary etiology of acromegaly is the fact that peripheral concentrations of GHRH are low, although this finding does not exclude the possibility that hypothalamic GHRH excess or somatostatin deficiency is the cause in some patients. Abnormal GH pulsations in some surgically "cured" acromegalics could be due to an underlying hypothalamic disorder, residual tumor, or previous GH excess.

GHRH-induced acromegaly is rare (<1 percent in one series) but is clinically indistinguishable from acromegaly caused by pituitary adenomas. This diagnosis should be considered when pituitary somatotroph hyperplasia, rather than an adenoma, is diagnosed histologically. Bronchial carcinoids and pancreatic islet cell tumors are the ones most likely to secrete GHRH ectopically, but small cell carcinoma of the lung, medullary thyroid carcinoma, and carcinoids of the small intestine and thymus contain GHRH as well. Many of the tumors associated with GHRH production also cause ectopic ACTH production. Hypothalamic gangliocytomas, hamartomas, and gliomas can produce GHRH (as well as somatostatin) and cause somatotroph hyperplasia and acromegaly. GHRH is not routinely measured in acromegalic patients unless somatotroph hyperplasia is present or an appropriate nonpituitary tumor is discovered.

Isolated ectopic production of GH has been described in a patient with a pancreatic islet cell tumor; the tumor size in this instance

(420 g) suggests inefficient GH production, since GH-secreting pituitary tumors are usually small.

Diagnosis Patients with acromegaly have symptoms for an average of 9 years and often see several physicians before the diagnosis is made. Suspecting the diagnosis is the most difficult step in the process. Newly consulted physicians are more likely to make the diagnosis than is one who has watched the insidious progress of the disease. When suggestive facial features are noted, a comparison with old pictures may be helpful (Fig. 328-6).

Once the diagnosis is suspected, confirmation is straightforward. Because basal or random GH determinations can yield elevated values in normal persons, particularly in women and people with uncontrolled diabetes mellitus, renal failure, or stress, they should not be used to screen for acromegaly. Two diagnostic tests are available: measurements of glucose-suppressed GH concentrations and measurement of IGF-I concentrations. GH concentrations are measured 60 to 120 min after the oral administration of 100 g glucose. Although a serum GH concentration of <5 μg/L was previously accepted as normal, a postsuppression value of <2 μg/L is a more rigorous criterion and should now be applied. Acromegalics usually have a GH concentration after glucose administration of >10 μg/L; in some the value is suppressed to below 5 μg/L but it is rarely below 2 μg/L. IGF-I concentrations also provide an excellent screening test for acromegaly. Pitfalls include unreliable commercial assays, failure to use age-adjusted normal values (especially during puberty), and possible false-negative results with starvation. Measurements of serum IGF-I concentration correlate with disease activity even in patients with basal GH concentrations below 10 μg/L. As GH values rise to >20 μg/L, IGF-I concentrations plateau, probably explaining why dramatic falls in GH after therapy do not necessarily cause clinical improvement. Although GH concentrations decline, IGF-I may remain nearly maximal until GH falls below 20 μg/L.

GH concentrations in acromegaly may vary during the day, although they are never undetectable, as they are in normal persons. GH levels increase in response to insulin-induced hypoglycemia and arginine infusion, and the response to GHRH is enhanced in most acromegalics. Somatostatin infusion lowers GH concentration but usually not to a normal value. In addition, GH-secreting pituitary tumors respond to stimuli that do not affect normal somatotrophs: TRH increases GH in 80 percent, and LHRH increases GH in about 10 to 15 percent of acromegalics. Dopamine agonists stimulate GH release in normal persons but inhibit it in most acromegalics.

The IGF binding proteins (IGF-BPs) are a family of proteins that bind IGF-I and modulate its action at the cellular level. IGF-BP-3 is an integrated marker of somatotroph function, and its measurement may prove to be a useful test of growth hormone levels.

All patients with large pituitary adenomas should have measurements of IGF-I levels or GH response to glucose ingestion. In rare cases, patients with large pituitaries and elevated serum levels of GH and IGF-I do not have clinical evidence of acromegaly. This syndrome, called *silent somatotroph adenoma*, is unexplained.

Radiologic investigation is necessary once the laboratory tests confirm the clinical suspicion of acromegaly. Although conventional skull x-rays or coned-down views of the sella turcica are abnormal in 90 percent of patients with acromegaly, MRI provides better definition of tumor size and is necessary for therapeutic planning. Additional clues to the diagnosis on conventional skull x-rays include thickening of the skull with increased bone density, enlargement of the paranasal sinuses and proliferation of the mastoid air cells, and prognathism. On bone x-rays, one may see enlarged vertebral bodies with anterior lipping, tufting of the distal phalanges of the hands and feet, increased thickness and lengthening of the ribs and clavicles, and bowing of the femur, tibia, and fibula. Soft tissue x-rays demonstrate increased thickness of the heel pad (>18 mm in women and >21 mm in men).

Testing for hypopituitarism (due to compression of the normal pituitary tissue) and for increased prolactin levels (due either to stalk compression or to cosecretion of prolactin by the tumor) should be performed. Mass effects from large somatotroph adenomas can cause neurologic abnormalities (visual field defects or oculomotor or abducens nerve lesions). In addition, acromegaly may be associated with hyperparathyroidism and pancreatic islet cell tumors in the MEN 1 syndrome and rarely with pheochromocytomas or hyperaldosteronism (see Chap. 340). The α subunit of the glycoprotein hormones may be oversecreted in acromegaly and may serve as an additional marker of tumor regrowth.

℞ TREATMENT

The objectives of therapy are (1) return of GH and IGF-I levels to normal, (2) stabilization or decrease in tumor size, and (3) preservation of normal pituitary function. Although GH values of <5 μg/L were formerly considered to indicate cure, a value of <2 μg/L with a normal IGF-I level is a better criterion; patients with GH values between 2 and 5 μg/L may have persistent symptoms and increased IGF-I concentrations.

Surgery Transsphenoidal surgery has the advantage of producing a rapid therapeutic response; it is potentially curative and is the treatment of choice. Anesthesiologists should be alerted to the potential of a difficult intubation due to anatomic changes in the jaw, tongue, epiglottis, and larynx. GH concentrations may fall to normal within hours, and soft tissue (but not bony) enlargement may melt away, even before the patient has been discharged from the hospital. The success of this procedure depends on the completeness of the resection and hence on the size of the tumor. Cure rates vary from 80 percent for microadenomas to less than 50 percent for tumors larger than 1 cm in diameter. Preoperative GH levels are also of predictive value. In expert hands, apparent cure rates (GH below 5 μg/L) average 75 percent in patients with preoperative GH levels of <40 μg/L but only 35 percent in those with preoperative GH levels >40 μg/L. More stringent criteria, such as a GH level of <2 μg/L and a normal IGF-I level, are rarely used in surgical series; the cure rate is probably closer to 20 to 40 percent when these criteria are applied. This may explain why tumor regrowth and recurrent acromegaly are more common than previously appreciated. Persistent GH response to TRH stimulation may have predictive value in assessing risk of relapse, even in those patients with "normal" postoperative GH concentrations. Postoperative hypopituitarism occurs in 10 to 20 percent of patients with large tumors, but up to 10 percent of patients with pituitary insufficiency prior to surgery regain normal function.

Radiation Heavy-particle pituitary irradiation is successful in lowering GH levels in acromegaly but is slow to accomplish this goal. Patients with suprasellar extension of the pituitary adenoma are generally excluded from this therapy. The Harvard cyclotron uses the Bragg peak with proton irradiation, achieving delivery of up to 12,000 cGy (12,000 rad) to the center of the pituitary adenoma. In patients with mean pretherapy GH concentration of 60 μg/L, GH concentrations are <5 μg/L in 29 percent of patients at 2 years, in 40 percent at 4 years, in 75 percent at 10 years, and in 92 percent by 20 years. The risk of hypopituitarism is at least 20 percent.

Conventional pituitary irradiation [4500 cGy (4500 rad) over 5 weeks] can cause a lowering of GH levels, but the effect may take years to develop. GH generally falls 50 percent after 2 ± 1 years. GH concentrations of <5 μg/L occur in 50 percent of patients at 5 years and in 70 percent at 10 years (after a mean pretherapy GH level of 60 μg/L). GH concentrations of <2.5 μg/L occur in 40 percent of patients, and values <1 μg/L are seen in 20 percent at 10 to 15 years. Hypopituitarism is a common sequela of radiation treatment, and up to 50 percent of patients require hormone replacement. The hypopituitarism is probably due to hypothalamic damage, which is possibly less common with focused heavy particles or gamma radiation. Higher doses of focused radiation [4000 to 7000 cGy (4000 to 7000 rad)] can be delivered with the cobalt 60 gamma unit ("gamma knife"), which delivers collimated radiation through multiple portals (over 200 in some units) that converge on the target. The radiation is delivered in a single session; radiation delivery to the tumor is the equivalent of two to three times the dosage of conventional radiation treatment. Reports to date do not suggest an advantage (apart from convenience) over conventional radiation treatment in terms of either efficacy or of the risk of hypopituitarism; however, the data are still preliminary. Rare complications of pituitary irradiation include development of malignancies in the radiation field, damage to the visual apparatus, brain necrosis, and cognitive impairment. Radiation treatment is advised for patients who have failed surgery and medical therapy, for tumors in an inoperable location, and when surgery is contraindicated or is refused by the patient. Because of the long delay between irradiation of the pituitary and response, medical therapy should be given in the interim.

Medical Treatment Bromocriptine is a useful adjunct to other modalities of therapy but rarely is successful alone. Clinical improvement is reported in up to 90 percent of patients with dosages of 20 to 60 mg/d. Objective decrease in hand and ring size as well as improvement in diabetes mellitus may occur in the absence of decreasing GH values. However, GH concentrations fall to <10 μg/L in only 35 percent of patients, and values of <5 μg/L are achieved in only 21 percent; IGF-I levels return to normal in only 8 percent. Tumor size decreases rarely.

The long-acting somatostatin analogue octreotide lowers GH to <5 μg/L and IGF-I to normal in half of acromegalics. Modest tumor regression occurs in 30 to 50 percent of patients. The drug must be administered subcutaneously several times a day. Dosages average 100 to 200 μg every 8 h but range from 50 to 250 μg every 6 to 12 h to a maximum of 1500 μg/d. Constant subcutaneous pump therapy also has been employed to prevent the rise in GH between injections. Temporary side effects are minimal and include local pain, steatorrhea, and abdominal cramps; the risk of cholelithiasis is substantial and may be due to decreased gallbladder contractility. Octreotide is 2000 times as potent as somatostatin in inhibiting GH secretion but only 1.5 to 2 times as potent an inhibitor of insulin secretion. Although impairment of glucose tolerance or worsening of diabetes mellitus may occur, the GH-lowering effects of the drug may improve glucose tolerance. Inhibition of TSH does not result in hypothyroidism. Headaches disappear quickly, possibly due to an effect on cerebral blood flow. The role of this agent as a primary treatment for acromegaly remains to be defined, but some patients have been treated successfully for over 5 years. It is likely that octreotide will be most useful as adjunctive therapy after unsuccessful surgery and/or radiation therapy. Studies suggesting that the success rate of surgery in acromegalic patients with invasive macroadenomas is higher after octreotide pretreatment have not been confirmed.

All acromegalic patients require long-term follow-up and evaluation for recurrent disease. Interlaboratory variation in GH determinations may be considerable; whenever possible, serial GH levels should be measured by the same laboratory. False elevations of GH concentrations in some acromegalics may be due to antibodies that displace GH in the radioimmunoassays used. Surveillance for colonic polyps and/or colon cancer, including colonoscopy, may be appropriate for all acromegalics; other workers advocate such surveillance only for those at higher risk: subjects over age 50, those with more than 10 years of acromegaly, and those with more than three skin tags.

GH DEFICIENCY AND PITUITARY DWARFISM GH is often the first hormone to be lost in pituitary and hypothalamic disorders. In adults, GH deficiency is usually cryptic and can only be diagnosed on the basis of stimulation tests for GH release. The consequences of GH deficiency and replacement in adults are being explored. GH deficiency may contribute to the increased cardiovascular mortality in hypopituitary adults; conversely, these patients have a decreased cancer mortality. Diabetics with GH deficiency show a reduction in insulin requirements and may develop hypoglycemia. In children GH deficiency leads to impaired growth and short stature and is often a consequence of hypothalamic GHRH deficiency (see Chap. 329). Short-term replacement therapy in GH-deficient adults results in improved exercise tolerance, decreased body fat, and increased lean body

mass. Long-term studies of the benefits, risks, and optimal dosing of GH in adults are under way.

GONADOTROPINS

PHYSIOLOGY The gonadotropins, LH and FSH, are secreted by the gonadotrophs (see also Chaps. 336 and 337). These cells make up about 10 percent of the anterior pituitary and are dispersed throughout the lobe, often situated close to the lactotrophs. Most gonadotrophs produce both LH and FSH, although a few cells produce only one hormone.

LH and FSH are glycoproteins of similar size (about 30,000 mol wt) which share a common α subunit [also present in TSH and human chorionic gonadotropin (hCG)] but have unique β subunits. The α and β chains are encoded by separate genes, and α chains are often produced in excess. The carbohydrate components of the molecules influence the biologic behavior and duration of action and may vary during the menstrual cycle. Although both FSH and LH are secreted in pulsatile fashion, FSH has a longer half-life, so that FSH levels fluctuate less throughout the day. FSH and LH regulate ovarian and testicular function. hCG is also produced in the normal pituitary.

FSH stimulates the growth of the granulosa cells of the ovarian follicle and controls the aromatase responsible for estradiol formation in these cells. LH stimulates the ovarian theca cells to produce androgens, which diffuse to the granulosa cells, where they are converted to estrogens. The level of estradiol, the principal estrogen, peaks about 1 day prior to the LH surge, which, in turn, triggers ovulation. After ovulation LH contributes to corpus luteum formation. Once conception has occurred, pituitary gonadotropin function is no longer necessary to sustain pregnancy.

In the testis LH controls testosterone production by the Leydig cells. FSH, in conjunction with intratesticular testosterone, stimulates the seminiferous tubules to produce sperm. Thus, LH and FSH both are necessary for normal spermatogenesis, whereas testosterone production requires only LH.

Luteinizing hormone–releasing hormone [LHRH, also known as gonadotropin-releasing hormone (GnRH)], a decapeptide produced by the arcuate nuclei of the hypothalamus, is responsible for the release of both LH and FSH. Extrahypothalamic LHRH is present in other areas of the brain as well. Noradrenergic agonists appear to facilitate, whereas endogenous opioids inhibit, LHRH release.

LHRH acts on high-affinity pituitary receptors to stimulate LH and FSH production and release. The pituitary response to LHRH varies greatly throughout life. LHRH and the gonadotropins first appear in the fetus at about 10 weeks of gestation. During the first 3 months after birth, LHRH elicits a brisk gonadotropin rise. The sensitivity to LHRH then declines until the onset of puberty. Before puberty FSH levels increase to a greater extent after LHRH administration than does LH. With the onset of puberty, sensitivity to LHRH increases, and pulsatile LH secretion is first apparent during sleep. Later in puberty and during the reproductive years, pulsations are present throughout the day, with LH being more responsive to LHRH than is FSH. After menopause, FSH and LH levels rise, and postmenopausal FSH levels are higher than those of LH.

Pulsatile LHRH release results in pulsatile LH and FSH release. However, sustained infusion of LHRH and its analogues results in inhibition of LH and FSH release. This phenomenon has been used successfully in the treatment of gonadotropin-mediated precocious puberty by the sustained administration of LHRH or its analogues. Conversely, in people with LHRH deficiency, the pulsatile administration of LHRH can restore ovarian or testicular function.

The feedback relationship between the gonadal steroids and the hypothalamus and pituitary is detailed in Chaps. 336 and 337. Low doses of estrogens decrease the frequency of LHRH pulses and, more important, decrease the pituitary response to LHRH; this phenomenon is seen most clearly in postmenopausal women with elevated gonadotropin levels. However, sustained elevation of estrogens results in a positive-feedback signal that stimulates LHRH and LH release; this phenomenon is responsible, in part, for the LH surge that precedes ovulation. The sensitivity of LHRH to this positive feedback by estrogen increases during middle to late puberty. Although progesterone decreases LHRH pulse frequency, the progesterone rise in the late follicular phase augments the pituitary LH response to LHRH and contributes to the LH surge. In castrated men, testosterone administration usually suppresses LH to undetectable levels and less often lowers FSH to normal (but not undetectable) concentrations. Inhibin, a peptide hormone produced by the testicular Sertoli cell and ovarian granulosa cell, is a potent inhibitor of FSH (but not LH) release. Its physiologic role is under investigation. Testosterone decreases the frequency of LH pulsations, probably by a direct effect on LHRH release and is converted in many tissues, including the brain, to estradiol, which inhibits the pituitary response to LHRH.

Gonadotropin Measurements   In evaluating gonadal failure associated with low testosterone concentrations in men or low estradiol levels in women, gonadotropin measurements help separate primary from central (secondary, hypogonadotropic) hypogonadism. High gonadotropin concentrations are indicative of primary gonadal failure; low or normal gonadotropin concentrations suggest hypothalamic or pituitary disease (see Chap. 330). Primary gonadal failure, as in women at menopause or after oophorectomy or in men with testicular failure, causes a marked increase in FSH and LH levels. Such elevated gonadotropin concentrations ensure the adequacy of pituitary gonadotroph function and establish that the disorder is at the gonadal level. On the other hand, gonadotropin measurements are rarely indicated in a woman with ovulatory menses and in men with normal sperm counts.

HYPOGONADOTROPIC (CENTRAL, SECONDARY) HYPOGONADISM   Isolated gonadotropin deficiency may be a congenital or hereditary disorder. Kallmann's syndrome is a heterogeneous genetic disorder afflicting 1 in 10,000 to 60,000 individuals; X-linked as well as autosomal inheritance has been described. Kallmann's syndrome is characterized by gonadotropin deficiency due to LHRH deficiency in association with anosmia and midline anatomic defects. LHRH-secreting neurons migrate from the olfactory placode into the brain, along with the olfactory and other nerves. The mutation in X-linked Kallmann's syndrome results in a defect in neuronal migration. Most patients with Kallmann's syndrome secrete gonadotropins in response to LHRH administration after suitable priming. Mutations in the β subunit of LH are another cause of hypogonadism.

Acquired defects of LHRH production are common. Hyperprolactinemia causes amenorrhea due to inhibition of LHRH release, possibly mediated by increased hypothalamic dopamine. Amenorrhea that occurs with anorexia nervosa, starvation, intense exercise, and "stress" appears to be due to inhibition of LHRH release as well. Gonadotropin deficiency may be a relatively early defect in patients with large pituitary adenomas. Gonadotropin deficiency also occurs in patients with polyglandular endocrine deficiencies, presumably on an autoimmune basis (see Chap. 340), and in patients with hemochromatosis.

Patients with LHRH deficiency who desire fertility may respond to pulsatile therapy with LHRH or its agonists. When gonadotropin deficiency is due to pituitary disease, injections of FSH (menotropin) and chorionic gonadotropin (a hormone with LH-like activity) are necessary to achieve fertility.

ECTOPIC GONADOTROPIN SECRETION   Ectopic gonadotropin production (usually of hCG) can be associated with germinomas of the nonseminoma type (see Chap. 98), lung carcinomas, hepatomas, and other tumors. Children may develop precocious puberty, and men may develop gynecomastia. No distinct clinical syndrome occurs in women.

GONADOTROPIN-SECRETING PITUITARY TUMORS
Gonadotropin-secreting pituitary tumors, like other pituitary adenomas, are monoclonal in origin, implying that a somatic mutation in a single gonadotrope is responsible. The inhibin subunits that make up

activin, a member of the transforming growth factor β family of peptides, are produced by these tumors and may play a role in their growth. Gonadotroph adenomas are generally large and are most commonly diagnosed in men with decreased libido, decreased serum testosterone levels, and normal or slightly elevated prolactin levels. Although 20 to 25 percent of pituitary macroadenomas are considered nonfunctioning (i.e., they do not cause a clinical syndrome of hormone overproduction), many of these tumors produce gonadotropin. Some produce high levels of intact gonadotropins (usually FSH or FSH in conjunction with LH, rarely LH alone), with or without a clinical syndrome. Testicular enlargement due to FSH excess and testosterone elevation due to elevated LH levels occur but are rare. The finding of an increased FSH concentration may be misinterpreted as primary hypogonadism if a pituitary adenoma is not suspected. Inhibin levels may be increased (as a consequence of FSH increase) in contrast to low inhibin levels in patients with primary hypogonadism. In some, the FSH has enhanced biologic activity, possibly because of altered glycosylation. In others, normal amounts of intact gonadotropins are associated with unbalanced production of gonadotropin subunits, particularly the α subunit of FSH or the LH β subunit. Although LH concentrations are often normal or elevated, testosterone levels are often low and respond normally to hCG administration. This suggests that the LH is biologically inactive (possibly because of abnormal glycosylation) or that the measured LH value represents immunologic cross-reactivity due to LH subunit overproduction. Some tumors secrete normal amounts of intact gonadotropins and gonadotropin subunits but demonstrate abnormal responses to TRH stimulation. FSH increase in response to TRH (e.g., 400 μg intravenously) occurs in 40 percent of patients with gonadotropin-secreting tumors but not in normal individuals, hypogonadal men, or postmenopausal women; an increased response of gonadotropin α and LH β subunits is common as well. Some tumors express gonadotropin gene mRNA and/or hormone production in vitro but do not cause in vivo abnormalities.

In postmenopausal women with macroadenomas, it may be difficult to ascertain whether a gonadotropin elevation is due to normal menopause or to a gonadotropin-secreting adenoma. TRH testing may provide a partial answer. Most such tumors produce increased LH β, FSH, or LH in response to TRH administration.

The therapy of nonfunctioning pituitary macroadenomas and gonadotropin-secreting adenomas is the same: surgery and/or radiation therapy. The response to bromocriptine, somatostatin analogues, or LHRH analogues is disappointing in terms of tumor shrinkage even when a hormonal response is achieved.

Men with primary hypogonadism (low testosterone level, elevated LH and FSH levels) are occasionally investigated for the presence of a gonadotropin-secreting tumor. There is no simple way of differentiating these two clinical situations. Primary hypogonadism is common; gonadotropin-secreting tumors are rare. The tumors are almost always large, but radiographic procedures may be necessary to exclude a tumor. A normal testicular response to hCG administration points toward a gonadotropin-secreting adenoma, but this test is cumbersome and poorly standardized.

THYROTROPIN

PHYSIOLOGY   TSH is a glycoprotein hormone (28,000 mol wt) composed of an α subunit which it shares with LH, FSH, and hCG and a unique β subunit that confers specificity (also see Chap. 331). The individual subunits have no intrinsic biologic activity. TSH is produced by thyrotrophs, which constitute about 5 percent of the cells of the anterior pituitary. TSH regulates the biosynthesis, storage, and release of thyroid hormones and determines thyroid gland size. TSH first appears in the fetal pituitary at about 10 weeks of gestation. TSH levels in normal subjects average 0.5 to 5.0 mU/L, with a slight increase in the nocturnal hours. The nocturnal TSH rise is absent in patients with central hypothyroidism.

Thyrotropin-releasing hormone (TRH), the major hypothalamic mediator of TSH release, is a tripeptide found in highest concentrations in the medial division of the hypothalamic paraventricular nuclei and in the median eminence. Extrahypothalamic TRH is found in the posterior pituitary, in other parts of the brain and spinal cord, and in the gastrointestinal tract. TRH stimulates TSH secretion by increasing cytoplasmic free calcium; phosphatidylinositol and membrane phospholipids probably participate in TRH-stimulated TSH secretion. TRH stimulation increases the glycosylation and hence the biologic activity of secreted TSH. TRH stimulates the release of prolactin as well as that of TSH. The prolactin response is enhanced in hypothyroidism and diminished in hyperthyroidism. TRH-induced GH stimulation may occur in acromegaly, renal failure and depression; it also occurs in many normal children and in occasional normal adults.

The thyroid hormones thyroxine (T_4) and triiodothyronine (T_3) inhibit TSH production directly at the pituitary level. Both T_3 and T_4 bind to receptors on pituitary nuclei, but T_3 has a 40-fold greater affinity for these receptors than does T_4. Nevertheless, exogenous T_4 is more potent than T_3 in inhibiting TSH release because circulating T_4 is a more effective means of delivering T_3 to the pituitary than is T_3 itself. Half of intrapituitary T_3 is derived from T_4 conversion within the pituitary. The effects of T_4 and T_3 on hypothalamic TRH release in humans are unknown, but in animals they cause inhibition of TRH synthesis and release. In the usual causes of hyperthyroidism, TSH is suppressed, and the TSH response to TRH is absent; in primary hypothyroidism, the basal TSH concentration is elevated, and the response to TRH is exaggerated.

Somatostatin decreases basal TSH release, the TSH response to TRH, and the nocturnal TSH peak. Dopamine and glucocorticoids decrease the basal TSH concentration and the TSH response to TRH. Patients with untreated primary adrenal insufficiency may have slightly elevated TSH levels. TSH levels decline with severe illness.

TSH concentrations can be interpreted only when serum thyroid hormone concentrations are known (see Chap. 327). In the usual cases of hyperthyroidism, thyroid hormone levels are elevated, and TSH release is inhibited. TSH-induced hyperthyroidism is rare. Only sensitive TSH assays can differentiate between low and normal concentrations. A detectable serum TSH concentration by a sensitive assay excludes the common causes of hyperthyroidism. Low thyroid hormone and elevated serum TSH concentrations are characteristic of primary hypothyroidism. Low thyroid hormone concentrations with a "normal" or "low" TSH concentration are found in central (secondary) hypothyroidism. The TRH stimulation test (no TSH response in hyperthyroidism, exaggerated TSH response in primary hypothyroidism) has largely been supplanted by sensitive TSH measurements. The TRH stimulation test is also not useful in the diagnosis of secondary hypothyroidism or in differentiating pituitary from hypothalamic disease.

PRIMARY HYPOTHYROIDISM Thyroid gland failure (primary hypothyroidism) leads to compensatory hypertrophy of the thyrotrophs. With thyroid failure of long duration, the pituitary gland and the sella turcica may enlarge, occasionally causing visual field defects. Although TSH-secreting tumors may develop in animals after thyroid gland removal, the increased TSH and pituitary size in human hypothyroidism is not autonomous and decreases with thyroid hormone replacement. Since hyperprolactinemia also may occur in patients with primary hypothyroidism, pituitary enlargement (hyperplasia) may be incorrectly diagnosed as a prolactinoma; however, the return to normal of prolactin concentrations with thyroid hormone therapy excludes that diagnosis. Severe primary hypothyroidism occasionally causes impaired release of GH and ACTH after appropriate stimuli (so-called pituitary myxedema), and hypothyroid children may develop precocious puberty. These abnormalities are all corrected with thyroid hormone therapy.

SECONDARY HYPOTHYROIDISM Hypothyroidism due to pituitary or hypothalamic disease may be difficult to diagnose. With primary hypothyroidism, serum TSH commonly rises before thyroid hormone concentrations decline below the normal range. No similar early laboratory clue exists in secondary hypothyroidism. Patients with central hypothyroidism usually do not have goiter, and many have deficiencies of other pituitary trophic hormones.

Some patients with hypothalamic hypothyroidism have mild TSH elevations, rather than normal or low concentrations, as expected.

Although the TSH elevations rarely exceed 10 mU/L, they are above the expected range for hypothyroidism due to TSH deficiency. Biologically inactive but immunologically active thyrotropin is present in such cases. After TRH injection, the TSH concentration rises, and the biologic potency of the TSH is increased. This suggests an additional role for TRH in controlling the biologic activity of the TSH molecule by controlling its rate of glycosylation. Although subclinical primary hypothyroidism is also characterized by mild TSH elevations, serum T_4 levels differ in the two states. Patients with central hypothyroidism and associated TSH elevations have very low T_4 concentrations; patients with subclinical hypothyroidism have normal or near-normal T_4 concentrations. TSH concentrations must not be used to guide replacement therapy in central hypothyroidism, because TSH concentrations fall before full replacement is achieved; rather, peripheral levels of T_4 and free T_4 should be monitored. Severe illness may cause laboratory changes indistinguishable from those of central hypothyroidism, part of the so-called euthyroid sick syndrome.

PITUITARY (TSH-INDUCED) HYPERTHYROIDISM Hyperthyroidism is not usually a disease of TSH overproduction. However, the following two types of TSH-mediated hyperthyroidism are recognized.

Pituitary Tumors These are usually macroadenomas with autonomous TSH secretion, unresponsive to thyroid hormone suppression or TRH stimulation. Patients with these tumors may appear to have Graves' disease with high free thyroxine levels and diffuse goiters with high radioiodine uptakes. However, they do not have the eye or skin changes of Graves' disease and do not have suppressed TSH levels. A hallmark of such tumors is overproduction of the glycoprotein hormone α subunit with a molar ratio of α to intact TSH of greater than 1:1 in serum. The free α subunit may be an important tumor marker and differs from the native α subunit in that one of its amino acids is carbohydrate-blocked and hence cannot combine with β subunits. These tumors may produce other pituitary hormones in addition to TSH, most commonly GH. In some patients TSH levels are within normal limits; increased TSH bioactivity is believed to explain the hyperthyroidism in such patients. Therapy is generally transsphenoidal surgery to remove the tumor, but control of hyperthyroidism may require radioactive iodine or antithyroid drugs. Octreotide may lower TSH levels when complete tumor removal is not possible.

Pituitary Resistance to Thyroid Hormone In this situation, thyroid hormone fails to inhibit TSH secretion appropriately in the absence of a pituitary adenoma. Since TSH secretion is not inhibited, TSH rises and stimulates thyroid hormone overproduction. The peripheral tissues are not resistant to thyroid hormone, and clinical hyperthyroidism results. The pituitary resistance to thyroid hormone is incomplete, since TSH can be suppressed with supraphysiologic levels of thyroid hormone and stimulated further with TRH; bromocriptine or octreotide may lower TSH as well. Pituitary resistance is usually diagnosed after thyroid gland ablation, when TSH cannot be lowered to normal values with the usual therapeutic doses of thyroid hormone. However, once the hyperthyroidism has been treated, pituitary resistance is of no clinical consequence, although the TSH measurements cannot be utilized to monitor adequacy of hormone replacement. In some patients the molecular defect in the thyroid hormone β receptor is the same as that in generalized resistance to thyroid hormone (see Chap. 331).

ADRENOCORTICOTROPIN

PHYSIOLOGY ACTH is produced by corticotrophs, which constitute about 15 percent of anterior pituitary cells and are located principally in the central portion of the gland. ACTH is synthesized as part of a large precursor molecule termed *pro-opiomelanocortin* (POMC, 265 amino acids). ACTH contains 39 amino acids, with nearly complete biologic activity residing in the *N*-terminal 26 amino acids. In the anterior pituitary, POMC is cleaved to yield ACTH, β-lipotropin, and an *N*-terminal precursor.

ACTH controls the release of cortisol from the adrenal cortex. Although aldosterone is primarily controlled by the renin-angiotensin system, ACTH also stimulates aldosterone release acutely. Other derivatives of the POMC molecule, such as γ melanocyte-stimulating hormone (γ-MSH), also influence aldosterone production and are found in increased levels in the plasma of patients with idiopathic hyperaldosteronism. Patients with ACTH deficiency have near-normal aldosterone production and do not require mineralocorticoid replacement.

Corticotropin-releasing hormone (CRH) is the major but not exclusive regulator of ACTH release. CRH contains 41 amino acids in a single polypeptide chain. It is synthesized primarily by neurons of the paraventricular nuclei of the hypothalamus but is also present in other areas of the brain, including the limbic system and cortex, and in the placenta, pancreas, gut, and adrenal medulla. Circulating CRH, which is largely of nonhypothalamic origin, is bound to a high-affinity binding protein. CRH stimulates cyclic AMP production, regulates intracellular calcium, and increases the concentration of POMC mRNA. Vasopressin potentiates the release of ACTH by CRH through a cyclic AMP–independent mechanism and may play a physiologic role in ACTH release. Naloxone, an opiate antagonist, causes release of CRH (and hence ACTH) in humans.

ACTH is released in pulses with an overriding circadian rhythm. With a normal sleeping pattern, ACTH concentration is highest in the early morning (around 4 A.M.) and lowest in late evening. The normal diurnal rhythm of plasma cortisol occurs in response to these ACTH changes. In primary adrenal insufficiency (Addison's disease), cortisol concentrations fall, and ACTH concentrations rise. This results in hyperpigmentation owing to the melanocyte-stimulating properties of ACTH. Cortisol administration inhibits ACTH release, a phenomenon dependent on both the rate of rise of cortisol and its absolute concentration. Increased plasma cortisol inhibits CRH-induced ACTH release and also may inhibit CRH release. When pharmacologic doses of glucocorticoids are given for prolonged periods, the hypothalamic-pituitary–adrenal cortex axis may remain suppressed for months after the drugs are stopped, probably as the result of prolonged hypothalamic CRH suppression (see Chap. 332).

Stress, including hypoglycemia, surgery, and psychic distress, stimulates ACTH release, in part via increased CRH release, but the magnitude of the ACTH release is greater than can be achieved with maximal doses of CRH. With severe illness, the requirements for cortisol may increase significantly; failure of cortisol secretion to be enhanced during such periods may cause clinical adrenal insufficiency when adrenal reserve is impaired.

The immune system is tightly linked to the hypothalamic-pituitary-adrenal (HPA) axis. Glucocorticoids inhibit immune function, and immune mediators such as interleukin 1 are potent stimulators of ACTH secretion. These mediators may explain at least part of the link between "stress" and activation of the HPA axis, the subsequent cortisol response serving to limit the immune response.

ACTH is present at low levels in normal serum [2 to 18 pmol/L (10 to 80 pg/mL)]. It is difficult to measure ACTH in plasma and often not possible to separate low from normal values using commercial assays. Random ACTH measurements have little clinical significance. Tests for adrenal insufficiency and excess rely primarily on measurements of cortisol and its metabolites rather than on measurement of ACTH.

ACTH EXCESS (CUSHING'S DISEASE AND NELSON'S SYNDROME) Clinical Features Cortisol excess is characterized by a central distribution of adipose tissue, muscle weakness, purplish striae, hypertension, amenorrhea, decreased libido, impotence, osteoporosis, fatigue, and psychiatric abnormalities. This syndrome may be caused by pituitary or ectopic ACTH overproduction, adrenal tumors, or exogenous glucocorticoid administration.

The presence of cortisol excess is suggested by the failure to suppress an 8 A.M. cortisol level to <140 nmol/L (<5 μg/dL) after an overnight dexamethasone suppression test (1 mg by mouth at mid-

night). Because there are many causes of false-positive failure of suppression, the diagnosis must be confirmed by the finding of increased excretion of urine free cortisol and/or 17-hydroxycorticosteroids that fails to decrease appropriately after 2-day low-dose dexamethasone administration (0.5 mg every 6 h for eight doses). Additional suppression (and occasionally stimulation) tests are required to determine whether the Cushing's syndrome is due to a pituitary lesion (Cushing's disease) or to some other cause. In patients with pituitary ACTH hypersecretion, high-dose overnight dexamethasone administration (8 mg at midnight) results in greater than 50 percent reduction in the 8 A.M. plasma cortisol level, and two-day dexamethasone administration (2 mg every 6 h for eight doses) should result in greater than 60 percent suppression of urine 17-hydroxycorticosteroids and more than 90 percent suppression of urine free cortisol. Urine 17-hydroxycorticosteroids increase after metyrapone administration in Cushing's disease. In contrast, most adrenal and ectopic tumors that produce cortisol and/or ACTH autonomously do not demonstrate suppression with dexamethasone or stimulation with metapyrone.

Plasma ACTH levels are normal or high-normal in Cushing's disease and show an exaggerated increase after CRH administration. ACTH levels are low in adrenal Cushing's disease and do not increase with CRH. In ectopic Cushing's disease ACTH levels can be extremely high but are often high normal, overlapping the levels in pituitary Cushing's disease. However, most patients with ectopic Cushing's disease do not exhibit a rise in ACTH with CRH administration. Pituitary Cushing's disease is caused by a corticotroph microadenoma in 90 percent of patients and by a macroadenoma in most of the rest. The microadenomas are often small (3 to 6 mm or less) and may be difficult to find even with the use of gadolinium-enhanced MRI. Corticotroph hyperplasia has been documented in a few cases. Previously, pituitary surgery was often recommended on the basis of dynamic testing alone. However, some ACTH-producing tumors, particularly bronchial carcinoids, give dynamic hormone test results similar to those in Cushing's disease, leading to misdiagnosis and inappropriate surgery. The technique of bilateral inferior petrosal sinus catheterization to localize the site of ACTH production is a major advance for confirming the pituitary source of ACTH production and for localizing adenomas when imaging studies are negative.

Nelson's syndrome (characterized by hyperpigmentation and high plasma ACTH levels despite adequate glucocorticoid replacement) is caused by growth of the residual pituitary tumor after bilateral adrenalectomy in patients with pituitary Cushing's disease. These tumors can cause mass effects such as bitemporal hemianopsia from optic chiasm compression or oculomotor nerve palsy from cavernous sinus invasion. The tumors are usually identified on MRI and may exhibit aggressive growth patterns.

℞ **TREATMENT**

Transsphenoidal microsurgery is successful in treating microadenomas in more than 80 percent of patients. When surgery is successful, plasma cortisol concentrations fall almost to zero and often remain low for many months owing to delayed recovery of CRH and ACTH secretion by the hypothalamus and normal remaining pituitary. Thus, glucocorticoid replacement is necessary until the hypothalamic-pituitary-adrenal axis recovers. Cushing's syndrome may recur, and long-term follow-up is important. Prior to the development of transsphenoidal surgery, bilateral adrenalectomy was the therapy of choice for pituitary Cushing's disease. Unfortunately, after this procedure Nelson's syndrome develops in 10 to 30 percent of patients, particularly in younger individuals.

Ectopic ACTH production is the cause of 10 to 15 percent of cases of Cushing's syndrome and may be difficult to diagnose (see Chaps. 102 and 332). When ACTH production is caused by a rapidly growing tumor such as small cell carcinoma of the lung, many of the symptoms of Cushing's syndrome may be absent. Rather, patients have hypokalemia, muscle weakness, weight loss, and hyperpigmentation. ACTH concentrations often exceed 66 pmol/L (300 pg/mL) and do not change with dexamethasone administration. ACTH concentrations may be lower in immunoradiometric assays that do not measure larger fragments of the POMC molecule. When slow-growing tumors such as thymic carcinoids, bronchial carcinoids, medullary carcinoma of the thyroid, and pancreatic islet cell tumors produce ACTH, the features of Cushing's syndrome are present. In the latter group, ACTH measurements and cortisol response to dexamethasone administration may mimic those found in patients with pituitary adenomas. When it is unclear whether ACTH production is pituitary or ectopic, bilateral inferior petrosal sinus catheterization for measurement of ACTH is necessary. Cushing's syndrome can rarely be caused by ectopic production of CRH itself.

ACTH DEFICIENCY (SECONDARY ADRENAL INSUFFICIENCY)   ACTH deficiency may be isolated or occur in association with other anterior pituitary hormone deficiencies. Reversible isolated ACTH deficiency is common after long-term glucocorticoid administration. If glucocorticoids are withdrawn suddenly in this situation or continued at physiologic doses when severe illness is present, adrenal insufficiency may occur (see Chap. 332). Symptoms include nausea, vomiting, fatigue, joint discomfort, and dizziness, and there may be fever, hypotension, hyponatremia, and hypoglycemia. Reversible dementia may occur in the elderly. Although cortisol is necessary for free water excretion, it is not needed for potassium excretion. Hence, patients with ACTH deficiency are hyponatremic but not hyperkalemic, in contrast to patients with primary adrenal insufficiency. Hyperpigmentation does not occur. These factors make diagnosis of secondary adrenal insufficiency more difficult than that of primary adrenal insufficiency. Isolated ACTH deficiency may occur without prior glucocorticoid therapy and may be of hypothalamic or pituitary origin. The diagnosis is often missed.

In general, patients undergoing pituitary surgery need to be treated with "stress" doses of glucocorticoids until normal adrenal function can be demonstrated postoperatively. All patients with pituitary macroadenomas or hypothalamic disease require testing of the pituitary-adrenal axis, but when pituitary surgery is planned, testing can be limited in focus until after surgery is completed.

THE ENDOGENOUS OPIOID PEPTIDES

The endogenous opioid peptides bind to a family of opioid receptors. The endorphins, enkephalins, and dynorphins, although chemically related, arise by different biosynthetic pathways. In the pituitary, β-endorphin, the most abundant endorphin, is synthesized as part of a larger precursor molecule (proopiomelanocortin, POMC) that also contains the full sequences of ACTH, γ-MSH, β-MSH, and β-lipotropin (β-LPH) (Fig. 328-7). This biosynthetic pathway represents the

FIGURE 328-7   Biosynthetic pathway for β-endorphin in the pituitary gland. A single precursor protein, pro-opiomelanocortin (POMC) (molecular weight of approximately 31,000), is initially synthesized from translation of a gene that encodes the structure of adrenocorticotropin (ACTH), β-lipotropin (β-LPH), and β-endorphin. Prohormone-type cleavages can generate other hormones from the same precursor, although this occurs in tissues other than the pituitary. Abbreviations: MSH, melanocyte-stimulating hormone; LPH, lipotropin; CLIP, corticotropin-like intermediate peptide; ACTH, adrenocorticotropin.

only pathway for pituitary ACTH synthesis. In adrenal insufficiency and Nelson's syndrome and after CRH administration, plasma levels of ACTH and β-endorphin are elevated in parallel. Ectopic production of ACTH by tumors is also accompanied by β-endorphin and β-LPH excess. Unfortunately, differential processing of POMC by tumors does not usually allow separation of pituitary from ectopic ACTH production by analysis of metabolites. Production of "big" and "big-big" ACTH by tumors reflects the incomplete processing of the POMC precursor; the detection of higher ACTH levels by radioimmunoassay than by immunoradiometric assay also reflects this incomplete processing. The increased ratio of β-LPH to ACTH may be due to increased processing of ACTH to corticotropin-like intermediate lobe peptide (CLIP) by the tumor. Alternative processing of POMC occurs within other tissues. For example, hypothalamic neurons produce POMC, which serves as a precursor of β-endorphin in the brain; ACTH is not an end-product of POMC metabolism in these cells.

Two other opioid precursors give rise to potent endogenous opioids, including the enkephalins, dynorphins, and neoendorphins. These opioid precursors are produced in many parts of the brain, including various hypothalamic nuclei. Dynorphin often colocalizes with vasopressin in neurons.

The pituitary is the richest site of endorphin. ACTH- and endorphin-containing cells are found in the anteromedial region of the anterior lobe, at the posterior boundary of the anterior lobe, and in nerve fibers of the posterior lobe. The limbic system contains substantial quantities of immunoreactive endorphin, suggesting a role in memory, learning, and emotion.

Neurons containing the enkephalins are widely distributed in the central nervous system. Levels are particularly high in the dorsal horn of the spinal cord, a region that contains opiate receptors and is involved in the transmission of pain (see Chap. 12). Enkephalins may act at this location to inhibit pain transmission by sensory nerves. Euphoria produced by morphine may be related to enkephalin production in the locus coeruleus. Enkephalin concentrations are higher in the myenteric plexus of the longitudinal muscles of the gastrointestinal tract than in the brain. Enkephalin is released together with epinephrine and norepinephrine as part of the sympathetic response to stress and in patients with pheochromocytoma.

Two approaches have been employed to define the physiologic role of the endogenous opiates: assessment of the effects of administration of morphine or endogeneous opiate peptides and study of the effects of antagonists. Five opiate receptor types have been identified, making it difficult to draw general conclusions from the use of antagonists. Naloxone blocks the effects of endogenously secreted opiates on mu and epsilon receptors, revealing a tonic or physiologic role of opiate peptides. Endogenous opioids and exogenous opiates stimulate the release of GH and prolactin and inhibit the release of TSH and gonadotropin. Hence, amenorrhea is common in narcotic addicts. Opiates decrease the function of the pituitary-adrenal axis. Naloxone may prevent the stress-mediated rise in prolactin, stimulates LH and FSH release, and may reinitiate menses in some patients with hypothalamic amenorrhea. ACTH and cortisol are elevated only after high doses of naloxone. Naloxone may inhibit vasopressin release in some patients with the syndrome of inappropriate vasopressin secretion (SIADH).

Physiologic actions for these hormones may include (1) morphine-like analgesic properties, (2) euphoria and other behavioral effects, and (3) neurotransmitter and neuromodulator functions. The peptides may play a role in memory, learning, response to stress, reproduction, pain transmission, and regulation of appetite, temperature, and respiration. In addition, the placebo response, acupuncture-mediated analgesia, stress-induced amenorrhea, and the pathogenesis of shock may be mediated in part by enkephalins and the endorphins. Tranquilization, irritability, agitation, violent behavior, catalepsy, narcolepsy, catatonia, the smoking habit, alcoholism, and drug addiction may all be due to biochemical abnormalities of this system.

DISEASES OF THE HYPOTHALAMUS AND PITUITARY

Diseases that affect the hypothalamus and pituitary can have both endocrine and nonendocrine manifestations.

HYPOTHALAMUS The human hypothalamus weighs about 4 g; hypothalamic dysfunction occurs only when disease is bilateral. Tumors in this region are often slow-growing and may achieve large size before symptoms appear. Signs of hydrocephalus due to third ventricle obstruction may coexist with hypopituitarism and hypothalamic dysfunction. Neurologic symptoms and signs may be caused by compression of the optic nerve, chiasm, or tract. Large tumors may affect frontal or temporal lobe function.

Nonendocrine functions of the hypothalamus include the following:

1. *Food intake and feeding behavior.* The basal hypothalamus controls maintenance of a stable weight. Several regions of the hypothalamus are implicated in hunger and satiety. The ventromedial nucleus is thought to be involved in satiety, and there is a hunger center in the lateral hypothalamus. Stimulation of appetite and termination of food ingestion are affected by many neuropeptides and neurotransmitters. Appetite is stimulated by γ-aminobutyric acid (GABA), dopamine, β-endorphin, enkephalin, and neuropeptide Y; appetite is inhibited by serotonin, norepinephrine, cholecystokinin, neurotensin, TRH, bombesin, naloxone, somatostatin, and VIP. Hypothalamic obesity in humans is usually associated with lesions in the vicinity of the ventromedial nucleus; this obesity appears to involve a resetting of the weight set-point. With lesions in this area, aggressive behavior and marked hyperphagia (possibly related to rapid gastric emptying) occur until the new weight set-point is reached, at which time patients often demonstrate decreased activity and finicky eating. Animal models of obesity include the *ob/ob* mouse, in which deficiency of leptin prevents satiety, and the *db/db* mouse, in which the leptin receptor is deficient. Other factors, including thyroid and adrenal hormones, also influence feeding behavior. Acute hypothalamic damage often causes hyperglycemia, whereas chronic damage may rarely cause hypoglycemia.

2. *Temperature regulation.* The anterior hypothalamus contains warm- and cold-sensitive neurons that respond to local and environmental thermal gradients (see Chaps. 17 and 19). Serotonin released in this area stimulates hypothalamic heat production, an effect blocked by norepinephrine and epinephrine. The posterior hypothalamus, in response to input from the anterior hypothalamus, conserves heat by inducing shivering and vasoconstriction and controls heat dissipation by inducing vasodilation and sweating. Acetylcholine injection in this region results in hypothermia. The temperature increase associated with infections is generated by the hypothalamus. Phagocytic cells throughout the body produce a number of pyrogenic cytokines (including interleukin 1 and tumor necrosis factor) which stimulate the anterior hypothalamus to produce prostaglandin E_2. Prostaglandin E_2 raises the thermostat set point, leading to heat conservation and increased heat production until blood and core temperatures match the new hypothalamic set point.

Abnormalities of temperature regulation may occur with hypothalamic disease. Poikilothermia (a change in body temperature of >1°C with change in enviromental temperature) is usually due to large posterior hypothalamic lesions. Hypothermia is a rare consequence of diffuse hypothalamic disease (see Chap. 19). Paroxysmal hypothermia due to sweating and vasodilation is accompanied by fatigue, decreased alertness, hypoventilation, and arrhythmias. This rare syndrome may be associated with agenesis of the corpus callosum; the therapeutic response to anticonvulsants, clonidine, and cyproheptadine is variable. Severe, acute hyperthermia may accompany acute pathologic processes such as hemorrhage into the third ventricle, hypothalamic surgery, or hypothalamic infarction. Such fever rarely lasts longer than 2 weeks. Paroxysmal hyperthermia with episodic shaking chills, spiking fevers, and autonomic phenomena is uncommon but may respond to anticonvulsants. It is important to remember that adrenal insufficiency can cause fever or hypothermia and that hypothyroidism can cause hypothermia.

3. *Sleep-wake cycle.* Lesions in the sleep center of the anterior hypothalamus result in insomnia and agitation, as in some patients with encephalitis. The posterior hypothalamus is important for arousal and maintenance of the waking state; posterior hypothalamic destruction due to ischemia, encephalitis, or trauma can result in a hypersomnolent state from which arousal is possible. Larger lesions extending to the reticular formation of the rostral midbrain cause coma (see Chap. 24).

4. *Memory and behavior.* Lesions of the ventromedial hypothalamus and premammillary region result in loss of short-term memory, often with Korsakoff's syndrome. However, dorsomedial thalamic lesions correlate best with memory loss (see Chap. 380). Longer-term memory is often intact. Large hypothalamic lesions also may cause symptoms and signs of dementia. The role of ACTH, ACTH fragments, vasopressin, and oxytocin in memory integration is under investigation. Rage reactions may result with ventromedial lesions, and lateral hypothalamic destruction may cause an apathetic state.

5. *Thirst.* The hypothalamus is the center for vasopressin production and for the control of thirst by serum osmolality. Impaired thirst may occur with hypothalamic lesions; rarely, primary polydipsia without diabetes insipidus is a consequence of hypothalamic lesions (see Chap. 330).

6. *Autonomic nervous system function.* Parasympathetic outputs are organized in the anterior hypothalamus; sympathetic pathways in the posterior hypothalamus. Subarachnoid hemorrhage may cause hypotension, bradycardia, electrocardiographic abnormalities and myocardial necrosis; the latter changes may be prevented by sympathetic blockade. Diencephalic epilepsy is a rare syndrome associated with paroxysms of autonomic hyperactivity. This syndrome is not clearly epileptic in nature and does not usually respond to anticonvulsants. The clinical picture may mimic that of pheochromocytoma.

A diencephalic syndrome in children, characterized by emaciation, hyperkinesis, and inappropriate affect, often with a cheerful disposition, is usually caused by gliomas of the anterior hypothalamus. Most of these children die by the age of 2 years, but in those who survive, the clinical picture changes to one of increased appetite with obesity, irritability, and rage reactions.

In general, slow-growing tumors produce dementia, disturbances of food intake (obesity or emaciation), and endocrine dysfunction. Acute destructive processes are more likely to cause coma or disturbances of the autonomic nervous system.

Diseases of the anterior hypothalamus include craniopharyngiomas, gliomas of the optic nerve, sphenoid ridge meningiomas, granulomatous disease (including sarcoidosis), germinomas, and aneurysms of the internal carotid artery. Suprasellar pituitary adenomas and tuberculum sella meningiomas may grow into the hypothalamus as well. Lesions of the posterior hypothalamus include gliomas, hamartomas, ependymomas, germinomas, and teratomas.

Precocious puberty, particularly in males, can be associated with "pinealomas." However, these tumors actually are germinomas, and the precocious puberty appears to result from the ectopic production of hCG by the tumors rather than from an effect on pituitary gonadotropins.

Craniopharyngiomas Craniopharyngiomas arise from remnants of Rathke's pouch and constitute 3 to 5 percent of all intracranial neoplasms. Most of these tumors are suprasellar, but about 15 percent are intrasellar. The tumors are usually cystic or partially cystic, often contain calcium, and are lined with stratified squamous epithelium. Although craniopharyngiomas are usually manifested in childhood,

45 percent of patients are over age 20, and 20 percent are over age 40 at the time of diagnosis.

Children usually present with signs of increased intracranial pressure due to hydrocephalus (80 percent), including headache, vomiting, and papilledema. Visual abnormalities such as loss of vision and field cuts occur in 60 percent. Short stature is found in 7 to 40 percent, and retarded bone age is even more common. Delayed sexual development occurs in about 20 percent, and diabetes insipidus may be present.

About 80 percent of adults present with visual complaints, and an additional 10 percent have visual abnormalities on careful testing. Papilledema is present in about 15 percent of adults. Headaches (40 percent), mental deterioration or personality change (26 percent), and hypogonadism (35 percent) are relatively common. Hyperprolactinemia is present in one-third to one-half of patients, but prolactin levels rarely exceed 100 to 150 μg/L. Diabetes insipidus (15 percent), weight gain (15 percent), and panhypopituitarism (7 percent) may occur as well. Rarely, the cyst contents spill into the cerebrospinal fluid, causing aseptic meningitis, and an inflammatory hypophysitis may occur when craniopharyngiomas extend into the sella. Craniopharyngiomas may enlarge and become symptomatic during pregnancy.

Suprasellar calcification (see Fig. 328-15) in a flocculent, granular, or curvilinear pattern is present on skull x-rays in most children and in some adults with craniopharyngioma. Calcification is evident on CT in most of these adults, however. Hypothalamic germinomas may calcify as well. Skull x-ray abnormalities include calcification, sellar enlargement, and signs of increased intracranial pressure in 90 percent of children and 60 percent of adults.

Therapy of craniopharyngiomas is often unsatisfactory. Total removal often results in major functional deficits. We generally favor biopsy and partial resection followed by conventional radiation therapy as a more conservative approach. Tumors less than 3 cm in diameter have a better prognosis.

Germ Cell Tumors Germinomas originate in the posterior third ventricle, in the anterior third ventricle (supra- or intrasellar), or in both locations (see also Chap. 98). Germinomas (also known as *atypical teratomas*) were previously confused with parenchymal tumors of the pineal (pinealomas); when located in the anterior third ventricle, they were known as "ectopic pinealomas." Germinomas often infiltrate the hypothalamus and occasionally metastasize to the cerebrospinal fluid or distant sites.

Most patients have diabetes insipidus and variable anterior pituitary insufficiency. Precocious puberty in boys is probably due to hCG production by these tumors. Diplopia, headache, vomiting, lethargy, weight loss, and hydrocephalus are common. The tumors begin in childhood but may be diagnosed in young adults. Because germinomas are radiosensitive, early recognition is important. Germinomas of the nonseminoma type may produce hCG and/or alpha fetoprotein, whereas pure seminomas rarely produce tumor markers (see Chap. 375). Elevated cerebrospinal fluid levels of hCG or alpha fetoprotein are virtually diagnostic; when elevated, a biopsy is generally unnecessary. When tumor markers are absent, a biopsy should be considered. When the tumor is located in the anterior third ventricle, biopsy by the transsphenoidal route is often possible. Tumors in the pineal region are more difficult to biopsy, leading some authors to recommend empirical radiation therapy or chemotherapy, whereas others prefer surgical biopsy or debulking followed by radiation and chemotherapy (see Chap. 375).

PITUITARY ADENOMAS Pituitary adenomas account for about 10 to 15 percent of intracranial neoplasms. They can cause either excess or deficiency of anterior pituitary hormones or structural problems related to invasion of surrounding structures. Small pituitary tumors are present in 6 to 24 percent of adults at autopsy. These incidental pituitary tumors (pituitary "incidentalomas") are recognized with increasing frequency now that cranial MRI and CT scans are commonly performed. Pituitary adenomas are monoclonal in origin. The mechanisms of tumorigenesis are unknown except for G protein mutations in some somatotroph adenomas and rare *ras* mutations in invasive pituitary adenomas.

Pathology Pituitary tumors were previously classified as basophilic, acidophilic, or chromophobic on the basis of hematoxylin and eosin staining. Corticotroph adenomas are generally basophilic; the more densely granulated prolactin-secreting tumors are acidophilic; the majority of prolactinomas, sparsely granulated GH-secreting tumors, TSH-secreting and gonadotropin-secreting tumors, and nonsecreting tumors are chromophobic. Because this classification provides little insight into hormone production, it has been abandoned. Many nonfunctioning pituitary tumors, however, are still referred to as "chromophobes." The current classification is based on immunohistochemical staining: corticotroph (ACTH and POMC), somatotroph (GH), thyrotroph (TSH), gonadotroph (LH, FSH, and their subunits), lactotroph (prolactin), and null cell.

Pituitary tumors have also been classified by Kovacs and Horvath according to size and invasive characteristics: Microadenomas are <10 mm, and macroadenomas are ≥10 mm in greatest diameter. Microadenomas may cause hormone overproduction but do not cause hypopituitarism, structural problems, or sellar enlargement. Intrapituitary adenomas are contained within the substance of the pituitary gland; intrasellar adenomas are confined to the sella. Diffuse adenomas may fill the sella and cause focal sellar wall erosions and be difficult to distinguish from intrasellar adenomas. Invasive adenomas erode through the sella into surrounding tissues, including but not limited to the sphenoid bone, cavernous sinuses, optic chiasm, third ventricle, and brain. Pituitary carcinomas are rare and are diagnosed when distant metastases are present.

Endocrine Manifestations Anterior pituitary hormone overproduction is suspected on clinical grounds and confirmed by appropriate laboratory evaluation (see Table 328-5). The most common secretory pituitary tumors are prolactinomas. They cause galactorrhea and hypogonadism, including amenorrhea, infertility, and impotence. GH-secreting tumors cause acromegaly or gigantism. Corticotroph adenomas cause cortisol excess (Cushing's disease). Although glycoprotein hormone–secreting pituitary adenomas are the second most common type, clinical syndromes of excess LH, FSH, or TSH are rare. Most patients with gonadotropin-secreting adenomas have clinically nonfunctioning tumors with hypogonadism, although testicular enlargement or testosterone excess may occur. TSH-secreting adenomas are a rare cause of hyperthyroidism.

About 15 percent of patients with tumors that come to surgery have adenomas that secrete more than one pituitary hormone. The most common combination is GH and prolactin, and other common patterns are GH-TSH, GH-prolactin-TSH, and ACTH-prolactin. Most of these tumors have one type of cell that secretes two hormones (unimorphous), but some tumors have two or more cell types, each producing a single hormone (polymorphous).

Prolactinomas in women and corticotroph adenomas in both sexes are usually microadenomas. In contrast, most patients with acromegaly and most men with prolactinomas have macroadenomas at diagnosis. Glycoprotein hormone–secreting tumors are also usually large at the time of diagnosis.

About 30 to 40 percent of pituitary adenomas that come to surgery are apparently nonsecretory, although most stain immunohistochemically for pituitary hormones. These statistics are influenced by the fact that most prolactinomas do not require surgery. In some cases, particularly with gonadotropin-secreting tumors, hormone secretion is overlooked. Some "nonfunctioning" pituitary tumors, as well as some functional ones, secrete part of the glycoprotein hormone molecule, most commonly the α subunit. An α subunit excess is a frequent finding in patients with TSH-secreting adenomas, and FSH α and β may be hypersecreted in patients with gonadotropin-secreting tumors.

Null cell tumors (no specific hormones identified by immunostaining) also are generally large when diagnosed, since no hormonal overproduction provides early clues to diagnosis. As with the glycoprotein-secreting tumors that are also clinically nonfunctioning, the presenting features usually relate to mass effects. Oncocytomas are nonsecretory pituitary adenomas with abundant mitochondria, commonly found in older men.

Pituitary adenomas are occasionally part of the MEN 1 syndrome (see Chap. 340). This dominantly inherited disease causes adenomas of the pituitary gland, secretory tumors of the endocrine pancreas, and hyperparathyroidism involving multiple parathyroid glands. Pituitary adenomas may be of any cell type. Insulinomas and gastrinomas are the most common pancreatic tumors in MEN-1. Pancreatic GHRH-secreting tumors can cause acromegaly and pituitary hyperplasia.

Mass Effects of Pituitary Tumors *Visual field defects* The optic chiasm lies anterior and superior to the pituitary, usually 8 to 13 mm above the diaphragma sella. In 80 percent of normal persons the chiasm overlies the pituitary fossa, in about 15 percent it is anterior to the tuberculum sella (prefixed), and in 5 percent it overlaps the dorsum sella posteriorly (postfixed). Since 90 percent of chiasmal axons originate in the macula, central vision is lost early. Foggy or dim vision is also described by many patients.

The most common visual field defect with pituitary adenomas is a bitemporal hemianopsia; about 8 percent of patients develop complete loss of vision in one eye and have a temporal defect in the other eye. Alternatively, patients may have bitemporal scotomas rather than hemianopsia, particularly with a rapidly growing lesion in a patient with a prefixed chiasm. For this reason, visual field examinations must assess more than the lateral fields of vision. Of those patients with visual field defects, about 9 percent have a single eye defect, most commonly a superior temporal defect. Occasionally, there is a monocular field loss, such as a central scotoma, that mimics a nonpituitary lesion. Pituitary adenomas causing visual field defects are macroadenomas with sellar enlargement and suprasellar extension.

Oculomotor palsies Pituitary adenomas may extend laterally, invade the cavernous sinuses, and cause oculomotor palsies. When this occurs, visual field defects are usually not present. Involvement of the third cranial nerve is most common and may mimic diabetic third nerve neuropathy in that pupillary reactivity is usually preserved. Additional findings with lateral extension of the adenoma may include involvement of the fourth and sixth cranial nerves, pain or numbness in the distribution of the fifth cranial nerve, and compression or obstruction of the carotid artery.

Headaches are common with larger tumors and are present in most patients with acromegaly. Headaches may be exacerbated by coughing. Headaches are thought to be due to stretching of the diaphragma sella but may be vascular in origin and can be referred to several locations, including the vertex of the skull and retroorbital, frontooccipital, frontotemporal, or occipital-cervical areas.

Very large pituitary tumors may invade the hypothalamus and cause hyperphagia, abnormal temperature regulation, loss of consciousness, and loss of hormonal input from the hypothalamus. Obstructive hydrocephalus that involves the third ventricle or causes diabetes insipidus is less common with pituitary adenomas than with craniopharyngiomas and other extrapituitary masses. Tumor invasion

Table 328-5

Pituitary Hormone Evaluation

Hormone	Excess	Deficiency

Growth hormone	A. Measurement of plasma growth hormone 1 h after glucose PO
	B. Measurement of IGF-I
		A. Measurement of plasma growth hormone 30, 60, and 120 min after one of the following:
		  1. Regular insulin 0.1 to 0.15 unit/kg IV
		  2. Levodopa 10 mg/kg PO
		  3. L-Arginine 0.5 mg/kg intravenously over 30 min
		B. Measurement of IGF-I

Prolactin	A. Measurement of basal serum prolactin, preferably fasting	A. Measurement of serum prolactin 10 to 20 min after one of the following:
		  1. TRH 200 to 500 μg IV
		  2. Chlorpromazine 25 mg IM

TSH	A. Measurement of T_4, free T_4 index, T_3, TSH, TSH α	A. Measurement of T_4, free T_4 index, TSH
Gonadotropins	A. Measurement of FSH, LH, LH β, testosterone, FSH β, FSH response to TRH	A. Measurement of basal LH, FSH in postmenopausal women; no measurements in menstruating, ovulating women B. Testosterone, FSH, and LH in men

ACTH	A. Measurement of urine free cortisol*
	B. Dexamethasone suppression by one of the following:
	  1. Measurement of 8 A.M. plasma cortisol after administration of 1 mg dexamethasone at midnight
	  2. Measurement of 8 A.M. plasma cortisol or 24-h urine 17-hydroxysteroids or free cortisol after 0.5 mg dexamethasone PO q 6 h for 8 doses
	C. High-dose dexamethasone suppression by one of the following:
	  1. Measurement of plasma cortisol after 8 mg dexamethasone PO at midnight
	  2. Measurement of 8 A.M. plasma cortisol or 24-h urine 17-hydroxysteroids or free cortisol after 2 mg dexamethasone q 6 h for 8 doses
	D. Metyrapone response (same protocol as for deficiency testing)†
	E. Response of plasma ACTH and cortisol to ovine corticotropin releasing hormone (1 μg/kg body wt)
		A. Measurement of serum cortisol at 30 and 60 min after regular insulin 0.05 to 0.15 units per kilogram IV
		B. Metyrapone response by one of the following:
		  1. Measurement of plasma 11-deoxycortisol at 8 A.M. after 30 mg/kg body wt metyrapone at midnight (maximal dose 2 g)†
		  2. Measurement of 24-h urinary 17-hydroxycorticoids or plasma 11-deoxycortisol day of and day after 750 mg metyrapone q 4 h for 6 doses†
		  3. Measurement of 24-h urinary 17-hydroxycorticoids day of and day after 500 mg metyrapone q 2 h for 12 doses†
		C. ACTH stimulation test: Measurement of plasma cortisol and aldosterone at 0, 30, and 60 min after IM or IV administration of 0.25 mg cosyntropin
		D. ?Response of plasma ACTH and cortisol to ovine corticotropin-releasing hormone (1 μg/kg body weight)

Arginine vasopressin (AVP)	A. Measurement of serum sodium and osmolality, urine osmolality in presence of normal renal, adrenal, thyroid function B. Simultaneous measurement of serum osmolality and ADH levels	A. Comparison of urine osmolality and serum osmolality under conditions of increased AVP secretion‡ B. Simultaneous measurement of serum osmolality and AVP levels

* Tests 1 and 2 establish the diagnosis of Cushing's syndrome. Tests 3, 4, and 5 localize the Cushing's disease to the pituitary gland. Often bilateral inferior petrosal sinus catheterization will be necessary.
† Give food with metyrapone.
‡ May be achieved by water deprivation or saline administration.

of the temporal lobe may cause complex partial seizures; invasion of the posterior fossa may be associated with brainstem dysfunction; and invasion into the frontal lobes causes alterations in mental state and frontal release signs.

Pituitary apoplexy   Acute hemorrhagic infarction of a pituitary adenoma may cause a dramatic syndrome including severe headache, nausea, vomiting, and depression of consciousness. Ophthalmoplegia, visual and pupillary disturbances, and meningismus may be present. Most of these symptoms are caused by direct pressure from the tumor, whereas meningismus results from blood in the cerebrospinal fluid. The syndrome may either evolve slowly over a period of 24 to 48 h or may lead to sudden death.

Pituitary apoplexy occurs most commonly in patients with somatotroph or corticotroph adenomas, but it may be the first clinical manifestation of a pituitary tumor; the diagnosis is often missed initially. Both anticoagulation and radiotherapy predispose to hemorrhagic infarction. Rarely, pituitary apoplexy produces "autohypophysectomy" with "cure" of acromegaly, Cushing's disease, or hyperprolactinemia. Hypopituitarism is a common sequela; although hormonal measurements may be normal acutely, cortisol deficiency can develop rapidly. Some of the morbidity and mortality with pituitary apoplexy is due to failure to recognize and treat acute adrenal insufficiency. Gonadal steroid levels decline over days, and thyroxine concentrations fall over weeks. Diabetes insipidus is rare.

It is important to differentiate between pituitary apoplexy and a leaking aneurysm; MRI may allow this distinction to be made, but angiography may be necessary. Acute pituitary apoplexy is usually a neurosurgical emergency and often requires acute decompression of the pituitary, generally via the transsphenoidal route. Many pituitary tumors contain small hemorrhagic foci that are clinically silent.

℞ TREATMENT

Ideal therapy for pituitary adenomas permanently corrects hormonal hypersecretion without causing hypopituitarism and shrinks or removes the tumor mass without morbidity or mortality. Therapy for microadenomas may achieve both these goals, whereas therapy for macroadenomas is usually less successful. In considering therapy, it is critical to weigh the disability caused by the tumor against the disability that could arise from the treatment. Regardless of tumor size, the therapy should not be worse than the disease. Potentially serious diseases such as Cushing's disease or acromegaly may require more aggressive treatment than do prolactinomas. (See also the sections on individual pituitary hormones in this chapter.)

Medical Treatment   Bromocriptine, a dopamine agonist, is the therapy of choice in the United States for most patients with microprolactinomas who require therapy. Bromocriptine corrects hyperprolactinemia in most patients with microprolactinomas; however, when the drug is stopped, prolactin levels often return to pretreatment levels. More potent dopamine agonists are available outside the United States. Cabergoline, a dopamine agonist administered once or twice weekly, is under investigation in the United States.

The side effects of nausea, gastric irritation, and postural hypotension produced by bromocriptine can be minimized by initially giving a low dose (0.625 to 1.25 mg) at bedtime with a snack. Other side effects include headache, fatigue, abdominal cramps, nasal congestion, and constipation. The dosage is gradually increased to a twice-daily schedule (most commonly 2.5 mg bid) until prolactin levels and/or symptoms return to normal. In some patients, control can be achieved with a single bedtime dose. Vaginal administration of bromocriptine is better tolerated by some patients.

Bromocriptine is also effective for large prolactin-secreting macroadenomas. (Nonfunctioning macroadenomas causing minimal prolactin elevation must be excluded.) The prolactin level is lowered by at least 80 percent in 90 percent of patients, and normal values are achieved in about 40 percent of patients. Abnormal visual fields return to normal in most patients; the tumor shrinks by 50 percent in about 40 percent of patients within 3 months. Tumor shrinkage may be accompanied by reversal of hypopituitarism. With giant adenomas, bromocriptine-induced tumor shrinkage rarely causes a

devastating intracranial hemorrhage or a cerebrospinal fluid leak. Prolactin levels quickly rise when bromocriptine is stopped; however, tumor regrowth may be delayed.

Surgery is required when visual field defects do not rapidly return to normal (e.g., after 1 to 3 months of bromocriptine). Symptomatic hyperprolactinemia with an inadequate response to bromocriptine requires further therapy with surgery and/or radiation. Additional indications for surgery include patients with cystic or hemorrhagic tumors and patients who require neuroleptic agents (bromocriptine may counteract the effectiveness of such drugs). In the United States, bromocriptine is usually stopped at the onset of pregnancy and reinstituted if tumor regrowth is symptomatic; alternatively, bromocriptine can be continued throughout pregnancy, although it is not licensed for this indication in the United States.

The somatostatin analogue octreotide is the most effective adjunctive therapy in acromegaly. IGF-I levels return to normal in more than half of treated patients. Bromocriptine is an effective adjunct in some patients with acromegaly, particularly those with coexisting hyperprolactinemia. GH and IGF-I levels rarely return to normal, but symptomatic improvement and tumor shrinkage may occur. While less effective bromocriptine is often tried in patients with persistent acromegaly after transsphenoidal surgery because it can be taken by mouth. Bromocriptine or octreotide can also be given to acromegalic subjects while waiting for radiation treatment to take effect. Octreotide also may be a useful adjunctive agent in patients with TSH-secreting adenomas. Nonfunctioning and gonadotropin-secreting adenomas usually shrink by 10 percent or less in response to high doses of octreotide or bromocriptine; the one instance in which medical therapy may be effective for these tumors may be tumors that secrete the α subunit.

Surgery   Transsphenoidal surgery of pituitary microadenomas is safe and frequently corrects hormonal oversecretion. Hormonal overproduction is corrected within 24 h in over 75 percent of patients with Cushing's disease due to corticotroph microadenomas, acromegaly with GH levels of <40 μg/L, and microprolactinomas with serum prolactin levels of <200 μg/L. The surgical cure rate depends on the experience and skill of the neurosurgeon. Transsphenoidal surgery is the treatment of choice for Cushing's disease with high cure rates in many centers; when Cushing's disease is not cured by an initial operation, a second operation has a 75 percent cure rate. If the second operation is unsuccessful, additional options include bilateral adrenalectomy, radiation therapy, and/or medical therapy. Surgery is also the first line of therapy for acromegaly. The initial success rate for microprolactinomas varies among institutions from 50 to 95 percent. Unfortunately, after initially successful surgery, hyperprolactinemia recurs in about 17 percent of patients followed for 3 to 5 years, and possibly in 50 percent after 5 to 10 years. The recurrence rates after initially successful surgery in acromegaly and Cushing's disease are not well established.

We treat most patients with microadenomas with bromocriptine but recommend surgery for those patients who are intolerant of dopamine agonists. Surgery does not generally result in hypopituitarism. Surgery is also our treatment of choice in acromegaly and in Cushing's disease.

The mortality rate for transsphenoidal surgery of microadenomas is 0.27 percent, and the morbidity rate is about 1.7 percent. Major complications include cerebrospinal fluid rhinorrhea, oculomotor palsy, and visual loss.

Pituitary surgery is less successful at correcting hormonal hypersecretion with larger secretory tumors. In patients with serum prolactin levels of >200 μg/L, the levels return to normal in only 30 percent, and recurrence rates may be as high as 80 percent. These patients should be treated with a dopamine agonist. Surgery is successful in 40 to 60 percent of patients with Cushing's disease due to macroadenoma and 30 percent of acromegalics with GH levels of >40 μg/L. Whether pretreatment of patients with acromegaly due to invasive macroadenomas with octreotide improves the outcome is under study.

Patients with nonfunctioning macroadenomas require surgery if the tumor is symptomatic, is located near the optic chiasm, or is continuing to grow. In such cases the goal may be decompression of adjacent structures regardless of whether complete tumor resection is possible.

Although visual field abnormalities are usually reversible with surgery for macroadenomas, cure of the tumor is less likely than with microadenomas. The intrasellar portion of tumors invading the cavernous sinus may be debulked, but parasellar extension remains. Early series noted an 85 percent recurrence of symptoms (due to structural problems such as visual field defects) over 10 years in patients treated with surgery alone. When radiation therapy was used in combination with surgery, the 10-year recurrence rate was 15 percent. These series antedated modern radiologic techniques, hormone measurements, and medical therapy. Recurrence rates are now much lower, and in some patients with late recurrence a second operation may be successful.

Surgery for macroadenomas has a mortality rate of around 0.86 percent and a morbidity rate of about 6.3 percent. Hypopituitarism occurs in about 10 percent of patients, transient diabetes insipidus occurs in about 5 percent, and permanent diabetes insipidus occurs in 1 percent. Other complications of surgery for macroadenoma include cerebrospinal fluid rhinorrhea (3.3 percent), permanent visual loss (1.5 percent), permanent oculomotor palsy (0.6 percent), and meningitis (0.5 percent).

Radiation Conventional radiation therapy is effective in preventing tumor growth (70 to 90 percent) but is unsatisfactory in the acute management of pituitary hyperfunction. Therapy generally consists of 4500 cGy (4500 rad) at 1.8 Gy (180 rad) per day over 5 weeks using rotational techniques. GH values of <5 μg/L are achieved in half of acromegalics after 5 years and in 70 percent after 10 years; values of <2.5 μg/L are achieved in 40 percent, and values of <1 μg/L are achieved in only 20 percent by 10 to 15 years. Data on IGF-I are not readily available. Conventional radiation therapy alone is rarely successful in treating corticotroph adenomas in adults. The major complications of conventional radiation treatment are hypopituitarism in up to 50 percent of patients and post-therapy lassitude and fatigue lasting many months in the majority. Whether subtle cognitive defects occur is less certain. We generally use radiation treatment as an adjunct to surgery and medical therapy for patients with continued symptomatic hormonal oversecretion and for those with substantial residual tumor after surgery or when tumor regrowth is rapid. Slow tumor regrowth over 5 or 6 years is usually treated with repeat surgery.

The "gamma knife" delivers 4000 to 10,000 cGy (4000 to 10,000 rad) through several hundred portals in a single session, a dose thought to be equivalent to two to three times the total dose given by conventional radiation treatment. Preliminary results using 4000 to 7000 cGy for acromegaly are comparable to those achieved with conventional radiation treatment. Therapy for Cushing's disease with 7000 to 10,000 cGy is apparently successful in up to 75 percent of adults; this rate is comparable to that achieved with heavy-particle therapy (see below) and apparently represents a better result than achieved with conventional radiation therapy.

Heavy-particle therapy with proton beam or alpha particles is effective in treating secretory adenomas, but response is slow. Tumors with suprasellar extension or tissue invasion are generally excluded from such series. With proton beam therapy at the Harvard cyclotron, radiation doses of up to 14,000 cGy (14,000 rad) can be given safely without damage to surrounding structures. At 2 years, 28 percent of acromegalics achieve GH values of <5 μg/L; this response rate increases to 56 percent at 5 years and to 75 percent by 10 years. Values of IGF-I are not reported. With Cushing's disease proton beam irradiation corrects the hypercortisolism in 55

percent of patients at 2 years and in 80 percent by 5 years. Proton beam therapy effectively lowers ACTH and stops the growth of most corticotroph adenomas in patients with Nelson's syndrome, with the exception of adenomas that are invasive at the time of therapy. Long-term results for treatment of other tumors with proton beam therapy are not available.

Complications of heavy-particle therapy include hypopituitarism in at least 20 percent of patients, although the exact long-term prevalence of this complication is uncertain. Visual field defects and oculomotor dysfunction, usually temporary, have been reported in about 1.5 percent of patients. The major drawback of all forms of radiotherapy is the long delay before hormonal hypersecretion is corrected. Rare complications include malignancies in the radiation field, damage to the visual apparatus, cognitive impairment, and brain necrosis. Radiotherapy is an effective alternative to surgery in patients with acromegaly, Cushing's disease, or large intrasellar nonfunctioning tumors who have contraindications to or refuse surgery.

Pituitary adenomas may be discovered during MRI or CT scanning of the brain for other purposes (pituitary "incidentaloma"). With pituitary microadenomas, hormonal overproduction must be identified and treated; hypopituitarism and structural symptoms do not occur. If no hormone abnormalities are found in a patient with an incidentally discovered microadenoma, long-term monitoring for tumor growth is necessary. A follow-up scan at 6 months, then one yearly for 2 years, and subsequently one every 2 to 5 years seems reasonable.

Pituitary macroadenomas, however discovered, need to be evaluated for hormonal over- and underproduction and for mass effects, including visual field abnormalities. The approach to the hormonally active tumor has been described above. Should nonfunctioning tumors be treated with bromocriptine? Is prophylactic surgery or radiation therapy indicated? How often should the MRI and endocrine evaluations be repeated? The answers are unknown. We tend to recommend surgery for tumors directly abutting the optic chiasm. For other tumors, MRI scans should be repeated at 6 and 12 months and yearly thereafter. If growth occurs, surgery or radiation treatment with conventional radiation, the gamma knife, or protons may be indicated. Ten to fifteen percent of tumors shrink with bromocriptine therapy; how many stabilize without therapy is unknown.

HYPOPITUITARISM *Hypopituitarism* refers to deficiency of one or more pituitary hormones and has many causes (Table 328-6). Pituitary hormone deficiency may be congenital or acquired (see Chap. 329). Isolated GH or gonadotropin deficiency is common. Temporary ACTH deficiency as a consequence of long-term glucocorticoid therapy is also common, but permanent isolated deficiency of ACTH or TSH is rare. Deficiency of any of the anterior pituitary hormones may occur at the level of the pituitary gland or the hypothalamus. Mutations in Pit-1, a pituitary-specific transcription factor, cause a combined deficiency of GH, prolactin, and TSH. When diabetes insipidus is present, the primary defect is almost invariably in the hypothalamus or high in pituitary stalk; the diabetes insipidus often is accompanied by mild hyperprolactinemia and anterior pituitary hypofunction.

The manifestations of hypopituitarism depend on the specific pituitary hormones that are lacking. Growth failure due to GH deficiency is a common presenting complaint in children. GH deficiency in adults causes more subtle manifestations, such as fine wrinkling around the eyes and mouth and, in subjects with diabetes mellitus, increased sensitivity to insulin. Subcutaneous fat may be increased, and muscle mass is decreased. The mortality of GH-deficient individuals from cardiovascular disease is increased. Symptoms of gonadotropin deficiency include amenorrhea and infertility in women and testosterone deficiency and decreased libido, decreased beard and body hair, and preservation of a youthful scalp hairline in men. TSH deficiency causes hypothyroidism with fatigue, cold intolerance, and puffy skin in the absence of goiter. ACTH deficiency results in cortisol deficiency, manifested by fatigue; decreased appetite; weight loss; decreased skin and nipple pigmentation; an abnormal response to stress characterized

Table 328-6

CHAPTER 328
Neuroendocrine Regulation

1993

Causes of Hypopituitarism

Isolated hormone deficiencies
   Congenital or acquired deficiencies including mutations in Pit-1
Tumors
   Large pituitary adenomas
   Pituitary apoplexy
   Hypothalamic tumors, e.g., craniopharyngiomas, germinomas, chordomas, meningiomas, gliomas, and others
   Metastatic carcinoma
Inflammatory diseases
   Granulomatous disease, e.g., sarcoidosis, tuberculosis, syphilis, granulomatous hypophysitis
   Eosinophilic granuloma
   Lymphocytic hypophysitis (autoimmune)
Vascular diseases
   Sheehan's postpartum necrosis
   ? Diabetic peripartum necrosis
   Carotid aneurysm
Destructive-traumatic events
   Surgery
   Stalk section
   Radiation (conventional—hypothalamus; heavy-particle—pituitary)
   Trauma
Developmental anomalies
   Pituitary aplasia
   Basal encephalocoele
Infiltration
   Hemochromatosis
   Amyloidosis
"Idiopathic" causes
   ? Autoimmune disease

by fever, hypotension, and hyponatremia; and a high mortality rate. Unlike primary adrenal insufficiency ACTH deficiency does not cause hyperpigmentation, hyperkalemia, or salt loss. With combined ACTH and gonadotropin deficiency, axillary and pubic hair may be lost. Children with combined GH and cortisol deficiency often develop hypoglycemia. Prolactin deficiency causes failure to lactate postpartum. AVP deficiency causes diabetes insipidus with polyuria and increased thirst. When pituitary adenomas impair anterior pituitary function, GH is often the first hormone to be compromised, followed by deficiencies of gonadotropins, TSH, and ACTH. Panhypopituitarism may be accompanied by inappropriate secretion of vasopressin (see Chap. 330).

Etiology Damage to the anterior pituitary can be due to a pituitary adenoma (with or without infarction), pituitary surgery or irradiation, closed head trauma, or infarction during the postpartum period (Sheehan's syndrome). Postpartum pituitary infarction occurs in the setting of hemorrhage with systemic hypotension; vasospasm is thought to mediate the pituitary destruction that ensues. The enlarged pituitary gland of pregnancy may be more vulnerable to ischemia. Inability to lactate is the most common initial clinical clue, and other symptoms of hypopituitarism may unfold over months or years. The condition is sometimes diagnosed years after the primary event. Although clinical diabetes insipidus is rare in this setting, a decreased vasopressin response to appropriate stimuli is common. Patients with diabetes mellitus are also prone to develop hypopituitarism late in pregnancy.

Lymphocytic hypophysitis that causes hypopituitarism is primarily a disease of women during pregnancy or in the postpartum period but occurs rarely in men and postmenopausal women. In this syndrome, a mass lesion is often seen on MRI or CT scanning which, when biopsied, consists of lymphocytic infiltration. Lymphocytic hypophysitis is due to autoimmune pituitary destruction and often occurs with other autoimmune diseases such as Hashimoto's (autoimmune) thyroiditis and gastric atrophy (see Chaps. 331 and 340). Circulating antibodies to lactotrophs have been identified in some patients. It is not clear whether autoimmune hypophysitis is a common cause of "idiopathic" hypopituitarism in adults.

Hypothalamic or pituitary stalk damage has many causes (Table 328-6). Certain lesions in this region, such as sarcoidosis, metastatic

carcinoma, germinomas, histiocytosis, and craniopharyngiomas, commonly cause diabetes insipidus along with hypofunction of the anterior pituitary. Necrotizing infundibular hypophysitis is a rare entity associated with necrosis of the pituitary and stalk. Pituitary insufficiency, resulting from conventional radiation treatment to the brain or pituitary, is thought to be largely hypothalamic in origin, although diabetes insipidus generally does not occur.

"Functional" hypopituitarism is common. Anorexia nervosa, severe stress, and major illness are all associated with reversible LHRH deficiency. Emotional stress in children may cause GH deficiency and cessation of growth (*psychosocial dwarfism*). Severe illness may be associated with TSH and free T_4 deficiency (part of the "euthyroid sick" syndrome). ACTH deficiency occurs after long-term suppression of the hypothalamic-pituitary-adrenal axis.

Diagnosis (See Table 328-5) To diagnose GH deficiency, the most reliable GH stimulus is insulin-induced hypoglycemia in which the blood sugar declines to less than 2.2 pmol/L (40 mg/dL) (Fig. 328-8). Other pharmacologic agents that cause a rise in GH include arginine, which decreases the inhibitory effects of somatostatin, and levodopa and clonidine, which increase endogenous GHRH levels. A GH concentration of >10 µg/L after stimulation with hypoglycemia, levodopa, or arginine effectively excludes GH deficiency; it is unclear whether a cutoff point of 5 or 7 µg/dL should be used. Measurement of the basal GH or serum IGF-I level is a less reliable indicator,

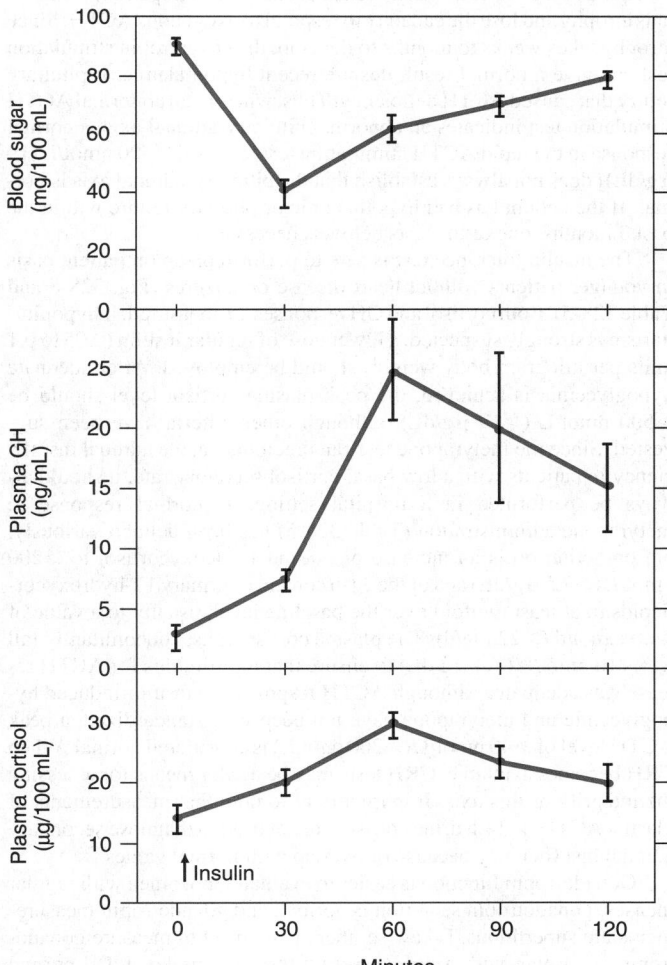

FIGURE 328-8 The insulin tolerance test. After an intravenous injection of regular insulin (0.1 unit per kilogram body weight) a fall in blood sugar and a rise in plasma GH and cortisol is expected. This test permits evaluation of both GH and ACTH in patients with pituitary disease. (*After KJ Catt, Lancet 1:933, 1970.*)

because GH levels are undetectable in normal persons for much of the day and because IGF-I levels in GH deficiency may overlap the normal range. Integrated 24-h GH secretion is low in some short children with a normal response to GH provocative stimuli. Few data are available about the best way to diagnose GH deficiency in adults; there is substantial overlap in the response to GH-provocative stimuli between normal and GH-deficient men.

ACTH deficiency results in cortisol deficiency and is potentially life-threatening. Basal cortisol function may be preserved in the face of extensive pituitary destruction; consequently, it is necessary to assess the ability of pituitary ACTH secretion to increase in response to "stress." A morning serum cortisol level of <3 μg/dL in this setting is always diagnostic of adrenal insufficiency; a level of >19 μg/dL establishes adequacy of the hypothalamic-pituitary-adrenal axis. Morning cortisol levels between these values mandate further testing. If chronic adrenal insufficiency is suspected, a rapid cosyntropin stimulation test is the best screening test. If hypothalamic or pituitary injury has occurred within a few months, an insulin tolerance test or metyrapone test is required.

The rapid ACTH stimulation test (Table 328-5) is the safest and most convenient screening test for determining the adequacy of the pituitary-adrenal axis if chronic deficiency is suspected. Although this test directly measures only the functional integrity of the adrenals, it indirectly assesses hypothalamic and pituitary function, because the adrenals depend on endogenous ACTH. When ACTH production is impaired, the adrenals atrophy and lose the capacity to respond to exogenous ACTH. Since atrophy takes weeks to months to develop, the cosyntropin stimulation test can give a normal result despite recent hypothalamic or pituitary injury that caused ACTH deficiency. Thus, whereas an abnormal ACTH stimulation test indicates an abnormal pituitary-adrenal axis, a normal response in the rapid ACTH stimulation test [cortisol >500 nmol/L (19 μg/dL)] does not always establish that the pituitary-adrenal axis is normal. If the patient has had hypothalamic or pituitary failure within the past 3 months, one of the tests below is necessary.

The insulin tolerance test is safe to perform on an outpatient basis in younger patients without heart disease or seizures (Fig. 328-8 and Table 328-5). Both cortisol and GH responses are measured. If hypopituitarism is strongly suspected, a lower dose of regular insulin (0.05 to 0.1 units per kilogram body weight) should be employed. After adequate hypoglycemia is achieved, the peak plasma cortisol level should be >500 nmol/L (>19 μg/dL), although other criteria have been suggested. Since the metyrapone test can precipitate acute adrenal insufficiency in patients with a low basal cortisol secretory rate, it should always be performed in a hospital setting. A normal response to metyrapone administration (Table 328-5) has been defined variously, but one criterion is an increase of plasma 11-deoxycortisol to >200 nmol/L (>7.5 μg/dL) and of the 24-h content of urinary 17-hydroxycorticoids to at least twofold over the baseline level, usually to a value of >60 μmol/d (>22 mg/d). The plasma cortisol must concomitantly fall to <110 nmol/L (<4 μg/dL) to ensure that the stimulus for ACTH release was adequate. Although ACTH responses to insulin-induced hypoglycemia and metyrapone have not been well standardized, a peak ACTH level of >40 pmol/L (>200 pg/mL) is considered normal. When CRH becomes available, CRH tests may be a safer means for assessing the integrity of this axis. It is important to note that measurements of plasma ACTH or 24-h urine cortisol are not used to diagnose secondary adrenal insufficiency because of overlap with normal values.

Gonadotropin function is easier to evaluate. In women with regular menses, gonadotropin secretion is normal, and gonadotropin measurements are superfluous. Likewise, there is no need to measure gonadotropins in a man with a normal serum testosterone level and normal spermatogenesis. In postmenopausal women, gonadotropin levels are elevated (the menopausal state effectively being an endogenous stimulation test); "normal" levels suggest gonadotropin deficiency. Estrogen deficiency in women and testosterone deficiency in men in the absence of elevated gonadotropins imply gonadotropin deficiency.

To diagnose central hypothyroidism (thyrotropin deficiency), the serum T_4 and free T_4 levels (or the free T_4 index) should first be measured. If these are in the mid-normal range, TSH function is likely to be normal. If the T_4 and free T_4 levels are low and the serum TSH level is not elevated, central hypothyroidism is present. Minimal TSH elevation (with bioinactive TSH) can occur in hypothalamic hypothyroidism, usually with low free T_4 concentrations. Mild central hypothyroidism, a consideration in patients with known pituitary disease who have low-normal serum T_4 and free T_4 concentrations, remains a clinical diagnosis. Before considering the diagnosis of isolated TSH deficiency in patients with the biochemical features of central hypothyroidism without evidence of other pituitary hormone deficiencies, it is important to exclude the syndrome of thyroxine-binding globulin (TBG) deficiency (low T_4, increased T_3 resin uptake, low to low-normal free T_4 index, normal TSH) and the "euthyroid sick" syndrome (low T_4, low free T_4 or free T_4 index, normal or low TSH) (see Chap. 331).

Several diagnostic tests utilize hypothalamic-releasing hormones to assess pituitary reserve. While these tests are generally *not helpful* in assessing the adequacy of anterior pituitary function, they can be useful in certain situations. In patients with isolated gonadotropin deficiency, the gonadotropin response to gonadorelin (synthetic LHRH) may be useful in predicting which patients will respond to therapy with gonadorelin. CRH testing may be useful in the differential diagnosis of Cushing's syndrome and has been suggested as a test for the pituitary-adrenal response to stress. TRH stimulation testing is useful in some patients in supporting a diagnosis of hyperthyroidism, recurrent acromegaly, or gonadotropin-secreting tumor and in those cases in which documentation of prolactin deficiency is necessary to support a diagnosis of more generalized anterior pituitary hormone deficiency (e.g., mild central hypothyroidism). TRH testing is not necessary in the evaluation of central hypothyroidism and cannot reliably separate pituitary from hypothalamic hypothyroidism. "Mega" tests with multiple releasing hormones have little clinical utility.

℞ TREATMENT

Multiple hormones must be replaced in patients with panhypopituitarism, but cortisol replacement is most important. We prefer using prednisone for reasons of convenience and cost, but many physicians use cortisone acetate or hydrocortisone (cortisol). Prednisone (5 to 7.5 mg) or cortisone acetate (20 to 37.5 mg) can be given to some patients as a single morning dosage, whereas others require divided doses (two-thirds at 8 A.M. and one-third at 3 P.M.). Hypopituitary patients may require lower daily glucocorticoid dosages than do patients with Addison's disease and do not require mineralocorticoid replacement. In stress situations or when these patients are being prepared for pituitary or other surgery, higher doses of glucocorticoids should be administered (e.g., for major surgery, hydrocortisone hemisuccinate 50 to 75 mg intramuscularly or intravenously every 6 h or methyl prednisolone sodium succinate 15 mg intramuscularly or intravenously every 6 h). Levothyroxine is the therapy of choice in central hypothyroidism (0.05 to 0.15 mg/d). The free T_4 level should be monitored, rather than the TSH level. Since thyroxine accelerates the degradation of cortisol and can precipitate adrenal crisis in patients with limited pituitary reserve, glucocorticoid replacement should always precede levothyroxine therapy in panhypopituitarism. Hypogonadism is treated in women with estrogen-progestogen combinations and in men with testosterone esters by injection or transdermal testosterone patch. To achieve fertility, gonadotropins must be administered by injection in patients with pituitary disease, whereas gonadorelin may be successful in those with hypothalamic disease. Therapy of GH deficiency in adults is under investigation; in children GH administration usually is required, but GHRH injections may be effective in those with hypothalamic disease (see Chap. 329). Diabetes insipidus is treated with nasal desmopressin (usually 0.05 to 0.1 mL twice a day) (see Chap. 330).

RADIOLOGY OF THE PITUITARY Conventional postero-anterior and lateral skull x-rays define the contours of the sella turcica (Fig. 328-9). Abnormalities that may be identified on these films

FIGURE 328-9 X-ray of the sella, lateral view. Note (1) planum sphenoidale, (2) limbus sphenoidale, (3) sulcus chiasmaticus, (4) tuberculum sellae, (5) sella floor with distinct lamina dura, (6) dorsum sellae, (7) anterior clinoid, and (8) sphenoid sinus. *[From SM Wolpert, in The Pituitary Adenoma, KD Post et al (eds). New York, Plenum, 1980.]*

include enlargement, erosions, hyperostosis, and calcification in the region of the sella. However, detailed study of pituitary and hypothalamic lesions requires MRI or CT scanning (Fig. 328-10). Anterior tomograms of the sella may be required to delineate the bony anatomy before transsphenoidal surgery; however, the high radiation doses and the limited information provided make routine tomography obsolete for diagnostic purposes. Angiography may be required when an aneurysm or vascular malformation is suspected as a cause of an enlarged sella; MRI often obviates the need for this study.

MRI (usually before and after intravenous injection of the contrast agent gadolinium; see Chap. 362) is the imaging study of choice for pituitary and hypothalamic abnormalities. Details of the optic chiasm, pituitary stalk, pituitary gland itself, intracavernous portion of the carotid artery, and relation to the cavernous sinus can be delineated on MRI (Figs. 328-10 and 328-11). Advantages over CT include lack of radiation, lack of iodinated contrast material, better tissue contrast, and direct multiplanar capability. MRI is clearly superior to CT in delineating microadenomas, visualizing the optic chiasm, and detecting cavernous sinus invasion. Patients with severe claustrophobia, those unable to remain still, and those with metallic implants (including ferrometallic aneurysm clips, pacemakers, and ossicular implants) require CT imaging. The use of sedatives and a prone position may allow patients with mild claustrophobia to tolerate MRI. MRI is less useful when details of bony erosion or calcification are desired. Specific problems with CT in this location include radiation to the lens of the eye, difficulty in obtaining direct coronal views, artifacts due to bone and dental amalgam, and limited soft tissue density resolution.

The normal pituitary has an appearance similar to brain white matter on most MR images; it has a height of 3 to 7 mm, although values up to 9 mm can be found, particularly in young women. The upper aspect is flat, concave, or, in younger patients, convex. The stalk is located in the midline and usually is less than 2 mm in diameter. The posterior pituitary usually has a bright signal on T1-weighted images; 10 percent of normal individuals lack this intense signal. Cerebrospinal fluid appears dark on T1-weighted images and bright on T2-weighted images and is easily visualized within the sella in patients with the empty sella syndrome (Fig. 328-12). The normal pituitary gland, stalk, and cavernous sinus all show an enhanced signal on T1-weighted images after intravenous gadolinium administration. Microadenomas do not enhance or have delayed enhancement, allowing improved resolution of these lesions (Fig. 328-11). Five minutes after gadolinium administration, this contrast may no longer be evident. Stalk deviation and upward bulging of the pituitary suggest a microadenoma but are not specific. Up to 20 percent of normal persons show pituitary abnormalities on contrast-enhanced CT scan or MRI. In random autopsies, up to one-fourth of individuals have

small pituitary abnormalities (e.g., microadenomas, cysts, metastatic tumors, pituitary infarcts), but it is unclear whether such abnormalities correspond to the focal abnormalities on CT and MRI scanning.

Localization of corticotroph adenomas in patients with Cushing's disease may be helpful in directing the surgical approach. MRI in this situation may be negative in 30 percent or more of patients, and incidental nonfunctioning adenomas may be present in some patients with pituitary Cushing's disease. Bilateral inferior petrosal sinus catheterization for measuring ACTH (preferably with CRH administration) is useful when the MRI is negative and when the question of ectopic versus pituitary Cushing's disease is unresolved. Whether it is necessary in all cases of presumed pituitary Cushing's disease is uncertain. In patients with modest prolactin elevations, the purpose of pituitary and hypothalamic imaging is to exclude larger pathologic entities. Whether a microprolactinoma is actually visualized is less important, since this disorder is generally treated medically.

Pituitary macroadenomas causing sellar enlargement with or without bony erosion may be suspected on the basis of conventional radiography. However, these findings are not specific. Additional findings on skull x-rays in acromegaly may include prognathism, enlarged paranasal sinuses, hyperostosis of the external occipital protuberance, increased density of the central bone of the sella, and an enlarged, square sella with a tapered tuberculum. GH-secreting adenomas may calcify and regress to leave a calculus or stone.

Macroadenomas are well delineated on MRI. Coronal views are best (Fig. 328-13) for visualizing optic chiasm compromise, invasion of the cavernous sinus, vascular encasement, and invasion of the base of the skull. The medial wall of the cavernous sinus is thin and is not directly visualized. The lateral wall of the cavernous sinus is an important landmark; the presence of tissue between the lateral wall of the cavernous sinus and the internal carotid artery is a reliable sign of invasion. Macro-

FIGURE 328-10 Coronal T1-weighted MRI scan through the posterior portion of the supraoptic hypothalamus (*). Note the anterior pituitary (1), cavernous sinus with internal carotid artery (5), proximal optic tracts (14), pituitary stalk (17), medial temporal lobes (24), and third ventricle (III). *(From DJ Quint, 1992.)*

FIGURE 328-11 *A.* Coronal noncontrast T1-weighted MRI scan demonstrates pituitary gland asymmetry (*arrow*) compatible with a pituitary microadenoma. Cavernous internal carotid artery (5), optic chiasm (13), sphenoid sinus (21), and temporal lobe (24). *B.* Coronal gadolinium-enhanced T1-weighted MRI scan identifies a 4-mm right paramidline microadenoma (*arrows*). *(From DJ Quint, 1992.)*

adenomas are hyperdense on T2-weighted images in one-third to one-half of patients; in the remainder they are isointense. Old hemorrhage or cyst formation results in a focally hyperintense signal and may be seen in up to 22 percent of macroadenomas (see below). With hemorrhage, the signal is bright on T1 and T2; with fluid, the signal is of low intensity on T1 and bright on T2. Approximately one-fifth of patients

with macroadenomas have a partially empty sella due to tumor degeneration or necrosis and the presence of cerebrospinal fluid density within the sella. The enlargement of the residual pituitary distinguishes this entity from the primary empty sella (see below), where the residual pituitary is normal in size. Pituitary hyperplasia (e.g., thyrotroph hyperplasia in primary hypothyroidism or lactotroph hyperplasia in pregnancy) appears as a symmetrically enlarged pituitary.

Pituitary apoplexy is caused by a sudden increase in the size of a pituitary macroadenoma due to hemorrhage or infarction; enlargement of the sella is almost always evident on plain films. Acute hemorrhage (<7 days) is hypointense or isointense to brain on T1- and T2-weighted images. During the subacute stage (7 to 14 days), signal intensity is increased in the periphery of the hematoma (owing to hemoglobin breakdown products such as methemoglobin), with the center remaining hypointense. After 14 days (chronic stage), the entire hematoma appears bright on T1- and T2-weighted images.

Craniopharyngiomas can often be suspected on the basis of nodular or curvilinear calcification in the suprasellar region on x-ray (Fig. 328-14). This calcification is visible in 80 to 90 percent of children and in about half of adults. On CT scanning, cystic components are present with ring or nodular calcification in most children and in 80 percent of adults. The findings on MRI are variable; some cysts resemble cerebrospinal fluid (CSF) in their behavior; some are less intense than CSF on T1 images but brighter than CSF on T2 images; and some mimic subacute hemorrhage, being hyperintense on T1 and T2 images. Calcification is usually not seen on MRI unless it is present in large amounts. Some craniopharyngiomas are primarily solid.

Most meningiomas of the sellar region cause abnormalities on routine skull films, including calcifications of the tumor and hyperostosis of the planum sphenoidale or of the chiasmatic sulcus. Meningiomas also may cause sella enlargement and thereby mimic pituitary adenomas. Meningiomas may be difficult to see on MRI without enhancement because they are isodense to gray matter. Almost all enhance with gadolinium, as they do on CT scans with iodine contrast. Delayed scanning (after 45 min) may be necessary with MRI to allow the normal enhancement of the pituitary gland and mucosal surfaces to

FIGURE 328-12 Empty sella. Coronal contrast-enhanced T1-weighted MRI scan through the pituitary region demonstrates an enlarged sella turcica (*arrows*) with normally enhancing pituitary tissue (16) displaced inferiorly. Note the optic chiasm (13) and intracavernous carotid artery (5). *(From DJ Quint, 1992.)*

FIGURE 328-13 Macroadenoma. MRI scan through the pituitary region demonstrates a large sellar mass (*arrows*) elevating the optic chiasm (13) and invading the right cavernous sinus (*arrowheads*). The contrast-enhanced study differentiates the nonenhancing optic chiasm (13) from the enhancing tumor. (*From DJ Quint, 1992.*)

FIGURE 328-14 Lateral skull x-ray in a patient with a craniopharyngioma. Note dense calcification in suprasellar region (*arrow*).

dissipate. Vascular encasement of the carotid artery is common with meningiomas but rare with other sella-region tumors.

Aneurysms in the region of the sella contain concentric calcifications demonstrable on plain skull films in about 30 percent of patients. Aneurysms can cause sella enlargement, usually with lateral depression and erosion of the sella floor. On MRI, many aneurysms have the dark appearance of a flow void owing to blood flow through the lumen. Multilamellated thrombi appear as a high-intensity signal on T1 images; adjacent brain may show a low-intensity signal on T2 owing to hemosiderin deposition. In difficult cases, especially those with complete thrombosis, additional studies may be required, such as digital subtraction angiography, conventional angiography, and/or magnetic resonance angiography.

Other pathologic entities in the sellar region may be noted with MRI or CT. In hemochromatosis, the pituitary is dark, particularly on T2-weighted images, owing to iron deposition. Additional suprasellar masses include optic chiasm or hypothalamic gliomas, metastases to the hypothalamus or pituitary stalk, germinomas, sarcoid granulomas, histiocytosis, dermoid tumors, epidermoid tumors, and arachnoid cysts.

THE ENLARGED SELLA– EMPTY SELLA SYNDROME

Enlargement of the sella can be caused by pituitary adenomas, hypothalamic masses and cysts, aneurysms, primary hypothyroidism or hypogonadism, and increased intracranial pressure. It also can occur in patients with the primary empty sella syndrome (Fig. 328-15). In this situation, the sella tends to be symmetrically ballooned without bony ero-

sion. The suprasellar subarachnoid space herniates through an incomplete diaphragma sella (Fig. 328-15) so that the sella is filled with CSF within an arachnoid-lined sac. An incomplete diaphragma sella is thought to be a prerequisite. It is not clear whether transiently or persistently increased CSF pressure is necessary to produce sella enlargement in these patients, but CSF pressure is generally normal when measured. The pituitary is flattened and pushed to one side but tends to function normally. The fact that CSF fills the sella can be demonstrated best with MRI scanning (see Fig. 328-12).

It is important to differentiate a primary empty sella from the enlarged, partially empty sella caused by a degenerated pituitary adenoma. In the former the pituitary volume is usually normal, whereas in the latter the pituitary volume is generally increased.

Most patients with the primary empty sella syndrome are obese, multiparous women with headaches; about 30 percent have hypertension. It is of interest that multiparity, obesity, and hypertension are associated with increases in CSF pressure. Selection bias cannot be excluded in case reports, since skull x-rays may be obtained in patients with headaches, which, in turn, uncovers the enlarged sella. Endocrine

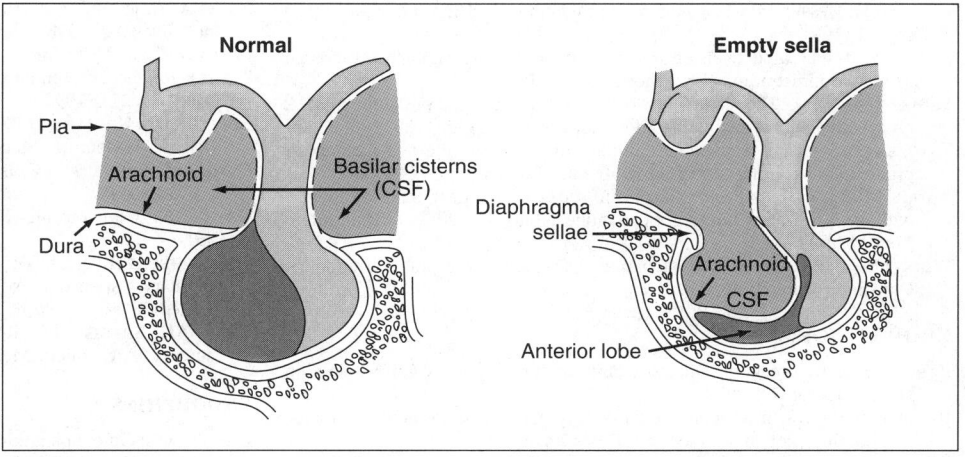

FIGURE 328-15 The findings in patients with the empty sella syndrome. *Left panel:* the normal anatomic relationships. With the empty sella syndrome *(right panel)*, ballooning of the sella results when an arachnoid diverticulum herniates through an incompetent diaphragma sellae. (*After RM Jordan et al, 1977.*)

abnormalities are uncommon. The report that antipituitary antibodies are present in 70 percent of these patients is therefore difficult to understand. Hyperprolactinemia occurs on occasion, possibly owing to stalk stretching or coincidental microprolactinomas. The GH secretory reserve is often abnormal in these patients, probably as a result of obesity. Spontaneous CSF rhinorrhea and pseudotumor cerebri have each been reported in about 10 percent of cases, but this association may represent an ascertainment bias. CSF rhinorrhea often necessitates surgical correction. Visual field defects have been reported and are thought to be caused by herniation of the optic chiasm into the sella turcica. Once the diagnosis of the empty sella syndrome is established by MRI or CT, further diagnostic studies should be performed to exclude hormone excess or deficiency; when hormone levels are normal, the therapy is reassurance.

Please refer to Chap. 55, Adenohypophyseal hormones and their hypothalamic releasing factors, in Goodman & Gilman's The Pharmacological Basis of Therapeutics, *9th ed, New York, McGraw-Hill, 1996.*

BIBLIOGRAPHY

GENERAL

BURKE CW: The pituitary megatest: Outdated. Clin Endocrinol 36:133, 1992

CROWLEY WR, ARMSTRONG WE: Neurochemical regulation of oxytocin secretion in lactation. Endocrinol Rev 13:33, 1992

HERMAN V et al: Clonal origin of pituitary adenomas. J Clin Endocrinol Metab 71:1427, 1990

JENKINS JS, NUSSEY SS: The role of oxytocin: Present concepts. Clin Endocrinol 34:515, 1991

JONES A: Radiation oncogenesis in relation to the treatment of pituitary tumours. Clin Endocrinol 35:379, 1991

JUNEAU P et al: Malignant tumors of the pituitary gland. Arch Neurol 49:555, 1992

KLIBANSKI A: Editorial: Further evidence for a somatic mutation theory in the pathogenesis of human pituitary tumors. J Clin Endocrinol Metab 71:1415, 1990

——, ZERVAS NT: Diagnosis and management of hormone-secreting pituitary adenomas. N Engl J Med 324:822, 1991

LAMBERTS SWJ: The role of somatostatin and its analogues in the diagnosis and treatment of tumors. Endocrinol Rev 12:450, 1991

MOTLICH ME, RUSSELL EJ: The pituitary "incidentaloma." Ann Intern Med 112:925, 1990

SCHEITHAUER BW et al: The pituitary gland in pregnancy: A clinicopathologic and immunohistochemical study of 69 cases. Mayo Clin Proc 65:461, 1990

PROLACTIN

BEVAN JS et al: Dopamine agonists and pituitary tumor shrinkage. Endocrinol Rev 13:220, 1992

CUNNAH D, BESSER M: Management of prolactinomas. Clin Endocrinol (Oxf) 34:231, 1991

KATZ E et al: Increased levels of bromocriptine following vaginal as compared to oral administration. Fertil Steril 55:882, 1991

SCHLECTE J et al: The natural history of untreated hyperprolactinemia: A prospective analysis. J Clin Endocrinol Metab 68:412, 1989

TSAGARAKIS S et al: Megavoltage pituitary irradiation in the management of prolactinomas: Long-term follow up. Clin Endocrinol 34:399, 1991

VANCE ML et al: Treatment of prolactin-secreting pituitary macroadenomas with the long-acting non-ergot dopamine agonist CV 205-502. Ann Intern Med 112:668, 1990

WOOD DF et al: Dopamine, the dopamine D2 receptor and pituitary tumours. Clin Endocrinol 35:455, 1991

GROWTH HORMONE

BARKAN AL: Acromegaly: Diagnosis and treatment. Endocrinol Metab Clin North Am 18:277, 1989

BAUMANN G: Growth hormone heterogeneity: Genes, isohormones, variants, and binding proteins. Endocrinol Rev 12:424, 1991

EZZAT S, MELMED S: Are patients with acromegaly at increased risk of neoplasia? J Clin Endocrinol Metab 72:245, 1991

FROHMAN LA: Therapeutic options in acromegaly. J Clin Endocrinol Metab 72:1175, 1991

HO KKY et al: Impact of octreotide, a long-acting somatostatin analogue, on glucose tolerance and insulin sensitivity in acromegaly. Clin Endocrinol 36:271, 1992

MARCUS R et al: Effects of short-term administration of recombinant human growth hormone to elderly people. J Clin Endocrinol Metab 70:519, 1990

MELMED S: Acromegaly. N Engl J Med 322:966, 1990

MURUAIS C et al: Corticosteroid-induced growth hormone secretion in normal and obese subjects. Clin Endocrinol 35:485, 1991

ROSS DA, WILSON CB: Results of transsphenoidal microsurgery for growth hormone-secreting pituitary adenomas in a series of 214 patients. J Neurosurg 68:854, 1988

RUDMAN D et al: Effects of human growth hormone in men over 60 years old. N Engl J Med 323:1, 1990

SANO T et al: Growth hormone–releasing hormone–producing tumors: Clinical, biochemical and morphological manifestations. Endocrinol Rev 9:357, 1988

THORNER MO, VANCE ML: Growth hormone 1988. J Clin Invest 82:745, 1988

—— et al: Stereotactic radiosurgery with the cobalt-60 gamma unit in the treatment of growth hormone–producing pituitary tumors. Neurosurgery 29:663, 1991

TSH

BECK-PECCOZ P et al: Treatment of hyperthyroidism with the somatostatin analogue SMS 201-995. J Clin Endocrinol Metab 68:208, 1989

FAGLIA G et al: Inappropriate secretion of thyrotropin by the pituitary. Horm Res 26:79, 1987

MAGNER JA: Thyroid-stimulating hormone: Biosynthesis, cell biology and bioactivity. Endocrinol Rev 11:354, 1990

GONADOTROPINS AND α SUBUNITS

DANESHDOOST L et al: Recognition of gonadotroph adenomas in women. N Engl J Med 324:589, 1991

HESELTINE DM et al: Testicular enlargement and elevated serum inhibin concentrations occur in patients with pituitary macroadenomas secreting follicle-stimulating hormone. Clin Endocrinol 31:411, 1989

KATZNELSON L et al: Imbalanced follicle-stimulating hormone β-subunit hormone biosynthesis in human pituitary adenomas. J Clin Endocrinol Metab 74:1343, 1992

MOGHISSI KS: Clinical applications of gonadotropin-releasing hormones in reproductive disorders. Endocrinol Metab Clin North Am 21:125, 1992

OPPENHEIM DS, KLIBANSKI A: Medical therapy of glycoprotein hormone–secreting pituitary tumors. Endocrinol Metab Clin North Am 18:339, 1989

—— et al: Prevalence of alpha-subunit hypersecretion in patients with pituitary tumors. J Clin Endocrinol Metab 64:1187, 1990

SNYDER PJ: Gonadotroph cell adenomas of the pituitary. Endocrinol Rev 6:552, 1985

TSATSOULIS A et al: Bioactive gonadotrophin secretion in man. Clin Endocrinol 35:193, 1991

WEISS J et al: Hypogonadism caused by a single amino acid substitution in the β-subunit of luteinizing hormone. N Engl J Med 326:179, 1992

WHITCOMB RW, CROWLEY WF JR: Clinical review 4: Diagnosis and treatment of isolated gonadotropin-releasing hormone deficiency in men. J Clin Endocrinol Metab 70:3, 1990

ACTH

BATEMAN A et al: The immune-hypothalamic-pituitary-adrenal axis. Endocrinol Rev 10:92, 1989

FLACK MR et al: Urine free cortisol in the high-dose dexamethasone suppression test for the differential diagnosis of the Cushing syndrome. Ann Intern Med 116:211, 1992

LORIAUX DL, NIEMANN L: Corticotropin-releasing hormone testing in pituitary disease. Endocrinol Metab Clin North Am 20:363, 1991

ORME SM, BELCHETZ PE: Isolated ACTH deficiency. Clin Endocrinol (Oxf) 35:213, 1991

ORTH DN: Corticotropin-releasing hormone in humans. Endocrinol Rev 13:164, 1992

SCHLAGHECKE R et al: The effect of long-term glucocorticoid therapy on pituitary response to exogenous corticotropin-releasing hormone. N Engl J Med 326:226, 1992

TAHIR AH, SHEELER LR: Recurrent Cushing's disease after transsphenoidal surgery. Arch Intern Med 152:977, 1992

ENDORPHINS

DELITALA G: Opioid peptides and pituitary function: Basic and clinical aspects, in *Brain Endocrinology*, 2d ed, M Motta (ed). New York, Raven, 1991, p 217

KROMER W: Endogenous and exogenous opioids in the control of gastrointestinal motility and secretion. Pharmacol Rev 40:121, 1989

LUNDBLAD JR, ROBERTS JL: Regulation of pro-opiomelanocortin gene expression in the pituitary. Endocrinol Rev 9:135, 1988

HYPOTHALAMUS

DINARELLO CA: Interleukin 1 and the pathogenesis of the acute phase response. N Engl J Med 54:301, 1984
PLUM F, VAN UITERT R: Nonendocrine disease and disorders of the hypothalamus, in *The Hypothalamus*, S Reichlin et al (eds). New York, Raven, 1978, pp 415–473

CRANIOPHARYNGIOMAS

BANNA M: Craniopharyngioma: Based on 160 cases. Br J Radiol 49:206, 1976
FISCHER EG et al: Treatment of craniopharyngiomas in children, 1971–1980. J Neurosurg 62:486, 1985

HYPOPITUITARISM

ABBOUD CF: Laboratory diagnosis of hypopituitarism. Mayo Clin Proc 61:35, 1986
ARAFAH BM: Reversible hypopituitarism in patients with large nonfunctioning pituitary adenomas. J Clin Endocrinol Metab 62:1173, 1986
EDWARDS OM, CLARK JDA: Post-traumatic hypopituitarism. Medicine 62:281, 1986
MUIR A, MACLAREN NK: Autoimmune diseases of the adrenal glands, parathyroid glands, gonads and hypothalamic-pituitary axis. Endocrinol Metab Clin North Am 20:619, 1991
ROSEN T, BENGTSSON BA: Premature mortality due to cardiovascular disease in hypopituitarism. Lancet 336:285, 1990

RADIOLOGY

CHAKERES DW et al: Magnetic resonance imaging of pituitary and parasellar abnormalities. Radiol Clin North Am 27:265, 1989
CONSTINE LS et al: Hypothalamo-pituitary dysfunction after radiation for brain tumors. N Engl J Med 328:87, 1993
GLICK RP, TIESI JA: Subacute pituitary apoplexy: Clinical and magnetic resonance imaging characteristics. Neurosurgery 27:214, 1990
JOHNSON MR et al: The evaluation of patients with a suspected pituitary microadenoma: Computed tomography compared to magnetic resonance imaging. Clin Endocrinol 36:335, 1992
QUINT DJ: Hypothalamic, pituitary, and pineal imaging, in *Endocrine Imaging*, MP Sandler et al (eds). Norwalk, CT, Appleton & Lange, 1992

FIGURE 329-1 Nomogram for height of boys and girls.

single cell becomes a complex organism in which billions of cells work in harmonious concert. The growth rate is astounding; the most rapid growth rate occurs during the second trimester. Prenatal growth is controlled by different mechanisms than those that act in the postnatal period. Prenatal growth rates are dependent on uterine blood flow and other maternal influences and less on the factors that determine ultimate stature; growth hormone and thyroid hormone have relatively minor effects on prenatal growth. The correlation between body length at birth and adult height is weak ($r = 0.3$); by 2 years of age, the correlation between body length and adult height is stronger ($r = 0.7$), indicating that the factors influencing adult stature begin operating early in postnatal life.

Genetic Factors Stature is a polygenic trait (see Chap. 65), so there is no simple method of predicting the adult height of any given child. However, there is a correlation between the mean height of parents and the mean heights attained by their children.

Nutrition The next most important factor affecting growth is nutrition. Severe nutritional deprivation, as in marasmus or kwashiorkor (see Chap. 74), impairs growth, as may subclinical deficiencies of nutrients and selective deficiencies of vitamins and minerals. The trend toward increased adult stature over the last century may be due

---

329	*Raymond L. Hintz*

DISORDERS OF GROWTH

NORMAL GROWTH Children can grow rapidly over short periods of time, and the physician must be aware of normal standards for growth and development as a function of age. A record of these changes provides a sensitive indication of general health. Minimal aberrations in health may be reflected first in a deviation from the normal growth rate; conversely, an actively growing child seldom has a serious systemic disease. Thus, height and growth rate provide important information.

Both longitudinal and cross-sectional studies indicate that differences exist in growth among different ethnic groups. However, normal, well-nourished children have remarkably similar growth patterns. For example, the average length of children, which at birth is about 50 cm, increases by about 25 cm in the first year of life, 12.5 cm in the second year, and 6.0 cm per year thereafter until puberty. This formula can be used to estimate average height up to about age 10. Nomograms have been constructed to give a more accurate picture of average growth and the range of normal deviations from the mean (Figs. 329-1 and 329-2).

CONTROL OF GROWTH Growth involves an increase in both the number of cells and the size of individual cells. The relative importance of these processes varies from organ to organ and with age. The control and integration of growth also vary among tissues and with the stage of development.

Prenatal Growth Prenatal development exemplifies the complexities of the integration and control of growth. During this time, a

FIGURE 329-2 Nomogram for growth rate in boys and girls.

to improvement in diet, especially to an increase in protein intake during the period of rapid growth in infancy.

Hormones *Growth hormone* Growth hormone (GH, or somatotropin) plays the central role in the modulation of growth from birth until the completion of puberty. In the total absence of GH, linear growth occurs at about half to a third the normal rate. GH also plays a role in the control of body anabolism throughout life.

GH is a member of a family of hormones that includes pituitary prolactin and human placental lactogen (hPL) (see Chap. 328). The most common form of GH in the pituitary and in the circulation is the 22-kDa ("22K") form. This is the hormone that was purified and sequenced from human pituitary glands. The second most abundant form is a 20-kDa ("20K") form. This variant is coded by the same gene sequence as the 22K growth hormone, but a segment of one coding exon in the gene is not transcribed, resulting in a shorter hormone. Whether this variant serves some specific function is not clear; the 20K form seems to have equivalent growth-promoting activity but may have less effect on carbohydrate function than the 22K form.

GH secretion is under both positive and negative hypothalamic control (see Chap. 328). The somatotropin release-inhibiting factor (SRIF, somatostatin) is a 14-amino-acid peptide that is synthesized in the hypothalamus and is widely distributed in other tissues as well; it is a potent inhibitor of the secretion of many hormones, including insulin, glucagon, and gastrin.

The biologic action of GH-releasing hormone (GRH, somatocrinin) is contained in the first 29 amino acids of the 44-amino-acid peptide, and the amino-terminal amino acid is crucial for its biologic action. Patients with idiopathic GH deficiency may have a deficiency of GRH rather than an inability to make GH in the pituitary. Indeed, half or more of individuals with GH deficiency respond to prolonged pulsatile administration of GRH with an increase in plasma GH and an accelerated growth rate.

The secretion of somatostatin and GRH, and hence the release of GH, is under the influence of several factors (Fig. 329-3). Higher centers in the central nervous system have axons that terminate on hypothalamic cells that secrete somatostatin and GRH and exert both positive and negative effects. In addition, both GH and the GH-controlled insulin-like growth factors (IGFs) influence the secretion or action of GRH and somatostatin. The secretion of GH is episodic, and the hormone has a relatively short half-life (10 to 15 min) in plasma. A significant proportion of GH in serum is bound to a GH-binding protein (GHBP) that is structurally related to the GH receptor. Although small amounts of GH are secreted during waking periods, most GH secretion occurs during sleep, especially during third- and fourth-stage sleep.

Insulin-like growth factors Although GH may exert some direct effects on growth, most of its growth-promoting actions are mediated by the IGF or somatomedin peptides. Two human IGF peptides, IGF-I and IGF-II, have about 50 percent structural homology with human insulin and 70 percent homology with each other. Somatomedin C (SM-C) and IGF-I are structurally and functionally equivalent. The IGF peptides are bound tightly to six specific plasma IGF-binding proteins (IGFBPs) and have half-lives of hours rather than minutes. Levels of IGF-I and IGFBP-3 are dependent on GH secretion and consequently are high in acromegaly and low in hypopituitarism. Levels are also age-dependent, being low in early childhood, peaking during adolescence, and declining after age 50. The plasma levels of IGF-II also depend on the presence of a minimal amount of GH, but supraphysiologic levels of GH do not result in a further increase in IGF-II. Thus, the values of IGF-II are low in hypopituitarism but are not elevated in acromegaly. Plasma levels of IGF-II are constant from 1 year of age to beyond the eighth decade of life.

Thyroid hormone Unlike the pattern of growth with GH deficiency, the total absence of thyroid hormone causes an almost complete cessation of linear growth. Thus, adequate thyroid hormone appears to be an absolute prerequisite for normal growth. There are several potential mechanisms for this phenomenon. Thyroid hormones exert direct effects on cell metabolism, and thyroid hormone deficiency also results in diminished GH secretion in response to stimulation. In addition, the action of IGF-I on cartilage cells may be dependent on thyroid hormone.

Gonadal steroids Androgens and estrogens exert their major stimulation of growth at puberty. Much of the pubertal growth spurt is due to these hormones. Androgens directly stimulate the growth and maturation of bone, cartilage, and muscle. Estrogens appear to have a biphasic action, stimulating growth at low levels and inhibiting growth at high levels. In addition, estrogens are responsible for the closure of the epiphyses and the cessation of linear growth.

Insulin Insulin has anabolic actions that are separate from its effects on carbohydrate metabolism. These actions include stimulation of protein synthesis and cell division. The large size of infants of diabetic mothers may be the consequence of high levels of plasma insulin in the fetus. The close structural relationship of insulin to the IGF group of growth factors and the ability of insulin to bind to the IGF-I receptor may explain some of these effects of insulin at high levels. However, insulin also stimulates growth directly in some cell types.

Other factors Nerve growth factor, which is structurally related to the insulin-IGF family of peptides, has actions on the development of sympathetic neurons and possibly on the maintenance and repair of other neurons. Epidermal growth factor controls the maturation of the skin and also acts on other cell types. Platelet-derived growth factor is released from platelets upon clotting and is also a potent mitogen for many cells. The plasma levels, control mechanisms, interactions with other growth-stimulating peptides, and physiologic roles of these growth factors remain to be elucidated.

DIAGNOSIS OF GROWTH DISORDERS Most short people do not have a disease in the usual sense but exhibit some deviation from the normal growth pattern (Table 329-1). Thus, the first step in evaluating growth disorders is to identify those individuals with a normal variation in stature who presumably do not require treatment.

FIGURE 329-3 Feedback control of growth hormone secretion. GH, growth hormone; GHRH, growth hormone–releasing hormone; SM, somatomedins (insulin-like growth factors). Stimulating influences are shown by arrows in color. Inhibitory influences are shown in black.

Table 329-1

Causes of Short Stature

Diagnosis	Usual Practice, %	Referral Center, %
Constitutional growth delay	98	80
GH deficiency	0.1	10
Hypothyroidism	0.2	4
Systemic disease	0.3	3
Chromosomal disorders	0.1	1
Bone-cartilage dysplasia	0.3	1
Psychosocial disorders	1	1

SOURCE: Modified from Horner et al.

Table 329-2

CHAPTER 329
Disorders of Growth

2001

Physical Findings in Syndromes of Short Stature

Syndrome	Specific Physical Findings
GH deficiency	Frontal bossing, central obesity, high-pitched voice
Hypothyroidism	Dry skin, coarse hair, immature facies
Cushing's syndrome	Central obesity, striae, hypertension
Gonadal dysgenesis	Webbed neck, multiple pigmented nevi, shield chest, delayed sexual development
Pseudohypoparathyroidism	Moon facies and obesity, short metacarpals, mental retardation
Bone-cartilage dysplasia	Abnormal proportions, macrocephaly
Russell-Silver dwarfism	Small at birth, "pointed" facies, asymmetry

Height and Growth Rate   An important factor in the differential diagnosis of short stature is the height percentile of the patient relative to others of the same age. This factor is determined using a nomogram such as the one shown in Fig. 329-1. A straightedge is placed on the points representing the patient's age and height. The value of the intercept with the right-hand scale is an estimate of the number of standard deviations (SDs) from the mean height for age. In general, the further the patient is from the mean height for age, the more likely it is that short stature is due to disease. A height above the −2-SD level indicates that the patient is likely normal. The growth rate also should be determined, if possible, either from existing growth data or by observation (see Fig. 329-2). A growth rate consistently below the mean is a cause for concern.

Because short stature is common, clinical judgment plays a large role in the approach to this problem. Individuals with severely short stature (−3 SD or greater for age) should undergo immediate evaluation, while those with a less severe abnormality may be observed serially so that the growth rate can be assessed. A consistently low growth rate should prompt further investigation. The diagnosis of constitutional delay is one of exclusion. In general, if hypothyroidism, GH deficiency, and the more common systemic diseases have been excluded, it is reasonable to observe the patient. However, the boundaries between "normal" and "disease" may be blurred, and the indications for treatment may change. Furthermore, continued failure to maintain a normal growth rate is an indication for reinvestigation.

History   Important features in the history include the weight and gestational age at birth, growth and development in early infancy, and the presence of systemic disease. It is also crucial to assess the stature of the parents and first- and second-degree relatives and to review the growth and pubertal development patterns of parents, siblings, and other relatives. A family history of late pubertal development may be diagnostically helpful.

Physical Examination   The body proportions must be evaluated. Limbs that are short relative to the trunk suggest either long-standing hypothyroidism or one of the chondrodystrophies, such as achondro-

Table 329-3

Screening Laboratory Investigations in Short Stature

Test or X-Ray	Disorder
Serum thyroxine	Hypothyroidism
IGF-I and IGFBP-3	GH deficiency
GHBP	GH insensitivity syndromes
Bone age	Constitutional delay, hypothyroidism, GH deficiency
Magnetic resonance imaging	Craniopharyngioma or other central nervous system lesions
Serum calcium	Pseudohypoparathyroidism
Serum phosphate	Vitamin D–resistant rickets
Serum bicarbonate	Renal tubular acidosis
Blood urea nitrogen	Renal failure
Complete blood count	Anemia, nutritional disorder
Erythrocyte sedimentation rate	Inflammatory disease of bowel
Chromosomal karyotype	Gonadal dysgenesis or other abnormality

plastic dwarfism; subtle forms of chondrodystrophy may be difficult to recognize (see also Chap. 348). It is also important to note the height-to-weight ratio. A short child who is underweight for height may have malnutrition or a systemic disease. On the other hand, a child who is short but overweight is more likely to have an endocrine disease. Patients with Cushing's syndrome, GH deficiency, or hypothyroidism may be overweight for their height. Specific physical findings may suggest specific syndromes (Table 329-2).

Laboratory Evaluation   Assessment of bone age is useful to indicate possible pathology and to estimate final adult height. Because the manifestations of hypothyroidism may be minimal, thyroid function should be assessed routinely. Measurements of IGF-I and IGFGP-3 are also useful screening procedures, since most patients with GH deficiency have low values. Syndromes of GH resistance, such as Laron dwarfism, are characterized by low IGF-I levels, low GHBP levels, and high GH levels. Appropriate tests may be ordered to screen for other disease states (as summarized in Table 329-3). Any girl with unexplained short stature should have a chromosomal karyotype.

Testing of GH secretion   Because GH secretion is episodic and therefore variable, random measurements of plasma GH are not an adequate test of GH deficiency. Some GH stimulation tests for screening for GH deficiency are summarized in Table 329-4 (also see Chap. 328). Because of the long half-life of IGF-I and IGFBP-3, a random measurement during the day is an accurate reflection of the mean

Table 329-4

Screening Tests for Assessing GH Secretion

IGF-I RADIOIMMUNOASSAY*

Age, years	Male Range, μg/L	Female Range, μg/L
1–2	31–160	11–206
3–4	45–230	75–320
5–6	51–288	70–320
7–8	157–385	125–396
9–10	136–308	123–330
11–12	180–440	191–462
13–14	220–616	286–660
15–16	200–836	242–660
17–18	286–627	240–506

IGFBP-3 RADIOIMMUNOASSAY*

Age	Range, mg/L	Mean, mg/L
1–12 months	0.5–1.2	1.3
1–5 years	1.4–3.0	2.1
5–7 years	1.5–3.4	2.4
7–9 years	2.1–4.2	3.0
9–11 years	2.0–4.8	3.3
11–13 years	2.1–6.2	3.8
13–15 years	2.2–5.9	4.2
15–18 years	2.5–4.8	3.8
Adults, 20–30 years	2.0–4.2	3.0

CLONIDINE TEST OF GH RELEASE

NPO after midnight
Administration of clonidine by mouth:

Body Weight, kg	Dose, mg
5–15	0.05
15–25	0.10
25–35	0.15
35–50	0.20
>50	0.25

Samples for measurement of GH at 0, 60, and 90 min
Side effects: Postural hypotension and somnolence
Keep patient supine until after postural hypotension is gone
Normal response: Greater than or equal to 10 μg/L (10 ng/mL) on any sample

* Values for age-related normal individuals (may vary with assay).

plasma concentration. If care is taken to use age-related standards, measurement of IGF-I and IGFBP-3 provide a reasonable screen for GH deficiency. Low levels of IGF-I or IGFBP-3 should prompt more extensive evaluation. The other tests listed are indirect and largely nonphysiologic ways of provoking the release of GH. In our clinic, a GH level of 10 μg/L (10 ng/mL) after a clonidine test is considered a normal response. If that level is not achieved, more definitive testing of the GH reserve should be carried out, as described in Chap. 328.

TREATMENT

GH Deficiency The only established use of human GH is in the treatment of children who are GH-deficient. Between 1 in 4000 and 1 in 20,000 children have a GH deficiency; about half these cases are due to idiopathic GH deficiency, and the other half are secondary to tumor and/or radiation therapy. In approximately one-third of the latter cases, GH deficiency is isolated, and in the other two-thirds, there are multiple pituitary hormone deficiencies. Short stature due to chronic renal failure or gonadal dysgenesis is also an indication for GH treatment. If short stature is due to a systemic disease, treatment is directed toward the underlying disease state. Similarly, short stature due to hypothyroidism or cortisol excess is managed by treatment of the primary disorder. In general, the earlier the disorder is diagnosed and treated, the more successful is the growth response; if treatment of the underlying disease is delayed until after puberty, little or no improvement in stature can be expected.

Unlike the broad species specificity of peptide hormones such as insulin, GH exhibits a narrow species specificity. Human GH stimulates linear growth in children with GH deficiency, whereas the bovine hormone is ineffective in humans. The preparation of human GH from pituitary glands obtained from autopsy material did not supply enough hormone for the treatment of all children who had GH deficiency, let alone for the evaluation of the usefulness of GH treatment for other conditions. Furthermore, the distribution of human pituitary GH in the United States and several other countries was discontinued in 1985 because of the development of Creutzfeldt-Jakob disease in some patients who had been treated with human GH. The availability since 1985 of synthetic GH has relieved the supply problem. Hormone is readily available for patients with GH deficiency, and the potentially unlimited supply has allowed exploration of other therapeutic uses of GH, including the treatment of gonadal dysgenesis.

Most children with GH deficiency respond to GH treatment with an acceleration of growth to normal or above-normal rates. As with other hormones, there is a dose-response curve for GH administration. The doses that have been tested range from 0.01 to 0.1 mg per kilogram body weight as a subcutaneous injection daily. There is a wide variation in response, but the higher dosages usually result in higher average growth rates. Indeed, daily doses of 0.025 or 0.050 mg/kg cause a good growth response in most GH-deficient patients. If the patient fails to show an adequate growth rate, the dose can be increased until an adequate growth response is obtained or until the upper limit of 0.50 mg/kg per week is reached. GH doses above this level are associated with an increased risk of glucose intolerance and other complications.

An alternative method under study for the treatment of GH deficiency is the use of either GH-releasing hormone (GHRH) or GH-releasing peptide (GHRP). Since at least half of children with GH deficiency are able to secrete GH in response to GHRH, this approach may ultimately be useful for those patients.

Short Stature Of Other Causes IDIOPATHIC SEVERE SHORT STATURE Growth hormone has been given to some patients with growth failure not due to GH deficiency. Some children with severe short stature (more than 2.5 SDs below the mean for age) do not have GH deficiency but are responsive to GH treatment. Many of these patients have low IGF-I, IGFBP-3, and/or GHBP levels and

may have a partial defect in the control of GH secretion. Many such children show a short-term increase in growth rate in response to GH therapy; whether their final height is greater than it would have been without GH treatment is not established. Furthermore, it is not known whether there are serious long-term side effects from GH treatment in this situation.

Gonadal Dysgenesis GH also may have a role in the treatment of gonadal dysgenesis (see Chap. 66). Most women with gonadal dysgenesis have an average adult height between 135 and 142 cm. Treatment with androgens can cause a short-term increase in the rate of growth of girls with this disorder but does not result in a greater final adult stature. The use of GH at modest doses is also associated with an increase in the rate of growth. Results of multicenter group studies in which synthetic GH was administered either alone or in combination with androgens are encouraging in terms of both initial growth response and increases in final height.

Skeletal Disorders Growth hormone also has been used to treat small numbers of subjects with a wide variety of other growth disorders, including bone-cartilage dysplasias and other genetic syndromes associated with short stature. It is not clear whether GH is of use in any of these disorders.

Please refer to Chap. 55 in Goodman & Gilman's The Pharmacological Basis of Therapeutics, *9th ed, McGraw-Hill, New York, 1996.*

BIBLIOGRAPHY

BAUMANN G: Growth hormone heterogeneity: Genes, isohormone, variants and binding proteins. Endocr Rev 12:424, 1991

BLUM WF et al: A specific radioimmunoassay for the growth hormone–dependent somatomedin binding protein: Its use for diagnosis of growth hormone deficiency. J Clin Endocrinol Metab 70:1291, 1990

BROWN P: Potential epidemic Creutzfeldt-Jakob disease from human growth hormone therapy. N Engl J Med 313:728, 1985

FRASIER SD: A review of growth hormone stimulation tests in children. Pediatrics 53:929, 1974

GRUMBACH M: Growth hormone therapy and the short end of the stick. N Engl J Med 319:238, 1988

HINDMARSH PC et al: Wider indications for treatment with biosynthetic human growth hormone in children. Clin Endocrinol 34:417, 1991

HINTZ RL: Growth factors. Curr Opin Pediatr 2:786, 1990

———: Untoward events in patients treated with GH in the USA. Horm Res 38(Suppl 1):44, 1992

——— et al: Efficacy of growth hormone therapy in patients without classically defined growth hormone deficiency. Growth Genet Horm 8(Suppl 1):10, 1992

———: The prismatic case of Creutzfeldt-Jakob disease associated with pituitary growth hormone treatment. J Clin Endocrinol Metab 80:2298, 1995.

HOPWOOD NJ et al: Growth response of non-growth hormone deficient children with marked short stature during three years of growth hormone therapy. J Pediatr 123:215, 1993

HORNER JM et al: Growth deceleration patterns in constitutional short stature: An aid to diagnosis. Pediatrics 62:529, 1978

LANTOS J et al: Ethical issues of growth hormone therapy. JAMA 261:1020, 1989

LEE PDK et al: Efficacy of insulin-like growth factor I levels in predicting the response to provocative growth hormone testing. Pediatr Res 27:45, 1990

ROSENFELD RG et al: Six-year results of a randomized, prospective trial of human growth hormone and oxandrolone in Turner's syndrome. J Pediatr 49:121, 1992

——— et al: The diagnosis of childhood growth hormone deficiency revisited. J Clin Endocrinol Metab 80:1532, 1995

TANNER JM, DAVIS PSW: Clinical longitudinal standards for height and height velocity for North American children. J Pediatr 107:317, 1985

———, ISREALSOHN WJ: Parent-child correlations for body measurements of children between the ages of one month and 7 years. Ann Hum Genet 26:245, 1963

——— et al: Effect of human growth hormone treatment for 1 to 7 years on growth of 100 children with growth hormone deficiency, inherited smallness, Turner's syndrome, and other complaints. Arch Dis Child 46:317, 1985

THORNER MO et al: Growth hormone–releasing hormone and growth hormone–releasing peptide as potential therapeutic modalities. Acta Paediatr Scand (Suppl) 376:29, 1990

VIPANI OV et al: Prevalence of severe growth hormone deficiency. Br Med J 2:427, 1977

DISORDERS OF THE NEUROHYPOPHYSIS

Axons from two largely independent hypothalamic-neurohypophyseal systems in the supraoptic and paraventricular nuclei extend through the pituitary stalk to the posterior pituitary. The hormones vasopressin and oxytocin are formed in separate ganglion cells and migrate down the axons as parts of precursor proteins. They are stored in secretory granules in the nerve terminals in the neurohypophysis and are released by exocytosis into the bloodstream in response to appropriate stimuli. Vasopressin (AVP; also called antidiuretic hormone, ADH) controls water conservation, and its release is coordinated with the activity of the thirst center that regulates fluid intake. Oxytocin stimulates uterine contractions and milk ejection.

VASOPRESSIN SYNTHESIS, RELEASE, AND ACTION

SYNTHESIS AVP is synthesized in the magnocellular neurons of the anterior hypothalamus as a preprohormone and is altered in the Golgi apparatus to form a prohormone that is packaged into neurosecretory vesicles. While it is being transported to axonal terminals, the prohormone is cleaved into AVP, a protein called *neurophysin* with a molecular weight of 10,000, and a 39-amino-acid glycopeptide. All three products are released into the peripheral circulation.

ACTIONS AVP initiates its action to conserve water and concentrate the urine by binding to the V_2 receptor on the basolateral surface of the principal cell of the renal conducting duct. AVP enhances the hydrosmotic flow of water from the lumen of the duct through the cell to the medullary interstitium and peritubular capillaries. AVP also increases the permeability of the collecting duct to urea and increases sodium absorption in the thick ascending limb of the loop of Henle. High concentrations of AVP acting on V_1 receptors can also cause vasoconstriction, as in response to severe hypotension or after infusion of vasopressin for treatment of bleeding esophageal varices.

AVP, perhaps from axons that terminate in the cerebrum, may play a role in learning and memory, and AVP from fibers in the median eminence participates in the stimulation of corticotropin secretion in response to stress.

NORMAL HORMONE LEVELS AVP concentrations in plasma and urine can be measured by radioimmunoassay. The results may be expressed either as units based on pressor activity in the rat or in terms of weight of purified vasopressin. Arginine vasopressin has a biologic activity of approximately 400 units/mg (1 mU = 2.5 ng = 2.3 pmol). The neurohypophysis under conditions of random fluid intake contains approximately 8 units of AVP. Under the same conditions, peripheral plasma AVP concentration ranges from 1.4 to 5.6 pmol/L (1.5 to 6 ng/L). At the latter plasma level and above, urine osmolality is maximal. The AVP concentration in plasma fluctuates, with a maximum late at night and in the early morning and a minimum in the early afternoon. Under conditions of normal hydration, healthy subjects release approximately 370 to 1400 pmol (400 to 1500 ng) from the pituitary and excrete 23 to 80 pmol (25 to 90 ng) AVP in urine in 24 h. During 24 to 28 h of dehydration, the amount released increases three to five times.

METABOLISM Inactivation of AVP occurs largely in liver and kidneys through cleavage of the terminal glycinamide to produce a biologically inactive substance. Approximately 7 to 10 percent of secreted AVP is excreted in the urine as active hormone.

CONTROL OF AVP RELEASE *Osmoregulation* Under normal conditions, AVP release is regulated primarily by osmoreceptors in the hypothalamus. Changes in the concentrations of plasma solutes to which the cellular membrane is impermeable cause alterations in the volume of the osmoreceptor cells, which in turn alter the electric activity of the neurons and control both the synthesis and

release of AVP. As a consequence of this servomechanism between effective plasma osmolality and AVP release, plasma osmolality is normally maintained within a very narrow range. The mean plasma osmolality in a group of normal subjects following a water load of 20 mL/kg of body weight was 281.7 mmol/kg plasma water, and the osmolality that initiated AVP release following infusion of hypertonic saline solution into water-loaded subjects was 287.3 mmol/kg. Thus, the increase in plasma osmolality between full diuresis and the initiation of antidiuresis by hypertonic saline solution is only 5.6 mmol/kg or 2 percent.

The infusion of hypertonic saline solution into water-loaded subjects causes a linear rise in plasma osmolality with time. After an interval, there is an abrupt, progressive fall in free water clearance without a significant change in solute or creatinine excretion. We defined the osmotic threshold for AVP release as the plasma osmolality at the onset of antidiuresis under these conditions, which occurred at a mean plasma osmolality of 287 mmol/kg. The osmotic threshold for AVP release also may be determined, with very similar results, by constructing a linear regression line between simultaneously obtained plasma osmolality and either plasma or urine AVP concentration during hypertonic saline infusion and extrapolating the regression line to the *x*-axis intercept (plasma osmolality).

Volume Regulation Decreases in plasma volume, through effects on stretch receptors in the left atrium and perhaps in the pulmonary veins, stimulate the release of AVP by reducing the tonic inhibitory impulses from the left atrium to the hypothalamus. The neural impulses travel via the vagi to the reticular formation of the midbrain and diencephalon and then to the supraoptic and paraventricular nuclei, where they are integrated with the other stimuli that affect AVP release. Positive-pressure breathing, quiet standing, and vasodilation may activate this mechanism, which serves to restore plasma volume, even at times overriding osmotic inhibition of AVP release. Following volume contraction, plasma AVP levels may reach 10 times the levels induced by hypertonicity. Increased plasma volume inhibits AVP release by the reverse mechanisms, leading to a diuresis and correction of the hypervolemia. Negative-pressure breathing, recumbency, lack of gravitational force (as in space travel), submersion in water, and exposure to cold can activate this mechanism.

Baroreceptor Regulation Activation of carotid and aortic baroreceptors in response to hypotension causes release of AVP. Hypotension due to blood loss is the most potent stimulus and may at times raise plasma levels of AVP to 560 pmol/L (600 ng/L). These concentrations of AVP may cause vasoconstriction, which probably plays a role in the restoration of blood pressure.

Neural Regulation Several hypothalamic neurotransmitters and neuropeptides influence the release of AVP. Acetylcholine stimulates AVP release by its nicotinic action on supraoptic neurons. Angiotensin II, histamine, bradykinin, and neuropeptide Y probably stimulate AVP release. Norepinephrine, prostaglandins, and dopamine stimulate or inhibit AVP release, depending on the experimental conditions. Gamma-aminobutyric acid appears to act as an inhibitory neurotransmitter; serotonin and substance P are also present in the supraoptic nucleus, but their influence on AVP release is not clear. The regulatory action of opioid peptides on AVP release is also unclear, with reports indicating stimulation, inhibition, or no effect. Though the roles of these and other transmitters and peptides are incompletely defined, the antidiuretic actions of stress, emesis, and pain and the diuretic actions of hypnosis, psychological conditioning, and inhalation of carbon dioxide indicate that higher centers have an important influence on the release of AVP.

Aging Aging is associated with enhanced AVP release in response to a rising plasma osmolality and a progressive increase in plasma AVP concentration. These changes appear to place the older individual at greater risk of developing water retention and hyponatremia, despite a concomitant decline in maximal renal concentrating capacity in response to AVP, which is usually manifest after age 60.

Pharmacologic Influences   Nicotine, morphine, vincristine, vinblastine, cyclophosphamide, clofibrate, chlorpropamide, and some tricyclic anticonvulsants and antidepressants stimulate AVP release. Ethanol exerts diuretic properties by inhibiting neurohypophyseal function under a variety of conditions. Some narcotic antagonists also inhibit AVP release. Experimentally, chlorpromazine, reserpine, and phenytoin all inhibit the secretion of AVP by the pituitary and the rise in urinary excretion of AVP after water deprivation. In humans, phenytoin and chlorpromazine may inhibit AVP release and produce diuresis.

AVP RESPONSE TO WATER DEPRIVATION AND TO WATER LOADING   Water deprivation provides both an osmotic and a volume stimulus for vasopressin release by increasing plasma osmolality and decreasing plasma volume, but the maximum urinary osmolality after water deprivation depends on renal medullary osmolality and other intrarenal factors. In response to fluid deprivation for 18 to 24 h, plasma osmolality rarely rises above 292 mmol/kg in normal individuals. The resultant stimulation of AVP release increases plasma AVP concentration to 7.4 to 14 pmol/L (8 to 15 ng/L).

The administration of water lowers plasma osmolality and expands blood volume, inhibiting the release of AVP via both osmoreceptor and atrial volume receptor mechanisms. An oral water load of 20 mL/kg in normal adults causes a fall in plasma osmolality to a mean of 281.7 mmol/kg and a maximum diuresis in 1 to 1½ h with free water clearance rising to approximately 12 mL/min and urine osmolality falling to 40 to 60 mmol/kg. The delay in reaching maximal diuresis is accounted for by the time required for absorption of water from the gut, for metabolism of previously secreted vasopressin, and for renal recovery from the action of vasopressin.

INTERACTION OF OSMOTIC AND VOLUME INFLUENCES   Under conditions of water deprivation and of water loading, volume and osmotic influences act in parallel to influence AVP release. In other circumstances, volume and osmotic influences may be competitive, and changes in plasma volume can modify the effects of hypertonic stimuli on AVP release. Osmotic factors ordinarily predominate to maintain plasma osmolality within a narrow range. Larger changes in blood volume, such as those induced by hemorrhage, may blunt and eventually overcome the osmotic influences, and hypotension can stimulate AVP secretion and override simultaneous inhibiting influences.

RELATION BETWEEN AVP RELEASE AND THIRST-INDUCED WATER INTAKE   Under normal conditions, there is close coordination between AVP release and thirst, both of which are regulated by small changes in plasma osmolality. The perception of thirst generally becomes apparent when plasma osmolality exceeds 292 mmol/kg. Thus, thirst occurs only when the urine is maximally concentrated. Angiotensin II increases thirst and AVP release under conditions of extracellular volume depletion. Normally, therefore, water losses lead to slight hypernatremia, which increases thirst and fluid intake to restore and maintain normal plasma osmolality. In contrast, when thirst perception is impaired (adipsia), fluid losses are uncorrected, and hypernatremia occurs even though AVP release is adequate to concentrate the urine maximally.

EFFECTS OF GLUCOCORTICOIDS   Glucocorticoids and the posterior pituitary have antagonistic effects on water excretion. Cortisol elevates the osmotic threshold for AVP release elicited by hypertonic saline infusion in water-loaded normal subjects and protects against water intoxication and overcomes the impaired response to water loading in adrenal insufficiency.

Although the impaired ability to dilute the urine in adrenal insufficiency may be due in part to excessive plasma AVP, glucocorticoids also can act directly on the renal tubules to decrease water permeability and increase free water excretion in the absence of AVP.

ANTIDIURETIC ACTION OF AVP   The mechanism of action of AVP is demonstrated in Fig. 330-1: (1) AVP binds to a receptor (V_2) on the basolateral surface of the principal cell of the medullary collecting duct. This V_2 receptor has seven transmembrane domains.

FIGURE 330-1   Schematic representation of the cellular mechanism for the antidiuretic action of vasopressin in the principal cell of the renal collecting duct. See text for the description of the mechanism. (*Modified from H Valtin, JA Schafer, Renal Function 3d ed, Boston, Little, Brown, 1955, with permission.*)

(2) The receptor-hormone complex activates a guanine nucleotide binding stimulatory protein (G_s). (3) This protein in turn activates adenylate cyclase in the membrane, which increases the concentration of cyclic AMP in the cytosol. AVP also stimulates prostaglandin E_2 production, which, in turn, acts as a feedback inhibitor of adenylate cyclase activity. (4) Cyclic AMP activates protein kinase A. (5) The activated protein kinase A causes the phosphorylation of unidentified proteins. (6) The phosphorylated protein stimulates exocytosis which causes the insertion of water channels, composed of proteins called aquaporins, into the apical membrane of the cell. This event coincides with the appearance of particle aggregates (Fig. 330-2). (7) As a consequence, the membrane becomes water permeable. (8) When AVP is removed, the water channels are reinternalized back into the cell, and the membrane particle aggregates disappear. Consequently, the membrane is again impermeable to water. (9) The basolateral membrane remains permeable to water, allowing water that has entered the cell under the influence of AVP to exit the cell along osmotic gradients into the medullary insterstitium and peritubular capillaries.

A variety of cations and drugs influence the action of AVP. Calcium and lithium inhibit the adenylate cyclase response to AVP. Lithium also interferes with a subsequent biochemical action, as does potassium deficiency. Demeclocycline inhibits adenylate cyclase stimulation by AVP and also inhibits the cyclic AMP–dependent protein kinase. In contrast, chlorpropamide increases AVP-induced activation of adenylate cyclase.

DEFICIENCY OF VASOPRESSIN: DIABETES INSIPIDUS

Diabetes insipidus refers to the passage through the body of a large quantity of dilute fluid. This state of excessive water intake and hypotonic polyuria may be due to failure of AVP release in response to normal physiologic stimuli (central or neurogenic diabetes insipidus) or failure of the kidney to respond to AVP (nephrogenic diabetes insipidus).

PATHOPHYSIOLOGY   Deficiency of vasopressin release in response to the appropriate stimuli can result from lesions at several functional sites in the physiologic chain of events that regulates hor-

FIGURE 330-2 *Top*: Virtual absence of particle clusters in renal collecting duct luminal membrane obtained from untreated Brattleboro (congenital diabetes insipidus) rat. *Bottom*: Appearance of particle clusters (*arrows*) after treatment with AVP. The appearance of clusters coincides with the insertion of water channels into the cell membrane. (*From MC Harmanci et al, Am J Physiol 235:F440, 1978.*)

mone release. Four types of central diabetes insipidus can be defined. Patients with the first type show very little rise in urine osmolality, even with a marked increase in plasma osmolality (Fig. 330-3, line 1) and no evidence of AVP release during hypertonic saline infusion. They are essentially devoid of releasable AVP. In patients with the second type, there is an abrupt increase in urine osmolality during dehydration (Fig. 330-3, line 2), but there is no evidence of an osmotic threshold during saline infusion. These patients have a defective osmoreceptor mechanism but can release AVP in response to the hypovolemia of severe dehydration. Patients with the third type of disease have some rise in urine osmolality with increasing plasma osmolality (Fig. 330-3, line 3) and have an elevated osmotic threshold for AVP release. These patients have a sluggish release mechanism due to a high-set osmoreceptor. In patients with the fourth type of disease, urine and plasma osmolality coordinates are shifted to the right of normal (Fig. 330-3, line 4). AVP release in these patients is initiated at a normal plasma osmolality but is subnormal in amount.

Patients with the second to fourth types of disease may develop a good antidiuresis in response to nausea, nicotine, methacholine, chlorpropamide, or clofibrate, indicating that AVP formation is sufficient to allow for adequate urinary concentrating ability in the presence of an appropriate stimulus to release. In rare instances, patients with the second to fourth types of disease present with asymptomatic hypernatremia associated with mild or no polyuria.

ETIOLOGY The causes of central diabetes insipidus in 135 patients who satisfied the criteria described under "Diagnostic Tests" (below) and who had had the disorder for at least 6 months are shown

FIGURE 330-3 Relation of plasma and urinary osmolality during hydration and dehydration in normal adult subjects (*shaded area*) and in four types of patients with diabetes insipidus.

in Table 330-1. Diabetes insipidus frequently starts in childhood or early adult life (median age of onset, 24 years) and is more common in males than females. The major causes include the following: (1) *Neoplastic* or *infiltrative lesions* of the hypothalamus or pituitary, including pituitary adenomas, craniopharyngiomas, germinomas, pinealomas, metastatic tumors, leukemia, Langerhans cell granulomatosis (histiocytosis X), and sarcoidosis, caused diabetes insipidus in 37 patients. In approximately 60 percent of these patients partial or complete loss of anterior pituitary function was evident. (2) *Pituitary* or *hypothalamic surgery* caused diabetes insipidus in 32 patients and was usually associated with anterior hypopituitarism. Surgically induced diabetes insipidus usually develops 1 to 6 days after surgery and often disappears after a few days. It may recur and become chronic after an "interphase" of 1 to 5 days. Removal of the posterior lobe of the pituitary induces permanent diabetes insipidus only if the pituitary stalk is sectioned high enough to induce retrograde degeneration of most neurons of the supraoptic nucleus. (3) *Severe head injuries,*

Table 330-1

Characteristics of 135 Cases of Long-Standing* Central Diabetes Insipidus Diagnosed by the Authors at SUNY Health Science Center, Syracuse. Categories Are Arranged in Order of Increasing Median Age of Onset.

	Age of Onset, Years				Percent of Cases
Cause	**Median†**	**Range**	**Males**	**Females**	
Langerhans cell granulomatosis	2	1–30	3	2	4
Primary brain tumor					
Postoperative‡	15	6–50	9	11	15
Preoperative§	18	7–58	17	3	15
Idiopathic	20	<1–66	20	14	25
Head trauma	22	5–48	15	9	18
Nontraumatic encephalomalacia	43	15–73	3	4	5
Ruptured cerebral aneurysm	39		1	0	1
Post-hypophysectomy	42	24–68	4	8	9
Sarcoidosis	42		0	1	1
Metastatic cancer	56	32–72	6	5	8
			(58%)	(42%)	

* Longer than 6 months or until death.
† Median age of entire group = 24 years.
‡ 16 cases were of craniopharyngioma.
§ 5 cases were glioma, 7 germinoma, and 4 craniopharyngioma.

usually associated with fractures of the skull, caused diabetes insipidus in 24 patients and were associated with anterior hypopituitarism in about one-sixth of patients. Spontaneous remissions of traumatic diabetes insipidus may occur even after 6 months, presumably because of regeneration of disrupted axons within the pituitary stalk. (4) *Idiopathic diabetes insipidus* (in 34 patients) usually starts in childhood and is seldom (<20 percent of patients) associated with anterior pituitary dysfunction. This diagnosis can be made only after a careful search has failed to reveal a tumor, infiltrative or vascular lesion, or other presumptive cause of AVP deficiency. The presence of anterior hypopituitarism or hyperprolactinemia or radiologic evidence of lesions in or above the sella should stimulate a continuing search for a causative lesion at 3- to 12-month intervals. The diagnosis of idiopathic diabetes insipidus is made with increasing confidence as the duration of negative findings on follow-up increases. The number of neurons in the supraoptic and paraventricular nuclei may be decreased in idiopathic diabetes insipidus, and circulating antibodies to hypothalamic nuclei may be present. In rare instances, diabetes insipidus may be inherited as an isolated autosomal dominant defect or as part of an autosomal recessive syndrome (DIDMOAD) consisting of diabetes insipidus (DI), diabetes mellitus (DM), optic atrophy (OA), and deafness (D) (also called the *Wolfram syndrome*; see Chap. 340). (5) Seven patients had nontraumatic encephalomalacia from a variety of causes, including shock, cardiopulmonary arrest, hypertensive encephalopathy, poisoning, and meningitis; each was brain dead and maintained on total life support systems. Central diabetes insipidus has also been reported in patients with lymphocytic hypophysitis and AIDS. The diabetes insipidus in the latter group can be due to central nervous system (CNS) infection with herpes simplex virus, *Toxoplasma gondii*, or cytomegalovirus; lymphoma of the CNS has also been reported.

Diabetes insipidus may appear during pregnancy and cease a few days after delivery, or it may commence after parturition in women with Sheehan's syndrome, especially when cortisol deficiency is treated. Mild symptoms of diabetes insipidus may either worsen or improve during pregnancy. AVP-resistant diabetes insipidus also may develop during pregnancy, perhaps owing to increased circulating levels of placental vasopressinase. Fortunately, such patients respond to treatment with desmopressin.

CLINICAL MANIFESTATIONS *Polyuria, excessive thirst*, and *polydipsia* are invariably present in diabetes insipidus. Characteristically, these symptoms are sudden in onset, both when the disorder first becomes manifest and when the effects of administered vasopressin disappear during long-term therapy. In severe cases, the urine is pale in color, and the volume may be immense (up to 16 to 24 L/d), requiring micturition every 30 to 60 min throughout the day and night. More frequently, however, urine volume is only moderately increased (2.5 to 6 L/d) and causes no complaints in subjects who become accustomed to excessive water turnover. Urinary concentration of less than 290 mmol/kg (specific gravity less than 1.010) is usual, but the concentration may be higher than that of serum when subjects with mild disease are deprived of fluids.

The slight rise in serum osmolality resulting from hypotonic polyuria stimulates thirst. Large volumes of fluid are imbibed, and cold drinks are preferred, patients often going to great trouble to secure cold fluids. Although thirst is probably secondary to loss of water, the administration of vasopressin may relieve or reduce thirst, even in the absence of fluid intake.

Normal function of the thirst center ensures that polydipsia closely matches polyuria, so dehydration is seldom detectable except by a mild elevation of serum sodium. However, when replenishment of excreted water is inadequate, severe dehydration may cause weakness, fever, psychic disturbances, hypotension, tachycardia, prostration, and death. These features are associated with a rising serum osmolality and serum sodium concentration, the latter sometimes exceeding 175 mmol/L. Adipsia does not occur in idiopathic diabetes insipidus, but it may result from impairment of the hypothalamic thirst center because

of extension of the same process that caused the diabetes insipidus. Alternatively, dehydration can occur during unconsciousness produced by surgical anesthesia, head trauma, or other causes.

Hydronephrosis and renal failure may complicate polyuria, especially in patients who fail to empty their bladders adequately because of bladder atony, urethral strictures, or other causes.

DIAGNOSTIC TESTS The cause of hypotonic polyuria can usually be recognized by a pragmatic clinical approach. Even though stimuli such as nausea, nicotine administration, hypoglycemia, and hypotension may release AVP, the results are clinically irrelevant. It is of little consequence to the patient with symptomatic diabetes insipidus that one or more nonosmotic stimuli retain their capacity to release AVP. Procedures that utilize plasma and urine osmolality determinations are readily available, reliable, and safe, and they allow the physician to establish the diagnosis and to initiate therapy rapidly. Measurements of plasma or urine AVP are expensive and time-consuming and are only occasionally needed, when osmolality measurements are inconclusive (Fig. 330-4). Diagnostic tests should not be performed in the presence of untreated thyroid or adrenocortical deficiency or when there is an osmotic diuresis (e.g., uncontrolled diabetes mellitus).

Assessment of the Relation of Plasma to Urine Osmolality The normal relationship between plasma osmolality (assuming no increase in blood urea or glucose) and urine osmolality is indicated in Fig. 330-3. If several simultaneously determined plasma and urine osmolalities in a patient with polyuria fall substantially to the right of the shaded area, the patient has central or nephrogenic diabetes insipidus. The latter diagnosis can be made if the response to injected vasopressin is subnormal (see "Dehydration Test," below) or if the plasma or urinary AVP concentration is increased. The practice of relating plasma to urine osmolality is useful, particularly in postoperative neurosurgical patients or after head trauma, where its use can permit quick differentiation of diabetes insipidus from parenteral fluid excess. If necessary, intravenous hydration can be slowed temporarily, and repeated plasma and urine osmolalities can be plotted as in Fig. 330-3, to determine whether the relationship is normal.

Dehydration Test Comparison of the urinary osmolality after dehydration with that after vasopressin administration is a simple and reliable way of diagnosing diabetes insipidus and of differentiating vasopressin deficiency from other causes of polyuria. This test should be combined with an assessment of the relationship between plasma and urine osmolality.

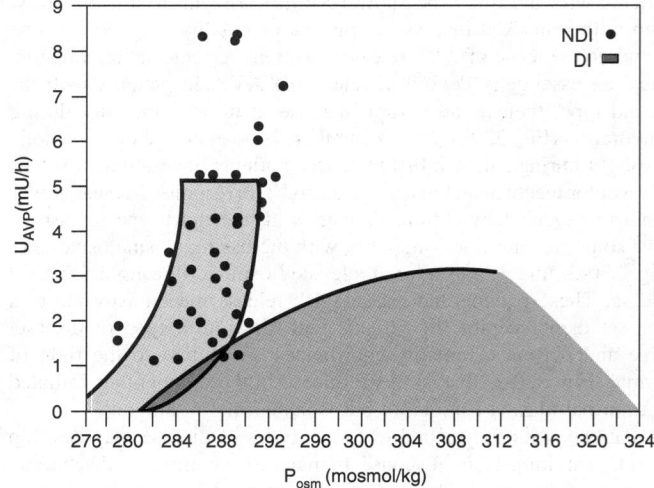

FIGURE 330-4 Relation between plasma osmolality (P_{osm}) and urinary AVP excretion (U_{AVP}) in normal subjects (*shaded area on left*), patients with central diabetes insipidus (*shaded area on right*), and patients with nephrogenic diabetes insipidus (*individual data points*). Correlates in patients with SIADH and with some other types of hyponatremia fall to the left of the normal range. [*From AM Moses, in Frontiers of Hormone Research, vol 13: Diabetes Insipidus in Man, P Czernichow, AG Robinson (eds). Basel, Karger, 1985.*]

The maximal urinary concentrating capacity varies among individuals, and no absolute lower limits of "normal" can be defined in patients with nonspecific illnesses in whom AVP is produced in adequate amounts. It is impossible to distinguish between deficiency and sufficiency of AVP release solely by the level of the urinary osmolality attained after specified periods of water deprivation. On the other hand, if after prolonged dehydration vasopressin administration induces a further rise in urinary osmolality, there is a strong implication that vasopressin deficiency exists.

Procedure

1. Fluids are withheld long enough to result in stable hourly urinary osmolalities (an hourly increase of <30 mmol/kg for at least three successive hours). This goal is usually associated with a loss in body weight of at least 1 kg. In patients whose daily urinary volume exceeds 10 liters, the fluid deprivation should begin between 4 A.M. and 6 A.M. so that the patient can be carefully watched and the test terminated if weight loss exceeds 2 kg or the clinical condition deteriorates. In patients whose urinary volumes are only mildly increased or who are hyponatremic, water deprivation may be started about midnight.
2. Urine specimens are collected hourly for osmolality measurements from 6 A.M. at least until noon and preferably until the osmolality remains stable for three consecutive hours.
3. After the third hour of stable urinary osmolality, the patient is given vasopressin as 5 units of aqueous arginine vasopressin or 1 μg of desmopressin by subcutaneous injection or 10 μg of desmopressin by nasal spray.
4. Plasma osmolality is determined immediately before the injection of vasopressin, and urinary osmolality is measured on the specimen collected between 30 and 60 min after the injection.

Vital signs should be monitored during the procedure, but when the test is performed as described adverse effects are rare.

Interpretation In subjects with normal pituitary function, urinary osmolality does not rise by more than 9 percent after the injection of vasopressin, whatever the maximal urinary osmolality achieved after dehydration alone. In central diabetes insipidus, the rise in urinary osmolality after vasopressin administration exceeds 9 percent. To ensure adequacy of dehydration, plasma osmolality before the vasopressin injection should be above 288 mmol/kg. Patients who have polyuria from renal diseases, potassium depletion, or nephrogenic diabetes insipidus (see below) usually show little rise in urinary osmolality with dehydration and no further rise after vasopressin injection. Patients with compulsive water drinking (primary polydipsia) often require prolonged water deprivation before plasma osmolality reaches 288 mmol/kg and before a plateau in urinary osmolality is reached; urinary osmolality rises by <9 percent after the administration of exogenous vasopressin.

Hypertonic Saline Infusion This test is sometimes necessary to differentiate between primary polydipsia and partial central diabetes insipidus. In the former condition the osmotic threshold is low, normal, or slightly increased, while in the latter it is substantially increased or absent. The saline infusion test is more precise and gives more quantitative data than dehydration. However, some patients cannot tolerate the saline, and the procedure is technically demanding. (See the bibliography for sources giving details.)

DIFFERENTIAL DIAGNOSIS Diabetes insipidus must be distinguished from other types of hypotonic polyuria (primary polydipsia and nephrogenic diabetes insipidus) and from states of osmotic diuresis (Table 330-2). Several types are recognizable by the history (e.g., types that occur following lithium or mannitol administration, surgery under methoxyflurane anesthesia, or renal transplantation). In other types, the physical examination or simple laboratory procedures will indicate the diagnosis (evidence of glycosuria, renal disease, sickle cell anemia, hypercalcemia, or potassium depletion, including primary aldosteronism).

Congenital nephrogenic diabetes insipidus is an X-linked recessive disorder resulting from mutations in the V_2 (antidiuretic) receptor gene

Table 330-2

Major Polyuric Syndromes

Primary disorders of water intake or output
A. Excessive water intake
  1. Psychogenic polydipsia
  2. Hypothalamic disease: histiocytosis X, sarcoidosis, trauma
  3. Drug-induced polydipsia
    a. Thioridazine
    b. Chlorpromazine
    c. Anticholinergic drugs (dry mouth)
B. Inadequate tubular reabsorption of filtered water
  1. Vasopressin deficiency
    a. Central diabetes insipidus
    b. Drug-induced inhibition of AVP release
      (1) Narcotic antagonists
  2. Renal tubular unresponsiveness to AVP
    a. Nephrogenic diabetes insipidus (congenital and familial)
    b. Nephrogenic diabetes insipidus (acquired)
      (1) Several chronic renal diseases, after obstructive uropathy, unilateral renal arterial stenosis, after renal transplantation, after acute tubular necrosis
      (2) Potassium deficiencies, including primary aldosteronism
      (3) Chronic hypercalcemias, including hyperparathyroidism
      (4) Drug-induced: lithium, methoxyflurane anesthesia, demeclocycline
      (5) Various systemic disorders: multiple myeloma, amyloidosis, sickle cell anemia, Sjögren's syndrome

Primary disorders of renal absorption of solutes (osmotic diuresis)
A. Glucose: diabetes mellitus
B. Salts, especially sodium chloride
  1. Various chronic renal diseases, especially chronic pyelonephritis
  2. After various diuretics, including mannitol

located at the q28 region of the X chromosome. More than 50 V_2 receptor mutations have been characterized. Affected males are totally resistant to vasopressin, while heterozygote females are usually asymptomatic but may have varying degrees of polyuria, rarely severe. Females with severe symptoms are thought to have skewed X chromosome inactivation resulting in predominant expression of the mutant allele. Nephrogenic diabetes insipidus may also be inherited as an autosomal recessive defect due to mutations in the aquaporin gene that result in an absent or defective water channel resistant to the action of AVP. Some women with sporadic nephrogenic diabetes insipidus (defect unknown) respond to large doses of vasopressin. V_1 receptor–mediated functions are normal in patients with congenital nephrogenic diabetes insipidus.

When patients with nephrogenic and central diabetes insipidus cannot be differentiated by simpler means, the documentation of a plasma or urinary AVP concentration that is elevated relative to plasma osmolality (Fig. 330-4) or of an AVP concentration that is high relative to urine osmolality will allow the diagnosis of nephrogenic diabetes insipidus.

Primary Polydipsia Primary or psychogenic polydipsia may be difficult to differentiate from diabetes insipidus when the polydipsia and polyuria are sustained throughout the day and night. At the other extreme, polydipsia may occur at intervals of weeks or months, a condition referred to as PIP (psychosis intermittent polydipsia). Between these extremes are individuals with various degrees of excessive water turnover. When polydipsia is extreme, dilution hyponatremia may occur even when urinary diluting capacity is normal. However, this phenomenon is rare because normal persons can excrete between 10 and 14 mL/min of solute-free water. Hyponatremia is more common when diluting capacity is impaired either by renal disease or by drugs such as nonsteroidal anti-inflammatory agents or thiazide diuretics.

We evaluated 22 women and 14 men (median age, 38) with symptomatic primary polydipsia. In 13 there was no definable cause, and 12 had a variety of psychiatric illnesses, often treated with medications having anticholinergic side effects such as dry mouth. Two had CNS

FIGURE 330-5   Approach to hypotonic polyurias.

sarcoidosis, two had antecedent head trauma, and two developed symptoms after becoming toxic from vitamin A or tretinoin. The disease in four was related to prolonged lactation, lithium therapy, chronic stomatitis, and hypertension. One was the sister of a subject with congenital nephrogenic diabetes insipidus.

The diagnosis of primary polydipsia is usually evident from the combination of low plasma and urinary osmolalities. The relationship between urine and plasma osmolality during water deprivation is typically normal or supranormal (to the left of normal in Fig. 330-3). There is little or no rise in urine osmolality after injection of vasopressin at the plateau of urine osmolality during dehydration. However, chronic overingestion of water may suppress release of AVP, and chronic polyuria may cause a wash-out of the medullary osmotic gradient, so that urine osmolality may be subnormal in relation to plasma osmolality (to the right of normal in Fig. 330-3). Therefore, it may be difficult, if not impossible, to differentiate primary polydipsia from partial central diabetes insipidus. Indeed, patients may have both problems. Treatment of these patients with vasopressin, even under close supervision, usually results in water intoxication.

A simple diagnostic approach to patients with hypotonic polyuria is shown in Fig. 330-5.

Determination of the Cause of Hypotonic Polyuria   Once the type of the hypotonic polyuria is established, the cause must be determined (see "Etiology," above). Although treatment of the underlying disease rarely causes the polyuria to regress, the underlying disease may be treated with success (e.g., germinoma). In this sense, the development of the polyuria can be considered a tumor marker.

The history can reveal important clues, such as the age of onset and duration of disease, its presence in other members of the family, the constancy of symptoms, a preference for cold or lukewarm fluids, head trauma, evidence of anterior pituitary deficiency, or symptoms suggesting a space-occupying lesion. Examination may reveal evidence of endocrine deficiency or excess (particularly hyperprolactinemia) or of malignant, granulomatous, or infectious disease. Routine laboratory tests and chest radiographs may provide important information.

Most patients with newly diagnosed central diabetes insipidus and primary polydipsia should have a magnetic resonance imaging study of the pituitary-hypothalamic area. In addition to providing insight into the underlying pathologic abnormality, the presence or absence of the posterior pituitary hyperintense signal with appropriate T1-weighted imaging may confirm the diagnosis, since the signal is absent in central diabetes insipidus and present in primary polydipsia. Information obtained from lumbar puncture or even, at times, hypothalamic biopsy may diagnose lesions observed by magnetic resonance imaging. If magnetic resonance imaging is negative in patients with central diabetes insipidus, it should be repeated at increasing time intervals.

℞ **TREATMENT**
(See Table 330-3.) Aqueous arginine vasopressin may be administered subcutaneously in doses of 5 to 10 units and usually has a duration of action of 3 to 6 h. The main use of this preparation is in initial management of unconscious patients with acute onset of diabetes insipidus following head trauma or a neurosurgical procedure. The short duration of action of this agent allows recognition of the recovery of neurohypophyseal function and minimizes the development of water intoxication in patients receiving intravenous fluids.

Desmopressin has a prolonged antidiuretic activity and is almost completely devoid of pressor effects. When used intranasally in amounts between 10 and 20 μg (0.1 to 0.2 mL) or by subcutaneous or intravenous injection (1 to 4 μg), it exerts an antidiuretic action for 10 to 24 h in most patients. This analogue is the drug of choice in the treatment of most patients with diabetes insipidus. Lypressin is a nasal spray; a single application may result in an antidiuresis lasting approximately 4 to 6 h. Nasal absorption of both analogues may be decreased in the presence of an upper respiratory infection or allergic rhinitis. In such circumstances and in unconscious or uncooperative patients with diabetes insipidus, desmopressin should be given by subcutaneous or intravenous injection.

Patients with diabetes insipidus who have some residual releasable AVP (types 2 to 4 disease) may respond to oral treatment

Table 330-3

Agents Used in Treatment of Central Diabetes Insipidus

Route of Administration	Product Description	Chemical Composition	Concentration	Amount Administered and Mean Duration of Activity, h*
Intranasal	DDAVP or desmopressin acetate by rhinal tube or nasal spray	Desmopressin acetate	100 μg/mL	10 μg (0.1 mL) → 12 15 μg (0.15 mL) → 16 20 μg (0.2 mL) → 20
	Diapid nasal spray	Lypressin (lysine vasopressin)	50 USP units (185 μg)/mL	2–4 U → 4–6
Subcutaneous or intravenous	DDAVP injectable	Desmopressin acetate	4 μg/mL	0.5 μg → 10 1.0 μg → 14 2.0 μg → 18 4.0 μg → 22
Subcutaneous	Pitressin (aqueous)	Arginine vasopressin	50 μg (20 USP units)/mL	12.5 μg (5 U) → 4
Oral nonhormonal agents	Chlorpropamide		100- and 250-mg tablets	200–500 mg → 12–24
	Clofibrate		500-mg capsules	500 mg qid → 24 or more
	Carbamazepine		200-mg tablets	400–600 mg → 24

* All the listed durations of action are variable between patients but quite consistent in individual patients. Desmopressin acetate is also marketed in far higher concentrations (1.5 mg/mL) as Stimate for treatment of bleeding disorders.

with chlorpropamide, clofibrate, or carbamazepine. Chlorpropamide stimulates AVP release and potentiates the antidiuretic action of submaximal amounts of AVP. Doses of 200 to 500 mg, usually taken once daily, are sufficient for an antidiuretic response. The action of this agent starts within several hours of administration and usually lasts for 24 h. Chlorpropamide also may restore thirst perception and thus be useful in patients with thirst center defects. Oral agents are used rarely because of hypoglycemia and other undesirable side effects.

Primary polydipsia can be treated effectively only by eliminating the underlying problem. However, clozapine may improve the PIP syndrome in the subset of polydipsia patients with schizophrenia.

The only way to treat most patients with nephrogenic diabetes insipidus is by solute restriction and the administration of thiazides or other diuretics. The resulting sodium depletion causes a fall in glomerular filtration rate with enhanced reabsorption of fluid in the proximal portion of the nephron and decreased delivery of sodium to the ascending limb of the loop of Henle and consequently reduced capacity to dilute the urine. Some women with congenital nephrogenic diabetes insipidus and some patients with lithium-induced polyuria have been treated effectively by injecting large doses of desmopressin.

When antidiuretic therapy is initiated in patients with long-standing diabetes insipidus, care must be taken to avoid excessive drinking, which could result in water intoxication. Education about drinking water and other liquids according to thirst must be reinforced constantly in some patients. Excessive fluid intake may be more common and severe in subjects whose diabetes insipidus is due to sarcoidosis or lymphoma. Adipsic patients with diabetes insipidus are difficult to manage. Intake and output of fluids, body weight, vital signs, serum sodium, and renal function must be monitored closely. Fluid intake must approximate urine volume and fluid losses by other routes. Otherwise, such individuals can develop hypernatremia and circulatory collapse without becoming thirsty. Patients who are confused, obtunded, or unconscious must be monitored in the same way. Special care must be taken when patients with treated diabetes insipidus are subjected to procedures that require fluid restriction, as in preparation for an intravenous pyelogram, or hydration, as after administration of chemotherapy. In the former situation, fluid intake must be restricted to conform to urine output. In patients receiving antidiuretic therapy, fluids should not be administered beyond the amounts determined by thirst or urine output. If high urine flow rates are necessary, antidiuretic therapy can be discontinued, or furosemide may be administered while antidiuretic therapy is continued.

SYNDROMES ASSOCIATED WITH VASOPRESSIN EXCESS

Excessive blood levels or actions of vasopressin are associated with and probably cause water retention in several circumstances:

1. As a mechanism for *prevention of a rise in plasma osmolality*, which would otherwise result from sodium retention in edema associated with congestive heart failure, cirrhosis with ascites, nephrosis, orthostatic edema, myxedema, and treatment with sodium-retaining drugs (fludrocortisone, nonsteroidal anti-inflammatory agents, and others)
2. As a mechanism of *defense against hypovolemia and/or hypotension* in subjects with adrenal insufficiency, excessive fluid loss (from vomiting, diarrhea, drug-induced diuresis, or excessive sweating), fluid deprivation, and probably positive-pressure respiration
3. As a consequence of *drug- or disease-induced release of vasopressin from the neurohypophysis* caused by
   a. *Central nervous system disorders*: head trauma, subdural hematoma, subarachnoid hemorrhage, cerebral vascular thrombosis, brain tumor, cerebral atrophy, acute encephalitis, acute psychosis, tuberculous and other meningitides

Table 330-4

Causes of SIADH

Malignant neoplasms with autonomous AVP release	Cerebral atrophy
Small cell carcinoma of lung	Acute encephalitis
Carcinoma of pancreas	Tuberculous meningitis
Lymphoma, lymphocytic	Purulent meningitis
lymphoma, Hodgkin's disease	Guillain-Barré syndrome
Carcinoma of duodenum	Lupus erythematosus
Thymoma	Acute intermittent porphyria
Nonmalignant pulmonary diseases	**Drugs**
Tuberculosis	Chlorpropamide
Lung abscess	Vincristine
Pneumonia	Vinblastine
Viral pneumonitis	Cyclophosphamide
Empyema	Carbamazepine
Chronic obstructive airways	Oxytocin
disease	General anesthesia
Central nervous system disorders	Narcotics
Skull fracture	Tricyclic antidepressants
Subdural hematoma	**Miscellaneous causes**
Subarachnoid hemorrhage	Hypothyroidism
Cerebral vascular thrombosis	Positive pressure respiration

   b. *Drugs that release or potentiate the action of AVP*: chlorpropamide, vincristine, vinblastine, cyclophosphamide, carbamazepine, general anesthetics, tricyclic antidepressants
4. *In ectopic AVP production and release*:
   a. *From neoplastic tissue*: small cell carcinoma of lung, pancreatic carcinoma, lymphoma, Hodgkin's disease, lymphocytic lymphoma, thymoma, carcinoma of duodenum or bladder
   b. *From inflammatory lung diseases*: tuberculosis, lung abscess, pneumonias, empyema
5. *Other conditions*: Guillain-Barré syndrome, lupus erythematosus, acute intermittent porphyria, severe renovascular hypertension, and old age

SYNDROME OF INAPPROPRIATE AVP SECRETION The syndrome of inappropriate AVP secretion [commonly termed the syndrome of inappropriate antidiuretic hormone (SIADH)] is applied to vasopressin excess of types 3 to 5 listed above, which are associated with hyponatremia without edema (Table 330-4). In these patients, the AVP excess is considered to be inappropriate because it occurs in the presence of plasma hyposmolality. SIADH is analogous to abnormalities produced by administration of vasopressin and water to normal subjects. Although it may be conceptually valid to consider the AVP excess to be inappropriate in adrenal insufficiency and in the edematous, hypovolemic, and hypotensive disorders listed in entries 1 and 2 above, the different pathogenic mechanisms and treatments make it advisable not to consider these disorders as variants of SIADH.

Pathogenesis of SIADH The ectopic origin of authentic AVP from neoplasms and pulmonary tissue of the types listed above has been documented by tissue analysis. Neoplastic cells obtained from the tumors of patients with SIADH can synthesize, store, and release AVP. Both AVP and its associated neurophysin are elevated in the plasma of over 60 percent of patients with small cell carcinoma of the lung. There is an excellent correlation between the increases in plasma AVP and neurophysin concentrations on the one hand and the clinical responses to treatment or the recurrences of disease on the other. Vasopressin also has been demonstrated in tuberculous lung tissue. Intracranial lesions (meningitis, encephalitis, trauma, vascular accidents) probably stimulate release of AVP from the neurohypophysis, possibly acting through cytokine-mediated mechanisms. Some drugs, such as vincristine, chlorpropamide, and carbamazepine, stimulate release of AVP from the neurohypophyseal system, and others (e.g., chlorpropamide and nonsteroidal anti-inflammatory agents) potentiate the antidiuretic action of secreted AVP.

Excessive release or an excessive renal tubular effect of vasopressin results in the excretion of a concentrated urine (with a urinary osmolality usually over 300 mmol/kg) despite a subnormal plasma osmolality and serum sodium concentration. Sodium excretion in the urine is maintained (usually above 20 mmol/L) by hypervolemia, suppression of the renin-angiotensin-aldosterone system, and an increased plasma concentration of atrial natriuretic peptide. However, the urinary sodium concentration may be below 20 mmol/L if sodium intake is low but is higher if sodium intake is unrestricted. Blood urea nitrogen and uric acid concentrations tend to fall because of plasma dilution and increased excretion of nitrogenous compounds. Because of the hypervolemia blood pressure shows no orthostatic fall, but in spite of hypervolemia there is no recumbent hypertension (except when plasma angiotensin II is simultaneously elevated) and no peripheral edema (for unknown reasons). The extracellular hypotonicity leads to intracellular swelling, and severe symptoms may result from cerebral edema.

Clinical Manifestations of SIADH   In general, the rate of fall in serum sodium concentration is more important in producing the neurologic features of SIADH than the absolute magnitude of the fall. When SIADH is mild, with serum Na concentrations of 130 to 135 mmol/L, or develops gradually over several weeks, symptoms may be absent or limited to anorexia, nausea, and vomiting, as in other forms of hyponatremia. When hyponatremia is severe or acute in onset, body weight increases, and the symptoms of cerebral edema are predominant, including restlessness, irritability, confusion, coma, and convulsions associated with nonspecific electroencephalographic changes. Pitting edema is almost always absent.

Diagnosis   SIADH should be suspected in patients who have hyponatremia and a concentrated urine (osmolality >300 mmol/kg) associated with lethargy and in the absence of edema, orthostatic hypotension, and features of dehydration. The diagnosis of SIADH is made when other causes of enhanced AVP release are excluded. The diagnosis is supported by the finding of blood urea nitrogen, serum uric acid, creatinine, and albumin concentrations in the low-normal or subnormal range. However, it is essential in making the diagnosis to differentiate SIADH from (1) the *dilutional hyponatremias* listed in entry 2 above, particularly adrenocortical insufficiency, in which orthostatic hypotension, tachycardia, and an elevated or high-normal blood urea nitrogen are characteristic; (2) the *edematous states* listed in entry 1 above, particularly hypothyroidism and congestive heart failure with hyponatremia; (3) *hypertensive states* associated with hyponatremia caused by renovascular stenosis or diuretic therapy; (4) *primary polydipsia*, which is always associated with a dilute urine (osmolality <150 mmol/kg); (5) *pseudohyponatremia* associated with excessive plasma glucose, triglyceride, or protein concentrations; and (6) the *"sick-cell" syndrome*, in which hyponatremia is due to a subnormal setting of the hypothalamic osmoreceptors, associated usu-

ally with a chronic, debilitating disease. Conditions (1) through (5) in this list are easily recognizable by the associated plasma abnormalities.

When the diagnosis of SIADH is not obvious after other causes of hyponatremia have been excluded, a positive diagnosis can usually be made with a *water-load test*. The water-load test is particularly useful in differentiating patients with a low-set osmoreceptor (who excrete the water normally) from all other hyponatremic states associated with a concentrated urine. This test should not be performed unless or until the serum sodium concentration has been elevated to a safe level (above 125 mmol/L) by restriction of water intake and/or, if necessary, by saline administration. The patient is asked to drink the water load (20 mL/kg of body weight up to 1500 mL) in 10 to 20 min, and urine is collected in hourly samples, with the patient recumbent between voidings, for 4 to 5 h in the morning. At least 65 percent of the water load should be excreted in 4 h or 80 percent in 5 h, and the lowest urinary osmolality, usually reached in the second hour, should be below 100 mmol/kg. It is essential to restrict further water intake for the rest of the day to prevent water intoxication in patients who fail to excrete the water load normally. Failure to excrete the water load may occur in adrenal insufficiency or renal insufficiency, as well as in SIADH. It is important to appreciate, too, that SIADH cannot be diagnosed in the presence of severe pain, nausea, "stress," hypovolemia, hypotension, or other conditions that can stimulate AVP release even in the presence of plasma hypotonicity.

Measurements of plasma or urinary AVP (P_{AVP}, U_{AVP}) are useful adjuncts in establishing the diagnosis of SIADH. Plasma AVP is often unmeasurable in hyponatremic states but is detectable, even after a water load, in SIADH. The correlates of plasma osmolality (P_{osm}) versus P_{AVP} or U_{AVP} concentration fall to the left of the normal values in SIADH (Fig. 330-4) and in the other hyponatremic states associated with a concentrated urine. Thus, in most patients with SIADH, P_{AVP} and U_{AVP} concentrations, which may fluctuate widely, are unrelated to concomitant changes in P_{osm} Occasionally, this lack of correlation between P_{osm} and P_{AVP} or U_{AVP} may be inconsistent. Rarely, for instance, the baseline, unstimulated AVP level may be inappropriately elevated and may fail to change as P_{osm} is raised until the P_{osm} reaches the normal range. Further increases in P_{osm} induced by hypertonic saline infusion or water deprivation may then result in normal or subnormal increases in P_{AVP} or U_{AVP}. This unusual phenomenon may reflect uncontrolled "leakage" of AVP into the circulation.

The diagnostic approach to SIADH is depicted in Fig. 330-6.

℞ TREATMENT

Restriction of fluid intake to 800 to 1000 mL daily is essential. Since this intake is almost always exceeded by urinary output plus insensible fluid loss, a negative water balance ensues that results in gradual, daily reduction in weight, a progressive rise in serum Na concentration and osmolality, and symptomatic improvement. It is useful to verify the effectiveness of fluid restriction by documenting the changes in weight and serum Na concentration daily, until serum Na exceeds 135 mmol/L.

Unless and until the underlying cause of the SIADH can be corrected, fluid intake should be restricted continuously, to maintain

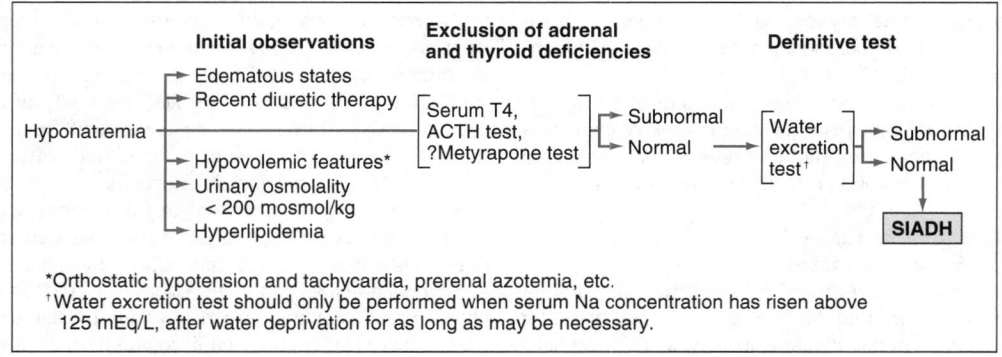

FIGURE 330-6   Approach to diagnosis of SIADH in patients with hyponatremia.

normonatremia. In addition to restriction of fluid intake, 200 to 300 mL of 3% or 5% sodium chloride solution should be infused intravenously over 3 to 4 h in patients with severe confusion, convulsions, or coma. To avoid the possibility of inducing pontine myelinosis, the serum Na concentration should not be raised too rapidly. The possibility of causing congestive heart failure by infusing hypertonic saline is remote as long as fluid is restricted and may be further reduced by the simultaneous intravenous administration of furosemide.

Attempts should be made to identify and correct the cause of the SIADH as soon as possible. The administration of water-retaining drugs should be stopped. Treatment of hypothyroidism should be initiated. Pulmonary tuberculosis and other pulmonary infections should be treated appropriately, and meningitis or other CNS disorders should be treated, if present. When a malignant tumor is the source of autonomous AVP release and SIADH, surgery, radiation, and/or chemotherapy is often beneficial even if the underlying neoplasm cannot be cured.

Antagonism of the release or action of AVP is seldom successful. Although phenytoin inhibits AVP release, it is seldom effective in SIADH. Drugs that block the effect of AVP on the renal tubule are occasionally useful. Demeclocycline is the most potent inhibitor of AVP action available for chronic administration, in doses of 900 to 1200 mg/d. Patients receiving demeclocycline should be followed carefully to detect any evidence of renal failure, bacterial superinfection, or excessive drug-induced water loss. Lithium salts interfere with the action of AVP on tubular water reabsorption and can cause polyuria by this mechanism. Unfortunately, lithium can cause serious side effects in hyponatremic patients and, for this reason, is not recommended for treatment of SIADH.

Prognosis The prognosis of SIADH depends on the cause. Drug-induced SIADH is rapidly and completely corrected by withdrawal of the causative agent. Similarly, treatment of pulmonary or CNS infections can result in improvement and eventual cure of SIADH. Although SIADH resulting from small cell carcinoma of the lung or other malignancies can often be controlled with rigorous restriction of fluid intake, the underlying malignancy determines the prognosis.

PARAVENTRICULAR-NEUROHYPOPHYSEAL SYSTEM AND OXYTOCIN

CHEMISTRY AND PHYSIOLOGY Oxytocin, a nonapeptide that differs by two amino acids from vasopressin, is produced in the cell bodies of the paraventricular nuclei and to a lesser extent in those of the supraoptic nuclei. It is synthesized and transported in neurosecretory granules by way of neuronal axons to the neurohypophysis, where it is stored or released, in conjunction with an oxytocin-specific neurophysin. Oxytocin release is stimulated by nerve impulses from the hypothalamus that cause depolarization of the neurosecretory terminals of the posterior pituitary and subsequent release of oxytocin through a calcium-dependent process, similar to the mechanism for vasopressin release. Estrogen stimulates release of oxytocin and its neurophysin. The secretion of oxytocin, as well as of vasopressin, is inhibited by ethanol. Some stimuli such as pain apparently cause simultaneous release of oxytocin and vasopressin but most stimuli cause the two hormones to be released independently. Oxytocin is liberated during suckling, whereas vasopressin is released in much greater quantities than is oxytocin after an osmotic stimulus or hemorrhage. Manipulation or distention of the female genital tract, artificially or during parturition, is a more effective stimulus of oxytocin release than suckling.

Oxytocin acts on the membranes of myometrial and myoepithelial cells to cause an increased force of contraction. The sensitivity of the myometrium to oxytocin increases with the duration of pregnancy, and a role for oxytocin in the initiation and maintenance of labor is probable. Oxytocin may have survival value to the offspring, since it may hasten the final stages of birth and lessen the chances of anoxia. Oxytocin also exerts a contractile action on the myometrium post

partum and causes contraction of the myoepithelial cells of the mammary alveoli, causing them to expel milk from the secretory tissue to the nipple. In the human oxytocin is 100 times more potent than vasopressin in its milk-ejecting activity. In contrast, the antidiuretic potency of oxytocin is about 200 times less than that of vasopressin. Oxytocin probably does not exert any significant physiologic effects other than those on the uterus and breast.

One milligram of a purified oxytocin preparation contains 450 IU of hormone, and the amount of oxytocin in the posterior pituitary is similar to that of vasopressin. Even though oxytocin has no known role in the male, the male neural lobe stores oxytocin in amounts similar to those in the female. The plasma oxytocin concentration in both men and women exhibits episodic increases, with values ranging from about 1 to 4 pmol/L (1.25 to 5 ng/L) but with no diurnal variation. In normal women, there is a midcycle increase in plasma oxytocin concentration from a preovulatory value of about 2 pmol/L (2.5 ng/L) to a peak value of 4 to 8 pmol/L (5 to 10 ng/L) at the time of ovulation. During labor, plasma oxytocin concentrations increase and then fall rapidly after delivery to prepartum levels. During suckling, the plasma oxytocin levels of the mother are usually about 10 to 20 pmol/L (12 to 25 ng/L). The half-life of oxytocin in plasma is about 3 to 5 min. Oxytocin is removed from the circulation mainly by the kidneys and liver, although the uterus and mammary gland may remove some.

CLINICAL USE OF OXYTOCIN The clinical use of oxytocin is limited to the induction of labor, control of hemorrhage following incomplete abortion and curettage, and treatment of impaired milk ejection. For discussion of the obstetric uses of oxytocin, the reader is referred to textbooks on obstetrics. Care must be taken because oxytocin may cause uterine rupture and fetal death. The antidiuretic action of oxytocin can be elicited with single intravenous doses of as little as 100 mU. Maximal antidiuresis is reached with 40 to 50 mU/min. Since 10 to 40 units of oxytocin per liter of intravenous fluid may be used in obstetric practice, water intoxication may result. The vasodilatory action of oxytocin may cause hypotension, tachycardia, arrhythmias, and sudden death in obstetric patients with heart disease. Anesthetics may modify the cardiovascular responses to oxytocin. For instance, in patients under cyclopropane anesthesia, oxytocin causes more hypotension but less tachycardia than in unanesthetized subjects. The vasodilatory effect of oxytocin can be blocked by vasopressin.

Please refer to Chap. 30 in Goodman & Gilman's The Pharmacological Basis of Therapeutics, *9th ed, McGraw-Hill, New York, 1996.*

BIBLIOGRAPHY

CROSS BA, LENG G: *Progress in Brain Research*, vol 60: *The Neurohypophysis: Structure, Function and Control*. Amsterdam, Elsevier, 1983

CZERNICHOW P, ROBINSON AG: *Frontiers of Hormone Research*, vol 13: *Diabetes Insipidus in Man*. Basel, Karger, 1985

DURR JA: Diabetes insipidus in pregnancy. Am J Kidney Dis 9:276, 1987

KNOERS NVAM et al: Inheritance of mutations in the V₂ receptor gene in thirteen families with nephrogenic diabetes insipidus. Kidney Int 46:170, 1994

LEADBETTER RA, SHUTTY MS JR: Differential effects of neuroleptics and clozapine on polydipsia and intermittent hyponatremia. J Clin Psychiatry 55:9(Suppl B), 1994

MCLEOD JF et al: Familial neurohypophyseal diabetes insipidus associated with a signal peptide mutation. J Clin Endocrinol Metab 77:599, 1993

MILLER M et al: Recognition of partial defects in antidiuretic hormone secretion. Ann Intern Med 73:721, 1970

MOSES AM: Osmotic thresholds for AVP release using plasma and urine AVP and free water clearance. Am J Physiol 256:R892, 1989

———, CLAYTON B: Impairment of osmotically stimulated AVP release in patients with primary polydipsia. Am J Physiol 265:R1247, 1993

———, STREETEN DHP: Pathophysiologic and pharmacologic alterations in the release and action of ADH. Metabolism 25:697, 1976

——— et al: Marked hypotonic polyuria resulting from nephrogenic diabetes insipidus with partial sensitivity to vasopressin. J Clin Endocrinol Metab 59:1044, 1984

—— et al: Two distinct pathophysiological mechanisms in congenital nephrogenic diabetes insipidus. J Clin Endocrinol Metab 66:1259, 1988

—— et al: The use of T_1-weighted magnetic resonance imaging to differentiate between primary polydipsia and central diabetes insipidus. Am J Neuroradiol 13:1273, 1992

REICHLIN S: *The Neurohypophysis. Physiological and Clinical Aspects.* New York, Plenum, 1984

ROBERTSON GL: The regulation of vasopressin function in health and disease. Recent Prog Hormone Res 33:333, 1977

331 *Leonard Wartofsky*

DISEASES OF THE THYROID*

Normal function of the thyroid gland is directed to the secretion of L-thyroxine (T_4) and 3,5,3'-triiodo-L-thyronine (T_3), the active thyroid hormones that influence a diversity of metabolic processes (Fig. 331-1). Diseases of the thyroid are manifested by qualitative or quantitative alterations in hormone secretion, enlargement of the thyroid (goiter), or both. Insufficient hormone secretion results in *hypothyroidism* or *myxedema*, in which decreased caloric expenditure (hypometabolism) is a principal feature. Conversely, excessive secretion of hormone results in hypermetabolism and other features, together termed *hyperthyroidism* or *thyrotoxicosis*. Enlargement of the thyroid gland (which normally weighs 15 to 18 g in adults) may be generalized or focal. Generalized enlargements may not be symmetric, the right lobe tending to enlarge more than the left. Goiters may be associated with increased, normal, or decreased hormone secretion, depending on the underlying disturbance. Focal enlargement usually reflects neoplastic disease, either benign or malignant; the former sometimes is responsible for hypersecretion of hormone and hyperthyroidism, whereas the latter rarely causes hyperthyroidism. Any goiter may compress adjacent structures in the neck or mediastinum.

EMBRYOLOGY, ANATOMY, AND HISTOLOGY

The thyroid originates embryologically from an evagination of the pharyngeal epithelium with some contribution from the lateral pharyn-

* Revision and update of work by the late Sidney Ingbar.

geal pouches. Progressive descent of the midline thyroid anlage gives rise to the thyroglossal duct, which extends from the foramen cecum near the base of the tongue to the isthmus of the thyroid. Remnants of tissue may persist along the course of this tract as "lingual thyroid," thyroglossal cysts or nodules, or a structure contiguous with the thyroid isthmus called the *pyramidal lobe*. The latter is usually not discernible except when the remainder of the gland is enlarged. Rarely, lingual thyroid may be the sole functioning thyroid tissue. In such cases, its output may or may not be sufficient to maintain a normal metabolic (euthyroid) state. Thyroid aplasia and functional failure of ectopic thyroid tissue are causes of sporadic neonatal hypothyroidism (1 in every 4000 or 5000 newborns), which responds to early treatment.

The fetal thyroid acquires the capacity to concentrate and organify iodine at about 10 weeks of gestation. Both T_4 and thyroid-stimulating hormone (TSH, thyrotropin) are detectable in the blood soon thereafter and increase in concentration during the second trimester. The increase in serum T_4 is due both to increasing thyroid secretion and to the appearance in plasma of thyroxine-binding globulin (TBG), and the increase in TSH is a reflection of the maturation of the fetal hypothalamus with resulting secretion of thyrotropin-releasing hormone (TRH). Maternal TRH readily crosses the placenta and may play a role in the development of the fetal pituitary-thyroid axis. Maternal TSH, by contrast, does not cross the placenta. T_3 is detectable in the blood later during the second trimester, but its concentration in blood and amniotic fluid remains low until shortly after parturition. By contrast, the concentration of its analogue, 3,3',5'-triiodo-L-thyronine (reverse T_3, rT_3), is increased in fetal blood and amniotic fluid relative to that in maternal blood (see Fig. 331-1). These differences are due to qualitative alterations in T_4 metabolism in the fetus. The low level of T_3 in fetal blood and amniotic fluid in the face of a high maternal concentration indicates that maternal-fetal transfer of T_3, while it occurs, is minimal, and the same is true for T_4. Hence T_4 from the fetal thyroid is the major thyroid hormone available to the fetus. Except for the possible effect of maternal TRH, therefore, the fetal pituitary-thyroid axis is a functional unit distinct from that of the mother.

The normal adult thyroid consists of two lobes joined by an isthmus and lies just anterior and caudal to the cartilages of the larynx. Fibrous septa divide the gland into pseudolobules which, in turn, are composed of vesicles, called *follicles* or *acini*, surrounded by a capillary network. Normally, the follicle walls are composed of cuboidal epithelium. The lumen is filled with a proteinaceous *colloid*, which contains a unique protein, *thyroglobulin*, within the peptide sequence of which T_4 and T_3 are synthesized and stored. The thyroid also contains a second, smaller population of cells, the C cells. They are the source of calcitonin and give rise to medullary thyroid carcinoma when they undergo malignant transformation.

FIGURE 331-1 Structural formulas of thyroxine, its precursors, and certain of its metabolites.

THYROID HORMONE ECONOMY: NORMAL PHYSIOLOGY

The term *thyroid hormone economy* denotes the processes involved in the synthesis of hormones in the thyroid gland, their transport in the circulation, their action and metabolism in the peripheral tissues, and the regulatory mechanisms that maintain a normal supply of thyroid hormones.

TSH AND THE TSH RECEPTOR

The pituitary hormone thyrotropin (TSH) controls thyroid function and acts by binding to TSH receptors (TSH-R) on the basolateral membrane of thyroid follicular cells. Binding to TSH-R leads to activation of the adenylate cyclase and phospholipase C pathways of intracellular signaling that regulate thyroid function and growth. TSH-R is a member of the G protein–coupled receptor family and is organized into three domains: an extracellular domain of 398 amino acids, a membrane-spanning domain of 266 amino acids, and an 83-amino-acid intracellular carboxy-terminal domain. This protein is encoded by a single gene more than 60 kilobases long. Somatic mutations and clonal expansion of the TSH-R gene appear to account for chronic stimulation of the cyclic adenosine monophosphate (AMP) cascade leading to toxic follicular adenomas.

HORMONE SYNTHESIS AND SECRETION The synthesis of thyroid hormone depends on entry into the thyroid of adequate quantities of iodine, a constituent of T_4 and T_3; on normal iodine metabolism in the gland; and on the synthesis of thyroglobulin, a receptor protein for iodine. The structure of thyroglobulin favors iodination and particularly the formation of T_4 and T_3. Secretion of normal quantities of hormone requires both a normal rate of hormone synthesis and hydrolysis of thyroglobulin to liberate active hormones. Iodine enters the thyroid in the form of inorganic or ionic iodide, whose source is iodide derived either from the deiodination of thyroid hormones or from iodide ingested in food, water, or medication. Formerly, a dietary iodine intake of approximately 0.2 mg/d was considered normal in the United States, and this was sufficient to sustain a plasma iodide concentration of approximately 40 nmol/L (0.5 µg/dL). However, owing to iodine contamination of some foods and to the widespread use of iodine in drugs, vitamin preparations, and antiseptic agents, the average iodine intake has increased to about 0.5 to 1.0 mg/d, with corresponding increases in plasma iodide concentration. Iodide is removed from the plasma by the thyroid, kidneys, and salivary and gastrointestinal glands, but since iodide that enters gastrointestinal secretions is reabsorbed, net clearance is effected by the thyroid and kidneys. In effect, the thyroid and kidneys compete for plasma iodide. Renal clearance is largely a function of glomerular filtration rate and is not influenced by humoral factors or plasma iodide concentration. Hence, adjustments in the rate of iodide uptake by the thyroid relative to the rate of urinary excretion are mediated by changes in thyroid rather than renal avidity.

The synthesis and secretion of the active thyroid hormones can be divided into four sequential steps, each of which is under the control of TSH (Fig. 331-2). The first involves active transport of iodide into the thyroid cell, a process mediated by a protein in the plasma membrane of these cells termed the Na^+/I^- symporter. The rate of active iodide transport exceeds the rate of passive diffusion of iodide out of the gland, so that the thyroid maintains a concentration gradient for iodide (thyroid/plasma concentration ratio), which is usually around 25 but can be 500 or more under certain conditions. Energy for iodide transport depends on oxidative metabolism in the gland.

The second step involves oxidation of iodide to a higher-valence form that is capable of iodinating tyrosyl residues in thyroglobulin, a glycoprotein of approximately 660,000 mol wt that is synthesized in the follicular cell. Oxidation of iodide is effected by a peroxidase, which uses hydrogen peroxide generated during the course of oxidative metabolism in the gland. Organic iodinations occur at the cell-colloid interface, taking place largely in newly synthesized thyroglobulin undergoing exocytosis into the follicular lumen. The consequence is the

formation of the peptide-bound precursors monoiodotyrosine (MIT) and diiodotyrosine (DIT).

In the third step, the iodotyrosines undergo oxidative condensation, again through the mediation of peroxidase. This coupling reaction occurs within the thyroglobulin molecule and yields a variety of iodothyronines, including T_4 and T_3. Although minute quantities of thyroglobulin are detectable in the blood, most thyroglobulin is retained for a time in the gland, serving as a storage vehicle for the thyroid hormones. Liberation of the active hormones into the blood involves pinocytosis of follicular colloid at the apical margin of the cells to form colloid droplets. The droplets fuse with thyroid lysosomes to form "phagolysosomes," in which thyroglobulin is hydrolyzed by proteases. The final step is release of the free iodothyronines T_4 and T_3 into the blood. The thyroid is the only source of endogenous T_4; in contrast, only about 20 percent of T_3 is produced in the thyroid, the remainder being generated in extraglandular tissues by the enzymatic removal of the 5′-iodine from the outer ring of T_4. Inactive iodotyrosines liberated by the hydrolysis of thyroglobulin are stripped of their iodine by an intrathyroid enzyme, iodotyrosine dehalogenase. Most iodide so liberated is reused in the synthesis of hormone, but a small proportion is lost into the blood (iodide leak); iodide leakage may become large under certain circumstances.

The thyroid also concentrates other monovalent anions such as pertechnetate, which is available as the radioactive isotope sodium [^{99m}Tc]pertechnetate. Unlike iodide, little pertechnetate is organically bound; hence, its duration of stay in the thyroid is short. This property, together with its short physical half-life, makes pertechnetate a valuable radionuclide for imaging the thyroid by scintillation scanning.

The foregoing reactions are subject to inhibition by a variety of agents, which are called *goitrogens* because their ability to inhibit hormone synthesis and indirectly stimulate TSH secretion enables them to induce goiter formation. Inorganic anions such as perchlorate and thiocyanate inhibit iodide transport and thereby reduce the supply of substrate for hormone formation. The goiter and hypothyroidism that follow, however, can be prevented or relieved by an amount of

FIGURE 331-2 Schema depicting pathways in the synthesis and secretion of thyroid hormones and mechanisms for the suprathyroid and intrathyroid regulation of thyroid function. *Small, solid arrows* indicate pathways of iodine metabolism; *open arrows* indicate stimulation; *cross-hatched arrows* indicate inhibitory influences. TRH, thyrotropin-releasing hormone; TSH, thyroid-stimulating hormone; IPO, iodide peroxidase; prot., thyroid protease; peptid., thyroid peptidase; MIT, monoiodotyrosine; DIT, diiodotyrosine; T_4, thyroxine; T_3, 3,5,3′-triiodothyronine.

iodide large enough to enable adequate quantities to enter the gland by passive diffusion. The commonly employed antithyroid agents, such as the derivatives of thiourea and mercaptoimidazole, exert more complex actions on hormone biosynthesis. These agents inhibit the initial oxidation (organic binding) of iodide, decrease the proportion of DIT relative to MIT, and block coupling of iodotyrosines to form the hormonally active iodothyronines. The latter reaction is the most sensitive. Thus, the synthesis of hormonally active iodothyronines may be decreased, although the total incorporation of iodine by the thyroid is affected minimally. The goitrogenic action of thioureas is not overcome by large quantities of iodine. Indeed, certain weak goitrogens, such as sulfonamides and antipyrine, are more potent when given with iodide, an effect not understood. Iodine itself, when given acutely in large doses, blocks the organic binding and coupling reactions. This action (the Wolff-Chaikoff effect) is normally transient, but prolonged administration of iodide may be associated with continued inhibition of hormone synthesis and development of goiter, with or without hypothyroidism (iodide myxedema). Many patients with Graves' disease, especially after treatment with radioiodine or surgery, or with Hashimoto's disease are sensitive to the blocking effect of iodide and develop hypothyroidism when given iodides chronically. The fetal thyroid is similarly sensitive, and pregnant women should not ingest iodide in large amounts because of the danger of inducing goitrous hypothyroidism in the fetus. Iodide in large doses is capable of inhibiting proteolysis of thyroglobulin and hormone release, an effect responsible for the ameliorative action of iodides in hyperthyroidism. Excess iodide also may induce thyrotoxicosis in susceptible individuals, as discussed below. Lithium has several effects on intrathyroidal iodine metabolism, one of which is to inhibit hormone release. Glucocorticoids causes a decrease in serum thyroid hormone levels due to inhibition of TSH secretion and decreased binding of T_4 to TBG. Serum T_3 is also decreased, in part because of inhibition of the conversion of T_4 to T_3. A direct inhibitory action of glucocorticoids on the thyroid may occur in Graves' disease, possibly by inhibition of thyroid-stimulating immunoglobulins. Dexamethasone, in conjunction with iodide, can effect a rapid reduction in the degree of thyrotoxicosis.

HORMONE TRANSPORT AND METABOLISM

HORMONE TRANSPORT   In the blood, T_4 and T_3 are almost entirely bound to plasma proteins. T_4 is bound, in decreasing order of intensity, to thyroxine-binding globulin (TBG), to a T_4-binding prealbumin (transthyretin, TTR), and to albumin. High-density lipoproteins transport about 3 percent of circulating T_4 and 6 percent of T_3. By virtue of its intense affinity for T_4, TBG is the major determinant of normal binding. T_4 interacts with its binding proteins in a reversible binding equilibrium in which most of the hormone is bound and only about 0.03 percent is free. While TTR transports only about 15 percent of circulating T_4, its contribution to free hormone is comparable to that from TBG owing to its higher dissociation constant. T_3 is not bound significantly by TTR and is bound 10 to 20 times less firmly by TBG than is T_4. As a consequence, the normal proportion of free T_3 (approximately 0.3 percent) is 8 to 10 times greater than that of T_4. Only the free or unbound hormone is available to tissues; therefore, the metabolic state correlates more closely with the concentration of free hormone than total hormone in plasma, and homeostatic regulation of thyroid function is directed toward maintenance of a normal concentration of free hormone. Moreover, the relatively weak binding of T_3 accounts for its more rapid onset and offset of action.

Disturbances of thyroid hormone–plasma protein interaction are of two general types (Table 331-1). In the first, the thyroid-pituitary axis is intrinsically normal, and the homeostatic control of thyroid hormone secretion is intact. In this situation, disordered binding interactions result from alterations in thyroid hormone binding. For example, an increase in the TBG concentration initially lowers the concentration of free hormone and thus diminishes the quantity of hormone

Table 331-1

Classification of the Varieties of Disordered Thyroid Hormone–Plasma Protein Interactions

Type of Abnormality	Serum T_4 and T_3 Levels	Percent FT_4 and FT_3 or RT_3U	FT_4 and FT_3 Levels or FT_4I and FT_3I
PRIMARY ABNORMALITY IN TBG			
Increased concentration	↑	↓	N
Decreased concentration	↓	↑	N
PRIMARY DISORDER OF THYROID FUNCTION			
Hypothyroidism	↓	↓	↓
Hyperthyroidism	↑	↑	↑

NOTE: FT_4, free T_4; FT_3, free T_3; FT_4I, free T_4 index; FT_3I, free T_3 index; N, normal; RT_3U, resin T_3 uptake; TBG, thyroid-binding globulin.

available to tissues. The total hormone concentration in serum then increases until the concentration of free hormone is restored to normal. The increase in total hormone concentration counterbalances the decrease in the free proportion; as a result, the absolute concentration of free hormone is normal, and the metabolic state of the patient is normal. Opposite changes occur when the concentration of TBG declines. Table 331-2 summarizes the states associated with primary alterations in the concentration of TBG. Primary disturbances in thyroid hormone binding also occur when other binding proteins in blood are increased or when abnormal binding proteins appear. These are discussed below.

The second type of disturbance of thyroid hormone binding interactions results from a primary alteration in the concentration of thyroid hormones in the blood, as in hypothyroidism or thyrotoxicosis. Here, normal homeostatic control of thyroid hormone secretion is lost, either because of disease in the control mechanism or because an intact control mechanism is incapable of overcoming the effects of disease elsewhere. Under these circumstances, the concentration of TBG is changed little, if at all, and the concentration of free hormone varies directly with the total concentration of hormone. Since homeostatic mechanisms cannot restore the concentration of free hormone to normal, primary changes in thyroid function cause persistent changes in the concentration of total and free hormone and, consequently, alterations in the metabolic state.

HORMONE METABOLISM   Following penetration into the cell, T_4 and T_3 undergo reactions that lead ultimately to their excretion or inactivation. Thyroid hormones undergo sequential removal of single iodine atoms (monodeiodinations), which ultimately yields the thyronine nucleus stripped of iodine. Deiodinative pathways account for approximately 70 percent of T_4 and T_3 disposal. In the case of T_4, the most important of these is the 5′-monodeiodination that leads to the generation of T_3. Since approximately 30 percent of T_4 is converted to T_3, and since T_3 has approximately three times the metabolic potency of T_4, virtually all the metabolic action of T_4 can be ascribed to the action of the T_3 that it gives rise to. Normally, extraglandular formation

Table 331-2

Circumstances Associated with Altered Concentrations of TBG

Increased TBG	Decreased TBG
Pregnancy	Androgen use
Newborn state	Use of large doses of glucocorticoid
Use of oral contraceptives and other sources of estrogen	Chronic liver disease
Use of tamoxifen	Severe systemic illness
Infectious and chronic active hepatitis	Active acromegaly
Biliary cirrhosis	Nephrosis
Acute intermittent porphyria	Genetic determination
Perphenazine	
Genetic determination	

accounts for about 80 percent of the T_3 in the blood and of overall T_3 production, the remainder coming from thyroid secretion. As a consequence, abnormal states and pharmacologic agents that impair T_3 formation lower the serum T_3 concentration (Table 331-3). When patients with thyroid hypofunction are treated with synthetic T_4 (levo-thyroxine) to sustain normal serum T_4 concentrations, normal or nearly normal serum T_3 concentrations are maintained. The generalization that the thyroid secretes relatively little T_3 does not apply when the thyroid is hyperfunctioning or is under increased stimulation by TSH. Under these conditions, the T_3/T_4 ratios of the secretory product and of the serum hormones are increased. In addition, when T_4 production is decreased, as in early thyroid failure or iodine deficiency, the T_3/T_4 concentration ratio in blood is increased still further by an autoregulatory mechanism that leads to an increase in the efficiency of T_3 formation.

Approximately 40 percent of T_4 disposal is accounted for by mono-deiodination at the 5 position of its inner ring to yield reverse T_3 (rT_3); this process accounts for nearly all rT_3 produced. rT_3 has little, if any, metabolic potency; therefore, the relative rates of outer- and inner-ring monodeiodination of T_4 determine the availability of metabolically active hormone. Factors that impair T_3 formation almost invariably increase the serum rT_3 concentration. This increase is due not to an increase in the production of rT_3 from T_4, but rather to a decrease in the 5'-mono-deiodination of rT_3 to yield 3,3'-diiodothyronine (3,3'T_2); i.e., both the decreased conversion of T_4 to T_3 and the decreased degradation of rT_3 result from a selective impairment of 5'-monodeiodination. There are two 5'-deiodinases. Most T_4 to T_3 conversion is effected by the type I isoenzyme in liver and kidney. The type II enzyme is localized in the pituitary, central nervous system, placenta, and brown fat and generates T_3 in these tissues. The type I enzyme is inactive during systemic illness and during normal fetal life, leading to low serum levels of T_3. An increase in type II activity in hypothyroidism allows continued T_3 formation in brain and pituitary as T_4 levels fall.

A second major pathway of metabolism of T_4, T_3, and their metabolites is conjugation in the liver, principally with glucuronate and sulfate. Conjugates either undergo deiodination locally or are secreted into the bile. The magnitude of the enterohepatic circulation of these compounds in humans is unknown. Reabsorption is incomplete at best, since the fecal excretion of T_4, T_3, and their iodine-containing metabolites accounts for approximately 20 percent of overall T_4 disposal. About 20 percent of T_4 and T_3 undergoes oxidative deamination and decarboxylation of the alanine side chain to yield tetraiodo- and triiodo-thyroacetic acid (*tetrac* and *triac*, respectively).

Both phenobarbital and phenytoin increase the metabolic clearance of thyroid hormones without increasing the proportion of free hormone in the blood. Indeed, in the case of phenytoin, both total and free T_4 concentrations are diminished. Nevertheless, in the presence of an intact thyroid gland a normal metabolic state is maintained, possibly because of an increase in T_3 formation.

HORMONE ACTION Thyroid hormones influence the growth and maturation of tissues, cell respiration and total energy expenditure, and the turnover of essentially all substrates, vitamins, and hormones, including the thyroid hormones themselves. Some actions of these hormones on cell metabolism may be mediated at the level of the mitochon-

Table 331-3

States Associated with Decreased Peripheral Conversion of T_4 to T_3

Physiologic
  Fetal and early neonatal life
  ? Old age
Pathologic
  Fasting
  Malnutrition
  Systemic illness
  Physical trauma
  Postoperative state
  Drugs (propylthiouracil, dexamethasone, propranolol, amiodarone)
  Radiographic contrast agents (ipodate, iopanoate)

drion to influence oxidative metabolism or at the level of the plasma membrane and endoplasmic reticulum to influence the activity of Ca^{2+}-ATPase and the transcellular flux of substrates and cations. However, the primary action of the hormone is exerted via binding to one or more intracellular receptor complexes, which, in turn, bind to specific regulatory sites in the chromosomes to influence genomic expression (see Chap. 327). Two classes of thyroid hormone receptor (TR), TRα and TRβ, are encoded by genes on chromosomes 17 and 3, respectively. By alternative splicing, these two genes generate additional isoforms (α_1, α_2, β_1, β_2, etc.). The TR proteins are part of a superfamily of genes encoded by mRNAs of cellular (c) homologues of the avian retroviral v-*erb* A proto-oncogene. The TR genes, c-*erb*-A-α (TRα) and c-*erb*-A-β (TRβ), encode receptor proteins with a T_3-binding domain and a DNA-binding domain. The DNA-binding domain attaches to regulatory sequences in those target genes with T_3-regulated transcription (e.g., the TSH, prolactin, and growth hormone genes). In an interaction stabilized by TR auxiliary proteins (TRAPs), the activation and modulation of rates of transcription are mediated by regulatory sequences called *thyroid response elements* (TREs). Thus, in the pituitary, the binding of T_3-TR complexes to TREs serves to inhibit the expression of genes for the synthesis of the α and β subunits of TSH. While the pituitary may contain the highest concentrations of TR, all tissues with high-affinity nuclear T_3 binding express TRα and TRβ receptors. High concentrations of c-*erb*-A-β_1 are found in brain, liver, heart, and kidney. The variable lack of T_3 responsiveness in different tissues ("resistance") is due to point mutations in the T_3-binding domain of the TRβ (see below).

THYROID HORMONE RESISTANCE Generalized thyroid hormone resistance (GTHR) is a syndrome characterized by reduced responsiveness to elevated levels of thyroid hormone. The resistance to thyroid hormone action is associated with elevated circulating levels of free T_4 and free T_3, inappropriately normal or elevated (i.e., nonsuppressed) serum TSH, and intact TSH responsiveness to TRH. Kindreds have been described whose members express variable patterns of resistance, and the responsiveness of target tissues may vary within the same individual. The varied phenotypes are due to a heterogeneous series of mutations of the TRβ. Clinical features include short stature, hyperactivity, attention deficits with mental deficiency or learning disability, and goiter. While GTHR patients are either euthyroid or hypothyroid, the differential diagnosis includes isolated pituitary resistance to thyroid hormone and a TSH-secreting pituitary tumor, disorders usually associated with hyperthyroidism. Indications for treatment of GTHR vary depending on the clinical features, but the presence of increased serum TSH reflects the need for supplemental thyroid hormone, the dosage requirement depending on parameters of tissue responses to thyroid hormone.

REGULATION OF THYROID FUNCTION Thyroid function is regulated by suprathyroid and intrathyroid mechanisms (Fig. 331-2). The mediator of suprathyroid regulation is TSH, a glycoprotein secreted by basophilic (thyrotropic) cells in the anterior pituitary. TSH stimulates thyroid hypertrophy and hyperplasia; accelerates most aspects of intermediary metabolism in the thyroid; enhances the synthesis of nucleic acids and proteins, including thyroglobulin; and stimulates the synthesis and secretion of thyroid hormones.

Regulation of TSH secretion, in turn, is controlled by two opposing influences at the level of the thyrotropic cell. Thyrotropin-releasing hormone (TRH), a tripeptide of hypothalamic origin, stimulates the secretion and synthesis of TSH, whereas thyroid hormones both inhibit the TSH secretory mechanism directly and antagonize the action of TRH. Thus, homeostatic control of TSH secretion is exerted in a negative-feedback manner by thyroid hormones, and the threshold for feedback inhibition is apparently set by TRH. TRH reaches the pituitary via the hypophyseal portal blood system and binds to specific high-affinity receptors on the plasma membrane of the thyrotropic cell. Either activation of the adenylate cyclase system or a concomitant translocation of extracellular calcium into the cell initiates release of

TSH. In addition to stimulating release of stored TSH, TRH enhances the synthesis of TSH via transcription and translation of the gene for the β subunit. TRH also plays a role in posttranslational processing of TSH, as indicated by the fact that TSH in patients with hypothalamic hypothyroidism has reduced biologic activity. The negative-feedback effect of the thyroid hormones appears to take place entirely at the level of the thyrotropic cell. Experimentally, thyroid hormones both inhibit production of TRH mRNA and TRH prohormone and reduce the number of TRH receptors on the thyrotropic cell, thus impairing the cell's responsiveness to TRH. The major negative-feedback action of the thyroid hormones is at the pituitary level, mediated by binding of the hormones to TR in the nucleus of the thyrotropic cell, resulting in reduced expression of the genes for the α and β subunits of TSH. The principal arbiter of thyroid hormone action in the pituitary is T_3, both that generated in the pituitary from T_4 and that derived from plasma. To what extent T_4 itself is effective in the pituitary is uncertain, but other factors also modify the secretion of TSH and its response to TRH. Both somatostatin and dopamine appear to be physiologic inhibitors of TSH secretion. Estrogens enhance responsiveness to TRH, whereas glucocorticoids inhibit this function. Catecholamines also play a role, with alpha$_1$-adrenergic pathways being inhibitory and alpha$_2$ pathways being stimulatory. Experimentally, tumor necrosis factor and interleukin 1 inhibit TSH secretion; these effects possibly play a role in the sick euthyroid syndrome.

Intrathyroid regulation of thyroid function is also important. In some manner, changes in glandular organic iodine content cause reciprocal changes in thyroid iodide transport activity and regulate growth, amino acid uptake, glucose metabolism, and nucleic acid synthesis. These influences are evident in the absence of TSH stimulation and hence may be termed *autoregulatory*, but their most important role is to modify the response to TSH (iodine-enrichment inhibiting and iodine-depletion enhancing), probably by influencing the generation of cyclic AMP consequent to TSH stimulation. Cytokines may exert stimulatory or inhibitory effects on thyroid hormone synthesis or secretion and on interactions with TSH, but the physiologic and pathophysiologic significance of these substances (e.g., atrial natriuretic peptide, tumor necrosis factor, transforming growth factor, epidermal growth factor, and endothelin) remains to be clarified.

LABORATORY TESTS

Laboratory tests of thyroid hormone economy can be divided into five general categories: direct tests of thyroid function, tests related to the concentration and binding of thyroid hormones in blood, metabolic indexes, tests of the homeostatic control of thyroid function, and miscellaneous tests.

DIRECT TESTS OF THYROID FUNCTION Those tests that involve in vivo administration of radioactive iodine test glandular function per se. Measurement of the *thyroid radioactive iodine uptake* (RAIU) is the most common of these. [131]I has been used for this purpose, but ^{123}I is preferable because it allows the use of a lower radiation dose. The administered radioiodine mixes uniformly with the endogenous iodide pool and, in the steady state, can be used to assess what percentage of the iodide entering and leaving the extracellular space per unit time is accumulated by the thyroid. The RAIU is measured 24 h after administration of the isotope, since it usually reaches a plateau value at this time, but in cases of severe thyroid hyperfunction it may peak early. The RAIU varies inversely with the plasma iodide concentration and directly with the functional state of the thyroid. At levels of iodine intake usual in the United States (up to 1 mg/d), the normal 24-h RAIU is approximately 10 to 30 percent of the administered dose. Consequently, this test discriminates poorly between normal and hypothyroid states. Values above the normal range, however, usually indicate thyroid hyperfunction and are useful in the diagnosis of hyperthyroidism. Measurement of the RAIU is also a part of the thyroid suppression test (see below).

One valuable application of the RAIU test occurs when thyrotoxicosis is associated with a low RAIU. Causes include iodine-induced hyperthyroidism, thyrotoxicosis factitia, inadvertent ingestion of ground meat containing thyroid glands ("hamburger toxicosis"), and the spontaneously resolving thyrotoxicosis associated with painless chronic thyroiditis, postpartum thyroiditis, or subacute thyroiditis.

TESTS RELATED TO HORMONE CONCENTRATION AND BINDING OF HORMONE IN BLOOD Prior to the evolution of highly sensitive assays for TSH, measurement of the concentration of T_4 and/or T_3 in serum, in conjunction with some assessment of hormone binding, was the traditional means of confirming a clinical diagnosis of hyperthyroidism or hypothyroidism. Highly specific and sensitive radioimmunoassays are used to measure *serum T_4 and T_3* concentrations and rarely for the measurement of *serum rT_3* concentration. The approximate normal ranges are 60 to 150 nmol/L (5 to 12 μg/dL) for T_4, 1 to 3 nmol/L (70 to 190 ng/dL) for T_3, and 0.2 to 0.6 nmol/L (10 to 40 ng/dL) for rT_3.

As mentioned above, alterations in hormone binding by plasma proteins, as well as alterations in the rate of hormone secretion, influence the concentration of hormone in the blood. However, only alterations in hormone secretion lead to steady-state alterations in free hormone levels. Because they most consistently reflect the rate of hormone production, free hormone concentrations usually correlate better with the metabolic state than do total levels. The free T_4 concentration (FT$_4$) can be measured directly by equilibrium dialysis of serum enriched with a tracer quantity of labeled T_4. The percent of T_4 that is dialyzable or free is thereby determined, and the product of this value and the total T_4 is the FT$_4$. However, since the dialysis technique is cumbersome, it has been replaced by indirect assays. The expression "free T_4 estimate" (FT$_4$E) may refer to a free T_4 fraction determined from equilibrium dialysis, to a derived free T_4 estimate, or to any other indirectly measured or calculated free T_4 concentration. One traditional indirect method, the in vitro uptake test, represents an assessment of hormone binding in which the serum is enriched with labeled T_4 or labeled T_3 and is then incubated with an insoluble particulate material, such as resin or charcoal, that binds free hormone (resin T_3 uptake, RT$_3$U). The percent of labeled hormone taken up by the particulate material varies inversely with both the concentration of unoccupied sites among the serum proteins and their affinity for the particular hormone being used. The RT$_3$U may be expressed as a thyroid hormone binding ratio (THBR), which serves to lessen confusion of the T_3 uptake with assays for T_3. Under most clinical conditions, values of the RT$_3$U, THBR, or FTE are proportionate to those of the percent of FT$_4$ and percent of free T_3 (FT$_3$). This proportionality reflects the fact that, in normal serum, T_4 and T_3 are mainly bound by a common binding site on TBG. Therefore, alterations in binding produced by an excess or deficiency of TBG or by an excessive or insufficient supply of T_4 do not seriously disturb the relationship between the intensity of T_4 binding and that of T_3. Under these conditions, therefore, one may calculate a *free T_4 index* (FT$_4$I) and a *free T_3 index* (FT$_3$I) as the product of the RT$_3$U and the total T_4 and T_3 concentrations, respectively; these quantities are proportional to the actual FT$_4$ and FT$_3$ concentrations.

Primary alterations in plasma TBG concentration (see Table 331-2) produce changes in the RT$_3$U that are inverse and approximately proportional to the changes in the serum T_4 and serum T_3 levels; as a result, the FT$_4$I and FT$_3$I remain normal. By contrast, alterations in T_4 secretion cause changes in the percent FT$_4$ and in the RT$_3$U that are in the same direction as those in serum T_4. As a result, the FT$_4$ and FT$_4$I deviate from normal values more markedly than do the percent FT$_4$ and RT$_3$U alone. Immunoradiometric assay (IRMA) and chemiluminescent assay methods for the direct measurement of FT$_4$ provide reliable results in a wide range of disorders and may replace measurement of total T_4, RT$_3$U, and FT$_4$I in the diagnosis of thyrotoxicosis and hypothyroidism. In spite of improvements in free T_4 assays, the highly sensitive TSH assay is the most sensitive test of thyroid function. The measurement of a TSH level and a FT$_4$E or FT$_4$I will provide effective diagnosis and management of most patients with thyroid disease.

As noted earlier, several disorders are characterized by increased plasma binding of T_4 in which, because the protein involved is not TBG, the intensity of T_4 binding relative to that of T_3 is abnormal. Most commonly, binding of T_4 is enhanced, while that of T_3 is increased little if at all. Included among these disorders is *familial dysalbuminemic hyperthyroxinemia* (FDH), inherited as an autosomal dominant trait, in which the plasma concentration of an albumin variant with an unusually high affinity for T_4 is increased. As a result, the serum T_4 is markedly elevated, but, in keeping with the euthyroid state, the FT_4 is normal. Because the RT_3U does not reflect the increase in the intensity of T_4 binding, calculated values of the FT_4I are increased, often leading to a mistaken diagnosis of thyrotoxicosis. Similar findings occur when there is *increased T_4 binding by transthyretin* or when *circulating antibodies* against T_4 are present.

In the foregoing disorders, serum T_4 is increased owing to an increase in T_4 binding, and the FT_4 and metabolic state are normal. These disorders therefore are classified among those that lead to a state of *euthyroid hyperthyroxinemia*, a term that implies the presence of hyperthyroxinemia not caused by intrinsic thyroid disease (Table 331-4). The mechanisms responsible are variable and in some cases uncertain. The increases in total T_4 do not appear to affect the metabolic state, but hyperthyroidism may be mistakenly diagnosed.

Some states are associated with an increased thyroid secretion of T_3, at least relative to the secretion of T_4. As a result, the serum T_3 concentration is disproportionately high relative to that of T_4. This situation apparently is caused by hyperfunction of the follicular cell, since it occurs in all varieties of hyperthyroidism and in early thyroid failure, when the gland is exposed to elevated TSH levels. Accordingly, the serum T_3 concentration and the derived value FT_3I are generally better for the diagnosis of hyperthyroidism than measurement of the T_4 concentration. In *early* hyperthyroidism, by contrast, the serum T_3 concentration and the FT_3I are often normal despite subnormal values for the serum T_4 and FT_4I. Consequently, the serum T_3 concentration is not reliable for the diagnosis of hypothyroidism.

Measurement of the serum rT_3 concentration is valuable in differentiating the "low T_3 syndrome" (see below) from intrinsic hypothyroidism; in the former the serum rT_3 concentration is increased, whereas in the latter it is usually subnormal.

METABOLIC INDEXES Although measurements of the metabolic impact of thyroid hormones have value in the investigative setting, none is sufficiently sensitive, specific, and easily performed for routine use. Measurements of oxygen consumption in the basal state (basal metabolic rate, BMR) were once a mainstay in the diagnosis of thyroid disease but are now of historic interest. Several blood

tests may yield abnormal results in patients with thyroid disease. For example, serum concentrations of creatine phosphokinase and, less frequently, lactate dehydrogenase and aspartate aminotransferase are increased in hypothyroidism and may be slightly decreased in hyperthyroidism. The changes are nonspecific, and the reason to be aware of them is to avoid making the inference that other diseases that produce similar changes are present. The concentrations in serum of testosterone-binding globulin (TeBG), the iron storage protein ferritin, and angiotensin-converting enzyme are thyroid hormone–dependent and are, therefore, increased in thyrotoxicosis, but they are of no value in the diagnosis of thyroid disease. Increases in the *serum cholesterol concentration* are common in hypothyroidism of thyroid origin, and decreases in serum cholesterol are common in thyrotoxicosis. *Systolic time indexes*, such as the preejection period and pulse-wave arrival time, are prolonged in hypothyroidism and shortened in hyperthyroidism. They may be of value in monitoring thyroid replacement therapy in elderly patients or in patients with coexisting heart disease.

TESTS OF HOMEOSTATIC CONTROL Measurement of the basal *serum TSH concentration* is useful in the diagnosis of both advanced and subclinical hypothyroidism. The latter state represents a stage in the evolution of hypothyroidism, in which a structural or functional abnormality that impairs hormone synthesis is compensated for by hypersecretion of TSH. In thyrotoxic states, the serum TSH concentration is almost always low or undetectable. While the original radioimmunoassays (RIAs) could not distinguish between normal and subnormal values, immunoradiometric or chemiluminescent techniques employing monoclonal antibodies now provide exquisite sensitivity. Thyrotoxic patients tend to have undetectable levels (<0.1 mU/L), while values in most normal subjects range between 0.3 and 3.0 mU/L in these assays (Fig. 331-3). Thus, these assays offer advantage over conventional RIAs and may be useful in the diagnosis of hyperthyroidism and hypothyroidism. Serum TSH concentrations are absolutely or inappropriately elevated relative to serum FT_4 and FT_3 values in patients with TSH-induced hyperthyroidism. This rare syndrome results either from a TSH-secreting pituitary adenoma or resistance of the TSH secretory mechanism to feedback inhibition by T_4 and T_3. Measurement of serum TSH is the best means of distinguishing between untreated hypothyroidism of thyroid origin, in which the values are invariably increased, and pituitary or hypothalamic hypothyroidism, in which the values are usually low or within the normal range. Occasional patients with hypothalamic or pituitary

Table 331-4

States Associated with Euthyroid Hyperthyroxinemia

Disorder	FT_4	FT_4I	T_3	TSH	Comments
Increased T_4 binding					
Increased TBG level	N	N	↑	N	See Tables 331-1 and 331-2
FDH	N	↑	N,	N	Autosomal dominant inheritance
Increased TBPA binding	N	↑	Sl↑	N	Increased concentration (islet cell tumor) or affinity
Anti-T_4 antibody	N	↑	N N	N	Anti-T_3 antibody may be present
Pituitary and peripheral thyroid					
hormone resistance	↑	↑	↑	↑	If only pituitary is resistant, patient will be thyrotoxic
Various disorders					
Sick euthyroid syndrome	↑, N	↑	↓	N,↓	Uncommon; poorly understood
Acute psychiatric illness	↑, N	↑	N,↑	N,↑	Remits without treatment in several weeks
Hyperemesis gravidarum	↑	↑	N	↓	Remits in several weeks
Drugs					
Inhibitors of T_3 formation	↑	↑	↓	↑	Particularly ipodate and iopanoate
Radiographic contrast agents					
Propranolol	↑	↑	↓	N,↑	Especially with large doses
Amiodarone	↑	↑	↓	↑	Increased TSH during first several months
Heparin	↑	↑	N	—	Requires only small intravenous doses
Levothyroxine	↑	↑	N	↓	Hyperthyroxinemia in about 50% of cases

NOTE: FDH, familial dysalbuminemic hyperthyroxinemia; FT_4, free T_4 concentration; FT_4I, free T_4 index calculated from an in vitro T_3 uptake test; TBPA, thyroxine-binding prealbumin; TSH, basal serum TSH concentration and response to TRH; N, normal; Sl, slightly.

hypothyroidism secrete a form of TSH that is immunoactive but not bioactive. Here, serum TSH concentrations may be elevated rather than depressed.

The *thyrotropin-releasing hormone stimulation test* assesses the TSH-secretory mechanism and has diagnostic value in diverse circumstances. Following the intravenous injection of TRH in normal subjects, the serum TSH level increases, reaches a maximum between 20 and 45 min, and then rapidly declines. The pituitary feedback mechanism is such that, when hypothalamic-pituitary function is normal, one would expect an increased response to TRH when the thyrotropic cell senses a deficiency of thyroid hormone, particularly T_3, and a decreased or absent response when thyroid hormone is in excess. Thus, except in the rare case of pituitary resistance to thyroid hormone, in which responses are usually normal, thyrotoxicosis is invariably accompanied by a blunted or absent TSH response to TRH. Owing to the extreme sensitivity of the TSH-secretory mechanism to feedback inhibition, diminished responses to TRH commonly occur in apparently euthyroid patients with serum T_4 or T_3 levels within the normal range but with marginally increased T_4 or T_3 output from autonomously functioning toxic adenomas or toxic multinodular goiters. Blunted TRH responses also may be seen in some patients with euthyroid Graves' disease. In addition, responses to TRH are often decreased in elderly individuals, especially men. Despite these exceptions, a subnormal or absent response to TRH is a useful confirmatory test for thyrotoxicosis. With the availability of highly sensitive TSH assays, the TRH test is rarely used for this purpose. TRH tests are of even less value in the diagnosis of hypothyroidism. Responses are increased in patients with primary hypothyroidism, but the magnitude of the increase is generally proportional to the extent of increase in basal serum TSH. Some patients with pituitary hypothyroidism have subnormal responses, and some with TRH deficiency due to hypothalamic disease have a near-normal response. Further, in about one-fourth of patients with hypothyroidism due to hypothalamic-pituitary disease, basal serum TSH levels are normal or slightly elevated, and the response to TRH is exaggerated, although some of this TSH may not be bioactive.

The *thyroid suppression test* is used to assess the homeostatic control of thyroid function. Normally, exogenous thyroid hormone suppresses pituitary TSH secretion, resulting in a decrease in the RAIU. Since liothyronine is usually employed for the test (100 µg/d for 7 to 10 days), the resulting decline in serum T_4, as well as in the RAIU, can serve as an index of suppression. A normal suppressive response is a decrease of the RAIU to less than half the control value and a decline of the serum T_4 to low-normal or subnormal values. A normal suppression test is incompatible with and excludes a diagnosis of hyperthyroidism, because liothyronine suppresses TSH rather than the thyroid directly and because TSH is unmeasurable in most hyperthyroid states. The suppression test always gives an abnormal result in hyperthyroidism, irrespective of the underlying cause; this finding usually indicates either autonomy of thyroid function or the presence of an abnormal (non-TSH) thyroid stimulator or, rarely, unremitting hypersecretion of TSH. An abnormal suppression test result is not pathognomonic of hyperthyroidism, however, since it may persist after treatment of hyperthyroidism in Graves' disease and is seen in about half the euthyroid patients with the ophthalmopathy of Graves' disease.

Because of the risk of adverse effects from exogenous thyroid hormone, especially liothyronine, in elderly patients and in those with cardiovascular disease, highly sensitive TSH measurements have almost entirely supplanted the thyroid suppression test in the diagnosis of hyperthyroidism.

MISCELLANEOUS TESTS Various tests that do not assess thyroid function are of value in defining the nature of the thyroid disorder or in planning therapy. For example, high titers of *antithyroid peroxidase* (anti-TPO or antimicrosomal) *antibodies* or *antithyroglobulin antibodies* are found in the serum of most patients with Hashimoto's disease and in many with primary thyroprivic hypothyroidism or Graves' disease. In the latter states, the serum also contains antibodies against the TSH receptor that are capable of inhibiting the receptor binding of TSH (TSH-binding inhibitory immunoglobulins, TBII) or of stimulating the production of cyclic AMP therein [thyroid-stimulating antibodies (TSAb) or thyroid-stimulating immunoglobulins (TSI)], respectively. The clinical utility of tests for TSI stems from the fact that the disappearance of these factors from the serum during a course of antithyroid therapy implies the likelihood of a long-term remission of hyperthyroidism when therapy is withdrawn. The analogous TBII antibodies have no intrinsic stimulatory effect but block the response to endogenous TSH and produce nongoitrous hypothyroidism. Both stimulatory and blocking anti-TSH receptor antibodies have the ability to cross the placenta and produce transient hyperthyroidism (neonatal Graves' disease) or hypothyroidism, respectively, in the newborn. Measurement of these antibodies during the last months of pregnancy makes it possible to assess the likelihood that these disorders will develop in the neonate.

Some patients, most commonly those with autoimmune thyroid disease, develop *circulating antibodies* against T_3, T_4, or both. In RIAs for these hormones, because the endogenous antibody competes with the exogenous antibody for binding of the added labeled ligand, spuriously high or low values for the concentration of the hormone are obtained, depending on the technique of RIA used. The true concentration of the hormone, as determined in extracts of the serum, is increased owing to the additional binding sites provided by the antibody, but antibody-bound hormone is unavailable for metabolic action. In the case of anti-T_3 antibodies, the usual values of the RT_3U are low because endogenous antibody competes with the resin for binding of the added labeled T_3. Such antibodies can be detected by adding labeled hormone to serum and demonstrating that immunoglobulins bind the labeled hormone.

Along with several other thyroid disorders, differentiated carcinomas of the thyroid release thyroglobulin into the bloodstream. As a consequence, measurements of the *serum thyroglobulin* by RIA have value not in the initial diagnosis of thyroid carcinoma but in assessing the adequacy of initial therapy and in monitoring for recurrence or dissemination of the disease; endogenous antithyroglobulin antibodies

FIGURE 331-3 Utility of sensitive TSH assay in evaluation of suspected thyroid dysfunction in ambulatory patients.

can cause falsely low values. In patients with thyrotoxicosis, subnormal serum thyroglobulin concentrations together with decreased values of the RAIU suggest thyrotoxicosis factitia.

Imaging by *scintiscanning* permits localization of sites of accumulation of radioiodine or sodium [^{99m}Tc]pertechnetate. This technique is useful for defining areas of increased or decreased function within the thyroid and for detecting retrosternal goiter, ectopic thyroid tissue, hemiagenesis of the thyroid, and functioning metastases of thyroid carcinoma. Ultrasonic examination of the thyroid is also useful for differentiating cystic from solid nodules. Since ultrasonic scans provide an accurate indication of size, are noninvasive, and apparently have no injurious effects, sequential scans can be employed to assess changes in the size of the thyroid as a whole or of discrete nodules over time or in response to treatment.

SICK EUTHYROID SYNDROME

Severe illness, physical trauma, or physiologic stress can induce changes in one or more aspects of thyroid hormone economy, leading to findings referred to as the *sick euthyroid syndrome* (SES). Abnormalities in SES include alterations in the peripheral transport and metabolism of the thyroid hormones, in the regulation of TSH secretion, and, in some cases, in thyroid function itself. Acting alone or together, these alterations lead to changes in the concentrations of the circulating thyroid hormones, both total and free, which serve to define the several variants of SES. Because of the frequency and nonspecificity of the disorders that cause it, SES is probably a more common cause of abnormalities in the concentration of thyroid hormones in the blood than is intrinsic thyroid disease.

NORMAL-T$_4$ VARIANT OF SES Decreased production of T$_3$ owing to inhibition of the peripheral 5'-monodeiodination of T$_4$ is a consistent feature of SES. This effect is reflected in a decrease in the serum total T$_3$ concentration, which varies in severity with that of the illness. In moderately ill patients, serum total T$_4$ concentration is within the normal range. A decrease in the intensity of protein binding, greater for T$_4$ than for T$_3$, is also present. As a result, values of the RT$_3$U are moderately increased, and the percent FT$_4$ is increased to a proportionately greater extent. As a consequence, the values of the FT$_4$I and of the FT$_4$ concentration are often increased. Serum rT$_3$ concentrations are increased, owing to a decrease in the plasma clearance of rT$_3$ secondary to inhibition of the 5'-monodeiodination of T$_3$. The plasma clearance rate of T$_4$ is increased, probably as a result of decreased T$_4$ binding, and this alteration, in the face of normal T$_4$ concentrations, indicates that the overall rate of T$_4$ degradation and production is increased. Production rates for T$_3$ are decreased, and those for rT$_3$ are normal. The serum TSH concentration and the response of serum TSH to TRH are generally normal, although they may increase and then return to normal as recovery from the illness takes place. Despite the reduction in the serum T$_3$ level, this variant of SES can be separated from intrinsic thyroid disease because the serum T$_4$ and TSH levels are normal and because the serum T$_3$ level is not useful for diagnosing hypothyroidism.

LOW-T$_4$ VARIANT OF SES In more seriously ill patients, T$_3$ production rates and serum total and free T$_3$ concentrations decrease still further, and abnormalities in hormone binding increase in severity. As a consequence, serum T$_4$ concentrations decrease into the hypothyroid range. This effect is partly but not entirely due to decreased T$_4$ binding, since the FT$_4$ concentration is frequently subnormal. These changes are probably the result of decreased T$_4$ production in the most severely ill patients and are secondary to decreased secretion of TSH. Serum TSH concentrations appear normal by conventional assay but are low with sensitive TSH assays, and TRH responses are often blunted. Hence, in this variant of SES, there is an inappropriate hyposecretion of TSH, considering the low serum total and free T$_4$ and T$_3$ concentrations, and a diagnosis of pituitary hypothyroidism may be suggested. While the cause is unknown, the low TSH level may be due to the effects of somatostatin or cytokines such as interleukin 1 and tumor necrosis factor on the pituitary. With resolution of the underlying illness, TSH levels rise and may be transiently elevated

until T$_4$ and T$_3$ levels return to normal. Production rates for rT$_3$ are diminished owing to the decreased availability of the precursor T$_4$; nonetheless, serum rT$_3$ concentrations are increased due to slowing of rT$_3$ degradation, providing an important means of differentiating SES from pituitary hypothyroidism, in which serum rT$_3$ levels are low. In patients with primary hypothyroidism who have associated illness, serum TSH levels remain elevated, although generally they are lower than they otherwise would be.

HIGH-T$_4$ VARIANT OF SES An unusual variant of SES (approximately 1 percent of sick patients) is associated with increased serum total and free T$_4$ concentrations. This variant is most often seen in elderly women, many of whom have received medications that contain iodine. The principal source of diagnostic confusion is with the syndrome of "T$_4$ toxicosis," i.e., true thyrotoxicosis on which illness has been superimposed, so that serum T$_4$ levels are increased and serum T$_3$ concentrations are normal. In thyrotoxicosis, however, serum rT$_3$ concentrations are higher, the values of the serum total T$_3$ and of FT$_3$I are higher, TSH is usually undetectable, and TRH responses are blunted or absent.

ABNORMALITIES IN HORMONE BINDING IN SES Multiple factors are responsible for the decreased binding of T$_4$ and T$_3$ in SES. Illness is associated with decreased synthesis of TTR and a decrease in its serum concentration, but the extent to which this effect contributes to decreased T$_4$ binding is uncertain. In chronically ill patients, the serum TBG concentration is subnormal. Most often, however, the extent of decreased T$_4$ binding cannot be explained by decreases in serum TTR and TBG, and an inhibitor of hormone binding may be present. Its nature is uncertain, but one or more fatty acids may be responsible and may also cause diminished conversion of T$_4$ to T$_3$.

The importance of SES is that the changes in circulating thyroid hormone concentrations should not be confused with those due to intrinsic thyroid or pituitary disease. It is unclear whether the metabolic impact of thyroid hormone in peripheral tissues is decreased in SES and whether the syndrome is a beneficial or adverse response to illness. However, patients with low T$_4$ and T$_3$ levels due to SES do not appear to benefit from treatment with thyroid hormones.

AIDS AND THYROID FUNCTION Patients with AIDS may exhibit abnormal results on thyroid function tests that vary with the course of the illness. All but the most severely ill patients maintain normal levels of serum T$_4$ and T$_3$ (representing the normal-T$_4$ variant of SES). With falling CD4 counts and increasing frequency of systemic infections, serum T$_3$ falls in tandem with progressive cachexia (the low-T$_4$ variant of SES). Levels of rT$_3$ and serum TSH may remain normal. Rarely, AIDS patients develop hypothyroidism due to *Pneumocystis carinii* thyroiditis or involvement of the thyroid by Kaposi's sarcoma.

SIMPLE (NONTOXIC) GOITER

Endemic goiter has been defined as the presence of generalized or localized thyroid enlargement in more than 10 percent of the population. *Sporadic* goiter arises in nonendemic areas as a result of factors that do not affect the population generally. Since these terms fail to define the causes of goiter, and since thyroid enlargement of diverse etiologies may exist in both endemic and nonendemic regions, it is prudent to employ a general term such as *simple* or *nontoxic goiter*, which can be defined as any enlargement of the thyroid gland that does not result from an inflammatory or neoplastic process and that is not initially associated with thyrotoxicosis or myxedema.

ETIOLOGY AND PATHOGENESIS Simple goiter is sometimes due to a definable cause of impaired thyroid hormone synthesis, such as iodine deficiency, ingestion of a goitrogen, or a defect in a hormone biosynthetic pathway, but the cause is usually unknown. Whatever the cause, the clinical manifestations reflect the operation of a common pathophysiologic mechanism. Simple goiter occurs when one or more factors impair the capacity of the thyroid to secrete sufficient hormones to meet the needs of the peripheral tissues. Although this situation has been presumed to lead to increased secretion of TSH, concentrations of TSH in the serum of patients with established simple goiter are usually normal. Hence, other mechanisms of goitrogenesis may be operative. For example, depletion of organic iodine accompanying impaired hormone synthesis may increase the responsiveness to normal levels of TSH. The resulting increase in the functioning mass of the thyroid overcomes mild impairment of hormone synthesis, and the patient is metabolically normal, though goitrous. When the underlying disorder is severe, compensatory responses, now including hypersecretion of TSH, are inadequate to overcome the impairment, and the patient is both goitrous and hypothyroid. Thus, simple goiter cannot be clearly separated in the pathogenic sense from goitrous hypothyroidism. Specific causes of simple goiter may produce hypothyroidism in some cases (Table 331-5). Defective iodination of thyroglobulin may be a cause in many patients. Goiter may also be due to antibodies that stimulate the growth but not the function of the thyroid.

PATHOLOGY The histopathology of simple goiter varies with the etiology and the stage at which the examination is made. Initially, the gland exhibits a uniform hypertrophy, hyperplasia, and hypervascularity. As the disorder persists or undergoes exacerbations and remissions, the thyroidal architecture loses uniformity. Occasionally, most of the gland displays a uniform involution or hyperinvolution with colloid accumulation. More often, areas of involution are interspersed with areas of focal hyperplasia. Fibrosis may demarcate hyperplastic or involuted nodules, which may resemble true neoplasms (adenomas). Areas of hemorrhage and irregular calcification may be present. The evolution of the multinodular stage is usually accompanied by the development of functional autonomy. Indeed, heterogeneity of structure and function and a degree of functional autonomy are the hallmarks of the mature stage of this disorder.

CLINICAL MANIFESTATIONS In simple goiter, the manifestations arise solely from enlargement of the thyroid, since the metabolic state is normal. In goitrous hypothyroidism, symptoms caused by thyromegaly are accompanied by signs and symptoms of hormonal insufficiency. Mechanical sequelae include compression and displacement of the trachea or esophagus, occasionally with obstructive symptoms if the goiter becomes sufficiently large. Superior mediastinal obstruction may occur with large retrosternal goiters. Signs of compression can be induced with large retrosternal goiters when the patient's arms are raised above the head; they may include suffusion of the face, giddiness, and syncope (Pemberton's sign). Hoarseness due to compression of the recurrent laryngeal nerve is rare in simple goiter, and its presence suggests a neoplasm. Sudden hemorrhage into a nodule may lead to an acute, painful swelling in the neck and may produce or enhance compressive symptoms. Hyperthyroidism may supervene in long-standing multinodular goiter (toxic multinodular goiter). In both endemic and sporadic cases of multinodular goiter, the ingestion of excess iodide may result in the development of thyrotoxicosis (jodbasedow phenomenon).

In regions where iodine deficiency is severe, goitrous enlargement also may be associated with varying degrees of hypothyroidism. Cretinism, both goitrous and nongoitrous, occurs with increased frequency in the children of goitrous parents in many countries with endemic goiter. Although iodine deficiency is a factor in the etiology of endemic goiter, the frequency of goiter differs among persons with equally severe iodine deficiency. In such instances, dietary or waterborne goitrogens appear to be important conditioning factors. In some areas, goitrogens may cause goiter in the absence of iodine deficiency.

DIAGNOSIS The diagnosis of simple goiter requires demonstration of a euthyroid state and demonstration of normal serum T_4 and T_3 concentrations. The euthyroid state may be difficult to document because manifestations of thyrotoxicosis may be subtle or atypical, especially among the elderly (see the section "Toxic Multinodular Goiter"). Furthermore, serum T_4 and T_3 concentrations may be near the upper limit of the normal range, and the fact that serum T_3 concentrations may decrease in euthyroid elderly persons complicates the interpretation of this test. The RAIU is usually normal but may be increased in the presence of iodine deficiency or a biosynthetic defect. Thus, the presence of measurable concentration of TSH by a highly sensitive technique is the best index of euthyroidism. Indeed, subclinical thyrotoxicosis may be secondary to the functional autonomy of the goiter and consequently may cause a decrease in both the basal TSH level and the TSH response to TRH. Differentiation of nontoxic goiter from Hashimoto's disease is facilitated by the greater frequency of multinodularity in the former and by the presence of high titers of circulating antimicrosomal or antithyroglobulin antibodies in the latter. In some instances, emergence of a strongly dominant nodule may suggest the presence of a carcinoma, especially if bleeding has caused it to increase in size rapidly and to lose the ability to accumulate iodine or pertechnetate. Appropriate radiographic studies (computed tomography, magnetic resonance imaging) and respiratory flow measurements should be obtained when substernal extension has the potential to cause upper airway obstruction.

℞ **TREATMENT**

The object of treatment is to reduce the size of the goiter, either by relieving external encumbrances to hormone formation or by providing enough exogenous hormone to inhibit TSH secretion and thereby put the thyroid gland at rest. In disorders characterized by decreased thyroid iodide stores, such as iodine deficiency or impairment of the thyroid iodide-concentrating mechanism, small doses of iodide may prove effective. Occasionally, a known extrinsic goitrogen can be withdrawn. Most commonly, however, no specific etiologic factor can be detected, and thyroid hormone therapy is required. For this purpose, levothyroxine (L-thyroxine) is the agent of choice. In the younger patient with the early diffuse stage of simple goiter, treatment is instituted with 100 μg of levothyroxine daily, and the dose is increased over the next month or so to a maximum of 150 or 200 μg/d (the average dose being 1.7 μg/kg body weight per day). Complete suppression would imply reduction of serum TSH to levels of <0.1 mU/L as determined by an ultrasensitive assay. In patients at risk for loss of bone mineral (e.g., postmenopausal women not on estrogen replacement, patients with prior Graves' disease) thyroxine therapy should be titrated to slightly less than a fully suppressive dose. Adequacy of suppression also may be assessed by measuring the RAIU, which should decrease to less

Table 331-5

Classification of the Causes of Hypothyroidism

Thyroid
  Thyroprivic
    Congenital development defect
    Primary idiopathic
    Postablative (radioiodine, surgery)
    Postradiation (e.g., for lymphoma)
  Goitrous
    Heritable biosynthetic defects
    Maternally transmitted (iodides, antithyroid agents)
    Iodine deficiency
    Drug-elicited (aminosalicylic acid, iodides, phenylbutazone, iodoantipyrine, lithium)
    Chronic thyroiditis (Hashimoto's disease)
    Interleukin 2 and lymphokine-activated killer cells
Suprathyroid (Trophoprivic)
  Pituitary
    Panhypopituitarism
    Isolated TSH deficiency
  Hypothalamic
    Congenital defects
    Infection (encephalitis)
    Neoplasm
    Infiltrative (sarcoidosis)
Self-limited
  Following withdrawal of suppressive thyroid therapy
  Subacute thyroiditis and chronic thyroiditis with transient hypothyroidism (usually after a phase of thyrotoxicosis)

than 5 percent of the administered dose at 24 h. Lesser decreases indicate that suppression is only partial, which may reflect the presence of autonomous foci demonstrable by scanning techniques. In the elderly or in patients with long-standing multinodular goiter, TSH should be measured by an ultrasensitive assay before treatment with levothyroxine is initiated to determine whether significant functional autonomy is present. If such is indicated by the absence of a detectable basal TSH level, suppressive therapy with levothyroxine is contraindicated, as such patients are or will become thyrotoxic. Rather, consideration should be given to radioiodine ablation of the autonomous foci (see "Toxic Multinodular Goiter"). On the other hand, if the basal TSH level is normal (excluding autonomous hyperfunction) treatment with levothyroxine can be initiated. In elderly patients the initial dose should not exceed 50 μg/d, and the dosage should be increased gradually, the end point being partial rather than complete suppression of basal TSH and/or the RAIU. It is the usual practice to obtain a thyroid scan as part of the initial evaluation of all patients with multinodular goiter. In those patients in whom full suppressive doses of thyroxine are indicated, it is desirable to repeat the RAIU measurement and scan (suppression scan), when practical, to ascertain the efficacy of suppression and/or the presence of autonomous foci.

Results of therapy vary widely. Early diffuse, hyperplastic goiters respond well, with regression or disappearance in 3 to 6 months. In the author's experience, the later, nodular stage responds less well, and significant reduction in gland size is achieved only in about one-third of cases; however, in the remainder, suppressive treatment may forestall further glandular growth. Internodular tissue regresses more often than do nodules themselves. The latter may therefore appear to become more prominent during treatment. After maximum regression of the goiter has occurred, suppressive medication may be maintained for a prolonged period, reduced to a minimal level, or, in some cases, withdrawn. The goiter may stay regressed or may recur unpredictably. In the latter situation, if malignancy is ruled out by fine-needle biopsy, suppressive therapy should be reinstituted and continued indefinitely. In areas of endemic iodine deficiency, the size and prevalence of goiter and the frequency of cretinism can be reduced by the provision of iodized salt or water or the periodic injection of iodized oil.

Surgical therapy of simple goiter is physiologically unsound but may occasionally be necessary to relieve obstruction. Large substernal goiters with partial upper airway obstruction also have been treated by radioactive iodine with moderate success. Surgical exploration of nodular goiter also may be indicated in some individuals when evidence suggests carcinoma. However, the idea that subtotal resection of a multinodular nontoxic goiter affords effective prophylaxis against the development of thyroid carcinoma is unsound. If for some reason subtotal thyroidectomy has been performed, levothyroxine in a usual dose of about 1.7 μg/kg body weight per day is recommended to inhibit regenerative hyperplasia and further goitrogenesis.

HYPOTHYROIDISM

Hypothyroidism results from abnormalities that lead to insufficient synthesis of thyroid hormone. Hypothyroidism dating from birth and resulting in developmental abnormalities is termed *cretinism*. The term *myxedema* connotes severe hypothyroidism in which there is accumulation of hydrophilic mucopolysaccharides in the ground substance of the dermis and other tissues, leading to thickening of the facial features and doughy induration of the skin.

ETIOLOGY AND PATHOGENESIS A classification of hypothyroidism is presented in Table 331-5. The primary thyroid varieties account for the vast majority of cases, only 5 percent or fewer being suprathyroid in origin. In thyroprivic hypothyroidism, loss of thyroid tissue leads to inadequate synthesis of thyroid hormone, despite maximum stimulation of any thyroid remnant by TSH. The most common cause is surgical or radioiodine ablation of the thyroid gland for the treatment of Graves' disease. Thyroprivic hypothyroidism also may

occur as a primary idiopathic disorder, which is usually due to autoimmunity and is associated with circulating cytotoxic antithyroid antibodies or, in some cases, antibodies that block the TSH receptor. This disorder may coexist with diabetes mellitus and other diseases in which circulating autoantibodies are found, such as pernicious anemia, systemic lupus erythematosus, rheumatoid arthritis, Sjögren's syndrome, and chronic hepatitis. In addition, hypothyroidism can be one manifestation of a polyglandular endocrine deficiency state in which autoantibodies cause variable insufficiency of thyroid, adrenal, parathyroid, and gonadal function (see Chap. 340). All these diseases, including isolated primary hypothyroidism, are associated with an increased frequency of specific HLA haplotypes. Finally, a developmental defect may result in failure of the gland to function adequately, leading to sporadic nongoitrous cretinism or juvenile hypothyroidism. A self-limited period of hypothyroidism is common in the course of subacute thyroiditis and in the syndrome of "painless thyroiditis," including the postpartum variant, and usually occurs after a temporary period of thyrotoxicosis. Owing to a persisting lack of TSH stimulation, intrinsically euthyroid subjects from whom chronic suppressive therapy is abruptly withdrawn experience a several-week period of thyroid hypofunction.

Inability to synthesize enough thyroid hormone leads to hypersecretion of TSH and hence goiter. If the compensatory response is inadequate, goitrous hypothyroidism ensues. The most common cause of goitrous hypothyroidism in North America is Hashimoto's disease, in which defective organic binding of iodide and abnormal secretion of iodoproteins are frequent. Iodide-induced goiter with or without hypothyroidism appears to arise from an intrinsic defect in the organic binding mechanism, which permits a persistent Wolff-Chaikoff effect. Euthyroid patients with Graves' disease, especially after surgery or radioiodine treatment, patients with Hashimoto's disease, and normal fetuses are particularly susceptible to iodide-induced goiter. In view of the susceptibility of the fetal thyroid to iodide, iodine in large doses should not be given during pregnancy. Less common causes of goitrous hypothyroidism are hereditary defects in hormone biosynthesis and ingestion of drugs that induce defects in hormone biosynthesis, such as aminosalicylic acid and lithium. Finally, in areas of environmental iodine deficiency, goitrous cretinism and hypothyroidism can be endemic. Diminished thyroid reserve occurs as a stage in the evolution of hypothyroidism.

Rarely, long-standing hypothyroidism leads to diffuse, nodular, or adenomatous thyrotroph hyperplasia. These patients may present with headache, visual field defects, abnormal pubertal development, galactorrhea, and pituitary enlargement, all of which disappear with levothyroxine therapy. Such patients have marked elevations in serum TSH levels, whereas in hypothyroidism of suprathyroid origin, the thyroid is intrinsically normal but is deprived of stimulation by TSH. Deprivation of TSH, most commonly the result of postpartum pituitary necrosis or a tumor of the pituitary, results in pituitary hypothyroidism. Hypothalamic hypothyroidism is less common and results from inadequate secretion of TRH.

CLINICAL PICTURE The manifestations of hypothyroidism in children depend on the age at which the deficiency began and the promptness with which replacement therapy is instituted. Cretinism may be manifest at birth but usually becomes evident within the first several months after birth, depending on the extent of thyroid failure. Hypothyroidism is present in approximately 1 in every 5000 neonates and manifests itself as persistence of physiologic jaundice, a hoarse cry, constipation, somnolence, and feeding problems; since clinical diagnosis is difficult and early treatment is crucial for normal intellectual development, all neonates should be screened for hypothyroidism with measurements of the serum T₄ or TSH. Later, delay in reaching the normal milestones of development becomes evident, and the physical characteristics of the cretin appear. These include short stature; coarse features with a protruding tongue, broad, flat nose, and widely set eyes; sparse hair; dry skin; a protuberant abdomen with an umbilical hernia; impaired mental development; retarded bone age; epiphyseal dysgenesis; and delayed dentition.

In the older child, the clinical manifestations of hypothyroidism include retardation of linear growth and delayed puberty. Poor performance at school may call attention to the diagnosis. Variable manifestations of adult hypothyroidism are present. X-ray examination reveals delayed union of the epiphyses.

In the adult, early symptoms of hypothyroidism are nonspecific and insidious in onset. In the elderly, symptoms may be erroneously attributed to aging itself, Parkinson's disease, depression, or Alzheimer's disease. They may include fatigue, lethargy, constipation, cold intolerance, stiffness and cramping of the muscles, carpal tunnel syndrome, and menorrhagia. Intellectual and motor activity slows, appetite declines, and weight increases. The hair becomes dry and tends to fall out, and the skin becomes dry. The voice becomes deeper and hoarse, and auditory acuity may deteriorate. Obstructive sleep apnea may occur. Ultimately, the clinical picture of florid myxedema appears, with a dull, expressionless facies, sparse hair, periorbital puffiness, large tongue, and pale, cool skin that feels rough and doughy. Thyroid tissue is usually not palpable, except in the goitrous variety. The heart is enlarged owing to both dilation and pericardial effusion; if the heart is small, pituitary hypothyroidism (with secondary adrenal insufficiency) or coincident primary adrenal insufficiency (Schmidt's syndrome) should be considered. Adynamic ileus may cause megacolon or intestinal obstruction. Rarely, psychiatric symptoms or cerebellar ataxia may dominate the clinical picture. The relaxation phase of the deep tendon reflexes is characteristically prolonged, the so-called hung-up reflex. If left untreated, the patient with long-standing hypothyroidism may pass into a hypothermic, stuporous state (*myxedema coma*) that may be fatal. Respiratory depression is an important component of this state, and hence arterial P_{CO_2} may be increased. Factors that predispose to myxedema coma include cold exposure, trauma, infection, and administration of central nervous system depressants. Hyponatremia may result from impaired water excretion and from disordered regulation of vasopressin secretion.

LABORATORY TESTS The single most useful measurement is the serum TSH, which is increased in the thyroprivic and goitrous varieties and is usually normal or undetectable in pituitary or hypothalamic hypothyroidism (see Fig. 331-3). In the latter instances, hyposecretion of TSH is usually accompanied by hyposecretion of other pituitary hormones (see Chap. 328). Decreases in serum T_4 and in the FT_4I are common to all varieties of hypothyroidism. In the primary varieties, the serum T_3 may be decreased less than the serum T_4, presumably because the compensatory hypersecretion of TSH leads to a relative preponderance of T_3 secretion. In thyroprivic hypothyroidism, the decreased RAIU is of limited diagnostic utility because of the low value for the lower limit of the normal range. In goitrous hypothyroidism, the RAIU may range from low to increased.

Manifestations of the hypothyroid state include an increased serum cholesterol level in hypothyroidism of thyroid (but not pituitary) origin and increased serum levels of creatine phosphokinase, aspartate transaminase, and lactate dehydrogenase. Systolic time intervals are altered in that the preejection period is prolonged and the ratio of the preejection period to the left ventricular ejection time is increased. Electrocardiographic changes include bradycardia, low-amplitude QRS complexes, and flattened or inverted T waves. In primary thyroprivic hypothyroidism, pernicious anemia occurs in about 12 percent of patients; histamine-fast achlorhydria and circulating antigastric parietal cell antibodies are more common.

Some patients who appear clinically euthyroid display laboratory evidence of early thyroid failure (subclinical hypothyroidism). In mild cases, serum TSH and its response to TRH administration are increased, while serum T_4 and T_3 levels are normal. When thyroid failure is more advanced, the serum T_4 concentration is decreased, but the serum T_3 concentration is normal or nearly so owing to TSH-induced hypersecretion of T_3 relative to T_4 and perhaps to more efficient conver-

sion of T_4 to T_3. Subclinical hypothyroidism is most often seen in patients with Hashimoto's disease or those with Graves' disease who have been treated with ^{131}I or surgery; in the latter, subclinical hypothyroidism usually represents a stage in the evolution of frank hypothyroidism.

DIFFERENTIAL DIAGNOSIS It is not difficult to diagnose the classic picture of cretinism or juvenile and adult hypothyroidism. Occasionally, an infant with Down's syndrome may be confused with a cretin. Chronic nephritis and the nephrotic syndrome may simulate myxedema, particularly because of the facial puffiness and pallor. The nephrotic patient may have anemia, hypercholesterolemia, and anasarca, and the serum T_4 may be decreased if TBG is lost into the urine. However, the FT_4I is normal or increased, the serum T_3 concentration is often subnormal (as in any severe systemic illness, owing to impaired peripheral generation from T_4), and the serum TSH concentration is normal.

℞ **TREATMENT**

Hormones available for the treatment of hypothyroidism (Table 331-6) include the synthetic hormones levothyroxine (L-thyroxine), liothyronine (L-triiodothyronine), and liotrix (a combination of the two). A preparation of natural origin still occasionally used is thyroid extract, USP. Because of their uniform potency, the author prefers the synthetic preparations, specifically levothyroxine. Unlike liothyronine, liotrix, and even thyroid extract, ingestion of levothyroxine does not lead to an abrupt increase in serum T_3 level, which can cause adverse and sometimes dangerous effects in the older patient or the patient with coexisting heart disease. Rather, a stable T_3 concentration is attained through continuous generation from administered levothyroxine.

In most instances, a normal metabolic state should be restored gradually, especially in the elderly and in patients with heart disease, since a sudden increase in metabolic rate may tax cardiac or coronary reserve. In adults, an initial daily dose of 25 μg levothyroxine can be increased by 25- to 50-μg increments at 4-week intervals until a normal metabolic state is attained. Patients on levothyroxine who have autoimmune thyroid disease tend to require less levothyroxine than patients who have had total thyroidectomy, because some functioning tissue usually persists in the former group. Such patients require about 1.7 μg levothyroxine per kilogram body weight per day, whereas totally thyroidectomized patients require approximately 2.1 μg per kilogram body weight per day. Because of its long half-life, levothyroxine is administered as a single daily dose. While the serum T_3 may be superior to the serum T_4 as an indicator of the metabolic state in patients receiving levothyroxine, the optimal dose is best determined by clinical criteria and measurement of TSH by an ultrasensitive assay. An elevated TSH indicates that treatment is insufficient, and an elevated T_3 indicates that it is excessive. Serum T_3 is a particularly useful parameter in patients with pituitary or hypothalamic disease, in whom interpretation of serum TSH levels is more difficult.

In some circumstances a previously stable dosage of levothyroxine may need to be increased or decreased. Increases of 25 to 50 μg per day may be required during pregnancy, as evidenced by increases in serum TSH. Progressive increases in dose may be required as further atrophy of the gland occurs in patients with Hashi-

Table 331-6

Approximate Therapeutic Equivalence of Various Thyroid Hormone Preparations

Preparation	Average Daily Oral Maintenance Dose	Serum (T_4)	Undesirable Lability in Serum (T_3)
Levothyroxine	125 μg	Slightly increased	−
Liothyronine	50 μg	Decreased	+ +
Liotrix ($T_4/T_3 = 4:1$)	2 units	Normal	+
Thyroid extract, USP	120–180 mg	Normal	+

Table 331-7

Reasons for Changing Levothyroxine Requirements in Patients on a Previously Stable Dosage*

Requirement for increased dose
  Pregnancy
  Further decrease in thyroid function due to
    Graves' disease after radioiodine administration
    Hashimoto's thyroiditis
  Impaired levothyroxine absorption due to
    Cholestyramine, colestipol
    Iron sulfate
    Sucralfate
    Aluminum hydroxide
    Short bowel syndromes
  Augmented levothyroxine metabolism due to
    Phenytoin
    Rifampin
    Carbamazepine
Requirement for decreased dose
  Spontaneous recovery from Hashimoto's thyroiditis due to disappearance
    of TSH receptor–blocking antibodies
  Reactivation of Graves' disease
  Emergence of autonomous nodules
  Advanced age
  Factitious ingestion of levothyroxine

* Exclusive of poor compliance

Table 331-8

Varieties of Thyrotoxicosis

Associated with thyroid hyperfunction*
  Excess production of TSH (rare)
  Abnormal thyroid stimulator
    Graves' disease
    Trophoblastic tumor
  Intrinsic thyroid autonomy
    Hyperfunctioning adenoma
    Toxic multinodular goiter
Not associated with thyroid hyperfunction†
  Disorders of hormone storage
    Subacute thyroiditis
    Chronic thyroiditis with transient thyrotoxicosis
  Extrathyroid source of hormone
    Thyrotoxicosis factitia
    "Hamburger toxicosis"
  Ectopic thyroid tissue
    Struma ovarii
    Functioning follicular carcinoma

* Associated with increased RAIU unless body iodine burden is excessive.
† Associated with decreased RAIU.

moto's disease or in patients with Graves' disease who have been treated with surgery or radioiodine. A number of drugs may interfere with gastrointestinal absorption or enhance the metabolic clearance of levothyroxine (Table 331-7). Similarly, decreases in dosage may be required with spontaneous disappearance of TSH receptor blocking antibodies in Hashimoto's disease, with increases in stimulatory antibodies to the TSH receptor causing reactivation of Graves' disease, or with the emergence of autonomy and hyperfunction in uninodular or multinodular goiter.

In neonatal, infantile, and juvenile hypothyroidism, full replacement therapy should be begun as soon as possible; otherwise, the chances of normal intellectual development and growth are poor. Infants and children require doses of levothyroxine that are disproportionately large in relation to body size. *In known or strongly suspected cases of pituitary and hypothalamic hypothyroidism, thyroid replacement should not be instituted until treatment with hydrocortisone has been initiated*, since acute adrenocortical insufficiency may be precipitated by an increase in metabolic rate and increased clearance of glucocorticoids.

In some adults, hypothyroidism should be treated rapidly. These include patients with myxedema coma and, because of the extreme sensitivity to central nervous system depressants, hypothyroid patients being prepared for emergency surgery. In these patients, intravenous administration of levothyroxine, in conjunction with the use of hydrocortisone, is indicated.

Patients with myxedema coma and associated systemic illness may have a reduced ability to convert T_4 to T_3, as in the sick euthyroid syndrome. Consequently, supplementary doses of liothyronine may be warranted, even though sole therapy with full doses of liothyronine is not recommended in view of the cardiovascular risk. For comatose patients, parenteral forms of both levothyroxine and liothyronine are available. A combined approach allows initial administration of 3 to 4 μg of levothyroxine per kilogram body weight intravenously followed by 100 μg/d thereafter, along with 10 μg of liothyronine every 8 h. Both parenteral preparations are discontinued when the patient becomes able to take oral medications.

THYROTOXICOSIS

The term *thyrotoxicosis* denotes the clinical, physiologic, and biochemical findings that result when the tissues are exposed to, and respond to, excess thyroid hormone. Rather than being a specific disease, thyrotoxicosis can originate in a variety of ways (Table 331-8). The most important of these disorders are those that lead to sustained overproduction of hormone by the thyroid gland itself. Rarely, this hyperfunction results from excessive secretion of TSH by a pituitary tumor or as a result of resistance to thyroid hormone in the pituitary but not in peripheral tissues. Other causes are the action of a homeostatically unregulated thyroid stimulator of extrapituitary origin, as in Graves' disease, Hashimoto's disease, and trophoblastic tumors, and the development of one or more areas of autonomous hyperfunction within the gland itself. Thyrotoxicosis not associated with thyroid hyperfunction includes that associated with subacute thyroiditis and the syndrome called chronic thyroiditis with transient thyrotoxicosis. In these disorders, an excess of preformed hormone leaks from the gland owing to the presence of inflammatory disease. New hormone formation is decreased because of the suppression of TSH secretion by the hormone excess and, in some cases, because of the inflammatory injury itself. Since the inflammatory disorders are transitory and since stores of preformed hormone are eventually depleted, the thyrotoxicosis in these disorders is self-limited and is often followed by a transient period of thyroid hormone insufficiency. Thyrotoxicosis can also occur when the source of excess hormone is outside of the thyroid gland, as in thyrotoxicosis factitia, the ingestion of meat contaminated with animal thyroids ("hamburger toxicosis"), the rare functioning metastatic thyroid carcinoma, and struma ovarii.

Not all of the foregoing disorders are associated with *hyperthyroidism*, a term that should be used to denote only those conditions in which sustained hyperfunction of the thyroid leads to thyrotoxicosis. This distinction has implications for diagnosis and for treatment. In hyperthyroidism, hyperfunction of the thyroid is reflected in an increased RAIU, whereas in the nonhyperthyroid thyrotoxic states, thyroid function (as reflected in the RAIU) is subnormal. Further, treatment of thyrotoxicosis by means intended to decrease hormone synthesis (antithyroid agents, surgery, or radioiodine) is appropriate in hyperthyroidism but is inappropriate and ineffective in other forms of thyrotoxicosis.

Although the diseases that cause thyrotoxicosis make their own imprint on the clinical picture, the manifestations of the thyrotoxic state are largely the same. For this reason, the common manifestations of thyrotoxicosis are described in relation to Graves' disease.

GRAVES' DISEASE

Graves' disease, also known as Parry's or Basedow's disease, is a disorder with three major manifestations: hyperthyroidism with diffuse goiter, ophthalmopathy, and dermopathy. These manifestations need not appear together. Indeed, one or two need never appear, and the three may run largely independent courses.

PREVALENCE Graves' disease is a relatively common disorder that can occur at any age but is especially common in the third and fourth decades. The disease is more frequent in women. In nongoitrous areas, the ratio of predominance in women may be as high as 7:1. In areas of endemic goiter, the ratio is lower. Genetic factors play an important role; there is an increased frequency of haplotypes HLA-B8 and -DRw3 in Caucasian, HLA-Bw36 in Japanese, and HLA-Bw46 in Chinese patients with the disease. Not surprisingly, there is a familial predisposition. In addition, among family members, a clinical and immunologic overlap exists with respect to Hashimoto's disease, primary thyroprivic hypothyroidism, and pernicious anemia and probably with respect to other autoimmune disorders as well. In occasional patients, the picture may change from Graves' disease to Hashimoto's disease or vice versa, and, rarely, patients with primary myxedema later become hyperthyroid. Thus, it is proper to consider Graves' disease, Hashimoto's disease, and primary myxedema as closely related autoimmune thyroid diseases.

ETIOLOGY AND PATHOGENESIS The cause of Graves' disease is unknown. In view of the variety of manifestations and courses, it is possible that no single factor is responsible for the entire syndrome. With respect to hyperthyroidism, the central disorder is a disruption of homeostatic mechanisms that normally control hormone secretion. This disruption results from the presence in plasma of thyroid-stimulating immunoglobulins (TSIs) of the IgG class that are elaborated by lymphocytes. When human thyroid tissue is used as the assay system, the end points are stimulation of colloid droplet or cyclic AMP generation (for thyroid-stimulating antibodies, TSAbs) and inhibition of the binding of TSH to its receptors in human thyroid tissue (TSH-binding inhibitory immunoglobulins, TBIIs). These factors represent antibodies against the thyroid TSH receptor (TRAbs). Activities of this type are also found in the serum of some patients with euthyroid ophthalmic Graves' disease, occasional patients with Hashimoto's disease, and some euthyroid relatives of patients with Graves' disease. Presumably, the absence of thyrotoxicosis in such instances reflects the predominance of blocking over stimulatory TRAbs or intrinsic thyroid disease that prevents a hyperthyroid response. Disappearance of stimulatory factors from the serum during antithyroid treatment augurs well for long-term remission after treatment is withdrawn. Thus, while the basic cause of Graves' disease is not understood, an immunoglobulin or family of immunoglobulins directed against the TSH receptor mediates the thyroid stimulation. An inherited abnormality in immune surveillance may permit particular lymphocytes to survive, proliferate, and secrete the stimulatory immunoglobulins in response to precipitating factors.

The pathogenesis of the ophthalmic component is more enigmatic. An antigen in orbital tissues that cross-reacts with the thyroid has been postulated, and fibroblasts from orbital tissues contain a material that reacts with antibodies to the TSH receptor. Both cellular and humoral immunity may play a role in the ophthalmopathy. Cytokines and/or growth factors released by T cells may lead to production of an inflammatory reaction with proliferation of more fibroblasts and glycosaminoglycan production, thereby initiating the edema and increase in muscle volume and retroorbital fat. Even less is known about the pathogenesis of the dermopathy.

PATHOLOGY The *thyroid gland* is diffusely enlarged, soft, and vascular. There is parenchymatous hypertrophy and hyperplasia, characterized by increased height of the epithelium and redundancy of the follicular wall, causing papillary infoldings, and cytologic evidence of increased activity. Such hyperplasia is usually accompanied by lymphocytic infiltration that reflects the immune nature of the disease and correlates with levels of antithyroid antibodies in the blood. Following iodine medication, there is colloid storage, which sometimes causes enlargement and increased firmness of the gland. Graves' disease is associated with generalized lymphoid hyperplasia

and infiltration and occasionally with enlargement of the spleen or thymus. Thyrotoxicosis may lead to degeneration of skeletal muscle fibers, enlargement of the heart, fatty infiltration or diffuse fibrosis of the liver, decalcification of the skeleton, and loss of body tissue (including fat deposits, osteoid, and muscle).

The *ophthalmopathy* is characterized by an inflammatory infiltrate of the orbital contents, exclusive of the globe, with lymphocytes, mast cells, and plasma cells. The orbital musculature is often enlarged owing to infiltration with lymphocytes, mucopolysaccharides, and edema, which with fat largely account for the increased volume of the orbital contents that causes the globe to protrude. Muscle fibers show degeneration and loss of striations, with ultimate fibrosis.

The *dermopathy* of Graves' disease is characterized by thickening of the dermis, which is infiltrated with lymphocytes and with hydrophilic, metachromatically staining mucopolysaccharides.

CLINICAL MANIFESTATIONS The manifestations include those that reflect the associated thyrotoxicosis and those specifically related to Graves' disease.

Manifestations of Thyrotoxicosis Common manifestations include nervousness, emotional lability, inability to sleep, tremors, frequent bowel movements, excessive sweating, and heat intolerance. Weight loss is usual despite a well-maintained or increased appetite. Proximal muscle weakness with loss of strength is often manifested by difficulty in climbing stairs. In premenopausal women, oligomenorrhea and amenorrhea tend to occur. Dyspnea, palpitations, and, in older patients, enhancement of angina pectoris or cardiac failure may be present. In general, nervous symptoms dominate the clinical picture in younger individuals, whereas cardiovascular and myopathic symptoms predominate in older subjects.

Usually, the patient appears anxious, restless, and fidgety. The skin is warm and moist with a velvety texture, and palmar erythema is present. Separation of the fingernail from the nailbed (onycholysis; Plummer's nail) is common, especially on the ring finger. The hair is fine and silky. A fine tremor of the fingers and tongue, together with hyperreflexia, is characteristic. *Ocular signs* include a characteristic stare with widened palpebral fissures, infrequent blinking, lid lag, and failure to wrinkle the brow on upward gaze. These signs result from sympathetic overstimulation and usually subside when the thyrotoxicosis is corrected. They are to be distinguished from the *infiltrative ophthalmopathy* characteristic of Graves' disease, discussed below.

Cardiovascular features include a wide pulse pressure, sinus tachycardia, atrial arrhythmias (especially atrial fibrillation), systolic murmurs, increased intensity of the apical first sound, cardiac enlargement, and, at times, overt heart failure. A to-and-fro, high-pitched sound may be audible in the pulmonic area and may simulate a pericardial friction rub (Means-Lerman scratch).

Manifestations of Graves' Disease The distinctive manifestations—diffuse hyperfunctioning goiter, ophthalmopathy, and dermopathy—appear in varying combinations and in varying frequencies, goiter being the most common. Premature graying of the hair and patchy vitiligo are not specific for Graves' disease and are common in other autoimmune disorders.

The *diffuse toxic goiter* may be asymmetric and lobular. The presence of a bruit over the gland usually signifies that the patient is thyrotoxic, but this sign is present rarely in other forms of thyroid hyperplasia. Venous hums and carotid souffles should be distinguished from true thyroid bruits. An enlarged pyramidal lobe of the thyroid may be palpable.

The signs associated with the *ophthalmopathy* of Graves' disease may be divided into two components: the spastic and the mechanical. The former includes the stare, lid lag, and lid retraction that accompany thyrotoxicosis and account for the "frightened" facies and eye signs previously described. These findings need not be associated with proptosis, may be ameliorated by adrenergic antagonists, and usually return to normal after correction of thyrotoxicosis. The mechanical component includes proptosis of varying degrees with ophthalmoplegia and congestive oculopathy characterized by chemosis, conjunctivitis, periorbital swelling, and the potential complications of corneal ulceration, optic neuritis, and optic atrophy. When exophthalmos progresses rapidly and becomes the major concern in Graves' disease, it is termed *progressive* and, if severe, *malignant exophthalmos*. The term *exophthalmic ophthalmoplegia* refers to the ocular muscle weakness that results in impaired upward gaze and convergence and strabismus with varying degrees of diplopia. Exophthalmos may be unilateral early but usually becomes bilateral with time.

The *dermopathy* usually occurs over the dorsum of the legs or feet and is termed *localized* or *pretibial myxedema*. It is usually a late phenomenon but is not a manifestation of hypothyroidism. About half of cases occur during the active stage of thyrotoxicosis, and virtually all have ophthalmopathy. The affected area is usually demarcated from normal skin by being raised and thickened and having a *peau d'orange* appearance; it may also be pruritic and hyperpigmented. The most common presentation is a nonpitting edema, but the lesions may be plaquelike, nodular, or polypoid in configuration. Clubbing of the fingers and toes with bony changes that differ from those of hypertrophic pulmonary osteoarthropathy may accompany the dermal changes (*thyroid acropachy*).

DIAGNOSIS When severe, Graves' disease presents little difficulty in diagnosis. Florid thyrotoxicosis is manifested by weakness, weight loss despite a good appetite, nervous instability, tremor, intolerance to heat, sweating, palpitations, and hyperdefecation. When associated with diffuse thyroid enlargement, often accompanied by a bruit, and particularly when associated with ophthalmopathy, the clinical picture is virtually unique. In such instances, laboratory tests documenting undetectable TSH and increased values of the RAIU, of serum T_4 and T_3 levels, of the RT_3U, and of the FT_4I serve as baselines for evaluation of therapy rather than necessary diagnostic aids. Occasionally, laboratory tests reveal a normal RAIU, a normal serum T_4 level and RT_3U, and an elevated serum T_3 level and FT_3I (T_3 toxicosis).

In less severe cases, particularly when ophthalmopathy is lacking, the diagnosis may be more difficult, since the symptoms of mild thyrotoxicosis are similar to those of other disorders (see "Differential Diagnosis," below). The presence of a goiter makes the diagnosis of hyperthyroidism likely, but careful palpation is necessary to determine whether toxic multinodular goiter, toxic adenoma, or subacute thyroiditis is present. Absence of thyroid enlargement makes the diagnosis of Graves' disease less likely but does not exclude it. In mild cases, confirmatory laboratory tests assume great importance. Unfortunately, mild thyrotoxicosis is often associated with marginal abnormalities in serum T_4 and T_3 values. In such instances, an ultrasensitive TSH assay or the TRH stimulation test assumes crucial importance.

In a few (usually older) patients, the clinical picture is one of apathy rather than hyperactivity, and evidence of hypermetabolism may be slight (*apathetic thyrotoxicosis*). In such patients, myopathic features may be pronounced. More often, cardiovascular manifestations predominate, since mild hyperthyroidism may produce severe disability in patients with underlying heart disease. Hence, *all patients with unexplained cardiac failure or atrial arrhythmias should be evaluated for thyrotoxicosis*.

DIFFERENTIAL DIAGNOSIS Signs and symptoms of several nonthyroid disorders may simulate certain aspects of the thyrotoxic syndrome. Anxiety is a prominent feature of thyrotoxicosis, and there is overlap in the symptomatology of thyrotoxicosis and of anxiety states. Tachycardia, tremulousness, irritability, weakness, and fatigue are common to both disorders. In anxiety, however, the peripheral manifestations of excessive thyroid hormones are absent; the skin is usually cold and clammy rather than warm and moist. Weight loss, when present in emotional anxiety, is characteristically accompanied by anorexia, whereas in thyrotoxicosis the appetite is increased. Thyrotoxicosis can occasionally be confused with such disorders as metastatic carcinoma, cirrhosis of the liver, hyperparathyroidism, sprue, myasthenia gravis, and muscular dystrophy. Hypokalemic periodic paralysis is more common in thyrotoxic patients, especially in Asian and Latin American men. Signs and symptoms of thyrotoxicosis may overlap with those of pheochromocytoma, which can cause heat intolerance, sweating, tachycardia with palpitations, and a hypermetabolic state. Laboratory tests usually make it possible to differentiate these various disorders from thyrotoxicosis.

When bilateral ophthalmopathy is accompanied by goiter and thyrotoxicosis, the diagnosis of Graves' ophthalmopathy is virtually certain. The presence of unilateral ophthalmopathy, even when associated with thyrotoxicosis, raises the possibility of some other intraorbital or intracranial disease. In the euthyroid patient with either unilateral or bilateral ophthalmopathy, other causes that must be excluded are cavernous sinus thrombosis, sphenoidal ridge meningioma, retrobulbar tumors, including leukemic deposits, and the rare granulomatous disorder pseudotumor oculi. Exophthalmos also may be seen in certain systemic disorders, such as uremia, accelerated hypertension, chronic alcoholism, chronic obstructive pulmonary disease, superior mediastinal obstruction, and Cushing's syndrome. Ophthalmoplegia in the absence of infiltrative manifestations can be confused with that in diabetes mellitus, myasthenia gravis, and myopathies. When doubt exists about the cause of ophthalmopathy, the demonstration of significant titers of TSI or TBII or of an abnormal result on a TRH stimulation or thyroid suppression test suggests that the cause is Graves' disease, though not all patients with "euthyroid Graves' disease" demonstrate abnormal responses. In such cases, ultrasonography, magnetic resonance imaging, or computed tomography of the orbits is valuable in demonstrating characteristic thickening of the extraocular muscles.

When a thyrotoxic state occurs in a patient lacking the ophthalmopathy of Graves' disease, other causes of thyrotoxicosis must be considered. Careful palpation of the thyroid and studies with radioactive iodine are important in this regard. A symmetric, diffuse goiter of moderate or large size suggests the diagnosis of Graves' disease, especially if a bruit is present. However, the uncommon patient whose hyperthyroidism is secondary to an excess of TSH (associated with a *pituitary tumor* or resistance to feedback suppression of TSH secretion) or an abnormal stimulator of trophoblastic origin (*hydatidiform mole* or *choriocarcinoma of the uterus* or *testis;* see Chap. 102) may present in this way. A single, prominent thyroid nodule or multiple nodules suggest *toxic adenoma* or *toxic multinodular goiter*, respectively. Tenderness of the thyroid associated with firm nodularity suggests *subacute thyroiditis*, while a small, firm, nontender goiter is consistent with chronic thyroiditis with spontaneously resolving thyrotoxicosis. The foregoing disorders are discussed in later sections. Absence of a palpable thyroid gland suggests an extrathyroid source of hormone, such as ectopic thyroid tissue (*struma ovarii*) or, more commonly, self-administration of hormone (*thyrotoxicosis factitia*). Studies with radioactive iodine are also helpful. Except when hormone overproduction is secondary to increased iodine intake, values of the RAIU are increased in all disorders producing hyperthyroidism. Conversely, thyrotoxicosis that is not the result of hyperthyroidism is characterized by subnormal values of the RAIU. Subacute thyroiditis and chronic thyroiditis with spontaneously resolving thyrotoxicosis are the most common. Ectopic thyroid tissue producing thyrotoxicosis is rare. Here, the RAIU, as measured over the thyroid, is low, since TSH secretion is suppressed, but urinary excretion of radioactive iodine is slowed, owing to accumulation by the ectopic tissue. Functioning ectopic tissue can be located by scintillation scanning.

Thyrotoxicosis factitia most frequently occurs in medical or paramedical personnel or in those who have easy access to thyroid hormone. The disorder resembles thyrotoxicosis caused by ectopic thyroid tissue in that the patient's thyroid is suppressed. Consequently, the RAIU is very low, and most of administered radioactive iodine is excreted promptly in the urine. When the disorder is caused by ingestion of preparations containing T_4, such as levothyroxine or thyroid extract, the serum T_4 is increased. On the other hand, when it is caused by liothyronine, the serum T_4 is subnormal. Irrespective of the preparation, the serum T_3 is increased, but more so when liothyronine is the offending agent. Measurement of serum thyroglobulin is useful to confirm thyrotoxicosis factitia. Levels are elevated in Graves' disease and thyroiditis but are subnormal with exogenous thyroid hormone suppression. The demonstration of elevated titers of thyroid-stimulating immunoglobulins in the blood also provides strong evidence that Graves' disease is the cause of thyrotoxicosis.

℞ TREATMENT

Hyperthyroidism Hyperthyroidism is often characterized by cyclic phases of exacerbation and remission, which are of unpredictable onset and duration. Moreover, long-standing disease may be associated with progressive thyroid failure, probably consequent to chronic thyroiditis, with the supervention of hypothyroidism or decreased thyroid reserve. These characteristics have important implications for the choice of and response to therapy.

The major treatments are directed to limiting the quantity of thyroid hormones the gland can produce. Antithyroid agents chemically block hormone synthesis—an effect that persists only as long as the drug is administered—and they may also enhance evolution to remission through their anti-immune effects. Their principal use is to control active thyrotoxicity while remission is awaited. The second major approach to limiting hormone production is ablation of thyroid tissue, either by surgery or by the use of radioactive iodine. Since these procedures permanently alter the thyroid anatomy, they can control the active phase of the disease and are more likely to prevent later exacerbation or recurrence. On the other hand, surgery or radiation is more likely to lead to hypothyroidism, either shortly after treatment or with the passage of years.

Each type of therapy has advantages and disadvantages, indications and contraindications, both relative and absolute. In general, a trial of long-term antithyroid therapy is desirable in children, adolescents, young adults, and pregnant women but also may be employed in older patients. Indications for ablative procedures include relapse or recurrence following drug therapy, a large goiter, drug toxicity, failure to follow a medical regimen, or failure to return for periodic examinations. Subtotal thyroidectomy may be elected for patients under the age of 30 in whom ablative therapy is required; however, opinions differ, and some authorities employ radioactive iodine in the treatment of patients in the second or third decade. Surgery is also preferable in patients with very large goiters or with a coincident nonfunctioning nodule, especially if there is a history of radiation to the head and neck. Radioactive iodine is the ablative procedure of choice in older patients, in patients with previous thyroid surgery, and in those in whom systemic disease contraindicates elective surgery.

In patients selected for *long-term antithyroid therapy*, satisfactory control can almost always be achieved if sufficient drug is administered. Most patients can be managed with propylthiouracil, 100 to 150 mg every 6 or 8 h. Larger doses may be required for initial control. Methimazole is at least as effective as propylthiouracil when administered at one-tenth the dosage. However, propylthiouracil has the advantage of inhibiting the peripheral conversion of T_4 to T_3, thereby bringing about more rapid symptomatic improvement. Once euthyroidism is achieved, the daily dosage may be reduced to the smallest amount that controls the thyrotoxicosis. In some clinics, the initial dose is continued and is supplemented with levothyroxine. This regimen avoids the risk of hypothyroidism from overdosage of antithyroid drugs and thus may forestall the undesirable consequences of hypothyroidism, such as enhancement of ophthalmopathy and enlargement of the goiter. The duration of antithyroid drug therapy is difficult to predict in the individual patient and may be a function of the natural course of the disease. The longer the course of therapy, the more likely it is that the patient will remain well when the drug is discontinued. In general, a 12- to 24-month course is employed, after which one-third to one-half of patients remain well for a prolonged period or indefinitely. The likelihood of a prolonged remission is increased by a decrease in goiter size, reversion of the results of the thyroid suppression test and TRH stimulation test to normal, or disappearance of TRAbs from the serum during treatment.

Leukopenia is the principal undesirable side effect of antithyroid drugs. A complete blood count should be obtained prior to initiating therapy to identify those patients with leukopenia related to Graves' disease. Mild transient leukopenia with antithyroid drugs may occur in an additional 10 percent of patients and is not necessarily an indication for discontinuing therapy. When the absolute number of polymorphonuclear leukocytes reaches $\leq 1500/\mu L$, antithyroid medication should be discontinued. Allergic rashes and drug sensitivity also occur on occasion. These may disappear with antihistamine therapy at the same or a reduced dosage of antithyroid agent, but when sensitivity reactions occur it is preferable to change to another drug. On rare occasions (in fewer than 0.2 percent of cases), agranulocytosis occurs. It may be sudden in onset. Hepatitis, drug fever, and arthralgias can also occur. In the author's view, severe sensitivity reactions, including agranulocytosis, mandate the abandonment of antithyroid therapy rather than recourse to an alternative drug.

Iodide inhibits the release of hormones from the hyperfunctioning thyroid gland, and its ameliorative effects occur more rapidly than those of agents that inhibit hormone synthesis. Hence, its main use is in patients with actual or impending thyrotoxic crisis and in patients with severe cardiac disease. The response to iodide alone is often incomplete and transient. Furthermore, by expanding the thyroid store of hormone, iodide may prolong the latency of response to antithyroid therapy. Therefore, iodide is safely used only in conjunction with the antithyroid agents. If the clinical course is sufficiently severe to require iodide administration, antithyroid drugs are usually the primary therapeutic agents and should be given in large doses prior to iodide. Iodide is also useful in controlling thyrotoxicosis following ^{131}I administration, during the period in which the therapeutic effect of radioiodine has not yet taken place. Large doses of *glucocorticoids* (2 mg dexamethasone every 6 h) reduce the serum T_4 concentration when relief of thyrotoxicosis is urgent. The iodinated x-ray contrast agent sodium ipodate has a similar effect. Iodine liberated from this agent inhibits thyroid secretion of T_4 and T_3, and serum T_3 is further reduced by the inhibition by ipodate of peripheral T_3 formation. Daily doses of 1 g orally are effective, but the same precautions that apply to the use of iodine therapy apply to ipodate.

Owing to the adrenergic component in thyrotoxicosis, various *adrenergic antagonists* have been employed in its management. Of these, propranolol is the agent of choice because of its relative freedom from side effects. In doses of 40 to 120 mg/d, propranolol alleviates such adrenergic manifestations as sweating, tremor, and tachycardia and may reduce to some extent the conversion of T_4 to T_3. However, propranolol should be used only as adjunctive therapy, since the underlying metabolic abnormalities are not affected. Moreover, although the diminution in heart rate and cardiac work may be beneficial, the blocking of adrenergic support of myocardial contractility necessitates caution in the use of this agent in patients with coexisting heart failure, unless the latter is rate- or rhythm-related. As an adjunctive agent, propranolol is useful while the response to conventional antithyroid agents or to radioiodine therapy is awaited and in the management of thyrotoxic crisis. It has been employed as the sole agent in preparation for thyroidectomy, but its use in this setting is not recommended, since it does not render the patient euthyroid, and thus probably does not minimize the risk of surgically induced crisis.

Radioactive iodine (^{131}I) affords a relatively simple, effective, and economical means of treating thyrotoxicosis. It can produce the ablative effects of surgery without the operative and postoperative complications. The principal disadvantage of ^{131}I therapy, in the dosage usually employed, is its tendency to produce hypothyroidism with a frequency that increases with time. As many as 40 to 70 percent of patients may develop this complication within 10 years after treatment. Although hypothyroidism is treatable once diagnosed, the insidious onset may obscure the diagnosis until serious complications develop. Hence, some workers recommend that all patients be treated with relatively large doses of ^{131}I to ensure relief of thyrotoxicosis and then placed on permanent physiologic replacement doses of thyroid hormone.

There is no evidence that radioiodine has carcinogenic or leuke-mogenic effects when given to adults in the doses commonly used in treating hyperthyroidism. However, the susceptibility to carcinogenesis may be increased in the thyroids of children. Mutagenic effects have not been reported and would be difficult to document. For these reasons, many physicians prefer to reserve radioiodine therapy for patients over 30 years of age or those unlikely to have children afterward. Moreover, the longer the life expectancy after ^{131}I therapy, the greater the likelihood that hypothyroidism will develop. Among younger patients, therefore, only those with recurrent thyrotoxicosis following surgery, those who refuse surgery, and those with a complicating illness that contraindicates surgery are candidates for radioiodine therapy. In elderly patients, treatment with large doses of radioiodine is the general method of choice, so that the undesirable effects of incomplete treatment or recurrence can be avoided. It is controversial whether radioiodine therapy worsens ophthalmopathy, but in patients with significant ophthalmopathy, it may be prudent to administer glucocorticoids for approximately 2 weeks before and 6 weeks after the ^{131}I dose to reduce the likelihood of exacerbation of eye disease. Other possible risk factors for worsening opthalmopathy include smoking and more severe thyrotoxicosis.

The usual therapeutic dose of [131]I [approximately 5.9 MBq (160 μCi) per gram of estimated gland weight] leads to a high frequency of hypothyroidism. As a result, some authorities who continue to use this dose regularly administer prophylactic replacement doses of thyroid hormone. Others have administered smaller doses [approximately 3.0 MBq/g (80 μCi/g)]. However, these smaller doses do not diminish the frequency of late hypothyroidism but merely delay its onset. Moreover, they are less likely to relieve thyrotoxicosis within a relatively short period. Antithyroid agents can be employed, however, to speed the attainment of a eumetabolic state, and propranolol can be given to relieve symptoms while the effect of the ^{131}I is taking hold. There is general agreement that patients with coexisting cardiac disease should receive ^{131}I in large doses in view of the hazard of persistent or recurrent thyrotoxicosis.

Radiation thyroiditis is an occasional early complication of ^{131}I therapy. It commonly appears within 7 to 10 days and is associated with accelerated release of hormone into the blood. Rarely, radiation thyroiditis causes thyrotoxic crisis (see below), most commonly in elderly thyrotoxic patients with other systemic illness. For these reasons, patients with severe hyperthyroidism or underlying heart disease should be rendered eumetabolic with antithyroid agents before ^{131}I is administered. Interruption of antithyroid therapy for 3 to 4 days before and after ^{131}I treatment suffices to permit adequate accumulation and retention of administered [131]I. Propranolol may be used as an adjunct both before and after ^{131}I administration but should not be relied on to provide adequate prophylaxis if given alone. The swelling that accompanies radiation thyroiditis may contraindicate the use of large doses of ^{131}I in patients with large retrosternal goiters.

Before radioactive iodine was introduced, *subtotal thyroidectomy* was the standard ablative therapy, and it is still employed in younger patients in whom antithyroid therapy is unsuccessful. Although precise preoperative programs differ, several general principles should be emphasized. Patients should first be rendered euthyroid by means of antithyroid agents. Only then should iodide (five drops of Lugol's solution a day for approximately 10 days) be administered concomitantly to effect an involutional response in the gland. Antithyroid drugs should not be discontinued merely because treatment with iodide is instituted. The response of the patient, and not the calendar, should dictate when surgery is performed.

Hazards of subtotal thyroidectomy include immediate complications, such as anesthetic accidents, hemorrhage sometimes leading to respiratory obstruction, and damage to the recurrent laryngeal nerve leading to vocal cord paralysis. Later complications include wound infection, hemorrhage, hypoparathyroidism, and hypothyroidism. Subtotal thyroidectomy should be performed by a surgeon experienced in this procedure; under this condition, surgery is effec-tive and relatively safe. Postoperative recurrences are uncommon. However, carefully conducted follow-up studies reveal that hypothyroidism follows surgery more frequently than previously suspected, although not as often as with conventional doses of [131]I.

The *treatment of hyperthyroidism during pregnancy* is a subject of some disagreement. Most physicians believe that antithyroid therapy is preferable to surgery, which should not be performed in any event during the first and third trimesters. Antithyroid agents carry less risk to the patient and the pregnancy. Further, since they traverse the placental barrier, they have the theoretical advantage of preventing fetal and neonatal hyperthyroidism when maternal titers of TRAbs are high. As a clue to the risk of fetal hyperthyroidism, assays of such stimulators should be conducted in the third trimester in pregnant women with a history of Graves' disease, whether treated or not. On the other hand, the major disadvantage of antithyroid therapy is the possibility of inducing hypothyroidism in the fetus. T_4 and T_3 traverse the human placenta from mother to fetus only slowly, and simultaneous administration of thyroid hormone and antithyroid drugs to the mother will not protect the fetus from hypothyroidism. Hence, the cardinal rule in using the antithyroid agents in pregnancy is that the dosage should be the smallest necessary to control hyperthyroidism in the mother. From the laboratory standpoint, the physician should aim to keep the serum TSH and FT_4 concentrations within the normal limits, remembering that pregnancy is normally associated with some elevation of the serum total T_4 owing to an increase in serum TBG concentration. Since pregnancy appears to attenuate the severity of hyperthyroidism, control can often be achieved with maintenance doses of 200 mg of propylthiouracil daily or less. At this dose, fetal goiter and hypothyroidism have not been a problem. Patients who require doses of 300 mg/d or more during the first trimester should probably be treated by subtotal thyroidectomy during the middle trimester. The author believes that patients carried through pregnancy on antithyroid agents should not be given propranolol as adjunctive treatment, in view of reports that the agent may cause fetal growth retardation and neonatal respiratory depression. Propylthiouracil tends to be favored over methimazole, even though earlier reports of fetal anomalies with the latter agent have not been confirmed. Advantages of propylthiouracil include its effect on inhibiting conversion of T_4 to T_3 and its higher degree of protein binding, which retards its excretion into breast milk. Radioiodine should never be administered to a pregnant woman, and all women of childbearing age who are about to receive ^{131}I should have a pregnancy test performed first.

Ophthalmopathy, Dermopathy Severe and progressive ophthalmopathy is the most difficult component of Graves' disease to treat satisfactorily. Fortunately, in most patients the disorder runs a benign course that is largely independent of the hyperthyroidism, and even moderately severe disease usually improves with time, although some exophthalmos and ophthalmoplegia may persist. In mild disease, considerable benefit may be obtained from simple measures, such as elevating the head at night, administering diuretics to reduce edema, and providing tinted glasses for protection from sun, wind, and foreign bodies. A 1% solution of methylcellulose or plastic shields may prevent corneal drying in patients unable to close the lids during sleep. In more severe cases with progressive exophthalmos, chemosis, ophthalmoplegia, or loss of vision, large doses of prednisone (100 to 120 mg/d) are usually effective in reducing the edematous and infiltrative components. With improvement, the dosage is reduced to the lowest effective level to minimize glucocorticoid excess. Orbital radiation may be helpful in some patients with acute, severe infiltrative manifestations, particularly when administered concomitantly with glucocorticoids. In cases that progress despite these measures, orbital decompression—i.e., removal of part of the bony orbit—is required to relieve intraorbital pressure. The management must always be conducted in concert with an ophthalmologist.

Severe dermopathy can be alleviated by the topical application of glucocorticoids; only 10 percent of patients achieve complete remission, and 40 to 50 percent achieve partial remission.

TOXIC MULTINODULAR GOITER

Toxic multinodular goiter is an occasional consequence of long-standing simple goiter, although the frequency with which this complication arises is uncertain. In areas where goiter is not endemic, the cause of nontoxic multinodular goiter is usually indeterminate. Hence, it is unclear whether a specific factor underlies those cases of nontoxic multinodular goiter that progress to the thyrotoxic phase. A common feature of many nontoxic multinodular goiters, even in areas of iodine sufficiency, is a decreased iodine content of thyroglobulin, a finding that suggests either a conditioned deficiency of iodine or an impairment of the normal incorporation of iodine into the protein. There is no pathologic feature to distinguish nontoxic from toxic multinodular goiter. However, the transition from nontoxic to toxic nodular goiter involves the development of functional autonomy, i.e., independence from TSH stimulation in one or more areas of the gland. Scattered foci of functional autonomy are demonstrable early in the disease process, and they increase in size and number with time so that about a fourth of seemingly euthyroid patients with nontoxic nodular goiter display, as evidence of functional autonomy, subnormal or absent responses to TRH administration. As judged from scintillation scanning, functional patterns may be of two types. In the more common type, iodine accumulation occurs diffusely in patchy foci throughout the gland, whereas in the less common pattern, iodine accumulates in one or more discrete nodules within the gland, the remainder of the gland appearing to be essentially nonfunctional. Histologic and autoradiographic studies reveal marked heterogeneity of structure and function, the two being poorly correlated. In both endemic and sporadic nontoxic multinodular goiter, administration of iodides may lead to the development of thyrotoxicosis (jodbasedow), a complication consonant with the functional autonomy of this disorder.

Because it arises on a background of long-standing simple goiter, toxic multinodular goiter is a disease of the aging or elderly. For this reason, and because of the nature of the underlying disease, the clinical presentation differs from that of Graves' disease. Ophthalmopathy is rare and would signal the emergence of Graves' disease superimposed on simple goiter. Some patients have typical thyrotoxicosis. Often, however, the thyrotoxicosis is less severe than that in Graves' disease, although its physiologic impact on specific organ systems may be great. Notable among these is the cardiovascular system, in which arrhythmias or congestive failure may be precipitated or accentuated by thyrotoxicosis that may be manifested elsewhere by only subtle findings (apathetic hyperthyroidism). Weakness and wasting may predominate, frequently with loss of appetite rather than hyperphagia, suggesting the presence of malignancy.

In some patients, a definitive diagnosis of toxic nodular goiter is difficult to establish. On the one hand, enlargement or nodularity of the gland may escape detection because the patient has a short neck or is kyphotic or because the thyroid is substernal. When this is the case, and when the clinical findings suggest thyrotoxicosis, RAIU determination and scintiscan are particularly helpful. On the other hand, even when a nodular goiter is palpable, the presence of mild but clinically significant thyrotoxicosis may be difficult to confirm, since values of the serum total T_4 and T_3, the FT_4, and FT_4I are often only slightly above normal. For example, a serum T_3 value that would be normal for a young adult may represent an increase in the elderly patient, since serum T_3 usually declines with age. Despite their value in situations such as this, thyroid suppression tests should rarely be undertaken in elderly patients because of the hazard of adverse cardiovascular responses. Unfortunately, although a normal response to TRH would exclude a diagnosis of thyrotoxicosis in a patient with a nodular goiter, subnormal responses do not establish the diagnosis. Responses

to TRH decline in the elderly, especially in men, and seemingly euthyroid patients with nodular goiter may respond subnormally to TRH as a reflection of at least partial functional autonomy of the gland. An undetectable basal TSH and absent response to TRH by an ultrasensitive assay imply thyrotoxicosis (see Fig. 331-3). When laboratory and clinical findings do not permit a clear diagnosis of thyrotoxicosis, a therapeutic trial of antithyroid drugs may be useful.

Radioactive iodine is the treatment of choice for toxic multinodular goiter. In contrast to Graves' disease, large doses [740 to 1110 MBq (20 to 30 mCi)] are usually required, owing to the generally lower RAIU and the variable degree of function throughout the gland. Moreover, the physiologic instability of the elderly patient makes definitive treatment urgent. For the same reason, it is usually wise to initiate therapy with antithyroid agents, withholding radioiodine until a euthyroid state is achieved, thereby forestalling an exacerbation of thyrotoxicosis should radiation thyroiditis occur. Unless contraindicated, propranolol is often useful in controlling manifestations of thyrotoxicosis both before and after radioiodine therapy, while its therapeutic effect is awaited. Hypothyroidism is an uncommon consequence of radioiodine treatment of toxic multinodular goiter owing to the variable activity of differing portions of the gland, which permits previously quiescent areas to function in place of those destroyed by ^{131}I.

UNUSUAL VARIETIES OF THYROTOXICOSIS

Thyrotoxicosis is also seen in other disorders, including follicular adenoma of the thyroid and various forms of thyroiditis, which are discussed in later sections. This section will consider still other unusual causes of thyrotoxicosis and unusual ways in which thyrotoxicosis may present.

UNUSUAL CAUSES OF THYROTOXICOSIS Rarely, hyperthyroidism and thyrotoxicosis are the result of sustained hypersecretion of TSH either from a *TSH-secreting pituitary adenoma* or owing to a selective *resistance of the TSH-secretory mechanism* to feedback inhibition by thyroid hormones. The various syndromes in which both the pituitary and peripheral tissues are relatively resistant to thyroid hormones are discussed above. TSH-secreting pituitary adenomas can be distinguished, in many cases, by radiologic evidence of a pituitary tumor, by the fact that the concentration of free α subunits of TSH in serum is elevated, and by the fact that the response of the serum TSH to TRH is negligible. In the variant caused by pituitary resistance, subunit concentrations are not grossly elevated, and the TSH response to TRH is usually normal.

Patients with *trophoblastic tumor*, either choriocarcinoma or hydatidiform mole, frequently display elevations, sometimes marked, of serum total and free T_4 and T_3 concentrations. In addition to signs of pregnancy, the usual manifestations of thyrotoxicosis may be present, but ophthalmopathy is absent. Thyroid hyperfunction is caused by a circulating thyroid stimulator of trophoblastic origin, which is human chorionic gonadotropin (hCG), and the diagnosis may be confirmed by the finding of extremely high blood or urine levels of βhCG. Abnormal thyroid function tests remit promptly after removal of the tumor.

Thyrotoxicosis factitia is a form of thyrotoxicosis without hyperthyroidism that results from purposeful or inadvertent ingestion of large amounts of thyroid hormone. The syndrome is usually a form of malingering and occurs most commonly in women with an underlying psychiatric disorder, usually paramedical personnel, or in patients who have taken thyroid hormones in the past or who have relatives who take thyroid hormones. In such patients, endogenous thyroid function is suppressed, as evidenced by subnormal values of the RAIU and serum thyroglobulin concentration. Serum TSH is suppressed, and both serum T_4 and T_3 concentrations are increased if the patient is taking a preparation that contains T_4, whereas the serum T_3 concentration is elevated and the serum T_4 depressed in patients taking T_3 alone. Factitious hyperthyroidism also has been described in people who ingest ground meats contaminated with thyroid tissue.

Very rarely, thyrotoxicosis with a low RAIU is the result of excess hormone secretion by *ectopic thyroid tissue*, either widespread functioning metastases of thyroid carcinoma or struma ovarii.

The *jodbasedow phenomenon* refers to the induction of thyrotoxicosis in a previously euthyroid patient as a result of exposure to iodine. It typically occurs in areas of endemic iodine deficiency when measures to increase iodine intake are implemented. The presumption is that the supplemental iodine permits functionally autonomous thyroid tissue to produce and secrete excessive hormone. A similar phenomenon can occur in patients with nontoxic multinodular goiter who receive large doses of iodide. Since such patients tend to be elderly, with the danger of serious cardiovascular manifestations should thyrotoxicosis ensue, large doses of iodine should not be given to those with multinodular goiter. Similarly, in such patients, pharmaceuticals containing iodine, such as x-ray contrast media, should be used only when indicated and with consideration of the possible hazard of the jodbasedow phenomenon. When a contrast study is indicated under these conditions, it may be judicious to administer large doses of propylthiouracil (450 to 600 mg/d) prior to and for a week after the procedure. Some patients develop hyperthyroidism following exposure to large quantities of iodine despite the fact that after the iodine is withdrawn, they recover, thyroid function appears to be entirely normal, and there is no evidence of functional autonomy.

The antiarrhythmic drug amiodarone has multiple effects on thyroid function, including inhibition of the deiodination of T_4 to T_3, induction of hypothyroidism, and induction of hyperthyroidism. The drug contains 37 percent iodine, and amiodarone-induced thyrotoxicosis in patients with underlying Graves' disease or autonomous adenomas is consistent with the jodbasedow phenomenon; this disorder is associated with goiter, measurable RAIU, and normal to slightly elevated interleukin-6 (IL-6) levels and is managed like other forms of jodbasedow. In contrast, a variant of amiodarone-induced thyrotoxicosis in nongoitrous individuals is a type of "chemical" thyroiditis marked by very low RAIU and high IL-6 levels. The latter disorder may require treatment with perchlorate and glucocorticoids in addition to symptomatic management.

UNUSUAL PRESENTATIONS OF THYROTOXICOSIS
T_3 Toxicosis   Thyrotoxicosis in which serum T_4 is normal or low in the absence of a deficiency of TBG, while the serum T_3 is increased, is termed *T_3 toxicosis*. Although the production rate of T_3 is increased disproportionately relative to that of T_4 in all forms of hyperthyroidism, in some patients with Graves' disease, multinodular goiter, or hyperfunctioning adenoma this discrepancy is exaggerated. The diagnosis should be suspected in a patient with clinical manifestations of thyrotoxicosis in whom the serum T_4 and FT_4 are normal or low and the RAIU is normal or increased. These features, together with the goiter, serve to differentiate this disorder from liothyronine-induced thyrotoxicosis factitia. In contrast to nonthyroidal disorders that mimic thyrotoxicosis, patients with this disorder have nonsuppressible thyroid function in response to exogenous T_3, undetectable serum TSH, and absent responses to TRH. In many patients, thyrotoxicosis with increased serum T_3 and normal serum T_4 precedes emergence of typical increases in both, either during an initial episode of hyperthyroidism or, more commonly, during recurrence after previous treatment. In some patients in whom symptoms of thyrotoxicosis fail to regress during antithyroid therapy despite return of the serum T_4 level to normal, the serum T_3 concentration is persistently elevated. Such patients are likely to experience a recurrence of thyrotoxicosis when antithyroid therapy is withdrawn.

T_4 Toxicosis   In most patients with hyperthyroidism, the serum T_3 is increased relatively more than is the serum T_4. This fact reflects the fact that in hyperthyroidism T_3 generated from T_4 peripherally is supplemented by release of substantial quantities of T_3 from the thyroid. However, thyrotoxicosis sometimes is associated with a clear elevation of serum T_4 and a seemingly normal serum T_3 concentration. This syndrome of *T_4 toxicosis* occurs most commonly in the setting of prior excess iodine exposure in patients who are elderly, ill, or both. Increased iodine intake favors T_4 biosynthesis. In the absence of a history of excess iodine, the combination of a high serum T_4 concentration and a normal serum T_3 concentration presumably reflects inhibition of peripheral generation of T_3 from T_4 combined with persistence of T_3 and T_4 secretion from the thyroid.

MAJOR COMPLICATIONS OF THYROTOXICOSIS

CARDIAC DISEASE   Thyrotoxicosis causes increases in both systolic and diastolic cardiac function, probably secondary to effects on the expression of genes for the contractile protein myosin. Untreated, the increased work eventually progresses to decompensation. The increased cardiac output and the peripheral effects of thyroid hormone impose a variety of burdens on the heart. Hypermetabolism of the peripheral tissues increases both the metabolic and the nonmetabolic (heat-loss) circulatory load, while direct effects of thyroid hormone on the myocardium cause rapid filling and increase the force, velocity, and rate of ventricular contraction. As a result, cardiac work and cardiac output are increased. Moreover, atrial irritability is enhanced, leading to arrhythmias, most importantly atrial fibrillation. In patients with a normal heart, these burdens are usually tolerated. When there is underlying heart disease, however, cardiac insufficiency may be precipitated or aggravated. These complications are more common in elderly patients and in patients with toxic multinodular goiter and sometimes are the most prominent manifestation of the thyrotoxic state. In patients with cardiac insufficiency, clues to the presence of thyrotoxicosis include atrial fibrillation, relatively rapid circulation time, increased cardiac output (high-output failure), and resistance to the usual therapeutic doses of digitalis. In a 10-year follow-up of older individuals in the Framingham Heart Study, a low serum TSH level ("subclinical hyperthyroidism") was associated with a threefold increase in the risk of developing atrial fibrillation.

 TREATMENT
Treatment is directed at rapid alleviation of thyrotoxicosis and restoration of cardiac compensation. The former objective is best met by administration of large doses of an antithyroid agent, followed by iodine if the clinical situation is urgent. In less severe cases, radioiodine treatment is preceded by antithyroid drug treatment alone. The cardiac decompensation is managed in the usual manner, employing larger than usual doses of digitalis but with care to avoid digitalis intoxication as thyrotoxicosis is alleviated. Adrenergic antagonists should be used with caution in the presence of cardiac failure, unless failure is the consequence primarily of a disturbance of cardiac rate or rhythm.

THYROTOXIC CRISIS   Thyrotoxic crisis, or storm, involves a fulminating increase in the signs and symptoms of thyrotoxicosis. In the past, this disturbance usually occurred postoperatively in patients poorly prepared for surgery. However, with the preoperative use of antithyroid drugs and iodide and with appropriate therapy to control metabolic factors, weight, and nutritional status, postoperative thyrotoxic crisis should not occur. Now, so-called medical storm is more common and occurs in untreated or inadequately treated patients. It is precipitated by surgical emergency or complicating illness, usually sepsis. The syndrome is characterized by extreme irritability, delirium or coma, fever to 41°C or more, tachycardia, restlessness, hypotension, vomiting, and diarrhea. Rarely, the picture may be more subtle, with apathy, prostration, and coma, but with only slight elevation of temperature. Such postoperative complications as sepsis, septicemia, hemorrhage, and transfusion or drug reactions may mimic thyrotoxic crisis. The physiologic factor(s) that initiates thyrotoxic crisis is unknown. It does not appear to be an acute increase in the severity of thyroid hyperfunction. Rather, it may represent a shift from protein-bound to free hormone secondary to circulating inhibitors to binding in systemic illness.

 TREATMENT
Treatment consists of providing supportive therapy while undertaking measures to alleviate thyrotoxicosis as rapidly as possible. Supportive therapy includes treatment of dehydration and the intravenous

administration of glucose and saline, vitamin B complex, and glucocorticoids. The latter are indicated because of the increased glucocorticoid requirements in thyrotoxicosis and because adrenal reserve may be reduced. Patients should be placed in a cooled, humidified oxygen tent, and if hyperpyrexia is present a cooling blanket should be used. Digitalization is required to control ventricular rate in those with atrial fibrillation. If shock exists, intravenous pressor agents should be employed. Therapy of the hyperthyroidism consists of blockade of hormone synthesis by the immediate and continued administration of large doses of an antithyroid agent (e.g., 100 mg propylthiouracil every 2 h). If the patient is unable to swallow the medication, the tablets should be triturated and given by nasogastric tube or per rectum, since parenteral preparations are unavailable. Following initiation of antithyroid therapy, hormone release is inhibited through the administration of large doses of iodine intravenously or by mouth. The iodinated x-ray contrast agent sodium ipodate can be administered instead of iodine and has the added action of inhibiting the peripheral conversion of T_4 to T_3. Doses of 1 g/d are effective. Adrenergic antagonists are an important, and perhaps critical, part of the therapeutic regimen in the absence of cardiac failure. Propranolol can be administered in doses of 40 to 80 mg every 6 h. If medications cannot be taken orally, 2 mg propranolol may be given intravenously, with careful electrocardiographic monitoring. Large doses of dexamethasone (e.g., 2 mg every 6 h) also should be administered, since they inhibit hormone release, impair the peripheral generation of T_3 from T_4, and provide adrenal support. Indeed, with the combined use of propylthiouracil, iodine, and dexamethasone, the serum T_3 concentration generally returns to normal within 24 to 48 h. Dexamethasone may be tapered thereafter, while antithyroid therapy and iodine must be continued until a normal metabolic state is approached, at which time iodine is progressively withdrawn and plans are made for definitive treatment.

NEOPLASMS

The prevalence of solitary nodules of the thyroid gland increases with age, averaging 6.4 percent of women and 1.5 percent of men. Many palpable thyroid nodules thought to be solitary are actually part of a multinodular thyroid gland. High-resolution ultrasound identifies nodules in a third of patients being evaluated for nonthyroid indications, and autopsy studies reveal thyroid nodules in as many as 50 percent of necropsies. In general, a nodule must reach a size of 1 cm in diameter to be detectable by palpation. In addition to thyroid neoplasms, the differential diagnosis of apparent thyroid nodules includes cysts, adenopathy, cystic hygroma, parathyroid tumors, and laryngocele. True intrathyroidal nodules usually represent colloid adenomas or simple follicular adenomas.

THYROID ADENOMAS True adenomas, as opposed to localized adenomatous areas, are encapsulated and compress contiguous tissue. Adenomas vary in size and are classified into three histologic types: papillary, follicular, and Hürthle cell. The follicular adenomas can be subdivided according to the size of the follicles into colloid or macrofollicular, fetal or microfollicular, and embryonal varieties. Adenomas vary in physiologic differentiation, as judged by their ability to concentrate radioiodine. The more highly differentiated adenomas (follicular) are the most common and are the most likely to mimic the function of normal thyroid tissue. Though the function may be responsive to TSH stimulation, it usually differs from that of normal thyroid tissue in being autonomous; i.e., the basal activity is independent of TSH stimulation. Adenomas of this type are usually unifocal, presenting as a single nodule. Often the patient reports that the nodule has grown slowly over many years. Initially, its function is insufficient to disturb hormonal equilibrium, although its capacity to accumulate radioiodine is evident in scintiscans as an area of increased density within the still-functioning extranodular tissue (a *"warm" nodule*). At this stage, demonstration of inherent autonomy requires scintiscanning

while the patient is receiving suppressive doses of exogenous thyroid hormone (suppression scan). With time, the nodule grows larger, its function increasing until it is sufficient to suppress TSH secretion. Consequently, the remainder of the gland undergoes relative atrophy and loss of function, and the scintiscan reveals radioiodine accumulation only in the region of the nodule (a *"hot" nodule*). At this time, TSH is suppressed ("chemical" thyrotoxicosis), but the patient may or may not be overtly thyrotoxic. Frank thyrotoxicosis usually supervenes eventually (*toxic adenoma*) and may be precipitated by iodine exposure, such as from radiographic contrast dyes. Hyperfunctioning adenomas are a relatively frequent cause of T_3 toxicosis. They are amenable to ablation by surgery or by treatment with ^{131}I. Large doses of the latter are usually required to bring about a prompt cure. Although it has been thought that radiation damage would be confined solely to the hyperfunctioning nodule being treated with ^{131}I, the remaining tissue being spared, this may not always be the case, since some patients with hyperfunctioning adenoma become euthyroid after treatment with ^{131}I, only to become hypothyroid years later.

Although hyperfunctioning nodules are rarely the seat of carcinoma, one advantage of surgical excision (usually lobectomy) is the acquisition of definitive histologic diagnosis. Nevertheless, surgery is recommended infrequently for hyperfunctioning nodules because of its associated risks, the low incidence of cancer, and the efficacy of radiodine. One exception may be nodules >4 cm in diameter, for which the required dose of radiation is so large as to create a risk of radiation-induced neoplasia in the contralateral lobe.

Hyperfunctioning adenomas may undergo hemorrhagic necrosis. The resulting pain and nodularity may suggest subacute thyroiditis. With infarction of the hyperfunctioning nodule, the subsequent loss of function causes TSH levels to return to normal and the previously suppressed extranodular thyroid tissue to resume functioning. The previously hyperfunctioning nodule may then appear as a *"cold" nodule* on scintiscanning, which, together with the history of pain, could be misinterpreted to represent a carcinoma. Indeed, hypofunctioning, hemorrhagic adenomas and thyroid cysts account for most of the cold nodules initially suspected of being carcinoma.

MALIGNANT TUMORS OF THE THYROID Owing to its rich vascular supply, the thyroid is a common site of secondary or metastatic cancers from primary tumors elsewhere. Some common sources include malignant melanoma and carcinomas of the lung, breast, and esophagus. The thyroid also may be the site of lymphoproliferative disease, namely *thyroid lymphoma*, which constitutes about 5 percent of all thyroid malignancies. Of the latter, large cell histocytic (or immunoblastic) lymphoma is the most common and typically occurs in women between the ages of 55 and 75, who often have chronic lymphocytic thyroiditis with positive serum antithyroglobulin or anti-TPO antibodies. Indeed, the risk of this tumor is so much higher in elderly patients with Hashimoto's thyroiditis that an enlarging thyroid mass should be considered to be thyroid lymphoma until an appropriate evaluation rules out the diagnosis. The prognosis depends on the cell type and the extent of disease beyond the neck. Variable success rates have been reported with combinations of surgery, radiation, and chemotherapy.

Primary thyroid carcinomas may be classified into two varieties depending on whether the lesion arises in thyroid follicular epithelium or from the parafollicular or C cells. The latter disorder, *medullary thyroid carcinoma* (MTC), may occur in four presentations: a sporadic form, which accounts for 80 percent of cases, and three familial forms, which account for the remaining 20 percent. Two of these familial forms occur as part of types 2A and 2B, respectively, of the multiple endocrine neoplasia (MEN) syndrome, and the third occurs in a non-MEN setting. In familial forms, the disease may be diagnosed early in family members by means of screening measurements of serum calcitonin. This assay is not recommended for the routine evaluation of thyroid nodules, because MTC occurs in <0.5 percent of thyroid nodules. Calcitonin measurement may be useful when the diagnosis of carcinoma is suggested by fine-needle aspiration. The MEN syndromes are discussed in detail in Chap. 340. In brief, MEN 2A is characterized by MTC with pheochromocytoma and in some cases hyperparathyroidism. The MTC of MEN 2A is often preceded by C cell hyperplasia and contains multifocal tumors. MEN 2B includes MTC, pheochromocytoma, and mucosal neuromata. The *RET* proto-oncogene is responsible for MEN 2A and 2B, and heterogeneous mutations in *RET* have also been identified in sporadic MTC.

The incidence of the sporadic form peaks in the sixth and seventh decades of life, and patients usually have cervical lymph node metastases at presentation. The tendency of the tumor and involved lymph nodes to calcify may provide a clue to the diagnosis when calcification is noted on x-rays of the neck. Serum calcitonin serves as a tumor marker for residual disease after treatment, and the serum levels correlate with tumor burden. The status of the *RET* gene can be assessed in samples obtained by fine-needle aspiration of a thyroid nodule; differentiation between the mutations known for sporadic versus familial MTC makes it possible to decide whether preoperative screening for pheochromocytoma is necessary. The mainstay of therapy is surgical excision. Preoperative diagnosis of MTC will prepare the surgeon to search for metastases and perform extensive lymph node dissection. External radiation therapy and chemotherapy have a palliative role for recurrent or residual disease.

Carcinomas of Follicular Epithelium Of the three general histologic types, *papillary* and *follicular carcinomas*, which tend to be slow growing, account respectively for 70 and 15 percent of all thyroid cancers, while *anaplastic carcinoma* is the least common, constituting approximately 5 percent of thyroid cancers. *Anaplastic carcinoma* usually occurs in the sixth or seventh decade of life. The tumor is histologically undifferentiated, composed largely of spindle and giant cells, fast-growing, and highly malignant. Despite radical surgery, the prognosis is dismal, with survival in months rather than years, although survival is better in younger patients with early disease. The rapidly fatal character of the lesion is due to extensive local invasion that is refractory to both external radiation therapy and radioiodine therapy (because the tumor does not concentrate iodine). The fact that many patients have coexisting differentiated carcinoma suggests that anaplastic tumors arise from the former, and metastases of papillary or follicular carcinoma can undergo late malignant dedifferentiation. Anaplastic thyroid carcinoma may be confused with lymphoma or sarcoma, and positive immunocytochemical stains for keratin or the cytoskeletal protein vimentin help to confirm the diagnosis. While thyroglobulin staining may be positive owing to entrapped follicular cells or colloid, measurements of serum thyroglobulin are of no diagnostic value as a tumor marker for this tumor in contrast to the situation in well-differentiated thyroid cancer. The lack of calcitonin immuno-reactivity differentiates anaplastic carcinoma from undifferentiated medullary thyroid carcinoma.

Follicular carcinoma tends to occur in older individuals, resembles normal thyroid epithelium histologically, is encapsulated, and differs from benign follicular adenoma only by the presence of capsular and/or vascular invasion. These tumors can be classified as minimally, moderately, or highly invasive, and prognosis varies accordingly. One subtype of follicular carcinoma, the Hürthle cell tumor, tends to be more invasive, to metastasize frequently to bone, and to have an unfavorable clinical course. Follicular carcinoma undergoes early hematogenous spread, and the patient may present with a distant metastasis, usually in lung, bone, or the central nervous system. Lesions in bone are osteolytic. As for papillary carcinoma, large primary lesions are associated with worse prognosis, but even small lesions may metastasize widely. Rarely, the functioning mass of metastatic follicular carcinoma is great enough to cause increased serum levels of T_4 and/or T_3 and clinical thyrotoxicosis. Follicular carcinoma or follicular elements in papillary carcinoma are responsible for the instances in which thyroid carcinoma, in situ or metastatic, accumulates significant quantities of ^{131}I. The third and most common type of tumor, *papillary carcinoma*, has a bimodal frequency—i.e., peaks occur in the second and third decades and again in later life. This lesion is slow-growing and usually unencapsulated, and it may spread through the thyroid capsule to structures in the surrounding neck, especially the regional lymph nodes, where it may remain indolent for many years. The prognosis depends on the size of the original lesion, with tumors less

than 2 cm in diameter having a potentially excellent outcome. The presence of involved lymph nodes may be associated with a greater risk of recurrence but not, apparently, with increased mortality. Acceleration of the disease may take place at any time. Follicular elements are usually present in both the primary lesion and its metastases. Papillary carcinoma is the most common thyroid malignancy to develop after exposure of the head and neck to radiation in childhood. Tumors in this setting are usually multicentric, thereby meriting more extensive thyroidectomy, but they are associated with a good prognosis.

Diagnosis and treatment The diagnosis and treatment of thyroid carcinoma are interwoven with the management of the nodular goiter. In the past, there were a wide variety of views on this subject, stemming from seemingly contradictory data. On the one hand, surgically excised specimens of thyroid nodules, particularly solitary nodules, revealed a high frequency of carcinoma (as much as 20 percent in some series). On the other hand, despite the incidence of nodular goiter in the general population (approximately 4 percent), the frequency of thyroid carcinoma, either newly diagnosed or as a cause of death, is low. These two lines of data led to either vigorous or conservative approaches to the management of nodular goiter. The discordance can be explained by the ability of the physician to select for surgery those patients who are at high risk of harboring thyroid carcinoma, with consequent weighting of statistics from surgical series. With the advent of fine-needle aspiration biopsy, this capability has increased, bringing us closer to the as yet unrealized aim of operating only on those patients whose thyroids harbor carcinoma and avoiding surgery in patients whose thyroids do not.

Several features suggest the presence of carcinoma. Recent growth of a thyroid nodule or mass, especially if rapid and unaccompanied by tenderness and hoarseness, should prompt suspicion. Of particular importance is a history of radiation to the head or neck or upper mediastinum in infancy or childhood, because it is associated with a high incidence of thyroid disease, including carcinoma, later in life. Nodular disease develops in approximately 20 percent of patients so exposed and may not be apparent until 30 years or more after the exposure. Among patients in this group who have palpable nodules, approximately one-third have thyroid carcinoma at surgery, often multicentric and sometimes metastatic. The risk for neoplasia correlates directly with younger age at exposure, female sex, and radiation dose. Patients who do not undergo surgery should be followed indefinitely and may be candidates for levothyroxine therapy.

Skillful palpation of the thyroid provides important information. A nodule in an otherwise normal gland (a solitary nodule) should raise more suspicion of thyroid tumor than does one nodule among many, since the latter is likely to be part of a diffuse process, such as simple goiter. In addition, carcinomas are usually firm or hard in consistency and nontender. Fixation to surrounding structures and lymphadenopathy are late features, although patients may present with a midline mass above the thyroid isthmus (a Delphian node) or lateral cervical adenopathy. Since purely cystic lesions, especially cysts less than a few centimeters in diameter, are less likely to reflect malignancy than solid lesions, transillumination and/or ultrasonography is sometimes helpful. The age and sex of the patient also influence the clinical decision. Benign nodular lesions are more common in women than in men; malignant nodular lesions less so. Hence, nodular lesions create more suspicion of carcinoma in men than in women.

Laboratory tests are of little assistance in differentiating between malignant and nonmalignant thyroid nodules. Overall thyroid function is usually normal. Except in patients with medullary thyroid carcinoma, in whom serum calcitonin concentrations may be elevated, tumor markers are of little value. Serum thyroglobulin is elevated in many patients with differentiated thyroid carcinoma, but this feature is not useful in the initial diagnosis, as it may be present in patients with benign adenoma, simple goiter, or Graves' disease. Soft tissue x-rays of the neck may be of assistance, since finely stippled calcification in the thyroid suggests the presence of psammoma bodies within a papillary carcinoma, and more dense calcifications may signify medullary carcinoma.

Fine-needle aspiration for cytology is the initial procedure of choice in the evaluation of most patients (Fig. 331-4). The technique is simple to learn, free of complications, and applicable to most nodules. Success depends on obtaining a satisfactory specimen and on expert histopathologic interpretation. When the latter is available, aspiration biopsy provides a reliable means of differentiating between benign and malignant nodules in all except highly cellular lesions or follicular lesions, where evidence of vascular invasion may be required to differentiate benign from malignant forms. Needle aspirates of papillary carcinoma may reveal psammoma bodies, lymphocytes suggestive of Hashimoto's disease, and large pink follicular cells with large pale nuclei ("Orphan Annie cells") and numerous nucleoli. Despite the occasional occurrence of false-positive and false-negative results, the procedure can reduce the number of operations performed for nodules that prove to be benign. Further, a diagnosis of carcinoma permits the surgery to be planned preoperatively.

While fine-needle aspiration for cytology is the keystone of the approach to the management of the patient with nodular goiter, less specific measures such as ultrasonography or scintillation scanning also may be useful. Although only approximately 20 percent of nonfunctioning thyroid nodules prove to be malignant, the demonstration that a nodule is "cold" on scintiscan adds substantial weight to other factors suggesting carcinoma. Hyperfunctioning nodules are rarely malignant. Ultrasonograms of the thyroid have value in demonstrating whether nodules are cystic, solid, or a mixture of the two. Cystic nodules can be aspirated, a procedure that is often curative, and their contents should be subjected to cytopathologic examination. Solid or mixed lesions are consistent with tumor but may be either benign or malignant.

When the cytologic results are equivocal, the physician must decide whether to continue to observe the patient; to administer suppressive doses of thyroid hormone in the expectation that the suspect nodule will shrink or disappear—a hope that in the author's experience is usually unrealized; or to proceed to excisional biopsy and thyroidectomy. Patients in whom the author chooses the latter course include those with a history of radiation to the thyroid and one or more clearly palpable nodules, as well as young men and women with solitary cold nodules, particularly nodules that are hard, nontender, and changing rapidly in size. In the remainder, thyroid hormone therapy with repeat aspiration cytology in 3 to 6 months is recommended.

Regardless of the operative procedure planned, surgery for thyroid carcinoma should be performed by a surgeon experienced in the procedure. Should surgery be delayed, suppressive therapy with levothyroxine is often recommended preoperatively to facilitate the operative procedure and perhaps decrease the likelihood of tumor dissemination. In patients in whom a definitive preoperative diagnosis has not been made, the suspected lesion is removed en bloc with a wide margin of surrounding tissue and is examined by frozen section. Opinions vary as to the preferable procedure when carcinoma is found. For lesions 2 cm or less in size that are not multicentric and have not metastasized, some recommend ipsilateral lobectomy, isthmectomy, and possibly contralateral partial lobectomy. Despite its higher rate of morbidity, the author prefers a near-total thyroidectomy, especially for lesions >2 cm in size, in view of the frequency with which tumor is seeded throughout the gland by transglandular lymphatic spread and of evidence that both recurrence rates and subsequent mortality are lower after the more extensive operation. Regional lymph nodes should be explored and removed if there is evidence of involvement, but radical neck dissection is not justified. If permanent sections reveal carcinoma when frozen sections had failed to do so and the initial procedure was limited, secondary surgery should be undertaken to remove residual thyroid tissue, preferably within a few days. A more complete thyroidectomy is warranted for follicular carcinoma in view of its tendency to metastasize to distant sites. This is so because the metastases do not concentrate adequate ^{131}I in the presence of residual normal thyroid tissue, which both competes for the ^{131}I and prevents the increase in serum TSH required to stimulate uptake by tumor cells.

The need for postoperative ablation of the thyroid remnant with radioiodine and for subsequent periodic radioisotopic scanning for residual or recurrent disease varies with the histologic type of cancer, size of lesion, presence of metastases, and other indications of invasiveness or aggressiveness. Radioiodine treatment of known residual disease is associated with clinical improvement and reduced recurrence rates, but it is not clear whether mortality rates are improved by prophylactic postoperative ablation. Papillary cancers that are <1.5 cm in size and are unaccompanied by nodal metastases tend to have an excellent prognosis, and it is questionable whether ablation of the residual normal thyroid bed and subsequent scanning are necessary. The author favors a more conservative approach in such cases, only administering levothyroxine suppression with periodic follow-up determinations of serum thyroglobulin levels.

Total-body scintiscanning with ^{131}I is the method employed to evaluate for residual normal or malignant thyroid tissue in the neck and for distant metastases. Postoperatively, if replacement therapy is

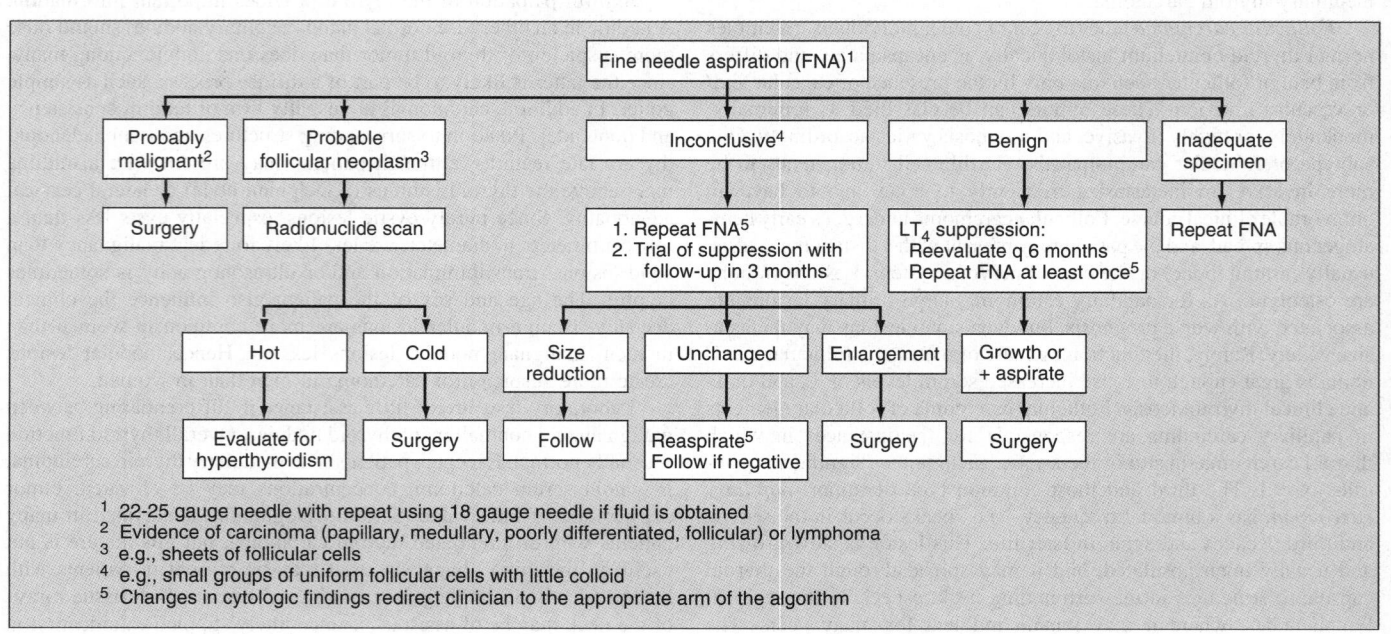

¹ 22-25 gauge needle with repeat using 18 gauge needle if fluid is obtained
² Evidence of carcinoma (papillary, medullary, poorly differentiated, follicular) or lymphoma
³ e.g., sheets of follicular cells
⁴ e.g., small groups of uniform follicular cells with little colloid
⁵ Changes in cytologic findings redirect clinician to the appropriate arm of the algorithm

FIGURE 331-4 Diagnostic approach to the solitary nodule.

initiated with liothyronine (50 to 75 μg) rather than levothyroxine, a more rapid increase in TSH secretion is seen when the liothyronine is withdrawn some 3 weeks later. After an additional 2 or 3 weeks without any thyroid hormone replacement, when the serum TSH concentration has risen to the range of 50 mU/L, a large scanning dose of ^{131}I [185 to 370 MBq (5 to 10 mCi)] is administered and whole-body scans are obtained at 72 h. If residual thyroid tissue is found, as is usually the case, a thyroid-ablating dose of 1850 to 2220 MBq (50 to 60 mCi) of ^{131}I is administered; if functioning metastases are present, the dose is doubled. Suppressive therapy with levothyroxine is reinstituted 24 to 48 h later. Approximately 1 week after administration of the second (treatment) dose of ^{131}I, whole-body scans are repeated, since the larger dose of radioiodine may permit demonstration of functioning metastases not seen after the smaller initial dose. When metastases are found, some clinics withdraw suppressive therapy, administer an additional 3700 MBq (100 mCi) of ^{131}I, and then reinstitute suppressive therapy with levothyroxine. The future availability of recombinant human TSH for parenteral injection promises to make it unnecessary to discontinue thyroid hormone therapy for scanning. In some patients, only measurements of serum thyroglobulin before and after TSH injection might be performed, with follow-up scanning solely in those in whom a significant rise in thyroglobulin is seen. A practical consideration is whether the high doses of ^{131}I (a β-particle emitter) used for diagnostic scanning may have an adverse effect on the subsequent uptake of the therapeutic dose, a phenomenon that has been called "stunning." Pending an answer to this question, some centers employ ^{123}I (a pure γ-ray emitter) for initial scans and ^{131}I only when the ^{123}I scan is negative but residual disease is suspected on the basis of elevated serum thyroglobulin levels.

Patients are reexamined approximately 6 months after the initial operation and at least every 6 months for several years thereafter. At these examinations, the neck is palpated for evidence of recurrence of metastases, which often can be treated with selective surgical removal. Blood is drawn for a serum thyroglobulin measurement, since elevated values in patients receiving suppressive therapy signal the presence of metastatic disease. At the initial 6-month examination, patients in whom metastases had previously been found are prepared for a whole-body scan as described above. Those in whom no metastases have been demonstrated by earlier scans are not rescanned unless the serum thyroglobulin is elevated but are rescanned approximately 1 year after the initial surgery. Patients in whom whole-body scans are positive are reentered into the therapeutic algorithm, as described above. Those in whom scans are negative continue to be reexamined and have measurements of serum thyroglobulin concentrations at regular intervals. If both serum thyroglobulin concentrations and scans are unrevealing, patients are scanned for the last time after approximately 3 years, unless serum thyroglobulin concentrations rise. In some patients, serum thyroglobulin may be elevated despite the absence of demonstrable functioning metastases. Some patients treated with high-dose ^{131}I, irrespective of the fractional uptake, are said to exhibit a reduction in serum thyroglobulin, ostensibly reflecting therapeutic benefit. Alternatively, the patients can be imaged by CT or MRI to ascertain the site of the thyroglobulin-secreting metastases and to determine whether they may be amenable to external radiation.

A program of this nature, involving near-total thyroidectomy, long-term suppressive therapy, and treatment of functioning metastases with radioiodine, reduces the recurrence rate and prolongs survival in patients with papillary carcinoma of the thyroid. Follicular carcinoma should be treated with even greater vigor, since the results are generally less favorable. Because follicular carcinoma metastasizes to lung and bone, appropriate follow-up x-rays and measurements of serum thyroglobulin should be performed. Mixed differentiated tumors with both follicular and papillary elements tend to behave biologically as papillary tumors and should be so managed. Radioiodine treatment of medullary thyroid carcinoma is usually not successful; the cases that show some reduction in serum calcitonin possibly represent a rare variant of mixed medullary and follicular cancer. Treatment of anaplastic carcinoma is largely palliative; most patients die within 6 months of diagnosis.

THYROIDITIS

The term *thyroiditis* embraces disorders of differing etiology. *Pyogenic thyroiditis* and *chronic fibrosing (Riedel's) thyroiditis* are rare. Pyogenic thyroiditis is usually preceded by infection elsewhere and is characterized by tenderness and swelling of the thyroid, redness and warmth of the overlying skin, and constitutional signs of infection. Treatment consists of antibiotic therapy and incisional drainage of any fluctuant areas in the thyroid. Patients with AIDS may present with thyroiditis due to unusual organisms such as *Pneumocystis carinii*. Riedel's thyroiditis is a disorder in which intense fibrosis of the thyroid and surrounding structures causes induration of the neck and may be associated with mediastinal and retroperitoneal fibrosis. This disorder must be differentiated from thyroid neoplasia. The other forms of thyroiditis—subacute thyroiditis, chronic thyroiditis with transient thyrotoxicosis, and Hashimoto's thyroiditis—are more common. They are notable for their different clinical courses and for the fact that each can be associated, at one time or another, with a euthyroid, thyrotoxic, or hypothyroid state.

SUBACUTE THYROIDITIS This disorder, also termed *granulomatous, giant cell,* or *de Quervain's thyroiditis*, is viral in origin. Symptoms of thyroiditis usually follow those of an upper respiratory infection and include pronounced asthenia, malaise, and symptoms referable to stretching of the thyroid capsule, principally pain over the thyroid or pain referred to the lower jaw, ear, or occiput. Referred pain may predominate. These symptoms may smolder for weeks before the diagnosis is suspected. Less commonly, the onset is acute, with severe pain over the thyroid, fever, and occasionally symptoms of thyrotoxicosis. Physical findings include exquisite tenderness and nodularity of the thyroid, which may be unilateral but usually involves other areas of the gland. Although local or referred pain is usual, occasional patients have other features typical of the disease but no pain.

Two laboratory findings are characteristic: a high erythrocyte sedimentation rate (ESR) and a depressed RAIU. Values for the remaining tests depend on the stage of the disease at which they are obtained. Early, many patients are mildly thyrotoxic owing to leakage of hormone from the gland. The serum T_4 and T_3 are high, and TSH is undetectable. Later, as glandular hormone is depleted, the patient may pass through a hypothyroid phase, in which serum T_4 and T_3 are low and TSH is increased. Serum levels of the cytokine IL-6 increase during the thyrotoxic phase and return to normal with recovery. This phenomenon is presumed to relate to thyroid destruction; IL-6 levels are also elevated in amiodarone-induced thyroiditis, after radioiodine therapy, and after the therapeutic injection of ethanol into toxic adenomas. Diagnosis of the thyrotoxic phase is especially troublesome in the painless variant because the patient may be thought to have Graves' disease or toxic nodular goiter, and therapy inappropriate for subacute thyroiditis may be instituted. Demonstration of a low RAIU usually serves to differentiate subacute thyroiditis from these other causes of hyperthyroidism. Differentiation of painless subacute thyroiditis from chronic thyroiditis with transient thyrotoxicosis is discussed below.

The disorder may smolder for months but eventually subsides with a return of normal thyroid function. In mild cases, aspirin suffices to control the symptoms. In more severe cases, glucocorticoids (prednisone, 20 to 40 mg/d) are generally effective. Propranolol can be used to control associated thyrotoxicosis. When the RAIU and serum T_4 return to normal, therapy can be withdrawn without recurrence of symptoms.

CHRONIC THYROIDITIS WITH TRANSIENT THYROTOXICOSIS This term denotes a disorder in which a self-limited episode of thyrotoxicosis is associated with a histologic picture of chronic lymphocytic thyroiditis that differs from that of Hashimoto's disease. This syndrome has been variously designated as *painless thyroiditis, silent thyroiditis, hyperthyroiditis, chronic thyroiditis with spontaneously resolving hyperthyroidism*, or, as the author prefers, *chronic thyroiditis with transient thyrotoxicosis* (CT/TT). Designations that imply the existence of hyperthyroidism are inappropriate, since ongoing production of thyroid hormone is negligible and the RAIU is decreased.

The syndrome occurs in patients of any age and mainly in women. Manifestations of thyrotoxicosis are usually mild but may be severe. The thyroid is nontender, firm, symmetric, and slightly or moderately enlarged. Findings include elevations of the serum T_4 and T_3 levels consonant with the thyrotoxicosis and a depressed RAIU. The ESR is normal or slightly elevated, rarely exceeding 50 mm/h, and antithyroid antibodies, when present, are low in titer.

The etiology, pathogenesis, and pathophysiology of this disorder are unclear. Viral antibody titers show no characteristic patterns. It is presumed that thyrotoxicosis results from leakage of hormone from the gland, as in subacute thyroiditis. Low values for the RAIU, in turn, reflect hormonal suppression of TSH secretion and not increased plasma iodine, since urinary iodine excretion is not greatly elevated. Some degree of thyroid malfunction is indicated by failure of the RAIU to respond briskly to exogenous TSH stimulation.

Thyrotoxicosis in CT/TT usually abates within 2 to 5 months, and the thyrotoxic phase may be followed by a hypothyroid phase. The latter is usually self-limited and may be the only component of the disease recognized if the thyrotoxic phase is brief. Most patients recover completely; some have recurrent episodes.

A variant of CT/TT after pregnancy is termed *postpartum thyroiditis*. This disorder develops within 2 to 6 months after delivery in 5 to 6 percent of otherwise normal women and in about one-fourth of women with insulin-dependent diabetes mellitus. Such patients usually have a small goiter and a family history of thyroid disease and may have postpartum depression. Within the first 2 to 3 months post partum, transient symptoms of thyrotoxicosis, such as fatigue, palpitations, emotional lability, and heat intolerance, are likely. Laboratory findings include elevated serum levels of T_4 and T_3, suppressed TSH, elevated titers of antithyroid antibodies, and a low RAIU. Patients may undergo a subsequent hypothyroid phase (from 4 to 8 months post partum) associated with a low serum T_4 level, elevated TSH, and high titers of autoantibodies. These patients require symptomatic management with levothyroxine until the thyroid recovers. Women who become pregnant again are at risk for recurrent postpartum thyroiditis.

In the thyrotoxic phase, this disorder can be differentiated from Graves' disease by demonstration of a depressed RAIU and the absence of increased urinary iodine excretion. The latter finding also excludes the jodbasedow syndrome. When these data are available, the disorder must be differentiated from other causes of thyrotoxicosis with a low RAIU, principally subacute thyroiditis. Lack of tenderness or nodularity of the thyroid and absence of marked elevation of the ESR tend to exclude the latter diagnosis. Patients with either functioning ectopic thyroid tissue or thyrotoxicosis factitia characteristically respond to exogenous TSH stimulation with a brisk increase in RAIU. Definitive diagnosis of CT/TT can be made by thyroid biopsy.

Since the thyroid is not hyperfunctioning in this disorder, measures used in the treatment of hyperthyroidism are useless. Propranolol may be administered until the thyrotoxicosis abates.

HASHIMOTO'S THYROIDITIS   This disorder, also termed *lymphadenoid goiter*, is a common chronic inflammatory disease of the thyroid in which autoimmune factors play a prominent role. It occurs most frequently in women of middle age and is the most common cause of sporadic goiter in children. Evidence of the participation of autoimmune factors includes the lymphocytic infiltration of the gland and the presence in the serum of increased concentrations of immunoglobulins and antibodies against several components of thyroid tissue. Of these, the most important from the clinical standpoint are the antithyroglobulin antibody, detected by the tanned red cell agglutination test, and antithyroid peroxidase (anti-TPO or antimicrosomal) antibody, detected by immunofluorescence, complement fixation, or the more sensitive enzyme-linked immunosorbent assay (ELISA). These autoantibodies probably reflect but do not cause the thyroid destruction noted in autoimmune thyroid disease. The cloning and sequencing of the genes that encode

the three major thyroid antigens—thyroglobulin, thyroid peroxidase, and the TSH receptor—have made possible detailed characterization of these autoantibodies. Hashimoto's thyroiditis also coexists with some frequency with other diseases of an autoimmune nature, including pernicious anemia, Sjögren's syndrome, chronic active hepatitis, systemic lupus erythematosus, rheumatoid arthritis, adrenal insufficiency, diabetes mellitus, and Graves' disease itself (see Chap. 340). These disorders, as well as Hashimoto's disease, also occur frequently in family members of patients with Hashimoto's disease. An association of HLA-DR3 and -DR5 with the atrophic and goitrous forms of Hashimoto's disease, respectively, has been noted. It is unclear whether Hashimoto's thyroiditis is a frequent precursor of the atrophic thyroid of primary hypothyroidism. The prevalence of Hashimoto's thyroiditis appears to be increasing, and the disorder is more common in the United States than in Europe. Increased iodine ingestion has been proposed as an explanation.

In the usual presentation of the disease, goiter is the outstanding feature. The enlargement involves the entire gland, but not necessarily symmetrically. Typically, the consistency is rubbery, the margins are scalloped, and the general outline of the gland is preserved. The pyramidal lobe may be prominent. Early in the disease the patient is metabolically normal; even then decreased thyroid reserve is often manifest in an increase in serum TSH. The RAIU may be elevated early, reflecting the secretion of physiologically inactive iodoproteins, but the serum T_4 and T_3 are normal, and the patient is euthyroid. As the disease progresses, thyroid failure, at first subclinical, may supervene owing to progressive replacement of thyroid parenchyma by lymphocytes or fibrous tissue. The thyroid failure is manifested first by a rise in serum TSH concentration. With time, the serum T_4 level declines, though the serum T_3 level remains normal. Eventually, the serum T_3 level falls, and frank hypothyroidism supervenes. Autoimmune thyroiditis, including Hashimoto's disease, may account for as many as 90 percent of cases of hypothyroidism. High titers of anti-TPO antibody are almost always present. High titers also may occur in other thyroid disorders, particularly primary thyroprivic hypothyroidism and Graves' disease, but with lesser frequency. Although the foregoing findings usually suffice to permit a diagnosis, histologic confirmation may be obtained by needle biopsy. An elevated serum TSH dictates that levothyroxine therapy be given. Treatment is probably also indicated in patients with marginally elevated TSH levels and positive antibody titers, in view of the frequency with which hypothyroidism eventually develops. In some patients, replacement therapy is associated with regression of goiter. Pregnant women with high antibody titers may be at a higher risk for miscarriage, independent of the thyroid status.

Occasional patients present with hyperthyroidism in association with a thyroid gland that is unusually firm and with high titers of circulating antithyroid antibodies, a combination that suggests, probably correctly, the concurrence of Graves' disease and Hashimoto's thyroiditis ("Hashitoxicosis"). In others, hyperthyroidism supervenes in a patient known to have Hashimoto's thyroiditis, presumably owing to the emergence of clones of lymphocytes that produce stimulatory anti-TSH receptor antibodies. Hyperthyroidism in association with Hashimoto's thyroiditis is treated in a conventional manner, but ablative therapy is less commonly employed, since the associated chronic thyroiditis tends to limit the duration of thyroid hyperfunction and also predisposes the patient to the development of hypothyroidism after surgical or radioiodine treatment.

Please refer to Chap. 57 in Goodman & Gilman's The Pharmacological Basis of Therapeutics, *9th ed, McGraw-Hill, New York, 1996.*

BIBLIOGRAPHY

AIN KB: Papillary thyroid carcinoma: Etiology, assessment, and therapy. Endocrin Metab Clin North Am 24:711, 1995

AYALA A, WARTOFSKY L: Minimally symptomatic (subclinical) hypothyroidism. The Endocrinologist 7:44, 1997

BRUCKER-DAVIS F et al: Genetic and clinical features of 42 kindreds with resistance to thyroid hormone. Ann Intern Med 123:572, 1995

BURCH HB: Evaluation and management of the solid thyroid nodule. Endocrin Metab Clin North Am 24:663, 1995

————, WARTOFSKY L: Graves' ophthalmopathy: Current concepts regarding pathogenesis and management. Endocr Rev 14:747, 1993

BURROW GN: Thyroid function and hyperfunction during gestation. Endocr Rev 14:194, 1993

DEGROOT LJ et al: Therapeutic controversies: Radiation and Graves' ophthalmopathy. J Clin Endocrinol Metab 80:339, 1995

FATOURECHI V et al: Dermopathy of Graves' disease (pretibial myxedema). Medicine 73:1, 1994

FRANKLIN JA: The management of hyperthyroidism. N Engl J Med 330:1731, 1994

GREBE SKG, HAY ID: Follicular thyroid cancer. Endocrin Metab Clin North Am 24:761, 1995

HADEN ST et al: Subclinical hyperthyroidism. The Endocrinologist 6:322, 1996

LEVETAN C, WARTOFSKY L: A clinical guide to the management of Graves' disease with radioactive iodine. Endocrine Practice 1:205, 1995

MAHONEY KM, WARTOFSKY L: Significance of alterations in thyroid function tests in the critical care setting. J Intens Care Med 7:318, 1992

MARSH DJ et al: Medullary thyroid carcinoma: Recent advances and management update. Thyroid 5:407, 1995

MASTERS PA, SIMONS RJ: Clinical use of sensitive assays for thyroid-stimulating hormone. J Gen Intern Med 11:115, 1996

MAZZAFERRI EL, JHIANG SM: Long-term impact of initial surgical and medical therapy on papillary and follicular thyroid cancer. Am J Med 97:418, 1994

OERTEL YC: Fine-needle aspiration and the diagnosis of thyroid cancer. Endocrin Metab Clin North Am 25:69, 1996

OPPENHEIMER JH et al: A therapeutic controversy. Thyroid hormone therapy: When and what? J Clin Endocrinol Metab 80:2873, 1995

REFETOFF S et al: The syndromes of resistance to thyroid hormone. Endocr Rev 14:348, 1993; Update 1994, Endocr Rev Monographs 3:336, 1994

SARNE DH, SCHNEIDER AB: External radiation and thyroid neoplasia. Endocrin Metab Clin North Am 25:181, 1996

SINGER PA: Thyroiditis: Acute, subacute, and chronic. Med Clin North Am 75:61, 1991

———— et al: Treatment guidelines for patients with hyperthyroidism and hypothyroidism. JAMA 273:808, 1995

SMALLRIDGE RC: Postpartum thyroid dysfunction: A frequently undiagnosed endocrine disorder. The Endocrinologist 6:44, 1996

SURKS MI et al: American Thyroid Association guidelines for use of laboratory tests in thyroid disorders. JAMA 263:1529, 1990

————, SIEVERT R: Drugs and thyroid function. N Engl J Med 333:1688, 1995

TOFT AD: Thyroxine therapy. N Engl J Med 331:174, 1994

TORRENS JI, BURCH HB: Serum thyroglobulin measurement: Utility in clinical practice. Endocrinologist 6:125, 1996

VAN SANDE J et al: Somatic and germline mutations of the TSH receptor gene in thyroid diseases. J Clin Endocrinol Metab 80:2577, 1995

WARTOFSKY L: Myxedema coma, in The Thyroid, 7th ed, LE Braverman, RD Utiger (eds). Philadelphia, Lippincott, 1996, p 871

————: Thyrotoxic storm, in The Thyroid, 7th ed, LE Braverman, RD Utiger (eds). Philadelphia, Lippincott, 1996, p 701

WEETMAN AP, MCGREGOR AM: Autoimmune thyroid disease: Further developments in our understanding. Endocr Rev 15:788, 1994

WOHLLK N et al: Application of genetic screening information to the management of medullary thyroid carcinoma and multiple endocrine neoplasia Type 2. Endocrin Metab Clin North Am 25:1, 1996

FIGURE 332-1 Basic steroid structure and nomenclature.

C_{21} steroid that acts predominantly on intermediary metabolism; a *mineralocorticoid* is a C_{21} steroid that acts predominantly on the metabolism of sodium and potassium.

BIOSYNTHESIS OF ADRENAL STEROIDS Cholesterol, derived from the diet and from endogenous synthesis, is the substrate for steroidogenesis. Uptake of cholesterol by the adrenal cortex is mediated by the low-density lipoprotein (LDL) receptor. With long-term stimulation of the adrenal cortex by adrenocorticotropic hormone (ACTH), the number of LDL receptors increases. The three major adrenal biosynthetic pathways lead to the production of glucocorticoids (cortisol), mineralocorticoids (aldosterone), and adrenal androgens (dehydroepiandrosterone). Separate zones of the adrenal cortex synthesize specific hormones; this facts reflects the enzymatic capacity of each zone to carry out certain transformations and hydroxylations (Fig. 332-2). The outer (glomerulosa) zone contains the enzymes for aldosterone biosynthesis, and the inner (fasciculata-reticularis) zone is the site of cortisol and androgen biosynthesis.

STEROID TRANSPORT Some steroid hormones, e.g., testosterone and cortisol, circulate bound to a considerable extent to plasma proteins. Cortisol occurs in the plasma in three forms: free cortisol, protein-bound cortisol, and cortisol metabolites. *Free cortisol* is physiologically active hormone that is not protein-bound and, therefore, that can act directly on tissue sites. Normally, less than 5 percent of circulating cortisol is free. Only the unbound cortisol and its metabolites are filterable at the glomerulus. Increased quantities of free steroid are excreted in the urine in states characterized by hypersecretion of cortisol, because the unbound fraction of plasma cortisol rises. *Protein-bound cortisol* is bound reversibly to circulating plasma proteins. Plasma has two cortisol-binding systems. One is a high-affinity, low-capacity alpha$_2$ globulin termed *transcortin* or *cortisol-binding globulin* (CBG), and the other is a low-affinity, high-capacity protein, *albumin*. The binding affinity of CBG for cortisol is reduced in areas of inflammation, thus increasing the local concentration of free cortisol. CBG in normal human plasma can bind approximately 700 nmol of cortisol per liter (25 μg/dL). When the concentration of cortisol exceeds this level, part of the excess binds to albumin, and a greater proportion than usual circulates unbound. For example, when the total cortisol level is 1400 nmol/L (50 μg/dL), 25 percent is free. The CBG level is increased in high-estrogen states (e.g., pregnancy, oral

332 *Gordon H. Williams, Robert G. Dluhy*

DISEASES OF THE ADRENAL CORTEX

BIOCHEMISTRY AND PHYSIOLOGY

STEROID NOMENCLATURE Steroids contain as their basic structure a cyclopentenoperhydrophenanthrane nucleus consisting of three 6-carbon hexane rings and a single 5-carbon pentane ring (Fig. 332-1). The carbon atoms are numbered in a sequence beginning with ring A. Adrenal steroids contain either 19 or 21 carbon atoms. The C_{19} steroids have methyl groups at C-18 and C-19. C_{19} steroids with a ketone group at C-17 are termed *17-ketosteroids*. The C_{19} steroids have predominantly androgenic activity. The C_{21} steroids have a 2-carbon side chain (C-20 and C-21) attached at position 17 and methyl groups at C-18 and C-19. C_{21} steroids with a hydroxyl group at position 17 are termed *17-hydroxycorticosteroids*. The C_{21} steroids have either glucocorticoid or mineralocorticoid properties. A *glucocorticoid* is a contraceptive administration). The rise in CBG is accompanied by a parallel rise in protein-bound cortisol, with the result that the plasma cortisol concentration is elevated. However, the free cortisol level probably remains normal, and manifestations of glucocorticoid excess are absent. Most synthetic glucocorticoid analogues bind less efficiently to CBG (approximately 70 percent binding). This may explain the propensity of some synthetic analogues to produce cushingoid effects at low doses. *Cortisol metabolites* are biologically inactive and bind only weakly to circulating plasma proteins.

Aldosterone is bound to proteins to a smaller extent than either testosterone or cortisol, and an ultrafiltrate of plasma contains as much as 50 percent of the circulating concentration of aldosterone. This limited binding by plasma protein influences aldosterone metabolism.

STEROID METABOLISM AND EXCRETION **Glucocorticoids** The daily secretion of cortisol ranges between 40 and 80

μmol (15 and 30 mg), with a pronounced circadian cycle. Cortisol is distributed in a volume of body fluids approximating the total extracellular fluid space, with more than 90 percent in the protein-bound fraction. The plasma concentration of cortisol is determined by the rate of secretion, the rate of inactivation, and the rate of excretion of free cortisol. The liver is the major organ responsible for steroid inactivation. The major pathway is reduction of ring A and conjugation of the reduced products with glucuronic acid at position C-3 to form water-soluble compounds. The enzyme 11β-hydroxysteroid dehydrogenase converts cortisol to the inactive metabolite cortisone in the kidney. The activity of this enzyme is influenced by the level of circulating thyroid hormone, the oxidative reaction being increased in hyperthyroidism.

Mineralocorticoids In normal subjects with a normal salt intake, the average daily secretion of aldosterone ranges between 0.1 and 0.7 μmol (50 and 250 μg). Since aldosterone binds only weakly to proteins, its volume of distribution is larger than that of cortisol, being approximately 35 L. During a single passage through the liver, more than 75 percent of circulating aldosterone is normally inactivated by ring A reduction and conjugation with glucuronic acid. However, under certain conditions, such as congestive failure, this rate of inactivation is reduced.

From 7 to 15 percent of aldosterone is excreted in the urine as a glucuronide conjugate, from which free aldosterone is released on standing at pH 1. This *acid-labile conjugate* is formed in the liver and kidney. For persons with an average salt intake, the 24-h urine excretion of the acid-labile conjugate ranges from 15 to 50 nmol (5 to 19 μg), that of the reduced derivative ranges from 70 to 100 nmol (25 to 35 μg), and that of the nonconjugated, nonreduced free aldosterone ranges from 0.5 to 2 nmol (0.2 to 0.6 μg).

Adrenal Androgens The major androgen secreted by the adrenal is dehydroepiandrosterone (DHEA) and its C-3 sulfuric acid ester. From 15 to 30 mg of these compounds is secreted daily. Smaller amounts of androstenedione, 11β-hydroxyandrostenedione, and testosterone are secreted. DHEA is the major precursor of the urinary 17-ketosteroids. Two-thirds of the urine 17-ketosteroids in the male are derived from adrenal metabolites, and the remaining one-third comes from testicular androgens. In the female, almost all urine 17-ketosteroids are derived from the adrenal.

Steroids diffuse passively through the cell membrane and bind to intracellular receptors (see Chap. 327). These receptors are part of a superfamily of transcription regulatory factors that includes the thyroid hormone receptor. Glucocorticoid receptors are of two types: I and II. The type I receptor is the same as the mineralocorticoid receptor. Mineralocorticoids do not bind to the type II receptor, but most glucocorticoids bind to either receptor, although with different affinities. After the steroid binds to the receptor, the steroid-receptor complex is transported to the nucleus, where it binds

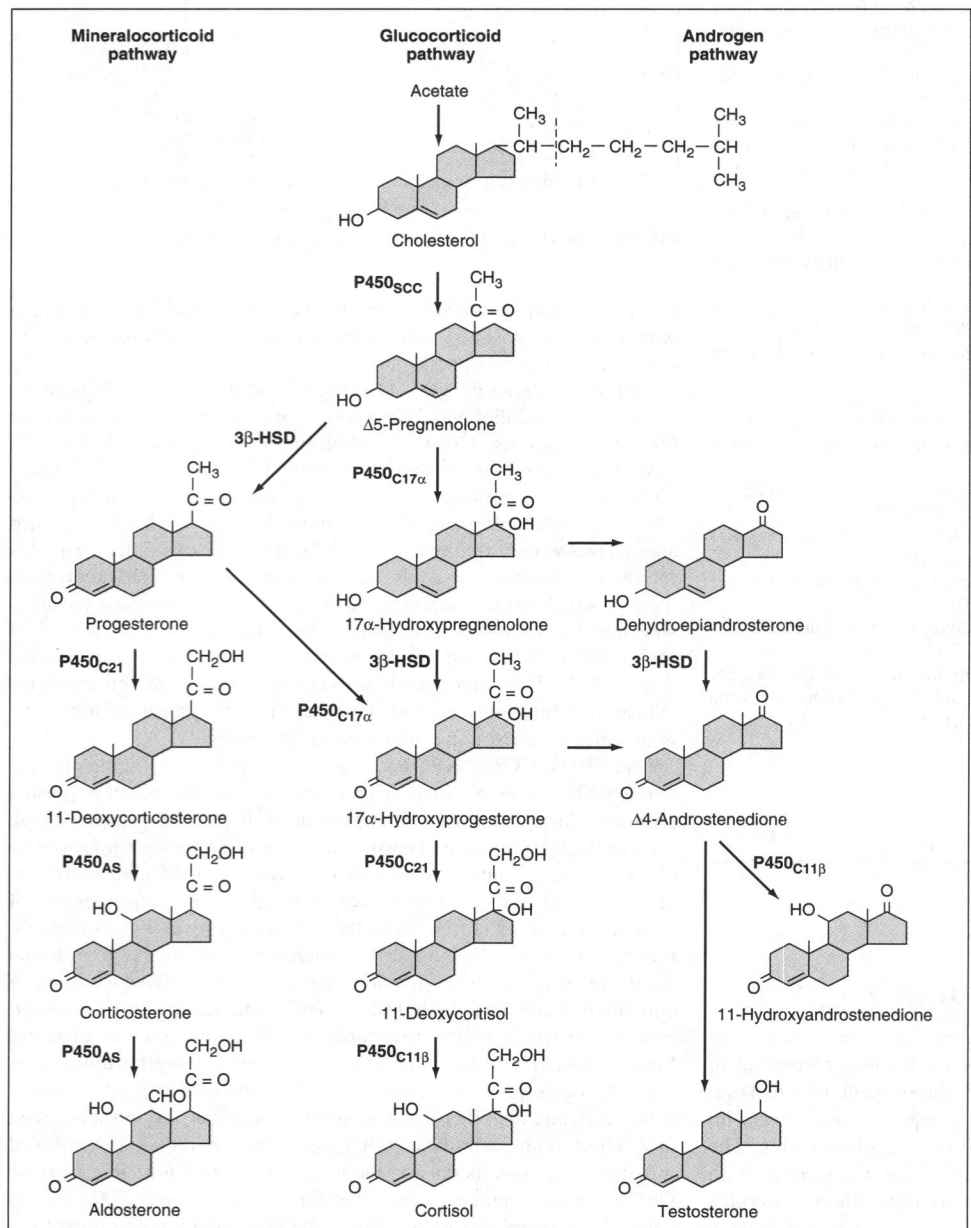

FIGURE 332-2 Biosynthetic pathways for adrenal steroid production; major pathways to mineralocorticoids, glucocorticoids, and androgens. Circled letters and numbers denote specific enzymes: P450$_{SCC}$, cholesterol side chain cleavage enzyme; 3β-HSD, 3β-hydroxysteroid dehydrogenase; P450$_{C11β}$, C-11 hydroxylase; P450$_{C17α}$, C-17 hydroxylase; P450$_{C21}$, C-21 hydroxylase; P450$_{AS}$, aldosterone synthase.

to specific sites on steroid-regulated genes, modifying mRNA and protein synthesis. Because cortisol binds to the mineralocorticoid (type I glucocorticoid) receptor with the same affinity as aldosterone, mineralocorticoid specificity is achieved by local metabolism of cortisol to the inactive compound cortisone by 11β-hydroxysteroid dehydrogenase. Cortisone binds only minimally to the type I receptor. The glucocorticoid effects of other steroids, such as high-dose progesterone, correlate with their relative binding affinities for the type II glucocorticoid receptor. Inherited defects in the glucocorticoid receptor cause glucocorticoid resistance states. Individuals with type II receptor defects have high levels of cortisol but do not have manifestations of hypercortisolism.

ACTH PHYSIOLOGY ACTH (see Chap. 328) is an unbranched polypeptide containing 39 amino acids. ACTH and a number of other peptides (lipotropins, endorphins, and melanocyte-stimulating hormones) are processed from a larger precursor molecule of 31,000 mol wt—pro-opiomelanocortin (POMC) (see Chap. 328). POMC is made in a variety of tissues, including brain, anterior and posterior pituitary, and lymphocytes. The actual peptide secreted depends on the tissue. In the anterior pituitary, ACTH is synthesized and stored in basophilic cells. The basophilic staining of the corticotrophs is the result of the glycosylation of ACTH and related peptides. The N-terminal 18-amino-acid fragment of ACTH has full biologic potency, and shorter N-terminal fragments have partial biologic activity. Release of ACTH and related peptides from the anterior pituitary gland is governed by a "corticotropin-releasing center" in the median eminence of the hypothalamus, which, on stimulation, releases a 41-amino-acid peptide (corticotropin-releasing hormone, CRH) that travels via the portal vessels of the pituitary stalk to the anterior pituitary, where it stimulates the release of ACTH (Fig. 332-3). Some related peptides such as β-lipotropin (β-LPH) are released in equimolar concentrations with ACTH, suggesting that they are cleaved enzymatically from the parent POMC before or during the secretory process. However, β-endorphin levels may or may not correlate with circulating levels of ACTH, depending on the nature of the stimulus. The functions and regulation of secretion of the related peptides derived from POMC are poorly understood.

The major factors controlling ACTH release include CRH, the free cortisol concentration in plasma, stress, and the sleep-wake cycle (see Fig. 332-3). The plasma level of ACTH varies during the day as a result of its pulsatile secretion, and it follows a circadian pattern with a peak just prior to waking and a nadir before retiring. If a new sleep-wake cycle is adopted, the pattern changes over several days to conform to it. ACTH and cortisol levels also increase in response to eating. Stress (e.g., pyrogens, surgery, hypoglycemia, exercise, and severe emotional trauma) causes the release of CRH and arginine vasopressin (AVP) and activation of the sympathetic nervous system. These changes in turn enhance ACTH release, acting individually or in concert. For example, AVP release acts synergistically with CRH to amplify ACTH secretion; CRH also stimulates the locus coeruleus/sympathetic system. Stress-related secretion of ACTH abolishes the circadian periodicity of ACTH levels but is, in turn, suppressed by prior high-dose glucocorticoid administration. The normal pulsatile, circadian pattern of ACTH release is regulated by CRH; this mechanism is the so-called open feedback loop. CRH secretion, in turn, is influenced by hypothalamic neurotransmitters. For example, serotoninergic and cholinergic systems stimulate the secretion of CRH and ACTH; there is contradictory evidence regarding the inhibitory effects of alpha-adrenergic agonists and γ-aminobutyric acid (GABA) on CRH release. In addition, there may be direct pituitary effects of these neurotransmitters. There is also evidence for peptidergic regulation of ACTH release. For example, β-endorphin and enkephalin inhibit the secretion of ACTH, whereas vasopressin and angiotensin II augment it. The immune system also influences the hypothalamic-pituitary-adrenal axis (Fig. 332-4). For example, inflammatory cytokines [tumor necrosis factor (TNF)-α, interleukin (IL)-1α, IL-1β, and IL-6] produced by monocytes increase ACTH release by stimulating secretion of CRH and/or AVP. Finally, ACTH release is regulated by the level of free cortisol in plasma. Cortisol decreases the responsiveness of

FIGURE 332-3 The hypothalamic-pituitary-adrenal axis. The main sites for feedback control by plasma cortisol are the pituitary gland (1) and the hypothalamic corticotropin-releasing center (2). Feedback control by plasma cortisol also occurs at the locus coeruleus/sympathetic system (3) and may involve higher nerve centers (4) as well. There also may be a short feedback loop involving inhibition of CRH by ACTH (5). Hypothalamic neurotransmitters influence CRH release; serotoninergic and cholinergic systems stimulate the secretion of CRH and ACTH; alpha-adrenergic agonists and γ-aminobutyric acid (GABA) probably inhibit CRH release. The opioid peptides β-endorphin and enkephalin inhibit, and vasopressin and angiotensin II augment, the secretion of CRH and ACTH. CRH, corticotropin-releasing hormone; β-LPH, β-lipotropin; POMC, pro-opiomelanocortin; LC, locus coeruleus; NE, norepinephrine.

pituitary corticotropic cells to CRH; that is, in the presence of cortisol, more CRH is required to produce a given increment of ACTH. The response of the POMC mRNA to CRH is also inhibited by glucocorticoids. In addition, glucocorticoids inhibit the locus coeruleus/sympathetic system and CRH release. The latter servomechanism establishes the primacy of cortisol in the control of ACTH secretion. The inhibition of ACTH occurs in two phases: (1) an early fast feedback, mediated via the type I glucocorticoid receptor, which lasts less than 10 min and depends on both the rate of increase of glucocorticoid levels and the specific glucocorticoid administered; and (2) a time-dependent, delayed feedback, likely mediated by the type II glucocorticoid receptor, which is probably due to inhibition of synthesis of the precursor protein. The suppression of ACTH secretion that results in adrenal atrophy following *prolonged* glucocorticoid therapy may be related primarily to suppression of hypothalamic CRH release, since exogenous CRH administration in this circumstance produces a rise in plasma ACTH. Cortisol also exerts feedback effects on higher brain centers (hippocampus, reticular system, and septum) and perhaps on the adrenal cortex (see Fig. 332-4).

The biologic half-life of ACTH in the circulation is less than 10 min. The action of ACTH is also rapid; within minutes of its release,

FIGURE 332-4 The immune-adrenal axis. Cortisol has anti-inflammatory properties that include effects on the microvasculature, cellular actions, and the suppression of inflammatory cytokines (the so-called immune-adrenal axis). A stress such as sepsis increases adrenal secretion, and cortisol in turn suppresses the immune response via this system. −, suppression; +, stimulation; CRH, corticotropin-releasing hormone; ACTH, adrenocorticotropin; IL, interleukin; TNF, tumor necrosis factor; PAF, platelet activating factor.

the concentration of steroids in the adrenal venous blood increases. ACTH stimulates steroidogenesis via activation of the membrane-bound adenyl cyclase. Adenosine-3',5'-monophosphate (cyclic AMP), in turn, activates protein kinase enzymes, thereby resulting in the phosphorylation of proteins that activate steroid biosynthesis.

RENIN-ANGIOTENSIN PHYSIOLOGY (See also Chap. 246) Renin is a proteolytic enzyme that is produced and stored in the granules of the juxtaglomerular cells surrounding the afferent arterioles of glomeruli in the kidney. Renin exists in both active and inactive forms. Whether the inactive form is a precursor ("prorenin") or is a product formed after release is uncertain. The juxtaglomerular apparatus consists of both the juxtaglomerular cells and the cells of the macula densa. Renin acts on the basic substrate angiotensinogen (a circulating alpha$_2$ globulin made in the liver) to form the decapeptide angiotensin I (Fig. 332-5). Angiotensin I is then enzymatically transformed by angiotensin converting enzyme (converting enzyme), which is present in many tissues (particularly the pulmonary vascular endothelium), to the octapeptide angiotensin II by the removal of the two

C-terminal amino acids. Angiotensin II is a potent pressor agent and exerts its action by a direct effect on arteriolar smooth muscle. In addition, angiotensin II stimulates production of aldosterone by the zona glomerulosa of the adrenal cortex; the heptapeptide angiotensin III also may stimulate aldosterone production. The two major classes of angiotensin receptors are termed AT1 and AT2; AT1 may exist as two subtypes α and β. Most of the effects of angiotensins II and III are mediated by the AT1 receptor. Angiotensinases rapidly destroy angiotensin II (half-life, approximately 1 min), while the half-life of renin is more prolonged (10 to 20 min). In addition to circulating renin-angiotensin, many tissues have a local renin-angiotensin system and the ability to produce angiotensin II. These tissues include the uterus, placenta, vascular tissue, heart, brain, and, particularly, the adrenal cortex and kidney. While the role of locally generated angiotensin II is not established, it may be involved in the growth and modulation of function of the adrenal cortex and vascular smooth muscle.

Renal renin release is controlled by four interdependent factors, and the amount of renin released reflects the combined effects of all four factors. The *juxtaglomerular cells*, which are specialized myoepithelial cells that cuff the afferent arterioles, act as miniature pressure transducers, sensing renal perfusion pressure and corresponding changes in afferent arteriolar perfusion pressures. For example, under conditions of a reduction in circulating blood volume, there is a corresponding reduction in renal perfusion pressure and, therefore, in afferent arteriolar pressure (see Fig. 332-5). This change is perceived by the juxtaglomerular cells as a decreased stretch exerted on the afferent arteriolar walls. The juxtaglomerular cells then release more renin into the kidney circulation. This results in the formation of angiotensin I, which is converted in the kidney and peripherally to angiotensin II by converting enzyme. Angiotensin II influences sodium homeostasis via two major mechanisms: it changes renal blood flow so as to maintain a constant glomerular filtration rate, thereby changing the filtration fraction of sodium, and it stimulates the adrenal cortex to release aldosterone. Increasing plasma levels of aldosterone lead to increasing renal sodium retention and thus result in expansion of the extracellular fluid volume, which, in turn, dampens the initiating signal for renin release. In this context, the renin-angiotensin-aldosterone system regulates volume by modifying renal hemodynamics and tubular sodium transport.

A second control mechanism for renin release is centered in the *macula densa* cells, a group of distal convoluted tubular epithelial cells directly apposed to the juxtaglomerular cells. They may function as chemoreceptors, monitoring the sodium (or chloride) load presented to the distal tubule, and such information may be conveyed to the juxtaglomerular cells, where appropriate modifications in renin release take place. Under conditions of increased delivery of filtered sodium to the macula densa, increasing release of renin is capable of decreasing the glomerular filtration rate, thereby reducing the filtered load of sodium.

The *sympathetic nervous system* regulates the release of renin in response to assumption of the upright posture. The mechanism is either a direct effect on the juxtaglomerular cell to increase adenyl cyclase activity or an indirect effect on either the juxtaglomerular or the macula densa cells via vasoconstriction of the afferent arteriole.

Finally, circulating factors influence renin release. Increased dietary intake of *potassium* decreases, and decreased potassium intake increases, renin release. The significance of these effects is unclear. *Angiotensin II* exerts negative feedback control on renin release that is independent of alterations in renal blood flow, blood pressure, or aldosterone secretion. *Atrial natriuretic peptides* also inhibit renin release. Thus, the control of renin release involves both *intrarenal* (pressor receptor and macula densa) and *extrarenal* (sympathetic nervous system,

FIGURE 332-5 The interrelationship of the volume and potassium feedback loops on aldosterone secretion. Integration of signals from each loop determines the level of aldosterone secretion.

potassium, angiotensin, etc.) mechanisms. Steady-state renin levels reflect all these factors, with the intrarenal mechanism predominating.

GLUCOCORTICOID PHYSIOLOGY The division of adrenal steroids into glucocorticoids and mineralocorticoids is arbitrary in that most glucocorticoids have some mineralocorticoid-like properties. The descriptive term *glucocorticoid* is used for adrenal steroids whose predominant action is on intermediary metabolism. The principal glucocorticoid is cortisol (hydrocortisone). The effect of glucocorticoids on intermediary metabolism is mediated by the type II glucocorticoid receptor. Physiologic effects of glucocorticoids include the regulation of protein, carbohydrate, lipid, and nucleic acid metabolism. Glucocorticoids raise the blood glucose level by acting as an insulin antagonist and by suppressing the secretion of insulin, thereby inhibiting peripheral glucose uptake, which promotes hepatic glucose synthesis (gluconeogenesis) and increases hepatic glycogen content. The actions on protein metabolism are mainly catabolic in effect, resulting in an increase in protein breakdown and nitrogen excretion. In large part, these actions reflect a mobilization of glycogenic amino acid precursors from peripheral supporting structures, such as bone, skin, muscle, and connective tissue, due to protein breakdown and inhibition of protein synthesis and amino acid uptake. Hyperaminoacidemia also facilitates gluconeogenesis by stimulating glucagon secretion. Glucocorticoids act directly on the liver to stimulate the synthesis of certain enzymes, such as tyrosine aminotransferase and tryptophan pyrrolase. Glucocorticoids inhibit the synthesis of nucleic acids in most body tissues, but in the liver, RNA synthesis is stimulated. Glucocorticoids regulate fatty acid mobilization by enhancing the activation of cellular lipase by lipid-mobilizing hormones (e.g., catecholamines and pituitary peptides).

The actions of cortisol on protein and adipose tissue differ in different parts of the body. For example, pharmacologic doses of cortisol can deplete the protein matrix of the vertebral column (trabecular bone), but long bones (which are primarily compact bone) are affected only minimally; similarly, peripheral adipose tissue mass decreases, whereas abdominal and interscapular fat expand.

Glucocorticoids have anti-inflammatory properties, which are probably related to effects on the microvasculature and to suppression of inflammatory cytokines. In this sense, glucocorticoids modulate the immune response via the so-called immune-adrenal axis. This "loop" is one mechanism by which a stress, such as sepsis, increases adrenal hormone secretion, and the elevated cortisol level in turn suppresses the immune response. For example, cortisol maintains vascular responsiveness to circulating vasoconstrictors and opposes the increase in capillary permeability during acute inflammation. Glucocorticoids cause a leukocytosis due to release from the bone marrow of mature cells as well as to inhibition of their egress through the capillary wall. Glucocorticoids produce a depletion of circulating eosinophils and of lymphoid tissue, specifically T cells, by causing a redistribution from the circulation into other compartments. Thus, cortisol impairs cell-mediated immunity. Glucocorticoids also inhibit the production and action of the mediators of inflammation, such as the lymphokines and prostaglandins. These actions occur via the type II glucocorticoid receptor and are blocked by inhibitors of RNA and protein synthesis. Glucocorticoids inhibit the production and action of interferon by T lymphocytes and the production of IL-1 and IL-6 by macrophages. The antipyretic action of glucocorticoids may be explained by the effect on IL-1, which appears to be an endogenous pyrogen. Glucocorticoids also inhibit the production of T cell growth factor (IL-2) by T lymphocytes. Glucocorticoids reverse macrophage activation and antagonize the action of migration-inhibiting factor (MIF), leading to reduced adherence of macrophages to vascular endothelium. Glucocorticoids inhibit prostaglandin and leukotriene production by inhibiting the activity of phospholipase A_2, thus blocking release of arachidonic acid from phospholipids. Finally, glucocorticoids inhibit the production and inflammatory effects of bradykinin, platelet activating factor, and serotonin. It is probably only at pharmacologic dosages that antibody production is reduced and lysosomal membranes are stabilized, the latter effect suppressing the release of acid hydrolases.

Cortisol levels respond within minutes to stress, whether physical (trauma, surgery, exercise), psychological (anxiety, depression), or physiologic (hypoglycemia, fever). The reasons why elevated glucocorticoid levels protect the organism under stress are not understood, but in conditions of glucocorticoid deficiency, such stresses may cause hypotension, shock, and death. Consequently, in individuals with adrenal insufficiency, glucocorticoid administration should be increased during stress.

Cortisol has major effects on body water. It helps regulate the extracellular fluid volume by retarding the migration of water into cells and by promoting renal water excretion, the latter effect mediated by suppression of vasopressin secretion, by an increase in the rate of glomerular filtration, and by a direct action on the renal tubule. The consequence is to prevent water intoxication by increasing solute-free water clearance. Glucocorticoids also have weak mineralocorticoid-like properties, and high doses promote renal tubular sodium reabsorption and increased urine potassium excretion. Glucocorticoids also can influence behavior; emotional disorders may occur with either an excess or a deficit of cortisol. Last, cortisol suppresses the secretion of pituitary POMC and its derivative peptides (ACTH, β-endorphin, and β-lipotropin) and the secretion of hypothalamic CRH and vasopressin.

MINERALOCORTICOID PHYSIOLOGY The major mineralocorticoid, aldosterone, has two important actions: It is a major regulator of extracellular fluid volume and a major determinant of potassium metabolism. These effects are mediated by the binding of aldosterone to the type I glucocorticoid (mineralocorticoid) receptor in target tissues (see Chap. 327). Volume is regulated through a direct effect on the collecting duct, where aldosterone causes a decrease in sodium excretion and an increase in potassium excretion. The reabsorption of sodium ions causes a fall in the transmembrane potential, thus enhancing the flow of positive ions, such as potassium, out of the cell into the lumen. The reabsorbed sodium ions are transported out of the tubular epithelium into the renal interstitial fluid and from there into the renal capillary circulation. Water passively follows the transported sodium.

Since the concentration of hydrogen ion is greater in the lumen than in the cell, hydrogen ion also is actively secreted. Mineralocorticoids also act on the epithelium of the salivary ducts, sweat glands, and gastrointestinal tract to cause reabsorption of sodium in exchange for potassium.

When normal individuals are given aldosterone, an initial period of sodium retention is followed by natriuresis, and sodium balance is reestablished after 3 to 5 days. As a result, edema does not develop. This process is referred to as the *escape phenomenon*, signifying an "escape" by the renal tubules from the sodium-retaining action of aldosterone. While renal hemodynamic factors may play a role in the escape, the level of atrial natriuretic peptide also increases. However, it is important to realize that there is no escape from the potassium-losing effects of mineralocorticoids. Aldosterone can also interact with a cell surface receptor, thereby possibly acting by a nongenomic mechanism.

Three primary mechanisms control aldosterone release—the renin-angiotensin system, potassium, and ACTH (Table 332-1). The renin-angiotensin system controls extracellular fluid volume via regulation of aldosterone secretion (see Fig. 332-1). In effect, the renin-angiotensin system maintains the circulating blood volume constant by causing aldosterone-induced sodium retention during volume deficiency and by decreasing aldosterone-dependent sodium retention when volume is ample.

Potassium ion directly regulates aldosterone secretion, independently of circulating renin-angiotensin (see Fig. 332-5). However, potassium stimulates the adrenal production of angiotensin II, and converting-enzyme inhibitors block the synthesis of angiotensin II and reduce the acute aldosterone response to potassium. Oral potassium loading increases aldosterone secretion, excretion, and plasma levels. In addition, an increase in serum potassium of as little as 0.1 mmol/L increases plasma aldosterone levels under certain circumstances.

Physiologic amounts of ACTH stimulate aldosterone secretion acutely, but this action is not sustained if ACTH is infused for longer

Table 332-1

Factors Regulating Aldosterone Biosynthesis

Factor	Effect
Renin-angiotensin system	Stimulation
Sodium ion	Inhibition (?physiologic)
Potassium ion	Stimulation
Neurotransmitters	
Dopamine	Inhibition
Serotonin	Stimulation
Pituitary hormones	
ACTH	Stimulation
Non-ACTH pituitary hormones (e.g., growth hormone)	Permissive (for optimal response to sodium restriction)
β-Endorphin	Stimulation
γ-MSH	Permissive
Atrial peptide	Inhibition
Ouabain-like factors	Inhibition

than 10 to 12 h. Most studies relegate ACTH to a minor role in the control of aldosterone. For example, subjects receiving high-dose glucocorticoid therapy and with presumed complete suppression of ACTH have normal aldosterone secretion in response to sodium restriction.

Prior dietary intake of both potassium and sodium can alter the magnitude of the aldosterone response to acute stimulation. This effect results from a change in aldosterone synthase. Increasing potassium intake or decreasing sodium intake sensitizes the response of the glomerulosa cells to acute stimulation by ACTH, angiotensin II, and/or potassium. Thus, regulation of aldosterone secretion occurs both early and late in the synthetic pathway.

Neurotransmitters (dopamine and serotonin) and some peptides, such as atrial natriuretic peptide, γ-melanocyte-stimulating hormone (γ-MSH), and β-endorphin, also participate in the regulation of aldosterone secretion (see Table 332-1). Thus, the control of aldosterone secretion involves both stimulatory and inhibitory factors.

ANDROGEN PHYSIOLOGY Androgens regulate male secondary sexual characteristics and can cause virilizing symptoms in women. Steroids with predominantly androgenic activity have 19 carbon atoms (see Fig. 332-1). The principal adrenal androgens are dehydroepiandrosterone (DHEA), androstenedione, and 11-hydroxyandrostenedione. DHEA and androstenedione are weak androgens and exert their effects via conversion to the potent androgen testosterone in extraglandular tissues. DHEA also has poorly understood effects on the immune and cardiovascular systems. Adrenal androgen formation is regulated by ACTH, not by gonadotropins. It follows that adrenal androgens are suppressed by exogenous glucocorticoid administration.

LABORATORY EVALUATION OF ADRENOCORTICAL FUNCTION

The basic assumption is that measurements of the plasma or urinary level of a given steroid reflects the rate of adrenal *secretion* of that steroid. However, urine *excretion* values may not truly reflect the secretion rate because of improper collection or altered metabolism. Measurement of the actual adrenal secretory rate of a given steroid is difficult, involving isotope dilution techniques following administration of a radioactive steroid. Plasma levels reflect the level of secretion only at the time of measurement. The plasma level (PL) depends on two factors: the secretion rate (SR) of the hormone and the rate at which it is metabolized, i.e., its metabolic clearance rate (MCR). These three factors can be related as follows:

$$PL = \frac{SR}{MCR} \quad \text{or} \quad SR = MCR \times PL$$

BLOOD LEVELS (See Table 332-2) **Peptides** The plasma levels of ACTH and angiotensin II can be measured by immunoassay

techniques. ACTH levels fluctuate from moment to moment, and basal ACTH secretion shows a circadian rhythm, with lower levels in the early evening than in the morning. Angiotensin II levels also vary diurnally and are influenced by dietary sodium intake and posture. Both upright posture and sodium restriction elevate angiotensin II levels.

Most clinical determinations of the renin-angiotensin system, however, involve measurements of peripheral *plasma renin activity* (PRA) in which the renin activity is gauged by the generation of angiotensin I during a standardized incubation period. This method depends on the presence of sufficient angiotensinogen in the plasma as substrate. The generated angiotensin I is measured by radioimmunoassay. The plasma renin activity depends on the dietary sodium intake and on whether the patient is ambulatory. In normal humans, the PRA shows a diurnal rhythm characterized by peak values in the morning and decreases in activity in the afternoon.

Steroids Cortisol and aldosterone are both secreted episodically, and levels generally vary during the day, with peak values in the morning and low levels in the evening. In addition, the plasma level of aldosterone, but not of cortisol, is increased by dietary potassium loading, by sodium restriction, or by assumption of the upright posture. Measurement of the sulfate conjugate of DHEA may be a useful index of adrenal androgen secretion, since little DHEA sulfate is formed in the gonads and since the half-life of DHEA sulfate is 7 to 9 h. However, DHEA sulfate levels reflect both DHEA production and sulfatase activity.

URINE LEVELS For the assessment of glucocorticoid secretion, the urine *17-hydroxycorticosteroid* assay has been replaced largely by measurement of urinary free cortisol. Elevated levels of urinary free cortisol correlate with states of hypercortisolism, reflecting changes in the levels of unbound, physiologically active circulating cortisol. Normally, the rate of excretion is higher in the daytime (7 A.M. to 7 P.M.) than at night (7 P.M. to 7 A.M.).

Urinary *17-ketosteroids* contain a ketone group at C-17 (see Fig. 332-1). They originate in either the adrenal gland or the gonad. In normal women, 90 percent of urinary 17-ketosteroids is derived from the adrenal, and in men 60 to 70 percent is of adrenal origin. Urine 17-ketosteroid values are highest in young adults and decline with age.

Table 332-2

Range of Normal Values for Tests of Adrenal Function

Test	Normal Value, Range
Plasma cortisol, nmol/L (μg/dL):	
8 A.M.	140–690 (5–24)
4 P.M.	80–330 (3–12)
Cortisol secretory rate, μmol/d (mg/d)	14–69 (5–25)
Urinary free cortisol, nmol/d (μg/d)	55–275 (20–100)
17-Hydroxycorticosteroids, μmol/d (mg/d)	5.5–28 (2–10)
Plasma testosterone, nmol/L (ng/mL):	
Men	10–35 (3–10)
Women	<3.5 (<1)
Plasma dehydroepiandrosterone (DHEA), nmol/L (μg/L)	7–31 (2–9)
Plasma DHEA sulfate, μmol/L (μg/L)	1.3–6.7 (500–2500)
Plasma 11-deoxycortisol (S), nmol/L (μg/dL)	<30 (<1)
Plasma 17OH progesterone, nmol/L (μg/L):	
Women	
Follicular phase	0.6–3 (0.2–1)
Luteal phase	1.5–10.6 (0.5–3.5)
Men	0.2–9 (0.06–3)
Plasma aldosterone, pmol/L (ng/dL) (100 mmol Na$^+$, 60–100 mmol K$^+$, supine, 8 A.M.)	<240 (<8)
Aldosterone secretion, nmol/d (μg/d) (100 mmol Na$^+$, 60–100 mmol K$^+$)	140–690 (50–250)
Aldosterone excretion, nmol/d (μg/d) (100 mmol Na$^+$, 60–100 mmol K$^+$)	14–53 (5–19)
Plasma renin activity (μg/L)/h [(ng/mL)/h] (100 mmol Na$^+$, 60–100 mmol K$^+$, supine, 8 A.M.)	1–2.5 (1–2.5)
Plasma angiotensin II, ng/L (pg/mL) (100 mmol Na$^+$, 60–100 mmol K$^+$, supine, 8 A.M.)	10–30 (10–30)
Plasma ACTH, pmol/L (pg/mL) (8 A.M.)	2–14 (10–60)

A carefully timed urine collection is a prerequisite for all excretory determinations. Urinary creatinine should be measured simultaneously to determine the accuracy and adequacy of the collection procedure.

STIMULATION TESTS   Stimulation tests are useful in the diagnosis of hormone deficiency states. A standardized and specific stimulus for the production and release of a given hormone is applied, and the amount of hormone released is then measured.

Tests of Glucocorticoid Reserve   Within minutes after administration of ACTH, cortisol levels increase in adrenal venous blood. This responsiveness can be used as an index of the functional reserve of the adrenal gland for production of cortisol. Under maximal ACTH stimulation, cortisol secretion increases tenfold, to 800 μmol/d (300 mg/d), but maximal stimulation can be achieved only with prolonged ACTH infusions. For example, in normal subjects, cortisol levels exceed 1100 nmol/L (40 μg/dL) following a 24-h infusion of cosyntropin at a rate of 0.02 mg/h. In patients with secondary adrenal insufficiency, the maximal plasma cortisol value at 24 h ranges between 280 and 1100 nmol/L (10 and 40 μg/dL). Patients with primary adrenal insufficiency have smaller responses.

A screening test (the so-called rapid ACTH stimulation test) involves the administration of 25 units (0.25 mg) of cosyntropin intravenously or intramuscularly and measurement of plasma cortisol levels before and 30 and 60 min after administration; the test can be performed at any time of the day. The most clear-cut criterion for a normal response is a stimulated cortisol level of >500 nmol/L (>18 μg/dL), and the minimal stimulated normal increment of cortisol is >200 nmol/L (>7 μg/dL) above baseline. Severely ill patients with elevated basal cortisol levels may show no further increases following acute ACTH administration.

Tests of Mineralocorticoid Reserve and Stimulation of the Renin-Angiotensin System   Stimulation tests use protocols designed to create a programmed volume depletion, such as sodium restriction, diuretic administration, or upright posture. A simple, potent test consists of severe sodium restriction and upright posture. After 3 to 5 days of a 10-mmol/d sodium intake, rates of aldosterone secretion or excretion should increase two- to threefold over the control values. Supine morning plasma aldosterone levels are usually increased three- to sixfold, and they increase a further two- to fourfold in response to 2 to 3 h of upright posture.

When the dietary sodium intake is normal, stimulation testing requires the administration of a potent diuretic, such as 40 to 80 mg furosemide, followed by 2 to 3 h of upright posture. The normal response is a two- to fourfold rise in plasma aldosterone levels.

SUPPRESSION TESTS   Suppression tests to document hypersecretion of adrenal hormones involve measurement of the target hormone response after standardized suppression of its tropic hormone.

Tests of Pituitary-Adrenal Suppressibility   The ACTH release mechanism is sensitive to the circulating glucocorticoid level. When blood levels of glucocorticoid are increased in normal individuals, less ACTH is released from the anterior pituitary, and less steroid is produced by the adrenal gland. The integrity of this feedback mechanism can be tested clinically by giving a glucocorticoid and judging the suppression of ACTH secretion by analysis of urine steroid levels and/or plasma cortisol and ACTH levels. A potent glucocorticoid such as dexamethasone is used, so that the agent can be given in an amount small enough not to contribute significantly to the pool of steroids to be analyzed.

The best *screening* procedure is the overnight dexamethasone suppression test. This involves the measurement of plasma cortisol levels at 8 A.M. following the oral administration of 1 mg dexamethasone the previous midnight. The 8 A.M. value for plasma cortisol in normal subjects should be less than 140 nmol/L (5 μg/dL).

The definitive test of adrenal suppressibility consists in administering 0.5 mg dexamethasone every 6 h for two successive days while collecting urine over a 24-h period for determination of creatinine and free cortisol and/or measuring plasma cortisol levels. In a patient with a normal hypothalamic-pituitary ACTH release mechanism, a fall in the urine free cortisol to less than 80 nmol/d (30 μg/d) or of plasma cortisol to less than 140 nmol/L (5 μg/dL) is seen on the second day of administration.

A normal response to either suppression test implies that the ACTH control of the adrenal glands is physiologically normal. However, an isolated abnormal result, particularly to the overnight suppression test, does not in itself imply pituitary and/or adrenal disease.

Tests of Mineralocorticoid Suppressibility   These tests rely on an expansion of extracellular fluid volume, which should result in a decrease in renal renin release, a decrease in circulating plasma renin activity, and a decrease in the secretion and/or excretion of aldosterone. Various tests differ in the rate at which extracellular fluid volume is expanded. One convenient suppression test involves the intravenous infusion of 500 mL/h of normal saline solution for 4 h, which normally suppresses plasma aldosterone levels to <220 pmol/L (<8 ng/dL) on a sodium-restricted diet or to <140 pmol/L (<5 ng/dL) on a normal sodium intake. This test should not be performed in potassium-depleted subjects.

TESTS OF PITUITARY-ADRENAL RESPONSIVENESS Stimuli such as insulin hypoglycemia, arginine vasopressin, and pyrogens cause the release of ACTH from the pituitary by an action on higher neural centers or on the pituitary itself. Insulin-induced hypoglycemia is particularly useful, because it stimulates the release of both growth hormone and ACTH. In this test, 0.05 to 0.1 unit of regular insulin per kilogram body weight is given intravenously as a bolus to reduce the fasting glucose level to at least 50 percent below basal. The normal cortisol response is a rise to more than 500 nmol/L (18 μg/dL).

One of the best ways to test the integrity of the pituitary-adrenal axis is the metyrapone test. Metyrapone inhibits 11β-hydroxylase in the adrenal. As a result, the conversion of 11-deoxycortisol (compound S) to cortisol is impaired, causing 11-deoxycortisol to accumulate in the blood and the blood level of cortisol to decrease (see Fig. 332-2). The hypothalamic-pituitary axis responds to the declining cortisol blood levels by releasing more ACTH. *Note that assessment of the response depends on both an intact hypothalamic-pituitary axis and an intact adrenal gland.*

While modifications of the original metyrapone test have been described, we believe the best involves administering 750 mg of the drug by mouth every 4 h over a 24-h period and comparing the control and postmetyrapone plasma levels of 11-deoxycortisol, cortisol, and ACTH. In normal individuals, plasma 11-deoxycortisol levels should exceed 290 nmol/L (10 μg/dL) following metyrapone administration. The metyrapone test does not accurately reflect ACTH reserve if subjects are ingesting exogenous glucocorticoids or drugs that accelerate the metabolism of metyrapone (e.g., phenytoin).

A direct and selective test of the pituitary corticotrophs can be achieved with the investigational agent corticotropin-releasing hormone (CRH). The bolus injection of 1 μg of ovine CRH per kilogram of body weight stimulates secretion of ACTH and β-lipotropin in normal human subjects within 60 to 180 min. However, the magnitude of the ACTH response is less than that produced by the insulin tolerance test, which implies that additional factors (such as vasopressin) augment stress-induced increases in ACTH secretion.

Although the rapid ACTH stimulation test is useful for the diagnosis of primary adrenal insufficiency, normal cortisol responsiveness may be seen in some patients with a partial ACTH deficit and absence of adrenal atrophy. These patients have an inadequate pituitary ACTH reserve and fail to increase ACTH secretion in response to a stress such as surgery or hypoglycemia. Since the use of a bolus of exogenous ACTH does not invariably exclude a diagnosis of secondary adrenocortical insufficiency, direct tests of pituitary ACTH reserve (metyrapone test, insulin tolerance testing) may be required in the appropriate clinical setting. On the other hand, the rapid ACTH test can distinguish between primary and secondary adrenal insufficiency, because aldosterone secretion is preserved in secondary adrenal failure by the renin-angiotensin system and potassium. Cosyntropin (25 units) is given intravenously or intramuscularly, and plasma cortisol and aldosterone levels are measured before and 30 and 60 min after administration.

The cortisol response is abnormal in both groups, but patients with secondary insufficiency show an increase in aldosterone levels by at least 140 pmol/L (5 ng/dL). No aldosterone response is seen in patients in whom the adrenal cortex is destroyed.

HYPERFUNCTION OF THE ADRENAL CORTEX

Excess cortisol is associated with Cushing's syndrome; excess aldosterone causes aldosteronism; and excess adrenal androgens cause adrenal virilism. These syndromes do not always occur in the "pure" form but may have overlapping features.

CUSHING'S SYNDROME **Etiology** Cushing described a syndrome characterized by truncal obesity, hypertension, fatigability and weakness, amenorrhea, hirsutism, purplish abdominal striae, edema, glucosuria, osteoporosis, and a basophilic tumor of the pituitary. As awareness of this syndrome has increased, the diagnosis of Cushing's syndrome has been broadened into the classification shown in Table 332-3. Regardless of etiology, all cases of endogenous Cushing's syndrome are due to increased production of cortisol by the adrenal. In most cases the cause is *bilateral adrenal hyperplasia* due to hypersecretion of pituitary ACTH or production of ACTH by a nonendocrine tumor. The incidence of pituitary-dependent adrenal hyperplasia is three times greater in women than in men, and the most frequent age of onset is the third or fourth decade. The cause of the hypersecretion of pituitary ACTH is still debated. Some workers speculate that the primary defect is the de novo development of a pituitary adenoma, since in some reports tumors are found in over 90 percent of patients with pituitary-dependent adrenal hyperplasia. Alternatively, the defect may reside in the hypothalamus or in higher neural centers, leading to release of CRH inappropriate to the level of circulating cortisol. The consequence would be that a higher level of cortisol is required to reduce ACTH secretion to normal. This primary defect leads to hyperstimulation of the pituitary, resulting in hyperplasia or tumor formation. With time the pituitary tumor may become independent of the regulating influence of the central nervous system and/or circulating cortisol levels. In surgical series, most individuals with hypersecretion of pituitary ACTH are found to have a microadenoma (<10 mm in diameter; 50 percent are 5 mm or less in diameter), but a pituitary macroadenoma (>10 mm) or diffuse hyperplasia of the corticotropic cells may be found. The finding of a microadenoma in pituitary-dependent adrenal hyperplasia does not rule out dysregulation of hypothalamic CRH as the defect in Cushing's disease. Long-term follow-up to determine the rate of recurrence following successful surgical resection is necessary to answer this issue. In some studies, the recurrence rate is greater than 20 percent. Unfortunately, it may be difficult to distinguish between recurrence and inadequate primary therapy. Traditionally, only an individual who has an ACTH-producing pituitary tumor is defined as having *Cushing's disease*, but in some centers this designation is used for anyone who has

hypersecretion of pituitary ACTH, regardless of whether a tumor is identified by radiography. In this chapter we will use the traditional definition, although these definitions may become less distinct as small tumors are more easily diagnosed by high-resolution scanning.

Nonendocrine tumors may secrete polypeptides that are biologically, chemically, and immunologically indistinguishable from either ACTH or CRH and that cause bilateral adrenal hyperplasia (see also Chap. 102). The ectopic production of CRH results in clinical, biochemical, and radiologic features indistinguishable from those caused by hypersecretion of pituitary ACTH. The typical signs and symptoms of Cushing's syndrome may be absent or minimal with ectopic ACTH production, and hypokalemic alkalosis is the prominent manifestation. Most of these cases are associated with the primitive small cell (oat cell) type of bronchogenic carcinoma or with tumors of the thymus, pancreas, or ovary; medullary carcinoma of the thyroid; or bronchial adenomas. The onset of Cushing's syndrome may be sudden, particularly in patients with carcinoma of the lung, and this feature accounts in part for the failure of these patients to exhibit the classic manifestations. On the other hand, patients with carcinoid tumors or pheochromocytomas have longer clinical courses and usually exhibit the typical cushingoid features. The secretion of ACTH by nonendocrine tumors is also accompanied by the accumulation of ACTH fragments in plasma and by elevated plasma levels of ACTH precursor molecules. Since such tumors may produce large amounts of ACTH, baseline steroid values are usually markedly elevated, and increased skin pigmentation may be present. Indeed, hyperpigmentation in patients with Cushing's syndrome almost always points to an extraadrenal tumor, either in an extracranial location or within the cranium.

Approximately 20 to 25 percent of patients with Cushing's syndrome have an adrenal neoplasm. These tumors are usually unilateral, and about half are malignant. Occasionally, patients have biochemical features both of hypersecretion of pituitary ACTH and of an adrenal adenoma. These individuals usually have micro- or macronodularity of both adrenal glands resulting in *nodular hyperplasia*. Two specific entities cause nodular hyperplasia: a familial autoimmune disorder in children or young adults (so-called pigmented multinodular cortical dysplasia) and hypersensitivity to gastric inhibitory polypeptide, probably secondary to enhanced expression of receptors for this peptide in the adrenal cortex.

The most common cause of Cushing's syndrome is *iatrogenic* administration of steroids for a variety of reasons. While the clinical features bear some resemblance to those seen with adrenal tumors, these patients are usually distinguishable on the basis of history and laboratory studies.

Clinical Signs, Symptoms, and Laboratory Findings Many of the signs and symptoms of Cushing's syndrome follow logically from the known action of glucocorticoids (Table 332-4). Mobilization of peripheral supportive tissue causes muscle weakness and fatigability, osteoporosis, cutaneous striae, and easy bruisability. The latter signs are secondary to weakening and rupture of collagen fibers in the dermis. Osteoporosis may cause collapse of vertebral bodies and pathologic fractures of other bones. Increased hepatic gluconeogenesis

---

Table 332-3

Causes of Cushing's Syndrome

Adrenal hyperplasia
  Secondary to pituitary ACTH overproduction
    Pituitary-hypothalamic dysfunction
    Pituitary ACTH-producing micro- or macroadenomas
  Secondary to ACTH or CRH-producing nonendocrine tumors (bronchogenic carcinoma, carcinoid of the thymus, pancreatic carcinoma, bronchial adenoma)
Adrenal nodular hyperplasia
Adrenal neoplasia
  Adenoma
  Carcinoma
Exogenous, iatrogenic causes
  Prolonged use of glucocorticoids
  Prolonged use of ACTH

Table 332-4

Frequency of Signs and Symptoms in Cushing's Syndrome

Sign or Symptom	Percent of Patients
Typical habitus	97
Increased body weight	94
Fatigability and weakness	87
Hypertension (blood pressure >150/90)	82
Hirsutism	80
Amenorrhea	77
Cutaneous striae	67
Personality changes	66
Ecchymoses	65
Edema	62
Polyuria, polydipsia	23
Hypertrophy of clitoris	19

and insulin resistance can cause impaired glucose tolerance. Overt diabetes mellitus occurs in fewer than 20 percent of patients, who probably are individuals with a predisposition to this disorder. Hypercortisolism promotes the deposition of adipose tissue in characteristic sites, notably the upper face (producing the typical "moon" facies), the interscapular area (producing the "buffalo hump"), and the mesenteric bed (producing "truncal" obesity) (Fig. 332-6). Rarely, episternal fatty tumors and mediastinal widening secondary to fat accumulation occur. The reason for this peculiar distribution of adipose tissue is not known, but it is associated with insulin resistance and/or elevated insulin levels. The face appears plethoric, even in the absence of any increase in red blood cell concentration. Hypertension is common, and emotional changes may be profound, ranging from irritability and emotional lability to severe depression, confusion, or even frank psychosis. In women, increased levels of adrenal androgens can cause acne, hirsutism, and oligomenorrhea or amenorrhea. Some signs and symptoms in patients with hypercortisolism—i.e., obesity, hypertension, osteoporosis, and diabetes—are nonspecific and therefore are less helpful in diagnosing the condition. On the other hand, easy bruising, typical striae, myopathy, and virilizing signs (although less frequent) are, if present, more suggestive of Cushing's syndrome.

Except in iatrogenic Cushing's syndrome, plasma and urine cortisol levels are variably elevated. Occasionally, hypokalemia, hypochloremia, and metabolic alkalosis are present, particularly with ectopic production of ACTH.

Diagnosis   The diagnosis of Cushing's syndrome depends on the demonstration of increased cortisol production and failure to suppress cortisol secretion normally when dexamethasone is administered. Once the diagnosis is established, further testing is designed to determine the etiology (Fig. 332-7 and Table 332-5).

For initial screening, the overnight dexamethasone suppression test is recommended (see above). In difficult cases (e.g., in obese patients), measurement of a 24-h urine free cortisol also can be used as a screening test. A level greater than 275 nmol/d (100 μg/d) is suggestive of Cushing's syndrome. The definitive diagnosis is then established by failure of urinary cortisol to fall to less than 80 nmol/d (30 μg/d) or of plasma cortisol to fall to less than 140 nmol/L (5 μg/dL) after a standard low-dose dexamethasone suppression test (0.5 mg every 6 h for 48 h). Owing to circadian variability, plasma cortisol and, to a certain extent, ACTH determinations are not meaningful when performed in isolation, but demonstration that the

FIGURE 332-6   A woman with Cushing's syndrome due to a right adrenal cortical adenoma. *A.* Two years prior to surgery, age 18. *B.* One month prior to surgery, age 20. *C.* One year after surgery, age 21.

FIGURE 332-7   Diagnostic flowchart for evaluating patients suspected of having Cushing's syndrome. *This group probably includes some patients with pituitary-hypothalamic dysfunction and some with pituitary microadenomas. In some instances, a pituitary microadenoma may be visualized by MRI scanning of the sella turcica.

normal fall in evening levels of plasma cortisol does not occur may be useful.

The task of determining the etiology of Cushing's syndrome is complicated by the fact that all the available tests lack specificity and by the fact that the tumors producing this syndrome are prone to spontaneous and often dramatic changes in hormone secretion (periodic hormonogenesis). No test has a specificity greater than 95 percent, and it may be necessary to use a combination of tests to arrive at the correct diagnosis. A useful step to distinguish patients with an ACTH-secreting pituitary microadenoma or hypothalamic-pituitary dysfunction from those with other forms of Cushing's syndrome is to determine the response of cortisol output to administration of high-dose dexamethasone (2 mg every 6 h for 2 days). Indeed, when the diagnosis of Cushing's syndrome is clear-cut on the basis of baseline urinary and plasma assays, the high-dose dexamethasone suppression test may

Table 332-5

Diagnostic Tests to Determine the Type of Cushing's Syndrome

Test	Pituitary Macro-adenoma	Pituitary-Hypothalamic Dysfunction or Micro-adenoma	Ectopic ACTH or CRH Pro-duction	Adrenal Tumor
Plasma ACTH level	↑ to ↑↑	N to ↑	↑ to ↑↑↑	↓
Percent who respond to high-dose dexamethasone	<10	95	<10	<10
Percent who re-spond to CRH	>90	>90	<10	<10

NOTE: N, normal; ↑, elevated; ↓, decreased. See text for definition of a response.

be used without performing the preliminary low-dose suppression test. The high-dose suppression test provides close to 100 percent specificity if the criterion used is suppression of urinary free cortisol by greater than 90 percent. Occasionally, in individuals with bilateral nodular hyperplasia and/or ectopic CRH production, steroid output is also suppressed. Failure of low- and high-dose dexamethasone administration to suppress cortisol production (see Table 332-5) is usual in patients with adrenal hyperplasia secondary to an ACTH-secreting pituitary macroadenoma or an ACTH-producing tumor of nonendocrine origin and in those with adrenal neoplasms.

Plasma ACTH levels can be useful in distinguishing the various causes of Cushing's syndrome, particularly in separating ACTH-dependent from ACTH-independent causes. In general, measurement of plasma ACTH is useful in the diagnosis of ACTH-independent etiologies of the syndrome, since most adrenal tumors cause low or undetectable ACTH levels. Furthermore, ACTH-secreting pituitary macroadenomas and ACTH-producing nonendocrine tumors usually result in elevated ACTH levels. In the ectopic ACTH syndrome, ACTH levels may be elevated above 110 pmol/L (500 pg/mL), and in most patients the level is above 40 pmol/L (200 pg/mL). In Cushing's syndrome as the result of a microadenoma or pituitary-hypothalamic dysfunction, ACTH levels range from 6 to 30 pmol/L (30 to 150 pg/mL) [normal, <14 pmol/L (<60 pg/mL)], with half of values falling in the normal range. However, the main problem with the use of ACTH levels in the differential diagnosis of Cushing's syndrome is that ACTH levels may be similar in individuals with hypothalamic-pituitary dysfunction, pituitary microadenomas, ectopic CRH production, and ACTH production from some nonendocrine tumors (especially carcinoid tumors) (see Table 332-5).

Because of these difficulties, several additional tests have been advocated, such as the metyrapone and CRH infusion tests. The rationale underlying these tests is that steroid hypersecretion by an adrenal tumor or the ectopic production of ACTH will suppress the hypothalamic-pituitary axis so that inhibition of pituitary ACTH release can be demonstrated by either test. Thus, most patients with pituitary-hypothalamic dysfunction and/or a microadenoma have an increase in steroid or ACTH secretion in response to metyrapone or CRH administration, while most patients with ectopic ACTH-producing tumors do not. Most pituitary macroadenomas also respond to CRH, while their response to metyrapone is variable. The usefulness of the CRH infusion test, however, is uncertain because only a limited number of studies have been performed and because CRH is not readily available. In addition, false-positive and false-negative CRH tests can occur in patients with nonendocrine and pituitary tumors.

The main diagnostic dilemma in Cushing's syndrome is to distinguish those instances due to microadenomas of the pituitary and/or pituitary-hypothalamic dysfunction from those due to tumors (e.g., carcinoids or pheochromocytoma) that produce CRH and/or ACTH

ectopically. The clinical manifestations are similar unless the ectopic tumor produces other symptoms, such as diarrhea and flushing from a carcinoid tumor or episodic hypertension from a pheochromocytoma. Sometimes, one can distinguish between ectopic and pituitary ACTH production by using metyrapone or CRH tests, as noted above. In these situations, computed tomography (CT) of the pituitary gland is usually normal. Magnetic resonance imaging (MRI) with the enhancing agent gadolinium may be better than CT for this purpose but demonstrates pituitary microadenomas in only half of patients with Cushing's disease. In subjects with negative imaging studies, selective venous sampling for ACTH is employed in some centers. Demonstration of an ACTH gradient between the petrosal sinus and peripheral blood localizes the source of ACTH overproduction to the pituitary gland but does not distinguish pituitary-dependent adrenal hyperplasia from pituitary hyperplasia secondary to a tumor producing CRH. CRH levels should be measured in the peripheral blood prior to petrosal sinus sampling. No reliable test is available to make this distinction if the ectopic tumor is not seen or if it produces no other hormones.

The diagnosis of a *cortisol-producing adrenal adenoma* is suggested by disproportionate elevations in baseline urine free-cortisol levels with only modest changes in urinary 17-ketosteroids or plasma DHEA sulfate. Adrenal androgen secretion is usually reduced in these patients owing to the cortisol-induced suppression of ACTH and subsequent involution of the androgen-producing zona reticularis.

The diagnosis of *adrenal carcinoma* is suggested by a palpable abdominal mass and by *markedly* elevated baseline values of *both* urine 17-ketosteroids and plasma DHEA sulfate. Plasma and urine cortisol levels are variably elevated. Adrenal carcinoma is usually resistant to both ACTH stimulation and dexamethasone suppression. Elevated adrenal androgen secretion often leads to virilization in the female. Estrogen-producing adrenocortical carcinoma usually presents with gynecomastia in men and dysfunctional uterine bleeding in women. These adrenal tumors secrete increased amounts of androstenedione, which is converted peripherally to the estrogens estrone and estradiol (see Chap. 338). Adrenal carcinomas that produce Cushing's syndrome are most often associated with elevated levels of the intermediates of steroid biosynthesis (especially 11-deoxycortisol), suggesting inefficient conversion of the intermediates to the final product. Approximately 20 percent of adrenal carcinomas are not associated with endocrine syndromes and are presumed to be nonfunctioning or to produce biologically inactive steroid precursors. In addition, the excessive production of steroids is not always clinically evident (e.g., androgens in adult men).

Differential Diagnosis *Pseudo-Cushing's syndrome* Problems in diagnosis include patients with obesity, chronic alcoholism, depression, and acute illness of any type. Extreme *obesity* is uncommon in Cushing's syndrome; furthermore, with exogenous obesity, the adiposity is generalized, not truncal. On adrenocortical testing, abnormalities in patients with exogenous obesity are usually modest. Basal urine steroid excretion levels in obese patients are also either normal or slightly elevated. Some patients have elevated conversion of secreted cortisol into excreted metabolites. Urinary and blood cortisol levels are usually normal, and the diurnal pattern in blood and urine levels is normal. Patients with *chronic alcoholism* and those with *depression* share similar abnormalities in steroid output: modestly elevated urine cortisol, absent circadian rhythm of cortisol levels, and resistance to suppression with dexamethasone (particularly in the overnight and low-dose tests). In contrast to alcoholic subjects, depressed patients do not have signs and symptoms of Cushing's syndrome. Following discontinuation of alcohol and/or improvement in the emotional status, results of steroid testing usually return to normal. A normal cortisol response to insulin-induced hypoglycemia may distinguish these patients from subjects with Cushing's syndrome. *Acutely ill* patients often have abnormal results on laboratory tests and fail to exhibit pituitary-adrenal suppression in response to dexamethasone, since major stress (such as pain or fever) interrupts the normal regulation of ACTH secretion. A rare cause of hypercortisolism without cushingoid stigmata is *primary cortisol resistance* due to mutations in the type I glucocorticoid receptor; the resistance is incomplete because patients do not exhibit signs of adrenal insufficiency. *Iatrogenic Cushing's syndrome*, induced by the administration of glucocorticoids or other steroids such as megestrol that bind to the glucocorticoid receptor, is indistinguishable by physical findings from endogenous adrenocortical hyperfunction. The distinction can be made, however, by measuring blood or urine cortisol levels in a basal state; in the iatrogenic syndrome these levels are low secondary to suppression of the pituitary-adrenal axis. The severity of iatrogenic Cushing's syndrome is related to the total steroid dose, the biologic half-life of the steroid, and the duration of therapy. Also, individuals taking afternoon and evening doses of glucocorticoids develop Cushing's syndrome more readily and with a smaller total daily dose than do patients taking morning doses only. The enzymatic disposition and binding of administered steroids differ among patients.

Radiologic Evaluation for Cushing's Syndrome   The preferred radiologic study for visualizing the adrenals is a CT scan of the abdomen (Fig. 332-8). CT is of value both for localizing adrenal tumors and for diagnosing bilateral hyperplasia. All patients believed to have hypersecretion of pituitary ACTH should have a pituitary MRI scan with the contrast agent gadolinium. Even with this technique, small microadenomas may be undetectable; alternatively, false-positive masses due to nonsecretory variations of the normal pituitary

anatomy may be imaged. In patients with ectopic ACTH production, chest tomography is a useful first step.

Evaluation of Asymptomatic Adrenal Masses   With abdominal CT scanning, many incidental adrenal masses (so-called incidentalomas) are discovered. This is not surprising, since 10 to 20 percent of subjects at autopsy have adrenocortical adenomas. The first step in evaluating such patients is to determine whether the tumor is functioning by means of appropriate screening tests, e.g., measurement of 24-h urine catecholamines and metabolites and serum potassium and assessment of adrenal cortical function by dexamethasone suppression testing. However, 90 percent of incidentalomas are nonfunctioning. If an extraadrenal malignancy is present, there is a 30 to 50 percent chance that the adrenal tumor is a metastasis. If the primary tumor is being treated and there are no other metastases, it is prudent to obtain a fine-needle aspirate of the adrenal mass to establish the diagnosis. In the absence of a known malignancy the next step is unclear. The probability of adrenal carcinoma is less than 0.01 percent, the vast majority of adrenal masses being benign adenomas. Features suggestive of malignancy include large size (a size greater than 4 to 6 cm

FIGURE 332-8   Computed tomography is the preferred method for visualizing the adrenal glands (*arrows*). *A.* The normal right adrenal gland is adjacent to the inferior vena cava (V) where it emerges from the liver. Approximately 90 percent of the right adrenal glands appear as linear structures extending posteriorly from the inferior vena cava into the space between the right lobe of the liver and the crus of the diaphragm. The normal left adrenal gland is lateral to the left crus of the diaphragm and below the stomach. Most left adrenal glands are shaped like an inverted V or Y. *B.* Adrenal CT scan of a patient with ectopic ACTH production. Both adrenal glands (*arrows*) are enlarged (compare with *A*). In contrast, only 50 percent of patients with bilateral adrenal hyperplasia secondary to pituitary ACTH hypersecretion show enlargement of the adrenals when imaged by CT scan. *C.* CT scan of a patient with Cushing's syndrome with biochemical evidence only of cortisol overproduction. The left adrenal has been replaced by a racquet-shaped 2-cm tumor (*arrow*). Attenuation of the tumor is low because of its high lipid content. *D.* CT scan in a patient with Cushing's syndrome and biochemical evidence of an adrenal carcinoma. In contrast to the tumor in *C*, the right-sided mass in this patient is large and has a heterogeneous appearance—usual characteristics of an adrenal carcinoma.

suggests carcinoma); irregular margins; and inhomogeneity, soft tissue calcifications visible on CT (see Fig. 332-8), and findings characteristic of malignancy on a chemical-shift MRI image. If surgery or fine-needle aspiration is not performed, a repeat CT scan should be obtained in 3 to 6 months.

℞ **TREATMENT**

Adrenal Neoplasm When an adenoma or carcinoma is diagnosed, adrenal exploration is performed with excision of the tumor. Because of the possibility of atrophy of the contralateral adrenal, the patient is treated pre- and postoperatively as if for total adrenalectomy, even when a unilateral lesion is suspected, the routine being similar to that for an Addisonian patient undergoing elective surgery (see Table 332-11).

Despite operative intervention, most patients with adrenal carcinoma die within 3 years of diagnosis. Metastases occur most often to liver and lung. The principal drug for the treatment of adrenocortical carcinoma is mitotane (*o,p'*-DDD), an isomer of the insecticide DDT. This drug suppresses cortisol production and decreases plasma and urine steroid levels. Although its cytotoxic action is relatively selective for the glucocorticoid-secreting zone of the adrenal cortex, the zona glomerulosa also may be inhibited. Because mitotane also alters the extraadrenal metabolism of cortisol, plasma and urinary cortisol levels must be assessed to titrate the effect. The drug is usually given in divided doses three to four times a day, with the dose increased gradually to 8 to 10 g daily. At higher doses, almost all patients experience side effects, which may be gastrointestinal (anorexia, diarrhea, vomiting) or neuromuscular (lethargy, somnolence, dizziness). All patients treated with mitotane should receive long-term glucocorticoid maintenance therapy, and, in some, mineralocorticoid replacement is appropriate. In approximately one-third of patients, both tumor and metastases regress, but long-term survival is limited. In many patients, mitotane only inhibits steroidogenesis and does not cause regression of tumor metastases. Osseous metastases are usually refractory to the drug and should be treated with radiation therapy. Mitotane also can be given as adjunctive therapy after surgical resection of an adrenal carcinoma, although there is no evidence that this improves survival.

Bilateral Hyperplasia Patients with hyperplasia have a relative or absolute increase in ACTH levels. Since therapy would logically be directed at reducing ACTH levels, the ideal primary treatment for ACTH- or CRH-producing tumors, whether pituitary or ectopic, is surgical removal. Occasionally (particularly with ectopic ACTH production) surgical excision is not possible because the disease is far advanced. In this situation, "medical" or surgical adrenalectomy may correct the hypercortisolism.

Controversy exists as to the proper treatment for bilateral adrenal hyperplasia when the source of the ACTH overproduction is not apparent. In some centers, these patients (especially those who suppress after the administration of a high-dose dexamethasone) undergo surgical exploration of the pituitary via a transsphenoidal approach in the expectation that a microadenoma will be found. However, in most circumstances selective petrosal sinus venous sampling is recommended, and the patient is referred to an appropriate center if the procedure is not available locally. If a microadenoma is not found at the time of exploration, total hypophysectomy may be needed. Complications of transsphenoidal surgery include cerebrospinal fluid rhinorrhea, diabetes insipidus, panhypopituitarism, and optic or cranial nerve injuries. Furthermore, these pituitary neoplasms may recur if the primary abnormality actually resides in the hypothalamus.

In other centers, total adrenalectomy is the treatment of choice. The cure rate with this procedure is close to 100 percent. The adverse effects include the certain need for lifelong mineralocorticoid and glucocorticoid replacement and a 10 to 20 percent probability of a pituitary tumor developing over the next 10 years (Nelson's syn-

drome; see Chap. 328). Many of these tumors require surgical therapy. It is uncertain whether they arise de novo in these patients or were present prior to adrenalectomy but were too small to be detected. Periodic radiologic evaluation of the pituitary gland by MRI as well as serial ACTH measurements should be performed in all individuals after bilateral adrenalectomy for Cushing's syndrome. Such pituitary tumors may become locally invasive and impinge on the optic chiasm or extend into the cavernous or sphenoid sinuses.

Except in children, pituitary irradiation is rarely used as primary treatment, being reserved rather for postoperative tumor recurrences. In some centers, high levels of gamma radiation can be focused on the desired site with less scattering to surrounding tissues by using stereotactic techniques. Side effects of radiation include ocular motor palsy and hypopituitarism. There is a long lag time between treatment and remission, and the remission rate is usually less than 50 percent.

Finally, in occasional patients in whom a surgical approach is not feasible, "medical" adrenalectomy may be indicated (Table 332-6). Inhibition of steroidogenesis also may be indicated in severely cushingoid subjects prior to surgical intervention. Chemical adrenalectomy may be accomplished by the administration of the inhibitor of steroidogenesis ketoconazole (600 to 1200 mg/d). In addition, mitotane (2 or 3 g/d) and/or the blockers of steroid synthesis aminoglutethimide (1 g/d) and metyrapone (2 or 3 g/d) may be effective either alone or in combination. Mitotane is slow to take effect (weeks). Mifepristone, a competitive inhibitor of the binding of glucocorticoid to its receptor, may be a treatment option. Adrenal insufficiency is a risk with all these agents, and replacement steroids may be required.

ALDOSTERONISM Aldosteronism is a syndrome associated with hypersecretion of the mineralocorticoid aldosterone. In *primary* aldosteronism the cause for the excessive aldosterone production resides within the adrenal gland; in *secondary* aldosteronism the stimulus is extraadrenal.

Primary Aldosteronism In the original case of excessive and inappropriate aldosterone production, the disease was the result of an *aldosterone-producing adrenal adenoma* (Conn's syndrome). Most cases involve a unilateral adenoma, which usually is small and may occur on either side. Rarely, primary aldosteronism is due to an adrenal carcinoma. Aldosteronism is twice as common in women as in men, usually occurs between the ages of 30 and 50, and is present in approximately 1 percent of unselected hypertensive patients. In many cases with clinical and biochemical features of primary aldosteronism, a solitary adenoma is not found at surgery. Instead, these patients have *bilateral cortical nodular hyperplasia*. In the literature, this disease is also termed pseudoprimary aldosteronism, idiopathic hyperaldosteronism, and nodular hyperplasia. The cause is unknown.

Signs and symptoms Hypersecretion of aldosterone increases the renal distal tubular exchange of intratubular sodium for secreted potassium and hydrogen ions, with progressive depletion of body potassium and development of hypokalemia. Most patients have diastolic hypertension, usually not very severe, and headaches. The hypertension is probably due to the increased sodium reabsorption and extracellular volume expansion. *Potassium depletion* is responsible for the muscle weakness and fatigue and is due to the effect of potassium depletion on the muscle cell membrane. The polyuria results from impairment of urinary concentrating ability and is often associated with polydipsia.

Table 332-6

Treatment Modalities for Patients with Adrenal Hyperplasia Secondary to Pituitary ACTH Hypersecretion

Treatments to reduce pituitary ACTH production
  Transsphenoidal resection of microadenoma
  Radiation therapy
Treatments to reduce or eliminate adrenocortical cortisol secretion
  Bilateral adrenalectomy
  Medical adrenalectomy (metyrapone, mitotane, aminoglutethimide, ketoconazole)*

* Not curative but effective as long as chronically administered in selected patients.

Electrocardiographic and roentgenographic signs of left ventricular enlargement are secondary to the hypertension. Electrocardiographic signs of potassium depletion include prominent U waves, cardiac arrhythmias, and premature contractions. In the absence of associated congestive heart failure, renal disease, or preexisting abnormalities (such as thrombophlebitis), edema is characteristically absent. In cases of long duration, nephropathy with azotemia may be associated with congestive heart failure and edema.

Laboratory findings Laboratory findings depend on both the duration and the severity of potassium depletion. An overnight concentration test often reveals impaired ability to concentrate the urine, probably secondary to the hypokalemia. Urine pH is neutral to alkaline because of excessive secretion of ammonium and bicarbonate ions to compensate for the metabolic alkalosis.

Hypokalemia may be severe (less than 3 mmol/L) and reflects body potassium depletion, usually in excess of 300 mmol. *Hypernatremia* is due to sodium retention, a concomitant water loss from polyuria, and a resetting of the osmostat. Metabolic alkalosis and elevation of serum bicarbonate are a result of hydrogen ion loss into the urine and migration into potassium-depleted cells. The alkalosis is perpetuated by potassium deficiency, which increases the capacity of the proximal convoluted tubule to reabsorb filtered bicarbonate. If hypokalemia is severe, serum magnesium levels are also reduced.

Total-body sodium content and total exchangeable sodium are usually increased, while total exchangeable body potassium is reduced. The expanded extracellular fluid volume may be responsible for the reversed circadian excretory pattern for salt and water, with salt and water excretion occurring predominantly during the night.

Diagnosis The diagnosis is suggested by persistent hypokalemia in a nonedematous patient with a normal sodium intake who is not receiving potassium-wasting diuretics (furosemide, ethacrynic acid, thiazides). If hypokalemia occurs in a hypertensive patient taking a potassium-wasting diuretic, the diuretic should be discontinued and the patient should be given potassium supplements. After 1 to 2 weeks, the potassium level should be remeasured, and if hypokalemia persists the patient should be evaluated for a mineralocorticoid excess syndrome (Fig. 332-9).

The criteria for the diagnosis of primary aldosteronism are (1) diastolic hypertension without edema, (2) hyposecretion of renin (as judged by low plasma renin activity levels) that fails to increase appropriately during volume depletion (upright posture, sodium depletion), and (3) hypersecretion of aldosterone that does not suppress appropriately in response to volume expansion (salt loading).

Patients with primary aldosteronism characteristically *do not have edema*, since they exhibit an "escape" phenomenon from the sodium-retaining aspects of mineralocorticoids. Rarely, pretibial edema is present in patients with associated nephropathy and azotemia.

The estimation of plasma renin activity is of limited value in separating patients with primary aldosteronism from those with hypertension of other causes. While failure of plasma renin activity to rise normally during volume-depletion maneuvers is a criterion for a diagnosis of primary aldosteronism, suppressed renin activity also occurs in about 25 percent of patients with essential hypertension.

Since the determination of plasma renin responsiveness is not sufficient, the demonstration of lack of suppression of aldosterone secretion is necessary to diagnose primary aldosteronism (see Fig. 332-9). The autonomy exhibited by aldosterone tumors in these patients refers only to the resistance to suppression of secretion during volume expansion; such tumors can and do respond in a normal or above-normal fashion to the stimulus of potassium loading or ACTH infusion.

Once hyposecretion of renin and failure of aldosterone secretion suppression are demonstrated, aldosterone-producing adenomas should be localized by abdominal CT scan, using a spiral, thin-slice technique since many aldosteronomas are less than 1 cm in size. If the CT scan is negative, percutaneous transfemoral bilateral adrenal vein catheterization with adrenal vein sampling may demonstrate a two- to threefold increase in plasma aldosterone concentration on the involved side. In cases of hyperaldosteronism secondary to cortical

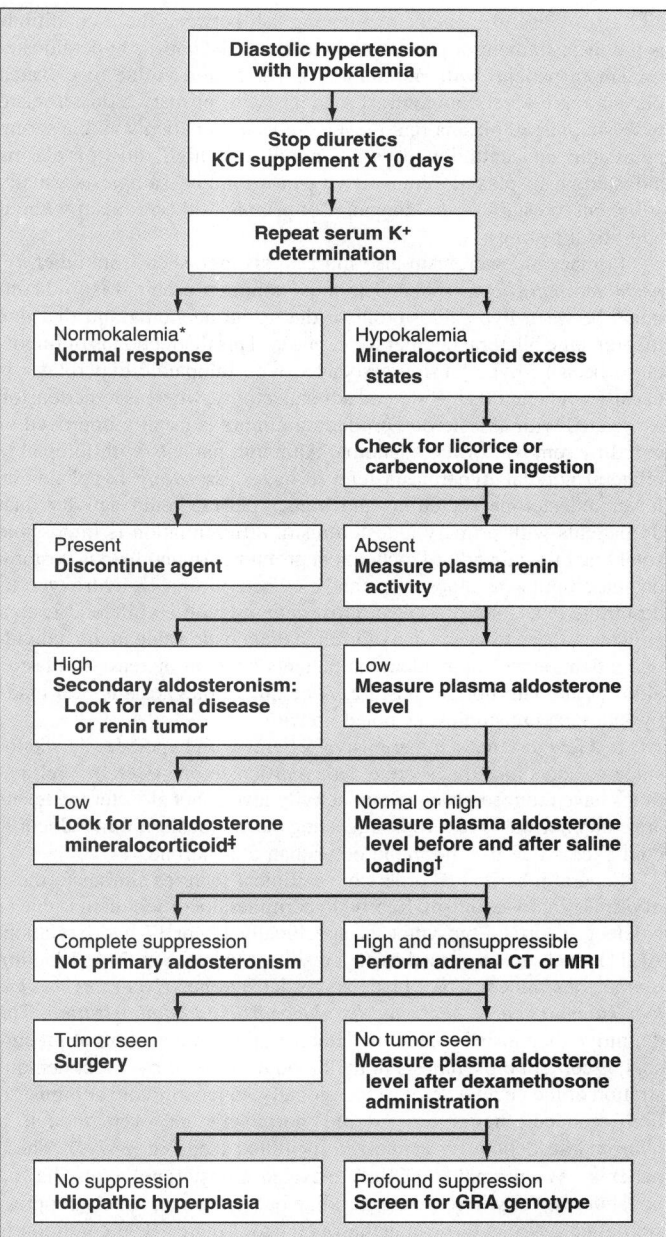

FIGURE 332-9 Diagnostic flowchart for evaluating patients with suspected primary aldosteronism. *Serum K^+ may be normal in some patients with hyperaldosteronism who are taking potassium-sparing diuretics (spironolactone, triamterene) or who have a low sodium intake and a high potassium intake. †This step should not be taken if hypertension is severe (diastolic pressure >115 mmHg) or if cardiac failure is present. Also, serum potassium levels should be corrected before the infusion of saline solution. Alternative methods that produce comparable suppression of aldosterone secretion include oral sodium loading (200 mmol/d for 3 days) or administration of 10 mg deoxycorticosterone acetate (DOCA) intramuscularly every 12 h for 3 days. (GRA, glucocorticoid-remediable aldosteronism.) ‡For example, Liddle's syndrome, apparent mineralocorticoid excess syndrome, or a deoxycorticosterone-secreting tumor.

nodular hyperplasia, no localization is found. It is important for samples to be obtained simultaneously if possible and for cortisol levels to be measured to ensure that false localization does not reflect an ACTH- or stress-induced rise in aldosterone levels.

Differential diagnosis Patients with hypertension and hypokalemia may have either primary or secondary hyperaldosteronism (Fig.

332-10). A useful maneuver to distinguish between these conditions is the measurement of plasma renin activity. Secondary hyperaldosteronism in patients with accelerated hypertension is due to elevated plasma renin levels; in contrast, patients with primary aldosteronism have suppressed plasma renin levels. Indeed, in patients with a serum potassium concentration of <2.5 mmol/L, a high ratio of plasma aldosterone to plasma renin activity in a random sample is usually sufficient to establish the diagnosis of primary aldosteronism without additional testing.

Primary aldosteronism also must be distinguished from other *hypermineralocorticoid states*. The most common problem is to distinguish between hyperaldosteronism due to an adenoma and that due to idiopathic bilateral nodular hyperplasia. This distinction is of importance because hypertension associated with idiopathic hyperplasia is usually not benefited by bilateral adrenalectomy, whereas hypertension associated with aldosterone-producing tumors is usually improved or cured by removal of the adenoma. Although patients with idiopathic bilateral nodular hyperplasia tend to have less severe hypokalemia, lower aldosterone secretion, and higher plasma renin activity than do patients with primary aldosteronism, differentiation is impossible solely on clinical and/or biochemical grounds. An anomalous postural decrease in plasma aldosterone and elevated plasma 18-hydroxycorticosterone levels are present in most patients with a unilateral lesion. However, these tests are also of limited diagnostic value in the individual patient, since some adenoma patients have an increase in plasma aldosterone with upright posture. A definitive diagnosis is best made by radiographic studies, as noted above.

In a few instances, hypertensive patients with hypokalemic alkalosis have adenomas that secrete deoxycorticosterone (DOC). Such patients have reduced plasma renin activity levels, but aldosterone levels are either normal or reduced, suggesting the diagnosis of mineralocorticoid excess due to a hormone other than aldosterone.

Several inherited disorders have clinical features similar to those of primary aldosteronism. Rarely, hypermineralocorticoidism is due to a defect in cortisol biosynthesis, specifically 11- or 17-hydroxylation. ACTH levels are increased, with a resultant increase in the production of the mineralocorticoid 11-deoxycorticosterone. *Hypertension and hypokalemia can be corrected by glucocorticoid administration.* The definitive diagnosis is made by demonstrating an elevation of precursors of cortisol biosynthesis in the blood or urine or by direct demonstration of the genetic defect. Occasionally, glucocorticoid administration produces normotension and normokalemia even though a hydroxylase deficiency cannot be identified (see Fig. 332-9). These patients have normal to slightly elevated aldosterone levels that do not suppress fully in response to saline but that usually show suppression after 2 weeks of dexamethasone (1 to 2 mg/d). The condition is inherited as an autosomal dominant trait and is termed *glucocorticoid-remediable aldosteronism* (GRA). This entity is secondary to a chimeric gene duplication whereby the 11β-hydroxylase gene promoter

(which is under the control of ACTH) is fused to the aldosterone synthase coding sequence. Thus, aldosterone synthase activity is expressed in the zona fasciculata and is regulated only by ACTH, in a fashion similar to the regulation of cortisol secretion. Screening for this defect is best performed by assessing the presence or absence of the chimeric gene. Since the abnormal gene may be present in the absence of hypokalemia, its frequency as a cause of hypertension is unknown. Individuals with suppressed plasma renin levels and juvenile-onset hypertension or a history of early-onset hypertension in first-degree relatives should be screened for this disorder.

Liddle's syndrome is a rare autosomal dominant disorder that mimicks hyperaldosteronism. The defect is in the gene encoding the β subunit of the epithelial sodium channel. Both renin and aldosterone levels are low, owing to the continuously activated sodium channel and the resulting excess sodium reabsorption in the renal tubule.

A rare autosomal recessive cause of hypokalemia and hypertension is 11β-hydroxysteroid dehydrogenase deficiency, in which cortisol cannot be converted to cortisone and hence binds to the glucocorticoid type I (mineralocorticoid) receptor and acts as a mineralocorticoid. This condition, also termed *apparent mineralocorticoid excess syndrome*, is caused by a defect in the gene encoding the renal isoform of this enzyme. Patients can be identified either by documenting an increased ratio of cortisol to cortisone in the urine or by genetic analysis.

The ingestion of candies or chewing tobacco containing certain forms of licorice produces a syndrome that mimics primary aldosteronism. The component of such agents that causes sodium retention is glycyrrhizinic acid, which inhibits the 11β-hydroxysteroid dehydrogenase and hence allows cortisol to act as a mineralocorticoid and cause sodium retention, expansion of the extracellular fluid volume, hypertension, depressed plasma renin levels, and suppressed aldosterone levels. The diagnosis is established or excluded by a careful history.

℞ TREATMENT

Primary aldosteronism due to an adenoma is usually treated by surgical excision of the adenoma. Where possible a laparoscopic approach is favored. However, dietary sodium restriction and the administration of an aldosterone antagonist (spironolactone) are effective in many cases. Hypertension and hypokalemia are usually controlled by doses of 25 to 100 mg spironolactone every 8 h. In some patients medical management has been successful for years, but chronic therapy in men is usually limited by side effects of spironolactone such as gynecomastia, decreased libido, and impotence.

When idiopathic bilateral hyperplasia is suspected, surgery is indicated only when significant, symptomatic hypokalemia cannot be controlled with medical therapy, e.g., by spironolactone, triamterene, or amiloride. Hypertension associated with idiopathic hyperplasia is usually not benefited by bilateral adrenalectomy.

Glucocorticoid-remediable hyperaldosteronism documented by genetic analysis may be treated with glucocorticoid administration or antimineralocorticoids, e.g., spironolactone, triamterene, or amiloride. Glucocorticoids should be used only in small doses to avoid inducing iatrogenic Cushing's syndrome. A combination approach is often necessary. Patients with the 11β-hydroxysteroid dehydrogenase deficiency syndrome can be treated with small doses of dexamethasone. Although dexamethasone is a potent glucocorticoid that suppresses ACTH and endogenous cortisol production, it binds less well to the mineralocorticoid receptor than does cortisol.

Secondary Aldosteronism *Secondary aldosteronism* refers to an appropriately increased production of aldosterone in response to activation of the renin-angiotensin system (see Fig. 332-10). The production rate of aldosterone is often higher in patients with secondary aldosteronism than in those with primary aldosteronism. Secondary aldosteronism usually occurs in association with the accelerated phase of hypertension or on the basis of an underlying edema disorder. Secondary aldosteronism in pregnancy is a normal physiologic response to estrogen-induced increases in circulating levels of renin substrate and plasma renin activity and to the antialdosterone actions of progestogens.

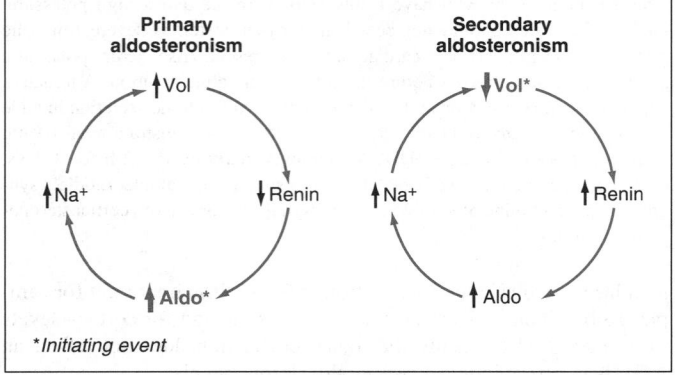

FIGURE 332-10 Responses of the renin-aldosterone volume control loop in primary versus secondary aldosteronism.

Secondary aldosteronism in hypertensive states is due either to a primary overproduction of renin (primary reninism) or to an overproduction of renin secondary to a decrease in renal blood flow and/or perfusion pressure (see Fig. 332-10). Secondary hypersecretion of renin can be due to a narrowing of one or both of the major renal arteries by atherosclerosis or by fibromuscular hyperplasia. Overproduction of renin from both kidneys also occurs in severe arteriolar nephrosclerosis (malignant hypertension) or with profound renal vasoconstriction (the accelerated phase of hypertension). The secondary aldosteronism is characterized by hypokalemic alkalosis, moderate to severe increases in plasma renin activity, and moderate to marked increases in aldosterone levels (see Chap. 246).

Secondary aldosteronism with hypertension also can be caused by rare renin-producing tumors (primary reninism). These patients have the biochemical characteristics of renal vascular hypertension, but the primary defect is renin secretion by a juxtaglomerular cell tumor. The diagnosis can be made by demonstration of normal renal vasculature and/or demonstration of a space-occupying lesion in the kidney by radiographic techniques and documentation of a unilateral increase in renal vein renin activity. Rarely, these tumors arise in tissues such as the ovary.

Secondary aldosteronism is present in many forms of *edema*. The rate of aldosterone secretion is usually increased in patients with edema caused by either cirrhosis or the nephrotic syndrome. In congestive heart failure, elevated aldosterone secretion varies depending on the severity of cardiac failure. The stimulus for aldosterone release in these conditions appears to be *arterial hypovolemia* and/or hypotension. Thiazides and furosemide often exaggerate secondary aldosteronism via volume depletion; hypokalemia and, on occasion, alkalosis can then become prominent features.

On occasion secondary hyperaldosteronism occurs without edema or hypertension (Bartter's syndrome). This syndrome is characterized by severe hyperaldosteronism (hypokalemic alkalosis) with moderate to marked increases in renin activity but normal blood pressure and no edema. Renal biopsy shows juxtaglomerular hyperplasia. The pathogenesis may involve a defect in the renal conservation of sodium or chloride and/or an increased production of prostaglandins. The renal loss of sodium is thought to stimulate renin secretion and aldosterone production. Hyperaldosteronism produces potassium depletion, and hypokalemia further elevates prostaglandin production and plasma renin activity. In some cases, the hypokalemia may be potentiated by a defect in renal conservation of potassium. Increased production of prostaglandins is probably not a primary abnormality, since administration of inhibitors of prostaglandin synthesis reverses the features only temporarily (see Chap. 278).

SYNDROMES OF ADRENAL ANDROGEN EXCESS Adrenal androgen excess results from excess production of dehydroepiandrosterone and androstenedione, which are converted to testosterone in extraglandular tissues; elevated testosterone levels account for most of the virilization. Adrenal androgen excess may be associated with the secretion of greater or smaller amounts of other adrenal hormones and may, therefore, present as "pure" syndromes of virilization or as "mixed" syndromes associated with excessive glucocorticoids and Cushing's syndrome.

Clinical Signs and Symptoms The manifestations can be divided into four types: hirsutism, oligomenorrhea, acne, and virilization. Clinically, it is important to distinguish between hypertrichosis, simple hirsutism, and hirsutism associated with virilization. Hypertrichosis is an increased growth of hair in males or females anywhere on the body. In contrast, hirsutism is limited to females and is hair growth in a male pattern of distribution. Most cases of simple hirsutism have no known cause. However, if the patient is virilized as well as hirsute, increased levels of androgens are usually present (see Chap. 53). In general, the degree of virilization reflects both the duration and the degree of excess androgen secretion, although significant virilization can result from minimal changes in testosterone production, and a significant increase in testosterone production can cause minimal signs of virilization. The occurrence of oligomenorrhea in a hirsute patient increases the probability that androgen production is increased. Thus,

the evaluation of the hirsute patient should include a careful history of the onset of menarche, past and present menstrual history, and reproductive capacity and examination for signs and symptoms of androgen excess.

Etiology As in other states of adrenocortical hyperfunction, the syndromes associated with androgen excess may result from hyperplasia, adenoma, or carcinoma (the latter two are discussed above). *Congenital adrenal hyperplasia* is the consequence of enzymatic defects. In these patients, increased adrenal androgen production is associated with either excessive or decreased secretion of mineralocorticoids or decreased production of glucocorticoids. Since cortisol is the principal adrenal steroid regulating ACTH elaboration and since ACTH stimulates production of both cortisol and adrenal androgen, a block in cortisol synthesis may result in the enhanced secretion of adrenal androgens. In severe congenital virilizing hyperplasia, the adrenal output of cortisol may be so compromised as to cause adrenal deficiency despite adrenal hyperplasia.

Congenital adrenal hyperplasia is the most common adrenal disorder of infancy and childhood and is the consequence of any of several autosomal recessive mutations (see Chap. 339). Partial enzyme deficiencies can be expressed after adolescence, predominantly in women with hirsutism and oligomenorrhea but minimal virilization. Late-onset adrenal hyperplasia may account for 5 to 25 percent of cases of hirsutism and oligomenorrhea in women, depending on the population.

Defects have been described in the $P450_{C21}$, $P450_{C18}$, $P450_{C17\alpha}$, and $P450_{C11\beta}$ hydroxylases and in 3β-hydroxysteroid dehydrogenase (3β-HSD) (see Fig. 332-2). While the cDNAs for these enzymes have been cloned, the diagnosis of specific enzyme deficiencies with genetic techniques is not practical for routine use. $P450_{C21}$ deficiency is closely linked to the histocompatibility leukocyte antigen (HLA)-B locus of chromosome 6 so that HLA typing and/or DNA polymorphism can be used to detect the heterozygous carriers and to diagnose affected individuals in some families (see Chap. 306). The clinical expression in the different disorders is variable, ranging from virilization of the female ($P450_{C21}$) to feminization of the male (3β-HSD) (see also Chap. 339).

Adrenal virilization in the female at birth is associated with ambiguous external genitalia (*female pseudohermaphroditism*). Virilization probably begins after the fifth month of intrauterine development. At birth there may be enlarged genitalia in the male infant and enlargement of the clitoris, partial or complete fusion of the labia, and sometimes a urogenital sinus in the female. If the labial fusion is nearly complete, the female infant has external genitalia resembling a penis with hypospadias. In the *postnatal* period, congenital adrenal hyperplasia is associated with virilization in the female and isosexual precocity in the male. The excessive androgen levels result in accelerated growth, so that bone age exceeds chronologic age. Since epiphyseal closure is hastened by excessive androgens, growth stops, but truncal development continues, the characteristic appearance being a short child with a well-developed trunk.

The most common form of congenital adrenal hyperplasia (95 percent of cases) is a result of impairment of $P450_{C21}$. In addition to cortisol deficiency, aldosterone secretion is decreased in approximately one-third of the patients. Thus, with $P450_{C21}$ deficiency, adrenal virilization occurs with or without a salt-losing tendency due to aldosterone deficiency (see Fig. 332-2).

$P450_{C11\beta}$ deficiency causes a "hypertensive" variant of congenital adrenal hyperplasia. Hypertension and hypokalemia occur because of the impaired conversion of 11-deoxycorticosterone to corticosterone, resulting in the accumulation of 11-deoxycorticosterone, a potent mineralocorticoid. The degree of hypertension is variable. Increased shunting again occurs into the androgen pathway.

$P450_{C17\alpha}$ deficiency is characterized by hypogonadism, hypokalemia, and hypertension. This rare disorder causes decreased production of cortisol and shunting of precursors into the mineralocorticoid pathway with hypokalemic alkalosis, hypertension, and suppressed plasma renin activity. Usually, 11-deoxycorticosterone production is elevated. Because $P450_{C17\alpha}$ hydroxylation is required for biosynthesis of both adrenal androgens and gonadal testosterone and estrogen, this defect is associated with sexual immaturity, high urinary gonadotropin levels, and low urinary 17-ketosteroid excretion. Female patients have primary amenorrhea and lack of development of secondary sexual characteristics. Because of deficient androgen production, male patients have either ambiguous external genitalia or a female phenotype *(male pseudohermaphroditism)*. Exogenous glucocorticoids can correct the hypertensive syndrome, and treatment with appropriate gonadal steroids results in sexual maturation.

With 3β-HSD deficiency, conversion of pregnenolone to progesterone is impaired, so that the synthesis of both cortisol and aldosterone is blocked, with shunting into the adrenal androgen pathway via 17α-hydroxypregnenolone and DHEA. Because DHEA is a weak androgen, and because this enzyme deficiency is also present in the gonad, the genitalia of the male fetus may be incompletely virilized or feminized. Conversely, in the female, overproduction of DHEA may produce partial virilization.

Diagnosis The diagnosis of *congenital adrenal hyperplasia* should be considered in infants having episodes of acute adrenal insufficiency or salt wasting or with hypertension. The diagnosis is further suggested by the finding of hypertrophy of the clitoris, fused labia, or a urogenital sinus in the female or of isosexual precocity in the male. In infants and children with a *P450$_{C21}$ block*, increased urine 17-ketosteroid excretion and increased plasma DHEA sulfate levels are typically associated with an increase in the blood levels of 17-hydroxyprogesterone and the excretion of its urinary metabolite pregnanetriol. Demonstration of elevated levels of 17-hydroxyprogesterone in amniotic fluid at 14 to 16 weeks of gestation allows prenatal detection of affected female infants.

The diagnosis of a *salt-losing form of congenital adrenal hyperplasia* due to defects in P450$_{C21}$ is suggested by episodes of acute adrenal insufficiency with hyponatremia, hyperkalemia, dehydration, and vomiting. These infants and children often crave salt and have laboratory findings indicating deficits in both cortisol and aldosterone secretion.

With the *hypertensive form of congenital adrenal hyperplasia* due to P450$_{C11\beta}$ deficiency, 11-deoxycorticosterone and 11-deoxycortisol accumulate. The diagnosis is confirmed by demonstrating increased levels of 11-deoxycortisol in the blood or increased amounts of tetrahydro-11-deoxycortisol in the urine. Elevation of 17-hydroxyprogesterone levels does not imply a coexisting P450$_{C21}$ deficiency.

Very high levels of urine dehydroepiandrosterone with low levels of pregnanetriol and of cortisol metabolites in urine are characteristic of children with 3β-HSD deficiency. Marked salt wasting may also occur.

Adults with *late-onset adrenal hyperplasia* (partial deficiency of P450$_{C21}$, P450$_{C11\beta}$, or 3β-HSD) are characterized by normal or moderately elevated levels of urinary 17-ketosteroids and plasma DHEA sulfate. A high basal level of a precursor of cortisol biosynthesis (such as 17-hydroxyprogesterone, 17-hydroxypregnenolone, or 11-deoxycortisol), or elevation of such a precursor after ACTH stimulation, confirms the diagnosis of a partial deficiency. Measurement of steroid precursors 60 min after bolus administration of ACTH is usually sufficient. Adrenal androgen output is easily suppressed by the standard low-dose (2 mg) dexamethasone test.

Differential Diagnosis The causes of hirsutism can be divided into four broad categories: familial, idiopathic, androgen excess, and drugs. In general, hirsutism of the first two types is not associated with other signs of androgen excess (i.e., oligomenorrhea, significant acne, or virilization). Likewise, drug-induced hirsutism is usually not associated with other signs and symptoms of androgen excess, unless the drug is an androgen. The drugs that produce an increase in body hair include phenothiazines, minoxidil, and phenytoin. Each of these drugs, particularly minoxidil, produces a generalized increase in hair growth, not just an increase in male-pattern hair. The mechanism may be related to the ability of these drugs to convert vellus into terminal hair follicles.

If drugs are excluded, the only known cause of hirsutism amenable to treatment is excess production of androgens by either the adrenal or the ovary.

In the female, the differential diagnosis of hirsutism and virilization is between adrenal and ovarian etiologies (Table 332-7). *Sudden onset of progressive hirsutism and virilization* suggests an adrenal or ovarian neoplasm. *Adrenal adenomas and carcinomas* may cause a pure or mixed virilizing syndrome. Since adrenal androgens are weak androgens, adrenal virilization is characterized by a *markedly elevated urine 17-ketosteroid excretion*. Virilizing adrenal adenomas are rare. *Virilizing adrenal carcinomas*, the most common adrenal tumors causing virilization, are associated with high plasma levels of DHEA sulfate and high rates of urinary excretion of 17-ketosteroids; as a rule, the tumors exceed 6 cm in size. Cortisol levels in blood and urine are normal or moderately elevated. Failure of urinary 17-ketosteroid levels and plasma DHEA sulfate levels to fall to normal in response to dexamethasone suppression (0.5 mg given orally every 6 h for 2 days) supports a diagnosis of virilizing adrenal tumor and excludes congenital adrenal hyperplasia.

The most common virilizing *ovarian tumor* is the arrhenoblastoma, but other ovarian tumors, such as adrenal rest tumor, granulosa cell tumor, hilar cell tumor, and Brenner tumor, can be responsible. Virilization due to ovarian tumors is usually characterized by normal levels of urinary 17-ketosteroids and DHEA sulfate, since the neoplasm usually secretes the potent androgen testosterone. Increases in 17-ketosteroid excretion occur in some patients with ovarian neoplasms, but an excretion rate in excess of 100 μmol/d (30 mg/d) is rare, except in the case of adrenal rest tumors. As with adrenal neoplasms, steroid production by ovarian tumors is not suppressed by dexamethasone. With the exception of adrenal rest tumors, these tumors are largely independent of ACTH stimulation. Elevations of plasma testosterone do not localize the neoplasm to the ovary, since testosterone can be elevated owing to peripheral conversion of adrenal precursors, such as DHEA (see Chap. 337).

The most common ovarian cause of excess androgen production is ovarian hyperthecosis or polycystic ovaries (see Chap. 337). Virilization is less common with polycystic ovaries than with ovarian or adrenal tumors, whereas hirsutism is quite frequent. Many patients with this condition are obese and have hyperinsulinemia, glucose intolerance, and acanthosis nigricans. The rate of 17-ketosteroid excretion may be partially reduced by dexamethasone. Plasma levels and production rates of androstenedione and, to a lesser extent, testosterone are usually increased. Follicle-stimulating hormone (FSH) levels tend to be low, and luteinizing hormone (LH) levels may be tonically elevated, leading to an increased LH/FSH ratio. The laboratory findings in patients with hirsutism-virilizing syndromes are summarized in Table 332-8.

 TREATMENT

Treatment of adrenal virilism is dictated by the type of lesion. Patients with *congenital adrenal hyperplasia* have a fundamental defect of cortisol deficiency with resultant excessive ACTH secretion, producing hyperplasia of the adrenal glands and causing additional shunting into the adrenal androgen pathway. Therapy in these patients consists of daily administration of glucocorticoids to suppress pituitary ACTH secretion. Because of its cost and intermediate

Table 332-7

Causes of Hirsutism in Women

Familial
Idiopathic
Ovarian
   Polycystic ovaries; hilus cell hyperplasia
   Tumor: arrhenoblastoma, hilus cell, adrenal rest
Adrenal
   Congenital adrenal hyperplasia
   Noncongenital adrenal hyperplasia (Cushing's)
   Tumor: virilizing carcinoma or adenoma

half-life, prednisone is the drug of choice except in infants, in whom hydrocortisone is usually used. In adults with late-onset adrenal hyperplasia, the smallest single bedtime dose of a long- or intermediate-acting glucocorticoid that suppresses pituitary ACTH secretion should be administered. The amount of steroid required by children with congenital adrenal hyperplasia is approximately 1 to 1.5 times the normal cortisol production rate of 27 to 35 μmol (10 to 13 mg) of cortisol per square meter of body surface per day and is given in divided doses two or three times per day. The dosage schedule is governed by repetitive analysis of the urinary 17-ketosteroids, plasma DHEA sulfate, and/or precursors of cortisol biosynthesis. Skeletal growth and maturation also must be monitored closely, since overtreatment with glucocorticoid replacement therapy retards linear growth.

Table 332-8

Laboratory Evaluation of Hirsutism-Virilizing Syndromes

	Ovarian		Adrenal			
	PCO	Ovarian Tumor	CAH	Adrenal Neoplasm	Cushing's Syndrome	Idiopathic
Urinary 17-ketosteroids, plasma DHEA sulfate	N↑	N	N↑	↑↑↑	N↑	N
Plasma testosterone	N↑	↑↑	N↑	N↑	N↑	N
LH/FSH ratio	N↑	N	N	N	N	N
Precursors of cortisol biosynthesis:						
Basal	N	N	N↑	N↑	N	N
Following ACTH infusion	N	N	↑↑	N↑	N	N
Cortisol following overnight dexamethasone suppression test	N	N	N	↑	↑	N

NOTE: CAH, congenital adrenal hyperplasia; PCO, polycystic ovary syndrome; N, normal; ↑, elevated.

HYPOFUNCTION OF THE ADRENAL CORTEX

Cases of adrenal insufficiency can be divided into two general categories: (1) those associated with primary inability of the adrenal to elaborate sufficient quantities of hormone and (2) those associated with a secondary failure due to inadequate ACTH formation or release (Table 332-9).

PRIMARY ADRENOCORTICAL DEFICIENCY (ADDISON'S DISEASE) The original description of Addison's disease—"general languor and debility, feebleness of the heart's action, irritability of the stomach, and a peculiar change of the color of the skin"—summarizes the dominant clinical features. Advanced cases are usually easy to diagnose, but recognition of the early phases can be a real challenge.

Incidence Primary insufficiency is relatively rare, may occur at any age, and affects both sexes equally. Because of the common therapeutic use of steroids, secondary adrenal insufficiency is relatively common.

Etiology and Pathogenesis Addison's disease results from progressive destruction of the adrenals, which must involve more than 90 percent of the glands before adrenal insufficiency appears. The adrenal is a frequent site for chronic granulomatous diseases, predominantly tuberculosis but also histoplasmosis, coccidioidomycosis, and cryptococcosis. In early series, tuberculosis was responsible for 70 to 90 percent of cases, but the most frequent cause now is *idiopathic* atrophy, and an autoimmune mechanism is probably responsible. Rarely, other lesions are encountered, such as adrenoleukodystrophy, bilateral hemorrhage, tumor metastases, amyloidosis, adrenomyeloneuropathy, familial adrenal insufficiency, or sarcoidosis.

Half of patients have circulating adrenal antibodies. Specific adrenal antigens to which autoantibodies may be directed include P450$_{C21}$. While most antibodies cause adrenal destruction, some antibodies cause adrenal insufficiency by blocking the binding of ACTH to its receptors. Some patients also have antibodies to thyroid, parathyroid, and/or gonadal tissue (see also Chap. 340). There is also an increased incidence of chronic lymphocytic thyroiditis, premature ovarian failure, type I diabetes mellitus, and hypo- or hyperthyroidism. The presence of two or more of these autoimmune endocrine disorders in the same person defines the polyglandular autoimmune syndrome type II. Additional features include pernicious anemia, vitiligo, alopecia, nontropical sprue, and myasthenia gravis. Within families, multiple generations are affected by one or more of the above diseases. Type II polyglandular syndrome is the result of a mutant gene on chromosome 6 and is associated with the HLA alleles B8 and DR3.

The combination of parathyroid and adrenal insufficiency and chronic mucocutaneous moniliasis constitutes type I polyglandular autoimmune syndrome. Other autoimmune diseases in this disorder include pernicious anemia, chronic active hepatitis, alopecia, primary hypothyroidism, and premature gonadal failure. There is no HLA association; this syndrome is inherited as an autosomal recessive trait. The type I syndrome usually presents during childhood, whereas the type II syndrome is usually manifested in adulthood. The mechanisms by which genetic predisposition and/or autoimmunity interact in the pathogenesis of these disorders are unknown.

Clinical suspicion of adrenal insufficiency should be high in patients with AIDS (see Chap. 308). Cytomegalovirus regularly involves the adrenal glands [so-called cytomegalovirus (CMV) necrotizing adrenalitis], and involvement with *Mycobacterium avium-intracellulare*, *Cryptococcus*, and Kaposi's sarcoma has been reported. Adrenal insufficiency in AIDS patients may not be manifest, but tests of adrenal reserve frequently give abnormal results. When interpreting tests of adrenocortical function, it is important to remember that medications such as rifampin, phenytoin, ketoconazole, and opiates may cause or potentiate adrenal insufficiency.

Adrenoleukodystrophy causes severe demyelination and early death in children, and adrenomyeloneuropathy is associated with a mixed motor and sensory neuropathy with spastic paraplegia in adults; both disorders are associated with elevated circulating levels of very long chain fatty acids and cause adrenal insufficiency. Familial adrenal insufficiency is an autosomal recessive disorder that causes unresponsiveness to ACTH secondary to mutations in the ACTH receptor. Adrenal hemorrhage and infarction occur in patients on anticoagulants and in those with circulating anticoagulants and hypercoagulable states, such as the antiphospholipid syndrome.

Clinical Signs and Symptoms Adrenocortical insufficiency caused by gradual adrenal destruction is characterized by an insidious onset of fatigability, weakness, anorexia, nausea and vomiting, weight

Table 332-9

Classification of Adrenal Insufficiency

PRIMARY ADRENAL INSUFFICIENCY

Anatomic destruction of gland (chronic or acute)
  "Idiopathic" atrophy (autoimmune, adrenoleukodystrophy)
  Surgical removal
  Infection (tuberculous, fungal, viral—especially in AIDS patients)
  Hemorrhage
  Invasion: metastatic
Metabolic failure in hormone production
  Congenital adrenal hyperplasia
  Enzyme inhibitors (metyrapone, ketoconazole, aminoglutethimide)
  Cytotoxic agents (mitotane)
ACTH-blocking antibodies
Mutation in ACTH receptor gene

SECONDARY ADRENAL INSUFFICIENCY

Hypopituitarism due to hypothalamic-pituitary disease
Suppression of hypothalamic-pituitary axis
  By exogenous steroid
  By endogenous steroid from tumor

loss, cutaneous and mucosal pigmentation, hypotension, and occasionally hypoglycemia (Table 332-10). Depending on the duration and degree of adrenal hypofunction, the manifestations vary from mild chronic fatigue to fulminating shock associated with acute destruction of the glands, as described by Waterhouse and Friderichsen.

Asthenia is the cardinal symptom. Early it may be sporadic, usually most evident at times of stress; as adrenal function becomes more impaired, the patient is continuously fatigued, and bed rest is necessary.

Hyperpigmentation may be striking or absent. It commonly appears as a diffuse brown, tan, or bronze darkening of parts such as the elbows or creases of the hand and of areas that normally are pigmented such as the areolae about the nipples. Bluish-black patches may appear on the mucous membranes. Some patients develop dark freckles, and irregular areas of vitiligo may paradoxically be present. As an early sign, tanning following sun exposure may be persistent.

Arterial hypotension with postural accentuation is frequent, and blood pressure may be in the range of 80/50 or less.

Abnormalities of gastrointestinal function often are the presenting complaint. Symptoms vary from mild anorexia with weight loss to fulminating nausea, vomiting, diarrhea, and ill-defined abdominal pain, which may be so severe as to be confused with an acute abdomen. Patients may have personality changes, usually consisting of excessive irritability and restlessness. Enhancement of the sensory modalities of taste, olfaction, and hearing is reversible with therapy. Axillary and pubic hair may be decreased in women due to loss of adrenal androgens.

Laboratory Findings In the early phase of gradual adrenal destruction, there may be no demonstrable abnormalities in the routine laboratory parameters, but adrenal reserve is decreased—that is, while basal steroid output may be normal, a subnormal increase occurs after stress. Adrenal stimulation with ACTH uncovers abnormalities in this stage of the disease, eliciting a subnormal increase of cortisol levels or no increase at all. In more advanced stages of adrenal destruction, serum sodium, chloride, and bicarbonate levels are reduced, and the serum potassium level is elevated. The hyponatremia is due both to loss of sodium into the urine (due to aldosterone deficiency) and to movement into the intracellular compartment. This extravascular sodium loss depletes extracellular fluid volume and accentuates hypotension. Elevated plasma vasopressin and angiotensin II levels may contribute to the hyponatremia by impairing free water clearance. Hyperkalemia is due to a combination of aldosterone deficiency, impaired glomerular filtration, and acidosis. Basal levels of cortisol and aldosterone are subnormal and fail to increase following ACTH administration. Mild to moderate hypercalcemia occurs in 10 to 20 percent of patients for unclear reasons. The electrocardiogram may show nonspecific changes, and the electroencephalogram exhibits a generalized reduction and slowing. There may be a normocytic anemia, a relative lymphocytosis, and a moderate eosinophilia.

Diagnosis The diagnosis of adrenal insufficiency should be made only with ACTH stimulation testing to assess adrenal reserve capacity

Table 332-10

Frequency of Symptoms and Signs in Adrenal Insufficiency

Sign or Symptom	Percent of Patients
Weakness	99
Pigmentation of skin	98
Weight loss	97
Anorexia, nausea, and vomiting	90
Hypotension (<110/70)	87
Pigmentation of mucous membranes	82
Abdominal pain	34
Salt craving	22
Diarrhea	20
Constipation	19
Syncope	16
Vitiligo	9

for steroid production (see above for ACTH test protocols). In *severe adrenal insufficiency*, the rate of cortisol secretion is markedly decreased, which may be ascertained indirectly by the finding of low to absent 24-h urine cortisol. With *mild adrenal insufficiency* (decreased adrenal reserve) urine and blood steroid values overlap the normal range; thus, the diagnosis of adrenal insufficiency should never be excluded solely on the basis of normal basal urine steroid determinations. Plasma cortisol values vary from zero to the lower range of normal and therefore have little diagnostic value. Aldosterone secretion is usually low, resulting in salt wasting and increases in plasma renin levels. In primary adrenal insufficiency, plasma ACTH and associated peptides (β-lipotropin) are elevated because of loss of the usual cortisol-hypothalamic-pituitary feedback relationship, whereas in secondary adrenal insufficiency, plasma ACTH values are low or "inappropriately" normal (Fig. 332-11).

Differential Diagnosis Since weakness and fatigue are common, diagnosis of early adrenocortical insufficiency may be difficult. However, the combination of mild gastrointestinal distress, weight loss, anorexia, and a suggestion of increased pigmentation makes it mandatory to perform ACTH stimulation testing to rule out adrenal insufficiency, particularly before steroid treatment is begun. Weight loss is useful in evaluating the significance of weakness and malaise. Racial pigmentation may be a problem, but a *recent* and progressive *increase* in pigmentation is usually reported by the patient with gradual adrenal destruction. Hyperpigmentation is usually absent when adrenal destruction is rapid, as in bilateral adrenal hemorrhage. The fact that hyperpigmentation occurs with other diseases also may present a problem, but the appearance and distribution of pigment in adrenal insufficiency are usually characteristic. When doubt exists, measurement of ACTH levels and testing of adrenal reserve with the infusion of ACTH provide clear-cut differentiation.

℞ TREATMENT

All patients with adrenal insufficiency should receive specific hormone replacement. Like diabetics, these patients require careful education about the disease. Replacement therapy should correct

FIGURE 332-11 Diagnostic flowchart for evaluating patients with suspected adrenal insufficiency. Plasma ACTH levels are low in secondary adrenal insufficiency. In adrenal insufficiency secondary to pituitary tumors or idiopathic panhypopituitarism, other pituitary hormone deficiencies are present. On the other hand, ACTH deficiency may be isolated, as seen following prolonged use of exogenous glucocorticoids. Since the isolated blood levels obtained in these screening tests may not be definitive, the diagnosis may need to be confirmed by a continuous 24-h ACTH infusion. Normal subjects and patients with secondary adrenal insufficiency may be distinguished by insulin tolerance or metyrapone testing.

both glucocorticoid and mineralocorticoid deficiencies. Hydrocortisone (cortisol) is the mainstay of treatment. The dose for most adults (depending on size) is 20 to 30 mg/d. Patients are advised to take glucocorticoids with meals or, if that is impractical, with milk or an antacid, because the drugs may increase gastric acidity and exert direct toxic effects on the gastric mucosa. To simulate the normal diurnal adrenal rhythm, two-thirds of the dose is taken in the morning, and the remaining one-third is taken in the late afternoon. Some patients exhibit insomnia, irritability, and mental excitement after initiation of therapy; in these, the dosage should be reduced. Other situations that may necessitate smaller doses are hypertension and diabetes mellitus. Obese individuals and those on anticonvulsive medications may require increased dosages. Measurements of plasma ACTH or cortisol or of urine cortisol levels do not appear to be useful in determining optimal glucocorticoid dosages.

Since the replacement dosage of hydrocortisone does not replace the mineralocorticoid component of the adrenal hormones, mineralocorticoid supplementation is usually needed. This is usually accomplished by the administration of 0.05 to 0.1 mg fludrocortisone per day by mouth. Patients also should be instructed to maintain an ample intake of sodium (3 to 4 g/d).

The adequacy of mineralocorticoid therapy can be assessed by measurement of blood pressure and serum electrolytes. Blood pressure should be normal and without postural changes; serum sodium, potassium, creatinine, and urea nitrogen levels also should be normal. Measurement of plasma renin levels may also be useful in titrating the dose.

Complications of glucocorticoid therapy, with the exception of gastritis, are *rare* at the dosages recommended for treatment of adrenal insufficiency. Complications of mineralocorticoid therapy include hypokalemia, hypertension, cardiac enlargement, and even congestive heart failure due to sodium retention. Periodic measurements of body weight, serum potassium level, and blood pressure are useful. All patients with adrenal insufficiency should carry medical identification, should be instructed in the parenteral self-administration of steroids, and should be registered with a medical alerting system.

Special Therapeutic Problems During periods of intercurrent illness, especially in the setting of fever, the dose of hydrocortisone should be doubled. With severe illness it should be increased to 75 to 150 mg/d. When oral administration is not possible, parenteral routes should be employed. Likewise, before surgery or dental extractions, supplemental glucocorticoids should be administered. Patients also should be advised to increase the dose of fludrocortisone and to add salt to their otherwise normal diet during periods of strenuous exercise with sweating, during extremely hot weather, and with gastrointestinal upsets. A simple strategy is to supplement the diet one to three times daily with salty broth (1 cup of beef or chicken bouillon contains 35 mmol of sodium). For a representative program of steroid therapy for the patient with adrenal insufficiency who is undergoing major surgery, see Table 332-11. This schedule is designed so that on the day of surgery it will mimic the output of cortisol in normal individuals undergoing prolonged major stress (10 mg/h, 250 to 300 mg/d). Thereafter, if the patient is improving and is afebrile, the dose of hydrocortisone is tapered by 20 to 30 percent daily. Parenteral mineralocorticoid administration is unnecessary at hydrocortisone doses greater than 100 mg/d because of the mineralocorticoid effects of hydrocortisone at such dosages.

SECONDARY ADRENOCORTICAL INSUFFICIENCY

ACTH deficiency causes *secondary* adrenocortical insufficiency; it may be a selective deficiency, as is seen following prolonged administration of excess glucocorticoids, or it may occur in association with deficiencies of multiple pituitary hormones (panhypopituitarism) (see Chap. 328). Patients with secondary adrenocortical hypofunction have many symptoms and signs in common with those having primary disease but are *characteristically not hyperpigmented*, since ACTH and related peptide levels are low. In fact, plasma ACTH levels distinguish between primary and secondary adrenal insufficiency, since they are

Table 332-11

Steroid Therapy Schedule for a Patient with Adrenal Insufficiency Undergoing Surgery*

	Hydrocortisone Infusion, Continuous, mg/h	Hydrocortisone (Orally)		Fludrocortisone (Orally),
		8 A.M.	4 P.M.	8 A.M.
Routine daily medication		20	10	0.1
Day before operation		20	10	0.1
Day of operation	10			
Postoperative				
Day 1	5–7.5			
Day 2	2.5–5			
Day 3	2.5–5 *or*	40	20	0.1
Day 4	2.5–5 *or*	40	20	0.1
Day 5		40	20	0.1
Day 6		20	20	0.1
Day 7		20	10	0.1

* All steroid doses are given in milligrams. An alternative approach is to give 100 mg hydrocortisone as an intravenous bolus injection every 6 h on the day of the operation (see text).

elevated in the former and decreased to absent in the latter. Patients with total pituitary insufficiency have manifestations of multiple hormone deficiencies. An additional feature distinguishing primary adrenocortical insufficiency is the *near-normal level of aldosterone secretion* seen in pituitary and/or isolated ACTH deficiencies (see Fig. 332-11). Patients with pituitary insufficiency may have hyponatremia, which can be dilutional or secondary to a subnormal increase in aldosterone secretion in response to severe sodium restriction. However, severe *dehydration, hyponatremia,* and *hyperkalemia* are characteristic of severe mineralocorticoid insufficiency and favor a diagnosis of primary adrenocortical insufficiency.

Patients receiving long-term steroid therapy, despite physical findings of Cushing's syndrome, develop adrenal insufficiency because of prolonged pituitary-hypothalamic suppression and adrenal atrophy secondary to the loss of endogenous ACTH. These patients have two deficits, a loss of adrenal responsiveness to ACTH and a failure of pituitary ACTH release. They are characterized by low blood cortisol and ACTH levels, a low baseline rate of steroid excretion, and abnormal ACTH and metyrapone responses. Most patients with steroid-induced adrenal insufficiency eventually recover normal hypothalamic-pituitary-adrenal responsiveness, but recovery time varies from days to months. The rapid ACTH test provides a convenient assessment of recovery of hypothalamic-pituitary-adrenal function. Since the plasma cortisol concentrations after injection of cosyntropin and during insulin-induced hypoglycemia usually are similar, the rapid ACTH test assesses the integrated hypothalamic-pituitary-adrenal function (see "Tests of Pituitary-Adrenal Responsiveness," above). Additional tests to assess pituitary ACTH reserve include the standard metyrapone and insulin tolerance tests.

Glucocorticoid therapy in patients with secondary adrenocortical insufficiency does not differ from that for the primary disorder. Mineralocorticoid therapy is usually not necessary, since aldosterone secretion is preserved.

ACUTE ADRENOCORTICAL INSUFFICIENCY Acute adrenocortical insufficiency may result from several processes. On the one hand, *adrenal crisis* may be a rapid and overwhelming intensification of chronic adrenal insufficiency, usually precipitated by sepsis or surgical stress. Alternatively, acute hemorrhagic destruction of both adrenal glands can occur in previously well subjects. In children, this event is usually associated with septicemia with *Pseudomonas* or meningococcemia (Waterhouse-Friderichsen syndrome). In adults, anticoagulant therapy or a coagulation disorder may result in bilateral adrenal hemorrhage. Occasionally, bilateral adrenal hemorrhage in the newborn results from birth trauma. Hemorrhage has been observed during pregnancy, following idiopathic adrenal vein thrombosis, and as a complication of venography (e.g., infarction of an adenoma). The third and most frequent cause of acute insufficiency is the rapid withdrawal of steroids from patients with adrenal atrophy owing to chronic steroid administration. Acute adrenocortical insufficiency also may occur in patients with congenital adrenal hyperplasia or those with decreased adrenocortical reserve when they are given drugs capable of inhibiting steroid synthesis (mitotane, ketoconazole) or of increasing steroid metabolism (phenytoin, rifampin).

Adrenal Crisis The long-term survival of patients with adrenocortical insufficiency depends largely on the prevention and treatment of adrenal crisis. Consequently, the occurrence of infection, trauma (including surgery), gastrointestinal upsets, or other stresses necessitates an immediate increase in hormone. In untreated patients, preexisting symptoms are intensified. Nausea, vomiting, and abdominal pain may become intractable. Fever may be severe or absent. Lethargy deepens into somnolence, and hypovolemic vascular collapse ensues. In contrast, patients previously maintained on chronic glucocorticoid therapy may not exhibit dehydration or hypotension until they are in a preterminal state, since mineralocorticoid secretion is usually preserved. In all patients in crisis, a precipitating cause should be sought.

℞ **TREATMENT**

Treatment is directed primarily toward repletion of circulating glucocorticoids and replacement of the sodium and water deficits. Hence an intravenous infusion of 5% glucose in normal saline solution should be started with a bolus intravenous infusion of 100 mg hydrocortisone followed by a continuous infusion of hydrocortisone at a rate of 10 mg/h. An alternative approach is to administer a 100-mg bolus of hydrocortisone intravenously every 6 h. However, only continuous infusion maintains the plasma cortisol constantly at stress levels [>830 nmol/L (30 μg/dL)]. Effective treatment of hypotension requires glucocorticoid replacement and repletion of sodium and water deficits. If the crisis was preceded by prolonged nausea, vomiting, and dehydration, several liters of saline solution may be required in the first few hours. Vasoconstrictive agents (such as dopamine) may be indicated in extreme conditions as adjuncts to volume replacement. With large doses of steroid, e.g., 100 to 200 mg hydrocortisone, the patient receives a maximal mineralocorticoid effect, and supplementary mineralocorticoid is superfluous. Following improvement, the steroid dosage is tapered over the next few days to maintenance levels, and mineralocorticoid therapy is reinstituted if needed (see Table 332-11).

HYPOALDOSTERONISM

Isolated aldosterone deficiency accompanied by normal cortisol production occurs in association with hyporeninism, as an inherited biosynthetic defect, postoperatively following removal of aldosterone-secreting adenomas, during protracted heparin or heparinoid administration, in pretectal disease of the nervous system, and in severe postural hypotension.

The feature common to all forms hypoaldosteronism is the inability to increase aldosterone secretion appropriately in response to salt restriction. Most patients have unexplained hyperkalemia, which often is exacerbated by restriction of dietary sodium intake. In severe cases, urine sodium wastage occurs at a normal salt intake, whereas in milder forms, excessive loss of urine sodium occurs only with salt restriction.

Most cases of isolated hypoaldosteronism occur in patients with a deficiency in renin production (so-called hyporeninemic hypoaldosteronism), most commonly in adults with diabetes mellitus and mild renal failure and in whom hyperkalemia and metabolic acidosis are out of proportion to the degree of renal impairment. Plasma renin levels fail to rise normally following sodium restriction and postural changes. The pathogenesis is uncertain. Possibilities include renal disease (the most

likely), autonomic neuropathy, extracellular fluid volume expansion, and defective conversion of renin precursors to active renin. Aldosterone levels also fail to rise normally after salt restriction and volume contraction; this effect is probably related to the hyporeninism, since biosynthetic defects in aldosterone secretion usually cannot be demonstrated. In these patients, aldosterone secretion increases promptly after ACTH stimulation, but it is uncertain whether the magnitude of the response is normal. On the other hand, the level of aldosterone appears to be subnormal in relationship to the hyperkalemia.

Hypoaldosteronism also can be associated with high renin levels. In many patients with this condition, the transformation of the C-18 methyl of corticosterone to the C-18 aldehyde of aldosterone is impaired, probably owing to a defect in corticosterone methyloxidase. These patients have low to absent aldosterone secretion, elevated plasma renin levels, and elevated levels of the intermediates of aldosterone biosynthesis (corticosterone and 18-hydroxycorticosterone). Severely ill patients also may have hyperreninemic hypoaldosteronism; such patients have a high mortality rate (80 percent). Hyperkalemia is not present. Possible explanations for the hypoaldosteronism include adrenal necrosis (uncommon) or a shift in steroidogenesis from mineralocorticoids to glucocorticoids, possibly related to prolonged ACTH stimulation.

Before the diagnosis of isolated hypoaldosteronism is considered for a patient with hyperkalemia, "pseudohyperkalemia" (e.g., hemolysis, thrombocytosis) should be excluded by measuring the plasma potassium level. The next step is to demonstrate a normal cortisol response to ACTH stimulation. Then, the response of renin and aldosterone levels to stimulation (upright posture, sodium restriction) should be measured. Low renin aldosterone levels establish the diagnosis of hyporeninemic hypoaldosteronism. A combination of high renin levels and low aldosterone levels is consistent with an aldosterone biosynthetic defect or a selective unresponsiveness to angiotensin II. Finally, elevated renin and aldosterone levels suggest primary renal unresponsiveness to aldosterone, so-called pseudohypoaldosteronism.

℞ **TREATMENT**

The treatment is to replace the mineralocorticoid deficiency. For practical purposes, the oral administration of 0.05 to 0.15 mg fludrocortisone daily should restore electrolyte balance if salt intake is adequate (e.g., 150 to 200 mmol/d). However, patients with hyporeninemic hypoaldosteronism may require higher doses of mineralocorticoid to correct hyperkalemia. This need poses a potential risk in patients with hypertension, mild renal insufficiency, or congestive heart failure. An alternative approach is to reduce salt intake and to administer furosemide, which can ameliorate acidosis and hyperkalemia. Occasionally, a combination of these two approaches is efficacious.

NONSPECIFIC CLINICAL USE OF ADRENAL STEROIDS

The widespread use of glucocorticoids emphasizes the need for a thorough understanding of the metabolic effects of these agents. Before adrenal hormone therapy is instituted, the expected gains should be weighed against undesirable effects.

HOW SERIOUS IS THE DISORDER? In a patient who has unexplained shock or in whom other measures have failed, the physician need not hesitate to employ high-dose steroid therapy. In contrast, one should exercise restraint in administering steroids to a patient with early rheumatoid arthritis for whom physiotherapy, analgesics, and general medical care have not been tried.

HOW LONG WILL GLUCOCORTICOID THERAPY BE REQUIRED? The use of intravenous steroids for 24 to 48 h for a life-threatening situation such as status asthmaticus or pseudotumor cerebri has few or no contraindications, in contrast to the initiation of chronic steroid therapy for asthma, arthritis, or psoriasis. In the latter instances, the almost certain development of some degree of Cushing's syndrome must be weighed against the potential benefit. These side effects should be minimized by a careful choice of steroid preparations, alternate-day or interrupted therapy, and the judicious use of supplementary adjuvants.

WHICH PREPARATION IS BEST? Several considerations should be taken into account in deciding which steroid preparation to use.

1. *The biologic half-life.* The rationale behind alternate-day therapy is to decrease the metabolic effects of the steroids for a significant part of each 48 h period while still producing a pharmacologic effect durable enough to be effective. Too long a half-life would defeat the first purpose, and too short a half-life would defeat the second. In general, the more potent the steroid, the longer its biologic half-life.

2. *The importance of the mineralocorticoid effects of the steroid.* Most synthetic steroids have less mineralocorticoid effect than hydrocortisone (Table 332-12).

3. *The biologically active form of the steroid.* Cortisone and prednisone have to be converted to biologically active metabolites before anti-inflammatory effects can occur. Because of this, in a condition for which steroids are known to be effective and when an adequate dose has been given without response, one should consider substituting hydrocortisone or prednisolone for cortisone or prednisone.

4. *The cost of the medication.* This is a serious consideration if chronic administration is planned. Prednisone is the least expensive of available steroid preparations.

5. *The type of formulation.* This factor may modify absorption, and patients whose steroid dosage has been standardized should use the same preparation consistently to avoid relapse or overdosage.

EVALUATION OF PATIENTS PRIOR TO INITIATING STEROID THERAPY (See Table 332-13) **Chronic Infection** Three issues demand attention: (1) Any active infection, particularly tuberculosis, should be identified. (2) If tuberculosis is present, steroid therapy should be employed only in conjunction with antituberculous chemotherapy. The chest film and tuberculin test provide baseline information for future comparison. Since high-dose steroids may impair the tuberculin reaction, serial chest roentgenograms may be necessary. (3) Infection due to opportunistic pathogens should be constantly considered in patients on steroid therapy, especially when combined with other immunosuppressive agents.

Diabetes Mellitus Prolonged glucocorticoid therapy may unmask or aggravate diabetes mellitus. The presence of diabetes mellitus or the demonstration of impaired glucose tolerance may affect the decision to institute adrenal hormone therapy.

Table 332-12

Glucocorticoid Preparations

Commonly Used Name*	Estimated Potency†	
	Glucocorticoid	Mineralocorticoid
SHORT-ACTING		
Hydrocortisone	1	1
Cortisone	0.8	0.8
INTERMEDIATE-ACTING		
Prednisone	4	0.25
Prednisolone	4	0.25
Methylprednisolone	5	<0.01
Triamcinolone	5	<0.01
LONG-ACTING		
Paramethasone	10	<0.01
Betamethasone	25	<0.01
Dexamethasone	30–40	<0.01

* The steroids are divided into three groups according to the duration of biologic activity. Short-acting preparations have a biologic half-life of less than 12 h; long-acting, greater than 48 h; and intermediate, between 12 and 36 h. Triamcinolone has the longest half-life of the intermediate-acting preparations.

† Relative milligram comparisons with hydrocortisone, setting the glucocorticoid and mineralocorticoid properties of hydrocortisone as 1. Sodium retention is insignificant for commonly employed doses of methylprednisolone, triamcinolone, paramethasone, betamethasone, and dexamethasone.

Table 332-13

A Checklist for Use Prior to the Administration of Glucocorticoids in Pharmacologic Doses

1. Presence of tuberculosis or other chronic infection (chest x-ray, tuberculin test)
2. Evidence of glucose intolerance or history of gestational diabetes mellitus
3. Evidence of preexisting osteoporosis (bone density assessment in postmenopausal patients)
4. History of peptic ulcer, gastritis, or esophagitis (stool guaiac test)
5. Evidence of hypertension or cardiovascular disease
6. History of psychological disorders

Osteoporosis Patients receiving long-term steroid therapy are at risk for osteoporosis. Indeed, osteoporosis with vertebral fractures or compression is a dreaded complication for patients at high risk (postmenopausal women, elderly men, and patients with restricted physical activity). Alternate-day or interrupted steroid therapy minimizes the risk of this complication (Table 332-14), and adjunctive therapies may be effective in treating the osteoporosis (see Chap. 355). Spine density should be assessed periodically with CT or digital radiography.

Peptic Ulcer, Gastric Hypersecretion, or Esophagitis In conventional doses (equivalent to 15 mg prednisone per day or less), glucocorticoids probably do not cause peptic ulceration; whether higher doses cause ulcer disease is not established and probably depends on duration and dose of treatment and predisposing factors such as hypoalbuminemia or cirrhosis. However, even at conventional doses, patients with a history of ulcer may experience aggravation of symptoms while receiving glucocorticoids. Consequently, all individuals with a positive history or with known risk factors should be managed with a vigorous antiulcer program (antacids, H_2 receptor antagonists, or ATPase inhibitors) along with glucocorticoids. *The development of anemia in a patient receiving glucocorticoids should suggest gastrointestinal bleeding as a cause.*

Hypertension or Cardiovascular Disease The capacity of many adrenal steroid preparations to promote sodium retention makes it necessary to exercise caution when using them in patients with preexisting hypertension or cardiovascular or renal disease. The use of preparations with minimal sodium-retaining activity, restriction of dietary sodium intake, and the use of diuretic agents and supplementary potassium salts minimize the mineralocorticoid effects of steroids. However, hypertension may be exacerbated by steroid-induced in-

Table 332-14

Supplementary Measures to Minimize Undesirable Metabolic Effects of Glucocorticoids

A. Monitor caloric intake to prevent weight gain.
B. Restrict sodium intake to prevent edema and minimize hypertension and potassium loss.
C. Provide supplementary potassium if necessary.
D. Provide antacid, H_2 receptor antagonist, and/or H^+,K^+-ATPase inhibitor therapy.
E. Institute alternate-day steroid schedule if possible. Patients receiving steroid therapy over a prolonged period should be protected by an appropriate increase in hormone level during periods of acute stress. A rule of thumb is to *double* the maintenance dose.
F. Minimize osteopenia by
   1. Administering gonadal hormone replacement therapy: 0.625–1.25 mg conjugated estrogens given cyclically with progesterone, unless the uterus is absent; testosterone replacement for hypogonadal men
   2. Ensuring high calcium intake (should be approximately 1200 mg/d)
   3. Administering supplemental vitamin D if blood levels of calciferol or 1,25(OH)$_2$ vitamin D are reduced
   4. Administering calcitonin or diphosphonate if fractures occur even with the above treatments

creases in renin substrate and angiotensin II levels and by reduction in vasodilator prostaglandin production. Steroids also accelerate atherogenesis by induction of hypertension, glucose intolerance, and unfavorable lipid profiles. Glucocorticoid-associated lipid abnormalities include hypertriglyceridemia, hypercholesterolemia, and increased LDL cholesterol levels.

Psychological Difficulties Steroid therapy may cause psychological disturbances. In general, these disturbances correlate better with the patient's personality than with the dose of hormone, although larger doses cause more serious reactions. There is no reliable method of predicting the psychological reaction to steroid therapy; moreover, previous tolerance of steroids does not necessarily ensure immunity to subsequent courses. Likewise, untoward psychological reactions on one occasion do not invariably mean that the patient will respond unfavorably to a second course. However, patients with depressive symptoms during a first course of steroids may benefit from prophylactic lithium treatment prior to a second course.

Sleeplessness is common and can be minimized by using the shorter-acting steroids and by prescribing the total daily amount as a single early-morning dose.

ALTERNATE-DAY STEROID THERAPY The most effective way to minimize the cushingoid effects of glucocorticoids is to administer the total 48-h dose as a *single* dose of *intermediate-acting steroid* in the morning, *every other day*. If symptoms of the underlying disorder can be controlled by this technique, it offers distinct advantages. Three considerations deserve mention: (1) The alternate-day schedule may be approached through transition schedules that allow the patient to adjust gradually. (2) Supplementary nonsteroid medications may be needed on the "off" day to minimize symptoms of the underlying disorder. (3) Many symptoms that occur during the off day (e.g., fatigue, joint pain, muscle stiffness or tenderness, and fever) may represent relative adrenal insufficiency rather than exacerbation of the underlying disease.

The alternate-day approach capitalizes on the fact that cortisol secretion and plasma levels normally are highest in the early morning and lowest in the evening. The normal pattern is mimicked by administering an intermediate-acting steroid in the morning (7 to 8 A.M.) (see Table 332-12).

Initially, the steroid program often requires daily or more frequent doses of steroid to achieve the desired anti-inflammatory or immunity-suppressing action. *Only after this desired effect is achieved is an attempt made to switch to an alternate-day program.* A number of schedules can be used for transferring from a daily to an alternate-day program. The key points to be considered are flexibility in arranging a program and the use of supportive measures on the off day. One may attempt a gradual transition to the alternate-day schedule rather than an abrupt changeover. One approach is to keep the steroid dose constant on one day and gradually reduce it on the alternate day. Alternatively, the steroid dose can be increased on one day and reduced on the alternate day. In any case, it is important to anticipate that some increase in pain or discomfort may occur in the 36 to 48 h following the last dose.

The general principles advocated for the long-term use of steroids and for implementing an alternate-day schedule are as follows:

1. Utilize intermediate-acting steroids, such as prednisone or prednisolone.
2. Give the total daily amount of steroid as a single morning dose.
3. Begin a transition program as soon as the manifestations of the diseases are under reasonable control.
4. If possible, eliminate steroid medication on the alternate day.

WITHDRAWAL OF GLUCOCORTICOIDS FOLLOWING LONG-TERM USE It is possible to reduce gradually and eventually to discontinue a daily steroid dose, but under most circumstances withdrawal of steroids should be initiated by first implementing an alternate-day schedule. Patients who have been on an alternate-day

program for a month or more experience less difficulty during termination regimens. The dosage is gradually reduced and finally discontinued after a replacement dosage has been reached (e.g., 5 to 7.5 mg prednisone). Complications rarely ensue unless undue stress is experienced, and patients should understand that for 1 year or longer after withdrawal from long-term high-dose steroid therapy, supplementary hormone should be given in the event of a serious infection, operation, or injury. A useful strategy in patients with symptoms of adrenal insufficiency on a tapering regimen is to measure plasma cortisol levels prior to the steroid dose. A level less than 140 nmol/L (5 μg/dL) indicates continuing suppression of the pituitary-adrenal axis and implies that a more cautious tapering of steroids is indicated.

In patients on high-dose daily steroid therapy, it is advised to reduce dosage to approximately 20 mg prednisone daily as a single morning dose before beginning the transition to alternate-day therapy. If a patient cannot tolerate an alternate-day program, consideration should be given to the possibility that the patient has developed primary adrenal insufficiency.

See Chap. 59, Adrenocorticotropic hormone; adrenocortical steroids and their synthetic analogs; inhibitors of the synthesis and actions of adrenocortical hormones, in Goodman & Gilman's The Pharmacological Basis of Therapeutics, *9th ed, New York, McGraw-Hill, 1996.*

BIBLIOGRAPHY

AZZIZ R et al: Nonclassic adrenal hyperplasia: Current concepts. Clinical review 56. J Clin Endocrinol Metab 78:810, 1994

BAMBERGER CM et al: The glucocorticoid receptor and RU 486 in man. Ann NY Acad Sci 761:296, 1995

BECKER M et al: Ectopic ACTH syndrome and CRH-mediated Cushing's syndrome. Endocrinol Metab Clin North Am 23:585, 1994

BERTAGNA X: Proopiomelanocortin-derived peptides. Endocrinol Metab Clin North Am 23:467, 1994

BONCHICCHIO D et al: Factors influencing the immediate and late outcome of Cushing's disease treated by transsphenoidal surgery: A retrospective study by the European Cushing's Disease Survey Group. J Clin Endocrinol Metab 80:3114, 1995

BRAVO EL: Primary aldosteronism. Issues in diagnosis and management. Endocrinol Metab Clin North Am 23:271, 1994

CONLIN PR et al: Disorders of the renin-angiotensin-aldosterone system, in *Renal and Electrolyte Disorders, 5th ed*, Schrier RW (ed). Boston, Little, Brown, 1997

DLUHY RG et al: Glucocorticoid-remediable aldosteronism. Endocrinol Metab Clin North Am 23:285, 1994

FERNANDEZ-REAL JM et al: Pre-clinical Cushing's syndrome: Report of three cases and literature review. Horm Res 41:230, 1994

GORDON RD et al: Primary aldosteronism—some genetic, morphological, and biochemical aspects of subtypes. Steroids 60:35, 1995

HATTNER RS: Practical considerations in the scintigraphic evaluation of endocrine hypertension. The adrenal cortex and medulla. Radiol Clin North Am 31:1029, 1993

HORTON R et al: Hypoaldosteronism. Curr Ther Endocrinol Metab 5:146, 1994

JORGE P et al: X-linked adrenoleukodystrophy in patients with idiopathic Addison disease. Eur J Pediatr 153:594, 1994

KATER GE et al: Disorders of steroid 17 alpha-hydroxylase deficiency. Endocrinol Metab Clin North Am 23:341, 1994

KONG MF et al: Eighty-six cases of Addison' disease. Clin Endocrinol 41:757, 1994

McCANCE DR et al: Bilateral adrenalectomy: Low mortality and morbidity in Cushing's disease. Clin Endocrinol 39:315, 1993

MORTENSEN RM, WILLIAMS GH: Aldosterone action (physiology), in *Endocrinology*, 3d ed, DeGroot LJ et al (eds). Philadelphia, Saunders, 1994, p 1668

MUNE T et al: Human hypertension caused by mutations in the kidney isozyme of 11 beta-hydroxysteroid dehydrogenase. Nat Genet 10:394, 1995

NEW MI: Steroid 21-hydroxylase deficiency (congenital adrenal hyperplasia). Am J Med 98:2S, 1995

ORTH DN: Cushing's syndrome. N Engl J Med 332:791, 1995

OSELLA G et al: Endocrine evaluation of incidentally discovered adrenal masses (incidentalomas). J Clin Endocrinol Metab 79:1532, 1994

QUINN SJ, WILLIAMS GH: Regulation of aldosterone secretion, in *The Adrenal Gland*, 2d ed, VHT James (ed). New York, Raven, 1992, p 152

RAFF H: Interactions between neurohypophysial hormones and the ACTH adrenocortical axis. Ann NY Acad Sci 689:411, 1993

SAMBROOK P et al: Prevention of corticosteroid osteoporosis. A comparison of calcium, calcitriol, and calcitonin. N Engl J Med 328:1747, 1993

SAVASTANO S et al: Hypothalamic-pituitary-adrenal axis and immune system. Acta Neurol 16:206, 1994

SHIMKET RA et al: Liddle's syndrome: Heritable human hypertension caused by mutations in the beta subunit of the epithelial sodium channel. Cell 79:407, 1994

STAREN E et al: Selection of patients with adrenal incidentalomas for operation. Surg Clin North Am 75:499, 1995

UIBO R et al: Autoantibodies to cytochrome P450 enzymes P450scc, P450c17, and P450c21 in autoimmune polyglandular disease types I and II and in isolated Addison's disease. J Clin Endocrinol Metab 78:323, 1994

UR E et al: Corticotropin-releasing hormone in health and disease: An update. Acta Endocrinol 127:193, 1992

WHITE PC et al: Steroid 11 beta-hydroxylase deficiency and related disorders. Endocrinol Metab Clin North Am 23:325, 1994

WILLIAMS GH: Hirsutism, in: Office Practice of Medicine, 3d ed, Branch WT (ed). Philadelphia, Saunders, 1994, p 505

333 Lewis Landsberg, James B. Young

PHEOCHROMOCYTOMA

Pheochromocytomas produce, store, and secrete catecholamines. They are usually derived from the adrenal medulla but may develop from chromaffin cells in or about sympathetic ganglia (extraadrenal pheochromocytomas or paragangliomas). Related tumors that secrete catecholamines and produce similar clinical syndromes include chemodectomas derived from the carotid body and ganglioneuromas derived from the postganglionic sympathetic neurons.

The clinical features are due predominantly to the release of catecholamines and to a lesser extent to the secretion of other substances. Hypertension is the most common sign, and hypertensive paroxysms or crises, often spectacular and alarming, occur in over half the cases.

Pheochromocytoma occurs in approximately 0.1 percent of the hypertensive population but is, nevertheless, an important correctable cause of high blood pressure. Indeed, it is usually curable if properly diagnosed and treated, but it may be fatal if undiagnosed or mistreated. Postmortem series indicate that most pheochromocytomas are unsuspected clinically even when the tumor is related to the fatal outcome.

PATHOLOGY **Location and Morphology** In adults, approximately 80 percent of pheochromocytomas are unilateral and solitary, 10 percent are bilateral, and 10 percent are extraadrenal. In children, a fourth of tumors are bilateral, and an additional fourth are extraadrenal. Solitary lesions inexplicably favor the right side. Although pheochromocytomas may grow to large size (over 3 kg), most weigh less than 100 g and are less than 10 cm in diameter. The tumors are highly vascular.

The tumors are made up of large, polyhedral, pleomorphic chromaffin cells. Less than 10 percent of these tumors are malignant. As with other endocrine tumors, malignancy cannot be determined from the histologic appearance; tumors that contain large numbers of aneuploid or tetraploid cells, as determined by flow cytometry, are more likely to recur. Local invasion of surrounding tissues or distant metastases indicate malignancy.

Familial pheochromocytoma In approximately 5 percent of cases, pheochromocytoma is inherited as an autosomal dominant trait either alone or in combination with other abnormalities such as multiple endocrine neoplasia (MEN) type 2a (Sipple's syndrome) or type 2b (mucosal neuroma syndrome) (see Chap. 340), von Recklinghausen's neurofibromatosis, or von Hippel–Lindau's retinal cerebellar hemangioblastomatosis. Bilateral adrenal pheochromocytomas are common in the familial syndromes; within MEN kindreds, over half of pheochromocytomas are bilateral. A familial syndrome should be suspected in any patient with bilateral pheochromocytomas.

Extraadrenal pheochromocytomas Extraadrenal pheochromocytomas usually weigh 20 to 40 g and are less than 5 cm in diameter. Most are located within the abdomen in association with the celiac,

superior mesenteric, and inferior mesenteric ganglia. Approximately 1 percent are in the thorax, 1 percent are within the urinary bladder, and less than 1 percent are in the neck, usually in association with the sympathetic ganglia or the extracranial branches of the ninth or tenth cranial nerves.

Catecholamine Synthesis, Storage, and Release Pheochromocytomas synthesize and store catecholamines by processes resembling those of the normal adrenal medulla (see Chap. 70). Little is known about the mechanisms of catecholamine release from pheochromocytomas, but changes in blood flow and necrosis within the tumor may be the cause in some instances. These tumors are not innervated, and catecholamine release does not result from neural stimulation. Pheochromocytomas also store and secrete a variety of peptides, including endogenous opioids, adrenomedullin, endothelin, erythropoietin, parathyroid hormone–related protein, neuropeptide Y, and chromagranin A (see Chap. 70). These peptides contribute to the clinical manifestations in selected cases, as noted below.

Epinephrine, norepinephrine, and dopamine Most pheochromocytomas contain and secrete both norepinephrine and epinephrine, and the percentage of norepinephrine is usually greater than in the normal adrenal. Most extraadrenal pheochromocytomas secrete norepinephrine exclusively. Rarely, pheochromocytomas produce epinephrine alone, particularly in association with MEN. Although epinephrine-producing tumors may cause a preponderance of metabolic and beta-receptor effects, in general the major catecholamine secreted cannot be predicted from the clinical presentation. Increased production of dopamine and homovanillic acid (HVA) is uncommon with benign lesions but may occur with malignant pheochromocytoma.

CLINICAL FEATURES Pheochromocytoma occurs at all ages but is most common in young to midadult life. Some series show a slight female preponderance. Most patients come to medical attention as a result of hypertensive crisis, paroxysmal symptoms suggestive of seizure disorder or anxiety attacks, or hypertension that responds poorly to conventional treatment. Less commonly, unexplained hypotension or shock in association with surgery or trauma will suggest the diagnosis. Most patients have hypertension in association with headaches, excessive sweating, and/or palpitations.

Hypertension Hypertension is the most common manifestation. In approximately 60 percent of cases the hypertension is sustained, although significant blood pressure lability is usually present, and half of patients with sustained hypertension have distinct crises or paroxysms. The other 40 percent have blood pressure elevations only during an attack. The hypertension is often severe, occasionally malignant, and may be resistant to treatment with standard antihypertensive drugs.

Paroxysms or Crises The paroxysm or crisis occurs in over half of patients. In an individual patient, the symptoms are often similar with each attack. The paroxysms may be frequent or sporadic, occurring at intervals as long as weeks or months. With time, the paroxysms usually increase in frequency, duration, and severity.

The attack usually has a sudden onset. It may last from a few minutes to several hours or longer. Headache, profuse sweating, palpitations, and apprehension, often with a sense of impending doom, are common. Pain in the chest or abdomen may be associated with nausea and vomiting. Either pallor or flushing may occur during the attack. The blood pressure is elevated, often to alarming levels, and the elevation is usually accompanied by tachycardia.

The paroxysm may be precipitated by any activity that displaces the abdominal contents. In some cases a particular stimulus may induce an attack in a characteristic fashion, but in others no clearly defined precipitating event can be found. Although anxiety may accompany the attacks, mental or psychological stress does not usually provoke a crisis.

Other Distinctive Clinical Features Symptoms and signs of an increased metabolic rate, such as profuse sweating and mild to moderate weight loss, are common. Orthostatic hypotension is a consequence of diminished plasma volume and blunted sympathetic reflexes. Both these factors predispose the patient with unsuspected pheochromocytoma to hypotension or shock during surgery or trauma. Secretion of the hypotensive peptide adrenomedullin may contribute to the hypotension in some patients.

Cardiac manifestations   Sinus tachycardia, sinus bradycardia, supraventricular arrhythmias, and ventricular premature contractions all have been noted. Angina and acute myocardial infarction may occur even in the absence of coronary artery disease. A catecholamine-induced increase in myocardial oxygen consumption and, perhaps, coronary spasm may play a role in these ischemic events. Electrocardiographic changes, including nonspecific ST-T wave changes, prominent U waves, left ventricular strain patterns, and right and left bundle branch blocks may be present in the absence of demonstrable ischemia or infarction. Cardiomyopathy, either congestive with myocarditis and myocardial fibrosis or hypertrophic with concentric or asymmetric hypertrophy, may be associated with heart failure and cardiac arrhythmias. Multiorgan system failure with noncardiogenic pulmonary edema may be the presenting manifestation. Elevated levels of amylase, originating from damaged pulmonary endothelium, and abdominal pain may suggest acute pancreatitis, although serum lipase levels are normal.

Carbohydrate intolerance   Over half of patients have impaired carbohydrate tolerance due to suppression of insulin and stimulation of hepatic glucose output. The impaired glucose tolerance rarely requires treatment with insulin and disappears after removal of the tumor.

Hematocrit   The elevated hematocrit is secondary to diminished plasma volume. Rarely, production of erythropoietin by the tumor may cause a true erythrocytosis.

Other manifestations   Hypercalcemia has been attributed to the ectopic secretion of parathyroid hormone–related protein. Fever and an elevated erythrocyte sedimentation rate have been reported in association with the production of interleukin 6. Elevated temperature more commonly reflects catecholamine-mediated increases in metabolic rate and diminished heat dissipation secondary to vasoconstriction. Polyuria is an occasional finding, and rhabdomyolysis with myoglobinuric renal failure may result from extreme vasoconstriction with muscle ischemia.

Pheochromocytoma of the urinary bladder   Pheochromocytoma in the wall of the urinary bladder may result in typical paroxysms in relation to micturition. The location in the bladder wall is responsible for the occurrence of symptoms while the tumors are quite small, and, consequently, catecholamine excretion may be normal or minimally elevated. Hematuria is present in over half of patients, and the tumor can often be visualized at cystoscopy.

Adverse Drug Interactions   Severe and occasionally fatal paroxysms have been induced by opiates, histamine, adrenocorticotropin, saralasin, and glucagon. These agents appear to release catecholamines directly from the tumor. Indirect-acting sympathomimetic amines, including methyldopa (when administered intravenously), may cause an increase in blood pressure by releasing catecholamines from the augmented stores within nerve endings. Drugs that block neuronal uptake of catecholamines, such as tricyclic antidepressants or guanethidine, may enhance the physiologic effects of circulating catecholamines. Indeed, all medications should be considered carefully and administered cautiously in patients with known or suspected pheochromocytoma.

Associated Diseases   Pheochromocytoma is associated with medullary carcinoma of the thyroid in the MEN syndrome types 2a and 2b and with hyperparathyroidism in MEN 2a (see Chap. 340). Hypercalcemia, resolving after tumor resection, also has been described in the absence of parathyroid disease, as described above. Individuals at risk for MEN 2a and 2b should be screened periodically for pheochromocytoma by assay of a 24-h urine sample for catecholamines, including measurement of epinephrine. Pheochromocytoma should be excluded or removed before thyroid or parathyroid surgery.

The association of pheochromocytoma and neurofibromatosis is not common. Nevertheless, since incomplete forms of neurofibromatosis may be associated with pheochromocytoma, minor manifestations such as café au lait spots, vertebral abnormalities, or kyphoscoliosis should increase the suspicion of pheochromocytoma in a patient with hypertension. The incidence of pheochromocytoma in some kindreds with von Hippel–Lindau disease may be as high as 10 to 25 percent. Many of these are unsuspected clinically and diagnosed on a computed tomography (CT) scan or at postmortem.

The incidence of cholelithiasis is 15 to 20 percent. Cushing's syndrome is a rare association, usually a consequence of ectopic secretion of adrenocorticotropic hormone by the pheochromocytoma or, less commonly, by a coexistent medullary carcinoma of the thyroid.

Diagnosis   The diagnosis is established by the demonstration of increased excretion of catecholamines or catecholamine metabolites. The diagnosis can usually be made by the analysis of a single 24-h urine sample, provided the patient is hypertensive or symptomatic at the time of collection.

Biochemical Tests   The assays employed include those for vanillylmandelic acid (VMA), the metanephrines, and unconjugated or "free" catecholamines (see Chap. 70). The VMA assay is both less sensitive and less specific than assays of metanephrines or catecholamines. Accuracy of diagnosis is improved when two of the three determinations are employed. The following considerations apply to all the urinary tests: (1) Despite claims for the adequacy of determinations made on random urine samples, analysis of a full 24-h urine sample is preferable. Creatinine should be determined as well to assess the adequacy of collection. (2) Where possible, the collection should be made when the patient is at rest, on no medication, and without recent exposure to radiographic contrast media. When it is not practical to discontinue all medications, drugs known specifically to interfere with these assays (as noted below) should be avoided. (3) The urine should be acidified and refrigerated during and after collection. (4) With high-quality assays, dietary restrictions are minimal and should be specified by the laboratory performing the analyses. (5) Although most patients with pheochromocytoma excrete increased amounts of catecholamines and catecholamine metabolites, the yield is increased in patients with paroxysmal hypertension if a 24-h urine collection is initiated during a crisis.

Free catecholamines   The upper limit of normal for total urinary catecholamines is between 590 and 885 nmol (100 and 150 μg) per 24 h. In most patients with pheochromocytoma, values in excess of 1480 nmol (250 μg) per day are obtained. Measurement of epinephrine is often of value, since increased epinephrine excretion [over 275 nmol (50 μg) per 24 h] is usually due to an adrenal lesion and may be the only abnormality in cases associated with MEN. False-positive increases in catecholamine excretion result from exogenous catecholamines and related drugs such as methyldopa, levodopa, labetalol, and sympathomimetic amines, which may elevate catecholamine excretion for up to 2 weeks. Endogenous catecholamines from stimulation of the sympathoadrenal system also may increase urinary catecholamine excretion. Relevant clinical situations that cause such increases include hypoglycemia, strenuous exertion, central nervous system disease with increased intracranial pressure, and clonidine withdrawal.

Metanephrines and VMA   In most laboratories, the upper limit of normal is 7 μmol (1.3 mg) of total metanephrine and 35 μmol (7.0 mg) of VMA excretion per 24 h. In most patients with pheochromocytoma, the increase in these urinary metabolites is considerable, often to more than three times the normal range. Metanephrine excretion is increased by exogenous and endogenous catecholamines and by treatment with monoamine oxidase inhibitors; propranolol may cause a spurious increase in metanephrine excretion, since a propranolol metabolite interferes in the commonly used spectrophotometric assay. VMA is less affected by endogenous and exogenous catecholamines but is spuriously increased by a variety of drugs, including carbidopa. VMA excretion is decreased by monoamine oxidase inhibitors.

Plasma catecholamines   Measurement of plasma catecholamines has a limited application. The care required in obtaining basal levels (see Chap. 70) and the satisfactory results with urinary determinations make measurement of plasma catecholamines unnecessary in most cases. Plasma catecholamine levels are affected by the same drugs and physiologic perturbations that increase urinary catecholamine excretion. In addition, alpha- and beta-adrenergic receptor blocking agents may elevate plasma catecholamines by impairing clearance.

When the clinical features suggest pheochromocytoma and the urinary assay results are borderline, measurement of plasma catecholamines may be worthwhile. Markedly elevated basal levels of total catecholamines support the diagnosis, although approximately one-third of patients with pheochromocytoma have normal or slightly elevated basal values. The usefulness of plasma catecholamine determinations may be increased by agents that suppress sympathetic nervous system activity. Clonidine and ganglionic blocking agents (see Chap. 70) reduce plasma catecholamine levels in normal subjects and in patients with essential hypertension. These drugs have little effect on catecholamine levels in patients with pheochromocytoma. In patients with elevated or borderline basal catecholamine values, failure to suppress plasma or urinary levels with clonidine supports the diagnosis of pheochromocytoma.

Pharmacologic Tests Reliable methods for the measurement of catecholamines and catecholamine metabolites in urine have rendered obsolete both the provocative and adrenolytic tests, which are nonspecific and entail considerable risk. A modified version of the adrenolytic test may be of some use, however, as a therapeutic trial in a patient in hypertensive crisis with features suggestive of pheochromocytoma. A positive response to phentolamine (5-mg bolus following a test dose of 0.5 mg) is a reduction in blood pressure of at least 35/25 mmHg that peaks after 2 min and persists for 10 to 15 min. The pharmacologic response is never diagnostic, and biochemical confirmation is essential. Provocative tests in normotensive patients are potentially dangerous and rarely indicated. However, a glucagon provocative test may be of use in patients with paroxysmal hypertension and nondiagnostic basal catecholamine levels. Glucagon has a negligible effect on blood pressure or plasma catecholamine levels in normal or hypertensive subjects. In patients with pheochromocytoma, on the other hand, glucagon may increase both blood pressure and circulating catecholamine levels. The elevation in plasma catecholamine concentration, moreover, may occur without a blood pressure response. It must be emphasized, however, that life-threatening pressor crises have occurred after administration of glucagon to patients with pheochromocytoma, so the test should never be performed casually. Careful continuous monitoring of the blood pressure is required, intravenous access must be adequate, and phentolamine must be at hand to terminate the test if a significant pressor reaction ensues.

Differential Diagnosis Since the manifestations of pheochromocytoma can be protean, the diagnosis must be considered and excluded in many patients with suggestive clinical features. In patients with essential hypertension and "hyperadrenergic" features such as tachycardia, sweating, and increased cardiac output, and in patients with anxiety attacks associated with blood pressure elevations, analysis of a 24-h urine collection is usually decisive in excluding the diagnosis. Repeated determinations on urine collected during attacks may be necessary, however, before the diagnosis can be excluded with certainty. The clonidine suppression and glucagon stimulation tests may be helpful in excluding the diagnosis in difficult cases. Pressor crises associated with clonidine withdrawal and the use of cocaine or monoamine oxidase inhibitors (Chap. 70) may mimic the paroxysms of pheochromocytoma. Factitious crises may be produced by self-administration of sympathomimetic amines in psychiatrically disturbed patients.

Intracranial lesions, particularly posterior fossa tumors or subarachnoid hemorrhage, may cause hypertension and increased excretion of catecholamines or catecholamine metabolites. While this is most common in patients with an obvious neurologic catastrophe, the possibility of subarachnoid or intracranial hemorrhage secondary to pheochromocytoma should be considered. Diencephalic or autonomic epilepsy may be associated with paroxysmal spells, hypertension, and increased plasma catecholamine levels. This rare entity may be difficult to distinguish from pheochromocytoma, but an aura, an abnormal electroencephalogram, and a beneficial response to anticonvulsant medications will often suggest the proper diagnosis.

 TREATMENT

Preoperative Management The induction of stable alpha-adrenergic blockade is the basis of preoperative management and provides the foundation for successful surgical treatment. Once the diagnosis is established, the patient should be placed on phenoxybenzamine to induce a long-lived, noncompetitive alpha-receptor blockade. The usual initial dose is 10 mg every 12 h with increments of 10 to 20 mg added every few days until the blood pressure is controlled and the paroxysms disappear. Because of the long duration of action, the therapeutic effects are cumulative, and the optimal dose must be achieved gradually with careful monitoring of supine and upright blood pressures. Most patients require between 40 and 80 mg phenoxybenzamine per day, although 200 mg or more may be necessary. Phenoxybenzamine should be administered for at least 10 to 14 days prior to surgery. Over this time, the combination of alpha-receptor blockade and a liberal salt intake will restore the contracted plasma volume to normal. Before adequate alpha-adrenergic blockade with phenoxybenzamine is achieved, paroxysms may be treated with intravenous phentolamine. Selective alpha$_1$ antagonists have been employed preoperatively, but their role in management has not been established. They may be useful as antihypertensive agents in patients with suspected pheochromocytoma while workup is in progress, since they are usually better tolerated than phenoxybenzamine and will prevent serious pressor crises if pheochromocytoma is present. Nitroprusside, calcium channel blocking agents, and possibly angiotensin converting enzyme inhibitors reduce blood pressure in patients with pheochromocytoma. Nitroprusside may be useful on occasion in the treatment of pressor crises.

Beta-adrenergic receptor blocking agents should be given only after alpha blockade has been induced, since administration of such agents by themselves may cause a paradoxic increase in blood pressure by antagonizing beta-mediated vasodilation in skeletal muscle. Beta blockade is usually initiated when tachycardia develops during the induction of alpha-adrenergic blockade. Low doses often suffice, and a reasonable starting dose is 10 mg propranolol three to four times per day, increased as needed to control the pulse rate. Beta blockade is effective for catecholamine-induced arrhythmias, particularly those potentiated by anesthetic agents.

Preoperative Localization of the Tumor Surgical removal of pheochromocytoma is facilitated if the location of the tumor or tumors can be established preoperatively. Once pheochromocytoma is diagnosed, localization should be undertaken while the patient is being prepared for surgery. CT or magnetic resonance imaging (MRI) of the adrenals is usually successful in identifying intraadrenal lesions. Extraadrenal tumors within the chest can frequently be identified by conventional chest films or CT. MRI is useful in identifying extraadrenal tumors in the abdomen. If these studies are negative, abdominal aortography (once alpha-adrenergic blockade is complete) may identify extraadrenal pheochromocytomas in the abdomen, since these lesions are often supplied by a large aberrant artery. If aortography and CT fail to localize the lesion, venous sampling at different levels of the inferior and superior vena cava may reveal catecholamine gradients in the region drained by the tumor; this area may then be restudied by selective angiography or scanning by CT or MRI. An additional localization technique involves a radionuclide scintiscan after administration of the radiopharmaceutical [131I]metaiodobenzylguanidine (MIBG). This agent is concentrated by the amine uptake process and produces an external scintigraphic image at the site of the tumor. This type of scanning may be useful in characterizing lesions discovered by CT when biochemical confirmation is indeterminate, as well as in localizing extraadrenal pheochromocytomas. Percutaneous fine-needle aspiration of chromaffin tumors is contraindicated; indeed, pheochromocytoma should be considered before adrenal lesions are aspirated.

Surgery Surgical treatment of pheochromocytoma is best performed in centers with experience in the preoperative, anesthetic, and intraoperative management of pheochromocytoma. In experienced hands surgical mortality is 2 or 3 percent.

Monitoring during the surgical procedure should include continuous recording of arterial pressure and central venous pressure as well as electrocardiography; in the presence of cardiac disease or if congestive failure has been present, pulmonary capillary wedge pressure should be monitored. Adequate fluid replacement is crucial. Intraoperative hypotension responds better to volume replacement than to vasoconstrictors. Hypertension and cardiac arrhythmias are most likely during induction of anesthesia, intubation, and manipulation of the tumor. Intravenous phentolamine is usually sufficient to control the blood pressure, but nitroprusside may be required. Propranolol may be given in the treatment of tachycardia or ventricular ectopy.

PHEOCHROMOCYTOMA IN PREGNANCY Spontaneous labor and vaginal delivery in unprepared patients are usually disastrous for mother and fetus. In early pregnancy, the patient should be prepared with phenoxybenzamine, and the tumor should be removed as soon as the diagnosis is confirmed. The pregnancy need not be terminated, but the operative procedure itself may result in spontaneous abortion. In the third trimester treatment with adrenergic blocking agents should be undertaken; when the fetus is of sufficient size, cesarean section may be followed by extirpation of the tumor. Although the safety of adrenergic blocking drugs in pregnancy is not established, these agents have been administered in several cases without obvious adverse effect. Antepartum diagnosis and treatment lowers the maternal death rate, sometimes to zero, although fetal death still occurs on occasion.

UNRESECTABLE AND MALIGNANT TUMORS In cases of metastatic or locally invasive tumor or in patients with intercurrent illness that precludes surgery, long-term medical management is required. When the manifestations cannot be adequately controlled by adrenergic blocking agents, the concomitant administration of metyrosine may be required. This agent inhibits tyrosine hydroxylase, diminishes catecholamine production by the tumor, and often simplifies chronic management. Malignant pheochromocytoma frequently recurs in the retroperitoneum, and it metastasizes most commonly to bone and lung. Although these malignant tumors are resistant to radiotherapy, combination chemotherapy has had limited success in controlling them. Use of MIBG has had limited success in the treatment of malignant pheochromocytoma.

PROGNOSIS AND FOLLOW-UP The 5-year survival rate after surgery is usually over 95 percent, and the recurrence rate is less than 10 percent. After successful surgery, catecholamine excretion returns to normal in about 1 week and should be measured to ensure complete tumor removal. Catecholamine excretion should be assessed at the reappearance of suggestive symptoms or yearly for several years, if the patient remains asymptomatic. For malignant pheochromocytoma, the 5-year survival rate is less than 50 percent.

Complete removal cures the hypertension in approximately three-fourths of patients. In the remainder hypertension recurs but is usually well controlled by standard antihypertensive agents. In this group either underlying essential hypertension or irreversible vascular damage induced by catecholamines may cause the persistence of the hypertension.

See Chap. 10, Catecholamines, sympathomimetic drugs, and adrenergic receptor antagonists, in Goodman & Gilman's The Pharmacological Basis of Therapeutics, 9th ed, New York, McGraw-Hill, 1996.

BIBLIOGRAPHY

AVERBUCH SD et al: Malignant pheochromocytoma: Effective treatment with a combination of cyclophosphamide, vincristine, and dacarbazine. Ann Intern Med 109:267, 1988

DALY PA, LANDSBERG L: Phaeochromocytoma: Diagnosis and management. Baillieres Clin Endocrinol Metab 6:143, 1992

FUDGE TL et al: Current surgical management of pheochromocytoma during pregnancy. Arch Surg 115:1224, 1980

FUKUMOTO S et al: Pheochromocytoma with pyrexia and marked inflammatory signs: A paraneoplastic syndrome with possible relation to interleukin-6 production. J Clin Endocrinol Metab 73:877, 1991

GAGNER M et al: Early experience with laparoscopic approach for adrenalectomy. Surgery 114:1120, 1993

GAN TJ et al: Phaeochromocytoma presenting as acute hyperamylasemia and multiple organ failure. Can J Anaesth 41:244, 1994

GRAHAM PE et al: Laboratory diagnosis of pheochromocytoma: Which analyses should we measure? Ann Clin Biochem 30:129, 1993

HORTON WA et al: von Hippel–Lindau disease: Clinical and pathological manifestations in nine families with 50 affected members. Arch Intern Med 136:769, 1976

KREMPF M et al: Use of m-(^{131}I) iodobenzylguanidine in the treatment of malignant pheochromocytoma. J Clin Endocrinol Metab 72:455, 1991

LANDSBERG L: Pheochromocytoma complicating pregnancy. Eur J Endocrinol 130:215, 1994

MACDOUGALL IC et al: Overnight clonidine suppression test in the diagnosis and exclusion of pheochromocytoma. Am J Med 84:993, 1988

McCORKELL SJ, NILES NL: Fine-needle aspiration of catecholamine-producing adrenal masses: A possibly fatal mistake. Am J Roentgenol 145:113, 1985

MERIGIAN KS et al: Adrenergic crisis from crack cocaine ingestion: Report of five cases. J Emerg Med 12:485, 1994

NEUMANN HPH et al: Pheochromocytomas, multiple endocrine neoplasia type 2, and von Hippel-Lindau disease. N Engl J Med 329:1531, 1993

OISHI S et al: Elevated immunoreactive endothelin levels in patients with pheochromocytoma. Am J Hypertension 7:717, 1994

PANG L-C et al: Flow cytometric DNA analysis for the determination of malignant potential in adrenal and extra-adrenal pheochromocytomas or paragangliomas. Arch Pathol Lab Med 117:1142, 1993

PERRIER NA et al: Malignant pheochromocytoma masquerading as acute pancreatitis—a rare but potentially lethal occurrence. Mayo Clin Proc 69:366, 1994

REINIG JW, DOPPMAN JL: Magnetic resonance imaging of the adrenal. Radiologe 26:186, 1986

SANTIAGO JA et al: Synthetic human adrenomedullin and adrenomedullin 15-52 have potent short-lived vasodilator activity in the hindlimb vascular bed of the cat. Life Sci 55:Pl85, 1994

SHEMIN D et al: Pheochromocytoma presenting as rhabdomyolysis and acute myoglobinuric renal failure. Arch Intern Med 150:2384, 1990

STEWART AF et al: Hypercalcemia in pheochromocytoma. Ann Intern Med 102:776, 1985

334 ***Daniel W. Foster***

DIABETES MELLITUS

Diabetes mellitus, the most common endocrine disease, is characterized by metabolic abnormalities and by long-term complications involving the eyes, kidneys, nerves, and blood vessels. The disorder is not homogeneous, and several distinct diabetic syndromes have been delineated.

DIAGNOSIS The diagnosis of symptomatic diabetes is not difficult. When a patient presents with signs and symptoms attributable to an osmotic diuresis and has hyperglycemia, the diagnosis is unequivocal. There is likewise no disagreement about an asymptomatic patient with persistently elevated fasting plasma glucose concentrations. The problem arises with the asymptomatic patient who for one reason or another is considered to be a potential diabetic but has a normal fasting glucose concentration in plasma. Such patients are often given an oral glucose tolerance test and, if abnormal values are found, are diagnosed as having impaired glucose tolerance or diabetes. There seems to be little question that normal glucose tolerance is strong evidence against the presence of diabetes; the predictive value of an abnormal test is less certain. Much evidence suggests that the standard oral glucose tolerance test overdiagnoses diabetes, probably because a variety of stresses can cause an abnormal response. The operative mechanism is thought to be epinephrine discharge. Epinephrine blocks insulin secretion, stimulates glucagon release, activates glycogen breakdown, and impairs insulin action in target tissues, so that hepatic glucose production is increased and the capacity to dispose of exogenous glucose is impaired. Even anxiety over venipunctures may generate enough epinephrine to produce an abnormal test. Coexisting illness, inadequate diet, and lack of physical exercise also contribute to false-positive tests.

In an attempt to deal with these problems, the National Diabetes Data Group of the National Institutes of Health in 1979 revised the criteria for the diagnosis of diabetes:

1. *Fasting (overnight):* Venous plasma glucose concentration ≥ 7.8 mmol/L (140 mg/dL) on at least two separate occasions.[1]
2. *Following ingestion of 75 g of glucose:* Venous plasma glucose concentration ≥ 11.1 mmol/L (200 mg/dL) at 2 h and on at least one other occasion during the 2-h test; i.e., *two* values ≥ 11.1 mmol/L (200 mg/dL) must be obtained for diagnosis.

If the 2-h value is between 7.8 and 11.1 mmol/L (140 and 200 mg/dL) and one other value during the 2-h test period is equal to or greater than 11.1 mmol/L (200 mg/dL), a diagnosis of "impaired glucose tolerance" is suggested. Persons in this category are at increased risk for the development of fasting hyperglycemia or symptomatic diabetes, but such progression is not predictable in an individual patient.

CLASSIFICATION A classification of diabetes is given in Table 334-1. The basic categories are those recommended by the National Diabetes Data Group, except for the division into primary and secondary types. *Primary* implies that no associated disease is present, while in the *secondary* category, some identifiable condition causes or allows a diabetic syndrome to develop. Insulin dependence in this classification is not equivalent to insulin therapy. Rather, the term means that the patient is at risk for diabetic ketoacidosis (DKA) in the absence of insulin. Many patients classified as non-insulin-dependent require insulin for control of hyperglycemia, although they do not become ketoacidotic if insulin is withdrawn.

The term *type 1 diabetes* is often used as a synonym for insulin-dependent diabetes mellitus (IDDM), and *type 2 diabetes* is considered equivalent to non-insulin-dependent diabetes mellitus (NIDDM). This linkage is not ideal, because a subset of patients with apparent non-insulin-dependent diabetes later become fully insulin-dependent and prone to ketoacidosis. These patients are nonobese and usually express HLA antigens associated with susceptibility to insulin-dependent diabetes and have evidence of an immune response to islet cell antigens (see "Pathogenesis," below). For this reason, it has been suggested that the classification shown in Table 334-1 be modified so that the terms *insulin-dependent* and *non-insulin-dependent* describe physiologic states (ketoacidosis-prone and ketoacidosis-resistant, respectively), while the terms *type 1* and *type 2* refer to pathogenetic mechanisms (immune-mediated and non-immune-mediated, respectively). Using such a classification, three major forms of primary diabetes would be recognized: (1) type 1 IDDM, (2) type 1 NIDDM, and (3) type 2 NIDDM. Category 2 is an intermediate stage of autoimmune destruction in which the capacity to produce insulin is sufficient to prevent ketoacidosis but not to maintain normal blood glucose; this variant likely occurs when the autoimmune process begins at an older age and progresses more slowly than usual. It is uncommon when IDDM appears in childhood or early adolescence. A subset of obese people with apparent non-insulin-dependent diabetes can become transiently insulin dependent and develop DKA. Such individuals do not have markers of autoimmunity suggestive of type 1 disease and may not require insulin permanently after recovery from DKA. Presumably, diminution of insulin reserve renders such subjects vulnerable to stress-induced metabolic decompensation and causes transient insulin dependence.

There are several secondary forms of diabetes. *Pancreatic disease*, particularly chronic pancreatitis in alcoholics, is a common cause. Destruction of the beta cell mass is the etiologic mechanism. *Hormonal* causes include pheochromocytoma, acromegaly, Cushing's syndrome, and administration of steroid hormones. "Stress hyperglycemia," associated with severe burns, acute myocardial infarctions, and other life-threatening illnesses, is due to endogenous release of glucagon and catecholamines. Hormonal hyperglycemia results from varying combinations of impairment of insulin release and induction of insulin resistance. A large number of *drugs* can lead to impaired glucose tolerance or hyperglycemia. Hyperglycemia and even ketoacidosis can be due to quantitative or qualitative defects in the *insulin receptor* or to antibodies directed against it. The mechanism is essentially pure insulin resistance. *Genetic syndromes* associated with impaired glucose tolerance or hyperglycemia include the lipodystrophies, myotonic dystrophy, and ataxia-telangiectasia. The final category, *other*, is poorly defined and is meant to include any condition that does not fit elsewhere in the etiologic scheme. The appearance of abnormal carbohydrate metabolism in association with any of these secondary causes does not necessarily indicate the presence of underlying diabetes, although, in some cases, mild, asymptomatic primary diabetes is made overt by the secondary illness.

PREVALENCE The prevalence of diabetes is difficult to determine because various standards, many no longer acceptable, have been used in diagnosis. If fasting hyperglycemia is the diagnostic standard, the prevalence in the United States is probably 1 to 2 percent. Using data from the National Health Interview Surveys, an estimate of 3.1 percent was made in 1993; the National Diabetes Data Group, using the response to a 75-g oral glucose tolerance test as the diagnostic criterion, estimated the prevalence of diabetes at 6.6 percent, with 11.2 percent of the population having impaired glucose tolerance. These figures are almost certainly too high. Most subjects who are diagnosed as having impaired glucose tolerance or diabetes on the basis of oral glucose tolerance testing never develop fasting hyperglycemia or symptomatic diabetes when followed longitudinally. For example, in a massive screening program (more than 300,000 subjects) carried out in Cleveland, Ohio, only 31 percent of persons who had 2-h glucose values of 10 mmol/L (180 mg/dL) or higher in the glucose tolerance test progressed to overt diabetes after 5 years. Other studies confirm the imprecision of oral glucose challenges in predicting or diagnosing diabetes—hence the estimates of 1 to 2 percent prevalence used here. Similar conclusions have been reached in Sweden, where the prevalence is around 1.5 percent. Estimates for IDDM are more reliable than for the NIDDM because most patients are diagnosed

---

Table 334-1

Classification of Diabetes Mellitus

PRIMARY

Autoimmune (type 1) diabetes mellitus
   Non-insulin-dependent diabetes mellitus (type 1 NIDDM—*transient*)
   Insulin-dependent diabetes mellitus (type 1 IDDM)
Non-autoimmune (type 2) diabetes mellitus
   Insulin-dependent diabetes mellitus (type 2 IDDM—*transient*)
   Non-insulin-dependent diabetes mellitus (type 2 NIDDM)
   Maturity-onset diabetes of the young (MODY)

SECONDARY

Diabetes caused by pancreatic disease
Diabetes caused by hormonal abnormalities
Drug- or chemical-induced diabetes
Diabetes caused by insulin receptor abnormalities
Diabetes associated with genetic syndromes
Diabetes of other causes

---

[1] Venous whole blood concentrations of glucose are 15 percent lower than plasma values. Capillary whole blood, utilized in patient self-monitoring, is equivalent to venous plasma.

after the abrupt appearance of symptoms. In England, the prevalence of the type 1 disorder is estimated to be 0.22 percent by age 16, and a study in the United States suggested a prevalence of 0.26 percent by age 20. If the prevalence of diabetes is about 2 percent, it follows that NIDDM is seven to eight times more common than IDDM. The ratio of the frequency of IDDM to that of NIDDM varies with age, being higher if a young population is studied and lower in the older age range. The cited prevalences are for populations as a whole. Certain subsets have different rates. For example, more than 40 percent of Pima Indians in the United States have type 2 NIDDM.

The fact that persons with asymptomatic, undiagnosed diabetes occasionally develop complications despite the absence of fasting hyperglycemia has led to suggestions that large-scale screening with glucose tolerance tests be instituted. For the reasons given above, this course seems unwise.

PATHOGENESIS OF IDDM   By the time IDDM appears, most of the beta cells in the pancreas have been destroyed. The destructive process is almost certainly autoimmune in nature, although details remain obscure. Pathogenesis begins with a genetic susceptibility to the disease, and some environmental event initiates the process in such susceptible individuals. Viral infection is one triggering mechanism, but noninfectious agents also may be involved. The best evidence that an environmental insult is required comes from studies in monozygotic twins, in whom the concordance rate for diabetes is less than 50 percent. If diabetes were a purely genetic illness, concordance rates should approximate 100 percent. Autoimmune attack then follows. Although the process is clinically silent, the islets become infiltrated by monocytes/macrophages and activated cytotoxic T cells. This infiltration is usually designated *insulitis* but is sometimes called *isletitis*. Multiple antibodies against beta cell antigens are present in blood. The patient's state while the immune attack is underway but unrecognized is termed *prediabetes*. The prediabetic state may be brief or prolonged and may be progressive and uninterrupted or intermittent. What is clear is that the insulin reserve steadily diminishes until it is insufficient to maintain blood glucose within normal bounds. At this point the diagnosis is diabetes.

Rarely, type 1 diabetes develops exclusively from an environmental insult, as from the ingestion of Vacor, a rat poison. It is also possible that autoimmune diabetes can develop in the absence of an environmental trigger, i.e., can be purely genetic. Usually, however, the pathogenetic sequence is genetic predisposition → environmental insult → autoimmune destruction of the beta cells → diabetes mellitus.

Genetics   The mechanism of inheritance of IDDM is unclear. At various times, transmission has been postulated to be autosomal dominant, autosomal recessive, and mixed. While IDDM occurs with increased frequency in some families, familial aggregation is uncommon, so deduction of the mechanism of inheritance is difficult. The genetic predisposition is probably permissive and not causal.

Analysis of pedigrees shows a low prevalence of direct vertical transmission. In 493 families selected by the presence of a proband with IDDM, only 79 (16 percent) had a parent or sibling with diabetes. The risks for siblings is higher if the proband develops disease before age 10. Overall, the chance of a child developing type 1 diabetes when another first-degree relative has the disease is only 5 to 10 percent (Table 334-2). HLA identity in a sibling (see below) increases the risk; HLA nonidentity decreases it; and haploidentity (sharing of one HLA genotype) carries an intermediate risk. The presence of NIDDM in a parent increases the risk for IDDM in the offspring. It is not known whether the intermixing of IDDM and NIDDM in the same family represents the operation of a single genetic trait (i.e., the apparent NIDDM is really type 1 NIDDM) or whether two common genetic predispositions coexist in the family by chance, each perhaps influencing the expression of the other. While the low rates of transmission of IDDM make it difficult to discern mechanisms of inheritance through study of families, they are reassuring to diabetics who wish to have children.

Table 334-2

Relative Risk of Developing IDDM

Group	Percent Risk
US population	0.4
Relative of proband with IDDM	
Parent	3
Child	6
With affected father	8
With affected mother	3
Sibling	5
Identical twin	33
HLA-identical	15
HLA-haploidentical	5
HLA-nonidentical	1

SOURCE: Estimates from Atkinson and MacLaren.

Type 1 diabetes appears to be a disease in which *sexual imprinting* plays a role. The risk of diabetes is up to five times higher when the father has the disease than when the mother is diabetic. This paternity-related increased risk appears to be limited to fathers carrying an HLA DR4 susceptibility gene.

Genetic susceptibility to IDDM probably involves more than one gene. Candidate loci have been proposed on chromosomes 2, 6, 11, and 15. In NOD mice, which have an autoimmune form of diabetes resembling human IDDM, the number of susceptibility genes may be as high as 16. One (possibly the only) primary genetic site in humans is believed to be located in the major histocompatibility locus on the short arm of the 6th chromosome. There are strong associations between IDDM and certain human leukocyte antigens encoded by the major histocompatibility region. Four loci designated by the letters A, B, C, and D are recognized, with alleles at each site identified by numbers (e.g., HLA-DR3). A lowercase w indicates that identification is provisional. Gene products of the A, B, and C regions are called *class I molecules*, while D region products are called *class II molecules*. A map of the human major histocompatibility complex (MHC) is shown in Fig. 334-1. HLA gene products are glycoproteins located in the plasma membranes of cells and are believed to be recognition and/or programming signals for the initiation and amplification of immune responses in the body. These are two-chain molecules; the light chain in class I HLA is β_2-microglobulin, and the D region light chain encoded on chromosome 15 is a dimer composed of α and β chains. Class I molecules are present on all nucleated cells and function to defend against infections (especially viruses) and in immune surveillance against malignancy. Class II molecules are normally present on circulating and tissue macrophages, endothelial cells, B lymphocytes, and activated T lymphocytes. They function in the presentation of antigen to the regulatory T cell system. Activation of the immune system is "MHC-restricted," meaning that antigens are recognized only if they reach the cell surface in association with a "self" HLA allele that "fits" the receptor on the responding T cell. Thus, activation of cytotoxic T lymphocytes to fight a viral infection requires that a viral antigen be presented by a class I molecule recognized by the responding cytotoxic T cell. A similar restriction applies to antigen presentation by macrophages to helper T cells.

While definite associations exist between class I alleles and type 1 diabetes (B8, B15), the D locus is considered of primary importance. Class I loci are involved through nonrandom associations with D alleles (*linkage disequilibrium*). Because about 95 percent of white type 1 IDDM patients express either DR3 or DR4 or the heterozygous DR3/DR4 configuration, it was thought initially that a susceptibility gene might be located nearby. The focus has since shifted to the DQ locus. Typing of D regions is now carried out by analyzing DNA with allele-specific oligonucleotide probes. For example, DQβ_1*0301 and DQβ_1*0302 identify DR4 haplotypes, and DQβ_1*0201 segregates with DR3 haplotypes. DQβ_1*0502 and DQβ_1*0602 are associated with DR2 haplotypes. Some class II alleles predict susceptibility to IDDM, and others predict protection against it. Still others are apparently neutral. Susceptibility appears to be primarily vested in DQβ_1*0201 and DQβ₁*0302, with DQβ₁*0201/0302 heterozygosity portending a particularly high risk. DQβ₁*0602 is rarely present in persons with IDDM and is considered to be protective; i.e., it cancels the effects of a susceptibility gene when both are present. The DR2 allele, with which it is associated, is known to be protective. When IDDM occurs in a DR2/DR2 individual, it is due to a recombination event resulting in the presence of a susceptibility gene such as DQβ₁*0302. Terminology in the HLA field changes rapidly. DQβ₁*0301 was formerly known as DQw7 or DQw3.1; DQβ₁*0302 was previously known as DQw8 or DQw3.2; and DQβ₁*0602 was known as DQw1.2.

How might HLA alleles predispose to or protect from IDDM? Probably by exhibiting different affinities for diabetogenic peptides presented to the immune system. Thus HLA DQβ₁*0302 might bind a diabetogenic peptide with greater affinity for presentation on the cell surface than DQβ₁*0301. Conversely, a dominant protective allele (which presumably would not present antigen in such a way as to activate the immune system) might bind the diabetogenic peptide with such high affinity as to effectively "steal" it from a susceptibility gene even when both are present, thereby preventing the disease. Although the DQβ-chain alleles appear to predict risk for diabetes most precisely, they may well be influenced by interaction with α chains. Thus, T cell recognition of a DQβ₁*0302 chain is modified by the associated DQα chain. The situation is further complicated by the fact that α and β chains from different HLA molecules may interact to form new dimers, a process called *transcomplementation*. Susceptibility to autoimmune diabetes may be linked to decreased expression of class I HLA molecules on splenocytes and lymphocytes in NOD mice (which get autoimmune diabetes) and in humans. The meaning of this finding and its reproducibility are not clear.

Environmental Event   As noted earlier, the fact that a significant proportion of monozygotic twins remains discordant for diabetes suggests that nongenetic factors are required for development of diabetes. Similarly, HLA identity or haploidentity does not ensure concordance.

The environmental factor in many cases is believed to be a viral infection of the beta cell. A viral etiology was originally suggested by seasonal variations in the onset of the disease and by what appeared to be more than a chance relationship between the appearance of diabetes and preceding episodes of mumps, hepatitis, infectious mononucleosis, congenital rubella, and coxsackievirus infections. Furthermore, certain strains of encephalomyocarditis virus cause diabetes in genetically susceptible mice. The isolation of a coxsackievirus B4 from the pancreas of a previously healthy boy who died after an episode of ketoacidosis, and the induction of diabetes in animals inoculated with the isolated virus, also suggested a viral etiology, and the fact that the titer of neutralizing antibody to coxsackievirus rose in this patient during the weeks prior to death indicated that the infection was recently acquired. Further support for the viral theory comes from the observation that about one-fifth of individuals with congenital rubella develop IDDM. The presence of an HLA susceptibility allele in the fetus may double the risk. Cytomegalovirus genes are present in the genome of one-fifth of patients with type 1 diabetes, and retroviral genes are present in the beta cells of NOD mice. Presumably, viral infections of the pancreas could induce diabetes by two mechanisms: direct inflammatory disruption of islets or induction of an immune response.

Despite its attractiveness, the viral theory should be treated with consider-

able caution. Serologic studies seeking evidence of recent viral infection in patients with new-onset IDDM are inconclusive at best.

It has been suggested that exposure to cow's milk or milk products early in life predisposes to autoimmune diabetes. The proposed environmental trigger is bovine albumin, operating through the mechanism of molecular mimicry. In the initial study, diabetic subjects were found to have antibodies to bovine albumin, and an antibody subset specific for a 17-amino-acid epitope showed the strongest association with the disease. The latter antibodies bind to a 69-kDa protein (p69) on the surface of the pancreatic beta cell. Exposure to cow's milk is presumed to induce an immune response to the 17-amino-acid fragment in some infants, and cross-reactivity of the antibody would destroy beta cells expressing the p69 antigen. Not universally present on beta cells, p69 can be induced through the action of interferon γ produced by intermittent viral infections. This hypothesis has not received wide support.

Insulitis/Isletitis   In animals, macrophages and activated T lymphocytes infiltrate the pancreatic islets prior to or simultaneously with development of diabetes. Lymphocytes are also found in the islets of young persons dying from new-onset diabetes, and radioactively labeled lymphocytes localize in the pancreas in humans with IDDM. These findings are in accord with the fact that immune endocrinopathies are associated with lymphocytic infiltration of the affected tissue. It is not clear, however, that insulitis is central to the destructive sequence in autoimmune diabetes; the cellular infiltration may be an epiphenomenon.

Conversion of the Beta Cell from Self to Nonself and Activation of the Immune System   There seems to be little doubt that the immune system mediates destruction of the beta cells in type 1 diabetes. The disease is frequently associated with other autoimmune endocrinopathies such as adrenal insufficiency and Hashimoto's thyroiditis; pancreatic tissue transplanted from a nondiabetic monozygotic twin into the diabetic twin is rapidly destroyed in the absence of immunosuppression, and temporary reversal of clinical symptoms occurs with early use of cyclosporine. Moreover, most patients have antibodies directed against insulin and other beta cell antigens. Since the immune

FIGURE 334-1   Schematized map of the human major histocompatibility complex. Primary sites of association with IDDM are shown as stippled bars. A1, A2, B1, and B2 in the DP and DQ regions refer to α and β chains. The top line (0 to 1000) represents the class II region; the middle line (1100 to 2000) represents the class III region (genes for some complement factors, heat shock protein 70S, and tumor necrosis factor), and the bottom line (2100 to 4000) represents the class I region. Unlabeled bars are pseudogenes. (*Map provided courtesy of Dr. Peter Stasny.*)

system normally does not attack self tissues, IDDM can be viewed as an autoimmune disease.

The mechanism behind this autoimmune destruction is not known. As noted earlier, an environmental trigger appears to be involved frequently. The putative environmental agent could be a virus, a toxin, or a food and might act in one of several ways. Direct destruction of beta cells by a virus or toxin might expose cryptic antigens to the immune system, evoking an immune response. Alternatively, destructive cytokines might be released by viruses to kill beta cells, or programmed cell death (apoptosis) might be induced. A relative deficiency of early complement components might impair the clearing of islet cell viruses (a mechanism analogous to the one responsible for persistent hepatitis B infection in some patients with chronic active hepatitis), thereby prolonging stimulation of the immune system by cryptic antigens. Another hypothesis is the aforementioned molecular mimicry, in which there is a chance homology between a foreign antigen and amino acid sequences in normal tissue. The best-known example occurs in acute rheumatic fever, where the immune response to group A streptococci results in cross-reacting attack on the heart. Once cytotoxic T cells and plasma cells are activated against a particular antigenic epitope (armed), they seek and destroy any cell bearing the epitope. The bovine milk albumin hypothesis presumes molecular mimicry, and homology exists between a coxsackievirus protein and glutamic acid decarboxylase (GAD). Antibodies against GAD are common in young people with type 1 diabetes.

A third possibility, currently less popular, is that viral infection, via cytokine release, induces expression of HLA D region molecules in the pancreas (where they are not normally present), converting one or more cell types into antigen-presenting cells.

Some patients may have a purely genetic form of the disease. In neonatal life, autoreactive T cells are normally destroyed in the thymus ("clonal deletion"). Any cells escaping the thymus are rendered anergic or suppressed in the periphery by regulatory T cells. Failure of either process could leave a repertoire of cells capable of responding to self antigens following cell injury. In support of the possibility that a contributing factor in autoimmune disease is suboptimal removal or regulation of autoreactive T cells, intrathymic injection of islets prevents autoimmune diabetes in the BB rat. Presumably, the presence of additional beta cell antigens in the thymus allows the removal of autoreactive lymphocytes capable of responding to islet tissue.

In summary, the precise mechanisms remain a mystery, but immune attack is believed to be the fundamental cause of IDDM.

Destruction of Beta Cells and Development of IDDM Because insulin-dependent diabetes often begins with an abrupt onset of symptomatic hyperglycemia, polyuria, and/or ketoacidosis, it was long assumed that beta cell damage occurred rapidly. It is now believed that loss of insulin reserve occurs over a few to many years. This insight came from studies of discordant monozygotic diabetic twins and triplets in whom one twin or triplet developed diabetes long after the index case. In the slow course, the earliest sign of abnormality is the development of islet cell antibodies when blood sugar and glucose tolerance are normal and when insulin responses to a glucose load are intact. A phase then ensues in which the only metabolic abnormality is decreased glucose tolerance. Fasting blood sugar remains normal. This is the last prediabetic phase. In the third stage, fasting hyperglycemia develops, but ketosis does not occur even when the diabetes is poorly controlled. The clinical appearance is that of NIDDM. Continued destruction of beta cells then leads to the insulin-dependent stage and a propensity for ketoacidosis, especially during stress. Once this stage is reached, the patient ordinarily requires lifelong insulin therapy unless a pancreatic transplant is performed. However, a few patients, after immunosuppression with cyclosporine, become insulin independent for months or years.

The immune-directed destruction of beta cells probably involves both humoral and cell-mediated mechanisms, the latter being more important. Islet cell antibodies include antibodies to insulin, proinsulin,

two forms of glutamic acid decarboxylase (GAD 65 and GAD 67), carboxypeptidase H, two ganglioside antigens (GT3 and GM2-1), ICA 69 (the antigen that cross-reacts with antibody against bovine albumin), and ICA 512 (which may be a protein phosphatase). The presence of anti-GAD antibody may have modest predictive value for subsequent development of IDDM in persons who are at potential risk because of disease in a first-degree relative, but it does not definitively predict overt disease. A subset of anti-GAD antibodies appears to react with human and rat but not mouse islets. These "restricted" islet cell antibodies appear to be linked to the protective HLA allele $DQ\beta_1*0602$ and thus may protect against development of diabetes rather than predict its development.

Cells involved in the attack on the beta cell include natural killer cells, activated cytotoxic T lymphocytes (CD8 +), and macrophages. Cell destruction may be at least partially due to release of cytokines such as interleukin 1 (IL-1) and tumor necrosis factor α (TNFα) from activated macrophages. Experimentally, mixtures of cytokines (IL-1, TNFα, interferon γ, and lymphotoxin) are more potent than single agents. Cytokines may work through induction of nitric oxide or of superoxide. Beta cells have a low capacity for free radical destruction and are especially vulnerable to oxygen toxicity.

By the time overt diabetes appears, most insulin-producing cells have disappeared. In one study, pancreatic weight at autopsy averaged 40 g in persons with type 1 diabetes versus 82 g in control individuals. Endocrine cell mass in subjects with IDDM decreased from 1395 mg to 413 mg, and the beta cell mass, which averaged 850 mg in normal individuals, was unmeasurable. Since alpha cells remained essentially intact, the ratio of glucagon- to insulin-producing cells approached infinity.

PATHOGENESIS OF NIDDM Although NIDDM is more common than IDDM and more frequently exhibits familial aggregation, its pathogenesis is less well understood. Nevertheless, both beta cell defects and insulin resistance are present in overt disease, and the major enviromental factor is obesity. The relation between the beta cell abnormality and insulin resistance is not resolved.

Genetics Although NIDDM occurs in families, modes of inheritance are not known except for the variant termed maturity-onset diabetes of the young (MODY). MODY is usually manifested by mild hyperglycemia in young persons who are resistant to ketosis. Three lines of evidence suggest transmission as an autosomal dominant trait. First, three-generation direct transmission has been demonstrated in over 20 families. Second, a 1:1 ratio of diabetic to nondiabetic children is found when one parent has the disease. Third, about 90 percent of obligate carriers have diabetes. Three different mutations can cause MODY. The gene for MODY 1 is located on the long arm of chromosome 20, and that for MODY 3 is on the long arm of chromosome 12. MODY 2 is due to mutations in the glucokinase gene located on the short arm of chromosome 7.

It is highly likely that ordinary NIDDM is polygenic. Much effort has been spent in evaluating candidate genes, with emphasis on molecules involved in glucose metabolism in the pancreatic beta cell, liver, muscle, and fat. A few cases of NIDDM appear to be associated with mutations in genes coding for insulin, mitochondrial components, the insulin receptor, glucokinase, and glycogen synthase. At best these account for only a fraction of NIDDM cases. More than 250 candidate genes have been examined by various groups, but none is established to be relevant to ordinary NIDDM. Whatever its nature, the genetic influence is powerful, since the concordance rate for diabetes in monozygotic twins with type 2 disease may be as high as 80 percent. Risk to offspring and siblings of patients with NIDDM is higher than in type 1 diabetes. Nearly four-tenths of siblings and one-third of offspring eventually develop abnormal glucose tolerance or frank diabetes.

Pathophysiology Patients with type 2 NIDDM have two physiologic defects: abnormal insulin secretion and resistance to insulin action in target tissues. Which of the abnormalities is primary is not known. Descriptively, three phases can be recognized in the usual clinical sequence. In the first phase, the plasma glucose remains normal despite demonstrable insulin resistance, because insulin levels are elevated. In the second phase, insulin resistance tends to worsen, so that postprandial hyperglycemia develops despite elevated insulin concentrations. In the third phase, insulin resistance does not change, but declining insulin secretion causes fasting hyperglycemia and overt diabetes. Most authorities believe that insulin resistance is primary and that hyperinsulinemia is secondary; i.e., insulin secretion increases to compensate for the resistance state. However, hypersecretion of insulin (and amylin?) may cause insulin resistance; i.e., a primary islet cell defect causes insulin hypersecretion, and insulin hypersecretion, in turn, leads to insulin resistance. Explanatory hypotheses involve increased fat synthesis in the liver and enhanced fat transport [via very low density lipoprotein (VLDL)] leading to secondary fat storage in muscle. Increased fat oxidation would impair glucose uptake and glycogen synthesis. Most patients with NIDDM are obese, and obesity per se causes insulin resistance. However, nonobese relatives of persons with NIDDM may have hyperinsulinemia and diminished insulin sensitivity, proving that obesity is not the sole cause of resistance. This statement is not to diminish the importance of excess fat, since a modest reduction in weight often results in major improvement in blood sugar control in obese subjects with NIDDM. The late decline in insulin release could be due to the underlying genetic defect or to metabolic toxicity in the beta cell. High levels of glucose or increased tissue levels of long-chain fatty acids ("lipotoxicity") could be the damaging molecules.

In summary, it is likely that an insulin secretory defect and insulin resistance are both required for diabetes to be expressed, since massively obese persons with marked insulin resistance may have normal glucose tolerance. Presumably, the beta cell lesion is not present in such persons. This fact might suggest that the primary defect resides in the insulin-producing cells. Beta cell mass is intact in type 2 NIDDM, in contrast to the situation with type 1 IDDM. The alpha cell population is increased, resulting in an elevated ratio of alpha to beta cells and in the excess of glucagon relative to insulin that characterizes all hyperglycemic states, including NIDDM.

Although insulin resistance in type 2 NIDDM is associated with decreased numbers of insulin receptors, most of the resistance is postreceptor in nature (see below). It has long been known that deposits of amyloid are found in the pancreas of patients with type 2 diabetes. This material is a 37-amino-acid peptide termed *amylin*. Amylin is normally copackaged with insulin in secretory granules and is released simultaneously with insulin in response to insulin secretagogues. In animals, amylin has been reported to induce insulin resistance, but in diabetic subjects an amylin derivative has hypoglycemic effects, apparently because it causes delayed absorption of nutrients from the gastrointestinal tract. Amylin deposition in the islets may be the consequence of overproduction secondary to the insulin resistance to which it contributes. Alternatively, accumulation of amylin in the islets might contribute to the late failure of insulin production with long-standing NIDDM. A definitive role for amylin is not established.

Regardless of the mechanism, the physiologic consequences of insulin resistance are clear. There is no major abnormality in either glucose uptake by the cell or its oxidative metabolism to CO_2, water, and lactate. Rather, the major metabolic block is in glycogen synthesis ("nonoxidative metabolism"). Impaired glycogen synthesis, like hyperinsulinemia and insulin resistance, may be seen in nonobese, normoglycemic relatives of subjects with NIDDM.

A rare form of type 2 NIDDM, clinically mild, is due to production of an abnormal insulin that does not bind well to insulin receptors. Persons with this variant of the disease respond normally to exogenous insulin.

CLINICAL FEATURES The manifestations of symptomatic diabetes mellitus vary from patient to patient. Most often, symptoms are due to hyperglycemia (polyuria, polydipsia, polyphagia), but the first event may be an acute metabolic decompensation resulting in diabetic coma. Occasionally, the initial expression is a degenerative complication, such as neuropathy, in the absence of symptomatic hyperglycemia. The metabolic derangements of diabetes are due to a relative or absolute deficiency of insulin and a relative or absolute excess of glucagon. Normally, a rise in the molar ratio of glucagon to insulin leads to metabolic decompensation. Changes in this ratio

can be caused by a fall in insulin or a rise in glucagon concentration, separately or together. Alteration in the biologic response to either hormone would have the same effect. Thus, insulin resistance could cause the metabolic effects expected of an elevated glucagon/insulin ratio, even if the ratio found by immunoassay of the two hormones in plasma were normal or even decreased (the glucagon being biologically active, the insulin relatively inactive). The relationship between metabolic abnormalities and degenerative complications will be discussed subsequently. Typically, the clinical features of IDDM and NIDDM are distinctive.

Insulin-Dependent Diabetes IDDM usually begins before age 40; in the United States, peak incidence is around age 14. Some patients develop type 1 diabetes late in life, with a first episode of ketoacidosis occurring at age 50 or even later in rare instances. The author has seen one patient with typical diabetic ketoacidosis as the initial event of IDDM at the age of 80. These patients, who on the basis of age should have type 2 NIDDM, are usually not obese. Onset of symptoms may be abrupt, with thirst, excessive urination, increased appetite, and weight loss developing over several days. In some cases, the disease is heralded by the appearance of ketoacidosis during an intercurrent illness or following surgery. As outlined in Table 334-3, type 1 patients may have normal weight or may be wasted, depending on the length of time between onset of symptoms and start of treatment. Characteristically, the plasma insulin level is low or unmeasurable. Glucagon levels are elevated but are suppressed by insulin administration. Once symptoms develop, insulin therapy is required. Occasionally, an initial episode of ketoacidosis is followed by a symptom-free interval (the "honeymoon" period), during which no treatment is required. The likely explanation for this phenomenon is shown in Fig. 334-2.

Non-Insulin-Dependent Diabetes NIDDM usually begins in middle life or later. The typical patient is overweight. Symptoms begin gradually, and the diagnosis is frequently made when an asymptomatic person is found to have an elevated plasma glucose level on routine laboratory examination. In contrast to IDDM, plasma insulin levels are normal to high in absolute terms, although they are lower than predicted for the level of the plasma glucose; i.e., relative insulin deficiency is present. Stated in another way, if plasma glucose concentrations in nondiabetic subjects were raised to levels equivalent to those found in NIDDM patients, insulin values would be higher in the normal group. This relative deficiency reflects the previously mentioned insulin secretory defect in NIDDM. Glucagon metabolism in NIDDM is complex. While the elevated fasting plasma concentrations can be lowered by large amounts of insulin, the exaggerated glucagon response to ingested nutrients cannot be suppressed; i.e., alpha cell function remains abnormal. For unknown reasons, patients with NIDDM do not develop ketoacidosis but are susceptible to development of hyperosmolar, nonketotic coma. One hypothesis to explain the absence of ketoacidosis during stress is that the liver is resistant

Table 334-3

General Characteristics of IDDM and NIDDM

Characteristic	IDDM	NIDDM
Genetic locus*	Chromosome 6	Unknown
Age of onset†	Usually <40	>40
Body habitus	Normal to wasted	Obese
Plasma insulin	Low to absent	Normal to high
Plasma glucagon	High, suppressible	High, resistant
Acute complication	Ketoacidosis	Hyperosmolar coma
Insulin therapy	Responsive	Responsive to resistant
Response to sulfonylurea therapy	Unresponsive	Responsive

* Both IDDM and NIDDM are polygenic (see text).
† Most cases of IDDM appear before age 20, but onset can be late in life.

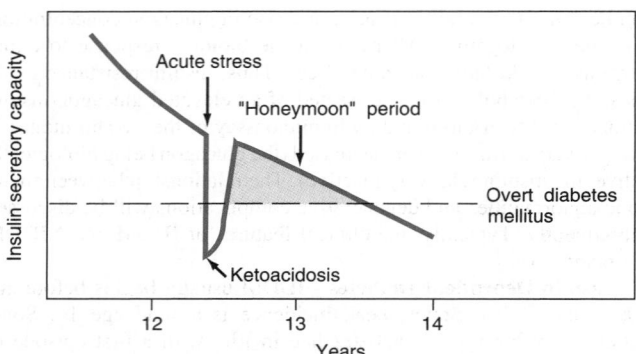

FIGURE 334-2 Schematic representation of the "honeymoon" period. The insulin secretory capacity is shown gradually decreasing in a patient destined to develop diabetes. At approximately 13½ years, insulin would become insufficient to maintain plasma glucose in the normal range. An initial episode of ketoacidosis—for example, in association with acute appendicitis—is shown occurring in the twelfth year. Presumably, stress-induced epinephrine release blocks insulin secretion and causes the syndrome. In normal subjects, insulin reserve is such that hormone release is adequate even in the face of stress. Following recovery from the stressful episode, insulin secretory capacity returns to the previous level and remains sufficient for an additional year, as indicated by the shaded area—the "honeymoon" period.

to glucagon, so that malonyl-CoA levels remain high, inhibiting the fatty acid oxidation–ketogenic pathway (see below). If weight loss can be induced, patients may be managed by diet alone. Most patients who fail dietary therapy respond to sulfonylureas or to combinations of sulfonylureas plus metformin, but, in many, the resulting improvement of hyperglycemia is not sufficient for control of diabetes. For this reason, a high percentage of patients with NIDDM are treated with insulin.

℞ TREATMENT

Diet For many years, dietary prescriptions for patients with diabetes were rigid and difficult to follow. "Exchange" lists of major foods were provided, listing calories and composition, and diets were constructed using the exchanges, such as the precalculated diets provided by the American Diabetes Association (ADA). This approach has now been abandoned by the ADA, whose policy for diet/nutrition is now as follows:

Today there is no ONE 'diabetic' or 'ADA' diet. The recommended diet can only be defined as a dietary prescription based on nutrition assessment and treatment goals. Medical nutrition therapy for people with diabetes should be individualized, with consideration given to eating habits and other lifestyle factors. Nutrition recommendations are then developed to meet treatment goals and desired outcomes. Monitoring metabolic parameters, including blood glucose, glycated hemoglobin, lipids, blood pressure, and body weight, as well as quality of life, is crucial to ensure successful outcomes.

Flexibility in use of ordinary foods is important for patients and families. The first decision is the caloric content of the diet, based on the need to gain, lose, or maintain current weight. Caloric recommendations from the Food and Nutrition Board for adults carrying out "average" activity decrease with age and range from 175 kJ/kg of body weight (42 kcal/kg) in 18-year-old men to 140 kJ/kg (33 kcal/kg) for 75-year-old women. Intakes slightly less than the official recommendations are usually preferable; 150 kJ/kg (36 kcal/kg) for men and 140 kJ/kg (34 kcal/kg) for women are reasonable initial values in most patients.

The minimal protein requirement for good nutrition is about 0.9 g/kg of body weight per day, and the acceptable range is 1.0 to 1.5 g/kg per day. Since very low protein diets may slow the progression

of nephropathy, protein content should probably be limited to 0.8 g/kg per day, or about 10 percent of daily calories, when this complication develops.

The distribution of calories between carbohydrate and fat must be determined individually. Restriction of fat is usually prudent if weight loss is desired because of the high energy content of fat relative to protein and carbohydrate. An average recommendation for nonobese patients and those without hyperlipidemias is that fat should make up 30 percent or less of total calories, with less than 10 percent as saturated fat. In hypercholesterolemic subjects, saturated fat should be lowered to less than 7 percent of calories, and cholesterol intake should be below 200 mg/day. An increase in polyunsaturated fats is usually recommended. Fat restriction is not recommended by all authors. For example, a 50 percent fat diet with 33 percent monounsaturated fatty acids and 35 percent carbohydrates was reported to lower glucose levels, insulin requirements, and VLDL levels while increasing the concentrations of high-density lipoprotein (HDL). Some authors recommend the addition of fish oils containing omega-3 fatty acids as beneficial, but this is not standard practice.

After the protein and fat content is chosen, the remaining calories are assigned to carbohydrate. Sucrose can be allowed in moderation as part of the carbohydrate component. Increasing the fiber content of the diet may be helpful. As in any dietary regimen, it is the long-term, overall dietary pattern that counts. Deviation for one or two meals does not matter much. Thus, a teenage diabetic may be allowed to eat a high-sugar, high-fat dessert, ordinarily forbidden, as a special treat with the understanding that resumption of the diet will be necessary the next day. Even in adults the "treat" technique often ensures better dietary cooperation than more rigid demands. Ideally, patients should be trained by dieticians in a formal teaching program. Such classes are available in most large hospitals. If a patient is from a smaller community, it will probably be helpful to refer him or her to a larger center for initial training.

In insulin-requiring patients, the distribution of calories is also important if hypoglycemia is to be avoided. A typical pattern might include 20 percent of the total for breakfast, 35 percent for lunch, 30 percent for dinner, and 15 percent as a late-evening feeding. Often, a midmorning and a midafternoon snack are necessary as well. Different distributions may be required for different life-styles; i.e., a person employed on a late-evening or night shift would not eat the major meal at noon. When regimes of meticulous control are attempted using multiple injections of insulin or insulin pumps, more frequent feedings are often prescribed. Thus one might recommend 20 percent of energy intake at both breakfast and lunch, 30 percent at dinner, and the remaining 30 percent as midmorning, midafternoon, and late-evening snacks, depending on the pattern of plasma glucose level during the day.

The importance of diet in the management of diabetes varies with the type of disease. In insulin-dependent patients, particularly those on intensive insulin regimens, the composition of the diet is not of critical importance, since adjustment of insulin can cover wide variations in food ingestion. In non-insulin-dependent patients not treated with exogenous insulin, more rigorous adherence to diet is required, since the endogenous insulin reserve is limited. Such patients cannot respond to the increased demand produced by excess calories or increased intake of rapidly absorbed carbohydrate.

Insulin Insulin is required for treatment of all patients with IDDM and many patients with NIDDM. If the physician does not use oral agents (see below), all diet-unresponsive NIDDM subjects must be given the hormone. It is fairly easy to control the symptoms of diabetes with insulin, but it is difficult to maintain a normal blood sugar throughout 24 h, even with the use of multiple injections of regular insulin or infusion pumps. In the Diabetes Control and Complications Trial (see below), where teams of health care workers attempted to return the blood glucose level to normal or near normal with much more frequent professional input than is usual in clinical situations, blood glucose levels and hemoglobin A_{1c} concentrations remained above normal in most subjects. It is even more difficult to maintain normal blood sugars by means of traditional insulin therapy given as one or two injections a day. Nondiabetic subjects maintain the plasma glucose concentration within a narrow range at all times despite episodic food intake. When a meal is eaten, a prompt rise in insulin release occurs, such that absorbed carbohydrate is rapidly taken up by the liver and other tissues. Even after meals, therefore, the plasma glucose level in normal subjects does not rise into the hyperglycemic or glycosuric range. As the plasma glucose level falls under the influence of insulin, release of the hormone is damped, and counterregulatory hormones enter the circulation to prevent hypoglycemia, ensuring smooth control of plasma glucose throughout the absorptive process. The patient treated with insulin by injection cannot reproduce these physiologic responses. If enough insulin is given to keep the postprandial glucose normal, too much insulin will inevitably be present during the postabsorptive phase, and hypoglycemia will result.

No single standard exists for patterns of administration of insulin, and treatment plans vary from physician to physician and, with a given physician, for different patients. Three treatment regimes will be described: conventional, multiple subcutaneous injections (MSI), and continuous subcutaneous insulin infusion (CSII). MSI or CSII is required in intensive treatment schedules designed to protect against complications. *Conventional insulin therapy* involves the administration of one or two injections a day of intermediate-acting insulin such as zinc insulin (lente insulin) or isophane insulin (NPH insulin) with or without the addition of small amounts of regular insulin. If the newly diagnosed subject is not in acute distress, therapy can be started on an outpatient basis, provided the patient has been instructed adequately on diet, insulin use, and monitoring and the physician or nurse-clinician can be reached by telephone for consultation. Adults of normal weight may be started on 15 to 20 units a day. (The estimated daily insulin production rate in nondiabetic subjects of normal size is about 25 units a day.) Obese patients, because of insulin resistance, may be started on 25 to 30 units a day. It is preferable to use the same quantity of insulin for several days before changing, the one exception being in a hypoglycemic patient, whose dose should be decreased immediately unless a nonrecurrent cause of hypoglycemia (such as excessive exercise) is present. Generally, changes should be no more than 5 or 10 units per step. It is probable that a single daily injection of insulin provides adequate control only in patients who have some residual capacity for insulin secretion. Patients with poorly controlled disease should be placed on split therapy, with about two-thirds of the total insulin given before breakfast and the remainder before supper. Two injections are almost always used when the total dose reaches 50 or 60 units a day but are helpful at smaller doses as well, since the peak action of intermediate insulins appears to be dose-related; i.e., a low dose may exhibit maximal activity earlier and disappear sooner than a large dose. Many physicians routinely add regular insulin to the intermediate dose even at initiation of therapy. Thus, in a single-dose schedule, one might begin with 20 units of intermediate and 5 units of regular insulin rather than 25 units of intermediate alone. This practice is based on the concept that the regular insulin lowers the plasma glucose level rapidly, after which the more slowly absorbed insulin maintains the lowered level. Most patients on twice-daily insulin injections are also treated with a mixture of intermediate and regular insulin; e.g., 25 units NPH plus 10 units of regular before breakfast and 10 units of NPH plus 5 units of regular before supper. Commercial premixed insulin (70/30 intermediate/regular) is acceptable and convenient for many patients. All patients should be taught to decrease insulin when significant extra activity or exercise is anticipated. The proper decrement must be determined by trial and error, although a reduction of 5 to 10 units is a reasonable first step. The blood glucose–lowering effect of exercise is due primarily to increased energy demands in previously noncontracting muscle. Extra regular insulin can be taken before a meal that contains extra calories or food ordinarily not allowed (e.g., when the diabetic must eat out at a banquet or the teenager goes out on a date). For patients willing to self-monitor plasma glucose level, an algorithm for ad-

justing insulin can be provided. A typical protocol is shown in Table 334-4. Patients with complicated control problems may require hospitalization, where frequent plasma glucose determinations can guide therapy.

The *multiple subcutaneous insulin injection technique* most commonly involves administration of intermediate- or long-acting insulin in the evening as a single dose together with regular insulin prior to each meal. Home glucose monitoring by the patient is necessary if the goal is the return of the plasma glucose level to normal. One approach to initiation of therapy involves administration of 25 percent of the previous daily insulin dose in the patient's conventional regimen at bedtime as intermediate insulin (NPH or lente insulin), with the other 75 percent given as regular insulin divided such that 40, 30, and 30 percent is given 30 min before breakfast, lunch, and supper, respectively. Alternatively, a three-injection schedule can be created by omitting the night intermediate insulin and giving a long-acting insulin, such as insulin zinc extended (ultralente insulin) or protamine zinc insulin (PZI insulin), before the evening meal. Adjustments of dosage depend on response of the plasma glucose. A number of different protocols have been used, all of which represent sliding scales of insulin based on the plasma glucose level. A typical schedule based on home monitoring of the plasma glucose level is shown in Table 334-5. Individual patients may require different dosages. For specific details, the reader should consult one of the published papers on the use of the technique (e.g., Schriffrin and Belmonte; Campbell and May). MSI can be effective in controlling the plasma glucose level, and in some studies it appears to match goals achieved with CSII.

Continuous subcutaneous insulin infusion involves the use of a small battery-driven pump that delivers insulin subcutaneously into the abdominal wall, usually through a 27-gauge butterfly needle. With CSII, insulin is delivered at a basal rate continuously throughout the day, with increases in rate programmed prior to meals. Adjustments in dosage are made in response to measured capillary glucose values in a fashion similar to that used in MSI. Ordinarily, about 40 percent of the total daily dose is given at the basal rate, the remainder being administered as preprandial boluses. There is little question that CSII can give better diabetic control than conventional therapy. Most patients report positive feelings of well-being as control improves. The danger of hypoglycemia is real, especially during the night in patients who maintain the plasma glucose consistently below 5.5 mmol/L (100 mg/dL). A fall in plasma glucose of 2.7 mmol/L (50 mg/dL) may not be important if the starting value is 8.3 mmol/L (150 mg/dL) but may be fatal if it occurs against a steady-state level of 3.3 mmol/L (60 mg/dL). Several deaths from hypoglycemia have occurred in pump users. There is also an increased frequency of diabetic ketoacidosis in persons using CSII.

Table 334-4

Adjusting Insulin Dosage in Conventional Insulin Therapy*

Blood Glucose		Regular Insulin, units	
		Breakfast	**Supper**
		(To Be Mixed with Intermediate Dosage)	
mmol/L	**mg/dL**		
2.8–5.5	51–100	8	4
5.6–8.3	101–150	10	5
8.4–11.1	151–200	12	6
11.2–13.9	201–250	14	7
14.0–16.6	251–300	16	8
>16.6	>300	20	10

* Once the patient's blood sugar level is in the reasonable range at most measurements, a prescription can be written for varying the regular insulin dosage as illustrated. The prescription in this case was for a patient in reasonable control on 25 units of NPH insulin plus 10 units of regular insulin before breakfast and 10 units of NPH insulin plus 5 units of regular insulin before supper. Change in metabolic status may require adjustments in both intermediate insulin and the sliding scale of regular insulin.

Table 334-5

Adjusting Insulin Dosage in a Multiple-Injection Schedule*

INITIATION OF THERAPY

1. 0.6 to 0.7 units insulin per kilogram body weight
2. 25% NPH insulin at 9 P.M.; 75% regular insulin in divided doses (40% before breakfast, 30% before lunch, 30% before supper)
3. Adjust NPH insulin every 48 h based on fasting blood glucose
   <3.3 mmol/L (<60 mg/dL):   − 2 units
   >5.0 mmol/L (>90 mg/dL):   + 2 units
4. Adjust regular insulin every 48 h based on 1-h postprandial glucose
   <3.3 mmol/L (<60 mg/dL):   − 2 units
   >7.8 mmol/L (>140 mg/dL):   + 2 units

DAILY THERAPY

Preprandial Glucose		
mmol/L	mg/dL	Regular Insulin, units
<3.3	<60	−2
3.4–5.0	61–90	No change
5.1–6.7	91–120	+1
6.8–8.3	121–150	+2
8.4–11.0	151–200	+3
11.1–13.9	201–250	+4
>13.9	>250	+6

* During the initiation of therapy, the insulin dosage is changed until the target range is reached (see Table 334-6). After initial stabilization, a variable insulin schedule is prescribed to maintain tight control. For example, if after initiation the patient is found generally to require 12 units of regular insulin before breakfast but has a prebreakfast blood sugar level of 8.9 mmol/L (160 mg/dL), 15 units of regular insulin instead of the usual 12 would be taken.

SOURCE: Adapted from Schiffrin and Belmonte.

Pumps should be prescribed only in disciplined and motivated patients who are under the care of a physician with extensive experience in their use.

In some centers, the catheters for insulin infusion pumps have been placed intravenously rather than subcutaneously. While few difficulties have been reported, this procedure appears unwise for routine use. Intraabdominal insulin pumps with reservoirs that are refillable from outside the body have been tried on experimental protocols. At present, no advantage is apparent except that a pump does not have to be worn externally.

For surgical procedures in diabetic patients, intermediate insulin is omitted, and treatment is carried out with regular insulin alone. An effective method is to add 10 to 20 units of insulin to a liter of 5% glucose in water with infusion at a rate of 100 to 150 mL/h. Measurement of plasma glucose in capillary blood allows the rate to be changed to avoid significant hypo- or hyperglycemia. It is also possible to administer 10 units of regular insulin subcutaneously and infuse 5% or 10% glucose at rates sufficient to avoid major changes in glucose concentration. Following surgery, a sliding scale can be constructed for use in postoperative management.

Types of Insulin   A variety of insulins are available for use in the treatment of diabetes. Rapid-acting preparations are used in diabetic emergencies and in CSII and MSI programs. Intermediate-acting preparations are used in conventional and MSI regimens. Long-acting formulations are used almost exclusively in three-injection MSI schedules. Peak effects and duration vary from patient to patient and depend not only on route of administration but on dose. In patients treated for long periods, insulin action appears to be delayed, probably because of the presence of anti-insulin antibodies in plasma. In one study in diabetic subjects, the action of regular insulin given subcutaneously had its onset at about 1 h, reached a peak at 6 h, and remained measurable on average for 16 h, whereas in normal persons onset is within minutes, action peaks at around 2 h, and duration is only 6 to 8 h. With NPH insulin, diabetic patients exhibited an onset of action at 2.5 h, a peak at 11 h, and a total

period of action of 25 h, more closely approximating values in normal subjects.

Commercial insulins are prepared in concentrations of 100 U/mL (U100), although higher concentrations can be obtained (e.g., U500). All animal insulins are purified so that proinsulin contamination is extremely low. Most patients are now treated with synthesized "human" insulin. The amino acid sequence is identical to that of the human hormone, and biologic activity appears to be equivalent. Complications of insulin therapy, such as insulin allergy, fat atrophy, and fat hypertrophy, are less common than with animal insulins but still occur.

Lente and NPH insulin are used in most conventional therapy and are roughly equivalent in biologic effects, although lente appears to be slightly more immunogenic and to mix less well with regular insulin than does NPH.

Self-Monitoring of Glucose Level   For many years, the effectiveness of treatment for diabetes was followed by reviewing symptoms (such as frequency of nocturia) and measuring the glucose in urine by semiquantitative techniques. Since the renal threshold for glucose in normal persons is in the range of 10 to 11 mmol/L (180 to 200 mg/dL) plasma glucose and may increase with the appearance of renal disease, assessment of glycosuria is of little value. Most insulin-requiring patients now monitor control and alter therapy based on self-measurement of the capillary blood sugar. In addition to the fact that such measurements are necessary in all treatment schedules involving variable insulin dosage, the ability to assess the blood glucose as needed has other positive benefits. It gives the patient a sense of confidence and independence, has a reinforcing effect on therapeutic goals (e.g., the effect of dietary indiscretion can be immediately seen), serves to give early warning of incipient hypoglycemia, and allows verification of hypoglycemia when suggestive symptoms are present.

Although the blood glucose level can be estimated visually with the use of reagent strips, it is generally preferable to use an instrument for readings. This is so because it is difficult for many patients to extrapolate accurately between the color changes and because subjective wishes may influence the extrapolation. It is harder to ignore a number appearing in a machine. A variety of glucose analyzers are available. The cost of equipment is reasonable, and many insurance carriers reimburse for its purchase. The patient needs to have supervised training in the technique, and simultaneous checks of the blood sugar in a laboratory should be done periodically to test the accuracy of the self-analysis. Repeated studies show that patients can measure blood glucose accurately using these techniques.

Although urine testing for glucose is now rarely used to follow diabetes, the measurement of ketones in the urine remains important.

Goals of Therapy   Intensive insulin therapy designed to keep the blood glucose level as near normal as possible has for many years been considered mandatory during pregnancy and after renal transplantation. Maintenance of a normal blood glucose level during pregnancy prevents fetal macrosomy, respiratory distress syndrome, and perinatal mortality. Prevention of congenital malformations probably requires that the blood glucose level be near normal at the time of conception, although one multicenter trial concluded that no relationship existed between control of diabetes and malformed fetuses. For maximal safety, however, intensive therapy should be started prior to conception, if at all possible. The issue of gestational diabetes, defined as carbohydrate intolerance first recognized in pregnancy, is controversial. Some authorities recommend screening of all women, while others test only those at high risk. Treatment is by diet, and insulin is rarely required.

The conclusion of the NIH-sponsored multicenter Diabetes Control and Complication Trial (DCCT) required broadening of the recommendation for intensive insulin therapy. This very large trial, involving more than 1400 patients with IDDM followed for 7 to 10 years, established that degenerative complications of diabetes are diminished by better control of the blood glucose level, although, as mentioned earlier, return of blood glucose level to normal was not achieved. Protection rates as high as 70 percent were seen in the case of retinopathy. It follows that many more patients and their physicians will desire intensive insulin therapy than has been the case in the past. To meet this demand will not necessarily be easy. It is clear from the DCCT that even with health care teams staffed with physicians, nutritionists, and experienced nurse-clinicians and with a dedicated group of participating volunteers, treatment goals were not met. Furthermore, there was a significant increase in the frequency and severity of hypoglycemia, so the therapy was not without risk. Patients with NIDDM were not studied. It thus remains to be seen whether the results of the DCCT can be applied widely under ordinary clinical circumstances.

If an experienced health care team familiar with both MSI and CSII is available and if the patient is physically, emotionally, intellectually, and financially able to undergo the rigors of intensive therapy, it should be tried. Intensive therapy should not be offered for patients under the age of 7 because of the danger of impairment of brain development by hypoglycemia. Older persons and those with comorbidity such as coronary artery disease or stroke should be excluded. Although subjects with NIDDM were not studied in the DCCT, it is likely that lowering the blood glucose level would be beneficial in the prevention of complications in these patients as well. Insulin resistance may prove a problem in NIDDM, especially if hyperinsulinemia proves to be a risk factor for atherosclerosis and hypertension, as some investigators believe. The treatment group in the DCCT also had significant weight gain, which likely will be a greater problem in NIDDM, since most patients are significantly overweight or obese. In short, persons with NIDDM should not be excluded, but considerable caution is required, especially in older persons with the disease.

Goals of therapy have not been defined. One set of standards for blood glucose is listed in Table 334-6. The "acceptable" category would apply in conventional therapy using a two-dose schedule of intermediate and regular insulin. The upper limit of 11.1 mmol/L (200 mg/dL) postprandially is arbitrary but is based on the finding in the Pima Indian population that complications of diabetes are rare if the 2-h value in the oral glucose tolerance test is less than 11.1 mmol/L. The "ideal" column represents values targeted in meticulous control regimens. Although some authors are more stringent and prefer the 1-h postprandial value to be no more than 7.8 mmol/L (140 mg/dL), the risk of hypoglycemia is greater under these circumstances. In general, avoidance of serious hypoglycemia is more important than avoidance of hyperglycemia, because the former has immediate consequences that may threaten the life of the patient or others (e.g., through an automobile accident), while the detrimental effects of hyperglycemia are long-term and less certain.

Hypoglycemia, the Somogyi Effect, and the Dawn Phenomenon (See also Chap. 335) The problem of hypoglycemia is common in insulin-dependent diabetics, particularly when aggressive efforts are made to keep both the fasting plasma glucose level and postprandial hyperglycemia within the normal range. Hypoglycemia may be caused by missing a meal or doing unexpected exercise but can occur in the absence of known precipitating events. Daytime episodes of hypoglycemia are usually recognized by autonomic symptoms, such as sweating, nervousness, tremor, and hunger. Hypoglycemia during sleep may produce no symptoms or cause night

sweats, unpleasant dreams, and early-morning headache. In one study of insulin-dependent diabetic children monitored throughout 24 h, 18 percent had asymptomatic nocturnal hypoglycemia. If hypoglycemia is not aborted by counterregulatory hormone response or by ingestion of carbohydrate, central nervous system symptoms ensue: confusion, abnormal behavior, loss of consciousness, or convulsions.

As blood glucose concentrations fall, protection against hypoglycemia is normally provided by two mechanisms: cessation of insulin release and mobilization of counterregulatory hormones. The latter increase hepatic glucose production and decrease glucose utilization in nonhepatic tissues. Glucagon is the primary counterregulatory hormone, while epinephrine and norepinephrine released from the adrenal medulla and the sympathetic nervous system serve as the major backup. Catecholamines are not required for maintenance of the blood glucose level, provided glucagon is available, but they become critical in the absence of glucagon. Cortisol and growth hormone do not function acutely but come into play with prolonged fasting or sustained hypoglycemia. Diabetic patients are vulnerable to hypoglycemia because of both insulin excess and counterregulatory failure. Since insulin is given by injection or infusion, the body does not have the capacity to decrease plasma concentrations of insulin as glucose levels fall. Very early on, patients with type 1 IDDM lose the capacity to increase glucagon release in response to hypoglycemia. Protection thus depends on epinephrine. Unfortunately, many patients subsequently also lose the capacity to release epinephrine and norepinephrine in response to hypoglycemia. Since the initial clinical signals of hypoglycemia are dependent on epinephrine (the other counterregulatory hormones are clinically silent), the loss of the catecholamine response results in the syndrome of *hypoglycemia unawareness*. This syndrome originally was thought to be due solely to autonomic neuropathy in patients with long-standing diabetes. It is now recognized that the syndrome may be *caused* by low blood glucose in the absence of neuropathy, with even a single episode of afternoon hypoglycemia having discernible effects the next day. Previous hypoglycemia does not prevent epinephrine release but lowers the level of glucose required to trigger the response. The end result is that potentially dangerous hypoglycemia is unrecognized, and the defense against hypoglycemia is impaired.

Both the hormonal defense against hypoglycemia and its warning symptoms are thought to originate in the hypothalamus. One explanation for the unawareness syndrome is an adaptive response to hypoglycemia that allows the brain to continue taking up a normal amount of glucose despite low glucose levels in the blood. Presumably, this effect is due to an increase in brain glucose transporter (GLUT 1) units. While there is evidence to support this concept in patients with IDDM, it would not explain the induction of next-day unawareness by a single episode of hypoglycemia. Hypoglycemia unawareness induced by hypoglycemia (as opposed to unawareness due to autonomic neuropathy) can be reversed by avoidance of hypoglycemia. Most patients with this syndrome are receiving intensive insulin therapy and have nearly normal hemoglobin A_{1c} levels. Relaxation of therapy sufficient to raise hemoglobin A_{1c} into the range of 7.0 to 7.5 percent is usually sufficient to restore warning signals in the absence of autonomic neuropathy.

An important question is whether hypoglycemic symptoms can occur in the absence of low plasma glucose levels. It was believed traditionally that counterregulatory hormone release and autonomic symptoms are not triggered until the plasma glucose level approaches 3 mmol/L (50 to 55 mg/dL). Careful studies in humans using auditory or visual evoked potentials as a measure of cortical function in the brain have shown that abnormalities can occur at a glucose level of 4 mmol/L (70 to 72 mg/dL). A drop in glucose level of only 0.5 mmol/L (10 mg/dL) resulted in a delay of the evoked potential and, with time, release of counterregulatory hormones. Thus, neuroglyco-

Table 334-6

Goals for Blood Glucose Levels in the Control of Diabetes*

Goal	Acceptable		Ideal	
	mmol/L	mg/dL	mmol/L	mg/dL
Fasting	3.3–7.2	60–130	3.9–5.6	70–100
Preprandial	3.3–7.2	60–130	3.9–5.6	70–100
Postprandial (1 h)	<11.1	<200	<8.9	<160
3 A.M.	>3.6	>65	>3.6	>65

* Values for healthy patients below the age of 65. Goals may be shifted upward in older patients. *Acceptable* refers to goals for conventional therapy, while *ideal* indicates goals with intensive insulin therapy.

penic symptoms may occur in the presence of blood glucose levels not considered hypoglycemic.

From time to time, patients with diabetes report symptoms suggestive of catecholamine release in the presence of documented hyperglycemia. The cause is unknown, but possibilities include simple anxiety, insulin-induced vascular permeability with a hypotensive response, and activation of the sympathetic nervous system by insulin-enhanced carbohydrate utilization. Patients with poorly controlled disease release counterregulatory hormones at higher concentrations of blood glucose than do normal subjects or patients with tightly controlled diabetes. Thus, insulin treatment affects the counterregulatory response in two ways. With intensive therapy and tight control, especially with intermittent hypoglycemia, epinephrine release is impaired, and hypoglycemia unawareness may ensue. When control is less rigorous or is poor, symptoms of hypoglycemia may occur in the presence of normal blood glucose values, because of a shift upward in the counterregulatory glucose threshold.

Hypoglycemia can result from other mechanisms. Diabetic renal disease may be accompanied by diminished insulin requirements and may lead to frank hypoglycemia if adjustments in dosage are not made. The mechanism is not known. Although half-times for insulin in plasma are increased in such patients, other factors doubtless play a role. The impairment of gluconeogenesis by uremia may play a role.

Hypoglycemia may be due to the development of autoimmune adrenal insufficiency as part of polyglandular autoimmune deficiency (see Chap. 340), which is more frequent in persons with diabetes than in the population as a whole. Hypoglycemia can develop in association with high levels of circulating insulin antibodies. The exact mechanism is not known, but one possibility is dissociation of insulin from the antibody during the overnight fast. Occasionally, an insulinoma may develop in a diabetic patient. Very rarely, permanent remission of apparently typical diabetes occurs. The reason is not known, but the initial sign may be frequent hypoglycemia in a patient with previously well-controlled disease.

It must be emphasized that hypoglycemic attacks are dangerous and, if frequent, portend a serious or even fatal outcome. If the patient is conscious, sugar, candy, or a sugar-containing beverage can be given. If the patient is unarousable or unconscious, intravenous glucose is required. Patients should have a vial of glucagon available as well. If access to medical care is delayed, administration of 1 mg glucagon intramuscularly frequently aborts the attack.

The *Somogyi phenomenon* refers to rebound hyperglycemia following an episode of hypoglycemia due to counterregulatory hormone release. It should be suspected whenever wide swings in the plasma glucose occur over short time intervals, even if symptoms are not reported. Such rapid changes contrast with the changes after insulin withdrawal in previously well-controlled diabetic patients, in whom hyperglycemia and ketosis develop gradually and smoothly over a 12- to 24-h period. Excessive hunger and weight gain in the context of worsening hyperglycemia are clues that the insulin dosage may be too high, since poor control due to underinsulinization usually results in weight loss (because of osmotic diuresis and glucose wastage). If the Somogyi phenomenon is suspected, the insulin dose should be decreased as a trial, even when specific symptoms of overinsulinization are absent. The Somogyi phenomenon is probably rare in adults but may be more frequent in children.

The *dawn phenomenon* refers to an early morning rise in plasma glucose requiring increased amounts of insulin to maintain euglycemia. Although similar early morning hyperglycemia may result from hypoglycemia, as just described, the dawn phenomenon itself is thought to be independent of the Somogyi mechanism. The nocturnal surge of growth hormone release may be a factor. Increased clearance of insulin also occurs in the early morning hours, but the changes are probably not of major importance. Usually, the dawn phenomenon can be differentiated from posthypoglycemic hyperglycemia by

measuring the blood glucose at 3 A.M. It is important to make this distinction, because the Somogyi phenomenon is avoided by decreasing insulin dosages for the critical time period, while the dawn phenomenon usually requires increased insulin to maintain glucose in the normal range.

Oral Agents NIDDM that cannot be controlled by dietary management often responds to sulfonylureas. The drugs are easy to use and appear to be safe. Nevertheless, use of oral agents has decreased in response to the emphasis on better control as a means of slowing the development of late complications. These drugs can bring plasma glucose back to normal in some patients with relatively mild disease, but in patients with significant hyperglycemia, plasma glucose tends to improve but not to approach the normal range in response to these agents. Thus, a high percentage of patients with NIDDM are now treated with insulin.

Sulfonylureas act primarily by stimulating release of insulin from the beta cell. The cDNA for the sulfonylurea receptor has been cloned and appears to be a subunit of the K_{ATP} channel that controls membrane potential in the beta cell. Binding of sulfonylureas to the receptor causes the channel to close and causes depolarization, calcium influx, and insulin secretion. Extrapancreatic actions of sulfonylureas include increasing the number of insulin receptors and enhancing the insulin-mediated glucose transport independent of increased insulin binding. The extrapancreatic effects are probably physiologically unimportant. Mean levels of plasma insulin do not increase following treatment with sulfonylureas, despite significantly improved mean plasma glucose concentrations. The paradox of improved glucose metabolism in the absence of higher steady state levels of insulin is explained by the fact that elevation of plasma glucose to pretreatment values results in a rise of plasma insulin to levels higher than those seen before treatment. Thus, the initial action of the drugs is to increase insulin release with lowering of the blood glucose level. As glucose levels fall, insulin levels also decrease, since blood glucose is the major stimulus to insulin release, thereby masking the initial stimulation of insulin secretion. The insulinogenic effect can then be unmasked by raising the blood glucose. The fact that sulfonylureas are ineffective in IDDM, where beta cell mass is diminished, supports the idea that the pancreatic effect is primary, although, as noted, extrapancreatic mechanisms may play a minor role.

The characteristics of the sulfonylureas are summarized in Table 334-7. Second-generation drugs, such as glipizide and glyburide, are effective in smaller doses but otherwise differ little from agents in long use, such as chlorpropamide and tolbutamide. First-generation agents are now infrequently prescribed, although in generic form they are less expensive. In patients with significant renal disease, it is preferable to use tolbutamide or tolazamide, since these agents are metabolized and inactivated exclusively by the liver. Chlorpropamide has the capacity to sensitize the renal tubule to antidiuretic hormone. It thus is helpful in some patients with partial diabetes insipidus but may cause water retention in patients with diabetes mellitus. Hypoglycemia occurs less often with oral agents than with insulin, but, when it occurs, it tends to be severe and prolonged. Some patients have required massive glucose infusions for days following the last dose of sulfonylurea. For this reason, hospitaliza-

Table 334-7

The Sulfonylureas*

Agent	Dose, mg/d	Doses per Day	Duration of Hyperglycemic Action, h	Metabolism/ Excretion
Chlorpropamide	100–500	1	60	Kidney
Tolazamide	100–1000	1–2	12–14	Liver
Tolbutamide	500–3000	2–3	6–12	Liver
Glyburide	1.25–20	1–2	To 24	Liver/kidney
Glipizide	2.5–40	1–2	To 24	Liver/kidney

* Metformin, a biguanide, may be administered in combination with sulfonylureas (see text). The dose varies from 500 to 2500 mg/d.

tion is mandatory in patients with sulfonylurea-induced hypoglycemia.

Metformin, a biguanide useful in NIDDM patients who are not responsive to diet and exercise, may be prescribed as monotherapy in obese diabetics but is usually added as an adjunctive agent in patients whose disease is not controlled by maximal doses of sulfonylureas. The primary action of metformin is thought to be inhibition of hepatic gluconeogenesis, and it also may enhance glucose disposal in muscle and adipose tissue. In contrast to sulfonylureas, metformin does not cause hypoglycemia. Metformin can cause lactic acidosis, like the earlier biguanides, although it does so much less frequently. To avoid this complication, the drug should not be given to patients with renal disease. It should be stopped at once if nausea, vomiting, diarrhea, or intercurrent illness appears.

Thiazolidine derivatives are under study for the treatment of NIDDM. Pioglitazone, a prototype of the class, lowers the blood levels of glucose, free fatty acids, and triglycerides and appears to reduce insulin resistance, possibly by increasing insulin receptor kinase activity.

Two peptides are under evaluation as adjunct treatments for NIDDM. Both insulin-like growth factor 1 (IGF-1, somatomedin C) and glucagon-like peptide 1 (GLP-1), a peptide derived from the proglucagon molecule, lower blood glucose levels in normal subjects and in patients with diabetes. GLP-1 (7-36) and (7-37) amides are the lead agents under trial. Their usefulness is not established.

Monitoring the Control of Diabetes As mentioned earlier, patients on intensive insulin therapy who keep accurate records of capillary blood glucose levels can easily monitor the adequacy of control of their disease and detect changing trends. It is also standard practice to measure hemoglobin A_{1c} levels quarterly in all patients. This step is particularly important in patients who do not measure glucose values frequently at home. Hemoglobin A_{1c} is an electrophoretically fast-moving hemoglobin component that is present in normal persons and increases in amount in the presence of hyperglycemia. It is formed by the nonenzymatic glycation of the amino acids valine and lysine on the beta chain of hemoglobin A. Some laboratories also report the level of total glycated hemoglobin. However, this quantity includes the level of the reversible Schiff base, which can change rapidly with alterations in blood glucose. Only hemoglobin A_{1c}, which is irreversibly glycated and thus stable, should be used for the assessment of glucose control. When properly assayed, the level of glycated hemoglobin gives an estimate of diabetic control for the preceding 3-month period. Normal values must be established for each laboratory; on average, nondiabetic subjects have hemoglobin A_{1c} values of less than 6 percent, while levels in patients with poorly controlled diabetes may be considerably above 10 percent. Measurement of glycated hemoglobin gives an objective assessment of metabolic control. Discrepancies between reported plasma glucose values and hemoglobin A_{1c} concentrations suggest that either the measurement or the reporting of the former is not accurate.

ACUTE METABOLIC COMPLICATIONS In addition to hypoglycemia, patients with diabetes are susceptible to two major acute metabolic complications: diabetic ketoacidosis and hyperosmolar, nonketotic coma. The former is a complication of IDDM, while the latter usually occurs in the setting of NIDDM. Ketoacidosis is rare in true NIDDM, although it can occur in that setting.

Diabetic Ketoacidosis Diabetic ketoacidosis appears to require insulin deficiency coupled with a relative or absolute increase in glucagon concentration. It is often caused by cessation of insulin intake, but it may result from physical (e.g., infection, surgery) or emotional stress despite continued insulin therapy. In the former case, the concentration of glucagon rises secondary to insulin withdrawal, while in stress, the stimulus for glucagon release is probably epinephrine. In addition to stimulating glucagon secretion, epinephrine presumably blocks the release of the small amount of residual insulin present in some subjects with IDDM and inhibits insulin-induced glucose transport in peripheral tissues. These hormonal changes have two critical effects: (1) They induce maximal gluconeogenesis and impair peripheral utilization of glucose, causing severe hyperglycemia. Glucagon facilitates gluconeogenesis by inducing a fall in fructose-2,6-bisphosphate, an intermediate that stimulates glycolysis and blocks gluconeogenesis. When fructose-2,6-bisphosphate levels fall, glycolysis is inhibited and gluconeogenesis is enhanced. The resulting hyperglycemia induces an osmotic diuresis that leads to the volume depletion and dehydration that characterize the ketoacidotic state. (2) They activate the ketogenic process and thus initiate the development of metabolic acidosis. For ketosis to occur, changes must be produced in both adipose tissue and the liver. Free fatty acids from adipose stores are the primary substrate for ketone body formation, and plasma levels of free fatty acids must rise if ketogenesis is to proceed at a high rate. However, fatty acids delivered to the liver are reesterified and stored as hepatic triglyceride or converted into VLDL and transported back into the circulation unless the hepatic oxidation of fatty acids is activated. While the release of free fatty acids is enhanced by insulin deficiency, accelerated fatty acid oxidation in the liver is induced primarily by glucagon, via its action on the carnitine palmitoyltransferase system of enzymes responsible for the transport of fatty acids into the mitochondria. When long-chain fatty acids reach the liver, they are first esterified to coenzyme A (CoA). The fatty acyl CoA cannot traverse the mitochondrial membranes until it is transesterified with carnitine. As shown in Fig. 334-3, carnitine palmitoyltransferase I transesterifies fatty acyl-CoA to fatty acylcarnitine, which then traverses the inner mitochondrial membrane via translocase. In the matrix the reverse reaction is then catalyzed by carnitine palmitoyltransferase II. In the fed state, carnitine palmitoyltransferase I is inactive, and, as a consequence, long-chain fatty acids cannot reach the β-oxidative enzymes for ketone body production. During starvation or uncontrolled diabetes, the system is activated; under these circumstances, the rate

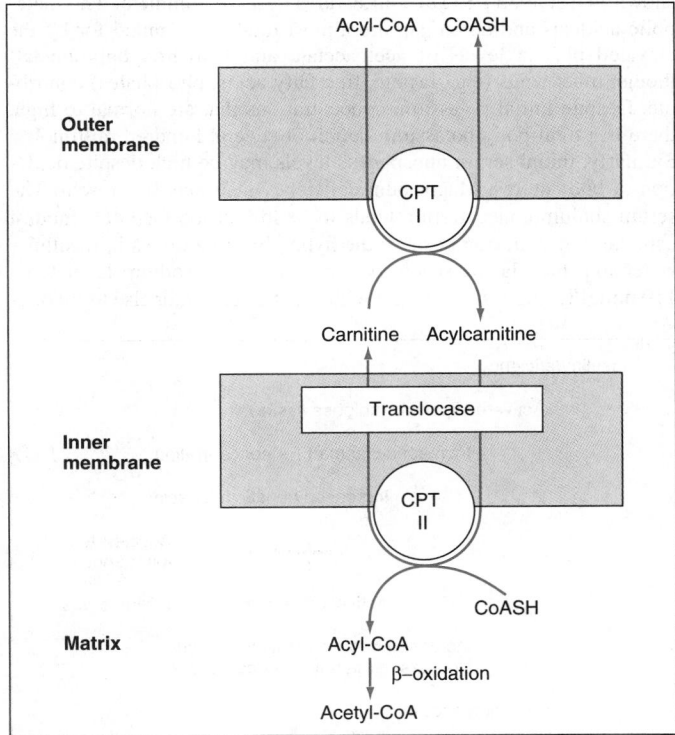

FIGURE 334-3 The carnitine palmitoyltransferase system. Long-chain fatty acyl-CoA molecules require transesterification to carnitine to traverse the inner mitochondrial membrane. Once across, the transesterification is reversed, and the fatty acyl-CoA is oxidized to either ketone bodies (liver) or CO_2 and water with the generation of ATP (nonhepatic tissues). CPT 1 is the rate-limiting step, controlled by malonyl-CoA levels in tissue. CPT 1, carnitine palmitoyltransferase 1; CPT II, carnitine palmitoyltransferase II.

of ketogenesis is a first-order function of the concentration of fatty acids reaching carnitine palmitoyltransferase I.

Glucagon (or a change in the glucagon/insulin ratio) activates the transport system in two ways. First, it causes a rapid fall in hepatic malonyl-CoA content by interrupting the sequence glucose-6-phosphate → pyruvate → citrate → acetyl-CoA → malonyl-CoA by means of the previously mentioned decrease in fructose-2,6-bisphosphate. Glucagon also inhibits acetyl-CoA carboxylase, the enzyme that converts acetyl-CoA to malonyl-CoA. Malonyl-CoA, the first committed intermediate in the synthesis of fatty acids from glucose, is a competitive inhibitor of carnitine palmitoyltransferase I, and a fall in its concentration activates the enzyme. Second, glucagon causes a rise in hepatic carnitine concentration, which then drives the reaction toward fatty acylcarnitine formation by mass action. These events are summarized schematically in Fig. 334-4. At high plasma fatty acid concentrations, hepatic uptake of fatty acids is sufficient to saturate both oxidative and esterifying pathways, resulting in fatty liver, hypertriglyceridemia, and ketoacidosis. Overproduction of ketones by the liver is the primary event in ketotic states, but peripheral utilization is impaired at high levels of acetoacetate and β-hydroxybutyrate.

Clinically, ketoacidosis begins with anorexia, nausea, and vomiting, coupled with an increased rate of urine formation. Abdominal pain may be present. If the condition is not treated, altered consciousness or frank coma may occur. The initial examination usually shows Kussmaul respiration together with signs of volume depletion. Rarely, the latter is sufficient to cause vascular collapse and renal shutdown. Body temperature is normal or below normal in uncomplicated ketoacidosis; therefore, fever suggests the presence of infection. Leukocytosis, frequently very marked, is a feature of diabetic acidosis per se and may not indicate infection.

The characteristic metabolic abnormalities of diabetic coma are shown in Table 334-8. Several features deserve comment. The metabolic acidosis and anion gap are almost totally accounted for by the elevated plasma levels of acetoacetate and β-hydroxybutyrate, although other acids (e.g., lactate, free fatty acids, phosphates) contribute. Despite initial potassium concentrations that are normal to high, there is a total-body potassium deficit of several hundred millimoles. Similarly, initial serum phosphorus levels may be high despite depletion of body stores. Magnesium deficiency also may be present. The serum sodium concentration tends to be low in the face of a modest osmolar concentration because the hyperglycemia draws intracellular water into the plasma space. A very low serum sodium level (e.g., 110 mmol/L) suggests vomiting with water drinking, or else pseudohy-

FIGURE 334-4 The regulation of ketogenesis. Significant production of acetoacetate and β-hydroxybutyrate by the liver requires provision of adequate free fatty acid substrate and activation of fatty acid oxidation. Lipolysis is increased primarily by insulin deficiency, while the fatty acid oxidative series activated primarily by glucagon. The immediate signal for oxidation in malonyl-CoA content. (*After JD McGarry, DW Foster, Am J Med 76.*)

Table 334-8

Initial Laboratory Findings in Diabetic Ketoacidosis

Series:	Dallas*	Los Angeles†	Washington‡
Age, years:	38	36	43
Glucose, mmol/L (mg/dL)	26(475)	37(675)	41(733)
Sodium, mmol/L	132	131	132
Potassium, mmol/L	4.8	5.3	6.0
Bicarbonate, mmol/L	<10	6	10
BUN, mmol/L (mg/dL)	9(25)	11(32)	15(42)
Acetoacetate, mmol/L	4.8	—	—
β-Hydroxybutyrate, mmol/L	13.7	—	—
Free fatty acids, mmol/L	2.1	—	2.3
Lactate, mmol/L	4.6	—	—
Osmolality, mosmol/L	310	323	331

* Eighty-eight consecutive episodes of ketoacidosis at Parkland Memorial Hospital (DW Foster, unpublished observations).
† Mean data from 308 episodes of nonfatal ketoacidosis (PM Beigelman, Diabetes 20:490, 1971).
‡ Mean data from 10 episodes of ketoacidosis (JE Gerich et al, Diabetes 20:228, 1971).

ponatremia due to severe hypertriglyceridemia if the assays were done in autoanalyzers that do not remove fat prior to assay. Hypertriglyceridemia is common in ketoacidosis and is due both to impaired activity of lipoprotein lipase (a disposal defect) and to hepatic overproduction of VLDL. If a fatty meal has been ingested prior to the onset of ketoacidosis, chylomicrons may make up a major portion of the circulating fat. Hyperlipidemia is usually visible if the triglyceride concentration is above 4.5 mmol/L (400 mg/dL). Prerenal azotemia, reflecting volume depletion, is usually modest in degree and reverses with treatment. The serum amylase level may be elevated, and frank pancreatitis can occur.

The diagnosis of ketoacidosis in a patient known to have insulin-dependent diabetes is not difficult. Its appearance in a patient not known to be diabetic requires differentiation from the other common causes of metabolic acidosis with an anion gap: lactic acidosis, uremia, alcoholic ketoacidosis, and certain poisonings. The first step is to test the urine for glucose and ketones. If the urine is negative for ketones, another cause for the acidosis is likely. If it is positive, plasma examination is required to be certain that something more than starvation ketosis is present. Since quantitative assays of acetoacetate and β-hydroxybutyrate are not routinely available, semiquantitative tests must be done using ketone reagent strips. Serial dilutions of plasma can be made and tested. Undiluted plasma may give a strongly positive result when starvation alone is the problem; a strong reaction at a dilution exceeding 1:1 is presumptive evidence for ketoacidosis. Apart from diabetes, the only other common ketoacidotic state is alcoholic ketoacidosis. This syndrome, which by definition occurs in chronic alcoholics, usually follows a binge, but the patient may not have had alcohol for 24 h or longer. It never occurs in the absence of starvation and frequently is associated with severe vomiting and abdominal pain. Pancreatitis is present in up to 75 percent of patients. A plasma glucose level of less than 8.3 mmol/L (150 mg/dL) was found in three-fourths of cases in one series, and in 15 percent the level was less than 2.8 mmol/L (50 mg/dL) on arrival at the hospital. Hyperglycemia may occur but is usually mild and rarely, if ever, exceeds 17 mmol/L (300 mg/dL). Plasma free fatty acid concentrations are higher (mean, 2.9 mmol/L) than in normal starvation (range, 0.7 to 1.0 mmol/L), reaching levels seen in diabetic ketoacidosis. Presumably, the liver is activated for ketogenesis by starvation in these patients and is driven to maximal rates of ketone formation by the high fatty acid levels. Why some alcoholics mobilize fatty acids excessively is not known. In contrast to diabetic acidosis, the syndrome is rapidly reversed by the intravenous administration of glucose. As in all alcoholics given glucose, thiamine should be supplied to avoid precipitation of acute beriberi. (Other water-soluble vitamins, although not as critical, also should be infused.) Insulin is required only if hyperglycemia persists during therapy. True ketoacidosis can develop with fasting during the third trimester of pregnancy and in nursing mothers who do not eat, but the complication is rare.

Diabetic ketoacidosis cannot be reversed without insulin. For decades, 50 or more units of insulin was given per hour until ketosis was reversed, but now most patients are treated by "low-dose" insulin schedules in which 8 to 10 units of insulin are infused intravenously each hour. Most cases of diabetic acidosis can be reversed adequately with low-dose treatment, but some patients do not respond. Presumably, the insulin resistance that is characteristic of diabetic ketoacidosis is more pronounced in these patients than in responsive subjects. The problem is that resistant subjects cannot be identified prospectively. For this reason, it is probably preferable to give 25 to 50 units of insulin as an initial intravenous bolus, followed by an infusion of 15 to 25 units an hour until ketoacidosis is reversed. There are no known toxic effects of larger insulin doses, since the maximal physiologic response is obtained once the insulin receptors are saturated, regardless of how much insulin is given. The advantage of the higher dosage schedule is that it ensures saturation of the receptors in the face of competing antibodies or other resistance factors. High concentrations of insulin probably accelerate the reversal of ketoacidosis by acting via the IGF-1 receptor. Hormonal interaction with this receptor can lower the blood glucose level by a mechanism independent of the insulin receptor. Diabetic ketosis has been reversed by IGF-1 therapy in a patient with severe insulin resistance. If physicians choose to use the low-dose insulin schedule, they should be alert to the possibility of resistance. Should acidosis persist unabated after several hours of treatment, larger amounts of insulin are clearly indicated. Ketoacidosis also can be treated adequately with intramuscular (but not subcutaneous) insulin.

Therapy of ketoacidosis also requires intravenous fluids. The usual fluid deficit is 3 to 5 L, and both salt solutions and free water are needed. Between 1 and 2 L of isotonic saline or Ringer's lactate should be given rapidly intravenously on arrival, with additional amounts determined by urine output and clinical assessment of the fluid state. When the plasma glucose level falls to about 17 mmol/L (300 mg/dL), 5% glucose solutions should be added, both as a source of free water and as a prophylactic measure to prevent the late cerebral edema syndrome. The latter is a rare complication of ketoacidosis, occurring most often in children. It is suspected when the patient remains comatose or lapses into coma following reversal of acidosis.

Potassium replacement is always necessary, but the time of administration will vary. The initial potassium level is often high despite a total-body deficit because of the severe acidosis. In this case, the cation will ordinarily not be needed until 3 to 4 h after initiation of therapy, when reversal of acidosis and the action of insulin cause a shift of K^+ into intracellular water. On the other hand, if the admission value is normal or low, potassium should be given early, since plasma concentrations fall rapidly during therapy, predisposing the patient to cardiac arrhythmias or paralysis of the respiratory muscles. If the potassium is very low, insulin should be withheld for 60 to 90 min until 40 to 50 mmol of potassium can be given. In view of the phosphate depletion of ketoacidosis, potassium may be administered initially as the phosphate salt rather than as potassium chloride.

Bicarbonate therapy may be indicated in severely acidotic patients (pH 7.0 or below), especially if hypotension is present (acidosis itself can cause vascular collapse). It is not used routinely in less acutely ill subjects because rapid alkalinization may have detrimental effects on oxygen delivery to tissues. The hemoglobin-oxygen dissociation curve is normal in diabetic ketoacidosis because of the opposing effects of acidosis and deficiency of red blood cell 2,3-bisphosphoglycerate (2,3-BPG). If the acidosis is rapidly reversed, the deficiency of 2,3-BPG becomes manifest, increasing the avidity with which hemoglobin binds oxygen and impairing the release of oxygen in peripheral tissues. In a volume-depleted patient with poor tissue perfusion, such a change theoretically could predispose to the development of lactic acidosis. It is also thought that bicarbonate may impair left ventricular function through paradoxical acidification due to more rapid entry of CO_2 than bicarbonate into intracellular water. If bicarbonate is given, the infusion should be stopped when the pH reaches 7.2 to minimize possible detrimental side effects and to prevent metabolic alkalosis as circulating ketones are metabolized to bicarbonate with reversal of ketoacidosis.

Two points about following the response to treatment should be emphasized. (1) The plasma glucose level invariably falls more rapidly than the plasma ketone level. Insulin administration should not be stopped because glucose concentrations approach normal; rather, as mentioned, glucose should be infused and insulin continued until the ketosis has cleared. (2) Plasma ketone values are not very helpful in assessing clinical response. The testing materials measure acetoacetate and acetone but not β-hydroxybutyrate. Since β-hydroxybutyrate must be oxidized to acetoacetate prior to utilization, it is characteristic for the level of the plasma ketones measured by reagent strip to remain stable or even rise early in therapy at a time when total ketone concentration (acetoacetate plus β-hydroxybutyrate) is falling. Because β-hydroxybutyrate and acetoacetate represent a redox couple in equilibrium with mitochondrial NADH/NAD concentrations, vascular collapse or severe hypoxia may mask the presence of ketoacidosis because acetoacetate is reduced to β-hydroxybutyrate. Under these circumstances, the β-hydroxybutyrate/acetoacetate ratio, normally about 3:1, may reach 7:1 or 8:1. Paradoxically, in such a situation ketosis may seem to worsen as the patient gets better because of conversion of β-hydroxybutyrate to acetoacetate when the circulation is reestablished and tissue oxygenation is restored. The key parameters to follow are the pH and the calculated anion gap, since these give a more accurate assessment of response. The usual picture is for the pH to rise and the anion gap to narrow even though the plasma bicarbonate level remains low. The persistently low bicarbonate level is the consequence of hyperchloremia, which develops because of rapid infusion of sodium chloride, the loss of potential bicarbonate from the body in urine as ketones, and exchanges with intracellular buffers. Some patients demonstrate a persistent anion gap despite clinical improvement and a rising pH. Presumably, the unmeasured anion derives from tissue buffers. An anion gap that remains elevated and a pH that is persistently low indicate insulin resistance and mandate an aggressive increase in the amount of insulin administered. On the other hand, persistence of the anion gap does not indicate resistance when accompanied by clinical improvement, a rising pH, and clearing of urine ketones.

All patients should be followed with a flow sheet outlining amounts and timing of insulin and fluids together with a record of vital signs, urine volume, and blood chemistries. Without such a record, therapy tends to become chaotic.

Most patients with diabetic ketoacidosis recover when properly treated. While the mortality rate in large series is reported to be around 10 percent, most deaths result from late complications of ketoacidosis rather than from ketoacidosis itself. The major causes are myocardial infarction and infection, particularly pneumonia. Poor prognostic signs on admission include hypotension, azotemia, deep coma, and associated illness. In children, cerebral edema is a common cause of death (less frequent in adults). The cause of the brain swelling is not known. Theories include osmotic disequilibrium between brain and plasma as glucose is rapidly lowered, decreased plasma oncotic pressure due to infusion of large amounts of saline, and insulin-induced ion flux across the blood-brain barrier. Whatever the mechanism, mortality rates are high. Diagnosis is usually made by computed tomography. Treatment involves the bolus infusion of 1 g mannitol per kilogram of body weight in the form of a 20% solution. Although of questionable benefit, dexamethasone is also usually given: 12 mg initially, then 4 mg every 6 h. If there is no response, an anesthesiologist or pulmonary specialist should induce hyperventilation to an arterial P_{CO_2} of about 28 mmHg.

Other acute complications of ketoacidosis include vascular thrombosis and the adult respiratory distress syndrome. The former is induced by volume depletion, hyperosmolality, increased viscosity of blood, and changes in clotting factors favoring thrombosis. The cause of the pulmonary lesion is not known; it is probably not related to the metabolic acidosis, since respiratory distress syndrome occurs in hyperosmolar coma as well. Acute gastric dilation is another rare complication. An unusual infection associated with ketoacidosis is mucormycosis (see below). Table 334-9 summarizes the complications of diabetic ketoacidosis and their treatment.

Hyperosmolar Coma Hyperosmolar, nonketotic diabetic coma is usually a complication of NIDDM. It is a syndrome of profound dehydration resulting from a sustained hyperglycemic diuresis under circumstances in which the patient is unable to drink enough water to keep up with urinary fluid losses. Commonly, an elderly diabetic patient—often living alone or in a nursing home—develops a stroke or infection that worsens hyperglycemia and prevents adequate water intake. The full-blown syndrome probably does not occur until volume depletion is severe enough to decrease urine output. Hyperosmolar coma also can be precipitated by peritoneal dialysis or hemodialysis, tube feeding of high-protein formulas, high-carbohydrate infusion loads, and the use of osmotic agents such as mannitol and urea. Phenytoin, glucocorticoids, immunosuppressive agents, and diuretics also have been reported to initiate the disorder.

The absence of ketoacidosis is important in the pathophysiology of this condition. When ketoacidosis develops, nausea, vomiting, and air hunger bring the patient to the physician before extreme dehydration can occur. Such a protective mechanism is not operative in ketoacidosis-resistant, maturity-onset diabetes. Interestingly, hyperosmolar coma can occur in insulin-dependent diabetic patients who are given enough insulin to prevent ketosis but not enough to control hyperglycemia. Although it is unusual, the same person may present on one occasion with ketoacidosis and on the next with hyperosmolar coma.

The reason for the absence of ketoacidosis in maturity-onset diabetes is not known. The hepatic ketogenic machinery is not impaired, since the patients frequently have ketone concentrations in the starvation range (2 to 4 mmol/L). Free fatty acid levels are lower in hyperosmolar coma than in ketoacidosis, and substrate deficiency may limit ketone formation. However, some patients with hyperosmolar coma have high levels of free fatty acids in plasma. A more likely explanation is that insulin levels in the portal vein in IDDM are higher than those of insulin-dependent subjects and prevent full activation of the hepatic carnitine palmitoyltransferase system. Other possibilities include glucagon resistance, previously mentioned, and maintenance of high malonyl-CoA levels via increased Cori cycle activity. The *Cori cycle*

consists in the conversion of circulating glucose to lactate by peripheral tissues and the return of lactate to the liver for gluconeogenesis.

Clinically, patients present with extreme hyperglycemia, hyperosmolality, volume depletion, and central nervous system signs ranging from a clouded sensorium to coma. Seizure activity—sometimes Jacksonian in type—is not unusual, and transient hemiplegia may be seen. Infections, particularly pneumonia and gram-negative sepsis, are common and indicate a grave prognosis. Pneumonia is often due to gram-negative organisms. A high index of suspicion for infection should be maintained, and the blood and spinal fluid should be cultured. Because of the extreme dehydration, plasma viscosity is high, and widespread in situ thrombosis has been found at postmortem. Bleeding, probably caused by disseminated intravascular coagulation, and acute pancreatitis may occur.

The laboratory findings in two large series are shown in Table 334-10. Plasma glucose is generally around 55 mmol/L (1000 mg/dL), about twice the value seen in ketoacidosis. The serum osmolality is high, but because of the hyperglycemia, the absolute serum sodium concentration is often not elevated.[2] Prerenal azotemia causes marked elevation of blood urea nitrogen (BUN) and creatinine. Metabolic acidosis is mild, plasma bicarbonate on average being about 20 mmol/L. The acidosis is due to a combination of starvation ketosis, retention of inorganic acids secondary to renal hypoperfusion, and elevation of plasma lactate, the latter due to volume depletion. If the bicarbonate level is less than 10 mmol/L and plasma ketones are not elevated, lactic acidosis is assumed to be present.

The mortality rate in hyperosmolar coma is high (>50 percent). As a consequence, immediate treatment is urgent. The most important measure is rapid administration of large amounts of intravenous fluids to reestablish the circulation and urine flow. The average fluid deficit is 10 to 11 L. While free water is ultimately needed, initial therapy should be with isotonic salt solutions, and 2 to 3 L should be given over the first 1 to 2 h. Subsequently, half-strength saline can be used. As the glucose level approaches normal, 5% dextrose can be given as a vehicle for free water. While hyperosmolar coma may be reversed by fluids alone, insulin should be given to control the hyperglycemia more rapidly. Many authors recommend small doses of insulin, but larger amounts may be necessary, particularly in the obese patient. Potassium salts are usually required earlier in the treatment of hyperosmolar coma than in ketoacidosis because the intracellular shift of plasma K^+ during therapy is accelerated in the absence of acidosis. If lactic acidosis is present, sodium bicarbonate should be given until tissue perfusion can be reestablished. Antibiotics are required if infection is present.

LATE COMPLICATIONS OF DIABETES The diabetic patient is susceptible to a series of complications that cause morbidity and premature mortality. While some patients never develop these problems and in others they begin early, on average, symptoms develop 15 to 20 years after the appearance of overt hyperglycemia. Rare patients have complications at the time of diagnosis. A given patient may experience several complications simultaneously, or a single problem may dominate the picture.

Circulatory Abnormalities Atherosclerosis is more extensive and occurs earlier than in the general population. The cause of this accelerated course is not known, although, as discussed below, nonenzymatic glycation of lipoproteins may be important. The atherosclerotic lesion appears to be initiated by oxidized low-density lipoprotein (LDL) (not by native LDL) in a complicated cascade that operates through the acetyl-LDL or scavenger receptor. Both HDL and antioxi-

Table 334-9

Clues to Complications in Diabetic Ketoacidosis

Complication	Clues
Acute gastric dilatation or erosive gastritis	Vomiting of blood or "coffee-ground" material
Cerebral edema	Obtundation or coma with or without neurologic signs, especially if occurring after initial improvement
Hyperkalemia	Cardiac arrest
Hypoglycemia	Adrenergic or neurologic signs; rebound ketosis
Hypokalemia	Cardiac arrhythmias
Infection	Fever
Insulin resistance	Unremitting acidosis after 4–6 h of adequate therapy
Myocardial infarction	Chest pain, appearance of heart failure; appearance of hypotension despite adequate fluids
Mucormycosis	Facial pain, bloody nasal discharge, blackened nasal turbinates, blurred vision, proptosis
Respiratory distress syndrome	Hypoxemia in the absence of pneumonia, chronic pulmonary disease, or heart failure
Vascular thrombosis	Strokelike picture or signs of ischemia in nonnervous tissue

SOURCE: Adapted from DW Foster, in *Current Therapy in Endocrinology and Metabolism 1985–1986*, DT Krieger, CW Bardin (eds), Toronto/Philadelphia, Decker, 1985.

---

[2] Serum osmolality can be estimated from the following formula: Serum osmolality (mosmol/L) = 2([Na$^+$] + [K$^+$]) + [glucose] (mmol/L) + BUN (mmol/L). Glucose and blood urea nitrogen (BUN) values in conventional units can be converted to mmol/L by dividing concentrations in milligrams per deciliter by 18 and 2.4, respectively. In practice, the contribution of the BUN is often ignored, since it contributes to total osmolality but does not reflect the free-water deficit. Situations in which an increased osmolality is not equivalent to dehydration include severe alcohol intoxication, the ethanol itself providing the unmeasured osmolyte.

Table 334-10

CHAPTER 334
Diabetes Mellitus

2075

Initial Laboratory Findings in Hyperosmolar Coma

Series:	Brooklyn*	Washington†
Age, years:	**60**	**57**
Glucose, mmol/L (mg/dL)	65(1166)	54(976)
Sodium, mmol/L	144	142
Potassium, mmol/L	5	5
Chloride, mmol/L	99	98
Bicarbonate, mmol/L	17	22
BUN, mmol/L (mg/dL)	31(87)	23(65)
Creatinine, mmol/L (mg/dL)	490(5.5)	—
Free fatty acids, mmol/L	0.73	0.96
Osmolarity, mosmol/L	384	374

* Mean data from 33 episodes of hyperosmolar coma (AA Arieff, HJ Carroll, Medicine 51:73, 1972).

† Mean data from 20 episodes of hyperosmolar coma (JE Gerich et al, Diabetes 20:228, 1971).

dants have the capacity to impair LDL oxidation, thereby exerting an antiatherogenic action. In experimental animals, diabetes accelerates the oxidative process. Although lipoproteins are often in the normal range, HDL levels tend to be low, while LDL levels are high normal or high. A low HDL/LDL ratio favors atherosclerosis, presumably because reverse cholesterol transport out of arteries is impaired and because diminished antioxidant activity by the HDL-associated enzyme paraoxonase accelerates foam cell/plaque formation. Lipoprotein (a) levels are elevated in IDDM but not in NIDDM.

Other factors of potential importance are increased platelet adhesiveness, possibly due to enhanced thromboxane A_2 synthesis, and decreased prostacyclin synthesis. Hyperglycemia has been reported to increase secretion of endothelin-1 in vitro, and production of nitric oxide is diminished in aortas of diabetic rats and the coronary microvasculature of humans. Endothelin is a powerful vasoconstrictor and is mitogenic for vascular smooth muscle, while nitric oxide is a vasodilator, is antimitogenic in vascular smooth muscle, and inhibits platelet aggregation. Diabetes appears to be a procoagulant state with increased levels of tissue factor and deficiency of tissue factor pathway inhibitor type 1 playing major roles. Levels of factor VIII and von Willebrand factor are elevated. Fibrinolysis is impaired, probably due to elevated levels of tPA inhibitor, type 1.

Atherosclerosis produces symptoms in a variety of sites. Peripheral deposits may cause intermittent claudication, gangrene, and, in men, organic impotence on a vascular basis. Surgical repair of large-vessel lesions may be unsuccessful because of the simultaneous presence of widespread disease of the small vessels.

Coronary artery disease and stroke are common. Silent myocardial infarction occurs with increased frequency in diabetes and should be suspected whenever symptoms of left ventricular failure appear suddenly. Diabetes also may be associated with the clinical picture of cardiomyopathy, in which heart failure occurs in the face of apparently normal coronary arteries and in the absence of other identifiable causes of heart disease. As in nondiabetic subjects, smoking is a major risk for both coronary and peripheral vascular disease and should be avoided. Hypertension is a significant risk in many diabetic patients. An unusual ischemic lesion is focal infarction of muscle that causes painful lesions but not gangrene. This lesion may be confused with abscess.

Retinopathy Diabetic retinopathy is a leading cause of blindness in the United States. On the other hand, most diabetic patients never become blind. Retinopathic lesions are divided into two large categories, *simple* (background) and *proliferative* (Table 334-11). The earliest sign of retinal change is an increased capillary permeability that is evidenced by leakage of dye into the vitreous humor after fluorescein injection. Occlusion of retinal capillaries follows, with subsequent formation of saccular and fusiform aneurysms. Arteriovenous shunts also occur. The vascular lesions are accompanied by proliferation of lining endothelial cells and a loss of the pericytes that surround and support the vessels. Hemorrhages into the inner retinal areas are dot-shaped, while bleeding into the more superficial nerve fiber layer causes flame-shaped, blot-shaped, or linear lesions. Preretinal hemorrhages characteristically have a boat-shaped appearance. Exudates are of two types. Cotton-wool spots can be shown by angiography to be microinfarcts—nonperfused areas surrounded by a ring of dilated capillaries. A sudden increase in the number of cotton-wool spots is an ominous prognostic sign and may herald rapidly advancing retinopathy. Hard exudates are more common than cotton-wool spots and probably represent leakage of protein and lipids from damaged capillaries. Retinal edema due to the previously mentioned increase in vascular permeability is most often seen in the posterior pole of the eye, often in association with hard exudates. If the edema is in the macular region, visual acuity may be seriously and permanently impaired. Macular edema should be suspected when loss of visual acuity is not corrected by glasses, especially if posterior-pole exudates are seen. Edema is difficult to recognize without slit-lamp examination or stereoscopic fundal photographs. Consultation with a retinal surgeon should be sought early, since vision may be spared by laser therapy of the macular edema.

The fundamental characteristics of proliferative retinopathy are new vessel formation and scarring. The stimulus for neovascularization may be retinal hypoxia secondary to capillary or arteriolar occlusion. The primary angiogenic stimulus appears to be vascular endothelial growth factor (VEGF). Two serious complications of proliferative retinopathy are vitreal hemorrhage and retinal detachment. Either may cause a sudden loss of vision in one eye.

The frequency of diabetic retinopathy appears to vary with the age of onset as well as the duration of the disease. Approximately 85 percent of patients eventually develop the complication, but some never develop lesions even after 30 years of disease. Retinopathy appears to develop earlier in older patients, but proliferative retinopathy is less common. Some 10 to 18 percent of patients with simple retinopathy progress to proliferative disease in a 10-year period. About half of patients with proliferative disease progress to blindness within 5 years. Proliferative retinopathy appears to be more common in insulin-treated patients than in those not treated with insulin.

The treatment for diabetic retinopathy is photocoagulation. This treatment decreases the incidence of hemorrhage and scarring and is always indicated when new vessel formation occurs. Photocoagulation is also useful in treatment of microaneurysms, hemorrhages, and macular edema even if the proliferative stage has not begun. Panretinal photocoagulation is often used to diminish retinal demands for oxygen in the hope that the stimulus for neovascularization will be decreased. In this technique, several thousand lesions are produced over a 2-week period. Complications of photocoagulation are within the acceptable range. Some loss of peripheral vision is inevitable with extensive burns. Another surgical technique, pars plana vitrectomy, is used for treatment of nonresolving vitreal hemorrhage and retinal detachment. Postoperative complications are more frequent than with photocoagulation and include retinal tears, retinal detachment, cataracts, recurrent vitreal hemorrhage, glaucoma, infection, and loss of the eye. Hypophysectomy, once performed for diabetic retinopathy, is no longer recommended. There is hope that inhibition of angiogenesis by drugs such as the experimental heparin analogue beta-cyclodextrin tetradecasulfate

Table 334-11

Lesions of Diabetic Retinopathy

Background	Proliferative
Increased capillary permeability	New vessels
Capillary closure and dilatation	Scar (retinitis proliferans)
Microaneurysms	Vitreal hemorrhage
Arteriovenous shunts	Retinal detachment
Dilated veins	
Hemorrhages (dot and blot)	
Cotton-wool spots	
Hard exudates	

may prevent proliferative retinopathy. All patients with diabetic retinopathy should be followed by retinal specialists.

Diabetic Nephropathy   Renal disease is a leading cause of death
and disability in diabetes. About half of the cases of end-stage renal
disease in the United States are now due to diabetic nephropathy.
Approximately 35 percent of patients with IDDM develop this complication. The prevalence in NIDDM varies from 15 to 60 percent depending on ethnic background. Pima Indians have the highest rates,
while Europeans have the lowest. Nephropathy, like other complications, is probably influenced by the genetic background of the patient.
Some families with multiple diabetic members rarely have renal disease, while in others, more than 80 percent of persons at risk have
nephropathy.

Diabetic nephropathy involves two distinct pathologic patterns,
which may or may not coexist: diffuse and nodular. The former, which
is more common, consists of widening of the glomerular basement
membrane together with generalized mesangial thickening. In the nodular form, large accumulations of periodic acid–Schiff-positive material are deposited at the periphery of the glomerular tufts, the Kimmelstiel-Wilson lesion. In addition, there may be hyalinization of afferent
and efferent arterioles, "drops" in Bowman's capsule, fibrin caps, and
occlusion of glomeruli. Deposition of albumin and other proteins
occurs in both glomeruli and tubules. The most specific lesions of
diabetic glomerulosclerosis are hyalinization of afferent glomerular
arterioles and the Kimmelstiel-Wilson nodules. Clinical renal dysfunction in diabetes does not correlate well with the histologic abnormalities.

Diabetic nephropathy may be functionally silent for long periods
(10 to 15 years). At onset, the kidneys are usually enlarged and show
"superfunction" (i.e., glomerular filtration rates may be 40 percent
above normal). The next stage is the appearance of *microproteinuria*
(microalbuminuria), the excretion of albumin in the range of 30 to 300
mg/d. Normal persons excrete less than 30 mg/d. Microalbuminuria is
not detected by reagent sticks for urinary protein, which generally
become positive only when proteinuria is greater than 550 mg/d, a
degree of leakage termed *macroproteinuria*. Microalbuminuria appears to be due primarily to decreased concentration of anionic heparan
sulfate–proteoglycan in the glomerular basement membrane. Since
microalbuminuria is initially transient and can be induced by mechanisms other than diabetes, diagnosis requires an excretion rate of
albumin greater than 30 mg/d in two of three samples collected in a
6-month period. Persistent leakage of protein greater than 50 mg/d is
predictive of subsequent macroproteinuria. Interestingly, microalbuminuria also appears to predict cardiovascular mortality in diabetes.
Once the macroproteinuric phase begins, there is a steady decline in
renal function, with glomerular filtration rate falling, on average, by
about 1 mL/min per month. A plot of the reciprocal of the serum
creatinine level against time usually yields a straight line and allows
prediction of the rate of deterioration. Ordinarily, azotemia begins
about 12 years after diagnosis of diabetes. The nephrotic syndrome
may occur prior to azotemia. Progression of renal disease is accelerated
by hypertension.

There is no specific treatment for diabetic nephropathy. Meticulous
control of diabetes can reverse microalbuminuria in some patients,
and the progression of diabetic nephropathy may be slowed, as shown
in the intensive treatment group of the DCCT. Hypertension must be
treated aggressively whenever present. Angiotensin-converting enzyme inhibitors appear to slow progression of diabetic nephropathy.
They should be used in hypertensive patients with diabetes and may
have a role in normotensive subjects with microalbuminuria. Experimental studies in animals and humans indicate that low-protein diets
may be useful. Once the azotemic phase is reached, treatment does
not differ from that for other forms of renal failure. Chronic dialysis
and renal transplantation are routine in patients with renal failure due
to diabetes. Hyporeninemic hypoaldosteronism, which is associated
with renal tubular acidosis, may require alkalinizing solutions (sodium

bicarbonate or Shohl's solution) and avoidance of external potassium
loads. Potassium tends to rise in parallel with hyperglycemia in the
syndrome, since in the absence of aldosterone potassium loads must
be disposed of intracellularly under the influence of insulin. Hyperglycemia, reflecting insulin deficiency, indicates impairment of the disposal pathway. Rarely, fludrocortisone may be required to control
hyperkalemia.

Diabetic Neuropathy   Diabetic neuropathy may affect every part
of the nervous system, with the possible exception of the brain. While
rarely a direct cause of death, neuropathy is a major cause of morbidity.
Several distinct syndromes are recognized, and more than one type
may be present in the same patient. The most common picture is that
of *peripheral polyneuropathy*. Usually bilateral, the symptoms include
numbness, paresthesias, severe hyperesthesias, and pain. The pain,
which may be deep-seated and severe, is often worse at night. It is
occasionally lancinating or lightning in type, resembling tabes dorsalis
(pseudotabes). Fortunately, extreme pain syndromes are usually self-
limited, lasting from a few months to a few years. Involvement of
proprioceptive fibers leads to abnormalities of gait and development
of typical Charcot joints, particularly in the feet. Loss of arch with
multiple fractures of tarsal bones is a common finding by x-ray. On
physical examination, absent stretch reflexes and loss of vibratory
sense are early signs. Diabetic neuropathy also may cause delay in
return of the ankle reflex identical to that seen in hypothyroidism.
Mononeuropathy, though less common than polyneuropathy, also may
occur. Characteristically, there is a sudden wrist drop, foot drop, or
paralysis of the third, fourth, or sixth cranial nerves. Other single
nerves, including the recurrent laryngeal, have been reported to be
involved. Mononeuropathy is characterized by a high degree of spontaneous reversibility, usually over a several-week period. *Radiculopathy*
is a sensory syndrome in which pain occurs over the distribution of
one or more spinal nerves, usually in the chest wall or abdomen. The
severe pain may mimic herpes zoster or an acute surgical abdomen.
Like mononeuropathy, the lesion is usually self-limited. *Autonomic
neuropathy* may present in a variety of ways. The gastrointestinal tract
is a prime target, and there may be esophageal dysfunction with
difficulty in swallowing, delayed gastric emptying, constipation, or
diarrhea. The latter symptom is often nocturnal. Incompetence of
the internal anal sphincter may mimic diabetic diarrhea. Orthostatic
hypotension and frank syncope may occur. Cardiorespiratory arrest
and sudden death, thought to be due solely to autonomic neuropathy,
have been reported. Bladder dysfunction or paralysis is particularly
distressing and often leads to the necessity of chronic catheter drainage.
Impotence and retrograde ejaculation are additional manifestations in
men. Erectile dysfunction is associated with a failure of nitric oxide
generation in the penile vasculature. Deficiency of vasoactive intestinal
polypeptide (VIP) may also be involved. Clues to autonomic neuropathy can be obtained by clinical tests such as measuring response of
the heart rate to the Valsalva maneuver or standing. In both tests the
subject has an electrocardiograph running for assessment of heart
rate. In the former, the subject blows against an anaeroid or mercury
manometer to 40 mmHg pressure for 15 s. The test is performed three
times with a rest period of 1 min in between. Normally the heart rate
speeds during Valsalva such that the ratio of the longest interval
between beats after release to the shortest interval during the test is
greater than 1.2. In autonomic neuropathy involving the parasympathetic system the ratio is less than 1.1. Similarly, the ratio at the
thirtieth beat after standing relative to that at the fifteenth beat should
be greater than 1.0. It is less than 1.0 in autonomic neuropathy. Diabetic
amyotrophy is likely a form of neuropathy, although atrophy and
weakness of the large muscles in the upper leg and pelvic girdle
resemble primary muscle disease. Anorexia and depression may accompany amyotrophy. Because of the weight loss, such patients are
often thought to have a paraneoplastic neuropathy.

Treatment of diabetic neuropathy is unsatisfactory in most respects. When pain is severe, it is easy for the patient to become
habituated or addicted to narcotics or powerful nonnarcotic analgesics
such as pentazocine. If the pain requires something stronger than
aspirin, acetaminophen, or other nonsteroidal anti-inflammatory

agents, codeine is the drug of choice. Phenytoin is used by some physicians, but others have not found it helpful. Combination therapy with amitriptyline and fluphenazine causes relief of pain in some patients and is worth trying. The recommended dosage is 75 mg amitriptyline at bedtime and 1 mg fluphenazine three times a day. Desipramine is as effective as amitriptyline; fluoxetine is no better than placebo. Mononeuropathies and radiculopathies usually require no specific therapy because they are self-limited. Diabetic diarrhea often responds to treatment with diphenoxylate and atropine or loperamide. Orthostatic hypotension is best treated by having the patient sleep with the head of the bed elevated, avoid sudden assumption of the upright position, and use full-length elastic stockings. Occasionally, volume expansion with fludrocortisone is required, as in other forms of orthostatic hypotension.

Experimental therapy with aldose reductase inhibitors and myoinositol has failed to provide significant clinical benefit, although enhanced regeneration of nerves has been reported in humans treated with an aldose reductase antagonist. Topical application of capsaicin is occasionally helpful with burning pain syndromes and hyperesthesia.

Diabetic Foot Ulcers A special problem in the diabetic patient is the development of ulcers of the feet and lower extremities. The ulcers appear to be due primarily to abnormal pressure distribution secondary to diabetic neuropathy. The problem is accentuated when there is bony distortion in the feet. Callus formation is usually the initial abnormality. Alternatively, the ulcer may be initiated by ill-fitting shoes that cause blister formation in patients whose sensory deficits preclude recognition of pain. Cuts and punctures from foreign bodies such as needles, tacks, and glass are common, and a foreign body of which the patient is unaware may be found in the soft tissue. For this reason, all patients with ulcers should have x-rays of the feet. Vascular disease with diminished blood supply contributes to development of ulcers, and infection is common, often with multiple organisms. While no specific therapy is available for diabetic ulcers, supportive treatment that minimizes weight bearing may make it possible to save the leg. One approach is simply to put the patient to bed, using hydrotherapy and debridement to remove nonviable tissue. Others recommend casting the leg with plaster to redistribute weight bearing and protect the lesion. Pending culture results, the initial antibiotic therapy for infected ulcers without systemic signs might be cefoxitin or ampicillin-sulbactam. If signs of sepsis are present, ampicillin-sulbactam plus gentamicin or aztreonam may be prescribed.

All patients should be instructed about proper foot care in an attempt to prevent ulcers. Feet should be kept clean and dry at all times. Patients with neuropathy should not walk barefoot, even in the home. Properly fitted shoes are essential. This is a particular problem with women, since an adequate shoe is not often stylish. The feet should be carefully inspected daily for callus, infection, abrasions, or blisters and the physician consulted about any potentially troublesome lesion. Transforming growth factor beta (TGFβ) improves the healing of decubitus ulcers and presumably would help for diabetic ulcers as well; it is not approved for clinical use.

What Causes the Complications of Diabetes? The cause of diabetic complications is not known and may be multifactorial. Major emphasis has been placed on the polyol pathway, wherein glucose is reduced to sorbitol by the enzyme aldol reductase. Sorbitol, which appears to function as a tissue toxin, has been implicated in the pathogenesis of retinopathy, neuropathy, cataracts, nephropathy, and aortic disease. The mechanism is perhaps best worked out in experimental diabetic neuropathy, where sorbitol accumulation is associated with a decrease in myoinositol content, abnormal phosphoinositide metabolism, and a decrease in Na^+,K^+-ATPase activity. In experimental models, the primacy of the polyol pathway in initiating neuropathy was proven by showing that inhibition of aldol reductase prevented the fall in tissue myoinositol content and the decrease in ATPase activity. Myoinositol deficiency was not found in sural nerve biopsy specimens from humans with diabetic neuropathy, in contrast to animals. Aldol reductase inhibition also has been shown to prevent experimental cataracts and retinopathy. It thus seems possible that neuropathy

and retinopathy are due primarily to activation of the polyol pathway. This pathway also may play a role in diabetic nephropathy.

A second mechanism of potential pathogenetic importance is glycation of proteins. (Current terminology uses *glycation* for nonenzymatic addition of hexoses to proteins and *glycosylation* for enzymatic addition.) The effect of such glycation on hemoglobin has been mentioned, but multiple proteins in the body are altered in the same way, often with disturbance of their function. Examples include plasma albumin, lens protein, fibrin, collagen, lipoproteins, and the glycoprotein recognition system of hepatic endothelial cells. Particularly intriguing is the effect of glycation on lipoproteins. Glycated LDL is not recognized by the normal LDL receptor, and its plasma half-life is increased. Conversely, glycated HDL turns over more rapidly than native HDL. It also has been reported that glycated collagen traps LDL at rates two to three times that of normal collagen.

Glycated collagen is less soluble and more resistant to degradation by collagenase than native collagen, but it is not clear that these changes are related either to the basement membrane thickening or to the tight, waxy skin syndrome with limited joint mobility (scleroderma-like) seen in some patients with IDDM (see "Miscellaneous Abnormalities," below). However, evidence that nonenzymatic glycation of protein plays a role in some degenerative complications is less direct than with the polyol pathway. Linkage between the polyol pathway and the glycation sequence occurs as a result of the glycation of collagen and other proteins by fructose generated from sorbitol. The rate of glycation with fructose is seven or eight times that with glucose.

Glycated proteins also form cross-linked proteins termed *advanced glycation end products* (AGE) through a series of biochemical reactions that are poorly understood. An intermediate in the cross-linking is 3-deoxyglucose, which can be derived from either glucose or fructose. Receptors for AGE are present on macrophages and endothelial cells. Binding of AGE to its receptors may induce the synthesis or release of cytokines, vascular adhesion molecules, endothelin-1, and tissue factor. The latter plays a preeminent role in the initiation of coagulation, as mentioned earlier. The AGE also destroy endothelial-derived nitric oxide. Experimentally, AGE formation may be impaired or prevented by aminoguanidine, an agent currently in clinical trials. In animals, it has a beneficial effect in prevention of retinopathy, nephropathy, and neuropathy. In the past it has been common to attribute *microvascular complications* (retinopathy, nephropathy, neuropathy) to the polyol pathway and *macrovascular complications* (stroke, gangrene, myocardial infarction) to glycation and AGE. However, both pathways contribute to both sets of complications.

Increased blood flow may play an initiating role in diabetic complications, possibly by increasing the filtration of macromolecules that function as tissue toxins. There is supportive evidence for a role of hyperperfusion in diabetic nephropathy, but the hemodynamic hypothesis does not appear as attractive as the first two.

Can Diabetic Complications Be Prevented by Meticulous Control of Diabetes? As mentioned earlier, the strongest evidence that the answer is yes comes from the DCCT. Additional clinical evidence supports the view that metabolic environment per se influences or causes complications independent of genetic factors. For example, kidneys from donors who have neither diabetes nor a family history of diabetes develop characteristic lesions of diabetic nephropathy within 3 to 5 years after transplantation into a diabetic recipient. In contrast, diabetic nephropathy did not develop when a kidney was transplanted into a diabetic subject whose disease had been reversed by pancreatic transplantation prior to renal transplantation. It also has been reported that kidneys manifesting diabetic nephropathy demonstrated reversal of the lesion when transplanted into normal recipients. All these findings suggest that hyperglycemia or some other aspect of the abnormal metabolism of diabetes causes or influences the development of complications; additional factors, probably genetic, must also play a role. This follows from the fact that diabetic subjects with decades of poor control may escape the ravages of the late complications and from the fact that typical diabetic complications may be found in patients at the time of diagnosis of diabetes or even in the absence of fasting hyperglycemia.

Meticulous control with insulin infusion pumps has been reported to decrease microalbuminuria, improve motor nerve conduction velocity, lower plasma lipoproteins, and decrease capillary leakage of fluorescein in the retina. The width of the capillary basement membrane in skeletal muscle also has been decreased. The changes are small in general, however, and of questionable biologic significance. Thus, firm evidence does not exist to show that late complications can be *reversed* by long-term return of the plasma glucose to near-normal levels. Retinopathy can progress despite successful reversal of diabetes by pancreatic transplantation. The progression of diabetic complications after the return of the plasma glucose level to normal or near normal has been termed *hyperglycemic memory*. The mechanism may be formation of advanced glycation end products during hyperglycemia, which, being irreversible, continue their effects over the long term.

The question of intensive therapy for all patients with diabetes remains open, because it is uncertain that the results achieved in the DCCT can be matched in the general population. Persons with diabetes are often cared for by nonspecialists who do not have access to teams of support personnel like the ones used in the DCCT. There is no question, however, but that the thrust of treatment should be toward tighter control.

Miscellaneous Abnormalities of Diabetes   Diabetes affects almost every system in the body. Space limitations preclude discussion of all associated features, but several deserve comment. *Infections* in persons with diabetes may not occur more frequently than in nondiabetics, but they tend to be more severe, possibly because of impaired leukocyte function, a frequent accompaniment of poor control. In addition to common infections of the skin, urinary tract, lungs, and bloodstream, four unusual infections appear to have a specific relationship with diabetes. *Malignant external otitis*, usually due to *Pseudomonas aeruginosa*, tends to occur in older patients and is characterized by severe pain in the ear, drainage, fever, and leukocytosis. Soft tissues around the ear are swollen and tender. A mound of granulation tissue is characteristically present internally at the junction of the osseous and cartilaginous portions of the ear. The facial nerve becomes paralyzed in half the cases, and other cranial nerves also may be involved. Facial nerve paralysis is a poor prognostic sign, and the mortality rate approximates 50 percent in this subset of patients. A 6-week course of ticarcillin or carbenicillin together with tobramycin is the treatment of choice. Ciprofloxacin, imipenem + cilastin, or third-generation parenteral antipseudomonal cephalosporin also may be used. Surgical debridement is often necessary. *Rhinocerebral mucormycosis* is a rare fungal infection that usually develops during or following an episode of diabetic ketoacidosis. Organisms are from the genera *Mucor, Rhizopus*, and *Absidia*. Onset is sudden, with periorbital and perinasal swelling, pain, bloody nasal discharge, and increased lacrimation. The nasal mucosa and underlying tissues become black and necrotic. Cranial nerve palsies and thrombosis of the internal jugular vein or sinuses of the brain may occur. Proptosis, chemosis, and retinal vein engorgement indicate cavernous sinus thrombosis. If the condition is untreated, death usually occurs in a week to 10 days. Amphotericin B and aggressive debridement are the indicated therapies. *Emphysematous cholecystitis* tends to affect diabetic men (in contrast to ordinary cholecystitis, a disease predominantly present in women). Gangrene of the gallbladder is 30 times more frequent than in the usual forms and accounts for high rates of perforation and higher mortality rates than in ordinary cholecystitis. Diagnosis is made when gas is seen in the gallbladder wall on plain films of the abdomen. Clostridial species are frequently cultured from bile, but other organisms may be present. Treatment is cholecystectomy and use of broad-spectrum antibiotics. Mezlocillin plus metronidazole provides adequate initial coverage. *Emphysematous pyelonephritis* is signaled by detection of gas in the kidney or perirenal space. Antibiotic therapy is usually ineffective,

and nephrectomy may be required. Mortality rates of 80 percent have been reported.

Hypertriglyceridemia is common in diabetes and is due both to overproduction of VLDL in the liver and to a disposal defect in the periphery. The latter is a consequence of a deficiency of lipoprotein lipase, an insulin-dependent enzyme. Some patients exhibit hyperlipidemia even when diabetic control is adequate; these patients likely have a primary familial hyperlipoproteinemia that is independent of diabetes. Patients who do not respond to insulin and dietary therapy should be treated for hypertriglyceridemia and hypercholesterolemia with drugs, as in nondiabetic subjects (see Chap. 341).

A variety of skin lesions occur in diabetes. *Necrobiosis lipoidica diabeticorum* is a plaquelike lesion with a central yellowish area surrounded by a brownish border. It is usually found over the anterior surfaces of the legs. Ulceration may occur. *Diabetic dermopathy* ("shin spots") is also usually located over the anterior tibial surface. The lesions are small, rounded plaques with a raised border; they may crust at the edges and ulcerate centrally. Several plaques may be arranged in linear fashion. Pigmentation is not prominent early, but as the lesion heals, a depressed scar occurs with diffuse brown discoloration. A rarer abnormality is *bullosis diabeticorum*. The bullae may be superficial, with mildly hemorrhagic or clear serum. The cause is unknown. *Infestations of the skin* with *Candida* and dermatophytes are common, and bacterial infections of a variety of types occur. In women, *vaginal moniliasis* may be troublesome during hyperglycemic-glycosuric periods. While the symptoms respond to nystatin or gentian violet, recurrence is inevitable unless glycosuria is reversed. *Atrophy of adipose tissue* may occur at the site of insulin injections, even with recombinant human insulin. *Hypertrophy* of fat also may occur, producing a lipoma-like lesion visible on physical examination.

Hyperviscosity occurs in diabetes, and *platelet aggregation* is enhanced, possibly owing to increased thromboxane synthesis. *Wound healing* is impaired in experimental diabetes, but this effect probably is not a major factor clinically. An interesting accompaniment of IDDM is the presence of *joint contractures* (Dupuytren's contractures) coupled with *tight, waxy skin* over the dorsum of the hands. The hands resemble those in patients with scleroderma. The cause of the tendon contractures is unknown, although alterations of cross-linking in collagen has been proposed. Patients with the syndrome of joint contractures and waxy skin appear to have accelerated development of other diabetic complications. *Scleredema* is a common finding in diabetes. This benign lesion is a thickening of the skin over the shoulders and upper back that resembles scleroderma.

Patients with diabetes may have additional illnesses. For example, there is a significant prevalence of eating disorders in young women with IDDM.

NONROUTINE THERAPIES   Transplantation with whole pancreas or pancreatic segments has cured diabetes but is usually performed only when kidney transplantation is required. There is no question that successful transplantation can return the blood glucose level to normal. If the kidney is transplanted simultaneously, immunosuppression is required, and the pancreatic transplantation is simply piggy-backed. The question of whether better diabetic control is worth the risks of immunosuppression when the pancreas alone is transplanted has not been addressed in clinical trials. Transplantation of islet cells (as opposed to whole pancreas) also has been attempted, but the results are poor. The use of nonpancreatic cells that have been genetically engineered to produce human insulin under glucose control is being studied.

Prevention of autoimmune diabetes by immunosuppressant agents is a desirable goal. Reversal of hyperglycemia without the need for insulin has been achieved in humans with new-onset diabetes using powerful drugs such as cyclosporine. The reversal is not permanent, however, and most physicians believe that prophylactic treatment with potent immunosuppressant agents is not warranted; i.e., the potential dangers are too great. Preventive trials are under way in which insulin is used as prophylaxis in subjects predicted to develop diabetes in the near future based on the presence of islet cell antibodies and diminished insulin response to an intravenous glucose load. Scattered positive results have been reported. Other trials are testing the effect of nicotinamide as a possible protective and repair agent.

INSULIN RESISTANCE Insulin resistance is defined arbitrarily as the requirement of 200 or more units of insulin per day to control hyperglycemia and prevent ketosis. Relative insulin resistance is present in most persons with diabetes when carefully sought using the glucose clamp technique. It is the consequence of near-complete insulin deficiency in IDDM, whereas in NIDDM the major cause is obesity.

The normal anabolic metabolism mediated by insulin requires the secretion of adequate amounts of insulin in response to meals. Insulin must then bind to a specific insulin receptor in target tissues (see Chap. 327). The insulin receptor is a tetrameric glycoprotein consisting of two α and two β subunits linked by disulfide bonds. The β subunit is a tyrosine kinase that is activated when insulin binds to the α subunit. The tyrosine kinase autophosphorylates the insulin receptor and initiates subsequent intracellular phosphorylations that mediate the multiple actions of insulin. The only such action that is reasonably understood is glucose transport. Glucose enters the cell by facilitated diffusion mediated by glucose transporter molecules. While some transporters are always present in the plasma membrane, the binding of insulin to the receptor initiates a rapid mobilization of intracellular stores of the transporter to the plasma membrane and activates units already in place. In poorly controlled diabetes, the number of stored transporters appears to be deficient.

Insulin resistance is characterized as *prereceptor* (abnormal insulin or anti-insulin antibodies), *receptor* (decreased receptor number or diminished binding of insulin), or *postreceptor* (abnormal signal transduction, especially failure to activate the receptor tyrosine kinase). Combinations may exist. The nature of the molecular defect is known in some forms of insulin resistance but has not been identified in many.

With full-blown insulin resistance (>200 units of insulin required per day), the problem is usually prereceptor resistance due to anti-insulin antibodies. Anti-insulin antibodies of the IgG class are present in most subjects within 60 days of the initiation of insulin therapy. The titer of these antibodies fluctuates for reasons that are not clear. Although the correlation between antibody titer and functional resistance is not close, binding of insulin by antibody is presumed to be the primary mechanism in most cases. Probably fewer than 0.1 percent of insulin-treated patients ever have significant resistance. The problem may appear within a few weeks of the start of therapy or many years later. The onset may be abrupt, resulting in ketoacidosis, but usually it is gradual, with uncontrollable hyperglycemia being the major problem. About 20 to 30 percent of patients have accompanying insulin allergy. Treatment requires glucocorticoids in large amounts—80 to 100 mg prednisone per day initially. Response often occurs in 48 to 72 h but may take longer. If no improvement has resulted after 3 to 4 weeks, it can be assumed that steroids will not be effective. Once insulin requirements begin to fall, the prednisone dosage can be decreased rapidly (by 10 to 20 mg every 3 to 7 days) until a maintenance level of 5 to 10 mg/d is reached. Maintenance therapy may be required for many months. Whether remission has occurred and therapy can be discontinued must be determined by trial. Sulfated insulin may be of benefit.

On rare occasions, insulin resistance appears to be due to enhanced destruction of the hormone at the subcutaneous injection site. Such patients tend to respond normally to insulin given intravenously or intraperitoneally. In some patients, addition of a protease inhibitor (aprotinin) to the insulin mixture is helpful. When resistance is extreme, U500 regular insulin should be used in order to control the volume of the injection.

Insulin resistance also occurs in the absence of overt diabetes. In such disorders, *acanthosis nigricans* is a physical sign of its presence. Acanthosis nigricans is a brown to black, velvety hyperpigmentation of the skin, usually present in the posterior and lateral folds of the neck, the axilla, groin, umbilicus, and other areas. Acanthosis nigricans occurred in about 7 percent of children in one study. The prevalence is higher in Hispanics and blacks than in whites. Although acanthosis nigricans may be a sign of occult malignancy, it is not associated with

neoplasia in the insulin-resistance states. A list of the major syndromes of insulin resistance is given in Table 334-12.

Obesity is the most common cause of insulin resistance. It is associated with decreased receptor number, but the major problem is at the postreceptor level, where there is apparently a failure to activate the tyrosine kinase. *Werner's syndrome* is an autosomal recessive illness with a high incidence of hyperglycemia despite elevated concentrations of plasma insulin. There is little response to exogenous hormone. Other features include growth retardation, alopecia or premature graying of the hair, cataracts, hypogonadism, leg ulcers, atrophy of muscle, fat, and bone, soft tissue calcification, and a high frequency of sarcomas and meningiomas.

Of the rare conditions associated with acanthosis nigricans, the variants associated with *insulin receptor abnormalities* have attracted the greatest interest. Type A patients are tall young women with a tendency to hirsutism and abnormalities of the reproductive tract who have polycystic ovaries or other causes of ovarian androgen excess. Many mutations in the insulin receptor have been found in patients with the type A syndrome, most of them interfering with the activity of the receptor by blocking or diminishing its tyrosine kinase activity. Type B subjects are older women with immunologic disease. The clinical picture includes arthralgias, alopecia, enlarged salivary glands, proteinuria, leukopenia, and antinuclear and anti-DNA antibodies. Insulin resistance in these patients is due to blocking antibodies directed against the insulin receptor (not against insulin itself). Interestingly, antireceptor antibodies on occasion may cause hypoglycemia. Whether agonist (hypoglycemia) or antagonist (insulin resistance) activity occurs presumably depends on the site of binding to the insulin receptor. Both A and B patients have high plasma insulin concentrations.

Generalized and *partial lipodystrophies* are fat depletion syndromes that differ primarily in the extent of fat atrophy (see Chap. 352). In the generalized form, essentially all body fat is missing, while the more common partial type exhibits atrophy of fat in the face and trunk with normal or increased adiposity in the lower half of the body. The disease can be either congenital or acquired. Typically, the patients develop hyperglycemia at puberty, but ketoacidosis never occurs. Marked hypertriglyceridemia with eruptive xanthoma is common. Characteristic features are hepatomegaly, splenomegaly, cardiomegaly, hirsutism, lymphadenopathy, hypertrophy of the external genitalia, varicose veins, and (in the congenital forms) muscle hypertrophy. Mental retardation is common, and renal disease may develop. The term *lipoatrophic diabetes* is synonymous with total lipodystrophy. All patients have elevated plasma insulin levels. Resistance may be due to a decreased number of receptors, diminished affinity of the receptor for insulin, or a postreceptor defect.

The *pineal hypertrophy syndrome* is characterized by insulin resistance, early dentition with malformed teeth, dry skin, thick nails, hirsutism, and a peculiar sexual precocity with enlargement of the external genitalia. The latter may reach near adult size by age 3 or 4.

Table 334-12

Insulin-Resistant States

Prereceptor Resistance
  Mutated insulins
Anti-insulin antibodies
Receptor and Postreceptor Resistance
  Obesity
  Type A syndrome (absent or dysfunctional receptor)
  Type B syndrome (antibody to insulin receptor)
  Lipodystrophic states (partial or generalized)
  Leprechaunism
  Ataxia-telangiectasia
  Rabson-Mendenhall syndrome
  Werner syndrome
  Alström syndrome
  Pineal hyperplasia syndrome

The insulin resistance is severe, and ketoacidosis may occur despite high endogenous insulin levels. The *Alström syndrome* is a rare autosomal recessive disease characterized by childhood blindness due to retinal degeneration, nerve deafness, vasopressin-resistant diabetes insipidus, and, in males, hypogonadism with high plasma gonadotropin levels. The patients thus appear to have end organ resistance to multiple hormones. Other features include baldness, hyperuricemia, hypertriglyceridemia, and aminoaciduria. Superficially, the patients may resemble subjects with the Laurence-Moon-Biedl syndrome but can be differentiated on initial examination by the absence of polydactyly and mental deficiency. Insulin resistance in the Alström syndrome is mild. *Ataxia-telangiectasia* is characterized by cerebellar ataxia, telangiectasia, a predisposition to breast cancer, and a variety of abnormalities in the immune system in addition to insulin resistance. The *Rabson-Mendenhall syndrome* consists of dental dysplasia, dystrophic nails, premature puberty, and acanthosis nigricans. The insulin resistance is probably due to an insulin receptor abnormality. *Leprechaunism* is characterized by an elfin appearance of the face, hirsutism, absence of subcutaneous fat, thickened skin, and insulin resistance. Defects are found in both the α and the β subunits of the insulin receptor, causing expression in plasma membranes to be markedly diminished. Not listed in Table 334-12 is insulin resistance due to hormone excess (acromegaly, Cushing's syndrome), myotonic dystrophy, and thalassemia major. The insulin resistance in these conditions usually is not clinically significant.

INSULIN ALLERGY Insulin allergy is due to IgE antibodies to insulin. Manifestations include immediate reactions with local stinging or itching, delayed local reactions with brawny swelling lasting up to 30 h, and generalized urticaria or frank anaphylaxis. Systemic reactions are usually seen in patients who have stopped insulin therapy for one reason or another and have then resumed treatment. The allergic reaction may occur as early as the second injection on resumption of therapy. Mild reactions can be treated with antihistamines. If the problem is severe, desensitization procedures are required. A 1-day insulin desensitization procedure is shown in Table 334-13. Once the patient is desensitized, insulin therapy should not be interrupted.

THE EMOTIONAL RESPONSE TO DIABETES It is difficult to accept that one has a chronic disease that requires a change in life-style. This is particularly true in the case of diabetes, since patients are usually aware that they are vulnerable to late complications and that their life expectancy is shortened. It is not surprising that the emotional response to diabetes often hampers treatment. The primary reaction can range from denial with an accompanying refusal to cooperate to excessive preoccupation with the illness. The physician should make every effort to bring the patient to a middle ground of acknowledging the disease and responding prudently without becoming obsessed. The goal is to live with diabetes, not for it. Patients with diabetes are no different from other patients, in that they may use their disease manipulatively with both family and physician. These problems are particularly acute with children and adolescents. While the psychiatric aspects of diabetes are not discussed here, most problems can be anticipated and handled if common sense is coupled with sympathy and firmness. It is also appropriate to offer cautious hope that the disease will be handled better in the future than is possible now.

Please refer to Chap. 60, Insulin, oral hypoglycemic agents, and the pharmacology of the endocrine pancreas, in Goodman & Gilman's The Pharmacological Basis of Therapeutics, *9th ed., New York, McGraw-Hill.*

BIBLIOGRAPHY

GENERAL REVIEW

UNGER RH, FOSTER DW: Diabetes mellitus, in *Williams' Textbook of Endocrinology*, 9th ed, JD Wilson, DW Foster (eds). Philadelphia, Saunders, 1997 (in press)

GENETICS AND PATHOGENESIS

ATKINSON MA, MACLAREN NK: The pathogenesis of insulin-dependent diabetes mellitus. N Engl J Med 331:1428, 1994

BINGLY PJ et al: Can we really predict IDDM? Diabetes 42:213, 1993

COUSTAN DR et al: Gestational diabetes: Predictors of subsequent disordered glucose metabolism. Am J Obstet Gynecol 168:1139, 1993

GHOSH S, SCHORK NJ: Genetic analysis of NIDDM. The study of quantitative traits. Diabetes 45:1, 1996

HAGOPIAN WA et al: Glutamate decarboxylase-, insulin-, and islet cell-antibodies and HLA typing to detect diabetes in a general population-based study of Swedish children. J Clin Invest 95:1505, 1995

HARRISON LC et al: MHC molecules and β-cell destructive immune and nonimmune mechanisms. Diabetes 38:815, 1989

HYÖTY H et al: A prospective study of the role of coxsackie B and other enterovirus infections in the pathogenesis of IDDM. Diabetes 44:652, 1995

PALMER JP, MCCULLOCH DK: Prediction and prevention of IDDM—1991. Diabetes 40:943, 1991

PERMUTT MA et al: Glucokinase and NIDDM: A candidate gene that paid off. Diabetes 41:1367, 1992

POLONSKY KS et al: Non-insulin-dependent diabetes mellitus—a genetically programmed failure of the beta cell to compensate for insulin resistance. N Engl J Med 334:777, 1996

PUGLIESE A et al: HLA-DQB1*0602 is associated with dominant protection from diabetes even among islet cell antibody-positive first-degree relatives of patients with IDDM. Diabetes 44:608, 1995

THAI AC, EISENBARTH GS: Natural history of IDDM. Diabetes Rev 1:1, 1993

UMPIERREZ GE et al: Diabetic ketoacidosis in obese African-Americans. Diabetes 44:790, 1995

DIABETIC COMPLICATIONS

AIELLO LP et al: Vascular endothelial growth factor in ocular fluid of patients with diabetic retinopathy and other retinal disorders. N Engl J Med 331:1480, 1994

BEISSWENGER PJ et al: Formation of immunochemical advanced glycosylation end products precedes and correlates with early manifestations of renal and retinal disease in diabetes. Diabetes 44:824, 1994

BORG WP et al: Local ventromedial hypothalamus glucopenia triggers counterregulatory hormone release. Diabetes 44:180, 1995

BOYLE PJ et al: Brain glucose uptake and unawareness of hypoglycemia in patients with insulin-dependent diabetes mellitus. N Engl J Med 333:1726, 1995

BROWNLEE M: Glycation products and the pathogenesis of diabetic complications. Diabetes Care 15:1835, 1992

FOSTER DW, MCGARRY JD: The metabolic derangements and treatment of diabetic ketoacidosis. N Engl J Med 309:159, 1983

KROLEWSKI AS et al: Glycosylated hemoglobin and the risk of microalbuminuria in patients with insulin-dependent diabetes mellitus. N Engl J Med 332:1251, 1995

LEURS PB et al: Tissue factor pathway inhibitor activity in patients with IDDM. Diabetes 44:80, 1995

PARTANEN J et al: Natural history of peripheral neuropathy in patients with non-insulin-dependent diabetes mellitus. N Engl J Med 333:89, 1995

SEQUIST ER et al: Familial clustering of diabetic renal disease: Evidence for genetic susceptibility and diabetic nephropathy. N Engl J Med 320:1161, 1989

SIPERSTEIN MD: Diabetic ketoacidosis and hyperosmolar coma. Endocrinol Metab Clin North Am 21:915, 1992

TOWLER DA et al: Mechanism of awareness of hypoglycemia. Perception of neurogenic (predominantly cholinergic) rather than neuroglycopenic symptoms. Diabetes 42:1791, 1993

Table 334-13

Insulin Desensitization*

Time, h	Dose, U	Route	Time, h	Dose, U	Route
0	0.001	Intradermal	3.5	0.2	Subcut.
0.5	0.002	Intradermal	4	0.5	Subcut.
1	0.004	Subcut.	4.5	1	Subcut.
1.5	0.01	Subcut.	5	2	Subcut.
2	0.02	Subcut.	5.5	4	Subcut.
2.5	0.04	Subcut.	6	8	Subcut.
3	0.1	Subcut.			

* Following desensitization, use 2 to 10 U of regular insulin every 4 to 6 h for 24 to 36 h after the 6-h injection before switching to intermediate-acting insulin.

SOURCE: *Schedule of JA Galloway.* For detailed information see JA Galloway, R Bressler, Med Clin North Am 62:663, 1978.

Viberti J et al: Diabetic nephropathy: Future avenue. Diabetes Care 15:1216, 1992

TREATMENT

AMERICAN DIABETES ASSOCIATION: Clinical Practice Recommendations 1996. Nutrition recommendations and principles for people with diabetes mellitus. Diabetes Care 19(Suppl 1):S16, 1996

BAILEY CJ et al: Metformin. N Engl J Med 334:574, 1996

CAMPBELL PJ, MAY ME: A practical guide to intensive insulin therapy. Am J Med Sci 310:24, 1995

RAVID M et al: Long-term stabilizing effect of angiotensin-converting enzyme inhibition on plasma creatinine and on proteinuria in normotensive type II diabetic patients. Ann Intern Med 118:577, 1993

ROBERTSON RP: Pancreatic and islet transplantation for diabetes—cures or curiosities? N Engl J Med 327:1861, 1992

SANTIAGO JV: Intensive management of insulin dependent diabetes: Risks, benefits, and unanswered questions. J Clin Endocrinol Metab 75:977, 1992

SKYLER JS: Insulin pharmacology. Med Clin North Am 72:1337, 1988

INSULIN RESISTANCE

FLIER JS: Syndromes of insulin resistance: From patient to gene and back again. Diabetes 41:1207, 1992

TAYLOR SI: Molecular mechanisms of insulin resistance: Lessons from patients with mutations in the insulin receptor gene. Diabetes 41:1473, 1992

335 *Daniel W. Foster, Arthur H. Rubenstein*

HYPOGLYCEMIA

Maintenance of the plasma glucose concentration within narrow bounds is essential for health. Hypoglycemia is dangerous (in the short run more so than hyperglycemia) because glucose is the primary energy substrate of the brain. Its absence, like that of oxygen, produces deranged function, tissue damage, and death if the deficit is prolonged. The brain is vulnerable to hypoglycemia because it cannot utilize circulating free fatty acids as an energy source, in contrast to other tissues. The short-chain fatty acid metabolites acetoacetate and β-hydroxybutyrate (*ketone bodies, ketoacids*) are oxidized by the brain and can protect it from damage by hypoglycemia when present at moderate concentrations in plasma. However, development of ketosis requires a number of hours so that ketogenesis is ineffective in protecting against acute hypoglycemia. Preservation of central nervous system function in the early phases of fasting and during hypoglycemia thus requires a prompt increase in the production of glucose by the liver. At the same time, glucose utilization by other tissues is diminished by the availability of free fatty acids as an alternative substrate. These adaptive mechanisms are hormonally controlled and are effective under ordinary circumstances. When the system breaks down or is overwhelmed, hypoglycemia occurs.

DEFENSE AGAINST HYPOGLYCEMIA   The hypoglycemic states can best be understood as derangements of normal fuel metabolism. Under ordinary circumstances, energy needs are met by exogenous substrate in the form of food. Oxidation of the constituent molecules of food to carbon dioxide and water generates adenosine triphosphate (ATP), the principal high-energy compound of the body. In one sense, life can be defined as the generation of ATP (and related high-energy nucleotides) for the preservation of cellular integrity. When caloric intake is greater than immediate oxidative needs, as after the usual meal, excess substrate is stored as fat, protein, and glycogen. In this *anabolic* phase of metabolism, the flux of substrate is from intestine to liver to utilization and storage sites. Insulin is the primary hormone mediating the anabolic phase, and counterregulatory hormone levels are suppressed.

The *catabolic* phase of metabolism begins about 5 to 6 h after a meal. Normally, the only significant catabolic period in the day is during the overnight fast, but under some circumstances, particularly serious illness, catabolic periods may be longer. During fasting/catabolism, the liver is activated to produce glucose and to maintain the plasma glucose level in a range safe for central nervous system func-

tion, and free fatty acids are mobilized to provide substrate for most other tissues of the body. Initially, glucose from the liver is derived almost exclusively from hepatic glycogen. However, since only about 70 g of glycogen are stored in the human liver, glycogenolysis ordinarily can sustain the plasma glucose only for 8 to 10 h. Exercise and the stress of severe illness may shorten this protective period. To compensate for glycogen depletion, gluconeogenesis increases early, with a flux of substrate from muscle and adipose tissue stores to liver and then to utilization sites.

The precursors for hepatic glucose synthesis (gluconeogenesis) are lactate/pyruvate and amino acids (primarily alanine and glutamine) derived from muscle and glycerol released from adipose tissue by lipolysis. Amino acids constitute the primary substrate for gluconeogenesis. Most of the lactate is recycled from preformed glucose (the *Cori cycle*), the only net contribution coming from the breakdown of muscle glycogen. Glycerol is initially a minor substrate but increases in importance with time. The liver is the primary source of glucose production after an overnight fast, but the kidney may contribute as much as half of glucose production in a prolonged fast, accounting for the frequent occurrence of hypoglycemia in renal failure. The rate of glucose production in the kidney is hormonally regulated, like that in the liver, and appears to be especially responsive to epinephrine. Proteolysis to provide amino acids for gluconeogenesis causes the negative nitrogen balance of starvation. The same mechanism is operative in the stress of trauma, surgery, and severe infection. In quantitative terms, the liver produces about 11 μmol/kg per minute (2 mg/kg per minute) of glucose in the initial phases of fasting. Higher rates of glucose production indicate increased utilization of glucose, an important consideration in the differential diagnosis of hypoglycemia.

The switch to fat metabolism is accomplished by activation in adipose tissue of the hormone-sensitive lipase, which hydrolyzes stored triglycerides to long-chain fatty acids and glycerol. The released fatty acids have two fates. Most (normally about 120 g/d) is used directly, and the remainder (about 40 g/d) is oxidized in the liver to acetoacetic and β-hydroxybutyric acids. Ketoacids can be used efficiently as an energy source by most tissues (liver uses them only minimally), but their primary importance is as backup substrate for the brain, as noted above. The shift of most tissues to lipid metabolism is important because the preferential oxidation of free fatty acids and ketones in place of glucose spares the latter for utilization by the central nervous system.

Catabolic metabolism is initiated by a fall in the concentration of insulin in plasma and secretion of the five counterregulatory hormones: glucagon, epinephrine, norepinephrine, cortisol, and growth hormone. Norepinephrine is released both from sympathetic neurons and from the adrenal medulla. Glucagon is the primary hormone of glucose maintenance, and epinephrine and norepinephrine play important backup roles. This backup function is particularly important in the defense against hypoglycemia in diabetes mellitus, where the glucagon response is lost early (see Chap. 334). Cortisol and growth hormone antagonize the action of insulin and promote the mobilization of substrate and activation of gluconeogenesis.

The anabolic and catabolic phases of metabolism are summarized in Table 335-1. Breakdown in any of the adaptive mechanisms can lead to hypoglycemia.

SYMPTOMATOLOGY   Symptoms of hypoglycemia fall into two main categories: those induced by *excessive secretion of epinephrine/norepinephrine (autonomic response)* and those due to *dysfunction of the central nervous system (neuroglycopenia)*. Rapid epinephrine release causes sweating, tremor, tachycardia, anxiety, and hunger. Central nervous system (CNS) symptoms worsen in severity with severe or prolonged hypoglycemia and include dizziness, headache, clouding of vision, blunted mental acuity, loss of fine motor skill, confusion, abnormal behavior, convulsions, and loss of consciousness. When the onset of hypoglycemia is gradual, the autonomic response may be masked so that CNS symptoms dominate the clinical picture. With a more rapid drop in plasma glucose (as in insulin reactions),

Table 335-1

The Feeding-Fasting Cycle

Phase	Primary Hormone	Plasma Substrates	Substrate Flux	Active Process
Anabolic*	Insulin	↑ Glucose ↑ Triglycerides ↑ Branched-chain amino acids ↓ Free fatty acids ↓ Ketones	Splanchnic bed → storage and utilization sites	Glycogen storage Protein synthesis Triglyceride formation
Catabolic†	Glucagon	↓ Glucose ↓ Triglycerides ↑ Alanine and glutamine‡ ↑ Free fatty acids ↑ Ketones	Storage sites → liver and utilization sites	Glycogenolysis Gluconeogenesis Proteolysis Lipolysis Ketogenesis

* Expected findings during the first several hours after ingestion of a mixed meal of fat, carbohydrate, and protein.
† The major daily catabolic phase occurs during the overnight fast, although partial catabolic cycles occur between meals.
‡ Arrows indicate plasma concentrations except for alanine and glutamine. While arterial concentrations of these amino acids are relatively constant, uptake by the liver and intestine is increased in the catabolic phase.

autonomic symptoms are prominent. In the diabetic subject, autonomic symptoms may not be manifest if severe neuropathy is present or if the syndrome of hypoglycemia unawareness is present.

The literature concerning the level of plasma glucose required to activate hormonal defenses and to produce symptoms is confusing because in many experimental studies, glucose is measured in "arterialized" venous blood samples (drawn from a hand vein in a heated box), while in clinical practice, glucose ordinarily is measured in plain venous blood, where its level may be as much as 1 mmol/L (18 mg/dL) lower than in an equivalent arterialized sample. Recognizable symptoms occur in persons without diabetes when the venous plasma glucose concentration falls below 2.5 mmol/L (45 mg/dL) if the plasma glucose is lowered acutely, as by insulin injection. With acute hypoglycemia, progressive defense responses occur as the glucose level falls. In one study (using arterialized venous samples), insulin secretion ceased at 4.6 mmol/L glucose (83 mg/dL), and glucagon and epinephrine were released at 3.8 mmol/L (68 mg/dL), growth hormone at 3.7 mmol/L (67 mg/dL), and cortisol at 3.2 mmol/L (58 mg/dL). Thus, protective mechanisms are activated before the symptomatic threshold is reached. Although overt symptoms are not present, CNS function may be impaired with minimal decrements of plasma glucose. In a study utilizing auditory evoked potentials as a sensitive indicator of CNS function, abnormalities were seen in normal persons with a drop of glucose in arterialized venous blood from 4.8 to 4.0 mmol/L (87 to 72 mg/dL). When blood glucose was sustained at 4.0 mmol/L (72 mg/dL), counterregulatory release eventually occurred (at 2 to 3 h) despite the fact that no symptoms were produced. Major CNS dysfunction may not develop until plasma glucose concentrations approximate 1 mmol/L (20 mg/dL) because cerebral blood flow increases enough to deliver some glucose to the brain even when glucose levels are low. Cerebral atherosclerosis, which reduces the elasticity of the nonelastic blood vessels, compromises this protective mechanism so that symptomatic distress occurs at higher glucose levels. Symptoms (autonomic or neuroglycopenic) due to hypoglycemia are unlikely to occur at a plasma glucose level above 2.8 mmol/L (50 mg/dL) in nondiabetic persons. As noted above, subtle CNS dysfunction occurs at higher glucose levels. Patients with poorly controlled diabetes mellitus appear to develop hypoglycemic symptoms at higher glucose concentrations than nondiabetic individuals, and patients with meticulously controlled diabetes have a lower symptomatic threshold and may exhibit the syndrome of *hypoglycemia unawareness* (see Chap. 334). In hypoglycemia unawareness the thresholds are reversed so that the autonomic response is not activated before the onset of neuroglycopenic symptoms. Some patients with insulinoma also have a lowering of the glucose threshold at which release of counterregulatory hormones is induced and thus experience hypoglycemia unawareness.

A rare syndrome that mimics the CNS manifestations of hypoglycemia has been described in which blood glucose is normal but the glucose level in cerebrospinal fluid (CSF) is low, presumably owing to a defect in the glucose transporter molecule GLUT 1. Seizures may result.

CLASSIFICATION It is traditional to classify hypoglycemia as either *postprandial* (reactive) or *fasting*. Pathologically low plasma glucose concentrations occur in the former type only in response to meals, while in the latter type they occur only after hours of fasting. Patients with fasting hypoglycemia (particularly those with insulinomas) may exhibit a reactive component, but reactive patients do not have symptoms when food is withdrawn. Fasting hypoglycemia usually means that a disease process is responsible, but symptoms suggestive of postprandial hypoglycemia may occur in the absence of recognizable disease.

CAUSES OF HYPOGLYCEMIA

Postprandial Hypoglycemia The most common cause of postprandial hypoglycemia is alimentary hyperinsulinism (Table 335-2). Patients who have undergone gastrectomy, gastrojejunostomy, pyloroplasty, or vagotomy are subject to hypoglycemia after meals, presumably because of rapid gastric emptying, brisk absorption of glucose, and excessive insulin release. Glucose levels fall more rapidly than insulin levels under these circumstances, and insulin-glucose imbalance leads to hypoglycemia. Ingestion of fructose or galactose causes hypoglycemia in children with fructose intolerance or galactosemia. Leucine intake rarely causes the syndrome in susceptible infants. The early phase of diabetes mellitus is usually listed as a cause of reactive hypoglycemia, but in our experience symptomatic hypoglycemia as a premonitory symptom of diabetes is uncommon. Prediabetics, who by definition are normoglycemic, may have a late fall in plasma glucose after oral glucose tolerance testing, but this pattern is similar to that frequently present in asymptomatic, healthy individuals (see below).

Idiopathic alimentary hypoglycemia consists of two syndromes: *true hypoglycemia* and *pseudohypoglycemia*. In the former, adrenergic symptoms appear postprandially and are accompanied by a low plasma glucose level. Symptoms appear spontaneously during everyday life and are relieved by ingestion of carbohydrate, which raises the plasma glucose. Such patients are rare. The mechanism of this disorder is unknown, although subtle dysfunction of the gastrointestinal tract might be operative. Some patients with true postprandial hypoglycemia turn out to have insulinomas (see below).

In pseudohypoglycemia, adrenergic symptoms suggestive of hypoglycemia appear 2 to 5 h after a meal, but plasma glucose concentrations are normal when symptoms are present. The condition is often self-diagnosed and "confirmed" when a 5-h glucose tolerance test reveals a lower than "normal" plasma glucose between 2 and 5 h.

Two questions have to be asked about pseudohypoglycemia. First, what causes the symptoms (which may be incapacitating)? Second, can a valid diagnosis of hypoglycemia be made by a glucose tolerance test? The symptoms of nervousness, weakness, tremor, tachycardia, dizziness, and sweating in this disorder are probably due to epinephrine release. Many normal people experience similar symptoms at some time in their lives and may even have gained relief by eating. Patients with pseudohypoglycemia, in contrast, develop the symptoms regularly and repetitively. In one study, 80 consecutive subjects with reproducible postprandial symptoms were studied by 5-h glucose tolerance testing. Hypoglycemia was considered to be present if (1) the plasma glucose fell below 3.3 mmol/L (60 mg/dL) during the test; (2) symptoms or signs compatible with hypoglycemia were present; and (3) at least a doubling of the plasma cortisol level occurred 30 to 90 min

Table 335-2

Causes of Postprandial (Reactive) Hypoglycemia

Alimentary hyperinsulinism	Leucine sensitivity
Hereditary fructose intolerance	Idiopathic
Galactosemia	

after the nadir of plasma glucose (indicating hypoglycemia severe enough to activate the hypothalamic-pituitary-adrenal axis). Only 18 of the 80 (23 percent) subjects whose history suggested postprandial hypoglycemia fulfilled these criteria. Twenty-five percent of asymptomatic matched normal controls also met all three criteria. When the patients and controls were tested after a mixed meal, no subject in either group had a plasma glucose below 3.3 mmol/L (60 mg/dL), yet 14 of the 18 patients (78 percent) had symptoms typical of those after glucose tolerance testing. The absence of hypoglycemia after mixed meals despite the presence of typical symptoms has been observed in other studies. *Pseudohypoglycemia* appears to be an accurate descriptive term for the syndrome and is preferable to "idiopathic postprandial syndrome," which also has been used. Many such patients are thought to have stress or anxiety as a predisposing factor. Presumably they have enhanced catecholamine release following a meal, or they may be abnormally sensitive to normal postprandial norepinephrine/epinephrine release. Insulin can stimulate epinephrine release in humans even if hypoglycemia is prevented. Whether enhanced insulin release plays a role in the pseudohypoglycemia syndrome is not known.

Fasting Hypoglycemia The causes of fasting hypoglycemia are many, but in all instances there is an imbalance between the production of glucose by the liver and its utilization in peripheral tissues. In some patients, hypoglycemia is due primarily to a defect in glucose production, while in others, the problem is excess glucose utilization. Both defects may be present. For example, with insulin excess enhanced glucose utilization is coupled with blunted hepatic glucose production. The latter is caused by blockade by insulin of the glycogenolytic/gluconeogenic effects of the counterregulatory hormones. Dual defects are probably operative in disorders of fat oxidation and non-insulin-producing tumors as well.

Supply-side hypoglycemia (*impaired production of glucose*) characteristically requires much less glucose during therapy than does demand-side hypoglycemia (*overutilization of glucose*) (Table 335-3). As noted above, in normal people glucose production during a fast approximates 11 μmol/kg per minute (2 mg/kg per minute), but with insulin-induced hypoglycemia, glucose utilization increases to about 67 μmol/kg per minute (12 mg/kg per minute). Thus, if more than 56 mmol (10 g) of glucose per hour is required to prevent or reverse hypoglycemia, it can be assumed that overutilization is present.

Underproduction of glucose As discussed earlier, the production of glucose by the liver initially involves breakdown of stored glycogen and subsequent gluconeogenesis, the synthesis of glucose from precursors delivered to the liver from peripheral tissues. Inadequate production of glucose during fasting can be due to five causes: (1) hormone deficiency, (2) defects in glycogenolytic or gluconeogenic enzymes, (3) inadequate substrate delivery, (4) liver disease, and (5) drugs. Hypopituitarism and adrenal insufficiency are the common hormonal causes of hypoglycemia. Defects in catecholamine or glucagon release are rare. Enzymatic abnormalities causing hypoglycemia are usually seen in children and not adults. Glucose-6-phosphatase deficiency is the classic example of a defect in glycogen breakdown, but hypoglycemia may occur in young children with deficiencies of hepatic glycogen phosphorylase and in other forms of glycogen storage disease (Chap. 347). The inability to make glycogen because of inadequate glycogen synthase activity also renders infants susceptible to fasting hypoglycemia. In addition to glucose-6-phosphatase, three other enzymes are necessary for gluconeogenesis: pyruvate carboxylase, phosphoenolpyruvate carboxykinase, and fructose-1,6-bisphosphatase (fructose-1,6-diphosphatase) (Fig. 335-1). Hypoglycemia can occur when any of these enzymes is deficient, often with associated lactic acidosis. The cause of lactic acidosis in this situation is not known, although impaired hepatic lactate uptake due to the gluconeogenic defect probably plays a role. Substrate deficiency appears to be one of the causes of ketotic hypoglycemia of infancy, since alanine turnover in such patients is low. Inadequate substrate supply also may contribute to hypoglycemia in malnutrition, muscle-wasting states, chronic renal failure, and late pregnancy. Acquired liver disease can cause serious hypoglycemia. Hepatic congestion due to right-sided heart failure is particularly troublesome, and severe viral hepatitis or cirrhosis also

can cause hypoglycemia. Hypothermia, especially in association with alcohol ingestion, may cause very low levels of plasma glucose. Slowed enzymatic activity of the liver is the likely mechanism. The hypoglycemia of renal failure has multiple causes. Some patients have diminished release of alanine (and possibly of glutamine) from muscle, and uremic toxins may suppress hepatic gluconeogenesis. With end-stage renal disease, diminished kidney mass decreases the capacity for renal gluconeogenesis. Decreased insulin clearance, although present, is not thought to play a major role.

A number of drugs, in addition to insulin and sulfonylureas, cause hypoglycemia. Alcohol induces hypoglycemia only after a period of fasting sufficient to deplete liver glycogen stores. In this circumstance, hepatic glucose production is dependent on gluconeogenesis. The oxidation of ethanol in the liver generates high concentrations of NADH, the reduced form of nicotinamide adenine dinucleotide (NAD). The increased NADH/NAD ratio diverts oxaloacetate into malate formation, diminishing its availability to the gluconeogenic sequence via the action of phosphoenolpyruvate carboxykinase (see Fig. 335-1). Gluconeogenesis from pyruvate is thus blocked, leading to decreased hepatic glucose output and hypoglycemia. Large amounts of ethanol are not required to produce this syndrome, and plasma alcohol concentrations may be as low as 5.4 mmol/L (25 mg/dL) when symptoms occur. Ethanol-induced hypoglycemia usually occurs in adults but can occur in children who drink alcohol unknowingly. Many reports of the association between hypoglycemia and drugs are probably due to chance occurrence. Pentamidine, sulfonamides, salicylates (usually in children), propranolol, and quinine probably do cause hypoglycemia rarely. Pentamidine (no longer used commonly for prevention of *Pneumocystis* pneumonia in AIDS patients) induces β-cell cytolysis ("insulin leak"). The mechanism by which sulfonamides and salicylates induce hypoglycemia is unclear but may involve interaction of the agents with the sulfonylurea receptor (see below). Quinine has been reported to cause hyperinsulinemic hypoglycemia, but the issue

Table 335-3

Major Causes of Fasting Hypoglycemia

PRIMARILY DUE TO IMPAIRED PRODUCTION OF GLUCOSE

Hormone deficiencies	**Liver disease**
Hypopituitarism	Hepatic congestion
Adrenal insufficiency	Severe hepatitis
Catecholamine deficiency	Cirrhosis
Glucagon deficiency	Uremia (probably multiple
Enzyme defects	mechanisms)
Glucose-6-phosphatase	Hypothermia
Liver phosphorylase	**Drugs**
Pyruvate carboxylase	Alcohol
Phosphoenolpyruvate carboxykinase	Propranolol
Fructose-1,6-bisphosphatase	Salicylates
Glycogen synthetase	
Substrate deficiency	
Ketotic hypoglycemia of infancy	
Severe malnutrition, muscle wasting	
Late pregnancy	

PRIMARILY DUE TO OVERUTILIZATION OF GLUCOSE

Hyperinsulinism
Insulinoma
Exogenous insulin
Sulfonylureas
Immune disease with insulin or insulin receptor antibodies
Drugs: quinine in falciparum malaria, disopyramide, pentamidine
Sepsis
Appropriate insulin levels
Extrapancreatic tumors
Systemic carnitine deficiency
Deficiency in enzymes of fat oxidation
3-Hydroxy-3-methylglutaryl-CoA lyase deficiency
Cachexia with fat depletion

FIGURE 335-1 Scheme of hepatic carbohydrate metabolism. Only the sequences for gluconeogenesis, glycogen synthesis, and glycogenolysis are shown.

is clouded, because hypoglycemia also occurs in untreated malaria, possibly owing to malnutrition, liver involvement, or cytokine release.

Overutilization of glucose Overutilization of glucose occurs in two settings: when hyperinsulinism is present and when plasma insulin concentrations are low. There are four causes of hyperinsulinemic hypoglycemia: insulinoma, administration of exogenous insulin or of sulfonylureas, and a peculiar form of insulin autoimmunity. *Insulinoma* is used generically here to include single solid tumors, microadenomatosis, and islet cell hyperplasia (nesidioblastosis), a rare syndrome in adults. Familial hyperinsulinemic hypoglycemia of infancy is due to a gain-of-function mutation in the sulfonylurea receptor that causes constitutive, unregulated insulin secretion. Hypoglycemia in a diabetic taking prescribed insulin or oral agents is not a diagnostic problem. The difficulty occurs when a nondiabetic individual induces hypoglycemia deliberately and surreptitiously because of psychiatric disturbance, raising the possibility of an insulin-producing tumor. The diagnostic differentiation of insulinoma and factitious hypoglycemia is considered below. Rarely, hypoglycemia with hyperinsulinism is due to antibodies to endogenous insulin. The mechanisms underlying hypoglycemia in the latter condition are not well understood, although the most important is probably dissociation of free insulin from hormone-antibody complexes at inappropriate times. Idiotypic antibodies (antibodies against the anti-insulin antibodies) also might function as insulin agonists with the insulin receptor. By binding insulin, the antibodies also may induce excessive release of insulin from the pancreas. Some patients have alternating insulin resistance/hyperglycemia and hypoglycemia. Insulin autoantibodies have been seen most frequently in subjects with hyperthyroidism treated with methimazole but presumably can occur in any autoimmune syndrome. Antibodies directed against the insulin receptor, usually a cause of insulin resistance, also may induce hypoglycemia with high plasma insulin levels. Under these circumstances, the configuration of the antibody is thought to allow it to activate the insulin receptor, simultaneously blocking the clearance of insulin.

Sepsis with endotoxinemia causes hyperglycemia followed by hypoglycemia in experiment animals. Enhanced insulin release is thought to be caused by sepsis-associated cytokine release, probably acting directly on the β cells.

Hypoglycemia in the context of glucose overutilization and appropriately low plasma insulin concentrations occurs in two situations. The first is in association with solid extrapancreatic tumors, usually fibromas and sarcomas of large size but occasionally hepatomas, carcinomas of the gastrointestinal tract, renal cell carcinomas, or adrenal cancers. The mechanism of the hypoglycemia is not clear, although high levels of insulin-like growth factor (IGF)-2 are believed to play a role. The physiologic role of IGF-2 is not completely understood, although it is associated with organ hypertrophy (e.g., Beckwith-Wiedemann syndrome) and appears to function as an oncogene in Wilms' tumor of the kidney. IGF-2 could cause hypoglycemia through its own receptor or by interacting with the insulin receptor. One patient with tumor-associated hypoglycemia was reported to have an increased number of insulin receptors in liver, muscle, and circulating mononuclear cells, but the significance of the finding is not clear.

Hypoglycemia due to overutilization also may occur when fatty acids and ketones are not available for oxidation in muscle and other tissues. Patients with *systemic carnitine deficiency* can have severe hypoglycemia. In this condition, the level of carnitine, a metabolite that is necessary for the transportation of fatty acids into mitochondria for oxidation, is low in plasma, muscle, liver, and other tissues. As a consequence, peripheral tissues cannot utilize fatty acids for energy production, and the liver cannot make ketone bodies as alternative substrate. The result is that all tissues become glucose-dependent, and the liver's capacity to meet the demand is exceeded. Other features of systemic carnitine deficiency include nausea, vomiting, elevated blood ammonia levels, and hepatic encephalopathy. The illness thus constitutes one form of the Reye syndrome. (In *myopathic carnitine deficiency*, only muscle is involved, and a polymyositis-like syndrome without hypoglycemia is produced.) Nonketotic (or hypoketotic) hypoglycemia with secondary systemic carnitine deficiency and the Reye syndrome also accompany *deficiencies of medium- and long-chain acyl-CoA dehydrogenases and 3-hydroxy-3-methylglutaryl-CoA (HMG-CoA) lyase*. The first two enzymes operate in the fatty acid oxidative sequence, while HMG-CoA lyase catalyzes the conversion of HMG-CoA to acetoacetate and acetyl-CoA in the ketogenic cycle. Any time there is a block in fatty acid oxidation or ketone formation, a secondary carnitine deficiency may develop. Accumulated acyl-CoA is transesterified to form acyl carnitine, which is then lost in the urine. Systemic carnitine deficiency in the absence of an enzymic defect probably is due to a primary renal leak. It is not known whether the block in ketone production per se leads to hypoglycemia or whether secondary carnitine deficiency is required. If the former is the case, ketones must become a primary (necessary) substrate during an extended fast. Hypoglycemia is less common with deficiency of *carnitine palmitoyltransferases*. Presumably, the defect is not complete in most patients, so that some fatty acid oxidation occurs, and the tendency to hypoglycemia is minimized. The clinical picture is that of an exercise-induced myopathy with myoglobinuria. Hypoglycemia also occurs in patients with cachexia due to advanced cancer. At autopsy, no recognizable triglyceride stores are present in adipose tissue, suggesting that free fatty acid deficiency is the primary mechanism.

Hypoglycemia in Hospitalized Patients The frequency of this diagnosis varies in different series of hospitalized patients. Drugs are the most common cause, the three drugs most frequently implicated being insulin, sulfonylureas, and alcohol. It has been estimated that one of these three agents is involved in about 60 percent of the instances in which hypoglycemia is diagnosed in this population. Other causes include renal failure (about 15 percent), liver disease (about 15 percent), malnutrition (about 10 percent), and sepsis (about 5 percent). The finding of hypoglycemia in nondiabetic persons without uremia, liver disease, cachexia, or a history of alcohol intake should raise a high index of suspicion for insulinoma, solid tumors, enzymatic defects, or hormonal deficiencies.

DIAGNOSIS Fasting Hypoglycemia If a person with diabetes mellitus presents with symptoms of hypoglycemia, it is usually safe to conclude that no special diagnostic tests are needed because such hypoglycemia is almost always related to therapy. If a nondiabetic develops similar symptoms—particularly if confusion, loss of consciousness, or convulsions are present—a diagnostic workup is required. If the patient is seen in the office or emergency room with symptoms compatible with hypoglycemia, blood should be drawn for a glucose and hormone assay before intravenous glucose is administered. *The ideal time for a diagnosis is during an episode of spontaneous hypoglycemia.* The goal is to assess the plasma insulin level and the counterregulatory hormone response while the plasma glucose level is low. Assays should be carried out for glucose, insulin, insulin-connecting peptide (C peptide), cortisol, drugs, and toxins, especially sulfonylureas and alcohol. It is often wise to freeze a separate sample of plasma for subsequent tests (for example, for proinsulin, carnitine, insulin antibodies, or lactate) should the diagnosis not be clear from the initial evaluation. Demonstration that hypoglycemia is accompanied by inappropriate insulin levels sharply narrows the clinical possibilities.

If the patient is not seen during a hypoglycemic episode, the approach is somewhat different. The pattern of symptomatic episodes should be ascertained with an emphasis on the relation to food intake and the timing of symptom development (namely, during or after the overnight fast or after daytime meals). Obtaining a medication history is essential. Signs of heart failure and hepatic congestion should be sought, and the presence and thickness of the adipose tissue mass should be noted. Pigmentation of the skin may suggest adrenal insufficiency. The workup includes liver function studies and computed tomography (CT) or abdominal sonography (to look for solid tumors in the retroperitoneal space or abdominal cavity). Patients with enzyme defects and rare hormonal deficiencies (epinephrine, glucagon) usually require evaluation in referral centers, since assays for these hormones and enzymes are not routinely available. If hypoglycemia is severe or prolonged in a hospitalized patient, it is important to quantitate the amount of glucose required to prevent recurrent hypoglycemia during acute-phase therapy; if 8 to 10 g of glucose per hour is sufficient to prevent hypoglycemia, diminished glucose production is probably operative. A requirement for infusion rates higher than that suggests enhanced glucose utilization.

If the patient has a history compatible with recurrent unexplained hypoglycemia but does not have symptoms at the time of examination, hospitalization for fasting has traditionally been required. The fast should be carried out for at least 72 h unless symptoms develop. Plasma glucose, insulin, C peptide, and cortisol should be measured every 6 h. Occasionally, quantitation of plasma free fatty acids, glucagon, and total ketones is helpful. (For the glucagon assay, a protease inhibitor such as aprotinin must be added.) Two points are at issue. First, does the patient have fasting hypoglycemia? Second, is the hypoglycemia associated with hyperinsulinism? Neither question is easy to answer. There is no definitive lower limit of plasma glucose that unequivocally defines pathologic hypoglycemia during a 72-h fast. Values of the nadir in one study are shown in Table 335-4. Women usually develop lower levels than men. Another series reported mean minimal levels of 3.4 mmol/L (62 mg/dL) in men and 2.9 mmol/L (52 mg/dL) in women during a 72-h fast. However, values as low as 1.2 mmol/L (22 mg/dL) may occur in normal women without symptoms. On balance, a presumptive diagnosis of hypoglycemia is probably justified if the plasma glucose falls below 2.5 mmol/L (45 mg/dL) in venous blood at any time during the fast, provided typical symptoms are induced. The diagnosis of hypoglycemia is strengthened if symptoms are rapidly relieved by administration of glucose. If symptoms do not occur during a 72-h fast, the diagnosis of hypoglycemia should be made with caution.

Insulin measurements are not always helpful in diagnosing hyperinsulinism. In normal subjects when glucose concentrations rise, insulin levels also increase, and when plasma glucose concentrations fall, insulin release is inhibited. This relationship means that plasma insulin concentrations must be interpreted in the light of the simultaneously determined glucose value. Thus, a "nor-mal" insulin level may be abnormal in the face of hypoglycemia, while high levels may be appropriate if the glucose level is elevated.

Plasma insulin levels generally reach background values for the assay when the plasma glucose falls below about 4.6 mmol/L (83 mg/dL), as noted earlier. While some studies have shown lower cutoff points, any measurable insulin level should probably be considered suspicious if the venous plasma glucose is below 2.5 mmol/L (45 mg/dL). If hyperinsulinism is not present, another cause of fasting hypoglycemia must be sought.

Some investigators screen for insulinoma in the outpatient setting. The C peptide suppression test is based on the fact that suppression of the release of endogenous insulin and C peptide during insulin infusion is impaired in persons with insulinomas. The results are influenced by age and obesity. Less well standardized tests involve intravenous tolbutamide infusion and rigorous exercise in the fasted state. However, the 72-h fast remains the gold standard when the patient cannot be studied during a spontaneous episode of hypoglycemia.

If hypoglycemia does not develop during fasting, an insulinoma or other hypoglycemia-producing organic disease is unlikely, although in rare cases (<2 percent) an insulinoma does not cause hypoglycemia during a prolonged fast. Insulinomas rarely cause only postprandial hypoglycemia. The diagnosis usually is suspected in such cases because insulin levels are inappropriately high during the postmeal episodes.

Postprandial Hypoglycemia In patients presumed to have postprandial hypoglycemia, the most widely used test in the past was the 5-h oral glucose tolerance test. Since normal persons may have chemical hypoglycemia without symptoms in the glucose tolerance test and since subjects with pseudohypoglycemia have symptoms in the absence of hypoglycemia following meals, the 5-h glucose tolerance test should be abandoned as a tool for diagnosis. The only unequivocal diagnostic test for true pseudohypoglycemia is the demonstration of a low plasma glucose concentration (less than 2.5 mmol/L, or 45 mg/dL) during the occurrence of spontaneous symptoms. Some physicians use a home glucose analyzer in diagnosis. If no hypoglycemia is demonstrated during 1 week of testing (on arising, 2 h after each meal, at bedtime, and during symptoms), the diagnosis of true postprandial hypoglycemia is rejected. Most authors consider home testing unreliable because of measurement inaccuracies in the hypoglycemic range. Patients with pseudohypoglycemia usually have slightly elevated glucose concentrations during spontaneous attacks because of the hyperglycemic action of epinephrine, the stress hormone that induces the symptoms.

Insulinoma versus Factitious Hypoglycemia The self-induction of hypoglycemia by the injection of insulin or the ingestion of sulfonylureas is probably as common as insulinoma. Therefore, the demonstration of hyperinsulinism during hypoglycemia is not definitive evidence for an islet cell tumor. Factitious disease should be suspected when hypoglycemic symptoms appear in medical personnel or relatives of diabetic patients. Several tests are helpful in distinguishing insulinoma from factitious hypoglycemia once hyperinsulinism is established. Patients with insulinoma tend to have high concentrations of proinsulin in plasma (>20 percent of total insulin). Plasma proinsulin is not elevated by the administration of insulin or sulfonylureas.

Table 335-4

Mean Plasma Glucose and Insulin during Fasting in Normal Individuals

Assay	Subjects	Hours of Fast				
		0*	24	36	48	72
Glucose, mmol/L (mg/dL)	Men	4.7 (85)	4.6 (83)	4.3 (78)	4.3 (78)	3.9 (71)
	Women	4.6 (83)	3.5 (63)	2.8 (50)	2.6 (46)	2.7 (48)
Insulin, pmol/L (μU/mL)	Men	100 (14)	64 (9)	57 (8)	57 (8)	43 (6)
	Women	86 (12)	43 (6)	29 (4)	21 (3)	29 (4)

* Zero values were obtained after overnight fast. Results are mean values for 20 normal men and 60 normal women.
SOURCE: TJ Merimee, JE Tyson, Diabetes 26:161, 1977.

Table 335-5

Differential Diagnosis of Insulinoma and Factitious Hyperinsulinism

Test	Insulinoma	Exogenous Insulin	Sulfonylurea
Plasma insulin	High	Very high*	High
Insulin/glucose ratio	High	Very high	High
Proinsulin	Increased	Normal or low	Normal
C peptide	Increased	Normal or low†	Increased
Insulin antibodies	Absent	± Present‡	Absent
Plasma or urine sulfonylurea	Absent	Absent	Present

* Total plasma insulin in patients with insulinoma is rarely above 1435 pmol/L (200 μU/mL) in the basal state and often is much lower. Values greater than 7175 pmol/L (1000 μU/mL) are highly suggestive of exogenous insulin injection.
† C-peptide level may be normal in absolute terms but low in relation to the increased insulin value. See text for C-peptide suppression test.
‡ Insulin antibodies may not be present if only a few injections have been given, especially with purified insulin.

Measurement of the C-peptide level will indicate whether plasma insulin is of endogenous or exogenous origin. When insulin is cleaved from its precursor proinsulin molecule, C peptide is released into the portal vein in a 1:1 ratio with insulin. Thus, in patients with insulinoma, C-peptide levels should parallel plasma insulin values. The characteristic pattern in factitious hypoglycemia due to insulin injection is a high level of plasma insulin and a low plasma level of C peptide, because exogenous insulin, which does not contain C peptide, suppresses endogenous insulin release in normal persons, as described earlier. Antibodies to insulin are helpful if present because they usually indicate chronic insulin injection. Sulfonylureas elevate the concentrations of both C peptide and insulin in plasma. Therefore, factitious hypoglycemia due to oral agents can only be diagnosed by a high index of suspicion coupled with assay of the drug in plasma or urine. The features of insulinoma and the two types of factitious hypoglycemia are shown in Table 335-5.

℞ TREATMENT

The initial treatment of serious hypoglycemia (producing confusion or coma) is the intravenous administration of a bolus of 25 or 50 g glucose as a 50% solution followed by constant infusion of glucose until the patient is able to eat a meal. The importance of eating is due to the fact that repletion of hepatic glycogen is ineffective with small quantities of intravenous glucose. Patients in the overutilization-category may require large amounts of intravenous glucose to maintain consciousness. It is not enough to infuse 5% dextrose at a rate of 1 to 2 mL/min and assume the patient is protected (20% to 30% dextrose solutions may be required in some cases). Capillary glucose levels should be measured frequently during the acute treatment phase. Intravenous glucose usually can be stopped once the patient has eaten, but that can only be determined by trial. Adrenergic reactions without central nervous system abnormalities can be treated with oral carbohydrate and do not require parenteral therapy.

Hypoglycemia caused by sulfonylureas may last for prolonged periods (days) (Fig. 335-2), and patients may lapse back into coma if glucose infusions are stopped too soon. The reason for the prolonged effect is not always clear, though drug interactions, hepatic disease, and renal failure may play a role in some cases.

Surgery is the treatment of choice for insulinoma. The tumor is best localized by endoscopic ultrasonography. Intraoperative ultrasound may be useful if preoperative localization was unsuccessful. CT, magnetic resonance imaging, and arteriography are not as reliable. If the tumor cannot be found in the pancreas or in an extrapancreatic site at the time of surgery, stepwisepancreatectomy (from tail to head) should be carried out

with examination of frozen sections of sequential slices. Capillary glucose should be measured at each stage of the resection if the tumor is not obvious. A rise in plasma glucose may indicate removal of a small, nonpalpable lesion. In general, resection is stopped with an 85 percent pancreatectomy, even if the tumor is not found, to avoid malabsorption. While most patients are cured by surgery, as many as 15 percent have persistent hypoglycemia. Postoperative complications include acute pancreatitis, peritonitis, fistulas, pseudocyst formation, and diabetes mellitus.

Medical treatment for insulinoma is indicated only in preparation for surgery or after failure to find the tumor at operation. Two drugs are available, diazoxide and octreotide, an analogue of somatostatin. Diazoxide can be given intravenously or orally in doses of 300 to 1200 mg/d. Because of its salt-retaining properties, it must be accompanied by a diuretic. Octreotide is given subcutaneously in divided doses of 100 to 600 μg/d. Chronic use may cause nausea and diarrhea and predispose to cholelithiasis. Treatment of insulin-producing carcinomas is unsatisfactory. It has been reported that streptozocin plus doxorubicin is superior to streptozocin plus fluorouracil (median survival 2.2 and 1.4 years, respectively). The use of chlorozotocin is currently under study; this agent appears to produce fewer toxic side effects than streptozocin. Despite the poor prognosis, occasional patients with islet cell carcinomas survive for long periods.

Therapy of other forms of recurrent hypoglycemia, apart from hormone replacement in cases of pituitary or adrenal insufficiency, is dietary. In most cases, avoidance of fasting is all that is required. This measure is critical in diseases of fat oxidation or ketone synthesis. If intercurrent illness prevents eating, hospitalization for intravenous glucose administration is absolutely required. A high-protein, low-carbohydrate diet may relieve symptoms in patients with pseudohypoglycemia. The most effective agents for pseudohypoglycemia are beta-adrenergic blockers, propranolol probably being the most effective. With true alimentary hypoglycemia, the size of the individual meals should be small. The practice of giving massive amounts of vitamin E, crude adrenocortical extract, and trace metals to patients with pseudohypoglycemia is useless even if harmless (which has not been established).

BIBLIOGRAPHY

BRACKETT JC et al: A novel mutation in medium chain acyl-CoA dehydrogenase causes sudden neonatal death. J Clin Invest 94:1477, 1994

CHARLES MA et al: Comparison of oral glucose tolerance tests and mixed meals in patients with apparent idiopathic postabsorptive hypoglycemia: Absence of hypoglycemia after meals. Diabetes 30:465, 1981

FIGURE 335-2 Prolonged and refractory hypoglycemia in factitious hypoglycemia due to chlorpropamide in an alcoholic. Note continued hypoglycemia despite the infusion of glucose at rates up to 50 g/h. (*From RM Jordan et al, Arch Intern Med 137:390, 1977. Copyright 1977, American Medical Association. Used by permission.*)

CRYER PE: Glucose counterregulation: Prevention and correction of hypoglycemia in humans. Am J Physiol 264:E149, 1993

——— et al: Hypoglycemia. Diabetes Care 17:734, 1994

DAUGHADAY WH: The pathophysiology of IGF-II hypersecretion in non-islet tumor hypoglycemia. Diabetes Rev 3:62, 1995

DE FEO P et al: Modest decrements in plasma glucose concentration cause early impairment in cognitive function and later activation of glucose counterregulation in the absence of hypoglycemic symptoms in normal man. J Clin Invest 82:436, 1988

GRUNBERGER G et al: Factitious hypoglycemia due to surreptitious administration of insulin: Diagnosis, treatment, and long-term follow-up. Ann Intern Med 108:252, 1988

KLONOFF DC et al: Hypoglycemia following inadvertent or factitious sulfonylurea overdosage. Diabetes Care 18:563, 1995

MERIMEE TJ: Insulin-like growth factors in patients with nonislet cell tumors and hypoglycemia. Metabolism 35:360, 1986

MOERTEL CG et al: Streptozocin-doxorubicin, streptozocin-fluorouracil, or chlorozotocin in the treatment of advanced islet-cell carcinoma. N Engl J Med 326:519, 1992

MORISON IM et al: Somatic overgrowth associated with overexpression of insulin-like growth factor II. Nature Med 2:321, 1996

PANDIT MK et al: Drug-induced disorders of glucose tolerance. Ann Intern Med 118:529, 1993

PHILIPSON LH, STEINER DF: Pas de deux or more: The sulfonylurea receptor and K+ channels. Science 268:372, 1995

SERVICE FJ et al: C-peptide suppression test: Effects of gender, age, and body mass index; implications for the diagnosis of insulinoma. J Clin Endocrinol Metab 74:204, 1992

———: Hypoglycemic disorders. N Engl J Med 332:1144, 1995

normal young men (Fig. 336-2). Testosterone is transported in plasma bound to protein, largely to albumin and to a specific transport protein, testosterone-binding globulin (TeBG, also called sex hormone–binding globulin, SHBG). The bound and unbound fractions in plasma are in dynamic equilibrium, only about 1 to 3 percent being unbound. The fraction of circulating testosterone available for entry into tissues approximates the sum of the free and albumin-bound fractions or about half the total plasma testosterone.

Peripheral Metabolism of Androgens   Testosterone serves as a circulating precursor (or prohormone) for the formation of two other hormones that mediate many of the physiologic processes involved in androgen action (see Fig. 336-1). Testosterone can be 5α-reduced to dihydrotestosterone, which is responsible for many of the differentiative, growth-promoting, and functional aspects of male sexual differentiation and virilization. Circulating testosterone (and androstenedione) also can be converted to estrogens in extraglandular tissues. In males estrogens act in some instances in concert with androgens, but they also can have effects independent of or opposite to those of androgens. Thus the physiologic effects of testosterone are the result of the combined effects of testosterone itself plus those of the active androgen and estrogen metabolites of the parent molecule. (In normal men, small amounts of estradiol and dihydrotestosterone are also de-

336

James E. Griffin, Jean D. Wilson

DISORDERS OF THE TESTES

The testes produce sperm and the steroid hormones that regulate male sexual function. Both processes are under complex feedback control by the hypothalamic-pituitary system so that the testes have biosynthetic and regulatory features similar to those of the ovary and the adrenal. Testicular hormones are also responsible for the formation of the basic male phenotype during embryogenesis. The function of the embryonic testis and the disorders of sexual differentiation are described in Chap. 339.

PHYSIOLOGY AND REGULATION OF TESTICULAR FUNCTION   The testis consists of two components—clusters of interstitial or Leydig cells, where androgenic steroids are synthesized, and a system of spermatogenic tubules for the production and transport of sperm.

THE LEYDIG CELL   Testosterone Synthesis   The biochemical pathway by which the 27-carbon sterol cholesterol is converted to androgens and estrogens is depicted in Fig. 336-1. Cholesterol can either be synthesized de novo in the Leydig cell or derived from plasma lipoproteins. Five enzymatic transformations are required for the conversion of cholesterol to testosterone. In this process, the side chain of cholesterol is cleaved in two steps to reduce the size of the molecule from 27 to 19 carbons, and the A ring of the steroid is converted to the Δ^4-3-keto configuration. The five enzyme reactions are cholesterol side chain cleavage (P450$_{SCC}$), 3β-hydroxysteroid dehydrogenase/isomerase (3β-HSD), 17α-hydroxylase (P450$_{17\alpha}$), 17,20-lyase (P450$_{17\alpha}$), and 17β-hydroxysteroid dehydrogenase (17β-HSD). Both the 17α-hydroxylase and the 17,20-lyase activities are present in a single cytochrome P450$_{17\alpha}$. The first four reactions take place in the adrenal as well as the testis.

The rate-limiting process in testosterone synthesis is the conversion of cholesterol to pregnenolone by P450$_{SCC}$; luteinizing hormone (LH) from the pituitary regulates the activity of this enzyme and of other enzymes in the pathway. Additional steroids including estradiol are synthesized in small amounts in the Leydig cell.

Testosterone Secretion and Transport   Only about 70 nmol (20 μg) of testosterone is stored in the normal testes, so the total hormone content turns over about 200 times each day to provide the average of 17 to 20 μmol (5 to 6 mg) that is secreted into plasma in

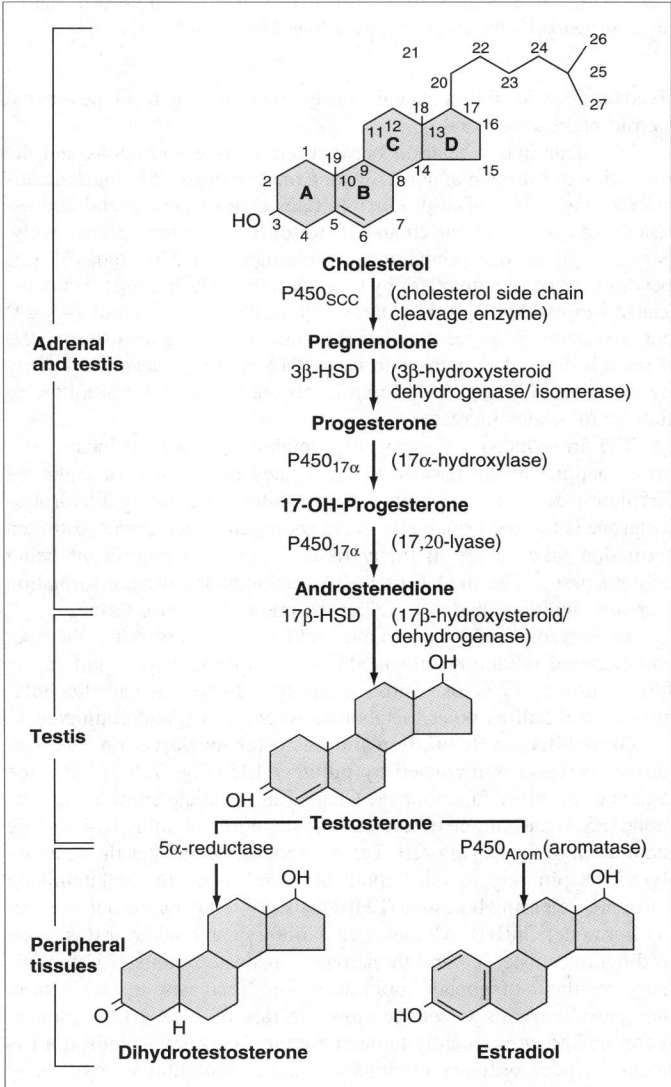

FIGURE 336-1   Pathways of androgen formation in the testis and the conversion of androgens to other active hormones in peripheral tissues.

FIGURE 336-2 Androgen and estrogen production in normal young men. The average production of androstenedione and testosterone is shown in the top boxes, and the mean daily production of estrone and estradiol is shown in the lower boxes. Estrogen is formed by extraglandular aromatization (*braces*) or is secreted directly by the testes. *Vertical arrows* indicate the rates of extraglandular aromatization of androgens, and *horizontal arrows* indicate the interconversion of androgen and estrogens by 17β-hydroxysteroid dehydrogenase. Thus, estradiol arises from plasma testosterone, from estrone, and by direct secretion by the testes. *(Adapted from MacDonald et al.)*

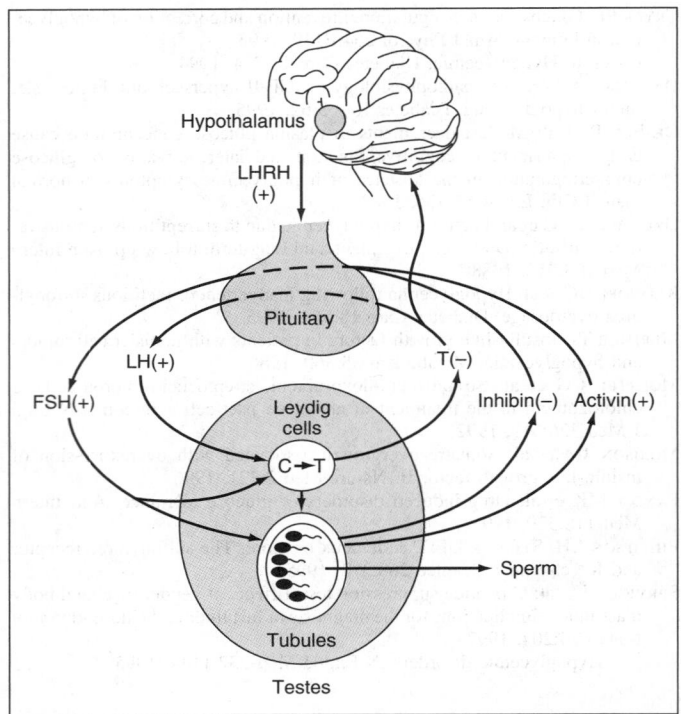

FIGURE 336-3 Regulation of testosterone and sperm production by LH and FSH. (C, cholesterol; T, testosterone.)

rived by direct secretion from the testes and indirectly from the adrenal steroid androstenedione.)

The quantitative relation between circulating androgens and the formation of estrogen in normal young men is illustrated diagrammatically in Fig. 336-2. The production rates of testosterone and androstenedione average about 20 and 10 μmol (6 and 3 mg), respectively, per day. All estrone production [averaging about 240 nmol (66 μg) per day] can be accounted for by formation from circulating precursors. The mean estradiol production is approximately 170 nmol (45 μg) per day; about 35 percent is derived from circulating testosterone, 50 percent is derived from the estrone, and 15 percent is secreted directly by the testes. When gonadotropin levels are elevated, estradiol secretion by the testes increases.

The 5α-reduced and estrogenic metabolites can exert local (paracrine) actions in the tissues in which they are formed or enter the circulation and act as hormones at other sites. Circulating dihydrotestosterone is formed principally in the androgen target tissues; estrogen formation takes place in many tissues, the most significant being adipose tissue. The overall rate of extraglandular estrogen formation increases with age and with increased mass of adipose tissue.

Testosterone and its active metabolites are catabolized in the liver and excreted predominantly in the urine, approximately half in the form of urinary 17-ketosteroids (primarily androsterone and etiocholanolone) and half as polar metabolites (diols, triols, and conjugates).

Gonadotropin Regulation and Testosterone Secretion Testosterone secretion is regulated by pituitary LH (Fig. 336-3). (For the details of pituitary function, see Chap. 328.) Follicle-stimulating hormone (FSH) may augment testosterone secretion, possibly by inducing maturation of the Leydig cell. Testosterone also regulates the sensitivity of the pituitary to the hypothalamic-releasing factor luteinizing hormone–releasing hormone (LHRH, also called gonadotropin-releasing hormone, GnRH). Although the pituitary can convert testosterone to dihydrotestosterone and to estrogens, testosterone itself is the primary regulator of gonadotropin secretion. Testosterone also acts in the central nervous system to slow the rate of LHRH formation or secretion and consequently to decrease the frequency of pulsatile LH release. Under ordinary circumstances, LH secretion is exquisitely sensitive to the feedback effects of testosterone, with complete suppression after the administration of amounts of exogenous androgen that approximate the normal daily secretory rate of testosterone (about 20

μmol or 6 mg). However, prolonged elevation of plasma LH (as in testicular deficiency) renders the pituitary less sensitive to negative feedback control by androgen.

The plasma concentration of neither testosterone nor LH is constant, each fluctuating in a pulsatile manner that reflects changes in secretory rates (Fig. 336-4). Major sleep-related surges in the pulsatile secretion of both LH and testosterone signal the beginning of male puberty. In young adults the magnitude of episodic secretion of LH and testosterone varies diurnally, so that peak levels of testosterone are about 25 to 30 percent higher in the morning than in late afternoon.

Androgen Action The major functions of androgen are regulation of LH secretion, formation of the male phenotype during sexual differentiation, and induction of sexual maturation at puberty. The cellular process by which androgens perform these functions is schematized in Fig. 336-5. Testosterone enters the cell by passive diffusion and can be converted to dihydrotestosterone by either 5α-reductase 1 or 2; 5α-reductase 2 is responsible for dihydrotestosterone formation in most androgen target tissues. Testosterone or dihydrotestosterone is then bound to the androgen-receptor protein in the nucleus. The hormone-receptor complex attaches to specific chromosomal sites and regulates the transcription of messenger RNA and, ultimately, the

FIGURE 336-4 The 24-h pattern of plasma LH and testosterone in a normal man, as sampled every 20 min. *(From Griffin and Wilson.)*

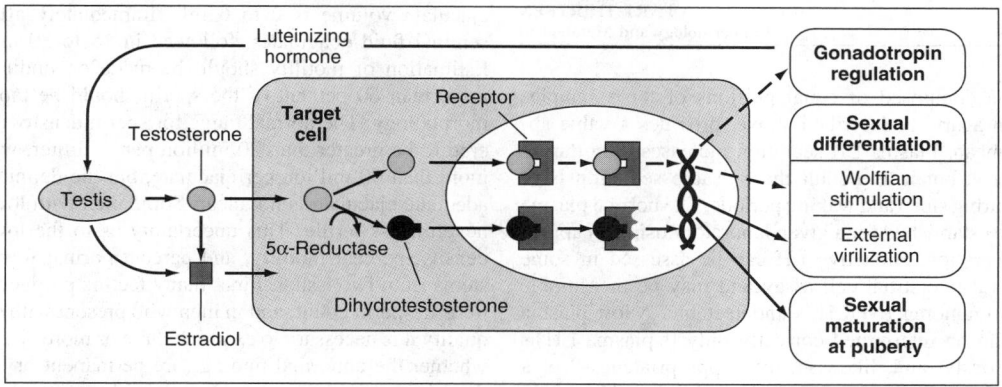

FIGURE 336-5 Current concepts of androgen action.

synthesis of cellular proteins. The androgen receptor is encoded by a gene on the long arm of the X chromosome; it contains 917 amino acids and has a molecular mass of about 110 kDa. It is similar in structure to other steroid hormone receptors and has distinct hormone-binding, DNA-binding, and functional domains (see Chap. 327). Estradiol acts by a mechanism similar to that of androgens but involving its own receptor (see Chap. 337).

Although testosterone and dihydrotestosterone bind to the same receptor, their physiologic roles differ. The testosterone-receptor complex regulates gonadotropin secretion, spermatogenesis, and the virilization of the wolffian ducts during sexual differentiation (see Chap. 339), whereas the dihydrotestosterone-receptor complex is responsible for external virilization during embryogenesis and for most androgen actions during sexual maturation and adult sexual life. The mechanism by which two hormones can interact with the same receptor but have different physiologic effects is also not well understood. Dihydrotestosterone binds to the receptor much more tightly than does testosterone, and hence its formation serves to amplify the hormonal signal.

THE SEMINIFEROUS TUBULE AND SPERMATOGENESIS Normal function of the seminiferous tubule is dependent on the pituitary and on the adjacent Leydig cells, both FSH and androgen being essential for spermatogenesis (see Fig. 336-3). The major site of FSH action is the Sertoli cell in the seminiferous tubules, and the seminiferous tubules also contain androgen receptors. Androgen appears to be essential for spermatogenesis, and FSH is required for spermatid maturation. Several cytokines and growth factors are also thought to be involved in the regulation of spermatogenesis by paracrine and autocrine mechanisms. The normal adult testes produce more than 100 million sperm per day.

The Sertoli cell cannot synthesize steroid hormones de novo and is dependent on testosterone that diffuses in from adjacent Leydig cells. Sertoli cells can convert testosterone to estradiol and to dihydrotestosterone. The seminiferous tubules also produce the peptide hormones inhibin, which exerts a negative feedback control, and activin, which feeds back positively on FSH secretion by the pituitary (see Fig. 336-3). Testosterone and estradiol also can inhibit FSH secretion.

The interlocking system in which two pituitary hormones regulate testicular function provides a precise dual-control mechanism in which hormonal signals from Leydig cells and the spermatogenic tubules feed back on the hypothalamic-pituitary system to regulate their own function (see Fig. 336-3).

ASSESSMENT OF TESTICULAR FUNCTION

LEYDIG CELL FUNCTION   History and Physical Examination The assessment of Leydig cell function and androgen status should include inquiry about the presence of developmental abnormalities of the urogenital tract, the timing and extent of sexual maturation at puberty, the rate of beard growth, and the current libido, sexual function, strength, and energy. Inadequate Leydig cell function or androgen action during embryogenesis may cause hypospadias, cryptorchidism, or microphallus. If Leydig cell failure occurs prior to pu-

berty, sexual maturation will not occur, and the individual will develop the features termed *eunuchoidism*, including an infantile amount and distribution of body hair, poor development of skeletal muscles, and failure of closure of the epiphyses, so that the arm span is more than 5 cm greater than the height and the lower body segment (heel to pubic bone) is more than 5 cm longer than the upper body segment (pubic bone to crown). Detection of postpubertal Leydig cell failure requires a high index of suspicion and appropriate laboratory assessment. One reason is that decreased sexual function in adult men may be caused by nonendocrine as well as endocrine factors. The second is that certain functions that require androgens for initiation continue unabated when Leydig cell failure occurs, and functions that eventually regress may do so very slowly. For example, the frequency of shaving may not decrease for months or years because of slow decline in the rate of beard growth once established.

Plasma Testosterone and Dihydrotestosterone Levels Plasma testosterone is measured by radioimmunoassay. Testosterone is secreted into plasma in a pulsatile fashion every 60 to 90 min (see Fig. 336-4); a single random sample provides a result within ±20 percent of the true mean value only two-thirds of the time, while three equally spaced samples 15 to 20 min apart provide a more accurate assessment. The samples do not need to be assayed separately, and aliquots of the three samples should be pooled for a single determination. The range of plasma testosterone in normal adult men is 10 to 35 nmol/L (3 to 10 ng/mL). In adult men, the plasma values vary somewhat throughout the day and at different times of the year. In young adult men the level of plasma testosterone is about 30 percent higher in the morning than in the evening. Estimation of TeBG concentration by radioimmunoassay is sometimes useful in the interpretation of total plasma testosterone levels. Bioavailable testosterone in plasma can be estimated by measuring the non-TeBG-bound fraction of testosterone.

The plasma testosterone value is slightly higher in prepubertal boys than in girls, the range in both being 0.2 to 0.7 nmol/L (0.05 to 0.2 ng/mL). The rise in plasma testosterone at the start of male puberty begins as a result of sleep-related nocturnal gonadotropin surges, so that plasma testosterone and LH are initially higher at night than during the day. Random daytime levels of plasma testosterone increase gradually as puberty progresses and reach adult levels at about age 17.

Dihydrotestosterone is also measured by radioimmunoassay. In young men the plasma dihydrotestosterone level is about one-tenth the value for testosterone and averages around 2 nmol/L (0.6 ng/mL). In older men with benign prostatic hyperplasia, plasma dihydrotestosterone levels average about 3 nmol/L (0.9 ng/mL).

Urinary 17-Ketosteroids The measurement of urinary 17-ketosteroids is not a valid way to assess testicular function because testosterone contributes only about 40 percent of urinary 17-ketosteroids in men, the bulk being derived from adrenal androgens.

Plasma LH Plasma LH is also measured by immunoassay. Dual-site immunometric assays have largely replaced competitive radioimmunoassays. LH is secreted in a pulsatile fashion and fluctuates widely so that in adult men a random plasma LH value is likely to be within ±20 percent of true mean value only a third of the time. Again, assay of a pool of plasma composed of equal portions of three samples drawn 15 to 20 min apart, as described above, provides a value approaching the true mean. Plasma LH secretion increases only during sleep in early puberty, but in the adult the pulsatile secretion is of similar magnitude during sleep and waking periods. The normal plasma LH values should be established for a given laboratory using an appropriate standard preparation. Bioactive LH can be assessed in some laboratories by the rat interstitial cell assay and may be measurable at times when the immunoreactive LH is undetectable. A low plasma testosterone level can be interpreted correctly only if plasma LH is measured simultaneously, and, likewise, the "appropriateness" of a given plasma LH value must be interpreted in relation to the plasma testosterone value. For example, a low plasma testosterone level coupled with a low LH level implies hypothalamic or pituitary disease, whereas the finding of a low plasma testosterone level and a high LH level suggests primary testicular insufficiency (see Chap. 327).

Response to Gonadotropin Stimulation Leydig cell function is difficult to assess prior to puberty when both LH and testosterone levels are low, and it is common to measure response of plasma testosterone to gonadotropin stimulation as an index of Leydig cell capacity. Normal prepubertal boys respond to 3 to 5 days of injection of 1000 to 2000 IU of human chorionic gonadotropin (hCG) with an increase in plasma testosterone to about 7 nmol/L (2 ng/mL); the response increases with the initiation of puberty and peaks in early puberty.

Response to Luteinizing Hormone–Releasing Hormone Prior to puberty, quantitative responses of plasma LH and FSH to the administration of LHRH are similar. With pubertal development, the LH response to acute administration of LHRH increases, while the FSH response remains the same. The amount of LH released following acute administration of LHRH probably reflects the amount of stored hormone in the pituitary. When 100 μg LHRH is given subcutaneously or intravenously to normal men, LH levels usually increase four- to fivefold, with the peak level at 30 min. However, the range of response is broad, some normal men having less than a doubling of LH levels. In primary testicular failure, measurement of basal LH is usually sufficient, and measurement of LHRH response is of little aid in diagnosis. Furthermore, since men with either pituitary or hypothalamic disease can have a normal or an abnormal LH response to acute administration of LHRH, a normal response is of no diagnostic value. A subnormal response is of value in establishing that an abnormality exists, even though the site is not determined. The LHRH test is most useful in men with secondary hypogonadism and subnormal LH response to acute administration of LHRH; if daily infusions of LHRH for a week lead to the development of a normal acute LH response, a hypothalamic etiology is likely. This test is rarely performed.

SEMINIFEROUS TUBULE FUNCTION **Examination of the Testes** Evaluation of the testes is an essential portion of the physical examination. The seminiferous tubules account for about 60 percent of testicular volume. The prepubertal testis measures about 2 cm in length and 2 mL in volume and grows during puberty to reach the adult proportions by age 16. When damage to the seminiferous tubules occurs prior to puberty, the testes are small and firm, whereas the testes are usually small and soft following postpubertal damage (the capsule, once enlarged, does not contract to its previous size). Testes in adults average 4.6 cm in length (range, 3.5 to 5.5 cm), corresponding to a volume of 12 to 25 mL. Advanced age does not influence testicular size, so the significance of small testes is the same at all ages in the adult. Testis size varies among ethnic groups. Asian men have smaller testes than western Europeans, independent of differences in body size. Because of its possible causal role in infertility, the presence of varicocele should be sought by palpation with the patient standing.

Semen Analysis Seminal fluid analysis is performed on samples obtained by masturbation into a glass container after 24 to 36 h of abstinence. Analysis should be performed within an hour. The normal ejaculate volume is 2 to 6 mL. Immediately after ejaculation, the seminal fluid coagulates, followed in 15 to 30 min by liquefaction. Estimation of motility should be made on undiluted seminal fluid; more than 60 percent of the sperm should be motile and of normal morphology. The normal range for sperm density is generally considered to be greater than 20 million per milliliter, with a total count of more than 60 million per ejaculate, but the definition of a minimally adequate ejaculate is not clear. Some men with low sperm counts are nevertheless fertile. This uncertainty as to the lower level of sperm density, percent motility, and percent normal forms in fertile semen stems from two issues. First, many factors produce temporary aberrations in sperm count, and in men who present with semen of equivocal quality it is necessary to examine three or more ejaculates to determine whether the abnormal findings are permanent or temporary. Second, the seminal fluid is routinely evaluated by tests that do not assess the functional capacity of sperm.

Plasma FSH Plasma FSH, as measured by immunoassay, usually correlates inversely with spermatogenesis. When damage to the germinal epithelium is severe, plasma levels of inhibin B fall, and plasma levels of FSH increase.

Testicular Biopsy Testicular biopsy is useful in some patients with oligospermia and azoospermia both as an aid in diagnosis and as an indication of the feasibility of treatment. For example, normal findings on testicular biopsy and a normal FSH level in an azoospermic man suggest obstruction of the vas deferens, which may be correctable surgically.

ESTROGENIC FUNCTION **Examination of the Breasts** Breast enlargement (gynecomastia) is the most consistent feature of feminizing states in men (see Chap. 338). Gynecomastia is due to an increase in both glandular and adipose tissue. The presence of gynecomastia should be sought by examining the sitting patient, using the fingers to grasp glandular tissue. Palpation with the flat of the hand while the patient is supine may result in failure to detect early or minimal breast enlargement. In obese men it is important to try to define the rim of the glandular tissue where it meets the adipose tissue of the chest wall.

Plasma Estrogen As discussed above, most of the estradiol and all of the estrone produced in normal men is formed by extraglandular aromatization of circulating androgens. The plasma level of estradiol is usually less than 180 pmol/L (50 pg/mL) in normal men; the plasma estrone level is somewhat higher but usually is less than 300 pmol/L (80 pg/mL). Elevations in estrogen production and estrogen plasma levels can be due to elevations in plasma precursors (liver or adrenal disease), to increases in extraglandular aromatization (obesity), or to increased production by the testes (testicular tumors or androgen resistance).

PHASES OF NORMAL TESTICULAR FUNCTION

The phases of male sexual life can be defined in terms of the plasma testosterone value (Fig. 336-6). In the male embryo the production of testosterone by the testes commences at about 7 weeks of gestation. Shortly thereafter, plasma testosterone attains a high value that is maintained until late in gestation. The level then falls so that at the time of birth plasma testosterone is only slightly higher in males than in females. Shortly after birth, plasma testosterone in the male infant again begins to rise and remains elevated for approximately 3 months, falling to low levels by age 6 months to 1 year. The concentration then remains low (but slightly higher in boys than in girls) until the onset of puberty, when it begins to rise in boys, reaching adult levels by about age 17. The level of bioavailable testosterone remains constant until the 40s when it begins to decline at a rate of about 1.2 percent per year; the level of TeBG increases by about 1.2 percent per year so that there is little decline in total testosterone until the later decades of life. During the third, or adult, phase of male sexual life, sperm production becomes sufficient to allow reproduction to take place. The physiologic events during these various phases differ, as do the pathologic consequences of derangements in testicular func-

FIGURE 336-6 Phases of male sexual life. *(From Griffin and Wilson.)*

tion. Male sexual differentiation during embryogenesis is considered in Chap. 339. The role of the surge of testosterone formation during the first year of life is not certain. However, in primates, neonatal activation of the hypothalamic-pituitary-testicular axis is important for subsequent normal pubertal development. The focus of this chapter is on testicular pathophysiology during puberty, adulthood, and old age.

ABNORMALITIES OF TESTICULAR FUNCTION

PUBERTY The control of puberty is poorly understood and may reside in the hypothalamic-pituitary system, the testes, or the adrenals. Prior to the onset of puberty, gonadotropin secretion by the pituitary is low, but prepubertal castration results in a rise in plasma gonadotropin levels. This suggests that prior to puberty the negative feedback control of gonadotropin secretion is exquisitely sensitive to the small amount of circulating testosterone. The onset of puberty is heralded by sleep-associated surges in gonadotropin secretion. Later in puberty the rises in LH and FSH levels persist throughout the day. Thus, with maturation, the hypothalamic-pituitary system becomes less sensitive to negative feedback control, and the consequences are a higher mean plasma testosterone level, maturation of the testes, and the onset of spermatogenesis. The rise in gonadotropin secretion is the consequence of both an increase in LHRH secretion and an increase in the sensitivity of the pituitary to LHRH. Plasma levels of bioactive LH increase even more than those of immunoreactive hormone. The somatic changes at the time of puberty are secondary to the rise in plasma testosterone. Growth of the accessory organs of male reproduction (the penis, the prostate, the seminal vesicles, and the epididymides) accounts for about one-fourth of androgen-mediated nitrogen retention during puberty. Accelerated linear growth is accompanied by growth of muscle and connective tissue, accounting for the major portion of nitrogen retention at puberty. The principal androgen-sensitive muscles are those of the pectoral region and the shoulder. The characteristic hair growth of male puberty involves development of mustache and beard; regression of the scalp line; appearance of body, extremity, and perianal hair; and extension of the pubic hair upward into a diamond-shaped pattern. Growth of axillary and pubic hair is initiated under the control of adrenal androgens and is promoted by testicular androgens. The larynx enlarges, and the vocal cords thicken, resulting in a lowering of the pitch of the voice. Hemoglobin levels increase by about 10 g/L. These various androgen-mediated growth and maturation processes reach some limiting value so that once puberty is completed the administration of pharmacologic doses of androgen has no further effect. The entire process is heralded by testicular enlargement beginning at age 11 to 12 and is usually completed within 5 years, although some aspects of virilization, such as growth of the chest hair, may continue over a decade or more.

The events of normal male puberty are variable in onset, duration, and sequence. The central issue in dealing with disorders of puberty is separating true absence or precocity from the extremes of normal variation. The use of staging criteria that correlate developmental and anatomic landmarks with chronologic age is useful in making this distinction (see Marshall and Tanner).

Sexual Precocity Premature development of sexual characteristics that are phenotypically appropriate—i.e., virilization in boys—is termed *isosexual precocity. Heterosexual precocity* refers to feminizing syndromes in boys.

Isosexual precocity Sexual development prior to age 9 in boys is generally considered abnormal. *True precocious puberty* or *complete isosexual precocity* occurs when both virilization and spermatogenesis are premature, and *precocious pseudopuberty* or *incomplete isosexual precocity* refers to virilization unaccompanied by spermatogenesis. This distinction is blurred in practice, because pure virilizing syndromes may cause activation of gonadotropin secretion secondarily and thus be followed by development of spermatogenesis. Furthermore, local androgen production in the testis, as in Leydig cell tumors, can cause local areas of spermatogenesis and limited sperm production around the tumor. We therefore prefer a two-part classification: virilizing syndromes (in which hypothalamic-pituitary activity is appropriate for age) and premature activation of the hypothalamic-pituitary system.

Virilizing syndromes can result from Leydig cell tumors, hCG-secreting tumors, adrenal tumors, congenital adrenal hyperplasia (most commonly 21-hydroxylase deficiency), androgen administration, or Leydig cell hyperplasia. In these disorders plasma testosterone levels are inappropriately elevated for the age. Leydig cell tumors are rare in children but should be suspected when the testes are asymmetric in size (see Chap. 98). Virilizing adrenal tumors mainly secrete androstenedione and dehydroepiandrosterone, some of which is converted to testosterone; consequently, they cause elevated 17-ketosteroid excretion. Glucocorticoid administration does not suppress 17-ketosteroid excretion to normal in patients with testicular or adrenal tumors, in contrast to the prompt decrease that occurs after such treatment in congenital adrenal hyperplasia. Congenital adrenal hyperplasia leads to elevated 17-hydroxyprogesterone levels and, as a consequence, elevated androgen levels (see Chaps. 332 and 339). When this disorder is treated with glucocorticoids, true precocious puberty can then result if the increased androgen levels have caused sufficient hypothalamic maturation.

Gonadotropin-independent sexual precocity in boys may occur as a result of autonomous Leydig cell hyperplasia in the absence of a Leydig cell tumor. The disorder is inherited as a male-limited autosomal disorder either from affected fathers or from mothers who are unaffected carriers and is due to point mutations in the LH receptor that cause constitutive activation of the receptor in the absence of LH. Virilization begins usually by age 2. Testosterone levels are elevated, often to the adult male range; however, immunoreactive and bioactive LH levels and the LH response to LHRH are prepubertal. In the past many of these boys were mistakenly thought to have true precocious puberty because spermatogenesis may be present.

Premature activation of the hypothalamic-pituitary system may be "idiopathic" or due to central nervous system (CNS) tumors, infections, or injuries. Early hypothalamic-pituitary activation typically is associated with features of normal puberty, i.e., sleep-related gonadotropin secretion, elevated plasma bioactive LH, and enhanced gonadotropin response to LHRH. Since the diagnosis of idiopathic true precocious puberty is one of exclusion, patients may later prove to have been misclassified and to have a CNS abnormality. With improved means of diagnosis, such as magnetic resonance imaging, delays in diagnosis will probably be less frequent.

Management of sexual precocity due to steroid- or gonadotropin-producing tumors, congenital adrenal hyperplasia, or CNS abnormality is directed toward the primary disease. In boys with Leydig cell hyperplasia, attempts have been made to lower plasma testosterone with medroxyprogesterone acetate or ketoconazole, but the long-term effectiveness of these agents is unknown. Idiopathic true precocious puberty and true precocious puberty due to inoperable CNS lesions are treated with LHRH analogue therapy, which causes reversal of the pubertal maturation, including a decrease in the rate of skeletal development.

Heterosexual precocity Feminization in prepubertal boys can result from absolute or relative increases in estrogen due to a variety of causes (see Chap. 338).

Delayed or Incomplete Puberty The separation of failure of puberty from variants of normal development is one of the most difficult problems in endocrinology. Some boys fail to show the normal spurt of growth and sexual development at the usual time but eventually commence puberty by age 16 or older. Adolescence may then either progress rapidly, or a slow development and growth may continue until age 20 to 22. Many men with delayed onset of puberty attain heights within the normal adult range. At times the history reveals that a parent or sibling had a similar pattern of development. The major problem is to separate this group of boys with delayed puberty from those with organic disorders that impair puberty. Panhypopituitarism and hypothyroidism can cause pubertal failure (see Chaps. 328 and 331). Absent puberty also can result from primary testicular disease; this diagnosis is suspected on the basis of low plasma testosterone and elevated FSH and LH levels. Hereditary androgen resistance (in which plasma testosterone and LH levels are both high) usually causes male pseudohermaphroditism but in mild form may be manifested by absent or incomplete puberty (see Chap. 339).

Most boys with absent puberty have low plasma levels of both testosterone and gonadotropins; in these boys it is necessary to distinguish delayed puberty from isolated gonadotropin deficiency or idiopathic *hypogonadotropic hypogonadism* (*Kallman syndrome*). The manifestations of isolated gonadotropin deficiency vary from boys with eunuchoidal features and testes of prepubertal size to those with partial LH and/or FSH deficiency and some degree of testicular enlargement and pubertal development. Anosmia or hyposmia and cryptorchidism are common. The disorder is inherited as an X-linked recessive trait or as an autosomal dominant trait with variable expressivity. Serum FSH and LH levels are usually below the normal male range, and plasma testosterone levels are low for age. The secretion of other pituitary hormones is usually normal. The defect appears to be in the synthesis or release of LHRH. Defects have been identified in a neural cell adhesion molecule (KAL) involved in the migration of LHRH neurons into the olfactory bulb. The administration of synthetic LHRH corrects the endocrine abnormalities and initiates spermatogenesis. If untreated, these patients usually remain in the prepubertal state indefinitely. A prepubertal manifestation is microphallus, in which the size of the penis is below the fifth percentile for the age. Indeed, one-fourth or more of cases of isolated prepubertal microphallus are due to hypogonadotropic hypogonadism. Distinguishing between this disorder and delayed puberty is particularly difficult in patients of early or midpubertal age; the presence of microphallus, anosmia, or a family history of hypogonadotropic hypogonadism may suggest the diagnosis. In the absence of such evidence, it may take several years of observation before it becomes clear which of these states a patient has. Since delayed puberty is associated with a decreased bone mass, therapy should not be delayed too long. In some cases the response of plasma LH to LHRH stimulation may be helpful in suggesting that puberty is imminent.

ADULT ABNORMALITIES OF TESTICULAR FUNCTION At the completion of puberty, plasma testosterone levels reach the adult level of 10 to 35 nmol/L (3 to 10 ng/mL) throughout the day, plasma gonadotropins are in the normal adult range, and sperm production is sufficient to allow reproduction. The adult set of the complex regulatory system (see Fig. 336-3) is sustained in the normal man for more than 40 years. However, the system is subject to a variety of influences, at the level of both the testes and the hypothalamic-pituitary system. Spermatogenesis is exquisitely sensitive to alterations in temperature, and brief increases in either systemic or local temperature (as in a hot bath) can be followed by temporary decreases in sperm production. The system also is influenced by diet,

drugs, alcohol, environmental agents, and psychological stress, any of which may cause temporary decreases in sperm count.

Persistent abnormalities of testicular function in adults can be due to hypothalamic-pituitary disorders (see Chap. 328), testicular defects, or abnormalities of sperm transport. Certain of these conditions tend to affect Leydig cell function or spermatogenesis selectively, but most impair both androgenization and fertility (Table 336-1). The interlocking of Leydig cell function and fertility is due to the dependence of spermatogenesis on androgen. Even a partial decrease in testosterone production can cause infertility. Certain conditions (hyperprolactinemia, radiation therapy, cyclophosphamide therapy, autoimmunity, paraplegia, androgen resistance) can cause either isolated infertility or a combined defect in testicular function.

Hypothalamic-Pituitary Disorders Disorders of the hypothalamus and pituitary can impair the secretion of gonadotropins either as one manifestation of a generalized disease of the anterior pituitary (see Chap. 328) or as an isolated defect. In the latter case the cause is usually hypogonadotropic hypogonadism, in which secretion of both LH and FSH are impaired. This disorder usually is congenital but rarely is an acquired defect. Alternatively, gonadotropin secretion can be altered by factors other than hypothalamic-pituitary pathology. For example, elevation of plasma cortisol in the *Cushing syndrome* can depress LH secretion independent of a space-occupying lesion of the pituitary. Some patients with *congenital adrenal hyperplasia* have suppressed gonadotropin secretion and consequent infertility. *Hyperprolactinemia* (as the consequence either of pituitary adenomas or of

Table 336-1

Abnormalities of Adult Testicular Function

Infertility with Underandrogenization	Infertility with Normal Virilization
HYPOTHALAMIC-PITUITARY	
Panhypopituitarism	
Isolated gonadotropin deficiency	Isolated FSH deficiency
Cushing's syndrome	Congenital adrenal hyperplasia
Hyperprolactinemia	Hyperprolactinemia
Hemochromatosis	Androgen use
TESTICULAR	
Developmental and structural defects	
Klinefelter's syndrome*	Germinal cell aplasia
XX male	Cryptorchidism
	Varicocele
	Immotile cilia syndrome
Acquired defects	
Viral orchitis*	*Mycoplasma* infection
Trauma	
Radiation	Radiation
Drugs	Drugs
(spironolactone, alcohol,	(cyclophosphamide)
ketoconazole,	
cyclophosphamide)	
Environmental toxins	Environmental toxins
Autoimmunity	Autoimmunity
Granulomatous disease	
Associated with systemic diseases	
Liver disease	Febrile illness
Renal failure	Celiac disease
Sickle cell disease	
Immune disease (AIDS,	
rheumatoid arthritis)	
Neurologic disease (myotonic	Neurologic disease (paraplegia)
dystrophy, spinobulbar muscular	
atrophy, and paraplegia)	
Androgen resistance	Androgen resistance
SPERM TRANSPORT	
	Obstruction of the epididymis or
	vas deferens (cystic fibrosis,
	diethylstilbesterol exposure,
	congenital absence)

* The common testicular causes of underandrogenization and infertility in adults—Klinefelter's syndrome and viral orchitis—are associated with small testes.

drugs such as phenothiazines) can cause combined Leydig cell and seminiferous tubule dysfunction, presumably due to inhibition of LH and FSH secretion by prolactin. Occasionally, impaired fertility in hyperprolactinemia is associated with normal gonadotropin and androgen levels and is presumed to result from direct inhibition of spermatogenesis by prolactin. *Hemochromatosis* usually impairs testicular function as the result of effects on the pituitary; less often it affects the testis directly (see Chap. 342). The use of *androgens* for purposes other than replacement therapy is often associated with impaired sperm production (see below). In some conditions, testosterone levels may be decreased in association with normal LH levels, and the mechanism is less clear. Men with massive obesity have decreased levels of TeBG and of total and bioavailable testosterone, which return toward normal with weight loss. Obesity may be part of the mechanism for decreased testosterone levels in the subset of such men with Pickwickian syndrome (see Chap. 263). Some men with temporal lobe seizures also have hypogonadotropic hypogonadism.

Testicular Defects Abnormalities of testicular function in the adult can be grouped into several categories: developmental and structural defects of the testes, acquired testicular defects, and disorders secondary to systemic disease.

Developmental abnormalities The *Klinefelter syndrome* (both the classic and the mosaic forms) and the *XX male syndrome* are usually not recognized until after the time of expected puberty (see Chap. 339). Some developmental defects cause infertility in the presence of normal androgen production. These include varicocele, germinal cell aplasia, and cryptorchidism. *Varicocele* may be of etiologic importance in as much as one-third of all cases of male infertility. It is caused by retrograde flow of blood into the internal spermatic vein that eventuates in progressive, often palpable dilation of the peritesticular pampiniform plexus of veins. Varicocele occurs in about 10 to 15 percent of men in the general population and in 20 to 40 percent of men with infertility and is thought to result from incompetence of the valve between the internal spermatic vein and the renal vein. It is more common on the left side (85 percent). Unilateral varicocele increases the blood flow and the temperature of both testes as a result of the extensive anastomoses of the venous systems. The increased scrotal (and testicular) temperature is believed to be the cause of the poor-quality semen and infertility (the testes no longer are 2°C cooler than the abdominal cavity, as they normally are). The findings on semen analysis are usually nonspecific, with all parameters showing some abnormality. Surgical resection results in fertility in about half of men, with the best results (70 percent pregnancy rate) in those whose preoperative sperm counts are over 10 million per milliliter.

Some patients with *germinal cell aplasia* (the Sertoli cell–only syndrome) have a positive family history and may constitute a specific group in whom the germinal epithelium is missing with resulting azoospermia; plasma testosterone and LH values are normal, and plasma FSH levels are elevated. Other patients with identical histologic and clinical findings have androgen resistance or a history of viral orchitis or cryptorchidism; as many as 18 percent of men with idiopathic azoospermia or severe oligospermia have microdeletions in the Yq interval 6 region, and more than one gene has been proposed as an azoospermia factor (AZF) gene.

Unilateral *cryptorchidism*, even when corrected prior to puberty, is associated with abnormal semen in many individuals. This observation suggests that even in unilateral cryptorchidism the testicular abnormality is usually bilateral.

The *immotile cilia syndrome* is an autosomal recessive defect characterized by immotility or poor motility of the cilia of the airways and of the sperm. Kartagener's syndrome is a subgroup of the immotile cilia syndrome associated with situs inversus, chronic sinusitis, and bronchiectasis (see Chap. 256). The immotile sperm cannot fertilize. The structural abnormality leading to impaired motility of cilia can usually be defined by the electron-microscopic appearance. The specific defects that are known to cause the syndrome include defects in the dynein arms, spokes, or microtubule doublets. Cilia from epithelia and sperm tails from the same individual exhibit the same defects,

but the pulmonary manifestations may be minor. *Other less well understood structural defects of sperm* can cause immotility without involvement of cilia in the lung.

Acquired testicular defects Acquired testicular failure in the adult can be due to *viral orchitis*. The responsible viruses include mumps virus, echovirus, lymphocytic choriomeningitis virus, and group B arboviruses. The orchitis is due to actual infection of the tissue by virus rather than to indirect effects of infection. Orchitis occurs in as many as one-fourth of adult men with mumps; in about two-thirds the orchitis is unilateral, and in the remainder it is bilateral. Orchitis usually develops a few days after the onset of parotitis but may precede it. The testis may return to normal size and function or undergo atrophy. Atrophy is believed to be due both to direct effects of the virus on the seminiferous tubules and to ischemia secondary to pressure and edema within the taut tunica albuginea. Semen analysis returns to normal in three-fourths of men with unilateral involvement and in only one-third of men with bilateral orchitis. Atrophy is usually perceptible within 1 to 6 months after the acute illness, and the degree of atrophy is not necessarily proportional to the severity of the acute orchitis. Unilateral atrophy occurs in about one-third of patients, and bilateral atrophy occurs in about one-tenth.

Trauma can also cause secondary atrophy of the testes. The exposed position of the testes in the scrotum renders them susceptible to both thermal and physical trauma—particularly in individuals with hazardous occupations.

The testes are sensitive to *radiation damage;* decreased secretion of testosterone appears to be a consequence of diminished testicular blood flow. Doses higher than 200 mGy (20 rad) cause increases in plasma FSH and LH levels and damage to the spermatogonia. After about 800 mGy (80 rad), oligospermia or azoospermia develops, and higher doses may obliterate the germinal epithelium, except for occasional stem and Sertoli cells. Fractionated radiation may have a more profound effect than single-dose radiation. Recovery of sperm density occurs in a dose-related fashion, and complete recovery of sperm density may require as long as 5 years. Permanent infertility can occur after radiation therapy for malignant lymphoma despite shielding of the testes. Permanent androgen deficiency in adult men is uncommon after therapeutic radiation; however, most boys given direct testicular radiation therapy for acute lymphoblastic leukemia have permanently low plasma testosterone levels.

In general, *drugs* interfere with testicular function in one of four ways—inhibition of testosterone synthesis, blockade of androgen action, enhancement of estrogen levels, or direct inhibition of spermatogenesis. Some drugs have multiple effects, and agents such as guanethidine that block the sympathetic nervous system can impair sexual function in men whose pituitary-testicular axis is normal.

Spironolactone and ketoconazole block the synthesis of androgen by interfering with the late steps in androgen biosynthesis. Spironolactone and cimetidine compete with androgen for binding to the androgen receptor and thus block androgen action in target cells. Testosterone levels may be low, and estradiol levels may be elevated in persons using marijuana, heroin, or methadone, although the exact reasons are unclear. Alcohol, when consumed in excess for prolonged periods, causes decreased plasma testosterone, independent of liver disease or malnutrition. Elevated plasma estradiol and decreased plasma testosterone levels have been reported in men taking digitalis.

Antineoplastic and chemotherapeutic agents commonly interfere with spermatogenesis. Cyclophosphamide causes azoospermia or extreme oligospermia within a few weeks after the initiation of therapy. Cessation of therapy is followed by a return of spermatogenesis within 3 years in about half of patients. Combination chemotherapy for acute leukemia, Hodgkin's disease, and other malignancies also may impair Leydig cell function. In pubertal boys this is manifested by decreased serum testosterone and elevated LH levels; in adult men, testosterone levels do not decline, and the impaired Leydig cell function may only be detected as an enhanced LH response to LHRH. The alkylating agents in the chemotherapeutic regimens seem to be responsible for Leydig cell toxicity.

Because of the potentially toxic effects of many physical and chemical agents on spermatogenesis, the occupational and recreational history should be carefully evaluated in all men with infertility. Known environmental hazards include microwaves and ultrasound and chemicals such as the nematocide dibromochloropropane, cadmium, and lead. In some populations, sperm density is said to have declined by as much as 40 percent in the past 50 years, and it has been postulated that environmental estrogens or antiandrogens may be responsible.

Testicular failure also occurs as a part of *polyglandular autoimmune insufficiency* (see Chap. 340). Sperm antibodies are also a cause of isolated male infertility. In some instances, such antibodies may be secondary phenomena resulting from duct obstruction or vasectomy. *Granulomatous diseases* such as leprosy can destroy the testes, and testicular atrophy occurs in 10 to 20 percent of men with lepromatous leprosy owing to direct invasion of the tissue by the mycobacteria. The tubules are involved initially, followed by endarteritis and destruction of Leydig cells.

Testicular abnormalities associated with systemic disease The common systemic diseases that cause underandrogenization and infertility are liver disease and renal failure. In *cirrhosis of the liver*, a combined testicular and pituitary abnormality leads to decreased testosterone production independent of the direct toxic effects of ethanol. Although plasma LH is elevated, the level may be below the expected range given the degree of androgen deficiency. This situation most likely results from the inhibition of LH secretion by estrogen in patients with chronic liver disease. Increased estrogen production results from impaired hepatic extraction of adrenal androstenedione and subsequent increased extraglandular conversion to estrone and estradiol. In effect, estrogen precursors are shunted to sites of extraglandular aromatization. Testicular atrophy and gynecomastia are present in about half of men with cirrhosis, and many such men are impotent. Successful liver transplantation reverses the effects of cirrhosis on the pituitary-testicular axis.

In chronic *renal failure*, androgen synthesis and sperm production decrease in the setting of elevated plasma gonadotropins. The elevated LH level is due to increased production and reduced clearance but is incapable of effecting normal testosterone production. In addition, about one-fourth of men with renal failure have hyperprolactinemia; the role of hyperprolactinemia in decreasing testosterone production is unclear. Low testosterone coupled with normal or increased plasma estrogen levels cause gynecomastia in about half of men on chronic hemodialysis, and about half of men on dialysis have decreased libido and/or impotence. The etiology of the testicular abnormalities in renal failure is not well understood. Improvement in testosterone production with hemodialysis is incomplete, but successful transplantation may return testicular function to normal.

Men with *sickle cell anemia* usually have impaired secondary sexual development, and testicular atrophy is present in one-third of them. The defect may be at either the testicular or the hypothalamic-pituitary level. Abnormalities in Leydig cell function, frequently accompanied by decreased sperm density, have been noted in a variety of chronic systemic diseases, including protein-energy *malnutrition*, advanced *Hodgkin's disease* and *cancer* prior to chemotherapy, and *amyloidosis*. Most of these disorders cause a lowered plasma testosterone level coupled with a normal to increased plasma LH level, suggesting combined hypothalamic-pituitary and testicular defects. Similar hormone changes occur following *surgery, myocardial infarction*, and severe *burns* and thus may be a nonspecific effect of illness. Men with AIDS may have decreased testosterone levels without an appropriate elevation of gonadotropins; although human immunodeficiency virus (HIV) may infect the testes, the hormonal changes are likely nonspecific and related to severe illness. Whether testosterone deficiency contributes to muscle wasting in this disorder is unclear.

The temporary decrease in sperm density after *acute febrile illness* usually occurs in the absence of any changes in testosterone production. Infertility in men with *celiac disease* is associated with a hormonal pattern typical of androgen resistance, namely elevated testosterone and LH levels. *Neurologic diseases* associated with altered testicular function include myotonic dystrophy, spinobulbar muscular atrophy, and paraplegia. In myotonic dystrophy, small testes may be associated with abnormalities of both spermatogenesis and Leydig cell function. Men with spinobulbar muscular atrophy often have as a late manifestation underandrogenization and infertility and the hormonal features of androgen resistance (see Chap. 339). Expansion of the glutamine repeat sequences in the amino-terminal region of the androgen receptor impairs its function, but it is unclear whether altered androgen receptor function is related to the neurologic disorder. Spinal cord lesions that cause paraplegia lead to a temporary decrease in testosterone levels and persistent defects in spermatogenesis; some patients retain the capacity to obtain erection and to ejaculate.

Androgen resistance Defects of the androgen receptor cause resistance to the action of androgen, usually associated with defective male phenotypic development, infertility, and underandrogenization (see Chap. 339). A less severe form of androgen resistance, associated with infertility due to oligo- or azoospermia in otherwise phenotypically normal men, may be the cause of a significant fraction of cases of infertility previously classified as idiopathic azoospermia. Point mutations in the hormone-binding domain of the androgen receptor have been reported in idiopathic infertility.

Impairment of Sperm Transport Disorders of sperm transport may cause infertility in as many as 6 percent of infertile men with normal virilization. The obstruction may be unilateral or bilateral, congenital or acquired. In men with unilateral obstruction of sperm transport, the infertility may result from antisperm antibodies. Obstructive azoospermia at the level of the epididymis also occurs in association with chronic infections of the paranasal sinuses and lungs. Tuberculosis, leprosy, and gonorrhea are rare causes of acquired obstruction of ejaculatory structures. Congenital defects of the vas deferens can occur as an isolated abnormality associated with absence of the seminal vesicles (and consequently absence of fructose in the ejaculate), in men whose mothers received *diethylstilbestrol* during pregnancy, and in patients with *cystic fibrosis*. Furthermore, congenital bilateral absence of the vas deferens can be due to mutations in the cystic fibrosis conductance regulator different than the mutations that cause full-blown cystic fibrosis. Thus, isolated congenital absence of the vas and cystic fibrosis represent a spectrum of defects that have a similar molecular basis.

Empirical Therapy of Male Infertility The management of male infertility is usually unsatisfactory. Disorders for which there are logical or effective treatments (genital tract obstruction, sperm autoimmunity, gonadotropin deficiency) account for only 10 percent of infertile men, and pregnancies are infrequent with genital tract obstruction or sperm autoimmunity. Severe oligospermia/azoospermia of other causes accounts for about a fourth of cases of male infertility and has largely been considered untreatable. The other two-thirds of infertile men have a partial reduction in semen parameters and subfertility of a variable degree, and in this group spontaneous fertility may occur in untreated men (as high as 25 percent in one year). In the past a variety of empirical therapies (e.g., testosterone rebound, gonadotropins, antiestrogens) have been unsuccessful. The only successful empirical therapy for men with mild to moderate defects in semen quality is in vitro fertilization. However, standard in vitro fertilization does not provide a good outcome with severely abnormal semen parameters, such as a sperm density of <5 million/mL, poor motility, and many abnormal forms. For such men the technique of intracytoplasmic sperm injection makes in vitro fertilization more successful; indeed fertilization and pregnancy rates with this technique are similar to those for standard in vitro techniques in couples with fallopian tube pathology, i.e., a 50 to 70 percent fertilization rate and a 30 percent pregnancy rate per cycle.

Fertility Control in Men A variety of approaches to fertility control in men have been tried, including use of the condom as an effective barrier that also prevents sexually transmitted diseases. Another widely used technique is ligation of the vas deferens, a procedure that has been successful in large numbers of men and can be performed on an outpatient basis. The time required for azoospermia to occur following the operation depends on the number of sperm in the terminal vas deferens and ejaculatory ducts at the time of surgery but is usually less than 40 days. Azoospermia should be documented in each case to prove effectiveness. No deleterious effects on either testosterone production or the hypothalamic-pituitary axis have been documented. Despite reports of immune-complex–associated accelerated atherosclerosis in vasectomized nonhuman primates, there does not appear to be any association between vasectomy and atherosclerosis in men. Vasectomy should only be recommended for men requesting permanent sterilization. Only about 30 to 40 percent of men subjected to vasovasostomy for reanastomosis of the vas subsequently achieve fertility.

OLD AGE Beginning at about age 40, mean plasma bioavailable testosterone concentrations decline gradually, and about 40 percent of elderly men have low bioavailable testosterone levels. Nevertheless, although statistically lower than the levels in young men, the concentrations of total testosterone even in elderly men usually remain within the normal range. The cause of the decreased testosterone level is likely a decreased number of Leydig cells in the testes. There is also a decline in seminiferous tubule function and decreased sperm production in older men. Plasma LH and FSH levels are usually increased in elderly men, and an increase in the rate of conversion of androgen to estrogen in peripheral tissues results in a decrease in the effective ratio of androgen to estrogen. These latter endocrine changes may play a role in the development of prostatic hyperplasia and possibly in the development of gynecomastia in aging men (see Chaps. 97 and 338). Male sexual function gradually declines after early adulthood, but there is no convincing evidence that hormonal changes have any direct bearing on changes in sexual function with age in healthy men.

Prostatic Hyperplasia See Chap. 97
Cancer of the Prostate See Chap. 97
DISORDERS OF ALL AGES Testicular Tumors (See Chap. 98) Chorionic gonadotropin is present in normal testes, and it is not surprising that plasma gonadotropins may be elevated in persons with testicular tumors. Indeed, an elevated plasma level of the β subunit of human chorionic gonadotropin (hCG-β) is a sensitive and specific marker of tumor activity in some men with germ cell tumors. Plasma levels of hCG-β are elevated in all men with choriocarcinoma, in one-third of those with embryonal carcinomas and teratocarcinomas, and rarely in those with seminomas. Changes in hCG-β levels correlate with response to therapy.

Testicular tumors can give rise to elevated estradiol and testosterone levels by at least two mechanisms. Trophoblastic tumors and Leydig and Sertoli cell tumors produce both hormones autonomously; plasma gonadotropin levels and hormone production by the uninvolved portions of the testes are depressed, and azoospermia is common. However, secretion of gonadotropins by the tumor increases estradiol and testosterone production in the unaffected areas of the testes, and azoospermia is uncommon with such tumors. When estrogens and androgens are formed (directly or indirectly) by the tumors, feminization, virilization, or no obvious change may result, depending on the hormones produced and the age of the patient. Other cellular markers of testicular tumor activity include alpha fetoprotein.

Gynecomastia See Chap. 338

℞ **TREATMENT**

Androgens PHARMACOLOGIC PREPARATIONS When testosterone itself is ingested, it is absorbed into the portal blood and degraded promptly by the liver, so that only insignificant amounts reach the systemic circulation; when administered parenterally, testosterone is rapidly absorbed from the injection vehicle and rapidly degraded. As a consequence, effective androgen therapy requires either the administration of a slowly absorbed form of testosterone (dermal patches or micronized oral preparation) or the administration

of modified analogues. Such chemical modifications either retard absorption or catabolism, so as to sustain effective blood levels, or enhance the androgenic potency of each molecule, so that full effects can be achieved at a lower blood level of drug. Three types of modification have had widespread clinical application (Fig. 336-7): esterification of the 17β-hydroxyl group, alkylation at the 17α position, and alteration of the ring structure, particularly by substitutions at the 2, 9, and 11 positions. Most agents actually have combinations of ring structure alterations and either 17α-alkylation or esterification of the 17β-hydroxyl group. Esterification serves to decrease the polarity of the molecule so that the steroid is more soluble in the fat vehicles used for injection and is released into the circulation more slowly. Most esters must be injected parenterally. The larger the acid esterified, the more prolonged is the action. Esters such as testosterone cypionate and testosterone enanthate can be injected every 1 to 3 weeks. Because the esters are hydrolyzed before the hormones act, the effectiveness of therapy can be monitored by assaying plasma testosterone level with time after administration.

The oral effectiveness of 17α-alkylated androgens (such as methyltestosterone and methandrostenolone) is due to slower hepatic catabolism, which allows the alkylated derivatives to escape degradation by the liver and reach the systemic circulation. For this reason, 17α-methyl or -ethyl substitution is a feature of most orally active androgens. Unfortunately, all 17α-alkylated steroids can cause abnormal liver function, and for this reason they have a limited role in medicine.

Other alterations of the ring structure have been adopted empirically; some slow the rate of inactivation, others enhance the potency of a given molecule, and some alter the conversion to other active metabolites. For example, the potency of fluoxymesterone may be due to the fact that, unlike most androgens, it is a poor precursor for conversion to estrogens in peripheral tissues. Two transdermal preparations in which a testosterone-loaded patch is applied each day are available. One is a single scrotal patch applied each morning;

FIGURE 336-7 Some of the androgen preparations available for pharmacologic use.

the other system involves two nonscrotal patches applied at bedtime. Both preparations produce physiologic testosterone levels and avoid the wide swings in serum testosterone values that occur between injections of testosterone esters.

SIDE EFFECTS OF ANDROGENS   All androgens carry the risk of inducing virilization in women. Early manifestations include acne, coarsening of the voice, hirsutism, and menstrual irregularities. If treatment is discontinued as soon as these effects develop, the manifestations may slowly subside. Long-term side effects such as male-pattern baldness, worsening of the hirsutism and voice changes, and hypertrophy of the clitoris are largely irreversible. At physiologic replacement doses, testosterone esters have no known toxic effects in mature men. At supraphysiologic doses, however, gonadotropin secretion is inhibited, the testes shrink, and the sperm count falls (indeed, low sperm counts may persist for as long as 9 months after cessation of androgen abuse).

The so-called toxic side effects differ among the different agents and with the clinical setting in which they are used. Retention of a limited amount of sodium is an inevitable consequence of androgen therapy, but in patients with underlying heart disease or renal failure or when androgens are administered in enormous amounts, sodium retention may lead to edema. Although androgens do not cause malignancy, they may promote the growth of and intensify pain from carcinomas of the prostate and breast in men.

The feminizing side effects of androgen therapy in men are poorly understood. Testosterone (but not 5α-reduced androgens) can be converted (aromatized) in extraglandular tissues to estradiol. The most common manifestation of feminization is the development of gynecomastia. Such breast enlargement is common in children given androgens, possibly because of a greater capacity to convert androgens to estrogens in childhood. The administration of testosterone esters to men results in an increase in plasma estrogen levels, but in men with normal liver function gynecomastia usually develops only after use of high doses.

All 17α-alkylated androgens can produce liver function abnormalities such as elevation of plasma levels of alkaline phosphatase and conjugated bilirubin. The incidence of clinical liver disease probably depends on the previous integrity of the liver, but jaundice may occur in the absence of preexisting liver disease. 17α-Alkylated drugs also cause an increase in the levels of a variety of plasma proteins that are synthesized in the liver. The most serious complications of use of 17α-alkylated androgens are peliosis hepatis (blood-filled cysts in the liver) and hepatoma. These disorders were initially described in patients with aplastic anemia, many of whom had Fanconi anemia, itself a predisposing factor for the development of malignancy. However, both lesions also have been reported in patients who received substituted androgens for other indications, including use by athletes. These tumors may either follow a benign course after discontinuation of the drugs or be rapidly fatal.

One indication for 17α-alkylated androgens is in the treatment of hereditary angioedema in which the desired therapeutic benefit (increase in the level of the inhibitor of the first component of complement) may actually be an effect of the 17-alkylated side chain rather than of the parent androgen. As a consequence, weak androgens such as danazol are effective in this disorder (see Fig. 336-7). Danazol is also used in the management of endometriosis (see Chap. 52).

REPLACEMENT THERAPY   The aim of androgen therapy in hypogonadal men is to restore or bring to normal male secondary sexual characteristics (beard, body hair, external genitalia) and male sexual behavior and to mimic the hormonal effects on somatic development (hemoglobin, muscle mass, nitrogen balance, and epiphyseal closure). Since an assay for plasma testosterone is available for monitoring therapy, the treatment of androgen deficiency is almost universally successful. The parenteral administration of a long-acting testosterone ester such as 100 to 200 mg testosterone enanthate at

1- to 2-week intervals results in a sustained increase in plasma testosterone to the normal male range. Such esters act only through the release of testosterone itself into the circulation. Alternatively, testosterone may be administered transdermally. If the hypogonadism is primary and of long duration (as in the Klinefelter syndrome), suppression of plasma LH to the normal range may not occur for many weeks, if at all. There is considerable variability in the relation between plasma testosterone and male sexual behavior, but in cases of postpubertal testicular failure (even of many years duration), normal sexual activity usually is resumed after adequate replacement. Androgen administration does not restore spermatogenesis in hypogonadal states, but the volume of the ejaculate (derived largely from the prostate and seminal vesicles) and other male secondary sex characteristics return to normal. The effects of endogenous androgen on hemoglobin, nitrogen retention, and skeletal development are also reproduced.

In men of all ages in whom hypogonadism developed prior to expected puberty (such as men with isolated gonadotropin deficiency), it is appropriate to bring plasma testosterone slowly into the adult range. When therapy is commenced at the time of expected puberty in such men, the normal events of puberty proceed in the usual fashion. If therapy is delayed until after the time of usual puberty, the degree to which normal virilization will occur is variable, but many patients undergo a relatively complete anatomic and functional maturation. Intermittent low-dose androgen therapy is indicated in prepubertal hypogonadal boys with microphallus to bring the external genitalia into the normal range. If such patients are monitored closely and given androgens only for short periods, such therapy usually has no adverse effects on somatic growth.

In boys of pubertal age with either isolated gonadotropin deficiency or primary testicular disease, the usual practice is to institute androgen therapy between the ages of 12 and 14 years, depending on the subjective need for sexual development. The initial administration of small doses of testosterone esters followed by a gradual increase to 100 to 150 mg/m^2 of body surface area every 1 to 3 weeks should result in a normal pubertal growth spurt. The time from the start of treatment to the appearance of secondary sex characteristics is variable. Penile development, deepening of the voice, and the appearance of other secondary sexual characteristics usually commence during the first year of treatment. In normal boys, puberty extends over several years, and treatment designed to replicate normal development does not shorten the process greatly.

Testosterone exerts its full action only in the presence of a balanced hormonal environment and, particularly, in the presence of adequate levels of growth hormone. Consequently, prepubertal boys with coexisting growth hormone and androgen deficiency respond poorly to androgens unless growth hormone is given simultaneously.

PHARMACOLOGIC USES   Androgens have been used for a variety of disorders unassociated with hypogonadism, in the hope that potential benefits from the nonvirilizing actions of the agents (such as increase in nitrogen retention and muscle mass, increased hemoglobin, etc.) would outweigh any deleterious actions of the drugs. The most common nonreplacement uses of androgen have been attempts to improve nitrogen balance in catabolic states, self-administration by athletes in the belief that muscle mass and/or athletic performance will be improved, attempts to enhance erythropoiesis in refractory anemias (including the anemia of renal failure), treatment of hereditary angioedema and endometriosis, and management of growth retardation of various etiologies. Most of the expected benefits in these disorders did not materialize, for two reasons. First, modest pharmacologic doses of androgens do little, if anything, in men beyond the normal testicular androgen, and in women the virilizing side effects of androgens are formidable. Second, no androgen has been devised that exhibits only the nonvirilizing effects of the hormone. This is not surprising in view of the fact that the physiologic actions of androgens are mediated by a single, high-affinity receptor protein in the cytoplasm (see Fig. 336-5).

The most pervasive form of androgen abuse is by male athletes in the expectation that muscle development and athletic performance will be improved. In controlled studies using modest pharmacologic doses (two to four times the usual replacement doses), these agents do not improve performance consistently. However, at the doses frequently taken by athletes (which sometimes exceed 10 times the replacement dose), these agents do enhance nitrogen balance and muscle mass; since the drugs have multiple side effects at high doses, these putative benefits do not outweigh the risks associated with androgen abuse, a practice that cannot be condemned too harshly. The only established indications for androgen therapy outside of male hypogonadism are in selected patients with anemia due to bone marrow failure or hereditary angioedema and as an adjunct to growth hormone therapy.

Gonadotropins Gonadotropin therapy is used to establish or restore fertility in patients with gonadotropin deficiency of any cause. Two gonadotropin preparations are available: human menopausal gonadotropins (hMG) (purified from the urine of postmenopausal women) and human chorionic gonadotropin (hCG) (purified from the urine of pregnant women). hMG contains 75 IU FSH and 75 IU LH per vial. hCG has little FSH activity and resembles LH in its ability to stimulate testosterone production by Leydig cells. Because of the expense of hMG, treatment is usually begun with hCG alone, and hMG is added later to promote the FSH-dependent stages of spermatid development. A high ratio of LH to FSH activity and a long duration of treatment (3 to 6 months) are necessary to bring about maturation of the prepubertal testes. Once spermatogenesis is restored in hypophysectomized patients or initiated in hypogonadotropic hypogonadal men by combined therapy, it can usually be maintained with hCG alone.

The dosage of hCG required to maintain a normal testosterone level varies from 1000 to 5000 IU weekly. A number of regimens have been used to induce maturation of spermatogenesis. Most involve starting with 2000 IU hCG three or more times a week until most of the clinical parameters, including plasma testosterone levels, are normal. hMG (usually one ampul) is then added three times a week to complete the development of spermatogenesis. After spermatogenesis has regressed, the length of therapy required to restore spermatogenesis may be as long as 12 months.

Luteinizing Hormone–Releasing Hormone And LHRH Analogues LHRH (gonadorelin) is available for endocrine testing. LHRH therapy is used by some physicians for chronic therapy of the infertility of hypogonadotropic hypogonadism. It is necessary to administer LHRH in frequent boluses (25 to 200 ng/kg of body weight every 2 h), which necessitates the use of portable infusion pumps. In general, LHRH does not appear to be more efficacious than gonadotropin in returning sperm counts to normal. LHRH analogues (leuprolide and nafarelin) are available for the suppression of gonadotropin secretion and the induction of hypogonadism. In prostatic cancer, testicular androgen production can be blocked by monthly injection of 7.5 mg leuprolide in depot form.

See Chap. 58, Androgens, in Goodman & Gilman's The Pharmacological Basis of Therapeutics, *9th ed, New York, McGraw-Hill, 1996.*

BIBLIOGRAPHY

Baker HWG: Male infertility, in *Endocrinology*, 3d ed, LLJ deGroot (ed). Philadelphia, Saunders, 1995, pp 2404–2433

Carr BR, Griffin JE: Fertility control and its complications, in *Williams Textbook of Endocrinology*, 8th ed, JD Wilson, DW Foster (eds). Philadelphia, Saunders, 1992, pp 1007–1031

———, Robertson DM: The isolation and physiology of inhibin and related proteins. Biol Reprod 40:33, 1989

Chillon M et al: Mutations in the cystic fibrosis gene in patients with congenital absence of the vas deferens. N Engl J Med 332:1475, 1995

de Kretser DM: Declining sperm counts. BMJ 312:457, 1996

Goldzieher JW et al: Improving the diagnostic reliability of rapidly fluctuating plasma hormone levels by optimized multiple-sampling techniques. J Clin Endocrinol Metab 43:824, 1976

Gray A et al: Age, disease and changing sex hormone levels in middle-aged men: Results of the Massachusetts male aging study. J Clin Endocrinol Metab 73:1016, 1991

Griffin JE, Wilson JD: Disorders of the testes and male reproductive tract, in *Williams Textbook of Endocrinology*, 8th ed, JD Wilson, DW Foster (eds). Philadelphia, Saunders, 1992, pp 799–852

Grumbach MM, Styne DM: Puberty: Ontogeny, neuroendocrinology, physiology, and disorders, in *Williams Textbook of Endocrinology*, 8th ed, JD Wilson, DW Foster (eds). Philadelphia, Saunders, 1992, pp 1139–1221

Handlesman DJ: Testicular dysfunction in systemic disease. Endocrinol Metab Clin North Am 23:839, 1994

Illingworth PJ et al: Inhibin-B: A likely candidate for the physiologically important form of inhibin in men. J Clin Endocrinol Metab 81:1321, 1996

Laue L et al: Treatment of familial male precocious puberty with spironolactone and testolactone. N Engl J Med 320:496, 1989

MacDonald PC et al: Origin of estrogen in normal men and in women with testicular feminization. J Clin Endocrinol Metab 49:905, 1979

Marshall WA, Tanner JM: Variation in the pattern of pubertal changes in boys. Arch Dis Child 45:13, 1970

Meikle AW et al: Enhanced transdermal delivery of testosterone across non-scrotal skin produces physiological concentrations of testosterone and its metabolites in hypogonadal men. J Clin Endocrinol Metab 74:623, 1992

Najmabadi H et al: Substantial prevalence of microdeletions of the Y-chromosome in infertile men with idiopathic azoospermia and oligospermia detected using a sequence-tagged site-based mapping strategy. J Clin Endocrinol Metab 81:1347, 1996

Palermo GD et al: Intracytoplasmic sperm injection: A novel treatment for all forms of male factor infertility. Fertil Steril 63:1231, 1995

Pescovitz OH et al: Paracrine control of spermatogenesis. Trends Endocrinol Metab 3:126, 1994

Poretsky L et al: Testicular dysfunction in human immunodeficiency virus-infected men. Metabolism 44:946, 1995

Rugarli EI, Ballabio A: Kallmann syndrome. JAMA 270:2173, 1993

Snyder PJ: Hypogonadotropic hypogonadism: Gonadotropin therapy, in *Current Therapy in Endocrinology and Metabolism*, 5th ed, CW Bardin (ed). St Louis, Mosby, 1994, pp 300–303

Snyder PF, Lawrence DA: Treatment of male hypogonadism with testosterone enanthate. J Clin Endocrinol Metab 51:1335, 1980

Whitcomb RW, Crowley WF Jr: Hypogonadotropic hypogonadism: Gonadotropin-releasing hormone therapy, in *Current Therapy in Endocrinology and Metabolism*, 5th ed, CW Bardin (ed). St Louis, Mosby, 1994, pp 303–305

337

Bruce R. Carr, Karen D. Bradshaw

DISORDERS OF THE OVARY AND FEMALE REPRODUCTIVE TRACT

The ovary is the source of ova for reproduction and of the hormones that regulate female sexual life. The anatomic structure, response to hormonal stimuli, and secretory capacity of the ovary differ at different periods of life. This chapter will review normal ovarian physiology as a background for understanding ovarian abnormalities and will consider other disorders of the female reproductive tract.

DEVELOPMENT, STRUCTURE, AND FUNCTION OF THE OVARY

EMBRYOLOGY During the third week of gestation, the primordial germ cells differentiate from the endoderm lining the yolk sac at the caudal end of the embryo. The germ cells migrate to the genital ridge adjacent to the mesonephric kidney by the fifth week of gestation and undergo mitotic division. The gonads exist in an undifferentiated state until the seventh week of fetal life, at which time the primitive ovary can be distinguished from the testis (see Chap. 339). Estrogen formation in the ovary commences between weeks 8 and 10, and by 10 to 11 weeks of gestation, oogonia in the ovarian cortex begin developing into primary oocytes. The ovary contains a finite number of germ cells, the number peaking at about 7 million oogonia by the fifth to sixth month of gestation. Subsequently, the germ cells decrease in number through a process of atresia so that only 1 million remain at birth, 400,000 are present at menarche, and only a few remain at menopause. Two X chromosomes are required for normal development of the ovary; in individuals with a 45,X karyotype, ovarian development occurs, but the rate of atresia is accelerated so that only a fibrous streak remains at birth (see Chap. 339).

After the oogonia cease to proliferate, meiosis commences, continues until the diplotene stage of the first meiotic division is completed and then is arrested until the onset of ovulation at puberty. From the fifth month of fetal life, the primordial follicle consists of the primary oocyte arrested in meiosis, a single surrounding layer of granulosa cells, and a basement membrane that separates the primordial follicle from surrounding stromal (interstitial) tissues.

PUBERTAL MATURATION The final maturation of ovarian follicles commences during puberty. The two major hormones that regulate follicular development are the pituitary gonadotropins—follicle-stimulating hormone (FSH) and luteinizing hormone (LH) (Fig. 337-1). During the second trimester of fetal development, the plasma gonadotropins rise to levels similar to those at menopause. This peak in gonadotropin levels may be responsible for the simultaneous peak in oocyte replication. After the second trimester, the hypothalamic-pituitary axis (the so-called gonadostat) becomes functional and is sensitive to negative feedback by steroid hormones, particularly estrogen and progesterone produced in the placenta. The levels of circulating gonadotropins consequently decrease, and gonadotropins are almost undetectable at the time of birth. In the neonate, concomitant with the decrease in estrogen and progesterone levels caused by separation from the placenta, there is a rebound increase in gonadotropin secretion for the first few months of life. With continued maturation of the hypothalamic-pituitary system, the gonadostat becomes sensitive to negative feedback by low levels of circulating steroid hormones, and plasma gonadotropins again decrease.

As the time of puberty nears, a decrease in the sensitivity of the gonadostat allows for increased secretion of FSH and LH, possibly secondary to increased episodic or pulsatile secretion of luteinizing hormone–releasing hormone (LHRH) by the hypothalamus (see Chap. 328). A sleep-induced, pulsatile pattern of LH secretion then ensues,

the first step in the development of a cyclic pattern of gonadotropin secretion (see Fig. 337-1). The increase in estrogen secretion exerts a positive feedback, which leads to an exaggeration of the pulsatile release of LH and eventually to ovulation and the menarche, after which plasma gonadotropin concentrations reach adult values in which day and night levels are similar. After the menopause, plasma gonadotropin levels rise, then plateau 5 to 10 years after menopause and remain fairly constant until the eighth to ninth decade of life when the levels may fall. Although ovarian function is regulated primarily by LH and FSH, the ovary is a source of peptide and protein hormones and growth factors that may play a role in ovarian function.

With puberty the sensitivity of the hypothalamic-pituitary centers to circulating steroid hormones is decreased, LHRH release by the hypothalamus increases, gonadotropin secretion by the pituitary is enhanced, ovarian estrogen secretion increases, and the anatomic changes of puberty ensue. At age 10 to 11, the first secondary sexual characteristics begin to appear in girls, namely, development of the breast buds (thelarche), followed by the development of pubic hair (pubarche), and later by the development of axillary hair (adrenarche). Pubic and axillary hair are believed to be controlled by adrenal androgens, the levels of which begin to rise at approximately 6 to 8 years of age. A growth spurt ensues, and peak growth rate is attained by age 12.

The culmination of puberty is the onset of predictable, cyclic menses. The average time between the beginning of breast development and the onset of menses (menarche) is 2 years. During the first few years after menarche, menstrual cycles are often irregular and unpredictable due to anovulation. The age of menarche is variable and is influenced by socioeconomic and genetic factors and by general health. In the United States, the mean age of menarche is believed to have decreased at a rate of 3 to 4 months per decade over the past 100 years and is now around 13 years, a change believed to be due to improved nutrition. A body weight of around 48 kg or some critical combination of weight, body water, and body fat is associated with development of hypothalamic insensitivity to feedback by steroids that leads to increased secretion of gonadotropins and finally to menarche. Obese girls have earlier menarche than girls with normal weights. In contrast, participation in sports or ballet, malnutrition, and chronic debilitating disease can delay menarche.

MATURE OVARY **Morphology** The anatomic components and function of the adult ovary are illustrated schematically in Fig. 337-2. Under the influence of gonadotropins, a group of primary follicles are recruited, and by day 6 to 8 of the menstrual cycle, one

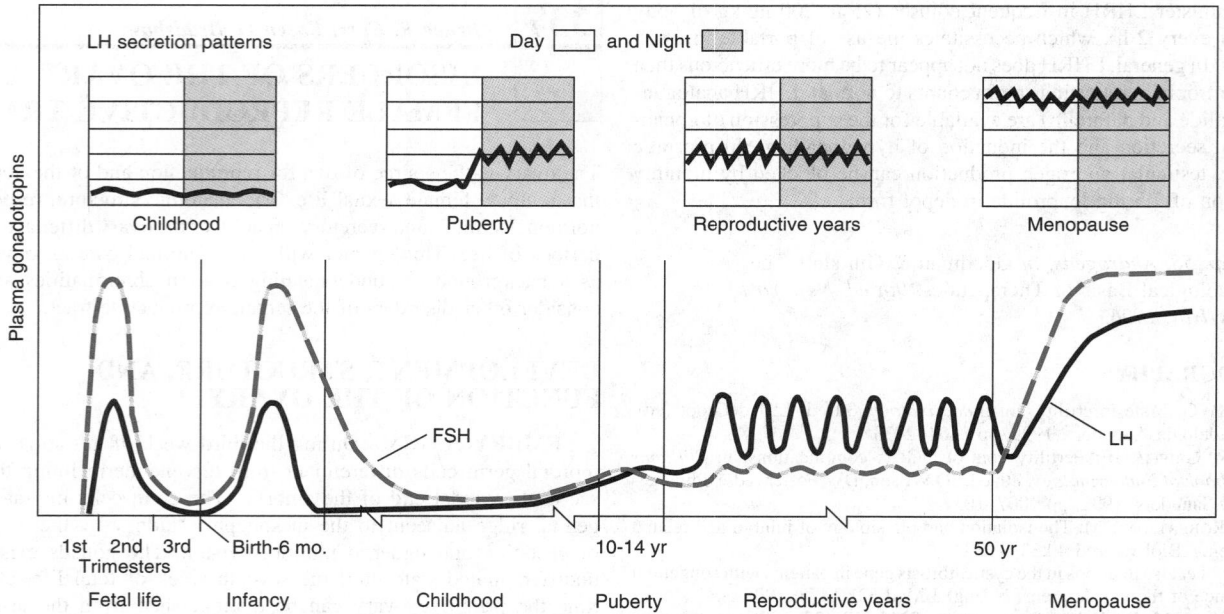

FIGURE 337-1 Pattern of gonadotropin secretion during different stages of life in women. FSH, follicle-stimulating hormone; LH, luteinizing hormone. The secretory patterns of LH during the waking hours (clear area) and night (stippled area) for each stage are indicated in the upper insets. (*After Faiman et al.*)

follicle becomes mature or "dominant," a process characterized by accelerated growth of granulosa cells and enlargement of the fluid-filled antrum. The recruited follicles not destined to ovulate undergo degeneration, similar to the atresia that occurs in other follicles during embryogenesis. Just prior to ovulation, meiosis resumes in the ovum of the dominant follicle, and the first meiotic division results in formation of the first polar body. The antrum rapidly enlarges (up to 10 to 25 mm in size), follicular fluid increases in amount, and the follicular surface thins and forms a conical stigma. Ovulation from the dominant follicle occurs some 16 to 23 h after the LH peak and some 24 to 38 h after the onset of the LH surge as the result of rupture of the follicular wall at the area of the stigma. The ovum is then expelled together with a mass of surrounding granulosa cells called *cumulus cells*. The rupture is believed to result from the action of hydrolytic enzymes on the surface of the follicle, possibly under the control of prostaglandins. The second meiotic division occurs after the egg is fertilized by a sperm, and the second polar body is then extruded. The formation of the corpus luteum begins in the retained remnant of the ovulated follicle; the remaining granulosa and theca cells increase in size and accumulate lipids and a yellow pigment, lutein, to become "luteinized." The basement membrane that separated the granulosa cells from the stroma and blood vessels breaks, and capillaries, fibroblasts, and lymphatics from the theca invade the granulosa cells and reach the central cavity, thereby filling it with blood. After a period of 14 ± 2 days (the functional life of the corpus luteum), vessels regress, and the corpus luteum begins to atrophy, to be replaced in time by a fibrous scar, the corpus albicans. The factors that limit the life span of the human corpus luteum are not known, but if pregnancy occurs, the corpus luteum persists under the influence of placental or chorionic gonadotropins, and progesterone is produced by the corpus luteum for the support of pregnancy.

Hormone Formation *Steroid hormones* Like other steroid hormones, ovarian steroids are derived from cholesterol (Fig. 337-3). The ovary can synthesize cholesterol de novo and also can utilize cholesterol obtained from circulating lipoproteins as substrate for steroid hormone formation (Fig. 337-4). Virtually all ovarian cells are believed to possess the complete complement of enzymes required for the synthesis of estradiol from cholesterol (see Fig. 337-3); however, different cell types in the ovary contain different amounts of these enzymes so that the main steroids produced differ in different compartments. For example, the corpus luteum forms mainly progesterone and 17-hydroxyprogesterone, whereas theca and stromal cells convert cholesterol to androstenedione and testosterone. Granulosa cells are particularly rich in the aromatase responsible for estrogen synthesis and utilize as substrates for this process androgens synthesized in the granulosa cells and the adjacent theca cells.

The principal sites of action of LH and FSH are also illustrated in Figs. 337-3 and 337-4. LH acts primarily to regulate the first step in steroid hormone biosynthesis, namely, the conversion of cholesterol to pregnenolone, and also induces subsequent enzymes in the pathway. FSH acts to regulate the final process by which androgens are aromatized to estrogens. As a consequence, LH enhances substrate flow and the formation of androgens and/or progesterone in the absence of FSH, whereas FSH action is impeded in the absence of LH because of diminished substrate for aromatization.

ESTROGENS   Naturally occurring estrogens are 18-carbon steroids characterized by an aromatic A ring, a phenolic hydroxyl group at C-3, and either a hydroxyl group (estradiol) or a ketone (estrone) at C-17 (see Fig. 337-3). (For the numbering of the steroid ring, see Fig. 336-1.) The principal estrogen secreted by the ovary and the most potent estrogen is estradiol. Estrone is also secreted by the ovary, but most estrone is formed by extraglandular conversion of androstenedione in peripheral tissues. Estriol (16-hydroxyestradiol), the main estrogen in urine, arises from the 16-hydroxylation of estrone and estradiol. Catechol estrogens are formed by hydroxylation of estrogens at the C-2 or C-4 position and may act as the intracellular mediators of some estrogen action. Estrogens promote development of the secondary sexual characteristics in women and cause uterine growth, thickening of the vaginal mucosa, thinning of the cervical mucus, and development of the ductule system of the breasts. The mechanism of estrogen action in target tissues is similar to that for other steroid hormones and involves binding to a nuclear steroid receptor and enhancement of the transcription of messenger RNA, which in turn causes increased protein synthesis in the cell cytoplasm (see Chap. 327).

FIGURE 337-2 Developmental changes in the adult ovary during a complete 28-day cycle.

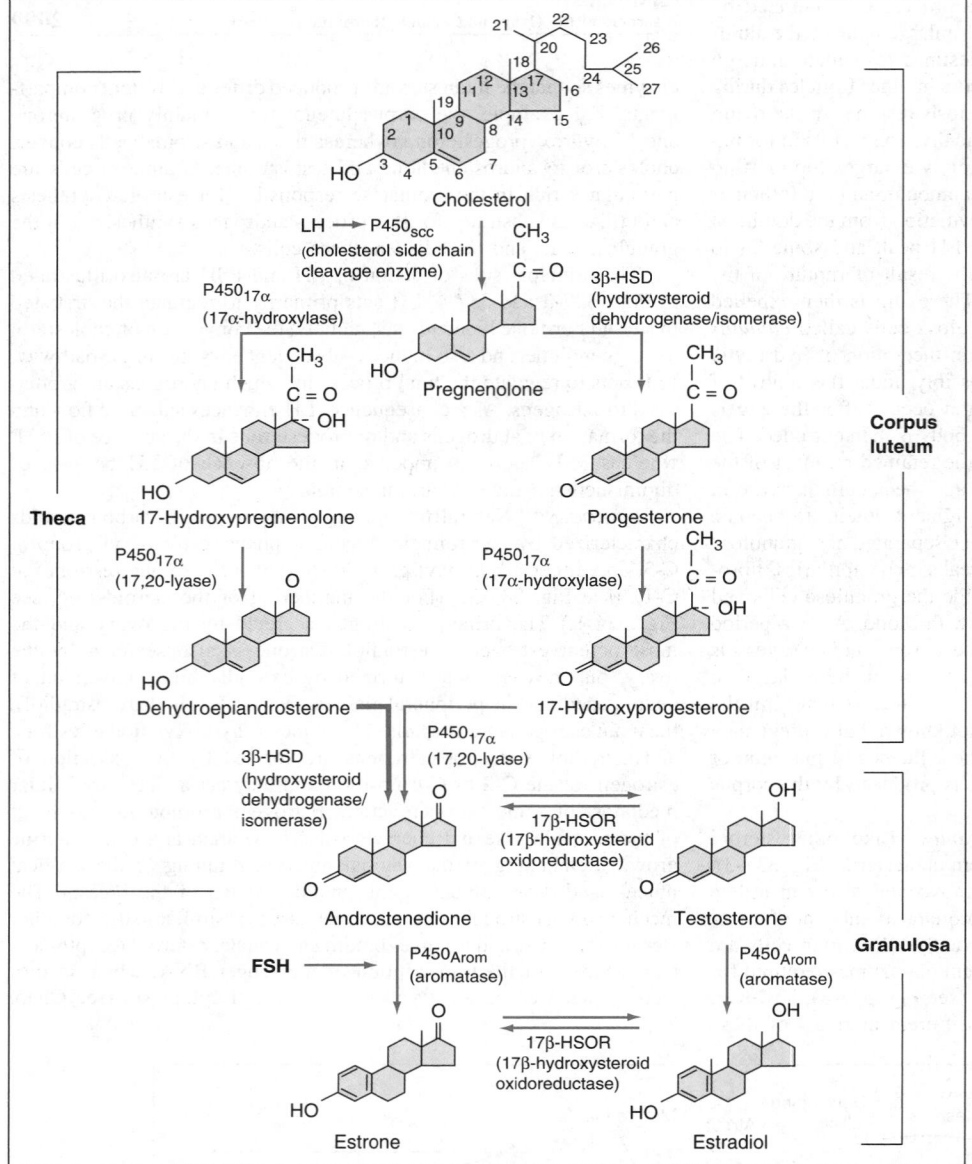

FIGURE 337-3 The principal pathway of steroid hormone biosynthesis in the ovary. Although every ovarian cell probably contains the complete enzyme complement required for the formation of estradiol from cholesterol, the amounts of the various enzymes and consequently the predominant hormones formed differ among the various cell types. The major enzyme complements for the corpus luteum, stroma, and granulosa cells are shown by the brackets; as a consequence, these cells produce predominantly progesterone and 17-OH progesterone, androgen, and estrogen, respectively. The major sites of action of LH and FSH in mediating this pathway are shown in the horizontal arrows. The dotted line emphasizes that the metabolism of 17-hydroxyprogesterone is limited in the human ovary. *(From Carr, 1992.)*

tium. Androstenedione also can be converted to testosterone and estrogens in peripheral tissues. Only testosterone and dihydrotestosterone are true androgens that interact with the androgen receptor and induce virilizing signs in women (see Chaps. 53 and 336).

Other hormones Some ovarian hormones play an uncertain role in human physiology. *Relaxin*, a polypeptide hormone produced by the human corpus luteum and by the decidua, causes softening of the cervix and loosening of the symphysis pubis in preparation for parturition in animals. *Oxytocin, vasopressin*, and other hypothalamic and pituitary hormones are also present in granulosa and/or luteal cells, but their function in these cells is unknown. *Follicular inhibin*, or *folliculostatin* (the equivalent of testicular inhibin), is secreted by the follicle and is believed to inhibit the release of FSH by the hypothalamic-pituitary unit. *Activin* is also secreted by the follicle and may enhance FSH secretion. *Follicle regulatory protein* (FRP), found in human follicular fluid, inhibits granulosa secretion and growth. *Gonadocrinins*, peptides purified from rat follicular fluid, stimulate the release of both FSH and LH from the pituitary in vitro and in vivo. Granulosa cells secrete *oocyte maturation inhibitor* (OMI), a factor that prevents premature ovulation. In addition, in the gonads of both sexes a *meiosis-inducing substance* (MIS) triggers the onset of meiosis, an event that occurs earlier in ovarian than in testicular development. Local growth factors [including insulin-like growth factors (IGFs) 1 and 2 and transforming growth factors (TGFs) α and β] may also influence steroid secretion by the ovary.

The Normal Menstrual Cycle
The menstrual cycle is divided into a follicular or proliferative phase and a luteal or secretory phase (Fig. 337-5). The secretion of FSH and LH is fundamentally under negative feedback control by ovarian steroids (particularly estradiol) and probably by inhibin, but the response of gonadotropins to different levels of estradiol varies. FSH secretion is inhibited progressively as estrogen levels increase—typical negative feedback. In contrast, LH secretion is suppressed maximally by low levels of estrogen and is enhanced by a rising and sustained elevation of estradiol—positive feedback. Negative feedback of estrogen involves both the hypothalamus and pituitary, whereas positive feedback operates primarily at the level of the pituitary.

The length of the menstrual cycle is defined as the time from the onset of one menstrual bleeding episode to onset of the next. In women of reproductive age, the cycle averages 28 ± 3 days, and the mean duration of flow is 4 ± 2 days. Longer menstrual cycles (usually characterized by anovulation) occur at menarche and prior to menopause. At the end of a cycle plasma levels of estrogen and progesterone fall, and circulating levels of FSH increase. Under the influence of FSH, follicular recruitment results in development of the follicle that will be dominant during the next cycle.

PROGESTERONE Progesterone, a 21-carbon steroid (see Fig. 337-3), is the principal hormone secreted by the corpus luteum and is responsible for progestational effects, namely, induction of secretory activity in the endometrium of the estrogen-primed uterus in preparation for implantation of the fertilized egg. Progesterone also induces a decidual reaction in endometrium. Other effects include inhibition of uterine contractions, an increase in the viscosity of cervical mucus, glandular development of the breasts, and an increase in basal body temperature (thermogenic effect).

ANDROGENS The ovary synthesizes a variety of 19-carbon steroids, including dehydroepiandrosterone, androstenedione, testosterone, and dihydrotestosterone, principally in stromal and thecal cells. The major ovarian 19-carbon steroid is androstenedione (see Fig. 337-3), part of which is secreted into the plasma and part of which is converted to estrogen in granulosa cells or to testosterone in the intersti-

FIGURE 337-4 Cellular interactions in the ovary during the follicular phase (*top*) and luteal phase (*bottom*). LDL, low-density lipoprotein; FSH, follicle-stimulating hormone; LH, luteinizing hormone. (*From Carr et al, 1982.*)

After the onset of menses, follicular development continues, but FSH levels decrease. Approximately 8 to 10 days prior to the midcycle LH surge, plasma estradiol levels begin to rise as the result of estradiol formation by the granulosa cells of the dominant follicle. During the second half of the follicular phase, LH levels also begin to rise (owing to positive feedback). Just before ovulation, estradiol secretion reaches a peak and then falls. Immediately thereafter, a further rise in the plasma level of LH mediates the final maturation of the follicle, followed by follicular rupture and ovulation 16 to 23 h after the LH peak. The rise in LH is accompanied by a smaller increase in the level of plasma FSH, the physiologic significance of which is unclear. The plasma progesterone level also begins to rise just prior to midcycle and facilitates the positive feedback action of estradiol on LH secretion.

At the onset of the luteal phase, plasma gonadotropins decrease, and plasma progesterone increases. A secondary rise in estrogens causes further gonadotropin suppression. Near the end of the luteal phase, progesterone and estrogen levels fall, and FSH levels begin to rise to initiate the development of the next follicle (usually in the contralateral ovary) and the next menstrual cycle.

The endometrium lining the uterine cavity undergoes marked alterations in response to the changing plasma levels of ovarian hormones (see Fig. 337-5). Concurrent with the decrease in plasma estrogen and progesterone and the decline of corpus luteum function in the late luteal phase, intense vasospasm occurs in the

spiral arterioles supplying blood to the endometrium, causing ischemic necrosis, endometrial desquamation, and bleeding. This vasospasm is caused by locally synthesized prostaglandins. The onset of bleeding marks the first day of the menstrual cycle. By the fourth to fifth day of the cycle, the endometrium is thin. During the proliferative phase, glandular growth of the endometrium is mediated by estrogen. After ovulation, increased progesterone levels lead to further thickening of the endometrium, but the rapid growth slows. The endometrium then enters the secretory phase, characterized by tortuosity of the glands, curling of the spiral arterioles, and glandular secretion. As corpus luteum function begins to wane in the absence of conception, the sequence of events leading to menstruation is again set into action.

Biphasic changes in basal body temperature are characteristic of the ovulatory cycle and are mediated by alterations in progesterone levels (see Fig. 337-5). An increase in basal body temperature by 0.3 to 0.5°C begins after ovulation, persists during the luteal phase, and returns to the normal baseline (36.2 to 36.4°C) after the onset of the subsequent menses.

Cellular Interactions in the Ovary during the Normal Cycle LH stimulates thecal cells surrounding the follicle to form androgens, and androstenedione diffuses across the basement membrane of the follicle into granulosa cells, where it is aromatized to estrogen (see Figs. 337-3 and 337-4).

The increase of FSH late in the preceding menstrual cycle stimulates growth and recruitment of the primary follicles by enhancing granulosa cell proliferation, resulting ultimately in the formation of the dominant follicle. In the granulosa cells, FSH also stimulates estrogen synthesis. Enhanced secretion of estradiol causes an increase in the number of estradiol receptors and further proliferation of granulosa cells. In the late follicular phase, FSH, in concert with estradiol, causes induction of LH receptors on the granulosa cells. LH acts via these receptors to increase progesterone secretion at midcycle. The amount of progesterone formed by the follicle is believed to be limited by the availability of cholesterol to serve as substrate for steroidogene-

FIGURE 337-5 The hormonal, ovarian, endometrial, and basal body temperature changes and relationships throughout the normal menstrual cycle.

sis and by the fact that most of the progesterone is converted to androstenedione by thecal cells. Prior to ovulation, the granulosa cells of the follicle are bathed in follicular fluid but have limited access to circulating blood and consequently to plasma low-density lipoprotein (LDL). As depicted in Fig. 337-4, the granulosa cells become vascularized after ovulation, and plasma cholesterol is made available to serve as the major substrate for progesterone synthesis by the corpus luteum. Thus, increased progesterone synthesis by the corpus luteum is the consequence of increased substrate availability. The peak in progesterone secretion by the corpus luteum occurs 8 days after ovulation at the time of maximal vascularization of the granulosa cells.

MENOPAUSE The *menopause* is defined as the final episode of menstrual bleeding in women. However, the term is used commonly to refer to the period that encompasses the transitional period between the reproductive years up to and after the last episode of menstrual bleeding. During this period, there is a progressive loss of ovarian function and a variety of endocrine, somatic, and psychological changes.

The median age of women at the time of cessation of menstrual bleeding is 50 to 51 years. Since the life expectancy of women is close to 80 years, approximately one-third of life occurs after cessation of reproductive function. Preceding the menopause, the pattern of menstrual cycles is variable, but the interval between menses usually becomes longer. In addition, there is an increase in the mean levels of plasma FSH and LH, despite the continuation of ovulatory cycles. Thus, the ovary appears to become less responsive to gonadotropins prior to the menopause.

The menopause is the consequence of the exhaustion of ovarian follicles. The decrease in the number of ova begins in intrauterine life; by the time of the menopause, few ova remain, and these appear to be nonfunctional. Only a small number of ova are lost as the result of ovulation during reproductive life; the majority are lost by atresia. The cessation of follicular development results in decreased production of estradiol and other hormones, which, in turn, causes a loss of negative feedback on the hypothalamic-pituitary centers. In turn, the levels of plasma gonadotropins increase, with FSH levels rising earlier and higher than LH levels (Figs. 337-1 and 337-6). The higher concentration of FSH than LH in postmenopausal women may result from the decrease in inhibin secretion by the ovary, from the fact that FSH is cleared from plasma less rapidly than LH, and possibly from the loss of positive feedback on LH production by estradiol. Intravenous

administration of LHRH to menopausal women results in a pronounced increase in the secretion of both FSH and LH, consistent with the enhanced hypothalamic-pituitary secretory activity in other forms of primary ovarian failure.

The ovaries of postmenopausal women are small, and the residual cells are predominantly stromal. Estrogen and androgen levels in plasma are reduced but not absent (see Fig. 337-6). Prior to the menopause, plasma androstenedione is derived almost equally from the adrenals and the ovaries; after menopause the ovarian contribution ceases so that the plasma levels of androstenedione fall by 50 percent (see Fig. 337-6). However, the menopausal ovary continues to secrete testosterone, presumably formed in stromal cells.

Circulating estrogens in the ovulating woman are derived from two sources. Sixty percent of mean estrogen formation during the menstrual cycle is in the form of estradiol, formed primarily by ovaries, and the remainder is estrone, formed mainly in extraglandular tissues from androstenedione. After menopause, extraglandular estrogen formation is the major pathway for estrogen synthesis. Estrogen production by the menopausal ovary is minimal, and oophorectomy does not cause a further decrease in estrogen levels. Plasma levels of estradiol, the principal estrogen secreted by the follicle, are lower in postmenopausal women than levels of estrone. The rate of peripheral formation of estrone increases somewhat in menopausal women so that estrone production is usually only slightly less than it was prior to the menopause despite the fall in plasma androstenedione. Because adipose tissue is a major site of extraglandular estrogen production, peripheral estrogen formation may actually be enhanced in obese postmenopausal women, so that total estrogen production rates may be as great or greater than in premenopausal women. The predominant estrogen formed is estrone rather than estradiol.

The most common menopausal symptoms are vasomotor instability (hot flashes), atrophy of the urogenital epithelium and skin, decreased size of the breasts, and osteoporosis. Approximately 40 percent of menopausal women develop symptoms serious enough to seek medical assistance.

The pathogenesis of the hot flash is uncertain. There is a close temporal relationship between the onset of the hot flash and pulses of LH secretion; however, hot flashes occur in women with hypopituitarism and after treatment with LHRH analogues, when LH levels are absent or low. Alterations in catecholamine, prostaglandin, endorphin, or neurotensin metabolism may play a role in conjunction with low estrogen production. Symptoms associated with the hot flash, including nervousness, anxiety, irritability, and depression, may or may not be due to estrogen deficiency.

The decrease in size of the tissues of the female reproductive tract and breasts in the menopause is due to estrogen deficiency. The vaginal mucosa and the endometrium usually become thin and atrophic (although endometrial hyperplasia occurs in one-fifth of postmenopausal women).

Osteoporosis is one of the dread afflictions of aging, and there is a close relationship between estrogen deprivation and its development. Approximately one-fourth of aging women and one-tenth of elderly men sustain a vertebral or hip fracture between the ages of 60 and 90, and the incidence is highest in elderly white women. Such fractures are a major cause of death and morbidity, and the fracture-related mortality increases from less than 10 percent in the 60- to 64-year age group to 30 percent or more in patients over 80 (see Chap. 355). Many factors affect the development of osteoporosis, including diet, activity, smoking, and general health, and estrogen deprivation is of particular importance. White postmenopausal women are more predisposed to osteoporosis and its consequences because bone density in this group is lower prior to menopause, so loss in bone density has more severe consequences. Further evidence that osteoporosis is a disease of estrogen deprivation is suggested by the early development of osteoporosis in women with premature menopause due to either natural causes or surgical castration. After the menopause women experience an increase in the incidence of cardiovascular disease, possibly as the result of a decrease in the level of high-density lipoprotein (HDL) cholesterol.

FIGURE 337-6 Differences in hormone concentration in women during the reproductive years and in women during the menopause. FSH, follicle-stimulating hormone; LH, luteinizing hormone; E_2, estradiol-17β; E_1, estrone; Δ^4-A, androstenedione; T, testosterone. *[From SSC Yen, RB Jaffe (eds), Reproductive Endocrinology. Philadelphia, Saunders, 1986; and from DR Mishell Jr, V Dajavan (eds), Reproductive Endocrinology, Infertility, and Contraception, 2d ed, Philadelphia, Davis, 1986.]*

LABORATORY AND CLINICAL ASSESSMENT OF HORMONAL STATUS

The hormonal status of women can usually be assessed by history and physical examination. In general, the presence of secondary sexual characteristics such as normal female breast development indicates adequate estrogen secretion in the past, and the presence of regular, predictable, cyclic menses implies that ovulation and the production of gonadotropins, estrogen, progesterone, and androgens are adequate and that the outflow tract is intact. Such a history may be more valuable than laboratory tests in evaluating ovarian hormone status. However, laboratory tests provide valuable ancillary information in the workup of women with endocrine dysfunction or infertility.

PITUITARY GONADOTROPINS   Plasma gonadotropins are assessed by radioimmunoassay (RIA), fluoroimmunoassay (FIA), or enzyme-linked immunosorbent assay (ELISA). Because both FSH and LH are secreted in a pulsatile manner, the results obtained from a single serum sample may be difficult to interpret. Consequently, multiple samples taken at 20-min intervals over 2 h may be pooled to obtain a mean value. Serum gonadotropin measurements are of the most use in evaluating women with suspected ovarian failure and in supporting the diagnosis of polycystic ovarian disease and hypogonadotropic hypogonadism. The normal ranges for serum LH and FSH in ovulating women are 0.8 to 57 and 1.4 to 21 IU/L, respectively. FSH levels that are persistently above 34 IU/L are diagnostic of ovarian failure, and an LH value of less than 0.8 IU/L suggests hypogonadotropic hypogonadism. In practice, however, gonadotropin values may be equivocal and must be interpreted in light of the remainder of the findings.

OVARIAN HORMONES   The mean plasma levels and production rates of the principal ovarian hormones are presented in Table 337-1. The production rate of a hormone is the sum of the amount of hormone formed by direct glandular secretion and by extraglandular conversion of prohormones.

Estrogen   The presence of normal secondary sexual characteristics implies that estrogen production was adequate in the past. The current estrogen status can be estimated by pelvic examination. The presence of a moist, rugated vagina with copious, clear, thin cervical mucus that can be stretched and that exhibits arborization or ferning when spread on a slide is strong evidence of adequate estrogen production. Cytologic demonstration of mature vaginal epithelial cells and abundant cornified squamous epithelial cells with pyknotic nuclei confirms the presence of adequate estrogen levels.

The progesterone-withdrawal test provides a functional assessment of estrogen status. If menses appear within a week to 10 days after the end of a trial of medroxyprogesterone acetate (10 mg by mouth once or twice a day for 5 days) or after a single intramuscular injection of progesterone (100 mg), then prior estrogen priming was adequate to allow withdrawal bleeding.

Owing to its variable level in plasma during the normal cycle and the difficulty of estimating the day of the cycle in women with abnormal cycles, the measurement of estrogen levels in plasma or urine is of little use in the routine assessment of estrogen status. Measurement of plasma estradiol is useful during attempts to induce ovulation with human menopausal gonadotropins to prevent the development of the ovarian hyperstimulation syndrome and is used along with ultrasound assessment to monitor follicular growth in women who are to undergo in vitro fertilization.

Progesterone   Cyclic, predictable menses also imply that adequate progesterone is secreted during the luteal phase of the menstrual cycle. Assessment of progesterone is useful to detect ovulation, to evaluate the adequacy of the luteal phase in infertile women, and to distinguish women with müllerian agenesis from those with testicular feminiza-

tion. Several functional assays of progesterone can be used. The least expensive and most useful is the daily measurement of basal body temperature throughout a cycle. Owing to the thermogenic properties of progesterone, a normal biphasic monthly curve showing a temperature elevation lasting for approximately 2 weeks after ovulation is a valid indication of progesterone secretion during the luteal phase (see Fig. 337-5). The presence of viscous cervical mucus that does not stretch or fern and of predominantly intermediate cells on vaginal cytology or demonstration of a secretory epithelium in an endometrial biopsy during the luteal phase on days 20 to 22 of the cycle provides additional assessment of progesterone secretion. In addition, serum progesterone can be measured by RIA, FIA, or ELISA to assess the function of the corpus luteum.

Androgen   Under normal conditions, the ovary secretes androstenedione, testosterone, and dehydroepiandrosterone. In conditions of androgen excess, hirsutism and/or virilization are common. The evaluation of androgen excess is discussed in Chap. 53.

DIAGNOSIS OF PREGNANCY   Pregnancy is usually recognized on the basis of the history and physical examination. That is, a woman with previously cyclic, predictable menses develops amenorrhea accompanied by breast tenderness, malaise, lassitude, and nausea, and on physical examination the uterus is soft and enlarged.

Assays of placental products facilitate the diagnosis of pregnancy. Human chorionic gonadotropin (hCG) is secreted by the trophoblastic cells of the placenta into the maternal plasma and excreted in the urine. Assays of the hCG content of serum or urine use either antibody against hCG or the LH/hCG receptor and make it possible to detect pregnancies 8 to 10 days after ovulation, before the first missed menstrual period and long before pregnancy can be diagnosed by clinical assessments. Assay of the β subunit of hCG in serum or urine makes it possible to differentiate between excess LH and hCG, an important distinction in evaluating women with trophoblastic disease such as hydatidiform mole or choriocarcinoma.

DISORDERS OF OVARIAN FUNCTION

PREPUBERTAL YEARS   Puberty is said to be *precocious* if breast budding begins before age 8 or if menarche occurs before age 9. Those disorders in which the developing sexual characteristics are appropriate for the genetic and gonadal sex—i.e., feminization in girls or virilization in boys—are termed *isosexual precocity*, whereas *heterosexual precocity* occurs when sexual characteristics are not in accord with the genetic sex, namely, virilization in girls or feminization in boys. Pubertal disorders of boys are described in Chap. 336.

Isosexual Precocious Puberty   Isosexual precocious puberty in girls can be divided into three major categories (Table 337-2).

True precocious puberty   True precocious puberty is characterized by an early but otherwise normal sequence of pubertal development, including increased secretion of gonadotropins and ovulatory

Table 337-1

Concentrations, Metabolic Clearance Rates, and Production Rates of the Major Ovarian Steroid Hormones in Blood of Ovulatory Women

Steroid	Binding*	Phase of Menstrual Cycle	Plasma Concentration, nmol/L, ng/ml	Production Rate, μmol/d, mg/d
Estradiol	TeBG and albumin	Follicular	0.07–2.6 (0.02–0.7)	0.3–3.6 (0.08–1.0)
		Luteal	0.7 (0.2)	0.9 (0.25)
Estrone	Albumin	Follicular	0.2–1.1 (0.05–0.3)	0.4–2.6 (0.1–0.7)
		Luteal	0.4 (0.1)	0.9 (0.24)
Progesterone	CBG and albumin	Follicular	3 (1)	6.4 (2)
		Luteal	16–80 (5–25)	80 (25)
Androstenedione	Albumin	—	5.6 (1.6)	10 (3)
Testosterone	TeBG and albumin	—	1.4 (0.4)	0.9 (0.25)

* TeBG, testosterone-binding globulin; CBG, cortisol-binding globulin.
SOURCE: Modified from MB Lipsett, in *Reproductive Endocrinology*, SSC Yen, RB Jaffe (eds). Philadelphia, Saunders, 1986.

Differential Diagnosis of Sexual Precocity

Isosexual precocity
  A. True precocious puberty
    1. Constitutional
    2. Organic brain disease
    3. Congenital adrenal hyperplasia
  B. Precocious pseudopuberty
    1. Ovarian tumors
    2. Adrenal tumors
    3. McCune-Albright syndrome
    4. Hypothyroidism
    5. Russell-Silver syndrome
    6. Estrogen-containing medications
  C. Incomplete sexual precocity
    1. Premature thelarche
    2. Premature adrenarche
    3. Premature pubarche
Heterosexual precocity
  A. Ovarian tumors
  B. Adrenal tumors
  C. Congenital adrenal hyperplasia

menstrual cycles. Constitutional or idiopathic precocious puberty accounts for 90 percent of cases. In these individuals, no cause for the premature maturation of the central nervous system–hypothalamic-pituitary axis can be identified, and the diagnosis is one of exclusion. As many as half these individuals have abnormal findings on electroencephalograms. Premature appearance of secondary sexual characteristics and of ovulatory cycles with the accompanying risk of fertility may cause significant emotional disturbance. Therefore, prompt initiation of therapy is imperative. LHRH analogues inhibit estrogen synthesis and thus reverse precocious puberty; they may also prevent premature closure of the epiphyses and the resulting short stature.

About 10 percent of cases are due to organic brain diseases, including brain tumors (hypothalamic gliomas, astrocytomas, ependymomas, germinomas, and hamartomas), encephalitis, meningitis, hydrocephalus, head injury, tuberous sclerosis, and neurofibromatosis. It is essential to distinguish this group of patients from those with the idiopathic disorder, and patients whose disorder is designated as idiopathic occasionally prove to have such tumors. Fortunately, most patients with organic lesions serious enough to cause precocious puberty have obvious neurologic signs and symptoms. Evaluation of all patients with precocious puberty should include, at a minimum, skull films and computed tomography (CT) or magnetic resonance imaging (MRI) of the brain. The success of treatment depends on the nature of the lesion, but surgical and radiation treatment of well-localized tumors is occasionally successful.

A rare cause of isosexual precocity is congenital adrenal hyperplasia due to 21-hydroxylase deficiency in girls in whom treatment is delayed until 4 to 8 years of age. After initiation of glucocorticoid replacement, such individuals may undergo isosexual precocious puberty (see Chap. 332).

Precocious pseudopuberty Precocious pseudopuberty occurs when girls undergo feminization as a consequence of enhanced estrogen formation but do not ovulate or develop cyclic menses. Ovarian cysts or tumors that secrete estrogen (granulosa-theca cell tumors) are the most frequent cause of precocious pseudopuberty. Granulosa-theca cell tumors associated with intestinal polyps and pigmentation of the mucous membranes occur in the Peutz-Jeghers syndrome. Other ovarian tumors that secrete estrogens (or androgens that can be converted to estrogens at extraglandular sites) include dysgerminomas, teratomas, cystadenomas, and ovarian carcinomas (also see Chap. 99). Ovarian tumors usually can be detected by rectoabdominal examination or by sonography, CT, MRI, and/or laparoscopy. Ovarian teratomas and choriocarcinomas and other carcinomas that secrete hCG do not cause precocious puberty in girls unless they also secrete estrogen (hCG or

LH in the absence of FSH does not induce ovarian estrogen production). Rarely, feminizing tumors of the adrenal cause isosexual precocious puberty by direct formation of estrogens or by secretion of weak androgens, which are converted to estrogens in extraglandular tissues.

Other causes of precocious pseudopuberty include the following:

1. The McCune-Albright syndrome (polyostotic fibrous dysplasia) is due to a G-protein defect that causes gonadotropin receptor activation in the absence of ligand, leading to autonomous ovarian follicle development and estrogen formation. It is characterized by café au lait spots, cystic fibrous dysplasia of bones, and sexual precocity. Occasionally, this disorder leads to true precocious puberty (see Chap. 340).
2. Primary hypothyroidism is associated with enhanced secretion of thyrotropin-releasing hormone (TRH) and, occasionally, of other hypothalamic hormones as well, leading to increased FSH levels and ovarian estrogen secretion, frequently with galactorrhea.
3. The Russell-Silver syndrome, or congenital asymmetry, is associated with short stature and precocious feminization.
4. Estrogen-containing medications, including use of estrogen-containing creams for diaper rash or the ingestion of meat from estrogen-treated animals or poultry or of any estrogen by mouth, can cause this disorder.

Incomplete isosexual precocity This term is used to describe the premature development of a single pubertal event and encompasses several entities. Breast budding prior to age 8 (*premature thelarche*) without other evidence of estrogen secretion and without premature bone maturation is believed to be due to a transient increase in estrogen secretion or to a temporary increase in sensitivity to the small amounts of circulating estrogens formed prior to puberty. Usually, the disorder is self-limited and resolves spontaneously. Occasionally, axillary hair and/or pubic hair (*premature adrenarche* and *pubarche*) appear without any other secondary sexual development. The phenomenon is associated with adrenal androgen secretion in the range of normal puberty and can be distinguished from syndromes of virilization by the absence of clitoromegaly. It requires no treatment, and patients enter puberty at about the average time.

Heterosexual Precocity Virilization in a prepubertal female is usually due to congenital adrenal hyperplasia or to androgen secretion by an ovarian or adrenal tumor. The manifestations of virilization are described in Chaps. 53 and 332. Virilization in girls with congenital adrenal hyperplasia usually takes place in a background of variable sexual ambiguity (see Chap. 339).

Evaluation of Sexual Precocity The evaluation of sexual precocity involves a careful history and physical examination, including rectoabdominal examination, abdominal sonography, determination of bone age, and measurement of thyroid hormones, thyroid-stimulating hormone (TSH), and gonadotropins (and androgen or estrogen levels when appropriate). MRI and/or CT scans should be obtained if a neurologic disorder is suspected and no evidence of ovarian or adrenal tumor is found.

REPRODUCTIVE YEARS Disorders of the Menstrual Cycle *Abnormal uterine bleeding* Between menarche and the menopause, almost every woman experiences one or more episodes of abnormal uterine bleeding, here defined as any bleeding pattern that differs in frequency, duration, or amount from the pattern observed during a normal menstrual cycle. A variety of descriptive terms (such as *menorrhagia*, *metrorrhagia*, and *menometrorrhagia*) have been used to characterize patterns of abnormal uterine bleeding. A more logical approach is to divide abnormal uterine bleeding into those patterns associated with ovulatory cycles and those associated with anovulatory cycles.

Ovulatory cycles Normal menstrual bleeding with ovulatory cycles is spontaneous, regular, cyclic, and predictable and frequently is associated with discomfort (dysmenorrhea). Deviations from this pattern associated with cycles that are still regular and predictable are most often due to organic disease of the outflow tract. For example, regular but prolonged and excessive bleeding episodes unassociated with bleeding dyscrasias (hypermenorrhea or menorrhagia) can result from abnormalities of the uterus such as submucous leiomyomas, adenomyosis, or endometrial polyps. Regular, cyclic, predictable menstruation characterized by spotting or light bleeding is termed *hypomenorrhea* and is due to obstruction of the outflow tract as from intrauterine synechiae or scarring of the cervix. Intermenstrual bleeding between episodes of regular, ovulatory menstruation is also often due to cervical or endometrial lesions. An exception to the association between organic disease and abnormal uterine bleeding is the occurrence of regular menstruation more frequently than 21 days apart (polymenorrhea). Such cycles may be a normal variant.

Anovulatory cycles Uterine bleeding that is unpredictable with respect to amount, onset, and duration and is usually painless is described as *dysfunctional uterine bleeding*. This disorder is not due to abnormalities of the uterus but rather to chronic anovulation and occurs when there is interruption of the normal sequence of follicular and luteal phases under the influence of a dominant follicle and its resulting corpus luteum. As discussed above, uterine bleeding in ovulatory cycles is due to progesterone withdrawal and requires that the endometrium first be primed with estrogen. (When castrates or postmenopausal women are given progesterone, withdrawal bleeding usually does not occur.)

Dysfunctional uterine bleeding can occur in women who have a transient disruption of the synchronous hypothalamic-pituitary-ovarian patterns necessary for ovulatory cycles, most often at the extremes of the reproductive life—in the early menarche and in the perimenopausal period—but also after temporary stress or intercurrent illness.

Primary *dysfunctional uterine bleeding* can result from three disorders.

1. *Estrogen withdrawal bleeding* occurs when estrogen is given to a castrated or postmenopausal woman and then withdrawn. As in other types of dysfunctional uterine bleeding, this form of menstrual bleeding is usually painless.
2. *Estrogen breakthrough bleeding* occurs when there is continuous estrogen stimulation of the endometrium not interrupted by cyclic progesterone secretion and withdrawal. This is the most common type of dysfunctional uterine bleeding and is usually due to anovulation associated with chronic acyclic estrogen production, as in women with polycystic ovarian disease. Such women may have histories of irregular, unpredictable menses, oligomenorrhea, or amenorrhea (see below). Alternatively, estrogen breakthrough bleeding can occur in hypogonadal women given estrogens chronically rather than intermittently and in women with estrogen-secreting tumors of the ovary. Estrogen breakthrough bleeding may be profuse and is unpredictable with respect to duration, amount of flow, and time of occurrence. The endometrium is typically thin because its repair between episodes of bleeding is incomplete.
3. *Progesterone breakthrough bleeding* occurs in the presence of abnormally high ratios of progesterone to estrogen, e.g., in women using continuous low-dose oral contraceptives.

The approach to a patient with dysfunctional uterine bleeding begins with a careful history of menstrual patterns and prior hormonal therapy. Since not all urogenital tract bleeding is from the uterus, rectal, bladder, and vaginal or cervical sources must be excluded by physical examination. If the bleeding is from the uterus, a pregnancy-related disorder such as abortion or ectopic pregnancy must be ruled out. Once the diagnosis of dysfunctional uterine bleeding is established, a rational approach to management is as follows: During a first episode of dysfunctional bleeding the patient can simply be observed, provided the bleeding is not copious and no evidence of bleeding dyscrasia is present. If bleeding is moderately severe, control can be achieved with relatively high dose estrogen oral contraceptives for 3 weeks. Alternatively, a regimen of three or four low-dose oral contraceptive pills per day for 1 week followed by tapering to the usual dosage for up to 3 weeks is also effective. If uterine bleeding is more severe, hospitalization, bed rest, and intramuscular injections of estradiol valerate (10 mg) and hydroxyprogesterone caproate (500 mg) or intravenous or intramuscular conjugated estrogens (25 mg) usually control

the bleeding. After initial treatment, iron replacement should be instituted, and recurrence can be prevented by cyclic oral contraceptives for 2 to 3 months (or more if pregnancy is not desired). Alternatively, menses can be induced every 2 to 3 months with medroxyprogesterone acetate, 10 mg by mouth once or twice a day for 10 days. If hormone therapy fails to control uterine bleeding, an endometrial biopsy, hysteroscopy, or dilatation and curettage may be required for diagnosis and therapy. Indeed, uterine sampling should be performed prior to hormone therapy in women at risk for endometrial cancer (i.e., in women who are approaching the age of menopause or are massively obese); endometrial cancer is rare in ovulatory women of reproductive age.

Amenorrhea An acceptable definition of amenorrhea is failure of menarche by age 16, irrespective of the presence or absence of secondary sexual characteristics, or the absence of menstruation for 6 months in a woman with previous periodic menses. However, women who do not fulfill these criteria should be evaluated if (1) the subject and/or her family are greatly concerned, (2) no breast development has occurred by age 14, or (3) any sexual ambiguity or virilization is present (Chap. 339). Amenorrhea is commonly categorized as either primary (the woman has never menstruated) or secondary (when menstruation has been present for a variable period of time in the past and has ceased). However, some disorders can cause either primary or secondary amenorrhea. For example, most women with gonadal dysgenesis have primary amenorrhea, but some have some follicles and ovulate for short periods so that pregnancy occurs rarely. Furthermore, patients with chronic anovulation (polycystic ovarian disease) usually have secondary amenorrhea but on occasion have primary amenorrhea. For these reasons, categorization of amenorrhea into primary and secondary types is less helpful than a classification based on the underlying physiologic derangements: (1) anatomic defects, (2) ovarian failure, and (3) chronic anovulation with or without estrogen present.

ANATOMIC DEFECTS Anatomic or structural defects of the genital tract can preclude menstrual bleeding. Starting from the caudal end of the female genital tract, labial agglutination or fusion is often associated with disorders of sexual development, particularly female pseudohermaphroditism (congenital adrenal hyperplasia or exposure to maternal androgens in utero) (see Chap. 339). Congenital defects of the vagina, imperforate hymen, and transverse vaginal septae also can cause amenorrhea. These women frequently have accumulation of menstrual blood behind the obstruction and may have cyclic, predictable episodes of abdominal pain.

More severe müllerian anomalies include müllerian agenesis (the Mayer-Rokitansky-Küster-Hauser syndrome; see Chap. 339), second in frequency only to gonadal dysgenesis as a cause of primary amenorrhea. Women with this syndrome have a 46,XX karyotype, female secondary sex characteristics, and normal ovarian function, including cyclic ovulation, but have absence or hypoplasia of the vagina. The uterus usually consists of only rudimentary bicornuate cords, but if the uterus contains endometrium, cyclic abdominal pain and accumulation of blood may occur, as in other forms of outlet obstruction. One-third of women with this syndrome have abnormalities of the urogenital tract, and one-tenth have skeletal anomalies, usually involving the spine. The major diagnostic problem is distinguishing müllerian agenesis from complete testicular feminization, in which 46,XY genetic males with testes differentiate as phenotypic women but with a blind vaginal pouch and no uterus. Women with testicular feminization have feminized breasts but a paucity of pubic and axillary hair. The disorder is due to a defect in the androgen receptor that causes profound resistance to the action of testosterone (see Chap. 339). Testicular feminization can be diagnosed by demonstrating a male level of serum testosterone or a 46,XY karyotype, whereas demonstration of a 46,XX karyotype, the biphasic basal body temperature curve characteristic of ovulation, and elevated levels of progesterone during the luteal phase establish the diagnosis of müllerian agenesis.

A rare cause of absence of the uterus in 46,XY phenotypic women who are sexually infantile is the so-called testicular regression syndrome or testicular agenesis (see Chap. 339).

Other abnormalities of the uterus that cause amenorrhea include obstruction due to scarring or stenosis of the cervix, often resulting from surgery, electrocautery, laser therapy, or cryosurgery. Such destruction of the endometrium (Asherman's syndrome) usually follows vigorous curettage for postpartum hemorrhage or after therapeutic abortion complicated by infection. This diagnosis is confirmed by hysterosalpingography or by direct visual examination of the endometrial scarring or synechiae using a hysteroscope.

Treatment of disorders of the outflow tract is surgical.

OVARIAN FAILURE   Primary ovarian failure is associated with elevated plasma gonadotropin levels and can result from several causes. The most frequent cause is *gonadal dysgenesis*, in which the germ cells are absent and the ovary is replaced by a fibrous streak (also see Chaps. 65 and 339). Women with gonadal dysgenesis can be divided into two broad groups on the basis of chromosomal karyotype. The most common type is due to deletion of genetic material in the X chromosomes and accounts for about two-thirds of cases of gonadal dysgenesis. A 45,X karyotype is found in about half of women with this disorder, and most have somatic defects, including short stature, webbed neck, shield chest, and cardiovascular defects, collectively termed the *Turner phenotype*. The remainder of women with X chromosome abnormalities have chromosomal mosaicism with or without associated structural abnormalities of the X. The most common form of mosaicism is 45,X/46,XX. Gonadal tumors are rare in 45,X patients, but gonadal malignancies may occur in women with chromosomal mosaicism involving the Y chromosome. Therefore, chromosomal analysis should be performed in all cases of amenorrhea associated with ovarian failure, and the streak gonad should be removed if a Y chromosome is present. One means of identifying the presence of a Y chromosome is to amplify the sex-determining regions of the Y chromosome (SRY) by means of the polymerase chain reaction (see Chap. 339). Approximately 90 percent of women with gonadal dysgenesis due to partial or complete deletion of the X never have menstrual bleeding, and the remaining 10 percent have sufficient follicles to experience menses and, rarely, fertility; the menstrual and reproductive lives of such individuals are invariably brief.

One-tenth of individuals identified as having bilateral streak gonads have a normal 46,XX or 46,XY karyotype and are said to have *pure gonadal dysgenesis*. These individuals have either normal or above-average stature, owing to failure of estrogen-mediated epiphyseal closure in the presence of a normal chromosomal constitution. Pure gonadal dysgenesis does not constitute a phenotypic or chromosomally homogeneous disorder (see Chap. 339). Occasional women with a 46,XY karyotype develop signs of virilization, including clitoromegaly, and have an increased incidence of tumors in the gonadal streaks; as a consequence, gonadal streaks should be removed prophylactically, as discussed above, when a Y chromosome is present. Approximately two-thirds of women with 46,XX gonadal dysgenesis experience no menses, while the remainder have one or more menstrual episodes and are occasionally fertile.

Other causes of ovarian failure and amenorrhea include deficiency of the $P450_{17\alpha}$ gene that encodes 17α-hydroxylase and 17,20-lyase activities, premature ovarian failure, the resistant-ovary syndrome, and ovarian failure secondary to chemotherapy or radiation therapy for malignancy. *17α-Hydroxylase deficiency* is characterized by primary amenorrhea, sexual infantilism, and hypertension, the latter due to increased production of desoxycorticosterone (DOC); whereas women with *17,20-lyase deficiency* have primary amenorrhea and sexual infantilism with normal blood pressure (see Chaps. 332 and 339). The diagnosis of *premature ovarian failure* or *premature menopause* is applied to women who cease menstruating prior to age 40. The ovaries in such women are similar to the ovaries of postmenopausal women, containing few or no follicles as the result of accelerated follicular

atresia. Premature ovarian failure due to ovarian antibodies may be one component of polyglandular failure, together with adrenal insufficiency, hypothyroidism, and other autoimmune disorders (see Chap. 340). A rare form of ovarian failure is the *resistant-ovary syndrome*, in which the ovaries contain many follicles that are arrested in development prior to the antral stage, possibly because of resistance to the action of FSH in the ovary. To differentiate this disorder from the 46,XX variety of pure gonadal dysgenesis, which also is associated with sexual immaturity, it is necessary to perform ovarian biopsy. However, it is not clinically useful to make this distinction, since the conventional treatment of infertility in both conditions is usually unsuccessful. Women with ovarian failure who desire pregnancy have been treated with hormone replacement and transfer of donor embryos to the uterine cavity or fallopian tubes.

Chronic anovulation   At least 80 percent or more of gynecologic endocrine disorders result form chronic anovulation. Women with chronic anovulation fail to ovulate spontaneously but may ovulate with appropriate therapy. The ovaries of such women do not secrete estrogen in a normal cyclic pattern; it is clinically useful to differentiate those women who produce enough estrogen to have withdrawal bleeding after progestogen therapy from those who do not; the latter often have hypothalamic-pituitary dysfunction.

CHRONIC ANOVULATION WITH ESTROGEN PRESENT   Women with chronic anovulation who experience withdrawal bleeding after progestogen administration are said to be in a state of "estrus" due to the acyclic production of estrogen, largely estrone, by extraglandular aromatization of circulating androstenedione. This disorder is commonly termed *polycystic ovarian disease* (PCOD) and is characterized by infertility, hirsutism, obesity, and amenorrhea or oligomenorrhea. When spontaneous uterine bleeding occurs in women with PCOD, it is unpredictable as to time of onset, duration, and amount; on occasion the bleeding can be severe. The dysfunctional uterine bleeding is usually due to estrogen breakthrough (see above).

The disorder, as originally described by Stein and Leventhal, was characterized by enlarged, polycystic ovaries, but it is now known to be associated with a variety of pathologic findings in the ovaries, only some of which result in enlargement and none of which are pathognomonic. The most common finding is a white, smooth, sclerotic ovary with a thickened capsule, multiple follicular cysts in various stages of atresia, a hyperplastic theca and stroma, and rare or absent corpora albicans. Other ovaries have hyperthecosis in which the ovarian stroma is hyperplastic and may contain lipid-laden luteal cells. Thus, the diagnosis of PCOD is a clinical one, based on the coexistence of chronic anovulation and varying degrees of androgen excess.

In most women with PCOD, menarche occurs at the expected time, but uterine bleeding is unpredictable in onset, duration, and amount. Amenorrhea ensues after a variable period, although primary amenorrhea occurs in some women. Signs of androgen excess (hirsutism) usually become evident around the time of menarche. One scenario suggests that this disorder originates as an exaggerated adrenarche in obese girls (Fig. 337-7). The combination of elevated levels of adrenal androgens and obesity leads to increased formation of extraglandular estrogen. This estrogen exerts a positive feedback on LH secretion and negative feedback on FSH secretion, resulting in a ratio of LH to FSH levels in plasma that is characteristically greater than 2. The increased LH levels can then lead to hyperplasia of the ovarian stroma and theca cells and increased androgen production, which in turn provides more substrate for peripheral aromatization and perpetuates the chronic anovulation. In the advanced stage of the disorder, the ovary is the major site of androgen production, but the adrenal may continue to secrete excess androgen as well. The greater the obesity, the more strongly this sequence would be perpetuated because more androgen is converted to estrogen by adipose tissue stromal cells, which in turn exaggerates inappropriate LH release by positive feedback.

Thus, the fundamental defect in PCOD is viewed as inappropriate signals to the hypothalamus and pituitary. In turn, the hypothalamic-pituitary axis responds appropriately to high levels of estrogen, and ovulation can be induced with antiestrogen agents such as clomiphene

FIGURE 337-7 Proposed mechanism for the initiation and perpetuation of chronic anovulation in polycystic ovarian disease (PCOD). This cycle may be entered or initiated via adrenal androgen excess or obesity, both of which result in enhanced extraglandular formation of estrogens. The therapy of PCOD involves interruption of the cycle at any of several steps. *[From SSC Yen, RB Jaffe (eds), Reproductive Endocrinology. Philadelphia, Saunders, 1986; and from U Goebelmann, in Reproductive Endocrinology, Infertility, and Contraception, 2d ed, DR Mishell Jr, V Davajan (eds), Philadelphia, Davis, 1986.]*

citrate. Increased levels of plasma endorphins and inhibin may contribute to the perpetuation of the defect. The concept that the fundamental defect is one of inappropriate signals is supported by the findings in the ovary itself. Ovarian follicles from women with PCOD have low aromatase activity, but normal aromatase can be induced by treatment with FSH. In short, the anovulation is not due to an intrinsic abnormality in the ovary but rather results from a deficiency of FSH and an excess of LH. An association exists between PCOD/hyperthecosis, virilization, acanthosis nigricans, and insulin resistance; in the ovary, insulin may interact via the insulin-like growth factor receptors to enhance androgen synthesis in insulin-resistant states.

℞ **TREATMENT**

Treatment of PCOD is directed toward interrupting the self-perpetuating cycle and can be accomplished in several ways, such as by decreasing ovarian androgen secretion (by wedge resection or the use of oral contraceptive agents), decreasing peripheral estrogen formation (by weight reduction), or enhancing FSH secretion [by administration of clomiphene, human menopausal gonadotropin (hMG), LHRH (gonadorelin) by portable infusion pump, or purified FSH (urofollitropin)]. The choice of therapy depends on the clinical findings and the needs of the patient. An attempt at weight reduction is appropriate in all who are obese. If the woman is not hirsute and does not desire pregnancy, periodic withdrawal menses can be induced with medroxyprogesterone acetate 10 days per month; such treatment prevents the development of endometrial hyperplasia. If the woman is hirsute and does not desire pregnancy, the ovarian (and possibly the adrenal) component of androgen production can be suppressed with combined estrogen-progestogen oral contraceptive agents. Combined oral contraceptives are also indicated if prolonged or excessive menstrual bleeding is present. Once androgen excess is controlled, treatment of previously existing hair growth by shaving, depilatories, or electrolysis may be indicated (see Chap. 53). If pregnancy is desired ovulation must be induced. The drug of choice for this purpose is clomiphene, which promotes ovulation in three-fourths of cases, or hMG, urofollitropin, or gonadorelin. Pretreatment with LHRH analogues prior to use of hMG, urofollitropin, or gonadorelin may improve the rates of ovulation and pregnancy. An alternative therapy is ovarian drilling by laser or cautery performed at laparoscopy in women in whom hormonal therapy is not effective; however, the procedure is associated with a high incidence of ovarian adhesions.

Chronic anovulation with estrogen present also may occur with tumors of the ovary. These include granulosa-theca cell tumors, Brenner tumors, cystic teratomas, mucous cystadenomas, and Krukenberg tumors (also see Chap. 99). Such tumors can either secrete excess estrogen themselves or produce androgens that are aromatized in extraglandular sites. Chronic anovulation and the clinical features of PCOD result. Occasionally, areas of the ovary not involved with tumors show the characteristic histologic changes of PCOD. Other causes of chronic anovulation with estrogen present include adrenal production of excess androgen (usually adult-onset adrenal hyperplasia due to partial $P450_{C21}$ deficiency) and various thyroid disorders.

CHRONIC ANOVULATION WITH ESTROGEN ABSENT Women with chronic anovulation who have low or absent estrogen production and do not experience withdrawal bleeding after progestogen treatment usually have hypogonadotropic hypogonadism due to disease of either the pituitary or the central nervous system.

Isolated hypogonadotropic hypogonadism associated with defects of smell (olfactory bulb defects) is known as the *Kallmann syndrome* (see Chaps. 328 and 336). Affected women are sexually infantile and have a defect in the synthesis and/or release of LHRH. Hypothalamic lesions that impair LHRH production and cause hypogonadotropic hypogonadism include craniopharyngioma, germinoma (pinealoma), glioma, Hand-Schüller-Christian disease, teratomas, endodermal-sinus tumors, tuberculosis, sarcoidosis, and metastatic tumors that cause suppression or destruction of the hypothalamus. Central nervous system trauma and irradiation also can cause hypothalamic amenorrhea and deficiencies in secretion of growth hormone, adrenocorticotropic hormone (ACTH), vasopressin, and thyroid hormone.

More commonly, gonadotropin deficiency leading to chronic anovulation is believed to arise from functional disorders of the hypothalamus or higher centers. A history of a stressful event in a young woman is frequent. For example, chronic anovulation can begin suddenly in a woman who leaves home for the first time or experiences the death of a loved one. Gonadotropin and estrogen levels are in the low to low-normal range as compared with normal women in the early follicular phase of the cycle. In addition, rigorous exercise such as jogging or ballet and diets that result in excessive weight loss may lead to chronic anovulation, particularly in girls with a history of prior menstrual irregularity. The amenorrhea in these women does not appear to be due to weight loss alone but to a combination of a decrease in body fat and chronic stress. An extreme form of weight loss with chronic anovulation occurs in anorexia nervosa. Anorexia nervosa is characterized by the development in a young woman of amenorrhea with associated severe weight loss, distorted attitudes toward eating and weight gain, self-induced vomiting, extreme emaciation, and distorted body image. In anorexia nervosa amenorrhea can precede, follow, or coincide with weight loss (see Chap. 76). During successful therapy, gonadotropin changes recapitulate those observed during normal puberty (see Fig. 337-1).

In addition, chronic debilitating diseases such as end-stage kidney disease, malignancy, and malabsorption are believed to lead to development of hypogonadotropic hypogonadism via a hypothalamic mechanism.

Treatment of chronic anovulation due to hypothalamic disorders includes ameliorating the stressful situation, decreasing exercise, and correcting weight loss if appropriate. These women appear to be susceptible to the development of osteoporosis; estrogen replacement therapy is recommended to induce and maintain normal secondary sexual characteristics and prevent bone loss in those who do not desire pregnancy, and gonadotropin or gonadorelin therapy is indicated when pregnancy is desired (see "Treatment," below). When appropriate, therapy is directed at the primary disease of the hypothalamus.

Disorders of the pituitary can lead to the estrogen-deficient form of chronic anovulation by at least two mechanisms—direct interference with gonadotropin secretion by lesions that either obliterate or interfere with the gonadotropic cells (chromophobe adenomas, Sheehan's syndrome) or inhibition of gonadotropin secretion in association with excess prolactin (prolactinoma). *Pituitary tumors* make up approximately 10 percent of all intracranial tumors and may secrete no hormone, one hormone, or more than one hormone (see Chap. 328). Prolactin levels are elevated in 50 to 70 percent of patients with pituitary tumors, either because of prolactin secretion by the tumor itself (in the case of prolactinomas) or because the tumor mass interferes with the normal hypothalamic inhibition of prolactin secretion.

Prolactinomas can be divided into microadenomas (less than 10 mm in diameter) and macroadenomas (greater than 10 mm). Prolactin excess associated with low levels of LH and FSH constitutes a specific subtype of hypogonadotropic hypogonadism. One-tenth or more of amenorrheic women have increased levels of serum prolactin, and more than half of women with both galactorrhea and amenorrhea have elevated prolactin levels. The amenorrhea is most often associated with decreased or absent estrogen production, but prolactin-secreting tumors on occasion are associated with normal ovulatory menses or chronic anovulation with estrogen present. Most prolactin-secreting adenomas grow slowly, and some cease to grow after attaining a certain size. The increased frequency of diagnosis of prolactin-secreting adenomas is probably due to several factors, including increased awareness, improved radiographic detection methods, and availability of radioimmunoassays for prolactin. Since in older autopsy series a 9 to 23 percent prevalence of pituitary adenomas was observed in asymptomatic women, the clinical and prognostic significance of small microadenomas in asymptomatic individuals is unclear. However, when tumors of any size are associated with symptoms of amenorrhea or galactorrhea, particularly when visual field defects or severe headaches are present, bromocriptine therapy or neurosurgical evaluation is indicated. The evaluation, differential diagnosis, and management of hyperprolactinemia are described in Chap. 328. In the latter half of pregnancy, prolactin-secreting pituitary tumors may expand, leading to headaches, compression of the optic chiasm, and blindness. Therefore, before inducing ovulation for the purposes of achieving pregnancy, it is mandatory to exclude the presence of a pituitary tumor.

Large pituitary tumors such as null cell adenomas—whether or not hyperprolactinemia is present—are likely to be associated with deficiency of hormones in addition to gonadotropins (Chap. 328).

Craniopharyngiomas, which are thought to arise from remnants of Rathke's pouch, account for 3 percent of intracranial neoplasms, occur most frequently in the second decade of life, and may extend into the suprasellar region. Many of these tumors calcify and can be diagnosed by conventional skull films. Patients often present with sexual infantilism, delayed puberty, and amenorrhea due to gonadotropin deficiency; secretion of TSH, ACTH, growth hormone, and vasopressin may also be impaired.

Panhypopituitarism can occur spontaneously, result from surgical or radiation treatment of pituitary adenomas, or develop after postpartum hemorrhage (Sheehan's syndrome). Patients with the latter disorder characteristically have failure to lactate or ovulate, loss of genital and axillary hair, hypothyroidism, and adrenal insufficiency (see Chap. 328).

Evaluation of amenorrhea A general scheme for the evaluation of women with amenorrhea is given in Fig. 337-8. On physical examination, attention should be given to three features: (1) the degree of maturation of the breasts, pubic and axillary hair, and external genitalia; (2) the current estrogen status; and (3) the presence or absence of a uterus. All women with amenorrhea should be assumed to be pregnant until proven otherwise; it is prudent to exclude pregnancy by a suitable screening test even when the history and physical examination are not suggestive. Once that is done, the cause of amenorrhea can frequently be diagnosed clinically. For example, Asherman's syndrome is suggested by a history of curettage in a woman who previously menstruated; in women with primary amenorrhea and sexual infantilism, the essential differential diagnosis is between gonadal dysgenesis and hypopituitarism, and the diagnosis of gonadal dysgenesis (Turner's syndrome) or of anatomic defects of the outflow tract (müllerian agenesis, testicular feminization, and cervical stenosis) is frequently suggested on the basis of physical findings. When a specific cause is suspected, it is appropriate to proceed directly to confirm the diagnosis (as by obtaining a chromosomal karyotype or measurement of plasma gonadotropins). It is also useful to measure serum prolactin and FSH levels during the initial evaluation.

Estrogen status is evaluated by determining if the vaginal mucosa is moist and rugated and if the cervical mucus can be stretched and shown to fern upon drying. If these criteria are indeterminate, a progestational challenge is indicated, most often the administration of 10 mg medroxyprogesterone acetate by mouth once or twice daily for 5 days or 100 mg progesterone in oil intramuscularly. (It should be emphasized that progestogen should never be administered until pregnancy is excluded.) If estrogen levels are adequate (and the outflow tract is intact), menstrual bleeding should occur within 1 week of ending the progestogen treatment. If withdrawal bleeding occurs, the diagnosis is chronic anovulation with estrogen present, usually caused by polycystic ovarian disease.

If no withdrawal bleeding or only minimal vaginal spotting occurs, the nature of the subsequent workup depends on the results of the initial prolactin assay. If plasma prolactin is elevated, or if galactorrhea is present, radiography of the pituitary should be undertaken. When the plasma prolactin level is normal in an anovulatory woman with estrogen absent and with elevated FSH levels, the diagnosis is ovarian failure. If the gonadotropins are in the low or normal range, the diagnosis is either hypothalamic-pituitary disorder or an anatomic defect of the outflow tract. As indicated previously, the diagnosis of outflow tract disorder is usually suspected or established on the basis of the history and physical findings. When the physical findings are not clear-cut, it is useful to administer cyclic estrogen plus progestogen (1.25 mg oral conjugated estrogens per day for 3 weeks, with 10 mg medroxyprogesterone acetate added for the last 7 to 10 days of estrogen treatment), followed by 10 days of observation. If no bleeding occurs, the diagnosis of Asherman's syndrome or another anatomic defect of the outflow tract is confirmed by hysterosalpingography or hysteroscopy. If withdrawal bleeding occurs following the estrogen-progestogen combination, the diagnosis of chronic anovulation with estrogen absent (functional hypothalamic amenorrhea) is suggested. Radiologic evaluations of the pituitary-hypothalamic areas may be indicated in the latter cases—irrespective of the prolactin level—because of the danger of overlooking a pituitary-hypothalamic tumor and because the diagnosis of functional hypothalamic amenorrhea is one of exclusion (see Chap. 328).

Infertility Infertility, the failure to become pregnant after 1 year of unprotected intercourse, affects approximately 10 to 15 percent of couples and is a common reason for seeking gynecologic assistance. Male factors account for 40 percent of infertility problems (see Chap. 336). In women, failure of ovulation accounts for 30 percent of cases; pelvic factors, such as tubal disease or endometriosis, account for half; and a cervical factor is implicated in about one-tenth. In 10 to 20 percent of infertile women no etiology is found. An immunologic cause may underlie some of these cases. Finally, infertility in women may be due to *luteal-phase dysfunction*, in which ovulation is assumed to occur but progesterone formation is insufficient to allow preparation of the endometrium for implantation; the disorder is believed to be due to inadequate secretion or action of FSH and consequent inadequate formation of estrogen by the dominant follicle during the follicular phase.

The first diagnostic step in evaluation of the infertile couple is to determine whether the man or woman is the infertile partner, ordinarily by first performing a semen analysis in the man (see Chap. 336) and looking for signs of presumed ovulation in the woman. Documentation of ovulatory cycles is obtained by daily measurement of basal body temperatures throughout the month. Occasionally, accurate basal body temperature records are not obtained, and demonstration of elevated serum progesterone levels during the luteal phase may be used as evidence of ovulation. Dating of endometrium by histologic examination of a biopsy sample is also useful for establishing ovulation or luteal phase dysfunction.

If the infertility is associated with amenorrhea, then the workup is that described in Fig. 337-8. If polycystic ovarian disease is the basis for infertility, ovulation can be induced with clomiphene, gonadotropins, gonadorelin, or, on occasion, ovarian drilling. Bromocriptine is used to induce ovulation in cases of hyperprolactinemia. The appropriate therapy for prolactinomas in women who do not desire pregnancy is discussed in Chap. 328.

To evaluate the fallopian tubes and uterine cavity, hysterosalpingograms may be obtained, followed when appropriate by diagnostic laparoscopy and the demonstration of dye spillage from the fimbria after transcervical injection of dye during laparoscopy. Microsurgical repair of damaged or previously ligated fallopian tubes is followed by an apparent increase in pregnancy rates. Removal of peritubular and fimbrial adhesions by means of laparoscopic surgery plus laser beam therapy is an alternative treatment. Endometriosis can be diagnosed by laparoscopy, and treatment includes surgical resection of the endometrial implants or temporary gonadotropin suppression using danazol (400 to 800 mg orally in divided doses for 4 to 6 months), LHRH analogues given by nasal spray or subcutaneous or depot injection, or continuous low-dose oral contraceptive agents to promote regression of the implants.

The cervical factor in infertility is evaluated by study of cervical mucus at an appropriate time after coitus, preferably just prior to ovulation (day 12 to 13) when cervical mucus is thin and stretchy; such an examination provides information as to the penetration and survival of the sperm in the female genital tract. The preferred treatment of infertility due to such abnormality is intrauterine insemination with washed sperm.

When other treatment modalities are unsuccessful, in vitro fertilization and embryo transfer (IVF-ET) may be tried. Indications for the use of IVF-ET in infertile couples include tubal obstructive disease, cervical factors, endometriosis, oligospermia, and unexplained infertility. Multiple follicles are induced with clomiphene and/or gonadotropins, and follicles are usually obtained by transvaginal aspiration with ultrasound monitoring. After fertilization and cleavage, embryos are transferred to the uterine cavity. Although pregnancy rates vary, successful pregnancy has been reported in as many as 30 percent of cases after IVF-ET. Other techniques include a modification of IVF-ET known as *gamete-intrafallopian transfer* (GIFT), in which a mixture of sperm and ova are introduced into the end of the fallopian tube at laparoscopy, and intrauterine insemination after gonadotropin stimulation.

Medical Aspects of Pregnancy The possibility of pregnancy should be considered in all women of reproductive age who are evaluated for medical illness or considered for surgery. Procedures such as x-ray exposure, drugs, and anesthetics may be harmful to the developing fetus, and a variety of medical problems may worsen during pregnancy, including hypertension; diseases of the heart, lungs, kidney, and liver; and metabolic and endocrine disorders. Indeed, all women who present with abnormal vaginal bleeding or amenorrhea during the reproductive years should be assumed to have a complication of pregnancy, such as incomplete abortion, ectopic pregnancy, or trophoblastic disease (hydatidiform mole or choriocarcinoma). Women who present with these complications of pregnancy often have histories of abdominal pain and vaginal bleeding and may have evidence of intraabdominal hemorrhage.

Choriocarcinoma is a particular problem because of its protean manifestations. Half these malignancies follow pregnancies complicated by hydatidiform mole, and the remainder occur after spontaneous abortion, ectopic pregnancy, or normal deliveries. Patients may present with intraabdominal bleeding due to rupture of the uterus, liver, or

FIGURE 337-8 Flow diagram for the evaluation of women with amenorrhea. The most common diagnosis for each category is shown in parentheses. The dotted lines indicate that in some instances a correct diagnosis can be reached on the basis of history and physical examination alone.

ovary, with pulmonary manifestations (cough, hemoptysis, pleuritic pain, dyspnea, and respiratory failure) or gastrointestinal symptoms, usually chronic blood loss or melena. In addition, patients can present with cerebral metastases or renal involvement. The diagnosis can be established by demonstrating an elevated level of the β subunit of hCG in plasma. Treatment and cure are possible with chemotherapeutic agents (dactinomycin and/or methotrexate). →*For manifestations of choriocarcinoma in men, see Chap. 98.*

Ovarian Tumors   See Chap. 99

℞ **TREATMENT**

Progestogens   The major use of progestogens is in conjunction with estrogen to ensure the full maturation of the endometrium, both in combination birth control pills and in the therapy of hypogonadal states. In certain circumstances, however, progestogen therapy is appropriate by itself—to induce a progestational effect on the estrogen-primed endometrium (in diagnostic tests for the evaluation of amenorrhea), to inhibit pituitary gonadotropins for contraception (the progestogen-only birth control pill or progestogen-containing implants), for prophylaxis to prevent hyperplasia in PCOD, for palliation in cases of endometrial and breast carcinoma, and for treatment of endometriosis. Even when a direct progestational effect is desired, the available oral drugs substitute a synthetic derivative for the naturally occurring hormone. Oral progestogens include medroxyprogesterone acetate, megestrol acetate, norethindrone, norgestrel, and micronized progesterone. Parenteral agents include progesterone in oil, medroxyprogesterone acetate suspension, and 17-hydroxyprogesterone caproate. Vaginal progesterone suppositories are used for treatment of luteal-phase defects, and progestogen implants are available for long-term contraception.

The most common undesirable side effect is breakthrough bleeding, which occurs when progestogens are used continuously. Other complications include nausea, vomiting, and hirsutism. Abnormal liver function is a side effect of those derivatives with alkyl substitution in the 17α position. Synthetic progestogens are contraindicated if pregnancy is known or suspected, because of the risk of birth defects.

Estrogens   Estrogens are used for the treatment of gonadal failure, the control of fertility, the management of dysfunctional uterine bleeding, and the treatment of carcinoma of the breast. (Carcinoma of the breast is discussed in Chap. 91.) However, none of the available oral or parenteral hormones replaces the pattern of circulating estradiol levels characteristic of the normally cycling, premenopausal woman (see Fig. 337-5). Estrogens that can be given by mouth are either nonsteroidal agents (such as diethylstilbestrol) that mimic the action of estradiol, estrogen conjugates that must be hydrolyzed before they become active (usually estrone sulfate from pregnant mare's urine), or estrogen analogues that cannot be metabolized to estradiol (mestranol, quinestrol) (Fig. 337-9). Even when micronized estradiol is given orally, it is rapidly converted in the body to estrone. Because oral therapy neither replaces nor mimics the daily secretory pattern of the lost hormone, such therapy must be viewed as a pharmacologic substitution rather than a physiologic replacement. Likewise, the use of parenteral estrogens rarely mimics the physiologic situation. Parenteral preparations of conjugated estrogens, like the oral derivatives, are poor precursors of estradiol, and estradiol esters (estradiol benzoate and valerate) rarely result in plasma estradiol levels that mimic the normal monthly secretory cycle of the hormone. Transdermal estradiol results in constant levels of blood estradiol and is effective in the treatment of menopausal symptoms. The side effects of estrogen substitution differ at various times of life.

HYPOESTROGENISM   In women with decreased estrogen production, whether due to disease of the ovaries (gonadal dysgenesis) or to hypogonadotropic hypogonadism, treatment with cyclic estrogens should be instituted at the time of expected puberty to induce the development and maintenance of female secondary sexual character-

istics and to prevent osteoporosis. The most commonly used medications are conjugated estrogens (0.625 to 1.25 mg/d by mouth) together with medroxyprogesterone acetate (2.5 mg/d or 5 to 10 mg during the last several days of monthly estrogen treatment to prevent development of endometrial hyperplasia). Alternatively, oral contraceptives may be given. Abnormal bleeding in women receiving estrogen replacement mandates histologic evaluation of the endometrium. Such substitution therapy or the use of oral contraceptives (see below) also may be used for the purpose of suppressing pituitary gonadotropins, as in women with PCOD, in whom the major therapeutic aim is suppression of ovarian androgen production prior to the time when fertility is desired.

Temporary administration of estrogens in larger quantities (up to two times the usual adult maintenance dose) may be necessary to induce the full development of secondary sexual characteristics in girls and for the control of menopausal symptoms. Even larger doses of parenteral estrogens (10 mg estradiol valerate or 25 mg conjugated estrogen) in conjunction with progestogen may be required in some instances of dysfunctional uterine bleeding. In addition to the potential long-term side effects of all estrogens (see below), high doses may cause nausea, vomiting, and edema.

Fertility Control   An understanding of the use, mechanisms of actions, and consequences of contraceptive agents is important to all physicians. Furthermore, since pregnancy may aggravate a variety of chronic illnesses, fertility control is an essential feature of the management of many disorders.

To be effective, fertility control requires patient compliance. Widely used methods include (1) rhythm and withdrawal techniques; (2) barrier methods, including the condom, jellies, foam, suppositories, and diaphragms; (3) intrauterine devices (IUDs); (4) hormonal contraceptives; (5) sterilization; and (6) abortion.

The rhythm and withdrawal techniques and the barrier methods are effective if used correctly and consistently, but in practice they have high failure rates because of imperfect compliance. Nevertheless, these methods carry the lowest incidence of side effects, and the side effects, when produced, are minor except for local allergic reactions. When the rhythm method is combined with self-evaluation of the preovulatory part of the menstrual cycle (i.e., evaluation of cervical mucus) plus home LH testing, it is an effective method of contraception. Use of these methods should be recommended when there is a relative or absolute contraindication to other methods.

Barrier methods are among the oldest, simplest, and most widely used forms of birth control. The term *barrier* originally implied a

FIGURE 337-9   The circulating forms of administered estrogenic drugs.

physical barrier that prevents the sperm from reaching the egg, but the definition has been broaded to include biologic, chemical, and physical means of preventing fertilization. Barrier contraceptives are often underutilized, but if used correctly and continuously they provide adequete contraception and some protection against sexually transmitted diseases. All barrier methods require prior planning and motivation.

The most widely used nonsurgical methods of contraception, the IUD and oral contraceptive agents, are effective but may be associated with significant side effects.

IUD The success rates of most IUDs are 95 to 98 percent. Only two devices are marketed in the United States. Both are T-shaped, cause minimal pain at insertion, and are associated with low expulsion rates. One contains copper, which enhances effectiveness, and is replaced at 8-year intervals. The other contains slow-release progesterone, which makes annual replacement necessary. The IUD is believed to prevent pregnancy by inducing a chronic inflammatory reaction in the endometrium, resulting in an unfavorable environment for the implantation of the blastocyst, although some evidence suggests that IUDs prevent fertilization.

Once the IUD is inserted, it is necessary to check periodically to be certain that the device is in place. Both minor and serious side effects can occur. Intermenstrual spotting and increased bleeding and pain or cramps at the time of menses are frequent causes of discontinuation of IUD use. In addition, the device may be expelled spontaneously during a menstrual period without the user noticing. The most serious side effect is pelvic infection, occasionally leading to the development of tuboovarian abscess and subsequent infertility. Pelvic infection is more frequent than in users of oral or barrier contraceptives but no more common than in women using no contraception. Women with multiple sex partners are at the greatest risk for pelvic infection. For this reason, use of IUDs by nulligravid women is not advocated by many gynecologists. In addition, pregnancy with an IUD in place is more likely to be ectopic, because intrauterine but not extrauterine pregnancies are inhibited. Because of the increased incidence of spontaneous and septic abortions when IUDs are in place, the device should be removed if pregnancy is detected. When persistent, severe bleeding, lower abdominal pain, fever, or discharge develops, the IUD should be removed.

ORAL CONTRACEPTIVES Oral contraceptive agents have been used by over 200 million women worldwide and by 1 of 4 women in the United States under age 45. The agents are popular because of ease of administration, low pregnancy rates (less than 1 percent), and relatively infrequent side effects.

The most widely used oral contraceptives are either combination tablets or triphasic formulations. A list of oral contraceptives marketed in the United States is given in Table 337-3. Combination oral contraceptive tablets contain one of two synthetic estrogens (mestranol or ethinyl estradiol) and one of seven synthetic progestogens (norethindrone, norethindrone acetate, norethynodrel, norgestrel, ethynodiol diacetate, desogestrel, and norgestimate). The available agents contain no more than 50 μg of ethinyl estradiol or its equivalent. The combination or triphasic tablets are taken for 21 consecutive days followed by 7 days of rest. Progestogen-only tablets are taken continuously on a daily basis. Presumably, the best contraceptive— i.e., one that is effective while producing the fewest side effects— is the one that contains the lowest amount of steroid that is sufficient to prevent pregnancy or breakthrough bleeding. The triphasic tablets,

Table 337-3

Composition of Currently Marketed Oral Contraceptives

Name	Estrogen	μg	Progestogen	mg
COMBINATION-TYPE				
Fixed type				
Estrogen content = 50 μg:				
Ortho-Novum 1/50	Mestranol	50	Norethindrone	1.0
Norinyl 1/50	Mestranol	50	Norethindrone	1.0
Ovcon 50	Ethinyl estradiol	50	Norethindrone	1.0
Ovral	Ethinyl estradiol	50	Norgestrel	0.5
Demulen	Ethinyl estradiol	50	Ethynodiol diacetate	1.0
Norlestrin 2.5/50	Ethinyl estradiol	50	Norethindrone acetate	2.5
Norlestrin 1/50	Ethinyl estradiol	50	Norethindrone acetate	1.0
Estrogen content <50 μg:				
Ortho-Novum 1/35	Ethinyl estradiol	35	Norethindrone	1.0
Norinyl 1+35	Ethinyl estradiol	35	Norethindrone	1.0
Modicon	Ethinyl estradiol	35	Norethindrone	0.5
Brevicon	Ethinyl estradiol	35	Norethindrone	0.5
Ovcon 35	Ethinyl estradiol	35	Norethindrone	0.4
Demulen 1/35	Ethinyl estradiol	35	Ethynodiol diacetate	1.0
Loestrin 1.5/30	Ethinyl estradiol	30	Norethindrone acetate	1.5
Loestrin 1/20	Ethinyl estradiol	20	Norethindrone acetate	1.0
Nordette	Ethinyl estradiol	30	Levonorgestrel	0.15
Lo-Ovral	Ethinyl estradiol	30	Norgestrel	0.3
Desogen	Ethinyl estradiol	30	Desogestrel	0.15
Ortho-cept	Ethinyl estradiol	30	Desogestrel	0.15
Ortho-cyclen	Ethinyl estradiol	35	Norgestamate	0.25
Biphasic type				
Ortho-Novum 10/11				
First 10 days	Ethinyl estradiol	35	Norethindrone	0.5
Next 11 days	Ethinyl estradiol	35	Norethindrone	1.0
Triphasic type				
Ortho-Novum 7/7/7				
First 7 days	Ethinyl estradiol	35	Norethindrone	0.5
Second 7 days	Ethinyl estradiol	35	Norethindrone	0.75
Third 7 days	Ethinyl estradiol	35	Norethindrone	1.0
Tri-Norinyl				
First 7 days	Ethinyl estradiol	35	Norethindrone	0.5
Next 9 days	Ethinyl estradiol	35	Norethindrone	1.0
Next 5 days	Ethinyl estradiol	35	Norethindrone	0.5
Triphasil				
First 6 days	Ethinyl estradiol	30	Levonorgestrel	0.05
Second 5 days	Ethinyl estradiol	40	Levonorgestrel	0.075
Third 10 days	Ethinyl estradiol	30	Levonorgestrel	0.125
Tri-Levein				
First 6 days	Ethinyl estradiol	30	Levonorgestrel	0.05
Second 5 days	Ethinyl estradiol	40	Levonorgestrel	0.075
Third 10 days	Ethinyl estradiol	30	Levonorgestrel	0.125
Ortho Tri-Cyclen				
First 7 days	Ethinyl estradiol	35	Norgestimate	0.18
Second 7 days	Ethinyl estradiol	35	Norgestimate	0.215
Third 7 days	Ethinyl estradiol	35	Norgestimate	0.25
PROGESTOGEN ONLY				
Micronor	None		Norethindrone	0.35
Nor Q.D.	None		Norethindrone	0.35
Ovrette	None		Norgestrel	0.075

containing 35 μg or less of estrogen and less than 1 mg progestogen, come closest to this goal.

Oral contraceptives inhibit ovulation by suppressing FSH and LH secretion. In consequence, the secretion of all ovarian steroids, including estrogen, progesterone, and androgen, is also suppressed (Fig. 337-10). These agents also exert minor direct inhibitory effects on the reproductive tract, altering the cervical mucus and thereby decreasing sperm penetration, and decreasing the motility and secretions of the fallopian tubes and uterus.

The death rates associated with oral contraceptives and other forms of birth control are summarized in Table 337-4. Up to age 40, the mortality rates in women using oral contraceptives and IUDs are lower than in women using no contraception (this difference results from the increased risk of death with pregnancy). The decrease in death rate below age 40 is even more striking in nonsmokers than in smokers using contraceptives. In fact, the death rates in nonsmoking women aged 15 to 24 who use oral agents are lower than those with other forms of fertility control. The increased death rates in women using rhythm or barrier techniques probably results from the higher failure rate and the consequent risk of pregnancy in such women. Oral contraceptive agents are not recommended for

smoking women after age 35 and for women of any ages who are at increased risk for myocardial infarction.

Despite the overall safety of these agents, users are at risk for serious side effects. In most retrospective and prospective studies, there is an increased incidence of *deep vein thrombosis* and *pulmonary embolism.* The increased risk varies from two- to twelvefold and is greater for women taking tablets containing more than 50 μg estrogen. The use of oral contraceptives is also associated with an increased risk of thromboembolism after surgery, and for this reason, the agents should be discontinued at least 1 month prior to elective surgery. In retrospective studies there is a three- to ninefold increase in the risk for *thromboembolic stroke* and a twofold increase in the risk for *hemorrhagic stroke* in oral contraceptive users. However, three large prospective studies of contraceptive use demonstrated only a slight increase in the rate of hemorrhagic stroke. Nevertheless, the drugs should be discontinued in women who experience visual complaints or severe headaches. Smoking and age increase the risk for stroke and the frequency of death from deep venous thrombosis, pulmonary emboli, and myocardial infarction.

A small rise in blood pressure is common, and 5 percent of women develop significant *hypertension* (blood pressure greater than 140/90) after 5 years of oral contraceptive use. Estrogens induce the synthesis of a variety of proteins by the liver, including the renin substrate angiotensinogen. The resulting increased formation of angiotensin is believed to be involved in the development of hypertension. Alternatively, the progestogen component of oral contraceptives may be associated with increased risk of hypertension. In most cases, blood pressure returns to normal when the agents are discontinued.

Serum lipids and lipoproteins are altered in women on oral contraceptives, the nature of the change depending on the specific contraceptive. In general, estrogens increase serum levels of HDL and of very low density lipoprotein (VLDL), and progestogens decrease the concentration of HDL. However, with oral contraceptives containing less than 35 μg estrogen, lipoprotein levels change little if at all.

A few women taking oral contraceptives develop *impairment of glucose tolerance* as manifested by abnormal glucose levels and elevated plasma insulin levels after an oral glucose load; both indices usually return to normal after discontinuing the agents. Because juvenile-onset and adult-onset diabetes may be associated with increased incidence of cardiovascular disease, it is preferable to use other forms of contraception in these individuals.

Oral contraceptives should not be used by women with abnormal results on liver function tests or with acute or chronic liver disease. A rare complication is the development of peliosis hepatis, which can cause death due to sudden rupture and hemorrhage of the liver. Cholestatic jaundice may occur in those women predisposed to the development of the recurrent jaundice of pregnancy.

Oral contraceptives cause an increased concentration of cholesterol in the bile, which is probably the cause for the twofold increase in *cholelithiasis* and cholecystitis in women on oral contraceptives.

Estrogens induce elevated levels of a variety of proteins secreted by the liver, including cortisol-binding globulin (CBG), testosterone-binding globulin (TeBG), and thyroxine-binding globulin (TBG). Consequently, results of various laboratory tests of adrenal and thyroid function may be altered, and these tests must be interpreted with caution (see Chap. 331). Oral contraceptives also slightly lower plasma ACTH levels possibly owing to an inhibitory effect on ACTH secretion or cortisol catabolism. Finally, serum prolactin levels are slightly elevated in women using oral contraceptives, but such treatment is not believed to play a role in the development of pituitary prolactinomas.

Other effects of oral contraceptive pills include minor dyspepsia, breast discomfort, weight gain, development of pigmentation of the face (chloasma), which is augmented by exposure to the sun, and a variety of psychological effects, such as depression and changes in libido. There is no convincing evidence that oral contraceptive use is associated with a significant increase in the incidence of cancer

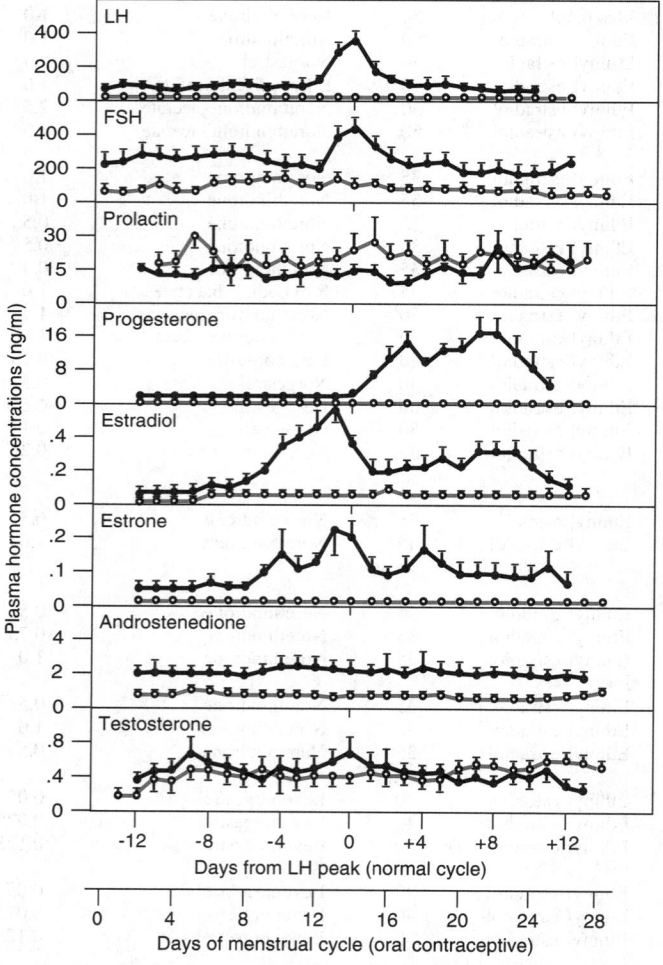

FIGURE 337-10 The mechanism of action of oral contraceptives. Mean daily plasma hormone concentrations during the ovarian cycle are shown for four ovulating women and four women treated with combination-type oral contraceptives. Data for the normal ovarian cycle are presented in relationship to the day of the LH peak; day 1 of the contraceptive cycle corresponds to the first day of uterine bleeding. The values are the mean ± SE obtained from four women. *(From Carr et al, 1979.)*

of the uterus, cervix, or breast. In fact, oral contraceptives have many beneficial effects including control of dysmenorrhea and anovulatory bleeding, prevention of sexually transmitted diseases, and a decreased incidence of endometrial and ovarian cancer.

The absolute contraindications to the use of oral contraceptives include previous thromboembolic disorders, cerebral vascular or coronary artery disease, known or suspected carcinoma of the breast or estrogen-dependent neoplasia, undiagnosed abnormal genital bleeding, or known or suspected pregnancy. Relative contraindications must be weighed against the potential benefits and include hypertension, migraine headaches, diabetes mellitus, uterine leiomyomas, sickle cell anemia, hyperlipidemia, and elective surgery.

OTHER STEROID CONTRACEPTIVES Types of steroid contraception other than the conventional oral contraceptives include injectable steroids, such as progestogen-containing implants and depot medroxyprogesterone acetate (150 mg by injection every 3 months). Alternatively, postcoital contraception can be effective, such as ingestion of high-dose estrogen for 5 days during the fertile part of the cycle (the morning-after pill) but is associated with significant side effects, particularly nausea.

Estrogen Treatment of the Menopause   The rationale for use of estrogens in postmenopausal women is the belief that such therapy may relieve some of the complications of the postmenopausal state, including osteoporosis, and some manifestations of aging itself. In some parts of the United States, by the mid-1970s as many as half of women in the menopausal age group used one or more forms of estrogen replacement for a median period of 5 years, accounting for more than 30 million prescriptions per year.

The menopause is not a state of simple estrogen deprivation, since some estrogens continue to be produced but is instead a state of altered estrogen metabolism; the predominant estrogen becomes estrone, which is formed by extraglandular conversion of prehormone, rather than estradiol secreted by the ovary. As is true for all estrogen therapy, the estrogen treatment of the menopause is actually a pharmacologic substitution of one or another estrogen analogue for estradiol rather than a physiologic replacement of the missing steroid. The estrogens available for replacement therapy include conjugated estrogens, estrogen substitutes (diethylstilbestrol), synthetic estrogen (ethinyl estradiol or derivatives), micronized estradiol, estrogen-containing vaginal creams, and estrogen-containing dermal patches. Regimens associated with a low risk of complications include (1) cyclic estrogen therapy in the lowest effective dose for 25 days per month or continuous estrogens given each day of the month and (2) estrogens plus the addition of progestogen during the last 10 to 14 days of estrogen therapy, or low-dose continuous progestogen plus estrogen given daily.

The most clear-cut early benefit of estrogen therapy in the menopause is the relief of vasomotor instability (hot flashes) and of atrophy of the urogenital epithelium and skin. Estrogen therapy ameliorates these symptoms in most cases. When estrogen therapy is intended to treat hot flashes alone, it should be continued for only a few years, since hot flashes tend to diminish after 3 to 4 years in untreated women.

Several lines of evidence indicate that routine estrogen therapy is beneficial in preventing the complications of menopausal osteoporosis, especially in high-risk women (i.e., thin white women). First, in women undergoing premature menopause, the incidence and complication rates of osteoporosis are increased, and long-term estrogen replacement appears to be beneficial. Second, estrogen therapy has short-term positive effects on calcium balance and long-term beneficial effects on bone density. Third, in women given estrogen therapy, the incidence of fractures is decreased.

Of the potential side effects, the possibility of an increased risk of endometrial carcinoma is perhaps most worrisome. The relative risk of developing endometrial adenocarcinoma in estrogen users is between six and eight times the risk in nonusers. This risk increases with increasing duration and dosage of estrogen but is smaller in women given combination estrogen-progestogen therapy.

Despite the large body of evidence linking endometrial carcinoma and estrogen use, doubts have been raised about the clinical significance of the association. First, some epidemiologists have argued that the increased risk associated with estrogens has been exaggerated because of problems inherent in inadequate controls in retrospective analyses. Second, despite the increased incidence of endometrial carcinoma in the United States, there was no concomitant increased mortality from this disease. In fact, the increased incidence apparently involves low-grade malignancies that may be difficult to distinguish histologically from hyperplasia. These forms of malignancy have little effect on life expectancy.

Apprehension concerning worsening of hypertension and thromboembolic disease appears to be due to reports of the effects of estrogen-progestogen oral contraceptives during the reproductive years and not to estrogen use in postmenopausal women. There is no conclusive evidence that low-dose estrogen therapy after menopause increases the incidence or the severity of thromboembolic disease, breast cancer, or hypertension. Low-dose estrogen treatment after menopause does not appear to influence the development of atherosclerosis, myocardial infarction, or stroke. Strong evidence suggests that, in fact, estrogens may decrease the incidence of death from myocardial infarction. There is a slightly increased risk for the development of gallbladder disease with postmenopausal estrogen use.

A reasonable approach to the postmenopausal use of estrogens is as follows: (1) For long-term use, estrogens should be given in the minimal effective doses (0.625 mg conjugated estrogen orally or 1.0 mg micronized estradiol or transdermal estradiol 0.05 to 1.0 mg in a formulation that is changed every 3.5 days or every week). For women with an intact uterus, it is the practice in some clinics to give estrogens alone for 15 days and estrogen plus a daily progestogen dose for the remainder of the month. The most common regimens involve continuous estrogen plus low-dose continuous progestogen. (2) Such replacement therapy is indicated routinely in women undergoing premature menopause (surgically induced or spontaneous). (3) Estrogen therapy is also indicated routinely in women of all ages who have severe hot flashes or symptomatic atrophy of the urogenital epithelium. Hot flashes rarely persist for longer than 7 years, so, if therapy is given for this purpose, its duration can be limited. (4) In women who have had a hysterectomy, the potential benefits of treatment appear to outweigh the dangers, and in such women cyclic or continuous estrogen without progestogen is recommended. Whether estrogens should be given routinely to all women with intact uteri is an unsettled question, but the authors prescribe it routinely in the absence of contraindications in hopes of ameliorating

Table 337-4

Annual Death Rates Associated with Fertility Control per 100,000 Women

	Age Group					
Contraceptive Techniques	15–19	20–24	25–29	30–34	35–39	40–44
None (birth-related)	7.0	7.4	9.1	14.8	25.7	28.2
Oral contraceptives						
Smokers	2.4	3.6	6.8	13.7	51.4	117.6
Nonsmokers	0.5	0.7	1.1	2.1	14.1	32.0
IUD	1.3	1.1	1.3	1.3	1.9	2.1
Abortion	0.5	1.1	1.3	1.9	1.8	1.1
Barrier methods (birth-related)	1.5	1.4	1.0	0.8	1.3	7.6

SOURCE: Adapted from HW Ory, Fam Plann Perspect 15:57, 1983.

osteoporosis. (5) Each woman receiving estrogens must be monitored indefinitely at yearly intervals.

Induction of Ovulation The most common treatment for ovulation induction in women with PCOD is *clomiphene*. This agent is believed to act as an antiestrogen in the hypothalamus and thus to allow FSH levels to rise, stimulating follicular development and resulting in ovulation. Clomiphene therapy is usually begun with a dose of 50 mg by mouth daily for 5 days commencing on the fifth day of progestogen-induced uterine bleeding. If ovulation does not occur, the dose may be increased to 100 or 150 mg/d. Such treatment results in ovulatory cycles in 60 percent of women with PCOD. Additional regimens include clomiphene in combination with human menopausal gonadotropins (hMG), glucocorticoids, or human chorionic gonadotropin (hCG).

The most commonly used gonadotropins for induction of ovulation are hMG, urofollitropin, and hCG. These agents are indicated in women who fail to ovulate on clomiphene. (For women with hypogonadotropic hypogonadism, urofollitropin is not recommended.) The usual treatment regimen requires 1 to 3 ampuls of hMG or urofollitropin per day over an 8- to 12-day period to achieve adequate follicular stimulation and growth, followed by a single injection of 10,000 units of hCG 12 to 24 h after the last injection of hMG. For women with PCOD, pretreatment with LHRH analogues prior to hMG or urofollitropin appears to improve ovulation and pregnancy rates. Ovulation is successful in 90 percent of women, and pregnancy rates exceed 50 to 60 percent. Measurement of daily estrogen levels and frequent evaluation of ovarian size by ultrasound are indicated to prevent ovarian hyperstimulation. Ovarian hyperstimulation syndrome results from excessive stimulation of ovarian follicles with resulting enlargement of the ovaries; it may progress to the development of ascites, hypotension, and shock. Therapy using hMG, urofollitropin, and hCG also carries a 20 percent risk of multiple pregnancies.

Bromocriptine is a dopamine agonist that is effective in inducing ovulation in women with elevated prolactin levels. Treatment is instituted at a usual dosage of 2.5 mg by mouth two or three times a day. Treatment should be discontinued as soon as pregnancy is diagnosed. → *The management of prolactin-secreting pituitary tumors is discussed in Chap. 328.*

LUTEINIZING HORMONE–RELEASING HORMONE (GONADORELIN) AND ANALOGUES Gonadorelin has been used successfully to induce ovulation in infertile women. The agent is infused subcutaneously or intravenously by a portable infusion pump which administers pulses at 90- to 120-min intervals for 10 to 20 days. After ovulation has occurred, hCG is given to maintain corpus luteum function.

LHRH analogues that block ovulation have been used to treat a variety of gynecologic disorders; ovulation and ovarian steroidogenesis are inhibited owing to the down-regulation of LHRH receptors with a resulting decreased release of gonadotropins. Conditions for which these agents are under trial include fertility control, true precocious puberty, endometriosis, uterine leiomyomas, hirsutism, and, in combination with gonadotropins, ovulation induction and in vitro fertilization.

OTHER DISORDERS OF THE FEMALE REPRODUCTIVE TRACT

VULVA Most disorders of the vulva are due to venereal disease, most commonly syphilis (painless chancre), condylomata acuminata (venereal warts), and herpes vulvitis (painful ulcers) (see Chap. 129). All other lesions of the vulva, particularly in older women, must be biopsied. Early biopsy of cancer of the vulva is mandatory, because when it becomes symptomatic (pruritus and bleeding), it has often progressed to an advanced stage.

VAGINA Infections of the vagina usually present as vaginal discharge and pruritus. The most frequent organisms are *Trichomonas*,

Candida albicans, and *Gardnerella vaginalis* (see also Chap. 129). The diagnosis is made by microscopic examination of the discharge, and appropriate therapy can be instituted using vaginal or oral antibiotics.

Abnormalities of the vagina and cervix in female offspring of women given diethylstilbestrol during pregnancy include adenosis of the vagina and structural abnormalities of the vagina, cervix, and uterus; the risk of developing a rare vaginal cancer (adenocarcinoma, clear cell type) is increased (2 per 10,000 exposed women). Periodic examination of women at risk should begin at age 12 to 14, and reexamination should be done after any episode of abnormal bleeding.

CERVIX Preinvasive lesions of the cervix (also known as *cervical intraepithelial neoplasia*) and invasive carcinoma of the cervix can be detected reliably by obtaining a Papanicolaou smear (Pap smear).

Evaluation of the Pap Smear The incidence of invasive cervical cancer has declined as a result of Pap smear screening. In the United States, approximately 2 to 3 million abnormal Pap smears are found each year. Most represent low-grade lesions but require appropriate follow-up. The follow-up of abnormal Pap smears requires an understanding of the Bethesda System for evaluating such smears and of the limitations of cytologic screening systems. Further evaluation may require repeat cytologic examination, colposcopy, or both.

Current Screening Recommendations Risk factors for cervical neoplasia include a history of multiple sexual partners, coitus beginning at an early age, a history of infection with human papillomavirus, infection with human immunodeficiency virus (HIV) or another immunosuppressed state, and a history of cancer of the lower genital tract. Cervical cancer screening is recommended annually beginning at 18 years of age or when the woman becomes sexually active, if earlier than age 18. "Less frequent" screening is performed when three consecutive, negative, satisfactory annual Pap smears have been obtained or if the woman is in a low-risk category. There is no upper age limit for screening, because the prevalence of invasive cancer shows a linear increase with age, most of these cancers being diagnosed after age 50. Even after hysterectomy, annual screening should be performed if there is a history of abnormal Pap smears or other lower genital tract neoplasia.

The Bethesda System of Cytologic Examination Pap smears are evaluated in regard to the adequacy of the specimen (satisfactory for evaluation, satisfactory but limited, or unsatisfactory for evaluation because of a stated reason), the general diagnosis (normal or abnormal), and a descriptive diagnosis if the smear is abnormal. The descriptive diagnoses include benign cellular changes, reactive cellular changes, and epithelial cell abnormalities, the latter including (1) atypical squamous cells of undetermined significance (ASCUS); (2) low-grade squamous intraepithelial lesion (LSIL), which is further categorized to include human papillomavirus (HPV) infection, cervical intraepithelial neoplasia (CIN 1), and high-grade squamous intraepithelial lesion (HSIL, which is itself subdivided into CIN 2 and CIN 3); and (3) squamous cell carcinoma.

Guidelines for the Management of Women with Abnormal Pap Smears For ASCUS smears that are unqualified or suggest a reactive process, a repeat smear should be obtained every 4 to 6 months for 2 years until three consecutive negative smears have been obtained. For ASCUS smears that are unqualified but have severe inflammation, any specific cause should be treated, and the smear should be repeated in 2 to 3 months; because invasive carcinoma can be obscured by severe inflammation, clinical evaluation is mandatory. For postmenopausal women not using hormone replacement, a course of topical estrogen should be given before the test is repeated. For LSIL smears, the Pap test is repeated every 4 to 6 months for 2 years until three consecutive negative smears have been obtained; treatment of HPV is of no established benefit, and there is a high rate of regression of LSIL, so that in compliant, low-risk individuals, the outcome is usually favorable. If LSIL is persistent, colposcopy with directed biopsy is performed, and endocervical curettage is undertaken if a specific diagnosis is made by biopsy. Cervical cone biopsy or loop electrosurgical excision procedures are performed for higher-grade lesions such as HSIL. If cervical cancer is diagnosed by biopsy, clinical staging is performed, and the patient is treated with radiation therapy or surgery.

UTERUS   Only 40 percent of cases of endometrial adenocarcinoma are detected by Pap smear. In women at high risk for endometrial carcinoma (because of obesity, a history of chronic anovulatory cycles, diabetes mellitus, hypertension, or estrogen treatment), yearly endometrial sampling should be performed. Low-dose oral estrogen therapy rarely causes breakthrough or withdrawal bleeding in postmenopausal women. Therefore, irrespective of whether the patient is using estrogen therapy, the occurrence of postmenopausal bleeding makes it mandatory to obtain a tissue diagnosis by either endometrial sampling or curettage to exclude endometrial cancer.

One of the most common disorders of the uterus and the most frequent tumor of women (one of four women affected) is the uterine leiomyoma, or fibroid tumor. Three-fourths of women with leiomyoma are asymptomatic, and the diagnosis is made on routine pelvic examination. When the tumor is associated with excessive menstrual blood loss, is large or fast-gowing, or causes significant pelvic pain (see Chap. 52), the preferred treatment is hysterectomy if there is no desire for further childbearing. In young women, myomectomy is sometimes indicated when infertility or repeated fetal wastage is a manifestation or where future childbearing is desired.

FALLOPIAN TUBES AND OVARIES   Infectious pelvic inflammatory disease is a common disorder of the fallopian tubes and usually becomes symptomatic after a menstrual period; the symptoms include fever, chills, abdominal pain, and vaginal discharge, and pelvic tenderness on physical examination is common. The initiating organism most often is *Chlamydia trachomatis* or *Neisseria gonorrhoeae*, but tuboovarian abscess and sterility are probably caused by mixed aerobic and anaerobic superinfections and require wide-spectrum antibiotic treatment (see Chap. 130).

Endometriosis is a benign disorder characterized by the presence and proliferation of endometrial tissue (stroma and glands) outside the endometrial cavity. The clinical manifestations are variable. Endometriosis occurs most commonly between the ages of 30 and 40 and is found incidentally at the time of surgery in approximately one-fifth of all gynecologic operations. The fertility rate is reduced in affected women. The disorder usually involves the posterior cul-de-sac or the ovaries and can give rise to ovarian enlargement (endometriomas), although it may involve distant sites (lung, umbilicus). The major symptom is pelvic pain, characteristically dysmenorrhea (see Chap. 52). However, the frequency and severity of symptoms correlate poorly with the extent of disease. Other manifestations include dyspareunia, pain with defecation, and infertility. The characteristic physical findings are multiple tender nodules palpable along the uterosacral ligament at the time of rectal-vaginal examination, a posteriorly fixed uterus, or enlarged, cystic ovaries. The diagnosis can only be confirmed by direct visualization, usually at diagnostic laparoscopy. Treatment depends on the degree of involvement and the desires of the patient and includes observation for mild disease with no associated infertility or pain, hormonal suppressive therapy (see "Infertility," above), conservative surgery if fertility is desired, or removal of the uterus, tubes, and ovaries in severe disease. Endometriosis is rare after the menopause.

Any adnexal mass that persists for more than 6 weeks or is larger than 6 cm must be evaluated. Although ovarian cysts and neoplasms are the most common pelvic adnexal masses (see above), tumors of the fallopian tubes, uterus, gastrointestinal tract, or urinary tract also should be considered. Sonography or radiographic evaluation is often helpful in identifying the nature of the adnexal mass prior to surgical exploration.

See Chap. 57, Estrogens and progestins, in Goodman & Gilman's The Pharmacological Basis of Therapeutics, *9th ed, New York, McGraw-Hill, 1996.*

BIBLIOGRAPHY

ADASHI EV, LEUNG PCK: *The Ovary*. New York, Raven Press, 1993
CARR BR: Disorders of the ovary and reproductive tract, in *Williams Textbook of Endocrinology*, 8th ed, JD Wilson, DW Foster (eds). Philadelphia, Saunders, 1992, pp 733–798

————, BLACKWELL RE (eds): *Textbook of Reproductive Medicine*. Norwalk, CT, Appleton & Lange, 1993
————, GRIFFIN JE: Fertility control and its complications, in *Williams Textbook of Endocrinology*, 8th ed, JD Wilson, DW Foster (eds). Philadelphia, Saunders, 1992, pp 1007–1031
CUNNINGHAM FG et al: *Williams' Obstetrics*, 19th ed. Norwalk, CT, Appleton & Lange, 1993
FUTTERWEIT W: *Polycystic Ovarian Disease*. New York, Springer-Verlag, 1984
GRAVE GD, CUTLER GB: *Sexual Precocity*. New York, Raven Press, 1993
GRUMBACH MM, CONTE FA: Disorders of sex differentiation, in *Williams Textbook of Endocrinology*, 8th ed, JD Wilson, DW Foster (eds). Philadelphia, Saunders, 1992, pp 853–952
————, STYNE DM: Puberty: Ontogeny, neuroendocrinology, physiology and disorders, in *Williams Textbook of Endocrinology*, 8th ed, JD Wilson, DW Foster (eds). Philadelphia, Saunders, 1992, pp 1139–1222
HATCHER RA et al: *Contraceptive Technology 1994–1996*. New York, Irvington, 1996
HERBST AL et al: *Comprehensive Gynecology*, 2d ed. St. Louis, Mosby, 1992
KAPLAN SA (ed): *Clinical Pediatric Endocrinology*. Philadelphia, Saunders, 1990
KNOBIL E, NEILL JD (eds): *The Physiology of Reproduction,* 2d ed. New York, Raven Press, 1994
LOBO RA: *Treatment of the Menopausal Woman*. New York, Raven Press, 1993
ROCK JA et al: *Female Reproductive Surgery*. Baltimore, Williams & Wilkins, 1992
SEIBEL MM: A new era in reproductive technology. N Engl J Med 318:828, 1988
SODERSTROM RM: *Operative Laparoscopy*. New York, Raven Press, 1993
SPEROFF L et al: *Clinical Gynecologic Endocrinology and Infertility*, 5th ed. Baltimore, Williams & Wilkins, 1994
STUDD JWW, WHITEHEAD MI (eds): *The Menopause*. Oxford, Blackwell, 1988
STYNE DM, GRUMBACH MM: Disorders of puberty in the male and female, in *Reproductive Endocrinology*, SSC Yen, RB Jaffe (eds). Philadelphia, Saunders, 1991, pp 11–54
THOMPSON JD, ROCK JA: *Te Lindes Operative Gynecology*. Philadelphia, Lippincott, 1992
YEN SSC, JAFFE RB (eds): *Reproductive Endocrinology*, 3d ed. Philadelphia, Saunders, 1991

338   *Jean D. Wilson*

ENDOCRINE DISORDERS OF THE BREAST

Examination of the breasts is an important part of the physical examination. The breasts are the site of fatal and preventable disease in women and provide clues to underlying systemic illness in both men and women. It is the duty of every physician to distinguish the abnormal from the normal at the earliest possible stage and to call for assistance if there is any doubt. → *For further discussion of cancer of the breast, see Chap. 91*

ENDOCRINE CONTROL OF THE BREAST   There is no histologic or functional difference in the breasts of boys and girls prior to the onset of puberty, but a profound sexual dimorphism in breast development ensues at the time of puberty. The endocrine control of female breast development is illustrated in Fig. 338-1. The pubertal growth of the female breast is dependent primarily on the action of estradiol, which induces the growth, division, and elongation of the tubular duct system and maturation of the nipples. In men the administration of estrogen is equally effective in this regard. To produce true alveolar development at the ends of the ducts, however, the synergistic action of progesterone is required, a ratio of estrogen to progesterone of 1:20 to 1:100 being optimal. Within the gland a variety of mediators influence cell division and differentiation, including stimulatory factors such as the insulin-like growth factors and epidermal growth factor and inhibitory factors such as transforming growth factor beta. Once the anatomic development of the ducts and alveoli is complete, the continued action of estrogen and progesterone is not required for lactation itself.

The endocrine control of milk formation is complex, requiring, in addition to appropriate priming by estrogen and progesterone, specific lactogenic hormone and the permissive action of glucocorticoid, insulin, thyroxine, and, in some species, growth hormone. There are two lactogenic hormones. Human placental lactogen (hPL, or chorionic somatomammotropin) is secreted in large amounts by the placenta during the latter part of gestation and prepares the breast for milk production. hPL disappears from the maternal (and fetal) circulation shortly after termination of pregnancy. The secretion of pituitary prolactin (see Chap. 328) rises during pregnancy and plays the critical role in the initiation and maintenance of lactation in the puerperium; during late pregnancy and lactation, 60 to 80 percent of the anterior pituitary may consist of prolactin-secreting cells.

Unlike most pituitary hormones, the predominant regulation of prolactin secretion is negative, i.e., under ordinary basal conditions inhibitory hypothalamic hormones, the most important being dopamine, are delivered from the central nervous system to the pituitary via the hypothalamic portal system and inhibit the release of prolactin into the blood (see Chap. 328). Most factors that influence prolactin secretion do so by affecting the synthesis or release of the inhibitory factor(s). Basal prolactin levels fall following delivery, but prolactin secretion is enhanced by stimulation of the breasts, such as the act of nursing (the so-called sucking reflex), a phenomenon that is probably mediated by the reflex release of oxytocin. Prolactin binds to a specific receptor on the cell surface of the breast acinar cells to enhance the synthesis of milk constituents via a tyrosine kinase–mediated process. In the postgestational state, the normal lactating woman forms about a liter of milk per day containing 38 g fat, 70 g lactose, and 12 g protein. Lactation can be suppressed by the administration of estrogens or diethylstilbestrol, which inhibit milk production by direct effects on the breast, or dopaminergic agents such as bromocriptine, which inhibit prolactin secretion by the pituitary. Alternatively, if a woman does not nurse or empty her breasts postpartum, lactation usually ceases in 1 to 2 weeks.

GALACTORRHEA Exactly what constitutes nonpuerperal or inappropriate lactation is not always clearly defined in the literature. According to the studies of Friedman and Goldfein, no breast secretions whatsoever are detectable in normal, regularly menstruating nulligravid women, but breast secretions can be demonstrated in a fourth of normal women who have been pregnant in the past; thus breast secretions in small amounts may be of no clinical significance in these instances. Spontaneous leakage of milk from the breasts is usually of more importance than milk that must be expressed. A second problem

is related to the composition of the breast secretions. When the secretion is milky or white, it is safe to assume that it contains fat, casein, and lactose and is in fact milk; however, when the secretion is brown or greenish, it rarely contains normal milk constituents and consequently may not result from an underlying endocrinopathy. Milk also must be distinguished from blood or bloody discharges that may be due to neoplasms of the breast. It also should be remembered that the composition of milk constituents may increase upon repeated sampling, from low, colostrum-like values to those typical of milk. With these problems in mind, galactorrhea can be defined as inappropriate production of milk that is persistent or worrisome to the patient, recognizing that in some instances no underlying pathology may be demonstrated.

Since the action of a lactogenic hormone is necessary for the initiation of milk production, it is logical to consider galactorrhea as a consequence of deranged prolactin physiology. However, as indicated above, a complex endocrinologic milieu is necessary for lactation, and in many instances in which prolactin is elevated, both in women who have not been appropriately primed and in men, no production of milk takes place. As a consequence, hyperprolactinemia is more common than galactorrhea. Furthermore, while enhanced prolactin secretion is necessary for the initiation of lactation, continued production can be maintained in the presence of minimally or intermittently elevated prolactin levels so that basal plasma prolactin levels are not always elevated in patients with galactorrhea. In some such women prolactin levels may be elevated only during sleep; in others, hyperprolactinemia is believed to have been present transiently. Perhaps the strongest evidence for a critical role for prolactin in galactorrhea is the fact that administration of dopaminergic agents that suppress plasma prolactin levels causes a disappearance of galactorrhea even when the basal plasma prolactin levels are normal.

Differential Diagnosis Galactorrhea is due either to a failure of the normal hypothalamic inhibition of prolactin release, to increased prolactin-releasing factor(s), or to autonomous prolactin secretion by tumors (Table 338-1). Pituitary stalk section results in a striking increase in prolactin secretion, as the result of the interruption of the delivery of prolactin inhibitory factors to the pituitary. Likewise, many drugs that influence the central nervous system (including virtually all psychotropic agents, methyldopa, reserpine, and antiemetics) cause enhanced prolactin release, presumably by inhibiting synthesis or release of prolactin inhibitory factors such as dopamine. Estrogens on the one hand increase prolactin secretion, and on the other estrogen withdrawal (as in the discontinuation of oral contraceptives) may trigger the onset of galactorrhea. Central nervous system diseases outside the pituitary presumably cause galactorrhea by interfering with delivery of the inhibitory factors to the pituitary (central nervous system sarcoidosis, craniopharyngioma, pinealoma, encephalitis, meningitis, hydrocephalus, hypothalamic tumors).

Stage	Duct system	Major hormones	Permissive hormones
Prepubertal		None	Unknown
Adult		Estrogen (progesterone)	
Pregnancy		Estrogen Progesterone Prolactin Human placental lactogen	Insulin Thyroxine Glucocorticoids Growth hormone
Lactation		Prolactin Oxytocin	

FIGURE 338-1 Endocrine control of female breast development and function at various stages of life.

Table 338-1

Classification of Galactorrhea

A. Failure of normal hypothalamic inhibition of prolactin release
  1. Pituitary stalk section
  2. Drugs (phenothiazines, butyrophenones, methyldopa, tricyclic antidepressants, opiates, reserpine, verapamil)
  3. Central nervous system disease, including extrapituitary tumors and null cell adenomas of the pituitary
B. Enhanced prolactin-release
  1. Hypothyroidism
  2. Sucking reflex and breast trauma
C. Autonomous prolactin release
  1. Pituitary tumors
    a. Prolactin-secreting tumors
    b. Mixed growth hormone and prolactin-secreting tumors
    c. Null cell adenomas
  2. Ectopic production of human placental lactogen and/or prolactin
    a. Hydatidiform moles and choriocarcinomas
    b. Bronchogenic carcinoma and hypernephroma
D. Idiopathic

In primary hypothyroidism, galactorrhea results from enhanced prolactin-releasing activity. Thyrotropin-releasing hormone (TRH) stimulates prolactin release, and thyroid hormone replacement cures the galactorrhea. A similar mechanism, as the result of enhanced secretion of oxytocin, may cause the galactorrhea that follows breast surgery or breast trauma.

Enhanced prolactin release also can occur from pituitary or nonpituitary tumors. Three types of pituitary tumors (see Chap. 328) may be associated with galactorrhea: pure prolactin-secreting tumors (micro- or macroadenomas), mixed tumors that secrete both growth hormone and prolactin and cause acromegaly with galactorrhea, and some null cell adenomas. The latter may interfere with the delivery of inhibitory factors to the pituitary. Excess growth hormone secretion in the absence of hyperprolactinemia may on occasion cause galactorrhea. Prolactin also can be secreted by other malignancies such as bronchogenic carcinoma, and hydatidiform moles and choriocarcinomas may secrete placental lactogen.

In series involving several hundred patients, a pituitary tumor was identified in about one-fourth, other known causes could be identified in another fourth or fifth, and the remaining half fell into the idiopathic category. Many of the latter group ultimately developed prolactin-secreting pituitary tumors, some probably had subtle disorders of hypothalamic function, and in others a drug-related cause may have been missed; but the fact remains that no satisfactory diagnosis is reached in many patients. When normal menses and galactorrhea coexist, the likelihood of establishing a diagnosis is poor.

Galactorrhea is unusual in men, even in the presence of profound elevations of plasma prolactin; when it does occur, it is usually upon the background of a feminizing state (see below).

Diagnostic Evaluation If hyperprolactinemia is present, the workup is fundamentally that of a pituitary tumor once drug causes and hypothyroidism are excluded (see Chap. 328). Even when a specific cause cannot be identified and the diagnosis of idiopathic galactorrhea is made by exclusion, it is necessary to remember that pituitary tumors may subsequently become manifest. The higher the prolactin values and the more persistent the galactorrhea, the greater is the likelihood of such a development.

℞ **TREATMENT**

Breast binders can be effective in patients with mild galactorrhea of unknown etiology, presumably by preventing stimulation of the nipple and the consequent perpetuation of lactation. The aim of treatment in other instances is to correct the elevated prolactin, and treatment of a pituitary tumor, cessation of causative drugs, or correction of hypothyroidism is often followed by the disappearance of galactorrhea. Dopaminergic agents that suppress plasma prolactin have been used to treat idiopathic hyperprolactinemia, prolactin-secreting tumors of the pituitary (see Chap. 328), and even normoprolactinemic galactorrhea. These drugs not only suppress lactation but also may cause resumption of menstrual cycles (and even fertility) in patients with amenorrhea and galactorrhea.

GYNECOMASTIA A central issue in the evaluation of breast tissue in adult men is the separation of the normal from the abnormal. The incidence of active gynecomastia in autopsy series is between 5 and 9 percent, but Nuttall and colleagues have reported that approximately 40 percent of normal men and up to 70 percent of hospitalized men have palpable breast tissue. The reason for this discrepancy is not clear. On the one hand, it may be difficult to distinguish true breast tissue from masses of adipose tissue without true breast enlargement (lipomastia); in such cases, true gynecomastia can be separated from lipomastia by mammography or ultrasonography. Alternatively, the incidence of gynecomastia may have increased (possibly due to exposure to environmental or plant estrogens), or the autopsy data may underestimate the frequency of palpable breast tissue. Regardless, we are left with major uncertainties; the finding of gynecomastia (distinct from lipomastia) may indicate underlying pathology or a normal variant. In this discussion, we shall assume that any palpable breast tissue in men (except for the three physiologic states; see below) can be

due to an underlying endocrinopathy and deserves, at a minimum, a limited evaluation.

Early gynecomastia is characterized by proliferation in the breast of both the fibroblastic stroma and the duct system, which elongates, buds, and duplicates. As gynecomastia persists, progressive fibrosis and hyalinization are associated with regression of epithelial proliferation and, eventually, a decrease in the number of ducts. When the cause of the gynecomastia is corrected early in the course, resolution occurs by reduction in size and epithelial content with gradual disappearance of the ducts, leaving hyaline bands that eventually disappear.

Growth of the breast in men, as in women, is mediated by estrogen and results from disturbances of the normal ratio of active androgen to estrogen. As described in Chap. 336, estradiol formation in normal men occurs principally by the conversion of circulating androgen to estrogen in extraglandular tissues; the normal ratio of production of testosterone to estradiol in adult men is approximately 100:1 (6 mg versus 45 μg/day), and the normal ratio of the two hormones in plasma is about 300:1. Growth of the breast ensues in men when the normal ratio decreases as the result of diminished testosterone production or action, enhanced estrogen formation, or both processes occurring simultaneously.

Enlargement of the male breast can be a normal physiologic phenomenon at certain times of life or the result of several pathologic states (Table 338-2).

Table 338-2

Differential Diagnosis of Gynecomastia

PHYSIOLOGIC GYNECOMASTIA

Newborn
Adolescence
Aging

PATHOLOGIC GYNECOMASTIA

A. Deficient production or action of testosterone
   1. Congenital anorchia
   2. Androgen resistance (testicular feminization and Reifenstein syndrome)
   3. Defects of testosterone synthesis
   4. Klinefelter syndrome
   5. Viral orchitis
   6. Trauma
   7. Castration
   8. Neurologic and granulomatous diseases
   9. Renal failure
B. Increased estrogen production
   1. Increased estrogen secretion
      a. Testicular tumors
      b. True hermaphroditism
      c. Carcinoma of the lung and other tumors producing hCG
   2. Increased substrate for extraglandular aromatase
      a. Adrenal disease
      b. Liver disease
      c. Malnutrition
      d. Hyperthyroidism
   3. Increase in extraglandular aromatase
C. Drugs
   1. Estrogens (diethylstilbestrol, birth control pills, digitalis, estrogen-containing cosmetics, estrogen-contaminated foods, phytoestrogens)
   2. Drugs that enhance endogenous estrogen secretion (gonadotropins, clomiphene)
   3. Inhibitors of testosterone synthesis and/or action (ketoconazole, metronidazole, alkylating agents, cisplatin, spironolactone, cimetidine, flutamide, etomidate)
   4. Unknown mechanisms (busulfan, isoniazid, methyldopa, tricyclic antidepressants, penicillamine, diazepam, omeprazole, calcium channel blockers, angiotensin-converting enzyme inhibitors, marijuana, heroin, finasteride)
D. Idiopathic

Physiologic Gynecomastia In the *newborn*, transient enlargement of the breast is due to the action of maternal and/or placental estrogens. The enlargement usually disappears in a few weeks but may persist longer. *Adolescent* gynecomastia is common at some time during puberty. The median age of onset is 14; it is often asymmetric, occasionally unilateral for a portion of its course, and frequently tender, and it regresses so that by age 20 only a small number of men have palpable vestiges of gynecomastia in one or both breasts. Although the origin of the excess estrogen has not been identified, the onset of gynecomastia correlates with transient elevations of plasma estradiol prior to the completion of puberty so that the androgen/estrogen ratio is low. *Gynecomastia of aging* also occurs in otherwise healthy men. Forty percent or more of aged men have gynecomastia. A likely explanation is the increase with age in the conversion of androgens to estrogens in extraglandular tissues. Abnormal liver function or drug therapy may be contributing causes in such men.

Pathologic Gynecomastia Pathologic gynecomastia can result from one of three basic mechanisms: deficiency in testosterone production or action (with or without a secondary increase in estrogen production), increase in estrogen production, or drugs (Table 338-2). Most of the individual disorders that cause primary and secondary testicular failure are discussed in Chap. 336. The fact that a deficiency in testosterone production by itself can cause gynecomastia is illustrated by the syndrome of congenital anorchia in which normal (or slightly low) estradiol production in the presence of profoundly decreased testosterone production results in florid gynecomastia. Decreased testosterone production is also responsible in some patients with Klinefelter syndrome and in men with testicular failure from other causes. In the disorders of androgen resistance, such as testicular feminization, deficient androgen action and increased testicular estrogen production are both present.

A primary increase in estrogen production can result from a variety of causes. Increased secretion of testicular estrogen may result from elevations in plasma gonadotropins, for example, in cases of aberrant production of chorionic gonadotropin by testicular tumors or by bronchogenic carcinoma, from the ovarian elements in the gonads of men with true hermaphroditism, or as the result of formation by testicular tumors (particularly Leydig cell and Sertoli cell tumors). Increased conversion of androgen to estrogens in extraglandular tissues can be due either to increased availability of substrate for extraglandular estrogen formation, for example, from increased production of androstenedione (congenital adrenal hyperplasia, hyperthyroidism, and most feminizing adrenal tumors), or to diminished catabolism of androstenedione (liver disease). Increased amounts of extraglandular aromatase can be caused by a rare hereditary abnormality or by tumors of the liver or adrenal gland.

Drugs can cause gynecomastia by several mechanisms. Many drugs either act directly as estrogens or cause an increase in plasma estrogen activity, for example, in men receiving diethylstilbestrol for prostatic carcinoma and in transsexuals in preparation for sex-change operations. Boys and young men are particularly sensitive to estrogen and can develop gynecomastia after the use of dermal ointments containing estrogen or after the ingestion of milk or meat from estrogen-treated animals. The gynecomastia of digitalis ingestion is usually attributed to an estrogen-like side effect of the drug, but in the experience of the author it usually occurs in men with abnormal liver function. A second mechanism of drug-induced gynecomastia is illustrated by clomiphene and human chorionic gonadotropin (hCG), which cause enhanced testicular secretion of estrogen. Other drugs cause gynecomastia by interfering with testosterone synthesis (ketoconazole and alkylating agents) and/or testosterone action, for instance, by blocking the binding of androgen to its receptor protein in target tissues (spironolactone and cimetidine). Finally, drugs that cause gynecomastia by mechanisms that have not been defined include busulfan, ethionamide, isoniazid, methyldopa, tricyclic antidepressants, penicillamine, omeprazole, calcium channel blocking agents, angiotensin-converting en-

zyme inhibitors, diazepam, marijuana, and heroin. In some instances, the feminization is due to effects of drugs on liver function.

Diagnostic Evaluation The evaluation of patients with gynecomastia should include: (1) a careful drug history; (2) measurement and examination of the testes (if both are small, a chromosomal karyotype should be obtained; if they are asymmetric, a workup for testicular tumor should be instituted); (3) evaluation of liver function; and (4) endocrine evaluation to include measurement of serum androstenedione or 24-h urinary 17-ketosteroids (usually elevated in feminizing adrenal states), measurement of plasma estradiol and hCG (helpful if elevated but usually normal), and measurement of plasma luteinizing hormone (LH) and testosterone. If LH is high and testosterone is low, the diagnosis is usually testicular failure; if LH and testosterone are both low, the diagnosis is most likely increased primary estrogen production (e.g., a Sertoli cell tumor of the testis); and if both LH and testosterone are elevated, the diagnosis is either an androgen-resistance state or a gonadotropin-secreting tumor.

A satisfactory diagnosis can be made in only half or fewer of patients referred for gynecomastia. This implies either that the diagnostic techniques are not sufficiently refined to recognize mild disturbances, that many causes of gynecomastia are as yet undefined, that the causes may be transient and difficult to diagnose, or, as suggested by Nuttall, that gynecomastia may in some instances be normal rather than due to a pathologic state. Because of the problem of separating the normal from the abnormal, gynecomastia should probably be routinely worked up only if the drug history is negative, the breast is tender (indicating rapid growth), or the breast mass is larger than 4 cm in diameter. In other instances, a decision to perform an endocrine evaluation depends on the clinical context. For example, gynecomastia associated with signs of underandrogenization should always be evaluated.

℞ TREATMENT

When the primary cause can be identified and corrected, the breast enlargement usually subsides promptly and eventually disappears. For example, androgen replacement therapy may produce dramatic improvement in men with testicular insufficiency. However, if the gynecomastia is of long duration (and fibrosis has replaced the original ductal hyperplasia), correction of the primary defect may not be followed by resolution. In such instances and when the primary cause cannot be corrected, surgery is the only effective therapy. Indications for surgery include several psychologic and/or cosmetic problems, continued growth, or a suspected malignancy. Although the relative risk of carcinoma of the breast is increased in men with gynecomastia, it is rare nevertheless. Prophylactic radiation of the breasts prior to the institution of diethylstilbestrol therapy is effective in preventing gynecomastia and has a low complication rate in elderly men. In rare patients who have painful gynecomastia and who are not candidates for other therapy, treatment with antiestrogens such as tamoxifen may be indicated.

BIBLIOGRAPHY

GALACTORRHEA

ABDEL GADIN A et al: The etiology of galactorrhea in women with regular menstruation and normal prolactin levels. Human Reprod 7:912, 1992

BENJAMIN F: Normal lactation and galactorrhea. Clin Obstet Gynecol 37:887, 1994

CAVANAUGH J et al: Gynecomastia and cirrhosis of the liver. Arch Intern Med 150:563, 1990

CHOTINER HC et al: Lactose and casein content of nonpuerperal breast secretion. J Reprod Med 22:267, 1979

FRANTZ AG, WILSON JD: Endocrine disorders of the breast, in *Williams Textbook of Endocrinology*, 8th ed, JD Wilson, DW Foster (eds). Philadelphia, Saunders, 1992, p 593

FRIEDMAN S, GOLDFEIN A: Breast secretions in normal women. Am J Obstet Gynecol 104:846, 1969

JOHNSON DG et al: Prolactin secretion and biological activity in females with galactorrhoea and normal circulating prolactin concentrations at rest. Clin Endocrinol 22:661, 1985

KLEINBERG DL: Galactorrhea. Curr Ther Endocrinol Metab 5:360, 1994

KOPPELMAN MCS et al: Hyperprolactinemia, amenorrhea, and galactorrhea. A retrospective assessment of twenty-five cases. Ann Intern Med 100:115, 1984

KULSKI JK et al: Changes in the milk composition of nonpuerperal women. Am J Obstet Gynecol 139:597, 1981

LAMBERTS SW, QUIK RF: A comparison of the efficacy and safety of pergolide and bromocriptine in the treatment of hyperprolactinemia. J Clin Endocrinol Metab 72:635, 1991

LAURENCE DJ, MONAGHAN P, GUSTERSON BA: The development of the normal human breast. Oxf Rev Reprod Biol 13:149, 1991

RUIZ-VELASCO V: Hyperprolactinemia and mammary prostheses. A report of eight cases. J Reprod Med 31:267, 1986

SAUER HJ: Physiology of lactation and factors affecting lactation. Obstet Gynecol Clin North Am 14:615, 1987

TURKSOY RN et al: Diagnostic and therapeutic modalities in women with galactorrhea. Obstet Gynecol 56:323, 1980

YAMAGUCHI M et al: Effects of nocturnal hyperprolactinemia on ovarian luteal function and galactorrhea. Eur J Obstet Gynecol 39:187, 1991

GYNECOMASTIA

ANDERSON JA, GROOM JB: Male breast at autopsy. Acta Pathol Microbiol Immunol Scand 90:191, 1982

CIMORA GA et al: Percutaneous oestrogen-induced gynecomastia: A case report. Br J Plast Surg 35:209, 1982

DE GASPARO M et al: Antialdosterones: Incidence and prevention of sexual side effects. J Steroid Biochem 32:223, 1989

FASS D et al: Radiotherapeutic prophylaxis of estrogen-induced gynecomastia: A study of late sequela. Int J Radiat Oncol Biol Phys 12:407, 1986

FELDMAN D: Ketoconazole and other imidazole derivatives as inhibitors of steroidogenesis. Endocr Rev 7:409, 1986

FRANTZ AG, WILSON JD: Endocrine disorders of the breast, in *Williams Textbook of Endocrinology*, 8th ed, JD Wilson, DW Foster (eds). Philadelphia, Saunders, 1992, p 953

GEORGIADIS E et al: Incidence of gynaecomastia in 954 young males and its relationship to somatometric parameters. Ann Hum Biol 21:579, 1994

KORENMAN SG: The endocrinology of the abnormal male breast. Ann NY Acad Sci 464:400, 1986

MABUCHI K et al: Risk factors for male breast cancer. J Natl Cancer Inst 74:371, 1985

MAHONEY CP: Adolescent gynecomastia: Differential diagnosis and management. Pediatr Clin North Am 37:1389, 1990

MCDERMOTT MT et al: Tamoxifen therapy for painful idiopathic gynecomastia. South Med J 83:1283, 1990

NIEWOEHNER CV, NUTTALL FQ: Gynecomastia in a hospitalized male population. Am J Med 77:633, 1984

NUTTALL FQ: Gynecomastia as a physical finding in normal men. J Clin Endocrinol Metab 48:338, 1979

ROSE DP: Endocrine epidemiology of male breast cancer (review). Anticancer Res 8:845, 1988

THOMPSON DF, CARTER R: Drug-induced gynecomastia. Pharmacotherapy 13:37, 1993

339

Jean D. Wilson, James E. Griffin

DISORDERS OF SEXUAL DIFFERENTIATION

Sexual differentiation is a sequential and ordered process. *Chromosomal sex*, established at the moment of fertilization, determines *gonadal sex*, and gonadal sex, in turn, causes the development of *phenotypic sex*, in which the male or female urogenital tract is formed (Table 339-1). A disturbance of any step in this process during embryogenesis may impair sexual differentiation. Known causes of such disorders include environmental insults as in the ingestion of a virilizing drug during pregnancy, nonfamilial aberrations of the sex chromosomes as in 45,X gonadal dysgenesis, birth defects of multifactorial etiology as in most cases of hypospadias, and disorders due to single gene mutations as in the testicular feminization syndrome.

Limitations of knowledge make it necessary to make empirical assignments as to the nature of the derangement in certain disorders, but specific diagnoses usually can be made as the result of genetic, endocrine, phenotypic, and chromosomal assessment. As a consequence, appropriate gender assignment can be made, even in extreme instances of ambiguous genitalia, and tailoring of the phenotype can be undertaken when appropriate.

NORMAL SEXUAL DIFFERENTIATION

The first event in sexual differentiation is the establishment of chromosomal sex, the heterogametic sex (XY) being male and the homogametic sex (XX) female. The embryos of both sexes then develop in an identical fashion until approximately 40 days of gestation. The second phase of sexual differentiation is the conversion of the indifferent gonad into a testis or an ovary. No matter how many X chromosomes are present (as in 47,XXY, 48,XXXY, etc.), a testis will develop as long as a normal Y chromosome is present. Differentiation of the indifferent gonad into a testis is mediated by a single gene on the short arm of the Y chromosome (SRY); insertion of a transgene containing this gene into female mice causes them to develop as males. The gene encodes a DNA-binding protein, but the mechanism by which it promotes testicular development is unknown. The final process, the translation of gonadal sex into phenotypic sex, is the consequence of the type of gonad formed and the endocrine secretions of the fetal gonads and results in the formation of the male and female urogenital tracts.

The internal urogenital tract is derived from the wolffian and müllerian ducts that exist side by side in early embryos of both sexes (Fig. 339-1A). In the male the wolffian ducts give rise to the epididymides, vasa deferentia, and seminal vesicles, and the müllerian ducts disappear. In the female the fallopian tubes, uterus, and upper vagina are derived from the müllerian ducts, and the wolffian ducts regress. The external genitalia and urethra in the two sexes develop from common anlage—the urogenital sinus and the genital tubercle, folds, and swellings (Fig. 339-1B). The urogenital sinus gives rise to the prostate and prostatic urethra in the male and to the urethra and lower portion of the vagina in the female. The genital tubercle gives rise to the glans penis in the male and the clitoris in the female. The urogenital swellings become the scrotum or the labia majora, and the urethral folds develop into the labia minora or fuse to form the shaft of the penis and the male urethra.

In the absence of the testis, as in the normal female or in the male embryo castrated prior to the onset of gonadal differentiation, phenotypic sex develops along female lines. Thus, masculinization of the fetus is induced by hormones from the fetal testes, whereas female development does not require the presence of the ovary. Phenotypic sex normally conforms to chromosomal sex. That is, chromosomal sex determines gonadal sex, and gonadal sex, in turn, controls phenotypic sex.

Table 339-1

Classification of Disorders of Sexual Development

Disorders of Chromosomal Sex
   Klinefelter syndrome
   XX male
   Gonadal dysgenesis
   Mixed gonadal dysgenesis
   True hermaphroditism
Disorders of Gonadal Sex
   Pure gonadal dysgenesis
   Absent testis syndrome
Disorders of Phenotypic Sex
   Female pseudohermaphroditism
      Congenital adrenal hyperplasia
      Nonadrenal female pseudohermaphroditism
      Developmental disorders of müllerian ducts
   Male pseudohermaphroditism
      Abnormalities in androgen synthesis
      Abnormalities in androgen action
      Persistent müllerian duct syndrome
      Development defects of male genitalia

The formation of the male phenotype is vested in the action of three hormones. Two—müllerian duct inhibitor and testosterone—are secreted by the fetal testis. Müllerian duct inhibitor [(MDI), also termed müllerian-inhibiting substance or antimüllerian hormone] is a protein that suppresses the müllerian ducts and prevents development of the uterus and fallopian tubes in the male. Testosterone acts directly to virilize the wolffian duct and is the precursor for the third embryonic male hormone, dihydrotestosterone (see Chap. 336), which promotes development of the male urethra and prostate and formation of the penis and scrotum. Testosterone and dihydrotestosterone induce formation of the male urogenital tract during fetal life by the same intracellular machinery by which they act in postembryonic life (Chap. 336).

The secretion of testosterone by the fetal testes approaches a maximum by the tenth week of gestation, and formation of the sexual phenotypes is largely completed by the end of the first trimester. During the latter phases of gestation, the ovarian follicles develop and the vagina matures in the female, and descent of the testes and growth of the external genitalia take place in the male.

DISORDERS OF CHROMOSOMAL SEX

Disorders of chromosomal sex (Table 339-2) occur when the number or structure of the X or Y chromosomes is abnormal (see Chap. 66).

KLINEFELTER SYNDROME Clinical Features Klinefelter syndrome is characterized by small, firm testes, azoospermia, gynecomastia, and elevated levels of plasma gonadotropins in men with two or more X chromosomes. The common karyotype is either a 47,XXY chromosomal pattern (the classic form) or 46,XY/47,XXY mosaicism. It is the most frequent major abnormality of sexual differentiation, the incidence being around 1 in 500 men.

Prepubertally, the testes are small but otherwise appear normal. After puberty, the disorder is manifest as infertility, gynecomastia, or occasionally underandrogenization (Table 339-3). Hyalinization of the seminiferous tubules and azoospermia are consistent features of the 47,XXY variety. The small, firm testes are usually <2 cm and always <3.5 cm in length (corresponding to 2- and 12-mL volume, respectively). The increased mean body height results from longer legs. Gynecomastia ordinarily develops during adolescence, is generally bilateral and painless, and may become disfiguring (see Chap. 338). Obesity and varicose veins occur in one-third to one-half, and mild mental deficiency, social maladjustment, abnormalities of thyroid function, diabetes mellitus, and pulmonary disease may be present. The risk of breast cancer is 20 times that of normal men (but only about a fifth that in women). Most have male psychosexual orientation and function sexually as normal men.

The mosaic variant comprises about 10 percent of the patients, as estimated by chromosomal karyotypes on peripheral blood leukocytes. The frequency of this variant may be underestimated, since chromosomal mosaicism may be present in the testes when the peripheral leukocyte karyotype is normal. The mosaic form is usually not as severe as the 47,XXY variety, and the testes may be normal in size (see Table 339-3). The endocrine abnormalities are less severe, and gynecomastia and azoospermia are less common. Indeed, occasional mosaic individuals are fertile. In some the diagnosis may not even be suspected because of the minor manifestations.

Approximately 30 additional variants of Klinefelter syndrome have been described, including those with uniform cell lines (such as 48,XXYY, 48,XXXY, and 49,XXXXY) and a variety of mosaicisms of the X chromosome with or without associated structural abnormalities of the X. In general, the greater the chromosomal abnormality the more severe are the manifestations.

Pathophysiology The classic form is due to meiotic nondisjunction of the chromosomes during gametogenesis (Fig. 339-2). About 40 percent of the responsible meiotic nondisjunctions occur during spermatogenesis, and 60 percent occur during oogenesis. Advanced maternal age is a predisposing factor. The mosaic form is thought to result from chromosomal mitotic nondisjunction after fertilization of the zygote and can take place in either a 46,XY zygote (see Fig. 339-2) or a 47,XXY zygote. The latter situation, double nondisjunction (meiotic and mitotic), may be the usual cause and thus explain why the mosaic form is less frequent than the classic disorder.

Plasma follicle stimulating hormone (FSH) and luteinizing hormone (LH) levels are usually high; FSH shows the best discrimination, little overlap occurring with normal individuals, because of the consistent damage to the seminiferous tubules. The plasma testosterone level averages half normal but may overlap the normal range. Mean plasma estradiol levels are elevated; early, estradiol secretion by the testes may be increased in response to the elevated plasma LH level, but the testicular secretion of estradiol and testosterone eventually declines. Elevated plasma estradiol late in the course is probably due both to decreased metabolic clearance rate and to increased conversion of testosterone to estradiol in extragonadal tissues. The net result both early and late is a variable degree of feminization and virilization. The feminization, including gynecomastia, depends

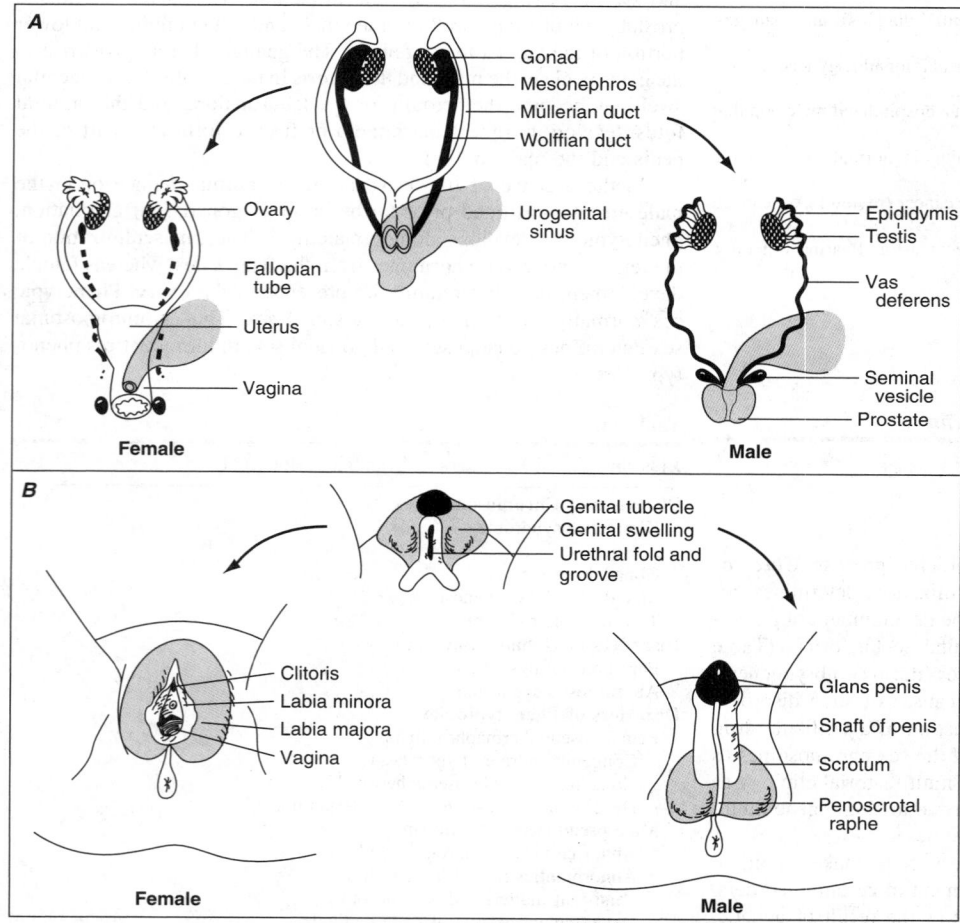

FIGURE 339-1 Normal sexual differentiation. *A.* Internal urogenital tract. *B.* External genitalia.

Table 339-2

Clinical Features of the Disorders of Chromosomal Sex

Disorder	Common Chromosomal Complement	Gonadal Development	External Genitalia	Internal Genitalia	Breast Development	Comment
Klinefelter syndrome	47,XXY *or* 46,XY/47,XXY	Hyalinized testes	Normal male	Normal male	Gynecomastia	Most common disorder of sexual differentiation; tall stature.
XX male	46,XX	Hyalinized testes	Normal male	Normal male	Gynecomastia	Shorter than normal men; increased incidence of hypospadias. Similar to Klinefelter syndrome. May be familial.
Gonadal dysgenesis (Turner syndrome)	45,X *or* 46,XX/45,X	Streak gonads	Immature female	Hypoplastic female	Immature female	Short stature and multiple somatic abnormalities. May be 46,XX with structurally abnormal X chromosome.
Mixed gonadal dysgenesis	46,XY/45,X *or* 46,XY	Testis and streak gonad	Variable but almost always ambiguous; 60% reared as female	Uterus, vagina, and one fallopian tube	Usually male	Second most common cause of ambiguous genitalia in the newborn; tumors common.
True hermaphroditism	46,XX *or* 46,XY *or* mosaics	Testis and ovary or ovotestis	Variable but usually ambiguous; 60% reared as males	Usually a uterus and urogenital sinus; ducts correspond to gonad	Gynecomastia in 75%	May be familial.

on the ratio of circulating estrogen to androgen (relative or absolute), and individuals with lower plasma testosterone and higher plasma estradiol levels are more likely to develop gynecomastia (see Chap. 338). The normal feedback inhibition of testosterone on pituitary LH secretion is diminished. Men with untreated Klinefelter syndrome may have enlarged or abnormal sella turcicas, presumably due to hyperplasia of the gonadotrophs because of inadequate testosterone feedback.

℞ TREATMENT

In men with some sperm production fertility might be achieved with in vitro fertilization (see Chap. 336). Gynecomastia should be treated surgically. Some underandrogenized patients benefit from supplemental androgen, but such treatment may worsen the gynecomastia, presumably by providing increased substrate estrogen formation in peripheral tissues. Testosterone should be injected in the form of testosterone cypionate or testosterone enanthate or administered via the transdermal route (see Chap. 336). Following the administration of testosterone, the plasma LH level returns to normal only after several months, if at all.

XX MALE SYNDROME A 46,XX karyotype is found in approximately 1 in 20,000 phenotypic males. The findings resemble

Table 339-3

Characteristics of Patients with Classic versus Mosaic Klinefelter Syndrome*

	47,XXY, %	46,XY/47,XXY, %
Abnormal testicular histology	100	94†
Decreased length of testis	99	73†
Azoospermia	93	50†
Decreased testosterone	79	33
Decreased facial hair	77	64
Increased gonadotropins	75	33†
Decreased sexual function	68	56
Gynecomastia	55	33†
Decreased axillary hair	49	46
Decreased length of penis	41	21

* Table based on 519 XXY patients and 51 XY/XXY patients.
† Significantly different at $p < .05$ or better.
SOURCE: After Gordon et al.

those in Klinefelter syndrome: the testes are small and firm (generally less than 2 cm), gynecomastia is frequent, the penis is normal to small in size, azoospermia and hyalinization of the seminiferous tubules are usual, no female urogenital structures are present, psychosexual identification is male, mean plasma testosterone level is low, plasma estradiol level is elevated, and plasma gonadotropin levels are high. Affected individuals differ from typical Klinefelter patients only in that average height is less than in normal men, the incidence of cognitive problems is not increased, and the incidence of hypospadias is increased.

The majority of XX males whose DNA is probed with Y-chromosome DNA fragments containing the SRY gene are positive for Y-related DNA; thus an X-Y or Y-autosome translocation appears to be the common cause. Some 46,XX males are negative for all Y-specific DNA, suggesting that the disorder is due to mutation in a downstream, autosomal or X-linked gene involved in development of the testes. The management is similar to that of Klinefelter syndrome.

GONADAL DYSGENESIS (TURNER SYNDROME) **Clinical Features** Gonadal dysgenesis is characterized by primary amenorrhea, sexual infantilism, short stature, multiple congenital anomalies, and bilateral streak gonads in phenotypic women with any of several defects of the X chromosome. This condition should be distinguished from (1) mixed gonadal dysgenesis in which a unilateral testis and a contralateral streak gonad may be present; (2) pure gonadal dysgenesis in which bilateral streak gonads are associated with a normal 46,XX or 46,XY karyotype, normal stature, and primary amenorrhea; and (3) the Noonan syndrome, an autosomal dominant disorder in both sexes characterized by webbed neck, short stature, congenital heart disease, cubitus valgus, and other congenital defects despite normal karyotypes and normal gonads.

The incidence is estimated at 1 in 3000 newborn females; the prenatal incidence may be as high as 2 percent of all human conceptuses, only a small fraction of whom survive to term. The diagnosis is made either at birth because of the associated anomalies or at puberty when amenorrhea and failure of sexual development are noted in conjunction with the associated anomalies. Gonadal dysgenesis is the most common cause of primary amenorrhea, accounting for a third of such patients. The external genitalia are unambiguously female but remain immature, and there is no breast development unless exogenous estrogen is given. The fallopian tubes and uterus are immature, and bilateral streak gonads are present in the broad ligaments. Primordial germ cells are present transiently during embryogenesis but disappear because of an accelerated rate of atresia (see Chap. 337). After the age of expected puberty, these streaks lack identifiable follicles and ova and consist of fibrous tissue that is indistinguishable from normal ovarian stroma.

The associated somatic anomalies primarily involve the skeleton and connective tissue. Lymphedema of the hands and feet, webbing of the neck, low hairline, redundant skin folds on the back of the neck, a shieldlike chest with widely spaced nipples, and growth retardation are features that suggest the diagnosis in infancy. Micrognathia, epicanthal folds, prominent low-set or deformed ears, a fishlike mouth, and ptosis may be present. Short fourth metacarpals are present in half, and 10 to 20 percent have coarctation of the aorta. In adults, the average height rarely exceeds 150 cm. Associated conditions include renal malformations, pigmented nevi, hypoplastic nails, tendency to keloid formation, perceptive hearing loss, unexplained hypertension, glucose intolerance, and autoimmune thyroid disease.

Pathophysiology About half have a 45,X karyotype, approximately one-fourth have mosaicism with no structural abnormality (46,XX/45,X), and the remainder have a structurally abnormal X chromosome with or without mosaicism (see Chap. 66). The mechanism of chromosome loss is unknown but may occur during gametogenesis in either parent or as a mitotic error during one of the early cleavage divisions of the fertilized zygote (see Fig. 339-2). Short stature and other somatic features result from loss of genetic material on the short arm of the X chromosome. Streak gonads result when genetic material is missing from either the long or short arm of the X. In individuals with mosaicism or structural abnormalities of the X, phenotypes on average are intermediate in severity between that seen in the 45,X variety and the normal. In some patients with hypertrophy of the clitoris, there is an unidentified fragment of a chromosome present in addition to the X chromosome, assumed to be an abnormal Y; gonadoblastoma may develop in the streak gonads in this subset of patients. The Y-linked genes that predispose to gonadoblastoma are believed to be distinct from SRY because XY women with SRY deletions or mutations are at risk. Rarely, familial transmission of gonadal dysgenesis can be the result of a balanced X-autosome translocation (see Chap. 66). Analysis of chromosomal karyotype is necessary to establish the diagnosis and to identify the group with Y chromosomal elements and a high chance of developing malignancy in the streak gonads.

After the time of expected puberty pubic and axillary hair remain sparse, the breasts are infantile, and no menses occur. Serum FSH is elevated in infancy, falls during midchildhood to the normal range, and increases to castrate levels at the age of 9 or 10. At this time, the serum LH level is also elevated, and plasma estradiol levels are low [<40 pmol/L (<10 pg/mL)]. Approximately 2 percent of 45,X and 12 percent of mosaic women have sufficient residual follicles to allow some menstruation. Indeed, occasionally minimally affected women become pregnant; the reproductive life in such individuals is brief.

℞ **TREATMENT**

At the anticipated time of puberty, replacement therapy with estrogen should be instituted to induce maturation of the breasts, labia, vagina, uterus, and fallopian tubes (see Chap. 337). Linear growth and bone maturation rates are approximately doubled during the first year of treatment with estradiol, but the eventual height rarely approaches the predicted level. Combination therapy with oxandrolone and/or growth hormone accelerates growth and increases final height (see Chap. 329).

Gonadal tumors are rare in 45,X patients but do occur in women carrying Y chromosome fragments or with mosaicism of the Y chromosome; consequently, streak gonads should be removed in all women with evidence of virilization or with Y-chromosome sequences.

MIXED GONADAL DYSGENESIS **Clinical Features** Mosaicism for a Y-bearing cell line, usually the 45,X/46,XY karyotype, is responsible for most instances of mixed gonadal dysgenesis. Affected individuals usually have a testis on one side and a streak gonad on the other, but bilateral dysgenetic testes or bilateral streak gonads may be present. The incidence is unknown, but in most hospitals the disorder is the second most common cause of ambiguous genitalia in the neonate after congenital adrenal hyperplasia.

The phenotype varies depending on the proportion of XY cells and their distribution. About two-thirds of such children are reared as females. Many have ambiguous genitalia, including phallic enlargement, a urogenital sinus, and some labioscrotal fusion. In most the testis is located intraabdominally; individuals with a testis in the inguinal or scrotal position are usually reared as males. A uterus, vagina, and at least one fallopian tube are almost invariably present.

The prepubertal testis appears relatively normal. The postpubertal testis contains abundant Leydig cells, but the seminiferous tubules lack germinal elements and contain only Sertoli cells. The streak gonad, a thin, pale, elongated structure located either in the broad ligament or along the pelvic wall, is composed of ovarian stroma. At puberty the testis secretes androgen, causing virilization and phallic enlargement. Feminization is rare; when it occurs, estrogen secretion from a gonadal tumor should be suspected.

Approximately a third of such individuals exhibit somatic features of 45,X gonadal dysgenesis, i.e., low posterior hairline, shield chest, multiple pigmented nevi, cubitus valgus, webbing of the neck, and short stature (height less than 150 cm).

Approximately two-thirds have the 45,X/46,XY karyotype, and the remainder have a 46,XY karyotype or a variant mosaicism. The origin of 45,X/46,XY mosaicism is best explained by the loss of a Y chromosome during an early mitotic division of an XY zygote similar to the postulated loss of the X chromosome in the 46,XY/47,XXY mosaicism shown in Fig. 339-2.

Pathophysiology It is assumed (but has been difficult to prove) that the 46,XY cell line stimulates testicular differentiation, whereas the 45,X stem leads to the development of the contralateral streak gonad.

FIGURE 339-2 Schema for normal spermatogenesis and fertilization showing effects of meiotic and mitotic nondisjunction leading to classic Klinefelter syndrome, Turner syndrome, and mosaic Klinefelter. The schema would be similar if the abnormal events took place during oogenesis.

Both masculinization and müllerian duct regression in utero are incomplete. Since Leydig cell function is normal at puberty, inadequate virilization in utero may be due to delayed development of a testis that is ultimately capable of normal Leydig cell function.

℞ **TREATMENT**

For the older child or adult in whom gender is fixed prior to diagnosis, the central issue in management is the possibility of tumor development in the gonads, which may occur prior to puberty. The overall incidence of seminomas and gonadoblastomas may be as high as 25 percent. Such tumors occur most frequently in subjects with a female phenotype who lack the somatic features of 45,X gonadal dysgenesis and are more common in testes than in the streak gonad. When the diagnosis is established in phenotypic females, prophylactic gonadectomy should be performed because gonadal tumors may occur in childhood and because the testes secrete androgen at puberty and thus cause virilization. Such women, like those with gonadal dysgenesis, are then given estrogen to induce and maintain feminization.

When the diagnosis is established in phenotypic males during late childhood or in adults, the management is more complicated. Men with mixed gonadal dysgenesis are infertile (no germinal elements are present in the testes) and have a high risk of developing gonadal tumors. In deciding which testes can be safely conserved the following observations apply: (1) tumors develop in scrotal streak gonads but not in scrotal testes, (2) tumors that develop in intraabdominal testes are always associated with ipsilateral müllerian duct structures, and (3) tumors in streak gonads are always associated with tumors in the contralateral abdominal testis. Based on these observations, it is recommended that (1) all streak gonads should be removed, (2) scrotal testes should be preserved, and (3) intraabdominal testes should be excised unless they can be relocated in the scrotum and are not associated with ipsilateral müllerian duct structures. Reconstructive surgery of the phallus should be performed when appropriate.

When the diagnosis is established in early infancy and the genitalia are ambiguous, gender assignment is usually female, and resection of the phallus and gonadectomy can be performed in infancy, sometimes in one procedure. If the decision is for male gender assignment, the same criteria apply as to which testes should be removed as in older males.

TRUE HERMAPHRODITISM **Clinical Features** True hermaphroditism is a condition in which both an ovary and a testis or one or more gonads with features of both (ovotestis) are present. To justify the diagnosis, both types of gonadal epithelium must be documented histologically, the presence of ovarian stroma without oocytes not being sufficient. The incidence is unknown, but more than 400 cases have been reported. Three categories are recognized: (1) one-fifth are bilateral—testicular and ovarian tissue (ovotestes) on each side, (2) two-fifths are unilateral—an ovotestis on one side and an ovary or a testis on the other, and (3) the remainder are lateral—a testis on one side and an ovary on the other.

The external genitalia exhibit all gradations of the male-to-female spectrum. Two-thirds are sufficiently masculinized to be reared as males, but less than one-tenth have normal male external genitalia; most have hypospadias and incomplete labioscrotal fusion. Two-thirds of phenotypic females have an enlarged clitoris, and most have a urogenital sinus. Differentiation of the internal ducts usually corresponds to the adjacent gonad. Although an epididymis usually develops adjacent to a testis, the vas deferens is complete in only one-third. Of the patients with an ovotestis, three-fourths have an epididymis, two-thirds have a fallopian tube, one-tenth have a vas deferens, and one-tenth have both a vas deferens and a fallopian tube. The uterus may be hypoplastic or unicornuate. The ovary is usually in the normal position, but the testis or ovotestis may be found at any level along the route of embryonic testicular descent, frequently associated with an inguinal hernia. Testicular tissue is present in the scrotum or the labioscrotal fold in one-third, in the inguinal canal in one-third, and in the abdomen in one-third.

Variable feminization and virilization ensue at puberty, three-fourths develop gynecomastia, and about half menstruate. In phenotypic men, menstruation may cause cyclic hematuria. Ovulation occurs in approximately one-fourth and is more common than spermatogenesis. In men, ovulation may cause testicular pain. Fertility has been reported in women and more rarely in men. Congenital malformations of other systems are rare.

Pathophysiology About two-thirds of individuals have a 46,XX karyotype, a tenth have a 46,XY karyotype, and the remainder are chimeras or mosaics in whom a Y cell line is present. The mechanism responsible for the gonadal development is unknown. Only 10 percent of 46,XX true hermaphrodites are SRY positive and are believed to have either mosaicism or translocation involving a portion of the Y chromosome; the remainder are believed to result from gain of function mutations in downstream genes involved in SRY action. In rare instances, multiple sibs with a 46,XX karyotype are affected, possibly the result of an autosomal or X-linked mutation.

Because corpora lutea are frequently present in the ovaries, it is presumed that the female neuroendocrine axis functions normally in such individuals. Feminization (gynecomastia and menstruation) is the result of secretion of estradiol by ovarian tissue. In masculinized patients, secretion of androgen predominates, and some produce sperm.

℞ **TREATMENT**

When the diagnosis is made in early infancy, gender assignment depends on the anatomic features. In older children and adults, gonads and internal duct structures that are contradictory to the predominant phenotype (and the gender of rearing) should be removed, and the external genitalia should be modified when appropriate. Gonadal tumors are rare but have been reported in true hermaphrodites who carry Y chromosome sequences. Consequently, the possibility of future tumor development must be taken into account when the decision regarding conservation of gonadal tissue is made.

DISORDERS OF GONADAL SEX

Disorders of gonadal sex result when chromosomal sex is normal, but for one of several reasons differentiation of the gonads is abnormal. Thus, gonadal sex does not correspond to chromosomal sex.

PURE GONADAL DYSGENESIS **Clinical Features** Pure gonadal dysgenesis is a disorder in which phenotypic females with gonads and genitalia characteristic of gonadal dysgenesis (bilateral streaks, infantile uterus and fallopian tubes, and sexual infantilism) have normal height, few if any somatic anomalies, and either a normal 46,XX or 46,XY karyotype. This disorder is about one-tenth as common as gonadal dysgenesis. It is genetically distinct but cannot be distinguished clinically from those instances of gonadal dysgenesis with minimal somatic abnormalities. The height is normal or greater than normal, some individuals being over 170 cm. Estrogen levels vary from profound deficiency typical of 45,X gonadal dysgenesis to some breast development and menses that terminate in an early menopause. About 40 percent have some feminization. Axillary and pubic hair are scanty, and the internal genitalia consist of müllerian derivatives only.

Tumors may develop in the streak gonads, particularly dysgerminoma or gonadoblastoma in the 46,XY disorder. Such tumors may be heralded by the development of virilizing signs or a pelvic mass.

Pathophysiology Although chromosomal mosaicisms have been described under this nosology, the designation here is restricted to women with uniform 46,XX or 46,XY karyotypes. (Those with mosaicism are variants of gonadal dysgenesis or mixed gonadal dysgenesis, as described above.) The rationale for this restricted definition is based on the fact that both the XX and XY varieties can result from single gene mutations that are presumed to involve gene(s) essential for gonadal development. Several sibships have been reported in which more than one individual is affected with the 46,XX disorder, frequently the result of consanguineous matings, suggesting an autosomal recessive inheritance. Familial occurrence of the 46,XY variety also has been described; in some the disorder appears to be inherited as an X-linked trait, and in others the pattern suggests a male-limited autosomal recessive inheritance. About 15 percent of the 46,XY women have either a deletion or a mutation in the SRY coding sequence. Other instances could be due to mutations in SRY outside the coding sequence, in the downstream genes that are controlled by SRY, or in other genes that influence SRY expression. One of these downstream genes is the SOX 9 gene; mutations of this gene are associated with 46,XY gonadal dysgenesis and skeletal abnormalities (campomelic dysplasia). In both the 46,XX and the 46,XY forms the disorder prevents differentiation of ovary or testis, respectively; the development of the female phenotype and the elevation of gonadotropin secretion are due to failure of gonadal development.

 TREATMENT

The management of the estrogen deficiency is identical to that in gonadal dysgenesis; namely, appropriate estrogen replacement therapy is initiated at the time of expected puberty and maintained in adult life (see Chap. 337). Because of the high frequency of gonadal tumors in the 46,XY variety, the streak gonads should be removed once the diagnosis is made; development of virilizing signs is indication for immediate surgery. The natural history of the gonadal tumors is uncertain, but the prognosis after surgical removal is usually good.

THE ABSENT TESTES SYNDROME (ANORCHIA, TESTICULAR REGRESSION, GONADAL AGENESIS, AGONADISM) Clinical Features A spectrum of phenotypes occurs in 46,XY males with absent or rudimentary testes but in whom unequivocal evidence exists that endocrine function of the testis (e.g., consistent müllerian duct regression and variable testosterone synthesis) was present at some time during embryonic life. In pure gonadal dysgenesis, in contrast, no evidence can be inferred for gonadal function during embryonic development. The manifestations vary from complete failure of virilization to incomplete virilization of the external genitalia to otherwise normal men with bilateral anorchia.

The purest form is represented by 46,XY females with absent testes, sexual infantilism, and absence of both müllerian duct derivatives and accessory organs of male reproduction. Such individuals differ from those with 46,XY pure gonadal dysgenesis in that no gonadal remnant can be identified, including no streak gonad and no müllerian derivatives. Testicular failure must have occurred between the onset of MDI synthesis and the onset of testosterone secretion, i.e., after development of Sertoli cells but before the onset of Leydig cell function.

In others, testicular failure occurred later in gestation, and these individuals may constitute problems in gender assignment. In some, failure of müllerian regression is more pronounced than failure of testosterone secretion, but none exhibit normal müllerian development. In those with more extensive virilization, the external genitalia are phenotypically male, but rudimentary oviducts and vasa deferentia may coexist internally.

At the final extreme is the syndrome of bilateral anorchia in which phenotypic men have absence of müllerian structures and gonads but male wolffian duct derivatives and external genitalia. Microphallus implies that failure of testosterone secretion occurred late in embryogenesis after anatomic development of the male urethra was complete. Gynecomastia may or may not be present.

Pathophysiology The pathogenesis is not understood. Testicular regression could be the result of mutant genes, teratogen, or trauma, and the disorder may well be heterogeneous in origin. Sibships with multiple affected individuals have been described, and several instances of agonadism have occurred in the same family, some unilateral and others bilateral. Some subjects in whom no testes can be identified at laparotomy have blood testosterone values above the castrate range, presumably derived from remnant testes.

The management of the two extremes is clear-cut. Sexually infantile, phenotypic females should be given adequate estrogen to ensure appropriate feminization, and any coexisting vaginal agenesis should be treated by surgical or medical means. Likewise, phenotypic males with anorchia should be given androgen replacement to allow normal male secondary sexual development. Individuals with incomplete virilization or ambiguous external genitalia demonstrate a more complex problem and require careful assessment to determine appropriate gender assignment, hormonal therapy at the time of expected puberty, and surgical correction of the external genitalia when appropriate.

DISORDERS OF PHENOTYPIC SEX

FEMALE PSEUDOHERMAPHRODITISM Congenital Adrenal Hyperplasia *Clinical features* The pathways by which glucocorticoids are synthesized in the adrenal gland and androgens are formed in the testis and adrenal are summarized in Fig. 339-3. Three reactions are common to both pathways (cholesterol side chaincleavage, 3β-hydroxysteroid dehydrogenase/isomerase, and 17α-hydroxylase); impairment of any of these reactions results in deficiency of glucocorticoid and androgen synthesis and consequently in both congenital adrenal hyperplasia (due to enhanced ACTH levels) and defective virilization of the male embryo (male pseudohermaphroditism). Two reactions are involved exclusively in androgen synthesis (17,20-lyase and 17β-hydroxysteroid dehydrogenase); deficiency in either results in pure male pseudohermaphroditism with normal glucocorticoid synthesis. Deficiency of either of the terminal two enzymes of glucocorticoid synthesis (21-hydroxylase and 11β-hydroxylase) impairs formation of hydrocortisone; the compensatory increase in ACTH secretion causes adrenal hyperplasia and a secondary increase in androgen formation that causes virilization in the female and precocious masculinization in the male.

The major features of congenital adrenal hyperplasia are listed in Table 339-4. The *adrenal insufficiency* can be equally severe and lifethreatening in both sexes and is described in Chap. 332. From the standpoint of *abnormal sexual development*, some defects in steroidogenesis result in female pseudohermaphroditism, and some cause male pseudohermaphroditism. (3β-Hydroxysteroid dehydrogenase/isomerase deficiency can cause either male or female pseudohermaphroditism, but since incomplete virilization of the male is more common, the disorder will be discussed under male pseudohermaphroditism.)

Congenital adrenal hyperplasia due to classic 21-hydroxylase deficiency is the most common cause of ambiguous genitalia in the newborn, with an incidence of between 1 in 5000 and 1 in 15,000 live births in Europe and the United States; it may or may not be associated with mineralocorticoid deficiency (salt loss) (see Table 339-4). Virilization is usually apparent at birth in the female and within the first 2 to 3 years of life in the male. Manifestations in females include hypertrophy of the clitoris with ventral binding (chordee), partial fusion of the labioscrotal folds, and variable virilization of the urethra. The uterus, fallopian tubes, and ovaries are normal, and the wolffian ducts do not virilize, probably because adrenal function begins relatively late in embryogenesis. The external appearance of an affected female newborn is similar to that of a male with bilateral cryptorchidism and hypospadias. The labioscrotal folds are bulbous and rugated and resemble a scrotum. Rarely, the virilization is so severe that development of a complete penile urethra and prostate results in errors in sex assignment at birth. Radiography following the injection of radiopaque dye into the external genital orifice is helpful in demonstrating the presence of vagina, uterus, and (sometimes) fallopian tubes. Occasionally, virilization of the female is slight or absent at birth and becomes evident in later infancy, adolescence, or adulthood (the socalled nonclassic or late-onset form of the disorder). In both sexes, rapid somatic maturation results in premature epiphyseal closure and a short adult height. The untreated female with the classic disorder grows rapidly during the first year of life and has progressive virilization. At the time of expected puberty there is a failure of normal female sexual development and absence of menstruation.

Since male phenotypic differentiation is normal, the condition is usually not recognized at birth in boys in the absence of adrenal insufficiency. However, early maturation of the external genitalia, development of secondary sex characteristics, coarsening of the voice, frequent erections, and excessive muscular development are noticeable during the first few years of life. Virilization in the male can follow two patterns. Excessive adrenal androgens can inhibit gonadotropin production so that the testes remain infantile in size despite the acceleration of masculinization. Such untreated adult men are capable of erection and ejaculation but have no spermatogenesis. Alternatively, adrenal androgen secretion can induce premature maturation of the hypothalamic-pituitary axis and initiate a true precocious puberty including early maturation of spermatogenesis (see Chap. 336). The untreated male is also subject to the development of ACTH-dependent "tumors" of the adrenal rest cells of the testes.

In classic 21-hydroxylase deficiency, which accounts for about 95 percent of congenital adrenal hyperplasia, decreased production of hydrocortisone leads to increased release of ACTH, enlargement of the adrenal glands, and partial or complete compensation of the defect in the secretion of hydrocortisone. In about half, the enzyme defect appears to be partial, and cortisol secretion is normal. This form is termed *simple virilizing*. When deficiency of the enzyme is more complete, the so-called salt-losing form of 21-hydroxylase deficiency, production of cortisol and aldosterone is inadequate, and severe salt wastage with anorexia, vomiting, volume depletion, and collapse occurs within the first few weeks of life. In untreated patients, overproduction of the cortisol precursors prior to the 21-hydroxylase step leads to increase in plasma progesterone and 17-hydroxyprogesterone. These steroids are weak aldosterone antagonists at the receptor level, and in the compensated state aldosterone production increases to attempt to maintain normal sodium balance. Increased substrate availability is also responsible for the increase in androgen synthesis and hence for the virilization.

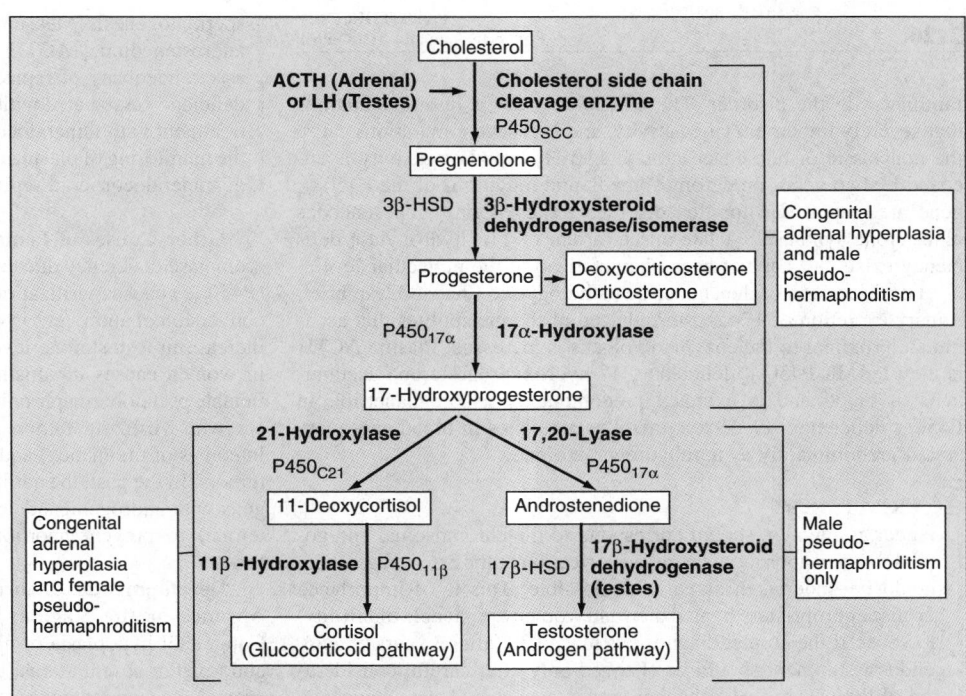

FIGURE 339-3 Pathways of glucocorticoid and androgen synthesis. Note abnormal conditions corresponding to impaired enzyme reactions.

Female pseudohermaphroditism also occurs in 11β-hydroxylase deficiency. In this disorder, a block in hydroxylation at the 11 carbon results in the accumulation of 11-deoxycortisol and deoxycorticosterone (DOC), a potent salt-retaining hormone that causes hypertension rather than salt loss. The clinical features that stem from glucocorticoid deficiency and androgen excess are similar to those in 21-hydroxylase deficiency.

Pathophysiology Both disorders are due to autosomal recessive mutations. The carrier frequency for P450$_{C21}$ deficiency is about 1 in 50. Because the gene is located on the sixth chromosome close to the HLA-B locus, carriers of the disorder (as well as homozygotes) within a given family can be identified on the basis of the HLA haplotype. At the molecular level the mutations that give rise to 21-hydroxylase deficiency are even more polymorphic; indeed, deletions of portions of the gene (10 to 30 percent), conversion of the gene from a functional state to a form that is not transcribed normally (10 percent), and point mutations (60 to 75 percent) have been characterized in different

Table 339-4

Forms of Congenital Adrenal Hyperplasia

Deficiency	Cortisol	Aldosterone	Degree of Virilization of Females	Failure of Virilization in Males	Dominant Steroid Secreted	Comment
Classic 21-hydroxylase: Partial (simple virilizing or compensated)	Normal	↑	+ + + +	0	17-Hydroxy-progesterone	Most common type (95% of total); from one- to two-thirds salt losers
Severe (salt-losing)	↓	↓	+ + + +	0	17-Hydroxy-progesterone	
11β-Hydroxylase (hypertension)	↓	↓	+ + + +	0	11-Deoxycortisol and 11-deoxy-corticosterone	Hypertension
3β-Hydroxysteroid dehydrogenase/isomerase	0	0	+	+ + + +	Δ⁵-3β-OH compounds (dehydroepiandrosterone)	Probably second most common, usually salt loss
17α-Hydroxylase	↓	↓	0	+ + + +	Corticosterone and 11-deoxy-corticosterone	No feminization of female, hypertension
Cholesterol side chain cleavage	0	0	0	+ + + +	Cholesterol(?)	Rare, usually salt loss

families with the disorder. The classic disorder is due to mutations that severely impair enzyme activity, and less severe mutations cause the nonclassic or late-onset variety. 11β-Hydroxylase activity is encoded by two genes on chromosome 8, and mutations of the $P450_{11\beta1}$ gene are responsible for this disorder. (The $P450_{11\beta2}$ gene encodes aldosterone synthase.) A late-onset variant of 11β-hydroxylase deficiency exists but has not been characterized at the molecular level.

For discussion of the endocrine pathology see Chap. 332. In brief, urinary excretion of 17-ketosteroids and of the metabolites that accumulate proximal to the enzymatic blocks is increased. Plasma ACTH is elevated. In $P450_{C21}$ deficiency, 17-hydroxyprogesterone accumulates in blood and is excreted predominantly as pregnanetriol. In $P450_{11\beta}$ deficiency, 11-deoxycortisol accumulates in blood and is excreted predominantly as tetrahydrocortexolone.

℞ TREATMENT

Gender assignment should correspond to the chromosomal and gonadal sex, and appropriate surgical correction of the external genitalia should be undertaken as early as possible. This is of importance because appropriately treated men and women are capable of fertility. However, if the correct diagnosis is made late (after 3 years of age), gender assignment should be changed only after careful consideration of the psychosexual background.

Treatment with appropriate glucocorticoids prevents the consequences of hydrocortisone deficiency, arrests the rapid virilization, and prevents premature somatic and epiphyseal maturation. The suppression of the abnormal steroid secretion corrects the hypertension in $P450_{11\beta}$ deficiency and in both disorders allows normal onset of menses and development of female secondary sex characteristics. In males, glucocorticoid therapy suppresses adrenal androgens and results in normal gonadotropin secretion, testicular development, and spermatogenesis. Measurements of plasma 17-hydroxyprogesterone, androstenedione, ACTH, and renin levels have all been used to assess adequacy of replacement therapy. In severe 21-hydroxylase deficiency associated with salt loss or elevated plasma renin activity, treatment with mineralocorticoids is also indicated. In such patients, the monitoring of plasma renin is useful for determining the adequacy of mineralocorticoid replacement.

Other Causes of Female Pseudohermaphroditism Placental aromatase deficiency due to mutations in the gene encoding aromatase ($P450_{arom}$) causes virilization of female embryos because of defective conversion of androgens to estrogens in the placenta and the secondary increase in testosterone levels; in postnatal life aromatase deficiency in women causes hirsutism and development of polycystic ovaries. Female pseudohermaphroditism can also occur in babies born to mothers with virilizing tumors of the ovary (e.g., arrhenoblastomas or luteomas of pregnancy) and, rarely, to mothers with virilizing adrenal tumors. In the past, the administration to pregnant women of progestogens with androgenic side effects (such as 17α-ethinyl-19-nor-testosterone) to prevent abortion resulted in masculinization of female fetuses.

Developmental Disorders of Müllerian Ducts (Congenital Absence of the Vagina, Müllerian Agenesis) *Clinical features* Congenital hypoplasia or absence of the vagina in combination with abnormal or absent uterus (the Mayer-Rokitansky-Kuster-Hauser syndrome) is second to gonadal dysgenesis as a cause of primary amenorrhea. Most patients are ascertained after the time of expected puberty because of failure to menstruate. The height is normal, and the breasts, axillary and pubic hair, and habitus are feminine in character. The uterus can vary from almost normal, lacking only a conduit to the introitus, to the characteristic rudimentary bicornuate cords with or without a lumen. In some patients cyclic abdominal pain indicates that sufficient functional endometrium is present to result in retrograde menstruation and/or hematometra.

Table 339-5

Anatomic, Genetic, and Endocrine Profile of Hereditary Male Pseudohermaphroditism

Disorder	Inheritance	Phenotype					
		Müllerian Ducts	Wolffian Ducts	Spermatogenesis	Urogenital Sinus	External Genitalia	Breast
DEFECTS IN TESTOSTERONE SYNTHESIS							
Five enzyme deficiencies	Autosomal or X-linked recessive	Absent	Variable development	Normal or decreased	Variable from male to female	Generally female	Usually male
DEFECTS IN ANDROGEN ACTION							
Steroid 5α-reductase 2 deficiency	Autosomal recessive	Absent	Male	Normal or decreased	Female	Clitoromegaly	Male
Receptor disorders:							
Complete testicular feminization	X-linked recessive	Absent	Absent	Absent	Female	Female	Female
Incomplete testicular feminization	X-linked recessive	Absent	Male	Absent	Female	Clitoromegaly and posterior fusion	Female
Reifenstein syndrome	X-linked recessive	Absent	Variable development	Absent	Variable from male to female	Incomplete male development	Female
Infertile male syndrome	X-linked recessive	Absent	Male	Absent or decreased	Male	Male	Usually male
Undervirilized fertile male	X-linked recessive	Absent	Male	Normal or decreased	Male	Male	Usually male
DEFECTS IN MÜLLERIAN REGRESSION							
Persistent müllerian duct syndrome	Autosomal or X-linked recessive	Rudimentary uterus and fallopian tubes	Male	Normal	Male	Male	Male

About one-third have abnormal kidneys, most commonly agenesis, ectopy, fused kidneys of the horseshoe type, or solitary ectopic kidneys in the pelvis. Skeletal abnormalities are present in one-tenth; most involve the spine, and limb and rib defects account for the rest. Specific abnormalities include wedge vertebrae, fused rudimentary or asymmetric vertebral bodies, supernumerary vertebrae, and the Klippel-Feil syndrome (congenital fusion of the cervical spine, short neck, low posterior hairline, and painless limitation of cervical movement).

Pathophysiology The karyotype is 46,XX. Familial occurrence has been described, and the pattern of inheritance in most is consistent with a sex-limited autosomal dominant mutation. Sporadic cases may represent new mutations of the type responsible for the familial disorder or be multifactorial in etiology. In the familial cases, expressivity is variable; some have skeletal or renal abnormalities only, and some have other abnormalities of müllerian derivatives such as a double uterus. Bilateral renal aplasia in stillborn infants is commonly associated with absence of the uterus and vagina. Thus, the family history should be probed for isolated skeletal and renal abnormalities and for stillbirths that might result from congenital absence of both kidneys. Ovarian function is normal, and successful pregnancies have occurred after corrective vaginal surgery in patients with a normal uterus.

℞ TREATMENT

Vaginal agenesis can be treated by surgical or nonsurgical means. Surgical repair generally utilizes a split-thickness skin graft around a solid rubber mold to create an artificial vagina. Medical therapy involves the repeated application of pressure against the vaginal dimple with a simple dilator to force development of adequate vaginal depth. In view of complication rates of 5 to 10 percent in surgical series, surgery should be reserved for patients in whom a well-formed uterus is present and the possibility of fertility exists. Frequent coitus or instrumental dilatation is essential for maintaining patency of neovaginas formed by either technique.

Endocrine Profile Relative to Normal Male		
Testosterone Production	Estrogen Production	LH
Normal to decreased	Variable	High
Normal	Normal	Normal or increased
High	High	High
High	High	High
High	High	High
Normal or high	Normal or high	Normal or high
Normal or high	Normal or high	Normal or high
Normal	Normal	Normal

MALE PSEUDOHERMAPHRODITISM Defective virilization of the male embryo (male pseudohermaphroditism) can result from defects in androgen synthesis, defects in androgen action, defects in müllerian duct regression, and uncertain causes.

Abnormalities in Androgen Synthesis *Clinical features* Enzymatic defects that result in defective testosterone synthesis (see Fig. 339-3) account for only about a fifth of cases of male pseudohermaphroditism (Tables 339-4 and 339-5). Each of the defects blocks a step in the synthesis of other adrenal hormones as well: cholesterol side chain cleavage, 3β-hydroxysteroid dehydrogenase/isomerase, and 17α-hydroxylase or P450$_{17\alpha}$. Consequently, their deficiency results in congenital adrenal hyperplasia (see Table 339-4) as well as male pseudohermaphroditism. Two others (17,20-lyase and 17β-hydroxysteroid dehydrogenase) are unique to the pathway of androgen synthesis, and their deficiency results only in male pseudohermaphroditism. Since androgens are obligatory precursors of estrogens, synthesis of estrogen is also low in all but the terminal defect (17β-hydroxysteroid dehydrogenase deficiency).

The adrenal dysfunction is described in Chap. 332, and the present discussion concerns the abnormal sexual development. In genetic males with defective testosterone synthesis, absence of the uterus and fallopian tubes indicates that müllerian duct inhibition was normal during embryogenesis. Masculinization of the urogenital tract and external genitalia and virilization at puberty vary from almost normal to absent, and, therefore, the manifestations vary from men with mild hypospadias to phenotypic women who prior to puberty resemble patients with complete testicular feminization. This variability is the consequence of varying severity of the enzymatic defects, varying effects of the steroids that accumulate proximal to the various metabolic blocks, and the presence of alternative enzymatic pathways in some disorders. In patients with partial defects in whom the plasma testosterone level is normal, the diagnosis can only be made by measuring the steroids that accumulate proximal to the metabolic block.

Cholesterol side chain cleavage deficiency (lipoid adrenal hyperplasia) is an autosomal recessive disorder in which virtually no urinary steroids (either 17-ketosteroids or 17-hydroxycorticoids) can be detected. The defect is an inability to convert cholesterol to pregnenolone, a step catalyzed by a single cholesterol side chain cleavage enzyme (P450$_{SCC}$). Manifestations of this disorder include salt wasting and profound adrenal insufficiency, and most affected individuals die during infancy. At autopsy, the adrenals and testes are enlarged and infiltrated with lipid. Affected males are incompletely masculinized, whereas affected female infants have normal genital development. The coding sequence of the P450$_{SCC}$ gene is normal in several affected individuals, and the nature of the molecular defect is unknown.

3β-Hydroxysteroid dehydrogenase/isomerase deficiency causes varying failure of masculinization and development of a vagina in male infants. Female infants may be modestly virilized at birth due to the weak androgenic potency of dehydroepiandrosterone, the major steroid secreted. If the enzyme is absent in both the adrenal and testis, no urinary steroids contain a Δ⁴-3-keto configuration, whereas in patients in whom the defect is partial or affects only the testis, the urine may contain normal or elevated levels of Δ⁴-3-ketosteroids. Most patients have marked salt wasting and profound adrenal insufficiency, and long-term survival in untreated cases occurs only in states of partial deficiency. Minimally affected males may experience an otherwise normal male puberty except for profound gynecomastia. In these boys, a low-normal blood testosterone level is accompanied by elevated Δ⁵ precursors. 3β-Hydroxysteroid dehydrogenase is catalyzed by more than one isoenzyme. The type 1 gene is expressed in many tissues, and type 2 is expressed in adrenals and gonads. The human deficiency is due to any of several mutations in the type 2 enzyme, but the coding sequence of this gene is said to be normal in several individuals with the late-onset variant of the disease.

17α-Hydroxylase-17,20-lyase (P450$_{17\alpha}$) deficiency impairs the introduction of the 17-hydroxyl and the scission of the C-17,20 carbon bond that convert pregnenolone and progesterone to dehydroepiandros-terone and androstenedione, respectively, which are mediated by a single enzyme, $P450_{17\alpha}$, encoded on chromosome 10; it is unclear why both reactions occur in the ovary and testis, whereas in the adrenal 17-hydroxyprogesterone is largely converted to glucocorticoids and mineralocorticoids rather than the 19-carbon steroids. Likewise, it is unclear why some patients appear to have selective impairment of either 17α-hydroxylase or 17,20-lyase activity; the distinction between these activities must be functional and may involve the relative concentration of steroid substrates and competing enzymes. Whatever the explanation, the consequences of 17α-hydroxylase and 17,20-lyase deficiencies are different.

17α-Hydroxylase deficiency is characterized by hypogonadism, absence of secondary sex characteristics, hypokalemic alkalosis, hypertension, and virtually undetectable hydrocortisone secretion in phenotypic women. Formation of both corticosterone and DOC by the adrenal is elevated, and urinary 17-ketosteroids are low. Aldosterone secretion is low due to high plasma DOC and depressed angiotensin levels and returns to normal after suppressive doses of glucocorticoids. In 46,XX individuals, amenorrhea, absent sexual hair, and hypertension are common, but the phenotype is that of a normal prepubertal woman. In males, the deficiency results in defective virilization that varies from complete male pseudohermaphroditism to ambiguous genitalia with perineoscrotal hypospadias and, in some, gynecomastia. Adrenal insufficiency does not develop, since the secretion of both corticosterone (a weak glucocorticoid) and DOC (a mineralocorticoid) is elevated. Hypertension and hypokalemia are prominent (even in the neonatal period) and remit after suppression of the DOC secretion by glucocorticoid replacement. A variety of point mutations, deletions, and insertions in the $P450_{17\alpha}$ gene on chromosome 10 have been characterized in affected individuals.

17,20-Lyase deficiency in males is associated with normal function of the adrenal cortex and a variable pattern of male pseudohermaphroditism. In the majority there is genital ambiguity at birth, with some virilization at the time of expected puberty. Rare 46,XY patients have had a female phenotype and no virilization at the time of expected puberty. The disorder has been recognized in one 46,XX woman with sexual infantilism. The molecular defect in this disorder has not been described but is presumed to involve less severe mutations of the $P450_{17\alpha}$ gene.

17β-Hydroxysteroid dehydrogenase (17β-HSD-3) *deficiency* involves the final step in testosterone biosynthesis, reduction of the 17-keto group of androstenedione. This is the most common enzymatic defect in testosterone synthesis. Affected 46,XY males usually have a female phenotype with a blind-ending vagina and absence of müllerian derivatives, but inguinal or abdominal testes and virilized wolffian duct structures are present. At the time of expected puberty, both virilization (with phallic enlargement and development of facial and body hair) and a variable degree of feminization take place. In some untreated patients, reversal of gender behavior from female to male occurs at puberty. Plasma testosterone level may be in the low-normal range, making it essential to document elevation in plasma androstenedione to make the diagnosis. Isoenzymes encoded by several different genes possess 17β-hydroxysteroid dehydrogenase activity, but the isoenzyme 3 is expressed in the testes. A variety of mutations have been characterized in the 17β-HSD-3 gene in affected individuals.

Pathophysiology These various disorders are inherited as autosomal recessive traits. The pattern of steroid secretion and excretion depends on the site of the various metabolic blocks (see Fig. 339-3). In general, gonadotropin secretion is high, and many individuals with incomplete defects are able to compensate so that the steady state levels of testosterone may be normal or almost normal.

In rare cases of male pseudohermaphroditism, testosterone formation is deficient for reasons other than a single enzyme defect in androgen synthesis. These include disorders in which Leydig cell agenesis is due to autosomal recessive loss-of-function mutations of the LH receptor or to the secretion of a biologically inactive LH

molecule. In addition, as described above, several disorders, including familial 46,XY pure gonadal dysgenesis, sporadic dysgenetic testes, and the absent testis syndrome, are characterized by deficient testosterone production due to abnormal gonadal development.

℞ **TREATMENT**

Therapy with glucocorticoids and in some instances mineralocorticoids is indicated in those disorders causing adrenal hyperplasia. The management of the genital abnormalities depends on the individual case. Fertility has not been reported, and its consideration does not enter into sex assignment. In genetic females there is no problem (except in diagnosis), in that affected individuals are raised appropriately as females and estrogen therapy is begun at the time of expected puberty to promote development of female secondary sex characteristics. Whether newborn males with ambiguous genitalia should be raised as males or females depends on the anatomic defect; in general, the more severely affected should be raised as females, and corrective surgery of the genitalia and removal of the testes should be undertaken as early as possible. In such women estrogen therapy is begun at the appropriate age to allow development of normal female secondary sex characteristics. In individuals raised as males, corrective surgery is indicated for any coexisting hypospadias, and plasma androgens should be monitored at the time of expected puberty to determine whether testosterone therapy is appropriate.

Abnormalities in Androgen Action Several disorders of male phenotypic development result from abnormalities of androgen action. The spectrum of phenotypes is described in Tables 329-4 and 329-5. In these disorders, testosterone formation and müllerian regression are normal, but male development is impaired because of resistance to androgen action in target tissues.

Steroid 5α-reductase 2 deficiency This autosomal recessive disorder is characterized by (1) severe perineoscrotal hypospadias; (2) a blind vaginal pouch of variable size opening either into the urogenital sinus or into the urethra; (3) testes with normal epididymides, vasa deferentia, and seminal vesicles, and termination of the ejaculatory ducts in the blind-ending vagina; (4) a female habitus with normal axillary and pubic hair but without female breast development; (5) the absence of uterus and fallopian tubes; (6) normal male plasma testosterone; and (7) masculinization to a variable degree at the time of puberty.

The realization that virilization during embryogenesis is defective only in the urogenital sinus and the external genitalia provided insight into the fundamental abnormality. Testosterone, the androgen secreted by the fetal testis, is responsible for conversion of the wolffian duct into the epididymis, vas deferens, and seminal vesicle, whereas dihydrotestosterone mediates virilization of the urogenital sinus and the external genitalia. Consequently, impairment of dihydrotestosterone formation in a male embryo would be expected to cause the phenotype in this disorder—normal male wolffian duct derivatives with defective masculinization of the external genitalia and urogenital sinus. Since testosterone itself regulates LH secretion (see Chap. 336), plasma LH level is normal or minimally elevated. As a result, testosterone and estrogen production rates are those of normal men, and gynecomastia does not develop.

The fact that 5α-reductase 2 enzyme is deficient in this disorder was established by assay of biopsied tissues and cultured fibroblasts from affected individuals. Deletions or point mutations in the gene encoding steroid 5α-reductase 2 have been identified in most families studied. Approximately 40 percent are compound heterozygotes.

Receptor disorders The androgen receptor is a typical member of the steroid/thyroid family of receptors with steroid-binding, DNA-binding, and functional domains and is encoded by a gene on the long arm of the X chromosome. Mutations of this gene impair receptor function and hence impair male phenotypic differentiation and/or virilization.

CLINICAL FEATURES *Complete testicular feminization* is a common form of male pseudohermaphroditism; estimates of frequency vary from 1 in 20,000 to 1 in 64,000 male births. It is the third most common cause of primary amenorrhea after gonadal dysgenesis and congenital absence of the vagina. The features are characteristic. Namely, a woman is ascertained either because of inguinal hernia (prepubertal) or primary amenorrhea (postpubertal). The development of the breasts, the habitus, and the distribution of body fat are female in character so that most have a truly feminine appearance. Axillary and pubic hair is absent or scanty, but some vulval hair is usually present. Scalp hair is that of a normal woman, and facial hair is absent. The external genitalia are unambiguously female, and the clitoris is normal. The vagina is short and blind-ending and may be absent or rudimentary. All internal genitalia are absent except for testes that contain normal Leydig cells and seminiferous tubules without spermatogenesis. The testes may be located in the abdomen, along the course of the inguinal canal, or in the labia majora. Occasionally, remnants of müllerian or wolffian duct origin are present in the paratesticular fascia or in fibrous bands extending from the testis. Patients tend to be rather tall, and bone age is normal. Psychosexual development is unmistakably female with regard to behavior, outlook, and maternal instincts.

The major complication of undescended testes in this disorder, as in all forms of cryptorchidism, is the development of tumors (Chap. 98). Since affected individuals undergo normal pubertal growth and feminize at the time of expected puberty and since testicular tumors rarely develop until after puberty, it is usual to delay castration until after the time of expected puberty. Prepubertal castration is indicated if the testes are present in the inguinal region or labia majora and result in discomfort or hernia formation. (If hernia repair is indicated prepubertally, most physicians prefer to remove the testes at the same time to limit the number of operative procedures.) If the testes are removed prepubertally, estrogen therapy is required at the appropriate age to ensure normal growth and breast development. When castration is performed postpubertally, menopausal symptoms and other evidence of estrogen withdrawal supervene, and suitable estrogen replacement is indicated (see Chap. 337).

Incomplete testicular feminization is about one-tenth as frequent as the complete form. In this disorder there is minor virilization of the external genitalia (partial fusion of the labioscrotal folds and/or some degree of clitoromegaly), normal pubic hair, and mixed virilization and feminization at the time of expected puberty. The vagina is short and blind-ending, but in contrast to the complete form, the wolffian duct derivatives are often partially developed. Since women with the incomplete disorder virilize at the time of expected puberty, gonadectomy should be performed before the expected time of puberty in all prepubertal patients with clitoromegaly or posterior labial fusion.

Reifenstein syndrome is the term applied to forms of incomplete male pseudohermaphroditism initially described by a number of eponyms (Reifenstein syndrome, Gilbert-Dreyfus syndrome, Lubs syndrome). These syndromes are mutations that partially impair the function of the androgen receptor. The most common phenotype is a man with perineoscrotal hypospadias and gynecomastia, but the spectrum of defective virilization in affected families ranges from men with azoospermia to phenotypic women with pseudovaginas. Axillary and pubic hair is normal, but chest and facial hair is scanty. Cryptorchidism is common, the testes are small, and azoospermia is present. Some have defects in wolffian duct derivatives such as absence or hypoplasia of the vas deferens. Since the psychological development in most is unequivocally male, the hypospadias and cryptorchidism should be corrected surgically. The treatment of the gynecomastia is surgical removal.

The *infertile male syndrome* may be the most common disorder of the androgen receptor and is not actually a form of male pseudohermaphroditism. Some such individuals are minimally affected subjects in families with Reifenstein syndrome in whom azoospermia is the only manifestation of the receptor defect. More commonly, subjects with negative family histories present with male infertility. The *undervirilized fertile male* is another manifestation of an androgen receptor defect. In these families, affected men have gynecomastia and undervirilization, and some are fertile.

PATHOPHYSIOLOGY   The karyotype is 46,XY, and the mutation is X-linked. The frequency of a positive family history varies from about two-thirds of patients with testicular feminization and Reifenstein syndrome to only occasional patients with the infertile male syndrome.

The patients with a negative family history are believed to be the result of new mutations.

Hormone dynamics are similar in all disorders of the androgen receptor. Plasma testosterone levels and rates of testosterone production by the testes are normal or high. Elevated testosterone production is caused by the high mean plasma level of LH, which, in turn, is due to defective feedback regulation caused by resistance to the action of androgen at the hypothalamic-pituitary level. Elevated LH concentration is responsible also for the increased estrogen production by the testes (see Chap. 338). (In normal men, most estrogen is derived from peripheral formation from circulating androgens, but when the plasma LH level is elevated, the testes secrete increased amounts of estrogen into the circulation.) Thus resistance to the feedback regulation of LH secretion by circulating androgen results in elevated plasma LH levels, and this, in turn, results in the enhanced secretion of both testosterone and estradiol by the testes. Gonadotropin levels rise even higher (and menopausal symptoms may develop) when the testes are removed, indicating that gonadotropin secretion is under partial feedback control. Presumably, in the steady state and in the absence of an androgen effect, estrogen alone regulates LH secretion, a control purchased at the expense of an elevated plasma estrogen concentration for a male. The hormonal changes in the infertile male syndrome are similar to those in the other receptor disorders but less marked. Some men with this syndrome do not have an elevation of plasma LH or plasma testosterone level.

Feminization in these disorders is the result of two interlocking phenomena. First, androgens and estrogens have antagonistic effects, and in the absence of androgen action, the cellular effect of estrogen is unopposed. Second, the testicular production of estradiol is greater than that of the normal male (although less than that of the normal female). Variable degrees of androgen resistance and enhanced estradiol production result in different degrees of defective virilization and enhanced feminization in the four clinical syndromes.

Each of these syndromes is the result of defects in the androgen receptor. In most families, the fundamental defect is due to point mutations in the coding sequence leading to premature termination codons or to amino acid substitutions in the hormone-binding domain. Such mutations impair receptor function to variable degrees. Some families with clinical syndromes typical of an androgen receptor disorder have normal androgen binding in fibroblasts; in most, point mutations in the DNA-binding domain of the androgen receptor are responsible for the androgen resistance.

℞ TREATMENT

Individuals with 5α-reductase deficiency who are raised as females but elect at the time of expected puberty to change social sex to male or who are raised from the first as males should be monitored carefully and given supplemental androgens, preferably androgens such as nandrolone decanoate that do not require 5α-reduction for activation, when virilization is incomplete. Fertility has been reported in such an individual. Subjects with 5α-reductase deficiency who continue to function as females should be gonadectomized, given feminizing doses of estrogens indefinitely, and receive surgical correction of the introitus when appropriate. The management of subjects with androgen receptor defects depends on the phenotypic manifestations. Women with testicular feminization should be castrated (preferably after the completion of the pubertal growth spurt and the feminization of the breasts) to prevent tumor development in the testes, receive estrogen replacement to maintain feminization, prevent hot flashes, and protect the bones; shallow vaginal depth can usually be treated medically with the Frank technique. Men with the Reifenstein phenotype should have surgical correction of the hypospadias and may require surgery for gynecomastia; supplemental androgen therapy in these men rarely improves the incomplete virilization.

Persistent Müllerian Duct Syndrome   Men with this uncommon disorder have testes and male phenotypic development and in addition have fallopian tubes and a uterus. In some, one or both testes are descended and the uterus and ipsilateral fallopian tube are in the inguinal canal or scrotum; both testes and fallopian tubes may be present in the hernia sac or can be drawn into it. In others, the testes are located high in the abdomen and hernias are not present. In both types, the vasa deferentia are embedded in the wall of the uterus, a feature that complicates surgical procedures designed to preserve potential fertility. Most patients have uninformative family histories, but in some the condition is inherited as an autosomal recessive trait. Because the external genitalia are well developed and the patients masculinize normally at puberty, it is assumed that during the critical stage of embryonic differentiation the fetal testes produce a normal amount of androgen. However, müllerian regression does not occur. Two types of mutations have been described in this disorder. In one the gene that encodes MDI is defective, and blood levels of MDI are usually low or undetectable; in the other the MDI receptor is defective, and blood levels of MDI are elevated. To minimize the chance of tumor development and to maintain virilization, orchiopexy should be performed. Malignancy in the uterus or vagina has not been described, and because the vasa deferentia are closely associated with the broad ligaments, the uterus and vagina should be left in place to avoid disruption of the vasa deferentia during removal and consequently to preserve possible fertility.

Developmental Defects of the Male Genitalia *Hypospadias* Hypospadias is a congenital anomaly in which the urethra terminates in an abnormal position along the ventral midline of the penis at some site between the normal urethral meatus and the perineum. This malformation occurs in 0.5 to 0.8 percent of male births in the United States and is often associated with ventral contraction and bowing of the penis (chordee). It is common to categorize hypospadias as glandular (involving the glans penis), penile, or perineoscrotal. Since androgens control penile development, hypospadias is generally assumed to result from some unidentified defect in androgen formation or action during embryogenesis. Indeed, hypospadias occurs in most disorders of male sexual differentiation, and a rare cause of hypospadias is maternal ingestion of progestational agents early in pregnancy. However, the known causes (single-gene defects, chromosomal abnormalities, and maternal drug ingestion) account for only about one-fourth of cases, and the etiology of most is unknown. The management is surgical.

Cryptorchidism The control of testicular descent is poorly understood, both in regard to the nature of the forces that cause the movement and to the hormonal factors that regulate the process. In anatomic terms, testicular descent can be divided into three phases: (1) transabdominal movement of the testis from its site of origin above the kidney to the inguinal ring, (2) formation of the opening in the inguinal canal (processus vaginalis) through which the testis exits the abdominal cavity, and (3) actual movement of the testis through the inguinal canal to its permanent site in the scrotum. This process occurs over a 6- to 7-month period during gestation, beginning at about the sixth week and not completed in some until after birth. Impairment at any stage in this process can impair descent of one or both testes. About 3 percent of full-term and 30 percent of premature male infants have at least one cryptorchid testis at birth, but descent is usually completed within the first few weeks of life, so that the incidence of failure of descent by 6 to 9 months of age is only 0.6 to 0.7 percent. It is this latter category of maldescent that requires intervention.

Permanent cryptorchidism can be classified as intraabdominal (10 percent), canalicular (in the inguinal canal) (20 percent), high scrotal (40 percent), or obstructed (30 percent), in which maldescent is due to a physical barrier between the inguinal pouch and the inlet of the scrotum. These disorders must be distinguished from the temporarily retracted normal testis.

The cryptorchid testis functions poorly after puberty, but the extent to which maldescent is the result of an abnormality of the testis or the cause of abnormal function is unknown. Two general theories have been advanced as to the etiology—inadequate intraabdominal pressure and deficient endocrine function of the testis either because

of deficient testosterone synthesis or inadequate formation of MDI. Indeed, defects that result in inadequate development of intraabdominal pressure or inadequate development of the testes can cause cryptorchidism. As in hypospadias, however, the known causes of cryptorchidism constitute only a small fraction of the cases, and the etiology in most remains to be identified. Two complications of cryptorchidism are important; spermatogenesis cannot occur at the temperature of the abdominal cavity, and it is necessary to correct the process as early as possible to allow possible fertility. The fact that infertility is common in men who have been treated for unilateral as well as bilateral cryptorchidism suggests that maldescent is usually the consequence rather than the cause of the testicular malfunction. There is also a greater frequency of malignancy in undescended testes, and all should be surgically corrected for this reason (see Chap. 98).

BIBLIOGRAPHY

AFFARA NA et al: Analysis of the SRY gene in 22 sex-reversed XY females identifies four new point mutations in the conserved DNA binding domain. Am J Hum Genet 2:785, 1993

ANDERSSON S et al: 17β-Hydroxysteroid dehydrogenase 3 deficiency. Trends Endocrinol Metab 7:121, 1996

BEHRINGER RR et al: Müllerian-inhibiting substance function during mammalian sexual development. Cell 79:415, 1994

BERTA P et al: Genetic evidence equating SRY and the testis-determining factor. Nature 348:448, 1990

BOUCEKKINE C et al: Clinical and anatomical spectrum in XX sex reversed patients. Relationship to the presence of Y-specific DNA sequences. Clin Endocrinol 40:733, 1994

CONTE FA et al: A syndrome of female pseudohermaphroditism, hypergonadotropic hypogonadism, and multicystic ovaries associated with missense mutations in the gene encoding aromatase (P450$_{arom}$). J Clin Endocrinol Metab 78:1287, 1994

DE LA CHAPELLE A: The etiology of maleness in XX men. Hum Genet 58:105, 1981

DONAHOE PK et al: Mixed gonadal dysgenesis, pathogenesis and management. J Pediatr Surg 14:287, 1979

——— et al: Congenital adrenal hyperplasia, in *The Metabolic and Molecular Bases of Inherited Disease*, 7th ed, CR Sriver et al (eds). New York, McGraw-Hill, 1995, p 2929

EDMAN CD et al: Embryonic testicular regression: A clinical spectrum of XY agonadal individuals. Obstet Gynecol 49:208, 1977

FOSTER JW et al: Campomelic dysplasia and autosomal sex reversal caused by mutations in an SRY-related gene. Nature 372:525, 1994

GEORGE FW, WILSON JD: Sex determination and differentiation, in *The Physiology of Reproduction*, 2d ed, E Knobil, JD Neill (eds). New York, Raven Press, 1994, vol 1, pp 3–28

GORDON DL et al: Pathologic testicular findings in Klinefelter's syndrome. 47,XXY vs 46,XY/47,XXY. Arch Intern Med 130:726, 1972

GRIFFIN JE, WILSON JD: Disorder of sexual differentiation, in *Campbell's Textbook of Urology*, 6th ed, PC Walsh et al (eds). Philadelphia, Saunders, 1992, pp 1509–1542

——— et al: Congenital absence of the vagina. The Mayer-Rokitansky-Kuster-Hauser syndrome. Ann Intern Med 85:224, 1976

——— et al: The androgen resistance syndromes: 5α-Reductase deficiency, and related disorders, in *The Metabolic and Molecular Bases of Inherited Disease*, 7th ed, CR Scriver et al (eds). New York, McGraw-Hill, p. 2967, 1995

GRUMBACH MM, CONTE FA: Disorders of sexual differentiation, in *Williams Textbook of Endocrinology*, 8th ed, JD Wilson, DW Foster (eds). Philadelphia, Saunders, 1992, pp 853–951

IMBEAUD S et al: Insensitivity to anti-Müllerian hormone due to a mutation in the human anti-Müllerian hormone receptor. Nat Genet 11:679, 1995

JOSSO N et al: Anti-müllerian hormone and intersex states. Trends Endocrinol Metabol 2:227, 1991

LATRONICO AC et al: Testicular and ovarian resistance to luteinizing hormone caused by inactivating mutations of the luteinizing hormone-receptor gene. N Engl J Med 334:507, 1996

LEONARD JM et al: The classification of Klinefelter's syndrome, in *Genetic Mechanism of Sexual Development*, HL Vallet, IH Porter (eds). New York, Academic Press, 1979, p 407

MILLER WL: Molecular biology of steroid hormone synthesis. Endocrinol Rev 9:295, 1988

RAMSAY M et al: XX True hermaphroditism in Southern African blacks: An enigma of primary sexual differentiation. Am J Hum Genet 43:4, 1988

RHEAUME E et al: Molecular basis of congenital adrenal hyperplasia in two siblings with classical nonsalt-losing 3β-hydroxysteroid dehydrogenase deficiency. J Clin Endocrinol Metab 79:1012, 1994

Sakai Y et al: No mutation in cytochrome P450 side chain cleavage in a patient with congenital lipoid adrenal hyperplasia. J Clin Endocrinol Metab 79:1198, 1994

Simpson JL: Gonadal dysgenesis and sex chromosome abnormalities: Phenotypic-karyotypic correlations, in *Genetic Mechanisms of Sexual Development,* HL Vallet, IH Porter (eds). New York, Academic Press, 1979, p 365

Wilson JD et al: Steroid 5α-reductase 2 deficiency. Endocrinol Rev 14:577, 1993

Yanase T et al: 17α-Hydroxylase/17,20-lyase deficiency: From clinical investigation to molecular definition. Endocrinol Rev 12:91, 1991

340 Steven I. Sherman, Robert F. Gagel

DISORDERS AFFECTING MULTIPLE ENDOCRINE SYSTEMS

NEOPLASTIC DISORDERS AFFECTING MULTIPLE ENDOCRINE ORGANS

In several familial disorders, neoplasia of multiple endocrine organs causes syndromes of hormone excess. Management of these disorders requires an understanding of endocrine neoplasia and of the unique features associated with the manifestations of multiple hormone excess in a single patient. Genetic loci for the two major syndromes and several others have been identified, and DNA-based genetic screening is now available for these disorders.

MULTIPLE ENDOCRINE NEOPLASIA (MEN) TYPE 1 Clinical Manifestations MEN 1, or Wermer's syndrome, is characterized by neoplasia of parathyroid, pituitary, and pancreatic islet cells (Table 340-1). The syndrome is inherited as an autosomal dominant trait so that each child of an affected parent has a 50 percent chance of inheriting the predisposing gene.

Several features of this syndrome have an impact on management. First, the disease process within a single organ is multicentric. Each of the tumors is derived from a single cell, and any endocrine cell within the affected organs can become transformed. Second, hyperplasia is the initiating lesion, followed later by adenomatous or carcinomatous changes. Third, neoplasia in one organ may affect the progression of disease in another organ. For example, hormone production by a pancreatic tumor may stimulate growth of a pituitary tumor. Fourth, this syndrome generally evolves over a 30- to 40-year period, and the manifestations depend in part on when the disorder is identified.

Hyperparathyroidism is the most common manifestation. Hypercalcemia may be present during the teenage years, and most individuals are affected by age 40. Screening for hyperparathyroidism involves measurement of either an albumin-adjusted or ionized serum calcium level. The diagnosis is established by demonstrating elevated levels of serum calcium and intact parathyroid hormone. Manifestations of hyperparathyroidism in MEN 1 do not differ substantially from those in sporadic hyperparathyroidism and include calcium-containing kidney

stones, bone abnormalities, and gastrointestinal and musculoskeletal complaints (see Chap. 354).

Other familial disorders associated with hypercalcemia include familial parathyroid hyperplasia, familial adenomatous hyperparathyroidism, and familial hypocalciuric hypercalcemia (FHH). Calcium excretion is usually elevated in the patient with MEN 1 or other forms of primary hyperparathyroidism and low in FHH. Another distinguishing feature is that the serum calcium level is rarely elevated at birth in patients with MEN 1 and frequently elevated at birth in patients with FHH. Differentiation of hyperparathyroidism of MEN 1 from other forms of familial primary hyperparathyroidism is usually based on family history, histologic features of resected parathyroid tissue, and, sometimes, long-term observation to determine whether other manifestations of MEN 1 develop. FHH is due to inactivating mutations of the calcium sensor, a transmembrane G-protein normally present in parathyroid tissue and kidney (see Chap. 354).

Parathyroid hyperplasia is the common cause of hyperparathyroidism in MEN 1, although single and multiple adenomas have been described. Hyperplasia of one or more parathyroid glands is common in younger patients; adenomas are usually found in older patients or those with long-standing disease.

Neoplasia of the pancreatic islets is the second most common manifestation of MEN 1 and tends to occur in parallel with hyperparathyroidism. The syndromes of pancreatic islet cell hormone excess cause increases in levels of pancreatic polypeptide (75 to 85 percent), gastrin (60 percent, Zollinger-Ellison syndrome), insulin (25 to 35 percent), vasoactive intestinal peptide (VIP) (3 to 5 percent, Verner-Morrison or watery diarrhea syndrome), glucagon (5 to 10 percent), and somatostatin (1 to 5 percent). The tumors rarely produce adrenocorticotropin (ACTH), corticotropin-releasing hormone (CRH), growth hormone–releasing hormone (GHRH), calcitonin gene products, neurotensin, gastric inhibitory peptide, and others. Many of the tumors produce more than one peptide. The pancreatic neoplasms differ from the other components of MEN 1 in that approximately one-third of the tumors display malignant features, including hepatic metastases.

Pancreatic islet cell tumors are diagnosed by identification of a characteristic clinical syndrome, hormonal assays with or without provocative stimuli, or radiographic techniques. One approach involves annual screening of people at risk with measurement of basal and meal-stimulated levels of pancreatic polypeptide to identify the tumors as early as possible; the rationale of this screening strategy is the concept that surgical removal of islet cell tumors at an early stage will be curative. Other approaches to screening include measurement of serum gastrin and pancreatic polypeptide levels every 2 to 3 years, with the rationale that pancreatic neoplasms will be detected at a later stage but can be managed medically, if possible, or by surgery. High resolution computed tomography (CT) scanning provides the best noninvasive technique for identification of these tumors, but intraoperative ultrasonography is the most sensitive method for detection of small tumors.

Table 340-1

Disease Associations in the Multiple Endocrine Neoplasia (MEN) Syndromes

| MEN 1 | MEN 2 | | Mixed Syndromes |
	MEN 2A	MEN 2B	
Parathyroid hyperplasia or adenoma	MTC	MTC	Familial pheochromocytoma and islet cell tumor
Islet cell hyperplasia, adenoma, or carcinoma	Pheochromocytoma	Pheochromocytoma	von Hippel–Lindau syndrome, pheochromocytoma, and islet cell tumor
Pituitary hyperplasia or adenoma	Parathyroid hyperplasia or adenoma	Mucosal and gastrointestinal neuromas	Neurofibromatosis with features of MEN 1 or 2
Other less common manifestations: foregut carcinoid, pheochromocytoma, subcutaneous or visceral lipomas	With cutaneous lichen amyloidosis	Marfanoid features	Myxomas, spotty pigmentation, and generalized endocrine overactivity in a single family
	With Hirschsprung disease		
	FMTC		

NOTE: MTC, medullary thyroid carcinoma; FMTC, familial MTC.

Zollinger-Ellison syndrome (ZES) is caused by excessive gastrin production and occurs in more than half of MEN 1 patients with pancreatic islet cell tumors (see Chap. 95). Clinical features include increased gastric acid production, recurrent peptic ulcers, diarrhea, and esophagitis. The ulcer diathesis is refractory to conservative therapy such as antacids. The diagnosis is made by finding increased gastric acid secretion, elevated basal gastrin levels in serum [generally >115 pmol/L (200 pg/mL)], and an exaggerated response of serum gastrin to either secretin or calcium. Other causes of elevated serum gastrin levels, such as achlorhydria, treatment with H_2 receptor antagonists or omeprazole, retained gastric antrum, small-bowel resection, gastric outlet obstruction, and hypercalcemia, should be excluded. Gastrin-producing carcinoid-like tumors may be present in the duodenal wall.

Insulinoma causes hypoglycemia in about one-third of MEN 1 patients with pancreatic islet cell tumors (see Chap. 335). The tumors may be benign or malignant (25 percent). On occasion, the diagnosis can be established by documenting hypoglycemia during a short fast with simultaneous inappropriate elevation of serum insulin and C-peptide levels. More commonly, it is necessary to subject the patient to a supervised 72-h fast to provoke hypoglycemia (see Chap. 335). Large insulin-secreting tumors may be localized by CT scanning, and small tumors not detected by radiographic techniques may be localized by selective arteriographic injection of calcium into each of the arteries that supply the pancreas and sampling the hepatic vein to determine the anatomic region containing the tumor. Intraoperative ultrasonography can also be used to localize these tumors, but preoperative calcium injection data are helpful in guiding the subtotal pancreatectomy if multiple or no abnormalities are detected by intraoperative ultrasonography.

Glucagonoma in occasional MEN 1 patients causes a syndrome of hyperglycemia, skin rash (necrolytic migratory erythema), anorexia, glossitis, anemia, depression, diarrhea, and venous thrombosis. In about half of these patients the plasma glucagon level is high, leading to its designation as the *glucagonoma syndrome*, although elevation of plasma glucagon level in MEN 1 patients is not necessarily associated with these symptoms. The glucagonoma syndrome may represent a complex interaction between glucagon overproduction and the nutritional status of the patient, although continuous infusion of glucagon sometimes reproduces the syndrome.

The *Verner-Morrison* or *watery diarrhea syndrome* consists of watery diarrhea, hypokalemia, hypochlorhydria, and metabolic acidosis. The diarrhea can be voluminous and is almost always found in association with an islet cell tumor, prompting use of the term *pancreatic cholera*, although the syndrome is not restricted to pancreatic islet tumors and has been observed with carcinoids or other tumors. This syndrome is believed to be due to overproduction of VIP, although plasma VIP levels may not be elevated. Hypercalcemia is believed to be caused by the effects of VIP on bone.

Pituitary tumors occur in more than half of MEN 1 patients and tend to be multicentric, making them difficult to resect (see Chap. 328). The most common tumors are prolactinomas, which are diagnosed by finding serum prolactin levels >200 μg/L with or without a pituitary mass evident by magnetic resonance imaging (MRI). Values less than 200 μg/L may be due to a prolactin-secreting neoplasm or to compression of the pituitary stalk. Acromegaly due to excessive growth hormone production is the second most common syndrome caused by pituitary tumors in MEN 1 (see Chap. 328) but can rarely be due to production of GHRH by an islet cell tumor. Cushing's disease can be caused by ACTH-producing pituitary tumors or by ectopic production of ACTH or CRH by other tumors in the MEN 1 syndrome. Diagnosis of pituitary Cushing's disease is generally best accomplished by a high-dose dexamethasone suppression test or by petrosal venous sinus sampling for ACTH after intravenous injection of CRH (see Chap. 328). Differentiation of a primary pituitary tumor from an ectopic CRH-producing tumor may be difficult because the pituitary is the source of ACTH in both disorders; documentation of CRH production

by a pancreatic islet or carcinoid tumor may be the only method of proving ectopic CRH production.

Unusual manifestations of MEN 1 The rare carcinoid tumors in MEN 1 are of the foregut type and are derived from thymus, lung, stomach, or duodenum; they may metastasize or be locally invasive. These tumors usually produce serotonin, calcitonin, or CRH; the typical carcinoid syndrome with flushing, diarrhea, and bronchospasm is rare (see Chap. 95). Subcutaneous or visceral lipomas and cutaneous leiomyomas also may be present but rarely undergo malignant transformation.

Genetics and Pathophysiology The mutation responsible for MEN 1 is believed to involve a *tumor suppressor gene* that plays an important role in the regulation of cell growth. The disorder is inherited as an autosomal dominant trait, and the responsible gene on chromosome 11q13 encodes a protein termed menin. A second possible mechanism for development of MEN 1 tumors is that elevated levels of fibroblast growth factor may stimulate epithelial growth in the parathyroid glands.

℞ **TREATMENT**

Almost everyone who inherits a mutant MEN 1 gene develops at least one of the manifestations. Most develop hyperparathyroidism, 80 percent develop pancreatic islet cell tumors, and more than half develop pituitary tumors. In most cases, surgery is not curative; most patients require surgery on two or more endocrine glands during a lifetime, and many require multiple surgical procedures. For this reason, it is essential to establish clear goals for management of these patients rather than to recommend surgery casually each time a tumor is discovered. Ranges for acceptable management are discussed below.

Hyperparathyroidism Hyperparathyroid individuals with serum calcium levels >3.0 mmol/L (12 mg/dL), evidence of calcium nephrolithiasis or renal dysfunction, neuropathic or muscular symptoms, or bone involvement (including osteopenia) should undergo parathyroid exploration. In MEN 1 an additional criterion for parathyroid surgery is hypercalcemia associated with elevated gastrin levels, because elevated serum calcium may stimulate gastrin production and ZES, a condition that may be reversed by return of calcium levels to normal. There is less agreement regarding the necessity for parathyroid exploration in individuals who do not meet these criteria, and observation may be appropriate in the MEN 1 patient with asymptomatic hyperparathyroidism.

When parathyroid surgery is indicated in MEN 1, all parathyroid tissue should be identified and removed at the time of primary operation, and parathyroid tissue should be implanted in the nondominant forearm. If reoperation is necessary, transplanted tissue can be resected under local anesthesia with titration of tissue removal to return the serum calcium level to normal. A less desirable approach is to remove 3 to 3½ parathyroid glands from the neck, carefully marking the location of residual tissue so that the remaining tissue can be located easily during subsequent surgery.

Pancreatic Islet Tumors (See Chap. 95 for discussion of pancreatic islet tumors not associated with MEN 1.) Two features of pancreatic islet cell tumors in MEN 1 complicate the management. First, the pancreatic islet cell tumors are multicentric, malignant about a third of the time, and cause death in 10 to 20 percent of patients. Second, removal of all pancreatic islets to prevent malignancy causes diabetes mellitus, a disease with severe long-term complications. These features make it difficult to formulate clear-cut guidelines, but some general concepts appear to be valid. First, islet cell tumors producing insulin, glucagon, VIP, GHRH, or CRH should be resected because medical therapy is ineffective. Second, gastrin-producing islet cell tumors that cause ZES are frequently multicentric, and the surgical cure rate is low. If a single tumor can be identified, a surgical approach seems reasonable, and duodenal wall carcinoid tumors that cause ZES can also be successfully resected in most cases. Treatment with H_2 receptor antagonists (cimetidine or ranitidine) and the H^+,K^+-ATPase inhibitor omeprazole provides an effective alternative to surgery for control of the ulcers in patients with multicentric tumors or with hepatic metastases. Third, in families in which there is a high incidence of malignant islet cell tumors that cause death, total pancreatectomy at an early age may be justified to prevent malignancy.

Management of metastatic islet cell carcinoma is unsatisfactory. Hormonal abnormalities can sometimes be controlled. For example, ZES can be treated with H$_2$ receptor antagonists or omeprazole, and the somatostatin analogue octreotide is useful in the management of carcinoid and the watery diarrhea syndrome. Bilateral adrenalectomy may be required for ectopic ACTH syndrome if medical therapy is ineffective (see Chap. 332). Islet cell carcinomas frequently metastasize to the liver but may grow slowly. Hepatic artery embolization or chemotherapy (5-fluorouracil, streptozocin, chlorozotocin, doxorubicin, or dacarbazine) may reduce tumor mass, control symptoms of hormone excess, and prolong life but are never curative.

Pituitary Tumors Treatment of prolactinomas with bromocriptine usually returns the serum prolactin level to normal and prevents further tumor growth (see Chap. 328). Surgical resection of a prolactinoma is rarely curative but may relieve mass effects. Transsphenoidal resection is appropriate for neoplasms that secrete ACTH, growth hormone (GH), or the α-subunit of the pituitary glycoprotein hormones. Octreotide reduces tumor mass in one-third of tumors and reduces GH and insulin-like growth factor I levels in more than 75 percent of patients with postoperative elevations in GH levels. Radiation therapy may be useful for large or recurrent tumors.

MULTIPLE ENDOCRINE NEOPLASIA TYPE 2 Clinical Manifestations
Thyroid carcinoma and pheochromocytoma are associated in two major syndromes (see Table 340-1). MEN type 2A is the combination of medullary thyroid carcinoma, hyperparathyroidism, and pheochromocytoma. Three subvariants of MEN 2A are familial medullary thyroid carcinoma (FMTC), MEN 2A with cutaneous lichen amyloidosis, and MEN 2A with Hirschsprung disease. MEN type 2B is the combination of medullary thyroid carcinoma, pheochromocytoma, mucosal neuromas, intestinal ganglioneuromatosis, and marfanoid-like features.

Multiple endocrine neoplasia type 2A Medullary thyroid carcinoma is the most common manifestation. The fully developed neoplasm is typically located at the junction of the upper one-third and lower two-thirds of each lobe of the thyroid and appears grossly as chalky white to yellow lesions; tumors greater than 1 cm in size are frequently associated with local or distant metastases. This tumor usually develops in childhood, beginning as hyperplasia of the calcitonin-producing cells (C cells) of the thyroid. Measurement of the serum calcitonin level after injection of a stimulator of release such as calcium or pentagastrin makes it possible to diagnose this disorder when the likelihood of metastasis is low.

Pheochromocytoma occurs in approximately 50 percent of MEN 2A patients and causes palpitations, nervousness, headaches, and sometimes sweating. About half the tumors are bilateral, and more than 50 percent of patients who have had unilateral adrenalectomy develop a pheochromocytoma in the contralateral gland within a decade. A second feature of these tumors is a disproportionate increase in the secretion of epinephrine relative to norepinephrine. Patients with minimal abnormalities of epinephrine secretion may be asymptomatic. Capsular invasion is common, but malignant behavior is uncommon.

Hyperparathyroidism occurs in 15 to 20 percent of patients, with the peak incidence in the third or fourth decade. Hyperparathyroidism may occur early. The manifestations of hyperparathyroidism do not differ from those in other forms of primary hyperparathyroidism (see Chap. 354), with nephrolithiasis being common. Diagnosis is established by finding hypercalcemia, hypophosphatemia, hypercalciuria, and an inappropriately high serum level of intact parathyroid hormone. Multiglandular parathyroid hyperplasia is the most common histologic finding, although withlong-standing disease adenomatous changes may be superimposed on hyperplasia.

Multiple endocrine neoplasia type 2B The association of medullary thyroid carcinoma, pheochromocytoma, mucosal neuromas, and a marfanoid habitus in the absence of hyperparathyroidism is designated MEN 2B. Medullary thyroid carcinoma in MEN 2B develops earlier and is more aggressive than in MEN 2A. Metastatic disease has been described prior to 1 year of age, and death commonly occurs in the second or third decade of life. However, the prognosis is not invariably bad even in patients with metastatic disease, as evidenced by a number of multigenerational families with this disease.

Pheochromocytoma occurs in more than half of MEN 2B patients and does not differ from that in MEN 2A. Hypercalcemia is rare in MEN 2B, and there are no well-documented examples of hyperparathyroidism.

The mucosal neuromas and marfanoid body habitus are the most distinctive features and are recognizable in childhood. Neuromas are present on the tip of the tongue, under the eyelids, and throughout the gastrointestinal tract and are true neuromas, distinct from neurofibromas. Children may present with gastrointestinal symptoms, including increased gas, intermittent obstruction, and diarrhea caused by neuromas.

Genetics and Pathophysiology Mutations of the *c-ret* proto-oncogene have been identified in 93 to 95 percent of patients with MEN 2. Two regions of the Ret tyrosine kinase receptor are mutated (Fig. 340-1). The first is a cysteine-rich extracellular domain; point mutations in the coding sequence for one of five cysteines (codons 609,

FIGURE 340-1 Schematic diagram of the *c-ret* proto-oncogene showing mutations found in multiple endocrine neoplasia type 2 and sporadic medullary thyroid carcinoma. The *c-ret* proto-oncogene is located on the proximal arm of chromosome 10q (10q11.2). Activating mutations of two functional domains of Ret tyrosine kinase receptor have been identified. The first affects a cysteine-rich (Cys-Rich) region in the extracellular portion of the receptor. Each germline mutation changes a cysteine at codons 609, 611, 618, 620, or 634 to another amino acid. The second region is the intracellular tyrosine kinase (TK) domain. Germline mutations of codons 768, 804, and 918 have been identified. Codon 634 mutations account for approximately 80 percent of all germline mutations. Mutations of codons 630, 768, 883, and 918 have been identified as somatic (nongermline) mutations that occur in a single parafollicular or C cell within the thyroid gland in sporadic medullary thyroid carcinoma. A codon 918 mutation is the most common somatic mutation. Abbreviations: MEN 2, multiple endocrine neoplasia type 2; CLA, cutaneous lichen amyloidosis; FMTC, familial medullary thyroid carcinoma; Signal, the signal peptide; Cadherin, a cadherin-like region in the extracellular domain; TM, transmembrane domain; TK, tyrosine kinase domain; MTC, medullary thyroid carcinoma.

611, 618, 620, or 634) cause amino acid substitutions that activate the receptor and initiate transformation. Codon 634 mutations occur in 80 to 90 percent of MEN 2A kindreds and are most commonly associated with classic MEN 2A features (Figs. 340-1 and 340-2); an arginine substitution at this codon accounts for half of all MEN 2A mutations. All reported families with MEN 2A and cutaneous lichen amyloidosis have a codon 634 mutation (Fig. 340-1). Mutations of codons 609, 611, 618, or 620 occur in 10 to 15 percent of MEN 2A kindreds and are more commonly associated with FMTC (Fig. 340-2). Mutations in codons 609, 618, and 620 have also been identified in the MEN 2A and Hirschsprung variant (Fig. 340-1). Although a codon 634 mutation is most commonly associated with classic MEN 2A and mutations in codons 609, 611, 618, or 620 with FMTC, overlap exists (Fig. 340-2).

The second region of the Ret tyrosine kinase that is mutated in MEN 2 is in the substrate recognition pocket at codon 918 (Fig. 340-1). This activating mutation is present in approximately 95 percent of MEN 2B patients and accounts for 10 to 15 percent of all *c-ret* proto-oncogene mutations in MEN 2.

Approximately 5 percent of kindreds with FMTC have no identifiable mutation of either of these regions. In a few such kindreds a point mutation of codon 768 or 804 has been identified. The glial-cell-line–derived neurotropic factor is a ligand for the Ret tyrosine kinase receptor, and it seems likely that mutations of this peptide might also cause either MEN 2 or Hirschsprung disease.

Somatic mutations (mutations found only in the tumor and not transmitted in the germline) of the *c-ret* proto-oncogene have been identified in sporadic medullary thyroid carcinoma; 25 to 50 percent of sporadic tumors have codon 918 mutations, and a few somatic codon 630, 768, and 804 mutations have been identified (Fig. 340-1). Germline mutations of the *c-ret* proto-oncogene are present in about 6 percent of patients with apparent sporadic medullary thyroid carcinoma, indicating that other family members may be at risk for development of this disease. This finding suggests that all patients with sporadic medullary thyroid carcinoma should have a peripheral blood *c-ret* proto-oncogene analysis.

R̲x̲ **TREATMENT**

Screening for Multiple Endocrine Neoplasia Type 2   Death from medullary thyroid carcinoma can be prevented by early thyroidectomy. The identification of *c-ret* proto-oncogene mutations and the application of DNA-based molecular diagnostic techniques to identify these mutations has simplified the screening process. During the initial evaluation of a kindred, a *c-ret* proto-oncogene analysis should be performed on an individual with proven MEN 2A. Establishment of the specific mutation in a kindred facilitates the subsequent analysis of other family members. Each family member at risk should be tested twice for the presence of the specific mutation, and the second analysis should be performed on a second sample and in a second laboratory to exclude sample mixup or technical error.[1] Individuals in a kindred with a known mutation who have two normal analyses can be dropped from further screening.

Two approaches have evolved for management of potential thyroid malignancy in individuals with mutations of codons 609, 611, 620, or 634. The first is to perform a total thyroidectomy in early childhood, usually before the age of 6 years. More than 90 percent of affected individuals will develop medullary thyroid carcinoma (Fig. 340-2), and metastases have occurred in MEN 2A by age 6. This approach eliminates the need for annual pentagastrin screening. Risks of thyroidectomy include hypoparathyroidism and recurrent laryngeal nerve damage, although the frequency of these complications is no greater in children.

---

[1] A list of laboratories that perform *c-ret* proto-oncogene testing can be found on the University of Texas M.D. Anderson Cancer Center Web site at: http://endrcr06.mda.uth.tmc.edu. A pamphlet for patients with MEN 2A and FMTC that provides a description of clinical features and diagnostic testing is also available at the same Web site.

A second approach, based on many years of experience in MEN 2A screening, is to measure each year the release of calcitonin into the bloodstream after the administration of pentagastrin or combined pentagastrin-calcium to carriers of the mutations to identify medullary thyroid carcinoma or its precursor lesion, C-cell hyperplasia, before development of metastatic disease. Screening of individuals at risk should begin in early childhood, preferably before age 5. The

FIGURE 340-2   Clinical features associated with mutations of specific codons of the cysteine-rich region of the Ret tyrosine kinase receptor. A compilation of clinical features found in kindreds with mutations of codons 609, 611, 618, 620, and 634. Classic multiple endocrine neoplasia type 2A, the association of medullary thyroid carcinoma, pheochromocytoma, and parathyroid neoplasia, is most commonly found in association with a codon 634 mutation. However, this compilation clearly makes the point that parathyroid neoplasia has been identified in 10 to 20 percent of kindreds with mutations of codons 609, 611, 618, and 620, and pheochromocytoma has been identified in 20 to 40 percent of kindreds with codon 611, 618, and 620 mutations. Pheochromocytoma has not been identified in a kindred with a codon 609 mutation, although the infrequency of this mutation (fewer than 10 reported kindreds) suggests additional experience is needed. The data in this figure have been accumulated from published information from over 300 kindreds.

pentagastrin test involves measurement of serum calcitonin basally and 2, 5, 10, and 15 min after bolus injection of 5 μg pentagastrin/kg body weight. Patients should be warned before injection of epigastric tightness, nausea, warmth, and tingling of extremities and reassured that the symptoms will last approximately 2 min. Thyroidectomy should be performed when an abnormal pentagastrin test is identified. A follow-up of children identified with this approach indicates that 90 percent have no recurrence of disease 15 to 20 years later. The advantage of this approach is a delay of thyroidectomy, on average, until 10 years of age. The disadvantages include the cost and discomfort of annual testing and the small possibility that metastases could occur before thyroidectomy is performed.

There is no consensus on which of these approaches is better, although the excellent results with early thyroidectomy; the potential for improvement of cure rate; and the avoidance of the cost, discomfort, and parental anxiety associated with annual pentagastrin testing suggest that early total thyroidectomy will become accepted with time.

The *c-ret* proto-oncogene analysis should be performed in patients with suspected MEN 2B to detect codon 918 mutations, especially in newborn children where the diagnosis is suspected but the clinical phenotype not fully developed. Other family members at risk may also be tested if the diagnosis is not clear because the mucosal neuromas can be subtle and not always identified. In the occasional families with proven germline transmission of medullary thyroid carcinoma but no identifiable *c-ret* proto-oncogene mutation, annual pentagastrin or calcium-pentagastrin testing should be performed on members at risk.

Annual screening for pheochromocytoma in subjects with germline *c-ret* mutations should be performed by measuring basal plasma or 12-h urine catecholamines. The goal is to identify a pheochromocytoma before it causes significant symptoms or is likely to cause sudden death, an event most commonly associated with large tumors. Radiographic studies, such as MRI or CT scans, are generally reserved for individuals with abnormal screening tests or with symptoms suggestive of pheochromocytoma (see Chap. 333). Women should be tested during pregnancy because undetected pheochromocytoma can cause maternal death during childbirth.

Measurement of serum calcium and parathyroid hormone levels every 2 to 3 years provides an adequate screen for hyperparathyroidism, except in those families in which hyperparathyroidism is a prominent component, where measurements should be made annually.

Treatment of Medullary Thyroid Carcinoma FMTC is a multicentric disorder. Total thyroidectomy with a central lymph node dissection should be performed in children who carry the mutant genes. Long-term follow-up studies indicate an excellent outcome with approximately 90 percent of children free of disease 15 to 20 years after surgery. In contrast, 15 to 25 percent of patients in whom the diagnosis is made on the basis of a palpable thyroid nodule die from the disease within 15 years.

In adults with medullary thyroid cancer greater than 1 cm in size, metastases to regional lymph nodes are common. Total thyroidectomy with central lymph node dissection and selective dissection of other regional chains provides the best chance for cure. In patients with extensive local metastatic disease in the neck, external radiation may prevent local recurrence or reduce tumor mass but is not curative. Chemotherapy with combinations of adriamycin, vincristine, cyclophosphamide, and dacarbazine may provide palliation.

Treatment of Pheochromocytoma The long-term goal for management of pheochromocytoma is to prevent death and cardiovascular complications. Improvements in radiographic imaging of the adrenals make direct examination of the apparently normal contralateral gland during surgery less important, making a posterior approach practical for unilateral adrenalectomy. The major question is whether to remove both adrenal glands or to remove only the affected adrenal at the time of primary surgery. Issues to be considered in making this decision include the possibility of malignancy (fewer than 15 reported cases), the likelihood of development of pheochromocytoma in the apparently unaffected gland over an 8- to 10-year period, and the risks of adrenal insufficiency caused by

removal of both glands (two deaths related to adrenal insufficiency in MEN 2 patients). Most but not all clinicians recommend removal only of the affected gland and leave the contralateral gland. If both adrenals are removed, glucocorticoid and mineralocorticoid replacement is mandatory. An alternative approach is to remove the pheochromocytoma and adrenal medulla, leaving the adrenal cortex behind. If successful, this approach eliminates the necessity for steroid hormone replacement, although the pheochromocytoma recurs in some.

Treatment of Hyperparathyroidism Hyperparathyroidism has been managed by one of two approaches. Removal of 3½ glands with maintenance of the remaining half gland in the neck is the usual procedure. In families in whom hyperparathyroidism is a prominent manifestation and recurrence is common, total parathyroidectomy with transplantation of parathyroid tissue into the nondominant forearm is preferred. This approach is discussed above in the context of hyperparathyroidism associated with MEN 1.

OTHER GENETIC TUMOR SYNDROMES A number of mixed syndromes exist in which the neoplastic associations differ from those in MEN 1 or 2 (see Table 340-1).

von Hippel–Lindau (VHL) syndrome, the association of central nervous system tumors, renal cell carcinoma, pheochromocytoma, and islet cell neoplasms, is caused by mutations in a tumor-suppressor gene. Germline-inactivating mutations of the VHL gene cause tumor formation when there is additional loss or somatic mutation of the normal VHL allele in brain, kidney, pancreatic islet, or adrenal medullary cells. A specific subset of mutations is more common in families with pheochromocytomas.

The molecular defect in type 1 neurofibromatosis inactivates neurofibromin, a cell membrane–associated protein that normally activates a GTPase. Inactivation of this protein impairs GTPase and causes continuous activation of p21 Ras and its downstream tyrosine kinase pathway.

IMMUNOLOGIC SYNDROMES AFFECTING MULTIPLE ENDOCRINE ORGANS

When immune dysfunction affects two or more endocrine glands and other nonendocrine immune disorders are present, the polyglandular autoimmune (PGA) syndromes should be considered. These syndromes are designated PGA types I, II, and III (Table 340-2). The type I syndrome starts in childhood and is characterized by mucocutaneous candidiasis, hypoparathyroidism, and adrenal insufficiency. Patients with the type II (or Schmidt) syndrome are more likely to present as adults and typically have adrenal insufficiency, thyroiditis, and type 1 diabetes mellitus. The type III syndrome is heterogeneous and consists of autoimmune thyroid disease along with any autoimmune glandular dysfunction other than adrenal insufficiency.

POLYGLANDULAR AUTOIMMUNE SYNDROME TYPE I PGA type I usually is recognized in the first decade of life and requires two of three components for diagnosis: mucocutaneous candi-

Table 340-2

Disease Associations in Polyglandular Autoimmune (PGA) Syndromes

PGA I	PGA II	PGA III
Mucocutaneous candidiasis	Adrenal insufficiency	Type 1 diabetes and autoimmune thyroid disease or adrenal insufficiency and autoimmune thyroid disease
Hypoparathyroidism	Hypothyroidism	
Adrenal insufficiency	Graves' disease	
Hypogonadism	Type 1 diabetes	
Alopecia	Hypogonadism	
Hypothyroidism	Myasthenia gravis	
Malabsorption	Vitiligo	
Chronic active hepatitis	Alopecia	
Vitiligo	Pernicious anemia	
Pernicious anemia	Celiac disease	

diasis, hypoparathyroidism, and adrenal insufficiency. Mineralocorticoids and glucocorticoids may be lost simultaneously or sequentially. This disorder is also called *autoimmune polyendocrinopathy-candidiasis-ectodermal dystrophy* (APECED). Other endocrine defects can include gonadal failure, hypothyroidism, and, less commonly, destruction of the β cells of the pancreatic islets and development of insulin-dependent (type 1) diabetes mellitus. Additional features include hypoplasia of the dental enamel, ungual dystrophy, tympanic membrane sclerosis, vitiligo, keratopathy, and gastric parietal cell dysfunction resulting in pernicious anemia. Some patients develop autoimmune hepatitis, malabsorption (variably attributed to intestinal lymphangiectasia, IgA deficiency, bacterial overgrowth, or hypoparathyroidism), asplenism, achalasia, and cholelithiasis. At the outset, only one organ may be involved, but the number increases with time so that patients eventually manifest two to five components of the syndrome. In one variant among Iranian Jews, hypoparathyroidism frequently occurs by itself.

In a Finnish series, 78 percent of patients had a nonendocrine presentation, most commonly oral candidiasis. Although candidiasis occurs in most patients, is poorly responsive to treatment, and relapses frequently, the symptoms are often mild and can easily be missed. Involvement of the parathyroid glands usually occurs before adrenal insufficiency develops. More than 60 percent of postpubertal women develop premature hypogonadism. The endocrine components, including adrenal insufficiency and hypoparathyroidism, may not develop until the fourth decade, making continued surveillance necessary.

POLYGLANDULAR AUTOIMMUNE SYNDROME TYPE II Lymphocytic infiltration of the adrenal and thyroid glands along with type 1 diabetes mellitus and hypogonadism are characteristic of PGA type II, or Schmidt, syndrome. Type 1 diabetes mellitus occurs in approximately half of affected families. The autoimmune thyroid disease causes either Hashimoto's thyroiditis or hyperthyroidism; however, many patients with antimicrosomal and antithyroglobulin antibodies never develop abnormalities of thyroid function. Thus these antibodies alone are poor predictors of future disease. Dermatologic manifestations include vitiligo, caused by antibodies against the melanocyte, and alopecia and are less common than in the type I syndrome. Mucocutaneous candidiasis does not occur. A few patients develop a late-onset, usually transient hypoparathyroidism caused by antibodies that compete with parathyroid hormone for binding to the parathyroid hormone receptor. Up to 25 percent of patients with myasthenia gravis and an even higher percentage who have myasthenia and a thymoma have PGA type II (see Chap. 382).

POLYGLANDULAR AUTOIMMUNE SYNDROME TYPE III In rare families, hereditary abnormalities of the thyroid and adrenal or the thyroid and pancreatic islets occur in the absence of other autoimmune disorders. These families either have diabetes mellitus and autoimmune thyroid disease or adrenal insufficiency and Hashimoto's thyroiditis.

GENETICS AND PATHOGENESIS The underlying defects in these disorders are unknown but probably include inherited and acquired components. Type I PGA syndrome shows no HLA associations and is inherited as an autosomal recessive trait. The Finnish variant of PGA type I is linked to chromosome 21q22.3 and has been mapped to a 500 kb segment. The type II and III syndromes are usually associated with the DR3 or DR4 HLA haplotypes, or both, and are inherited as autosomal dominant traits with variable expressivity. Epidemiologic studies of twins with either type 1 diabetes mellitus or Graves' disease showed development of disease in both twins only about half of the time. Thus, additional factors must contribute to the immune dysregulation. Putative precipitants for either type 1 diabetes mellitus or thyroiditis include viral infections (rubella, Coxsackie B, mumps, and cytomegalovirus) and dietary antigens such as milk proteins.

Patients with the PGA syndromes may have a variety of autoantibodies directed against organ-specific antigens. Some of the antibodies are specific markers of autoimmunity and recognize cytoplasmic components of various endocrine cells, e.g., antibodies against thyroid peroxidase, adrenal side chain cleavage enzyme, or pancreatic glutamic acid decarboxylase. Other antibodies may interact directly with cell-surface receptors such as those for thyroid-stimulating hormone (TSH), adrenocorticotropin, or insulin and impair normal function. Still others bind to complement and lead to cytotoxicity. The role of cytokines such as interferon and of impairment of cell-mediated immunity in the pathogenesis of the PGA syndromes is unclear.

DIAGNOSIS The clinical manifestations of adrenal insufficiency often develop slowly, may be difficult to detect, and can be fatal if not diagnosed and treated appropriately. Thus, prospective screening should be performed routinely in all patients and family members at risk for PGA I and II. The most effective screening test for adrenal disease is a cosyntropin stimulation test (see Chap. 332). A fasting blood glucose level can be obtained to screen for hyperglycemia. Additional screening tests should include measurements of TSH, luteinizing hormone, follicle-stimulating hormone, and, in men, testosterone levels. In families with suspected type I PGA syndrome, calcium and phosphorus levels are also measured. These screening studies should be performed every 1 to 2 years up to about age 50 in families with PGA type II and III syndrome and until about age 40 in patients with type I syndrome. Screening measurements of autoantibodies against potentially affected endocrine organs are of uncertain prognostic value. The differential diagnosis of PGA should include the DiGeorge syndrome (hypoparathyroidism due to glandular agenesis and mucocutaneous candidiasis), Kearns-Sayre syndrome (hypoparathyroidism, primary hypogonadism, type 1 diabetes mellitus, and panhypopituitarism), Wolfram's syndrome (congenital diabetes insipidus and diabetes mellitus), and congenital rubella (type 1 diabetes mellitus and hypothyroidism).

℞ TREATMENT

With the exception of Graves' disease, the management of each of the endocrine components of the disease involves hormone replacement and is covered in detail in the chapters on adrenal, thyroid, gonadal, and parathyroid disease (Chaps. 332, 331, 336, 337, and 354). One aspect of therapy deserves special emphasis. Namely, primary hypothyroidism can mask adrenal insufficiency by prolonging the half-life of cortisol, and consequently administration of thyroid hormone to a patient with unsuspected adrenal insufficiency can precipitate adrenal crisis. Thus, all patients with hypothyroidism in the context of PGA should be screened for adrenal disease and, if present, be treated with glucocorticoids prior to or concurrently with thyroid hormone therapy.

OTHER AUTOIMMUNE ENDOCRINE SYNDROMES   Insulin Receptor Antibodies Insulin resistance, defined as a decrease in the biologic response to a given amount of insulin, occurs commonly in patients with obesity, severe infections, trauma, or surgery, as well as in individuals with acromegaly or Cushing's syndrome, in whom growth hormone or cortisol excess can antagonize the action of insulin. Rare insulin-resistance syndromes occur in patients who develop spontaneous antibodies directed against insulin receptor, thereby preventing interaction of insulin with the insulin receptor. Conversely, other classes of anti-insulin receptor antibodies can activate the receptor and can cause hypoglycemia and must be considered in the differential diagnosis of fasting hypoglycemia (see Chap. 335).

Patients with insulin receptor antibodies and acanthosis nigricans are often middle-aged women who acquire insulin resistance in association with other autoimmune disorders such as systemic lupus erythematosus or Sjögren's syndrome. Vitiligo, alopecia, Raynaud's phenomenon, and arthritis also may be seen. Other autoimmune endocrine disorders, including thyrotoxicosis, hypothyroidism, and hypogonadism, occur rarely. Acanthosis nigricans, a velvety, hyperpigmented, thickened skin lesion, is prominent on the dorsum of the neck and other skin fold areas in the axillae or groin and often heralds the diagnosis in these patients. However, acanthosis nigricans also occurs in patients with obesity or polycystic ovarian syndrome, in which insulin resistance appears to be due to a postreceptor defect, and thus acanthosis nigricans itself is not diagnostic of the immunologic form of insulin resistance. This syndrome is called the *type B insulin resistance syndrome* and must be differentiated from type A insulin resistance syndromes, which are secondary to mutations in the gene that encodes the insulin receptor and impair insulin receptor signaling.

Anti-insulin receptor antibodies block the interaction of the hormone with its receptor and impair its action to varying degrees. Activation of the receptor by the antibodies also may result in receptor downregulation and desensitization. The degree of insulin resistance can be quite variable. Some patients with acanthosis nigricans show normal to mild glucose intolerance, with a compensatory increase in insulin secretion that is only detected when insulin levels are measured. Others have severe diabetes mellitus requiring massive doses of insulin (several thousand units per day) to lower the blood glucose levels. The nature of the antibodies determines the manifestations. Although insulin resistance is more common, fasting hypoglycemia can be the presenting symptom or develop during the course of the disease. The hypoglycemia results from the interaction of insulinomimetic antibodies with insulin receptor.

Ataxia telangiectasia is an autosomal recessive disorder with insulin-resistant diabetes mellitus, ataxia, telangiectasia, immune abnormalities, and an increased incidence of malignancies. This disorder is also associated with anti-insulin antibodies.

Autoimmune Insulin Syndrome with Hypoglycemia In this disorder polyclonal insulin-binding autoantibodies, typically found in patients with other autoimmune disorders, bind to endogenously synthesized insulin. If the insulin dissociates from the antibodies several hours or more after a meal, hypoglycemia can result. Most cases of the syndrome have been described from Japan, and there may be a genetic component. The anti-insulin antibodies may interfere in the insulin assay and falsely elevate measured insulin levels. A finding of normal C-peptide levels in this situation suggests a false-positive insulin measurement. In plasma cell dyscrasias such as multiple myeloma, the plasma cells may produce monoclonal antibodies against insulin and cause hypoglycemia by a similar mechanism.

Antithyroxine Antibodies and Hypothyroidism Circulating autoantibodies against thyroid hormones in patients with both immune thyroid disease and plasma cell dyscrasias such as Waldenström's macroglobulinemia can bind thyroid hormones, decrease their biologic activity, and result in primary hypothyroidism. In other patients the antibodies simply interfere with thyroid hormone immunoassays and cause false elevations or decreases in measured hormone levels.

Crow-Fukase Syndrome The features of this syndrome are highlighted by an acronym that emphasizes its important features: *p*olyneuropathy, *o*rganomegaly, *e*ndocrinopathy, *M*-proteins, and *s*kin changes (POEMS). The most important feature is a severe, progressive sensorimotor polyneuropathy associated with a plasma cell dyscrasia. Localized collections of plasma cells (plasmacytomas) can cause sclerotic bone lesions and produce monoclonal IgG or IgA proteins. Endocrine manifestations include amenorrhea in women and impotence and gynecomastia in men, hypogonadism, hyperprolactinemia, type 2 diabetes mellitus, primary hypothyroidism, and adrenal insufficiency. Skin changes include hyperpigmentation, thickening of the dermis, hirsutism, and hyperhidrosis. Hepatomegaly and lymphadenopathy occur in about two-thirds of patients, and splenomegaly is seen in about one-third. Other manifestations include increased cerebrospinal fluid pressure with papilledema, peripheral edema, ascites, pleural effusions, glomerulonephritis, and fever.

Table 340-3

Other Disorders with Common Polyglandular Manifestations

Condition	Clinical Features	Type of Endocrine Involvement						Inheritance/ Molecular Defect
		Hypothalamic-Pituitary	Thyroid	Parathyroid	Pancreas	Adrenal	Gonads	
Ataxia-telangiectasia	Early ataxia Oculocutaneous telangiectasia Immunologic deficiency	Occasional diminished pituitary reserve			Diabetes mellitus	Cortical hypoplasia	Dysgenetic gonads: gonadoblastomas later in females	Autosomal recessive
Pseudo-hypoparathyroidism	Short stature Short metacarpals and metatarsals Round facies Ectopic calcification	Variable deficiency of all pituitary hormones including prolactin	Hypo- or hyper-thyroidism	Elevated parathyroid hormone levels with normo- or hypocalcemia	Diabetes mellitus		Ovarian failure	Mutation of the $G_{\alpha s}$
Myotonic dystrophy	Muscular dystrophy Premature baldness Mental retardation	Gonadotropin and growth hormone abnormalities, ? related to central integrative defect	Hypo-thyroidism		Diabetes mellitus		Primary gonadal failure	Insertion of unstable CTG repeat in myotonic dystrophy gene on chromosome 19
Noonan syndrome	Short stature Ptosis Webbed neck Pulmonary stenosis	Gonadotropin deficiency	Thyroiditis				Primary gonadal failure	Autosomal dominant
Fanconi syndrome	Short stature Bone marrow hypoplasia Abnormal skin pigmentation Radius malformations	Panhypo-pituitarism			Diabetes mellitus	Adrenal atrophy	Gonadal atrophy	Autosomal recessive
Werner syndrome	Premature aging Atropic skin Cataracts Early osteopenia		Papillary thyroid carcinoma		Diabetes mellitus		Gonadal atrophy	Autosomal recessive

The systemic nature of the disorder may cause confusion with other connective tissue diseases. The endocrine manifestations suggest an autoimmune basis of the disorder, but circulating antibodies against endocrine cells have not been demonstrated. Increased serum and tissue levels of interleukin 6 are present, but the pathophysiologic basis for the POEMS syndrome is uncertain. Therapy directed against the plasma cell dyscrasia such as local radiation of bony lesions or chemotherapy may result in endocrine improvement.

MISCELLANEOUS DISORDERS WITH ENDOCRINE MANIFESTATIONS

A variety of other clinical and genetic disorders are associated with multiple endocrine manifestations (Table 340-3). The molecular and genetic defects for several of these disorders are now known. One example is the McCune-Albright syndrome, in which a constitutively activating mutation of the α subunit of the stimulatory G-protein causes overactivity of adenyl cyclase in a variety of glands. The clinical syndrome can include precocious puberty, acromegaly, thyrotoxicosis, and Cushing's syndrome, all reflecting autonomous hyperfunction of glands usually regulated by a G protein–dependent receptor.

BIBLIOGRAPHY

AALTONEN J et al: An autosomal locus causing autoimmune disease: Autoimmune polyglandular disease type I assigned to chromosome 21. Nat Genet 8:83, 1994

AHONEN P et al: Clinical variation of autoimmune polyendocrinopathy-candidiasis-ectodermal dystrophy (APECED) in a series of 68 patients. N Engl J Med 322:1829, 1990

BARDWICK PA et al: Plasma cell dyscrasia with polyneuropathy, organomegaly, endocrinopathy, M protein, and skin changes: The POEMS syndrome. Medicine 59:311, 1980

CHANDRASEKHARAPPA SC et al: Positional cloning of the gene for multiple endocrine neoplasia-type 1. Science 276:404, 1997

DURBEC P et al: GDNF signalling through the Ret receptor tyrosine kinase. Nature 381:789, 1996

GAGEL RF: Multiple endocrine neoplasia, in *Williams Textbook of Endocrinology*, 9th ed, JD Wilson, DW Foster (eds). Philadelphia, Saunders, in press
—— et al: The clinical outcome of prospective screening for multiple endocrine neoplasia type 2a. An 18-year experience. N Engl J Med 318:478, 1988

KAHN CR et al: The syndromes of insulin resistance and acanthosis nigricans: Insulin-receptor disorders in man. N Engl J Med 294:739, 1976

LATIF F et al: Identification of the von Hippel-Lindau disease tumor suppressor gene. Science 260:1317, 1993

LIPS CJM et al: Clinical screening as compared with DNA analysis in families with multiple endocrine neoplasia type 2A. N Engl J Med 331:828, 1994

MULLIGAN LM et al: Germline mutations of the RET proto-oncogene in multiple endocrine neoplasia type 2A (MEN 2A). Nature 363:458, 1993

NEUFELD M et al: Two types of autoimmune Addison's disease associated with different polyglandular autoimmune (PGA) syndromes. Medicine 60:355, 1981

RIZZOLI R et al: Primary hyperparathyroidism in familial multiple endocrine neoplasia type I. Long-term follow-up of serum calcium levels after parathyroidectomy. Am J Med 78:467, 1985

SHERMAN SI, LADENSON PW: Octreotide therapy of growth hormone excess in the McCune-Albright syndrome. J Endocrinol Invest 15:185, 1992

SKOGSEID B et al: Multiple endocrine neoplasia type 1: A 10-year prospective screening study in four kindreds. J Clin Endocrinol Metab 73:281, 1991

THAKKER RV: Multiple endocrine neoplasia type 1, in *Endocrinology*, 3d ed, LJ DeGroot (ed). Philadelphia, Saunders, 1995, pp 2815–2831

WELLS SA JR et al: Predictive DNA testing and prophylactic thyroidectomy in patients at risk for multiple endocrine neoplasia type 2A. Ann Surg 220:237, 1994

WOHLLK N et al: Application of genetic screening information to the management of medullary thyroid carcinoma and multiple endocrine neoplasia type 2. Endocrinol Metab Clin North Am 25:1, 1996

SECTION 2

DISORDERS OF INTERMEDIARY METABOLISM

341

Henry N. Ginsberg, Ira J. Goldberg

DISORDERS OF LIPOPROTEIN METABOLISM

Lipoproteins are macromolecular complexes that carry hydrophobic plasma lipids, particularly cholesterol and triglyceride, in the plasma. More than half of the coronary heart disease (CHD) in the United States is attributable to abnormalities in the levels and metabolism of plasma lipids and lipoproteins. Some premature CHD is due to mutations in major genes involved in lipoprotein metabolism, but elevated lipoprotein levels in most patients with CHD reflect the adverse impact of a sedentary lifestyle, excess body weight, and diets high in total and saturated fat on a less-than-perfect genetic background. Primary care providers and subspecialists need to understand the pathophysiology of and available therapies for these disorders. This chapter is focused on the major lipid disorders, both the dyslipoproteinemias caused by single-gene defects and the disorders that are likely to be polygenic in origin. We will then provide a practical approach to assist in the identification, evaluation, and treatment of patients with increased risk of CHD.

LIPID AND LIPOPROTEIN TRANSPORT

LIPOPROTEIN STRUCTURE Lipoproteins are spherical particles made up of hundreds of lipid and protein molecules. They are smaller than red blood cells and visible only by electron microscopy. However, when the larger, triglyceride-rich lipoproteins are present in high concentration, plasma can appear turbid or milky to the naked eye. The major lipids of the lipoproteins are cholesterol, triglycerides, and phospholipids. Triglycerides and the esterified form of cholesterol (cholesteryl esters) are nonpolar lipids that are insoluble in aqueous environments (hydrophobic) and comprise the core of the lipoproteins. Phospholipids and a small quantity of free (unesterified) cholesterol, which are soluble in both lipid and aqueous environments (amphipathic), cover the surface of the particles, where they act as the interface between the plasma and core components. A family of proteins, the apolipoproteins, also occupies the surface of the lipoproteins to serve as an additional interface between lipid and aqueous environments. These proteins play crucial roles in the regulation of lipid transport and lipoprotein metabolism.

Lipoproteins have been classified on the basis of their densities into five major classes: chylomicrons, very low density lipoproteins (VLDL), intermediate-density lipoproteins (IDL), low-density lipoproteins (LDL), and high-density lipoproteins (HDL). The physical-chemical characteristics of the major lipoprotein classes are presented in Table 341-1.

APOLIPOPROTEINS The apolipoproteins (apos) provide structural stability to the lipoproteins and determine the metabolic fate of the particles upon which they reside. They were named in an arbitrary alphabetical order and, for the purposes of this discussion, will be described in relation to their association with lipoprotein classes (Table 341-2.)

There are two forms of apo B—apo B100 and apo B48. Apo B100 is the major apolipoprotein of VLDL, IDL, and LDL, comprising approximately 30, 60, and 95 percent of the proteins in these lipoproteins respectively. Apo B100 has a molecular mass of about 545 kDa and is synthesized in the liver. It is essential for the assembly and secretion of VLDL from the liver and is the ligand for the removal of LDL by the LDL receptor. The LDL receptor is a cell-surface protein that binds and internalizes lipoproteins that contain apo B100 or apo E. The LDL receptor binding domain of apo B100 is the sequence between amino acids 3200 and 3600, a region that is absent in apo B48.

Apo B48 is essential for the assembly and secretion of chylomicrons. Apo B48 is encoded by the same gene and the same messenger ribonucleic acid (mRNA) as Apo B100, but in the intestine the mRNA is edited in an unusual way: A cytidine deaminase in the intestine changes a cytidine to a uridine in base 6666 of the apo B100 mRNA to produce a nonsense codon so that apo B48 contains only the N-terminal 48 percent of the full-length apo B100. In contrast, the apo B100 mRNA in human liver is not edited. The role of apo B48 in the metabolism of chylomicrons in plasma is unclear. Individuals with mutations that interfere with the normal synthesis of apo B have absent or very low levels of chylomicrons, VLDL, IDL and LDL.

The apolipoproteins of the C series are synthesized in the liver and are present in all plasma lipoproteins (trace amounts in LDL). Individual apo C's have different metabolic roles, but all inhibit the removal of plasma chylomicrons and VLDL remnants by the liver. Overexpression of apo CI in transgenic mice inhibits the uptake of chylomicron and VLDL remnants by the liver. Apo CI under- or overexpression has not been described in humans. Apo CII is an essential activator of the enzyme lipoprotein lipase (LPL), which hydrolyzes triglycerides in chylomicrons and VLDL, and individuals lacking apo CII have severe hypertriglyceridemia. Apo CIII inhibits LPL, and apo CIII overexpression in transgenic mice causes severe hypertriglyceridemia. Two humans who lacked apo CIII had accelerated rates of lipolysis of VLDL triglyceride.

Apo E is synthesized mainly in hepatocytes but is also made in other cells, including macrophages, neurons, and glial cells. It is found in chylomicrons, IDL, VLDL, and HDL and mediates the uptake of these lipoproteins in liver both by the LDL receptor and by the LDL receptor–related protein (LRP). Apo E can also bind to heparin-like proteoglycan molecules on the surface of all cells. Three major alleles of the apo E gene encode E2, E3, and E4, isoforms that differ in sequence at two positions and have frequencies of about 0.12, 0.75,

and 0.13 in the general population. Apo E2 binds to the LDL receptor with lower affinity than apo E3 or E4. Individuals who are homozygous for apo E2 may develop severe hyperlipidemia (type III dyslipoproteinemia), and complete absence of apo E causes elevations of plasma levels of chylomicron and VLDL remnants and early atherosclerosis.

Apo AI, apo AII, and apo AIV are found primarily on HDL. Apo AI and apo AII are synthesized in the small intestine and the liver; apo AIV is made only in the intestine. Apo AI comprises about 70 to 80 percent of the protein of HDL and plays a critical role in maintaining the integrity of HDL particles. Individuals with a profound deficiency of apo AI also lack HDL. Apo AI also activates the enzyme lecithin:cholesterol acyltransferase (LCAT), which esterifies free cholesterol in plasma. Plasma levels of HDL cholesterol and apo AI are inversely related to risk for CHD, and some patients with apo AI deficiency develop early, severe atherosclerosis. Transgenic mice overexpressing human apo AI are resistant to atherosclerosis. Apo AII is the second most abundant apoprotein in HDL, and its function has not been determined; transgenic mice that overexpress apo AII have high plasma levels of both HDL cholesterol and triglycerides and may be susceptible to atherosclerosis. Apo AII knockout mice have low levels of HDL, indicating that apo AII is also necessary for the integrity of HDL particles. Apo AIV, a minor component of HDL and chylomicrons, may play a role in the activation of LCAT.

Apoprotein(a), a large glycoprotein that shares a high degree of sequence homology with the plasma zymogen plasminogen, is made by hepatocytes and is secreted into plasma where it forms a covalent linkage with the apo B100 of LDL to form lipoprotein(a). The physiologic role of lipoprotein(a) is not known, but elevated levels are associated with an increased risk for atherosclerosis.

LIPOPROTEIN METABOLISM LPL is synthesized in fat and muscle, secreted into the interstitial space, transported across endothelial cells, and binds to proteoglycans on the luminal surfaces in the adjacent capillary beds. LPL mediates the hydrolysis of the triglycerides of chylomicrons and VLDL to generate free fatty acids

Table 341-1

Physical-Chemical Characteristics of the Major Lipoprotein Classes

Lipoprotein	Density, g/dL	Molecular Mass, kDa	Diameter, nm	Lipid, %		
				TG	Chol	PL
Chylomicrons	0.95	400×10^3	75–1200	80–95	2–7	3–9
VLDL	0.95–1.006	$10–80 \times 10^3$	30–80	55–80	5–15	10–20
IDL	1.006–1.019	$5–10 \times 10^3$	25–35	20–50	20–40	15–25
LDL	1.019–1.063	2.3×10^3	18–25	5–15	40–50	20–25
HDL	1.063–1.210	$1.7–3.6 \times 10^2$	5–12	5–10	15–25	20–30

NOTE: TG, triglyceride; Chol, the sum of free and esterified cholesterol; PL, phospholipid. The remaining percent composition is made up of the apoproteins.

Table 341-2

Characteristics of the Major Apolipoproteins

Apolipoprotein	Molecular Mass, Da	Lipoproteins	Metabolic Functions
Apo AI	28,016	HDL, chylomicrons	Structural component of HDL; LCAT activator
Apo AII	17,414	HDL, chylomicrons	Unknown
Apo AIV	46,465	HDL, chylomicrons	Unknown: possibly facilitates transfer of other apos between HDL and chylomicrons
Apo B48	264,000	Chylomicrons	Necessary for assembly and secretion of chylomicrons from the small intestine
Apo B100	540,000	VLDL, IDL, LDL	Necessary for assembly and secretion of VLDL from the liver; structural protein of VLDL, IDL, LDL; ligand for LDL receptor
Apo CI	6630	Chylomicrons, VLDL, IDL, HDL	May inhibit hepatic uptake of chylomicron and VLDL remnants
Apo CII	8900	Chylomicrons, VLDL, IDL, HDL	Activator of lipoprotein lipase
Apo CIII	8800	Chylomicrons, VLDL, IDL, HDL	Inhibitor of lipoprotein lipase; may inhibit hepatic uptake of chylomicron and VLDL remnants
Apo E	34,145	Chylomicrons, VLDL, IDL, HDL	Ligand for binding of several lipoproteins to the LDL receptor, to LRP, and possibly to a separate hepatic apo E receptor

and glycerol. The free fatty acids diffuse into adjacent tissues to be burned for energy or stored as fat. Most circulating LPL is associated with LDL. Insulin stimulates the synthesis and secretion of LPL, and reduced LPL activity in diabetes mellitus can lead to impaired triglyceride clearance. Homozygotes for mutations that impair LPL have severe hypertriglyceridemia that is usually manifested in childhood (type I hyperlipidemia), and heterozygotes for LPL defects have mild to moderate fasting hypertriglyceridemia but may have marked hypertriglyceridemia after consuming a high-fat meal. LPL is also expressed in macrophages, including cholesteryl ester–laden macrophages (foam cells) in atherosclerotic lesions. In this setting, secreted LPL may associate with LDL, causing retention of the lipoprotein in the subendothelial space.

Hepatic triglyceride lipase (HTGL), a member of a family of enzymes that includes LPL and pancreatic lipase, is synthesized in the liver and interacts with lipoproteins in hepatic sinusoids. HTGL can remove triglycerides from VLDL remnants (IDL), thus promoting the conversion of VLDL to LDL, and may also play a role in the clearance of chylomicron remnants and in the conversion of HDL_2 to HDL_3 in the liver by hydrolyzing the triglyceride and phospholipid in HDL (see below). Severe hypertriglyceridemia in individuals with genetic deficiency of HTGL is due to accumulation of chylomicron and VLDL remnants in plasma. In contrast to most patients with hypertriglyceridemia, however, subjects with HTGL deficiency have normal levels of HDL.

LCAT is synthesized in the liver and secreted into plasma where it is bound predominantly to HDL. LCAT mediates the transfer of linoleate from lecithin to free cholesterol on the surface of HDL to form cholesteryl esters that are then transferred to VLDL and eventually LDL. Apo AI is a cofactor for esterification of free cholesterol by LCAT.

Cholesteryl ester transfer protein (CETP) is synthesized primarily in the liver and circulates in plasma in association with HDL. CETP mediates the exchange of cholesteryl esters from HDL with triglyceride from chylomicrons or VLDL. LDL cholesteryl ester can also be exchanged with triglyceride from chylomicrons and VLDL, leading to small, dense LDL. Individuals who are homozygotes for mutations in the CETP gene have marked elevations of HDL cholesterol and apo AI, and heterozygotes for these mutations have slight elevations of HDL, indicating that CETP plays an important role in the removal of cholesteryl esters from HDL.

TRANSPORT OF EXOGENOUS (DIETARY) LIPIDS
Exogenous lipid transport in chylomicrons and chylomicron remnants is depicted in Fig. 341-1A. In western societies, where individuals ordinarily consume 50 to 100 g of fat and 0.5 g of cholesterol during three or four meals, transport of dietary fats is essentially continual. Normolipidemic individuals dispose of most dietary fat in the bloodstream within 8 h of the last meal, but some individuals with dyslipidemia, particularly those with elevated fasting levels of VLDL triglyceride, have measurable levels of intestinally derived lipoproteins in the circulation as long as 24 h after the last meal.

In the intestinal mucosa dietary triglyceride and cholesterol are incorporated into the core of nascent chylomicrons. The surface coat of the chylomicron is composed of phospholipid, free cholesterol, apo B48, apo AI, apo AII, and apo AIV. The chylomicron, essentially a fat droplet containing 80 to 95 percent triglycerides, is secreted into lacteals and transported to the circulation via the thoracic duct. In the plasma, apo C proteins are transferred to the chylomicron from HDL. Apo CII is required for hydrolysis of triglycerides by LPL on capillary endothelial cells in fat and muscle, and apo CIII may modulate core triglyceride hydrolysis by regulating LPL activity. The addition of apo E allows the chylomicron remnant to bind to hepatic LDL receptors and/or LRP after the triglyceride core has been hydrolyzed and after apo CII and apo CIII have recirculated back to HDL. As a consequence, dietary triglyceride is delivered to adipocytes and muscle cells as fatty acids, and dietary cholesterol is taken up by the liver where it can be used for bile acid formation, incorporated into membranes, resecreted

as lipoprotein cholesterol back into the circulation, or excreted as cholesterol into bile. Dietary cholesterol also regulates endogenous hepatic cholesterol synthesis.

Abnormal transport and metabolism of chylomicrons may predispose to atherosclerosis, and postprandial hyperlipidemia may be a risk

FIGURE 341-1 *A.* Transport of endogenous hepatic lipids via VLDL, IDL, and LDL. Note the relative and absolute changes in apoproteins, other than apo B100, as VLDL is converted to IDL and LDL. The sites of action of the two lipases, LPL and HTGL, are denoted as well, although the role of HTGL has not been completely defined. *B.* A schematic depiction of the transport of exogenously derived lipids from the intestine to peripheral tissues and liver via the chylomicron system. The cyclic movement of several apoproteins between HDL and chylomicrons is represented also. *C.* Simplified representation of HDL metabolism and the role of HDL in reverse cholesterol transport. Free cholesterol is accepted from peripheral tissues by HDL_3 and, after esterification, may be transferred to apo B100 lipoproteins. Cholesteryl ester also may be delivered to the liver by HDL itself. The significance of each of the three possible transport systems for cholesterol in overall reverse cholesterol transport is unknown. CETP, cholesteryl ester transfer protein; FFA, free fatty acids; HDL, high-density lipoprotein; HTGL, hepatic triglyceride lipase; IDL, intermediate-density lipoprotein; LDL, low-density lipoprotein; LPL, lipoprotein lipase; PL, phospholipase; TG, triglyceride; VLDL, very low density lipoprotein. *[From HN Ginsberg, Endocrinol Metab Clin North Am 19(2): 211, 1990.]*

factor for CHD. Chylomicrons and their remnants can be taken up by cells of the vessel wall, including monocyte-derived macrophages that migrate into the vessel wall from plasma. Cholesteryl ester accumulation by these macrophages transforms them into foam cells, the earliest cellular lesion of the atherosclerotic plaque. If the postprandial levels of chylomicrons or their remnants are elevated or if their removal from plasma is prolonged, cholesterol delivery to the artery wall may be increased.

TRANSPORT OF ENDOGENOUS LIPIDS The endogenous lipid transport system, which conveys lipids from the liver to peripheral tissues and from peripheral tissues back to the liver, can be separated into two subsystems: the apo B-100 lipoprotein system (VLDL, IDL, and LDL) and the apo AI lipoprotein system (HDL).

The apo B100 Lipoprotein System (See Fig. 341-1*B*) In the liver, triglycerides are made from fatty acids that are either taken up from plasma or synthesized de novo within the liver. Cholesterol can also be synthesized by the liver or delivered to the liver via chylomicron remnants. These core lipids are packaged together with apo B100 and phospholipids into VLDL and secreted into plasma where apos CI, CII, CIII, and E are added to the VLDL particles. Triglycerides make up the bulk of the VLDL (55 to 80 percent by weight), and the size of the VLDL is determined by the amount of triglyceride available. Hence, very large triglyceride-rich VLDL is secreted in situations where excess triglycerides are synthesized, such as in states of caloric excess, in diabetes mellitus, and with alcohol consumption. Small VLDL is secreted when fewer triglycerides are available. Although VLDL is normally the principal hepatic lipoprotein secreted by most individuals, VLDL and cholesteryl ester–enriched IDL and/or LDL-like particles may be secreted by the liver in individuals with combined hyperlipidemia (see below).

In the plasma, VLDL interacts with LPL, and as the triglycerides are hydrolyzed, VLDL particles become smaller and more dense and are converted to VLDL remnants (IDL). In contrast to chylomicron remnants, VLDL remnants can either enter the liver or give rise to LDL. Larger VLDL particles carry more triglycerides and are likely to be removed directly from plasma without being converted to LDL; apo E in the VLDL remnants is the ligand that binds the remnants to the LDL receptor for removal from the plasma. Smaller, more dense VLDL particles are efficiently converted to LDL, and apo E and HTGL play important roles in this process. Individuals with deficiency of either apo E2 or HTGL accumulate IDL in plasma. Apo B100 is the only protein remaining on the surface of the LDL particle.

The half-life of LDL in plasma is determined principally by the availability (or "activity") of LDL receptors. Most plasma LDL is taken up by the liver, and the remainder is delivered to peripheral tissues, including the adrenals and gonads, which utilize cholesterol as a precursor for steroid hormone synthesis. The adrenals have the highest concentration of LDL receptors per cell in the body. Overall, about 70 to 80 percent of LDL catabolism occurs via LDL receptors, and the remainder is removed by fluid endocytosis and possibly by other receptors.

The LDL receptor, a glycoprotein with a molecular mass of approximately 160 kDa, is present on the surfaces of nearly all cells in the body. Goldstein and Brown characterized the molecular genetics and cell biology of the LDL receptor and defined its role in cholesterol metabolism by showing that cholesterol delivered to the cytoplasm by LDL regulates both the rate of cholesterol synthesis in the liver and the number of LDL receptors on the surface of hepatocytes. These feedback mechanisms allow cells to maintain cholesterol homeostasis. While the LDL receptor is a major factor in determining plasma LDL cholesterol levels, the rates of entry of VLDL into plasma and the efficiency with which VLDL is converted to LDL also influence steady-state LDL concentrations in plasma.

Increased levels of plasma LDL cholesterol and apo B100 are risk factors for atherosclerosis. Normal LDL does not cause foam cell formation when incubated with cultured macrophages or smooth-muscle cells, but when LDL undergoes lipid peroxidation it becomes a ligand for an alternative, scavenger receptor pathway. Scavenger receptors are present on endothelial cells and macrophages, and uptake

of modified (oxidized) lipoproteins by these receptors in macrophages results in formation of cholesterol-laden foam cells. In addition to inducing foam cell formation, oxidized LDL acts in the vessel wall to stimulate the secretion of cytokines and growth factors by endothelial cells, smooth-muscle cells, and monocyte-derived macrophages. The consequence is recruitment of more monocytes to the lesion and proliferation of smooth-muscle cells, which synthesize and secrete increased amounts of extracellular matrix, such as collagen. The critical role of LDL in atherosclerosis has been confirmed in genetically altered mice. Although mice are normally resistant to atherosclerosis, increased plasma levels of remnant lipoproteins or LDL lead to atherosclerosis in this species.

The role of VLDL in atherogenesis is uncertain. The major reason for this uncertainty derives from the inverse relationship between elevated levels of triglyceride-rich lipoproteins and reduced levels of the antiatherogenic HDL cholesterol, and it is possible that hypertriglyceridemia may not be directly atherogenic but the surrogate of other lipoprotein abnormalities. Hence, if postprandial hyperlipidemia is a risk factor for CHD, individuals who have normal fasting plasma triglyceride levels but develop postprandial hypertriglyceridemia after consumption of a fat load would be misclassified as normal in studies in which only fasting blood samples are analyzed. It is clear that cholesteryl ester–enriched VLDL, isolated from cholesterol-fed animals, can be taken up by receptors on macrophages and smooth-muscle cells and cause foam cell formation. These cholesteryl ester–rich VLDL are enriched in apo E and are probably representative of VLDL remnants. Thus, the risk of atherosclerosis from hypertriglyceridemia and elevated VLDL levels may be determined by the level of cholesteryl ester–enriched VLDL remnants within the plasma VLDL. The atherogenic potential of IDL is probably similar to that of VLDL remnants.

Apo AI–Containing Lipoproteins (See Fig. 341-1*C*) In contrast to atherogenic apo B lipoproteins, the apo AI–containing HDL appear to be antiatherogenic. In fact, in some studies, HDL cholesterol levels are as strong an indicator of protection from CHD as LDL cholesterol levels are an indicator of risk. Although a great deal is known about the HDL transport system, the mechanism by which these lipoproteins protect against atherosclerosis is poorly defined.

HDL particles are formed in plasma from the coalescence of individual phospholipid-apolipoprotein complexes. Apo AI appears to be the crucial, structural apoprotein for HDL, and apo AI/phospholipid complexes probably fuse with other phospholipid vesicles containing apo AII and apo AIV to form the various types of HDL. The C apoproteins can be added to HDL after their secretion as phospholipid complexes or by transfer from triglyceride-rich lipoproteins. These small, cholesterol-poor nascent HDL particles are heterogeneous in size and content and are referred to as HDL_3. Free cholesterol is transferred from cell membranes to HDL_3 and converted by LCAT to cholesteryl ester, which moves into the core of the particle. Formation of cholesteryl ester increases the capacity of the HDL_3 to accept more free cholesterol and enlarge to form the more buoyant class of HDL particles termed HDL_2. HDL_2 can be metabolized by two pathways: (1) cholesteryl esters can be transferred from HDL_2 to apo B lipoproteins or cells, or (2) the entire HDL_2 particle can be removed from plasma. The transfer of cholesteryl ester from HDL to triglyceride-rich, apo B lipoproteins (chylomicrons and VLDL in the fed and fasted states, respectively) is mediated by CETP. Triglyceride is transferred to HDL in this process and is a substrate for lipolysis by LPL and/or HTGL. As a result, HDL_2 is converted back into HDL_3. HDL-mediated reverse cholesterol transport (from peripheral tissues to the liver) is thought to be the primary mechanism by which HDL protects against atherosclerosis. When the apo B lipoproteins are removed by the liver, reverse cholesterol transfer is complete. HDL cholesteryl ester may also be transferred selectively to cells via interaction of HDL with cell membranes. Alternatively, the subset of HDL particles that contains apo E can be taken up in toto via LDL receptors or LRP.

In rare cases low plasma HDL is due to a genetic deficiency of one of the structural components of HDL (such as apo AI), but low HDL cholesterol levels are usually the secondary consequence of increased plasma levels of VLDL and IDL (or chylomicrons and their remnants). Low levels of HDL cholesterol and apo AI may increase atherosclerosis risk by any of several mechanisms. HDL could remove cholesterol from foam cells in atherosclerotic lesions or protect LDL from oxidative-modification. Alternatively, the atherosclerotic risk of low HDL may be due to the commonly associated elevations of apo B–containing lipoproteins, which both accept HDL cholesteryl ester and deliver cholesteryl esters to the vessel wall.

THE HYPERLIPOPROTEINEMIAS (See Table 341-3)

HYPERCHOLESTEROLEMIA Elevated levels of fasting plasma total cholesterol in the presence of normal levels of triglycerides are almost always associated with increased concentrations of plasma LDL cholesterol (type IIa), since LDL carries about 65 to 75 percent of total plasma cholesterol. The rare patient with markedly elevated HDL cholesterol may also have increased plasma total cholesterol levels. Elevations of LDL cholesterol can result from single-gene defects, polygenic disorders, and secondary effects of other disease states.

Familial Hypercholesterolemia FH is a codominant genetic disorder that occurs in the heterozygous form in approximately 1 in 500 individuals. FH is due to mutations in the gene for the LDL receptor and is genetically heterogeneous, more than 200 different mutations in the gene having been described. Plasma levels of total and LDL cholesterol are elevated at birth and remain so throughout life. In untreated adults, total cholesterol levels range from 7 to 13 mmol/L (275 to 500 mg/dL). Plasma triglyceride levels are typically normal, and HDL cholesterol levels are normal or reduced. As would be expected with a decreased number of LDL receptors, the fractional clearance of LDL apo B is decreased. LDL production is increased because more VLDL and more IDL are secreted by the liver and more IDL particles are converted to LDL rather than taken up by the hepatic LDL receptors. *Tendon xanthomas*, which are due to both intracellular and extracellular deposits of cholesterol, most commonly involve the Achilles tendons and the extensor tendons of the knuckles and are found in about 75 percent of adults with FH. *Tuberous xanthomas*, which are softer, painless nodules on the elbows and buttocks, and *xanthelasmas*, which are barely elevated deposits of cholesterol on the eyelids, are common in heterozygous FH. In men CHD develops by the fourth decade of life (or earlier).

The homozygous form of FH occurs in one out of 1 million individuals and is associated with plasma cholesterol levels >13 mmol/L (>500 mg/dL), large xanthelesmas, and prominent tendon and planar xanthomas. These individuals have an aggressive, premature CHD that can be manifested in childhood.

Familial Defective Apo B100 This autosomal dominant disorder is a phenocopy of FH and is due to a missense mutation at amino acid 3500 that reduces the affinity of LDL for the LDL receptor and thus impairs LDL catabolism. The prevalence and manifestations of both the heterozygous and homozygous forms are similar to those produced by mutations of the LDL receptor.

Polygenic Hypercholesterolemia Most moderate hypercholesterolemia [plasma cholesterol levels between 6.5 and 9 mmol/L (240 and 350 mg/dL)] is polygenic in origin. Multiple genes interact with environmental factors to contribute to the hypercholesterolemia, and both overproduction and reduced catabolism of LDL are thought to play roles in the pathophysiology. The severity is probably affected by the consumption of saturated fat and cholesterol, by age, and by the level of physical activity. Plasma triglyceride and HDL cholesterol levels are usually normal. Tendon xanthomas are not present. Genes involved in cholesterol and bile acid metabolism may be involved in the pathogenesis.

HYPERTRIGLYCERIDEMIA The diagnosis of hypertriglyceridemia is made by determining levels of plasma lipids after an overnight fast. Because of the less certain association of triglycerides with CHD (compared to LDL cholesterol), plasma concentrations

Table 341-3

Characteristics of Common Hyperlipidemias

| Lipid Phenotype | Plasma Lipid Levels, mmol/L (mg/dL) | Lipoproteins | | Clinical Signs |
		Elevated	Phenotype	
ISOLATED HYPERCHOLESTEROLEMIA				
Familial hypercholesterolemia	Heterozygotes: total chol = 7–13 (275–500)	LDL	IIa	Usually develop xanthomas in adulthood and vascular disease at 30–50 years
	Homozygotes: total chol > 13 (>500)	LDL	IIa	Usually develop xanthomas and vascular disease in childhood
Familial defective apo B100	Heterozygotes: total chol = 7–13 (275–500)	LDL	IIa	
Polygenic hypercholesterolemia	Total chol = 6.5–9.0 (250–350)	LDL	IIa	Usually asymptomatic until vascular disease develops; no xanthomas
ISOLATED HYPERTRIGLYCERIDEMIA				
Familial hypertriglyceridemia	TG = 2.8–8.5 (250–750) (plasma may be cloudy)	VLDL	IV	Asymptomatic; may be associated with increased risk of vascular disease
Familial lipoprotein lipase deficiency	TG > 8.5 (>750) (plasma may be milky)	Chylomicrons	I, V	May be asymptomatic; may be associated with pancreatitis, abdominal pain, hepatosplenomegaly
Familial apo CII deficiency	TG > 8.5 (>750) (plasma may be milky)	Chylomicrons	I, V	As above
HYPERTRIGLYCERIDEMIA AND HYPERCHOLESTEROLEMIA				
Combined hyperlipidemia	TG = 2.8–8.5 (250–750) Total chol = 6.5–13.0 (250–500)	VLDL, LDL	IIb	Usually asymptomatic until vascular disease develops; familial form may also present as isolated high TG or an isolated high LDL cholesterol
Dysbetalipoproteinemia	TG = 2.8–5.6 (250–500) Total chol = 6.5–13.0 (250–500)	VLDL, IDL; LDL normal	III	Usually asymptomatic until vascular disease develops; may have palmar or tuboeruptive xanthoma

NOTE: total chol, the sum of free and esterified cholesterol; LDL, low-density lipoprotein; TG, triglycerides; VLDL, very low density lipoproteins; IDL, intermediate-density lipoprotein.

greater than the 90th or 95th percentile for age and sex have been used to define hypertriglyceridemia. Isolated elevations of plasma triglycerides can be due to increased levels of VLDL (type IV) or combinations of VLDL and chylomicrons (type V). Rarely, only chylomicron levels are elevated (type I). Plasma is usually clear when triglyceride levels are <4.5 mmol/L (<400 mg/dL) and becomes cloudy when levels are higher and VLDL (and/or chylomicron) particles become large enough to diffuse light. When chylomicrons are present, a creamy layer floats to the top of plasma after storage in the cold for several hours. Tendon xanthomas and xanthelasma do not occur with isolated hypertriglyceridemia, but eruptive xanthomas, small orange-red papules, can appear on the trunk and extremities when triglyceride levels are >11 mmol/L (>1000 mg/dL) (i.e., when chylomicronemia is present). At these high levels of triglycerides, the retinal vessels can appear to be orange-yellow in color (lipemia retinalis). Pancreatitis is the major risk associated with plasma triglyceride concentrations >11 mmol/L (>1000 mg/dL).

Elevations in plasma triglycerides are usually associated with increased synthesis and secretion of VLDL triglycerides by the liver. Hepatic triglyceride synthesis is regulated by substrate flow (the availability of free fatty acids), energy balance (the level of glycogen stores in the liver), and hormonal status (the balance between insulin and glucagon). Obesity, excessive consumption of simple sugars and saturated fats, inactivity, alcohol consumption, and insulin resistance are commonly associated with hypertriglyceridemia. In most of these situations, increased free fatty acid flux from adipose tissue to the liver stimulates the assembly and secretion of VLDL. When VLDL triglyceride levels are markedly elevated [>11 mmol/L (>1000 mg/dL)], LPL may be saturated so that even if there is no underlying genetic disorder an acquired LPL deficiency develops during the postprandial period. The addition of chylomicrons to the circulation may cause dramatic increases in plasma triglycerides.

Familial Hypertriglyceridemia Familial hypertriglyceridemia appears to be transmitted as an autosomal dominant disorder, but the underlying mutation(s) have not been identified. The pathophysiology is complex; both reduced catabolism of triglyceride-rich lipoproteins and overproduction of VLDL have been reported. Elevated levels of fasting plasma triglycerides in the range of 2.3 to 8.5 mmol/L (200 to 750 mg/dL) are usually associated with increased levels of VLDL triglycerides only. When VLDL triglyceride levels are markedly elevated (regardless of etiology), chylomicron triglycerides can also be present, even after a 14-h fast. This disorder does not appear to increase risk for CHD, either because large triglyceride-rich lipoproteins are not atherogenic or because only normal amounts of LDL can be generated.

Familial Lipoprotein Lipase Deficiency This autosomal recessive disorder is due to the impairment or absence of LPL, as a consequence of which chylomicrons accumulate to massive levels in plasma. Manifestations begin in infancy and include pancreatitis, eruptive xanthomas, hepatomegaly, splenomegaly, foam cell infiltration of the bone marrow, and, when the level of triglycerides is greater than 11 mmol/L (1000 mg/dL), lipemia retinalis. Atherosclerosis is not accelerated. The diagnosis is suspected by finding a layer of cream (chylomicrons) at the top of plasma that has incubated overnight at 4°C and confirmed by demonstrating that LPL levels in plasma do not increase after the administration of heparin (which normally releases LPL from endothelial surfaces). Manifestations recede dramatically when patients are placed on fat-free diets.

LPL levels are within the normal range in most patients with moderate hypertriglyceridemia [2.8 to 5.6 mmol/L (250 to 500 mg/dL)], but heterozygous mutations in the LPL gene are present in 5 to 10 percent of hypertriglyceridemic individuals; LPL activity may be reduced by 20 to 50 percent in these heterozygotes.

Familial Apoprotein CII Deficiency This rare autosomal recessive disorder causes a functional deficiency of LPL and clinical manifestations that are similar to those of familial LPL deficiency. Deficiency of apoprotein CII impairs hydrolysis of chylomicrons and VLDL so that either or both lipoproteins accumulate in blood. The diagnosis is suspected in children or adults with recurrent attacks of pancreatitis and confirmed by demonstrating absence of apo CII on

gel electrophoresis and demonstrating that the transfusion of plasma (which contains abundant apo CII) causes a dramatic fall in plasma triglycerides. Heterozygotes have half normal levels of apo CII, may have mild elevations of triglycerides, and are asymptomatic. Dietary fat restriction should be life-long.

Hepatic Lipase Deficiency Total deficiency of HTGL is a rare autosomal recessive disorder that impairs the final catabolism and/or remodeling of small VLDL and IDL. Subjects with HTGL deficiency often have elevated levels of VLDL remnants, and HDL_2 levels may be elevated since HTGL participates in the conversion of HDL_2 to HDL_3. HTGL activity is frequently elevated in hypertriglyceridemic subjects, but the meaning of this association is unclear.

HYPERCHOLESTEROLEMIA WITH HYPERTRIGLYCERIDEMIA Concomitant hypercholesterolemia and hypertriglyceridemia occurs in two disorders.

Familial Combined Hyperlipidemia (FCHL) FCHL is inherited as an autosomal dominant disorder, and probands (the initial case discovered within a family) may have combined hyperlipidemia, isolated hypertriglyceridemia, or isolated elevated levels of LDL cholesterol. The diagnosis requires documentation at some time of combined hyperlipidemia in the proband or, if the proband has isolated hypercholesterolemia or hypertriglyceridemia, the various lipid phenotypes in first-degree relatives at risk. In affected individuals the lipoprotein phenotype may change with time. The underlying defect in this disorder is not known, although mutations or polymorphisms in the gene for LPL and in the gene cluster for apo AI, apo CIII, and apo AIV may contribute to the disorder in some families. Insulin resistance is present in many individuals with FCHL; the link may be via increased free fatty acid flux driving assembly and secretion of apo B100 lipoproteins.

FCHL is associated with increased secretion of VLDL particles, as determined by the flux of VLDL apo B. The lipoprotein patterns associated with the disorder are most likely determined by genetic polymorphisms in genes that regulate the metabolism of VLDL. For example, if the affected individual also has a defect in LPL, hypertriglyceridemia will be present. Since the hydrolysis of VLDL triglycerides also regulates the generation of LDL in plasma, individuals with FCHL who have inefficient catabolism of VLDL may have reduced levels of LDL cholesterol and high VLDL cholesterol. Finally, individuals with FCHL who synthesize normal quantities of triglycerides and secrete VLDL that carries normal amounts of triglyceride generate increased numbers of LDL particles and present with isolated elevations of plasma LDL cholesterol. These variations in VLDL catabolism, together with additional genetic heterogeneity and environmental variability, are the basis for the variable phenotype in this disorder. FCHL may occur in as many as 0.5 to 1.0 percent of Americans and is the most common familial lipid disorder in survivors of myocardial infarction. The increased risk for atherosclerosis is due to the presence of increased numbers of small, atherogenic VLDL and the conversion of VLDL to the more atherogenic IDL and LDL. Subjects with FCHL usually have clear plasma and do not have xanthomas or xanthelasma.

Dysbetalipoproteinemia This rare disorder affects 1 in 10,000 persons and is due to homozygosity for apo E2, the binding-defective form of apo E. Because apo E plays a crucial role in the catabolism of chylomicron and VLDL remnants, affected individuals have elevations in both VLDL triglyceride and VLDL cholesterol, and chylomicron remnants are present in fasting plasma. The ratio of total cholesterol to triglyceride approximates 1.0 and the ratio of VLDL cholesterol to triglyceride is greater than 0.25. LDL and HDL cholesterol levels are usually low. Although 1 percent of the population is homozygous for apo E2, most have normal plasma triglyceride and cholesterol levels. Thus, a second defect in lipid metabolism must be present in the 0.01 percent of individuals with dysbetalipoproteinemia. These individuals can have tuberous xanthomas and deposits of cholesterol in the palmar creases (striae palmaris); the latter, appearing as yellow-orange lines, are specific for dysbetalipoproteinemia. Risk for athero-sclerosis and its complications is increased, with onset in the fourth and fifth decades. The incidence of peripheral vascular disease is higher than in familial hypercholesterolemia.

REDUCED HDL CHOLESTEROL Low levels of HDL cho-lesterol can be defined as <0.9 mmol/L (<35 mg/dL) in men and <1 to 1.2 mmol/L (<40 to 45 mg/dL) in women. Low concentrations of HDL cholesterol are usually associated with coexistent hypertriglyc-eridemia, although "primary hypoalphalipoproteinemia" has been identified in both individuals and families. The relationship between hypertriglyceridemia and low HDL levels probably derives from (1) CETP-mediated transfer of cholesteryl ester from the core of HDL to VLDL; (2) shift of surface components, particularly phospholipids, apo C-II, and apo C-III, from HDL to VLDL; and (3) increased fractional catabolism of the cholesteryl ester–poor HDL that results from the first two processes. The complexity of the relationship be-tween HDL and triglyceride levels is highlighted by the fact that HDL levels do not return to normal when fasting plasma triglycerides are reduced in most persons with hypertriglyceridemia and low HDL cholesterol levels. Low HDL is clinically silent, and the plasma is usually clear (it can be cloudy or creamy if there is concomitant hypertriglyceridemia).

Primary hypoalphalipoproteinemia refers to the state where HDL cholesterol concentrations are markedly reduced but plasma triglyc-eride concentrations are normal. Although this disorder certainly exists,

many individuals with this phenotype have had hypertriglyceridemia in the past or have an older (or more obese) first-degree relative who has both low HDL and increased triglyceride levels. Hence, both family studies and long-term follow-up may be required to identify individuals with primary reductions in HDL cholesterol. Rare muta-tions have been described in the apo AI gene that lead to reductions in apo AI synthesis or increases in catabolism. One mutation that is common in Italy, apo AI-Milano, is associated with a high fractional clearance rate of apo AI but is not associated with increased risk for atherosclerosis.

Some rare genetic disorders of lipid metabolism are summarized in Table 341-4.

SECONDARY CAUSES OF HYPERLIPOPROTEINEMIA
(See Table 341-5) **Diabetes Mellitus** Diabetes can affect lipid and lipoprotein metabolism through several mechanisms. In insulin-depen-dent diabetes mellitus (IDDM), plasma lipids are usually normal when control of diabetes with insulin is adequate. In diabetic ketoacidosis, hypertriglyceridemia can be severe due to increases in both VLDL and chylomicrons; these abnormalities are associated with overproduc-tion of VLDL and LPL deficiency secondary to insulinopenia and usually improve with tight control of the diabetes. In non-insulin-dependent diabetes mellitus (NIDDM), insulin resistance and obesity combine to cause mild to moderate hypertriglyceridemia and low HDL cholesterol levels. In general, this pattern of dyslipidemia is due to overproduction of VLDL. LDL cholesterol is usually normal in NIDDM, although the LDL are small, dense, and perhaps more athero-genic. Treatment of NIDDM and weight reduction improve but usually do not cure the dyslipidemia, particularly the low HDL cholesterol

Table 341-4

Rare Genetic Disorders of Lipid Metabolism

Disorder	Typical Age of Onset	Plasma Lipid Abnormality	Major Clinical Manifestations	Pathogenesis	Treatment
Hypobetalipopro-teinemia, Abetalipoproteinemia	Early childhood	Very low cholesterol and triglyceride levels	Malabsorption of fat, ataxia, neuropathy, retinitis pigmentosa, acanthocytosis	Defective synthesis or secretion of apopro-tein B leads to low or absent chylomicrons, VLDL, and LDL in plasma	Vitamin E
Tangier disease	Childhood	Low cholesterol; tri-glycerides, normal to slightly elevated	Large orange tonsils, corneal opacities, re-lapsing polyneu-ropathy No premature athero-sclerosis	Abnormal cholesterol uptake into and/or efflux from macro-phages; increased Apo AI clearance	None
Lecithin:cholesterol acyltransferase (LCAT) deficiency (fish-eye disease)	Young adult	Total plasma choles-terol level variable with marked decrease in esterified choles-terol and increase in unesterified choles-terol; elevated VLDL level; structure of all lipoproteins is ab-normal	Corneal opacities, he-molytic anemia, renal insufficiency, prema-ture atherosclerosis	Decreased LCAT activ-ity in plasma leads to accumulation of ex-cess unesterified cho-lesterol in plasma and body tissues	Fat-restricted diet, kidney trans-plantation
Cerebrotendinous xanthomatosis	Young adult	None	Progressive cerebellar ataxia, dementia and spinal cord paresis, subnormal intelli-gence, tendon xantho-mas, cataracts	Defective synthesis of primary bile acids in liver leads to in-creased hepatic synthe-sis of cholesterol and cholestanol, which ac-cumulate in brain, ten-dons, and other tissues	None
Sitosterolemia	Childhood	Elevated levels of plant sterols in plasma, elevated or normal levels of cho-lesterol, normal tri-glyceride levels	Tendon xanthomas	Increased intestinal ab-sorption of dietary cho-lesterol, sitosterol, and other plant sterols with accumulation in plasma and tendons	Diet low in plant sterols and cho-lesterol

NOTE: VLDL, very low density lipoprotein; LDL, low-density lipoprotein; HDL, high-density lipoprotein; LCAT, lecithin:cholesterol acyltransferase.

SOURCE: Modified from MS Brown and JL Goldstein in *Harrison's Principles of Internal Medicine,* 13th ed, KJ Isselbacher et al (eds), New York, McGraw-Hill, 1994.

levels. Therapy of hyperlipidemia should not be delayed in patients with NIDDM, who are at increased risk for CHD.

Hypothyroidism Hypothyroidism accounts for about 2 percent of all cases of hyperlipidemia and is second only to diabetes mellitus as a cause of secondary hyperlipidemia. Levels of LDL cholesterol can be elevated, even in patients with subclinical disease in whom thyroid-stimulating hormone (TSH) levels are elevated but other thyroid function tests are normal. Hypertriglyceridemia can occur if obesity is also present. Hypothyroidism is also associated with increased levels of HDL cholesterol, probably because of reduced HTGL activity. Correction of hypothyroidism reverses the lipid abnormalities.

Renal Disease Renal disease causes a wide range of lipid abnormalities. The nephrotic syndrome can be accompanied by elevations in LDL, VLDL, or both, the severity of the hyperlipidemia correlating with the degree of hypoproteinemia. Renal failure is associated with hypertriglyceridemia and low HDL cholesterol concentrations.

Ethanol The metabolism of ethanol enhances the level of NADH in the liver, which in turn stimulates the synthesis of fatty acids and their incorporation into triglycerides. Moderate ethanol consumption raises plasma VLDL levels, with the degree of elevation dependent on the baseline level. Severe hypertriglyceridemia and pancreatitis usually develop on the background of a genetic hyperlipidemia and heavy alcohol intake. Because ethanol also stimulates the synthesis of apo AI and inhibits CETP, ethanol-associated hypertriglyceridemia is usually accompanied by normal or elevated levels of HDL cholesterol.

Liver Disease Primary biliary cirrhosis and extrahepatic biliary obstruction can cause hypercholesterolemia and elevated levels of plasma phospholipids associated with elevated levels of an abnormal lipoprotein (lipoprotein X) (see Chap. 293). Severe liver injury often leads to a decrease in levels of both cholesterol and triglyceride. Acute hepatitis can cause elevated levels of VLDL and impairment of LCAT formation.

DIAGNOSIS Although the initial indication of an abnormality in lipoprotein metabolism is via blood measurements of triglyceride and cholesterol, the disorders are due to abnormalities of specific lipoproteins. Thus, lipoprotein analysis should assess VLDL, LDL, and HDL levels. Direct measurements of plasma LDL require laborious centrifugation techniques, but LDL cholesterol concentrations can be

estimated indirectly in individuals with triglyceride levels <4.5 mmol/L (<400 mg/dL) by subtracting the HDL and VLDL cholesterol from the total plasma cholesterol. HDL cholesterol is determined after chemical precipitation of VLDL and LDL. VLDL cholesterol is estimated to be the plasma triglyceride level divided by five. Therefore

$$\text{LDL cholesterol} = \text{total cholesterol} - (\text{HDL} + \text{triglycerides}/5)$$

where all values are measured in milligrams per deciliter.

In subjects with triglyceride levels >4.5 mmol/L (>400 mg/dL), the ratio of triglyceride to cholesterol in VLDL is >5 so this equation cannot be used to calculate the plasma LDL cholesterol level. The other disorder that is not detected with this method is dysbetalipoproteinemia, because the ratio of triglyceride to cholesterol in the VLDL is <<5. In these two situations, direct measurement of LDL cholesterol must be performed in ultracentrifuged plasma.

Since plasma triglyceride levels rise and since both HDL and LDL cholesterol levels fall modestly (due to the action of CETP) after a fat-containing meal, it is preferable to measure plasma lipids after a 12-h fast. Since measuring only cholesterol levels will not detect individuals with isolated low HDL, screening for CHD should include measurement of HDL. Since serum lipid levels vary from day to day, at least two to three measurements should be made days or weeks apart before initiating therapy. Some experts advocate the use of total cholesterol/HDL ratios as a better assessment of individual risk, a reasonable approach provided both the patient and physician are aware that the treatment goal is to reduce LDL. In addition, physicians must be aware of the absolute values of each because rare patients with very high or very low levels of both LDL and HDL have ratios that are not interpretable on the basis of population studies. Although research and clinical laboratories often offer measurements of individual apoproteins, e.g., apo B-100 and apo AI, this information is generally not helpful in decision-making. Lipoprotein electrophoresis is also not useful except for the diagnosis of dysbetalipoproteinemia, which otherwise requires ultracentrifugation methods. Genotyping of apo E is available in some laboratories and is helpful in the diagnosis of dysbetalipoproteinemia (although rarely the disorder can be due to other defects in the apo E gene).

Both LDL and HDL cholesterol levels are temporarily decreased for several weeks after myocardial infarction or acute inflammatory states but can be accurately measured if blood is obtained within 8 h of the event.

℞ **TREATMENT**

Elevated LDL Cholesterol Treatment can have either of two aims—primary prevention of the complications of atherosclerosis or secondary treatment after complications have occurred. The rationale for primary prevention is based on the large body of data linking elevated levels of LDL cholesterol with increased CHD risk and an impressive body of clinical and experimental data demonstrating that reducing LDL cholesterol slows progression and may actually induce regression of CHD. Both primary and secondary intervention trials indicate that total mortality can be reduced when the LDL cholesterol is lowered.

For primary prevention the National Cholesterol Education Program (NCEP) Adult Treatment Panel recommends aggressive therapy for patients with multiple risk factors. Risk factors include family history of premature CHD (below the age of 55 years in a male parent or sibling or below 65 in female relatives), hypertension (even if it is controlled with medications), cigarette smoking (>10 cigarettes per day), diabetes mellitus, and low HDL [<0.9 mmol/L (<35 mg/dL)]. In addition, since CHD is more prevalent in older individuals, age (men >45 years, women >55 years, or younger women with premature menopause without estrogen replacement) are also at risk. HDL cholesterol >1.6 mmol/L (>60 mg/dL) is a negative risk factor, i.e., one other risk factor can be negated by a high HDL cholesterol level.

Table 341-5

Secondary Causes of Lipoprotein Abnormalities

HYPERCHOLESTEROLEMIA

Hypothyroidism	Acute intermittent porphyria
Obstructive liver disease	Drugs: progestogens, cyclosporine,
Nephrotic syndrome	thiazides
Anorexia nervosa	

HYPERTRIGLYCERIDEMIA

Obesity	Pregnancy
Diabetes mellitus	Drugs: estrogen, isotretinoin, beta
Chronic renal failure	blockers, glucocorticoids, bile
Lipodystrophy	acid–binding resins, thiazides
Glycogen storage disease	Acute hepatitis
Alcohol	Systemic lupus erythematosus
Ileal bypass surgery	Monoclonal gammopathy: multiple
Stress	myeloma, lymphomas
Sepsis	

HYPOCHOLESTEROLEMIA

Malnutrition	Monoclonal gammopathy
Malabsorption	Chronic liver disease
Myeloproliferative diseases	
Chronic infectious diseases: AIDS,	
tuberculosis	

LOW HDL

Malnutrition	Beta blockers
Obesity	Anabolic steroids
Cigarette smoking	

NOTE: HDL, high-density lipoprotein.

Table 341-6

LDL Cholesterol Treatment Guidelines

	Levels of LDL for Beginning Therapy, mmol/L (mg/dL)		
	Diet	Drugs	Goal
No CHD and less than two risk factors	≥4.1(≥160)	≥4.9(≥190)	<4.1(<160)
No CHD but two or more risk factors	≥3.4(≥130)	≥4.1(≥160)	<3.4(<130)
Presence of CHD	>2.6(>100)	>3.4(>130)	<2.6(<100)

The NCEP guidelines are stringent for the secondary treatment of patients with CHD. Patients with CHD should be screened for lipid abnormalities during and after their initial diagnoses. A goal of lowering plasma LDL concentrations to <2.6 mmol/L (<100 mg/dL) is advocated for such individuals (Table 341-6).

ALTERATIONS IN LIFE-STYLE The typical American diet derives about 35 percent of its calories from fat (14 to 15 percent from saturated fat) and contains 400 to 500 mg/d of cholesterol. Individuals with hyperlipidemia should be encouraged to eat a diet lower in cholesterol and saturated fat. The NCEP Step 1 diet, which is recommended for all Americans above age 2, provides 30 percent of calories from fat, fewer than 10 percent calories from saturated fat, and less than 300 mg/d of cholesterol. Carbohydrate is the typical nutrient used to replace fat in patients with isolated hypercholesterolemia. In general, whole-milk dairy products, egg yolks, meats, palm oil, and coconut oil should be replaced with fresh fruits and vegetables, complex carbohydrates (especially whole-grain products), and

Table 341-7

The Two-Step Approach to Treating Hypercholesterolemia*

Nutrient	Step 1 Diet	Step 2 Diet
Total fat	<30% calories	<30% calories
Fatty acids		
Saturated	<10% calories	<7% calories
Polyunsaturated	≤10% calories	≤10% calories
Monounsaturated	10–15% calories	10–15% calories
Carbohydrates	50–60% calories	50–60% calories
Protein	10–20% calories	10–20% calories
Cholesterol	<300 mg/d	<200 mg/d

* Total calories: to achieve and maintain desirable body weight.

low-fat dairy products. Shellfish are low in fat content and, except for shrimp, also have low cholesterol levels; shrimp, in moderation, is acceptable. Portion size needs to be stressed; the protein and fat-rich portion of meat in a given meal should be less than 115 g (4 oz), the size of a deck of cards. Substitutions with any food low in saturated fat such as bran, nuts, and olive oil will have positive effects on LDL. Hydrogenation of vegetable oils increases the saturation of the fatty acids and is not advantageous. In particular, trans-fatty acids, mainly found in commercially hydrogenated vegetable oils, raise LDL and can lower HDL cholesterol levels. When further diet therapy is indicated, the NCEP Step 2 diet provide 30 percent calories as fat but fewer than 5 percent calories from saturated fat, and less than 200 mg/d of cholesterol. The NCEP recommendations for the Step 1 and Step 2 diets are presented in Table 341-7. (See also Chap. 77.) The response in LDL cholesterol upon changing from the average American diet to the Step 1 diet is a drop of 8 to 10 percent; an additional reduction of 5 to 7 percent can be achieved by moving to the Step 2 diet. There is, however, great individual variability in diet responsiveness, and several values should be obtained before judging efficacy of any diet treatment.

The decision as to how long diet therapy be attempted as the sole form of therapy should be based on the severity of the hyperlipidemia and the goals of treatment as determined by the risk factors for CHD. If a patient with CHD has only a modestly elevated LDL cholesterol level [i.e., <3.4 mmol/L (<130 mg/dL)] and the goal is an LDL cholesterol level <2.6 mmol/L (<100 mg/dL), a 4- to 6-week period of Step 1 diet therapy can precede the addition of drugs. If the patient is elderly, has no CHD, and has only one other risk factor besides a high LDL level, long-term diet therapy alone may be sufficient. In such a patient, moving to the Step 2 diet, which provides the same total fat but fewer than 5 percent of calories from saturated fat, can be useful. If, however, the LDL cholesterol is very high, if multiple risk factors are present, or if CHD is documented, drug therapy should be instituted along with diet therapy.

DRUG THERAPY (See Table 341-8) Three classes of lipid-lowering agents are recommended as first-line therapy against hypercholesterolemia: the bile acid sequestrants or –binding resins; niacin; and the 3-hydroxy-3-methylglutaryl-coenzyme A (HMG-CoA) reductase inhibitors. Fibric acid derivatives such as gemfibrozil are second-line agents for hypercholesterolemia and are most effective for lowering of triglycerides.

1. *Bile acid–binding resins.* The bile acid–binding resins cholestyramine and colestipol have been in use as lipid-lowering agents for almost three decades. These drugs interfere with reabsorption of bile acids in the intestine, resulting in a compensatory increase in bile acid synthesis and upregulation of LDL receptors in hepatocytes. The bile acid sequestrants are primary agents in the treatment

Table 341-8

Hypolipidemic Agents

Class	Mode of Action	Lipoprotein Class Affected	Dose
Bile acid–binding resins	Interrupts enterohepatic circulation of bile acids; ↑ Synthesis of new bile acids and LDL receptors	↓ LDL cholesterol 20–30% ↑ HDL cholesterol and triglycerides	Cholestyramine 8–12 g bid or tid Colestipol 10–15 g bid or tid
Nicotinic acid	↓ Synthesis of VLDL and LDL	↓ Triglycerides 25–85% ↓ VLDL cholesterol 25–35% ↓ LDL cholesterol 15–25% HDL may ↑	Niacin 50–100 mg tid initially then increase to 1.0–2.5 g tid
HMG-CoA reductase inhibitors	↓ Cholesterol synthesis ↑ LDL receptors	↓ LDL cholesterol 25–40% ↓ VLDL	Lovastatin 10–80 mg/d Pravastatin 10–40 mg/d Simvastatin 5–40 mg/d Fluvastatin 20–40 mg/d Atorvastatin 10–80 mg/d
Fibric acid derivatives	↑ LPL and ↑ triglyceride hydrolysis ↓ VLDL synthesis ↑ LDL catabolism	↓ Triglycerides 25–40% ↑ or ↓ LDL cholesterol ↑ HDL	Gemfibrozil 600 mg bid

NOTE: LDL, low-density lipoprotein; HMG-CoA, 3-hydroxy-3-methylglutaryl-coenzyme A; HDL, high-density lipoprotein; VLDL, very low density lipoprotein; LPL, lipoprotein lipase.

of patients with elevated levels of LDL cholesterol and normal triglycerides. Sequestrants produce dose-dependent decreases on the order of 15 to 25 percent in total cholesterol and of 20 to 35 percent in LDL cholesterol. The agents cause modest increases in HDL cholesterol. A limitation of the sequestrants is their tendency to raise triglyceride levels through compensatory increases in hepatic synthesis of VLDL, and they should not be given to hypertriglyceridemic individuals. Bile acid–binding resins are efficacious and safe and are recommended for young adult men and premenopausal women with moderate cholesterol elevations. Patient compliance is low, in part because of the need to dissolve these powdered agents in fluid; the availability of colestipol as a tablet may alleviate this problem. Gastrointestinal side effects include constipation, bloating, and gas.

2. *Niacin.* The mechanism of action of niacin is not fully understood, but it appears to inhibit the secretion of lipoproteins containing apo B100 from the liver. Niacin decreases both total and LDL cholesterol approximately 15 to 25 percent, reduces VLDL levels by 25 to 35 percent, and raises HDL cholesterol levels by as much as 15 to 25 percent. Thus, on the basis of its effects on three major lipoproteins, VLDL, LDL, and HDL, niacin would appear to be an optimal agent. Efficacy of monotherapy was confirmed in a long-term secondary prevention trial in which niacin significantly reduced the incidence of myocardial infarction. An even longer-term follow-up of that study (15 years total) showed an 11 percent decrease in all-cause mortality among patients randomized to niacin. Like the bile acid–binding resins, niacin is safe, having been in use for almost 30 years. Niacin, however, has unpleasant side effects that limit patient acceptability, including uncomfortable and potentially dose-limiting cutaneous flushing with or without pruritus. However, the cutaneous symptoms tend to subside after several weeks and may be minimized by initiating therapy at low doses. Less common adverse effects include elevations of liver enzymes, gastrointestinal distress, impaired glucose tolerance, and elevated serum uric acid levels with or without gouty arthritis. Liver enzymes may be elevated in 3 to 5 percent of patients on full doses of niacin (>2 g/d).

3. *HMG-CoA reductase inhibitors.* HMG-CoA reductase inhibitors, which include lovastatin, simvastatin, pravastatin, fluvastatin, and atorvastatin inhibit the rate-limiting step in hepatic cholesterol biosynthesis (the conversion of HMG-CoA to mevalonate), which causes a rise in LDL receptor levels in hepatocytes and enhanced receptor-mediated clearance of LDL cholesterol from the circulation. At usual doses, the HMG-CoA reductase inhibitors decrease total cholesterol by 20 to 30 percent and LDL cholesterol by 25 to 40 percent. Larger reductions may be achieved with higher doses. Treatment with reductase inhibitors often produces reductions in triglycerides of 10 to 20 percent, possibly due to reduced secretion of VLDL by the liver. HDL cholesterol levels rise about 5 to 10 percent. In comparison with other lipid-lowering agents, HMG-CoA reductase inhibitors are relatively free of side effects, which have been reported by fewer than 5 percent of patients. Mild, transient elevations in liver enzymes occur with all of the agents at the highest doses, but elevations in serum aminotransferases to more than three times the upper limits of normal occur in fewer than 2 percent of patients. Therapy should be discontinued when elevations of this magnitude occur. A rare but potentially serious adverse effect of HMG-CoA reductase inhibitors is myopathy, with elevations of serum creatine phosphokinase (CPK) more than 10 times the upper limit of normal; this occurs in fewer than 1 percent of patients treated with reductase inhibitors alone but is more common (about 5 percent) when used in combination with gemfibrozil, niacin, or cyclosporine.

4. *Combination therapy.* Combinations of bile acid–binding resins and reductase inhibitors are effective for the treatment of severe, isolated elevations of LDL cholesterol. Combinations of either resins and niacin or reductase inhibitors and niacin are useful for the treatment of high LDL and low HDL cholesterol levels, although the latter combination carries an increased risk of myositis (2 to 3 percent). If triglyceride and LDL levels are both elevated (HDL is usually reduced as well), resins and niacin are an excellent combination, with resins and gemfibrozil as an alternative. The combination of a reductase inhibitor and gemfibrozil can be useful when LDL cholesterol is very high in the face of concomitant hypertriglyceridemia, but the risk of myositis (about 5 percent) must be considered. Combinations of reductase inhibitors with either niacin or gemfibrozil might best be reserved for patients with CHD and combined hyperlipidemia.

5. *LDL apheresis.* In patients with homozygous FH and in ordinary FH patients who respond poorly to diet and drug therapy or who cannot tolerate drugs, apheresis at 7- to 14-day intervals can cause profound lowering of LDL cholesterol levels. Diet and drug regimens are continued during treatment. The long-term efficacy/safety of such therapy is not established, but the therapy should be considered for patients with few therapeutic options.

High Triglycerides and Low HDL The evidence that treatment to reduce plasma triglyceride levels or increase levels of HDL cholesterol leads to long-term health benefits is less compelling than that for treatment of high LDL levels. There have been no intervention trials in which only increases in HDL cholesterol concentrations have been achieved. However, treatment of hypercholesterolemic patients with gemfibrozil led to a decrease in CHD events that was greater than that expected with the observed decreases in LDL. Beneficial effects of niacin have been attributed, in part, to its HDL-raising action as well as the lowering of triglycerides and LDL. Even with drugs that primarily

Side Effects	Contraindications	Drug Interactions	Combined Use with
Constipation, gastric discomfort, nausea, hemorrhoidal bleeding	Biliary track obstruction, gastric outlet obstruction, hypertriglyceridemia	↓ Absorption of phenylbutazone, phenobarbital, thyroid hormones, digitalis, warfarin, thiazide diuretics, some antibiotics	Nicotinic acid, HMG-CoA reductase inhibitors, gemfibrozil
Flushing, tachycardia, atrial arrhythmias, pruritus, dry skin, nausea, diarrhea, hyperuricemia, peptic ulcer disease, glucose intolerance, hepatic dysfunction	Peptic ulcer disease, cardiac arrhythmias, liver disease, gout, diabetes mellitus	Synergistic with ganglionic blocking agents	Bile acid–binding resins, HMG-CoA reductase inhibitors, gemfibrozil
Abnormal liver function, myositis	↑ Myositis in patients with renal failure and in patients on gemfibrozil, nicotinic acid, or cyclosporine	Gemfibrozil, ketoconazole, cyclosporine, warfarin, niacin	Bile acid–binding resins
↑ Lithogenicity of bile, nausea, abnormal liver functions, myositis	Hepatic or biliary disease; ↓ dose in renal insufficiency	↑ Anticoagulant activity of warfarin	Bile acid–binding resins

affect LDL cholesterol levels, such as bile acid–binding resins and HMG-CoA reductase inhibitors, some of the benefits achieved may be related to increases in HDL cholesterol levels.

Efforts should be made to reduce triglycerides when they are at levels that may precipitate pancreatitis. Thus, triglyceride levels >5.6 mmol/L (>500 mg/dL) are generally treated whereas lower levels [2.2 to 5.6 mmol/L (200 to 500 mg/dL)] are not treated unless other CHD risk factors are present.

ALTERATIONS IN LIFESTYLE (See above under "Hypercholesterolemia"). In patients with isolated elevations of triglyceride levels or with hypertriglyceridemia and high LDL cholesterol, weight reduction should be strongly encouraged if obesity is present. Also, fat intake should be decreased, but the concomitant increase in the intake of carbohydrate may raise triglyceride and lower HDL cholesterol levels. If this occurs, replacing some of the saturated fat with monounsaturated fat, which will not raise LDL cholesterol, may be valuable. Severe hypertriglyceridemia and hyperchylomicronemia require very low fat diets, avoidance of free sugars, and decreased alcohol intake. Patients with genetic LPL deficiency are instructed to prepare their food using medium-chain triglycerides, which are not incorporated into chylomicrons. Fish oils decrease triglyceride synthesis and in high doses may be used for severe hypertriglyceridemia.

DRUG THERAPY The recommendations for evaluating and treating hypertriglyceridemia focus on the associated LDL and HDL concentrations as guidelines for therapy. Thus, the overall risk profile can be used to set goals for LDL cholesterol, using a low HDL level (commonly associated with hypertriglyceridemia) as a concomitant major risk factor for atherosclerosis. However, when triglyceride levels are >5.6 mmol/L (>500 mg/dL), the risk of developing pancreatitis increases, and a direct focus on lowering triglycerides is recommended.

1. *Niacin.* Niacin is a first-line drug for hypertriglyceridemia. The positive and negative characteristics of niacin were outlined above, but it is relevant to note that since LDL cholesterol is the target of intervention in many patients with elevated plasma triglyceride levels, the potency of niacin against both triglycerides and LDL cholesterol makes it a top choice. The ability of niacin to raise HDL cholesterol further enhances its usefulness. Because of its propensity to worsen the control of blood sugar, niacin should be used with caution in patients with diabetes mellitus.

2. *Gemfibrozil.* The only fibric acid derivative widely used in the United States is gemfibrozil. The mechanism of action of the fibrates is only partially understood, but they appear to stimulate the enzyme LPL, probably the basis for much of the triglyceride-lowering effect. However, fibrates may also reduce VLDL triglyceride entry into plasma and reduce synthesis of apo CIII by impairing gene transcription, which might improve LPL-induced lipolysis or reduce VLDL secretion. Stimulation of peroxisomal fatty acid oxidation by fibrates may also contribute to the triglyceride-lowering actions. In any event, gemfibrozil treatment is associated with 25 to 40 percent reductions in plasma triglyceride levels. Postprandial triglyceride levels, which are linked to fasting concentrations, are also reduced. Gemfibrozil and a low-fat diet are particularly useful in the treatment of dysbetalipoproteinemia and are the first line of therapy for this disorder except in postmenopausal women, who should initially be given estrogen replacement.

Significant increases in LDL cholesterol can accompany otherwise potentially beneficial falls in triglycerides and increases in HDL cholesterol during fibrate therapy. Such rises may require a change to another drug or addition of a second agent.

In the short term, these drugs are well tolerated, with mild gastrointestinal distress in the form of epigastric pain as the major side effect. Mild elevations of liver enzymes occur in 2 to 3 percent of patients but do not usually require cessation of treatment. Rarely, hepatitis can occur. Fibrates appear to make the bile more lithogenic, and long-term use is probably associated with a twofold increase in gallstone formation. Myopathy with myositis is a rare occurrence with the fibrates, alone or in combination. The long-term safety issues have been the source of controversy; in a meta-analysis of several studies in which fibrates were used, overall mortality was slightly increased despite reductions in CHD events and CHD deaths.

3. *Combination therapy.* (See above)

HYPOCHOLESTEROLEMIA

A low total cholesterol concentration [<2.6 mmol/L (<100 mg/dL)] in an adult can be due to rare hereditary traits or secondary to a number of diseases. As described earlier, mutations in the gene for apo B100 that disrupt synthesis or produce truncated forms of apo B100 are associated with hypobetalipoproteinemia. These mutations are inherited as codominant traits, and heterozygotes have plasma cholesterol levels in the range of 1.3 to 2.6 mmol/L (50 to 100 mg/dL), with reduced LDL cholesterol levels but normal plasma HDL cholesterol levels. Heterozygotes are asymptomatic, whereas hypolipoproteinemia homozygotes (or compound heterozygotes) have even lower total and LDL cholesterol concentrations and may have malabsorption of fats and fat-soluble vitamins similar to that in abetalipoproteinemia.

Abetalipoproteinemia (Table 341-4) is a rare, autosomal recessive disorder in which the microsomal triglyceride transfer protein (MTP) is absent because of mutations in the MTP gene. Individuals who are homozygous for this disorder have total cholesterol levels <1.3 mmol/L (<50 mg/dL) and essentially no VLDL, IDL, LDL, or chylomicrons. Because dietary fat as well as vitamins A and E are transported from the intestine in chylomicrons, these patients may have malabsorption of fat and fat-soluble vitamins. Vitamin E deficiency in infancy and early childhood can result in neurologic problems (see also Chap. 79). If vitamin replacement is adequate, individuals with abetalipoproteinemia can live normal, healthy lives.

Moderately low levels of total cholesterol may also be associated with extreme reductions in HDL cholesterol; as noted above, these are almost always secondary to mutations in the gene for apo AI and a lack of apo AI in plasma.

A number of systemic diseases can cause low cholesterol concentrations. Malnutrition, often associated with alcoholism or gastrointestinal disease, can cause low levels of total and LDL cholesterol. Patients with AIDS may have total cholesterol levels <2.1 mmol/L (<80 mg/dL), usually associated with severe wasting, diarrhea, and a poor prognosis. Several neoplasms, particularly those involving the hematopoietic system, are associated with hypocholesterolemia. Patients with acute and chronic myelogenous leukemia and myeloid metaplasia with splenomegaly can have severe reductions in both LDL and HDL levels. Other diseases with concomitant splenomegaly, including lipid storage diseases such as Gaucher's disease and Niemann-Pick disease, can cause very low LDL and HDL cholesterol concentrations due to increased lipoprotein catabolism.

See Chap. 36, Drugs used in the treatment of hyperlipoproteinemia, in Goodman & Gilman's The Pharmacological Basis of Therapeutics, 9th ed, New York, McGraw-Hill, 1996.

BIBLIOGRAPHY

FRUCHART JC, SHEPHERD J: *Human Plasma Lipoproteins: Clinical Biochemistry, Principles, Methods, Applications.* Berlin, Walter De Gruyter, 1989

GINSBERG HN: Treatment of hypertriglyceridemia, in *Lipoproteins and Coronary Artery Disease*, RA Kreisberg, JA Segrest (eds). Cambridge, MA, Blackwell Scientific, 1992, pp 331–356

GOLDBERG IJ: American College of Physicians Medical Knowledge Self-Assessment Program 10. Endocrinology and Metabolism Syllabus. Philadelphia, American College of Physicians, 1994, pp 1075–1079

GOLDSTEIN JL et al: Familial hypercholesterolemia, in *The Metabolic and Molecular Bases of Inherited Disease*, 7th ed, CR Scriver et al (eds). New York, McGraw-Hill, 1995, p 1981

GORDON BR et al: Treatment of refractory familial hypercholesterolemia by low-density lipoprotein apheresis using an automated dextran sulfate cellulose absorption system. Am J Cardiol 70:1010, 1992

HUNNINGHAKE D (ed): Lipid disorders. Med Clin North Am vol 78, no. 1, January 1994

REPORT OF THE NATIONAL CHOLESTEROL EDUCATION PROGRAM EXPERT PANEL ON DETECTION, EVALUATION AND TREATMENT OF HIGH BLOOD CHOLESTEROL IN ADULTS. Arch Intern Med 148:36, 1988
SUMMARY OF THE SECOND REPORT OF THE NATIONAL CHOLESTEROL EDUCATION PROGRAM EXPERT PANEL ON DETECTION, EVALUATION, AND TREATMENT OF HIGH BLOOD CHOLESTEROL IN ADULTS. JAMA 269:3015, 1993

CHAPTER 342
Hemochromatosis

2149

342 — HEMOCHROMATOSIS

Lawrie W. Powell, Kurt J. Isselbacher

DEFINITION   Hemochromatosis is a common disorder of iron storage in which inappropriate increase in intestinal iron absorption results in deposition of excessive amounts of iron in parenchymal cells with eventual tissue damage and impaired function of organs, especially the liver, pancreas, heart, and pituitary. The disease was termed *hemochromatosis* and the iron-storage pigment was called *hemosiderin* because it was believed that the pigment was derived from the blood. The terms *hemosiderosis* and *siderosis* are often used to describe the presence of stainable iron in tissues, but tissue iron must be quantified to assess body iron status (see below and Chap. 106). *Hemochromatosis* implies present or potentially severe progressive iron overload leading to fibrosis and organ failure. Cirrhosis of the liver, diabetes mellitus, arthritis, cardiomyopathy, and hypogonadotrophic hypogonadism are common manifestations. Although there is debate about definitions, it seems logical to use the following terminology: (1) *hereditary* or *genetic hemochromatosis*—the disorder due to the inheritance of a mutant gene that is tightly linked to the HLA-A6 locus of the major histocompatibility complex on chromosome 6p, and (2) *secondary iron overload*—with tissue injury usually secondary to an iron-loading anemia such as thalassemia or sideroblastic anemia, in which increased erythropoiesis is ineffective. In the acquired iron-loading disorders, massive iron deposits in parenchymal tissues can lead to the same clinical and pathologic features as in hemochromatosis.

The metabolic defect leading to increased iron absorption in hemochromatosis is unknown. The genetic disease can be recognized during its early stages when the iron overload and organ damage are minimal. At this stage the disease is best referred to as *early* or *precirrhotic hemochromatosis* (see Fig. 342-1).

PREVALENCE   Hemochromatosis is one of the most common autosomal recessive disorders. The mutation is believed to be of Celtic origin. In European populations, approximately 1 in 10 persons is a heterozygous carrier, and 0.3 percent of persons are homozygotes. However, expression of the disease is modified by several factors, especially dietary iron intake, blood loss associated with menstruation and pregnancy, and blood donation. The clinical expression is 5 to 10 times more frequent in men than in women. Nearly 70 percent of patients develop the first symptoms between ages 40 and 60. The disease is rarely evident below age 20, although with family screening (see below) and periodic health examinations asymptomatic subjects with iron overload can be identified, including young menstruating women.

GENETICS AND MODE OF INHERITANCE   The gene for hemochromatosis is closely linked to the HLA-A locus on chromosome 6. Discovery of this linkage made it possible to clarify the mode of inheritance and prevalence of the disorder. For example, the fact that siblings with hemochromatosis usually share the same HLA haplotypes implied that they are homozygotes for the same autosomal recessive mutation. A candidate gene in this region of chromosome 6 termed HLA-H encodes a 343 amino acid MHC class 1 protein, and 83 percent of affected subjects have a homozygous Cys281Tyr substitution in the protein. The role in the remainder of the patients of a second variant in the HLA-H protein His63Asp is unclear. The function of the normal HLA-H protein in iron metabolism is also not known.

PATHOGENESIS   Normally, the body iron content of 3 to 4 g is maintained such that intestinal mucosal absorption of iron is equal to iron loss. This amount is approximately 1 mg/d in men and 1.5 mg/d in menstruating women. In hemochromatosis, mucosal absorption is inappropriate to body needs and amounts to 4 mg/d or more. The resulting progressive accumulation of iron causes an early elevation in plasma iron, an increased saturation of transferrin, and progressive elevation of plasma ferritin level. The basic defect causing increased iron absorption is unknown. In hemochromatosis the coordinate regulation of the synthesis of ferritin and the transferrin receptor is intact and responds normally to the usual influences, e.g., blood loss. An abnormally fast transport of iron out of intestinal and reticuloendothelial cells has been postulated, but the mechanism is not known. Either the demonstration of normal function or location of the encoding genes on chromosomes other than chromosome 6 makes it possible to exclude a primary role in the pathogenesis for ferritin, the transferrin receptor, and the iron regulatory protein involved in the coordinate regulation of ferritin and the transferrin receptor.

In advanced disease the body may contain 20 g or more of iron deposited mainly in parenchymal cells of the liver, pancreas, and heart. Iron in the liver and pancreas may increase 50 to 100 times and in the heart 5 to 25 times. Iron deposition in the pituitary causes hypogonadotrophic hypogonadism in both men and women. Tissue injury may result from disruption of iron-laden lysosomes, from lipid peroxidation of subcellular organelles by excess iron, or from stimulation of collagen synthesis by activated stellate cells.

Parenchymal iron overload leading to *secondary iron overload* occurs in chronic disorders of erythropoiesis, particularly in those due to defects in hemoglobin synthesis or ineffective erythropoiesis such as sideroblastic anemia and thalassemia. In these disorders, the absorption of iron is increased, and such patients are also frequently treated with iron and blood transfusions. Porphyria cutanea tarda (PCT), a disorder characterized by a defect in porphyrin biosynthesis (Chap. 343), is also sometimes associated with excessive parenchymal iron deposits; however, the magnitude of the iron load is usually insufficient to produce tissue damage. The exact relationship between these two disorders is unclear, although iron may accentuate the inherited enzyme deficiency in PCT. Another cause of hepatic parenchymal iron overload is hereditary aceruloplasminemia. In this disorder impairment of iron

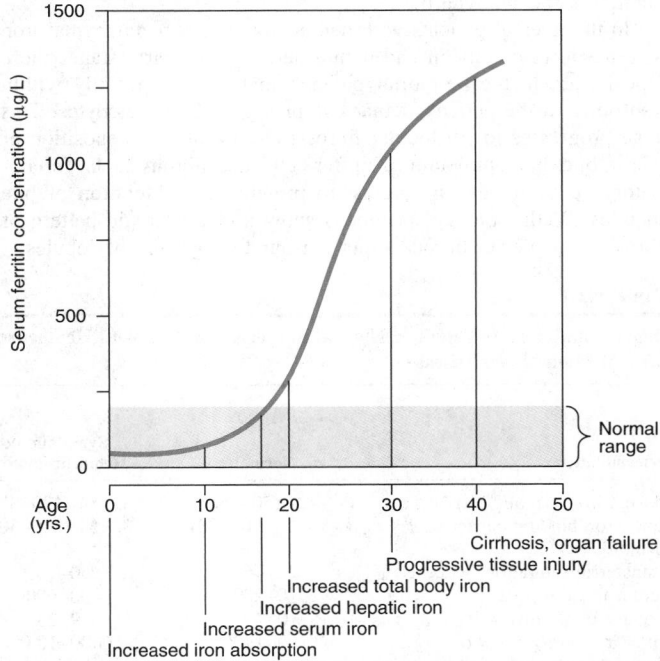

FIGURE 342-1   Sequence of events in genetic hemochromatosis and their correlation with the serum ferritin concentration. Increased iron absorption is present throughout life. Overt, symptomatic disease usually develops between ages 40 and 60, but latent precirrhotic disease can be detected long before this.

mobilization due to deficiency of ceruloplasmin (a ferroxidase) causes iron overload in hepatocytes.

Alcoholic subjects with chronic liver disease and increased tissue iron stores can be divided into two groups. The first comprises patients with a moderate increase in stainable hepatic iron but relatively normal body iron. These patients have alcoholic liver disease (usually cirrhosis) but not hemochromatosis. The increased iron may be due in part to cell death and uptake of released iron. The second (less common) group of alcoholics with increased hepatic iron have gross iron deposition and increased body iron stores and usually prove to have hemochromatosis with or without superimposed alcoholic liver disease. Hemochromatosis in a heavy drinker may be distinguished from alcoholic liver disease in two ways: (1) measurement of hepatic iron concentration and hepatic iron index (see below and Table 342-1) and (2) studying relatives for evidence of the disease, including HLA typing.

Excessive iron ingestion over many years rarely, if ever, results in hemochromatosis. The one important exception is South African blacks, in whom the intake of excessive iron in an alcoholic beverage has been due to the practice of brewing fermented beverages in vessels made of iron. In other populations hemochromatosis has on occasion been described in apparently normal subjects who have taken medicinal iron over many years, but such individuals probably have the genetic disorder. Family studies may be helpful.

The common denominator in all patients with hemochromatosis is *excessive amounts of iron in parenchymal tissues*. Parenteral administration of iron in the form of blood transfusions or iron preparations results predominantly in *reticuloendothelial cell* iron overload. This appears to lead to less tissue damage than iron loading of parenchymal cells.

PATHOLOGY At autopsy, the enlarged, nodular liver and pancreas are rusty in color. Histologically, iron is increased in amount in many organs, particularly in the liver, heart, and pancreas and to a lesser extent in the endocrine glands. The epidermis of the skin is thin, and *melanin* is increased in the cells of the basal layer. Deposits of iron are present around the synovial lining cells of the joints, and calcium pyrophosphate crystals may be present within deposits of calcium in the synovial tissue.

In the liver of patients with hemochromatosis, parenchymal iron is in the form of ferritin and hemosiderin. In the early stages these deposits are in the periportal parenchymal cells, especially within lysosomes in the pericanalicular cytoplasm of the hepatocytes. This stage progresses to perilobular fibrosis and eventually deposition of iron in bile duct epithelium, Kupffer cells, and fibrous septa. Inflammatory cells are few in contrast to prominent proliferation of bile ductules. Wedge biopsy specimens show a characteristic pattern of fibrosis with dense fibrous septa surrounding groups of lobules—

somewhat analogous to the findings in the liver in chronic biliary tract disease. In the advanced stage, a macronodular or mixed macro- and micronodular cirrhosis develops.

CLINICAL MANIFESTATIONS The symptoms and signs include skin pigmentation, diabetes mellitus, liver and cardiac impairment, arthropathy, and hypogonadism. Initial symptoms include weakness, lassitude, weight loss, change in skin color, abdominal pain, loss of libido, and symptoms of diabetes mellitus. Hepatomegaly, pigmentation, spider angiomas, splenomegaly, arthropathy, ascites, cardiac arrhythmias, congestive heart failure, loss of body hair, testicular atrophy, and jaundice are prominent in advanced disease.

The *liver* is usually the first organ to be affected, and hepatomegaly is present in more than 95 percent of symptomatic patients. Hepatic enlargement may exist in the absence of symptoms or of abnormal liver function tests. Indeed, over half the patients with symptomatic hemochromatosis have little laboratory evidence of functional impairment of the liver, in spite of hepatomegaly and fibrosis. Loss of body hair, palmar erythema, testicular atrophy, and gynecomastia are common. Manifestations of portal hypertension and esophageal varices occur less commonly than in cirrhosis from other causes. *Hepatocellular carcinoma* develops in about 30 percent of patients with cirrhosis. Its incidence increases with age, and it is the most common cause of death in treated patients. However, it occurs almost exclusively in cirrhotic patients; hence the importance of early diagnosis and therapy. Splenomegaly occurs in approximately half of symptomatic cases.

Excessive *skin pigmentation* is present in over 90 percent of symptomatic patients at the time of diagnosis due to melanin deposition in the skin; this usually gives rise to bronzing. The characteristic metallic or slate gray hue is believed to result from increased melanin or of both melanin and iron in the dermis. Pigmentation usually is diffuse and generalized, but it may be more pronounced on the face, neck, extensor aspects of the lower forearms, dorsa of the hands, lower legs, genital regions, and in scars. In rare cases pigmentation is demonstrable in the oral mucosa.

Diabetes mellitus occurs in about 65 percent of patients and is more likely to develop in those with a family history of diabetes. The genetic predisposition and direct damage to the pancreas by iron deposition both contribute to the development of diabetes. The management is similar to that of other forms of diabetes except for a higher incidence of insulin resistance. Late degenerative sequelae are the same as in ordinary diabetes mellitus.

Arthropathy develops in 25 to 50 percent of patients. It usually occurs after age 50 but may occur as a first manifestation or long after therapy. The joints of the hands, especially the second and third metacarpophalangeal joints, are usually the first joints involved, a feature that helps to distinguish this chondrocalcinosis from the idiopathic form. A progressive polyarthritis involving wrists, hips, ankles, and knees also may ensue. Acute brief attacks of synovitis may be associated with deposition of calcium pyrophosphate (chondrocalcinosis or pseudogout), chiefly in the knees. Radiologic manifestations

Table 342-1

Representative Iron Values in Normal Subjects, Patients with Hemochromatosis, and Patients with Alcoholic Liver Disease

Determination	Normal	Symptomatic Hemochromatosis	Homozygotes with Early, Asymptomatic Hemochromatosis	Heterozygotes	Alcoholic Liver Disease
Plasma iron, μmol/L (μg/dL)	9–27 (50–150)	32–54 (180–300)	Usually elevated	Elevated or normal	Often elevated
Total iron-binding capacity, μmol/L (μg/dL)	45–66 (250–370)	36–54 (200–300)	36–54 (200–300)	Elevated or normal	45–66 (250–370)
Transferrin saturation, percent	22–46	50–100	50–100		27–60
Serum ferritin, μg/L	10–200	900–6000	200–500	Usually <500	10–500
Urinary iron,* mg/24 h	0–2	9–23	2–5	2–5	Usually <5
Liver iron, μg/g dry wt	300–1400	6000–18,000	2000–4000	300–3000	300–2000
Hepatic iron index (μg/g dry wt) 56 × age	<1.0	>2	Usually >2	<2	<2

* After intramuscular administration of 0.5 g deferoxamine.

include cystic changes of sclerosis of the subchondral bones, loss of articular cartilage with narrowing of the joint space, diffuse demineralization, hypertrophic bone proliferation, and calcification of the synovium. The arthropathy tends to progress despite removal of iron by phlebotomy. Although the relation of these abnormalities to iron metabolism is not known, the fact that similar changes occur in other forms of iron overload suggests that iron is a critical factor.

Cardiac involvement is the presenting manifestation in about 15 percent of patients, the most common manifestation being congestive heart failure in about 10 percent of young adults with the disease. Symptoms of congestive failure may develop suddenly, with rapid progression to death if untreated. The heart is diffusely enlarged and may be misdiagnosed as idiopathic cardiomyopathy if other overt manifestations are absent. Cardiac arrhythmias include premature supraventricular beats, paroxysmal tachyarrhythmias, atrial flutter, atrial fibrillation, and varying degrees of atrioventricular block.

Hypogonadism occurs in both sexes and may antedate other clinical features. Manifestations include loss of libido, impotence, amenorrhea, testicular atrophy, and sparse body hair. Gynecomastia is less common than in other forms of cirrhosis. These changes are due to the decreased production of gonadotropins due to impairment of hypothalamic-pituitary function by iron deposition. Adrenal insufficiency, hypothyroidism, and hypoparathyroidism occur on occasion.

DIAGNOSIS The association of (1) hepatomegaly, (2) skin pigmentation, (3) diabetes mellitus, (4) heart disease, (5) arthritis, and (6) hypogonadism should suggest the diagnosis. However, a parenchymal iron overload of comparatively short duration or modest degree may exist with none or only some of these manifestations [e.g., in young subjects (see Fig. 342-1)]. Therefore, a high index of suspicion is needed to make the diagnosis early, and hemochromatosis should be considered in any patient with unexplained hepatomegaly, cardiomyopathy, abnormal skin pigmentation, loss of libido, diabetes mellitus, or arthritis. This is particularly important because treatment before there is permanent organ damage can reverse the iron toxicity and restore life expectancy to normal (see below).

The history should be particularly detailed in regard to disease in other family members, alcohol ingestion, iron intake, and ingestion of large doses of ascorbic acid, which promotes iron absorption. Appropriate tests should be performed to exclude the iron deposition of hematologic disease. The presence of liver, pancreatic, cardiac, and joint disease should be confirmed by physical examination, roentgenography, and standard function tests of these organs. Then it must be demonstrated that there is an increase in total-body iron stores and, in particular, an increase in parenchymal iron concentration with or without tissue damage.

The methods available for assessing parenchymal iron stores include (1) measurement of serum iron and the percent saturation of transferrin, (2) measurement of serum ferritin concentration, (3) liver biopsy with measurement of the iron concentration and calculation of the hepatic iron index (Table 342-1), (4) estimation of chelatable iron stores following the administration of deferoxamine, and (5) computed tomography and/or magnetic resonance imaging of the liver. Each has its advantages and limitations. The serum iron level and percent saturation of transferrin are elevated early in the course, but their specificity is reduced by significant false-positive and false-negative rates. For example, serum iron concentration may be increased in patients with alcoholic liver disease without iron overload; in this situation, however, the hepatic iron index is usually not increased as in hemochromatosis (Table 342-1). In otherwise healthy persons, a fasting serum transferrin saturation greater than 62 percent suggests homozygosity for hemochromatosis.

The serum ferritin concentration is usually a good index of body iron stores, whether decreased or increased. In fact, an increase of 1 μg/L in serum ferritin level reflects an increase of some 65 mg in body stores. In most untreated patients with hemochromatosis, the serum ferritin level is greatly increased (Fig. 342-1 and Table 342-1).

These tests have generally replaced the more cumbersome screening tests involving measurement of urinary iron excretion after the administration of the iron chelator deferoxamine. However, in patients with inflammation and hepatocellular necrosis, serum ferritin levels may be elevated out of proportion to body iron stores due to increased release from tissues. A repeat determination of serum ferritin should therefore be carried out when any concurrent acute hepatocellular damage has subsided, e.g., in alcoholic liver disease. Ordinarily, the *combined measurements* of the percent transferrin saturation and serum ferritin level provide a simple and reliable screening test for hemochromatosis, including the precirrhotic phase of the disease. If either of these tests is abnormal, liver biopsy should be performed, since it is the *definitive* diagnostic test. It permits histochemical estimation of tissue iron, measurement of hepatic iron concentration, and the presence or absence of cirrhosis. In addition, calculation of the hepatic iron index (hepatic iron concentration ÷ age in years) helps to distinguish early homozygous subjects from heterozygotes and from patients with alcoholic liver disease (see Table 342-1). Increased density of the liver due to iron deposition can be demonstrated by computed tomography. Magnetic resonance imaging also may detect increased tissue iron, but its sensitivity requires further evaluation. A retrospective assessment of body iron storage is also provided by performing *weekly phlebotomy* and calculating the amount of iron removed before iron stores are exhausted (1 mL blood = approximately 0.5 mg iron).

When the diagnosis of hemochromatosis is established, it is of importance to examine family members. Asymptomatic as well as symptomatic family members with the disease usually have an increased saturation of transferrin and an increased serum ferritin concentration. These changes occur even before the iron stores are greatly increased (see Fig. 342-1). A liver biopsy should then be performed, since it is imperative to confirm the diagnosis, confirm or exclude the presence of cirrhosis, and begin therapy as early as possible. As stated above, HLA typing is helpful in evaluating families with the disease. Affected siblings (homozygotes) usually have both HLA haplotypes identical with those of the proband. When children of a proband are affected, a homozygote-heterozygote mating has probably occurred. Siblings sharing only one HLA haplotype with a patient (heterozygotes) will probably not develop progressive iron overload. Thus HLA typing helps in predicting the probability of a sibling later developing the disease and therefore in determining the desirable frequency of screening.

The distinction between hemochromatosis and alcoholic cirrhosis with increased tissue iron is usually not difficult if liver iron concentration and hepatic iron index are measured (Table 342-1). Where biopsy is not possible, the deferoxamine excretion test can provide diagnostic information. It should be reemphasized that subjects with a history of excessive alcohol consumption and who have increased hepatic iron concentration are usually homozygous for hemochromatosis.

℞ **TREATMENT**

The therapy of hemochromatosis involves removal of the excess body iron and supportive treatment of damaged organs. Iron removal is best begun by weekly or twice-weekly phlebotomy of 500 mL. Although there is an initial modest decline in the volume of packed red blood cells to about 35 mL/dL, the level stabilizes after several weeks. The plasma transferrin saturation remains increased until the available iron stores are depleted. In contrast, the plasma ferritin concentration falls progressively, reflecting the gradual decrease in body iron stores. Since one 500-mL unit of blood contains from 200 to 250 mg iron and about 25 g iron should be removed, weekly phlebotomy may be required for 1 or 2 years. When the transferrin saturation and ferritin level become normal, phlebotomies are performed at intervals as required to maintain levels within the normal range. The measurements promptly become abnormal with iron reaccumulation. Usually one phlebotomy every 3 months will suffice.

Chelating agents such as deferoxamine, when given parenterally, remove 10 to 20 mg iron per day, a fraction of that mobilized by once weekly phlebotomy. Phlebotomy is also less expensive, more convenient, and safer for most patients. However, chelating agents are indicated when anemia or hypoproteinemia is severe enough to preclude phlebotomy. Subcutaneous infusion of deferoxamine using a portable pump is the most effective means of administration.

The management of the hepatic failure, cardiac failure, and diabetes mellitus is similar to conventional therapy for these conditions. Loss of libido and change in secondary sex characteristics are partially relieved by parenteral testosterone or gonadotropin therapy (see Chap. 336).

PROGNOSIS The principal causes of death in *untreated* patients are cardiac failure (30 percent), hepatocellular failure or portal hypertension (25 percent), and hepatocellular carcinoma (30 percent).

Life expectancy is improved by removal of the excessive stores of iron and maintenance of these stores at near-normal levels. The 5-year survival rate with therapy increases from 33 to 89 percent. With repeated phlebotomy, the liver and spleen decrease in size, liver function improves, pigmentation of skin decreases, and cardiac failure may be reversed. Diabetes improves in about 40 percent, but removal of excess iron has little effect on hypogonadism or arthropathy. Hepatic fibrosis may decrease, but cirrhosis is irreversible. End-stage liver disease can be treated with orthotopic liver transplantation, but the results are suboptimal unless excess iron stores are first corrected. Hepatocellular carcinoma occurs as a late sequela in about one-third of patients who are cirrhotic at presentation despite adequate iron removal. The apparent increase in its incidence in treated patients is probably related in part to the increased life span. Hepatocellular carcinoma does not appear to develop if the disease is treated in the precirrhotic stage. Indeed, the life expectancy of homozygotes treated before the development of cirrhosis is normal.

The importance of family screening and early therapy cannot be emphasized too strongly. Asymptomatic subjects detected by family studies should have phlebotomy therapy if iron stores are moderately to severely increased. Assessment of iron stores at appropriate intervals is also important. With this management approach, most manifestations of the disease can be prevented.

BIBLIOGRAPHY

BROCK J et al: *Iron Metabolism in Health and Disease.* London, Saunders, 1994
EDWARDS CQ et al: Prevalence of hemochromatosis among 11,065 presumably healthy blood donors. N Engl J Med 318:1355, 1988
FEDER JN et al: A novel MHC class I-like gene is mutated in patients with hereditary hemochromatosis. Nat Gen 13:399, 1996
GUALDI R et al: Excess iron into hepatocytes is required for activation of collagen Type 1 gene during experimental siderosis. Gastroenterology 107:1118, 1994
HARRIS ZL et al: Aceruloplasminemia: Molecular characterization of this disorder of iron metabolism. Proc Natl Acad Sci USA 92:2539, 1995
JAZWINSKA EC et al: Localization of the hemochromatosis gene close to D6S105. Am J Hum Genet 53:347, 1993
KLAUSNER RD, HARFORD JB: Cis-trans models for post-transcriptional gene regulation. Science 246:870, 1989
NEIDERAU C et al: Long-term survival in patients with hereditary hemochromatosis. Gastroenterology, 110:1107, 1996
RAMM GA et al: Chronic iron overload causes activation of rat lipocytes in vivo. Am J Physiol 268:G451, 1995

343 *Robert J. Desnick*

THE PORPHYRIAS

The porphyrias are inherited or acquired disorders of specific enzymes in the heme biosynthetic pathway (Fig. 343-1). These disorders are classified as either *hepatic* or *erythropoietic* depending on the primary site of overproduction and accumulation of the porphyrin precursor or porphyrin (Tables 343-1 and 343-2), but some have overlapping features. The major manifestations of the hepatic porphyrias are neurologic, including abdominal pain, neuropathy, and mental disturbances, whereas the erythropoietic porphyrias characteristically cause cutaneous photosensitivity. The reason for neurologic involvement in the hepatic porphyrias is poorly understood. Cutaneous sensitivity to sunlight is due to the fact that excitation of excess porphyrins in the skin by long-wave ultraviolet light leads to cell damage, scarring, and deformation. Steroid hormones, drugs, and nutrition influence the production of porphyrin precursors and porphyrins, thereby precipitating or increasing the severity of some porphyrias. Thus, the porphyrias are actually *ecogenic* disorders, in which environmental, physiologic, and genetic factors interact to cause disease.

Many symptoms of the porphyrias are nonspecific, and diagnosis is often delayed. Laboratory testing can confirm or exclude the diagnosis of a porphyria. Table 343-2 summarizes the major metabolites that accumulate in each porphyria. Urinary δ-aminolevulinic acid (ALA) and porphobilinogen (PBG) are easily quantitated by chemical methods, and the urinary porphyrin isomers can be separated and quantitated by high-performance liquid chromatography. The diagnostic profile of accumulated precursors and/or porphyrins in each disorder can also be defined by extraction and thin-layer chromatography of fecal porphyrins. However, a definite diagnosis requires demonstration of the specific enzyme deficiency. The isolation and characterization of the cDNAs encoding the heme biosynthetic enzymes have permitted the definition of the molecular lesions that cause each porphyria. Molecular analyses that take advantage of this information make it possible to provide prenatal diagnoses in families with known mutations or with informative polymorphisms.

HEME BIOSYNTHESIS The first and last three enzymes in the heme biosynthetic pathway are located in the mitochondrion, whereas the other four are in the cytosol (see Fig. 343-1). The first enzyme, δ-aminolevulinate synthase (ALA synthase), catalyzes the condensation of glycine, activated by pyridoxal phosphate and succinyl coenzyme A, to form ALA. In the liver, this rate-limiting enzyme can be induced by a variety of drugs, steroids, and other chemicals. Distinct erythroid-specific and nonerythroid (i.e., housekeeping) forms of ALA synthase are encoded by separate genes. The two ALA synthase genes provide the basis for tissue-specific regulation of this pathway.

The second enzyme, δ-aminolevulinate dehydratase (ALA dehydratase), catalyzes the condensation of two molecules of ALA to form PBG. Four molecules of PBG condense to form the tetrapyrrole uroporphyrinogen III by a two-step process catalyzed by hydroxymethylbilane (HMB) synthase (also known as PBG deaminase or uroporphyrinogen I synthase) and uroporphyrinogen III (URO) synthase. HMB synthase catalyzes the head-to-tail condensation of four PBG molecules by a series of deaminations to form the linear tetrapyrrole hydroxymethylbilane. URO synthase catalyzes the rearrangement and rapid cyclization of HMB to form the asymmetric, physiologic, octacarboxylate porphyrinogen uroporphyrinogen III.

The fifth enzyme in the pathway, uroporphyrinogen decarboxylase (URO decarboxylase), catalyzes the sequential removal of the four carboxyl groups from the acetic acid side chains of uroporphyrinogen III to form coproporphyrinogen III, a tetracarboxylate porphyrinogen. This compound then enters the mitochondrion, where coproporphyrinogen (COPRO) oxidase, the sixth enzyme, catalyzes the decarboxylation of two of the four propionic acid groups to form the two vinyl groups of protoporphyrinogen IX, a dicarboxylate porphyrinogen. Next, protoporphyrinogen (PROTO) oxidase oxidizes protoporphyrinogen IX to protoporphyrin IX by the removal of six hydrogen atoms. The product of the reaction is a porphyrin (oxidized form), in contrast to the preceding tetrapyrrole intermediates, which are porphyrinogens (reduced forms). Finally, ferrous iron is inserted into protoporphyrin IX to form heme, a reaction catalyzed by the eighth enzyme in the pathway, ferrochelatase (also known as heme synthetase or protoheme ferrolyase).

Each of the heme biosynthetic enzymes is encoded by a separate gene. Full-length human cDNAs for each of the enzymes, including those for both forms of ALA synthase, have been isolated and se-

quenced, and the chromosomal locations of the genes have been identified (Table 343-3).

CHAPTER 343
The Porphyrias

2153

REGULATION OF HEME BIOSYNTHESIS   About 85 percent of the heme produced in the body is synthesized in erythroid cells to provide heme for hemoglobin, and most of the remainder is produced in the liver, where the biosynthetic pathway is under negative feedback control. "Free" heme in the liver regulates the synthesis and mitochondrial translocation of the housekeeping form of ALA synthase. Heme represses the synthesis of the ALA synthase mRNA and interferes with the transport of the enzyme from the cysotol into mitochondria. ALA synthase is inducible by many of the same chemicals that induce the cytochrome P450 enzymes in the endoplasmic reticulum of the liver. Because most of the heme in the liver is used for the synthesis of cytochrome P450 enzymes, hepatic ALA synthase and the cytochrome P450s are regulated in a coordinated fashion.

Different regulatory mechanisms control production of heme for hemoglobin. The erythroid-specific ALA synthase encoded on the X chromosome is expressed at higher levels than the hepatic enzyme, and an erythroid-specific control mechanism regulates iron transport into erythroid cells. During erythroid differentiation, the activities of the heme biosynthetic enzymes increase in a coordinated fashion.

THE HEPATIC PORPHYRIAS

The acute hepatic porphyrias are characterized by the rapid onset of neurologic manifestations. During the acute attack, individuals have

FIGURE 343-1   The human heme biosynthetic pathway.

Table 343-1

Classification of the Human Porphyrias

Type/Porphyria	Deficient Enzyme	Inheritance*	Photosensitivity	Neurovisceral Symptoms
HEPATIC PORPHYRIAS				
ALA dehydratase deficiency	ALA dehydratase	AR	−	+
Acute intermittent porphyria (AIP)	HMB synthase	AD	−	+
Hereditary coproporphyria (HCP)	COPRO oxidase	AD	+	+
Variegate porphyria (VP)	PROTO oxidase	AD	+	+
Porphyria cutanea tarda (PCT)	URO decarboxylase	AD	+	−
ERYTHROPOIETIC PORPHYRIAS				
X-linked sideroblastic anemia (XLSA)	ALA synthase	XLR	−	−
Congenital erythropoietic porphyria (CEP)	URO synthase	AR	+ + +	−
Erythropoietic protoporphyria (EPP)	Ferrochelatase	AD	+	−

* AR, autosomal recessive; AD, autosomal dominant; XLR, X-linked recessive.

markedly elevated plasma and urinary concentrations of the porphyrin precursors ALA and PBG, which originate from the liver.

ALA DEHYDRATASE–DEFICIENT PORPHYRIA This disease is a rare autosomal recessive trait that has been described in four unrelated males in Europe. Onset and severity of the disease are variable, presumably depending on the amount of residual ALA dehydratase activity. Treatment and prevention of the neurologic complications are the same as for other acute porphyrias (see below).

Clinical Features The clinical presentation is variable. The first reported cases were in two unrelated German men who had the onset during adolescence of abdominal pain and neuropathy, resembling acute intermittent porphyria (AIP; see below). The third patient, a Swedish infant, presented with failure to thrive and required transfu-

Table 343-2

The Major Metabolites Accumulated in the Human Porphyrias

Type/Porphyria	Increased Erythrocyte Porphyrins	Porphyrin Excretion*	
		Urine	Stool
HEPATIC PORPHYRIAS			
ALA dehydratase deficiency	—	ALA, COPRO III	—
Acute intermittent porphyria (AIP)	—	ALA, PBG	—
Hereditary coproporphyria (HCP)	—	ALA, PBG, COPRO III	COPRO III
Variegate porphyria (VP)	—	ALA, PBG COPRO III	COPRO III, PROTO IX
Porphyria cutanea tarda (PCT)	—	URO I, 7-carboxylate, porphyrin	ISOCOPRO
ERYTHROPOIETIC PORPHYRIAS			
X-linked sideroblastic anemia (XLSA)	—	—	—
Congenital erythropoietic porphyria (CEP)	URO I	URO I	COPRO I
Erythropoietic protoporphyria (EPP)	PROTO IX	—	PROTO IX

* ALA, δ-aminolevulinic acid; PBG, porphobilinogen; COPRO I, coproporphyrin I; COPRO III, coproporphyrin III; ISOCOPRO, isocoproporphyrin; URO I, uroporphyrin I; URO III, uroporphyrin III; PROTO, protoporphyrin IX

sions and parenteral nutrition. Presumably, the earlier age of onset and more severe manifestations reflect a more complete enzyme deficiency. The fourth patient, a Belgian man, developed an acute motor polyneuropathy and polycythemia at age 63.

Diagnosis All four patients had increased urinary levels of ALA and coproporphyrin. ALA dehydratase activity in erythrocytes was <5 percent of normal. Both succinylacetone (which accumulates in hereditary tyrosinemia and is structurally similar to ALA) and lead can inhibit ALA dehydratase, increase urinary excretion of ALA, and cause manifestations that resemble those of the acute porphyrias. Therefore, lead intoxication and hereditary tyrosinemia (fumarylacetoacetase deficiency) should be considered in the differential diagnosis of the dehydratase–deficient porphyria. Immunologic studies in the four reported cases demonstrated the presence of nonfunctional enzyme proteins that cross-reacted with anti–ALA dehydratase antibodies. DNA analysis revealed different missense mutations that resulted in the amino acid substitutions G133R and V275M in the infantile-onset case and R240W and A274T in one of the juvenile-onset cases.

Heterozygotes are clinically asymptomatic and do not excrete increased levels of ALA, but they can be detected by demonstration of intermediate levels of erythrocyte ALA dehydratase activity or by demonstrating a specific mutation in the ALA dehydratase gene. Prenatal diagnosis of this disorder has not been achieved but should be possible by determination of the ALA dehydratase activity in cultured chorionic villi or amniocytes.

℞ **TREATMENT**

Treatment is similar to that of AIP (see below). The severely affected infant was supported by hyperalimentation and periodic blood transfusions. Continued failure to thrive led to a liver transplant, which did not improve the hematologic manifestations.

ACUTE INTERMITTENT PORPHYRIA This hepatic porphyria is an autosomal dominant condition resulting from the half-normal level of HMB synthase activity. The disease is widespread but is especially common in Scandinavia and perhaps Great Britain. The enzyme deficiency can be demonstrated in most heterozygous individuals, but clinical expression is highly variable. Activation of the disease is related to ecogenic factors, such as drugs, diet, and steroid hormones, which can precipitate the manifestations. Attacks can be prevented by avoiding known precipitating factors.

Table 343-3

The Heme Biosynthetic Genes and Their Chromosomal Locations

Structural Gene	cDNA and Genomic Sequences Characterized	Chromosomal Assignment
ALA synthase		
Housekeeping	+	3p21
Erythroid	+	Xp11.21
ALA dehydratase	+	9q34
HMB synthase	+	11q23 → qter
URO synthase	+	10q25.3 → 26.3
URO decarboxylase	+	1p34
COPRO oxidase	−	3q12
PROTO oxidase	−	1q32
Ferrochelatase	+	18q21.3

Table 343-4

CHAPTER 343
The Porphyrias

2155

Categories of Unsafe and Safe Drugs in AIP, HCP, and VP

Unsafe	Safe
Barbiturates	Narcotic analgesics
Sulfonamide antibiotics	Aspirin
Meprobamate	Acetaminophen
Glutethimide	Phenothiazines
Methyprylon	Penicillin and derivatives
Ethchlorvynol	Streptomycin
Mephenytoin	Glucocorticoids
Succinimides	Bromides
Carbamazepine	Insulin
Valproic acid	Atropine
Pyrazolones	
Griseofulvin	
Ergots	
Synthetic estrogens and progestogens	
Danazol	
Alcohol	

Clinical Features Most heterozygotes remain clinically asymptomatic (latent) unless exposed to factors that increase the production of porphyrins. Endogenous and exogenous gonadal steroids, porphyrinogenic drugs, alcohol ingestion, and low-calorie diets, usually instituted to produce weight loss, are common precipitating factors. Table 343-4 lists the major drugs that are harmful in AIP [and also in hereditary coproporphyria (HCP) and variegate porphyria (VP)] and some drugs and anesthetic agents known to be safe. More extensive lists of drugs considered harmful or safe are available (see the bibliography), but information is incomplete for many of them. Attacks also can be provoked by infections and by surgery.

Because the neurovisceral symptoms rarely occur before puberty and are often nonspecific, a high index of suspicion is required to make the diagnosis. The disease can be disabling but is rarely fatal. Abdominal pain, the most common symptom, is usually steady and poorly localized but may be cramping. Ileus, abdominal distention, and decreased bowel sounds are common. However, increased bowel sounds and diarrhea may occur. Abdominal tenderness, fever, and leukocytosis are usually absent or mild because the symptoms are neurologic rather than inflammatory. Nausea, vomiting, constipation, tachycardia, hypertension, mental symptoms, pain in the limbs, head, neck, or chest, muscle weakness, sensory loss, dysuria, and urinary retention are characteristic. Tachycardia, hypertension, restlessness, tremors, and excess sweating are due to sympathetic overactivity.

The peripheral neuropathy is due to axonal degeneration (rather than demyelination) and affects primarily motor neurons. Significant neuropathy does not occur with all acute attacks; abdominal symptoms are usually more prominent. Motor neuropathy affects the proximal muscles initially, more often in the shoulders and arms. The course and degree of involvement are variable. Deep tendon reflexes may be normal or hyperactive but are usually decreased or absent with advanced neuropathy. Motor weakness can be asymmetric and focal and may involve cranial nerves. Sensory changes such as paresthesias and loss of sensation are less prominent. Progressive muscle weakness can lead to respiratory and bulbar paralysis and death when diagnosis and treatment are delayed. Sudden death may result from sympathetic overactivity and cardiac arrhythmia.

Mental symptoms such as anxiety, insomnia, depression, disorientation, hallucinations, and paranoia can occur

in acute attacks. Seizures can be due to neurologic effects or to hyponatremia. Treatment of seizures is difficult because virtually all antiseizure drugs (except bromides) may exacerbate AIP (clonazepam may be safer than phenytoin or barbiturates). Hyponatremia results from hypothalamic involvement and inappropriate vasopressin secretion or from electrolyte depletion due to vomiting, diarrhea, poor intake, or excess renal sodium loss. Persistent hypertension and impaired renal function may occur. When an attack resolves, abdominal pain may disappear within hours, and paresis begins to improve within days and may continue to improve over several years.

Diagnosis ALA and PBG levels are increased in plasma and urine during acute attacks. Urinary PBG excretion is usually 220 to 880 μmol/d (50 to 200 mg/d) [normal, 0 to 18 μmol/d (0 to 4 mg/d)], and urinary ALA excretion is 150 to 760 μmol/d (20 to 100 mg/d) (normal, 8 to 53 μmol/d [1 to 7 mg/d]). The excretion of these compounds generally decreases with clinical improvement, particularly after hematin infusions (see below). A normal urinary PBG level effectively excludes AIP as a cause for current symptoms. Fecal porphyrins are usually normal or minimally increased in AIP, in contrast to HCP and VP. Most asymptomatic ("latent") heterozygotes with HMB synthase deficiency have normal urinary excretion of ALA and PBG. Therefore, measurement of HMB synthase in erythrocytes is useful to confirm the diagnosis and to screen asymptomatic family members.

The enzyme deficiency is detectable in erythrocytes from most AIP heterozygotes (*classic AIP*). However, the activity is higher in young erythrocytes and may increase into the normal range in AIP when erythropoiesis is increased due to a concurrent condition. However, patients with the rare erythroid form of AIP (*erythroid AIP*) have normal enzyme levels in erythrocytes and deficient activity in nonerythroid tissues (see below). The erythroid and housekeeping forms of HMB synthase are encoded by a single gene, which has two promoters. One promotes transcription of messenger RNA for the housekeeping form found in all tissues, and the other promotes formation of the erythroid-specific transcript. Several deletions and over 45 different point mutations in the coding region of the gene have been found in unrelated AIP families (Fig. 343-2). These mutations alter the kinetic properties and/or stability of the mutant enzymes or create premature termination codons. Mutations that cause erythroid AIP variants with half-normal enzyme in nonerythroid tissues but normal activity in erythrocytes include point mutations in the initiation methionine codon (that prevent translation) or in the 5' splice site

FIGURE 343-2 Mutations in the HMB synthase gene causing AIP. Mutation nomenclature: letters, one-letter code for amino acids; numbers, codon positions.

of intron 1 (that cause abnormal splicing of the HMB synthase transcript).

Heterozygotes can be identified by restriction fragment length polymorphism (RFLP) studies in informative families using various polymorphic sites in the HMB synthase gene. Efforts are now under way to identify the specific mutations in the HMB synthase gene in all AIP families; this information will make it possible to identify all heterozygotes in affected families and to advise them to avoid the factors known to cause acute attacks. The prenatal diagnosis of a fetus at risk can be made with cultured amniotic cells or chorionic villi.

℞ TREATMENT

During acute attacks, narcotic analgesics may be required for abdominal pain, and phenothiazines are useful for nausea, vomiting, anxiety, and restlessness. Chloral hydrate can be given for insomnia, and benzodiazepines in low doses are probably safe if a minor tranquilizer is required. Although intravenous glucose (at least 300 g/d) has been given for acute attacks of porphyria, a more complete parenteral nutritional regimen may be beneficial if oral feeding is not possible for a prolonged period. However, intravenous heme is more effective than glucose in reducing porphyrin precursor excretion and probably leads to more rapid recovery. The response to heme therapy is reduced if therapy is delayed. Therefore, 3 to 4 mg of heme, in the form of hematin (Abbott Laboratories), heme albumin, or heme arginate (Leiras Oy, Turku, Finland), may be infused daily for 4 days beginning as soon as possible after onset of an attack. Heme arginate and heme albumin are chemically stable and are less likely than hematin to produce phlebitis or an anticoagulant effect. The rate of recovery from an acute attack depends on the degree of neuronal damage and may be rapid (1 to 2 days) with prompt therapy. Recovery from severe motor neuropathy may continue for months or years. Identification and avoidance of inciting factors can hasten recovery from an attack and prevent future attacks. Multiple inciting factors may contribute to a symptomatic episode. Frequent clear-cut cyclical attacks occur in some women and can be prevented with a luteinizing hormone–releasing hormone analogue (this indication is not approved by the U.S. Food and Drug Administration).

PORPHYRIA CUTANEA TARDA Porphyria cutanea tarda (PCT), the most common of the porphyrias, can be sporadic (type I) or familial (types II and III) and also can develop after exposure to halogenated aromatic hydrocarbons. Hepatic URO decarboxylase is deficient in all types of PCT. In type I PCT, URO decarboxylase activity is normal in erythrocytes. In type II PCT, an autosomal dominant trait, the enzyme is deficient in erythrocytes and other tissues. In type III PCT, deficiency of the enzyme is limited to the liver. Deficient hepatic URO decarboxylase and a porphyrin pattern resembling PCT can be produced by exposure of normal individuals to a number of halogenated aromatic hydrocarbons. Hepatoerythropoietic porphyria (HEP) is an autosomal recessive form of porphyria that results from deficiency of URO decarboxylase.

Clinical Features Cutaneous photosensitivity is the major clinical feature. Neurologic manifestations are not observed. Fluid-filled vesicles and bullae develop on sun-exposed areas such as the face, the dorsa of the hands and feet, the forearms, and the legs. The skin in these areas is friable, and minor trauma may lead to the formation of bullae. The appearance of small white plaques, termed *milia*, may precede or follow vesicle formation. Bullae and denuded skin heal slowly and are subject to infection. Other features include hypertrichosis and hyperpigmentation, especially of the face, and thickening, scarring, and calcification resembling the cutaneous changes of systemic sclerosis.

A number of factors contribute to the development of hepatic URO decarboxylase deficiency, including excess alcohol, iron, and estrogens. PCT also can be induced by various chemicals; an epidemic

of PCT occurred in eastern Turkey in the 1950s as a result of consumption of wheat contaminated with the fungicide hexachlorobenzene. Hexachlorobenzene produces a disorder similar to PCT and induces hepatic URO decarboxylase deficiency in animals. PCT in humans has occurred after exposure to other chemicals, including di- and trichlorophenols and 2,3,7,8-tetrachlorodibenzo-(p)-dioxin (TCDD, dioxin). Patients with PCT characteristically have liver damage and are at risk for hepatocellular carcinoma. These carcinomas do not produce porphyrins.

Hepatoerythropoietic porphyria (HEP) resembles congenital erythropoietic porphyria (CEP) but also has erythropoietic features and usually presents with blistering skin lesions, hypertrichosis, scarring, and red urine in infancy or childhood.

Diagnosis Porphyrins are increased in the liver, plasma, urine, and stool. The urinary ALA level may be slightly increased, but the PBG level is normal. Urinary porphyrins consist mostly of uroporphyrin and 7-carboxylate porphyrin, with lesser amounts of coproporphyrin and 5- and 6-carboxylate porphyrins. Plasma porphyrins also are increased in a pattern that resembles that in urine. Isocoproporphyrins are increased in feces and sometimes also in plasma and urine. The finding of increased isocoproporphyrins is diagnostic for a deficiency of hepatic URO decarboxylase.

Type II PCT and HEP can be distinguished by finding low activity of URO decarboxylase in erythrocytes. URO decarboxylase activity in liver, erythrocytes, and cultured skin fibroblasts in type II PCT is approximately 50 percent of normal in affected individuals and in family members with latent disease. In HEP, the URO decarboxylase activity is 3 to 28 percent of normal. Several point mutations have been identified in the coding region of the URO decarboxylase gene from unrelated type II PCT and HEP patients (Fig. 343-3). Hepatic iron contributes to development of sporadic and familial forms of PCT. In the familial forms (types II and III), iron inhibits the residual normal enzyme, so that enzymatic activity in liver is less than 50 percent of normal. In type I PCT the decreased hepatic URO decarboxylase activity is not accompanied by a decrease in the amount of enzyme protein, suggesting that the enzyme is present in an inactive form, and hepatic URO decarboxylase activity gradually increases after a remission is induced by phlebotomy.

℞ TREATMENT

Alcohol, estrogens, iron supplements, and, if possible, any drugs that may exacerbate the disease should be discontinued, but this step does not always lead to improvement. A complete response can almost always be achieved by repeated phlebotomy to reduce hepatic iron. A unit (450 mL) of blood can be removed every 1 to 2 weeks. Because iron overload is not marked in most cases, remission may occur after only five or six phlebotomies. Hemoglobin levels or hematocrits and serum ferritin should be followed closely to prevent development of iron deficiency and anemia. After remission, continued phlebotomy may not be needed even if ferritin levels return to normal. Relapses are treated by additional phlebotomy.

PCT also can be treated with chloroquine or hydroxychloroquine, both of which complex with the excess porphyrins and promote their excretion. Small doses (e.g., 125 mg chloroquine phosphate

FIGURE 343-3 Mutations in the URO synthase gene causing familial PCP and HEP. Mutation nomenclature as in Fig. 343-2.

twice weekly) should be given, because standard doses can induce transient, sometimes marked increases in photosensitivity and hepatocellular damage. Hepatic imaging may be advisable to exclude complicating hepatocellular carcinoma. Treatment of PCT in patients with end-stage renal disease is facilitated by administration of erythropoietin.

HEREDITARY COPROPORPHYRIA   Hereditary coproporphyria (HCP) is an autosomal dominant form of hepatic porphyria that results from deficiency of COPRO oxidase. Photosensitivity may occur. A few cases of homozygous HCP have been reported.

Clinical Features   HCP is influenced by the same factors that cause attacks in AIP. The disease is latent before puberty, and symptoms are more common in women. Neurovisceral symptoms and other manifestations are virtually identical to those of AIP. Photosensitivity may resemble that in PCT and VP. Cutaneous lesions may begin in childhood in homozygous cases.

Diagnosis   Coproporphyrin is markedly increased in the urine and feces in symptomatic disease and sometimes when there are no symptoms. Urinary ALA and PBG levels are increased during acute attacks but may return to normal when symptoms resolve. Although the diagnosis can be confirmed by measuring COPRO oxidase activity, these assays are not widely available and require cells other than erythrocytes.

℞ TREATMENT

Neurologic symptoms are treated as in AIP (see above). Phlebotomy and chloroquine are ineffective when cutaneous lesions are present.

VARIEGATE PORPHYRIA   VP is a hepatic porphyria that results from the deficient activity of PROTO oxidase, is inherited as an autosomal dominant trait, and can present with neurologic symptoms, photosensitivity, or both.

Clinical Features   Neurovisceral signs and symptoms develop after puberty and are similar to those of AIP or HCP (see above). Attacks are provoked by the same drugs, steroids, and nutritional factors that are detrimental in AIP. Skin manifestations are more common than in HCP but usually occur apart from the neurovisceral symptoms. Since the skin lesions in VP, HCP, and PCT are not distinguishable by clinical examination or biopsy, these conditions must be diagnosed by assay of porphyrins and porphyrin precursors in blood, urine, and feces.

VP is particularly common in South Africa, where 3 of every 1000 whites have the disorder. Most are descendants of a couple who emigrated from Holland to South Africa in 1688. Homozygous VP is associated with photosensitivity, neurologic symptoms, and developmental disturbances, including growth retardation, in infancy or childhood; all cases had increased erythrocyte levels of zinc protoporphyrin, a characteristic finding in all homozygous porphyrias so far described.

Dual porphyria, the simultaneous occurrence of VP and familial PCT, has been documented in several kindreds. *Chester porphyria* was described in a large British family in which individuals had acute porphyric attacks and deficiency of both PROTO oxidase and HMB synthase. Photosensitivity was not observed. It is unclear whether Chester porphyria is a variant of VP or AIP.

Diagnosis   When VP is symptomatic, levels of fecal protoporphyrin and coproporphyrin and of urinary coproporphyrin are increased. Urinary ALA and PBG levels are increased during acute attacks. Plasma levels of porphyrins are increased, particularly when there are cutaneous lesions. VP can be distinguished rapidly from all other porphyrias by examining the fluorescence emission spectrum of porphyrins in plasma at neutral pH. This test is particularly useful for differentiating VP from PCT.

Assays of PROTO oxidase activity in cultured fibroblasts or lymphocytes are not widely available. Some latent cases of VP can be diagnosed by measurement of fecal porphyrins in relatives of VP patients.

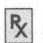 TREATMENT

Acute attacks are treated with hematin as in AIP. Other than avoiding sun exposure, there are few effective measures for treating the skin lesions. β-Carotene, phlebotomy, and chloroquine are not helpful.

THE ERYTHROPOIETIC PORPHYRIAS

In the erythropoietic porphyrias, porphyrins from bone marrow erythrocytes and plasma are deposited in the skin and lead to cutaneous photosensitivity.

X-LINKED SIDEROBLASTIC ANEMIA   X-linked sideroblastic anemia (XLSA) results from the deficient activity of the erythroid form of ALA synthase and is associated with ineffective erythropoiesis, weakness, and pallor.

Clinical Features   Males with XLSA develop refractory hemolytic anemia, pallor, and weakness during infancy. They have secondary hypersplenism, become iron overloaded, and can develop hemosiderosis. The severity depends on the level of residual erythroid ALA synthase activity and on the responsiveness of the specific mutation to pyridoxal 5′-phosphate supplementation (see below). Peripheral blood smears reveal a hypochromic, microcytic anemia with striking anisocytosis, poikilocytosis, and polychromasia; the leukocytes and platelets appear normal. Hemoglobin content is reduced, and the mean corpuscular volume and mean corpuscular hemoglobin concentration are decreased.

Diagnosis   Bone marrow examination reveals a hypercellular marrow with a left shift and megaloblastic erythropoiesis with an abnormal maturation. A variety of Prussian blue–staining sideroblasts are observed. Levels of urinary porphyrin precursors and of both urinary and fecal porphyrins are normal. The level of erythroid ALA synthase is decreased in bone marrow, but this enzyme is difficult to measure in the presence of the normal housekeeping enzyme. Definitive diagnosis requires the demonstration of mutations in the erythroid ALA synthase gene.

℞ TREATMENT

The severe anemia may respond to pyridoxine supplementation. This cofactor is essential for ALA synthase activity, and mutations in the pyridoxine binding site of the enzyme have been found in several responsive patients. Cofactor supplementation may make it possible to eliminate or reduce the frequency of transfusion. Unresponsive patients may be transfusion-dependent and require chelation therapy.

CONGENITAL ERYTHROPOIETIC PORPHYRIA   Congenital erythropoietic porphyria (CEP) is an autosomal recessive disorder, also known as *Gunther's disease*, that is due to deficiency of URO synthase activity and is associated with hemolytic anemia and cutaneous lesions. CEP is characterized by accumulation of the type I isomers of uroporphyrin and coproporphyrin.

Clinical Features   Severe cutaneous photosensitivity begins in early infancy. The skin over sun-exposed areas is friable, and bullae and vesicles are prone to rupture and infection. Skin thickening, focal hypo- and hyperpigmentation, and hypertrichosis of the face and extremities are characteristic. Secondary infection can lead to disfiguring of the face and hands. Porphyrins are deposited in teeth and in bones. As a result, the teeth are reddish brown and fluoresce on exposure to long-wave ultraviolet light. Hemolysis is probably due to the marked increase in erythrocyte porphyrins and leads to splenomegaly. A milder form of the disease begins in adulthood.

Diagnosis   Uroporphyrin and coproporphyrin (mostly isomer I) accumulate in the bone marrow, erythrocytes, plasma, urine, and feces. The diagnosis should be confirmed by demonstration of markedly deficient URO synthase activity. The disease can be detected in utero by measuring porphyrins in amniotic fluid and URO synthase activity in cultured amniotic cells or chorionic villi. Molecular analyses of the mutant alleles from over 20 unrelated patients have revealed the presence of gene rearrangements, an mRNA processing defect, and several point mutations that cause amino acid substitutions.

 TREATMENT

The transfusion of sufficient blood to suppress erythropoiesis is effective but results in iron overload. Splenectomy may reduce hemolysis and decrease transfusion requirements. Protection from sunlight and from minor skin trauma is important. β-Carotene may be of some value. Complicating bacterial infections should be treated promptly. Bone marrow transplantation was tried in one patient, who died from transplant complications.

ERYTHROPOIETIC PROTOPORPHYRIA Erythropoietic protoporphyria (EPP) is due to the partial deficiency of ferrochelatase and is inherited as an autosomal dominant trait. Protoporphyrin accumulates in erythroid cells and plasma and is excreted in bile and feces. EPP is the most common erythropoietic porphyria and, after PCT, the second most common porphyria.

Clinical Features Skin photosensitivity usually begins in childhood. The skin manifestations differ from those of other porphyrias. Vesicular lesions are uncommon. Redness, swelling, burning, and itching can develop within minutes of sun exposure and resemble angioedema. Symptoms may seem out of proportion to the visible skin lesions. Sparse vesicles and bullae occur in 10 percent of cases. Chronic skin changes may include lichenification, leathery pseudovesicles, labial grooving, and nail changes. Severe scarring is rare, as are pigment changes, friability, and hirsutism.

The primary source of excess protoporphyrin is the bone marrow reticulocyte. Erythrocyte protoporphyrin is free (not complexed with zinc) and is mostly bound to hemoglobin. In plasma protoporphyrin is bound to albumin. Hemolysis and anemia are usually absent or mild.

Liver function is usually normal, but in some patients accumulation of protoporphyrin causes chronic liver disease that can progress to liver failure and death. The hepatic complications are often preceded by increasing levels of erythrocyte and plasma protoporphyrin and probably result, in part, from protoporphyrin accumulation in the liver. Protoporphyrin is insoluble, forms crystalline structures in liver cells, and can decrease hepatic bile flow. Gallstones composed at least in part of protoporphyrin occur in some patients.

Some obligate heterozygotes are asymptomatic and have little or no increase in erythrocyte protoporphyrin. Thus there is phenotypic variation in this disease.

Diagnosis Protoporphyrin levels are increased in bone marrow, circulating erythrocytes, plasma, bile, and feces. Urinary levels of porphyrin and porphyrin precursors are normal. Ferrochelatase activity in cultured lymphocytes or fibroblasts is decreased.

 TREATMENT

Oral β-carotene (Hoffmann-LaRoche) (120 to 180 mg/d) improves tolerance to sunlight in many patients. The dosage may need to be adjusted to maintain serum carotene levels in the recommended range of 10 to 15 μmol/L (600 to 800 μg/dL). Mild skin discoloration due to carotenemia is the only significant side effect. The beneficial effects of β-carotene may involve quenching of singlet oxygen or free radicals. Unfortunately, this drug is less effective in other forms of porphyria associated with photosensitivity.

Treatment of hepatic complications is difficult. However, cholestyramine and other porphyrin absorbents such as activated charcoal may interrupt the enterohepatic circulation of protoporphyrin and promote its fecal excretion, leading to some improvement. Splenectomy may be helpful when the disease is accompanied by hemolysis and significant splenomegaly. Caloric restriction and drugs or hormones that may induce the heme pathway or impair hepatic excretory function should be avoided. Iron deficiency should be prevented or treated. Transfusions or intravenous heme therapy

may suppress erythroid and hepatic protoporphyrin production and are sometimes beneficial. Liver transplantation has been carried out in some patients with severe liver complications.

BIBLIOGRAPHY

ANDERSON KE et al: A GnRH analogue prevents cyclical attacks of porphyria. Arch Intern Med 150:1469, 1990

ASTRIN KH, DESNICK RJ: Molecular basis of acute intermittent porphyria. Hum Mutation 4:243, 1994

COTTER PD et al: Enzymatic defect in "X-linked" sideroblastic anemia: Molecular evidence for erythroid δ-aminolevulinate synthase deficiency. Proc Natl Acad Sci USA 89:4028, 1992

DESNICK RJ, ANDERSON KE: Heme biosynthesis and its disorders: Porphyrias and sideroblastic anemias, in *Hematology: Basic Principles and Practices,* 2d ed, R Hoffman et al (eds). New York, Churchill Livingstone, 1995, pp 523–545

KAPPAS A et al: The porphyrias, in *The Metabolic and Molecular Bases of Inherited Disease,* 7th ed, CR Scriver et al (eds). New York, McGraw-Hill, 1995, pp 2103–2159

MOORE MR et al: *Disorders of Porphyrin Metabolism.* New York, Plenum, 1987

MUSTAJOKI P, NORDMANN Y: Early administration of heme arginate for acute porphyric attacks. Ann Intern Med 153:2004, 1993

PLEWINSKA M et al: δ-Aminolevulinate dehydratase deficient porphyria: Identification of the molecular lesions in a severely affected homozygote. Am J Hum Genet 49:167, 1991

XU W et al: Congenital erythropoietic porphyria: Identification and expression of 10 mutations in the uroporphyrinogen III synthase gene. J Clin Invest 95:905, 1995

344 *Robert L. Wortmann*

GOUT AND OTHER DISORDERS OF PURINE METABOLISM

Gout encompasses a group of disorders that occur alone or in combination and include (1) hyperuricemia, (2) attacks of acute, typically monarticular, inflammatory arthritis, (3) tophaceous deposition of urate crystals in and around joints, (4) interstitial deposition of urate crystals in renal parenchyma, and (5) urolithiasis. *Hyperuricemia,* the cardinal feature and prerequisite for gout, is defined as a plasma urate level greater than 420 μmol/L (7.0 mg/dL) and indicates that total-body urate is increased. Hyperuricemia can result from increased production or decreased excretion of uric acid or from a combination of the two processes. When hyperuricemia exists, plasma and extracellular fluids are supersaturated with respect to urate, and conditions favor crystal formation and tissue deposition. These conditions cause the clinical manifestations included in the term *gout.*

URIC ACID METABOLISM Uric acid is the final breakdown product of purine degradation in humans. It is a weak acid with pK_as of 5.75 and 10.3. Urates, the ionized forms of uric acid, predominate in plasma, extracellular fluid, and synovial fluid, with approximately 98 percent existing as monosodium urate at pH 7.4. Monosodium urate is easily ultrafiltered and dialyzed from plasma. Binding of urate to plasma proteins has little physiologic significance.

Plasma is saturated with monosodium urate at a concentration of 415 μmol/L (6.8 mg/dL) at 37°C. At higher concentrations, plasma is therefore supersaturated, and potential exists for urate crystal precipitation. However, precipitation does not occur even at plasma urate concentrations as high as 4800 μmol/L (80 mg/dL), perhaps because of the presence of solubilizing substances in plasma.

Uric acid is more soluble in urine than in water, possibly because of the presence of urea, proteins, and mucopolysaccharides. The pH of urine greatly influences its solubility. At pH 5.0, urine is saturated with uric acid at concentrations ranging from 360 to 900 μmol/L (6 to 15 mg/dL). At pH 7.0, saturation is reached at concentrations between 9480 and 12,000 μmol/L (158 and 200 mg/dL). Ionized forms of uric acid in urine include mono- and disodium, potassium, ammonium, and calcium urates.

Although purine nucleotides are synthesized and degraded in all tissues, urate is produced only in tissues that contain xanthine oxidase, primarily liver and small intestine. The amount of urate in the body is the net result of the amount produced and the amount excreted (Fig. 344-1). Urate production varies with the purine content of the diet and the rates of purine biosynthesis, degradation, and salvage. Normally, two-thirds to three-fourths of urate is excreted by the kidneys, and most of the remainder is eliminated through the intestines. A three-component model that includes glomerular filtration and both tubular secretion and reabsorption is proposed for the renal handling of uric acid in humans (Fig. 344-2). Approximately 8 to 12 percent of urate filtered by the glomeruli is excreted in the urine as uric acid. After filtration, 98 to 100 percent of the urate is reabsorbed, about half the reabsorbed urate is secreted back into the proximal tubule, and about 40 percent of that is again reabsorbed.

Serum urate levels vary with age and sex. Most children have serum urate concentrations of 180 to 240 μmol/L (3.0 to 4.0 mg/dL). Levels begin to rise during puberty in males but remain low in females until menopause. Although the cause of this gender variation is not completely understood, it is in part due to higher excretion of urate in females and is attributable to hormonal influences. Mean serum urate values for adult men and premenopausal women are 415 and 360 μmol/L (6.8 and 6.0 mg/dL), respectively. After menopause, values for women increase to approximate those of men. Adult concentrations rise steadily over time and vary with height, body weight, blood pressure, renal function, and alcohol intake.

HYPERURICEMIA

Hyperuricemia may be defined as a plasma (or serum) urate concentration greater than 420 μmol/L (7.0 mg/dL). This definition is based on physicochemical, epidemiologic, and disease-related criteria. Physicochemically, hyperuricemia is the concentration of urate in the blood that exceeds the solubility limits of monosodium urate in plasma, 415 μmol/L (6.8 mg/dL). In epidemiologic studies, hyperuricemia is defined as the mean plus 2 standard deviations of values determined from a randomly selected healthy population. When measured in unselected individuals, 95 percent have serum urate concentrations below 420 μmol/L (7.0 mg/dL). Finally, hyperuricemia can be defined in relation to the risk of disease. The risk of developing gout or urolithiasis increases with urate levels greater than 420 μmol/L (7.0 mg/dL) and escalates in proportion to the degree of elevation. Hyperuricemia is present in between 2.0 and 13.2 percent of ambulatory adults and somewhat more frequently in hospitalized individuals.

FIGURE 344-2 Schematic for handling of uric acid by the kidney. Components are illustrated with the percentage of filtered urate.

CAUSES OF HYPERURICEMIA It is useful to classify hyperuricemia in relation to the underlying physiology, i.e., whether the hyperuricemia results from increased production, decreased excretion, or a combination of the two (Fig. 344-1, Table 344-1).

Increased Urate Production Diet provides an exogenous source of purines and, accordingly, contributes to the serum urate in proportion to its purine content. Strict restriction of purine intake reduces the mean serum urate level by as little as 60 μmol/L (1.0 mg/dL) and urinary uric acid excretion by approximately 1.2 mmol/d (200 mg/d). Because about 50 percent of ingested RNA purine and 25 percent of ingested DNA purine appear in the urine as uric acid, foods high in nucleic acid content have a significant effect on the serum urate level. Such foods include liver, "sweetbreads" (i.e., thymus and pancreas), kidney, and anchovy.

Endogenous sources of purine production also influence the serum urate level (Fig. 344-3). De novo purine biosynthesis, the formation of a purine ring from nonring structures, is an 11-step process that results in formation of inosine monophosphate (IMP). The first step combines phosphoribosylpyrophosphate (PRPP) and glutamine and is catalyzed by amidophosphoribosyltransferase (amidoPRT). The rates of purine biosynthesis and urate production are determined, for the most part, by this enzyme. AmidoPRT is regulated by the substrate PRPP, which drives the reaction forward, and by the end products of biosynthesis (IMP and other ribonucleotides), which provide feedback inhibition. A second regulatory pathway is the salvage of purine bases by hypoxanthine phosphoribosyltransferase (HPRT). HPRT catalyzes the combination of the purine bases hypoxanthine and guanine with PRPP to form the respective ribonucleotides IMP and guanosine mono-

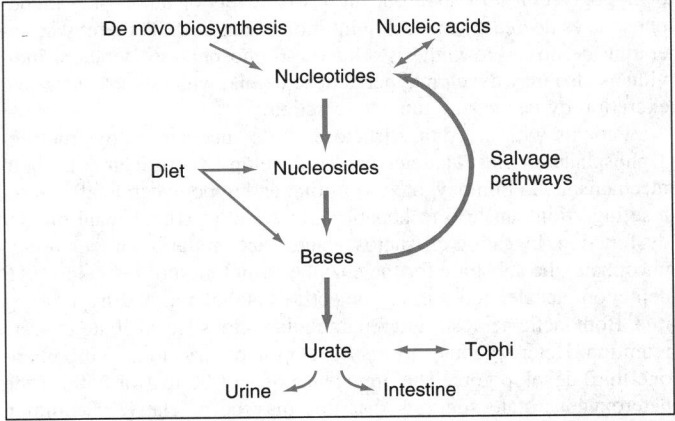

FIGURE 344-1 The total-body urate pool is the net result between urate production and excretion. Urate production is influenced by dietary intake of purines and the rates of de novo biosynthesis of purines from nonpurine precursors, nucleic acid turnover, and salvage by phosphoribosyltransferase activities. The formed urate is normally excreted by urinary and intestinal routes. Hyperuricemia can result from increased production, decreased excretion, or a combination of both mechanisms. When hyperuricemia exists, urate can precipitate and deposit in tissues as tophi.

Table 344-1

Classification of Hyperuricemia

URATE OVERPRODUCTION		
Primary idiopathic	Myeloproliferative diseases	Rhabdomyolysis
HPRT deficiency		Exercise
PRPP synthetase overactivity	Polycythemia vera	Alcohol
	Psoriasis	Obesity
Hemolytic processes	Paget's disease	Purine-rich diet
Lymphoproliferative diseases	Glycogenosis III, V, and VII	

DECREASED URIC ACID EXCRETION		
Primary idiopathic	Starvation ketosis	Drug ingestion
Renal insufficiency	Berylliosis	Salicylates (>2 g/d)
Polycystic kidney disease	Sarcoidosis	Diuretics
Diabetes insipidus	Lead intoxication	Alcohol
Hypertension	Hyperparathyroidism	Levodopa
Acidosis	Hypothyroidism	Ethambutol
Lactic acidosis	Toxemia of pregnancy	Pyrazinamide
Diabetic ketoacidosis	Bartter's syndrome	Nicotinic acid
	Down syndrome	Cyclosporine

COMBINED MECHANISM		
Glucose-6-phosphatase deficiency	Fructose-1-phosphate aldolase deficiency	Alcohol
		Shock

FIGURE 344-3 Abbreviated scheme of purine metabolism. (1) Phosphoribosylpyrophosphate (PRPP) synthetase, (2) amidophosphoribosyltransferase (amidoPRT), (3) adenylosuccinate lyase, (4) adenylate (AMP) deaminase, (5) 5′-nucleotidase, (6) adenosine deaminase, (7) purine nucleoside phosphorylase, (8) hypoxanthine phosphoribosyltransferase (HPRT), (9) adenine phosphoribosyltransferase (APRT), and (10) xanthine oxidase. PRPP, phosphoribosylpyrophosphate; PRA, phosphoribosylamine; SAICAR, succinylaminoimidazole carboxamide ribotide; AICAR, aminoimidazole carboxamide ribotide; GMP, guanylate; IMP, inosinate; AMP, adenylate.

phosphate (GMP). Increased salvage activity thus retards de novo synthesis by reducing PRPP levels and increasing concentrations of inhibitory ribonucleotides.

Serum urate levels are closely coupled to the rates of de novo purine biosynthesis. An X-linked disorder that causes an increase in activity of the enzyme PRPP synthetase causes increased PRPP production and accelerated de novo biosynthesis. PRPP is a substrate and allosteric activator of amidoPRT, the first enzyme in the de novo pathway. Individuals with this inborn error of metabolism have overproduction of purines, hyperuricemia, and hyperuricaciduria and develop uric acid calculi and gout before age 20.

Similarly, individuals deficient in HPRT have hyperuricemia, hyperuricaciduria, uric acid calculi, and gout because of urate overproduction. HPRT deficiency is also X-linked. A complete deficiency of HPRT, the Lesch-Nyhan syndrome, is also associated with self-mutilation, choreoathetosis, and other neurologic problems. Individuals with partial HPRT deficiency, the Kelley-Seegmiller syndrome, develop gout and renal calculi only. HPRT deficiency enhances urate biosynthesis in two ways. PRPP is accumulated as a result of decreased utilization in the salvage pathway and, in turn, provides increased substrate for amidoPRT and de novo biosynthesis. In addition, decreased formation of the nucleoside monophosphates IMP and GMP via the salvage pathway impairs feedback inhibition on amidoPRT, further enhancing de novo biosynthesis.

Accelerated purine nucleotide degradation also can cause hyperuricemia, e.g., with conditions of rapid cell turnover, proliferation, or cell death, as in leukemic blast crises, cytotoxic therapy for malignancy, hemolysis, or rhabdomyolysis. Nucleic acids released from cells are hydrolyzed by the sequential activities of nucleases and phosphodiesterases, forming nucleoside monophosphates, and then are degraded to nucleosides, bases, and urate. Hyperuricemia can result from excessive

degradation of skeletal muscle ATP after strenuous physical exercise or status epilepticus and in glycogen storage diseases types III, V, and VII (see Chap. 347). The hyperuricemia of myocardial infarction, smoke inhalation, and acute respiratory failure also may be related to accelerated breakdown of ATP.

Decreased Uric Acid Excretion As many as 98 percent of individuals with primary hyperuricemia and gout have a defect in the renal handling of uric acid. This is evidenced as a lower than normal ratio of urate clearance to glomerular filtration rate (or urate to inulin clearance rate) over a wide range of filtered loads. As a result, gouty individuals excrete approximately 40 percent less uric acid than nongouty individuals for any given plasma urate concentration. Uric acid excretion increases in gouty and nongouty individuals when plasma urate levels are raised by purine ingestion or infusion, but in those with gout, plasma urate concentrations must be 60 to 120 μmol/L (1 to 2 mg/dL) higher than normal to achieve equivalent uric acid excretion rates.

Altered uric acid excretion could theoretically result from decreased glomerular filtration, decreased tubular secretion, or enhanced tubular reabsorption. Decreased urate filtration does not appear to cause primary hyperuricemia but does contribute to the hyperuricemia of renal insufficiency. Although hyperuricemia is invariably present in chronic renal disease, the correlation between serum creatinine, urea nitrogen, and urate concentration is poor because although uric acid excretion per unit of glomerular filtration rate increases progressively with chronic renal insufficiency, tubular secretory capacity tends to be preserved, tubular reabsorptive capacity is reduced, and extrarenal clearance of uric acid increases as renal damage becomes more severe.

Decreased proximal tubular secretion of urate may cause the hyperuricemia in individuals with gout and no evidence of urate overproduction. Decreased tubular secretion of urate also causes the secondary hyperuricemia of acidosis. Diabetic ketoacidosis, starvation, ethanol intoxication, lactic acidosis, and salicylate intoxication are accompanied by accumulations of organic acids (β-hydroxybutyrate, acetoacetate, lactate, or salicylates) that compete with urate for tubular secretion. In some individuals with gout, hyperuricemia may be due to enhanced reabsorption of uric acid distal to the site of secretion, a mechanism known to be responsible for the hyperuricemia of extracellular volume depletion such as with diabetes insipidus or diuretic therapy.

Combined Mechanisms Both increased urate production and decreased uric acid excretion may contribute to hyperuricemia. Individuals with a deficiency of glucose-6-phosphatase, the enzyme that hydrolyzes glucose-6-phosphate to glucose, are hyperuricemic from infancy and develop gout early in life (see Chap. 347). Increased urate production results from accelerated ATP degradation during fasting or hypoglycemia. In addition, the lower levels of nucleoside monophosphates decrease feedback inhibition of amidoPRT, thereby accelerating de novo biosynthesis. Glucose-6-phosphatase–deficient individuals also may develop hyperlacticacidemia, which blocks uric acid excretion by decreasing tubular secretion.

Patients with hereditary fructose intolerance caused by fructose-1-phosphate aldolase deficiency also develop hyperuricemia by both mechanisms. In homozygotes, vomiting and hypoglycemia after fructose ingestion can lead to hepatic failure and proximal renal tubular dysfunction. Ingestion of fructose causes accumulation of fructose-1-phosphate, the substrate for the enzyme, which in turn results in ATP depletion, accelerated purine nucleotide catabolism, and hyperuricemia. Both lactic acidosis and renal tubular acidosis contribute to urate retention. Heterozygous carriers develop hyperuricemia, and perhaps one-third develop gout. The prevalence of 1 of 80 to 1 of 250 for the heterozygous state suggests that this may be a relatively common cause of familial gout.

Alcohol also promotes hyperuricemia by both mechanisms. Excessive alcohol consumption causes accelerated hepatic breakdown of ATP and increased urate production and may cause hyperlacticacidemia, which blocks uric acid secretion. The higher purine content in some alcoholic beverages such as beer may be a factor.

EVALUATION OF HYPERURICEMIA Hyperuricemia does not necessarily represent a disease, nor is it a specific indication for therapy. Rather, the finding of hyperuricemia is an indication to determine its cause. The decision to treat depends on the cause and the potential consequences of the hyperuricemia in each individual.

Quantification of the uric acid excretion can be used to determine whether hyperuricemia is caused by overproduction or decreased excretion. On a purine-free diet, men with normal renal function excrete less than 3.6 mmol/d (600 mg/d). Thus, the hyperuricemia of individuals who excrete more uric acid while on a purine-free diet is due to purine overproduction, and that in those excreting less is due to decreased excretion. If the assessment is performed while the patient is on a regular diet, the level of 4.2 mmol/d (800 mg/d) can be used as the discriminating value. With renal insufficiency, less urate is filtered in the glomeruli and less uric acid appears in the urine. Consequently, a lower 24-h urinary uric acid value in the presence of renal insufficiency does not necessarily rule out urate overproduction, but an elevated value provides strong evidence of urate overproduction. Spuriously high values can occur if a uricosuric agent is being taken at the time of urine collection. Glucocorticoids, ascorbic acid, salicylates in doses greater than 2 g/d, and other agents that promote urate excretion interfere with the interpretation of results.

Assessment of the ratio of uric acid to creatinine (or the ratio of uric acid clearance to creatinine clearance) in spot or random urine samples is not a reliable method to screen for urate overproduction. However, this is a useful tool for evaluating individuals with acute renal failure suspected of having acute uric acid nephropathy (see below).

COMPLICATIONS OF HYPERURICEMIA   Although the manifestations of gout can occur in almost any combination, the typical sequence involves progression through asymptomatic hyperuricemia, acute gouty arthritis, interval or intercritical gout, and chronic or tophaceous gout. Nephrolithiasis can occur before or after the first attack of gouty arthritis.

The prevalence of hyperuricemia ranges between 2.0 and 13.2 percent, and the prevalence of gout is between 1.3 and 3.7 percent of the general population. The higher the serum urate level, the more likely an individual is to develop gout. In one study, the incidence of gout was 4.9 percent for individuals with serum urate concentrations of 540 μmol/L (9.0 mg/dL) or more compared with 0.5 percent for those with values between 415 and 535 μmol/L (7.0 and 8.9 mg/dL). The complications of gout correlate with both the duration and severity of hyperuricemia. Most first attacks of gouty arthritis follow 20 to 40 years of sustained hyperuricemia; the peak age of onset is between 40 and 60 years for men and after menopause for women.

Gouty Arthritis   The benchmark feature of gout is acute monarticular arthritis. The first attack begins explosively and is very painful. Occasionally, individuals report a prodrome or previous episodes of milder pain lasting hours. The agonizing pain of acute gout is accompanied by signs of intense inflammation: swelling, erythema, warmth, exquisite tenderness, and on occasion low-grade fever. If untreated, the attack usually peaks 24 to 48 h after the first symptoms and subsides within 7 to 10 days. The skin over the involved part may desquamate as the episode resolves.

The initial attack usually affects a single joint, although polyarticular onsets occur and may be more common in women. Gouty arthritis primarily affects peripheral joints, particularly those of the lower extremities, but periarticular sites such as plantar fascia, Achilles tendon insertions, Heberden's nodes, or other tenosynovia can be affected. The first metatarsophalangeal joint is involved in over 50 percent of first attacks and in 90 percent of individuals at some time. Sacroiliac, sternomanubrial, and spinal involvement is rare.

Any factor that causes either an abrupt increase or decrease in the serum urate level may provoke an acute attack, the best correlations being with factors that cause a rapid fall. In theory, sudden increases in urate concentration may cause new crystals to form, whereas a drop in serum and extracellular urate concentrations may lead to partial dissolution and shedding of previously formed crystals. Other provocative factors include stress, trauma, infection, hospitalization, surgery, starvation, weight reduction, hyperalimentation, excessive food intake, alcohol, and medications (Table 344-2). Of these, hospitalization and medications are probably the most significant. Acute gouty attacks

Table 344-2

Medications with Uricosuric Activity

Acetohexamide	Glyceryl guaiacolate
ACTH	Glycopyrrolate
Ascorbic acid	Halofenate
Azauridine	Meclofenamate
Benzbromarone	Phenolsulfonphthalein
Calcitonin	Phenylbutazone
Chlorprothixene	Probenecid
Citrate	Radiographic contrast agents
Dicumarol	Salicylates (>2 g/2d)
Diflunisal	Sulfinpyrazone
Estrogens	Tetracycline that is outdated
Glucocorticoids	Zoxazolamine

occur in 20 to 86 percent of individuals with a history of gout when they are hospitalized for medical or surgical reasons. The stress of a severe illness, changes in medication, shifts in fluid status or electrolytes, and general anesthesia probably contribute to the exacerbations. Attacks can follow the use of thiazide diuretics that cause hyperuricemia or after initiation of allopurinol or other therapies to lower serum urate.

Occasional attacks of acute gouty arthritis occur in the absence of hyperuricemia. Presumably most such attacks can be explained by factors that lower serum concentrations, temporarily altering the usual hyperuricemic state (and that perhaps triggered the attack). Occasionally, hyperuricemia cannot be documented despite repeated attempts. Gout could theoretically develop anytime synovial fluid is supersaturated with urate. Free water is cleared from the joint space more rapidly than urate, and if the amount of synovial fluid containing a normal level of urate increases because of trauma or edema, then the urate level within the joint would temporarily increase as the problem resolved and the water was more rapidly cleared. Supersaturated concentrations of urate could cause the formation of crystals and precipitate an attack.

Some individuals have only a single gouty attack in their lifetime; others experience recurrence. Although the interval between first and second attacks may be over 40 years, three-fourths have a second attack within 2 years. The terms *interval gout* or *intercritical gout* describe the periods between attacks of acute arthritis when the individual has no joint complaints. In severe cases, unless therapeutic intervention occurs, chronic gouty arthritis develops with time. The pain-free intercritical periods shorten, and acute attacks occur with increased frequency, last longer, and involve more joints. The intensity of attacks may lessen somewhat, and involvement becomes polyarticular. Chronic gout is characterized by persistent polyarticular low-grade pain with acute or subacute inflammation. During this stage, tophi become apparent on physical examination (Fig. 344-4). The rates of urate deposition in joint tissues and of articular destruction correlate with the duration and severity of hyperuricemia. Approximately 10 years usually elapse between the first attack of arthritis and appearance of tophi. During the interim, however, destruction of cartilage and bone occurs, as evidenced by the radiographic changes (Fig. 344-5).

Pathogenesis   Acute gout results from the interaction between urate crystals and polymorphonuclear leukocytes (Fig. 344-6) and involves activation of humoral and cellular inflammatory mechanisms. Urate crystals activate complement through both the classic and alternate pathways. Factor XII (Hageman factor) and the contact system of coagulation are also activated and result in generation of bradykinin, kallikrein, and plasmin. Urate crystals interact with neutrophils to cause the release of lysosomal enzymes, oxygen-derived free radicals, leukotriene and prostaglandin metabolites, collagenase, and protease. Phagocytosis of crystals by neutrophils causes release of crystal-induced chemotactic factor. Chemotactic factor, leukotriene B$_4$, and the activated complement component C5a are all chemotactic and contribute to the marked polymorphonuclear leukocyte response in the initial phase of acute arthritis. With time, phagocytic mononuclear cells replace the

FIGURE 344-4 Chronic tophaceous gout. The left panel shows deformities of the foot in a 65-year-old man with a long history of gouty arthritis. On the right are tophi in an olecranon bursa and in the fingers of a 25-year-old man with Kelley-Seegmiller syndrome (partial HPRT deficiency).

FIGURE 344-5 Radiographic changes in gout are the result of urate deposition. At first deposits are microscopic and are undetectable by x-ray. With persistent hyperuricemia, tophi enlarge to involve juxtaarticular bone and are apparent radiographically but not on physical examination. If unaltered by therapy, tophi continue to enlarge and become obvious in physical examination. The classic radiographic change of gout is a bony erosion. The location can be intraarticular, paraarticular, or at a distance from the joint. The erosions tend to be round and surrounded by a sclerotic border, giving a "punched out" appearance. There may be an "overhanging margin or lip." Nodular soft tissue prominence develops as the tophi enlarge. Joint spaces are typically preserved until late in the disease when secondary degenerative changes may occur. The left panel shows classic advanced changes of tophaceous gout including soft tissue distortion and erosion with sclerotic margins and overhanging edges. The right panel shows an erosive lesion in the interphalangeal joint in a patient with no tophi found on physical examination.

polymorphonuclear cells. Urate crystals cause these cells to release prostaglandins (PGE_2), lysosomal enzymes, tumor necrosis factor α, and interleukin (IL) 1 and IL-6. Synovial lining cells participate in the inflammation by releasing inflammatory mediators such as IL-8.

The inflammatory potential of urate crystals is affected by the presence of absorbed proteins. Absorbed purified IgG causes enhanced crystal-induced platelet secretion, increased superoxide generation, and increased lysosomal enzyme release from polymorphonuclear leukocytes. On the other hand, apoprotein B, a component of very low density, low-density, and intermediate-density lipoproteins, inhibits urate crystal–induced stimulation of neutrophils. Apoprotein B is not normally present in synovial fluid and probably does not have access to that compartment under normal conditions because of its size. When synovitis develops, larger molecules, including lipoproteins, enter the joint space, bind to urate crystals, and, perhaps, play a role in terminating the attack.

Tophi are aggregates of monosodium urate monohydrate crystals and are generally surrounded by a giant cell, foreign body–type mononuclear cell inflammatory reaction. They can form in extraarticular and articular structures and cause deformity and destruction of hard and soft tissues. In joints, they lead to destruction of cartilage and bone, triggering secondary degeneration.

Renal Disease Despite the invariable hyperuricemia in renal failure, gouty arthritis occurs in fewer than 1 percent of patients with chronic renal failure. Since most gouty arthritis follows many years of sustained hyperuricemia, most patients with renal failure are probably not hyperuricemic long enough to accumulate the necessary urate load. In addition, individuals with chronic renal insufficiency have diminished inflammatory responses to urate crystals injected subcutaneously. Polycystic disease of the kidneys is an exception, with a prevalence of gout between 24 and 36 percent. The mechanism for this association is unknown.

Chronic renal failure patients on long-term hemodialysis can experience recurrent acute arthritis or periarthritis. Some of these attacks are gout due to urate crystal deposition, and others are caused by crystals of calcium phosphate (apatite) or calcium oxalate.

Gout is an important cause of morbidity in recipients of renal allografts. From 7 to 12 percent of individuals who receive cyclosporine and glucocorticoids for immunosuppression develop acute gouty arthritis, an occurrence that is even more common when diuretics are given concomitantly; there is a mean duration of about 17 months between transplantation and first attack. In contrast, gouty attacks are rare in transplant recipients maintained with azathioprine and glucocor-

ticoids. In cyclosporine-treated transplant recipients, urate synthesis is normal, and urate clearance is decreased compared with azathioprine-treated controls.

Hyperuricemia causes several renal problems: (1) nephrolithiasis; (2) urate nephropathy, a rare cause of renal insufficiency attributed to monosodium urate crystal deposition in the renal interstitium; and (3) uric acid nephropathy, a reversible cause of acute renal failure resulting from deposition of large amounts of uric acid crystals in the renal collecting ducts, pelvis, and ureters.

Nephrolithiasis Nephrolithiasis may precede the onset of gouty arthritis in 40 percent of individuals with both conditions. In gout, the prevalence of nephrolithiasis correlates with the serum and urinary uric acid levels, reaching approximately 50 percent with serum urate levels of 770 μmol/L (13 mg/dL) or urinary uric acid excretion over 6.5 mmol/d (1100 mg/d).

Not all kidney stones in individuals with gout are composed of uric acid. Stones of calcium oxalate, calcium phosphate, or those salts combined with uric acid occur in approximately 15 percent of cases. Uric acid may act as a nidus on which calcium oxalate can precipitate or lower the formation product for calcium oxalate crystallization. Furthermore, uric acid stones can develop in individuals with no other manifestations of gout, only 20 percent of whom are hyperuricemic. Some nongouty individuals with calcium oxalate stones have hyperuricemia or hyperuricaciduria.

Urate nephropathy Urate nephropathy, sometimes referred to as *urate nephrosis*, is a late manifestation of severe gout and is characterized histologically by deposits of monosodium urate crystals surrounded by a giant cell inflammatory reaction in the medullary intersti-

FIGURE 344-6   Crystals of monosodium urate in polymorphonuclear leukocytes and synovial fluid.

tium and pyramids and can cause chronic renal insufficiency. The disorder is now rare and cannot be diagnosed in the absence of gouty arthritis. The lesions may be clinically silent or cause proteinuria, hypertension, and renal insufficiency.

Prior to the advent of antihyperuricemic agents and aggressive treatment for asymptomatic hypertension, renal failure was the cause of death in up to 25 percent of individuals with gout. Postmortem evaluations of kidneys from patients with gout frequently revealed urate crystals, pyelonephritis, and vascular changes. At present, aging or coexisting diseases that cause nephropathy, such as cardiovascular disease, hypertension, or independently occurring renal disease, are usually responsible for decreased renal function in gout.

Uric acid nephropathy   This reversible cause of acute renal failure is due to precipitation of uric acid in renal tubules and collecting ducts that causes obstruction to urine flow. Uric acid nephropathy develops following sudden urate overproduction and marked hyperuricaciduria. Factors that favor uric acid crystal formation include dehydration and acidosis. This form of acute renal failure occurs most often during an aggressive "blastic" phase of leukemia or lymphoma prior to or coincident with cytolytic therapy but also has been observed in individuals with other neoplasms, following epileptic seizures, and after vigorous exercise with heat stress. Autopsy studies have demonstrated intraluminal precipitates of uric acid, dilated proximal tubules, and normal glomeruli. The initial pathogenic events are believed to include obstruction of collecting ducts with uric acid and obstruction of distal renal vasculature.

If recognized, uric acid nephropathy is potentially reversible. Appropriate therapy has reduced the mortality from about 50 percent to practically nil. Serum levels cannot be relied on for diagnosis because this condition has developed in the presence of urate concentrations varying from 720 to 4800 μmol/L (12 to 80 mg/dL). The distinctive feature is the urinary uric acid concentration. In most forms of acute renal failure with decreased urine output, urinary uric acid content is either normal or reduced, and the ratio of uric acid to creatinine is less than 1. In acute uric acid nephropathy the ratio of uric acid to creatinine in a random urine sample or 24-h specimen is greater than 1, and a value that high is essentially diagnostic.

℞ TREATMENT

Asymptomatic Hyperuricemia   For many years, fear of adverse outcomes caused physicians to prescribe urate-lowering agents for asymptomatic hyperuricemia. Today, treatment of asymptomatic hyperuricemia is not generally cost-effective or beneficial. The excep-

tion is in individuals with neoplastic disease who are about to receive cytolytic therapy and are at risk for acute uric acid nephropathy.

Although hyperuricemic individuals are at risk for gouty arthritis, especially those with higher serum urate levels, treatment of asymptomatic hyperuricemia to prevent the first attack of gouty arthritis is not appropriate because most hyperuricemic people never develop gout. Furthermore, neither structural kidney damage nor tophi are identifiable before the first attack. Reduced renal function cannot be attributed to asymptomatic hyperuricemia, and treatment of asymptomatic hyperuricemia does not alter the progression of renal dysfunction in patients with renal disease. Although nephrolithiasis is common in gouty patients and although a number of individuals with nephrolithiasis are hyperuricemic, the risk of stone formation in people with asymptomatic hyperuricemia is not established. Nor is hyperuricemia an independent risk factor for atherosclerotic cardiovascular disease.

Thus, because treatment with antihyperuricemic agents entails inconvenience, cost, and potential toxicity, routine treatment of asymptomatic hyperuricemia cannot be justified other than for prevention of acute uric acid nephropathy. In addition, routine screening for asymptomatic hyperuricemia is not recommended. If hyperuricemia is diagnosed, however, the cause should be determined. Causal factors should be corrected if the condition is secondary, and associated problems such as hypertension, hypercholesterolemia, diabetes mellitus, and obesity should be treated.

Symptomatic Hyperuricemia   Initially, therapy should be directed toward relieving symptoms. Both gouty arthritis and nephrolithiasis are excruciatingly painful. Once the presenting symptoms are controlled, a decision must be made whether to initiate antihyperuricemic therapy.

Acute Gouty Arthritis   As with any disease, appropriate and effective treatment requires accurate diagnosis. Few conditions can be diagnosed with more certainty or treated more successfully than gout. A definitive diagnosis requires aspiration of the involved joint or tissue and demonstration of intracellular monosodium urate crystals in synovial fluid polymorphonuclear leukocytes or in tophaceous aggregates. Using polarized light microscopy with a first-order red compensator, the strong negative birefringence of the needle-shaped crystals can be demonstrated easily. The triad of acute monarticular arthritis, hyperuricemia, and a dramatic response to colchicine provides presumptive evidence for gouty arthritis. These criteria, however, are a poor substitute for crystal identification, because some patients with gout are not hyperuricemic at the time of the attack. In addition, colchicine may be effective for other disorders, especially pseudogout (calcium pyrophosphate dehydrate crystal deposition disease) and calcific (basic calcium phosphate or apatite) tendinitis. These diseases that mimic acute gout may occur in individuals who happen to be hyperuricemic. Finally, acute gouty arthritis can coexist with septic arthritis, psoriatic arthritis, systemic lupus erythematosus, rheumatoid arthritis, osteoarthritis, and pseudogout.

Once the diagnosis of gouty arthritis is secure, the choice of therapeutic agents includes colchicine, nonsteroidal anti-inflammatory drugs (NSAIDs), or intraarticular glucocorticoids. Regardless of the choice, the effectiveness of the agent is dependent on when it is used. Each will work if started early; none works quickly if initiated late in the attack.

Colchicine, the traditional agent used, inhibits neutrophil activation by inhibiting crystal-induced protein tyrosine phosphorylation. Oral doses of 0.6 mg are given every hour until improvement occurs, gastrointestinal side effects develop, or 10 doses have been taken without relief (in which case the diagnosis may be questioned). Although highly effective, oral colchicine cannot be tolerated by up to 80 percent of people because of abdominal pain, diarrhea, and nausea. Colchicine also can be given intravenously, but administration by this route is potentially dangerous and should be used with extreme caution despite the fact that this route of administration can eliminate the gastrointestinal side effects (provided the drug is not also being taken orally). A single dose of 1 or 2 mg diluted in 20 mL normal saline is usually adequate. A second dose of 1 mg can be repeated 6 to 12 h later. Absolute contraindications for intravenous colchicine include depressed bone marrow function, renal disease (creatinine clearance less than 10 mL/min, oliguria, or anuria), liver disease (liver function tests over twice the upper limit of normal), and sepsis.

Because of its relative specificity for acute gouty arthritis, oral colchicine is the agent of choice for the ambulatory patient in whom the diagnosis is not certain. If the diagnosis is certain, NSAIDs may be more appropriate because of better tolerance. Indomethacin is the usual agent, but ibuprofen, naproxen, tolmetin, sulindac, piroxicam, ketoprofen, flurbiprofen, and other NSAIDs have been effective. These agents are less specific for gout than colchicine, but they are effective, especially if used early in the attack. Treatment is begun with the highest approved dose of the selected agent and is continued until 3 to 4 days after all signs of inflammation have resolved. These agents are contraindicated in patients with active peptic ulcer disease; should be used with caution in patients with heart failure, other edematous states, or hypertension because of potential problems from sodium retention; and may precipitate hyperkalemia and renal insufficiency.

Intraarticular injection of glucocorticoids also may be used for acute gout. This is most useful when the patient cannot take oral medications, when colchicine and NSAIDs are contraindicated, or in refractory cases. A single intramuscular injection of ACTH (40 or 50 units) has also been employed for acute gouty arthritis.

INTERCRITICAL AND CHRONIC GOUT The term *intercritical* (or *interval*) *gout* applies to the period after the acute gouty attack when the patient is asymptomatic. At that time the decision must be made whether to initiate antihyperuricemic therapy. All authors agree that hyperuricemia should be treated in patients with recurrent attacks, those with chronic gout or evidence of tophi, and those with gouty arthritis and nephrolithiasis. Some maintain that the first attack of acute gouty arthritis alone is sufficient indication. Others argue that first attacks are easily, inexpensively, and effectively treated and postpone urate-lowering therapy until one or more additional attacks occur.

Sustained hyperuricemia provides a definite risk to bone and cartilage for those with gouty arthritis. If hyperuricemia is not controlled, urate deposits enlarge and become radiographically evident before subcutaneous tophi develop. In a study of patients with intercritical gout, 42 percent had radiographic changes characteristic of bony tophi despite no evidence of tophi on physical examination (see Fig. 344-5). One cannot predict from the frequency of acute attacks, the history of therapy, or the serum urate levels at the time of evaluation which patients will show bony changes.

Before starting treatment with urate-lowering agents, the patient should be free of all signs of inflammation and have begun colchicine for prophylaxis. The sudden drop in serum urate with the initiation of allopurinol or uricosuric therapy may prolong or precipitate an acute attack. Colchicine, at a dose of 0.6 mg orally one to three times a day, is about 90 percent effective in preventing subsequent gout attacks. Rarely, a reversible colchicine-induced toxicity may be manifested by subacute myopathy and axonal neuropathy with elevated serum creatinine kinase levels. This toxicity is most common in individuals with renal insufficiency and is reversible when colchicine is discontinued.

Once antihyperuricemic therapy is initiated, the dosage used should maintain the serum urate at or below 300 μmol/L (5.0 mg/dL). Extracellular fluid is saturated with urate at a concentration of approximately 415 μmol/L (6.8 mg/dL). If the serum urate remains above this level, tissue deposition of urate crystals will continue. A reduction of the serum urate concentration from 600 to 480 μmol/L (10 to 8 mg/dL), for example, will not reduce the total-body urate pool but will slow the rate at which the pool increases. If, on the other hand, the urate concentration is reduced below 415 μmol/L (6.8 mg/dL), urate crystals can dissolve, and the urate pool will decrease. Successful therapy will prevent future attacks of gout and cause resolution of tophi.

Treatment of hyperuricemia includes diet and specific urate-lowering agents. Diet now plays a minor role in the treatment of hyperuricemia because modern therapeutic agents are so effective, but dietary counseling is important and should address obesity, hyperlipidemia, diabetes mellitus, hypertension, and the use of alcohol.

Allopurinol, a substrate and competitive inhibitor of xanthine oxidase, is the most widely used antihyperuricemic agent. Oxypurinol, the major metabolite of allopurinol, is also an effective inhibitor of xanthine oxidase. Allopurinol is efficiently absorbed from the gastrointestinal tract and has a half-life of 3 h. Oxypurinol excretion is enhanced by uricosuric agents and is reduced in renal insufficiency. Allopurinol is effective in the treatment of all types of hyperuricemia but is specifically indicated for the following: (1) Patients with gout and (a) evidence of urate overproduction [24-h urinary uric acid greater than 4.8 mmol (800 mg) on a general diet or greater than 3.6 mmol (600 mg) on a purine-restricted diet], (b) nephrolithiasis, (c) renal insufficiency (creatinine clearance less than 80 mL/min), (d) tophaceous deposits, (e) age over 60 years, or (f) inability to take uricosuric agents because of ineffectiveness or intolerance; (2) patients with nephrolithiasis of any type plus urinary uric acid excretion greater than 3.6 mmol/d (600 mg/d); (3) patients with renal calculi composed of 2,8-dihydroxyadenine; and (4) patients with, or at risk for, acute uric acid nephropathy

Allopurinol administration decreases the serum urate concentration and the urinary excretion of uric acid in the first 24 h, with a maximum reduction occurring within 2 weeks. The average effective dose of allopurinol is 300 mg/d. However, the dosage required to control the serum urate concentration depends on the severity of the tophaceous disease and on renal function. Failure of a 400-mg dose to produce an adequate antihyperuricemic effect is rare and suggests noncompliance. Allopurinol can be given once a day because of the long half-life (18 h) of its active metabolite oxypurinol. The drug is effective in patients with renal insufficiency, but the dose should be reduced.

Side effects, serious complications, and toxicity of allopurinol are unusual. The most frequent side effects are skin rash, gastrointestinal distress, diarrhea, and headache. The rash is usually maculopapular and erythematous, but exfoliative dermatitis and toxic epidermal necrolysis may occur. Desensitization with low doses of allopurinol may be useful in individuals with demonstrated hypersensitivity.

Serious adverse effects include alopecia, fever, lymphadenopathy, bone marrow suppression, hepatic toxicity, interstitial nephritis, renal failure, hypersensitivity vasculitis, and death. Such toxicity is fortunately rare but does occur in patients with renal insufficiency or in those taking thiazide diuretics.

Potential drug interactions must be considered when allopurinol is prescribed. Because 6-mercaptopurine and azathioprine are inactivated by xanthine oxidase, allopurinol prolongs the half-life of these agents and thus potentiates their therapeutic and toxic effects. Cyclophosphamide toxicity also may be enhanced by concomitant use. A threefold increase in ampicillin- and amoxicillin-related skin rashes has been reported in patients taking allopurinol.

Uricosuric agents also can effectively lower serum urate concentrations by the partial inhibition of proximal tubular reabsorption of filtered and secreted urate from the luminal side of the tubule at a site distal to the point of uric acid secretion. Candidates for these agents are gouty patients who meet all the following criteria: (1) hyperuricemia attributable to decreased uric acid excretion [less than 4.8 mmol (800 mg) urinary uric acid per day while taking a regular diet or less than 3.6 mmol (600 mg) with a purine-restricted diet], (2) age under 60 years, (3) satisfactory renal function (a creatinine clearance greater than 80 mL/min), and (4) no history of nephrolithiasis.

Uricosuric agents are effective in 70 to 80 percent of patients. Failure to control the serum urate concentration may be attributed to drug intolerance, poor compliance, concomitant salicylate ingestion, or impaired renal function. Salicylates block the uricosuric effects of these agents, probably by inhibiting urate secretion. Uricosuric agents lose effectiveness as the creatinine clearance falls and are ineffective when glomerular filtration falls below 30 mL/min. The most commonly used uricosuric agents are probenecid and sulfinpyrazone. Probenecid therapy is begun at 250 mg twice a day and is increased as necessary up to 3.0 g/d. Because the half-life is 6 to 12 h, probenecid should be taken in two to three evenly spaced doses. Sulfinpyrazone therapy is initiated at a dose of 50 mg twice a day. The usual maintenance level is 300 to 400 mg/d in three or four divided doses.

By promoting uric acid excretion, uricosuric agents may precipitate nephrolithiasis. This rare complication can occur early in the course of treatment and may be prevented by initiating therapy at low doses, forcing hydration, and, possibly, alkalinizing the urine. Hypersensitivity, skin rash, and gastrointestinal complaints are the major side effects. Serious toxicity is rare, but hepatic necrosis and the nephrotic syndrome have been reported.

Nephrolithiasis Antihyperuricemic therapy is recommended for the individual who has both gouty arthritis and either uric acid– or calcium-containing stones, both of which may occur in association with hyperuricaciduria. Regardless of the nature of the calculi, fluid ingestion should be sufficient to produce a daily urine volume greater than 2 L. Alkalinization of the urine with sodium bicarbonate or acetazolamide may be justified to increase the solubility of uric acid. Specific treatment of uric acid calculi requires reducing the urine uric acid concentration with allopurinol. Allopurinol is also useful in reducing the recurrence of calcium oxalate stones in gouty subjects and in nongouty individuals with hyperuricemia or hyperuricaciduria. Potassium citrate (30 to 80 mmol/d orally in divided doses) is an alternative therapy for patients with uric acid stones alone or mixed calcium/uric acid stones. Allopurinol is also indicated for the treatment of 2,8-dihydroxyadenine kidney stones.

Uric Acid Nephropathy Uric acid nephropathy is often preventable, and immediate, appropriate therapy has reduced the mortality rate to practically nil. Vigorous intravenous hydration and diuresis with furosemide dilute the uric acid in the tubules and promote urine flow to 100 mL/h or more. The administration of acetazolamide, 240 to 500 mg every 6 to 8 h, and sodium bicarbonate, 89 mmol/L, intravenously enhances urine alkalinity and thereby solubilizes more uric acid. It is important to ensure that the urine pH remains above 7.0 and to watch for circulatory overload. In addition, antihyperuricemic therapy in the form of allopurinol in a single dose of 8 mg/kg is administered to reduce the amount of urate that reaches the kidney. If renal insufficiency persists, subsequent daily doses should be reduced to 100 to 200 mg because oxypurinol, the active metabolite of allopurinol, accumulates in renal failure. Despite these measures, hemodialysis may be required.

HYPOURICEMIA

Hypouricemia, defined as a serum urate concentration less than 120 µmol/L (2.0 mg/dL), can result from decreased production of urate, increased excretion of uric acid, or a combination of both mechanisms. It occurs in fewer than 0.2 percent of the general population and fewer than 0.8 percent of hospitalized individuals. Hypouricemia causes no symptoms or pathology and therefore requires no therapy. It is, however, a sign of potential pathology, and its cause should be determined.

Most hypouricemia results from increased renal uric acid excretion. The finding of normal amounts of uric acid in a 24-h urine collection in an individual with hypouricemia is evidence for a renal cause. Medications with uricosuric properties (see Table 344-2) include aspirin (at doses over 2.0 g/d), x-ray contrast materials, and glycerylguaiacholate. Total parenteral hyperalimentation also can cause hypouricemia, possibly a result of the high glycine content of the infusion formula. Other causes of an increased urate clearance include neoplastic disease, hepatic cirrhosis, diabetes mellitus, inappropriate secretion of vasopressin, and defects in renal tubular transport such as primary Fanconi syndrome and Fanconi syndromes caused by Wilson's disease, cystinosis, multiple myeloma, and heavy metal toxicity, and as isolated congenital defects in the bidirectional transport of uric acid.

Hypouricemia from decreased production of urate is accompanied by very low urinary uric acid levels. Accumulation of other purine nucleosides and bases may occur depending on the specific defect. Individuals treated with allopurinol and some subjects with neoplastic disease or severe hepatic dysfunction are hypouricemic and excrete increased quantities of hypoxanthine and xanthine in the urine. Xanthine oxidase deficiency can be inherited or acquired. Inherited forms include isolated xanthine oxidase deficiency and combined xanthine oxidase and sulfite oxidase deficiencies. Both cause hypouricemia and xanthinuria. Affected individuals excrete essentially no uric acid and may develop xanthine nephrolithiasis. Individuals with purine nucleoside phosphorylase deficiency, an inborn error of metabolism causing T cell–deficient immune dysfunction, are hypouricemic and excrete increased quantities of guanosine, deoxyguanosine, inosine, and deoxyinosine in the urine.

INBORN ERRORS OF PURINE METABOLISM
(See also Table 344-3, Fig. 344-3)

HPRT DEFICIENCY A complete deficiency of HPRT, the Lesch-Nyhan syndrome, is characterized by hyperuricemia, self-mutilative behavior, choreoathetosis, spasticity, and mental retardation. A partial deficiency of HPRT, the Kelley-Seegmiller syndrome, is associated with hyperuricemia but no central nervous system manifestations. In both disorders, the hyperuricemia results from urate overpro-

Table 344-3

Inborn Errors of Purine Metabolism

Enzyme	Activity	Inheritance	Clinical Features
Hypoxanthine phosphoribosyltransferase	Complete deficiency	X-linked	Self-mutilation, choreoathetosis, hyperuricemia, gout, and uric acid lithiasis
	Partial deficiency	X-linked	Hyperuricemia, gout, and uric acid lithiasis
Phosphoribosylpyrophosphate synthetase	Overactivity	X-linked	Hyperuricemia, gout, uric acid lithiasis, and deafness
Adenine phosphoribosyltransferase	Deficiency	Autosomal recessive	2,8-Dihydroxyadenine lithiasis
Xanthine oxidase	Deficiency	Autosomal recessive	Xanthinuria and xanthine lithiasis
Adenylosuccinate lyase	Deficiency	Autosomal recessive	Autism and psychomotor retardation
Myoadenylate deaminase	Deficiency	Autosomal recessive	Myopathy with exercise intolerance or asymptomatic
Adenosine deaminase	Deficiency	Autosomal recessive	Severe combined immunodeficiency disease and chrondro-osseous dysplasia
Purine nucleoside phosphorylase	Deficiency	Autosomal recessive	T cell–mediated immunodeficiency

duction and can cause uric acid crystalluria, nephrolithiasis, obstructive uropathy, and gouty arthritis. Early diagnosis and appropriate therapy with allopurinol can prevent or eliminate all the problems attributable to hyperuricemia but have no effect on the behavioral or neurologic abnormalities.

HPRT catalyzes the reaction that combines PRPP and the purine bases hypoxanthine and guanine to form the respective nucleoside monophosphate IMP or GMP and pyrophosphate. The enzyme is encoded by a single gene located on the X chromosome. Consequently, affected males are hemizygous for the trait and inherit the mutant allele from their asymptomatic mother, who is a carrier, or are the result of spontaneous gene mutations. The deficiency state is generally the result of point mutations, deletions, insertions, or endoduplication of exons rather than major gene alterations.

INCREASED PRPP SYNTHETASE ACTIVITY   Cells from individuals with increased PRPP synthetase activity contain elevated levels of PRPP. The high substrate content drives de novo purine synthesis causing overproduction of uric acid. Similar to the HPRT deficiency states, PRPP synthetase overactivity is X-linked and results in gouty arthritis and uric acid nephrolithiasis. Nerve deafness occurs in some families.

ADENINE PHOSPHORIBOSYLTRANSFERASE (APRT) DEFICIENCY   Individuals with a deficiency of APRT develop kidney stones composed of 2,8-dihydroxyadenine. APRT catalyzes the conversion of adenine to adenosine monophosphate (AMP). In the absence of APRT, adenine is converted by xanthine oxidase to 2,8-dihydroxyadenine, which is insoluble in urine. Reports of 2,8-dihydroxyadenine stones are rare, most likely because of its chemical similarity to uric acid. Analysis by x-ray powder diffraction is necessary for correct identification. Because this technique is rarely employed, many 2,8-dihydroxyadenine stones are incorrectly called uric acid. The consequence of this misidentification is not too severe, because allopurinol therapy is the correct treatment for each type of stone.

APRT deficiency is inherited as an autosomal recessive trait. Caucasians with the deficiency have a complete deficiency (type I), whereas Japanese subjects have some measurable enzyme activity (type II). Expression of the defect is similar in the two populations, as is the frequency of the heterozygous state (0.4 to 1.1 per 100).

HEREDITARY XANTHINURIA   A deficiency of xanthine oxidase causes all purine in the urine to occur in the form of hypoxanthine and xanthine. About two-thirds of deficient individuals are asymptomatic. The remainder develop kidney stones composed of xanthine. A very small number of symptomatic individuals also have myopathy or recurrent polyarteritis. Xanthinuria appears to be inherited in an autosomal recessive pattern.

In a second form of inherited xanthinuria, the deficiency of xanthine oxidase is associated with a deficiency of sulfite oxidase. Neurologic symptoms attributable to the sulfite oxidase deficiency predominate over those of xanthinuria in individuals with the combined deficiency.

MYOADENYLATE DEAMINASE DEFICIENCY   Adenylate deaminase (AMP deaminase) catalyzes the conversion of AMP to IMP with the release of ammonia and is an integral component of the purine nucleotide cycle, which plays an important role in skeletal muscle energy metabolism. A deficiency of myoadenylate deaminase, the isoform of AMP deaminase in skeletal muscle, is associated with myopathic syndromes.

Both primary (inherited) and secondary (acquired) forms of myoadenylate deaminase deficiency have been described. Myoadenylate deaminase is the only activity affected in the inherited form, whereas other muscle enzymes (creatine kinase and myokinase) are also decreased in the acquired deficiencies. Inherited deficiency is probably the result of point mutations, small deletions, or rearrangements. A single nonsense mutation has been identified in 11 unrelated families. In contrast, mRNA abundance is low in muscle from patients with acquired deficiencies, suggesting a different molecular basis for this form. The primary form is inherited as an autosomal recessive trait. Clinically, this form tends to be a relatively benign disorder characterized by easy fatigability and postexercise cramps and myalgias. Most individuals with this defect may be asymptomatic, and some believe that other explanations for the myopathy should be sought in symptomatic patients.

The acquired deficiency occurs in association with a wide variety of neuromuscular diseases, including muscular dystrophies, neuropathies, inflammatory myopathies, and collagen vascular diseases. Measurement of plasma lactate and ammonia levels after ischemic exercise of the forearm can be used to screen for this disorder. Under these conditions, subjects deficient in myoadenylate can generate lactate but not ammonia. The diagnosis can be made only by documenting the enzyme deficiency in a muscle biopsy specimen.

ADENYLOSUCCINATE LYASE DEFICIENCY   Adenylosuccinate lyase participates in the synthesis of purine nucleotides in two ways. It catalyzes the conversion of succinylaminoimidazole carboxamide ribotide (SAICAR) to aminoimidazole carboxamide ribotide (AICAR) in the de novo pathway and in the conversion of AMP succinate to AMP in the purine nucleotide cycle. Deficiency of this enzyme is due to an autosomal recessive trait and causes profound psychomotor retardation, seizures, and other movement disorders. All individuals with this deficiency are mentally retarded, and most are autistic.

ADENOSINE DEAMINASE DEFICIENCY AND PURINE NUCLEOSIDE PHOSPHORYLASE DEFICIENCY   See Chap. 307.

See Chap. 27, Drugs used in the treatment of gout, in Goodman & Gilman's The Pharmacological Basis of Therapeutics, *9th ed. New York, McGraw-Hill, 1996.*

BIBLIOGRAPHY

BECKER MA et al: Purines and pyrimidines, in *The Molecular and Metabolic Bases of Inherited Disease,* 7th ed, CR Scriver et al (eds). New York, McGraw-Hill, 1995, pp 1655–1841

KELLEY WN, WORTMANN RL: Gout and hyperuricemia, in *Textbook of Rheumatology,* 5th ed, WN Kelley et al (eds). Philadelphia, Saunders, 1996, p 1313

MCCARTHY GM et al: Influence of antihyperuricemic therapy on the clinical and radiographic progression of gout. Arthritis Rheum 34:1489, 1991

ROSENTHAL AK, RYAN LM: Treatment of refractory crystal-associated arthritis. Rheum Clin North Am 21:151, 1995

WORTMANN RL: Management of hyperuricemia, in *Arthritis and Allied Conditions,* 13th ed, DJ McCarty, WJ Koopman (eds). Philadelphia, Lea & Febiger, 1996, p 1807

WYNGAARDEN JB, KELLEY WN: *Gout and Hyperuricemia.* New York, Grune & Stratton, 1976

| 345 | *I. Herbert Scheinberg* |

WILSON'S DISEASE

Wilson's disease is an inherited disorder of copper metabolism in individuals with two mutant ATP7B genes. Impairment of the normal excretion of hepatic copper results in toxic accumulations of the metal in liver, brain, and other organs. The disease occurs in every ethnic and geographic population, with a worldwide prevalence of about 1 in 30,000, and the frequency of heterozygous carriers of the mutation is about 1 in 90.

NATURAL HISTORY   The average low concentration of ceruloplasmin and high concentration of hepatic copper in normal neonates are indistinguishable from the concentrations exhibited by neonates with Wilson's disease. In normal infants, the ceruloplasmin concentration increases and the hepatic copper concentration falls to adult levels during the first year of life. However, in infants with Wilson's disease, the neonatal deficiency of ceruloplasmin and excess of hepatic copper persist indefinitely. Clinical manifestations are rare before age 6, occur most frequently in mid-adolescence, and eventually develop in all untreated patients.

In about half of patients any of four types of hepatic disturbances may herald the clinical onset. *Acute hepatitis* is usually self-limited and often mistaken for viral hepatitis or infectious mononucleosis. It may be overlooked later in life when a diagnosis of Wilson's disease is entertained unless the patient is carefully questioned. *Parenchymal liver disease* may persist after acute hepatitis or develop insidiously without prior acute disease into a histologic and clinical picture indistinguishable from chronic active hepatitis and cirrhosis. In other patients *cirrhosis* may develop insidiously after a lapse of decades with no sign or symptom of liver disease. *Fulminant hepatitis*, generally fatal, is characterized by progressive jaundice, ascites, encephalopathy, hypoalbuminemia, hypoprothrombinemia, moderately elevated plasma levels of liver enzymes, and Coombs-negative hemolytic anemia.

In most other patients neurologic or psychiatric disturbances are the first clinical signs and are always accompanied by Kayser-Fleischer rings (**see Plate III-16**). These golden deposits of copper in Descemet's membrane of the cornea do not interfere with vision but indicate that copper has been released from the liver and has probably caused brain damage. If a patient with frank neurologic or psychiatric disease does not have Kayser-Fleischer rings when examined by a trained observer using a slit lamp, the diagnosis of Wilson's disease can be excluded. Rarely, Kayser-Fleischer rings may be accompanied by sunflower cataracts.

The neurologic manifestations include resting and intention tremors, spasticity, rigidity, chorea, drooling, dysphagia, and dysarthria. Babinski responses may be present, and abdominal reflexes are often absent. Inexplicably—in view of the ubiquity of copper excess in the brain—sensory changes, save for headache, never occur.

Psychiatric disturbances are present in most patients with neurologic symptoms. Schizophrenia, manic-depressive psychoses, and classic neuroses may occur, but the commonest disturbances are bizarre behavioral patterns that defy classification. Improvement in the psychiatric state can occur with pharmacologic reduction of the copper excess, but psychotherapy and additional pharmacotherapy may be required.

In about 5 percent of patients the clinical onset reflects neither a hepatic nor a central nervous system disturbance. The first manifesta-

FIGURE 345-2 Electron micrograph of a liver biopsy sample from a 6-year-old asymptomatic boy. There are prominent vacuoles, containing granular material, in mitochondria (M). P, peroxisome; PM, plasma membrane.

tion may be primary or secondary amenorrhea or repeated and unexplained spontaneous abortions, perhaps due to excess free copper in intrauterine secretions. Kayser-Fleischer rings may occasionally first be discovered during routine ophthalmologic examination.

PATHOGENESIS The metabolic defect in Wilson's disease is an inability to maintain a near-zero balance of copper. Dietary copper is generally in excess of the small amount that is essential to life. Normally any excess copper that is absorbed is excreted by the liver, but in patients with Wilson's disease copper accumulates in the liver.

Fatty infiltration of the hepatic parenchyma and nuclear glycogen deposits are the earliest findings by light microscopy (Fig. 345-1). With electron microscopy, characteristic mitochondrial abnormalities appear to be specific for Wilson's disease (Fig. 345-2). Later, necrosis, inflammation, fibrosis, bile duct proliferation, and cirrhosis ensue. Abnormalities in liver chemistries, particularly elevations in aminotransferases, may be seen at any stage. The capacity of hepatocytes to store copper is eventually exceeded, and copper is released into blood and taken up into extrahepatic tissues with disastrous effects in the brain (Table 345-1).

With magnetic resonance imaging, the effects of copper toxicity in the brain are seen most frequently in the lenticular nuclei and less commonly in the pons, medulla, thalamus, cerebellum, and cerebral cortex. Opalski and Alzheimer type II cells are present early in the course, although neither is specific for Wilson's disease, and neuronal necrosis and cavitation develop later.

Increased copper in the kidney produces little, if any, structural change and usually does not alter renal function. Microscopic hematuria and/or minimal proteinuria occur occasionally, and nephrocalcinosis, renal calculi, and renal tubular acidosis are rare. Pathologic effects in other organs and tissues are minor.

GENETICS The ATP7B gene on chromosome 13 that is mutated in this disease has been cloned and sequenced, and the protein product has been identified as a P type, copper-transporting ATPase.

FIGURE 345-1 Macro- and microvesicular fatty changes, glycogen deposits in nuclei, and cellular infiltrates in a hematoxylin- and eosin-stained section of liver from an asymptomatic boy with Wilson's disease.

Table 345-1

Summary of Analytic Data in Patients with Wilson's Disease,
Heterozygous Carriers, and Control Subjects

Group	Serum Ceruloplasmin		Hepatic Copper Concentration	
	No. of Patients	Mean ± SD, mg/L	No. of Patients	Mean ± SD, μg/g Dry Weight
Wilson's disease:				
Asymptomatic	31	36 ± 53	36	983.5 ± 368
Symptomatic	84	59 ± 71	33	588.3 ± 304
Heterozygous carriers	95*	284 ± 85	14	117.0 ± 51
Normal subjects	180	307 ± 35	16	31.5 ± 6.8

* 71 parents of patients with Wilson's disease and 24 children, each of whom had one
parent with Wilson's disease.
SOURCE: Sternlieb and Scheinberg, 1968.

More than 40 mutant forms of the normal gene have been identified,
and the disease can develop either in homozygotes or individuals who
are compound heterozygotes for these mutant genes. As a consequence,
molecular diagnosis is only practical in family members of patients
in whom the genetic defect has already been identified. The mechanism
by which the normal ATP7B protein promotes the excretion of hepatic
copper is not yet established, nor is it clear whether the secondary
decrease in ceruloplasmin in this disorder plays a role in the pathogenesis of the disease.

DIAGNOSIS *The diagnosis is easy provided it is suspected.*
Wilson's disease should be considered in any patient under the age
of 40 with an unexplained disorder of the central nervous system,
signs or symptoms of hepatitis, chronic active hepatitis, unexplained
persistent elevations of serum aminotransferase, hemolytic anemia in
the presence of hepatitis, or unexplained cirrhosis and in any patient
who has a near blood relative with Wilson's disease.

The diagnosis is confirmed by the demonstration of either: (1) a
serum ceruloplasmin level less than 200 mg/L *and* Kayser-Fleischer
rings or (2) a serum ceruloplasmin level less than 200 mg/L *and* a
concentration of copper in liver biopsy greater than 250 μg/g dry
weight. Most symptomatic patients excrete more than 100 μg copper
per day in urine and have histologic abnormalities on liver biopsy.

About 5 percent of patients have a serum ceruloplasmin level
greater than 200 mg/L, and some patients with other hepatic disorders,
usually primary biliary cirrhosis, have elevated hepatic copper levels
and, rarely, Kayser-Fleischer rings. In either circumstance, measurement of the ability to incorporate isotopic copper into ceruloplasmin
is useful as a discriminating test. Even in the presence of a normal
concentration of ceruloplasmin, patients with Wilson's disease incorporate little or no isotope into the protein, while patients with other
liver disorders incorporate the isotope normally.

℞ **TREATMENT**
Treatment consists of removing and detoxifying the deposits of
copper as rapidly as possible and must be instituted once the diagnosis is secure whether the patient is ill or asymptomatic. Penicillamine
is administered orally in an initial dose of 1 g daily in a single or
divided doses at least 30 min before and 2 h after eating. Because
penicillamine has an antipyridoxine effect, 25 mg/d of pyridoxine is
also given. In about 10 percent of patients sensitivity to penicillamine
develops early, making it necessary to monitor the body temperature
and skin daily and to assess white blood cell and platelet counts and
perform urinalysis several times during the first month of treatment.
Penicillamine should be discontinued if rash, fever, leukopenia,
thrombocytopenia, lymphadenopathy, or proteinuria develops. After
subsidence of the reaction, the drug can usually be resumed in small
and gradually increasing dosage. Reactions are less likely to recur
if 20 mg/d of prednisone is given during the first 2 weeks after

penicillamine therapy is reinstituted, but prednisone should not be
used for isolated leukopenia. Allergic reactions requiring a desensi-
tizing regimen may recur several times before penicillamine can be
administered without a glucocorticoid.

After therapy with penicillamine has been successfully instituted,
the patient should be seen at 1- to 3-month intervals to assess the
effectiveness of therapy and monitor for late drug toxicity. The
history and the physical examination should focus on hepatic, neurologic, and psychiatric signs and symptoms; slit-lamp examination
of the cornea should be performed by an ophthalmologist at least
yearly. White blood cell and platelet counts, transaminase levels,
albumin, bilirubin, and free serum copper (total serum copper minus
ceruloplasmin-bound copper) should be measured, the aim being a
concentration of free copper less than about 2 μmol/L (10 μg/
dL). A persistent concentration greater than 4 μmol/L (20 μg/dL)
indicates that the dose of penicillamine is too low or that the patient
is noncompliant. In patients who are asymptomatic or who have
improved maximally after several years on 1 g/d of penicillamine,
the usual effective maintenance dose is 0.75 g/d taken 45 min before breakfast.

At any time, even after years of uneventful penicillamine administration, granulocytopenia, thrombocytopenia, the nephrotic syndrome, Goodpasture's syndrome, systemic lupus erythematosus, severe arthralgias, myasthenia, mammary gigantism, or elastosis
perforans serpiginosa may supervene. The toxicity is sometimes
dose-related, and it may be possible to reduce the dose to a level that
is effective but nontoxic. Glucocorticoids may control penicillamine-
associated lupus or arthralgias.

In two situations penicillamine should be replaced by trientine.
First, although irreversible intolerance to penicillamine is rare, some
types of toxicity such as significant, persistent proteinuria may make
discontinuation necessary. Second, in occasional patients the com-
mencement of penicillamine treatment may cause the appearance or
worsening of neurologic manifestations. Substitution of trientine for
penicillamine is indicated if neurologic symptoms persist or worsen
over a 4- to 6-week period.

The dose of trientine is 1g/d in divided doses given on an empty
stomach. Pyridoxine need not be given. Although the only reported
toxic reaction to trientine is sideroblastic anemia, the same parameters should be followed during its administration as with penicillamine therapy. Except for systemic lupus and elastosis perforans
serpiginosa, the other late penicillamine-induced toxic reactions disappear or improve with trientine therapy. Moreover, trientine appears
to be as effective as penicillamine.

Zinc salts are effective at doses of 150 mg/d of elemental zinc
in patients whose copper stores have been reduced by penicillamine
or trientine. Zinc must *not*, however, be given together with penicillamine or trientine since zinc can chelate either drug and form complexes that are ineffective.

Treatment must be continual and lifelong. Inadequate treatment
or interruption of therapy can be fatal or cause irreversible relapse.
Indeed, of 11 patients who voluntarily discontinued penicillamine
after years of successful treatment, 8 died after an average of 2.6
years of noncompliance. In contrast, of 13 patients in whom trientine
was substituted because of an adverse reaction to penicillamine, 1
died accidentally, 5 were lost to follow-up, and 7 are alive and well
11 to 23 years later.

Prophylactic treatment of more than 100 asymptomatic patients
with a documented diagnosis of Wilson's disease has shown that
continual therapy with penicillamine or trientine can maintain the
asymptomatic state indefinitely; several such patients having been
followed for over 30 years.

Patients with severe neurologic disease who do not improve on
penicillamine or trientine therapy that has reduced serum free copper
to less than 2 μmol/L (10 μg/dL) may benefit from treatment with
dimercaprol. Intramuscular injections of 3 mL of the drug are given
on five successive days. Therapy is interrupted for 2 to 3 weeks,
and if neurologic improvement occurs during this intermission, the
courses should be repeated until no further improvement is noted.

The simultaneous occurrence of fulminant hepatitis and Coombs-negative hemolytic anemia may be the initial clinical manifestation of Wilson's disease or may occur in a noncompliant patient. The syndrome is almost always fatal, usually within a week or two, unless liver transplantation is performed. Of 55 patients who received liver transplants, 43 had survived for from 3 months to 20 years at last follow-up.

BIBLIOGRAPHY

BREWER GJ et al: Treatment of Wilson's disease with zinc: XI. Interaction with other anticopper agents. J Am Coll Nutr 12:26, 1993

HOOGENRAAD TU et al: Management of Wilson's disease with zinc sulfate: Experience in a series of 27 patients. J Neurol Sci 77:137, 1987

PETRUKHIN K et al: Mapping, cloning and genetic characterization of the region containing the Wilson disease gene. Nature (Genetics) 5:338, 1993

SCHEINBERG IH, STERNLIEB I: Wilson's disease, in *Major Problems in Internal Medicine.* Philadelphia, Saunders, 1984

——, ——— 1994.: Treatment of the neurological manifestations of Wilson's disease. Arch Neurol 52:339, 1995

——— et al: The use of trientine in preventing the effects of interrupting penicillamine therapy in Wilson's disease. N Engl J Med 317:209, 1987

——— et al: Penicillamine may detoxify copper in Wilson's disease. Lancet 2:95, 1987

SCHILSKY ML et al: Liver transplantation for Wilson's disease: Indications and outcome. Hepatology 19:583, 1994

STERNLIEB I: Evolution of the hepatic lesion in Wilson's disease (hepatolenticular degeneration), in *Progress in Liver Diseases*, H Popper et al (eds). New York, Grune & Stratton, 1972, vol IV, pp 511–526

——, SCHEINBERG IH: Prevention of Wilson's disease in asymptomatic patients. N Engl J Med 278:352, 1968

——, ———: Chronic hepatitis as a first manifestation of Wilson's disease. Ann Intern Med 76:59, 1972

WALSHE JM: Wilson's disease, in *Handbook of Clinical Neurology*, PJ Vinken et al (eds). New York, American Elsevier, 1986, vol 5 (49)

346 *Margaret M. McGovern*

LYSOSOMAL STORAGE DISEASES

GENERAL FEATURES

DEFINITION The lysosomal storage diseases are a family of over 30 disorders that result from different defects in lysosomal function. Lysosomes are cytoplasmic organelles containing acid hydrolases that degrade macromolecules to their basic building blocks: peptides, amino acids, monosaccharides, nucleic acids, and fatty acids (Fig. 346-1). Lysosomal enzymes are synthesized in the endoplasmic reticulum, usually as precursor forms that undergo posttranslational processing (proteolytic cleavage, the addition of N-linked oligosaccharide chains, and the synthesis of recognition markers such as mannose-6-phosphate) prior to packaging in primary lysosomes. The primary lysosomes may fuse with other vesicles, including phagosomes or autophagosomes that contain macromolecules, cell debris, and cellular organelles to form secondary lysosomes where degradation of macromolecules occurs. Through absorptive endocytosis, lysosomes also function in the uptake of vitamin B_{12}, lipoproteins, peptide hormones, and growth factors.

Disorders of lysosomal function are traditionally classified according to the nature of the primary stored material and include mucopolysaccharidoses, lipid storage diseases, mucolipidoses, glycoprotein storage diseases, and others (Table 346-1). The first delineation of the pathophysiology of a lysosomal disorder came from the observation that accumulation of glycogen in lysosomes in Pompe's disease [glycogen storage disease (GSD) type II] is due to deficiency of a specific enzyme, α-glucosidase. Based on this finding and observations in other disorders, Hers defined the lysosomal storage diseases as disorders characterized by deficiency of a single lysosomal enzyme and the consequent accumulation of its substrates in lysosomes. Subsequently, the definition was expanded to include disorders such as the mucoli-

pidoses and multiple sulfatase deficiency, in which single-gene defects impair the function of more than one lysosomal enzyme, and the deficiency of other proteins required for normal lysosomal function such as cofactors or protective proteins.

The clinical features of the lysosomal storage diseases can be predicted by knowing the normal site of degradation of the deficient enzyme's substrate and are dependent on the rate and magnitude of accumulation of undegraded material. Thus, defects of myelin degradation cause white matter disease; defective glycolipid degradation causes organomegaly; and defects in the degradation of mucopolysaccharides, which are ubiquitous, cause abnormalities in numerous tissues. The disorders are progressive, and most affected individuals appear normal at birth and develop manifestations after months or years. Many of the disorders are fatal in childhood or adolescence, although there is extensive phenotypic variability.

DIAGNOSIS The lysosomal storage diseases should be included in the differential diagnosis for any patient with progressive neurologic dysfunction, hepatosplenomegaly, and/or skeletal dysostosis. In particular, progression of disease and neurologic degeneration suggest a storage disease. The evaluation of a patient suspected of having one of these disorders should include a three-generation pedigree to detect consanguinity and/or the presence of an X-linked pattern of inheritance and determination of the ethnic background, because there is an increased frequency of Tay-Sachs disease, Niemann-Pick disease (NPD), and Gaucher's disease in Ashkenazi Jews; mannosidosis and aspartylglucosaminuria in Scandinavians; and the juvenile form of sialidosis in Japanese. The history should include the developmental milestones, which may be characterized by a period of normal development followed by slowing of development and then regression. Particular attention should be given to neurologic symptoms including seizures, visual loss and auditory impairment, the presence of umbilical hernias, a delayed or aberrant growth pattern, and joint limitations or pain.

Physical findings include coarse features, enlarged tongue, corneal clouding, exaggerated startle response (hyperacusis), hepatosplenomegaly, limited joint mobility and contractures, and umbilical hernias. Gigantism is a feature early in the course for the mucopolysaccharide and glycoprotein storage diseases, whereas short stature is characteristic for many of the other disorders. Neurologic examination should focus on determining the extent of involvement of gray matter, white matter, and peripheral nerves. Cutaneous features, when present, are distinctive and include angiokeratomas in Fabry's disease and fucosidosis, ichthyosis in multiple sulfatase deficiency, and papular, pebbly lesions of the shoulders and trunk in Hunter's syndrome. Funduscopic and slit-lamp examinations may reveal corneal clouding or the presence of a cherry red macule. Laboratory evaluation should include examination of the peripheral smear for vacuolated lymphocytes, analysis of the urine for mucopolysaccharides, and radiography of the spine and tubular bones to determine skeletal involvement. In some patients light- and electron-microscopic examination of biopsies of skin, conjunctivae, rectum, bone marrow, liver, or peripheral nerves may demonstrate engorgement of lysosomes. However, on the basis of clinical findings, skeletal survey, and the analysis of mucopolysaccharides in urine, it is usually possible to select a small number of enzyme assays in serum, leukocytes, or cultured skin fibroblasts to provide a definitive diagnosis.

GENETICS AND HETEROGENEITY The lysosomal storage diseases are inherited as autosomal recessive traits, with the exceptions of Hunter's syndrome [mucopolysaccharidosis (MPS) type II, or MPS II] and Fabry's disease, which are X-linked. Most of the conditions are characterized by clinical, biochemical, and genetic heterogeneity. In some cases, different mutations in the lysosomal structural genes account for the observed heterogeneity. For example, one mutation in a gene that encodes a lysosomal enzyme may cause total loss of the enzyme activity, whereas another mutation in the same gene may result in only partial impairment of enzyme activity and a less severe clinical course. Other mutations alter posttransitional modification or the affinity for various substrates. Heterogeneity in these disorders is further increased by the fact that patients with autosomal recessive traits are frequently compound heterozygotes and inherit two different mutant alleles, one from each carrier parent. The different mutant alleles may cause different properties, further increasing biochemical diversity among affected individuals. A typical example of heterogeneity among the lysosomal storage diseases is MPS I, which is discussed in detail below. A different type of genetic heterogeneity is demonstrated by the Sanfilippo syndromes (MPS III A, B, C, and D), in which similar phenotypes are caused by mutations in different genes.

The molecular pathology and specific mutations have been elucidated for many of the lysosomal diseases, and in some instances informative correlations can be made between genotype and the resulting phenotype. For example, in Gaucher's disease one mutation in the β-glucosidase gene, N370S, is protective against the development of neurologic disease. Similarly, in NPD the 608 mutation does not occur in patients with neurologic disease but is associated with variable somatic manifestations including organomegaly. Such genotype-phenotype correlations, when informative, are useful in prognosis and permit genetic counseling that allows families to make decisions about future pregnancies.

MANAGEMENT AND PREVENTION Most lysosomal storage diseases are characterized by a progressive course with severe morbidity and early mortality. Treatment is largely symptomatic, a notable exception being Gaucher's disease which is amenable to therapy with recombinantly produced acid β-glucosidase. However, such therapy has not been evaluated in patients with Gaucher's disease who have central nervous system (CNS) involvement. There is also a limited experience with bone marrow transplantation in the mucopolysaccharidoses, NPD, and Gaucher's disease. The results have been variable but with no appreciable effect on CNS involvement.

Because of the lack of effective therapy, prevention is of central importance. Couples who have had one affected child should be offered prenatal diagnosis in future pregnancies, since all the lysosomal storage diseases in which the enzymatic deficiency is known can be diagnosed in utero. Heterozygote identification for at-risk family members is also available for many of these disorders, both by enzymatic assays and by the identification of specific alleles in families that have been genotyped. Another approach to prevention is by the prospective identification of carrier couples at risk through heterozygote screening programs, such as the one for Tay-Sachs disease. However, these programs require the availability of a rapid and inexpensive carrier detection method and are usually targeted at populations known to be at increased risk, such as Ashkenazi Jews in whom Tay-Sachs disease, Gaucher's disease, and NPD occur with increased frequency. In other groups carrier screening would be less cost effective because of the low frequency of the mutant alleles in the general population.

SPECIFIC DISORDERS

The Mucopolysaccharidoses MPS results from the deficiency of one of the lysosomal enzymes required for glycosaminoglycan (GAG) catabolism. GAGs, which are major constituents of connective tissue, are long-chain, complex carbohydrates that are usually linked to proteins to form proteoglycans and include chondroitin-4-sulfate, chondroitin-6-sulfate, heparan sulfate, dermatan sulfate, keratan sulfate, and hyaluronic acid. The clinical features of the mucopolysaccharidoses result from the lysosomal accumulation of partially degraded or undegraded GAGs and typically include coarse facies, corneal clouding, organomegaly, joint stiffness, bony abnormalities, hernias, short stature, and, in some disorders, mental retardation. The phenotype of each disorder is determined by the specific enzymatic deficiency and the resultant pattern of accumulation of GAG degradation products; dermatan, keratan, and chondroitin sulfate degradation products are associated with visceral manifestations, and accumulation of heparan sulfate degradation products causes mental deficiency.

Laboratory findings include the presence of vacuolated lymphocytes in the peripheral smear and the presence of GAGs in urine. Since some features of the mucopolysaccharidoses also occur with the mucolipidoses, glycoprotein storage diseases, and other lysosomal storage diseases, definitive diagnosis is made by specific enzyme assays in leukocytes and/or cultured skin fibroblasts. Prenatal diagnosis by enzyme assays in fetal cells and/or by isotopic studies of GAG formation in cultured amniotic cells is avail-

FIGURE 346-1 Biology of lysosomes. Lysosomal enzymes are synthesized in the endoplasmic reticulum and undergo posttranslational processing in the Golgi prior to packaging in the primary lysosome. Primary lysosomes can then participate in the process of autophagy or form secondary lysosomes as depicted. E, precursor and mature forms of lysosomal enzymes. [*From A Beaudet: Liposomal storage diseases, in KJ Isselbacher et al (ed), Harrison's Principles of Internal Medicine, 13th ed. New York, McGraw-Hill, p 2091, 1994.*]

able for each MPS, and carrier identification is possible in individuals with a positive family history by appropriate enzyme assay in leukocytes or serum. In addition, molecular identification of carriers is possible after the mutant alleles have been characterized in the family.

MPS IH (Hurler's disease) is one of the more severe forms and results from the deficiency of α-L-iduronidase. It is characterized by progressive organ involvement and mental retardation and causes death, usually in the first decade. Patients appear normal at birth and have accelerated growth in the first year, followed by slowing of growth and eventual short stature. The diagnosis is usually made by 2 years of age when organomegaly, corneal clouding, coarse features, large tongue, and joint stiffness are apparent. Developmental delay appears between 12 and 28 months, and subsequently there is regression in mental function. Other features include hearing loss, chronic respiratory infections, valvular heart disease, and increased intracranial pressure. MPS IS (Scheie's disease) and MPS I H/S (Hurler-Scheie disease) result from allelic mutations in the α-L-iduronidase gene and are characterized by a less severe clinical course, presumably due to the presence of residual α-L-iduronidase activity.

MPS II (Hunter's syndrome) is inherited as an X-linked recessive trait and is notable for the absence of corneal clouding and the presence of severe and mild forms with and without mental impairment. MPS IIIA, IIIB, IIIC, and IIID (the Sanfilippo syndromes) result from one of four enzymatic deficiencies and are characterized by behavioral problems and seizures, moderately severe somatic manifestations, and survival into the third decade. Individuals with MPS IV (Morquio's syndrome) have normal intelligence and severe skeletal findings sometimes confused with the spondyloepiphyseal dysplasias. The most serious complication is upper cervical spinal cord compression due to atlantoaxial instability. Patients with MPS VI (Maroteaux-Lamy disease) have a phenotype similar to Hurler's disease but with normal intelligence.

Treatment of the mucopolysaccharidoses is symptomatic and may include corneal transplantation, correction of nerve entrapments in the hands, and heart valve replacement. In MPS III, control of the behavioral problems may require psychotropic medications. For patients with MPS IV, cervical myelopathy should be prevented by surgery of the cervical spine. Attempts at enzyme replacement in various forms of MPS have not been successful, and bone marrow transplantation has produced variable results.

The GM₂ Gangliosidoses The GM_2 gangliosidoses include Tay-Sachs disease and Sandhoff's disease, each of which results from deficiency of hexosaminidase and the accumulation in lysosomes of GM_2 gangliosides, particularly in the CNS. Both disorders have infantile, juvenile, and adult-onset forms, depending on the age of onset and clinical features. Hexosaminidase A is composed of one α and one β subunit, and hexosaminidase B has two β subunits. Hexosaminidase A deficiency (Tay-Sachs disease) results from mutations in the α subunit, and mutations in the β subunit gene result in the deficiency of both hexosaminidase A and B and cause Sandhoff's disease. Both disorders are inherited as autosomal recessive traits; the carrier frequency of Tay-Sachs disease in Ashkenazi Jews is known 1 in 25.

The cDNAs for both the α and β subunits of hexosaminidase have been cloned. To date, over 50 mutations have been identified, most associated with the infantile forms of disease. Three mutations account for over 95 percent of mutant alleles among Ashkenazi Jews, including one allele associated with the adult-onset form. Mutations that cause the subacute or chronic forms have resulted in higher residual enzymatic activity levels that correlate with the severity of the disease.

The infantile form of Tay-Sachs disease causes loss of motor skills, increased startle reaction, and macular pallor (cherry red spot) on slit-lamp examination; it causes death by age 4. The juvenile-onset form is associated with ataxia and dementia and progresses to death by age 10 to 15. The adult-onset disorder is characterized by clumsiness in childhood and motor weakness in adolescence. Although spinocerebellar and lower motor neuron symptoms predominate in the adult form, some patients are psychotic. Intelligence and vision are typically normal. The infantile form of Sandhoff's disease is nearly identical in course to infantile Tay-Sachs, but two distinguishing features are the presence of organomegaly and occasional bony changes. Treatment is supportive.

The diagnosis of infantile Tay-Sachs and Sandhoff's disease is usually suspected during infancy on the basis of neurologic features and the finding of a cherry red spot and is confirmed by measurement of hexosaminidase levels in blood leukocytes. Future at-risk pregnancies can be monitored by prenatal diagnosis by amniocentesis or chorionic villus sampling, and identification of carriers within the family can be by hexosaminidase assays. Indeed, carrier screening of all couples in whom at least one member is an Ashkenazi Jew is recommended prior to the beginning of pregnancy to identify couples at risk. Since the introduction of such carrier screening programs for Ashkenazi Jews, the incidence of Tay-Sachs disease in this population has decreased.

The Lipid Storage Disorders The lipid storage diseases include Fabry's disease, Gaucher's disease, and NPD. For each of these disorders affected individuals may survive into adulthood.

Fabry's disease Fabry's disease is an inborn error of glycosphingolipid metabolism characterized by angiokeratomas (telangiectatic skin lesions), hypohidrosis, corneal and lenticular opacities, acroparesthesia, and vascular disease of the kidney, heart, and/or brain. The disease is an X-linked recessive trait that is manifested in affected hemizygous males and has an estimated prevalence of 1 in 40,000. Atypical hemizygous males with residual α-galactosidase A activity may be asymptomatic or have late-onset, mild manifestations, usually limited to the heart. Heterozygous females are usually asymptomatic or exhibit mild manifestations.

The disease results from the deficient activity of α-galactosidase A, which is encoded by a gene on the long arm of the X chromosome (Xq22). The defect leads to the accumulation of neutral glycosphingolipids, primarily globotriaosylceramide, in the plasma and lysosomes of vascular endothelial and smooth-muscle cells. The progressive deposition of glycosphingolipid in vessel walls results in ischemia and infarction, the major disease manifestations. Affected males who have blood group B or AB have a more severe course due to accumulation of blood group B substance, which is normally degraded by α-galactosidase A. The cDNA and genomic sequences encoding α-galactosidase A have been characterized, and known mutations responsible for this disease include amino acid substitutions, gene rearrangements, and mRNA splicing defects.

The angiokeratomas in Fabry's disease usually appear in childhood and may lead to early diagnosis. The lesions are punctate, dark red to blue-black, and flat or slightly raised. They do not blanch with pressure, and the larger ones may show slight hyperkeratosis. They increase in size and number with age and range from barely visible to several millimeters in diameter. Characteristically, the lesions are most dense between the umbilicus and knees, in the "bathing trunk area," but may occur anywhere, including the oral mucosa. The hips, thighs, buttocks, umbilicus, lower abdomen, scrotum, and penis are common sites, and there is a tendency toward bilateral symmetry. Skin lesions are not invariably present. Sweating is usually decreased or absent. Corneal opacities and characteristic lenticular lesions, observed in slit-lamp examination, are present in affected men and in about 70 percent of asymptomatic heterozygotes. Tortuosity of the conjunctival and retinal vessels is common.

Pain is the most debilitating symptom in childhood and adolescence. Fabry crises, lasting from minutes to days, consist of agonizing, burning pain in the hands, feet, and proximal extremities and are usually precipitated by exercise, fatigue, or fever. These painful acroparesthesias usually become less frequent in the third and fourth decades of life but on occasion become more frequent and more severe. Abdominal or flank pain may simulate appendicitis or renal colic.

With age the major morbidity is caused by progressive involvement of the vascular system. Early in the course casts, red cells, and lipid inclusions with characteristic birefringent "Maltese crosses" appear in the urinary sediment. Proteinuria, isosthenuria, and deterioration of

Table 346-1

Summary of Lysosomal Storage Diseases

Disorder	Enzyme Deficiency	Stored Material	Clinical Subtypes (Onset)	Inheritance	Neurologic
MUCOPOLYSACCHARIDOSES (MPS)					
MPS I H, Hurler (78) MPS I H/S, Hurler/Scheie MPS I S, Scheie	α-L-Iduronidase	Dermatan sulfate Heparan sulfate	Infantile Intermediate Adult	AR	Mental retardation, except in Scheie
MPS II, Hunter (78)	Iduronate sulfatase	Dermatan sulfate Heparan sulfate	Severe infantile Mild juvenile	X-linked	Mental retardation, less in mild form
MPS III A, Sanfilippo A (78)	Heparan-N-sulfatase	Heparan sulfate	Late infantile	AR	Severe mental retardation
MPS III B, Sanfilippo B	N-Acetyl-α-glucosaminidase	Heparan sulfate	Late infantile	AR	Severe mental retardation
MPS III C, Sanfilippo C	Acetyl-CoA: α-glucosaminide N-acetyltransferase	Heparan sulfate	Late infantile	AR	Severe mental retardation
MPS III D, Sanfilippo D	N-Acetylglucosamine-6-sulfate sulfatase	Heparan sulfate	Late infantile	AR	Severe mental retardation
MPS IV, Morquio (78)	N-Acetylgalactosamine-6-sulfate sulfatase	Keratan sulfate Chondroitin-6 sulfate	Childhood	AR	0
MPS VI, Maroteaux-Lamy (78)	Arylsulfatase B	Dermatan sulfate	Late infantile	AR	0
MPS VII (78)	β-Glucuoronidase	Dermatan sulfate Heparan sulfate	Neonatal Infantile Adult	AR	Mental retardation, absent in some adults
GM₂ GANGLIOSIDOSES					
Tay-Sachs' disease (92)	Hexosaminidase A	GM₂ gangliosides	Infantile Juvenile	AR	Mental retardation, seizures, later juvenile form
Sandhoff's disease (92)	Hexosaminidases A and B	GM₂ gangliosides	Infantile	AR	Mental retardation, seizures
LIPID STORAGE DISORDERS					
Fabry's disease (89)	α-Galactosidase A	Trihexosylceramide	Childhood	X-linked	Painful neuropathy
Gaucher's disease (86)	Acid β-Glucosidase	Glucosylceramide	Adult, type 1 Infantile, type 2 Juvenile, type 3	AR	Mental retardation in infantile, ataxia in juvenile, no symptoms in adult
Niemann-Pick's disease (84)	Sphingomyelinase	Sphingomyelin	Infantile neuronopathic, type A Nonneuronopathic, type B	AR	Mental retardation and seizures in type A
GLYCOPROTEINOSES					
Fucosidosis (81)	α-Fucosidase	Glycopeptides, oligosaccharides	Infantile Juvenile	AR	Mental retardation
α-Mannosidosis (81)	α-Mannosidase	Oligosaccharides	Infantile Milder variant	AR	Mental retardation
β-Mannosidosis (81)	β-Mannosidase	Oligosaccharides		AR	Seizures, mental retardation
Aspartylglucosaminuria (81)	Aspartylglucosaminidase	Aspartylglucosamine, glycopeptides	Young adult onset	AR	Mental retardation
Sialidosis (81)	Neuraminidase	Sialyloligosaccharides	Type I, congenital Type II, infantile and juvenile forms	AR	Myoclonus, mental retardation
MUCOLIPIDOSES (ML)					
ML-II, I-cell disease (78)	UDP-N-Acetylglucosamine-1-phosphotransferase	Glycoprotein, glycolipids	Infantile	AR	Mental retardation
ML-III, pseudo-Hurler polydystrophy (79)	UDP-N-Acetylglucosamine-1-phosphotransferase	Glycoprotein, glycolipids	Late infantile	AR	Mild mental retardation
LEUKODYSTROPHIES					
Krabbe's disease (87)	Galactosylceramidase	Galactocerebroside	Infantile	AR	Mental retardation
Metachromatic leukodystrophy (88)	Arylsulfatase A	Cerebroside sulfate	Infantile Juvenile Adult	AR	Mental retardation, dementia, and psychosis in adult
Multiple sulfatase deficiency (88)	Arylsulfatases A, B, and C	Sulfatides, mucopolysaccharides	Late infantile	AR	Mental retardation
Wolman's disease (82)	Acid lipase	Cholesterol ester, triglycerides	Infantile	AR	Mild mental retardation
Cholesterol ester storage disease (82)	Acid lipase	Cholesterol ester, triglycerides	Adult	AR	0
Farber's disease (83)	Acid ceramidase	Ceramide	Infantile Juvenile	AR	Occasional mental retardation

NOTE: Numbers in parentheses refer to the chapters in Scriver et al, 7th edition, in which the disorders are discussed.

Liver and/or Spleen Enlargement	Skeletal Dysplasia	Clinical Features Ophthalmologic	Hematologic	Unique Features
+++	++++	Corneal clouding	Vacuolated lymphocytes	Coarse facies, cardiovascular involvement, joint stiffness
+++	++++	Retinal degeneration, no corneal clouding	Granulated lymphocytes	Coarse facies, cardiovascular, joint stiffness, distinctive pebbly skin lesions
+	+	0	Granulated lymphocytes	Mild coarse facies
+	+	0	Granulated lymphocytes	Mild coarse facies
+	+	0	Granulated lymphocytes	Mild coarse facies
+	+	0	Granulated lymphocytes	Mild coarse facies
+	++++	Corneal clouding	Granulated neutrophils	Distinctive skeletal deformity, odontoid hypoplasia, aortic valve disease
++	++++	Corneal clouding	Granulated neutrophils and lymphocytes	Coarse facies, valvular heart disease
+++	+++	Corneal clouding	Granulated neutrophils	Coarse facies, vascular involvement, hydrops fetalis in neonatal form
0	0	Cherry red spot in infantile form	0	Macrocephaly, hyperacusis in infantile
0	0	Cherry red spot	0	Macrocephaly, hyperacusis
0	0	Corneal dystrophy, vascular lesions	0	Cutaneous angiokeratoses, hypohydrosis
++++	++	0	Foam cells	Adult form includes pathologic fractures
++++	0	Macular degeneration and cherry red spot in type A	Foam cells	Pulmonary infiltrates
++	++	0	Vacuolated lymphocytes, foam cells	Coarse facies, angiokeratomas in juvenile form
+++	++	Cataracts, corneal clouding	Vacuolated lymphocytes, granulated neutrophils	Coarse facies, enlarged tongue
	++	0	Vacuolated lymphocytes, foam cells	Angiokeratomas
0	++	0	Vacuolated lymphocytes, foam cells	Coarse facies
++, less in type I	++ less in type I	Cherry red spot	Vacuolated lymphocytes	MPS phenotype in type II
0/+	++++	Corneal clouding	Vacuolated and granulated neutrophils	Coarse facies, absence of mucopolysacchariduria, gingival hypoplasia
0	+++	Corneal clouding, mild retinopathy, hyperopic astigmatism		Coarse facies, stiffness of hands and shoulders
0	0	0	0	White matter globoid cells
0	0	Optic atrophy	0	Gait abnormalities in late infantile
+	++	Retinal degeneration	Vacuolated and granulated cells	Ichthyosis
+++	0	0		Adrenal calcification
0	0	0		Premature atherosclerosis
+/−	0	Macular degeneration	0	Arthropathy, subcutaneous nodules

renal function are apparent by the second to fourth decades of life. Cardiovascular manifestations may include hypertension, left ventricular hypertrophy, anginal chest pain, myocardial ischemia or infarction, and congestive heart failure, frequently due to mitral insufficiency. Electrocardiographic and echocardiographic abnormalities are common. Cerebrovascular manifestations are due to multifocal small vessel involvement. Other features include chronic bronchitis and dyspnea, lymphedema of the legs without hypoproteinemia, episodic diarrhea, osteoporosis, growth retardation, and delayed puberty. Death is due to renal failure or vascular disease of the heart or brain. Prior to hemodialysis or renal transplantation, the mean age of death was 41 years. Atypical patients with residual α-galactosidase A activity may be asymptomatic or mildly affected, and patients with no early manifestations can develop late-onset cardiac or cardiopulmonary disease. In these "cardiac variants," cardiomegaly usually involves the left ventricular wall and interventricular septum, and electrocardiographic abnormalities are consistent with cardiomyopathy. Hypertrophic cardiomyopathy and/or myocardial infarction have been described.

The diagnosis is typically made from the history of painful acroparesthesias and the presence of hypohidrosis, characteristic skin lesions, and typical corneal opacities and lenticular lesions. The disorder is often misdiagnosed as rheumatic fever, erythromyalgia, or neurosis. The skin lesions must be differentiated from the benign angiokeratomas of the scrotum (Fordyce's disease) and from angiokeratoma circumscriptum. Angiokeratomas identical to those of Fabry's disease have been reported in fucosidosis, aspartylglycosaminuria, late-onset GM_1 gangliosidosis, galactosialidosis, α-N-acetylgalactosaminidase deficiency, and sialidosis. The diagnosis of the mild cardiac variants should be considered in individuals with left ventricular hypertrophy and/or cardiomyopathy of unknown etiology. The diagnosis is confirmed by demonstration of decreased α-galactosidase A activity in plasma, leukocytes, or cultured lymphoblasts or skin fibroblasts.

Heterozygous females may have corneal opacities, isolated skin lesions, and intermediate levels of α-galactosidase A in plasma or cells. Rare heterozygous women have manifestations as severe as those in men. Even asymptomatic at-risk women in families with Fabry's disease should be diagnosed by the direct analysis of the specific family mutation. Affected males can be diagnosed prenatally by demonstration of deficient α-galactosidase A activity or of the specific family mutation in chorionic villi in the first trimester or in cultured amniocytes in the second trimester of pregnancy.

Phenytoin and carbamazepine decrease the frequency and severity of the chronic acroparesthesias and of the periodic crises of excruciating pain. Otherwise, treatment is supportive and nonspecific. Renal transplantation and chronic hemodialysis can be lifesaving. Replacement therapy using partially purified human enzyme has been biochemically effective in short-term pilot trials, but sufficient enzyme is not available to evaluate the clinical effectiveness of long-term therapy. The availability of the cDNA encoding human α-galactosidase A may make possible the production of recombinant enzyme for long-term trials.

Gaucher's disease Gaucher's disease is a multisystemic lipidosis characterized by hematologic problems, organomegaly, and skeletal involvement, usually manifested as bone pain and pathologic fractures. It is the most common lysosomal storage disease and the most common genetic defect in Ashkenazi Jews. The three clinical subtypes are delineated by the absence or presence and progression of neurologic manifestations: type 1, the adult, nonneuronopathic form; type 2, the infantile or acute neuronopathic form; and type 3, the juvenile or Norrbotten form. All three are inherited as autosomal recessive traits. Type 1, which accounts for 99 percent of cases, has an incidence of about 1 in 1000 and a carrier frequency of 1 in 18 in Ashkenazi Jews.

Gaucher's disease results from deficiency of the lysosomal hydrolase, acid β-glucosidase, which is encoded by a gene on chromosome 1 (q21 to q31). The defect causes progressive accumulation of undegraded glycolipid substrates, particularly glucosylceramide, in reticu-

loendothelial cells and results in infiltration of the bone marrow, hepatosplenomegaly, and skeletal complications. The cDNA for acid β-glucosidase has been cloned, and the more than 35 identified mutant alleles include missense, insertion, and deletion mutations. Four of these mutations, N370S, L444P, 84insG, and IVS2, account for 90 to 95 percent of mutations among Ashkenazi Jews, making screening practical in this population. The molecular basis of the clinical heterogeneity in Gaucher's disease type 1 is partially understood. For example, homozygotes for the N370S mutation tend to have later onset of manifestations and a more indolent course than patients with one copy of N370S and another common allele.

Manifestations of Gaucher's disease type 1 have a variable age of onset, from early childhood to late adulthood, but most patients are symptomatic by adolescence; manifestations include easy bruisability due to thrombocytopenia, chronic fatigue secondary to anemia, hepatomegaly with or without elevated liver function tests, splenomegaly, bone pain, and occasional pulmonary involvement. Patients presenting in the first decade are frequently non-Jewish, have growth retardation, and have a more malignant course. Other patients are discovered fortuitously and have a benign course. In symptomatic patients, splenomegaly is progressive and can become massive. Bone involvement, which occurs in over 20 percent of patients, can cause pain or pathologic fractures or be manifested only by radiologic findings, including Erlenmeyer flask deformities of the distal femur. With symptomatic bone disease, lytic lesions in the femur, ribs, and pelvis and osteosclerosis may be evident at an early age, and bone crises with pain and swelling can be severe. Bleeding secondary to thrombocytopenia may manifest as epistaxis and bruising and is frequently overlooked until other symptoms become apparent. With the exception of the child with severe growth retardation and developmental delay secondary to the effects of chronic disease, development and intelligence are normal. The pathologic hallmark of the disease is the Gaucher cell in the reticuloendothelial system, particularly in the bone marrow. These cells are 20 to 100 μm in diameter and have a characteristic "wrinkled paper" appearance resulting from intracytoplasmic inclusions of substrate. The cytoplasm of the Gaucher cell reacts strongly positive with the periodic acid Schiff stain, and the presence of this cell in bone marrow and tissue biopsy specimens is suggestive of Gaucher's disease, although similar cells may be found in patients with granulocytic leukemia and myeloma.

Gaucher's disease type 2 is less common, does not have a striking ethnic predilection, and is characterized by a rapid neurodegenerative course with extensive visceral involvement and death within the first 2 years. It presents in infancy with increased tone, strabismus, organomegaly, failure to thrive, and stridor due to laryngospasm. After a period of psychomotor retrogression, death is usually due to respiratory complications. Gaucher's disease type 3 has clinical manifestations that are intermediate to those in types 1 and 2; they begin in childhood and cause death by age 10 to 15. Type 3 disease has a predilection for the Swedish Norbotten population where the incidence is 1 in 50,000. Neurologic involvement begins later and is less severe than in type 2 disease. Type 3 is further classified as type 3a and 3b, based on whether there is progressive myotonia and dementia (type 3a) or isolated supranuclear gaze palsy (type 3b).

The diagnosis should be considered in any patient with unexplained organomegaly, easy bruisability, and/or bone pain. Bone marrow examination usually reveals the presence of Gaucher cells, but the diagnosis should be confirmed by measurement of acid β-glucosidase activity in isolated leukocytes or cultured fibroblasts. Heterozygous carriers can be identified by enzyme and/or by molecular testing in many families. Testing should be offered to all family members, recognizing that heterogeneity even among members of the same kindred can be so great that asymptomatic affected individuals may be diagnosed during such testing. Prenatal diagnosis is available by determination of enzyme activity in chorionic villi or cultured amniotic fluid cells.

In the past, symptomatic management included blood transfusions for anemia, partial or total splenectomy for mechanical cardiopulmonary compromise or hypersplenism, analgesics for bone pain, and orthopedic procedures or joint replacement for severe bony involvement. A small number of patients have been cured by bone marrow transplantation, but the morbidity and mortality of the procedure limit its usefulness. It is now established that enzyme replacement with purified placental acid β-glucosidase is safe and efficacious. Most extraskeletal manifestations are reversed by administration of 30 to 60 IU/kg of enzyme intravenously every other week. The effectiveness of this therapy in reversing and preventing bony manifestations is under study, but some data suggest that it is efficacious in this regard as well. An enzyme made by recombinant DNA technology is being studied in clinical trials. Once the efficacy of the recombinant enzyme is documented, enzyme therapy for Gaucher's disease will be implemented more widely.

Niemann-Pick disease   The original report of NPD described what is now known as type A NPD, a fatal disorder of infancy characterized by failure to thrive, hepatosplenomegaly, a rapidly progressive neurodegenerative course, and death by 2 to 3 years of age. Six subtypes of NPD are now recognized, including type B, which is a nonneuronopathic form in adults, and other, rarer forms that result from defects in cholesterol metabolism. All six subtypes are inherited as autosomal recessive traits and display variable clinical features.

Types A and B NPD result from the deficient activity of sphingomyelinase, a lysosomal enzyme encoded by a gene on chromosome 11 (11p15.1 to p15.4). The defect results in accumulation of sphingomyelin, a ceramide phospholipid, and other lipids in the monocyte-macrophage system. The progressive deposition of sphingomyelin in the CNS causes the neurodegenerative manifestations in type A and in the systemic manifestations of type B, including progressive lung disease in some. The sphingomyelinase gene has been sequenced, and 12 mutations that cause types A and B NPD have been identified, including 9 single-base substitutions and 3 small deletions.

The manifestations and course of type A NPD are relatively uniform and are characterized by normal appearance at birth (although the newborn period is sometimes complicated by prolonged jaundice); hepatosplenomegaly, moderate lymphadenopathy, and psychomotor retardation are evident by 6 months of age, followed thereafter by regression. The loss of motor function and the deterioration of intellectual capabilities become progressively debilitating and eventuate in spasticity, rigidity, and loss of contact with the environment. In contrast, the manifestations and course of type B disease are more variable. Most patients are diagnosed in infancy or childhood when enlargement of the liver and/or spleen is detected during a routine physical examination, and evidence of mild pulmonary involvement is usually evident as a diffuse reticular or finely nodular infiltrate on the chest roentgenogram. Although hepatosplenomegaly is prominent in childhood, the abdominal protuberance decreases and becomes less conspicuous with time. In mildly affected patients, the splenomegaly may not be noted until adulthood, and disease manifestations may be minimal.

In most type B patients, pulmonary diffusion is decreased due to alveolar infiltration during childhood and worsens with age. Pulmonary compromise may be severe by 15 to 20 years of age. Such patients have low P_{O_2} levels and dyspnea on exertion. Bronchopneumonia and cor pulmonale may occur. Liver involvement can lead to cirrhosis of the liver, portal hypertension, and ascites. Pancytopenia due to secondary hypersplenism may respond to partial or complete splenectomy. Type B patients usually do not have neurologic involvement and are intellectually intact.

Type C NPD patients may have prolonged neonatal jaundice, appear normal for 1 to 2 years, and then undergo a slowly progressive and variable neurodegeneration. The hepatosplenomegaly is less severe than with types A or B NPD, and these patients may survive into adulthood. The underlying biochemical defect in type C NPD is an abnormality in cholesterol transport, leading to the accumulation of sphingomyelin and cholesterol in lysosomes and a secondary reduction in sphingomyelinase activity. Type D NPD patients develop neurologic symptoms later in childhood and have a slower course of neurodegeneration than type C patients. Most individuals with type D disease share a common ancestry traceable to Acadians from Yarmouth County, Nova Scotia. These patients also have an abnormality in cholesterol metabolism, and the defect may be allelic to the defect in type C NPD.

In type B NPD patients, splenomegaly is usually noted in early childhood, but in mild cases detection of splenic enlargement may be delayed into adolescence or adulthood. The presence of the characteristic NPD cells in the bone marrow aspirates supports the diagnosis of type B NPD. However, patients with types C and D NPD also have NPD cells in the bone marrow, and the suspected diagnosis should be confirmed by measuring sphingomyelinase in peripheral leukocytes, cultured fibroblasts, and/or lymphoblasts. Patients with types A and B NPD have markedly decreased levels (1 to 10 percent), whereas patients with types C and D NPD have intermediate levels and patients with Gaucher's disease and other storage disorders that cause hepatosplenomegaly and/or neurologic involvement have normal or near-normal levels of sphingomyelinase. The enzymatic identification of NPD carriers is problematic, but in families in whom the specific molecular defect has been identified, heterozygotes can be identified by DNA analysis. Prenatal diagnosis of NPD can be made by measurement of sphingomyelinase in cultured amniocytes or chorionic villi, and molecular studies of fetal DNA can provide the diagnosis or serve as a confirmatory test.

There is no specific treatment for NPD. Orthotopic liver transplantation in an infant with type A disease and amniotic cell transplantation in several type B NPD patients have had little or no success. Bone marrow transplantation in one type B NPD patient reduced the spleen and liver volumes, the sphingomyelin content in the liver, the number of NPD cells in the marrow, and the radiologic infiltration of the lungs, but the patient died 3 months after transplantation. To date, lung transplantation has not been performed.

The Glycoproteinoses   The glycoproteinoses, or oligosaccharidoses, are disorders of impaired glycoprotein degradation and include fucosidosis, mannosidosis, sialidosis, and aspartylglucosaminuria. These disorders, each of which is inherited as an autosomal recessive trait, share features with both the mucopolysaccharidoses and the sphingolipidoses and are characterized by neurologic manifestations and varying somatic features. *Fucosidosis* is a rare disorder that results from the deficient activity of α-fucosidase. Although the disorder is panethnic, most described patients have been from Italy or the United States. Within the first year it causes developmental delay, somatic features similar to those in MPS, sweat electrolyte abnormalities, and development of angiokeratomas. Most severely affected patients have a relentless neurodegenerative course with death in childhood, although a mild variant is compatible with longer survival. *Mannosidosis*, resulting from α-mannosidase deficiency, includes a severe infantile form characterized by progressive mental retardation, facial coarsening, dysostosis multiplex, and organomegaly with death in childhood. A juvenile–adult-onset phenotype with survival into adulthood is characterized by normal early development and the later appearance of neurologic symptoms and mental retardation in childhood or adolescence. *Aspartylglucosaminuria*, which has its highest incidence in Finland, presents later in childhood with progressive mental deterioration, coarsening of the facies, and behavioral problems. The deficiency of aspartylglucosaminidase results in the excretion of aspartylglucosamine in urine in diagnostic quantities. *Sialidosis* results from sialidase deficiency and includes a neonatal form that presents with hydrops and an infantile form characterized by glomerular nephropathy. A childhood form shares somatic features with Hurler's syndrome, including coarse facies; the juvenile form (the cherry red spot myoclonus syndrome) is characterized by the development of ocular cherry red spots and generalized myoclonus in the second decade. Combined deficiencies of sialidase and β-galactosidase are due to defects in a glycoprotein required for the protection of both enzymes from degradation.

No treatment is available for the glycoproteinoses, although one patient with α-mannosidosis had some improvement in somatic manifestations after bone marrow transplantation. Prenatal diagnosis is available for each disorder using either chorionic villi or cultured amniocytes, and molecular identification of the specific mutation in some of these disorders makes prenatal diagnosis and carrier detection possible.

The Leukodystrophies The leukodystrophies are disorders of the white matter of the brain and include Krabbe's disease (or globoid cell leukodystrophy) and metachromatic leukodystrophy (MLD). Krabbe's disease, a rapidly progressive, fatal disorder of infancy that results from galactosylceramidase deficiency, is characterized by the presence of multinucleated globoid cells, almost complete loss of myelin, and astrocytic gliosis in the white matter. Manifestations are confined to the nervous system, and patients rarely survive beyond the second year. Diagnosis is by the demonstration of the enzymatic defect, and treatment is supportive. In contrast, MLD may present at any age and has been divided into late infantile, juvenile, and adult forms. The disease results from the deficient activity of arylsulfatase A and the accumulation of galactosyl sulfatide in the white matter of the CNS and peripheral nervous system. The infantile form typically presents in the second year and is fatal, whereas the juvenile and adult forms are more variable and include gait disturbances, mental regression, peripheral neuropathy, seizures, and, in adults, behavioral disturbances and dementia. Treatment of late-onset disease by bone marrow transplantation has yielded variable results. Each of these disorders can be detected by prenatal diagnosis.

Glycogen Storage Disease Type II (See also Chap. 347) GSDII or Pompe's disease is due to deficiency of acid α-glucosidase and the accumulation of glycogen in lysosomes, particularly in cardiac and skeletal muscle. The infantile form is a rapidly fatal disorder associated with cardiomegaly, macroglossia, and hypotonia. The juvenile form is characterized by progressive proximal muscle weakness, including impairment of respiratory function. Electromyography can be helpful in making the diagnosis, but in adult patients the abnormalities vary among different muscles. Treatment is supportive. Prenatal diagnosis is available.

The Mucolipidoses The mucolipidoses include I-cell disease or mucolipidosis (ML) II and pseudohurler polydystrophy or ML-III. I-cell disease shares many phenotypic features with Hurler's syndrome, whereas ML-III is a milder disorder that presents later. Both disorders result from abnormal transport of the lysosomal enzymes, which results in decreased levels of several enzymes in the cell and excretion of the enzymes into the extracellular compartment. The specific defect is in the lysosomal enzyme *N*-acetylglucosamine-1-phosphotransferase, an essential enzyme for the synthesis of a mannose-6-phosphate recognition marker that targets lysosomal enzymes to the lysosome. The diagnosis is by demonstrating elevated serum levels of the lysosomal enzymes or by demonstration of the phosphotransferase deficiency. Treatment is supportive, and carrier identification and prenatal diagnosis are possible.

BIBLIOGRAPHY

BEIGHTON P (ed): *Heritable Disorders of Connective Tissue*, 5th ed. St. Louis, Mosby, 1993

HERS HG, VAN HOOF F (eds): *Lysosomes and Storage Diseases*. New York, Academic Press, 1973

SCRIVER CR et al (eds): *The Metabolic and Molecular Bases of Inherited Diseases*, 7th ed. New York, McGraw-Hill, 1995

WATTS RWE, GIBBS DA (eds): *Lysosomal Storage Diseases: Biochemical and Clinical Aspects*. Philadelphia, Taylor and Francis, 1986

347 *Yuan-Tsong Chen*

GLYCOGEN STORAGE DISEASES

Glycogen, the storage form of glucose in animal cells, is composed of glucose residues joined in straight chains by α1-4 linkages and branched at intervals of 4 to 10 residues with α1-6 linkages. The treelike molecule can have a molecular weight of many millions and may aggregate to form structures recognizable by electron microscopy. In muscle, glyco-

gen forms β particles, which are spherical and contain up to 60,000 glucose residues. Each β particle contains a covalently linked protein called *glycogenin*. Liver contains β particles and rosettes of glycogen called α *particles*, which appear to be aggregated β particles.

The primary function of glycogen varies in different tissues. In skeletal muscle, stored glycogen is a source of fuel that is used for short-term, high-energy consumption during muscle activity; in the brain, the small amount of stored glycogen is used during brief periods of hypoglycemia or hypoxia as an emergency supply of energy. In contrast, the liver takes up glucose from the bloodstream after a meal and stores it as glycogen. When blood glucose levels start to fall, the liver converts glycogen back into glucose and releases it into the blood for use by tissues such as brain and erythrocytes that cannot store significant amounts of glycogen.

Glycogen storage diseases are inherited disorders that affect glycogen metabolism. Disorders in virtually every enzyme involved in the synthesis or degradation of glycogen and its regulation cause some type of glycogen storage disease (Fig. 347-1) in which glycogen is abnormal in quantity, quality, or both. Excluded from this chapter are those conditions in which tissue glycogen accumulation is secondary, such as overtreatment of diabetes mellitus with insulin or administration of pharmacologic amounts of glucocorticoids.

Historically, the glycogen storage diseases were categorized numerically in the order in which the enzymatic defects were identified, up to number VII. They can also be classified by the organs involved and clinical manifestations, the system followed in this chapter (Table 347-1).

Because liver and muscle have abundant glycogen, they are the most commonly and seriously affected tissues. The hepatic glycogen storage diseases can be divided into two groups, with some overlap. The first is characterized by hepatomegaly and hypoglycemia. Because carbohydrate metabolism in the liver controls plasma glucose levels, the disorders of hepatic glycogen degradation and glucose release cause fasting hypoglycemia. Diseases in this group include glucose-6-phosphatase deficiency (type I), debranching enzyme deficiency (type III), liver phosphorylase deficiency (type VI), and phosphorylase kinase deficiency (formerly type VIa or IX). The second group, characterized by cirrhosis of the liver and hepatomegaly, is associated with accumulation of abnormal forms of glycogen, which may be the cause of the hepatocellular injury. This group includes branching enzyme deficiency (type IV) and debranching enzyme deficiency (type III).

The role of glycogen in muscle is to provide substrates for the generation of sufficient ATP for muscle contraction. The muscle glycogen storage diseases can also be divided into two groups. The first is a muscle-energy disorder characterized by muscle pain, exercise intolerance, myoglobinuria, and susceptibility to fatigue. This group includes type V (McArdle disease), a muscle phosphorylase deficiency, and deficiencies of phosphofructokinase (type VII), phosphoglycerate kinase, phosphoglycerate mutase, or lactate dehydrogenase. Some of these latter enzyme deficiencies are associated with a compensated hemolysis, suggesting a more generalized defect in glucose metabolism. The second group of muscle disorders is characterized by progressive skeletal muscle weakness and atrophy and/or cardiomyopathy and includes a lysosomal enzyme deficiency (acid α-glucosidase, type II), muscle debranching enzyme deficiency (type IIIa), a form of branching enzyme deficiency (type IV), and deficiency of cardiac-specific phosphorylase kinase.

The overall frequency of all forms of glycogen storage disease is approximately 1 in 20,000 to 25,000 live births. The most common childhood disorders are glucose-6-phosphatase deficiency (type I), lysosomal acid α-glucosidase deficiency (type II), debrancher deficiency (type III), and liver phosphorylase kinase deficiency (formerly type VIa or IX). The most common adult disorder is myophosphorylase deficiency (type V, or McArdle disease). In the past, the prognosis for many glycogen storage diseases was guarded. Early diagnosis and better management have improved the survival rates, and many affected children are now adults.

The majority of the glycogen storage diseases are inherited as autosomal recessive traits, but phosphoglycerate kinase deficiency and

FIGURE 347-1 Metabolic pathways related to glycogen storage disease. A hypothetical composite cell is shown depicting both hepatic and muscle pathways. The shaded areas depict pathways that are blocked in the hepatic-hypoglycemic diseases or in the muscle-energy diseases. Nonstandard abbreviations are as follows: GS$_a$, active glycogen synthase; GS$_b$, inactive glycogen synthase; P$_a$, active phosphorylase; P$_b$, inactive phosphorylase; P$_a$P, phosphorylase a phosphatase; P$_b$K$_a$, active phosphorylase b kinase; P$_b$K$_b$, inactive phosphorylase b kinase. [*From AR Beaudet: Glycogen storage diseases, in KJ Isselbacher et al. (ed): Harrison's Principles of Internal Medicine, 13th ed., New York, McGraw-Hill, 1994, p 1855.*]

Table 347-1

Glycogen Storage Diseases by Organ Involvement and Clinical Features

Type	Basic Defect	Clinical Features	Comments
LIVER GLYCOGENOSES			
Disorders with hepatomegaly and hypoglycemia			
Ia	Glucose-6-phosphatase	Growth retardation, enlarged liver and kidney, hypoglycemia, elevated blood lactate, cholesterol, triglycerides, and uric acid	Common, severe hypoglycemia
Ib	Glucose-6-phosphate translocase	As for Ia, with additional findings of neutropenia and neutrophils dysfunction	~10% of type Ia
IIIa	Liver and muscle debranching enzyme	Childhood: Hepatomegaly, growth retardation, muscle weakness, hypoglycemia, hyperlipidemia, elevated liver transaminases; liver symptoms improve with age Adulthood: muscle atrophy and weakness; onset: third to fourth decades; variable cardiomyopathy	Common, intermediate severity of hypoglycemia See below for liver cirrhosis and myopathy
IIIb	Liver debranching enzyme deficiency, normal muscle debrancher activity	Liver symptoms same as in type IIIa; no muscle symptoms	~15% of type III
VI	Liver phosphorylase	Hepatomegaly, mild hypoglycemia, hyperlipidemia and ketosis; symptoms improve with age	Rare, "benign" glycogenosis.
Formerly VIa or IX	Liver phosphorylase kinase α subunit	As for VI	Common, "benign glycogenosis," X-linked
Disorders with liver cirrhosis			
IIIa and IIIb	Debranching enzyme	Elevated transaminases in childhood, improve with age; periportal fibrosis to micronodular cirrhosis, mostly nonprogressive, rare overt cirrhosis	Overt cirrhosis frequently seen in Japanese patients
IV	Branching enzyme	Failure to thrive, hypotonia, hepatomegaly, splenomegaly, progressive liver cirrhosis and failure (death usually before fifth year); some without progression	One of the rarer glycogenoses; other neuromuscular variants exist, see below
MUSCLE GLYCOGENOSES			
Disorders with muscle-energy impairment			
V	Muscle phosphorylase	Exercise intolerance, muscle cramps, myoglobinuria on strenuous exercise, increased CK	Common, male predominance
VII	Phosphofructokinase—M subunit	As for type V, with additional findings of a compensated hemolysis	Prevalent in Japanese and Ashkenazi Jews
	Phosphoglycerate kinase	As for type V, with additional findings of a hemolytic anemia and CNS dysfunction	Rare, X-linked
	Phosphoglycerate mutase—M subunit	As for type V	Rare; majority of patients are African-American
	Lactate dehydrogenase—M subunit	As for type V, with additional findings of erythematous skin eruption and uterine stiffness resulting in childbirth difficulty in female	Rare
	Muscle-specific phosphorylase kinase	As for type V, some patients may have muscle weakness and atrophy	Rare, autosomal recessive
Disorders with progressive skeletal muscle weakness, atrophy, and/or cardiomyopathy			
II	Lysosomal acid α-glucosidase	Infantile: hypotonia, muscle weakness, cardiac enlargement and failure, fatal early Juvenile and adult: progressive skeletal muscle weakness and atrophy, proximal muscle and respiratory muscle are seriously affected	Common, undetectable, or very low level of enzyme activity in infantile form; residual enzyme activity in late-onset
IIIa	Debranching enzyme	Muscle weakness and atrophy; onset third to fourth decades; both proximal and distal muscles involved; variable cardiomyopathy	Only in patients with debranching enzyme deficiency in muscle
IV	Branching enzyme	Neonatal severe hypotonia, muscle atrophy, and neuronal involvement; death in neonatal period Childhood presentation with myopathy or cardiomyopathy Adult with central and peripheral nervous system dysfunction	Very rare
	Cardiac-specific phosphorylase kinase	Severe cardiomyopathy and failure; fatal early	Very rare

NOTE: CK, creatine kinase; M, muscle; CNS, central nervous system.

one form of phosphorylase kinase deficiency are X-linked disorders. For most glycogen storage diseases, the genes that encode the defective enzymes have been characterized at the molecular level, including genes for glucose-6-phosphatase, lysosomal α-1,4-glucosidase, debrancher enzyme, branching enzyme, phosphorylase, phosphorylase kinase, phosphofructokinase, phosphoglycerate mutase, phosphoglycerate kinase, and lactate dehydrogenase—muscle subunit. Genetic heterogeneity is present at the protein, mRNA, and DNA levels. Advances in understanding the molecular basis of the disease are being used to improve the diagnosis and management of the disorders, and some are candidates for early trials of gene therapy.

LIVER GLYCOGENOSES

DISORDERS WITH HEPATOMEGALY AND HYPOGLYCEMIA   Type I Glycogen Storage Disease (Glucose-6-Phosphatase or Translocase Deficiency, von Gierke Disease)   Type I glycogen storage disease is due to a defect in glucose-6-phosphatase in liver, kidney, and intestinal mucosa. It can be divided into two subtypes: type Ia, in which the glucose-6-phosphatase enzyme is defective, and type Ib, which is due to a defect in the translocase that transports glucose-6-phosphate across the microsomal membrane. The defects in both type Ia and Ib lead to inadequate conversion in liver of glucose-6-phosphate to glucoses and thus make affected individuals susceptible to fasting hypoglycemia.

Clinical and laboratory findings   Patients with type I disease may develop hypoglycemia and lactic acidosis during the neonatal period but more commonly present at 3 to 4 months of age with hepatomegaly and/or hypoglycemia. These children may have doll-like faces with fat cheeks, relatively thin extremities, short stature, and a protuberant abdomen that is due to massive hepatomegaly; the kidneys are enlarged, and the spleen and heart are of normal size.

The hallmarks of the disease are hypoglycemia, lactic acid acidosis, hyperuricemia, and hyperlipidemia. Hypoglycemia and lactic acid acidosis can develop after a short fast. Hyperuricemia is present in young children, but gout rarely develops before puberty. Despite hepatomegaly, liver enzymes are usually normal or near normal. Intermittent diarrhea may occur (the mechanism is not known). Easy bruising and epistaxis are associated with a prolonged bleeding time as a result of impaired platelet aggregation/adhesion.

Hypertriglyceridemia may cause the plasma to appear "milky," and cholesterol and phospholipids are also elevated. The lipid abnormality resembles type IV hyperlipidemia and is characterized by increased levels of very low density lipoprotein (VLDL); low-density lipoprotein (LDL); increased levels of apoliproteins B, C, and E; and normal or reduced levels of apoliproteins A and D. The hepatocytes are distended by glycogen and fat with large and prominent lipid vacuoles. There is no associated fibrosis.

All these findings apply to both type Ia and Ib glycogen storage diseases, but type Ib has the additional feature of recurrent bacterial infections due to neutropenia and impaired neutrophil function. Oral and intestinal mucosa ulcerations are common, and inflammatory bowel disease may occur.

Long-term complications   Although type I glycogen storage disease mainly affects the liver, multiple organ systems are also involved. Gout usually becomes symptomatic around puberty as a result of the long-term hyperuricemia. Puberty is often delayed, but fertility appears to be normal. Hypertriglyceridemia causes an increased risk of pancreatitis, but premature atherosclerosis has not been documented. Impaired platelet aggregation may reduce the risk of atherosclerosis.

By the second or third decade of life, most patients with type I glycogen storage disease develop hepatic adenomas that can hemorrhage and, in rare cases, may become malignant. Other complications include pulmonary hypertension and osteoporosis.

Renal disease is a late complication, and almost all patients above age 20 have proteinuria. Many have hypertension, kidney stones, nephrocalcinosis, and altered creatinine clearance. Glomerular hyperfiltration, increased renal plasma flow, and microalbuminuria can occur before the onset of gross proteinuria. In young patients, hyperfiltration and hyperperfusion may be the only signs of renal abnormalities. With advanced renal disease, focal segmental glomerulosclerosis and interstitial fibrosis are evident on biopsy. In some patients, renal function deteriorates and progresses to failure, requiring dialysis or transplantation. Other abnormalities in renal function include amyloidosis, Fanconi-like syndrome, and distal renal tubular acidification defect. The increases in renal perfusion and maternal blood volume that normally occur in pregnancy can exacerbate renal problems. In addition, hypoglycemia may also become more difficult to control.

Diagnosis   The diagnosis of type I disease can be suspected on the basis of clinical presentation and abnormal plasma lactate and lipid values. In addition, administration of glucagon or epinephrine causes little or no rise in blood glucose but increases lactate levels significantly. A definitive diagnosis, however, requires a liver biopsy to demonstrate a deficiency of either glucose-6-phosphatase or translocase. Molecular diagnoses can now be made for the majority of type Ia glycogen storage disease patients.

℞ **TREATMENT**

Treatment is designed to maintain normal blood glucose levels and is achieved by continuous nasogastric infusion of glucose or oral administration of uncooked cornstarch. Nasogastric drip feeding in early infancy may consist of an elemental enteral formula or may contain only glucose to maintain normoglycemia during the night; frequent feedings with a high-carbohydrate content are given during the day.

Uncooked cornstarch acts as a slow-release form of glucose and can be given at a dose of 1.6 g/kg every 4 h for infants under the age of 2 years. As the child grows older, the cornstarch regimen can be changed to every 6 h, and it can be given by mouth as a liquid (1:2, weight:volume) at a dose of 1.75 to 2.5 g/kg of body weight. Because fructose and galactose cannot be converted to free glucose, their dietary intake should be restricted, and dietary supplements of multivitamins and calcium are required. Allopurinol is given to lower the levels of uric acid. In patients with type Ib glycogen storage disease, granulocyte and granulocyte-macrophage colony stimulating factors have been used successfully to correct the neutropenia, decrease the severity of bacterial infection, and improve the chronic inflammatory bowel disease.

Prior to surgery, the bleeding status should be evaluated, and good metabolic control should be established. Prolonged bleeding time can be corrected by the administration of a constant intravenous glucose infusion for 24 to 48 h prior to surgery. Vasopressin can be given during surgery to reduce bleeding complications, and normal glucose levels should be maintained throughout surgery.

Prognosis   In the past, many patients with type I glycogen storage disease died, and the prognosis was guarded for those who survived. The long-term complications discussed above occur mostly in adults whose disease was not adequately treated during childhood. Early diagnosis and initiation of effective treatment have improved the outcome, but it is not known if all long-term complications can be avoided through good metabolic control.

Genetics   Type I glycogen storage disease is an autosomal recessive disorder. Both type Ia and Ib diseases have been reported in many ethnic groups, but type Ia is rarely seen in blacks. The structural gene for glucose-6-phosphatase is located on chromosome 17; three common mutations (R83C, 130X, Q347X) are responsible for 70 percent of the known disease alleles. Carrier detection and prenatal diagnosis are possible with the use of molecular techniques.

Type III Glycogen Storage Disease (Debrancher Deficiency, Limit Dextrinosis)   Type III glycogen storage disease is caused by a deficiency of glycogen debranching enzyme. Debranching enzyme and phosphorylase are responsible for complete degradation of glycogen; when debranching enzyme is defective, glycogen breakdown is incomplete, and an abnormal glycogen that has short outer chains and that resembles limit dextrin accumulates.

Clinical and laboratory findings Deficiency of glycogen debranching enzyme causes hepatomegaly, hypoglycemia, short stature, variable skeletal myopathy, and cardiomyopathy. The disorder usually involves both liver and muscle and is termed *type IIIa glycogen storage disease*. However, in about 15 percent of patients, the disease appears to involve only the liver and is classified as *type IIIb*.

During infancy and childhood, the disease may be almost indistinguishable from type I disease because hepatomegaly, hypoglycemia, hyperlipidemia, and growth retardation are common features of both. Splenomegaly may be present, but kidneys are not enlarged in type III. Remarkably, hepatomegaly and hepatic symptoms in most of type III patients improve with age and usually disappear after puberty. Overt liver cirrhosis is rare except in Japanese patients.

In patients with muscle involvement (type IIIa), muscle weakness is usually minimal during childhood but can become severe during the third or fourth decade of life, as evidenced by slowly progressive weakness and muscle wasting. Electromyographic (EMG) changes are consistent with a widespread myopathy, and nerve conduction may be abnormal. Ventricular hypertrophy is frequent, but overt cardiac dysfunction is rare. Hepatic symptoms may be so mild that the diagnosis is not made until adulthood, when neuromuscular disease becomes manifest.

Hypoglycemia, hyperlipidemia, and elevated liver transaminases occur in childhood. In contrast to type I disease, fasting ketosis is prominent, and blood lactate and uric acid concentrations are usually normal. The administration of glucagon 2 h after a carbohydrate meal causes a normal rise of blood glucose, but after an overnight fast glucagon may provoke no change in blood glucose. Serum creatine kinase levels can sometimes be used to identify patients with muscle involvement, but normal levels do not rule out muscle enzyme deficiency.

The histology of the liver is characterized by a universal distention of hepatocytes by glycogen and by the presence of fibrous septa. The fibrosis and the paucity of fat distinguish type III from type I glycogenosis. The fibrosis can range from minimal periportal fibrosis to micronodular cirrhosis and appears, in most cases, to be nonprogressive.

Diagnosis In glycogen storage disease type IIIa, deficient debranching enzyme activity can be demonstrated in liver, skeletal muscle, and heart. In contrast, type IIIb patients have debranching enzyme deficiency only in the liver and not in muscle. Definitive diagnosis and assignment of subtype in this disorder require enzyme assays in both liver and muscle.

℞ **TREATMENT**

Dietary management of type III disease is less demanding than in type I. If hypoglycemia is present, frequent high-carbohydrate meals with cornstarch supplements or nocturnal gastric drip feedings are usually effective. A high-protein diet during the daytime plus overnight protein enteral infusion may be tried in patients with myopathy, but it is not established whether such a regimen is effective. Patients do not need to restrict dietary intake of fructose and galactose, as do those with type I disease.

Prognosis Liver symptoms improve with age and usually disappear after puberty. Cirrhosis of the liver is rare. In type IIIa disease muscle weakness and atrophy worsen during adulthood.

Genetics The type III glycogenoses are inherited as autosomal recessive traits. The disease has been reported in many different ethnic groups, and the frequency is relatively high in non-Ashkenazi Jews of North African descent. The gene for debranching enzyme is located on chromosome 1p21. Carrier detection and prenatal diagnosis are possible using DNA-based linkage or mutation analysis.

Type VI Glycogen Storage Disease [Liver Phosphorylase Deficiency (Hers Disease) and Phosphorylase Kinase Deficiency] Defects of the phosphorylase system cause a heterogeneous group of glycogenoses. The heterogeneity is due to the complexity of the reactions involved in glycogenolysis. A cascade of enzymatic reactions, involving adenylate cyclase, cyclic adenosine monophosphate–dependent protein kinase (protein kinase A), and phosphorylase kinase, activate phosphorylase, the rate-limiting enzyme of glycogenolysis. Theoretically, glycogen storage disease can result from any enzyme deficiency along this pathway, but phosphorylase kinase deficiency is the most common. Phosphorylase kinase has four subunits (α, β, γ, and δ), each encoded by different genes and differentially expressed in various tissues.

The numerical classification of this group of glycogenoses is confusing, ranging from type VI, VIa, to IX. It is advisable to refrain from such a designation and to classify the various disorders according to organ involvement and mode of inheritance.

Clinical and laboratory findings LIVER PHOSPHORYLASE DEFICIENCY Liver phosphorylase deficiency has been documented in only a small number of patients. It appears to be a benign disorder. The patients present with hepatomegaly and growth retardation early in childhood. Hypoglycemia, hyperlipidemia, and hyperketosis are usually mild, if present. Lactate and uric acid levels are normal. The heart and skeletal muscles are not involved. The hepatomegaly improves with age and usually disappears around puberty. The liver phosphorylase gene has been cloned and mapped to chromosome 14.

X-linked liver phosphorylase kinase deficiency X-linked liver phosphorylase kinase deficiency is one of the most common liver glycogenoses. Phosphorylase kinase activity may also be deficient in erythrocytes and leukocytes but is normal in muscle. Typically, a child between the ages of 1 and 5 years presents with growth retardation and hepatomegaly. Levels of cholesterol, triglycerides, and liver enzymes are mildly elevated. Ketosis may occur after fasting. Lactate and uric acid levels are normal. Hypoglycemia is mild, if present. The rise in blood glucose following the administration of glucagon is normal. Hepatomegaly and abnormal blood chemistries gradually return to normal with age. Most adults achieve a normal final height and are practically asymptomatic, despite a persistent phosphorylase kinase deficiency.

Liver histology shows glycogen-distended hepatocytes. The accumulated glycogen (α particles, rosette form) has a frayed or burst appearance and is less compact than in type I or III disease. Fibrous septae and low-grade inflammatory changes may be present.

The structural gene for the liver isoform of the phosphorylase kinase α-subunit is located on chromosome Xp22, and mutations of this gene have been found in the disorder.

AUTOSOMAL LIVER AND MUSCLE PHOSPHORYLASE KINASE DEFICIENCY An autosomal recessive form of liver and muscle phosphorylase kinase deficiency has been reported in several patients. As in the X-linked form of the disorder, hepatomegaly and growth retardation are the predominant symptoms in early childhood. Some patients also exhibit muscle hypotonia and have reduced activity of phosphorylase kinase in muscle. Because of the autosomal recessive mode of inheritance, mutations are likely to be found in the genes that encode the β and/or γ subunits of the phosphorylase kinase.

MUSCLE-SPECIFIC PHOSPHORYLASE KINASE DEFICIENCY Muscle-specific phosphorylase kinase deficiency causes cramps and myoglobinuria on exercise or progressive muscle weakness and atrophy. The activity of the enzyme is decreased in muscle but (when determined) normal in liver and blood cells. There is no hepatomegaly or cardiomegaly. The disorder is presumed to be an autosomal recessive trait.

CARDIAC-SPECIFIC PHOSPHORYLASE KINASE DEFICIENCY Phosphorylase kinase deficiency limited to the heart has been reported in only two cases. Both patients died during infancy from cardiac failure due to massive glycogen deposition in the myocardium.

Diagnosis Definitive diagnosis of phosphorylase kinase deficiency requires demonstration of the enzymatic defect in affected tissues. Although phosphorylase kinase can be measured in leukocytes and erythrocytes, the enzyme has many tissue-specific isozymes, and the diagnosis can be missed without studies of the liver, muscle, or heart.

TREATMENT

The treatment for liver phosphorylase or phosphorylase kinase deficiency is based on symptoms. A high-carbohydrate diet and frequent feedings are effective in preventing hypoglycemia, but most patients require no specific treatment. Prognosis is usually good; adult patients have normal stature and minimal hepatomegaly. There is no treatment for the fatal form of isolated cardiac phosphorylase kinase deficiency.

Genetics Carrier detection is possible using DNA-based linkage or mutation analysis for the common form of X-linked phosphorylase kinase deficiency.

DISORDERS WITH LIVER CIRRHOSIS Type IV Glycogen Storage Disease (Branching Enzyme Deficiency, Amylopectinosis, or Andersen Disease) Deficiency of branching enzyme activity results in accumulation of an abnormal glycogen with poor solubility. The disease is referred to as *type IV glycogen storage disease* or *amylopectinosis*, because the abnormal glycogen has fewer branch points, more α1-4 linked glucose units, and longer outer chains, resulting in a structure resembling amylopectin.

Clinical and laboratory findings This disorder is clinically variable. The most common form is characterized by progressive cirrhosis of the liver and is manifest in the first 18 months of life as hepatosplenomegaly and failure to thrive. The cirrhosis progresses to cause portal hypertension, ascites, esophageal varices, and liver failure that leads to death by age 5. Rare patients survive without progression of liver disease.

Tissue deposition of amylopectin-like materials can be demonstrated in liver, heart, muscle, skin, intestine, brain, spinal cord, and peripheral nerve. The histologic findings in the liver are characterized by both micronodular cirrhosis and faintly stained basophilic inclusions in the hepatocytes. The inclusions consist of coarsely clumped, stored material that is periodic acid Schiff–positive and partially resistant to diastase digestion. Electron microscopy shows, in addition to the conventional α and β glycogen particles, an accumulation of fibrillar aggregations typical of amylopectin. Definitive diagnosis requires demonstration that branching enzyme activity is deficient in liver, muscle, cultured skin fibroblasts, or leukocytes.

A neuromuscular form of type IV glycogen storage disease has also been reported. These patients may (1) present at birth with severe hypotonia, muscle atrophy, and neuronal involvement and die during the neonatal period; (2) present in late childhood with myopathy or cardiopathy; or (3) present as adults with diffuse central and peripheral nervous system dysfunction accompanied by accumulation of polyglucosan bodies in the nervous system (so-called adult polyglucosan body disease). Definitive diagnosis of the adult disease requires assay of branching enzyme in leukocytes or nerve biopsy, as the deficiency is limited to those tissues.

 TREATMENT

There is no specific treatment for type IV glycogen storage disease. For progressive hepatic failure, liver transplantation has been performed, but because it is a multisystem disorder the long-term success of liver transplantation is not known.

Genetics Type IV glycogen storage disease is a rare autosomal recessive disease. Prenatal diagnosis is available by using cultured aminocytes or chorionic villi to measure the level of enzymatic activity. The glycogen branching enzyme gene is located on chromosome 3p14. Mutations responsible for type IV glycogen storage disease have been identified, and their characterization in individual patients may be useful in predicting the clinical course.

MUSCLE GLYCOGENOSES

DISORDERS WITH MUSCLE-ENERGY IMPAIRMENT Type V Glycogen Storage Disease (Muscle Phosphorylase Deficiency, McArdle Disease) Deficiency of muscle phosphorylase is the prototype muscle-energy disorder. Deficiency of this enzyme in muscle limits ATP generation by glycogenolysis and results in glycogen accumulation.

Clinical and laboratory findings Symptoms usually develop first in adulthood and are characterized by exercise intolerance with muscle cramps. Two types of activity tend to cause symptoms: (1) brief exercise of great intensity, such as sprinting or carrying heavy loads; and (2) less intense but sustained activity, such as climbing stairs or walking uphill. Moderate exercise, such as walking on level ground, can be performed by most patients for long periods. Many patients experience a characteristic "second wind" phenomenon; if they rest briefly at the first appearance of muscle pain, they can resume exercise with more ease. About half report burgundy-colored urine after exercise, the consequence of myoglobinuria secondary to the rhabdomyolysis. Intense myoglobinuria after vigorous exercise may cause renal failure. Although most patients are diagnosed in the second or third decade, many report weakness and lack of endurance since childhood. In rare cases, EMG findings may suggest an inflammatory myopathy, and the diagnosis can be confused with polymyositis.

The level of serum creatine kinase is usually elevated at rest and increases more after exercise. Exercise also increases the levels of blood ammonia, inosine, hypoxanthine, and uric acid. The latter abnormalities are attributed to accelerated recycling of muscle purine nucleotides in the face of insufficient ATP production.

Clinical heterogeneity is not common, but late-onset disease with no symptoms as late as the eighth decade and an early-onset, fatal form with hypotonia, generalized muscle weakness, and progressive respiratory insufficiency have been reported.

Diagnosis Lack of an increase in blood lactate and exaggerated blood ammonia elevations after an ischemic exercise test are indicative of muscle glycogenosis and suggest a defect in the conversion of glycogen or glucose to lactate. The abnormal exercise response, however, is not limited to type V disease and can occur with other defects in glycogenolysis or glycolysis, such as deficiencies of muscle phosphofructokinase or debranching enzyme (when the test is done after fasting). Definitive diagnosis is made by enzymatic assay of muscle.

 TREATMENT

Exercise tolerance can be augmented by oral administration of glucose or fructose or by injection of glucagon. A high-protein diet may increase exercise endurance in some patients. In general, avoidance of strenuous exercise prevents the symptoms, and there is no need for a specific therapy. Longevity does not appear to be affected.

Genetics Type V glycogen storage disease is an autosomal recessive disorder that does not appear to have ethnic predilection. The gene for muscle phosphorylase is located on chromosome 11q13-qter. The most common mutation in U.S. patients is a nonsense mutation that changes an arginine to a stop at codon 49 (R49X), and the most common mutation in the Japanese is deletion of a single codon (ΔF708). This allows DNA-based diagnosis and carrier detection for the two populations.

Type VII Glycogen Storage Disease (Muscle Phosphofructokinase Deficiency, Tarui Disease) Type VII disease is caused by a deficiency of muscle phosphofructokinase, which catalyzes the conversion of fructose-6-phosphate to fructose-1,6-diphosphate and is a key regulatory enzyme of glycolysis.

Phosphofructokinase is composed of three isozyme subunits (M, muscle; L, liver; and P, platelet), which are encoded by different genes and are differentially expressed in tissues. Skeletal muscle contains only M subunit, and red blood cells contain a hybrid of L and M forms. Type VII disease is due to defective M isoenzyme, which causes complete enzyme deficiency in muscle and partial deficiency in red blood cells.

Clinical and laboratory findings The features are similar to those in type V disease, namely, early onset of fatigue and pain with exercise.

Vigorous exercise causes severe muscle cramps and myoglobinuria. However, several features of type VII disease are distinctive. (1) Exercise intolerance is usually evident in childhood, is more severe than in type V disease, and may be associated with nausea and vomiting. (2) A compensated hemolysis occurs as evidenced by an increased level of serum bilirubin and reticulocyte count. (3) Hyperuricemia is common and becomes more marked after exercise. (4) An abnormal glycogen resembling amylopectin is present in muscle fibers; it is periodic acid Schiff–positive and resistant to diastase digestion. (5) Exercise intolerance is particularly acute following meals rich in carbohydrate because glucose cannot be utilized in muscle and because the ingested glucose inhibits lipolysis and thus deprives muscle of fatty acid and ketone substrates. In contrast, patients with type V disease can metabolize glucose derived from either liver glycogenolysis or exogenous glucose. Indeed, glucose infusion improves exercise tolerance in type V patients.

Two rare type VII variants have been reported. One presents in infancy with hypotonia and limb weakness, and a rapidly progressive myopathy leads to death by age 4. The other presents in adults and is characterized by a slowly progressive, fixed muscle weakness rather than by cramps and myoglobinuria.

Diagnosis The M isoenzyme defect must be demonstrated in muscle, red blood cells, or cultured skin fibroblasts by biochemical or histochemical techniques.

℞ TREATMENT

There is no specific treatment. Avoidance of strenuous exercise prevents acute attacks of muscle cramps and myoglobinuria.

Genetics Type VII glycogen storage disease is inherited as an autosomal recessive trait. The disease appears to be rare, and most reported patients are either Japanese or Ashkenazi Jews. The gene for the M isoenzyme is located on chromosome 1 cen-1q32. In Ashkenazi Jews 95 percent of mutant alleles are either a splicing defect or a nucleotide deletion.

Other Muscle Glycogenoses with Muscle-Energy Impairment Three additional enzyme defects produce muscle glycogenoses, namely, deficiencies in phosphoglycerate kinase, phosphoglycerate mutase, and lactate dehydrogenase. All three enzymes affect terminal glycolysis, and deficiency causes muscle-energy impairment similar to that in type V and VII disease. The failure of blood lactate to increase in response to exercise can be used to separate muscle glycogenoses from disorders of lipid metabolism, such as carnitine palmitoyl transferase II deficiency and very long chain acyl–coenzyme A dehydrogenase deficiency, which also cause muscle cramps and myoglobinuria. Muscle glycogen levels may be normal in the disorders affecting terminal glycolysis, and definitive diagnosis is made by assaying the enzymatic activity in muscle.

DISORDERS WITH PROGRESSIVE SKELETAL MUSCLE WEAKNESS, ATROPHY, AND/OR CARDIOMYOPATHY Glycogen Storage Disease Type II (α1,4-Glucosidase Deficiency, Pompe Disease) (See also Chap. 346) GSD II is caused by a deficiency of lysosomal acid α1,4 glucosidase (acid maltase), an enzyme responsible for the degradation of glycogen in lysosomal vacuoles. This disease is characterized by accumulation of glycogen in lysosomes as opposed to its accumulation in cytoplasm in the other glycogenoses.

Clinical and laboratory findings The disorder encompasses a range of phenotypes, each including myopathy but differing in age of onset, organ involvement, and clinical severity. The most severe is the infantile-onset disease with cardiomegaly, hypotonia, and death prior to 2 years of age. Infants appear normal at birth but soon develop generalized muscle weakness with feeding difficulties, macroglossia,

hepatomegaly, and congestive heart failure due to a hypertrophic cardiomyopathy. Electrocardiographic findings include a high-voltage QRS complex and a shortened PR interval. Death usually occurs from cardiorespiratory failure or aspiration pneumonia.

The juvenile or late-childhood form is characterized by skeletal muscle manifestations, usually without cardiac involvement, and a slowly progressive course. The juvenile form typically presents as delayed motor milestones (if age of onset is early enough) and difficulty in walking and is followed by swallowing difficulties, proximal muscle weakness, and respiratory muscle involvement; it can cause death before the end of the second decade.

An adult form of type II disease presents as a slowly progressive myopathy without cardiac involvement and has its onset between the second and seventh decades. The clinical picture is dominated by slowly progressive proximal muscle weakness with truncal involvement and greater involvement of the lower than the upper limbs. Pelvic girdle, paraspinal muscle, and diaphragm are most seriously affected. The initial symptoms may be respiratory insufficiency manifested by somnolence, morning headache, orthopnea, and exertional dyspnea.

Laboratory findings include elevated levels of serum creatine kinase, aspartate transaminase, and lactate dehydrogenase, particularly in infants. Muscle biopsy shows the presence of vacuoles that stain positively for glycogen, and muscle acid phosphatase is increased, presumably from a compensatory increase of lysosomal enzymes. Electron microscopy reveals the glycogen accumulation. EMG reveals myopathic features with irritability of muscle fibers and pseudomyotonic discharges. Serum creatine kinase is not always elevated in adults, and, depending on the muscle biopsied or tested, muscle histology or EMG may not be abnormal. It is prudent to examine affected muscle.

Diagnosis Diagnosis can be established by demonstration of absence or reduced levels of acid α-glucosidase activity in muscle or cultured skin fibroblasts. Deficiency is usually more severe in the infantile form than in the juvenile and adult disorders.

℞ TREATMENT

No effective treatment for the infantile form is available. A high-protein diet may be useful for the juvenile and adult forms. Nocturnal ventilatory support in adults may improve the quality of life and have dramatic effects during respiratory decompensation.

Genetics Pompe disease is an autosomal recessive disorder and does not appear to have an ethnic predilection. The gene for acid α-glucosidase is on chromosome 17q23. A splice site mutation (IVS1-13T→G) is commonly seen in patients with adult-onset disease. Prenatal diagnosis using amniocytes or chorionic villi is available in the fatal infantile form.

BIBLIOGRAPHY

CHEN Y-T, BURCHELL A: Glycogen storage diseases, in *The Metabolic and Molecular Bases of Inherited Disease*, 7th ed, CR Scriver et al (eds). New York, McGraw-Hill, 1995, pp 935–965

———— et al: Renal disease in Type I glycogen storage disease. N Engl J Med 318:7, 1988

FERNANDEZ J et al: Glycogen storage disease. Recommendations for treatment. Eur J Pediatr 147:226, 1988

HIRSCHHORN R: Glycogen storage disease type II: Acid α-glucosidase (acid maltase) deficiency, in *The Metabolic and Molecular Bases of Inherited Disease*, 7th ed, CR Scriver et al (eds). New York, McGraw-Hill, 1995, pp 2243–2464

LEI K-J et al: Mutations in the glucose-6-phosphatase gene that cause glycogen storage disease type Ia. Science 262:580, 1993

TALENTE GM et al: Glycogen storage disease in adults: A retrospective study of clinical and laboratory findings in types Ia, Ib, and III. Ann Intern Med 120:218, 1994

TSUJINO S et al: Molecular genetic heterogeneity of myophosphorylase deficiency (McArdle's disease). N Engl J Med 329:241, 1993

INHERITED DISORDERS OF CONNECTIVE TISSUE

Heritable disorders that involve the major connective tissues of the body such as bone, skin, cartilage, blood vessels, and basement membranes are among the most common genetic diseases in human beings. Such diseases include many clinical entities that were not previously recognized either as involving specific components of connective tissue or being inherited. Here we will focus primarily on those disorders that can have severe manifestations, are relatively common, and are sufficiently understood at the molecular level to provide useful paradigms: osteogenesis imperfecta (OI), the Ehlers-Danlos syndrome (EDS), chondrodysplasias (CDs), the Marfan syndrome (MS), epidermolysis bullosa (EB), and the Alport syndrome (AS).

THE CHALLENGE OF CLASSIFYING THE DISEASES The first comprehensive effort to classify diseases of connective tissue was made by McKusick in a series of reports and then in the monograph *Heritable Disorders of Connective Tissue*, in which he drew attention to patients and families with connective tissue disorders in whom the changes appeared to be inherited as single-gene traits. He subsequently expanded the classification to include more than 12 major diseases of connective tissue that were likely to be caused by single-gene defects on the basis of the pattern of inheritance, the cluster of signs and symptoms, the histologic changes in tissues, and limited information about the molecular defects involved. This classification was extended by other investigators so that about a dozen types and subtypes were defined for OI, about the same number for the EDS, and over 150 for the CDs.

For some of the original disease categories, most patients with the classic features of the disease have a mutation in a gene or genes coding for a single protein. For example, the majority of patients with OI have a mutation in one of the two genes coding for type I procollagen. Similarly, most patients with MS have mutations in a gene for fibrillin. For other disease categories, the situation is more complex. In EDS, for example, the type IV variant is usually due to mutations in the gene for type III procollagen, the type VI variant to defects in the gene for lysyl hydroxylase, and the type VII variant to defects that impair the processing of type I procollagen to type I collagen.

Several limitations in the original classifications are now apparent. One is that the same mutation does not always produce the same disease phenotype in terms of severity of the condition or its clinical course. Such phenotypic variation occurs in many genetic diseases, including the connective tissue disorders, in which some members of a family are severely affected, whereas others with the same mutation have a mild disorder.

Classifications of these disorders also tend to overemphasize the etiologic differences between severe genetic diseases that are apparent in infants and the more common diseases that appear much later in life. Single-gene defects can cause subsets of late-onset diseases such as osteoporosis, aneurysms, and osteoarthritis. For example, a small subset of patients with postmenopausal osteo-porosis have mutations in the genes for procollagen I similar to the mutations in the same genes that produce lethal variants of OI. Likewise, a subset of patients with familial aortic aneurysms have mutations in the gene for procollagen III similar to the mutations in the same gene that cause lethal variants of type IV EDS, and occasional patients with osteoarthritis have mutations in the gene for procollagen II similar to the mutations in the same gene that cause lethal CDs. There is disagreement as to the best diagnosis for such patients in that some investigators feel that after a mutation similar to those seen in the early-onset diseases is identified, the patients should be reclassified as having mild forms of OI, EDS, or CD, even though they do not have definitive evidence of the early-onset diseases or seek medical attention until adulthood. The debate is fueled by the fact that many of the classification systems are based on clusters of signs and symptoms for which there are few objective criteria. However, some patients with late-onset diseases of connective tissue such as osteoporosis, osteoarthritis, and aneurysms inherit the disorders in a manner suggesting single-gene defects. Therefore, the category of diseases referred to as *inherited disorders of connective tissue* may have to be expanded.

DEFINITION AND COMPOSITION OF CONNECTIVE TISSUES Connective tissues are composed of specific macromolecules, many of which are also constituents of the lung, the kidney, the walls of blood vessels, the vitreous gel of the eye, and the synovial fluid. Indeed, most organs and tissues contain small amounts of the same macromolecules assembled into membranes and septa. Therefore, virtually all structures contain connective tissue.

The distinguishing feature of connective tissues is that the component macromolecules are assembled into an insoluble extracellular matrix (Table 348-1). The macromolecules include at least 19 different

Table 348-1

Constituents of Various Connective Tissues

Connective Tissue	Known Constituents	Approximate Amounts, % dry wt	Characteristics or Functions
Skin, ligaments, tendons	Type I collagen	80	Bundles of fibrils
	Type III collagen	5–15	Thin fibrils
	Type IV collagen, laminin, nidogen	<5	In basal laminae under epithelium and in blood vessels
	Types V, VI, and VII collagens	<5	Functions unclear
	Elastin, fibrillin	<5	Provide elasticity
	Fibronectin	<5	Associated with collagen fibers and cell surfaces
	Proteoglycans* and hyaluronate	0.5	Provide resiliency
Bone (demineralized)	Type I collagen	90	Complex fibril network
	Type VI collagen	1–2	Function unclear
	Proteoglycans	1	Function unclear
	Osteonectin, osteocalcin, osteopontin, α2-glycoprotein, sialoproteins	1–5	Probably initial or regulate mineralization
Aorta	Type I collagen	20–40	Fibril network
	Type III collagen	20–40	Thin fibrils
	Elastin, fibrillin	20–40	Provide elasticity
	Type IV collagen, laminin, nidogen	<5	Form basal lamina
	Types V and VI collagens	<2	Functions unclear
	Proteoglycans	<3	Provide resiliency
Cartilage	Type II collagen	40–50	Arcades of thin fibrils
	Type IX collagen	5–10	Links type II fibrils
	Type X collagen	5–10	Surrounds hypertrophic cells
	Type XI collagen	<10	Function unclear
	Proteoglycans and hyaluronate	15–50	Provide resiliency

* As discussed in text, at least five proteoglycans have now been identified. They differ in the structures of their core proteins and their contents of mucopolysaccharide side chains of chondroitin-4-sulfate, chondroitin-6-sulfate, dermatan sulfate, and keratan sulfate. Basil lamina contain a proteoglycan with a side chain of heparan sulfate that resembles heparin.

types of collagens, the related fibrous proteins known as *elastin* and *fibrillin*, a series of proteoglycans, and components whose structure and function are only partially defined.

Differences in the connective tissues of bone, skin, and cartilage are in part explained by differences in the content of specific components (see Table 348-1). For example, tendons and ligaments consist primarily of type I collagen fibrils and small amounts of other components that help organize the type I fibrils into fibers and fiber bundles. Cartilage consists primarily of fibrils of type II collagen in the form of arcades that are distended by highly charged proteoglycans. The extracellular matrix of the aorta contains collagens that provide tensile strength and elastin that provides elasticity. Differences among the connective tissues also depend on the three-dimensional organization of the molecular components. The type I collagen fibrils in tendon are packed into thick, parallel bundles of fibers, whereas type I collagen fibrils in skin are randomly oriented. In cortical bone, helical arrays of type I collagen fibrils are deposited around haversian canals.

BIOSYNTHESIS OF CONNECTIVE TISSUE Connective tissues largely form by self-assembly, in which a molecule of the correct size, shape, and surface properties binds to other molecules with the same or similar structure in a spontaneous but ordered manner. The molecular mechanisms and driving forces are similar to those involved in crystal formation.

The self-assembly of connective tissue is illustrated by the assembly of collagen into fibrils. The fibril that forms collagen is a long, thin rod consisting of three polypeptide α chains wrapped into a rigid, ropelike triple helix (Fig. 348-1). The fibril has a triple-helical conformation, because each of the three α chains has a simple, repetitive amino acid sequence of about 1000 amino acids in which glycine (Gly) appears as every third amino acid. Therefore, the sequence of

each α chain can be designated as $(-Gly-X-Y-)_{333}$, where X and Y represent amino acids other than glycine. To fold into a triple helix, every third amino acid in an α chain must be glycine, the smallest amino acid, since this residue must fit in a sterically restricted space where the three chains of the triple helix come together. Many of the X- and Y-position amino acids are proline and hydroxyproline, which provide rigidity to the triple helix. The remaining amino acids form clusters of hydrophobic and charged regions on the surface of the molecule that direct how one molecule spontaneously binds to other collagen molecules and thereby self-assembles into the large collagen fibrils in tissues (see Fig. 348-1).

More than 19 different collagens have been identified. Most are minor constituents that probably have highly specialized functions. The fibrillar collagens are found in tissues as long, highly ordered fibrils with a characteristic banding pattern by electron microscopy. Type I collagen, the most abundant, is found as cross-striated fibrils in a large number of tissues (see Table 348-1). It is composed of two identical α chains called α1(I) and one α2(I) chain. Type II collagen, a fibrillar collagen of cartilage, is composed of three identical α chains called α1(II). Type III collagen is found in small amounts in many tissues that contain type I collagen and in large amounts in large blood vessels; it is composed of three identical chains called α1(III). The nonfibrillar collagens are similar to the fibrillar collagens in that they contain -Gly-X-Y- sequences of amino acids that form triple-helical domains, but they also contain large globular domains. Self-assembly of most of the nonfibrillar collagens usually involves binding between the globular domains to form networks. For example, the type IV collagen in basement membranes self-assembles into a complex three-dimensional network that provides a diffusion barrier in the renal glomerulus and pulmonary alveolus and provides support for epithelial and endothelial cells in these tissues and in skin, the gastrointestinal tract, and blood vessels. Some nonfibrillar collagens bind to the surface of fibrils formed by the more abundant collagens and alter the lateral growth of the fibrillar collagens or prevent the fibrils from coalescing into fiber bundles.

Because fibrillar collagens spontaneously self-assemble into fibrils, they are first synthesized as larger and more soluble precursors called *procollagens*. The procollagen forms of type I, II, and III collagens are 1.5 times the mass of the mature collagens because of the presence of amino acid sequences (*propeptides*) located at both the N and C termini of the proα chains of the procollagens.

The biosynthesis of procollagens involves complex intracellular processing (see Fig. 348-1) and an unusual self-assembly whereby the three chains fold into a triple helix. As the proα chains of procollagen are synthesized on ribosomes, the free ends move into the cisternae of the rough endoplasmic reticulum. Hydrophobic signal peptides at the N terminus are cleaved, and additional posttranslational reactions begin. Proline residues in the Y position of the repeating -Gly-X-Y- sequences are converted to hydroxyproline by prolyl hydroxylase in a reaction requiring ascorbic acid. Lysine residues in the Y position are similarly hydroxylated to hydroxylysine by lysyl hydroxylase. Many of the hydroxylysine residues are glycosylated with galactose or with galactose and glucose. A large mannose-rich oligosaccharide is assembled on the C-terminal propeptide of each chain. As

FIGURE 348-1 Schematic representation of synthesis of a type I collagen fibril by a fibroblast. *A.* Intracellular steps in the assembly of the procollagen molecule. Hydroxylations and glycosylations of the proα chains begin soon after the amino termini pass into the cisternae of the rough endoplasmic reticulum and continue after the three chains associate through their carboxy-terminal propeptides and become disulfide linked. *B.* Cleavage of procollagen to collagen, self-assembly of the collagen molecule into quarter-staggered fibrils, and cross-linking of the molecules in the fibrils. Cleavage of the propeptides may occur within crypts of the fibroblast, as shown here, or some distance from the cell. (*From DJ Prockop and KI Kivirikko, N Engl J Med 311:376, 1984, with permission.*)

the last amino acids are incorporated into the proα chains, they are released into the cisternae of the rough endoplasmic reticulum. At this stage two proα1(I) and one proα2(I) chains are associated through their C-propeptides. The association of the proα chains is directed by the structure and the surface properties of the globular C-propeptides. After the C-propeptides assemble correctly, the structure is locked in place by the formation of interchain disulfide bonds. Posttranslational modifications of the proα chains continue until each chain acquires about 100 hydroxyproline residues. Then a few of the hydroxyproline-rich -Gly-X-Y- sequences at the C terminus of the protein fold into a triple helix. The short region of triple helix becomes a nucleus for self-assembly of the triple helix of the whole protein, much like a nucleus for crystallization, in that the triple-helical conformation in one -Gly-X-Y- sequence induces the next -Gly-X-Y- sequence to fold into the same conformation. As a result, the conformation is propagated in a zipper-like fashion from the C terminus to the N terminus of the molecule, and the entire α-chain domain becomes a continuous triple helix. The protein then passes from the rough endoplasmic reticulum to other compartments and is secreted. The requirement for ascorbic acid in the hydroxylation of prolyl residues explains why wounds fail to heal in scurvy (see Chap. 79). If sufficient proline residues are not converted to hydroxyproline, collagen cannot fold into a triple helix that is stable at body temperature. The abnormal protein accumulates in the cisternae of the rough endoplasmic reticulum and is slowly degraded.

After secretion, procollagen is processed to collagen by cleavage of the N-propeptides by procollagen N-proteinase and of the C-propeptides by procollagen C-proteinase. The processing of type I procollagen by the two proteinases converts the soluble precursor to type I collagen, whose solubility is less than 1 μg/mL under the same conditions. The 1000-fold decrease in solubility as procollagen is converted to collagen provides the entropic energy that drives the spontaneous self-assembly of the collagen into fibrils, a process that is again similar to crystal formation. Collagen monomers first assemble into a nucleus that grows by addition of monomers as determined by the structure of the nucleus. The initial nucleus for fibril assembly probably involves few molecules and has been difficult to define. However, structures intermediate between the initial nucleus and the final fibrils have pointed and highly symmetrical tips and grow by addition of monomers to the pointed tips. The nucleus, the intermediate structures, and the final fibril can all be assembled spontaneously from a single kind of collagen such as type I or type II, but other fibrils are assembled as copolymers in which two or more collagens are incorporated into the same fibril simultaneously. Alternatively, a second collagen or a proteoglycan can bind to the surface of a growing fibril or to a fully formed fibril and thereby influence the final structure and the functional properties of the fibrils. The final structure of the fibrils in tissues is also influenced by the pressure and tensions on the fibrils, particularly after their tips are inserted into muscle and bone. The tension on tendons, for example, probably makes the initial thin fibrils coalesce into large fiber bundles. The initial self-assembly of collagen into fibrils, however, involves a large number of specific interactions along the surface of each rodlike molecule and therefore can only be altered by molecules that bind either to the surface of the large, rodlike monomer or to the surfaces of the growing fibrils.

Self-assembled collagen fibers have considerable tensile strength, which is increased by cross-linking reactions that form covalent bonds between α chains in one molecule and α chains in adjacent molecules. The first step in cross-linking is oxidation by lysyl oxidase of amino groups on a few lysine or hydroxylysine residues to form aldehydes. The aldehydes then interact to form stable covalent bonds that may or may not involve enzymic reactions.

Collagen fibers in most tissues of normal adults undergo very little metabolic turnover. One exception to this is the collagen fibrils that are degraded and resynthesized as part of the continual remodeling of bone. During growth and development the collagen fibrils in all tissues undergo repeated synthesis, degradation, and resynthesis. The degradation of collagen fibers in tissues is initiated by specific collagenases in leukocytes, fibroblasts, synovial cells, or related cell types.

The collagenases cleave the collagen molecule at a point about three-quarters of the distance from its N terminus. The cleavage apparently triggers unfolding of the molecules on the surface of a fibril and further degradation by other proteinases.

Although the collagen in many adult tissues is metabolically stable, the rate of turnover changes under some circumstances. In starvation, a large fraction of the collagen in skin and other connective tissues is degraded, thus providing amino acids for gluconeogenesis. Large losses of collagen also occur in most connective tissues during immobilization or prolonged periods of low-gravitational stress. In rheumatoid arthritis, pannus invasion causes a rapid degradation of collagen in the articular cartilage, and glucocorticoid excess decreases the collagen content of most connective tissues, including bone, by decreasing the rate of collagen synthesis. Decrease in collagen weakens the tissues. In many pathologic states, however, collagen is deposited in excess. With injury to tissue, inflammation is usually followed by increased deposition primarily of type I collagen fibrils in the form of fibrotic tissue and scars. The deposition of collagen fibrils during the repair process is largely irreversible and is a major feature of the pathologic changes in hepatic cirrhosis, pulmonary fibrosis, atherosclerosis, and nephrosclerosis and in the scarring in skin and ligaments after surgery or trauma.

The biosynthesis of all collagens involves essentially the same steps of assembly and processing. Assembly of nonfibrillar collagens such as the type IV of basement membranes does not, however, involve cleavage of the globular domains at the ends of the protein, since the globular domains are required for the self-assembly of the proteins. Elastin assembly appears to be closely related to that of collagen, since a few of the prolines in the protein are hydroxylated to hydroxyproline by prolyl hydroxylase. The elastin monomer, however, is a single polypeptide that does not fold into a defined three-dimensional structure and is not synthesized as a larger precursor molecule. Instead, it is slowly secreted from cells into extracellular compartments, where it forms amorphous deposits around previously deposited microfibrils. The elastin deposits then become covalently cross-linked through oxidation of lysine residues to aldehydes by the lysyl oxidase that initiates the cross-linking of collagen. The microfibrils in elastin deposits are largely composed of fibrillin, a large protein that forms beadlike strands. The amorphous deposits of elastin and fibrillin also may contain additional components that have not been identified.

The synthesis of proteoglycans begins in the cisternae of the rough endoplasmic reticulum with assembly of a core protein that then undergoes modification by sugar and sulfate transferases that generate large side chains of glycosaminoglycans. At least five proteoglycans have been identified by differences in the structures of their core proteins. The major proteoglycan of cartilage, called *aggrecan*, has a core protein of about 2000 amino acids to which are bound multiple side chains of chondroitin sulfate and keratin sulfate, mucopolysaccharides consisting of highly charged and repetitive disaccharide sequences. After secretion from cells, the aggrecan monomer binds to a smaller protein called a *link protein*. The complex of core protein and link protein then spontaneously binds to a long chain of hyaluronic acid to form a huge copolymer called a *proteoglycan aggregate*. The highly charged proteoglycan aggregate binds water and small ions and thereby provides a large swelling pressure and resiliency to cartilage. Smaller proteoglycans such as decorin, biglycan, and fibromodulin have smaller core proteins with different mucopolysaccharide side chains. They do not form large aggregates with hyaluronate but bind to fibrils of collagen or fibronectin and may thereby help regulate the assembly or spatial orientation of fibrils. One group of small proteoglycans known as *syndecans* binds to the plasma membranes of cells and may have a role in cell migration along fibrils or in signal transduction.

The assembly of bone follows much the same principles as the assembly of other connective tissues (see also Chap. 353). The first step is deposition of osteoid tissue that consists largely of type I collagen fibrils (see Fig. 348-1). Mineralization of osteoid occurs by steps that are still incompletely defined; proteins such as osteopontin and osteocalcin probably bind to the collagen fibrils and chelate calcium to initiate mineralization. Small proteoglycans such as decorin or fibromodulin also may play a role.

MUTATIONS THAT PRODUCE DISEASES OF CONNECTIVE TISSUES Because of the large number of tissue-specific macromolecules present in connective tissues, a large number of gene-protein systems are candidates for mutations that might cause disease. The situation is somewhat simplified by the fact that most of the disease-causing mutations identified to date are in genes that encode collagen or collagen-associated proteins. Therefore, the molecular mechanisms by which the mutations cause their deleterious effects can be related to a single paradigm. However, achondroplasia is caused by mutations in a fibroblast growth factor receptor, and mutations in genes involved in embryonic patterning such as homeo box genes may cause abnormalities of the skeletal system. Therefore, the number of mutant genes that can cause connective tissue diseases is likely to increase.

The most complete data on mutations causing heritable disorders of connective tissue are available on OI. Most patients with severe OI (types II and III) have mutations in either the gene for the proα1(I) chain or the gene for the proα2(I) chain of type I procollagen (the COL1A1 and COL1A2 genes). In patients with mild disease, some of the mutations decrease expression of protein from one allele of the genes. Most of the mutations in patients with severe OI cause synthesis of a structurally abnormal but partially functional proα chain (Figs. 348-2 and 348-3). Mutations that cause synthesis of structurally abnormal proα chains include partial gene deletions, partial gene duplications, and RNA splicing mutations. The most common mutations, however, cause the substitution of single amino acids with bulky side chains for the glycine residues that appear as every third amino acid in the triple helix of a proα chain (Fig. 348-4). The structurally abnormal proα chains exert their effects primarily through one of three mechanisms (see Fig. 348-2). First, the presence of an abnormal proα

FIGURE 348-3 Space-filling model showing a cysteine substitution of glycine α1-748 of type I procollagen (*on the left*) and dark-field light micrographs (*on the right*) of fibrils formed from control type I collagen at 32°C (*A*) and from the mixture of normal and mutated type I collagen containing the same cysteine substitution (*B*). (*From A Vogel et al, J Biol Chem 263:19249, 1988; and KE Kadler et al, Biochemistry 30:5081, 1991, with permission.*)

chain in a procollagen molecule containing two normal proα chains can prevent folding of the protein into a triple-helical conformation and lead to degradation of the whole molecule in a process called *procollagen suicide*. Similar dominant negative mutations are seen with other multisubunit proteins. The net result of procollagen suicide is a reduction in the amount of collagen available for fibril assembly. Second, the presence of one abnormal proα chain in a procollagen molecule can interfere with cleavage of the N-propeptide from the protein. The persistence of the N-propeptide on a fraction of the molecules interferes with the self-assembly of normal collagen so that thin and irregular collagen fibrils are formed. Third, the substitution of a bulkier amino acid for glycine can produce a change in the conformation of the molecule and result in the assembly of collagen fibrils that are abnormally branched (see Fig. 348-3) or abnormally thick and short. Also, copolymerization of the mutated collagen with normal collagen can slow fibril assembly and decrease the total amount of collagen incorporated into fibrils.

There are several reasons why most of the mutations that cause OI are in the type I procollagen genes. One, because collagen fibrils are a principal source of the strength of bone, the structure is weakened by any mutation that reduces the amount or distorts the normal geometry of collagen. The self-assembly of collagen fibrils is easily disrupted when a defective subunit can participate in the assembly process but has the wrong structure. For example, the substitution of a bulky amino acid for a single glycine in one proα chain can interfere with the zipper-like formation of the triple helix and trigger degradation of both the normal and abnormal proα chains. In a similar manner, the presence of a few incompletely processed or flawed collagen monomers can interfere with the self-assembly of normal collagen into fibrils. Hence a mutation at any one of a large number of different sites can either decrease the amount of collagen available for fibril assembly or interfere with the process of fibril assembly so as to markedly decrease the strength of bone and other connective tissues.

Over 150 mutations in the two genes for type I procollagen have been found in patients with OI (see Fig. 348-4). Initially, there was concern

Procollagen suicide

Dendritic fibrils

FIGURE 348-2 Schematic summary of three mechanisms (see text) whereby mutations that cause biosynthesis of structurally abnormal proα1(I) or proα2(I) chains of type I procollagen interfere with either the assembly of the protein (*A*) or its processing to normal collagen fibrils (*B*). (*From DJ Prockop et al, Am J Med Genet 34:60, 1989, with permission.*)

that many of the mutations might be neutral variations in the structure of the genes and not the cause of the disease phenotypes. However, the causal relationship between most of the mutations and the disease has been established by several kinds of evidence: (1) DNA linkage studies in families with mild variants of OI showed that specific mutated alleles were coinherited with the disease phenotypes. (2) Probands with lethal variants of OI were shown to have new mutations not found in the normal parents or in only a few cells from a mosaic parent (see below). (3) Studies with cultured skin fibroblasts from patients demonstrated that the mutations either produced specific disruptions in the biosynthesis of type I procollagen or caused synthesis of a type I procollagen that formed abnormal collagen fibrils (see Fig. 348-2). (4) The mutations in probands with OI were not found in normal alleles for the genes. (5) Expression

FIGURE 348-4 Single-base mutations found in type I procollagen in patients with OI and osteoporosis. Mild refers to type I OI, severe to type II OI, and moderate to type III or type IV OI.

of several of the mutated genes for type I procollagen in transgenic mice generates disease phenotypes similar to those seen in patients who inherited the mutated genes (Fig. 348-5).

The data on mutations in type I procollagen that cause OI have been used as a paradigm for defining other mutations in collagen and procollagen genes that cause other disorders of connective tissue. For example, similar mutations in the gene for type III procollagen occur in patients with the type IV variant of EDS, which causes early death because of rupture of the aorta or other hollow organs (Fig. 348-6). Also, similar mutations in the gene for type II procollagen (COL2A1) are found in about half of patients with the CDs (Fig. 348-7). In addition, transgenic mice expressing mutated genes for type II procollagen develop phenotypes resembling the CDs. Similar mutations in the gene for type VII collagen (COL7A1) are found in patients with the dystrophic form of EB, and mutations in the genes for type IV collagen are found in many patients with AS. As discussed below, the paradigm for defining the consequences of mutations in procollagen genes also helps explain findings on mutations in a fibrillin gene that cause MS and mutations in keratin genes that cause the simplex variant of EB.

Several generalizations can be made about mutations in collagen genes. One is that unrelated patients rarely have the same mutation in the same gene. Another is that mutations that cause the most severe disease are usually new mutations in one allele that occur either during the generation of the germline in one of the parents or during meiosis in the fertilized egg. Still another is that most mild variants are caused by mutations that are specific or "private" to a given family. Indeed, the number of recurrent mutations in structural genes are so infrequent that there are, in effect, no common mutations responsible for the disorders in unrelated patients and no "hot spots" that contain most of the mutations.

Another general trend is that similar mutations in the same gene can produce different disease syndromes in terms of both severity and the major tissues involved. One reason for heterogeneity in pathologic manifestations is that different regions of a large molecule may be more important for its function in some connective tissues than in others. For example, some regions of the type I collagen molecule may be essential for the binding of mineralizing proteins in bone so that mutations in these regions cause fragile bones but do not impair function in skin and other nonmineralizing tissues. It is more difficult, however, to explain how the same mutation can produce a severe phenotype in some and a mild phenotype in other members of the same family. Such phenotypic variation appears to be characteristic of OI, where some subjects are short and have multiple fractures from minor trauma, whereas others in the same family can be of normal stature and free of fractures. In the past, such phenotypic variation

was explained by undefined variations in the genetic background of different family members. Studies in transgenic mice, however, demonstrated similar phenotypic variation with expression of a mutated collagen gene in an inbred strain of mice in whom the genetic background is uniform. Therefore, the phenotypic variation is probably caused by undefined stochastic or chance events during embryonic and fetal development. Although dramatic phenotypic variation is relatively rare in OI and related disorders, it is important to consider in counseling families about the consequences of inherited mutations.

OSTEOGENESIS IMPERFECTA OI is an inherited disorder that causes a generalized decrease in bone mass (osteopenia) and makes the bones brittle. The disorder is frequently associated with blue sclerae, dental abnormalities (dentinogenesis imperfecta), progressive hearing loss, and a positive family history. The most severe forms cause death in utero, at birth, or shortly thereafter. The course of mild and moderate forms is more variable. Some patients appear normal at birth and become progressively worse. Some have multiple fractures in infancy and childhood, improve after puberty, and fracture more frequently later in life. Women are particularly prone to fracture during pregnancy and after menopause. A few women from families with mild variants of OI do not develop fractures until after menopause, and their disease may be difficult to distinguish from postmenopausal osteoporosis.

Classification The most common classification for OI was developed by Sillence (Table 348-2). Type I, the mildest form, is inherited as an autosomal dominant trait. Most patients have distinctly blue

FIGURE 348-5 Similarities of the phenotypes in transgenic mice with mutated type I procollagen and in an OI child. Note in both pictures the waviness of the ribs due to fractures in utero.

FIGURE 348-6 Mutations in the gene for the proα1(III) chain of type III procollagen that cause EDS IV and familial aneurysms.

FIGURE 348-7 Mutations in the gene for the proα1(II) chain of type II procollagen that cause CD and related disorders.

sclerae. Type I is subdivided into types IA and IB depending on whether or not dentinogenesis imperfecta is present. Type II is lethal in utero or shortly after birth. Radiographic criteria can be used to subdivide type II into five groups, with subgroup 1 showing the most severe changes and subgroup 5 the least. Types III and IV OI are intermediate in severity between types I and II. They differ from type I because of lesser severity and because the sclerae are only slightly bluish in infancy and white in adulthood. Type III differs from type IV in that it tends to become more severe with age. Also, type III can be inherited either as an autosomal recessive or autosomal dominant trait, whereas type IV is always dominant. The clinical courses are variable, and the mode of inheritance in types III and IV may be difficult to ascertain because many patients have sporadic mutations and because many couples with one severely affected OI child do not have additional children. For these and related reasons, the distinction between type IV OI and other severe variants of OI may not be helpful. Therefore, it may be sufficient to classify patients simply as mild (type I), lethal (type II), and moderately severe (type III).

Incidence Type I OI has a frequency of about 1 in 30,000. Type II OI has a reported incidence at birth of about 1 in 60,000, but the incidence of the three severe forms recognizable at birth (types II, III, and IV) may be as high as 1 in 20,000.

Skeletal Changes In type I OI, the fragility of bones may be severe enough to limit physical activity or so mild that individuals are unaware of any disability. Radiographs of the skull of patients with mild disease may show a mottled appearance, because of small islands of irregular ossification. In type II OI bones and other connective tissues are so fragile that massive injuries can occur in utero or during delivery (see Fig. 348-5). Ossification of many bones is frequently incomplete. Continuously beaded or broken ribs and crumpled long bones (accordina femora) may be present. For unclear reasons, the long bones may be either thick or thin. In types III and IV, multiple fractures from minor physical stress can produce severe deformities. Kyphoscoliosis can impair respiration, cause cor pulmonale, and predispose to pulmonary infections. The appearance on radiographs of "popcorn-like" deposits of mineral on the ends of long bones is an ominous sign. Progressive neurologic symptoms may result from basilar compression and communicating hydrocephalus.

In all forms of OI, bone mineral density in unfractured bone is decreased.

However, the degree of osteopenia may be difficult to evaluate because recurrent fractures limit exercise and thereby worsen the decrease in bone mass. Surprisingly, fractures appear to heal normally.

Ocular Changes The sclerae can be normal, slightly bluish, or bright blue. The color is probably caused by a thinness of the collagen layers of the sclerae that allows the choroid layers to be seen. Blue sclerae, however, are an inherited trait in some families who do not have increased bone fragility.

Dentinogenesis Imperfecta The teeth may be normal, moderately discolored, or grossly abnormal. The enamel generally appears normal, but the teeth may have a characteristic amber, yellowish brown, or translucent bluish gray color because of improper deposition or deficiency of dentin. The deciduous teeth are usually smaller than normal, whereas permanent teeth are frequently bell-shaped and restricted at the base. In some patients, the teeth readily fracture and need to be extracted. The defect in dentin is directly attributable to the fact that normal dentin is rich in type I collagen. Similar tooth defects, however, can occur without any evidence of OI.

Hearing Loss Hearing loss usually begins during the second decade of life and occurs in 90 percent of subjects over age 30. The loss can be conductive, sensorineural, or mixed and varies in severity. The middle ear usually exhibits maldevelopment, deficient ossification, persistence of cartilage in areas that are normally ossified, and abnormal calcium deposits.

Associated Features Other connective tissue involvement can include thin skin that scars extensively, joint laxity with permanent

Table 348-2

Classification of Osteogenesis Imperfecta (OI)

Type	Bone Fragility	Blue Sclerae	Abnormal Dentition	Hearing Loss	Inheritance*
I	Mild	Present	Absent in IA, present in IB	Present in most	AD
II	Extreme	Present	Present in some	Unknown	S, rarely AR
III	Severe	Bluish at birth	Present in some	High incidence	AR or AD
IV	Variable	Absent	Absent in IVA, present in IVB	High incidence	AD

* AD, autosomal dominant; AR, autosomal recessive; S, sporadic.

dislocations indistinguishable from those of EDS, and, occasionally, cardiovascular manifestations such as aortic regurgitation, floppy mitral valves, mitral incompetence, and fragility of large blood vessels. For unknown reasons, some patients develop a hypermetabolic state with elevated serum thyroxine levels, hyperthermia, and excessive sweating.

Molecular Defects Most patients with OI have mutations in one of the two genes that encode type I procollagen. A third or more of the patients with type I OI have as yet undefined mutations in the proα1(I) gene that decrease the steady-state levels of the mRNA for proα1(I) chains and decrease the rates of synthesis of proα1(I) chains relative to those for proα2(I) chains. In more severe forms (types II, III, and IV), the effects of mutations that cause synthesis of abnormal proα chains are amplified by the three mechanisms discussed above (see Fig. 348-2). Mutations that change the structure of the protein near the N-proteinase cleavage site cause accumulation of a partially processed procollagen and produce lax joints similar to those in type VII EDS. Mutations that change the structure in the middle or near the C terminus of the molecule tend to cause severe or lethal variants of OI. It is difficult, however, to correlate the site or nature of the mutation and the clinical phenotype (see Fig. 348-4). Rare patients are homozygotes with two mutated alleles for proα1(I) or proα2(I) chains.

Mosaicism in Germ Line Cells and in Somatic Cells Most lethal OI is the result of new autosomal dominant mutations. The frequency of a second child with lethal OI in the same family, however, is about 7 percent because of germ line mosaicism in one of the parents. The presence of germ line mosaicism has been demonstrated in several fathers of patients with type II OI by demonstrating the mutated gene in a fraction of their sperm. Apparently normal parents of children with severe OI also may have somatic cell mosaicism in which the mutated allele is present in a fraction of somatic cells such as fibroblasts, leukocytes, and hair root cells. Because of the possibility of germ line mosaicism, asymptomatic parents of a child with severe OI should be counseled that recurrence can occur.

Diagnosis The diagnosis is usually made on the basis of clinical criteria. The presence of fractures together with blue sclerae, dentinogenesis imperfecta, or family history of the disease is usually sufficient to make the diagnosis. Other causes of pathologic fractures must be excluded, including the battered child syndrome, nutritional deficiencies, malignancies, and other inherited disorders such as CDs and hypophosphatasia (Table 348-3). X-rays usually reveal a decrease in bone density that can be verified by photon or x-ray absorptiometry. There is no consensus, however, as to whether the diagnosis can be made by microscopy of bone. With research procedures, a molecular defect in type I procollagen can be demonstrated in half or more of patients by incubating skin fibroblasts with radioactive amino acids and then analyzing the proα chains by polyacrylamide gel electrophoresis. The analysis detects decreases in the rate of synthesis of proα1(I) chains relative to proα2(I) chains, abnormally long proα chains, abnormally short proα chains, and proα chains with abnormal posttranslational modification because of an amino acid substitution that impairs folding of the triple helix. The mutations themselves can be defined in most patients by sequencing of cDNA or genomic DNA. Because each proband and family usually has a "private" mutation, extensive analysis of 5000 or more bases in each of the two genes is required to identify the exact mutation. After a mutation in a type I procollagen gene is identified, a test based on the polymerase chain reaction can be used to screen family members at risk and for prenatal diagnosis.

℞ TREATMENT

Treatment is ineffective, but many subjects have successful careers despite severe deformities. Those with mild disorder may need little treatment when fractures decrease after puberty, but women require special attention during pregnancy and after menopause, when fractures again increase. More severely affected children require a comprehensive program of physical therapy, surgical management of fractures and skeletal deformities, and vocational education.

Many of the fractures are only slightly displaced and have little soft tissue swelling. Therefore, they can be treated with minimal support or traction for a week or two followed by a light cast. If fractures are relatively painless, physical therapy can be initiated early. A judicious amount of exercise prevents loss of bone mass secondary to physical inactivity. Some physicians advocate insertion of steel rods into long bones to correct limb deformities; the risk/benefits and cost/benefits of such procedures are difficult to evaluate. Aggressive conventional intervention is usually warranted for pneumonia and cor pulmonale. For severe hearing loss, stapedectomy or replacement of the stapes with a prosthesis may be successful. Moderately to severely affected patients should be evaluated periodically to anticipate possible neurologic problems. About half of children have a substantial increase in growth when given growth hormone. Treatment with bisphosphorates to decrease bone loss has been discussed, but no controlled studies have been reported.

A program for careful orthotic management developed by Bleck and a program for compressive management developed by Marini are useful. Counseling and emotional support is important for patients and parents, and lay organizations in some countries provide help in these areas. Prenatal ultrasonography will detect severely affected fetuses at about 16 weeks of pregnancy. Diagnosis by demonstrating synthesis of abnormal proα chains or by DNA sequencing can be carried out in chorionic villa biopsies at 8 to 12 weeks of pregnancy.

EHLERS-DANLOS SYNDROME EDS is characterized by hyperelasticity of the skin and hypermobile joints (Fig. 348-8).

Classification Beighton initially identified five types of EDS based primarily on the extent to which the skin, joints, and other tissues are involved, but the classification has now been extended (Table 348-4). Type I is the classic, severe form of the disease, with both severe joint hypermobility and skin that is velvety in texture, hyperextensible, and easily scarred. Type II is similar to type I but milder. In type III joint hypermobility is more prominent than skin changes, and the skin changes in type IV are more prominent than joint changes. However, type IV patients are predisposed to sudden death from rupture of large blood vessels or the large bowel. Type V is similar to type II but is inherited as an X-linked trait. Type VI is characterized by scoliosis, ocular fragility, and a cone-shaped deformity of the cornea (keratoconus). Type VII is characterized by marked joint hypermobility that is difficult to distinguish from type III except by the specific molecular defects in the processing of type I procollagen to collagen. Type VIII is distinguished by periodontal changes. Types IX, X, and XI were defined on the basis of preliminary biochemical

Table 348-3

Differential Diagnosis of OI

Age	Diagnosis	Distinguishing Features
At birth	Hypophosphatasia	Unmineralized skull
	Achondrogenesis	Unmineralized vertebrae
	Thanatophoric dwarfism	H-shaped vertebrae
	Asphyxiating thoracic dystrophy	Cylindrical thorax
	Achondroplasia	Large head, short, tubular bones
Infancy	Battered child syndrome	Skull and rib fractures more common
	Immobilization osteogenesis	
	Scurvy	
	Congenital syphilis	
Childhood	Homocystinuria	Marfanoid appearance and mental deficiency
	Celiac disease	Steatorrhea, anemia
	Adrenal cortical tumor	
	Glucocorticoid therapy	

SOURCE: After R Smith et al, *The Brittle Bone Syndrome: Osteogenesis Imperfecta*, London, Butterworth, 1983, p 128.

FIGURE 348-8 Schematic representation of the skin and joint changes in EDS. Girl in upper right has type VII EDS with dislocations of both hips that were not correctable by surgery. *[From DJ Prockop and NA Guzman, Hosp Pract 12(12):61, 1977, with permission.]*

and clinical data, but these classifications have not proven useful. Because of overlapping signs and symptoms, many patients and families cannot be assigned to any of the defined types.

Incidence The incidence of EDS is difficult to establish, largely because patients with mild skin or joint symptoms rarely seek medical attention. It is also difficult to define the normal range of variation for joint mobility or skin elasticity. The incidence may be about 1 in 5000 births, although a higher value has been reported for blacks. Types I, II, and III account for most diagnoses.

Skin The changes vary from thin and velvety skin to skin that is either dramatically hyperextensible ("rubber man" syndrome) or easily torn or scarred. Type I patients develop characteristic "cigarette-paper" scars. In type IV extensive scars and hyperpigmentation develop over bony prominences, and the skin may be so thin that subcutaneous blood vessels are visible. In type VIII the skin is more fragile than

hyperextensible, and it heals with atrophic, pigmented scars. Easy bruisability occurs in several types of EDS.

Ligament and Joint Changes Laxity and hypermobility of joints vary from mild to unreducible dislocations of hips and other large joints. In mild forms patients learn to reduce dislocations themselves and to avoid them by limiting physical activity. In more severe forms, surgical repair may be required. Some patients have progressive difficulty with age, but severe joint laxity is compatible with a normal life span.

Associated Changes Mitral valve prolapse and hernias occur, particularly in type I. Pes planus and mild to moderate scoliosis are common. Extreme joint laxity and repeated dislocations may lead to degenerative arthritis. In type VI the eye may rupture with minimal trauma, and kyphoscoliosis can cause respiratory impairment. Sclerae may be blue in type VI.

Molecular Defects The molecular defects in most patients with the type I, II, and III forms of EDS are unknown, but the responsible gene has been identified in three families. In one there is a mutation in the COL5A1 gene for the $\alpha1(V)$ chain of type V collagen, a collagen found in small amounts in association with type I collagen. Linkage to the same gene was present in a second family with type II EDS, but mutation in this gene has been excluded in other families with types I or II EDS. One type III EDS family had a mutation in the COL3A1 gene that caused replacement of an obligate glycine in type III procollagen. Electron microscopy of skin from some patients with types I, II, or III EDS are consistent with mutations in a low-abundance collagen such as types III or V that either copolymerize with or bind to the surface of type I fibrils. However, irregular fibrils are not seen in all patients, and similar irregular fibrils can be seen in normal skin.

Most patients with type IV EDS have a defect either in the synthesis or structure of type III procollagen, a finding consistent with the fact that these patients are prone to spontaneous rupture of the aorta and intestines, tissues rich in type III collagen. The thinness and scarring of skin are more difficult to explain, since type III constitutes a small fraction of the collagen in skin (see Table 348-1). The more than 50 mutations identified in the type III procollagen gene include partial gene deletions, RNA splicing mutations, and single-base mutations that cause substitution of amino acids with bulkier side chains for glycine (see Fig. 348-6). In brief, most of the mutations lead to synthesis of abnormal but partially functional pro$\alpha1(III)$ chains that produce procollagen suicide or alter fibril formation by the same mechanisms that amplify the effects of mutations in the genes for type I procollagen. Similar mutations in type III procollagen can cause aortic aneurysms in some individuals without other evidence of EDS type IV, MS, or other inherited disorders of connective tissue.

Type VI EDS is caused by a deficiency of lysyl hydroxylase. Mutations in the gene for this enzyme have been defined in several patients. One was a compound heterozygote, and two probands were homozygotes for the same large deletion and rearrangement of the gene; the mutations in the four alleles from these two patients were identical even though the parents were not thought to be related. Both types of mutation caused profound deficiency of lysyl hydroxylase, a decrease in the hydroxylysine content of collagen, and a decrease in the cross-links in collagen fibers.

Type VII EDS is due to a defect in the conversion of procollagen to collagen caused either by mutations that make type I procollagen resistant to cleavage by procollagen N-proteinase or by mutations that decrease the activity of the enzyme. The type VIIA mutations alter the cleavage site in the pro$\alpha1(I)$ chain, and the type VIIB mutations alter the cleavage site in the pro$\alpha2(I)$ chain. Both types are dominantly inherited. Type VIIC is caused by mutations that decrease the activity of procollagen N-proteinase and is inherited as an autosomal recessive trait. In all three forms of type VII EDS, the persistence of the N-propeptide causes the formation of collagen fibrils that are thin and irregular. Since most patients do not have clinical osteopenia, the thin and irregular fibrils apparently suffice for the mineralization of bone but do not provide the necessary tensile strength for ligaments and joint capsules.

The cause of type VIII EDS is unknown. Type IX is a disorder of copper transport. The syndrome, also referred to as *Menkes' syn-*

drome, is due to an X-linked defect and is associated with cutis laxa, hypopigmentation, unusual hair ("kinky"), vascular aneurysms, neurologic degeneration, and mental retardation. Mutations in a gene coding for a copper-transporting ATPase cause the disease. Type X EDS may be caused by defects in fibronectin, but no specific mutations have been defined. (See also Chaps. 80 and 350.)

Diagnosis The diagnosis is based on clinical criteria. Biochemical assays and gene analyses for known molecular defects in EDS are difficult and time-consuming, but specific diagnostic tests should be available in the future for families in which the mutations have been defined.

℞ **TREATMENT**

There is no specific therapy. Surgical repair and tightening of joint ligaments require careful evaluation of individual patients, since the ligaments frequently do not hold sutures. Patients with easy bruisability should be evaluated for other bleeding disorders. Patients with type IV EDS and members of their families probably should be evaluated at regular intervals by sonography and related techniques for early detection of aneurysms. Surgical repair of aneurysms may be difficult because of increased friability of tissues, and there is limited experience with elective surgery in such patients. Also, women with type IV EDS should be counseled about the increased risk of uterine rupture, bleeding, and other complications of pregnancy.

CHONDRODYSPLASIAS The chondrodysplasias are inherited skeletal disorders that cause dwarfism and abnormal body proportions. The category also includes some individuals with normal stature and body proportions who have features such as typical ocular changes or cleft palate that are common in more severe CDs. Many patients develop degenerative joint changes, and mild CD in adults may be difficult to differentiate from primary generalized osteoarthritis. Some authors refer to the disorders as "skeletal dysplasias," but CD is a more widely used term.

Classification Over 150 distinct types and 8 major subtypes have been defined (Table 348-5) based on criteria such as "bringing death" (thanatophoric), causing "twisted" bones (diastrophic), affecting metaphyses (metaphyseal), affecting epiphyses (epiphyseal), and producing histologic changes such as an apparent increase in the fibrous material in the epiphyses (fibrochondrogenesis). Also, a number of eponyms are based on the first or most comprehensive case reports. Severe forms of the diseases produce gross distortions of most cartilaginous structures and of the eye (see Table 348-1). Mild forms are more difficult to classify. Among the features are cataracts, degeneration of the vitreous and retinal detachment, high forehead, hypoplastic facies, cleft palate, short and thin extremities, and gross distortions of the epiphyses, metaphyses, and joint surfaces.

Incidence Data on the frequency of most CDs are not available, but the incidence of the Stickler syndrome may be as high as 1 in 10,000. Therefore, the diseases are probably among the more common heritable disorders of connective tissue.

Molecular Defects The first mutations shown to cause CDs were in the COL2A1 gene for type II collagen, the most abundant protein in cartilage. Over

40 mutations in this gene have now been reported in variants of CD ranging from mild to lethal (Fig. 348-7). About 20 percent of patients with severe or moderate CD and about 2 percent of families with early-onset generalized osteoarthritis have mutations in the same gene. However, similar phenotypes can also be caused by mutations in other genes, including genes for three other collagens, additional components of the cartilage matrix, growth factors, growth factor receptors, and transcription factors (Table 348-6). The number of mutated genes reported does not necessarily reflect the incidence of such mutations in the diseases themselves but rather the complexity of the genes and the technical difficulties in searching the complete gene for mutations. Also, it reflects the availability of large families for DNA linkage analysis and the vigor with which investigators have pursued their interest in a given gene. It is likely that mutations in additional genes will be found.

Most of the 40 or so mutations identified in the COL2A1 gene are in patients with severe CD and cause gross deformities of bones and cartilage such as hypochondrogenesis/achondrogenesis II and the Kniest syndrome. However, mutations in the COL2A1 gene have been found in a few families in which few if any symptoms are present in childhood but in which joint stiffness, joint pain, and degenerative changes of osteoarthritis develop in midlife. The mutations in the COL2A1 gene are similar to the mutations in the genes for types I and III procollagens (Fig. 348-7), and the correlations between genotype and phenotype are equally difficult. However, the first four mutations identified to cause premature termination signals for a collagen gene were in the COL2A1 gene and were in patients with the Stickler syndrome. In addition, mutations that change a codon for a Y-position amino acid in the -Gly-X-Y- repeat sequence from an arginine to

Table 348-4

Clinical Features, Mode of Inheritance, and Biochemical Defects in EDS

Type	Clinical Features	Inheritance*	Biochemical Defect
I, gravis	Soft, velvety, hyperextensible skin; easy bruising; "cigarette paper" scars; hypermobile joints; varicose veins; prematurity	AD	Some in type V collagen
II, mitis	Similar to EDS type I but less severe	AD	Some in type I collagen
III, familial hypermobility	Soft skin, no scarring, marked hypermobility	AD	Some in type II procollagen
IV, acrogeric, ecchymotic, vascular	Thin, translucent skin with visible veins; increased bruisability, skin and joints have normal extensibility; arterial, bowel, and uterine rupture	AD	Mutations in type III procollagen (see Fig. 348-6)
V, X-linked	Similar to EDS type II	XLR	Not known
VI, ocular-scoliotic	Soft, velvety, hyperextensible skin; hypermobile joints; scoliosis; ocular fragility and keratoconus	AR	Lysyl hydroxylase deficiency
VII, arthrochalasis multiplex congenita	Marked joint hypermobility, soft skin with normal scarring	AD	A. Structural defect in the proα1(I) chain
		AD	B. Structural defect in the proα2(I) chain
		AR	C. Procollagen *N*-proteinase deficiency
VIII, periodontal	Generalized periodontitis, skin similar to EDS type II	AD	Not known
IX, cutis laxa occipital horn syndrome	Vacant, now recategorized as a disorder of copper transport		
X	Similar to EDS type II	AR	Possible defect in fibronectin
XI, familial joint instability	Vacant, now recategorized with familial articular hypermobility syndromes		

* AD, autosomal dominant; AR, autosomal recessive; XLR, X-linked recessive.

SOURCE: After PH Byers, in *Clinical Medicine*, Philadelphia, Harper & Row, 1983, p. 1; and P Beighton et al, Am J Med Genet 29:581, 1988.

Table 348-5

Classifications of Chondrodysplasias

Achondrodysplasia family
    Achondroplasia
    Hypochondroplasia
    Thanatophoric dysplasia
Spondyloepiphyseal dysplasia (SED) family
    Achondrogenesis type IA
    Achondrogenesis type IB
    Achondrogenesis type II
    Hypochondrogenesis
    SED congenita
    Strudwick syndrome
    Stickler syndrome
    Kniest dysplasia
Chondrodysplasia punctata family
    Rhizomelic chondrodysplasia punctata
    Conradi-Hünermann disease
    X-linked dominant chondrodysplasia punctata
    Chondrodysplasia punctata associated with Xp
Short rib (-polydactyly) family
    Ellis–van Creveld syndrome
    Asphyxiating thoracic dysplasia
    Short rib–polydactyly syndrome type I
    Short rib–polydactyly syndrome type II
Metatropic dysplasia family
    Metatropic dysplasia
    Metatropic-like dysplasia
Metaphyseal chondrodysplasia family
    Metaphyseal chondrodysplasia, Jansen type
    Metaphyseal chondrodysplasia, Schmid type
    Metaphyseal chondrodysplasia, McKusick type
Brachyolmia family
    Brachyolmia, Hobaek type
    Brachyolmia, Maroteaux type
    Brachyolmia, autosomal dominant type
Acromelic dysplasia family
    Peripheral dysostosis
    Achodysplasia
    Trichorhinophalangeal syndrome type I
    Trichorhinophalangeal syndrome type II

SOURCE: After J Spranger, Eur J Pediatr 151:407, 1992; WA Horton and JT Hecht.

cystine were found in families with early-onset osteoarthritis and minimal evidence of CDs.

Many individuals with the Schmid metaphyseal CD, characterized by short stature, *coxa vara*, flaring metaphyses, and waddling gait, have mutations in the gene for the type X collagen, a short, network-forming collagen found primarily in the hypertrophic zone of endochondral cartilage. A few patients with the nonocular variants of the Stickler syndrome have mutations in the gene for the α2(XI) chain of type XI collagen, a low-abundance collagen in cartilage and other tissues.

Mutations in the receptor for fibroblast growth factor (FGFR) 3 are present in most patients with achondroplasia, the most common cause of short-limbed dwarfism accompanied by macrocephaly and dysplasias of the metaphyses of long bones. The same single-base mutation in the gene that converts glycine to arginine at position 380 is present in more than 90 percent of patients. Most patients represent sporadic new mutations, and this nucleotide change must be one of the most common recurring mutations in the human genome. The mutation causes unregulated signal transduction through the receptor and inappropriate development of cartilage. Mutations that alter other domains of FGFR-3 have been found in patients with the more severe disorders hypochondroplasia and thanatophoric dysplasia and in a few families with a variant of craniosynostosis. However, most patients with craniosynostosis appear to have mutations in the related gene FGFR-2.

Mutations in the gene for the cartilage oligomeric matrix protein (COMP) have been found in patients with multiple epiphyseal dysplasia or pseudoachondroplasia, related syndromes characterized by short limbs and degenerative arthritis. However, one family with multiple epiphyseal dysplasia had a mutation in the gene for the α2(IX) chain of type IX collagen (COL9A1).

Diagnosis   The diagnosis of severe forms of CD is made on the basis of analysis of the physical appearance, x-ray findings, histologic changes, and clinical course (Table 348-5).

Ⓡ TREATMENT

No definitive therapy is available. Symptomatic treatment is directed to secondary features such as degenerative arthritis. Many patients require joint replacement surgery and corrective surgery for cleft palates. The eyes should be monitored carefully for the development of cataracts and for the need for laser therapy to prevent retinal detachment. Patients probably should be advised to avoid obesity and contact sports. Counseling for the psychological problems of short stature is critical, and support groups have formed in many countries. Ultrasonography is sometimes successful for prenatal diagnosis but less frequently than with OI. Specific tests should be available in the future for the CDs caused by mutations in the COL2A1 gene.

MARFAN SYNDROME   Severe MS is characterized by a triad of features: (1) long, thin extremities frequently associated with other skeletal changes; (2) reduced vision as the result of dislocations of the lenses (ectopia lentis); and (3) aortic aneurysms that typically begin at the base of the aorta. Mild forms of the disorder, particularly those with only the skeletal changes, are difficult to classify.

Classification   The severe form is usually caused by a mutation in a single allele of the fibrillin gene (FBN1). At the same time, MS must be distinguished from related syndromes: (1) homocystinuria, which can cause ectopia lentis and the same skeletal changes as MS; (2) congenital contractural arachnodactyly that causes similar skeletal changes but none of the other features of MS and is caused by mutations in a related fibrillin gene (FBN2); (3) familial ectopia lentis not associated with other features of MS; and (4) familial aortic aneurysms that result from a more common autosomal dominant disorder not associated with other features of MS, type IV EDS, or other known disorders of connective tissue.

Incidence and Inheritance   MS has an incidence of about 1 in 10,000 in most racial and ethnic groups. The disorder is inherited as an autosomal dominant trait; at least one-fourth of patients do not have an affected parent, and their cases are probably due to new mutations.

Skeletal Changes   Patients are usually tall compared with other members of the same family and have long limbs. The ratio of the upper segment (top of the head to top of the pubic ramus) to the lower segment (top of the pubic ramus to the floor) is usually 2 standard deviations below mean for age, race, and sex. The fingers and hands are long and slender and have a spider-like appearance (arachnodactyly). Many patients have severe chest deformities, including depression (pectus excavatum), protrusion (pectus carinatum), or asymmetry. Scoliosis is usually accompanied by kyphosis. High-arched palate and high pedal arches or pes planus are common. A few patients have joint hypermobility similar to that in mild EDS, but joint mobility is usually normal.

Cardiovascular Changes   Cardiovascular abnormalities are the major source of morbidity and mortality. Mitral valve prolapse develops early in life and in about one-quarter progresses to mitral valve regurgitation of increasing severity because of redundancy of the leaflets, stretching of the chordae tendineae, and dilatation of the valvulae annulus. Dilatation of the root of the aorta and the sinuses of Valsalva may be detected by echocardiography in utero. The rate of dilatation is unpredictable, but the dilatation can cause aortic regurgitation, dissection of the aorta, and rupture. Dilatation is probably accelerated by physical and emotional stress, as well as by pregnancy.

Ocular Changes   The dislocation of the lens may be readily apparent, but diagnosis usually requires pupillary dilatation and slit-lamp examination. The displacement is usually not progressive but may contribute to the formation of cataracts. The ocular globe is frequently elongated, most patients are myopic, and some develop retinal detachment. A few patients have lattice degeneration and retinal tears; most have adequate vision.

Associated Changes Striae may occur over the shoulders and buttocks. Otherwise the skin is normal. A number of patients develop spontaneous pneumothorax. Inguinal and incisional hernias are common. Marked dilatation of the dural sac is seen frequently in computed tomography scans, but the condition is usually asymptomatic. Patients are typically thin with little subcutaneous fat, but adults may develop centripetal obesity.

Molecular Defects Most patients with the classic features of MS are heterozygotes for mutations in a gene on chromosome 15 that encodes fibrillin, a glycoprotein of 350 kDa that is a major component of elastin-associated microfibrils. These microfibrils are abundant in large blood vessels and the suspensory ligaments of the lens. About one-third of the mutations cause premature termination of translation, and most of the remainder cause single amino acid substitutions in the epidermal growth factor–like domains of the molecule that may be involved in calcium binding. The function of fibrillin has not been defined, but the data suggest that fibrillin self-assembles into a fibrillar structure and that the conformation and surface properties of the entire molecule are critical for normal assembly. Therefore, the functional consequences of mutations that change the amino acid sequence of fibrillin may be similar to the effects of mutations that change the conformation of a fibrillar collagen (see Figs. 348-2, 348-4, 348-6, and 348-7). DNA linkage studies indicate that the gene that causes familial ectopia lentis without any other signs of MS is also located on chromosome 15, but it is unclear whether the gene is identical with FBN1. Several families with a Marfan-related syndrome characterized by congenital contractural arachnodactyly demonstrate linkage to a second fibrillin gene located on chromosome 5 (FBN2). A third fibrillin gene (FBN3) is present on chromosome 17, but no defect has yet been linked to the gene. Also, two patients with atypical forms of MS have defects in the proα2(I) chain of type I procollagen.

Diagnosis The diagnosis is easily established if the patient and other members of the family have dislocated lenses, aortic dilatation, and long and thin extremities together with kyphoscoliosis or other chest deformities. The diagnosis is frequently made if ectopia lentis and an aneurysm of the ascending aorta occur in the absence of a Marfan habitus or a positive family history. All patients in whom the diagnosis is suspected should have a slit-lamp examination and an echocardiogram. Also, homocystinuria (see Table 348-3) should be ruled out by a negative cyanide-nitroprusside test for disulfides in the urine. A few patients with types I, II, and III EDS have ectopia lentis but lack the Marfan habitus and instead have characteristic skin changes not present in MS. Patients with familial aortic aneurysms tend to develop aneurysms at the base of the abdominal aorta. The location of the aneurysms, however, is variable, and the high incidence of aortic aneurysms (1 in 100) makes the differential diagnosis difficult unless other features of MS are clearly present. A few families with familial aortic aneurysms have mutations in the gene for type III procollagen (see Fig. 348-6).

℞ **TREATMENT**

There is no established treatment, but several investigators have recommended use of propranolol or other beta-adrenergic blocking agents to delay or prevent aortic dilatation. Surgical replacement of the aorta, aortic valve, and mitral valve has been successful in some patients, and all patients should be followed carefully with echocardiography and other techniques for evaluation of cardiovascular changes. Patients probably should be advised of the risks of severe physical and emotional stress and of pregnancy.

The scoliosis tends to be progressive and should be treated by mechanical bracing and physical therapy if greater than 20 degrees or by surgery if it progresses to greater than 45 degrees. Estrogen has been tried in girls with scoliosis, but the results are inconclusive. Dislocated lenses rarely require surgical removal, but patients should be followed closely for retinal detachment. Pyeritz has summarized current protocols for the management of patients.

Diagnostic tests based on detection of fibrillin defects in cultured skin fibroblasts or DNA analysis of the gene may be available in the near future.

EPIDERMOLYSIS BULLOSA Epidermolysis bullosa (EB) is the name given to a group of disorders in which the skin and related epithelial tissues break and blister as the result of minor trauma. As with most heritable disorders of connective tissues, the clinical manifestations range from lethal to mild disorders.

Classification Three categories are defined on the basis of the level at which blistering occurs: EB simplex for blistering in the epidermis, EB junctional for blistering in the dermal-epidermal junction, and EB dystrophica for blistering in the dermis. More than 20 subtypes have been separated on the basis of the clinical findings together with ultrastructural and immunohistologic changes in skin.

Incidence The incidence of EB in the United States is estimated to be 1 in 50,000.

Molecular Defects The molecular basis of several specific variants of EB has been defined. Some of the first information came from experiments with transgenic mice in which mice expressing a gene for a truncated keratin (keratin 14) developed intraepidermal blistering similar to that seen in patients with EB simplex. Subsequently, a series of patients with EB simplex were found to have mutations in either keratin 14 or keratin 5, two of the major keratins in basal epithelial cells. Patients with the related syndrome, epidermolytic icthyosis, have mutations in keratin 1 and keratin 10. Some patients with the more severe dystrophic EB have mutations in type VII collagen (COL7A1),

Table 348-6

Reported Gene Mutations in Chondrodysplasias*

Disease	Mutated Gene (Number Reported)					
	COL2A1	COL9A2	COL10A1	COL11A2	FGFR-3	COMP
Achondrodysplasia family						
Achondrodysplasia					>250	
Hypochondroplasia					3	
Thanatophoric dysplasia					9	
SED family						
Achondrogenesis II/ hypochondrogenesis	13					
SED congenita	11					
Stickler syndrome						
Classic	6					
Nonocular				2		
Kniest dysplasia	5					
Metaphyseal CD family						
Schmid type			17			
Multiple epiphyseal dysplasia or pseudo-chondroplasia		1				23
Osteoarthritis with mild CD	3					

* Additional mutations reported: A series of patients with craniosynostoses (Crouzon, Apert, Jackson-Weiss, and Pfeiffer syndromes) had mutations in the FGFR-2 gene, but three families with the Crouzon syndrome and acanthosis nigricans had mutations in the FGFR-3 gene.

NOTE: FGFR, fibroblast growth factor; COMP, cartilage oligomeric matrix protein; SED, spondyloepiphyseal dysplasia.

the collagen that forms strandlike fibrils that anchor the basal lamina to the type I collagen and other collagens of the dermis. Patients with junctional EB have mutations in the gene for laminin 5, one of a family of large, cross-shaped proteins in basal membranes.

Diagnosis   The diagnosis is based on skin that readily breaks and forms blisters. EB simplex, which affects only the epidermis, is generally milder than EB junctional or EB dystrophica. EB dystrophica variants usually cause large and prominent scars. Classification within subtypes usually requires electron microscopy.

℞ TREATMENT

The treatment is symptomatic. Bruckner-Tuderman has reviewed the diagnostic criteria and management.

ALPORT SYNDROME (See also Chap. 275)   AS is an inherited disorder characterized by hematuria. Four forms of the disease are now recognized: (1) classic AS, which is inherited as an X-linked disorder with hematuria, sensorineural deafness, and conical deformation of the anterior surface of the lens (lenticonus); (2) a second X-linked form associated with diffuse leiomyomatosis; (3) an autosomal recessive form; and (4) an autosomal dominant form. The two autosomal forms can cause renal disease without deafness or lenticonus.

Incidence   The incidence of AS is about 1 in 10,000 in the general population and as high as 1 in 5000 in some ethnic groups.

Molecular Defects   Electron microscopy of kidneys from patients with classic AS demonstrated that the glomerular basement membrane was up to five times thicker than normal and that the lamina densa was distorted and split. The X-linked and autosomal recessive forms are caused primarily by mutations in genes for the $\alpha2(IV)$, $\alpha4(IV)$, $\alpha5(IV)$, or $\alpha6(IV)$ chains of type IV collagen, a major component of basement membranes. The type IV collagen in most membranes consists primarily of $\alpha1(IV)$ and $\alpha2(IV)$ chains folded into a large, rodlike molecule with globular ends and a long triple-helical domain that is interrupted by short sequences that do not form triple helices. The molecules self-assemble through both the globular ends and the long triple-helical domain to form a complex three-dimensional network. The four additional α chains of type IV collagen are similar in structure and are probably incorporated into the same or similar molecules. The six genes for the proteins are arranged in tandem pairs on different chromosomes in a head-to-head orientation and with overlapping promoters, i.e., the $\alpha1(IV)$ and $\alpha2(IV)$ genes are head-to-head on chromosome 13q34, the $\alpha3(IV)$ and $\alpha4(IV)$ genes are on chromosome 2q35-37, and the $\alpha5(IV)$ and $\alpha6(IV)$ genes are on chromosome Xq22. An X-linked variant is caused by mutations in the COL4A6 gene, and the X-linked variant associated with leiomyomatosis is caused by deletions that involve both the COL4A5 gene and the nearby COL4A6 gene. The autosomal recessive variants are caused by mutations in either the COL4A3 or COL4A4 genes, and the mutations responsible for the autosomal dominant variants are still unknown.

Diagnosis   The diagnosis of classic AS is based on X-linked inheritance of hematuria, sensorineural deafness, and lenticonus. Because of the X-linked transmission, women are usually less severely affected than men and are generally underdiagnosed. The hematuria progresses to nephritis and may cause renal failure in late adolescence in affected males and at older ages in some women. The sensorineural deafness is primarily in the high-tone range. It frequently can be detected only by an audiogram and usually is not progressive. The lenticonus rarely occurs without nephritis and is considered to be pathognomonic of classic AS.

℞ TREATMENT

There is no known treatment.

BIBLIOGRAPHY

BRUCKNER-TUDERMAN L: Epidermolysis bullosa, in *Connective Tissue and Its Heritable Disorders*, PM Royce, B Steinmann (eds). New York, Wiley-Liss, 1993, p 507

BYERS PH: Osteogenesis imperfecta, in *Connective Tissue and Its Heritable Disorders*, PM Royce, B Steinmann (eds). New York, Wiley-Liss, 1993, p 317

CHRISTIANO AM, UITTO J: Molecular complexity of the cutaneous basement membrane zone. Revelations from the paradigms of epidermolysis bullosa. Exp Dermatol 5:1, 1996

DIETZ HC, PYERITZ RE: Mutations in the human gene for fibrillin-1 (FBN1) in the Marfan syndrome and related disorders. Hum Mol Genet 4:1799, 1995

FLINTER FA et al: Genetics of classic Alport's syndrome. Lancet 2:1005, 1988

HORTON WA, HECHT JT: The chondrodysplasias, in *Connective Tissue and Its Heritable Disorders*, PM Royce, B Steinmann (eds). New York, Wiley-Liss, 1993, p 641

KASHTAN CE: Clinical and molecular diagnosis of Alport syndrome. Proc Assoc Am Physicians 107:306, 1995

KUIVANIEMI H et al: Mutations in the fibrillar collagens (types I, II, III, IX and XI), and fibril-associated collagen, and the network-forming collagen (type X) cause a spectrum of diseases of bone, cartilage and blood vessels. Hum Mutat, 1997

MARINI JC: Osteogenesis imperfecta. Comprehensive management. Adv Pediatr 35:391, 1988

———— et al: Evaluation of growth hormone axis and responsiveness to growth stimulation of short children with osteogenesis imperfecta. Am J Med Genet 45:261, 1993

McKUSICK VA: *Heritable Disorders of Connective Tissue*, 4th ed. St Louis, Mosby, 1972

MEYERS GA: FGFR2 exon IIIa and IIIc mutations in Crouzon, Jackson-Weiss, and Pfeiffer syndromes: Evidence for missense changes, insertions, and a deletion due to alternative RNA splicing. Am J Med Genet 58:491, 1996

PROCKOP DJ: Mutations in collagen genes as a cause of connective-tissue diseases. N Engl J Med 326:540, 1992

————, KIVIRIKKO KI: Collagen: Molecular biology, diseases and potentials for therapy. Annu Rev Biochem 64:403, 1996

PYERITZ RE: The Marfan syndrome, in *Connective Tissue and Its Heritable Disorders*, PM Royce, B Steinmann (eds). New York, Wiley-Liss, 1993, p 437

SILLENCE DO: Osteogenesis imperfecta: An expanding panorama of variance. Clin Orthop 191:11, 1981

STEINMANN et al: The Ehlers-Danlos syndrome, in *Connective Tissue and Its Heritable Disorders*, PM Royce, B Steinmann (eds). New York, Wiley-Liss, 1993, p 351

Louis J. Elsas, Nicola Longo, Leon E. Rosenberg

INHERITED DISORDERS OF AMINO ACID METABOLISM AND STORAGE

All polypeptides and proteins are polymers of amino acids. Eight amino acids, referred to as *essential*, cannot be synthesized by humans and must be obtained from dietary sources. The others are formed endogenously. Although most of the body's amino acids are "tied up" in proteins, small intracellular pools of *free* amino acids are in equilibrium with extracellular reservoirs in plasma, cerebrospinal fluid, and the lumina of the gut and kidney. Physiologically, amino acids are more than mere "building blocks." Some (glycine, glutamate, gamma-aminobutyric acid) are neurotransmitters. Others (phenylalanine, tyrosine, tryptophan, glycine) are precursors of hormones, coenzymes, pigments, purines, or pyrimidines. Each has a unique degradative pathway by which its nitrogen and carbon components are used for the synthesis of other amino acids, carbohydrates, and lipids.

More than 70 disorders of amino acid metabolism are now known, the catabolic and storage defects (approximately 60) discussed in this chapter far outnumbering the transport abnormalities (approximately 10) considered in Chap. 350. Each of these disorders is rare—the incidences range from 1 in 10,000 for cystinuria or phenylketonuria to 1 in 200,000 for homocystinuria or alkaptonuria. Collectively, however, they occur in perhaps 1 in 500 to 1 in 1000 live births.

The features of inherited disorders of amino acid catabolism are summarized in Table 349-1. In general, these disorders are named for the compound that accumulates to highest concentration in blood (*-emias*) or urine (*-urias*). For many conditions (often called *amino-*

Table 349-1

Inherited Disorders of Amino Acid Catabolism

Amino Acid(s) Affected	Disorder or Condition	Enzyme Defect	Clinical Manifestations*						Inheritance Pattern†
			Mental Retardation	Neuro-psychiatric Dysfunction	Protein Intolerance	Metabolic Ketoacidosis	Ammonia Intoxication	Other	
AROMATIC—HETEROCYCLIC									
Phenylalanine	Phenylketonuria type I (severe to mild)	Phenylalanine hydroxylase	+	+	−	−	−	Hypopigmented skin and hair, eczema	AR
	Phenylketonuria type II	Dihydropteridine reductase	+	+	−	−	−		AR
	Phenylketonuria type III	Dihydrobiopterin synthesis	+	+	−	−	−		AR
	Malignant hyperphenylalaninemia	GTP cyclohydrolase	+	+	−	−	−		AR
Tyrosine	Tyrosinemia type I (hepatorenal)	Fumarylacetoacetate hydrolase	−	−	±	−	−	Cirrhosis, hepatic failure, renal tubular defects, rickets	AR
	Tyrosinemia type II (oculocutaneous)	Tyrosine transaminase	±	−	−	−	−	Palmoplantar keratosis, painful corneal erosions with photophobia	AR
	Tyrosinemia type III	4-Hydroxyphenylpyruvate dioxygenase	−	−	−	−	−		AR
	Hawkinsinuria	4-Hydroxyphenylpyruvate dioxygenase	−	−	−	−	−	Failure to thrive, metabolic acidosis in infancy, fine hairs	AD
	Alkaptonuria	Homogentisic acid oxidase	−	−	−	−	−	Ochronosis, arthritis	AR
	Albinism (oculocutaneous)	Tyrosinase	−	−	−	−	−	Hypopigmentation of hair, skin, and optic fundus	AR
	Albinism (ocular)	Unknown	−	−	−	−	−	Hypopigmentation of optic fundus	XL, AR
Tryptophan	Tryptophanuria	Unknown	+	+	−	−	−	Photosensitive skin rash	AR
	Xanthurenic aciduria	Kynureninase	?	−	−	−	−		?
Histidine	Histidinemia	Histidine-ammonia lyase	±	±	−	−	−	Hearing and speech deficit	AR
	Urocanic aciduria	Urocanase	+	+	−	−	−		?
	Formiminoglutamic aciduria	Formiminotransferase	?	+	−	−	−		(AR)
GLYCINE-IMINO ACIDS									
Glycine	Hyperglycinemia	Glycine cleavage	+	+	−	−	−		AR
	Sarcosinemia	Sarcosine dehydrogenase	−	−	−	−	−		AR
	Hyperoxaluria (type I)	Alanine: glyoxylate amino-transferase	−	−	−	−	−	Calcium oxalate nephrolithiasis, renal failure	AR
	Hyperoxaluria (type II)	D-Glyceric acid dehydrogenase/glyoxylate reductase	−	−	−	−	−	Calcium oxalate nephrolithiasis, renal failure	AR
Imino acids	Hyperprolinemia (type I)	Proline oxidase	−	−	−	−	−		AR
	Hyperprolinemia (type II)	Δ'-Pyrroline dehydrogenase	−	−	−	−	−		AR
	Hyperhydroxyprolinemia	Hydroxyproline reductase	−	−	−	−	−		AR
	Iminopeptiduria	Prolidase	+	−	−	−	−	Crusting erythematous, ecchymotic dermatitis, recurrent infections	AR

(continued)

Table 349-1—(*Continued*)

Inherited Disorders of Amino Acid Catabolism

Amino Acid(s) Affected	Disorder or Condition	Enzyme Defect	Clinical Manifestations*						Inheritance Pattern†
			Mental Retardation	Neuro-psychiatric Dysfunction	Protein Intolerance	Metabolic Ketoacidosis	Ammonia Intoxication	Other	
SULFUR-CONTAINING									
Methionine	Hypermethioninemia	Methionine adenosyltransferase	−	−	−	−	−		?
Homocystine	Homocystinuria	Cystathionine β-synthase	±	±	−	−	−	Dislocated lenses, osteoporosis, thrombotic vascular disease	AR
	Homocystinuria	5,10-Methylene-tetrahydrofolate reductase	+	+	−	−	−		AR
	Homocystinuria and methylmalonic acidemia (cblC, -D)‡	Cobalamin (vitamin B_{12}) reductase (cytosol)	+	+	−	−	−	Megaloblastic anemia	AR
	Homocystinuria and methylmalonic acidemia (cblF)	Lysosomal efflux	+	+	−	−	−		(?)
	Homocystinuria (cblE, -G)	Methyltransferase-associated cobalamin reductase (?)	+	+	−	−	−	Megaloblastic anemia	AR
Cystathionine	Cystathioninuria	Cystathionase	−	−	−	−	−		AR
Cystine	Cystinosis	Lysosomal efflux	−	−	−	−	−	Fanconi syndrome, renal failure, photophobia	AR
S-Sulfo-L-cysteine	S-Sulfo-L-cysteine, sulfite, and thiosulfaturia	Sulfite oxidase	+	+	−	−	−	Dislocated lenses	AR
CATIONIC									
Lysine	Hyperlysinemia	α-Aminoadipic semialdehyde synthase			−	−	−		AR
	Saccharopinuria	δ-Aminoadipic semialdehyde synthase	−	−	−	−	−		?
	α-Ketoadipic aciduria	α-Ketoadipic acid dehydrogenase			−	−	−		?
	Glutaric aciduria (type I)	Glutaryl CoA dehydrogenase	−	+	−	−	−	Progressive dystonia and athetosis	AR
	Glutaric aciduria (type II)	Electron transfer flavoprotein; or ETF-ubiquinone oxidoreductase	−	+	−	+	−	Hypoglycemia, acidosis, "sweaty feet" odor, hypotonia, fatty degeneration of liver and kidney	AR
Ornithine	Hyperornithinemia, hyperammonemia, homocitrullinuria	Mitochondrial ornithine translocator (?)	+	+	+	−	+		AR
	Hyperornithinemia	Ornithine-D-aminotransferase	−	−	−	−	−	Gyrate atrophy of choroid and retina	AR
UREA CYCLE									
Carbamylphosphate	Hyperammonemia (type I)	Carbamylphosphate synthetase I	+	+	+	−	+		AR
N-acetylglutamate	Hyperammonemia (type IA)	N-acetylglutamate synthetase	?	+	+	−	+		AR
Ornithine	Hyperammonemia (type II)	Ornithine transcarbamylase	±	+	+	−	+		XL
Citrulline	Citrullinemia	Argininosuccinate synthetase	+	+	+	−	+		AR
Argininosuccinic acid	Argininosuccinic aciduria	Argininosuccinase	+	+	+	−	+		AR
Arginine	Argininemia	Arginase	+	+	+	−	+		AR

(*continued*)

Table 349-1—*(Continued)*

Inherited Disorders of Amino Acid Catabolism

Amino Acid(s) Affected	Disorder or Condition	Enzyme Defect	Clinical Manifestations*						Inheritance Pattern†
			Mental Retardation	Neuro-psychiatric Dysfunction	Protein Intolerance	Metabolic Ketoacidosis	Ammonia Intoxication	Other	
BRANCHED-CHAIN									
Valine	Hypervalinemia	Valine aminotransferase	+	+	+	−	−		AR
Leucine, isoleucine	Hyperleucine-isoleucinemia	Leucine-isoleucine aminotransferase	+	+	+	−	−		?
Valine, leucine, isoleucine	Classic branched-chain ketoaciduria	Branched-chain ketoacid dehydrogenase	+	+	+		−	"Maple syrup" odor	AR
	Intermittent branched-chain ketoaciduria	Branched-chain ketoacid dehydrogenase	±	−	+	+	−		AR
Leucine	Isovaleric acidemia	Isovaleryl CoA dehydrogenase	±	±	+	+	±	"Sweaty feet" odor	AR
	β-Methylcrotonyl glycinuria	β-Methylcrotonyl CoA carboxylase	+	+	−	+	−	"Cat's urine" odor	AR
	β-Hydroxy-β-methylglutaric aciduria	β-Hydroxy-β-methylglutaryl CoA lyase	−	+	+	+	−		?
Isoleucine, valine	α-Methylacetoacetic aciduria	β-Ketothiolase	±	±	+	+	+		AR
	Propionic acidemia (pcc A, B, C)‡	Propionyl CoA carboxylase	±	±	+	+	+		AR
	Propionic acidemia (bio)‡	Holocarboxylase synthetase; biotinidase	+	±	+	+	−		AR
	Methylmalonic acidemia (mut)‡	Methylmalonyl CoA mutase	±	±	+	+	+		AR
	Methylmalonic acidemia (cbl A)‡	Cobalamin (vitamin B$_{12}$) reductase (mitochondrial) (?)	±	±	+	+	+		AR
	Methylmalonic acidemia (cbl B)‡	Cobalamin (vitamin B$_{12}$): ATP adenosyltransferase	±	±	+	+	+		AR

* +, Regularly present; ±, sometimes present; −, absent; ?, uncertain; all designations refer to manifestations in untreated disorder.
† AR, autosomal recessive; XL, X-linked; (AR), probably autosomal recessive.
‡ Designations in parentheses refer to complementation groups assigned by genetic analysis with cultured cells.

acidopathies), the parent amino acid is found in excess; for others, generally referred to as *organic acidemias*, products in the catabolic pathway accumulate. Which compound(s) accumulates depends, of course, on the site of the enzymatic block, the reversibility of the reactions proximal to the lesion, and the availability of alternative pathways of metabolic "runoff." For some amino acids, such as the sulfur-containing or branched-chain molecules, defects have been described at nearly each step in the catabolic pathway. For others, only small numbers of defective reactions have been described. Biochemical and genetic heterogeneity is common. Four distinct forms of hyperphenylalaninemia, seven forms of homocystinuria, and seven types of methylmalonic acidemia are recognized. Such heterogeneity reflects the presence of an even larger array of molecular defects.

The manifestations of these conditions differ widely (see Table 349-1). Some, such as sarcosinemia or hyperprolinemia, produce no clinical consequences. At the other extreme, complete deficiency of ornithine transcarbamylase or of branched-chain keto acid dehydrogenase is lethal in the untreated neonate. Central nervous system (CNS) dysfunction, in the form of developmental retardation, seizures, alterations in sensorium, or behavioral disturbances, is present in more

than half the disorders. Protein-induced vomiting, neurologic dysfunction, and hyperammonemia occur in many disorders of urea cycle intermediates. Metabolic ketoacidosis, often accompanied by hyperammonemia, is a frequent presenting finding in the disorders of branched-chain amino acid metabolism. Occasional disorders produce focal tissue or organ involvement such as liver disease, renal failure, cutaneous abnormalities, or ocular lesions.

The clinical manifestations in many of these conditions can be prevented or mitigated if diagnosis is achieved early and appropriate treatment (i.e., dietary protein or amino acid restriction or vitamin supplementation) is instituted promptly. For this reason, several aminoacidopathies and organic acidemias are screened for in mass newborn surveys that analyze blood or urine with an array of chemical and microbiologic techniques. Once a presumptive diagnosis is made, confirmation can be provided by direct enzyme assay on extracts of leukocytes, erythrocytes, or cultured fibroblasts. DNA-based diagnostic capability is possible for several disorders. For example, substitutions, deletions, and insertions can be utilized to diagnose and characterize phenylketonuria, ornithine transcarbamylase deficiency, citrullinemia, gyrate atrophy of the retina, propionic acidemia, and methylmalonic acidemia (see also Chap. 65). As additional mutations are defined, DNA-based analysis will be used to predict outcome and the therapeutic plan.

Several of these disorders (including branched-chain ketoaciduria, isovaleric acidemia, propionic acidemia, methylmalonic acidemia, homocystinuria, cystinosis, phenylketonuria, ornithine transcarbamylase deficiency, citrullinemia, argininosuccinic aciduria) can be diagnosed prenatally by chemical analysis of amniotic fluid or by chemical, enzymatic, or DNA-based studies of fresh or cultured amniotic fluid cells. In addition to predicting genotype and alleviating parental anxiety, prenatal diagnosis has led to improved treatment of affected newborns.

The focus in this chapter is on selected disorders that illustrate the principles, properties, and problems presented by the disorders of amino acid metabolism.

THE HYPERPHENYLALANINEMIAS

DEFINITION   The hyperphenylalaninemias (see Table 349-1) result from impaired conversion of phenylalanine to tyrosine. The most common and clinically important is phenylketonuria, which is characterized by an increased concentration of phenylalanine in blood, increased concentrations of phenylalanine and its by-products (notably phenylpyruvate, phenylacetate, phenyllactate, and phenylacetylglutamine) in urine, and severe mental retardation if untreated in infancy.

ETIOLOGY AND PATHOGENESIS   Each of the hyperphenylalaninemias results from reduced activity of *phenylalanine hydroxylase*. In humans, the complete enzyme system is expressed only in liver. Phenylalanine and molecular oxygen are substrates, and a reduced pteridine, tetrahydrobiopterin, is cofactor (Fig. 349-1). Tyrosine and dihydrobiopterin are the products of this catalytic system, the latter being reconverted to tetrahydrobiopterin by a second enzyme, dihydropteridine reductase. In the most severe forms of phenylketonuria type I, activity of the hydroxylase apoenzyme, encoded by a gene on chromosome 12q22-q24.1, is almost totally deficient. More than 200 mutations in this gene have been identified in patients with phenylketonuria. The prevalence of these mutations varies widely among different ethnic groups. Mutations causing a complete impairment of enzyme activity, such as the R408W, are associated with more severe outcome, requiring stringent dietary restriction of phenylalanine. Mutations causing a less complete deficiency of the enzyme, such as the I65T, are associated with milder forms of type I phenylketonuria. Transient hyperphenylalaninemia (sometimes called *transient phenylketonuria*)

is caused by a delayed maturation of the hydroxylase apoenzyme. In "malignant" hyperphenylalaninemia, however, persistent impairment of hydroxylating activity results not from abnormality in the apohydroxylase but from tetrahydrobiopterin deficiency due to blocks in the pathway by which tetrahydrobiopterin is synthesized from GTP (phenylketonuria type III and malignant hyperphenylalaninemia) or deficiency of dihydropteridine reductase (phenylketonuria type II), the enzyme that regenerates tetrahydrobiopterin from dihydrobiopterin (see Fig. 349-1). Tyrosine hydroxylase and tryptophan hydroxylase also require tetrahydrobiopterin, and their products (L-dopa and 5-hydroxytryptophan) are essential for the synthesis of neurotransmitters.

Abnormalities in phenylalanine metabolism are autosomal recessive traits that occur in about 1 in 10,000 births. Phenylketonuria type I, which accounts for nearly two-thirds of these, is widely distributed among whites and Asians. It is rare in blacks. Phenylalanine hydroxylase activity in obligate heterozygotes is low but higher than in affected homozygotes. Adult heterozygous carriers are clinically well but can be identified by an increased ratio of phenylalanine/tyrosine in plasma in the semifasting state. They may have transient cognitive impairment after phenylalanine loads.

Phenylalanine accumulation in blood and urine and reduced tyrosine formation are direct consequences of the impaired hydroxylation. In untreated phenylketonuria and in its tetrahydrobiopterin-deficient variants, plasma concentrations of phenylalanine become sufficiently high [>1 mmol/L (16 mg/dL)] to activate alternative pathways of metabolism and lead to formation of phenylpyruvate, phenylacetate, phenyllactate, and other derivatives that are rapidly cleared by the kidney and excreted in urine. Plasma concentrations of several other amino acids are moderately reduced, probably secondary to inhibition of gastrointestinal absorption or impairment of renal tubular reabsorption by excess phenylalanine. The severe brain damage is due to several consequences of phenylalanine accumulation: competitive inhibition of transport of other amino acids required for protein synthesis, impaired polyribosome formation or stabilization, reduced synthesis and increased degradation of myelin, and inadequate formation of norepinephrine and serotonin. Phenylalanine is a competitive inhibitor of tyrosinase, a key enzyme in the pathway of melanin synthesis. This block, plus reduced availability of the melanin precursor tyrosine, accounts for the hypopigmentation of hair and skin.

CLINICAL MANIFESTATIONS   No abnormalities are apparent at birth, but untreated children with classic phenylketonuria fail to attain early developmental milestones, develop microcephaly, and demonstrate progressive impairment of cerebral function. Hyperactivity, seizures, and severe mental retardation are major clinical problems later in life. Electroencephalographic abnormalities, "mousy" odor of skin, hair, and urine (due to phenylacetate accumulation), and a tendency to hypopigmentation and eczema complete the devastating clinical picture. In contrast, affected children who are detected at birth and treated promptly show none of these abnormalities. Children with tetrahydrobiopterin deficiency, however, are the most unfortunate. Seizures appear early, followed by progressive cerebral and basal ganglia dysfunction (rigidity, chorea, spasms, hypotonia). Most succumb to secondary infection within a few years despite early diagnosis and vigorous treatment.

A number of women with phenylketonuria who have been treated since infancy have reached adulthood and become pregnant. If phenylalanine levels are not strictly controlled before and during pregnancy, the offspring is at risk from *maternal phenylketonemia*. At birth, such children have microcephaly and an increased risk of congenital defects. After birth, these children have severe neurodevelopmental delay and growth retardation. Since these children are heterozygous, not homozygous, carriers of a mutation in the phenylalanine hydroxylase gene, the clinical manifestations must be attributed to damage produced by the elevated maternal concentrations of phenylalanine to which they have been exposed in utero.

DIAGNOSIS   Plasma phenylalanine concentrations are usually normal at birth in the hyperphenylalaninemias but rise rapidly after institution of protein feedings. To prevent mental retardation, diagnosis

FIGURE 349-1   Pathways, enzymes, and coenzymes involved in the hyperphenylalaninemias. Blocked-in symbols highlight points of etiologic or therapeutic significance to the various genetic defects underlying these disorders. Abbreviations: GTP, guanosine triphosphate; GTP-CH, guanosine triphosphate cyclohydrolase; DNT, dihydroneopterin triphosphate; 6-PTS, 6-pyruvoyltetrahydropterin synthase; BH$_4$, tetrahydrobiopterin; BH$_2$, dihydrobiopterin; DHPR, dihydropteridine reductase; PAH, phenylalanine hydroxylase.

and initiation of dietary treatment of classic phenylketonuria must occur before the child is 3 weeks of age. For this reason, most newborns in North America and Europe are screened by determinations of blood phenylalanine concentration using the Guthrie bacterial inhibition assay. Abnormal values are confirmed with more quantitative fluorometric or chromatographic assays. In newborns with type I phenylketonuria, plasma levels depend on the amount of phenylalanine to which the infant has been exposed and the degree of impaired phenylalanine hydroxylase. Dietary phenylalanine restriction is usually instituted if blood phenylalanine levels are above 250 μmol/L (4 mg/dL). Careful monitoring of these infants reveals the degree of phenylalanine hydroxylase impairment and dictates the degree of dietary phenylalanine restriction. Deficiency of tetrahydrobiopterin, which occurs in 1 to 5 percent of newborns with increased blood phenylalanine, is excluded by screening the urinary pteridine profile and by assay of dihydropteridine reductase activity on dried blood specimens. Tetrahydrobiopterin deficiency manifests with hyperphenylalaninemia and progressive neurologic impairment despite prompt restriction of dietary phenylalanine. Prenatal diagnosis of type I phenylketonuria is now feasible using DNA-based tests capable of detecting specific mutations or restriction fragment length polymorphisms of the phenylalanine hydroxylase gene. Dihydropteridine reductase deficiency and the blocks in tetrahydrobiopterin synthesis also can be detected in utero using assays on cultured amniocytes.

℞ TREATMENT

Phenylketonuria is the first inherited metabolic disease in which prevention of the accumulation of the offending metabolite prevented the dire clinical consequences. This was accomplished by a special diet low in phenylalanine and supplemented with tyrosine. Tyrosine becomes an essential amino acid in phenylalanine hydroxylase deficiency. Sufficient phenylalanine is provided for new protein synthesis and normal growth. This amount varies with age and requires frequent adjustments, especially early in life. Ordinarily, plasma phenylalanine concentrations are maintained between 120 and 360 μmol/L (2 and 6 mg/dL).

Such diet therapy must be instituted during the first 3 weeks of life. Even then, modest CNS dysfunction may occur with more deleterious mutations or after excess protein intake. Because uncontrolled hyperphenylalaninemia results in brain damage throughout childhood (and perhaps in adults), dietary restriction should usually be continued and monitored indefinitely, recognizing that transient phenylketonuria may not require lifelong therapy. Children with tetrahydrobiopterin deficiency deteriorate despite dietary phenylalanine restriction; efficacy of pteridine cofactor replacement is under study. Such patients may be helped, however, by a regimen in which dietary phenylalanine restriction is combined with supplements of levodopa and 5-hydroxytryptophan. Finally, the deleterious consequences of maternal phenylketonuria can be minimized by continuing lifelong phenylalanine-restricted diets in females with phenylketonuria and assuring even stricter phenylalanine restriction prior to conception and throughout gestation.

THE HOMOCYSTINURIAS (HYPERHOMOCYSTEINEMIAS)

The homocystinurias are seven biochemically and clinically distinct disorders (see Table 349-1), each characterized by increased concentration of the sulfur-containing amino acid homocystine in blood and urine. The most common form results from reduced activity of cystathionine β-synthase, an enzyme in the transsulfuration pathway that converts methionine to cysteine (Fig.

349-2). The other forms are the result of impaired conversion of homocysteine to methionine, a reaction catalyzed by homocysteine:methyltetrahydrofolate methyltransferase and two essential cofactors, methyltetrahydrofolate and methylcobalamin (methyl-vitamin B$_{12}$). Depending on the underlying disorder, some patients show chemical and, in some instances, clinical improvement following administration of specific vitamin supplements (pyridoxine, folate, or cobalamin). In classic homocystinuria, the levels of free homocystine in plasma increase and result in homocystinuria. Hyperhomocysteinemia refers to increased total plasma concentration of homocysteine and homocystine, free and protein-bound. Hyperhomocysteinemia in the absence of significant homocystinuria is found in heterozygotes and homozygotes for variant forms involving impaired folate or vitamin B$_{12}$ metabolism and cystathionine synthase deficiency. Elevation of total plasma homocysteine is an independent risk factor for premature vascular disease.

CYSTATHIONINE β-SYNTHASE DEFICIENCY Definition Deficiency of this enzyme leads to increased concentrations of methionine and homocystine in body fluids and to decreased concentrations of cysteine and cystine. Clinical hallmarks include dislocation of optic lenses (usually downward and medially), mental retardation, marfanoid habitus, osteoporosis, and thrombotic vascular disease.

Etiology and Pathogenesis The sulfur atom of the essential amino acid methionine is transferred ultimately to cysteine by the transsulfuration pathway (Fig. 349-2). In one of these steps, homocysteine condenses with serine to form cystathionine. This reaction is catalyzed by the pyridoxal phosphate–dependent enzyme cystathionine β-synthase. The gene for this homodimeric enzyme has been mapped to chromosome 21q22.3. Heterogeneous mutations in this gene are present in different families. The G307S mutation is associated with lack of response to pyridoxine, while the I278T mutation correlates with pyridoxine-responsiveness and a milder clinical phenotype. Homocystinuria is relatively common in Ireland (1 in 60,000 births) but rare elsewhere (less than 1 in 200,000 births).

Homocysteine and methionine accumulate in cells and body fluids; cysteine synthesis is impaired, resulting in reduced concentrations of this amino acid and its disulfide form cystine. In approximately half of patients, synthase activity in liver, brain, leukocytes, and cultured fibroblasts is undetectable. In the remaining patients, tissues retain 1 to 5 percent of normal activity, and this residual activity often can be stimulated by pyridoxine supplementation. Heterozygosity for cystathionine β-synthase deficiency is a cause of hyperhomocyst(e)inemia, which increases the risk for thrombotic vascular disease.

Homocysteine interferes with the normal cross-linking of collagen, an effect that likely plays an important role in the ocular, skeletal, and vascular complications. Altered collagen in the suspensory ligament of

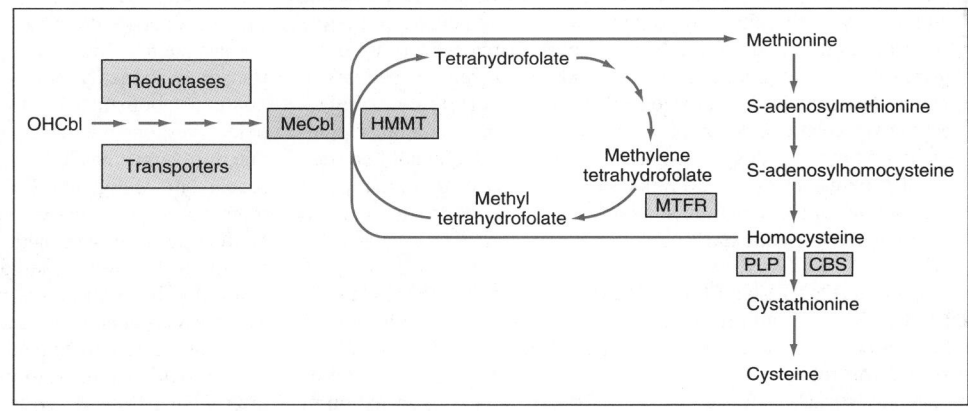

FIGURE 349-2 Pathways, enzymes, and coenzymes involved in the homocystinurias. Blocked-in symbols highlight specific moieties of particular etiologic or therapeutic significance to the various genetic defects underlying these disorders. Abbreviations: OHCbl, hydroxocobalamin (hydroxo B$_{12}$); MeCbl, methylcobalamin; MTFR, methylene tetrahydrofolate reductase; PLP, pyridoxal phosphate; CBS, cystathionine β-synthase.

the optic lens and in bone matrix may account for the dislocated lenses and osteoporosis. Similarly, interference with normal ground substance metabolism in vascular walls may predispose to the arterial and venous thrombotic diathesis. Increased platelet adhesiveness may result from homocysteine accumulation, thereby contributing to the thrombotic occlusive disease so often observed. Recurrent cerebrovascular accidents secondary to thrombotic disease may account for the mental retardation, but direct chemical effects on cerebral cell metabolism have not been excluded.

Clinical Manifestations More than 80 percent of homozygotes for complete cystathionine synthase deficiency develop dislocated optic lenses. This abnormality usually appears by 3 to 4 years of age and often results in glaucoma and impaired visual acuity. Mental retardation occurs in about half of such patients, often accompanied by ill-defined behavioral disturbances. Osteoporosis is a common radiologic finding (seen in two-thirds of patients by age 15) but rarely causes clinical disease. Life-threatening vascular complications, probably initiated by damage to vascular endothelium, are the major cause of morbidity and mortality. Occlusion of coronary, renal, and cerebral arteries with attendant tissue infarction can occur during the first decade of life. Nearly a fourth of patients die of vascular disease before age 30. These vascular complications seem to be exacerbated by angiographic procedures. Importantly, pyridoxine-responsive patients have milder clinical manifestations and may escape newborn screening and present with ectopia lentis or premature vascular occlusion. Heterozygous carriers for synthase deficiency (about 1 in 70 in the population) and others with high concentrations of plasma homocystine are at increased risk for premature coronary, peripheral, and cerebral vascular disease.

Diagnosis The cyanide-nitroprusside test is a simple way of demonstrating increased excretion of sulfhydryl-containing compounds in urine. The diagnosis is confirmed by measurement of free plasma methionine and homocystine. Plasma methionine tends to be increased in synthase-deficient patients and normal or low in those with other causes of homocystinuria and impaired methionine formation (see below). Diagnostic confirmation depends on measurements of cystathionine β-synthase activity in tissue extracts or cells cultured from patients. Heterozygotes can be identified by measurement of peak serum homocystine after an oral methionine load and by measurement of tissue synthase activity.

℞ TREATMENT

As with classic phenylketonuria, effective treatment depends on early diagnosis. A number of infants diagnosed in the newborn period have been treated successfully with methionine-restricted, cystine-supplemented diets. Their clinical course is benign compared with that of untreated affected siblings. In approximately half of patients, oral pyridoxine (25 to 500 mg/d) produces a fall in plasma and urinary methionine and homocystine and an increase in cystine concentration in body fluids. This effect probably reflects a modest increase in cystathionine β-synthase activity in cells of patients in whom the defect is characterized either by reduced affinity for cofactor or by accelerated degradation of mutant enzyme. Vitamin supplementation at these doses is apparently harmless and should be tried in all patients. There are no reports of the effect of the initiation of pyridoxine supplementation soon after birth. Similarly, there are no data regarding pyridoxine supplements in heterozygous carriers.

5,10-METHYLENETETRAHYDROFOLATE REDUCTASE DEFICIENCY

Definition Hyperhomocysteinemia with normal or decreased methionine levels is caused by deficiency of 5,10-methylenetetrahydrofolate reductase, the enzyme involved in the synthesis of 5-methyltetrahydrofolate, a cofactor in the enzymatic formation of methionine from homocysteine (Fig. 349-2). CNS dysfunction and premature vascular occlusion may occur.

Etiology and Pathogenesis 5-Methyltetrahydrofolate:homocysteine methyltransferase catalyzes the conversion of homocysteine to methionine. The methyl group transferred in this reaction comes from 5-methyltetrahydrofolate, which is converted to tetrahydrofolate in the process. 5-Methyltetrahydrofolate, in turn, is synthesized enzymatically from 5,10-methylenetetrahydrofolate by 5,10-methylenetetrahydrofolate reductase. Thus reductase activity controls both methionine synthesis and tetrahydrofolate generation. This series of reactions is critical to normal DNA and RNA synthesis. A primary defect in the reductase activity results, secondarily, in deficient methyltransferase activity and impaired conversion of homocysteine to methionine. Methionine deficiency and impaired nucleic acid synthesis may contribute to the CNS dysfunction, while homocystine accumulation may predispose to thrombosis. The disorder appears to be inherited as an autosomal recessive trait. The gene for methylenetetrahydrofolate reductase maps to chromosome 1p36.3, and mutations have been identified in patients with hyperhomocysteinemia due to deficiency of this gene. A thermolabile variant form of this enzyme has reduced activity and may be a common cause of hyperhomocysteinemia associated with increased risk of vascular disease in young adults.

Clinical Manifestations More than 25 children with homocystinuria due to methylenetetrahydrofolate reductase deficiency have been reported. The most severely affected have developmental retardation and cerebral atrophy early in life. Others have behavioral disturbances (catatonia) during the second decade or mild retardation. The severity of the clinical manifestations reflects the severity of the reductase deficiency.

Diagnosis Increased concentrations of free homocystine in body fluids with normal or decreased concentrations of methionine should suggest severe methylenetetrahydrofolate reductase deficiency. Total plasma homocysteine levels slightly above the normal range suggest milder dysfunction of this enzyme. Serum folate concentrations are low in some patients. Confirmation requires direct assay of methylenetetrahydrofolate reductase in tissue extracts (brain, liver, cultured fibroblasts).

℞ TREATMENT

Therapeutic experience is limited. Folate, methionine, or betaine supplementation decreases urinary homocystine excretion and improves the clinical manifestations in some patients.

DEFICIENCY OF COBALAMIN (VITAMIN B₁₂) COENZYME SYNTHESIS

Definition Five other forms of homocystinuria also reflect impaired conversion of homocysteine to methionine. The primary defects in these entities, however, are in the synthesis of methylcobalamin, a cobalamin (vitamin B_{12}) coenzyme required by methyltetrahydrofolate:homocysteine methyltransferase (see Fig. 349-2). In some, methylmalonic acid accumulates in body fluids because of impaired synthesis of a second coenzyme, adenosylcobalamin, required for isomerization of methylmalonyl coenzyme A (CoA) to succinyl CoA. These disorders are designated cblC, -D, -E, -F, and -G.

Etiology and Pathogenesis As with 5,10-methylenetetrahydrofolate reductase deficiency, each disorder impairs remethylation of homocysteine. Since methylcobalamin is required for methyl-group transfer from methyltetrahydrofolate to homocysteine, impaired cobalamin metabolism leads to deficient methyltransferase activity. The defects responsible for impaired synthesis of methylcobalamin involve one of several steps in lysosomal or cytosolic activation of the vitamin precursor (see Fig. 349-2). In the cblF disorder, the transport of cobalamins out of lysosomes is impaired. In cblC and -D, a reductase needed for formation of both methylcobalamin and adenosylcobalamin is deficient. In cblE and -G, some component required to maintain a reduced form of cobalamin on the methyltransferase apoenzyme is impaired. Somatic cell genetic studies indicate that each of these abnormalities is distinct and imply that all are inherited as autosomal recessive traits.

Clinical Manifestations More than 45 patients—mostly children—have been described. Although clinical manifestations vary, abnormalities include developmental delay, dementia, spasticity, megaloblastic anemia, and pancytopenia. It is not possible to define a specific clinical syndrome for each of the defects in cobalamin metabolism.

Diagnosis Homocystinuria, homocystinemia, and hypomethioninemia are the chemical hallmarks. Methylmalonic acidemia, too, has been noted in those defects resulting from defective synthesis of both cobalamin coenzymes. These findings also may be present in juvenile- or adult-onset pernicious anemia in which intestinal cobalamin absorption is impaired. Measurement of serum cobalamin concentrations, low in pernicious anemia and normal in patients with defective conversion of cobalamin vitamin to coenzymes, helps in the differential diagnosis. Definitive diagnosis depends on demonstrating impaired coenzyme synthesis in cultured cells.

TREATMENT
Treatment of affected children with cobalamin supplements (1 to 2 mg/d) causes homocystine and methylmalonate excretion to fall to near normal values; the hematologic and neurologic deficits also improve to a variable degree in some patients. Intervention early in life seems to offer the best long-term prognosis.

ALKAPTONURIA

DEFINITION Alkaptonuria is a rare disorder of tyrosine catabolism in which deficiency of homogentisic acid oxidase leads to excretion of large amounts of homogentisic acid in urine and accumulation of oxidized homogentisic acid pigment in connective tissues (*ochronosis*). After many years, ochronosis produces a distinctive form of degenerative arthritis.

ETIOLOGY AND PATHOGENESIS Homogentisic acid is an intermediate in the catabolism of tyrosine. Activity of homogentisic acid oxidase, the enzyme that catalyzes the opening of the phenolic ring yielding maleylacetoacetic acid, is deficient in the liver and kidneys of patients with alkaptonuria, and homogentisic acid accumulates in cells and body fluids. The gene for this enzyme has been mapped to chromosome 3q2. Patients have minimally increased concentrations of homogentisic acid in blood because it is rapidly cleared by the kidney. The excretion of as much as 3 to 7 g of homogentisic acid in the urine per day is of little pathophysiologic significance. However, homogentisic acid and its oxidized polymers bind to collagen, leading to the progressive deposition of a gray to bluish-black pigment. The mechanism(s) by which this deposition causes degenerative changes in cartilage, intervertebral disks, and other connective tissues is unknown but may involve direct chemical irritation, impaired collagen cross-linking, disturbed articular chondrocyte metabolism, or some combination of factors.

Alkaptonuria was the first human disease shown to be inherited as an autosomal recessive trait. Affected homozygotes occur with a frequency around 1 in 200,000. Heterozygous carriers are clinically well and excrete no homogentisic acid in urine, even after loading doses of tyrosine.

CLINICAL MANIFESTATIONS Alkaptonuria may go unrecognized until middle life when degenerative joint disease develops. Prior to this time, the tendency of the patient's urine to darken on standing may go unnoticed, as may slight discoloration of the sclerae and ears. The latter manifestations are generally the earliest external evidence of the disorder and develop after age 20 to 30. Foci of gray-brown scleral pigment and generalized darkening of the concha, anthelix, and finally, helix of the ear are typical. Ear cartilages may be irregular and thickened. *Ochronotic arthritis* is heralded by pain, stiffness, and some limitation of motion of the hips, knees, and shoulders. Acute arthritis may resemble rheumatoid arthritis, but small joints are usually spared. Limitation of motion and ankylosis of the lumbosacral spine are common late manifestations. Pigmentation of heart valves, larynx, tympanic membranes, and skin occurs, and occasional patients develop pigmented renal or prostatic calculi. Degenerative cardiovascular disease may be increased in older patients.

DIAGNOSIS A patient whose urine darkens to blackness on standing must be suspected of having alkaptonuria but, because of modern plumbing conditions, this change is not often observed. The diagnosis is usually made from the triad of degenerative arthritis, ochronotic pigmentation, and urine that turns black upon alkalinization.

Homogentisic acid in urine may be identified presumptively by other tests: upon addition of ferric chloride, a purple-black color is observed; treatment with Benedict's reagent yields a brown color; addition of a saturated silver nitrate solution produces an intermediate black color. These screening tests can be confirmed by chromatographic, enzymatic, or spectrophotometric determinations of homogentisic acid. X-rays of the lumbar spine are virtually pathognomonic. They show degeneration and dense calcification of the intervertebral disks and narrowing of the intervertebral spaces.

TREATMENT
There is no specific treatment for ochronotic arthritis. Joint manifestations might be mitigated if homogentisic acid accumulation and deposition could be curbed by dietary restriction of phenylalanine and tyrosine, but the long-term course of the disease discourages such therapeutic attempts. Ascorbic acid impedes oxidation and polymerization of homogentisic acid in vitro, but the efficacy of this form of treatment has not been established. Symptomatic treatment is similar to that for osteoarthritis (Chap. 322).

CYSTINOSIS

DEFINITION Cystinosis is a rare disorder characterized by the intralysosomal accumulation of free cystine in body tissues. This results in the appearance of cystine crystals in the cornea, conjunctiva, bone marrow, lymph nodes, leukocytes, and internal organs. Three variants have been identified: an infantile (nephropathic) form leading to the Fanconi syndrome and renal insufficiency in the first decade, a juvenile (intermediate) form in which renal disease is manifest during the second decade, and an adult (benign) form characterized by deposition of cystine in the cornea but not in the kidney.

ETIOLOGY AND PATHOGENESIS The basic defect involves impaired efflux of cystine from lysosomes rather than an abnormality in cystine catabolism. Lysosomal cystine efflux is an active, ATP-dependent process. The cystine content of tissues may be more than 100 times normal in the infantile form and more than 30 times normal in the adult form. Intracellular cystine in lysosomes does not exchange with other intracellular or extracellular pools of this amino acid. Neither plasma nor urinary concentrations of cystine are particularly elevated.

The extent of crystal deposition varies from patient to patient, depending on the form of the disease and on the methods used to prepare pathologic specimens. Cystine accumulation in the kidney causes renal insufficiency in the infantile and juvenile forms. The kidneys are pale and shrunken, the capsule is adherent, and the corticomedullary junction is obscured. Microscopically, nephron organization is interrupted, glomeruli are hyalinized, connective tissue is increased, and the normal epithelium of the tubules is replaced by cuboidal cells. Narrowing and shortening of the proximal tubule produce the swan-neck deformity that is characteristic of but not specific for cystinosis. Patchy depigmentation and degeneration of the peripheral retina occur in the infantile and juvenile forms. Cystine crystals also may be deposited in the cornea, ocular conjunctiva, or uvea.

All types of the disorder are inherited as autosomal recessive traits. In 24 families with infantile and juvenile forms of cystinosis, the mutant gene was mapped to chromosome 17p. Obligate heterozygotes have intracellular cystine concentrations intermediate between those of normal persons and affected patients but are free of clinical abnormalities.

CLINICAL MANIFESTATIONS In the infantile form, abnormalities are usually apparent by 4 to 6 months of age. Growth retardation, vomiting, fever, vitamin D–resistant rickets, polyuria, dehydration, and metabolic acidosis are prominent. Generalized proximal tubular dysfunction (the Fanconi syndrome) leads to hyperphosphaturia and hypophosphatemia, renal glycosuria, generalized amino aciduria, hypouricemia, and often hypokalemia. Pyelonephritis may contribute, along with interstitial fibrosis, to progressive glomerular insufficiency. Death due to uremia or intercurrent infection usually occurs before age 10. Ocular manifestations are prominent. Photophobia is usually demonstrable within the first years of life due to cystine deposits in the cornea, and retinal degeneration may appear even earlier.

In contrast, patients with the adult form have only ocular abnormalities. Photophobia, headache, and burning or itching of the eyes are major complaints. Glomerular and tubular function and the integrity of the retina are preserved. The findings in the juvenile variant fall between these extremes. Ocular and renal manifestations do not become significant until the second decade. The renal lesion, albeit milder than that in the infantile form, eventually leads to renal insufficiency.

DIAGNOSIS Cystinosis must be considered in any child with vitamin D–resistant rickets, the Fanconi syndrome, or glomerular insufficiency. Hexagonal or rectangular cystine crystals can be detected in the cornea (by slit-lamp examination), in leukocytes from peripheral blood or bone marrow, or in biopsies of rectal mucosa. Diagnosis can be confirmed by quantification of cystine in peripheral blood leukocytes or cultured fibroblasts. The infantile form has been diagnosed prenatally by the demonstration of increased cystine content in cultured amniotic fluid cells.

℞ TREATMENT

The adult form is benign and requires no treatment. Treatment of renal disease in the infantile or juvenile form does not differ from that of other forms of chronic renal failure: maintenance of adequate fluid intake to prevent dehydration; correction of the metabolic acidosis; and administration of supplementary calcium, phosphate, and vitamin D to heal the rickets. Such measures are effective in maintaining growth, development, and well-being in affected children for a time. One specific therapy has been useful. Administration of the free thiol cysteamine slows the progression of renal dysfunction, improves growth, and dissolves corneal cystine crystals. This compound acts in lysosomes by forming a mixed disulfide with cysteine that can be transported out of the organelle by a different transporter than the one deficient in the disease. Although cysteamine causes a definite improvement during the first few years, gradual loss of kidney function continues.

Children with nephropathic cystinosis and end-stage renal disease benefit from kidney transplantation. Those patients who tolerated the procedure and do not develop immunologic problems have return of kidney function toward normal. The transplanted kidneys have not developed the functional abnormalities typical of cystinosis (i.e., the Fanconi syndrome or glomerular insufficiency). However, patients may continue to accumulate cystine in the cornea and other ocular tissues. Because the usual life span of a transplanted kidney is generally 15 to 20 years, some patients with the infantile form of cystinosis have received two or more transplanted kidneys.

PRIMARY HYPEROXALURIA

DEFINITION Primary hyperoxaluria is the designation for two rare disorders characterized by chronic excessive urinary excretion of oxalic acid and by calcium oxalate nephrolithiasis and nephrocalcinosis. Typically, patients with both forms develop renal insufficiency early in life and die of uremia. At postmortem examination, calcium oxalate deposits are widespread in renal and extrarenal tissues, a condition referred to as *oxalosis*.

ETIOLOGY AND PATHOGENESIS The metabolic basis for the primary hyperoxalurias involves pathways of glyoxylate metabolism. In type I hyperoxaluria, urinary excretion of oxalate and of the oxidized and reduced forms of glyoxylate is increased. The excessive synthesis of these substances results from a block in glyoxylate metabolism. The primary defect in most patients is deficiency of the hepatic

peroxisomal enzyme alanine:glyoxylate amino transferase. The gene for this enzyme maps to chromosome 2q36→37, and several distinct mutations have been defined in patients with type I hyperoxaluria. Some of these mutations misdirect the enzyme to mitochondria and render it nonfunctional. Expansion of the glyoxylate pool leads to enhanced oxidation of glyoxylate to oxalate and to enhanced reduction of glyoxylate to glycolate. Each of these 2-carbon acids is then excreted in excess in the urine. In type II hyperoxaluria, L-glyceric acid is excreted in excess along with oxalate. In this condition, activity of D-glyceric acid dehydrogenase, which catalyzes the reduction of hydroxypyruvate to D-glyceric acid in the catabolic pathway of serine metabolism, is absent in leukocytes (and presumably other tissues). The accumulated hydroxypyruvate is instead reduced by lactic dehydrogenase to the L-isomer of glycerate, which is excreted in the urine. The same enzyme possesses glyoxylate reductase activity, and its deficiency promotes the oxidation of glyoxylate to oxalate, thus causing the formation of increased oxalate. Both disorders are inherited as autosomal recessive traits. Heterozygotes are asymptomatic.

Stone formation, nephrocalcinosis, and oxalosis are due to insolubility of calcium oxalate. Extrarenal deposits of oxalate are prominent in the heart, walls of arteries and veins, male urogenital tract, and bone, particularly in type I hyperoxaluria.

CLINICAL MANIFESTATIONS Nephrolithiasis and oxalosis may be manifest during the first year of life. Most patients experience renal colic or hematuria between ages 2 and 10 and succumb to uremia before age 20. With the onset of uremia, patients may develop severe peripheral arterial spasm and necrosis with resulting vascular insufficiency. Oxalate excretion falls as renal failure worsens. In patients with delayed onset of symptoms, survival to age 50 or 60 has been reported, despite recurrent nephrolithiasis. Type II hyperoxaluria is a milder disease with less involvement of extrarenal organs and delayed impairment of kidney function.

DIAGNOSIS Oxalate excretion in normal children or adults is less than 0.5 mmol (60 mg) per 1.73 m^2 surface area per day. Patients with type I or type II hyperoxaluria excrete two to four times this amount. Distinction between the two types depends on the identification of the other organic acids that identify them: glycolic acid in type I and L-glyceric acid in type II. Since patients with pyridoxine deficiency or chronic ileal disease may excrete excessive amounts of oxalate, these conditions must be excluded.

℞ TREATMENT

There is no satisfactory treatment. Urinary oxalate concentration can be transiently reduced by increasing the urinary flow rate. Large doses of pyridoxine (100 mg/d) may reduce urinary oxalate in some patients, but long-term effects are not dramatic. A diet high in phosphate content seems to reduce the frequency of renal colic, but oxalate excretion is unaffected. Combined liver-kidney transplantation can correct the enzyme deficiency and replace the damaged organs and warrants further study.

BIBLIOGRAPHY

BOUSHLEY CJ et al: A quantitative assessment of plasma homocysteine as a risk factor for vascular disease. Probable benefit of increasing folic acid intakes. JAMA 274:1049, 1995

DANPURE CJ, PURDUE PE: Primary hyperoxaluria, in *The Molecular and Metabolic Bases of Inherited Disease*, 7th ed, CR Scriver et al (eds). New York, McGraw-Hill, 1995, p 2385

ELSAS LJ, ACOSTA PB: Nutritional support of inherited metabolic diseases, in *Modern Nutrition in Health and Disease*, 8th ed, ME Shils et al (eds). Philadelphia, Lea & Febiger, 1994, p 1147

FENTON WA, ROSENBERG LE: Inherited disorders of cobalamin transport and metabolism, in *The Molecular and Metabolic Bases of Inherited Disease*, 7th ed, CR Scriver et al (eds). New York, McGraw-Hill, 1995, p 3129

FROSST P et al: A candidate genetic risk factor for vascular disease: A common mutation in methylenetetrahydrofolate reductase. Nature (Genetics) 10:111, 1995

GAHL WA et al: Lysosomal transport disorders: Cystinosis and sialic acid storage disorders, in *The Molecular and Metabolic Bases of Inherited Disease*, 7th ed, CR Scriver et al (eds). New York, McGraw-Hill, 1995, p 3763

LA DU BN: Alkaptonuria, in *The Molecular and Metabolic Bases of Inherited Disease*, 7th ed, CR Scriver et al (eds). New York, McGraw-Hill, 1995, p 1371

MUDD SH et al: Disorders of transsulfuration, in *The Molecular and Metabolic Bases of Inherited Disease*, 7th ed, CR Scriver et al (eds). New York, McGraw-Hill, 1995, p 1279

ROSENBERG LE, SCRIVER CR: Disorders of amino acid metabolism, in *Metabolic Control and Disease*, 8th ed, PK Bondy, LE Rosenberg (eds). Philadelphia, Saunders, 1980, p 583

ROSENBLATT DS: Inherited disorders of folate transport and metabolism, in *The Molecular and Metabolic Bases of Inherited Disease*, 7th ed, CR Scriver et al (eds). New York, McGraw-Hill, 1995, p 3111

SCRIVER CR et al: The hyperphenylalaninemias, in *The Molecular and Metabolic Bases of Inherited Disease*, 7th ed, CR Scriver et al (eds). New York, McGraw-Hill, 1995, p 1015

350

Louis S. Elsas, Nicola Longo, Leon E. Rosenberg

INHERITED DEFECTS OF MEMBRANE TRANSPORT

The passage of many molecules across plasma cell membranes depends on transport systems that owe their specificity to membrane receptor and "carrier" proteins. These membrane constituents recognize individual molecules or structurally related substances and catalyze their transmembrane movement. The disorders considered in this chapter have three features in common: each is characterized by a specific defect in the transport of one or more compounds; each is inherited as a dominant or recessive trait, implying that variation in a single genetic locus is involved; and each is presumed to reflect a primary alteration in a specific membrane protein. Some of these defects have been well characterized physiologically and genetically, and the genes and/or cDNAs encoding several of these transporters have been identified.

More than 20 inherited disorders of membrane transport have been described (Table 350-1). Most affect the gut and/or kidney only. Classes of substrates represented include amino acids, sugars, cations, anions, vitamins, and water. Some are discussed elsewhere in this text. Those impairing the transport of amino acids, hexoses, urate, and chloride are discussed here as examples of the abnormalities encountered.

DISORDERS OF AMINO ACID TRANSPORT

As noted in Table 350-1, ten disorders of amino acid transport have been described. Five (cystinuria, dibasicaminoaciduria, Hartnup disease, iminoglycinuria, and dicarboxylicaminoaciduria) show transport abnormalities for structurally related amino acids, thereby implying the existence of group-specific membrane receptors or carriers. With the exception of iminoglycinuria and dicarboxylicaminoaciduria, the defects have important clinical consequences. The remaining five disorders affect the transport of only one amino acid, implying the existence of substrate-specific transport systems. Each of these conditions affects transport in the kidney, gut, or both; none has been shown to alter transport in other tissues.

CYSTINURIA   Definition   Cystinuria, the most common inborn error of amino acid transport, is characterized by impaired tubular reabsorption and excessive urinary excretion of the dibasic amino acids lysine, arginine, ornithine, and cystine. A similar transport defect exists in the intestinal mucosa. Because cystine is the least soluble of the naturally occurring amino acids, its overexcretion predisposes to the formation of renal, ureteral, and bladder stones. Such stones are responsible for the signs and symptoms of the disorder.

Etiology and Pathogenesis   Massive excretion of cystine and the other dibasic amino acids occurs in homozygotes for classic cystinuria. The disorder, inherited as an autosomal recessive trait, results from impaired function of membrane carrier proteins essential for transport of this group of amino acids in the apical brush border of proximal renal tubule and small intestinal cells. Although the renal clearance of all four amino acids is increased in homozygotes, the presence of some residual transport capacity for these compounds plus the existence of three other disorders marked by selective excretion of members of this group (dibasicaminoaciduria, hypercystinuria, lysinuria) argues for the existence of at least three discrete renal transport systems for these amino acids: one for each amino acid alone; one shared by lysine, arginine, and ornithine; and one for all four amino acids.

Whereas urinary excretion patterns and renal clearance abnormalities in all homozygotes are similar, evidence for three variants has come from studies of intestinal transport in homozygotes and of urinary excretion in heterozygotes. Type I homozygotes lack mediated intestinal transport of cystine, lysine, arginine, and ornithine; heterozygotes have normal urinary amino acid excretion patterns. Type II homozygotes lack mediated lysine transport in the gut but retain some capacity for cystine transport; heterozygotes have moderately increased urinary excretion of each of the four amino acids. Type III homozygotes retain some capacity for mediated intestinal transport of the four involved substrates; heterozygotes have modestly increased urinary lysine and cystine. The gene for type I cystinuria, solute carrier family 3 (SLC3A1), has been mapped to 2p16.3. Heterogeneous mutations in this gene cause the type I disorder. Some of the mutations virtually abolish cystine transport when the mutant cDNAs are expressed in reporter cells.

Clinical Manifestations   Cystinuria is among the most common inborn errors, with a frequency of 1 in 10,000 to 1 in 15,000 in many ethnic groups. Two-thirds of adults with cystinuria are type I homozygotes. Cystine stones account for 1 to 2 percent of all urinary tract calculi but are the most common cause of stones in children. The maximum solubility of cystine in the physiologic urinary pH range of 4.5 to 7.0 is about 1200 μmol/L (300 mg/L). Since affected homozygotes regularly excrete 2400 to 7200 μmol (600 to 1800 mg) daily, crystalluria and stone formation are a constant threat. Stone formation usually becomes manifest in the second or third decade but may occur in the first year of life or as bladder calculi in the newborn. Symptoms and signs are those typical of urolithiasis: hematuria, flank pain, renal colic, obstructive uropathy, and infection (see Chap. 279). Recurrent urolithiasis may lead to progressive renal insufficiency.

Diagnosis   The presence of cystine in a urinary tract stone is pathognomonic of cystinuria. However, since half the stones in cystinuric subjects are of mixed composition and since as many as 10 percent may have a cystine core that is not detected, a urinary nitroprusside test should be done on all patients with urolithiasis to exclude this diagnosis. The nitroprusside test is also positive (appearance of a cherry red color) in some heterozygotes for cystinuria and in patients with hypercystinuria, homocystinuria, and mercaptolactate-cystine disulfiduria. When cystine content exceeds 1000 μmol/L (250 mg/L), cystine crystals may be seen in the sediment of acidified, concentrated, chilled urine. These hexagonal crystals are pathognomonic of cystine overexcretion in patients not taking sulfonamides.

Diagnostic confirmation of cystinuria depends on demonstration of the characteristic amino acid excretion pattern in the urine. Selective overexcretion of cystine, lysine, arginine, and ornithine can be demonstrated by qualitative and quantitative chromatography. Quantitation is important for differentiating some heterozygotes from homozygotes and for following free cystine excretion during therapy.

℞ **TREATMENT**

Management is aimed at preventing cystine crystal formation by reducing the concentration of cystine in urine. This aim is accomplished by increasing urinary volume and by maintaining an alkaline urine pH. Fluid ingestion in excess of 4 L/d is essential, and 5 to 7 L/d is optimal. Urinary cystine concentration should be less than 1000 to 1200 μmol/L (250 to 300 mg/L). The daily fluid ingestion necessary to maintain this dilution of excreted cystine should be

Table 350-1

Genetic Disorders of Membrane Transport

Class of Substance and Disorder	Individual Substrates	Tissues Manifesting Transport Defect	Proposed Molecular Basis of Defect	Major Clinical Manifestations	Mode of Inheritance	Location of Discussion
AMINO ACIDS						
Classic cystinuria	Cystine, lysine, arginine, ornithine	Proximal renal tubule, jejunal mucosa	Mutation of shared dibasic-cystine transport protein	Cystine nephrolithiasis	Autosomal recessive	Chap. 350
Dibasicamino-aciduria	Lysine, arginine, ornithine	Proximal renal tubule, jejunal mucosa	Mutation of dibasic transport protein	Type I: Benign Type II: Protein intolerance, hyperammonemia, retardation	Autosomal recessive	Chap. 350
Hypercystinuria	Cystine	Proximal renal tubule	Mutation of cystine transport protein	Some risk of cystine nephrolithiasis	Autosomal recessive	Chap. 350
Lysinuria	Lysine	Proximal renal tubule, jejunal mucosa	Mutation of lysine transport protein	Seizures, physical and mental retardation	Possible autosomal recessive	Chap. 350
Hartnup disease	Neutral amino acids	Proximal renal tubule, jejunal mucosa	Mutation of shared neutral amino acid transport protein	Constant neutral aminoaciduria, intermittent symptoms of pellagra	Autosomal recessive	Chap. 350
Tryptophan malabsorption	Tryptophan	Jejunal mucosa	Mutation of tryptophan transport protein	Indoluria, ?hypercalcemia, ?nephrocalcinosis	Probable autosomal recessive	Chap. 350
Methionine malabsorption	Methionine	Jejunal mucosa	Mutation of methionine transport protein	α-Hydroxybutyricaciduria, white hair, mental retardation, convulsions, hyperpneic attacks, edema	Probable autosomal recessive	Chap. 350
Histidinuria	Histidine	Proximal renal tubule, jejunal mucosa	Mutation of histidine transport protein	Mental retardation	Autosomal recessive	Chap. 350
Iminoglycinuria	Glycine, proline, hydroxyproline	Proximal renal tubule, jejunal mucosa	Mutation of shared glycine–imino acid transport protein	None	Autosomal recessive	Chap. 350
Dicarboxylic-aminoaciduria	Glutamic acid, aspartic acid	Proximal renal tubule, jejunal mucosa	Mutation of shared dicarboxylic amino acid transport protein	None	Probable autosomal recessive	Chap. 350
Cystinosis	Cystine	Lysosomal membranes	Mutation of cystine transport protein	Renal failure, hypothyroidism, blindness	Autosomal recessive	Chap. 349
HEXOSES						
Renal glycosuria	D-Glucose	Proximal renal tubule	Mutation of D-glucose transport protein	Glycosuria with normal blood glucose	Autosomal recessive	Chap. 350
Glucose-galactose malabsorption	D-Glucose D-Galactose	Jejunal mucosa, proximal renal tubule	Mutation of shared Na^+-dependent glucose-galactose transport protein	Watery diarrhea on feeding glucose, lactose, sucrose, or galactose	Autosomal recessive	Chaps. 285, 350
LIPIDS						
Familial hypercholesterolemia	Cholesterol	Fibroblasts, lymphoid lines, leukocytes	Mutation of membrane LDL–cholesterol receptor protein	Hypercholesterolemia, tendon xanthomas, arcus corneae, coronary artery atherosclerosis	Autosomal dominant	Chap. 341
URATE						
Hypouricemia	Uric acid	Proximal renal tubule	Mutation of urate transport protein	Hypouricemia, hyperuricosuria, ?hypercalcinuria	Autosomal recessive	Chap. 350

(continued)

Table 350-1—*(Continued)*

Genetic Disorders of Membrane Transport

Class of Substance and Disorder	Individual Substrates	Tissues Manifesting Transport Defect	Proposed Molecular Basis of Defect	Major Clinical Manifestations	Mode of Inheritance	Location of Discussion
ANIONS						
Familial hypophosphatemic rickets	Inorganic phosphate	Proximal renal tubule, jejunal mucosa	Mutation of inorganic phosphate transport protein	Hypophosphatemia, phosphaturia, phosphatopenic rickets/osteomalacia	X-linked dominant	Chap. 355
Congenital chloridorrhea	Chloride	Ileal and colonic mucosa	Mutation of Cl^-/H^+ uptake pump of Cl^-/HCO_3^- exchange pump carrier protein	Hydramnios, watery diarrhea, elevated fecal chloride, achloriduria, metabolic alkalosis with volume depletion, hyperaldosteronism	Autosomal recessive	Chaps. 285, 350
Cystic fibrosis	Chloride	Lung, pancreas, sweat gland	Mutation of ion channel protein	Pulmonary, pancreatic destruction	Autosomal recessive	Chap. 257
Familial goiter	Inorganic iodide	Thyroid gland, salivary gland, gastric mucosa	Mutation of iodide transport protein	Congenital hypothyroidism (cretinism), goiter	Probable autosomal recessive	Chap. 331
CATIONS						
Distal renal tubular acidosis (type I—gradient)	Hydrogen ion	Distal renal tubule	Mutation of distal tubule H^+ pump carrier protein	Hyperchloremic acidosis, hypokalemia, acquired nephrocalcinosis, and hypercalcinuria	Autosomal dominant	Chap. 278
Proximal renal tubular acidosis (type II—HCO_3^- wasting)	Hydrogen ion	Proximal renal tubule	Mutation of proximal tubule H^+ pump carrier protein	Hyperchloremic acidosis, bicarbonate wasting	Probable autosomal recessive	Chap. 278
Menkes' disease	Copper	Most tissues except liver	Mutation of copper-transporting ATPase (ATP7B)	Severe mental retardation, pili torti (kinky hair), typical facies, arterial tortuosity, excess Wormian bones, thermal instability	X-linked recessive	Chap. 80
Wilson's disease	Copper	Liver and kidney	Mutation in copper-transporting ATPase (ATP7B)	Motor and psychiatric disturbances, hepatolenticular degeneration	Autosomal recessive	Chap. 345
Lethal diarrhea	Sodium ion	Jejunal intestinal cells	Mutation of Na^+/H^+ proton exchange pump	Watery diarrhea, severe sodium depletion, and acidosis	Recessive?	Chap. 285
WATER						
Nephrogenic diabetes insipidus (AVP-resistant)	Water	Distal renal tubule	Lack of activation of AVP-responsive luminal membrane adenylate cyclase, possible defect in receptor or enzyme protein	Polyuria, polydipsia, hyposthenuria	X-linked recessive	Chap. 278
VITAMINS						
Juvenile pernicious anemia	Cobalamin (vitamin B_{12})	Ileal mucosa	Mutation of receptor for intrinsic factor–cobalamin complex	Megaloblastic anemia	Autosomal recessive	Chap. 108
Folate malabsorption	Folic acid	Small bowel	Mutation of folate transport protein	Megaloblastic anemia	Autosomal recessive	Chap. 108
OTHER						
Sialic acid storage	Sialic acid (monosaccharide)	Lysosomes	Mutation of sialic acid transport protein	Retardation	Autosomal recessive	Chap. 346
Carnitine transport	Carnitine	Muscle, kidney leukocytes, fibroblasts	Mutation of high-affinity carnitine transporter	Hypoketotic hypoglycemia, cardiomyopathy, hypotonia	Autosomal recessive	Chap. 335

spaced over 24 h, with one-third of the total volume ingested between bedtime and 2 to 3 A.M. Stones can be prevented and even dissolved by such hydration. It must be made clear to cystinuric subjects that for them water is a necessary drug. Solubility of cystine rises sharply in urine above pH 7.5, and urinary alkalinization can be therapeutic in some situations. Vigorous administration of sodium bicarbonate, acetazolamide, and polycitrates is required to maintain a persistently alkaline pH, but this measure introduces the danger of inducing formation of calcium oxalate, calcium phosphate, and magnesium ammonium phosphate stones and of producing nephrocalcinosis.

Another treatment involves administration of penicillamine, which undergoes sulfhydryl-disulfide exchange with cystine to form the mixed disulfide of penicillamine and cysteine. Since this disulfide is more than 50 times as soluble as cystine, penicillamine (in doses of 1 to 3 g/d) reduces free cystine excretion markedly, thereby preventing new stone formation and promoting dissolution of existing calculi. Unfortunately, side effects include acute serum sickness, agranulocytosis, pancytopenia, immune glomerulitis, and the Goodpasture syndrome. Thus its use should be reserved for patients who fail to respond to hydration alone or who are in a high-risk category (one remaining kidney, renal insufficiency). Those patients unable to tolerate penicillamine may benefit from α-mercaptopropionylglycine, an experimental drug whose mechanism of action is similar to that of penicillamine but whose structure, and hence toxicity, is different. As many as two-thirds of patients unable to tolerate penicillamine may take α-mercaptopropionylglycine without ill effects. Captopril, a sulfhydryl-containing antihypertensive agent, is ineffective in reducing cystine excretion. When medical management fails, urologic surgery is required but should be considered a last resort since cystine stones reform more easily in scarred epithelium. Lithotripsy is not useful and may produce smaller fragments that cause severe colic. Occasional patients may require renal transplantation.

DIBASICAMINOACIDURIA   This disorder is characterized by a defect in renal tubular reabsorption of lysine, arginine, and ornithine but *not* of cystine. The disorder almost surely reflects mutations in the gene(s) coding for a widely distributed transport protein used solely by the three dibasic amino acids. Two variants are each apparently inherited as an autosomal recessive trait. Manifestations are related to the losses of ornithine, arginine, and perhaps lysine.

In the common form of dibasicaminoaciduria (type II), also known as *lysinuric protein intolerance* and more common in Finland (1 in 60,000) than elsewhere, homozygotes show defective intestinal transport of dibasic amino acids as well as exaggerated renal losses. The transport defect affects basolateral rather than luminal membrane transport and is associated with impairment of the urea cycle. Affected individuals present in childhood with hepatosplenomegaly, protein intolerance, and episodic ammonia intoxication. Older subjects may present with severe osteoporosis, impairment of kidney function, or interstitial changes in the lungs. Plasma concentrations of lysine, arginine, and ornithine are reduced, and urinary excretion of lysine is increased. Hyperammonemia may develop after the ingestion of protein loads or with infections and is believed to be due to insufficient amounts of arginine and ornithine to maintain proper function of the urea cycle. The clinical features have been attributed to the hyperammonemia and to insufficient amounts of lysine to support synthesis of protein and carnitine during growth. Obligate heterozygotes are healthy and show no excess urinary loss of dibasic amino acids.

Type I dibasicaminoaciduria has been described in a large French-Canadian kindred. These patients have profound mental retardation without hyperammonemia or protein intolerance. The condition also differs from type II by the presence of modest excesses of dibasic amino acids in urine of asymptomatic heterozygotes. Type I disease may involve the same transport system as that impaired in the more common type II disorder.

Treatment includes dietary protein restriction and supplementation with citrulline, a neutral amino acid whose intestinal and hepatic transport are unimpaired, and which, when metabolized to arginine and ornithine, fuels the urea cycle. With 2.0 to 8.0 g of oral citrulline daily, dietary protein intake can be increased and growth improved in children. Carnitine supplements may improve growth by sparing lysine and by enhancing fatty acid oxidation.

HARTNUP DISEASE   Pellagra-like skin lesions, variable neurologic manifestations, and neutral or aromatic aminoaciduria characterize this disease. Alanine, serine, threonine, valine, leucine, isoleucine, phenylalanine, tyrosine, tryptophan, glutamine, asparagine, and histidine are excreted in urine in quantities 5 to 10 times normal, and intestinal transport for these same amino acids is defective. The clinical manifestations result from nutritional deficiency of the essential amino acid tryptophan, caused by intestinal and renal malabsorption. Manifestations are episodic, related, at least in part, to metabolic demands for tryptophan. Only a small fraction of patients with the chemical findings of this disorder develop a pellagra-like syndrome, implying that manifestations depend on factors over and above the transport defect.

The major pathway of tryptophan metabolism leads to the synthesis of niacin and nicotinamide-adenine dinucleotide. This pathway supplies about half the daily niacin needs. In patients with Hartnup disease, the renal and intestinal transport defect for tryptophan leads to niacin deficiency. The transport defect likely reflects abnormalities of a group-specific system for neutral amino acids. Some residual reabsorptive capacity persists for each involved amino acid. This suggests that they are transported by other carrier systems as well, a conclusion supported by the identification of patients with substrate-specific transport errors for tryptophan, methionine, and histidine.

Hartnup disease is inherited as an autosomal recessive trait. Homozygotes occur with a frequency of about 1 in 24,000 births. Heterozygotes exhibit no clinical or chemical abnormalities.

Pellagra is the clinical syndrome produced by dietary niacin deficiency, and its features are those of Hartnup disease (see Chap. 79). The diagnosis of Hartnup disease should be suspected in any patient with pellagra without a history of dietary niacin deficiency. The neurologic and psychiatric manifestations range from attacks of cerebellar ataxia with mild emotional lability to frank delirium and usually accompany exacerbations of the erythematous, eczematoid skin rash. Fever, sunlight, stress, and sulfonamide therapy provoke clinical relapses. Diagnosis is made by detection of the neutral aminoaciduria that does not occur in dietary niacin deficiency. Treatment is directed at niacin repletion and includes a high-protein diet and daily nicotinamide supplementation (50 to 250 mg). Tryptophan ethyl esters also can bypass the absorption defect.

IMINOGLYCINURIA   This benign autosomal recessive trait is characterized by excessive urinary excretion of glycine and the imino acids proline and hydroxyproline. Homozygotes occur with a frequency of about 1 in 16,000. The enhanced excretion of glycine, proline, and hydroxyproline reflects a defect in the tubular transport system shared by these three compounds. An intestinal transport defect also may be present. This suggests that more than one mutation may lead to iminoglycinuria, a thesis corroborated by the demonstration that obligate heterozygotes from some but not all families have glycinuria. No consistent clinical abnormalities have been reported in homozygotes, who are usually detected by urinary amino acid screening programs.

DICARBOXYLICAMINOACIDURIA   Selective urinary loss and exaggerated endogenous renal clearance of glutamic and aspartic acids have been described in two unrelated children. Intestinal absorption of these dicarboxylic amino acids was impaired in one. This child had recurrent hypoglycemia; the other was asymptomatic.

SUBSTRATE-SPECIFIC DEFECTS IN AMINO ACID TRANSPORT   Rare pedigrees exist in which individuals have defective renal tubular reabsorption and/or impaired intestinal absorption of a single free amino acid. These disorders, each apparently inherited as an autosomal recessive trait, suggest that transport of amino acids is catalyzed by substrate-specific as well as group-specific transport mechanisms.

Hypercystinuria Two siblings exhibited modest cystinuria without excessive urinary excretion of lysine, arginine, or ornithine. Fractional tubular reabsorption of cystine was reduced to about 80 percent of the filtered load, and up to 250 mg/d was excreted in the urine. Intestinal absorption of cystine was normal. Both were clinically well, although the cystine excretion places them at risk for cystine urolithiasis. Cystine excretion by the parents was normal.

Lysinuria A child with selective impairment of renal tubular reabsorption of lysine has been described. Endogenous lysine clearance was increased; intestinal transport was impaired; plasma lysine was reduced. Mental and growth retardation and seizures were present. A lysine-supplemented diet stimulated growth. Carnitine requires lysine for biosynthesis and may be deficient in this condition.

Histidinuria Two siblings, each with mental retardation, exhibited a selective renal transport defect for histidine. Urinary loss of histidine approached 40 to 50 percent of the filtered load, and intestinal transport of histidine also was defective. The clinically normal parents had normal urinary excretion but a modest defect in intestinal absorption of histidine. In two additional cases of isolated histidinuria myoclonic seizures occurred.

Methionine Malabsorption Children from two pedigrees have shown an intestinal transport defect for methionine. One may have had a renal transport defect as well. This disorder was detected because of urinary excretion of α-hydroxybutyric acid, a by-product of the intestinal bacterial breakdown of the unabsorbed methionine. This compound, which gives an odor resembling malt or dried celery to the urine, appears to be responsible for the white hair, attacks of hyperpnea, convulsions, edema, and mental retardation. Treatment of one of these children with a methionine-restricted diet caused improvement in all clinical manifestations. Transient methioninuria in early childhood has been associated with colic that improved with dietary methionine restriction.

Tryptophan Malabsorption An isolated defect in intestinal absorption of tryptophan has been described in two siblings. The renal tubular reabsorption of tryptophan was normal. A number of indoles were excreted in stool and urine. These compounds result from chemical degradation of unabsorbed tryptophan by intestinal bacteria and may be present in patients with Hartnup disease as well. Because of concomitant renal disease, hydrolytic enzymes were released into the urine, acted on the indoles found there, and led to the formation of a blue pigment, indigotin. This sequence of events earned this condition the sobriquet "blue-diaper syndrome." No pellagra-like symptoms were described. The mother also excreted indole compounds, suggesting that she is a carrier of this trait.

DISORDERS OF HEXOSE TRANSPORT

Nondiabetic melituria occurs in a number of conditions. Pentoses, hexoses, heptoses, and disaccharides have been identified in the urine; all except sucrose yield a positive test for reducing substances. Some meliturias result from diffuse renal injury, others from ingestion of nonmetabolizable sugars. In still others the sugars accumulate in blood owing to deficient activity of catabolizing enzyme systems and "spill" into the urine. Only among the hexoses have specific inherited disorders of sugar transport been identified. The existence of renal glycosuria and intestinal glucose-galactose malabsorption as heritable, autosomal recessive disorders points to the existence of at least two specific carrier proteins for hexoses in human jejunal and renal brush border membranes: one for glucose and one shared by glucose and galactose.

RENAL GLYCOSURIA Renal glycosuria is characterized by the urinary excretion of glucose at normal concentrations of blood glucose. The renal tubular malabsorption is specific for glucose. Unlike generalized tubular dysfunction, other compounds such as phosphate and amino acids are transported normally. The condition is benign, but occasionally glycosuria may be great enough to cause polyuria

and polydipsia. Even more rarely, dehydration or ketosis may develop under conditions of stress such as pregnancy or starvation.

In normal persons, glucose is present in the glomerular filtrate at a concentration equal to that in plasma water and is reabsorbed throughout the proximal renal tubule by a sodium-dependent, phlorizin-inhibitable transport process. Reabsorptive capacity exceeds normal plasma glucose concentration. Thus glucose does not appear in the urine until the threshold for reabsorption is reached. The plasma concentration at which filtered glucose begins to escape proximal tubular reabsorption is usually around 10 mmol/L (200 mg/dL). Maximal renal reabsorptive capacity is exceeded at a filtered load of around 2 mmol (325 mg)/min per 1.73 m^2 body surface area, and this value is defined as the tubular maximum for glucose (TmG).

Two patterns of glycosuria are recognized: type A, characterized by a reduced tubular maximum reabsorptive capacity, and type B, showing a reduced threshold for glycosuria, an increased "splay" in the titration curve, and a normal TmG. Renal glycosuria occurs in homozygotes for either of these recessively inherited mutations and in compound heterozygotes for these presumably allelic mutations. Modest reduction in renal threshold or TmG is present in heterozygotes in some families; modest glycosuria occurs in such family members when plasma glucose is elevated. In the few patients studied, renal glycosuria was not associated with impaired intestinal transport.

GLUCOSE-GALACTOSE MALABSORPTION In this condition, infants develop a profuse, watery diarrhea when fed milk or foods containing lactose, sucrose, glucose, or galactose. Fructose or carbohydrate-free formulas are well tolerated. A specific defect in intestinal absorption of glucose and galactose can be demonstrated by oral tolerance tests that produce little or no increase in plasma glucose or galactose. The primary defect involves the sodium/hexose cotransporter in the intestinal and renal brush border. Active D-glucose and D-galactose transport is absent in affected children, and intermediate transport capacity is present in their parents. These findings confirm the specificity and the autosomal recessive inheritance of the disorder. Treatment with a glucose- and galactose-free diet leads to resolution of symptoms in childhood. Although the basic transport defect is present throughout life, most patients show an improved tolerance for glucose and galactose with age.

A number of these patients have renal glycosuria at normal plasma glucose concentrations. Renal titration studies generally demonstrate a reduced threshold for glucose reabsorption (type B renal glycosuria) and a normal TmG. Urinary glucose loss is not as severe as in isolated renal glycosuria. This finding suggests the presence of multiple glucose transport proteins in the kidney. One, whose gene remains to be identified, is responsible for the bulk of glucose reabsorption, is located in the proximal convoluted tubule, and is believed to be abnormal in renal glycosuria. Another (SGLT1) is shared by glucose and galactose and is responsible for the reabsorption of the last traces of glucose in the late proximal straight tubule. SGLT1 is abnormal in glucose-galactose malabsorption, and heterogeneous mutations have been demonstrated in the encoding gene on chromosome 22q. In glucose-galactose malabsorption, as in renal glycosuria, transport of sugars in other tissues is normal, reflecting the multiplicity and tissue specificity of hexose transporters.

DEFECTIVE URATE TRANSPORT: HYPOURICEMIA

Individuals with a selective defect in renal tubular reabsorption of sodium urate have marked hypouricemia with serum urate levels ranging from 12 to 110 μmol/L (0.2 to 1.8 mg/dL). Moderate uricosuria is present, and 25 percent of patients have renal calculi, which is the only known adverse manifestation of this condition.

Renal urate clearance normally averages 15 percent of glomerular filtration rate, and the excreted urate is composed both of filtered urate that has escaped reabsorption and of secreted urate. Subjects with isolated hypouricemia have urate clearances averaging from 33 to 85 percent of the filtration rate; in some, urate clearance exceeds the glomerular filtration rate. Studies with probenecid, which blocks tubular reabsorption of urate, and pyrazinamide, which blocks tubular secretion, reveal that 11 of the 16 families described have a presecretory urate reabsorptive defect, and 5 have defective transport affecting the entire tubule. In four families hypercalciuria due to enhanced intestinal calcium absorption is also present, but in others only uricosuria has been demonstrated. The defect is inherited as an autosomal recessive trait. Urate transport appears to be normal in nonrenal tissue. Obligate heterozygotes have moderately increased urate clearance. The defect is presumed to reflect mutation of one or both of the proximal renal tubular membrane proteins that transport sodium urate. The findings in these families support the hypothesis that renal urate reabsorption is controlled by more than one transport protein.

DEFECTIVE ANION TRANSPORT: CHLORIDORRHEA

This rare, autosomal recessive disease results from impairment of active transport of chloride in the ileum and colon. Absence of chloride-bicarbonate ion exchange causes profound symptoms even before birth (polyhydramnios and absence of meconium). Massive watery diarrhea is apparent from the first days of life. This fluid loss, with its attendant impairment of electrolyte homeostasis, is life-threatening. A hypokalemic, hypochloremic, hyponatremic metabolic alkalosis develops with dehydration and secondary hyperaldosteronism. Fecal fluid contains an excess of chloride ion over the sum of the accompanying cations sodium and potassium. Fecal chloride concentration always exceeds 90 mmol/L when volume and serum electrolyte disturbances are corrected, and this chloridorrhea is diagnostic. Renal chloride transport is normal. Decreased urine chloride results from the kidney's attempts to conserve salt and water. The gene for this condition maps to chromosome 7q and is distinct from the gene that is mutated in cystic fibrosis.

℞ TREATMENT

Treatment requires adequate, lifelong repletion of electrolyte and fluid losses. Exact replacement of water, sodium chloride, and potassium chloride can prevent the growth and psychomotor retardation and the development of progressive renal damage. The renal lesion, with hyalinized glomeruli, juxtaglomerular hyperplasia, calcifications, and arteriolar changes, is probably a result of chronic volume depletion. Treatment of hyperreninemia and hypokalemia with prostaglandin inhibitors may reduce renal damage but does not alter intestinal symptoms or the need for chronic sodium chloride repletion.

BIBLIOGRAPHY

DESJEUX JF: Congenital selective Na⁺ D-glucose cotransport defects leading to renal glycosuria and congenital selective intestinal malabsorption of glucose and galactose, in *The Molecular and Metabolic Bases of Inherited Disease*, 7th ed, CR Scriver et al (eds). New York, McGraw-Hill, 1995, p 3563

ELSAS LJ, ROSENBERG LE: Renal glycosuria, in *Strauss and Welt's Diseases of the Kidney*, 3d ed, LE Earley, CW Gottschalk (eds). Boston, Little, Brown, 1979, pp 1021–1028

———, LONGO N: Glucose transporters: Human disorders and insulin receptor regulation. Int Pediatr l0:57,1995

GASPARINI P et al: Molecular genetics of cystinuria: Identification of four new mutations and seven polymorphisms and evidence for genetic heterogeneity. Am J Hum Genet 57:781, 1995

LEVY HL: Hartnup disorder, in *The Molecular and Metabolic Bases of Inherited Disease*, 7th ed, CR Scriver et al (eds). New York, McGraw-Hill, 1995, p 3629

SEGAL S, THIER SO: Cystinuria, in *The Molecular and Metabolic Bases of Inherited Disease*, 7th ed, CR Scriver et al (eds). New York, McGraw-Hill, 1995, p 3581

SHORT EM, ROSENBERG LE: Renal aminoaciduria, in *Strauss and Welt's Diseases of the Kidney*, 3d ed, LE Earley, CW Gottschalk (eds). Boston, Little, Brown, 1979, pp 975–1020

SIMELL O: Lysinuric protein intolerance and other cationic aminoacidurias, in *The Molecular and Metabolic Bases of Inherited Disease*, 7th ed, CR Scriver et al (eds). New York, McGraw-Hill, 1995, p 3603

SPERLING O: Hereditary renal hypouricemia, in *The Molecular and Metabolic Bases of Inherited Disease*, 7th ed, CR Scriver et al (eds). New York, McGraw-Hill, 1995, p 3747

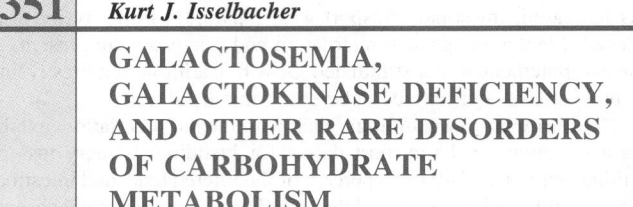

351   *Kurt J. Isselbacher*

GALACTOSEMIA, GALACTOKINASE DEFICIENCY, AND OTHER RARE DISORDERS OF CARBOHYDRATE METABOLISM

DEFINITION   *Galactosemia* refers to any of three inborn errors of galactose metabolism. *Classic galactosemia* is due to the deficiency of galactose-1-phosphate uridyl transferase (GALT) and is typically associated with cataract formation, mental retardation, and cirrhosis. The second disorder, *galactokinase deficiency*, leads primarily to cataract formation. The third, *UDP-galactose-4-epimerase deficiency*, is the rarest of the group; few cases have been described, and the eventual outcome is uncertain.

PATHOGENESIS   Lactose, the main carbohydrate in milk, is a disaccharide containing galactose and glucose; when ingested, it is hydrolyzed by intestinal lactase. Normally, the absorbed galactose is converted to glucose in the liver. The first reaction in this pathway is the phosphorylation of galactose to galactose-1-phosphate by galactokinase (specified by a gene on chromosome 17):

$$\text{Galactose} + \text{ATP} \xrightarrow{\text{galactokinase}} \text{galactose-1-phosphate}$$

The next step involves the conversion of galactose-1-phosphate to glucose-1-phosphate by GALT (the gene for which is on chromosome 9):

$$\text{Galactose-1-phosphate} + \text{UDP-glucose}$$

$$\xrightarrow{\text{GALT}} \text{UDP-galactose} + \text{glucose-1-phosphate}$$

The uridine diphosphate (UDP) sugars can be reversibly interconverted by an epimerase reaction (UDP-galactose-4-epimerase):

$$\text{UDP-galactose} \rightleftharpoons \text{UDP-glucose}$$

Galactose also can be metabolized by alternative pathways. It can be converted (reduced) in the presence of NADPH (or NADH) to galactitol (dulcitol) by aldose reductase. It also can be oxidized to a limited extent by galactose dehydrogenase, leading to the formation of galactonic acid, xyulose, and CO_2. These pathways account for limited galactose metabolism in patients with galactosemia.

In galactokinase deficiency, galactose accumulates in the blood and tissues. In the lens, galactose is converted by aldose reductase to galactitol, a sugar to which the lens is impermeable. As a consequence, excessive hydration occurs which, together with a decrease in glutathione in the lens, leads to cataract formation.

In classic galactosemia, GALT deficiency results in tissue accumulation of galactose-1-phosphate and galactose. As in galactokinase deficiency, cataracts develop secondary to galactitol accumulation in the lens. It is assumed that the cirrhosis and mental retardation of classic galactosemia are related to increased amounts of galactose-1-phosphate in these tissues. Elevated blood galactose levels may lead to a decreased hepatic output of glucose and hence to hypoglycemia. In the kidney and intestine, accumulation of galactose and galactose-1-phosphate appears to lead to an inhibition of amino acid transport. In female homozygotes there is an increased incidence of hypergonadotrophic hypogonadism in which ovarian failure develops at an early age, and this complication may persist despite dietary therapy.

Both galactokinase and GALT deficiencies are transmitted as autosomal recessive traits. Heterozygotes for these disorders have half-normal enzyme levels but are asymptomatic. Maternal deficiency of galactokinase, together with lactose intake during pregnancy, may contribute to cataract formation during fetal development. However, not all persons with decreased GALT enzyme activity in their cells are carriers of classic galactosemia. GALT is a polymorphic enzyme, and the most common variant, called the *Duarte variant* (D), has reduced activity. In addition, the D allele has numerous isoforms.

The most common mutation of the GALT gene that causes classic galactosemia is the Q188R substitution (G); the homozygous form of this disorder (GG) has a frequency of about 1 per 40,000 births in the white population. The Duarte phenotypes (D/N, D/D, and D/G) have approximately 75, 50, and 25 percent of normal GALT activity, respectively, and occur with an overall prevalence of about 6 percent in whites. Such individuals are clinically asymptomatic.

CLINICAL FEATURES   Symptoms of classic galactosemia usually begin within days to weeks after birth. The infant usually is reluctant to ingest breast milk or milk formulas, develops vomiting, shows poor nutrition, and fails to thrive. Jaundice, hepatomegaly, and evidence of liver disease may develop. Cataracts are usually not present at birth but develop gradually over weeks to months. Mental retardation becomes evident after 6 to 12 months and is usually not reversible. Infants with classic galactosemia are subject to bacterial sepsis (especially with *Escherichia coli*), and this may be the leading cause of death in the neonatal period. The only consistent feature of galactokinase deficiency is cataract formation.

DIAGNOSIS   Galactokinase deficiency should be suspected in infants or children with cataract formation who have non-glucose-reducing substances in the urine. The diagnosis is made by demonstrating the deficiency of galactokinase in red blood cells.

Classic galactosemia must be considered when one or more of the clinical features described above are found. If the patient is ingesting milk, reducing sugar is present in the urine but gives a negative glucose oxidase reaction (i.e., is not glucose) and is identified as galactose by other techniques, such as chromatography. If the child is vomiting, has a poor food intake, or is on intravenous glucose feedings, galactose may not be present in the urine. The definitive diagnosis is made by demonstrating a lack or deficiency of red cell GALT by one of several techniques. The disease also can be diagnosed prenatally by enzyme studies on cultured amniocentesis cells or by demonstrating increased galactitol in amniotic fluid. A nonenzymatic glycosylation of hemoglobin, analogous to that in diabetes mellitus, can be detected in patients with galactosemia as manifested by increased concentrations in the blood of Hb A_{lab} rather than Hb A_{lc}.

In the neonatal period galactosemia needs to be differentiated from primary liver disease. With liver damage, galactose removal from the blood is impaired, and elevated blood galactose levels and galactosuria may be present. However, GALT levels are normal in patients with liver damage.

℞ TREATMENT

The treatment of galactosemia consists of the removal of galactose-containing foods from the diet, especially milk. Milk substitutes such as Nutramigen are often used. Although soybean preparations contain polysaccharide-bound galactose, they appear to be well tolerated because the bound galactose is not readily liberated. In general, the red cell levels of galactose-1-phosphate are not increased in affected infants fed soybean formulas.

The institution of a galactose-free diet usually leads to a dramatic improvement in all clinical features except for mental retardation. Patients should be kept on galactose-free diets indefinitely or at least until they have attained adequate physical and neurologic development.

OTHER DISORDERS OF CARBOHYDRATE METABOLISM   Features of hereditary fructose intolerance and fructose-1,

Table 351-1

Some Other Disorders of Carbohydrate Metabolism

Metabolic Defect	Manifestations
HEREDITARY FRUCTOSE INTOLERANCE	
Deficiency of fructose-1-phosphate aldolase leads to accumulation of fructose-1-PO$_4$ in tissues.	Liver disease, renal tubular damage, and hypoglycemia.
FRUCTOSE-1,6-DIPHOSPHATASE DEFICIENCY	
Deficiency of the enzyme prevents gluconeogenesis from its normal precursors, lactate, glycerol, and alanine. Thus maintenance of blood sugar is dependent on exogenous glucose.	Lactic acidosis leads to hyperventilation, somnolence, and coma, usually with hypoglycemia and ketosis.

6-diphosphatase deficiency, two autosomal recessive disorders of fructose metabolism that lead to hypoglycemia, are summarized in Table 351-1 (also see Chaps. 335 and 347).

BIBLIOGRAPHY

BEUTLER E: Galactosemia: Screening and diagnosis. Clin Biochem 24:293, 1991

ELIAS LJ et al: A common mutation associated with the Duarte galactosemia allele. Am J Hum Genet 54:1030, 1994

GITZELMANN R et al: Disorders of fructose metabolism, in *The Metabolic and Molecular Bases of Inherited Disease*, 7th ed, CR Scriver et al (eds). New York, McGraw-Hill, 1995, p 905

KAUFMAN FR et al: Correlation of ovarian function with galactose-1-phosphate uridyl transferase levels in galactosemia. J Pediatr 112:754, 1988

NG WG et al: Biochemical and molecular studies of 132 patients with galactosemia. Hum Genet 94:359, 1994

REICHARDT JKV, WOO SLC: Molecular basis of galactosemia: Mutations and polymorphisms in the gene encoding human galactose-1-phosphate uridyl-transferase. Proc Natl Acad Sci USA 88:2633, 1991

SEGAL S, BERRY GT: Disorders of galactose metabolism, in *The Metabolic and Molecular Bases of Inherited Disease*, 7th ed, CR Scriver et al (eds). New York, McGraw-Hill, 1995, p 967

WAGGONER D et al: Long-term prognosis in galactosemia: Results of a survey of 350 cases. J Inherited Metab Dis 13:802, 1990

352   *Daniel W. Foster*

THE LIPODYSTROPHIES AND OTHER RARE DISORDERS OF ADIPOSE TISSUE

This chapter is concerned with rare abnormalities in adipose tissue. In most instances, the pathophysiology is not clear.

THE LIPODYSTROPHIES

The lipodystrophies are characterized by generalized or partial loss of body fat and metabolic abnormalities, including insulin resistance, hyperglycemia, and hypertriglyceridemia. A classification is shown in Table 352-1. In *generalized lipodystrophy* essentially all body fat is lost, while in *partial lipodystrophy* fat atrophy is limited. The common acquired form of partial lipodystrophy ordinarily involves the upper half of the body, whereas dominantly transmitted partial lipodystrophy tends to spare the face. One variant is associated with eye and tooth malformations, the Rieger anomaly. *Localized lipodystrophy* may be either inflammatory or noninflammatory. The best-studied localized disorder is *centrifugal lipodystrophy*, in which fat atrophy begins in

Table 352-1

The Lipodystrophies

I. Generalized lipodystrophy
   A. Congenital (familial or sporadic)
   B. Acquired (sporadic)
II. Partial lipodystrophy
   A. Common (sporadic)
   B. Dominant (familial)
      1. Limb and trunk
      2. With Rieger anomaly

III. Localized lipodystrophy
   A. Inflammatory
   B. Noninflammatory

the groins or axillae of children under the age of 3 and spreads centrally to involve the entire abdomen. Occasionally, the disorder begins outside the abdomen. The edge of the lesion is red and scaly, with an inflammatory infiltrate demonstrable on histologic examination. Fat atrophy usually disappears spontaneously by about 13 years of age.

GENERALIZED LIPODYSTROPHY Generalized lipodystrophy (also called *lipoatrophic diabetes*) may be either congenital or acquired. The congenital form is an autosomal recessive disorder that affects both sexes equally. Parental consanguinity is common. Loss of fat is usually obvious at birth, but other manifestations may not appear until later (up to 30 years). The acquired form often develops after some other illness such as measles, chicken pox, whooping cough, and infectious mononucleosis; hypothyroidism, hyperthyroidism, and pregnancy have also been implicated. Some cases begin with painful nodular swellings of adipose tissue that resemble acute panniculitis (see below). The manifestations of the congenital and acquired forms are similar (Table 352-2).

Fat Atrophy Loss of body fat is the central feature. In congenital cases the skin of the face is tightly drawn, and the entire body appears to be devoid of adipose tissue on physical examination. However, with whole-body magnetic resonance imaging (MRI) some fat can be demonstrated in the orbits, palms, soles, and juxtaarticular and epidural regions where the cushioning functions of adipose tissue are critical. Thus, mechanical (supportive or cushioning) fat is spared while metabolic fat disappears. In the acquired form the face may be spared. In atrophic areas adipocytes devoid of triglyceride stores can be identified microscopically. Paradoxically, the liver is engorged with fat, and the reticuloendothelial system contains lipid-laden macrophages (foam cells). The cause of the fat atrophy is not known. Fat-mobilizing polypeptides have been described in the urine of patients with generalized lipodystrophy, but their role in the disease is uncertain.

A candidate molecule for the induction of lipodystrophy would be a compound similar to tumor necrosis factor α (TNFα), a potent inhibitor of lipoprotein lipase that causes fat depletion and hypertriglyceridemia when injected into animals. Lipoprotein lipase activity is low in generalized lipodystrophy, as would be predicted if TNFα or a similar cytokine were the cause. However, plasma levels of TNF

were normal in two of the author's patients. Hepatic lipase is not impaired. Since triglyceride content of the adipocyte is the result of a balance between fat synthesis and fat breakdown, an alternative mechanism might involve activation of the hormone-sensitive lipase that catalyzes hydrolysis of triglycerides in the fat cell. For example, a defect in a natural inhibitor of the lipase, such as adenosine, could enhance the response to normal levels of lipolytic hormones. Enhanced lipolysis also could be due to sympathetic nervous system activity. Release of free fatty acids into plasma following norepinephrine infusion is impaired, but this may simply reflect the depleted triglyceride stores.

A mutation or deletion of an adipocyte developmental gene might also be involved. For example, the transcription factor PPARγ2 (peroxisome proliferator activated receptor-γ2) can transform fibroblasts to fat cells in tissue culture and, if mutated, might thwart adipocyte development. In the acquired form, one would have to postulate another mechanism that could cause dedifferentiation of the adipocyte, perhaps the indirect consequence of a viral infection or other insult.

Growth and Maturation Linear growth is accelerated in the first few years of life in the congenital disorder and in acquired disease that begins early in childhood. Epiphyses close early, however, so that the final height is usually normal. Muscular hypertrophy is present, and patients may have an acromegalic appearance with coarse facial features and large hands and feet. The ears tend to be prominent in the congenital form. Many viscera are enlarged, and generalized lymphadenopathy may be present. The cause of the growth disorder is not known. Levels of growth hormone and insulin-like growth factor (IGF) I are normal or low. IGF-II has not been systematically assessed. Abnormal growth and pseudoacromegaly might be due to high concentrations of insulin in plasma secondary to insulin resistance (see below). Insulin binds to the IGF-I receptor and at high concentrations could cause acromegalic features by activating the IGF-I receptor.

Liver Fatty engorgement of the liver causes protuberance of the abdomen and may progress to cirrhosis, especially in the acquired disorder. Portal hypertension can cause splenomegaly and bleeding esophageal varices.

Kidneys The kidneys are usually enlarged. Subjects with the acquired disorder may have proteinuria and the nephrotic syndrome, although not as frequently as in partial lipodystrophy. Moderate hypertension is common.

Genitalia The external genitalia (penis and testes in males, clitoris and labia majora in females) are usually enlarged in children with the congenital disease. In women, polycystic ovaries can cause the clinical picture of Stein-Leventhal syndrome. The cause of the genital abnormalities is not known.

Skin Acanthosis nigricans is present in most. Hypertrichosis of face, neck, trunk, and limbs is frequent. Scalp hair is usually thick and curly, particularly early in life.

Central Nervous System Mental retardation is present in about half the congenital cases. It appears to be less common in the acquired form. Early studies suggesting that structural abnormalities are present in brain have not been confirmed by computed tomography (CT) and MRI studies.

Table 352-2

Characteristics of the Lipodystrophies

Feature	Congenital General	Acquired General	Acquired Partial	Dominant Partial
Inheritance	Autosomal recessive	Sporadic	Usually sporadic	Autosomal dominant
Age of onset	Infancy	Childhood to adult	Childhood to adult	Puberty
Sex incidence	Males and females equal	Female preponderance	Female preponderance	Female preponderance
Lipoatrophy	Face, trunk, limbs	Face, trunk, limbs	Face, upper trunk, upper limbs	Trunk and limbs
Liver involvement	+	+ +	Rare	0
Renal disease	+	+	+ +	0
Insulin resistance	+	+	+	+
Hyperglycemia	+	+	+	+
Hypertriglyceridemia	+	+	+	+
Acanthosis nigricans	+	+	Rare	+
Genital hypertrophy	+	+	Rare	+
Bone age	Accelerated	Normal to accelerated	Normal	Normal

Other Abnormalities Osteolytic lesions may cause bone cysts, and the skeleton occasionally appears sclerotic. Cystic bone lesions also occur in membranous lipodystrophy (Nasu disease), which is associated with presenile dementia; despite its name, membranous lipodystrophy is associated with fat necrosis and is actually a form of panniculitis (see below). Cardiomegaly is common but rarely leads to heart failure. Goiter is frequent. The associated abnormalities in generalized lipodystrophy are summarized in Table 352-3.

Metabolic and Endocrine Abnormalities Three major metabolic disturbances are characteristic.

1. *Insulin-resistant diabetes mellitus (lipoatrophic diabetes).* Insulin resistance may be mild or severe, and, when severe, the diabetes may be difficult to control. Insulin and C-peptide concentrations are relatively or absolutely elevated, and response to exogenous insulin is impaired. The cause of the insulin resistance is not known, but mutations in the insulin receptor gene have been excluded as a major factor. It is possible that elevated levels of free fatty acids may induce insulin resistance in muscle and fat and stimulate insulin secretion; increased free fatty acid turnover is believed to cause insulin resistance by impairing glucose transport into cells. Insulin in the plasma of affected individuals is biologically active. Although glucagon levels are high (indicating insulin resistance in the alpha cell of the islets of Langerhans) and free fatty acid concentrations are elevated, ketoacidosis is unusual.

True ketoacidosis may be infrequent because insulin resistance is less severe in liver and skeletal muscle than in adipose tissue. Glycogen levels in the liver are high (insulin stimulates glycogen synthesis), and levels of branched-chain amino acids fall normally in response to injected insulin. Elevated insulin levels in portal vein plasma would counteract the actions of glucagon in the insulin-responsive hepatocyte (see Chap. 335), prevent activation of ketone body synthesis in liver, and ensure utilization of fatty acids for triglyceride/very low density lipoproteins (VLDL) synthesis. The long-chain fatty acids in the plasma are of dietary origin and fall toward normal with restriction of dietary fat. Diabetes mellitus of lipodystrophy appears to be typical apart from insulin resistance, including a propensity to develop late degenerative complications. High levels of insulin in plasma and resistance to ketoacidosis distinguish this condition from type I (autoimmune) insulin-dependent diabetes mellitus, although both conditions begin in childhood or early adult life.

2. *Hypertriglyceridemia with accumulation of both chylomicrons and VLDL in the blood.* Eruptive xanthomas, lipemia retinalis, and recurrent pancreatitis may be seen. Although lipoprotein lipase is low and the disposal of triglycerides in the atrophied fat tissue is defective, the major cause for the hypertriglyceridemia is overproduction of VLDL in the liver, probably driven by the elevated free fatty acids in blood, since dietary fat restriction returns VLDL production rates toward normal. Hyperinsulinemia may contribute by enhancing hepatic fat synthesis.

3. *High metabolic rate despite normal thyroid function.* Basal metabolic rates are usually elevated, although thyroid function is normal. Patients do not gain weight with excessive caloric intake, indicating a facile capacity to waste calories as heat. Daily food intakes as high as 21,000 kJ (5000 kcal) are not unusual. One 16-month-old child ate 10,000 kJ (2400 kcal) daily. Following thyroidectomy in one patient, the basal metabolic rate decreased but did not return to normal;

symptomatic hypothyroidism developed and required treatment with thyroid hormone despite continued high metabolic rates. It thus seems clear that hypermetabolism is not due to hyperthyroidism. There is also no evidence of mitochondrial defects. The most likely explanation for the increased metabolic rate is enhanced "futile" cycles with wastage of ATP, possibly due to increased sympathetic nervous system activity. Function of the adrenal medulla is normal.

Course Patients with generalized lipodystrophy may die at an early age from hepatic failure, hemorrhage from esophageal varices, renal failure, or recurrent pancreatitis. Despite longstanding hypertriglyceridemia, symptomatic coronary artery disease is rare.

℞ TREATMENT

There is no specific treatment for lipodystrophy, although dietary fat restriction is generally recommended. Medium-chain triglyceride supplementation has been reported to be of benefit. Because of insulin resistance, large amounts of insulin are often required to control the plasma glucose. Gemfibrozil is usually prescribed to lower triglycerides but is often ineffective. In patients with recurrent pancreatitis, nicotinic acid may lower triglycerides.

ACQUIRED PARTIAL LIPODYSTROPHY This is the most common of the lipodystrophies and usually affects women. The cause is unknown. Transplantation of tissue from atrophic areas to unaffected areas is said to restore the retention of triglycerides, whereas transplantation of normal tissue to atrophic areas causes atrophy of adipocytes, suggesting a local lesion as the cause of fat atrophy. Fat atrophy occurs in the upper half of the body, including the face, and spares the lower extremities. Rarely, the lower half of the body is affected, and the upper torso is intact. Occasionally, the lesion is unilateral. The anatomic features of generalized lipodystrophy are usually absent, and liver disease is unusual. Proteinuria, with or without the nephrotic syndrome, occurs more frequently than in other forms. The complement system is abnormal, and C3 levels tend to be low. C3 nephritic factor, a polyclonal IgG immunoglobulin that interacts with alternative pathway convertase (C3bBb) to augment C3 activation, is present in serum, and lupus erythematosus can develop after many years. In unaffected first-degree relatives C3 levels may be low, but C3 nephritic factor is not present. Complement abnormalities disappeared after renal transplantation in one subject. Dermatomyositis and Sjögren's syndrome may occur. Rarely, partial lipodystrophy progresses to the generalized form of the disease.

An unusual form of partial lipodystrophy is mandibuloacral dysplasia, a syndrome with typical features of lipodystrophy, including insulin resistance, hypermetabolism, and increased glucose production. Other features include hypoplasia of the mandibles and clavicles with lytic bone lesions, wrinkled skin, and joint contractures. Some patients have hypogonadism, short stature, and alopecia.

LIPODYSTROPHY WITH DOMINANT TRANSMISSION This variant is characterized by fat atrophy of the limbs and trunk and with sparing of the face, which may actually be rounded, and neck. The disease usually begins at puberty but may not appear until middle age. Males are rarely affected. In families with the Rieger anomaly, onset tends to be in infancy. Insulin resistance and hyperglycemia are usual, and severe hypertriglyceridemia may cause eruptive xanthomas. The labia majora are hypertrophied, and polycystic ovaries may be seen. Acanthosis nigricans is usually present, but liver and renal disease do not occur.

LOCALIZED LIPODYSTROPHY Localized lipodystrophy takes several patterns. Centrifugal lipodystrophy (*lipodystrophia centrifugalis abdominalis infantilis*) has been mentioned. *Annular lipoatrophy* is a bandlike ring of fat atrophy encircling a limb or the ankles. Occasionally, only half the limb is involved, in which case the term often used is *lipoatrophia semicircularis*. On biopsy, inflammatory infiltrates in the areas of fat atrophy suggest that this condition is actually a form of panniculitis. Localized lipodystrophy also may occur

Table 352-3

Accompanying Abnormalities of Lipodystrophy

Bone	Sclerosis, cystic angiomatosis
Brain	Mental retardation, third ventricle dilatation
Genitalia	Clitoromegaly, polycystic ovaries, penile hypertrophy
Heart	Cardiomegaly
Kidneys	Hypertrophy without renal failure
Liver	Hepatomegaly, fatty liver, cirrhosis, hepatic failure
Lymph nodes	Generalized lymphadenopathy
Skin	Acanthosis nigricans, hypertrichosis
Thyroid	Goiter, euthyroid state

secondary to injection of insulin, iron dextrans, triamcinolone, and diphtheria/pertussis/tetanus vaccine.

DIAGNOSIS The diagnosis of the lipodystrophies is clinical. Taut stretching of the skin of the face may suggest scleroderma. The hypertrophied muscles appear "cleaved" as in body builders, because of absence of the usual fat between muscles. The finding of fat atrophy together with acanthosis nigricans, eruptive xanthomas, and typical laboratory findings usually render diagnosis straightforward.

MULTIPLE SYMMETRIC LIPOMATOSIS

Multiple symmetric lipomatosis usually occurs in men and is characterized by formation of nonencapsulated lipomas in two patterns of distribution: In the *type I* variant, lipomas are primarily in the nape of the neck and in the supraclavicular and deltoid regions, resulting in an extraordinary bull-necked appearance (*Madelung collar*). Extension of the lipomas into the mediastinum may obstruct the trachea or vena cava. Fat over the remainder of the body appears normal. In the *type II* pattern, lipomas extend over the body, giving the appearance of simple obesity. Diagnosis requires recognition that the fat masses are symmetric and that the distal arms and legs are spared. Deep lipomatosis is absent in type II disease, and vena caval and tracheal compression do not occur.

Multiple symmetric lipomatosis may occur sporadically or in families. Autosomal dominant transmission has been postulated in the latter. Alcoholism is common and may cause coexisting folate deficiency, macrocytic anemia, and abnormal liver function. Neuropathy may be sensory, motor, or autonomic, and neuropathic foot ulcers can develop. Histologic evidence from sural nerve biopsies suggests that neuropathy is integral to the disease, namely, a chronic distal atrophy without the axonal degeneration and demyelination of alcohol injury. Central nervous system abnormalities include defects in evoked potentials.

Metabolic abnormalities include hyperuricemia, hypertriglyceridemia (VLDL, chylomicrons), and paradoxically, elevated high-density lipoproteins (HDL). Diabetes mellitus has not been reported, although hyperinsulinism may be present. Renal tubular acidosis has occurred.

The cause is not known. The lipomas do not contain brown fat, and the fat cells are slightly smaller than normal, suggesting hyperplasia. Isolated adipocytes have increased lipoprotein lipase activity and a defect in adrenergic lipolysis. Lipolytic response to cyclic AMP is intact, suggesting an abnormality at the hormone receptor/adenylate cyclase unit. The biochemical abnormalities are not present in all cases.

There is no treatment except for surgical removal of lipomas that cause compression or for cosmetic reasons.

OTHER LIPOMATOSES

MEDIASTINOABDOMINAL This disorder may be a variant of multiple symmetric lipomatosis. The syndrome comprises (1) exertional dyspnea due to compression of airways by lipomas of the mediastinum, (2) massive enlargement of the abdomen (pseudoascites) due to intraperitoneal and retroperitoneal fat, and (3) abnormal glucose tolerance or diabetes mellitus. The metabolic abnormalities and enzymic changes in adipocytes are identical with those in multiple symmetric lipomatosis except that HDL levels are not elevated.

PELVIC Pelvic lipomatosis is characterized by overgrowth of dense, unencapsulated fat in pelvic spaces enveloping the pelvic viscera. The male-to-female ratio is 18:1. Symptoms include bladder dysfunction (frequency, dysuria, hematuria), constipation, and vague abdominal pain. Bilateral ureteral obstruction may cause hydronephrosis and renal failure. Hypertension is common. Radiographic studies show a deformed bladder, deviation of the ureters, displacement of rectosigmoid junction, and hydronephrosis in advanced cases. MRI or CT defines the compressing fat. There is no treatment except surgery to remove the fat and relieve upper urinary tract obstruction.

EPIDURAL Epidural lipomatosis is a syndrome of spinal cord compression due to adipose tissue. It causes back pain, radicular pain, or compression of the cord. The disorder is most often seen with chronic glucocorticoid therapy and may occur in Cushing's syndrome. Cord compression requires laminectomy, but otherwise a trial of decreased steroid dosage should be undertaken.

ACUTE PANNICULITIS (NODULAR FAT NECROSIS)

The appearance of single or multiple crops of tender nodules in subcutaneous fat with a histologic picture of fat cell necrosis, infiltration of inflammatory cells, and development of fat-filled macrophages (foam cells) is the hallmark of acute panniculitis. The nodules range in size from 0.5 to 10 cm and may be firm or fluctuant. They are usually tender. On occasion they drain an oily solution, and suppuration may occur. Individual lesions last from 1 to 8 weeks before disappearing, sometimes leaving a pigmented depressed area at the involved site. While some patients have only panniculitis, which may or may not be relapsing, others develop fever, abnormal liver function, a leukemoid white blood cell response, bleeding tendencies, nodular lung lesions, and pancreatic dysfunction with elevated amylase and lipase levels. In the past this constellation of findings was called *Weber-Christian disease*. However, painful or nonpainful panniculitis may result from a variety of conditions, and the term should probably be abandoned.

It is not possible to develop a firm classification of acute panniculitis since the lesions may appear in sporadic fashion with many conditions. One classification system is given in Table 352-4.

Panniculitis without systemic disease is usually due to trauma (sometimes factitiously induced) or cold. For example, in equestrian cold panniculitis the lesions appear in the outer thighs of persons riding horseback for several hours in cold weather. Subcutaneous fat necrosis of the newborn may be due to a combination of obstetric trauma and hypothermia.

Panniculitis with systemic disease can be divided into several large categories. Collagen vascular diseases such as lupus and scleroderma are a frequent cause. Indeed, nodular fat necrosis occurs in about 2 to 3 percent of patients with lupus and is more common in discoid than in systemic lupus. Lymphomas and histiocytosis represent a second category. Histiocytic cytophagic panniculitis (HCP) is characterized by fever, pleural effusions, hepatosplenomegaly, panniculitis, anemia, leukopenia, thrombocytopenia, and coagulation defects. The characteristic lesion is the "beanbag" histiocyte containing ingested lymphocytes, red cells, and platelets. While some patients have a benign course, most die from hemorrhagic complications. Malignant T cell lymphoma may involve subcutaneous tissue directly and can mimic HCP. Infiltrating T lymphocytes in HCP are of clonal origin, suggesting that subcutaneous T cell lymphomas are a malignant, late transformation phase of HCP. Panniculitis with systemic symptoms also occurs in lymphoplasmatic lymphoma with crystal-laden histiocytes. Deficiencies of α_1-antitrypsin have been found in a number of patients with acute panniculitis. It is postulated that the α_1-antitrypsin deficiency

Table 352-4

Causes of Panniculitis

Panniculitis without systemic disease
   Trauma
   Cold
   Subcutaneous fat necrosis of the newborn
Panniculitis with systemic disease
   Connective tissue disorders (lupus erythematosus, scleroderma)
   Lymphoproliferative disease (lymphoma, histiocytosis)
   α_1-Antitrypsin deficiency
   Pancreatic disease (cancer, pancreatitis)
   Generalized lipodystrophy
   Paraproteinemia with C1 inhibitor deficiency
   Fasciitis-panniculitis syndrome
   Miscellaneous (see text)

predisposes to panniculitis after trauma and induces a hyperactive immune response. Panniculitis with systemic symptoms, including fever and hepatitis, also occurs with light chain paraproteinemia and acquired deficiency of C_1 inhibitor in the classic complement-generating sequence. Severe pancreatic disease also can cause acute panniculitis. One variant, *disseminated fat necrosis,* is described below. Panniculitis rarely may be associated with generalized lipodystrophy, especially the acquired type. Other rare causes of panniculitis include gout, familial Mediterranean fever, Nasu disease (see above), drugs (glucocorticoids, aspartame), renal failure, atheromatous emboli, and infection. Eosinophilic panniculitis may occur with vasculitis, parasitic infestation, lymphomas, and atopic dermatitis. Eosinophilic panniculitis can also be a variant of the fasciitis-panniculitis syndrome characterized by chronic inflammation, induration of the skin, and eosinophilic fasciitis, resulting in fibrosis of subcutaneous and muscle septae, and may follow Sweet's syndrome.

Acute panniculitis can only be diagnosed histologically, and then a search for the cause must be made. If systemic symptoms are present and the course is rapidly downhill, the primary differential diagnosis is between collagen vascular disease, lymphoproliferative disorder, and pancreatitis or pancreatic cancer. Milder cases raise the possibility of α_1-antitrypsin deficiency.

℞ TREATMENT

Treatment is often unsatisfactory. Some patients with histiocytic cytophagic panniculitis respond to combined chemotherapy with cyclophosphamide, bleomycin, and prednisone. Patients with α_1-antitrypsin deficiency may respond to dapsone and may be given α_1-antiprotease concentrate (60 mg/kg body weight weekly) if this fails.

DISSEMINATED FAT NECROSIS

Disseminated fat necrosis (also called *metastatic fat necrosis*) is a disorder in which patients with pancreatitis (two-thirds) or carcinoma of the pancreas (one-third) develop lesions that are characteristic of nodular panniculitis and that have a predilection for periarticular sites. Fever is usual. Arthritis occurs in about 60 percent of cases and may cause joint destruction. Sinus tracts may extend from the site of subcutaneous fat necrosis to the joint space, leading to deposition of necrotic material. Lytic bone lesions may underlie the site of fat necrosis. Polyserositis and vasculitis may be present. Since complement levels are low and immunofluorescent staining shows deposition of complement and IgG, the syndrome resembles, in some respects, lupus-associated panniculitis. Serologic studies for lupus have not been reported systematically, but antinuclear antibody (ANA) and rheumatoid factor have been undetectable in some patients.

Release of pancreatic enzymes into blood may cause disseminated fat necrosis at distal sites in some patients. Presumably, free fatty acids released by pancreatic lipase and phospholipase A_2, both of which may be elevated in serum, induce tissue necrosis, with trypsin playing an ancillary role. Experimentally, necrosis can be induced in pericardial, subpleural, and subcutaneous fat by ligation of pancreatic ducts. Amylase and lipase levels may be elevated in pleural, pericardial, and ascitic fluid. These enzymes also have been found in fluid aspirated from subcutaneous nodules. The possibility that release of pancreatic enzymes is causal is supported by the occurrence of disseminated fat necrosis in patients with pancreatic–portal vein fistulas. The relation of pancreatic enzyme leakage to autoimmune mechanisms, if any, and the meaning of the eosinophilia that frequently accompanies disseminated fat necrosis are not known.

Mortality rates are high (even in the absence of pancreatic carcinoma), and death may occur in weeks to months. No treatment is known. Infusion of the protease inhibitor aprotinin appeared to have beneficial effects in one patient.

ADIPOSIS DOLOROSA

Adiposis dolorosa (Dercum's disease) occurs in women (30:1) and is characterized by painful circumscribed adipose tissue deposits in

subcutaneous tissues of the extremities and of other parts of the body. Juxtaarticular areas, particularly the knees, are the most common sites. Lesions vary from 0.5 to 5.0 cm. Pain and paresthesia may occur spontaneously or result from pressure. Affected individuals are usually obese. The disorder is associated with weakness, fatigue, emotional instability, and occasional dementia and rarely begins before menopause. Most cases are sporadic, but familial occurrence has been noted with a presumed dominant inheritance. Most reported associations are probably chance phenomena. Autopsy reports from early in the century suggested abnormalities of the pituitary and other endocrine glands, but modern endocrinologic evaluations have not been undertaken.

Biopsy of affected sites may show no abnormalities, but granulomas with giant cell formations are usually seen. Fat necrosis is rare, thus separating the condition from acute panniculitis.

Treatment is unsatisfactory, although intravenous lidocaine, glucocorticoids, surgical excision, and liposuction have been tried.

BIBLIOGRAPHY

LIPODYSTROPHY

CHANDALIA M et al: Postmortem findings in congenital generalized lipodystrophy. J Clin Endocrinol Metab 80:3077, 1995

CHUN SI et al: Membranous lipodystrophy: Primary idiopathic type. J Am Acad Dermatol 24:844, 1991

CUTLER DL et al: Insulin-resistant diabetes mellitus and hypermetabolism in mandibulo-acral dysplasia: A newly recognized form of partial lipodystrophy. J Clin Endocrinol Metab 73:1056, 1991

DESBOIS-MOUTHOU C et al: Lipoatrophic diabetes: Genetic exclusion of the insulin receptor gene. J Clin Endocrinol Metab 80:314, 1995

GARG A et al: Peculiar distribution of adipose tissue in patients with congenital generalized lipodystrophy. J Clin Endocrinol Metab 75:358, 1991

KLEIN S et al: Generalized lipodystrophy: In vivo evidence for hypermetabolism and insulin-resistant lipid, glucose, and amino acid kinetics. Metabolism 41:893, 1992

MORISON IM et al: Somatic overgrowth associated with overexpression of insulin-like growth factor II. Nature Med 2:321, 1996

SEIP M: Generalized lipodystrophy, in *Ergebnisse der Inneren Medizin und Kinderheilkunde,* P Frick et al (eds). Berlin, Springer-Verlag, 1971, pp 59–95

MULTIPLE SYMMETRIC LIPOMATOSIS

ENZI G: Multiple symmetric lipomatosis: An updated clinical report. Medicine 63:56, 1984

KAZUMI T et al: Failure to detect brown adipose tissue uncoupling protein mRNA in benign symmetric lipomatosis (Madelung's disease). Endocr J 41:315, 1994

NAUMANN M et al: Neurological multisystem manifestation in multiple symmetric lipomatosis: A clinical and electrophysiological study. Muscle Nerve 18:693, 1995

MEDIASTINOABDOMINAL LIPOMATOSIS, PELVIC LIPOMATOSIS, AND EPIDURAL LIPOMATOSIS

FESSLER RG et al: Epidural lipomatosis in steroid-treated patients. Spine 17:183, 1992

HEYNS CF: Pelvic lipomatosis: A review of its diagnosis and management. J Urol 146:267, 1991

ACUTE PANNICULITIS

ALEGRE VA, WINKELMANN RK: Histiocytic cytophagic panniculitis. J Am Acad Dermatol 20:177, 1989

ATTIAS D et al: Acute neutrophilic myositis in Sweet's syndrome: Late transformation into fibrosing myositis and panniculitis. Hum Pathol 26:687, 1995

HARADA M et al: Crystal-storing histiocytosis associated with lymphoplasmacytic lymphoma mimicking Weber-Christian disease: Immunohistochemical, ultrastructural and gene-rearrangement studies. Hum Pathol 27:84, 1996

HYTIROGLOU P et al: Histiocytic cytophagic panniculitis: Molecular evidence for a clonal T-cell disorder. J Am Acad Dermatol 27:333, 1992

NASCHITZ JE et al: The fasciitis-panniculitis syndromes. Clinical and pathologic features. Medicine 75:6, 1996

PETERS MS, SU WPD: Panniculitis. Dermatol Clin 10:37, 1992

SMITH KC et al: Panniculitis associated with severe α_1-antitrypsin deficiency: Treatment and review of the literature. Arch Dermatol 123:1655, 1987

DISSEMINATED FAT NECROSIS

POTTS JR: Pancreatic–portal vein fistula with disseminated fat necrosis treated by pancreaticoduodenectomy. South Med J 84:632, 1991

WILSON HA et al: Pancreatitis with arthropathy and subcutaneous fat necrosis. Evidence for the pathogenicity of lipolytic enzymes. Arthritis Rheum 26:121, 1983

ADIPOSIS DOLOROSA

BRODOVSKY J et al: Adiposis dolorosa (Dercum's disease): 10 year follow-up. Ann Plast Surg 33:664, 1994

SECTION 3

DISORDERS OF BONE AND MINERAL METABOLISM

353

Michael F. Holick, Stephen M. Krane, John T. Potts, Jr.

CALCIUM, PHOSPHORUS, AND BONE METABOLISM: CALCIUM-REGULATING HORMONES

BONE STRUCTURE AND METABOLISM (See also Chap. 355) Bone is a dynamic tissue that is remodeled constantly throughout life. The arrangement of compact and cancellous bone provides a strength and density suitable for mobility. In addition, bone provides a reservoir for calcium, magnesium, phosphorus, sodium, and other ions necessary for homeostatic functions. The skeleton is highly vascular and receives about 10 percent of the cardiac output.

The properties of bone are a function of its extracellular components. The structure consists of a solid mineral phase in close association with an organic matrix, of which 90 to 95 percent is type I collagen (see Chap. 348). The noncollagenous portion of the organic matrix contains proteins derived from serum (albumin and α_2-HS glycoproteins), proteins containing α-carboxyglutamic acid (GLA) [*bone GLA protein* (BGP), *osteocalin*, and a matrix GLA protein], the glycoprotein *osteonectin*, the phosphoprotein *osteopontin*, sialoproteins, *thrombospondin*, and other less well characterized proteins. Some of these proteins may function in initiating mineralization and in binding of the mineral phase to the matrix. The mineral phase is made up of calcium and phosphate and is best characterized as a poorly crystalline hydroxyapatite, although the calcium/phosphate molar ratio is less than the 1.67 molar ratio of hydroxyapatite [empirical formula $Ca_{10}(PO_4)_6(OH)_2$]. Additional ions are present, particularly in the surface layers. The mineral phase of bone is deposited initially in intimate relation to the collagen fibrils and is found in specific locations in the "holes" between the collagen fibrils. This architectural arrangement of mineral and matrix results in a two-phase material well suited to withstand mechanical stresses. The formation and localization of the inorganic phase are determined in part by the organic matrix.

Cells of mesenchymal origin—*osteoblasts*—synthesize and secrete the organic matrix. Mineralization of the matrix, largely in *osteons* (haversian systems), begins soon after the matrix is secreted (primary mineralization) but is not completed until after several weeks (secondary mineralization). Osteoblasts are characterized by their location and morphology, the presence of a specific skeletal form of alkaline phosphatase, the presence of receptors for parathyroid hormone (PTH) and 1,25-dihydroxyvitamin D [$1,25(OH)_2D$], and the ability to synthesize specific matrix proteins, such as type I collagen, osteocalcin, and osteopontin. As an osteoblast secretes matrix, which is then mineralized, the cell becomes surrounded by matrix and becomes an *osteocyte*, still connected with its blood supply through a series of canaliculi. Resorption of bone is carried out mainly by *osteoclasts*, multinucleated cells that are formed by fusion of hematopoietic stem cells related to the mononuclear phagocyte series. Resorption of bone takes place in scalloped spaces (Howship's lacunae) where the osteoclasts are attached through a specific $\alpha v \beta 3$ integrin to components of the bone matrix such as osteopontin. This zone (clear zone) contains contractile proteins. The resorbing end of the cell forms a specialized ruffled border. Mineral and matrix are removed in this space where the ruffled border is folded and is in contact with the bone. Proteins, including a specialized proton-pump ATPase, are found in the ruffled border membrane, which contributes to the production in the enclosed extracellular compartment of an acid environment, which solubilizes the mineral phase. This area is also rich in protein encoded by the oncogene c-*src* and in the Src phosphorylation substrate p80/85. In addition to the proton pump, carbonic anhydrase (type II isoenzyme) is required to maintain the acid pH. Other features of osteoclasts include the presence of tartrate-resistant acid phosphatase, cell-surface receptors for calcitonin, sodium pumps of the kidney type, a bicarbonate/chloride exchanger of the band 3 family, and an ability to resorb mineralized bone. The bone matrix is resorbed in the acid environment adjacent to the ruffled border by acid hydrolyases following solubilization of the mineral phase. Several soluble ligands modulate the differentiation of osteoblasts or osteoclasts from precursor cells and modulate the function of the differentiated cells; prominent among these substances are the colony stimulating factors and interleukins (ILs) 6 and 11. Bone is a storehouse for growth-regulatory factors. Some that affect osteoblast function include transforming growth factor (TGF) β types I and II, acidic fibroblast growth factor (aFGF) and basic fibroblast growth factor (bFGF), platelet-derived growth factor (PDGF), and insulin-like growth factors (IGFs) I and II. In addition, several proteins that induce ectopic bone formation may have a role in bone remodeling, e.g., osteoinductive factor, osteogenin, and bone morphogenic proteins. Other cytokines modulate resorption through effects on osteoclasts, e.g., IL-1, tumor necrosis factor (TNF), interferon γ, and colony stimulating factors (CSFs). Some of these effects on osteoclasts are mediated by osteoblasts and adjacent stromal fibroblasts in the marrow. For example, PTH receptors are not found on mature osteoclasts, and PTH increases osteoclastic bone resorption by first acting on osteoblasts or stromal fibroblasts. $1,25(OH)_2D$ receptors are found in precursor cells that can differentiate into monocytes or osteoclasts, and $1,25(OH)_2D$ promotes differentiation along the osteoclast pathway. Some cytokines, such as IL-1 and TGFα, may induce local production of prostaglandins and other cytokines, such as IL-6 and CSFs. What was initially termed *osteoclast-activating factor* is currently thought to reflect the presence of cytokines such as IL-1, TNFα, TNFβ (lymphotoxin), and probably others as well.

In the embryo and in the growing child, bone develops by remodeling and replacing previously calcified cartilage (endochondral bone formation) or is formed without a cartilage matrix (intramembranous bone formation). New bone, whether formed in infants or in adults during repair, has a relatively high ratio of cells to matrix and is characterized by coarse fiber bundles of collagen that are interlaced and randomly dispersed (woven bone). In adults, the more mature bone is organized with fiber bundles regularly arranged in parallel or concentric sheets (lamellar bone). In long bones, deposition of lamellar bone in a concentric arrangement around blood vessels forms the haversian systems. Growth in length of bones is dependent on proliferation of cartilage cells and on the endochondral sequence at the growth plate. Growth in width and thickness is accomplished by formation of bone at the periosteal surface and by resorption at the endosteal surface, with the rate of formation exceeding that of resorption. In adults, after the epiphyses close, growth in length and endochondral bone formation cease, except for some activity in the cartilage cells beneath the articular surface. Even in adults, however, remodeling of bone (remodeling of haversian systems as well as trabecular bone) continues through life. Newly forming surfaces are characterized by smooth character, by uptake of tetracycline, and by relatively low mineral density and are covered by active osteoblasts. The osteoid seam that results from the lag in mineralization of the newly formed organic matrix is about 12 μm in width. An index of the rate of bone formation can be obtained by examination of undemineralized sections of bone biopsy specimens from individuals who have received tetracycline for two periods separated by a drug-free interval. The distance between the fluorescent bands on the sections reflects the amount of new bone formed. Resorption areas are characterized by irregular configurations and the presence of osteoclasts (Fig. 353-1). Resorption precedes formation and is more intense, but it does not persist as long as formation. In adults, approximately 4 percent of the surface of trabecular bone (such as iliac crest) is involved in active resorption, whereas 10 to 15 percent of trabecular surfaces is covered with osteoid. Radioisotope studies indicate that as much as 18 percent of the total skeletal calcium is deposited and removed each year. Thus, bone is an active metabolizing tissue that requires an intact blood supply. The remodeling of bone is somehow related to the mechanical stresses to which it is subjected. Bone also serves as an important reservoir of mineral ions such as calcium, which are critical for a variety of processes.

The response of bone to fractures, infection, and interruption of blood supply and to expanding lesions is relatively limited. Dead bone must be resorbed, and new bone must be formed, a process carried out in association with growth of new blood vessels into the involved area. In injuries that disrupt the organization of the tissue, such as a fracture in which apposition of fragments is poor and motion exists at the fracture site, the progenitor stromal cells differentiate into cells with functional capacities different from those of osteoblasts, and varying amounts of fibrous tissue and cartilage are formed. When there is good apposition with fixation and little motion at the fracture

site, repair occurs predominantly by formation of new bone without other scar tissue. Remodeling of this bone occurs along lines of force determined by mechanical stresses that are somehow translated into biologic response.

Expanding lesions in bone, such as tumors, induce resorption at the surface in contact with the tumor. A bowing deformity causes increased new bone formation at the concave surface and resorption at the convex surface, all seemingly designed to produce the strongest mechanical structure. Even in a disorder as architecturally disruptive as Paget's disease, remodeling is dictated by mechanical forces. Thus, the plasticity of bone is due to the interaction of cells with each other and with the environment.

Mechanisms of Bone Formation and Resorption   Bone formation is an orderly process in which deposition of inorganic mineral is controlled by an organic matrix. The mineral phase is composed of calcium and phosphorus, and the concentration of these ions in the plasma and extracellular fluid (ECF) influences the rate at which mineral is formed. In vitro, mineralization can proceed, and crystals of hydroxyapatite can grow, at concentrations of calcium and phosphorus similar to those in an ultrafiltrate of plasma. However, the concentration of these ions at the sites of mineralization is unknown, and the cells involved (osteoblasts, osteocytes) may influence the local ion concentrations. Collagens from a variety of sources can catalyze the nucleation of a mineral phase of calcium and phosphorus from solutions of these ions, and the initial mineral phase is deposited in specific locations in the "holes" produced by the packing arrangement of the collagen molecules. The organization of collagen probably influences the amount and type of mineral phase formed in bone. The primary structures of type I collagen in skin and bone tissues are similar. There are differences, however, in posttranslational modifications of type I collagen, such as hydroxylations, glycosylations, and the type, number, and distribution of intermolecular cross-links. In addition, the holes in the packing structure of the collagen are larger in mineralized collagen of bone and dentin than in unmineralized collagens such as tendon. The fact that single-amino-acid substitutions in the helical portion of either the α1 or α2 chain of type I collagen due to mutations in the *COL*1A1 or *COL*1A2 genes in osteogenesis imperfecta disrupt the organization of bone indicates the importance of the fibrillar matrix in the structure of bone (see also Chap. 348). The noncollagenous organic components such as osteocalcin, osteonectin, and osteopontin also may play a role in the mineralization of bone. Alkaline phosphatase is a marker for osteoblasts, and cellular levels of this enzyme correlate with mineralization potential of osteoblasts. Although mineralization defects occur in individuals with mutations that cause decreased alkaline phosphatase activity (hypophosphatasia), the function of alkaline phosphatase in mineralization is not completely understood. Inorganic pyrophosphate is a potent inhibitor of mineralization at levels below those necessary to bind calcium ions. Since alkaline phosphatase in osteoblasts and other cells can catalyze the hydrolysis of inorganic pyrophosphate at neutral pH, this enzyme could regulate mineralization by controlling the concentrations of pyrophosphate. In addition, macromolecular inhibitors such as proteoglycan aggregates also may influence mineralization. In cartilage undergoing calcification, mineralization may be initiated in membrane-bound vesicles outside the cells.

In bone, the calcium phosphate solid phase at the inception of mineralization is brushite ($CaHPO_4 \cdot 2H_2O$). As mineralization progresses, the solid phase is a poorly crystalline hydroxyapatite with a relatively low (~1.2) calcium/phosphate molar ratio. With age and maturation, the perfection of the crystals and the calcium/phosphate ratio increase. Fluoride ions, when incorporated into the mineral phase, decrease the proportion of amorphous calcium phosphate and enhance the crystal structure.

There is a limit for the concentration of calcium and phosphorus ions in the ECF below which mineralization does not occur. A "solubility product" for bone mineral is difficult to calculate because the

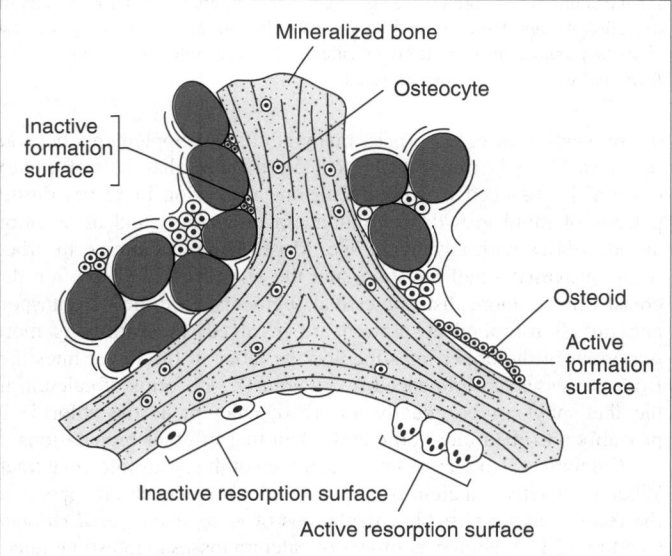

Mineralized bone

Osteocyte

Inactive formation surface

Osteoid

Active formation surface

Inactive resorption surface

Active resorption surface

FIGURE 353-1   Schematic representation of bone remodeling surfaces in trabecular bone. Most bone surfaces in adults are involved in neither formation nor resorption. Such surfaces are usually smooth, have no osteoid seam, and are covered either by no visible cells or by flattened cells. Active formation surfaces are smooth and covered by osteoblasts which have an osteoid seam (*solid blue*), normally no thicker than 12 μm. The calcification front is located at the junction of the osteoid seam and mineralized bone (*stippled*). Inactive formation surfaces are not covered by osteoblasts but by only a few flattened cells. Active resorption surfaces are irregular or scalloped and contain multinucleated osteoclasts. The latter are not seen on inactive resorption surfaces.

mineral phase itself is of variable composition and because the various components in ECF that regulate this solubility product are not known. Nevertheless, when the concentrations of calcium and phosphorus in ECF are excessive, a mineral phase may form in areas that are not normally mineralized.

When bone is resorbed, calcium and phosphorus ions are released into the ECF, and the organic matrix is resorbed. The fact that bone resorption takes place in the region of the osteoclast adjacent to the bone surface, where the extracellular pH is low, suggests that an acid environment is required for solubilization of bone mineral. The alkaline phosphatase of bone cells is an ectoenzyme that is released into the ECF. Increased circulating levels of the bone-derived enzyme are correlated with rates of bone formation. Other circulating markers of bone formation include osteocalcin and type I procollagen carboxy-terminal peptides. Urinary markers for bone resorption are hydroxyproline, hydroxylysine and its glycosides, and the bone-specific hydroxy-pyridinium collagen cross-links.

CALCIUM METABOLISM A total of 1 to 2 kg of calcium is present in the average adult, over 98 percent of it in the skeleton. The calcium of the mineral phase at the surface of the crystals is in equilibrium with that in the ECF, but only a minor fraction of the total pool (about 0.5 percent) is exchangeable. The calcium in ECF is critical for a variety of functions and is remarkably constant. In normal adults plasma levels range from 2.2 to 2.6 mmol/L (8.8 to 10.4 mg/dL). The calcium in plasma is present as three forms: free ions, ions bound to plasma proteins, and, to a small extent, diffusible complexes. The concentration of free calcium ions, averaging 1.2 mmol/L (4.8 mg/dL), influences many cellular functions and is subjected to tight hormonal control, especially through PTH, as described below. The concentration of serum proteins is an important determinant of calcium ion concentration; most calcium ion is bound to albumin. Ionized calcium can be measured directly with the use of calcium-specific electrodes. If ionized calcium cannot be measured, certain approximations can be used to distinguish the protein-bound and ionized fractions. One formula that approximates the amount of calcium bound to protein is

$$\% \text{ protein-bound Ca} = 0.8 \times \text{albumin (g/L)} \\ + 0.2 \times \text{globulin (g/L)} + 3$$

A simplified correction is sometimes used to indicate whether a stated total serum calcium concentration is abnormal when serum proteins are low. The correction is to add 1 mg/dL to the serum calcium level for every 1 g/dL by which the serum albumin level is below 4.0 g/dL. If the serum calcium level, for example, is 7.8 mg/dL (a subnormal value) and the serum albumin level is only 3.0 mg/dL, then the stated serum calcium level is corrected by adding 1 mg/dL; the corrected value of 8.8 mg/dL is within the normal range. These rough approximations generally agree with measurements of ionized calcium in patients with subnormal serum proteins.

Calcium ions inside the cell mediate a variety of cellular functions. Most intracellular calcium is in the form of insoluble complexes. The level of free calcium in the cell, which is critical for functional regulation, is low, approximately 0.1 μmol/L; thus, the gradient between plasma and intracellular free calcium is about 10,000 to 1. This gradient is tightly regulated. The concentration of calcium ions in the ECF is kept constant by processes that constantly add and remove calcium. Calcium enters the plasma via absorption from the intestinal tract and resorption of ions from the bone mineral. Calcium leaves the ECF via secretion into the gastrointestinal tract (~100 to 200 mg/d), urinary excretion (~50 to 300 mg/d), deposition in bone mineral, and losses in sweat (up to 100 mg/d). Bone resorption and formation are tightly coupled, approximately 12 mmol (500 mg) calcium entering and leaving the skeleton daily (Fig. 353-2).

The average dietary calcium intake for most adults in the United States is approximately 15 to 20 mmol/d (0.6 to 0.8 g/d). However, with heightened awareness of the role of adequate calcium intake for

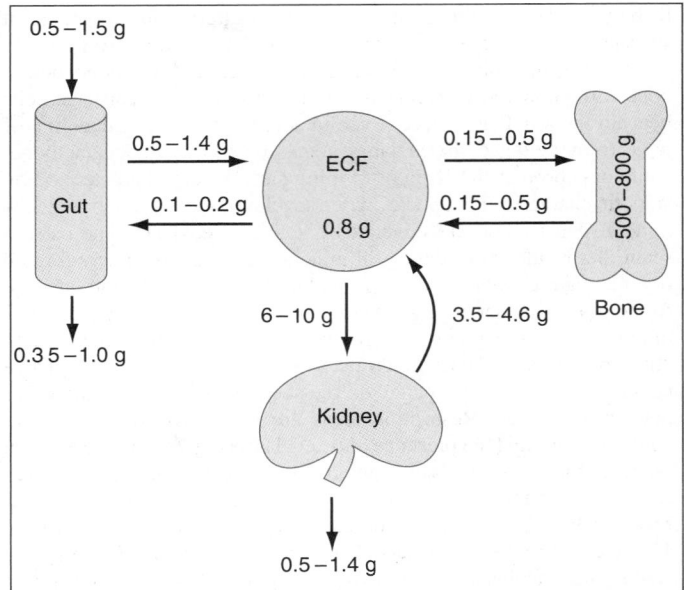

FIGURE 353-2 Calcium homeostasis. Schematic illustration of calcium content of extracellular fluid (ECF) and bone as well as of diet and feces; magnitude of calcium flux per day as calculated by various methods is shown at sites of transport in intestine, kidney, and bone. Ranges of values shown are approximate and chosen to illustrate certain points discussed in text. In intestine, absorption efficiency varies inversely with dietary calcium (chronic adaptation). This is reflected in typical quantities absorbed and excreted in feces; with 0.5-g intake, 50 percent absorption is depicted to occur (0.25 g), but at 1.5 g, only 30 percent (0.5 g). Endogenous fecal calcium, the 0.1 to 0.2 g secreted into the intestinal lumen daily, is constant and does not vary with calcium intake or absorption. Quantities of calcium depicted as filtered, reabsorbed, and excreted at the kidney are chosen arbitrarily to indicate that at lower rates of filtration of calcium (expected at lower glomerular filtration rates), most is reabsorbed (e.g., 5.85 of 6 g), leading to urinary excretion of 150 mg; at higher rates of filtration (at high dietary calcium intake), slightly less is reabsorbed (e.g., 9.7 of 10 g), leading to a higher urinary excretion, 300 mg. In all situations, renal calcium reabsorption exceeds 95 percent of filtered load. Urinary calcium excretion is seen, therefore, to increase by only 150 mg despite a 1-g increase in dietary intake. In conditions of calcium balance, rates of calcium release from and uptake into bone are equal.

the prevention of osteoporosis, many adults on supplements have an intake of 20 to 37 mmol/d (0.8 to 1.5 g/d). Less than half of dietary calcium is absorbed in adults. Calcium absorption increases during periods of rapid growth in children, in pregnancy, and in lactation and decreases with advancing age. Most of the calcium is absorbed in the proximal small intestine, and the efficiency of absorption decreases in the more distal intestinal segments. Both active transport and diffusion-limited absorption are involved; the former is more important in the upper intestine and the latter in the lower intestine. Both processes are influenced by vitamin D. All forms of calcium in the diet may not be equally absorbed; calcium as the chloride is probably absorbed more efficiently than that in other preparations.

Calcium is also secreted into the lumen of the gastrointestinal tract. When radioactive calcium is administered intravenously, it appears in the feces, making possible calculations of *endogenous fecal calcium* (see Fig. 353-2). Higher estimates of calcium losses in intestinal juices have been made by other techniques. Secretion of calcium into the intestinal lumen is constant and independent of absorption. If calcium availability in the diet is low [<12 mmol/d (500 mg/d)], a positive calcium balance requires an efficiency of absorption greater than 30 to 40 percent.

The urinary calcium excretion of normal adults having an average calcium intake ranges between 2.5 and 10 mmol/d (100 and 400 mg/d). When the dietary calcium level is below 5 mmol/d (200 mg/d), urinary calcium excretion is usually less than 5 mmol/d (200 mg/d). However, in most normal individuals, wide variations in dietary intake have little effect on urinary calcium. Hence, when the diet is low in calcium, the relative inefficiency of renal calcium conservation leads to a negative calcium balance unless calcium absorption is maximal (see Fig. 353-2).

The amount of calcium in the urine is small compared with that filtered by the glomerulus [about 150 to 250 mmol/d (6 to 10 g/d)] because the rates of reabsorption of the filtered calcium are high. Reabsorption takes place predominantly in the proximal tubule (~60 percent) and in Henle's loop (~25 percent) and to a small extent in the distal tubule. It is not clear whether non-protein-bound, nonionic calcium such as calcium citrate is cleared at different rates. The excretion of other electrolytes affects the urinary excretion of calcium. For example, urinary calcium is usually proportional to urinary sodium; sulfate also increases calcium excretion.

Maintenance of the calcium balance depends on the efficiency of intestinal absorption (see Fig. 353-2). A deficiency of PTH or vitamin D, intestinal disease, or severe dietary calcium deprivation may provide challenges to calcium homeostasis that cannot be compensated adequately by renal calcium conservation, resulting in a negative calcium balance. Increased bone resorption may protect against ECF calcium depletion even in states of chronic negative calcium balance but only at the expense of progressive bone loss.

Pathophysiology A decrease in the concentration of free calcium ions in plasma results in increased neuromuscular irritability and tetany. This syndrome is characterized by peripheral and perioral paresthesias, carpal spasm, pedal spasm, anxiety, seizures, bronchospasm, laryngospasm, Chvostek's, Trousseau's, and Erb's signs, and lengthening of the QT interval of the electrocardiogram. In infants tetany may be manifested only by irritability and lethargy. The level of calcium ions that determines which features of tetany will be manifested varies among individuals. Tetany is also influenced by other components of the ECF. For example, hypomagnesemia and alkalosis lower whereas hypokalemia and acidosis raise the threshold for tetany.

Increases in total serum calcium are usually accompanied by increases in free calcium levels and may be associated with anorexia, nausea, vomiting, constipation, hypotonia, depression, and occasionally lethargy and coma. Persistent hypercalcemia, especially when accompanied by normal or elevated levels of serum phosphate, may cause ectopic deposition of a solid phase of calcium and phosphate in walls of blood vessels, connective tissue about the joints, gastric mucosa, cornea, and renal parenchyma. Hypercalcemia per se alters renal function in addition to the pathologic effects of calcium phosphate deposition.

PHOSPHORUS METABOLISM Phosphorus is a major component of bone and of all other tissues and in some form is involved in almost all metabolic processes. About 32 mol (1 kg) of phosphorus is present in the normal adult, of which about 85 percent is in the skeleton.

In fasting plasma, most of the phosphorus is present as inorganic orthophosphate in concentrations of approximately 0.9 to 1.3 mmol/L (2.8 to 4 mg/dL). In contrast to calcium, of which about 50 percent is bound, only about 12 percent of the phosphorus in plasma is bound to proteins. Free HPO_4^{2-} and $NaHPO_4^-$ normally accounts for about 75 percent of the total phosphorus, and free $H_2PO_4^-$ accounts for 10 percent. Since so many species are present, depending on pH and other factors, concentrations are usually expressed in terms of elemental phosphorus, in units of mmol/L or mg/dL. Total phosphorus levels are higher in children and in women after menopause. There is a circadian variation in phosphorus levels even during a 24-h fast, mediated in part by the adrenal cortex. The nadir occurs between 9 A.M. and 12 noon, followed by an increase to a plateau in the afternoon and another small peak after midnight. The magnitudes of the peaks and troughs vary with phosphorus intake but occur regardless of whether the intake is high or low. Dietary restriction of phosphorus that only modestly decreases the morning fasting levels may abolish the afternoon rise. Even with twofold changes in serum phosphorus levels, levels of serum ionized calcium do not change significantly.

During phosphate depletion, phosphaturia decreases before serum phosphorus declines. This adaptive response of increasing tubular transport when luminal concentrations are decreasing is an intrinsic property of tubular cells. There is also heterogeneity of phosphorus transport among different segments of proximal renal tubules. Tubular fluxes of phosphorus, rather than hypophosphatemia per se, may be critical in modulating effects of hypophosphatemia such as the stimulation of 25(OH)D-1α-hydroxylase. Conversely, increased phosphorus loads and increased renal tubular phosphorus fluxes result in decreased renal tubular reabsorption and increased clearance of phosphorus and suppress the activity of 25(OH)D-1α-hydroxylase (see below). Ingestion of carbohydrate depresses serum phosphorus acutely by 0.3 to 0.5 mmol/L (1 to 1.5 mg/dL), presumably owing to cellular uptake and formation of phosphate esters. Ingestion of phosphorus per se increases serum levels. Therefore, for the interpretation of serum levels and urinary clearances, samples should be obtained in the fasting state. Decreases in plasma phosphorus also occur during induction of alkalosis.

Whereas dietary calcium is absorbed inefficiently from the intestine, phosphorus absorption is remarkably efficient. At levels of intake less than 2 mg/kg of body weight per day, 80 to 90 percent of ingested phosphorus is absorbed. Even with levels of intake greater than 10 mg/kg of body weight per day in the form of dairy products, cereals, eggs, and meat, absorption is about 70 percent. Hypophosphatemia due to deficient intestinal absorption is unusual except when nonabsorbable antacids are administered; the antacids bind phosphorus and prevent absorption from the intestinal lumen.

The major control of phosphorus economy is exerted at the level of the kidney. Phosphorus filtered through the glomerulus is reabsorbed largely in the proximal tubule (there is homeostatically important distal reabsorption as well) so that only about 10 to 15 percent of the filtered load is normally excreted. When filtered loads of phosphorus decrease, proximal tubular reabsorption increases. Conversely, when phosphorus loads are increased, tubular reabsorption decreases, and clearance rises. Thus, the urinary excretion of phosphorus normally reflects dietary intake, and conservation or elimination of excessive amounts depends on adequate renal handling (Fig. 353-3). There is no good evidence for renal tubular phosphate secretion. Proximal reabsorption of phosphorus is dependent on parallel sodium reabsorption, but whereas the sodium rejected by the proximal tubule may be reabsorbed distally, the rejected phosphorus is not. Therefore, volume expansion and decreased sodium reabsorption increase phosphorus clearance; similarly, diuretics that act proximally, such as acetazolamide, are phosphaturic to a degree that parallels the degree to which they are natriuretic.

Pathophysiology No direct symptoms result from hyperphosphatemia. When high levels are maintained for long periods, however, mineralization is enhanced, and calcium phosphate may be deposited in abnormal sites. Ectopic calcification occurs in untreated chronic renal failure, with severe hypercalcemia, and in vitamin D intoxication. *Tumoral calcinosis* is a rare heritable disorder in which ectopic calcification is associated with hyperphosphatemia and a normal glomerular filtration rate (GFR). The disorder is characterized by a high ratio of phosphorus tubule maximum (TmP) to GFR and increased serum levels of 1,25(OH)₂D. The latter is a paradoxical finding and presumably is related to the abnormal renal tubular phosphate fluxes. In contrast, severe acute hypophosphatemia may cause anorexia, dizziness, bone pain, proximal muscular weakness, and waddling gait. Significant hypophosphatemia is encountered in severe alcoholics and may be aggravated after repletion of nutrients, in the course of therapy of diabetic ketoacidosis, and for various reasons in severely ill, hospitalized elderly patients (see also Chap. 356). Myopathy in hypophosphatemia may be accompanied by elevations in serum creatinine kinase levels and by rhabdomyolysis. Severe congestive cardiomyopathy can occur with chronic hypophosphatemia, and restoration of phosphorus deficits leads to prompt reversal. Respiratory muscle weakness in severe hypophosphatemia also may improve with phosphate repletion. The bone pain and waddling gait are attributed to the osteomalacia that occurs with phosphate depletion. The muscular weakness may be due either to direct effects of hypophosphatemia on nerves and muscle

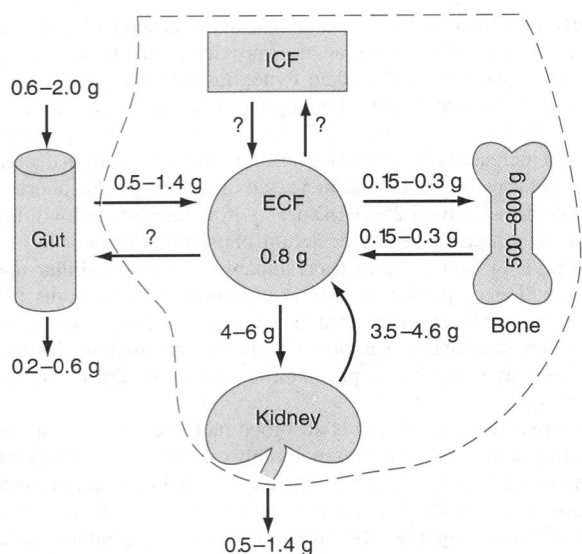

FIGURE 353-3 Phosphate homeostasis. Schematic illustration of inorganic phosphorus content (termed here *phosphate*) in extracellular fluid (ECF) and bone as well as diet and feces; magnitude of phosphorus flux per day as estimated by various methods is shown at transport sites in intestine, kidney, and bone. Range of values shown illustrates special features of phosphorus metabolism discussed in text. Intestinal phosphorus absorption is highly efficient, 85 percent at a lower intake (0.5 g of a 0.6-g intake) and 70 percent at a higher intake (1.4 g of a 2.0-g intake). Estimates of magnitude of endogenous fecal phosphate are less well established than for calcium. Contribution of at least 0.15 g is estimated to be added to the nonabsorbed phosphorus to provide a total of 0.2 g fecal phosphorus at the low intake level. At high phosphorus dietary intakes, no correction for endogenous fecal phosphate is calculated. Higher quantities of phosphorus are excreted in urine at all levels of dietary intake than for corresponding intakes of calcium; quantities excreted match closely the quantities absorbed, thereby maintaining phosphorus balance (no correction in this illustration is made for endogenous fecal phosphorus). Note that renal phosphorus reabsorption, in contrast to high and relatively invariant renal calcium reabsorption, varies from a low of 75 percent of filtered load to greater than 85 percent. The compartment labeled ICF refers to intracellular phosphorus, both organic and inorganic; rapid shifts of phosphorus into cells (and corresponding, possibly slower, efflux of phosphorus from cells) contribute to changes in ECF phosphorus. These shifts between ECF and ICF and phosphorus release from and uptake by bone are equal in conditions of phosphorus balance.

or, occasionally, to the effects of hyperparathyroidism (either primary or secondary), which may have a role in the etiology of the hypophosphatemia. Phosphorus depletion in children may impair growth. Hypophosphatemia causes decreased levels of 2,3-diphosphoglyceric acid and ATP in erythrocytes, which in turn alter the dissociation of oxyhemoglobin so that less oxygen is delivered to tissues. Hemolytic anemia may result from impairment of the ability of erythrocytes to deform in small vessels.

VITAMIN D

Vitamin D is a hormone rather than a vitamin. With adequate exposure to sunlight, no dietary supplements are needed. The active principle of vitamin D is synthesized under metabolic control via successive hydroxylations in the liver and kidney and is transported through the blood to its target tissues (the small intestine and bone), where it regulates calcium homeostasis. Calcium and phosphate ions, parathyroid hormone, and possibly other peptide and steroid hormones regulate the renal metabolism of vitamin D. Analysis of hereditary and acquired defects in these processes has provided new insights into the pathophysiology of several disorders involving calcium, phosphorus,

and bone metabolism. These discoveries culminated in the chemical synthesis of active vitamin D metabolites and analogues, the clinical use of 1,25-dihydroxyvitamin D, [1,25(OH)$_2$D] (calcitriol) in many vitamin D–resistant states, and the development of assays for measuring vitamin D metabolites in blood to define abnormalities in vitamin D metabolism.

PHOTOBIOGENESIS OF VITAMIN D Vitamin D$_3$ is a derivative of 7-dehydrocholesterol (provitamin D$_3$), the immediate precursor of cholesterol. When skin is exposed to sunlight or certain artificial light sources, the ultraviolet radiation enters the epidermis and causes transformation of 7-dehydrocholesterol to vitamin D$_3$. Wavelengths between 290 and 315 nm are absorbed by the conjugated double bonds at C$_5$ and C$_7$ of 7-dehydrocholesterol and fragment the B ring between C$_9$ and C$_{10}$ to yield a 9,10-secosterol (*seco* means "split"), previtamin D$_3$ (Fig. 353-4). Previtamin D$_3$ is biologically inert but undergoes a spontaneous temperature-dependent molecular rearrangement of its conjugated triene system (three double bonds) to form the thermally stable 9,10-secosterol, vitamin D$_3$ (see Fig. 353-4). At body temperature it takes approximately 24 h for previtamin D$_3$ to convert completely into vitamin D$_3$. Wide changes in skin surface temperature do not affect the rate of this conversion because the process occurs in the actively growing layers of the epidermis, where the temperature is relatively constant; changes in the core body temperature also have little effect on this reaction. Once vitamin D$_3$ is synthesized, it is translocated from the epidermis into the circulation by the vitamin D–binding protein. Thus, vitamin D is made in the skin from the previtamin for many hours after a single sun exposure (see Fig. 353-4). Although melanin in the skin competes with 7-dehydrocholesterol for ultraviolet photons and thus can limit the synthesis of previtamin D$_3$, the photochemical isomerization of previtamin D$_3$ and vitamin D$_3$ to biologically inert products appears to be more important in preventing excessive production of previtamin D$_3$ and vitamin D$_3$ during prolonged exposure to the sun.

Aging decreases the capacity of the skin to produce vitamin D$_3$; this capacity is reduced more than fourfold after age 70. Topical sunscreens can reduce or prevent cutaneous production of vitamin D$_3$ by absorbing the solar radiation responsible for previtamin D$_3$ synthesis in the skin. Other factors that affect the cutaneous synthesis of vitamin D$_3$ include altitude, geographic location, time of day, and area exposed. Latitude has profound effects on the cutaneous synthesis of vitamin D$_3$. As the zenith angle of the sun increases with approaching winter, more of the high-energy ultraviolet photons responsible for formation of the previtamin are absorbed by the ozone layer. In Boston (42°N) and in Edmonton (52°N), the absorption of these photons is so complete that essentially no vitamin D$_3$ is made in the skin between the months of November through February and October through March, respectively. When the entire body is exposed to sufficient sunlight to cause mild erythema, the increase in the blood vitamin D is about equivalent to consuming an oral dose of 10,000 to 25,000 international units (1 IU = 0.025 μg) of vitamin D. Only when skin irradiation is insufficient to produce the required quantities of vitamin D$_3$ is dietary supplementation needed to prevent skeletal mineralization defects. Fish liver oils, a natural source of vitamin D, were used widely for the treatment of rickets early in this century. The fortification of milk and some cereals with either crystalline vitamin D$_2$ (see Fig. 353-4) or vitamin D$_3$ prevents rickets and osteomalacia. However, a survey of the vitamin D content in milk from the United States and western Canada revealed that 71 percent did not contain 80 to 120 percent of the amount of vitamin D on the label and that approximately 15 percent of skim milk did not contain detectable vitamin D. Although the National Research Council of the United States recommends an intake of 200 IU/d for adults, this amount may be inadequate if there is little cutaneous production of vitamin D$_3$. In the absence of sunlight, between 400 and 600 IU of vitamin D is required to satisfy the daily requirement.

METABOLISM OF VITAMIN D Once vitamin D enters the circulation, either by absorption from the diet or through synthesis in the skin, it is transported to the liver bound to a specific alpha$_1$ globulin (vitamin D–binding protein). In the liver, vitamin D is metabolized to 25-hydroxyvitamin D [25(OH)D] by hepatic mitochondrial and/or microsomal enzyme(s) (see Fig. 353-4). 25(OH)D is one of the major circulating metabolites, and its half-life is about 21 days. The concentrations of 25(OH)D and some of its metabolites in the serum are measured using competitive binding assays. The normal serum 25(OH)D concentration varies among different laboratories from 20 to 200 nmol/L (8 to 80 ng/mL). Individuals exposed to excessive sunlight may have concentrations of 25(OH)D up to 250 nmol/L (100 ng/mL) without adverse effects on calcium metabolism. The normal range is lower in Great Britain, where additions of vitamin D to foods are not routine and where exposure to sunlight is less than in most regions of the United States. The serum 25(OH)D levels usually reflect both 25-hydroxyvitamin D_2 [25(OH)D_2] and 25-hydroxyvitamin D_3 [25(OH)D_3]. The ratio of these two 25-hydroxylated derivatives depends on the relative amounts of vitamins D_2 or D_3 present in the diet and the amount of previtamin D_3 produced by exposure to sunlight.

The hepatic 25-hydroxylation of vitamin D is regulated by a product feedback mechanism. This regulation, however, is not tight; an increase in dietary intake or endogenous production of vitamin D_3 causes increases in 25(OH)D levels in the serum. The levels can rise to greater than 1200 nmol/L (500 ng/mL) when the intake of vitamin D is excessive. Serum 25(OH)D levels are reduced in severe chronic liver disease (Table 353-1).

25(OH)D is not biologically active at physiologic levels in vivo but is active in vitro at high concentrations. After formation in the liver, 25(OH)D is bound by the vitamin D–binding protein and transported to the kidney for an additional stereospecific hydroxylation on either C_1 or C_{24} (see Fig. 353-4). The kidney plays a pivotal role in the metabolism of 25(OH)D to the biologically active metabolite. The renal mitochondrial 25(OH)D-1-hydroxylase activity is enhanced by hypocalcemia, so that hypocalcemia causes the rate of conversion of 25(OH)D to 1,25(OH)$_2$D to increase. Hypocalcemia may not control this hydroxylation directly, however. Any decrease in the serum concentration of calcium below normal is a stimulus for increased secretion of PTH, which increases the synthesis of 1,25(OH)$_2$D in the renal proximal convoluted tubule. The renal production of 1,25(OH)$_2$D enhances the effects of PTH in lowering circulating concentrations (and presumably renal intracellular concentrations) of phosphate (Fig. 353-5). 1,25(OH)$_2$D also influences the renal metabolism of 25(OH)D by diminishing 25(OH)D-1α-hydroxylase activity and enhancing the metabolism of 25(OH)D to 24R,25-dihydroxyvitamin D [24,25(OH)$_2$D].

24,25(OH)$_2$D is normally present in serum at a concentration of 1 to 10 nmol/L (0.5 to 5.0 ng/mL). 24,25(OH)$_2$D is also a substrate for renal 25(OH)D-1α-hydroxylase and is converted to 1α,24R,25-trihydroxyvitamin D [1,24,25(OH)$_3$D], which, in turn, is metabolized to the biologically inactive substance calcitroic acid (see Fig. 353-4). Cultured cells that possess nuclear receptors for 1,25(OH)$_2$D, such as chondrocytes, skin keratinocytes and fibroblasts, and intestinal and melanoma cells, also metabolize 25(OH)D to 24,25(OH)$_2$D. Although 24,25(OH)$_2$D may play a role in the expression of vitamin D action, it is more likely that the C_{24} hydroxylation is the first step in the degradation of both 25(OH)D and 1,25(OH)$_2$D to water-soluble inactive metabolites, including cal-

citroic acid; 25(OH)D and 1,25(OH)$_2$D are converted to more than 35 metabolites, most of which appear to be degradation products.

PHYSIOLOGY OF VITAMIN D

1,25(OH)$_2$D, produced by the kidney and the placenta, is the only known important metabolite of vitamin D; the potential roles of other metabolites have not been clarified. 1,25(OH)$_2$D bound to a vitamin D–binding protein is deliv-

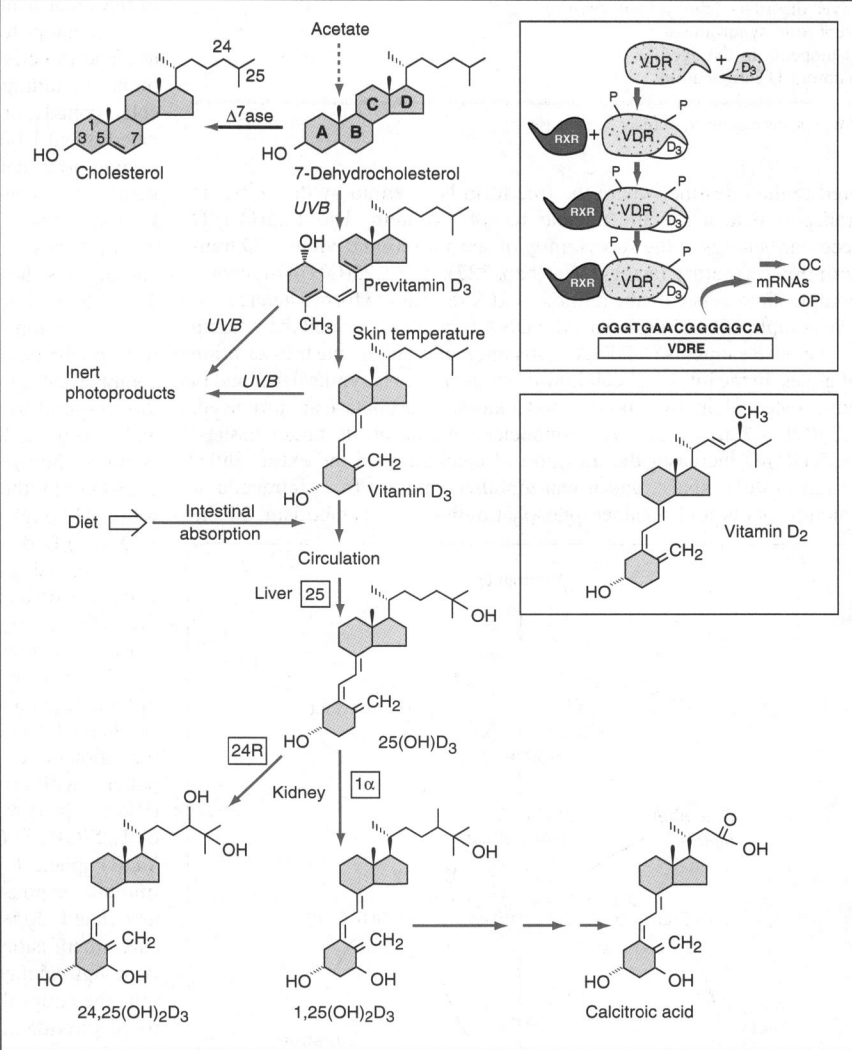

FIGURE 353-4 The photobiogenesis and metabolism of vitamin D. 7-Dehydrocholesterol either can be reduced by 7-dehydrocholesterol reductase ($Δ^7$ase) to cholesterol or photolyzed in the skin by solar ultraviolet B radiation (UVB) to previtamin D_3. Once formed, previtamin D_3 thermally isomerizes to vitamin D_3. Exposure of previtamin D_3 and vitamin D_3 to UVB radiation results in the generation of a variety of biologically inert photoproducts. Vitamin D_3 enters the circulation and is hydroxylated by the hepatic vitamin D-25-hydroxylase (step 25) to 25-hydroxyvitamin D_3, shown as 25(OH)D_3. 25-Hydroxyvitamin D_3 can be metabolized by a 25(OH)D-24-hydroxylase (step 24R) to 24,25-dihydroxyvitamin D_3, i.e., 24,25-(OH)$_2$$D_3$. 25-Hydroxyvitamin D_3 is converted in the kidney by the 25-OH-D-1α-hydroxylase (step 1α) to its biologically active form, 1,25-dihydroxyvitamin D_3, i.e., 1,25(OH)$_2$$D_3$. This form enters the circulation and is ultimately recognized by target tissues that possess a specific nuclear receptor (VDR) for it.

As shown in the top two inserts, the VDR, a member of the steroid superfamily of receptors, interacts with 1,25(OH)$_2$$D_3$ (identified as D_3), resulting in the phosphorylation of the 1,25(OH)$_2$$D_3$–VDR complex. This complex interacts with the retinoic acid X receptor (RXR) to form a heterodimer which, in turn, interacts with the vitamin D–responsive element (VDRE) in the targeted nuclei. In the bone, this interaction increases the expression of mRNAs for osteocalcin (OC) and osteopontin (OP).

1,25-Dihydroxyvitamin D_3 can undergo multiple hydroxylations in its side chain that may ultimately result in the formation of the water-soluble biologically inactive calcitroic acid.

The lower insert is the structure for vitamin D_2. It is structurally different from vitamin D_3 in having a double bond between C_{22} and C_{23} and a methyl group on C_{24}.

Table 353-1

Serum Concentrations of 25(OH)D in Disorders of Calcium, Phosphorus, and Bone Metabolism

Disease States	Serum 25(OH)D
Vitamin D deficiency	↓
Intestinal malabsorption syndromes	↓
Liver disorders (chronic and severe)	↓
Nephrotic syndrome	↓
Osteopenia in the aged	N or ↓
Vitamin D intoxication	↑

NOTE: ↓, decreased; N, normal; ↑, increased.

ered to the intestine, where the free form is taken up by the cells and transported to a specific nuclear receptor protein. The 1,25(OH)$_2$D receptor belongs to the superfamily of steroid-retinoid-vitamin D transcription regulatory factors (see Chap. 327). The 1,25(OH)$_2$D-receptor complex interacts with the retinoic acid X receptor to form a heterodimeric complex that binds to specific DNA sequences, termed the vitamin D response elements (VDREs). This interaction alters the transcription of genes; in the intestine, calcium-binding protein is synthesized, and in bone, osteocalcin, osteopontin, and alkaline phosphatase are produced. 1,25(OH)$_2$D also may have nonnuclear effects on its target tissues; 1,25(OH)$_2$D increases the transport of calcium from the extracellular to intracellular space, and it can mobilize calcium from intracellular calcium pools and enhance phosphatidylinositol metabolism. In the

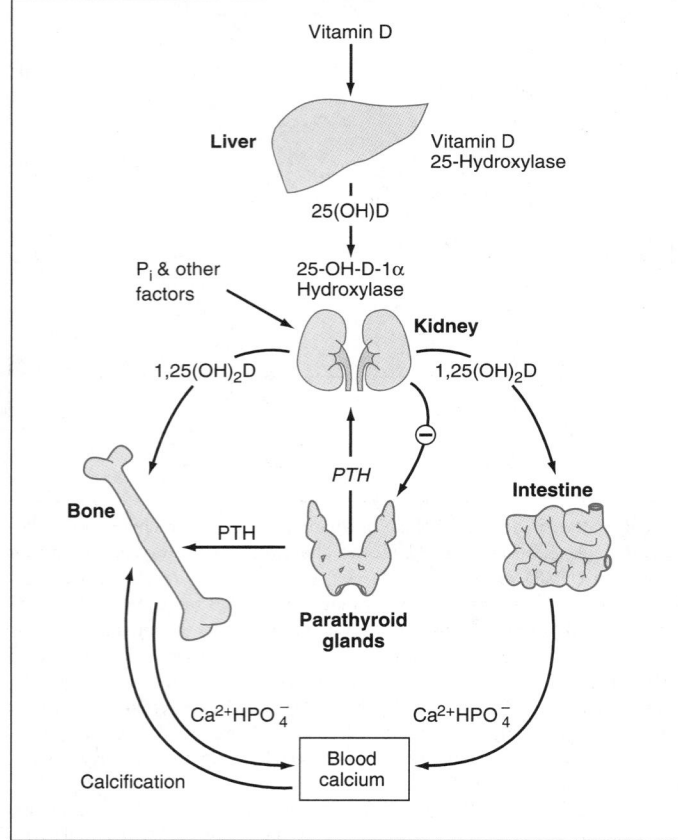

FIGURE 353-5 Schematic representation of the hormonal control loop for vitamin D metabolism and function. A reduction in the serum calcium below approximately 2.2 mmol/L (8.8 mg/dL) prompts a proportional increase in the secretion of PTH and so mobilizes additional calcium from the bone. PTH promotes the synthesis of 1,25(OH)$_2$D in the kidney, which, in turn, stimulates the mobilization of calcium from bone and intestine and regulates the synthesis of PTH by negative feedback.

intestine, the net effect of 1,25(OH)$_2$D is to stimulate calcium and phosphate transport from the lumen of the small intestine into the circulation (see Fig. 353-5). The effect of 1,25(OH)$_2$D on the enhancement of bone resorption is believed to be synergistic with that of PTH. Mature osteoclasts do not possess receptors either for PTH or for 1,25(OH)$_2$D, and the two hormones may increase bone resorption activity by stimulating immature osteoclastic precursors that possess receptors for both to become mature osteoclasts and/or by interacting with osteoblasts and bone marrow stromal cells to produce cytokines that enhance the activity of mature osteoclasts. The role of 1,25(OH)$_2$D in the renal handling of calcium and phosphorus remains uncertain.

Receptors for 1,25(OH)$_2$D are present in intestine, bone, and kidney and in cells not classically considered target organs for this hormone, including skin, breast, pituitary, parathyroids, pancreatic beta cells, gonads, brain, skeletal muscle, circulating monocytes, and activated B and T lymphocytes. Although its physiologic role in these cells remains to be determined, in vitro, 1,25(OH)$_2$D inhibits proliferation of keratinocytes and fibroblasts, stimulates terminal differentiation of keratinocytes, induces monocytes to produce IL-1 and to mature into macrophages and osteoclast-like cells, inhibits the production of PTH, and inhibits the production of IL-2 and immunoglobulin by activated T and B lymphocytes, respectively.

In addition, a variety of tumor cell lines, including lines derived from breast carcinomas, melanomas, and promyeloblasts, possess receptors for 1,25(OH)$_2$D. Tumor cell lines that have 1,25(OH)$_2$D receptors respond to the hormone by decreasing the rate of proliferation and enhancing differentiation. For example, when malignant receptor-positive human promyelocytic cells (HL-60) are exposed to 1,25(OH)$_2$D, the cells mature into functioning macrophages within 1 week. Although the mechanism of induction of maturation is unknown, 1,25(OH)$_2$D decreases the expression of c-*myc* oncogene coincident with decreasing replication. This effect, however, is not a lasting one; when the metabolite is removed from maturing HL-60 promyelocytes, the cells revert to their original malignant state, and expression of c-*myc* oncogene is no longer suppressed.

The role of 1,25(OH)$_2$D in the regulation of differentiation and immunoregulation is also unknown. However, it may regulate PTH synthesis by negative feedback (see Fig. 353-5). This possibility is the rationale for giving 1,25(OH)$_2$D$_3$ intravenously to suppress PTH in patients with chronic renal failure. Patients with vitamin D–dependent rickets type II who are unable to respond to physiologic concentrations of 1,25(OH)$_2$D (because of mutations that impair the function of the VDR) appear to have no demonstrable in vivo defects in the cellular immune response and in the growth of skin (with the exception of the associated alopecia) and other tissues. Administration of intravenous calcium infusions to these patients reverses the metabolic bone disease. Although calcitriol [1,25(OH)$_2$D] is not useful for the treatment of leukemia, the antiproliferative effects of calcitriol and its analogue calcipotriene provide the rationale for their use in the treatment of psoriasis.

Most measurements of circulating 1,25(OH)$_2$D in various physiologic or pathologic states utilize a receptor/competitive binding assay (Table 353-2). Serum levels of vitamin D and 25(OH)D vary with the season and with vitamin D intake, whereas levels of 1,25(OH)$_2$D appear to be unaltered by seasonal variation, by increases in dietary vitamin D, or by exposure to sunlight (Table 353-2); as long as vitamin D supplies and circulating concentrations of 25(OH)D are sufficient, metabolic influences control the renal 25(OH)D-1α-hydroxylase to ensure a closely regulated circulating concentration of 1,25(OH)$_2$D. The serum concentration of 1,25(OH)$_2$D ranges from 40 to 160 pmol/L (16 to 65 pg/mL), and its serum half-life is from 3 to 6 h.

The principal physiologic mechanism regulating the production of 1,25(OH)$_2$D appears to involve changes in serum extracellular calcium concentrations that result in reciprocal changes in secretion of PTH, the latter controlling, possibly through actions on serum or tissue phosphorus levels, the rate of 1,25(OH)$_2$D production. Other factors that enhance 1,25(OH)$_2$D production include estrogen, prolactin, and growth hormone. Humans adapt to increased calcium requirements during growth, pregnancy, and lactation by increasing the efficiency of intestinal calcium absorption, possibly by enhancing 25(OH)D-1-

Serum Concentrations of 1,25(OH)$_2$D in Disorders of Calcium, Phosphorus, and Bone Metabolism

Disease States	Serum 1,25(OH)$_2$D
Vitamin D deficiency	↓*
Renal failure:	
GFR > 30 (mL/min)/1.7 m^2	↓ or N
GFR < 30 (mL/min)/1.7 m^2	↓
Hypoparathyroidism	↓ or N
Pseudohypoparathyroidism	↓ or N
Vitamin D–dependent rickets:	
Type I	↓
Type II	↑
X-linked vitamin D–resistant rickets	↓ or N
Tumor-induced osteomalacia	↓
Oncogenic hypercalcemia	↓
Some lymphomas	↑
Hyperparathyroidism	↑
Sarcoidosis, tuberculosis, silicosis	↑
Idiopathic hypercalciuria	N or ↑
Williams' syndrome	↑
Vitamin D intoxication	N or ↑

* Serum 1,25(OH)$_2$D concentrations are normal or elevated in occasional patients with biopsy-proven osteomalacia and undetectable or low circulating concentrations of 25(OH)D. These patients also have secondary hyperparathyroidism, and they may represent a partially treated state; if a small amount of vitamin D is obtained from the diet or generated in the skin in these patients, the vitamin is efficiently converted to 1,25(OH)$_2$D. The net effect is low or undetectable circulating concentrations of 25(OH)D along with normal or elevated concentrations of 1,25(OH)$_2$D. However, in extreme vitamin D deficiency, circulating concentrations of 1,25(OH)$_2$D are low or undetectable.

NOTE: ↓, decreased; N, normal; ↑, increased; GFR, glomerular filtration rate.

hydroxylase activity. During the first two trimesters of pregnancy, the levels of 1,25(OH)$_2$D increase in proportion to the concentration of the vitamin D–binding protein; levels of free 1,25(OH)$_2$D do not change. During the last trimester, the need for calcium for mineralization of the fetal skeleton is met by an increase in the concentrations of free 1,25(OH)$_2$D and enhanced maternal intestinal calcium absorption.

PATHOPHYSIOLOGY OF DISORDERS OF VITAMIN D NUTRITION AND METABOLISM *Hypovitaminosis D* results from inadequate endogenous production of vitamin D$_3$ in the skin, from insufficient dietary supplementation, and/or from an inability of the small intestine to absorb adequate amounts of the vitamin from the diet. Resistance to the effects of vitamin D can result from (1) use of drugs that antagonize vitamin D action, (2) alterations in the metabolism of vitamin D, or (3) deficient or defective receptors for 1,25(OH)$_2$D. The consequences of hypovitaminosis D include (1) disturbances of mineral ion metabolism and secretion of PTH and (2) mineralization defects in the skeleton (e.g., rickets in children, osteomalacia in adults). The changes in the skeleton are described in Chap. 355. With regard to calcium metabolism, lack of vitamin D action leads to insufficient intestinal calcium absorption and hypocalcemia. The latter stimulates the secretion of PTH (secondary hyperparathyroidism), which enhances calcium release from bone and decreases calcium clearance by the kidney and tends to blunt the hypocalcemia; as a consequence most patients have a normal or low-normal serum calcium level. (Late in the course of untreated hypovitaminosis D, severe hypocalcemia develops.) Hypophosphatemia is more marked than hypocalcemia, especially in early stages of the deficiency. The efficiency of intestinal phosphate absorption is also decreased. The increased secretion of PTH, although partially effective in minimizing hypocalcemia, leads to urinary phosphate wasting through decreases in renal tubular reabsorption. This latter effect is the most significant factor in causing hypophosphatemia. With an adequate GFR, the main changes are hypophosphatemia, normal or near-normal serum calcium levels, increased levels of PTH, and low levels of 25(OH)D (see Table 353-1). As discussed in Chap. 355, defects in skeletal mineralization may accompany these disturbances in mineral ion metabolism.

Although the conversion of vitamin D to 25(OH)D is impaired in severe chronic liver disease, there is no strong correlation between low serum 25(OH)D levels and osteopenia. Patients with nephrotic syndrome with more than 4 g/d of proteinuria may have low 25(OH)D levels owing to loss in the urine of the vitamin D–binding protein with its associated tightly bound 25(OH)D. Circulating levels of 25(OH)D also may be decreased when the metabolism of 25(OH)D to 1,25(OH)$_2$D is increased, as in sarcoidosis and hyperparathyroidism. Chronic anticonvulsant therapy also can cause the development of osteomalacia or rickets; mineralization defects are worse in patients receiving multiple drug therapy and when vitamin D intake or exposure to sunlight is inadequate. Anticonvulsant drugs have multiple effects on calcium metabolism. Phenobarbital induces hepatic microsomal enzymes, alters the kinetics of the vitamin D-25-hydroxylase, and stimulates bile secretion, resulting in decreased serum concentrations of vitamin D and 25(OH)D. Phenytoin and phenobarbital inhibit intestinal calcium transport and bone mineral mobilization, independent of effects of vitamin D metabolism.

Glucocorticoids in high doses cause osteoporosis but do not induce osteomalacia and rickets. Glucocorticoids directly inhibit vitamin D–mediated intestinal calcium absorption and bone mineral mobilization and enhance the sensitivity of bone cells to 1,25(OH)$_2$D by stabilizing the 1,25(OH)$_2$D receptor or by increasing the affinity or number of receptors. Patients receiving glucocorticoids chronically may have depressed circulating levels of 1,25(OH)$_2$D; the mechanism(s) is unknown.

A genetic defect in the hepatic 25-hydroxylation of vitamin D has not been described, but in one inherited disorder of calcium and bone metabolism renal production of 1,25(OH)$_2$D is defective. In the syndrome of pseudovitamin D–deficient rickets (also known as vitamin D–dependent rickets type I; see Chap. 355), renal production of 1,25(OH)$_2$D is impaired, circulating levels of 1,25(OH)$_2$D are low, but the therapeutic response to physiologic doses of calcitriol (0.25 to 1.0 μg/d) is normal. These findings are accounted for by a deficiency in renal 25(OH)D-1α-hydroxylase activity. In patients with a similar phenotype, pseudovitamin D–resistant rickets (vitamin D–dependent rickets type II), mutations impair the function of the 1,25(OH)$_2$D receptor by altering the binding of the hormone to the receptor or the binding of the hormone-heterodimer complex to DNA. Individuals with this disorder have high circulating levels of 1,25(OH)$_2$D; administration of high doses of vitamin D produces further increases in the levels of 1,25(OH)$_2$D.

In patients with X-linked hypophosphatemic rickets, serum concentrations of 1,25(OH)$_2$D are normal or low. Since hypophosphatemia is a potent stimulator of the renal 25(OH)D-1α-hydroxylase, levels of 1,25(OH)$_2$D should be high. In this syndrome there is a functional defect in the 25(OH)D-1-hydrolase. Therefore, the combination of calcitriol and phosphate supplements is more effective than therapy with phosphate supplements alone (Chap. 355). In patients with mild to moderate chronic renal failure [GFR > 0.5 mL/s (> 30 mL/min)] and decreased phosphate clearance, hyperphosphatemia and acidosis play important roles in suppressing the renal production of 1,25(OH)$_2$D despite high circulating concentrations of PTH. With progressive destruction of the renal cortex, the reserves of the 25(OH)D-1α-hydroxylase are depleted to a point at which the kidney is unable to produce sufficient 1,25(OH)$_2$D to maintain calcium homeostasis, even when serum phosphorus concentrations are normal. Under these circumstances, replacement therapy with calcitriol is most beneficial (Chap. 355). Aging decreases the responsiveness of the renal 25(OH)D-1-hydroxylase to PTH, results in small decreases in circulating levels of 1,25(OH)$_2$D, and may contribute to decreased calcium absorption in the elderly.

Patients with hypocalcemia due to hypoparathyroidism or pseudohypoparathyroidism have lower-than-normal mean serum concentrations of 1,25(OH)$_2$D, although individual values may be in the normal range. In these patients, small replacement doses of calcitriol (0.25 to 1.0 μg/d; see Chap. 354) are effective even when the serum 25(OH)D concentrations are elevated. These observations suggest that absent or ineffective action of PTH decreases the activity of renal 25(OH)D-1-

hydroxylase. It is not known whether serum $1,25(OH)_2D$ levels would be restored if the hyperphosphatemia were controlled.

Patients with tumor-induced (oncogenic) osteomalacia have low levels of serum phosphorus and $1,25(OH)_2D$. These tumors presumably secrete a substance(s) that causes renal phosphorus wasting and inhibits the synthesis of $1,25(OH)_2D$; after removal of the tumor, the serum phosphorus and $1,25(OH)_2D$ levels return to normal.

In disorders such as sarcoidosis (and other chronic granulomatous disorders), lymphomas, idiopathic hypercalciuria, and Williams' syndrome there is enhanced synthesis of $1,25(OH)_2D$ from $25(OH)D$ (see Table 353-2). Hypercalcemia and hypercalciuria in sarcoidosis are associated with elevated circulating concentrations of $1,25(OH)_2D$; granulomas and pulmonary alveolar macrophages from patients with sarcoidosis synthesize $1,25(OH)_2D$. Normal pulmonary macrophages also can be induced to metabolize $25(OH)D$ to $1,25(OH)_2D$ in vitro when exposed to lipopolysaccharides from the cell wall of gram-negative bacteria or to interferon γ. Most patients with tumor-induced hypercalcemia have low circulating levels of $1,25(OH)_2D$ (see Table 353-2). The exceptions are patients with several types of lymphoma (including T cell, mixed histiocytic-lymphocytic, and B cell immunoblastic lymphomas) where hypercalcemia is associated with elevated concentrations of $1,25(OH)_2D$. In one report, surgical excision of a solitary splenic lymphoma resulted in rapid return of elevated serum $1,25(OH)_2D$ and calcium levels to normal, suggesting that the lymphoma metabolized $25(OH)D$ to $1,25(OH)_2D$ in an unregulated manner. Patients with hypercalcemia and elevated blood levels of $1,25(OH)_2D$ due to unregulated extrarenal production of the hormone respond to glucocorticoids with a decrease in the circulating concentrations of $1,25(OH)_2D$ and calcium. Patients with primary hyperparathyroidisim, hypercalciuria, and renal stones usually have elevated circulating levels of $1,25(OH)_2D$. Similarly, in some instances of idiopathic hypercalciuria, intestinal calcium absorption is increased inappropriately. Approximately one-third of these patients have high-normal or elevated circulating $1,25(OH)_2D$. These findings are consistent with the hypothesis that excessive $1,25(OH)_2D$ production is responsible for the hyperabsorption of calcium by the small intestine. Infants with hypercalcemia associated with supravalvular aortic stenosis, mental retardation, and elfin facies (*Williams' syndrome*) also have elevated serum concentrations of $1,25(OH)_2D$. It is not clear whether the increased levels result from abnormal synthesis or degradation of $1,25(OH)_2D$.

It has been suggested that alteration of vitamin D receptor levels in target tissues (such as intestine) could affect calcium and bone metabolism, and bone mineral density appears to be associated with specific polymorphism of the VDR gene. These polymorphisms affect the noncoding intervening DNA sequences (introns) or the coding sequence in a way that does not alter the amino acid sequence of the VDR; specifically, polymorphisms involving the endonucleases Bsm-I and Taq-I (bb, TT) have been associated with higher bone mineral density.

PHARMACOLOGY AND SOURCES OF VITAMIN D AND ITS METABOLITES Casual exposure to sunlight provides most humans with their vitamin D requirement. For the elderly who wish to take advantage of this natural source of vitamin D, exposure of hands, face, and arms to a suberythemal dose of sunlight two to three times a week is usually adequate. If the patient plans to remain outdoors in sunlight after the initial exposure, a sunscreen with a protection factor of at least 15 (SPF-15) should be applied to help prevent the damaging effects caused by excessive chronic overexposure to sunlight. A variety of over-the-counter vitamin preparations contain 400 IU of either vitamin D_2 or vitamin D_3. More potent preparations of vitamin D (calciferol) are available in capsule and tablet form (50,000 IU), as oil (500,000 IU/mL), and in oral solution (8000 IU/mL). A single oral dose of 50,000 IU of vitamin D_2 increases the circulating concentrations of vitamin D from less than 25 nmol/L (10 ng/mL) to 130 to 260 nmol/L (50 to 100 ng/mL) within 12 to 24 h; the plasma half-life is about 2 d. Serum concentrations of $25(OH)D$ and $1,25(OH)_2D$ are

not changed by these doses of vitamin D. For treatment of vitamin D deficiency, 50,000 IU of vitamin D once a week for 8 weeks raises the circulating concentration of $25(OH)D$ into the normal range; in the presence of secondary hyperparathyroidism, the circulating concentrations of $1,25(OH)_2D$ can increase to supranormal levels [up to 600 pmol/L (250 pg/mL)]. $25(OH)D_2$ (calcifediol) is available in capsules containing either 20 or 50 μg. This drug may be useful in treating vitamin D deficiency [low $25(OH)D$ concentrations] in patients with severe liver dysfunction. Pharmacologic doses are used to treat disorders of $25(OH)D$ metabolism; in pharmacologic doses, $25(OH)D_3$ is believed to act via interaction with the VDR. Calcitriol is available in capsules containing 0.25 or 0.5 μg and as a solution for intravenous use (1.0 and 2.0 $\mu g/mL$). Calcitriol is efficacious in a variety of disorders (see Chap. 354). 1α-Hydroxyvitamin D_3 [$1(OH)D_3$] is a potent $1,25(OH)_2D_3$ agonist that is used in Europe and Japan. The structure of this analogue is identical to that of the natural renal hormone with the exception that it lacks a C_{25} OH (Fig. 353-6). In humans, this analogue is rapidly metabolized by the liver to $1,25(OH)_2D_3$. Topical preparations of calcitriol (3 $\mu g/g$) in Europe and calcipotriene (50 $\mu g/g$) in Europe and the United States are used for the treatment of psoriasis. When used over a large surface area, both potentially could cause hypercalcemia and hypercalciuria. Oral calcitriol is also effective for psoriasis and psoriatic arthritis.

When vitamin D is chemically manipulated to rotate the A ring through 180 degrees, the C_3 β-OH assumes a geometric position that mimics the C_1 α-OH (see Fig. 353-6). These compounds, called *pseudo-1α-hydroxyvitamin D analogues*, include the clinically useful dihydrotachysterol (DHT). This analogue is less effective in stimulating intestinal calcium transport on a weight basis than either vitamin

FIGURE 353-6 Structure of 1,25-dihydroxyvitamin D_3, i.e., $1\alpha,25(OH)_2D_3$, and some of its clinically important analogues. When vitamin D_3 is hydrogenated, its A ring is rotated 180°, placing the 3β-OH in a pseudo 1α spatial orientation. This analogue, dihydrotachysterol (DHT$_3$) is metabolized by a liver 25-hydroxylase (step 25) to 25-hydroxydihydrotachysterol, i.e., $25(OH)DHT_3$. It is believed that $25(OH)DHT_3$ is the biologically active form that mimics $1,25(OH)_2D_3$ in its activity. Two clinically important analogues of $1\alpha,25(OH)_2D_3$ include its 25-deoxy derivative 1α-hydroxyvitamin D_3, i.e., $1\alpha(OH)D_3$, and calcipotriene. $1\alpha(OH)D_3$ is metabolized in the liver by 25-hydroxylase to $1\alpha,25(OH)_2D_3$. Calcipotriene is an analogue that is currently being used in Europe for the topical treatment of psoriasis.

D or 1,25(OH)$_2$D, but because it does not require 1-hydroxylation to be active on intestinal calcium transport, it is 3 to 10 times more potent than vitamin D in disease states that impair renal 25(OH)D-1-hydroxylase, such as hypoparathyroidism and chronic renal failure. Dihydrotachysterol is efficiently metabolized in the liver to 25-hydroxy-DHT, which is the biologically active form.

PARATHYROID HORMONE **Physiology** The function of PTH is to maintain the ECF calcium concentration. The hormone acts directly on bone and kidney and indirectly on intestine through its effects on synthesis of 1,25(OH)$_2$D to increase serum calcium concentrations; in turn, PTH production is closely regulated by the concentration of serum ionized calcium. This feedback system is the critical homeostatic mechanism for maintenance of ECF calcium. Any tendency toward hypocalcemia, as might be induced by calcium-deficient diets, is counteracted by an increased secretion of PTH. This in turn (1) acts to increase the rate of dissolution of bone mineral, thereby increasing the flow of calcium from bone into blood; (2) reduces the renal clearance of calcium, returning more of the calcium filtered at the glomerulus into ECF; and (3) increases the efficiency of calcium absorption in the intestine. The relative physiologic importance in minute-to-minute calcium homeostasis of stimulation of calcium transport in bone, kidney, and intestine is not established, but immediate control of blood calcium is probably due to effects of the hormone on bone and, to a lesser extent, on renal calcium clearance. Maintenance of steady-state calcium balance, on the other hand, probably results from the effects of the hormone on 1,25(OH)$_2$D levels and hence on the efficiency of intestinal calcium absorption. As much as 12 mmol (500 mg) calcium is transferred between the ECF and bone each day (a large amount in relation to the total ECF calcium pool), and PTH has a major effect on this transfer. The homeostatic role of the hormone serves to preserve calcium concentration in blood acutely at the cost of bone destruction. The action of PTH on kidney to increase the reabsorption of filtered calcium also may contribute to rapid regulation of blood calcium concentration.

PTH has multiple actions on bone, some direct and some indirect. There is an increased rate of release of calcium from bone into blood after administration of PTH, the time needed to observe the change varying with the dose of hormone and the overall metabolic status (influenced by age, diet, etc.). Usually 30 min to 1 h is required to detect a significant increase in blood calcium, but with the use of radioisotopes, changes in bone calcium release can be seen within minutes. When the phenomenon is studied carefully, there is even a rapid efflux of calcium out of blood into bone, presumably into bone cells, that precedes the release of calcium from bone. The chronic effects of PTH cause an increase in the number of bone cells, especially osteoclasts, and an increase in the remodeling of bone; these effects are apparent within hours after the hormone is given and persist for hours after PTH is withdrawn. Continuous exposure to elevated levels of PTH for days (as in hyperparathyroidism or the long-term infusions in animals) leads to osteoclast-mediated bone resorption. However, the administration of PTH intermittently over days in animals leads to a net stimulation of bone formation rather than bone breakdown. Studies in humans confirm that chronic *intermittent* hormone administration can lead to anabolic actions in skeleton rather than merely increased turnover. This skeletal anabolic action of PTH is being evaluated in clinical trials (see Chap. 355). Osteoblasts are thought to be crucial to this bone-forming effect of PTH, and osteoclasts are thought to mediate bone breakdown. Osteoblasts, which have PTH receptors, stimulate osteoclasts indirectly. Osteoclasts are believed to lack PTH receptors.

The action of PTH on osteoclasts is believed to be indirect, through cytokines released from osteoblasts to activate osteoclasts; in experimental studies of bone resorption in vitro osteoblasts must be present along with osteoclasts for PTH to activate osteoclasts to resorb bone. The nature of the cytokines that stimulate osteoclasts is a subject of major interest. IGF-1, interleukin-6, granulocyte-macrophage colony stimulating factor (GM-CSF), and possibly other agents are candidates, but the definitive messenger(s) has not been determined.

Chemistry The complete amino acid sequences of PTH from cow, pig, rat, and human have been defined. The peptides consist of a single-chain structure composed of 84 amino acids. The molecules lack cysteine or cystine; the sequences of the four forms of the hormone are similar. The sequence of chicken PTH has been deduced from the nucleotide sequence of the cloned cDNA. This molecule differs from the mammalian hormones. One large sequence deletion in the middle of the molecule and a larger addition near the carboxyl terminus result in a molecule of 88 rather than 84 amino acids. There is, however, marked conservation in the amino-terminal portion needed for biologic actions of the molecule.

Some structural requirements for the binding of the hormone to receptors and hence for its biologic activity have been defined. Synthetic fragments containing the amino-terminal sequence residues 1–34 (or even shorter sequences, 2–26 being minimally active) exert the known biologic actions of the hormone on mineral ion transport in kidney and bone and, by stimulating the renal 25-hydroxyvitamin D-1α-hydroxylase, stimulate intestinal calcium absorption. The biologic role of the carboxyl-terminal region of PTH is under investigation; a separate receptor may exist for this region of the molecule.

Fragments shortened at the amino terminus bind to the PTH receptor but have lost the capacity to stimulate biologic response. The peptide composed of sequences 7–34 is a competitive inhibitor of the binding of active hormone to receptors in vitro but is a weak inhibitor in vivo.

Biosynthesis, Secretion, and Metabolism and Mode of Action Several larger molecular forms have been identified in the biosynthetic sequence leading from gene transcription and translation to final packaging of the 84-amino-acid peptide in secretory granules prior to secretion. The earliest detected precursor, *preproparathyroid hormone*, consists of 115 amino acids; this molecular form is converted to an intermediate form of 90 amino acids termed *proparathyroid hormone* and then to the secreted product of 84 amino acids, PTH. PTH shares with other polypeptides and proteins destined for secretion from cells this complex pattern of initial synthesis as a larger molecule, which is then reduced in size by several cleavages prior to secretion; there is close analogy with the regulatory steps in biosynthesis, transport, and packaging of other proteins destined for secretion. The hydrophobic regions of the preproparathyroid hormone are similar to preprotein-specific regions of other cell-secreted proteins and serve a role in guiding transport of the polypeptide from sites of synthesis on polyribosomes through the endoplasmic reticulum to secretory granules. The degree and nature of the regulation of these sequential steps in PTH biosynthesis is poorly understood. In one kindred with hypoparathyroidism, a mutation in the preprotein region of the gene disrupts the critical hydrophobic sequence and interferes with hormone secretion.

The genes for bovine, rat, and human PTH have been cloned, and the gene structures from these three species are highly homologous. Studies with cloned and expressed PTH genes in vitro have demonstrated regions for control of gene expression at the transcriptional level, including sites for interaction and regulation by 1,25(OH)$_2$D and its receptor and "upstream" silencer elements as well as sites in which ambient calcium concentration regulates transcription. These in vitro observations are not well understood in terms of physiologic regulation of PTH biosynthesis and secretion; the rate of processing of hormone precursors and the proteolytic destruction and turnover of the hormone itself (posttranslational regulation of hormone production) may be more central to hormone availability than changes in rates of transcription. It does not appear that changes in transcriptional activity of the PTH gene in the normal physiologic range of levels of blood calcium and 1,25(OH)$_2$D nor in short-term environmental stresses (e.g., fasting for 24 h) are important in control of blood levels of the hormone. Control over hormone stores is exerted by variation in the rates of proteolytic destruction of preformed hormone under the control of ECF calcium; high calcium increases and low calcium inhibits the proteolytic destruction of hormone stores.

Blood calcium concentration over wide ranges controls the secretion of PTH; the ionized fraction of blood calcium is the important determinant of hormone secretion. Hormone secretion increases steeply to a maximum value of five times the basal rate of secretion as calcium concentration falls from normal to the range of 1.9 to 2.0 mmol/L (7.5 to 8.0 mg/dL) (measured as total calcium). Beta-adrenergic agonists such as epinephrine and H_2 agonists also may increase hormone secretion, but the physiologic significance of these secretagogues is not established. Furthermore, drugs such as propranolol or cimetidine do not reproducibly decrease circulating PTH levels.

Magnesium may influence hormone secretion in the same direction as calcium but is a less potent secretagogue. It is unlikely that physiologic variations in magnesium concentration affect PTH secretion, but severe intracellular magnesium deficiency impairs PTH secretion.

ECF calcium level controls PTH secretion by interaction with a calcium sensor, a G protein–linked receptor for which Ca^{2+} ions act as the ligand. Stimulation of the receptor by high calcium levels leads to a suppression of the rate of PTH secretion via intracellular signals generated by the active receptor. The intracellular signals appear to be inositol triphosphate and diacylglycerol formed by activation of phospholipase by the calcium sensor. This receptor is a member of a subfamily of the G protein receptor superfamily that is characterized by a large extracellular domain suitable for "clamping" the small-molecule ligand. The receptor is present in parathyroid glands, the calcitonin-secreting cells (C cells) of the thyroid, brain, and kidney. The biologic role of the receptor in tissues other than the parathyroid gland is not known. As discussed in Chap. 354, the physiologic role of the calcium sensor as the mediator of the response of the gland was substantiated by demonstrating that point mutations that impair function of the receptor lead to distinctive phenotypes, hyperparathyroidism or hypoparathyroidism.

The hormone secreted in vivo by normal bovine and human parathyroid glands and from parathyroid adenomas is indistinguishable by immunologic criteria and by molecular size from the 84-amino-acid peptide (molecular weight 9500) extracted from glands. However, much of the immunoreactive material found in the circulation of humans and animals (cow, dog) is smaller than the extracted or secreted hormone. The principal circulating fragments of immunoreactive hormone (approximate molecular weight 7000) lack a portion of the critical amino-terminal sequence required for biologic activity and, hence, may be biologically inactive fragments (so-called middle- and carboxyl-terminal fragments). Study of these fragments suggests that an endopeptidase cleaves the molecule into at least two types of pieces. Much of the proteolysis of hormone occurs in the liver and kidney.

The proteolytic process should result in formation of a second fragment (molecular weight 2000 to 3000) representing the amino-terminal, biologically active portion of the hormone. Hormone fragments as well as intact hormone are also released from the gland. However, fragments corresponding only to the middle- and carboxyl-terminal portions have been detected so far in effluent blood. If biologically active fragments do actually survive hormone proteolysis within the gland or in peripheral sites, such amino-terminal fragments could be alternative active hormonal species. After much study, certain conclusions can be drawn. There is no convincing evidence for circulating amino-terminal fragments. Circulating biologically active fragments are also not detected after analysis of products produced by peripheral metabolism. Peripheral metabolism of PTH does not appear to be regulated by physiologic states (high versus low calcium, etc.); hence peripheral metabolism of hormone, although responsible for rapid clearance of secreted hormone, appears to be a high-capacity, metabolically invariant catabolic process.

The rate of clearance of the secreted 84-amino-acid peptide from blood is more rapid than the rate of clearance of the biologically inactive fragment(s) corresponding to the middle- and carboxyl-terminal regions of the molecules that result from peripheral metabolism or glandular secretion. Hence measurements of PTH in blood by most earlier immunoassays provided only an overall index of parathyroid gland activity rather than a direct measure of biologically active hormone. Changes in the rate of production or clearance of fragments can change the concentration of immunoreactive hormone without influencing the rate of hormone secretion. Such discordance between concentrations of immunoreactive hormone and biologically active peptide occurs, for example, in renal failure, since the kidney seems to be the principal route of excretion of inactive hormone fragments. The problems inherent in accurate measurements of PTH in blood due to the heterogeneity of circulating forms of the molecule are circumvented by use of double-antibody assays that detect only the intact molecule. → *This is discussed in Chap. 354).*

Parathyroid Hormone–Related Protein The hormone termed parathyroid hormone–related protein (PTHrP) is responsible for hypercalcemia in cancer patients, a syndrome that resembles hyperparathyroidism. This hormone, now appreciated to be principally a paracrine or autocrine factor, plays a role both in fetal development and in adult physiology. Many different cell types produce PTHrP, including brain, pancreas, heart, lung, mammary tissue, placenta, endothelial cells, and smooth muscle.

PTH and PTHrP, although distinctive proteins and products of different genes, share considerable functional and structural homology (Fig. 353-7) and may have evolved from an ancestral gene. The structure of the gene for human PTHrP, however, is more complex than that of PTH, containing multiple exons and multiple sites for alternate splicing patterns during formation of the messenger RNA. Protein products of 141, 139, and 173 amino acids are produced. The varying molecular forms have multiple potential internal cleavage sites, and the biologic roles of these various molecular species and the nature of the circulating forms of PTHrP are unclear. The assays currently available are based on a variety of immunologic methods. Furthermore, multiple PTHrP products are synthesized, and other molecular forms

FIGURE 353-7 Schematic diagram to illustrate similarities and differences in structure of human PTH and human PTHrP. Close structural (and functional) homology exists between the first 30 amino acids of hPTH and hPTHrP. The PTHrP sequence may be 144 amino acid residues in length or longer. PTH is only 84 residues long; after residue 30, there is little structural homology between the two. Dashed lines in the PTHrP sequence indicate homology; underlined residues, although different from those of PTH, still represent conservative changes (charge or polarity preserved). Eleven amino acids are identical, and a total of 21 of 30 are homologues.

may result from tissue-specific degradation at accessible internal cleavage sites. In fact, it is uncertain whether PTHrP circulates at all in normal human adults; as a paracrine factor, PTHrP may be produced, act within, and be destroyed locally within tissues.

In adults PTHrP may have little to do with calcium homeostasis, except in disease states (Chap. 354), when large tumors, especially of the squamous cell type, lead to massive overproduction of PTHrP, which then circulates. PTHrP (see Fig. 353-7) shares a significant homology with PTH in the critical amino terminus that allows it to bind to the PTH receptor; synthetic molecules corresponding to the first 34 amino acids of PTHrP bind to and activate the PTH receptor indistinguishably from effects seen with PTH.

PTHrP exerts important developmental influences in calcium and bone biology. Homozygous knockout of the PTHrP gene in mice causes a lethal deformity in which animals are born with severe skeletal deformities resembling chondrodysplasia. In fetal animals, PTHrP directs transplacental calcium transfer, and high concentrations of PTHrP are produced in mammary tissue and secreted into milk. Human and bovine milk, for example, contain very high concentrations of the hormone. The biologic significance of the latter is unknown. PTHrP also may play a role in uterine contraction.

Hormone Action The action of PTH at the biochemical level involves receptor-mediated effects on second messengers in target cells. Stimulation of enzyme activity (adenyl cyclase, phospholipase C) during hormone–target cell membrane interaction leads to an increase in second messengers, including intracellular cyclic AMP, products of polyphosphoinositol metabolism, and transmembrane and intracellular fluxes of calcium. PTH interacts with a specific receptor/adenylate cyclase complex on plasma membranes of target cells consisting of hormone receptor, enzyme catalytic unit (adenylate cyclase), and a guanyl nucleotide (GTP or GDP)–binding regulatory protein (G protein). The latter protein consists of α subunits that bind GTP and dissociate from the remainder of the G protein complex. The α subunit with bound GTP complexes with adenylate cyclase, thereby activating the enzyme to increase the rate of cyclic AMP production from ATP. Hydrolysis of the GTP to GDP on the α subunit leads to reassociation of the G units and reduction in adenylate cyclase activity. The receptor, when activated by hormone binding, drives the G protein cycle by binding the α subunit portion and catalyzing the GDP/GTP exchange. Other G proteins link hormone action to phospholipase C; rapid changes in intracellular calcium concentrations within cells may be independent of phospholipase C stimulation.

The multiplicity of PTH actions on target cells in kidney and bone and the variety of second messengers—cyclic AMP, inositol 1,4,5-triphosphate (IP$_3$), diacylglycerol (DAG), and Ca^{2+}—raise obvious questions as to the mechanism whereby specific responses are mediated. With many other hormonal systems, different receptor subtypes modulate different hormone responses.

However, only one species of PTH receptor (PTH2 receptor) has been detected so far in PTH target cells in kidney and bone in human, rat, and other animal species; studies involving the cloned PTH receptor indicate that a single PTH receptor (Fig. 353-8*B*) can be coupled to more than one G protein second-messenger kinase pathway. The receptors for PTH and calcitonin (the two receptors share close homology) are polypeptides of 500 to 600 amino acids. These receptors belong to a family of structurally related receptors that includes those for glucagon, secretin, and vasoactive intestinal peptide. Receptors of this type share limited amino acid sequence homology (Fig. 353-9) but no sequence homology with other membrane receptors. The primary amino acid sequence predicts the structures illustrated in Fig. 356-9: an extracellular domain, seven hydrophobic membrane-spanning domains connected by three extracellular and three intracellular loops, and a carboxyl-terminal intracellular domain. The extracellular regions are involved in hormone binding, and the intracellular domains, after hormone activation, bind G protein subunits to transduce hormone signaling into cellular responses through stimulation of second messengers by activated G protein subunits.

A second PTH receptor (PTH2 receptor) is expressed in brain. Its amino acid sequence and the pattern of its binding and stimulatory

FIGURE 353-8 Schematic model of PTH action. Only one PTH receptor has been identified in bone and kidney. Different G proteins—G$_s$, G$_q$, etc.—activate a cellular second messenger pathway involving either an effect on adenyl cyclase (AC) to enhance cyclic AMP (cAMP) or phospholipase C (PL-C) activation of diacylglycerol (DAG) and inositol triphosphate (IP$_3$). These second messengers then activate protein kinase A (PK-A) or protein kinase C (PK-C). Phosphorylation of specific proteins mostly still unidentified leads to distal biologic responses. Cellular specificity or other factors, such as hormone levels, receptor expression levels, must determine which pathway is activated predominantly in a given cell type. Although only one form of receptor appears to be present in kidney and bone, another receptor (PTH2 receptor) has been described in brain, and others may exist.

response to PTH and PTHrP indicate that it is structurally distinct from the PTH1 receptor. The tissue distribution of PTH2 receptor is also different. The endogenous ligand and the physiologic significance of this receptor are not defined.

The details of the biochemical steps by which an increased intracellular concentration of cyclic AMP, IP$_3$, or DAG lead to changes in calcium and phosphate ion translocation are unknown. Stimulation of protein kinases (protein kinase A, cyclic AMP; protein kinase C, DAG) and calcium transport channels is associated with a variety of hormone-specific tissue responses, some of which are cyclic AMP–dependent and others cyclic AMP–independent. These responses include inhibition of phosphate and bicarbonate transport and stimulation of calcium transport and renal 1α-hydroxylase in the kidney. The responses in bone include effects on collagen synthesis; alkaline phosphatase activity; ornithine decarboxylase, citrate decarboxylase, and glucose-6-phosphate dehydrogenase activity; DNA, protein, and phospholipid synthesis; and calcium and phosphate transport. Ultimately, these cellular biochemical events lead to an integrated hormonal response in bone turnover and calcium homeostasis.

Pathophysiology In hyperparathyroidism, PTH is overproduced by tumors of the parathyroid or by hyperplasia involving all glands. The excess hormone results in hypercalcemia secondary to increased intestinal calcium absorption [increased synthesis of 1,25(OH)$_2$D], reduced renal calcium clearance, and increased bone calcium release. Bone turnover increases in all patients, and resorption exceeds formation in many. Individual patients respond to the excess hormone variably at intestinal, renal, and bone target sites; the factors influencing the response from patient to patient are not known.

Hypophosphatemia results from the actions of the excessive PTH on renal tubular phosphate reabsorption. Hypophosphatemia in turn aggravates the hypercalcemia by increasing the synthesis of 1,25(OH)$_2$D and by increasing the sensitivity of the bone to PTH. Hypophosphatemia also may interfere with the normal mineralization of bone, leading to a mixed picture of increased resorption and deficient mineralization in adjacent skeletal sites.

Hypoparathyroidism causes hypocalcemia and hyperphosphatemia, a reversal of the response seen with hormone excess. See Chap. 354 for details of the clinical syndromes.

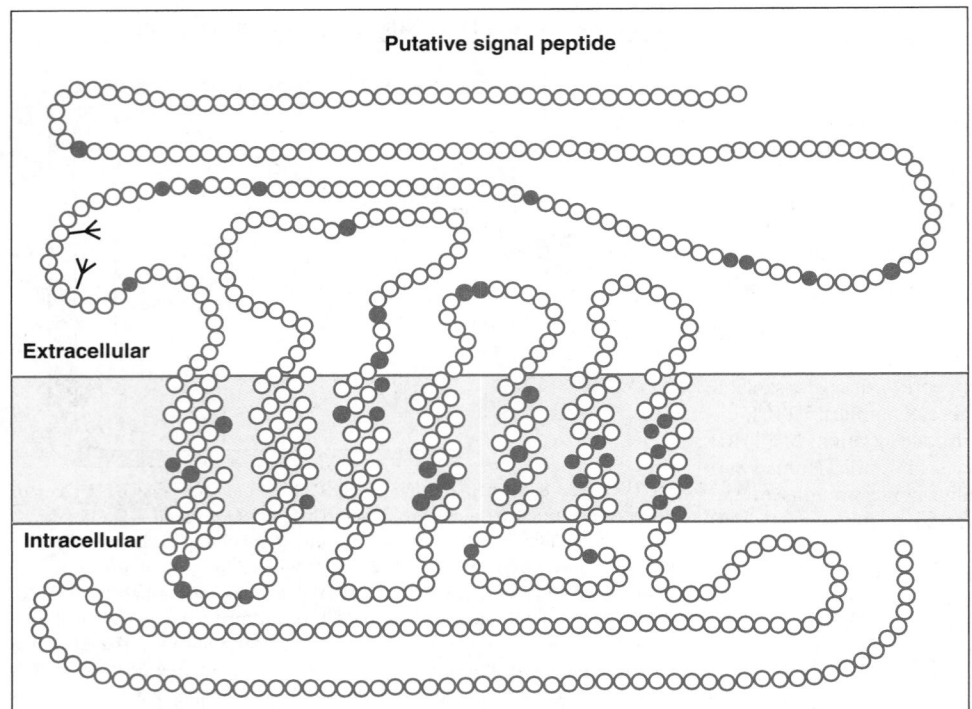

FIGURE 353-9 Schematic illustration of predicted structure of the PTH and calcitonin receptors contains one large extracellular domain, seven membrane-spanning domains, three extracellular loops connecting the membrane-spanning domains on the cell surface, one large intracellular domain, and three intracellular loops. Backbone structure is of the PTH receptor; solid residues are common between PTH and the CT receptor.

CALCITONIN (See also Chap. 340)   Calcitonin is a hypocalcemic peptide hormone that, in many ways, acts as the physiologic antagonist to parathyroid hormone. The hypocalcemic activity is accounted for primarily by inhibition of osteoclast-mediated bone resorption and secondarily by stimulation of renal calcium clearance. These effects are mediated by receptors on osteoclasts and renal tubular cells. Calcitonin exerts additional effects presumably through binding to receptors present in brain, gastrointestinal tract, and the immune system (Fig. 353-9). The hormone, for example, exerts analgesic effects directly on cells in the hypothalamus and related structures, possibly by interacting with receptors for related peptide hormones, such as calcitonin gene–related peptide (CGRP) or amylin. The latter ligands have specific high-affinity receptors and also can bind to and trigger calcitonin receptors. The calcitonin receptors, as deduced from the nucleotide sequences of the cDNA, contain seven transmembrane α-helical domains, like G protein–coupled receptors. The calcitonin, PTH, and PTHrP receptors are sufficiently different from other G protein–coupled receptors to constitute a distinct subfamily. Other members of this subfamily include receptors for secretin, vasoactive intestinal peptide, growth hormone–releasing hormone, and gastric inhibitory peptide. Interaction of calcitonin with its receptors activates signal transduction pathways that, like those for PTH, involve distinct G proteins. Thus calcitonin can stimulate adenylyl cyclase and protein kinase A as well as protein kinase C and can induce calcium transients a well. These specific G protein interactions probably involve distinct amino acid sequences in a single receptor protein.

The thyroid is the major source of the hormone, and the cells involved in calcitonin synthesis arise from neural crest tissue. During embryogenesis, these cells migrate into the ultimobranchial body, derived from the last branchial pouch. In submammalian vertebrates, the ultimobranchial body constitutes a discrete organ, anatomically separate from the thyroid gland, but in mammals the ultimobranchial gland fuses with and is incorporated into the thyroid gland.

The naturally occurring calcitonins consist of a peptide chain of 32 amino acids. There is considerable sequence variability among species. The entire chain of 32 amino acids appears to be required for biologic activity in the intact animal, although fragments function in in vitro systems. Calcitonin from salmon is 10 to 100 times more potent than mammalian forms in lowering serum calcium in animals; eel calcitonin is also potent. Slow turnover may in part explain the greater potency of salmon calcitonin, but the hormone binds more tightly to receptor sites as well. Calcitonin is synthesized as a precursor molecule that is four times larger than calcitonin itself. Analysis of the sequence of the coding portions of the gene for rat calcitonin indicates that at least two peptides flank calcitonin, from which they are separated by basic residues. It is likely (by analogy with the common precursor for adrenocorticotropic hormone and endorphin) that these peptides are released along with calcitonin. They have no known biologic function.

There are two calcitonin genes, α and β, located on chromosome 11 in the general region of the β globulin and parathyroid hormone genes. The two genes are sometimes called calcitonin/CGRP-1 and /CGRP-2. The transcription of these genes is complex. Two different messenger RNA molecules are transcribed from the α gene; one is translated into the precursor for calcitonin, and the other message is transcribed into an alternative product, CGRP. CGRP is synthesized wherever the calcitonin message is expressed, e.g., in medullary carcinoma of the thyroid. The β, or CGRP-2, gene is transcribed into the messenger RNA for CGRP in the central nervous system (CNS) in animals; this gene is silent for calcitonin production. CGRP has cardiovascular actions and may serve a neurotransmitter or developmental role in CNS.

The secretion of calcitonin is under the direct control of blood calcium: An increase in the blood calcium level causes an increase in the calcitonin level, and a decrease in the blood calcium level causes a decrease in the calcitonin level. Once secreted, calcitonin disappears from the circulation with a half-life of 2 to 15 min.

The circulating level of calcitonin in humans is lower than that in many other species. Basal and stimulated immunoreactive calcitonin levels are lower in women than in men and tend to decrease with age to a greater extent in women.

In animals calcitonin acts to lower both blood calcium and blood phosphate levels by inhibiting bone resorption and by increasing urinary calcium and phosphate clearance. The actions of calcitonin on kidney and bone are in turn modulated by the regulation of calcitonin production by serum calcium. The view that calcitonin serves to protect against hypercalcemia is thus explained by the hypocalcemic effects of calcitonin triggered in response to hypercalcemia.

In humans changes in calcium and phosphate metabolism are not seen despite extreme variations in calcitonin production; no definite effects are attributable to calcitonin deficiency (totally thyroidectomized patients receiving only replacement thyroxine) or excess (patients with medullary carcinoma of the thyroid, a calcitonin-secreting tumor) (see Chap. 340). Although there are no obvious abnormalities in calcium metabolism in patients with elevated calcitonin levels, bone remodeling is chronically suppressed. Calcitonin is a useful pharmacologic agent to suppress bone resorption in Paget's disease (Chap. 358) and osteoporosis (Chap. 355).

BIBLIOGRAPHY

CALCIUM, PHOSPHOROUS, AND BONE METABOLISM

ANDERSON JB: Nutritional biochemistry of calcium and phosphorus. J Nutr Biochem 2:300, 1991

AVIOLI LV, KRANE SM (eds): *Metabolic Bone Disease and Clinically Related Disorders.* Philadelphia, Saunders, 1990

BRINGHURST FR: Calcium and phosphate distribution, turnover, and metabolic actions, in *Endocrinology*, 3d ed, LJ DeGroot et al (eds). Philadelphia, Saunders, 1995, p 1015

CANALIS E et al: Growth factors and cytokines in bone cell metabolism. Annu Rev Med 42:17, 1991

COHN DV et al (eds): *Calcium Regulating Hormones and Bone Metabolism: Bone and Clinical Aspects.* Amsterdam, Excerpta Medica, 1992

DELMAS PD: Clinical use of biochemical markers of bone remodeling in osteoporosis. Bone 13:S17, 1992

HEANEY RP: Thinking straight about calcium. N Engl J Med 328:503, 1993

HOROWITZ MC: Cytokines and estrogen in bone: Anti-osteoporotic effects. Science 260:626, 1993

MATKOVIC V: Calcium intake and peak bone mass. N Engl J Med 327:119, 1992

PORTALE AA et al: Physiologic regulation of the serum concentration of 1,25-dihydroxyvitamin D by phosphorus in normal men. J Clin Invest 83:1494, 1989

ROODMAN GD: Interleukin-6: An osteotropic factor? J Bone Miner Res 7:474, 1992

SAGE EH, BORNSTEIN P: Extracellular proteins that modulate cell-matrix interactions. SPARC, tenascin, and thrombospondin. J Biol Chem 266:14831, 1991

SLAVKIN H, PRICE P (eds): *Chemistry and Biology of Mineralized Tissues.* Amsterdam, Excerpta Medica, 1992

SORIANO P et al: Targeted disruption of the c-*src* proto-oncogene leads to osteopetrosis in mice. Cell 64:693, 1991

SUDA T et al: Modulation of osteoclast differentiation. Endocr Rev 13:66, 1992

UEBELHART D et al: Urinary excretion of pyridinium crosslinks: A new marker of bone resorption in metabolic bone disease. Bone Miner 8:87, 1990

VITAMIN D

DARWIN H, DELUCA H: Vitamin D-regulated gene expression. Crit Rev Eukaryotic Gene Expr 3:89, 1993

DEMAY M: Hereditary defects in vitamin D metabolism and vitamin D receptor defects, in *Endocrinology*, 3d ed, LJ DeGroot et al (eds). Philadelphia, Saunders, 1995, p 1173

HOLICK MF: McCollum Award Lecture 1994: Vitamin D—new horizons for the 21st century. Am J Clin Nutr 60:617, 1994

————: Vitamin D: Biosynthesis, metabolism, and mode of action, in *Endocrinology*, 3d ed, LJ DeGroot et al (eds). Philadelphia, Saunders, 1995 p 990

PIKE JW: Vitamin D_3 receptors: Structure and function in transcription. Annu Rev Nutr 11:189, 1991

TILYARD MW et al: Treatment of postmenopausal osteoporosis with calcitriol or calcium. N Engl J Med 326:356, 1992

PARATHYROID HORMONE AND CALCITONIN

ABOU-SAMRA AB et al: Expression cloning of a common receptor for parathyroid hormone and parathyroid hormone–related peptide from rat osteoblast-like cells: A single receptor stimulates intracellular accumulation of both cAMP and inositol triphosphates and increases intracellular free calcium. Proc Natl Acad Sci USA 89:2732, 1992

ARNOLD A et al: Mutation of the signal peptide-encoding region of the preproparathyroid hormone gene in familial isolated hypoparathyroidism. J Clin Invest 86:1094, 1990

DEMAY MB et al: Sequences in the human parathyroid hormone gene that bind the 1,25-dihydroxyvitamin D_2 receptor and mediate transcriptional repression in response to 1,25-dihydroxyvitamin D_3. Proc Natl Acad Sci USA 89:8097, 1992

FITZPATRICK LA, ARNOLD A: Hypoparathyroidism, in *Endocrinology*, 3d ed, LJ DeGroot et al (eds). Philadelphia, Saunders, 1995, p 1123

GORN AH et al: The cloning characterization and expression of a human calcitonin receptor from an ovarian carcinoma cell line. J Clin Invest 90:1726, 1992

KARAPLIS AC et al: Disruption of parathyroid hormone–related peptide gene leads to a multitude of skeletal abnormalities and perinatal mortality. J Bone Miner Res 7(Suppl 1):abst 1, 1992

LEVINE MA, SPIEGEL AM: Pseudohypoparathyroidism, in *Endocrinology*, 3d ed, LJ DeGroot et al (eds). Philadelphia, Saunders, 1995, p 1136

MACINTYRE I: Calcitonin: Physiology, biosynthesis, secretion, metabolism, and mode of action, in *Endocrinology*, 3d ed, LJ DeGroot et al (eds). Philadelphia, Saunders, 1995, p 1123

MARTIN TJ, MOSELEY JM: Parathyroid hormone-related protein, in *Endocrinology*, 3d ed, LJ DeGroot et al (eds). Philadelphia, Saunders, 1995, p 967

MIRIC A et al: Heterogenous mutations in the gene encoding the alpha subunit of the stimulating G protein of adenylyl cyclase in Albright hereditary osteodystrophy. J Clin Endocrinol Metab 76:1560, 1993

POTTS JT JR et al: Parathyroid hormone: Physiology, chemistry, biosynthesis, secretion, metabolism, and mode of action, in *Endocrinology*, 3d ed, LJ DeGroot et al (eds). Philadelphia, Saunders, 1995, p 920

SCHIPANI E et al: Identical complementary deoxyribonucleic acids encode a human renal and bone parathyroid hormone (PTH)/PTH–related peptide receptor. Endocrinology 132:2157, 1993

USDIN TB et al: Identification and functional expression of a receptor selectively recognizing parathyroid hormone, the PTH2 receptor. J Biol Chem 270:15455, 1995

354	*John T. Potts, Jr*

DISEASES OF THE PARATHYROID GLAND AND OTHER HYPER- AND HYPOCALCEMIC DISORDERS

HYPERCALCEMIA

Hypercalcemia can be a manifestation of a serious illness such as malignancy or can be detected coincidentally by laboratory testing in a patient with no obvious illness. The number of patients recognized with asymptomatic hypercalcemia has increased severalfold in the past 25 years, and management is a particular problem in the asymptomatic patient.

Whenever hypercalcemia is confirmed, a definitive diagnosis must be established. Although hyperparathyroidism, a frequent cause of asymptomatic hypercalcemia, is a chronic disorder in which manifestations, if any, may be expressed only over months or years, hypercalcemia also can be the earliest manifestation of malignancy, the second most common cause of hypercalcemia in the adult. The causes of hypercalcemia are numerous (Table 354-1), but hyperparathyroidism and cancer account for 90 percent of cases. Diagnosis can usually be established, but the appropriate management of hypercalcemia is sometimes unclear. Whether all asymptomatic hyperparathyroidism should be corrected surgically is unsettled, but there is now a consensus that simple medical surveillance is appropriate for patients over age 50 when bone and renal status are satisfactory.

Before undertaking a workup, it is essential to be sure that true hypercalcemia, not a false-positive laboratory test, is present. Hypercalcemia is a chronic problem, and it is cost-effective to obtain several

Table 354-1

Classification of Causes of Hypercalcemia

I. Parathyroid-related
   A. Primary hyperparathyroidism
      1. Solitary adenomas
      2. Multiple endocrine neoplasia
   B. Lithium therapy
   C. Familial hypocalciuric hypercalcemia
II. Malignancy-related
   A. Solid tumor with metastases (breast)
   B. Solid tumor with humoral mediation of hypercalcemia (lung, kidney)
   C. Hematologic malignancies (multiple myeloma, lymphoma, leukemia)
III. Vitamin D–related
   A. Vitamin D intoxication
   B. ↑ $1,25(OH)_2D$; sarcoidosis and other granulomatous diseases
   C. Idiopathic hypercalcemia of infancy
IV. Associated with high bone turnover
   A. Hyperthyroidism
   B. Immobilization
   C. Thiazides
   D. Vitamin A intoxication
V. Associated with renal failure:
   A. Severe secondary hyperparathyroidism
   B. Aluminum intoxication
   C. Milk-alkali syndrome

serum calcium measurements; these tests need not be in the fasting state. False-positive hypercalcemia is usually the result of inadvertent hemoconcentration during blood collection or elevation in serum proteins such as albumin. There is no advantage, except in research applications, to measurement of ionized rather than total calcium.

Clinical features are helpful in differential diagnosis. Hypercalcemia in an adult who is asymptomatic is usually due to primary hyperparathyroidism. In malignancy-associated hypercalcemia the disease is usually not occult; rather, symptoms of malignancy bring the patient to the physician, and hypercalcemia is discovered during the workup. In such patients the interval between detection of hypercalcemia and death is often less than 6 months. Accordingly, if an asymptomatic individual has had hypercalcemia or some manifestation of hypercalcemia, such as kidney stones, for more than 1 or 2 years, it is unlikely that malignancy is the cause. Nevertheless, differentiating primary hyperparathyroidism from *occult* malignancy can occasionally be difficult, and careful evaluation is required, particularly when the duration of the hypercalcemia is unknown.

Hypercalcemia not due to hyperparathyroidism or malignancy can result from excessive vitamin D action, high bone turnover from any of several causes, or from renal failure (Table 354-1). The sensitivity and specificity of various diagnostic tests for the differential diagnosis previously were not optimal, but parathyroid hormone (PTH) immunoassays based on double-antibody methods are reliable. Dietary history and a history of ingestion of vitamins and drugs are often helpful in diagnosing some of the less frequent causes. Except in malignancy-associated hypercalcemia, acute management of the hypercalcemia is usually successful prior to definitive therapy. The type of treatment is based on the severity of the hypercalcemia and the nature of associated symptoms.

Hypercalcemia from any cause can result in fatigue, depression, mental confusion, anorexia, nausea, vomiting, constipation, reversible renal tubular defects, increased urination, a short QT interval in the electrocardiogram, and, in some patients, cardiac arrhythmias. There is a variable relation from one patient to the next between the severity of hypercalcemia and the symptoms. Generally, symptoms are more common at calcium levels above 2.9 to 3 mmol/L (11.5 to 12.0 mg/dL), but some patients, even at this level, are asymptomatic. When calcium exceeds 3.2 mmol/L (13 mg/dL), calcification in kidneys, skin, vessels, lungs, heart, and stomach and renal insufficiency may develop, particularly if blood phosphate levels are normal or elevated due to impaired renal function. Severe hypercalcemia, usually defined as 3.7 mmol/L (15 mg/dL) or above, is a medical emergency. When serum calcium is 3.7 to 4.5 mmol/L (15 to 18 mg/dL) or higher, coma and cardiac arrest can occur.

PARATHYROID-RELATED HYPERCALCEMIA Primary Hyperparathyroidism *Natural history and incidence* Primary hyperparathyroidism is a generalized disorder of calcium, phosphate, and bone metabolism due to an increased secretion of parathyroid hormone. The elevation of circulating hormone usually leads to hypercalcemia and hypophosphatemia. There is great variation in the manifestations. Patients may present with multiple signs and symptoms, including recurrent nephrolithiasis, peptic ulcers, mental changes, and, less frequently, extensive bone resorption. However, with greater awareness of the disease and wider use of multiphasic screening tests, including blood calcium assays, the diagnosis is frequently made in patients who have no symptoms and minimal, if any, signs of the disease other than hypercalcemia and elevated levels of parathyroid hormone. The annual incidence of the disease is estimated to be as high as 0.2 percent in patients over age 60, with an estimated prevalence including undiscovered asymptomatic patients of 1 percent or higher. The manifestations may be subtle, and the disease may have a benign course for many years or a lifetime. Rarely, the disease develops or worsens abruptly and causes severe complications, such as marked dehydration and coma, so-called hypercalcemic parathyroid crisis. The disease has a peak incidence between the third and fifth decades but occurs in young children and in the elderly.

Etiology and pathology SOLITARY ADENOMAS The cause of hyperparathyroidism is one or more hyperfunctioning glands. The traditional view has been that a single abnormal gland is the cause in approximately 80 percent of patients; the abnormality in the gland is usually a benign neoplasm or adenoma and rarely a parathyroid carcinoma. In approximately 15 percent all glands are hyperfunctioning; this is termed *chief cell parathyroid hyperplasia* and is usually hereditary and frequently associated with other endocrine abnormalities. Some surgeons and pathologists report that the enlargement of multiple glands is common.

MULTIPLE ENDOCRINE NEOPLASIA Hereditary hyperparathyroidism can occur without other endocrine abnormalities but is usually part of a multiple endocrine neoplasia (MEN) (see Chap. 340). MEN 1 (Wermer's syndrome) consists of hyperparathyroidism and tumors of the pituitary and pancreas, often associated with gastric hypersecretion and peptic ulcer disease (Zollinger-Ellison syndrome). MEN 2A consists of hyperparathyroidism, pheochromocytoma, and medullary carcinoma of the thyroid. Both disorders are inherited as autosomal dominant defects. Since the various endocrine tumors can develop at widely separated intervals, management of these patients is a formidable challenge, and in MEN 2A a screening technique makes it possible to identify (or exclude) first-degree relatives at risk.

MOLECULAR DEFECTS IN HYPERPARATHYROIDISM Analyses of kindreds with MEN 1 and MEN 2A and cytogenetic studies of tumor tissue from patients with solitary adenomas have documented that at least two molecular defects are involved in the hyperparathyroid state, namely, overactivity of a proto-oncogene, or growth-promoting gene, and loss of function of a growth-regarding gene, or antioncogene.

A gene locus on chromosome 11 appears to be responsible for MEN 1, and the normal allele of this gene may be an antioncogene. The loss of one allele is inherited as an autosomal trait, and loss of the other allele via somatic cell mutation leads to monoclonal expansion and tumor development in tissues such as the parathyroids. In approximately 25 percent of sporadic parathyroid adenomas, the same locus on chromosome 11 appears to be lost, implying that the same defect responsible for MEN 1 can also cause the common disease. In MEN 1 there is a defect in one allele at birth, and in patients with sporadic adenomas one copy is lost as a silent somatic mutation; in both disorders, the second allele becomes mutated or deleted in some cell, resulting in a monoclonal outgrowth (Fig. 354-1A).

In other parathyroid adenomas, a second mechanism of abnormal growth is operative, namely, activation of a proto-oncogene (Fig. 354-1B). The synthesis of parathyoid hormone is under the control of a promoter that, in the presence of a reciprocal translocation involving chromosome 11, can also drive the expression of a gene product termed PRAD-1, a D-cyclin protein that plays a role in cell division. If overexpressed (or mutated), cyclins contribute to abnormal cell replication. This translocation is found in 5 percent or more of parathyroid adenomas, usually in larger glands. These findings also explain why hyperparathyroidism develops earlier in the MEN syndromes (germ line defect) than with parathyroid adenomas (two somatic mutations required). Proliferation of parathyroid cells may favor such somatic mutations because more than 60 percent of patients operated on for secondary hyperparathyroidism due to renal failure appear to have monoclonal proliferation associated with loss of a portion of the X chromosome.

Additional genetic abnormalities are probably involved in the etiology of hyperparathyroidism, because allelic loss of a portion of chromosome 1 is found in 40 percent of parathyroid adenomas. Still different mechanisms appear to be operative in parathyroid carcinoma, namely, loss of both copies of the retinoblastoma gene. Hence, unlike the situation with some cancers in which there appears to be progression from benign to malignant neoplasms as cellular genetic defects accumulate, parathyroid adenomas do not seem to be precursors of parathyroid carcinoma.

In MEN 2A the frequency of hyperparathyroidism is less common than in MEN 1 and varies within families and between families. The mutation in MEN 2A is one of several activating mutations in a tyrosine kinase–type proto-oncogene RET (see Chap. 340). The mutation is carried in all cells as a germ line defect and can be detected by diagnostic genetic techniques. The principal practical utility of this assay is that it makes it possible to make the diagnosis and operate early to prevent development of medullary thyroid cancer.

Adenomas are most often located in the inferior parathyroid gland, but in 6 to 10 percent of patients, parathyroid adenomas may be located in the thymus, the thyroid, the pericardium, or behind the esophagus. Adenomas are usually 0.5 to 5 g in size but may be as large as 10 to 20 g (normal glands weigh 25 mg on average). Chief cells are predominant in both hyperplasia and adenoma. The adenoma is sometimes encapsulated by a rim of normal tissue. With chief cell hyperplasia, the enlargement may be so asymmetric that some involved glands appear grossly normal. If hyperplasia is present, histologic examination reveals a uniform pattern of chief cells and disappearance of fat even in the absence of an increase in gland weight. Thus, microscopic examination of biopsy specimens of several glands is essential to interpret findings at surgery. When an adenoma is present, the other glands are usually normal and contain a normal distribution of all cell types (rather than only chief cells) and normal amounts of fat.

Parathyroid carcinoma is usually not aggressive in character. Long-term survival without recurrence is common if at initial surgery the entire gland is removed without rupture of the capsule. Even recurrent parathyroid carcinoma is usually slow-growing with local spread in the neck, and surgical correction of recurrent disease may be feasible. Occasionally, however, parathyroid carcinoma is more aggressive, with distant metastases (lung, liver, and bone) found at the time of initial operation. It may be difficult to appreciate initially that a primary tumor is carcinoma; increased numbers of mitotic figures and increased fibrosis of the gland stroma may precede invasion. The diagnosis of carcinoma is often made in retrospect. Hyperparathyroidism from a parathyroid carcinoma may be indistinguishable from other forms of primary hyperparathyroidism; a potential clue to the diagnosis, however, is provided by the degree of calcium elevation. Calcium values of 3.5 to 3.7 mmol/L (14 to 15 mg/dL) are frequent with carcinoma and may alert the surgeon to remove the abnormal gland with care to avoid capsular rupture.

Signs and symptoms Half or more of patients with hyperparathyroidism are asymptomatic. In series in which patients are followed without operation, as many as 80 percent are classified as without symptoms; the number may be smaller if mild manifestations, such as silent bone deterioration or reduced renal function, are included. Manifestations of hyperparathyroidism involve primarily the kidneys and the skeletal system. Kidney involvement, due either to deposition of calcium in the renal parenchyma or to recurrent nephrolithiasis, was present in 60 to 70 percent of patients prior to 1970. With earlier detection, renal complications are less common.

Renal stones are usually composed of either calcium oxalate or calcium phosphate. In occasional patients repeated episodes of nephrolithiasis or the formation of large calculi may lead to urinary tract obstruction, infection, and loss of renal function. Nephrocalcinosis also may cause decreased renal function and phosphate retention.

The unique bone manifestation of hyperparathyroidism is osteitis fibrosa cystica, which in the past occurred in 10 to 25 percent of patients. Histologically, the pathognomonic features are a reduction in the number of trabeculae, an increase in the giant multinucleated osteoclasts in scalloped areas on the surface of the bone (Howship's lacunae), and a replacement of the normal cellular and marrow elements by fibrous tissues. Other bone changes include resorption of the phalangeal tufts and replacement of the usually sharp cortical outline of the bone in the digits by an irregular outline (subperiosteal resorption). Loss of the lamina dura of the teeth is less specific. Tiny "punched-out" lesions may cause the so-called salt-and-pepper appearance in the skull.

Osteitis fibrosa cystica is now uncommon, even though hyperparathyroidism may be of long standing. The reduced frequency is unexplained. Other bone disorders, however, are frequent. The rate of bone mineral turnover is enhanced in most patients, even in those who do not have a decrease in bone mass; in such patients, rates of bone formation and bone restoration must be increased but balanced. In some patients, however, rates of formation and resorption are not

FIGURE 354-1 *A*. Schematic diagram indicating concept of autosomal recessive rather than autosomal dominant inheritance of tumor susceptibility. The patient with the hereditary abnormality (multiple endocrine neoplasia, or MEN) is envisioned as having one defective gene (mutant receptor) inherited from the affected parent on chromosome 11, but one copy of the normal gene is present from the other parent. In the monoclonal tumor (benign tumor), a somatic event, here partial chromosomal deletion, removes the normal gene from a cell. The cell, deprived of growth-regulating influence from this gene, has unregulated growth and becomes a tumor. A different genetic locus also involving loss of an anti-oncogene, or growth-regulating gene, on chromosome 13 is involved in the pathogenesis of parathyroid carcinoma. *B*. Schematic illustration of the mechanism and consequences of gene rearrangement and overexpression of the PRAD 1 proto-oncogene (pericentromeric inversion of chromosome 11) in parathyroid adenomas. The excessive expression by the highly active PTH gene promoter in the parathyroid cell of PRAD 1, which is a cell cycle control protein, contributes to excess cellular proliferation, thereby activating the receptor, increasing activity of PLC through Gq. *(From Habener et al, with permission.)*

balanced so that a progressive loss of bone mineral mass causes osteopenia. There are no pathognomonic criteria to separate unequivocally parathyroid-dependent osteopenia from "high-turnover" osteoporosis, as can occur in patients who are not hyperparathyroid.

Improved techniques are now available for monitoring bone mineral density. Computed tomography (CT) and quantitative digital radiography (DEXA) of the spine provide reproducible quantitative estimates (within a few percent) of spinal bone density. Similarly, cortical bone density in the extremities can be quantified by single-photon densitometry. Serial measurements with these techniques can provide early evidence as to whether osteopenia is progressive. Most studies indicate that in hyperparathyroidism cortical rather than trabecular bone tends to be lost selectively.

In symptomatic patients, dysfunctions of the central nervous system, peripheral nerve and muscle, the gastrointestinal tract, and the joints also occur. An awareness of the signs and symptoms of hyperparathyroidism may give the initial clue to the diagnosis. It has been reported that severe neuropsychiatric manifestations may be reversed by parathyroidectomy; it is not clear that this improvement is a defined cause-and-effect relationship in the absence of controlled studies, however. Generally, the fact that hyperparathyroidism is common in elderly patients, in whom there are often other problems, suggests the possibility that such coexisting problems as hypertension, renal deterioration, and depression may not be parathyroid-related and suggests caution in recommending parathyroid surgery as a cure for these conditions. It is not apparent why some patients with hyperparathyroidism have no symptoms, while others with similar biochemical abnormalities develop symptomatic disease.

Neuromuscular manifestations may include proximal muscle weakness, easy fatigability, and atrophy of muscles and may be so striking as to suggest a primary neuromuscular disorder. The distinguishing feature is the complete regression of neuromuscular disease after surgical correction of the hyperparathyroidism.

Gastrointestinal manifestations are sometimes subtle and include vague abdominal complaints and disorders of the stomach and pancreas. Again, cause and effect are unclear, except in certain situations such as the multiple endocrine syndromes. In MEN 1 patients with hyperparathyroidism, duodenal ulcer is a result of the associated pancreatic tumors that secrete excessive quantities of gastrin (the Zollinger-Ellison syndrome). Pancreatitis has been reported in association with hyperparathyroidism, but the incidence and the mechanism are not established.

Chondrocalcinosis and pseudogout are said to be sufficiently frequent in hyperparathyroidism that screening of such patients is warranted. Occasionally, pseudogout is the initial manifestation.

Diagnosis   The diagnosis is made primarily on clinical grounds. The newer immunoassays for PTH are reliable and cost-effective. Since hypercalcemia can be the presenting evidence for malignancy or other serious disease, a thorough evaluation of possible etiologies, including hyperparathyroidism, is indicated even in asymptomatic subjects.

Hypercalcemia is the most common manifestation—either sustained or intermittent hypercalcemia. Careful consideration must be given to the justification for surgical exploration in the absence of hypercalcemia. So-called normocalcemic hyperparathyroidism, i.e., surgically proven hyperparathyroidism accompanied by a normal calcium level but elevated values of immunoreactive PTH (iPTH), is rare in the absence of renal failure or vitamin D deficiency. If normocalcemic patients have coexisting conditions that interfere with the calcium-elevating actions of PTH, such as chronic renal failure, severe malabsorption, or vitamin D deficiency, then the lack of calcium elevation need not mitigate against the presence of hyperparathyroidism. Confusing situations can arise, however, in patients with recurrent kidney stones who are suspected of having hyperparathyroidism because of elevated iPTH levels but who have normal serum calcium. These patients may have true normocalcemic hyperparathyroidism. In such situations in which the symptoms call for early definitive diagnosis and treatment, it may be useful to search for postabsorptive hypercalcemia (detectable in certain patients when fasting hypercalcemia is absent) or to use a provocative test with benzothiadiazides (see below).

Hypercalciuria is common in hyperparathyroidism. However, PTH actually reduces calcium clearance, and the daily excretion of calcium in urine is lower than in patients with equivalent degrees of hypercalcemia from nonparathyroid causes.

Serum phosphate is usually low but may be normal, especially if renal failure has developed. Hypophosphatemia is a less specific diagnostic finding than hypercalcemia for two reasons. First, phosphate levels are influenced by dietary intake, diurnal variations, and other factors; to be useful, samples must be obtained in the morning under fasting conditions. Second, patients with severe hypercalcemia of any cause may have a low serum phosphate.

Many tests based on renal responses to excess parathyroid hormone (renal calcium and phosphate clearance; blood phosphate, chloride, magnesium; urinary or nephrogenous cyclic AMP) have been used in the past. These tests have low specificity for hyperparathyroidism, are not cost-effective, and have been replaced by PTH immunoassays.

℞ TREATMENT

Medical Treatment   Management of hyperparathyroidism involves two separate issues. The critical question is whether the disease should be treated surgically (see below). If surgery is indicated, the serum calcium may need to be lowered prior to surgery. However, since surgery is the quickest method of lowering serum calcium in hyperparathyroidism, operation should be performed promptly when hypercalcemia is severe. Hypercalcemia is not symptomatic in most patients with hyperparathyroidism, and it is usually not difficult to control the hypercalcemia. Simple hydration often suffices to lower the calcium concentration to values below 2.9 mmol/L (11.5 mg/dL). There have been discussions in the past as to whether the hypercalcemia of hyperparathyroidism should be treated chronically with oral phosphate. Lowering the calcium level by phosphate is accompanied by an increase in iPTH levels in blood; it is unclear whether the increased PTH levels would cause more or less organ deterioration. There have been no controlled trials to evaluate medical therapy for hyperparathyroidism, but in postmenopausal women with hyperparathyroidism who are unwilling or unable to undergo surgery, estrogen therapy may retard demineralization of the skeleton and reduce blood and urinary calcium levels.

Several hundred patients have been followed in attempts to define the natural history of the disease and to define the benefits of surgery versus the risks of medical observation. Large-scale randomized, prospective clinical trials have not been undertaken, however. Rather, the long-term effects of hyperparathyroidism have been assessed in patients who do not have kidney stones, osteitis fibrosa cystica, or other clear-cut symptoms. Of principal concern is the possibility of progressive loss of bone density, a worrisome problem in women who face the problem of age-dependent and estrogen-deficient bone loss in the absence of hyperparathyroidism. The concern is that such patients, even though asymptomatic, will suffer sufficient bone loss due to PTH excess to make them more vulnerable to developing symptomatic osteoporosis.

The National Institutes of Health held a Consensus Conference on Management of Asymptomatic Hyperparathyroidism in 1991. *Asymptomatic hyperparathyroidism* was defined as documented (presumptive) hyperparathyroidism without signs or symptoms attributable to the disease. It was concluded that surgery to correct the hyperparathyroidism is always an acceptable approach, if feasible medically, but surveillance may be justified in patients over the age of 50 with minimal calcium elevation when renal function and bone mass are close to normal and remain so during careful monitoring.

The recommendation was that the diagnosis of primary hyperparathyroidism can best be established by demonstrating persistent hypercalcemia (artifactual elevation in serum calcium concentration must be excluded) and an elevated serum iPTH level. The panel agreed that the PTH assay is now sensitive, specific, and reliable and that other tests are usually unnecessary.

As to which asymptomatic patients should be followed medically, the consensus was that a subgroup of patients over age 50 is appropriate for medical monitoring if certain criteria are met and the patients wish to avoid surgery.

Patients under age 50 should be routinely operated on, given the long surveillance that would be required. Other guidelines for recommending surgery in patients with asymptomatic hyperparathyroidism include the following:

1. Elevation of serum calcium, more than 0.25 to 0.40 mmol/L (1 to 1.6 mg/dL) above the upper limit of normal for the laboratory.
2. History of an episode of life-threatening hypercalcemia, such as an episode induced by dehydration and recurring illness.
3. Reduction of creatinine clearance by greater than 30 percent compared with age-matched controls (the author finds it difficult to use this criterion as an absolute, given the multiplicity of factors that affect creatinine clearance with age).
4. Presence of kidney stones detected by abdominal radiograph even if they are asymptomatic.
5. Elevation of 24-h urinary calcium excretion above 400 mg.
6. Reduction of bone mass more than 2 standard deviations below normal by one of several noninvasive methods of measuring bone mass.

Other considerations that favor surgery include concern that consistent follow-up would be unlikely or that coexistent illness would complicate management. Asymptomatic patients should be monitored regularly. Surgical correction of hyperparathyroidism can always be undertaken when indicated, since the success rate is high (>90 percent), mortality is low, morbidity is minimal, and cure is common. The goals of monitoring are early detection of worsening hypercalcemia, deteriorating bone or renal status, or other complications of hyperparathyroidism. Cortical bone mass is principally at risk in untreated primary hyperparathyroidism. Indeed, reports that vertebral bone fractures are increased in patients with untreated hyperparathyroidism have been challenged, and cancellous bone loss may be a problem only when vitamin D and calcium intakes are low.

Although patients have reduced bone mass at the time of initial detection, there may be little further loss over years of subsequent follow-up. The use of single-photon absorptiometry to follow cortical bone mass is relatively easy and inexpensive; increased loss of cancellous bone and increased risk of vertebral fractures are unusual, and the monitoring of spinal bone mass by dual-energy x-ray absorptiometry need not be undertaken. The consensus panel did not make a recommendation as to estrogen use in patients for whom surgery was not elected because there was insufficient cumulative experience with such therapy. It has been reported that untreated hyperparathyroidism is a risk factor for increased cardiovascular mortality, leading some to recommend surgery for all patients. The majority view is that medical surveillance is justified since the reports of increased cardiovascular risk are retrospective in nature.

Surgical Treatment Parathyroid exploration is best undertaken by an experienced surgeon with the help of an experienced pathologist. Certain features help in predicting the pathology; for example, in familial cases multiple abnormal glands are likely. However, some critical decisions regarding management can be made only during the operation. The examination by frozen section of tissue removed at surgery helps direct the subsequent course of the operation.

As discussed under "Etiology and Pathogenesis," there are many unresolved issues to consider in surgery for this disease. At the extreme of conservatism, the surgical approach is based on the view that typically only one gland (the adenoma) is abnormal. If an enlarged gland is found, a normal gland should be sought. If a biopsy of a normal-sized second gland confirms its histologic (and presumed functional) normality, no further exploration, biopsy, or excision is needed. At the other extreme is the minority viewpoint that all four glands be sought and that most of the total parathyroid tissue mass should be removed.

The concern with the former approach is that the rate of recurrence of hyperparathyroidism may be high if a second abnormal gland is missed; the latter approach could involve unnecessary surgery and an unacceptable rate of hypoparathyroidism.

The majority viewpoint, judged by surgical reviews, is in favor of conservative surgery, i.e., removal of what is usually only one enlarged gland but only after four-gland exploration to eliminate the possibility that more than one gland is abnormal. When normal glands are found in association with one enlarged gland, excision of the single adenoma usually leads to cure or symptom-free disease, although long-term follow-up studies are limited.

Multiple gland hyperplasia, as predicted in familial cases, poses more difficult questions of surgical management. Once a diagnosis of hyperplasia is established, all the glands must be identified, and two schemes have been proposed for surgical management. One is that three glands be totally removed and the fourth gland be partially excised; care is taken to leave a good blood supply for the remaining gland. Other surgeons advocate total parathyroidectomy with immediate transplantation of a portion of a removed, minced parathyroid gland into the muscles of the forearm with the view that even if recurrence of residual gland enlargement and hyperfunction is seen, surgical excision is easier from the ectopic site in the arm. When parathyroid carcinoma is encountered, the tissue should be widely excised; care must be taken to avoid rupture of the capsule to prevent local seeding of tumor cells.

If no abnormal parathyroid glands are found in the neck, the issue of further exploration must be decided. There are documented cases of five or six parathyroid glands and, therefore, of unusual locations for adenomas. A variety of techniques have been developed to aid in the preoperative localization of the abnormal parathyroid tissue. Noninvasive or minimally invasive techniques include ultrasound, CT of the neck and mediastinum, and differential scanning after technetium-sestamibi administration. Usually these techniques are recommended only in patients with initial unsuccessful neck explorations, since the combined success of the localization techniques is not better than that of an experienced parathyroid surgeon in finding the abnormal tissue at the first operation.

When a second parathyroid exploration is indicated, the minimally invasive techniques such as ultrasound, CT, and isotope scanning should probably be combined with selective digital arteriography in one of the centers specializing in these techniques. At one center, long-term cures have been achieved with selective embolization or injection of large amounts of contrast material into the endarterial circulation feeding the parathyroid tumor.

A decline in serum calcium occurs within 24 h after successful surgery; usually blood calcium falls to low-normal values for 3 to 5 days until the remaining parathyroid tissue resumes hormone secretion. Intraoperative monitoring of PTH levels by rapid PTH immunoassays may be useful in guiding the surgery, especially in patients who are reexplored after an initial unsuccessful operation. Severe postoperative hypocalcemia is likely only if osteitis cystica is present or if injury to all the normal parathyroid glands occurs during surgery.

In general, patients who do not have symptomatic bone disease or a large deficit in bone mineral and who have good renal and gastrointestinal function have few problems with postoperative hypocalcemia. The extent of postoperative hypocalcemia varies with the surgical approach. If all glands are biopsied, hypocalcemia may be transiently symptomatic and more prolonged. Hypocalcemia is more likely to be symptomatic after second parathyroid explorations, particularly when normal parathyroid tissue was removed at the initial operation and when the manipulation and/or biopsy of the remaining normal glands is more extensive in the search for the missing adenoma. Patients with hyperparathyroidism have efficient intestinal calcium absorption due to the increased levels of 1,25-dihydroxyvitamin D $[1,25(OH)_2D]$ stimulated by parathyroid excess. Once hypocalcemia signifies successful surgery, patients can be put on a high-calcium intake or be given oral calcium supplements. Despite mild hypocalcemia, most patients do not require parenteral therapy. If the serum calcium falls below 2 mmol/L (8 mg/dL), *in particular if the phosphate level simultaneously rises*, the possibility that surgery has caused hypoparathyroidism must be considered. Coexistent hypomagnesemia should be checked for, since it interferes with PTH secretion and causes a relative hypoparathyroidism. Parenteral calcium replacement at a low level should be instituted when hypocalcemia is symptomatic. Such indications include a general sense of anxiety and positive Chvostek and Trousseau signs coupled with serum calcium consistently below 2 mmol/L (8 mg/dL). For parenteral therapy, calcium (gluconate or chloride) solutions are prepared at a concentration of 1 mg/mL in 5% dextrose in water. The rate and duration of intravenous therapy are determined by the severity of the symptoms and the response of the serum calcium. A rate of infusion of 0.5 to 2 (mg/kg)/h or 30 to 100 mL/h of a 1-mg/mL solution usually suffices to relieve symptoms. Usually, parenteral therapy is required for only a few days. If symptoms worsen or if parenteral calcium is needed for more than 2 to 3 days, therapy with a vitamin D analogue and/or oral calcium (2 to 4 g/d) should be started (see below). It is cost-effective to use calcitriol (doses of 0.5 to 1.0 μg/d) because of the rapidity of onset and rapidity of cessation of action, in contrast to vitamin D per se (see below). A sudden rise in blood calcium after several months of vitamin D replacement may indicate restoration of parathyroid function to normal. It is also appropriate to monitor serum PTH serially to estimate gland function in such patients.

Magnesium deficiency also may complicate the postoperative course. Magnesium deficiency impairs the secretion of PTH, and therefore, hypomagnesemia should be corrected whenever detected. Magnesium chloride is effective by mouth, but this compound is not widely available. Accordingly, repletion is usually parenteral. Since the depressant effect of magnesium on central and peripheral nerve functions does not occur below 2 mmol/L (normal range 0.8 to 1.2 mmol/L), parenteral replacement can be given rapidly. A cumulative dose as great as 0.5 to 1 mmol/kg of body weight can be administered if severe hypomagnesemia is present; often, however, total doses of 20 to 40 mmol are sufficient. The magnesium is given either as an intravenous infusion over 8 to 12 h or in divided doses intramuscularly (magnesium sulfate, USP).

Lithium Therapy Lithium, used in the management of bipolar depression and other psychiatric disorders, causes hypercalcemia in approximately 10 percent of patients. The parathyroids are involved in mediation of the hypercalcemia, and PTH levels may be elevated. The hypercalcemia is dependent on continued lithium treatment, remitting and recurring when lithium is stopped and restarted. In a few patients, parathyroid adenomas were present. Histologic findings in the remaining parathyroid glands in these patients have not been described, but the implication is that there is a single abnormal gland.

The presence of hypercalcemia does not correlate with plasma lithium level, but the frequency with which hypercalcemia occurs is sufficiently high to support a causal relationship between lithium and the hypercalcemia, particularly the dependence of the hypercalcemia on the continuation of the lithium. It is presumed that in most cases an adenoma is not present, merely hyperfunctioning glands. Lithium, at the levels achieved in blood in treated patients, can be shown in vitro to shift the curve describing PTH secretion by parathyroid glands as a function of calcium level to the right; i.e., higher calcium levels are required to lower PTH secretion. It is logical to assume that this effect can cause elevated PTH levels and consequent hypercalcemia in otherwise normal individuals. If careful studies were done, elevated PTH levels might be found in even more patients treated with lithium than the 10 percent in whom hypercalcemia is symptomatic. The adenomas reported in some hypercalcemic patients with lithium ther-

apy may reflect the presence of an independently occurring parathyroid tumor; a permanent effect of lithium on parathyroid gland growth need not be implicated since most patients have complete reversal of hypercalcemia when lithium is stopped. However, long-standing stimulation of parathyroid cell replication may predispose to development of adenomas such as those seen in primary hyperparathyroidism, and it is possible that chronic lithium stimulation of the parathyroids may be a risk factor for adenoma formation. Some hypercalcemic patients are continued on lithium because of psychiatric indications. These patients are presumably best managed according to the principles used in asymptomatic hypercalcemia independent of lithium administration. If troubling symptoms or signs such as rising blood calcium levels, progressive bone demineralization, or kidney stones develop, it may be necessary to try alternative psychotropic medication. Parathyroid surgery should not be recommended unless hypercalcemia and elevated PTH levels persist after lithium is discontinued.

Familial Hypocalciuric Hypercalcemia (FHH) FHH (also called familial benign hypercalcemia) is inherited as an autosomal dominant trait. Affected individuals are discovered because of asymptomatic hypercalcemia. This disorder and Jansen's disease (discussed below) are variants of hyperparathyroidism. FHH involves excessive secretion of parathyroid hormone, and Jansen's disease excessive biological activity of the parathyroid hormone receptor in target tissues. Neither disorder, however, involves a primary growth disorder of the parathyroid glands and hence cannot be cured by parathyroidectomy.

The pathophysiology of FHH is now understood. The primary defect is abnormal sensing of the blood calcium by the parathyroid gland and renal tubule, causing inappropriate secretion of parathyroid hormone and excessive renal reabsorption of calcium (Fig. 354-2*A*). As discussed in Chap. 353, the calcium sensor consists of a member of the G protein family of receptor proteins tightly coupled to a transmembrane calcium channel. More than a dozen different point mutations in the calcium-sensing receptor have been identified in patients with FHH (Fig. 354-2*B*). These mutations lower the capacity of the sensor to bind calcium, and the mutant receptors function as though blood calcium were low; excessive secretion of parathyroid hormone occurs from an otherwise normal gland. The mutations act in a dominant negative fashion so that one abnormal copy of the receptor impairs the function of the normal allele. Other affected individuals and kindreds do not appear to have mutations in the coding sequence of this gene but may have mutations outside the coding sequence or mutations in other components of the calcium sensor.

Prior to the elucidation of the pathophysiology, abundant clinical evidence served to separate FHH from primary hyperparathyroidism. Most patients with primary hyperparathyroidism have less than 99 percent renal calcium reabsorption, and most patients with FHH exceed 99 percent reabsorption. The hypercalcemia in FHH is often detectable in affected members of the kindreds in the first decade of life, whereas hypercalcemia rarely occurs in patients with primary hyperparathyroidism and the MEN syndromes under the age of 10 years. The iPTH values may be elevated in FHH, but the values are usually normal or lower for the same degree of calcium elevation than in patients with primary hyperparathyroidism. Parathyroid surgery in a few patients led to permanent hypoparathyroidism, but hypocalciuria persisted nevertheless; the hypocalciuria, therefore, is not PTH-dependent but due to the abnormal calcium sensor in the kidney. Serum magnesium levels are, on average, higher in FHH than in primary hyperparathyroidism.

Few clinical signs or symptoms are present in patients with FHH. Unlike the MEN syndromes, other endocrine abnormalities are not present in FHH kindreds. Most patients are detected as a result of family screening after the diagnosis of hyperparathyroidism is made in one member of the kindred. All too commonly, the initial patient is operated on, and extensive parathyroid resection does not result in reversal of the hypercalcemia. At operation, the parathyroids appear normal or moderately hyperplasic. No patient has had reversal of hypercalcemia by surgery unless all the parathyroid tissue has been inadvertently removed, rendering the patient hypoparathyroid, a most undesirable outcome. The natural history of this disorder is not clear, but since the parathyroid glands are permissive rather than responsible

FIGURE 354-2   A. The calcium sensor's role in PTH secretion and calcium homeostasis. The extracellular domain is shown closing upon binding to calcium. PLC, phospholipase C; the G protein is shown as Gq (the subclass of G protein thought to activate PLC). When calcium in the blood is low, the sensor is less active and suppression of PTH secretion is lowered (i.e., more PTH is secreted). *(From Conklin and Bourne, with permission.)* B. Schematic two-dimensional diagram illustrating multiple points in the amino acid sequence

for the syndrome, parathyroid surgery is not appropriate, nor, in view of the lack of symptoms, does medical treatment seem needed to lower the calcium. Organic compounds that bind to and activate the calcium sensor (calcimimetic agents) are under trial.

The characteristic mild elevation in blood calcium reflects a moderate excess in PTH levels; the hormone acts on target cells in bone and elsewhere to increase blood calcium levels until a new steady state is achieved between blood calcium and PTH secretion. A homozygous offspring of a consanguineous marriage has been identified in one FHH kindred, resulting in a profound neonatal hyperparathyroidism.

Jansen's Disease   Children with this rare disorder often do not survive to adulthood. There are multiple developmental defects of the skeleton, including short stature, bowed legs, and multiple cystic resorptive areas in bones, associated with hypercalcemia and hypophosphatemia. PTH levels are undetectable, and the disorder is due to mutations that cause constitutive activation of the PTH receptor; two principle mutations have been identified in patients (Fig. 354-3). When these mutant receptors are expressed in vitro, they exhibit high levels of PTH-independent activity, indicating that the disease is due to excessive biological effects mimicking those of the hormone itself.

MALIGNANCY-RELATED HYPERCALCEMIA   Clinical Syndromes and Mechanisms of Hypercalcemia   Hypercalcemia due to malignancy is common (occurring with 10 to 15 percent of certain types of tumor, such as lung carcinoma), often severe and difficult to manage, confusing as to etiology, and sometimes difficult to distinguish from primary hyperparathyroidism. Traditionally, hypercalcemia in malignancy was thought to be due to a local invasion and destruction of bone by tumor cells; many cases are now known to result from the elaboration by the malignant cells of humoral mediators of hypercalcemia.

Although malignancy is often clinically obvious, hypercalcemia can occasionally be due to an occult tumor. With occult malignancy, diagnosis and definitive treatment must be accomplished quickly if the patient is to be protected from the complications of the underlying malignancy.

of the calcium sensor (receptor) due to point mutations in the gene. The identified sequence alterations (X) cause loss of function and lead to inadequate suppression of PTH release and, therefore, mild hypercalcemia (FHH); ✸, a gain-of-function mutation that causes hypocalcemia; S, a stop codon that is a loss of function mutation; ●, conserved residues; ▲, acidic residues. *(From Brown et al, with permission.)*

Humoral hypercalcemia of malignancy occurs with certain types of cancer of the lung and kidney, in which bone metastases are absent, minimal, or not detectable clinically. The clinical picture resembles primary hyperparathyroidism (hypophosphatemia accompanies hypercalcemia), and elimination or regression of the primary tumor leads to disappearance of the hypercalcemia. The disorder is due to secretion by the tumors of parathyroid hormone–like factors chemically distinct from PTH.

Many patients with the humoral hypercalcemia of malignancy have elevated urinary nephrogenous cyclic AMP excretion, hypophosphatemia, and increased urinary phosphate clearance, findings compatible with the actions of a humoral agent that emulates PTH action. However, with second-generation immunoassays, patients with the hypercalcemia of malignancy have either undetectable or suppressed immunoreactive PTH levels, making the differential diagnosis easier. Other features of the disorder differ from true hyperparathyroidism.

FIGURE 354-3   Pathogenesis of hypercalcemia in Jansen's disease is due to mutations at two sites in the PHT receptor, illustrated schematically with seven transmembrane-spanning domains. Histidine (H) found invariably in all members of the receptor family to which the PTH receptor belongs is mutated to arginine (R) in one locus; in the other, threonine (T) is mutated to proline (P). The resulting mutated receptors are constantly (constitutively) active without requiring PTH for simulation, thereby causing hypercalcemia and a condition simulating hyperparathryoidism. *(From Schipani et al, with permission.)*

Patients may have high, rather than low, renal calcium clearance (relative to serum calcium when compared to true hyperparathyroidism), levels of serum chloride <103 mmol/L, and low to normal levels of $1,25(OH)_2D$, all consistent with mediation by humoral factors distinct from PTH. The reason that the humoral syndrome differs from hyperparathyroidism in these parameters is unclear since the biological actions of PTH and the humoral mediator in cancer hypercalcemia are similar.

The histologic character of the tumor is more important than the extent of skeletal metastases in predicting hypercalcemia. Small cell carcinoma (oat cell) and adenocarcinoma of the lung, although the most common lung tumors associated with skeletal metastases, rarely cause hypercalcemia. By contrast, as many as 10 percent of patients with squamous cell carcinoma of the lung develop hypercalcemia. Histologic studies of bone in patients with squamous cell or epidermoid carcinoma of the lung, in sites invaded by tumor as well as areas remote from tumor invasion, reveal bone remodeling, including osteoclastic and osteoblastic activity. In contrast, minimal skeletal metabolic activation occurs despite extensive skeletal metastases of small cell (oat cell) carcinoma.

At least two mechanisms of hypercalcemia are operative in cancer hypercalcemia. Many solid tumors associated with hypercalcemia, particularly squamous cell and renal tumors, produce and secrete humoral factors that cause increased bone resorption and mediate the hypercalcemia through systemic actions on the skeleton. Alternatively, direct bone marrow invasion occurs with hematologic malignancies such as leukemia, lymphoma, and multiple myeloma and with solid tumors such as breast carcinoma. Lymphokines and cytokines produced by cells involved in the marrow response to the tumors promote resorption of bone through local destruction.

Disorders of the latter class include myeloma and other hematologic malignancies involving the bone marrow that cause bone destruction and hypercalcemia through local mechanisms of malignant cells in the marrow spaces. Breast carcinoma is typical of solid tumors that cause hypercalcemia through *localized osteolytic destruction*, probably mediated by locally secreted tumor products that may differ from those involved in multiple myeloma or lymphoma.

In some patients with the humoral hypercalcemia of malignancy, osteoclastic resorption is unaccompanied by an osteoblastic or bone-forming response to bone resorption, implying some inhibition of the normal coupling of formation and resorption. Thus the interaction of more than one substance may determine whether hypercalcemia develops in a particular patient.

Several hormones, hormone analogues, cytokines, and growth factors have been implicated as the result of clinical assays, in vitro tests, or chemical isolation. In some lymphomas, typically B cell lymphomas, there is an increased blood level of $1,25(OH)_2D$, which is probably produced by lymphocytes. The etiologic factor produced by activated normal lymphocytes and by myeloma and lymphoma cells, termed *osteoclast activation factor*, now appears to represent the biologic action of several different cytokines, probably interleukin 1 and lymphotoxin or tumor necrosis factor.

As discussed in Chap. 353, *parathyroid hormone–related protein* (PTHrP), which resembles but is distinct from PTH, fulfills the criteria for a humoral agent in the hypercalcemia syndrome. This factor binds to the PTH receptor and activates the receptor in a manner indistinguishable from PTH itself. As discussed in Chap. 353, immunoassays for PTHrP are complicated by the heterogeneity of the circulating forms of the peptide, but nonetheless, elevated levels of PTHrP are present in patients with the typical syndrome of humoral hypercalcemia of malignancy. The complexity of the etiologic mechanisms in cancer hypercalcemia are illustrated by the fact that some breast carcinoma cells and a distinctive type of T cell lymphoma/leukemia due to human T cell lymphotropic virus I infection produce PTHrP so that these tumors may produce hypercalcemia both by humoral and local mechanisms. Breast carcinoma cells also produce and secrete prosta-

glandins of the E series, which are potent local stimulators of bone resorption.

Several aspects of the hypercalcemia of malignancy remain unclear. Levels of urinary cyclic AMP rise in test animals treated with synthetic PTHrP, but $1,25(OH)_2D$ levels also rise, which is at variance with the fact that many patients with the humoral hypercalcemic syndrome have normal or depressed levels of $1,25(OH)_2D$. Tumor-derived growth factors, believed to act as autocrine regulators to maintain the transformation and growth of tumor cells, and cellular growth factors produced by nonmalignant cells are also potent bone-resorbing agents in vitro. Several of these factors stimulate production of prostaglandins of the E_2 type.

Assays to detect PTHrP using different approaches (single-antibody, double-antibody, different epitopes) give similar results. Most data indicate that levels are undetectable (or low) in normal subjects, elevated in many cancer patients with the humoral syndrome, and high in human milk. Thus, identification of PTHrP represents a singular advance.

Diagnostic Issues Ordinarily, the diagnosis of cancer hypercalcemia is not difficult because tumor symptoms are prominent when hypercalcemia is detected. Indeed, hypercalcemia may be noted incidentally during the workup of a patient with known or suspected malignancy. Patients with malignancy and hypercalcemia may also have a coexistent parathyroid adenoma.

Laboratory testing is critical to exclude occult carcinoma. Levels of iPTH by the double-antibody technique are undetectable or extremely low in tumor hypercalcemia, as would be expected with the mediation of the hypercalcemia by a factor other than PTH (the hypercalcemia suppressing the normal parathyroid glands). Improvement in the usefulness of the PTH assay is a significant advance in laboratory diagnosis. (Earlier assays gave equivocal results.) Assays for PTHrP should be helpful; low or undetectable PTH and elevated PTHrP would focus attention on occult malignancy.

Clinical suspicion that malignancy is the cause of the hypercalcemia is heightened when symptoms associated with neoplasia, such as weight loss, fatigue, muscle weakness, and unexplained skin rash, or symptoms specific for a particular tumor are present. Squamous cell tumors are most frequently associated with hypercalcemia, particularly tumors of the lung, kidney, and urogenital tract. Radiologic examinations can focus on these areas when clinical evidence is unclear. Bone scans with technetium-labeled bisphosphonate are useful for detection of osteolytic metastases; the sensitivity is high, but specificity is low; results must be confirmed by conventional x-rays to be certain that areas of increased uptake are due to osteolytic metastases per se. Bone marrow biopsies are helpful in patients with anemia or abnormal peripheral blood smears.

℞ TREATMENT

Treatment of the hypercalcemia of malignancy is directed to control of the tumor, and reduction of tumor mass usually corrects hypercalcemia. If a patient has severe hypercalcemia yet has an excellent chance for effective tumor therapy, treatment of the hypercalcemia should be vigorous while awaiting the results of definitive therapy. If hypercalcemia, on the other hand, occurs in the late stages of a tumor that is resistant to therapy, the treatment of the hypercalcemia should be judicious, since hypercalcemia can have a mild sedating effect. Standard therapies for hypercalcemia (discussed below) are applicable to patients with malignancy.

VITAMIN D–RELATED HYPERCALCEMIA Hypercalcemia related to abnormal vitamin D action can be due to *excessive ingestion* of vitamin D or *abnormal metabolism* of the vitamin. Abnormal metabolism of the vitamin is usually acquired in association with some widespread granulomatous disorder, but one rare hereditary form of vitamin D sensitivity in infants is associated with other developmental anomalies. As discussed in Chap. 353, vitamin D metabolism is carefully regulated, particularly the activity of the renal 1α-hydroxylase responsible for the production of $1,25(OH)_2D$. The regulation of 1α-hydroxylase and the normal feedback suppression by $1,25(OH)_2D$

on the kidney enzyme seem to work less well in infants than in adults and to operate poorly, if at all, in sites other than the renal tubule; these phenomena explain the occurrence of hypercalcemia secondary to excessive $1,25(OH)_2D_3$ production in infants with Williams' syndrome and adults with sarcoidosis or lymphoma.

Vitamin D Intoxication   The chronic ingestion of 50 to 100 times the normal physiologic requirement of vitamin D (amounts in excess of 50,000 to 100,000 U/d) is required to produce hypercalcemia in normal individuals. In animals, vitamin D intoxication causes increased bone resorption and increased intestinal calcium absorption. In humans, vitamin D excess increases intestinal calcium absorption, but it is not known whether bone resorption is increased.

The mechanism for the hypercalcemia is an excessive production of $1,25(OH)_2D$ as a consequence of an increase in the substrate for the renal 1α-hydroxylase, namely, $25(OH)D$. The production of $25(OH)D$ is less tightly regulated than is the production of $1,25(OH)_2D$. Hence concentrations of $25(OH)D$ are elevated 5- to 10-fold on average in patients on high-dose vitamin D. $25(OH)D$ has a definite, if low, biologic activity in intestine and bone, and part of vitamin D intoxication may be due to high levels of both $25(OH)D$ and $1,25(OH)_2D$.

The diagnosis is substantiated by documenting elevated levels of $25(OH)D$. Hypercalcemia is usually controlled by restriction of dietary calcium intake and appropriate attention to hydration. These measures, plus discontinuation of vitamin D, usually lead to resolution of hypercalcemia. However, vitamin D stores in fat may be substantial, and vitamin D intoxication may persist for weeks after vitamin D ingestion is terminated. Such patients are responsive to glucocorticoids, which in doses of 100 mg of hydrocortisone per day, or its equivalent, usually return serum calcium levels to normal over several days; severe intoxication may require intensive therapy.

Sarcoidosis and Other Granulomatous Diseases   In patients with sarcoidosis, $1,25(OH)_2D$ is believed to be synthesized in macrophages or other cells in the granulomas. Indeed, hypercalcemia has been reported in an anephric sarcoidosis patient in association with increased $1,25(OH)_2D$ levels. Macrophages obtained from granulomatous tissue convert $25(OH)D$ to $1,25(OH)_2D$ at an increased rate. There is a positive correlation in patients with sarcoidosis between $25(OH)D$ levels (reflecting vitamin D intake) and the circulating concentrations of $1,25(OH)_2D$, whereas normally there is no increase in $1,25(OH)_2D$ with increasing $25(OH)D$ levels due to multiple feedback controls on the renal 1α-hydroxylase (see Chap. 353). The usual regulation of active metabolite production by calcium or PTH does not operate in these patients; hypercalcemia does not lead to a reduction in the blood levels of $1,25(OH)_2D$ in patients with sarcoidosis. The PTH independence of $1,25(OH)_2D$ production in this disorder is indicated by reports of normal $1,25(OH)_2D$ production in a patient with sarcoidosis and hypoparathyroidism. Clearance of $1,25(OH)_2D$ from blood may be decreased in sarcoidosis as well.

Even normocalcemic patients with sarcoidosis have unregulated production of $1,25(OH)_2D$ in response to vitamin D loading. Exposure to sunlight or administration of as little as 9000 units of vitamin D daily is followed by increased levels of the active metabolite. Administration of moderate doses of glucocorticoids leads to a reversal of the hypercalcemia, as in other cases of excessive vitamin D action such as vitamin D intoxication, and reversal of the abnormal responsiveness of $1,25(OH)_2D$ levels to vitamin D challenge. Presumably, glucocorticoids have multiple effects in the disease and block both excessive production of the metabolite and the response to it in target organs.

Variation in reported frequency of hypercalcemia in sarcoidosis (10 percent or less in recent reports, 60 percent or more in older reports) is probably explained in part by the common use of glucocorticoids to control pulmonary complications and other manifestations of the granulomatous disease. Lytic lesions also occur in bone so that increased bone resorption may play a role in some cases. In most, however, hypercalcemia is directly related to an increased intestinal calcium absorption. Hypercalcemia is usually a manifestation of disseminated disease. Hence pulmonary involvement is usually evident; chest x-ray may reveal a diffuse fibronodular infiltrate and/or prominent hilar adenopathy. Levels of angiotensin-converting enzyme are

elevated; blood gamma globulin also may be elevated. The most useful diagnostic procedure is demonstration of noncaseating granulomas in liver or lymph node biopsy. Hypercalcemia due to sarcoidosis can be elusive when the typical features of the disease are lacking (see "Differential Diagnosis: Special Tests").

Management of the hypercalcemia can be accomplished by avoiding excessive sunlight exposure and by limiting vitamin D and calcium intake; glucocorticoids in the equivalent of 100 mg hydrocortisone per day or less usually are sufficient to control hypercalcemia. Presumably, however, the abnormal sensitivity to vitamin D and abnormal regulation of $1,25(OH)_2D$ synthesis will persist as long as the disease is active. PTH levels are usually low and $1,25(OH)_2D$ levels are elevated, but primary hyperparathyroidism and sarcoidosis may coexist in some patients.

Idiopathic Hypercalcemia of Infancy   This rare disorder, also referred to as *Williams' syndrome*, consists of multiple congenital development defects, including supravalvular aortic stenosis, mental retardation, and an elfin facies, in association with hypercalcemia due to abnormal sensitivity to vitamin D. The syndrome was first recognized in England after the fortification of milk with vitamin D. Hypercalcemia develops with vitamin D intakes as small as 2000 to 4000 U/d. Levels of $1,25(OH)_2D$ are elevated, ranging from 46 to 120 nmol/L (150 to 500 pg/mL). The mechanism of the abnormal sensitivity to vitamin D and of the increased circulating levels of $1,25(OH)_2D$ is unclear. Hypercalcemia is due to excessive intestinal calcium absorption. The abnormality in vitamin D metabolism and the increased sensitivity to vitamin D intake disappear after the first year of life. Treatment is restriction of calcium intake. When the hypercalcemia is severe, glucocorticoids in the doses used for vitamin D intoxication or sarcoidosis, adjusted for body weight, are effective.

HYPERCALCEMIA ASSOCIATED WITH HIGH BONE TURNOVER   **Hyperthyroidism**   As many as 20 percent of hyperthyroid patients have high-normal or mildly elevated serum calcium concentrations; hypercalciuria is even more common. The hypercalcemia is due to increased bone turnover, with bone resorption exceeding bone formation. Severe calcium elevations are not typical, and the presence of such suggests a concomitant disease such as hyperparathyroidism. Indeed, patients with thyrotoxicosis are more sensitive to the hypercalcemic effects of PTH. Usually, the diagnosis is obvious, but signs of hyperthyroidism may occasionally be occult, particularly in the elderly. Hypercalcemia is managed by treatment of the hyperthyroidism.

Immobilization   Immobilization is a rare cause of hypercalcemia in adults in the absence of an associated disease but may cause hypercalcemia in children and adolescents, particularly after spinal cord injury and paraplegia or quadriplegia. With resumption of some ambulation, the hypercalcemia in children usually returns to normal.

The mechanism appears to involve a disproportion between bone formation and bone resorption. Hypercalciuria and increased mobilization of skeletal calcium can develop in normal volunteers subjected to extensive bed rest, although hypercalcemia is unusual. Immobilization of an adult with a disease associated with high bone turnover, such as Paget's disease, may cause hypercalcemia.

Thiazides   Administration of benzothiadiazines (thiazides) can cause hypercalcemia in patients with high rates of bone turnover, such as patients with hypoparathyroidism treated with high doses of vitamin D. Traditionally, thiazides are associated with aggravation of hypercalcemia in primary hyperparathyroidism, but this effect can be seen in other high-bone-turnover states as well. The mechanism of action of thiazides is complex, but the result seems to be to impose a challenge to calcium homeostasis by actions on renal calcium excretion, bone-calcium turnover, and parathyroid action. Thiazide administration to normal individuals causes a transient increase in blood calcium (usually within the high-normal range) that reverts to preexisting levels after a week or more of continued administration. If hormonal function and calcium and bone metabolism are normal, homeostatic controls are reset to counteract the calcium-elevating effect of the thiazides. In the presence of hyperparathyroidism or increased bone turnover from another cause, homeostatic mechanisms are ineffective. The abnormal effects of the thiazide on calcium metabolism disappear within days of cessation of the drug.

Many aspects of thiazide action on calcium metabolism are unclear. The drugs augment PTH responsiveness of bone and renal tubule. Chronic thiazide administration leads to reduction in urinary calcium; the hypocalciuric effect appears to reflect the enhancement of proximal tubular resorption of sodium and calcium in response to sodium depletion. Some of this renal action is due to augmentation of PTH action and is more pronounced in individuals with intact parathyroid secretion. However, thiazides cause hypocalciuria in hypoparathyroid patients on high-dose vitamin D and oral calcium replacement if sodium intake is restricted. This finding is the rationale for the use of thiazides as an adjunct to therapy in hypoparathyroid patients as discussed below.

Vitamin A Intoxication Vitamin A intoxication is a rare cause of hypercalcemia. Most vitamin A intoxication is a side effect of dietary faddism (see Chap. 79). Calcium levels can be elevated into the 3 to 3.5 mmol/L (12 to 14 mg/dL) range after the ingestion of 50,000 to 100,000 units of vitamin A daily (10 to 20 times the minimum daily requirement). Typical features of severe hypercalcemia include fatigue, anorexia, and in some severe muscle and bone pain. Vitamin A intake excess is presumed to increase bone resorption.

Diagnosis can be established by history and by measurement of vitamin A levels in serum, which may be severalfold above normal. Occasionally, skeletal x-rays reveal periosteal calcifications, particularly in the hands. Withdrawal of the vitamin is usually associated with the prompt disappearance of the hypercalcemia and reversal of the skeletal changes. As in vitamin D intoxication, administration of 100 mg/d hydrocortisone or its equivalent leads to a rapid return of the serum calcium to normal.

HYPERCALCEMIA ASSOCIATED WITH RENAL FAILURE Severe Secondary Hyperparathyroidism Secondary hyperparathyroidism occurs when partial resistance to the metabolic actions of the hormone leads to excessive PTH production. Parathyroid gland hyperplasia occurs because resistance to the normal level of the hormone leads to hypocalcemia, which, in turn, is a stimulus to enlargement of the parathyroid glands with resultant increased secretion of PTH. This concept is based on studies in experimental animals with renal failure and phosphate retention and studies of the treatment of patients with bisphosphonates that block skeletal resorptive response. When the parathyroid secretory reserve is tested by deliberately lowering blood calcium, the extent of rise in PTH for each decrement of plasma calcium is greater with hyperplastic than with normal parathyroids. There is, therefore, a higher concentration of iPTH at any given level of calcium concentration. Since a portion of PTH secretion by each parathyroid cell is not suppressible by any degree of elevation of blood calcium, larger glands (more cells) have a higher hormone output at the hypercalcemic end of the dose-response curve.

Secondary hyperparathyroidism occurs in patients with renal failure, osteomalacia (vitamin D deficiency), and pseudohypoparathyroidism (deficient response to PTH at the level of the receptor). The clinical manifestations of secondary hyperparathyroidism vary in these states. Hypocalcemia seems to be the common denominator in secondary hyperparathyroidism. Primary and secondary hyperparathyroidism can be distinguished conceptually by the autonomous growth of the parathyroid glands in primary hyperparathyroidism (presumably irreversible) and the adaptive growth of the parathyroids in secondary hyperparathyroidism (presumably reversible). In fact, reversal over weeks from an abnormal pattern of secretion, presumably accompanied by involution of parathyroid gland mass to normal, occurs in patients who have been treated medically to reverse the resistance to PTH.

In progressive renal failure, the initial tendency to hypocalcemia is attributable to phosphate retention due to the reduced excretion of phosphate and reduced production of $1,25(OH)_2D$ by the failing kidney.

The net consequence is reduced skeletal responsiveness to PTH. $1,25(OH)_2D$ deficiency also interferes with calcium absorption from the intestine, already impaired in uremia. The consequence in any given patient with chronic renal failure represents the outcome of competing physiologic adaptations, stimuli that cause parathyroid gland hyperplasia (tendency toward hypercalcemia and excessive bone resorption) versus those that modify the responsiveness of the end organs—bone, gut, and residual renal tubules (tendency toward hypocalcemia, hyperphosphatemia, and reduced bone resorption). Typically patients with renal failure exhibit hyperphosphatemia (renal retention and increased bone breakdown) and a low-normal or moderately low blood calcium level (calcium-lowering action of the phosphate level and reduced availability of calcium from bone and gut). In patients with severe secondary hyperparathyroidism, hypercalcemia and hyperphosphatemia both develop due to an increase in bone resorption; parathyroid hypersecretion "overshoots" the degree of resistance to hormone action; monoclonal expansion of parathyroid gland mass may contribute to the "overshoot" and hypercalcemia.

In addition to hypercalcemia and hyperphosphatemia, patients with secondary hyperparathyroidism may develop bone pain, ectopic calcification, and pruritus. The bone disease in patients with secondary hyperparathyroidism and renal failure is usually termed *renal osteodystrophy*. Concomitant osteomalacia (vitamin D and calcium deficiency) and osteitis fibrosa cystica (excessive PTH action on bone) may occur. In fact, osteitis fibrosa cystica is now more common in untreated renal failure than in primary hyperparathyroidism.

Two other skeletal disorders are associated with long-term dialysis in patients with renal failure. Aluminum deposition (see below) is associated with an osteomalacia-like picture. The other entity is a low bone turnover state termed "aplastic" or "adynamic" bone disease; PTH levels are lower than in typical secondary hyperparathyroidism. The adynamic state responds to measures that stimulate PTH secretion, implying that the cause is excessive involution of the hyperparathyroidism by calcium carbonate.

℞ TREATMENT

Medical therapy to reverse secondary hyperparathyroidism includes reduction of excessive blood phosphate by restriction of dietary phosphate, the use of nonabsorbable antacids, and careful, selective addition of calcitriol (0.25 to 2.0 µg/d); calcium carbonate is preferred over aluminum-containing antacids to prevent aluminum toxicity. Intravenous administration of calcitriol, sometimes administered as several pulses each week, has been reported to cause long-term involution of secondary hyperparathyroidism. Involution of the parathyroids often occurs; reduction of the increased parathyroid mass causes the exaggerated secretory response to return to normal. The level of PTH at any given level of blood calcium is now more appropriate, and excessive parathyroid action is reversed. Somewhat paradoxically, during successful medical reversal of secondary hyperparathyroidism, elevated serum calcium (and phosphate) levels may return to normal despite the administration of increased amounts of calcium and vitamin D metabolites that might have been expected to aggravate the hypercalcemia.

Occasional patients develop severe manifestations of secondary hyperparathyroidism, including hypercalcemia, pruritus, extraskeletal calcifications, and painful bones, despite aggressive medical efforts to suppress the hyperparathyroidism. Parathyroid surgery may be necessary to control the condition. Since one or more of the enlarged glands may be monoclonal in nature, this phenomenon must be due to conversion of the parathyroids from a state of reversible hyperplasia to an irreversible growth defect and state of PTH hypersecretion no longer responsive to medical therapy. This state of severe hyperparathyroidism in patients with renal failure that requires surgery has been referred to as *tertiary hyperparathyroidism*.

Aluminum Intoxication Aluminum intoxication may occur in patients on chronic dialysis; manifestations include acute dementia and unresponsive and severe osteomalacia. Bone pain, multiple nonhealing fractures, particularly of the ribs and pelvis, and a proximal myopathy may occur. Hypercalcemia develops when these patients are treated with vitamin D or calcitriol, as in the typical patient with severe secondary hyperparathyroidism and renal osteodystrophy, as discussed above. Acute hypercalcemia occurs after administration of vitamin D because of impaired skeletal responsiveness. Aluminum is present at the site of osteoid mineralization, osteoblastic activity is minimal, and calcium incorporation into the skeleton is impaired. Prevention is accomplished by avoidance of aluminum excess in the dialysis regimen; treatment involves mobilizing aluminum through the use of the chelating agent deferoxamine. Aluminum is mobilized from bone and, being tightly bound to the chelating agent, can be removed via dialysis. After aluminum toxicity is reversed, patients may show typical features of renal osteodystrophy and secondary hyperparathyroidism and are managed like other patients with secondary hyperparathyroidism due to renal disease. Failure to recognize the syndrome is associated with persistence of the disabling bone disease and with hypercalcemia inadvertently induced by treatment with vitamin D. The iPTH levels may not increase to the normal hyperparathyroid range as a result of the aluminum toxicity.

Milk-Alkali Syndrome The milk-alkali syndrome can cause several clinical presentations—acute, subacute, and chronic—all of which feature hypercalcemia, alkalosis, and renal failure. The disorder is due to an excessive ingestion of calcium and absorbable antacids such as milk or calcium carbonate and is less frequent since nonabsorbable antacids and other treatments became available for peptic ulcer disease.

Individual susceptibility must be important in the pathogenesis, since many patients are treated with calcium carbonate without developing the syndrome. One variable is the fractional calcium absorption as a function of calcium intake. Some individuals absorb a high fraction of calcium, even with intakes as high as 2 g and more of elemental calcium per day, instead of reducing calcium absorption with high intake, as occurs in most normal individuals. Resultant mild hypercalcemia after meals in such patients is postulated to contribute to the generation of alkalosis. Development of hypercalcemia causes increased sodium excretion and some depletion of total-body water. These phenomena and perhaps some suppression of endogenous PTH secretion due to mild hypercalcemia lead to increased bicarbonate resorption and to alkalosis in the face of continued calcium carbonate ingestion. Alkalosis per se selectively enhances calcium resorption in the distal nephron, thus aggravating the hypercalcemia. The cycle of mild hypercalcemia $\rightarrow$ bicarbonate retention $\rightarrow$ alkalosis $\rightarrow$ renal calcium retention $\rightarrow$ severe hypercalcemia perpetuates and aggravates hypercalcemia and alkalosis as long as calcium and absorbable alkali are ingested.

Acute hypercalcemia and alkalosis occurring within days of beginning calcium and alkali ingestion, *acute milk-alkali syndrome*, is manifested by weakness, myalgia, irritability, and apathy. The impairment of renal function, including reduced renal concentrating ability and tubular dysfunction, hypercalcemia, and alkalosis reverse rapidly upon stopping the intake of calcium and alkali.

The far-advanced milk-alkali syndrome, sometimes referred to as *Burnett's syndrome*, is due to long-standing calcium and alkali ingestion. Severe hypercalcemia, irreversible renal failure, and phosphate retention may be accompanied by ectopic calcification. Some improvement may result when the ingestion of calcium and alkali is reduced, but prior to the availability of renal dialysis renal failure led to death. There is an intermediate or subacute form in which the renal failure is reversible over a period of weeks after withdrawal of excessive calcium and alkali intake.

DIFFERENTIAL DIAGNOSIS: SPECIAL TESTS Differential diagnosis of hypercalcemia is best achieved by using clinical criteria, but the radioimmunoassay for PTH is useful in distinguishing among major causes. The clinical features that deserve major emphasis are the presence or absence of symptoms or signs of disease and evidence of chronicity. If one discounts fatigue or depression, more than 90 percent of patients with *asymptomatic hypercalcemia* have primary hyperparathyroidism; symptoms of malignancy are usually present in cancer hypercalcemia. Disorders other than hyperparathyroidism and malignancy cause no more than 10 percent of cases of

Table 354-2

Differential Diagnosis of Hypercalcemia

Criterion	Conclusion
Clinical issues alone	
>90% caused by hyperparathyroidism or cancer	
If asymptomatic or chronic:	Hyperparathyroidism most likely
Level of PTH measured by PTH assay	
Increased or normal (despite hypercalcemia):	Hyperparathyroidism confirmed
Decreased or undetectable:	Acute presentation with or without symptoms—screen carefully for malignancy
	Chronic—malignancy unlikely, sarcoidosis or other rarer cause

hypercalcemia, and some of the nonparathyroid causes are associated with clear-cut manifestations such as renal failure.

Chronicity is the second most important clinical criterion. If hypercalcemia has been manifest for more than 1 year, malignancy can usually be excluded as the cause. A striking feature of malignancy-associated hypercalcemia is the rapidity of the course, whereby signs and symptoms of the underlying malignancy are evident within months of the detection of hypercalcemia. Hyperparathyroidism is the likely diagnosis in patients with *chronic hypercalcemia*. Diseases such as sarcoidosis are rare causes of chronic hypercalcemia. A careful *history* of dietary supplements and drug use may suggest intoxication with vitamins D or A or the use of thiazides.

Although clinical considerations are helpful in arriving at the correct diagnosis of the cause of hypercalcemia, appropriate laboratory testing is essential for definitive diagnosis (Table 354-2). Theoretically, the radioimmunoassay for PTH should separate hyperparathyroidism from all other causes of hypercalcemia, those with hyperparathyroidism having elevated levels of iPTH despite hypercalcemia and patients with malignancy and the other causes of hypercalcemia (except for disorders mediated by PTH such as lithium-induced hypercalcemia) having levels of hormone below normal or undetectable. Assays based on the double-antibody method separate those with primary hyperparathyroidism from the hypercalcemia of malignancy (Fig. 354-4 and Table 354-2). 1,25(OH)$_2$D levels are elevated in many (but not all) patients with primary hyperparathyroidism and are increased in states of vitamin D intoxication, particularly sarcoidosis. In other disorders associated with hypercalcemia, concentrations of 1,25(OH)$_2$D are low or, at the most, normal. Since not all patients with hyperparathyroidism have elevated 1,25(OH)$_2$D levels, and since not all nonparathyroid hypercalcemic patients have suppressed 1,25(OH)$_2$D, the test is of low specificity and not cost-effective in differential diagnosis; measurement of 1,25(OH)$_2$D is of critical value in establishing the cause of hypercalcemia in sarcoidosis and certain B cell lymphomas.

PTH levels are elevated in chronic renal failure; the elevation seen in early assays reflects, in part, accumulation of fragments secondary to renal failure rather than true parathyroid oversecretion. Results with the double-antibody assay correlate well with independent evidence for parathyroid gland overactivity. Patients with sarcoidosis have low or undetectable levels of iPTH. No systematic surveys have been reported of the results of double-antibody PTH radioimmunoassays in many of the other non-parathyroid-related causes of hypercalcemia largely because of the infrequency of the disorders, but it is predicted that they will be low or undetectable.

In summary, iPTH values are elevated in more than 90 percent of parathyroid-related causes of hypercalcemia, undetectable or low in malignancy-related hypercalcemia, and undetectable or normal in vitamin D–related and high-bone-turnover causes of hypercalcemia (although there is little data for these latter categories).

FIGURE 354-4 Levels of iPTH detected in patients with primary hyperparathyroidism, hypercalcemia of malignancy, and hypoparathyroidism. Boxed area represents the upper and normal limits of blood calcium and/or iPTH. *(From Nussbaum and Potts, with permission.)*

Measurements of nephrogenous cyclic AMP are of limited value in distinguishing primary hyperparathyroidism and malignancy because nephrogenous cyclic AMP is elevated in some patients with malignancy as well as in most patients with primary hyperparathyroidism. Specific laboratory tests are of utility in diagnosing particular disorders (such as thyrotoxicosis), and the newer immunoassays for PTH-rP are helpful in diagnosing certain types of malignancy-associated hypercalcemia.

Some general conclusions are warranted as to the differential diagnosis of hypercalcemia. Two independent causes of hypercalcemia in the same person, although reported, are rare. If a specific disease traditionally associated with hypercalcemia is clinically evident, it is reasonable to assume that the disease is responsible for the hypercalcemia. In view of the specificity of the PTH immunoassay and the high frequency of hyperparathyroidism in hypercalcemic patients, it is cost-effective to measure the iPTH level in all hypercalcemic patients unless malignancy or a specific nonparathyroid disease is obvious. If hypercalcemia disappears in response to control of hyperthyroidism or after reduction of excessive intake of fat-soluble vitamins or alkali and calcium, in the cases of vitamin D intoxication and milk-alkali syndrome, respectively, there is no need to search for a second cause of hypercalcemia. If specific treatment does not lead to a reversal of the hypercalcemia, a search for an additional cause must be undertaken. It also follows that the management of the hypercalcemia of malignancy focuses on treatment of the malignancy.

When the diagnosis is unclear, either because the patient is asymptomatic or because chronic illness obscures manifestations that might indicate the presence of malignancy, the following general approach can be used: If the patient is *asymptomatic* and there is evidence by history of *chronicity* to the hypercalcemia, hyperparathyroidism is almost certainly the cause. If iPTH levels (usually measured at least twice) are elevated, little additional evaluation is necessary. Hyperparathyroidism is never confirmed until abnormal parathyroid tissue is removed surgically and hypercalcemia is corrected, but the presumptive diagnosis can be made in patients with asymptomatic hypercalcemia on the basis of elevated concentration of iPTH. If there is a family history suggestive of other endocrine abnormalities, screening for MEN should be undertaken in the patient and family.

If the patient does not have clear-cut symptoms and there is only a short history or no clue as to the duration of the hypercalcemia, *occult malignancy* must be considered. If the iPTH levels with the double-antibody technique are increased, the diagnosis of asymptomatic hyperparathyroidism is established.

If patients with recent-onset hypercalcemia have clear-cut systemic symptoms and/or the iPTH levels are not elevated, then a thorough workup must be undertaken for malignancy, including chest x-ray, CT of chest and abdomen, and bone scan. Attention also should be paid to clues for underlying hematologic disorders such as anemia, increased plasma globulin, and abnormal serum immunoelectrophoresis; bone scans can be negative in patients with multiple myeloma.

Finally, if a patient with *chronic hypercalcemia* is *asymptomatic* but iPTH values are not elevated, and if malignancy seems unlikely on clinical grounds (chronicity), it is useful to search for other chronic causes of hypercalcemia, such as occult sarcoidosis. Table 354-2 summarizes the approach.

℞ TREATMENT

Hypercalcemic States The acute treatment of hypercalcemia is usually successful. The serum calcium concentration can be decreased by 0.7 to 2.2 mmol/L (3 to 9 mg/dL) within 24 to 48 h in most patients, enough to relieve acute symptoms, prevent death from hypercalcemic crisis, and permit diagnostic evaluation. However, the chronic medical management of hypercalcemia is less satisfactory unless the underlying cause can be corrected because available therapies are inconvenient and may be toxic.

Hypercalcemia develops because of excessive skeletal calcium release, increased intestinal calcium absorption, or inadequate renal calcium excretion. Understanding the particular pathogenesis helps guide therapy. For example, hypercalcemia in patients with osteolytic metastases or acute immobilization is primarily due to excessive skeletal calcium release and is, therefore, minimally improved by restriction of dietary calcium. On the other hand, patients with vitamin D hypersensitivity or vitamin D intoxication have excessive intestinal calcium absorption, and restriction of dietary calcium is beneficial. Decreased renal function or extracellular fluid depletion decreases urinary calcium excretion. If additional abnormalities, such as increased bone breakdown, are present, hypercalcemia will develop. This may happen, for example, when patients with resorptive bone disease become dehydrated. In such situations, rehydration may rapidly reduce or reverse the hypercalcemia, even though bone resorption and urinary calcium excretion are increased.

HYDRATION, INCREASED SALT INTAKE, MILD AND FORCED DIURESIS The first principle of treatment is to restore *normal hydration*. Many hypercalcemic patients are dehydrated because of vomiting, inanition, and/or hypercalcemia-induced defects in urinary concentrating ability. The resultant drop in glomerular filtration rate is accompanied by an additional decrease in renal tubular sodium and calcium clearance. Restoring a normal extracellular fluid volume corrects these abnormalities and increases urine calcium excretion by 2.5 to 7.5 mmol/d (100 to 300 mg/d). Increasing urinary sodium excretion to 400 to 500 mmol/d increases urinary calcium excretion even further than simple rehydration. After rehydration has been achieved, saline can be administered or furosemide or ethacrynic acid can be given twice daily to depress the tubular reabsorptive mechanism for calcium (care must be taken to prevent dehydration). The combined use of these therapies can increase urinary calcium excretion to 12.5 mmol/d (500 mg/d) or higher in most hypercalcemic patients. Since this is a substantial percentage of the exchangeable calcium pool, the serum calcium concentration usually falls 0.25 to 0.75 mmol/L (1 to 3 mg/dL) within 24 h. Precautions should be taken to prevent potassium and magnesium depletion; calcium-containing renal calculi are a potential complication.

Under life-threatening circumstances, the preceding approach can be pursued more aggressively, giving as much as 6 L isotonic saline (900 mmol sodium) daily plus furosemide or equivalent in doses up to 100 mg every 1 to 2 h or ethacrynic acid in doses to 40 mg every 1 to 2 h. Urinary calcium excretion may exceed 25 mmol/d (1000 mg/d), and the serum calcium may decrease by 1 mmol/L (4 mg/dL) or more within 24 h. Depletion of potassium and magnesium is inevitable unless replacements are given; pulmonary edema can be precipitated. The potential complications can be reduced by careful monitoring of central venous pressure and plasma or urine electrolytes; catheterization of the bladder may be necessary. This treatment approach should be supplemented with agents to block bone resorption that become effective within a few days, since forced diuresis is difficult to sustain even in patients with good cardiopulmonary and renal function.

BISPHOSPHONATES The bisphosphonates are analogues of pyrophosphate, with high affinity for bone, especially in areas of increased bone turnover. These bone-seeking compounds are stable in vivo because phosphatase enzymes cannot hydrolyze the central carbon-phosphorus-carbon bond. The bisphosphonates are concentrated in areas of high bone turnover and are taken up by and inhibit osteoclast action; the mechanism of action is not well understood. Bisphosphonates may alter proton pump function or impair the release of acid hydrolases into the extracellular lysosomes contiguous with mineralized bone. They also may inhibit the differentiation of monocyte-macrophage precursors into osteoclasts and possibly have effects on osteoblasts as well.

Etidronate, a first-generation bisphosphonate, is poorly absorbed and, like most bisphosphonates, generally must be given intravenously to be effective. At times, the continuation of oral etidronate after intravenous therapy may be useful to control hypercalcemia.

A newer class of bisphosphonates has more favorable efficacy and longer duration of action (Table 354-3). Pamidronate is a potent inhibitor of osteoclast-mediated skeletal resorption yet does not cause mineralization defects at ordinary doses. Several additional bisphosphonates (alendronate, tiludronate, and risedronate) are highly potent and have a favorable ratio of blocking resorption over inhibiting bone formation. The potency of the compounds for inhibition of bone resorption varies a thousandfold in the order of etidronate, tiludronate, pamidronate, alendronate, and risedronate. Oral alendronate is approved for the therapy of osteoporosis in the United States, and in Europe oral preparations of these bisphosphonates are used in the chronic treatment of hypercalcemia. Only the intravenous use of pamidronate is approved for this purpose in the United States; between 60 and 90 mg pamidronate, given as a single intravenous dose, returns serum calcium to normal for weeks in 80 to 100 percent of patients.

While the bisphosphonates have similar structures, efficacy, toxicity, and side effects vary. Etidronate causes hyperphosphatemia, through a direct renal mechanism, whereas hypophosphatemia is seen following therapy with other bisphosphonates. Pamidronate causes low-grade fever in as many as 20 percent of patients, likely related to release of cytokines from osteoclasts, monocytes, and macrophages (Table 354-3). Overall, second-generation bisphosphonates are now the agents of choice in severe hypercalcemia, particularly that associated with malignancy.

CALCITONIN Calcitonin acts within minutes of its administration, through receptors on osteoclasts, to decrease the release of skeletal calcium, phosphorus, and hydroxyproline. In addition, inhibition of renal tubular calcium reabsorption may, in part, contribute to its rapid onset of action. In various reports, however, the adminis-

Table 354-3

Therapies for Severe Hypercalcemia

Treatment	Onset of Action	Duration of Action	Advantages	Disadvantages
MOST USEFUL THERAPIES				
Hydration with saline	Hours	During infusion	Rehydration invariably needed	
Forced diuresis; saline + loop diuretic	Hours	During treatment	Rapid action	Cardiac decompensation, intensive monitoring electrolyte disturbance, hypokalemia, hypomagnesemia
Bisphosphonates				
1st generation: etidronate	1–2 days	5–7 days in doses used	First available bisphosphonate; intermediate onset of action	Hyperphosphatemia; 3-day infusion
2d generation: pamidronate	1–2 days	10–14 days after high dose	High potency; intermediate onset; prolonged duration of action	Fever in 20%; hypophosphatemia, hypocalcemia, hypomagnesemia
Calcitonin	Hours	2–3 days	Rapid onset of action; useful as adjunct in severe hypercalcemia	Often limited calcium lowering, rapid tachyphylaxis
OTHER THERAPIES				
Gallium nitrate	Day after 5-day administration	7–10 days	High potency	Length of IV administration; cannot be used with renal failure
Plicamycin	3–4 days	Days	Potent antiresorptive	Liver, kidney, and marrow toxicity; bleeding
Phosphate				
Oral	24 h	During use	Low toxicity if P < 4 mg/dL	Limited use except as adjuvant or chronic therapy
Intravenous	Hours	During use and 24–48 h afterward	Rapid action, highly potent	Ectopic calcification; severe hypocalcemia
Glucocorticoids	Days	Days, weeks	Oral therapy, antitumor agent	Active only in certain malignancies; glucocorticoid side effects
Dialysis	Hours	During use and 24–48 h afterward	Useful in renal failure; onset of effect in hours; can immediately reverse life-threatening hypercalcemia	Complex procedure, reserved for extreme or special circumstances

tration of 2 to 8 U/kg of body weight intravenously, subcutaneously, or intramuscularly every 6 to 12 h caused variable and minimal lowering of calcium in some patients. Tachyphylaxis, a known phenomenon with this drug, may explain the variable results. This escape from the hypocalcemic effects of calcitonin can be prevented by glucocorticoids in vitro. In vivo in humans, administration of glucocorticoids in combination with calcitonin may augment or prolong the action of calcitonin; in some patients, particularly those with lymphoproliferative malignancies, lowering of calcium may persist for as long as 10 days. In other studies, however, glucocorticoids did not prevent tachyphylaxis. Calcitonin therapy with the salmon, porcine, and human sequences, as currently used, rarely returns serum calcium to normal and can best be viewed as a nontoxic therapy with a very rapid onset of action and limited efficacy. However, in life-threatening hypercalcemia, calcitonin can be used while waiting for more sustained effects from plicamycin, gallium, or bisphosphonate. Calcitonin therapy may be associated with transient nausea, cramping, abdominal pain, and flushing.

PLICAMYCIN For the acute management of hypercalcemia, plicamycin (mithramycin), which inhibits bone resorption, has been a useful therapeutic agent. Plicamycin must be given intravenously, either as a bolus injection or by slow infusion. The usual dose is 25 μg/kg of body weight. In some patients, 10 μg/kg of body weight can be given twice a week for chronic therapy. Treatment should not be repeated until hypercalcemia recurs, because toxicity is dependent on the frequency of treatment and the total dosage. Careful monitoring is needed if repeated doses are used. The major side effects are thrombocytopenia, hepatocellular necrosis with increased lactic acid dehydrogenase (LDH) and aspartate aminotransferase (AST) levels, and decreased levels of clotting factors with resultant epistaxis, bruising, hemorrhage, and bleeding gums. Azotemia, proteinuria, hypocalcemia, hypophosphatemia, hypokalemia, nausea, vomiting, stomatitis, and facial swelling may occur. Toxicity is rare when only one or two doses are used and can be minimized by repeating single doses only when hypercalcemia recurs. Toxic effects other than hemorrhage can usually be reversed by stopping the drug. Use of plicamycin has been largely replaced by the less toxic second-generation bisphosphonates.

GALLIUM NITRATE Gallium nitrate exerts a hypocalcemic action by inhibiting bone resorption and altering the structure of bone crystals. Major disadvantages include the 5-day duration of infusion and the potential for nephrotoxicity. Alternative, shorter-dosage regimens have not been reported. (Its use is approved by the FDA for the treatment of hypercalcemia; further experience should define its ultimate role.)

OTHER THERAPIES Glucocorticoids increase urinary calcium excretion and decrease intestinal calcium absorption when given in pharmacologic doses (e.g., 40 to 200 mg prednisone daily in divided doses), but they also cause negative skeletal calcium balance. In normal subjects and in patients with primary hyperparathyroidism, glucocorticoids neither increase nor decrease the serum calcium concentration. In patients with hypercalcemia due to certain osteolytic malignancies, however, glucocorticoids may be effective as a result of antitumor effects. The malignancies in which hypercalcemia responds to glucocorticoids include multiple myeloma, leukemia, Hodgkin's disease, other lymphomas, and carcinoma of the breast, at least early in the course. Glucocorticoids are also effective in treating hypercalcemia due to vitamin D intoxication and sarcoidosis. In all the preceding situations, the hypocalcemic effect develops over several days, and the usual glucocorticoid dosage is 40 to 100 mg prednisone (or its equivalent) daily in four divided doses. The side effects of chronic glucocorticoid therapy may be acceptable in some circumstances.

Hypercalcemia complicated by renal failure is difficult to manage; dialysis is often the treatment of choice. Peritoneal dialysis with calcium-free dialysis fluid can remove 5 to 12.5 mmol (200 to 500 mg) of calcium in 24 to 48 h and lower the serum calcium concentration by 0.7 to 3 mmol/L (3 to 12 mg/dL). Large quantities of phosphate are lost during dialysis, and serum inorganic phosphate concentrations usually fall, thus aggravating hypercalcemia. Therefore, the serum inorganic phosphate concentration should be measured after dialysis, and phosphate supplements should be added to the diet or to dialysis fluids if necessary.

Phosphate therapy, oral or intravenous, has a role in certain circumstances. Patients with primary hyperparathyroidism are frequently hypophosphatemic, and hypercalcemia of other causes also may be complicated by hypophosphatemia. Hypophosphatemia decreases the rate of calcium uptake into bone, increases intestinal calcium absorption, and directly and indirectly stimulates bone breakdown. These effects aggravate hypercalcemia, and correcting hypophosphatemia lowers the serum calcium concentration. The usual treatment is 1 to 1.5 g phosphorus per day for several days, given in four divided doses to minimize the chances of developing hyperphosphatemia. Such therapy has been administered for prolonged periods in selected patients. It is generally believed but not established that toxicity does not occur if therapy is limited to restoring serum inorganic phosphate concentrations to normal.

Raising the serum inorganic phosphate concentration above normal does decrease serum calcium levels, sometimes strikingly. Intravenous phosphate is one of the most dramatically effective treatments available for severe hypercalcemia but is toxic and even dangerous so that it is used rarely and only in severely hypercalcemic patients with cardiac or renal failure. A dose of 1500 mg phosphate phosphorus or more intravenously over 6 to 8 h leads to a prompt decrease in serum calcium of as much as 1.2 to 2.5 mmol/L (5 to 10 mg/dL) in patients with initially normal serum inorganic phosphate concentrations. This therapy should be employed only in extreme emergencies for two reasons. First, fatal hypocalcemia can be produced by excessive dosage; serum calcium should be measured frequently if intravenous phosphate is administered. Second, unlike sodium chloride, sodium phosphate does not remove calcium from the body. In fact, urine calcium generally declines, and fecal calcium declines or remains the same. The decline in serum calcium reflects a redistribution of calcium within the body. There is a rapid efflux of calcium with no change in calcium influx to the circulation, findings indicative of precipitation of calcium phosphate salt. The calcium precipitates in bone, and metastatic calcification also may occur in patients receiving oral or intravenous phosphate therapy for hypercalcemia. Indeed, hyperphosphatemia can cause metastatic calcification in normocalcemic animals. Thus administration of intravenous phosphate in patients with compromised renal function who cannot have diuretic therapy is justifiable only as an emergency treatment.

Inorganic phosphate is commercially available for oral use in liquid, powder, and capsule form and as a liquid for intravenous use. It is important to calculate doses in terms of phosphate phosphorus.

SUMMARY The various therapies for hypercalcemia are listed in Table 354-3. The choice depends on the underlying disease, the severity of the hypercalcemia, the serum inorganic phosphate level, and the renal, hepatic, and bone marrow function. Mild hypercalcemia [3 mmol/L (12 mg/dL) or less] can usually be managed by the sequence of hydration followed by intravenous sodium chloride and, if needed, small doses of furosemide or ethacrynic acid. Severe hypercalcemia [3.7 mmol/L (15 mg/dL)] requires rapid correction. Calcitonin should be given for its rapid, albeit short-lived, blockade of bone resorption, and intravenous pamidronate should be administered, although its onset of action is delayed for 1 to 2 days. Hence aggressive sodium-calcium diuresis with intravenous saline and large doses of furosemide and ethacrynic acid works but should be initiated only if appropriate monitoring is available and cardiac function is adequate.

There is a role for oral phosphate therapy in chronic management of hypercalcemia, but its utility may be superseded by the bisphosphonates. Phosphate should only be given if hyperphosphatemia is not present.

Dietary calcium should be restricted and glucocorticoids should be administered if intestinal absorption is enhanced (in sarcoidosis, vitamin D intoxication). Dialysis is appropriate for hypercalcemia complicating acute or chronic renal failure.

Chronic therapy of hypercalcemia poses greater problems of toxicity. One satisfactory regimen for chronic use is a combination of dietary calcium restriction, administration of sodium chloride with or without furosemide or ethacrynic acid to maintain high urinary calcium, and moderate-dose oral phosphate (the patient is kept normophosphatemic). Some of the effective remedies (plicamycin, glucocorticoids, high-dose oral phosphate) may have significant toxicity when used chronically. Oral bisphosphonates, if proven nontoxic, may become the chronic treatment of choice in hypercalcemia where increased bone resorption is present.

HYPOCALCEMIA

PATHOPHYSIOLOGY OF HYPOCALCEMIA: CLASSIFICATION BASED ON MECHANISM *Chronic hypocalcemia* is less common than hypercalcemia; causes include chronic renal failure, hereditary and acquired hypoparathyroidism, vitamin D deficiency, pseudohypoparathyroidism (PHP), and hypomagnesemia.

Critically ill patients may have transient hypocalcemia with severe sepsis, burns, acute renal failure, and extensive transfusions with citrated blood. Acute hypocalcemia with certain medications is also usually transient and may have no symptoms. Although as many as half of patients in an intensive care setting are reported to have calcium concentrations below 2.1 mmol/L (8.5 mg/dL), fewer than 10 percent have a reduction in ionized calcium. Patients with severe sepsis may have a decrease in ionized calcium (true hypocalcemia), but in other severely ill subjects, hypoalbuminemia is the cause of the reduced total calcium concentration. Alkalosis increases calcium binding to proteins, and in this setting direct measurements of ionized calcium should be made.

Medications such as protamine, heparin, and glucagon may cause transient hypocalcemia. These forms of hypocalcemia are usually not associated with tetany and resolve with improvement in the overall medical condition. The hypocalcemia after repeated transfusions of citrated blood also usually resolves quickly.

Patients with acute *pancreatitis* have hypocalcemia that persists during the acute inflammation and varies in degree with the severity of the pancreatitis. The cause of hypocalcemia remains unclear. PTH values are reported to be low, normal, or elevated, and both resistance to PTH and impaired PTH secretion have been postulated. Occasionally, a chronic low total-blood calcium and low ionized calcium concentration are detected in an elderly patient without obvious cause and with a paucity of symptoms; the pathogenesis is unclear.

Chronic hypocalcemia, however, is usually symptomatic and requires treatment. Neuromuscular and neurologic manifestations of chronic hypocalcemia include muscle spasms, carpopedal spasm, facial grimacing, and, in extreme cases, laryngeal spasm and convulsions. Respiratory arrest may occur. Increased intracranial pressure occurs in some patients with long-standing hypocalcemia, often in association with papilledema. Mental changes include irritability, depression, and psychosis. The QT interval on the electrocardiogram is prolonged, in contrast to its shortening with hypercalcemia. Arrhythmias occur, and digitalis effectiveness may be reduced. Intestinal cramps and chronic malabsorption may occur. Chvostek's or Trousseau's sign can be used to confirm latent tetany.

The classification of hypocalcemia shown in Table 354-4 is based on the premise that PTH is responsible for minute-to-minute regulation of plasma calcium concentration within narrow limits and, therefore, that the occurrence of hypocalcemia must mean a failure of the homeostatic action of PTH. Failure of the PTH response can occur due to hereditary or acquired parathyroid gland failure, if PTH is ineffective in target organs, or if the action of the hormone is overwhelmed by the loss of calcium from the extracellular fluid at a rate faster than it can be replaced.

PTH ABSENT Hypoparathyroidism, whether hereditary or acquired, has a number of common components. Acute and chronic symptoms of untreated hypocalcemia are shared by both types of

Table 354-4

Functional Classification of Hypocalcemia (Excluding Neonatal Conditions)

PTH ABSENT	
Hereditary hypoparathyroidism	Hypomagnesemia
Acquired hypoparathyroidism	
PTH INEFFECTIVE	
Chronic renal failure	Active vitamin D ineffective
Active vitamin D lacking	Intestinal malabsorption
↓ Dietary intake or sunlight	Vitamin D–dependent rickets
Defective metabolism:	type II
Anticonvulsant therapy	Pseudohypoparathyroidism
Vitamin D–dependent rickets	
type I	
PTH OVERWHELMED	
Severe, acute hyperphosphatemia	Osteitis fibrosa after
Tumor lysis	parathyroidectomy
Acute renal failure	
Rhabdomyolysis	

hypoparathyroidism, although typically the onset of hereditary hypoparathyroidism is more gradual and hereditary hypoparathyroidism is associated with developmental defects. In earlier decades, acquired hypoparathyroidism secondary to surgery in the neck was more common than hereditary hypoparathyroidism, but the frequency of surgically induced parathyroid failure has diminished as a result of improved surgical techniques that spare the parathyroid glands and increased use of nonsurgical therapy for hyperthyroidism. Basal ganglia calcification and extrapyramidal syndromes are more common and earlier in onset in hereditary hypoparathyroidism. PHP, an example of ineffective PTH action rather than a failure of parathyroid gland production, shares several features with hypoparathyroidism, including extraosseous calcification and extrapyramidal manifestations such as choreoathetotic movements and dystonia. Papilledema and raised intracranial pressure occur in both states, as do chronic changes in fingernails and hair and lenticular cataracts, the latter usually reversible with treatment of hypocalcemia. Certain skin manifestations, including alopecia and candidiasis, occur exclusively in hereditary hypoparathyroidism.

Hypocalcemia associated with hypomagnesemia is associated with both deficient PTH release and impaired responsiveness to the hormone (see also Chap. 357). Patients with hypocalcemia secondary to hypomagnesemia have absent or low levels of circulating PTH, indicative of diminished hormone release despite maximum physiologic stimulus by hypocalcemia. Plasma PTH levels return to normal with correction of the hypomagnesemia. Thus hypoparathyroidism with low levels of PTH in blood can be due to hereditary gland failure, acquired gland failure, or acute but reversible gland dysfunction (hypomagnesemia). Patients with acquired or hereditary hypoparathyroidism also have hyperphosphatemia and absent or low levels of 1,25(OH)$_2$D.

Hereditary Hypoparathyroidism Hereditary hypoparathyroidism can occur as an isolated entity without other endocrine or dermatologic manifestations (idiopathic hypoparathyroidism) or, more typically, in association with other abnormalities such as defective development of the thymus or failure of function of other endocrine organs such as the adrenal thyroid or ovary (see also Chap. 340). Idiopathic and hereditary hypoparathyroidisms are often manifest within the first decade but may appear later.

A rare form of hypoparathyroidism associated with defective development of both the thymus and the parathyroid glands is termed the *DiGeorge syndrome*, or the *third and fourth branchial pouch syndrome*. Congenital cardiovascular and other developmental defects are present, and most patients die in early childhood with severe infections, hypocalcemia and seizures, or cardiovascular complications. Some survive into adulthood, and milder, incomplete forms occur. Most cases are sporadic, and cytogenetic abnormalities involving chromosome 22 are reported.

Hypoparathyroidism can occur in association with other diverse developmental defects or as part of a complex hereditary autoimmune syndrome involving failure of the adrenals, the ovaries, and the parathyroids in association with recurrent mucocutaneous candidiasis, alopecia, vitiligo, and pernicious anemia (see Chap. 340). In many cases, antibodies to endocrine organs are present; there is, in addition, a failure of cell-mediated immunity. The autoimmune disorder is inherited as an autosomal recessive trait, and some unaffected family members show antibodies to endocrine tissue without evidence of endocrine failure. The disorder is usually referred to as *autoimmune polyglandular deficiency*.

Hereditary hypoparathyroidism occurs also as an isolated entity without any other defects. The pattern of inheritance varies from one kindred to another, including autosomal dominant, autosomal recessive, and X-linked inheritance patterns. In one family in which the disorder was transmitted as an autosomal dominant trait, a structural abnormality in the PTH gene has been identified. The defect in the signal sequence needed for processing of the hormone before secretion impairs PTH secretion. In another kindred with autosomal recessive inheritance, the mutant allele in the first intron of the PTH gene causes a splicing defect in mRNA production. Gain-of-function mutations in the calcium sensor are the cause of autosomal dominant hypoparathyroidism in at least three families; the exaggerated responsiveness of the calcium sensor to calcium causes inappropriate suppression of PTH secretion. In most kindreds, however, the genetic basis of the hypoparathyroidism is not known.

Acquired Hypoparathyroidism *Acquired chronic hypoparathyroidism* is usually the result of inadvertent surgical removal of all the parathyroid glands; in some instances, not all the tissue is removed, but the remainder undergoes compromise of vascular supply secondary to fibrotic changes in the neck after surgery. In the past, the most frequent cause of acquired hypoparathyroidism was surgery for hyperthyroidism. Hypoparathyroidism now usually occurs after surgery for hyperparathyroidism when the surgeon, facing the dilemma of removing too little tissue and thus not curing the hyperparathyroidism, removes too much.

Parathyroid function may not be totally absent in all patients with postoperative hypoparathyroidism, but suitable therapy varies greatly from patient to patient irrespective of the type of hypoparathyroidism or the question of residual parathyroid activity.

Even rarer causes of acquired chronic hypoparathyroidism include radiation-induced damage subsequent to radioiodine therapy of hyperthyroidism and glandular damage in patients with hemochromatosis or hemosiderosis after repeated blood transfusions. Infection may involve one or more of the parathyroids but usually does not cause hypoparathyroidism because all four glands are rarely involved.

Transient hypoparathyroidism is frequent following surgery for hyperparathyroidism. After a variable period of hypoparathyroidism, normal parathyroid function may return due to hyperplasia or recovery of remaining tissue. Occasionally, recovery occurs months after surgery. The management of transient postoperative hypoparathyroidism is discussed under the surgical treatment of hyperparathyroidism. The treatment of chronic acquired hypoparathyroidism is similar to that of idiopathic hypoparathyroidism: replacement with calcitriol and oral calcium.

 TREATMENT

Treatment of acquired and hereditary hypoparathyroidism is similar to that for PHP, although specific features of each disease require specific treatments. Replacement therapy with vitamin D or calcitriol combined with a high oral calcium intake usually suffices to regulate blood calcium and phosphate levels satisfactorily. Oral calcium and vitamin D restore the overall calcium-phosphate balance but do not reverse the lowered urinary calcium reabsorption typical of hypoparathyroidism. Therefore, care must be taken to avoid excessive urinary calcium ex-

cretion after vitamin D and calcium replacement therapy; otherwise, kidney stones can develop. Thiazide diuretics lower urine calcium by as much as 100 mg/d in hypoparathyroid patients on vitamin D, provided they are maintained on a low-sodium diet. Use of thiazides seems to be of benefit in mitigating hypercalciuria.

Hypomagnesemia Severe hypomagnesemia is associated with severe hypocalcemia (see also Chap. 357). Restoration of the total-body magnesium deficit leads to rapid reversal of hypocalcemia. There are at least two causes of the hypocalcemia—impaired PTH secretion and reduced responsiveness to PTH.

Hypomagnesemia is generally classified as primary or secondary; primary hypomagnesemia is due to hereditary defects in intestinal absorption or renal reabsorption of magnesium. Secondary hypomagnesemia, a more common condition, occurs on a nutritional basis or as a result of acquired intestinal or renal disorders. The most common causes of the secondary disorder are chronic alcoholism with poor nutritional intake, intestinal malabsorption syndromes, and parenteral nutrition when magnesium replacement is omitted.

The effects of magnesium on PTH secretion are similar to those of calcium; hypermagnesemia suppresses and hypomagnesemia stimulates PTH secretion. The effects of magnesium on PTH secretion are normally of little significance, however, because the calcium effects dominate. Greater change in magnesium than in calcium is needed to influence hormone secretion. Nonetheless, hypomagnesemia might be expected to increase hormone secretion. It is therefore surprising to find that severe hypomagnesemia is associated with blunted secretion of PTH. The explanation for the paradox is that severe, chronic hypomagnesemia reflects intracellular magnesium deficiency, which interferes with secretion and peripheral responses to PTH. The mechanism of the cellular defects of hypomagnesemia is unknown, although a defective adenylate cyclase (for which magnesium may serve as a cofactor) has been proposed.

In most cases in which hypomagnesemia is associated with hypocalcemia, serum magnesium is below 0.4 mmol/L (1.0 mg/dL). PTH levels are usually undetectable or inappropriately low despite the stimulus of severe hypocalcemia, and acute repletion of magnesium leads to a rapid increase in PTH level. Since PTH secretion is blunted in virtually all patients with severe hypomagnesemia, absolute or relative hypoparathyroidism is present in most patients with hypocalcemia secondary to hypomagnesemia.

In addition, diminished peripheral responsiveness to administered PTH occurs in some patients, as manifested by subnormal response in urinary phosphorus and urinary cyclic AMP excretion after administration of exogenous PTH to patients who are hypocalcemic and hypomagnesemic. Both blunted PTH secretion and lack of renal response to administered PTH can occur in the same patient. When acute magnesium repletion is undertaken, the restoration of PTH levels to normal or supranormal may precede by several days restoration of normal serum calcium.

Blunted PTH secretory response in hypomagnesemia seems the main cause of hypocalcemia. The fact that impaired peripheral responsiveness, particularly renal response, is more variable from patient to patient suggests that an even greater degree of magnesium deficiency is required to induce end-organ resistance than to impair hormone secretion.

Several other features have been noted. The brisk increase in PTH secretion following magnesium repletion, sometimes demonstrable within minutes of giving parenteral magnesium, indicates that hormone biosynthesis is not impaired, only secretion. Serum phosphate levels are often not elevated, in contrast to the situation with acquired or idiopathic hypoparathyroidism, probably because phosphate deficiency is a frequent accompaniment of hypomagnesemia. Magnesium wasting may occur in chronic renal disease; magnesium may be elevated in acute renal failure but is usually normal in chronic renal failure.

 TREATMENT

Repletion of magnesium cures the condition, and attention must be given to restoring the intracellular deficiency, which may be considerable. After intravenous magnesium administration, serum magnesium may return transiently to the normal range, but unless replacement therapy is adequate serum magnesium will again fall. If renal function is normal, a useful indicator of restoration of magnesium deficiency is the urinary magnesium excretion; magnesium is retained by the kidney until magnesium deficiency is repleted. Intracellular deficits can be as great as 50 mmol or more. Parenteral administration of 10 to 14 mmol magnesium usually reverses the signs of magnesium deficiency. If the cause of the hypomagnesemia is renal magnesium wasting, magnesium may have to be given chronically to prevent recurrence.

PTH INEFFECTIVE   PTH is considered ineffective when the hormone receptor–guanyl nucleotide–binding protein complex is defective, when PTH action to promote calcium absorption from the diet is impaired because of vitamin D deficiency or because vitamin D is ineffective (receptor or synthesis defects), or in chronic renal failure in which the calcium-elevating action of PTH is impaired.

Despite diverse pathophysiologic mechanisms, these latter conditions involving ineffectiveness of PTH (excluding the rare condition of defective PTH-receptor response) often involve the unavailability of vitamin D as a cofactor for PTH. Hypocalcemia is usually mild and is accompanied by hypophosphatemia. Typically, hypophosphatemia is more severe than hypocalcemia because of the increased secretion of PTH, which is only partly effective in elevating blood calcium but is capable of promoting renal phosphate excretion in vitamin D deficiency, so that phosphaturia leads to hypophosphatemia. Varying degrees of bone disease with impaired mineralization and/or frank osteomalacia are the consequence of chronic renal failure and/ or impairment of vitamin D action by the hypophosphatemia.

PHP, on the other hand, has a pathophysiology different from the other disorders of ineffective PTH action. PHP resembles conditions in which PTH synthesis is deficient and is manifested by hypocalcemia and hyperphosphatemia. The cause of the disorder is defective hormone binding to the receptor or deficient activation of guanyl nucleotide–binding proteins, resulting in failure of PTH to increase intracellular cyclic AMP (see below).

Chronic Renal Failure   Severe abnormalities in mineral and bone metabolism occur in chronic renal failure, and improved medical management of chronic renal failure and/or a more indolent course of the renal disease allow many patients to survive long enough for renal osteodystrophy, the bone disease associated with renal failure, to become manifest. Phosphate retention and impaired production of $1,25(OH)_2D$ are the principal factors that cause calcium deficiency, secondary hyperparathyroidism, and bone disease. The uremic state also causes impairment of intestinal absorption by mechanisms other than defects in vitamin D metabolism. Nonetheless, treatment with supraphysiologic amounts of vitamin D or calcitriol corrects the calcium absorption.

Hyperphosphatemia in renal failure lowers blood calcium levels by several mechanisms, including extraosseous deposition of calcium and phosphate, impairment of the bone-resorbing action of PTH, reduction in $1,25(OH)_2D$ production by surviving renal tissue, and reduction in calcium absorption due to trapping of calcium in insoluble form as calcium phosphate complexes. In animals, prevention of hyperphosphatemia by dietary means can block the development of secondary hyperparathyroidism, emphasizing the importance of phosphate retention in the pathogenesis of secondary hyperparathyroidism and the associated disorders of mineral and bone metabolism in renal failure. Low levels of $1,25(OH)_2D$ are due to hyperphosphatemia and to destruction of renal tissue and are critical in the hypocalcemia.

℞ **TREATMENT**

Therapy of chronic renal failure (see Chaps. 271 and 272) involves appropriate management of patients prior to dialysis and adjustment of regimens once dialysis becomes necessary. Attention should be paid to restriction of phosphate in the diet; use of phosphate-binding antacids such as those based on aluminum hydroxide or calcium-containing salts, which avoid the problem of aluminum intoxication;

provision of an adequate calcium intake by mouth, usually 1 to 2 g/d; and supplementation with 0.25 to 1.0 μg/d calcitriol. Each patient must be monitored closely. The aim of therapy is to restore normal calcium balance to prevent osteomalacia and secondary hyperparathyroidism. Reduction of hyperphosphatemia and restoration of normal intestinal calcium absorption by calcitriol can improve blood calcium levels and reduce the manifestations of secondary hyperparathyroidism. Since adynamic bone disease can occur in association with low PTH levels, it is important to avoid excessive suppression of the parathyroid glands while recognizing the beneficial effects of controlling the secondary hyperparathyroidism.

Vitamin D Deficiency Due to Inadequate Diet and/or Sunlight
Vitamin D deficiency is more common in the United States than previously recognized. Biopsies of bone in elderly patients with hip fracture (documenting osteomalacia) and abnormal levels of vitamin D metabolites, PTH, calcium, and phosphate indicate that vitamin D deficiency may occur in as many as 25 percent of elderly patients, particularly in areas where there is little ambient sunlight. Concentrations of 25(OH)D are low or low normal in these patients. Quantitative histomorphometry of bone biopsy specimens reveals widened osteoid seams consistent with osteomalacia. PTH hypersecretion compensates for the tendency for the blood calcium to fall but also induces renal phosphate wasting and results in osteomalacia.

The genesis of vitamin D deficiency is inadequate intake of dairy products enriched with vitamin D, lack of vitamin supplementation, and reduced sunlight exposure in the elderly, particularly during winter in northern latitudes.

Treatment involves the administration of vitamin D and provision of 1 to 1.5 g calcium in the diet. Vitamin D supplementation should aim to provide several times the recommended daily requirement in younger people; a dosage of 1000 to 2000 units of vitamin D per day is satisfactory. Vitamin D is usually not available in small-dose forms. Hence the administration of a capsule containing 50,000 units of vitamin D once monthly is safe in elderly patients who have osteomalacia. The increased awareness of the importance of calcium supplementation, particularly in women, even without supplementation of vitamin D, may lessen the frequency of this problem. Severe hypocalcemia rarely occurs in moderately severe vitamin D deficiency of the elderly, but vitamin D deficiency must be considered in the differential diagnosis of mild hypocalcemia.

Defective Vitamin D Metabolism   *Anticonvulsant therapy* Anticonvulsant therapy with any of several agents induces acquired vitamin D deficiency by increasing the conversion of vitamin D to inactive compounds. The more marginal the vitamin D intake in the diet, the more likely that anticonvulsant therapy will lead to abnormal mineral and bone metabolism. Manifestations may include severe rickets with bone fractures, hypocalcemia, hypophosphatemia, and, on occasion, proximal myopathy. More often, hypocalcemia is minimal, and mild osteomalacia is the only sign. In other patients on long-term anticonvulsant therapy, no symptoms or signs are present, but bone density is low and responds to vitamin D supplementation.

Anticonvulsants stimulate the hepatic microsomal mixed-oxidase enzymes and hence increase the rate of clearance of vitamin D and its metabolites. Phenytoin also impairs intestinal calcium absorption independent of effects on vitamin D and has deleterious effects on bone cell function in vitro, including inhibition of collagen synthesis.

Although $1,25(OH)_2D$ levels are lower in patients treated with chronic anticonvulsants than in the normal population, there is a great deal of variation. The greater prevalence of the disorder in some European populations and in the mentally retarded probably reflects the lower vitamin D intake of those groups. Restoration of bone mineral mass and reversal of hypocalcemia can be accomplished with vitamin D replacement plus oral calcium. Adjustments in dose are indicated depending on the age and size of the patient, but approximately 50,000 units of vitamin D weekly plus 1 g elemental calcium per day for several months is usually sufficient. Alternatively, administration of administration of 50,000 units of vitamin D monthly may be preventive if anticonvulsant therapy is given chronically.

Vitamin D–dependent rickets type I Rickets can be due to *resistance to the action* of vitamin D as well as to vitamin D deficiency. Vitamin D–dependent rickets type I, previously termed *pseudo-vitamin D–dependent rickets*, differs from vitamin D–resistant rickets in that it is less severe and the biochemical and radiographic abnormalities can be reversed with large doses of the vitamin.

Clinical features include hypocalcemia, often with tetany or convulsions, hypophosphatemia, secondary hyperparathyroidism, and osteomalacia, often associated with skeletal deformities and increased alkaline phosphatase. Doses of vitamin D or calcifediol, 100 to 1000 times above the usual amounts, are required to heal the bone disease, whereas physiologic amounts of calcitriol cure the disease. This finding fits with the pathophysiology. The disorder is due to an autosomal recessive defect in conversion of 25(OH)D to 1,25(OH)$_2$D. Plasma levels of 1,25(OH)$_2$D are low or undetectable even after administration of large doses of vitamin D or calcifediol. Response to high doses of vitamin D or calcifediol is probably due to direct effects of 25(OH)D at high levels. Treatment requires careful adjustment of calcitriol dose, particularly during growth periods.

Vitamin D Ineffective *Intestinal malabsorption* Mild hypocalcemia, secondary hyperparathyroidism, severe hypophosphatemia, and a variety of nutritional deficiencies occur with gastrointestinal diseases. Hepatocellular dysfunction can lead to reduction in 25(OH)D levels, as in portal or biliary cirrhosis of the liver, and malabsorption of vitamin D and its metabolites, including 1,25(OH)$_2$D, may occur in a variety of bowel diseases, hereditary or acquired. Hypocalcemia itself can lead to steatorrhea, due to deficient production of pancreatic enzymes and bile salts. Depending on the disorder, vitamin D or its metabolites can be given parenterally, guaranteeing adequate blood levels of active metabolites.

Vitamin D–dependent rickets type II Pseudo-vitamin D–dependent rickets can be due to defective response to 1,25(OH)$_2$D. This disorder, vitamin D–dependent rickets type II, results from any of several types of end-organ resistance to the active metabolite, including absence or qualitative defects of the intracellular vitamin D receptor and postreceptor blocks in hormone action (see Chap. 327). The clinical features resemble those of the type I disorder and include hypocalcemia, hypophosphatemia, secondary hyperparathryoidism, and rickets. Plasma levels of 1,25(OH)$_2$D are at least three times normal, in keeping with the refractoriness of the end organs. Alopecia totalis may be severe early in life. Patients require much higher doses of vitamin D or vitamin D metabolites than with the type I disorder.

Pseudohypoparathyroidism PHP is a hereditary disorder characterized by symptoms and signs of hypoparathyroidism, typically in association with distinctive skeletal and developmental defects. The hypoparathyroidism is due to a deficient end-organ response to PTH. Hyperplasia of the parathyroids, a response to the resistance to hormone action, causes elevation of PTH levels. Studies, both clinical and basic, have clarified some aspects of this syndrome, including the variable spectrum of the clinical features, the pathophysiology, the genetic defects, and the inheritance.

Most patients show a characteristic phenotype termed *Albright's hereditary osteodystrophy* (AHO), consisting of short stature, round face, skeletal anomalies (brachydactyly), and heterotopic calcification. Patients have low calcium and high phosphate levels, as with true hypoparathyroidism. PTH levels, however, are elevated, and resistance to hormone action can be demonstrated by defective urinary cyclic AMP response to

PTH administration. The disorder is usually familial; some kindreds do not show the AHO phenotype but only abnormal mineral metabolism. A few patients are resistant to PTH but have normal urinary cyclic AMP response (responses in calcium and phosphate seemingly blocked after the adenyl cyclase step).

At least part of the defect in most patients (those with the AHO phenotype) is due to inheritance of one defective allele that encodes the α subunit of the guanyl nucleotide–binding protein (G$_{sα}$). This defect causes a diminished response to PTH (approximately 50 percent of normal, consistent with one defective allele). However, in some kindreds individuals with a distinctive AHO phenotype who, while unaffected with symptoms or signs of defective mineral metabolism, still have a demonstrable 50 percent reduction in assays of G$_{sα}$ subunits (so-called pseudopseudohypoparathyroidism). Hence the defective guanyl nucleotide subunit is not itself sufficient to explain the pathophysiology. Perhaps another independently inherited allelic defect so far undetected is needed to provide full expression of the disordered mineral metabolism.

Since the defective G$_{sα}$ subunit function was recognized, attention has focused on the molecular mechanism of the defective guanyl nucleotide–binding protein function. The gene encoding this subunit has been cloned (chromosome 20); multiple defects have now been identified, including abnormalities in splice junctions associated with deficient mRNA production and point mutations that result in a protein unit with defective function. The view that the disease is an X-linked disorder has given way, with a combination of careful family and molecular genetic studies, to recognition that the subset with hereditary osteodystrophy is due to an autosomal dominant mode of inheritance (chromosome 20). The inheritance of the variant disorder in which individuals do not have hereditary osteodystrophy is not understood.

A working classification of the various forms of PHP is given in Table 354-5. The classification scheme is based on the signs of ineffective PTH action (low calcium and high phosphate), urinary cyclic AMP response to exogenous PTH, the presence or absence of AHO, and assays of the concentration of the G$_{sα}$ subunit of the adenylate cyclase enzyme. Using these criteria, there are four types: PHP type I, subdivided into a and b categories; PHP-II; and pseudopseudohypoparathyroidism (PPHP). Individuals with PHP-I, the most common of the disorders, show a deficient response in urinary cyclic AMP to administration of exogenous PTH. PHP-II refers to patients with hypocalcemia and hyperphosphatemia who have a normal urinary cyclic AMP response to PTH. These patients are assumed to have a defect in the response to PTH at a lcous beyond that of cyclic AMP production, although at least some patients may instead have occult vitamin D deficiency. It is disputed whether PHP-II is a discrete phenotypic and genotypic entity because vitamin D deficiency and an associated hypocalcemia can cause an enhanced cyclic AMP response yet a blunted phosphatemic response to administered PTH (the hallmark of PHP-II). Patients with PHP-I are divided into type a, who have reduced amounts of G$_{sα}$ in in vitro assays, and type b, with normal amounts of G$_{sα}$ in erythrocytes. Subjects with PHP-Ia have shortened metacarpals and metatarsals and the other features of AHO and commonly show resistance to hormones in addition to PTH. Patients with PHP-Ib have a normal phenotype without the AHO syndrome. Fibroblasts cultured from the skin of some patients with PHP-Ib show a much reduced response of cyclic AMP accumulation to PTH, consistent with the presence of a defective receptor. A subset of these patients,

Table 354-5

Classification of Pseudohypoparathyroidism (PHP) and Pseudopseudohypoparathyroidism (PPHP)

Type	Hypocalcemia, Hyperphosphatemia	Response of Urinary cAMP to PTH	Serum PTH	G$_{sα}$ Subunit Deficiency	AHO	Resistance to Hormones in Addition to PTH
PHP-Ia	Yes	↓	↑	Yes	Yes	Yes
PHP-Ib	Yes	↓	↑	No	No	No
PHP-II	Yes	Normal	↑	No	No	No
PPHP	No	Normal	Normal	Yes	Yes	±

NOTE: ↓, decreased; ↑, increased; AHO, Albright's hereditary osteodystrophy.

however, has a normal response to cyclic AMP production fibroblasts in vitro, and no structural defects in the PTH receptor have been identified in these patients to date.

Patients with PHHP have typical features of the hereditary osteodystrophy syndrome despite normal serum calcium levels and normal response of urinary cyclic AMP to exogenous PTH. These individuals are usually first-degree relatives of patients with PHP-Ia, and patients initially classified as having PHHP occasionally develop mild hypocalcemia. Patients with PPHP on average have levels of $G_{s\alpha}$ subunits that are half normal, suggesting that PPHP is a mild variant of PHP-Ia.

The mineral deposits in ectopic sites may include true bone, whereas bone formation never occurs in ectopic sites in idiopathic hypoparathyroidism. Amorphous deposits of calcium and phosphate are found in the basal ganglia in about half of patients. The defects in metacarpal and metatarsal bones are sometimes accompanied by short phalanges as well, possibly reflecting premature closing of the epiphyses. The typical findings are short fourth and fifth metacarpals and metatarsals. The defects are usually bilateral. Exostoses and radius curvus are frequent. Impairments in olfaction and taste and unusual dermatoglyphic abnormalities have been reported. There is little improvement in mental status even after adequate therapy with calcium and vitamin D.

The diagnosis can usually be made without difficulty. Positive family history for developmental defects and/or the presence of developmental defects characteristic of PHP-Ia, including brachydactyly, in association with the signs of hypoparathyroidism, low calcium, and high phosphate, make the diagnosis likely on clinical grounds. However, patients with PHP-Ib or PHP-II do not have phenotypic abnormalities but have hypocalcemia with high PTH levels. In PHP-Ib, the response of urinary cyclic AMP to the administration of exogenous PTH is blunted; such tests are useful to confirm the diagnosis even in PHP-Ia. Low levels of $G_{s\alpha}$ subunits in erythrocyte membranes can also distinguish patients with PHP-Ia from those with PHP-Ib. In both categories serum PTH levels are elevated, particularly in hypocalcemic patients. The diagnosis of PHP-II is more complex, in that cyclic AMP responses in urine are, by definition, normal. Since vitamin D deficiency itself can result in dissociation between phosphaturic and urinary cyclic AMP responses to exogenous PTH, vitamin D deficiency must be excluded before diagnosis of PHP-II can be made.

℞ TREATMENT

Treatment of PHP is similar to that of hypoparathyroidism, except that the doses of vitamin D and calcium are usually lower than those required in true hypoparathyroidism, presumably because the defect in PHP is only partial (a 50 percent reduction in $G_{s\alpha}$). Variability in response makes it necessary to establish the optimal regimen for each patient, based on maintaining the appropriate blood calcium level and urinary calcium excretion.

PTH Overwhelmed Occasionally, loss of calcium from the extracellular fluid is so severe that PTH cannot compensate. Such situations include acute pancreatitis and severe, acute hyperphosphatemia, often in association with renal failure, conditions in which there is rapid efflux of calcium from extracellular fluid. Severe hypocalcemia can occur quickly; PTH rises in response to hypocalcemia but does not return blood calcium to normal. The chance of hypocalcemia is enhanced when renal failure is present.

Severe, Acute Hyperphosphatemia Severe hyperphosphatemia is associated with extensive tissue damage or cell destruction (see Chap. 356). The combination of increased release of phosphate from muscle and impaired ability to excrete phosphorus because of renal failure causes moderate to severe hyperphosphatemia, the latter causing calcium loss from the blood and mild to moderate hypocalcemia. Hypocalcemia is usually reversed with tissue repair and restoration of renal function as phosphorus and creatinine values return to normal. There may even be a mild hypercalcemic period in the oliguric phase of recovery of renal function. This sequence, severe hypocalcemia followed by mild hypercalcemia, reflects widespread deposition of

calcium in muscle and subsequent redistribution of some of the calcium to the extracellular fluid after return of phosphate levels to normal.

Other causes of hyperphosphatemia include hypothermia, massive hepatic failure, and hematologic malignancies, either because of high cell turnover of malignancy or because of cell destruction with chemotherapy.

℞ TREATMENT

Treatment is directed toward lowering of blood phosphate by the administration of phosphate-binding antacids or dialysis, often needed for the management of renal failure. Although calcium replacement may be necessary if hypocalcemia is severe and symptomatic, calcium administration during the hyperphosphatemic period tends to increase extraosseous calcium deposition and aggravate tissue damage. Although the levels of $1,25(OH)_2D$ may be low during the hyperphosphatemic phase and return to normal during the oliguric phase of recovery, mineral ion imbalance per se seems to be the principal pathophysiologic mechanism.

Osteitis Fibrosis after Parathyroidectomy Severe hypocalcemia after parathyroid surgery is less common now that osteitis fibrosa cystica is an infrequent manifestation of hyperparathyroidism. When osteitis fibrosa cystica is severe, however, bone mineral deficits can be large, and after parathyroidectomy hypocalcemia can persist for days if calcium replacement is inadequate. The mechanism of the hypocalcemia is complex. Increased cellularity of bone in osteitis fibrosa cystica involves both osteoblasts and osteoclasts, but high levels of PTH enhance resorption more than formation; an abrupt decrease in PTH levels with surgery leaves bone formation favored over resorption. Calcium loss from blood is increased, and temporary hyporesponsiveness of bone to the bone-resorbing actions of PTH (lowered hormone levels after parathyroid surgery in the presence of receptor down-regulation) may add to the imbalance between bone resorption and bone formation. Treatment may require parenteral administration of calcium; addition of calcitriol and oral calcium supplementation make it possible to discontinue parenteral calcium and/ or reduce the amount.

DIFFERENTIAL DIAGNOSIS Care must be taken to ensure that true hypocalcemia is present; in addition, acute transient hypocalcemia can be a manifestation of a variety of severe, acute illnesses, as discussed above. *Chronic hypocalcemia*, however, can usually be ascribed to a few disorders associated with absent or ineffective PTH. Important clinical criteria include the duration of the illness, signs or symptoms of associated disorders, and the presence of features that suggest a hereditary abnormality. A nutritional history can be helpful in recognizing a low intake of vitamin D and calcium in the elderly, and a history of excessive alcohol intake can be the clue to magnesium deficiency.

Hypoparathyroidism and PHP are typically lifelong illnesses; hence a recent onset of hypocalcemia in an adult is usually due to nutritional deficiencies, renal failure, or intestinal disorders that result in deficient or ineffective vitamin D. A history of seizure disorder raises the issue of anticonvulsive medication. Neck surgery, even long past, can be associated with a delayed onset of postoperative hypoparathyroidism. Developmental defects, particularly in childhood and adolescence, may point to the diagnosis of PHP. Rickets and a variety of neuromuscular syndromes and deformities may indicate ineffective vitamin D action, either due to defects in vitamin D metabolism or to vitamin D deficiency.

A pattern of *low calcium with high phosphorus* in the absence of renal failure or massive tissue destruction almost invariably means hypoparathyroidism or PHP. A *low calcium and low phosphorus* points to absent or ineffective vitamin D, thereby impairing the action of PTH on calcium metabolism. The relative ineffectiveness of PTH in vitamin D deficiency, anticonvulsant therapy, gastrointestinal disorders, and hereditary defects in vitamin D metabolism leads to secondary hyperparathyroidism as a compensation. The relatively unopposed action of the excess PTH on renal tubule phosphate transport, which is less dependent on vitamin D than calcium transport, accounts for renal phosphate wasting and hypophosphatemia.

Exceptions to these patterns may occur. Most forms of hypomagnesemia are due to long-standing nutritional deficiency, and despite the fact that the hypocalcemia is due principally to an acute absence of PTH, phosphate levels are usually low rather than elevated as in hypoparathyroidism. Chronic renal failure is often associated with hypocalcemia and hyperphosphatemia, despite secondary hyperparathyroidism.

Diagnosis is usually established by application of the PTH radioimmunoassay, tests for vitamin D metabolites, and measurements of the urinary cyclic AMP response to exogenous PTH. In hereditary and acquired hypoparathyroidism and in severe hypomagnesemia, PTH is either undetectable or in the normal range, and this finding in a hypocalcemic patient is supportive of hypoparathyroidism, as distinct from ineffective PTH action, in which even mild hypocalcemia is associated with elevated PTH levels. Hence a failure to detect elevated PTH levels establishes the diagnosis of hypoparathyroidism; elevated levels suggest the presence of secondary hyperparathyroidism, as found in many of the situations in which the hormone is ineffective due to associated abnormalities in vitamin D action. Assays for 25(OH)D and 1,25(OH)$_2$D can be helpful. Low or low normal 25(OH)D indicates vitamin D deficiency due to lack of sunlight, inadequate vitamin D intake, or intestinal malabsorption. A low level of 1,25(OH)$_2$D in the presence of elevated concentrations of PTH suggests ineffective PTH action; include the causes chronic renal failure, severe vitamin D deficiency, vitamin D–dependent rickets type I, and PHP. Recognition that mild hypocalcemia, rickets, and hypophosphatemia are due to anticonvulsant therapy is made by history.

℞ TREATMENT

Hypocalcemic States The management of hypoparathyroidism, PHP, chronic renal failure, and hereditary defects in vitamin D metabolism involves the use of vitamin D or vitamin D metabolites and calcium supplementation. Vitamin D itself is the least expensive form of vitamin D replacement and is frequently used in the management of uncomplicated hypoparathyroidism and disorders associated with ineffective vitamin D action. When vitamin D is used prophylactically, as in the elderly or in those with chronic anticonvulsant therapy, there is a wider margin of safety than with the more potent metabolites. However, most of the conditions in which vitamin D is administered chronically for hypocalcemia require amounts 50 to 100 times the daily replacement dose because the formation of 1,25(OH)$_2$D is deficient. In such situations, vitamin D is no safer than the active metabolite because intoxication can occur with high-dose therapy. Calcitriol is more rapid in onset of action and also has a short biologic half-life; in high doses, vitamin D is stored in body tissues and is cleared slowly.

From 1 to 5 μg/d of vitamin D or calcifediol and lower doses of calcitriol (0.25 to 1.0 μg/d) are required to prevent rickets in normal subjects. In contrast, 500 to 3000 μg of vitamin D$_2$ or D$_3$ is typically required in hypoparathyroidism; doses of calcifediol are also high (several hundred micrograms per day). The dose of calcitriol is unchanged in hypoparathyroidism, since the defect is in hydroxylation by the 1α-hydroxylase.

The greater therapeutic efficacy of calcifediol than vitamin D$_3$ when the metabolism of the vitamin is impaired may be due to superior metabolic availability for the renal 1α-hydroxylase or to direct action directly by 25(OH)D at receptors in target tissues. Vitamin D is metabolized to a variety of compounds other than the principal product, 25(OH)D. Calcifediol bypasses these alternative pathways and is directly available for metabolism to 1,25(OH)$_2$D. In hypoparathyroidism and in hereditary defects in renal 1α-hydroxylase, the formation of 1,25(OH)$_2$D from 25(OH)D is impaired, but

some formation occurs at high substrate levels. Calcifediol has about 1 percent of the potency of calcitriol in vivo and in vitro.

Unless a loading dose is given, 2 to 4 weeks or even longer are required to achieve the maximum calcium replacement action of vitamin D or calcifediol; the onset of action of calcifediol is more rapid. Calcitriol can be given for hypoparathyroidism at the same dose required for the prevention of rickets in euparathyroid individuals, 0.2 to 1.0 μg/d. Its onset of action is days rather than weeks. When vitamin D or calcifediol is withdrawn, weeks are required for the disappearance of the biologic effects, compared with a few days for calcitriol.

Patients with hypoparathyroidism should be given 2 to 3 g elemental calcium by mouth each day. The two agents, vitamin D (or vitamin D metabolites) and oral calcium, can be varied independently. Higher doses of vitamin D or its metabolites increase the efficiency of intestinal calcium absorption; higher intakes of oral calcium permit adequate calcium assimilation despite a lower efficiency of intestinal calcium absorption. When hypercalcemia occurs during the treatment of chronic hypocalcemia, discontinuation of the calcium lowers calcium within 24 h, even more rapidly than withdrawal of calcitriol. Most patients with hypoparathyroidism can be managed with high-dose vitamin D therapy and 2 to 3 g oral calcium per day. If hypocalcemia alternates with episodes of hypercalcemia, administration of calcitriol often makes management easier.

The administration of thiazide diuretics in the usual antihypertensive doses and sodium restriction in patients with hypoparathyroidism lowers urinary calcium excretion and makes it possible to reduce the doses of calcium and vitamin D. Patients have a lower urinary calcium excretion at any given level of blood calcium on thiazides. Thiazides also may protect against the development of kidney stones, a potential complication of the management of hypoparathyroidism. If on dialysis, patients with chronic renal failure and hypocalcemia can have adjustments in dialysate calcium concentrations as an alternative to vitamin D and calcium supplementation. The doses of vitamin D and calcium required for the management of PHP are usually lower than those required for hypoparathyroidism, reflecting incomplete resistance to the action of PTH in PHP. The acute treatment of hypomagnesemia is discussed above.

BIBLIOGRAPHY

AHN TG et al: Familial isolated hypoparathyroidism: A molecular genetic analysis of 8 families with 23 affected persons. Medicine 65:73, 1986

ARNOLD A et al: Monoclonality of parathyroid tumors in chronic renal failure and in primary parathyroid hyperplasia. J Clin Invest 95:2047, 1995

BENSON L et al: Hyperparathyroidism presenting as the first lesion in multiple endocrine neoplasia type 1. Am J Med 82:731, 1987

BROWN EM et al: The cloning of extracellular Ca^{2+}-sensing receptors from parathyroid and kidney: Molecular mechanisms of extracellular Ca^{2+}-sensing. J Nutr 125:1965S, 1995

CHOU Y-H W et al: Mutations in the human Ca^{2+}-sensing-receptor gene that cause hypocalciuric hypercalcemia. Am J Hum Genet 56:1075, 1995

CONKLIN BR, BOURNE HR: Marriage of the flytrap and the serpent. Nature 367:22, 1994

CRYNS VL et al: Frequent loss of chromosome arm Ip DNA in parathyroid adenomas. Genes Chromosom Cancer 13:9, 1995

DIRKS JH: The kidney and magnesium regulation. Kidney Int 23:771, 1983

FIBISON WJ et al: Molecular studies of DiGeorge syndrome. Am J Hum Genet 46:888, 1990

FITCH N: The identification and inheritance of Albright's hereditary osteodystrophy. Am J Med Genet 11:11, 1982

FITZPATRICK LA, ARNOLD A: Hypoparathyroidism in *Endocrinology*, L DeGroot et al (eds). Philadelphia, Saunders, 1995, p 1123

FLEISCH H: Bisphosphonates: Pharmacology and use in the treatment of tumor-induced hypercalcemia and metastatic bone disease. Drugs 42:919, 1991

FRIEDMAN E et al: Clonality of parathyroid tumors in familial multiple endocrine neoplasia type 1. N Engl J Med 321:213, 1989

FUKAGAWA M et al: Suppression of parathyroid gland hyperplasia by 1,25(OH)$_2$D$_3$ pulse therapy. N Engl J Med 315:421, 1990

GRILL V et al: PTH-related protein: Elevated levels in both humoral hypercalcemia of malignancy and hypercalcemia complicating metastatic breast cancer. J Clin Endocrinol 73:1309, 1991

GUISE TA, MUNDY GR: Breast cancer and bone. Curr Opin Endocrinol Diab 2:548, 1995

HABENER J et al: Hyperparathyroidism, in *Endocrinology*, L DeGroot et al (eds). Philadelphia, Saunders, 1995, p 1044

HINDIE E et al: Primary hyperparathyroidism: Is technetium-99m–sestamibi/iodine-123 subtraction scanning the best procedure to locate enlarged glands before surgery? J Clin Endocrinol Metab 80:302, 1994

HOWE JR et al: Prevalence of pheochromocytoma and hyperparathyroidism in multiple endocrine neoplasia type 2A: Results of long-term follow-up. Surgery 114:1070, 1993

JAMESON JL, ARNOLD A: Recombinant DNA strategies for determining the molecular basis of endocrine disorders. J Endocrinol Metab 70:301, 1990

KRUSE K, SCHÜTZ C: Calcium metabolism in the Jansen type of metaphyseal dysplasia. Eur J Pediatr 152:912, 1993

LEDGER GA et al: Genetic testing in the diagnosis and management of multiple endocrine neoplasia type II. Ann Intern Med 122:118, 1995

LEVINE MA, SPIEGEL AM: Pseudohypoparathyroidism, in *Endocrinology*, L DeGroot et al (eds). Philadelphia, Saunders, 1995, p 1136

LIPS CJM et al: Clinical screening as compared with DNA analysis in families with multiple endocrine neoplasia type 2A. N Engl J Med 331:828, 1994

MALLETTE LE, EICHORN E: Effects of lithium carbonate on human calcium metabolism. Arch Intern Med 146:770, 1986

MARCUS R: Editorial: Bones of contention: The problem of mild hyperparathyroidism. J Clin Endocrinol Metab 80:720, 1995

MARX SJ: Familial hypocalciuric hypercalcemia, in *Primer on the Metabolic Bone Diseases and Disorders of Mineral Metabolism*, MJ Favus (ed). Richmond, VA, William Byrd Press, 1990, p 113

MAYNARD FM: Immobilization hypercalcemia following spinal cord injury. Arch Phys Med Rehabil 67:41, 1986

MITCHELL BK et al: Primary hyperparathyroidism: Preoperative localization using technetium-sestamibi scanning. J Clin Endocrinol Metab 80:7, 1995

MOTOKURA T et al: Cloning and characterization of human cyclin D3, a cDNA closely related in sequence to the PRAD1/cyclin D1 proto-oncogene. J Biol Chem 267:20412, 1992

MUDDE AH et al: Ectopic product of 1,25-dihydroxyvitamin D by B-cell lymphoma as a cause of hypercalcemia. Cancer 59:1543, 1987

NEMETH EF, HEATH H III: The calcium receptor and familial benign hypocalciuric hypercalcemia. Curr Opin Endocrinol Diab 2:556, 1995

NEUFELD M et al: Autoimmune polyglandular syndromes. Pediatr Ann 9:43, 1980

NUSSBAUM SR, POTTS JT JR: Immunoassays for parathyroid hormone 1-84 in the diagnosis of hyperparathyroidism. J Bone Miner Res 6 (Suppl 2):S43, 1991

——— et al: Medical management of hyperparathyroidism and hypercalcemia, in *Endocrinology*, DeGroot L et al (eds). Philadelphia, Saunders, 1995, p 1094

O'RIORDAN DS et al: Surgical management of primary hyperparathyroidism in multiple endocrine neoplasia types 1 and 2. Surgery 114:1031, 1993

ORWOLL ES: The milk-alkali syndrome: Current concepts. Ann Intern Med 97:242, 1982

PARFITT AM et al: Asymptomatic primary hyperparathyroidism discovered by multichannel biochemical screening: Clinical course and considerations bearing on the need for surgical intervention. J Bone Miner Res 6 (Suppl 2):S97, 1991

PARKINSON DB, THAKKER RV: A donor splice site mutation in the parathyroid hormone gene is associated with autosomal recessive hypoparathyroidism. Nature Genet 1:149, 1992

PATTEN JL: Mutation in the gene encoding the stimulatory G protein of adenylyl cyclase in Albright's hereditary osteodystrophy. N Engl J Med 322:1412, 1990

POLLAK MR et al: Mutations in the human Ca^{2+}-sensing receptor gene cause familial hypocalciuric hypercalcemia and neonatal severe hyperparathyroidism. Cell 75:1297, 1993

POTTS JT JR et al (eds): Proceedings of the NIH Consensus Development Conference on Diagnosis and Management of Asymptomatic Primary Hyperparathyroidism. J Bone Miner Res 6 (Suppl 2):S1, 1991

RALSTON SH et al: Cancer-associated hypercalcemia: Morbidity and mortality. Ann Intern Med 12:499, 1990

RATCLIFFE WA et al: Immunoreactivity of plasma parathyrin-related peptide. Clin Chem 37:1781, 1991

ROSENBERG CL et al: Coding sequence of the overexpressed transcript of the putative oncogene PRAD1/cyclin D1 in two primary human tumors. Oncogene 8:519, 1993

SALUSKY IB et al: The renal osteodystrophies, in *Endocrinology*, L DeGroot et al (eds). Philadelphia, Saunders, 1995, p 1151

SCHIPANI E et al: A constitutively active mutant PTH-PTHrP receptor in Jansen-type metaphyseal chondrodysplasia. Science 268:98, 1995

SEGRE GV, POTTS JT JR: Differential diagnosis of hypercalcemia, in *Endocrinology*, DeGroot L et al (eds). Philadelphia, Saunders, 1995, p 1075

SILVERBERG SJ et al: Longitudinal measurements of bone density and biochemical indices in untreated primary hyperparathyroidism. J Clin Endocrinol Metab 80:723, 1995

——— et al: Increased bone mineral density after parathyroidectomy in primary hyperparathyroidism. J Clin Endocrinol Metab 80:729, 1995

STEFENELLI T et al: Primary hyperparathyroidism: Incidence of cardiac abnormalities and partial reversibiity after successful parathyroidectomy. Am J Med 95:197, 1993

STEWART AF et al: Malignancy-associated hypercalcemia, in *Endocrinology*, DeGroot L et al (eds). Philadelphia, Saunders, 1995, p 1061

STUCKEY BGA et al: Fasting calcium excretion and parathyroid hormone together distinguish familial hypocalciuric hypercalcaemia from primary hyperparathyroidism. Clin Endocrinol 27:525, 1987

THAKKER RV et al: Association of parathyroid tumors in multiple endocrine neoplasia type 1 with loss of alleles on chromosome 11. N Engl J Med 321:218, 1989

——— et al: Mapping the gene causing X-linked recessive idiopathic hypoparathyroidism to Xq26–Xq27 by linkage studies. J Clin Invest 86:40, 1990

WARRELL RP et al: A randomized double-blind study of gallium nitrate compared with etidronate for acute control of cancer related hypercalcemia. J Clin Oncol 9:1467, 1991

WILSON DI et al: A prospective cytogenetic study of 36 cases of DiGeorge syndrome. Am J Hum Genet 51:957, 1992

 Stephen M. Krane, Michael F. Holick

355 METABOLIC BONE DISEASE

OSTEOPOROSIS

GENERAL CONSIDERATIONS *Osteoporosis* is the term used for diseases that cause a reduction in the mass of bone per unit volume. It is used to define any degree of skeletal fragility sufficient to increase the risk of fracture. The reduction in mass results from an imbalance in the processes that influence the acquisition and maintenance of skeletal mass and is not accompanied by a change in the ratio of the mineral phase to the organic phase or by any abnormality in bone mineral or organic matrix. Histologically, the disorder is characterized by a decrease in cortical thickness and in the number and size of the trabeculae of cancellous bone. Individual trabecular plates are abnormally perforated and may be fractured, and trabecular connectivity is reduced. The osteoid seams, however, are of normal width. Osteoporosis, the most common of the metabolic bone diseases (disorders in which all the skeleton is involved), is an important cause of morbidity in the elderly.

The remodeling of bone (its formation and resorption) is a continuous process. Since the bone mass is decreased in osteoporosis, the affected individual either failed to attain optimal skeletal mass during the first 3 decades of life, and/or the rate of bone resorption exceeded that of bone formation after peak skeletal mass was attained. Bone formation is higher in cortical than in cancellous bone. This difference is exaggerated by the normal menopause and exaggerated further in patients with osteoporosis, because rates of formation of cancellous bone tend to be lower in patients with osteoporosis, particularly in women after the menopause. The fact that about a third of postmenopausal women have high skeletal turnover, as assessed by histomorphometry, retention of bone-seeking markers such as ^{99m}Tc-methylene diphosphonate, and biochemical markers, could reflect the greater relative contribution of cortical remodeling in these women. After closure of epiphyses and cessation of longitudinal growth, there is a period of consolidation with a decrease in cortical porosity. When peak adult bone mass is reached at about age 30 to 35 for cortical bone and probably earlier for trabecular bone, rates of bone formation and resorption are relatively low (compared with the period of growth spurt) and approximately equal. The normal balance between bone formation and bone resorption maintains skeletal mass. The rates of remodeling differ, however, not only between cortical and trabecular bone but also in individual bones or portions of bones. Most of the bone surfaces are "inactive" and not involved at any given time either in formation or resorption. Active surfaces may be distributed randomly, but formation and resorption are locally coupled as units. Resorption areas are covered by osteoclasts if active; bone formation surfaces are characterized by the presence of osteoid seams and are covered by active osteoblasts. Resorption precedes formation and is probably more intense, but it does not last as long as formation. As a consequence, there are more sites of active formation than of resorption. Bone turnover is high when many units are active and low when few are active. Unless formation compensates for resorption, bone mass decreases. After age 40 to 50, cortical bone is lost at a rate of about 0.3 to 0.5 percent per year in both sexes. Around the menopause in women, an accelerated loss of cortical bone is superimposed on the age-related loss. Loss of trabecular bone begins at an earlier age in both sexes but is probably greater in women. The cumulative losses of bone mass range from 20 to 30 percent in men and 40 to 50 percent in some women. Bone loss involves predominantly trabecular bone in the spine and distal radius in women and the spine and hip in both women and men. The fact that loss is not uniform has been documented with techniques such as single- and dual-photon absorptiometry, quantitative computed tomography, dual-energy x-ray densitometry (DEXA), and neutron activation analysis of total-body calcium. For example, the rate of loss is greater in the metacarpals, the femoral neck, and the vertebral bodies than in the midshaft of the femur, the tibia, and the skull.

Remodeling activity is increased in most women with postmenopausal osteoporosis as compared with age-matched controls. These differences are even more marked when the comparison is with healthy premenopausal women in whom rates of remodeling are lower than in healthy postmenopausal women. Even in those individuals with increased bone resorption, however, bone formation does not compensate. At some critical point if the difference between rates of formation and resorption is maintained, loss of bone substance may become so marked that the bone can no longer resist the normal mechanical forces to which it is subjected, and fracture results. The template for formation of new bone is lost, and loss of bone accelerates as bone resorption continues and is even more uncoupled from formation. Osteoporosis may only be recognized as a clinical problem when fractures occur. Although the level of reduction in bone mass required to cause fractures after minimal trauma varies, the bone mineral density as measured by DEXA is an excellent predictor of fracture risk. The strength of bones such as vertebrae depends on "quality" (e.g., trabecular connectivity and arrangement) and on mineral density. For example, the horizontal trabeculae of the cancellous bone of vertebrae are preferentially lost in osteoporosis. Additional factors that influence the susceptibility to fracture include the adequacy of ligamentous support and age-related changes in the intervertebral disks. Microfractures are frequent. Age- or drug-related impairments of vision, hearing, and other neurologic and intellectual functions are additional contributors to the occurrence of fractures.

In the remodeling of lamellar bone in adults, most of the net resorption occurs at the corticoendosteal surface. The abnormal remodeling in osteoporosis follows the same pattern; the loss of cancellous bone, cortical bone at the endosteal surface, and intracortical bone results in enlargement of the medullary cavity and thinning of the cortex. Since bone formation at the periosteum continues at a slow rate, the diameter of the bone does not decrease, and the periosteal surface remains smooth. The cancellous bone also undergoes progressive resorption, some trabeculae being resorbed faster than others, particularly horizontal vertebral trabeculae.

The age-related loss of bone begins earlier and proceeds more rapidly in women and tends to accelerate before the menopause. All the factors responsible for bone loss with age are not known, although some risk factors have been identified. In general, white women have a greater risk than black women, and white men have a greater risk than black men. One explanation for these ethnic differences is that the bone mass at skeletal maturity is one determinant of the bone mass at subsequent ages. The lower incidence of osteoporosis and hip fracture in black men and women has been attributed to a higher bone mineral content in blacks than in whites, despite the fact that bone formation is lower in blacks. Since formation and resorption are usually coupled and since bone mass is increased, bone resorption (and turnover) also must be reduced. Osteoporotic subjects are frequently less muscular and have lower average body weight, and exercise may have a beneficial effect in maintaining bone mass. Patients who are kept at complete bed rest and astronauts in microgravity can lose approximately 1 percent of the bone mass each month. The facts that accelerated bone loss accompanies the menopause in some women and that premature osteoporosis occurs after premature surgical menopause suggest that estrogens play a major role in preventing bone loss. Osteoporotic women also have a higher incidence of cigarette smoking, which might affect bone remodeling directly or have secondary effects on ovarian function. Excessive alcohol consumption can decrease bone formation and is a risk factor for osteoporosis. Dietary calcium intake during the first 3 decades of life influences the ultimate peak bone mass, and calcium intake during adult life also has a small effect on bone mass and risk of fracture. Inability to synthesize adequate amounts of $1\alpha,25$-dihydroxyvitamin D $[1,25(OH)_2D]$ may play a role in the decreased calcium absorption, possibly because of decreased sensitivity of the $25(OH)D$-1α-hydroxylase to parathyroid hormone or impaired activity of the renal $25(OH)D$-1α-hydroxylase.

Genetic factors influence bone mass. Indeed, in identical twins, as much as 80 percent of age-specific variation in bone mass can be accounted for on a genetic basis. Several reports suggest that the presence of a specific polymorphism (termed *b* and *B*) in the vitamin D receptor correlates with bone mineral density in some populations; specifically, the homozygous *bb* genotype is associated with higher lumbar and femoral bone mineral density than the *Bb* or *BB* genotypes. Other gene loci also probably influence bone density and strength.

Local production of cytokines appears to mediate the enhanced osteoclast-mediated bone resorption of estrogen deficiency. Peripheral blood monocytes from patients with osteoporosis secrete more interleukin (IL) 1, and the increased production of IL-1 in women with postmenopausal osteoporosis is suppressed by estrogen treatment. IL-1 and other cytokines such as tumor necrosis factor α (TNFα) stimulate production of IL-6 by osteoblasts and other mesenchymal cells. IL-6 is probably the most important cytokine in the recruitment of osteoclasts in the abnormal bone remodeling in postmenopausal osteoporosis. Although osteoporosis occurs with Cushing's syndrome, there is no established role for adrenal steroids in the osteoporosis associated with the menopause or advanced age.

Excessive acid intake, particularly in the form of high-protein diets, may contribute to "dissolution" of bone as the body attempts to buffer the extra acid. Acidosis also may increase osteoclast function directly. Prolonged use of heparin as an anticoagulant is also associated with osteoporosis, and heparin potentiates bone resorption in vitro. The bone marrows of subjects with osteoporosis have increased numbers of mast cells, which presumably are capable of producing heparin and other substances that modulate bone cell function. Circumscribed and diffuse areas of osteoporosis occur in patients with systemic mastocytosis.

As mentioned earlier, the remodeling of bone is responsive to mechanical forces. Immobilization initially causes an increase in bone resorption, while bone formation remains normal or is decreased; later, there is a compensatory increase in bone formation. In osteoporosis, immobilization tends to aggravate the defect by increasing the gap between formation and resorption. A sedentary life-style may reduce mechanical forces exerted on the skeleton and increase the tendency to bone loss.

CLASSIFICATION (See Table 355-1) In some instances, osteoporosis is a manifestation of another disease, such as Cushing's syndrome or osteogenesis imperfecta (see Chap. 348). In most cases of osteoporosis, however, no other disease is apparent. One form occurs in children or young adults of both sexes and with normal gonadal function and is frequently termed *idiopathic osteoporosis*, although most of the other forms are also of unknown pathogenesis. *Type I osteoporosis* occurs in a subset of postmenopausal women who are between 51 and 75 years of age and is characterized by an acceler-

Table 355-1

CHAPTER 355
Metabolic Bone Disease   **2249**

Classification of Osteoporosis

Common forms, unassociated with other disease
   Idiopathic osteoporosis (juvenile and adult)
   Type I osteoporosis
   Type II osteoporosis
Disorders in which osteoporosis is a common feature
   Hypogonadism
   Hyperadrenocorticism
   Chronic glucocorticoid administration
   Hyperparathyroidism
   Thyrotoxicosis
   Malabsorption
   Scurvy
   Calcium deficiency
   Immobilization
   Chronic heparin administration
   Systemic mastocytosis
   Adult hypophosphatasia
   Other metabolic bone diseases
Heritable disorders of connective tissue in which osteoporosis is a feature
   Osteogenesis imperfecta
   Homocystinuria due to cystathionine synthase deficiency
   Ehlers-Danlos syndrome
   Marfan's syndrome
Disorders in which the pathogenesis of associated osteoporosis is not understood
   Rheumatoid arthritis
   Malnutrition
   Alcoholism
   Epilepsy
   Primary biliary cirrhosis
   Chronic obstructive pulmonary disease
   Menkes' syndrome

ated and disproportionate loss of trabecular bone. Fractures of vertebral bodies and the distal forearm are common complications. Decreased parathyroid gland function may be compensatory to increased bone resorption. *Type II osteoporosis* occurs in women and men over the age of 70 and is associated with fractures of the femoral neck, proximal humerus, proximal tibia, and pelvis, sites that contain both cortical and trabecular bone. Circulating levels of parathyroid hormone (PTH) tend to be high. Both groups have decreased mean circulating levels of $1,25(OH)_2D$.

GENERAL CLINICAL FEATURES   Although osteoporosis is a generalized disorder of the skeleton, the major sequelae result from fractures of the vertebrae, wrist, hip, humerus, and tibia. The most frequent symptoms from vertebral body fractures are pain in the back and deformity of the spine. Pain usually results from collapse of the vertebrae, especially in the dorsal and lumbar regions, is typically acute in onset, and often radiates around the flank into the abdomen. Such episodes may occur after sudden bending, lifting, or jumping movements that may have seemed trivial; on some occasions they cannot be related to trauma. The pain may be increased with even slight movements such as turning in bed or the Valsalva maneuver. Bed rest may relieve the pain temporarily, only for it to recur in spasms of variable duration. Radiation of pain down one leg is uncommon, and symptoms or signs of spinal cord compression are rare. The acute episodes of pain also may be accompanied by abdominal distention and ileus, thought to be due to retroperitoneal hemorrhage, but the use of narcotics also contributes to the ileus. Loss of appetite and muscular weakness also may be present. Episodes of pain usually subside after several days to a week, and by 4 to 6 weeks patients may be fully ambulatory and able to resume normal activities. Although acute pain may be minimal, nagging, deep, dull, uncomfortable sensations may be localized to the area of fracture and brought about by straining or sudden changes in position. Patients may be unable to sit up in bed and may have to arise by rolling over on the side and then propping themselves up, but the pain usually disappears or decreases between episodes of vertebral body collapse. Other patients do not have acute episodes but complain of backache that is made

worse by standing or sudden movement. Tenderness is common over involved areas of the spinous processes or rib cage. Some patients have an associated disease such as osteoarthritis of facet joints to account for chronic back pain. Vertebral bodies usually collapse anteriorly, producing a wedge-shaped deformity and contributing to loss in height. This is particularly common in the middorsal region, where collapse may not be associated with pain but may result in a dorsal kyphosis and exaggerated cervical lordosis described as a "dowager's" or "widow's" hump. Postural slumping with increase in existing curves contributes to the loss of height. Scoliosis is also common. Generalized skeletal pain is uncommon, and between fractures most patients are free of pain. Although recurrent episodes of vertebral collapse, increasing spine deformity, and loss of height are common, the course in any one person is not predictable, and there may be intervals of several years between fractures.

Hip fractures are the most severe complication. They may be the consequence of trauma, most resulting from a fall from standing height. The likelihood of fracture in a particular location is related in part to the site where the bond density is most reduced, such as the femoral neck or intertrochanteric region. The incidence of hip fractures in both men and women increases with age.

RADIOLOGIC FEATURES   Prior to fracture and collapse, the osteoporotic vertebral body shows a decrease in mineral density, an increase in the prominence of vertical striations due to a relatively greater loss of the horizontally oriented trabeculae, and prominence of the end plates. The bodies may become increasingly biconcave because of weakening of the subchondral plates, microfractures, and expansion of the intervertebral disks, resulting in so-called codfish vertebrae. When collapse occurs, it usually produces a decrease in the anterior height of the vertebral body and irregularity in the anterior cortex (Fig. 355-1). Older compression fractures may show reactive changes and osteophytes about the anterior margins. Most osteoporotic fractures occur in the middle and lower thoracic and upper lumbar

FIGURE 355-1   Lateral views of the lumbar spine of a 54-year-old man with idiopathic osteoporosis. A typical anterior compression fracture is indicated by the arrow.

vertebral bodies. Fractures of isolated vertebral bodies at T4 or higher suggest malignancy. Although the cortices of long bones may be thin because of excessive endosteal resorption, the outer margins are sharp, in contrast to the typical effects of the subperiosteal resorption of hyperparathyroidism. Pseudofractures or Looser's zones do not occur in the absence of osteomalacia, but it may be impossible to distinguish osteoporosis from osteomalacia on radiologic grounds alone. In the absence of fractures, standard roentgenograms are insensitive indicators of bone loss, since a decrease by as much as 30 percent in bone mass may not be appreciated. Other procedures are required to establish whether a given individual has a sufficient decrease in bone mass to be at risk for fracture. DEXA is an excellent technique because of its sensitivity, ability to scan the entire skeleton, low radiation exposure, and short scanning time. Single- and dual-photon absorptiometry and quantitative computed tomography (CT) also can detect small (1 to 2 percent) changes in the bone mineral density of the hip and lumbar spine.

LABORATORY FINDINGS The concentrations of calcium and inorganic phosphorus in the blood are usually normal. Slight hyperphosphatemia occurs in women who are past the menopause. The alkaline phosphatase level in uncomplicated instances is normal, but it may increase after fractures. About 20 percent of postmenopausal women with osteoporosis have hypercalciuria. Biochemical indices of bone resorption are, on the average, increased. Immunoassays for urinary excretion of type I collagen–derived pyridinoline cross-links such as free and total pyridinolines and N-telopeptide cross-links are better than assays of hydroxyproline. Such assays and serum assays of bone-specific alkaline phosphatase, osteocalcin, and C-terminal procollagen peptides are particularly useful in monitoring the effects of therapy.

DIFFERENTIAL DIAGNOSIS Since decrease in skeletal mass is a universal feature of aging, it is difficult to evaluate asymptomatic decreased bone density, determined radiographically, in older women, especially when not accompanied by marked increase in biconcavity of vertebral bodies or fractures. Quantitative measurement of bone mass is, however, a predictor of future fractures, and measurements of vertebral height may reveal the presence of asymptomatic fractures. In the presence of bone pain with or without fracture or deformity, it is important to establish the presence or absence of known causes of osteoporosis as listed in Table 355-1 and to be certain that osteoporosis is the correct diagnosis. Malignancies of various types, particularly *multiple myeloma, lymphoma, leukemia,* and *metastatic carcinoma,* may result in diffuse loss of bone, especially the trabecular bone of the vertebral column, even in the absence of hypercalcemia. The absence of anemia, elevated erythrocyte sedimentation rate, abnormal electrophoretic patterns of serum proteins, and Bence Jones proteinuria is helpful in eliminating the possibility of multiple myeloma. However, needle bone biopsy or marrow aspiration may be appropriate in instances of severe osteoporosis with fractures. Quantitative histomorphometry on standard biopsy samples from the iliac crest is a research tool but is available in some referral laboratories. Bone biopsy samples must be properly fixed, not demineralized, and embedded in plastic to rule out osteomalacia, however.

Radiologic evidence of osteoporosis is common in patients with primary *hyperparathyroidism,* who may not have osteitis fibrosa (discrete lytic lesions of varying size and subperiosteal resorption) and elevation of serum alkaline phosphatase. Although asymptomatic primary hyperparathyroidism is not a major risk factor in osteoporosis, it does contribute to accelerated bone loss. An element of secondary hyperparathyroidism may be present in some elderly patients with type II osteoporosis and in others with impairment of renal function, inadequate oral calcium intake, or decrease of intestinal calcium absorption. Increased numbers of osteoclasts may be present in bone biopsy specimens from such patients.

Osteomalacia may mimic osteoporosis or coexist with it, yet specific radiologic signs of osteomalacia are not always present. Although the presence of abnormalities such as low or undetectable circulating levels of 25-hydroxyvitamin D[25(OH)D] and PTH with or without hypophosphatemia suggests the possibility of osteomalacia, bone biopsy may be essential for diagnosis, as discussed below. Since osteomalacia is more responsive to therapy (e.g., vitamin D in hypovitaminosis D or phosphate supplements in phosphate depletion) than in the usual case of osteoporosis, such diagnostic procedures are often warranted. Subclinical vitamin D deficiency with associated secondary hyperparathyroidism may be more common in elderly women than previously recognized, and treatment of postmenopausal women with small doses of vitamin D (20 μg or 800 IU daily) may reduce the risk of hip fractures and other nonvertebral fractures.

In an occasional patient with *Paget's disease,* pure lytic radiologic features may be confused with osteoporosis. High alkaline phosphatase levels and increased urinary excretion of pyridinoline cross-links are clues to the presence of Paget's disease. Scanning procedures with bone-seeking isotopes are not helpful in differential diagnosis if fractures are present because fractures cause preferential uptake of isotope. In the absence of fractures "hot spots" are more suggestive of tumor or early Paget's disease, particularly if present in the appendicular skeleton.

IDIOPATHIC OSTEOPOROSIS *Idiopathic osteoporosis* occurs in younger men and in premenopausal women in whom no other etiologic factor is detected. These patients probably have a number of different disorders with superficial resemblances. Occasionally, osteoporosis appears in young women during or shortly after pregnancy. Such women have decreases in trabecular bone, and bone mass may remain low for many years. The etiology is unknown. Some patients have low levels of serum alkaline phosphatase, though not low enough to fulfill diagnostic criteria for *hypophosphatasia.* Estrogens are ineffective in this form of osteoporosis. Losses of calcium and phosphorus are probably excessive, and it is unwise to permit women with osteoporosis to breast-feed, because calcium losses via lactation are appreciable. Some patients have a disorder similar to mild forms of osteogenesis imperfecta and may thus have defects in type I collagen genes, although such features as family history, blue sclerae, and deafness are lacking. The course is variable; although recurrent episodes of fractures are characteristic, progressive deterioration does not occur in all patients, and in some the clinical problem is benign. Juvenile osteoporosis is a rare disorder, with onset usually between the ages of 8 and 14 years; it is characterized by the abrupt appearance of bone pain and fractures after minimal trauma. In many cases the disorder is self-limited, and recovery takes place spontaneously within 4 or 5 years.

GLUCOCORTICOID EXCESS Glucocorticoid excess does not appear to be involved in idiopathic osteoporosis or in the type I or II disorder. Osteoporosis, however, commonly accompanies Cushing's syndrome, both endogenous and exogenous, and in some instances is rapidly progressive, especially in children and in women over age 50. Bone loss is usually most rapid in the first 6 to 12 months of therapy with glucocorticoids but continues indefinitely with prolonged therapy. The skeletal pathophysiology is probably accounted for by a combination of low rates of bone formation (depressed osteoblastic function) and high rates of bone resorption reflected in the hypercalciuria that accompanies increased activation frequency of bone remodeling units. A part of the latter may be the result of glucocorticoid-induced secondary hyperparathyroidism, although increases in circulating PTH are not found consistently. Glucocorticoids, however, potentiate the effects of PTH and 1,25(OH)$_2$D on bone cells in vitro. Glucocorticoids depress collagen synthesis in many tissues, as evidenced by delayed wound healing, thinning of the dermis, striae, and tendency to blue sclerae. In some disorders in which glucocorticoids are administered in pharmacologic doses, such as rheumatoid arthritis, a tendency to osteoporosis is present beforehand, and the skeletal effects of the glucocorticoids may be particularly severe. Even low doses of glucocorticoids can accelerate bone loss in postmenopausal women and men with rheumatoid arthritis. Blood levels of 25(OH)D are normal or slightly decreased, and blood levels of 1,25(OH$_2$)D are usually normal. Glucocorticoids inhibit intestinal calcium absorption by a direct, vitamin D–independent action on the intestine, but osteomalacia does not occur. Once osteoporosis develops in adults with Cushing's syndrome, the abnormality may persist indefinitely following alleviation of the glucocorticoid excess. In children, however, cure of the Cushing's syndrome can result in striking improvement in the appearance of the spine due to new endochondral bone formation around the less dense, older osteoporotic bone. Likewise, increase in bone mass, increase in serum osteocalcin levels (indicative of increased osteoblastic function), and decrease in urinary excretion of markers of bone resorption may occur in young adults following treatment of Cushing's syndrome. Withdrawal of glucocorticoids or a decrease of the dose by use of an alternate-day schedule is important to halt progression of the osteoporosis. Anabolic steroids are not effective in this regard. The defect in intestinal calcium absorption may be overcome by administering calcitriol [1,25(OH)$_2$D] in oral doses of 0.5 to 1.0 μg/d plus 1 g supplemental oral calcium daily. Such regimens with or without calcitonin (e.g., 400 IU/d intranasally) are effective in preventing glucocorticoid-induced bone loss. Vitamin D metabolites such as calcifediol [25(OH)D] also may be effective. It is important to monitor serum and urinary calcium levels at intervals of 2 to 4 months. In Cushing's syndrome, spontaneous, symptomless fractures may occur in ribs and pubic and ischial rami even in the absence of marked osteoporosis of the spine. These fractures often heal partially with an exuberant calcified callus surrounding a radiolucent zone of nonunion, superficially resembling the pseudofractures of osteomalacia. If they appear in the thorax superimposed on the lungs, they may be confused with nodules suggesting primary or metastatic tumor.

GONADAL DEFICIENCY Osteoblasts have receptors for estrogens, and estrogens may function in these cells by stimulating production of substances that are anabolic for bone such as insulin-like growth factor I or by reducing the production of catabolic cytokines by osteoblasts and mononuclear phagocytes. Estrogen is deficient in the postmenopausal woman, and the administration of estrogen to such an individual reduces the negative calcium balance and decreases urinary excretion of markers of bone resorption. Estrogens are particularly useful in retarding the bone loss in women who have oophorectomy at an early age and in preventing the development of osteoporosis following the menopause. Bone mass is also decreased in women athletes who are amenorrheic, such as marathon runners. Such women are particularly prone to tibial stress fractures. In patients of either sex castrated at an early age, the adult skeleton is smaller to begin with, and, therefore, age-related losses are more significant. Bone density is also decreased in women with hyperprolactinemia and in men with hypogonadism of all types. Estrogens also play a critical role in skeletal growth and the attainment and maintenance of peak bone mass, as evidenced by the presence of severe osteopenia in a man with tall stature, marked osteoporosis, and increased urinary excretion of the markers of bone resorption associated with a loss-of-function mutation in the estrogen receptor.

THYROTOXICOSIS In many patients with hyperthyroidism, including some with mild or subclinical hyperthyroidism, excessive bone resorption, occasionally marked in degree and far exceeding that in the usual patient with osteoporosis, can be associated with increased excretion of calcium and phosphorus in urine and feces. The excessive bone resorption is usually accompanied by a compensatory increase in bone formation. PTH secretion is decreased, intestinal calcium absorption is low, and levels of 1,25(OH)$_2$D are normal or low. If the hyperthyroidism is of short duration, skeletal losses are inconsequential. In patients with chronic hyperthyroidism, however, especially in women after the menopause, this accelerated bone loss becomes significant, and it is important to eliminate hyperthyroidism as a contributing cause of osteoporosis. Mild or subclinical hyperthyroidism due to the use of excessive replacement doses of levothyroxine causes decrease in cortical bone, particularly in estrogen-deficient women. The treatment of hypothyroid patients with replacement doses of levothyroxine decreases bone mass to values found in normal individuals, and excessive doses of levothyroxine in these patients can result in accelerated bone loss. Although typical osteitis fibrosa (resorption lacunae containing osteoclasts and a fibrous stroma) may be seen on biopsy, the skeletal lesions have the radiologic appearance of osteoporosis.

ACROMEGALY Hypercalciuria and overall net negative calcium balance occur in acromegaly, and, occasionally, osteoporosis is

an associated finding. The secondary panhypopituitarism and the associated gonadal insufficiency may be factors in production of the osteoporosis. In adult animals, growth hormone decreases endosteal resorption and stimulates bone formation, and it is therefore unlikely that excessive secretion of growth hormone in itself produces osteoporosis.

DIABETES MELLITUS Individuals with juvenile or adult-onset diabetes mellitus have a decreased bone mass. In some series, the incidence of hip fractures is increased, but studies of large groups of diabetic subjects have not revealed abnormal calcium metabolism or significant bone disease specifically attributable to the diabetes.

CALCIUM DEFICIENCY AND MALABSORPTION Adequate calcium intake is an important influence in the attainment of peak bone mass. Calcium deficiency is not a major factor in the pathogenesis of postmenopausal osteoporosis or the osteoporosis of aging in both sexes. However, osteoporosis is present in many patients with steatorrhea, prolonged obstructive jaundice, and lactose intolerance and in patients following gastrectomy. Other patients may have a specific defect in calcium absorption or a failure to adapt adequately to a low-calcium diet either by increasing the percentage of dietary calcium absorbed or by decreasing urinary calcium excretion. Presumably, vitamin D is adequate in these instances to prevent osteomalacia.

HERITABLE DISORDERS OF CONNECTIVE TISSUE In the strict sense, the bone disease of osteogenesis imperfecta is osteoporosis (see Chap. 348). *Osteogenesis imperfecta* is clinically, genetically, and biochemically heterogeneous. Type I osteogenesis imperfecta is the autosomal dominant form, characterized by mild to moderate bone fragility, blue sclerae, and premature deafness. The frequency of fractures tends to decrease around puberty, and another period of increased incidence occurs in women after the menopause. Type II is the lethal perinatal disorder. Type III is characterized by severe bone fragility, progressive bone deformity, and white sclerae. In type IV, sclerae are white, but other features are similar to those of type I disease. Many instances of osteogenesis imperfecta of all types have been linked to mutations in the *COL*1A1 and *COL*1A2 genes that encode type I collagen. It is unlikely, however, that mutations in the coding region of the type I collagen genes are important in controlling bone mass in individuals with postmenopausal osteoporosis. Osteoporosis also occurs in patients with *homocystinuria* due to cystathionine synthase deficiency, an autosomal recessive trait associated with ectopia lentis, various deformities of the extremities, mental retardation, decreased pigmentation of hair and skin, and thromboembolism. The diagnosis is established by the finding of homocystine in urine. Homocystine has effects on the cross-linking of collagen, but it is not known how homocystinuria causes osteoporosis.

℞ **TREATMENT**

Potent agents are now available for preventing bone loss and for treating established osteoporosis. The ability to measure bone density and predict fracture in osteoporosis has changed the approach to treatment. Clinical benefit can be documented not only in the form of improved bone mass but as a decreased incidence of fractures. Although most available drugs are inhibitors of bone resorption, some agents, such as sodium fluoride, increase bone formation.

General Measures After Fractures Have Occurred Patients with acute pain secondary to fracture of vertebral bodies frequently require rest in bed in a position of maximum comfort, local heat, adequate analgesics, and avoidance of constipation. Use of traction or plaster jacket splints is not indicated. As soon as pain permits, the patient should attempt to move out of bed, slowly at first, perhaps with the support of a walker or crutches. Braces are commonly employed, but their efficacy in preventing progression of spinal deformity is not established. A well-made corset may provide support and comfort. Exercises to correct postural deformity and increase muscle tone are useful. Patients should be taught to avoid sudden painful movements such as jumping, and how to lift and carry objects with minimal back strain. After the fractures have healed, a supervised exercise program that includes daily walking may be helpful in preventing further skeletal losses.

Acute mortality after hip fracture is relatively low (around 3 to 4 percent), but mortality within a year is relatively high (20 to 25 percent). Morbidity is also high; only about one-half of patients return to prefracture activity levels within a year.

Estrogens and Androgens The administration of estrogens to postmenopausal women causes a decrease in urinary excretion of calcium and markers of bone resorption, especially during the first few months of treatment (see Chap. 337). Estrogens may have direct effects on osteoblasts and mononuclear phagocytes and can decrease the rate of bone resorption, but bone formation usually does not increase and eventually decreases. Nevertheless, estrogens produce significant calcium retention, decrease the difference between the rates of bone formation and resorption, and retard bone loss. Although any restoration of skeletal mass is minimal, the use of estrogens effectively prevents bone loss following castration and after the menopause and decreases the incidence of osteoporotic fracture in postmenopausal women. The major role of estrogens is in preventing osteoporosis in menopausal women rather than treating clinical disease already developed, although they also may be effective in mild or moderate disease during the first 10 years following cessation of ovarian function. The common dosage is 0.625 mg/d as conjugated estrogens, usually given in a cyclic fashion for the first 25 days of each month. (Lower doses are usually ineffective.) Estradiol also can be administered in a percutaneous patch or gel for transdermal absorption (see Chap. 337). In women after hysterectomy, progestogens are not necessary, but in women with a uterus, a progestogen (e.g., medroxyprogesterone, 5 mg/d) may be added for the last 12 days of estrogen administration (see Chap. 337). Estrogen (e.g., conjugated estrogens, 0.625 mg/d) and a progestogen (e.g., medroxyprogesterone, 2.5 mg/d) also may be administered continuously and will prevent the menstrual cycle. Patient compliance is a major problem in the use of estrogens in postmenopausal women. Many women are reluctant to use estrogens to prevent bone loss and/or treat established osteoporosis because of issues such as return of menstrual bleeding and fear of breast cancer. The estrogen antagonist tamoxifen retains agonist activity in the skeleton and prevents bone loss in the spine and femoral neck. Unfortunately, tamoxifen can also induce uterine bleeding. Testosterone preparations are useful in the treatment of osteoporotic men with gonadal deficiency, but there is no evidence of efficacy in men with normal gonadal function. There is also no proven advantage to combinations of estrogens and androgens in either sex.

Calcium Supplements, Vitamin D Metabolites, and Thiazide Diuretics Women who are estrogen-deprived require an average oral intake of 1500 mg/d of elemental calcium to remain in calcium equilibrium. The recommendation of the National Institutes of Health of 1000 mg elemental calcium per day for women on estrogen replacement and for men is reasonable. In postmenopausal women unable to take estrogens, the use of 1500 mg/d of oral calcium may have a minor benefit in preserving cortical bone but has no effects on trabecular bone mass. Adequate calcium intake before age 30 to 35 may enhance peak bone mass, however. The content of elemental calcium of available preparations varies depending on the accompanying anion and the composition (Table 355-2). Vitamin D preparations have been used in osteoporosis because calcium absorption is impaired and serum levels of $1,25(OH)_2D$ are marginally low.

Subclinical vitamin D deficiency and associated secondary hyperparathyroidism are common in elderly women, particularly those confined to nursing homes. In these women, low doses of vitamin D (20 µg or 800 IU daily) combined with calcium supplements (1 to 1.5 g elemental calcium daily) are effective in maintaining bone mass and decreasing the incidence of hip fractures. Oral administration of calcitriol also may improve intestinal calcium absorption, suppress bone resorption, and prevent bone loss in post-

Table 355-2

Elemental Calcium Content of Various Oral Calcium Preparations

Calcium Preparation	Elemental Calcium Content
Calcium citrate	40 mg/300 mg
Calcium lactate	80 mg/600 mg
Calcium gluconate	40 mg/500 mg
Calcium carbonate	400 mg/g
Calcium carbonate + 5 µg vitamin D_2 (OsCal 250)	250 mg/tablet
Calcium carbonate (Tums 500)	500 mg/tablet

menopausal osteoporosis. Bone formation is not increased, however, and at the doses suggested (an average of 0.8 µg/d) hypercalcemia and hypercalciuria may occur. Thiazide diuretics are useful in patients with high-turnover osteoporosis associated with hypercalciuria and secondary hyperparathyroidism. In the absence of secondary hyperparathyroidism, the thiazide diuretics lower urinary calcium excretion, suppress parathyroid gland function, inhibit the synthesis of $1,25(OH)_2D$, and reduce intestinal calcium absorption.

Calcitonin Calcitonin decreases bone resorption, and the use of salmon calcitonin in established osteoporosis has been recommended in doses of 50 U subcutaneously every other day. Patients with high-turnover osteoporosis (elevated levels of serum osteocalcin, increased urinary excretion of markers of bone absorption, and increased total-body retention of ^{99m}Tc-methylene diphosphonate) appear to respond best with improvement in bone mass. Calcitonin can also be administered by nasal spray (200 U/d) to avoid parenteral administration. Calcitonin may have beneficial effects on bone pain owing to a central analgesic effect.

Bisphosphonates The first bisphosphonate approved as an antiresorptive agent was etidronate, which was administered cycically in alternation with calcium and vitamin D supplements, to prevent mineralization defects. This regimen caused increases in the density of spinal bone and possibly decreases in the incidence of fractures.

Newer bisphosphonates such as alendronate, pamidronate, and tiludronate are more potent inhibitors of bone resorption and therefore do not cause osteomalacia at effective antiresorptive doses. In two large multicenter studies alendronate at a dose of 10 mg/d was effective over a 3-year period at increasing the mineral density of spinal bone by about 10 percent, increasing the density of femoral neck bone by about 5 percent, and decreasing the incidence of spine and hip fracture by about one-half. The agent is approved for use in the United States for established osteoporosis. Although there was no increased incidence of gastrointestinal side effects during the trials, it was recommended that to reduce the potential for esophageal irritation the agent be taken first thing on arising with a full glass of water [180 to 240 mL (6 to 8 oz)] at least 30 min before the first meal or beverage and that the patient should avoid lying down for at least 30 min after ingesting the medication. Esophagitis has been reported in postmarketing surveillance, and strict adherence to the dosing recommendations is essential to reduce the risk of this complication.

Fluoride Fluoride ions are deposited in the skeleton, where they are incorporated into the crystal lattice of hydroxyapatite, substituting for hydroxyl ions. This process results in a mineral phase of greater crystallinity. Sodium fluoride or intermittent low doses of PTH (currently in therapeutic trials) are the only agents that can stimulate osteoblastic proliferation and function and increase bone formation. Indeed, chronic ingestion of high amounts of fluoride, usually in areas where the fluoride content of drinking water is high, produces a form of hyperostosis, with dense bones, exostoses, neurologic complications due to bony overgrowth, and ligament ossification. An increased amount of bone with excessive osteoid is evidence of stimulation of bone formation. When sodium fluoride is used to treat osteoporosis, there is a continuous increase in the bone mass of the spine. In some series this increase in bone mass is accompanied by a decreased incidence of spinal fractures, but the therapy may result in an increased risk of fractures of the hip as well as other nonvertebral fractures. Even in series in which a satisfactory effect of sodium fluoride is observed, some patients do not respond at all. Some patients develop side effects, including knee, foot, and ankle pain attributed to microfractures; other patients cannot tolerate the drug because of nausea.

Parathyroid Hormone PTH stimulates bone resorption, but under some circumstances PTH is anabolic. Whereas high-dose, continuous administration results in lower bone mass, low-dose, intermittent administration can increase bone mass. In several studies, PTH prevented bone loss in young women treated with a luteinizing hormone–releasing hormone analogue for endometriosis and increased trabecular bone mass in postmenopausal women. Although not approved for use, this regimen may provide an additional approach for therapy.

RICKETS AND OSTEOMALACIA

Rickets and *osteomalacia* are disorders in which mineralization of the organic matrix of the skeleton is defective (Table 355-3). In *rickets* the growing skeleton is involved; defective mineralization occurs both in bone and in the cartilaginous matrix of the growth plate. The term *osteomalacia* is usually reserved for the disorder in the adult, in whom the epiphyseal growth plates are closed. A number of conditions result in rickets and/or osteomalacia, such as inadequate dietary intake of vitamin D, inadequate exposure to solar ultraviolet radiation with resulting inadequate formation of endogenous vitamin D, intestinal malabsorption of vitamin D, acquired and inherited disorders of vitamin D metabolism, inherited defects in the receptor for 1,25(OH)$_2$D in target tissues, chronic acidosis, renal tubular defects that produce hypophosphatemia or acidosis, aluminum intoxication, and chronic administration of anticonvulsants. In the renal tubular disorders, rickets and osteomalacia develop in the presence of normal intestinal function and are not cured by treatment with doses of vitamin D adequate to cure deficiency rickets. Thus, the term *vitamin D–resistant* (or *refractory*) *rickets* has been applied in these instances. Renal insufficiency, especially in children, and chronic hemodialysis per se are also associated with rickets or osteomalacia.

PATHOGENESIS AND HISTOPATHOLOGY For skeletal mineralization, sufficient calcium and phosphate must be present at the mineralization sites. Other conditions required for normal mineralization include intact metabolic and transport functions of osteoblasts and chondrocytes, adequate collagen matrix, possibly phosphorylation or other modifications of matrix components, and low concentrations of inhibitory substances such as proteoglycan aggregates or inorganic pyrophosphate. A specific function in the mineralization process for the noncollagenous matrix proteins synthesized by bone cells (e.g., osteocalcin, osteonectin, and phosphosialoproteins) has not been demonstrated, although they bind calcium ions. In cartilage the initial mineral phase is enclosed in membrane-bound extracellular vesicles. If the osteoblast continues to produce matrix components that cannot be mineralized adequately, rickets and osteomalacia result. If calcification continues to be inadequate, the production of organic matrix (osteoid) also gradually decreases. In bone there will be an increase in the fraction of the forming surface covered by incompletely mineralized osteoid, an increase in osteoid volume and thickness (the latter being normally less than 12 to 14 μm), and a decrease in the calcification or mineralization front. The latter is detected in undemineralized sections by the fluorescence of previously ingested tetracycline or by special stains. There is a marked decrease in the rate of apposition of mineralized bone. A number of methods are available to measure the thickness of the osteoid seams and the calcification front. In histologic sections stained with hematoxylin and eosin, the more heavily mineralized areas tend to appear violet or blue, whereas the osteoid seams appear pink. Subtle degrees of osteomalacia may not be appreciated with routine preparations, and undecalcified, thin sections (3 to 5 μm) stained, for example, with Goldner's trichrome method are necessary to establish its presence (Fig. 355-2). Rickets is also characterized by inadequate mineralization of the matrix of cartilage in the growing

Table 355-3

Classification of Rickets and Osteomalacia

Vitamin D deficiency
  Dietary deficiency
  Deficient endogenous synthesis
Gastrointestinal disorders
  Small-intestinal diseases with malabsorption
  Partial or total gastrectomy
  Hepatobiliary disease
  Chronic pancreatic insufficiency
Disorders of vitamin D metabolism
  Hereditary: pseudovitamin D deficiency or vitamin D dependency types I
    and II
  Acquired
    Anticonvulsants
    Chronic renal failure
    Tumor-associated (oncogenic) rickets and osteomalacia
Acidosis
  Distal renal tubular acidosis (classic or type I)
  Secondary forms of renal acidosis
  Ureterosigmoidostomy
  Drug-induced disease
    Chronic acetazolamide ingestion
    Chronic ammonium chloride ingestion
Chronic renal failure
Phosphate depletion
  Dietary: low phosphate intake plus ingestion of nonabsorbable antacids
  Impaired renal tubular phosphate reabsorption
    Hereditary
      X-linked hypophosphatemic rickets (vitamin D–resistant rickets)
      Adult-onset vitamin D–resistant hypophosphatemic osteomalacia
    Acquired
      Sporadic hypophosphatemic osteomalacia (phosphate diabetes)
      Tumor-associated (oncogenic) rickets and osteomalacia
      Neurofibromatosis
      Fibrous dysplasia
Generalized renal tubular disorders (Fanconi's syndrome)
  Primary renal
  Associated with systemic metabolic abnormality
    Cystinosis
    Glycogenosis
    Lowe's syndrome
  Systemic disorder with associated renal disease
    Hereditary
      Inborn errors
        Wilson's disease
        Tyrosinemia
      Neurofibromatosis
    Acquired
      Multiple myeloma
      Nephrotic syndrome
      Transplanted kidney
    Intoxications
      Cadmium
      Lead
      Outdated tetracycline
Primary mineralization defects
  Hereditary: hypophosphatasia
  Acquired
    Disodium etidronate treatment (Note: Of the bisphosphonates, only
      etidronate has this effect)
    Fluoride treatment
**States of rapid bone formation with or without a relative defect in bone
resorption**
  Postoperative hyperparathyroidism with osteitis fibrosa cystica
  Osteopetrosis
Defective matrix synthesis: fibrogenesis imperfecta ossium
Miscellaneous
  Magnesium-dependent conditions
  Axial osteomalacia
  Parenteral alimentation
  Aluminum intoxication

FIGURE 355-2 Photomicrograph of an undemineralized section stained with Goldner method of an iliac crest bone biopsy from a 45-year-old man with chronic renal failure maintained on hemodialysis. Almost the entire surface is covered by osteoid (O), which is readily distinguished from mineralized bone (MB). The thickness of the osteoid seams exceeds 100 μm in several areas.

epiphyseal plate. Calcification in the interstitial regions of the hypertrophic zone is defective, the growth plate increases in thickness, the columns of cartilage cells (which normally are highly ordered) are disorganized, and there is a variable cupping of the epiphyses. The rachitic bones are often incapable of withstanding usual mechanical stresses and tend to undergo bowing deformities. If rickets is untreated, growth at the epiphyseal plates is slowed, and the eventual length of the long bones is diminished.

It is not known whether vitamin D, through one of its metabolites, has a major direct effect on mineralization as long as the supply of mineral ions is adequate. Its primary roles after metabolic conversion to 25(OH)D and 1,25(OH)$_2$D are to regulate and enhance absorption of calcium ions from the intestinal lumen and, possibly, to enhance differentiation of stem cells to form osteoclasts. Insufficiency of the active metabolites of vitamin D leads to decreased intestinal absorption of calcium and decreased mobilization of calcium from bone, resulting in hypocalcemia. This stimulates increased synthesis and secretion of PTH and hyperplasia of the parathyroid glands. The increased circulating concentration of PTH tends to increase plasma levels of calcium to normal and to enhance renal phosphate clearance, which, in turn, produces hypophosphatemia. When the concentration of phosphorus in the extracellular fluid falls below a critical level, mineralization cannot proceed normally. In severe vitamin D deficiency, normal levels of serum calcium cannot be maintained, and the driving force for mineralization is further decreased. The absence of a metabolite of vitamin D such as 24,25(OH)$_2$D that acts directly on the skeleton also may play a role in the defective mineralization of rickets and osteomalacia.

Phosphate depletion alone can produce osteomalacia, as in patients consuming large amounts of nonabsorbable antacids and in persons with excessive renal loss of phosphate due to decreased tubular reabsorption. Secondary hyperparathyroidism is usually not present in these patients. Hypophosphatemia per se produces mineralization defects despite its effect of increasing the activity of the renal 25(OH)D-1α-hydroxylase, but it cannot account for the osteomalacia in all the disorders listed in Table 355-3. In chronic renal failure, for example, plasma phosphate levels are not decreased and usually are increased. Similarly, plasma phosphorus levels are not depressed in infants and children with osteomalacia secondary to hypophosphatasia, a hereditary deficiency in alkaline phosphatase. Osteomalacia in some patients with chronic renal failure is associated with accumulation of aluminum in bone, and the aluminum probably plays a role in production of the mineralization defect.

CLINICAL FINDINGS The clinical manifestations of rickets are the result of skeletal deformities, susceptibility to fractures, weakness and hypotonia, and disturbances in growth. In extreme instances of vitamin D–deficiency rickets, hypocalcemia causes tetany, which, when severe, may be accompanied by laryngeal spasm and seizures. In infants and young children, features include listlessness, irritability, and often profound hypotonia and muscular weakness. As the disorder progresses, children become unable to walk without support. Abnormal parietal flattening and frontal bossing develop in the skull. The calvariae are softened (craniotabes), and sutures may be widened. Prominence of the costochondral junctions is called the "rachitic rosary," and the indentation of the lower ribs at the site of attachment of the diaphragm is known as *Harrison's groove*. If untreated, deformities of the pelvis and extremities progress, with bowing being particularly common in the tibia, femur, radius, and ulna. Fractures are frequent, dental eruption is often delayed, and enamel defects are common.

The presentation of osteomalacia in adults is usually more insidious. The skeletal deformities may be overlooked, and the features of the underlying disorder may dominate, as, for example, in the vitamin D deficiency of adult celiac disease. Symptoms, when they occur, include diffuse skeletal pain and bony tenderness. Pain about the hips may result in an antalgic gait. Muscular weakness may be difficult to distinguish from hesitancy to move because of skeletal pain. Proximal weakness may mimic that of primary muscle disorders and contribute to the waddling gait. Pain and weakness may cause patients to be confined to bed and chair. Many factors, including secondary hyperparathyroidism, contribute to the myopathy. Clinical improvement in the myopathy usually results from specific therapy such as vitamin D repletion in nutritional osteomalacia, phosphate replacement in renal hypophosphatemia, or correction of acidosis. Fractures of the involved bones may occur with minimal trauma. When the ribs are involved, severe deformities may develop in the thoracic cage, and the collapse of vertebral bodies may produce loss of height.

RADIOLOGIC FEATURES In rickets, radiologic alterations are most evident at the epiphyseal growth plate, which is increased in thickness, cupped, and hazy at the metaphyseal border owing to decreased calcification of the hypertrophic zone and inadequate mineralization of the primary spongiosa. The trabecular pattern of the metaphyses is abnormal, the cortices of the diaphyses may be thinned, and the shafts may be bowed.

In osteomalacia, a decrease in bone density is usually associated with loss of trabeculae and thinning of the cortices. The radiologic changes may be indistinguishable from those in osteoporosis. Trabecular patterns may be blurred, producing a homogeneous ground glass appearance. The specific finding that suggests osteomalacia is the presence of radiolucent bands ranging from a few millimeters to several centimeters in length, usually oriented perpendicular to the surface of the bones. They are particularly common at the inner aspects of the femur, especially near the femoral neck, in the pelvis, in the outer edge of the scapula, in the upper fibula, and in the metatarsals (Figs. 355-3 and 355-4). These radiolucent bands, called *pseudofractures* or *Looser's zones*, occur most often at sites where major arteries cross the bones and are thought to be due to the mechanical stress of the pulsation of these vessels. On radionuclide bone scans, the pseudofractures appear as hot spots. Subperiosteal erosions along the diaphyseal cortices are sometimes seen in secondary hyperparathyroidism.

Increased rather than decreased density of bones may be observed in patients who have renal tubular disorders rather than vitamin D deficiency and may produce a striking thickening of the cortices and trabeculae of spongy bone. Despite the increase in bone mass per unit volume, the trabeculae are covered with thickened osteoid seams typical of osteomalacia. Similar findings may occur in patients with chronic renal failure. The reason for the hyperostosis is unknown; the bone is architecturally abnormal and is subject to fracture with minimal trauma.

FIGURE 355-3 Radiographs of the scapula of a 58-year-old woman with phosphate diabetes. The presence of a pseudofracture or Looser's zone is indicated by the arrow.

LABORATORY FINDINGS Changes in serum concentrations of calcium, inorganic phosphorus, 25(OH)D, and 1,25(OH)$_2$D vary with the different disorders (see Chap. 353). In vitamin D deficiency, whether due to dietary lack, inadequate sunlight exposure, or intestinal malabsorption, serum calcium levels are normal or low, whereas phosphorus and 25(OH)D levels are consistently low, the latter usually <20 nmol/L (<8 ng/mL) depending on the assay used. In contrast, levels of 1,25(OH)$_2$D may be normal or elevated owing to secondary hyperparathyroidism. Eventually, when levels of 25(OH)D become so low that there is inadequate substrate for the renal 25(OH)D-1α-hydroxylase, then the serum level of 1,25(OH)$_2$D also declines. In adults, the lower limit of serum phosphorus concentration is around

FIGURE 355-4 Radiograph of the femurs of a 47-year-old woman with Fanconi's syndrome of adult onset. The presence of multiple pseudofractures is indicated by the arrows.

0.9 mmol/L (2.8 mg/dL); in children, the lower limit of normal is closer to 1.3 to 1.5 mmol/L (4.0 to 4.5 mg/dL). In *severe* vitamin D depletion, hypocalcemia may be sufficient to produce tetany. Mild acidosis and generalized aminoaciduria result from secondary hyperparathyroidism. As a rule, patients with renal tubular disorders have normal serum calcium levels and hypophosphatemia. Other laboratory findings, such as glucosuria, aminoaciduria, acidosis, and hypouricemia, reflect variable degrees of disturbance of proximal tubular function or are features of the underlying disease (e.g., low plasma ceruloplasmin in Wilson's disease or abnormalities of immunoglobulins in multiple myeloma). In chronic renal failure, hyperphosphatemia and hypocalcemia are usually accompanied by normal 25(OH)D and low 1,25(OH)$_2$D levels. In nephrotic syndrome, serum 25(OH)D levels can be low owing primarily to urinary losses of protein-bound 25(OH)D. Serum phosphorus levels are also normal or elevated in hypophosphatasia. Increased urinary excretion of markers of bone resorption occurs when secondary hyperparathyroidism and excessive bone resorption are associated with the defect in mineralization. Alkaline phosphatase levels in plasma are usually elevated in rickets or osteomalacia, but typical and even severe osteomalacia, especially that due to renal tubular disorders, may be accompanied by normal levels or borderline elevations. Levels may increase during the early phases of therapy.

DIETARY VITAMIN D DEFICIENCY AND INADEQUATE ENDOGENOUS SYNTHESIS Most foods unfortified with vitamin D contain too little of the vitamin to prevent rickets in growing children or osteomalacia in adults living in temperate-zone cities. As discussed in Chap. 353, in the absence of supplements, vitamin D must be formed endogenously through the ultraviolet irradiation of precursor 7-dehydrocholesterol in the skin. Many factors decrease the formation of vitamin D$_3$ from its precursor: increased melanin pigmentation, hyperkeratosis, sunscreens, limited exposure of the body, increase in the angle of sunlight, especially during the winter, and factors in the atmosphere, such as smog, which prevent adequate penetration of solar ultraviolet radiation. Since fortification of milk and routine use of vitamin D supplements for infants have been in effect, deficiency is unusual in the United States. Poor, dark-skinned infants living in crowded northern cities are most susceptible. Furthermore, elderly individuals with insufficient sun exposure, particularly those who are housebound or in nursing homes, drink no milk, and receive no vitamin D supplements, may have low serum levels of 25(OH)D, secondary hyperparathyroidism, and increased frequency of hip fractures. Intestinal absorption of vitamin D is normal in the elderly.

VITAMIN D LOSS AND INTESTINAL MALABSORPTION Osteomalacia may occur with intestinal malabsorption, as in adult celiac disease and regional enteritis. Prior to the discovery of gluten sensitivity in some of these cases, celiac disease was among the more common disorders underlying osteomalacia. Vitamin D absorption, which normally occurs via chylomicrons, is impaired in diseases that cause steatorrhea, such as chronic biliary obstruction. Patients with cholestatic liver disease or extrahepatic biliary obstruction may have low serum levels of 25(OH)D and osteomalacia owing not only to poor vitamin D absorption but also to decreased hepatic production of 25(OH)D. Osteomalacia is less frequent in chronic pancreatic insufficiency. Patients who have had gastric surgery for peptic ulcer disease or gastric bypass for obesity also may develop osteomalacia, possibly owing to malfunction of the proximal small bowel. Additional factors may contribute to the osteomalacia in patients with small-bowel disease, such as inadequate absorbing surface and failure of intestinal cells to respond to the active metabolites of vitamin D. Secondary hyperparathyroidism is usually present in patients with intestinal malabsorption and in those with a dietary lack of vitamin D and may be particularly severe in patients who develop osteomalacia following intestinal bypass surgery. Some patients who lack vitamin D, usually owing to intestinal malabsorption, have normal circulating levels of 1,25(OH)$_2$D despite low or undetectable levels of 25(OH)D.

In these individuals the normal levels of 1,25(OH)$_2$D may be accounted for by ingestion of sufficient vitamin D in hospital diets to produce substrate 25(OH)D for 1α-hydroxylation by the renal enzyme, the activity of which is increased owing to secondary hyperparathyroidism. In other patients circulating 1,25(OH)$_2$D levels may not reflect levels at critical target cells.

ABNORMAL METABOLISM OF VITAMIN D Serum 25(OH)D levels are reduced in some instances of parenchymal and obstructive liver disease, but these findings have not been correlated with quantitative histologic studies of bone. Patients consuming anticonvulsant drugs such as phenobarbital, phenytoin, or carbamazepine may develop rickets or osteomalacia. The problem is most severe in patients taking multiple anticonvulsant drugs and in those who are institutionalized, not ambulatory, or confined indoors. The major laboratory abnormality is a low or undetectable serum level of 25(OH)D. Treatment with vitamin D (1000 IU/d) will return the serum level of 25(OH)D to normal. As discussed in Chap. 353, the anticonvulsant drugs have multiple actions on calcium homeostasis.

Two autosomal recessive syndromes associated with rickets have been termed *vitamin D–dependent rickets* (see also Chap. 353). Features of *type I vitamin D–dependent rickets* include hypocalcemia, hypophosphatemia, short stature, skeletal deformities of rickets, dental enamel hypoplasia, frequently marked elevations of serum alkaline phosphatase activity, generalized aminoaciduria, and secondary hyperparathyroidism. Circulating levels of 1,25(OH)$_2$D are low or undetectable. Treatment with massive doses of vitamin D or small doses of calcitriol reverses the abnormal biochemical findings, induces healing of the rickets, and restores the rate of skeletal growth. The abnormalities are due to mutations that impair the renal 25(OH)D-1α-hydroxylase. By linkage analysis, the disorder has been mapped to chromosome 12q14. Lifelong replacement therapy with calcitriol is required. *Type II vitamin D–dependent rickets*, also termed *hereditary resistance to 1,25(OH)$_2$D*, has many clinical features of the type I syndrome. Rickets is usually of early onset but varies in severity in different kindreds. Distinguishing features include alopecia, which may develop during the first few months of life, and multiple milia and epidermal cysts. The type II disorder is due to mutations that impair the structure and function of the 1,25(OH)$_2$D receptor. Different molecular abnormalities in different kindreds include mutations that impair binding of the receptor to DNA, mutations that cause the formation of incomplete receptor molecules, and mutations that cause single amino acid substitutions in the protein. This disorder also maps by linkage analysis to chromosome 12 in a locus close to but distinct from that for type I vitamin D–dependent rickets.

Both osteomalacia and acquired abnormalities in vitamin D metabolism may develop in patients receiving long-term total parenteral nutrition. Some of these individuals have secondary hypoparathyroidism, but hypoparathyroidism cannot account for the osteomalacia. Serum levels of 25(OH)D are normal, although levels of 1,25(OH)$_2$D may be low. Aluminum has been detected in increased amounts in plasma, urine, and bone and may play a role in the genesis of the osteomalacia similar to its postulated role in patients with renal failure on chronic hemodialysis.

RENAL TUBULAR DISORDERS Rickets and osteomalacia occur in association with a variety of disorders of proximal renal tubular function. These disorders have in common increased renal clearance of inorganic phosphorus and hypophosphatemia with a normal or near-normal glomerular filtration rate. Increased phosphate clearance with resultant hypophosphatemia is usually an isolated defect accompanied by no other abnormalities except for increased urinary glycine excretion (hyperglycinuria). X-linked hypophosphatemia (also called *phosphate diabetes* or *vitamin D–resistant rickets*) is an X-linked dominant disorder characterized by rickets in an otherwise well-nourished, healthy-appearing child. When the child begins to walk and bear weight, lower limb deformities appear and become progressively worse. The rate of linear growth is at first normal and then slowed.

Many of these individuals develop a unique disorder of tendons, ligaments, and joint capsules characterized by calcification or, more probably, ossification of insertions of tendons and ligaments and joint capsules (enthesopathy). In some patients, spontaneous remissions may be followed by recurrences in adult life, for example, with pregnancy and lactation. Hypophosphatemia is due to defective renal conservation of phosphate, which in turn is due to defective phosphate transport across the luminal membrane of proximal renal tubular cells, but the defect cannot be due to an intrinsic defect in the sodium-dependent phosphate transporter because the gene that encodes this protein maps to chromosome 5 and not to the X chromosome. (A model of the human disease occurs in a strain of hypophosphatemic mice designated Hyp). On the basis of analysis of restriction fragment polymorphism studies in several kindreds of X-linked hypophosphatemia, the mutant human gene has been mapped to the short arm of the X chromosome (Xp22.1). A candidate gene, called *PEX*, that exhibits homology to a family of endopeptidase genes has been identified, and several mutations, including deletions, frameshifts, and splice-junction defects, have been identified in kindreds with vitamin D–resistant rickets. In affected individuals, the serum levels of 25(OH)D are normal, and the levels of 1,25(OH)$_2$D are in the low-normal range. Whereas the induction of hypophosphatemia in normal individuals results in stimulation of 25(OH)D-1α-hydroxylase and an increase in the levels of 1,25(OH)$_2$D, altered renal tubular cellular phosphate fluxes in X-linked hypophosphatemia fail to stimulate the hydroxylase. Thus levels of 1,25(OH)$_2$D, although in the normal range, are inappropriately low relative to the degree of phosphate depletion. The skeletal mineralization defect is due both to the low ambient phosphate levels and to an intrinsic defect in osteoblast function, possibly related to that in the renal tubular cells. Effective therapy therefore requires both phosphate repletion with large amounts of oral phosphate and treatment with calcitriol (see below). Such combined therapy reverses the osteomalacia of trabecular bone surfaces, corrects the microscopic periosteocytic mineralization defects, and results in improvement in longitudinal growth. The patients who are shortest at the inception of therapy tend to have the poorest growth response to therapy. After the rickets is healed, defects in phosphate clearance and hypophosphatemia persist, and medical therapy is still required. The effects of excessive calcitriol administration, such as nephrocalcinosis and nephrolithiasis, must be avoided. Adults with X-linked hypophosphatemia frequently have pseudofractures; osteoarthritis in the sacroiliac joints, wrists, knees, hips, and feet; and marked enthesopathy. Another variant of hereditary rickets has been termed *hereditary hypophosphatemic rickets with hypercalciuria*. Muscular weakness, not a feature of X-linked hypophosphatemia, may be present. These individuals, whose disorder is probably inherited as an autosomal recessive trait, have normocalcemia, hypophosphatemia, and striking absorptive hypercalciuria; the latter disappears after fasting and returns after oral calcium loading. Levels of 1,25(OH)$_2$D in serum are elevated, in contrast to the low-normal levels found in X-linked hypophosphatemia. These elevations of serum 1,25(OH)$_2$D are an appropriate response of the 25(OH)D-1α-hydroxylase to phosphate depletion. Phosphate replacement induces healing of the rachitic lesions.

Sporadic cases of hypophosphatemia also have been described in adults in whom family histories are negative and proximal muscle weakness is a prominent feature (see also Chap. 356). These patients also are best treated with a combination of calcitriol and inorganic phosphorus. As mentioned above, secondary hyperparathyroidism is not present in most untreated patients with renal tubular disorders associated with rickets and osteomalacia.

In other patients the disorder in tubular function may be more widespread, involving (besides phosphorus) glucose, potassium, amino acids, and uric acid; the various combinations are termed the *de Toni-Debré-Fanconi syndrome*. The more complete renal tubular defects may occur sporadically or in families. In some instances, the lesion is part of a more widespread disorder, as in Wilson's disease and cystinosis. Fanconi's syndrome also may be a feature of plasma cell myeloma, where it is attributed to toxic effects of deposited Bence Jones protein. Similarly, osteomalacia and renal tubular acidosis have been observed in Sjögren's syndrome with increased urinary excretion of beta$_2$-microglobulin and retinol-binding protein. The acidosis of proximal tubular defects also plays a role in the development of osteomalacia, possibly by altering the metabolism of vitamin D or the renal handling of calcium and phosphorus. In this regard, osteomalacia has accompanied the hyperchloremic acidosis or ureterocolic anastomosis.

TUMOR-ASSOCIATED (ONCOGENOUS) OSTEOMALACIA Osteomalacia and hypophosphatemia with high renal phosphate clearance occur with a variety of mesenchymal tumors, including giant cell tumors (benign or malignant), reparative granulomas, hemangiomas, fibromas, and other mesenchymal neoplasms. A similar syndrome occurs in patients with prostatic carcinoma. In some instances, removal of the tumor resulted in return of renal phosphorus clearance to normal, a rise in serum phosphorus levels, and healing of the osteomalacia (or rickets in children). Serum 1,25(OH)$_2$D levels are low or undetectable, although chronic administration of sufficient calcitriol to raise circulating levels of this metabolite to normal does not alter renal phosphorus clearance or serum phosphorus concentrations. Humoral factors released by these tumors may impair proximal tubular functions such as 1α-hydroxylation of 25(OH)D *and* act as inhibitors of phosphate transport.

CHRONIC RENAL FAILURE Osteomalacia is common in patients with chronic renal failure; it tends to be the predominant type of renal osteodystrophy in younger patients and is more frequent in those with the lower plasma levels of calcium and phosphorus. A component of secondary hyperparathyroidism and osteitis fibrosa is almost always present. The defect itself probably involves a decreased conversion of 25(OH)D to 1,25(OH)$_2$D either because of insufficient viable renal cortical tissue or the inhibitory effect of hyperphosphatemia on renal 25(OH)D-1α-hydroxylase activity. In addition, there may be a primary defect in intestinal calcium absorption. Part of the secondary hyperparathyroidism also may be due to decreased phosphate clearance and subsequent hyperphosphatemia. Under circumstances of hyperphosphatemia and a near-normal plasma concentration of calcium, the presence of inhibitors probably causes the defective mineralization. In some patients, the osteomalacia responds to large doses of vitamin D or dihydrotachysterol or to small doses of calcitriol or calcifediol. In some patients, however, renal osteodystrophy does not respond to pharmacologic doses of vitamin D or to calcitriol. In others, accumulation of aluminum in the bone accounts for the vitamin D–refractory osteomalacia. Aluminum deposits can be identified at the mineralization fronts, and bone apposition rates are low. These individuals have high levels of aluminum and uncoupling of matrix deposition and mineralization. Individuals with lower amounts of aluminum develop a form of "aplastic" bone disease in which matrix deposition and mineralization are more closely coupled. Deferoxamine can mobilize aluminum from bone and other tissues and is effective therapy. In some patients with renal osteodystrophy, the total bone mass may be increased (osteosclerosis), resulting in increased density of bone. This is particularly evident in the spine, where a characteristic appearance is that of dense bone at the superior and inferior margins of the vertebral bodies with more radiolucent central portions ("rugger jersey sign"). Histologically, although there is more bone per unit area, each trabecula is covered by a wide osteoid seam.

HYPOPHOSPHATASIA Rickets is a feature of a deficiency of alkaline phosphatase in infants and children termed *hypophosphatasia*. There are four forms of hypophosphatasia: lethal perinatal, infantile, childhood, and adult. Rickets occurs in the infantile and childhood forms. In adults, the disorder may not be recognized until middle age, but there is frequently a history of early loss of deciduous or permanent teeth. Osteomalacia and calcium pyrophosphate deposition disease occur in the adult form. The severe perinatal and infantile forms are inherited as autosomal recessive traits; the pattern of inheritance in the other forms is uncertain. The low levels of circulating alkaline phosphatase activity are explained by a deficiency of the tissue-nonspecific enzyme (bone-liver-kidney). Missense mutations have been demonstrated in the alkaline phosphatase gene.

Although alkaline phosphatase is abundant in osteoclasts, its function in mineralization is not established. In hypophosphatasia, there is increased urinary excretion of phosphoethanolamine and increased circulating levels of pyridoxal-5'-phosphate. The metabolic origin of the phosphoethanolamine is not established. Concentrations of pyridoxal-5'-phosphate are not elevated intracellularly, and the extracellular increases are consistent with the function of alkaline phosphatase as an ectoenzyme; whether alterations of pyridoxal-5'-phosphate metabolism contribute to the clinical abnormalities is not known. Inorganic pyrophosphate (PPi) is a substrate for alkaline phosphatase, which accounts for increased levels of PPi in urine and plasma and for the increased incidence of calcium pyrophosphate deposition disease in hypophosphatasia. Since PPi also can function to inhibit growth of the calcium-phosphate mineral phase, excessive concentrations of PPi may cause the rickets and osteomalacia. There is no effective therapy.

OTHER DISORDERS ASSOCIATED WITH DEFECTIVE MINERALIZATION Disturbances in mineralization may be seen in patients consuming high doses of fluoride ion and in patients with Paget's disease treated with etidronate. Some decrease in mineralization of newly forming matrix, increase in surface covered by osteoid, and increase in the width of the osteoid seams may occur in conditions that are not usually considered as osteomalacia except by these criteria. Examples include patients with the osteitis fibrosa of hyperparathyroidism following surgical cure. In these circumstances, there is a temporary imbalance between the rate at which mineral is supplied to bone and the rate at which bone matrix is formed. Biopsies in some of these conditions show a normal calcification front. Wide osteoid seams and hypophosphatemia are also seen in children with osteopetrosis, in whom there is inadequate resorption of bone and calcified cartilage but active bone formation.

A condition that resembles osteomalacia and is associated with a coarsened, mottled bony trabecular pattern, pseudofractures, and bone pain but normal plasma levels of calcium and phosphorus is *fibrogenesis imperfecta ossium*. The bone has a distinctive histologic appearance, with wide osteoid seams, distortion of the birefringent pattern of normal bone, and abnormal collagen fibers by electron microscopy. The nature of the abnormality is not known.

℞ **TREATMENT**

In rickets and osteomalacia due to dietary absence of vitamin D or inadequate exposure to sunlight, vitamin D$_2$ (ergocalciferol) or vitamin D$_3$ (cholecalciferol) is given orally in doses of 800 to 4000 IU (0.02 to 0.1 mg) daily for 6 to 12 weeks, followed by daily supplements of 200 to 400 IU, which are adequate to prevent the development of the disorder in otherwise normal persons. In elderly persons with vitamin D deficiency, the administration of vitamin D, 50,000 IU by mouth once each week for 8 weeks, raises the serum levels of 25(OH)D into the mid-normal range. In infants and children, such treatment causes improvement in muscle tone and strength, an increase in serum calcium and phosphorus levels, and a decrease in alkaline phosphatase levels after several weeks. Radiologic evidence of healing appears within weeks, and healing may be complete by a few months. Calcium supplements and larger initial doses of vitamin D may be necessary in infants and children with tetany. In adults with nutritional osteomalacia, healing of pseudofractures may be evident within 3 to 4 weeks after therapy with as little as 2000 IU (0.5 mg) vitamin D daily. Healing is complete usually by 6 months.

Patients with osteomalacia due to intestinal malabsorption do not respond to small doses of vitamin D. In the presence of active steatorrhea, daily oral doses of vitamin D of 50,000 to 100,000 IU (1.25 to 2.5 mg) and large doses of calcium (e.g., 15 g calcium lactate or 4 g calcium carbonate orally per day) may be required. In some instances, oral vitamin D is ineffective, and the parenteral route is required (e.g., 10,000 IU/d intramuscularly). Another approach is the use of artificial ultraviolet B radiation or exposure to sunlight in addition to supplemental calcium. Small doses of calcitriol (0.5 to 1.0 μg daily) are also usually effective in this form of osteomalacia. Inorganic phosphate therapy is not indicated either in deficiency or in intestinal malabsorption of the vitamin, since hypocalcemia will develop and intestinal calcium absorption will remain inadequate. In all patients in whom large doses of vitamin D are used, serum calcium and 25(OH)D levels should be monitored periodically. Semiquantitative urinary calcium measurements are inadequate.

In patients treated with multiple anticonvulsant agents, it is usually necessary to continue the drugs while adding 1000 IU/d of vitamin D and to monitor levels of serum calcium and serum 25(OH)D until a therapeutic response (evidence of radiologic healing, improvement in symptoms) is obtained.

Treatment of rickets and osteomalacia in the presence of renal tubular disorders is more difficult. In the past, the X-linked form of hypophosphatemic osteomalacia was treated with large doses of vitamin D (from 50,000 to several hundred thousand IU per day), but skeletal responses were rarely complete. Currently, oral supplements of inorganic phosphate in divided doses of phosphorus, 1.0 to 3.6 g/d (50 mg/kg body weight per day for children), and calcitriol, 0.5 to 2.0 μg/d (30 ng/kg body weight per day for children), constitute the best regimen to restore skeletal growth and heal the bone disease. In some adults, therapy with inorganic phosphate alone abolishes muscle weakness and bone pain and produces radiologic and histologic healing. The addition of calcitriol improves calcium balance and helps decrease secondary hyperparathyroidism and maintain a sufficient level of serum phosphorus to permit complete healing. In some patients there may be a temporary increase in bone pain and rise in serum alkaline phosphatase during the early phases of treatment. In the osteomalacia associated with the chronic acidosis of renal tubular disorders, the use of alkali may be of value in supplementing therapy with phosphate and calcitriol. In patients with ureterosigmoidostomy, oral sodium bicarbonate can reverse acidosis, improve the serum phosphate level, and heal the bone disease; with maintenance doses of alkali, recurrence of symptoms can be prevented.

Patients with nephrotic syndrome and low serum 25(OH)D levels benefit from modest vitamin D supplementation (800 to 1000 IU/d). Small doses of calcitriol are equally effective in treating hypocalcemia and osteodystrophy resulting from chronic renal failure. The recommended initial dose of calcitriol is 0.25 μg/d. If after 2 to 4 weeks on this dose the biochemical parameters are unaltered, the dose is increased by 0.25 μg/d every 2 to 4 weeks until a satisfactory clinical biochemical response (including elevation of serum calcium levels and decrease in PTH levels) is obtained. The usual dose is 0.5 to 1.0 μg/d. Calcitriol also may be administered intravenously (1.0 to 2.5 μg three times weekly) in patients on dialysis, particularly to treat refractory osteitis fibrosa. Because there are no regulatory mechanisms to control the biologic responses to calcitriol, there is a high incidence of transient hypercalciuria and hypercalcemia, especially initially. Thus, serum calcium levels should be monitored frequently during the first 1 to 2 months of therapy and less frequently once a stable dose has been established. Some patients treated with calcitriol have an apparent increase in serum creatinine levels and a decrease in creatinine clearance; these changes are due to altered metabolism of creatinine rather than a decrease in renal function. Since calcitriol has a short duration of action and is not stored in fat depots, hypercalcemia usually resolves in 2 to 7 days after the dose is discontinued or decreased. Phosphate supplements are, of course, contraindicated in the usual patient with chronic renal failure. Occasionally, however, hypophosphatemia may result from the excessive use of nonabsorbable antacids or from excessive removal of phosphate through hemodialysis.

In patients who have had rickets in childhood, the abnormal mechanical stress of severe deformities may contribute to the development of degenerative joint disease, particularly in the hips and knees. Osteotomies at the proper time after healing may prevent this complication and the requirement for more extensive arthroplasties later in life.

See Chap. 61, Agents affecting calcification and bone turnover, in Goodman & Gilman's The Pharmacological Basis of Therapeutics, *9th ed, New York, McGraw-Hill, 1996.*

BIBLIOGRAPHY

OSTEOPOROSIS

ALOIA JF et al: Calcium supplementation with and without hormone replacement therapy to prevent postmenopausal bone loss. Ann Intern Med 120:97, 1994

AVIOLI LV, KRANE SM(eds): *Metabolic Bone Disease and Clinically Related Disorders.* Philadelphia, Saunders, 1990

BACHRACH LK et al: Osteopenia in adults with cystic fibrosis. Am J Med 96:27, 1994

CALVO MS et al: Molecular basis and clinical application of biological markers of bone turnover. Endocr Rev 17:333, 1996

CANALIS E: Insulin-like growth factors and their role in osteoporosis. Calcif Tissue Int 58:133, 1996

CHAPUY MC et al: Vitamin D_3 and calcium to prevent hip fractures in elderly women. N Engl J Med 327:1637, 1992

COLLINS JA: Hormone replacement therapy and breast cancer: What is happening? J Surg Obstet Gynecol Can 17:837, 1995

COSMAN F et al: Estrogen protection against bone resorbing effects of parathyroid hormone infusion. Ann Intern Med 118:337, 1993

CUMMINGS SR et al: Risk factors for hip fracture in white women. N Engl J Med 332:767, 1995

DE GROEN PC et al: Esophagitis associated with the use of alendronate. N Engl J Med 335:1016, 1996

DEMPSTER DW, LINDSAY R: Pathogenesis of osteoporosis. Lancet 341:797, 1993

EISMAN JA: Vitamin D receptor gene alleles and osteoporosis: An affirmative view. Editorial. J Bond Miner Res 10:1289, 1995

EPSTEIN FH: Mechanisms of disease. N Engl J Med 332:305, 1995

FINKELSTEIN JS et al: Parathyroid hormone for the prevention of bone loss induced by estrogen deficiency. N Engl J Med 331:1618, 1994

GREENSPAN SL et al: Fall severity and bone mineral density as risk factors for hip fracture in ambulatory elderly. JAMA 271:128, 1994

GREY AB et al: The effect of the antiestrogen tamoxifen on bone mineral density in normal late postmenopausal women. Am J Med 99:636, 1995

HEANEY RP: Fluoride and osteoporosis. Ann Intern Med 120:689, 1994

HOPPER JL et al: The bone density of female twins discordant for tobacco use. N Engl J Med 330:387, 1994

KRALL EA et al: Walking is related to bone density and rates of bone loss. Am J Med 96:20, 1994

LANDMAN JO et al: Skeletal metabolism in patients with osteoporosis after discontinuation of long term treatment with oral pamidronate. J Clin Endocrinol Metab 80:3465, 1995

LEE AH et al: Osteoporosis and bone morbidity in cardiac transplant recipients. Am J Med 96:35, 1994

LIBERMAN UA et al: Effect of oral alendronate on bone mineral density and the incidence of fractures in postmenopausal osteoporosis. N Engl J Med 333:1437, 1995

LINDSAY R: Prevention and treatment of osteoporosis. Lancet 341:801, 1993

MARCUS R et al: (eds): *Osteoporosis.* San Diego, Academic Press, 1996

NABULSI AA et al: Association of hormone-replacement therapy with various cardiovascular risk factors in postmenopausal women. N Engl J Med 328:1069, 1993

PAK CYC et al: Treatment of postmenopausal osteoporosis with slow-release sodium fluoride. Final report of a randomized controlled trial. Ann Intern Med 123:401, 1995

PEACOCK M: Vitamin D receptor gene alleles and osteoporosis: A contrasting view. Editorial. J Bone Miner Res 10:1294, 1995

REID IR et al: Effect of calcium supplementation of bone loss in postmenopausal women. N Engl J Med 328:460, 1993

RIGOTTI NA et al: The clinical course of osteoporosis in anorexia nervosa. A longitudinal study of cortical bone mass. JAMA 265:1133, 1991

RIGGS BL, MELTON LJ III: The prevention and treatment of osteoporosis. N Engl J Med 327:620, 1992

ROSEN HN et al: Specificity of urinary excretion of cross-linked N-telopeptides of type I collagen as a marker of bone turnover. Calcif Tissue Int 54:26, 1994

RYAN PJ et al: Osteoporosis and chronic back pain: A study with single-photon emission computed tomography bone scintigraphy. J Bone Miner Res 7:1455, 1992

SAMBROOK P et al: Prevention of corticosteroid osteoporosis: A comparison of calcium, calcitriol, and calcitonin. N Engl J Med 328:1747, 1993

SMITH EP et al: Estrogen resistance caused by a mutation in the estrogen-receptor gene in a man. N Engl J Med 331:1056, 1994

STEPAN JJ et al: Castrated men exhibit bone loss: Effect of calcitonin treatment on biochemical indices of bone remodeling. J Clin Endocrinol Metab 69:523, 1989

STEWART AF: PTHrP(1-36) as a skeletal anabolic agent for the treatment of osteoporosis. Bone 19:303, 1996

TILYARD MW et al: Treatment of postmenopausal osteoporosis with calcitriol or calcium. N Engl J Med 326:357, 1992

YAMAMOTO N et al: Bone mineral density and bone histomorphometric assessments of postpregnancy osteoporosis: A report of five patients. Calcif Tissue Int 54:20, 1994

OSTEOMALACIA

BONKOVSKY HL et al: Prevalence and prediction of osteopenia in chronic liver disease. Hepatology 12:273, 1990

CHINES A, PACIFICI R: Antacid and sucralfate-induced hypophosphatemic osteomalacia: A case report and review of the literature. Calcif Tissue Int 47:291, 1990

COLLINS N et al: A prospective study to evaluate the dose of vitamin D required to correct low 25-hydroxyvitamin D levels, calcium, and alkaline phosphatase in patients at risk of developing antiepileptic drug-induced osteomalacia. Q J Med 78:113, 1991

DAWSON-HUGHES B et al: Effect of vitamin D supplementation on wintertime and overall bone loss in healthy postmenopausal women. Ann Intern Med 115:505, 1991

FEDDE KN et al: Aberrant properties of alkaline phosphatase in patient fibroblasts correlate with clinical expressivity in severe forms of hypophosphatasia. J Clin Endocrinol Metab 81:2587, 1996

FRIEDMAN NE et al: Effects of calcitriol and phosphorus therapy on the growth of patients with X-linked hypophosphatemia. J Clin Endocrinol Metab 76:839, 1993

GALLAGHER JC: Vitamin D metabolism and therapy in elderly subjects. South Med J 85:2S43, 1992

GLORIEUX FH: Rickets, the continuing challenge. N Engl J Med 325:1875, 1991

HENDERSON JB et al: Blunted seasonal variation in serum 25-hydroxy vitamin D and increased risk of osteomalacia in vegetarian London Asians. Eur J Clin Nutr 46:509, 1992

HENTHORN PS et al: Different missense mutations at the tissue-nonspecific alkaline phosphatase gene locus in autosomal recessively inherited forms of mild and severe hypophosphatasia. Proc Natl Acad Sci USA 89:9924, 1992

HRUSKA KA et al: X-linked hypophosphatemic rickets and the murine Hyp homologue. Editorial. Am J Physiol 268:F357, 1995

HUTCHISON FN, BELL NH: Osteomalacia and rickets. Semin Nephrol 12:127, 1992

KLEIN GL, COLVURN JW: Bone disease in burn patients. J Bone Miner Res 8:337, 1993

KONISHI K et al: Hypophosphatemic osteomalacia in von Recklinghausen neurofibromatosis. Am J Med Sci 301:322, 1991

KUMAR R et al: Inhibitors of renal epithelial phosphate transport in tumor-induced osteomalacia and uremia. Proc Assoc Am Physicians 107:296, 1995

LABUDA M et al: Two hereditary defects related to vitamin D metabolism map to the same region of human chromosome 12q13-14. J Bone Miner Res 7:1447, 1992

LEICHT E et al: Tumor-induced osteomalacia: Pre- and postoperative biochemical findings. Horm Metab Res 22:640, 1990

MONTE NESTO JT et al: Osteomalacia secondary to renal tubular acidosis in a patient with primary Sjögren's syndrome. Clin Exp Rheumatol 9:625, 1991

NIJHAWAN R et al: Antiepileptic drugs, hepatic enzyme induction and raised serum alkaline phosphatase isoenzymes. Int J Clin Pharmacol Res 10:319, 1990

PETERSON DJ et al: X-linked hypophosphatemic rickets: A study (with literature review) of linear growth response to calcitrol and phosphate therapy. J Bone Miner Res 7:583, 1992

SCRIVER CR et al: X-linked hypophosphatemia: An appreciation of a classic paper and a survey of progress since 1958. Medicine 70:218, 1991

STONE MD et al: A neuroendocrine cause of oncogenic osteomalacia. J Pathol 167:181, 1992

SULLIVAN W et al: A prospective trial of phosphate and 1,25-dihydroxyvitamin D3 therapy in symptomatic adults with x-linked hypophosphatemic rickets. J Clin Endocrinol Metab 75:879, 1992

THE HYP CONSORTIUM: A gene (PEX) with homologies to endopeptidases is mutated in patients with X-linked hypophosphatemic rickets. Nature Genet 11:130, 1995

VILLAREAL DT et al: Subclinical vitamin D deficiency in postmenopausal women with low vertebral bone mass. J Clin Endocrinol Metab 72:6281, 1991

WEIDNER N: Review and update: Oncogenic osteomalacia-rickets. Ultrastruct Pathol 15:317, 1991

WHYTE MP: Hypophosphatasia, in The Molecular and Metabolic Bases of Inherited Disease, 7th ed, CR Scriver et al (eds). New York, McGraw-Hill, 1995, p 4113

356 James P. Knochel

DISORDERS OF PHOSPHORUS METABOLISM

Phosphorus is the most abundant intracellular anion and is critical for membrane structure, transport, and energy storage. The role of phosphate ions in tissues explains the systemic nature of cellular injury consequent to phosphorus deficiency.

At a plasma pH of 7.4, inorganic phosphate in plasma is a 4:1 mixture of HPO_4^{2-} and $H_2PO_4^{2-}$. The sum of the products of the valences of these ions ($4 \times 2^- + 1 \times 1^-$) divided by the sum of the ions ($4 + 1$) is equal to 9/5, or an average valence of 1.8. Of the average 700 g of phosphorus in the body, 85 percent is in the skeleton, about 15 percent is in soft tissues, and 0.1 percent is in extracellular fluid. The phosphorus in extracellular fluid is in a freely diffusible form that (1) permits excretion of hydrogen ions as phosphate buffer into the urine and (2) is in diffusion equilibrium with cytosolic inorganic phosphate in cells.

A normal adult consumes approximately 1 g phosphorus each day. Soluble phosphates in dairy products and meat are almost completely absorbed, predominantly in the midjejunum. Insoluble phosphates, in vegetables and seeds, are absorbable provided the phosphate can be digested from its ligand. For example, phosphorus in corn and oats is partly in the form of phytic acid; these foods contain little phytase, which splits phytic acid (inositol hexaphosphate) into phosphate and inositol, and hence phosphorus from this source may be poorly absorbed. Thus corn and oats may be rachitogenic in children if they are the major components of the diet. Addition of rye bran, which contains phytase, to the diet increases the bioavailability of phosphorus from these sources.

Phosphorus absorption is under the influence of vitamin D, and phosphorus excretion is under the control of parathyroid hormone (PTH). PTH decreases tubular phosphate reabsorption and increases excretion into the urine. The effect of vitamin D on phosphate reabsorption by the kidney is relatively minor. The quantity of soluble phosphorus available for absorption from the diet varies, and excretion of phosphorus in the urine on a given day depends directly on absorption. Accordingly, the range for phosphorus excretion in health is very broad.

HYPOPHOSPHATEMIA

CAUSES Hypophosphatemia has many causes (Table 356-1). The finding of hypophosphatemia is not always a reliable indicator of deficiency, since a total-body deficit of phosphorus may exist in the face of hyperphosphatemia, such as, for example, in diabetic ketoacidosis.

Hypophosphatemia can be moderate or severe. Decreased dietary intake is an unusual cause of hypophosphatemia because of the ubiquitous and abundant distribution of the mineral in foods. Decreased absorption of phosphorus from the small intestine occurs in a variety of malabsorptive states, but simple diarrhea is usually not a cause. One of the most common causes of hypophosphatemia is respiratory alkalosis. Indeed, discovery of hypophosphatemia should lead to a search for potentially serious causes of hyperventilation such as sepsis or otherwise unsuspected alcohol withdrawal. Reduction of intracellular PCO_2 and elevation of pH increase the activity of phosphofructokinase, the rate-limiting enzyme of glycolysis. Phosphorylation of glucose intermediates causes cellular uptake of phosphorus and hypophosphatemia. Administration of insulin and consumption of nutrients that stimulate insulin release are also common causes of hypophosphatemia. Insulin stimulates phosphorus uptake by cells. Cellular phosphorus uptake also occurs in patients recovering from hypothermia as a result of reactivation of metabolism. Certain rapidly growing

Table 356-1

Causes of Hypophosphatemia

I. Decreased dietary intake
II. Decreased intestinal absorption
   A. Vitamin D deficiency
   B. Malabsorption
   C. Steatorrhea
   D. Secretory diarrhea
   E. Vomiting
   F. PO$_4$-binding antacids
III. Shifts from extracellular fluid into cells
   A. Respiratory alkalosis
      1. Sepsis
      2. Alcohol withdrawal
      3. Heat stroke
      4. Neuroleptic malignant syndrome
      5. Hepatic coma
      6. Salicylate poisoning
      7. Gout
      8. Panic attacks
      9. Psychiatric depression
   B. Hormone effects
      1. Insulin
      2. Glucagon
      3. Epinephrine
      4. Androgens
      5. Glucocorticoids
      6. Oral contraceptives
   C. Nutritional effects
      1. Glucose
      2. Fructose
      3. Glycerol
      4. Lactate
      5. Amino acids
      6. Xylitol
   D. Cellular uptake syndromes
      1. Recovery from hypothermia
      2. Burkitt's lymphoma

      3. Histiocytic lymphoma
      4. Acute myelomonocytic leukemia
      5. Acute myelogenous leukemia
      6. Treatment of pernicious anemia
      7. "Hungry bone" syndrome
         a. Following parathyroidectomy
         b. Acute leukemia
IV. Increased excretion into the urine
   A. Hyperparathyroidism
   B. Renal tubular defects
      1. Renal rickets
         a. Fanconi syndrome
         b. Familial hypophosphatemia
      2. Polyostotic fibrous dysplasia
      3. Metaphyseal chondrodysplasia
      4. After kidney transplantation
      5. Oncogenic osteomalacia
      6. Recovery from hemolytic uremic syndrome
   C. Aldosteronism
   D. Licorice ingestion
   E. Volume expansion
   F. Inappropriate secretion of vasopressin
   G. Mineralocorticoid administration
   H. Glucocorticoid administration
   I. Diuretic therapy

Table 356-2

Causes of Severe Hypophosphatemia

Chronic alcoholism and alcohol withdrawal
Dietary deficiency
Ingestion of phosphate-binding antacids
Severe burns
Recovery from diabetic ketoacidosis
Hyperalimentation
Nutritional recovery syndrome
Respiratory alkalosis
Therapeutic hyperthermia
Neuroleptic malignant syndrome
Recovery from exhaustive exercise
Renal transplantation
Acute renal failure

content of skeletal muscle may occur because of the toxic effects of alcohol per se or because of a renal phosphate leak. In the case of ethanol, it is possible that negatively charged acetate ions, produced in the metabolism of ethanol, may enter the muscle cell and displace negatively charged phosphate ions from the cell. This, in conjunction with reduced capacity to reabsorb phosphate in the renal tubule, could well result in net phosphorus loss into the urine. The resulting phosphorus deficiency may cause a reduction of muscle magnesium and potassium and accumulations of calcium, sodium, chloride, and water. These findings are not necessarily associated with elevations of creatine phosphokinase activity that would reflect acute muscle damage. However, during withdrawal from alcohol, phosphorus is often taken up rapidly into skeletal muscle or liver, resulting in severe hypophosphatemia, and in this instance hypophosphatemia may precipitate acute rhabdomyolysis.

Most patients with diabetic ketoacidosis are not severely depleted of phosphorus. Although, on the one hand, metabolic acidosis and insulin deficiency mobilize intracellular phosphate stores and lead to their excretion into the urine, most patients have not been sick long enough for severe phosphorus deficiency to occur. On the other hand, patients with hypophosphatemia and hypokalemia, in the presence of severe diabetic ketoacidosis, are likely severely depleted of phosphorus and potassium and require treatment. The history usually shows that this type of patient with diabetic ketoacidosis has been sick for many days, has not had significant vomiting, has maintained a good intake of fluids, and has excreted phosphorus briskly for a period of many days, thus establishing severe deficiency. Such patients probably represent no more than 5 percent of cases of diabetic ketoacidosis.

MANIFESTATIONS The manifestations of phosphorus deficiency are listed in Table 356-3; many of these can occur simultaneously.

Phosphate trapping is an acute disorder resulting from reduction of intracellular inorganic phosphate concentration. The most common cause is administration of intravenous fructose. Fructose is metabolized by only three tissues in the body—the liver, the small bowel epithelium, and the proximal tubule of the kidney. When glucose is taken up into liver cells and phosphorylated by hexokinase, the resulting glucose-6-phosphate inhibits hexokinase, producing a smoothly regulated uptake of glucose that does not deplete or trap stores of inorganic phosphate. When fructose is administered intravenously, it is taken up into liver cells, where it is converted to fructose-1-phosphate by the enzyme fructokinase. Fructose-1-phosphate does not inhibit fructokinase, thus permitting rapid uptake of fructose into liver cells and consumption or trapping of available stores of inorganic phosphate.

malignancies may take up enough phosphate to cause hypophosphatemia. Deposition of bone mineral following parathyroidectomy also may be a cause (the "hungry bone syndrome"). Certain tumors secrete a substance that not only reduces renal tubular reabsorption of phosphorus but also reduces production of 1,25-dihydroxy vitamin D [1,25(OH)$_2$D] by the kidney, resulting in a condition called *oncogenic osteomalacia*. Reduction of vitamin D synthesis is paradoxical since hypophosphatemia usually increases D production. Benign, often small, mesenchymal tumors have usually been responsible. Fibrosarcomas, prostatic cancers, and possibly small cell cancers of the lung have been reported as additional causes. Removal of the tumor may be curative. Hypocalcemia consequent to saline infusion causes release of PTH. Thus volume expansion and PTH both reduce tubular reabsorption of phosphorus. A number of other conditions associated with chronic volume expansion may cause hypophosphatemia.

Severe hypophosphatemia is defined as phosphorus levels in serum below 0.3 mmol/L (1.0 mg/dL). Many of the conditions that result in such low levels are associated with prolonged hyperventilation with respiratory alkalosis or reflect rapid cellular uptake (Table 356-2). Respiratory alkalosis does not cause phosphorus deficiency but may reduce serum phosphorus values to 0.1 mmol/L (0.3 mg/dL) and urinary phosphorus excretion to virtually undetectable levels. Severe hypophosphatemia and severe total-body deficiency of phosphorus occur in patients with poor dietary intake who consume phosphate-binding antacids. Similarly, treatment of diabetic ketoacidosis results in hypophosphatemia. Reduction of serum phosphorus below 0.3 mmol/L (1.0 mg/dL) suggests, but does not prove, the existence of serious phosphorus depletion. In chronic alcoholics, reduction of phosphorus

Table 356-3

Hypophosphatemic Syndromes

Phosphate trapping	Leukocyte dysfunction
Rhabdomyolysis	Skeletal demineralization
Cardiomyopathy	Metabolic acidosis
Respiratory insufficiency	Nervous system dysfunction
Erythrocyte dysfunction	

Reduced intracellular phosphate concentration activates AMP deaminase and nucleotidase. The consequent reduction of adenylate compounds is reflected by increased uric acid production and hyperuricemia. Acute reduction of ATP, which is bound to magnesium, is heralded by a modest rise of magnesium in serum. Acute liver cell damage may occur. Disturbances of renal function also may occur after intravenous fructose. Hepatic and renal metabolic disturbances that follow fructose administration are preventable by infusing inorganic phosphate. Whether oral fructose affects intestinal epithelium in a similar manner is not known.

Rhabdomyolysis predictably occurs in chronic alcoholics who become acutely hypophosphatemic during the course of alcohol withdrawal. Hypophosphatemic rhabdomyolysis also occurs rarely during treatment for diabetic ketoacidosis, during the course of hyperalimentation, or while refeeding patients with malnutrition. In normal individuals, in contrast, acute hypophosphatemia does not appear to damage skeletal muscle, and rhabdomyolysis only occurs if there is preexisting muscle damage. Virtually all severe, chronic alcoholics have a subclinical myopathy characterized by biochemical abnormalities and ultrastructural damage. In these patients, the incidence and severity of rhabdomyolyis appear to be reduced if hypophosphatemia is prevented during realimentation.

Cardiomyopathy occurs in severe phosphorus depletion. The manifestations include reduction in cardiac output, hypotension, impaired pressor responsiveness to catecholamines, and a reduced threshold to ventricular arrhythmias. Patients in septic shock treated with catecholamines showed a 22 percent elevation of left ventricular stroke work index and a 12 percent elevation of systolic blood pressure without change of filling pressure when their hypophosphatemia [serum phosphorus below 0.6 mmol/L (2.0 mg/dL)] was treated by infusing 20 mmol (0.62 g) of elemental phosphorus over 60 min.

Respiratory insufficiency occurs in malnourished patients receiving intravenous nutrients with inadequate phosphorus who become progressively hypophosphatemic over 8 or 10 days. Profound weakness causes failure of diaphragm function, hypoxia, and respiratory acidosis. Despite severe hypophosphatemia, these patients rarely develop rhabdomyolysis, presumably because they had no preexistent muscle damage. The initial clue may be an inability to extubate a patient from a ventilator at the anticipated time. This syndrome is seldom seen in chronic alcoholics because rhabdomyolysis in such patients may correct hypophosphatemia spontaneously. Rapid correction of chronic respiratory acidosis also may cause hypophosphatemia and diaphragm weakness. In these patients, administration of phosphorus rapidly corrects muscle weakness and respiratory insufficiency. Fifty percent of patients with chronic obstructive pulmonary disease show abnormally low phosphorus content in both intercostal and peripheral skeletal muscle. This can be explained by chronic respiratory acidosis and/or the combined effects of treatment with glucocorticoids, xanthine derivatives, and diuretics.

Erythrocyte dysfunction is due to a decrease in 2,3-bisphosphoglycerate (2,3-BPG) content. The red cell is the only tissue in the body that produces this substance. Both 2,3-BPG and ATP facilitate dissociation of oxyhemoglobin and promote oxygen delivery to tissue. Reduced 2,3-BPG and ATP both enhance affinity of oxygen for hemoglobin and reduce tissue oxygenation. This mechanism may explain central nervous system dysfunction in hypophosphatemia. Hemolysis due to phosphorus deficiency probably does not occur.

Leukocyte dysfunction due to phosphorus deficiency results in impaired phagocytosis and opsonization. As a result, chronic hypophosphatemia increases susceptibility to bacterial and fungal infections.

Skeletal demineralization is an important effect of phosphorus deficiency, especially in patients with poor dietary intake who simultaneously ingest phosphate-binding antacids. Under conditions of increased bone turnover, in normal children or in adults with Paget's disease, hyperparathyroidism, or bony metastases, demineralization may occur at such a rate as to cause hypercalcemia. Osteopenia, bone pain, and a syndrome resembling osteomalacia occur in chronic phosphorus deficiency.

Phosphorus deficiency normally causes increased production of 1,25(OH)$_2$D by the kidney, which serves to increase intestinal absorption of phosphorus. In phosphorus-deficient normal volunteers, the normal rise of plasma 1,25(OH)$_2$D levels is reduced by superimposed metabolic acidosis by about 50 percent. One-half of the reduction is explained by increased metabolism of 1,25(OH)$_2$D and the remaining one-half by decreased vitamin D synthesis.

Metabolic acidosis may occur in children or adults with phosphorus deficiency due to vitamin D deficiency. Reduced phosphorus intake results in mobilization of hydroxyapatite from bone that serves to maintain normal levels of serum phosphorus. Hypercalciuria occurs normally as a result of phosphorus deprivation, which is also explained by hydroxyapatite mobilization. Severe hypophosphatemia has three important metabolic effects on the kidney. First, as hypophosphatemia becomes severe, inorganic phosphate excretion into the urine falls so that hydrogen excretion as NaH$_2$PO$_4$ into the urine is eliminated. Second, based upon experimental evidence, there is a marked reduction of the Na$^+$/H$^+$ antiporter activity in the proximal tubule, which by reducing H$^+$ secretion into the tubular lumen, prevents reabsorption of filtered HCO$_3$$^-$ ions. Third, phosphorus deficiency also decreases ammonia production. The reduction in ammonia production eliminates hydrogen excretion as ammonium ions (NH$_4$$^+$). Since excretion of hydrogen as phosphate buffer or ammonium accounts for nearly all the kidney's capacity to secrete acid, it is surprising that phosphorus deficiency is only rarely associated with metabolic acidosis. The explanation lies in the fact that mobilization of hydroxyapatite from bone provides carbonate ions, which, in turn, buffer the retained hydrogen ions that otherwise would be excreted in the urine. Under conditions in which hydroxyapatite cannot be mobilized during phosphorus deprivation (e.g., vitamin D deficiency, severe magnesium deficiency, perhaps aluminum poisoning, and experimentally by administration of colchicine), buffer cannot be mobilized adequately, and metabolic acidosis ensues.

Nervous system dysfunction is a distinctive and predictable feature of severe hypophosphatemia and phosphorus deficiency. This syndrome usually occurs in the setting of refeeding or hyperalimentation-induced hypophosphatemia that develops over the course of 8 to 10 days. Such patients become irritable and apprehensive and hyperventilate sufficiently to cause paresthesia and numbness. Profound muscular weakness is followed by dysarthria, confusion, obtundation, convulsive seizures, coma, and death. Alternatively, ascending motor paralysis with or without sensory disturbances may resemble the Guillain-Barré syndrome. In such cases, the cerebrospinal fluid is normal. Ophthalmoplegia, diplopia, and dysphagia suggest botulism, and poorly defined defects in color perception (metachromatopsia) suggests cerebral cortical dysfunction. In these patients, as in those with respiratory failure, spontaneous rhabdomyolysis does not occur despite severe hypophosphatemia.

Compared to normal persons of advanced age, patients with multiinfarct dementia or Alzheimer's type dementia show reduced concentrations of phosphorus and ionized calcium in cerebrospinal fluid. There is no known explanation for this observation.

℞ **TREATMENT**

Before initiating treatment for hypophosphatemia, the cause should be ascertained. Measurement of arterial pH and and blood gases of phosphorus concentration in the urine is helpful.

Milk is an excellent source of phosphorus, containing 33 mmol/L (100 mg/dL). Phosphate salts are also available for oral use. They are less likely to cause diarrhea in phosphorus-deficient patients than in a normal person. Phosphorus salts cannot be given by intramuscular or subcutaneous injection, but sodium phosphate and potassium phosphate are available for intravenous use. Intravenous sodium or potassium phosphate, 15 mmol (0.465 g of elemental phosphorus), given in 100 ml of 0.9% saline over 60 min elevated serum phosphorus from an average value of 0.6 to 1.2 mmol/L (1.75 to 3.8 mg/dL). The potassium salt should be given when hypokalemia and hypophosphatemia coexist. A safe dosage regimen for treatment of alcoholics who are hypophosphatemic, hypokalemic, and hypomagnesemic is the infusion each 8 to 12 h of 1 L of 0.5 normal NaCl in 5% glucose containing 9 mmol of potassium phosphate and 4.2 mmol $MgSO_4$ (2.0 mL of 50% $MgSO_4$ solution). Serum concentrations of potassium, magnesium, and phosphate should be monitored closely. Such infusions should be stopped when oral intake becomes possible.

PTH reduces renal tubular reabsorption of phosphorus by stimulating degradation of cyclic AMP to adenosine. Adenosine, in turn, inhibits Na^+/P_i transport. Dipyridamole inhibits adenosine uptake by the cell and reduces phosphaturia. Preliminary studies suggest that dipyridamole may be of use in treatment of PTH-mediated phosphaturia and familial hyperphosphaturic hypophosphatemia.

During treatment of hypophosphatemia, hyperphosphatemia should be avoided because it can cause severe hypocalcemia and crystal deposition in important structures, including blood vessels of the eye, lung, heart, and kidney. Fatal alveolar diffusion block has occurred, especially if the patient is alkalotic.

HYPERPHOSPHATEMIA

CAUSES   Defined in adults as an elevation of serum phosphorus above 1.67 mmol/L (5 mg/dL), hyperphosphatemia is a common finding with many causes (Table 356-4). Spurious hyperphosphatemia may occur in patients with thrombocytosis when blood is allowed to clot to obtain serum. Undelayed collection of plasma from heparinized samples will show lower values. Certain autoanalyzers cause spurious hyperphosphatemia because of chemical interference. Abnormal positively charged serum proteins, as in plasma cell dyscrasias, may cause marked elevations of phosphorus. In one instance, the serum concentration was 4.5 mmol/L (13.5 mg/dL), and each millimole of myeloma protein bound 15 molecules of phosphate.

Decreased renal excretion of phosphorus is the most common cause of hyperphosphatemia. Since PTH is phosphaturic, hyperphosphatemia is a cardinal feature of hypoparathyroidism, either as a primary disorder or in patients whose renal cyclic AMP response to PTH is abnormal (pseudohypoparathyroidism type I) or those whose phosphaturic response to PTH is suppressed (pseudohypoparathyroidism type II).

Of interest, severe hypomagnesemia causes marked suppression of PTH in plasma despite hypocalcemia but does not cause hyperphosphatemia. Hyperphosphatemia occurs in tumoral calcinosis, pseudoxanthoma elasticum, infantile hypophosphatasia, and hyperostosis because of decreased renal excretion. Untreated severe hyperthyroidism apparently increases cellular catabolism sufficiently to elevate serum phosphorus despite increased phosphorus loss in the urine. Acromegaly or administration of growth hormone causes modest hyperphosphatemia. Presumably, the higher phosphorus levels in children partly reflect growth hormone activity. Hyperphosphatemia occurs in untreated adrenal insufficiency because of volume contraction, metabolic acidosis, and possibly reduced glomerular permeability. Mild hyperphosphatemia may occur with bisphosphonate therapy because of increased tubular reabsorption of phosphorus.

Hyperphosphatemia, sometimes with levels up to 15 mmol/L (46 mg/dL), has occurred secondary to increased absorption from the gut following administration of excess phosphate salts by mouth or from the colon as a result of enemas that contain phosphorus. Overmedication with vitamin D and production of vitamin D by granulomatous tissue in diseases such as sarcoidosis and tuberculosis can cause hyperphosphatemia. Both acute metabolic and acute respiratory acidosis may decompose cellular organic phosphates, reduce phosphorylation, and result in diffusion of phosphorus from the cell and hyperphosphatemia. Lactic acidosis is especially important as a cause of hyperphosphatemia. Reduced insulin levels or clonidine administration also can cause hyperphosphatemia. Cellular release of phosphorus may cause hyperphosphatemia, particularly in rhabdomyolysis, infarction of other tissues, or hemolysis. The tumor lysis syndrome, usually seen in patients whose tumor responds briskly to chemotherapy, consists of hyperphosphatemia, hypocalcemia, hyperkalemia, metabolic acidosis, hyperuricemia, and, in many cases, acute renal failure. Severe hyperphosphatemia after intravenous infusion of phosphate salts is a particular danger in patients who are acidotic or oliguric. Finally, infusion of compounds containing phospholipids for parenteral nutrition has caused hyperphosphatemia.

Ⓡ TREATMENT

Hyperphosphatemia is potentially dangerous because of metastatic calcification. Before initiating treatment the cause should be identified and corrected whenever possible. Although only an approximate guide, a calcium-phosphorus product [serum Ca (mg/dL) X serum P (mg/dL)] greater than 70 indicates a potential threat of calcification. Calcification is more likely to occur in the presence of an elevated blood pH or an elevated level of serum PTH.

In the absence of renal insufficiency, hydration or volume expansion by the infusion of hypotonic saline increases the fractional clearance of phosphorus by the kidney. Aluminum-based antacids bind phosphorus in the lumen of the gastrointestinal tract and prevent its absorption. Although long-term use of these compounds may cause aluminum toxicity, short-term use may be very helpful in acute hyperphosphatemia. Hyperphosphatemia in the presence of renal insufficiency usually requires either peritoneal dialysis or hemodialysis.

Table 356-4

Causes of Hyperphosphatemia

Binding to serum proteins	**Internal redistribution**
Plasma cell dyscrasias	Acute metabolic acidosis
Decreased renal excretion	Lactic acidosis
Renal insufficiency	Acute respiratory acidosis
Hypoparathyroidism	Lactic acid infusion
Pseudohypoparathyroidism, types I	Reduced insulin level
and II	Clonidine administration
Tumoral calcinosis	**Cellular release**
Pseudoxanthoma elasticum	Rhabdomyolysis
Infantile hypophosphatasia	Organ infarction
Hyperostosis	Tumor lysis
Hyperthyroidism	Burkitt's lymphoma
Growth hormone activity	Lymphoblastic lymphoma
Adrenal insufficiency	Metastatic small cell carcinoma
Bisphosphonate therapy	Thyrotoxicosis
Increased intestinal absorption	Acute hemolysis
Phosphorus-containing cathartics	**Parenteral administration**
Vitamin D ingestion	Intravenous phosphate salts
Granulomatous diseases producing	Lipid (phospholipid) infusion
vitamin D	**Spurious hyperphosphatemia**
Sarcoidosis	Thrombocytosis
Tuberculosis	Hyperlipidemia

BIBLIOGRAPHY

AGARWAL R, KNOCHEL JP: Fluid and electrolyte disorders associated with alcoholism and liver disease, in *Fluid and Electrolytes*, 3d ed, JP Kokko, R Tannen (eds). Philadelphia, Saunders, 1996, p 449

BOLLAERT PE et al: Hemodynamic and metabolic effects of rapid correction of hypophosphatemia in patients with septic shock. Chest 107:1698, 1995

CAI Q et al: Brief report: Inhibition of renal phosphate transport by a tumor product in a patient with oncogenic osteomalacia. N Engl J Med 330:1645, 1994

DEMARCHI S et al: Renal tubular dysfunction in chronic alcohol abuse—effects of abstinence. N Engl J Med 329:1927, 1993

EMMETT M et al: The pathophysiology of acid-base changes in chronically phosphate-depleted rats. J Clin Invest 59:291, 1977

FERGUSON ER et al: Derangements of muscle composition, ion transport, and oxygen consumption in chronically alcoholic dogs. Am J Physiol 246:F700, 1984

FIACCADORI E et al: Hypophosphatemia and phosphorus depletion in respiratory and peripheral muscles of patients with respiratory failure due to COPD. Chest 105:1392, 1994

FULLER TJ et al: Reversible depression in myocardial performance in dogs with experimental phosphorus deficiency. J Clin Invest 62:1194, 1978

GREEN J et al: Acute phosphate depletion inhibits the Na$^+$/H$^+$ antiporter in a cultured renal cell line. Am J Physiol 265:F440, 1993

JOHNSON MA et al: Adenosine triphosphate turnover in humans. J Clin Invest 84:990, 1989

KNOCHEL JP: Central nervous system manifestations of hypophosphatemia and phosphorus depletion, in *Metabolic Brain Dysfunction in System Disorders*, AC Arieff, RC Griggs (eds). Boston, Little, Brown, 1992, chap 10, p 183

————: Hypophosphatemia and rhabdomyolysis. Am J Med 92:455, 1992

———— et al: Hypophosphatemia and phosphorus deficiency, in *The Kidney*, 5th ed, B Brenner, F Rector (eds). Philadelphia, Saunders, 1996, chap 25, p 1086

KOTANKO P: Hyperphosphatemia in multiple myeloma. N Engl J Med 326:1781, 1992

LEVI M et al: Disorders of phosphate and magnesium metabolism, in *Disorders of Bone and Mineral Metabolism*, FC Coe, MJ Favus (eds). New York, Raven Press, 1992, chap 28, p 587

LUTOMSKI DM et al: The effect of thrombocytosis on serum potassium and phosphorus concentrations. Am J Med Sci 307:255, 1994

MICHAUT P et al: Dipyridamole for renal phosphate leak? N Engl J Med 331:58, 1994

OSTER JR et al: Pathogenesis of hyperphosphatemia in lactic acidosis: Disparate effects of racemic (DL-) and levo (L-) lactic acid on plasma phosphorus concentration. Can J Physiol Pharmacol 63:1599, 1985

PORTALE AA et al: Metabolic acidosis reverses the increase in serum 1,25(OH)2D in phosphorus-restricted normal men. Am J Physiol 263:E1164, 1992

ROSEN GH et al: Intravenous phosphate repletion regimen for critically ill patients with moderate hypophosphatemia. Crit Care Med 23:1204, 1995

SUBHASH MN et al: Calcium and phosphorus levels in serum and CSF in dementia. Neurobiol Aging 12:267, 1991

THATTE L et al: Review of the literature: Severe hyperphosphatemia. Am J Med Sci 310:167, 1995

VEECH RL et al: Cystolic phosphorylation potential. J Biol Chem 254:6538, 1979

———— et al: Metabolic hyperpolarization of liver by ethanol: The importance of Mg^{2+} and H$^+$ in determining impermeant intracellular anionic charge and energy of metabolic reactions. Alcohol Clin Exper Res 18:1040, 1994

| 357 | *James P. Knochel* |

DISORDERS OF MAGNESIUM METABOLISM

Magnesium is the most abundant intracellular divalent cation. The total magnesium content of a normal man is 12.4 mmol (0.3 g) per kilogram of body weight. Of this, 1 percent is extracellular, 31 percent is in cells, and 67 percent is in bone. Serum magnesium ranges between 0.7 and 1.0 mmol/L (1.8 and 2.5 mg/dL). Of this, the unbound diffusible fraction is about 0.6 mmol/L (1.4 mg/dL). It exists in two forms in cells, one in solution in equilibrium with the diffusible form in plasma and a larger quantity bound to organic components. Since most magnesium inside cells is bound to ATP, MgATP is in equilibrium with free magnesium ions. Thus, shifts in free magnesium concentration may help regulate stores of ATP. From the opposite viewpoint, when the ATP concentration in cells is acutely reduced, e.g., by infusion of intravenous fructose, magnesium ions diffuse from the cell, and serum magnesium rises. Since ATP is critical to nearly all metabolic transformations, normal stores of magnesium are essential to sustain life.

The optimal intake of magnesium for an adult is 15 to 20 mmol/d (36 to 48 mg/d). Foods rich in magnesium include green vegetables, seed grains, nuts, peas, beans, and coca derivatives. Fresh meat, fish, and most fresh fruits contain relatively small amounts of magnesium. Magnesium is absorbed primarily in the jejunum and ileum, and healthy persons absorb about 30 to 40 percent of dietary magnesium. Absorption may increase to 70 percent when intake is low or magnesium deficiency exists. Vitamin D plays a minor role in magnesium absorption. When magnesium intake is restricted, fecal excretion becomes negligible, and urinary excretion decreases. Thus, magnesium retention by the kidney is very efficient. Magnesium excretion depends on glomerular filtration of the unbound fraction, of which 25 percent is reabsorbed in the proximal tubule and 50 to 60 percent is reabsorbed in the loop of Henle. Loop diuretics, such as ethacrynic acid, bumetanide, or furosemide, cause greater excretion of magnesium than do diuretics, such as thiazides, that act on the distal tubule. Magnesium excretion is increased when extracellular fluid volume is expanded by ingestion of water and salt, and aldosterone decreases reabsorption of magnesium by the renal tubule. Magnesium excretion increases sharply when the concentration in serum exceeds 0.8 mmol/L (2 mg/dL).

Slight hypomagnesemia occurs in athletically trained individuals, in hypermetabolic states such as pregnancy and cold acclimatization, and after administration of thyroid hormone.

MAGNESIUM DEFICIENCY

When any of the three major intracellular elements—magnesium, potassium, or phosphorus—is deprived or lost, deficiencies of the others usually follow. For this reason, deficiency of a single intracellular component almost never occurs. A diet devoid of magnesium causes depletion of phosphorus and potassium in skeletal muscle. Selective potassium deficiency may cause reductions in magnesium and phosphorus. Phosphorus deficiency may cause reductions in potassium and magnesium contents of tissue. The usual somatic responses to selective deprivation of one major intracellular element are anorexia, cellular atrophy, a negative nitrogen balance, and net loss of the other two major intracellular elements. Shrinkage of cell mass and expulsion of the elements not deprived help to maintain a normal intracellular composition.

During hyperalimentation a different situation prevails. Provision of a diet that is otherwise replete but deficient in one major intracellular element promotes an anabolic state, and newly synthesized protoplasm will be deficient in the deprived ion. Serious derangements of cellular composition ensue, including accumulations of sodium, chloride, calcium, and water. Indeed, elevation of cellular calcium may be an important cause of cellular injury in this situation by activating proteases and phospholipases.

As in deficiencies of other major intracellular elements, deficiency of body magnesium can be present when serum values are normal. In addition, certain tissues become deficient before others. The definition of a true deficit of an intracellular element is reduction of its ratio to nitrogen in the tissue. In muscle, this ratio is about 0.3 mmol (7 mg) magnesium per gram of nitrogen. Red cell magnesium content decreases consistently in magnesium deficiency, whereas muscle magnesium content may remain normal.

THE CLINICAL PHYSIOLOGY OF MAGNESIUM DEFICIENCY Within 3 to 7 days after reducing dietary magnesium intake to less than 0.5 mmol/d (12 mg/d), renal excretion of magnesium decreases to <0.5 mmol/d (12 mg/d). Anorexia, nausea, vomiting, lethargy, and weakness develop within weeks. Symptoms of severe magnesium deficiency, including paresthesia, muscular cramps, irritability, decreased attention span, and mental confusion, may require months to appear.

The physical findings are largely due to the associated hypocalcemia and include positive Trousseau and Chvostek signs, peculiar movements of the fingers best described as athetoid tetany, and, on occasion, convulsions. Fasciculations may be precipitated by a tap to muscle with a neurologic hammer. About half of patients with selective magnesium depletion become hypokalemic, the etiology of which is poorly understood. Aldosterone production may be enhanced, thus increasing potassium excretion into the urine. It is difficult to correct the potassium deficiency with supplemental potassium salts. However, correction of hypomagnesemia promptly reduces potassium excretion and corrects the hypokalemia. For this reason, it should be kept in mind that hypokalemia refractory to potassium supplements may be due to magnesium deficiency. Cardiac arrhythmias, disturbances of conduction, ventricular fibrillation, and cardiac arrest can occur in patients with coexisting hypokalemia and hypomagnesemia. Magnesium plays a critical role in maintenance of intracellular potassium concentration by regulating potassium movement through myocardial cell membranes. This property is known as *inward rectification*. In the sinus and atrioventricular nodule tissue, magnesium ions also affect transsarcolemmal calcium inflow and modulate intracellular handling of calcium in the sarcoplasmic reticulum. Indeed, the actions of magnesium resemble those of calcium channel blocking agents. Levels of magnesium below 0.7 mmol/L cause electrocardiographic changes similar to those of hypokalemia, including depression of ST segments, flattening of T waves, QT/QT$_c$ prolongation, and enhanced atrial and ventricular excitability; these changes in magnesium deficiency may be secondary to intracellular potassium deficiency. Either magnesium or potassium deficiency can cause a substantial reduction in myocardial Na,K-Mg-dependent ATPase. Since this enzyme is the site of digitalis binding, reduction in ATPase may explain the propensity for digitalis poisoning in both magnesium and potassium deficiency. In addition, magnesium deficiency itself increases the liklihood of cardiac arrhythmias. Because of QT prolongation, potentially dangerous arrhythmias, in particular torsade de pointes, are more likely to occur. The causes of magnesium deficiency are summarized in Table 357-1.

Hypocalcemia usually does not develop until serum magnesium falls below 0.5 mmol/L (1.2 mg/dL). Although mild magnesium deficiency may enhance release of parathyroid hormone (PTH), severe hypomagnesemia [levels below 0.4 mmol/L (1 mg/dL)] blocks release of PTH. In addition, magnesium deficiency impairs the normal calcemic response to PTH at the level of the skeleton. Hypocalcemia can become sufficiently severe to cause tetany. Although tetany has been reported in hypomagnesemia independently of hypocalcemia, both conditions usually coexist with this finding. In most cases the tetany with hypomagnesemia does not respond to infusions of calcium alone and requires correction of magnesium levels. In addition, the hypocalcemia may respond only to magnesium replacement, usually requiring 2 to 7 days for correction. When hypomagnesemia is caused by steatorrhea, administration of magnesium salts intravenously can cause prompt and sometimes marked release of PTH. In rare instances, acute hypercalcemia can occur.

GASTROINTESTINAL CAUSES OF MAGNESIUM DEFICIENCY Familial hypomagnesemia is manifested during childhood and is due to diminished absorption of dietary magnesium. The most common cause of magnesium deficiency in adults is intestinal malabsorption and steatorrhea, as in nontropical sprue, the short bowel syndrome, chronic pancreatic insufficiency, or biliary diversion. Because of unabsorbed fat, nonabsorbable magnesium–fatty acid soaps form in the intestinal lumen. When long-standing, hypomagnesemia is often associated with hypocalcemia, hypokalemia, and hypophosphatemia. Because of steatorrhea, malabsorption of fat-soluble vitamins, especially vitamins K, A, and D, may coexist. Vitamin D deficiency and osteomalacia can cause weakness due to proximal myopathy in association with pain in the lower back and hips. Secondary hyperparathyroidism, sometimes severe, almost always coexists.

Magnesium deficiency can also occur after ingestion of cellulose phosphate to reduce calcium absorption or after prolonged nasogastric suction in patients who have not received adequate magnesium supplementation. Acute hypomagnesemia, along with acute hypocalcemia, can occur in acute hemorrhagic pancreatitis when magnesium– and calcium–fatty acid soaps form in sites of tissue necrosis.

ENDOCRINE CAUSES OF HYPOMAGNESEMIA Hypomagnesemia occurs in poorly controlled diabetes mellitus and may be more severe after diabetic ketoacidosis. Moderate hypomagnesemia may occur in hyperparathyroidism, hypoparathyroidism, hyperthyroidism, and primary hyperaldosteronism. In primary hyperaldosteronism, aldosterone acts both directly and via volume expansion to enhance magnesium excretion. These effects can be reversed by spironolactone, triamterene, or amiloride. Hypomagnesemia may occur in patients

Table 357-1

Causes of Hypomagnesemia

I. Primary nutritional disturbances
   A. Inadequate intake
   B. Total parenteral nutrition
   C. Refeeding syndrome
II. Gastrointestinal disorders
   A. Specific absorptive defects
   B. Malabsorption syndromes
     1. Enteric fistulas
     2. Nontropical sprue
     3. Whipple's disease
     4. Intestinal lymphoma
     5. Chronic pancreatic insufficiency
     6. Biliary diversion
     7. Giardiasis
     8. Short bowel syndrome
   C. Prolonged diarrhea
   D. Prolonged nasogastric suction
   E. Pancreatitis
   G. Cellulose phosphate ingestion
III. Endocrine disorders
   A. Hyperparathyroidism
   B. Hypoparathyroidism
   C. Hyperthyroidism
   D. Primary hyperaldosteronism
   E. Bartter's syndrome
   G. Gitelman's syndrome
   H. Diabetic ketoacidosis
   I. Alcoholic ketoacidosis
IV. Cellular uptake or redistribution
   A. Administration of epinephrine
   B. Acute pancreatitis
   C. Following correction of respiratory acidosis
   D. "Hungry bone" syndrome after parathyroidectomy
   E. Massive blood transfusions
V. Chronic alcoholism, alcoholic withdrawal
VI. Increased renal excretion
   A. Ethanol ingestion
   B. Idiopathic
   C. Following renal transplantation
   D. Cyclosporine therapy
   E. Cisplatin therapy
   F. Aminoglycoside therapy
   G. Amphotericin B therapy
   H. Capreomycin therapy
   I. Viomycin therapy
   J. Syndrome of inappropriate vasopressin secretion (SIADH)
   K. Diuretic administration
     1. Furosemide
     2. Ethacrynic acid
     3. Bumetanide
     4. Acetazolamide
     5. Thiazides
     6. Chlorthalidone
     7. Osmotic agents
   J. Recovery phase of acute tubular necrosis
   K. Pentamidine therapy
   L. Theophylline toxicity
   M. Colony stimulating factor therapy

with the syndrome of inappropriate vasopressin secretion (commonly termed the syndrome of inappropriate antidiuretic hormone, SIADH) (see Chap. 330), presumably the result of increased aldosterone production and overexpansion of extracellular volume. Epinephrine and other potent beta agonists may cause transient hypomagnesemia as the result of uptake of magnesium into adipose tissue as fatty acids are released. Furthermore, release of fatty acids into the blood can cause the formation of insoluble fatty acid–magnesium and –calcium complexes in serum. If serum is centrifuged, the precipitates settle to the bottom of the tube, and spurious hypomagnesemia and hypocalcemia can be diagnosed. Hypomagnesemia has also been observed after multiple blood transfusions, possibly secondary to complex formation with sodium citrate. Transient hypomagnesemia occurs commonly after cardiopulmonary bypass surgery.

HYPOMAGNESEMIA ASSOCIATED WITH ALCOHOL- ISM Ethanol causes a transient loss of magnesium into the urine. Alcoholics with a reasonably normal nutrient intake and normal intestinal function usually have normal or only slightly depressed magnesium levels in blood. The total-body deficit of magnesium in chronic alcoholics is modest, amounting to 100 to 150 mmol (2.4 to 3.6 g). However, during alcohol withdrawal, hypomagnesemia may occur in association with acute hypophosphatemia and acute hypokalemia. Simultaneously, urinary excretion of magnesium, phosphate, and potassium decreases. Thus, hypomagnesemia occurs both because of net deficit and because of a shift into cells during withdrawal. In animals, sustained ethanol administration in intoxicating doses causes severe depletion of phosphorus, moderate depletion of magnesium and potassium, and increases in intracellular sodium, chloride, water, and calcium. Selective depletion of phosphorus also causes magnesium wasting and muscle magnesium deficiency. The same findings occur in muscle of severely alcoholic humans. In acute alcohol withdrawal, respiratory alkalosis and insulin release stimulated by administration of nutrients act in concert to move phosphate into cells. Increased ATP synthesis as a result of phosphate movement into cells may cause increased magnesium binding and worsen hypomagnesemia.

In alcoholic patients with intestinal malabsorption and steatorrhea, severe hypomagnesemia can be associated with hypocalcemia, hypophosphatemia, and hypokalemia. Although a relationship between hypomagnesemia and alcohol withdrawal seizures has been suggested, alcoholics in a withdrawal state also have prominent respiratory alkalosis, which lowers the threshold for seizure activity. Thus, the relationship of hypomagnesemia to seizures in this setting is not clear. Furthermore, correction of hypomagnesemia appears to have no favorable effect on the course of the alcohol withdrawal syndrome.

However, magnesium deficiency may play a role in the temporary hypertension that occurs during alcohol withdrawal. Independently of alcohol, magnesium deficiency causes accumulation of calcium in smooth muscle and increases vascular tone. Magnesium salts reduce arteriolar tone by reducing cytosolic calcium. Accumulation of calcium potentiates the pressor response to circulating catecholamines. Withdrawing alcoholics usually have elevations of circulating catecholamines and enhanced sympathetic nerve activity. Thus, the combined effects of magnesium depletion, calcium accumulation in cells, and elevated levels of catecholamines may cause the hypertension and explain the favorable effect of calcium channel blocking drugs under such circumstances.

MAGNESIUM DEFICIENCY DUE TO INCREASED RENAL EXCRETION Hypomagnesemia also can result from impaired renal tubular reabsorption, usually in association with renal potassium wasting and hypokalemia. Some patients, especially those with Bartter's syndrome, may be hypercalciuric. Gitelman's syndrome, resembling Bartter's syndrome, is also associated with hypokalemic metabolic alkalosis, hypermagnesuria, and hypomagnesemia, but calcium excretion is low. However, in these patients, calcium excretion is abnormally low. Transient hypomagnesemia due to reduced renal tubular reabsorption may follow renal transplantation.

Aminoglycosides, cisplatin, diuretics, foscarnet, and cyclosporine can cause magnesium wasting in the urine. Hypomagnesemia and hypokalemia as a result of impaired tubular reabsorption occur after prolonged aminoglycoside treatment, usually in patients who have received more than 8.0 g of the drug. Total recovery is the rule after the drug is stopped. Hypomagnesemia in patients treated with cisplatin can be severe; hypokalemia is less common. Renal tubular mitochondrial injury may be responsible. Even after cisplatin is withdrawn, the renal defect may persist indefinitely. Of interest, calcitriol may enhance magnesium wasting in patients with cisplatin nephrotoxicity who are also hypomagnesemic and hypocalcemic. About a fourth of patients treated with cyclosporine and prednisone after renal transplantation develop serum magnesium levels below 0.5 mmol/L (1.2 mg/dL). Although loop diuretics are potent magnesuric agents, hypomagnesemia is infrequent except in patients who receive large doses or who receive two or more diuretics that act at different sites in the nephron. Treatment with pentamidine, theophylline, and granulocyte-macro-

phage colony stimulating factor can on occasion cause hypermagnesuria and hypomagnesemia.

 TREATMENT

Treatment of hypomagnesemia should focus on correcting the cause. Hypomagnesemia due to inadequate dietary intake or to disorders that reduce intestinal absorption or cause excessive losses into the urine can often be corrected by oral administration of magnesium salts. Patients with potentially serious cardiac arrhythmias or with nausea and vomiting should be given intravenous magnesium sulfate. One mL of 50% magnesium sulfate heptahydrate ($MgSo_4\cdot 7\ H_2O$) contains 2.1 mmol (50 mg) of magnesium. The usual adult dose of magnesium sulfate is 2 mL of a 50% solution by mouth every 6 h on the first day and half this quantity for the following 3 to 4 days. Magnesium sulfate may be given intramuscularly, but this is painful and may cause elevation of creatine phosphokinase levels, reflecting muscle damage and thus blunting the value of measurements of the enzyme to detect rhabdomyolysis. When parenteral administration is indicated it is preferable to infuse magnesium in a dose of 4.2 mmol magnesium sulfate (1 g) every 6 h. Patients who require intravenous magnesium are often hypokalemic and hypophosphatemic. Potassium phosphate and potassium chloride may be included with magnesium sulfate in 0.5 N saline containing 5% glucose. The total potassium content in each infusion bottle should represent one-fourth of the daily requirement. In patients with adequate urine flow, such solutions can be given in a quantity of 750 mL every 6 h until nausea and vomiting cease and oral intake becomes possible. In patients with tetany due to magnesium deficiency, although hypocalcemia coexists, calcium is generally ineffective, and infusions of magnesium salts usually require 2 h or more to relieve the tetany. Up to a full day may be required for all signs of latent tetany, such as Chvostek and Trousseau signs, to disappear completely. Several oral preparations of magnesium salts are available. Thus, 5 mL of magnesium hydroxide–containing antacids (Maalox, Gelusil, Mylanta) contains 14 mmol (340 mg) of magnesium. However, there are two theoretical objections to the use of these preparations: they contain aluminum salts that may be hazardous if renal impairment is present, and they bind phosphate in the gut, which by itself promotes loss of magnesium. Other preparations include magnesium chloride tablets, magnesium gluconate tablets, and commercially available magnesium oxide powder. Since both spironolactone and triamterene cause retention of magnesium and potassium, these drugs may be useful adjuncts to maintain normal serum magnesium balance in patients taking diuretics.

The recommended dose of magnesium salts for treatment of torsade de pointes or ventricular arrhythmias is unsettled. In general, 4.0 mL of 50% $MgSO_4\cdot 7H_2O$ (8 mmol) may be safely infused over 1 to 2 min, which results in a serum magnesium concentration of 1.0 to 1.7 mmol/L (2.4 to 4.1 mg/dL). This is followed by infusions of 8 to 12 mmol/h (200 to 300 mg/h) for 4 to 8 h and smaller doses thereafter. Although this regimen may cause transient facial flushing and warmth, the resulting concentration in serum does not exceed 1.8 mmol/L (4.4 mg/dL). Magnesium salts should be administered with great caution in patients with renal insufficiency.

Several studies suggest that administration of magnesium salts to patients with acute myocardial infarction who are neither hypomagnesemic nor hypokalemic causes a reduction in mortality. However, in a more recent prospective study (ISIS-4) involving 58,050 patients who were given a loading dose of 8 mmol (200 mg) of magnesium followed by an additional 72 mmol (1800 mg) over the following 24 h, no benefit was observed. Thus, in the patient with uncomplicated myocardial infarction, there is no clear indication to administer magnesium.

Magnesium salts have also been proposed as an adjunct in the treatment of asthma to relax bronchial smooth muscle. There is not sufficient evidence at this time to establish efficacy of this treatment.

HYPERMAGNESEMIA

Patients with end-stage renal disease frequently have modest hypermagnesemia that is aggravated by ingesting magnesium-containing compounds such as antacids or cathartics. Surreptitious ingestion of magnesium salts as a cathartic can be diagnosed by demonstration of hypermagnesemia in serum and of fecal magnesium concentrations above 25 mmol/L (60 mg/dL). Rhabdomyolysis causes hypermagnesemia because of release from injured muscle. Adrenal insufficiency may cause hypermagnesemia. Half of patients with familial benign hypocalciuric hypercalcemia have hypermagnesemia. Pronounced hypermagnesemia [>6.5 mmol/L (16 mg/dL)] has been described in patients with near-drowning in the Dead Sea in Jordan or Basque Lake in British Columbia. Magnesium levels in water from these sources average 164 and 178 mmol/L (400 and 435 mg/dL), respectively. Survival in many near-drowning victims in the Dead Sea has been attributed to pronounced hypercalcemia because of the high calcium levels in this water.

Symptomatic hypermagnesemia is uncommon and is usually precipitated by inadvertent overdosage with magnesium salts or is deliberately induced to treat patients with eclampsia. Infants born of eclamptic mothers treated with magnesium may be hypermagnesemic. Magnesium can reduce neuromuscular transmission and act as a central nervous system depressant. Symptoms of hypermagnesemia correspond poorly to serum levels. However, the toxicity of any given level will be exaggerated in the presence of hypocalcemia, hyperkalemia, and uremia. Nausea and facial paresthesia usually appear between 2 and 4 mmol/L (5 and 10 mg/dL). Sedation, hypoventilation with respiratory acidosis, decreased deep tendon reflexes, and muscle weakness may appear at levels above 5 mmol/L (12 mg/dL). Hypotension, bradycardia, and diffuse vasodilatation appear at levels of 7.5 mmol/L. Areflexia, coma, and respiratory paralysis occur at higher levels. Patients treated for eclampsia must be observed very carefully for signs of magnesium intoxication. If this occurs, symptoms and findings can generally be reversed promptly by infusion of calcium salts, since these ions electrically oppose one another at their sites of action. Administration of saline and furosemide may help promote excretion of magnesium. Hemodialysis is also effective.

BIBLIOGRAPHY

ALFREY AC et al: Evaluation of body magnesium stores. J Lab Clin Med 84:153, 1974

AL-GHAMDI S et al: Magnesium deficiency: Pathophysiologic and clinical overview. Am J Kid Dis 24:737, 1994

ANDERSON R et al: Skeletal muscle phosphorus and magnesium deficiency in alcoholic myopathy. Miner Electrolyte Metab 4:106, 1980

BRITTON J: Dietary magnesium, lung function, wheezing, and airway hyperreactivity in a random adult population sample. Lancet 344:357, 1994

CLAUSEN T: Correlation between magnesium and potassium contents in muscle: Role of Na$^+$-K$^+$ pump. Am J Physiol 264:C457, 1993

CRONIN RE et al: Skeletal muscle injury after magnesium depletion in the dog. Am J Physiol 243:F113, 1982

D'ANGELO EKG et al: Magnesium relaxes arterial smooth muscle by decreasing intracellular Ca^{2+} without changing intracellular Mg^{2+}. J Clin Invest 89:1988, 1992

FAZEKAS T et al: Magnesium and the heart: Antiarrhythmic therapy with magnesium. Clin Cardiol 16:768, 1993

FERGUSON ER et al: Derangements of muscle composition, ion transport, and oxygen consumption in chronically alcoholic dogs. Am J Physiol 246:F700, 1984

FINE KD et al: Diagnosis of magnesium-induced diarrhea. N Engl J Med 324:1012, 1991

HAMPTON E et al: Intravenous magnesium therapy in acute myocardial infarction. Ann Pharmacother 28:212, 1994

ISIS-4 (FOURTH INTERNATIONAL STUDY OF INFARCT SURVIVAL) COLLABORATIVE GROUP: A randomised factorial trial assessing early oral captopril, oral mononitrate, and intravenous magnesium sulphate in 58,050 patients with suspected acute myocardial infarction: ISIS-4. Lancet 345:669, 1995

KNOCHEL JP: Hypophosphatemia in the alcoholic. Arch Intern Med 140:613, 1980

————: Hypophosphatemia and rhabdomyolysis. Am J Med 92:455, 1992

KROENKE K et al: The value of serum magnesium determination in hypertensive patients receiving diuretics. Arch Intern Med 147:1553, 1987

MCLEAN RM: Magnesium and its therapeutic uses: A review. Am J Med 96:63, 1994

PORATH A et al: Dead Sea water poisoning. Ann Emerg Med 18:121, 1989

RALSTON MA et al: Serum and tissue magnesium concentrations in patients with heart failure and serious ventricular arrhythmias. Ann Intern Med 113:841, 1990

SHILS ME: Experimental human magnesium depletion. Medicine 48:61, 1969

VICTOR M: The role of hypomagnesemia and respiratory alkalosis in the genesis of alcohol withdrawal symptoms. Ann NY Acad Sci 215:235, 1973

WEISS M et al: Should magnesium therapy be considered for the treatment of coronary heart disease? I. A critical appraisal of current facts and hypotheses. Magnesium Res 7:135, 1994

WHANG R: Magnesium homeostasis and clinical disorders of magnesium deficiency. Ann Pharmacother 28:220, 1994

---

358   *Stephen M. Krane*

PAGET'S DISEASE OF BONE

Paget's disease of bone (osteitis deformans) is usually focal but may be widespread. The initial event is excessive resorption of bone by osteoclasts, followed by the replacement of normal marrow by vascular, fibrous connective tissue. At some stage and to a variable degree, the resorbed bone is replaced by coarse-fibered, dense trabecular bone organized in haphazard fashion. The irregular and often rapid deposition of this new bone, to a great extent still lamellar, results in an increase in the number of prominent, irregular cement lines that give the bone its characteristic "mosaic" pattern. Most lesions show both excessive resorption and chaotic new bone formation.

INCIDENCE The prevalence is difficult to determine because the disease is often asymptomatic and is frequently detected when roentgenograms are obtained for other reasons or because of a high level of alkaline phosphatase on routine blood screening. On the basis of autopsy examination, the incidence is estimated to be about 3 percent in individuals over age 40; the likelihood of occurrence increases with age. The incidence varies in different parts of the world. Radiologic surveys indicate that the frequency in adults is less than 1 percent in the United States, Great Britain, and Australia. In India, Japan, the Middle East, and Scandinavia, the disease is rare.

ETIOLOGY The cause is unknown. No convincing evidence of endocrine abnormality has been produced. Likewise, although pagetic bone can be exceedingly vascular, the vascular abnormality may not be primary. Some of the manifestations can be suppressed with glucocorticoids, salicylates, and cytotoxic drugs, but there is no convincing evidence that the fundamental lesion is inflammatory. Intranuclear inclusions have been found by electron microscopy in osteoclasts in pagetic bone but not in osteoclasts or other bone cells in normal persons or patients with other bone diseases with the exception of pyknodysostosis. Some of the inclusions resemble nucleocapsids of viruses belonging to the measles group. Indirect immunofluorescence and immunoperoxidase studies using antibodies to measles virus suggest that the inclusions are indeed measles virus nucleocapsids. Measles virus nucleocapsid mRNA has been detected in some but not all in situ hybridization studies of bone cells from patients with Paget's disease, and measles virus nucleocapsid mRNA has been identified in bone marrow mononuclear cells using the polymerase chain reaction. The presence of mutations in specific regions of the viral genome is consistent with persistent infection. In some individuals with Paget's disease, osteoclasts and bone marrow mononuclear cells contain nucleocapsids of respiratory syncytial virus alone or in addition to nucleocapsids of measles virus, and in some areas of Britain canine distemper virus sequences have been identified in pagetic bone cells. Thus, different paramyxoviruses may have roles in the initiation or propagation of Paget's disease.

PATHOPHYSIOLOGY The characteristic feature is increased resorption of bone accompanied by an increase in bone formation, which is usually adequate to compensate. In the early phase bone resorption predominates (e.g., in the variant *osteoporosis circumscripta*), and the bones are very vascular. This has been termed the *osteoporotic, osteolytic,* or *destructive phase* of disease in which body calcium balance may be negative. Commonly, the excessive resorption is followed closely by formation of new pagetic bone. In this so-called mixed phase of the disease, the rate of bone formation is so geared to that of bone resorption that the magnitude of the increase in bone turnover is not reflected in the overall calcium balance.

As the activity decreases, the resorptive rate may decline progressively relative to formation, eventually leading to development of hard, dense, less vascular bone (the so-called *osteoplastic* or *sclerotic phase*) and a positive calcium balance. The rates of bone turnover may be increased enormously in the early phases of the disease, occasionally more than 20 times normal. Quantitative histomorphometry of bone biopsies confirms the extent of remodeling with marked increase in resorption surfaces and deep scalloped lacunae containing osteoclasts and increased numbers of osteoblasts lining the edges. Increased generation and overactivity of osteoclasts are considered the major abnormality. The osteoclasts are larger than normal and contain multiple pleomorphic nuclei. Increased numbers of osteoclast-like multinucleated cells are generated from hematopoietic precursors in long-term marrow cultures from individuals with Paget's disease compared with normal individuals. Production of the cytokine interleukin (IL) 6 by the pagetic bone and marrow cells is increased, and levels of the IL-6 receptor are high. Thus, IL-6 could act locally to contribute to the increased osteoclast formation. The calcification rate is also increased. The normal hematopoietic marrow is replaced by a loose stroma which may be highly vascular. The increase in bone turnover varies with the extent and activity of the disease. Bone turnover correlates with the increased plasma levels of bone alkaline phosphatase, which are higher in Paget's disease than in any other condition except for hereditary hyperphosphatasia. Although increased bone resorption enhances release of calcium and phosphate ions from bone, utilization of these ions for new bone formation and, presumably, feedback control of parathyroid hormone secretion usually maintain the concentration of calcium ions in the plasma at normal levels. The concentration of phosphate in the plasma is normal or slightly elevated. When the imbalance between bone formation and resorption favors resorption, as after prolonged immobilization or fractures, urinary calcium excretion may be increased, and on occasion hypercalcemia may occur. If, on the other hand, bone formation exceeds resorption (relatively uncommon), circulating levels of parathyroid hormone may be increased. Significant increases in trabecular bone resorption and osteoid surfaces in normal bone from patients with Paget's disease may be due to compensatory, secondary hyperparathyroidism. Resorption involves both the organic and mineral phases of bone. While the inorganic ions of the mineral phase are reutilized for bone formation, amino acids such as hydroxyproline and hydroxylysine and the hydroxypyridinium cross-link compounds are released during resorption of the collagen matrix of bone and are not reutilized for collagen biosynthesis. The increased urinary excretion of small peptides containing hydroxyproline reflects increased bone resorption. The pyridinium cross-link compounds pyridinoline (Pyr) and deoxypyridinoline (D-Pyr) are released from bone collagen during osteoclastic bone resorption and can be measured in urine by high-performance liquid chromatography and immunoassays. In some of the immunoassays the reacting antigen includes peptide sequences, whereas in others free Pyr or D-Pyr are measured. In Paget's disease measurement of the excretion of the bound forms correlates better with the extent and activity of the disease, and changes in excretion of the bound form are better indicators of responses to therapy than free Pyr or D-Pyr.

RADIOLOGIC CHANGES The radiologic findings reflect the underlying pathology and the phase of the disease that predominates at the time of the examination. The pelvic bones are most commonly involved, followed by the femur, skull, tibia, lumbosacral spine, dorsal spine, clavicles, and ribs; small bones are not as frequently diseased.

The lytic phase of the disease may be overlooked except when it occurs in the skull as osteoporosis circumscripta, with areas of sharply demarcated radiolucency in the frontal, parietal, and occipital bones. In the long bones, the lytic areas are usually first seen at one end and progress toward the other end with a V-shaped advancing edge. The lesion may cause expansion of the cortex and exhibit features suggesting malignancy. Usually lysis is followed by a zone of increased density, representing the new bone formation of the mixed phase of the disease. In general, the bone enlarges with an irregularly widened cortex in a coarse, striated pattern and with increased density, occasionally focal in distribution. Perpendicular lines of radiolucency (cortical infractions) are frequent and occur on the convex side of bowed long bones, particularly the femur and tibia. Transverse fractures may occur, some at the sites of these cortical infractions. The remodeling of the pagetic bone usually follows the lines of stress produced by muscle pull or gravity, accounting for the characteristic lateral bowing of the femur or anterior bowing of the tibia and the tendency for most of the dense bone to be deposited on the concave side of the bowed bone. In the mixed stage, there is enlargement and thickening of the skull, especially of the outer table, with irregular areas of increased density, often spotty (Fig. 358-1). Basilar invagination is common with involvement of the base of the skull. The changes in the pelvis reflect the varying degrees of bone resorption and new bone formation and are frequently accompanied by a characteristic thickening of the pelvic brim. In the sclerotic phase of the disease, the bone may show uniform increase in density, often in the absence of striations. This is common in the facial bones but occasionally occurs in the vertebrae, where a homogeneous, dense pattern gives an "ivory" appearance similar to that typical of Hodgkin's disease, although the involved vertebrae in Hodgkin's disease are not enlarged. Computed tomography and magnetic resonance imaging are useful in defining atypical lesions, particularly where neoplastic involvement is suspected. Technetium 99m diphosphonate bone scans are useful in documenting the extent of disease when therapy is contemplated or to confirm the diagnosis when radiologic findings are inconclusive.

CLINICAL PICTURE The clinical presentation is a function of the extent of the disease, the particular bones involved, and the presence of complications. Many patients are asymptomatic. In these

FIGURE 358-1 Lateral roentgenogram of the skull from a 58-year-old woman with Paget's disease of bone.

individuals the disorder is discovered during radiologic examination of the pelvis or spine for an unrelated disease or complaint or because of the finding of an elevated level of plasma alkaline phosphatase. Other individuals may gradually become aware of a swelling or deformity of a long bone or develop a disturbance in gait due to unequal length of the lower extremities. Enlargement of the skull is often not noticed by the patients, except by awareness of increasing hat size. Facial pain and headache are initial complaints in some; backache and leg pain are common. The pain is usually dull but may be shooting or knifelike. Back pain is most common in the lumbar region and may radiate into the buttocks or lower extremities. This pain can be due to the pagetic process itself, to distortion of articular facets, or to secondary osteoarthritis. Pain in the lower extremities may be associated with the transverse cortical infractions along the convex lateral surface of the femur or the anterior surface of the tibia. New lytic lesions detected on bone scan may be the most painful. Pain also may be due to involvement of the hip joint resembling degenerative joint disease and characterized by narrowing of the joint space, bony lipping at the margin of the acetabulum, and deepening of the acetabulum. Angioid streaks may be present in the retina. Hearing loss is due to direct involvement of the ossicles of the inner ear or of bone in the region of the cochlea or to impingement by bone on the eighth cranial nerve in the auditory foramen. More serious neurologic complications can result from overgrowth of bone at the base of the skull (platybasia) and compression of the brainstem. Compression of the spinal cord can cause paraplegia, particularly with involvement of the middorsal spine. Pathologic fractures of vertebrae also may produce spinal cord lesions.

COMPLICATIONS   Blood flow may be markedly increased in extremities involved with Paget's disease. There is proliferation of blood vessels in pagetic bone, but anatomic and functional studies have not confirmed the presence of arteriovenous fistulas. Although blood flow is increased in bone, cutaneous vasodilatation in the pagetic extremities accounts for the increased warmth noted clinically. When the disease is widespread, involving one-third or more of the skeleton, the increased blood flow may be associated with *high cardiac output* and rarely with high-output heart failure. However, heart disease in individuals with Paget's disease is usually due to the same conditions that occur in other patients of similar age. *Pathologic fracture* may occur at any stage but is more common in the destructive phase of the disease. In the weight-bearing bones fractures are often incomplete, multiple, and on the convex side of the bone. They may occur spontaneously or follow slight trauma; the lesions are painful but heal with no major disability. More serious fractures also may occur. Complete fractures are often transverse as if the bone were snapped like a piece of chalk. Under these circumstances the fracture may upset the delicate balance between bone formation and resorption in favor of resorption; the imbalance may cause increased urinary calcium excretion and in rare instances increased serum calcium level.

There is no characteristic level of urinary calcium excretion, although calcium excretion tends to be higher when the resorptive phase predominates, possibly accounting for the somewhat higher incidence of *urinary stones* in these patients. Secondary changes in the cartilage of the hip joints and knees may cause articular symptoms. Hyperuricemia and gout are common in men with Paget's disease, and calcific periarthritis may occur.

Sarcoma is the dread complication. The incidence is probably no greater than 1 percent, although higher incidence has been noted in series that include many patients with polyostotic involvement. The sarcomas most frequently arise in the femur, humerus, skull, facial bones, and pelvis and rarely in the vertebrae. Pagetic osteosarcomas are lytic in appearance on radiographs in contrast to the sclerotic appearance of radiation-induced osteosarcomas. In about 20 percent the tumors are multicentric. Fibrosarcomas and chondrosarcomas also have been found. Pain and swelling are the common complaints that lead to recognition of the sarcomas. The extent and character of the neoplastic involvement are established by computed tomography and/

or magnetic resonance imaging. The level of alkaline phosphatase in the serum of patients with sarcomas usually reflects the activity and extent of the Paget's disease. In occasional patients, an "explosive rise" of the phosphatase level may accompany the growth of the sarcoma, whereas in patients with limited Paget's disease, phosphatase levels may be only slightly elevated and give no clue to the development of the malignant lesion. The prognosis is poor following the development of sarcomas, and ablative surgery is rarely successful. In contrast to the successful treatment of some osteosarcomas in children, chemotherapy has little effect on survival of patients with pagetic osteosarcomas. Reparative granulomas resembling giant cell tumors may cause local destruction, but they do not metastasize.

℞ **TREATMENT**
Most patients require no treatment, since the disease is localized and does not cause symptoms. Indications for therapy include persistent pain in involved bones, neural compression, rapidly progressive deformity resulting in disabling disturbance of posture and/or gait, high-output congestive heart failure, hypercalcemia, severe hypercalciuria with or without formation of renal stones, repeated fractures or nonunion, and preparation for major orthopedic surgery. Nonsteroidal anti-inflammatory drugs such as *indomethacin*, 25 mg three or four times daily, may relieve pain, especially in the presence of hip involvement. Patients with severe hip or knee pain, unrelieved by analgesics and not responsive to therapy with agents that inhibit bone resorption, are candidates for total joint replacement. Results of the latter procedures are often excellent, although patients with Paget's disease have an increased risk of ectopic bone formation around the operative site. Osteotomies are also useful in patients with bowing deformities of the tibia. In patients who have undergone surgical procedures, early ambulation and adequate fluid intake are important to prevent the development of hypercalciuria and hypercalcemia.

Potent bisphosphonates can inhibit bone resorption and are safe and usually well tolerated. Cytotoxic drugs such as plicamycin and dactinomycin no longer have a place in therapy. Of the bisphosphonates etidronate, in dosages up to 20 mg/kg body weight per day, is moderately effective in reducing bone resorption and producing clinical improvement, but in many patients responses are incomplete. Furthermore, osteomalacia may occur as a complication of therapy. Etidronate is no longer the bisphosphonate of choice. The newer bisphosphonates such as alendronate, pamidronate, risendronate, and tiludronate are more potent than etidronate and do not produce mineralization defects. Two of these compounds, pamidronate for intravenous use and alendronate for oral administration, are approved for use in the United States. Alendronate is approximately 700-fold more potent than etidronate. All bisphosphonates act to inhibit bone resorption, possibly by adsorbing to the surface of the calcium/phosphate mineral phase of bone and inhibiting osteoclast function. Alternatively, the bisphosphonates may inhibit osteoclasts indirectly through actions on osteoblasts.

The bisphosphonates as a class are poorly absorbed from the gastrointestinal tract, and alendronate should be given orally with water after an overnight fast 30 to 60 min before breakfast; the dose is 40 mg/d for 6 months. Gastric irritability and rarely esophageal ulcerations may occur. Pamidronate is given intravenously at a dose of 30 mg/d as an infusion in 5% glucose in water or normal saline over 4 h on three successive days. Responses are usually rapid with decreases in urinary excretion of hydroxyproline and pyridinium cross-link compounds within days to weeks, followed by a fall in levels of serum alkaline phosphatase. Flulike symptoms accompanied by fever may occur but usually subside rapidly.

Patients given bisphosphonates should also be given daily calcium supplements of 1 to 1.5 g and approximately 400 IU of vitamin D. Clinical and biochemical improvement often lasts for more than a year after bisphosphonate therapy. Clinical evaluation and assessment of alkaline phosphatase levels at 3-month intervals are useful for assessing the need for retreatment. Radiographs at 6-month intervals may be indicated for evaluation of lytic lesions, which usually heal with these agents.

It is almost certain that calcitonin has been or will be replaced by bisphosphonates such as alendronate or pamidronate for primary treatment of severe disease, but calcitonin may still be useful in patients who cannot tolerate alendronate because of gastrointestinal side effects or who prefer to avoid intravenous therapy with pamidronate. The administration of porcine, salmon, and human *calcitonins* for prolonged periods to pagetic patients causes a decrease in plasma alkaline phosphatase and in urinary hydroxyproline excretion. Treatment with calcitonin causes variable decrease in bone pain due to suppression of the pagetic lesion, replacement of pagetic bone with normal lamellar bone, and an independent, centrally mediated analgesic effect. Calcitonin also induces improvement in neurologic symptoms and a decrease in elevated cardiac output. Some patients have not continued to respond to porcine and salmon calcitonins, possibly because of the development of neutralizing antibodies. These individuals usually continue to exhibit a satisfactory response to human calcitonin. In others, the development of secondary hyperparathyroidism has been postulated as the cause for a diminished response, although this cannot account for resistance in all cases. The calcitonins are probably most useful in patients with pain in areas of pagetic involvement not due to associated joint disease. The dose of salmon calcitonin is 50 to 100 MRC units daily given subcutaneously. In most cases, it is possible to reduce the dose to three times weekly. In severe cases, alkaline phosphatase levels decrease, but not to the normal range. The disorder relapses after weeks or months when the calcitonin is discontinued. Some patients develop a sensation of warmth and/or nausea 30 min to several hours after injection. This may occur after initiating treatment or after months or years of therapy. The etiology is unknown, but the symptoms may be severe enough to discontinue the medication. Nasal spray formulations of calcitonin can be administered at doses of 200 IU/d.

Although the bisphosphonates and calcitonins act primarily to decrease bone resorption, the rate of new bone formation subsequently falls. As a result, the state of high bone turnover is shifted to a state of lower turnover, where rates of formation and resorption are still apparently geared to each other. In this lower turnover state, collagen fibers of the bone matrix are deposited in a more orderly fashion similar to normal bone.

See Chap 61, Agents affecting calcification and bone turnover, in Goodman & Gilman's The Pharmacological Basis of Therapeutics, 9th ed, New York, McGraw-Hill, 1996.

BIBLIOGRAPHY

BONE HG, KLEEREKOPER M: Clinical review 39: Paget's disease of bone. J Clin Endocrinol Metab 75:1179, 1992

GARNERO P et al: Different effects of bisphosphonate and estrogen therapy on free and peptide-bound bone cross-links excretion. J Bone Mineral Res 10:641, 1995

HARINCK HIJ et al: Relation between signs and symptoms in Paget's disease of bone. Q J Med 226:133, 1986

HEALEY JH, BUSS D: Radiation and pagetic osteogenic sarcoma. Clin Orthop Rel Res 270:128, 1991

HUVOS AG et al: Osteogenic sarcoma associated with Paget's disease of bone: A clinicopathologic study of 65 patients. Cancer 52:1489, 1983

KHAN SA et al: Paget's disease of bone and unvaccinated dogs. Bone 19:47, 1996

LIN JH: Bisphosphonates: A review of their pharmacokinetic properties. Bone 18:75, 1996

MCDONALD DJ, SIM FH: Total hip arthroplasty in Paget's disease. J Bone Joint Surg 69A:766, 1987

MEE AP et al: Generation of multinucleated osteoclast-like cells from canine bone marrow: Effects of canine distemper virus. Bone 17:47, 1995

NAGANT DE DEUXCHAISNES C, KRANE SM: Paget's disease of bone: Clinical and metabolic observations. Medicine 43:233, 1964

REBEL A(ed): Symposium on Paget's disease. Clin Orthop 217:1, 1987

ROODMAN GR et al: Interleukin 6: A potential autocrine/paracrine factor in Paget's disease of bone. J Clin Invest 89:46, 1992

SINGER FR, KRANE SM: Paget's disease of bone, in Metabolic Bone Disease, LV Avioloi, SM Krane (eds). Philadelphia, Saunders, 1990, pp 546–615

SIRIS E et al: Comparative study of alendronate versus etidronate for the treatment of Paget's disease of bone. J Clin Endocrinol Metab 81:961, 1996

WALLACH S (ed): Paget's Disease of Bone. New York, Elsevier 1991, pp 1–313

359 *Stephen M. Krane, Alan L. Schiller*

HYPEROSTOSIS, FIBROUS DYSPLASIA, AND OTHER DYSPLASIAS OF BONE AND CARTILAGE

HYPEROSTOSIS

A number of disease states have in common an increase in the mass of bone per unit volume (hyperostosis) (Table 359-1). Such increase in bone mass is detected radiologically as increased density of the bone, often associated with disturbance in the architecture of the tissue. In the absence of quantitative histomorphometric data, it is usually not possible to distinguish an increase in bone mass due to excessive formation of new bone from that due to decreased resorption of bone already formed. When bone deposition is rapid, the new bone may be of the woven type, but if the process is more chronic, true lamellar bone is formed. The additional bone may be located at the periosteum, within the compact bone of the cortex, or in the trabeculae of the cancellous regions. In the medullary area, the new bone is deposited on and between the trabeculae and encroaches on the medullary spaces. Such responses are seen in areas adjacent to tumors or in association with infection. In some diseases, the increase in bone mass may be spotty, as in osteopoikilosis, whereas in others, most of the skeleton may be involved, as in the malignant form of osteopetrosis in children. The increase in mass usually is not due to an excessive amount of

Table 359-1

Causes of Hyperostosis

Endocrine disorders
  Primary hyperparathyroidism
  Hypothyroidism
  Acromegaly
Radiation osteitis
Chemical poisoning
  Fluoride
  Elemental phosphorus
  Beryllium
  Arsenic
  Vitamin A intoxication
  Lead
  Bismuth
Osteomalacia
  Renal tubular osteomalacia (vitamin D resistance or phosphate diabetes)
  Chronic renal glomerular failure
Osteosclerosis (localized) associated with chronic infection
Osteosclerotic phase of Paget's disease
Osteosclerosis associated with carcinomatous metastases, malignant lymphoma, and hematologic disorders (myeloproliferative disorders, sickle cell disease, leukemia, multiple myeloma, systemic mastocytosis)
Osteosclerosis of erythroblastosis fetalis
Osteopetrosis
  Infantile (malignant, autosomal recessive form)
  Adult (benign, dominant form)
  Intermediate form with carbonic anhydrase II deficiency and renal tubular acidosis
Unclassified disorders
  Pyknodysostosis
  Osteomyelosclerosis
  Hyperostosis corticalis generalisata
  Hyperostosis generalisata with pachydermia
  Hereditary hyperphosphatasia
  Progressive diaphyseal dysplasia (osteopathia hyperostotica multiplex infantilis; Camurati-Engelmann disease)
  Melorheostosis
  Osteopoikilosis
  Hyperostosis frontalis interna

mineral relative to matrix, except in disorders where islands of calcified cartilage may persist such as osteopetrosis. (The mineral density of calcified cartilage is greater than that of bone.) In some diseases, such as the osteosclerosis of untreated renal insufficiency, the bone mass and radiodensity may be increased, even though the new bone formed is poorly mineralized and contains widened osteoid seams. Although hyperostosis usually is due to decreased osteoclast function, dysfunction of osteoblasts can also occur. For example, an engineered null mutation of the osteocalcin gene in mice results in a higher bone mass due to increased bone formation without change in bone resorption. It is also of interest that infection of newborn mice produces an osteopetrosis-like phenotype in which osteoblast progenitors appear to induce increased bone formation. In human osteopetrosis of the relatively benign and sporadic type, viral nucleocapsid particles have been found in osteoclasts, and it is possible that viral infection accounts for the excessive bone mass.

Several of these conditions are discussed in more detail in other chapters, although some generalizations are pertinent. Bone that is denser than normal may be seen in the osteitis fibrosa associated with hyperparathyroidism. When the hyperparathyroidism is successfully treated, an abrupt decrease in the rate of bone resorption may lead to the development of areas of bone density greater than in the surrounding skeleton, especially in the healing of brown tumors. In addition, intermittent low levels of parathyroid hormone act directly on osteoblasts to increase bone formation. In hypothyroidism, the rates of both bone formation and resorption may be decreased, but when the balance is in favor of formation bones are of increased density but normal architecture. Increased bone density also occurs in some instances of osteomalacia associated with disturbances in renal tubular function. The increased mass of bone is accompanied by widened osteoid seams, as in untreated chronic renal glomerular insufficiency. In the vertebral bodies the bone appears denser in transverse bands at the upper and lower margins, with a relatively radiolucent center. This "sandwich" appearance is similar to that in osteopetrosis and has been termed by the British the *rugger jersey sign*. Skeletal hyperostosis, including cortical hyperostoses, periostitis, and tendon and ligament ossification, is also a complication of long-term therapy with synthetic retinoids such as isotretinoin.

OSTEOPETROSIS Osteopetrosis (Albers-Schönberg or marble bone disease) is clinically, biochemically, and genetically heterogeneous. Although osteopetrosis has many causes, a defect in bone resorption is always the underlying mechanism. Several inherited forms of osteopetrosis occur in rodents, some of which can be cured by bone marrow transplantation from a normal littermate and are probably due to stem cell defects. The osteopetrosis in *op/op* mice and in *tl/tl* toothless rats is not cured by bone marrow transplantation, however. These animals have few osteoclasts, and those that are present appear to be defective. The *op/op* mice have a defect in the coding region of the gene for colony stimulating factor 1 (CSF-1, also known as M-CSF, the M standing for macrophage), and the skeletal defects in these animals and in *tl/tl* rats can be reversed by treatment with CSF-1. Another form of osteopetrosis has been produced in mice by targeted disruption of the *c-src* gene, which is normally expressed at high levels in osteoclasts; these *src −/−* mice have osteoclasts on bone surfaces but fail to form a ruffled border at the bone-resorbing surface of the cells. Disruption of the c-*fos* gene results in osteopetrosis in which osteoclasts are absent. Human homologues of these rodent diseases have not been described, but the most severe osteopetrosis in human infants is also due to defects in the formation and/or function of osteoclasts. Infantile osteopetrosis is an autosomal recessive trait that is manifested in utero and progresses after birth with anemia, hepatosplenomegaly, hydrocephalus, cranial nerve involvement, and death, often due to infections. Transplantation of bone marrow from normal donors to provide normal osteoclast precursor cells has been successful in several patients, in whom osteopetrotic bone was repopulated with donor osteoclasts that produced radiologic and/or bone-biopsy evidence

of bone resorption. One infant received a bone marrow transplant from a brother and had a successful response lasting more than 4 years, although vision was not restored. In other individuals with osteopetrosis, peripheral blood monocyte function is defective. Attempts to stimulate osteoclast formation and/or activity with calcitriol or recombinant interferon γ have resulted in some clinical improvement.

Less fulminant forms of osteopetrosis occur in older children and adults. In some the disorder appears to be sporadic, and in others the osteopetrosis is inherited as an autosomal dominant trait and progresses with age; anemia is not as severe, neurologic abnormalities are not as frequent, and recurrent pathologic fractures are the main feature. Although most common in infants and children, the diagnosis may be made in adults when roentgenograms are obtained because of fractures or unrelated diseases. There is no sex predilection. The inherited adult disorder is heterogeneous. Type I is characterized by increased thickness of the cranial vault, whereas the rugger jersey sign and "endo bones" in the pelvis are features of type II. A defect in modeling of endosteal bone is present in both types, and the remodeling of trabecular bone is also defective in type II osteopetrosis.

An "intermediate" form of autosomal recessive osteopetrosis has been described in kindreds in which the skeletal abnormality is associated with renal tubular acidosis and cerebral calcification. This form is compatible with long survival and is associated with profound impairment of one of the isoenzymes of carbonic anhydrase (carbonic anhydrase II). Carbonic anhydrase II is a major component of the system that generates the acid environment adjacent to the ruffled border of the osteoclast, and deficiency of the enzyme impairs bone resorption. In some instances islands of unresorbed calcified cartilage are encased in bone. The defect in remodeling results in disorganization of bone structure, with thickened cortices and lack of funnelization of metaphyses. Despite increased density, the bone may be abnormal mechanically and can fracture readily. Osteomalacia or rickets is sometimes a component of osteopetrosis in children (Fig. 359-1).

The histologic changes are reflected in roentgenograms (Fig. 359-2), which reveal uniformly dense, sclerotic bone, often with no distinction between the cortical and cancellous regions. In the severe infantile form, there is persistence of the primary spongiosa with central calcified cartilage cores surrounded by woven bone. Osteoclasts may be increased in number but apparently do not function properly. Osteoclasts may be morphologically normal or have loss of the ruffled borders, suggesting that a spectrum of changes may occur. The variability may reflect heterogeneity in this syndrome, as in the osteopetrosis in rodents. The long bones are usually involved, with increased density along the entire shaft. Foci of increased density in the epiphyses may correspond to regions of unresorbed calcified cartilage. The metaphyses have a characteristic clubbed or splayed appearance. Alternating horizontal bands of increased and decreased density in the long bones and vertebrae suggest that the defect is intermittent during periods of growth. The skull, pelvis, ribs, and other bones may be involved. The phalanges and the distal humerus are usually spared.

Encroachment of bone on the marrow cavity, particularly in the severe infantile disorder, is associated with anemia of the myelo-

FIGURE 359-1 Lateral roentgenogram of the thorax of a 9-month-old boy with the "malignant" form of osteopetrosis. Note the uniform increase in mineral density of the vertebral bodies and the marked flaring of the ends of the ribs (*arrows*), indicative of rickets.

FIGURE 359-2 Roentgenogram of the spine and pelvis of a 55-year-old man with the more benign, dominant form of osteopetrosis.

phthisic type with extramedullary hematopoiesis in liver, spleen, and lymph nodes and enlargement of these organs. Neurologic abnormalities caused by encroachment on cranial nerves include optic atrophy, nystagmus, papilledema, exophthalmos, and impairment of extraocular muscles. Facial paralysis and deafness are frequent; trigeminal lesions and anosmia are less common. In infants, macrocephaly, hydrocephalus, and convulsions may occur, and infections such as osteomyelitis are frequent. Renal tubular acidosis is a feature of the osteopetrosis associated with a deficiency in carbonic anhydrase II.

In the less severe forms, about half of patients have no symptoms, and the disorder is discovered incidentally on roentgenograms. Others present with fractures, bone pain, osteomyelitis, and cranial nerve palsies.

Fractures may occur with trivial trauma. Healing of such fractures is usually slow but satisfactory. When the disease is manifested first in adult life, fractures may be the only clinical problem. Levels of calcium and alkaline phosphatase in the plasma are usually normal in adults, but hypophosphatemia and moderate hypocalcemia may occur in children. Serum acid phosphatase levels are usually increased.

The skeletal defect is not the same in all forms of osteopetrosis, and genetic and biochemical heterogeneity are common. As mentioned, in children with severe osteopetrosis, bone marrow transplantation from HLA-identical siblings has resulted in histologic and radiologic increases in bone resorption and variable improvement in anemia, vision, hearing, and growth and development.

Unfortunately, it is not always possible to find appropriate donors, or patients may not be good candidates for bone marrow transplantation. In patients with the lethal forms of the disorder, calcitriol therapy is associated with the appearance of osteoclasts with normal ruffled borders and other evidence for increased bone resorption.

PYKNODYSOSTOSIS *Pyknodysostosis* is an autosomal recessive form of osteosclerosis that superficially resembles osteopetrosis. It is one of the types of short-limbed dwarfism associated with bone fragility and a tendency to fracture with minimal trauma. Nevertheless, life span is usually normal. In addition to a generalized increase in bone density, features include short stature, separated cranial sutures, hypoplasia of the mandible, kyphoscoliosis and deformities of the trunk, persistence of deciduous teeth, progressive acroosteolysis of the terminal phalanges, high, arched palate, proptosis, blue sclerae,

and a pointed, beaked nose. Patients usually present because of frequent fractures. The responsible gene is located on chromosome 1q21 and encodes cathepsin K, a cysteine proteinase that is expressed in normal osteoclasts and that is mutated in patients with pynknodystostosis.

OSTEOMYELOSCLEROSIS *Osteomyelosclerosis* is a disorder in which the marrow cells are replaced by diffuse fibroplasia, occasionally accompanied by osseous metaplasia and increased skeletal density on roentgenograms. In early stages woven bone may be found in intratrabecular locations, whereas in more advanced stages, woven bone is observed in the medulla. The disorder is probably a phase in the course of the myeloproliferative disorders and is characteristically accompanied by extramedullary hematopoiesis.

Hyperostosis corticalis generalisata (van Buchem's disease) is characterized by osteosclerosis of the skull (base and calvaria), lower jaw, clavicles, and ribs and thickening of the diaphyseal cortices of the long and short bones. Alkaline phosphatase levels in the serum are elevated, and the disorder may be due to increased formation of bone of normal structure. The major manifestations are due to neural compression and consist of optic atrophy, facial paralysis, and perception deafness. In *hyperostosis generalisata with pachydermia* (Uehlinger), the sclerosis is due to increased formation of subperiosteal spongy bone and involves the epiphyses, metaphyses, and diaphyses. Pain, swelling of joints, and thickening of the skin of the lower arms are common.

HEREDITARY HYPERPHOSPHATASIA This disorder is characterized by structural deformities of the skeleton with increased thickness of the calvaria, increased density at the base of the skull, and widening and loss of normal architecture of the shafts and the epiphyses of the long and short bones. The failure to deposit normal bone and the haphazard orientation of lamellae suggest active remodeling that resembles that of Paget's disease. Osteoclasts with multiple nuclei characteristic of Paget's disease and the typical "mosaic" pattern of faceted units of lamellar bone are not found, however. Levels of plasma alkaline phosphatase and urinary excretion of hydroxyproline peptides and other collagen degradation products are increased. The disorder is apparently inherited as an autosomal recessive trait. Calcitonin therapy may be of value.

PROGRESSIVE DIAPHYSEAL DYSPLASIA A disorder in which a symmetric thickening and increased diameter of the diaphyses of long bones occurs, particularly in femurs, tibias, fibulas, radii, and ulnas, has been termed *progressive diaphyseal dysplasia* (Camurati-Engelmann disease). Pain over affected areas, fatigue, abnormal gait, and muscle wasting are the major manifestations. Serum alkaline phosphatase levels may be elevated, and, on occasion, hypocalcemia and hyperphosphatemia may be found. Other abnormalities include anemia, leukopenia, and an elevated erythrocyte sedimentation rate. Clinical and biochemical improvement may result from the use of glucocorticoids.

MELORHEOSTOSIS This rare condition usually begins in childhood and is characterized by a slowly progressive linear hyperostosis in one or more bones of one limb, usually in a lower extremity. All segments of the bone may be involved, with sclerotic areas that have a "flowing" distribution. The involved limb is often extremely painful. Soft tissue masses, not connected to bone, are often mineralized and are composed of osseous or cartilaginous tissue. Other types of soft tissue masses are associated with joint contractures or consist of fibrofatty, lymphatic, or vascular tissue.

OSTEOPOIKILOSIS This benign autosomal dominant trait is usually discovered by chance. It is characterized by dense spots of trabecular bone less than a centimeter in diameter, usually of uniform density, located in the epiphyses and adjacent parts of the metaphyses. All bones may be involved except the skull, ribs, and vertebrae.

HYPEROSTOSIS FRONTALIS INTERNA *Hyperostosis frontalis interna* is an abnormality of the inner table of the frontal bones of the skull consisting of smooth, rounded enostoses covered by dura and projecting into the cranial cavity. These enostoses are usually less than 1 cm at their greatest diameter and usually do not extend posteriorly beyond the coronal suture. The abnormality is found almost exclusively in women, who are frequently obese, hirsute, and have a variety of neuropsychiatric complaints (Morgagni-Stewart-Morel syndrome). The disorder also occurs in women with no obvious illness or particular associated disease. The finding in the skull may be a manifestation of a generalized metabolic disorder.

FIBROUS DYSPLASIA (McCUNE-ALBRIGHT SYNDROME)

The bony lesions of fibrous dysplasia are characterized by proliferation of fibroblast-like cells that in some areas have features of osteoblasts, with production of an extracellular matrix that may be calcified and have the appearance of woven bone. In other areas the cells have features of chondrocytes and produce a cartilage-like extracellular matrix. The lesions of fibrous dysplasia are usually focal and have a radiolucent appearance; they may be monostotic or polyostotic. The disorder occurs with equal frequency in both sexes. Some individuals have distinctive areas of skin pigmentation and precocious puberty (McCune-Albright syndrome). These diverse manifestations are the consequence of postzygotic mutations in the gene encoding the regulatory $G_{\alpha s}$ proteins.

Incidence The monostotic form is the most common type of fibrous dysplasia. The lesions can be asymptomatic, can be associated with local pain, or can predispose to pathologic fracture. Most of the lesions are in the ribs or in the craniofacial bones, especially the maxillas. Other bones that may be affected include metaphyseal or diaphyseal portions of the proximal femurs or tibias. Monostotic fibrous dysplasia is most often diagnosed between 20 and 30 years of age. There are usually no associated skin lesions. Approximately one-quarter of the individuals with the polyostotic form have more than half the skeleton involved by disease. One side of the body may be affected, and the lesions may be distributed segmentally in a limb, particularly in the lower extremities. Craniofacial lesions are present in approximately half of patients with the polyostotic form. Whereas the monostotic form is usually detected in young adults, fractures and skeletal deformities occur in childhood in the polyostotic form; early-onset disease is generally more severe. Lesions, especially monostotic lesions, can become quiescent at puberty and worsen during pregnancy. McCune-Albright syndrome (polyostotic fibrous dysplasia, multiple café au lait spots, and sexual precocity) is more common (10:1) in females. Short stature is due to premature closure of the epiphyses.

Pathology The skeletal lesions of the various forms of fibrous dysplasia are similar, although cartilaginous elements are more common in the polyostotic form. The marrow cavity is filled by gritty, gray-pink, rubbery tissue that replaces the normal cancellous bone. Often, the endosteal cortical surface is scalloped. Histologically, the lesions contain benign-appearing fibroblastic tissue arranged in a loose whorled pattern (Fig. 359-3). The grittiness is due to the presence in the fibrous tissue of irregularly arranged woven bone spicules, most of which lack osteoblastic palisading or rimming but which may contain prominent cement lines. In approximately 10 percent of cases islands

FIGURE 359-3 Photomicrograph of the lesion of fibrous dysplasia. Note spicules of dark-staining woven bone (WB) surrounded by loose fibroblastic tissue.

FIGURE 359-4 Roentgenogram of the upper extremity from a 33-year-old woman with fibrous dysplasia of bone. Typical lesions involve the entire humerus as well as the scapula and proximal ulna.

of hyaline cartilage are present, and myxoid tissue may predominate in young patients. Examination by polarized light and with the use of special stains indicates a contiguity of collagen fibers of the osseous and marrow tissue. In the polyostotic form, cystic degeneration may be characterized by the presence of hemorrhage, with hemosiderin-containing macrophages and osteoclast-type giant cells in the periphery of the cyst. Malignant transformation of either monostotic or polyostotic fibrous dysplasia occurs with a frequency of less than 1 percent. The malignant change is usually detected in the third or fourth decade in individuals who have had lesions first identified in childhood. In about one-third of the cases the neoplasms arise in previously irradiated lesions. Ossifying fibroma of long bones is a peculiar fibroosseous cortical lesion that may be a variant of fibrous dysplasia. It is most common in the tibial shaft in teenagers. Although benign, the lesion has a tendency to recur if not adequately excised.

Radiologic Changes The roentgenographic appearance of the lesions is that of a radiolucent area with a well-delineated, smooth or scalloped border, typically associated with focal thinning of the cortex of the bone (Fig. 359-4). Fibrous dysplasia and Paget's disease of bone can cause bones to become larger than normal. The lesions of fibrous dysplasia are not usually cysts in the strict sense, since they are not fluid-filled cavities. They occasionally appear multiloculated. The ground-glass appearance is due to the thin spicules of calcified woven bone. Deformities can include coxa vara, shepherd's-crook deformity of the femur, bowing of the tibia, Harrison's grooves, and protrusio acetabuli. Involvement of facial bones, usually with lesions of increased radiodensity, may create a leonine appearance (leontiasis ossea). Fibrous dysplasia of the temporal bones can cause progressive loss of hearing and obliteration of the external ear canal. Advanced skeletal age in girls is correlated with sexual precocity but can occur in boys without sexual precocity. The lesions tend to spare the epiphyseal regions before puberty, but in older individuals fibrous dysplasia may develop in the epiphyses. Occasionally, a focus of fibrous dysplasia may undergo cystic degeneration with an enormous distortion of the shape of the bone and mimic the so-called aneurysmal bone cyst.

Clinical Picture The clinical course is variable. Skeletal lesions are usually detected because of localized pain, deformities, or fractures. Other symptoms ascribable to bone involvement are headache, seizures, cranial nerve abnormalities, hearing loss, narrowing of the external ear canal, or even spontaneous scalp hemorrhages if there is craniofacial bone disease. On rare occasions the onset of sexual precocity is the first clinical manifestation of the McCune-Albright syndrome. Serum calcium and phosphorus values are usually normal. In approximately one-third of patients with the polyostotic form, bone turnover is increased, as reflected in high levels of serum alkaline phosphatase and increased urinary excretion of collagen breakdown products. In some subjects high cardiac output resembles that in extensive Paget's disease. Widespread disease is usually evident when the disorder is detected, whereas widespread disease usually does not develop when the disease is mild at the outset.

The cutaneous pigmentation in most patients with McCune-Albright syndrome consists of isolated dark-brown to light-brown macules that tend to be located on one side of the midline (Fig. 359-5). The border is usually, although not always, irregular or jagged ("coast of Maine"), in contrast to the smooth borders of the pigmented macules of neurofibromatosis ("coast of California"). As a rule, there are fewer than six of the lesions, which range in size from 1 cm to very large lesions, covering areas such as the back, buttocks, or sacral regions. When the lesions are in the scalp, the overlying hair may be more deeply pigmented than the other hair. Localized alopecia is associated with osteomas of the skin, and such lesions tend to overly skeletal lesions. The pigmentation also tends to be on the same side as the skeletal lesions and actually to overlie them. Occasionally, neurofibromatosis and fibrous dysplasia coexist.

Sexual precocity occurs more commonly in girls than in boys (see also Chaps. 336 and 337). Premature vaginal bleeding and development of axillary and pubic hair and of breasts are the usual features. In the few ovaries that have been examined, no corpora lutea have been seen. When measurements have been reported, the girls have high estrogen levels and low or undetectable gonadotropins. Estrogen receptors have been detected in the bone lesions, and it is therefore not surprising that precocious puberty is not limited to patients with cranial involvement. The characteristic pigmented macules are usual but not invariable. Hyperthyroidism occurs with increased frequency, and rare associations include Cushing's syndrome, acromegaly, hypogonadotropic hypogonadism, and soft tissue myxomas. Hypophosphatemic osteomalacia also may accompany fibrous dysplasia and resembles the disorder associated with other skeletal and nonskeletal tumors. Sexual precocity and adrenal and thyroid hyperfunction in association with fibrous dysplasia are due to autonomous end-organ activity, not to pituitary or hypothalamic dysfunction. Thus, luteinizing hormone (LH) and follicle-stimulating hormone (FSH) levels are low, do not show the expected early pubertal nocturnal rise, and are not responsive to luteinizing hormone–releasing hormone (LHRH). Furthermore, continuous treatment with LHRH agonists does not suppress gonadal steroid secretion or reverse sexual precocity.

As mentioned earlier, this disorder is due to postzygotic mutations in the genes encoding $G_{\alpha s}$ proteins. These mutations cause constitutive activation of the cyclic AMP–protein kinase A signal transduction pathway. Such postzygotic mutations are mosaic and are not present in all cells. In the monostotic disorder, the $G_{\alpha s}$ mutations are present only in the skeletal lesions, whereas with more extensive disease, the mosaicism is more generalized. It has been proposed that the constitutively activated $G_{\alpha s}$ proteins trigger increased expression of the c-*fos* proto-oncogene in bone cells. Animals that overexpress a c-*fos* transgene develop skeletal lesions that resemble those of fibrous dysplasia. It is of interest that the error in Albright's hereditary osteodystrophy (pseudohypoparathyroidism) is the opposite of that found in the McCune-Albright syndrome (fibrous dysplasia). In the former, inactivating mutations in $G_{\alpha s}$ proteins result in *deficient* activity and decreased responsiveness to hormones that function through cyclic AMP–mediated signal transduction pathways.

Although the lytic lesions of fibrous dysplasia resemble the brown tumors of hyperparathyroidism, the age of the patient, normal calcium levels, increased density of bone in the skull, and areas of cutaneous pigmentation identify the former condition. Fibrous dysplasia and hyperparathyroidism may coexist, however. Neurofibromas may involve bone and produce cutaneous pigmentation as well as nodules in the skin. The pigmented macules of neurofibromatosis are more numerous and more widely distributed than in fibrous dysplasia, usually have smooth borders, and tend to involve areas such as the axillary folds. Other lesions that have roentgenographic features similar to those of isolated fibrous dysplasia are unicameral bone cysts, aneurysmal bone cysts, and nonossifying fibromas. Leontiasis ossea is most often due to fibrous dysplasia, although other disorders also may produce this appearance, such as craniometaphyseal dysplasia, hyperphosphatasia, and, in adults, Paget's disease.

℞ TREATMENT

Fibrous dysplasia is not curable. The skeletal lesions, however, can be improved by orthopedic procedures such as casting, osteotomy with internal fixation, curettage, and bone grafting, depending on the lesion and the age of the patient. Indications for such procedures include progressive deformity, nonunion of fractures, and pain unresponsive to conservative treatment. Calcitonin may be effective in treatment of widespread disease associated with bone pain and high serum alkaline phosphatase levels (see Chap. 358).

OTHER DYSPLASIAS OF BONE AND CARTILAGE

A variety of diseases of bone and cartilage have been called *dystrophies* or *dysplasias*. The *osteochondrodysplasias* are heritable disorders of connective tissue that are characterized by primary abnormalities of cartilage that lead to disturbances in cartilage and bone growth and development. They comprise several hundred distinct entities, which can be distinguished on the basis of clinical, genetic, and radiologic features. The molecular defects in a number of these disorders have been identified utilizing positional cloning and screening of candidate genes. Several of the disorders are due to mutations in collagen genes (see also Chap. 348). For example, mutations in *COL2A1*, the gene that encodes type II collagen, have been identified in Stickler syndrome, Kniest dysplasia, chondrodysplasias associated with osteoarthritis, and spondyloepiphyseal dysplasia. A deletion in *COL10A1*, the gene that encodes type X collagen, has been identified in the Schmid form of metaphyseal chondrodysplasia. A mutation in *COL9A2*, the gene that encodes one chain of the type IX collagen heterotrimer, has been identified in another variant of the Stickler syndrome. Mutations in genes that encode other extracellular matrix proteins can also cause chondrodysplasia. For example, the gene that encodes cartilage oligomeric matrix protein (COMP), a relative of thrombospondin, is the site of mutations in pseudochondrodysplasia. In the Jansen type of chondrodysplasia, a mutation in the PTH receptor gene causes constitutive activity of the receptor, manifested by disordered growth plates and hypercalcemia. Eventually, it should be possible to classify these

FIGURE 359-5 Typical pigmented café au lait lesion of the skin in an 11-year-old boy with polyostotic fibrous dysplasia. The border has the jagged "coast of Maine" appearance that is characteristic of McCune-Albright's syndrome. Note that the lesion is limited to one side (left) of the body.

disorders on the basis of the genetic and biochemical defects. At present, however, a useful clinical classification has been formulated by Rubin based on the consideration of errors in modeling of bone and cartilage (Table 359-2). Other clinical and genetic features form the basis of a classification by Rimoin. Pathologic processes in the skeletal dysplasias may be expressed as a deficiency (hypoplasia) or excess (hyperplasia) in relation to normal development.

SPONDYLOEPIPHYSEAL DYSPLASIA The *spondyloepiphyseal dysplasias* are disorders in which abnormalities of growth occur in various bones, including the vertebrae, pelvis, carpal and tarsal bones, and the epiphyses of tabular bones. On the basis of roentgenographic findings, this group can be divided into (1) those with generalized platyspondyly, (2) those with multiple epiphyseal dysplasias, and (3) those with epiphysometaphyseal dysplasias. *Morquio's syndrome*, in which there is a defect in degradation of glycosaminoglycans (therefore, a "mucopolysaccharidosis"), is inherited as an autosomal recessive trait and is associated with corneal opacities, dental defects, variable disturbances in intellect, and increased urinary excretion of keratosulfate; it belongs in the first group (see also Chap. 347). Other forms of spondyloepiphyseal dysplasia, some of which are accounted for by defects in type II collagen, may not be recognized until late in childhood or young adult life. Flat vertebral bodies are associated with other abnormalities in shape and alignment. The disordered development of the capital femoral epiphyses leads to irregularities in shape and flattening of the femoral heads and early onset of osteoarthritis of the hips.

ACHONDROPLASIA *Achondroplasia* is a physeal dysplasia in which dwarfism results from a decrease in the proliferation of cartilage in the growth plate. This disorder is among the more common types of dwarfism and is inherited as an autosomal dominant trait, although most cases are sporadic and due to new mutations. Histologic sections through the growth plate show a thin zone of cartilage cells with absence or abbreviation of the normal columnar arrangement and

Table 359-2

Working Classification of Bone Dysplasias

Epiphyseal dysplasias
  Epiphyseal hypoplasias
    Failure of articular cartilage: spondyloepiphyseal dysplasia congenita and tarda
    Failure of ossification of center: multiple epiphyseal dysplasia congenita and tarda
  Epiphyseal hyperplasia
    Excess of articular cartilage: dysplasia epiphysialis hemimelica
Physeal (growth plate) dysplasias
  Cartilage hypoplasias
    Failure of proliferating cartilage: achondroplasia congenita and tarda
    Failure of hypertrophic cartilage: metaphyseal dysostosis congenita and tarda
  Cartilage hyperplasias
    Excess of proliferating cartilage: hyperchondroplasia
    Excess of hypertrophic cartilage: enchondromatosis
Metaphyseal dysplasias
  Metaphyseal hypoplasias
    Failure to form primary spongiosa: hypophosphatasia congenita and tarda
    Failure to absorb primary spongiosa: osteopetrosis congenita and tarda
    Failure to absorb secondary spongiosa: craniometaphyseal dysplasia congenita and tarda
  Metaphyseal hyperplasia
    Excessive spongiosa: familial exostosis
Diaphyseal dysplasias
  Diaphyseal hypoplasias
    Failure of periosteal bone formation: osteogenesis imperfecta congenita and tarda
    Failure of endosteal bone formation: idiopathic osteoporosis
  Diaphyseal hyperplasias
    Excessive periosteal bone formation: Engelmann's disease
    Excessive periosteal bone formation: hyperphosphatasia

zone of provisional calcification, although endochondral ossification may not be completely disorganized. Formation of the primary spongiosa is reduced, since there is often a transverse bar of bone sealing off the plate from further endochondral ossification. Formation and maturation of the secondary ossification centers and articular cartilage are not disturbed. Appositional growth at the metaphysis continues, with resulting flare in this region of the bone; intramembranous bone formation at the periosteum is normal. The abnormal proliferation at the growth plate, leaving other areas relatively unaffected in the tubular bones, causes production of short bones that are proportionately thick. The length of the spine is almost always normal. The appearance of short limbs, particularly the proximal portions, with a normal trunk is characteristically accompanied by a large head, a saddle nose, and an exaggerated lumbar lordosis. The disease is usually recognized at birth. Those who survive infancy usually have normal mental and sexual development, and life span may be normal. Spinal deformity nevertheless may lead to a cord compression and nerve root encroachment, especially in those with kyphoscoliosis. Homozygous achondroplasia is a more serious disorder and a cause of neonatal death.

The gene for achondroplasia has been mapped to chromosome 4p, and the responsible gene encodes the fibroblast growth factor (FGF) receptor 3 (FGFR3). The responsible mutation causes the substitution of an arginine for a glycine in the transmembrane domain of FGFR3 and is believed to cause a gain of function, implying that FGF normally acts via the FGFR3 to inhibit chondrocyte proliferation in the growth plate. Indeed, construction of a null mutation in the *FGFR3* gene in mice causes increased growth in the physis. Mutations in other domains of the *FGFR3* gene have been described in lethal thanaphoric dwarfism. In several types of the so-called craniosynostosis syndromes (Pfeiffer, Crouzon, Jackson-Weiss, and Apert syndromes), mutations have been identified in the *FGFR1* or *FGFR2* genes.

ENCHONDROMATOSIS (DYSCHONDROPLASIA, OLLIER'S DISEASE) This is also a disorder of the growth plate in which the hypertrophic cartilage is not resorbed and ossified normally. It results in masses of cartilage with disorderly arrangement of the chondrocytes showing variable proliferative and hypertrophic changes. These masses are located in the metaphyses in close association with the growth plate in children but may be diaphyseal in teenagers and young adults. The disorder is usually recognized in childhood by the appearance of deformities or retardation in growth. The most common sites of involvement are the ends of long bones, usually in the region where rate of growth is most marked. The pelvis is often involved, but ribs, sternum, and skull are seldom affected. There is also a tendency toward unilateral involvement. Chondrosarcoma develops occasionally in the enchondromata. Granulosa cell tumors of the ovary may occur. The association of enchondromatosis and cavernous hemangiomata in the soft tissues including the skin is known as *Maffucci's syndrome*.

MULTIPLE EXOSTOSES (DIAPHYSEAL ACLASIS OR OSTEOCHONDROMATOSIS) This is a disorder of the metaphysis, inherited as an autosomal dominant character, in which areas of the growth plate become displaced, presumably by growing through a defect in the perichondrium or so-called ring of Ranvier. The spongiosa forms within the mass as vessels invade the cartilage. Therefore, the diagnostic radiographic finding is the direct continuity of the mass to the marrow cavity of the parent bone with absence of underlying cortex. Usually the growth of these exostoses ceases when growth of the adjacent plate ceases. The lesions may be solitary or multiple and are usually located in the metaphyseal areas of long bones, with the apex of the exostosis directed toward the diaphysis. Often the lesions produce no symptoms, but occasionally, interference with the function of a joint or tendon or compression of nerves may result. Dwarfism may occur. The metacarpals may be shortened, resembling those seen in Albright's hereditary osteodystrophy. Multiple exostoses are sometimes seen in patients with pseudohypoparathyroidism.

An exostosis may suddenly begin to enlarge long after growth should have ceased, and rarely, chondrosarcomas may develop from the cartilage cap of an exostosis. Although pregnancy may stimulate growth of an exostosis that clinically may mimic malignancy, the lesion merely undergoes exuberant endochondral ossification and cartilage hyperplasia without malignant changes.

A gene that covers a chromosomal breakpoint has been identified in two families with multiple exostoses. The *EXT* gene probably functions normally as a tumor suppressor, and mutations in *EXT* could contribute both to the development of the exostoses and to malignant transformation to chondrosarcoma that sometimes occurs.

RELAPSING POLYCHONDRITIS   See Chap. 326.
TIETZE'S SYNDROME (COSTOCHONDRAL SYNDROME)   See Chap. 326.

BIBLIOGRAPHY

HYPEROSTOSIS

BENLI IT et al: Epidemiological, clinical and radiological aspects of osteopoikilosis. J Bone Joint Surg 74B:504, 1992

BOLLERSLEY J et al: Structural and histomorphometric studies of iliac crest trabecular and cortical bone in autosomal dominant osteopetrosis: A study of two radiological types. Bone 10:19, 1989

BYERS PH et al: Research perspectives in heritable disorders of connective tissue. Matrix 12:333, 1992

CAUDLE RJ et al: Melorheostosis of the hand: A case report with long-term follow-up. J Bone Joint Surg 69A:1229, 1987

CHAN Y-L et al: Dialysis osteodystrophy: A study involving 94 patients. Medicine 64:296, 1985

COINDRE JM et al: Histomorphometric analysis of sclerotic bone from idiopathic myeloid metaplasia (nine cases). J Pathol 144:163, 1984

CRISP AJ, BRENTON DP: Engelmann's disease of bone—a systemic disorder? Ann Rheum Dis 41:183, 1982

DiGIOVANNA JJ et al: Extraspinal tendon and ligament calcification associated with long-term therapy with etretinate. N Engl J Med 315:1177, 1986

EDELSON JG et al: Pycnodysostosis: Orthopedic aspects with a description of 14 new cases. Clin Orthop 280:263, 1992

EINHORN TA et al: Hyperphosphatasemia in an adult: Clinical, roentgenographic, and histomorphometric findings and comparison to classical Paget's disease. Clin Orthop 204:253, 1986

GENANT HK et al: Osteosclerosis in primary hyperparathyroidism. Am J Med 59:104, 1975

GOLDMAN AB et al: Case report 778. Skeletal Radiol 22:206, 1993

JACCOBSON HG: Dense bone—too much bone: Radiological considerations and differential diagnosis, part II. Skeletal Radiol 13:97, 1985

JOHNSON CC et al: Osteopetrosis: A clinical, genetic, metabolic and morphologic study of the dominantly inherited benign form. Medicine 47:149, 1968

KAPLAN FS et al: Successful treatment of infantile malignant osteopetrosis by bone-marrow transplantation. J Bone Joint Surg 70A:617, 1988

KRAEMER KH et al: Prevention of skin cancer in xeroderma pigmentosum with the use of oral isotretinoin. N Engl J Med 318:1633, 1988

KUIVANIEMI H et al: Mutations in collagen genes; causes of rare and some common diseases in humans. FASEB J 5:2052, 1991

SHAPIRO F et al: Variable osteoclast appearance in human infantile osteopetrosis. Calcif Tissue Int 43:67, 1988

SHELDON J et al: Engelmann's disease (progressive diaphyseal dysplasia): A review and presentation of two cases with abnormal phosphate retention. Metab Bone Dis Rel Res 2:307, 1981

SILVE C: Hereditary hypophosphatasia and hyperphosphatasia. Curr Opin Rheumatol 6:336, 1994

SINGER FR: Osteopetrosis. Semin Nephrol 12:191, 1992

SLY WS et al: Carbonic anhydrase II deficiency in 12 families with the autosomal recessive syndrome of osteopetrosis with renal tubular acidosis and cerebral calcification. N Engl J Med 313:139, 1985

THOMPSON RC JR et al: Hereditary hyperphosphatasia. Am J Med 47:209, 1969

VAN BUCHEM FSP et al: Hyperostosis corticalis generalisata. Am J Med 33:387, 1962

WHYTE MP, MURPHY WA: Osteopetrosis and other sclerosing bone disorders, in *Metabolic Bone Disease*, LV Avioloi, SM Krane (eds). Philadelphia, Saunders, 1990, pp 616–658

WULFSBERG EA et al: Chondrodysplasia punctata: A boy with X-linked recessive chondrodysplasia punctata due to an inherited X-Y translocation with a current classification of these disorders. Am J Med Genet 43:823, 1992

FIBROUS DYSPLASIA

ALBRIGHT FA et al: Syndrome characterized by osteitis fibrosa disseminata, areas of pigmentation and endocrine dysfunction, with precocious puberty in females. Report of five cases. N Engl J Med 216:727, 1937

BENEDICT PH et al: Melanotic macules in Albright's syndrome and in neurofibromatosis. JAMA 205:618, 1968

CANDELIERE GA et al: Increased expression of the c-fos proto-oncogene in bone from patients with fibrous dysplasia. N Engl J Med 332:1546, 1995

GRABIAS SL, CAMPBELL CJ: Fibrous dysplasia. Orthop Clin North Am 8:771, 1977

HARRIS WH et al: The natural history of fibrous dysplasia: An orthopaedic, pathological and roentgenographic study. J Bone Joint Surg 44A:207, 1962

RINGEL MD et al: Clinical implications of genetic defects in G proteins. The molecular basis of McCune-Albright syndrome and Albright hereditary osteodystrophy. Medicine 75:171, 1996

STEPHENSON RB et al: Fibrous dysplasia. An analysis of options for treatment. J Bone Joint Surg 69A:409, 1987

WEINSTEIN LS et al: Activating mutations of the stimulatory G protein in the McCune-Albright syndrome. N Engl J Med 325:1688, 1991

YABUL SM et al: Malignant transformation of fibrous dysplasia. A case report and review of the literature. Clin Orthop 281, 1988

OTHER DYSPLASIAS OF BONE AND CARTILAGE

AHN J et al: Cloning of the putative tumour suppressor gene for hereditary multiple exostoses (EXT1). Nature Genet 2:137, 1995

AKESON WH et al: *Symposium on Heritable Disorders of Connective Tissue.* St. Louis, Mosby, 1982

ERLEBACHER A et al: Toward a molecular understanding of skeletal development. Cell 80:371, 1995

GELB BD et al: Pycnodysostosis, a lysosomal disease caused by cathepsin K deficiency. Science 273:1236, 1996

LEE B et al: Identification of the molecular defect in a family with spondyloepiphyseal dysplasia. Science 244: 978, 1989

MULVIHILL JJ: Craniofacial syndromes: No such thing as a single gene disease. Nature Genetics 9:101, 1995

RIMOIN DL: The chondrodystrophies. Adv Hum Genet 5:1, 1975

RUBIN P: *Dynamic Classification of Bone Dysplasias.* Chicago, Year Book, 1964

SAMBROOK PN et al: Synovial complications of spondylepiphyseal dysplasia of late onset. Arthritis Rheum 31:282, 1988

SHIANG R et al: Mutations in the transmembrane domain of FGFR 3 cause the most common genetic form of dwarfism, achondroplasia. Cell 78:335, 1994

SILLENCE DO et al: Neonatal dwarfism. Pediatr Clin North Am 25:431, 1978

WICKLUND CL et al: Natural history study of hereditary multiple exostoses. Am J Med Genet 55:43, 1995

COLOR ATLASES

I. Atlas of Dermatology

    A. Common Skin Diseases and Lesions

    B. Cutaneous Neoplasms

    C. Pigmented Lesions—Benign and Malignant

    D. Infectious Disease and the Skin

    E. Immunologically Medicated Skin Disease

    F. Skin Manifestations of Internal Disease

II. Atlas of Endoscopic Findings

III. Atlas of Funduscopic Examination

IV. Atlas of Hematology

I. Atlas of Dermatology

Stephen F. Templeton / Thomas J. Lawley

A. Common Skin Diseases and Lesions

IA-1 **Acne vulgaris** with inflammatory papules, pustules, and comedones

IA-2 **Acne rosacea** with prominent facial erythema, telangiectasias, scattered papules, and small pustules

IA-3 **Psoriasis** is characterized by small and large erythematous plaques with adherent silvery scale.

IA-4 **Atopic dermatitis** with excoriated, lichenified plaques in the popliteal fossa

IA-5 **Dyshidrotic eczema,** characterized by deep-seated vesicles and scaling on palms and lateral fingers, is often associated with an atopic diathesis.

IA-6 **Seborrheic dermatitis** showing central facial erythema with overlying greasy, yellowish scale

IA-7 **Stasis dermatitis** showing erythematous, scaly, and oozing patches over the lower leg. Several stasis ulcers are also seen in this patient.

IA-8 **Allergic contact dermatitis,** acute phase, with sharply demarcated, weeping, eczematous plaques in a perioral distribution

IA-9 **Lichen planus** showing multiple flat-topped, violaceous papules and plaques. Nail dystrophy as seen in this patient's thumbnail may also be a feature.

IA-10 **Pityriasis rosea** Multiple round to oval erythematous patches with fine central scale are distributed along the skin tension lines on the trunk.

IA-11 **Vitiligo** in a typical acral distribution demonstrating striking cutaneous depigmentation, as a result of loss of melanocytes

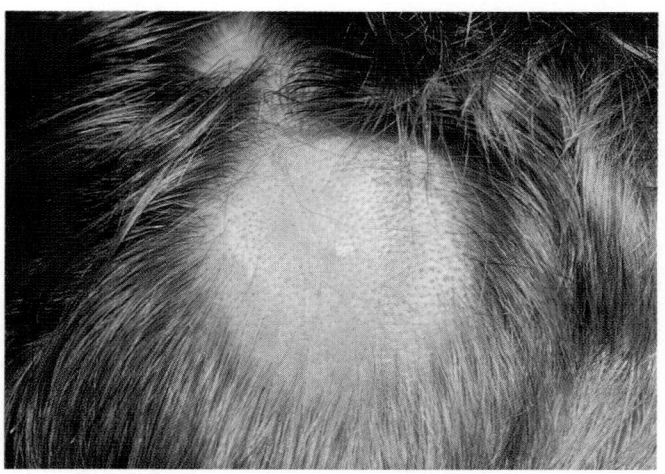

IA-12 **Alopecia areata** characterized by a sharply demarcated circular patch of scalp completely devoid of hairs. Follicular orifices are preserved, indicating a nonscarring alopecia.

IA-13 **Urticaria** showing characteristic discrete and confluent, edematous, erythematous papules and plaques

IA-14 **Epidermoid cysts** Several inflamed and noninflamed firm, cystic nodules are seen in this patient. Often a patulous follicular punctum is observed on the overlying epidermal surface.

IA-15 **Seborrheic keratoses** are seen as "stuck on," waxy, verrucous papules and plaques with a variety of colors ranging from light tan to black.

IA-16 **Keloids** resulting from ear piercing, with firm exophytic flesh-colored to erythematous nodules of scar tissue.

IA-17 **Cherry hemangiomas** are very common and arise in middle-aged to older adults. They are characterized by multiple erythematous to dark-purple papules usually located on the trunk.

B. Cutaneous Neoplasms

IB-18 **Actinic keratoses** consist of hyperkeratotic erythematous papules and patches on sun-exposed skin. They arise in middle-aged to older adults and have some potential for malignant transformation.

IB-19 **Keratoacanthoma** is a low-grade squamous cell carcinoma that presents as an exophytic nodule with central keratinous debris.

IB-20 **Basal cell carcinoma** showing central ulceration and a pearly, rolled, telangiectatic tumor border

IB-21 **Squamous cell carcinoma** seen here as a hyperkeratotic crusted and somewhat eroded plaque on the lower lip. Sun-exposed skin such as the head, neck, hands, and arms are other typical sites of involvement.

IB-22 **Kaposi's sarcoma** in a patient with AIDS demonstrating patch, plaque, and tumor stages

IB-23 **Mycosis fungoides** is a cutaneous T cell lymphoma, and plaque stage lesions are seen in this patient.

IB-24 **Non-Hodgkin's lymphoma** involving the skin with typical violaceous, "plum-colored" nodules

IB-25 **Metastatic carcinoma** to the skin is characterized by inflammatory, often ulcerated dermal nodules.

IC-26 **Nevus**   Nevi are benign proliferations of nevomelanocytes characterized by regularly shaped hyperpigmented macules or papules of a uniform color.

IC-27 **Dysplastic nevi** are irregularly pigmented and shaped nevomelanocytic lesions that may be associated with familial melanoma.

IC-28 **Superficial spreading melanoma** is the most common type of malignant melanoma and demonstrates color variegation (black, blue, brown, pink, and white) and irregular borders.

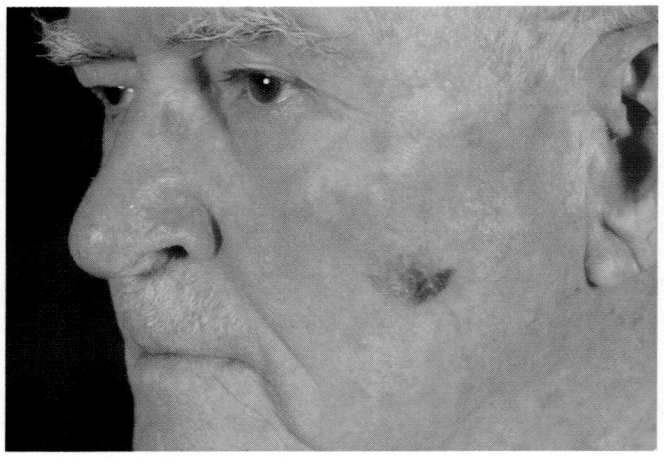

IC-29 **Lentigo maligna melanoma** occurs on sun-exposed skin as a large, hyperpigmented macule or plaque with irregular borders and variable pigmentation.

IC-30 **Nodular melanoma** most commonly manifests itself as a rapidly growing, often ulcerated or crusted black nodule.

IC-31 **Acral lentiginous melanoma** is more common in blacks, Asians, and Hispanics and occurs as an enlarging hyperpigmented macule or plaque on the palms and soles. Lateral pigment diffusion is present.

D. Infectious Disease and the Skin

ID-32 **Impetigo contagiosa** is a superficial streptococcal or *S. aureus* infection consisting of honey-colored crusts and erythematous weeping erosions. Occasionally bullous lesions may be seen.

ID-33 **Folliculitis** is a bacterial infection of hair follicles and is seen as erythematous follicular papules and pustules.

ID-34 **Erysipelas** is a streptococcal infection of the superficial dermis and consists of well-demarcated, erythematous, edematous, warm plaques.

ID-35 **Herpes simplex** Grouped vesiculopustules on an erythematous base characterize primary HSV infections.

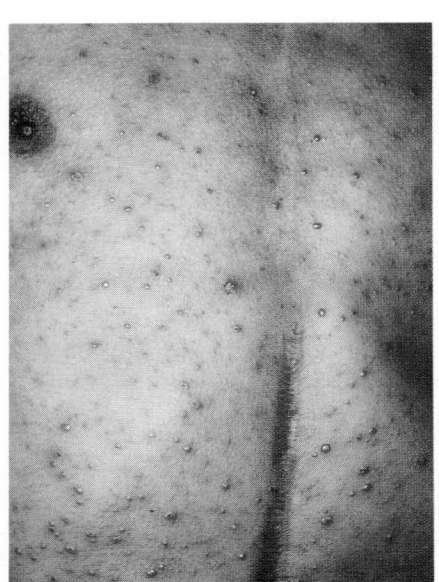

ID-36 **Varicella** showing numerous lesions in various stages of evolution: vesicles on an erythematous base, umbilicated vesicles, and crusts

ID-37 **Herpes zoster** is seen in this HIV-infected patient as hemorrhagic vesicles and pustules on an erythematous base grouped in a dermatomal distribution.

A. The patient reported external ear pain. A vesicular rash on the concha and antihelix suggested Ramsay Hunt syndrome.

B. After chemotherapy for prostate cancer, the patient developed disseminated zoster, which was eventually controlled with acyclovir.

ID-39 **Verrucae** characterized as multiple hyperkeratotic verrucous papules

ID-40 **Molluscum contagiosum** is a cutaneous poxvirus infection characterized by multiple umbilicated flesh-colored or hypopigmented papules.

ID-41 **Oral hairy leukoplakia** often presents as white plaques on the lateral tongue and is associated with Epstein-Barr virus infection.

ID-42 **Pseudomembranous oral candidiasis** Adherent white, mucoid plaques with an erythematous halo seen here on the palate often indicate an immunocompromised state.

ID-43 **Tinea corporis** is a superficial fungal infection seen here as an erythematous annular scaly plaque with central clearing.

ID-44 **Tinea cruris** is a superficial dermatophyte infection with bilateral scaly, erythematous, annular plaques extending from the inguinal crease to the upper thighs.

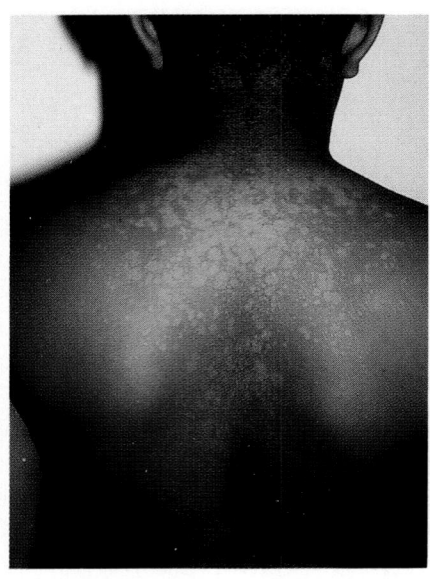

ID-45 **Tinea versi-color** is a superficial cutaneous fungal infection showing a wide variety of lesions. Finely scaling patches may be small or large, hyperpigmented or hypopigmented.

ID-46 **Scabies** showing typical scaling erythematous papules and few linear burrows

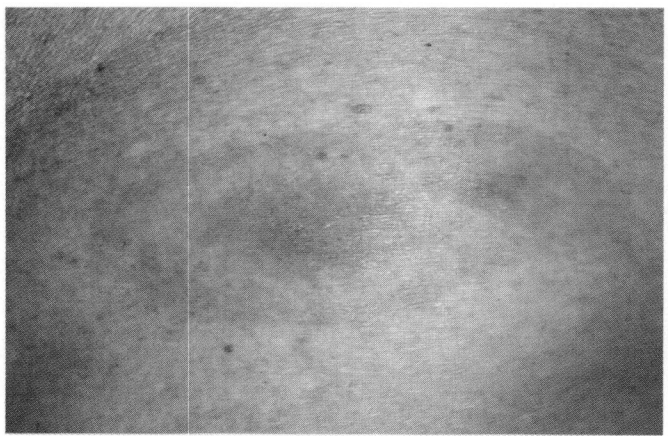

ID-47 **Erythema chronicum migrans** is the early cutaneous manifestation of Lyme disease and is characterized by erythematous annular patches, often with a central erythematous papule at the tick bite site.

ID-48 **Rocky Mountain spotted fever** demonstrating faint erythematous palmar macules in the early phase of the disease. Lesions may become hemorrhagic (purpuric) as the disease progresses.

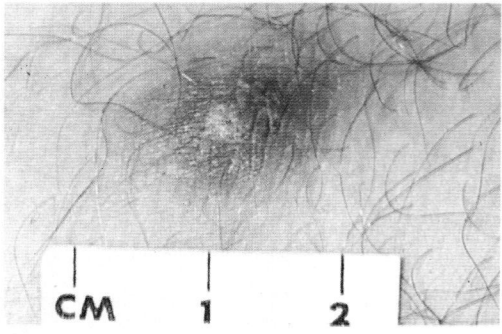

ID-49 **Disseminated gonococcemia** in the skin is seen as hemorrhagic papules and pustules with purpuric centers in an acral distribution.

ID-50 **Fulminant meningococcemia** with extensive angular purpuric patches

ID-51 **Primary syphilis** with a firm, nontender chancre

ID-53 **Secondary syphilis** commonly affects the palms and soles with scaling, firm, red-brown papules.

ID-52 **Secondary syphilis** demonstrating the papulosquamous truncal eruption

ID-54 **Condylomata lata** are moist, somewhat verrucous intertriginous plaques seen in secondary syphilis.

ID-55 **Chancroid** with characteristic penile ulcers and associated left inguinal adenitis (bubo)

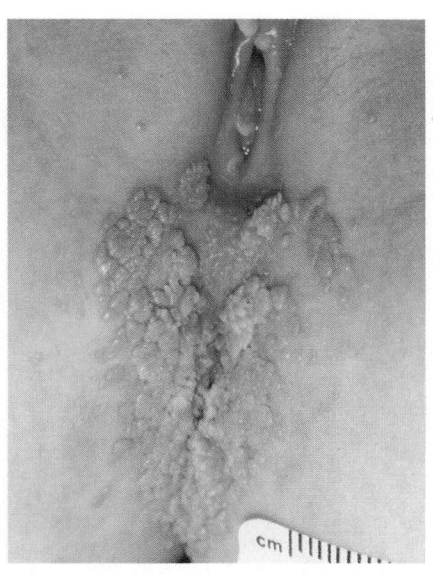

ID-56 **Condylomata acuminata** are lesions induced by human papillomavirus (HPV) and in this patient are seen as multiple verrucous papules coalescing into plaques.

ID-57 **Skin lesions of neutropenic patients**
A. Papules related to *Escherichia coli* bacteremia in a neutropenic patient with acute lymphocytic leukemia. *B.* The same papule 2 h later. *C.* The same lesion the following day. *D.* Ecthyma gangrenosum in a neutropenic patient with *Pseudomonas aeruginosa* bacteremia. *E.* Papule in a neutropenic patient with *Candida tropicalis* fungemia.

E. Immunologically Mediated Skin Disease

IE-58 **Systemic lupus erythematosus** showing prominent, scaly, malar erythema. Involvement of other sun-exposed sites is also common.

IE-59 **Discoid lupus erythematosus** Violaceous, hyperpigmented, atrophic plaques, often with evidence of follicular plugging, which may result in scarring, are characteristic of this cutaneous form of lupus.

IE-60 **Dermatomyositis** Periorbital violaceous erythema characterizes the classic heliotrope rash.

IE-61 **Dermatomyositis** often involves the hands as erythematous flat-topped papules over the knuckles (Gottron's sign) and periungal telangiectasias.

IE-62 **Scleroderma** showing acral sclerosis and focal digital ulcers

IE-63 **Scleroderma** is characterized by typical expressionless, mask-like facies.

IE-64 **Erythema multiforme** is characterized by multiple erythematous plaques with a target or iris morphology and usually represents a hypersensitivity reaction to drugs or infections (especially herpes simplex virus).

IE-65 **Erythema nodosum** is a panniculitis characterized by tender deep-seated nodules and plaques usually located on the lower extremities.

IE-66 **Vasculitis** Palpable purpuric papules on the lower legs are seen in this patient with cutaneous small vessel vasculitis.

IE-68 **Dermatitis herpetiformis** manifested by pruritic, grouped vesicles in a typical location. The vesicles are often excoriated and may occur on knees, buttocks, and posterior scalp.

IE-67 **Pemphigus vulgaris** demonstrating flaccid bullae that are easily ruptured, resulting in multiple erosions and crusted plaques

IE-69 **Bullous pemphigoid** with tense vesicles and bullae on an erythematous, urticarial base

F. Skin Manifestations of Internal Disease

IF-70 **Acanthosis nigricans** demonstrating typical hyperpigmented axillary plaques with a velvet-like, verrucous surface

IF-71 **Pretibial myxedema** manifesting as waxy, infiltrated plaques in a patient with Graves' disease

IF-72 **Sarcoid**   Infiltrated papules and plaques of variable color are seen in a typical paranasal and periorbital location.

IF-73 **Neurofibromatosis** demonstrating numerous flesh-colored cutaneous neurofibromas

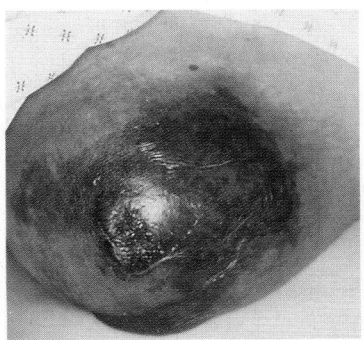

IF-74 **Coumarin necrosis** showing cutaneous and subcutaneous necrosis of a breast. Other fatty areas such as buttocks and thighs are also common sites of involvement.

IF-75 **Pyoderma gangrenosum** showing a somewhat purulent ulcer with violaceous and undermined wound edges

IF-76 **Plaques of Sweet's syndrome** in a patient with acute myelocytic leukemia.

II. Atlas of Endoscopic Findings

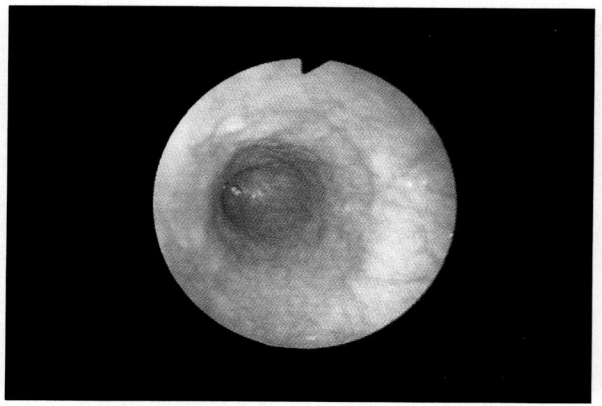

II-1 **Normal esophagus**   Fine vasculature can be seen

II-2 **Peptic regurgitant esophagitis**   Linear red streaks with a central white streak extend up the esophagus

II-3 **Ulcerated squamous cell carcinoma,** with a depressed center, involving one wall of the esophagus

II-4 **Moniliasis of the esophagus**   A white exudate is seen with underlying erythematous mucosa

II-5 **Barrett's metaplasia of the esophagus with an adeno-carcinoma**   The squamocolumnar junction is noted in the proximal esophagus. A mucosal irregularity in the center of the photograph was an adenocarcinoma.

II-6 **Normal body of the stomach with rugal folds**

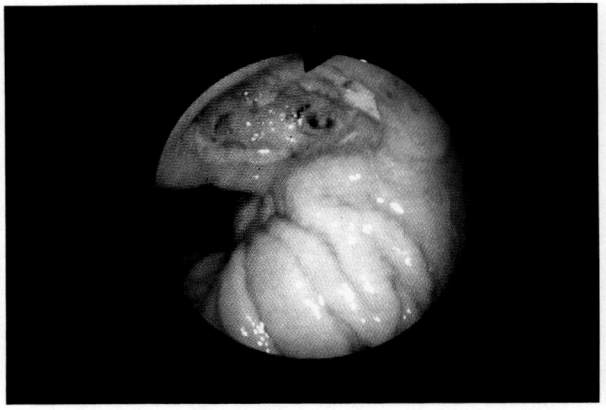

II-7 **Large, benign, lesser curve gastric ulcer**   The folds end at the ulcer margin.

II-8 **Gastric polyp**   The histologic type must be determined by excision and pathologic examination.

II-9 **Arteriovenous malformation of the gastric mucosa**

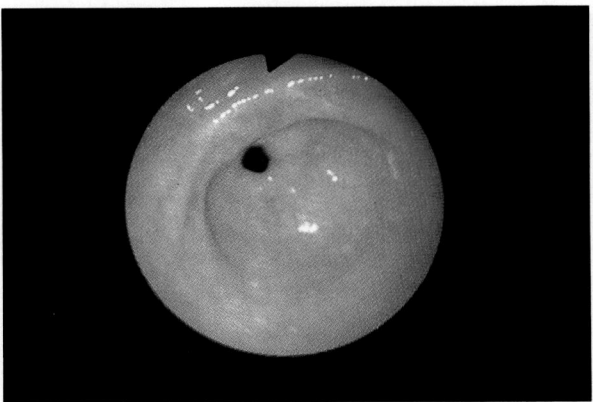

II-10 **Normal pylorus**   Note the absence of gastric rugal folds in the antrum proximal to the pylorus.

II-11 **Normal duodenal bulb**

II-12 **Duodenal ulcer**   A typical ulcer with a clean base is seen on the anterior surface of the duodenal bulb.

II-13 **Normal papilla of Vater** The fold pattern surrounding the papilla is normal; bile is seen adjacent to the papilla.

II-14 **Periampullary carcinoma** The mass at the papilla of Vater has been catheterized during ERCP.

II-15 **Endoscopic papillotomy** A papillotome has been passed into the papilla, the wire bowed, and an incision made, with electrosurgical current, in the superior aspect of the papilla.

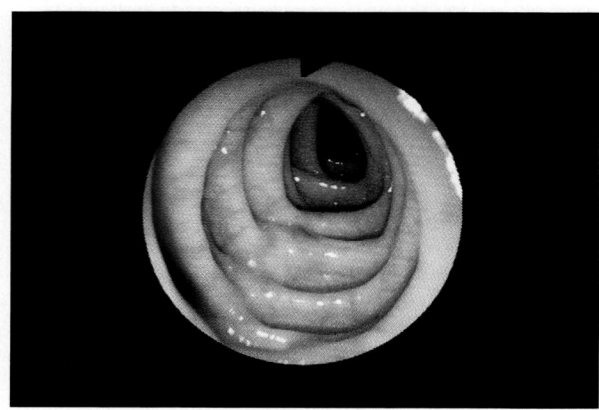

II-16 **Normal colon** Typical folds and vascular pattern can be seen.

II-17 **Colonic adenomatous polyp** The polyp is erythematous; a stalk is seen covered with normal mucosa.

II-18 **Multiple, small, colonic adenomatous polyps** in a case of familial polyposis coli. This colon must be removed to prevent the development of cancer.

II-19 **Colon adenocarcinoma**   The cancer is multilobed and growing into the lumen.

II-20 **Crohn's colitis** with linear, serpiginous, white-based ulcers surrounded by colonic mucosa that is relatively normal

II-21 **Severe ulcerative colitis** with diffuse ulceration, bleeding, and exudation

II-22 **Kaposi's sarcoma involving the colon** in a patient with AIDS. The erythematous lesions involve most of the colonic mucosa in the photograph.

II-23 **Colonic varices**   Multiple, serpiginous, subepithelial structures impinge on the colonic lumen.

II-24 **Ileal pouch**   The mucosa appears normal in this pouch reconstructed from ileum to provide a reservoir after total proctocolectomy and ileoanal anastomosis.

III. Atlas of Funduscopic Examination

III-1 **Cytomegalovirus** in a patient with AIDS appears as an arcuate zone of retinitis with hemorrhages and optic disc swelling. Often CMV is confined to the retinal periphery, beyond view of the direct ophthalmoscope.

III-2 **Hollenhorst plaque** lodged at the bifurcation of a retinal arteriole proves that a patient is shedding emboli from either the carotid artery, great vessels, or heart.

III-3 **Hypertensive retinopathy** with scattered flame (splinter) hemorrhages and cotton wool spots (nerve fiber layer infarcts) in a patient with headache and a blood pressure of 234/120

III-4 **Central retinal vein occlusion** can produce massive retinal hemorrhage ("blood and thunder"), ischemia, and vision loss.

III-5 **Anterior ischemic optic neuropathy** from temporal arteritis in a 78-year old woman with pallid disc swelling, hemorrhage, visual loss, myalgia, and an erythrocyte sedimentation rate of 86 mm/h

III-6 **Retrobulbar optic neuritis** is characterized by a normal fundus examination initially, hence the rubric, "the doctor sees nothing, and the patient sees nothing." Optic atrophy develops after severe or repeated attacks.

III-7 **Optic atrophy** is not a specific diagnosis but refers to the combination of optic disc pallor, arteriolar narrowing, and nerve fiber layer destruction produced by a host of eye diseases, especially optic neuropathies.

III-8 **Papilledema** means optic disc edema from raised intracranial pressure. This obese young woman with pseudotumor cerebri was misdiagnosed as a migraineur until fundus examination was performed, showing optic disc elevation, hemorrhages, and cotton wool spots.

III-9 **Optic disc drusen** are calcified deposits of unknown etiology within the optic disc. They are sometimes confused with papilledema.

III-10 **Retinal detachment** appears as an elevated sheet of retinal tissue with folds. In this patient the fovea was spared, so acuity was normal, but a superior detachment produced an inferior scotoma.

III-11 **Glaucoma** results in "cupping" as the neural rim is destroyed and the central cup becomes enlarged and excavated. The cup-to-disc ratio is about 0.7/1.0 in this patient.

III-12 **Age-related macular degeneration** begins with the accumulation of drusen within the macula. They appear as scattered yellow subretinal deposits.

III-13 **Diabetic retinopathy** results in scattered hemorrhages and yellow exudates. This patient has neovascular vessels proliferating from the optic disc, requiring urgent pan retinal laser photocoagulation.

III-14 **Retinitis pigmentosa** with black clumps of pigment in the retinal periphery known as "bone spicules." There is also atrophy of the retinal pigment epithelium, making the vasculature of the choroid easily visible.

III-15 **Melanoma** of the choroid, appearing as an elevated dark mass in the inferior temporal fundus, just encroaching upon the fovea.

III-16 **Kayser-Fleischer ring** develops in Wilson's disease from copper deposition in Descemet's membrane, producing brownish discoloration of the peripheral cornea. It should not be confused with the yellow-white lipid ring of arcus senilis, which is common in the elderly and occasionally signifies hyperlipidemia, especially when it appears at a young age.

IV. Atlas of Hematology

IV-1 **Normal blood smear** Normal red blood cells are round, possess an area of central pallor, appear slightly smaller than the nucleus of a mature lymphocyte, and vary little in size (anisocytosis) or in shape (poikilocytosis).

IV-2 **Megaloblastic anemia** Oval macrocytes, well filled with hemoglobin, are admixed with lesser numbers of small teardrop-shaped red blood cells. Note also hypersegmented granulocyte.

IV-3 **Liver disease** Round macrocytes of rather uniform size are seen. Many of the macrocytes are also target cells.

IV-4 **Iron-deficiency anemia** In severe iron deficiency, the red blood cells are smaller than normal (microcytosis), and their central area of pallor is expanded (hypochromia) so that the cells appear to have only a thin rim of hemoglobin.

IV-5 **ß Thalassemia intermedia** Microcytic and hypochromic red blood cells are seen that resemble the red blood cells of severe iron deficiency anemia shown in Fig. IV-4. Many elliptical and teardrop-shaped red blood cells are noted.

IV-6 **Sickle cell anemia** The elongated and crescent-shaped red blood cells seen on this smear represent circulating irreversibly sickled cells. Target cells and a nucleated red blood cell are also seen.

IV-7 **Traumatic hemolysis** The helmet-shaped red blood cell and the small triangular-shaped red blood cells seen on this smear represent morphologic evidence of mechanical damage to red blood cells within the blood vessels.

IV-8 **Spur cell anemia** Spur cells are recognized as distorted red blood cells containing several irregularly distributed thornlike projections. Cells with this morphologic abnormality are also called acanthocytes.

IV-9 **Uremia** The red blood cells in uremia may acquire numerous, regularly spaced, small spiny projections. Such cells, called burr cells or echinocytes, are readily distinguishable from the irregularly spiculated acanthocytes shown in Fig. IV-8.

IV-10 **Hereditary spherocytosis** Small, densely staining red blood cells are seen that have lost their central area of pallor (microspherocytes). Microspherocytes may also be found in other hemolytic disorders (Fig. IV-11).

IV-11 **Immunohemolytic anemia** Microspherocytes are seen on this blood smear along with several macrocytes with a slight purple tinge (polychromasia). The latter represent new red blood cells released early from the bone marrow. The microspherocytes seen in immunohemolytic anemia may be indistinguishable from the microspherocytes seen in hereditary spherocytosis (Fig. IV-10).

IV-12 **Leukoerythroblastic smear** Teardrop-shaped red blood cells indicative of membrane damage from collagen fibers, a nucleated red blood cell indicative of premature release of erythroid precursors, and immature myeloid cells indicative of extramedullary hematopoiesis are noted. This peripheral blood smear is related to marrow fibrosis, either primary myelofibrosis or secondary myelophthisis.

A   *B*

IV-13 A. **Normal granulocyte** The normal granulocyte has a segmented nucleus with heavy, clumped chromatin; fine neutrophilic granules are dispersed throughout its cytoplasm.

B. **Normal monocyte and lymphocyte** The normal monocyte is a large cell with an indented or folded nucleus containing loose, strand-like chromatin; the cytoplasm is a blue-gray color and usually contains fine azurophilic granules. The normal lymphocyte is a smaller cell. Its nucleus is usually round but may be indented, as in the cell shown in this plate. The nuclear chromatin has a smudgy appearance; the cytoplasm is blue.

IV-15 **Normal granulocyte precursors in marrow** The earliest granulocytic precursor (myeloblast) possesses a round nucleus with fine, punctate chromatin and one or more nucleoli; the cytoplasm is blue. As nuclear differentiation proceeds, the nucleoli disappear, the chromatin coarsens, and the nucleus becomes increasingly indented and finally segmented. As cytoplasmic differentiation proceeds, azurophilic granules appear and the cytoplasm changes color from blue to the yellow-pink-gray hue of the mature granulocyte, and as this occurs the azurophilic granules become obscured by fine neutrophilic granules.

A   *B*

IV-14 A. **Normal eosinophil** The eosinophil contains large, bright-orange granules; the nucleus is bilobed.

B. **Basophil** The basophil contains large purple-black granules that fill the cell and obscure the nucleus.

IV-16 **Neutrophils with toxic granulation** In infection and other toxic states, azurophilic granules may become visible in mature granulocytes as coarse, dark-staining cytoplasmic granules.

IV-17 **Band with Döhle body** *(center)* Döhle bodies are discrete, blue-staining non-granular areas found in the periphery of the cytoplasm of the neutrophil in infections and other toxic states. They represent aggregates of rough endoplasmic reticulum.

IV-18 **Hypersegmentation** Frequent five-lobed granulocytes on a blood smear or granulocytes with more than five lobes are evidence of hypersegmentation, an important clue to the diagnosis of megaloblastic anemia.

A   *B*

IV-19 A. **Chédiak-Higashi anomaly** In this ultimately fatal disorder, the granulocytes contain huge cytoplasmic granules, formed from aggregation and fusion of azurophilic and specific granules. Large, abnormal granules are found in other granule-containing cells throughout the body. *B.* **Pelger-Hüet anomaly** In this benign disorder, the majority of granulocytes are bilobed. The nucleus frequently has a spectacle-like or "pince-nez" configuration.

IV-20 **Reactive lymphocytes** (infectious mononucleosis) Reactive lymphocytes are usually large, and contain abundant cytoplasm. The nucleus may be eccentrically placed and may have irregular borders and indentations (not seen on this plate). The cytoplasm contains areas that stain a darker blue due to their increased content of RNA. The cytoplasm may be indented where it abuts against a red blood cell.

IV-21 **Chronic granulocytic leukemia** The peripheral WBC count is high due to increased numbers of granulocytes and their precursors. The majority of the WBCs are segmented granulocytes or band forms, but myelocytes (as seen on this plate) and promyeloblasts (not seen on this plate) may also be found on review of the blood smear.

IV-22 **Leukemic cell in acute promyelocytic leukemia** Note multiple Auer rods.

IV-23 **Chronic lymphocytic leukemia** The peripheral WBC count is high due to increased numbers of small, well-differentiated lymphocytes. However, the leukemic lymphocytes are fragile, and substantial numbers of broken, smudged cells are usually also present on the blood smear.

IV-24 **Leukemic cells in acute lymphoblastic leukemia** characterized by round or convoluted nuclei, high nuclear/cytoplasmic ratio and absence of cytoplasmic granules

IV-25 **Hodgkin's disease, mixed cellularity** A Reed-Sternberg cell is present near the center of the field; a large cell with a bilobed nucleus and prominent nucleoli. The majority of the cells are normal lymphocytes, neutrophils, and eosinophils that form a pleiomorphic cellular infiltrate.

IV-26 **Follicular lymphoma** The normal nodal architecture is effaced by nodular expansions of tumor cells. Nodules vary in size and mimic normal lymphoid follicles.

IV-27 **Multiple myeloma** (marrow) The cells bear the characteristic morphologic features of plasma cells, round or oval cells with an eccentric nucleus composed of coarsely clumped chromatin, a densely basophilic cytoplasm, and a perinuclear clear zone (hof) containing the Golgi apparatus. Binucleate and multinucleate malignant plasma cells also can be seen.

IV-28 **Diffuse large B cell lymphoma** The neoplastic cells are large with vesicular nuclear chromatin and prominent nucleoli.

IV-29 **Burkitt's lymphoma** The neoplastic cells are homogeneous, medium-sized B cells with frequent mitotic figures, a morphologic correlate of high growth fraction. Reactive macrophages are scattered through the tumor and their pale cytoplasm in a background of blue-staining tumor cells gives the tumor a so-called "starry sky" appearance.

IV-30 **Acute myelocytic leukemia** This marrow section shows sheets of primitive myeloblasts with numerous large nucleoli.

IV-31 **Auer rod** This peripheral blood smear shows a myeloblast with a single Auer rod in the cytoplasm. Auer rods, when present, are usually seen in acute myelocytic leukemia.

IV-32 **Normal bone marrow biopsy** This is a low power view of an H&E-stained section of normal marrow. Note that the nucleated cellular elements account for about 40 to 50 percent and the fat *(clear areas)* accounts for about 50 to 60 percent of the area.

IV-33 **Aplastic anemia** This marrow section shows only fat with nearly complete absence of hematopoietic tissue.

IV-34 **Marrow fibrosis** This marrow section shows the marrow cavity replaced by fibrous tissue composed of reticulin fibers and collagen. When this fibrosis is due to a primary hematologic process, it is called *myelofibrosis*. When the fibrosis is secondary to a tumor or a granulomatous process, it is called *myelophthisis*.

IV-35 **Erythroid hyperplasia** This marrow section shows an increase in the fraction of cells in the erythroid lineage as might be seen in a healthy marrow compensating for acute blood loss or hemolysis. The E/G ratio is greater than 1/1.

IV-36 **Granulocytic hyperplasia** This marrow section shows an increase in the fraction of cells in the myeloid or granulocytic lineage as might be seen in a healthy marrow responding to infection. The E/G ratio is less than 1/3.

IV-37 **Megaloblastic erythropoiesis** This marrow section demonstrates so-called nuclear-cytoplasmic dissociation; the cytoplasm of erythroblasts is filled with hemoglobin demonstrating nearly complete maturation while the nuclei have loose chromatin characteristic of more immature erythroid cells. The slow nuclear maturation is related to a decrease in DNA synthesis related to an insufficient supply of reduced folate to synthesize thymidylate. DNA synthesis inhibitors can produce this picture, as can folate and B_{12} deficiency.

IV-38 **Marrow iron stores** This marrow section is stained with Prussian blue. Iron takes up the stain and is concentrated in reticuloendothelial cells. This picture shows normal iron stores. In iron deficiency states, no stainable iron is detectable. In the anemia of chronic disease, iron is present but cytokines prevent its mobilization and utilization in heme synthesis.

IV-39 **Ringed sideroblast** Refractory anemia with ringed sideroblasts (RARS) is in the spectrum of myelodysplastic syndromes. This marrow Prussian blue stain shows an orthochromatic normoblast with a collar of blue granules surrounding the nucleus. The blue granules represent iron-laden mitochondria.

SOURCES OF PHOTOGRAPHS

I. DERMATOLOGY

Robert Swerlick, M.D.   IA-1 Acne rosacea; IA-9 Lichen planus; IA-12 Alopecia areata; ID-33 Folliculitis; IE-65 Erythema nodosum; IE-66 Vasculitis

S. Wright Caughman, M.D.   IC-30 Nodular melanoma; ID-35 Herpes simplex; ID-50 Fulminant meningococcemia; ID-58 Condylomata acuminatum

Alvin Solomon, M.D.   IC-29 Lentigo maligna melanoma; ID-53 Secondary syphilis of the palms

Mary Spraker, M.D.   ID-32 Impetigo contagiosa

Kim Yancey, M.D.   IF-74 Coumarin necrosis

John Greenspan, Ph.D.   ID-41 Oral hairy leukoplakia; ID-42 Pseudo-membranous oral candidiasis

Gregory Cox, M.D.   ID-51 Primary syphilis

Marilynne McKay, M.D.   IE-59 Discoid lupus erythematosus

James Krell, M.D.   IE-60 Dermatomyositis

Yale Resident's Slide Collection   ID-40 Molluscum contagiosum; ID-48 Rocky Mountain spotted fever; ID-69 Bullous pemphigoid; ID-47 Erythema chronicum migrans; ID-54 Condylomata lata; ID-64 Erythema multiforme

Kalman Watsky, M.D.   IA-1 Acne vulgaris

Jean Bolognia, M.D.   IA-6 Seborrheic dermatitis; IB-24 Non-Hodgkin's lymphoma

Robert Hartman, M.D.   ID-36 Varicella

Irwin Braverman, M.D.   IA-4 Atopic dermatitis

II. ENDOSCOPIC FINDINGS

FE Silverstein and **GN Tytgat**   *Atlas of Gastrointestinal Endoscopy,* New York, Gowen Medical Publishing, 1987   All photographs except II-12, II-23, II-24

GN Tytgat   II-12, II-23, II-24

III. FUNDUSCOPIC FINDINGS

Jonathan C. Horton, M.D., Ph.D.   All photographs, III-1 to III-16

IV. HEMATOLOGY

Elaine Jaffe, M.D.   IV-25 to IV-29

Robert S. Hillman, M.D., and **Kenneth A. Ault, M.D.**   *Hematology in General Practice,* New York, McGraw-Hill, 1995. Courtesy of the American Society of Hematology Slide Bank. IV-30 to IV-39

360 *Joseph B. Martin, Stephen L. Hauser*

APPROACH TO THE PATIENT WITH NEUROLOGIC DISEASE

Neurologic disorders are frequent in clinical medicine, yet many physicians are uncomfortable with the diagnosis of nervous system disease and unprepared to manage neurologic conditions efficiently. Neurologic disorders may produce a bewildering array of symptoms and signs or disturb a patient's ability to communicate normally with the examiner. The examination may be time-consuming, and correct diagnosis requires a working knowledge of relevant neuroanatomic principles. Finally, many physicians are disadvantaged by limited formal training in neurology, due to the growth of the field as an independent specialty with separate clinical services that sequester neurologic problems from general medical services.

Most patients with neurologic symptoms seek care from internists and other generalists rather than neurologists. This situation is likely to continue in the future as primary care–based health care systems become increasingly prevalent and the number of specialists, including neurologists, is reduced. For all practitioners, the importance of a level of competence in neurology cannot be overstated, as the explosive increase in the number of useful therapies for many neurologic disorders makes correct diagnosis an ethical imperative. In subsequent chapters, various algorithms are presented as aids to diagnosis and therapy of various neurologic disorders. Appropriate use of these algorithms requires that the physician first correctly assess and interpret the presenting symptoms and signs of these conditions.

The goal of the neurologic method is to define the patient's illness, first in anatomic and then in pathophysiologic terms. Arrival at a diagnosis permits the physician to institute therapy and to inform and counsel patients and their families as to the expected disease course.

THE NEUROLOGIC METHOD OF CLINICAL EVALUATION

The strategy used in evaluating a patient with neurologic illness is to begin with the question, "What portion of the neural axis is likely to be involved in causing the neurologic symptoms?" The first clues to defining the anatomic area of involvement appear in the history, and the examination is then directed to confirm or rule out these impressions and to clarify uncertainties suggested by the history. A more detailed examination of a particular region of the central nervous system (CNS) or peripheral nervous system is often indicated. For example, optokinetic nystagmus may be an important part of the examination in a patient with a left hemiparesis and dressing apraxia but irrelevant to the examination of a patient complaining of burning feet. In a patient who presents with a history of ascending paresthesia and weakness, the examination should be *directed* toward deciding, among other things, if the location of the lesion is the spinal cord or peripheral nerves. Notations regarding muscle stamina or endurance might be crucial to the examination of a patient with myasthenia gravis, as opposed to the usual tests of peak muscle power. What one does in the neurologic examination depends on what the questions are; the questions are formulated by a properly taken history.

Deciding "where the lesion is" accomplishes the task of delimiting the number of possible etiologies to a manageable, finite size. In addition, this strategy safeguards against making really tragic errors.

Symptoms of recurrent vertigo, diplopia, and nystagmus should not trigger "multiple sclerosis" as an answer (etiology) but "brainstem" or "pons" (location); then a diagnosis of brainstem arteriovenous malformation will not be missed because it is not considered. Similarly, the combination of optic neuritis and spastic ataxic paraparesis should not suggest only multiple sclerosis; CNS syphilis and vitamin B_{12} deficiency (both treatable) also can cause these findings. When the question, "Where is the lesion?" is answered, then the question, "What is the lesion?" can be addressed.

THE NEUROLOGIC HISTORY Careful attention to the description of the symptoms as experienced by the patient and substantiated by family members or friends permits, in many instances, an accurate localization and determination of the probable cause of the complaints even before the neurologic examination is undertaken. Two principles should be followed. First, each complaint should be pursued as far as possible in an effort to delineate where the lesion might be or, more important, *to formulate a set of questions to be answered by the examination.* A patient complains of weakness of the right arm. What are the associated features? Is this weakness for brushing the hair or opening a twist-top bottle? Second, in neurology—where many of the diseases are due to *anatomically restricted* lesions—*negative* associations may be crucial. A patient with a right hemiparesis without a language deficit likely has a different lesion (and likely etiology) than a patient with a right hemiparesis and aphasia. Additional important factors that aid in defining the nature of the neurologic disorder include the following:

1. *Temporal course of the illness.* It is important to ascertain the precise time of appearance and rate of progression of the symptoms experienced by the patient. The rapid onset of a neurologic complaint, occurring within seconds or minutes, usually indicates a vascular event or a seizure. Attention to the temporal march of symptoms may help define a focal seizure, a cerebral transient ischemic attack (TIA), or the onset of a migraine. For example, the onset of sensory symptoms located in one extremity that spread over a few seconds to adjacent portions of that extremity and then to the other limb or to the face suggests a seizure. A more gradual onset involving less discrete regions of the extremities points to the possibility of a TIA. A similar but slower progression of sensory change occurring in a young person together with other symptoms of headache, nausea, or visual disturbance suggests migraine. In general, the march of a migraine is slower than that of seizure, and a TIA tends to be more generalized in location on the side of the body or extremities. The presence of "positive" sensory symptoms (e.g., buzzing) or motor movements suggests a seizure; in contrast, transient loss of a function (negative symptom) suggests a TIA. A stuttering onset where symptoms appear, stabilize, and then progress over hours or days also suggests the presence of cerebrovascular disease. In acute vascular disease, a history of transient remission or regression indicates that the process is likely ischemic and not hemorrhagic. In some cases, a demyelinating process may also produce new symptoms that evolve rapidly over the course of a few hours. Progressing symptoms associated with the systemic manifestations of fever, stiff neck, and altered level of consciousness or awareness suggest the possibility of an infectious process. The course of the illness over years in terms of remissions and exacerbations offers additional clues to the nature of the process. Recurrent neurologic symptoms involving different levels of the neuraxis with partial or complete recovery suggest the possibility of multiple sclerosis. Slowly progressive symptoms without remissions tend to be characteristic of a neurodegenerative disorder.

2. *Subjective descriptions of the complaint.* This will be influenced by the patient's sophistication, familiarity with medical terminology, and general level of comfort with the physician. The same words often mean different things to individual patients. "Dizziness" may imply impending syncope, a sense of giddiness, or true spinning vertigo. "Numbness" may mean a complete loss of feeling, a positive sensation of tingling, or paralysis. "Blurring of vision" may be used to describe unilateral visual loss, as in transient monocular blindness, or diplopia. It is important to determine the patient's level of understanding with respect to the complaint in order to assess its significance accurately.

3. *Corroboration of the history by others.* It is often useful to obtain additional information from family, friends, or observers to corroborate or expand the patient's description. Memory loss, personality change, drug abuse, excess alcohol intake, and other factors may impair the patients' capacity to describe their subjective experiences or prevent them from being open and forthright about factors that have contributed to the illness. Episodes of loss of consciousness that may be due to syncope or seizures necessitate that details be sought from observers to ascertain the exact circumstances. Manifestations of depression and anxiety may mask or color the presentation given by the patient. Failure to note these underlying factors that interfere with the patient's performance may result in an incorrect interpretation of the presenting complaints.

4. *Family history.* Many neurologic disorders, particularly those presenting in childhood or early adulthood, are inherited conditions. It is essential to inquire about the existence of similar symptoms in other family members and also of the possibility of parental consanguinity. These may provide clues to a propensity toward a hereditary neurologic condition. It is critical to distinguish between a *negative* family history and an *incomplete* family history. It is insufficient to simply ask, Is there any similar illness in any member of your family? A negative response to such an inquiry may mean that there is, in fact, no such illness in the patient's family, but it also may mean that the patient is unfamiliar with relatives or their medical histories. It is wise to elicit specific positive or negative data about relatives as follows: Are your parents living? If so, are they well? If not, what illness did they have, and how did they die? It should always be remembered that maternity is a fact, but paternity is only an assumption.

It is also important to elicit family history data regarding all illnesses rather than just neurologic and psychiatric disorders. A familial propensity to hypertension or heart disease may be relevant to a patient who presents with a stroke. Many inherited neurologic illnesses are associated with signs and symptoms in other systems that may provide clues to the correct diagnosis (e.g., the phakomatoses, hepatocerebral disorders, neuroophthalmic syndromes).

5. *Medical illnesses.* Many neurologic illnesses occur in the context of systemic disorders. A history of allergy and asthma may suggest the onset of polyarteritis, with mononeuritis multiplex. Previous or current medical illnesses such as diabetes mellitus, hypertension, and abnormalities of blood lipids may be relevant to evolving symptoms that affect the nervous system. Similarly, the presence of systemic diseases that are associated with peripheral neuropathy should be explored. Most patients with coma in a hospital setting can be shown to have a metabolic, toxic, or infectious process.

6. *The patient's perception of the disease.* It is frequently helpful to ask patients what they perceive to be wrong. Patients who complain of failing memory are often concerned that they have early symptoms of Alzheimer's disease. Patients with headaches may fear that a tumor or an impending stroke is a possibility. Patients with sensory symptoms frequently are concerned about the possibility of multiple sclerosis. The patient may seek medical attention because a relative or friend has been diagnosed with a serious neurologic illness.

7. *Drug use and abuse and toxin exposure.* It is essential to inquire about the history of drug use, both prescribed and illicit.

Complaints of yellow vision may occur with digitalis administration. Excessive vitamin ingestion may lead to disease; for example, vitamin A and pseudotumor cerebri, or pyridoxine and peripheral neuropathy. Aminoglycoside antibiotics may exacerbate symptoms of weakness in patients with disorders of neuromuscular transmission, such as myasthenia gravis. Dizziness may be secondary to ototoxicity caused by the aminoglycosides. In eliciting a history of drug use it is often necessary to be specific and to use lay terminology. Many patients are unaware that over-the-counter sleeping pills, cold preparations, and diet pills are actually drugs. Alcohol, the most prevalent neurotoxin, is often not recognized as such by patients. History of environmental or industrial exposure to neurotoxins may provide the essential clue; consultation with the patient's family or employer may be required.

8. *History of malignancy.* Patients with prior malignancy can present with unexpected and unusual neurologic complications. Malignant tumors may present with nervous system metastases or occasionally with a paraneoplastic syndrome (see Chap. 103). In a patient with a history of malignancy, it is important to ask whether chemotherapy or radiotherapy was given.

9. *Formulating an impression of the patient.* Use the opportunity while taking the history to form an impression of the patient. Is there evidence of anxiety, depression, hypochondriasis? Are there any clues to defects of language, memory, inappropriate behavior, or secondary gain? The neurologic assessment begins as soon as the patient walks into the room and the first introduction is made.

THE NEUROLOGIC EXAMINATION   A systematic neurologic examination should encompass a survey of all functions from the cerebrum to peripheral nerve and muscle, i.e., from the mental status examination to the simplest reflexes. Physicians should acquire skills that come only from the repeated use of the same techniques and instruments on a large number of normal and abnormal individuals. Errors and serious omissions are avoided if the examination procedure is orderly and systematic, beginning with mental (cerebral) functions and continuing with cranial nerves; then with motor, reflex, and sensory functions of the arms, trunk, and legs; and finishing with an analysis of posture and gait.

Mental Status Examination (See also Chaps. 24 to 26)   These tests are designed to evaluate attention, orientation, memory, insight, judgment, and grasp of general information. A series of numbers can be recited and the patient asked to respond every time a specific item recurs (attention). The patient can be asked his or her name, the place, the day, and date. Retentive memory and immediate recall can be tested by determining the number of digits that can be repeated in sequence. Recent memory is evaluated by testing recall of a series of objects after defined times (e.g., 5 and 15 min). More remote memory is evaluated by assessment of the patient's ability to provide a coherent chronologic history of his or her illness or personal life events. Recall of major historical or current events can be used to assess the fund of general knowledge. If answers suggest that there may be a problem with insight, the patient should be asked whether anything is wrong with his or her health. Interpretation of proverbs (e.g., "People who live in glasshouses . . ."; A bird in the hand. . . .") can provide information relative to judgment and capacity to reason in an abstract manner.

Specific higher cortical functions can be tested when clinical circumstances suggest that deficits may be present. Evaluation of language function should include assessment of spontaneous speech, naming, repetition, reading, writing, and comprehension. Calculations, identification of right from left, identification of fingers, praxis (whistling, brushing teeth, combing hair, saluting), and ability to draw and copy figures may also be assessed.

Cranial Nerve (CN) Examination (See also Chaps. 28, 29, and 372)   *CN I*   Occlude each nostril sequentially. Use a mild test stimulus such as soap, toothpaste, coffee, or lemon oil. With the eyes closed, the patient sniffs and tries to identify the stimulus.

CN II   Check visual acuity (with eyeglasses or pinhole correction) using a Snellen chart (distance) or Jaeger's test type (near). Map visual fields by confrontation testing in each quadrant of the visual field for each eye individually. The best method is to sit facing the patient [0.6 to 1.0 m (2 to 3 ft) apart] and ask him or her to gently cover one eye and fix the uncovered eye on the examiner's nose. A small object (e.g., a white hatpin or cotton-tipped applicator) is then moved from the periphery of the field toward the center until appreciated by the patient. The patient's visual field should be mapped against the examiner's for comparison. The size of the blind spot can also be estimated in this manner; for central vision, use of a red pin will improve sensitivity of the study. Formal perimetry and tangent screen examinations may be required to identify and delineate small defects. Optic fundi should be examined with an ophthalmoscope, and the color, size, and degree of swelling or elevation of the optic disc recorded. The retinal vessels should be checked for size, regularity, arterial-venous nicking at crossing points, hemorrhage, exudates, aneurysms, etc. Normally, 8 to 12 vessels course over the disc margin, and the darker arterioles are approximately two-thirds the size of the lighter colored venules.

CN III, IV, VI Describe the size and shape of pupils and direct and consensual pupillary reaction to light. Check for pupillary accommodation with convergence (ask the patient to follow a small object as it moves towards the bridge of the nose). Check for lid droop, lag, or retraction. Ask the patient to follow a small object (e.g., a hatpin) at a distance of 0.6 m (2 ft). Move the target slowly in both horizontal and vertical planes; observe any paresis, nystagmus, or abnormality of smooth pursuit (saccades, oculomotor ataxia, etc.). Horizontal nystagmus is best assessed at 45° and not at extreme lateral gaze. If eye movements are incomplete, this may result from a nuclear or supranuclear cause; a supranuclear cause is present if full eye movements are present with doll's-head maneuver (gentle, rapid side-to-side or up-and-down movements of the neck).

CN V Feel the masseter and temporalis muscles as the patient bites down. Test jaw opening, protrusion, and lateral motion against resistance. Examine sensation over the entire face and corneals using a light wisp of cotton.

CN VII Look for asymmetry of face at rest and with spontaneous movements. Test eyebrow elevation, forehead wrinkling, eye closure, smiling, frowning, cheek puff, whistle, lip pursing, and chin muscle contraction. Look in particular for differences in strength of the lower versus upper facial muscles. Taste on the anterior two-thirds of the tongue may be impaired by lesions of the nerve proximal to the chordi tympani. Test taste for sweet (sugar), salt, sour (lemon), and bitter (quinine) using cotton-tipped applicators moistened in the appropriate solution and placed on the lateral margin of the protruded tongue halfway back from the tip.

CN VIII Check the ability to hear a tuning fork, finger rub, watch tick, and whispered voice with each ear. Check for air versus mastoid bone conduction (Rinne) and lateralization of a tuning fork placed on the center of the forehead (Weber). Examine the tympanic membranes. Accurate, quantitative testing of hearing requires formal audiometry.

CN IX, X Check for symmetric elevation of the palate-uvula with phonation ("aah") as well as the position of the uvula and palatal arch at rest. Sensation in the region of the tonsils, posterior pharynx, and tongue may also require testing in some patients. Pharyngeal ("gag") reflex is evaluated by stimulating the posterior pharyngeal wall on each side with a blunt object (e.g., tongue blade). Direct examination of vocal cords by laryngoscopy may be necessary in some situations.

CN XI Check shoulder shrug (trapezius muscle) and head rotation to each side (sternocleidomastoid muscle) against resistance.

CN XII Examine the bulk and power of the tongue. Look for atrophy, deviation from midline with protrusion, tremor, and small flickering or twitching movements (fibrillations, fasciculations).

Motor Examination (See also Chaps. 21 and 22) Muscles are examined for evidence of atrophy or hypertrophy. Fasciculations (involuntary contractions of a group of muscle fibers innervated by a single motor neuron) may be observed as fine twitching that occurs spontaneously or is induced by light percussion. Involuntary movements may be present, occurring either at rest (e.g., tics, myoclonus, choreoathetosis, ballismus), during maintained posture (three to five per second pill-rolling tremor of Parkinson's disease), or with voluntary action [intention tremors of cerebellar disease (7 per second) or familial tremor (8 to 12 per second)].

Muscle tone is tested by assessment of resistance to passive motion of a relaxed limb. During testing, it is useful to distract the patient from the examination to minimize active movements. In the upper limbs, tone is assessed by repetitive pronation and supination of the forearm and by rolling the hand at the wrist. In the lower limbs, the examiner's hands are placed behind the thighs and rapidly raised; with normal tone the ankles drag along the table surface for a variable distance before rising, whereas increased tone results in an immediate lift of the heel off the surface. Decreased tone is most commonly due to lower motor neuron, peripheral nerve, or cerebellar system disorders. Increased tone may be evident as spasticity (resistance determined by the angle and direction of motion), rigidity (similar resistance at all angles of motion), or paratonia/Gegenhalten (fluctuating changes in resistance to repetitive passive movements). Spasticity occurs with upper motor neuron/pyramidal tract disease, rigidity with extrapyramidal disease, and paratonia with frontal lobe or thalamic disorders. One frequently observed type of rigidity is the cogwheel rigidity of Parkinson's syndrome, in which passive motion elicits jerky interruptions in resistance.

Power should be tested for major movements at each joint (e.g., flexion, extension, adduction, and abduction). Strength is recorded using the following scale from 0 to 5:

0 = no movement
1 = flicker or trace of contraction but no associated movement at a joint
2 = movement with gravity eliminated
3 = movement against gravity but not against resistance
4− = movement against a mild degree of resistance
4 = movement against moderate resistance
4+ = movement against strong resistance
5 = full power

Reflexes The muscle stretch reflexes most commonly tested are the biceps, brachioradialis, and triceps reflexes in the upper limbs and the patellar (quadriceps) and Achilles reflexes in the lower limbs (Table 360-1). Stretch reflexes are best elicited in a relaxed limb. It is sometimes useful to use conversation to distract the patient during reflex testing. Reflexes may also be facilitated by asking the patient to voluntarily contract other, distant muscle groups (Jendrassik maneuver). For example, upper limb reflexes may be reinforced by voluntary teeth-clenching, and the Achilles reflex by hooking the flexed fingers of the two hands together and by attempting to pull them apart. For each reflex tested, left and right limbs should be similarly positioned and the two sides tested sequentially. It is more useful to determine the smallest stimulus required to elicit a reflex rather than the maximum response that can be obtained. For the biceps, brachioradialis, or patellar reflexes, it may be adequate to passively drop the head of the hammer from a distance of several inches away to elicit the reflex. Reflexes are commonly graded by the following scale:

0 = absent
1 = present but diminished
2 = normoactive
3 = exaggerated
4 = clonus

Clonus refers to repetitive rhythmic contractions evoked by a stretch stimulus; when present, it is most commonly noted at the

Table 360-1

Spinal Cord Levels for Deep Tendon Reflexes

Reflex	Level
Biceps	**C5**, C6
Brachioradialis	C5, **C6**
Triceps	**C7**, C8
Patellar	**L3**, L4
Ankle	**S1**, S2

Achilles tendon. Occasional normal individuals will have two or three beats of physiologic ankle clonus, but sustained ankle clonus is an abnormal finding that signifies hyperactivity of the motor unit resulting from an upper motor neuron lesion.

In addition to the stretch reflexes, assessment of the superficial cutaneous reflexes provides confirmatory and localizing data. The plantar reflex is elicited by stroking, with a blunt object (i.e., a key or tongue blade), the lateral surface of the foot beginning near the heel and moving toward the toes. The normal reflex consists of plantar flexion of the toes. With upper motor neuron lesions above the S1 level of the spinal cord, a paradoxical extension of the great toe is noted, associated with fanning and extension of the other toes (extensor plantar response or Babinski sign); a prominent extensor plantar response may be accompanied by triple flexion at the ankle, knee, and hip. In some patients with corticospinal tract lesions, the great toe on the involved side may assume an extensor posture at rest or following movement of the foot. Some patients may voluntarily withdraw from the plantar stroke, simulating an extensor response. In these situations, the direction of the plantar response may be determined by pressure applied to the anterior tibia, stroking towards the ankle (Oppenheim sign), pressure applied to the calf (Gordon sign) or ankle (Schaefer sign), or pricking of the dorsum of the great toe (Bing sign).

Superficial abdominal reflexes are often neglected but can be of diagnostic value, particularly in localization of spinal cord disease. These are elicited by lightly stroking the abdominal wall with a sharp object (e.g., a pin) and observing movement of the umbilicus. The upper abdominal reflex (spinal cord level T9) is elicited by stroking the lateral upper corner of the abdomen towards the umbilicus, whereas the lower abdominal reflex (T12) is stimulated by a stimulus beginning at the lower lateral abdomen. The normal response consists of diagonal deviation of the umbilicus toward the origin of the stimulus. With upper motor neuron lesions, these reflexes are absent. They are most helpful when there is preservation of upper but not lower abdominal reflexes, indicating a spinal lesion between T9 and T12, or when the response is asymmetric. Obese individuals or multiparous women may not have visible superficial abdominal reflexes. Many other useful cutaneous reflexes have been described, including the sacral cremasteric (ipsilateral elevation of the testicle following stroking of the medial thigh), anal (contraction of the anal sphincter following pinprick stimulation of the perianal region), and bulbocavernosus (contraction of urethra and anal sphincter following a stimulus to the glans penis) reflexes.

Finally, in patients with suspected frontal lobe disease, hydrocephalus, or dementia, several primitive reflexes, not normally present in the adult, may appear. These include the suck, root, grasp, and palmomental reflexes. The suck response is elicited by lightly touching the center of the lips, and the root reponse the corner of the lips, with a tongue blade; the patient will move the lips to suck or root in the direction of the stimulus. The grasp reflex is elicited by touching the palm, and in particular the area between the thumb and index finger, with the examiner's fingers; a positive (abnormal) response consists of a forced grasp of the stimulated hand. The palmomental response consists of contraction of the chin ipsilateral to a scratch stimulus diagonally applied to the palm.

Sensory Examination (See also Chap. 23) Five primary sensory modalities—vibration, joint position, light touch, pinprick, and temperature—are routinely tested in each limb. Unlike reflex testing, the evaluation of sensation requires cooperation and concentration by the patient. The examiner should provide a brief introduction to the purpose and methods of each sensory test prior to performing the examination. Assessment of vibration and position sense is usually performed first. Vibration testing generally utilizes a 128-Hz weighted tuning fork, but some physicians prefer the smaller 256-Hz fork. The vibrating tuning fork is applied to the terminal phalynx of the great toe or middle finger just below the nail bed. The examiner compares the patient's threshold of vibration perception with his or her own or compares

distal and proximal thresholds in the patient. For joint position testing, the examiner grasps the limb laterally and distal to the joint to be assessed. Light touch is best assessed with a wisp of cotton, pinprick with a clean pin (compare sharp versus blunt end), and temperature initially with a tuning fork immersed in cold and hot water. Patients with lesions above the level of the thalamus may have disorders of "discriminative sensation," resulting in an inability to perceive double simultaneous stimuli, to localize stimuli accurately, to identify closely approximated stimuli as separate (two-point discrimination), to identify objects by touch alone (stereognosis), or to judge weights, evaluate texture, or identify letters or numbers written on the skin surface (graphesthesia). Although difficult to master, facility with sensory examination skills is of great value in many clinical situations. In peripheral neuropathy, a gradient of distal more than proximal sensory loss may be present. In early stages of spinal cord disease, a sensory level may be detected to pinprick and temperature as the examiner moves up and down each side of the back. A tumor of the conus medullaris may present with focal sensory loss in a sacral distribution. In systemic vasculitis, identification of a mononeuropathy may signal involvement of the vasa nervorum (mononeuritis multiplex).

Coordination (See also Chap. 21) The patient is asked to touch his or her index finger repetitively to the nose and then to the examiner's outstretched finger; the examiner's finger can be moved with each repetition. Another useful test is to ask the patient to alternate tapping the palm then the back of one hand on the thigh. To test coordination in the legs, in the supine position the patient is asked to slide the heel (not the arch!) of each foot from the knee down the shin of the other leg, and to raise the leg and touch with the great toe the examiner's index finger. For all these movements, the accuracy, speed, and rhythm are noted.

Gait (See also Chap. 21) Gait is easily tested and highly informative, and observation of gait is an essential component of the neurologic examination. Unexpected abnormalities may be detected that prompt the examiner to return, in more detail, to other aspects of the examination. Normal gait requires that multiple systems—including power, sensation, coordination, and praxis—function in a coordinated fashion. The ability to rise from the sitting or lying position, to stand with eyes closed and feet together (Romberg test), and to walk, turn, and heel-toe walk along a straight line should be noted. The examination may reveal decreased arm swing on one side (corticospinal tract disease), a stooped posture and short-stepped gait (Parkinson's syndrome), a broad-based unstable gait (ataxia), scissoring (spasticity), or a high-stepped, slapping gait (posterior column or peripheral nerve disease) or the patient may appear to be stuck in place (apraxia).

This detailed neurologic examination is undertaken only if there are symptoms of disturbed nervous system functioning. If none are present, it suffices to do an abbreviated examination that includes evaluation only of pupils, ocular movements, optic fundi, facial movements, speech, strength of arm and leg muscles, tendon and plantar reflexes, pain and vibratory sensation in hands and feet, and gait. All this can be completed in 3 to 5 min. The findings, even in the short examination, should be recorded in the patient's record for future reference.

Two additional points about the examination are worth noting. First, in recording observations, it is important for the physician to describe what is found rather than to apply a poorly defined medical term (i.e., "patient groans to sternal rub" rather than "obtunded"). Second, if the patient's complaint is brought out by some activity, reproduce the activity in the office. If the complaint is of dizziness when raising the right arm and turning the head to the left, have the patient do it. If pain occurs after walking two blocks, have the patient demonstrate it, and repeat the examination.

Experience teaches that the neurologic examination may be normal even in patients with a serious neurologic disease, such as one that causes seizures or syncope. Or the patient may arrive in a coma with no available history, and the examination proceeds along the lines described in Chap. 24. An inadequate history may be compensated to some extent by a succession of examinations from which the course of the illness may be plotted.

FORMULATION OF THE PROBLEM AND ESTABLISHMENT OF AN ETIOLOGIC DIAGNOSIS   The clinical data obtained from the history and the examination are assembled into one of the known syndromes and are interpreted and translated in terms of neuroanatomy and neurophysiology. From the syndrome the physician should be able to determine the anatomic localization(s) that best explains the clinical findings. The anatomic localization, mode of onset and course of illness, other medical data, and laboratory findings are then integrated. Finally, the etiologic diagnosis is reached, and therapy appropriate for the disorder is proposed.

LABORATORY TESTS   The proper selection of tests is important to arrive at an anatomic, but more particularly an etiologic, diagnosis. The laboratory assessment of a patient with positive neurologic findings may include (1) serum electrolytes, complete blood count, and renal, liver, and endocrine studies; (2) cerebrospinal fluid (CSF) examination; (3) imaging studies of the CNS (see Chap. 362); or (4) electrophysiologic studies (see Chap. 361).

LUMBAR PUNCTURE   The clinical indications for lumbar puncture are listed in Table 360-2. In experienced hands, lumbar puncture is a safe procedure. It should always be performed under sterile conditions. The patient is asked to lie on his or her side facing away from the examiner. The back is positioned at the edge of the bed or table near the examiner. The patient is asked to "roll up into a ball"—the neck is gently flexed and the knees drawn up to the abdomen. Proper positioning is essential for success; the examiner should ensure that the shoulders and pelvis are aligned in a perfect vertical position without forward or backward tilt. A pillow is placed under the neck for comfort and a blanket offered for warmth. Because the spinal cord terminates at approximately the L1 vertebral level, the puncture is performed below this level; i.e., at or below the L2–L3 interspace. A useful anatomic guidepost is the posterior iliac crest that corresponds to the L3–L4 interspace. The interspace is chosen following gentle palpation to identify the spinous processes at each lumbar level. The area is draped and cleansed by multiple washings with antiseptic ointment and alcohol. Local anesthetic, typically 1% lidocaine, is injected into the subcutaneous tissue; a topical anesthetic cream (lidocaine 2.5%/prilocaine 2.5%) applied 90 min prior to the procedure can eliminate pain associated with injection. About 5 min after the lidocaine injection, the lumbar puncture needle (typically 22 gauge) is inserted in the midline between two spinous processes and slowly advanced at a slightly caudal angle aiming at the umbilicus. It is important that the bevel of the needle be maintained in a horizontal position, parallel to the direction of the dural fibers; this minimizes injury to the fibers as the dura is penetrated. In most adults, the needle is advanced 4 to 5 cm (1 1/2 to 2 in.) before the subarachnoid space is reached, and the examiner usually recognizes entry as a sudden release of resistance. Some examiners prefer to remove the stylet periodically as the needle is advanced to look for CSF flow. If the needle cannot be advanced because bone is hit, if the patient experiences sharp radiating pain down one leg, or if the tap is "dry," the needle is removed completely and repositioned.

Once the subarachnoid space is reached, a manometer is attached to the needle and pressure measured. The examiner should look for normal oscillations in CSF pressure associated with pulse and respirations. Depending on the clinical indication, fluid is then obtained for studies including: (1) cell count, differential, and presence of microorganisms—it is often useful to repeat the cell count in the first and last tube; (2) protein, sugar, and other chemical measurements; (3) cytology; (4) VDRL, cryptococcal antigen, and serologic and genetic tests for other microorganisms as appropriate; (5) immunoelectrophoresis for determination of gamma globulin level (paired serum sample essential), oligoclonal banding, and other special biochemical tests (for NH_3, pH, CO_2, enzymes, etc.); and (6) bacteriologic cultures and virus isolation. Normal values of CSF constituents are shown in Appendix A. Under most conditions, the physician should not be concerned about removing too large a quantity of CSF. A sufficient volume to obtain all the data required is essential. In particular, adequate volumes for cytology, when indicated, should be removed.

Failure to enter the lumbar subarachnoid space after two or three trials can usually be corrected by repositioning patients in the sitting position and then assisting them to lie on their side for pressure measurements and fluid removal. The "dry tap" is more often due to an improperly placed needle than to a pathologic obliteration of subarachnoid space by a compressive lesion of the spinal cord or by chronic adhesive arachnoiditis. A bloody tap due to penetration of a meningeal vessel may result in confusion with subarachnoid hemorrhage. In these situations it is essential that a specimen of CSF be centrifuged immediately after it is obtained; clear supernatant CSF following centrifugation supports the diagnosis of a bloody tap, whereas xanthochromic supernatant suggests subarachnoid hemorrhage. In general, bloody CSF due to a meningeal vessel puncture clears gradually in successive tubes, whereas blood due to a subarachnoid hemorrhage does not. Xanthochromic CSF not due to blood products may also be present in patients with liver disease or when the level of CSF protein is elevated [>1.5 to 2.0 g/L (150 to 200 mg/dL)].

There are several absolute or relative contraindications to lumbar puncture. Lumbar puncture should be undertaken with particular care in patients with thrombocytopenia or disorders of blood coagulation because serious hemorrhage into the extradural or intradural space may occur. In these situations, it is prudent whenever possible to transfuse platelets, administer fresh frozen plasma, or reverse therapeutic anticoagulation prior to the procedure. The presence of local skin or soft tissue infections along the needle tract may result in spread of infection to the meninges; thus lumbar puncture at these sites should be avoided.

Lumbar puncture also carries a risk if the CSF pressure is high (evidenced by headache and papilledema), for it increases the possibility of fatal cerebellar or tentorial herniation. If this possibility exists and if CSF examination is required, it is wise first to obtain a computed tomography (CT) or magnetic resonance imaging (MRI) scan to exclude a mass lesion before proceeding to lumbar puncture. An exception to this rule is suspected meningitis, where CSF examination is always indicated. In this situation, the lumbar puncture may be performed with a fine-bore (24-gauge) needle. If the pressure is over 400 mmHg, the minimum required sample of fluid should be obtained, the needle removed, and, according to the suspected clinical disease and the patient's condition, mannitol administered in a dose of 0.75 to 1.0 mg/kg. Unless contraindicated, dexamethasone may be started in a dose of 4 to 6 mg every 6 h.

Cisternal puncture and lateral cervical puncture (C1–C2) are safe procedures in the hands of the expert but should not be performed by

Table 360-2

Indications for Lumbar Puncture

ABSOLUTE INDICATIONS

Meningitis
Encephalitis
Meningeal cancer
Acute inflammatory polyneuritis (Guillain-Barré syndrome)
Acute demyelinating disorders
    Acute disseminated encephalomyelitis
    Transverse myelitis
    Brainstem encephalomyelitis
Benign intracranial hypertension (pseudotumor cerebri)
Unexplained neurologic disorders
    Seizure
    Stroke
    Polyneuropathy
    Dementia
    Altered level of consciousness
Therapeutic administration of antibiotics or antineoplastic agents
Diagnostic injections of dyes (myelography) or radioisotopes (CSF leak)

POSSIBLE INDICATIONS (Depending on the Clinical Situation)

Multiple sclerosis
Subarachnoid hemorrhage

those without experience. Cisternal puncture is sometimes necessary in instances of spinal block to perform myelography above a lesion.

Following lumbar puncture, the patient should be positioned in a comfortable, recumbant position for 1 h before rising. The principal complication of lumbar puncture is a headache, occurring in 5 to 10 percent of patients, caused by a drop in CSF pressure related to persistent leakage of CSF. Such headaches typically begin 12 to 48 h after the procedure and may last from several days to 2 weeks. These headaches are strikingly positional in character; they are worsened by an upright posture and are relieved by lying flat. → *Therapy is discussed in Chap. 15.*

BIBLIOGRAPHY

ADAMS RD, VICTOR M: *Principles of Neurology*, 6th ed. New York, McGraw-Hill, 1997

FISHMAN RA: *Cerebrospinal Fluid in Diseases of the Nervous System*, 2d ed. Philadelphia, Saunders, 1992

HAERER AF: *DeJong's The Neurologic Examination*. Philadelphia, Lippincott, 1992

SWANSON PD: *Symptoms and Signs in Neurology*. Philadelphia, Lippincott, 1984

361	*Michael J. Aminoff*

ELECTROPHYSIOLOGIC STUDIES OF THE CENTRAL AND PERIPHERAL NERVOUS SYSTEMS

ELECTROENCEPHALOGRAPHY

The electrical activity of the brain [the electroencephalogram (EEG)] is easily recorded from electrodes placed on the scalp. The potential difference between pairs of electrodes on the scalp (bipolar derivation) or between individual scalp electrodes and a relatively inactive common reference point (referential derivation) is amplified and displayed on paper or the screen of an oscilloscope. The findings depend on the patient's age and level of arousal. The rhythmic activity normally recorded represents the postsynaptic potentials of vertically oriented pyramidal cells of the cerebral cortex and is characterized by its frequency. In normal awake adults lying quietly with the eyes closed, an 8- to 13-Hz alpha rhythm is seen posteriorly in the EEG, intermixed with a variable amount of generalized faster (beta) activity, and it is attenuated when the eyes are opened (Fig. 361-1). During drowsiness, the alpha rhythm is also attenuated; with light sleep, slower activity in the theta (4 to 7 Hz) and delta (<4 Hz) ranges becomes more conspicuous.

The EEG is best recorded from several different electrode arrangements (montages) in turn, and activating procedures are generally undertaken in an attempt to provoke abnormalities. Such procedures commonly include hyperventilation (for 3 or 4 min), photic stimulation, sleep, and the deprivation of sleep on the night prior to the recording. Electroencephalography is relatively inexpensive and may aid clinical management in several different contexts.

THE EEG AND EPILEPSY The EEG is most useful in evaluating patients with suspected epilepsy. The presence of *electrographic seizure activity*, i.e., of abnormal, repetitive, rhythmic activity having an abrupt onset and termination, clearly establishes the diagnosis. The absence of such electrocerebral accompaniment does not exclude a seizure disorder, however, because there may be no change in the scalp-recorded EEG during simple or complex partial seizures. It is often not possible to obtain an EEG during clinical events that may represent seizures, especially when such events occur unpredictably or infrequently. The development of portable equipment to record the EEG continuously on cassettes for 24 h or longer in ambulatory patients has made it easier to capture the electrocerebral accompaniments of such clinical episodes, and monitoring by this means is sometimes helpful in confirming that seizures are occurring, characterizing the nature of clinically equivocal episodes, and determining the frequency of epileptic events.

The EEG findings may also be helpful in the interictal period by showing certain abnormalities that are strongly supportive of a diagnosis of epilepsy. Such *epileptiform activity* consists of bursts of abnormal discharges containing spikes or sharp waves. The presence of epileptiform activity is not specific for epilepsy, but it has a much greater prevalence in epileptic patients than in normal individuals. When epileptiform activity is found in the EEG of a patient with episodic behavioral disturbances that clinically might be epileptic in nature, the likelihood that epilepsy is the correct diagnosis is markedly increased.

The EEG findings also have been used in classifying seizure disorders and selecting appropriate anticonvulsant medication for individual patients (Fig. 361-2). The episodic generalized spike-wave activity that occurs both during and between seizures in patients with typical absences (petit mal epilepsy) contrasts with the normal findings, focal interictal epileptiform discharges, or ictal patterns found in patients with complex partial seizures. These latter seizures may have no correlates in the scalp-recorded EEG or may be associated with abnormal rhythmic activity of variable frequency, a localized or generalized distribution, and a stereotyped pattern that varies with the patient. Focal or lateralized epileptogenic lesions are important to recognize, especially if surgical treatment is contemplated. Intensive long-term monitoring of clinical behavior and the EEG is required for operative candidates, however, and this generally also involves recording from intracranially placed electrodes (which may be subdural, extradural, or intracerebral in location).

The findings in the routine scalp-recorded EEG may indicate the prognosis of seizure disorders: in general, a normal EEG implies a better prognosis than otherwise, whereas an abnormal background or profuse epileptiform activity suggests a poor outlook. The EEG findings are not helpful in determining which patients with head injuries, stroke, or brain tumors will go on to develop seizures, because in such circumstances epileptiform activity is commonly encountered regardless of whether seizures occur. The EEG findings are sometimes used to determine whether anticonvulsant medication can be discontinued in epileptic patients who have been seizure-free for several years, but the findings provide only a general guide to prognosis: further seizures may occur after withdrawal of anticonvulsant medication despite a normal EEG or, conversely, may not occur despite a continuing EEG abnormality. The decision to discontinue anticonvulsant medication is made on clinical grounds, and the EEG does not have a useful role in this context except for providing guidance when there is clinical ambiguity or the patient requires reassurance about a particular course of action.

The EEG has no role in the management of tonic-clonic status epilepticus except when there is clinical uncertainty whether seizures are continuing in a comatose patient. In patients treated by pentobarbital-induced coma for refractory status epilepticus, the EEG findings are useful in indicating the level of anesthesia and whether seizures are occurring. During status epilepticus, the EEG shows repeated electrographic seizures or continuous spike-wave discharges. In nonconvulsive status epilepticus, a disorder that may not be recognized unless an EEG is performed, the EEG may also show continuous spike-wave activity ("spike-wave stupor") or, less commonly, repetitive electrographic seizures (complex partial status epilepticus).

THE EEG AND COMA The EEG tends to become slower as consciousness is depressed, regardless of the underlying cause (Fig. 361-1). Other findings may also be present and may suggest diagnostic possibilities, as when electrographic seizures are found or there is a focal abnormality indicating a structural lesion. The response of the EEG to external stimulation is helpful prognostically because electrocerebral responsiveness implies a lighter level of coma than a nonreactive EEG. Serial records provide a better guide to prognosis than a single record and supplement the clinical examination in following the course of events. As the depth of coma increases, the EEG becomes nonreactive and may show a burst-suppression pattern, with bursts of mixed-frequency activity separated by intervals of relative cerebral inactivity. In other instances there is a reduction in amplitude of the EEG until eventually electrocerebral activity cannot be detected. Such electrocerebral silence does not necessarily reflect irreversible brain damage, because it may occur in hypothermic patients or with drug overdose. The prognosis of electrocerebral silence, when recorded using an adequate technique, depends upon the clinical context in which it is found. In patients with severe cerebral anoxia, for example, electrocerebral silence in a technically satisfactory record implies that useful cognitive recovery will not occur.

The EEG is usually normal in patients with locked-in syndrome and helps in distinguishing this disorder from the comatose state with which it is sometimes confused clinically.

THE EEG IN OTHER NEUROLOGIC DISORDERS In the developed countries, computed tomography (CT) scanning and magnetic resonance imaging (MRI) have taken the place of EEG as a noninvasive means of screening for focal structural abnormalities of the brain, such as tumors, infarcts, or hematomas (Fig. 361-1). Nonetheless, the EEG is still used for this purpose in many parts of the world, although infratentorial or slowly expanding lesions may fail to cause any abnormalities. Focal slow-wave disturbances, a localized loss of electrocerebral activity, or more generalized electrocerebral disturbances are common findings but provide no reliable indication about the nature of the underlying pathology.

The EEG is also helpful for diagnostic purposes when it reveals the characteristic but nonspecific abnormalities found in certain neurologic disorders. The presence of complexes occurring with a regular repetition rate (so-called periodic complexes) in dementing disorders, for example, supports a diagnosis of Creutzfeldt-Jakob disease (Fig. 361-1) or subacute sclerosing panencephalitis, depending upon the appearance and frequency of the complexes and the clinical context. Focal or lateralized periodic slow-wave complexes, sometimes with a sharpened outline, in patients with an acute encephalopathy suggest a diagnosis of herpes simplex encephalitis, and periodic lateralized epileptiform discharges are commonly found with acute hemispheric pathology such as a hematoma, abscess, or rapidly expanding tumor.

The EEG generally slows in metabolic encephalopathies, and triphasic waves may be present. The findings do not permit differentiation of the underlying metabolic disturbance but help to exclude other encephalopathic processes by indicating the diffuse extent of cerebral dysfunction.

The EEG findings in dementia are nonspecific and usually do not distinguish between the different causes of cognitive decline except in rare instances when Creutzfeldt-Jakob disease or subacute sclerosing panencephalitis is responsible. The EEG may be normal or diffusely slowed, and the EEG findings alone cannot indicate whether a patient is demented or distinguish between dementia and pseudodementia.

EVOKED POTENTIALS

SENSORY EVOKED POTENTIALS The noninvasive recording of spinal or cerebral potentials elicited by stimulation of specific afferent pathways is an important means of monitoring the functional integrity of these pathways but does not indicate the pathologic basis of lesions involving them. Such evoked potentials

(EPs) are so small compared to the background EEG activity that the responses to a number of stimuli have to be recorded and averaged with a computer in order to permit their recognition and definition. The background EEG activity, which has no fixed temporal relationship to the stimulus, is averaged out by this procedure.

Visual evoked potentials (VEPs) are elicited by monocular stimulation with a reversing checkerboard pattern and are recorded from the occipital region in the midline and on either side of the scalp. The component of major clinical importance is the so-called P100 response, a positive peak having a latency of approximately 100 ms. Its presence, latency, and symmetry over the two sides of the scalp are noted. Amplitude may also be measured, but changes in size are much less helpful for the recognition of pathology. VEPs are most useful in detecting dysfunction of the visual pathways anterior to the optic chiasm. In patients with acute severe optic neuritis, the P100 is frequently lost or grossly attenuated; as clinical recovery occurs and visual acuity improves, the P100 is restored but with an increased latency that generally remains abnormally prolonged indefinitely. The VEP findings are therefore helpful in indicating previous or subclinical optic neuritis. They may also be abnormal with ocular abnormalities and with other causes of optic nerve disease, such as ischemia or compression by a tumor. Normal VEPs may be elicited by flash stimuli in patients with cortical blindness.

Brainstem auditory evoked potentials (BAEPs) are elicited by monaural stimulation with repetitive clicks and are recorded between the vertex of the scalp and the mastoid process or earlobe. A series of potentials, designated by roman numerals, occur in the first 10 ms after the stimulus and represent in part the sequential activation of different structures in the pathway between the auditory nerve (wave I) and the inferior colliculus (wave V) in the midbrain. The presence, latency, and interpeak latency of the first five positive potentials recorded at the vertex are

FIGURE 361-1 *A.* Normal EEG showing a posteriorly situated 9-Hz alpha rhythm that attenuates with eye opening. *B.* Abnormal EEG showing irregular diffuse slow activity in an obtunded patient with encephalitis. *C.* Irregular slow activity in the right central region, on a diffusely slowed background, in a patient with a right parietal glioma. *D.* Periodic complexes occurring once every second in a patient with Creutzfeldt-Jakob disease. Horizontal calibration: 1 s; vertical calibration: 200 μV in A, 300 μV in other panels. *(From Aminoff, 1992.)* In this and the following figure, electrode placements are indicated at the left of each panel and accord with the international 10:20 system. A, earlobe; C, central; F, frontal; Fp, frontal polar; P, parietal; T, temporal; O, occipital. Right-sided placements are indicated by even numbers, left-sided placements by odd numbers, and midline placements by Z.

FIGURE 361-2 Electrographic seizures. *A.* Onset of a tonic seizure showing generalized repetitive sharp activity with synchronous onset over both hemispheres. *B.* Burst of repetitive spikes occurring with sudden onset in the right temporal region during a clinical spell characterized by transient impairment of external awareness. *C.* Generalized 3-Hz spike-wave activity occurring synchronously over both hemispheres during an absence (petit mal) attack. Horizontal calibration: 1 s; vertical calibration: 400 μV in A, 200 μV in B, and 750 μV in C. *(From Aminoff, 1992.)*

evaluated. The findings are helpful in screening for acoustic neuromas, detecting brainstem pathology, and evaluating comatose patients. The BAEPs are normal in coma due to metabolic/toxic disorders or bihemispheric disease but abnormal in the presence of brainstem pathology.

Somatosensory evoked potentials (SEPs) are recorded over the scalp and spine in response to electrical stimulation of a peripheral (mixed or cutaneous) nerve. The configuration, polarity, and latency of the responses depend on the nerve that is stimulated and on the recording arrangements. SEPs are used to evaluate proximal (otherwise inaccessible) portions of the peripheral nervous system and the integrity of the central somatosensory pathways.

Clinical Utility of Sensory Evoked Potentials EP studies may detect and localize lesions in afferent pathways in the central nervous

system (CNS). They have been used particularly to investigate patients with suspected multiple sclerosis (MS), the diagnosis of which requires the recognition of lesions involving several different regions of the central white matter. In patients with clinical evidence of only one lesion, the electrophysiologic recognition of abnormalities in other sites helps to suggest or support the diagnosis but does not establish it unequivocally. In patients with suspected MS (or other neurologic disorders) who have vague, ill-defined complaints, the organic basis of symptoms may be supported by the presence of EP abnormalities in the appropriate afferent pathway. MRI is also helpful in detecting lesions in patients with possible MS, but electrophysiologic studies are cheaper and monitor the functional rather than anatomic status of the afferent pathways under study. Moreover, the electrophysiologic studies occasionally reveal abnormalities missed by MRI or vice versa. The two techniques therefore complement each other. Normal electrophysiologic (or imaging) findings do not exclude MS when this is a clinical possibility. In established MS, the use of EP studies to follow the disorder or its response to treatment is of uncertain value and unjustified at the present time.

EP abnormalities occur in disorders other than MS that involve the afferent pathways under test. Even multimodality EP abnormalities are not specific for MS; they may occur in AIDS, Lyme disease, systemic lupus erythematosus, neurosyphilis, spinocerebellar degenerations, familial spastic paraplegia, and deficiency of vitamin E or B_{12}. The diagnostic utility of the electrophysiologic findings therefore depends upon the circumstances in which they are found. Abnormalities may aid in the localization of lesions to broad areas of the CNS, but attempts at precise localization on electrophysiologic grounds are misleading because the generators of many components of the EP are unknown.

The EP findings are sometimes of prognostic relevance. Bilateral loss of those SEP components that are generated in the cerebral cortex implies that cognition may not be regained in posttraumatic or postanoxic coma, and EP studies may also be useful in evaluating patients with suspected brain death. In patients with spinal cord injuries, SEPs have been used to indicate the completeness of the lesion—the presence or early return of a cortically generated response to stimulation of a nerve below the injured segment of the cord indicates an incomplete lesion and thus a better prognosis for functional recovery than otherwise. Intraoperative monitoring of function in neural structures placed at risk by the surgical procedure may permit the early recognition of dysfunction. This may enable any permanent deficit to be averted or minimized by alteration of the responsible operative manipulation.

Visual and auditory acuity have been determined by ophthalmologists and audiologists using EP techniques in patients whose age or mental state precludes their cooperation for behavioral testing.

COGNITIVE EVOKED POTENTIALS Certain EP components depend upon the mental attention of the subject and the setting in which the stimulus occurs, rather than simply on the physical characteristics of the stimulus. Such "event-related" potentials (ERPs) or "endogenous" potentials are related in some manner to the cognitive aspects of distinguishing an infrequently occurring target stimulus from other stimuli occurring more frequently. For clinical purposes, attention has been directed particularly at the so-called P3 component of the ERP, which is also designated the P300 component because of its positive polarity and latency of approximately 300 to 400 ms after onset of an auditory target stimulus. The P3 component is prolonged in latency in many patients with dementia, whereas it is generally normal in patients with depression or other psychiatric disorders that might be mistaken for dementia. ERPs are therefore sometimes helpful in making this distinction when there is clinical uncertainty, although a response of normal latency does not exclude a dementing disorder.

MOTOR EVOKED POTENTIALS The electrical potentials recorded from muscle or the spinal cord following stimulation of the motor cortex or central motor pathways are referred to as motor evoked potentials. For clinical purposes such responses are recorded most often as the compound muscle action potentials elicited by transcutaneous magnetic stimulation of the motor cortex. A strong but brief magnetic field is produced by passing a current through a coil, and this induces stimulating currents in the subjacent neural tissue. The procedure is painless and apparently safe. Abnormalities have been described in several neurologic disorders with clinical or subclinical involvement of central motor pathways, including MS and motor neuron disease. The clinical utility of the technique is still being examined. In addition to a possible role in the diagnosis of neurologic disorders or in evaluating the extent of pathologic involvement, the technique may provide information of prognostic relevance (for example, in suggesting the likelihood of recovery of motor function after stroke) and may be useful as a means of monitoring intraoperatively the functional integrity of central motor tracts.

ELECTROPHYSIOLOGIC STUDIES OF MUSCLE AND NERVE

The motor unit is the basic element subserving motor function. It is defined as an anterior horn cell, its axon and neuromuscular junctions, and all the muscle fibers innervated by the axon. The number of motor units in a muscle ranges from approximately 10 in the extraocular muscles to several thousand in the large muscles of the legs. There is considerable variation in the average number of muscle fibers within the motor units of an individual muscle, i.e., in the innervation ratio of different muscles. Thus the innervation ratio is less than 25 in the human external rectus or platysma muscle and between 1600 and 1700 in the medial head of the gastrocnemius muscle. The muscle fibers of individual motor units are divided into two general types by distinctive contractile properties, histochemical stains, and characteristic responses to fatigue. Within each motor unit, all of the muscle fibers are of the same type.

ELECTROMYOGRAPHY The pattern of electrical activity in muscle [i.e., the *electromyogram* (EMG)], both at rest and during activity, may be recorded from a needle electrode inserted into the muscle. The nature and pattern of abnormalities relate to disorders at different levels of the motor unit.

Relaxed muscle normally is electrically silent except in the end-plate region, but abnormal spontaneous activity (Fig. 361-3) occurs in various neuromuscular disorders, especially those associated with denervation or inflammatory changes in affected muscle. Fibrillation potentials and positive sharp waves (which reflect muscle fiber irritability) and complex repetitive discharges are most often—but not always—found in denervated muscle and may also occur after muscle injury and in certain myopathic disorders, especially inflammatory disorders such as polymyositis. After an acute neuropathic lesion they are found earlier in proximal rather than distal muscles and sometimes do not develop distally in the extremities for 4 to 6 weeks; once present, they may persist indefinitely unless reinnervation occurs or the muscle degenerates so completely that no viable tissue remains. Fasciculation potentials (which reflect the spontaneous activity of individual motor units) are characteristic of slowly progressive neuropathic disorders, especially those with degeneration of anterior horn cells (such as amyotrophic lateral sclerosis). Myotonic discharges—high-frequency discharges of potentials derived from single muscle fibers that wax and wane in amplitude and frequency—are the signature of myotonic disorders such as myotonic dystrophy or myotonia congenita but occur occasionally in polymyositis or other, rarer, disorders.

Slight voluntary contraction of a muscle leads to activation of a small

number of motor units. The potentials generated by any muscle fibers of these units that are within the pick-up range of the needle electrode will be recorded (Fig. 361-3). The parameters of normal motor unit action potentials depend on the muscle under study and age of the patient, but their duration is normally between 5 and 15 ms, amplitude is between 200 μV and 2 mV, and most are bi- or triphasic. The number of units activated depends on the degree of voluntary activity. An increase in muscle contraction is associated with an increase in the number of motor units that are activated (recruited) and in the frequency with which they discharge. With a full contraction, so many motor units are normally activated that individual motor unit action potentials can no longer be distinguished, and a complete interference pattern is said to have been produced.

The incidence of small, short-duration, polyphasic motor unit action potentials (i.e., having more than four phases) is usually increased in myopathic muscle, and an excessive number of units is activated for a specified degree of voluntary activity. By contrast the loss of motor units that occurs in neuropathic disorders leads to a reduction in number of units activated during a maximal contraction and an increase in their firing rate, i.e., there is an incomplete or reduced interference pattern; the configuration and dimensions of the potentials may also be abnormal depending on the duration of the neuropathic process and on whether reinnervation has occurred. The surviving motor units are initially normal in configuration but, as reinnervation occurs, they increase in amplitude and duration and become polyphasic (Fig. 361-3).

Action potentials from the same motor unit sometimes fire with a consistent temporal relationship to each other, so that double, triple, or multiple discharges are recorded, especially in tetany, hemifacial spasm, or myokymia.

Electrical silence characterizes the involuntary, sustained muscle contraction that occurs in phosphorylase deficiency, which is designated a *contracture*.

EMG enables disorders of the motor units to be detected and characterized as either neurogenic or myopathic. In neurogenic disorders, the pattern of affected muscles may localize the lesion to the anterior horn cells or to a specific site as the axons traverse a nerve root, limb plexus, and peripheral nerve to their terminal arborizations.

FIGURE 361-3 Activity recorded during EMG. *A.* Spontaneous fibrillation potentials and positive sharp waves. *B.* Complex repetitive discharges recorded in partially denervated muscle at rest. *C.* Normal triphasic motor unit action potential. *D.* Small, short-duration, polyphasic motor unit action potential such as is commonly encountered in myopathic disorders. *E.* Long-duration polyphasic motor unit action potential such as may be seen in neuropathic disorders.

The findings do not enable a specific etiologic diagnosis to be made, however, except in conjunction with the clinical findings and results of other laboratory studies.

The findings may provide a guide to the severity of an acute disorder of a peripheral or cranial nerve (by indicating whether denervation has occurred and the completeness of the lesion), and whether the pathologic process is active or progressive in chronic or degenerative disorders such as amyotrophic lateral sclerosis. Such information is important for prognostic purposes.

Various quantitative EMG approaches have been developed. The most common is to determine the mean duration and amplitude of 20 motor unit action potentials using a standardized technique. The technique of macro-EMG provides information about the number and size of muscle fibers in a larger volume of the motor unit territory and has also been used to estimate the number of motor units in a muscle. Scanning EMG is a computer-based technique that has been used to study the topography of motor unit action potentials and, in particular, the spatial and temporal distribution of activity in individual units. Both of these latter approaches are of limited interest except to specialists and merit no further discussion. The technique of single-fiber EMG is of immediate clinical relevance, however, and is discussed separately below.

NERVE CONDUCTION STUDIES Recording of the electrical response of a muscle to stimulation of its motor nerve at two or more points along its course (Fig. 361-4) permits conduction velocity to be determined in the fastest-conducting motor fibers between the points of stimulation. The latency and amplitude of the electrical response of muscle (i.e., of the compound muscle action potential) to stimulation of its motor nerve at a distal site are also compared with

values defined in normal subjects. Sensory nerve conduction studies are performed by determining the conduction velocity and amplitude of action potentials in sensory fibers when these fibers are stimulated at one point and the responses are recorded at another point along the course of the nerve. In adults, conduction velocity in the arms is normally between 50 and 70 m/s, and in the legs is between 40 and 60 m/s.

Nerve conduction studies complement the EMG examination, enabling the presence and extent of peripheral nerve pathology to be determined. They are particularly helpful in determining whether sensory symptoms are arising from pathology proximal or distal to the dorsal root ganglia (in the former instance, peripheral sensory conduction studies will be normal) and whether neuromuscular dysfunction relates to peripheral nerve disease. In patients with a mononeuropathy, they are invaluable as a means of localizing a focal lesion, determining the extent and severity of the underlying pathology, providing a guide to prognosis, and detecting subclinical involvement of other peripheral nerves. They enable a polyneuropathy to be distinguished from a mononeuropathy multiplex when this is not possible clinically, an important distinction because of the etiologic implications. Nerve conduction studies provide a means of following the progression and therapeutic response of peripheral nerve disorders and may suggest the underlying pathologic basis in individual cases. Conduction velocity is often markedly slowed, terminal motor latencies are prolonged, and compound motor and sensory nerve action potentials may be dispersed in the demyelinative neuropathies (such as in chronic inflammatory polyneuropathy, metachromatic leukodystrophy, or certain hereditary neuropathies); conduction block is frequent in acquired varieties of these neuropathies (see Chap. 381). By contrast, conduction velocity is normal or slowed only mildly, sensory nerve action potentials are small or absent, and there is EMG evidence of denervation in axonal neuropathies such as occur in association with metabolic or toxic disorders.

The utility and complementary role of EMG and nerve conduction studies are best illustrated by reference to a common clinical problem. Numbness and paresthesia of the little finger and associated wasting of the intrinsic muscles of the hand may result from a spinal cord lesion, C8/T1 radiculopathy, brachial plexopathy (lower trunk or medial cord), or a lesion of the ulnar nerve. If sensory nerve action potentials can be recorded normally at the wrist following stimulation of the digital fibers in the affected finger, the pathology is probably proximal to the dorsal root ganglia, i.e., there is a radiculopathy or more central lesion; absence of the sensory potentials, by contrast, suggests distal pathology. EMG examination will indicate whether the pattern of affected muscles conforms to radicular or ulnar nerve territory, or is more extensive (thereby favoring a plexopathy); ulnar motor conduction studies will generally also distinguish between a radiculopathy (normal findings) and ulnar neuropathy (abnormal findings) and will often identify the site of an ulnar nerve lesion—the nerve is stimulated at several points along its course to determine whether the compound action potential recorded from a distal muscle that it supplies shows a marked alteration in size or area, or a disproportionate change in latency, with stimulation at a particular site. The electrophysiologic findings thus permit a definitive diagnosis to be made and specific treatment instituted in circumstances where there is clinical ambiguity.

F WAVE STUDIES Stimulation of a motor nerve causes impulses to travel antidromically toward the spinal cord (as well as orthodromically to the nerve terminals). Such antidromic impulses cause a few of the anterior horn cells to discharge, producing a small motor response that occurs considerably later than the direct response elicited by nerve stimulation. The F wave so elicited is sometimes abnormal (absent or delayed) with proximal pathology of the peripheral nervous system, such as a radiculopathy, and may therefore be helpful in detecting abnormalities when conventional nerve conduction studies are normal. In general, however, the clinical utility of F wave studies has been disappointing, except perhaps in Guillain-Barré syndrome, where they are often absent or delayed.

H REFLEX STUDIES The H reflex is easily recorded only from the soleus muscle in normal adults. It is elicited by low-intensity stimulation of the tibial nerve, and represents a monosynaptic reflex in which spindle (Ia) afferent fibers constitute the afferent arc and

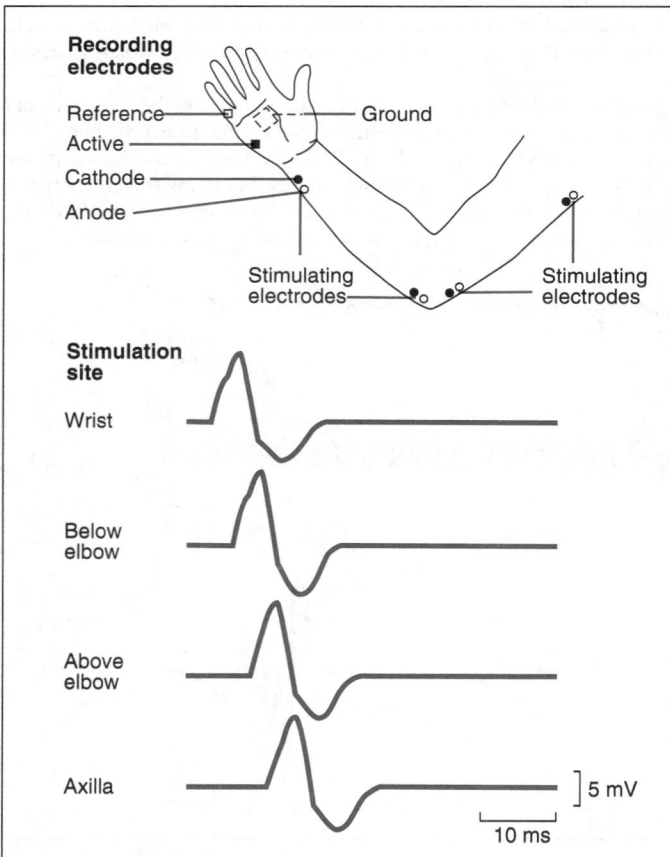

FIGURE 361-4 Arrangement for motor conduction studies of the ulnar nerve. Responses are recorded with a surface electrode from the abductor digiti minimi muscle to supramaximal stimulation of the nerve at different sites, and are shown in the lower panel. *(From Aminoff, 1987.)*

alpha motor axons the efferent pathway. The H reflexes are often absent bilaterally in elderly patients or with polyneuropathies and may be lost unilaterally in S1 radiculopathies.

MUSCLE RESPONSE TO REPETITIVE NERVE STIMU-LATION   The size of the electrical response of a muscle to supramaximal electrical stimulation of its motor nerve relates to the number of muscle fibers that are activated. Neuromuscular transmission can be tested by several different protocols, but the most helpful is to record with surface electrodes the electrical response of a muscle to supramaximal stimulation of its motor nerve by repetitive (2 to 3 Hz) shocks delivered before and at selected intervals after a maximal voluntary contraction.

There is normally little or no change in size of the compound muscle action potential following repetitive stimulation of a motor nerve at 2 to 3 Hz with stimuli delivered at intervals after voluntary contraction of the muscle for about 20 to 30 s, even though preceding activity in the junctional region influences the release of acetylcholine and thus the size of the endplate potentials elicited by a test stimulus. This is because more acetylcholine is normally released than is required to bring the motor endplate potentials to the threshold for generating muscle fiber action potentials. In disorders of neuromuscular transmission this safety factor is reduced. Thus, in myasthenia gravis repetitive stimulation, particularly at a rate of between 2 and 5 Hz, may lead to a depression of neuromuscular transmission, with a decrement in size of the response recorded from affected muscles. Similarly, immediately after a period of maximal voluntary activity, single or repetitive stimuli of the motor nerve may elicit larger muscle responses than before, indicating that more muscle fibers are responding. This postactivation facilitation of neuromuscular transmission is followed by a longer-lasting period of depression, maximal between 2 and 4 min after the conditioning period and lasting for as long as 10 min or so, during which responses are reduced in size.

Decrementing responses to repetitive stimulation at 2 to 5 Hz are common in myasthenia gravis but may also occur in the congenital myasthenic syndromes. In Lambert-Eaton myasthenic syndrome, in which there is defective release of acetylcholine at the neuromuscular junction, the compound muscle action potential elicited by a single stimulus is generally very small. With repetitive stimulation at rates of up to 10 Hz, the first few responses may decline in size, but subsequent responses increase. If faster rates of stimulation are used (20 to 50 Hz), the increment may be dramatic so that the amplitude of compound muscle action potentials eventually reaches a size that is several times larger than the initial response. In patients with botulism, the response to repetitive stimulation is similar to that in Lambert-Eaton syndrome, although the findings are somewhat more variable and not all muscles are affected.

SINGLE-FIBER ELECTROMYOGRAPHY   The technique of single-fiber EMG is particularly helpful in detecting disorders of neuromuscular transmission. A special needle electrode is placed within a muscle and positioned to record action potentials from two muscle fibers belonging to the same motor unit. The time interval between the two potentials will vary in consecutive discharges, and this is called the *neuromuscular jitter*. The jitter can be quantified as the mean difference between consecutive interpotential intervals and is normally between 10 and 50 μs. This value is increased when neuromuscular transmission is disturbed for any reason, and in some instances impulses in individual muscle fibers may fail to occur because of impulse blocking at the neuromuscular junction. Single-fiber EMG is more sensitive than repetitive nerve stimulation or determination of acetylcholine receptor antibody levels in diagnosing myasthenia gravis.

Single-fiber EMG can also be used to determine mean fiber density of motor units (i.e., mean number of muscle fibers per motor unit within the recording area) and to estimate the number of motor units in a muscle, but this is of less immediate clinical relevance.

BLINK REFLEXES   Electrical or mechanical stimulation of the supraorbital nerve on one side leads to two separate reflex responses of the orbicularis oculi—an ipsilateral R1 response having a latency of approximately 10 ms and a bilateral R2 response with a latency in the order of 30 ms. The trigeminal and facial nerves constitute the afferent and efferent arcs of the reflex, respectively. Abnormalities of either nerve or intrinsic lesions of the medulla or pons may lead to uni- or bilateral loss of the response, and the findings may therefore be helpful in identifying or localizing such pathology.

TESTS OF AUTONOMIC FUNCTION

Noninvasive tests of autonomic function are becoming increasingly important for the recognition of small-fiber peripheral neuropathies and in defining central dysautonomias, such as the Shy-Drager syndrome. Invasive tests, such as microneurography, provide information of considerable academic importance, but because of their specialized nature and limited clinical utility they are not discussed further. → *For further discussion, see Chap. 371.*

Heart-rate responses and the Valsalva maneuver are described in Chap. 371. Heart-rate increases with changes from a supine to erect posture are considered normal if the heart rate increases in the first 15 s or so and then slows. Assessment of sudomotor function is also discussed in Chap. 371.

BIBLIOGRAPHY

AMINOFF MJ: *Electromyography in Clinical Practice: Electrodiagnostic Aspects of Neuromuscular Disease*, 2d ed. New York, Churchill Livingstone, 1987
———— (ed): *Electrodiagnosis in Clinical Neurology*, 3d ed. New York, Churchill Livingstone, 1992
DALY DD, PEDLEY TA (eds): *Current Practice of Clinical Electroencephalography*, 2d ed. New York, Raven Press, 1990
DUMITRU D: *Electrodiagnostic Medicine*. Philadelphia, Hanley and Belfus, 1995
EBERSOLE JS (ed): *Ambulatory EEG Monitoring*. New York, Raven Press, 1988
KIMURA J: *Electrodiagnosis in Diseases of Nerve and Muscle*, 2d ed. Philadelphia, Davis, 1989
NIEDERMEYER E, LOPES DA SILVA F (eds): *Electroencephalography*, 3d ed. Baltimore, Urban & Schwarzenberg, 1993

---

362   *William P. Dillon*

NEUROIMAGING IN NEUROLOGIC DISORDERS

A dramatic increase in the role of imaging in diagnosis of neurologic diseases occurred with the development of computed tomography (CT) in the early 1970s and of magnetic resonance imaging (MRI) in the 1980s. MRI has gradually replaced CT for many indications and has also replaced many of the invasive neuroimaging techniques, such as myelography and angiography. Guidelines for the use of new imaging technologies are difficult to develop during a period of rapid advance. In general, MRI is more sensitive than CT for the evaluation of most lesions affecting the brain and spinal cord parenchyma. CT is more sensitive than MRI for visualizing osseous detail and brain hemorrhage (parenchymal or subarachnoid). Conventional angiography is reserved for cases in which small-vessel detail is essential for diagnosis (Table 362-1). Recent developments, such as helical CT, CT angiography (CTA), MR angiography (MRA), positron emission tomography, Doppler ultrasound, and interventional angiography have continued to advance diagnosis and therapy.

COMPUTED TOMOGRAPHY   Technique   The CT image is a computer-generated cross-sectional representation of anatomy created by an analysis of the attenuation of x-ray beams passed through various points around a section of the body. As the x-ray source, collimated to the desired slice thickness, rotates around the patient, sensitive x-ray detectors aligned 180° from the source detect x-rays attenuated by the patient's anatomy. A computer calculates a "back projection" image from the 360° x-ray attenuation profile. Greater x-ray attenuation, as caused by bone, results in areas of high "density," while soft tissue structures, which attenuate x-rays less, are lower in density. The resolution of an image depends on the radiation dose, the collimation (slice thickness), the field of view, and the matrix size of the display. A typical modern CT scanner is capable of obtaining sections 1 to 2, 5, and 10 mm thick at a speed of 1 to 3 s per section; complete studies of the brain can be completed in 2 to 3 min.

Intravenous contrast is often administered prior to or during a CT study to identify vascular structures and to detect defects in the blood-brain barrier (BBB) associated with pathologies such as tumors, infarcts, and infections. An intact BBB prevents contrast molecules, which are large, from exiting the intravascular compartment. In the normal central nervous system (CNS), only vessels and those structures not having a BBB (e.g., the pituitary gland, choroid plexus, and dura) enhance. The use of contrast agents carries a risk of allergic reaction, increases the dose of radiation when both noncontrast and contrast CT scans are to be obtained, adds expense, and may mask hemorrhage; thus before contrast is administered, the indication for its use should always be considered carefully.

Helical CT is a new technique in which continuous three-dimensional CT information is obtained. In the helical scan mode, the table moves continuously through the rotating x-ray beam, generating a "helix" of information which can be reformatted into various slice thicknesses. Advantages include shorter scan times, reduced patient and organ motion, and the ability to acquire images during the infusion of intravenous contrast. The contrast images can be used to construct CT angiograms of vascular structures. CTA images require a workstation to threshold and segment CT images for display (Fig. 362-1). CTA has proven useful in assessing the carotid bifurcation and intracranial arterial anatomy in selected instances in which a contraindication to MR angiography exists.

Indications The indications for CT have diminished since the development of MRI. While MRI gives greater soft tissue contrast and is more sensitive than CT in detecting early brain damage, CT is useful in imaging osseous structures of the spine, skull base, and temporal bones. CT is also more sensitive and specific than MRI for acute parenchymal and subarachnoid hemorrhage. In the spine, CT is often useful in evaluating patients with osseous spinal stenosis and spondylosis, but MRI is often preferred in those with neurologic deficits.

Complications CT is safe and reliable. Radiation levels are between 3 and 5 cGy per examination. The most frequent complications are associated with use of intravenous contrast agents. Two broad categories of contrast media, ionic and nonionic, are in use. Ionic agents are relatively safe and inexpensive but cause a higher incidence of toxicity reactions than nonionic agents.

Nephrotoxicity resulting from contrast administration (*contrast nephropathy*) may result from hemodynamic changes, tubular obstruction and cell damage, or immunologic reactions to contrast agents. A rise in serum creatinine of at least 1 mg/dL within 48 h of contrast administration is often used as a definition of contrast nephropathy, although other causes of acute renal failure must be excluded. The prognosis is usually favorable, with serum creatinine levels returning to baseline within 1 to 2 weeks. Risk factors for contrast nephropathy include advanced age, chronic renal insufficiency, diabetes, dehydration, and high contrast dose. Preexisting renal disease, diabetes, and cardiac disease indicate a worse prognosis. Diabetics and those with mild renal failure should be well hydrated prior to the administration of nonionic agents. Nonionic, low-osmolar media produce fewer abnormalities in renal blood flow and less endothelial cell damage than ionic agents (Table 362-2).

A sensation of heat, pain, nausea, and vomiting are well-known side effects following intravenous administration of ionic contrast media, and they become more important as studies require longer imaging times and repeated contrast injections. Pain and the sensation of heat are probably due to the osmolality of the agent and vasodilation. These side effects are less intense or nonexistent with nonionic contrast media.

Anaphylactoid reactions to intravenous contrast media range from mild hives to bronchospasm to acute anaphylaxis and death. The pathogenesis of these allergic reactions is not fully understood, but it is thought to include the release of mediators such as histamine, antibody-antigen reactions, and complement activation. Severe allergic

Table 362-1

Guidelines for the Use of CT, Ultrasound, and MRI

Condition	Recommended Technique
Hemorrhage	
Acute parenchymal	CT > MRI
Subacute/chronic	MRI
Subarachnoid hemorrhage	CT, lumbar puncture → angiography
Aneurysm	Angiography > ?MRA
Ischemic infarction	
Hemorrhagic infarction	CT or MRI
Bland infarction	MRI > CT
Carotid or vertebral dissection	MRI/MRA
Vertebral basilar insufficiency	MRI/MRA
Carotid stenosis	Doppler ultrasound, MRA
Suspected mass lesions	
Neoplasm, primary or metastatic	MRI + contrast
Infection/abscess	MRI + contrast
Immunosuppression with focal findings	MRI + contrast
Vascular malformations	MRI ± angiography
White matter disorders	MRI
Demyelinating disease	MRI ± contrast
Dementia	MRI or CT
Trauma	
Acute trauma	CT (noncontrast)
Shear injury/chronic hemorrhage	MRI
Headache/migraine	CT (noncontrast) or MRI
Seizure	
First time, no focal neurologic deficits	MRI > CT as screen
Partial complex/refractory	MRI + coronal T2W imaging
Cranial neuropathy	MRI + contrast
Meningeal disease	MRI + contrast
SPINE	
Low back pain	
No neurologic deficits	Conservative therapy, consider MRI or CT after 4 weeks
With focal deficits	MRI > CT
Spinal stenosis	MRI or CT
Cervical spondylosis	MRI or CT myelography
Infection	MRI + contrast, CT
Myelopathy	MRI + contrast, consider myelography if MRI negative
Arteriovenous malformations	MRI, myelography/angiography

FIGURE 362-1 CT angiography of middle cerebral aneurysm. A right middle cerebral aneurysm (*arrow*) is shown on CTA (*left image*) and confirmed by conventional internal carotid angiography (*right image*). CTA image is produced by helical scans or 1-mm CT scans performed during a rapid bolus infusion of intravenous contrast medium. Subtraction of background nonenhancing brain results in the CTA image. (*From RA Alberico et al, Am J Neuroradiol 16:1571, 1995.*)

Table 362-2

Guidelines for Use of Intravenous Contrast in Patients with Impaired Renal Function

Serum Creatinine Level, μmol/L (mg/dL)*	Guideline
<133 (<1.5)	Use either ionic or nonionic contrast at 2 mL/kg to 150 mL total
133–177 (1.5–2.0)	Use nonionic contrast; hydrate diabetics
>177 (>2.0)	Consider noncontrast CT or MRI; use nonionic contrast if required
177–221 (2.0–2.5)	Use nonionic contrast only if required (as above); contraindicated in diabetics
>265 (>3.0)	Nonionic contrast given only to patients undergoing dialysis within 24 h

* Note risk is greatest in patients with rising creatinine levels.

reactions occur in approximately 0.04 percent of patients receiving nonionic media, sixfold fewer than with ionic media. Risk factors include a history of prior contrast reaction, allergy (asthma and hay fever), and cardiac disease. In these patients, an alternative noncontrast CT or MRI procedure should be considered, or nonionic agents should be used in conjunction with pretreatment with glucocorticoids and antihistamines (Tables 362-3 and 362-4). Patients with allergic reactions to iodinated contrast material do not usually react against gadolinium-based MR contrast material, although it would be wise to pretreat in a similar fashion prior to MR contrast administration.

MAGNETIC RESONANCE IMAGING *Technique* The phenomenon of magnetic resonance is a complex interaction between protons in biologic tissues, a static and alternating magnetic field (the magnet), and energy in the form of radiofrequency waves of a specific frequency (Rf), introduced by coils placed next to the body part of interest. The energy state of the hydrogen protons is transiently excited. The subsequent return to equilibrium (relaxation) of the protons results in a release of Rf energy (the echo) which can be measured by the same surface coils that delivered the Rf pulses. The complex Rf signal or echo is transformed by Fourier analysis into the information used to form an MR image.

T1 and T2 relaxation times The rate of return to equilibrium of perturbed protons is called the *relaxation rate*. The relaxation rate is different for different normal and pathologic tissues. The relaxation rate of a hydrogen proton in a tissue is influenced by surrounding molecular environment and atomic neighbors. Two relaxation rates, the T1 and T2 relaxation times, are measurable. The T1 relaxation rate is the time for 63 percent of the protons to return to their normal equilibrium state, while the T2 relaxation rate is the time for 63 percent of the protons to become dephased owing to interactions among adjacent protons. The intensity of the signal and thus the image contrast can be modulated by altering certain parameters, such as the interval between Rf pulses (TR) and the time between the Rf pulse and the signal reception (TE). So-called T1-weighted (T1W) images are produced by keeping the TR and TE relatively short. Under these conditions, contrast between structures is based primarily on their T1 relaxation differences. T2-weighted (T2W) images are produced by using

Table 362-3

Indications for the Use of Nonionic Contrast Media

- Prior adverse reaction to contrast media, with the exception of heat, flushing, or an episode of nausea or vomiting
- Asthma or other serious lung disease
- History of atopic allergies (pretreatment with glucocorticoids and antihistamines recommended)
- Age under 2 years old
- Renal failure or a creatinine level >177 μmol/L (>2.0 mg/dL)
- Cardiac dysfunction, including cardiac failure, severe arrhythmias, unstable angina pectoris, recent myocardial infarction, or pulmonary hypertension
- Diabetes
- Severe debilitation

Table 362-4

Guidelines for the Premedication of Patients with Prior Allergic Reaction to Contrast Agents

12 h before examination
    Prednisone, 40 mg PO *or* methylprednisolone (Medrol), 32 mg PO

2 h before examination
    Prednisone, 40 mg PO *or* methylprednisolone (Medrol), 32 mg PO
        and
    Cimetidine, 300 mg PO *or* ranitidine, 150 mg PO

Immediately before examination
    Benadryl, 50 mg IV (alternatively, can be given PO 2 h before exam)

longer TR and TE times (Fig. 362-2). Fat and subacute hemorrhage have short T1 relaxation rates and have a high signal intensity on T1W images. Watery media, such as cerebrospinal fluid (CSF) and edematous tissue, have long T1 and T2 relaxation rates and have a low signal intensity on T1W images and a high signal intensity on T2W images (Table 362-5). Gray matter contains 10 to 15 percent more water than white matter, and white matter contains more lipid (due to myelin) than gray matter. These two chemical differences account for much of the contrast difference between gray and white matter on MRI (Fig. 362-2). T2W images are more sensitive than T1W images to edema or myelin destruction (see Fig. 376-2).

MR images can be generated in sagittal, coronal, axial, and oblique planes without changing the patient's position. Each plane obtained requires a separate sequence lasting 5 to 10 minutes. Unlike CT, movement of the patient during a sequence will distort *all* the images; therefore, patient cooperation is important. Approximately 5 percent of the population experience claustrophobia in the MR environment. This can be reduced by mild sedation. Three-dimensional volumetric imaging is also possible with MR, resulting in a volume of data that can be reformatted in any plane and manipulated in a real-time fashion to highlight certain disease processes.

Contrast material The heavy-metal element *gadolinium* forms the basis of all current intravenous MR contrast agents. Gadolinium is a paramagnetic substance, which means that it reduces the T1 and T2 relaxation times of nearby water protons, resulting in a high signal on T1W images. The metal is chelated to an agent such as DTPA, which allows renal excretion without toxicity. Approximately 0.2 mL/kg body weight is administered intravenously (10 to 15 mL for the average-sized adult); the cost is approximately $100. Gadolinium contrast does not cross a normal BBB, and thus it causes enhancement of brain tissue only at sites of abnormalities in the BBB (see Fig. 376-2C) and in areas of the brain that normally have no BBB, such as the pituitary gland. Allergic reactions are extremely rare; renal failure does not occur. These agents can be administered safely to children as well as adults.

MAGNETIC RESONANCE ANGIOGRAPHY Flowing blood exhibits complex MR signals that range from bright to dark relative to background stationary tissue (Fig. 362-2). Fast-flowing blood, such as arterial blood, shows no signal on routine MR images. Slower flow, as in veins or distal to arterial stenoses, may appear high in signal. It is possible, by varying the MR image parameters, to assess blood flow either qualitatively or quantitatively. This is the basis of

Table 362-5

Some Common Intensities on T1- and T2-Weighted MRI Sequences

Image	TR	TE	Signal Intensity CSF	Fat	Brain	Edema Fluid
T1W	Short	Short	Low	High	Low	Low
T2W	Long	Long	High	Low	High	High

ABBREVIATIONS: T1W, T1-weighted; T2W, T2-weighted.

MR angiography which capitalizes on the differences in signal between moving blood and stationary tissue on gradient echo images (Fig. 362-3). *Gradient echo images* differ from standard spin echo images in being more sensitive to blood products, calcification, and other susceptibility artifacts. The suppression of background signal achieved in short-flip-angle gradient echo images provides the contrast needed for flowing blood to appear bright in signal on MRA images.

It is important to understand that MRA provides a *vascular flow map* rather than the anatomic map given by conventional angiography. Two MRA techniques, time-of-flight (TOF) and phase-contrast, are currently used. TOF, currently the technique used most frequently, relies on the suppression of nonmoving tissue to provide a background for the high signal intensity of flowing blood. A typical TOF angiography sequence results in a series of contiguous thin MR sections (0.9 mm thick), which can be viewed as a stack to create an angiographic image data set that can be reformatted or viewed in various planes and angles to reveal the vascular relationships (Fig. 362-3). Either arterial or venous structures may be highlighted.

Phase-contrast MRA has a longer acquisition time than TOF MRA but reveals the velocity and direction of blood flow in addition to providing anatomic information similar to that of TOF imaging. Through the selection of different imaging parameters, differing blood velocities can be highlighted; selective venous and arterial MRA images thus can be obtained. One advantage of phase-contrast MRA is the excellent suppression of background signal.

MRA has lower resolution than conventional angiography and therefore cannot detect small-vessel detail, such as is needed in the workup of vasculitis. It is also less sensitive to slow flow and thus may not differentiate occlusive disease from near-occlusive disease. Motion, either by the patient or by anatomic structures, may distort the images, creating artifacts that may be misinterpreted as stenoses or occlusions. These limitations notwithstanding, MRA has proved useful in evaluation of the cervical carotid artery and larger-caliber intracranial arterial and venous structures. It has also proved useful in the noninvasive detection of intracranial aneurysms (Fig. 366-13) and vascular malformations.

ECHO-PLANAR MR IMAGING Recent improvements in gradients, software, and high-speed computer processors now permit MR imaging of the brain on the order of milliseconds. With echo-planar MRI (EPI), fast gradients are switched on and off at high speeds to create the information used to form an image. In routine spin echo imaging, images of the brain can be obtained in 5 to 10 min. With EPI, all of the information required for processing an image is accumulated in 50 to 150 ms, and the information for the entire brain is obtained in 5 to 10 s (Fig. 362-4A). EPI allows motion-free imaging, as well as perfusion imaging, diffusion imaging (Fig. 362-4B), functional MRI (Fig. 362-5), and kinematic motion studies.

EPI techniques are just now making their way into clinical practice. The hope for these techniques is that they can provide useful functional data in addition to exquisite anatomic images. Early indications suggest a possible role for EPI perfusion and diffusion imaging in early detection of ischemic injury of the brain and in the characterization of white matter tracts (Fig. 362-4B). *Functional MRI* of the brain is a technique that localizes regions of activity in the brain following task activation. EPI or gradient echo techniques can be used for somatosensory localization with tasks that alter the balance of oxyhemoglobin and deoxyhemoglobin. Repetitive actions such as finger tapping elicit an increase in the amount of blood flow delivered to a specific region of the brain, resulting in a slight increase in oxyhemoglobin and a 2 to 3 percent change in signal intensity (Fig. 362-5). Further work will determine whether these techniques are cost effective or clinically useful.

Complications of MRI and Patient Safety MRI is considered safe for patients at magnetic field levels up to 3 T. However, serious injuries have been caused by the high magnetic fields used. Ferromagnetic (metal) objects can be attracted to the magnet and act as missiles if brought into the magnet room. Likewise, ferromagnetic aneurysm clips may torque within the magnet, causing hemorrhage and even death. Metallic foreign bodies in the eye have moved and caused hemorrhage, so screening for ocular metallic fragments is indicated in those with a history of metalwork. Implanted cardiac pacemakers are a contraindication to MRI owing to the risk of induced arrhythmias. All personnel and patients must be screened thoroughly to prevent such disasters. Table 362-6 lists several of the more common contraindications for MRI.

POSITRON EMISSION TOMOGRAPHY Positron emission tomography (PET) relies on the detection of positrons emitted during the decay of a radionuclide that has been injected into a patient. The most frequently used moiety is 2-[^{18}F]fluoro-2-deoxy-D-glucose (FDG), which is an analogue of glucose and is taken up by cells competitively with 2-deoxyglucose. Multiple images of glucose uptake activity are formed after 45 to 60 min. Images reveal differences in regional glucose activity among normal and pathologic brain structures. FDG PET scanning has been used to assist in differentiating radiation necrosis from active neoplasm following therapy, in localizing temporal lobe

FIGURE 362-2 Normal MRI scans of the brain. *A, B.* Axial T2-weighted images through (*A*) the lateral ventricles and (*B*) the circle of Willis. Note that gray matter is slightly higher in signal intensity than white matter. CSF has a bright signal intensity owing to its free mobile water content. Moving protons in arterial structures demonstrate a signal void (*arrows*). *C.* T1-weighted image. Less contrast is visible between gray and white matter structures; however white matter appears slightly higher in signal intensity than gray matter owing to a shorter T1 relaxation time. Signal flow voids are seen in arterial structures and CSF spaces.

FIGURE 362-3 Use of MR angiography in cerebral ischemia. *A.* Axial proton density–weighted image demonstrates two focal areas of increased signal intensity in the right frontal lobe consistent with subcortical infarction (*arrows*). *B.* One of 90 sections from a 3-D time-of-flight gradient echo MR angiogram sequence in which flowing blood produces high signal intensity. The left internal carotid and basilar arteries show normal flow-related enhancement (*arrows*). The absence of signal in the right internal carotid artery (*arrowheads*) indicates either occlusion or high-grade stenosis with extremely slow flow in the internal carotid artery system. *C.* Maximum intensity projection, collapsed (submento-vertex) view, MRA. This image is obtained from the summation of the 90 partitions, one of which is shown in *B.* The left internal carotid artery is patent (*arrow*). Flow is absent in the right internal carotid artery. The right middle cerebral artery (*arrowheads*) is perfused by collateral flow across the anterior communicating artery as well as through the posterior communicating arteries. *D.* A 15° projection from a 2-D time-of-flight MR angiogram sequence through the cervical carotid arteries. The right internal carotid artery is occluded at the carotid bifurcation (*black arrow*). A high-grade (70 to 80 percent) stenosis is also present at the origin of the left internal carotid artery (*white arrow*).

tively high concentration and volume of contrast material and visualization by x-ray "spot films" and formal "overhead" plain films. The radiation exposure during conventional myelography is 4 to 8 cGy, making it one of the more radiation-intense procedures. The gonads should be shielded if possible, although doing so is sometimes difficult. CT scanning is often performed after myelography (*CT myelography*), in which case it demonstrates the spinal cord and roots as filling defects in the opacified subarachnoid space. CT myelography alone, in which CT is performed after the subarachnoid injection of a relatively small amount of relatively dilute contrast material, has replaced conventional myelography for many indications, thereby reducing exposure to radiation and contrast media. CT slices 3 to 5 mm thick are routinely obtained through the area of interest.

Indications For diagnosis of diseases of the spinal canal and cord, myelography has been largely replaced by CT, CT myelography, and MRI (Table 362-1). The remaining indications for conventional plain film myelography include the evaluation of suspected meningeal

FIGURE 362-4 Echo-planar imaging (EPI) of the brain. *A.* Axial T2-weighted, "single-shot," spin-echo EPI of the brain. The image is distorted by susceptibility effects near the calvaria and the aerated frontal sinuses. Otherwise, this image resembles a spin echo T2-weighted image of the brain, but was obtained in 100 ms. *B.* Sagittal echo planar diffusion-weighted image. Restriction of microscopic water motion, such as occurs within axons coursing in one plane, results in increased signal intensity. So-called diffusion anisotropy is demonstrated in the corpus callosum (*arrows*). Diffusion of water protons is restricted in the corpus callosum to the left-to-right direction along the axonal fibers. This technique is also very sensitive to early infarction.

epileptic foci, and in detecting metastatic disease and determining cardiac viability. A lower activity of FDG in the parietal lobes has been associated with Alzheimer's disease (see Fig. 367-1).

MYELOGRAPHY Technique Myelography involves the intrathecal instillation of 8 to 15 mL of water-soluble iodinated contrast medium (180 to 300 mg%) into the lumbar or cervical subarachnoid space via a percutaneously placed spinal needle (22 gauge or smaller). Contrast is maneuvered into the area of interest by fluoroscopic guidance and patient rotation. *Conventional myelography* involves a rela-

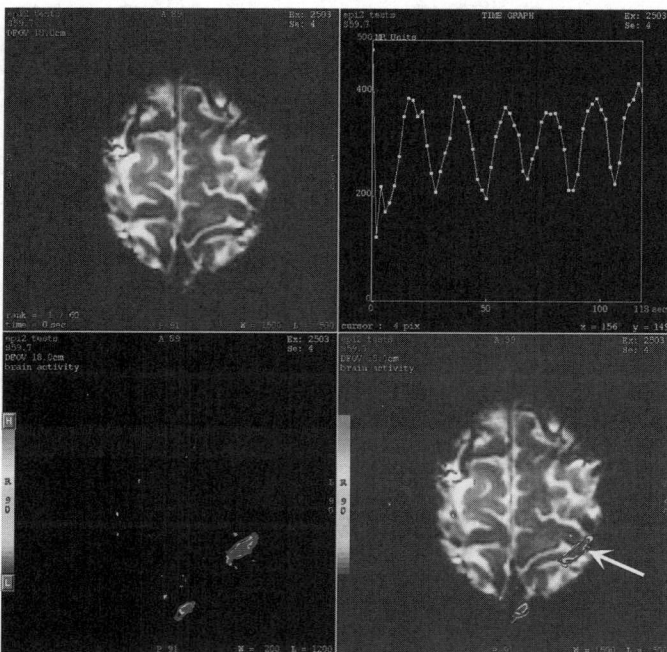

FIGURE 362-5 Functional EPI imaging with somatosensory localization. The patient was asked to repetitively touch his right index finger to thumb with a periodicity of 2 Hz for 10 s intervals alternating with rest periods of 10 s (*upper right image*). Echo planar images were obtained with a TE of 26 and 60 ms (*upper left image*). Subtraction of task-on and task-off images reveals changes in signal intensity related to increases in the level of oxyhemoglobin brought to the site of activation (*lower left image*). Superimposition shows that the increase in oxyhemoglobin during task activation overlies the anatomic region of the central sulcus corresponding to the right index finger and thumb regions (*arrow, lower right image*).

or arachnoid cysts and the localization of spinal dural arteriovenous fistulas and CSF fistulas. Conventional myelography and CT myelography provide the most precise information in patients with prior spinal fusion and spinal fixation hardware.

Contraindications Myelography is relative safe. However, it should be performed with caution in any patient with suspected herniation, elevated intracranial pressure, or a history of allergic reaction to intrathecal contrast media. In patients with a suspected spinal block, only a small amount of contrast medium should be instilled below

Table 362-6

Common Contraindications for MRI*

Cardiac pacemaker or permanent pacemaker leads
Internal defibrillatory devices
Cochlear prostheses
Bone growth stimulators
Implanted spinal cord stimulators
Electronic infusion devices
Intracranial aneurysm clips (some but not all)
Ocular implants (some) or ocular metallic foreign body
McGee stapedectomy piston prosthesis
Omniphase penile implant
Swan-Ganz catheter
Magnetic stoma plugs
Magnetic dental implants
Magnetic sphincters
Ferromagnetic IVC filters, coils, stents—considered safe at 6 weeks after implantation
Tattooed eyeliner (contains ferromagnetic material and may result in eye irritation)

* For a complete list, see Shellock and Kanal.

the level of the block to prevent deterioration. Lumbar puncture is to be avoided in patients with bleeding disorders, including patients receiving anticoagulant therapy.

Complications Complications resulting from myelography are related to the needle puncture and to reactions to intrathecal contrast material.

Vasovagal syncope may occur during lumbar puncture; it is accentuated by the upright position used during lumbar myelography. Adequate hydration before and after myelography will reduce the incidence of this complication.

Headache, nausea, and vomiting are the most frequent complications of dural puncture and myelography, occurring in up to 38 percent of patients. These symptoms are thought to result from neurotoxic effects of the contrast agent, persistent leakage of CSF at the puncture site, or psychological reactions to the procedure. The incidence of headache has been reduced with the use of smaller-gauge spinal needles and nonionic, water-soluble contrast agents.

Postural headache (post–lumbar puncture headache) is generally due to prolonged leakage of CSF from the puncture site, resulting in CSF hypotension. Intravenous hydration may be helpful, and an autologous epidural blood patch is indicated in patients with persistent headache 48 h after myelography (see also Chap. 15).

Hearing loss is a rare complication. It may result from a direct toxic effect of the contrast medium or from an alteration of the pressure equilibrium between CSF and perilymph in the inner ear.

Puncture of the spinal cord is a rare but serious complication of cervical (C1-2) and high lumbar puncture. The cervical approach requires proper alignment of the patient and is best performed in the prone position using fluoroscopy guidance. Direct puncture of the spinal cord, laceration of epidural and vertebral venous and arterial structures, and hyperextension of the neck are reported complications. Injection of contrast material into the spinal cord can precipitate acute neurologic decline or subacute hemorrhagic necrosis of the gray matter. The risk of cord puncture is greatest in patients with spinal stenosis or conditions that reduce CSF volume. In these settings, a low-dose lumbar injection followed by thin-section CT is a safer alternative to cervical puncture.

Intrathecal contrast reactions are rare, but aseptic meningitis and encephalopathy may occur. The latter is usually dose-related and associated with contrast entering the intracranial subarachnoid space. *Seizures* occur following myelography in 0.1 to 0.3 percent of patients. Risk factors include a preexisting seizure disorder and the use of a total iodine dose of >4500 mg. Other reported symptoms include headache, hyperthermia, hallucinations, depression, and anxiety states. These neurotoxic side effects have been reduced by the development of nonionic, water-soluble contrast agents, as well as by head elevation and generous hydration following myelography.

Arachnoiditis, or inflammation of the leptomeninges, has also been ascribed to the use of contrast agents for myelography. Pantopaque, an oil-soluble contrast agent no longer used, was first noted to cause arachnoiditis, especially in cases where myelography results in subarachnoid bleeding (i.e., traumatic tap). The incidence of arachnoiditis with new water-soluble, nonionic contrast agents is much lower than with Pantopaque and with ionic, water-soluble agents (metrizamide). Other variables that increase the likelihood of arachnoiditis include trauma, infection, and subarachnoid hemorrhage.

ANGIOGRAPHY Technique Angiography is essential in the diagnostic evaluation of many patients with vascular pathology. However, it carries the greatest risk of morbidity of all diagnostic imaging procedures, owing to the necessity of inserting a catheter into a blood vessel, directing the catheter to the required location, injecting contrast material to visualize the vessel, and removing the catheter while maintaining hemostasis. Therapeutic transcatheter procedures (see below) have become important options for the treatment of some cerebrovascular diseases. The decision to undertake a diagnostic or therapeutic angiographic procedure requires careful assessment of the goals of the investigation and its attendant risks.

Patients undergoing angiography should be well hydrated before and after the procedure to better tolerate the contrast agents. Since the femoral route is used most commonly, the femoral artery must be compressed after the procedure to prevent a hematoma from developing. The puncture site and distal pulses should be evaluated carefully after the procedure in search of complications such as thigh hematoma or distal emboli.

Indications   Table 362-1 lists some of the indications for conventional angiography. Over the past 20 years, angiography has been replaced for many indications by CT or MRI. However, it is still used today for evaluating intracranial small-vessel pathology, such as vasculitis, for assessing vascular malformations and aneurysms, and in intravascular therapeutic procedures.

Complications   The vast majority of aortic arch, carotid, and vertebral arteriograms are carried out via transfemoral arterial access. A common femoral arterial puncture provides retrograde access via the aorta to the aortic arch and great vessels. The most feared complication of cerebral angiography is stroke. Thrombus can form on or inside the tip of the catheter, and atherosclerotic thrombus or plaque can be dislodged by the catheter or guidewire or by the force of injection and can embolize distally in the cerebral circulation. The duration and extent of the resulting ischemic neurologic deficit depends on the size and length of the embolus, its composition (fresh thrombus is thought to fragment more readily), its location, and the available collateral circulation. Risk factors for ischemic complications include limited experience on the part of the angiographer, atherosclerosis, vasospasm, low cardiac output, decreased oxygen-carrying capacity, advanced age, and possibly migraine. The risk of a neurologic complication varies but is approximately 4 percent for transient ischemic attack and stroke, 1 percent for permanent deficit, and very low (<0.1 percent) for death.

Ionic contrast material injected into the cerebral vasculature can be neurotoxic if the BBB is breached, either by an underlying disease or by the injection of hyperosmolar contrast agent. Ionic contrast media are less well tolerated than nonionic media, probably because they can induce changes in cell membrane electrical potentials. Patients with dolichoectasia of the basilar artery can suffer reversible brainstem dysfunction and acute short-term memory loss during angiography owing to the slow percolation of the contrast material and the consequent prolonged exposure of the brain. Rarely, an intracranial aneurysm ruptures during an angiographic contrast injection, causing subarachnoid hemorrhage, perhaps as a result of injection under high pressure.

Spinal Angiography   Spinal angiography may be indicated to evaluate vascular malformations and tumors and to identify the artery of Adamkiewicz prior to aortic aneurysm repair. The procedure is lengthy and requires the use of relatively large volumes of contrast; the incidence of serious complications, including paraparesis, subjective visual blurring, and altered speech, is approximately 2 percent.

Interventional Neuroradiology   This rapidly developing field is providing new therapeutic options for patients with difficult neurovascular problems. Available procedures include detachable coil therapy for aneurysms, particulate or liquid adhesive embolization of arteriovenous malformations, balloon angioplasty of stenosis or vasospasm, transarterial or transvenous embolization of dural arteriovenous fistulas, balloon occlusion of carotid-cavernous and vertebral fistulas, endovascular treatment of vein of Galen malformations, preoperative embolization of tumors, and thrombolysis of acute arterial or venous thrombosis. Many of these diseases place the patient at high risk of cerebral hemorrhage, stroke, or death. The therapeutic risks are comparable to those of neurosurgery rather than radiology.

The highest complication rates are found with the therapies geared to treating the highest-risk diseases. In a large series of surgically difficult intracranial aneurysms treated with detachable balloons, Higashida and colleagues reported a 7.4 percent incidence of stroke and a 9.8 percent death rate. These figures must be considered in light of the high morbidity and mortality associated with untreated and surgically unapproachable aneurysms (Chap. 366). The advent of the electrolytically detachable coil may reduce these rates, but endovascular therapy is still reserved largely for treatment of aneurysms not amenable to standard craniotomy and surgical clipping.

BIBLIOGRAPHY

BERG KJ, JACOBSEN JA: Nephrotoxicity related to contrast media, in *Patient Safety and Adverse Events in Contrast Medium Examinations. International Congress Series 816,* I Enge, J Edgren (eds). Amsterdam, Excerpta Medica, 1989

DONAGHY M et al: Encephalopathy after iohexol myelography. Letter. Lancet 2:887, 1985

EARNEST F, 4th et al: Complications of cerebral angiography: Prospective assessment of risk. Am J Roentgenol 142:247, 1984

GAA J et al: Noninvasive perfusion imaging of human brain tumors with EPISTAR. Eur Radiol 6(4):518, 1996

GUGLIELMI G: Embolization of intracranial aneurysms with detachable coils and electrothrombosis, in *Interventional Neuroradiology: Endovascular Therapy of the Central Nervous System,* F Viñuela et al (eds). New York, Raven Press, 1992, p 63

———— et al: Electrothrombosis of saccular aneurysms via endovascular approach. Part 2: Preliminary clinical experience. J Neurosurg 75:8, 1991

HIGASHIDA RT et al: Intracranial aneurysms: Interventional neurovascular treatment with detachable balloons—results in 215 cases. Radiology 178:663, 1991

KATAYAMA H: Report of the Japanese Committee on Safety of Contrast Media. Presented at the Radiological Society of North America Meeting, Chicago, IL, November 1988

MANI RL, EISENBERG RL: Complications of catheter cerebral arteriography: Analysis of 5,000 procedures. II. Relation of complication rates to clinical and arteriographic diagnoses. Am J Roentgenol 131:867, 1978

MATTAY VS et al: Whole-brain functional mapping with isotropic MR imaging. Radiology 201(2):399, 1996

PAN XM et al: Assessment of carotid artery stenosis by ultrasonography, conventional angiography, and magnetic resonance angiography: Correlation with ex vivo measurement of plaque stenosis. J Vasc Surg 21(1):82, 88, 1995

RIEDERER SJ et al: New technical developments in magnetic resonance imaging of epilepsy. Magn Reson Imaging 13(8):1095, 1995

SHELLOCK FG, KANAL E: Policies, guidelines, and recommendations for MR imaging safety and patient management. SMRI Safety Committee. J Magn Reson Imaging 1:97, 1991

SORENSEN AG et al: Hyperacute stroke: Evaluation with combined multisection diffusion-weighted and hemodynamically weighted echo-planar MR imaging. Radiology 199(2):391, 1996

WILTON NC et al: Epidural blood patch for postdural puncture headache: It's never too late. Anesth Analg 65:895, 1986

363   *Joseph B. Martin, Frank M. Longo*

MOLECULAR DIAGNOSIS OF NEUROLOGIC DISORDERS

The accelerating progress in the Human Genome Project will continue to increase the rate at which genes responsible for neurologic disorders are discovered. The widespread availability of DNA testing has already changed traditional diagnostic approaches and raised novel ethical issues. For example, the discovery of "susceptibility" genes that do not directly cause disease but modify the age of disease onset or rate of disease progression creates complexity in the application of molecular diagnosis, particularly in guiding the use of preventative therapies. In this chapter we will review molecular diagnostic approaches relevant to neurologic disease and illustrate how they contribute to patient care.

DNA-BASED DIAGNOSIS OF NEUROLOGIC DISORDERS   As in other laboratory applications, appropriate use of DNA testing in the clinical setting requires that the clinician have a general understanding of the available molecular diagnostic approaches. The majority of disorders listed in Table 363-1 have been mapped to specific chromosomal regions, although for many the specific gene affected by mutations has not been identified. Presymptomatic testing or DNA diagnosis in some disorders is possible by family linkage

Table 363-1

Classification of Neurologic Disorders

Disorder	Chromosomal Localization	Principal Clinical Findings—Phenotype	Mode of Inheritance	Genotype/Gene Products/ Functions/Disease Mechanisms	Genetic Testing Available	Reference or Chapter
NEURODEGENERATIVE DISEASE						
Dementia						
Alzheimer's disease, early onset	AD4: 1q31-42	Dementia, memory loss, typical Alzheimer's disease	AD	Mutations in presenilin-2 gene (*SM2*); product is a putative membrane protein which may be involved in intracellular protein transport		367
Alzheimer's disease, early onset	AD3: 14q24.3	Dementia, memory loss, typical Alzheimer's disease; accounts for majority of familial Alzheimer's disease cases	AD	Mutations in presenilin-1 gene (*S182*); product is a putative membrane protein which may be involved in intracellular protein transport		367
Alzheimer's disease, late onset familial, and sporadic	AD2: 19q13.2	Memory loss, dementia	Codominant	Apolipoprotein E4 associated with increased risk and earlier age of onset; ApoE is secreted by astrocytes and internalized by neurons, where it supports cellular functions requiring lipoprotein mobilization	Yes	367
Familial Alzheimer's disease with amyloid precursor protein (APP) mutation	AD1: 21q21.3-22.05	Rare cause of early-onset Alzheimer's disease	AD	Point mutations in APP gene alter APP metabolism	Possible	367
Huntington's disease*	4p16.3	Chorea, depression, dementia; rigidity and epilepsy in juvenile patients	AD	CAG triplet repeats in gene that encodes a novel protein huntingtin → expanded polyglutamate tract in protein, which may cause gain of toxic functions	Yes	367
Familial Creutzfeldt-Jakob disease	20pter-p12	Spongiform encephalopathy with dementia, myoclonus	AD	Prion protein gene mutation		379
Fatal familial insomnia	20pter-p12	Adult-onset insomnia	AD	Prion protein gene mutation		27
Gerstmann-Sträussler-Scheinker disease	20pter-p12	Spongiform encephalopathy with dementia, myoclonus	AD	Prion protein gene mutation		379
Movement disorders						
Ataxia telangiectasia	11q22.3	Cerebellar degeneration, choreoathetosis, ocular apraxia, oculocutaneous telangiectasia, immunodeficiency, endocrinopathy	AR	Mutations in *ATM* gene, which codes for protein with domains similar to phosphatidylinositol 3′ kinase, an intracellular growth and differentiation factor signal transduction mediator, and rad3, a DNA repair monitor/cell cycle checkpoint regulator protein		369
Autosomal dominant cerebellar ataxia with pigmentary macular dystrophy (ADCAII)	3p12-21.1	Cerebellar ataxia, decreased vision, ophthalmoplegia, decreased vibration sense, increased deep tendon reflexes	AD	Unknown; mapped to within 8 cM		Holmberg et al.
Dentatorubral-pallidoluysian atrophy (DRPLA)	12p12.3-13.1	Ataxia, choreoathetosis, dementia, progressive myoclonus epilepsy (PME), psychiatric disorder	AD	CAG repeat expansions in DRPLA gene—unknown function; PME more common with larger expansions	Yes	369
Episodic ataxia type 1 (EA-1)	12p13	Ataxic episodes lasting seconds to minutes, myokymia, paroxysmal kinesogenic choreoathetosis, acetazolamide and phenytoin responsive	AD	Potassium channel (KCNA1) gene mutations		369

(*continued*)

Table 363-1—(Continued)

Classification of Neurologic Disorders

Disorder	Chromosomal Localization	Principal Clinical Findings—Phenotype	Mode of Inheritance	Genotype/Gene Products/ Functions/Disease Mechanisms	Genetic Testing Available	Reference or Chapter
Episodic ataxia type 2 (EA-2)	19p13	Ataxic episodes lasting hours to days, downgaze nystagmus, headache, progressive cerebellar signs and atrophy, acetazolamide responsive	AD	Unknown		369
Friedreich's ataxia	9q13-21.1	Onset during puberty; ataxia, dysarthria, absent reflexes, decreased vibration, joint position sense, cardiomyopathy, diabetes mellitus	AR	GAA repeat expansion of *X25* (*frataxin*) gene	Possible	369; Campuzano et al.
Ataxia with vitamin E deficiency, Friedreich-like (AVED)	8q13	Same as Friedreich's ataxia but with severe vitamin E deficiency	AR	Mutations in α-tocopherol transfer protein gene (α*TTP*) → impaired binding of vitamin E to VLDL		369
Hereditary progressive dystonia with marked diurnal fluctuation (HPD)	14q22.1-22.2	Distal lower extremity dystonia in first decade, spreads to other limbs over years; symptoms greatest in evening, decreased in morning; responds markedly to levodopa	AD? female predominance	Mutations in GTP cyclohydrolase I gene → biopterin deficiency → decreased tyrosine hydroxylase activity → decreased dopamine		Ichinose et al.
Machado-Joseph disease (MJD)	14q24.3-31	Ataxia, ophthalmoparesis, corticospinal signs, dystonia-rigidity, amyotrophy	AD	CAG repeat expansions in *MJD1* gene	Yes	369
Spinocerebellar ataxia-1 (SCA1)	6p22-23	Ataxia, progressive dementia, spasticity, onset 3d or 4th decade; anticipation in successive generations	AD	Expansion of trinucleotide repeat (CAG) in ataxin-1; *SCA1* gene encoding ataxin-1	Yes	369
Spinocerebellar ataxia-2 (SCA2)	12q23-24.1	Features extensively overlap with SCA1, but more common hypotonia and ophthalmoplegia	AD	Unknown; anticipation observed, suggesting possibility of trinucleotide repeat expansion		369
Spinocerebellar ataxia-3(SCA3)	14qter-24.3	Similar to MJD	AD	CAG repeat expansions in *MJD1* gene	Yes	369
Spinocerebellar ataxia-4(SCA4)	16qter-24	Ataxia, axonal neuropathy, corticospinal signs, normal eye movements	AD	Unknown		369
Spinocerebellar ataxia-5(SCA5)	11 centromeric	Ataxia, dysarthria	AD	Unknown		369
Torsion dystonia	9q34	Early onset, generalized dystonia, occurs in both Ashkenazi Jewish (AJ) and non-Jewish pedigrees	AD	DYT1 locus; unknown gene	Yes	367
Wilson's disease	13q14.3	Disorder of copper transport into liver: extrapyramidal signs, psychiatric disorders	AR	Mutations in gene *ATP7B*, encoding a putative copper-transporting P-type membrane ATPase, 57% similar to that associated with Menkes' syndrome (MNK)		345
Retinitis pigmentosa Retinitis pigmentosa-1	3q21-24	Night blindness, peripheral field loss, blindness, abnormal ERG	AD	Mutations in gene that encodes rhodopsin → interference in maturational processing of wild-type protein		28

(continued)

Table 363-1—*(Continued)*

Classification of Neurologic Disorders

Disorder	Chromosomal Localization	Principal Clinical Findings—Phenotype	Mode of Inheritance	Genotype/Gene Products/ Functions/Disease Mechanisms	Genetic Testing Available	Reference or Chapter
Retinitis pigmentosa, peripherin-related	6p21.1-cen	Night blindness, peripheral visual loss leading to blindness	AD	Mutations in RDS/peripherin gene, a rod photoreceptor membrane protein		28
Spastic paraplegia						
Autosomal dominant familial spastic paraplegia (SPG3, SPG4, SPG6)	SPG3: 14q SPG4: 2p21-24 SPG6: 15q11.1	Pure spastic paraplegia	AD	Unknown		370
Autosomal recessive familial spastic paraplegia	8q	Pure spastic paraplegia	AR	Unknown		370
X-linked familial spastic paraplegia-2 (SPG2)	Xq21-22	Initial pure spastic paraplegia; involvement of entire CNS over years	X-LR	Myelin proteolipid protein gene mutation; allelic with Pelizaeus-Merzbacher		367
Vascular diseases						
Cerebral autosomal dominant arteriopathy with subcortical infarcts (CADASIL)	19q12	Multiple subcortical infarcts, dementia	AD	Unknown		Tournier-Lasserve et al.
Familial cerebral amyloid angiopathy (Dutch type)	21q21.3-22.05	Cerebral hemorrhage	AD	Point mutations in APP gene	Possible	Levy et al.
Familial hemiplegic migraine	19p13	Onset 5–30 years, aura with unilateral paresis and other focal symptoms lasting 30–60 min; followed by headache, may have persistent cerebellar signs	AD	Unknown, may be related to episodic ataxia - type 2		364
Hereditary cystatin C amyloid angiopathy (HCCAA) (Icelandic)	20p11.2	Cerebral hemorrhage	AD	Mutations in cystatin C gene, product is a cysteine protease inhibitor; forms amyloid, which deposits in the walls of cerebral vessels		Levy et al.
Miscellaneous						
Abetalipoproteinemia (Bassen-Kornzwieg)	4q24	Vitamin E deficiency; neuropathy, ataxia, retinitis pigmentosa, acanthocytosis	AR	Mutations in gene coding large subunit of microsomal triglyceride transfer protein (MTP) → impairment of synthesis of VLDL		Narcisi et al.
Adrenoleukodystrophy	Xq28	Leukodystrophy, hypoadrenalism, mild neuropathy, baldness, hypogonadism	X-LR	Mutations in ALD protein gene, a peroxisomal membrane transporter; associated with impaired β-oxidation of unbranched saturated very long chain fatty acids in peroxisomes		380
Menkes' syndrome (kinky hair disease, steely hair disease)	Xq13.3	Abnormal whitish kinky hair, growth and mental retardation, spastic quadriparesis, seizures	X-LR	Mutations in *ATP7A*, encoding MNK, a protein very similar to P-type cation-transporting membrane ATPases; may be involved in copper transport across membranes; mutations may lead to copper deficiency.		Das et al.

EPILEPSY SYNDROMES

Disorder	Chromosomal Localization	Principal Clinical Findings—Phenotype	Mode of Inheritance	Genotype/Gene Products/ Functions/Disease Mechanisms	Genetic Testing Available	Reference or Chapter
Awakening grand mal (AGM)	6p	Adolescent onset, pure grand mal occurring on awakening	?	Also linked to EJM1—may be allelic with juvenile myoclonic epilepsy		365

(continued)

Table 363-1—*(Continued)*

Classification of Neurologic Disorders

Disorder	Chromosomal Localization	Principal Clinical Findings—Phenotype	Mode of Inheritance	Genotype/Gene Products/ Functions/Disease Mechanisms	Genetic Testing Available	Reference or Chapter
Benign neonatal epilepsy-1 (EBN1)	20q13.2-13.3	Generalized seizures, neonatal onset, benign course, usually resolving at 6–12 months, 10–15% have seizures later in life	AD	Mutations in the α-4 subunit of the neuronal nicotinic acetylcholine receptor gene		365
Benign neonatal epilepsy-2 (EBN2)	8q	Clinically indistinguishable from EBN1	AD	Unknown		365
Familial partial epilepsy	10q	Simple partial seizures, normal intelligence	AD, reduced penetrance	Unknown; mapped to within 10 cM		365
Juvenile myoclonic epilepsy (JME)	6p11-21.2	Onset in adolescence, myoclonic jerks, generalized tonic-clonic seizures	Uncertain	Gene locus named EJM1		365
Nocturnal frontal lobe epilepsy (ADNFLE)	20q13.2-13.3	Nocturnal seizures	AD	May be allelic with EBN1, also with a normal low voltage electroencephalogram variant		365
Progressive epilepsy with mental retardation (EPMR)	8pter-p22	Normal at birth, generalized seizures onset age 5–10 years, severe mental retardation 2–5 years after seizure onset	AR	Unknown; mapped to within 7 cM		365
Progressive myoclonus epilepsy, Unverricht-Lundborg type (EPM1)	21q22.3	Generalized seizures, stimulus-reactive myoclonus, onset age 6–15, progressive	AD	Unknown; EPM1 mapped to within about 300 kb		365

NEUROMUSCULAR DISORDERS

Motor neuron diseases

Disorder	Chromosomal Localization	Principal Clinical Findings—Phenotype	Mode of Inheritance	Genotype/Gene Products/ Functions/Disease Mechanisms	Genetic Testing Available	Reference or Chapter
Familial amyotrophic lateral sclerosis, adult, dominant (ALS1)	21q22.1	Weakness, muscle atrophy, spasticity, increased deep tendon reflexes; about 10% of cases are familial, indistinguishable clinically from sporadic form	AD	Point mutations in Cu, Zn-superoxide dismutase (SOD1) in some families (20%); heterogeneity exists → motor neuron injury possibly due to defective detoxification of reactive oxygen species	Yes	370
Familial amyotrophic lateral sclerosis, juvenile recessive (ALS2)	2q33-35	Earlier onset and slower progression than ALS1	AR	Unknown		370
Familial amyotrophic lateral sclerosis, adult, dominant (ALS3)	11	Similar to ALS1	AD	Mutations in neurofilament protein heavy chain gene → disruption of neurofilament crosslinking		370
Spinal muscular atrophy (SMA) I–III	5q11.2-13.3	SMA I: infantile (Werdnig-Hoffman) disease—present by 3 months, hypotonia, proximal limb weakness, areflexia. SMA II: childhood onset, limb/girdle weakness, areflexia, 70% never ambulate independently. SMA III: juvenile (Kugelberg-Welander) disease—onset after age 2, slowly progressive symmetric proximal muscle weakness sparing bulbar muscles	AR	Mapped to about 1 Mb region; region is unstable and highly polymorphic making reconciliation of mapping data difficult; two candidate genes have been identified: "neuronal apoptosis inhibitory protein" (NAIP) gene, with amino acid homology to baculovirus apoptosis inhibitory proteins and survival motor neuron (SMN) gene coding a novel 294 aa protein	Yes	370

(continued)

Table 363-1—*(Continued)*

Classification of Neurologic Disorders

Disorder	Chromosomal Localization	Principal Clinical Findings—Phenotype	Mode of Inheritance	Genotype/Gene Products/ Functions/Disease Mechanisms	Genetic Testing Available	Reference or Chapter
Spinobulbar muscular atrophy (Kennedy syndrome)	Xq12	Muscular weakness and atrophy	X-LR	Trinucleotide repeats in androgen receptor gene → expanded polyglutamate tract in protein may cause partial loss of some physiologic functions and gain of other functions	Yes	370
Muscle diseases						
Becker myotonia (recessive myotonia congenita)	7q35	Similar to myotonia congenita	AR	Known *CIC-1* mutations present in about 16% unrelated cases		383
Central core disease (CCD)	19q13.1	Nonprogressive primarily proximal myopathy, onset in infancy	AD	Mutation in ryanodine receptor gene (*RYR1*); allelic with MHS1		383
Congenital muscular dystrophy (merosin deficient) (CMD)	6q2	Weakness and hypotonia at birth, limb contractures at birth or later	AR	Probable mutations in merosin gene		383
Congenital myasthenic syndromes/ "slow-channel" syndrome (SCS)	2q,17p	Weakness, fatigability, hypotonia, muscle atrophy	AD (?)	Mutations in genes encoding subunits of the acetylcholine receptor → altered channel kinetics		Sine et al.
Duchenne/Becker muscular dystrophy (DMD/BMD)	Xp21.2	DMD: onset of muscular weakness early in life, progressive; BMD form is later onset, less severe	X-LR	Mutations in dystrophin gene resulting in complete absence or major deletions of dystrophin (DMD), or less severe derangements of dystrophin structure (BMD) → disruption of linkage between microfilaments and the trans-sarcolemmal glycoprotein complex mediating adhesion to the extracellular matrix protein merosin → may lead to membrane damage with contraction	Yes	383
Emery-Dreifuss muscular dystrophy	Xq28	Childhood onset, benign course with early contractures, progressive muscle wasting with humeral/peroneal predominance, cardiac conduction defects—arrhythmias, heart block	X-LR	Mutations in emerin gene; codes a 254 aa serine-rich protein which may be membrane-anchored and has unknown function		383
Facioscapulohumeral dystrophy	4q35	Weakness, atrophy; face and shoulder muscles	AD	Unknown; exhibits anticipation, which may be associated with successive deletions in a region of tandem repeats		383
Fukuyama-type congenital muscular dystrophy (FCMD)	9q31-33	Weakness and hypotonia at birth, cerebral and cerebellar polymicrogyria and cerebellar cysts, ocular anomalies; overlaps with Walker-Warburg syndrome	AR	Unknown; proposed allelic with Walker-Warburg syndrome		383
Hereditary myoglobinuria	1p32	Episodic myalgia, rhabdomyolysis, myoglobinuria presenting 2nd and 3rd decades	AR	Mutations in gene coding carnitine palmitoyltransferase II → diminished import of long-chain fatty acids into mitochondria → mitochondrial dysfunction		Taroni et al.

(continued)

Table 363-1—(*Continued*)

Classification of Neurologic Disorders

Disorder	Chromosomal Localization	Principal Clinical Findings—Phenotype	Mode of Inheritance	Genotype/Gene Products/ Functions/Disease Mechanisms	Genetic Testing Available	Reference or Chapter
Hyperkalemic periodic paralysis (HYPP)	17q23.1-25.3	Myotonia, periodic areflexic paralysis	AD	Point mutation in α subunit, sodium channel (SCN4A) $\rightarrow$ impairment of sodium current inactivation; normokalemic variants occur (normoPP)		383
Hypokalemic periodic paralysis (HOKPP)	1q32	Similar to HYPP, but attacks accompanied by hypokalemia, triggered by insulin and epinephrine, last longer and patients have no myotonia	AD	Loss of function mutations in α-1 subunit of the dihydropyridine (DHP) receptor gene, a slow voltage-gated L-type calcium channel $\rightarrow$? dominant negative disruption of channel function (decreased Ca^{2+} current); predominant expression in males may be hormone effect		383
Limb-girdle muscular dystrophy, autosomal dominant 1A (LGMD1A)	5q22.3-31.3	Late (third decade) onset muscular dystrophy, sparing the face; slow progression	AD	Unknown; mapped to within 7 cM		383
Limb-girdle muscular dystrophy, autosomal recessive 2A (LGMD2A)	15q15.1-21.1	Progressive symmetric atrophy of proximal limb muscles, beginning in first two decades	AR	Mutations in calcium-activated neutral protease 3 (CANP3) gene, large subunit gene important, but probably requires another as-yet-unidentified mutation for disease expression (digenic model)		383
Limb-girdle muscular dystrophy, autosomal recessive 2B (LGMD2B)	2p13-16	Pelvic girdle affected earliest; onset in late 2d decade	AR	Unknown		383
Malignant hyperthermia (MHS1) and central core disease (CCD)	19q13.1	Sensitivity to volatile anesthetics, muscle contraction	AD	Mutation in ryanodine receptor gene (*RYR1*) at 19q13.1 $\rightarrow$? disturbance of Ca^{2+} release; when mild $\rightarrow$ excessive contraction; when severe (as in CCD) $\rightarrow$ Ca^{2+} mediated mitochondrial toxicity		MacLennan
Malignant hyperthermia (MHS2,3,4)	MHS2: 17q11.2-24 MHS3: 7q21-22 MHS4: 3q13.1	Sensitivity to volatile anesthetics, muscle contraction	AD	Unknown		MacLennan
Myotonia congenita (dominant MC, Thomsen's disease)	7q35	Onset first decade, muscle stiffness/ myotonia, muscle hypertrophy without weakness	AD	Known mutations in the chloride channel gene (*ClC-1*) account for about 15% of MC cases. Mutations cause loss of function and functional channel is likely homooligomer $\rightarrow$ dominant-negative mechanism		383
Myotonic dystrophy	19q13.3	Multisystem disorder: cataracts, myotonia, weakness, frontal baldness, mental retardation	AD, anticipation	CTG repeats at 3′ end of myotonin protein kinase gene—product is membrane associated and localized primarily to neuromuscular and myotendinous junctions; expression of adjacent genes may also be affected	Yes	383

(*continued*)

Table 363-1—*(Continued)*

Classification of Neurologic Disorders

Disorder	Chromosomal Localization	Principal Clinical Findings—Phenotype	Mode of Inheritance	Genotype/Gene Products/ Functions/Disease Mechanisms	Genetic Testing Available	Reference or Chapter
Nemaline my-opathy	1p13-q25	Most commonly congenital non- or slowly progressive myopathy; forms range from severe congenital to mild adult	AD (other forms AR)	Dominant form associated with α-tropomyosin gene (*TPM3*) mutation. Met9Arg mutation may increase tropomyosin-actin affinity → rod body formation		383
Oculopharyngeal muscular dystrophy (OPMD)	14q11.2-13	Onset usually after age 50, ptosis, dysphagia	AD	Gene unknown; maps near cardiac β-myosin		383
Paramyotonia congenita (PC)	17q23.1-25.3	Cold-induced muscle stiffness (myotonia) and weakness, occasional periodic paralysis	AD	SCN4A mutations; allelic with HYPP		383
Potassium-aggravated myotonia (PAM)	17q23.1-25.3	Potassium-sensitive muscle stiffness (myotonia) and weakness, occasional periodic paralysis	AD	SCN4A mutations; allelic with HYPP [other variants occur ("sodium-channel myotonias")]		Hoffman et al.
Severe childhood autosomal recessive muscular dystrophy (SCARMD, LGMD2C, LGMD2D)	13q12, 17q21	Similar to DMD or BMD	AR	17q21-linked form: mutations of adhalin gene; adhalin is a component of the membrane glycoprotein complex noted above; 13q12-linked form: gene unknown		383
Startle disease (hyperekplexia)	5q21-31	Exaggerated startle, neonatal hypertonia, nocturnal myoclonus	AD, AR	Mutations in the α-1 subunit of the inhibitory glycine receptor → mechanisms unknown, though Arg271 mutations seen in some human cases causes decreased agonist sensitivity in a mouse model		22; Rees et al.
X-linked myotubular myopathy	Xq28	Severe neonatal hypotonia, apnea, common perinatal death	X-LR	Unknown		Wallgren-Pettersson et al.
Peripheral neuropathies						
Charcot-Marie-Tooth disease, type 1A (CMT1A)	17p11.2	HMSNI: Variable onset, motor > sensory neuropathy, distal muscle atrophy, absent reflexes, high arches in feet, decreased nerve conduction velocities, +/- nerve enlargement	AD	Mutations or 1.5 Mb duplication in peripheral myelin protein (PMP-22) gene, product is a component of compact myelin	Yes	381
Charcot-Marie-Tooth disease, type 1B (CMT1B)	1q22	HMSNI	AD	Mutations in P_o gene, product is a component of compact myelin		381
Charcot-Marie-Tooth disease, type 1, X-linked (CMTX1,2,3)	CMTX1: Xq13.1 CMTX2: Xp22.2 CMTX3: Xq26	HMSNI	X-linked dominant	CMTX1: mutations in connexin32 gene coding a gap junction protein localized to uncompacted peripheral myelin at the nodes of Ranvier and Schmidt-Lanterman clefts; CMTX2,3: genes unknown	Yes	381
Charcot-Marie-Tooth disease, type 2A (CMT2A)	1p35-36	HMSNII: Later onset, sensorimotor axonal neuropathy, near normal nerve conduction velocities	AD	Unknown		381

(continued)

Table 363-1—*(Continued)*

Classification of Neurologic Disorders

Disorder	Chromosomal Localization	Principal Clinical Findings—Phenotype	Mode of Inheritance	Genotype/Gene Products/ Functions/Disease Mechanisms	Genetic Testing Available	Reference or Chapter
Charcot-Marie-Tooth disease, type 4A (CMT4A)	8q13-21.1	HMSNI	AR	Unknown		381
Dejerine-Sottas disease, type A (DSDA)	17p11.2-12	HMSNIII: Onset birth/infancy, slowly progressive sensori-motor deficits, high arches, scoliosis, ataxia, enlarged nerves, markedly decreased conduction velocities	AD	*PMP-22* mutations (see above)		362
Dejerine-Sottas disease, type B (DSDB)	1q22-23	HMSNIII	?	P_o mutations (see above)		362
Familial amyloidotic polyneuropathy (FAP)	18q11.2-12.1	Sensory/autonomic peripheral neuropathy, cardiomyopathy	AD	Mutations in transthyretin gene → formation of amyloid	Yes	381
Hereditary neuropathy with pressure palsies, type A (HNPPA)	17p11.2	Recurrent entrapment/pressure neuropathies, segmental demyelination	?AD	*PMP-22* deletions; CMT1A and HNPPA may result from reciprocal products of unequal crossover	Yes	381

CENTRAL NERVOUS SYSTEM TUMORS

Disorder	Chromosomal Localization	Principal Clinical Findings—Phenotype	Mode of Inheritance	Genotype/Gene Products/ Functions/Disease Mechanisms	Genetic Testing Available	Reference or Chapter
Neurofibromatosis, type 1 (Von Recklinghausen) (NF1)	17q11.2	Multiple neurofibromas, 1:3500 individuals, café au lait spots, malignant gliomas, Lisch nodules in iris	AD	Disruption of *NF1* gene; encodes neurofibromin, a member of the Ras-GTPase activating protein (GAP) family		375
Neurofibromatosis, type 2 (NF2)	22q12.2	Acoustic neuromas, bilateral meningiomas	AD	Deletions in the *NF2* gene that encodes for merlin/schwannomin, a tumor suppressor protein with sequence similarity to tyrosine phosphatase and cytoskeleton linkage protein	Yes	375
Retinoblastoma	13q14.1-14.2	40% hereditary, 60% nonhereditary, multiple tumors in inherited form	AR	*Rb* gene mutations or deletions cause disease; Rb protein is 105-kDa tumor suppressor, DNA-binding protein	Possible	28, 65
Von Hippel-Lindau type 1, 2 (VHL1, VHL2)	3p25-26	Type 1: retinal angiomas, CNS hemangioblastomas, pancreatic cysts in some Type 2: identical to type 1 plus pheochromocytoma	AD	Type 1: 56% microdeletions, deletions, insertions, nonsense mutations in *VHL* gene, a tumor suppressor of otherwise unknown function Type 2: 96% missense mutations in *VHL* gene	Yes	375

DEFECTS OF NEURONAL MIGRATION AND DIFFERENTIATION

Disorder	Chromosomal Localization	Principal Clinical Findings—Phenotype	Mode of Inheritance	Genotype/Gene Products/ Functions/Disease Mechanisms	Genetic Testing Available	Reference or Chapter
Familial cavernous malformations of the brain	7q11.2-21	Seizures, headache, intracerebral hemorrhage, neurologic deficits	AD	Unknown		Dubovsky et al.
Fragile X syndrome-A (FRAXA)	Xq27.3	Mental retardation, decreased head size, large forehead, macroorchidism	X-LR	CGG trinucleotide repeat expansions in 5′ region of *FMR-1* gene → transcriptional inhibition of gene due to overmethylation, as well as translational inhibition. *FMR-1* product contains KH domains and RGG box, motifs found in RNA binding proteins	Yes	Feng et al.

(continued)

Table 363-1—*(Continued)*

Classification of Neurologic Disorders

Disorder	Chromosomal Localization	Principal Clinical Findings—Phenotype	Mode of Inheritance	Genotype/Gene Products/ Functions/Disease Mechanisms	Genetic Testing Available	Reference or Chapter
Fragile X syndrome-E (FRAXE)	Xq28	Mild mental retardation	X-LR	CGG/CCG repeat expansions, 600 kb distal to FRAXA site; developmentally regulated transcript recently found in region	Yes	Knight et al.
Hydrocephalus due to stenosis of the aqueduct of Sylvius (HSAS)	Xq28	Hydrocephalus with moderate to severe mental retardation, adducted hypoplastic thumbs (25% of cases), spastic paraparesis, aplasia or hypoplasia of the corticospinal tract and corpus callosum	X-LR	Mutations in L1 gene— product is a multifunctional/ multidomain cell adhesion molecule		Wong et al.
MASA syndrome (Gareis-Mason syndrome)	Xq28	Mental retardation, aphasia, shuffling gait (due to spastic paraparesis) and adducted thumbs (due to absent or hypoplastic extensor pollicis brevis and/or longus); may also have hydrocephalus	X-LR	L1 gene mutations		Wong et al.
Spastic paraplegia, X-linked, type 1 (SPXL or SPG1)	Xq28	Spastic paraplegia, ataxia, absent extensor pollicis longus	X-LR	L1 gene mutations		367; Wong et al.
Kallmann syndrome	Xp22.3	Anosmia with hypogonadism (GnRH deficiency); syndrome due to failure of olfactory neuronal migration	X-LR	Mutations in gene (*KALIG-1*) that encodes protein with homology to neural-cell adhesion (N-CAM) molecules		337
Miller-Dieker lissencephaly syndrome	17p13.3	Microcephaly, micrognathia, epilepsy, agyria due to failure of cortical neuronal migration	AD	Mutation in *LIS-1* gene coding the 45-kDa (regulatory) subunit of platelet-activating factor (PAF) acetylhydrolase; part of heterotrimeric enzyme which inactivates PAF; PAF proposed to modulate neuronal differentiation or migration; effect of mutation on PAF unknown	Yes	Hattori et al.
Norrie disease (ND)	Xp11.4	Retinal malformation, hearing loss, mental retardation	X-LR	Mutations in *ND*; sequence comparisons and modeling suggest similarity to transforming growth factor β family/ cysteine-knot motif growth factors		Chen et al; Berger
Tuberous sclerosis, type 1	9q34	1:10,000 births, mental retardation, seizures, adenoma sebaceum	AD	Unknown; may be a growth suppressor		White
Tuberous sclerosis, type 2	16p13.3	Hamartomas, epilepsy, mental retardation	AD	Gene encodes tuberin, which has homology to GTPase activating protein GAP3; effects of mutations on protein function unknown		Rouleau et al.

(continued)

Table 363-1—*(Continued)*

Classification of Neurologic Disorders

Disorder	Chromosomal Localization	Principal Clinical Findings—Phenotype	Mode of Inheritance	Genotype/Gene Products/ Functions/Disease Mechanisms	Genetic Testing Available	Reference or Chapter
Waardenburg syndrome-1 (WS1)	2q35	Deafness, white forelock, dystopia canthorum, pigmentary abnormalities	AD	Mutation in paired box-containing *(PAX-3)* gene; product is a transcription factor involved in embryonic patterning/neural crest migration; heterozygotes have WS1, homozygotes have WS3, which is more severe and includes upper limb abnormalities		Tassabehji
Waardenburg syndrome-2 (WS2)	3p12.3-14.1	Deafness, white forelock, dystopia canthorum, heterochromia irides, early graying	AD	Mutations in microphthalmia *(MITF)* gene encoding a putative basic helix-loop-helix-leucine-zipper transcription factor		Tassabehji
Walker-Warburg syndrome (WWS)	9q31-33	Lissencephaly, ocular anomalies, hydrocephalus, callosal hypoplasia, septal agenesis, congenital muscular dystrophy	AR	Unknown; proposed allelic with FCMD		Arahata et al.

* HD causes both dementia and movement disorder.

NOTE: AD, autosomal dominant; AR, autosomal recessive; CNS, central nervous system; ERG, electroretinogram; GnRH, gonadotropin-releasing hormone; HMSN, hereditary motor and sensory neuropathy; Rb, retinoblastoma; VLDL, very low density lipoprotein; X-LR, X-linked recessive.

analysis. Linkage analysis requires that family relationships (such as paternity) are correctly established, that the clinical status of family members is accurate, that informative markers are available, and that an adequate number of family members are genotyped. For many patients, these requirements often eliminate application of DNA diagnosis.

Direct DNA diagnosis can be used in a large number of disorders. Most disease-causing mutations consist of single base substitutions leading to amino acid substitutions (missense mutations), premature translation stop signals (nonsense mutations), or abnormal RNA transcript splicing. Other mutations result from DNA deletions or instability of trinucleotide repeats. For genetic diseases in which the pathologic phenotype is caused by only one or a small number of well-defined mutations within a given gene, detection of the mutation can be used for diagnosis. The ability to detect a mutation eliminates the need for diagnosis by physical examination and the need for linkage studies.

Approaches for Detection of DNA Mutations *Direct sequencing of patient DNA* These methods generally require amplification of DNA by the polymerase chain reaction (PCR). With most current methods, only 300 to 400 DNA bases are sequenced; therefore, sequencing-based strategies are best applied when a limited region contains the majority of potential mutation sites. Direct DNA sequencing allows novel mutations to be detected and decreases the chances of a "false-negative" result. In some cases, the significance of previously uncharacterized missense mutations will be difficult to interpret. They might code for harmless amino acid polymorphisms or in other cases constitute the cause of the disease. The segregation of the same mutation with the disease phenotype within a family or the substitution of nonconserved amino acids, especially in critical protein regions, would suggest the latter.

Allele-specific oligonucleotide hybridization This technique, in which sequence-specific oligonucleotides differentially recognize DNA segments with normal sequence or mutated sequence, is best suited for detecting known mutations and can be applied to a large number of samples.

Differential restriction endonuclease patterns of PCR-amplified DNA DNA is digested with restriction enzymes that recognize either normal or mutated DNA sequence; the size pattern of resulting DNA fragments indicates whether the DNA sample contains normal or variant sequence (see Chap. 65). This method is also directed toward detecting known mutations.

Analysis of single-stranded conformation polymorphisms Segments of the gene of interest of several hundred bases in length are PCR amplified and electrophoresed under denaturing conditions. Mutation-induced alterations of DNA structure lead to altered electrophoretic patterns. This approach can detect novel mutations directly. Large numbers of samples either covering many exons of a large gene or from many patients can be analyzed.

Detection of DNA deletions by fluorescence in situ hybridization DNA deletions are detected by hybridizing chromosomes with a fluorescent probe corresponding to the gene of interest. Fluorescence in situ hybridization (FISH) can detect deletions smaller than the 2000- to 3000-kb minimum detected by banding techniques.

Cytogenetic testing Chromosomes isolated from peripheral blood lymphocytes or tissue are stained allowing identification of insertions, deletions, other chromosome imbalances, and assessment of chromosomal number (see Chap. 66).

Some disorders such as muscular dystrophy (DM), neurofibromatosis (type 1 and 2), and familial amyotrophic lateral sclerosis (ALS) can be caused by dozens of different mutations within one gene. Genetic heterogeneity over a wide region of a given gene is common for many genes involved in metabolic diseases. Many methods of DNA analysis focus on recurring point mutations or relatively short segments of DNA. Using such focused DNA analysis, mutations are found in only about two-thirds of Duchenne muscular dystrophy (DMD), Becker muscular dystrophy (BMD), and neurofibromatosis type 2 patients and in less than half of those with neurofibromatosis type 1. Advances in multiplex PCR and single-strand chain polymorphism analysis have increased this yield, but the clinician should be aware of the "sensitivity" of each DNA analysis.

Detection of Protein Abnormalities   For some applications, diagnostic methods based on protein properties or function are more effective and efficient than DNA-based tests. Traditional enzyme activity–based assays continue to be useful for diagnosis of many metabolic diseases, and additional protein functions can be used to detect other disorders. For example, immunologic assays may reveal decreased protein levels or aberrant distribution of dystrophin in a muscle biopsy of a patient in whom no DNA mutations are detected.

COMPLICATIONS AND LIMITATIONS OF GENETIC TESTING   The limitations of DNA testing must also be considered. If the presumed diagnosis is in error or if the phenotype overlaps with other disorders, the detection of normal alleles of the gene tested is of limited value. Different mutations in the same gene can result in different phenotypes (*allelic heterogeneity*), and mutations in different genes can result in the same phenotype (*nonallelic genetic heterogeneity*). Other phenomena such as phenocopies, incomplete penetrance, age-dependent onset of phenotype, polygenic inheritance, imprinting mitochondrial inheritance, and dynamic mutations (trinucleotide repeats) may also make interpretation of genetic testing difficult.

Nonallelic Genetic Heterogeneity   Nonallelic genetic heterogeneity (also known as genetic heterogeneity) describes the occurrence of individuals or families with similar pathologic and/or clinical syndromes who have mutations in different genes, as in the multiple demyelinating forms of Charcot-Marie-Tooth disease (CMT; see Table 363-1). For CMT type 1A the locus is 17p11.2, and the affected gene encodes the peripheral myelin protein (PMP-22) gene. CMT type 1B, which is clinically similar to CMT 1A but less common, is caused by a mutation on chromosome 1q that results from a mutation in the gene for P$_o$, a component of compact myelin. Familial Alzheimer's disease (AD) is caused by mutations in genes located on chromosome 14 (*presenilin 1*, causing 70 to 80 percent of early-onset AD), chromosome 1 (*presenilin 2*), and chromosome 21 (*amyloid precursor protein*). Several forms of type I autosomal dominant spinocerebellar ataxias (SCA) including SCA1 and SCA3/Machado-Joseph disease (MJD) are caused by expansions of CAG repeats in genes located at 6p23 (*SCA1*) and 14q32 (*SCA3/MJD1*), respectively. Familial ALS can be caused by mutations in the gene encoding cytosolic copper/zinc superoxide dismutase 1 (SOD1) or, less commonly, the gene for the heavy neurofilament subunit, and retinitis pigmentosa can be caused by mutations in more than 10 different genes.

Allelic Heterogeneity   Different mutations in the same gene (allelic mutations) cause DMD and BMD (dystrophin gene, Xp21.2) and infantile and juvenile onset spinal muscular atrophies (5q11.2-13.3). Familial Creutzfeldt-Jakob disease, fatal familial insomnia, and Gerstmann-Sträussler-Scheinker disease are all caused by allelic mutations in the prion protein gene (20pter-p12), each of which results in distinct aberrant protein isoforms or alterations in expression.

Phenocopies   Patients may have a clinical presentation that resembles a disease phenotype but that has a nongenetic cause. Examples include vascular dementia appearing as familial AD, toxin- or drug-induced chorea mimicking Huntington's disease (HD), and vitamin E deficiency resembling Friedreich's ataxia.

Variable Expressivity   Variable expressivity occurs when the severity of a trait resulting from a mutant allele varies from mild to severe. Expression of the disease phenotype can be modified by other factors such as predisposing alleles of other genes, environmental agents, sex, and age. Variation in expression can also occur following somatic variations in trinucleotide repeats, as occurs in DM.

Incomplete Penetrance   Penetrance refers to the all-or-none expression of a mutant genotype. If a disease is expressed in fewer than 100 percent of individuals carrying the abnormal allele, it is said to have incomplete penetrance.

Polygenic Inheritance   Some diseases are caused by concomitant mutations in multiple genes. In one form of retinitis pigmentosa mutations are present in both the RDS/peripherin and *ROM1* genes.

Similarly, some forms of Hirschsprung disease may result from simultaneous mutations in loci at 13q22 and 21q22.

INFLUENCE OF GENETIC BACKGROUND   MJD and SCA3 are autosomal dominant ataxias originally described in different ethnic backgrounds and described as having distinct features. MJD occurs in families, often of Portuguese-Azorean origin, and is manifest as hereditary ataxia with dystonia, rigidity, faciolingual fasciculation, and bulging eyes. In French families with progressive ataxia and dysarthria, the SCA3 gene was mapped to a site on chromosome 14q near the MJD locus. It is now clear that MJD and SCA3 are both caused by expansion of the same tract of CAG repeats in the same gene (*MJD1*) at 14q32.1. Although expansions in *MJD1* are the most common mutations in German SCA patients, the diagnosis of MJD has not previously been considered in this population. The extent to which different genetic backgrounds causes phenotypical heterogeneity will require further studies.

SUSCEPTIBILITY GENES   Allelic variations or mutations can cause increased susceptibility to specific diseases. Detection of such DNA polymorphisms can influence differential diagnosis, as in the genotyping of *APOE* alleles in the diagnosis of AD. Apolipoprotein E (apoE) is a 299-amino-acid protein involved in mobilization and reutilization of lipoprotein cholesterol. ApoE secreted by astrocytes appears to be internalized by neurons via low-density, lipoprotein-related receptors where it contributes to neuronal function. The three isoforms of apoE (apoE2, apoE3, and apoE4) are derived from three corresponding alleles of the *APOE* gene located at 19q13.2; the apoE4 allele is overrepresented in sporadic and familial AD, and its presence is a significant risk factor for the disease. In contrast, the apoE2 allele is underrepresented and thus may have a "protective" effect (see Chap. 367).

The increased incidence of the *APOE4/4* genotype in AD patients has raised the possibility that ascertainment of *APOE* genotype might be useful in the diagnostic assessment of patients with dementia. For example, since AD accounts for some two-thirds of late-onset dementia, the prior probability of an elderly patient with dementia having AD is approximately 0.66. Based on preliminary studies, it appears that the probability of a demented patient with the *APOE4/4* genotype having AD increases to 0.94 and in a patient with *APOE3/4* to 0.81.

As a research tool, *APOE* genotyping is likely to contribute substantially to the neurobiologic understanding of AD and to be an important stratification variable for future clinical trials. On the other hand, current data do not, for several reasons, support its routine application in the clinical assessment of dementia. First, available *APOE* genotype data are not derived from age-specific epidemiologic studies. If a 25-year-old presents with dementia and has the *APOE4/4* genotype, it nevertheless is very unlikely that this patient has AD. Second, since individuals with all *APOE* genotypes can have AD, genotypes cannot absolutely rule in or rule out this diagnosis. Even if genotyping increases the odds that a given patient has AD, it does not rule out the possibility that a treatable cause of dementia is present. Since current diagnostic studies for demented patients are focused on detecting reversible causes of dementia, it can be argued that *APOE* genotype results would not change the diagnostic evaluation and therefore should not be ordered on a routine basis. Nevertheless, *APOE* genotyping might eventually be combined with other diagnostic tests such as cerebrospinal fluid β-amyloid or τ protein levels to form a "panel" of data with acceptable sensitivity and specificity for diagnosis (see Chap. 367).

The issue of predictive *APOE* genotyping for asymptomatic individuals must also be considered. Until genotyping can contribute to identifying individuals who might benefit from preventive therapy, many clinicians would consider predictive testing to be unethical. Moreover, useful predictions of age of onset based solely on *APOE* genotyping are not possible. For the 2 percent of the population with the high-risk *E4/E4* genotype, the period of risk extends from the fifties to beyond the nineties.

APPROACH TO GENETIC TESTING   One indication for DNA analysis is confirmatory diagnosis for a specific disease already suggested by clinical assessment. DNA testing can also be useful in narrowing a differential diagnosis in situations where multiple diagnostic possibilities are present. DNA testing for HD often allows patients to avoid neuroimaging and other diagnostic studies. Another application of genetic analysis is presymptomatic testing in members of families known or suspected to have a specific disorder. In these cases the most common reasons for individuals desiring testing are life management issues, reproductive planning decisions, and eliminating the stress of not knowing one's own carrier status. Development of new therapies that delay onset or progression of neurodegenerative diseases will provide additional indication for presymptomatic testing.

Genetic testing should be conducted only in the context of comprehensive genetic counseling, in which the implications of potential test results are fully understood and adequate support services are available. Clinicians ordering genetic studies should be familiar with issues regarding informed consent, suicide risk, ongoing patient support, insurance, employment discrimination, testing of minors, and testing of fetal tissue.

A computerized directory of laboratories offering DNA diagnostic services, known as Helix, is accessible to health care professionals, and information on access and/or listing of new laboratories can be obtained at the Helix office [(206) 527-5742]. Many university centers offer testing for multiple neurogenetic disorders.

CLINICAL AND GENETIC CLASSIFICATION OF GENE DISORDERS Neurogenetic disorders have traditionally been classified and subtyped on the basis of clinical and pathophysiologic concepts. The complexity, variability in phenotype, and overlapping features limit the resolution of phenotype-based classification and confound disease nosology. Identification of tightly linked disease markers and discovery of disease-causing mutations have provided a basis for refining such classifications. For example, the distinction between neurofibromatosis type 1 and type 2 has been upheld by the discovery that they are caused by mutations in different genes belonging to distinct gene families: GTPase-activating protein and the merlin (schwannomin) cytoskeletal protein, respectively. In contrast, the finding that DMD and BMD are caused by mutations in the same gene points to shared pathophysiologic mechanisms and blurs the distinctions between these disorders. Mutations in different genes can lead to overlapping clinical syndromes in the case of the inherited ataxias. In other instances, phenotypically dissimilar disorders are caused by mutations in the same gene; both X-linked spastic paraparesis and X-linked hereditary hydrocephalus are caused by mutations in the gene encoding the L1 cell adhesion molecule.

Neurogenetic disorders with known chromosomal gene localization are organized primarily by clinical-pathologic phenotype in Table 363-1. Neurogenetic diseases resulting from mutations in mitochondrial DNA are reviewed in Chap. 383. Chromosomal disorders involving gross structural aberrations or alterations in number (aneuploidy) cause a large number of syndromes, many of which include mental retardation (see Chap. 383).

In the classification used in Table 363-1, the first group is the neurodegenerative disorders, which implies that deterioration and death of neurons occurs after normal development. These diseases may affect any portion of the nervous system. The second group is the epilepsy syndromes. The third group is the neuromuscular diseases, which affect the peripheral nervous system, the neuromuscular junction, or muscle. The fourth group is tumors of the central nervous system. The fifth group is abnormalities of development characterized by defects in neuronal development and migration. The availability of testing by DNA diagnostic laboratories is indicated.

Different modes of inheritance occur in each of these categories. Neurologic genetic disorders inherited in Mendelian autosomal dominant mutations include HD, familial AD, ALS, DM, CMT, familial hyperkalemic periodic paralysis, SCA, and tuberous sclerosis. Autosomal recessive disorders include Friedreich's ataxia (FA), Wilson's disease, ataxia telangiectasia, Tay-Sach's disease, and other lysosomal disorders, whereas DMD, spinobulbar muscular atrophy (Kennedy syndrome), Kallmann's syndrome, and fragile X syndrome are X-linked recessive traits. Non-Mendelian patterns of transmission such

as maternal inheritance can result from mitochondrial mutations (see Chap. 383) and unstable trinucleotide repeats (see below).

The types of mutations causing neurologic genetic disorders include gene deletions (the most common finding in DMD), insertions (e.g., Von Hippel-Lindau, type 1), duplications (e.g., CMT1A), translocations that interrupt the gene (neurofibromatosis type 1), and point mutations (e.g., in the superoxide dismutase gene in ALS). Point mutations can substitute an alternative base and thereby alter the amino acid sequence (missense mutations) or introduce stop codons leading to premature truncation of protein translation (nonsense mutations). These DNA alterations are considered "static" mutations because they generally remain stable during meiosis and provide the basis for classic Mendelian inheritance. Unstable trinucleotide repeats cause "dynamic" mutations and account for the clinical phenomenon of anticipation.

GENETICALLY INDUCED MECHANISMS OF CELL DEATH Three general mechanisms for cell death in genetic disorders have been proposed: (1) loss of function, (2) dominant-negative effects, and (3) gain of function.

In *loss-of-function disorders*, the mutation causes a deficiency in an enzyme or protein resulting in cellular dysfunction. The best defined examples are the lysosomal storage disorders in which enzymatic deficiencies in complex lipid metabolism lead to accumulation of normal or abnormal cellular constituents. The mode of inheritance in these disorders is most often autosomal recessive, but it can also be X-linked or the result of a combined inherited germ cell mutation and an acquired somatic mutation ("second hit") that knocks out both alleles (such as the loss of a growth suppressor gene as occurs in tumors like retinoblastoma). It is less common for loss-of-function disorders to result from autosomal dominant mutations. One example is the mutation of one allele of the low-density lipoprotein receptor gene ("haplo-insufficiency") with insufficient compensation by the normal allele causing familial hypercholesterolemia.

In the case of a *dominant-negative effect*, the abnormal mutation competes with or abolishes the normal allelic function at either the DNA, RNA, or protein level. This mechanism has been postulated to be an important example of cellular dysfunction in osteogenesis imperfecta in which abnormal collagen protein causes destruction of collagen fibrils. A dominant-negative mechanism in DM has been suggested by observations that RNA transcripts with expanded CTG repeats precipitate normal RNA transcripts. True dominant disorders such as HD and SCA1, in which the heterozygote genotype elicits the full spectrum of the disease phenotype, could be the result of either dominant-negative or true toxic gain-of-function effects. In the former, proteins with expanded polyglutamine tracts would form oligomers with normal protein isoforms and thereby interfere with their function. In the case of *gain-of-function effects*, the abnormal cellular function exerted by the mutation at one allele would in some way render the cell susceptible to toxic effects, whether or not the normal allele is expressed.

DISORDERS ASSOCIATED WITH TRINUCLEOTIDE REPEATS At least 10 neurologic disorders are caused by abnormal expansions of trinucleotide repeats (Table 363-2). A useful way of organizing repeat diseases and understanding their mechanisms can be based on the location of the repeat expansions within the gene. Expansions can occur in the 5' untranslated region (UTR), within the open reading frame (translated portion of the gene), within the 3' UTR, or within introns.

Four fragile X sites located on the long arm of the X chromosome (FRAXA, FRAXE, FRAXF, and FRA16A) are associated with expansions of CGG or CCG trinucleotide repeats (see also Chap. 66). The FRAXA site is associated with the fragile X syndrome, the most common cause of inherited mental retardation. FRAXA is located in the 5' UTR of the *FMR1* gene, which encodes a protein identified as FMRP. Loss of FMRP is responsible for the fragile X phenotype. One proposed mechanism to account for the defect in fragile X syndrome is that expanded CGG repeats become methylated and become targets of methyl CpG binding proteins that act to inhibit transcription. A loss-of-function model is suggested by studies showing decreased *FMR1* RNA and FMRP protein in fragile X patients and by the identification of two patients with classic features of fragile X with intragenic loss-of-function deletions. In expansions of more than 200 repeats, inhibition of transcript translation also affects FMRP levels. Expansions at the FRAXE locus are associated with a mild form of mental retardation.

The second category of trinucleotide expansion diseases consists of six neurodegenerative disorders in which expansion of a CAG repeat in the open reading frame encodes an aberrant protein with an expanded polyglutamine tract. The stretches of CAG repeats, which vary between 5 and 37 in the normal alleles of each condition, are increased by two- to fourfold in the mutation. Earlier age of onset and increased severity of the neurologic disorder demonstrate a striking correlation with larger numbers of repeats. Normal alleles identified to date never contain more than 38 CAG repeats. One possible disease mechanism is that the expanded polyglutamine tract causes a loss of protein function. HD patients homozygous for the disease allele have phenotypes similar to heterozygous patients.

These observations suggest a model in which a gain of function is toxic to neurons. One possibility is that expanded polyglutamine tracts provide a substrate for transglutaminases causing abnormal cross-linking of proteins. Expanded polyglutamine tracts might also acquire the function of "polar zippers" via hydrogen bond formation between main-chain and side-chain amides of interacting proteins. In both models, loss of the function of a critical protein(s), inhibited or depleted by aberrant interaction with expanded polyglutamine tracts, would lead to neuronal degeneration. Several lines of evidence support such a protein-based hypothesis. Open reading frame CAG repeats are indeed translated into protein. Transgenic mice expressing a human

SCA1 gene with an expanded CAG repeat develop the characteristic phenotype only when the transgene is expressed. One study has suggested that polyglutamine tracts of the proteins that cause HD and dentatorubral-pallidoluysian atrophy (DRPLA) interact with glyceraldehyde-3-phosphate dehydrogenase and thereby might have a deleterious effect on neuronal energy metabolism.

Gain-of-function models of polyglutamine tract diseases must also reconcile the observations that each neurodegenerative disease affects only regionally specific populations of neurons, yet proteins associated with these disorders are widely expressed. One possibility is that each of these polyglutamine tract proteins interacts with yet-to-be discovered proteins that are indeed cell-type specific. The huntingtin-associated protein (HAP1) is one such candidate. HAP1 is selectively expressed in brain tissue and demonstrates enhanced association with forms of huntingtin protein with increased lengths of glutamine repeats. Another potential mechanism of cell-type specificity is that somatic instability of CAG repeats leads to greater expansions in specific cell populations. The relatively small variations of three to five in the number of triplet repeats in the HD gene in different regions of the brain makes this explanation less likely.

In the third category of trinucleotide repeat disorders, repeat expansion occurs in the 3' UTR. So far, only one disease demonstrates expansion in this region. In DM, a GTC (CAG in the antisense) repeat in the 3' UTR of the DM kinase gene expands manyfold from 5 to 40 repeats in normal alleles to several kilobases in severe cases. The repeat expansion is variable in different tissues, indicating that errors in DNA replication can occur during meiosis and during somatic cell mitosis. Since DNA sequence motifs in the 3' UTR of RNA transcripts regulate transcript stability and processing, expansions in this region might affect transcript levels and alter DM kinase protein levels. Quantitative analysis of messenger RNA in muscle biopsies demonstrated marked disease-specific decreases in DM kinase mRNA in adult-onset DM patients. Levels of normal DM transcripts as well as mutant transcripts were decreased, suggesting a novel mechanism of a dominant-negative mutation occurring at the RNA level.

A second potential mechanism in DM is that expansion of the GTC repeat could inhibit expression of nearby genes. The *DMR-N9* gene is located immediately upstream (telomeric) from the DM kinase gene and the highest expression of *DMR-N9* is in neural tissue and testis; therefore alterations in its expression might cause pathology at these sites. A novel homeodomain-encoding gene (DM-locus-associated homeodomain protein) is located immediately downstream (centromeric) of the GTC repeat. The disruption of adjacent chromatin structure by repeat expansion is one mechanism by which expression of adjacent genes could be inhibited. Alternatively, repeat expansions at one locus might affect expression of more than one gene by a *cis*-acting effect, and expansion-containing transcripts may alter levels of transcripts derived from a separate allele by a *trans*-acting effect.

A fourth category of trinucleotide repeat disease occurs with repeat expansion in an intron. FA is caused by the expansion of a GAA triplet in intron 1 of the *X25* gene. Decreased mRNA levels due to either inhibition of transcription or disrupted RNA splicing occurs. Consistent with an autosomal recessive pattern of inheritance and a loss-of-function disease mechanism, the majority of

Table 363-2

Neurologic Diseases Caused by Expansion of Trinucleotide Repeats

Disorders	Site of Repeat	Effect on Gene Expression
Fragile X-A	CGG repeat 5' to translation initiation site; point mutation identified in some patients	Failure of expression of FMR-1
Fragile X-E	CGG/CCG repeats; relationship to genes unknown	Unknown
Dentatorubral-pallidoluysian atrophy (DRPLA)	CAG repeat within ORF	Normal gene expression
Huntington's disease	CAG repeat within ORF	IT15 transcript shows normal expression without cellular selectivity; expanded polyglutamine tract may alter huntingtin protein intersection with huntingtin-associated protein-1 (HAP-1) or GAPDH
Kennedy syndrome	CAG repeat within ORF of androgen receptor gene	Normal gene expression; polyglutamine tract in androgen receptor
Spinocerebellar ataxia type 1 (SCA1)	CAG repeat within ORF	Normal gene expression
Spinocerebellar ataxia type 2 (SCA2)	CAG repeat within ORF	Normal gene expression
Spinocerebellar ataxia type 3 (SCA3): also called Machado-Joseph disease	CAG repeat within ORF	Normal gene expression
Myotonic dystrophy	CTG repeat in 3' untranslated region of *DM*-1 gene, 5' end of DM-associated homeodomain protein gene; cases without repeats also described	Gene expression decreased; possible dominant-negative effect at RNA level
Friedreich's ataxia	GAA repeat in intron 1 of *X25* gene	Decreased mRNA levels due to inhibition of transcription or disrupted RNA splicing

NOTE: ORF, open reading frame.

FA patients tested to date demonstrate homozygosity for expanded alleles, while some are heterozygous with a combination of one expanded allele and point mutations in the other allele. FA is not associated with anticipation (see below) and manifests more often during adolescence rather than middle age, characteristics that are different from other trinucleotide repeat diseases identified.

The discovery of triplet repeats has given molecular precision to old concepts such as *anticipation* (earlier onset of the disease in successive generations, which is associated with further expansion of the abnormal repeats in those individuals who are more severely affected) and has helped to account for variations in gene expression. Variations in trinucleotide repeats in HD (and particularly in DM) have given a molecular explanation for concepts of *variable expression* (where variations in repeats occurring among individual members of the family can lead to earlier onset or more severe symptoms and signs, as occurs in juvenile HD). Studies suggesting that other neurologic and psychiatric disorders involve anticipation raise the possibility that additional trinucleotide repeat diseases will be discovered.

ONLINE MENDELIAN INHERITANCE IN MAN (OMIM)
The OMIM catalogue contains a frequently updated listing of all genetic traits. For each disease one can obtain information on clinical manifestations, mapping studies and identity (if available) of the relevant gene, and status of genetic testing. OMIM is located at the National Center for Biotechnologic Information and can be accessed via the Internet. The OMIM Home Page is http://www3.ncbi.nlm.nih.gov/omim/.

BIBLIOGRAPHY

BIRD TD: Apolipoprotein E genotyping in the diagnosis of Alzheimer's disease: A cautionary view. Ann Neurol 38:2, 1995

———, BENNETT RL: Why do DNA testing? Practical and ethical implications of new neurogenetic tests. Ann Neurol 38:141, 1995

BURKE JR et al: Huntingtin and DRPLA proteins selectively interact with the enzyme GAPDH. Nat Med 2:347, 1996

CAMPUZANO V et al: Friedreich's ataxia: Autosomal recessive disease caused by an intronic GAA triplet repeat expansion. Science 271:1423, 1996

DAS S et al: Diverse mutations in patients with Menkes disease often lead to exon skipping. Am J Hum Genet 55:883, 1994

DOERFLINGER N et al: Ataxia with vitamin E deficiency: Refinement of genetic localization and analysis of linkage disequilibrium by using new markers in 14 families. Am J Hum Genet 56:1116, 1995

DUBOVSKY J et al: A gene responsible for cavernous malformations of the brain maps to chromosome 7q. Hum Mol Genet 4:453, 1995

FENG Y et al: Translational suppression by trinucleotide repeat expansion at *FMR1*. Science 268:731, 1995

FINK JK et al: Autosomal dominant, familial spastic paraplegia, type I: Clinical and genetic analysis of a large North American family. Neurology 45:325, 1995

FU Y-H et al: An unstable triplet repeat in a gene related to myotonic dystrophy. Science 255:1256, 1992

HARDING AE: Clinical features and classification of inherited ataxias. Adv Neurol 61:1, 1993

HOFFMAN EP et al: Overexcited or inactive: Ion channels in muscle disease. Cell 80:681, 1995

HOLMBERG M et al: Localization of autosomal dominant cerebellar ataxia associated with retinal degeneration and anticipation to chromosome 3p12-p21.1. Hum Mol Genet 4:1441, 1995

HUNTINGTON'S DISEASE COLLABORATIVE RESEARCH GROUP: A novel gene containing a trinucleotide repeat that is expanded and unstable on Huntington's disease chromosomes. Cell 72:971, 1993

ICHINOSE H et al: Hereditary progressive dystonia with marked diurnal fluctuation caused by mutations in the GTP cyclohydrolase I gene. Nat Genet 8:236, 1994

INTERNATIONAL HUNTINGTON ASSOCIATION (IHA) AND THE WORLD FEDERATION OF NEUROLOGY (WFN) RESEARCH GROUP ON HUNTINGTON'S CHOREA: Guidelines for the molecular genetics predictive test in Huntington's disease. Neurology 44:1533, 1994

KNIGHT SJL et al: Trinucleotide repeat amplification and hypermethylation of a CpG island in *FRAXE* mental retardation. Cell 74:127, 1993

LANDER ES, SCHORK NJ: Genetic dissection of complex traits. Science 265:2037, 1994

LA SPADA AR et al: Meiotic stability and genotype-phenotype correlation of the trinucleotide repeat in X-linked spinal and bulbar muscular atrophy. Nat Genet 2:301, 1992

LEVY E et al: Mutation of the Alzheimer's disease amyloid gene in hereditary cerebral hemorrhage, Dutch type. Science 248:1124, 1990

LONGO FM: Transgenic mice: What are we learning about gene function and neurological disease? Neuroscientist 1:309, 1995

MACLENNAN DH: Discordance between phenotype and genotype in malignant hyperthermia. Curr Opin Neurol 8:397, 1995

NARCISI TM et al: Mutations of the microsomal triglyceride-transfer-protein gene in abetalipoproteinemia. Am J Hum Genet 57:1298, 1995

REES MI et al: Evidence for recessive as well as dominant forms of startle disease (hyperekplexia) caused by mutations in the α1 subunit of the inhibitory glycine receptor. Hum Mol Genet 3:2175, 1994

ROSES AD: Apolipoprotein E genotyping in the differential diagnosis, not prediction, of Alzheimer's disease. Ann Neurol 38:6, 1995

SERVADIO A et al: Expression analysis of the ataxin-1 protein in tissues from normal and spinocerebellar ataxia type 1 individuals. Nat Genet 10:94, 1995

SINE SM et al: Mutation of the acetylcholine receptor alpha subunit causes a slow-channel myasthenic syndrome by enhancing agonist binding affinity. Neuron 15:229, 1995

TARONI F et al: Identification of a common mutation in the carnitine palmitoyl-transferase II gene in familial recurrent myoglobinuria patients. Nat Genet 4:314, 1993

TOURNIER-LASSERVE E et al: Cerebral autosomal dominant arteriopathy with subcortical infarcts and leukoencephalopathy maps to chromosome 19q12. Nat Genet 3:256, 1993

WALLGREN-PETTERSSON C et al: The myotubular myopathies: Differential diagnosis of the X-linked recessive, autosomal dominant, and autosomal recessive forms and present state of DNA studies. J Med Genet 32:673, 1995

WONG EV et al: Mutations in the cell adhesion molecule L1 cause mental retardation. Trends Neurosci 18:168, 1995

SECTION 2

DISEASES OF THE CENTRAL NERVOUS SYSTEM

---

364 *Neil H. Raskin*

MIGRAINE AND THE CLUSTER HEADACHE SYNDROME

MIGRAINE

The term *migraine* stems from Galen's usage of *hemicrania* to describe a periodic disorder consisting of paroxysmal blinding hemicranial pain, vomiting, photophobia, recurrence at regular intervals, and relief by dark surroundings and sleep. *Hemicrania* was later corrupted into low Latin as *hemigranea* and *migranea*; eventually the French cognate, *migraine*, gained acceptance in the eighteenth century and has prevailed ever since. Time has proved this to be a misleading designation

for the condition, however, as it is manifested by lateralized head pain in less than 60 percent of those affected. Furthermore, undue emphasis on the dramatic features of migraine has often led to the illogical conclusion that periodic headache lacking such features is not migrainous in mechanism. It has become clear that severe headache attacks, regardless of cause, are more likely to be described as throbbing and associated with vomiting and scalp tenderness. Milder headaches tend to be nondescript—tight, band-like discomfort often involving the entire head—the profile of "tension headache." These differing clinical profiles of headaches that are not caused by an intracranial structural anomaly or systemic disease probably represent different points on a continuum rather than disparate clinical entities. Whether a single common mechanism underlies these various headache profiles is currently not known. A working definition of migraine offered here is benign recurring headache and/or neurologic dysfunction usually attended by pain-free interludes and often provoked by stereotyped stimuli. Migraine may be identified by its activators (red wine, menses, hunger, lack of sleep, glare, perfumes, periods of letdown) and its deactivators (sleep, pregnancy, exhilaration, sumatriptan). It is by far more common in women; there is a hereditary predisposition toward attacks; and the cranial circulatory phenomena that attend attacks appear to be secondary to a primary central nervous system (CNS) disorder.

CLINICAL SUBTYPES The designation *classic migraine* (migraine with aura) denotes the syndrome of headache associated with characteristic premonitory sensory, motor, or visual symptoms; *common migraine* (migraine without aura) denotes one in which no focal neurologic disturbance precedes the headache. Common migraine is by far the more frequent clinical problem, and focal neurologic disturbances are more common during headache attacks than as prodromal symptoms. Focal neurologic disturbances without headache or vomiting have come to be known as *migraine equivalents* or *accompaniments* and appear to occur more commonly in patients between the ages of 40 and 70 years. The term *complicated migraine* has generally been used to describe migraine with dramatic focal neurologic features, thus overlapping with *classic migraine*; it has also been used to describe a migraine attack that leaves a persisting residual neurologic deficit.

Common Migraine Benign periodic headache of several hours' duration, often attributed to "tension" by its sufferers, is the most liberal definition of common migraine. Traditional definitions of migraine often identify only patients with severe attacks, not those with more modest head pain; thus, in various combinations, unilateral pain, attendant nausea or vomiting, a positive family history, responsiveness to ergotamine, and scalp tenderness have been considered necessary to establish a diagnosis of migraine. However, the validity of using such clinical features to diagnose migraine has never been formally established (Table 364-1). Common migraine is the most frequent headache type reported by patients.

Classic Migraine The most common premonitory symptoms reported by migraineurs are visual, arising from dysfunction of occipital lobe neurons. Scotomas and/or hallucinations occur in about one-third of migraineurs and usually appear in the central portions of the visual fields. A highly characteristic syndrome occurs in about 10 percent of patients; it usually begins as a small paracentral scotoma, which slowly expands into a "C" shape. Luminous angles appear at the enlarging outer edge, becoming colored as the scintillating scotoma expands and moves toward the periphery of the involved half of the visual field. It eventually disappears over the horizon of peripheral vision, the entire process taking 20 to 25 min. This phenomenon never occurs *during* the headache phase of an attack and is pathognomonic for migraine, never having been described in association with a cerebral structural anomaly. It is commonly referred to as a *fortification spec-*

trum because the serrated edges of the hallucinated "C" seemed to Dr. Hubert Airy to resemble a "fortified town with bastions all round it"; "spectrum" is used in the sense of an apparition or specter.

Basilar Migraine Symptoms referable to a disturbance in brainstem function, such as vertigo, dysarthria, or diplopia, occur as the only neurologic symptoms of the attack in about 25 percent of patients. Bickerstaff called attention to a stereotyped sequence of dramatic neurologic events, often comprising total blindness and sensorial clouding, that is common among but not restricted to adolescent women. These episodes begin with total blindness accompanied or followed by admixtures of vertigo, ataxia, dysarthria, tinnitus, and distal and perioral paresthesia. In about one-quarter of patients, a confusional state supervenes. The neurologic symptoms usually persist for 20 to 30 min and are generally followed by a throbbing occipital headache. This basilar migraine syndrome is now known also to occur in children and in adults over age 50. An altered sensorium may persist for as long as 5 days and may take the form of confusional states superficially resembling psychotic reactions. Full recovery after the episode is the rule.

Carotidynia The carotidynia syndrome, sometimes called *lower-half headache* or *facial migraine*, is most common among older patients, with the incidence peaking in the fourth through sixth decades. Pain is usually located at the jaw or neck, although sometimes periorbital or maxillary pain occurs; it may be continuous, deep, dull, and aching, and it becomes pounding or throbbing episodically. There are often superimposed sharp, ice pick–like jabs. Attacks occur one to several times per week, each lasting several minutes to hours. Tenderness and prominent pulsations of the cervical carotid artery, and soft tissue swelling overlying the carotid, usually are present ipsilateral to the pain; many patients also report throbbing ipsilateral headache concurrent with carotidynia attacks as well as between attacks. Dental trauma is a common precipitant of this syndrome. Carotid artery involvement appears also to be common in the more traditional forms of migraine; over 50 percent of patients with frequent migraine attacks are found to have carotid tenderness at several points on the side most often involved during their hemicranial migraine attacks.

PATHOGENESIS Modern orientations toward migraine began with the publication by Liveing in 1873 of the first major treatise devoted to the subject of migraine, *A Contribution to the Pathology of Nerve Storms*. Liveing believed that the analogy of migraine to epilepsy was obvious and that the clinically apparent circulatory phenomena that occurred during migrainous attacks were secondary to cerebral discharges, or "nerve storms." Attention was focused on the vascular features of migraine by Graham and Wolff in the 1930s, who showed that the administration of ergotamine reduced the amplitude of the pulsations of the temporal artery in patients with headache, and that this effect was often, although *not consistently*, associated with a decrease in head pain. Because of these observations and other less substantial lines of evidence, it was widely held for many years that the headache phase of migrainous attacks was caused by extracranial vasodilation and that the neurologic symptoms were produced by intracranial vasoconstriction, the "vascular" hypothesis of migraine.

K.S. Lashley, physiologic psychologist at Harvard, in 1941 was among the first to chart his own migrainous fortification spectrum in detail and at brief intervals. He was able to estimate that the evolution of his own scotoma proceeded across the occipital cortex at a rate of 3 mm/min. He speculated that a wavefront of intense excitation followed by a wave of complete inhibition of activity were propagated across the visual cortex. In 1944, the phenomenon that has come to be known as *spreading depression* was described by the Brazilian physiologist, Leão, in the cerebral cortex of laboratory animals. It is a slowly moving (2 to 3 mm/min), potassium-liberating depression of cortical activity, preceded by a wavefront of increased metabolic activity that can be produced by a variety of experimental stimuli, including hypoxia, mechanical trauma, and the topical application of potassium. These observations could not easily be integrated into a simple vascular model of migraine.

Current concepts of the pathogenesis of migraine focus on three mechanisms and anatomic regions. First, there is a vasomotor compo-

Table 364-1

Symptoms Accompanying Severe Migraine Attacks in a Group of 500 Patients

Symptom	Percent of Patients Affected
Nausea	87
Vomiting	56
Diarrhea	16
Photophobia	82
Visual disturbances	36
Fortification spectra	10
Photopsia	26
Paresthesia	33
Scalp tenderness	65
Lightheadedness	72
Vertigo	33
Alteration of consciousness	18
Seizure	4
Syncope	10
Confusional state	4

SOURCE: NH Raskin: *Headache*, 2d ed, New York, Churchill Livingstone, 1988.

nent mediated by constriction or dilation of arteries within and outside the brain. Second, there is a midbrain trigger, perhaps in serotonergic neurons of the dorsal raphe. Third, there is activation of a trigeminal-vascular system, consisting of medullary neurons in the trigeminal nucleus caudalis that terminate on the walls of arteries and release vasoactive neuropeptides. The role of each of these systems in the production of specific symptoms of migraine is unknown; it is possible that activation of any of the three may be *sufficient* for headache production, and that one mechanism may dominate in a particular migrainous syndrome. For example, the evolution of the fortification spectrum may be entirely neurogenic, requiring only activation of the dorsal raphe system.

Vasomotor Component   Regional cerebral blood flow studies have shown that in patients with classic migraine there is, during attacks, a modest cortical hypoperfusion that begins in the visual cortex and spreads forward at a rate of 2 to 3 mm/min. The decrease in blood flow averages 25 to 30 percent (insufficient to explain symptoms on the basis of ischemia) and progresses anteriorly in a wave-like fashion independent of the topography of cerebral arteries. The wave of hypoperfusion persists for 4 to 6 h, appears to follow the convolutions of the cortex, and does not cross the central or lateral sulcus, progressing to the frontal lobe via the insula. Perfusion of subcortical structures is normal. Contralateral neurologic symptoms appear during temporoparietal hypoperfusion; at times, hypoperfusion persists in these regions after symptoms cease. More often, frontal spread continues as the headache phase begins. A few patients with classic migraine show no flow abnormalities; an occasional patient has developed focal ischemia sufficient to cause symptoms. However, focal ischemia does not appear to be *necessary* for focal symptoms to occur. During common migraine, no flow abnormalities are usually seen.

Serotonergic Projections and the Dorsal Raphe   Taken together, the pharmacologic data on migraine point to involvement of serotonin receptors. About 35 years ago, methysergide was found to antagonize certain peripheral actions of serotonin [5-hydroxytryptamine (5-HT)] and was introduced as the first drug capable of preventing migraine attacks. Subsequently, it was found that platelet levels of serotonin fall consistently at the onset of headache and that migrainous episodes may be triggered by drugs that cause serotonin to be released. Such changes in circulating levels proved to be pharmacologically trivial, however, and interest in the humoral role of serotonin in migraine declined. Currently, there is renewed interest, due almost entirely to the introduction of the drug sumatriptan, which is remarkably effective for migraine attacks. Of still greater interest is the fact that sumatriptan is a designer drug, synthesized to activate selectively a particular subpopulation of serotonin receptors.

There are four main families of 5-HT receptors—types 1, 2, 3, and 4; receptor subtypes have been found for each type. Many of the drugs effective in migraine prophylaxis are type 2 antagonists, whereas the abortive agents are type 1 agonists. Sumatriptan is most potent as an agonist of 5-HT$_{1D}$ receptors, and is less potent at 5-HT$_{1A}$ and 5-HT$_{1B}$ receptors. By contrast, dihydroergotamine, another drug that is highly effective in aborting migraine attacks, is most potent as an agonist of 5-HT$_{1A}$ receptors and is an order of magnitude less potent at 5-HT$_{1D}$ receptors. After systemic administration, dihydroergotamine in the brain is found in the highest concentrations in the midbrain dorsal raphe. The dorsal raphe is a good candidate as a generator of migraine and as a site of antimigraine drug action; the highest concentration of serotonin receptors in brain tissue is found there. They are mainly of the 5-HT$_{1A}$ variety, but 5-HT$_{1D}$ receptors also are present.

Electrical stimulation near dorsal raphe neurons can result in migraine-like headaches (see also Chap. 15). Blood flow in the pons and midbrain increases focally during migraine headache episodes; this alteration probably results from increased activity of cells in the dorsal raphe and locus ceruleus. There are projections from the dorsal raphe that terminate on cerebral arteries and alter cerebral blood flow. There are also major projections from the dorsal raphe to important visual centers, including the lateral geniculate body, superior colliculus, retina, and visual cortex. These various serotonergic projections may represent the neural substrate for the circulatory and visual characteris-

FIGURE 364-1   The actions of the antimigraine drugs at brainstem and forebrain synapses. The solid arrows indicate stimulative or agonist properties, and the segmented arrows indicate inhibitory properties. 5-HIAA, 5-hydroxyindoleacetic acid. (*From NH Raskin: Headache, 2d ed, New York, Churchill Livingstone, 1988.*)

tics of migraine. The dorsal raphe cells stop firing during deep sleep, and sleep is known to ameliorate migraine; the antimigraine prophylactic drugs also inhibit activity of the dorsal raphe cells through a direct or indirect agonist effect (Fig. 364-1).

Trigeminal-Vascular System   Activation of cells in the trigeminal nucleus caudalis in the medulla (a pain processing center for the head and face region) results in the release of vasoactive neuropeptides, including substance P and calcitonin gene–related peptide, at vascular terminations of the trigeminal nerve. Moskowitz and colleagues have proposed that these peptide neurotransmitters induce a sterile inflammation that activates trigeminal nociceptive afferents originating on the vessel wall, further contributing to the production of pain. This mechanism also provides a potential mechanism for the soft tissue swelling and tenderness of blood vessels that attend migraine attacks.

The genetic basis of migraine is largely unknown. Family studies indicate that genetic heterogeneity—i.e., independent migraine genes—is likely to be present. Genetic linkage analysis has been successful in one rare migraine syndrome, autosomal dominant familial hemiplegic migraine (see Chap. 363). In this disorder, hemiplegia and hemisensory loss develop and persist for hours to days, after which headache supervenes. In approximately one-half of families, a mutation in a P/Q-type calcium channel α1-subunit gene located on chromosome 19 has been found.

℞ **TREATMENT**

The mainstay of therapy is the judicious use of one or more of the many drugs that are relatively specific for migraine.

Acute Treatment   In general, an adequate dose of whichever agent is chosen should be used at the onset of an attack. If additional medication is required in 30 to 60 min because symptoms return or have not abated, the initial dose should be increased for subsequent attacks. Drug absorption is impaired during migrainous attacks because of reduced gastrointestinal motility. Delayed absorption occurs in the absence of nausea and is related to the severity of the attack and not its duration. Therefore, when oral agents fail, alternative therapies, including rectal ergotamine, subcutaneous sumatriptan, parenteral dihydroergotamine, and intravenous chlorpromazine and prochlorperazine, should be tried.

For patients whose headaches have a prolonged buildup, oral agents may indeed suffice. When aspirin and acetaminophen alone fail, the addition of butalbital and caffeine to these analgesics is highly effective; ibuprofen (600 to 800 mg) and naproxen (375 to 750 mg) are often useful. Isometheptene compound, 1 to 2 capsules, is effective for mild to moderate "common migraine." When these measures fail, more aggressive therapy should be considered (Table 364-2).

A subnauseating dose of ergotamine should be sought; a dose that provokes nausea—probably a centrally mediated side effect—is too high and may intensify head pain. The average oral dose is 3 mg (three 1-mg ergotamine-caffeine tablets taken together). The drug also exists in suppository form (2 mg); the average dose is one-half of a suppository (1 mg), and many patients achieve an excellent result with one-quarter of a suppository (0.5 mg). Sumatriptan may be given as a 50-mg oral dose or a 6-mg subcutaneous dose; there is a high recurrence rate because of the short half-life of this drug (2 h), so that a second dose may be necessary.

Dihydroergotamine is available as a parenteral preparation and as a nasal spray. Peak plasma levels of dihydroergotamine are achieved 45 min after subcutaneous dosing, 30 min after intramuscular dosing, and 3 min after intravenous dosing. If an attack has not already peaked, subcutaneous or intramuscular administration of 1 mg suffices for about 90 percent of patients. The nasal spray results in substantial blood levels in 45 to 60 min. A common intravenous protocol is the administration over 2 min of a mixture of 5 mg of prochlorperazine and 0.5 mg of dihydroergotamine (they are miscible).

If a patient's headache profile transforms into a chronic daily headache syndrome, opiate-type analgesics should be restricted to 2 days out of 7. The mainstay of therapy for these patients is daily amitriptyline (30 to 100 mg) or nortriptyline (40 to 120 mg). If the syndrome is recalcitrant, valproic acid (500 to 2000 mg) or phenelzine (45 to 90 mg) may be necessary

Prophylaxis A substantial number of drugs are now available that have the capacity to stabilize migraine (Table 364-3). They must be taken daily. The decision of whether to use this approach depends on the frequency of attacks and on how well acute treatment is working. The occurrence of at least two or three attacks per month could be an indication for this approach. There is usually a lag of 2 weeks before an effect is seen. The major drugs and recommended daily doses are as follows: propranolol (60 to 320 mg), amitriptyline (10 to 175 mg), valproate (500 to 1500 mg), verapamil (160 to 480 mg), phenelzine (30 to 75 mg), and methysergide (2 to 8 mg). Phenelzine and methysergide are usually reserved for recalcitrant cases because of their serious potential side effects. Phenelzine is a monoamine oxidase inhibitor; therefore, tyramine-containing foods, decongestants, and meperidine are contraindicated. Methysergide may cause retroperitoneal or cardiac valvular fibrosis when it is used for more than 8 months, so monitoring is required for patients using this drug; the risk of the fibrotic complication is about 1:1500 and is likely to reverse after the drug is stopped.

The probability of success with any one of the antimigraine drugs is 60 to 75 percent; if one drug is assessed each month, there is a good chance that effective stabilization will be achieved within a few months. The large majority of patients are successfully managed with propranolol or amitriptyline; for more urgent resolution, valproate, methysergide, or phenelzine can be used. Once effective stabilization is achieved, the drug is continued for 5 to 6 months and then slowly tapered to assess the continued need for it. Many patients are able to discontinue medication and experience fewer

and milder attacks for long periods, suggesting that these drugs may alter the natural history of migraine.

Nonpharmacologic Approaches Patients with migraine do not encounter more stress than headache-free individuals; over-responsiveness to stress appears to be the issue. Since the stresses of everyday living cannot be eliminated, lessening one's response to stress by various techniques is helpful for many patients, as long as these methods are practiced continually. They include yoga, transcendental meditation, hypnosis, and conditioning techniques such as biofeedback. For most patients, this approach is, at best, an adjunct to pharmacotherapy.

CLUSTER HEADACHE

In the past, a variety of names have been used for this condition, including *Raeder's syndrome*, *histamine cephalalgia*, and *sphenopalatine neuralgia*. *Cluster headache* is now firmly established as a distinctive syndrome, whose recognition is important since it is likely to be responsive to treatment. The episodic type is most common, and is characterized by one to three short-lived attacks of periorbital pain per day over a 4- to 8-week period, followed by a pain-free interval that averages 1 year. The chronic form, which may begin de novo or several years after an episodic pattern has become established, is characterized by the absence of sustained periods of remission. Each type may transform into the other. Men are affected seven to eight times more often than women; hereditary factors are usually absent. Although the onset is generally between ages 20 and 50, it may occur as early as the first decade of life. Propranolol and amitriptyline are largely ineffective. Lithium is beneficial for cluster headache and ineffective in migraine. The cluster syndrome is thus clinically, genetically, and therapeutically different from migraine. Nevertheless, mixed features of the two disorders are occasionally present, suggesting some common elements to their pathogenesis.

CLINICAL FEATURES Periorbital, or, less commonly, temporal, pain begins without warning and reaches a crescendo within 5 min. It is often excruciating in intensity and is deep, nonfluctuating, and explosive in quality; only rarely is it pulsatile. Pain is strictly unilateral and usually affects the same side in subsequent months. Attacks last from 30 min to 2 h; there are often associated symptoms of homolateral lacrimation, reddening of the eye, nasal stuffiness, lid ptosis, and nausea. Alcohol provokes attacks in about 70 percent of patients but ceases to be provocative when the bout remits; this on-off vulnerability to alcohol is pathognomonic of cluster headache. Only rarely do foods or emotional factors precipitate pain, in contrast to migraine.

There is a striking periodicity of attacks in at least 85 percent of patients. At least one of the daily attacks of pain recurs at about the same hour each day for the duration of a cluster bout. Onset is nocturnal in about 50 percent of the cases, and in that case the pain usually awakens the patient within 2 h of falling asleep.

PATHOGENESIS No consistent cerebral blood flow changes accompany attacks of pain. Perhaps the strongest evidence for a central mechanism is the periodicity of attacks; the existence of a central mechanism also is suggested by the observation that autonomic symptoms that accompany the pain are bilateral and are more severe on the painful side. The hypothalamus may be the site of activation in this disorder. The posterior hypothalamus contains cells that regulate autonomic functions, and the anterior hypothalamus contains cells (in the suprachiasmatic nuclei) that constitute the principal circadian pacemaker in mammals. Activation of both is necessary to explain the symptoms of cluster headache. The pacemaker is modulated via serotonergic dorsal raphe projections. It can be concluded tentatively that both migraine and cluster headache result from abnormal serotonergic neurotransmission, albeit at different loci.

℞ **TREATMENT**
The most satisfactory treatment is the administration of drugs to prevent cluster attacks until the bout is over. Effective prophylactic drugs are prednisone, lithium, methysergide, ergotamine, and vera-

Table 364-2

Treatments Used to Abort Migraine Headaches

Time to Peak Head Pain,* h	Treatment Option 1	Treatment Option 2	Treatment Option 3
>3	Ergotamine tablets (Wigraine), 2–3 tablets	Isometheptene compound (Midrin), 1–2 capsules	Butalbital compound with aspirin or acetaminophen (Fiorinal, Floricet, Esgic), 1–2 tablets
1–3	Dihydroergotamine nasal spray (Migranal), one dose (2 mg)	1/2 ergotamine suppository (= 1 mg) (Cafergot, Wigraine)	Sumatriptan (Imitrex), 1 tablet, 25 or 50 mg
<1	Sumatriptan (Imitrex), 6 mg SC	Dihydroergotamine (DHE-45), 1 mg IM or SC	Nasal butorphanol (Stadol), 1–2 mg

* The time required for head pain to reach its peak intensity after first being perceived by the patient.

Table 364-3

Drugs Effective for the Prophylaxis of Migraine

Drug	Daily Dosage Range (mg)	Most Common Side Effects
Amitriptyline	10–175	Sedation, dry mouth, weight gain
Propranolol	60–320	
Nadolol	40–160	
Atenolol	50–200	Lethargy, insomnia, lightheadedness, impotence
Timolol	20–60	
Metoprolol	50–200	
Papaverine	300–900	Nausea
Cyproheptadine	8–32	Sedation, weight gain
Verapamil	160–480	Constipation, nausea, fluid retention, lightheadedness, hypotension
Phenelzine	30–75	Insomnia, lightheadedness, slowed bladder emptying, weight gain
Valproic acid	500–1500	Nausea, weight gain, tremor, hair loss
Methysergide	2–8	Nausea, muscle cramps, insomnia, weight gain, peripheral vasoconstriction; retroperitoneal fibrosis with prolonged use (>6 months)

pamil. Lithium (600 to 900 mg daily) appears to be particularly useful for the chronic form of the disorder. A 10-day course of prednisone, beginning at 60 mg daily for 7 days followed by a rapid taper, may interrupt the pain bout for many patients. When ergotamine is used, it is most effective when given 1 to 2 h before an expected attack; for patients who have a single nocturnal episode, 1 mg of ergotamine in suppository form taken at bedtime may be all that is necessary. Patients must be educated regarding the early symptoms of ergotism when ergotamine is used daily; a weekly limit of 14 mg should be adhered to.

For the attacks themselves, oxygen inhalation (9 L/min via a loose mask) is the most effective modality; 15 min of inhalation of 100% oxygen is often necessary. The self-administration of intranasal lidocaine, either 4% topical or 2% viscous, to the most caudal aspect of the inferior nasal turbinate can produce a sphenopalatine ganglionic block that is usually remarkably effective in terminating an attack. Sumatriptan, 6 mg subcutaneously, will usually shorten an attack to 10 to 15 min.

BIBLIOGRAPHY

BATES D et al: Subcutaneous sumatriptan during the migraine aura. Neurology 44:1587, 1994

DAVIDOFF RA: *Migraine*. Philadelphia, Davis, 1995

FERRARI MD, SAXENA PR: On serotonin and migraine; a clinical and pharmacological review. Cephalalgia 13:151, 1993

GOADSBY PJ, EDVINSSON L: Human in vivo evidence for trigeminovascular activation in cluster headache. Brain 117:427, 1994

JOUTEL A et al: Genetic heterogeneity of familial hemiplegic migraine. Am J Hum Genet 55:1166, 1994

KELLY K: Cardiac arrest following use of sumatriptan. Neurology 45:1211, 1995

LAURITZEN M: Pathophysiology of the migraine aura: The spreading depression theory. Brain 117:199, 1994

MCLACHLAN RS, GIRVIN JP: Spreading depression of Leão in rodent and human cortex. Brain Research 666:133, 1994

MOSKOWITZ MA: The visceral organ brain: Implications for the pathophysiology of vascular head pain. Neurology 41:182, 1991

OLESEN J: Cerebral and extracranial circulatory disturbances in migraine: Pathophysiological implications. Cerebrovasc Brain Metab Rev 3:1, 1991
——— et al (eds): *The Headaches*. New York, Raven, 1993

OPHOFF RA et al: Familial hemiplegic migraine and episodic ataxia type-2 are caused by mutations in the Ca^{2+} channel gene CACNL1A4. Cell 87:543, 1996

PLOSKER GL, MCTAVISH D: Sumatriptan: A reappraisal of its pharmacology and therapeutic efficacy in the acute treatment of migraine and cluster headache. Drugs 47:622, 1994

REPORT OF THE QUALITY STANDARDS SUBCOMMITTEE OF THE AMERICAN ACADEMY OF NEUROLOGY: Practice parameter: Appropriate use of ergotamine tartrate and dihydroergotamine in the treatment of migraine and status migrainosus. (Summary statement.) Neurology 45:585, 1995

WEILLER C et al: Brain stem activation in spontaneous human migraine attacks. Nature Med 1:658, 1995

WELCH KMA: Drug therapy of migraine. N Engl J Med 329:1476, 1993

WINNER P et al: A double-blind study of subcutaneous dihydroergotamine vs subcutaneous sumatriptan in the treatment of acute migraine. Arch Neurol 53:180, 1996

WOODS RP et al: Bilateral spreading cerebral hypoperfusion during spontaneous migraine headache. N Engl J Med 331:1689, 1994

365 Daniel H. Lowenstein

SEIZURES AND EPILEPSY

A *seizure* (from the Latin *sacire*, "to take possession of") is a paroxysmal event due to abnormal, excessive, hypersynchronous discharges from an aggregate of central nervous system (CNS) neurons. Depending on the distribution of discharges, this abnormal CNS activity can have various manifestations, ranging from dramatic convulsive activity to experiential phenomena not readily discernible by an observer. Although a variety of factors influence the incidence and prevalence of seizures, approximately 5 to 10 percent of the population will have at least one seizure during their lifetime, with the highest incidence occurring in early childhood and late adulthood. Because seizures are common, this clinical problem is encountered frequently during medical practice in a variety of settings.

The meaning of the term seizure needs to be carefully distinguished from that of epilepsy. *Epilepsy* describes a condition in which a person has *recurrent* seizures due to a chronic, underlying process. This definition implies that a person with a single seizure, or recurrent seizures due to correctable or avoidable circumstances, does not necessarily have epilepsy. Epilepsy refers to a clinical phenomenon rather than a single disease entity, since there are many forms and causes of epilepsy. However, among the many causes of epilepsy there are various *epilepsy syndromes* in which the clinical and pathologic characteristics are distinctive and suggest a specific underlying etiology.

Using the definition of epilepsy as two or more unprovoked seizures, the incidence of epilepsy is approximately 0.3 to 0.5 percent in different populations throughout the world, and the prevalence of epilepsy has been estimated at 5 to 10 people per 1000.

CLASSIFICATION OF SEIZURES

An essential step in the evaluation and management of a patient with a seizure is to determine the type of seizure that has occurred. The importance of this cannot be over emphasized—classifying the seizure is essential for focusing the diagnostic approach on particular etiologies, selecting the appropriate therapy, and providing potentially vital information regarding prognosis. In 1981, the International League Against Epilepsy (ILAE) published a modified version of the International Classification of Epileptic Seizures that has continued to be a useful classification system (Table 365-1). This system is based on the clinical features of seizures and associated electroencephalographic (EEG) findings. Other potentially distinctive features such as etiology or cellular substrate are not factored into the classification system, although this will probably change in the future as more is learned about the pathophysiologic mechanisms that underlie specific seizure types.

The main characteristic that distinguishes the different categories of seizures is whether the seizure activity is *partial* (synonymous with *focal*) or *generalized*. Partial seizures are those in which the seizure activity is restricted to discrete areas of the cerebral cortex. Generalized seizures involve diffuse regions of the brain simultaneously in a bilaterally symmetric fashion. As a rule, partial seizures are typically associated with structural abnormalities of the brain. In contrast, generalized seizures may result from cellular, biochemical, or structural abnormalities that have a more widespread distribution. Other aspects of seizure classification and semiology (phenomenology) continue to be debated among epileptologists, including the definition of altered consciousness, use of the terms "partial" versus "focal," and the concept of aura.

PARTIAL SEIZURES Partial seizures occur within discrete regions of the brain. If consciousness is fully preserved during the seizure, the clinical manifestations are considered relatively simple and the seizure is termed a *simple-partial seizure*. If consciousness is impaired, the symptomatology is more complex and the seizure is termed a *complex-partial seizure*. An important additional subgroup comprises those seizures that begin as partial seizures and then spread diffusely throughout the cortex, i.e., *partial seizures with secondary generalization*.

Simple-Partial Seizures Simple-partial seizures cause motor, sensory, autonomic, or psychic symptoms without an obvious alteration in consciousness. For example, a patient having a partial motor seizure arising from the right primary motor cortex in the vicinity controlling hand movement will note the onset of involuntary movements of the contralateral, left hand. These movements are typically clonic (i.e., repetitive, flexion/extension movements) at a frequency

of approximately 2 to 3 Hz; pure tonic posturing may be seen as well. Since the cortical region controlling hand movement is immediately adjacent to the region for facial expression, the seizure may also cause abnormal movements of the face synchronous with the movements of the hand. The EEG recorded with scalp electrodes during the seizure (i.e., an ictal EEG) may show abnormal discharges in a very limited region over the appropriate area of cerebral cortex if the seizure focus involves the cerebral convexity. Seizure activity occurring within deeper brain structures is often not recorded by the standard EEG, however, and may require intracranial electrodes for its detection.

Three additional features of partial motor seizures are worth noting. First, in some patients the abnormal motor movements may begin in a very restricted region such as the fingers and gradually progress (over seconds to minutes) to include a larger portion of the extremity. This phenomenon was originally described by Hughlings Jackson and is known as a "Jacksonian march," representing the spread of seizure activity over a progressively larger region of motor cortex. Second, patients may experience a localized paresis (Todd's paralysis) for minutes to many hours in the involved region following the seizure. Third, in rare instances the seizure may continue for hours or days. This condition, termed *epilepsia partialis continua*, is often quite refractory to medical therapy.

Other forms of simple-partial seizures include those that cause changes in somatic sensation (e.g., paresthesia), vision (flashing lights or formed hallucinations), equilibrium (sensation of falling or vertigo), or autonomic function (flushing, sweating, piloerection). Simple-partial seizures arising from the temporal or frontal cortex may also cause alterations in hearing, olfaction, or higher cortical function (psychic symptoms). This includes the sensation of unusual, intense odors (e.g., burning rubber or kerosene) or sounds (crude or highly complex sounds), or an epigastric sensation that rises from the stomach or chest to the head. Some patients describe odd, internal feelings such as fear, a sense of impending change, detachment, depersonalization, déja vu, or illusions that objects are growing smaller (micropsia) or larger (macropsia). When such symptoms precede a complex-partial or secondarily generalized seizure, these simple-partial seizures serve as a warning, or *aura*.

Complex-Partial Seizures Complex-partial seizures are characterized by focal seizure activity accompanied by a transient impairment of the patient's ability to maintain normal contact with the environment. Operationally this means that the patient is unable to respond to visual or verbal commands during the seizure and has impaired recollection or awareness of the ictal phase. The seizures frequently begin with an aura (i.e., a simple-partial seizure) that is stereotypic for the patient. The start of the ictal phase is often a sudden behavioral arrest or motionless stare, and this marks the onset of the event for which the patient will be amnestic. The behavioral arrest is usually accompanied by automatisms, which are involuntary, automatic behaviors that have a wide range of manifestations. Automatisms may consist of very basic behaviors such as chewing, lip smacking, swallowing, or "picking" movements of the hands, or more elaborate behaviors such as a display of emotion or running. The patient is typically confused following the seizure, and the transition to full recovery of consciousness may range from seconds up to an hour. Careful examination of the patient immediately following the seizure may show an anterograde amnesia or, in cases involving the dominant hemisphere, a postictal aphasia.

The routine, interictal (i.e., between seizures) EEG in patients with complex-partial seizures is often normal, or may show brief discharges termed *epileptiform spikes*, or *sharp waves*. Since complex-partial seizures often arise from the medial temporal lobe or inferior frontal lobe, i.e., regions distant from the scalp, the EEG recorded during the seizure may be non–localizing. However, the seizure focus is often detected using special electrodes such as sphenoidal or surgically-placed intracranial electrodes.

The range of potential clinical behaviors linked to complex-partial seizures is so broad that extreme caution is advised before concluding that stereotypic episodes of bizarre or atypical behavior are not due to seizure activity. In such cases it is imperative to consider more

Table 365-1

Classification of Seizures

1. Partial seizures
   A. Simple-partial seizures (with motor, sensory, autonomic, or psychic signs)
   B. Complex-partial seizures
   C. Partial seizures with secondary generalization
2. Primarily generalized seizures
   A. Absence (petit mal)
   B. Tonic-clonic (grand mal)
   C. Tonic
   D. Atonic
   E. Myoclonic
3. Unclassified seizures
   A. Neonatal seizures
   B. Infantile spasms

detailed EEG studies in order to determine whether the behaviors are caused by a seizure disorder.

CHAPTER 365
Seizures and Epilepsy   **2313**

Partial Seizures with Secondary Generalization Partial seizures can spread to involve both cerebral hemispheres and produce a generalized seizure, usually of the tonic-clonic variety (discussed below). Secondary generalization is observed frequently following simple-partial seizures, especially those with a focus in the frontal lobe, but may also be associated with partial seizures occurring elsewhere in the brain. A partial seizure with secondary generalization is often difficult to distinguish from a primarily generalized tonic-clonic seizure, since bystanders tend to emphasize the more dramatic, generalized convulsive phase of the seizure and overlook the more subtle, focal symptoms present at onset. In some cases, the focal onset of the seizure becomes apparent only when a careful history identifies a preceding aura (i.e., simple-partial seizure). Often, however, the focal onset is not clinically evident and may be established only through careful EEG analysis. Nonetheless, distinguishing between these two entities is extremely important, as there may be substantial differences in the evaluation and treatment of partial versus generalized seizure disorders.

GENERALIZED SEIZURES By definition, generalized seizures arise from both cerebral hemispheres simultaneously. However, it is currently impossible to exclude entirely the existence of a focal region of abnormal activity that initiates the seizure prior to rapid secondary generalization. For this reason, generalized seizures may be practically defined as bilateral clinical and electrographic events without any detectable focal onset. Fortunately, a number of the subtypes of generalized seizures have distinctive features that facilitate clinical diagnosis.

Absence Seizures (Petit Mal) Absence seizures are characterized by sudden, brief lapses of consciousness without loss of postural control. The seizure typically lasts for only seconds, consciousness returns as suddenly as it was lost, and there is no postictal confusion. Although the brief loss of consciousness may be clinically inapparent or the sole manifestation of the seizure discharge, absence seizures are usually accompanied by subtle, bilateral motor signs such as rapid blinking of the eyelids, chewing movements, or small-amplitude, clonic movements of the hands.

Absence seizures almost always begin in childhood (ages 4 to 8) or early adolescence and are the main seizure type in 15 to 20 percent of children with epilepsy. The seizures can occur hundreds of times per day, but the child may be unaware of or unable to convey their existence. This can lead to a situation in which the patient is constantly struggling to piece together experiences that have been interrupted by the seizures. Since the clinical signs of the seizures are subtle, especially to new parents, it is not surprising that the first clue to absence epilepsy is often unexplained "daydreaming" and a decline in school performance recognized by a teacher.

The electrophysiologic hallmark of typical absence seizures is a generalized, symmetric, 3 Hz spike-and-wave discharge that begins and ends suddenly on a normal EEG background. Periods of spike-and-wave discharges lasting more than a few seconds usually correlate with the clinical signs, but the EEG often shows many more periods of abnormal cortical activity than were suspected clinically. Hyperventilation tends to provoke these electrographic discharges and even the seizures themselves and is routinely used when recording the EEG.

Typical absence seizures are not associated with other neurologic problems and respond well to treatment with specific anticonvulsants. Although estimates vary, approximately 60 to 70 percent of such patients will have a spontaneous remission during adolescence. Unfortunately, a significant number of the nonremitting patients have associated generalized, tonic-clonic seizures and suffer from the problems of chronic epilepsy.

Atypical Absence Seizures Atypical absence seizures have features that deviate from both the clinical and EEG features of typical absence seizures. For example, the lapse of consciousness is usually of longer duration and less abrupt in onset and cessation, and the seizure is accompanied by more obvious motor signs that may include focal or lateralizing features. The EEG shows a generalized, slow spike-and-wave pattern with a frequency of 2.5 per second or less, as well as other abnormal activity. Atypical absence seizures are usually associated with diffuse or multifocal structural abnormalities of the brain and therefore may accompany other signs of neurologic dysfunction such as mental retardation. Furthermore, the seizures are less responsive to anticonvulsants compared to typical absence seizures.

Generalized, Tonic-Clonic Seizures (Grand Mal) Primarily generalized, tonic-clonic seizures are the main seizure type in approximately 10 percent of all persons with epilepsy. They are also the most common seizure type resulting from metabolic derangements and are therefore frequently encountered in many different clinical settings. The seizure usually begins abruptly without warning, although some patients describe vague premonitory symptoms in the hours leading up to the seizure. This prodrome should be distinguished from the stereotypic auras associated with focal seizures that secondarily generalize. The initial phase of the seizure is usually tonic contraction of muscles throughout the body, accounting for a number of the classic features of the event. Tonic contraction of the muscles of expiration and the larynx at the onset will produce a loud moan or cry. Respirations are impaired, secretions pool in the oropharynx, and the patient becomes cyanotic. Contraction of the jaw muscles may cause biting of the tongue. A marked enhancement of sympathetic tone leads to increases in heart rate, blood pressure, and pupillary size. After 10 to 20 s, the tonic phase of the seizure typically evolves into the clonic phase, produced by the superimposition of periods of muscle relaxation on the tonic muscle contraction. The periods of relaxation progressively increase until the end of the ictal phase, which usually lasts no more than 1 min. The postictal phase is characterized by unresponsiveness, muscular flaccidity, and excessive salivation that can cause stridorous breathing and partial airway obstruction. Bladder or bowel incontinence may occur at this point as well. Patients gradually regain consciousness over minutes to hours, and during this transition there is typically a period of postictal confusion. Patients will subsequently complain of headache, fatigue, and muscle ache that can last for many hours. The duration of impaired consciousness in the postictal phase can be extremely long, i.e., many hours, in patients with prolonged seizures or underlying CNS diseases such as alcoholic cerebral atrophy.

The EEG during the tonic phase of the seizure shows a progressive increase in generalized low-voltage fast activity, followed by generalized high-amplitude, polyspike discharges. In the clonic phase, the high-amplitude activity is typically interrupted by slow waves to create a spike-and-wave pattern. The postictal EEG shows diffuse slowing that gradually recovers as the patient awakens.

There are many variants of the generalized tonic-clonic seizure, including pure tonic and pure clonic seizures. Brief tonic seizures lasting only a few seconds are especially noteworthy since they are usually associated with known epileptic syndromes having mixed seizure phenotypes, such as the Lennox-Gastaut syndrome (discussed below).

Atonic Seizures Atonic seizures are characterized by sudden loss of postural muscle tone lasting 1 to 2 s. Consciousness is briefly impaired, but there is usually no postictal confusion. A very brief seizure may cause only a quick head drop or nodding movement, while a longer seizure will cause the patient to collapse. This can be quite dramatic and extremely dangerous, since there is a substantial risk of direct head injury with the fall. The EEG shows brief, generalized spike-and-wave discharges followed immediately by diffuse slow waves that correlate with the loss of muscle tone. Similar to pure tonic seizures, atonic seizures are usually seen in association with known epileptic syndromes.

Myoclonic Seizures Myoclonus is a sudden and brief muscle contraction that may involve one part of the body or the entire body. A normal, common physiologic form of myoclonus is the sudden jerking movement observed while falling asleep. Pathologic myoclonus is most commonly seen in association with metabolic disorders, degenerative CNS diseases, or anoxic brain injury (see Chap. 21).

Although the distinction from other forms of myoclonus is imprecise, myoclonic seizures are considered to be true epileptic events since they are caused by cortical (versus subcortical or spinal) dysfunction. The EEG shows bilaterally synchronous spike-and-wave discharges. Myoclonic seizures usually coexist with other forms of generalized seizure disorders but are the predominant feature of juvenile myoclonic epilepsy (discussed below).

UNCLASSIFIED SEIZURES Not all seizure types can be classified as partial or generalized. This appears to be especially true of seizures that occur in neonates (i.e., less than 1 month of age) and infants (younger than 1 year). The distinctive phenotypes of seizures at these early ages likely result, in part, from differences in neuronal function and connectivity in the immature versus mature CNS.

Neonatal Seizures Neonatal seizures are characteristically very subtle (especially to the nonneonatologist) and may consist of brief episodes of apnea, eye deviation, eye blinking, or repetitive movements of the arms and legs. An EEG is critical for diagnosis in such cases. Generalized tonic-clonic seizures, multifocal clonic seizures, and myoclonus can also be observed in some patients, but these are the exception rather than the rule.

Infantile Spasms Infantile spasms are usually seen in infants under 12 months of age and are characterized by abrupt movements of the head, trunk, or limbs that often occur in clusters of 10 to 20 movements per episode. The classic spasm is a sudden flexion of the neck and abdomen with extension of the limbs ("jackknife" seizure), although other combinations of flexion and extension are described. Infantile spasms are often quite subtle and can appear strikingly similar to the signs of discomfort in a baby with colic. The EEG usually shows *hypsarrythmia*, which consists of high-voltage slowing, multifocal spikes, and a variety of other pleiomorphic abnormalities. Infantile spasms are often seen in association with other signs of CNS dysfunction, including developmental delay and mental retardation.

EPILEPSY SYNDROMES

In addition to recognizing the patterns of different types of seizures, it is also useful to be familiar with some of the more common epilepsy syndromes, since this often helps in the determination of therapy and prognosis. Epilepsy syndromes are disorders in which epilepsy is a predominant feature, and there is sufficient evidence (e.g., through clinical, EEG, radiologic, or genetic observations) to suggest a common underlying mechanism. Some examples are listed below.

IDIOPATHIC (PRIMARY) EPILEPSY SYNDROMES **Benign Neonatal Convulsions** Benign neonatal convulsions is an idiopathic, generalized seizure disorder observed in otherwise normal newborn infants typically between the second to sixth day of life. The seizures are usually tonic or manifest as short apneic spells and spontaneously remit within days to weeks; the infants have no further problems. A subgroup of patients have an inherited form of this syndrome known as *benign familial neonatal convulsions*. A mutation in chromosome 20 has been shown to be associated with the disease in at least one family.

Juvenile Myoclonic Epilepsy Juvenile myoclonic epilepsy (JME) is a generalized seizure disorder of unknown cause that appears in early adolescence and is usually characterized by bilateral myoclonic jerks that may be single or repetitive. The myoclonic seizures are most frequent in the morning after awakening and can be provoked by sleep deprivation. Consciousness is preserved unless the myoclonus is especially severe. Many patients also experience generalized tonic-clonic seizures, and up to one-third have absence seizures. The condition is otherwise benign, and although complete remission is uncommon, the seizures respond well to appropriate anticonvulsant medication. There is often a family history of epilepsy, and genetic linkage studies suggest a polygenic cause (see Chap. 363).

Benign Childhood Epilepsy with Centrotemporal Spikes This is an idiopathic, focal epilepsy that appears in otherwise normal children between ages 3 and 13 and may account for 25 percent of all epilepsies in childhood. Patients have brief, simple-partial seizures characterized by hemifacial sensory or motor symptoms that can spread to the limbs or become generalized. Most seizures, especially those that generalize, occur during sleep. The interictal EEG shows a distinctive pattern of high-voltage spikes or sharp waves in the centrotemporal region that may shift from one side to the other. The seizures are easily treated with anticonvulsant medications and almost always remit by age 15. The disorder has an autosomal dominant inheritance pattern with variable penetrance, and many clinically unaffected family members are found to have the EEG abnormality.

SYMPTOMATIC (SECONDARY) EPILEPSY SYNDROMES **Lennox-Gastaut Syndrome** Lennox-Gastaut syndrome occurs in children (ages 1 to 8) and is defined by the following triad: (1) multiple seizure types (usually including generalized tonic-clonic, atonic, and atypical absence seizures); (2) an EEG showing slow (<3 Hz) spike-and-wave discharges and a variety of other abnormalities; and (3) impaired cognitive function in most but not all cases. Lennox-Gastaut syndrome is associated with CNS disease or dysfunction from a variety of causes, including developmental abnormalities, perinatal hypoxia/ischemia, trauma, infection, and other acquired lesions. The multifactorial nature of this syndrome suggests that it is a nonspecific response of the brain to diffuse neural injury. Unfortunately, many patients have a poor prognosis due to the underlying CNS disease and the physical and psychosocial consequences of severe, poorly controlled epilepsy. A similar syndrome in infancy that often evolves into Lennox-Gastaut syndrome is *West syndrome*, characterized by infantile spasms, other findings of cerebral dysfunction, and a characteristic EEG pattern.

Mesial Temporal Lobe Epilepsy Syndrome Mesial temporal lobe epilepsy (MTLE) is the most common syndrome associated with complex-partial seizures and is an example of a symptomatic, partial epilepsy. Distinctive clinical, electroencephalographic, and pathologic features define this syndrome (Table 365-2). High-resolution magnetic resonance imaging (MRI) can detect the characteristic hippocampal sclerosis that appears to be an essential element in the pathophysiology of MTLE for many patients (Fig. 365-1). Recognition of this syndrome is especially important because it tends to be refractory to treatment with anticonvulsants but responds extremely well to surgical interven-

Table 365-2

Characteristics of the Mesial Temporal Lobe Epilepsy (MTLE) Syndrome

HISTORY

History of febrile seizures	Seizures may remit and reappear
Positive family history of epilepsy	Seizures often intractable
Early onset	
Rare secondarily generalized seizures	

CLINICAL OBSERVATIONS

Aura common	Postictal disorientation, memory
Behavioral arrest/stare	loss, dysphasia (with focus in
Complex automatisms	dominant hemisphere)
Unilateral posturing	

LABORATORY STUDIES

Unilateral or bilateral anterior temporal spikes on EEG
Hypometabolism on interictal PET
Hypoperfusion on interictal SPECT
Material-specific memory deficits on intracranial amobarbital (Wada's) test
MRI findings:
    Small hippocampus with increased signal on T2-weighted sequences
    Small temporal lobe
    Enlarged temporal horn
Pathologic findings:
    Highly selective loss of specific cell populations within hippocampus in
      most cases

ABBREVIATIONS: PET, positron emission tomography; SPECT, single photon emission computed tomography

FIGURE 365-1 Mesial temporal lobe epilepsy. The EEG suggested a right temporal lobe focus. Coronal high-resolution T2-weighted fast spin echo magnetic resonance image obtained through the body of the hippocampus demonstrates abnormal high signal intensity in the right hippocampus (white arrows; compare with the normal hippocampus on the left, black arrows) consistent with mesial temporal sclerosis.

tion. Major advances in the understanding of basic mechanisms of epilepsy have come through studies of experimental models of MTLE, discussed below.

THE CAUSES OF SEIZURES AND EPILEPSY

Seizures are a result of a shift in the normal balance of excitation and inhibition within the CNS. Given the numerous properties that control neuronal excitability, it is not surprising that there are many different ways to perturb this normal balance, and therefore many different causes of both seizures and epilepsy. Our understanding of the basic mechanisms involved remains very limited, and consequently there is not a rigorous, mechanistic-based framework for organizing all the etiologies. Conceptually, however, three important clinical observations emphasize how a variety of factors determine why certain conditions may cause seizures or epilepsy in a given patient.

1. *The normal brain is capable of having a seizure under the appropriate circumstances, and there are differences between individuals in the susceptibility or threshold for seizures.* For example, seizures may be induced by high fevers in children who are otherwise normal and who never develop other neurologic problems, including epilepsy. However, febrile seizures occur only in approximately 3 to 5 percent of children. This implies there are various underlying, *endogenous factors* that influence the threshold for having a seizure. Some of these factors are clearly genetic, as it has been shown that a family history of epilepsy will influence the likelihood of seizures occurring in otherwise normal individuals. Normal development also plays an important role, since the brain appears to have different seizure thresholds at different maturational stages.

2. *There are a variety of conditions that have an extremely high likelihood of resulting in a chronic seizure disorder.* One of the best examples of this is severe, penetrating head trauma, which is associated with up to a 50 percent risk of leading to epilepsy. The high propensity for severe traumatic brain injury to lead to epilepsy suggests that the injury results in a long-lasting, pathologic change in the CNS that transforms a presumably normal neural network into one that is abnormally hyperexcitable. This process is known as *epileptogenesis*, and the specific changes that result in a lowered seizure threshold can be considered *epileptogenic factors*. Other processes associated with epileptogenesis include stroke, infections, and abnormalities of CNS development. Likewise, the genetic abnormalities associated with epilepsy, such as the gene mutations linked to benign familial neonatal

convulsions or JME, likely involve processes that trigger the appearance of specific sets of epileptogenic factors.

3. *Seizures are episodic.* Patients with epilepsy have seizures intermittently and, depending on the underlying cause, many patients are completely normal for months or even years between seizures. This implies there are important provocative or *precipitating factors* that induce seizures in patients with epilepsy. Similarly, precipitating factors are responsible for causing the single seizure in someone without epilepsy. Precipitants include those due to intrinsic physiologic processes, such as psychological or physical stress, sleep deprivation, or hormonal changes associated with the menstrual cycle. They also include exogenous factors such as exposure to toxic substances and certain medications.

These observations emphasize the concept that the many causes of seizures and epilepsy result from a dynamic interplay between endogenous factors, epileptogenic factors, and precipitating factors. The potential role of each needs to be carefully considered when determining the appropriate management of a patient with seizures. For example, the identification of predisposing factors (e.g., family history of epilepsy) in a patient with febrile seizures may increase the necessity for closer follow-up and a more aggressive diagnostic evaluation. Finding an epileptogenic lesion may help in the estimation of seizure recurrence and duration of therapy. Finally, removal or modification of a precipitating factor may be an effective and safer method for preventing further seizures than the prophylactic use of anticonvulsant drugs.

CAUSES ACCORDING TO AGE In practice, it is useful to consider the etiologies of seizures based on the age of the patient, as age is one of the most important factors determining both the incidence and likely causes of seizures or epilepsy (Table 365-3). During the *neonatal period and early infancy*, potential causes include hypoxic-ischemic encephalopathy, trauma, CNS infection, congenital CNS abnormalities, and metabolic disorders. Babies born to mothers using neurotoxic drugs such as cocaine, heroin, or ethanol are susceptible to drug-withdrawal seizures in the first few days after delivery. Hypoglycemia and hypocalcemia, which can occur as secondary complications of perinatal injury, are also causes of seizures early after delivery. Seizures due to inborn errors of metabolism usually present once regular feeding begins, typically 2 to 3 days after birth. Pyridoxine (vitamin B_6) deficiency, an important cause of neonatal seizures, can be effectively treated with pyridoxine replacement. The idiopathic or inherited forms of benign neonatal convulsions are also seen during this time period.

The most common seizures arising in *late infancy and early childhood* are febrile seizures, which are seizures associated with fevers but without evidence of CNS infection or other defined causes. The overall prevalence is 3 to 5 percent and even higher in some parts of the world, such as Asia. Patients often have a family history of febrile seizures or epilepsy. Febrile seizures usually occur between 3 months and 5 years of age and have a peak incidence between 18 and 24 months. The typical scenario is a child who has a generalized, tonic-clonic seizure during a febrile illness in the setting of a common childhood infection such as otitis media, respiratory infection, or gastroenteritis. The seizure is likely to occur during the rising phase of the temperature curve (i.e., during the first day) rather than well into the course of the illness. A *simple* febrile seizure is a single, isolated event, brief, and symmetric in appearance. *Complex* febrile seizures have repeated seizure activity, last more than 15 minutes, or have focal features. Approximately one-third of patients with febrile seizures will have a recurrence, but fewer than 10 percent have three or more episodes. Recurrences are much more likely when the febrile seizure occurs in the first year of life. Simple febrile seizures are not associated with an increase in the risk of developing epilepsy, while complex febrile seizures have a risk of 2 to 5 percent; other risk factors include the presence of preexisting neurologic deficits and a family history of nonfebrile seizures.

Table 365-3

The Causes of Seizures

Neonates (<1 month)	Perinatal hypoxia and ischemia
	Intracranial hemorrhage and trauma
	Acute CNS infection (bacterial and viral meningitis)
	Metabolic disturbances (hypoglycemia, hypocalcemia, hypomagnesemia, pyridoxine deficiency)
	Drug withdrawal
	Developmental disorders (acquired and genetic)
	Genetic disorders
Infants and children (>1 mo and <12 years)	Febrile seizures
	Genetic disorders (metabolic, degenerative, primary epilepsy syndromes)
	CNS infection
	Developmental disorders (acquired and genetic)
	Trauma
	Idiopathic
Adolescents (12–18 years)	Trauma
	Genetic disorders
	Infection
	Brain tumor
	Illicit drug use
	Idiopathic
Young adults (18–35 years)	Trauma
	Alcohol withdrawal
	Illicit drug use
	Brain tumor
	Idiopathic
Older adults (>35 years)	Cerebrovascular disease
	Brain tumor
	Alcohol withdrawal
	Metabolic disorders (uremia, hepatic failure, electrolyte abnormalities, hypoglycemia)
	Alzheimer's disease and other degenerative CNS diseases
	Idiopathic

Childhood marks the age at which many of the well-defined epilepsy syndromes present, including typical childhood absence epilepsy and benign childhood epilepsy with centrotemporal spikes. Some children who are otherwise normal develop idiopathic, generalized tonic-clonic seizures without other features that fit into specific syndromes. Temporal lobe epilepsy usually presents in childhood and may be related to mesial temporal lobe sclerosis (as part of the MTLE syndrome) or other focal abnormalities such as cortical dysgenesis. Other types of partial seizures, including those with secondary generalization, may be the relatively late manifestation of a developmental disorder, an acquired lesion such as head trauma, CNS infection (especially viral encephalitis), or very rarely a CNS tumor. This is also the period that Lennox-Gastaut syndrome is identified, almost always in the child who has other neurologic problems such as static encephalopathy.

The period of adolescence and early adulthood is one of transition during which the idiopathic or genetically based epilepsy syndromes, including JME and juvenile absence epilepsy, become less common, while epilepsies secondary to acquired CNS lesions begin to predominate. Seizures in patients in this age range can be associated with head trauma, CNS infections (including parasitic infections such as cysticercosis), brain tumors, congenital CNS abnormalities, illicit drug use, or alcohol withdrawal.

Head trauma is a common cause of epilepsy in adolescents and adults. The head injury can be caused by a variety of mechanisms, and the likelihood of developing epilepsy is strongly correlated with the severity of the injury. A patient with a penetrating head wound, depressed skull fracture, intracranial hemorrhage, or prolonged post-traumatic coma or amnesia has a 40 to 50 percent risk of developing

Table 365-4

Drugs and Other Substances that Can Cause Seizures

Antimicrobials	Radiographic contrast agents
β-lactam and related compounds	Theophylline
Quinolones	Sedative-hypnotic drug withdrawal
Isoniazid	Alcohol
Ganciclovir	Barbiturates
Anesthetic and antiarrhythmics	Benzodiazepines
Beta-adrenergic antagonists	Drugs of abuse
Local anesthetics	Amphetamine
Class 1B agents	Cocaine
Immunosuppressants	Phencyclidine
Cyclosporine	Methylphenidate
OKT3 (monoclonal antibodies to T cells)	
Psychotropics	
Antidepressants	
Antipsychotics	
Lithium	

epilepsy, while a patient with a closed head injury and cerebral contusion has a 5 to 25 percent risk. Recurrent seizures usually develop within 1 year after head trauma, although intervals of 10 years or longer are well known. In controlled studies, mild head injury, defined as a concussion with amnesia or loss of consciousness of less than ½ h, was not found to be associated with an increased likelihood of epilepsy. Nonetheless, most epileptologists know of patients who have partial seizures within hours or days of a mild head injury and subsequently develop chronic seizures of the same type; such cases may represent rare examples of chronic epilepsy resulting from mild head injury.

The causes of seizures in *older adults* include cerebrovascular disease, trauma (including subdural hematoma), CNS tumors, and degenerative diseases. Cerebrovascular disease may account for approximately 50 percent of new cases of epilepsy in patients older than 65. Acute seizures (i.e., occurring at the time of the stroke) are seen more often with embolic rather than hemorrhagic or thrombotic stroke. Chronic seizures typically appear months to years after the initial event and are associated with all forms of stroke.

Metabolic disturbances such as electrolyte imbalance, hypo- or hyperglycemia, renal failure, and hepatic failure may cause seizures at any age. Similarly, endocrine disorders, hematologic disorders, vasculitides, and many other systemic diseases may cause seizures over a broad age range. A wide variety of medications and abused substances are known to precipitate seizures as well (Table 365-4).

BASIC MECHANISMS

MECHANISMS OF SEIZURE INITIATION AND PROPAGATION Partial seizure activity can begin in a very discrete region of cortex and then spread to neighboring regions, i.e., there is a *seizure initiation* phase and a *seizure propagation* phase. Studies of experimental models of these phases suggest that the initiation phase is characterized by two concurrent events in an aggregate of neurons: (1) high-frequency bursts of action potentials, and (2) hypersynchronization. The bursting activity is caused by a relatively long-lasting depolarization of the neuronal membrane due to influx of extracellular calcium (Ca^{2+}), which leads to the opening of voltage-dependent sodium (Na^+) channels; influx of Na^+; and generation of repetitive action potentials. This is followed by a hyperpolarizing afterpotential mediated by γ-aminobutyric acid (GABA) receptors or potassium (K^+) channels, depending on the cell type. The synchronized bursts from a sufficient number of neurons result in a so-called spike discharge on the EEG.

Normally, the spread of the bursting activity is prevented by intact hyperpolarization and a region of surrounding inhibition created by inhibitory neurons. With sufficient activation there is a recruitment of surrounding neurons via a number of mechanisms. Repetitive discharges lead to the following: (1) an increase in extracellular K^+, which blunts the extent of hyperpolarization and depolarizes neighboring neurons; (2) accumulation of Ca^{2+} in presynaptic terminals, leading to enhanced neurotransmitter release; and (3) depolarization-induced activation of the *N*-methyl-D-aspartate (NMDA) subtype of the excitatory amino acid receptor, which causes more Ca^{2+} influx and neuronal activation. The recruitment of a sufficient number of neurons leads to a loss of the surrounding inhibition and propagation of seizure activity into contiguous areas via local cortical connections, and to more distant areas via long commissural pathways such as the corpus callosum.

Many factors control neuronal excitability, and thus there are many potential mechanisms for altering a neuron's propensity to have bursting activity. Examples of mechanisms *intrinsic* to the neuron include changes in the conductance of ion channels, response characteristics of membrane receptors, cytoplasmic buffering, second-messenger systems, and protein expression as determined by gene transcription, translation, and posttranslational modification. Mechanisms *extrinsic* to the neuron include changes in the amount or type of neurotransmitters present at the synapse, modulation of receptors by extracellular ions and other molecules, and temporal and spatial properties of both synaptic and nonsynaptic input. Nonneural cells, such as astrocytes and oligodendrocytes, have an important role in many of these mechanisms as well.

Certain known causes of seizures are explained by these mechanisms. For example, accidental ingestion of domoic acid, which is an analogue of glutamate (the principal excitatory neurotransmitter in the brain), causes profound seizures via direct activation of excitatory amino acid receptors throughout the CNS. Penicillin, which can lower the seizure threshold in humans and is a potent convulsant in experimental models, reduces inhibition by antagonizing the effects of GABA and its receptor. The basic mechanisms of other precipitating factors of seizures, such as sleep deprivation, fever, alcohol withdrawal, hypoxia, and infection, are not as well understood but presumably involve analogous perturbations in neuronal excitability. Similarly, the endogenous factors that determine an individual's seizure threshold may relate to these properties as well.

Knowledge of the mechanisms responsible for the initiation and propagation of most generalized seizures (including tonic-clonic, myoclonic, and atonic types) remains rudimentary and reflects the limited understanding of the connectivity of the brain at a systems level. Much more is understood about the origin of generalized spike-and-wave discharges in absence seizures. These appear to be related to oscillatory rhythms that are normally generated during sleep by circuits connecting the thalamus and cortex. This oscillatory behavior involves an interaction between $GABA_B$ receptors, T-type Ca^{2+} channels, and K^+ channels located within the thalamus. Pharmacologic studies indicate that modulation of these receptors and channels can induce absence seizures, and there is speculation that the genetic forms of absence epilepsy may be associated with mutations of components of this system.

MECHANISMS OF EPILEPTOGENESIS Epileptogenesis refers to the transformation of a normal neuronal network into one that is chronically hyperexcitable. For example, there is often a delay of months to years between an initial CNS injury such as trauma, stroke, or infection and the first seizure. The injury appears to initiate a process that gradually lowers the seizure threshold in the affected region until a spontaneous seizure occurs. In many genetic and idiopathic forms of epilepsy, epileptogenesis is presumably determined by developmentally regulated events.

Pathologic studies of the hippocampus from patients with temporal lobe epilepsy have led to the suggestion that some forms of epileptogenesis are related to *structural changes in neuronal networks*. For example, many patients with MTLE syndrome have a highly selective loss of neurons that has been proposed to contribute to inhibition of the main excitatory neurons within the dentate gyrus. There is also evidence that, in response to the loss of neurons, there is reorganization or "sprouting" of surviving neurons in a way that affects the excitability of the network. Some of these changes can be seen in experimental models of prolonged electrical seizures or traumatic brain injury. Thus, an initial injury such as head injury may lead to a very focal, confined region of structural change that causes local hyperexcitability. The local hyperexcitability leads to further structural changes that evolve over time until the focal lesion produces clinically evident seizures. Similar models have also provided strong evidence for long-term alterations in *intrinsic, biochemical properties of cells* within the network, such as chronic changes in glutamate receptor function. Recent studies of a rare childhood epilepsy syndrome (Rasmussen's syndrome) have also raised the possibility that some forms of epileptogenesis may be caused by an immune response in which autoantibodies against glutamate receptors lead to receptor activation, depolarization, seizures, and excitotoxic cell injury.

GENETIC CAUSES OF EPILEPSY The genetic causes of a few epilepsy syndromes have recently been discovered. Myoclonic epilepsy with ragged red fibers (MERRF) syndrome is associated with a mutation of mitochondrial tRNA-lysine. Mutations in the cystatin B gene may cause another form of progressive myoclonus epilepsy (Unverricht-Lundborg type), and a mutation within the gene encoding the β_4 subunit of the acetylcholine receptor appears responsible for a frontal lobe epilepsy syndrome consisting of nocturnal partial seizures (see Chap. 363). A number of other epilepsy syndromes have been mapped to chromosomal locations. Epilepsy has been produced in transgenic mice having a wide range of genetically engineered mutations, suggesting that many potential genetic abnormalities can result in a change in the seizure threshold.

MECHANISMS OF ACTION OF ANTIEPILEPTIC DRUGS Currently available antiepileptic drugs appear to act primarily by blocking the initiation or spread of seizures. Phenytoin, carbamazepine, valproic acid, and lamotrigine inhibit Na^+-dependent action potentials in a frequency-dependent manner, resulting in a preferential blockade of the sustained high-frequency activity that is characteristic of burst-firing neurons in a seizure focus. Phenytoin also appears to suppress seizure spread through inhibition of specific voltage-gated Ca^{2+} channels. Benzodiazepines and barbiturates augment inhibition by distinct interactions with GABA receptors. Valproic acid elevates the concentration of GABA in the brain, perhaps through interaction with enzymes involved in the synthesis (glutamic acid decarboxylase) and catabolism (GABA transaminase) of GABA. Gabapentin, which is a structural analogue of GABA, appears to increase GABA levels by enhancing GABA synthesis and release and may also cause a decrease in glutamate synthesis. The two most effective drugs for absence seizures, ethosuximide and valproic acid, probably act by inhibiting T-type Ca^{2+} channels in thalamic neurons.

In contrast to the relatively large number of antiepileptic drugs that can attenuate seizure activity, there are currently no drugs known to prevent the formation of a seizure focus following CNS injury in humans. The eventual development of such "antiepileptogenic" drugs will provide an important means of preventing the emergence of epilepsy following injuries such as head trauma, stroke, and CNS infection.

EVALUATION OF THE PATIENT WITH A SEIZURE

When a patient presents shortly after a seizure, the first priorities are attention to vital signs, respiratory and cardiovascular support, and treatment of seizures if they resume (see "Treatment"). Life-threatening conditions such as CNS infection, metabolic derangement or drug toxicity must be recognized and managed appropriately.

When the patient is not acutely ill, the evaluation will initially focus on whether or not there is a history of earlier seizures (Fig. 365-2). If this is the patient's first seizure, then the emphasis will be to (1) establish whether the reported episode was a seizure rather than another paroxysmal event, (2) determine the cause of the seizure by identifying risk factors and precipitating events, and (3) decide whether anticonvulsant therapy is required in addition to treatment for any underlying illness.

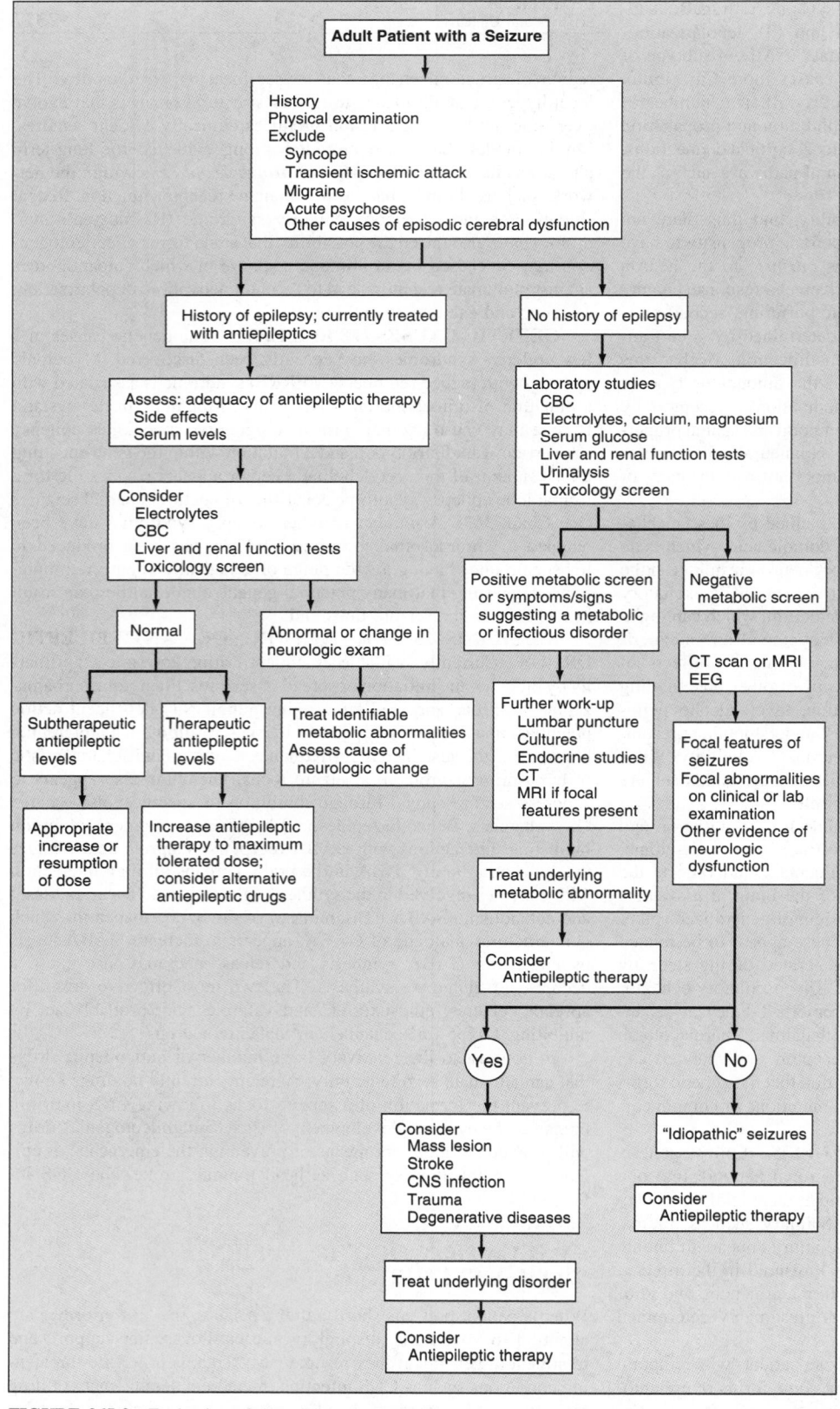

FIGURE 365-2 Evaluation of the adult patient with a seizure. CBC, complete blood count; CT, computed tomography; MRI, magnetic resonance imaging; EEG, electroencephalogram; CNS, central nervous system.

In the patient with prior seizures or a known history of epilepsy, the evaluation is directed toward (1) identification of the underlying cause and precipitating factors, and (2) determination of the adequacy of the patient's current therapy.

HISTORY AND EXAMINATION The history should first determine whether the event was truly a seizure. It is essential to take the time to gather an in-depth history, for *in many cases the diagnosis of a seizure is based solely on clinical grounds—the examination and laboratory studies are often normal.* Keeping in mind the characteristics of different seizure types, questions need to focus precisely on the symptoms before, during, and after the episode in order to discriminate a seizure from other paroxysmal events (see "Differential Diagnosis of Seizures"). Seizures frequently occur out-of-hospital, and the patient may be unaware of the ictal and immediate postictal phases; thus witnesses to the event should be interviewed carefully.

The history should also focus on risk factors and predisposing events. Clues for a predisposition to seizures include a history of febrile seizures, earlier auras or brief seizures not recognized as such, and a family history of seizures. Epileptogenic factors such as prior head trauma, stroke, tumor, or vascular malformation should be identified. In children, a careful assessment of developmental milestones may provide evidence for underlying CNS disease., Precipitating factors such as sleep deprivation, systemic diseases, electrolyte or metabolic derangements, acute infection, drugs that lower the seizurem threshold (see Table 365-4), or alcohol or illicit drug use should also be identified.

The general physical examination includes a search for signs of infection or systemic illness. Careful examination of the skin may reveal signs of tuberous sclerosis (adenoma sebaceum, "ash-leaf" spots), neurofibromatosis (café au lait spots, peripheral neurofibromas), Sturge-Weber syndrome (facial angioma), or chronic liver or renal disease. A finding of organomegaly may indicate a metabolic storage disease, and limb asymmetry may provide a clue for brain injury early in development. Signs of head trauma and use of alcohol or illicit drugs should be sought. Auscultation of the heart and carotid arteries may identify an abnormality that predisposes to cerebrovascular disease.

All patients require a complete neurologic examination, with particular emphasis on eliciting signs of cerebral hemispheric disease (see Chap. 360). Careful assessment of mental status (including memory, language function, and abstract thinking) may suggest lesions in the anterior frontal, parietal, or temporal lobes. Testing of visual fields will help screen for lesions in the optic pathways and occipital lobes. Screening tests of motor function such as pronator drift, deep tendon reflexes, gait, and coordination may suggest lesions in motor (frontal) cortex, and cortical sensory testing (e.g., double simultaneous stimulation) may detect lesions in the parietal cortex.

LABORATORY STUDIES Routine blood studies are indicated to identify the more common metabolic causes of seizures, such as abnormalities in electrolytes, glucose, calcium, or magnesium, and hepatic or renal disease. A screen for toxins in blood and urine should also be obtained from all patients in the appropriate risk groups, especially when no clear precipitating factor has been identified. A lumbar puncture is indicated if there is any suspicion of meningitis or encephalitis and is mandatory in all patients infected with the human immunodeficiency virus, even in the absence of symptoms or signs suggesting infection.

All patients who have a possible seizure disorder should be evaluated with an EEG (see Chap. 361) as soon as possible. The EEG may help to establish the diagnosis of epilepsy, classify the seizure type, and provide evidence for the existence of a particular epilepsy syndrome. If the patient is having frequent seizures, such as a child with absence epilepsy, the EEG may confirm the presence of seizures and help to identify the seizure type. In patients with infrequent seizures, the EEG may reveal potentially abnormal interictal activity that, when combined with clinical or radiologic data, aids in establishing the diagnosis. However, the existence of epileptiform patterns such as spikes or sharp waves are not diagnostic in themselves, since similar patterns can be seen in 1 to 2 percent of normal individuals. Ideally, the EEG should be performed after sleep deprivation to increase the potential diagnostic yield of the study.

Almost all patients with new-onset seizures should have a brain imaging study to determine whether there is an underlying structural abnormality that is responsible. The main exception to this rule is children who have an unambiguous history and examination suggestive of a benign, generalized seizure disorder such as absence epilepsy. MRI has been shown to be superior to computed tomography (CT) in scanning for the detection of cerebral lesions associated with epilepsy. In some cases MRI will identify lesions such as tumors, vascular malformations, or other pathologies that need immediate therapy. The use of newer MRI methods has increased the sensitivity for detection of abnormalities of cortical architecture, including hippocampal atrophy associated with mesial temporal sclerosis, and abnormalities of cortical neuronal migration. In such cases the findings may not lead to immediate therapy, but they do provide an explanation for the patient's seizures and point to the need for chronic anticonvulsant therapy or possible resective surgery.

In the patient with suspected CNS infection or mass lesions, CT scanning should be performed emergently when MRI is not immediately available. Otherwise, it is usually appropriate to obtain an MRI study within a few days of the initial evaluation. Functional imaging procedures such as positron emission tomography (PET) and single photon emission computed tomography (SPECT) are also used to evaluate certain patients with medically refractory seizures (discussed below).

DIFFERENTIAL DIAGNOSIS OF SEIZURES

The various disorders that may mimic seizures are listed in Table 365-5. In most cases seizures can be distinguished from these other conditions by meticulous attention to the history and relevant laboratory studies. On occasion, additional studies, such as video-EEG monitoring, sleep studies, tilt table analysis, or cardiac electrophysiology may be required to reach a correct diagnosis. Two of the more common syndromes in the differential diagnosis are detailed below.

Syncope The diagnostic dilemma encountered most frequently is the distinction between a generalized seizure and syncope. Observations by the patient and bystanders that can help discriminate between the two are listed in Table 365-6. Characteristics of a seizure include the presence of an aura, cyanosis, unconsciousness, motor manifesta-

Table 365-5

The Differential Diagnosis of Seizures

1. Syncope	5. Transient ischemic attack (TIA)
Vasovagal syncope	Basilar artery TIA
Cardiac arrhythmia	6. Sleep disorders
Valvular heart disease	Narcolepsy/cataplexy
Cardiac failure	Benign sleep myoclonus
Orthostatic hypotension	7. Movement disorders
2. Psychological disorders	Tics
Psychogenic seizure	Nonepileptic myoclonus
Hyperventilation	Paroxysmal choreoathetosis
Panic attack	8. Special considerations in
3. Metabolic disturbances	children
Alcoholic blackouts	Breath-holding spells
Delirium tremens	Migraine with recurrent
Hypoglycemia	abdominal pain and cyclic
Hypoxia	vomiting
Psychoactive drugs	Benign paroxysmal vertigo
(e.g., hallucinogens)	Apnea
4. Migraine	Night terrors
Confusional migraine	Sleepwalking
Basilar migraine	

tions lasting more than 30 s, postictal disorientation, muscle soreness, and sleepiness. In contrast, a syncopal episode is more likely if the event was provoked by acute pain or anxiety or occurred immediately after arising from the lying or sitting position. Patients with syncope often describe a stereotyped transition from consciousness to unconsciousness that includes tiredness, sweating, nausea, and tunneling of vision, and they experience a relatively brief loss of consciousness. Headache or incontinence may be observed following either a seizure or syncope and are thus not useful distinguishing features. A brief period (i.e., 1 to 10 s) of convulsive motor activity is frequently seen immediately at the onset of a syncopal episode, especially if the patient remains in an upright posture after fainting (e.g., in a dentist's chair) and therefore has a sustained decrease in cerebral perfusion. Rarely, a syncopal episode can induce a full tonic-clonic seizure. In such cases the evaluation must focus on both the cause of the syncopal event as well as the possibility that the patient has a propensity for recurrent seizures.

Psychogenic Seizures Psychogenic seizures are nonepileptic behaviors that resemble seizures. The behavior is often part of a conversion reaction precipitated by underlying psychological distress. Certain behaviors, such as side-to-side turning of the head, asymmetric and large amplitude shaking movements of the limbs, twitching of all four extremities without loss of consciousness, pelvic thrusting, and screaming or talking during the event, are more commonly associated

Table 365-6

Clinical Features of a Generalized Tonic-Clonic Seizure Versus Syncope

Features	Seizure	Syncope
Immediate precipitating factors	Usually none	Emotional stress, Valsalva, other specific causes
Premonitory symptoms	None or aura (e.g., odd odor)	Tiredness, nausea, diaphoresis, tunneling of vision
Posture at onset	Variable	Usually erect
Transition to unconsciousness	Often immediate	Gradual over seconds*
Duration of unconsciousness	Minutes	Seconds
Duration of tonic or clonic movements	30–60 s	Never more than 15 s
Facial appearance during event	Cyanosis, frothing at mouth	Pallor
Disorientation and sleepiness after event	Many minutes to hours	<5 min
Aching of muscles after event	Often	Sometimes
Biting of tongue	Sometimes	Rarely
Incontinence	Sometimes	Sometimes

* May be sudden with certain cardiac arrhythmias.

with psychogenic rather than epileptic seizures. However, the distinction is sometimes difficult on clinical grounds alone, and there are many examples of diagnostic errors made by experienced epileptologists. This is especially true for psychogenic seizures that resemble complex-partial seizures, since the behavioral manifestations of complex-partial seizures (especially of frontal lobe origin) can be extremely unusual, and in both cases the routine surface EEG may be normal. Video-EEG monitoring is often useful when the clinical observations are nondiagnostic. Generalized tonic-clonic seizures always produce marked EEG abnormalities during and after the seizure. For suspected complex-partial seizures of temporal lobe origin, the use of additional electrodes beyond the standard scalp locations (e.g., sphenoidal electrodes) may be required to detect a seizure focus. Measurement of serum prolactin levels may also help to discriminate between organic and psychogenic seizures, since most generalized seizures and many complex-partial seizures are accompanied by rises in serum prolactin (during the immediate 30-min postictal period), whereas psychogenic seizures are not. It is important to note that the diagnosis of psychogenic seizures does not exclude a concurrent diagnosis of epilepsy, since the two often coexist.

℞ TREATMENT

Therapy for a patient with a seizure disorder is almost always multimodal and includes treatment of underlying conditions that cause or contribute to the seizures, avoidance of precipitating factors, suppression of recurrent seizures by prophylactic therapy with antiepileptic medications or surgery, and addressing a variety of psychological and social issues. Treatment plans must be individualized, given the many different types and causes of seizures as well as the differences in efficacy and toxicity of antiepileptic medications for each patient. In almost all cases a neurologist with experience in the treatment of epilepsy should design and oversee implementation of the treatment strategy. Furthermore, patients with refractory epilepsy or those who require polypharmacy with antiepileptic drugs should remain under the regular care of a neurologist.

Treatment of Underlying Conditions If the sole cause of a seizure is a metabolic disturbance such as an abnormality of serum electrolytes or glucose, then treatment is aimed at reversing the metabolic problem and preventing its recurrence. Therapy with antiepileptic drugs is usually unnecessary unless the metabolic disorder cannot be corrected promptly and the patient is at risk of having further seizures. If the apparent cause of a seizure was a medication (e.g., theophylline) or illicit drug use (e.g., cocaine), then appropriate therapy is avoidance of the drug and there is usually no need for antiepileptic medications unless subsequent seizures occur.

Seizures caused by a structural CNS lesion such as a brain tumor, vascular malformation, or brain abscess may not recur after appropriate treatment of the underlying lesion. However, despite removal of the structural lesion, there is a risk that the seizure focus will remain in the surrounding tissue or develop *de novo* as a result of gliosis and other processes induced by surgery, radiation, or other therapies. Most patients are therefore maintained on an antiepileptic medication for at least 1 year, and an attempt is made to withdraw medications only if the patient has been completely seizure-free. If the seizures are refractory to medication, the patient may benefit from surgical removal of the epileptic brain region (see "Surgical Treatment of Refractory Epilepsy").

Avoidance of Precipitating Factors Unfortunately, little is known about the specific factors that determine precisely when a seizure will occur in a patient with epilepsy. Some patients can identify particular situations that appear to lower their seizure threshold; these situations should be avoided. For example, a patient who has seizures in the setting of sleep deprivation should be advised to maintain a normal sleep schedule. Many patients note an association between alcohol intake and seizures, and they should be encouraged to modify their drinking habits accordingly. There are also relatively rare cases of patients with seizures that are induced by highly specific stimuli such as a video game monitor, music, or an individual's voice ("reflex epilepsy"). If there is an association between stress and seizures, stress reduction techniques such as physical exercise, meditation, or counseling may be helpful.

Antiepileptic Drug Therapy Antiepileptic drug therapy is the mainstay of treatment for most patients with epilepsy. The overall goal is to completely prevent seizures without causing any untoward side effects, preferably with a single medication and a dosing schedule that is easy for the patient to follow. Seizure classification is an important element in designing the treatment plan, since some antiepileptic drugs have different activities against various seizure types. However, there is considerable overlap between many antiepileptic drugs, such that the choice of therapy is often determined more by specific needs of the patient, especially the patient's subjective assessment of side effects.

WHEN TO INITIATE ANTIEPILEPTIC DRUG THERAPY Antiepileptic drug therapy should be started in any patient with recurrent seizures of unknown etiology or a known cause that cannot be reversed. Whether to initiate therapy in a patient with a single seizure is controversial. Patients with a single seizure due to an identified lesion such as a CNS tumor, infection, or trauma, in which there is strong evidence that the lesion is epileptogenic, should be treated. The risk of seizure recurrence in a patient with an apparently unprovoked or idiopathic seizure is uncertain, with estimates ranging from 31 to 71 percent in the first 12 months after the initial seizure. This uncertainty arises from differences in the underlying seizure types and etiologies in various published epidemiologic studies. Generally accepted risk factors associated with recurrent seizures include the following: (1) an abnormal neurologic examination, (2) seizures presenting as status epilepticus, (3) postictal Todd's paralysis, (4) a strong family history of seizures, or (5) an abnormal EEG. Most patients with one or more of these risk factors should be treated. Issues such as employment or driving may influence the decision whether or not to start medications as well. For example, a patient with a single, idiopathic seizure and whose job depends on driving may prefer taking antiepileptic drugs rather than risking a seizure recurrence and the potential loss of driving privileges.

SELECTION OF ANTIEPILEPTIC DRUGS The choices of antiepileptic drugs in the United States for different seizure types are shown in Table 365-7, and the main pharmacologic characteristics of commonly used drugs are listed in Table 365-8. Older medications such as phenytoin, valproic acid, carbamazepine, and ethosuximide are

Table 365-7

Antiepileptic Drugs of Choice

Focal-Onset Seizures*	Generalized Seizures			
	Generalized Tonic-Clonic	Absence	Myoclonic	Atonic
FIRST-LINE				
Carbamazepine	Valproic acid	Ethosuximide	Valproic acid	Valproic acid
Phenytoin	Carbamazepine	Valproic acid		
Valproic acid	Phenytoin			
ALTERNATIVES				
Lamotrigine	Phenobarbital	Acetazolamide	Clonazepam	Clonazepam
Gabapentin	Primidone	Clonazepam	Acetazolamide	
Phenobarbital		Phenobarbital		
Primidone				

* Simple-partial, complex-partial, and secondarily generalized tonic-clonic seizures.

Table 365-8

Commonly Used Antiepileptic Drugs

Generic Name	Trade Name	Principal Uses	Typical Dosage and Dosing Intervals	Half-Life	Therapeutic Range	Adverse Effects Neurologic	Adverse Effects Systemic	Drug Interactions
Phenytoin (diphenyl-hydantoin)	Dilantin	Tonic-clonic (grand mal) Focal-onset	300–400 mg/d (3–6 mg/kg, adult; 4–8 mg/kg, child) qd-bid	24 h (wide variation, dose-dependent)	10–20 µg/mL	Ataxia Incoordination Confusion Cerebellar	Gum hyperplasia Lymphadenopathy Hirsutism Osteomalacia Facial coarsening Skin rash	Level increased by isoniazid, sulfonamides Level decreased by carbamazepine, phenobarbital Altered folate metabolism
Carbamazepine	Tegretol	Tonic-clonic Focal-onset	600–1800 mg/d (15–35 mg/kg, child) bid-qid	13–17 h	4–12 µg/mL	Ataxia Dizziness Diplopia Vertigo	Aplastic anemia Leukopenia Gastrointestinal irritation Hepatotoxicity	Level decreased by phenobarbital, phenytoin Level increased by erythromycin, propoxyphene, isoniazid, cimetidine
Valproic acid	Depakane Depakote	Tonic-clonic Absence Atypical absence Myoclonic Focal-onset	750–2000 mg/d (20–60 mg/kg) bid-qid	15 h	50–150 µg/mL	Ataxia Sedation Tremor	Hepatotoxicity Thrombocytopenia Gastrointestinal irritation Weight gain Transient alopecia Hyperammonemia	Level decreased by carbamazepine, phenobarbital, phenytoin
Phenobarbital	Luminol	Tonic-clonic Focal-onset	60–180 mg/d (1–4 mg/kg, adult); (3–6 mg/kg, child) qd	90 h (70 h in children)	10–40 µg/mL	Sedation Ataxia Confusion Dizziness Decreased libido Depression	Skin rash	Level increased by valproic acid, phenytoin Enhances metabolism of other drugs via liver enzyme induction
Primidone	Mysoline	Tonic-clonic Focal-onset	750–1000 mg/d (10–25 mg/kg) bid-tid	Primidone, 8–15 h Phenobarbital, 90 h	Primidone, 4–12 µg/mL Phenobarbital, 10–40 µg/mL	Same as phenobarbital		
Ethosuximide	Zarontin	Absence (petit mal)	750–1250 mg/d (20-40 mg/kg) qd-bid	60 h, adult 30 h, child	40–100 µg/mL	Ataxia Lethargy Headache	Gastrointestinal irritation Skin rash Bone marrow suppression	
Gabapentin	Neurontin	Focal-onset	900–2400 mg/d tid-qid	5–9 h	Not established	Sedation Dizziness Ataxia Fatigue	Gastrointestinal irritation	No known significant interactions
Lamotrigine	Lamictal	Focal-onset Lennox-Gastaut syndrome	150–500 mg/d bid	25 h 14 h (with enzyme-inducers) 59 h (with valproic acid)	Not established	Dizziness Diplopia Sedation Ataxia Headache	Skin rash Stevens-Johnson syndrome	Level decreased by carbamazepine, phenobarbital, phenytoin Level increased by valproic acid
Clonazepam	Klonopin	Absence Atypical absence Myoclonic	1–12 mg/d (0.1–0.2 mg/kg) qd-tid	24–48 h	10–70 ng/mL	Ataxia Sedation Lethargy	Anorexia	Level decreased by carbamazepine, phenobarbital
Felbamate	Felbatol	Focal-onset Lennox-Gastaut syndrome	2400–3600 mg/d, (45 mg/kg, child) tid-qid	16–22 h	Not established	Insomnia Dizziness Sedation Headache	Aplastic anemia Hepatic failure Weight loss Gastrointestinal irritation	Increases phenytoin, valproic acid, active carbamazepine metabolite

generally used as first-line therapy for most seizure disorders since, overall, they are as effective as recently marketed drugs and significantly less expensive. Experience with newer drugs such as gabapentin and lamotrigine is comparatively limited in the United States, and their use is predominantly as add-on or alternative therapy. Felbamate, introduced in 1993, was found to be associated with a relatively high incidence of irreversible aplastic anemia and hepatic

failure and is currently recommended only for medically refractory patients.

In addition to efficacy, other factors influencing the specific choice of an initial medication for a patient include the relative convenience of dosing schedule (e.g., once daily versus three or four times daily) and potential side effects. Almost all of the commonly used antiepileptic drugs can cause similar, dose-related side effects such as sedation, ataxia, and diplopia. Close follow-up is required to insure these are promptly recognized and reversed. Most of the drugs may also cause idiosyncratic toxicity such as rash, bone marrow suppression, or hepatotoxicity. Although rare, these side effects need to be carefully considered during drug selection, and patients require laboratory tests (e.g., complete blood count and liver function tests) prior to the institution of a drug (to establish baseline values) and during initial dosing and titration of the agent.

1. *Antiepileptic drug selection for partial seizures.* Carbamazepine or phenytoin is currently the initial drug of choice for the treatment of partial seizures, including those that secondarily generalize. Overall they have very similar efficacy, but differences in pharmacokinetics and toxicity are the main determinants for use in a given patient. Phenytoin has a relatively long half-life and offers the advantage of once or twice daily dosing compared to two or three times daily dosing for carbamazepine. An advantage of carbamazepine is that its metabolism follows first-order pharmacokinetics, and the relationship between drug dose, serum levels, and toxicity is linear. By contrast, phenytoin shows properties of saturation kinetics, such that small increases in phenytoin doses above a standard maintenance dose can precipitate marked side effects. This is one of the main causes of acute phenytoin toxicity. Long-term use of phenytoin is associated with untoward cosmetic effects (e.g., hirsutism, coarsening of facial features, and gingival hypertrophy), so it is often avoided in young patients who are likely to require the drug for many years. Carbamazepine can cause leukopenia, aplastic anemia, or hepatotoxicity and would therefore be contraindicated in patients with predispositions to these problems.

Valproic acid is an effective alternative for some patients with partial seizures, especially when the seizures secondarily generalize. Gastrointestinal side effects are fewer when using the valproate semisodium formulation (Depakote). Valproic acid also rarely causes reversible bone marrow suppression and hepatotoxicity, and laboratory testing is required to monitor toxicity. This drug should generally be avoided in patients with preexisting bone marrow or liver disease. Irreversible, fatal hepatic failure appearing as an idiosyncratic rather than dose-related side-effect is a relatively rare complication; its risk is highest in children younger than 2 years old, especially those taking other antiepileptic drugs or with inborn errors of metabolism. Valproic acid therapy should therefore only be used in infants and young children when the benefits clearly exceed this risk.

Lamotrigine, gabapentin, and phenobarbital are additional drugs currently used for the treatment of partial seizures with or without secondary generalization. Lamotrigine appears to have an overall efficacy profile similar to the more standard drugs but may cause severe rash or Stevens-Johnson syndrome, particularly in children. Lamotrigine must be started very slowly when used as add-on therapy with valproic acid, since its inhibition of lamotrigine metabolism causes a substantial prolongation of its half-life. Gabapentin is unique among the standard antiepileptic drugs in not having any significant drug interactions. This makes it potentially useful as add-on therapy, especially in patients who are particularly susceptible to side effects of other medications. Gabapentin is also useful in patients with severe liver disease since its clearance is exclusively renal. Until recently, phenobarbital and other barbiturate compounds were commonly used as first-line therapy for many forms of epilepsy. However, the barbiturates frequently cause sedation in adults, hyperactivity in children, and other more subtle cognitive changes; thus, their use should be limited to situations in which no other suitable treatment alternatives exist.

2. *Antiepileptic drug selection for generalized seizures.* Valproic acid is currently considered the best initial choice for the treatment of primarily generalized, tonic-clonic seizures, and carbamazepine and phenytoin are suitable alternatives. Valproic acid is also particularly effective in absence, myoclonic, and atonic seizures and is therefore the drug of choice in patients with epilepsy syn-

dromes having mixed seizure types. Ethosuximide remains the preferred drug for the treatment of uncomplicated absence seizures, but it is not effective against tonic-clonic or partial seizures. Ethosuximide rarely causes bone marrow suppression, so that periodic monitoring of blood cell counts is required. Clonazepam is an alternative for the treatment of myoclonic, atonic, and absence seizures, but it is not indicated for the treatment of most other seizure types. This is especially important since the drug is sometimes abused due to its sedative-hypnotic qualities rather than its antiepileptic effect. Although approved for use in partial seizure disorders, lamotrigine is proving to be effective in epilepsy syndromes with mixed, generalized seizure types such as JME and Lennox-Gastaut syndrome.

INITIATION AND MONITORING OF THERAPY Because the response to any antiepileptic drug is unpredictable, patients should be carefully educated about the approach to therapy. Patients need to understand that the goal is to prevent seizures and minimize the side effects of therapy; determination of the optimal dose is often a matter of trial and error. This process may take months or longer if the baseline seizure frequency is low. Most anticonvulsant drugs need to be introduced relatively slowly to minimize side effects, and patients should expect that minor side effects such as mild sedation, slight changes in cognition, or imbalance will typically resolve within a few days. Starting doses are usually the lowest value listed under the dosage column in Table 365-8. Subsequent increases should only be made after achieving a steady state with the previous dose (i.e., after an interval of five or more half-lives).

Monitoring of serum antiepileptic drug levels can be very useful for establishing the initial dosing schedule. However, the published therapeutic ranges of serum drug concentrations are only an approximate guide for determining the proper dose for a given patient. The key determinants are the clinical measures of seizure frequency and presence of side effects, not the laboratory values. Conventional assays of serum drug levels measure the total drug (i.e., both free and protein-bound), yet it is the concentration of free drug that reflects extracellular levels in the brain and correlates best with efficacy. Thus, patients with decreased levels of serum proteins (e.g., decreased serum albumin due to impaired liver or renal function) may have an increased ratio of free to bound drug, yet the concentration of free drug may be adequate for seizure control. These patients may have a "subtherapeutic" drug level, but the dose should be altered only if seizures remain uncontrolled, not just to achieve a "therapeutic" level. In practice, other than during the initiation or modification of therapy, monitoring of antiepileptic drug levels is most useful for documenting compliance.

If seizures continue despite gradual increases to the maximum tolerated dose and documented compliance, then it becomes necessary to switch to another antiepileptic drug. This is usually done by maintaining the patient on the first drug while a second drug is added. The dose of the second drug should be adjusted to decrease seizure frequency without causing toxicity. Once this is achieved, the first drug can be gradually withdrawn (usually over weeks unless there is significant toxicity). The dose of the second drug is then further optimized based on seizure response and side effects.

WHEN TO DISCONTINUE THERAPY Overall, about 70 percent of children and 60 percent of adults who have their seizures completely controlled with antiepileptic drugs can eventually discontinue therapy. Clinical studies suggest that the following patient profile yields the greatest chance of remaining seizure-free after drug withdrawal: (1) complete medical control of seizures for 1 to 5 years; (2) single seizure type, either partial or generalized; (3) normal neurologic examination, including intelligence; and (4) a normal EEG. The appropriate seizure-free interval is unknown and undoubtedly varies for different forms of epilepsy. However, it seems reasonable to attempt withdrawal of therapy after 2 years in a patient who meets all of the above criteria, is motivated to discontinue the medication, and clearly understands the potential risks and benefits. In most cases it is preferable to reduce the dose of the drug gradually over 2 to 3 months. Most recurrences occur in the first 3 months after discontinuing therapy, and patients should be advised to avoid potentially dangerous situations such as driving or unsupervised swimming during this period.

TREATMENT OF REFRACTORY EPILEPSY Approximately one-third of patients with epilepsy do not respond to treatment with a single antiepileptic drug, and it becomes necessary to try a combination of drugs to control seizures. Patients who have focal epilepsy related to an underlying structural lesion, or those with multiple seizure types and developmental delay are particularly likely to require multiple drugs. There are currently no clear guidelines for rational polypharmacy, but in most cases the initial combination therapy is with two of the three first-line drugs, i.e., carbamazepine, phenytoin, and valproic acid. If these drugs are unsuccessful, then the addition of a newer drug such as lamotrigine or gabapentin is indicated. Patients with myoclonic seizures resistant to valproic acid may benefit from the addition of clonazepam, and those with absence seizures may respond to a combination of valproic acid and ethosuximide. The same principles concerning the monitoring of therapeutic response, toxicity, and serum levels for monotherapy apply to polypharmacy, and potential drug interactions need to be recognized. If there is no improvement, a third drug can be added while the first two are maintained. If there is a response, the least effective of the first two drugs should be gradually withdrawn.

Surgical Treatment of Refractory Epilepsy Twenty percent of patients with epilepsy are resistant to medical therapy despite efforts to find an effective combination of antiepileptic drugs. For some, surgery can be extremely effective in substantially reducing seizure frequency and even providing complete seizure control. Understanding the potential value of surgery is especially important when, at the time of diagnosis, a patient has an epilepsy syndrome that is considered likely to be drug-resistant. Rather than submitting the patient to years of unsuccessful medical therapy and the associated psychosocial trauma of ongoing seizures, the patient should have an efficient but relatively brief attempt at medical therapy and then be referred for surgical evaluation.

The most common surgical procedure for patients with temporal lobe epilepsy involves resection of the anteromedial temporal lobe (temporal lobectomy) or a more limited removal of the underlying hippocampus and amygdala. Focal seizures arising from extratemporal regions may be suppressed by a focal neocortical resection or precise removal of an identified lesion (lesionectomy). When the cortical region cannot be removed, multiple subpial transection, which disrupts intracortical connections, is sometimes used to prevent seizure spread. Hemispherectomy or multilobar resection is useful for some patients with severe seizures due to hemispheric abnormalities such as hemimegaloencephaly or other dysplastic abnormalities, and corpus callosotomy has been shown to be effective for disabling tonic or atonic seizures, usually when they are part of a mixed-seizure syndrome (e.g., Lennox-Gastaut syndrome).

Presurgical evaluation is designed to identify the functional and structural basis of the patient's seizure disorder. Inpatient video-EEG monitoring is used to define the anatomic location of the seizure focus and to correlate the abnormal electrophysiologic activity with behavioral manifestations of the seizure. Routine scalp or scalp-sphenoidal recordings are usually sufficient for localization, and advances in neuroimaging have made the use of invasive electrophysiologic monitoring such as implanted depth electrodes or subdural electrodes much less common. A high-resolution MRI scan is routinely used to identify structural lesions. Functional imaging studies such as SPECT and PET are adjunctive tests that may help verify the localization of an apparent epileptogenic region with an anatomic abnormality. Once the presumed location of the seizure onset is identified, additional studies, including neuropsychological testing and the intracarotid amobarbital test (Wada's test) may be used to assess language and memory localization and to determine the possible functional consequences of surgical removal of the epileptogenic region. In some cases, the exact extent of the resection to be undertaken is determined by performing cortical mapping at the time of the surgical procedure. This involves electrophysiologic recordings and cortical stimulation in the awake patient to identify the extent of epileptiform disturbances and the function of cortical regions in question.

Advances in presurgical evaluation and microsurgical techniques have led to a steady increase in the success of epilepsy surgery. Clinically significant complications of surgery are less than 5 percent, and the use of functional mapping procedures has markedly reduced the neurologic sequelae due to removal or sectioning of brain tissue. For example, about 70 percent of patients treated with temporal lobectomy will become seizure-free, and another 15 to 25 percent will have at least a 90 percent reduction in seizure frequency. Marked improvement is also usually seen in patients treated with hemispherectomy for catastrophic seizure disorders due to large hemispheric abnormalities. Postoperatively, patients generally need to remain on antiepileptic drug therapy, but the marked reduction of seizures following surgery can have a dramatic, beneficial effect on their quality of life.

STATUS EPILEPTICUS Status epilepticus refers to continuous seizures or repetitive, discrete seizures with impaired consciousness in the interictal period. The duration of seizure activity sufficient to meet the definition of status epilepticus has traditionally been specified as 15 to 30 min. However, a more practical definition is to consider status epilepticus as a situation in which the duration of seizures prompts the acute use of anticonvulsant therapy, typically when seizures last beyond 5 min.

Status epilepticus is an emergency, since cardiorespiratory dysfunction, hyperthermia, and metabolic derangements can develop as a consequence of prolonged seizures, and these can lead to irreversible neuronal injury after approximately 2 h. Furthermore, CNS injury can occur even when the patient is paralyzed with neuromuscular blockade but continues to have electrographic seizures. The most common causes of status epilepticus are anticonvulsant withdrawal or noncompliance, metabolic disturbances, drug toxicity, CNS infection, CNS tumors, refractory epilepsy, and head trauma.

Generalized status epilepticus is obvious when the patient is having overt convulsions. However, after 30 to 45 min of uninterrupted seizures, the signs may become increasingly subtle. Patients may have mild clonic movements of only the fingers, or fine, rapid movements of the eyes. There may be paroxysmal episodes of tachycardia, hypertension, and pupillary dilation. In such cases, the EEG may be the only method of establishing the diagnosis. Thus, if the patient stops having overt seizures, yet remains comatose, an EEG should be performed to rule out ongoing status epilepticus.

The first step in the management of a patient in status epilepticus is to attend to any acute cardiorespiratory problems or hyperthermia, perform a brief medical and neurologic examination, establish venous access, and send samples for laboratory studies aimed at identifying metabolic abnormalities. Anticonvulsant therapy should then begin without delay; a suggested treatment approach is shown in Fig. 365-3.

BEYOND SEIZURES: OTHER MANAGEMENT ISSUES

Interictal Behavior The adverse effects of epilepsy often go beyond the occurrence of clinical seizures, and the extent of these effects depends largely upon the etiology of the seizure disorder, the degree to which the seizures are controlled, and the presence of side effects from antiepileptic therapy. Many patients with epilepsy are completely normal between seizures and able to live highly successful and productive lives. In contrast, patients with seizures secondary to developmental abnormalities or acquired brain injury may have impaired cognitive function and other neurologic deficits. Frequent interictal EEG abnormalities have been shown to be associated with subtle dysfunction of memory and attention. Patients with many seizures, especially those emanating from the temporal lobe, often note an impairment of short-term memory that may progress over time.

FIGURE 365-3 Pharmacologic treatment of generalized tonic-clonic status epilepticus in adults.

Patients with epilepsy are at risk of developing a variety of psychiatric problems including depression, anxiety, and psychosis. This risk varies considerably depending on many factors, including the etiology, frequency, and severity of seizures and the patient's age and previous history. Depression occurs in approximately 20 percent of patients, and the incidence of suicide is higher in epileptic patients than in the general population. Depression should be treated through counseling or antidepressant medication. The selective serotonin reuptake inhibitors typically have no effect on seizures, while the tricyclic antidepressants may lower the seizure threshold. Anxiety can appear as a manifestation of a seizure, and anxious or psychotic behavior can sometimes be observed as part of a postictal delirium. Interictal psychosis is a rare phenomenon that typically occurs after a period of increased seizure frequency. There is usually a brief lucid interval lasting up to a week, followed by days to weeks of agitated, psychotic behavior. The psychosis will usually resolve spontaneously but may require treatment with antipsychotic or anxiolytic medications.

There is ongoing controversy as to whether some patients with epilepsy (especially partial-complex epilepsy) have a stereotypical "interictal personality." The predominant view is that the unusual or abnormal personality traits observed in such patients are, in most cases, not due to epilepsy but result from an underlying structural brain lesion, the effects of antiepileptic drugs, or psychosocial factors.

Psychosocial Issues There continues to be a cultural stigma about epilepsy, although it is slowly declining in societies with effective health education programs. Because of this stigma, many patients with epilepsy harbor fears, such as the fear of becoming mentally retarded or dying during a seizure. These issues need to be carefully addressed by educating the patient about epilepsy and by ensuring that family members, teachers, fellow employees, and other associates are equally well informed. The Epilepsy Foundation of America (1-800-EFA-1000) is a patient advocacy organization and a useful source of educational material.

Employment and Driving Many patients with epilepsy face difficulty in obtaining or maintaining employment, even when their seizures are well controlled. Federal and state legislation is designed to prevent employers from discriminating against patients with epilepsy, and patients should be encouraged to understand and claim their legal rights. Patients in these circumstances also benefit greatly from the assistance of health providers who act as strong patient advocates.

Loss of driving privileges is one of the most disruptive social consequences of epilepsy. Physicians should be very clear about local regulations concerning driving and epilepsy, since the laws vary considerably among states and countries. In all cases, it is the physician's responsibility to warn patients of the danger imposed on themselves and others while driving if their seizures are uncontrolled (unless the seizures are not associated with impairment of consciousness or motor control). In general, most states allow patients to drive after a seizure-free interval (on or off medications) between 6 months and 2 years.

SPECIAL ISSUES RELATED TO WOMEN AND EPILEPSY

Catamenial Epilepsy Some women experience a marked increase in seizure frequency around the time of menses. This is thought to reflect either the effects of estrogen and progesterone on neuronal excitability or changes in antiepileptic drug levels due to altered protein binding. Acetazolamide (250 to 500 mg/d) has been found effective as adjunctive therapy when started 7 to 10 days prior to the onset of menses and continued until bleeding stops. Some patients may benefit from increases in antiepileptic drug dosages during this time or from control of the menstrual cycle through the use of oral contraceptives.

Pregnancy Most women with epilepsy who become pregnant will have an uncomplicated gestation and deliver a normal baby. However, epilepsy poses some important risks to a pregnancy. Seizure frequency during pregnancy will remain unchanged in approximately 50 percent of women, increase in 30 percent, and decrease in 20 percent. Changes in seizure frequency are attributed to endocrine effects on the CNS, variations in antiepileptic drug pharmacokinetics (such as acceleration of hepatic drug metabolism or effects on plasma protein binding), and changes in medication compliance. It is therefore useful to see patients at more frequent intervals during pregnancy and monitor serum antiepileptic drug levels. Measurement of the unbound drug concentrations may be useful if there is an increase in seizure frequency or worsening of side effects of antiepileptic drugs.

The overall incidence of fetal abnormalities in children born to mothers with epilepsy is 5 to 6 percent, compared to 2 to 3 percent in healthy women. Part of the higher incidence is due to teratogenic effects of antiepileptic drugs, and the risk increases with the number of medications used (e.g., 10 percent risk of malformations with three drugs). A syndrome comprising facial dysmorphism, cleft lip, cleft palate, cardiac defects, digital hypoplasia, and nail dysplasia was originally ascribed to phenytoin therapy, but it is now known to occur with other first-line antiepileptic drugs (i.e., carbamazepine and valproic acid) as well. Also, valproic acid and carbamazepine are associated with a 1 to 2 percent incidence of neural tube defects compared with a baseline of 0.5 to 1 percent. Little is currently known about the safety of newer drugs.

Since the potential harm of uncontrolled seizures on the mother and fetus is considered greater than the teratogenic effects of antiepileptic drugs, it is currently recommended that pregnant women be maintained on effective drug therapy. When possible, it seems prudent to have the patient on monotherapy at the lowest effective dose, especially during the first trimester. Patients should also take folate (1–4 mg), since the antifolate effects of anticonvulsants are thought to play a role in the development of neural tube defects, although the benefits of this treatment remain unproved in this setting.

Enzyme-inducing drugs such as phenytoin, phenobarbital, and primidone cause a transient and reversible deficiency of vitamin K–dependent clotting factors in approximately 50 percent of newborn infants. Although neonatal hemorrhage is uncommon, the mother should be treated with oral vitamin K (20 mg daily) in the last 2 weeks of pregnancy, and the infant should receive an intramuscular injection of vitamin K (1 mg) at birth.

Breast Feeding Antiepileptic medications are excreted into breast milk to a variable degree. The ratio of drug concentration in breast milk relative to serum is approximately 80 percent for ethosuximide, 40 to 60 percent for phenobarbital, 40 percent for carbamazepine, 15 percent for phenytoin, and 5 percent for valproic acid. Given the overall benefits of breast feeding and the lack of evidence for long-term harm to the infant by being exposed to antiepileptic drugs, mothers with epilepsy should not be discouraged from breast feeding. This should be reconsidered, however, if there is any evidence of drug effects on the infant, such as lethargy or poor feeding.

BIBLIOGRAPHY

Brodie MJ, Dichter MA: Antiepileptic drugs. N Engl J Med 334:168, 1996

Engel J Jr: *Seizures and Epilepsy.* Philadelphia, FA Davis, 1989

Engel J Jr: Surgery for seizures. N Engl J Med 334:647, 1996

Hopkins A, Shorvon S, Cascino G (eds): *Epilepsy,* 2d ed. London, Chapman and Hall Medical, 1995

McNamara JO: Cellular and molecular basis of epilepsy. J Neuroscience 14:3413, 1994

Noebels JL: Targeting epilepsy genes. Neuron 16:241, 1996

Sackellares JC, Berent S (eds): *Psychological Disturbances in Epilepsy.* Boston, Butterworth-Heinemann, 1996

Steinlein OK et al: A missense mutation in the neuronal nicotinic acetylcholine receptor alpha 4 subunit is associated with autosomal dominant nocturnal frontal lobe epilepsy. Nat Genet 11:201, 1995

Wyllie E (ed): *The Treatment of Epilepsy,* 2d ed. Baltimore, Williams & Wilkins, 1997

J. Donald Easton, Stephen L. Hauser, Joseph B. Martin

CEREBROVASCULAR DISEASES

Cerebrovascular diseases predominate in the middle and late years of life. They cause approximately 200,000 deaths in the United States each year as well as considerable neurologic disability. The incidence of stroke increases with age and affects many people in their "golden years," a rapidly growing segment of the population. These diseases cause either ischemia-infarction or intracranial hemorrhage (Table 366-1). Ischemia and infarction constitute 85 to 90 percent of the total group in western countries, while 10 to 15 percent are intracranial hemorrhages; hemorrhage constitutes a larger percentage in Asia. The morbidity and mortality from cerebrovascular diseases has been diminishing in recent years, due largely to better recognition and treatment of the underlying arterial and cardiac diseases, including hypertension.

Table 366-1

Classification of Cerebrovascular Diseases

Cerebral Ischemia-Infarction	Intracranial Hemorrhage
Thrombotic occlusion	Intracerebral
Embolic occlusion	Subarachnoid
Artery-to-artery	Subdural (usually traumatic)
Cardiogenic	Epidural (traumatic)

Most cerebrovascular diseases present as the abrupt onset of a focal neurologic deficit. The deficit may remain fixed, or it may rapidly improve or progressively worsen. It is this abrupt onset of a nonconvulsive and focal neurologic deficit that is referred to as a stroke, a cerebrovascular accident (CVA), or apoplexy. In the United States, the term *stroke* is generally used specifically to mean cerebral infarction. It is always preferable to use the more precise terms: cerebral ischemia, cerebral infarction, intracerebral hemorrhage, etc.

Cerebral ischemia is caused by a reduction in blood flow that lasts for several seconds or a few minutes. If the cessation of flow lasts for more than a few minutes, *infarction* of brain tissue results. A *generalized* reduction in cerebral blood flow due to systemic hypotension (e.g., cardiac arrhythmia, myocardial infarction, or hemorrhagic shock) usually produces syncope (see Chap. 20), infarction in the border zones between the major cerebral artery distributions, or widespread brain necrosis, depending on the duration of hypotension. *Focal* ischemia or infarction, on the other hand, is usually caused by disease in the cerebral vessels themselves or by emboli from a proximal arterial source or the heart.

Intracranial hemorrhage may occur into the brain parenchyma, the subarachnoid space, or the subdural or epidural space. Subdural and epidural hematomas are usually the result of trauma, not cerebrovascular disease, and are discussed elsewhere (see Chap. 374). The majority of intracerebral hemorrhages are associated with hypertension; spontaneous hemorrhage, arteriovenous malformation (AVM), and bleeding into a neoplasm are less common causes. Subarachnoid hemorrhage (SAH) is usually due to a ruptured saccular aneurysm or, less commonly, an AVM. Sometimes, no source for the hemorrhage can be found.

GENERAL PATHOPHYSIOLOGY OF CEREBRAL ISCHEMIA AND INFARCTION Within 10 s after cerebral blood flow ceases, metabolic failure of brain tissue occurs. The electroencephalogram shows slowing of electrical activity, and the brain dysfunction becomes clinically manifest. If the circulation is immediately restored, there is abrupt and complete recovery of function. If the perfusion abnormality persists for a few minutes, neuronal injury results. With restoration of flow, the recovery of function takes several minutes or hours and may be incomplete. In addition, during the circulatory failure, the blood elements may sludge, the capillary endothelium may swell, and the blood flow may not reestablish itself, even when the primary cause of the flow failure is corrected (the "no-reflow" phenomenon). More prolonged periods of ischemia result in frank tissue necrosis. Cerebral edema follows and progresses over the subsequent 2 to 4 days. If the region of infarction is large, the edema may produce considerable mass effect with all of its attendant consequences (see Chap. 374).

The commonest causes of cerebral ischemia and infarction are *atherosclerosis with thromboembolism* and *cardiogenic embolism* (see Table 366-2).

ATHEROSCLEROTIC ISCHEMIA AND INFARCTION

Ischemic cerebrovascular disease is divided into two broad categories: thrombotic and embolic. The precise cause of ischemia often cannot be determined. When it occurs in elderly patients, especially those with

Table 366-2

Causes of Ischemic Stroke

Thrombosis
  Atherosclerosis
  Vasculitis
    Collagen vascular diseases: temporal (giant cell) arteritis, polyarteritis
      nodosa, Wegener's granulomatosis, Takayasu's arteritis, syphilis
    Meningitis: tuberculosis, fungi, syphilis, bacteria, herpes zoster
  Arterial dissection: carotid, vertebral, intracranial arteries at the base of
    the brain (spontaneous or traumatic)
  Hematologic disorders: polycythemia, thrombocytosis, thrombotic
    thrombocytopenic purpura, disseminated intravascular coagulation,
    dysproteinemias, hemoglobinopathies (sickle cell disease)
  Miscellaneous: cocaine, amphetamines, moyamoya disease, fibromuscular
    dysplasia, Binswanger's disease
Embolism
  Cardiac source: see Table 366-4
  Atherothrombotic arterial source: bifurcation of common carotid artery,
    carotid siphon, distal vertebral artery, aortic arch
  Unknown source: may be associated with a hypercoagulable state
    secondary to systemic disease, carcinoma (especially pancreatic),
    eclampsia, oral contraceptives, lupus, factor C or S deficiency, factor V
    mutation, etc.
Vasoconstriction
  Vasospasm: cerebral vasospasm following subarachnoid hemorrhage
  Reversible cerebral vasoconstriction: idiopathic, migraine, eclampsia,
    trauma
Venous
  Dehydration, pericranial infection, postpartum and postoperative states,
    systemic cancer

---

other manifestations of atherosclerosis, the term *atherothrombotic*, or *atherothromboembolic*, is used when it seems likely that atherosclerosis-induced thrombosis occurred and the thrombus then lysed or embolized distally and fragmented. Thrombotic strokes occur without warning symptoms in 80 to 90 percent of patients. Between 10 and 20 percent are heralded by one or more transient ischemic attacks (TIAs). Thrombotic strokes often present with stuttering, fluctuating symptoms that worsen over several minutes or hours. Embolic strokes usually present with a neurologic deficit that is maximum at onset.

PATHOPHYSIOLOGY Atherosclerosis is usually maximal at arterial bifurcations, and it commonly affects the origin of the internal carotid artery in the neck and the origin of major and minor arterial branches inside the head. Although individuals with the most atherosclerosis are the ones most likely to have a stroke, the correlation is only approximate. Some patients with large infarcts have minimal disease, and others have no ischemic symptoms but one or more major cerebral artery occlusions. The integrity of the extracranial and intracranial collateral circulation, the state of systemic cardiovascular function, and, possibly, hematologic factors play a role in determining whether a given atherosclerotic lesion will cause ischemia or infarction.

Atherosclerotic plaques can cause an arterial stenosis that produces a *hemodynamic obstruction to flow*. If this regional decrease in cerebral blood flow falls below a critical level, it will cause a transient or permanent ischemic event. In addition, *artery-to-artery emboli* appear to be an important cause of retinal and hemispheric ischemia and infarction. When an atherosclerotic plaque on the arterial wall ulcerates, the necrotic material (cholesterol crystals, calcified connective tissue debris, etc.) may dislodge and serve as emboli or may provide a surface on which aggregation of platelets and coagulation of fibrin occurs. The resulting fibrin clot also may dislodge into the arterial circulation, or it may enlarge and produce thrombotic occlusion of the artery. The contribution of vasospasm in cerebral ischemia or infarction is not known. *Lacunar infarcts* are small infarcts in the deep white matter of the hemisphere or brainstem. They are usually

due to hypertension-induced lipohyalinosis or arteriosclerosis of small penetrating arteries, rather than to large artery atherosclerosis or cardioembolism.

Although the exact cause of ischemia or infarction in a given patient with atherosclerosis is not always known, the primary abnormality is clearly atherosclerosis with its complicating lesion, the fibrous plaque. The plaque contains various degrees of degeneration that may result in *stenosis* or *ulceration*, with subsequent *thrombosis* or *embolization*.

Frequently, however, cerebral infarction occurs in elderly people without an obvious source. The term *cerebral atherothromboembolism of unknown source* is used. Some authors presume the event is embolic when a sudden stroke occurs and cardiac monitoring, echocardiography, and carotid, vertebral, and transcranial Doppler studies fail to disclose an obvious source. About 40 percent of ischemic strokes fall into this category, one of the most perplexing problems in cerebrovascular disease. Sophisticated analyses of activity of the hemostatic system, blood coagulation factors, and autoantibodies show that patients with hypercoagulable states are prone to cerebral embolism. Hypercoagulability may be induced by antiphospholipid antibodies, factor V mutations, protein C deficiency, protein S deficiency, antithrombin III deficiency, systemic neoplasm, and traumatic and surgical tissue injury. These pathophysiologic conditions undoubtedly contribute to cerebral atherothromboembolism, but their importance is uncertain.

CEREBRAL EDEMA At the cellular level, several types of brain edema have been described: cytotoxic, vasogenic, interstitial and ischemic. The various types differ in cause, time of development, region of the brain affected, and response to various methods of prevention or treatment.

Cytotoxic edema is caused by swelling of glia, neurons, and endothelial cells and begins within minutes after an insult such as hypoxia. Because of failure of the energy-dependent sodium pump in the cellular membrane, sodium accumulates intracellularly, and water moves from the extracellular to the intracellular space to maintain osmotic equilibrium. Cytotoxic edema affects predominantly the gray matter.

Vasogenic edema, the most common type of brain edema, results from increased permeability of the capillary endothelial cells; the white matter is primarily affected. Breakdown in the blood-brain barrier allows movement of proteins from the intravascular space through the capillary wall into the extracellular space. This same mechanism permits the leakage of contrast agents which cause computed tomography (CT) and magnetic resonance (MR) brain scans to "contrast enhance." This is in contrast to cytotoxic edema, in which the permeability of the brain vasculature is unaltered.

Interstitial edema is seen in hydrocephalus when outflow of cerebrospinal fluid (CSF) is obstructed and intraventricular pressure increases. The result is movement of sodium and water across the ventricular wall into the paraventricular space.

Cerebral ischemia results initially in cytotoxic, and subsequently vasogenic, edema. The pathophysiology is sufficiently characteristic that many authors propose that it be designated "ischemic edema." Within several minutes of the onset of ischemia, cells begin to swell, particularly those surrounding capillaries. Swelling is more prominent in astrocytes than in neurons. If circulation is restored quickly, these changes may be reversible. If it is not, a series of additional changes is superimposed on the initial cytotoxic edema. As swelling occurs in the glia surrounding the capillaries and in the endothelial cells, the capillary lumen is progressively compressed. Thus, even if circulation is reestablished, the compressed capillaries may not perfuse. This no-reflow phenomenon may contribute to further development of ischemia and necrosis.

In the vasogenic phase, permeability of capillary membranes increases. Some studies indicate that this increased permeability is due both to enhanced pinocytotic transport across the endothelium and to disruption of the tight junctions between endothelial cells. Permeability of the blood-brain barrier tends to increase after return of flow to the ischemic area, and the rapidity with which edema occurs depends on the duration and severity of the ischemia. As in other forms of vasogenic edema, white matter is predominantly affected.

Necrosis develops simultaneously with cytotoxic and vasogenic edema. Glia and neurons are particularly susceptible to necrosis, whereas the capillary endothelium is relatively resistant. With degradation of these cellular elements, osmolarity increases, and this promotes the further accumulation of water.

Ischemic edema reaches its maximum 2 to 4 days after infarction and subsides by the end of the second week. If the infarction and edema are not sufficient to cause death, inflammatory changes and phagocytosis occur in the area of necrosis during the days and weeks that follow, resulting in removal of necrotic debris and resolution of the edema. It is possible that edema itself contributes to ischemia and, thus, to a progressively enlarging infarct.

CELLULAR MECHANISMS OF ISCHEMIC NEURONAL INJURY

Experimental studies of focal ischemic stroke support the concept that there is a core of severe ischemia, the "ischemic core," that is surrounded by an area of reduced perfusion, the "ischemic penumbra," where cells may remain viable for several hours. Within the ischemic core, failure of glucose and oxygen delivery leads to rapid depletion of energy stores and cell death. The etiology of progressive cell injury and death in the ischemic penumbra has been clarified to some extent. *Acidosis* results from the anaerobic metabolism of glucose into lactic acid; blood normally carries far more glucose than oxygen, hence in hypoxic tissue glucose delivery may still be adequate to support anaerobic metabolism. *Excitotoxicity* results from excessive release and impaired (astrocyte) uptake of the excitatory neurotransmitter glutamate (Chap. 380). Glutamate activates the *N*-methyl-D-aspartate (NMDA) receptor, increasing levels of intracellular calcium leading to activation of proteases, lipases, and other mediators of cell injury; it also results in membrane depolarization and spreading depression (Chap. 365), further increasing energy demands and levels of extracellular glutamate. *Free radicals* (partially reduced oxygen species) are generated that damage DNA, proteins, and fatty acids. Induction of *programmed cell death* (*apoptosis*) may also occur as a mechanism of cell death. Neuroprotective drugs that interfere with these processes of cell injury represent important potential new therapies for cerebrovascular disease.

CLINICAL MANIFESTATIONS OF ISCHEMIC STROKE

The typical ischemic stroke presents with the abrupt onset of a focal neurologic deficit and is characterized clinically by its mode of onset and subsequent course. A *TIA* is manifested by a neurologic deficit lasting less than 24 h (usually 5 to 20 min). It is often referred to as a mini-, warning, or transient stroke, because it quickly resolves but often portends an impending stroke. The deficit is focal and confined to an area of the brain perfused by a specific artery. This definition of TIA excludes presyncope and syncope, which are due to diffuse, not focal, cerebral ischemia.

The presumed pathophysiologic mechanisms responsible for TIAs are: (1) low flow in an artery due to tight stenosis or occlusion, or (2) embolism from the heart or proximal arterial or atherosclerotic plaque debris or thrombus. Any obstructive vascular process in the extra- or intracranial arteries can cause a low-flow TIA if collateral flow to the potentially ischemic brain is also impaired (see Figs. 366-1 and 366-2), and can lead to arterial thrombosis. If symptoms or signs persist beyond 24 h, infarction has occurred. Even symptoms that last only an hour or so may be associated with infarction.

Because presyncope and syncope often are confused with focal cerebral ischemia, it is necessary to distinguish these conditions and their pathophysiology from focal cerebral ischemia (see Chap. 20).

Reversible ischemic neurologic deficit is an infrequently used term that defines an ischemic event in which the deficit usually recovers over a 24- to 72-h period, but which may take as long as 1 week to resolve.

A *completed stroke*, or cerebral infarction, of the thrombotic type is generally nonhemorrhagic. It typically evolves to its maximal deficit within a few hours. Often, the patient awakens with a completed deficit. A completed stroke is sometimes heralded by one or more TIAs in the preceding days, weeks, or months. This is most likely when a tight arterial stenosis is causative. Ischemic strokes are produced by the same pathophysiologic mechanism responsible for TIAs. Thrombo-

sis complicating atherosclerosis accounts for most thrombotic strokes, and embolism from proximal atherosclerosis or the heart accounts for most embolic strokes.

In *progressing stroke*, or stroke-in-evolution, the focal ischemia worsens from minute to minute or hour to hour. There are usually stepwise incremental increases in neurologic deficit occurring over a several-hour period. In the posterior circulation, however, the stroke may evolve over 2, 3, or even several days. Many clinicians include *crescendo TIA*, i.e., the sudden onset of a series of ischemic attacks over a few hours or days, in this category. While there may be several pathogenic mechanisms producing a progressing stroke, one such appears to be a thrombus-in-evolution, with a thrombus extending from its site of origin in a primary artery and progressively obliterating collateral branches, thereby interfering with anastomotic vessels.

The symptoms and signs of an ischemic stroke vary depending on the location of the occlusion and the extent of the spared collateral flow. The hallmark presentation is the abrupt onset of a hemiparesis in an individual in the atherosclerotic age group. Virtually any symptom of brain dysfunction may occur, however. Symptoms and signs of carotid system disease most commonly affect the distribution of the middle cerebral artery, and the patient may exhibit a contralateral hemiparesis, hemisensory deficit, and hemianopia. If the dominant

FIGURE 366-1 Arrangement of the major arteries of the right side carrying blood from the heart to the brain. Also shown are vessels of collateral circulation that may modify the effects of cerebral ischemia (*A, B, C*). Not shown is the circle of Willis, which also provides a source for collateral circulation. *A.* The anastomotic channels between the distal branches of the anterior and middle cerebral artery, termed border-zone or watershed anastomotic channels. Note that they also occur between the posterior and middle cerebral arteries and the anterior and posterior cerebral arteries. *B.* Anastomotic channels occurring through the orbit between branches of the external carotid artery and ophthalmic branch of the internal carotid artery. *C.* Wholly extracranial anastomotic channels between the muscular branches of the ascending cervical arteries and muscular branches of the occipital artery that anastomose with the distal vertebral artery. Note that the occipital artery arises from the external carotid artery, thereby allowing reconstitution of flow in the vertebral from the carotid circulation. (*Courtesy of CM Fisher, M.D.*)

hemisphere is involved, there is usually some degree of aphasia. Lacunar infarction is common in the distribution of the lenticulostriate branches of the middle cerebral artery.

Either the anterior (carotid) or posterior (vertebrobasilar) circulation may be involved. The following descriptions apply to ischemia and infarction in specific arteries due to atherothrombosis, although similar syndromes may occur with other types of arterial pathology, after embolic stroke, and occasionally after intracerebral hemorrhage.

Atherothrombotic Disease of the Internal Carotid Artery and Its Branches *Pathophysiology* The origin of the internal carotid artery is the most common site of atherosclerosis and superimposed atherothrombosis that leads to TIA or stroke. Less often, disease at the siphon (S-shaped portion of the internal carotid artery in the cavernous sinus) or in the proximal segment of the middle or anterior cerebral arteries may be responsible. These intracranial sites predominate in African Americans and Asians. Rarely, the origin of the common carotid artery may be the site.

INTERNAL CAROTID ARTERY Atherosclerosis in the proximal internal carotid artery is usually most severe in the first 2 cm and arises from the posterior wall, often extending downward into the common carotid artery. Atherosclerosis at this site is often heralded by a TIA

or minor stroke, presumably caused by embolism or, less frequently, low flow.

Emboli arising from a stenotic or ulcerated atherosclerotic plaque at the origin of the internal carotid artery may cause occlusion of the ophthalmic artery, the proximal middle cerebral artery or one of its branches, or, less often, the anterior cerebral artery. Small platelet emboli that occlude the ophthalmic artery branches cause transient monocular blindness (TMB; amaurosis fugax). Larger emboli composed of platelet-fibrin thrombus may occlude the primary and secondary branches of the middle cerebral territory (e.g., lenticular nucleus, deep white matter, and cortical surface). In some instances, only deep infarction occurs because collateral flow through leptomeningeal artery collaterals over the cortical surface are sufficient (see Fig. 366-1A). Large emboli may partially occlude a major artery or may migrate or lyse and disperse, causing a neurologic deficit that fluctuates (stroke-in-evolution) or resolves.

In some patients, an ulcerated plaque may be the only lesion in the carotid bifurcation, but more often there is an accompanying stenosis of 50 percent or more. A nonstenotic or slightly stenotic carotid lesion in conjunction with a stroke or a single prolonged TIA suggests the heart as the source of the embolus. Atheromatous lesions at the origin of the great vessels in the aortic arch also can produce cerebral emboli that cause ischemia or infarction, but the incidence of this mechanism is thought to be low.

When *low flow* is the mechanism, there is presumably inadequate collateral flow through the circle of Willis.

INTRACRANIAL INTERNAL CAROTID ARTERY Although less common, lesions in the siphon can cause strokes and TIAs whose pathophysiologic and clinical features duplicate those discussed above.

MIDDLE CEREBRAL ARTERY In contrast to the internal carotid artery, occlusion of the proximal middle cerebral artery or one of its major branches is usually due to embolus (artery-to-artery, cardiac, or of unknown source) rather than intracranial atherothrombosis, though intracranial atherothrombosis is common in African Americans and Asians. Symptomatic atheroma are rarely located distal to the first bifurcation of the middle cerebral artery. Because the circle of Willis is proximal to the origin of the middle cerebral artery, collateral blood flow to the distal middle cerebral artery territory must arise from small cortical surface border zones and anastomotic (leptomeningeal) arteries of the anterior and posterior cerebral arteries.

ANTERIOR CEREBRAL ARTERY Atheromatous deposits in the proximal segment of the anterior cerebral artery rarely cause symptoms because the effects of occlusion are usually mitigated by collateral circulation through the anterior communicating artery. If the anterior communicating artery is congenitally atretic, or the atheromatous lesion occurs distal in the anterior cerebral artery, TIAs and stroke may occur.

Clinical manifestations MIDDLE CEREBRAL ARTERY The cortical branches of the middle cerebral artery supply the lateral surface of the hemisphere except for (1) the frontal pole and

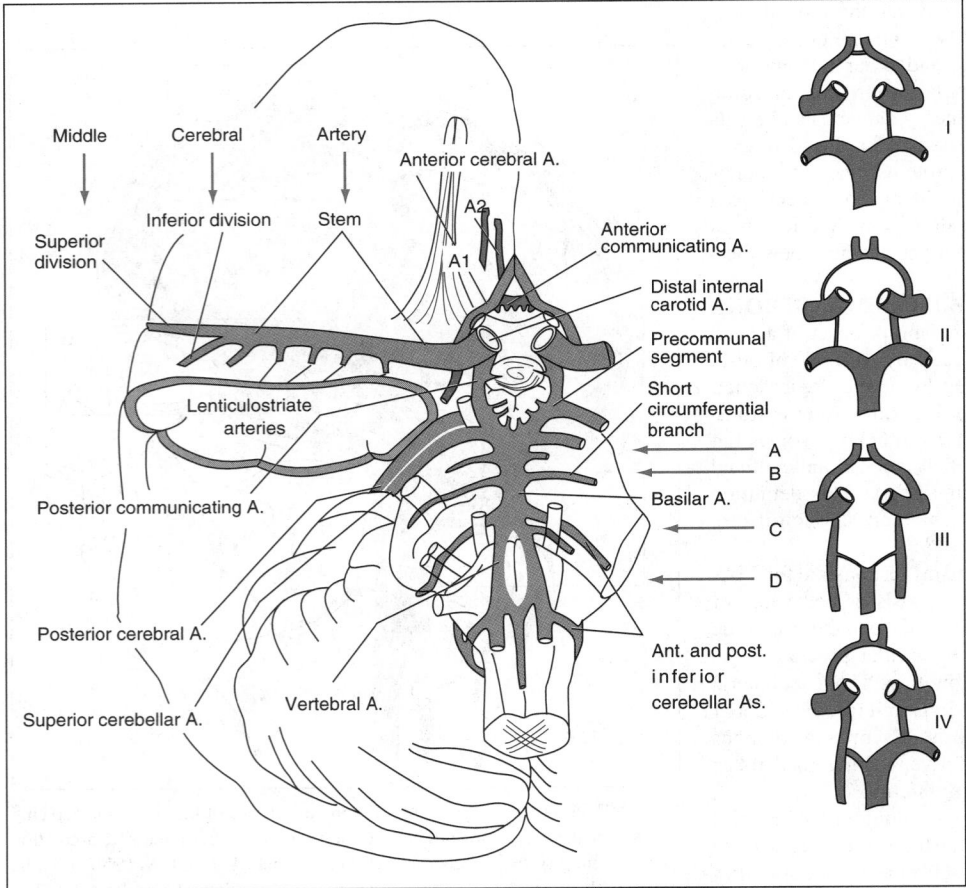

FIGURE 366-2 Diagram of the brainstem, cerebellum, inferior right frontal lobe, and transected temporal lobe. Principal branches of the vertebral basilar arterial system are pictured. The stem of the middle cerebral artery with its small, deep penetrating lenticulostriate arteries and the circle of Willis with its small, deep penetrating branches are shown. Roman numerals I, II, III, and IV represent some of the possible variations of the circle of Willis due to atresia of one or more of its arterial components. A, B, C, and D arrows point to the four cross sections of the brainstem diagrammed below (D, Fig. 366-7; A, Fig. 366-8; B, Fig. 366-9; C, Fig. 366-10). Although typical vascular syndromes of the pons and medulla have been designated by the shaded areas in Figs. 366-7 to 366-10, the shading is approximate only. Great variability in infarct size and location occurs when the basilar or vertebral arteries or one of their penetrating branches becomes occluded. This variability is because of variation in arterial anatomic location and available collateral circulation. Thus the stroke syndromes produced are often atypical, incomplete, or merge with one another. *(Courtesy of CM Fisher, M.D.)*

In the figure labels:
Middle — Cerebral — Artery
Anterior cerebral A.
Superior division
Inferior division — Stem
A2
A1
Anterior communicating A.
Distal internal carotid A.
Precommunal segment
Short circumferential branch
Lenticulostriate arteries
A
B
Basilar A.
C
Posterior communicating A.
D
III
Posterior cerebral A.
Ant. and post. inferior cerebellar As.
Superior cerebellar A.
Vertebral A.

a strip along the superomedial border of the frontal lobe supplied by the anterior cerebral artery, and (2) the lower temporal and occipital pole convolutions, which are in the territory of the posterior cerebral artery (Fig. 366-3).

The proximal middle cerebral artery gives rise to penetrating branches that supply the putamen, outer globus pallidus, posterior limb of the internal capsule above the plane of the upper border of the globus pallidus, the adjacent corona radiata, and the body and upper and lateral head of the caudate nucleus. In the sylvian fissure, the middle cerebral artery in most patients divides into *superior* and *inferior* divisions. Branches of the inferior division supply the inferior parietal and temporal cortex, and those from the superior division supply the frontal and superior parietal cortex (Fig. 366-4). There is considerable variability in the parietal lobe supply between the two divisions, with about two-thirds of individuals having an inferior division that supplies regions above the angular gyrus.

If the entire middle cerebral artery is occluded at its origin, blocking both its penetrating and cortical branches, and the distal collaterals are limited, the clinical findings are contralateral hemiplegia, hemianesthesia, and homonymous hemianopia. When the dominant hemisphere is involved, global aphasia is present also, and when the nondominant hemisphere is affected, apractagnosia and anosognosia are found (see Fig. 366-4). Dysarthria also may occur.

Complete middle cerebral territory syndromes occur most often when a thromboembolus occludes the stem of the artery. Cortical collateral blood flow and differing arterial configurations are probably responsible for the development of partial middle cerebral artery syndromes. Partial middle cerebral territory syndromes also may be due to an embolus that enters the proximal middle cerebral artery without complete occlusion or that lyses and moves distally. Symptoms and signs may fluctuate in such patients (stroke-in-evolution).

Partial syndromes resulting from embolic occlusion of a single branch include hand, or arm and hand, weakness alone (brachial syndrome) or facial weakness with motor aphasia, with or without arm weakness (frontal opercular syndrome). A combination of sensory disturbance, motor weakness, and motor aphasia suggests that an embolus has occluded the proximal superior division and infarcted large portions of the frontal and parietal cortices (see Fig. 366-4). If Wernicke's aphasia occurs without weakness, the inferior division of the middle cerebral artery supplying the posterior part (temporal cortex) of the dominant hemisphere is probably involved (see Fig. 366-4). Jargon speech and an inability to comprehend written and spoken language are prominent features, often accompanied by a contralateral, homonymous inferior quadrantanopia or hemianopia (see Chap. 25). Hemineglect or spatial agnosia without weakness indicates that the inferior division of the middle cerebral artery in the nondominant hemisphere is involved.

ANTERIOR CEREBRAL ARTERY The anterior cerebral artery is divided into two segments: the precommunal (A1) circle of Willis, or stem, which connects the internal carotid artery to the anterior communicating artery, and the postcommunal (A2) segment distal to the anterior communicating artery (see Fig. 366-2). The A1 segment of the anterior cerebral artery gives rise to several deep penetrating branches that supply the anterior limb of the internal capsule, the anterior perforate substance, amygdala, anterior hypothalamus, and the inferior part of the head of the caudate nucleus (see Fig. 366-3).

Occlusion of the proximal anterior cerebral artery is usually well tolerated because of collateral flow. Occlusion of a single A2 segment

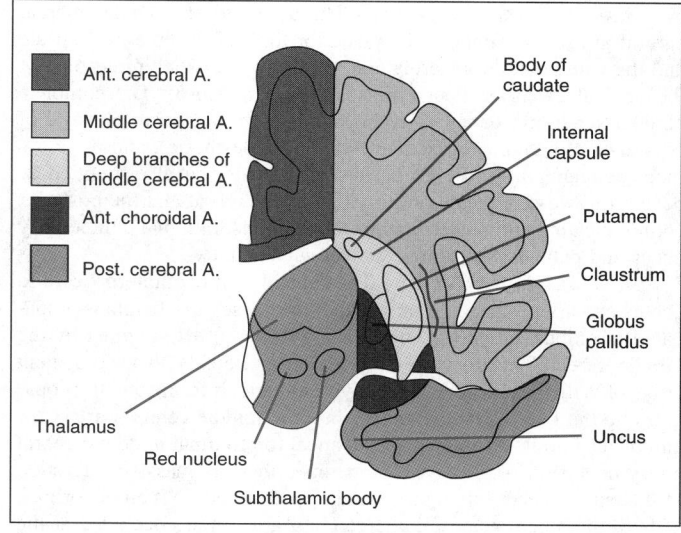

FIGURE 366-3 Diagram of a cerebral hemisphere in coronal section showing the territories of the major cerebral vessels. *(Courtesy of C M Fisher, M.D.)*

results in the contralateral symptoms noted in the legend of Fig. 366-5. If both A2 segments arise from a single anterior cerebral stem (contralateral A1 segment atresia), the occlusion affects both hemispheres. Profound abulia (a delay in verbal and motor response) and bilateral pyramidal signs with paraparesis and urinary incontinence result.

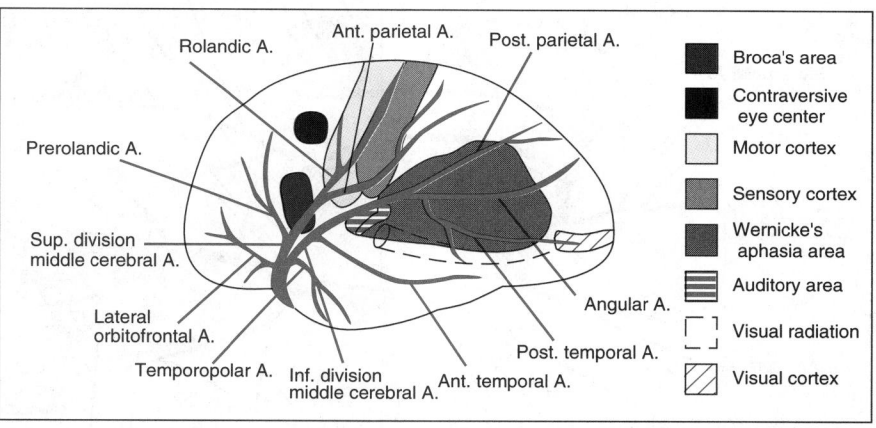

FIGURE 366-4 Diagram of a cerebral hemisphere, lateral aspect, showing the branches and distribution of the middle cerebral artery and the principal regions of cerebral localization. Note the bifurcation of the middle cerebral artery into a superior and inferior division. *(Courtesy of CM Fisher, M.D.)*

Signs and symptoms: *Structures involved*

Paralysis of the contralateral face, arm, and leg; sensory impairment over the same area (pinprick, cotton touch, vibration, position, two-point discrimination, stereognosis, tactile localization, barognosis, cutaneographia): *Somatic motor area for face and arm and the fibers descending from the leg area to enter the corona radiata and corresponding somatic sensory system*

Motor aphasia: *Motor speech area of the dominant hemisphere*

Central aphasia, word deafness, anomia, jargon speech, sensory agraphia, acalculia, alexia, finger agnosia, right-left confusion (the last four comprise the Gerstmann syndrome): *Central, suprasylvian speech area and parietooccipital cortex of the dominant hemisphere*

Conduction aphasia: *Central speech area (parietal operculum)*

Apractognosia of the minor hemisphere (amorphosynthesis), anosognosia, hemiasomatognosia, unilateral neglect, agnosia for the left half of external space, dressing "apraxia," constructional "apraxia," distortion of visual coordinates, inaccurate localization in the half field, impaired ability to judge distance, upside-down reading, visual illusions (e.g., it may appear that another person walks through a table): *Nondominant parietal lobe (area corresponding to speech area in dominant hemisphere); loss of topographic memory is usually due to a nondominant lesion, occasionally to a dominant one*

Homonymous hemianopia (often homonymous inferior quadrantonopia): *Optic radiation deep to second temporal convolution*

Paralysis of conjugate gaze to the opposite side: *Frontal contraversive field or projecting fibers*

ANTERIOR CHOROIDAL ARTERY This artery arises from the internal carotid artery and supplies the posterior limb of the internal capsule and the white matter posterolateral to it, through which pass some of the geniculocalcarine fibers (Figs. 366-3 and 366-6). The complete clinical syndrome of anterior choroidal artery occlusion consists of contralateral hemiplegia, hemianesthesia (hypesthesia), and homonymous hemianopia. However, because this territory is also supplied by penetrating vessels of the proximal middle cerebral and the posterior communicating and posterior choroidal arteries, minimal deficits may occur and patients frequently recover substantially.

INTERNAL CAROTID ARTERY The clinical picture of internal carotid occlusion varies depending on whether the cause of ischemia is propagated thrombus, embolism, or low flow. The cortex supplied by the middle cerebral territory is affected most often. With a competent circle of Willis, occlusion can be asymptomatic. If the thrombus propagates up the internal carotid artery into the middle cerebral artery, or embolizes into it, symptoms are identical to proximal middle cerebral artery occlusion (see above). Sometimes there is massive infarction of the entire deep white matter and cortical surface. When the origins of both the anterior and middle cerebral arteries are occluded at the top of the carotid artery, abulia or stupor occurs with hemiplegia, hemianesthesia, and aphasia or anosognosia. When the posterior cerebral artery arises from the internal carotid artery (an unusual configura-

tion called a *fetal posterior cerebral artery*), it also may become occluded and give rise to symptoms referable to its peripheral territory (see Figs. 366-5 and 366-6).

In addition to supplying the ipsilateral brain, the internal carotid artery perfuses the optic nerve and retina via the ophthalmic artery. In about 25 percent of symptomatic internal carotid disease, recurrent TMB warns of the lesion. Patients typically describe a shade that sweeps down or up across the field of vision. They also may complain that their vision was blurred in that eye or that the upper or lower half of vision disappeared. In most cases, these symptoms last only a few minutes. Rarely, ophthalmic or central retinal artery ischemia or infarction occurs at the time of cerebral TIA or infarction.

The natural history of asymptomatic atherosclerotic lesions of the carotid bifurcation that produce a bruit is uncertain. There is evidence that the tighter the stenotic lesion, the more likely symptoms are to occur over time. Patients with tightly stenotic lesions that are hemodynamically significant (approximately 75 percent diameter stenosis) are at higher risk of embolic stroke. Although such patients have reduced flow in the distal internal carotid artery, they remain asymptomatic because of adequate collateral flow in the circle of Willis. However, thrombus may form in the low-flow carotid and cause occlusion or artery-to-artery embolism.

A high-pitched prolonged carotid bruit fading into diastole is often associated with such tightly stenotic lesions. As the stenosis grows tighter and flow distal to the stenosis becomes reduced, the bruit becomes fainter and may disappear when occlusion is imminent.

COMMON CAROTID ARTERY All the neurologic symptoms and signs of internal carotid occlusion also may be present with occlusion of the common carotid artery. Bilateral common carotid artery occlusion at their origin may occur in Takayasu's arteritis or the aortic arch syndrome (see Chap. 319). An incomplete aortic arch syndrome has been reported consisting of various combinations of carotid, subclavian, or innominate stenosis or occlusion (see below).

Atherothrombotic Disease of the Vertebrobasilar–Posterior Cerebral Artery System The two vertebral arteries join to form the basilar artery at the pontomedullary junction. The basilar artery divides into two posterior cerebral arteries in the interpeduncular fossa (see Fig. 366-2). Each of these major arteries gives rise to long and short circumferential branches and to smaller deep penetrating branches that supply the cerebellum, medulla, pons, midbrain, subthalamus, thalamus, hippocampus, and medial temporal and occipital lobes. Atherosclerosis has a predilection for the origin and the distal segments of the vertebral arteries, the proximal basilar artery, and the origin of the major and minor branches of the vertebral, basilar, and posterior cerebral arteries. Predictably, atheromatous disease at each site produces its own clinical syndromes.

Pathophysiology POSTERIOR CEREBRAL ARTERY In 75 percent of patients, both posterior cerebral arteries arise from the bifurcation of the basilar artery; in 20 percent, one or the other comes from the ipsilateral internal carotid artery; in 5 percent, both come from the ipsilateral internal carotid artery via the

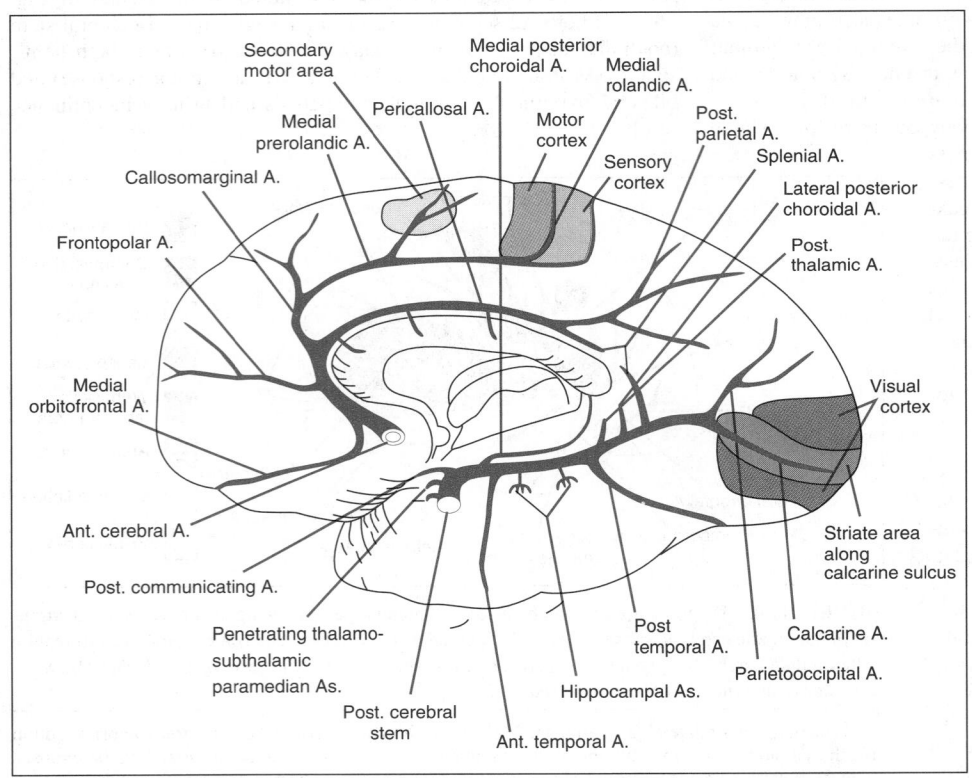

FIGURE 366-5 Diagram of a cerebral hemisphere, medial aspect, showing the branches and distribution of the anterior cerebral artery and the principal regions of cerebral localization. (*Courtesy of CM Fisher, M.D.*)

Signs and symptoms: *Structures involved*

Paralysis of opposite foot and leg: *Motor leg area*
A lesser degree of paresis of opposite arm: *Arm area of cortex or fibers descending to corona radiata*
Cortical sensory loss over toes, foot, and leg: *Sensory area for foot and leg*
Urinary incontinence: *Sensorimotor area in paracentral lobule*
Contralateral grasp reflex, sucking reflex, gegenhalten (paratonic rigidity): *Medial surface of the posterior frontal lobe (?) supplemental motor area*
Abulia (akinetic mutism), slowness, delay, intermittent interruption, lack of spontaneity, whispering, reflex distraction to sights and sounds: *Uncertain localization—probably cingulate gyrus and medial inferior portion of frontal, parietal, and temporal lobes*
Impairment of gait and stance (gait apraxia): *Frontal cortex near leg motor area*
Dyspraxia of left limbs, tactile aphasia in left limbs: *Corpus callosum*

posterior communicating arteries. The precommunal segment (mesencephalic portion) of the true posterior cerebral artery is atretic in such cases.

Atheroma formation at the top of the basilar artery or along the precommunal segment of the posterior cerebral artery may cause symptoms by narrowing one or more of the small brainstem-penetrating branches (see Figs. 366-2 and 366-6) that supply the middle cerebral peduncles, the substantia nigra, red nucleus, oculomotor nuclei, midbrain reticular formation, subthalamic nucleus, decussation of the superior cerebellar peduncles, the medial longitudinal fasciculus, and the medial lemniscus. The artery of Percheron (the posterior thalamosubthalamoparamedian artery) is a single artery that arises from either the right or the left precommunal segment of the posterior cerebral artery. It divides in the subthalamus to supply the inferomedial and anterior portions of the thalamus and subthalamus bilaterally. The thalamogeniculate branches, which also originate from the precommunal portion of the posterior cerebral artery, supply the dorsal, dorsomedial, anterior and inferior thalamus, and the medial geniculate body. The medial posterior choroidal artery supplies the superior dorsomedial and dorsoanterior thalamus and the medial geniculate body in addition to the tela choroidea of the third ventricle. The lateral posterior choroidal artery supplies the choroid plexus of the lateral ventricle.

Atheroma in the posterior cerebral artery distal to the junction with the posterior communicating artery (see Fig. 366-6) may occlude small circumferential branches that course around the midbrain to supply the lateral part of the cerebral peduncles, medial lemniscus, tegmentum of the midbrain, superior colliculi, lateral geniculate body and posterolateral nucleus of the thalamus, choroid plexus, and hippocampus. On the rare occasions when atheroma occur more distally in the posterior cerebral artery, occlusion may produce ischemia in the inferomedial temporal lobe, parahippocampal and hippocampal gyri, and occipital lobe—including the calcarine cortex and the visual association areas 18 and 19.

VERTEBRAL AND POSTERIOR INFERIOR CEREBELLAR ART- ERIES Each *vertebral artery* arises from the respective subclavian artery and divides into four anatomic segments. The first extends from its origin to its entrance into the sixth or fifth transverse vertebral foramen. The second transverses the vertebral foramina from C6 to C2. The third passes through the transverse foramen and circles around the arch of the atlas to pierce the dura at the foramen magnum. The fourth segment courses upward to join the other vertebral artery to form the basilar artery; only the fourth segment gives rise to branches that supply the brainstem and cerebellum. The *posterior inferior cerebellar artery* in its proximal segment supplies the lateral medulla and, in its distal branches, the inferior surface of the cerebellum. Anastomotic channels exist among the ascending cervical arteries, the thyrocervical arteries, the occipital artery (branch of the external carotid artery), and the second segment of the vertebral artery.

Atherothrombotic lesions have a predilection for the first and fourth segments of the vertebral artery. Although the atheromatous narrowing in the first segment may be significant, it seldom produces strokes. Collateral flow from the contralateral vertebral artery or the ascending cervical and ascending thyrocervical or occipital arteries is usually sufficient to prevent ischemia. When one vertebral artery is atretic and an atherothrombotic lesion threatens the origin of the other, the collateral circulation is through the ascending cervical artery, the thyrocervical artery, and the occipital artery or by retrograde flow down the basilar artery via the posterior communicating artery (see Figs. 366-2 and 366-6). In this setting, low flow in the verte-

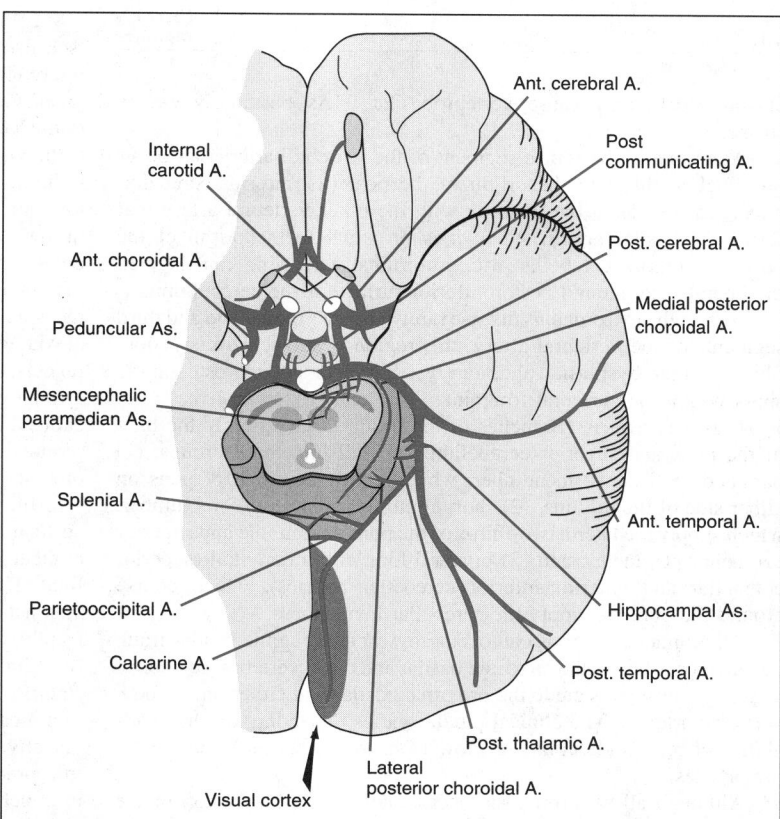

FIGURE 366-6 Inferior aspect of the brain with the branches and distribution of the posterior cerebral artery and the principal anatomic structures shown. *(Courtesy of CM Fisher, M.D.)*

Signs and symptoms: *Structures involved*

1. Peripheral territory (see also Fig. 366-5)
   Homonymous hemianopia (often upper quadrantic): *Calcarine cortex or optic radiation nearby*
   Bilateral homonymous hemianopia, cortical blindness, awareness or denial of blindness; tactile naming, achromatopsia (color blindness), failure to see to-and-fro movements, inability to perceive objects not centrally located, apraxia of ocular movements, inability to count or enumerate objects, tendency to run into things that the patient sees and tries to avoid: *Bilateral occipital lobe with possibly the parietal lobe involved*
   Verbal dyslexia without agraphia, color anomia: *Dominant calcarine lesion and posterior part of corpus callosum*
   Memory defect: *Hippocampal lesion bilaterally or on the dominant side only*
   Topographic disorientation and prosopagnosia: *Usually with lesions of nondominant, calcarine, and lingual gyrus*
   Simultagnosia, hemivisual neglect: *Dominant visual cortex, contralateral hemisphere*
   Unformed visual hallucinations, peduncular hallucinosis, metamorphopsia, teleopsia, illusory visual spread, paliopsia, distortion of outlines, central photophobia: *Calcarine cortex*
   Complex hallucinations: *Usually nondominant hemisphere*
2. Central territory
   Thalamic syndrome: sensory loss (all modalities), spontaneous pain and dysesthesias, choreoathetosis, intention tremor, spasms of hand, mild hemiparesis: *Posteroventral nucleus of thalamus; involvement of the adjacent subthalamus body or its afferent tracts*
   Thalamoperforate syndrome: crossed cerebellar ataxia with ipsilateral third nerve palsy (Claude's syndrome): *Dentatothalamic tract and issuing third nerve*
   Weber's syndrome: third nerve palsy and contralateral hemiplegia: *Third nerve and cerebral peduncle*
   Contralateral hemiplegia: *Cerebral peduncle*
   Paralysis or paresis of vertical eye movement, skew deviation, sluggish pupillary responses to light, slight miosis and ptosis (retraction nystagmus and "tucking" of the eyelids may be associated): *Supranuclear fibers to third nerve, interstitial nucleus of Cajal, nucleus of Darkschewitsch, and posterior commissure*
   Contralateral rhythmic, ataxic action tremor; rhythmic postural or "holding" tremor (rubral tremor): *Dentatothalamic tract (?)*

brobasilar system and TIAs may occur. In addition, thrombosis in the proximal basilar or distal vertebral system may occur. If the subclavian is blocked proximal to the origin of the vertebral artery, exercise of the left arm may draw blood in a retrograde fashion down the vertebral artery to the distal subclavian artery. This "subclavian steal" may cause vertebrobasilar TIAs but rarely causes stroke.

Atheroma in the fourth segment of the vertebral artery can occur proximal or distal to the origin of the posterior inferior cerebellar artery, as well as at the junction with the other vertebral artery that forms the basilar artery. When it is proximal to the origin of the posterior inferior cerebellar artery, a critical narrowing can threaten the lateral medulla and posteroinferior surface of the cerebellum.

Although atheromatous disease rarely narrows the second and third segments of the vertebral artery, this region is subject to dissection, fibromuscular dysplasia, and, rarely, encroachment by osteophytic spurs within the vertebral foramina.

BASILAR ARTERY Branches of the basilar artery supply the base of the pons and superior cerebellum and fall into three groups: (1) paramedian, 7 to 10 in number, which supply a wedge of pons on either side of the midline; (2) short circumferential, 5 to 7 in number, which supply the lateral two-thirds of the pons and middle and superior cerebellar peduncles; and (3) bilateral long circumferential (superior cerebellar and anterior inferior cerebellar arteries), which course around the pons to supply the cerebellar hemispheres.

Atheromatous lesions can occur anywhere along the basilar trunk but are most often in the proximal basilar and distal vertebral segments. Typically, lesions occlude the proximal basilar and either one or both vertebral arteries. The clinical picture varies depending on the availability of retrograde collateral flow from the posterior communicating arteries.

Although atherothrombosis occasionally occludes the top of the basilar artery, emboli from the heart or proximal vertebral or basilar segments are more common.

Clinical manifestations POSTERIOR CEREBRAL ARTERY The site of atheromas and the degree of narrowing determine the clinical syndrome. Although factors of collateral circulation or serum viscosity may play a role in some cases, embolic occlusion is the usual cause of stroke in this vascular territory. Two syndromes are commonly observed: (1) midbrain, subthalamic, and thalamic signs, which are due to disease of the precommunal segment or of its penetrating branches; and (2) cortical temporal and occipital lobe syndromes, due to occlusion of the postcommunal segment.

1. *Proximal precommunal syndromes (central territory).* If the proximal posterior cerebral artery is occluded, infarction usually occurs in the ipsilateral subthalamus, medial thalamus and midbrain (Fig. 366-6). Hemiplegia secondary to infarction of the cerebral peduncle may occur. Involvement of the red nucleus and/or dentatorubrothalamic tract can produce contralateral ataxia. A third nerve palsy may be combined with contralateral ataxia (Claude's syndrome) or with contralateral hemiplegia (Weber's syndrome). If the subthalamic nucleus is involved, contralateral hemiballismus may occur. Occlusion of the artery of Percheron produces paresis of upward gaze and drowsiness and is often associated with abulia. Extensive infarction in the midbrain and subthalamus occurring with bilateral proximal posterior cerebral artery occlusion is usually secondary to embolism. Coma, bilateral pyramidal signs, and decerebrate rigidity occur in this setting.

Atheromatous occlusion of the penetrating branches of thalamic and thalamogeniculate arteries produces less extensive thalamic and thalamocapsular lacunar syndromes. The *thalamic syndrome of Déjérine and Roussy* is the best known. Its main feature is contralateral hemisensory loss of both superficial sensation (pain and temperature) and deep sensation (touch and proprioception). Occasionally, it may affect only pain and temperature or vibration and joint position sense. After a few weeks or months, an agonizing, searing or burning pain may develop in the affected areas. It is persistent and responds poorly to analgesics. Anticonvulsants or tricyclic drugs may be beneficial. If the posterior limb of the internal capsule is involved, hemiparesis may accompany the hemisensory syndrome. Other associated motor signs include hemiballismus, choreoathetosis, intention tremor, incoordination, and posturing of the hand and arm, particularly while walking.

2. *Postcommunal syndromes (peripheral or cortical territory)* (see also Fig. 366-6). Occlusion of the posterior cerebral artery causes infarction of the cortical surface of the medial temporal and occipital lobes. Contralateral homonymous hemianopia is the usual manifestation. Occasionally, only the upper quadrant of visual field is involved. If the visual association areas are spared and only the calcarine cortex is involved, the patient is aware of visual defects. Medial temporal lobe and hippocampal involvement may cause an acute disturbance in memory, particularly if it occurs in the dominant hemisphere. The defect usually clears because memory has bilateral representation. If the dominant hemisphere is affected and the infarct extends to involve the splenium of the corpus callosum, the patient may demonstrate alexia without agraphia (see Chap. 25). Visual agnosia for faces, objects, mathematical symbols, and colors and anomia with paraphasic errors (amnestic aphasia) also may occur in this setting, even without callosal involvement. Occlusion of the posterior cerebral artery can produce *peduncular hallucinosis* (visual hallucinations of brightly colored scenes and objects).

Bilateral infarction in the distal posterior cerebral arteries produces cortical blindness. The patient is often unaware of the blindness. The clinical clue to the site is a finding of normal pupillary reaction to light. Tiny islands of vision may persist, and the patient reports that vision fluctuates as images are captured in the preserved portions. Rarely, only peripheral vision is lost and central vision is spared, resulting in "gun-barrel" vision. A constellation of symptoms termed *Balint's syndrome* can occur with unilateral or bilateral visual association area lesions (see Chap. 25). It includes optic ataxia, (inability to visually guide limb movements), ocular ataxia (inability to direct eyes to a precise point in the visual field), inability to enumerate objects in a picture or extract meaning from a picture, and inability to avoid objects seen in one's path. Balint's syndrome is seen most often with bilateral infarctions secondary to low flow in the "watershed" between the distal posterior and middle cerebral artery territories, as occurs after cardiac arrest. Embolic occlusion of the top of the basilar artery can produce a clinical picture that includes any or all of the central or peripheral territory symptoms; its hallmark is suddenness of onset and bilaterality of symptoms, including ptosis and somnolence (see above in the discussion of the artery of Percheron).

VERTEBRAL AND POSTERIOR INFERIOR CEREBELLAR ARTERIES TIAs resulting from vertebral artery insufficiency cause dizziness or vertigo, numbness of the ipsilateral face and contralateral limbs, diplopia, hoarseness, dysarthria, and dysphagia. Hemiparesis is rare.

When *infarction* ensues, it most often affects the lateral medulla with or without the posteroinferior cerebellum (Wallenberg's syndrome). Its features are listed in Fig. 366-7. In the majority of cases, the syndrome occurs after ipsilateral vertebral artery occlusion; in the remainder, it results from posterior inferior cerebellar artery occlusion. Atherothrombotic occlusion of the medullary penetrating branches of the vertebral or posterior inferior cerebellar artery results in partial syndromes of the ipsilateral medulla.

Rarely, a medial medullary syndrome occurs in which the pyramid becomes infarcted, causing a contralateral hemiparesis of the arm and leg and sparing the face. If the medial lemniscus and emerging hypoglossal nerve fibers are involved, contralateral loss of joint position sense and ipsilateral tongue weakness occur.

Cerebellar infarction with edema formation can lead to *sudden respiratory arrest* due to raised intracranial pressure in the posterior fossa. Drowsiness, Babinski signs, dysarthria, and bifacial weakness may be absent, or present only briefly, before respiratory arrest ensues. Gait unsteadiness, dizziness, nausea, and vomiting may be the only early symptoms and signs of this impending complication.

BASILAR ARTERY Because the brainstem contains many structures in close proximity, a diversity of clinical syndromes may emerge with ischemia. Involvement of the corticospinal tracts, corticobulbar tracts, and cranial nerve nuclei causes the common symptoms and signs (Figs. 366-8 to 366-10).

Unfortunately, the symptoms of transient ischemia or infarction in the territory of the basilar artery often do not indicate whether the basilar artery itself or one of its branches is diseased, yet the distinction has important implications for therapy. The picture of complete basilar insufficiency, however, is easy to recognize. A combination of bilateral long tract signs (sensory and motor) with signs of cranial nerve and cerebellar dysfunction suggests this diagnosis. A "locked-in" state of awake quadriplegia, bifacial and oropharyngeal palsy, and paralysis of horizontal gaze occurs with bilateral basis pontis infarction. Stupor indicates dysfunction of the reticular activating system, and when combined with third cranial nerve palsies it suggests devastating upper midbrain infarction (see Chap. 24). The therapeutic goal, however, is to recognize *impending* basilar occlusion before devastating infarction occurs. A series of TIAs or a slowly progressive, fluctuating stroke are extremely significant as they often herald an atherothrombotic occlusion of the distal vertebral or proximal basilar artery.

TIAs in the proximal basilar distribution may produce dizziness (often described by patients as "swimming," "swaying," "moving," "unsteadiness" or "light-headedness"). Other symptoms that warn of basilar thrombosis include diplopia, dysarthria, facial or circumoral numbness, and hemisensory symptoms. In general, symptoms of basilar branch TIAs affect one side of the brainstem, whereas symptoms of basilar artery TIAs usually affect both sides, though a "herald" hemiparesis has been emphasized as an initial symptom of basilar occlusion. Most often TIAs, whether due to impending occlusion of the basilar artery or a basilar branch, are short-lived (5 to 30 min) and repetitive, occurring several times a day. The pattern suggests intermittent reduction of flow.

Atherothrombotic occlusion of the basilar artery with *brainstem infarction* usually causes *bilateral* brainstem signs. For example, gaze paresis or internuclear ophthalmoplegia may be associated with ipsilateral hemiparesis. By contrast, occlusion of a branch of the basilar artery usually causes *unilateral* symptoms and signs involving motor, sensory, and cranial nerves.

SUPERIOR CEREBELLAR ARTERY Occlusion of this artery results in severe ipsilateral cerebellar ataxia, nausea and vomiting, dysarthria, and contralateral loss of pain and temperature sensation over the extremities, body, and face. Partial deafness, ataxic tremor of the ipsilateral upper extremity, Horner's syndrome, and palatal myoclonus may also occur. Partial syndromes are common (Fig. 366-8).

ANTERIOR INFERIOR CEREBELLAR ARTERY Occlusion produces variable degrees of infarction because the size of this artery and the territory it supplies vary inversely with those of the posterior inferior cerebellar artery. The principal symptoms include ipsilateral deafness, facial weakness, true vertigo (whirling dizziness), nausea and vomiting, nystagmus, tinnitus, cerebellar ataxia, Horner's syndrome, and paresis of conjugate lateral gaze. The opposite side of the body loses pain and temperature sensation. An occlusion close to the origin of the artery may cause corticospinal tract signs (see Fig. 366-10).

Occlusion of one of the five to seven short circumferential branches of the basilar artery affects the lateral two-thirds of the pons and middle or superior cerebellar pe-

duncle, whereas occlusion of one of the 7 to 10 paramedian branches affects a wedge-shaped area on either side of the medial pons (Figs. 366-8 to 366-10).

Lacunar Disease The term *lacunar infarction* refers to infarction following atherothrombotic or lipohyalinotic occlusion of one of the penetrating branches of the circle of Willis, middle cerebral artery stem, or vertebral and basilar arteries.

Pathophysiology The middle cerebral artery stem, the arteries comprising the circle of Willis (A1 segment of the anterior cerebral artery, anterior and posterior communicating arteries, precommunal segment of the posterior cerebral arteries), and the basilar and vertebral

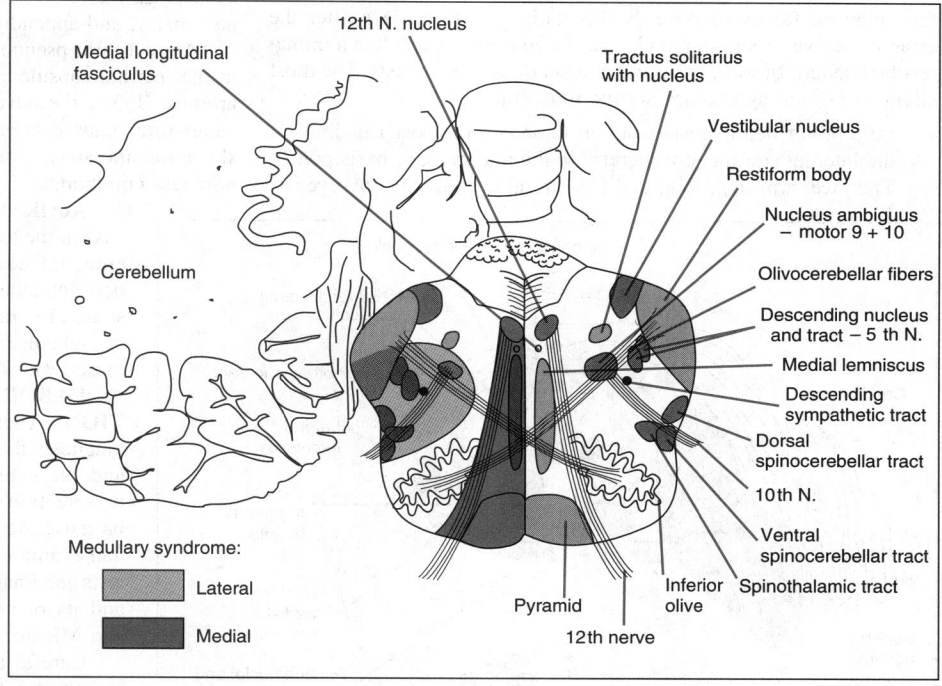

FIGURE 366-7 *(Courtesy of CM Fisher, M.D.)*
Signs and symptoms: *Structures involved*

1. Medial medullary syndrome (occlusion of vertebral artery or of branch of vertebral or lower basilar artery)
   On side of lesion
      Paralysis with atrophy of half the tongue: *Ipsilateral twelfth nerve*
   On side opposite lesion
      Paralysis of arm and leg sparing face; impaired tactile and proprioceptive sense over half the body: *Contralateral pyramidal tract and medial lemniscus*
2. Lateral medullary syndrome (occlusion of any of five vessels may be responsible—vertebral, posterior inferior cerebellar, superior, middle, or inferior lateral medullary arteries)
   On side of lesion
      Pain, numbness, impaired sensation over half the face: *Descending tract and nucleus fifth nerve*
      Ataxia of limbs, falling to side of lesion: *Uncertain—restiform body, cerebellar hemisphere, cerebellar fibers, spinocerebellar tract (?)*
      Nystagmus, diplopia, oscillopsia, vertigo, nausea, vomiting: *Vestibular nucleus*
      Horner's syndrome (miosis, ptosis, decreased sweating): *Descending sympathetic tract*
      Dysphagia, hoarseness, paralysis of palate, paralysis of vocal cord, diminished gag reflex: *Issuing fibers ninth and tenth nerves*
      Loss of taste: *Nucleus and tractus solitarius*
      Numbness of ipsilateral arm, trunk, or leg: *Cuneate and gracile nuclei*
   On side opposite lesion
      Impaired pain and thermal sense over half the body, sometimes face: *Spinothalamic tract*
3. Total unilateral medullary syndrome (occlusion of vertebral artery): Combination of medial and lateral syndromes
4. Lateral pontomedullary syndrome (occlusion of vertebral artery): Combination of lateral medullary and lateral inferior pontine syndromes
5. Basilar artery syndrome (the syndrome of the lone vertebral artery is equivalent): A combination of the various brainstem syndromes plus those arising in the posterior cerebral artery distribution
      Bilateral long tract signs (sensory and motor; cerebellar and peripheral cranial nerve abnormalities): *Bilateral long tract; cerebellar and peripheral cranial nerves*
      Paralysis or weakness of all extremities, plus all bulbar musculature: *Corticobulbar and corticospinal tracts bilaterally*

arteries all give rise to 100- to 300-μm diameter branches that penetrate the deep gray and white matter of the cerebrum or brainstem (see Fig. 366-2). Each of these small branches can thrombose either by atherothrombotic disease at its origin or by the development of lipohyalinotic thickening. Thrombosis of these vessels causes small infarcts that are referred to as *lacunes*. They range in size from as small as 3 or 4 mm to 1 or 2 cm. Hypertension is the principal risk factor for such small-vessel disease. Lacunar infarcts cause approximately 20 percent of all strokes.

Clinical manifestations Lacunar infarcts cause recognizable stroke syndromes. Transient symptoms (lacunar TIAs) may herald a lacunar infarct; they may occur several times a day and last only a few minutes. Recovery often begins within hours or days after the infarct, and over weeks or months may be complete or result in minimal residual deficit. In some cases, significant disability persists. The most common lacunar syndromes are the following:

1. Pure motor hemiparesis from an infarct in the posterior limb of the internal capsule, crus cerebri in the midbrain, or basis pontis. The face, arm, leg, foot, and toes are almost always involved.

2. Pure sensory stroke from an infarct in the ventrolateral thalamus.
3. Ataxic hemiparesis from an infarct in the base of the pons.
4. Dysarthria and a clumsy hand or arm due to infarction in the base of the pons or in the genu of the internal capsule.
5. Pure motor hemiparesis with "motor aphasia" due to thrombotic occlusion of a lenticulostriate branch supplying the genu and anterior limb of the internal capsule and adjacent white matter of the corona radiata.

Syndromes resulting from occlusion of the penetrating arteries of the proximal posterior cerebral artery were discussed above. Syndromes resulting from occlusion of the penetrating arteries of the basilar artery (see Figs. 366-8 to 366-10) include ipsilateral ataxia and crural (leg) paresis, pure motor hemiparesis with horizontal gaze palsy, and hemiparesis with a contralateral sixth nerve palsy. Lower basilar branch syndromes include sudden internuclear ophthalmoplegia, horizontal gaze palsy, and appendicular cerebellar ataxia.

An anarthric pseudobulbar syndrome due to bilateral infarctions in the internal capsule can occur from disease in the lenticulostriate arteries. Before the advent of antihypertensive therapy, multiple lacunes often caused pseudobulbar palsy with emotional instability, a slowed abulic state, and bilateral pyramidal signs; this syndrome is now less common.

Aortic Atheromatous Disease Atherosclerotic disease of the ascending aorta is a potential source of cerebral emboli. One study found a strong, independent association between atherosclerotic disease of the aortic arch, demonstrated by transesophageal echocardiography, and the risk of ischemic stroke. The incidence and natural history of these lesions are uncertain.

LABORATORY AND IMAGING EVALUATION Therapy in ischemic stroke is aided by a precise diagnosis that determines the primary vascular pathology and the extent and location of the stroke. The clinical presentation and temporal profile of a stroke often suggest its cause. Accurate diagnosis is based largely on the history and examination, supplemented by judicious use of blood tests and imaging of the brain [CT and MR imaging (MRI)] and its blood vessels (arterial Doppler ultrasonography, and MR and x-ray angiography).

Careful auscultation for bruits of the carotid arteries and their extracranial branches may add supporting evidence for a diagnosis. Ancillary diagnostic studies generally should be used to confirm or exclude other conditions, rather than to search for evidence of every possible diagnosis. Chest x-rays, urinalysis, complete blood count, erythrocyte sedimentation rate, serum electrolytes, blood urea nitrogen, blood sugar, serologic tests for syphilis, serum lipid profile, serum uric acid, blood clotting studies, and thyroid function studies all may be helpful in detecting precipitating causes of vascular thrombosis or intracranial hemorrhage. An electrocardiogram (ECG) may demonstrate conduction abnormalities and arrhythmias or reveal evidence of recent myocardial infarction. A CT scan will often demonstrate an area of infarction and will confirm or exclude the presence of an intracerebral, subdural, or epidural hemorrhage or other mass lesion. Moreover, it may demonstrate large aneurysms and AVMs and subarachnoid or intraventricular blood. A lumbar puncture (LP) will confirm or exclude subarachnoid hemorrhage or meningitis due to syphilis or other chronic infections. An LP should not be performed on patients with intracranial mass lesions (Chap. 360).

Atherothrombotic Disease of the Internal Carotid Artery and its Branches Several diagnostic techniques are available for evaluating patients with carotid bruits, TIA, and stroke. Positive findings must be interpreted in the appropriate clinical context. For example, a carotid artery bruit in the neck or an ulcerated plaque at the origin of the internal carotid artery detected by ultrasonography

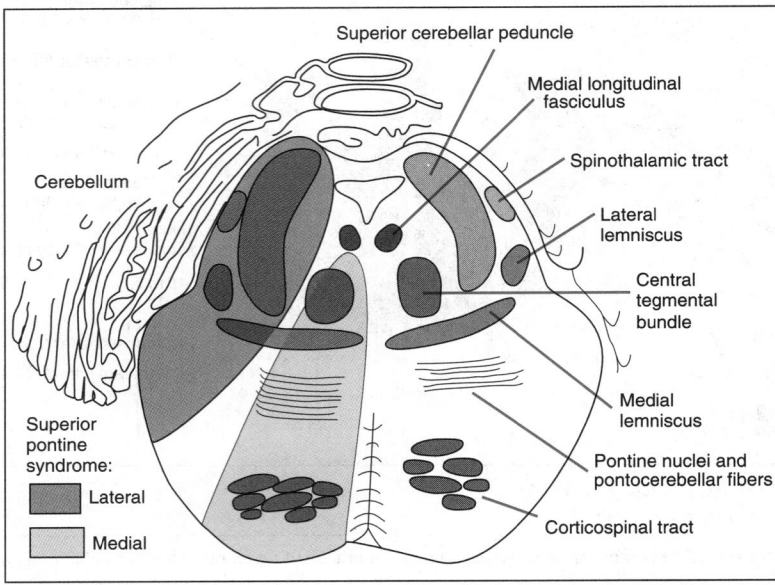

FIGURE 366-8 *(Courtesy of CM Fisher, M.D.)*
Signs and symptoms: *Structures involved*

1. Medial superior pontine syndrome (paramedian branches of upper basilar artery)
   On side of lesion
   Cerebellar ataxia (probably): *Superior and/or middle cerebellar peduncle*
   Internuclear ophthalmoplegia: *Medial longitudinal fasciculus*
   Myoclonic syndrome, palate, pharynx, vocal cords, respiratory apparatus, face, oculomotor apparatus, etc.: *Localization uncertain—central tegmental bundle (?), dentate projection (?), inferior olivary nucleus (?)*
   On side opposite lesion
   Paralysis of face, arm, and leg: *Corticobulbar and corticospinal tract*
   Rarely touch, vibration, and position are affected: *Medial lemniscus*
2. Lateral superior pontine syndrome (syndrome of superior cerebellar artery)
   On side of lesion
   Ataxia of limbs and gait, falling to side of lesion: *Middle and superior cerebellar peduncles, superior surface of cerebellum, dentate nucleus*
   Dizziness, nausea, vomiting; horizontal nystagmus: *Vestibular nucleus*
   Paresis of conjugate gaze (ipsilateral): *Pontine contralateral gaze*
   Skew deviation: *Uncertain*
   Miosis, ptosis, decreased sweating over face (Horner's syndrome): *Descending sympathetic fibers*
   Static tremor reported in one case: *Dentate nucleus (?), superior cerebellar peduncle (?)*
   On side opposite lesion
   Impaired pain and thermal sense on face, limbs, and trunk: *Spinothalamic tract*
   Impaired touch, vibration, and position sense, more in leg than arm (there is a tendency to incongruity of pain and touch deficits): *Medial lemniscus (lateral portion)*

or contrast angiography in a patient with dizzy spells or syncopal episodes is almost certainly an incidental finding. Inappropriate reliance on an isolated clinical finding (e.g., a bruit) or on a vascular abnormality detected in an ancillary study may result in incorrect diagnosis and inappropriate therapy.

Brain imaging (Figs. 366-11 and 362-3) Brain imaging is important in assessing the patient who has just experienced a TIA or stroke.

CT scans identify or exclude hemorrhage as the cause of stroke, and they identify extraparenchymal hemorrhages, neoplasms, abscesses, and other conditions masquerading as a stroke. Scans obtained in the first several hours after an infarction generally show no abnormality, and the infarct may not be seen reliably for 24 to 48 h (see Chap. 362). Even later, they may fail to show small ischemic strokes in the posterior fossa because of bone artifact. Also, they may miss small infarcts on the cortical surface. Contrast-enhanced CT scans add specificity by showing contrast enhancement of subacute infarcts.

MRI reliably documents the extent and location of infarction within 1 h of onset in all areas of the brain, including the posterior fossa and cortical surface. It also identifies intracranial hemorrhage and other abnormalities. The higher the field strength, the more reliable and precise the image.

Xenon-blood-flow and *positron emission tomography* (PET) can assess cerebral blood flow, and PET scanning can measure metabolism. These two methods are generally used for research (see Chap. 362).

Artery imaging X-RAY ANGIOGRAPHY Cerebral angiography, performed by injection of x-ray contrast dye into selected extracranial arteries after transfemoral catheterization, remains the most accurate method of assessing the cerebrovascular system. It can detect atherosclerotic plaque stenoses and ulcers, intralumenal thrombi, arterial dissections, arteritis and vasospasm, collateral circulation around the circle of Willis and on the cortical surface, and occlusion of large and small arteries.

The advantages of selective cerebral angiography must be balanced in each patient against complications that occur in 0.5 to 3 percent. The principal risks are stroke, allergic reactions to the dye, and renal failure. Because of the risks of invasive angiography, ultrasonography and MR angiography are supplanting it in many situations.

ULTRASONOGRAPHY Stenoses at the origin of the internal carotid artery can be reliably identified and quantified by ultrasonography, utilizing a B-mode ultrasound image combined with a Doppler ultrasound assessment of flow. Transcranial Doppler can also assess flow in middle, anterior, and posterior cerebral arteries and in the vertebrobasilar systems. It can detect stenotic lesions in the middle cerebral stem, the distal vertebral arteries, and the basilar artery because such lesions increase systolic flow velocity. When there is an occlusion or a hemodynamically significant stenosis at the origin of the internal carotid artery or in the carotid siphon, transcranial Doppler assesses collateral flow across the anterior or posterior circle of Willis. Ultrasound cannot distinguish reliably between complete and near-complete carotid occlusion, a very important distinction in some clinical situations. The distinction can be made reliably only by x-ray angiography.

Noninvasive techniques are increasingly used to evaluate asymptomatic patients found to have a carotid bruit in the neck on routine physical examination. The role of these techniques in the management of cerebral vascular disease is uncertain because the treatment for asymptomatic carotid artery stenosis is controversial (see below). Noninvasive carotid testing is a useful and risk-free method to document progression of stenosis.

MR ANGIOGRAPHY This rapidly developing and noninvasive technique provides images of arterial flow. It is particularly valuable for identifying lesions of the extracranial carotid circulation. These images tend to overestimate the degree of stenosis and also cannot distinguish reliably between complete and near-complete carotid occlusion. Using high field strengths (1.5 tesla) and different pulse sequencing, blood flow also may be imaged in the large intracranial arteries. MR angiography does not reliably detect carotid siphon and middle cerebral stem lesions.

In many cases, MR angiography combined with carotid and transcranial ultrasound studies eliminates the need for x-ray angiography in evaluating carotid artery lesions. The combination of the two studies is less expensive than x-ray angiography.

Atherothrombotic Disease of the Vertebrobasilar System CT scanning may detect a large cerebellar infarction in the territory of the posterior inferior cerebellar artery. MRI is more sensitive than CT; it detects cerebellar infarction earlier and can also detect lateral medullary infarction. MR angiography can detect patency of the vertebral artery and occasionally the posterior inferior cerebellar artery. Cerebral angiography is rarely necessary to evaluate stroke in this territory if MR angiography is available. Transcranial Doppler analysis of flow in the vertebral artery determines its patency, but its sensitivity in detecting distal vertebral artery stenotic lesions is limited.

Infarction in the peripheral territory of the posterior cerebral artery can be documented easily by CT or MRI. Infarction in the central territory of the posterior cerebral artery, particularly in territories supplied by the penetrating branches of the posterior cerebral artery, is not reliably detected by CT, but generally is with MRI. MR angiography and intracranial Doppler may identify atherosclerosis stenotic lesions in the proximal posterior cerebral artery.

MRI scanning can detect brainstem infarction due to either basilar artery or basilar branch occlusion. MR angiography combined with transcranial Doppler analysis may eventually replace conventional

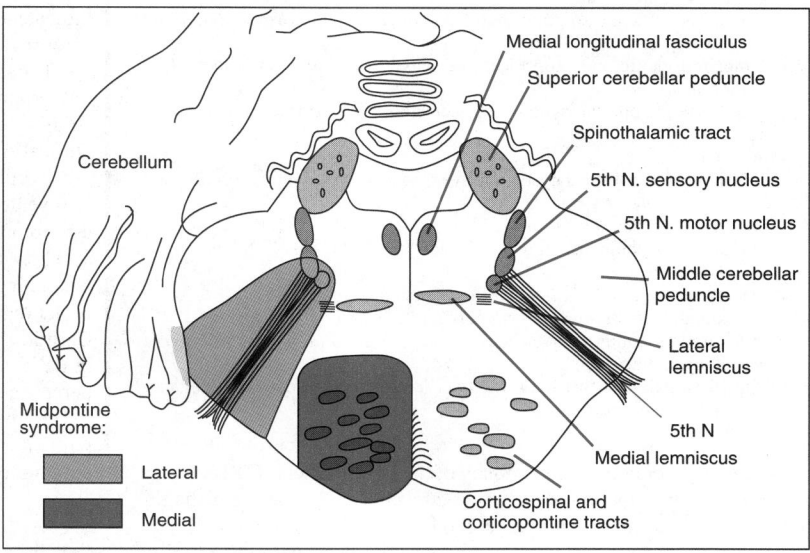

FIGURE 366-9 *(Courtesy of CM Fisher, M.D.)*
Signs and symptoms: *Structures involved*

1. Medial midpontine syndrome (paramedian branch of midbasilar artery)
   On side of lesion
      Ataxia of limbs and gait (more prominent in bilateral involvement): *Pontine nuclei*
   On side opposite lesion
      Paralysis of face, arm, and leg: *Corticobulbar and corticospinal tract*
      Variable impaired touch and proprioception when lesion extends posteriorly: *Medial lemniscus*
2. Lateral midpontine syndrome (short circumferential artery)
   On side of lesion
      Ataxia of limbs: *Middle cerebellar peduncle*
      Paralysis of muscles of mastication: *Motor fibers or nucleus of fifth nerve*
      Impaired sensation over side of face: *Sensory fibers or nucleus of fifth nerve*
   On side opposite lesion
      Impaired pain and thermal sense on limbs and trunk: *Spinothalamic tract*

FIGURE 366-10 *(Courtesy of CM Fisher, M.D.)*
Signs and symptoms: *Structures involved*

1. Medial inferior pontine syndrome (occlusion of paramedian branch of basilar artery)
   On side of lesion
     Paralysis of conjugate gaze to side of lesion (preservation of convergence): *"Center" for conjugate lateral gaze*
     Nystagmus: *Vestibular nucleus*
     Ataxia of limbs and gait: *Middle cerebellar peduncle (?)*
     Diplopia on lateral gaze: *Abducens nerve*
   On side opposite lesion
     Paralysis of face, arm, and leg: *Corticobulbar and corticospinal tract in lower pons*
     Impaired tactile and proprioceptive sense over half of the body: *Medial lemniscus*
2. Lateral inferior pontine syndrome (occlusion of anterior inferior cerebellar artery)
   On side of lesion
     Horizontal and vertical nystagmus, vertigo, nausea, vomiting, oscillopsia: *Vestibular nerve or nucleus*
     Facial paralysis: *Seventh nerve*
     Paralysis of conjugate gaze to side of lesion: *"Center" for conjugate lateral gaze*
     Deafness, tinnitus: *Auditory nerve or cochlear nucleus*
     Ataxia: *Middle cerebellar peduncle and cerebellar hemisphere*
     Impaired sensation over face: *Descending tract and nucleus fifth nerve*
   On side opposite lesion
     Impaired pain and thermal sense over half the body (may include face): *Spinothalamic tract*

angiography in documenting patency of the basilar artery. CT scanning is not reliable in detecting brainstem infarcts but can show hemorrhages and assess mass effect after large cerebellar infarctions.

Selective x-ray arteriography remains the best method to define atherothrombotic disease of the basilar artery. Arteriography entails potential morbidity and may precipitate the very stroke one is seeking to prevent. It is recommended only when MR angiography fails to detect the clinically suspected basilar arterial lesion that, if known, would influence patient management. Occasionally, injection of angiographic dye in the posterior circulation precipitates a delirious state sometimes associated with cortical blindness. This reversible state can last for 1 or 2 or, rarely, several days.

Lacunes The CT scan detects most supratentorial lacunar infarcts, and MRI detects both supratentorial and infratentorial infarctions when the lacunes are 5 mm or greater. Lacunar infarction can be diagnosed when the infarct size is less than 2 cm and its location is attributable to occlusion of a small penetrating arterial branch of a major parent vessel at the base of the brain.

FIGURE 366-11 MRI findings in acute cerebral infarction. Acute onset of right hemiparesis. The axial postcontrast T1-weighted image (*left*) demonstrates contrast enhancement within the vascular bed (*white arrows*) distal to a high-grade stenosis or occlusion. Gadolinium percolates slowly into these vessels through collaterals resulting in enhancement of vessels distal to the occlusion. 24 h later, abnormal prolongation of T2-weighted signal is seen in the cortex supplied by the middle cerebral occlusion (*right image, black arrows*).

℞ TREATMENT

Treatments for atherothrombotic stroke can be divided into those for prevention and those for acute management.

Prevention **GENERAL PRINCIPLES** Many means are now available for preventing stroke. Some can be applied widely across large populations of people because they are effective, cost little, and carry minimal risk. Other measures are expensive and carry substantial risk; these cannot be applied broadly across the population but may be valuable in selected high-risk patients for whom the benefits substantially outweigh the cost and risk. Some may be indicated only for secondary prevention in patients with preexisting cerebrovascular or cardiovascular disease.

The concept of a *clinical risk profile* is well known but often not articulated. One study analyzed data from pooled published studies to determine whether one can reliably predict, based on clinical manifestations of cerebrovascular atherosclerosis (e.g., cervical bruit, TIA, stroke), the annual risk of stroke (Table 366-3). It revealed that the annual stroke rates are low for patients with asymptomatic carotid stenosis and high for patients who have had a major stroke. The analysis suggested that a hierarchical profile of worsening clinical characteristics mirrors a hierarchical progression of increasing risk for stroke. The North American Symptomatic Carotid Endarterectomy Trial (NASCET; see below) found that even in patients with the same degree of carotid artery stenosis (70 to 99 percent), nine prospectively selected risk factors predicted stroke risk in the medically treated patients. In the high-risk group (those with more than six risk factors), 39 percent of medically treated patients experienced an ipsilateral stroke within 2 years. The rate

Table 366-3

Annual Vascular Event Rates for Individuals with Various Features of Atherothrombotic Cerebral Vascular Disease

Cerebrovascular Features	Annual Probability, %, of		
	Stroke	Vascular Death	All Death
Asymptomatic carotid disease	1.3	3.4	6.0
Transient monocular blindness	2.2	3.5	4.3
Transient ischemic attack	3.7	2.3	4.0
Minor stroke	6.1	3.2	4.9
Major stroke	9.0	3.5	7.6
>70% Symptomatic carotid stenosis	15.0	2.0	

NOTE: The annual probability of stroke in the general elderly male population is 0.6%.
SOURCE: Modified with permission from Wilterdink and Easton, 1992.

for the low-risk group (fewer than six risk factors) was less than half but was still 17 percent. Patients with six risk factors had an intermediate risk of 23 percent. These data support the view that there is a clinical risk profile, in addition to the conventional atherosclerosis risk factor profile, that estimates the likelihood of stroke.

ATHEROSCLEROSIS RISK FACTORS Chapter 242 describes the relationship of various factors to the risk of atherosclerosis. Older age, family history of thrombotic stroke, diabetes mellitus, hypertension, tobacco smoking, elevated blood cholesterol, and other factors are either proven or probable risk factors for ischemic stroke, largely by their link to atherosclerosis. Whether or not tight control of blood sugars in patients with diabetes and other general care measures lower stroke risk is uncertain. Tobacco smoking should be discouraged in everyone.

Of the atherosclerosis factors, hypertension is of the greatest importance. In general, all hypertension should be treated. The first lines of treatment are dietary and life-style modification. All stages of hypertension are associated with increased risk of nonfatal and fatal cardiovascular disease events and renal disease. The higher the blood pressure, the greater the risk. High blood pressure stage 1, previously termed "mild," is the most common form of high blood pressure in the adult population and is therefore responsible for a large proportion of the excess morbidity, disability, and mortality attributable to hypertension. The presence of cerebrovascular disease is not a contraindication to treatment aimed at achieving normotension. Also, the value of treating systolic hypertension in older patients has been clearly established. Care must be taken to avoid overtreatment of hypertension, as these patients may have focal vascular stenoses and impaired vasomotor reactivity. The treatment goal should be gradually to achieve normotension.

Recommendations regarding the treatment of hyperlipidemia are complicated. There are strong data regarding the value of treating hypercholesterolemia to prevent coronary artery disease and consequent myocardial infarction and vascular death. While the treatment benefits regarding stroke are less clear, coronary artery disease is the commonest cause of death in patients with cerebrovascular disease. As with treatment of hypertension, the first line of treatment is dietary and life-style modification. Drug treatment generally should be reserved for those at highest risk for coronary heart disease.

ANTIPLATELET AGENTS *Platelet antiaggregation agents* prevent atherothrombotic events, including TIA and stroke. They inhibit the formation of intraarterial platelet aggregates that can form on diseased arteries, induce thrombus formation, and occlude the artery or embolize into the distal circulation. Aspirin and ticlopidine are the antiplatelet agents used most for this purpose.

Aspirin is the most widely studied antiplatelet agent. Its antiplatelet effect is accomplished by acetylating the cyclooxygenase enzyme in platelets. This irreversibly inhibits the formation in platelets of thromboxane A_2, a platelet aggregating and vasoconstricting prostaglandin. This effect is permanent and lasts for the usual 8-d life of the platelet. Paradoxically, aspirin also inhibits the formation in endothelial cells of prostacyclin, an antiaggregating and vasodilating prostaglandin. This effect is transient. As soon as the aspirin is cleared from the blood, the nucleated endothelial cells again produce prostacyclin. Aspirin in low doses given once daily inhibits the production of thromboxane A_2 in platelets without substantially inhibiting prostacyclin formation. Therefore, many physicians recommend aspirin in doses of 300 mg or less per day.

Ticlopidine blocks the ADP receptor on platelets and thus prevents the cascade resulting in activation of the glycoprotein IIb/IIIa receptor that leads to fibrinogen binding to the platelet and consequent platelet aggregation (see Chap. 60). Ticlopidine is more effective than aspirin. However, it has the disadvantage of causing a small incidence of neutropenia, diarrhea, and skin rash. It commonly is recommended for use as an antiplatelet agent only if aspirin is contraindicated or fails. Dipyridamole is an antiplatelet agent that acts by inhibiting platelet phosphodiesterase, which is responsible for the breakdown of cyclic AMP. The resulting elevation in cyclic

AMP inhibits aggregation of platelets. Dipyridamole has not been proven more effective than aspirin, and there is no proof of an additional antiplatelet benefit when added to aspirin.

Many large clinical trials have demonstrated clearly that antiplatelet agents reduce vascular atherothrombotic events (ischemic stroke, myocardial infarction, and death due to all vascular causes) in at-risk patients. The overall *relative* reduction in risk of nonfatal stroke is 25 to 30 percent and of overall vascular events is 25 percent. The *absolute* reduction varies considerably depending on the particular patient's risk. Individuals at very low risk for stroke seem to experience the same relative reduction, but their risk may be so low that the "benefit" is meaningless. On the other hand, someone with a 10 to 15 percent risk per year can reduce the risk to between 7.5 and 11 percent.

Aspirin is inexpensive, can be given in low doses as infrequently as every other day, and could be recommended for all adults to prevent both stroke and myocardial infarction. However, it causes adverse effects including epigastric discomfort, gastric ulceration, and gastrointestinal hemorrhage. The gastric bleeding may be asymptomatic and detectable only by regular stool examinations. A life-threatening hemorrhage may occur without warning. Consequently, not every 20- or 30-year-old should be advised to take aspirin regularly because the risk of atherothrombotic stroke is extremely low and is outweighed by the risk of adverse side effects. Conversely, every patient who has experienced an atherothrombotic stroke and has no contraindication should be taking an antiplatelet agent regularly because the average annual risk of another stroke is 8 to 10 percent, and another few percent will experience a myocardial infarction or vascular death. In this setting, the likelihood of benefit far outweighs the risks of treatment.

The choice of antiplatelet agent, and dose, similarly must balance the risk of stroke against the benefit, risk, and cost of the treatments. These data are less definitive, and opinions therefore vary. Many authorities believe low-dose (30 to 75 mg daily) and high-dose (650 to 1300 mg daily) aspirin are equally effective. Most physicians in North America recommend 325 to 1300 mg daily, while most Europeans recommend 30 to 325 mg. Similarly, the choice of aspirin or ticlopidine must balance the fact that ticlopidine is more effective than aspirin but the cost and risk of adverse effects are higher.

ANTICOAGULATION THERAPY The role of anticoagulation in atherothrombotic cerebral disease is uncertain. Four randomized prospective studies comparing anticoagulant-treated patients with TIA to controls showed no significant difference in the incidence of stroke or death in the two groups. All of these early randomized trials involved inadequate numbers of patients to provide definitive results.

Heparin is widely used for "unstable TIA" (i.e., crescendo or recent-onset TIA). There are almost no data from controlled studies regarding the systematic use of heparin for these patients. It has been largely for theoretical reasons, and by extrapolation from the results of studies of anticoagulation for progressing stroke and myocardial infarction, that anticoagulation is used.

In progressing stroke, the focal ischemia worsens over several hours or a day or two. Progressing stroke is common; approximately 20 percent of carotid territory strokes, and a higher percentage of posterior circulation strokes, progress. For example, a few hours after the onset of a stroke a patient may appear to have a stable deficit such as a mild aphasia and right hemiparesis, but the following morning a severe aphasia and right hemiplegia are noted. It is difficult to predict or monitor for progression; thus many physicians heparinize all patients with recent mild ischemic stroke in order to prevent some of the worsening that will occur in 20 percent. Results of a recent small randomized, controlled trial of heparin for the prevention of progression in acute partial thrombotic stroke did not support the use of heparin. Nevertheless, heparin continues to be used for many of these patients. The bleeding complication rate for 7 days of heparin is about 10 percent, with a serious bleed rate of about 2 percent. Clearly the value of this approach must be clarified.

A recent study found a substantial reduction in death and disability from acute ischemic stroke with a new low-molecular-weight heparin, nadroparin, administered subcutaneously for 10 days. Confirmation will be required before the results are accepted and widely applied. The International Stroke Trial (IST) and Trial of Organon 10172 in Acute Stroke Treatment (TOAST) are two large trials currently addressing the role of heparin and a low-molecular-weight heparinoid in acute ischemic stroke.

When used, heparinization generally is accomplished by giving 3000 to 5000 units of heparin intravenously, followed with 600 to 1000 units per hour by intravenous drip infusion, monitored to maintain the activated partial thromboplastin time at approximately twice normal. This regimen is maintained for 2 to 5 days. During this time the patient is monitored for hemorrhagic complications and a decision is made regarding the need for carotid endarterectomy and long-term warfarin or antiplatelet therapy. If long-term anticoagulation is chosen, warfarin is administered. When the international normalized ratio (INR) (see Chap. 119) is about 3.0, the heparin is discontinued.

There also are few data to support the use of long-term warfarin for preventing atherothrombotic stroke. Two large trials in progress, The Stroke Prevention in Reversible Ischemia Trial (SPIRIT) and The Warfarin Aspirin Recurrent Stroke Study (WARSS), should clarify the role of anticoagulation in the prevention and progression of ischemic stroke. It may be some time before data become available to decide the optimal preventive treatment for specific groups of patients at risk.

SURGICAL THERAPY Surgery for atherosclerotic occlusive disease is largely limited to *carotid endarterectomy* for plaques located at the origin of the internal carotid artery in the neck. About 100,000 carotid endarterectomies are done annually in the United States. Surgery in the proximal common carotid, the subclavian, and the vertebral arteries is uncommon. Anastomosing extracranial scalp arteries to major intracranial arteries to bypass inoperable obstructions in the internal carotid artery is of no value.

Carotid endarterectomy is valuable for some individuals with carotid stenosis, but not all. The benefits vary greatly, depending on the clinical profiles of the patients and the operative complication rates of the surgeons. In many communities the perioperative stroke and death rates are as high as 6 to 8 percent and 1 to 3 percent respectively, in which case the operation is not beneficial.

1. *Symptomatic patients.* Both the NASCET and the European Carotid Surgery Trial (ECST) showed a substantial benefit for surgery in patients with a symptomatic carotid artery stenosis of greater than 70 percent. In NASCET, the average cumulative ipsilateral stroke rate at 2 years was 26 percent for patients treated medically and 9 percent for those receiving the same medical treatment plus a carotid endarterectomy, corresponding to a 65 percent *relative* risk reduction favoring surgery. For every 100 patients treated surgically, 17 were spared an ipsilateral stroke over the next 2 years. The perioperative stroke plus death rate was 5.8 percent in the surgical group and 3.3 percent in the medical group in the same 1-month period, in spite of optimal medical therapy. Thus the excess morbidity and mortality attributable to the surgery was 2.5 percent. If minor ischemic events are excluded from the analyses, the excess major stroke and death rate for the surgical patients was 1.2 percent (2.1 less 0.9 percent) and the excess fatality rate was 0.3 percent (0.6 less 0.3 percent). The NASCET and ECST investigators concluded that their patients with a 70 to 99 percent stenosis clearly benefited from carotid endarterectomy. Results in community hospitals should be similar if patients are properly selected and the perioperative morbidity and mortality are comparably low.

Analysis of several subgroups yielded important information. The cumulative risk of ipsilateral stroke correlated with the degree of stenosis. While the absolute risk reduction favoring the entire surgical group was 17 percent in NASCET, the risk reduction favoring those with a 90 to 99 percent stenosis was 26 percent, and this decreased to 12 percent for those with a 70 to 79 percent stenosis. The overall 26 percent cumulative risk of an ipsilateral stroke at 2 years for this group of patients with "high-grade" stenosis calculates to an annual risk of 13 percent. The operative morbidity and mortality were similar for patients with different degrees of stenosis.

The presence of retinal versus hemispheric symptoms, degree of arterial stenosis, extent of associated medical conditions, surgical morbidity and mortality in the patients' institution, and other factors are all important in estimating an individual patient's risk of stroke and therefore magnitude of benefit from surgery. A patient with multiple atherosclerosis risk factors, symptomatic hemispheric ischemia, very high grade stenosis in the appropriate internal carotid artery, and an institutional perioperative morbidity and mortality rate of less than 6 percent generally should undergo carotid endarterectomy. The spontaneous risk of stroke is much higher than the operative risk, and surgery confers a long-term benefit. On the other hand, a patient with few atherosclerosis risk factors, an asymptomatic moderate-grade stenosis in one internal carotid artery, and an institutional perioperative morbidity and mortality rate of 6 percent should not undergo carotid endarterectomy (see below).

In summary, it is now clear that about one in four recently symptomatic patients with a high-grade carotid stenosis will have an ipsilateral stroke in the next 2 years, even while receiving good risk factor management and aspirin. These patients clearly will benefit from carotid endarterectomy, provided it is done by a surgeon with proven good results. However, there are patients within this ≥70 percent stenosis group whose risk of stroke, and risk of surgical complications, is substantially higher or lower than the group's average.

The ECST additionally showed that patients with a 0 to 29 percent stenosis have a low risk of ipsilateral stroke and are not helped by surgery. The value of carotid endarterectomy for patients with a 30 to 69 percent carotid stenosis remains uncertain, and the NASCET and ECST are continuing to study this group.

2. *Asymptomatic patients.* The Asymptomatic Carotid Atherosclerosis Study (ACAS) demonstrated that asymptomatic people with internal carotid artery stenoses greater than 60 percent are at low risk for stroke. More than 1600 patients were randomized to treatment with the best medical therapies available versus the same medical treatment plus carotid endarterectomy. Patients in the nonsurgical group had a risk over 5 years for ipsilateral stroke (and any perioperative stroke or death) of 5.1 percent, whereas the risk for the nonsurgical group was 11 percent. While this demonstrates a 53 percent *relative* risk reduction, the *absolute* risk reduction is only 5.9 percent over 5 years, or 1.2 percent annually. If only major strokes and death are counted, the comparable numbers are 43 percent relative risk reduction, and an absolute risk reduction of only 2.6 percent over 5 years, or 0.5 percent annually. This latter result was not statistically significant. There was no clear difference in benefit for those with moderate (60 to 80 percent) compared with severe (80 to 99 percent) stenosis.

Many of the strokes in the surgery group were caused by preoperative angiograms. If carotid artery ultrasonography and MR angiography replace catheter angiography, this morbidity and mortality will be obviated.

While there are benefits for carotid endarterectomy in patients with asymptomatic carotid stenosis, the benefits are very small. Medical therapy for reduction of atherosclerosis risk factors in addition to aspirin (325 mg/d) generally are recommended for patients with asymptomatic carotid stenosis.

3. *Conclusions.* From a public health point of view, it is important to consider the magnitude of any benefits demonstrated in clinical trials, particularly if the intervention is costly. In the NASCET, there was a 17 percent absolute reduction in ipsilateral stroke, meaning that six endarterectomies need to be performed in order to prevent one ipsilateral stroke. There was a 10.1 percent

absolute reduction in the most significant outcomes of major stroke and death, meaning that 10 operations need to be performed in order to prevent 1 of these disasters. Most people probably find these trade-offs acceptable. However, at some point the cost may become too high. In the ACAS, surgery reduced the absolute risk of stroke by only 1.2 percent annually; thus 85 endarterectomies need to be performed to prevent 1 stroke annually in a group of patients with these characteristics. The same calculation for preventing 1 major or fatal stroke annually would require that 192 endarterectomies be performed.

As the average carotid endarterectomy in the United States likely costs more than $15,000, and about 100,000 are done annually, the total cost to the nation is about $1.5 billion. At some level, these costs must be considered in decisions regarding treatment of this common disease. Obviously, the higher the expected event rate and the lower the surgical morbidity, the fewer the number of patients who need to be treated to prevent one event. Additionally, the more serious the event and the cheaper the treatment, the greater the overall benefits.

Finally, the results of the carotid endarterectomy trials emphasize the fact that carotid artery disease is a marker for cardiovascular disease. One-half to two-thirds of all deaths in these patients are due to heart disease, and a much smaller proportion are due to stroke (about 5 percent in asymptomatic patients and nearly 20 percent in symptomatic patients). This is despite appropriate treatment for atherosclerotic risk factors and with aspirin. The optimal cardiac evaluation and management of these patients has not been determined.

ANGIOPLASTY Angioplasty is an experimental procedure in the prevention of stroke.

Acute Management ***GENERAL PRINCIPLES*** When cerebral infarction occurs, the immediate goal is to optimize cerebral perfusion of the ischemic area. Also, attention is directed toward preventing the common complications of bedridden patients, namely, infections (pneumonia, urinary tract, and skin) and deep venous thrombosis with pulmonary embolism.

Elevated blood pressure should not be lowered unless there is malignant hypertension (see Chap. 246). If the blood pressure is low, raising it is advisable. Fever is detrimental and should be avoided.

Between 5 and 10 percent of patients develop symptomatic cerebral edema, resulting in obtundation with its attendant consequences or brain herniation. Edema peaks on the second or third day but causes mass effect for 10 days. The larger the infarct, the more likely edema will be a problem. Even small amounts of edema from a cerebellar stroke can raise intracranial pressure in the posterior fossa. The resulting brainstem compression may result in coma and respiratory arrest requiring emergency surgical decompression. Restriction of free water and intravenous mannitol may be used to raise the serum osmolarity. Intravascular volume should be maintained.

Other treatments for cerebral ischemia-infarction have not been proved beneficial. These include use of mannitol and low-molecular-weight dextran to lower blood viscosity, vasodilating agents to increase cerebral blood flow, hypothermia and barbiturates to decrease the metabolic demands of ischemic tissue, and hyperoxygenation to reduce hypoxic damage.

THROMBOLYSIS The role of thrombolysis in acute cerebral infarction is not entirely clear. Several studies have shown that occlusions in arteries appropriate to the symptoms are very frequently found if angiography is carried out within a few hours of acute infarction. It is this association of atherothromboembolic arterial occlusion with acute neurologic symptoms that prompted the use of thrombolytic agents in stroke patients. In 1992, a meta-analysis reviewed the 60 published reports of thrombolytic therapy for stroke. It was not possible to conclude anything about benefit or safety because there were no controls. Nevertheless, the overall recanalization rate at 24 h reported in these limited studies was about 60 percent, as compared to the spontaneous rate of 20 percent. These results were encouraging, if tentative.

Three recent trials of streptokinase were stopped because of safety concerns in the streptokinase-treated patients. The death rate was higher in the thrombolysis groups, mainly due to symptomatic intracranial bleeds. In one trial, there was a significant increase in death and disability at 3 months, whereas in another moderate disability was reduced in a selected subgroup of patients.

The European Cooperative Acute Stroke Study (ECASS) reported results of a randomized trial using intravenous recombinant tissue plasminogen activator (rt-PA), alteplase, (1.1 mg/kg to a 100-mg maximum; 10 percent as a bolus, then the remainder over 60 min) versus placebo in patients with ischemic stroke within 6 h of onset. The median time to treatment was 4 h. Overall, thrombolysis was not beneficial because of an excess of cerebral hemorrhage. However, in those patients who had no signs of major infarction on the initial CT scan the functional outcome was improved. The investigators emphasized that identification of this subgroup is difficult and depends on recognition of early CT findings of major infarction.

The National Institute of Neurological Disorders and Stroke (NINDS) rt-PA Stroke Study showed a clear benefit for rt-PA in selected patients with acute stroke. The NINDS rt-PA trial used intravenous rt-PA alteplase (0.9 mg/kg to a 90-mg maximum; 10 percent as a bolus, then the remainder over 60 min) versus placebo in patients with ischemic stroke within 3 h of onset. Symptomatic intracerebral hemorrhage occurred in 6.4 percent of patients on rt-PA and 0.6 percent on placebo. There was a 4 percent reduction in mortality on rt-PA (21 percent on placebo and 17 percent on rt-PA), and a 12 percent increase in the number of patients with only minimal disability (32 percent on placebo and 44 percent on rt-PA). Thus, despite an increased incidence of symptomatic intracerebral hemorrhage, treatment with intravenous rt-PA within 3 h of the onset of ischemic stroke improved clinical outcome. A lower dose of rt-PA was used than in ECASS, and half of the patients were treated within 90 min of stroke onset and the other half between 90 and 180 min. These two features may account for much of the increase in benefit and decrease in bleeding hazard compared to the results seen in ECASS.

It seems clear that thrombolysis works. However, the therapeutic window is narrow, and the selection of patients and timing and dose of drug are key determinants of the therapeutic response. Thrombolysis should only be administered using the strict protocol of the NINDS rt-PA study, with adequate protection of patients by full disclosure of the possible risks. Additional trials in progress will further clarify the overall role for thrombolysis in acute ischemic stroke.

REHABILITATION Rehabilitation of the stroke patient is important, and it includes early physical, occupational, and speech therapy. It is directed toward educating the patient and family about the patient's neurologic deficit, preventing the complications of immobility (e.g., pneumonia, pressure sores of the skin, muscle contractures), and providing encouragement and instruction in overcoming the deficit.

CEREBRAL EMBOLISM

PATHOPHYSIOLOGY OF CARDIOGENIC CEREBRAL EMBOLISM Cardioembolism causes about 15 percent of all strokes. Stroke caused by heart disease is primarily due to embolism of thrombotic material forming on the atrial or ventricular wall or the left heart valves. These thrombi then detach and embolize into the arterial circulation where they may fragment or lyse, and the circulation may be restored quickly. Alternatively, the arterial occlusion may be permanent, and thrombosis distal to the obstruction may occur with consequent disruption of the distal collateral circulation.

Emboli from the heart most often lodge in the middle cerebral artery or one of its branches. They infrequently cause infarcts in the anterior cerebral artery territory. Emboli large enough to occlude the stem of the middle cerebral artery (3 to 4 mm) lead to a large stroke that involves both deep gray and white matter and some portions of the cortical surface and its underlying white matter. A smaller embolus may occlude a small cortical or penetrating arterial branch. The location and size of an infarct also depend on the extent of the spared collateral circulation.

Cardiogenic cerebral embolism is presumed to have occurred when cardiac arrhythmias or structural abnormalities are found or known to be present. The commonest causes of cardioembolic stroke are nonrheumatic (often called nonvalvular) atrial fibrillation (AF), myocardial infarction, prosthetic valves, rheumatic heart disease (RHD), and ischemic cardiopathy (see Table 366-4). Many clinical trials in recent years have evaluated treatments for stroke prevention in nonrheumatic AF. A smaller number of good studies in the treatment of prosthetic heart valves and myocardial infarction have been done. Most of the other conditions causing cardioembolic stroke have been less well studied.

Nonrheumatic AF is the commonest cause of cerebral embolism. Patients with AF have an average annual risk of stroke of about 5 percent. However, the risk varies according to the presence of certain risk factors, including old age, hypertension, poor left ventricular function, prior cardioembolism, and diabetes mellitus. Patients less than 60 years of age with none of these risk factors have an annual risk for stroke of about 0.5 percent. Those with most of these risks have a rate of about 15 percent. The presumed stroke mechanism is thrombus formation in the fibrillating atrium or atrial appendage, with subsequent embolization.

Recent *myocardial infarction*, especially when transmural and involving the anteroapical ventricular wall, is an important risk for embolus, particularly in the first few weeks.

Cardiomyopathies with poor left ventricular function are frequently associated with left ventricular thrombus formation.

Prosthetic heart valves, especially mechanical ones, are a common cause of cerebral embolism.

RHD usually causes ischemic stroke when there is prominent mitral stenosis or AF; left atrial enlargement and congestive heart failure are further risk factors for formation of atrial thrombi.

Mitral valve prolapse can be a source of emboli. This common disorder probably causes cerebral embolism only when severe.

Congenital septal defects are associated with cerebral embolism. Usually they are major defects, but a small foramen ovale or septal aneurysm may occasionally be causative. It is presumed that the deep peripheral venous system is usually the source of *paradoxical emboli*. Transesophageal and bubble echocardiographic techniques can demonstrate a patent foramen ovale. Other causes, such as fat and tumor in

Table 366-4

Causes of Cardiogenic Cerebral Embolism

Dysrhythmia
   Atrial fibrillation, sick sinus syndrome
Coronary heart disease
   Myocardial infarction
   Ischemic cardiomyopathy
Rheumatic heart disease
   Mitral stenosis with or without atrial fibrillation
Other
   Nonischemic cardiomyopathies
   Prosthetic valve
   Congenital heart disease: patent foramen ovale, mitral valve prolapse, etc.
   Septic endocarditis
   Mitral annulus calcification
   Atrial myxoma
   Fat emboli
   Nonbacterial thrombotic endocarditis
   Hypercoagulable states: cancer, systemic diseases, oral contraceptives

the blood, marantic endocarditis, and air and amniotic fluid emboli associated with parturition, may occasionally be responsible.

Infectious endocarditis (see Chap. 126) causes vegetations that give rise to multiple septic emboli. The appearance of multifocal or diffuse symptoms and signs in a patient with stroke should raise the possibility of underlying bacterial endocarditis. Infarcts may be microscopic in size or large, and septic emboli may produce brain abscess, mycotic aneurysms, and subarachnoid hemorrhage (SAH) or intracerebral hemorrhage.

Nonbacterial thrombotic (marantic) endocarditis, mitral annulus calcification, chronic sinoatrial disorder, systemic lupus erythematosus (Libman-Sacks vegetations), atrial myxoma, and thrombus in a pulmonary vein also increase the risk of cerebral embolism.

PATHOLOGY Cerebral infarcts may be pale (nonhemorrhagic) or red (hemorrhagic). Vascular congestion of varying degree is common in all infarcts, but extravasation of blood is usually associated with embolic infarcts. Because emboli migrate and lyse, recirculation into the infarcted brain may cause petechial hemorrhages. Sometimes there is enough seepage of blood into the infarct to cause visible *hemorrhagic infarction* on a CT scan. *Hemorrhagic transformation* of a pale infarct typically occurs from 12 to 36 h after embolization and is often asymptomatic. Frank hemorrhage into the infarct almost always causes clinical worsening. This is more likely to occur when the stem of the middle cerebral artery is occluded and a large infarct develops in the territory of the lenticulostriate arteries before recirculation occurs.

Infarcts in the distribution of small, penetrating arteries ultimately leave small cavities or lacunes (lacunar infarcts), whereas major arterial occlusions may produce a wide area of necrosis that ultimately leaves a large, fluid-filled cavity in the brain.

Edema invariably accompanies the tissue necrosis. In small infarcts it may be relatively insignificant. In large infarcts, however, massive edema compresses adjacent tissue and adds to the ischemic process; it also increases intracranial pressure and may cause herniation of the brain from one intracranial compartment to another.

CLINICAL MANIFESTATIONS An embolus to the brain usually causes the sudden onset of a focal neurologic deficit that is maximum at the onset. Deficits correspond to the areas of cerebral cortex supplied by the affected artery and resemble those caused by occlusive atheromatous lesions (see sections on atherothrombosis and lacunar stroke). Certain neurologic syndromes suggest embolism as their cause. In the middle cerebral artery territory these include the following: (1) the frontal opercular syndrome, in which there is facial weakness and severe aphasia or dysarthria; (2) the brachial or hand plegia syndrome, in which the arm or hand is paralyzed, with or without cortical sensory abnormalities; (3) Broca's or Wernicke's aphasia alone; or (4) left visual neglect, when the nondominant parietal lobe is involved. Sudden hemianopia suggests a posterior cerebral artery embolus, and sudden foot and shoulder weakness suggests an anterior cerebral artery embolus. Sudden sleepiness and inability to look up associated with bilateral ptosis suggest an embolus to the top of the basilar artery, specifically to the artery of Percheron (the small artery supplying both sides of the medial subthalamus and thalamus arising from the top of the basilar artery).

Seizures at the time of stroke occur in 3 to 5 percent of infarctions. They occur more often after embolism than thrombosis. They usually are associated with supratentorial cortical surface infarctions. Another 3 to 5 percent of patients develop epilepsy from 6 to 18 months after their stroke. Many cases of idiopathic epilepsy in the elderly are probably the result of silent cortical infarction.

LABORATORY AND IMAGING EVALUATION Although early CT scanning is usually negative in the first several hours after an embolic stroke, it excludes hemorrhage. Later it visualizes the location and extent of infarction, and it can support the diagnosis of embolism by demonstrating hemorrhagic infarction or multiple infarcts. However, embolic injury may appear as a single low-density area compatible with pale infarction. Petechial hemorrhages within the area may not visualize as increased tissue density because when superimposed on the low-density infarct, the average tissue density is near that of normal brain. MRI scanning is the most sensitive method to detect embolic infarction.

A thorough cardiac evaluation should be undertaken when embolism is suspected, including young patients and those with a history of heart disease, multifocal or hemorrhagic infarcts, or seizures at onset. Continuous ECG monitoring may demonstrate an intermittent arrhythmia. An echocardiogram may disclose mitral valve disease, an intracardiac thrombus or tumor, and akinetic myocardium. Transesophageal and bubble echocardiography can demonstrate a patent foramen ovale.

In patients with myocardial infarction, the clinical and ECG findings, together with echocardiography, may identify those patients with large anteroapical infarcts, ventricular aneurysms, mural thrombi, and other factors that predispose to peripheral embolism.

Cerebral angiography is rarely indicated. When performed in the first day or two it often shows occlusion of one or more vessels. Complete lysis of emboli often occurs, and angiography performed after several days may be normal.

CSF obtained immediately after a cerebral embolism is usually normal. The presence of more than a few white or red blood cells makes bacterial endocarditis more likely.

℞ TREATMENT

Treatment of patients with embolic infarction consists of managing the stroke itself, in both the acute and chronic phases, and of preventing further emboli.

Prevention Virtually every type of cardiac disease is associated with increased risk for stroke, and the best treatment for cerebral embolism is prevention. Consequently, prophylactic treatment of patients with thrombus-prone heart disease is indicated.

ANTICOAGULATION THERAPY Several recent clinical trials demonstrated that anticoagulation (INR of 2.0 to 3.0) in patients with chronic nonvalvular (nonrheumatic) AF prevents cerebral embolism and is safe. Anticoagulation with warfarin reduces the risk by about 65 percent and is generally recommended for these patients.

Anticoagulation also reduces the risk of embolism in acute myocardial infarction. Most clinicians recommend anticoagulation when there is substantial left ventricular dysfunction or a major, focal wall-motion abnormality.

Patients with prominent RHD are at risk of systemic embolism and should be anticoagulated indefinitely. This category includes mitral stenosis, a large left atrium, congestive heart failure, AF, and echocardiographically demonstrated atrial thrombi. Whether the benefit of long-term anticoagulation outweighs the risk in patients with lesser degrees of RHD is unclear.

Thromboembolism has been recognized as one of the most serious complications of prosthetic heart valve implantation since the procedure became feasible in 1960. Anticoagulation with warfarin has been proven effective for preventing strokes in this situation, while antiplatelet therapy alone has not; concomitant therapy with aspirin adds substantially to the beneficial effect of warfarin prophylaxis. Higher intensities of anticoagulation (INR of 3.5) are recommended for prosthetic heart valve patients compared to those with AF.

ANTIPLATELET AGENTS Warfarin is more effective than aspirin in preventing ischemic stroke associated with AF. However, some patients with AF have a low rate of ischemic stroke and do not need warfarin. Others have a high risk of hemorrhage and thus lose the benefit of anticoagulation. Still others are at such high risk for ischemic stroke that the benefits of warfarin override even the high hemorrhage rate. The use of any preventive treatment is based upon the relative risks and benefits for a particular patient.

Three clinical trials conducted in recent years systematically compared aspirin to placebo for prevention of cerebral infarction in patients with nonrheumatic AF. In aggregate, they showed about a 25 percent relative reduction in stroke with aspirin, compared to the reduction by warfarin of 65 percent. Still, not every patient with AF requires treatment with warfarin to prevent stroke. The Stroke Prevention in Atrial Fibrillation II trial showed that in low-risk patients (those without hypertension, recent heart failure, or prior thromboembolism) younger than 75 years old given aspirin, the thromboembolism rate was only 0.5 percent per year. Consequently, one could reasonably recommend that patients younger than 75 years old with no risk factors be treated with aspirin only.

Acute Management The acute management is basically the same as for thrombotic infarction. If the indications are appropriate, the patient should receive thrombolytic therapy. Since the embolic source generally persists at least temporarily, these patients are at substantial risk for early reembolization. For most of the causes, the risk is about 0.5 to 1 percent daily for the first week or two. Consequently, prompt anticoagulation is desirable. However, heparin is generally avoided for about a week when the infarct is large, as the risk of serious hemorrhage increases with increasing infarct size. It is also avoided if bacterial endocarditis is likely. The duration of anticoagulation is determined by the causative heart lesion and its associated continuing risk of future embolization. If the embolic source is self-limited or treatable, anticoagulation should be discontinued when the high-risk period has passed. For myocardial infarction, this is after 2 or 3 months; for a reversible cardiomyopathy it may be several weeks after cardiac function has recovered. After conversion of nonvalvular AF, the high-risk period may comprise the few weeks after the appearance of a stable sinus rhythm.

Generally, if the embolic source cannot be eliminated, anticoagulation should be continued indefinitely. This includes any patient with RHD, even if the mitral valve is replaced or the AF is successfully converted to normal sinus rhythm. It also includes the patient who has had one or more systemic emboli and who has nonvalvular AF, persistent cardiomyopathy with chronic ventricular failure, and, possibly, severe mitral valve prolapse.

OTHER CAUSES OF CEREBRAL INFARCTION

Dissection of the Cervicocerebral Arteries Dissection of the large extracranial arteries may cause cerebral infarction and is a frequent cause of stroke in children and young adults. A small tear in the intima allows blood to dissect into the media of the artery or separate the intima from the media. TIAs and infarction occur when the artery is critically narrowed or occluded or when thromboembolism results. Trauma, either severe or trivial, accounts for most cases.

The internal carotid artery high in the neck is the most common site. There are usually pain in the ipsilateral neck, face, or head and an oculosympathetic palsy (partial Horner's syndrome). A self-audible bruit may appear, and tenderness over the upper neck may be present. Dissection of a vertebral artery may produce posterior lateralized neck pain, accompanied by signs of lateral medullary ischemia or other brainstem syndromes.

TIAs, or TMB in carotid dissections, often precede infarction, leaving time for therapeutic intervention. When the patient has only oculosympathetic palsy, TIAs, or a minor stroke, anticoagulation with heparin is recommended. After the patient's symptoms have stabilized, anticoagulation with warfarin is recommended for 4 months. MR angiography with MRI of the dissection site often makes the diagnosis. X-ray angiography is sometimes required. Repeat imaging in 6 to 10 weeks often demonstrates a reestablished lumen in the formerly occluded vessel.

Fibromuscular Dysplasia Fibromuscular dysplasia rarely causes stroke. It affects the cervical arteries and occurs mainly in women. The carotid or vertebral arteries show multiple rings of segmental narrowing alternating with dilatation. Occlusion is usually incomplete. The process is often asymptomatic but occasionally is associated with an audible bruit, TIAs, or stroke. The cause and natural history of fibromuscular dysplasia is unknown (see Chap. 248). TIA or stroke generally occurs only when the artery is severely narrowed. Anticoagulation or antiplatelet therapy may be helpful.

Temporal Arteritis (Giant Cell Arteritis) This is a relatively common affliction of mainly elderly persons in which the external carotid system, particularly the temporal arteries, is the site of a subacute granulomatous inflammation with giant cells (Chap. 319). Occlusion of posterior choroidal branches of the ophthalmic artery results in blindness in one or both eyes in many patients. It rarely causes stroke.

Other Arteritides Arteritis due to bacterial or syphilitic infection is no longer a common cause of cerebral thrombosis in developed countries. Other arteritides are rare but can cause cerebral thrombosis (see below and Chaps. 312 and 319). Necrotizing or granulomatous arteritis, occurring alone or in association with generalized polyarteritis nodosa or Wegener's granulomatosis, involves the distal small branches (<2 mm diameter) of the main intracranial arteries and produces small ischemic infarcts in the brain, optic nerve, and spinal cord. The CSF often has inflammatory changes. Idiopathic giant cell arteritis involving the great vessels arising from the aortic arch (Takayasu's syndrome) may, on rare occasions, cause carotid or vertebral thrombosis. It is an infrequent cause of the aortic arch syndrome in the western hemisphere (see Chap. 319).

Moyamoya Disease Moyamoya disease is a poorly understood occlusive disease involving large intracranial arteries, especially the distal internal carotid artery and the stem of the middle and anterior cerebral arteries. The lenticulostriate arteries develop a rich collateral circulation around the middle cerebral occlusive lesion that on angiography gives the impression of a puff of smoke (*moyamoya*). Other collaterals include transdural anastomoses between the cortical surface branches of the middle cerebral artery and the scalp arteries. The disease mainly occurs in Asian children or young adults. Its etiology is unknown. Because of the occurrence of SAH from rupture of the transdural anastomotic channels, anticoagulation is risky.

Hypercoagulable States Certain diseases have been associated with ischemic infarction through a mechanism of a hypercoagulable state (see Chaps. 117 and 118). They include polycythemia vera, thrombotic thrombocytopenic purpura, idiopathic thrombocytosis, hyperproteinemia, sickle cell anemia, and inherited clotting abnormalities, e.g., protein C deficiency. Circulating antiphospholipid antibodies (including "lupus anticoagulants") have been associated with stroke in young adults.

Reversible Segmental Vasoconstriction Reversible, widespread cerebral segmental vasoconstriction occurs in patients with headache and fluctuating neurologic symptoms and signs. Sometimes cerebral infarction ensues. The cause is unknown. Head injury, migraine, sympathomimetic intoxication, eclampsia, and the postpartum period have all been associated with this entity. Angiography is the only means of establishing the diagnosis. The CSF is usually normal, but an elevated protein and slight lymphocytic pleocytosis occur. No effective therapy is known. Maintenance of normal systemic arterial pressure with adequate hydration seems prudent. Glucocorticoids and vasodilators may be considered.

Binswanger's Disease Binswanger's disease (diffuse white matter disease) is a rare condition in which infarction of the subcortical white matter occurs subacutely (see Chap. 367). CT or MRI scan detects periventricular areas of white matter disruption and gliosis. There is lipohyalinosis in the small arteries of the deep white matter, as in hypertension. There are usually associated lacunar infarcts. Binswanger's disease may represent a type of border-zone ischemic infarction in the deep white matter between the penetrating arteries of the circle of Willis and cortical vessels. The pathophysiologic basis of the disease is unclear, but it typically occurs in older patients with severe long-standing hypertension.

Oral Contraceptive Agents Oral contraceptives are associated with an increased incidence of stroke in young women, but the incidence is minimal unless there is associated hypertension, cigarette smoking, or migraine. Hypercoagulability may be the mechanism predisposing to thrombosis.

Venous Thrombosis Lateral or sagittal sinus thrombosis, or thrombosis of small cortical veins, occurs as a complication of pregnancy and the postpartum period, sepsis, intracranial infections (meningitis), and hypercoagulable states such as polycythemia and sickle cell anemia. Venous thrombosis may cause an increase in intracranial pressure, headaches, focal seizures, and infarction primarily affecting the parasagittal cortex. Paraparesis is common. Massive venous infarction with secondary edema may be fatal. The CT and MR scans show hemorrhagic infarction underlying the occluded veins and may show thrombus in the involved veins and sinuses. MR angiography makes the diagnosis. Because the primary abnormality is thrombosis, anticoagulation is recommended unless hemorrhage is prominent.

℞ TREATMENT

Anticoagulation is often recommended as preventive treatment in patients with extracranial cervicocerebral artery dissection, severe mitral valve prolapse, antiphospholipid antibody syndrome, cortical vein–dural sinus thrombosis, and other situations associated with stroke. It will be difficult to obtain definitive information about the proper preventive treatment of many of these conditions. Arterial dissections provide an example of the difficulty. Even if the stroke rate were as high as 5 percent after initiating treatment of a cervical dissection, a sample size of approximately 1600 patients would be required to compare two treatments with an 80 percent chance of detecting a 50 percent reduction in events ($\alpha = 0.05$; 2-tailed). It seems unlikely that such a definitive randomized trial will be carried out to evaluate the value of anticoagulation or any other treatment.

Antiplatelet therapy also is often recommended for patients with extracranial cervicocerebral artery dissection, mitral valve prolapse, vasculitis, and other conditions associated with arterial thromboembolism; definitive trials have not been conducted for any of these indications.

INTRACEREBRAL HEMORRHAGE

Intracerebral hemorrhage is the most common type of nontraumatic intracranial hemorrhage (Table 366-5). It is an important cause of stroke, especially in Asians and blacks. Hypertension and cerebral amyloid angiopathy cause the majority of these hemorrhages. Advanced age and heavy alcohol consumption increase the risk. Cocaine-induced hemorrhage is one of the most important causes in the young.

HYPERTENSIVE INTRACEREBRAL HEMORRHAGE Pathophysiology and Pathology Intracerebral hemorrhage usually results from spontaneous rupture of a small penetrating artery deep in the brain. The most common sites are (1) the basal ganglia (putamen, thalamus, and adjacent deep white matter), (2) the deep cerebellum, and (3) the pons. When hemorrhages occur in other brain areas or in nonhypertensive patients, greater consideration should be given to hemorrhagic disorders, neoplasms, and other causes. The small arteries in these areas seem most prone to hypertension-induced vascular injury. The leak may be small, or a large clot may form and compress adjacent tissue, causing herniation and death. Rupture or seepage into the ventricular system often occurs. Primary intraventricular hemorrhage is rare. If the patient survives, the clot liquefies, is absorbed, and leaves only a small residual cleft.

Most hypertensive intracerebral hemorrhages develop over 30 to 90 min, whereas those associated with anticoagulant therapy may evolve for as long as 24 to 48 h. Once bleeding stops, it generally

Table 366-5

Causes of Intracranial Hemorrhage

Spontaneous intracerebral hemorrhage	Ruptured arteriovenous malformation
Hypertensive	Cocaine, amphetamines
Amyloid angiopathy	Trauma (see Chap. 374)
Ruptured aneurysm	Bleeding with brain tumors
Saccular	Systemic bleeding disorders, including anticoagulation therapy
Mycotic	Hemorrhagic infarction

Table 366-6

CHAPTER 366
Cerebrovascular Diseases

2343

Common Symptoms and Signs of Intracerebral Hemorrhage

Location	Neurologic Signs
Basal ganglia	Contralateral hemiparesis, hemisensory loss, and homonymous hemianopia
	Aphasia with dominant hemisphere
	Conjugate deviation of eyes downward or toward the side of the hematoma
	Obtundation, stupor, or coma
Cerebellum	Vomiting and ataxia
	Skew deviation of eyes and small pupils
	Deviation of eyes toward the opposite side
	Obtundation, late-developing stupor, or coma
Pons	Abrupt onset of coma
	Pinpoint, reactive pupils
	Skew deviation of eyes and gaze paresis
	Decerebration or flaccidity
	Ataxic respiration

does not start again. Within 48 h macrophages begin to phagocytize the hemorrhage at its outer surface. After 1 to 6 months, the hemorrhage is generally resolved to a slitlike orange cavity lined with glial scar and hemosiderin-laden macrophages.

Clinical Manifestations Although not particularly associated with exertion, intracerebral hemorrhages almost always occur while the patient is awake and sometimes when stressed. The clinical presentation is generally that of an abrupt onset of a focal neurologic deficit that typically worsens steadily over 30 to 90 min. The common clinical presentations are shown in Table 366-6.

The putamen is the most common site for hypertensive hemorrhage, and the adjacent internal capsule is invariably damaged. Contralateral hemiparesis is therefore the sentinel sign. When mild, the face sags on one side, speech becomes slurred, the arm and leg gradually weaken, and the eyes deviate away from the side of the hemiparesis. The paralysis may worsen until the affected limbs become flaccid or extend rigidly with a Babinski sign on the same side. When hemorrhages are large, drowsiness gives way to stupor as signs of upper brainstem compression appear. Coma ensues, accompanied by deep, irregular, or intermittent respiration; a dilated and fixed ipsilateral pupil; bilateral Babinski signs; and decerebrate rigidity. In milder cases, edema in adjacent brain tissue may cause progressive deterioration over 12 to 72 h.

Thalamic hemorrhages also produce a hemiplegia or hemiparesis from pressure on, or dissection into, the adjacent internal capsule. A prominent sensory deficit involving all modalities is usually present. Aphasia, often with preserved verbal repetition, may occur after hemorrhage into the dominant (left) thalamus, and apractognosia or mutism occurs in some cases of nondominant hemorrhage. There also may be a transient homonymous visual field defect. Thalamic hemorrhages cause several typical ocular disturbances by virtue of extension medially into the upper midbrain. These include deviation of the eyes downward and inward so that they appear to be looking at the nose, unequal pupils with absence of light reaction, skew deviation with the eye opposite the hemorrhage displaced downward and medially, ipsilateral Horner's syndrome, absence of convergence, paralysis of vertical gaze, and retraction nystagmus. In pontine hemorrhages, deep coma with quadriplegia usually occurs over a few minutes. There is often prominent decerebrate rigidity and "pin-point" (1 mm) pupils that react to light. There is impairment of reflex horizontal eye

movements evoked by head turning (doll's-head or oculocephalic maneuver) or by irrigation of the ears with ice water (see Chap. 24). Hyperpnea, severe hypertension, and hyperhidrosis are common. Death usually occurs within a few hours, but there are exceptional survivors.

Cerebellar hemorrhages usually develop over several hours and are characterized by occipital headache, repeated vomiting, and ataxia of gait. In mild cases there may be no other neurologic signs; therefore it is imperative to test gait. Dizziness or vertigo may be prominent. There is often paresis of conjugate lateral gaze toward the side of the hemorrhage, forced deviation of the eyes to the opposite side, or an ipsilateral sixth nerve palsy. Less frequent ocular signs include blepharospasm, involuntary closure of one eye, ocular bobbing, and skew deviation. There may be little or no evidence of the usual signs of cerebellar disease, and only a minority of patients show nystagmus or limb ataxia. A mild ipsilateral facial weakness and a diminished corneal reflex are common. Dysarthria and dysphagia may occur. There are no Babinski signs until late in the evolution of the hemorrhage as it compresses or dissects into the ventral brainstem. As the hours pass, the patient often becomes stuporous and then comatose from brainstem compression.

In summary, ocular signs have been highlighted as a method of rapidly localizing hemorrhages. In putamenal hemorrhage, the eyes are deviated to the side opposite the paralysis; in thalamic hemorrhage, the eyes are deviated downward and the pupils may be 2 to 3 mm and minimally reactive; in pontine hemorrhage, the reflex lateral eye movements are impaired and the pupils are <1 mm yet reactive; and in cerebellar hemorrhage, the eyes may be deviated laterally (to the side opposite the lesion) in the absence of paralysis.

Laboratory and Imaging Evaluation The CT scan reliably detects acute focal hemorrhages of 1 cm or more in diameter (Fig. 366-12). Small pontine hemorrhages may not be identified because of motion and bone artifact that obscure structures in the posterior fossa. After the first 2 weeks, x-ray attenuation values of clotted blood diminish until they become isodense with surrounding brain. Mass effect and edema may remain. In some cases, a surrounding rim of contrast enhancement appears after 2 to 4 weeks and may persist for months. MRI, though more sensitive for delineating posterior fossa lesions, is not necessary in most instances. Images of flowing blood on MRI scan may identify AVMs as the cause of the hemorrhage. Angiography is used when the cause of intracranial hemorrhage is uncertain, particularly if the patient is not hypertensive and the hematoma is not in one of the four usual sites for hypertensive hemorrhage.

FIGURE 366-12 Acute onset of right hemiparesis. Transaxial noncontrast CT scans through the region of the basal ganglia reveals a hematoma involving the left putamen with extension into the left frontal horn of the lateral ventricle (B). This is a typical hypertensive hemorrhage.

For example, hemorrhage into the temporal lobe suggests rupture of a middle cerebral artery saccular aneurysm.

Since these patients typically have focal neurologic signs and obtundation, and often show signs of increased intracranial pressure, an LP should be avoided as it may induce cerebral herniation. Although the CSF usually will be bloody several hours after the hemorrhage, especially in large hemorrhages, it is sometimes normal initially. In either case, it does not provide definitive diagnostic information.

 TREATMENT

Prevention Hypertension is the leading cause of primary cerebral hemorrhage. Prevention is primarily aimed at reducing hypertension, excessive alcohol use, and use of illicit drugs such as cocaine and amphetamines.

Acute Management Approximately 75 percent of patients with a hypertensive intracerebral hemorrhage die. The size and location of the hematoma determine the prognosis. Supratentorial hematomas >5 cm in largest diameter have a poor prognosis, and infratentorial pontine hematomas >3 cm are usually fatal. Except possibly in patients with a bleeding disorder, nothing can be done about the hemorrhage itself. Treating severe hypertension seems reasonable, but harmful hypotension is a risk. Generally, the bleeding has stopped by the time the patient comes under medical care. General measures for treating intracranial hypertension secondary to mass effect are warranted.

Evacuation of the hematoma usually is not helpful, except in cerebellar hemorrhages. For cerebellar hemorrhages, a neurosurgeon should be consulted immediately to assist with the evaluation, with a view to possible surgery. Most hematomas >3 cm in diameter will require surgical evacuation. If the patient is alert without focal brainstem signs and if the hematoma is <1 cm in diameter, surgical removal usually will not be necessary. Patients with hematomas between 1 and 3 cm require careful observation for signs of impaired consciousness, which usually mean surgery is required.

If a patient survives the initial hemorrhage without signs of severe brain injury and subsequently fails to improve or insidiously worsens, surgical evacuation of the hematoma also should be considered.

Tissue surrounding hematomas is displaced and compressed but not necessarily infarcted. Hence, in survivors, major improvement commonly results as the hematoma is reabsorbed and the adjacent tissue regains its function. Careful management of the patient during the acute phase of the hemorrhage can lead to considerable recovery.

Mannitol and other osmotic agents reduce intracranial pressure that has been raised by the volume of the hematoma and edema (see Chap. 374). Glucocorticoids are not helpful for the edema from intracerebral hematoma. Both excessive hypo- and hypertension associated with acute hemorrhage should be treated cautiously to avoid excessive or precipitous blood pressure changes.

LOBAR INTRACEREBRAL HEMORRHAGE Pathophysiology and Pathology As control of hypertension in the general population has improved, the relative proportion of hemorrhages outside the basal ganglia and thalamus has increased. These "lobar hemorrhages" appear on CT scan as oval or circular clots in the subcortical white matter.

The role of chronic hypertension in their genesis is controversial, but many occur without a history of increased blood pressure. A number of other underlying conditions are found in many cases.

Cerebral *amyloid angiopathy* is a disease of the elderly in which arteriolar degeneration occurs and amyloid is deposited in the walls of the cerebral arteries, but not elsewhere in the body. Amyloid angiopathy causes both single and recurrent lobar hemorrhages and is probably the commonest cause of lobar hemorrhage in the elderly. This disorder can be diagnosed only by postmortem demonstration of Congo red staining of amyloid in cerebral vessels. Patients may have multiple hemorrhages over several months or years. Rarely, genetic causes are found as in mutation of the amyloid precursor peptide (see Chap. 363).

Other causes are bleeding diatheses (often associated with warfarin administration), AVM, aneurysm, and tumor (often a melanoma or glioma). Often the cause remains undetermined even after extensive study, though amyloid angiopathy can not be excluded in the absence of brain histology. Some lobar hemorrhages may result from AVMs or venous angiomas that are obliterated by the hemorrhage or are angiographically occult.

Clinical Manifestations The neurologic symptoms and signs of lobar hemorrhage appear over several minutes. Most hemorrhages are small and cause a restricted clinical syndrome that simulates an embolus to an artery supplying one lobe. For example, the major neurologic deficit of occipital hemorrhage is hemianopia; of left temporal hemorrhage, aphasia and delirium; of parietal hemorrhage, thalamic-like hemisensory loss; and of frontal hemorrhage, arm weakness. Large hemorrhages may be associated with stupor or coma if they secondarily compress the thalamus or midbrain. Most patients with lobar hemorrhages have focal headaches. More than half the patients vomit or are drowsy, while stiff neck and seizures are uncommon.

Laboratory and Imaging Evaluation CT scanning reliably detects all but the smallest lobar hemorrhages. MRI is more sensitive for delineating associated abnormalities, such as aneurysm, vascular malformation, and neoplasm. Angiography is used when the cause of intracranial hemorrhage is uncertain, especially in the young and the middle-aged in whom amyloid angiopathy is not a consideration.

 TREATMENT

The recommendations for management of hypertensive intracerebral hemorrhage generally apply in this condition. If a causative lesion is found, it is treated appropriately.

COCAINE-RELATED INTRACEREBRAL HEMORRHAGE Pathophysiology and Pathology Cocaine elevates the heart rate, blood pressure, body temperature, and metabolic rate and is associated with ischemia of the myocardium, kidney, intestines, and brain.

Cocaine-induced stroke is one of the most important causes of stroke in the young. Most cocaine-related strokes occur in individuals under 40 years of age. Intracerebral hemorrhage, ischemic stroke, and SAH are all associated with cocaine use; they occur with all routes of administration and in both first-time and chronic users. Hemorrhagic stroke occurs twice as often as ischemic stroke, especially with cocaine hydrochloride. With the use of crack cocaine, hemorrhagic and ischemic complications occur with nearly equal frequency.

The strokes typically occur within minutes to hours of cocaine administration. Angiographic findings vary from completely normal arteries to large vessel occlusion or stenosis, vasospasm, or changes consistent with vasculitis.

Slightly more than half of cocaine-related intracranial hemorrhages are intracerebral and the rest are subarachnoid. Cocaine enhances sympathetic activity causing acute, sometimes severe, hypertension, and this may lead to hemorrhage. In patients with intracranial hemorrhage, underlying lesions are found in approximately half. In cases of SAH, a saccular aneurysm is usually identified; presumably, acute hypertension causes aneurysmal rupture. In the patients in whom no underlying lesion is found, approximately half have lobar hemorrhages or hematomas localized to the subcortical white matter. This is atypical for hypertensive hemorrhages, yet hypertension may still be responsible. These patients may have undetected underlying lesions such as cryptic AVMs, and some may have ischemic infarcts secondary to vasospasm followed by reperfusion and bleeding.

It is unclear whether cocaine can induce vasculitis. While occasional arteriograms of patients with cocaine-associated stroke show arterial beading or irregularities consistent with vasculitis, these findings are nonspecific and may be seen with vasospasm, fibromuscular dysplasia, and other disorders

Amphetamines cause stroke on the basis of acute hypertension and drug-induced vasculitis. Other stimulant drugs, including phenylephrine and ephedrine, are also reported to rarely induce intracerebral hemorrhage.

SUBARACHNOID HEMORRHAGE

The commonest cause of spontaneous SAH is a ruptured saccular aneurysm. Other causes are bleeding from an AVM or extension into the subarachnoid space from a primary intracerebral hemorrhage. Some cases are idiopathic, and these are often localized to the perimesencephalic cisterns and have an excellent prognosis. They probably have a venous or capillary, rather than arterial, source.

SACCULAR ANEURYSM Autopsy studies have found that 3 to 4 percent of the population harbor aneurysms, for a prevalence of 8 to 10 million in the United States. The incidence of bleeding is only 25,000 to 30,000 cases per year. The mortality rate for patients who arrive alive at hospital is about 50 percent during the first month. Of those who survive, more than half are left with major neurologic deficits as a result of the initial hemorrhage, cerebral vasospasm with infarction, or hydrocephalus. If the patient survives but the aneurysm is not obliterated, the annual rebleed rate is about 3 percent. Given these alarming figures, the major therapeutic emphasis is on preventing the predictable early complications of the rupture. Also, studies are in progress to assess the value of identifying and treating incidentally discovered aneurysms before they rupture.

Pathophysiology and Pathology Saccular aneurysms occur at the bifurcations of the large arteries at the base of the brain and rupture into the subarachnoid space in the basal cisterns. Approximately 85 percent of aneurysms occur on the anterior circulation, mostly on the circle of Willis. The common sites include the junction of the anterior communicating artery with the anterior cerebral artery, the junction of the posterior communicating artery with the internal carotid artery, and the bifurcation of the middle cerebral artery. The top of the basilar artery, the junction of the basilar artery and the superior cerebellar artery or the anterior inferior cerebellar artery, and the junction of the vertebral artery and the posterior inferior cerebellar artery comprise most of the remainder. About 20 percent of patients have multiple aneurysms, many at mirror sites bilaterally. As an aneurysm develops, it often forms a neck with a dome. The arterial internal elastic lamina disappears at the base of the neck. The media thins, and connective tissue replaces smooth-muscle cells. At the site of rupture (most often the dome), the wall thins, and the tear that allows bleeding is often no more than 0.5 mm long.

It is not possible to predict which aneurysms are likely to rupture, but limited data suggest that most ruptured aneurysms are large, e.g., average 7 mm in diameter.

Clinical Manifestations Most aneurysms present without warning as sudden SAH.

Occasionally, prodromal symptoms suggest the location of a progressively enlarging unruptured aneurysm. A third cranial nerve palsy, particularly when associated with pupillary dilatation, loss of light reflex, and focal pain above or behind the eye, may occur with an expanding aneurysm at the junction of the posterior communicating artery and the internal carotid artery. A sixth nerve palsy may indicate an aneurysm in the cavernous sinus, and visual field defects can occur with an expanding supraclinoid carotid aneurysm. Occipital and posterior cervical pain may signal a posterior inferior cerebellar artery (PICA) or anterior inferior cerebellar artery (AICA) aneurysm. Pain in or behind the eye and in the low temple can occur with an expanding middle cerebral aneurysm. Head pains in the absence of neurologic symptoms and signs are rarely caused by growing aneurysms.

Aneurysms can undergo small ruptures and leaks of blood into the subarachnoid space, so-called warning leaks. Sudden unexplained headache at any location should raise suspicion of SAH and be investigated because a major hemorrhage may be imminent.

At the moment of aneurysmal rupture with major SAH, the intracranial pressure suddenly rises. Abrupt, severe, and generalized vasospasm may occur transiently. These events may account for the sudden transient loss of consciousness that occurs in nearly half of patients. Sudden loss of consciousness may be preceded by a brief moment of

excruciating headache, but most patients first complain of headache upon regaining consciousness. In 10 percent of patients, aneurysmal bleeding is severe enough to cause loss of consciousness for several days. In about 45 percent of cases, severe headache associated with exertion is the presenting complaint. The headache is often called by the patient "the worst headache of my life," even in those who do not lose consciousness. The headache is usually generalized. Vomiting is common and when coupled with sudden headache should always raise the suspicion of SAH.

Although sudden headache in the absence of focal neurologic symptoms is the hallmark of aneurysmal rupture, focal neurologic deficits may occur (in addition to direct cranial nerve compression by the enlarging aneurysm as noted above). Anterior communicating artery or middle cerebral bifurcation aneurysms may rupture into the adjacent brain and form a hematoma large enough to produce mass effect. The common deficits that result include hemiparesis, aphasia, and abulia.

Delayed neurologic deficits There are three major causes of delayed neurologic deficits: rerupture, hydrocephalus, and vasospasm.

Rerupture The incidence of rerupture in the first month following subarachnoid hemorrhage is about 30 percent, with the peak at 7 days. It is associated with a 60 percent mortality and poor outcome. Early surgery eliminates this risk.

Hydrocephalus Acute hydrocephalus can cause stupor and coma. More often, subacute hydrocephalus develops over a few days or weeks and causes progressive drowsiness or abulia with incontinence. Differentiating hydrocephalus from symptomatic cerebral vasospasm in the anterior communicating arteries is often difficult. Hydrocephalus may clear spontaneously or require temporary ventricular drainage. Chronic hydrocephalus may appear a few weeks to months after SAH. It presents with gait difficulty, incontinence, or slowed mentation (abulia). The clue to the diagnosis may be a lack of initiative in conversation or a failure to recover independence.

Vasospasm Narrowing of the arteries at the base of the brain following SAH regularly occurs. This vasospasm causes symptomatic ischemia and infarction in approximately 30 percent of patients and is the major cause of delayed morbidity or death. Signs of ischemia appear 4 to 14 days after the hemorrhage, most frequently at about 7 days. The severity and distribution of vasospasm determine whether infarction will occur.

Although the precise mechanism of delayed vasospasm is uncertain, it seems related to direct effects of clotted blood and its breakdown products on the artery. In general, the more blood there is surrounding the arteries, the more likely there will be symptomatic vasospasm.

Symptomatic severe vasospasm presents with symptoms referable to the specific arterial territories involved. However, even severe vasospasm may not produce ischemic symptoms if sufficient collateral blood flow develops through border zone anastomotic channels (see Fig. 366-1A). Spasm of the middle cerebral artery typically causes contralateral hemiparesis and dysphasia (dominant hemisphere). Proximal anterior cerebral artery vasospasm causes abulia and incontinence, while severe vasospasm of the posterior cerebral artery causes hemianopia. Severe spasm of the basilar or vertebral arteries occasionally produces focal brainstem ischemia. All these focal neurologic symptoms may develop over a few days, fluctuate, or present abruptly.

Severe cerebral edema in patients with infarction from vasospasm may increase the intracranial pressure enough to reduce cerebral perfusion pressure.

Laboratory and Imaging Evaluation (Figs. 366-13 and 362-1) The hallmark of aneurysmal rupture is blood in the CSF. About 80 percent have enough blood to be visualized on a noncontrast CT scan obtained within 72 h. A small hemorrhage may not be seen by CT scan. If the scan neither establishes the diagnosis of SAH nor demonstrates a mass lesion or obstructive hydrocephalus, an LP should be performed to establish the presence of subarachnoid blood.

The extent and location of subarachnoid blood on CT scan help locate the underlying aneurysm and identify the cause of any neurologic deficit. The clot also will help predict delayed vasospasm. A noncontrast CT scan should be done first, because on an enhanced scan normal arteries in the basal cisterns may be mistaken for clotted blood. A high incidence of symptomatic vasospasm in the middle and anterior cerebral arteries has been found when early CT scans show subarachnoid clots larger than 5 × 3 mm in the basal cisterns, or layers of blood more than 1 mm thick in the cerebral fissures. CT scans less reliably predict vasospasm in the vertebral, basilar, or posterior cerebral arteries.

LP prior to scanning is indicated only if a CT scan is not available at the time of the suspected SAH. Once the diagnosis of hemorrhage from ruptured saccular aneurysm has been established, four-vessel angiography (both carotids and vertebrals) is generally performed to localize and define the anatomic details of the aneurysm and to determine if other unruptured aneurysms exist.

The ECG frequently shows ST-segment and T-wave changes similar to those associated with cardiac ischemia. Prolonged QRS complex, increased QT interval, and prominent "peaked" or deeply inverted symmetric T waves, although suggesting primary cardiac disease, are usually secondary to the intracranial hemorrhage. The cause of these changes is debated, but there is evidence that structural myocardial lesions may occur after SAH.

Serum electrolyte levels should be measured because hyponatremia may develop.

Transcranial Doppler ultrasound assessment of proximal middle, anterior, and posterior cerebral and basilar artery flow is helpful in detecting the onset of vasospasm, even prior to symptoms, and following its course and response to therapy.

FIGURE 366-13 Cerebral aneurysm. *Top.* Sudden onset of headache and reduced mental status. Noncontrast CT scan at the level of the suprasellar cistern (*left*) and the third ventricle (*right*) revealed subarachnoid hemorrhage within the suprasellar cistern and middle cerebral cisterns also extending along the sylvian fissures bilaterally. Communicating hydrocephalus is present, indicated by dilation of the temporal horns of the lateral ventricle (*left image*). Angiography demonstrated an aneurysm of the anterior communicating artery, which had ruptured. *Bottom.* MR angiogram of an unruptured aneurysm demonstrates the anterior communicating artery aneurysm (*paired arrows*) as well as the internal carotid arteries and the anterior cerebral arteries.

 TREATMENT

Aneurysm rerupture is common in the early days after SAH and is associated with a 60 percent incidence of death or poor outcome. Consequently, patients who are alert or only mildly drowsy, have no major neurologic deficit, and have a surgically accessible aneurysm should undergo prompt microsurgical clipping of their aneurysm. Early aneurysm repair prevents future hemorrhage and allows the safe application of techniques to improve blood flow (e.g., induced hypertension and hypervolemia) should symptomatic vasospasm develop. Patients who are not candidates for early surgery should be managed medically to minimize the complications of obtundation, rebleeding, vasospasm, and hydrocephalus. Promising new techniques, such as endovascular placement of intraaneurysmal coils, are currently being evaluated in these patients.

Following aneurysmal rupture, intracranial hypertension can occur secondary to the presence of subarachnoid blood or parenchymal hematoma, acute hydrocephalus, or loss of vascular autoregulation. Emergency ventriculostomy is indicated for patients who are lethargic, have neurologic deficits, or have radiographic evidence of mass effect. Medical therapies to reduce intracranial pressure (e.g., mild hyperventilation, mannitol, and sedation) also can be used as needed.

Care is required to maintain adequate cerebral perfusion pressure while avoiding excessive elevation of arterial pressure. Occasionally an intracranial hematoma causing neurologic deterioration requires removal.

Because rebleeding is common, all patients who are not candidates for early surgical treatment are put on bed rest in a quiet, preferably darkened, room and are given adequate stool softeners to prevent constipation. If headache or neck pain is severe, mild sedation and analgesia are prescribed. Aspirin, an antiplatelet agent, is inappropriate, but acetaminophen may be used. Extreme sedation is generally avoided because it can obscure the assessment for neurologic deficits. Adequate hydration is necessary since patients with a decreased blood volume are especially prone to brain ischemia.

Seizures are uncommon at the onset of aneurysmal rupture. The quivering, jerking, and extensor posturing that often accompany loss of consciousness are probably related to the sharp rise in intracranial pressure and perhaps acute generalized vasospasm. However, phenytoin or phenobarbital are usually given as prophylactic therapy, since a seizure may promote rebleeding.

Glucocorticoids may help reduce the head and neck ache caused by the irritative effect of the subarachnoid blood. There is no good evidence that they reduce the cerebral edema that sometimes develops or are neuroprotective or reduce vascular injury, and their routine use therefore is controversial.

Antifibrinolytic agents may be used in patients in whom treatment is delayed. They are associated with a reduced incidence of aneurysmal rerupture but also are associated with an increased incidence of delayed cerebral infarction. This is especially true in patients who develop vasospasm and is presumably due to thrombosis induced by the antifibrinolytic agent. Because of the increased risk of ischemic complications, antifibrinolytics are not routinely given to patients who are at risk for developing vasospasm.

Although vasospasm remains the leading cause of morbidity and mortality following aneurysmal SAH, therapies to prevent or treat symptomatic arterial narrowing have been disappointing. Treatment with the calcium channel antagonist nimodipine has been reported to have beneficial effects, but the effect seems to be modest.

The most commonly accepted therapy for symptomatic cerebral vasospasm is to increase the cerebral perfusion pressure by raising mean arterial pressure through plasma volume expansion and the judicious use of pressor agents, ordinarily phenylephrine or dopamine. Raised perfusion pressure has been associated with symptomatic improvement in many patients, but high arterial pressure may promote rebleeding in unprotected aneurysms. Therefore, this treatment is reserved for patients whose aneurysm has been obliterated. Treatment with induced hypertension and hypervolemia generally requires monitoring the arterial and central venous pressure and, in severe cases, the intracranial and pulmonary artery wedge pressure. If symptomatic vasospasm persists despite optimal medical therapy, intraarterial papaverine and percutaneous intraarterial angioplasty are considered. They can relieve focal symptomatic vasospasm in the arteries at the base of the brain but also can precipitate further ischemia or arterial rupture.

Acute hydrocephalus can cause stupor or coma; it may clear spontaneously or require temporary ventricular drainage. When chronic hydrocephalus develops, ventricular shunting is the treatment of choice.

Giant aneurysms, those larger than 2.5 cm in diameter, occur at the same sites as small aneurysms and account for 5 percent of cases. The three most common locations are the terminal internal carotid, middle cerebral bifurcation, and top of the basilar arteries. Although they can bleed, they usually cause symptoms by compressing the adjacent brain or cranial nerves.

Incidentally discovered aneurysms that have not previously hemorrhaged have a 2 to 3 percent annual risk of bleeding. The risk of surgery, typically 5 percent morbidity and mortality, is modified by the patients' age and medical condition. The overall role of prophylactic surgical excision of incidentally discovered asymptomatic aneurysms and other lesions with potential for bleeding is being studied.

Mycotic aneurysms are located distal to the first bifurcation of major arteries of the circle of Willis. Most result from infected emboli due to bacterial endocarditis causing septic degeneration of arteries and subsequent dilatation and rupture. Whether these lesions should be sought and treated prior to rupture, or left to heal spontaneously, is controversial.

ARTERIOVENOUS MALFORMATION

Vascular malformations, or angiomas, may be tiny and cryptic or massive anomalies that cause headaches, brain damage, seizures, and hemorrhages. AVMs are the most important vascular malformations of the nervous system and consist of a tangle of abnormal vessels forming an abnormal communication between the arterial and venous systems. Most are developmental arteriovenous fistulas in which the involved vessels enlarge with the passage of time. AVMs vary in size from a small blemish a few millimeters in diameter to a huge mass of tortuous channels composing an arteriovenous shunt of sufficient magnitude to raise the cardiac output. Hypertrophic and dilated arterial feeders approach the main lesion, disappear below the cortex, and break up into a network of thin-walled blood vessels that connect directly with draining veins. These often form huge, dilated, pulsating channels carrying away arterial blood. The blood vessels forming the tangle interposed between arteries and veins are usually abnormally thin and do not have a normal structure. AVMs occur in all parts of the brain, brainstem, and spinal cord, but the largest ones are most frequently in the posterior half of the hemispheres, commonly forming a wedge-shaped lesion extending from the cortex to the ventricle.

AVMs are more frequent in men and may occur in more than one member of a family in the same or successive generations. Although the lesion is present from birth, bleeding or other problems are most common between the ages of 10 and 30, occasionally as late as the fifties.

The chief clinical symptoms and signs are headache, seizures, and those associated with rupture. When headache occurs (without bleeding), it may be hemicranial and throbbing, like migraine, or diffuse. Focal seizures, with or without generalization, occur in about 30 percent of cases. In half of patients, AVMs become evident as intracerebral hemorrhages, and in most of these patients, the hemorrhage is mainly intraparenchymal with a small amount of spillage into the subarachnoid space. Blood is usually not deposited in the basal cisterns, and symptomatic cerebral vasospasm is therefore rare. The threat of rerupture in the early weeks is low, so antifibrinolytic agents are not used. Hemorrhages may be massive, leading to death, or may be as small as 1 cm in diameter, leading to minor focal symptoms or no deficit. In either case, the hematoma may compress the AVM so completely that angiography cannot detect it. Hence, when an AVM is suspected, angiography is best postponed until the hematoma has resolved, i.e., after 6 to 8 weeks. Rarely the AVM is large enough to steal blood away from adjacent normal brain tissue, rendering the surrounding brain ischemic. This is seen most often when large AVMs in the middle cerebral territory extend from the cortical surface to the ventricular system. Hydrocephalus may result if the vein of Galen enlarges as a channel for drainage from the AVM.

Large AVMs of the carotid–middle cerebral system may be associated with systolic and diastolic bruits (sometimes self-audible) over the eye, forehead, or neck where a bounding carotid pulse may be perceived. Headache at the onset of AVM rupture is not generally as explosive as with aneurysmal rupture. Contrast CT scanning often detects the channels of an AVM prior to rupture, and new MRI techniques are even more sensitive.

AVMs less than 0.5 cm in diameter are usually low-pressure venous angiomas that bleed infrequently and minimally. If they bleed, surgical or gamma-knife resection or obliteration should be considered.

Most data suggest that patients with asymptomatic AVMs have a low risk for hemorrhage, which increases after a first hemorrhage to about 2 to 3 percent annually. Smaller lesions seem to have a higher hemorrhage rate, and the mortality rate with each bleed is about 15 percent.

The management of patients with arterial AVMs is best accomplished by a team approach. Surgical excision, interventional radiologic obliteration techniques, and radiotherapy all have a role. Intraarterial occlusion of feeding arteries is often used to shrink the lesion and make surgical excision less formidable.

OTHER CAUSES OF INTRACRANIAL HEMORRHAGE

Trauma Head injury often causes intracranial bleeding. The common sites are intracerebral (especially temporal and inferior frontal lobes), subarachnoid, subdural, and epidural. Trauma must be considered in any patient with an unexplained acute neurologic deficit (hemiparesis, stupor, or confusion), particularly if the deficit occurred in the context of a fall. These entities are discussed more fully in Chap. 374.

Hematologic Intracerebral hemorrhage associated with hematologic disorders (leukemia, aplastic anemia, thrombocytopenic purpura) can occur at any site and may present as multiple intracerebral hemorrhages. Skin and mucous membrane bleeding is usually evident and offers a diagnostic clue. Intracranial hemorrhage associated with anticoagulant therapy can occur at any location but is often lobar or subdural. Anticoagulant-related intracerebral hemorrhages may evolve slowly, over 24 to 48 h. Fresh frozen plasma and vitamin K may be required. When intracerebral hemorrhage is associated with platelet deficiencies, platelet transfusion may be required.

Brain Tumors Hemorrhage into a brain tumor may be the first manifestation of neoplasm (Chap. 375). Choriocarcinoma, malignant melanoma, renal cell carcinoma, and bronchogenic carcinoma are among the most common metastatic tumors associated with intracerebral hemorrhage. Glioblastoma multiforme in adults and medulloblastoma in children also may have areas of intracerebral hemorrhage.

Hypertensive Encephalopathy (See Chap. 246) Hypertensive encephalopathy is a complication of malignant hypertension. In this acute syndrome, severe hypertension is associated with headache, nausea, vomiting, convulsions, confusion, stupor, and coma. Focal or lateralizing neurologic signs, either transitory or lasting, may occur but are infrequent and therefore suggest some other vascular disease (hemorrhage, embolism, or atherosclerotic thrombosis). Retinal hemorrhages, exudates, papilledema (hypertensive retinopathy grade IV), and evidence of renal and cardiac disease may be present. In most cases the CSF pressure and protein levels are elevated. Lowering the blood pressure reverses the process, but permanent damage may have occurred. Neuropathologic examination reveals multifocal or diffuse cerebral edema with hemorrhages that vary in size from petechial to massive. Microscopically, necrosis of arterioles, minute cerebral infarcts, and hemorrhages are noted.

The term *hypertensive encephalopathy* should be reserved for this syndrome and not for chronic recurrent headaches, dizziness, epileptic seizures, recurrent TIAs, or small strokes that often occur in association with high blood pressure.

Other Causes Primary intraventricular hemorrhage is rare. It usually begins intraparenchymally and dissects into the ventricular system without leaving signs of intraparenchymal hemorrhage. Inflammatory disease of the arteries and veins, especially polyarteritis nodosa and lupus erythematosus, can produce hemorrhage into the central nervous system, most often in association with hypertension. Sepsis can cause small petechial hemorrhages throughout the cerebral white matter. There is no blood in the spinal fluid. Moyamoya disease most commonly causes ischemic symptoms but may on occasion produce multiple small aneurysms that rupture. Hemorrhages into the spinal cord are usually the result of an AVM or metastatic tumor (see Chap. 373).

BIBLIOGRAPHY

ANTIPLATELET TRIALISTS' COLLABORATION: Collaborative overview of randomised trials of antiplatelet therapy—I: Prevention of death, myocardial infarction, and stroke by prolonged antiplatelet therapy in various categories of patients. BMJ 308:81, 1994

ATRIAL FIBRILLATION INVESTIGATORS: Risk factors for stroke and efficacy of antithrombotic therapy in atrial fibrillation. Analysis of pooled data from five randomized controlled trials. Arch Intern Med 154:1449, 1994 [Erratum: ibid, p 2254]

EASTON JD, WILTERDINK JL: Carotid endarterectomy: Trials and tribulations. Ann Neurol 35:5, 1994

EUROPEAN CAROTID SURGERY TRIALISTS' COLLABORATIVE GROUP: MRC European Carotid Surgery Trial: Interim results for symptomatic patients with severe (70–99%) or with mild (0–29%) carotid stenosis. Lancet 337:1235, 1991

EXECUTIVE COMMITTEE FOR THE ASYMPTOMATIC CAROTID ATHEROSCLEROSIS STUDY: Endarterectomy for asymptomatic carotid artery stenosis. JAMA 273:1421, 1995

MOORE WS et al: Guidelines for carotid endarterectomy: A multidisciplinary consensus statement from the Ad Hoc Committee, American Heart Association. Stroke 26:188, 1995

NORTH AMERICAN SYMPTOMATIC CAROTID ENDARTERECTOMY TRIAL COLLABORATORS: Beneficial effect of carotid endarterectomy in symptomatic patients with high-grade carotid stenosis. N Engl J Med 325:445, 1991

STROKE PREVENTION IN ATRIAL FIBRILLATION INVESTIGATORS: Warfarin versus aspirin for prevention of thromboembolism in atrial fibrillation: Stroke Prevention in Atrial Fibrillation II Study. Lancet 343:687, 1994

THE EUROPEAN ATRIAL FIBRILLATION TRIAL STUDY GROUP: Optimal oral anticoagulant therapy in patients with nonrheumatic atrial fibrillation and recent cerebral ischemia. The European Atrial Fibrillation Trial Study Group. N Engl J Med 333:5, 1995

THE NATIONAL INSTITUTE OF NEUROLOGICAL DISORDERS AND STROKE rt-PA STROKE STUDY GROUP: Tissue plasminogen activator for acute ischemic stroke. N Engl J Med 333:1581, 1995

VAN GIJN J et al: Major ongoing stroke trials: Anticoagulants versus aspirin in patients with transient ischemic attacks or nondisabling ischemic stroke: SPIRIT (Stroke Prevention In Reversible Ischemia Trial) (in progress). Stroke 26:1140, 1995

WILTERDINK JL, EASTON JD: Vascular event rates in patients with atherosclerotic cerebrovascular disease. Arch Neurol 49:857, 1992

367 *Thomas D. Bird*

ALZHEIMER'S DISEASE AND OTHER PRIMARY DEMENTIAS

ALZHEIMER'S DISEASE Alzheimer's disease (AD) is the most common cause of dementia in western countries. Approximately 10 percent of all persons over the age of 70 have significant memory loss, and more than half is the result of AD. This translates into approximately 3 to 4 million persons with AD in the United States, with a total health care cost of more than 50 billion dollars per year. It is estimated that the annual total cost of caring for a single AD patient in an advanced stage of the disease is $47,000. The disease also exacts a heavy emotional toll on family members and caregivers. AD was first described in 1907 in a 55-year-old woman by Professor Alois Alzheimer in Germany. The condition was initially thought to represent a relatively uncommon form of presenile dementia. However, it has become clear that AD can occur in any decade of adulthood and is the most common cause of dementia in the elderly. The disease is defined as a clinical-pathologic entity. Clinically, AD most often presents with subtle onset of memory loss followed by a slowly progressive dementia that has a course of several years. Pathologically there is gross, diffuse atrophy of the cerebral cortex with secondary enlargement of the ventricular system. Microscopically there are neuritic plaques containing $A\beta$ amyloid, silver-staining neurofibrillary tangles in neuronal cytoplasm, and accumulation of $A\beta$ amyloid in arterial walls of cerebral blood vessels (see "Pathogenesis," below). The recent identification of four different susceptibility genes for AD has provided a foundation for rapid progress in understanding the biologic basis of the disease.

Clinical Manifestations In the early stages of the disease, the memory loss may go unrecognized or may be ascribed to benign forgetfulness. Slowly the cognitive problems begin to interfere with daily activities, such as keeping track of finances, following instructions on the job, driving, shopping, and housekeeping. Some patients are unaware of these difficulties (agnosognosia) and others have considerable insight, resulting in frustration and anxiety. These major differences in insight have no clear explanation. Change of environment may be bewildering, and the patient may become lost on walks or while driving an automobile. In the middle stages of the disease, the patient is unable to work, is easily lost and confused, and requires daily supervision. Social graces, routine behavior, and superficial conversation may be surprisingly retained. Language may be impaired, especially comprehension and naming of objects. In some patients, aphasia is an early and prominent feature. Word-finding difficulties and circumlocution may be a problem even when formal testing demonstrates intact naming and fluency. Although confrontation naming is frequently deficient, there are often other language deficits as well, including impairments in fluency, comprehension, and repetition. Various apraxias are also common, that is, deficits in performing sequential motor tasks such as dressing, eating, solving simple puzzles, and copying geometric figures. Patients may be unable to do simple calculations or tell time. Rarely, AD patients may have a form of cortical blindness in which they deny their inability to see. This correlates at autopsy with severe neuropathologic changes in the visual cortex. In the late stages of the disease, some persons remain ambulatory but wander aimlessly and may have complete loss of judgment, reason, and cognitive abilities. Hallucinations and delusions are common; they are usually concrete and not too complex or bizarre. For example, patients may falsely accuse a spouse of infidelity, not recognize an old friend, think a visitor is a burglar, or become frightened of their own image in a mirror. Loss of inhibitions and belligerence may occur and may even alternate with passivity and social withdrawal. Sleep-wake patterns may be disturbed, and nighttime wandering may be very disruptive to the household. Some patients develop a shuffling gait with generalized muscle rigidity associated with slowness and awkwardness of movement. The patients often look parkinsonian but rarely have a rapid, rhythmic, resting tremor. In end-stage AD, patients frequently, but not always, become rigid, mute, incontinent, and bedridden. Help may be needed with the simplest tasks, such as eating, dressing, and toilet function. They may show hyperactive tendon reflexes and primitive sucking and snouting reflexes. Myoclonic jerks (sudden brief contractions of various muscles or the whole body) may occur spontaneously or in response to physical or auditory stimulation. This phenomenon raises the possibility of Creutzfeldt-Jakob disease (CJD) (Chap. 379), but the course of AD is much more prolonged. Generalized seizures may also occur. Death usually results from malnutrition, secondary infections, or heart disease. The typical duration of AD is 8 to 10 years, but the course can range from 1 to 25 years. For unknown reasons, some AD patients show a steady downhill decline in function, while others have prolonged plateaus without major deterioration.

Differential Diagnosis Early in the disease course, other etiologies of dementia should be excluded. These include treatable entities such as thyroid disease, vitamin deficiencies, brain tumor, drug and medication intoxication, chronic infection, and severe depression (pseudodementia) (see Chap. 26). Neuroimaging studies [computed tomography (CT) and magnetic resonance imaging (MRI)] are not specific for AD and may be normal early in the course of the disease. However, neuroimaging helps to exclude other disorders, such as primary and secondary neoplasms, multi-infarct dementia, diffuse white matter disease, and normal-pressure hydrocephalus. As AD progresses, diffuse cortical atrophy becomes apparent, and detailed MRI scans show atrophy of the hippocampus (Fig. 367-1A). The electroencephalogram (EEG) in AD may be normal or show nonspecific slowing. Routine spinal fluid examination gives normal results. Research studies have indicated a general decrease in cerebrospinal fluid (CSF) acetylcholine and Aβ amyloid levels with an increase in tau protein. There is considerable overlap of these levels with those of the normal aged population, and the usefulness of these measurements in diagnosis

remains unclear. The use of blood apolipoprotein (Apo) E genotyping is discussed under "Pathogenesis," below. A report has appeared that the pupillary reaction in patients with AD is hypersensitive to tropicamide and that this response could form the basis of a diagnostic test. There has been no confirmation of the clinical utility of this phenomenon, and its use is not presently recommended. Slowly progressive decline, normal results on laboratory tests, and an MRI or CT scan showing only diffuse cortical atrophy including the hippocampus is highly suggestive of AD. A clinical diagnosis of AD reached after careful evaluation is confirmed at autopsy about 85 to 90 percent of the time. The misdiagnosed cases usually represent one of the other dementing disorders described later in this chapter. Relatively simple clinical clues are useful in the differential diagnosis. Early prominent gait disturbance with only mild memory loss suggests normal-pressure hydrocephalus (see below). Resting tremor with stooped posture, bradykinesia, and mask facies suggests Parkinson's disease (Chap. 368). Chronic alcoholism suggests vitamin deficiency. Loss of sensibility to position and vibration stimuli accompanied by Babinski responses suggests vitamin B$_{12}$ deficiency (Chaps. 373 and 380). Early onset of a seizure suggests a metastatic or primary brain neoplasm (Chap. 375). A past history of long-term depression suggests pseudodementia (see below). A history of treatment for insomnia, anxiety, psychiatric disturbance, or epilepsy suggests chronic drug intoxication. Rapid progression over a few weeks or months associated with rigidity and myoclonus suggests CJD (Chap. 379). A positive family history of dementia suggests either one of the familial forms of AD or one of the other genetic disorders associated with dementia, such as Huntington's disease (see below), Pick's disease (see below), familial forms of prion diseases (Chap. 379), or rare forms of hereditary ataxias (Chap. 369).

Pathogenesis The most important risk factors for AD are old age and a positive family history. The frequency of AD increases with each decade of adult life to reach 20 to 40 percent of the population over the age of 85. A positive family history of dementia suggests a genetic cause of AD, as discussed below. Female gender may also be a risk factor independent of the greater longevity of women. Unconfirmed studies have suggested that postmenopausal estrogen use is associated with a decreased frequency of AD. Some AD patients have a past history of head trauma with concussion, but this appears to be a relatively minor risk factor. There is some suggestion that AD is more common in groups with lower educational attainment, but education influences test-taking ability, and it is clear that AD can affect persons of all intellectual levels. A recent unconfirmed study found that the capacity to express complex written language in early adulthood correlated with a decreased risk for AD. Numerous environmental factors, including aluminum, mercury, viruses, and prions, have been proposed as causes of AD, but none has been proved to play a role. Preliminary studies have suggested that the use of nonsteroidal anti-inflammatory agents is associated with a decreased risk of AD. Such reports require careful confirmation. Vascular disease does not seem to be a direct cause of AD, even though there is an associated amyloid angiopathy.

Positron emission tomography (PET) has indicated that the earliest metabolic changes in AD occur in parietal cortex (Fig. 367-1B). At autopsy, the most severe pathology is usually seen in the hippocampus, temporal cortex, and nucleus basalis. The most important microscopic findings are neuritic "senile" plaques and neurofibrillary tangles (NFTs). These two lesions accumulate in small numbers during normal aging of the brain but occur in quantitative excess in the dementia of AD. The neuritic plaques contain a central core that includes Aβ amyloid, proteoglycans, Apo E, α$_1$ antichymotrypsin, and other proteins. Aβ amyloid is a 4.2 kDa protein of 39 to 42 amino acids that is derived proteolytically from a larger transmembrane protein (amyloid precursor protein, APP). The normal function of Aβ amyloid is unknown. APP has been shown to have neurotrophic and neuroprotective activities. The plaque core is surrounded by the debris of

FIGURE 367-1 Alzheimer's disease. *A.* Axial T1-weighted MR images through the midbrain of a normal 86-year-old athlete (*left*) and a 77-year-old male (*right*) with Alzheimer's disease. Note that both individuals have prominent sulci and slight dilatation of the lateral ventricles. However, there is a reduction in the volume of the hippocampus of the patient with Alzheimer's disease (*arrows*) compared with that of the normal-aged athlete. *B, C.* Fluorodeoxyglucose PET scans of a normal-aged control (*left*) and a patient with Alzheimer's disease (*right*). Note that the patient with Alzheimer's disease has decreased activity in the parietal lobes bilaterally (*arrows*), a typical finding in this condition. (Images courtesy of TF Budinger, University of California.)

degenerating neurons and macrophages. The accumulation of Aβ amyloid in cerebral arterioles is termed *amyloid angiopathy*. The NFTs were first noted by Alzheimer. They are silver-staining, twisted neurofilaments in neuronal cytoplasm that represent abnormally phosphorylated tau (τ) protein and appear as paired helical filaments by electron microscopy. Tau is a microtubule-associated protein that may function to assemble and stabilize the microtubules that convey cell organelles, glycoproteins, and other important materials through the neuron. The ability of tau protein to bind to microtubule segments is determined partly by the number of phosphate groups attached to it. Increased phosphorylation of tau protein may disturb this normal process. Biochemically, AD is associated with a decrease in the cerebral cortical levels of several proteins and neurotransmitters, especially acetylcholine, its synthetic enzyme choline acetyltransferase (CAT), and nicotinic cholinergic receptors. Reduction of acetylcholine may be related in part to degeneration in the nucleus basalis of Meynert of cholinergic neurons that project to many areas of cortex. There is also

reduction in norepinephrine levels in brainstem nuclei such as the locus coeruleus.

Several genetic factors are known to play important roles in the pathogenesis of at least some cases of AD. One is the amyloid precursor protein gene on chromosome 21. Adults with trisomy 21 (Down's syndrome) consistently develop the typical neuropathologic hallmarks of AD if they survive beyond age 40. Many also develop a progressive dementia superimposed on their baseline mental retardation. APP is a membrane-spanning protein that is subsequently processed into smaller units, including the Aβ amyloid that is deposited in the neuritic plaques of AD. Presumably the extra dose of the APP gene on chromosome 21 is the initiating cause of AD in adult Down's syndrome and eventually results in an excess of cerebral Aβ amyloid. Furthermore, a few families with early-onset familial AD (FAD) have been discovered to have point mutations in the APP gene. Although very rare, these families were the first indication of a single-gene autosomal dominant genetic transmission of AD. The most frequent of these APP mutations is substitution of valine for isoleucine at position 717.

Investigation of large families with multigenerational FAD led subsequently to the discovery of two additional AD genes, termed the *presenilins*. Presenilin-1 (*PS-1*) is on chromosome 14 and encodes a protein called S182. Mutations in this gene cause an early-onset AD (onset before age 60 and often before age 50) that is transmitted in an autosomal dominant, highly penetrant fashion. More than 20 different mutations have been found in the *PS-1* gene in families from a wide range of ethnic backgrounds. Presenilin-2 (*PS-2*) is on chromosome 1 and encodes a protein called STM2. A mutation in the *PS-2* gene was first found in a group of American families with Volga German ethnic background. The two genes (*PS-1* and *PS-2*) are highly homologous and encode similar proteins that at first appeared to have seven transmembrane domains (hence the designation *STM*, but subsequent studies have suggested eight such domains with a ninth submembrane region). The normal function of these proteins and the means by which mutations affecting them result in AD is unknown. Both S182 and STM2 are cytoplasmic neuronal proteins that are widely expressed throughout the nervous system. They are homologous to a cell-trafficking protein, sel 12, that is found in the nematode *Coenorhabditis elegans*. Patients with mutations in these genes have elevated plasma levels of Aβ41-42 amyloid, suggesting a possible link between the presenilins and APP. Mutations in the chromosome-14 gene have thus far proved to be the most common cause of early-onset FAD, representing perhaps 70 percent of this relatively rare syndrome. Mutations in *PS-1* tend to produce AD with an earlier age of onset (mean, 45 years) and a shorter, more rapidly progressive course (mean duration, 6 to 7 years) than the disease caused by mutations in *PS-2* (onset, 53 years; duration, 11 years). Some carriers of uncommon *PS-2* mutations have had onset of dementia after the age of 70. It is not yet clear whether presenilins are involved in the more common sporadic cases of late-onset AD occurring in the general population. Molecular DNA blood testing for these uncommon mutations is now possible on a research basis. Any testing of asymptomatic persons at risk must be done in the context of formal, thoughtful genetic counseling (see Chap. 363).

A discovery of great importance has implicated the Apo E gene on chromosome 19 in the pathogenesis of late-onset familial and sporadic forms of AD. Apo E is involved in cholesterol transport (Chap. 341) and has three alleles: ε2, ε3, and ε4. The ε4 allele of Apo E shows a strong association with AD in the general population, including sporadic and late-onset familial cases. Approximately 24 to 30 percent of the normal white population has at least one ε4 allele (12 to 15 percent allele frequency), and about 2 percent are ε4/4 homozygotes. In a group of AD patients, approximately 40 to 65 percent have at least one ε4 allele, a highly significant difference compared with controls. On the other hand, many AD patients have no ε4 allele, and individuals with ε4 may never develop AD. Therefore, ε4 is neither necessary nor sufficient as a cause of AD. Nevertheless, it is clear that the Apo E ε4 allele, especially in the homozygous 4/4 state, is an important risk factor for AD. It appears to act as a dose-dependent modifier of age of onset, with the earliest onset associated with the ε4/4 homozygous state. It is unknown how Apo E functions as a risk factor modifying age of onset. Apo E is present in the neuritic amyloid plaques of AD, and it may also be involved in neurofibrillary tangle formation, because it binds to tau protein. Apo E4 decreases neurite outgrowth in cultures of dorsal root ganglion neurons. There is some evidence that the ε2 allele may be "protective," but that remains to be clarified. Interesting but unconfirmed reports suggest that AD patients with an ε4 allele may be less responsive to tacrine. There is also preliminary evidence that the A allele of α₁ antichymotrypsin increases the risk of AD in carriers of the Apo E ε4 genotype. The use of Apo E testing in the diagnosis of AD is controversial. It is not indicated as a predictive test in normal persons, because its precise predictive value is unclear, and many individuals with the ε4 allele never develop dementia. However, some cognitively normal ε4/4 homozygotes have

been found by PET to have decreased cerebral cortical metabolic rates, suggesting possible presymptomatic abnormalities compatible with the earliest stage of AD. It has also been proposed that in elderly demented persons, the finding of the Apo E ε4/4 homozygous state strongly confirms the diagnosis of AD, at about the 96 to 98 percent certainty level. Unfortunately, only a minority of persons are ε4/4 homozygotes, and even they may have other causes of dementia, such that a search for treatable causes is still necessary. Nevertheless, Apo E remains the single most important biologic marker associated with risk for AD, and studies of its functional role and diagnostic usefulness are progressing rapidly. Its association (or lack thereof) with other dementing illnesses needs to be fully evaluated. The ε4 allele is not associated with the dementia of Parkinson's disease or CJD.

℞ TREATMENT

The management of Alzheimer's disease is difficult and frustrating, because there is no specific treatment and the primary focus is on long-term amelioration of associated behavioral and neurologic problems. Building rapport with the patient, family members, and other caregivers is essential to successful management.

Tacrine (tetrahydroaminoacridine), 80 to 160 mg/d, is the only drug presently approved by the Food and Drug Administration (FDA) for treatment of AD. Its pharmacologic action is presumed to be inhibition of cholinesterase, with a resulting increase in cerebral levels of acetylcholine. Double-blind, placebo-controlled, crossover studies with tacrine have shown its use to be associated with improved caregiver ratings of patients' functioning and with an apparent decreased rate of decline in cognitive test scores over periods of up to 2 years. Such studies are difficult to perform because of the subjective nature of many of the observations and the lack of a uniform rate of decline among patients. Nevertheless, a small but important minority of AD patients (approximately 10 to 20 percent) appear to show a modest response to tacrine and tolerate its side effects (which include dose-related nausea, vomiting, and diarrhea). Tacrine gives no benefit in the late stages of AD. The medication is expensive and hepatotoxic, necessitating frequent testing of liver function and adjustment of the dose. Numerous other drugs, such as estrogen, anti-inflammatory agents, and anti-cholinesterases, are currently undergoing therapeutic trials.

Mild to moderate depression is common in the early stages of AD and may respond to antidepressant medication. Selective serotonin reuptake inhibitors (SSRIs) are commonly used, as are tricyclic antidepressants with low anticholinergic side effects (desipramine and nortriptyline). Generalized seizures should be treated with an appropriate anticonvulsant, such as phenytoin or carbamazepine. Agitation, insomnia, hallucinations, and belligerence are especially troublesome characteristics of some AD patients and often are responsible for nursing home placement. Mild sedation with benadryl may help insomnia, and agitation has been variously treated with phenothiazines (such as thioridazine), haloperidol, and benzodiazepines (such as lorazepam). These medications frequently have untoward side effects, including sedation, confusion, increased muscle tone, and adventitious movements. Low-dose haloperidol (0.5 to 2 mg), trazodone, buspirone, and propranolol may be the most helpful and have the least side effects. The few controlled studies comparing drugs with behavioral intervention in the treatment of agitation suggest that both approaches are equally effective. However, careful, daily, non-drug behavior management is often not available, rendering medication necessary. In the early stages of AD, memory aids such as notebooks and posted daily reminders are helpful. Common sense and clinical studies have shown that family members should emphasize activities that are pleasant and deemphasize those that are unpleasant. Kitchens, bathrooms, and bedrooms need to be made safe, and patients eventually must stop driving. Loss of independence and change of environment may worsen confusion, agitation, and anger. Communication and repeated calm reassurance are necessary. Caregiver "burnout" is common, often resulting in nursing home placement of the patient, and respite breaks for the caregiver help to maintain successful long-term management of the patient. Use of adult daycare centers can be most helpful. Local and national support groups, such as the Alzheimer's Disease and Related Disorders Association, are valuable resources.

VASCULAR DEMENTIA   Dementia associated with cerebral vascular disease can be divided into two general categories: multi-infarct dementia and diffuse white matter dementia (also called subcortical arteriosclerotic encephalopathy or Binswanger's disease). Cerebral vascular disease appears to be a more common cause of dementia in Asia than in Europe and North America. Individuals who have had several strokes may develop chronic cognitive deficits, commonly called *multi-infarct dementia*. The strokes may be large or small (sometimes lacunar) and usually involve several different brain regions. The occurrence of dementia seems to depend partly on the total volume of damaged cortex, but it is also more common in individuals with left-hemisphere lesions, independent of any language disturbance. The patients give a history of episodes of sudden neurologic deterioration. Multi-infarct dementia patients usually also have a history of hypertension, diabetes, coronary artery disease, or other manifestations of diffuse atherosclerosis. Physical examination usually shows focal neurologic deficits such as hemiparesis, unilateral Babinski reflex, a visual field defect, or pseudobulbar palsy. The recurrent strokes result in a stepwise progression of disease. Neuroimaging studies clearly show the multiple areas of infarction. Thus, the history and neuroimaging findings differentiate this condition from AD. However, AD and multiple infarctions are both common and sometimes occur together. With normal aging, there is also an accumulation of amyloid in cerebral blood vessels, leading to a condition called *cerebral amyloid angiopathy of aging* (not associated with dementia), which predisposes older persons to hemorrhagic lobar stroke. AD patients with amyloid angiopathy and hypertension also appear to be at increased risk of cerebral infarction. Apo E ε4 has been reported to be a risk factor for amyloid angiopathy independent of AD.

Some persons with dementia are discovered on MRI studies to have bilateral abnormalities of subcortical white matter, termed diffuse white matter disease (or leukoaraiosis) (Fig. 367-2). The dementia may be of subtle onset and slow progression, features that distinguish it from multi-infarct dementia. (A few such patients have been described with apparently sudden onset of cognitive impairment.) Early symptoms are mild confusion, apathy, change in personality, and memory deficit. Marked difficulties in judgment and orientation and dependence on others for daily activities develop later. Euphoria, elation, or aggressive behavior are common. A mixed picture of pyramidal and cerebellar signs may be present in the same patient. Lateralizing motor signs are uncommon. A gait disorder appears in at least half the patients. In advanced cases, urinary incontinence and dysarthria with or without pseudobulbar features are frequent. Seizures and myoclonic jerks appear in a minority of patients. This disorder appears to be the result of chronic ischemia due to occlusive disease of small penetrating cerebral arteries and arterioles (microangiopathy). The patients usually, but not always, have a history of hypertension, but any disease causing stenosis of small cerebral vessels may be the critical underlying factor. Binswanger described several patients with this condition, but the term *Binswanger's disease* should be used with caution, because it does not really identify a single entity. Other rare causes of white matter disease may also present with dementia, such as adult metachromatic leukodystrophy and progressive multifocal leukoencephalopathy (papovavirus infection).

Treatment of vascular dementia must be focused on the underlying causes, such as hypertension, atherosclerosis, and diabetes. Recovery of lost cognitive function is not likely to occur.

FIGURE 367-2   Diffuse white matter disease (Binswanger's disease). Axial T2-weighted MR image through the lateral ventricles reveals multiple areas of abnormal high signal intensity involving the periventricular white matter as well as the corona radiata and lentiform nuclei (*arrows*). While seen in some individuals with normal cognition, this appearance is more pronounced in patients with dementia of a vascular etiology.

PICK'S DISEASE   Pick's disease is a commonly discussed disorder that is difficult to differentiate clinically from AD and is less well defined as a distinct entity. The major distinguishing hallmarks are marked symmetric lobar atrophy of temporal and/or frontal lobes, which can be visualized by neuroimaging studies and is readily apparent at autopsy. For this reason, the diagnosis of frontotemporal dementia overlaps with Pick's disease. The atrophy is sometimes asymmetric and may involve the basal ganglia. Microscopic findings include gliosis, neuronal loss, and swollen or ballooned neurons, which frequently contain silver-staining cytoplasmic inclusions referred to as *Pick bodies*. Pick bodies consist of straight and constricted fibrils that share antigenic determinants with the NFTs of AD, including the microtubule-associated protein tau, suggesting that Pick bodies derive from altered components of the neuronal cytoskeleton. Onset is usually in the fifth through seventh decades. Clinically, there is a slowly progressive dementia often associated with hyper-oral behavior, bulimia, language disturbance, emotional disinhibition, irritability, and persistent aimless wandering. The language disturbance may be aphasia or forced repetitive speech patterns, sometimes progressing to echolalia, language impoverishment, and mutism. Unfortunately, each of these clinical characteristics, as well as relative lobar atrophy, may occur in AD, so that the clinical diagnosis of Pick's disease is simply an educated guess that must be confirmed at autopsy. Furthermore, brains containing Pick bodies may also have varying quantities of amyloid plaques and neurofibrillary tangles, again blurring the distinction from AD. Examples of familial Pick's disease that display an autosomal dominant-like pattern of inheritance have been reported. There is no specific treatment.

DIFFUSE LEWY BODY DISEASE   Lewy bodies are intraneuronal cytoplasmic inclusions that stain with periodic acid–Schiff (PAS)

A

B

FIGURE 367-3 Normal pressure hydrocephalus. *A.* Sagittal T1-weighted MR image demonstrates dilatation of the lateral ventricle and stretching of the corpus callosum (*arrows*), depression of the floor of the third ventricle (*single arrowhead*), and enlargement of the aqueduct (*double arrowheads*). Note the diffuse dilatation of the lateral, third, and fourth ventricles with a patent aqueduct, typical of communicating hydrocephalus. *B.* Axial T2-weighted MR images demonstrate dilatation of the lateral ventricles. This patient underwent successful ventriculoperitoneal shunting.

and ubiquitin. They are composed of straight neurofilaments 7 to 20 nm long with surrounding amorphous material. They contain epitopes recognized by antibodies against phosphorylated and nonphosphorylated neurofilament proteins as well as ubiquitin. Lewy bodies are traditionally found in the substantia nigra of patients with idiopathic Parkinson's disease. Large numbers of such inclusions have also been discovered in cortical neurons in patients with dementia. In patients

without other pathologic features, the condition is referred to as *diffuse Lewy body disease*. In patients whose brains also contain amyloid plaques and neurofibrillary tangles, the condition is called the *diffuse Lewy body type of Alzheimer's disease*. The quantity of Lewy bodies required to establish the diagnosis is not agreed on. Nevertheless, the diagnosis is primarily a neuropathologic entity. However, there is some evidence that there is a characteristic clinical syndrome. In addition to chronic progressive dementia, these patients often also have Parkinsonian features, especially rigidity sometimes combined with an intention tremor. There may be frequent fluctuations of behavior, cognitive ability, and level of alertness. These fluctuations can be marked, with the occurrence of episodic confusion and lucid intervals suggesting delirium. However, despite the fluctuating pattern, the clinical features persist over a long period, unlike a typical transient delirium. Delusions and visual hallucinations are common, and auditory hallucinations may also occur. Repeated unexplained falls are often noted. Frequently there is an unusual sensitivity to neuroleptic medications and benzodiazepines, with exaggerated adverse responses to standard doses. In most patients, this condition is difficult to distinguish from AD or Parkinson's disease with dementia. The population prevalence of diffuse Lewy body disease is unclear, but it is more commonly diagnosed nowadays with the use of ubiquitin staining during neuropathologic studies. At autopsy, 10 to 30 percent of demented patients may show cortical Lewy bodies. It is not yet clear what role Apo E may play in Lewy body disease without AD changes. There is no specific treatment.

NORMAL-PRESSURE HYDROCEPHALUS Normal-pressure hydrocephalus (NPH) is a syndrome with several clinical, physiologic, and neuroimaging characteristics. The clinical triad includes an abnormal gait (ataxic or apractic), dementia (usually mild to moderate), and urinary incontinence. Neuroimaging studies of the brain reveal enlarged lateral ventricles (hydrocephalus) with little or no cortical atrophy. This is a communicating hydrocephalus with a patent aqueduct of Sylvius (Fig. 367-3). Lumbar puncture opening pressure is in the high normal range, and the CSF protein and sugar concentrations and cell count are normal. NPH is presumed to be caused by obstruction to normal flow of CSF over the cerebral convexity and delayed absorption into the venous system. The indolent nature of the process results in enlarged lateral ventricles but relatively little increase in CSF pressure. There is presumably stretching and distortion of white matter tracts in the corona radiata, but the exact physiologic cause of the clinical syndrome is unclear. Some patients with NPH have a history of conditions producing scarring of the basilar meninges (blocking upward flow of CSF) such as previous meningitis, subarachnoid hemorrhage, or head trauma. Most patients seem to have no pertinent past history. In contrast to patients with AD, the patient with NPH has an early and prominent gait disturbance and no evidence of cortical atrophy on CT or MRI. A number of attempts have been made to use various special studies to improve the diagnosis of NPH and predict the success of ventricular shunting. These include radionuclide cisternography (showing a delay in CSF absorption over the convexity) and various attempts to monitor and alter CSF flow dynamics, including a constant-pressure infusion test. None of these studies has proven to be specific or consistently useful. There is sometimes a transient improvement in gait or cognition following lumbar puncture (or serial punctures) with removal of 30 to 50 mL of CSF, but this finding also has not proved to be consistently predictive of post-shunt improvement. One study determined that no more than 1 to 2 percent of a large group of demented patients had NPH. AD often masquerades as NPH, because the gait may be abnormal in AD and cortical atrophy sometimes is difficult to determine by CT or MRI early in the disease. Hippocampal atrophy on MRI may be a clue favoring AD. Approximately 30 to 50 percent of patients identified by careful diagnosis as having NPH will show improvement with a ventricular shunting procedure.

Gait may improve more than memory. Transient, short-lasting improvement is common. Patients should be carefully selected for this operation, because subdural hematoma and infection are known complications.

HUNTINGTON'S DISEASE Huntington's disease (HD) is a genetic, autosomal dominant, degenerative brain disorder. It has a population frequency of about 10/100,000. The two clinical hallmarks of the disease are chorea and behavioral disturbance. The illness may begin with either or both of these symptoms predominating. Onset is usually in the fourth or fifth decade, but there is a wide range in age of onset, from childhood to greater than 70 years. The chorea begins as subtle fidgeting that may be unrecognized by the patient and family. However, the movement disorder is usually slowly progressive and eventually may become disabling. There are frequent, irregular, sudden jerks and movements of any of the limbs or trunk. Grimacing, grunting, and poor articulation of speech may be prominent. The gait is disjointed and poorly coordinated and has a so-called dancing (choreic) quality. Memory is frequently not impaired until late in the disease, but attention, judgment, and executive functions may be seriously deficient at an early stage. Depression, apathy, social withdrawal, irritability, and intermittent disinhibition are common. Delusions and obsessive-compulsive behavior may occur. Schizophrenia is occasionally the initial diagnosis. The disease duration is typically about 15 years but also shows a wide range. Early onset before the age of 20 (juvenile HD) is associated with rigidity, ataxia, cognitive decline, and more rapid progression, with a typical duration of about 8 years. Seizures are rare with adult-onset HD but more common with juvenile-onset disease. There is no specific treatment, but the adventitious movements and behavioral changes may partially respond to phenothiazines, haloperidol, or benzodiazepines.

Neuropathologically, the disease predominantly strikes the striatum. Atrophy of the caudate nuclei, which form the lateral margins of the lateral ventricles, can be visualized on neuroimaging studies in the middle and late stages of the disease (Fig. 367-4). Microscopically there are no dramatic pathologic characteristics, such as the plaques and tangles seen with AD. However, there is gliosis and neuronal loss, especially of medium-sized spiny neurons in the caudate and putamen. There is relative sparing of large cholinergic aspiny neurons. (Treatment with 3-nitroproprionic acid, a succinate dehydrogenase inhibitor, has produced HD-like pathologic changes in experimental animals). Neurochemically there is a marked decrease of gamma-aminobutyric acid (GABA) and its synthetic enzyme glutamic acid decarboxylase throughout the basal ganglia. The levels of other neurotransmitters, including substance P and enkephalins, are also reduced. Nuclear magnetic resonance (NMR) spectroscopy in living subjects with HD has shown elevated levels of lactate in the basal ganglia.

The HD gene, called *IT15*, is located on chromosome 4p, contains a CAG trinucleotide repeat expansion, and codes for a protein called huntingtin. The protein is found in neurons throughout the brain; its normal function is unknown. Inactivation of the homologous gene in mice causes embryonic death in homozygotes, but heterozygotes are phenotypically normal. Transgenic mice with an expanded CAG repeat in the HD gene develop a progressive movement disorder. The CAG repeat codes for a long polyglutamine domain in the expressed protein. The disease process may result from a toxic gain of function (Chap. 363). One hypothesis is that these polyglutamine tracts cause abnormal protein binding reactions which then interfere with other cell processes, such as mitochondrial activity. Abnormal binding of IT15 to glyceraldehyde 3-phosphate dehydrogenase has been reported. There is also evidence for inappropriate neuronal apoptosis in HD.

The DNA repeat expansion forms the basis of a diagnostic blood test for the disease gene. Persons having 38 or more CAG repeats in the HD gene have inherited the disease mutation and will even-

A

B

FIGURE 367-4 Huntington's disease *A.* Sagittal T1-weighted MRI shows enlargement of the lateral ventricles reflecting typical caudate atrophy (*arrows*). *B.* Axial T2-weighted image demonstrates abnormal high signal intensity in the putamen (*arrows*).

tually develop symptoms if they live to an advanced age. Each of their children has a 50 percent risk of also inheriting the abnormal gene. There is a rough correlation between a larger number of repeats and an earlier age of onset, but most patients fall into a range of intermediate repeat numbers (40 to 49 repeats) in which this correlation is not clinically useful. For unclear reasons, juvenile onset with a large repeat expansion most often occurs when the father is the affected parent (a form of genetic anticipation). Asymptomatic adult children at risk for HD should receive careful genetic counseling prior to DNA testing, because a positive result may have serious emotional and social consequences. Detailed testing and counseling protocols have been published. In addition to use in genetic counseling of persons at risk for HD, the DNA test can also be used in differential diagnosis. For example, some persons with late-onset, apparently sporadic "senile" chorea have been found to carry the HD mutation. Also, disorders that may mimic HD, such as schizophrenia, benign familial chorea, inherited ataxias, neural acanthocytosis and familial AD, will not show the CAG expansion in the HD gene.

OTHER DEGENERATIVE DEMENTIAS Several other primary neurologic disorders have been associated with dementia and are the result of various poorly understood degenerative neuronal processes. These conditions include so-called frontal lobe dementia, cortical basal degeneration, progressive supranuclear palsy, and primary progressive aphasia. These are progressive dementing illnesses of unknown cause whose names are descriptive of the typical clinical signs or the anatomic brain areas that are involved with nonspecific atrophy and neuronal degeneration.

One such condition is *progressive supranuclear palsy* (see also Chap. 368). This is a degenerative disease that involves both the brainstem and neocortex with diffuse NFTs. Clinically, this disorder begins with vertical supranuclear gaze paresis and progresses slowly to include rigidity and dementia. Stiff posture with hyperextension of the neck and slow gait with frequent falls are common. Early in the disease, the patients have difficulty with down-gaze and lose vertical opticokinetic nystagmus on downward movement of the target. Although the patients have very limited voluntary eye movements, their eyes still retain oculocephalic reflexes (doll's head maneuver). The dementia is considered to be of the subcortical type, with slowed thought processes, impaired verbal fluency, and difficulty with sequential actions and with shifting from one task to another. Seizures and sleep apnea may occur. There is only a limited response to L-dopa, and there is no other effective treatment. Death occurs within 5 to 10 years. At autopsy, the NFTs are found in multiple subcortical structures (including the subthalamus, globus pallidus, substantia nigra, locus coeruleus, periaqueductal gray, superior colliculi, and oculomotor nuclei) as well as in the neocortex. The NFTs have similar staining characteristics to those of AD, but on electron microscopy they generally are seen to consist of straight tubules rather than the paired helical filaments found in AD.

Progressive supranuclear palsy is often confused with idiopathic *Parkinson's disease*. Although elderly Parkinson's patients may have some difficulty with upgaze, they do not develop significant downgaze paresis or progressive supernuclear palsy. However, dementia does occur in approximately 20 percent of Parkinson's patients. The occurrence of dementia in Parkinson's disease is more likely with increasing age, increasing severity of extrapyramidal signs, and the presence of depression. These patients may also show cortical atrophy on brain imaging. Neuropathologically, there may be Alzheimer changes in the cortex (amyloid plaques and NFTs), neuronal Lewy body inclusions in both the substantia nigra and the cortex, or no specific microscopic changes other than gliosis and neuronal loss.

Some authors refer to a condition called *frontal lobe* or *frontotemporal dementia* (see Chap. 25). In addition to progressive memory loss and confusion, the patients are often irritable and have loss of inhibitions. These patients may do better than those with AD on construction and calculation tasks. Imaging studies reveal atrophy confined to the frontal or frontal and temporal lobes. The condition is not a specific entity, and the designation usually includes Pick's disease. Frontal lobe dementia represents as much as 10 percent of dementia cases in some autopsy series.

Cortical basal degeneration is a slowly progressive dementing illness associated with severe gliosis and neuronal loss in both the neocortex and basal ganglia (substantia nigra and striatum). There is often a unilateral onset with rigidity, dystonia, and apraxia of one arm and hand. Eventually the condition becomes bilateral and includes dysarthria, slow gait, action tremor, and dementia. The microscopic features include enlarged, achromatic neurons in the cortex, and there may also be NFTs and amyloid plaques. The condition is rarely familial; the cause is unknown; and there is no specific treatment.

Another entity is *primary progressive aphasia* (see Chap. 25).

Patients with this disorder have aphasia associated with asymmetric atrophy of the left hemisphere and occasionally go on to develop dementia. Neuroimaging studies show the left hemisphere atrophy. Some patients are nonfluent, with hesitant, telegraphic speech associated with impaired comprehension and naming. Neuropathologic studies have shown a heterogeneous group of abnormalities, including Pick's disease, AD, CJD, and nonspecific gliosis.

A rare degenerative disease has also occurred in the Chamorro natives on the island of Guam and is referred to as the *ALS/parkinsonian/dementia complex of Guam* (see Chap. 370). Individual patients may have any combination of parkinsonian features, dementia, and motor neuron disease. The most characteristic pathologic features are the presence of NFTs in degenerating neurons of the cortex and substantia nigra and loss of motor neurons in the spinal cord. Epidemiologic evidence supports a probable environmental cause, such as exposure to a neurotoxin with a long latency period. One interesting but unproven candidate neurotoxin occurs in the seed of the false palm tree, which Guamanians traditionally used to make flour. The ALS syndrome is decreasing in frequency on Guam, but a dementing illness continues to be seen.

Finally, a rare autosomal dominant genetic form of dementia with nonspecific neuropathologic findings has been linked to DNA markers on chromosome 17. The specific gene has not been identified. Some of these families have dementia associated with motor neuron disease, others with parkinsonian features. This condition is now referred to as frontotemporal dementia with parkinsonism linked to chromosome 17 (FTDP-17).

BIBLIOGRAPHY

AMERICAN COLLEGE OF MEDICAL GENETICS/AMERICAN SOCIETY OF HUMAN GENETICS WORKING GROUP ON APOE AND ALZHEIMER DISEASE: Consensus statement on use of apolipoprotein E testing for Alzheimer disease. JAMA 274:1627, 1995

BIRD TD, BENNETT RL: Why do DNA testing? Practical and ethical implications of new neurogenetic tests. Ann Neurol 38:141, 1995

CAPLAN LR: Binswanger's disease—revisited. Neurology 45:626, 1995

DANIEL SE et al: The clinical and pathological spectrum of Steele-Richardson-Olszewski syndrome (progressive supranuclear palsy): A reappraisal. Brain 118:759, 1995

DAVIS KL, POWCHIK P: Tacrine. Lancet 345:625, 1995

DEL SER T et al: Vascular dementia: A clinicopathological study. J Neurol Sci 96:1, 1990

KERTESZ A et al: The pathology and nosology of primary progressive aphasia. Neurology 44:2065, 1994

LEVY-LAHAD E et al: Candidate gene for the chromosome 1 familial Alzheimer's disease locus. Science 269:973, 1995

————, BIRD TD: Genetic factors in Alzheimer's disease: A review of recent advances. Ann Neurol 40:829, 1996

LYNCH T et al: Clinical characteristics of a family with chromosome 17-linked disinhibition-dementia-parkinsonism-amyotrophy complex. Neurology 44:1878, 1994

MALM J et al: The predictive value of cerebrospinal fluid dynamic tests in patients with the idiopathic adult hydrocephalus syndrome. Arch Neurol 52:783, 1995

MCKEITH IG et al: An evaluation of the predictive validity and inter-rater reliability of clinical diagnostic criteria for senile dementia of Lewy body type. Neurology 44:872, 1994

MENDEZ MF et al: Pick's disease versus Alzheimer's disease: A comparison of clinical characteristics. Neurology 43:289, 1993

RAFTOPOULOS C et al: Cognitive recovery in idiopathic normal pressure hydrocephalus: A prospective study. Neurosurgery 35:397, 1994

REIMAN EM et al: Preclinical evidence of Alzheimer's disease in persons homozygous for the ε4 allele for apolipoprotein E. N Engl J Med 334:752, 1996

SHERRINGTON R et al: Cloning of a gene bearing missense mutations in early-onset familial Alzheimer's disease. Nature 375:754, 1995

TATEMICHI TK et al: Dementia after stroke: Baseline frequency, risks, and clinical features in a hospitalized cohort. Neurology 42:1185, 1992

TERRY RD et al: *Alzheimer Disease.* New York, Raven Press, 1994

TISON F et al: Dementia in Parkinson's disease: A population-based study in ambulatory and institutionalized individuals. Neurology 45:705, 1995

VAN BROECKHOVEN CJ: Molecular genetics of Alzheimer disease: Identification of genes and gene mutations. Eur Neurol 35:8, 1995

VANNESTE JAL: Three decades of normal pressure hydrocephalus: Are we wiser now? J Neurol Neurosurg Psychiatr 57:1021, 1994

WIGGINS S et al: The psychological consequences of predictive testing for Huntington's disease. N Engl J Med 237:1401, 1992

368 *Michael J. Aminoff*

PARKINSON'S DISEASE AND OTHER EXTRAPYRAMIDAL DISORDERS

PARKINSON'S DISEASE Parkinsonism is a syndrome consisting of a variable combination of tremor, rigidity, bradykinesia, and a characteristic disturbance of gait and posture. Parkinson's disease is a chronic, progressive disorder in which idiopathic parkinsonism occurs without evidence of more widespread neurologic involvement.

Parkinson's disease generally commences in middle or late life and leads to progressive disability with time. The disease occurs in all ethnic groups, has an equal sex distribution, and is common, with a prevalence of 1 to 2 per 1000 of the general population and 1 per 100 among people older than 65 years. Signs of parkinsonism are extremely common in the elderly; a recent survey indicated that 15 percent of individuals between 65 and 74 years of age, and more than half of all individuals after age 85, have abnormalities on examination consistent with the presence of an extrapyramidal disorder.

Neuroanatomy Symptoms of Parkinson's disease are caused by loss of nerve cells in the pigmented substantia nigra pars compacta and the locus coeruleus in the midbrain. Cell loss also occurs in the globus pallidus and putamen. Eosinophilic intraneural inclusion granules (Lewy bodies) are present in the basal ganglia, brainstem, spinal cord, and sympathetic ganglia; they do not occur in other disorders in which parkinsonism is a feature.

The neural pathways that modulate motor activity are considered in detail in Chap. 21. Pars compacta neurons of the substantia nigra provide dopaminergic input to the striatum, which is part of the basal ganglia (Fig. 21-4A). These dopaminergic neurons, and also cholinergic striatal interneurons, modulate a monosynaptic gamma-aminobutyric acid (GABA-ergic) inhibitory output to the globus pallidus interna and pars reticulata of the substantia nigra, which project in turn by a GABA-ergic inhibitory pathway to the ventroanterior and ventrolateral nuclei of the thalamus. Stimulation of this "direct" pathway in the striatum disinhibits these thalamic nuclei so that their excitatory output to the motor region of the cerebral cortex is increased. An alternative, polysynaptic ("indirect") pathway from the striatum reduces the excitatory output from these thalamic nuclei to the motor cortex, as shown in Fig. 21-4A. This latter pathway involves striatal GABA-ergic inhibitory neurons that project to the globus pallidus externa, which has an inhibitory effect on the subthalamic nucleus. This nucleus has excitatory glutamatergic connections with the globus pallidus interna and pars reticulata of the substantia nigra.

In Parkinson's disease, loss of dopaminergic cells in the substantia nigra leads to striatal dopamine depletion. Because dopamine activates excitatory D1 receptors in the direct pathway and represses inhibitory D2 receptors in the indirect pathway, this depletion results in decreased activity of the direct pathway and increased activity of the indirect pathway and so in reduced thalamic excitation of the motor cortex (Fig. 21-4B). Other neurotransmitters, such as norepinephrine, are also depleted, with clinical consequences that are uncertain but perhaps contribute to depression.

Pathogenesis Parkinsonism can be induced in primates by exposure to 1-methyl-4-phenyl-1,2,3,6-tetrahydropyridine (MPTP), which is converted by monoamine oxidase B to *N*-methyl-4-phenylpyridinium (MPP$^+$), an active toxin. MPP$^+$ is taken up by dopaminergic nigral neurons through an active transport system that is normally involved in dopamine reuptake, and then inhibits oxidative phosphorylation, possibly at the level of complex I in the respiratory chain. This results in the death of nigrostriatal neurons, dopamine depletion in the basal ganglia, and parkinsonism. In addition to energy failure, MPP$^+$ may also generate free radicals and oxidative stress.

The cause of Parkinson's disease is unknown. One suggested cause is exposure to an unrecognized environmental toxin, perhaps structurally similar to MPTP. Such exposure may have occurred years before the onset of any clinical disturbance, because symptoms will not develop until the cumulative cell loss from toxin exposure and natural aging approximates 80 percent of the original cell population. Alternatively or additionally, endogenous toxins may be responsible. In particular, the normal neurotransmitter dopamine readily oxidizes to produce free radicals, which can cause cell death by oxidizing various cellular constituents. Although the precise role of dopamine itself remains unclear, the evidence relating Parkinson's disease to damage by free radicals remains compelling.

It is not clear whether there is a significant genetic component in the etiology of Parkinson's disease. Studies in monozygotic and dizygotic twins initially suggested that the disease rarely had a genetic basis. More recent work involving positron emission tomography (PET) studies have shown, however, that asymptomatic twins of parkinsonian patients commonly have abnormalities of striatal dopamine uptake; this suggests that genetic factors are important, although this finding was present equally in monozygotic and dizygotic twins. Attempts to identify the responsible gene or genes contributing to the development of Parkinson's disease are currently in progress; linkage to chromosome 4q21-23 was recently reported in a large Italian family with autosomal dominant parkinsonism.

Clinical Manifestations The 4- to 6-Hz tremor is typically most conspicuous at rest and worsens with emotional stress. It often begins with rhythmic flexion-extension of the fingers, hand, or foot, or with rhythmic pronation-supination of the forearm, and may be confined initially to one limb or to the two limbs on one side before becoming more generalized. It may also involve the mouth and chin. In 10 to 15 percent of patients, however, the tremor is faster (7 to 8 Hz) and postural, resembling essential tremor (see below) both clinically and in its response to pharmacotherapy.

Rigidity, defined as an increase in resistance to passive movement (Chap. 21), is a common clinical feature that accounts for the flexed posture of many patients. The most disabling feature, however, is bradykinesia (or, in its most severe form, akinesia), a slowness of voluntary movement and an associated reduction in automatic movements, such as swinging of the arms when walking. There is a fixity of facial expression, with widened palpebral fissures and infrequent blinking. There may be blepharoclonus (fluttering of the closed eyelids), blepharospasm (involuntary closure of the eyelids), and drooling of saliva from the mouth. The voice is hypophonic and poorly modulated. Power is preserved, but fine or rapidly alternating movements are impaired. The combination of tremor, rigidity, and bradykinesia results in small, tremulous, and often illegible handwriting. Patients have difficulty in rising from bed or an easy chair and tend to assume a flexed posture when erect. Walking is often difficult to initiate, and patients may have to lean forward increasingly until they can advance. They walk with small, shuffling steps, have no arm-swing, are unsteady (especially on turning), and may have difficulty in stopping. Some patients walk with a festinating gait, i.e., at an increasing speed to prevent themselves from falling because of their abnormal center of gravity.

The tendon reflexes are unaltered, and the plantar responses are flexor. Repetitive tapping (at about 2 Hz) over the glabella produces a sustained blink response (Myerson's sign), in contrast to the response of normal subjects. A depressed mood is common, and an impairment of cognitive function—sometimes amounting to a frank dementia— is frequently evident in advanced cases.

Differential Diagnosis Parkinsonism is simulated by certain disorders. *Depression* is associated with changes in the voice and facial appearance and a poverty of spontaneous activity, such as occur in Parkinson's disease. A trial of treatment with antidepressant drugs helps to clarify the diagnosis if uncertainty persists and other signs of parkinsonism are absent. *Essential (benign, familial) tremor* may be mistaken for parkinsonian tremor, but a family history of tremor is common; alcohol in small quantities may ameliorate the tremor, and other neurologic signs are lacking. Moreover, essential tremor commonly involves the head (with a nodding or no-no tremor), whereas parkinsonism spares the head but affects the face and lips. *Normal-pressure hydrocephalus* (see Chap. 367) causes an apraxic gait disturbance (sometimes resembling the gait of parkinsonism), urinary incontinence, and dementia. Imaging studies reveal dilation of the ventricular system without cortical atrophy, and surgical shunting procedures to bypass any obstruction to the flow of cerebrospinal fluid (CSF) may be helpful.

Parkinsonism may occur as part of various neurologic diseases that are important to distinguish from Parkinson's disease for prognostic and therapeutic purposes. In *Wilson's disease* (see Chap. 345), other abnormal movements are also usually present. The family history, early age of onset, associated Kayser-Fleischer rings, and low serum copper and ceruloplasmin levels distinguish it from Parkinson's disease. *Huntington's disease* (see Chap. 367) sometimes presents with rigidity and akinesia, but the family history and any accompanying dementia point to the correct diagnosis, which can be confirmed by genetic studies. The *Shy-Drager syndrome* (see also Chap. 371) is a degenerative disorder characterized by parkinsonism, impaired autonomic function (resulting in postural hypotension, abnormal thermoregulatory sweating, disturbances of bladder and bowel control, impotence, and gastroparesis) and by signs of more widespread neurologic involvement (pyramidal, cerebellar, or lower motor neuron signs). There is generally no treatment except for the postural hypotension, which may respond to the measures discussed in Chap. 371. The response to antiparkinsonian agents is usually disappointing. *Striatonigral degeneration* (see below) leads to bradykinesia and rigidity, but tremor is usually inconspicuous. Cerebellar deficits sometimes occur (multisystem atrophy), and there may be autonomic insufficiency (Shy-Drager syndrome). Antiparkinsonian drugs are generally ineffective. *Progressive supranuclear palsy* (discussed separately, below) causes bradykinesia and rigidity, but conspicuous abnormalities of voluntary eye movements (especially vertical gaze), dementia, pseudobulbar palsy, and axial dystonia distinguish it from Parkinson's disease. There is little or no response to antiparkinsonian drugs. *Cortical-basal ganglionic degeneration* may be mistaken for Parkinson's disease, but intellectual decline, aphasia, apraxia, sensory neglect, and other evidence of cortical dysfunction should suggest the correct diagnosis. In *diffuse Lewy body disease*, parkinsonism is joined with a conspicuous dementia and with evidence of more widespread neurologic involvement. In *Creutzfeldt-Jakob disease*, any parkinsonian features are overshadowed by the rapidly progressive dementia; myoclonus is common, ataxia or pyramidal signs may occur, visual disturbances are sometimes conspicuous, and the electroencephalographic findings are often characteristic. Similarly, in *Alzheimer's disease* there may be minor extrapyrami-

dal deficits, but these are generally inconsequential compared with the marked cognitive impairment that characterizes the disorder. → *Alzheimer's disease and diffuse Lewy body disease are considered in Chap. 367, and Creutzfeldt-Jakob disease is discussed in Chap. 379.*

Parkinsonism sometimes occurs as a consequence of a systemic disorder. Drug-induced *secondary parkinsonism* is especially common (discussed below). MPTP-induced parkinsonism has occurred in several humans who inadvertently took this meperidine analogue for recreational purposes. The mechanisms involved are discussed above, and the history of exposure, unusually early age of onset, and rapid progression should suggest the correct diagnosis. Exposure to various toxins, such as manganese dust or carbon disulfide, also causes parkinsonism, and the diagnosis is suggested by an accurate occupational history. Parkinsonism sometimes occurs as a result of severe carbon monoxide poisoning or develops after an encephalitic illness. Postencephalitic parkinsonism was especially common after the outbreak of encephalitis lethargica that occurred in an early part of the twentieth century.

℞ TREATMENT

Approaches to treatment are summarized in Fig. 368-1.

Symptomatic Pharmacologic Treatment   Nonselective muscarinic antagonists (*anticholinergic drugs*) are sometimes helpful, especially in relieving tremor. Various preparations are available, including trihexyphenidyl, benztropine, procyclidine, and orphenadrine. The usual starting and maintenance doses are shown in Table

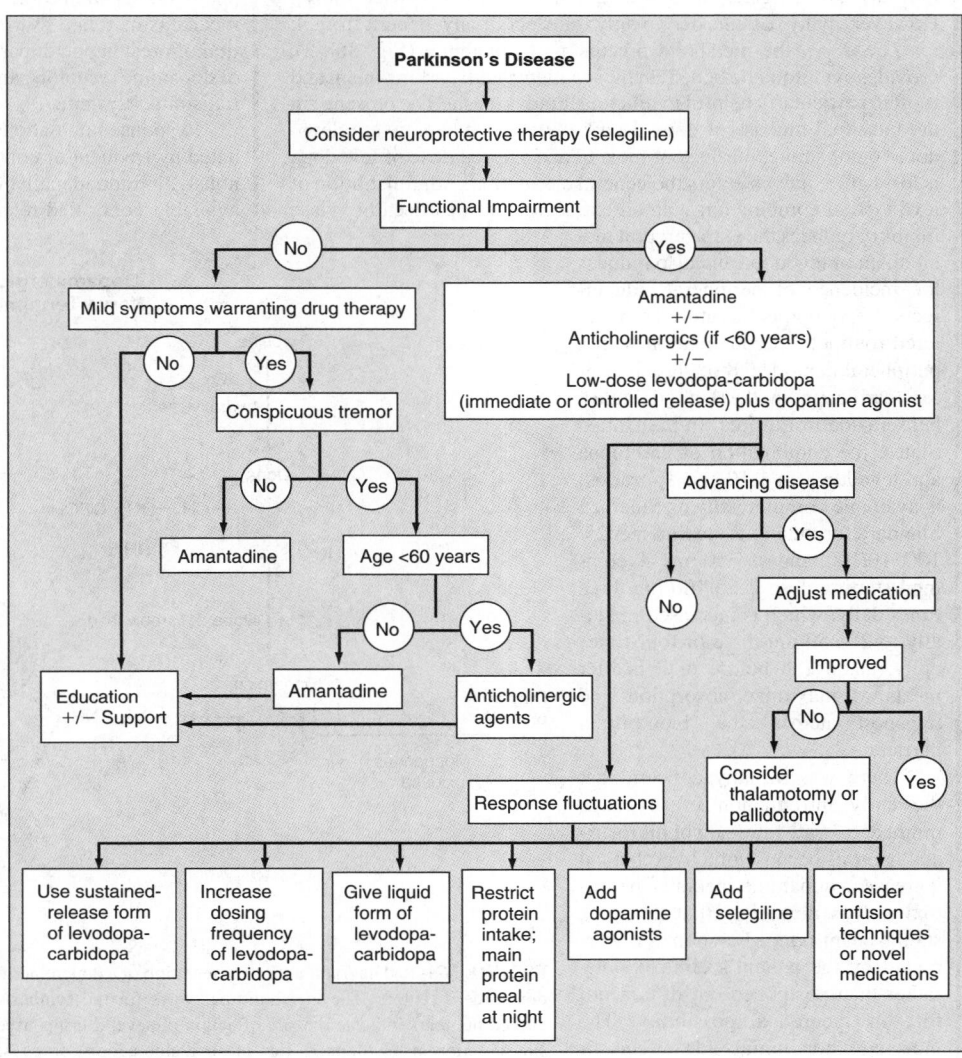

FIGURE 368-1   Algorithm for the management of patients with Parkinson's disease.

Table 368-1

Commonly Used Muscarinic Antagonists (Anticholinergic Drugs) for the Treatment of Parkinson's Disease

Generic Name	Proprietary Name	Tablet Strength	Usual Dose, mg
Benztropine	Cogentin	0.5, 1, 2	0.5–2 tid
Biperiden	Akineton	2	1–3 qid
Orphenadrine	Disipal	100	100 tid
Procyclidine	Kemadrin	5	2.5–10 tid
Trihexyphenidyl	Artane	2, 5	2–5 tid

368-1. Common side effects include dryness of the mouth, constipation, urinary retention, and blurred vision. Narrow-angle glaucoma may be aggravated. Confusion and hallucinations are especially troublesome in the elderly. Treatment is started with the preparation of choice in a small initial dose that is gradually increased depending on response and tolerance. If the drug is unhelpful, another anticholinergic preparation is substituted.

Amantadine, either alone or combined with an anticholinergic agent, is sometimes helpful for mild parkinsonism; it acts by potentiating the release of endogenous dopamine. It may improve all major clinical features of the disorder, has relatively uncommon side effects (restlessness, confusion, skin rashes, edema, disturbances of cardiac rhythm), and is given in a standard dose (100 mg twice daily). However, many patients derive only transient, if any, benefit from it.

Levodopa, the metabolic precursor of dopamine (Fig. 368-2), provides symptomatic benefit in most patients with parkinsonism and is often particularly helpful in relieving bradykinesia. The presence in the intestinal mucosa of dopa decarboxylase, which converts levodopa to dopamine, means that most of an ingested dose of levodopa is lost before it even enters the general circulation. Administration of levodopa in combination with an extracerebral dopa-decarboxylase inhibitor reduces the extracerebral metabolism of levodopa and also reduces the incidence of peripheral side effects. Levodopa is therefore administered routinely in combination with a peripheral dopa-decarboxylase inhibitor (carbidopa in the United States; benserazide in Europe). In the United States, the combination of carbidopa and levodopa (in 1:10 and 1:4 ratios) is available commercially as Sinemet. Standard formulations are Sinemet 25/100, 10/100, and 25/250 mg. A common starting dose is 25/100 mg three times daily, which is increased gradually to 25/250 mg three or four times daily, taken 1 h before or 2 h after meals to maximize absorption and transport across the blood-brain barrier.

There was initially concern that the early introduction of levodopa might accelerate the death of nigrostriatal neurons because of a hypothetical increase in dopamine-mediated neurotoxicity. It is now clear that levodopa should be introduced as soon as is warranted by the patient's clinical state, rather than postponed out of concern for this theoretical possibility. The most common initial side effects of levodopa are nausea, vomiting, pos-

tural hypotension, and, occasionally, cardiac arrhythmias. Abnormal movements (dyskinesias), restlessness (akathisia), and confusion tend to occur somewhat later and are dose-related. Dyskinesias probably result from denervation supersensitivity of postsynaptic dopamine receptors. They may be present during most of the day, occur only when plasma levodopa levels peak, or develop when the plasma levodopa concentration reaches a certain submaximal level. Management depends on distinguishing these possibilities by the temporal profile of the dyskinesia. When dyskinesias occur only at a certain submaximal blood level of levodopa, adjustment of the daily dose to produce higher or lower blood levels may alleviate them; dyskinesias related to peak blood levels of levodopa are helped by a reduction in dose.

Important late complications of levodopa therapy are the wearing-off effect (transient deterioration shortly before the next dose is due) and the "on-off" phenomenon—abrupt but transient fluctuations in clinical state that occur frequently during the day, without warning or an obvious relationship to dosing schedule, resulting in alternating periods of marked akinesia or greater mobility accompanied by iatrogenic dyskinesias. The on-off phenomenon can be controlled in part by reducing dosing intervals, administering levodopa 1 h before meals and restricting dietary protein intake (to reduce any competition by various amino acids with levodopa for the active carrier system that transports it into the blood and from the blood into the brain), or treatment with dopamine agonists. The addition of selegiline (5 mg at breakfast and lunch), a monoamine oxidase B inhibitor, reduces the metabolic breakdown of dopamine and may also be helpful (see "Neuroprotective Treatment" below). The pathogenesis of the on-off phenomenon is obscure, but proposed mechanisms relate to the pharmacokinetics of levodopa, degeneration of presynaptic dopaminergic nerve terminals, altered sensitivity of dopamine receptors, and abnormalities of nondopaminergic neurotransmitter systems.

Response fluctuations to oral levodopa may be reduced or eliminated by frequent or continuous administration of levodopa intravenously, intraduodenally, or by intragastric infusion. A commercially available controlled-release formulation of Sinemet (Sinemet CR

FIGURE 368-2 Diagrammatic representation of a dopaminergic nerve terminal and the associated postsynaptic dopamine receptors. The metabolic pathways for the synthesis and breakdown of dopamine are shown. The circled numbers indicate the site of action of several drugs used in the treatment of Parkinson's disease: *1*, the site of action of levodopa; *2*, that of dopamine agonist drugs, such as bromocriptine and pergolide; and *3*, that of selegiline. DA, dopamine.

25/100 or 50/200 mg) sometimes helps in reducing the dosing frequency and maintaining steady blood levels of levodopa, but it is of only limited benefit in reducing response fluctuations.

Dopamine agonist drugs, such as the ergot derivatives bromocriptine and pergolide, may produce symptomatic benefit by direct stimulation of dopamine receptors (Fig. 368-2), although the benefit may not be sustained unless levodopa is also taken. Their absorption and cerebral distribution are less erratic than those of levodopa, and they do not require enzymatic conversion to an active metabolite. Their early introduction in conjunction with low-dose Sinemet therapy (25/100 mg three times daily) yields sustained benefit and a lower incidence of late complications (such as response fluctuations and dyskinesias) than when levodopa is used alone and in a higher dose.

Bromocriptine, which stimulates dopamine D2 receptors, is introduced in a dose of 1.25 mg/d for one week and 2.5 mg/d for the next week, after which the daily dose is increased by 2.5-mg increments every 2 weeks, depending on response and tolerance. Maintenance doses range between 2.5 and 10 mg three times daily when the drug is taken with Sinemet. Pergolide activates both D1 and D2 dopamine receptors. It is introduced in a dose of 0.05 mg daily for 2 days; the dose is then increased by 0.1 to 0.15 mg/d every 3 days for 12 days and by 0.25 mg/d every 3 days thereafter. The usual maintenance dose is 1 mg three times daily. The side effects of these agonists are similar to those of levodopa, but psychiatric effects such as delusions or hallucinations are more common, and dyskinesias are less common, than with levodopa. Dopamine agonists are contraindicated in patients with psychotic disorders and are best avoided in those with recent myocardial infarction, severe peripheral vascular disease, or active peptic ulceration.

Various new dopamine agonists are being evaluated, and new means of administering them (e.g., by subcutaneous infusion pump or transdermally) may lead to a steadier clinical response.

Novel symptomatic therapies currently being evaluated or developed include selective catechol-*O*-methyltransferase (COMT) inhibitors, which may enhance the benefits of levodopa therapy by reducing the conversion of levodopa to 3-*O*-methyldopa (which competes with levodopa for an active carrier mechanism) and by increasing the availability in the brain of levodopa. Experimental studies suggest that glutamate antagonists may benefit patients with Parkinson's disease, and clinical studies of such agents are planned. G_{M1} ganglioside and various neurotrophic factors influence dopaminergic nigrostriatal cells, and work is in progress to develop delivery systems that will permit their use in the treatment of Parkinson's disease.

Surgical Treatment   Destructive neurosurgical procedures were used for some years to treat parkinsonism, but their use declined with the advent of levodopa. Unilateral posteroventral pallidotomy or thalamotomy has recently been resurrected as a therapeutic approach for relieving rigidity, bradykinesia, and tremor in patients with advanced disease in whom antiparkinsonian medication is ineffective or poorly tolerated. A positive (but incomplete) response to surgery is reported in preliminary studies to occur in more than 90 percent of patients; the beneficial effect predominates on the side contralateral to the procedure.

There has been recent interest in transplantation of fetal midbrain dopaminergic (nigral) cells into the putamen of patients with Parkinson's disease. Survival of engrafted cells has been documented by enhancement of fluorodopa uptake as visualized by PET, and in one autopsy study there was extensive striatal reinnervation by the transplanted cells. Fetal nigral transplantation remains an experimental procedure, and the nature of any long-term benefit is uncertain. Transplantation of autologous adrenal medullary tissue has also been attempted for Parkinson's disease, with mixed results; benefit seems most likely to occur in individuals younger than 50 years of age.

Neuroprotective Treatment   Selective inhibitors of monoamine oxidase B such as selegiline (Eldepryl; Deprenyl) may reduce oxidative damage and thus slow disease progression, but the evidence for this effect is incomplete. In a large multicenter study, treatment with selegiline delayed the need for symptomatic therapy in patients with untreated parkinsonism, suggesting that progression of the disease had been retarded, but it was subsequently found that selegiline itself has a mild effect on symptoms. Thus, the basis of the observed effect is uncertain. The use of selegiline for protective purposes should probably be discussed with all patients unless they have end-stage disease or are very elderly, but the uncertainty of any benefit should be indicated. Selegiline in a standard dose (5 mg with breakfast and 5 mg with lunch) is not associated with the hypertensive ("cheese") effect of nonselective monoamine oxidase inhibitors. Acute toxic interactions may, however, occur with meperidine, tricyclic drugs, or serotonin reuptake inhibitors, and selegiline should not be prescribed to patients receiving those medications. Selegiline is metabolized to amphetamine and methamphetamine, so some patients may experience anxiety or insomnia. Moreover, an increased mortality rate has recently been found among patients receiving selegiline, raising concerns about its long-term safety. Patients must understand that selegiline is not intended to relieve symptoms and that there is no means of determining whether it is affecting disease progression in individual cases. Other inhibitors of monamine oxidase B, such as lazabemide, are currently being evaluated for their effect on the natural history of Parkinson's disease and may clarify the issue.

Tocopherol (vitamin E) is an important scavenger of free radicals, but in a large study it failed to provide any protective benefit when taken in a dose of 2000 units daily. The extent to which it penetrates the brain, however, is not clear.

General Measures   Physical therapy and speech therapy may help patients with moderately severe parkinsonism. In advanced cases, the quality of life can be improved by certain aids to daily living, such as extra rails or banisters placed in the home, table cutlery with large handles, nonslip table mats, voice amplifiers, and chairs that can gently eject the occupant.

FAMILIAL OR BENIGN ESSENTIAL TREMOR   A postural tremor (Chap. 21) may develop in otherwise normal subjects, sometimes on a familial basis with autosomal dominant inheritance. The pathophysiologic basis of the disorder is unknown.

Symptoms can develop at any age but often do not appear until middle or later life. Typically one or both hands, the head, and the voice are affected in any combination; the legs are generally spared. Apart from the tremor, no other abnormalities are present on neurologic examination. The tremor may worsen with time and ultimately become an embarrassment, but it generally causes no disability except when it disturbs handwriting or performance of fine tasks with the hands. A small quantity of alcohol sometimes relieves the tremor for a short period.

℞ **TREATMENT**

Treatment is often unnecessary and is best delayed for as long as possible because, once initiated, it generally needs to be continued indefinitely. Propranolol, 40 to 120 mg orally twice daily, may reduce the amplitude of the tremor. A single oral dose (40 to 120 mg) may be taken in anticipation of known precipitating circumstances. Primidone is also effective but has to be introduced gradually.

PROGRESSIVE SUPRANUCLEAR PALSY   Progressive supranuclear palsy (also referred to as Steele-Richardson-Olszewski syndrome) is a sporadic degenerative disorder characterized pathologically by neuronal loss, gliosis, and neurofibrillary tangles in the midbrain, pons, basal ganglia, and dentate nuclei of the cerebellum. The neurofibrillary tangles of this disorder are distinct from those of Alzheimer's disease in that they are composed of straight filaments rather than paired helical filaments. There are decreased concentrations of dopamine and homovanillic acid in the caudate nucleus and putamen.

Clinical Manifestations   This uncommon disorder generally begins between the ages of 45 and 75 years; it affects men twice as frequently as women. Supranuclear ophthalmoplegia is characteristic. There is conspicuous failure of voluntary saccadic gaze (and of the fast phase of optokinetic nystagmus) in a vertical plane, especially downward, with later involvement of horizontal gaze. Eventually, smooth pursuit movements are also affected. Oculocephalic (e.g., doll's-head) and oculovestibular (caloric) reflexes are intact. Axial dystonia in extension, especially of the neck, is common and is frequently accompanied by limb rigidity and bradykinesia that may mimic Parkinson's disease. Tremor, however, is unusual. The combination of supranuclear ophthalmoplegia and axial rigidity accounts for the common presenting complaint of frequent falls. There may be facial weakness, dysarthria, dysphagia, and exaggerated jaw jerk and gag reflexes (pseudobulbar palsy) as well as exaggerated and inappropriate emotional responses (pseudobulbar affect). Brisk tendon reflexes, extensor plantar responses, and cerebellar signs are sometimes encountered. A global impairment of intellectual function is frequent, but focal cortical dysfunction is rare.

Progressive supranuclear palsy should be considered whenever a middle-aged or elderly person with repeated falls has an extrapyramidal syndrome accompanied by nuchal dystonia and paralysis of voluntary downgaze. The marked impairment of voluntary downward and horizontal gaze distinguishes this disorder from Parkinson's disease, as does the extended rather than flexed dystonic posturing of the axial musculature, the absence of tremor, and the poor response to antiparkinsonian medications.

℞ TREATMENT

The course is generally progressive, with aspiration or inanition leading to a fatal outcome within 10 years. The response to pharmacotherapy is usually disappointing. Dopaminergic preparations sometimes reduce rigidity and bradykinesia, and anticholinergic (trihexyphenidyl, 6 to 15 mg/d) or tricyclic drugs (amitriptyline, 50 to 75 mg at bedtime) may benefit speech, gait, and pseudobulbar affect.

CORTICAL-BASAL GANGLIONIC DEGENERATION

This rare sporadic disorder typically begins in middle or later life with functional impairment of one or more limbs. Examination reveals signs of parkinsonism, but the extrapyramidal abnormalities are generally insufficient to account for the clinical deficit, which results from apraxia. As the disorder progresses, other evidence of cortical dysfunction also appears, such as aphasia, agnosias, sensory inattention, and mild dementia. Pathologically there is cell loss and gliosis in the cerebral cortex as well as the substantia nigra. The response to antiparkinsonian medication is disappointing, and the course is generally progressive, with increasing disability and dependence leading ultimately to death.

STRIATONIGRAL DEGENERATION

In a few patients with seemingly classic Parkinson's disease, there is little or no response to dopaminergic medication, and pathologic study at autopsy reveals neuronal loss and gliosis in the putamen, globus pallidus, caudate and subthalamic nuclei, and substantia nigra. This disorder has therefore been called striatonigral degeneration. It has an age and gender distribution similar to those of Parkinson's disease. Clinical examination reveals the findings of parkinsonism, but tremor is usually relatively inconspicuous. Cognitive function is preserved.

There may be an accompanying impairment of autonomic function (Shy-Drager syndrome; Chap. 371), and examination in such cases often reveals that a combination of pyramidal and cerebellar signs is also present. Indeed, in some cases the cerebellar findings are so conspicuous that the disorder is more properly called spinocerebellar ataxia type 1 (olivopontocerebellar atrophy; Chap. 369).

The management of patients with striatonigral degeneration is difficult. Antiparkinsonian medications generally are prescribed but usually are ineffective.

MACHADO-JOSEPH DISEASE / SPINOCEREBELLAR ATAXIA TYPE 3

Machado-Joseph disease is an autosomal dominant form of striatonigral degeneration that generally begins in the third or fourth decade. Most affected individuals are of Portuguese ancestry. There may be only mild parkinsonian signs, whereas spasticity, hyperreflexia, extensor plantar responses, cerebellar findings, external ophthalmoplegia and, sometimes, peripheral neuropathy are conspicuous. Cognitive function is preserved. Pathologically the findings are similar to those of striatonigral degeneration, but the dentate nucleus of the cerebellum is also involved. There is no specific treatment. → *The different clinical subtypes of the disease, their genetic basis, and related autosomal dominant ataxias with some extrapyramidal features are discussed in Chap. 369.*

IDIOPATHIC TORSION DYSTONIA

The occurrence of dystonic movements and postures without other neurologic signs in patients with a normal birth and developmental history is designated *idiopathic torsion dystonia*. The pathophysiologic and biochemical basis of this entity is unknown. Pathologic examination reveals no specific abnormalities, but the disorder is attributed to basal ganglia dysfunction partly because of observations made in cases of secondary dystonia. Other possible causes of dystonia (Chap. 21) should be excluded before this diagnosis is made. The disorder may occur on a sporadic or hereditary basis. Inheritance can be either autosomal dominant (with the gene localized to 9q32-34 in some families), autosomal recessive, or X-linked recessive (Xq21.3). Onset in childhood is associated with a positive family history, symptoms that begin in the legs, and greater disability than with later onset. About one-third of patients eventually become chair- or bedbound.

Examination reveals the abnormal movements and sustained postures that characterize the disorder. There may be involvement of the neck, trunk, limbs, and face (blepharospasm or oromandibular dystonia). A description of these various motor abnormalities is provided in Chap. 21. Initially they may be brought out by voluntary activity, but eventually they are present constantly, leading to deformity and disability.

Occasional patients have *dopa-responsive dystonia*, which is inherited in an autosomal dominant manner with incomplete penetrance. The responsible gene maps to chromosome 14q. Onset is usually in childhood, and examination typically reveals associated bradykinesia and rigidity. The response to low-dose levodopa therapy is dramatic.

℞ TREATMENT

Treatment is purely symptomatic and is often unsatisfactory. Anticholinergic drugs in high doses (e.g., trihexyphenidyl, 40 to 50 mg/d) are probably the most effective means of providing some relief of the abnormal movements and postures. They are introduced in a low dose and built up gradually, depending on response and tolerance. Phenothiazines or haloperidol are sometimes helpful but usually cause mild parkinsonism. Diazepam, baclofen, and carbamazepine are helpful occasionally. Stereotactic thalamotomy may be beneficial when dystonia is predominantly unilateral and involves the limbs.

FOCAL TORSION DYSTONIA

Dystonia may occur as an isolated phenomenon affecting a discrete part of the body, rather than having the more generalized distribution described above. Such focal or segmental dystonias probably represent variants of idiopathic torsion dystonia. Both *blepharospasm* (spontaneous, involuntary forced closure of the eyelids) and *oromandibular dystonia* can occur as isolated focal dystonias. Oromandibular dystonia consists of involuntary contractions of the masticatory, lingual, and perioral muscles, leading to opening or closure of the mouth; pouting, pursing, or retraction of the lips; and roving or protruding movements of the tongue. The combination of blepharospasm and oromandibular dystonia is called *Meige syndrome*.

Spasmodic torticollis is characterized by a tendency for the head to turn to one side. The designation *anterocollis* indicates that the head is flexed forward, and *retrocollis* that it is pulled backward. These cervical dystonias are often intermittent initially, but eventually the head is held continuously in the abnormal position. Spontaneous remission occurs occasionally, especially in the first few months after onset, but thereafter the disorder is likely to be permanent and may worsen with time.

℞ TREATMENT

Pharmacotherapy is usually unrewarding, but the drugs used in treating idiopathic torsion dystonia are helpful in some patients. Local injection of botulinum toxin into the overactive muscles often produces a benefit lasting several weeks or months by producing a temporary presynaptic block of neuromuscular transmission, and injections can be repeated as needed. This is the most effective treatment available for most focal dystonias. Selective section of the spinal accessory nerve (cranial nerve XI) and the upper cervical nerve roots is sometimes helpful for patients with cervical dystonia unresponsive to other measures.

TASK-SPECIFIC FOCAL DYSTONIA Writer's cramp is a task-specific dystonia in which abnormal posturing of the hand and forearm occurs when the hand is used for writing. As the disorder worsens, abnormal posturing may also occur with other tasks, such as applying cosmetics, shaving, or using table cutlery. Drug treatment is usually unrewarding, and it is often necessary for patients to learn to use the other hand for these tasks. Injections of botulinum toxin into the involved muscles are sometimes helpful, but function usually remains impaired. Other task-specific dystonias include violinist's cramp, barber's cramp, and telegrapher's cramp, in each of which dystonic posturing occurs when the hand is used for a skilled, occupationally related function. The pathophysiologic basis of these disorders is uncertain, but recent work relates it to abnormal processing of sensory input from the affected extremity during the activity.

DRUG-INDUCED MOVEMENT DISORDERS **Parkinsonism** Parkinsonism is a frequent complication of treatment with dopamine-depleting agents such as reserpine or antipsychotic dopamine antagonists such as the phenothiazines or butyrophenones. The antipsychotic drugs most likely to cause parkinsonism are those that are potent D2 receptor antagonists having little anticholinergic effect, such as piperazine phenothiazines, haloperidol, and thiothixene. Women and the elderly have an increased risk of this complication. In comparison with Parkinson's disease, tremor is less common and bradykinesia is typically symmetric, but the two disorders are sometimes impossible to distinguish except by the history of drug ingestion. Signs usually develop within 3 months of starting the causal agent and may persist for several months (or longer) after its withdrawal. Drug-induced parkinsonism is best managed by discontinuing the antipsychotic drug when possible, substituting an antipsychotic with greater anticholinergic potency, or adding an anticholinergic drug such as trihexyphenidyl. Levodopa should not be prescribed—it is of no help if the offending neuroleptic agent is continued, and it may worsen the underlying psychotic disorder.

Acute Dystonia or Dyskinesia Acute dystonia (such as blepharospasm or torticollis) or dyskinesia (such as chorea or facial grimacing) may complicate treatment with a dopamine receptor antagonist. It typically commences within 1 week of the introduction of such medication, usually in the first 48 h, and is more common in young patients. Its pathophysiologic basis is uncertain. Treatment with an anticholinergic drug (e.g., benztropine, 2 mg, or diphenhydramine, 50 mg intravenously) is usually helpful.

Tardive Akathisia *Akathisia* denotes a motor restlessness. Patients are unable to sit still but feel obliged to move about. It is commonly induced by chronic antipsychotic drug treatment, especially in women, and is treated like drug-induced parkinsonism.

Tardive Dyskinesia or Dystonia Tardive dyskinesia or dystonia is a common complication of long-term antipsychotic drug treatment (with dopamine receptor antagonists). The risk of its development increases with advancing age, but its pathogenesis is unclear. One suggestion is that it is related to drug-induced supersensitivity of striatal dopamine receptors. However, although supersensitivity is an inevitable accompaniment of chronic antipsychotic drug treatment, tardive dyskinesia does not always occur. Moreover, the time courses of the two phenomena are different. Supersensitivity occurs relatively early during treatment and reverses when medication is withdrawn, whereas tardive dyskinesia usually requires exposure for at least 6 months before it develops and may persist indefinitely. Another suggestion is that it involves an abnormality of GABA-ergic neurons. This is supported by observations that GABA and glutamic acid decarboxylase (its synthesizing enzyme) are depleted in the basal ganglia by long-term administration of antipsychotic drugs to animals and that CSF levels of GABA are reduced in patients with tardive dyskinesia.

The clinical features of tardive dyskinesia include abnormal choreoathetoid movements, especially involving the face and mouth in adults and the limbs in children. Tardive dystonia may be focal, producing, for example, blepharospasm, torticollis, or oromandibular dystonia, or it may affect contiguous body parts (e.g., the face and neck or arm and trunk). Generalized dystonia is uncommon, especially in older patients. It may be impossible to distinguish these disturbances from those of Huntington's disease (Chap. 367), Sydenham's chorea (Chap. 236), or idiopathic torsion dystonia except by the history of drug exposure. The iatrogenic disorder often resolves spontaneously in children or young adults but frequently persists in middle-aged or older individuals.

℞ TREATMENT

Treatment of the established disorder is often unsatisfactory. It is therefore important that antipsychotic drugs be prescribed only when necessary and that their long-term use be accompanied by periodic drug holidays to determine whether treatment is still required. Drug holidays may actually unmask incipient dyskinesias, which often worsen on withdrawal of the causal agent. In such circumstances, permanent withdrawal of the antipsychotic medication, if this is possible, may lead to remission of the dyskinesia. Treatment with antidopaminergic agents such as haloperidol or phenothiazines (which cause the disorder) often suppresses the dyskinesias at least for a period, but these agents are best avoided, because they may exacerbate the underlying problem. Treatment with dopamine-depleting agents, such as reserpine, 0.25 mg gradually increased to 2 to 4 mg/d, or tetrabenazine (in countries where it is available), 12.5 mg gradually increased to as much as 200 mg/d, is sometimes worthwhile in reducing the severity of the dyskinesia. Other pharmacologic approaches are unrewarding in most instances. Tardive dystonia may respond to tetrabenazine (if available) or to anticholinergic drugs used as for idiopathic torsion dystonia.

Tardive tic resembles Gilles de la Tourette's syndrome (see below) and is best treated with clonidine or clonazepam.

Neuroleptic Malignant Syndrome Rigidity, hyperthermia, altered mental status resembling catatonia, labile blood pressure, and autonomic dysfunction characterize this serious complication of treatment with antipsychotic (neuroleptic) agents, especially haloperidol. Associated clinical features include tachycardia, tachypnea, metabolic acidosis, and myoglobinuria that may be fatal. The cause is unknown, but antagonism of dopamine is a likely contributor. The prevalence of this syndrome among patients receiving neuroleptics is less than 2 percent, with the disorder occurring must commonly in young adults. Symptoms evolve over 1 to 2 days. The syndrome can develop at any time during exposure to the medication, but usually it occurs within the first 30 days of use.

The differential diagnosis includes infection, malignant hyperthermia, and alcohol- or drug-withdrawal states. Drug-induced parkinsonism may be similar but is not associated with fever or the autonomic features described above.

℞ TREATMENT

Treatment includes immediate withdrawal of antipsychotic drugs and also of lithium and anticholinergic agents, which may increase the risk of developing the disorder. Symptomatic treatment is also necessary and includes antipyretics and artificial cooling, rehydration, and measures to maintain the blood pressure. Serum potassium should be monitored. Dantrolene, bromocriptine or another dopamine agonist, levodopa, amantadine, or benzodiazepines are sometimes helpful, but the mortality rate is on the order of 5 to 20 percent. Subcutaneous heparin administration reduces the risk of venous thrombosis. Most survivors recover completely, but potential complications include renal failure, pulmonary embolism, and a chronic cerebellar syndrome (related to the hyperthermia). Recovery generally occurs over 2 to 3 weeks.

Other Drug-Induced Movement Disorders Dyskinesia or dystonia may complicate therapy with levodopa or dopamine agonists as a dose-related phenomenon that is reversed by withdrawal of the medication or reduction of the dose. Reversible chorea may also complicate treatment with anticholinergic drugs, phenytoin, carbamazepine, amphetamines, lithium, and oral contraceptives; dystonia from lithium, carbamazepine, and metoclopramide; and postural tremor from theophylline, caffeine, lithium, thyroid hormone, tricyclic antidepressants, valproic acid, and isoproterenol.

GILLES DE LA TOURETTE'S SYNDROME Gilles de la Tourette's syndrome, which has a prevalence in the United States of approximately 0.05 percent, consists of chronic multiple motor and phonic tics that have no known cause. The disorder is not related to social or ethnic background or to perinatal abnormalities. Symptoms typically begin between 5 and 15 years of age and follow a relapsing and remitting course. A family history is sometimes obtained, and partial expression of the trait may occur in siblings or offspring of patients. In most families with chronic tic disorders, there is an autosomal dominant mode of inheritance with variable penetrance that is gender related. Boys are affected much more commonly than girls.

The pathophysiology is obscure, and no structural pathology has been recognized. A dopaminergic excess has been suggested by the clinical observation that the tics may respond to treatment with dopamine-blocking drugs.

Clinical Manifestations The first signs consist of single or multiple motor tics in 80 percent of cases and of phonic tics in 20 percent. Motor tics commonly affect the face and may consist of repetitive sniffing, winking, blinking, elevation of the eyelids, eye closure, pursing of the lips, or facial twitching. Patients eventually develop several different motor and phonic tics, the latter frequently taking the form of grunts, barks, hisses, sighs, throat-clearing, coughing, and verbal utterances that may involve coprolalia (involuntary and inappropriate swearing or obscene speech), echolalia (involuntary repetition of the phrases of others), and palilalia (repetition of words or phrases). The tics may change in location, severity, complexity, and character with time, are worsened by emotional stress, and can be suppressed voluntarily for short periods. In some cases, tics are complex (such as jumping up in the air) or involve repetitive self-mutilating activities (such as nail-biting, hair-pulling, or lip-biting). Tics that involve repetitive sensory phenomena, such as pressure, tickle, or thermal sensations, also occur. Many patients have associated behavioral abnormalities, especially obsessive-compulsive disorder and attention deficit hyperactivity disorder.

Apart from the presence of tics, physical examination typically reveals no other abnormalities, but the incidence of left-handedness or ambidexterity is greater than among normal persons, and many patients have nonspecific electroencephalographic abnormalities of no diagnostic significance.

The diagnosis is often delayed for years, the symptoms sometimes being attributed to psychiatric illness. Patients may be subjected to unnecessary and expensive treatment before the correct diagnosis is made. Depression, sometimes leading to suicide, may result from social embarrassment caused by the tics.

Differential Diagnosis Many children develop transient or chronic simple tics, and these have a benign prognosis and require no treatment. In some instances, simple or multiple tics persist for several years but resolve in late adolescence. Wilson's disease, a treatable cause of dyskinesias and tics, is generally associated with hepatic and renal involvement, Kayser-Fleischer corneal rings, low serum copper and ceruloplasmin levels, and increased 24-h urinary copper excretion (Chap. 345). The associated dementia, the character of the abnormal movements, and genetic studies distinguish Huntington's disease (Chap. 367). Sydenham's chorea (Chap. 236) may be confused with Gilles de la Tourette's syndrome when a history of rheumatic fever or polyarthritis is lacking and there is no cardiac involvement, but it usually resolves over 3 to 6 months. Tics may also occur in postencephalitic syndromes and as a side effect of stimulant or neuroleptic medication.

℞ TREATMENT

Treatment is symptomatic and may need to be continued indefinitely.

Clonidine alleviates motor and phonic tics in approximately 50 percent of children, possibly by reducing activity in noradrenergic neurons of the locus coeruleus. The initial dose is 2 to 3 g/kg per day, increased after 2 weeks to 4 g/kg per day and then, if required, to 5 g/kg per day. There may be a transient fall in blood pressure when this agent is introduced. Other side effects are sedation, reduced or excessive salivation, and diarrhea.

Haloperidol has been used widely for many years. It is introduced in a low daily dose (0.25 mg), which is gradually increased by 0.25 mg every 5 days, depending on response and tolerance. The optimal dose is usually 2 to 8 mg/d. Side effects include extrapyramidal movement disorders, sedation, xerostomia, blurred vision, and gastrointestinal disturbances. Pimozide, another dopaminergic-receptor antagonist, may be of benefit when haloperidol is unhelpful or poorly tolerated. It may produce widening of the QT interval and sudden death at high doses, so the electrocardiogram should be monitored routinely. Its long-term safety is unknown. It is introduced in a dose of 1 mg/d, and the dose is then increased by 2 mg every 10 days; most patients require 7 to 16 mg/d. The total dose should not exceed 0.3 mg/kg per day. Phenothiazines such as fluphenazine sometimes help, but patients unresponsive to haloperidol do not usually benefit from these drugs. Clonazepam or carbamazepine can also be tried. Family counseling and psychotherapy are sometimes helpful.

RESTLESS LEGS SYNDROME The restless legs syndrome is a common, chronic disorder that often has a familial basis, with evidence of autosomal dominant inheritance. It is characterized by a need to move because of unpleasant creeping sensations that arise deep within the legs and occasionally also in the arms, especially when patients are relaxed. For this reason, there is often difficulty in settling down to sleep at night. Periodic leg movements may also occur during sleep and can be documented by polysomnography. The cause is unknown, although the disorder is common during pregnancy and is sometimes associated with uremic or diabetic neuropathy, primary amyloidosis, or malignancy. Clinical examination may reveal evidence of underlying systemic disease or mild peripheral neuropathy but is more often normal. Symptoms may respond to correction of coexisting iron-deficiency anemia or to treatment with dopaminergic medication (such as levodopa or bromocriptine), benzodiazepines (diazepam or clonazepam), or opiates (codeine, propoxyphene, or oxycodone).

BIBLIOGRAPHY

AMINOFF MJ: Treatment of Parkinson's disease. West J Med 161:303, 1994

BENNETT DA et al: Prevalence of parkinsonian signs and associated mortality in a community population of older people. N Engl J Med 334:771, 1996

CLEETER MWJ et al: Irreversible inhibition of mitochondrial complex I by 1-methyl-4-phenylpyridinium: Evidence for free radical involvement. J Neurochem 58:786, 1992

DOGALI M et al: Stereotactic ventral pallidotomy for Parkinson's disease. Neurology 45:753, 1995

EDWARDS RH: Neural degeneration and the transport of neurotransmitters. Ann Neurol 34:638, 1993

GRATZ SS, SIMPSON GM: Neuroleptic malignant syndrome. Diagnosis, epidemiology and treatment. CNS Drugs 2:429, 1994

HYDE TM, WEINBERGER DR: Tourette's syndrome: A model neuropsychiatric disorder. JAMA 273:498, 1995

IANNACCONE S et al: Evidence of peripheral axonal neuropathy in primary restless legs syndrome. Mov Disord 10:2, 1995

KORDOWER JH et al: Neuropathological evidence of graft survival and striatal reinnervation after the transplantation of fetal mesencephalic tissue in a patient with Parkinson's disease. N Engl J Med 332:1118, 1995

LOZANO AM et al: Effect of GPi pallidotomy on motor function in Parkinson's disease. Lancet 346:1383, 1995

MOURADIAN MM et al: Modification of central dopaminergic mechanisms by continuous levodopa therapy for advanced Parkinson's disease. Ann Neurol 27:18, 1990

NYGAARD TG et al: Linkage mapping of dopa-responsive dystonia (DRD) to chromosome 14q. Nature Genet 5:386, 1993

PARKINSON STUDY GROUP: Effects of tocopherol and deprenyl on the progression of disability in early Parkinson's disease. N Engl J Med 328:176, 1993
———: Impact of deprenyl and tocopherol treatment on Parkinson's disease in DATATOP subjects not requiring levodopa. Ann Neurol 39:29, 1996

POLYMEROPOULOS MH et al: Mapping of a gene for Parkinson's disease to chromosome 4q21-q23. Science 274:1197, 1996

REMY P et al: Clinical correlates of [^{18}F]fluorodopa uptake in five grafted parkinsonian patients. Ann Neurol 38:580, 1995

QUINN N: Drug treatment of Parkinson's disease. BMJ 310:575, 1995

SCHULZER M et al: The antiparkinson efficacy of deprenyl derives from transient improvement that is likely to be symptomatic. Ann Neurol 32:795, 1992

WICHMANN T et al: Parkinson's disease and the basal ganglia: Lessons from the laboratory and from neurosurgery. Neuroscientist 1:236, 1995

369 *Roger N. Rosenberg*

ATAXIC DISORDERS

The inherited and acquired ataxic disorders comprise a series of clinical phenotypes that include ataxia, dysarthria, dysmetria, and intention tremor resulting from the involvement of the cerebellum and its afferent and efferent pathways.

Approach to the Patient

With Ataxic Disorders Ataxia is a common and important neurologic sign. Patients manifest symptoms and signs of ataxia with gait impairment, unclear speech, blurred vision, altered hand coordination, and tremor with movement. The rate and pattern of these cerebellar symptoms are important in determining the differential diagnostic possibilities (Table 369-1). A slow, regular, and progressive increase in symptoms with bilateral and symmetric involvement suggests a biochemical, metabolic, immunologic, or toxicity-induced cause of symptoms. Conversely, a focal, unilateral symptomatology with head-

ache and impaired level of consciousness, possibly accompanied by ipsilateral cranial nerve palsies and contralateral weakness, implies a space-occupying cerebellar lesion, such as a primary or metastatic cerebellar tumor, abscess, large infarction, hemorrhage, or subdural hematoma in the posterior fossa.

Progressive, symmetrical ataxia can be further classified as acute in onset (onset over hours or days), subacute in onset (weeks or months), or chronic, developing over months to years. The acute and reversible types of ataxia include those caused by intoxication with alcohol, diphenylhydantoin, barbiturates, and other agents. Intoxication caused by toluene exposure, gasoline sniffing, glue sniffing, spray painting, or exposure to mercury are examples. Children with a postinfectious syndrome can develop gait ataxia and mild dysarthria, which are both reversible. Subacute development of ataxia over weeks to months may be the combined direct effect of alcoholism and nutrition impairment, particularly for vitamins B_1 and B_{12}. A paraneoplastic syndrome, which may be associated with myoclonus and opsoclonus, is associated with incapacitating gait ataxia. Specific autoantibodies (Yo, Ri, and PCD) have been identified that are responsible for cerebellar degeneration involving principally the midline or vermis (see Chap. 103). Female patients may present with cerebellar ataxia prior to the identification of a breast or ovarian carcinoma. Removal of the tumor may prevent further progression of symptoms and in some patients results in gait improvement. Chronic gait ataxia of months' to years' duration suggests a metabolic or inherited ataxia. Hypothyroidism must be considered as a readily treatable and reversible form of gait ataxia.

In patients with focal, increasing signs of ataxia of an acute nature, it is important to consider vascular lesions, including acute cerebellar infarction with edema, cerebellar hemorrhage, and a posterior fossa subdural hematoma. Computed tomography (CT) will reveal clinically significant processes of this type, which may require surgical decompression. Similarly, a primary cerebellar glioma or a metastatic tumor to the cerebellar hemisphere may present with increasing focal deficits associated with an impaired level of consciousness. Herniation rostrally onto the brainstem or a sudden caudal herniation of cerebellar tonsils must be considered and an urgent evaluation implemented (see Chap. 366). A primary cerebellar abscess may present in a similar manner. Lymphoma or progressive multifocal leukoencephalopathy (PML) in a patient with AIDS may present with acute focal cerebellar signs. Patients with acute multiple sclerosis may present with significant focal and ipsilateral cerebellar deficits due to a large demyelinating plaque. A history of previous neurologic deficits and an examination of cerebrospinal fluid (CSF) may be highly diagnostic for multiple sclerosis.

Table 369-1

Etiology of Cerebellar Ataxia

Symmetrical and Progressive Signs			Focal and Ipsilateral Cerebellar Signs		
Acute (Hours to Days)	**Subacute** (Days to Weeks)	**Chronic** (Months to Years)	**Acute** (Hours to Days)	**Subacute** (Days to Weeks)	**Chronic** (Months to Years)
Alcohol, lithium, diphenylhydantoin, barbiturates (positive history and toxicology screen)	Intoxication: mercury, solvents, gasoline, glue; cytotoxic chemotherapeutic drugs	Paraneoplastic syndrome	Vascular: Cerebellar infarction, hemorrhage, or subdural hematoma	Neoplastic: cerebellar glioma or metastatic tumor (positive for neoplasm on MRI/CT)	Stable gliosis secondary to vascular lesion or demyelinating plaque (stable lesion on MRI/CT older than several months)
Acute viral cerebellitis (cerebrospinal fluid supportive of acute viral infection)	Alcoholic-nutritional (vitamin B_1 and B_{12} deficiency)	Hypothyroidism	Infectious: cerebellar abscess (positive mass lesion on MRI/CT, positive history in support of lesion)	Demyelinating: Multiple sclerosis (history, CSF and MRI are consistent)	Congenital lesion: Dandy-Walker or Arnold-Chiari malformations (malformation noted on MRI/CT)
Postinfection syndrome	Lyme disease	Inherited diseases Tabes dorsalis (tertiary syphilis)		AIDS-related progressive multifocal leukoencephalopathy (positive HIV test and CD4+ cell count for AIDS)	

ABBREVIATIONS: CSF, cerebrospinal fluid; CT, computed tomography; HIV, human immunodeficiency virus; MRI, magnetic resonance imaging.

True cerebellar ataxia needs to be separated from vertiginous ataxia, as the latter is a disorder of gait associated with a significant degree of dizziness, light-headedness, or the perception of movement (see Chap. 20). True cerebellar ataxia is devoid of these vertiginous complaints and is clearly an unsteady gait due to imbalance. Weakness of proximal leg muscles and a variant of acute idiopathic polyneuritis (Miller-Fisher syndrome) can simulate the imbalance of cerebellar disease.

ACQUIRED ATAXIAS

The cerebellar circuit comprising the cerebellum, spinocerebellar pathways, and the frontopontocerebellar pathway originating in the rostral frontal lobe (Brodmann's area 10) are also involved in a variety of acquired diseases. Cerebrovascular disease producing acute and subacute infarctions, hemorrhagic infarctions, and hemorrhages may result in an acute ataxic syndrome. Lesions of these types will result in cerebellar symptoms ipsilateral to the injured cerebellum and may be associated with impaired levels of consciousness due to increased intracranial pressure and ipsilateral pontine signs, including sixth and seventh nerve palsies due to direct pontine compression. Similarly, cerebellar tumors, demyelinating plaques of multiple sclerosis, and abscess formation produce progressive deficits ipsilateral to the cerebellar lesion. Two other important entities are paraneoplastic disease due to neoplasms outside the brain and causing acute bilateral cerebellar deficits by an antibody-mediated process (see Chap. 103) and subacute cerebellar degeneration of the vermis with gait ataxia, due to chronic alcoholism.

Patients with AIDS may develop an acute ataxic syndrome due to progressive multifocal leukoencephalopathy, which causes a rapid demyelinating process, as a result of the JC virus (see Chap. 379). Progressive ataxia of gait and extremities may also be caused by toxic or metabolic disorders, including hypothyroidism, hyponatremia, vitamin B_1 deficiency, vitamin B_{12} deficiency, toxic levels of phenytoin, lithium, bismuth, germanium, methyl mercury, and organic solvents, and treatment with cytotoxic chemotherapeutic drugs (see Chap. 380). Rarely, congenital lesions, such as the Chiari type I malformation with cerebellar tonsillar compression of the brainstem, and congenital dilation of the fourth ventricle into a large cyst owing to impaired drainage of CSF (Dandy-Walker syndrome), present in adults as a progressive diffuse ataxic syndrome. Specific infectious diseases that can present with ataxia are meningovascular syphilis in patients recently infected and tabes dorsalis due to degeneration of the spinocerebellar pathway in chronically infected patients. Lyme disease may cause ataxic symptoms.

Other rare infectious causes of acquired ataxia include poliovirus, coxsackievirus, echovirus, Epstein-Barr virus, toxoplasmosis, *Legionella*, and the prion protein mediating Creutzfeldt-Jakob disease (see Chaps. 153 and 379).

THE INHERITED ATAXIAS

Of the syndromes that constitute the inherited ataxias, some show autosomal dominant or autosomal recessive inheritance, and some are caused by mitochondrial mutations and thus show maternal inheritance. Significant progress has been made in recent years in identifying the molecular basis of these syndromes (Table 369-2), so that a genomic classification is superseding previous ones based on clinical expression alone.

Although the clinical manifestations and neuropathologic findings of cerebellar disease dominate the clinical picture, there may also be characteristic changes in the basal ganglia, brainstem, spinal cord, optic nerves, retina, and peripheral nerves. In large families with dominantly inherited disease, there are many gradations from purely cerebellar manifestations to mixed cerebellar and brainstem disorders,

cerebellar and basal ganglia syndromes, and spinal cord or peripheral nerve disease. Rarely, dementia is present as well. The clinical picture may be consistent within a family with dominantly inherited ataxia, but sometimes most affected family members show one characteristic syndrome, while one or several members have an entirely different phenotype.

The problem posed by dominantly inherited diseases of the nervous system, such as the inherited cerebellar degenerations, is the lack of a known primary metabolic clue, or primary storage product, to indicate a potential molecular basis for disease. In these cerebellar disorders, there is a patterned neuronal degeneration with variable secondary gliosis. Even the findings of specific protein abnormalities on two-dimensional gels or specific changes in messenger RNA on northern blots obtained from brain samples of patients having a dominantly inherited cerebellar disease do not warrant the conclusion that these products are due to primary gene mutations rather than being a result of the disease. Therefore, new research strategies must be employed to determine the molecular basis of autosomal dominant disorders and the molecular explanation for phenotypic variation within and between families. Linkage analysis has proved to be a powerful tool with which to map the chromosomal location of a series of dominantly inherited ataxic neurologic diseases for which no biochemical basis was known, and these new findings have aided the classification of the various clinical phenotypes (see Table 369-2).

AUTOSOMAL DOMINANT ATAXIAS As presented in Table 369-2, the new genomic classification of the dominantly inherited ataxias includes spinocerebellar ataxia (SCA) type 1, SCA2, SCA3/Machado-Joseph disease, SCA4, SCA5, dentatorubropallidoluysian atrophy (DRPLA), spinocerebellar degeneration with retinal degeneration (SCA7), and episodic ataxia (EA) types I and II (EA-1 and EA-2). The use of SCA6 has been for those autosomal dominant families with ataxia that have not been assigned a chromosomal locus.

SCA1 SCA1 was previously referred to as *olivopontocerebellar atrophy*, but the new genomic data has shown that that entity represents several different genotypes with overlapping clinical features.

Symptoms and signs The clinical syndrome of SCA1 is characterized by the development in adult or late middle life of progressive cerebellar ataxia of the trunk and limbs, impairment of equilibrium and gait, slowness of voluntary movements, scanning speech, nystagmoid jerks, and oscillatory tremor of the head and trunk. Dysarthria, dysphagia, and oculomotor and facial palsies may also occur. Extrapyramidal symptoms include rigidity, immobile facies, and parkinsonian tremor. The reflexes are usually normal, but knee and ankle jerks may be lost, and extensor plantar responses may occur. Dementia may occur but is usually mild. Impairment of sphincter function is common, with urinary and sometimes fecal incontinence.

Marked shrinkage of the ventral half of the pons, disappearance of the olivary eminence on the ventral surface of the medulla, and atrophy of the cerebellum are evident on gross postmortem inspection of the brain. Variable loss of Purkinje cells, reduction in the number of cells in the molecular and granular layer, demyelination of the middle cerebellar peduncle and the cerebellar hemispheres, and severe loss of cells in the pontine nuclei and olives are found on histologic examination. Degenerative changes in the striatum, especially the putamen, and loss of the pigmented cells of the substantia nigra may be found in cases with extrapyramidal features. More widespread degeneration in the central nervous system (CNS), including involvement of the posterior columns and the spinocerebellar fibers, is often present, especially in the cases with autosomal dominant inheritance.

Genetics SCA1 was mapped positionally to chromosome 6 (6p22-p23), and the causal gene was found to contain CAG expanded DNA repeats (see Chap. 363). The mutant allele has more than 43 CAG repeats, whereas alleles from control subjects have 36 or fewer repeats. There is a direct correlation between a larger number of repeats and a younger age of onset for SCA1. Juvenile cases have higher repeat numbers, and anticipation is present in subsequent generations. The SCA1 gene is 450 kilobases (kb) long and has nine exons, with the first seven exons located in a 5′ untranslated region and the last two exons containing the coding region. The SCA1 transcript contains

10,660 bases and is transcribed from both the wild-type allele and SCA1 alleles. The CAG repeat, which codes for a polyglutamine tract, lies within the coding region. The SCA1 gene product, called ataxin-1, is a novel protein of unknown function. It will be of great interest to discover how variable CAG repeat expansions, coding for polyglutamine tract lengths, can lead to selective neuronal degeneration accompanied by clinical anticipation (see Chap. 363).

SCA2 *Symptoms and signs* Another clinical phenotype, SCA2, has been described in Cubans. These patients probably are descendants of a common ancestor, and the population may be the largest homogeneous group of ataxic patients yet described. The age of onset ranges from 2 to 65 years, and there is considerable clinical variability within various families. Assuming these patients have a common ancestry, the frequency of the disease in the population represents a founder effect. Although neuropathologic and clinical findings are compatible with a diagnosis of SCA1 (including parkinsonian rigidity, optic disk pallor, spasticity, and retinal degeneration), it appears that SCA2 is a unique form of cerebellar degenerative disease.

Genetics The gene in SCA2 families has been mapped to 12q23-q24.1. Thus, the similar clinical phenotypes of SCA1 and SCA2,

mapped respectively to 6p and 12q, represent different genotypes. The gene has just been identified, and it also contains CAG repeat expansions. Dominant spinocerebellar atrophy with retinal disease is a separate genotype and maps to 3p12-p21.1.

Machado-Joseph Disease/SCA3 Machado-Joseph disease (MJD) is an autosomal dominant spinocerebellar degenerative disease first described among the Portuguese and their descendants in New England and California. Subsequently, MJD has been found in families from Portugal, Australia, Brazil, Canada, China, England, France, India, Israel, Italy, Japan, Spain, Taiwan, and the United States.

Symptoms and signs MJD has been classified into three clinical types. In type I MJD (amyotrophic lateral sclerosis–parkinsonism–dystonia type), neurologic deficits appear in the first two decades and involve weakness and spasticity of extremities, especially the legs, often with dystonia of the face, neck, trunk, and extremities. Patellar and ankle clonus are common, as are extensor plantar responses. The gait is slow and stiff, with a slightly broadened base and lurching

Table 369-2

Genotype Classification of the Spinocerebellar Ataxias

Name	Locus	Phenotype
SCA1 (autosomal dominant type 1)	6p22-p23 with CAG repeats	Ataxia with ophthalmoparesis, pyramidal and extrapyramidal findings
SCA2 (autosomal dominant type 2)	12q-23-24.1 with CAG repeats	Ataxia with slow saccades and minimal pyramidal and extrapyramidal findings
Machado-Joseph disease/SCA3 (autosomal dominant type 3)	14q24.3-q32 with CAG repeats in open reading frame	Ataxia with ophthalmoparesis and variable pyramidal, extrapyramidal, and amyotrophic signs
SCA4 (autosomal dominant type 4)	16q24-ter	Ataxia with normal eye movements, sensory axonal neuropathy, and pyramidal signs
SCA5 (autosomal dominant type 5)	Centromeric region of chromosome 11	Ataxia and dysarthria
SCA6 (autosomal dominant type 6)	Polymorphic CAG repeats in α_{1A}-voltage-dependent calcium channel	Ataxia, dysarthria, nystagmus, mild proprioceptive sensory loss
Dentatorubropallidoluysian atrophy (autosomal dominant)	12p12-ter with CAG repeats	Ataxia, choreoathetosis, dystonia, seizures, myoclonus, dementia
Spinocerebellar degeneration with retinal degeneration (autosomal dominant)	3p12-p21.1	Ataxia with retinal degeneration
Friedreich's ataxia (autosomal recessive)	9q with intronic GAA repeats	Ataxia, areflexia, extensor plantar responses, position sense deficits, cardiomyopathy, diabetes mellitus, scoliosis, foot deformities
Friedreich's ataxia (autosomal recessive)	8q13, α-TTP deficiency	Same as phenotype that maps to 9q but associated with vitamin E deficiency
Kearns-Sayre syndrome (sporadic)	mtDNA deletion and duplication mutations	Ptosis, ophthalmoplegia, pigmentary retinal degeneration, cardiomyopathy, diabetes mellitus, deafness, heart block, increased CSF protein, ataxia
Myoclonus epilepsy and ragged red fiber syndrome (MERRF) (maternal inheritance)	Mutation in mtDNA of tRNA^{lys} at 8344; also a mutation at 8356	Myoclonic epilepsy, ragged red fiber myopathy, ataxia
Mitochondrial encephalopathy, lactic acidosis, and stroke syndrome (MELAS) (maternal inheritance)	tRNA^{leu} mutation at 3243; also at 3271 and 3252	Headache, stroke, lactic acidosis, ataxia
Leigh's disease; subacute necrotizing encephalopathy (maternal inheritance or autosomal recessive)	mtDNA complex V defect (ATPase gene at 8993) or mitochondrial protein synthesis defect (both maternally inherited); or complex IV defect (autosomal recessive)	Obtundation, hypotonia, cranial nerve defects, respiratory failure, hyperintense signals on T2-weighted magnetic resonance images in basal ganglia, cerebellum, or brainstem; ataxia
Episodic ataxia, type I (EA-1) (autosomal dominant)	12p; potassium channel gene, KcNA1	Episodic ataxia for minutes; provoked by startle or exercise; with facial and hand myokymia; cerebellar signs are not progressive; responds to phenytoin
Episodic ataxia, type II (EA-2) (autosomal dominant)	19p; gene not known	Episodic ataxia for days; provoked by stress, fatigue; with down-gaze nystagmus; cerebellar atrophy results; progressive cerebellar signs; responds to acetazolamide
Ataxia telangiectasia (autosomal recessive)	11q22-23; *ATM* gene for regulation of cell cycle, mitogenic signal transduction, and meiotic recombination	Telangiectasia, ataxia, dysarthria, pulmonary infections, neoplasms of lymphatic system; IgA and IgG deficiencies; diabetes mellitus, breast cancer
Infantile-onset spinocerebellar ataxia of Nikali et al. (autosomal recessive)	10q23.3-q24.1	Infantile ataxia, sensory neuropathy; athetosis, hearing deficit, ophthalmoplegia, optic atrophy; primary hypogonadism in females

SOURCE: Modified from Rosenberg (1995).

from side to side; this gait results from spasticity, not true ataxia. There is no truncal titubation. Pharyngeal weakness and spasticity cause difficulty with speech and swallowing. Of note is the prominence of horizontal and vertical nystagmus, loss of fast saccadic eye movements, hypermetric and hypometric saccades, and impairment of upward vertical gaze. Facial fasciculations, facial myokymia, lingual fasciculations without atrophy, ophthalmoparesis, and ocular prominence are common and early manifestations.

In type II MJD (ataxic type), true cerebellar deficits appear, including dysarthria, gait, and extremity ataxia, beginning in the second to fourth decades, along with corticospinal and extrapyramidal deficits of spasticity, rigidity, and dystonia. Type II is the most common form of the disease. Ophthalmoparesis, upward vertical gaze deficits, and facial and lingual fasciculations are also present. Type II MJD must be distinguished from SCA1 and SCA2 degeneration, which share features with it.

Type III MJD (ataxic-amyotrophic type) presents in the fifth to the seventh decades with a pancerebellar disorder that includes dysarthria, gait, and extremity ataxia. Distal sensory loss involving pain, touch, vibration, and position senses and distal atrophy are prominent, indicating the presence of peripheral neuropathy. The deep tendon reflexes are depressed to absent, and no corticospinal or extrapyramidal findings occur.

The mean age of onset of symptoms in MJD is 25 years. Neurologic deficits invariably progress and lead to death from debilitation within 15 years of onset, especially in patients with types I and II disease. Patients retain full intellectual function.

The major pathologic findings are variable loss of neurons and glial replacement in the corpus striatum and severe loss in the zona compacta portion of the substantia nigra. A moderate loss of neurons occurs in the dentate nucleus of the cerebellum and in the red nucleus. Purkinje cell loss and granule cell loss is found in the cerebellar cortex. Cell loss also occurs in the dentate nucleus and in the cranial nerve motor nuclei. Sparing of the inferior olives distinguishes MJD from other dominantly inherited ataxias.

Genetics   The gene locus for MJD has been assigned to 14q24.3-q32 by genetic linkage. The genes from families with MJD in Japan and North and South America all map to the same chromosome locus. Unstable CAG repeat expansions are present in the MJD gene, and earlier age of onset is associated with longer repeats. Normal control subjects have between 12 and 37 CAG repeats, and MJD alleles have 62 to 84 CAG repeats.

SCA4   One family with progressive ataxia, pyramidal tract deficits, normal eye movements, and prominent sensory axonal neuropathy is described in which the trait has autosomal dominant transmission and is mapped to chromosome 16q24-ter.

SCA5   Finally, another family is reported (which has two major branches, both descended from the paternal grandparents of President Abraham Lincoln) in which dominantly inherited spinocerebellar ataxia (SCA5) is mapped to chromosome 11.

SCA6   Genomic screening for CAG repeats in other families with autosomal dominant ataxia have yielded another locus (see Table 369-2).

Dentatorubropallidoluysian Atrophy (DRPLA)   DRPLA is a disorder of variable clinical presentation that is characterized by progressive ataxia, choreoathetosis, dystonia, seizures, myoclonus, and dementia. The syndrome of DRPLA is due to unstable CAG triplet repeats in the open reading frame of a gene located on chromosome 12p12-ter. Larger expansions are found in patients with earlier onset. The number of repeats is ≥49 in patients with DRPLA; it is ≤26 in control individuals. Anticipation occurs; successive generations in individual families show progressively earlier onset of disease in association with an increasing CAG repeat number. Larger expansions occur in children who inherit the disease from their father.

SCA with Retinal Degeneration (SCA7)   Dominantly inherited spinocerebellar degeneration with associated pyramidal abnormalities

has also been described with retinal degeneration, including loss of color discrimination and macular degeneration. Anticipation is present in several families with this syndrome, suggesting that it may be due to a trinucleotide repeat expansion. This syndrome has been mapped to chromosome 3p12-p21.1, but the gene has not been cloned and identified.

EPISODIC ATAXIA TYPES 1 AND 2   These are two rare dominantly inherited disorders that have been mapped to chromosomes 12p (a potassium channel gene) for type 1 and to 19p for type 2. See Table 369-2 for more details.

AUTOSOMAL RECESSIVE ATAXIAS   Friedreich's Ataxia This is the most common form of inherited ataxia, comprising one-half of all hereditary ataxias. It can occur in a classic form or in association with a genetically determined vitamin E deficiency syndrome.

Symptoms and signs   Friedreich's ataxia presents before 25 years of age with progressive staggering gait, frequent falling, and titubation. The lower extremities are more severely involved than the upper ones. Dysarthria occasionally is the presenting symptom, and rarely progressive scoliosis, foot deformity, nystagmus, or cardiopathy are initial signs.

The neurologic examination reveals nystagmus, loss of fast saccadic eye movements, truncal titubation, dysarthria, dysmetria, and ataxia of extremity and truncal movements. Extensor plantar responses (with normal tone in trunk and extremities), absent deep tendon reflexes, and weakness (greater distally than proximally) are usually found. Loss of vibratory and proprioceptive sensation occurs. The median age of death is 35 years. Women have a significantly better prognosis, with 20-year survival being 100 percent in women versus 63 percent in men.

Cardiac involvement occurs in 90 percent of patients with Friedreich's ataxia. Cardiomegaly, symmetrical hypertrophy, murmurs, and conduction defects are reported. Moderate mental retardation or psychiatric syndromes are present in a small percentage of patients. An unusually high incidence of diabetes (20 percent) is found and is associated with insulin resistance, pancreatic beta-cell dysfunction, and type 1 diabetes. However, no linkage is reported between the Friedreich's ataxia gene and loci predisposing to diabetes mellitus. Musculoskeletal deformities are common and include pes cavus, pes equinovarus, and scoliosis.

The primary site of pathology is the spinal cord and the peripheral nerves. Slight atrophy of the cerebellum and cerebral gyri may occur. Sclerosis and degeneration are seen predominantly in the spinocerebellar tracts, lateral corticospinal tracts, and posterior columns. Degeneration of the glossopharyngeal, vagus, hypoglossal, and deep cerebellar nuclei is described. The cerebral cortex is histologically normal except for loss of Betz cells in the precentral gyri.

Peripheral nerves are extensively involved, with a loss of large myelinated fibers. The density of small myelinated fibers is normal, but axonal size and myelin thickness are diminished.

Cardiac pathology consists of myocytic hypertrophy and fibrosis, focal vascular fibromuscular dysplasia with subintimal or medial deposition of periodic acid–Schiff (PAS)-positive material, myocytopathy with unusual pleomorphic nuclei, and focal degeneration of myelinated and unmyelinated nerves and cardiac ganglia.

Genetics   The classic form of Friedreich's ataxia has been mapped to 9q13-q21, and the mutant gene contains expanded GAA triplet repeats in the first intron of the "frataxin gene." There is homozygosity for expanded GAA repeats in most patients. Normal persons have 7 to 22 GAA repeats and patients have 200 to 900 GAA repeats. Patients with Friedreich's ataxia have undetectable or extremely low levels of mRNA, as compared with carriers and unrelated controls, and thus, disease is caused by a loss of function of the frataxin protein. Classic Friedreich's ataxia must be compared and contrasted with Friedreich's ataxia associated with vitamin E deficiency. The clinical features of classic Friedreich's ataxia are indistinguishable from those of the form associated with vitamin E deficiency.

Two forms of hereditary ataxia associated with abnormalities in the interactions of vitamin E (α-tocopherol) with very-low-density lipoprotein (VLDL) have been delineated. Ataxia of the Friedreich's phenotype with vitamin E deficiency (AVED) and abetalipoproteinemia (Bassen-Kornzweig syndrome) have both been clarified at the molecular genetic level. Abetalipoproteinemia is caused by mutations in the gene coding for the larger subunit of the microsomal triglyceride transfer protein (MTP). Defects in MTP result in impairment of formation and secretion of VLDL in liver. This defect results in a deficiency of delivery of vitamin E to tissues, including the central and peripheral nervous system, as VLDL is the transport molecule for vitamin E and other fat-soluble substitutes. AVED is due to mutations in the gene for α-tocopherol transfer protein (α-TTP) on chromosome 8 (8q13). These patients have an impaired ability to bind vitamin E into the VLDL produced and secreted by the liver, resulting in a deficiency of vitamin E in peripheral tissues. Hence, either absence of VLDL (abetalipoproteinemia) or impaired binding of vitamin E to VLDL (AVED) causes an ataxic syndrome. The classic form of Friedreich's ataxia may also be related to impairment of VLDL or vitamin E metabolism. Once again, a genotype classification has proved to be essential in sorting out the various clinical forms of the Friedreich's disease syndrome.

Ataxia Telangiectasia *Symptoms and signs* Patients present in the first decade of life with progressive telangiectatic lesions associated with deficits in cerebellar function and nystagmus. The neurologic manifestations correspond to those seen in Friedreich's disease, and this entity should be included in that differential diagnosis. Truncal ataxia, extremity ataxia, dysarthria, extensor plantar responses, myoclonic jerks, areflexia, and distal sensory deficits may develop. There is a high incidence of recurrent pulmonary infections and neoplasms of the lymphatic and reticuloendothelial system in patients with ataxia-telangiectasia (AT). There is an increased incidence of cancer. Thymic hypoplasia with cellular and humoral (IgA and IgG2) immunodeficiencies, premature aging, and endocrine disorders such as insulin-dependent diabetes mellitus are described. There is an increased incidence of lymphomas, Hodgkin's disease, and acute leukemias. The acute leukemias are of T cell type. There is an increased incidence of breast cancer in women who are also heterozygous for AT.

The immunologic defects and increased susceptibility to cancer have been causally linked to cellular disorders in AT. Exposure of cultured cells to ionizing radiation slows the rate of DNA replication and increases the frequency of chromosomal aberrations.

The most striking neuropathologic changes include loss of Purkinje, granule, and basket cells in the cerebellar cortex as well as of neurons in the deep cerebellar nuclei. The inferior olives of the medulla also may have neuronal loss. There is a loss of anterior horn neurons in the spinal cord and of dorsal root ganglion cells associated with posterior column spinal cord demyelination. A poorly developed or absent thymus gland is the most consistent defect of the lymphoid system.

Genetics The gene for AT (the *ATM* gene) has been positionally mapped to chromosome 11q22-q23. *ATM*, which has a 12-kb transcript, was mutated in AT patients from all complementation groups described previously. A partial *ATM* cDNA clone of 5.9 kb encodes a protein that is similar to several yeast and mammalian phosphatidylinositol-3'-kinases involved in mitogenic signal transduction, meiotic recombination, and cell cycle control. The discovery of *ATM* will make possible the identification of heterozygotes who are at risk for cancer (e.g., breast cancer) and permit early diagnosis.

Mitochondrial Ataxias Spinocerebellar syndromes have been identified with mutations in mitochondrial DNA (mtDNA). Thirty pathogenic mtDNA point mutations and over 60 different types of mtDNA deletions are known, and several of these mutations cause or are associated with ataxia (see Chaps. 380 and 383).

Xeroderma Pigmentosum Xeroderma pigmentosum is a rare autosomal recessive neurocutaneous disorder caused by inability to repair damage to DNA, such as that produced by ultraviolet radiation. In addition to skin lesions, patients may show progressive mental deterioration, microcephaly, ataxia, spasticity, choreoathetosis, and hypogonadism. Nerve deafness, peripheral neuropathy (predominantly axonal), electroencephalographic abnormalities, and seizures are re-

ported. Neuronal death is noted in pyramidal cells, cerebellar Purkinje cells, the deep nuclei of the cerebellum, the brainstem, the spinal cord, and peripheral nerves.

Cockayne Syndrome This is a rare autosomal recessive disorder first described by Cockayne in 1936. Clinical features are mental retardation, optic atrophy, dwarfism, neural deafness, hypersensitivity of skin to sunlight, cataracts, and retinal pigmentary degeneration. Cerebellar, pyramidal, and extrapyramidal deficits and peripheral neuropathy may occur, with bird-headed facies and normal-pressure hydrocephalus. Skin fibroblasts show defective DNA repair when exposed to an ultraviolet light.

Marinesco-Sjögren Syndrome This rare syndrome, in which progressive cerebellar deficits begin early in childhood, is another rare example in which a Friedreich's syndrome is associated with additional specific features. In this case, cataracts, mental retardation, multiple skeletal abnormalities, hypogonadotropic hypogonadism, and severe cerebellar atrophy are associated. The syndrome is likely a lysosomal storage disorder caused by an enzymatic defect, but the pathophysiology is unknown.

℞ **TREATMENT**

There is no proven therapy for the dominant ataxias (SCA1-5). The physician's task is to identify treatable disease entities resembling these disorders. Malignancies may present with chronic progressive ataxia either directly with a mass effect in the posterior fossa or indirectly by paraneoplastic degeneration (see Chap. 103). Malabsorption syndromes leading to vitamin E deficiency may lead to ataxia. The vitamin E deficiency form of Friedreich's ataxia must be considered, and serum vitamin E levels measured. Vitamin E therapy is indicated for these rare patients. Vitamin B$_1$ and B$_{12}$ levels in serum must be measured, and the vitamin administered to patients having deficient levels. The deleterious effects of diphenylhydantoin and alcohol on the cerebellum are well known. Hypothyroidism may also produce ataxia. Aminoacidopathies, leukodystrophies, ureacycle abnormalities, and mitochondrial encephalomyopathies may produce ataxia, and some dietary or metabolic therapies are available (see Chap. 380). The cerebrospinal fluid should be tested for a syphilitic infection in patients with progressive ataxia and other features of tabes dorsalis. Similarly, antibody titers for Lyme disease and *Legionella* should be measured, and appropriate antibiotic therapy should be instituted in antibody-positive patients. The identification of gene defects will, it is hoped, lead to specific pharmacologic therapy. At present, identification of an at-risk person's genotype, together with appropriate family and genetic counseling, can reduce the incidence of these cerebellar syndromes (see Chap. 363).

BIBLIOGRAPHY

CONNER KE, ROSENBERG RN: The hereditary ataxias, in *The Molecular and Genetic Basis of Neurological Disease*, RN Rosenberg et al (eds). Boston, Butterworth-Heinemann, 1993, pp 697–736

DÜRR A et al: Clinical and genetic abnormalities in patients with Friedreich's ataxia. N Engl J Med 335:1169, 1996

HARDING AE: Clinical features and classification of inherited ataxias. Adv Neurol 61:1, 1993

KAWAGUCHI Y et al: CAG expansions in a novel gene for Machado-Joseph disease at chromosome 14q32.1. Nat Genet 8:221, 1994

MATILLA T et al: Molecular and clinical correlations in spinocerebellar ataxia type 3 and Machado-Joseph disease. Ann Neurol 38:68, 1995

ORR HT et al: Expansion of an unstable trinucleotide CAG repeat in spinocerebellar ataxia type 1. Nat Genet 4:221, 1993

OUAHCHI K et al: Ataxia with isolated vitamin E deficiency is caused by mutations in the alpha-tocopherol transfer protein. Nat Genet 9:141, 1995

SERVADIO A et al: Expression analysis of the ataxin-1 protein in tissues from normal and spinocerebellar ataxia type 1 individuals. Nat Genet 10:94, 1995

ROSENBERG RN: Autosomal dominant cerebellar phenotypes: The genotype has settled the issue. Neurology 45:1, 1995

———: DNA triplet repeats and neurologic disease. N Engl J Med 335:1222, 1996

————: The genetic basis of ataxia. Clin Neurosci 3:1, 1995

————: Spinocerebellar ataxias and ataxins. N Engl J Med 333:1351, 1995

————, IANNACCONE ST: The prevention of neurogenetic disease. Arch Neurol 52:356, 1995

TERRY JB, ROSENBERG RN: Frontal lobe ataxia. Surg Neurol 44:583, 1995

ZHUCHENKO O et al: Autosomal dominant cerebellar ataxia (SCA6) associated with small polyglutamine expansions in the α_{1A}-voltage-dependent calcium channel. Nat Genet 15:62, 1997

ZOGHBI H: Spinocerebellar ataxia and other disorders of trinucleotide repeats, in *Textbook of Molecular Medicine*, JL Jameson (ed). Cambridge, MA, Blackwell Science, 1997 (in press)

370

Robert H. Brown, Jr.

THE MOTOR NEURON DISEASES

AMYOTROPHIC LATERAL SCLEROSIS Amyotrophic lateral sclerosis (ALS) is the most common form of progressive motor neuron disease. It is a prime example of a neuronal system disease and is arguably the most devastating of the neurodegenerative disorders.

Pathology The pathology of motor neuron degenerative disorders involves lower motor neurons (consisting of anterior horn cells in spinal cord and their brainstem homologues innervating bulbar muscles) and upper or corticospinal motor neurons (emanating from layer five of motor cortex to descend via the pyramidal tract to synapse with lower motor neurons, either directly or indirectly via interneurons) (see Chap. 21). Although at its onset ALS may involve selective loss of function of only upper or lower motor neurons, it ultimately causes progressive loss of both categories of motor neurons (Tables 370-1 and 370-2). Indeed, in the absence of clear involvement of both motor neuron types, the diagnosis of ALS is questionable.

Other motor neuron diseases involve only particular subsets of motor neurons (Tables 370-1 and 370-2). Thus, in *bulbar palsy* and *spinal muscular atrophy* (also called progressive muscular atrophy), the lower motor neurons of brainstem and spinal cord, respectively, are most severely involved. By contrast, *pseudobulbar palsy*, *primary lateral sclerosis*, and *familial spastic paraplegia* affect only upper motor neurons innervating the brainstem and spinal cord.

In each of these diseases, the affected motor neurons undergo shrinkage, often with accumulation of the pigmented lipid (lipofuscin) that normally develops in these cells with advancing age. In ALS, the motor neuron cytoskeleton is typically affected early in the illness. Focal enlargements are frequent in proximal motor axons; ultrastructurally, these "spheroids" are composed of accumulations of neurofilaments. Beyond some astroglial proliferation, which is the inevitable accompaniment of all degenerative processes in the central nervous system (CNS), the interstitial and supportive tissues and the macrophage system remain largely inactive, and there is no inflammation.

The death of the peripheral motor neurons in the brainstem and spinal cord leads to denervation and consequent atrophy of the corresponding muscle fibers. Histochemical and electrophysiologic evidence indicates that in the early phases of the illness denervated muscle can be reinnervated by sprouting of nearby distal motor nerve terminals, although reinnervation in this disease is considerably less extensive than in most other disorders affecting motor neurons (e.g., poliomyelitis, peripheral neuropathy). As denervation progresses, muscle atrophy is readily recognized in muscle biopsies and on clinical examination. This is the basis for the term *amyotrophy* in the name for the disease. The loss of cortical motor neurons results in thinning of the corticospinal tracts that travel via the internal capsule and brainstem to the

lateral (and anterior) white matter columns of the spinal cord. The loss of fibers in the lateral columns and resulting fibrillary gliosis impart a particular firmness (*lateral sclerosis*) to the affected tissues (Fig. 370-1). A remarkable feature of the disease is the selectivity of neuronal cell death. By light microscopy, the entire sensory apparatus, the regulatory mechanisms for the control and coordination of movement, and the components of the brain that are needed for cognitive processes, remain intact. However, immunostaining indicates that neurons bearing ubiquitin, a marker for degeneration, are also detected in nonmotor systems. Moreover, studies of glucose metabolism early in the illness also indicate that there is neuronal dysfunction outside of the motor system. Within the motor system, there is some selectivity of involvement. Thus, motor neurons required for ocular motility remain unaffected, as do the parasympathetic neurons in the sacral spinal cord (the nucleus of Onufrowicz or Onuf) that innervate the sphincters of the bowel and bladder.

Clinical Manifestations The manifestations of ALS are somewhat variable depending on whether corticospinal or lower motor neurons in the brainstem and spinal cord are more prominently involved. With lower motor neuron dysfunction and early denervation, the first evidence of the disease typically is insidiously developing asymmetric weakness, usually first evident distally in one of the limbs. A detailed history often discloses recent development of cramping with volitional movements, typically in the early hours of the morning (e.g., while stretching in bed). Weakness caused by denervation is associated with progressive wasting and atrophy of muscles and, particularly early in the illness, spontaneous twitching of motor units, or fasciculations. In the hands, a preponderance of extensor over flexor weakness is common. When the initial denervation involves bulbar rather than limb muscles, the problem at onset is difficulty with chewing, swallowing, and movements of the face and tongue. Early involvement of the muscles of respiration may lead to death before the disease is far advanced elsewhere.

With prominent corticospinal involvement, there is hyperactivity of the muscle-stretch reflexes (tendon jerks) and, often, spastic resistance to passive movements of the affected limbs.

Patients with significant reflex hyperactivity complain of muscle stiffness often out of proportion to weakness. Degeneration of the corticobulbar projections innervating the brainstem results in dysarthria and exaggeration of the motor expressions of emotion. The latter leads to involuntary excess in weeping or laughing (so-called *pseudobulbar affect*).

Virtually any muscle group may be the first to show signs of the disease, but, as time passes, more and more muscles become involved until ultimately the disorder takes on a symmetric distribution in all regions. It is characteristic of ALS that, regardless of whether the initial disease involves upper or lower motor neurons, both will eventually be implicated. Even in the late stages of the illness, sensory, bowel and

Table 370-1

Sporadic Motor Neuron Diseases

CHRONIC

Upper and lower motor neurons
    Amyotrophic lateral sclerosis
Predominantly upper motor neurons
    Primary lateral sclerosis
Predominantly lower motor neurons
    Multifocal motor neuropathy with conduction block
    Motor neuropathy with paraproteinemia or cancer
    Motor-predominant peripheral neuropathies
Other
    Associated with other degenerative disorders
    Secondary motor neuron disorders (See Table 370-3)

ACUTE

Poliomyelitis
Herpes zoster
Coxsackie virus

Table 370-2

CHAPTER 370
The Motor Neuron Diseases

2369

Genetic Motor Neuron Diseases

Disease	Loci	Gene
I. Upper and lower motor neurons (familial ALS)		
A. Autosomal dominant	21q	Superoxide dismutase
	22q	Neurofilament heavy subunit
B. Autosomal recessive (juvenile)	2q	
II. Lower motor neurons		
A. Spinal muscular atrophies I, II, III	5q	Survival motor neuron
1. Infantile: Werdnig-Hoffmann disease, I		Neuronal apoptosis inhibitory protein
2. Childhood, II		
3. Adolescent: Kugelberg-Welander disease, III		
B. X-linked spinobulbar muscular atrophy	Xq	Androgen receptor
C. GM2 gangliosidosis		
1. Adult Tay-Sach's disease	15q	Hexosaminidase A
2. Sandhoff disease	5q	Hexosaminidase B
3. AB variant	5q	GM_2 activator protein
III. Upper motor neurons Familial spastic paraplegia (FSP)		
A. Autosomal dominant	2p, 14q	
B. Autosomal recessive	8p	
C. X-linked	Xq21	Proteolipid protein
	Xq28	*L1 CAM*

bladder, and cognitive functions are preserved. Dementia is not a component of sporadic ALS, although in some families with the inherited form dementia may be present. Similarly, even when there is severe brainstem disease, ocular motility is spared until the very late stages of the illness.

Epidemiology The illness is relentlessly progressive, leading to death from respiratory paralysis; the median survival is from 3 to 5 years. There are very rare reports of stabilization or even regression of ALS. In most societies there is an incidence of 1 to 3 per 100,000 and a prevalence of 3 to 5 per 100,000. Several endemic foci of higher prevalence exist in the western Pacific (e.g., in specific regions of Guam or Papua New Guinea). In the United States and Europe, males are somewhat more frequently affected than females. While ALS is overwhelmingly a sporadic disorder, some 5 to 10 percent of cases are inherited as an autosomal dominant trait.

Familial ALS Several forms of selective motor neuron disease are heritable (Table 370-2). Two involve both corticospinal and lower motor neurons. The most common is familial ALS (FALS). Apart from its inheritance as an autosomal dominant trait, it is clinically indistinguishable from sporadic ALS. Genetic studies have identified mutations in the gene encoding the cytosolic enzyme superoxide dismutase (SOD) 1 as the cause of one form of FALS. However, this accounts for only 20 percent of inherited cases of ALS; there clearly are other ALS genes to be identified. There is also a recessive form of hereditary ALS that, unlike sporadic or dominantly inherited ALS, begins in childhood and is associated with prolonged survival. A locus for this disease has been mapped to the long arm of chromosome 2. Another familial, adult-onset disorder that may mimic aspects of ALS is Kennedy's syndrome, described below.

Differential Diagnosis Because ALS is currently untreatable, it is imperative that potentially remediable causes of motor neuron

dysfunction be excluded (see Table 370-3). This is particularly true in cases that are atypical by virtue of (1) restriction to either upper or lower motor neurons, (2) involvement of neurons other than motor neurons, and (3) evidence of motor neuronal conduction block on electrophysiologic testing. Compression of the cervical spinal cord or cervicomedullary junction from tumors in the cervical regions or at the foramen magnum or from cervical spondylosis with osteophytes projecting into the vertebral canal can produce weakness, wasting, and fasciculations in the upper limbs and spasticity in the legs, closely resembling ALS. The absence of cranial nerve involvement may be helpful in differentiation, although some foramen magnum lesions may compress the twelfth cranial (hypoglossal) nerve, with resulting paralysis of the tongue. Absence of pain or of sensory changes, normal bowel and bladder function, normal roentgenographic studies of the spine, and normal cerebrospinal fluid (CSF) all favor ALS. Where doubt exists, magnetic resonance imaging (MRI) scans and contrast myelography should be performed to visualize the cervical spinal cord.

Another important entity in the differential diagnosis of ALS is *multifocal motor neuropathy with conduction block* (MMCB), discussed below. A diffuse, lower motor axonal neuropathy mimicking ALS sometimes evolves in association with hematopoietic disorders such as lymphoma. The underlying marrow pathology is often signaled by the presence of an M-component in serum which, in this clinical setting, should prompt consideration of a bone marrow biopsy. Lyme infection may also cause an axonal, lower motor neuropathy.

Other treatable disorders that occasionally mimic ALS are chronic lead poisoning and thyrotoxicosis. These disorders may be suggested by the patient's social or occupational history or by unusual clinical features. When the family history is positive, enzyme disorders involv-

FIGURE 370-1 Amyotrophic lateral sclerosis. Axial T2-weighted MRI scan through the lateral ventricles of the brain reveals abnormal high signal intensity within the corticospinal tracts (*arrows*). This MRI feature represents an increase in water content in myelin tracts undergoing Wallerian degeneration secondary to cortical neuronal loss. This finding is commonly present in ALS, but can also be seen in AIDS-related encephalopathy, infarction, or other disease processes that produce neuronal loss in a symmetric fashion.

ing SOD1, hexosaminidase A, or α-glucosidase deficiency must be excluded (see Chap. 346). These are readily identified by appropriate laboratory tests. Benign fasciculations are occasionally a source of concern because on inspection they resemble the fascicular twitchings that accompany motor neuron degeneration. The absence of weakness, atrophy, or denervation phenomena on electrophysiologic examination usually excludes ALS or other serious neurologic disease. Patients who have recovered from poliomyelitis may experience a delayed deterioration of motor neurons that presents clinically with progressive weakness, atrophy, and fasciculations. Its cause is unknown but is thought to reflect sublethal prior injury to motor neurons by poliovirus (see Chap. 379).

Rarely, ALS develops concurrently with features indicative of more widespread neurodegeneration. Thus, one infrequently encounters otherwise typical ALS patients with a Parkinsonian movement disorder or dementia. It remains unclear whether this reflects the unlikely simultaneous occurrence of two disorders or a primary defect triggering two forms of neurodegeneration. The latter is suggested by the observation that multisystem neurodegenerative diseases may

be inherited; rare families are reported with ALS and parkinsonism, or ALS and dementia with features of Pick's disease (see Chap. 368).

Pathogenesis   The cause of sporadic ALS is not well defined. Some data suggest that excitotoxic neurotransmitters such as glutamate may participate in the death of motor neurons in ALS. It is striking that one cellular defense against such excitotoxicity is the enzyme SOD1, which detoxifies the free radical superoxide anion. Because SOD1 is mutated in some familial cases of ALS, it may be that glutamate excitotoxicity and ALS result from free radical accumulations in motor neurons. Precisely why the SOD1 mutations are toxic to motor nerves is not established, although it is clear that the effect is not simply loss of normal scavenging of the superoxide anion.

℞ TREATMENT

There is no treatment capable of arresting the underlying pathologic process in ALS. Recently, the drug riluzole was approved for use in ALS because it produces a modest lengthening of survival. In one trial, the survival rate at 18 months with riluzole was similar to placebo at 15 months. The mechanism of this effect is not known with certainty; it may reduce excitotoxicity by diminishing glutamate release. There are encouraging preliminary results with other excitotoxin inhibitors or growth factors in ALS, and phase III clinical trials of several agents are in progress.

By contrast with ALS, several of the disorders (see Table 370-2) that bear some clinical resemblance to ALS are treatable; for this reason, a careful search for such forms of secondary motor neuron disease is warranted. In the absence of a primary therapy for ALS, a variety of rehabilitative aids may substantially assist ALS patients. Foot-drop splints facilitate ambulation by avoiding tripping on a floppy foot and obviating excessive hip flexion. Finger-extension splints can potentiate grip. Respiratory support may be life-sustaining. For patients electing against long-term ventilation by tracheostomy, positive-pressure ventilation by mouth or nose may provide transient (several weeks) relief from hypercarbia and hypoxia.

SELECTED LOWER MOTOR NEURON DISORDERS   In the varieties of motor neuron disease grouped under this heading, the peripheral motor neurons are affected without evidence of involvement of the corticospinal motor system (Table 370-1).

X-linked Spinobulbar Muscular Atrophy (Kennedy's Disease) This is an X-linked lower motor neuron disorder in which progressive weakness and wasting of limb and bulbar muscles begins in males in midadult life and is conjoined with androgen insensitivity manifested by gynecomastia and reduced fertility (see Chap. 336). In addition to gynecomastia, which may be subtle, two findings distinguishing this disorder from ALS are the absence of signs of pyramidal tract disease (spasticity) and the presence of a subtle sensory neuropathy in some patients. The underlying molecular defect is an expanded trinucleotide repeat (-CAG-) in the first exon of the androgen receptor gene on the X chromosome; this may be readily screened from DNA from blood. An inverse correlation appears to exist between the number of -CAG- repeats and the age of onset of the disease (see Chap. 363).

Adult Tay-Sach's Disease   Several reports have described adult-onset, predominantly lower motor neuropathies arising from deficiency of the enzyme β-hexosaminidase (hex A). These tend to be distinguishable from ALS because they are very slowly progressive; dysarthria and radiographically evident cerebellar atrophy may be prominent. In rare cases, spasticity may also be present, although it is generally absent (see Chap. 346).

Spinal Muscular Atrophy   The spinal muscular atrophies (SMAs) are a family of selective lower motor neuron diseases of early onset. Despite some phenotypic variability (largely in age of onset), the defect in the majority of families with SMA is genetically linked

Table 370-3

Etiology and Investigation of Motor Neuron Disorders

Diagnostic Categories	Investigations
Structural lesions	MRI scan of head (including
Parasagittal or foramen magnum tumors	foramen magnum), cervical spine
Cervical spondylosis	
Chiari malformation or syrinx	
Spinal cord arteriovenous malformation	
Infections	CSF exam, culture
Bacterial—tetanus, Lyme	Lyme antibody titer
Viral—poliomyelitis, herpes zoster	Antiviral antibody titers
Retroviral myelopathy	HTLV-1 titer
Intoxications, physical agents	
Toxins—lead, aluminum, other metals	24-h urine for heavy metals Serum and urine for lead, aluminum
Drugs—strychnine, phenytoin	
Electric shock, x-irradiation	
Immunologic mechanisms	Complete blood count
Plasma cell dyscrasias	Sedimentation rate
Autoimmune polyradiculoneuropathy	Immunoprotein electrophoresis Anti-GM1 antibodies
Paraneoplastic	Anti-Hu antibody
Paracarcinomatous/lymphoma	MRI scan, bone marrow biopsy
Metabolic	
Hypoglycemia	Fasting blood sugar (FBS), routine chemistries including calcium
Hyperparathyroidism	Thyroid functions
Hyperthyroidism	
Deficiency of folate, vitamins B₁₂, E, and folate	Vitamin B₁₂, folate levels
Malabsorption	24-h stool fat, carotene, prothrombin time
Hereditary biochemical disorders	
Superoxide dismutase 1 mutation	White blood cell DNA analysis
Androgen receptor defect (Kennedy's disease)	Abnormal CAG insert in androgen receptor gene
Hexosaminidase deficiency	Lysosomal enzyme screen
Infantile (-glucosidase deficiency (Pompe's disease)	
Hyperlipidemia	Lipid electrophoresis
Hyperglycinuria	Urine and serum amino acids
Methylcrotonylglycinuria	CSF amino acids

NOTE: CSF, cerebrospinal fluid; MRI, magnetic resonance imaging.

to a locus on the proximal long arm of chromosome 5. Two candidate genes have been identified at this locus: a putative motor neuron survival protein (SMN for *survival motor neuron*) and a protein that may be an inhibitor of apoptotic cell death (NAIP for *neuronal apoptosis inhibitory protein*). All types of SMA are transmitted as autosomal recessive traits. Neuropathologically these disorders are characterized by extensive loss of large motor neurons; muscle biopsy reveals evidence of denervation atrophy. Several clinical forms are described.

Infantile SMA (SMA I, Werdnig-Hoffmann Disease) has the earliest onset and most rapidly fatal course. In some instances it is apparent even before birth, as indicated by decreased fetal movements late in the third trimester. Though alert, afflicted infants are weak and floppy (hypotonic) and lack muscle stretch reflexes. Death generally ensues within the first year of life. When the family history is unclear, it is difficult in the early weeks and months to distinguish SMA I from benign congenital hypotonia. An electromyogram is often particularly helpful as SMA I usually demonstrates fulminant denervation, while in congenital hypotonia the electromyogram is often myopathic or normal.

Chronic childhood SMA (SMA II) begins later in childhood and evolves with a more slowly progressive course. *Juvenile SMA (SMA III, Wohlfart-Kugelberg-Welander disease)* manifests during late childhood and runs a slow, indolent course. Unlike most denervating diseases, in this chronic disorder weakness is greatest in the proximal muscles; indeed, the pattern of clinical weakness can suggest a primary myopathy such as limb-girdle dystrophy. Electrophysiologic and muscle biopsy evidence of denervation distinguish SMA III from the myopathic syndromes.

Multifocal Motor Neuropathy with Conduction Block In this disorder, lower motor neuron function is regionally and chronically disrupted by remarkably focal blocks in conduction. Many cases have elevated serum titers of mono- and polyclonal antibodies to ganglioside GM_1; it is hypothesized that the antibodies produce selective, focal, paranodal demyelination of motor neurons. MMCB is not typically associated with corticospinal signs. In contrast with ALS, MMCB may respond dramatically to therapy such as intravenous gamma globulin or chemotherapy; it is thus imperative that MMCB be excluded when considering a diagnosis of ALS.

Other Forms of Lower Motor Neuron Disease In individual families, other syndromes characterized by selective lower motor neuron dysfunction in an SMA-like pattern have been described. There are rare X-linked and autosomal dominant forms of apparent SMA. There is an ALS variant of juvenile onset, the Fazio-Londe syndrome, which involves mainly the musculature innervated by the brainstem. A component of lower motor neuron dysfunction is also found in some multisystem degenerative disorders such as Machado-Joseph disease and the related olivopontocerebellar degenerations (see Chap. 369).

SELECTED DISORDERS OF THE UPPER MOTOR NEURON Primary Lateral Sclerosis (PLS) This exceedingly rare disorder arises sporadically in adults in mid- to late life. Clinically it is characterized by progressive spastic weakness of the limbs, preceded or followed by spastic dysarthria and dysphagia, indicating combined involvement of the corticospinal and corticobulbar tracts. Fasciculations, amyotrophy, and sensory changes are absent; neither electromyography nor muscle biopsy shows denervation. On neuropathologic examination, there is selective loss of the large pyramidal cells in the precentral gyrus and degeneration of the corticospinal and corticobulbar projections. The peripheral motor neurons and other neuronal systems are spared. The course of PLS is variable; while long-term survival is documented, the course may be as aggressive as in ALS, with approximately 3-year survival from onset to death. Early in its course, PLS raises the question of multiple sclerosis or other demyelinating diseases such as adrenoleukodystrophy as diagnostic considerations. A myelopathy suggestive of PLS is infrequently seen with infection with the retrovirus HTLV-I (see Chap. 373). The clinical course and laboratory testing will distinguish these possibilities.

Familial Spastic Paraplegia (FSP) In its pure form, this disorder, usually transmitted in families as an autosomal dominant trait, is characterized by progressive spastic weakness beginning in the distal lower extremities. It arises in the third or fourth decade and typically has long survival, presumably because respiratory function is spared. Late in the illness there may be urinary urgency and incontinence, and sometimes fecal incontinence; sexual function tends to be preserved. In pure forms of FSP, ataxia, posterior column sensory loss, and amyotrophy are absent or minimal; however, in some patients, minor sensory changes (impaired vibration and position sense) may be observed in late stages. Some family members may show spasticity without clinical symptoms. Neuropathologically, in FSP there is degeneration of the corticospinal tracts, which appear nearly normal in the brainstem but show increasing atrophy at more caudal levels in the spinal cord. It is now apparent that defects at several different loci underlie both dominantly and recessively inherited forms of FSPs (Table 370-2). With one exception, the primary gene defects causing FSP have not been described. The exception is an infantile-onset form of X-linked, recessive FSP arising from mutations in the gene for proteolipid protein. This is an example of rather striking allelic variation, as most other mutations in the same gene cause not FSP but Pelizaeus-Merzbacher disease, a disorder of CNS myelin.

Rarely, FSP may arise concomitantly with significant involvement of other regions of the nervous system. Thus, it has been described concurrently with amyotrophy, mental retardation, mental retardation with skin thickening, optic atrophy, and sensory neuropathy. In some cases there is loss of fibers in the ascending posterior columns and the spinocerebellar tracts, features reminiscent of Friedreich's ataxia. These complicated forms of FSP emphasize the challenge inherent in classifying the neurodegenerative disorders; there may be considerable overlap of the clinical phenotypes in diseases otherwise classified as distinct. Fortunately, it is likely that increasingly available genetic testing will clarify these nosologic difficulties.

BIBLIOGRAPHY

BENSIMON G et al: A controlled trial of riluzole in amyotrophic lateral sclerosis. N Engl J Med 330:585, 1994

BROOKS BP, FISCHBECK KH: Spinal and bulbar muscular atrophy: A trinucleotide-repeat expansion neurodegenerative disease. Trends Neurosci 18:459, 1995

CRAWFORD TO: From enigmatic to problematic: The new molecular genetics of childhood spinal muscular atrophy. Neurology 46:335, 1996

DALAKAS MC: The post-polio syndrome as an evolved clinical entity. Definition and clinical description. Ann N Y Acad Sci 753:68, 1995

IKEDA M et al: Variable clinical symptoms in familial amyotrophic lateral sclerosis with a novel point mutation in the Cu/Zn superoxide dismutase gene. Neurology 45:2038, 1995

KUNST CB et al: Mutations in SOD1 associated with amyotrophic lateral sclerosis cause novel protein interactions. Nat Genet 15:91, 1997

LACOMBLEZ L et al: Dose-ranging study of riluzole in amyotrophic lateral sclerosis. Lancet 347:1425, 1996

LA SPADA AR et al: Androgen receptor gene mutations in X-linked spinal muscular atrophy. Nature 352:77, 1991

MARTIN JB: CNS genetic disorders: Loss of function, gain of function, or something else? Curr Opin Neurobiol 5:669, 1995

NAVON R et al: A new mutation in the HEXA gene associated with a spinal muscular atrophy phenotype. Neurology 45:539, 1995

PARANO E et al: Molecular basis of phenotypic heterogeneity in siblings with spinal muscular atrophy. Ann Neurol 40:247, 1996

ROSEN DR et al: Mutations in Cu/Zn superoxide dismutase gene are associated with familial amyotrophic lateral sclerosis. Nature 362:59, 1993

SMITH RA (ed): *Handbook of Amyotrophic Lateral Sclerosis.* New York, Marcel Dekker, 1992

VECHIO JD: Sequence variants in human neurofilament proteins: Absence of linkage to familial amyotrophic lateral sclerosis. Ann Neurol 40:603, 1996

371 John Engstrom, Joseph B. Martin

DISORDERS OF THE AUTONOMIC NERVOUS SYSTEM

The regulation of homeostatic functions is accomplished by the autonomic nervous system (ANS). An extensive peripheral innervation network combined with central vigilance provides rapid adjustments in vital physiologic mechanisms that are critical to survival. The importance of this regulation is emphasized by the extent and severity of disability resulting from compromised ANS function. This chapter describes the clinical manifestations, diagnosis, and treatment of ANS disorders. → *The functional anatomy and relevant pharmacology of the sympathetic and parasympathetic components of the ANS are discussed in Chap. 70. Hypothalamic disorders that cause disturbances in homeostasis are discussed in Chaps. 17 and 328.*

CLINICAL MANIFESTATIONS   Classification   Disorders of the ANS may result from central nervous system (CNS) or peripheral nervous system (PNS) causes; they may be generalized, segmental, or focal. In many instances, the clinical signs and symptoms are due to interruption of the reflex arc controlling autonomic responses. The interruption can occur in the afferent limb, CNS processing centers, or efferent limb of the reflex arc. For example, posterior fossa tumors and syringobulbia can produce lesions of the medulla that impair blood pressure (BP) responses to postural changes and result in orthostatic hypotension. Hypotension can also follow lesions of vasomotor nerve fibers to blood vessels (as in diabetes mellitus or spinal cord disease) or afferent connections (as in tabes dorsalis or Guillain-Barré syndrome). Segmental disorders or focal deficits occur in spinal cord disease, reflex sympathetic dystrophy (causalgia), and Horner's syndrome (Table 371-1). Diagnosis of the site of reflex interruption is dependent on associated clinical findings, autonomic nervous system tests, and neuroimaging.

Another approach to the classification of ANS disorders is based on the presence or absence of CNS signs. The primary value of this approach is that pathophysiology and prognosis differ between these two groups. Subcategories of disease are differentiated on the basis of characteristics such as the presence of a positive family history, pathologic findings, and the association with sensory or motor neuropathy. Unfortunately, some syndromes do not fit easily into any classification scheme and little is known about their causes, pathology, or treatment (see Table 371-1).

Symptoms of Autonomic Dysfunction   The clinical manifestations of autonomic lesions are influenced by the organ involved, the normal balance of sympathetic-parasympathetic innervation, the nature of the underlying illness, and the severity and stage of progression (Table 371-2). *Impotence* often heralds autonomic failure in men and may precede other symptoms by more than a decade, making its relevance apparent only in retrospect (see Chap. 51). A decrease in the frequency of spontaneous early morning erections may occur months before loss of nocturnal penile tumescence and development of total impotence. *Bladder dysfunction* also appears early in men and women, particularly in those with CNS involvement. Brain and spinal cord disease above the level of the lumbar spine (upper motor neuron or spastic bladder) results first in urinary frequency and small bladder volumes and eventually in incontinence. Disease of autonomic nerve fibers to the bladder (lower motor neuron bladder) or sensory denervation results in large bladder volumes, urinary frequency, and overflow incontinence. Measurements of bladder volume (postvoid residual volume) can be useful in distinguishing between upper and lower motor neuron bladder dysfunction. *Gastrointestinal dysfunction* is typically manifested as severe constipation. Diarrhea occurs occasionally (as in diabetes mellitus) due to rapid transit of contents or uncoordinated

small bowel motor activity, or on an osmotic basis from bacterial overgrowth associated with small bowel stasis. Impairment of glandular secretory function may cause difficulty with food intake (due to decreased salivation) and eye irritation (due to decreased lacrimation). Occasionally, temperature elevation and vasodilation can result from *anhidrosis*, since sweating is an important form of heat dissipation (see Chap. 17).

Orthostatic hypotension is the most disabling feature of autonomic dysfunction. Generally accepted criteria for diagnosis are a postural decrease from the supine to standing position of at least 20 mmHg in systolic or 10 mmHg in diastolic BP sustained for at least 3 min; the latter criterion differentiates autonomic failure from sluggish baroreflex responses that are common in the elderly. Postural hypotension can cause a variety of symptoms, including dimming or loss of vision, lightheadedness, diaphoresis, diminished hearing, pallor, and weakness. Syncope results when the drop in BP impairs cerebral perfusion and metabolism (see Chap. 20). Other manifestations of impaired cardiovascular control from baroreflex dysfunction include supine hypertension, a heart rate that is fixed regardless of posture, and postprandial hypotension.

Approach to the Patient

The most common, clinically significant autonomic disorders present with symptoms of orthostatic hypotension. Suggestive symptoms that may appear on standing include lightheadedness, dimming of vision, nausea, diminished hearing, sweating, pallor, and weakness. The results of the history and examination are essential to distinguish the types of syncope or near-syncope from each other—neurocardiogenic, cardiogenic, autonomic failure, and autonomic failure associated with neurologic disease (see Fig. 20-1). → *Neurocardiogenic and cardiac syncope are considered in Chap. 20.*

As a practical matter, the first step in the evaluation of symptomatic orthostasis is the exclusion of treatable causes for postural hypotension.

Table 371-1

Classification of ANS Disorders

Generalized ANS disorders
  With CNS signs
    Multiple system atrophy
      Shy-Drager syndrome
      Olivopontocerebellar degeneration
      Striatonigral degeneration
    Parkinson's disease
    Huntington's disease
    Hypothalamic disorders
  Without CNS signs
    Pure autonomic failure (as described by Bradbury and Eggleston)
    Guillain-Barré syndrome (occasionally accompanied by CNS signs)
    Chronic idiopathic anhidrosis
    Postural orthostatic tachycardia syndrome
    Raynaud's syndrome
    Familial dysautonomia—Riley-Day syndrome
Segmental or peripheral ANS disorders
  Diabetes mellitus
  Spinal cord and root disorders
  Peripheral neuropathy (amyloidosis, porphyria, alcoholism)
  Guillain-Barré syndrome
  Tabes dorsalis
  Lambert-Eaton syndrome
  Postprandial hypotension
Focal ANS disorders
  Complex regional pain syndrome type I (RSD)
    Shoulder–hand syndrome
  Complex regional pain syndrome type II (causalgia)
  Horner's syndrome
  Reinnervation anomalies
    "Crocodile" tears

The history should include an adequate review of patient medications (i.e., diuretics, antihypertensives, antidepressants, phenothiazines, ethanol, narcotics, insulin, barbiturates, and beta-adrenergic and calcium channel blockers), which may cause postural hypotension. Although medications may be responsible for symptoms, it is important to remember that exaggerated responses to medications may be the first sign of an underlying autonomic disorder. A complete list of patient medical problems may reveal a potential underlying cause for symptoms (i.e., diabetes, Parkinson's disease). The relationship of symptoms to meals (due to splanchnic shunting of blood) and awakening in the morning (due to relative intravascular volume depletion) should be sought.

The examination includes measurement of supine and standing pulse and blood pressure, with a gap of at least 2 min between positions. Sustained drops in systolic (>20 mmHg) or diastolic (>10 mmHg) blood pressure after standing for at least 2 min (unassociated with an appropriate increase in pulse rate) are suggestive of an autonomic deficit. Neurologic evaluation should include a mental status examination (to exclude neurodegenerative disorders), cranial nerve examination (to detect the impaired downgaze found with progressive supranuclear palsy), motor examination (for Parkinson's disease and parkinsonian syndromes), and sensory examination (for polyneuropathies). In patients without a clear initial diagnosis, follow-up neurologic evaluations performed at long intervals will often reveal an evolution of neurologic findings that makes it possible to reach a specific diagnosis. Autonomic function tests can be useful in selected circumstances to detect subclinical involvement, to evaluate the extent of abnormalities revealed by autonomic test results, and to monitor the effect of therapy on autonomic function.

Pharmacologic therapy is discussed below. It is helpful to remember that postural hypotension is a severely disabling disorder. Patients often lose their source of livelihood as a result, and families assume a tremendous burden for outpatient care. Adequate home health support for patients and psychological support for caregiving families is essential to maximize patient function.

Disorders of autonomic function need to be considered in the differential diagnosis of patients with symptoms of altered sweating (hyperhidrosis or hypohidrosis), constipation, impotence, or bladder dysfunction (urinary frequency, hesitancy, or incontinence). A review of concurrent medical illnesses, medications, and symptoms suggestive of autonomic or neurologic dysfunction will allow the examiner to decide which patients require further autonomic or neurologic evaluation.

Autonomic Testing (See also Chap. 361)   The functional characteristics of the ANS can be assessed by physiologic and pharmacologic tests. Commonly used physiologic tests primarily assess autonomic aspects of cardiovascular function. These tests are noninvasive, easy to use, and provide quantitative or regional information about autonomic function. Interpretation of results requires collection of data under controlled circumstances. Pharmacologic tests can elucidate pathophysiologic abnormalities and guide the development of rational therapy.

HEART RATE VARIATION WITH DEEP BREATHING   This is a test of parasympathetic influence on cardiovascular function. The test results are influenced by the subject's posture, rate and depth of respiration [5 to 6 breaths/min and a forced vital capacity (FVC) of >1.5 L are optimal], age, and medications and hypocapnea. Interpretation of results requires comparison of test data with results from normal control individuals collected under the same test conditions. For example, the lower limit of normal heart rate variation with deep breathing in persons younger than 20 years is more than 15 to 20 beats/min, but in persons over age 60 it is 5 to 8 beats/min. Heart rate variation with deep breathing (respiratory sinus arrhythmia) is abolished by the administration of atropine.

VALSALVA RESPONSE   This response assesses integrity of the afferent limb, central processing, and efferent limb of the baroreceptor reflex. The response is obtained with the subject sitting or supine. A constant expiratory pressure of 40 mmHg is maintained for 15 s while changes in heart rate and beat-to-beat BP are measured. There are four phases of BP and heart rate response to the Valsalva maneuver (Table 371-3). Phases I and III are mechanical, related to changes in intrathoracic and intraabdominal pressure, and will not be discussed further. In the first portion of phase II, reduced stroke volume and venous return results in a fall in BP, tachycardia, and increased total peripheral resistance. Increased total peripheral resistance arrests the BP drop approximately 5 to 8 s after the onset of the maneuver. The BP nadir normally is followed by a progressive rise in BP toward baseline by the end of the maneuver. Venous return and cardiac output return to normal in phase IV. Persistent peripheral arteriolar resistance results in the temporary BP overshoot and phase IV bradycardia (mediated by the baroreceptor reflex).

Autonomic function during the Valsalva maneuver can be measured in several ways. The *Valsalva ratio* is calculated from heart rate changes during the maneuver and is defined as the maximum phase II tachycardia divided by the minimum phase IV bradycardia. The ratio reflects the integrity of the entire baroreceptor reflex arc and of sympathetic efferents to blood vessels; sympathetic efferent function is assessed in the phase II BP response and the BP overshoot. Test results depend on the age and posture of the

Table 371-2

Major Clinical Manifestations in Some Generalized Autonomic Failure Syndromes*

Disorder	Postural Hypotension	Genitourinary Dysfunction	Gastrointestinal Involvement	Sweating Deficit	Other Manifestations
Aging	+ +	+	+	+/−	Postprandial hypotension
Alcoholism	+	+			Tachycardia
Amyloidosis	+ + +	+	+ +	+ +	Dissociated sensory loss
Diabetes mellitus	+ + +	+ +	+ + + +	+	Distal neuropathy
Familial dysautonomia	+ +	+	+ + +	+	Abdominal crises, fevers, reduced sensitivity to pain
Holmes-Adie syndrome	+ +		+ +	+	Tonic pupils, areflexia, supine hypertension
Multiple system atrophy	+ + + +	+ + +	+ + +	+ + +	Parkinsonian and/or cerebellar dysfunction
Parkinson's disease	+ +	+	+ +	+/−	Sweating may be increased
Progressive supranuclear palsy	+	+ +	+ + +	+	Rigidity, gaze palsies
Pure autonomic failure	+ + + +	+	+ + +	+ + +	

* Dr. Ronald Polinsky contributed to this table in the 13th edition.

ABBREVIATIONS: ±, inconsistent or minimal; +, mild; + +, moderate; + + +, severe; + + + +, disabling lack of adrenergic output. Also, insulin can cause profound hypotensive effects.

subject, the expiratory pressure, the duration of expiration, the FVC, and medications. Noninvasive recording of beat-to-beat BP changes provides a direct measure of sympathetic efferent input to blood vessels that does not depend on the presence of a normal baroreceptor reflex arc.

SUDOMOTOR FUNCTION The capacity to produce sweat can be assessed quantitatively or qualitatively. Sweating is induced by release of acetylcholine from sympathetic postganglionic fibers. The *quantitative sudomotor axon reflex test* (QSART) allows for quantification of acetylcholine-induced sweating. A reduced or absent response indicates a lesion of the postganglionic sudomotor axon. The test provides a *quantitative* measure of regional autonomic function. For example, sweating may be reduced in the legs as a result of peripheral neuropathy (e.g., in diabetes) before other signs of autonomic dysfunction emerge. The *thermoregulatory sweat test* (TST) is a *qualitative* measure of regional sweat production in response to an elevation of body temperature. An indicator powder placed on the anterior body surface changes color with sweat production during temperature elevation. The pattern of color changes is a measure of regional sweat secretion. The pattern of sweat abnormality may suggest a peripheral or central cause for the deficit. For example, a unilateral decrease over half the body suggests a central lesion. Measurement of galvanic skin responses in the limbs following an induced electrical potential is another qualitative test used for detecting the presence or absence of sweating. The response is simple to measure but habituates easily.

ORTHOSTATIC BLOOD PRESSURE RECORDINGS Beat-to-beat BP measurements determined in supine, 80° tilt, and tilt-back positions are useful to quantitate orthostatic failure in BP control. It is important to allow a 20-min period of supine rest before assessing changes in BP during tilting. The test can be useful for the evaluation of patients with unexplained syncope and to detect vagally mediated syncope.

COLD PRESSOR TEST The cold pressor test assesses sympathetic function by having the subject immerse one hand in ice water (1 to 4°C) and then measuring BP at 30 s and 1 min. The systolic and diastolic pressures normally rise by 10 to 20 mmHg. The afferent pathway is spinothalamic and thus is distinct from the afferent limb of the baroreceptor reflex arc. When spinothalamic pathways are intact, an abnormal response indicates an abnormality of autonomic central processing or sympathetic efferent function. When the response to cold pressor test is normal and the Valsalva response is abnormal, then the lesion is located in the afferent limb of the baroreceptor reflex arc.

PHARMACOLOGIC TESTS Pharmacologic assessments can help localize an autonomic defect to the central or peripheral nervous system. For example, very low supine plasma norepinephrine (NE) levels reflect postganglionic (PNS) involvement, as seen in diabetes mellitus and pure autonomic failure. Specific abnormalities in noradrenergic neuronal function can be defined by using drugs with pressor activity. Tyramine, an indirect sympathomimetic, increases BP if neuronal NE stores are adequate and uptake mechanisms are intact. Up-regulation of postsynaptic noradrenergic receptors, a manifestation of denervating lesions, can be demonstrated by measuring the BP response to NE. Denervation supersensitivity is reflected as a specific exaggerated pressor response to NE infusion (but not to tyramine), while a CNS lesion (decentralization) results in a nonspecific increase in BP responsiveness to sympathomimetic agents (i.e., to NE *and* tyramine).

SPECIFIC SYNDROMES OF ANS DYSFUNCTION Two neurodegenerative disorders, pure autonomic failure (PAF) and multiple system atrophy (MSA), have been studied intensively in an effort to clarify the distinction between central and peripheral ANS lesions (see Table 371-1).

Pure Autonomic Failure This syndrome of postural hypotension, impotence, bladder dysfunction, and defective sweating was described by Bradbury and Eggleston in 1925; it is also called *chronic postganglionic autonomic insufficiency*. The etiology is unknown. The disease is not inherited and occurs in the absence of peripheral neuropathy. The disorder generally begins insidiously in the middle decades and affects women more than men. The symptoms, particularly postural hypotension, can be disabling. The disease does not appear to shorten the life span. The clinical and neuropharmacologic characteristics suggest primary involvement of postganglionic sympathetic neurons. There is a severe reduction in the density of neurons within sympathetic ganglia. Low supine plasma NE levels, a reduced NE response to tyramine, decreased neuronal uptake of NE, and noradrenergic supersensitivity reflect the peripheral sympathetic noradrenergic dysfunction. The clinical diagnosis is tentative in the early stages because patients may present with just postural hypotension and only later develop signs of multiple system atrophy.

Multiple System Atrophy MSA comprises several overlapping clinical syndromes, including striatonigral degeneration, Shy-Drager syndrome, and olivopontocerebellar atrophy (see Chap. 370). The full clinical syndrome includes the postural hypotension, impotence, bladder and bowel dysfunction, and defective sweating seen in PAF; rigidity, tremor, loss of associative movements, or abnormal eye movements are additional clinical findings seen in MSA. The pathologic and neurochemical features of MSA differ also.

Shy-Drager syndrome is a well-characterized severe form of MSA that is accompanied by autonomic failure. Most patients present with autonomic dysfunction alone, and other neurologic manifestations usually develop within 5 years. Patients with the striatonigral variant exhibit a form of parkinsonism in which bradykinesia and rigidity are more prominent than tremor. Patients with either a pure cerebellar syndrome or striatonigral degeneration may also develop pyramidal tract involvement. Some patients have features of both subtypes (see Chap. 370).

These disorders progress relentlessly to death 7 to 10 years after onset. Normal or elevated plasma NE and low monoamine metabolite levels in cerebrospinal fluid (CSF) (norepinephrine/methoxyhydroxyphenylglycol, serotonin/5-hydroxyindoleacetic acid, and

Table 371-3

Normal Blood Pressure and Heart Rate Changes during the Valsalva Maneuver

Phase	Maneuver	Blood Pressure	Heart Rate	Comments
I	Onset of expiration against a partially closed glottis	Rises due to aortic compression	Decreases	
II*e**	Continued expiration	Falls due to decreased venous return	Increases	
II*l**	Continued expiration	Total peripheral vascular resistance increases (increased sympathetic discharge and plasma epinephrine)	Increases at slower rate	Requires efferent sympathetic response
III	End of expiration	Falls due to increased capacitance of pulmonary bed	Increases further	
IV	Recovery	Increases ("overshoot") due to vasoconstriction and increased cardiac output	Compensatory bradycardia	Requires efferent sympathetic response

* *e*, early; *l*, late.

dopamine/homovanillic acid) are consistent with CNS involvement in this syndrome. Neuropathologic changes include primary neuronal degeneration with loss of neurons and gliosis in many CNS regions, including the brainstem, the cerebellum, the striatum, and the intermediolateral cell column of the thoracolumbar spinal cord. Both PAF and MSA are relatively uncommon. Autonomic nervous system disorders occurring in Parkinson's disease, Huntington's disease, and progressive supranuclear palsy are more common (see Chap. 368).

Peripheral Nerve Disorders Peripheral neuropathies are the most common cause of chronic autonomic insufficiency (see Chap. 381). Neuropathies that affect small myelinated and unmyelinated fibers of the sympathetic and parasympathetic nerves occur in diabetes mellitus, amyloidosis, chronic alcoholism, porphyria, and Guillain-Barré syndrome.

Diabetes mellitus Autonomic involvement in diabetes may begin at any stage in the disease and often presents with asymptomatic abnormal vagal function (see Chap. 334) that can be detected as reduced heart rate variation with deep breathing. Loss of small myelinated and unmyelinated nerve fibers in the splanchnic distribution, carotid sinus, and vagus nerves characterize the disorder. Widespread enteric neuropathy can cause profound disturbances in gut motility (gastroparesis), nausea and vomiting, malnutrition, achlorhydria, and bowel incontinence. Other symptoms include impotence, urinary incontinence, pupillary abnormalities, and postural hypotension. Typical symptoms and signs of hypoglycemia may fail to appear because damage to the sympathetic innervation of the adrenal gland results in a lack of epinephrine release. Insulin excess may also cause profound hypotension. Autonomic dysfunction may lengthen the QT interval and enhance the risk of sudden death. The cause of the neuropathy in diabetes is unknown. Hyperglycemia appears to be one risk factor for autonomic involvement. Biochemical and pharmacologic studies in diabetic neuropathy are compatible with autonomic failure localized to the PNS and reveal low supine plasma NE levels, a decreased BP response to tyramine, and enhanced pressor responsiveness to phenylephrine.

Amyloid polyneuropathy Autonomic neuropathy occurs in both sporadic and familial forms of amyloidosis (see Chap. 381). Although patients usually present with a distal painful neuropathy accompanied by sensory loss, autonomic insufficiency can precede the development of the sensorimotor neuropathy. Cardiac and renal impairment are the usual causes of death. Postmortem studies reveal amyloid deposition in many organs, including two sites that contribute to autonomic failure: intraneural blood vessels and neurons in autonomic ganglia. Pathologic examination reveals a loss of unmyelinated and myelinated nerve fibers.

Alcoholic neuropathy Abnormal parasympathetic vagal and efferent sympathetic function occur in chronic alcoholics. Pathologic changes can be demonstrated in the vagus nerves, sympathetic fibers, and ganglia. Impotence is a major problem, but concurrent abnormalities in gonadal hormones may obscure the parasympathetic contribution to this symptom. Clinical symptoms of autonomic failure generally appear only when peripheral neuropathy is severe; however, orthostatic hypotension may be prominent in Wernicke's encephalopathy. Alcoholics with liver disease are more likely to develop autonomic neuropathy. Autonomic involvement may contribute to the high mortality rates associated with alcoholism.

Porphyria Although each of the porphyrias can cause autonomic dysfunction, the condition is most extensively documented in the acute intermittent type (see Chap. 343). Autonomic symptoms include tachycardia, sweating, urinary retention, hypertension, and, less commonly, hypotension. Other prominent symptoms include anxiety, abdominal pain, nausea, and vomiting. Abnormal autonomic function can occur both during acute attacks and during remissions. Elevated catecholamine levels during acute attacks correlate with the degree of tachycardia and hypertension. Interestingly, several heme precursors inhibit NE uptake in platelets from patients with acute porphyria.

Guillain-Barré syndrome Blood pressure fluctuation and arrhythmias can be severe in acute inflammatory demyelinating polyradi-

culoneuropathy. It is estimated that 2 to 10 percent of seriously ill patients with Guillain-Barré syndrome suffer fatal cardiovascular collapse. Abnormal sweating, sphincter disturbance, and pupillary dysfunction also occur. Demyelination has been described in the vagus and glossopharyngeal nerves, the sympathetic chain, and the white rami communicantes. The presence of autonomic involvement is not clearly related to the severity of motor or sensory involvement.

Spinal cord lesions Descending pathways from the brain normally coordinate organized patterns of sympathetic activity and modulate segmental autonomic reflexes necessary for homeostasis. Spinal cord transection may be attended by autonomic hyperreflexia affecting bowel, bladder, sexual, temperature-regulation, and cardiovascular functions. Dangerous increases or decreases in body temperature are the result of inability to experience the sensory accompaniments of heat or cold exposure below the level of the injury. Quadriparetic patients exhibit both orthostatic hypotension and supine hypertension after upward tilting. Markedly increased autonomic discharge (autonomic dysreflexia) can be elicited by bladder pressure or stimulation of the skin or muscles. This phenomenon affects 85 percent of patients with a spinal cord lesion above the C6 level. Suprapubic palpation of the bladder, catheter insertion, catheter obstruction, or urinary infection are common and correctable underlying causes. Blood pressure can often be lowered by tilting the head upward. Vasodilator drugs may be used to treat acute elevations in BP, and clonidine is used prophylactically to reduce the hypertension resulting from bladder stimulation. Sudden, dramatic increases in BP can lead to intracranial hemorrhage and death.

Multiple sclerosis The abnormalities in autonomic function that occur in patients with multiple sclerosis are the result of multifocal CNS disease. Abnormal sweating occurs in approximately 40 percent of cases. Impairment of cardiovascular control is less common (measured most consistently as reduced heart rate variation with deep breathing) and usually minor. There does not appear to be any relationship between the severity of the disease and the degree of autonomic involvement. However, the sympathetic nervous system can modulate immune mechanisms that could contribute to disease progression.

Reflex Sympathetic Dystrophy and Causalgia The role of the autonomic nervous system in the pathogenesis of these disorders is highly controversial. The lack of an accepted cause or mechanism to explain their cause has resulted in a change in nomenclature for reflex sympathetic dystrophy (RSD) and causalgia by the International Association for the Study of Pain. The terms *complex regional pain syndrome* (CRPS) *types I* and *II* are now substituted for *RSD* and *causalgia*, respectively.

CRPS type I (reflex sympathetic dystrophy) is a regional pain syndrome that usually develops after tissue trauma. Types of associated trauma include myocardial infarction, minor shoulder or limb injury, stroke, or medications. Spontaneous pain, *allodynia* (the perception of a nonpainful stimulus as painful), and *hyperpathia* (an exaggerated pain response to a mildly painful stimulus) are out of proportion to the initial trauma and are not confined to the distribution of a single peripheral nerve. CRPS type II (causalgia) is a regional pain syndrome that develops after injury to a peripheral nerve, as first described by the Civil War surgeon Weir Mitchell. Spontaneous pain develops in the territory of the affected nerve; it may spread beyond that region, but the initially affected area remains involved. Vasomotor abnormalities, sudomotor abnormalities, and focal edema may occur alone or in combination in both CRPS types I and II. Other conditions that can account for the observed degree of limb pain or dysfunction must be excluded before making the diagnosis of CRPS.

Pain is the primary clinical feature of CRPS. Vasomotor, sudomotor, or edematous changes must also be present to satisfy criteria for diagnosis. Limb pain syndromes that do not meet these criteria are best classified as "limb pain—not otherwise specified (NOS)" to avoid diagnostic and therapeutic confusion.

CRPS type I (RSD) is divided into three clinical phases. Phase I consists of pain and swelling in the distal extremity occurring within weeks to 3 months after the precipitating event. The pain is diffuse, spontaneous, and either burning, throbbing, or aching in quality. The involved extremity is warm and edematous, and the joints are tender. Increased sweating and hair growth are present. In phase II (3 to 6 months after injury), thin, shiny, cool skin appears. After 3 to 6 additional months (phase III), atrophy of the skin and subcutaneous tissue plus flexion contractures complete the clinical picture. A recent, large prospective study provides evidence for a more variable presentation and course.

Abnormalities of autonomic function are present in both CRPS types I and II. Autonomic dysfunction results in localized sweating (increased resting sweat output) and changes in blood flow that may result in temperature asymmetries between affected and unaffected limbs. The changes in blood flow and sweating may result from localized noradrenergic and cholinergic supersensitivity.

Therapy for both disorders is not entirely satisfactory. Limitations of treatment study designs include use of variable diagnostic criteria, lack of placebo-treated groups, failure to control for symptom duration, and small patient numbers. Despite these flaws, the desire to provide relief for these severely disabling pain syndromes has yielded a variety of surgical and medical treatments with conflicting reports of efficacy. Clinical trials suggest that early mobilization with physical therapy or a brief course of steroids may be helpful for CRPS type I (RSD). The long-term results of this treatment are unclear. Other medical treatments have included the use of adrenergic blockers, nonsteroidal anti-inflammatory drugs (NSAIDs), calcium channel blockers, phenytoin, opioids, and calcitonin. Stellate ganglion and regional intravenous blockade are commonly used invasive therapeutic techniques. A recent study found no difference in pain relief between patients with early RSD treated with placebo and those treated with intravenous regional blockade with guanethidine. Although stellate ganglion blocks often provide temporary pain relief, the efficacy of repetitive use of these blocks is controversial.

Postprandial Hypotension The importance of postprandial hypotension among healthy elderly persons, hypertensive patients, and elderly patients in nursing homes has probably been underestimated, as compared to the well-accepted association with diabetes, Parkinson's disease, renal failure treated with hemodialysis, cardiovascular disease, paraplegia, and autonomic failure. The wisdom of administering cardiovascular medications that have hypotensive effects at mealtimes to healthy and hypertensive elderly patients needs reassessment. Abnormally reduced peripheral vasoconstriction in response to shunting of blood to the splanchnic circulation after a meal often contributes to postprandial hypotension.

Inherited Disorders Riley-Day syndrome (familial dysautonomia) is an autosomal recessive disorder of infants and children which occurs among Ashkenazi Jews. The defective gene has not been identified. Decreased tearing, hyperhidrosis, reduced sensitivity to pain, areflexia, absent fungiform papillae on the tongue, and labile BP may be present. Episodic abdominal crises and fever are common. Increased sensitivity to intraocular methacholine and absent axon flare response to intradermal histamine injection are useful diagnostic markers. Normal resting plasma NE levels that do not increase upon standing are consistent with an afferent lesion. Pathologic examination of nerves reveals a loss of small myelinated and unmyelinated nerve fibers (see Chap. 363).

Miscellaneous Other conditions associated with autonomic failure include autoimmune disease, infections, exposure to toxins (botulinum), poisoning (organophosphates), malignancy, and aging. Disorders of the hypothalamus can affect autonomic function and produce abnormalities in temperature control, satiety, sexual function, and circadian rhythms (see Chap. 328).

 TREATMENT

In most conditions, management of autonomic failure is limited to alleviating the disability caused by the symptoms. If possible, the primary disorder should be treated, but that will not generally improve autonomic function. Treatment of orthostatic hypotension is important, because the hypotension can drastically impair function. The history is key to the identification of easily reversible conditions contributing to symptomatic hypotension. A review of patient medications, the relationship of symptoms to meals, medical illnesses, and other symptoms of possible autonomic origin is mandatory.

Orthostatic hypotension only requires treatment if it causes symptoms. In the early stages, patients can maintain normal function by using good judgment and a few precautions. For example, small meals are better tolerated by patients with postprandial hypotension. Alcohol intake and excessive environmental temperatures should be avoided, because vasodilation can precipitously lower BP in patients with deficient baroreflex activity. Drugs that affect BP should be used with caution; many nonprescription medicines contain sympathomimetic agents that may result in severe hypertension in the setting of autonomic failure accompanied by denervation supersensitivity.

Salt intake should be increased to the maximum tolerated. Sleeping in a reverse Trendelenburg position (head-up tilt) reduces nocturnal diuresis, morning postural hypotension, hypovolemia, and helps to minimize supine hypertension. Compressive garments are of questionable value but may be tried; they present a number of practical problems, particularly for individuals with neurogenic bladder and/or neurologic impairment.

Eventually, most patients require drug therapy for management of hypotension. Fludrocortisone, which enhances renal sodium conservation and increases the sensitivity of arterioles to norepinephrine, is the initial drug of choice; potassium supplements are often necessary with chronic administration. Inhibitors of prostaglandin synthesis (e.g., ibuprofen) have potent pressor effects in patients with autonomic dysfunction. Other pharmacologic agents have been used with variable success to elevate BP. These include beta-blockers (propranolol, pindolol, xamoterol), sympathomimetics (ephedrine, midodrine), dopamine antagonists (metoclopramide), and venoconstrictors (dihydroergotamine). The supine hypertension seen in many patients with autonomic failure often limits pharmacotherapy.

Other approaches include the vasopressin analogue desmopressin (DDAVP) and the somatostatin analogue octreotide. Long-term or short-term therapy with desmopressin minimizes fluid loss, which may play an important role in exacerbating the hypotension in patients with autonomic failure. Single intranasal doses at bedtime help prevent nocturia and morning postural hypotension. Octreotide is administered parenterally and inhibits release of gut peptides, some of which have profound vasodilator and hypotensive effects. Since these substances are typically released after a meal, octreotide is most effective in alleviating postprandial hypotension.

Novel approaches have been studied to treat orthostatic hypotension. A pilot study found that erythropoietin administration increased standing systolic pressure by 20 mmHg and improved orthostatic symptoms. Erythropoietin is administered subcutaneously or intravenously at doses of 25 to 75 U/kg three times a week. The hematocrit increases after 2 to 6 weeks. Moclobemide, a selective monoamine oxidase (MAO)-A inhibitor, has been combined with tyramine to provide a dose-dependent, graded activation of MAO-B receptors to treat orthostatic hypotension. Midodrine, an α_1 receptor agonist, has also been shown to be effective.

Many patients with ANS failure exhibit exaggerated sensitivity to various drugs. Compounds with hypotensive actions should generally be avoided. For example, anticholinergic agents are a better initial choice than dopaminergic compounds for parkinsonism. Anesthetic management poses unique problems since these patients may have abnormal baroreceptor reflexes, sympathetic innervation of peripheral arterioles, pharmacologic responses, abnormal fluid balance, and adrenal medullary insufficiency. More important than the choice of anesthetic is awareness by the physician of the implications autonomic failure may have for peri- and postoperative monitoring and management.

BIBLIOGRAPHY

BANNISTER R (ed): *Autonomic Failure*, 3d ed. London, Oxford University Press, 1992

BRAUS DF et al: The shoulder-hand syndrome after stroke: A prospective clinical trial. Ann Neurol 36:728, 1994

BRADBURY S, EGGLESTON C: Postural hypotension: A report of three cases. Am Heart J 1:73, 1925

DYCK P et al (eds): *Peripheral Neuropathy*, 3d ed. Philadelphia, Saunders, 1993

JANSEN RW, LIPSITZ LA: Postprandial hypotension: Epidemiology, pathophysiology, and clinical management. Ann Intern Med 122:286, 1995

KOZIN F et al: The reflex sympathetic dystrophy syndrome. I. Clinical and histological studies: Evidence for bilaterality, response to corticosteroids and articular involvement. Am J Med 60:321, 1976

LOW PA, PFEIFER MA: Standardization of autonomic function, in *Clinical Autonomic Disorders: Evaluation and Management*, PA Low (ed). Boston, Little, Brown, 1992

——— et al: Efficacy of midodrine vs. placebo in neurogenia orthostatic hypotension. JAMA 277:1046, 1997

MATHIAS CJ: Orthostatic hypotension: Causes, mechanisms, and influencing factors. Neurology 45(Suppl 5):S6, 1995

MCLEOD JG: Autonomic dysfunction in peripheral nerve disease. Invited review. Muscle Nerve 15:3, 1992

POLINSKY RJ: Clinical autonomic neuropharmacology. Neurol Clin 8:77, 1990

ROBERTSON D, DAVIS TL: Recent advances in the treatment of orthostatic hypotension. Neurology 45(Suppl 5):S26, 1995

SHY GM, DRAGER GA: A neurological syndrome associated with orthostatic hypotension. Arch Neurol 2:511, 1960

STANTON-HICKS M et al: Reflex sympathetic dystrophy: Changing concepts and taxonomy. Pain 63:127, 1995

VELDMAN PHJM et al: Signs and symptoms of reflex sympathetic dystrophy: Prospective study of 829 patients. Lancet 342:1012, 1993

372 *Joseph B. Martin, M. Flint Beal**

DISORDERS OF THE CRANIAL NERVES

The cranial nerves are susceptible to disorders that rarely affect the spinal peripheral nerves and, for this reason, deserve to be considered separately. This chapter describes the principal syndromes of disordered cranial nerve function and the diseases that cause them. → *Disorders of taste and smell, vision and ocular movement, and hearing and balance are discussed in Chaps. 20, 28, and 29.*

OLFACTORY NERVE See Chap. 29

OPTIC NERVE See Chap. 28

OCULOMOTOR, TROCHLEAR, AND ABDUCENS NERVES See Chap. 28

TRIGEMINAL NERVE

The trigeminal nerve supplies sensation to the skin of the face and anterior half of the head. Its motor part innervates the masseter and pterygoid masticatory muscles.

PAROXYSMAL FACIAL PAIN (TRIGEMINAL NEURALGIA, TIC DOULOUREUX) The most striking disorder of trigeminal nerve function is tic douloureux, a condition characterized by excruciating paroxysms of pain in the lips, gums, cheek, or chin and, very rarely, in the distribution of the ophthalmic division of the fifth nerve. The disorder occurs almost exclusively in middle-aged and elderly persons. The pain seldom lasts more than a few seconds or a minute or two but may be so intense that the patient winces, hence

* The authors acknowledge the contributions of Maurice Victor to this chapter in previous editions.

the term *tic*. The paroxysms recur frequently, both day and night, for several weeks at a time. Another characteristic feature is the initiation of pain by stimuli applied to certain areas on the face, lips, or tongue ("trigger zones") or by movement of these parts. Sensory loss cannot be demonstrated. The adequate stimulus to a trigger zone for precipitating an attack is a tactile one and possibly tickle, rather than a noxious or thermal stimulus. Usually a spatial and temporal summation of impulses is necessary to trigger an attack, which is followed by a refractory period of up to 2 or 3 min.

The *diagnosis* of this disorder rests on these strict clinical criteria, and the condition must be distinguished from other forms of facial and cephalic neuralgia and pain arising from diseases of the jaw, teeth, or sinuses (see Chap. 15). Tic douloureux is usually without assignable cause; occasionally, when it appears in younger adults, it may be due to a demyelinative plaque at the root entry zone of the fifth nerve. Very rarely it occurs with herpes zoster or a tumor. To a degree that remains uncertain, pain of tic douloureux may be caused by a redundant or tortuous blood vessel in the posterior fossa, causing an irritative lesion of the nerve or its root. Usually, however, lesions such as aneurysms, neurofibromas, or meningiomas affecting the nerve produce a loss of sensation (trigeminal neuropathy, see below).

℞ TREATMENT

The initial treatment of tic douloureux is pharmacologic. Carbamazepine is the drug of choice and is effective initially in 75 percent of patients. Carbamazepine should be started gradually, as a single daily dose of 100 mg taken with food, and increased to 200 mg qid. Doses greater than 1200 mg daily provide no additional benefit. Unfortunately, not all patients can tolerate the drug in the doses required to alleviate pain, in which case phenytoin, 300 to 400 mg daily, can be substituted. Baclofen may also be administered, either alone or in combination with carbamazepine or phenytoin. The initial dose is 5 to 10 mg tid gradually increasing as needed to 20 mg qid.

If drug treatment fails, surgical therapy should be offered. The most widely applied procedure is percutaneous retrogasserian rhizotomy accomplished by radiofrequency lesions. Injection of glycerol in Meckel's cave is a method preferred by some surgeons. Either procedure produces relief in more than 95 percent of patients. The pain recurs in 7 to 31 percent of patients. Complications and morbidity are infrequent in experienced hands. These procedures result in partial numbness of the face and carry a risk of corneal denervation with secondary keratitis when used for the rare instances of first-division trigeminal neuralgia.

A third treatment, microvascular decompression, requires a suboccipital craniectomy, a major procedure requiring several days of hospitalization. It has an 80 percent efficacy rate, but the pain may recur, and, in a small number of cases, there is damage to the eighth or seventh nerve.

TRIGEMINAL NEUROPATHY A variety of diseases in addition to those mentioned above may affect the trigeminal nerve. Most present with sensory loss on the face or with weakness of the jaw muscles. Deviation of the jaw on opening indicates weakness of the pterygoids on the side to which the jaw deviates. Tumors of the middle cranial fossa (meningiomas), of the trigeminal nerve (schwannomas), or of the base of the skull (metastatic tumors) may cause a combination of motor and sensory signs. Lesions in the cavernous sinus can affect the first and second divisions of the trigeminal nerve, and lesions of the superior orbital fissure can affect the first (ophthalmic) division. The accompanying corneal anesthesia increases the risk of ulceration (neurokeratitis).

Loss of sensation over the chin can be the only manifestation of systemic malignancy. Rarely, an idiopathic form of trigeminal neuropathy is observed. It is characterized by feelings of numbness and paresthesias, sometimes bilaterally, with loss of sensation in the territory of the trigeminal nerve but without weakness of the jaw. Recovery is the rule, but the symptoms may be troublesome for many months, or even years. Leprosy may involve the trigeminal nerves.

Tonic spasm of the masticatory muscles, known as *trismus*, is symptomatic of tetanus (see Chap. 146). It also may occur as an idiosyncratic reaction in patients treated with phenothiazine drugs; lesser degrees may be associated with disease of the pharynx, temporomandibular joint, teeth, and gums.

FACIAL NERVE

FACIAL PALSY AND FACIAL SPASM The seventh cranial nerve supplies all the muscles concerned with facial expression. The sensory component is small (the nervus intermedius of Wrisberg); it conveys taste sensation from the anterior two-thirds of the tongue and probably cutaneous impulses from the anterior wall of the external auditory canal. The motor nucleus of the seventh nerve lies anterior and lateral to the abducens nucleus. After leaving the pons, the seventh nerve enters the internal auditory meatus with the acoustic nerve. The nerve continues its course in its own bony channel, the facial canal, and exits from the skull via the stylomastoid foramen. It then passes through the parotid gland and subdivides to supply the facial muscles.

A complete interruption of the facial nerve at the stylomastoid foramen paralyzes all muscles of facial expression. The corner of the mouth droops, the creases and skin folds are effaced, the forehead is unfurrowed, and the eyelids will not close. Upon attempted closure of the lids, the eye on the paralyzed side is seen to roll upward (Bell's phenomenon). The lower lid sags also, and the punctum falls away from the conjunctiva, permitting tears to spill over the cheek. Food collects between the teeth and lips, and saliva may dribble from the corner of the mouth. The patient complains of a heaviness or numbness in the face, but sensory loss is rarely demonstrable and taste is intact.

If the lesion is in the middle ear portion, taste is lost over the anterior two-thirds of the tongue on the same side. If the nerve to the stapedius is interrupted, there is hyperacusis (painful sensitivity to loud sounds). Lesions in the internal auditory meatus also may affect the adjacent auditory and vestibular nerves, causing deafness, tinnitus, or dizziness. Intrapontine lesions that paralyze the face usually affect the abducens nucleus as well, and often the corticospinal and sensory tracts.

If the peripheral facial paralysis has existed for some time and recovery of motor function has begun but is incomplete, a kind of contracture (actually a continuous diffuse contraction) of facial muscles may appear. The palpebral fissure becomes narrowed, and the nasolabial fold deepens. With the passage of time, the face and even the tip of the nose become pulled to the unaffected side. Attempts to move one group of facial muscles may result in contraction of all of them (associated movements, or *synkinesis*). Facial spasms may develop and persist indefinitely, being initiated by every facial movement (*hemifacial spasm*). This condition may represent a transient or permanent sequela to a Bell's palsy but also may be due to an irritative lesion of the facial nerve (e.g., an acoustic neuroma, an aberrant artery that compresses the nerve and is relieved by surgery, or a basilar artery aneurysm). However, in the most common form of hemifacial spasm, the cause and pathology are unknown. Anomalous regeneration of the seventh nerve fibers may result in other troublesome phenomena. If fibers originally connected with the orbicularis oculi come to innervate the orbicularis oris, closure of the lids may cause a retraction of the mouth, or if fibers originally connected with muscles of the face later innervate the lacrimal gland, anomalous tearing ("crocodile tears") may occur with any activity of the facial muscles, such as eating. Yet another unusual facial synkinesia is one in which jaw opening causes a closure of the eyelids on the side of the facial palsy (jaw-winking).

BELL'S PALSY The most common form of facial paralysis is idiopathic, i.e., *Bell's palsy*. The incidence rate of this disorder is about 23 per 100,000 annually, or about 1 in 60 or 70 persons in a lifetime. The pathogenesis of the paralysis is unknown. The few autopsied cases of this disease have shown only nondescript changes in the facial nerve and not inflammatory changes, as is commonly presumed.

Clinical Manifestations The onset of Bell's palsy is fairly abrupt, maximal weakness being attained by 48 h as a general rule. Pain behind the ear may precede the paralysis for a day or two. Taste sensation may be lost unilaterally, and hyperacusis may be present. In some cases there is mild cerebrospinal fluid (CSF) lymphocytosis. Fully 80 percent of patients recover within a few weeks or months. Electromyography may be of value in distinguishing a temporary conduction defect from a pathologic interruption in the continuity of nerve fibers. Evidence of denervation after 10 days indicates that there has been axonal degeneration and that there will be a long delay (3 months, as a rule) before regeneration occurs and that it may be incomplete. The presence of incomplete paralysis in the first week is the most favorable prognostic sign.

℞ **TREATMENT**

Protection of the eye during sleep, massage of the weakened muscles, and a splint to prevent drooping of the lower part of the face are the measures generally employed in the management of such cases. A course of prednisone beginning with 60 to 80 mg daily during the first 5 days and then tapered over the next 5 days may be beneficial and appears to shorten the recovery period.

Differential Diagnosis There are many other causes of facial palsy. Tumors that invade the temporal bone (carotid body, cholesteatoma, dermoid) may produce a facial palsy, but the onset is insidious and the course progressive. The *Ramsay Hunt syndrome*, presumably due to herpes zoster of the geniculate ganglion, consists of a severe facial palsy associated with a vesicular eruption in the pharynx, external auditory canal, and other parts of the cranial integument; often the eighth cranial nerve is affected as well. *Acoustic neuromas* frequently involve the facial nerve by local compression. Infarcts and tumors are the common pontine lesions that interrupt the facial nerve fibers. Bilateral facial paralysis (facial diplegia) occurs in acute inflammatory polyradiculoneuritis (*Guillain-Barré syndrome*) and in a variety of sarcoidosis known as *uveoparotid fever* (*Heerfordt syndrome*). The patient should be screened for Lyme disease, which is a frequent cause of facial palsies in endemic areas. The *Melkersson-Rosenthal syndrome* consists of a rarely encountered triad of recurrent facial paralysis, recurrent—and eventually permanent—facial (particularly labial) edema, and less constantly, plication of the tongue; many causes of this rare syndrome have been suggested, but none has been established. Leprosy frequently involves the facial nerve.

A puzzling disorder is the *facial hemiatrophy of Romberg*. It occurs mainly in females and is characterized by a disappearance of fat in the dermal and subcutaneous tissues on one side of the face. It usually begins in adolescence or early adult years and is slowly progressive. In its advanced form, the affected side of the face is gaunt, and the skin is thin, wrinkled, and rather brown. The facial hair may turn white and fall out, and the sebaceous glands become atrophic. The muscles and bones are not involved as a rule. Sometimes the atrophy becomes bilateral. The condition is a form of lipodystrophy. There is no treatment other than transplantation of skin and subcutaneous fat by a plastic surgeon.

Facial myokymia refers to a fine rippling activity of the facial muscles; it may be caused by a plaque of multiple sclerosis. *Blepharospasm* is an involuntary recurrent spasm of both eyelids that occurs in elderly persons as an isolated phenomenon or with varying degrees of spasm of other facial muscles. Severe, persistent cases of blepharospasm or hemifacial spasm are now successfully treated by local injection of botulinus toxin into the orbicularis oculi; the spasms are relieved for 3 to 4 months, and the injections can be repeated without morbidity.

All these forms of nuclear or peripheral facial palsy must be distinguished from the supranuclear type. In the latter, the frontalis and orbicularis oculi muscles are involved less than those of the lower part of the face, since the upper facial muscles are innervated by corticobulbar pathways from both motor cortices, whereas the lower facial muscles are innervated only by the opposite hemisphere. In supranuclear lesions there may be a dissociation of emotional and voluntary facial movements, and often some degree of paralysis of the arm and leg or an aphasia (in dominant hemisphere lesions) is conjoined.

VESTIBULAR NERVE

The eighth cranial nerve has two components, vestibular and auditory. Symptoms and signs of involvement of the vestibular portion are discussed in Chap. 20 and in this section. The auditory nerve and its disorders are discussed in Chap. 29.

MÉNIÈRE'S SYNDROME Ménière's disease, or Ménière's syndrome, is the name applied to recurrent vertigo associated with tinnitus and progressive deafness. Tinnitus and/or deafness may be absent during the initial attack(s) of vertigo, but they invariably appear as the disease progresses and are increased in severity during an acute attack. With milder forms of the syndrome, the patient may complain more of head discomfort, slight instability, and difficulty in concentration than of vertigo and may be considered to be anxious or depressed. Provided that deafness is not complete, the recruitment phenomenon can be demonstrated (see Chap. 29).

Ménière's disease has its onset most frequently in the fifth decade of life, although younger adults and the elderly are not spared. The pathologic changes are said to consist of a dilation of the endolymphatic system that leads to a degeneration of the delicate vestibular and cochlear hair cells. The relation of these pathologic changes to the paroxysmal disorder of labyrinthine function is unknown.

℞ **TREATMENT**
During an acute attack, rest in bed is the most effective treatment, since the patient can usually find a position in which vertigo is minimal. Dimenhydrinate, cyclizine, or meclizine in doses of 25 to 50 mg tid is useful in treating more protracted attacks. A low-salt diet is still used in treatment, but its value is difficult to judge. Mild sedative drugs may help the anxious patient between attacks. Usually the deafness is unilateral and progressive, and when it is complete, the vertiginous attacks cease. However, the course is variable, and if the attacks persist in a severe manner, permanent relief can be obtained by surgical destruction of the labyrinth or section of the vestibular portion of the eighth nerve intracranially.

BENIGN POSITIONAL VERTIGO Another disorder of labyrinthine function is characterized by the occurrence of paroxysmal vertigo and nystagmus when the head assumes certain critical positions. This is the positional vertigo of Bárány, of the so-called benign paroxysmal type (see Chap. 20). In refractory cases, in which attacks continue, vestibular exercises may be beneficial.

DIFFERENTIAL DIAGNOSIS OF VERTIGO There are many other causes of acute vertigo, such as purulent labyrinthitis complicating meningitis, serous labyrinthitis due to infection of the middle ear, "toxic labyrinthitis" due to drug intoxication (e.g., with alcohol, quinine, streptomycin, gentamicin, and other antibiotics), motion sickness, trauma, and hemorrhage into the internal ear. In these instances, the attacks of vertigo tend to last longer than in the recurrent form, but in other respects the symptoms are similar. Aminoglycoside antibiotics may damage the fine hair cells of the vestibular end organs and cause a permanent disorder of equilibrium (as well as hearing), especially in older patients (see also Chap. 20).

There has been described a dramatic clinical syndrome, characterized by the abrupt onset of severe vertigo, nausea, and vomiting without tinnitus or hearing loss. The vertigo persists for several days or weeks, and labyrinthine function is permanently ablated on one side. Occlusion of the labyrinthine division of the internal auditory artery would logically explain this syndrome, but pathologic or angiographic confirmation of this hypothesis has so far not been obtained.

Vertigo of vestibular nerve origin may occur with diseases that involve the nerve in the petrous bone or the cerebellopontine angle.

Except that it is less severe and is less frequently paroxysmal, it has many of the characteristics of labyrinthine vertigo. The adjacent auditory division of the eighth cranial nerve also may be affected, which explains the frequent association of vertigo with tinnitus and deafness. The function of the eighth cranial nerve may be disturbed by tumors of the lateral recess (especially acoustic neuroma), less frequently by meningeal inflammation in this region and, rarely, by an abnormal vessel that compresses the nerve.

Vestibular neuronitis and *benign recurrent vertigo* are the names applied to a clinical syndrome that occurs mainly in middle-aged and young adults (sometimes in children) and is characterized by the abrupt onset of vertigo, nausea, and vomiting without impairment of hearing. The attacks are brief and leave the patient for some days with a mild positional vertigo. They may occur only once or recur in varying degrees of severity. The cause is unknown. The medical treatment is the same as for Ménière's disease.

GLOSSOPHARYNGEAL NERVE

GLOSSOPHARYNGEAL NEURALGIA This form of neuralgia resembles trigeminal neuralgia in many respects but is much less common. The pain is intense and paroxysmal; it originates in the throat, approximately in the tonsillar fossa. In some cases the pain is localized in the ear or may radiate from the throat to the ear because of involvement of the tympanic branch of the glossopharyngeal nerve. Spasms of pain may be initiated by swallowing. There is no demonstrable sensory or motor deficit. Cardiac symptoms—bradycardia, hypotension, and fainting—have been reported. A trial of carbamazepine or phenytoin is the recommended therapy, but if that is unsuccessful, division of the glossopharyngeal nerve near the medulla is the definitive treatment. Percutaneous rhizotomy of glossopharyngeal and vagal fibers in the jugular foramen alleviates pain in some patients.

Very rarely, herpes zoster involves the glossopharyngeal nerve. Glossopharyngeal neuropathy in conjunction with vagus and accessory nerve palsies may occur with a tumor or aneurysm in the posterior fossa or in the jugular foramen. Hoarseness due to vocal cord paralysis, some difficulty in swallowing, deviation of the soft palate to the intact side, anesthesia of the posterior wall of the pharynx, and weakness of the upper part of the trapezius and sternocleidomastoid muscles make up the syndrome (see Table 372-1, jugular foramen syndrome).

VAGUS NERVE

DYSPHAGIA AND DYSPHONIA Complete interruption of the intracranial portion of one vagus nerve results in a characteristic paralysis. The soft palate droops ipsilaterally and does not rise in phonation. There is loss of the gag reflex on the affected side, as well as of the "curtain movement" of the lateral wall of the pharynx, whereby the faucial pillars move medially as the palate rises in saying "ah." The voice is hoarse and slightly nasal, and the vocal cord lies immobile in the cadaveric position, i.e., midway between abduction and adduction. There also may be a loss of sensibility at the external auditory meatus and back of the pinna. Usually no change in visceral function can be demonstrated.

The pharyngeal branches of both vagi may be affected in diphtheria; the voice has a nasal quality, and regurgitation of liquids through the nose occurs during the act of swallowing.

The vagus nerve may be involved at the meningeal level by neoplastic and infectious processes and within the medulla by tumors, vascular lesions (e.g., the lateral medullary syndrome of Wallenberg), and motor neuron disease. This nerve may be involved by the inflammatory lesion of herpes zoster. Polymyositis and dermatomyositis, which cause hoarseness and dysphagia by direct involvement of laryngeal and pharyngeal muscles, may be confused with diseases of the vagus nerves. Also, dysphagia is a symptom in some patients with myotonic dystrophy. → *See Chap. 40 for discussion of nonneurologic forms of dysphagia.*

The recurrent laryngeal nerves, especially the left, are most often damaged as a result of intrathoracic disease. Aneurysm of the aortic arch, an enlarged left atrium, and tumors of the mediastinum and bronchi are much more frequent causes of an isolated vocal cord palsy than are intracranial disorders.

When confronted with a case of laryngeal palsy, the physician must attempt to determine the site of the lesion. If it is intramedullary, there are usually other signs, such as ipsilateral cerebellar dysfunction, loss of pain and temperature sensation over the ipsilateral face and contralateral arm and leg, and an ipsilateral Horner syndrome. If the lesion is extramedullary, the glossopharyngeal and spinal accessory nerves are frequently involved (see jugular foramen syndrome, Table 372-1). If it is extracranial in the posterior laterocondylar or retroparotid space, there may be a combination of ninth, tenth, eleventh, and twelfth cranial nerve palsies and a Horner syndrome. Combinations of these lower cranial nerve palsies have a variety of eponymic designations, listed in Table 372-1. If there is no sensory loss over the palate and pharynx and no palatal weakness or dysphagia, the lesion is below the origin of the pharyngeal branches, which leave the vagus nerve high in the cervical region; the usual site of disease is then the mediastinum.

Table 372-1

Cranial Nerve Syndromes

Site	Cranial Nerves Involved	Eponymic Syndrome	Usual Cause
Sphenoid fissure (superior orbital)	III, IV, first division V, VI	Foix	Invasive tumors of sphenoid bone; aneurysms
Lateral wall of cavernous sinus	III, IV, first division V, VI, often with proptosis	Foix Tolosa-Hunt	Aneurysms or thrombosis of cavernous sinus; invasive tumors from sinuses and sella turcica; benign granuloma responsive to steroids
Retrosphenoid space	II, III, IV, V, VI	Jacod	Large tumors of middle cranial fossa
Apex of petrous bone	V, VI	Gradenigo	Petrositis; tumors of petrous bone
Internal auditory meatus	VII, VIII		Tumors of petrous bone (dermoids, etc.); infectious processes; acoustic neuroma
Pontocerebellar angle	V, VII, VIII, and sometimes IX		Acoustic neuroma; meningioma
Jugular foramen	IX, X, XI	Vernet	Tumors and aneurysms
Posterior laterocondylar space	IX, X, XI, XII	Collet-Sicard	Tumors of parotid gland and carotid body and metastatic tumors
Posterior retroparotid space	IX, X, XI, XII and Horner syndrome	Villaret Mackenzie Tapia	Tumors of parotid gland, carotid body, lymph nodes; metastatic tumor; tuberculous adenitis

ACCESSORY NERVE

Isolated involvement of the accessory, or eleventh cranial, nerve can occur anywhere along its route, resulting in partial or complete paralysis of the sternocleidomastoid and trapezius muscles. More commonly, involvement occurs in combination with deficits of the ninth and tenth cranial nerves in the jugular foramen or after exit from the skull (see Table 372-1). An idiopathic form of accessory neuropathy, akin to Bell's palsy, has been described, and it may be recurrent in some cases. Most but not all patients recover.

HYPOGLOSSAL NERVE

The twelfth cranial nerve supplies the ipsilateral muscles of the tongue. The nucleus of the nerve or its fibers of exit may be involved by intramedullary lesions such as tumor, poliomyelitis, or most often motor neuron disease. Lesions of the basal meninges and the occipital bones (platybasia, invagination of occipital condyles, Paget's disease) may compress the nerve in its extramedullary course or in the hypoglossal canal. Isolated lesions of unknown cause can occur. Atrophy and fasciculation of the tongue develop weeks to months after interruption of the nerve.

MULTIPLE CRANIAL NERVE PALSIES

Several cranial nerves may be affected by the same disease process. In this situation, the main clinical problem is to determine whether the lesion lies within the brainstem or outside it. Lesions that lie on the surface of the brainstem are characterized by involvement of adjacent cranial nerves (often occurring in succession) and late and rather slight involvement of the long sensory and motor pathways and segmental structures lying within the brainstem. The opposite is true of intramedullary, intrapontine, and intramesencephalic lesions. The extramedullary lesion is more likely to cause bone erosion or enlargement of the foramens of exit of cranial nerves. The intramedullary lesion involving cranial nerves often produces a crossed sensory or motor paralysis (cranial nerve signs on one side of the body and tract signs on the opposite side).

Involvement of multiple cranial nerves outside the brainstem is frequently the result of diabetes or trauma (sudden onset), localized infections such as herpes zoster (acute onset), granulomatous disease such as Wegener's granulomatosis (subacute onset), Behçet's disease, or tumors and enlarging saccular aneurysms (chronic development). Of the tumors, lymphomas, neurofibromas, meningiomas, chordomas, cholesteatomas, carcinomas, and sarcomas have all been observed to involve a succession of lower cranial nerves. Owing to their anatomic relationships, the multiple cranial nerve palsies form a number of distinctive syndromes, listed in Table 372-1. Sarcoidosis has been found to be the cause of some cases of multiple cranial neuropathy, and chronic glandular tuberculosis (scrofula) the cause of a few others. Malignant granuloma of the nasopharynx also may affect multiple cranial nerves, as do nasopharyngeal tumors, platybasia, basilar invagination of the skull, and the Chiari malformation that becomes evident in adult life. A purely motor disorder without atrophy always raises the question of myasthenia gravis (see Chap. 382). Guillain-Barré syndrome commonly affects the facial nerves bilaterally (facial diplegia). In the Fisher variant of the Guillain-Barré syndrome, oculomotor paresis occurs with ataxia and areflexia in the limbs. Wernicke encephalopathy can cause a severe ophthalmoplegia combined with other brainstem signs.

An idiopathic form of multiple cranial nerve involvement on one or both sides of the face is occasionally seen (see Juncos and Beal). The syndrome consists of a subacute onset of boring facial pain, followed by paralysis of motor cranial nerves. The clinical features overlap those of the Tolosa-Hunt orbitocavernous sinus syndrome. The syndrome is frequently responsive to steroids.

BIBLIOGRAPHY

ADAMS RD, VICTOR M: *Principles of Neurology*, 6th ed. New York, McGraw-Hill, 1997, chap 47, pp 1370–1385

ADOUR KK: Medical management of idiopathic (Bell's) palsy. Otolaryngol Clin North Am 24:663, 1991

BECK RW et al: The effect of corticosteroids for acute optic neuritis on the subsequent development of multiple sclerosis. N Engl J Med 329:1764, 1993

BRODAL A: The cranial nerves, in *Neurological Anatomy in Relation to Clinical Medicine*, 3d ed. New York, Oxford, 1980, chap 7, pp 448–577

CHALK C, ISAACS H: Recurrent spontaneous accessory neuropathy. J Neurol Neurosurg Psychiatry 53:621, 1990

DALLESSIO DJ: Medical treatment of the major neuralgias. Semin Neurol 8:286, 1988

DURELLI L et al: The Melkersson-Rosenthal syndrome: A case with increased CNS IgG synthesis. Ann Neurol 18:623, 1985

FROMM GH et al: Baclofen in the treatment of refractory trigeminal neuralgia. Neurology 29:550, 1979

JANKOVIC J, BRIN MF: Therapeutic uses of botulinum toxin. N Engl J Med 324:1186, 1991

JUNCOS JL, BEAL MF: Idiopathic cranial polyneuropathy. Brain 110:197, 1987

KARNES WE: Diseases of the seventh cranial nerve, in *Peripheral Neuropathy*, 3d ed, PJ Dyck et al (eds). Philadelphia, Saunders, 1993, chap 43, pp 818–836

KEANE JR: Bilateral seventh nerve palsy: Analysis of 43 cases and review of the literature. Neurology 44:1198, 1994

———: Fourth nerve palsy: Historical review and study of 215 inpatients. Neurology 43:2439, 1993

KROENKE K et al: Causes of persistent dizzyness: A prospective study of 100 patients in ambulatory care. Ann Intern Med 117:898, 1992

LACHANCE DH et al: Primary leptomeningeal lymphoma: Report of 9 cases, diagnosis with immunocytochemical analysis, and review of the literature. Neurology 41:95, 1991

LECKY BRF et al: Trigeminal sensory neuropathy. Brain 110:1463, 1987

LOSSOS A, SIEGAL T: Numb chin syndrome in cancer patients: Etiology, response to treatment, and prognostic significance. Neurology 42:1181, 1992

MAYO CLINIC AND MAYO FOUNDATION: *Clinical Examinations in Neurology*, 6th ed. St. Louis, Mosby Year Book, 1991

SAWLE GV et al: The natural history of non-arteritic anterior ischemic optic neuropathy. J Neurol Neurosurg Psychiatry 53:830, 1990

SELBY G: Diseases of the fifth cranial nerve, in *Peripheral Neuropathy*, 3d ed, PJ Dyck et al (eds). Philadelphia, Saunders, 1993, chap 42, pp 801–817

SWEET WH: The treatment of trigeminal neuralgia (tic douloureux). N Engl J Med 315:174, 1986

———: Percutaneous methods for the treatment of trigeminal neuralgia and other faciocephalic pain; comparison with microvascular decompression. Semin Neurol 8:272, 1988

TROOST BT, PATTON JM: Exercise therapy for positional vertigo. Neurology 42:1441, 1992

Table 373-1

Some Treatable Spinal Cord Disorders

Compressive
  Epidural, intradural, or intramedullary neoplasm
  Epidural abscess
  Epidural hemorrhage
  Cervical spondylosis
  Herniated disc
  Posttraumatic compression by fractured or displaced vertebra or hemorrhage
Vascular
  Arteriovenous malformation
Inflammatory
  Transverse myelitis
  Multiple sclerosis
Infectious
  Herpes simplex virus type 2 infection
  Parasitic or bacterial infection
Developmental
  Syringomyelia
Metabolic
  Subacute combined degeneration

---

373 — Stephen L. Hauser

DISEASES OF THE SPINAL CORD

Diseases of the spinal cord are frequently devastating. They can produce quadriplegia, paraplegia, and sensory deficits far beyond the damage they would inflict elsewhere in the nervous system, because the spinal cord contains, in a small cross-sectional area, almost the entire motor output and sensory input systems of the trunk and limbs. Many spinal cord diseases are reversible if recognized and treated at an early stage (Table 373-1); thus, they are among the most critical of neurologic emergencies. The efficient use of diagnostic procedures, guided by a working knowledge of the relevant anatomy and clinical features of common spinal cord diseases, is often the key to a successful outcome.

Approach to the Patient

Spinal Cord Anatomy Relevant to Clinical Signs The spinal cord is a thin, tubular extension of the central nervous system contained within the bony spinal canal. It originates at the medulla and continues caudally to terminate at the filum terminale, a fibrous extension of the conus medullaris that terminates at the coccyx. The adult spinal cord is approximately 18 inches long, oval or round in shape, and enlarged in the cervical and lumbar regions, where neurons that innervate the upper and lower extremities, respectively, are located. The white matter tracts containing ascending sensory and descending motor pathways are located peripherally, whereas nerve cell bodies are clustered in an inner region shaped like a four-leaf clover that surrounds the central canal (anatomically an extension of the fourth ventricle). The membranes that cover the spinal cord—the pia, arachnoid, and dura—are continuous with those of the brainstem and cerebral hemispheres.

The spinal cord is somatotopically organized, consisting of 31 segments, each containing an exiting ventral motor root and entering dorsal sensory root (Fig. 373-1). During embryologic development, growth of the cord lags behind that of the vertebral column, and in the adult the spinal cord ends at approximately the first lumbar vertebral body. The lower spinal nerves take an increasingly downward course to exit via the appropriate intervertebral foramina. The first seven pairs of cervical spinal nerves exit above the same-numbered vertebral bodies, whereas all the subsequent nerves exit below the same-numbered vertebral bodies; this situation is due to the presence of eight cervical spinal cord segments but only seven cervical vertebrae. The approximate relationship between spinal cord segments and the corresponding vertebral bodies is shown in Table 373-2. These relationships assume importance for localization of lesions that cause spinal cord compression; a T10 spinal cord level, for example, indicates involvement of the cord adjacent to the seventh or eighth thoracic vertebral body.

LEVEL OF THE LESION The presence of a *level* below which sensory, motor, and/or autonomic function is disturbed is a hallmark of spinal cord disease. A sensory level is sought by asking the patient to identify as sharp a pinprick stimulus or as cool a cold stimulus (a dry tuning fork after immersion in cold water) applied to the low back and sequentially moved up toward the neck on each side. In general, a sensory level to pinprick or temperature, indicating damage to the spinothalamic tract, is located one to two segments below the actual level of a unilateral spinal cord lesion, but it may be at the level of

Table 373-2

Spinal Cord Levels Relative to the Vertebral Bodies

Spinal Cord Level	Corresponding Vertebral Body
Upper cervical	Same as cord level
Lower cervical	1 level higher
Upper thoracic	2 levels higher
Lower thoracic	2 to 3 levels higher
Lumbar	T10–T12
Sacral	T12–L1
Coccygeal	L1

the lesion when bilateral. That is because sensory fibers enter the cord at the dorsal root, synapse in the dorsal horn, and then ascend ipsilaterally for several segments before crossing just anterior to the central canal to join the opposite spinothalamic tract. Lesions that disrupt descending corticospinal and bulbospinal tracts cause paraplegia or quadriplegia, with increased muscle tone, exaggerated deep tendon reflexes, and extensor plantar signs. Such lesions also typically produce autonomic disturbances, with disturbed sweating and bladder, bowel, and sexual dysfunction. A sweat level may be determined by drawing a spoon up the torso. There will be little resistance to movement of the spoon along the dry, nonsweating skin; at the level at which sweating begins, resistance will suddenly increase.

The uppermost level of a spinal cord lesion is often localized by attention to *segmental signs* corresponding to disturbed motor or sensory innervation by an individual cord segment. A band of altered sensation (hyperalgesia or hyperpathia) at the upper end of the sensory disturbance, fasciculations or atrophy in muscles innervated by one or several segments, or a single diminished or absent deep tendon reflex may be noted. These signs may also occur with focal root or peripheral nerve disorders; thus, segmental signs are most useful when they occur with other signs of cord disease. With severe and acute transverse lesions, there may be flaccidity of the limbs rather than spasticity (so-called spinal shock). This state may last for several days, rarely for weeks, and may be initially mistaken for extensive damage to many segments of the cord (as in ascending necrotic myelopathy associated with cancer) or as polyneuropathy. Brief clonic or myoclonic movements of the limbs often precede paralysis in acute transverse lesions, particularly those due to cord infarction.

PATTERNS OF SPINAL CORD DISEASE The location of the major ascending and descending pathways of the spinal cord are shown in Fig. 373-1. Most fiber tracts—including the posterior columns and the spinocerebellar and pyramidal tracts—travel ipsilateral to the side of the body they innervate. As noted above, afferent fibers mediating pain and temperature sensation are unusual in that they ascend contralaterally as the spinothalamic tract. The anatomic relationships of these various fiber tracts and nuclei produce distinctive clinical syndromes that are pathognomonic of spinal cord disease and that often provide clues to the underlying disease process.

Brown-Sequard hemicord syndrome This syndrome consists of ipsilateral weakness (pyramidal tract) and loss of joint position and vibratory sense (posterior column), with contralateral loss of pain and temperature sense (spinothalamic tract) below the lesion. The sensory level for pain and temperature is one or two levels below the lesion. Segmental signs, such as radicular pain, muscle atrophy, or loss of a deep tendon reflex, when they occur, are unilateral. Pure examples of hemicord syndromes are rare; partial or bilateral forms are more common. Partial syndromes may involve the dorsal (posterior) quadrant, producing ipsilateral loss of vibration and position sense, or ventral (anterior) quadrant with ipsilateral paralysis and contralateral loss of pain and temperature sense.

Central cord syndrome The central cord syndrome results from disorders of gray matter nerve cells and crossing spinothalamic tracts near the central canal. In the cervical cord, the central cord syndrome produces arm weakness out of proportion to leg weakness and a "dissociated" sensory loss consisting of loss of pain and temperature sense in a cape distribution over the shoulders, lower neck, and upper trunk with intact light touch, joint position, and vibration sense. Trauma, syringomyelia, tumors, and anterior spinal artery ischemia are common causes of the central cord syndrome.

Anterior two-thirds syndrome This syndrome results from extensive bilateral disease of the spinal cord that spares the posterior columns. All spinal cord functions—motor, sensory and autonomic—are lost below the level of the lesion, with the striking exception of intact vibration and position sensation. The etiology is vascular, either thromboembolism of the anterior spinal artery or compression of this vessel by mass lesions within the spinal canal.

Intramedullary and extramedullary syndromes The diagnosis of spinal cord disorders frequently requires that *intramedullary* processes, which arise within the substance of the cord, be distinguished from *extramedullary* processes that compress the spinal cord or its vascular supply. Distinguishing features are relative and serve only as rough guides to clinical decision making. With extramedullary lesions, radicular pain is often prominent, and there is early sacral sensory loss (lateral spinothalamic tract) and spastic weakness in the legs (corticospinal tract) due to the superficial location of these fibers in the lateral spinal cord, which renders them susceptible to external compression. Intramedullary lesions tend to produce poorly localized burning pain rather than radicular pain and spare sensation in the perineal and sacral areas; corticospinal tract signs may appear late. With extramedullary lesions, the distinction between extradural and intradural masses is important, as the former are generally malignant and the latter benign; a long duration of symptoms favors an intradural origin.

SPECIFIC LOCALIZING SIGNS *Cervical cord* High cervical cord lesions are frequently life-threatening, producing quadriplegia and weakness of respiratory muscles innervated by the phrenic nerve (C3-C5). There is diaphragmatic paralysis, and breathing is possible only by use of accessory muscles of respiration. Extensive lesions near the junction of the cervical cord and medulla are usually fatal owing to involvement of adjacent medullary centers, which results in vasomotor and respiratory collapse. Partial lesions in this area, generally due to trauma, may interrupt decussating pyramidal tract fibers destined for the legs, which cross below those of the arms, resulting in a "crural paresis" of

FIGURE 373-1 Transverse section through the spinal cord, composite representation, illustrating the principal ascending (*left*) and descending (*right*) pathways. The lateral and ventral spinothalamic tracts (*dark blue*) ascend contralateral to the side of the body that is innervated. C, cervical; T, thoracic; L, lumbar; S, sacral; P, proximal; D, distal; F, flexors; E, extensors.

the lower limbs. Compressive lesions near the foramen magnum may produce weakness of the ipsilateral shoulder and arm followed by weakness of the ipsilateral leg, then the contralateral leg, and finally the contralateral arm; the patient may complain of suboccipital pain spreading to the neck and shoulders. Lesions at C4-C5 produce quadriplegia with preserved respiratory function. At the midcervical (C5-C6) level, there is relative sparing of shoulder muscles and loss of biceps and brachioradialis reflexes. Lesions at C7 spare the biceps but produce weakness of finger and wrist extensors and loss of the triceps reflex. Lesions at C8 paralyze finger and wrist flexion, and the finger flexor reflex is lost. In general, cervical cord disorders are best localized by the pattern of weakness that ensues, whereas sensory deficits have less localizing value. A Horner's syndrome (miosis, ptosis, and facial hypohidrosis) may also occur ipsilateral to cervical cord lesions at any level.

Thoracic cord　Lesions of the thoracic cord are best localized by identification of a sensory level on the trunk. Sensory dermatomes of the body are shown in Fig. 23-1; useful markers are at the nipples (T4) and umbilicus (T10). Weakness of the legs and disturbances of bladder, bowel, or sexual function may also accompany damage to the thoracic cord. The abdominal wall musculature, supplied by the lower thoracic cord, is observed during movements of respiration or coughing or by asking the patient to interlock the fingers behind the head in the supine position and attempt to sit up. Lesions at T9-T10 paralyze the lower, but spare the upper, abdominal muscles, resulting in upward movement of the umbilicus when the abdominal wall contracts (Beevor's sign) and in loss of lower, but not upper, superficial abdominal reflexes (see Chap. 360). With unilateral lesions, attempts to contract the abdominal wall produce movement of the umbilicus to the normal side; superficial abdominal reflexes are absent on the involved side. Midline back pain is a useful localizing sign in the thoracic region.

Lumbar cord　The lumbar and sacral cord segments progressively decrease in size, and focal lesions of these segments are less easily localized than in cervical and thoracic regions. Lesions at L2-L4 paralyze flexion and adduction of the thigh, weaken leg extension at the knee, and abolish the patellar reflex. Lesions at L5-S1 paralyze movements of the foot and ankle, flexion at the knee, and extension of the thigh, and abolish the ankle jerk (S1). A cutaneous reflex useful in localization of lumbar cord disease is the cremasteric reflex (see Chap. 360), which is segmentally innervated at L1-L2.

Sacral cord/conus medullaris　The conus medullaris is the tapered caudal termination of the spinal cord, comprising the lower sacral and single coccygeal segments. Isolated lesions of the conus medullaris spare motor and reflex functions in the legs. The conus syndrome is distinctive, consisting of bilateral saddle anesthesia (S3-S5), prominent bladder and bowel dysfunction (urinary retention and incontinence with lax anal tone), and impotence. The bulbocavernosus (S2-S4) and anal (S4-S5) reflexes are absent (see Chap. 360). Muscle strength is largely preserved. Lesions of the conus medullaris need to be distinguished from those of the cauda equina, the cluster of nerve roots derived from the lower cord as they descend to their exits in the intervertebral foramina. Cauda equina lesions are characterized by severe low back or radicular pain, asymmetric leg weakness or sensory loss, variable areflexia in the lower extremities, and relative sparing of bowel and bladder function. Mass lesions in the lower spinal canal may produce a mixed clinical picture in which elements of both cauda equina and conus medullaris syndromes coexist. → *Cauda equina syndromes are discussed in Chap. 16.*

ACUTE AND SUBACUTE SPINAL CORD DISEASES

Acute and subacute spinal cord disorders are commonly due to extramedullary compression (tumor, infection, spondylosis, or trauma), infarction or hemorrhage, or inflammation. In this category are some of the most dangerous—and treatable—disorders in clinical practice. Early recognition is the key to successful management. Epidural compression due to malignancy often presents with warning signs, generally neck or back pain, bladder disturbances, or sensory symptoms,

that precede the development of paralysis. Infarction, hemorrhage, or spinal subluxation is more likely to produce sudden "strokelike" myelopathy without antecedent symptoms.

NEOPLASTIC SPINAL CORD COMPRESSION Neoplasms of the spinal canal may be extramedullary (epidural or intradural) or intramedullary. In adults, the vast majority of neoplasms are epidural in origin, resulting from metastases to the adjacent vertebral body, spinous or transverse process, or pedicle. Vertebral metastases are essentially bone-marrow metastases, and the propensity of solid tumors to metastasize to the vertebral column probably reflects the high percentage of bone marrow located in the axial skeleton of older individuals. Retroperitoneal neoplasms (especially lymphomas or sarcomas) may enter the spinal canal through the intervertebral foramina; typically they produce radicular pain and other signs of root involvement prior to cord compression. Almost any malignant tumor can metastasize to the spinal canal, although breast, lung, prostate, kidney, lymphoma, and plasma cell dyscrasia are particularly frequent. The thoracic cord is most commonly involved; exceptions are metastases from prostate and ovarian cancer, which occur disproportionately in the sacral and lumbar vertebrae, perhaps resulting from spread through Batson's plexus, a network of veins along the anterior surface of the spinal cord in the epidural space.

Pain is the initial symptom; it may be either aching and localized or sharp and radiating in quality. Pain indicates displacement of pain-sensitive structures, especially periosteum and meninges. The pain worsens with movement, coughing, or sneezing and may awaken patients at night. The recent onset of back pain, particularly if in the thoracic spine (which is uncommonly involved by spondylosis), should prompt consideration of vertebral metastasis. Rarely, pain is mild or absent. Pain typically precedes signs of cord compression by weeks or even months, but once cord compression occurs, it is always progressive and may advance rapidly. Therapy is effective only if administered early, when signs of cord dysfunction are mild or absent; therapy will not reverse fixed paralysis of more than 48 h duration. These realities highlight the importance of prompt recognition and efficient management of epidural metastases.

Plain radiographs of the spine and radionucleotide bone scans have only a limited role in diagnosis because they fail to identify 15 to 20 percent of metastatic vertebral lesions and may miss paravertebral masses that reach the epidural space by growth through the intervertebral foramina. Magnetic resonance imaging (MRI) provides excellent anatomic resolution of the site and extent of the tumor (Fig. 373-2);

FIGURE 373-2　Epidural spinal cord compression due to breast carcinoma. Sagittal T1-weighted (*A*) and T2-weighted (*B*) MRI scans through the cervicothoracic junction reveal a compression fracture of the second thoracic vertebral body with posterior displacement and compression of the upper thoracic spinal cord. The low-intensity bone marrow signal in *A* signifies replacement by tumor.

at most centers, MRI has largely replaced computed tomography (CT) and myelography in the diagnosis of epidural masses. MRI can often distinguish between malignant lesions and other masses—epidural abscess, tuberculoma, or epidural hemorrhage, among others—that present in a similar fashion. Vertebral metastases are usually hypointense relative to a normal bone marrow signal on T1-weighted MR images; following the administration of gadolinium, contrast enhancement may "normalize" the appearance of the tumor by increasing its intensity to that of normal bone marrow. In contrast to infection, vertebral metastases typically do not cross the disk space. Nonetheless, it can be difficult to distinguish between infection and malignancy by MRI.

Because imaging resources are scarce, and both cancer and back pain are common, it is important to convey to the radiologist an estimate of the urgency of the imaging procedure requested. If signs of spinal cord involvement are present, imaging should be obtained on an emergent basis. If there are radicular symptoms but no evidence of myelopathy, it is usually safe to defer imaging for 24 to 48 h. With back or neck pain only, imaging studies should be obtained within a few days. Finally, up to 40 percent of patients who present with symptomatic disease at one level are found to have asymptomatic epidural disease elsewhere; thus, the entire spine should be imaged in all patients with epidural malignancy.

℞ TREATMENT

Management includes glucocorticoids to reduce interstitial edema, local radiotherapy (initiated as early as possible) to the symptomatic lesion, and specific therapy for the underlying tumor type. Glucocorticoids (dexamethasone, 40 mg daily) can be administered prior to the imaging study if the clinical suspicion is strong, and continued at a lower dose (20 mg daily in divided doses) until radiotherapy (a total of 3000 cGy administered in 15 daily fractions) is completed. Radiotherapy appears to be as effective as surgery, even for classically radioresistant metastases. Biopsy of the epidural mass is usually unnecessary in patients with known preexisting cancer, but biopsy is indicated if a history of underlying cancer is lacking. Surgery, either decompression or vertebral body resection, should be considered when signs of cord compression worsen despite radiotherapy, when the maximum tolerated dose of radiotherapy has been delivered previously to the site, or when a vertebral compression fracture contributes to cord compression. A good response to radiotherapy can be expected in individuals who are ambulatory at presentation; new weakness is prevented, and some recovery of motor function occurs in approximately half of treated patients. Fixed motor deficits—paraplegia or quadriplegia—do not usually respond to either radiotherapy or surgery.

In contrast to tumors of the epidural space, most intradural mass lesions are slow-growing and benign. Meningiomas and neurofibromas account for most of these lesions, with occasional cases representing chordoma, lipoma, dermoid, or sarcoma. Meningiomas (Fig. 373-3) are often located posterior to the thoracic cord or near the foramen magnum, although they can arise from the meninges anywhere along the spinal canal. Neurofibromas are benign tumors of the nerve sheath that typically arise near the posterior root; when multiple, neurofibromatosis (Chap. 375) is the likely etiology. Symptoms usually begin with radicular sensory symptoms followed by an asymmetric, progressive spinal cord syndrome. Therapy is surgical resection.

Primary intramedullary tumors of the spinal cord are uncommon. They typically present as central cord or hemicord syndromes, often in the cervical region; there may be poorly localized burning pain in the extremities and sparing of sacral sensation. In adults, most of these lesions are either ependymomas, hemangioblastomas, or low-grade astrocytomas (Fig. 373-4). Complete resection of an intramedullary ependymoma is often possible using microsurgical techniques. Debulking of an intramedullary astrocytoma can also be helpful, as these

FIGURE 373-3 MRI of a thoracic meningioma. Coronal T1-weighted post-contrast image through the thoracic spinal cord demonstrates intense enhancement of a well-circumscribed extramedullary mass (*arrows*) which displaces the spinal cord to the left, widening the cistern adjacent to the mass.

are often slowly growing lesions; the value of adjunctive radiotherapy is uncertain. Secondary (metastatic) intramedullary tumors are rare.

SPINAL CORD INFARCTION The spinal cord is supplied by three arteries that course vertically over its surface, a single anterior spinal artery, and paired posterior spinal arteries. At each segment, paired penetrators branching from the anterior spinal artery supply the anterior two-thirds of the spinal cord; the posterior spinal arteries, which often become less distinct below the midthoracic level, supply the posterior columns. Rostrally, the spinal arteries arise from the vertebral arteries. During embryogenesis, arterial feeders arise at each

FIGURE 373-4 MRI of an intramedullary astrocytoma. Sagittal T1-weighted postcontrast image through the cervical spine demonstrates expansion of the upper cervical spine by a mass lesion emanating from within the spinal cord at the cervicomedullary junction. Irregular peripheral enhancement occurs within the mass (*arrows*).

segmental level, but most involute before birth; generally, between three and eight major feeders remain, arising from the vertebral, subclavian, intercostal (off the aorta), iliac, and sacral arteries. In addition to the vertebral arteries, in adults, anterior spinal artery feeders often occur at C6, at an upper thoracic level, and at T11-L2 (artery of Adamkiewicz). Feeders from the aorta are more likely to arise from the left side.

Spinal cord ischemia can occur at any level. The signs are determined by the level of the lesion and by the individual vascular anatomy, including areas of watershed flow and potential for anastomosis. The anterior spinal artery is discontinuous in some individuals, increasing the importance of feeders to the lower cord. With systemic hypotension, cord infarction occurs at the level of greatest ischemic risk, often T3-T4, and also at boundary zones between the anterior and posterior spinal artery territories. The latter may result in an acute—or more commonly progressive—syndrome of weakness and spasticity with little sensory change resembling amyotrophic lateral sclerosis (ALS).

Acute infarction in the territory of the anterior spinal artery produces paraplegia or quadriplegia, dissociated sensory loss affecting pain and temperature sense but sparing vibration and position sense, and loss of sphincter control. Onset may be sudden and dramatic or progressive over minutes or hours. Sharp midline or radiating back pain localized to the area of ischemia is frequently noted. Partial infarction of one anterior hemicord (hemiplegia or monoplegia and crossed pain and temperature loss) may also occur. Areflexia due to spinal shock is often present initially; with time, hyperreflexia and spasticity appear.

The acute onset of pain, sparing of posterior column function, and sharply demarcated spinal cord level distinguish anterior spinal artery infarction from epidural spinal cord compression, in which pain is often chronic, posterior column sense is impaired, and a cord level is indistinct. An exception to this rule is when epidural tumors compress or invade vascular structures, resulting in an anterior spinal artery syndrome. Infarction in the territory of the posterior spinal arteries, resulting in loss of posterior column function, also occurs and may be underrecognized as a cause of loss of position and vibration sense.

Spinal cord infarction is associated with aortic atherosclerosis, dissecting aortic aneurysm (chest or back pain with diminished pulses in legs), or hypotension from any cause. Cardiogenic emboli, vasculitis related to collagen vascular disease, and surgical clipping of aortic aneurysms are other predisposing conditions. Occasional cases develop either during pregnancy or following acute back trauma or exercise that by an unknown mechanism leads to embolism of nucleus pulposus material into spinal vessels. In a substantial number of cases, no cause can be found, and thromboembolism in arterial feeders is suspected.

MRI is often normal but is useful to exclude other causes of acute myelopathy, in particular epidural compression, spinal cord hemorrhage (hematomyelia), infectious myelitis, or transverse myelitis. Lumbar puncture is indicated whenever the underlying cause has not been clarified by MRI. Other useful laboratory studies include a sedimentation rate to search for an underlying vasculitis, Venereal Disease Research Laboratories test, and evaluation for aortic or cardiac disease or for a hypercoagulable state.

Therapy is directed at treatment of any predisposing condition. In cord infarction due to presumed thromboembolism, anticoagulation is probably not indicated, with the exception of the unusual transient ischemic attack or incomplete infarction with a stuttering or progressive course.

HEMATOMYELIA Hemorrhage into the substance of the spinal cord is rare. It may result from trauma, an intraparenchymal vascular malformation (see below), vasculitis due to polyarteritis nodosa or lupus erythematosus, bleeding disorders, or spinal cord infection or neoplasm. Hematomyelia presents as an acute painful transverse myelopathy. With large lesions, extension into the subarachnoid space may occur, resulting in subarachnoid hemorrhage (Chap. 366). Diagnosis is best made by MRI. Therapy is supportive, and surgical intervention is generally not useful. An exception is hematomyelia due to an underlying vascular malformation; in such cases, selective spinal

angiography may be indicated, followed by acute surgical intervention to evacuate the clot and remove the underlying vascular lesion.

Hemorrhage into the subdural or epidural space can compress the spinal cord or roots. Presenting symptoms are the acute onset of focal or radicular pain followed by variable signs of a spinal cord or conus medullaris disorder. Trauma, tumor, or blood dyscrasias are predisposing conditions; rare cases complicate lumbar puncture or epidural anesthesia. MRI confirms the clinical suspicion and can delineate the extent of the bleed. Extrinsic spinal cord compression from any cause is a medical emergency, and appropriate treatment consists of prompt recognition, reversal of any underlying clotting disorder, and emergency surgical decompression. Surgery may be followed by substantial recovery, especially in patients with some preservation of motor function preoperatively. Because of the risk of hemorrhage, lumbar puncture should be avoided whenever possible in patients with thrombocytopenia or other coagulopathies (including those due to therapeutic anticoagulation) until the underlying bleeding disorder is reversed.

EPIDURAL ABSCESS Spinal epidural abscess presents as a clinical triad of pain, fever, and rapidly progressive weakness. Prompt recognition of this distinctive and treatable medical emergency will in most cases prevent severe and permanent sequelae. Epidural abscesses can form anywhere along the spinal canal. Pain is almost always present, either midline along the spine or radicular in type. The duration of pain prior to presentation is generally two weeks or less, but in some chronic cases it may be several months or longer. Fever is common, often accompanied by an elevated white blood cell count or sedimentation rate. As the abscess expands, spinal cord injury results from venous congestion and thrombosis, thrombophlebitis of the epidural space, spinal artery disease, or cord compression. Once weakness and other signs of myelopathy appear, progression is often rapid, although it may be gradual.

Risk factors include impaired immune status (diabetes mellitus, renal failure, alcoholism, malignancy), intravenous drug abuse, and infections of the skin or other tissues. Two-thirds of epidural infections result from hematogenous spread from the skin (furunculosis), soft tissue (pharyngeal or dental abscesses), or deep viscera (bacterial endocarditis). One-third result from direct extension of a local infection to the subdural space; examples of local predisposing conditions are vertebral osteomyelitis, decubitus ulcers, or iatrogenic complications of lumbar puncture, epidural anesthesia, or spinal surgery.

Most cases are due to *Staphylococcus aureus*; gram-negative bacilli, *Streptococcus*, anaerobes, and fungi can also cause epidural abscesses. Tuberculosis from an adjacent vertebral source remains an important cause in the underdeveloped world. As the population ages and the number of immunosuppressed individuals increases, an increase in the incidence of spinal epidural abscess (currently 2 per 1000 hospital admissions) has been noted.

MR images (Fig. 373-5) localize the abscess and exclude a primary intraparenchymal lesion, for example, transverse myelitis or hematomyelia. Lumbar puncture is often not required but may be indicated if encephalopathy or other clinical signs raise the question of associated meningitis, which is present in fewer than 25 percent of cases. In such situations, the level of the tap should be planned carefully to minimize the risk of inducing either meningitis by passage of the needle through infected tissue or herniation from decompression below an area of obstruction to the flow of cerebrospinal fluid (CSF). A high cervical tap is often the safest approach. CSF abnormalities in subdural abscess consist of pleocytosis with a preponderance of polymorphonuclear cells, an elevated protein level, and a reduced glucose level. Blood cultures are positive in fewer than 25 percent of cases.

℞ **TREATMENT**

Treatment is emergency decompressive laminectomy with debridement combined with long-term antibiotic treatment. Surgical evacuation will prevent development of paralysis and may improve or reverse paralysis in evolution, but it is unlikely to improve fixed

FIGURE 373-5 MRI of a spinal epidural abscess due to tuberculosis. *A.* Sagittal T2-weighted free spin-echo MR sequence. A hypointense mass replaces the posterior elements of C3 and extends epidurally to compress the spinal cord (*arrows*). *B.* Sagittal T1-weighted image following contrast administration reveals a diffuse enhancement of the epidural process (*arrows*) with extension into the epidural space.

neurologic deficits. Antibiotics should be started empirically before surgery, modified on the basis of culture results, and usually continued for at least 4 weeks. If surgery is contraindicated or if there is a fixed paraplegia or quadriplegia that is unlikely to improve following surgery, long-term administration of systemic and oral antibiotics can be used; in such cases, coverage may be guided by results of positive blood cultures. In medically treated patients, paralysis may develop or progress during antibiotic therapy; thus, initial surgical management remains the treatment of choice.

TRANSVERSE MYELITIS Transverse myelitis is an acute or subacute, generally monophasic, inflammatory disorder of the spinal cord. The initial symptom is focal neck or back pain, followed by various combinations of paresthesia, sensory loss, motor weakness, and sphincter disturbance evolving within hours to several days. There may be mild sensory symptoms only, or a devastating functional transection of the cord. Partial forms may selectively involve posterior columns, anterior spinothalamic tracts, or one hemicord. Dysesthesias may begin in the feet and ascend either symmetrically or asymmetrically, earlier in one leg than in the other; these symptoms may initially raise a question of Guillain-Barré syndrome, but involvement of the trunk with a sharply demarcated spinal cord level indicates the myelopathic nature of the process. In severe cases, areflexia indicating spinal shock may be present, but hyperreflexia soon supervenes; persistent areflexic paralysis indicates necrosis over multiple segments of the spinal cord.

Up to 40 percent of cases are associated with an antecedent infection or recent vaccination. Many infectious agents have been implicated, including influenza, measles, varicella, rubeola, mumps, and Epstein-Barr virus and cytomegalovirus, as well as *Mycoplasma*. As in the related disorder acute disseminated encephalomyelitis (Chap. 376), transverse myelitis often begins as the patient appears to be recovering from the infection, and infectious agents have not been isolated from the nervous system of affected individuals. These features suggest that transverse myelitis results from an autoimmune response triggered by infection and not from direct infection of the spinal cord.

Multiple sclerosis (MS) (see below) may present initially as transverse myelitis. MS-associated transverse myelitis usually is not associated with an antecedent infection or vaccination. Devic's disease

(Chap. 376) is a demyelinating disorder common in Asians that presents as transverse myelitis associated with optic neuritis that is typically bilateral. Transverse myelitis, at times recurrent, has also been associated with systemic lupus erythematosus and other collagen-vascular diseases, Sjögren's syndrome, and Behçet's disease; sarcoidosis may produce a subacute transverse myelopathy with severe cord swelling.

MRI findings in transverse myelitis consist of variable swelling of the cord and diffuse or multifocal areas of abnormal bright signal on T2-weighted sequences, often extending over several cord segments. Contrast enhancement, indicating disruption in the blood-brain barrier associated with perivenous inflammation, is also present in acute cases. MRI is also useful to exclude cord compression. A brain MRI should also be obtained in all cases to assess the likelihood that the transverse myelitis represents an initial attack of MS. A normal scan indicates that the risk of evolution to MS is low—approximately 5 percent over 3 to 5 years; by contrast, the finding of multiple periventricular T2-bright lesions indicates a risk of 50 percent or greater over the same time period. CSF findings in transverse myelitis may be normal, but more often there is pleocytosis, with up to several hundred mononuclear cells per microliter; in severe or rapidly evolving cases, polymorphonuclear cells may be present. CSF protein levels are normal or at most mildly elevated; oligoclonal banding is a variable finding but, when present, is associated with future evolution to MS.

There are no prospective trials of therapy. Glucocorticoids, consisting of intravenous methylprednisolone followed by oral prednisone (Table 376-4), is employed for treatment of moderate to severe symptoms.

ACUTE INFECTIOUS MYELOPATHIES These inflammatory disorders result from direct invasion of the spinal cord by infectious agents. Poliomyelitis is the prototypic virus that produces acute infection of the spinal cord. Herpes zoster is currently the most common viral cause of acute myelitis; cytomegalovirus, herpes simplex virus type 1, Epstein-Barr virus, and rabies virus have been identified in occasional cases. Herpes simplex virus type 2 may produce a recurrent sacral myelitis, which could be mistaken for MS, in association with outbreaks of genital herpes. → *Viral infections of the spinal cord are discussed in Chap. 379.*

Schistosomiasis (Chap. 224) is an important cause of parasitic myelitis worldwide. The myelitis is intensely inflammatory and granulomatous in nature, caused by a local response to tissue-digesting enzymes produced by ova from the parasite. Toxoplasmosis (Chap. 219) rarely causes a focal myelopathy, and this diagnosis should be considered in patients with AIDS owing to the high frequency of nervous system toxoplasmosis in this population.

CHRONIC MYELOPATHIES

SPONDYLITIC MYELOPATHY Cervical spondylosis and related degenerative diseases of the spine are discussed in Chap. 16. Neck and shoulder pain with stiffness are early symptoms; pressure on nerve roots results in radicular arm pain, most often in a C5 or C6 distribution. Compression of the cervical cord produces a slowly progressive spastic paraparesis, at times asymmetric, and often accompanied by paresthesia in the feet and hands. Vibratory sense is frequently diminished in the legs, and occasionally there is a sensory level for vibration on the upper thorax. Coughing or straining often produces leg weakness or radiating arm or shoulder pain. Dermatomal sensory loss in the arms, atrophy of intrinsic hand muscles, increased deep tendon reflexes in the legs, and extensor plantar responses are common. Urinary urgency or incontinence occur in advanced cases. Reflexes in the arms are often diminished at some level, often the biceps (C5-C6). In individual cases, radicular, myelopathic, or combined signs may predominate. The diagnosis should be considered in cases of progressive cervical myelopathy, paresthesia of the feet and hands, or wasting of the hands. Spondylitic myelopathy is also one of the most common causes of gait difficulty in the elderly.

Diagnosis is best made by MRI. Extrinsic compression is appreciated on axial views, and T2-weighted sequences may reveal abnormal areas of high signal intensity within the cord adjacent to the site of compression. Definitive therapy consists of surgical relief of the compression, generally by posterior laminectomy. When that is not feasible, an anterior approach with resection of the protruded disc material may be required.

Cervical spondylosis is both an under- and overdiagnosed disease. Many patients with intramedullary cord processes, particularly ALS (Chap. 370), have had cervical laminectomies in the incorrect belief that spondylosis might have been responsible.

VASCULAR MALFORMATIONS Although uncommon, these are important lesions because they represent a treatable cause of progressive myelopathy. Arteriovenous malformations (AVMs) are most often located posteriorly, within the dura or along the surface of the cord, at or below the midthoracic level. The typical presentation is a middle-aged man with a progressive myelopathy. The myelopathy may worsen slowly or rapidly or may have periods of apparent remission with superimposed worsenings resembling MS. Acute deterioration due to hemorrhage into the spinal cord or subarachnoid space may occur but is uncommon. At presentation, most patients have sensory, motor, and bladder disturbances. The motor disorder may predominate and produce a mixture of upper and lower motoneuron signs, simulating ALS. Pain, either dysesthesias or radicular pain, is also common. Other symptoms suggestive of AVM include intermittent claudication (symptoms that appear with exercise and are relieved by rest), or an effect of posture, menses, or fever on symptoms. A rare AVM syndrome presents as a progressive thoracic myelopathy with paraparesis developing over weeks or several months, associated with abnormally thick, hyalinized vessels (Foix-Alajouanine syndrome).

AVMs located at cervical or upper thoracic levels are distinctive; they occur equally in males and females, tend to be located anterior rather than posterior to the cord, often have an intramedullary component to the malformation, and may bleed (see "Hematomyelia," above).

A careful examination of the skin overlying the spine may reveal a vascular lesion, lipoma, or area of altered pigmentation, all clues to a spinal cord AVM. Bruits are rare but should be sought at rest or after exercise. High-resolution MRI with contrast administration will detect the vast majority of AVMs (Fig. 373-6). A small number of AVMs not detected by MRI may be visualized by CT myelography as enlarged vessels along the surface of the cord. Definitive diagnosis requires selective spinal angiography, which will also define the vascular feeders and extent of the malformation. Embolization with occlusion of the major feeding vessels may stabilize a progressive neurologic deficit or produce a gradual recovery.

RETROVIRUS-ASSOCIATED MYELOPATHIES The myelopathy associated with the human T cell lymphotropic virus type I (HTLV-I) presents as a slowly progressive spastic paraparesis with variable sensory and bladder disturbance. The myelopathy is typically thoracic. Approximately half of patients have back or leg pain. Signs may be asymmetric, may lack a well-defined sensory level, and may spare upper extremity function, although hyperreflexia in the arms is common. Onset is generally insidious, and the tempo of progression is variable, but most patients are nonambulatory within 10 years of onset. This presentation may resemble primary progressive MS or a thoracic AVM. Diagnosis is made by demonstration of HTLV-I–specific antibody in serum by enzyme-linked immunosorbent assay (ELISA), confirmed by radioimmunoprecipitation or Western blot analysis of specific antibody directed against protein products of the viral *gag* and *env* genes. There is no effective treatment; symptomatic therapy for spasticity and bladder symptoms may be helpful. → *HTLV-I infections of the nervous system are discussed in Chap. 379.*

A progressive myelopathy may also occur in AIDS, characterized by vacuolar degeneration of the posterior and lateral tracts resembling subacute combined degeneration (see below).

SYRINGOMYELIA Syringomyelia is a cavitary expansion of the spinal cord that may produce a progressive myelopathy. Syrinxes commonly occur in the lower cervical/high thoracic region or in the high cervical region, where they may extend rostrally to the medulla or pons (syringobulbia). Less commonly, the lumbar cord or the entire

spinal cord may be involved. Syringomyelia may result from developmental disorders of the posterior fossa and foramen magnum or from acquired disorders. More than half of all cases are associated with Chiari malformations. In the Chiari type 1 malformation, there is protrusion of the cerebellar tonsils through the foramen magnum and into the cervical spinal canal; when this abnormality is associated with protrusion of meninges (meningocele) or meninges and cord (meningomyelocele) through a spinal canal that has incompletely closed, it is designated a Chiari type 2 (or Arnold-Chiari) malformation. Other developmental disorders associated with syringomyelia are basilar skull impression (platybasia), atresia of the foramen of Magendie, or cysts of the posterior fossa (Dandy-Walker syndrome). Acquired cases result from intramedullary spinal cord tumors, trauma, or chronic arachnoiditis due to tuberculosis or other inflammatory conditions. Occasional cases are idiopathic.

Syringomyelia has been proposed to result from interference with the normal outflow of CSF from the fourth ventricle to the subarachnoid space due to obstruction of the foramina of Luschka and Magendie. This blockage leads to downward pressure on the cervical spinal cord and progressive syrinx formation. However, syringomyelia may occur without foraminal obstruction, indicating that other factors, for example, interference with normal upward CSF flow in the spinal canal, may also be important. Syrinxes associated with Chiari type 1 malformations generally communicate freely with the subarachnoid space, and the syrinx fluid resembles normal CSF; by contrast, in many acquired cases the syrinx cavities do not communicate, and the fluid is proteinaceous. The older literature distinguished between "true" syringomyelia, in which the cavity was separate from the central canal, and hydromyelia due to a primary enlargement of the central canal; this distinction is less useful than determination of whether the cavity communicates freely with the subarachnoid space.

FIGURE 373-6 Arteriovenous malformation. Sagittal MR scans of the thoracic spinal cord: T2 fast spin-echo technique (*left*) and T1 post-contrast image (*right*). On the T2-weighted image (*left*), abnormally high signal intensity is noted in the central aspect of the spinal cord (*arrowheads*). Numerous punctate flow voids indent the dorsal and ventral spinal cord (*arrow*). These represent the abnormally dilated venous plexus supplied by a dural arteriovenous fistula. Following contrast administration (*right*), multiple, serpentine, enhancing veins (*arrows*) on the ventral and dorsal aspect of the thoracic spinal cord are visualized, diagnostic of arteriovenous fistula. This patient was a 54-year-old man with a 4-year history of progressive paraparesis.

FIGURE 373-7 MRI of syringomyelia associated with Chiari malformation. Sagittal T1-weighted image through the cervical and upper thoracic spine demonstrates descent of the cerebellar tonsils and vermis below the level of the foramen magnum (*black arrows*). Within the substance of the cervical and thoracic spinal cord, a CSF collection dilates the central canal (*white arrows*).

The classic presentation is a central cord syndrome with dissociated sensory loss and areflexic weakness in the upper limbs. The sensory deficit consists of loss of pain and temperature sensation which is "suspended" over the nape of the neck, shoulders, and upper arms in a cape distribution or is in the hands; vibration and position sensation is largely preserved. Most cases begin asymmetrically with unilateral sensory loss. Muscle wasting in the lower neck, shoulders, arms, and hands with asymmetric or absent reflexes reflects extension of the cavity to the anterior horns. As the lesion enlarges, spasticity and weakness of the legs, bladder and bowel dysfunction, and, in some cases, a Horner's syndrome appear. Thoracic kyphoscoliosis is a frequent additional finding. Some patients develop numbness and sensory loss on the face from damage to the descending tract of the trigeminal nerve (C2 level or above). With Chiari malformations, cough headache, and neck, arm, or facial pain are common. Syringobulbia may present as palatal or vocal cord paralysis, dysarthria, horizontal or vertical nystagmus, episodic dizziness, and/or tongue weakness.

Symptoms typically begin insidiously in adolescence or early adulthood, progress irregularly, and may undergo spontaneous arrest for several years. Onset or sudden deterioration may follow trauma, neck manipulation or extension, or severe cough. Symptoms of syringobulbia may progress rapidly.

MRI scans accurately identify syrinx cavities and associated spinal cord enlargement (Fig. 373-7). In all cases, MRI scans of the brain and the entire spinal cord should be obtained to delineate the full extent of the syrinx, assess posterior fossa structures, and determine whether hydrocephalus is present. If a Chiari malformation is not found, a contrast-enhanced MRI scan should be obtained to search for abnormal enhancement from an associated spinal cord tumor.

℞ **TREATMENT**

Treatment is surgical. Syringomyelia associated with tonsillar herniation is treated with posterior fossa decompression, generally consisting of suboccipital craniectomy, upper cervical laminectomy, and placement of a dural graft. If obstruction of fourth ventricular outflow is present, flow is reestablished by enlargement of the opening. If the syrinx cavity is large, some surgeons recommend direct decompression of the fluid cavity, but the added benefit of this procedure is uncertain, and morbidity may occur. With Chiari malformations, shunting of hydrocephalus should generally precede any attempt to correct the syrinx. Surgical results are often excellent, with stabilization of the neurologic deficit in most cases; some patients have improvement postoperatively. Syringomyelia secondary to trauma or infection is treated with a decompression and drainage procedure in which a small shunt is inserted between the syrinx cavity and the subarachnoid space. Finally, syringomyelia due to an intramedullary spinal cord tumor is managed by resection of the tumor if feasible; decompression of the cyst cavity may produce temporary relief, but recurrence is common.

MULTIPLE SCLEROSIS The primary progressive form of MS may present as a progressive myelopathy. Involvement is typically asymmetric with resulting motor, sensory, and autonomic dysfunction. The diagnosis is made by recognition of other symptoms or signs typical for MS, by characteristic findings on brain MRI scans, by CSF analysis, and by exclusion of other conditions. Therapeutic efforts to reverse neurologic deficits or to stabilize the course of isolated progressive myelopathy due to MS have been disappointing. → *MS is discussed in Chap. 376.*

SUBACUTE COMBINED DEGENERATION (VITAMIN B$_{12}$ DEFICIENCY) This treatable myelopathy presents with parasthesia in the hands and feet, early loss of vibration and position sensation, and a progressive spastic and ataxic weakness. Loss of reflexes due to a superimposed peripheral neuropathy, present in many cases, is an important diagnostic clue. Optic atrophy and irritability and other mental changes may be prominent in advanced cases and on occasion are the presenting symptom (megaloblastic madness). The myelopathy of subacute combined degeneration tends to be diffuse rather than focal; signs are generally symmetric and reflect predominant involvement of the posterior and lateral tracts, and no focal spinal cord level is present. The diagnosis is confirmed by the finding of a low serum B$_{12}$ concentration and a positive Schilling test (Chap. 380).

TABES DORSALIS Tabes dorsalis and meningovascular syphilis of the spinal cord are presently rare but must be considered in the differential diagnosis of spinal cord syndromes, in particular those that arise in individuals infected with human immunodeficiency virus (HIV). The most common symptoms of tabes are characteristic fleeting and repetitive, lancinating pains, which occur mostly in the legs and less commonly in the back, thorax, abdomen, arms, and face. Ataxia of the legs and gait due to loss of position sense occurs in half of patients. Paresthesia, bladder disturbances, and acute abdominal pain with vomiting (visceral crisis) occur in 15 to 30 percent. The cardinal signs of tabes are loss of reflexes in the legs, impaired position and vibratory sense, Romberg's sign, and bilateral Argyll Robertson pupils, which fail to constrict to light but react with accommodation.

FAMILIAL SPASTIC PARAPLEGIA Occasional cases of progressive myelopathy occur on a familial basis. Most present with progressive spasticity and weakness in the legs. Sphincter disturbances and mild degrees of sensory loss may also be present. On examination, a sharply defined spinal cord level is not detected, in contrast to many focal spinal cord disorders. In some families, whose condition is referred to as "complicated" familial spastic paraplegia (FSP), additional neurologic signs, for example, nystagmus, ataxia, or optic atrophy, occur. Onset may be as early as the first year of life or as late as middle adulthood. The genetic basis of some forms of FSP is now known (Table 373-3). Adrenoleukodystrophy should be treated with steroid replacement if hypoadrenalism is present, and bone marrow transplantation, although experimental, has been attempted for this condition. No disease-modifying therapy exists for other forms of FSP.

→ *Traumatic spinal cord lesions are discussed in Chap. 374.*

MEDICAL REHABILITATION OF SPINAL CORD DISORDERS

Following an acute spinal cord lesion, the prospects for significant recovery fade after approximately 4 months. There are currently no effective means to promote repair of injured spinal cord tissue; promising experimental approaches include the use of factors that influence reinnervation by axons of the corticospinal tract or nerve graft bridges that promote reinnervation across spinal cord lesions. The disability associated with irreversible spinal cord damage is determined primarily by the level of the lesion and by whether the disturbance in function is complete or incomplete (Table 373-4). Even complete high cervical cord lesions may be compatible with a productive life. Development of a rehabilitation plan framed by realistic expectations, and attention to the neurologic, medical, and psychological complications that commonly arise, are primary goals of treatment.

The usual symptoms associated with medical illnesses may be lacking, because of the destruction of afferent pain pathways in the cord. Unexplained fever, worsening of spasticity, or deterioration in neurologic function should prompt search for an underlying cause such as infection, thrombophlebitis, or an intraabdominal pathology; these etiologies are far more likely to be responsible than primary neurologic events such as meningitis, secondary syringomyelia or chronic arachnoiditis. The loss of normal thermoregulation and inability to maintain normal body temperature can produce recurrent fever (*quadriplegic fever*), although most episodes of fever are due to infection of the urinary tract, lung, skin, or bone.

Bladder dysfunction generally results from loss of supraspinal innervation of the detrusor muscle of the bladder wall and the sphincter musculature. Detrusor spasticity is treated with anticholinergic drugs (oxybutinin, 2.5 to 5 mg qid) or tricyclic antidepressants with anticholinergic properties (imipramine, 25 to 200 mg/d). Failure of the sphincter muscle to relax during bladder emptying (urinary dyssynergia) may be managed with the alpha-adrenergic blocking agent terazosin hydrochloride (1 to 2 mg tid or qid), with intermittent catheterization, or, if that is not feasible, by use of a condom catheter in men or a permanent indwelling catheter. Surgical options include the creation of an artificial bladder by isolating a segment of intestine that can be catheterized intermittently (enterocystoplasty) or can drain continuously to an external appliance (urinary conduit). Bladder areflexia due to acute spinal shock or conus lesions is best treated by catheterization. The underlying pathophysiology of a bladder disorder correlates poorly with specific symptoms experienced by the patient, so urodynamic evaluation at intervals is required to assess detrusor and sphincter function.

Bladder dysfunction predisposes the patient to urinary tract infection. Bacteriuria due to asymptomatic colonization is extremely common and is generally not treated. Prophylaxis with antiseptics or antibiotics are of little value. Urinary tract infections may present only as foul-smelling urine or a change in voiding pattern; the development of high fever or other systemic signs often indicates pyelonephritis. Bowel regimens and disimpaction are necessary in most patients to ensure at least biweekly evacuation and avoid colonic distention or obstruction.

High cervical cord lesions cause various degrees of mechanical respiratory failure requiring artificial ventilation. In cases of incomplete respiratory failure, chest physical therapy is useful, and a negative-pressure cuirass may alleviate atelectasis, particularly if the major lesion is below C4. With severe respiratory failure, tracheal intubation, followed by tracheotomy, provides tracheal access for ventilation and suctioning. Phrenic nerve pacing may be useful in some patients with lesions at C5 or above.

Patients with acute cord injury are at high risk for venous thrombosis and pulmonary embolism. During the first two weeks, use of calf-compression devices and anticoagulation with heparin (5000 U subcutaneously every 12 h) or warfarin (INR, 2 to 3) are recommended. In cases of persistent paralysis, anticoagulation should probably be continued for 3 months.

Prophylaxis against decubitus ulcers should involve frequent changes in position in a chair or bed, the use of special mattresses, and cushioning of areas where pressure sores often develop, such as the sacral prominence and heels. Early treatment of ulcers with careful cleansing, surgical or enzyme debridement of necrotic tissue, and appropriate dressing and drainage may prevent infection of adjacent soft tissue or bone.

Spasticity (Chap. 21) is often a late manifestation of spinal cord disease, occurring weeks or even months after the initial insult. Stretching exercises are useful to maintain mobility of joints. Drug treatment is effective but may result in reduced function, as some patients use their spasticity as an aid to stand, transfer, or walk. Baclofen (20 to

Table 373-3

Inherited (Monogenic) Myelopathies*

Designation	Clinical Presentation	Genetics
Autosomal recessive	Early onset (age 1–20), progressive spasticity of legs, mild loss of vibration & position sense, bladder symptoms	Linked to chromosome 8; gene unknown
Autosomal dominant	Most common form; families have either early or late onset (before or after age 35)	Linkage to chromosome 2p for both early and late onset. Second locus at 14q.
X-linked	Early childhood onset as pure spastic paraplegia or "complicated" with nystagmus, ataxia, or other neurologic signs	"Complicated" form due to mutation of proteolipid protein gene (Xq21); differs from the dysmyelinating disorder Pelizaeus-Merzbacher disease in that the allelic protein DM20, essential for oligodendrocyte development, is normal
X-linked	Pure or "complicated"	Mutations in neural cell adhesion molecule L1CAM. Allelic disorders X-linked hydrocephalus and MASA syndrome (mental retardation, aphasia, shuffling gait, adducted thumbs)
X-linked	Adrenoleukodystrophy; may present as pure FSP beginning in early adulthood. Rare heterozygote females may present as FSP.	Accumulation of long-chain fatty acids due to defective peroxysomal degradation; linkage to Xq17-28

* See also Chap. 363.

ABBREVIATION: FSP, familial spastic paraplegia.

Table 373-4

Expected Neurologic Function Following Complete Cord Lesions

Level	Self-Care	Transfers	Maximum Mobility
High quadriplegia (C1-C4)	Dependent on others; requires respiratory support	Dependent on others	Motorized wheelchair
Low quadriplegia (C5-C8)	Partially independent with adaptive equipment	May be dependent or independent	May use manual wheelchair, drive an automobile with adaptive equipment
Paraplegia (below T1)	Independent	Independent	Ambulates short distances with aids

SOURCE: Adapted from Ditunno and Formal.

240 mg/d in divided doses) is the most effective drug available; it acts by facilitating GABA-mediated inhibition of motor reflex arcs. Diazepam acts by a similar mechanism and is useful for leg spasms that interrupt sleep (2 to 4 mg at bedtime). For nonambulatory patients, the direct muscle inhibitor dantrolene (25 to 100 mg qid) may be used, but it is potentially hepatotoxic. In severe cases, intrathecal baclofen administered via an implanted pump, botulinum toxin injections, or dorsal rhizotomy may be required to control spasticity.

Paroxysmal autonomic hyperreflexia may occur following lesions above the major splanchnic sympathetic outflow at T6. Headache, flushing, and diaphoresis above the level of the lesion, and hypertension with bradycardia or tachycardia, are the major symptoms. The trigger is typically a noxious stimulus—for example, bladder or bowel distention, a urinary tract infection, or a decubitus ulcer—below the level of the cord lesion. Ascending sensory fibers are thought to activate, via interneurons, sympathetic neurons of the intermediolateral nuclei in the thoracic spinal cord, producing vasoconstriction, tachycardia, and systemic hypertension. Reflex pathways, activated by carotid and aortic baroreceptors and projecting to the CNS via the vagus and glossopharyngeal nerves, then inhibit sympathetic activity above the cord lesion, producing vasodilation, but below the lesion, descending pathways are blocked and sympathetic hyperactivity continues. Treatment consists of removal of offending stimuli; ganglionic blocking agents (mecamylamine, 2.5 to 5 mg) or other short-acting antihypertensive drugs are useful in some patients (see review by Colachis).

BIBLIOGRAPHY

Blaivas JG: Bladder function in the SCI patient. J Neurol Rehab 8:47, 1994
Colachis SC: Autonomic hyperreflexia with spinal cord injury. J Am Paraplegia Soc 15(3):172, 1992
Cristante L, Herrmann H-D: Surgical management of intramedullary spinal cord tumors: Functional outcome and sources of morbidity. Neurosurgery 35:69, 1994
Darouiche RO et al: Bacterial spinal epidural abscess: Review of 43 cases and literature survey. Medicine 71:369, 1992
Ditunno JF, Formal CS: Chronic spinal cord injury. N Engl J Med 330:550, 1994
Jeffery DR et al: Transverse myelitis. Retrospective analysis of 33 cases, with differentiation of cases associated with multiple sclerosis and parainfectious events. Arch Neurol 50:532, 1993
Small JA, Sheridan PH: Research priorities for syringomyelia: A National Institute of Neurologic Disorders and Stroke workshop summary. Neurology 46:577, 1996
Young RR, Woolsey RM: *Diagnosis and Management of Disorders of the Spinal Cord.* Philadelphia, Saunders, 1995

374 Allan H. Ropper

TRAUMATIC INJURIES OF THE HEAD AND SPINE

Head injuries are frequent in industrialized countries, affecting many patients in the prime of life. The medical and social magnitude of this problem can be appreciated by recognizing that almost 10 million head injuries occur annually in the United States alone, about 20 percent of which are serious enough to cause brain damage. Among men under 35 years old, accidents, usually motor vehicle collisions, are the chief cause of death, and over 70 percent of these involve head injury. Minor head injuries are so common that almost all physicians encounter patients requiring immediate care or suffering from various sequelae. Traumatic spinal cord injuries often occur in conjunction with head injury. The two are best considered together in the context of trauma to the nervous system.

Declining mortality from head and spinal cord injuries can be attributed mainly to public health measures, such as use of seat belts

and motorcycle helmets, and the development of ambulance systems with trained personnel. A systematic approach to the evaluation of patients with head and spine trauma, beginning at the scene of the accident, has improved outcome. Understanding of the pathologic lesions produced by trauma, essential for diagnosis and management, has been revolutionized by the wide availability of computed tomography (CT).

TYPES OF HEAD INJURIES

SKULL FRACTURES A blow to the skull causes fractures if the elastic tolerance of the bone is exceeded. Significant intracranial lesions accompany two-thirds of skull fractures, and the presence of a skull fracture increases manyfold the chances of an underlying subdural or epidural hematoma. Consequently, fractures are important primarily as markers of the site and severity of injury. They also cause cranial nerve injuries and produce entry pathways to the cerebrospinal fluid (CSF) for bacteria (meningitis) and air (pneumocephalus) or for leakage of CSF. Fractures are classified as *linear, basilar, compound,* or *depressed*; linear fractures account for 80 percent of all skull fractures and are most often associated with subdural or epidural hematomas. Linear fractures usually extend from the point of impact toward the base of the skull.

Basilar skull fractures are often extensions of adjacent fractures over the convexity of the skull but may occur independently owing to stresses on the floor of the middle cranial fossa or occiput. They are usually located parallel to the petrous bone or along the sphenoid bone toward the sella turcica and ethmoidal groove. Most are uncomplicated, but they may cause CSF leakage, pneumocephalus, or cavernous-carotid fistula. Fractures of the basal skull bones are often accompanied by signs of hemotympanum (blood behind the tympanic membrane), delayed ecchymosis over the mastoid process (Battle's sign), or periorbital ecchymosis ("racoon sign"). Because routine x-ray examination can fail to disclose basilar fractures, they should be suspected if these clinical signs are present. Cerebrospinal fluid also may leak through the cribriform plate or the adjacent sinus and present as a watery discharge from the nose (CSF rhinorrhea). Persistence of rhinorrhea or recurrent meningitis is an indication for surgical repair of torn dura underlying the fracture. The site of the leak is often difficult to determine, but useful diagnostic tests include the instillation of water-soluble contrast into the CSF followed by CT, and injection of radionuclide compounds or fluorescein into the CSF followed by assessment of uptake by absorptive nasal pledgets. The site of intermittent leaks is rarely delineated, and most such leaks resolve spontaneously. Sellar fractures are sometimes radiologically occult, even ones associated with serious neuroendocrine dysfunction. Occasionally, fractures of the dorsum sella cause sixth or seventh nerve palsies or optic nerve damage. An air-fluid level in the sphenoid sinus suggests a fracture of the sellar floor.

About 20 percent of petrous bone fractures, usually ones oriented along the long axis of the bone, are associated with facial palsy. Disruption of ear ossicles and CSF otorrhea are other complications. Transverse petrous fractures are less common; they damage the cochlea or labyrinths almost always and the facial nerve often. External bleeding from the ear can result from petrous bone fractures, although local laceration of the external canal from abrasions is more common. Frontal bone fractures are often depressed, involving the frontal and paranasal sinuses and the orbits; anosmia results if the olfactory filaments in the cribriform plate are disrupted.

Depressed skull fractures are typically compound, but they are neurologically asymptomatic because the impact energy is dissipated in breaking the bone; however, some are associated with brain contusions and focal neurologic signs caused by damage to the underlying cortical area. Prompt debridement and exploration are required in order to avoid infection.

CRANIAL NERVE INJURIES Cranial nerves liable to injury with basilar skull fractures are the olfactory, optic, oculomotor, and trochlear nerves; the first and second branches of the trigeminal nerve; and the facial and auditory nerves. Anosmia and an apparent loss of taste (actually a loss of perception of aromatic flavors, with elementary tastes retained) occurs in approximately 10 percent of persons with serious head injuries, particularly with falls on the back of the head. This sequela results from displacement of the brain and shearing of the olfactory nerve filaments. Recovery usually occurs, leaving residual hyposmia, but if bilateral anosmia persists for several months, the prognosis is poor. Fractures of the sphenoid bone may bruise or transect the optic nerve, resulting in unilateral partial or complete blindness and an unreactive pupil, usually equal in size to that of the other side, with a preserved consensual light response. Partial optic nerve injuries from closed trauma result in blurring of vision, central or paracentral scotomas, or sector defects. Direct orbital injury may cause short-lived blurred vision for close objects because of reversible iridoplegia. Diplopia only on looking down, which suggests trochlear nerve damage from fracture of the lesser sphenoid wing, occurs as an isolated problem from minor injury and may be delayed for several days. Patients report that the diplopia can be corrected by tilting the head away from the affected eye. Direct facial nerve injury by a basal fracture is present immediately in 3 percent of severe injuries; it also may be delayed 5 to 7 days. Petrous fractures, particularly the less common transverse type, are liable to produce this injury. Delayed facial palsy has a good prognosis; its mechanism is not known. Injury to the eighth cranial nerve with fractures of the petrous bone causes loss of hearing, vertigo, and nystagmus immediately after injury; the nystagmus is frequently positional. Deafness due to nerve injury must be distinguished from that due to rupture of the eardrum, blood in the middle ear, or disruption of the ossicles from fracture through the middle ear. A high-tone hearing loss occurs with direct cochlear concussion.

CONCUSSION *Concussion* refers to an immediate but transient loss of consciousness, often described as dazed or "star struck," associated with a short period of amnesia. It typically occurs after a blunt impact to, or deceleration of, the frontal or occipital areas that creates a sudden movement of the brain within the skull. In severe cases, a brief convulsion or autonomic symptoms and signs such as facial pallor, bradycardia, faintness with mild hypotension, or sluggish pupillary reaction may occur, but most patients are neurologically normal. Higher primates are particularly susceptible to concussion; in contrast, billy goats, rams, and woodpeckers can tolerate impact velocity and deceleration a hundred times greater than that experienced by humans. The mechanism of loss of consciousness in concussion is believed to be a transient electrophysiologic dysfunction of the reticular activating system in the upper midbrain caused by rotation of the cerebral hemispheres on the relatively fixed brainstem. The mechanism of the associated amnesia is not known. Gross and light microscopic changes in the brain are usually absent after concussion, but biochemical and ultrastructural changes, such as mitochondrial ATP depletion and local disruption of the blood-brain barrier, suggest that complex abnormalities occur. The CT and magnetic resonance imaging (MRI) scans are usually normal. Approximately 3 percent of patients who have had concussions have an intracranial hemorrhage (subdural, epidural, or parenchymal); the presence of a skull fracture increases this risk.

Amnesia after concussion typically follows a few moments of unresponsiveness. Rarely, there is no loss of consciousness. The memory loss spans the time of, and moments before, mild impact injuries but may encompass previous weeks (rarely months) in cases of more severe trauma. Any anterograde amnesia is usually brief and disappears rapidly in alert patients. The extent of retrograde amnesia has been suggested as a rough measure of the severity of injury. Improvement usually occurs in an orderly progression from most distant to recent memories, with islands of amnesia occasionally remaining in severe cases. Hysterical posttraumatic amnesia is not uncommon and should be suspected when abnormalities of behavior occur, such as a tendency to recount events that cannot be recalled on later testing, bizarre affect, forgetting one's own name, or an anterograde deficit that is excessive in comparison with the degree of injury.

A single, uncomplicated head injury infrequently produces permanent neurobehavioral changes in patients who are free of preexisting psychiatric problems and substance abuse. However, there has been increasing attention to minor problems in memory and concentration that may have an anatomic correlate in small shearing or other microscopic lesions (see below).

CONTUSION, BRAIN HEMORRHAGES, AND SHEARING LESIONS **Hemispheral Lesions** Contusions on the surface of the brain and deeper hemorrhages result from mechanical forces that move the hemispheres relative to the skull. Deceleration of the brain against the inner skull causes contusions, either under a point of impact (coup lesion) or in the antipolar area (contrecoup lesion). Trauma sufficient to cause prolonged unconsciousness usually produces contusions varying from small superficial cortical petechiae to hemorrhagic and necrotic destruction of large portions of a hemisphere. Because the motion of the hemispheres brings them into contact with the prominences of the sphenoid and other frontal basal bones, blunt impact, as from an automobile dashboard or from falling forward while drunk, typically causes contusions on the orbital surfaces of the frontal lobes and the anterior and basal portions of the temporal lobes. With lateral forces, as from the doorframe of a car, contusions occur on the convexity of the hemispheres.

Contusions are visible on CT and MRI scans, appearing early as inhomogeneous hyperdensity on CT and hyperintensity on MR from scattered cortical and subcortical blood (Fig. 374-1); there is often an associated mass effect that distorts adjacent sulci and the lateral ventricles. In almost all cases there is also some degree of subarachnoid bleeding, which may be detected by scans or lumbar puncture. After several hours, the edematous tissue surrounding a contusion appears as a ring of lower density. Confluent, roughly spherical contusions can be distinguished from cerebral hemorrhages because they extend to the cortical surface. After a week, some contusions have a surrounding ringlike contrast enhancement that may be mistaken for tumor or abscess. Glial and macrophage reactions begin within 2 days and result years later in scarred, hemosiderin-stained depressions on the surface (*plaques jaunes*) that are one source of posttraumatic epilepsy.

The clinical signs produced by contusions vary with the location and size of the lesions; most often a hemiparesis or gaze preference is seen, similar to that caused by a middle cerebral artery stroke. Bilateral large contusions produce coma with extensor posturing; when contusions are limited to the frontal lobes, an abulic-taciturn state or inappropriate jocularity and indifference occur. Contusions of the

FIGURE 374-1 Temporal lobe contusion. Noncontrast CT scan demonstrates a hyperdense region in the anterior temporal lobe consistent with a hemorrhagic cerebral contusion, which typically occurs in the anterior temporal, frontal, and occipital regions.

temporal lobes may cause an aggressive, combative syndrome, described below. With large contusions, the secondary effect of progressive edema is the most threatening aspect of the injury. Coma and signs of secondary brainstem compression (pupillary enlargement) then dominate. Seizures soon after trauma are rare with contusions, as indeed they are for several weeks after most acute head injuries.

Deep hemorrhages in the central white matter may result from confluent contusions in the depths of a sulcus. However, ganglionic, diencephalic, and other deep hematomas due to torsion or shearing forces in the brain may occur independently of surface damage. The areas around these hematomas can become edematous, resulting in neural dysfunction in the affected region and progressively raised intracranial pressure. Large single hemorrhages after minor trauma may occur in patients with a bleeding diathesis or in the elderly, sometimes related to cerebrovascular amyloidosis. Another type of white matter, or "shearing," lesion consists of widespread acute disruption of axons at the time of impact. The affected areas of white matter are replaced by glial proliferation over a period of several months. In these cases, there are characteristically small areas of tissue disruption in the corpus callosum and dorsolateral pons, but these areas may not be appreciated in scans. There is apparently a continuum of traumatic deep tissue disruption that extends from the limited microscopic shearing lesions to large circumscribed clots within damaged tissue. The presence of widespread axonal shearing lesions in the deep white matter of both hemispheres, called *diffuse axonal injury*, has been proposed as the explanation of persistent coma or vegetative state, but small hemorrhages in the midbrain and low diencephalon are as often the cause. Only severe shearing lesions containing blood are visualized by CT, usually in the corpus callosum and centrum semiovale, but within days of the injury, MRI is able to show them throughout the white matter (Fig. 374-2) especially with the use of gradient echo MR sequences.

On occasion, especially in children, head trauma causes diffuse brain swelling within a few hours after injury, although CT fails to reveal focal lesions or hemorrhage. The swelling creates a mass effect with disastrous consequences. This problem is probably due to microvascular disruption and greatly increased cerebral blood flow.

Deep cerebral hemorrhages may be delayed until several days after severe injury. Sudden neurologic deterioration in an already

FIGURE 374-2 Shear hemorrhage due to head trauma following a motor vehicle accident. A coronal T2 gradient echo-weighted MRI scan demonstrates several foci of hypointense signal representing small shear hemorrhages at the gray/white junction in the right hemisphere (*arrows*). Foci punctate hemorrhages occur at zones of shearing forces between the gray and white matter of the brain.

comatose patient, or a sudden and unexplained rise in intracranial pressure, should therefore prompt a CT scan.

Residual symptoms and signs of primary or secondary compressive brainstem hemorrhages or ischemic lesions include cerebellar tremor, pupillary enlargement, eye movement abnormalities, or the "locked-in" syndrome (see Chap. 24). Midbrain or diencephalic hemorrhages are the only well-defined direct traumatic brainstem lesions responsible for coma. Most other lesions causing coma and subsequent persistent vegetative state that are unexplained by CT are probably due to diffuse axonal shearing injuries in the cerebral hemispheres or severe anoxia-ischemia at the time of trauma.

SUBDURAL AND EPIDURAL HEMATOMAS In severe head injury, hemorrhages beneath the dura (subdural) or between the dura and skull (epidural) may be combined with contusions and other injuries, making it difficult to determine their relative contribution to the clinical state. However, subdural and epidural hematomas often occur as the primary lesion, each with a characteristic clinical and radiologic appearance. Because the mass effect of the hemorrhage and the rise in intracranial pressure may be life-threatening, it is important to make an immediate diagnosis by CT or MRI scan (Fig. 374-2) and to carry out surgical evacuation.

Acute Subdural Hematoma Acute subdural hematomas become symptomatic minutes or hours after injury. Up to one-third of patients have a lucid interval before coma supervenes, but most are drowsy or comatose from the moment of injury. Arousable patients complain of unilateral headache and frequently have a slightly enlarged pupil on that side. Stupor or coma and unilateral pupillary enlargement are the major signs in larger hematomas. Pupillary dilation is usually ipsilateral, but 5 to 10 percent are contralateral to the hematoma. Signs such as a hemiparesis are also helpful but occasionally are ipsilateral to the clot. The CT scan shows the clot, allowing early evacuation. The degree of midline shift is often disproportionately greater than the apparent size of the clot in one axial CT scan, but, in general, the rules relating shift to the level of consciousness outlined in Chap. 24 remain useful. In an acutely deteriorating patient with diminished alertness and with pupillary enlargement, burr holes or an emergency craniotomy are appropriate at times without prior radiographic confirmation of subdural hematoma. A subacute syndrome with drowsiness, headache, confusion, or mild hemiparesis occurring days to 2 weeks after injury is seen in alcoholics and in the elderly.

Direct cranial trauma is not required for acute subdural hemorrhage to occur; acceleration forces alone, as from whiplash, are adequate, especially in the elderly. Most subdural hematomas are crescentic collections over the hemispheral convexity, adjacent to a variable degree of surface hemorrhagic contusion. Larger clots are thought to be primarily venous in origin, although additional arterial bleeding sites are often found, and some, when explored surgically, appear to be exclusively arterial. Most are located over the frontotemporal region, less often in the inferior middle fossa or over the occipital poles. Less common instances of interhemispheric, posterior fossa, or bilateral convexity clots are difficult to diagnose clinically, although drowsiness and the signs expected for each region can be detected. Small subdural hematomas may be asymptomatic and usually do not require therapy.

Acute Epidural Hematoma Epidural hematomas evolve more rapidly than subdural hematomas and therefore can be more treacherous. They occur in 1 to 3 percent of all head injuries, in up to 10 percent of severe cases, and are less often associated with underlying cortical damage than are subdural hematomas. Most patients are unconscious when first seen. A "lucid interval" of several minutes to hours before coma supervenes is said to be most characteristic of epidural hemorrhage, although it is not common, and epidural hemorrhage by no means is the only cause of this temporal profile.

The location of an epidural hematoma overlying the lateral temporal convexity is explained by its origin from torn dural vessels, most commonly the middle meningeal artery. Most patients have fractures of the squamous portion of the temporal bone, through the path of the torn vessel. Frontal, inferior temporal, or occipitoparietal epidural hematomas are less frequent, occurring when fractures disrupt branches of the middle meningeal artery. Epidural hematomas strip the tightly attached dura from the inner table of the skull, producing a characteristic lenticular clot on CT. They may be less frequent in the elderly because of the tighter attachment of dura to skull that occurs with aging. Posterior fossa epidural hematomas are rare and difficult to detect clinically; most result from surgery, such as resection of an acoustic neuroma.

Chronic Subdural Hematoma In chronic subdural hematoma, a preceding traumatic cause is less often clear; 20 to 30 percent of patients fail to give a history of injury, particularly elderly patients or those with a bleeding diathesis. The causative injury may be trivial (striking the head against the branch of a tree, a sudden stop in a car with lurching forward, or minor head contact during a fall or faint) and is often forgotten because it was remote in time. A period of weeks, or even months, follows when headaches (common but not invariable), slowed thinking, confusion, changes in personality, seizures, or a mild hemiparesis emerges. The headache typically fluctuates in severity, often with positional changes. Many chronic subdural hematomas are bilateral and give misleading clinical syndromes. The initial clinical impression is often of a stroke, brain tumor, or drug intoxication or of a depressive, senile, or other type of dementia, the latter because drowsiness, inattentiveness, or incoherence of thought is more prominent than focal signs such as hemiparesis. Hemianesthesia or hemianopia is seldom observed, probably because the anatomic structures subserving these functions are deep and not easily compressed. The diagnosis should be considered in dementias of rapid onset, particularly if headache is present.

Occasionally a chronic hematoma causes brief episodes of hemiparesis or aphasia, lasting more than 10 min, that are indistinguishable from transient ischemic attacks. Patients with undetected small bilateral subdural hematomas seem to have a low tolerance for surgery, anesthesia, and drugs that depress the nervous system, often remaining drowsy or confused for long periods postoperatively.

Skull x-rays are usually normal except for a shift of a calcified pineal body to one side or an occasional unexpected fracture. CT without contrast infusion typically shows a low-density mass over the convexity of the hemisphere, but between 2 to 6 weeks after the initial bleeding, CT may show only a shift of the midline structures and compression of the lateral ventricles because the clot is isodense to adjacent brain. Bilateral chronic hematomas may be missed because of the absence of lateral tissue shifts. A "hypernormal" CT scan with full cortical sulci and small ventricles in an older patient should suggest the diagnosis of bilateral isodense hematomas. Contrast infusion demonstrates a vascular fibrous capsule surrounding the clot. MRI is reliable in identifying a subacute or chronic clot (Fig. 374-3). Lumbar puncture is not recommended for diagnosis because of risk of worsening tissue shifts but, if performed, shows xanthochromia and a variable number of red blood cells. Chronic subdural hematomas can expand gradually and then behave clinically like a tumor. Treatment with glucocorticoids alone is sufficient in some cases, but surgical evacuation is most often successful. Fibrous membranes (pseudomembranes) that grow from the dura and encapsulate the region require surgical resection to prevent recurrent fluid accumulation. Small hematomas are largely resorbed, leaving only the organizing membranes, which become calcified after many years.

PENETRATING INJURIES, COMPRESSIONS, AND LACERATIONS Tangential scalp wounds from bullets can produce neurologic signs or delayed seizures due to small hemorrhages or contusions, even in the absence of missile penetration. Bullets en-

tering the brain cause considerable damage because of tremendous kinetic energy. A cylindrical area of necrosis surrounds the bullet track. Injuries differ for different projectiles; soft civilian bullets typically shatter on impact and leave a track of metallic fragments with moderate parenchymal damage, whereas military bullets, because of their high velocity and energy, disrupt tissue at great distances from the track and produce massive brain destruction.

Penetrating bullet injuries cause a rapid increase in intracranial pressure for several minutes followed by a drop depending on the volume of secondary hemorrhage and the degree of developing edema. Infection is a risk mainly from shell fragments, shrapnel, grenades, and mines, because such small projectiles carry surface bacteria and dirt into the brain. Most neurosurgeons administer systemic antibiotics prophylactically and perform local debridement for all types of penetrating injuries. Traumatic aneurysms can form as a result of disruption of vessel walls from the shock wave of the projectile; facial-orbital entrance wounds have the highest incidence of this complication. The aneurysms have an unpredictable course, but most that rupture do so in the first month. The prognosis for survival after missile injuries is good if consciousness is preserved and poor if coma is present from the outset.

Intracranial foreign bodies in injuries caused by knives, picks, studguns, or high-speed tool bits may be missed unless skull x-rays are taken after minor penetrating injuries. Surgical removal, debridement, and extensive exploration for hemorrhage and necrotic tissue are required.

TRAUMATIC VASCULAR OCCLUSION AND DISSECTION Minor, sometimes unnoticed, head or neck trauma can produce dissection (stripping of the intima or the media) of the internal carotid or vertebral arteries. Chiropractic neck manipulation accounts for some cases. Severe blunt trauma to the neck can initiate a dissection several centimeters above the origins of the internal carotid or vertebral arteries. In awake patients there is usually local neck pain over the affected carotid artery, a Horner's syndrome, and headache over the ipsilateral anterior cranium. Some patients with carotid dissection subsequently have large middle cerebral artery strokes with hemiplegia. In drowsy or comatose patients, evidence of dissection or subsequent stroke is difficult to determine, but its presence is suggested by unexplained hemiplegia, unilateral miosis, or appearance of cerebral infarction on CT scan. Angiography demonstrates either the typical "string sign," characterized by an elongated, narrowed lumen extending over 5 to 10 cm, or complete occlusion of the carotid artery beginning several centimeters distal to the bifurcation.

A

B

FIGURE 374-3 Acute and subacute subdural hematomas. *A*. Sagittal T1-weighted MRI scan of the brain without contrast demonstrates large fluid collections (*white arrows*) consistent with large subacute subdural hematomas. *B*. Axial T2-weighted MRI scan reveals hyperintense signal (*white arrows*) representing subacute blood and a hypointense signal (*black arrows*) representing more recent subdural hematoma.

Traumatic vertebral artery dissection can produce vertigo, vomiting, suboccipital or supraorbital headache, and other signs of lateral medullary or cerebellar ischemia. These symptoms may be attributed erroneously to vestibular concussion. In comatose patients, the only indication of vertebral artery occlusion may be inferior cerebellar infarction on the CT scan. Vasospasm from traumatic subarachnoid blood may also be involved in the development of infarction after head injury.

Cavernous sinus arteriovenous fistulas are serious complications in patients surviving severe head injury. They are first evident as a self-audible bruit (many are also audible to the examiner), proptosis, conjunctival injection, or visual impairment. Angiography shows early filling of the cavernous sinus and its draining tributaries. The fistula enlarges, causing increasingly severe local changes around the eye and orbit and decreased chances of visual recovery. About 10 percent, mostly small fistulas, resolve spontaneously. Many surgical approaches have been tried, including ligation of the carotid artery and direct obliteration of the fistula or cavernous sinus, but a detachable balloon technique has proved successful in many cases and is currently favored.

INTRACRANIAL PRESSURE AND CEREBRAL BLOOD FLOW

The regulation of intracranial pressure (ICP) and its relationship to cerebral blood flow (CBF), which are relevant to many pathologic processes including cerebral hemorrhage, encephalitis, and brain edema after stroke, is best presented and understood in the context of head trauma. The components of the intracranial compartment are brain, CSF, and blood. Because the skull limits the total intracranial volume, these compartments are compromised by expanding lesions within the cranial cavity. The brain is virtually incompressible; therefore, CSF and blood serve as the main buffers of increasing intracranial volume. The relationship between increments in intracranial volume and the associated rises in ICP, termed *compliance*, approximates an exponential function. ICP is normally between 2 and 12 mmHg. Raised ICP in the range 15 to 40 mmHg, while not harmful by itself, can rapidly progress to a state that causes secondary damage by precipitously decreasing cerebral perfusion when ICP approaches blood pressure (BP). As this is occurring, there are shifts of brain tissue due to compartmentalization of pressure between dural restrictions. These tissue shifts, not the raised ICP per se, compress the upper brainstem and account for the classic neurologic signs of an intracranial mass (see Chap. 24). The global damage from increased ICP is therefore ischemic in nature and related to the difference between ICP and BP in the major cerebral arteries. When this pressure difference, termed *cerebral perfusion pressure* (CPP), is below 20 to 30 mmHg, raised ICP becomes detrimental; therapy is therefore directed toward maintaining perfusion above this range. The rationale for keeping CPP even higher (i.e., bringing ICP below 15 to 20 mmHg) is to afford a margin of safety should transient increases in ICP occur. Physiologic changes or medications that increase BP do not necessarily improve CPP, because increased vascular pressures can exacerbate brain edema in damaged areas and raise cerebral blood volume, thereby resulting in further increases in ICP that ultimately lower perfusion.

The most important secondary nervous system complication of head injury is raised intracranial pressure arising from the added volume of contusions, hematomas, and the progressive edema surrounding them. At least 50 percent of patients who die as a result of head injury do so because of uncontrolled rises in ICP, and outcome is inversely related to the level of ICP after acute injury. Aggressive treatment of raised ICP in modern intensive care units is believed to improve survival after severe head injury, but the role of direct monitoring of ICP to guide therapy and improve outcome is controversial.

Resting ICP, CPP, and compliance are spontaneously interrupted by rises in ICP termed *plateau waves*. These may be precipitated by iatrogenic maneuvers such as suctioning, physical therapy, excess fluid administration, or pain. They are appreciated best by continuous trend recordings of ICP. Plateau waves are apparently due to a loss of cerebrovascular tone with a resultant increase in cerebral blood volume. Some spontaneous plateau waves are provoked by mild, often unnoticed hypotension that causes cerebrovascular dilation. Such episodes (lasting 1 to 10 min and ranging from 25 to 60 mmHg) are most pronounced in patients with diminished intracranial compliance. Signs of transtentorial herniation, such as pupillary enlargement, may occur after plateau waves (although more often they do not), and, occasionally, brain death ensues.

For several minutes to an hour after acute head injury, cerebral blood flow increases in some patients, although metabolic demands and oxygen consumption are diminished. Autoregulation—the ability of the cerebral vasculature to keep blood flow constant in response to decreased or increased perfusion pressure—is also impaired in damaged regions. Vascular factors have been found to account for approximately two-thirds of the rise in ICP after severe head injury. The blood-brain barrier also becomes more permeable after head injury in badly damaged regions, making edema formation more likely. Other secondary systemic phenomena after severe head injury cause brain damage and alter outcome.

CLINICAL SYNDROMES AND TREATMENT OF HEAD INJURY

MINOR INJURY　A patient who is fully alert and attentive after head injury and has one or more symptoms of headache, faintness, nausea, a single episode of emesis, difficulty with concentration, or slight blurring of vision has a good prognosis with little risk of subsequent deterioration. Such patients have sustained a concussion and have a brief amnestic epoch surrounding the moment of impact. Occasionally, vasovagal syncope occurs several minutes to an hour after the injury and causes concern. Constant generalized or frontal headache is common in the days following trauma; it is often throbbing and hemicranial in nature, like migraine. Children and young adults are particularly prone to drowsiness, vomiting, and irritability, which is sometimes delayed for several hours after apparently minor injuries. After several hours of observation, arrangements may be made for the patient to be accompanied home to be observed by family or friends. Most patients with a minor syndrome do not have a skull fracture on skull x-ray or hemorrhage on CT. The decision to perform these tests depends largely on clinical signs suggesting that the impact was severe (e.g., prolonged concussion, periorbital or mastoid hematoma, repeated vomiting).

Persistent severe headache and repeated vomiting in the context of normal alertness and no focal neurologic signs are usually benign, but radiologic studies should be obtained. Skull fractures increase the likelihood of a subdural or epidural hematoma. Patients with these exaggerated signs, even if they follow minor injury, deserve observation in the hospital. Clinical judgment, the presence of associated noncranial injuries, the availability of others at home, and the examiner's certainty of a normal neurologic examination should guide the decision regarding further surveillance.

INJURY OF INTERMEDIATE SEVERITY　Patients who are not comatose but who have persistent confusion, behavioral changes, subnormal alertness, extreme dizziness, or focal neurologic signs such as hemiparesis should be admitted to the hospital and soon thereafter have a CT scan. Usually a contusion or hematoma is found. The clinical syndromes most common in this group, in addition to postconcussive headache, dizziness, and vomiting of minor injury, include (1) delirium with a disinclination to be examined or moved, expletive speech, and resistance if disturbed (often associated with anterior temporal lobe contusions); (2) a quiet, disinterested, slowed mental state (abulia) with dull facial appearance and slight irascibility if bothered, the patient lying quietly with eyes closed when undisturbed (seen with inferior and frontopolar frontal contusions); (3) memory loss with poor retrograde and anterograde performance (from medial temporal lobe contusions or diffuse injury); (4) a focal deficit such as aphasia or mild hemiparesis (suggesting subdural hematoma or convexity contusion, or, rarely, stroke due to carotid artery dissection); (5) confusion with inattention, poor performance on simple mental tasks, and fluctuating or slightly erroneous orientation (associated with several types of injuries, including the first two described above as well as medial frontal contusions and interhemispheric subdural hematoma); (6) repetitive vomiting, nystagmus, drowsiness, and unsteadiness (usually from a labyrinthine concussion, but occasionally due to a posterior fossa subdural hematoma or vertebral artery dissection); and (7) diabetes insipidus with or without a frontal-temporal lobe syndrome (from damage to the median eminence or pituitary stalk and adjacent medial cortex). Many intermediate injuries are complicated by drug or alcohol intoxication.

Close clinical observation in a well-staffed setting is advisable to detect increasing drowsiness and a change in respiratory pattern or pupillary enlargement and to ensure restriction of free water (unless there is diabetes insipidus). Fully awake or slightly drowsy patients with small subdural hematomas may be treated with glucocorticoids and fluid restriction; those with larger clots, especially if there is fluctuating or worsening alertness, require surgery. Epidural hematomas causing compression of adjacent brain should be evacuated in patients who have a reasonable chance of recovery from other injuries. Free water intake should generally be limited, allowing serum osmolarity to rise spontaneously toward 290 mosmol/L. Fever must be treated assiduously with antipyretics or a cooling blanket, and its source (usually aspiration) must be identified. So-called central fever is rare. The routine administration of phenytoin is controversial; the best randomized trial has shown no benefit beyond the first week of drug administration. Glucocorticoids are of limited usefulness even if there is a contusion or edema on the CT scan; they complicate management and should be omitted.

Most patients with intermediate injury improve over 1 to 6 weeks. During the first week, alertness, irascibility, memory, and mental performance fluctuate. Behavioral changes such as agitation are most evident at night and sometimes seem to be worsened by large doses of glucocorticoids or drugs that depress the central nervous system. Haloperidol is useful when used sparingly. Subtle abnormalities of intellectual function, particularly attention, spontaneity, and memory, tend to return toward normal later, and sometimes do so abruptly. Persistent intellectual difficulties are discussed below.

SEVERE HEAD INJURY AND COMA   Patients who are stuporous or comatose from the outset require immediate neurologic attention and, often, resuscitation. Persistent unresponsiveness is a grave sign. After the patient is intubated and the BP is stabilized, attention is given to life-threatening noncranial injuries, followed by a survey neurologic examination. The possibility of cervical injuries should not be overlooked, and the cervical spine must be immobilized during the initial assessment. The depth of coma and the size of the pupils are most important. Extensor limb posturing and bilateral Babinski signs, combined with apparently purposeful movements, are common. Asymmetry in limb posture, limb movement, or gaze preference suggests a subdural or epidural hematoma or a large contusion.

As soon as vital functions permit and cervical spine x-rays and a CT scan have been obtained, the patient should be taken to a critical care unit. The finding of an epidural or subdural hematoma or large intracerebral hemorrhage is usually an indication for surgery and intracranial decompression. In one large series, the time between injury and evacuation of acute subdural hematomas was the major determinant of outcome. If such lesions are not present and the patient is still comatose and critically ill, attention is directed toward treating raised ICP. Patients with abnormal CT scans showing contusions, hemorrhages, or tissue shifts are the best candidates for direct monitoring of ICP. The practice in many head injury treatment centers is to use one of several devices inserted intracranially. The pressure can be monitored continuously; disturbances in compliance and falling cerebral perfusion pressure can be identified; and the appearance of plateau waves can be noted.

The treatment of raised ICP is best guided by direct measurement but may proceed on a presumptive basis using clinical status and CT scan as guides. All potentially exacerbating factors must be eliminated.

Hypoxia, hyperthermia, hypercarbia, awkward head positions, and high mean airway pressures from mechanical ventilation all increase cerebral blood volume and ICP. Many, but not all, patients will have lower ICP when the head and trunk are elevated. Active management of raised ICP includes induced hypocarbia to an initial level of 28 to 33 mmHg P_{CO_2} and hyperosmolar dehydration with 20% mannitol (0.25 to 1 g/kg every 3 to 6 h), preferably using directly measured ICP as a guide. Otherwise, a serum osmolality of 300 to 310 mosmol/L is desirable.

A persistently raised ICP after inception of this conservative therapy generally indicates a poor outcome. Although the addition of high-dose barbiturates may further lower ICP there is no beneficial effect on overall outcome. In many instances, barbiturates cause a parallel reduction in ICP and BP without resulting in net improvement in cerebral perfusion. Systolic BP should be maintained above 100 mmHg by vasopressor agents, if necessary. Mean BP levels above 110 to 120 mmHg may exaggerate brain edema, but some neurosurgeons allow the BP to rise above normal on the basis that this may abort plateau waves. A more conventional approach is to treat hypertension with diuretics and beta-adrenergic blocking agents, angiotensin-converting enzyme inhibitors, or intermittent doses of barbiturates. A number of other antihypertensive drugs, including some calcium-channel blockers, are relatively contraindicated because they raise ICP. Fluid must be administered cautiously, and free water intake should be limited. Antacids administered by nasogastric tube or direct-acting drugs should be given to keep gastric pH above 3.5 and prevent gastrointestinal bleeding. The use of large doses of glucocorticoids in severe head injury does not improve outcome. Several studies suggest that early nutritional support results in earlier neurologic recovery from head injury. If the patient remains comatose, it is worthwhile to repeat the CT or MRI scan to exclude a delayed surface or intracerebral hemorrhage. Intensive care salvages some critically ill head-injured patients by concentrating efforts on simple treatments that avoid medical complications, particularly pneumonia and sepsis and preventable increases in ICP. Whether more assiduous control of ICP and CPP produces better results remains to be proved.

ASSOCIATED DERANGEMENTS OCCURRING WITH SEVERE HEAD TRAUMA   Injuries outside the cranium should be searched for at the outset, because they are likely to be forgotten if not initially noted. In particular, associated spinal, long bone, and abdominal injuries may cause delayed difficulties in management. However, secondary medical complications dominate the intermediate-term intensive care of head trauma patients.

Fluids and Electrolytes   Over half of patients who persist in coma for 24 h after head injury develop abnormalities of electrolytes or fluid balance. Frequently these are a consequence of therapy, but the metabolic responses to head trauma are similar to those produced by trauma elsewhere and are important in planning treatment. Diabetes insipidus should be suspected if urine output increases and urine specific gravity is low. Replacement of water losses suffices for mild cases, but vasopressin may be required. Serum osmolality above approximately 320 mosmol/L should be avoided because of the associated decrease in cardiac output. Secretion of aldosterone and antidiuretic hormone (vasopressin, AVP) in response to stress favor the retention of sodium and free water, respectively. The latter usually predominates, leading to mild hypervolemic hyponatremia in untreated patients, but it is obscured by concomitant administration of osmotic agents. Severe hyponatremia results from excessive AVP secretion, which may occur with raised ICP, basilar skull fractures, and after prolonged mechanical ventilation.

Respiratory Complications   Some patients with head injuries have hypoxia acutely after injury without obvious pulmonary infiltrates. Aspiration pneumonia presents a great risk; lung injury from aspirated gastric contents, infection, and atelectasis may combine to produce the adult respiratory distress syndrome (ARDS) and severe arteriovenous shunting. There is some evidence that gastric coating agents, such as sucralfate, are associated with less aspiration pneumonia than are conventional prophylactic agents for gastric bleeding. ARDS also can occur owing to disseminated intravascular coagulopathy, fat embolism, or, rarely, "neurogenic" pulmonary edema (see below). Treatment is similar to that for ARDS in other settings, with positive end-expiratory pressure (PEEP) to allow lowered inspired oxygen concentrations and to prevent further atelectasis. The effect of PEEP on ICP is complex, but PEEP should not be withheld if necessary for oxygenation.

Atelectasis is common in all poorly responsive patients and is treated with chest physical therapy and adequate ventilator tidal volumes. Pulmonary embolism is also a major threat to bedridden patients, and intermittent pneumatic calf compression or modest doses of subcutaneous heparin may be useful prophylaxis. The latter has not predisposed to intracerebral or gastrointestinal bleeding. Early recognition of deep leg vein thrombosis and aggressive treatment by occlusion of the inferior vena cava may prevent later emboli.

Fat Embolism Patients with severe long bone injuries are subject to widespread cerebral fat embolism. This complication is seen less often than previously, perhaps owing to better fluid replacement. In the typical case, head injury is a minor part of the overall trauma; in a few, severe cranial injury masks the syndrome. Several days after the bone fractures occur, restlessness, delirium, or drowsiness progressing to coma in severe cases, seizures, generalized brain edema, and hypoxia develop. About half the patients have retinal and conjunctival punctate hemorrhages or visible fat in retinal vessels. A petechial rash, prominent in the anterior axillary folds and supraclavicular fossae, diffuse interstitial infiltrates on the chest x-ray, fat in the urine, and/or renal failure occurs in some patients. Severe reduction in arterial oxygen content is common from widespread lung injury (ARDS). Cerebral fat embolism causes a cerebral purpura, mainly in the white matter, due to capillary occlusion by fat globules. There is evidence that patients in whom this complication is recognized and treated early have a better prognosis. Massive doses of glucocorticoids and administration of positive-pressure ventilation with high end-expiratory pressures have been claimed to be useful. Heparin or intravenous alcohol are no longer recommended.

Gastrointestinal Hemorrhage Most patients with severe head injuries develop gastric erosions, but only a few have clinically significant hemorrhages. Gastrointestinal bleeding usually occurs in the first days to 1 week after injury. Unlike most patients in shock or with stress ulceration, head-trauma patients often have elevated gastric acidity. The synergistic effect of glucocorticoids in causing upper tract hemorrhage has been questioned, but the incidence of viscus perforation, particularly of the cecum, is elevated. Prophylactic treatment with gastric coating agents, as discussed above, with H_2 receptor blockers, or with frequent antacid administration to keep gastric pH high probably reduces gastric hemorrhage in other stress states and is commonly used in head trauma.

Cardiovascular Changes Acute head trauma may cause transient apnea and cardiac arrest. In the absence of overwhelming brain damage, recovery from the arrest is the rule. Subsequently, a sympathoadrenal discharge or raised ICP may cause systemic hypertension, either with the classically associated bradycardia (Cushing response) or, almost as frequently, with tachycardia. Cardiac arrhythmias are common, most notably sinus bradycardia, supraventricular tachycardias, nodal rhythm, and heart block. T-wave inversion and alterations in the ST segment may simulate subendocardial ischemia.

Neurogenic pulmonary edema is a form of ARDS in which the alveoli fill with fluid as they would in congestive heart failure, but left ventricular end-diastolic pressure (measured by pulmonary capillary wedge pressure) is normal. A pulmonary vascular leak may be produced when a sudden shift of intravascular volume occurs from the systemic to the pulmonary circulation, as occurs transiently with suddenly raised ICP, or there may be a direct neurogenic influence of hypothalamic function on the pulmonary microvasculature. Once the pulmonary vasculature has been damaged, an alveolar capillary leak may continue despite return of pulmonary vascular pressure to normal. The result is pulmonary edema with normal central venous and wedge pressures after the initial injury.

Hematologic Complications A large number of patients demonstrate a mild coagulopathy, and 5 to 10 percent have various degrees of disseminated intravascular coagulation, a harbinger of poor outcome. A correlation may exist between the severity of injury and the level of increased fibrin degradation products in blood. One cause of the coagulopathy is thought to be the release of highly thromboplastic material into the systemic circulation from the damaged brain.

PROGNOSIS Extensive work by Jennet's group in Glasgow and from the Traumatic Coma Data Bank has provided data on the outcome in severe head injury (Table 374-1). Verbal output, eye opening, and the best motor response are important predictors of ultimate outcome. Eighty-five percent of patients with aggregate Glasgow Coma Scale scores of 3 or 4 die 24 h after injury. Yet a number of patients with a poor initial prognosis, including absent pupillary light responses, survive, suggesting that aggressive management is justified in virtually all patients. Patients younger than approximately 20 years, particularly children, may make remarkable recoveries after having grave early neurologic signs. In one large study of severe head injury, 55 percent of children had a good outcome at 1 year, compared with 21 percent of adults. Increased intracranial pressure, older age, and signs of cisternal compression and midline shift on CT scan are all poor prognostic signs.

Evoked potentials also have prognostic value in head injury, similar to their use in ischemic-hypoxic brain injury, and their accuracy probably exceeds that of purely clinical methods. Somatosensory evoked potentials are the most useful, with bilaterally absent cortical potentials (with more caudal potentials present) being predictive of death or a vegetative state in 85 to 95 percent of patients. Prediction of a good functional outcome in the presence of normal or mildly abnormal test results is less certain.

NEUROPSYCHOLOGICAL OUTCOME AFTER HEAD INJURY

Traumatic damage and cognitive sequelae of head injury both constitute a continuum, but most patients recover to normal after mild injury. There is probably a high rate of temporary inattention and memory and other subtle deficits after all but the mildest injuries. Attention has recently been directed toward a structural basis for the fatigue, dizziness, headache, and difficulty in concentration after mild injury, termed the *postconcussion syndrome*. Based on experimental models,

Table 374-1

Glasgow Coma Scale for Head Injury

Eye opening (E)	
Spontaneous	4
To loud voice	3
To pain	2
Nil	1
Best motor response (M)	
Obeys	6
Localizes	5
Withdraws (flexion)	4
Abnormal flexion posturing	3
Extension posturing	2
Nil	1
Verbal response (V)	
Oriented	5
Confused, disoriented	4
Inappropriate words	3
Incomprehensible sounds	2
Nil	1

NOTE: Coma score = E + M + V. Patients scoring 3 or 4 have an 85 percent chance of dying or remaining vegetative, while scores above 11 indicate 5 to 10 percent likelihood of death or vegetative state and 85 percent chance of moderate disability or good recovery. Intermediate scores correlate with proportional chances of patients recovering.

some investigators believe that subtle axonal shearing lesions or bio-chemical alterations account for these symptoms despite normal findings on brain imaging, normal evoked potentials, and a normal electroencephalogram. In moderate and severe trauma, neuropsychological changes are found routinely; however, formal testing often shows deficits that are not important in daily functioning. This is partly due to the type of testing and the nature of the control groups. Test scores tend to improve rapidly during the first 6 months after injury, then more slowly for years.

SPINAL CORD TRAUMA

Approximately 10,000 patients a year in the United States, mostly young and otherwise healthy, become paraplegic or quadriplegic because of spinal cord injuries. There are an estimated 200,000 quadriplegics in the country. Most spinal cord injuries in civilian life result from damage to the surrounding vertebral column from fracture, dislocation, or both. Vertical compression with flexion is the main mechanism of injury in the thoracic cord, and hyperextension or flexion is the main cause of injury in the cervical cord. Preexisting spondylosis, a congenitally narrowed spinal canal, hypertrophied ligamentum flavum (see Chap. 373), and instability of the apophyseal joints of adjacent vertebrae from diseases such as rheumatoid arthritis predispose to severe spinal cord damage after minor degrees of injury.

PATHOPHYSIOLOGY AND PATHOLOGY OF SPINAL CORD INJURY Much damage to the spinal cord is due to secondary phenomena occurring in the minutes and hours following injury. Even when a complete transverse myelopathy is evident immediately after impact, some secondary changes are avoidable, and the resultant damage may be reversible. The immediate injury causes pericapillary hemorrhages that coalesce and enlarge, particularly in the gray matter. Infarction of gray matter and early white matter edema are evident within 4 h of experimental blunt injury. Eight hours after injury, there is global infarction at the injured level, and only at this point does necrosis of white matter and paralysis below the level of the lesion become irreversible. The necrosis and central hemorrhages enlarge to occupy one or two levels above and below the point of primary impact. Gliosis in these regions results in necrotic areas over several months and may cavitate causing a progressive syringomyelic syndrome.

The early phases of injury are associated with reduced regional blood flow from direct capillary damage and a more prolonged secondary ischemia. A number of interventions, including administration of opiate antagonists or thyrotropin-releasing hormone, local cord cooling, dextran infusion, adrenergic blockade, and hyperbaric oxygen, have been of uncertain clinical usefulness. A randomized trial has shown the benefit of high doses of methylprednisolone administered within 8 h of injury. This effect may result from inhibition of lipid peroxidation rather than from a direct anti-inflammatory action. The critical factor for recoverable function is the time from injury to institution of any therapy. Complete axonal disruption from the immediate trauma or from secondary phenomena precludes recovery.

TYPES OF SPINAL CORD INJURY AND THEIR MANAGEMENT Any patient with severe head injury potentially has an associated instability of the spinal column. The care of such patients begins at the scene of the accident. The neck should be immobilized to prevent spinal cord damage, and care should be taken during transport and during the physical and radiologic examinations to avoid extension or rotation of the neck and to prevent torsion-rotation of the thoracic spine. Most patients can be intubated, if necessary, by blind nasotracheal technique without neck extension. High thoracic or cervical cord trauma regularly causes mild hypotension and bradycardia because of functional sympathectomy, which responds to infusion of crystalloid or colloid (often corroborated by bilateral ptosis and miosis—Horner's syndrome). As noted, a study has demonstrated that acute administration of high doses of glucocorticoids improves functional outcome slightly, and this tactic has been adopted into practice.

The neurologic examination in the awake patient focuses on neck or back pain, diminished limb power, a sensory level on the trunk,

and deep tendon reflexes, usually absent below the level of an acute spinal cord injury. Injuries above C5 cause quadriplegia and respiratory failure. At C5 and C6 the biceps are also weak, and at C4 and C5 the deltoid and the supra- and infraspinatus are weak. C7 injuries cause weakness of the triceps, wrist extensors, and forearm pronators. Injuries at T1 and below cause paraplegia; the precise level can be determined from the level of sensory loss. Compression in the low thoracic and lumbar region causes a conus medullaris or cauda equina syndrome (see Chap. 373). Cauda equina injuries are usually incomplete, involving peripheral nerves rather than spinal cord, and therefore are surgically remediable for longer periods after injury than spinal cord compression. In a comatose patient, absent reflexes, especially with small pupils or paradoxical breathing, signify a high cervical cord injury.

The next priority is to exclude a surgically remediable and potentially reversible cord compression due to dislocation of a vertebral body. Many traumatic myelopathies have no clearly associated fracture or dislocation. If x-rays suggest any aberration in the position of vertebrae, then reduction should be undertaken quickly. The role of myelography is controversial, but many neurosurgeons instill a few drops of water-soluble contrast medium into the spinal subarachnoid space to demonstrate a block to the flow of CSF by CT or conventional myelography. Examination by MRI, when available, can be more useful. Decompression within 2 h of severe injury may lead to some recovery of spinal cord function. With incomplete myelopathies, especially if the limbs are becoming progressively weaker, early decompression is strongly recommended, even many hours after injury. The surgical approaches to decompressing the spinal column depend on the specific nature of the injury. In complete transverse myelopathies beyond 6 to 12 h after injury, decompressive laminectomies are usually unsuccessful in restoring function.

The concerns with spinal column fractures, with or without myelopathy, are threefold: (1) detection of vertebral dislocations causing cord compression, (2) instability caused by fractures that will lead to misalignment and cord compression in the future, and (3) the proper treatment of fractures through the pedicles, facets, or vertebral bodies. Some fractures heal with immobilizaton and time, usually 2 to 3 months; others require surgical fusion to ensure stability.

Atlantoaxial dislocations can cause immediate death from respiratory failure, an event that may occur with no other neurologic signs. Rheumatoid arthritis predisposes to this injury. Atlantooccipital dislocations occur predominantly in children and are almost always fatal. "Jefferson's fractures" are burst fractures of the ring of the atlas resulting from a force descending on the vertex of the skull as in diving accidents; they are usually asymptomatic. "Hangman's fractures" are produced by hyperextension and longitudinal distraction of the upper cervical spine, as occurs with penal hanging or striking the chin on a steering wheel in a head-on collision. These are usually fractures through the pedicles of C2 with subluxation anteriorly of C2 on C3. Traction reduction and immobilization allow proper healing.

Hyperflexion dislocation of the cervical vertebrae commonly causes traumatic quadriplegia. Occasionally, a markedly displaced injury is unassociated with neurologic dysfunction, presenting only with neck pain. In most cases, however, minor subluxation is associated with a severe neurologic deficit. Ligamentous disruption presumably allows compression of the cord at the moment of impact, but the vertebral bodies return closer to their original stations afterward. Therefore, any degree of subluxation must be treated as potentially unstable.

Compression fractures of the cervical spine can cause neurologic damage if a bone fragment is driven backward (burst fracture) into the spinal cord. "Teardrop fractures" with crushing of a vertebral body, leaving a fragment of bone anteriorly, are usually associated with ligamentous disruption and spinal instability. Single compression fractures of the thoracic spine are usually stable because the thoracic cage provides support, but they may be associated with anterior spinal cord compression and require decompression and stabilization with the insertion of metal rods.

Mild hyperextension injuries may cause only disruption of supporting ligamentous structures and can be well tolerated. More severe injuries cause vertebral displacement and cord compression. The "central cord syndrome" is produced by brief compression of the cervical cord and disruption of the central gray matter, and usually occurs in patients with an already narrow spinal canal, either congenitally or from cervical spondylosis. There is weakness of the arms, often with pinprick loss over the arms and shoulders, and relative sparing of leg power and sensation on the trunk and legs. Abnormality of bladder function is variable. The prognosis for recovery is good.

Thoracolumbar fractures are produced by impact in the high or middle back, usually while the patient is bent over. Impingement on the spinal canal results in a complex combination of cauda equina and conus medullaris dysfunction. Pure lumbar fractures produce cauda equina compression. Myelography, MRI, or CT allows precise localization, and surgical decompression is usually recommended, even with complete deficits, because the potential for recovery of peripheral nerves is great.

The subsequent care of patients with spinal cord injury is best undertaken in specialized centers. → *General principles of medical and urologic management are discussed in Chap. 373.*

BIBLIOGRAPHY

ADAMS JH et al: Diffuse brain damage of the immediate impact type. Brain 100:489, 1977

DACEY RG et al: Neurosurgical complications after apparently minor head injury. J Neurosurg 65:203, 1986

EISENBERG HM et al: Report of the Traumatic Coma Data Bank. J Neurosurg 75(Suppl)S1, 1991

GOLDSTEIN M: Traumatic brain injury: A silent epidemic. Ann Neurol 27:327, 1990

LANGFITT TW, GENARELLI TA: Can the outcome from head injury be improved? J Neurosurg 56:19, 1982

LEVIN HS et al: Neurobehavioral outcome following minor head injury: A three center study. J Neurosurg 66:234, 1987

REINUS WR et al: Practical selection criteria for noncontrast cranial computed tomography in patients with head trauma. Ann Emerg Med 22:1148, 1993

ROPPER AH (ed): *Neurological and Neurosurgical Intensive Care*, 3d ed. New York, Raven, 1993

ROSNER MJ et al: Cerebral perfusion pressure: Management protocol and clinical results. J Neurosurg 83:949, 1995

RUFF RM et al: Predictors of outcome following severe head trauma: Follow-up data from the Traumatic Coma Data Bank. Brain Inj 7:101, 1993

STEIN SC et al: Delayed and progressive brain injury in closed-head trauma: Radiological demonstration. Neurosurgery 32:25, 1993

| 375 | Stephen M. Sagar, Mark A. Israel |

TUMORS OF THE NERVOUS SYSTEM

Primary cancer of the brain and central nervous system (CNS) occurred in approximately 18,000 individuals and accounted for an estimated 13,300 deaths in the United States in 1996, a mortality rate of 2.6 per 100,000. Overall, CNS cancer is estimated to comprise 1.1 percent of newly occurring malignant tumors. CNS cancer is second only to leukemia as a cause of cancer-related deaths in children and young adults; it is the third leading cause between ages 15 and 34 and the fourth leading cause of cancer-related deaths in males aged 35 to 54. In older individuals, other diseases—especially cardiovascular and cerebrovascular disease and cancer of other organ systems—vastly exceed CNS tumors in prevalence. Among CNS tumors glial tumors are the most common, accounting for 50 to 60 percent of primary brain tumors. Meningiomas account for about 25 percent, schwannomas for

about 10 percent, and all other CNS tumors for the remainder. An increase in the incidence of gliomas in the elderly has been reported in recent years. It is unclear if this apparent increase is real or is the result of more frequent use of modern neuroimaging techniques.

Tumors that metastasize to the brain and vertebrae are more prevalent than primary CNS tumors. These tumors pose a major problem in the management of systemic cancer. About 15 percent of patients who die of cancer (80,000 individuals each year) have symptomatic brain metastases; an additional 5 percent suffer spinal cord involvement.

BRAIN TUMORS

Approach to the Patient

Clinical Features Brain tumors usually present with one of three syndromes: (1) subacute progression of a focal neurologic deficit; (2) seizure; or (3) nonfocal neurologic disorder such as headache, dementia, personality change, or gait disorder. The presence of systemic symptoms such as malaise, weight loss, anorexia, or fever suggests a metastatic rather than a primary brain tumor.

Focal neurologic deficits result from compression of neurons and white matter tracts by expanding tumor and accompanying edema. Although the mechanism of edema is unknown, tumor cells and infiltrating inflammatory cells may secrete cytokines and other factors that produce edema and may also directly affect neuronal and glial function. Venous or arterial compression may produce focal brain ischemia.

Seizures may result from stimulation of excitatory circuits or interference with inhibitory mechanisms by abnormal tissue. Tumors that invade or compress the cerebral cortex are more likely to be associated with seizures than subcortical neoplasms. Even small meningiomas that compress adjacent cerebral cortex may present with seizures.

Nonfocal neurologic dysfunction usually reflects increased intracranial pressure, hydrocephalus, or diffuse tumor spread. Multiple metastases or diffuse infiltration of the brain by glioma or lymphoma may present as dementia or a decline in level of alertness. Tumors arising in some areas of the brain may produce subtle deficits; for example, frontal lobe tumors may present with personality change or depression.

Headache may result from focal irritation or displacement of pain-sensitive structures (see Chap. 15), or from a generalized increase in intracranial pressure. In the former situation, the headache is typically localized and of constant intensity and may be strikingly positional. A headache that worsens rather than abates with recumbency is suggestive of a mass lesion. The headache of increased intracranial pressure has a characteristic pattern. Early on, as long as the elevated intracranial pressure is intermittent, headaches are primarily associated with *plateau waves* of increased intracranial pressure. These headaches are usually holocephalic and episodic, occurring more than once a day. They typically develop rapidly over several minutes, persist for 20 to 40 min, and subside quickly. They may awaken the patient from a sound sleep, generally 60 to 90 min after retiring, or may be precipitated by coughing, sneezing, or straining. Vomiting may occur with severe headaches. As elevated intracranial pressure becomes sustained, the headache becomes continuous but varying in intensity. The recent onset of a constant headache may require neuroimaging studies to distinguish brain tumor from benign etiologies, including the headache of depression. Elevated intracranial pressure may cause papilledema (see Chap. 28), although it is often not observed in patients over 55 years old.

Less commonly, brain tumor may present with a strokelike onset and focal neurologic deficit. This may be caused by hemorrhage into the tumor, but often no hemorrhage can be demonstrated and the mechanism is obscure. Tumors that often cause hemorrhage include high-grade astrocytomas and metastatic melanoma and choriocarcinoma. Rare brain tumor presentations include anosmia from a meningioma arising near the cribriform plates and olfactory tracts, and unilateral hearing loss from schwannomas of the eighth cranial nerve. Asymptomatic brain tumors, most often meningiomas, are commonly discovered incidentally on scans obtained for unrelated purposes.

The Karnofsky performance scale is useful in assessing and following brain tumor patients (see Chap. 81). A score of 70 or greater indicates that the patient is ambulatory and independent in self-care activities; it has often been taken as a level of function justifying aggressive therapy.

Laboratory Examination Primary brain tumors typically do not produce the serologic abnormalities such as an elevated sedimentation rate or tumor-specific antigens associated with other cancers. Metastases to the nervous system, depending on the type and extent of the primary tumor, may be associated with systemic features of malignancy (see Chap. 85). Lumbar puncture may precipitate brain herniation in patients with mass lesions; thus its indications are limited to the suspicion of meningitis or meningeal metastasis. Cerebrospinal fluid (CSF) findings in primary and metastatic nervous system tumors may include raised opening pressure, elevated protein level, and a mild lymphocytic pleocytosis. Astrocytomas that extend to the ventricular surface, or the rupture of an epidermoid cyst, can occasionally produce intense CSF inflammation simulating infectious meningitis. The CSF rarely contains malignant cells, with certain exceptions such as leptomeningeal metastases and primitive neuroectodermal tumors, including medulloblastoma.

Neuroimaging Computed tomography (CT) and magnetic resonance imaging (MRI) reveal mass effect and contrast enhancement. Mass effect reflects the volume of neoplastic tissue as well as surrounding edema. Brain tumors typically produce a *vasogenic* pattern of edema, with accumulation of excess water in white matter. Contrast enhancement reflects a breakdown in the blood-brain barrier, permitting leakage of intravascular contrast agent into the parenchyma. The normal blood-brain barrier results from tight junctions between endothelial cells and between endothelia and astrocytes that prevent entry of most charged molecules into the nervous system. Endothelia associated with malignant gliomas and other CNS tumors lack normal tight junctions and have abnormal passive diffusion and vesicular transport characteristics, all contributing to entry of solutes and edema. In planning therapy for malignant gliomas, the volume of enhancement observed following the intravenous administration of a contrast agent is assumed to represent the major tumor mass, but tumor cells typically extend beyond this boundary. Low-grade astrocytomas typically do not exhibit contrast enhancement.

Positron emission tomography (PET) scanning and single-photon emission tomography (SPECT) have ancillary roles in the imaging of brain tumors, primarily in distinguishing tumor recurrence from tissue necrosis that can occur following irradiation (see below). Electroencephalography (EEG) has a role in the evaluation of patients with possible seizures. Functional imaging with PET, MRI, or magnetoencephalography may be employed in surgical or radiosurgical planning to define the anatomic relationship of the tumor to critical brain regions such as the primary motor cortex.

 TREATMENT

Symptomatic Glucocorticoids decrease the volume of edema surrounding brain tumors and improve neurologic function; dexamethasone (12 to 20 mg/d in divided doses orally or intravenously) is employed because it has relatively little mineralocorticoid activity.

Tumors that involve the cerebral cortex or hippocampus may produce epilepsy and frequently present as a seizure. *Anticonvulsants* are therefore employed therapeutically and prophylactically; phenytoin, carbamazepine, and valproic acid are equally effective (Chap. 365). If the tumor is subcortical in location, prophylactic anticonvulsants are unnecessary.

Gliomas are associated with an increased risk for deep vein thrombosis and pulmonary embolism, probably because gliomas secrete procoagulant factors into the systemic circulation. Whether this risk extends to other brain tumors is unknown. Hemorrhage within gliomas is a frequent histopathologic finding, yet patients appear to be at no increased risk for intracranial bleeding following anticoagulation. Anticoagulation with low-dose subcutaneous heparin should be considered in glioma patients, especially those with lower limb weakness.

PRIMARY BRAIN TUMORS

ETIOLOGY Exposure to ionizing radiation is the only well-documented environmental risk factor for the development of brain tumors. A number of heritable syndromes, including several known to be caused by specific genetic alterations, are associated with an increased risk of brain tumors (Table 375-1). Genes that contribute to the development of brain tumors, as well as other malignancies, fall into two general classes. The first class, known as *tumor-suppressor genes*, functions physiologically to restrain cell proliferation. An *inactivating mutation* of a tumor-suppressor gene passed through the germline can predispose to the development of cancer. A single functioning copy of a tumor-suppressor gene is often sufficient to maintain normal function of the genetic locus; loss of both normal alleles is necessary to promote neoplasia. The second class of genes, *proto-oncogenes*, can contribute to tumor development by enhancing cellular proliferation. *Activating mutations* convert proto-oncogenes to oncogenes, which have a variety of functions that can promote the neoplastic phenotype. Proto-oncogenes typically encode proteins such as growth factors or growth factor receptors, mediators of signaling pathways, or regulators of gene expression. Epidermal growth factor receptor (*EGFR*) and c-*myc* are among the oncogenes that may be important for the development of brain tumors (Table 375-2).

Cytogenetic examination of chromosomes within brain tumor cells often reveals characteristic changes (Table 375-2). In astrocytic tumors, DNA is commonly lost on chromosomes 17p, 13q, and 9. In meningiomas portions of 22q are often lost. Less frequently there is evidence of amplification of specific genes, for example *EGFR* in some astrocytomas.

The particular constellation of genetic alterations varies among individual tumors, even those that appear to be histologically indistinguishable, particularly in astrocytomas. The accumulation of mutations is associated with increasingly aggressive malignant behavior.

ASTROCYTOMAS Tumors derived from astrocytes are the most com-

Table 375-1

Selected Hereditary Syndromes Associated with Brain Tumors

Syndrome	Gene	Chromosomal Location	Neoplastic Pathology of the CNS
von Hippel–Lindau syndrome*	VHL	3p	Retinal angioma, cerebellar hemangioblastoma
Li-Fraumeni syndrome*	P53	17p13	Glial tumors, medulloblastoma
Multiple endocrine neoplasia 1* (Werner's syndrome)	NK†	11q13	Pituitary adenomas, malignant schwannoma
von Recklinghausen's disease (neurofibromatosis type 1)*	NF1	17q	Neuroma, schwannoma, meningioma, optic glioma
Neurofibromatosis type 2*	NF2	22q12	Glial tumors
Retinoblastoma*	RB	13q14	Retinoblastoma, pinealoblastoma
Tuberous sclerosis	TSC1	9q	Astrocytoma
	TSC2	16p13	Astrocytoma
Turcot syndrome	APC	5q21	Astrocytomas, medulloblastoma
Werner's syndrome	WRN	8p12	Meningioma

* Genetic testing possible.
† Not known.

Table 375-2

Cytogenetic and Genetic Alterations in Brain Tumors

Tumor Type	Chromosomal Alteration	Genetic Changes
Astrocytoma	1p⁻, 9p⁻, del10, 13q⁻, 17p⁻, 17q⁻, 19q, 22q⁻, DMs*	P53, RB1, NF1, PTEN, *EGFR*, c-ros, *met, gli*, c-myc, cdk4, neu, ras
Medulloblastoma	17p,⁻ 6q⁻, 16q, DMs	
Meningioma	22q⁻	NF2
Oligodendroglioma	1p⁻, 9p⁻, 19q⁻	

* DMs, double minute chromosomes.

mon primary intracranial neoplasms (Fig. 375-1). Their neuropathologic appearance is highly variable, and numerous attempts have been made to devise histologic grading systems that accurately predict their clinical course. The traditional grading system of Kernohan and Sayre divided astrocytic tumors into grades I to IV, grade IV being the most malignant. Because of a number of limitations, this grading system has been abandoned in favor of two derivative systems, the most widely used of which is the World Health Organization (WHO) four-tiered grading system. Grade I is reserved for special histologic variants of astrocytoma that have an excellent prognosis following surgical excision. These include *juvenile pilocytic astrocytoma, subependymal giant cell astrocytoma* (which occurs in patients with tuberous sclerosis), and *pleiomorphic xanthroastrocytoma*. At the other extreme is grade IV, *glioblastoma multiforme*, a clinically aggressive tumor. In between are *astrocytoma* (grade II) and *anaplastic astrocytoma* (grade III). The defining features associated with aggressive behavior are hypercellularity, nuclear and cytoplasmic atypia, endothelial proliferation, mitotic activity, and necrosis. Endothelial proliferation and necrosis are widely regarded as important predictors of a tumor's potential for rapid growth and aggressive invasion of normal surrounding tissue. The WHO classification includes parallel grading systems for oligodendroglial and ependymal tumors. Another widely used grading system for astrocytic tumors, the Saint Anne–Mayo system, assigns a point for each of four histologic features: nuclear atypia, mitoses, endothelial proliferation, and necrosis. This produces a four-tiered grading scheme

FIGURE 375-1   Malignant astrocytoma (glioblastoma). Coronal proton density-weighted MR scan through the temporal lobes demonstrates a heterogeneous right temporal lobe mass (*arrows*) compressing the third and lateral ventricles. The area of hypointense signal (*double arrows*) indicates either hemorrhage or calcification. Heterogeneous MR signal intensity is typical of glioblastoma.

that correlates well with prognosis. A limitation of all grading schemes, especially when applied to a single biopsy, is that astrocytic tumors are histologically variable from region to region, and their histopathology may change over time. It is common for low-grade astrocytomas to recur with a higher histopathologic grade and more aggressive clinical course.

Quantitative measures of mitotic activity also correlate with clinical course. The *proliferation index* can be determined by measuring the uptake of the thymidine analogue bromodeoxyuridine (BUdR) into tumor tissue. BUdR is administered intravenously prior to surgery, and its uptake into the nuclei of tumor cells is assessed in biopsy specimens using a BUdR-specific monoclonal antibody. This provides a measure of DNA synthesis. Other methods of estimating mitotic activity include immunohistochemical staining with antibodies to the proliferating cell nuclear antigen (PCNA) or with a monoclonal antibody termed *Ki-67*, which recognizes a histone protein expressed in proliferating but not quiescent cells. These measures all correlate with malignant clinical behavior of the tumor.

The overall prognosis for patients with astrocytoma is poor. In a representative Finnish population, employing the WHO grading system, the median survival was 93.5 months for patients with grade I or II astrocytomas, 12.4 months for patients with grade III (anaplastic astrocytoma), and 5.1 months for patients with grade IV (glioblastoma) tumors. In the United States, the median survival of patients with high-grade brain tumors is approximately 12 months. In addition to histopathology, features that correlate with poor prognosis include age over 65 and a poor functional status, as defined by the Karnofsky performance scale (Table 81-2), at presentation.

Low-Grade Astrocytoma   Low-grade astrocytomas are more common in children than adults. Pilocytic astrocytoma of the cerebellum, named for its characteristic spindle-shaped cells, is the most common childhood brain tumor. Typically, this tumor is histologically benign, is well demarcated from adjacent brain, and may be cystic. Surgical excision is indicated, and long-term, disease-free survival is the rule.

The optimal management of other low-grade astrocytomas is controversial. For patients who are symptomatic, either from a focal neurologic deficit or poorly controlled epilepsy, surgical excision is the treatment of choice. Whether postoperative radiation should be administered routinely is uncertain. Although radiation may delay tumor recurrence, it is possible that radiation is best reserved for tumor recurrence, at which time the tumor may display a more malignant phenotype. When only a biopsy or partial resection is possible, postoperative external beam radiation therapy is usually administered. For patients who are asymptomatic or minimally symptomatic at presentation, a diagnostic biopsy should be performed or the tumor may be resected. There is no evidence that delaying definitive surgery and radiation therapy until the patient becomes more symptomatic is harmful. No role for chemotherapy in the management of low-grade astrocytoma has been defined.

High-Grade Astrocytoma   The overwhelming majority of astrocytomas arising in adults are high grade, supratentorial, and do not have a clear margin separating neoplastic and normal tissue. In such high-grade tumors, neoplastic cells migrate away from the main tumor mass and infiltrate otherwise-normal brain, often tracking along white matter fiber pathways. Imaging studies do not indicate the full extent of the tumor. These tumors are usually fatal, although prolonged survival occurs in a small minority of patients. Unlike systemic cancer, which is generally fatal when complications of metastases arise, gliomas cause fatal effects by local growth. Late in their course, gliomas, especially those located in the posterior fossa, can metastasize along CSF pathways to the spine. Metastases outside the CNS are rare.

High-grade astrocytomas are managed with glucocorticoids, surgery, radiation therapy, and chemotherapy. Therapy with dexamethasone is generally instituted at the time of diagnosis and continued for the duration of radiation therapy. After completion of radiotherapy, the dose is tapered to the lowest tolerated dose.

Because astrocytomas infiltrate adjacent normal tissue, total surgical resection is not possible. Surgery is indicated to obtain tissue for pathologic diagnosis and to control mass effect. In general, accessible astrocytomas are resected aggressively in patients younger than 65 years old who are in good general medical condition and in selected elderly patients. This practice is supported by retrospective studies demonstrating that the extent of tumor removal, as estimated by comparing preoperative and postoperative neuroimaging studies, correlates with survival. The extent to which selection bias influences these data is unknown. It is possible that younger, healthier patients in good neurologic condition are more likely to be offered aggressive surgery than older, sicker patients.

Postoperative radiation therapy prolongs survival and improves the quality of life of patients with high-grade astrocytomas, although the duration of benefit is only a few months. Treated with dexamethasone alone, the mean survival of patients under 65 years of age with glioblastoma is 7 to 9 months. Survival is prolonged to 11 to 13 months with radiation therapy. Focal brain irradiation is less toxic and as effective as whole-brain radiation in the treatment of primary glial tumors. It is generally administered to the tumor mass, as defined by contrast enhancement on a CT or MRI scan, plus a 3- to 4-cm margin. A total dose of 5000 to 7000 cGy is administered in 25 to 35 equal fractions, 5 days per week.

The roles of stereotaxic radiosurgery and interstitial brachytherapy are uncertain. *Stereotaxic radiosurgery* refers to the administration of a single, highly focused dose of radiation to a precisely defined volume of tissue. There are three methods of stereotaxic radiosurgery. The *gamma knife* is a series of gamma radiation sources arranged in a hemisphere around the patient's head. By controlling the dose administered from each source, a high dose of radiation can be administered to irregularly shaped tumors in a single sitting, with very low exposure of surrounding normal brain. Similar effects can be achieved with a modified linear accelerator or with a heavy particle source by rotating either the patient or the source. The latter are extremely expensive and available in only a few centers. Stereotaxic radiosurgery potentially can achieve tumor ablation without a craniotomy, and the entire procedure may be carried out in a single day. A major limitation of stereotaxic radiosurgery is that it can be used for only relatively small tumors, generally less than 3 cm in maximum diameter. *Interstitial brachytherapy*, the stereotaxic implantation of radioactive beads into the tumor mass, is generally reserved for tumor recurrence because of its associated toxicity—in particular, necrosis of normal brain tissue.

Chemotherapy is marginally effective in the treatment of high-grade astrocytoma and is often used as an adjuvant following surgery and radiation therapy. Nitrosoureas, including carmustine (BCNU) and lomustine (CCNU), are the most effective available agents. Since a typical glioma infiltrates normal brain where the blood-brain barrier is relatively intact, lipid-soluble agents such as the nitrosoureas, which cross the blood-brain barrier, may reach more malignant cells than water-soluble agents. Experimental approaches include intraarterial infusion of chemotherapy, administration of chemotherapy following osmotic disruption of the blood-brain barrier, and intensive chemotherapy regimens supported by autologous bone marrow transplantation.

Gliomatosis cerebri is a rare form of astrocytoma in which there is diffuse infiltration of the brain by malignant astrocytes without a focal enhancing mass. It generally presents as a multifocal CNS syndrome or a more generalized disorder including dementia, personality change, or seizures. Neuroimaging studies are often nonspecific, and biopsy is required to establish the diagnosis. Glio-

matosis is treated with whole-brain radiation therapy and, in selected patients, systemic chemotherapy.

OLIGODENDROGLIOMAS Oligodendrogliomas have a more benign course and are more responsive to treatment than astrocytomas. Five-year survival is greater than 50 percent, and 10-year survival is 25 to 34 percent.

Oligodendrogliomas occur chiefly in supratentorial locations; in adults about 30 percent are calcified (Fig. 375-2). Many gliomas contain mixtures of cells with astrocytic and oligodendroglial features. If this mixed histology is prominent, the tumor is termed a *mixed glioma* or an *oligoastrocytoma*. The greater the oligodendroglial component, the more benign the clinical course. As a rule, oligodendrogliomas are less infiltrative than astrocytomas, permitting more complete surgical excision. The histologic features of mitoses, necrosis, and nuclear atypia are associated with a more aggressive clinical course. If these features are prominent, the tumor is termed a *malignant oligodendroglioma*.

The optimal management of oligodendrogliomas has not been defined. Surgery, which may be limited to a stereotaxic biopsy, is necessary to establish a diagnosis. Many oligodendrogliomas are amenable to total surgical resection. In addition, oligodendrogliomas may respond dramatically to systemic combination chemotherapy with procarbazine, lomustine and vincristine administered before or after surgery. Chemotherapy may be employed as initial treatment, and residual tumor can be surgically excised or treated with stereotaxic radiosurgery. An alternative approach is to excise the accessible tumor mass initially, administer systemic chemotherapy following surgery, and employ stereotaxic radiosurgery or external beam radiation for residual tumor.

EPENDYMOMAS These tumors are derived from ependymal cells and occur in characteristic locations. In children, they occur within the ventricles, most often the fourth ventricle. Histologically, childhood tumors are highly cellular and may exhibit diagnostic ependymal rosettes. In adults they are located more often in the spinal canal, especially in the lumbosacral region, arising from the filum terminale of the spinal cord. Ependymomas arising in the sacral region of adults often have a *myxopapillary* histology, with a papillary arrangement of cells and mucin production. There is no generally accepted grading system for ependymomas, but ependymomas with his-

FIGURE 375-2 Oligodendroglioma. *A.* Noncontrast CT scan reveals a calcified mass involving the left temporal lobe (*arrows*) associated with mild mass effect but little edema. *B.* An MR T2-weighted image demonstrates a heterogeneous mass with hypointense signal (*black arrows*) surrounded by a zone of higher signal intensity (*white arrows*), consistent with a calcified temporal lobe mass. The tumor extends into the left medial temporal lobe and compresses the midbrain.

tologic signs of malignancy, including cellular atypia, frequent mitotic figures, or a high labeling index, virtually always recur. CT or MRI scans identify ependymomas as uniformly enhancing masses relatively well demarcated from adjacent neural tissue. Ependymomas may metastasize via CSF pathways: brain tumor metastases that spread to the spinal cord by this means are termed *drop metastases*.

Following total excision of an ependymoma the prognosis is excellent. The 5-year disease-free survival is over 80 percent. However, many ependymomas cannot be totally excised. In this situation, postoperative focal external beam radiation or stereotaxic radiosurgery is most often employed. Whether focal radiation is adequate or whether the entire neuraxis needs to be treated is not resolved. Prolonged survival is the rule, although the tumors generally recur.

GERMINOMAS These tumors most commonly present during the second decade of life, generally at sites within or adjacent to the third ventricle including the pineal region. Germinomas are the most frequent variety of *germ cell tumor*, a tumor type arising in midline structures and including *teratoma*, yolk sac tumor (*endodermal sinus tumor*), *embryonal carcinoma*, and *choriocarcinoma*. Germinomas of the CNS may be benign but are more often aggressive and invasive. Due to their location, patients frequently present with hypothalamic-pituitary dysfunction including diabetes insipidus, visual field deficits, disturbances of memory or mood, or hydrocephalus (see Chap. 328). On neuroimaging studies, germinomas are uniformly enhancing masses with or without well-defined borders. The treatment of choice is complete surgical resection. For unresectable tumors, a stereotaxic biopsy is performed for diagnosis, and focal radiation is given as primary therapy. When the extent of disease or very young age precludes the effective use of radiotherapy, platinum-based chemotherapeutic regimens can provide control, followed by irradiation of residual disease or irradiation of the tumor should it recur. Prognosis depends on the histology and surgical resectability of the tumor; these tumors are generally radiosensitive and chemosensitive, and 5-year survival is greater than 85 percent.

MEDULLOBLASTOMAS AND PRIMITIVE NEUROEC-TODERMAL TUMORS (PNET) These highly cellular malignant tumors are thought to arise from neural precursor cells. Medulloblastomas of the posterior fossa are the most frequent malignant brain tumor in children. If the tumor is not disseminated at presentation, prognosis is favorable; subsets of pediatric patients have 70 percent survival at

5 years, although fewer than 50 percent of children with medulloblastoma survive to adulthood. PNET is a term applied to tumors histologically indistinguishable from medulloblastoma but occurring either in adults or supratentorially in children. In adults, more than 50 percent present in the posterior fossa, but these tumors frequently disseminate along CSF pathways.

If possible, these tumors should be surgically excised, although outcome is not related to the extent of surgery. In children, the optimal use of radiation therapy and chemotherapy is currently under study; chemotherapy appears of benefit to children with high- but not low-stage disease. In adults, surgical excision of a PNET should be followed by chemotherapy and irradiation of the entire neuraxis, with a boost in radiation dose to the primary tumor. Aggressive treatment can be effective and may result in prolonged survival, although half of adult patients relapse within 5 years of treatment.

CNS LYMPHOMA Primary CNS Lymphoma This presents within the neuraxis without evidence of systemic lymphoma. While accounting for only a small proportion of total lymphomas, the incidence of primary CNS lymphoma is increasing in both immunocompetent and immunocompromised patients and may become the most common primary CNS tumor by the year 2000. Leptomeningeal involvement is present in approximately 15 percent of patients at presentation and in 50 percent at some time during the course of the illness. Histologically, primary CNS lymphomas are B cell malignancies of intermediate to high grade. They occur most frequently in immunosuppressed individuals, most often organ transplant recipients or AIDS patients (see Chap. 308). In these settings, CNS lymphomas are invariably associated with latent Epstein-Barr virus (EBV) infection of the tumor cells. Chromosomal translocations involving the c-*myc* gene occur in EBV-associated lymphomas that occur outside the CNS (Chap. 113) but not in primary CNS lymphoma.

In immunocompetent patients, neuroimaging studies most often reveal a uniformly enhancing mass lesion. In immunosuppressed patients, primary CNS lymphoma is likely to be multicentric and exhibit ring enhancement or to arise in the meninges (Fig. 375-3). Stereotaxic needle biopsy can be used to establish the diagnosis.

Prognosis is poor compared to histologically similar disease occurring elsewhere. Many patients experience a transient, at times dramatic, clinical and radiographic response to glucocorticoids. Radiotherapy is the mainstay of treatment, and systemic combination chemotherapy can provide additional benefit. Despite aggressive therapy, over 90 percent of patients develop recurrent CNS disease. In patients who do not receive systemic chemotherapy, intrathecal chemotherapy with

FIGURE 375-3 CNS lymphoma. *A.* Proton density–weighted MR image through the temporal lobe demonstrates a low signal intensity nodule (*small arrows*) surrounded by a ring of high signal intensity edema (*larger arrows*). *B.* Axial postcontrast T1-weighted MRI demonstrates ring enhancement surrounded by a nonenhanced rim of edema. In this patient with AIDS, a solitary lesion of this type suggests either lymphoma or toxoplasmosis; the presence of multiple lesions favors toxoplasmosis. *C.* In a different patient with lymphomatous meningitis, an axial postcontrast T1-weighted MRI through the midbrain demonstrates multiple areas of abnormal enhancement in periventricular and subependymal regions (*arrows*). Lymphoma tends to spread subependymally at interfaces of CSF and brain parenchyma.

methotrexate should be used if leptomeningeal disease is suspected. Historically, the survival of immunocompetent patients with CNS lymphoma has been approximately 18 months, and may now be longer with the use of systemic chemotherapy. In organ transplant recipients, reversal of the immunosuppressed state can improve outcome. AIDS-related primary CNS lymphoma has a very poor prognosis, generally 3 months or less; pretreatment performance status, the degree of immunosuppression, and the extent of CNS dissemination at diagnosis all appear to influence outcome.

Secondary CNS Lymphoma This almost always occurs in association with progressive systemic disease, generally in adults with B cell lymphoma or B cell leukemia who have tumor involvement of bone, bone marrow, testes, or the cranial sinuses. Leptomeningeal lymphoma is detected with contrast-enhanced CT or gadolinium-enhanced MRI of the brain and spine and by CSF examination. Treatment consists of systemic chemotherapy, intrathecal methotrexate, and CNS irradiation. It is usually possible to clear the leptomeningeal disease, although the overall prognosis is determined by the course of the systemic lymphoma.

PITUITARY ADENOMAS See Chap. 328.

MENINGIOMAS Meningiomas are derived from cells of the arachnoid granulations. These usually benign tumors are attached to the dura and may invade the skull but almost never invade the brain. They frequently occur along the sagittal sinus and over the cerebral convexities, in the cerebellar-pontine angle, and along the dorsum of the spinal cord. They are more frequent in women than men, with a peak incidence in middle age.

Meningiomas may be found incidentally on a CT or MRI scan or may present with a focal seizure, a slowly progressive focal deficit, or symptoms of raised intracranial pressure. The radiologic image of a dural-based, extraaxial mass with dense, uniform contrast enhancement is essentially diagnostic, although a dural metastasis must also be considered (Fig. 375-4). A meningioma may have a "dural tail," a streak of dural enhancement flanking the main tumor mass; however, this finding is not specific.

Total surgical resection of benign meningiomas is curative. If a total resection cannot be achieved, local external beam radiotherapy reduces the recurrence rate to less than 10 percent. For meningiomas that are not surgically accessible, targeted radiosurgery with the gamma knife or heavy particle radiation should be considered. Small asymptomatic, incidentally discovered meningiomas can safely be followed radiologically; these tumors grow at an average rate of only 0.24 cm in diameter per year and only rarely become symptomatic.

FIGURE 375-4 Meningioma. Coronal postcontrast T1-weighted MR image demonstrates an enhancing extraaxial mass arising from the falx cerebri (*arrows*).

Rare meningiomas have histologic evidence of malignancy such as nuclear pleomorphism and cellular atypia. A high mitotic index, as defined by BUdR labeling, is also predictive of aggressive behavior. *Hemangiopericytoma* is a morphologic variant of meningioma with an especially aggressive behavior. Meningiomas with features of aggressiveness, even if totally excised by gross inspection, should receive postoperative radiotherapy; chemotherapy has no benefit, and these tumors typically recur.

SCHWANNOMAS These tumors are also called *neuromas*, *neurinomas*, or *neurolemmomas*. They arise from Schwann cells of nerve roots, most frequently in the eighth cranial nerve (acoustic schwannoma). The fifth cranial nerve is the second most frequent site; however, schwannomas may arise from any cranial or spinal root, except the optic and olfactory nerves—myelinated by oligodendroglia rather than Schwann cells. Neurofibromatosis (NF) type II (see below) strongly predisposes to acoustic schwannoma, and schwannomas of spinal nerve roots are also seen in these patients.

Acoustic schwannomas are misnamed because they typically arise from the vestibular division of the eighth nerve rather than the acoustic division. Nevertheless, because the vestibular system adapts to slow destruction of the vestibular nerve, acoustic schwannomas characteristically present as progressive unilateral hearing loss rather than with dizziness or other vestibular symptoms. Unexplained unilateral hearing loss always merits evaluation, including audiometry and either brainstem auditory evoked potentials or an MRI scan (see Chap. 29). As an acoustic schwannoma grows, it can compress the cerebellum, pons, or facial nerve, producing corresponding symptoms. Schwannomas are with rare exceptions histologically and clinically benign. They are densely and uniformly enhancing on MRI (Fig. 375-5). Acoustic schwannomas enlarge the internal auditory meatus, an imaging feature that helps distinguish them from other cerebellopontine angle masses.

Whenever possible, schwannomas should be surgically excised. With small tumors, it is usually possible to preserve hearing in the involved ear. With large tumors, the patient is frequently deaf at presentation; nonetheless, surgery is indicated to prevent further compression of posterior fossa structures. Gamma knife treatment is also effective for acoustic schwannoma but is equivalent in cost and complication rate to surgery. Moreover, the long-term consequences of stereotaxic radiosurgery, including the possibility of secondary radiation-induced neoplasms, are unknown.

OTHER BENIGN BRAIN TUMORS *Epidermoid tumors* are thought to arise from embryonic epidermal rests within the cranium. They occur extraaxially near the midline, in the middle cranial fossa, the suprasellar region, or the cerebellopontine angle. Epidermal rests form cystic structures with the proliferative epidermal cells at the periphery, giving rise to more mature epidermal cells that migrate towards the center of the cyst. The mature cells desquamate into the liquid center of the cyst. If the cyst ruptures into the subarachnoid space, an intense chemical meningitis results. Epidermoid cysts are well-demarcated lesions that are amenable to complete surgical excision. Postoperative radiation therapy is unnecessary.

Dermoid cysts are thought to arise from embryonic rests of skin tissue trapped within the CNS during closure of the neural tube. The most frequent locations are in the midline supratentorially or at the cerebellopontine angle. Histologically, they are composed of all elements of the dermis, including epidermis, hair follicles, and sweat glands; they frequently calcify. Treatment is surgical excision.

Craniopharyngiomas are thought to arise from remnants of Rathke's pouch, the mesodermal structure from which the anterior pituitary gland is derived (see Chap. 328). Craniopharyngiomas typically present as suprasellar masses. Histologically, craniopharyngiomas resemble epidermoid tumors; they are usually cystic and in adults 80 percent are calcified. Because of their location, they may present as growth failure in children, endocrine dysfunction in adults, or visual loss in either age group. Treatment is surgical excision;

postoperative external beam radiation or stereotaxic radiosurgery is added if total surgical removal cannot be achieved.

Colloid cysts are benign tumors of unknown cellular origin that occur within the third ventricle. They can obstruct CSF flow. Intermittent obstruction can result in recurrent episodes of acute hydrocephalus, with headache and altered consciousness; sudden death rarely has been reported. Total surgical excision of a colloid cyst is usually possible.

Rare benign primary brain tumors include neurocytomas, subependymomas, and pleomorphic xanthoastrocytomas. Surgical excision is the primary treatment.

NEUROCUTANEOUS SYNDROMES

This group of genetic disorders, also known as the *phakomatoses*, produces a variety of developmental abnormalities that frequently involve skin, along with an increased risk of nervous system tumors (Table 375-1). These disorders are inherited as *autosomal dominant* conditions with variable penetrance.

NEUROFIBROMATOSIS TYPE 1 (VON RECKLING-HAUSEN'S DISEASE) NF1 is characterized by benign tumors of the peripheral nerves called *neurofibromas*, composed of Schwann cells and fibroblasts, and by pigmented lesions of the skin called *café au lait spots*. Neurofibromas frequently involve cutaneous nerves and present as multiple, palpable, rubbery, cutaneous tumors. They are generally asymptomatic; however, if they grow in an enclosed space, e.g., the intervertebral foramen, they may produce a compressive radiculopathy or neuropathy. The presence of at least six café au lait spots of more than 1.5 cm in diameter is diagnostic of NF1. Other features include hamartomas of the iris (*Lisch nodules*), axillary freckling, and pseudoarthrosis of the tibia. Hydrocephalus from aqueductal stenosis, scoliosis, short stature, hypertension, epilepsy, and mental retardation may also occur.

Mutation of the NF1 gene causes von Recklinghausen's disease. The NF1 gene on chromosome 17 encodes a protein, *neurofibromin*, which is a GTPase that modulates signal transduction through the *ras* pathway. NF1 is a tumor-suppressor gene. Patients with NF1 are at increased risk of developing nervous system neoplasms, including plexiform neurofibromas, optic gliomas, pheochromocytomas, ependymomas, meningiomas, and astrocytomas. Neurofibromas may undergo secondary malignant degeneration and become sarcomas.

NEUROFIBROMATOSIS TYPE 2 NF2 is characterized by the development of bilateral acoustic schwannomas in over 90 percent of gene carriers. Patients with NF2 have a predisposition for the development of meningiomas, gliomas, and schwannomas of cranial and spinal nerves. In addition, a characteristic type of cataract—juvenile posterior subcapsular lenticular opacity—occurs in NF2. Multiple café au lait spots and peripheral neurofibromas occur rarely.

In NF2 patients, acoustic schwannomas usually present with progressive unilateral deafness early in the third decade of life. At presentation, bilateral acoustic schwannomas may be detected on MRI (Fig. 375-5). Surgical management, designed to treat the underlying tumor and preserve hearing as long as possible, is difficult.

The NF2 gene on chromosome 22q has at different times been called *neurofibromin 2, schwannomin,* or *merlin,* with homology to a family of cytoskeletal proteins that includes moesin, ezrin, and radixin.

TUBEROUS SCLEROSIS (BOURNEVILLE'S DISEASE) Tuberous sclerosis is characterized by cutaneous lesions, seizures, and mental retardation. The cutaneous lesions include adenoma sebaceum (facial angiofibromas), ash leaf–shaped hypopigmented macules (best seen under ultraviolet illumination with a Wood's lamp), shagreen patches (yellowish thickenings of the skin over the lumbosacral region of the back), and depigmented nevi. Rhabdomyomas of the myocardium and angiomyomas of the kidney, liver, adrenals, and pancreas may also occur. Neurologic features may include epilepsy, mental retardation, and hydrocephalus. On neuroimaging studies, the presence of subependymal nodules, which may be calcified, is characteristic. Gene carriers are at increased risk of developing ependymomas and childhood astrocytomas, of which over 90 percent are *subependymal giant cell astrocytomas.* These are benign neoplasms that may develop in the retina or along the border of the lateral ventricles. They may obstruct the foramen of Monro and produce hydrocephalus.

Treatment is symptomatic. Anticonvulsants for seizures, shunting for hydrocephalus, and behavioral and educational strategies for mental retardation are the mainstays of management. Severely affected individuals generally die before age 30.

Mutations at both 9q (TSC-1) and 16p (TSC-2) are associated with tuberous sclerosis. The mutated genes code for *tuberins*, proteins that modulate the GTPase activity of other cellular proteins.

VON HIPPEL–LINDAU SYNDROME This syndrome consists of retinal angiomas and cerebellar hemangioblastomas, which are slowly growing cystic tumors that may present at any age. Hemangioma of the spinal cord; hypernephroma; renal cell carcinoma; pheochromocytoma; and cysts of the kidneys, pancreas, epididymis, or liver may also occur. Erythropoietin production by cerebellar hemangioblastomas may result in polycythemia. The von Hippel–Lindau (VHL) tumor suppressor gene has been identified on chromosome 3p; the normal VHL gene encodes a protein that appears to suppress transcription elongation by RNA polymerase II.

TUMORS METASTATIC TO BRAIN

MECHANISMS OF BRAIN METASTASES The large majority of brain metastases probably arise by hematogenous spread via the arterial circulation. The anatomic distribution of brain metastases parallels regional cerebral blood flow, with a predilection for the gray matter–white matter junction and for the border zone between middle cere-

FIGURE 375-5 Acoustic schwannoma (neuroma). *A.* Axial noncontrast T1-weighted MR scan through the cerebellopontine angle demonstrates an extraaxial mass that extends into a widened internal auditory canal, displacing the pons (*arrows*). *B.* Postcontrast T1-weighted image demonstrates intense enhancement of the acoustic schwannoma (*white arrow*). Abnormal enhancement of the left fifth nerve (*black arrow*) most likely represents another schwannoma in this patient with neurofibromatosis type II.

bral and posterior cerebral artery distributions. The lung is the most common origin of brain metastases; both primary lung cancer and cancers metastatic to the lung can metastasize to the brain. Breast cancer has a propensity to metastasize to the cerebellum and the posterior pituitary gland. This propensity could be explained by patterns of retrograde venous flow from the thorax into the skull or by an especially hospitable environment for breast cancer cells provided by the cerebellum and pituitary (the "seed and soil" hypothesis).

Invasion of the brain by a skull metastasis is rare. Although the skull is one of the most frequent bony sites of metastasis from systemic solid tumors, the dura is an effective barrier to tumor invasion of the brain. This same dural barrier also resists invasion by head and neck cancers. Skull metastases, however, can produce neurologic symptoms by compression of adjacent brain tissue or cranial nerves as they pass through skull foramina. They may also obstruct venous sinuses. Slow occlusion of venous sinuses by tumor growth may produce intracranial hypertension; however, hemorrhagic infarction of the brain generally does not occur as it does with acute venous sinus thrombosis (see Chap. 366).

In addition to lung cancer (adenocarcinoma and small cell lung cancer) and breast cancer (especially ductal carcinoma), gastrointestinal malignancies, and melanoma are other common tumors that metastasize to brain (Table 375-3). This reflects in part the high prevalence of these malignancies in the general population. Certain tumors, however, have a special propensity to metastasize to brain, including small cell lung cancer, melanoma, germ cell tumors, and thyroid cancer. By contrast, prostate cancer, ovarian cancer, and Hodgkin's disease rarely metastasize to the brain. Moreover, breast cancer that metastasizes to bone tends not to metastasize to the brain. Therefore, the cellular environment of the brain is hospitable to only a subset of systemic cancers. Parenchymal spinal cord metastases are rare.

EVALUATION OF METASTASES FROM KNOWN CANCER MRI scans reveal brain metastases as well-demarcated, approximately spherical lesions that are hypointense or isointense relative to brain on T1-weighted images, are bright on T2-weighted images, and enhance with gadolinium (Fig. 375-6). The administration of three times the usual dose of gadolinium is more sensitive than the standard protocol for detection of brain metastases. Small metastases often enhance uniformly. Larger metastases typically produce ring enhancement, representing extravasation of gadolinium through tumor vessels that lack a blood-tumor barrier, while the central area of nonenhancement represents a core of necrosis as the metastasis outgrows its blood supply. Metastases are variably surrounded by edema. Blood products may also be seen, reflecting hemorrhage of abnormal tumor vessels.

Table 375-3

Frequency of Primary Tumors that Metastasize to the Nervous System

Site of Primary Tumor	Brain Metastases, %	Leptomeningeal Metastases, %	Spinal Cord Compression, %
Lung	40	24	18
Breast	19	41	24
Melanoma	10	12	4
Gastrointestinal tract	7	13	6
Genitourinary tract	7		18
Other	17	10	30

The radiologic appearance of a brain metastasis is not specific. The differential diagnosis of ring-enhancement lesions includes brain abscess, radiation necrosis, toxoplasmosis, granulomas (tuberculosis, sarcoidosis), demyelinating lesions, primary brain tumors, primary CNS lymphoma, stroke, hemorrhage, and trauma. Prolonged focal seizures may produce MRI features of edema and contrast enhancement (resembling metastasis) at the site of the seizure focus. The contrast enhancement of a benign seizure focus, however, is generally patchy and not dense, only rarely forms a well-defined ring, and resolves 2 to 3 weeks after the seizures are brought under control.

Contrast-enhanced CT scanning is less sensitive than MRI for the detection of brain metastases. Moreover, in the presence of leaky tumor vessels there is some risk of precipitating a seizure by iodinated contrast material used for CT scanning. Pretreatment with intravenous diazepam (10 mg), or lorazepam (4 mg), 10 min before contrast administration may lessen the chance of provoking a seizure.

Cytologic examination of the CSF is not indicated, since intraparenchymal brain metastases almost never shed cells into CSF. Tumor markers such as carcinoembryonic antigen (CEA) are rarely helpful in management.

BRAIN METASTASES WITHOUT A KNOWN PRIMARY TUMOR In general hospital populations, up to one-third of patients presenting with brain metastases do not have a known underlying cancer. Lung cancer, particularly small cell lung cancer, and melanoma are the most frequent primary tumors responsible. No primary tumor can be identified even after extensive evaluation in 30 percent of patients.

The patient generally presents with either a seizure or a progressive neurologic deficit. Neuroimaging studies demonstrate one or multiple ring-enhancement lesions. In individuals who are not immunocompro-

FIGURE 375-6 Brain metastasis. *A.* Axial T2-weighted MRI through the lateral ventricles reveals two isodense masses, one in the subependymal region and one near the cortex (*arrows*). *B.* Postcontrast T1-weighted image at the same level as *A* reveals enhancement of the two masses seen on the T2-weighted image as well as a third mass in the left frontal lobe (*arrows*). *C.* Postcontrast T1-weighted axial image through the pons reveals at least four other enhancing metastatic lesions. Metastatic disease may not always produce vasogenic edema and may only be visible on postcontrast T-1 weighted images.

mised and not at risk for brain abscesses, this radiologic pattern is most likely due to brain metastasis. Diagnostic evaluation begins with a search for the primary tumor. Blood tests should include CEA and liver function tests. A careful examination of the skin for melanoma and the thyroid gland for masses should be carried out. Since most brain metastases arise from either lung cancer or malignancies that have metastasized to the lungs, a chest x-ray is the most important screening test. If the x-ray is negative, a CT scan of the chest is indicated. If these tests are still unrevealing, CT scan of the abdomen and pelvis should be obtained. If these are all negative, further imaging studies, including bone scan, other radionuclide scans, and upper and lower gastrointestinal series, are unlikely to be productive.

A tissue diagnosis is essential. After the above studies are completed, a decision must be made concerning the best site to biopsy. As a rule, the primary tumor will be more accessible to biopsy than any brain lesion. If a single brain lesion is found in a surgically accessible location without a primary tumor being discovered or with a primary tumor in a location difficult to biopsy, the brain metastasis should be approached surgically.

℞ **TREATMENT**

Once a systemic cancer metastasizes to the brain it is, with rare exception, incurable. Therapy is therefore palliative, designed to prevent disability and suffering and, if possible, to prolong life. Published outcome studies have focused on survival as the primary end point, leaving questions regarding quality of life unanswered. There is, however, widespread agreement that glucocorticoids, anticonvulsants, and radiation therapy improve the quality of life for many patients. The value of surgery and chemotherapy is less well established.

General Measures High-dose glucocorticoids frequently ameliorate symptoms of brain metastases. Improvement is often dramatic, occurs within 6 to 24 h, and is sustained with continued administration, although the toxicity of glucocorticoids is cumulative. Therefore, if possible, a more definitive therapy for metastases should be instituted to permit withdrawal of glucocorticoid therapy.

One-third of patients with brain metastases have one or more seizures. Anticonvulsants are empirically used for seizure prophylaxis when supratentorial metastases are present. There is a small risk of serious allergic reactions to phenytoin in patients undergoing cranial irradiation.

Specific Measures *RADIATION THERAPY* This is the primary treatment for brain metastases. It is assumed that there are multiple microscopic deposits of tumor cells throughout the brain in addition to metastases visualized by neuroimaging studies, thus whole-brain radiation is employed. Its benefit has been established in controlled studies, but no clear dose response has been shown. Standard protocol is to administer a total of 30 Gy in 10 to 15 fractions; an additional dose ("boost") of focal radiation to a single or large metastasis may also be administered.

SURGERY Up to 40 percent of patients with brain metastases have only a single tumor mass identified by CT scanning. Accessible single metastases are usually surgically excised as a palliative measure. Metastases are often sharply demarcated from surrounding normal brain, so they can be removed with minimal damage to functional nervous tissue. Patients frequently improve neurologically after surgery. If the systemic disease is under control, total resection of a brain lesion may improve survival and minimize disability. These expectations have been borne out in prospective and retrospective studies of lung cancer metastases.

CHEMOTHERAPY Some solid tumors that metastasize, for example, breast cancer, small cell lung cancer, and germ cell tumors, are potentially responsive to systemic chemotherapy. Although metastases frequently do not respond as well as the primary tumor, dramatic responses to systemic cytotoxic chemotherapy or hormonal therapy may occur in some cases. In patients who are neurologically

stable and in whom there is reason to expect the tumor to be sensitive to systemic therapy, hormonal therapy or two to four cycles of cytotoxic chemotherapy may be administered initially to reduce bulk disease and render the residual tumor more amenable to focal radiation therapy. Even if a complete radiologic remission is achieved, whole-brain radiation should then be administered.

EXPERIMENTAL THERAPIES These include stereotaxic radiosurgery, gene therapy, immunotherapy, intraarterial chemotherapy, and the chemotherapy administered with osmotic disruption of the blood-brain barrier.

LEPTOMENINGEAL METASTASES

Leptomeningeal metastases are also called *carcinomatous meningitis*, *meningeal carcinomatosis*, and, in the cases of specific tumors, *leukemic meningitis* and *lymphomatous meningitis*. Pathologically, three patterns of tumor involvement may be seen: (1) a diffuse coating of the leptomeninges by a thin layer of tumor cells, (2) nodular growth of macroscopic tumor metastases in meninges and on nerve roots, or (3) plaquelike metastases in the leptomeninges with many cells in the subarachnoid space and extension of tumor into Virchow-Robin spaces. Leptomeningeal metastases may coexist with parenchymal CNS metastases.

Cancers usually metastasize to the meninges via the bloodstream. Alternatively, a superficially located parenchymal metastasis may shed cells directly into the subarachnoid space. Some tumors, including squamous cell carcinoma of the skin and some non-Hodgkin's lymphomas, have a propensity to grow along peripheral nerves and may seed the meninges by that route.

Clinical evidence of leptomeningeal metastases is present in 8 percent of patients with metastatic solid tumors; at necropsy, the prevalence is as high as 19 percent. Among solid tumors, adenocarcinomas of the breast and lung and melanoma are most often responsible (Table 375-3). In one-quarter of patients the systemic cancer is under control; thus effective control of leptomeningeal disease can improve the quality and duration of life.

CLINICAL FEATURES Leptomeningeal metastases present with signs and symptoms at multiple levels of the nervous system, often in a setting of known systemic malignancy. Hydrocephalus, encephalopathy, or focal neurologic deficits from coexisting intra-parenchymal metastases may occur. Cranial nerve, spinal root, or spinal cord involvement may signify compression by bulky meningeal disease. Typically neurologic signs exceed the symptoms described by the patient.

LABORATORY EVALUATION Leptomeningeal metastases are diagnosed by cytologic examination of malignant cells in the CSF, by MRI demonstration of nodular tumor deposits in the meninges or diffuse meningeal enhancement (Fig. 375-7), or by meningeal biopsy. CSF findings are usually those of an inflammatory meningitis, consisting of lymphocytic pleocytosis, elevated protein levels, normal or low CSF glucose, and in some cases an oligoclonal increase of IgG.

A complete MRI examination of the neuraxis may demonstrate hydrocephalus due to obstruction of CSF pathways and identify bulky disease in the subarachnoid space.

℞ **TREATMENT**

Intrathecal chemotherapy and focal external beam radiotherapy to sites of leptomeningeal disease are the mainstays of management. Approximately 20 percent of patients aggressively treated for leptomeningeal metastases can expect a sustained response of approximately 6 months. Intrathecal therapy exposes meningeal tumor to high concentrations of chemotherapy with minimal systemic toxicity. Methotrexate can be safely administered intrathecally and is effective against leptomeningeal metastases from a variety of solid tumors and lymphoma; ara-C and thio-TEPA are alternative agents. Intrathecal chemotherapy may be administered either by repeated lumbar puncture or through an indwelling Ommaya reservoir, which consists of a catheter in one lateral ventricle attached to a reservoir implanted under the scalp.

FIGURE 375-7 Carcinomatous meningitis. Sagittal postcontrast MRI through the lower thoracic region demonstrates diffuse pial enhancement along the surface of the spinal cord (*arrows*), typical of CSF spread of neoplasm.

Large deposits of tumor on the meninges or along nerve roots are unlikely to respond to intrathecal chemotherapy, as the barrier to diffusion is too great. Therefore, external beam radiation is employed. Hydrocephalus is treated with a ventriculoperitoneal shunt; although seeding of the peritoneum by tumor is possible, it is rare in clinical practice.

MALIGNANT SPINAL CORD COMPRESSION

Spinal cord compression from solid tumor metastases usually results from expansion of a vertebral metastasis into the epidural space. Primary tumors that frequently metastasize to bone include lung, breast, and prostate cancer (Table 375-3). *Back pain* is usually the first symptom and is prominent at presentation in 90 percent of patients. The pain is typically dull, aching, and may be associated with localized tenderness. If a nerve root is compressed, radicular pain is also present. The neurologic signs that accompany spinal cord compression are determined by the level of the lesion; the thoracic cord is most often affected. Weakness, followed by *sensory loss* and *autonomic dysfunction* (urinary urgency and incontinence, fecal incontinence, and sexual impotence in men) are the hallmarks. Once signs of spinal cord compression appear they tend to progress rapidly. It is thus essential to recognize and treat this devastating complication of malignancy at the earliest possible time in order to prevent irreversible neurologic deficits. → *Diagnosis and management are discussed in Chap. 373.*

METASTASES TO THE PERIPHERAL NERVOUS SYSTEM

Systemic cancer may compress or invade peripheral nerves. Compression of the brachial plexus may occur by direct extension of Pancoast's tumors (cancer of the apex of the lung) or by extension of local lymph node metastases of breast or lung cancer or lymphoma. The lumbosacral plexus may be compressed by the retroperitoneal spread of prostate or ovarian cancer or lymphoma. Skull metastases may compress cranial nerve branches as they pass through the skull, and pituitary metastases may extend into the cavernous sinus. The epineurium generally provides an effective barrier to invasion of the peripheral nerves by solid tumors, but certain tumors have a special propensity to invade and spread along peripheral nerves. Squamous cell

carcinoma of the skin may spread along branches of the trigeminal nerve and extend intracranially. Non-Hodgkin's lymphoma may be neurotrophic and cause a syndrome resembling mononeuropathy multiplex. If the tumor is not sensitive to systemic chemotherapy or hormonal therapy, focal external beam radiation may reduce pain, prevent irreversible loss of peripheral nerve function, and possibly restore function.

In cancer patients with brachial or lumbosacral plexopathy, it may be difficult to distinguish tumor recurrence from radiation injury. High radiation dose or the presence of myokymia (rippling contractions of muscle) suggests radiation injury, whereas pain suggests tumor recurrence. Radiographic imaging studies may be equivocal, and surgical exploration is sometimes required.

COMPLICATIONS OF THERAPY

RADIATION TOXICITY The nervous system is vulnerable to injury by therapeutic radiation, although DNA synthesis, a primary target of radiation, occurs infrequently. The precise mechanism of injury is unknown, but the peroxidation of lipids in myelin and neuronal cell membranes following radiation-induced free radical production is probably contributory. Histologically, there is demyelination, hyaline degeneration of small arterioles, and eventually brain infarction and necrosis. However, radiation injury can occur without vasculopathy, suggesting that ischemia is a late manifestation and does not entirely account for the tissue damage.

Radiation injury to the brain is classified by the time of its occurrence. *Acute radiation injury* occurs during or immediately following therapy. It is rarely seen with current protocols of external beam radiation but may occur following stereotaxic radiosurgery. Manifestations include headache, sleepiness, and worsening of preexisting neurologic deficits. *Early delayed radiation injury* occurs within 4 months of therapy. It is associated with increased white matter T2 signal on MRI scans. In children, a common form of early delayed radiation injury is the *somnolence syndrome*, in which somnolence and ataxia develop after whole-brain radiation. Radiation to the cervical spine may cause Lhermitte's phenomenon, an electricity-like sensation evoked by neck flexion (see Chap. 373). Acute and early delayed radiation injury are steroid-responsive and self-limited disorders and do not appear to increase the risk of late radiation injury.

Late delayed radiation injury produces permanent damage to the nervous system. It occurs more than 4 months (generally 8 to 24 months) after completion of therapy; onset 15 years after therapy has been described. Following whole-brain irradiation, progressive dementia occurs, sometimes accompanied by gait apraxia. White matter signal abnormalities are present on MRI studies (Fig. 375-8). Following focal brain irradiation, radiation necrosis occurs within the radiation field, producing a contrast-enhanced mass, frequently with ring enhancement (Fig. 375-9). MRI or CT scans are often unable to distinguish radiation necrosis from recurrent tumor, but PET scans may demonstrate that glucose metabolism is increased in tumor tissue but decreased in radiation necrosis. Biopsy is frequently required to establish the correct diagnosis. *Peripheral nerves*, including the brachial and lumbosacral plexuses, may also develop late delayed radiation injury over a time span similar to that observed in the CNS.

If untreated, radiation necrosis of the CNS usually acts as an expanding mass lesion, although it may resolve spontaneously or after steroid treatment. Progressive radiation necrosis is best treated with surgical resection if the patient has a life expectancy of at least 6 months and a good Karnofsky performance score. There are anecdotal reports that anticoagulation with heparin or coumadin may be beneficial. Radiation injury also accelerates the development of atherosclerosis in large arteries, but an increase in the risk of stroke becomes significant only years following radiation treatment.

Endocrine dysfunction frequently follows exposure of the hypothalamus or pituitary gland to therapeutic radiation. Growth hormone is

FIGURE 375-8 Late delayed radiation injury 1 year following whole-brain radiation (5500 cGy). *A.* T2-weighted MRI image at the level of the temporal lobes reveals high signal intensity abnormality in periventricular white matter (*arrows*). *B.* Diffuse high signal intensity in pontine white matter (*arrows*) indicating demyelination or small vessel ischemic injury.

the pituitary hormone most sensitive to radiation therapy, and thyroid-stimulating hormone is the least sensitive; ACTH, prolactin, and the gonadotropins have an intermediate sensitivity.

Development of a second neoplasm is another risk of therapeutic radiation that generally occurs many years after radiation exposure. Depending on the radiated field, the risk of gliomas, meningiomas, sarcomas, and thyroid cancer is increased. With most high-grade gliomas and nervous system metastases, patients generally do not survive to experience these late complications of radiation therapy.

COMPLICATIONS OF CHEMOTHERAPY Chemotherapy regimens used for primary brain tumors are generally based on a nitrosourea and are well tolerated. Infrequently, nitrosoureas and other drugs used for CNS neoplasms cause altered mental states (e.g., confusion, depression), ataxia, and seizures. Chemotherapy employed for systemic malignancy is a more frequent cause of nervous system toxicity. Cisplatin commonly produces tinnitus and high-frequency bilateral hearing loss, especially in younger patients. At cumulative doses exceeding 450 mg/m², cisplatin can produce a symmetric, large fiber axonal neuropathy. Fluorouracil can cause cerebellar dysfunction that resolves following discontinuation of therapy; paclitaxel (Taxol) produces a similar picture. Vincristine, which is commonly used to treat lymphoma, may cause an acute ileus that requires discontinuation of the drug and is frequently associated with development of a progressive distal, symmetric sensory-motor neuropathy with foot drop and paresthesia.

BIBLIOGRAPHY

BIGNER SH: Cerebrospinal fluid cytology: Current status and diagnostic applications. J Neuropath Exp Neurol 51:235, 1992

BYRNE TN: Spinal cord compression from epidural metastases. N Engl J Med 327:614, 1992

FIGURE 375-9 Focal radiation necrosis 3 years after radiotherapy (7000 cGy) for carcinoma of the nasopharynx. *A.* Axial T2-weighted MRI demonstrates a mass in the right frontal lobe with surrounding vasogenic edema. Abnormal signal changes are also present on the left. *B.* T1-weighted postcontrast MRI reveals a heterogeneously enhancing mass in the right cingulate gyrus.

GLANTZ MJ et al: Treatment of radiation-induced nervous system injury with heparin and warfarin. Neurology 44:2020, 1994

KORI SH et al: Brachial plexus lesions in patients with cancer: 100 cases. Neurology 31:45, 1981

LI J et al: *PTEN*, a putative protein tyrasine phosphatase gene mutated in human brain, breast, and prostate cancer. Science 275:1943, 1997

LUNDBERG N: Continuous recording and control of ventricular pressure in neurosurgical practice. Acta Psychiatr Scand 36(Suppl 149):1, 1960

MCKUSICK VA (ed): *Online Mendelian Inheritance in Man.* URL: http://www3.ncbi.nlm.nih.gov80/Omim/. Washington, DC, National Library of Medicine, 1996

MECKLING S et al: Malignant supratentorial glioma in the elderly: Is radiotherapy useful? Neurology 47:901, 1996

MORANTZ RA, WALSH JW: *Brain Tumors.* New York, Marcel Dekker, 1994

PATCHELL RA et al: A randomized trial of surgery in the treatment of single metastases to the brain. N Engl J Med 322:494, 1990

PORTENOY RK et al: Back pain in the cancer patient: An algorithm for evaluation and management. Neurology 37:134, 1987

POSNER JB: *Neurologic Complications of Cancer.* Philadelphia, FA Davis, 1995

RUSSELL DS, RUBINSTEIN LJ: *Pathology of Tumors of the Nervous System,* 5th ed. Baltimore, Williams & Wilkins, 1989

SKLAR CA, CONSTINE LS: Chronic neuroendocrinological sequelae of radiation therapy. Int J Radiation Oncol Biol Phys 31:1113, 1995

WASSERSTROM WR et al: Diagnosis and treatment of leptomeningeal metastases from solid tumors. Cancer 49:759, 1982

WILSON CB: Meningiomas: Genetics, malignancy, and the role of radiation in induction and treatment. J Neurosurg 81:666, 1994

376	*Stephen L. Hauser, Donald E. Goodkin*

MULTIPLE SCLEROSIS AND OTHER DEMYELINATING DISEASES

The demyelinating diseases occupy a unique place in neurology owing to their frequency; their tendency to strike young adults; their diversity of manifestations, which challenges the most skilled clinician; and the range of fundamental questions in neurobiology, immunology, virology, and genetics that arise regarding their pathogenesis. These disorders share the common features of inflammation and selective destruction of central nervous system (CNS) myelin. Their course may be chronic (multiple sclerosis) or acute (acute disseminated encephalomyelitis and acute hemorrhagic leukoencephalitis). The peripheral nervous system (PNS) is generally spared. No specific tests for the demyelinating diseases exist, and diagnosis is based on recognition of the distinctive clinical patterns of CNS injury they produce.

MULTIPLE SCLEROSIS

Multiple sclerosis (MS) is characterized by chronic inflammation, demyelination, and gliosis (scarring). Lesions of MS are classically said to be disseminated in time and space. MS affects 350,000 Americans and is, with the exception of trauma, the most frequent cause of neurologic disability commencing in early to middle adulthood. Indirect evidence supports an autoimmune etiology for MS, likely triggered by an environmental exposure in a genetically susceptible host. As in other chronic inflammatory disorders, the manifestations of MS are variable and range from a benign illness to a rapidly evolving and incapacitating disease. Complications from MS may affect multiple body systems and require profound adjustments in life-style and goals for patients and their families; hence, a multidisciplinary approach is necessary to optimize clinical care.

PATHOLOGIC FEATURES   MS derives its name from the multiple scarred areas visible on macroscopic examination of the brain. These lesions, termed *plaques,* are well-demarcated gray or pink areas easily distinguished from surrounding white matter. Occasionally, plaques are also present in gray matter. Plaques vary in size from 1 or 2 mm to several centimeters. The acute MS lesion, rarely found at autopsy, is characterized by perivenular cuffing and tissue infiltration by mononuclear cells, predominantly T lymphocytes and macrophages. B cells and plasma cells are rarely found. The inflammatory infiltrates are associated with dissolution of the multilamellated myelin sheaths that surround axon cylinders. As the lesion evolves, large numbers of macrophages and microglial cells (specialized CNS phagocytes of bone marrow origin) scavenge the myelin debris, and proliferation of astrocytes (gliosis) occurs. Proliferation of oligodendrocytes, the myelin-producing cells, also occurs initially in some MS lesions, but these cells appear to be destroyed as the infiltration and gliosis progress. As a general rule, gliosis is more severe in MS lesions than in other neuropathologic conditions. Chronic MS lesions consist of complete or nearly complete demyelination, dense gliosis, and loss of oligodendroglia. In some plaques (chronic active lesions), gradations in histologic findings from the center to the lesion edge suggest that lesions expand by gradual concentric outward growth.

Lesions of MS are typically more numerous than anticipated on the basis of clinical criteria. Selective demyelination with sparing of axon cylinders is the hallmark of the disease, yet partial or total axonal destruction, and in extreme cases cavitation, may occur. Although partial remyelination (resulting in shadow plaques) is present in some lesions, more often significant remyelination does not occur. The correspondence between number and size of plaques ("plaque burden") and the severity of clinical symptoms is imprecise. Hence an extensive plaque burden may be associated with mild symptoms, or, conversely, seemingly minor pathologic changes may be present in some severely disabled individuals. Occasional cases either are clinically silent or produce "nonspecific" isolated symptoms such as facial pain, and evidence of MS is found unexpectedly at autopsy.

PATHOPHYSIOLOGY   Experimental studies indicate that demyelination may have either negative or positive effects on axonal conduction. Negative conduction abnormalities consist of slowed axonal conduction, variable conduction block that occurs in the presence of high- but not low-frequency trains of impulses, or complete conduction block. Conduction block in demyelinated fibers also may occur in response to raised temperature or with metabolic changes in the extracellular milieu of axons. Positive conduction abnormalities include ectopic impulse generation, spontaneously or following mechanical stress, and abnormal "crosstalk" between demyelinated axons. Conduction block may account for the fluctuations in function that vary from hour to hour and from day to day in MS and for the worsening that follows elevation in core body temperature. Ectopic impulse generation or "crosstalk" might give rise to Lhermitte's symptom, paroxysmal symptoms, or paresthesia (see below). Experimental therapies based on postulated conduction abnormalities in MS have included the use of calcium channel blockers to reduce the threshold for impulse generation and pharmacologic blockade (with 4-aminopyridine) of voltage-dependent potassium channels that are exposed in the internodal axon membrane following myelin loss.

PATHOGENESIS   **Epidemiology**   MS is approximately twice as common in females as in males. MS is unusual before adolescence; its incidence rises steadily from the teens to age 35 and declines gradually thereafter. The age of onset is slightly later in men than in women. MS beginning as early as age 2 or as late as the eighth decade of life is rare but well documented.

Different populations and ethnic groups have a markedly different prevalence of MS. The highest known prevalence (250 per 100,000) occurs in the Orkney islands, located north of the mainland of Scotland, and MS is also common in Scandinavia and throughout northern Europe. In the United States, the prevalence of MS is higher in Caucasians than in other racial groups, consistent with observations in other parts of the world. MS is extremely rare in Japan (2 per 100,000) and is essentially unknown in black Africans, yet Japanese Americans and African Americans are at significant risk of developing MS, with respective prevalence rates estimated at one-quarter and one-third that of Caucasian Americans.

MS is in general a disease of temperate climates. In both hemispheres, its prevalence increases with distance from the equator. Comparison of North American and European populations reveals similar prevalence rates and north-south gradients. Migration data in well-defined ethnic populations also support an effect of environment on risk. Numerous studies suggest that the prevalence of MS may be increasing, but it is possible that this finding represents an artifact due to improvements in diagnosis. Other evidence for an environmental effect on MS is derived from possible point epidemics that have occurred, e.g., the cluster of MS cases that appeared in the Faeroe Islands off the coast of Denmark following the British occupation during World War II.

Genetics Evidence for genetic susceptibility to MS has been identified in studies of ethnic groups and in family, adoption, and twin studies. Differences in the prevalence of MS among ethnic groups that reside in the same environment support an underlying genetic predisposition. Familial aggregation is also known to occur in MS, and first-, second-, and third-degree relatives of patients are at increased risk for the disease. Siblings of affected individuals have a lifetime risk for MS of 2 to 5 percent, whereas the risk for parents or to children of affected individuals is somewhat lower. Recent adoption and half-sibling studies from Canada support the concept that familial aggregation in MS is determined by genetics rather than environment. Perhaps the most compelling evidence for a genetic effect on MS is derived from twin studies, which demonstrate concordance rates of 25 to 30 percent in monozygotic twins and of only 2 to 5 percent in dizygotic twins.

A simple genetic model for the inheritance of MS is unlikely to be valid. A single-gene hypothesis is at odds with concordance estimates in twin and family studies and with the observed nonlinear decrease in disease risk as the genetic distance from the MS proband is increased. It is likely that susceptibility is determined by multiple independent genetic loci (polygenic inheritance), each with a relatively small contribution to the overall risk. It is also possible that different genetic causes of susceptibility to MS (genetic heterogeneity) may exist. Linkage and association studies have identified the major histocompatibility complex (MHC) on chromosome 6 as one genetic determinant for MS. This complex encodes the histocompatibility antigens (the HLA system) that present peptide antigens to T cells. The class II (HLA-D) region of the MHC is most strongly associated with MS, and susceptibility appears to result from the presence of the DR2 allele and its corresponding haplotype, defined by molecular criteria as DRB1 *1501, DQA1*0102, DQB1*0602. Attempts to further localize a susceptibility gene within the DR-DQ region have not provided consensus, owing to strong linkage disequilibrium across this region. In addition to the HLA region, some studies have implicated other genes, including the T cell receptor (TCR) β chain region on chromosome 7, the immunoglobulin heavy chain locus on chromosome 19, and, in a Finnish MS population but not other populations, a gene linked to myelin basic protein on chromosome 18.

Immunology MS appears to be an autoimmune disease mediated, at least in part, by T lymphocytes. In the laboratory model experimental allergic encephalomyelitis (EAE), an autoimmune disease resembling MS is induced by immunization with CNS antigens. Depending on the strain of animal or the immunization regimen used, antigens that can elicit EAE are the quantitatively major myelin proteins myelin basic protein (MBP) and proteolipid protein (PLP), the quantitatively minor protein myelin oligodendrocyte glycoprotein (MOG), and other myelin proteins or neural antigens. The sequence of immunopathogenic events in EAE is as follows. (1) Neural antigens are processed by antigen-presenting cells (APCs) in regional lymph nodes and presented to T cells capable of recognizing them. (2) Small numbers of sensitized memory T cells migrate to the CNS, where they are reactivated by antigen presented by macrophages or microglial

cells. (3) Proinflammatory cytokines, including interleukin (IL) 1, tumor necrosis factor (TNF) α, RANTES, and interferon (IFN) γ, are secreted that enhance expression of adhesion molecules by vascular endothelium, alter the permeability of the blood-brain barrier, and induce a second wave of inflammatory cell recruitment to the site. (4) Multiple effector mechanisms may contribute to the formation of EAE lesions, including autoantibodies, cytotoxicity mediated by T cells or natural killer cells, and cytokine-mediated injury to oligodendrocytes or myelin. In EAE, disease-inducing T cells most often recognize MBP or PLP, whereas autoantibodies appear to recognize MOG preferentially. The localization of MOG on the external surface of the myelin membrane probably facilitates its targeting by pathogenic antibody.

In MS, MBP-reactive T cells that carry mutations in a marker gene can be isolated from the peripheral blood. Presumably, these mutations result from chronic stimulation of MBP reactive T cells in vivo, and this finding appears to be specific for MS. The frequency of T cells reactive against either MBP or PLP is also higher in cerebrospinal fluid (CSF) than in peripheral blood in MS patients, indicating selective homing of autoreactive T cells to the CNS. Direct evidence that MBP reactive T cells are also present in MS lesions has been suggested based upon sequence analysis of the antigen-binding domain of TCR molecules expressed in brain lesions.

The diversity of the T cell response against MBP has been of considerable interest in MS. In rodents, EAE-inducing T cells recognize limited regions of the MBP molecule, termed *immunodominant regions*. These disease-inducing T cells may also express a limited repertoire of TCR genes. The limited heterogeneity of the T cell response in EAE has been exploited for therapeutic purposes, for example, by administration of synthetic peptides that resemble disease-inducing fragments of MBP but do not activate disease-inducing T cells or by immunization (vaccination) with synthetic peptides corresponding to TCR sequences present on pathogenic T cells. While effective against EAE, the usefulness of these and related approaches for the treatment of MS is uncertain. In MS, the repertoire of T cells capable of reacting against proteins of myelin appears to be heterogeneous as a rule, although immunodominant regions can be identified in some patients; for example, the region of MBP spanning amino acids 89 to 101 appears to be preferentially recognized in DR2-positive individuals.

Elevated levels of immunoglobulin in the CNS are also characteristic of MS. Membrane attack complexes can be detected in the CSF of MS patients, suggesting a role for complement-mediated antibody damage. Oligoclonal antibody—derived from expansion of a small number of different molecules—is also present in most cases. Oligoclonal Ig is also detected in other chronic inflammatory responses, including infections, and thus is not specific to MS. It is synthesized locally, and the specific pattern or fingerprint is unique to each patient. Attempts to identify an antigen against which most oligoclonal Ig is directed have been unsuccessful.

It is probable that cytokines regulate many of the cellular interactions that operate in MS. A large number of proinflammatory cytokines [IL-1, IL-2, IL-6, RANTES, macrophage inhibitory protein (MIP)-1α, TNFα, TNFβ, IFNγ] and regulatory cytokines [(IL-10, IL-4), transforming growth factor β (TGF-β)] have been detected in brain, CSF, and peripheral blood of MS patients. TNFα or IFNγ may contribute directly to tissue damage by injuring oligodendrocytes or the myelin membrane.

Patients with MS may experience relapses following nonspecific upper respiratory infections, suggesting that molecular mimicry between virus and myelin antigens may trigger attacks, or that some viruses may function as superantigens capable of activating disease-inducing T cells in MS.

Virology As noted above, epidemiologic evidence supports the role of an environmental exposure in MS. MS risk also correlates with high socioeconomic status, which may reflect improved sanitation and delayed initial exposures to infectious agents. Some viruses, e.g., poliomyelitis and measles viruses, produce neurologic sequelae that are more common when the age of initial infection is delayed.

Higher antibody titers against many viruses, including measles, herpes simplex, varicella, rubella, Epstein-Barr, and influenza-C viruses and some parainfluenza virus strains, have been detected in serum and CSF samples of MS patients compared to control individuals. In addition, a number of viruses or viral sequences have been recovered from MS tissues and fluids; recently, human herpes virus type 6 (HHV-6) antigen was reported to be commonly expressed in MS plaques. To date, no virus has been isolated consistently, nor viral material identified uniquely, from MS patients. In animals, the most widely studied model of virus-induced demyelinating disease has been infection with Theiler virus, a murine coronavirus similar to measles virus and canine distemper virus. Infection with some Theiler strains results in a chronic infection of oligodendrocytes with multifocal perivascular lymphocytic infiltration and demyelination.

CLINICAL MANIFESTATIONS (See Table 376-1)   The onset of MS may be dramatic or so mild as not to cause a patient to seek medical attention. In most published series, the most common initial symptoms were weakness in one or more limbs, visual blurring due to optic neuritis, sensory disturbances, diplopia, and ataxia.

Weakness of the limbs may appear insidiously as fatigue with exertion, a disturbance of gait, or loss of dexterity. Patients may report injury and stubbing of the great toe due to a subtle foot drop. At an early stage of the disease, weakness may not be detectable on testing. Increased motor tone (spasticity), hyperreflexia, an extensor plantar response, a Hoffmann reflex, and absence of the superficial abdominal reflex, all indicative of pyramidal tract disease, may be present. Occasionally, a tendon reflex, e.g., a triceps jerk, may be lost owing to a focal lesion in the dorsal root entry zone through which the afferent fibers of the motor reflex arc pass, simulating a radiculopathy.

Sensory symptoms include paresthesia (tingling, "pins and needles," or painful burning) or hypesthesia (numbness or a "dead" feeling). Sensory symptoms often begin in a focal area of a limb, the torso, or the head and spread over hours or days to adjacent ipsilateral or contralateral areas of the body. Involvement of segmental areas of the trunk with a "cord level" is diagnostically helpful because it distinguishes the spinal cord origin of the sensory attack from peripheral neuropathy due to the Guillain-Barré syndrome or other causes. In patients with established sensory deficits, complaints of unpleasant feelings of "swollen," "wet,", "raw", or "tightly wrapped" body parts are common.

Cerebellar involvement results in ataxia of gait and limbs. In advanced MS, cerebellar dysarthria (scanning speech) is common. In individual patients, the contribution of cerebellar involvement to specific symptoms may be difficult to define when motor and sensory deficits are also present.

Optic neuritis, common in MS, produces variable visual loss. It usually begins as blurring of the central visual field, which may remain mild or progress to severe visual loss, or, rarely, to complete loss of light perception. In mild cases, the patient may complain only of a subjective loss of brightness in the affected eye. Symptoms are generally monocular, but attacks may be bilateral. Pain, localized to the orbit or supraorbital area, is frequently present and may precede visual

loss. The pain typically worsens with eye movement. Diminished visual acuity can usually be documented on routine examination, and a scotoma (a focal area of visual loss) may be found. An afferent pupillary response (pupillodilation on exposure to direct light following constriction in response to indirect light) may be detected by a swinging flashlight test. In severe cases, the pupil on the affected side may be enlarged or irregular. Funduscopic examination may be normal or reveal swelling of the optic disc (papillitis). Venous sheathing of retinal vessels, due to the transendothelial migration of lymphocytes, is present in approximately 25 percent of cases. Pallor of the optic disc (optic atrophy) commonly follows bouts of optic neuritis. Rarely, uveitis also is present.

Visual blurring in MS may result from optic neuritis or diplopia. These two causes are distinguished by asking the patient to cover each eye sequentially and observing whether the visual difficulty clears. Diplopia in MS is often due to an internuclear ophthalmoplegia (INO) or to a sixth nerve palsy; ocular muscle palsies due to involvement of the third or fourth cranial nerve are rare. An INO consists of a delay or complete loss of adduction on attempted horizontal gaze to one side accompanied by nystagmus in the abducting eye. Convergence is preserved, which distinguishes INO from medial rectus palsy. An INO results from involvement of the crossed medial longitudinal fasciculus that connects contralateral third and sixth cranial nerve nuclei; involvement is usually on the side of the adducting eye. The finding of bilateral INO in an awake patient is highly suggestive of MS. Other gaze deficits include horizontal gaze palsy due to ipsilateral lesions of the lateral pontine tegmentum and the "one and a half" syndrome, consisting of a horizontal gaze palsy to one direction and an INO to the other.

Trigeminal neuralgia is a lancinating shocklike facial pain. In patients over 50 years of age, idiopathic trigeminal neuralgia is common and is only rarely due to MS (see Chap. 372). In patients with trigeminal neuralgia, clinical features that raise a question of underlying MS include onset at a young age, bilateral occurrence, objective facial sensory loss, and constant rather than paroxysmal pain.

Facial paralysis, resembling idiopathic Bell's palsy, may be due to MS. In MS, facial palsy is usually not associated with ipsilateral loss of taste sensation or retroaural pain, two characteristics of Bell's palsy. Chronic flickering contractions of the facial musculature, termed *facial myokymia*, is common in MS; it is thought to arise from involvement of corticobulbar tracts and deafferentation of the facial nucleus. Less commonly, facial hemispasm may occur.

Vertigo may appear suddenly and in dramatic fashion with gait unsteadiness and vomiting, resembling acute labyrinthitis. A brainstem rather than end-organ origin of vertigo is suggested by the presence of "neighborhood" signs, including trigeminal or facial nerve involvement, vertical nystagmus, or type 3 nystagmus on Bárány testing (i.e., no latency, no direction reversal, and no fatigue). Hearing loss also may occur in MS but is unusual.

Urinary bladder urgency, hesitancy, incomplete emptying, or incontinence occurs at some time in most MS patients and may be present at onset. Constipation, fecal urgency, or bowel incontinence also occur, especially in advanced MS.

Cognitive dysfunction is common in advanced MS and may also develop at an early stage or even at the onset of disease. Memory loss, impaired attention, problem-solving difficulties, slowed information processing, and difficulty in shifting between cognitive tasks are the most frequent cognitive changes observed. Impaired judgment or inappropriate jocularity may also be present. Pseudobulbar palsy consists of emotional lability, usually presenting as episodes of uncontrollable laughter or crying, associated with hyperactive facial reflexes, spastic dysarthria, and dysphagia. Depression is also common in MS.

Ancillary Symptoms   Lhermitte's symptom is a momentary electric-like sensation evoked by neck flexion, other neck movements, or coughing. The symptom typically is experienced as a shooting phenomenon that travels down the spine and into the legs. Variants

Table 376-1

Initial Symptoms of MS

Symptom	Percent of Cases	Symptom	Percent of Cases
Weakness	35	Lhermitte	3
Sensory loss	37	Pain	3
Paresthesias	24	Dementia	2
Optic neuritis	36	Visual loss	2
Diplopia	15	Facial palsy	1
Ataxia	11	Impotence	1
Vertigo	6	Myokymia	1
Paroxysmal attacks	4	Epilepsy	1
Bladder	4	Falling	1

SOURCE: After WB Matthews et al, *McAlpine's Multiple Sclerosis,* New York, Churchill Livingstone, 1991.

of Lhermitte's symptom include other tingling or painful sensations induced by neck movements, spread of the symptoms to the arms, and induction of the symptoms by movements of the lumbar spine. Lhermitte's symptom is common in MS but also occurs with many other disorders of the cervical spinal cord.

Heat sensitivity, i.e., the appearance or worsening of symptoms upon exposure to heat (typically a hot shower), occurs in most patients with MS. One characteristic form of heat sensitivity is Uhthoff's symptom, in which transient visual blurring, generally monocular, occurs with exercise or heat exposure.

Fatigue occurs in most MS patients. Fatigue is typically present in midafternoon and may consist of increased motor weakness, mental fatigue, or lassitude and sleepiness.

Paroxysmal attacks are brief, stereotyped, recurrent phenomena that frequently occur at the onset of MS or early in its course. Typical is the "tonic seizure," an unpleasant tingling or other sensation associated with tonic contraction of a limb, face, or trunk. Others consist of paroxysmal dysarthria and ataxia, diplopia, or transient unilateral paralysis, paresthesia, or pain. Attacks may be momentary or persist for 30 s or longer. They generally begin in clusters, occurring many times daily, and the patient may identify precipitating factors, such as hyperventilation or particular movements.

DISEASE COURSE   The various clinical courses of MS, illustrated in Fig. 376-1, may be grouped into four general categories. The first, *relapsing-remitting MS*, is characterized by unpredictable recurrent attacks of neurologic dysfunction. MS attacks generally evolve over days to weeks and may be followed by complete, partial, or no recovery. Recovery from attacks generally occurs within weeks to several months from the peak of symptoms, although rarely some recovery may continue for 2 or more years. Patients with a relapsing-remitting course experience no progression of neurologic impairment between attacks. This pattern characterizes the early course of the disease in most patients. In the second clinical pattern, *secondary progressive MS*, the disease has a relapsing-remitting pattern at first but evolves to be progressive. The progressive phase may begin shortly after disease onset or be delayed for several years or decades. The secondary progressive phase is distinguished from the relapsing-remitting phase by gradual progression of disability between attacks or gradual progression of disability after attacks are no longer evident.

A third pattern of MS, *primary progressive MS*, is characterized by gradual progression of disability from the onset of the disease. In some patients, periods of apparent clinical stability may occur, but there are no distinct relapses. *Primary progressive MS* affects fewer than 15 percent of all patients but is the most common form of MS in late-onset cases (i.e., after age 40). Occasionally, patients who appear to have primary progressive MS will experience superimposed relapses. This uncommon clinical course is known as *progressive-relapsing MS*.

Although the clinical course of MS is highly variable, some clinical and magnetic resonance imaging features appear to have prognostic value. Favorable prognostic factors include early onset (excluding childhood), visual or sensory symptoms alone at presentation, a relapsing-remitting course, and minimal neurologic impairment 5 years after onset. By contrast, poor prognosis is associated with truncal ataxia, severe action tremor, and a primary progressive disease course. In relapsing-remitting MS, disability results from poor or incomplete recovery from attacks in approximately half of patients and from an evolution to secondary progressive MS in the other half. In secondary or primary progressive MS, disability results from progressive spasticity, limb weakness, sphincter dysfunction, visual loss, or cognitive impairment. In general, the longer a cohort is followed, the smaller is the proportion of patients with mild disease. Fifteen years after diagnosis, approximately 20 percent of MS patients have no functional limitation, 70 percent are limited or unable to perform major activities of daily living, and 75 percent are not employed. In 1994, it was estimated that the total economic burden of MS in the United States was more than $9.7 billion.

In patients who experience a *first attack* of isolated optic neuritis, brainstem signs, or acute myelopathy, magnetic resonance imaging (MRI) of the head has been found to yield findings with some prognostic value. These patient groups are at high (50 to 65 percent) risk of developing clinically definite MS within 5 years if their brain MRI shows evidence of multiple T2-weighted lesions shortly after symptom onset. By contrast, patients with no evidence of disseminated disease by MRI at presentation have a low (5 percent) risk of developing MS over a 5 year period.

DIAGNOSIS   The diagnosis of MS is usually easily made in a young adult with relapsing and remitting symptoms referable to different areas of CNS white matter. Diagnosis is more difficult in a patient with the recent onset of neurologic complaints or with a primary progressive clinical course. In such situations, the patient should be questioned carefully for a history of prior attacks that may not be recalled initially. Other presentations that may cause diagnostic uncertainty include symptoms with a rapid or even explosive onset, suggesting a cerebrovascular accident; progressive brainstem syndromes, raising a question of brainstem glioma; cervical myelopathy in the setting of degenerative disk disease; or mild symptoms (for example sensory symptoms) unaccompanied by objective signs on examination. Rarely, a mass lesion resulting from intense inflammation and swelling may occur in MS and falsely suggest a primary or metastatic tumor.

Examination reveals evidence of neurologic disease in the great majority of patients. Abnormal signs are often more widespread than expected from the interview. For example, an MS patient may present with symptoms in one leg and signs in both. This type of finding is helpful when it permits exclusion of a single focal lesion as the source of a patient's symptoms. Other MS patients may experience symptoms unaccompanied by objective neurologic signs. They are frequently misdiagnosed as suffering from a conversion reaction, a label that should be avoided unless rigid diagnostic criteria for that condition are met.

The differential diagnosis of MS will vary depending on the specific clinical situation. Numerous diagnostic formulas have been proposed (Table 376-2); while they are useful, they cannot replace sound clinical judgment. No clinical sign or diagnostic test finding is unique to MS. However, the presence of features that are uncommon or rare in MS should call the diagnosis into question. These include aphasia, extrapyramidal syndromes suggesting Parkinson's disease, chorea, isolated dementia, amyotrophy with fasciculations, peripheral neuropa-

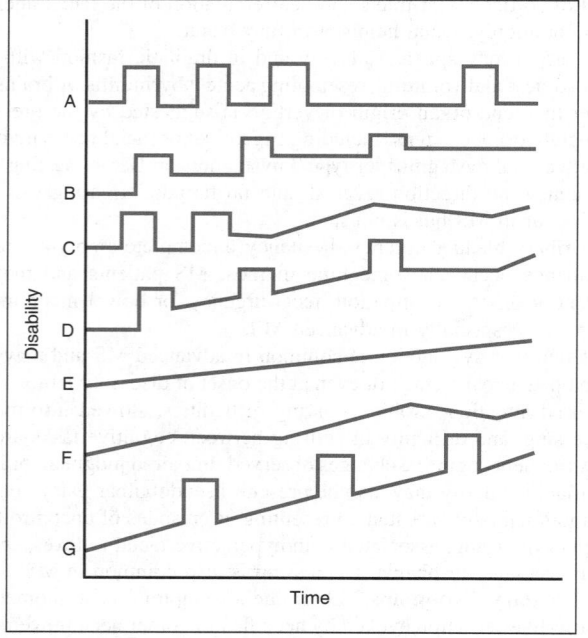

FIGURE 376-1   Clinical patterns of MS. A, B, relapsing-remitting; C, D, secondary-progressive; E, F, primary-progressive; G, progressive-relapsing.

thy, seizures, and coma. In patients with mild symptoms, there is often little to be gained by making a diagnosis of definite MS, and a wise course of action may be to exclude other, potentially treatable causes of the presenting symptoms.

Systemic lupus erythematosus (SLE) rarely produces a relapsing or progressive CNS disorder that mimics MS. Other signs of SLE are usually present, including an elevated erythrocyte sedimentation rate (ESR), autoantibodies, and evidence of systemic disease. Behçet's syndrome may produce a chronic illness with optic neuropathy and myelopathy but more often presents as an acute or subacute multifocal CNS disorder; the characteristic oral and genital lesions, associated uveitis, and elevated ESR are distinguishing features. Relapsing-remitting CNS disease also has been described in Sjögren's syndrome. Sarcoidosis may produce cranial nerve palsies (particularly of the seventh nerve), progressive optic atrophy, or myelopathy; lymphadenopathy, pulmonary or hepatic involvement, an elevated level of angiotensin-converting enzyme, and hypercalcemia may be present. Lyme borreliosis may involve the optic nerve, brainstem, or spinal cord in the absence of characteristic rash, fever, or meningoradiculitis. Other chronic infections, notably meningovascular syphilis, infection with human immunodeficiency virus (HIV) type 1, and infection with opportunistic pathogens, may need to be considered.

Human T lymphotropic virus (HTLV) type I–associated myelopathy (HAM; tropical spastic paraparesis) is characterized by back pain, progressive spasticity affecting predominantly the lower limbs, and bladder symptoms (see Chap. 379). Diagnosis is based on identification of specific antibody to HTLV-I in serum and CSF and by direct virus isolation. Infection with the HTLV-II retrovirus may cause a progressive myelopathy similar to that caused by HTLV-I.

Table 376-2

Diagnostic Criteria for MS

1. Examination must reveal *objective* abnormalities of the CNS.
2. Involvement must reflect predominantly disease of white matter long tracts, usually including (a) pyramidal pathways, (b) cerebellar pathways, (c) medial longitudinal fasciculus, (d) optic nerve, and (e) posterior columns.
3. Examination or history must implicate involvement of two or more areas of the CNS.
   a. MRI may be used to document a *second* lesion when only one site of abnormality has been demonstrable on examination. A confirmatory MRI must have either four lesions involving the white matter or three lesions if one is periventricular in location. Acceptable lesions must be greater than 3 mm in diameter. For patients older than 50 years, two of the following criteria must also be met: (a) lesion size >5 mm; (b) lesions abut the bodies of the lateral ventricles, and (c) lesion(s) present in the posterior fossa.
   b. Evoked response testing may be used to document a *second* lesion not evident on clinical examination.
4. The clinical pattern must consist of (a) two or more separate *episodes* of worsening involving different sites of the CNS, each lasting at least 24 h and occurring at least 1 month apart, or (b) gradual or stepwise *progression* over at least 6 months if accompanied by increased CSF IgG synthesis or two or more oligoclonal bands.
5. Age of onset between 15 and 60 years.
6. The patient's neurologic condition could not better be attributed to another disease. Laboratory testing that may be advisable in certain cases includes (a) CSF analysis, (b) MRI of the head or spine, (c) serum vitamin B_{12} level, (d) human T cell lymphotropic virus type I (HTLV-I) titer, (e) erythrocyte sedimentation rate, (f) rheumatoid factor, antinuclear, anti-DNA antibodies (SLE), (g) serum VDRL, (h) angiotensin-converting enzyme (sarcoidosis), (i) *Borrelia* serology (Lyme disease), (j) very long chain fatty acids (adrenoleukodystrophy), and (k) serum or CSF lactate, muscle biopsy, or mitochondrial DNA analysis (mitochondrial disorders).

DIAGNOSTIC CATEGORIES

1. *Definite MS:* All six criteria fulfilled.
2. *Probable MS:* All six criteria fulfilled except (a) only one objective abnormality despite two symptomatic episodes or (b) only one symptomatic episode despite two or more objective abnormalities.
3. *At risk for MS:* All six criteria fulfilled except only one symptomatic episode and one objective abnormality.

As noted above, the acute onset of a focal CNS disturbance in a previously healthy individual may suggest a stroke or migraine. Progressive focal deficits should always prompt consideration of a compressive lesion. Primary CNS lymphoma may produce solitary or multiple lesions that show contrast enhancement on MRI and may resemble acute lesions of MS. A progressive or relapsing brainstem disturbance may be due to a vascular malformation in the posterior fossa. Pontine glioma is distinguished from MS by its tendency to produce progressive deficits that involve contiguous structures. Chiari malformations presenting in adulthood may cause cerebellar ataxia, nystagmus, and spastic weakness of the limbs; headache, lower cranial nerve palsies, and a syringomyelic syndrome are useful distinguishing features. Progressive myelopathies may result from cervical spondylosis, spinal cord tumor, or arteriovenous malformation (see Chap. 373).

Subacute combined degeneration and two related inherited defects—cobalamin G mutation and plasma R binder deficiency—may produce MS-like syndromes in the absence of megaloblastic anemia. If a screening serum vitamin B_{12} level is low, biologically significant vitamin B_{12} deficiency is suggested by the finding of elevated serum methylmalonic acid and homocysteine levels. Mitochondrial disorders, including subacute necrotic encephalopathy (Leigh's disease), mitochondrial encephalopathy with acidosis and stroke (MELAS), and Leber's hereditary optic neuropathy, can be excluded by measurement of blood and CSF lactate levels, by muscle biopsy, and by biochemical or DNA identification of the specific deficit. Heredity ataxias produce progressive symmetric involvement of posterior columns and corticospinal and spinocerebellar tracts, with or without involvement of the peripheral nervous system. Other single-gene disorders that may resemble MS include the autosomal recessive disorders metachromatic leukodystrophy and Krabbe disease and the X-linked disorders Fabry disease and adrenoleukodystrophy. The latter is of particular interest because it is associated with an intense CSF inflammatory response.

Neuromyelitis optica (Devic's syndrome) is characterized by acute bilateral optic neuritis, followed within days to weeks by transverse myelitis. On occasion, optic neuritis may be unilateral or occur following an initial bout of myelitis. This form of demyelinating disease is unusual in Caucasians and is more common in Asians. CNS lesions may be necrotizing and severe. CSF findings may consist of polymorphonuclear pleocytosis and an increase in the protein content. Neuromyelitis optica is often a self-limited syndrome but may occur as an initial manifestation of MS or in association with SLE, or Behçet's disease.

Laboratory Diagnosis CSF abnormalities consist of mononuclear cell pleocytosis, an elevation in the level of total Ig, and the presence of oligoclonal Ig. In one large series, CSF mononuclear pleocytosis (>5 cells/µL) was present in 25 percent of MS patients. CSF cell counts are generally less than 20/µL in MS, and counts above 50/µL are unusual but may occur at the onset of disease. Pleocytosis of >75 cells/µL or a finding of polymorphonuclear leukocytes in CSF makes the diagnosis of MS unlikely. Pleocytosis is more common in young patients with relapsing-remitting MS than in older patients with progressive forms of MS. In approximately 80 percent of patients, CSF IgG is increased with a normal total protein level, due to the selective production of IgG within the CNS. Occasional MS patients exhibit mild elevations in the total CSF protein content. Various formulas are employed to distinguish local synthesized IgG from serum IgG that may have entered the CNS passively across a disrupted blood-brain barrier. One useful formula expresses the ratio of IgG to albumin in the CSF divided by the ratio in the serum ("the CSF IgG index").

Oligoclonal banding of CSF IgG is detected by agarose gel electrophoresis techniques. Two or more oligoclonal bands are found in 75 to 90 percent of MS patients. Oligoclonal banding may be absent at the onset of MS, and in individual patients the number of bands present may increase with time. It is important that paired serum samples be studied to exclude a systemic origin of the oligoclonal bands.

Paraclinical tests for MS include evoked response testing and MRI. Evoked response testing may detect slowed or abnormal conduction in visual, auditory, somatosensory, or motor pathways. These tests employ computer averaging techniques to record the electrical response evoked in the nervous system following repetitive sensory or motor stimuli. One or several evoked responses are abnormal in 80 to 90 percent of patients with MS. Testing is of greatest value when it provides evidence of a second lesion in a patient with a single clinically apparent lesion or when it demonstrates an objective abnormality in a patient with subjective complaints and normal findings on neurologic examination. Slowing of evoked response latencies in MS is thought to result from loss of saltatory conduction along the course of demyelinated axons. Nonetheless, these changes are etiologically nonspecific and are also present in other conditions, including vascular disease, in which selective demyelination does not occur.

Widespread availability of MRI has revolutionized the diagnostic approach to the patient with suspected MS. Disease-related changes are detected by MRI in more than 90 percent of patients who otherwise meet diagnostic criteria for definite MS (Fig. 376-2 and 376-3). On inversion-recovery or T1-weighted imaging sequences, the brain may appear normal or show darkened (hypointense) punctate foci in the white matter. Characteristic changes of MS are best appreciated with spin-echo (T2-weighted) and proton-density sequences, in which abnormal hyperintense areas stand out brightly from the surrounding brain substance. Some foci that are hyperintense on T2-weighted images may appear to extend outward from the ventricular surface, corresponding to a pattern of perivenous demyelination that is observed pathologically in MS (Dawson's fingers). Lesions are also commonly found within the brainstem, cerebellum, and spinal cord. The presence of lesions in the corpus callosum may also be useful, as the corpus callosum is frequently involved in MS but not in most vascular disorders.

Following administration of the contrast agent gadolinium DPTA, foci of white matter enhancement may be present, due to extravasation of the injected substance across a disrupted blood-brain barrier. New T2-weighted lesions are generally preceded or accompanied by transient gadolinium enhancement on T1-weighted scans, and histopathologic data indicate that gadolinium leakage in MS correlates with perivenous inflammation. Focal lesions that appear during or after gadolinium enhancement on T2-weighted and proton-density images are not histopathologically specific; they may reflect edema, inflammation, demyelination, gliosis, or axonal loss.

Serial MRI studies indicate that new abnormal foci appear far more frequently than anticipated by clinical criteria, suggesting that flares of subclinical disease activity occur commonly in MS. There is only a limited correlation between the total volume of lesions visible on

FIGURE 376-2 MRI findings in MS. *A, B.* Axial first-echo images from T2-weighted sequences demonstrate multiple bright signal abnormalities in white matter, typical for MS. *C.* Sagittal T2-weighted FLAIR (fluid attenuated inversion recovery) image in which the high signal of CSF has been suppressed. CSF appears dark, while areas of brain edema or demyelination appear high in signal as shown here in the corpus callosum (*arrows*). *D.* Sagittal T1-weighted image obtained after the intravenous administration of gadolinium DTPA reveals focal areas of blood-brain barrier disruption, identified as high-signal-intensity regions (*arrows*).

FIGURE 376-3 Spinal cord imaging in MS. Sagittal T2-weighted MRI scan (*left*) reveals multiple areas of bright signal abnormality (*black arrows*) within the spinal cord. In a T1 sequence (*right*), two discrete areas of contrast enhancement (*white arrows*) are present following administration of gadolinium EDTA.

T2-weighted scans and the clinical status of the patient. The correlation between MRI measures and clinical status may be improved by emerging imaging techniques, including magnetization transfer imaging, proton-magnetic resonance spectroscopy, and diffusion-weighted imaging, which better distinguish edema, demyelination, and axonal loss.

Criteria for use of MRI in support of a diagnosis of MS have been proposed. On T2-weighted or proton-density MRI brain scans, a finding of four or more focal lesions ≥3 mm in diameter or of three lesions of which one or more are periventricular in location strongly supports a diagnosis of definite MS in patients younger than 50 years. For patients older than 50 years, acceptable sensitivity and specificity are maintained by adding two of the following criteria: (1) lesion diameter greater than 5 mm, (2) the presence of lesion(s) abutting the bodies of the lateral ventricles, and (3) the presence of lesion(s) in the posterior fossa.

℞ TREATMENT

The treatment of MS may be divided into two categories: (1) treatment designed to arrest the disease process and (2) symptomatic management. The importance of longitudinal scoring of the functional consequences of MS cannot be overemphasized as an aid to decisions regarding therapy. The Kurtzke Expanded Disability Status Scale (EDSS) is the most widely used measure of neurologic impairment and disability in MS. It is based on composite scores of pyramidal, cerebellar, brainstem, sensory, bowel and bladder, visual, and mental functions (Table 376-3).

Disease Modifying Therapy (See Fig. 376-4) **PROPHYLAXIS AGAINST RELAPSES** Three treatments are available for patients with relapsing forms of MS: (1) IFNβ1b (Betaseron), (2) IFNβ1a (Avonex), and (3) copolymer 1 (Copaxone). There is a notion that patients with secondary progressive MS who experience frequent exacerbations may also benefit from these treatments. IFNβ1b, 8.0 million international units (MIU), is administered by subcutaneous injection every other day. IFNβ1a, 6.0 MIU, is administered by intramuscular injection once every week. Copolymer 1, 20 mg, is administered by subcutaneous injection every day. The mechanism of action of these treatments is not certain. IFNβ1b and -1a may act by down regulating the following: (1) the expression of MHC molecules on the surface of antigen presenting cells, (2) the actions of proinflammatory cytokines and, (3) the expression of vascular endothelial adhesion molecules that appear to mediate trafficking of activated lymphocytes and macrophages into the CNS. Copolymer 1 may act by (1) induction of antigen-specific suppressor T cells as a result of shared determinants between copolymer 1 and myelin basic protein and, (2) competitive binding to the MHC molecule on the surface of antigen-presenting cells. When compared to results in placebo recipients, each of these therapies reduces annual exacerbation rates by approximately one-third and IFNβ1b and -1a reduce the number of new lesions that are detected by monthly gadolinium-enhanced MRI scans. Of the three treatment options, IFNβ1a most convincingly delays the time to onset of sustained progression of disability. IFNβ1b and -1a and copolymer 1 are generally well tolerated. Erythematous injection site reactions are commonly experienced by IFNβ1b and copolymer 1 recipients. Approximately 15 percent of copolymer 1 recipients experience one or more episodes of flushing, chest tightness, dyspnea, palpitations, and anxiety following injection. This systemic reaction is unpredictable and generally lasts less than 1 h. Approximately 40 percent of IFNβ1b recipients and approximately 20 percent of IFNβ1a recipients develop neutralizing antibodies within 12 months of initiating therapy, and these patients may experience a return to their pretreatment attack rate. Treatment should probably be discontinued in IFNβ1b, -1a, and copolymer 1 recipients who continue to experience frequent attacks or gradual progression of disability for 6 or more months. It is unknown whether patients who fail treatment with one of these interventions will respond favorably to one of the alternatives or to combination therapy. Recently, intravenous immunoglobulin was also reported to be effective as prophylaxis against relapses, but confirmatory studies will be required before a role for this potential therapy is established.

ACUTE RELAPSES Acute relapses may be treated with a short course of intravenous methylprednisolone (MePDN) followed by oral prednisone (PDN) (Table 376-4). This combination has largely

FIGURE 376-4 Therapeutic decision making for MS.

replaced adrenocorticotropic hormone (ACTH) as the mainstay of treatment, but courses of ACTH may still be used in selected patients or in cases of MePDN/PDN treatment failure. Pulse therapy with these agents speeds recovery from acute relapses and may modestly improve the degree of recovery occurring over a short follow-up period.

MePDN/PDN is generally used to treat moderate or severe attacks that result in functional disability that can be measured by changes on the EDSS. Severe attacks that jeopardize patient safety are best treated in the hospital with intravenous methylprednisolone or intramuscular ACTH and coordinated efforts by experts in multidisciplinary rehabilitation. Mild attacks, for example, subjective sen-

sory symptoms unaccompanied by objective changes on examination, Lhermitte's symptom, or worsening of bladder function, are generally not treated.

When neurologic worsening occurs in patients with relapsing MS, it is useful to consider whether it reflects new inflammatory lesions in the CNS or whether it is a nonspecific consequence of infection (commonly a viral infection or urinary tract infection) or other intercurrent illness. MS typically worsens transiently following exposure of the patient to heat, stress, or infection. These "pseudoexacerbations" may consist only of recrudescences of old symptoms and may be short-lived (e.g., less than 48 h in duration). Patients with relapsing MS experience on average fewer than 1.0 true relapses per year.

Common side effects of short-term glucocorticoid therapy include fluid retention, potassium loss, weight gain, gastric distur-

---

Table 376-3

Scoring Systems for MS

KURTZKE EXPANDED DISABILITY SCORE (EDSS)

0.0 = Normal neurologic exam [all grade 0 in functional status (FS)]
1.0 = No disability, minimal signs in one FS (i.e., grade 1)
1.5 = No disability, minimal signs in more than one FS (more than one grade 1)
2.0 = Minimal disability in one FS (one FS grade 2, others 0 or 1)
2.5 = Minimal disability in two FS (two FS grade 2, others 0 or 1)
3.0 = Moderate disability in one FS (one FS grade 3, others 0 or 1) or mild disability in three or four FS (three/four FS grade 2, others 0 or 1) though fully ambulatory
3.5 = Fully ambulatory but with moderate disability in one FS (one grade 3) and one or two FS grade 2; or two FS grade 3; or five FS grade 2 (others 0 or 1)
4.0 = Ambulatory without aid or rest for ≥ 500 m
4.5 = Ambulatory without aid or rest for ≥ 300 m
5.0 = Ambulatory without aid or rest for ≥ 200 m
5.5 = Ambulatory without aid or rest for ≥ 100 m

6.0 = Unilateral assistance required to walk about 100 m with or without resting
6.5 = Constant bilateral assistance required to walk about 20 m without resting
7.0 = Unable to walk beyond about 5 m even with aid; essentially restricted to wheelchair; wheels self and transfers alone
7.5 = Unable to take more than a few steps; restricted to wheelchair; may need aid to transfer
8.0 = Essentially restricted to bed or chair or perambulated in wheelchair, but out of bed most of day; retains many self-care functions; generally has effective use of arms
8.5 = Essentially restricted to bed much of the day; has some effective use of arm(s); retains some self-care functions
9.0 = Helpless bed patient; can communicate and eat
9.5 = Totally helpless bed patient; unable to communicate or eat
10.0 = Death due to MS

FUNCTIONAL STATUS (FS) SCORE

A. Pyramidal functions
  0 = Normal
  1 = Abnormal signs without disability
  2 = Minimal disability
  3 = Mild or moderate paraparesis or hemiparesis, or severe monoparesis
  4 = Marked paraparesis or hemiparesis, moderate quadriparesis, or monoplegia
  5 = Paraplegia, hemiplegia, or marked quadriparesis
  6 = Quadriplegia
B. Cerebellar functions
  0 = Normal
  1 = Abnormal signs without disability
  2 = Mild ataxia
  3 = Moderate truncal or limb ataxia
  4 = Severe ataxia all limbs
  5 = Unable to perform coordinated movements due to ataxia
C. Brainstem functions
  0 = Normal
  1 = Signs only
  2 = Moderate nystagmus or other mild disability
  3 = Severe nystagmus, marked extraocular weakness, or moderate disability of other cranial nerves
  4 = Marked dysarthria or other marked disability
  5 = Inability to swallow or speak
D. Sensory functions
  0 = Normal
  1 = Vibration or figure-writing decrease only, in 1 or 2 limbs
  2 = Mild decrease in touch or pain or position sense, and/or moderate decrease in vibration in 1 or 2 limbs, or vibratory (c/s figure writing) decrease alone in 3 or 4 limbs
  3 = Moderate decrease in touch or pain or position sense, and/or essentially lost vibration in 1 or 2 limbs, or mild decrease in touch or pain, and/or moderate decrease in all proprioceptive tests in 3 or 4 limbs
  4 = Marked decrease in touch or pain or loss of proprioception, alone or combined, in 1 or 2 limbs or moderate decrease in touch or pain and/or severe proprioceptive decrease in more than 2 limbs

  5 = Loss (essentially) of sensation in 1 or 2 limbs or moderate decrease in touch or pain and/or loss of proprioception for most of the body below the head
  6 = Sensation essentially lost below the head
E. Bowel and bladder functions
  0 = Normal
  1 = Mild urinary hesitancy, urgency, or retention
  2 = Moderate hesitancy, urgency, retention of bowel or bladder, or rare urinary incontinence
  3 = Frequent urinary incontinence
  4 = In need of almost constant catheterization
  5 = Loss of bladder function
  6 = Loss of bowel and bladder function
F. Visual (or optic) functions
  0 = Normal
  1 = Scotoma with visual acuity (corrected) better than 20/30
  2 = Worse eye with scotoma with maximal visual acuity (corrected) of 20/30 to 20/59
  3 = Worse eye with large scotoma, or moderate decrease in fields, but with maximal visual acuity (corrected) of 20/60 to 20/99
  4 = Worse eye with marked decrease of fields and maximal acuity (corrected) of 20/100 to 20/200; grade 3 plus maximal acuity of better eye of 20/60 or less
  5 = Worse eye with maximal visual acuity (corrected) less than 20/200; grade 4 plus maximal acuity of better eye of 20/60 or less
  6 = Grade 5 plus maximal visual acuity of better eye of 20/60 or less
G. Cerebral (or mental) functions
  0 = Normal
  1 = Mood alteration only (does not affect EDSS score)
  2 = Mild decrease in mentation
  3 = Moderate decrease in mentation
  4 = Marked decrease in mentation
  5 = Chronic brain syndrome—severe or incompetent

SOURCE: After JF Kurtzke, Neurology 33:1444, 1983.

Therapeutic Regimens for Exacerbations of MS

Methylprednisolone-Prednisone

Inpatient administration: Methylprednisolone, 250 mg, is mixed in 250 mL D₅W and administered over 1–2 h IV q 6 h for 3 days, followed by oral prednisone (1 mg/kg/d as single A.M. dose) on days 4–17, 20 mg on day 18, and 10 mg on days 19–21

Outpatient administration: Methylprednisolone, 1000 mg slow IV push daily for 3 days, followed by oral prednisone (1 mg/kg/d) on days 4–17, 20 mg on day 18, and 10 mg on days 19–21

ACTH

1. Aqueous ACTH (20 U/mL), 80 U administered in 500 mL D₅W over 6–8 h for 3 days, followed by
2. ACTH gel (40 U/mL), 40 U administered IM bid for 7 days, followed by
3. ACTH gel (40 U/mL), tapered as follows: 35 U bid for 3 days; 30 U bid for 3 days; 50 U qd for 3 days; 40 U qd for 3 days; 30 U qd for 3 days; 20 U qd for 3 days; 20 U every other day for 3 doses

---

bances, acne, and emotional lability. Salt and fluid retention are managed with a low-salt, potassium-rich diet and avoidance of potassium-wasting diuretics. In patients who have heart disease or require concurrent diuretic therapy, oral potassium supplementation is advised. Lithium carbonate (300 mg orally bid) may provide effective prophylaxis for patients who experience emotional lability and insomnia associated with glucocorticoid therapy. In patients with a history of peptic ulcer disease, cimetidine (400 mg bid) or ranitidine (150 mg bid) is advised.

TREATMENT OF AN INITIAL ATTACK A modified approach is employed for treatment of an initial attack of demyelinating disease. In this setting, MS may be a diagnostic possibility, but recurrent signs and symptoms, required for a diagnosis of definite MS, have not occurred. In cases of moderate to severe acute optic neuritis, MePDN/PDN modestly speeds recovery but has little effect on the ultimate degree of recovery. It may also protect against evolution to clinically definite MS over a 2-year period in patients who have disseminated abnormalities detected by brain MRI. Oral PDN alone should probably not be used for treatment of uncomplicated optic neuritis, as its use in one study was associated with an increase in the frequency of subsequent relapses.

Treatment of other acute demyelinating disorders—including transverse myelitis and isolated brainstem syndromes—is largely empirical. It is reasonable to perform brain MRI on patients with all monosymptomatic presentations of demyelinating disease and to treat moderate to severe symptoms, or presumptive disseminated disease detected by MRI, with MePDN/PDN.

CHRONIC PROGRESSION There is a limited role for chronic immunosuppression in the specific treatment of progressive MS symptoms. These treatments should be administered only with the understanding that they carry both short- and long-term risks and that their efficacy in MS is modest. Monotherapy with either methotrexate or azathioprine given orally is a reasonable initial approach.

Methotrexate, 7.5 mg administered orally once each week for up to 2 years, reduces both disease activity as assessed by MRI and sustained progression of disability as measured by standardized tests of upper extremity function. An important practical advantage of methotrexate is the simplicity of a weekly dosing schedule. Most patients experience few or no side effects from low-dose methotrexate therapy. Nausea, diarrhea, headache, myalgia, or fever may require discontinuation of the drug, or these side effects may be treated symptomatically. Laboratory monitoring should include a complete blood count and tests of hepatic and renal function at 8-week intervals.

Chronic azathioprine therapy also has a small beneficial effect on the course of MS. It is administered orally as a single daily dose of 2 to 3 mg/kg. A complete blood count and tests of liver function should be performed initially at monthly intervals and then bimonthly in patients who receive azathioprine. In patients who experience a fall in the white blood cell count (WBC), the dosage is adjusted to

maintain the WBC between 3.5×10^3 and 4.0×10^3 cells/µL. The most frequent side effects of azathioprine therapy are nausea and abdominal pain that may require a lowering of the dose or cessation of therapy. The most serious long-term consequence of azathioprine is the development of hepatic toxicity, and liver function thus must be monitored closely. Other possible adverse effects include skin rash, susceptibility to opportunistic infection, and a possible increase in the frequency of non-Hodgkin's lymphoma.

Pulse therapy with the alkylating agent cyclophosphamide may slow disease progression in patients with secondary progressive MS. Benefits appear to be restricted to patients younger than 40 years who experience rapid progression of neurologic impairment. The side effects associated with treatment include nausea, hair loss, hemorrhagic cystitis, and temporary profound immunosuppression.

2-Chlorodeoxyadenosine (2-CDA; Cladribine) appears to reduce MRI activity and progression of disability in chronic progressive MS. 2-CDA is well tolerated when administered at a dose of 0.1 mg/kg body weight intravenously each day for 1 week each month for 4 months. Sustained lymphopenia, thrombocytopenia, and eruptions of herpes zoster are significant risks of this therapy. Uncontrolled studies suggest similar benefits when 2-CDA is administered subcutaneously at a dose of 0.07 mg/kg body weight for 5 consecutive days each month for 5 months. The results of a phase-III study of 2-CDA in patients with chronic progressive MS are expected in 1997 and will help clarify the role of this promising therapy.

The clinical efficacy of immunosuppression for progressive MS is modest and does not justify its use in all patients with progressive disease. Relative contraindications include age greater than 60 years, nonambulatory status, or a primary progressive course. Patients with secondary progressive MS who also experience frequent relapses may be best treated with IFNβ as initial therapy. If immunosuppression is undertaken, a yearly reevaluation of its value—its beneficial and deleterious effects—is required.

OTHER THERAPEUTIC CLAIMS Purported therapies of no proven value include megadose vitamins, calcium orotate, bee stings, cow colostrum, hyperbaric oxygen, and chelation. Patients should be discouraged from seeking out costly or potentially hazardous therapies carried out by well-meaning but naive practitioners. The National Multiple Sclerosis Society remains the best source for information on therapeutic options for MS.

Symptomatic Therapy Spasticity with stiffness, flexor spasms, and clonus can be disabling and painful. Acute worsening of spasticity may occur with underlying infection (frequently of the urinary tract), obstipation, bedsores, other painful lesions, or injuries. These precipitants should be sought out and treated specifically. All medications for spasticity have limited efficacy and may produce symptomatic worsening in patients who require stiffness in order to ambulate. Baclofen (15 to 80 mg/d in divided doses) is the most useful drug available. In refractory cases, oral baclofen in higher doses (up to 240 mg/d) or intrathecal administration via an indwelling catheter may be effective. Diazepam (2 mg bid or tid) is useful in patients who tolerate its sedative effect, and a single bedtime dose may be especially effective for nocturnal spasms. Cyclobenzaprine hydrochloride (5 to 10 mg bid or tid), clonazepam (0.5 to 1.0 mg tid, including a bedtime dose), tizanidine (2 to 8 mg tid, including a bedtime dose), and clonidine hydrochloride (0.1 to 0.2 mg tid, including a bedtime dose) may be useful in patients who fail to respond to baclofen. Dantrolene may produce unacceptable weakness, and its use is reserved for nonambulatory patients. A course of glucocorticoids may be given in exceptional cases where other agents have failed, but benefits seldom last more than 2 to 3 weeks.

Pain, including trigeminal neuralgia and painful dysesthesias, may respond to carbamazepine (100 to 1200 mg/d in divided, escalating doses), phenytoin (300 mg/d), or amitriptyline (50 to 200 mg/d). It may be difficult to distinguish dysesthesias due to MS from radiculopathy due to lumbar disk disease in patients with unilateral leg pain; nonsurgical therapy is justified in the absence of convincing signs of nerve root compression.

Paroxysmal symptoms respond to carbamazepine (up to 1200 mg in divided doses) or acetazolamide (125 to 250 mg tid). Although no treatment for tremor is satisfactory, slight improvement is occasionally seen with clonazepam (0.5 to 1.0 mg bid or tid), primidone (125 to 250 mg bid or tid), ondansetron (4 to 8 mg bid or tid), and isoniazid (up to 1200 mg in divided doses). Stereotaxic thalamotomy may be considered in rare cases of disabling tremor in which a unilateral reduction in symptoms is required, but the combined experience with this procedure has been disappointing.

Because specific symptoms of bladder dysfunction correlate poorly with physiologic findings, urodynamic evaluation is often required. The pathophysiology of abnormal micturition also may change over time in MS. Bladder hyperreflexia is treated with anticholinergics (oxybutynin, 5 mg bid or tid, or propantheline, 7.5 to 15 mg qid). Urinary retention due to bladder hyporeflexia may respond to the cholinergic drug bethanecol (10 to 50 mg tid or qid). Dyssynergia between detrusor and external sphincter muscles may be treated effectively with a combination of anticholinergic medication to decrease bladder contractions and intermittent catheterization. Terazosin hydrochloride (1 to 5 mg at bedtime) ameliorates dyssynergia but may result in urinary incontinence in occasional patients. Supravesical urinary diversion or a chronic indwelling catheter may be required in cases of severe bladder disturbance. Ascorbic acid may reduce the risk of urinary tract infections.

Bowel dysfunction, including constipation and urge incontinence, can be ameliorated by regimentation of bowel function with laxatives and enemas. A low-fiber diet to decrease bulk may be advised for incontinence. Sexual dysfunction may be treated in males by implantation of a penile prosthesis, or erections may be achieved pharmacologically using papaverine and phentolamine injections in the corpora cavernosa. Women may experience vaginismus, which may respond to antispasticity medications, or decreased vaginal lubrication leading to dyspareunia, which may be simply treated with lubricants.

Afternoon fatigue may benefit from a shift to an early work schedule or by a regular afternoon nap. Amantadine (100 mg bid), pemoline (37.5 mg bid), or fluoxetine hydrochloride (20 mg qd or bid) may prove useful in some patients with disabling fatigue. Emotional lability often responds to amitriptyline (25 to 75 mg/d) or fluoxetine (20 mg/d). It is essential to be vigilant for clinical evidence of depression, since suicide is an important cause of death in MS. Occupational counseling and other support services may assist patients and their families in coping with the effects of the disease. Health maintenance should be emphasized, including stress reduction, a balanced diet, avoidance of rapid weight loss, and adequate rest. There is little evidence linking vaccination with relapses of MS, yet it would be prudent to avoid unnecessary immunizations. Swimming is an ideal form of exercise for many patients because of the buoyant support and hypothermia that is achieved.

Pregnancy may affect the course of MS. Compared with nonpregnant MS patients, pregnant patients experience fewer attacks during gestation but more attacks in the first 3 months after parturition. The two effects appear to be roughly similar in magnitude; thus, no effect of pregnancy on disability or on the overall disease course has been identified. It is possible that high levels of prolactin induced in the postpartum period and maintained by breast feeding result in immune stimulation that predisposes to relapses of MS, but one retrospective study found no effect of breast feeding on attack frequency. The advisability of childbearing should be determined primarily by the patient's physical state and available family support.

ACUTE DISSEMINATED ENCEPHALOMYELITIS

DEFINITION AND PATHOGENESIS In contrast to the chronic disorder MS, acute disseminated encephalomyelitis (ADEM) is distinguished by a monophasic course and a frequent association with antecedent immunization (postvaccinal encephalomyelitis) or infection (postinfectious encephalomyelitis). The pathologic hallmark of ADEM is the presence of widely scattered small foci of perivenular inflammation and demyelination. The illness is sudden in onset and may be neurologically devastating or self-limited.

Postvaccinal encephalomyelitis may follow the administration of smallpox and certain rabies vaccines. Rabies vaccine complications result from the Semple vaccine, which uses phenol-inactivated virus propagated in brains of adult animals. The likelihood of ADEM from this vaccine has been variously estimated at between 1 in 400 and 1 in 5000. The introduction of rabies vaccine grown in duck embryo or human diploid tissue has largely eliminated this complication in developed countries, but use of the Semple vaccine continues in some parts of the world. ADEM also may complicate smallpox vaccination, but the worldwide disappearance of smallpox has eliminated the need for prophylaxis.

Postinfectious encephalomyelitis is most frequently associated with the viral exanthems of childhood. The neurologic syndrome generally begins late in the course of the viral illness as the exanthem is fading. Natural infection with measles virus is the most common antecedent (1 in 1000 cases). Worldwide, measles encephalomyelitis remains a common illness, but in developed countries, use of the live measles vaccine has dramatically reduced its incidence. An ADEM-like illness rarely follows vaccination with live measles vaccine (1 to 2 in 10^6 immunizations). ADEM is now most frequently associated with varicella-chickenpox infections (1 in 4000 to 10,000). It also may follow infection with rubella, mumps, influenza, parainfluenza, and infectious mononucleosis viruses and with *Mycoplasma*. In some patients, a nonspecific upper respiratory infection or no known antecedent illness is present.

An autoimmune response to MBP can be detected in the CSF from many patients with ADEM. This has been most clearly established following rabies vaccination and infection with measles virus. With measles infection, induction of immune responses to a variety of CNS antigens may occur, but only the response to MBP correlates with development of ADEM. As noted earlier, many cases of postvaccinal encephalomyelitis almost certainly result from sensitization with brain material that contaminates the viral vaccines. Many attempts to demonstrate direct viral invasion of the CNS have been unsuccessful. The molecular mechanism responsible for virus-induced triggering of an autoimmune response to MBP is not known but may include molecular mimicry due to antigens shared between the virus and host determinants or to virus-mediated CNS injury with secondary sensitization to MBP.

CLINICAL MANIFESTATIONS The severity of ADEM is variable. In severe cases, the onset is abrupt, and progression is rapid (hours to days). In postinfectious ADEM fever that may have faded reappears, and headache, meningismus, and lethargy progressing to coma may develop. Seizures are common. Signs of disseminated neurologic disease are consistently present. Motor findings may include hemiparesis or quadriparesis and extensor plantar responses. Tendon reflexes may be lost initially, later to become hyperactive. Variable degrees of sensory loss and of brainstem involvement may occur. In ADEM due to complications from chickenpox, cerebellar involvement is often prominent. CSF protein is modestly elevated (50 to 150 mg/dL). Lymphocytic pleocytosis, generally 200 cells per microliter or less, occurs in 80 percent of cases. Occasional patients have higher counts or a mixed polymorphonuclear-lymphocytic pattern during the initial days of the illness. Transient CSF oligoclonal banding has been reported in some patients. MRI scanning may reveal extensive gadolinium enhancement of white matter in brain and spinal cord. Electrophysiologic studies indicate involvement of the peripheral nervous system in a proportion of patients.

The prognosis reflects the severity of the underlying acute illness. Measles encephalomyelitis is associated with an estimated mortality of 5 to 20 percent, and most survivors have permanent neurologic sequelae. Children may recover but have persistent seizures and behavioral and learning disorders.

DIAGNOSIS The diagnosis is easily established when there is a history of recent vaccination or exanthematous illness. In severe cases with predominantly cerebral involvement, acute encephalitis due to infection with herpes simplex or other viruses may be difficult to exclude. In the absence of a specific viral prodrome or of immunization, it may not be possible to distinguish ADEM from acute MS. The simultaneous onset of disseminated symptoms and signs indicating optic nerve, brain, and spinal cord involvement is common in ADEM and rare in MS. Similarly, meningismus, drowsiness or coma, or seizures suggest ADEM. Optic nerve involvement is generally bilateral in ADEM and unilateral in MS, and transverse myelopathy is usually complete in the former and partial in the latter. The CSF protein level is normal in the great majority of MS patients; lymphocyte counts are rarely above 50 cells/μL, and polymorphonuclear leukocytes are not present. MRI findings that may support a diagnosis of ADEM include extensive and relatively symmetric white matter abnormalities and diffuse gadolinium enhancement of all abnormal areas, indicating active disease and a monophasic course. It is worth emphasizing that MS occasionally has an explosive presentation, particularly in children. The clinician is often best advised to classify such cases as acute demyelinating disease, reflecting this uncertainty.

TREATMENT

Treatment consists of intravenous methylprednisolone or methylprednisolone-prednisone as employed for MS (Table 376-4). Uncontrolled studies have found ACTH and plasmapheresis also to be of benefit. Occasional patients show evidence of relapse shortly after termination of therapy, and in such cases, reinstitution of therapy may be useful.

ACUTE HEMORRHAGIC LEUKOENCEPHALITIS

Acute hemorrhagic leukoencephalitis (AHL) of Weston Hurst is a rare, devastating, and hyperacute demyelinating disorder. CNS lesions of AHL are characterized by perivenous demyelination and intense infiltration by mononuclear and especially polymorphonuclear inflammatory cells. Vasculitis results in necrosis of the walls of venules, fibrin deposition, and innumerable small hemorrhages scattered throughout the white matter of the hemisphere, brainstem, and spinal cord. Large necrotic foci may form by coalescence of smaller lesions.

The clinical course resembles that of severe forms of ADEM but may be even more explosive in onset and progression. The CSF profile consists of marked pleocytosis (up to 3000 cells/μL), a variable number of red blood cells, and an elevated protein content. Peripheral blood may show an elevated ESR and leukocytosis. Occasional cases display mixed features of both ADEM and AHL or evolve from one form to the other during the course of the acute illness. As in ADEM, immune sensitization to MBP has been described in AHL. Thus, AHL may represent a form of ADEM in which a hyperacute inflammatory response is superimposed on lymphocyte-mediated perivenular demyelination.

The differential diagnosis of AHL includes viral encephalitis, acute bacterial cerebritis, venous thrombosis, and multiple embolic infarctions. The prognosis is generally poor, and death may occur within 2 to 4 days of onset. Therapy for AHL consists of methylprednisolone or methylprednisolone-prednisone regimens (see Table 376-4).

BIBLIOGRAPHY

BECK RW et al: A randomized, controlled trial of corticosteroids in the treatment of acute optic neuritis. N Engl J Med 326:581, 1992

FAZEKAS F et al: Randomized placebo-controlled trial of monthly intravenous immunoglobulin therapy in relapsing-remitting multiple sclerosis. Lancet 349:589, 1997

GOODKIN DE, RUDICK RA (eds): *Treatment of Multiple Sclerosis: Advances in Trial Design, Results and Future Perspectives.* London, Springer-Verlag, 1996

IFNβ MULTIPLE SCLEROSIS STUDY GROUP: Interferon beta-1b is effective in relapsing-remitting multiple sclerosis. I. Clinical results of a multicenter, randomized, double-blind, placebo-controlled trial. Neurology 43:655, 1993

JACOBS LD et al: Intramuscular interferon beta-1a for disease progression in relapsing multiple sclerosis. Ann Neurol 39:285, 1996

JOHNSON KP et al: Copolymer I reduces relapse rate and improves disability in relapsing-remitting multiple sclerosis. Results of a phase III multicenter, double-blind, placebo-controlled trial. Neurology 45:1268, 1995

JOHNSON RT et al: Measles encephalomyelitis: Clinical and immunologic studies. N Engl J Med 310:137, 1984

MATTHEWS WB et al: *McAlpine's Multiple Sclerosis.* New York, Churchill Livingstone, 1991

PATY DW et al: Interferon beta-1b is effective in relapsing-remitting multiple sclerosis. II. MRI analysis results of a multicenter, randomized, double-blind, placebo-controlled trial. Neurology 43:662, 1993

THE MULTIPLE SCLEROSIS GENETICS GROUP: A complete genomic screen for multiple sclerosis underscores a role for the major histocompatibility complex. Nature Genet 13:469, 1996

WAXMAN SG: Clinical course and electrophysiology of multiple sclerosis. Adv Neurol 47:1, 1988

---

377 *W. Michael Scheld*

BACTERIAL MENINGITIS, BRAIN ABSCESS, AND OTHER SUPPURATIVE INTRACRANIAL INFECTIONS

ACUTE BACTERIAL MENINGITIS

DEFINITION Bacterial meningitis may be defined as an inflammatory response to bacterial infection of the pia-arachnoid and the cerebrospinal fluid (CSF) of the subarachnoid space. Since the subarachnoid space is continuous over the brain, spinal cord, and optic nerves, infection in this space extends throughout the cerebrospinal axis unless there is obstruction of the subarachnoid space. Ventriculitis is nearly uniformly present in patients with bacterial meningitis.

EPIDEMIOLOGY Bacterial meningitis remains a common disease worldwide. Although precise figures are unavailable, the incidence of bacterial meningitis is between 3 and 5 per 100,000 people per year in the United States. More than 2000 deaths due to bacterial meningitis are reported annually in the United States. The disease is even more common in developing countries. The relative frequency

Table 377-1

Bacterial Etiologic Agents of Meningitis, by Patient Age

Organism	Neonates (≤1 month), %	Children (1 month to 15 years), %	Adults (>15 years), %
H. influenzae	0–3	40–60	1–3
S. pneumoniae	0–5	10–20	30–50
N. meningitidis	0–1	25–40	10–35
Gram-negative bacilli	50–60	1–2	1–10
Streptococci	20–40*	2–4	5
Staphylococci	5	1–2	5–15
Listeria species	2–10	1–2	5

* Nearly all isolates are group B streptococci.

SOURCE: After KL Roos et al: Acute bacterial meningitis in children and adults, in *Infections of the Central Nervous System,* WM Scheld et al (eds). New York, Raven Press, 1991, pp 335–409.

of isolation of various bacterial species as a cause of meningitis varies with age (Table 377-1). Gram-negative bacilli (principally *Escherichia coli*, of the K1 capsule type), other enteric bacilli, *Pseudomonas* sp., *Listeria monocytogenes*, and group B streptococci are the major causative agents during the neonatal period. *Haemophilus influenzae* and *Neisseria meningitidis* are the major causes in children beyond 1 month of age worldwide, although the proportion due to *H. influenzae* has declined dramatically in many geographic regions. Meningitis in adults is due primarily to meningococci and pneumococci, although disease due to aerobic gram-negative bacilli is observed with increasing frequency, especially in the elderly. *N. meningitidis* is the only major cause of epidemics of bacterial meningitis. Recent trends indicate an increase in the proportion of cases due to gram-negative bacilli and *L. monocytogenes*. The overall incidence per 100,000 population per year in the United States during 1986 was 2.9, 1.35, and 1.0 for meningitis due to *H. influenzae* (with significant variability by geographic region), *N. meningitidis*, and *Streptococcus pneumoniae*, respectively (Table 377-2). These most recent figures are derived from a prospective laboratory-based surveillance project in an area with a population of 34 million, 14 percent of the United States population. A similar overall incidence for neonatal meningitis of 2.8 cases per 100,000 population per year was observed in western Sweden during a comparable time period. A continued high incidence of *H. influenzae* meningitis was documented in a recent 3-year prospective nationwide study in Israel: 67.1 per 100,000 in the first year of life and 18.5 per 100,000 in children less than 5 years old. Nevertheless, there has been a profound reduction (by 76 to 90 percent) in the incidence of invasive *H. influenzae* infections in the United States in the past decade. This remarkable achievement has been attributed, in part, to the widespread use of *H. influenzae* conjugate vaccines, now licensed for use in children beginning at 2 months of age. Similar results have been observed in other areas, for example, Finland (from a peak of 43 cases per 100,000 population per year in the early 1970s to zero cases in 1991 in the greater Helsinki area) and in the United Kingdom (87 percent decline in cases between 1991 and 1993).

Meningitis is a major international health problem, as is evident by the recent experience in Africa and South America: explosive and highly fatal outbreaks may occur. At least 30 countries worldwide, including the United States, have reported serious outbreaks of meningococcal meningitis in recent years. More than 70,000 cases were reported from Africa in 1989 alone. During one decade (1973–1982), 4100 patients with meningitis were admitted to a single hospital in Salvador, Brazil, and this disease accounted for 27 percent of all admissions in this interval. The differences in etiology among various studies performed on four different continents are shown in Table 377-3. Worldwide, the three major meningeal pathogens (*H. influenzae*, *N. meningitidis*, and *S. pneumoniae*) account for approximately 75 to 80 percent of cases, but the proportion due to each organism varies among geographic regions.

ETIOLOGY Nearly all cases of *H. influenzae* meningitis occur in children under 6 years of age, and more than 90 percent are due to capsular type b strains (see Chap. 152). Meningitis usually follows nasopharyngeal acquisition of a virulent organism with subsequent systemic invasion. *H. influenzae* accounts for only about 0.5 percent of total CSF isolates in patients older than 6 years, and isolation of this organism in such a patient should suggest the presence of certain predisposing factors, such as sinusitis, epiglottitis, pneumonia, otitis media, head trauma with a CSF leak, diabetes mellitus, alcoholism, splenectomy or other asplenic states, and immune deficiency (including hypogammaglobulinemia and AIDS).

Meningitis due to *N. meningitidis* is most often encountered in children and young adults and may occur in epidemics (Chap. 149). Epidemic meningococcal meningitis is usually due to serogroups A or C, although the potential for epidemic spread of any serogroup exists. Type B strains are isolated most frequently in sporadic cases, accounting for approximately 50 percent of all isolates in the United States. A recent increase in the incidence of serogroup C meningococcal disease has been noted in North America, largely due to a clonal strain (ET-15) and related strains, which are associated with an increased number of outbreaks and a higher case-fatality rate. Type Y strains are associated with pneumonia. The meningococcus is isolated from approximately 20 percent of all patients with bacterial meningitis in the United States. Nasopharyngeal carriage of virulent organisms also can account for the initiation of infection. Infection is more likely in patients who have deficiencies in the terminal complement components (C5 to C8, and perhaps C9), the so-called membrane attack complex. Persons with these deficiencies have an 8000-fold increased risk of *Neisseria* infections, although the mortality rates appear to be lower than in patients with an intact complement system. Meningococcal meningitis also may occur in properdin-deficient individuals.

Pneumococcal meningitis is the most common type of meningitis in adults over age 30; it is much less common in children than in adults over age 60. It accounts for approximately 15 percent of the total cases of meningitis in the United States (see Chap. 141). In a recent review of 262 cases of community-acquired meningitis in adults reported from 1962 through 1988, the most common identified pathogens were *S. pneumoniae* (37 percent), *N. meningitidis* (13 percent) and *L. monocytogenes* (10 percent). Mortality rates for pneumococcal meningitis remain high in adults, in the 19 to 30 percent range. Pneumococcal infection of the meninges is often associated with distant foci such as pneumonia, otitis media, mastoiditis, sinusitis, or endocarditis. Serious pneumoccocal infections may be observed in patients with predisposing conditions, including splenectomy or asplenic states, multiple myeloma, hypogammaglobulinemia, alcoholism, cirrhosis, and the Wiskott-Aldrich syndrome. *S. pneumoniae* is the most common meningeal isolate in head trauma patients who have suffered a basilar skull fracture with subsequent CSF leak.

Although *L. monocytogenes* represents only a small minority of cases of bacterial meningitis in the United States, mortality remains high (see Table 377-2). *Listeria* infection is more likely in neonates, the elderly, alcoholics, diabetics, cancer patients, and immunosuppressed adults (e.g., renal transplant patients and patients with AIDS). The incidence of *Listeria* meningoencephalitis may be declining in renal transplant populations owing to the frequent use of trimethoprim-sulfamethoxazole prophylaxis. However, up to 30 percent of adults and 50 percent of children with listeriosis have no apparent underlying condition. Serious *Listeria* infections have been associated with several food-borne outbreaks involving contaminated cole slaw, milk, and cheese.

Meningitis due to aerobic gram-negative bacilli is unusual except at the extremes of life. *E. coli* is isolated from 30 to 50 percent of neonates with bacterial meningitis. *Klebsiella* sp., *E. coli*, and *Pseudomonas aeruginosa* also may be isolated following head trauma or neurosurgical procedures, in the elderly, in immunosuppressed patients, and in patients with gram-negative bacteremia or strongyloidiasis. Despite the relative low frequency of meningitis due to this group of microorganisms, the mortality rates remain high. Many of these infections are nosocomial in origin, although community-acquired gram-negative bacillary meningitis appears to be increasing in frequency, particularly among the elderly and in debilitated, alcoholic,

Table 377-2

Bacterial Meningitis in Five States and Los Angeles County, 1986

Organism	Percent of Total Cases	Case-Fatality Rate, %
H. influenzae	45	3
S. pneumoniae	18	19
N. meningitidis	14	13
Group B streptococci	5.7	12
L. monocytogenes	3.2	22
Other	15	18

SOURCE: After Wenger et al.

or diabetic adults. Staphylococcal meningitis is rare except in patients with indwelling CSF shunts, in whom *Staphylococcus epidermidis* is the most common organism. Meningitis due to *Staphylococcus aureus* is unusual and accounts for about 1 to 8 percent of cases in various surveys. *S. aureus* is the second most common cause of CSF shunt infections and is also a nosocomial pathogen. Although secondary meningitis in the setting of infective endocarditis is relatively uncommon, most of these infections are due to *S. aureus*. Other important associated conditions include head trauma, abscesses in other organs, neurosurgical procedures, sinusitis, osteomyelitis, pneumonia, cellulitis, decubitus ulcers, and infected intravascular grafts or shunts. Many patients have concomitant conditions, including diabetes mellitus, malignancy, renal failure, and immunosuppression. The mortality rate for staphylococcal meningitis remains high (about 50 percent in adults), although the prognosis for CSF shunt infections is more favorable.

Group B streptococci are an important cause of neonatal meningitis. These infections may occur either as early-onset septicemia associated with premature rupture of the membranes and low birth-weight or as late-onset meningitis appearing more than 7 days after birth. The early-onset form is acquired from the maternal genital tract, whereas the source of the group B streptococci in late-onset disease is more controversial; at least 40 percent of infected infants are born to culture-negative mothers. Rare cases of group B streptococcal meningitis have been reported in adults, including postpartum women after vaginal delivery. Bacteremic infections, unrelated to pregnancy, usually in older adults, occur in the setting of underlying risk factors: diabetes mellitus, malignancy, liver failure or a history of alcoholism, neurologic impairment, renal failure, collagen-vascular diseases, congestive heart failure, use of intravenous catheters, glucocorticoid administration, asplenia, and AIDS. Nevertheless, meningitis due to this organism is a rare disease in adults.

Meningitis due to anaerobic bacteria is rare, accounting for less than 1 percent of pyogenic cases. Recovery of anaerobic bacteria from CSF should suggest intraventricular rupture of a brain abscess. Most other cases arise from spread of infection secondary to a contiguous focus of disease and are seen in patients predisposed to focal suppurative intracranial processes.

A plethora of microorganisms have been documented as the cause of meningitis in isolated case reports or in small numbers of patients. Meningitis due to *Flavobacterium meningosepticum* may be a problem in certain neonatal intensive care units, and nosocomial meningitis due to other gram-negative bacilli or *Acinetobacter* sp. appears to be increasing in frequency. Polymicrobial bacterial meningitis, with simultaneous recovery of two or more bacterial species from CSF, is unusual, accounting for less than 1 percent of cases. Most cases occur in adults, and there is a wide spectrum of etiologic agents. Many patients have had either tumors close to the neuraxis, rectal carcinoma, or a fistulous communication with the central nervous system (CNS). Simultaneous isolation of viruses and bacteria from the CSF is rare. Nevertheless, CSF samples are not often cultured for both groups of microorganisms, so the number of reported cases may grossly underestimate the actual problem.

PATHOGENESIS AND PATHOPHYSIOLOGY Since most cases of bacterial meningitis are hematogenous in origin, pathogenesis involves sequential steps related to the expression of several different bacterial virulence factors that overcome host defense mechanisms and allow the pathogen to reach, invade, and replicate in the CSF. These pathogenic steps include (1) nasopharyngeal colonization, (2) nasopharyngeal epithelial cell invasion, (3) bloodstream invasion, (4) bacteremia with intravascular survival, (5) crossing of the blood-brain barrier and entry into CSF, and (6) survival and replication in the subarachnoid space.

Colonization and invasion of the nasopharyngeal mucosa by meningeal

pathogens require evasion of secretory IgA, avoidance of ciliary clearance mechanisms, adhesion to the apical epithelial cell membrane, and passage to the basolateral side of the cell. Virtually all clinical isolates of the three major meningeal pathogens secrete IgA proteases that cleave the hinge region of IgA and render it nonfunctional, thereby facilitating bacterial adhesion to the epithelium. Studies using a human nasopharyngeal organ culture model have elucidated the distinct mechanisms of adhesion and invasion by the human pathogens *H. influenzae* and *N. meningitidis*. Infection of human nasopharyngeal organ cultures with either organism results in injury to ciliated epithelial cells, with ciliostasis and selective adherence to nonciliated epithelial cells. Meningococcal binding is dependent on expression of cell-surface pili, and the organism interacts with epithelial cell microvilli. Meningococci enter nonciliated epithelial cells by an endocytotic process and proceed to the abluminal side by a transcellular route within membrane-bound vacuoles. *H. influenzae*, in contrast, creates separations between apical tight junctions of columnar epithelial cells and invades primarily via an intercellular route. After adhesion to and invasion of the nasopharyngeal epithelium, pathogenic bacteria must enter and survive within the intravascular space before penetrating the CNS. Evasion of the host's alternative complement pathway is an important strategy of meningeal pathogens for intravascular survival; this virulence property depends largely on expression of capsular polysaccharide. The actual molecular basis of this complement evasion strategy differs among the major meningeal pathogens. It has been attributed to the capsular sialic acid in group B streptococci, meningococci of serogroups B and C, and *E. coli*. The *H. influenzae* type b polysaccharide capsule (polyribosoyl ribose phosphate) helps evade complement by a somewhat different mechanism.

Once bacteremia occurs, the bacterial pathogens must invade the CNS. The site and mechanism of meningeal invasion by bacteria, however, are poorly understood. Early studies in an experimental infant rat model of *H. influenzae* meningitis suggested that the dural venous sinuses were the major route of CNS invasion. More recent studies, however, suggest that a nonspecific sterile focal inflammation above the cribriform plate facilitates CNS invasion at this site. Experimental studies also have demonstrated that bacteria may enter the CSF via the choroid plexus, a fact related to the exceptional high rate of blood flow and fenestrated capillaries of this structure. Three hypotheses are proposed to account for the observed neurotropism of meningeal pathogens and for their entry into the CNS: (1) Meningitis is secondary to a sustained bacteremia that must be of sufficient duration and magnitude; (2) adhesion to critical blood-brain barrier components may mediate CNS invasion, supported by the potential role of adhesion of *E. coli* strains to the luminal surface of microvascular cerebral endothelium and the epithelial lining of the choroid plexus and ventricles; and (3) microorganisms are carried in macrophages or other phagocytic cells, which enter the CNS by normal cellular trafficking pathways (as occurs in the case of *Streptococcus suis*).

Once bacteria cross the blood-brain barrier and enter the CNS, host humoral defense mechanisms, particularly those dependent on

Table 377-3

Etiology of Bacterial Meningitis in Four Geographic Areas (Percent of Total Cases)

Organism	United States, 1978–1981	United Kingdom, 1980–1984	Dakar, Senegal, 1970–1979	Salvador, Brazil, 1973–1982
H. influenzae	48	29	20	23
S. pneumoniae	13	20	29	17
N. meningitidis	20	25	11	32
Group B streptococcus	3	7	4	2
L. monocytogenes	2	2	<0.5	—
Other	8	16	9	8
Unknown	6	—	26	19

SOURCE: After KL Roos et al: Acute bacterial meningitis in children and adults, in *Infections of the Central Nervous System*, WM Scheld et al (eds). New York, Raven Press, 1991, pp 335–409.

immunoglobulin and complement activity, are virtually absent, so the pathogen has a significant advantage. Since opsonic activity is often undetectable even in infected CSF, phagocytosis of encapsulated bacterial pathogens in the fluid medium of the CSF is inefficient. Thus, bacterial meningitis represents an infection in an area of impaired host resistance; the bacteria commonly reach very high densities in CSF, and the use of bactericidal agents is a mandatory part of therapy.

Once bacteria enter and replicate in the CSF, the subarachnoid space becomes inflamed. This inflammation is largely responsible for the pathophysiologic consequences that contribute to the clinical syndrome of bacterial meningitis, including increased permeability of the blood-brain barrier, cerebral edema (vasogenic, interstitial, and cytotoxic in origin), increased outflow resistance to CSF, cerebral vasculitis, increased intracranial pressure, decreased cerebral blood flow and/or loss of autoregulation of cerebral blood flow, cortical hypoxia, and CSF acidosis.

CSF neutrophilic pleocytosis is a hallmark of subarachnoid-space inflammation. Nevertheless, the pathway by which neutrophils enter the CSF is largely unknown. Adhesion of neutrophils to vascular endothelial cells is a prerequisite. Pretreatment of endothelial cells in tissue culture with various inflammatory cytokines induces the formation of specific adhesion molecules [e.g., endothelial leukocyte adhesion molecule 1 (ELAM-1)], although some of these adhesion molecules have yet to be demonstrated in cerebral endothelium. Leukocyte endothelial cell adhesion is mediated by specific transmembrane glycoproteins expressed on the endothelial cells that interact with specific counterparts on neutrophils. Three families of adhesion molecules may mediate these important interactions: the immunoglobulin superfamily [e.g., intercellular adhesion molecules (ICAMs) 1 and 2], the integrin family (e.g., the CD11/CD18 subfamily), and the selectin family (ELAM-1). The complex interrelationships among these three families, including the inducibility of neutrophil adhesion, and the participation of multiple glycoproteins in diapedesis and the induction of inflammation are considered in greater detail in Chap. 120. In experimental animal models of meningitis, there is evidence that CSF pleocytosis is reduced by interventions designed to block the adhesion of neutrophils to endothelium—specifically, by the systemic administration of a monoclonal antibody (e.g., IB4) against the CD11/CD18 family of receptors, of monoclonal antibodies directed against ICAM-1, of peptides derived from *Bordetella pertussis* filamentous hemagglutinin (which mimic selectins), or of fucoidin, a homopolymer of sulfated L-fucose known to inhibit leukocyte "rolling receptor" L-selectin. These interventions prevent CSF pleocytosis from developing after challenge with live microorganisms or cell-wall components. Combination treatment with dexamethasone and monoclonal antibody IB4 is more effective than either agent alone in the prevention of CSF pleocytosis. Early in the disease, the adherence of leukocytes to cerebromicrovascular endothelium appears to occur preferentially in pial venules.

Subarachnoid-space inflammation is induced by constituents of bacteria. Capsular polysaccharides are remarkably noninflammatory, although the capsule is crucial for the survival of meningeal pathogens in the bloodstream and the subarachnoid space. Experimental animal studies have documented that the cell wall of gram-positive microorganisms and the endotoxin [lipopolysaccharide (LPS) or lipooligosaccharide] of gram-negative organisms induce subarachnoid space inflammation. In the case of pneumococcus, intracisternal injection of the major components of the cell wall—teichoic acid and peptidoglycan—induces inflammation. In gram-negative meningitis, the lipid A region of LPS is responsible for the induction of inflammation. Inflammatory changes in CSF are also elicited by the intracisternal inoculation of *H. influenzae* type b outer membrane vesicles, which may play a relevant role as a nonreplicating vehicle for the delivery of the toxic moieties of LPS to host cells in vivo. Pneumococcal cell wall and the LPS of *H. influenzae* type b elicit subarachnoid-space inflammation through the release of various inflammatory mediators within the CNS.

Both interleukin (IL) 1 and tumor necrosis factor (TNF) appear rapidly in CSF following the intracisternal inoculation of pneumococcal cell wall or of LPS from gram-negative bacteria. These proinflammatory cytokines induce subarachnoid-space inflammation independently and appear to act synergistically in this effect. In addition, increased concentrations of TNF in CSF may be specific for bacterial meningitis, as they are found in bacterial but not viral meningitis in both experimental animals and humans. The role of other inflammatory cytokines in the induction of subarachnoid-space inflammation is less clear. Although IL-6 and platelet-activating factor (PAF) are present in increased concentrations in the CSF during the disease, their role in the CNS is unknown. PAF appears to contribute directly to subarachnoid space inflammation during pneumococcal meningitis but to play only a supporting role when the inflammation is induced by *H. influenzae* LPS. Nevertheless, higher CSF concentrations of TNF and PAF are associated with more severe disease in children. IL-8 and IL-10 are also detected in the CSF of patients with bacterial meningitis; IL-10 may downregulate the inflammatory response in this disease.

One of the major pathophysiologic consequences of bacterial meningitis is an increase in the permeability of the blood-brain barrier, which leads to vasogenic cerebral edema. In experimental meningitis induced in animals by the intracisternal inoculation of bacterial pathogens, the cerebral capillary endothelium exhibits a uniform response, which is characterized morphologically by an early and sustained increase in pinocytotic vesicle formation and a progressive separation of intercellular tight junctions. These morphologic alterations correlate with the penetration of a marker protein (albumin) across the blood-brain barrier. CSF leukocytes augment these changes in permeability late in the disease course. When inoculated intracisternally, pneumococcal cell walls, *H. influenzae* type b LPS, outer membrane vesicles prepared from *H. influenzae*, and various proinflammatory cytokines all induce increased blood-brain permeability in vivo. Encapsulation of *H. influenzae* is not essential for blood-brain barrier injury, but it promotes this process in vivo by allowing the organism to escape host clearance mechanisms in the CSF. Studies that use in situ perfusion of albumin–colloidal gold as a tracer, as well as studies using complementary immunogold detection of perfused monomeric albumin, have identified the postcapillary venules as the site at which albumin enters the subarachnoid space during bacterial meningitis. Albumin crosses the blood-brain barrier primarily by a paracellular pathway through open intercellular junctions in venular segments, since transcytosis to the abluminal side of the endothelium is minimal. Although other gram-negative cell-wall components besides LPS (e.g., peptidoglycan) may induce subarachnoid-space inflammation, their effect is minimal compared to that of LPS. The primary and secondary messengers governing alterations in blood-brain barrier permeability and the paracellular leakage of albumin remain unknown, but ongoing development of in vitro systems of isolated cerebral microvascular endothelial cells may help in the delineation of the cellular mechanisms involved. Furthermore, the recent demonstration of elevated concentrations of excitatory amino acids in CSF during meningitis suggests that these substances may play a role in altered CNS homeostasis.

Another important pathophysiologic consequence of subarachnoid-space inflammation is an increase in intracranial pressure (ICP). This increase is caused primarily (but not exclusively) by cerebral edema, which may be vasogenic, cytotoxic, and/or interstitial in origin. Vasogenic cerebral edema results primarily from increased blood-brain barrier permeability. Cytotoxic cerebral edema results from the swelling of brain cells, most likely owing to the release of toxic factors from neutrophils and/or bacteria. Interstitial cerebral edema occurring during meningitis is due largely to obstruction of normal CSF pathways, with a resulting increase in the resistance to CSF outflow. Cerebral edema is always found in experimental animal models of meningitis, as measured by increased brain water content. The finding that administration of glucocorticoids to animals with experimental meningitis attenuated the cerebral edema, the increased ICP, and the increased CSF outflow resistance led to a reexamination of the potential adjunctive role of glucocorticoids in the treatment of this disease (see below). Cerebral blood flow alterations also have been found by multiple techniques in animal models and in patients with bacterial meningitis. In an infant rhesus monkey model of *H. influenzae* meningitis, certain areas of the cortex (postcentral, temporal, and occipital) were hypoperfused relative to the hypothalamus and midbrain, while the brainstem was hyperperfused. These findings suggest that cerebral cortical hypoperfusion with resulting relative cerebral anoxia may be an early physiologic change during *H. influenzae* meningitis. Loss of cerebral autoregulation has been documented in an experimental rabbit model of pneumococcal meningitis. It has been suggested that even minor fluctuations of mean arterial blood pressure may have adverse consequences for patients with meningitis, since autoregulation may be lost, resulting in an increased risk of brain injury from transient hypotension or hypertension. The blood flow alterations may lead to regional hypoxia, increased brain lactate concentrations secondary to utilization of glucose by anaerobic pathways, and CSF acidosis, which may be a precursor to encephalopathy. It is likely that the generation of reactive oxygen or nitrogen intermediates in the microvasculature potentiates these changes in regional cerebral blood flow. Infusion of superoxide dismutase, catalase, or deferoxime modifies the early alterations in cerebral blood flow in experimental models of pneumococcal meningitis. Elevated CSF concentrations of nitrite, a major metabolite of nitric oxide, have been observed in experimental animal models and patients with bacterial meningitis. Regional cerebral blood flow alterations, cerebral edema, blood-brain barrier permeability, and CSF pleocytosis are often reduced in animals receiving nitric oxide synthase inhibitors.

PATHOLOGY The pathologic hallmark of bacterial meningitis is an exudate in the subarachnoid space. On gross examination, the exudate has a typical grayish yellow or yellowish green appearance. It is most abundant in the cisterns at the base of the brain and over the convexities of the cerebral hemispheres in the rolandic and sylvian fissures. Purulent exudate accumulates in the basal cisterns and also, in the absence of obstruction, extends along the spinal cord and nerve sheaths and into the ventricular system. Microscopic examination of the subarachnoid exudate in the early stages of disease demonstrates large numbers of neutrophils and bacteria. Within 2 to 3 days of infection, evidence of inflammation in the wall of the small and medium-sized subarachnoid blood vessels appears. Subintimal infiltration of arterial walls by lymphocytes and neutrophils is relatively unique to infection of the meninges. The meningeal veins become distended and develop mural infection, which may be complicated by focal necrosis of the vessel wall, mural thrombus formation in the lumen, or involvement of the dural sinuses. Hemorrhagic cortical infarction may be the result of cortical venous and dural sinus thrombosis. By the end of the first week of meningeal inflammation, the cellular composition of the subarachnoid exudate changes. Neutrophils begin to degenerate and are removed by macrophages, which are derived from meningeal histiocytes. The nuclei of affected neurons and glial cells become shrunken, pyknotic, and darkly staining. Further infiltration of subependymal tissues and perivascular spaces by neutrophils and lymphocytes occurs. Blockage of normal CSF pathways, particularly of the midline foramen of Magendie and the lateral foramina of Luschka in the fourth ventricle, may result in noncommunicating or obstructive hydrocephalus. The absorption of CSF by the arachnoid villi may be impeded by accumulation of the fibrinopurulent exudate. Diffuse cerebral edema and/or increased ICP may lead to life-threatening brain herniation. Cranial and spinal nerve deficits, focal neurologic deficits, seizure disorders, encephalopathy, and subdural effusions are all recognized complications of meningitis.

CLINICAL MANIFESTATIONS The classic clinical presentation of adults with bacterial meningitis includes headache, fever, and meningismus, often with signs of cerebral dysfunction; these manifestations are found in more than 85 percent of patients. Nausea, vomiting, rigors, profuse sweating, weakness, myalgias, and photophobia are also common. The meningismus may be subtle or marked, accompanied by Kernig's and/or Brudzinski's signs. These signs are elicited in only about 50 percent of adults with bacterial meningitis, and their absence does not rule out this diagnosis. Cerebral dysfunction is manifested primarily by confusion, delirium, or a declining level

of consciousness ranging from lethargy to coma. Cranial nerve palsies, especially palsies involving cranial nerves IV, VI, and VII, are found in 10 to 20 percent of cases, occasionally in concert with focal neurologic deficits such as visual field defects, dysphasia, and hemiparesis. Seizures occur in about 40 percent of cases. Recurrent seizure activity and focal neurologic deficits are more common in the early stages of pneumococcal meningitis than in *H. influenzae* or meningococcal disease. The presence of bilateral sixth nerve palsies, manifested as weakness of the lateral rectus muscles, suggests a raised ICP. Papilledema is rare (<1 percent of patients) and should suggest a different diagnosis, such as an intracranial mass lesion. Later in the disease course, patients may develop other signs of increased ICP, including coma, hypertension, bradycardia, and third nerve palsy; these findings are ominous prognostic signs. Focal neurologic deficits, seizure activity, and encephalopathy may arise from cortical and/or subcortical ischemia and/or infarction, from increased ICP, or from the development of a subdural effusion.

Certain symptoms and/or signs may suggest a specific etiologic diagnosis in patients with meningitis. Meningococcemia with or without meningitis presents with a prominent rash, principally of the extremities, in about 50 percent of patients. Early in the disease process, the rash is often erythematous and macular, but typically it evolves quickly into a petechial phase with further coalescence into a purpuric form with gunmetal-gray necrosis in the center of the purpuric regions. This rash often matures rapidly, sometimes with the appearance of new petechial lesions during the performance of the physical examination. A similar rash may be seen in other forms of meningitis (e.g., meningitis due to echovirus type 9, *S. aureus*, *Acinetobacter* sp., and, rarely, *S. pneumoniae* or *H. influenzae*), in Rocky Mountain spotted fever and other rickettsioses, in *S. aureus* endocarditis, in rapid, overwhelming sepsis due to encapsulated bacteria in splenectomized patients, and in some noninfectious disorders such as vasculitis or thrombotic thrombocytopenic purpura. An additional suppurative focus of infection, typically otitis media, sinusitis, or pneumonia, is seen in approximately 30 percent of patients with pneumococcal or *H. influenzae* meningitis. Patients in whom meningitis develops in the wake of a CSF leak may have rhinorrhea or otorrhea due to a persistent defect.

Conversely, certain subgroups of patients may not manifest many of the classic signs and/or symptoms of bacterial meningitis. Meningismus and/or fever are commonly absent in neonates, and the only clinical clues may be listlessness, high-pitched crying, refusal to feed, irritability, or other nonspecific manifestations. In elderly patients, meningitis often has an insidious onset with lethargy or obtundation and with variable signs of meningeal inflammation and no fever. In this subgroup of patients, an altered mental status should not be ascribed to other causes until bacterial meningitis has been excluded by examination of CSF. Many of the signs of bacterial meningitis, including alteration in consciousness, are present in patients following neurosurgery or head trauma. Meningitis is difficult to spot in this situation, and the physician should have a low threshold for performing CSF examination if any clinical deterioration occurs.

DIAGNOSIS The diagnosis of bacterial meningitis rests on examination of the CSF, which is usually obtained by lumbar puncture. When papilledema and/or focal neurologic findings suggestive of an intracranial mass lesion are present, lumbar puncture should be deferred until computed tomography (CT) or magnetic resonance imaging (MRI) is performed. Nevertheless, if meningitis seems likely, blood should be drawn for culturing and empirical antimicrobial therapy started while the neuroimaging study is being carried out. Although empirical antibiotic therapy may render the CSF sterile (as determined by culturing), the CSF profile will still be suggestive of bacterial meningitis.

The typical CSF findings in acute bacterial meningitis consist of an elevated opening pressure, neutrophilic pleocytosis, elevated protein concentration, and hypoglycorrhachia. The opening pressure is elevated in virtually all cases. Values exceeding 600 mmH$_2$O suggest cerebral edema, communicating hydrocephalus, or the presence of intracranial suppurative foci. The gross appearance of the fluid may be cloudy or turbid if the white cell count is elevated. Occasionally, the fluid may appear turbid owing to the presence of microorganisms in the absence of significant CSF pleocytosis; this is an ominous prognostic sign. If the lumbar puncture is traumatic, the CSF may be bloody at first, but it should clear as flow continues. Although xanthochromia can occur during meningitis, this finding should suggest the possibility of subarachnoid hemorrhage, and in patients with heart valve disease it raises the possibility of ruptured mycotic aneurysm. The leukocyte concentration in CSF usually is elevated in untreated bacterial meningitis, with counts ranging from 1×10^3 to $>1 \times 10^6$/L. Values in the latter range are found in 60 to 70 percent of cases. The leukocytosis shows a neutrophilic predominance. A very low CSF white cell concentration in bacterial meningitis often has been associated with a poor outcome. Therefore, Gram's stain and culture should be performed on all CSF specimens, even in the absence of CSF pleocytosis. The CSF protein concentration is elevated in virtually all cases of bacterial meningitis, sometimes to an extreme degree when spinal block is present, presumably owing to disruption of the blood-brain barrier and/or generation of protein by leukocytes and/or microorganisms in the subarachnoid space. The CSF glucose concentration is less than <2.2 mmol/L (40 mg/dL) in approximately 60 percent of patients with bacterial meningitis, and the CSF-to-serum ratio of glucose concentrations is less than 0.31 in about 70 percent of patients. The CSF glucose concentration must be compared with a simultaneous serum glucose concentration for proper evaluation. A recent analysis found that each of the following criteria predicted the presence of bacterial as opposed to viral meningitis with a certainty of 99 percent or better: a CSF glucose level of less than 1.9 mmol/L (34 mg/dL), a CSF to blood glucose concentration ratio of less than 0.23, a CSF protein level of greater than 2.2 g/L (220 mg/dL), and more than 2000 $\times 10^6$ leukocytes per liter of CSF or more than 1180×10^6 neutrophils per liter of CSF.

Gram's staining should always be used in examining CSF, as it permits rapid and accurate identification of the etiologic agent in approximately 60 to 90 percent of cases of bacterial meningitis (the overall sensitivity is approximately 75 percent). The probability that the organism will be detected varies with the concentration of bacteria in CSF. False-positive findings may be caused by contamination of collection tubes or staining reagents. Negative CSF Gram's stains are usually related to prior antimicrobial therapy and low CSF concentrations of microorganisms. The CSF culture is positive in approximately 70 to 85 percent of patients with bacterial meningitis. The probability of identifying an organism decreases in patients who have received prior antimicrobial therapy. Blood cultures also should be obtained, because they are positive in a variable proportion of patients with bacterial meningitis, depending on the pathogen.

Many other rapid diagnostic tests have been developed to aid in the diagnosis of bacterial meningitis when Gram's staining gives negative results. Countercurrent immunoelectrophoresis (CIE) may be helpful in the detection of specific microbial antigens in CSF with a sensitivity of approximately 62 to 95 percent and with high specificity. Nevertheless, newer techniques employing staphylococcal coagglutination or latex agglutination are more rapid and sensitive than CIE, being able to detect bacterial antigen concentrations in CSF of approximately 1 ng/mL. It must be emphasized that a negative test result does not rule out infection with a particular meningeal pathogen. The limulus lysate test is highly sensitive at detecting LPS in CSF, although it does not distinguish among gram-negative organism, and its results often do not affect decisions regarding therapeutic regimen. Other tests may be useful in selected patients. Failure to find elevated CSF concentrations of C-reactive protein is strong evidence against bacterial meningitis. As noted above, increased CSF levels of TNF suggest a bacterial, not viral, etiology. The polymerase chain reaction (PCR) has been used to amplify bacterial DNA in CSF as an aid in the diagnosis of meningitis caused by *H. influenzae*, meningococci, strep-

tococci, and *Listeria*. Although problems with false-positive results have been noted, the specificity and sensitivity are both ~90 percent, and further refinements may facilitate diagnosis in cases that give negative results on Gram's staining and culture.

Neuroimaging techniques such as CT and MRI have little role in the diagnosis of acute bacterial meningitis, but they may detect complications and/or a parameningeal source of infection. CT or MRI may be useful in patients in whom fever still persists several days after initiation of antimicrobial therapy or who have prolonged obtundation or coma in the presence of new or recurrent seizure activity, signs of increased ICP, or focal neurologic deficits. MRI is more sensitive than CT for the evaluation of subdural effusions, cortical infarction, and cerebritis but is more difficult to perform in a critically ill patient. The vast majority of patients with suspected or proven bacterial meningitis do not require a neuroimaging study; if one is performed, its results usually will not affect decisions concerning therapy.

Most patients with suspected bacterial meningitis should undergo initial evaluation in an intensive care setting. Multiple complications may develop, including shock, disseminated intravascular coagulation, and the syndrome of inappropriate secretion of vasopressin (antidiuretic hormone). In addition to frequent monitoring, blood cultures and tests for coagulation factors and electrolytes, including indicators of renal function, are essential. A chest x-ray may reveal coexisting pneumonia. Staining of material from petechiae or purpuric lesions reveals intracellular cocci in approximately 70 percent of meningococcemia cases. In the presence of frank arthritis, arthrocentesis with culture and staining may reveal the etiologic agent.

DIFFERENTIAL DIAGNOSIS A variety of infectious and noninfectious processes can produce an acute meningitis syndrome and may be confused with acute bacterial meningitis. These entities include parameningeal foci of infection (e.g., brain abscess, subdural empyema, and epidural abscess; see below), viral meningitis or encephalitis, CNS syphilis, the neurologic manifestations of Lyme disease, tuberculous meningitis, fungal meningitis, bacterial endocarditis, rickettsial infections such as Rocky Mountain spotted fever, CNS neoplasms, cerebral vasculitis, granulomatous angiitis, sarcoidosis, cyst-related meningitis, subarachnoid hemorrhage, neuroleptic malignant syndrome, chemical meningitis due to drugs, radiocontrast agents or anesthetics, and various poorly understood chronic or recurrent meningeal syndromes.

 TREATMENT

Antimicrobial Therapy The initial procedure in a patient with suspected bacterial meningitis is a lumbar puncture to obtain CSF for analysis (Fig. 377-1). Patients should receive emergent empirical antimicrobial therapy based on age and underlying disease status if no etiologic agent is identified by Gram's staining or rapid diagnostic tests and if the diagnosis of bacterial meningitis is likely. In the few patients who present with focal signs on neurologic examination, a CT scan should be obtained prior to lumbar puncture. However, if meningitis is a strong possibility, empirical antimicrobial therapy should be instituted immediately after obtaining two blood samples for culturing. The empirical regimens for presumed bacterial meningitis are based primarily on the age of the host and the likely infecting pathogens. For neonates under 1 month of age, the most likely pathogens are *E. coli*, *Streptococcus agalactiae*, and *L. monocytogenes*. Empirical therapy commonly consists of ampicillin plus a third-generation cephalosporin, which is usually cefotaxime owing to the concerns of albumin binding by ceftriaxone and bilirubin metabolism in this age group. An alternative treatment regimen is ampicillin plus an aminoglycoside. In older infants (aged 4 to 12 weeks), infections with either *H. influenzae* or *S. pneumoniae* join the typical neonatal bacterial meningitides, and the regimen of choice is ampicillin plus a third-generation cephalosporin. From ages 3 months to 6 years, empirical therapy with a third-generation cephalosporin (and perhaps also with vancomycin; see below) may be used. Some authorities still recommend the use of ampicillin plus chloramphenicol or of chloramphenicol alone in this age group, but cefuroxime should be avoided. In young adults, most cases of meningitis are due to *N. meningitidis* or *S. pneumoniae*, and cefotaxime or ceftriaxone is often used. Because of the prevalence of gram-negative aerobic bacilli in older adults (over 50 years old) and the possibility of *L. monocytogenes* infection, the empirical regimen should consist of ampicillin in combination with a third-generation cephalosporin (and perhaps also with vancomycin). In postneurosurgical patients or in those with CSF shunts or foreign bodies in place, the likely infecting organisms include staphyloccocci, diphtheroids, and gram-negative bacilli, including *P. aeruginosa*. Empirical antimicrobial therapy in these situations should consist of vancomycin plus ceftazidime until culture results are available.

Once the infecting microorganism has been isolated in culture (or identified by other means), antimicrobial therapy can be modified on the basis of susceptibility results. For bacterial meningitis due to *N. meningitidis*, penicillin G or ampicillin remain the drugs of choice. The treatment of meningitis presumed or proved to be caused by *S. pneumoniae* has been markedly compromised by the global spread of penicillin-resistant pneumococci in recent years; penicillin alone can no longer be recommended as empirical therapy in any age group. Furthermore, before using penicillin against pneumococci, it is mandatory to test for susceptibility to this agent using pneumoccoccal isolates from sterile body fluids. Penicillin resistance is classified as being *relative* or *intermediate* if the minimum inhibitory concentration (MIC) is 0.1 to 1.0 μg/mL and as being *high* if the MIC is ≥2 μg/mL. While some areas (e.g., Spain, Hungary, and South Africa) reported a high proportion of penicillin-resistant isolates in the 1980s, in the United States, as of this writing, ~25 percent of pneumococcal isolates display intermediate resistance to penicillin, and ~5 to 7 percent display high-level resistance. Chloramphenicol is best avoided as an alternative, despite in vitro tests suggesting

susceptibility to this agent. Cefotaxime or ceftriaxone alone is recommended when relatively resistant strains are suspected or proved to be present. In contrast, in areas known to harbor isolates highly resistant to penicillin or to have a high proportion of isolates resistant to third-generation cephalosporins, the following regimens have been proposed: vancomycin plus either a third-generation cephalosporin or rifampin, or a third-generation cephalosporin with either ampicillin, vancomycin, or rifampin. No regimen has proven superiority. Care must be exercised when giving vancomycin to a patient who is also being treated with dexamethasone, as the latter agent reduces the penetrance of vancomycin into the CSF. Pending further data, the use of vancomycin plus a third-generation cephalosporin is reasonable. Repeat analysis of CSF after 24 to 48 h is also appropriate, especially if the patient is also receiving dexamethasone.

Meningococcal strains that are relatively resistant to penicillin also have been reported from several areas, particularly Spain, but patients harboring these strains have recovered with standard penicillin therapy. Penicillin resistance among meningococci remains stable at extremely low levels in the United States. Approximately 33 percent of *H. influenzae* isolates in the United States produce β-lactamase and are resistant to ampicillin. Fortunately, chloramphenicol resistance is rare in the United States, but it is found in more than 50 percent of CSF isolates in some countries.

The American Academy of Pediatrics has endorsed the use of the third-generation cephalosporins as empirical therapy in children with bacterial meningitis. Ceftriaxone is clearly superior to cefuroxime in this age group. The third-generation cephalosporins have revolutionized the treatment of gram-negative enteric bacillary meningitis. Cure rates of 78 to 94 percent have been achieved with these agents, and one, ceftazidime, may be used alone or as part of combination regimens for the care of patients with *Pseudomonas* meningitis. Intrathecal or intraventricular aminoglycoside administration should be considered for patients with gram-negative aerobic bacillary meningitis if there is no response to systemic therapy alone. The quinolone agents (e.g., ciprofloxacin, pefloxacin, and ofloxacin) have been used in some patients with gram-negative meningitis but should only be considered for adult patients with meningitis due to multidrug-resistant gram-negative bacilli or in patients failing conventional therapy. The third-generation cephalosporins are, however, inactive against *L. monocytogenes*; therefore, ampicillin is often added empirically for treatment of this organism. In documented *Listeria* meningitis, consideration should be given to a combination of an aminoglycoside and ampicillin to achieve synergy in vivo. In the penicillin-allergic patient, systemic trimethoprim-sulfamethoxazole, which is bactericidal against *Listeria* in vitro, can be used. Patients with *S. aureus* meningitis should be treated with nafcillin, oxacillin, or vancomycin. Since *S. epidermidis* is the most likely isolate in patients with a CSF shunt infection, vancomycin is the drug of choice; rifampin may be added if the patient fails to improve. Removal of the shunt often is necessary to optimize therapy.

The duration of therapy for bacterial meningitis is based largely on tradition, as rigorous scientific data are lacking. In general, the following treatment durations are recommended: for *N. meningitidis*, 7 days; for *H. influenzae*, 7 to 10 days; for *S. pneumoniae*, 10 to 14 days; and for gram-negative aerobic bacilli, 3 weeks. Therapy should be individualized and based on the clinical response; some patients require longer courses of treatment.

ADJUNCTIVE THERAPY Despite the availability of bactericidal antimicrobial therapy, the morbidity and mortality from bacterial meningitis remain unacceptably high. Recent studies have focused on the pathogenesis and pathophysiology of bacterial meningitis, since the simple introduction of newer antimicrobial agents may not improve the situation. However, rapid killing of bacteria—the desired effect of therapy with antimicrobial agents—may accelerate the release of proinflammatory bacterial cell-wall components into the CSF. Treatment with bacteriolytic agents in experimental menin-

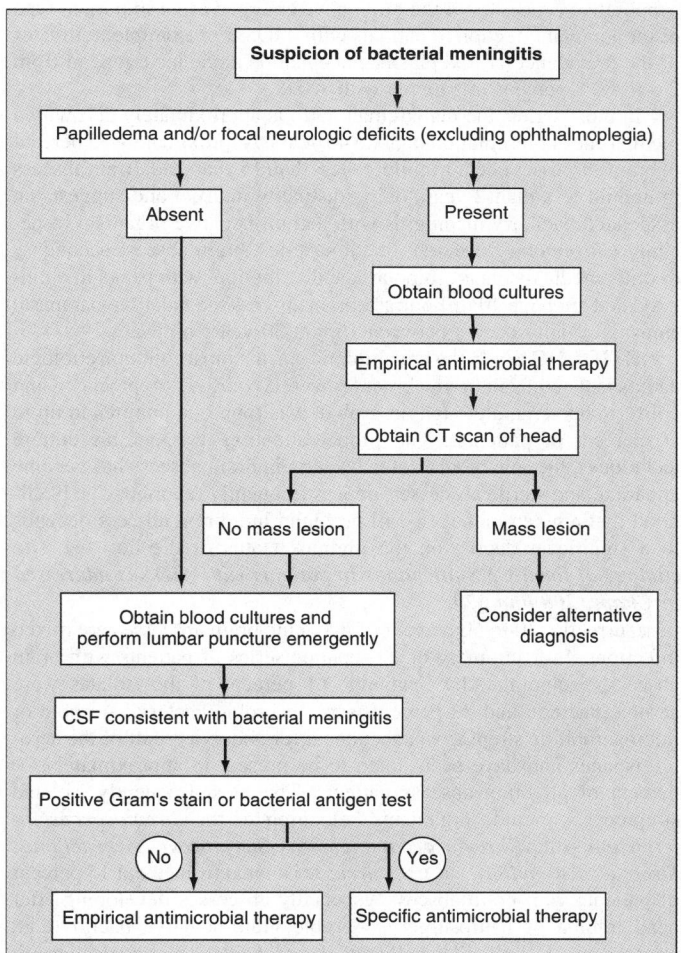

FIGURE 377-1 Algorithm for the initial management of patients with acute bacterial meningitis.

gitis often results in an increase in CSF leukocyte concentration. Antibiotic therapy also results in higher concentrations of free LPS in the CSF of children with *H. influenzae* meningitis during the first day of treatment. However, anti-inflammatory agents, particularly glucocorticoids, have been shown to decrease the inflammatory response in the subarachnoid space in experimental models of infection (as assessed by CSF pleocytosis), with resulting improvement in many of the pathophysiologic consequences, including increased permeability of the blood-brain barrier, cerebral edema, and increased ICP, On the basis of these studies and the known effects of glucocorticoids on cytokine generation, the use of glucocorticoids in patients with bacterial meningitis has been reevaluated. Several prospective, double-blind, randomized clinical trials have now evaluated dexamethasone as an adjunctive agent for children with meningitis. Most trials found no change in mortality rate, but CSF inflammatory indices normalized faster, fever disappeared more rapidly, and the incidence of moderate to severe bilateral sensorineural hearing loss and/or overall neurologic sequelae was reduced. Dexamethasone also reduced mortality in adults and children with pneumococcal meningitis in one Egyptian trial. Hearing impairment was reduced in children with pneumococcal meningitis in one recent trial reported from Turkey. Although concerns have been raised about the routine use of dexamethasone in all patients with bacterial meningitis, and virtually no information exists on the use of this treatment in neonates or older adults, adjunctive dexamethasone therapy is potentially beneficial in children, particularly those with proven or suspected *H. influenzae* disease. Close monitoring of the hematocrit and stool guaiac test for blood loss is essential during therapy. The mechanism of the beneficial effect of dexamethasone is not completely clear, but CSF concentrations of IL-1β fall more rapidly in children receiving dexamethasone than in children receiving a placebo. If dexamethasone is used, it should be administered shortly before or simultaneously with the first dose of antimicrobial agent to maximally attenuate the CSF inflammatory response. The recommended dose of dexamethasone is 0.15 mg/kg administered four times daily (a total of 0.6 mg/kg per day) for 4 days. Shorter courses of dexamethasone therapy (e.g., 2 days) may be appropriate, pending further data. The role of adjunctive dexamethasone in neonates and adults is unclear.

Other adjunctive treatments may be useful in critically ill patients with bacterial meningitis. Patients with signs of increased ICP may benefit from the insertion of an intracranial pressure monitoring device and vigorous treatment of raised ICP. Elevation of the head of the bed to 30°, hyperventilation to a Pa_{CO_2} of 27 to 30 mmHg, administration of hyperosmolar agents such as mannitol, use of intravenous lidocaine to reduce transient increases in ICP during endotracheal suctioning, and administration of glucocorticoids may be tried alone or in combination (see Chap. 374). Glycerol, which can be administered orally, may reduce auditory and/or neurologic sequelae regardless of dexamethasone use, but further data are needed before its routine use can be recommended in the care of patients with bacterial meningitis. To avoid status epilepticus, seizures should be treated promptly with appropriate agents, such as lorazepam or diazepam and/or phenytoin. Barbiturates occasionally are necessary to control seizure activity. Treatment of shock and/or disseminated intravascular coagulation may be necessary (see Chap. 124). Plasma exchange or plasmapheresis has proved life-saving in some patients with fulminant meningococcemia, but this treatment must be considered experimental.

PROGNOSIS Table 377-2 shows the overall case-fatality rates for meningitis caused by the major meningeal pathogens encountered in the United States in 1986. The mortality rate for *H. influenzae* meningitis is less than 5 percent, although it exceeds 20 to 25 percent in some developing countries. Meningococcemia without meningitis carries a worse prognosis than meningococcal meningitis alone. Pneumococcal meningitis has the highest mortality rate of the three major

types of bacterial meningitis. Gram-negative aerobic bacillary meningitis is often refractory to therapy, and relapses may occur. Permanent neurologic sequelae occur in approximately one-third to one-half of survivors of bacterial meningitis. The major sequelae include hearing loss or language delay, mental retardation, cerebral palsy, seizures, and behavioral problems. Prospective studies have documented persistent sensorineural hearing loss in approximately 10 percent of survivors of bacterial meningitis (and in approximately 31 percent of survivors of pneumococcal meningitis), a finding with critical implications for growth and educational development. Despite an apparent recent decline in the incidence of severe neurologic sequelae among children surviving bacterial meningitis, as measured by learning patterns upon school entry, the worldwide public health problems resulting from this disease are significant.

BRAIN ABSCESS

DEFINITION A brain abscess is a focal suppurative process in the brain parenchyma; the pathogenesis and etiology of the condition are diverse.

EPIDEMIOLOGY The incidence of brain abscess has remained relatively stable in the antibiotic era; nevertheless, it is generally regarded as a rare disease, with large autopsy series reporting an occurrence rate of 0.18 to 1.3 percent. It has been estimated that brain abscess accounts for approximately 1 out of every 10,000 general hospital admissions, and about 4 to 10 cases are seen yearly on active neurosurgical services in hospitals of developed countries. Although some series have noted a slightly increased incidence in recent years, this change may be an artifact due to more sensitive diagnostic techniques. In addition, brain abscess remains a significant problem in the developing world, particularly in children living in poverty. Focal suppurative processes of the brain have emerged as an important type of intracranial infection in patients with AIDS. For example, estimates of the prevalence of toxoplasma encephalitis alone have ranged from 2.6 to 30.8 percent in patients with AIDS.

In most series, the male/female ratio is approximately 2:1, with a median age at presentation of 30 to 45 years. Approximately 25 percent of brain abscesses occur in children less than 15 years old. Brain abscess in a child less than 2 years old is distinctly unusual and suggests an associated bacillary meningitis with a gram-negative organism (especially *Citrobacter diversus*). In some series, brain abscess secondary to otitis media displays a bipolar age distribution, with peaks in childhood and after age 40. In contrast, brain abscess secondary to paranasal sinusitis usually occurs between 10 and 30 years of age.

ETIOLOGY In the preantibiotic era, the most common etiologic agents isolated from brain abscesses were *S. aureus*, streptococci, and coliform bacteria, although no growth was found on cultures in up to 50 percent of patients. With proper attention to anaerobic culture techniques, the role of anaerobic bacteria in brain abscess has become apparent, and sterile abscesses are less frequently reported. The likelihood that a given pathogen will be found in a brain abscess depends to a significant degree on the immune status of the host. → *The etiology of focal CNS infections in patients with AIDS is addressed in Chaps. 308 and 379.*

Currently, 30 to 60 percent of pyogenic brain abscesses are mixed infections. In a summary of 12 separate series of patients with brain abscess, excluding AIDS patients, 61 percent of the isolates were aerobic bacteria and 32 percent were anaerobic bacteria. Aerobic or microaerophilic streptococci accounted for about one-half of the aerobic isolates and have been noted to be present in approximately 70 percent of all brain abscess patients. The most frequently isolated streptococci include organisms belonging to the *Streptococcus intermedius* group (*Streptococcus anginosus*, *Streptococcus constellatus*, *Streptococcus milleri*, etc.). *S. aureus* is isolated from about 15 percent of patients with brain abscess, especially abscesses developing after head trauma or neurosurgery. Aerobic gram-negative bacilli (e.g., *Proteus* sp., *E. coli*, *Klebsiella* sp., *Enterobacter* sp., and *P. aeruginosa*) have been observed with increased frequency in recent studies, often in mixed culture, and are isolated from 23 to 33 percent of patients. *Haemophilus* species other than *H. influenzae* are isolated in 5 to 10 percent of cases; *Haemophilus aphrophilus* is the most common of these. The anaerobes most recently encountered include *Bacteroides* sp. (including *Bacteroides fragilis*), *Fusobacterium* sp., *Prevotella* sp., anaerobic streptococci, and *Clostridium* sp. Anaerobic bacteria are particularly common pathogens in the setting of underlying chronic otitis or pulmonary disease.

The location of a brain abscess and its cause often suggest the most likely etiologic agent(s). Frontal lobe abscesses resulting from a preexisting sinusitis often yield an organism of the *S. intermedius* group in pure culture. Furthermore, brain abscess in association with chronic sinusitis is often a mixed infection, having an aerobic/anaerobic ratio of approximately 1 to 1.5 in most series. Posttraumatic or postoperative brain abscesses are usually caused by staphylococci. Temporal lobe abscesses are often a complication of otitis media and almost always yield multiple agents on culture, including streptococci, *Bacteroides* sp., and gram-negative aerobic bacilli. Approximately 33 percent of chronically infected ears yields anaerobes on culture. In contrast to the role of *S. pneumoniae*, *H. influenzae*, and *Moraxella catarrhalis* in acute otitis media, other streptococci, gram-negative aerobes including *P. aeruginosa*, anaerobic cocci, and *Bacteroides* sp. are the most common isolates from cases of chronic otitis media and its intracranial complications. Pneumococci, meningococci, and *H. influenzae* very rarely cause brain abscess, even in association with a purulent meningitis. Diagnosis of pneumococcal brain abscess should prompt consideration of infection with human immunodeficiency virus (HIV) as a predisposing factor.

In addition, the microbiology of a brain abscess is fundamentally influenced by the immune status of the host. Immunocompromised patients may develop brain abscess due to fungi, and *Toxoplasma gondii* is a major cause of focal CNS lesions in patients with AIDS. Brain abscess in neutropenic patients is usually due to aerobic gram-negative bacteria, *Candida* sp., *Aspergillus* sp., or zygomycosis. Approximately 50 percent of brain abscesses developing after bone marrow transplantation are due to *Aspergillus* sp.; survival is rare. Conversely, focal brain abscess in patients with abnormal cell-mediated immunity is commonly due to *T. gondii*, *Nocardia asteroides*, *L. monocytogenes*, *Mycobacterium* sp., or *Cryptococcus neoformans*. *Pseudallescheria boydii* abscess may follow a near-drowning episode. Multiple other fungi, protozoa, and helminths may cause brain abscess. *Xylohypha bantianum*, the most common agent of cerebral phaeohyphomycosis, shows a strong proclivity for causing brain abscesses.

PATHOGENESIS AND PATHOPHYSIOLOGY Most brain abscesses originate in association with one of three clinical settings: (1) the presence of a contiguous focus of infection, particularly otitis, sinusitis, or a dental infection; (2) the presence of a distant focus of infection (especially chronic pyogenic lung disease) with hematogenous spread; and (3) prior cranial trauma or surgery. The predisposing factor remains undefined in approximately 15 to 20 percent of cases.

A review of multiple series encompassing more than 3500 cases of brain abscess in the past half century reveals that about 45 percent of cases were associated with a contiguous focus of infection (predominantly otitis or sinusitis). Recent data suggest that otogenic brain abscesses are decreasing in frequency, perhaps owing to the availability and common use of antimicrobial agents for upper respiratory tract infections. Frequent but inadequate courses of antimicrobial agents for ear or sinus infections have, however, altered the natural history of brain abscess, resulting in puzzling or more subtle clinical presentations, often in association with cholesteatoma. Otogenic brain abscesses are most commonly located in the temporal lobe or cerebellum; conversely, 85 to 95 percent of cerebellar abscesses are associated with ear or mastoid infections. Usually these lesions are solitary. Sinusitis as a cause of brain abscess also appears to be decreasing in incidence. Rhinogenic abscesses are rare in children and in adults over the age of 60 years. Most brain abscesses in the setting of sinusitis are localized in the frontal lobe. Sphenoid sinusitis is notable for the frequency and severity of its intracranial complications. This form of sinusitis is often difficult to diagnose, which may lead to delay in instituting therapy. Cocaine inhalation is an additional risk factor for sphenoid sinusitis and subsequent

brain abscess development. Dental infections, often overlooked as a cause of brain abscess, have been implicated in about 10 percent of patients with brain abscess. Periapical abscesses surrounding the teeth are often detected in patients with "cryptogenic brain abscess." Brain abscesses rarely complicate the course of bacterial meningitis in adolescents or adults. However, the presence of a brain abscess should be strongly considered in neonates with gram-negative meningitis, particularly meningitis due to *Citrobacter* or *Proteus* sp.

Brain abscess is a rare complication of neurosurgical procedures or cranial trauma. CNS infections occur in only 0.6 to 1.7 percent of clean neurosurgical procedures, and brain abscess accounts for only 10 percent of these infections. Brain abscess may, however, complicate penetrating cranial injuries and is especially common in the setting of gunshot wound complications. Retained bone fragments have been noted consistently as an important risk factor.

About 25 percent of cases of brain abscess arise by hematogenous spread from a distant focus of infection. These lesions are associated most often with pulmonary infections and share the following characteristics: (1) location in the distribution of the middle cerebral artery, (2) initial location at the gray matter–white matter junction, (3) poor encapsulation, and (4) a higher rate of mortality than from other types of brain abscess. Hematogenous brain abscesses are most likely to present as multiple lesions. Multiple brain abscesses were reported in only 1 to 15 percent in older series; however, with the advent of CT scanning, multiple lesions are now detected in 10 to 50 percent of patients. Important preceding processes have included chronic lung infections (lung abscess, bronchiectasis, and empyema), osteomyelitis, cholecystitis, intraabdominal infection, and/or pelvic sources. Brain abscess has been observed following endoscopic sclerosis of esophageal varices or dilatation of esophageal strictures. Although a transient bacteremia may follow these procedures and is instrumental in the development of a brain abscess, macroscopic CNS lesions are rare as complications of bacterial endocarditis. *S. aureus* is the most common cause of endocarditis complicated by intracranial involvement. Hereditary hemorrhagic telangiectasia is an important risk factor for brain abscess, especially in affected patients with clubbing, cyanosis, and/or polycythemia. This condition (Osler-Rendu-Weber syndrome), as well as unrecognized asymptomatic pulmonary arteriovenous malformations, may be underrecognized in patients with brain abscess. Cyanotic heart disease is recognized in 3 to 14 percent of brain abscess cases and may be the most common underlying process found with brain abscess in children. Tetralogy of Fallot is the most commonly cited anomaly; however, brain abscess may complicate patent foramen ovale, ventricular septal defect, and transposition of the great vessels. The presence of a right-to-left shunt and hypoxia appears to be critical for the development of brain abscess in these patients.

Brain abscess development in any of the above-described clinical settings appears to require a compromised area of brain as the final common pathway. Experimental data suggest that the brain is remarkably resistant to infection. The development of a brain abscess from an area of contiguous infection usually occurs by one of two major mechanisms: (1) direct extension through areas of associated osteitis or osteomyelitis and (2) retrograde thrombophlebitic spread via diploic or emissary veins into the intracranial compartment. The polycythemia and systemic hypoxia observed in patients with cyanotic congenital heart disease and hereditary hemorrhagic telangiectasia increase blood viscosity, which may, in concert with a reduction in brain capillary blood flow, result in microinfarction or reduced tissue oxygenation in brain, which could serve as a nidus for ensuing infection.

PATHOLOGY A solitary brain abscess involves the following brain regions in approximate decreasing order of frequency: frontal ≥ temporal ≥ frontoparietal > parietal > cerebellar > occipital. This distribution reflects the associated, often contiguous foci of infection. Brainstem, intrasellar, basal ganglia, and thalamic abscesses are rare.

The pathologic evolution of brain abscess has been documented most convincingly in experimental models of infection and appears to involve four histopathologic stages. Importantly, the histopathologic features may correlate with specific findings on CT, a fact that has direct implications for subsequent therapy. The four stages are (1) early cerebritis (days 1 to 3 following intracerebral inoculation of animals), which is characterized by a perivascular inflammatory response surrounding a developing necrotic center, with profound edema; (2) late cerebritis, in which the well-formed necrotic center reaches its maximum size and fibroblasts and neovascularity appear in its periphery; (3) early capsule formation (days 10 to 13 following intracerebral inoculation of experimental animals), characterized by a well-developed layer of fibroblasts with persistent cerebritis, neovascularity, and reactive astrocytosis; and (4) late capsule formation, with thickening of the capsule and an abundance of reactive collagen. It should be noted, however, that this sequence is somewhat idealized; it is best described for abscesses following infection with alpha-hemolytic streptococci and may not represent the course of events in abscesses caused by other microorganisms. Encapsulation is frequently more complete on the cortical side of the abscess than on the ventricular side and is often less extensive in abscesses resulting from hematogenous spread than in those arising from a contiguous focus of infection. These observations may explain the propensity of abscesses to rupture medially into the ventricular system rather than peripherally into the subarachnoid space. Brain abscess formation represents a continuum from cerebritis to a well-encapsulated necrotic focus. The maturity of a given lesion depends on multiple factors, including local oxygen concentration, the offending microorganism, and the host immune response.

CLINICAL MANIFESTATIONS (See Table 377-4) The clinical course of a patient with a brain abscess may range from indolent to fulminant; however, the duration of symptoms is 2 weeks or less in about 75 percent of patients. In most cases, the prominent clinical manifestations of brain abscess reflect the expanding intracerebral mass rather than systemic signs of infection. Furthermore, the clinical manifestations are often nonspecific and depend on several variables (e.g., the virulence of the infecting organisms, the patient's immune status, the location of the abscess or abscesses, and the presence or absence of associated meningitis or ventricular rupture). Only a minority of patients display the classic triad of fever, headache, and focal neurologic deficits. Headache is most consistently observed (70 percent of patients). Fever is reported in only one-half of patients overall, but ≥80 percent of children are febrile. Focal neurologic deficits are encountered in about half the cases. The specific deficits present depend on the number and location of the brain abscesses and may include hemiplegia, hemianopia, cranial nerve abnormalities, and others. Cerebellar abscess often results in nystagmus, ataxia, vomiting, and dysmetria, whereas frontal lobe abscess is often dominated by headache, drowsiness, inattention, and a generalized deterioration in mental function. Hemiparesis with unilateral motor signs and/or a speech disorder are frequent findings. Seizures are observed in 25 to 45 percent of

Table 377-4

Clinical Manifestations of Brain Abscess

Symptom or Sign	Percent
Headache	50–75
Triad of fever, headache, focal deficit	<50
Fever	40–50
Focal neurologic deficit	~50
Seizures	25–40
Nausea/vomiting	22–50
Nuchal rigidity	~25
Papilledema	~25

NOTE: Other symptoms and signs are dependent on location.

SOURCE: After Wispelwey and Scheld.

patients and, when present, are usually generalized. The presence of nausea and vomiting correlates to some degree with the ICP. A change in mental status (lethargy to coma) occurs in most patients, but frank coma on presentation is now infrequent, a change that may reflect the availability of improved diagnostic modalities such as CT. Papilledema is observed with varying frequency; it does not correlate with the size of the abscess but appears to be associated closely with the presence of headache and vomiting. Nuchal rigidity (about 25 percent of patients) is observed more commonly with a shorter duration of illness and may lead to confusion with bacterial meningitis. Intrasellar abscess often simulates a pituitary tumor, presenting with headache, visual field defects, and endocrine disturbances.

Since the clinical presentation may be nonspecific and fever is often absent, brain abscess may be confused with several other processes, and the following should be considered in the differential diagnosis: pyogenic meningitis, subdural empyema, epidural abscess, encephalitis, mycotic aneurysm, complicated migraine headache, intracerebral or subarachnoid hemorrhage, cerebral infarction, cerebral venous sinus thrombosis, primary or metastatic malignancies of the CNS, and rarely, multiple sclerosis.

DIAGNOSIS Routine studies of the blood and urine are rarely helpful in the diagnosis of a brain abscess. A moderate peripheral blood leukocytosis may be present, but 40 percent of patients display a completely normal peripheral leukocyte count. The erythrocyte sedimentation rate is often elevated, but it may be normal in the setting of cyanotic congenital heart disease. The serum concentration of C-reactive protein has been used to differentiate brain abscess from intracranial neoplasms but is inadequate for this purpose. Blood cultures are only occasionally (≤10 percent) positive in patients with a brain abscess.

Although the CSF is often abnormal in patients with brain abscess, the findings are nonspecific, and lumbar puncture is usually contraindicated in a patient with a suspected parenchymal abscess. The diagnostic yield is poor, and the risk of herniation after the procedure has been reported to be as high as 20 percent. The poor diagnostic yield and significant morbidity of lumbar puncture in the presence of a brain abscess necessitate that this procedure be delayed in patients with a febrile CNS disorder with focal neurologic signs. However, if pyogenic meningitis is also a strong consideration, blood cultures should be obtained and appropriate antimicrobial agents started parenterally before a neuroradiologic study is performed. Although abnormalities may be noted, skull roentgenograms, electroencephalograms, arteriography, ventriculography, and/or technetium-99m brain scans are rarely necessary in the evaluation of a patient with a suspected brain abscess. Radionuclide brain scans are, however, useful in facilities lacking CT and MRI technology.

The introduction of CT and MRI has revolutionized the diagnostic and therapeutic approach to brain abscess. CT scans of the paranasal sinuses, mastoids, middle ear, and brain should be obtained, along with a chest roentgenogram, in all patients with suspected brain abscess. CT is sensitive (>95 percent) in the detection of a brain abscess, and it can give additional crucial information such as the extent of the surrounding edema, the presence of hydrocephalus and/or a midline shift, and the precise site of the lesion. On CT with contrast administration, a brain abscess typically appears as a hypodense lesion surrounded by a uniformly enhancing ring. A variable, hypodense area of edema extends beyond the ring. Unfortunately, this CT appearance is not specific for a brain abscess, and other processes, including neoplasm, granuloma, cerebral infarction, and resolving hematoma, may have similar appearance on CT. Furthermore, glucocorticoid use may alter the typical appearance on CT; only 40 to 60 percent of brain abscesses in patients receiving glucocorticoid therapy reveal ring enhancement on CT scan. Indium 111–labeled leukocyte scintigraphy may prove complementary to CT in the diagnosis of abscesses in the CNS. However, necrotic tumors may be confused with brain abscess by this technique, and the concomitant use of glucocorticoids also may produce a false-negative scan. A potentially exciting nuclear medicine modality in the evaluation of cerebral mass lesions was developed recently. Thallium-201 single photon emission CT (SPECT) may per-

FIGURE 377-2 MRI of brain abscess. Coronal T1-weighted spin-echo image following gadolinium-DTPA enhancement demonstrating large necrotic right frontal lobe mass with intense peripheral enhancement and surrounding edema. Multiple complications are also evident: ependymal enhancement in the lateral and third ventricles and enhancement of the subarachnoid space reflecting ventricular rupture, ventriculitis, and meningitis, and a mass effect with midline shift. Aspiration revealed pus and *S. milleri* in pure culture.

mit differentiation of CNS lymphoma from toxoplasmic encephalitis in AIDS patients (see Chap. 308), but its role in suspected pyogenic abscess is unsettled.

Data on the usefulness of MRI in the diagnosis and evaluation of patients with brain abscess continue to accumulate. MRI permits multiplanar imaging, is better than CT at distinguishing between gray and white matter, and affords a variety of imaging techniques to elucidate pathologic changes. In addition, bony artifact, which may hinder the interpretation of CT scans, is not a problem with MRI. MRI appears to be more sensitive than CT at detecting brain abscess in the cerebritis phase of its development as well as at detecting associated cerebral edema. Therefore, MRI may detect early satellite lesions not demonstrated by CT and is often more useful than CT for demonstration of extraparenchymal extension of an abscess (i.e., ventricular rupture) (Fig. 377-2). The lack of ionizing radiation, better tissue characterization, lack of bony artifact, increased sensitivity in follow-up evaluations, and less toxic contrast agents (e.g., gadolinium-DTPA) make MRI the procedure of choice in the evaluation of a patient with suspected brain abscess.

℞ TREATMENT

The optimal management of most patients with a bacterial brain abscess involves both administration of antimicrobial agents and surgical intervention. CT or MRI should be performed without delay in the patient with neurologic complaints and a predisposing condition suggesting brain abscess, as described above. Results in animal models and humans suggest that focal bacterial infections of the brain parenchyma can be "staged" by sequential CT scanning. Cerebritis is characterized by an area of low density surrounded by ring enhancement (often thick and diffuse) that is undecayed on repeat scans obtained 1 h later. In contrast, an encapsulated abscess is characterized by a faint ring on the unenhanced scan and ring enhancement

that is decayed on the repeat CT scan. These parameters may prove useful in planning a combined medical-surgical approach. Since 1971, it has been recognized that early antimicrobial therapy alone, in the absence of surgical intervention, could cure cerebritis and prevent the development of an encapsulated abscess. Subsequent cases in which the cure of an encapsulated abscess was claimed share many of the following features: (1) sequential CT scans were used to diagnose brain abscess and to follow the resolution of the lesion(s); aspiration biopsy and histopathologic analysis usually were not done; (2) prolonged courses (e.g., ≥8 weeks) of high-dose antibiotic therapy were administered; and (3) evidence of encapsulation often was lacking. Based on experimental animal models of brain abscess and the well-defined CT appearance of the cerebritis stage, medical "cures" of established brain abscess may represent successful resolution of bacterial cerebritis. In general, close cooperation between medical and surgical specialists is essential for the optimal management of a patient with suspected brain abscess.

The antimicrobial regimens recommended for the empirical (and specific) therapy of a brain abscess reflect considerations of the microbiology as well as evidence from both animal and human studies evaluating the penetration of a given antimicrobial agent into brain parenchyma and/or brain abscess pus. Unfortunately, no prospective, randomized clinical trials exist to guide the clinician in the choice of an optimal antimicrobial regimen. If CT suggests cerebritis and the patient is neurologically stable, antibiotics can be started and the patient observed. Since the early 1960s, a combination of penicillin G (20 to 24 million units per day intravenously) plus chloramphenicol (1.0 to 1.5 g intravenously every 6 h) has been advocated in adults. Penicillin remains a mainstay of therapy because of (1) excellent activity against streptococci, including the *S. intermedius* group, complicating contiguous foci of infection and pyogenic lung disease; (2) activity against most anaerobes encountered in brain abscess patients; (3) favorable results obtained in experimental animal models of brain abscess; and (4) a marked reduction in brain abscess mortality observed after the introduction of penicillin in the 1940s. Cefotaxime in high doses (e.g., 3 g intravenously every 8 h) is an acceptable substitute for penicillin in empirical combination regimens that include an antianaerobic agent, e.g., metronidazole. Chloramphenicol often has been administered concurrently with penicillin in the past because of its high lipid solubility, which results in brain tissue concentrations that often exceed the levels in plasma, and its good activity against anaerobic bacteria, including *B. fragilis*. The use of metronidazole for the therapy of brain abscess has increased greatly in recent years, and this agent has generally supplanted chloramphenicol because (1) metronidazole is bactericidal against *B. fragilis*, whereas chloramphenicol may be bacteriostatic; (2) metronidazole attains reproducibly excellent concentrations in brain abscess pus; (3) concomitant steroid treatment does not affect the entry of metronidazole into brain abscess pus, in contrast to its effect on several other antibiotics; (4) chloramphenicol may be degraded by desacetylation in pus, as shown in experimental intraabdominal abscess; and (5) use of metronidazole may reduce mortality rates, as suggested by several recent retrospective studies. Although use of metronidazole instead of chloramphenicol may lead to more rapid healing and a lower mortality rate, these two agents have never been compared in a prospective, randomized clinical trial. Nevertheless, an antianaerobic agent such as metronidazole (or, perhaps, ampicillin-sulbactam) is indicated for the treatment of brain abscess complicating otitis media, mastoiditis, or pyogenic lung abscess because anaerobes are often present. Metronidazole should never be used alone to treat a patient with suspected brain abscess. Antianaerobic therapy may not be necessary in addition to penicillin for patients with frontal or ethmoidal sinusitis and brain abscess, because *B. fragilis* is an uncommon isolate; however, empirical therapy with at least two agents is mandatory prior to culture confirmation. When the presence of staphylococci is proven or suspected, as in posttraumatic or postneurosurgical brain abscess, nafcillin or oxacillin (1.5 to 2 g intravenously every 4 h) is indicated. Vancomycin may be substituted if either the patient is allergic to penicillin or a methicillin-resistant strain is isolated. Fusidic acid is frequently employed in Europe, but it is not available in the United States. The frequent isolation of aerobic gram-negative bacilli from brain abscesses of otitic origin prompts many physicians to add a third-generation cephalosporin or trimethoprim-sulfamethoxazole to the antimicrobial regimen while awaiting culture results. Since *P. aeruginosa* is encountered in this setting of chronic middle ear infection, ceftazidime is a logical empirical choice. Recent data suggest that cefotaxime may be adequate for most streptococcal isolates as well, thereby replacing penicillin as the standard regimen (i.e., cefotaxime plus metronidazole as empirical therapy). It is unclear whether instillation of antibiotics into the abscess cavity during aspiration provides additional benefit.

The question of whether to use aspiration alone or total excision of a brain abscess in an individual patient remains problematic. Given the availability of stereotactic CT-guided aspiration, its low morbidity, and the chance it gives to obtain an accurate microbiologic and pathologic diagnosis, operative therapy should remain the definitive approach for most patients with brain abscess. If CT or MRI suggests the presence of cerebritis and the patient is neurologically stable, antibiotic therapy as previously outlined should be initiated and the patient observed. If the patient remains stable and the abscess or abscesses are accessible, CT-guided aspiration is then desirable to facilitate a specific pathologic and microbiologic diagnosis. This approach is advocated even if multiple lesions are present. Although this delay may render subsequent cultures negative, aspiration during the cerebritis stage may be associated with an unacceptable risk of hemorrhage, especially in children. If the lesion appears encapsulated by CT, antibiotic therapy should be started and aspiration for diagnosis and drainage performed immediately. Subsequent management will depend on both clinical and radiologic assessments. Multiple aspirations may be required to drain the abscess successfully, and this is a potential disadvantage relative to total excision. Neurologic deterioration, gas in the abscess cavity, or failure of the lesion to resolve on follow-up imaging studies is an indication for further surgery, often excision if feasible. The duration of antimicrobial therapy is empirical and also may relate to the initial surgical procedure used. Lesions treated by total excision may require a shorter duration of antimicrobial therapy than those treated with aspiration only. In general, most authorities recommend that patients be treated with at least 4 to 6 weeks of parenteral therapy. Metronidazole therapy may be an exception to this rule, because the high oral bioavailability of this agent facilitates the use of oral regimens. If a suitable oral agent or agents is available, a prolonged course of oral therapy, continuing for 2 to 6 months after the end of parenteral therapy, is often given, but it is of no proven benefit when compared with shorter treatment regimens. A cured brain abscess may continue to exhibit contrast enhancement on CT scans for from 4 to 10 weeks to up to 6 to 9 months after completion of successful therapy. The management of a focal CNS process in an HIV-infected patient requires a different approach and is discussed in Chap. 379. Empirical therapy for toxoplasmosis is often started if the CT appearance is characteristic in a seropositive patient. Brain biopsy for diagnosis may be considered in patients with a negative toxoplasmosis serology, atypical findings on CT, or evidence of a disseminated process due to another pathogen.

Adjunctive glucocorticoids are often employed during management of patients with brain abscess, but their role remains controversial. Glucocorticoids may reduce antibiotic entry into the CNS; they may decrease collagen formation and glial response and thereby lessen the degree of encapsulation of the brain abscess; and they may alter the CT appearance of ring enhancement as inflammation subsides, which may obscure information from sequential CT studies for the assessment of cure. Experimental animal models do not suggest that glucocorticoids alter the mortality rate. Glucocorticoids should be

employed in patients with proven or suspected elevation of ICP. In this circumstance, ICP monitoring may be advisable, and elevation may be controlled with steroids, hyperventilation, mannitol, or a combination of these methods. Anticonvulsants are frequently administered empirically to patients with suspected brain abscess.

PROGNOSIS The mortality rate of brain abscess was about 40 to 60 percent in the preantibiotic era and has remained high until relatively recently. The major reduction of the mortality rate (to about 10 percent) coincides with the advent of CT. The incidence of neurologic sequelae, however, ranges between 30 and 55 percent, and late seizures have been documented in as many as 90 percent of survivors. The relative uses of medical and surgical approaches for the individual patient continue to be elucidated. Earlier diagnosis through improved technology and an aggressive medical-surgical approach remain essential for the successful management of this unforgiving CNS infection.

SUBDURAL EMPYEMA

DEFINITION Subdural empyema is a collection of pus in the space between the dura mater and the arachnoid membrane. Subdural empyema accounts for about 20 percent of all localized intracranial infections. Prior to the advent of antimicrobial therapy, the disease was almost always fatal, but with current methods of diagnosis and treatment, mortality rates range from 10 to 40 percent.

EPIDEMIOLOGY Although precise incidence figures are unavailable, subdural empyemas are most often a complication of otorhinologic infection. Male patients predominate by a ratio of approximately 3:1, and about 70 percent of patients are in the second or third decade of life.

ETIOLOGY In most cases, a single microorganism is responsible for subdural empyema, but many cultures obtained at surgery are sterile because patients are often receiving antimicrobial therapy. In addition, the precise role of anaerobic bacteria in this infection has not been studied carefully because anaerobic techniques are often inadequate or not performed at surgery. Nevertheless, the major pathogens include aerobic and anaerobic streptococci (about 50 percent), staphylococci (about 12 to 16 percent), aerobic gram-negative bacilli (3 to 10 percent), and other anaerobic bacteria (about 5 percent). As with brain abscess, the causative organism is somewhat predictable based on the anatomic focus of contiguous infection. Otorhinogenic subdural empyemas are usually caused by streptococci (including members of the *S. intermedius* group), whereas staphylococci and anaerobes are unusual. Infections arising from head trauma, surgery, or indwelling foreign devices commonly involve staphylococci and/or aerobic gram-negative bacilli. Subdural empyema rarely complicates meningitis, but cases due to *S. pneumoniae* or *H. influenzae* have been described. Rare etiologic agents include *Salmonella* sp., *Campylobacter fetus*, *N. meningitidis*, *Pasteurella* sp., and *Actinomyces* sp.

PATHOGENESIS AND PATHOPHYSIOLOGY The subdural space, normally a potential rather than an actual space, is divided anatomically into several large compartments by the foramen magnum, tentorium cerebelli, base of the brain, and falx cerebri. Since these spaces are confined anatomically, a developing empyema can quickly evolve into a fatal expanding mass lesion. The pathogenesis usually involves spread of infection to the subdural space via valveless emissary veins in association with thrombophlebitis or by extension of an osteomyelitis of the skull with accompanying epidural abscess. Paranasal sinusitis predominates overwhelmingly as the precipitating factor. The frontal sinuses are almost always involved, often with other sinuses as well. The incidence of subdural empyema following frontal sinusitis is 1 to 2 percent. The frontal and sphenoid sinuses are intimately associated with the dura mater and are often separated from it by only a thin bony layer. Only about 10 percent of subdural empyemas are found infratentorially. The lesion may communicate with the contralateral side via the inferior free margin of the falx cerebri. The mastoid or middle ear is the source of subdural empyema in 10 to 20 percent of patients, especially in geographic areas (e.g., Sri Lanka) where delay in therapy of otitis media may be complicated by this event. Otitis or mastoiditis may extend directly into the subdural space via erosion of the tegmen tympani or bone adjacent to the dura mater and air cells or may spread indirectly by way of a progressive thrombophlebitis of the perforating veins. Otitis-induced subdural empyema is localized initially on or around the tentorium. Bacterial meningitis in adults is a very unusual cause of subdural empyema. Nevertheless, this lesion complicates about 2 percent of bacterial meningitis cases in infants and may follow an initially sterile subdural effusion. Other predisposing conditions include cranial trauma, use of cranial traction devices, neurosurgical or nasal procedures, and infection of a preexisting subdural hematoma. Subdural empyema is metastatic in origin in a small minority of cases (about 5 percent), arising principally from chronic infection in the chest. Once infection develops in the subdural space, spread along the falx and over the convexities may occur. Septic thrombophlebitis of the cortical veins and/or dural venous sinuses may evolve and lead to hemorrhage, cerebral infarction, brain edema, and fatal transtentorial herniation.

CLINICAL MANIFESTATIONS Subdural empyema may present as a rapidly progressive life-threatening condition. The symptoms and signs relate to the presence of increased ICP, meningeal irritation, or focal cortical inflammation. In addition, most patients (60 to 90 percent) have evidence of their antecedent infection (e.g., sinusitis or otitis). In general, patients often have a nonspecific illness for days to weeks prior to an acutely ill presentation. The most common symptoms and signs include headache, fever, stiff neck, and focal neurologic deficits. Headache, initially localized to the infected sinus or ear, is a prominent complaint and can become generalized as the infection progresses. Vomiting is common as ICP rises. Early during the course, about one-half of patients have altered mental status, which can progress to obtundation and/or coma in the absence of treatment. Fever above 39°C is present in most cases. Focal neurologic findings appear after 24 to 48 h of illness and progress rapidly to involvement of the entire cerebral hemisphere. Hemiparesis or hemiplegia is the most common focal finding; ocular palsy is common, and dysphasia, homonymous hemianopia, cerebellar signs, dilated pupils, and other focal presentations also have been observed. Seizures, either focal or generalized, are found in more than 50 percent of cases. Meningeal irritation (particularly meningismus) is found in 70 to 80 percent of patients, although Kernig's and/or Babinski's signs are less frequently noted. In the absence of treatment, neurologic deterioration occurs rapidly with signs of increased ICP and cerebral herniation. Papilledema develops in less than 50 percent of patients. Parafalcine subdural empyema characteristically produces contralateral leg symptoms, including weakness and focal seizures. This fulminant picture may not be seen in several clinical settings, including subdural empyema following cranial surgery and/or trauma, where the presentation may be subacute and subtle; subdural empyema affected by prior antimicrobial therapy; subdural empyema resulting from infection of a subdural hematoma; and metastatic infection of the subdural space from a chronic focus elsewhere. The clinical manifestations of subdural empyema in infants are similar to those found in adults, except that a bulging anterior fontanelle is a common finding.

DIAGNOSIS As with brain abscess, routine studies of blood, urine, and CSF are of limited value in the evaluation of patients with suspected subdural empyema. Most patients have a peripheral blood leukocytosis, and plain films of the skull may be useful in the demonstration of sinusitis or mastoiditis. Since a high degree of clinical suspicion and rapid diagnosis of this condition are critical for a successful outcome, subdural empyema should be suspected in any patient with a CNS syndrome with fever and focal neurologic findings. Lumbar puncture is contraindicated in this setting because of the risk of cerebral herniation. When it is performed, CSF findings are nonspecific and include an elevated opening pressure, a moderate neutrophilic pleocytosis, and an increased protein concentration. Unless the course is complicated by coexisting bacterial meningitis, Gram's staining and cultures of CSF are negative. Cerebral arteriography was the diagnostic procedure of choice prior to the development of CT.

Currently, CT with contrast enhancement and MRI are the diagnostic procedures of choice in patients with suspected subdural empyema.

The typical CT appearance is a crescentic or elliptical area of hypodensity below the cranial vault or adjacent to the falx cerebri. Loculations may be seen, and associated mass effect with displacement of midline structures is common. After the administration of contrast material, a fine, intense line of enhancement is seen between the subdural collection and the cerebral cortex. Gyral enhancement also is common. However, false-negative CT scans have been reported; MRI provides greater clarity for morphologic detail and may detect empyema not seen clearly on CT. MRI is of particular value in identifying subdural empyema located at the base of the brain, along the falx cerebri, or in the posterior fossa. On the basis of signal intensity, extraaxial empyemas can be differentiated from sterile effusions and/or chronic hematomas more readily by MRI than by CT. MRI is also better than CT for differentiating subdural empyema from epidural abscess and in delineating brain parenchymal abnormalities.

Both CT and MRI can be useful for the demonstration of sinusitis and otitis, although CT is better than MRI for bone imaging and should be used in cases of penetrating injury or when osteomyelitis is a consideration. Cerebral arteriography should be employed on an emergent basis when MRI is unavailable and subdural empyema is strongly suspected despite a normal CT appearance. Arteriography may establish the presence of a subdural avascular mass and detect spread of the lesion to the contralateral or parafalcine subdural space. As stated above, subdural empyema shows a striking predilection for young men in the second and third decades of life and should be strongly considered when a patient in this group has appropriate clinical findings.

℞ **TREATMENT**

Subdural empyema is a surgical emergency. While the patient is awaiting operative intervention, antibiotics should be chosen based on the suspected source of infection, the known organisms associated with that focus of infection, and the host immune status. A combined medical-surgical approach is optimal for the management of these patients. As with brain abscess, no controlled clinical trials have evaluated different antimicrobial regimens for the treatment of subdural empyema. Empirical therapy often includes penicillin G and/or chloramphenicol in the same doses as used for brain abscess (see above). If staphylococci are suspected, a β-lactamase–stable penicillin (e.g., nafcillin, 1.5 g intravenously every 4 h) should be used, with vancomycin (about 1 g intravenously every 12 h in adults) reserved for patients allergic to penicillin or when the presence of methicillin-resistant *S. aureus* is suspected. Metronidazole is often substituted for chloramphenicol at a loading dosage of 15 mg/kg, followed by 7.5 mg/kg intravenously every 6 h. Many authorities also add a third-generation cephalosporin (often cefotaxime or ceftriaxone) until culture results are available. Ceftazidime is useful in patients in whom *P. aeruginosa* is a consideration (e.g., in cases following neurosurgery or trauma). The duration of therapy is empirical; however, parenteral antibiotics should be continued for 3 to 4 weeks after drainage, depending on the patient's clinical response. Longer periods of intravenous therapy and/or continuation as an oral regimen may be required if an associated osteomyelitis is present.

Although case reports have suggested that subdural empyema may respond to antimicrobial agents alone, the optimal approach involves surgical drainage. The comparative efficacy of multiple burr holes versus an open craniotomy has not been subjected to rigorous clinical trial. All cases should involve close cooperation with a neurosurgical service. Previous reports of a lower mortality rate in studies of patients undergoing craniotomy may merely reflect the treatment of a larger percentage of gravely ill patients with burr hole drainage alone because of the greater surgical risk associated with an open craniotomy. Unfortunately, burr holes may be inadequate due to the thickened pus during the course of the infection. Craniotomy is often essential for posterior fossa subdural empyemas and is also needed in the 10 to 20 percent of patients who are initially treated with trephination. When craniotomy is performed, wide exposure should be obtained to allow adequate exploration of all areas where subdural pus is suspected. Although antibiotic irrigation at the time of surgery has become common, there are no data on the benefits of this practice. Drains or catheters are often left in the subdural space after the initial drainage, but this practice may increase the risk of nosocomial superinfection. Finally, surgical correction of the antecedent otorhinologic infection also may be necessary on an emergent basis. Adjunctive measures to control raised ICP are also essential. Preoperative use of mannitol, dexamethasone, and/or hyperventilation may be effective in controlling ICP. Glucocorticoids should, however, be tapered rapidly after surgical therapy because of the risk of secondary infection. Anticonvulsants are indicated in patients with seizures.

PROGNOSIS The overall mortality rate from subdural empyema averages 15 to 25 percent, with severe neurologic sequelae (chiefly disabling hemiparesis or aphasia) found in 5 to 25 percent of survivors. Seizures are documented on follow-up in 8 to 46 percent of patients. The presence of severe neurologic sequelae and of a more profound depression of consciousness at the time of presentation and/or initiation of therapy correlates directly with a higher mortality rate, a fact that underscores the need for rapid definitive diagnosis.

SPINAL SUBDURAL EMPYEMA This rare condition, with fewer than 50 cases reported in the literature, is far less common than spinal epidural abscess. The signs and symptoms include fever, back pain, and subsequent manifestations of spinal cord compression, but tenderness to palpation or percussion along the spine is often absent, in contrast to spinal epidural abscess. Most cases occur following hematogenous dissemination from a distant site of infection, and *S. aureus* is the most common etiologic agent. The presentation may resemble that of transverse myelitis. MRI is the diagnostic procedure of choice for suspected spinal subdural empyema, since it defines the extent of the lesion better than does CT. Spinal CT with metrizamide contrast is also useful in the diagnosis of this condition. Myelography should be performed when MRI and CT are not available. Myelography may not detect the entire length of the empyema if complete blocks are present in the spinal canal at multiple levels. Treatment should consist of empirical antibiotics directed initially at *S. aureus*. streptococci, and gram-negative enteric bacilli in association with prompt laminectomy for drainage of the empyema. The antimicrobial regimen is commonly administered for 2 to 4 weeks following surgical drainage.

EPIDURAL ABSCESS

SPINAL EPIDURAL ABSCESS This type of abscess possesses unique clinical features and constitutes an important neurologic and neurosurgical emergency. It is discussed in Chap. 373.

INTRACRANIAL EPIDURAL ABSCESS An *epidural abscess* is defined as a suppurative infection in the epidural space. This space is located between the dura mater and the overlying bone. Cranial epidural abscess often crosses the cranial dura along the emissary veins, so subdural empyema is also often present. Therefore, the etiology, pathogenesis, and bacteriology of intracranial abscess are usually similar to those described for subdural empyema, with an initial focus of infection in the paranasal sinuses, middle ear, or mastoids. The overall incidence of cranial epidural abscess is unknown. In general, it is the third most common localized intracranial infection, following brain abscess and subdural empyema in frequency. Only about 10 percent of all epidural abscesses arise in the intracranial epidural space. Unlike the striking sex and age distribution of subdural empyema, intracranial abscesses are rare in young children and have been reported over a wide age range, with a median in the sixth decade. Above the foramen magnum, the epidural space is only a potential space, since the dura is essentially adherent to the inner lining of the skull. Infections of the intracranial epidural space result primarily from an extension of

a contiguous focus of infection, such as sinusitis, mastoiditis, scalp or orbital cellulitis, and rhinocerebral mucormycosis, or as a result of an intracranial defect caused by a skull fracture or neurosurgical procedure, or as a complication of fetal monitoring. The risk of epidural abscess is increased if there has been more than one prior neurosurgical procedure or implantation of foreign material. In general, an epidural abscess is a slowly growing mass, a fact that accounts for its typically insidious clinical presentation. Intracranial abscesses rarely dissect beyond the base of the skull. As with subdural empyema, the organisms responsible for intracranial epidural abscesses depend on the underlying mechanism. Aerobic and microaerophilic streptococci predominate in cases derived from paranasal sinus infections, whereas *S. aureus* or *S. epidermidis* and aerobic gram-negative bacilli and/or anaerobes are associated with cranial trauma. Many other organisms have been isolated from localized intracranial abscesses, including *Salmonella* sp., *Eikenella corrodens*, *Aspergillus* sp., and the agents of mucormycosis. The onset of symptoms is often insidious and may be overshadowed by the primary focus of infection (e.g., sinusitis or otitis). Headache is a usual complaint, but the patient may otherwise be asymptomatic unless the clinical course is complicated by the development of subdural empyema or involvement of deeper intracranial structures, because the epidural abscess usually enlarges slowly and does not produce sudden major neurologic deficits unless complicated by deep extension. However, focal neurologic signs and/or focal generalized seizures, nausea, and vomiting may develop ultimately. Without treatment, papilledema or other signs of increased ICP develop as the abscess enlarges. An epidural abscess localized near the petrous bone may present as Gradenigo's syndrome, characterized by involvement of cranial nerves V and VI with unilateral facial pain and weakness of the lateral rectus muscle. If cranial osteomyelitis is present, edema and cellulitis of the face and/or scalp may be present. Attention may be focused on the primary process, such as sinusitis, cellulitis, or skull fracture, allowing a developing intracranial abscess to remain undetected. Thus, the striking manifestations of the complications, including an alteration in mental status and a declining level of consciousness (including coma and/or meningismus), may be the first indication of an intracranial process. Hyponatremia is found in ≥30 percent of cases. As with patients with suspected subdural empyema, CT scanning and MRI are the diagnostic procedures of choice for the detection of intracranial epidural abscess. Both studies usually demonstrate a superficial, circumscribed area of diminished density, often with a rim of contrast enhancement. This rim enhancement is usually thicker and more irregular with an epidural abscess than with subdural empyema. Subgaleal or subperiosteal abscesses, calvarial osteomyelitis, and frontal sinusitis are often associated with intracranial abscesses. MRI offers several advantages over CT scanning in the evaluation of patients with suspected intracranial epidural abscess. Small collections are often identified more accurately with MRI, and streak artifacts from bone are absent. In addition, MRI readily differentiates postoperative and posttraumatic abscesses from sterile effusions and/or chronic extraaxial hematomas; CT is far less accurate at making this distinction.

℞ **TREATMENT**

As is the case with other focal suppurative infections of the CNS, a combined medical-surgical therapeutic approach is optimal for management of intracranial epidural abscess. In adults, where 60 to 90 percent of intracranial abscesses are a direct result of extension from paranasal sinusitis or mastoiditis, empirical antimicrobial therapy should be directed against aerobic streptococci, staphylococci, and anaerobic bacteria and commonly involves a combination of agents. When cranial defects are suspected or proven, an antistaphylococcal agent such as a penicillinase-resistant penicillin or vancomycin should be added in the dosages discussed above. All intracranial epidural collections should be drained surgically. Furthermore, appropriate stains and cultures should be obtained at the time of surgery, including investigation for acid-fast bacteria and/or fungi if clinically warranted. The actual procedure employed, e.g., burr holes versus craniotomy or craniectomy, depends on the extent of the lesion and involvement of overlying bone. Dural grafting may be necessary if the dura has been breached by infection, and communications between sinus cavities and the epidural space may require surgical closure later. Perhaps owing to the insidious clinical presentation of intracranial epidural abscess, the high diagnostic accuracy of CT and MRI, and the availability of potent antimicrobial agents, the rates of morbidity and mortality from this condition are low. However, the prognosis is inversely related to the degree of encephalopathy at presentation.

SUPPURATIVE INTRACRANIAL THROMBOPHLEBITIS

EPIDEMIOLOGY AND ETIOLOGY Suppurative intracranial thrombophlebitis is defined by the simultaneous presence of venous thrombosis and suppuration in the intracranial compartment. The process may begin in veins and/or venous sinuses following infection of the paranasal sinuses, middle ear, mastoid, facial skin, or oropharynx and may involve additional vessels by propagation of clot or discontinuous spread. Septic intracranial thrombophlebitis also may complicate the presence of epidural abscess, subdural empyema, or bacterial meningitis. Occasionally, but rarely, metastatic spread of infection from a distant site leads directly to suppurative intracranial thrombophlebitis. Conditions that increase blood viscosity or coagulability, including dehydration, pregnancy, oral contraceptive use, sickle cell disease, polycythemia, malignancy, and trauma, all increase the likelihood of intracranial thrombosis and suppurative complications. Intracranial venous sinus thrombosis depends, to a large extent, on the close proximity of the dural venous sinuses to other structures involved by antecedent conditions. The usual predisposing conditions for the development of cavernous sinus thrombosis are paranasal sinusitis (especially of the frontal, ethmoidal, or sphenoidal sinuses) or infections of the face or mouth. The most common bacterial pathogens depend on the initial source of infection; with sinusitis, they are staphylococci, aerobic and/or microaerophilic streptococci, gram-negative bacilli, and/or anaerobes, whereas *S. aureus* predominates when a facial infection is the source. Otitis media or mastoiditis may be complicated by the development of lateral sinus thrombosis and/or infection of the superior and inferior petrosal sinuses. Infections of the face, scalp, subdural space, epidural space, or meninges are associated with suppurative thrombophlebitis of the superior sagittal sinus. Again, the most likely infecting microorganisms depend on the associated primary condition. *S. aureus* is the most important associated pathogen in patients with cavernous sinus thrombosis and is isolated in more than two-thirds of cases. This predominance reflects the importance of this organism in the associated infections of the face and scalp and in acute sphenoid sinusitis. Less common isolates in patients with cavernous sinus thrombosis include streptococci, pneumococci, gram-negative bacilli, and *Bacteroides* sp.

CLINICAL MANIFESTATIONS Not unexpectedly, the clinical presentation of suppurative cortical thrombophlebitis depends on the location of involvement. In addition, if the cortical venous system is involved, the likelihood of neurologic deficits depends on the adequacy of collateral venous drainage. Patients with inadequate collateral flow present with impairment of consciousness, focal or generalized seizures (often alternating in character), symptoms of increased ICP, and various focal neurologic findings (e.g., hemiparesis). Aphasia is common when the dominant cerebral hemisphere is involved. The most common complaints in patients with cavernous sinus thrombosis include periorbital swelling (73 percent) and headache (52 percent). Headache is more common when the antecedent condition is sinusitis rather than a facial cellulitis. Other prominent symptoms include diplopia, tearing, photophobia, drowsiness, and ptosis. Fever is present in over 90 percent of patients with cavernous sinus thrombosis. Upon examination, proptosis, chemosis, periorbital edema, and weakness of the extraocular muscles due to involvement of cranial nerves III, IV, or VI are common. Since the abducens nerve is the only cranial nerve traversing the inferior portion of the cavernous sinus, a lateral gaze palsy may be an early neurologic finding. Papilledema and/or retinal

hemorrhages, and venous engorgement with a change in mental status, are observed in approximately 65 and 55 percent of patients, respectively. Meningitis is present in about 40 percent of cases and often creates diagnostic confusion; it is usually secondary to retrograde spread of thrombophlebitis. About 25 percent of patients also have dilated or sluggishly reactive pupils, decreased visual acuity (frequently progressing to blindness), and dysfunction of cranial nerve V. With spread of the infection to the opposite cavernous sinus, these findings may be duplicated in the opposite eye. In addition, septic cavernous sinus thrombosis may present in two ways. In the acute presentation, the delay in onset between the primary infection (usually a facial cellulitis) and cavernous sinus thrombosis is less than 1 week. The patient appears seriously ill, with a rapid development of symptoms and signs described above and progression to bilateral eye signs. In contrast, some patients present with a more indolent form of cavernous sinus thrombosis, usually secondary to dental infections, otitis media, or paranasal sinusitis. The orbital manifestations are less impressive, and involvement of the contralateral eye is a late and inconsistent finding. Headache is the most prominent finding (>80 percent of cases) in patients with septic lateral sinus thrombosis, but earache, vomiting, nausea, and vertigo are often present, since otitis media is a common predisposing condition. Fever and abnormal ear findings are observed in most patients (about 80 and 98 percent, respectively); facial pain, altered facial sensation, papilledema, mild nuchal rigidity, and/or a sixth nerve palsy also may be present. Thrombosis of the superior sagittal sinus produces an abnormal mental status progressing to coma, motor deficits (bilateral leg weakness progressing to arm weakness), nuchal rigidity, and papilledema. Seizurs occur in more than 50 percent of patients. The onset may be subacute, particularly in patients with sinusitis. Involvement of the inferior petrosal sinus may produce ipsilateral facial pain and lateral rectus muscle weakness (Gradenigo's syndrome).

DIAGNOSIS MRI is the diagnostic procedure of choice for the evaluation of patients with suspected suppurative intracranial thrombophlebitis. MRI is far superior to CT in differentiating thrombosis from normally flowing blood and can be improved by use of magnetic resonance angiography. MRI also can reveal the evolution and resolution of the entire venoocclusive process. CT scanning, with and without intravenous contrast enhancement, also permits diagnosis of venous sinus thrombosis, but it is considerably less sensitive and reliable than MRI. The CT appearance usually consists of unilateral or bilateral multiple irregular filling defects in the enhancement of the cavernous sinus with or without orbital inflammatory changes. Both MRI and CT can reliably evaluate the paranasal sinuses and provide information concerning subdural and epidural infection, cerebral infarction, cerebritis, hemorrhage, and/or cerebral edema. In the unusual case in which MRI and CT are negative but suspicion of thrombophlebitis is high, carotid arteriography with venous phase studies should be performed. Arteriography reveals narrowing of the intracavernous segment of the carotid artery in cavernous sinus thrombosis. Orbital venography also may be useful and is the most definitive method of demonstrating cavernous sinus thrombosis. As with other focal suppurative intracranial processes, the lumbar puncture usually demonstrates a mild pleocytosis and an elevated protein concentration. In septic thrombosis of the superior sagittal sinus, however, the CSF findings may be consistent with a frank meningitis, and the causative organism is often isolated on CSF culture. Blood cultures may be positive, especially in patients with a rapidly progressing course. Chest radiographs may reveal evidence of septic pulmonary emboli following propagation of thrombus into the inferior petrosal sinus and the jugular vein.

℞ **TREATMENT**

As for subdural empyema and epidural abscess, empirical therapy should be directed at gram-positive organisms, including staphylococci, aerobic gram-negative bacilli, and anaerobes. In cavernous sinus thrombosis, a potent antistaphylococcal agent should always be included in the antimicrobial regimen. Nafcillin should be used, with vancomycin reserved for the penicillin-allergic patient and when methicillin-resistant organisms are suspected or proven. Combination regimens including nafcillin or vancomycin plus metronidazole plus a third-generation cephalosporin are often used. Surgical intervention may be required for optimal therapy. Surgical drainage of infected sinuses is necessary when antimicrobial therapy alone is ineffective. Operative intervention is often used for patients with cavernous sinus thrombosis, especially in the setting of sphenoid sinusitis. Internal jugular vein ligation and thrombectomy have been used in patients with lateral sinus vein thrombosis, but the efficacy of these procedures is poorly defined. Surgical therapy also may be necessary for other contiguous foci of infection, e.g., dental abscess. The role of anticoagulation is controversial. Although anticoagulation may prevent the spread of the thrombus, this benefit is most apparent when anticoagulation is started early in the course of disease. However, the hazards of intracranial hemorrhage, including bleeding from sites of cortical venous infarction, must be recognized. In the absence of definitive data and specific contraindications, anticoagulation is most likely to be useful early in the course of cavernous sinus thrombosis or when overt embolization has occurred. Anticoagulation is not recommended for septic lateral sinus thrombophlebitis, because the cortical veins overlying the infected mastoid may become occluded, resulting in small venous hemorrhagic infarcts and leading to intracerebral hemorrhage. The efficacy and safety of thrombolytic therapy (e.g., with urokinase), internal jugular vein ligation, or thrombectomy have not been determined for suppurative intracranial thrombophlebitis.

BIBLIOGRAPHY

BRADLEY JS, SCHELD WM: The challenge of penicillin-resistant *Streptococcus pneumoniae:* Current antibiotic therapy of meningitis in the 1990s. Clin Infect Dis 24 (Suppl 2):5213, 1997

DILL SR et al: Subdural empyema: Analysis of 32 cases and review. Clin Infect Dis 20:372, 1995

DINUBILE MJ et al: Septic cortical thrombophlebitis. J Infect Dis 161:1216, 1990

DURAND ML ET AL: Acute bacterial meningitis in adults. A review of 493 episodes. N Engl J Med 328:21, 1993

GELLIN BG et al: Epidural abscess, in *Infections of the Central Nervous System,* 2d ed, WM Scheld et al (eds). New York, Lippincott-Raven, 1997, pp 507–522

GREENLEE JE: Suppurative intracranial phlebitis, in *Mandell, Douglas and Bennett's Principles and Practices of Infectious Diseases,* 4th ed, Mandell GL et al (eds). New York, Churchill Livingstone, 1995, pp 907–909

HAGENSEE ME et al: Brain abscess following marrow transplantation: Experience at the Fred Hutchinson Cancer Research Center, 1984–1992. Clin Infect Dis 19:402, 1994

HELFGOTT DC et al: Subdural empyema, in *Infections of the Central Nervous System,* 2d ed, WM Scheld et al (eds). New York, Lippincott-Raven, 1997, pp 495–506

HLAVIN ML et al: Intracranial suppuration: A modern decade of postoperative subdural empyema and epidural abscess. Neurosurgery 34:974, 1994

LEBELL MH et al: Dexamethasone therapy for bacterial meningitis: Results of two double-blind, placebo-controlled trials. N Engl J Med 319:964, 1988

LEVY RM: Brain abscess and subdural empyema. Curr Opin Neurol 7:223, 1994

MAMELAK AN et al: Improved management of multiple brain abscesses: A combined surgical and medical approach. Neurosurgery 36:76, 1995

ODIO CM et al: The beneficial effects of early dexamethasone administration in infants and children with bacterial meningitis. N Engl J Med 324:1525, 1991

PARIS M et al: Management of meningitis caused by penicillin-resistant *Streptococcus pneumoniae.* Antimicrob Agents Chemother 39:2171, 1995

PFISTER HW et al: Spectrum of complications during bacterial meningitis in adults—results of a prospective clinical study. Arch Neurol 50:575, 1993

——— et al: Mechanisms of brain injury in bacterial meningitis: Workshop summary. Clin Infect Dis 19:463, 1994

PINNER RW et al: Meningococcal disease in the United States—1986. J Infect Dis 164:368, 1991

QUAGLIARELLO V, SCHELD WM: Bacterial meningitis: Pathogenesis, pathophysiology, and progress. N Engl J Med 327:864, 1992

———, ———: Drug therapy: Treatment of bacterial meningitis. N Engl J Med 336:708, 1997

ROOS KL et al: Acute bacterial meningitis in children and adults, in *Infections of the Central Nervous System,* 2d ed, WM Scheld et al (eds). New York, Lippincott-Raven, 1997, pp 335–402

ROSENFELD EA, BOWLEY AH: Infectious complications of sinusitis, other than meningitis in children: 12 year review. Clin Infect Dis 18:750, 1994

SAEZ-LLORENS X et al: Molecular pathophysiology of bacterial meningitis: Current concepts and therapeutic implications. J Pediatr 116:671, 1990

SEYDOUX CH, FRANCIOLI P: Bacterial brain abscesses: Factors influencing mortality and sequelae. Clin Infect Dis 15:394, 1992

SJOLIN J et al: Treatment of brain abscess with cefotaxime and metronidazole: Prospective study of 15 consecutive patients. Clin Infect Dis 17:857, 1993

SPANOS A et al: Differential diagnosis of acute meningitis. JAMA 262:2700, 1989

STEPHENS DS, FARLEY MM: Pathogenetic events during infection of the human nasal pharynx with *Neisseria meningitidis* and *Haemophilus influenzae.* Rev Infect Dis 13:22, 1991

TOWNSEND GC, SCHELD WM: Clinically important trends in bacterial meningitis. Infect Dis Clin Pract 4:423, 1995

TUNKEL AR, SCHELD WM: Pathogenesis and pathophysiology of bacterial meningitis. Ann Rev Med 44:103, 1993

———, ———: Acute bacterial meningitis. Lancet 346:1675, 1995

——— et al: Bacterial meningitis: Recent advances in pathophysiology and treatment. Ann Intern Med 112:610, 1990

WENGER JD et al: Bacterial meningitis in the United States, 1986: Report of a multistate surveillance study. J Infect Dis 162:1316, 1990

WISPELWEY B, SCHELD WM: Brain abscess, in *Infections of the Central Nervous System,* 2d ed, WM Scheld et al (eds). New York, Lippincott-Raven, 1997, pp 463–494

---

378 Walter J. Koroshetz, Morton N. Swartz

CHRONIC AND RECURRENT MENINGITIS

Chronic inflammation of the meninges (pia, arachnoid, and dura) can produce profound neurologic disability and may be fatal if not successfully treated. The condition is most commonly diagnosed when a characteristic neurologic syndrome exists for longer than 4 weeks and is associated with a persistent inflammatory response in the cerebrospinal fluid (CSF) (white blood cell count >5/μL). The causes are varied, and appropriate treatment depends on identification of the etiology. Five categories of disease account for most cases of chronic meningitis: (1) meningeal infections, (2) malignancy, (3) noninfectious inflammatory disorders, (4) chemical meningitis, and (5) parameningeal infections.

CLINICAL PATHOPHYSIOLOGY Neurologic manifestations of chronic meningitis (Table 378-1) are determined by the anatomic location of the inflammation and its consequences. Persistent headache with or without stiff neck and hydrocephalus, cranial neuropathies, radiculopathies, and cognitive or personality changes are the

Table 378-1

Symptoms and Signs of Chronic Meningitis

Symptoms	Signs
Chronic headache	+/− Papilledema
Neck or back pain	Brudzinski's or Kernig's sign of meningeal irritation
Change in personality	Altered mental status—drowsiness, inattention, disorientation, memory loss, frontal release signs (grasp, suck, snout), perseveration
Facial weakness	Peripheral seventh CN palsy
Double vision	Palsy of CNs III, IV, VI
Visual loss	Papilledema, optic atrophy
Hearing loss	Eighth CN palsy
Arm or leg weakness	Myelopathy or radiculopathy
Numbness in arms or legs	Myelopathy or radiculopathy
Sphincter dysfunction	Myelopathy or radiculopathy Frontal lobe dysfunction
Clumsiness	Ataxia

cardinal features. These can occur alone or in combination. When they appear in combination, widespread dissemination of the inflammatory process along CSF pathways has occurred. In some cases, the presence of an underlying systemic illness points to a specific agent or class of agents as the probable cause. The diagnosis of chronic meningitis is usually made when the clinical presentation prompts the astute physician to examine the CSF for signs of inflammation.

CSF is produced by the choroid plexus of the cerebral ventricles, exits through narrow foramina into the subarachnoid space surrounding the brain and spinal cord, circulates around the base of the brain and over the cerebral hemispheres, and is resorbed by arachnoid villi projecting into the superior sagittal sinus. CSF flow provides a pathway for rapid spread of infectious and malignant processes over the brain, spinal cord, and cranial and spinal nerve roots. Spread from the subarachnoid space into brain parenchyma may occur via the arachnoid cuffs that surround blood vessels that penetrate brain tissue (Virchow-Robin spaces).

Intracranial Meningitis Nociceptive fibers of the meninges (Chap. 15) are stimulated by the inflammatory process, resulting in headache, or neck or back pain. Obstruction of CSF pathways at foramina or arachnoid villi may produce hydrocephalus and symptoms of raised intracranial pressure, including headache, vomiting, apathy or drowsiness, gait instability, papilledema, visual loss, impaired upgaze, or palsy of the seventh cranial nerve (CN) (Chap. 28). Cognitive and behavioral changes during the course of chronic meningitis may also result from vascular damage, which may similarly produce seizures, stroke, or myelopathy.

Inflammatory deposits seeded via CSF circulation are often prominent around the brainstem and cranial nerves and along the undersurface of the frontal and temporal lobes. Such cases, termed *basal meningitis*, often present as multiple cranial neuropathies, with visual loss (CN II), facial weakness (CN VII), hearing loss (CN VIII), diplopia (CNs III, IV, and VI), sensory or motor abnormalities of the oropharynx (CNs IX, X, and XII), decreased olfaction (CN I), or facial sensory loss and masseter weakness (CN V).

Spinal Meningitis Injury may occur to motor and sensory roots as they traverse the subarachnoid space and penetrate the meninges. These cases present as multiple radiculopathies with combinations of radicular pain, sensory loss, motor weakness, and sphincter dysfunction. Meningeal inflammation can encircle the cord, resulting in myelopathy. Patients with slowly progressive involvement of multiple cranial nerves and/or spinal nerve roots are likely to have chronic meningitis. Electrophysiologic testing (electromyography, nerve conduction studies, and evoked response testing) may be helpful in determining whether there is involvement of cranial and spinal nerve roots.

Systemic Manifestations In some patients, evidence of systemic disease provides clues to the underlying cause of chronic meningitis. A careful history and physical examination is essential before embarking on a diagnostic workup, which may be costly, prolonged, and associated with risk from invasive procedures. A complete history of travel, sexual practice, and exposure to infectious agents should be sought. Infectious causes are often associated with fever, malaise, anorexia, and signs of localized or disseminated infection outside the nervous system. Infectious causes are of major concern in the immunosuppressed patient, especially in patients with AIDS, in whom chronic meningitis may present without headache or fever. Noninfectious inflammatory disorders often produce systemic manifestations, but meningitis may be the initial manifestation. Carcinomatous meningitis may or may not be accompanied by clinical evidence of the primary neoplasm.

Approach to the Patient

The occurrence of chronic headache, hydrocephalus, cranial neuropathy, radiculopathy, and/or cognitive decline in a patient should prompt consideration of a lumbar puncture for evidence of meningeal inflammation. On occasion the diagnosis is made when an imaging study [computed tomography (CT) or magnetic resonance imaging (MRI)] shows contrast enhancement of the meninges, always an abnormal finding except after a recent neurosurgical procedure. Once chronic meningitis is confirmed by CSF examination, effort is focused on identifying the cause (Tables 378-2 and 378-3) by (1) further analysis of the CSF, (2) diagnosis of an underlying systemic infection or noninfectious inflammatory condition, or (3) pathologic examination of meningeal biopsy specimens.

Two clinical forms of chronic meningitis exist. In the first, the symptoms are chronic and persistent, whereas in the second there are recurrent, discrete episodes of illness. In the latter group, all symptoms, signs, and CSF parameters of meningeal inflammation resolve completely between episodes without specific therapy. In such patients, the likely etiologies include infection with herpes simplex virus (HSV) type 2; chemical meningitis due to leakage into CSF of contents from an epidermoid tumor, craniopharyngioma, or cholesteatoma; primary inflammatory conditions, including Vogt-Koyanagi-Harada syndrome, Behçet's syndrome, Mollaret's meningitis, and systemic lupus erythematosus; and drug hypersensitivity with repeated administration of the offending agent. The duration of chronic meningitis may also be of value in diagnosis; for example, an untreated patient with tuberculous meningitis is unlikely to survive beyond 4 to 6 weeks.

The epidemiologic history is of considerable importance and may provide direction for selection of laboratory studies. Pertinent features include a history of tuberculosis or exposure to a likely case; past travel to areas endemic for fungal infections (the San Joaquin Valley in California and southwestern states for coccidioidomycosis; midwestern states for histoplasmosis, southeastern states for blastomycosis); travel to the Mediterranean region or ingestion of imported unpasteurized dairy products (*Brucella* infection); time spent in areas endemic for Lyme disease (e.g., Connecticut, New York, Massachusetts); exposure to sexually transmitted disease (syphilis); exposure of an immunocompromised host to pigeons and their droppings (*Cryptococcus*; Fig. 378-1); gardening (*Sporothrix schenkii*); ingestion of poorly cooked meat or contact with a household cat (*Toxoplasma gondii*); residence in Thailand or Japan (*Gnathostoma spinigerum*) or the South Pacific (*Angiostrongylus cantonensis*); rural residence and raccoon exposure (*Baylisascaris procyonis*); and residence in Latin America, the Philippines, or Southeast Asia when eosinophilic meningitis is present (*Taenia solium*).

The presence of focal cerebral signs in a patient with chronic meningitis suggests the possibility of a brain abscess or other parameningeal infection; identification of a potential source of infection (chronic draining ear, sinusitis, right-to-left cardiac or pulmonary shunt, chronic pleuropulmonary infection) supports this diagnosis. In some cases, diagnosis may be established by recognition and biopsy of unusual skin lesions (Behçet's syndrome, cryptococcosis, blastomycosis, lupus erythematosus, Lyme disease, intravenous drug use, sporotrichosis, trypanosomiasis) or enlarged lymph nodes [lymphoma, tuberculosis, sarcoid, infection with human immunodeficiency virus (HIV), secondary syphilis, or Whipple's disease]. A careful ophthalmologic examination may reveal uveitis [Vogt-Koyanagi-Harada syndrome, sarcoid, or central nervous system (CNS) lymphoma], keratoconjunctivitis sicca (Sjögren's syndrome), or iridocyclitis (Behçet's syndrome) and is essential to assess visual loss from hydrocephalus. Aphthous oral lesions, genital ulcers, and hypopyon suggest Behçet's syndrome. Hepatosplenomegaly suggests lymphoma, sarcoid, tuberculosis, or brucellosis. Herpetic lesions in the genital area or on the thighs suggests HSV-2 infection. A breast nodule, a suspicious pigmented skin lesion, or an abdominal mass directs attention to possible carcinomatous meningitis.

Imaging Once the clinical syndrome is recognized as a potential manifestation of chronic meningitis, proper analysis of the CSF is essential. However, if the possibility of raised intracranial pressure exists, a brain imaging study should be performed before lumbar puncture. In patients with communicating hydrocephalus caused by impaired resorption of CSF, lumbar puncture is safe and may lead to temporary improvement. However, if intracranial pressure is elevated because of a mass lesion or a block in ventricular CSF outflow (obstruc-

Table 378-2

Infectious Causes of Chronic Meningitis

Causative Agent	CSF Formula	Helpful Diagnostic Tests	Risk Factors and Systemic Manifestations
COMMON BACTERIAL CAUSES			
Partially treated suppurative meningitis	Mononuclear or mixed mononuclear-polymorphonuclear cells	CSF culture and Gram's stain	History consistent with acute bacterial meningitis and incomplete treatment
Parameningeal infection	Mononuclear or mixed mononuclear-polymorphonuclear cells	Contrast-enhanced MRI or CT to detect parenchymal, subdural, epidural, or sinus infection	Otitis media, pleuropulmonary infection, right-to-left cardiopulmonary shunt for brain abscess, focal neurologic signs; neck, back, ear, or sinus tenderness
Mycobacterium tuberculosis	Mononuclear cells except polymorphonuclear cells in early infection (leukocytes commonly <500/μL); low CSF glucose, elevated protein	Tuberculin skin test may be negative; AFB culture of CSF (sputum, urine, gastric contents if indicated); tuberculostearic acid detection in CSF; identify tubercle bacillus on acid-fast stain of CSF or protein pellicle; PCR	Exposure history; previous tuberculous illness; immunosuppressed or AIDS; young children; fever, meningismus, night sweats, miliary TB on x-ray or liver biopsy; stroke due to arteritis
Lyme disease (Bannwarth's syndrome): *Borrelia burgdorferi*	Mononuclear cells; elevated protein	Serum Lyme antibody titer; western blot confirmation; (patients with syphilis may have false-positive Lyme titer)	History of tick bite or appropriate exposure history; erythema chronicum migrans skin rash; arthritis, radiculopathy, Bell's palsy, meningoencephalitis–multiple sclerosis-like syndrome
Syphilis (secondary, tertiary): *Treponema pallidum*	Mononuclear cells; elevated protein	CSF VDRL; serum VDRL (or RPR); FTA or MHA-TP; serum VDRL may be negative in tertiary syphilis	Appropriate exposure history; HIV seropositive individuals at increased risk of aggressive infection; "dementia"; cerebral infarction due to endarteritis
UNCOMMON BACTERIAL CAUSES			
Actinomyces	Polymorphonuclear cells	Anaerobic culture	Parameningeal abscess or sinus tract (oral or dental focus); pneumonitis
Nocardia	Polymorphonuclear cells; occasionally mononuclear cells; often low glucose	Isolation may require weeks; weakly acid fast	Associated brain abscess may be present
Brucella	Mononuclear cells (rarely polymorphonuclear); elevated protein; often low glucose	CSF antibody detection; serum antibody detection	Intake of unpasteurized dairy products; exposure to goats, sheep, cows; fever, arthralgia, myalgia, vertebral osteomyelitis
Whipple's disease: *Tropherema whippelii*	Mononuclear cells	Biopsy of small bowel or lymph node; CSF PCR for *T. whippelii*; brain and meningeal biopsy (with PAS stain and EM examination)	Diarrhea, weight loss, arthralgias, fever; dementia, ataxia, paresis, ophthalmoplegia, oculomasticatory myoclonus
RARE BACTERIAL CAUSES			

Leptospirosis (occasionally if left untreated may last 3–4 weeks); *Pseudoallescheria boydii* (neutrophilic pleocytosis)

FUNGAL CAUSES

Causative Agent	CSF Formula	Helpful Diagnostic Tests	Risk Factors and Systemic Manifestations
Cryptococcus neoformans	Mononuclear cells; count not elevated in some patients with AIDS	India ink or fungal wet mount of CSF (budding yeast); blood and urine cultures; antigen detection in CSF	AIDS and immunosuppression; pigeon exposure; skin and other organ involvement due to disseminated infection
Coccidioides immitis	Mononuclear cells (sometimes 10–20% eosinophils); often low glucose	Antibody detection in CSF and serum	Exposure history—southwestern US; increased virulence in dark-skinned races
Candida sp.	Polymorphonuclear or mononuclear cells	Fungal stain and culture of CSF	IV drug abuse; recent surgery; prolonged intravenous therapy; disseminated candidiasis
Histoplasma capsulatum	Mononuclear cells; low glucose	Fungal stain and culture of large volumes of CSF; antigen detection in CSF, serum, and urine; antibody detection in serum, CSF	Exposure history—Ohio and central Mississippi River Valley; AIDS; mucosal lesions
Blastomyces dermatitidis	Mononuclear cells	Fungal stain and culture of CSF; biopsy and culture of skin, lung lesions; antibody detection in serum	Midwestern and southeastern US; usually systemic infection; abscesses, draining sinus, ulcers
Aspergillus sp.	Mononuclear or polymorphonuclear cells	CSF culture	Sinusitis; granulocytopenia or immunosuppression
Sporothrix schenckii	Mononuclear cells	Antibody detection in CSF and serum; CSF culture	Traumatic inoculation; IV drug use; ulcerated skin lesion
RARE FUNGAL CAUSES			

Cladophialophora bantiana (formerly *Cladosporium trichoides*) and other dark-walled (dematiaceous) fungi such as *Curvularia* and *Drechslera*; *Mucor*

(continued)

Table 378-2—(continued)

Infectious Causes of Chronic Meningitis

Causative Agent	CSF Formula	Helpful Diagnostic Tests	Risk Factors and Systemic Manifestations
PROTOZOAL CAUSES			
Toxoplasma gondii	Mononuclear cells	Biopsy or response to empirical therapy in clinically appropriate context (including presence of antibody in serum)	Usually with intracerebral abscesses; common in HIV-seropositive patients
Trypanosomiasis *Trypanosoma gambiense,* *Trypanosoma rhodesiense*	Mononuclear cells, elevated protein level	Elevated CSF IgM; identification of trypanosomes in CSF and blood smear	Endemic in Africa; chancre, lymphadenopathy; prominent sleep disorder
RARE PROTOZOAL CAUSES			
Acanthamoeba sp. causing granulomatous amebic encephalitis and meningoencephalitis in immunocompromised and debilitated individuals			
HELMINTHIC CAUSES			
Cysticercosis (infection with cysts of *Taenia solium*)	Mononuclear cells; may have eosinophils; glucose level may be low	Indirect hemagglutination assay in CSF; ELISA immunoblotting in serum	Usually with multiple cysts in basal meninges and hydrocephalus; cerebral cysts, muscle calcification
Gnathostoma spinigerum	Eosinophils, mononuclear cells	Peripheral eosinophilia	History of eating raw fish; common in Thailand and Japan; subarachnoid hemorrhage; painful radiculopathy
Angiostrongylus cantonensis	Eosinophils, mononuclear cells	Recovery of worms from CSF	History of eating raw shellfish; common in tropical Pacific regions; often benign
Baylisascaris procyonis (raccoon ascarid)	Eosinophils, mononuclear cells		Infection follows accidental ingestion of *B. procyonis* eggs from raccoon feces; fatal meningoencephalitis
RARE HELMINTHIC CAUSES			
Trichinella spiralis (trichinosis); *Echinococcus* cysts; *Schistosoma* sp. The first may produce a lymphocytic pleocytosis, whereas the latter two may produce an eosinophilic response in CSF associated with cerebral cysts (*Echinococcus*) or granulomatous lesions of brain or spinal cord			
VIRAL CAUSES			
Mumps	Mononuclear cells	Antibody in serum	No prior mumps or immunization; may produce meningoencephalitis; may persist for 3–4 weeks
Lymphocytic choriomeningitis	Mononuclear cells	Antibody in serum	Contact with rodents or their excreta; may persist for 3–4 weeks
Echovirus	Mononuclear cells; may have low glucose	Virus isolation from CSF	Congenital hypogammaglobulinemia; history of recurrent meningitis
HIV (acute retroviral syndrome)	Mononuclear cells	p24 antigen in serum and CSF; high level of HIV viremia	HIV risk factors; rash, fever, lymphadenopathy; lymphopenia in peripheral blood; syndrome may persist long enough to be considered chronic meningitis; or chronic meningitis may develop in later stages (AIDS) due to HIV
Herpes simplex	Mononuclear cells	PCR for HSV DNA; CSF antibody	Recurrent meningitis due to HSV-2 (rarely HSV-1) often associated with genital recurrences

ABBREVIATIONS: ELISA, enzyme-linked immunosorbent assay; EM, electron microscopy; FTA, fluorescent treponemal antibody absorption test; IV, intravenous; MHA-TP, microhemagglutination assay-*Treponema pallidum*; PAS, periodic acid–Schiff; PCR, polymerase chain reaction; RPR, rapid plasma reagin test; TB, tuberculosis.

tive hydrocephalus), then lumbar puncture carries the potential risk of brain herniation. Obstructive hydrocephalus usually requires direct ventricular drainage of CSF.

Contrast-enhanced MRI or CT studies of the brain and spinal cord can identify meningeal enhancement, parameningeal infections (including brain abscess), encasement of the spinal cord (malignancy or inflammation and infection), or nodular deposits on the meninges or nerve roots (malignancy or sarcoidosis). Imaging studies are also useful to localize areas of meningeal disease prior to meningeal biopsy.

Cerebral angiography may be indicated in patients with chronic meningitis and stroke to identify cerebral arteritis (granulomatous angiitis, infectious arteritis).

Cerebrospinal Fluid Analysis The CSF pressure should be measured and samples sent for bacterial culture, cell count and differential, Gram's stain, and measurement of glucose and protein. In cases without a known cause, CSF should be sent for the Venereal Disease Research Laboratories (VDRL) test, acid-fast bacillus (AFB) stain and culture, fungal wet mount and India ink preparation and culture, culture for

fastidious bacteria and fungi, assays for cryptococcal antigen and oligoclonal immunoglobulin bands, and cytology. Other specific CSF tests (Tables 378-2 and 378-3) or blood tests and cultures should be ordered as indicated on the basis of the history, physical examination, or preliminary CSF results (i.e., eosinophilic, mononuclear, or polymorphonuclear meningitis).

In most categories of chronic (not recurrent) meningitis, mononuclear cells predominate in the CSF. When neutrophils predominate after 3 weeks of illness, the principal etiologic considerations are *Nocardia asteroides, Actinomyces israelii, Brucella, Mycobacterium tuberculosis* (5 to 10 percent of early cases only), various fungi [*Blastomyces dermatitidis, Candida albicans, Histoplasma capsulatum, Aspergillus* species, *Pseudallescheria boydii, Cladophialophora bantiana*] and noninfectious causes [systemic lupus erythematosus (SLE), exogenous chemical meningitis]. When eosinophils predominate or are present in limited numbers in a primarily mononuclear cell response in the CSF, the differential diagnosis includes parasitic diseases (*A. cantonensis, G. spinigerum, B. procyonis,* or *Toxocara canis* infection, cysticercosis, schistosomiasis, echinococcal disease, *T. gondii* infection), fungal infections (6 to 20 percent eosinophils along with a predominantly lymphocyte pleocytosis, particularly with coccidioidal meningitis), neoplastic disease (lymphoma, leukemia, metastatic carcinoma), or other inflammatory processes (sarcoidosis, hypereosinophilic syndrome).

It is often necessary to broaden the number of diagnostic tests if the initial workup does not reveal the cause. In addition, repeated samples of large volumes of CSF may be required to diagnose certain infectious and malignant causes of chronic meningitis. For instance, lymphomatous or carcinomatous meningitis may be diagnosed by examination of sections cut from a cell block formed by spinning down the sediment from a large volume of CSF. The diagnosis of fungal meningitis may require large volumes of CSF for culture of sediment. If standard lumbar puncture is unrewarding, a cervical cisternal tap to sample CSF near to the basal meninges may be fruitful.

Laboratory Investigation In addition to the CSF examination, an attempt should be made to uncover pertinent underlying illnesses. Tuberculin skin test, chest radiograph, urine analysis and culture, blood count and differential, renal and liver function tests, and measurement of electrolytes (including calcium and phosphate), sedimentation rate, antinuclear antibody, and serum angiotensin-converting enzyme level are often indicated. Liver or bone marrow biopsy may be diagnostic in some cases of miliary tuberculosis, disseminated fungal infection, sarcoidosis, or metastatic malignancy. Abnormalities discovered on chest radiograph or chest CT can be pursued by bronchoscopy or transthoracic needle biopsy.

Meningeal Biopsy A diagnostic meningeal biopsy should be strongly considered in patients who are severely disabled, who need chronic ventricular decompression, or whose illness is progressing

Table 378-3

Noninfectious Causes of Chronic Meningitis

Causative Agents	CSF Formula	Helpful Diagnostic Tests	Risk Factors and Systemic Manifestations
Malignancy	Mononuclear cells, elevated protein, low glucose	Repeated cytologic examination of large volumes of CSF; CSF exam by polarizing microscopy; clonal lymphocyte markers; deposits on nerve roots or meninges seen on myelogram or contrast-enhanced MRI; meningeal biopsy	Metastatic cancer of breast, lung, stomach, or pancreas; melanoma, lymphoma, leukemia; meningeal gliomatosis; meningeal sarcoma; cerebral dysgerminoma; meningeal melanoma or B cell lymphoma
Chemical compounds	Mononuclear cells or PMNs, low glucose, elevated protein; xanthochromia from subarachnoid hemorrhage in week prior to presentation with "meningitis"	Contrast-enhanced CT scan or MRI; cerebral angiogram to detect aneurysm	History of recent injection into the subarachnoid space; history of sudden onset of headache; recent resection of acoustic neuroma or craniopharyngioma; epidermoid tumor of brain or spine, sometimes with dermoid sinus tract; pituitary apoplexy
Primary inflammation CNS sarcoidosis	Mononuclear cells; elevated protein; often low glucose	Serum and CSF angiotensin-converting enzyme levels; biopsy of extraneural affected tissues or brain lesion/meningeal biopsy	CN palsy, especially of CN VII; hypothalamic dysfunction, especially diabetes insipidus; abnormal chest radiograph; peripheral neuropathy or myopathy
Vogt-Koyanagi-Harada syndrome	Mononuclear cells		Recurrent meningoencephalitis with uveitis, retinal detachment, alopecia, lightening of eyebrows, and lashes, dysacusis, cataracts, glaucoma
Isolated granulomatous angiitis of the nervous system	Mononuclear cells, elevated protein	Angiography or meningeal biopsy	Subacute dementia; multiple cerebral infarctions; recent zoster ophthalmicus
Systemic lupus erythematosus	Mononuclear or polymorphonuclear cells	Anti-DNA antibody, antinuclear antibodies	Encephalopathy; seizures; stroke; transverse myelopathy; rash; arthritis
Behçet's syndrome	Mononuclear or polymorphonuclear cells, elevated protein		Oral and genital aphthous ulcers; iridocyclitis; retinal hemorrhages; pathergic lesions at site of skin puncture
Chronic benign lymphocytic meningitis	Mononuclear cells		Recovery in 2–6 months, diagnosis by exclusion
Mollaret's recurrent meningitis	Large endothelial cells and polymorphonuclear cells in first hours, followed by mononuclear cells	PCR for herpes; MRI/CT to rule out epidermoid tumor or dural cyst	Recurrent meningitis; exclude HSV-2; rare cases due to HSV-1; occasional case associated with dural cyst
Drug hypersensitivity	Polymorphonuclear cells; occasionally mononuclear cells or eosinophils		Exposure to ibuprofen, sulfonamides, isoniazid, tolmetin, ciprofloxacin, pyridium; improvement after discontinuation of drug; recurrent episodes with recurrent exposure
Wegener's granulomatosis	Mononuclear cells	Chest and sinus radiographs; urinalysis; ANCA antibodies in serum	Associated sinus, pulmonary, or renal lesions; CN palsies; skin lesions; peripheral neuropathy
Other: multiple sclerosis, Sjögren's syndrome, and rarer forms of vasculitis (e.g., Cogan's syndrome)			

ABBREVIATIONS: ANCA, anti-neutrophil cytoplasmic antibodies; PMN, polymorphonuclear neutrophil; PCR, polymerase chain reaction.

FIGURE 378-1 Cryptococcal disease. A 46-year-old woman presented with altered mental status, fever, and headache. She had many pigeons as pets and frequently cleaned their cage. CSF examination showed elevated protein and a lymphocytic pleocytosis. Cryptococcal antigen test was positive. Axial postcontrast T1-weighted MR image reveals multiple foci of abnormal contrast enhancement in the basal ganglia, internal capsule, and other sites (*arrows*).

rapidly. The activities of the surgeon, pathologist, microbiologist, and cytologist should be coordinated so that a large enough sample is obtained and the appropriate cultures and histologic and molecular studies, including electron microscopic and polymerase chain reaction studies, are performed. The diagnostic yield of meningeal biopsy can be increased by targeting regions that enhance with contrast on MRI or CT. With current microsurgical techniques, most areas of the basal meninges can be accessed for biopsy via a limited craniotomy. In a series from the Mayo Clinic reported by Cheng et al., MRI demonstrated meningeal enhancement in 47 percent of patients undergoing meningeal biopsy. Biopsy of an enhancing region was diagnostic in 80 percent of cases; biopsy of nonenhancing regions was diagnostic in only 9 percent; sarcoid (31 percent) and metastatic adenocarcinoma (25 percent) were the most common conditions identified.

Approach to the Enigmatic Case In approximately one-third of cases, the diagnosis is not known despite careful evaluation of CSF and potential extraneural sites of disease. A number of the organisms that cause chronic meningitis may take weeks to be identified by cultures. In enigmatic cases several options are available, determined by the extent of the clinical deficits and rate of progression. It is prudent to wait until cultures are finalized if the patient is asymptomatic or symptoms are mild and not progressive. Unfortunately, in many cases progressive neurologic deterioration occurs, and rapid treatment is required. Ventricular-peritoneal shunts may be placed to relieve hydrocephalus, but the risk of disseminating the undiagnosed inflammatory process into the abdomen must be considered.

Empirical Treatment Diagnosis of the causative agent is essential because effective therapies exist for many etiologies of chronic meningitis, but if the condition is left untreated, progressive damage to the CNS and cranial nerves and roots is likely to occur. Occasionally, empirical therapy must be initiated when all attempts at diagnosis fail. In general, empirical therapy in the United States consists of antimycobacterial agents, amphotericin for fungal infection, or glucocorticoids for noninfectious inflammatory causes. It is important to direct empirical therapy of lymphocytic meningitis at tuberculosis, particularly if the condition is associated with hypoglycorrhachia and sixth and other CN palsies, since untreated disease is fatal in 4 to 8 weeks. In the Mayo Clinic series, the most useful empirical therapy was administration of glucocorticoids rather than antituberculous therapy. Carcinomatous or lymphomatous meningitis may be difficult to diagnose initially, but the diagnosis becomes evident with time.

THE IMMUNOSUPPRESSED PATIENT Chronic meningitis is not uncommon in the course of HIV infection. Pleocytosis and mild meningeal signs often occur at the onset of HIV infection, and occasionally low-grade meningitis persists. Toxoplasmosis commonly presents as intracranial abscesses and may also be associated with meningitis. Other important causes of chronic meningitis in AIDS include infection with *Cryptococcus, Nocardia,* or other fungi; syphilis; and lymphoma. Toxoplasmosis, cryptococcosis, nocardiosis, and other fungal infections are important etiologic considerations in individuals with immunodeficiency states other than AIDS, including those due to immunosuppressive medications. Because of the increased risk of chronic meningitis and the attenuation of clinical signs of meningeal irritation in immunosuppressed individuals, CSF examination should be performed for any persistent headache or unexplained change in mental state.

BIBLIOGRAPHY

ANDERSON NE, WILLOUGHBY EW: Chronic meningitis without predisposing illness. A review of 83 cases. Q J Med 63:283, 1987
BOUZA E et al: Coccidioidal meningitis. Medicine 60:139, 1981
——— et al: Brucellar meningitis. Rev Infect Dis 9:810, 1987
BROSS JE, GORDON G: Nocardial meningitis. Rev Infect Dis 13:160, 1991
CHENG TM et al: Chronic meningitis: The role of meningeal or cortical biopsy. Neurosurgery 34:590, 1994
ELLNER JJ, BENNETT JE: Chronic meningitis. Medicine 55:341, 1976
HOPKINS AP, HARVEY PK: Chronic benign lymphocytic meningitis. J Neurol Sci 18:443, 1973
MAYER SA et al: Biopsy proven isolated sarcoid meningitis. J Neurosurgery 78:994, 1993
PEACOCK JE et al: Persistent neutrophilic meningitis. Medicine 63:379, 1984
PHILLIPS ME et al: Neoplastic versus inflammatory meningeal enhancement with Gd-DTPA. J Comput Assisted Tomogr 14:536, 1990
REIK L et al: Granulomatous angiitis presenting as chronic meningitis and ventriculitis. Neurology 33:1609, 1983
SCHELD WM et al: *Infections of the Central Nervous System.* New York, Raven Press, 1991
SMITH JE, AKSAMIT AJ: Outcome of chronic idiopathic meningitis. Mayo Clinic Proc 69:548, 1994
SWARTZ MN: "Chronic meningitis"—many causes to consider. N Engl J Med 317:957, 1987
WHEAT LJ et al: Histoplasma capsulatum infections of the central nervous system. Medicine 69:244, 1990

379 *Kenneth L. Tyler*

ASEPTIC MENINGITIS, VIRAL ENCEPHALITIS, AND PRION DISEASES

Hundreds of viruses have been reported to produce acute infection and injury to the central or peripheral nervous systems. Many aspects of the clinical characteristics of these diseases are determined by whether the infection is limited primarily to the meninges (*meningitis*) or extends to involve the parenchyma of the brain (*encephalitis*) and/ or spinal cord (*myelitis*). Although there are a number of similarities in the basic epidemiology and diagnostic approaches to these disorders, they are discussed separately. Viruses also can produce chronic or persistent infections of the central nervous system (CNS). These disorders are sufficiently different from acute viral infections and from each other as to merit separate consideration. Special emphasis is given to infection of the nervous system by human immunodeficiency virus (HIV), both because of its obvious epidemiologic importance and because of its capacity to produce myriad neurologic syndromes as it attacks virtually every part of the nervous system. An additional group of neurologic disorders, commonly discussed in the context of viral infections, are the human prion diseases. Recent evidence indicates that these disorders are caused by the accumulation and/or aberrant metabolism of abnormal isoforms of the prion protein.

ACUTE VIRAL INFECTIONS

VIRAL MENINGITIS   Clinical Manifestations   The syndrome of viral meningitis consists of fever, headache, and meningeal irritation coupled with an inflammatory cerebrospinal fluid (CSF) profile typically consisting of a lymphocytic pleocytosis, a slightly elevated protein level, and a normal glucose level. Fever may be accompanied by malaise, myalgia, anorexia, nausea and vomiting, abdominal pain, and/or diarrhea. It is not uncommon to see a mild degree of lethargy or drowsiness. The presence of more profound alterations in consciousness, such as stupor, coma, or marked confusion, should prompt consideration of alternative diagnoses. Similarly, the presence of seizures, cranial nerve palsies, or other focal neurologic signs or symptoms suggests parenchymal involvement and is not typical of uncomplicated viral meningitis. The headache associated with viral meningitis is typically frontal or retroorbital in location and often associated with photophobia and pain on moving the eyes. Nuchal rigidity is present in most cases but may be mild and present only near the limit of neck anteflexion. Evidence of severe meningeal irritation, such as Kernig's and Brudzinski's signs, are generally absent.

Etiology   Using routine serologic and culture techniques, a specific viral cause can be found in 30 to 70 percent of cases of viral meningitis. CSF polymerase chain reaction studies (see below) indicate that at least two-thirds of the cases of CSF culture-negative aseptic meningitis are due to enteroviruses, making this viral group by far the most important cause of viral meningitis (Table 379-1).

Epidemiology   It is impossible to determine the exact incidence of viral meningitis in the United States, since most cases go unreported to public health authorities. There is a striking increase in cases during the summer months, reflecting the seasonal predominance of enterovirus and arbovirus infections, with a peak monthly incidence of about 1 reported case per 100,000 population. The striking seasonal predilections of some of the viruses causing meningitis can provide a valuable clue to diagnosis (Table 379-2), although it is important to recognize that seasonal distributions are relative rather than absolute indicators of frequency.

Laboratory Diagnosis   *CSF examination*   The most important laboratory test in the diagnosis of meningitis is examination of the CSF. The typical profile in cases of viral meningitis is a lymphocytic pleocytosis, slightly elevated protein level, and normal glucose level. Organisms *cannot* be seen on Gram's or acid-fast stained smears or india ink wet mounts of CSF. Polymorphonuclear neutrophils (PMNs) may predominate in the first 48 h of illness, especially in some enteroviral infections, and may last longer when infection is due to echovirus 9 or Eastern equine virus. Patients with suspected viral meningitis and a PMN pleocytosis should have a follow-up CSF examination after 8 to 12 h to look for a shift toward mononuclear cells. The presence of a PMN pleocytosis always should prompt consideration of bacterial meningitis or parameningeal infections. The total CSF cell count per

Table 379-1

Viruses Causing Aseptic Meningitis

Common	Less Common	Rare
Enteroviruses	HSV-1	Adenoviruses
Arboviruses	LCMV	CMV
HIV	Mumps virus	EBV
HSV-2		Influenza A, B; measles; parainfluenza; rubella; VZV

ABBREVIATIONS: CMV, cytomegalovirus; EBV, Epstein-Barr virus; HIV, human immunodeficiency virus; HSV, herpes simplex virus; LCMV, lymphocytic choriomeningitis virus; VZV, varicella-zoster virus.

Table 379-2

Seasonal Prevalence of Viruses Commonly Causing Meningitis

Summer and Early Fall	Fall and Winter	Winter and Spring	Nonseasonal
Arboviruses	LCMV	Mumps	HIV
Enteroviruses			HSV

ABBREVIATIONS: As in Table 379-1.

microliter in viral meningitis rarely exceeds 1000. The CSF glucose level is typically normal in viral infections, although it may be decreased in cases due to mumps (10 to 30 percent), lymphocytic choriomeningitis virus (LCMV) and, less frequently, echovirus and other enteroviruses, herpes simplex virus (HSV) type 2, or varicella-zoster virus (VZV). As a rule, a lymphocytic pleocytosis with a low glucose level (≤25 mg/dL) should suggest the presence of fungal, listerial, or tuberculous meningitis or of noninfectious disorders (e.g., sarcoid, neoplastic meningitis).

A number of tests measuring levels of various CSF proteins, enzymes, and mediators, including C-reactive protein, lactic acid, lactate dehydrogenase, neopterin, quinolinate, interleukin (IL) 1β, IL-6, soluble IL-2 receptor, β$_2$-microglobulin, and tumor necrosis factor (TNF), have been proposed as potential discriminators between viral and bacterial meningitis or as markers of specific types of viral infection (e.g., infection with HIV), but are in limited general use. Patients with HIV CNS infection often have elevated CSF levels of p24 antigen, and this may be useful in diagnosis.

CSF culture   The overall results of CSF culture for the diagnosis of viral infection are disappointing (Table 379-3), presumably because of the generally low concentration of infectious virus present and the need to customize isolation procedures for individual viruses. For viral isolation, 2 mL of CSF should be obtained and brought promptly to the microbiology laboratory, where it should be refrigerated and processed as speedily as possible. As a general rule, CSF specimens for viral isolation should never be stored in a freezer (-20°C), since viruses are often unstable at this temperature, and most modern freezers have "frostfree" warmup cycles that are detrimental to viral stability. Storage for more than 24 h is probably best done in a -70°C freezer.

Other sources for viral isolation   It is important to remember that viruses also may be isolated from sites and body fluids other than CSF. Enteroviruses and adenoviruses may be found in feces; arboviruses, some enteroviruses, and LCMV, in blood; mumps and cytomegalovirus (CMV), in urine; and enteroviruses, mumps, and adenoviruses, in throat washings. During enteroviral infections, viral shedding in stool may persist for several weeks. The presence of enterovirus in stool is not diagnostic and may result from residual shedding from a previous enteroviral infection; it also occurs in some asymptomatic individuals during enteroviral epidemics.

Nucleic acid amplification   Amplification of viral-specific DNA or RNA from CSF using polymerase chain reaction (PCR) amplification has become an important method for diagnosing CNS viral infection. HSV-1 DNA is frequently amplified from the CSF of patients with herpes simplex encephalitis and recurrent (Mollaret) meningitis even when standard culture techniques are negative. PCR is also routinely used to diagnose CNS viral infections caused by CMV, Epstein-Barr virus (EBV), and VZV. Genomic amplification and detection of picornavirus (coxsackie, polio, echo, enterovirus) RNA in the

Table 379-3

Possibility of Culturing Specific Viruses from CSF

Excellent	Fair	Poor or None
Coxsackievirus, echovirus, LCMV, mumps virus	HIV, adenovirus, arboviruses (most), HSV-2, VZV, rabies virus	Poliovirus, HSV-1, EBV, CMV

ABBREVIATIONS: As in Table 379-1.

CSF of patients with meningitis is now the diagnostic procedure of choice for this group of viruses.

Serologic studies   In many cases, diagnosis of viral infection depends on documentation of seroconversion between acute-phase and convalescent sera (typically obtained after 2 to 4 weeks). Antiviral antibodies also may be measured in CSF (see below). The timing of the antibody response often means that serologic data are useful mainly for the retrospective establishment of a specific diagnosis, and their value in initial diagnosis and management is limited. Most viral infections of the CNS are associated with intrathecal synthesis of antiviral antibody. This results in an elevation in the CSF/serum antibody index, which can be calculated using the following formula:

$$\frac{(\text{CSF organism-specific Ig})/(\text{CSF total Ig})}{(\text{Serum organism-specific Ig})/(\text{Serum total Ig})}$$

An index value of ≥ 1.5 is suggestive of CSF infection, as it indicates that the CSF contains a relatively higher proportion of Ig specific for a particular organism than does the serum. This finding strongly suggests that CNS infection has resulted in intrathecal synthesis of organism-specific antibodies. Elevations in CSF Ig may occur as a result of breakdown in the blood-brain barrier, but this development typically is associated with elevation in the CSF/serum albumin ratio. Obtaining paired samples of CSF and serum for serologic testing may provide additional evidence that an antibody response is the result of CNS infection. The sensitivity of CSF/serum antibody index studies may be enhanced by correcting for breakdown of the blood-brain barrier using the CSF/serum albumin ratio or using CSF/serum antibody indexes of other viruses as controls. Although use of CSF/serum antibody index determinations may enhance the sensitivity of diagnosis, the technique still suffers from the delay between onset of infection and appearance of the host's antibody response.

Agarose electrophoresis or isoelectric focusing of CSF gamma globulins may reveal the presence of oligoclonal bands. These bands have been found in association with a number of viral infections, including infections with HIV, human T cell leukemia virus (HTLV) type I, and VZV, mumps, subacute sclerosing panencephalitis, and progressive rubella panencephalitis. The associated antibodies are often directed against viral proteins. The finding of oligoclonal bands may be of some diagnostic utility, since typically they are not seen with arbovirus, enterovirus, or HSV infections. It is important to recognize that oligoclonal bands are commonly encountered in certain noninfectious neurologic diseases (e.g., multiple sclerosis) and may be found in nonviral infections (e.g., syphilis, Lyme borreliosis).

Other laboratory studies   All patients with suspected viral meningitis should have a complete and differential blood count, a platelet count, liver function tests, and measurement of the hematocrit, erythrocyte sedimentation rate (ESR), blood urea nitrogen (BUN), and the plasma levels of electrolytes, glucose, creatinine, creatine kinase, aldolase, amylase, and lipase. Abnormalities in specific test results may suggest particular etiologic diagnoses. Magnetic resonance imaging (MRI), computed tomography (CT), electroencephalography (EEG), evoked response studies, electromyography (EMG), and nerve conduction studies are not necessary in most cases. They are best used selectively when atypical presentations or unusual features of particular cases present diagnostic problems.

Differential Diagnosis   Perhaps the most important issue in the differential diagnosis is the exclusion of nonviral causes that can mimic viral meningitis or encephalitis. The major categories of disease that should always be considered and excluded are (1) parameningeal infections or partially treated bacterial meningitis, (2) nonviral infectious meningitides where cultures may be negative (e.g., fungal, tuberculous, parasitic, or syphilitic disease), (3) infection with certain pathogens whose clinical presentation can resemble encephalitis (e.g., *Listeria, Brucella, Coxiella, Mycoplasma,* and *Rickettsia*), (4) neoplastic meningitis, and (5) meningitis secondary to noninfectious inflammatory diseases such as sarcoid, Behçet's disease, and the uveomeningitic syndromes. Although the diagnosis of a specific viral etiology in a particular case of viral meningitis can rarely be made on clinical grounds alone, proper attention to epidemiologic, clinical, and labora-

tory features may substantially narrow the diagnostic possibilities. Statistically, *enteroviruses* (see Chap. 195) are the most common cause of viral meningitis (>80 percent of cases with etiology identified) and should be considered the leading candidates when a typical case occurs in the summer months, especially in a child (<15 years of age) (Table 379-4). However, despite their summer prevalence, it is important to recognize that sporadic cases of enteroviral CNS infection are seen year-round. The physical examination should include a careful search for exanthemata, hand-foot-mouth disease, herpangina, pleurodynia, myopericarditis, and hemorrhagic conjunctivitis, which may be stigmata of enterovirus infections. PCR amplification of enteroviral RNA from CSF has become the diagnostic procedure of choice for these infections.

Mumps (see Chap. 198) should be considered when meningitis occurs in the late winter or early spring, especially in males (male/female ratio 3:1). With the widespread use of the live attenuated mumps vaccine in the United States since 1967, the incidence of mumps meningitis has fallen by more than 95 percent. Rare cases of mumps vaccine–associated meningitis have been reported, but they are not usually seen after vaccination with the attenuated Jeryl-Lynn strain of virus used in the United States. The presence of orchitis, oophoritis, parotitis, or pancreatitis or elevations in serum lipase and amylase are suggestive but can be found with other viruses, and their absence does not exclude the diagnosis. Clinical meningitis occurs in 5 percent of patients with parotitis, but only 50 percent of patients with meningitis have associated parotitis. Mumps infection confers lifelong immunity, so a documented history of previous infection excludes this diagnosis. The presence of hypoglycorrhachia (10 to 30 percent) may be an additional diagnostic clue, once other causes have been excluded (see above). Up to 25 percent of patients may have a PMN-predominant CSF pleocytosis, and CSF abnormalities may persist for months. Diagnosis is typically made by isolation of virus from CSF and/or demonstration of seroconversion between acute-phase and convalescent sera.

Development of meningitis in the late fall or winter associated with a history of exposure to house mice (*Mus musculus*), pet or laboratory rodents (e.g., hamsters), or their excreta should suggest the possibility of *LCMV infection* (see Chap. 201). Some patients have an associated rash, pulmonary infiltrates, alopecia, parotitis, orchitis, or myopericarditis. Laboratory clues to the diagnosis may include the presence of leukopenia, thrombocytopenia, abnormal liver function tests, or pulmonary infiltrates. Some cases present with a marked CSF pleocytosis (>1000 cells per microliter) and hypoglycorrhachia (<30 percent).

HSV-2 meningitis (see Chap. 184) occurs in approximately 35 percent of women and 11 percent of men at the time of an initial (primary) episode of genital herpes. Of these patients, 20 percent go on to have recurrent attacks of meningitis. Although HSV-2 can be cultured from CSF during a first episode of meningitis, cultures are invariably negative during recurrent episodes of HSV-2 meningitis. Diagnosis depends on amplification of HSV-2 DNA from CSF by PCR. Almost all cases of recurrent HSV meningitis are due to HSV-2, although rare cases due to HSV-1 have been reported. Most cases of benign recurrent lymphocytic meningitis, including those

Table 379-4

Serotypes of Enteroviruses Causing CNS Infections

Frequency as Cause of CNS Infections	Poliovirus	Coxsackievirus	Echovirus	Enterovirus
Frequent	—	B5	7, 9, 11, 30	70, 71
Common	—	A9, B3, B4	4, 6, 18	—
Rare	1–3	B1, B6	2, 3, 12, 22	—

SOURCE: After Rotbart.

meeting accepted diagnostic criteria for Mollaret's meningitis, appear to be due to HSV. Genital lesions may not be present, and most patients give no history of genital herpes. CSF cultures are negative, but HSV DNA can be amplified from CSF by PCR during attacks of meningitis but not during symptom-free intervals. *Epstein-Barr virus infections* also may produce aseptic meningitis, with or without accompanying evidence of the infectious mononucleosis syndrome. The diagnosis may be suggested by the presence of atypical lymphocytes in the CSF or an atypical lymphocytosis in peripheral blood. The demonstration of IgM antibody to viral capsid antigen (VCA), antibody to the diffuse (D) component of early antigen (EA), and a rising titer of antibody to nuclear antigen (EBNA) are indicative of acute EBV infection. EBV is almost never cultured from CSF, but nested PCR amplification of EBV DNA from CSF may be positive. HIV-infected patients may have positive CSF PCR for EBV DNA in the presence of primary CNS lymphoma, even when EBV-related meningoencephalitis is not present. *VZV meningitis* should be suspected in the presence of concurrent chickenpox or shingles. Some patients develop a distinctive syndrome of acute cerebellar ataxia. This typically occurs in children and presents with the abrupt onset of limb and truncal ataxia. VZV DNA can be amplified from CSF by PCR in many cases of meningitis and myelitis. The diagnosis of a VZV-related CNS infection is also supported by the demonstration of a VZV-specific intrathecal antibody response, or less frequently by positive culture of VZV from CSF. A similar syndrome occurs less commonly in association with EBV and enteroviral infection.

Arbovirus infections typically occur in the summer months, have clear geographic localization, and occur in epidemics, all factors reflecting the ecology of their transmission through infected insect vectors (see Fig. 379-1 and Table 379-6; see also Chap. 200). Arboviral meningitis should be considered when clusters of meningitis cases occur in a restricted geographic region during the summer or early fall. A history of tick exposure or travel or residence in the appropriate geographic area should suggest the possibility of Colorado tick fever virus or Powassan virus infection, although nonviral diseases producing meningitis (e.g., Lyme disease) or headache with meningismus (e.g., Rocky mountain spotted fever) also may present this way.

HIV infection is discussed more fully below and in Chap. 308. HIV meningitis should be suspected in any patient with known or identified risk factors for HIV infection. Aseptic meningitis is a common manifestation of primary exposure to HIV and occurs in 5 to 10 percent of cases (see Chap. 308). In some patients, seroconversion may be delayed for several months, and in seronegative patients, serology should be repeated after 3- and 6-month intervals. HIV can be cultured from CSF in some patients. Cranial nerve palsies are more common in HIV meningitis than in other viral infections, most commonly involving cranial nerves V, VII, or VIII.

Rx **TREATMENT**

In the usual case of viral meningitis, treatment is symptomatic, and hospitalization is not required. Exceptions to this rule include patients with deficient humoral immunity, neonates with overwhelming infection, and patients in whom the clinical or CSF profile suggests the possibility of a bacterial or other nonviral cause of infection. Patients with suspected bacterial meningitis should receive appropriate empirical therapy pending culture results (see Chap. 377). Patients with deficient humoral immunity should receive a trial of intravenous gamma globulin. Oral or intravenous acyclovir may help patients with meningitis caused by HSV-1 or HSV-2 and in cases of severe EBV or VZV infection. Zidovudine (AZT), didanosine (formerly dideoxyinosine; ddI) or dicalcitrine presumably would be of value in the treatment of HIV meningitis, although no clinical trials have been performed. Patients usually prefer to rest undisturbed in a quiet, darkened room. Analgesics can be used to relieve headache, which is often reduced by the initial diagnostic lumbar puncture. Antipyretics may help to reduce fever, which rarely exceeds

40°C. Hyponatremia may develop as a result of the syndrome of inappropriate vasopressin secretion (SIADH), so fluid and electrolyte status should be monitored. Repeat lumbar puncture is only indicated in patients whose fever and symptoms fail to resolve after a few days or if there is doubt about the initial diagnosis. Vaccination is an effective method of preventing the subsequent development of meningitis and other neurologic complications associated with poliovirus, mumps, and measles infection. A live attenuated VZV vaccine (Varivax) is now approved in the United States. Clinical studies indicate an effectiveness rate of 70 to 90 percent for this vaccine. Reduction in primary VZV infection would be expected to reduce the frequency and/or severity both of primary neurologic complications of varicella and of the consequences of later reactivation (e.g., shingles).

Prognosis In adults, the prognosis for full recovery from viral meningitis is excellent. Rare patients complain of persisting headache, mild mental impairment, incoordination, or generalized asthenia for weeks to months. The outcome in infants and neonates (<1 year of age) is less certain. Intellectual impairment, learning disabilities, hearing loss, and other lasting neurologic sequelae have been reported in some but not all studies; however, their frequency is uncertain.

VIRAL ENCEPHALITIS **Definition** In distinction to meningitis, where the infectious process and associated inflammatory response is limited largely to the meninges, in encephalitis the brain parenchyma also is involved.

Clinical Manifestations In addition to the acute febrile illness with evidence of meningeal involvement characteristic of meningitis, the patient with encephalitis commonly has an altered level of consciousness, an abnormal mental state, and evidence of either focal or diffuse neurologic signs and symptoms. All degrees of altered consciousness may occur, ranging from mild lethargy to deep coma. A patient with encephalitis is not mentally alert and is frequently confused, delirious, and disoriented. Mental aberrations may include hallucinations, agitation, personality change, behavioral disorders, and, at times, a frankly psychotic state. Focal or generalized seizures occur in more than 50 percent of patients with severe encephalitis. Virtually every possible type of focal neurologic disturbance has been reported in viral encephalitis, the signs and symptoms reflecting the sites of infection and inflammation. The most commonly encountered focal findings are aphasia, ataxia, hemiparesis (with hyperactive tendon reflexes and extensor plantar responses), involuntary movements (e.g., myoclonic jerks), and cranial nerve deficits (e.g., ocular palsies, facial weakness). Involvement of the hypothalamic-pituitary axis may result in temperature dysregulation, diabetes insipidus, or the development of SIADH. Despite the clear neuropathologic evidence that viruses differ in the regions of the CNS they injure, it is often impossible to reliably distinguish on clinical grounds alone one type of viral encephalitis (e.g., that caused by HSV) from others (see "Differential Diagnosis," below).

Etiology The number of viruses reported to cause encephalitis is legion. In the United States, there are approximately 20,000 reported cases per year. The same organisms responsible for aseptic meningitis are also responsible for encephalitis, although their relative frequencies differ (Table 379-5, Fig. 379-1).

Laboratory Diagnosis *CSF examination* CSF examination should be performed in all patients with suspected viral encephalitis unless contraindicated by the presence of severely increased intra-

Table 379-5

Viruses Causing Encephalitis

Common	Less Common	Rare
Arboviruses, enteroviruses, HSV-1, mumps	CMV, EBV, HIV, measles, VZV	Adenoviruses, CTFV, influenza A, LCMV, parainfluenza, rabies, rubella

ABBREVIATIONS: As in Table 379-1; also, CTFV, Colorado tick fever virus.

cranial pressure (ICP). The characteristic CSF profile is indistinguishable from that of viral meningitis and consists of a lymphocytic pleocytosis, a mildly elevated protein level, and a normal glucose level. A CSF pleocytosis (>5 cells per microliter) occurs in more than 95 percent of patients with documented viral encephalitis, and its absence should prompt a careful search for other causes of an encephalopathy. In rare cases, a pleocytosis may be absent on the initial lumbar puncture but present subsequently. Patients who are severely immunocompromised by radiation, chemotherapy, or certain lymphoreticular malignancies may fail to mount a CSF inflammatory response. The cell count exceeds 500/μL in only about 10 percent of patients. Infections with certain arboviruses (Eastern equine encephalitis or California encephalitis), mumps, and LCMV occasionally may result in more than 1000 cells per microliter, but this degree of pleocytosis should suggest the possibility of non-

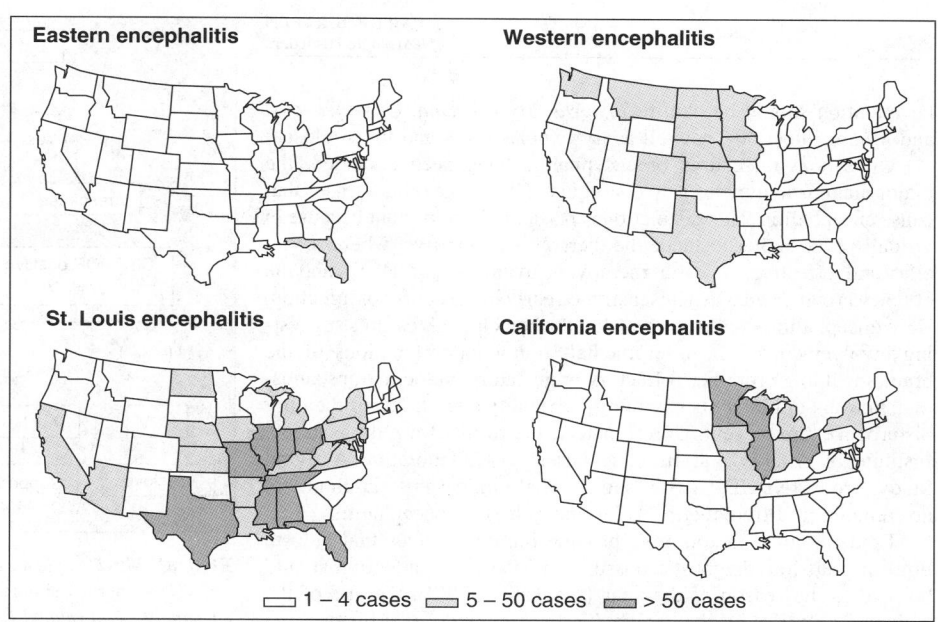

FIGURE 379-1 Geographic distributions of the most commonly encountered arbovirus encephalitides in the United States. *(From Johnson, with permission.)*

viral infections or other inflammatory processes. Atypical lymphocytes in the CSF may be seen in EBV infection and less commonly with other viruses, including CMV and HSV. The presence of substantial numbers of PMNs after the first 48 h should prompt consideration of bacterial infection, leptospirosis, amebic infection, and noninfectious processes such as acute hemorrhagic leukoencephalitis; however, large numbers of PMNs in the CSF are occasionally present with Eastern encephalitis, echovirus 9 infection, and other enteroviral infections. About 20 percent of patients with encephalitis will have a significant number of red blood cells (>500/μL) in the CSF in a nontraumatic tap. The pathologic correlate of this may be the presence of a hemorrhagic encephalitis of the type seen with HSV, Colorado tick fever virus, and occasionally California encephalitis virus. A decreased CSF glucose level is distinctly unusual in viral encephalitis and should suggest the possibility of fungal, tuberculous, parasitic, leptospiral, syphilitic, sarcoid, or neoplastic meningitis. Rare patients with mumps, LCMV, or advanced HSV encephalitis may have hypoglycorrhachia.

CSF culture Attempts to culture viruses from the CSF in cases of encephalitis are often disappointing (see Table 375-3). In particular, it should be noted that cultures are invariably negative in cases of HSV-1 encephalitis.

CSF nucleic acid amplification PCR amplification of viral nucleic acid has become the diagnostic procedure of choice for many types of viral encephalitis. Recent studies with HSV encephalitis indicate that the sensitivity and specificity of CSF PCR equals or exceeds that of brain biopsy. Although less detailed specificity and sensitivity data are available, PCR is now widely used as the primary diagnostic test for CNS infections caused by CMV, EBV, VZV, and enteroviruses (see "Viral Meningitis," above).

Serologic studies and antigen detection The basic approach to the serodiagnosis of viral encephalitis is identical to that discussed earlier for viral meningitis. In the case of HSV encephalitis, attention has focused on the detection of HSV antibodies in the CSF. In one large series, antibodies to HSV-1 glycoprotein B were found in 97 percent of biopsy-proven cases of HSV encephalitis. The specificity was 100 percent if the assay was corrected for leakage across the blood-brain barrier using adenovirus antibodies as a marker. In another study, virus glycoprotein antigens (gB, gC, gD, and gE) were found in the CSF of 92 percent of patients with biopsy-proven cases of HSV encephalitis and had a specificity of 82 percent. Unfortunately, the best results with these types of assays occur after the first week of illness. This limits their utility to retrospective diagnostic confirmation rather than acute diagnosis.

CT, MRI, EEG Patients with suspected encephalitis almost invariably undergo structural imaging studies and often EEG. The utility of these tests is to identify or help exclude alternative diagnoses and to help establish the existence of a focal, as opposed to a diffuse, encephalitic process. The presence of focal findings should always raise the possibility of HSV encephalitis. These are (1) periodic focal spikes on a background of slow or low-amplitude ("flattened") activity with a temporal predominance of EEG; (2) temporoparietal areas of low absorption, mass effect, and contrast enhancement on CT; or (3) areas of increased signal intensity in the frontotemporal, cingulate, or insular regions of the brain on T2-weighted spin-echo MRI images.

Brain biopsy Prior to the availability of PCR amplification of HSV DNA from CSF, the isolation of HSV from brain tissue obtained at biopsy was considered the gold standard for the diagnosis of HSV encephalitis. The need for brain biopsy to diagnose HSV and other forms of viral encephalitis has declined greatly with the widespread availability of CSF PCR diagnostic tests for HSV and many other viruses. When biopsy is performed, the tissue is cultured for virus and examined histopathologically and ultrastructurally. The biopsy is typically carried out under general anesthesia through a craniectomy. Tissue should be taken from a site that appears to be significantly involved on the basis of clinical and laboratory criteria. The sensitivity of brain biopsy exceeds 95 percent, and its specificity is probably greater than 99 percent. Although brain biopsy is not an innocuous procedure, the mortality rate is low (<0.2 percent). Potential morbidity, in addition to that related to general anesthesia, includes local bleeding and edema, the development of a seizure focus, and wound dehiscence or infection. From a practical viewpoint, the incidence of serious morbidity appears to be between 0.5 and 2 percent.

Patients suspected of having HSV encephalitis should be started on acyclovir (see below), and their CSF should be assayed for the presence of HSV DNA by PCR. A negative PCR test effectively excludes the diagnosis of HSV encephalitis and, except in rare circumstances, is sufficiently sensitive to allow discontinuation of acyclovir.

Differential Diagnosis The initial step in diagnosis is to exclude nonviral causes of encephalitis, including both infections and noninfectious diseases. Some of the most common illnesses masquerading as viral encephalitis, as identified in multicenter clinical trials using brain biopsy as a diagnostic standard, were vascular diseases; abscess and empyema; fungal, parasitic, rickettsial, and tuberculous infections; tumors; Reye's syndrome; toxic encephalopathy; subdural hematoma; and systemic lupus erythematosus. Of the nonviral infections, particular attention should be paid to *Listeria*, *Mycoplasma*, *Cryptococcus*, and *Mucor* infections, as well as to toxoplasmosis and tuberculosis.

Once nonviral causes of encephalitis have been excluded, the major diagnostic impetus is to distinguish HSV from other viruses that cause encephalitis. This distinction is particularly important because in virtually every other instance the therapy is supportive, whereas specific and effective antiviral therapy is available for HSV, and its efficacy is enhanced when it is instituted early in the course of infection. HSV encephalitis should be considered when clinical features suggesting involvement of the inferomedial frontotemporal regions of the brain, including prominent olfactory or gustatory hallucinations, anosmia, unusual or bizarre behavior or personality alterations, or memory disturbance, are present. Unfortunately, the results from the National Institute of Allergy and Immune Diseases–Collaborative Antiviral Study Group (NIAID-CASG) suggest that clinical criteria alone are not reliable in differentiating HSV and non-HSV encephalitis.

Epidemiologic factors may provide important clues that help to limit or focus the diagnostic possibilities. Particular attention should be paid to the season of the year (see Table 379-2), the age of the patient (Table 379-6), the geographic location and travel history (see Fig. 379-1 and Table 379-6), and possible exposure to animal bites, rodents, and ticks. *Morbidity and Mortality Weekly Reports* provides regular information about the prevalence of particular viruses causing encephalitis by season and region of the country. State public health authorities provide another valuable resource concerning isolation of particular agents in individual regions.

℞ TREATMENT

Specific antiviral therapy should be initiated when appropriate (Fig. 379-2, and see below). Vital functions, including respiration and blood pressure, should be monitored continuously and supported as required. In the initial stages of encephalitis, many patients will require care in an intensive care unit. Basic management and supportive therapy should include careful monitoring of ICP, fluid restriction and avoidance of hypotonic intravenous solutions, and suppression of fever. Seizures should be treated with standard anticonvulsant regimens, and prophylactic therapy is probably indicated in view of the high frequency of seizures in severe cases of encephalitis (>50 percent). Like all seriously ill, immobilized patients with altered consciousness, encephalitis patients are at risk for aspiration pneumonia, stasis ulcers and decubiti, contractures, deep venous thrombosis and its complications, and infections of indwelling lines and catheters.

Acyclovir (ACV) is of benefit in the treatment of HSV encephalitis and is also useful in selected cases of severe encephalitis due to infection with EBV or VZV (see Chap. 183). These viruses encode an enzyme, deoxypyrimidine (thymidine) kinase, that phosphorylates acyclovir to produce acyclovir-5′-monophosphate. Host cell enzymes then phosphorylate this compound to form a triphosphate derivative. It is the triphosphate that acts as an antiviral agent by inhibiting viral DNA polymerase and by causing premature termina-

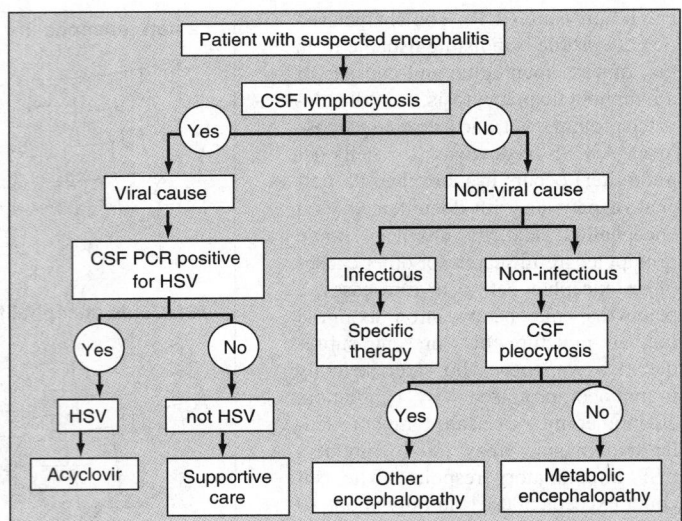

FIGURE 379-2 Scheme for the treatment of patients with suspected encephalitis. HSV, herpes simplex virus. *[Modified from DF Hanley et al: Viral encephalitis and related conditions, in TP Beck (ed): Atlas of Infectious Diseases. New York, Churchill Livingstone, 1995.]*

tion of nascent viral DNA chains. The specificity of action of acyclovir depends on the fact that uninfected cells do not phosphorylate significant amounts of acyclovir to acyclovir-5′-monophosphate. A second level of specificity is provided by the fact that the acyclovir triphosphate is a more potent inhibitor of viral DNA polymerase than of the analogous host cell enzymes.

Patients should receive a dose of 10 mg/kg of acyclovir intravenously every 8 h for a 14-day course. The drug should be diluted to a concentration not exceeding 7 mg/mL. (A 70-kg person would receive a dose of 700 mg, which would be diluted in a volume ≥100 mL.) Each dose should be infused slowly over 60 min rather than by rapid or bolus infusion, to minimize the risk of renal dysfunction. Care should be taken to avoid extravasation or intramuscular or subcutaneous administration. The alkaline pH of acyclovir can cause local inflammation and phlebitis (9 percent). Dose adjustment is required in patients with impaired renal glomerular filtration. Penetration into CSF is excellent, with average drug levels approximately 50 percent of serum levels. Complications of therapy include elevations in BUN and creatinine levels (5 percent), thrombocytopenia (6 percent), gastrointestinal toxicity (nausea, vomiting, diarrhea) (7 percent), and neurotoxicity (lethargy or obtundation, disorientation, confusion, agitation, hallucinations, tremors, seizures) (1 percent). Acyclovir resistance may be mediated by changes in either the viral deoxypyrimidine kinase or DNA polymerase. To date, acyclovir-resistant isolates have not been a significant clinical problem in immunocompetent individuals. However, there has been an increasing number of reports of clinically virulent acyclovir-resistant HSV isolates from immunocompromised individuals, including those with AIDS.

Table 379-6

Features of Selected Arbovirus Encephalitides

Feature	Virus				
	WEE	EEE	VEE	SLE	CE
Region	West, midwest	Atlantic and Gulf	South	All	East and north-central
Age	Infants, adults >50 years	Children	Adults	Adults >50 years	Children
Deaths	5–15 percent	50–75 percent	1 percent	2–20 percent	<1 percent
Sequelae	Low to moderate	80 percent	Rare	20 percent	Rare
Vector	Mosquito	Mosquito	Mosquito	Mosquito	Mosquito
Animal host	Birds	Birds	Horses, small mammals	Birds	Rodents

ABBREVIATIONS: CE, California encephalitis virus; EEE, Eastern equine encephalitis virus; SLE, St. Louis encephalitis virus; VEE, Venezuelan equine encephalitis virus; WEE, Western equine encephalitis virus.

SOURCE: After Whitley.

Both ganciclovir and foscarnet have been shown to be effective in the treatment of CMV-related CNS infections. Ganciclovir is a synthetic nucleoside analogue of 2′-deoxyguanosine. The drug is preferentially phosphorylated by virus-induced cellular kinases. Ganciclovir triphosphate acts as a competitive inhibitor of the CMV DNA polymerase, and its incorporation into nascent viral DNA results in premature chain termination. Following intravenous administration, CSF concentrations of ganciclovir are 25 to 70 percent of coincident plasma levels. The usual dose for treatment of severe neurologic illnesses is 5 mg/kg every 12 h given intravenously at a constant rate over 1 h. Induction therapy is followed by maintenance therapy of 5 mg/kg every day for an indefinite period. Doses need to be adjusted in patients with renal insufficiency. Treatment is often limited by the development of granulocytopenia and thrombocytopenia, which may require reduction in or discontinuation of therapy.

Foscarnet is a pyrophosphate analogue that inhibits viral DNA polymerases by binding to the pyrophosphate binding site. Following intravenous infusion, CSF concentrations are typically 15 to 100 percent of coincident plasma levels. The usual dose for serious CMV-related neurologic illness is 60 mg/kg every 8 h administered by constant infusion over 1 h. Induction therapy for 14 to 21 days is followed by maintenance therapy (60 to 120 mg/kg per day). Many patients develop renal impairment during treatment, which is reversible following discontinuation of therapy in most, but not all, cases. Reduction in serum calcium, magnesium, and potassium occur in approximately 15 percent of patients and may be associated with symptoms of tetany, cardiac rhythm disturbances, or seizures.

Sequelae There is considerable variation in the incidence and severity of sequelae in patients surviving viral encephalitis. In the case of Eastern equine encephalitis virus infection, nearly 80 percent of survivors have severe neurologic sequelae. At the other extreme are infections due to EBV, California encephalitis virus, and Venezuelan equine encephalitis virus, where sequelae are extremely rare. Detailed information about sequelae in patients with HSV encephalitis treated with ACV are available from the NIAID-CASG trials. Of 32 ACV-treated patients, 26 survived (81 percent). Of the 26 survivors, 12 (46 percent) had no or only minor sequelae, 3 (12 percent) were moderately impaired (gainfully employed but not functioning at their previous level), and 11 (42 percent) were severely impaired (requiring continuous supportive care). The incidence and severity of sequelae were directly related to the age of the patient and the level of consciousness at the time of initiation of therapy. Patients with severe neurologic impairment (Glasgow coma score ≤ 6) at initiation of therapy either died or survived with severe sequelae. Young patients (≤30 years old) with good neurologic function at initiation of therapy did substantially better (100 percent survival, 62 percent with no or mild sequelae) compared with their older counterparts (≥30 years); (64 percent survival, 57 percent no or mild sequelae).

MYELITIS AND RADICULITIS

The prototypical viral myelitis is the syndrome of acute anterior poliomyelitis caused by polioviruses and rarely by other enteroviruses and possibly EBV and mumps virus. A distinctive syndrome is produced by enterovirus 70. Patients develop acute hemorrhagic conjunctivitis, followed days to weeks later by a poliomyelitis-like syndrome (see below). Some cases of rabies present with an acute ascending paralysis with areflexia which can resemble poliomyelitis or the Guillain-Barré syndrome. Paralytic polio (see Chap. 195) is a rarity in the United States (<20 cases per year), although it remains a major problem in some other regions of the world. Most cases of paralytic polio in the United States occur as a result of the exceedingly rare reversion of vaccine strains to virulence. The cases are divided among those recently vaccinated and unvaccinated nonimmune adults exposed to recently vaccinated children. Occasional outbreaks have occurred in nonimmunized populations such as the Amish in Pennsylvania. Illness typically begins with prodromal symptoms, including fever, headache, myalgia, pharyngitis, nausea and vomiting, and meningeal signs. These

are associated with the typical CSF profile of aseptic meningitis. In some patients these symptoms are followed by the development of muscle weakness. The incidence, severity, and pattern of weakness are age-dependent, with more severe disease being seen with increasing age. Young children often develop weakness of one leg, older children weakness of both legs, and adults asymmetric quadriparesis often with associated urinary retention. Weakness is associated with fasciculations, loss of deep and superficial reflexes, and the development of atrophy. Involvement of the brainstem (bulbar polio) can result in dysphagia, dysarthria, respiratory impairment, and vasomotor disturbances. Although some patients complain of paresthesia, objective sensory loss is not present.

Viruses also may affect both the anterior and posterior portions of the spinal cord over a considerable longitudinal extent, producing the syndrome of "transverse" myelitis. The clinical syndrome is one of acutely developed muscle weakness, which may be of the flaccid hyporeflexic type initially but usually develops into spastic paralysis with hyperreflexia and extensor plantar responses. Sensory loss is almost invariably present and typically involves both pain-temperature and position-vibration, producing a sensory level. Urinary symptoms (retention, overflow incontinence, or in milder cases, hesitancy or decreased voiding sensation) and constipation or even fecal incontinence are present in virtually all patients. Although this syndrome can be caused by a variety of viruses, most cases are due to HSV-2, CMV, VZV, or EBV. Pathologic evidence of myelitis is commonly encountered in severe cases of St. Louis, Eastern, and Western encephalitis. A milder form of the syndrome may be encountered in patients with episodes of herpes genitalia. Especially during the primary outbreak, patients may develop an aseptic meningitis syndrome associated with urinary retention or other symptoms; dysesthesia, paresthesia, or neuralgia in the legs, buttocks, or genital area; and weakness in one or both legs. A chronic viral myelitis is associated with infection by HIV (vacuolar myelopathy) and by HTLV-I (tropical spastic paraparesis and HTLV-I–associated myelopathy) (see Chaps. 192 and 308).

HERPES ZOSTER (See Chap. 185) A distinctive clinical syndrome consisting of paresthesia or dysesthesia in a dermatomal distribution followed by a localized cutaneous eruption ("shingles," "zoster") is commonly associated with VZV infection and rarely may be produced by HSV. Zoster occurs in patients previously infected with chickenpox (varicella). During the initial varicella infection, virus in the skin travels up the sensory nerves to become latent in the sensory ganglia. The mechanisms that account for maintenance of latency and subsequent reactivation remain unknown. Reactivation results in active viral replication in sensory ganglia followed by spread of virus through nerves to the skin, where a dermatomal vesicular eruption occurs. The incidence of zoster increases with age and is higher in patients with compromised cellular immunity. The typical history is one of several days of itching, tingling, burning, or pain in a dermatomal distribution that is followed by a vesicular eruption consisting of clear vesicles on an erythematous base. The vesicles become cloudy, dry, and crust over after 1 to 2 weeks. The lesions are most commonly found in the thoracic dermatomes, with T5-T10 accounting for approximately two-thirds of cases. Most patients will have hypalgesia and hypesthesia in the affected dermatome. About 5 percent of patients develop motor weakness and atrophy (zoster paresis) in the associated myotome.

Three antiviral drugs, acyclovir, famciclovir, and valacyclovir, are available for treatment of herpes zoster (shingles). Both drugs result in more rapid resolution of cutaneous lesions and decreased duration of viral shedding compared to placebo if therapy is started within 72 h of rash onset (and preferably earlier). Antiviral treatment of herpes zoster has not been shown to result in a significant decrease in the incidence of postherpetic neuralgia. However, recent studies suggest that famciclovir may accelerate resolution of postherpetic neuralgia by a mean of twofold, reducing the duration of this debilitating problem by an average of 2 months. Adverse effects of typical oral doses of famciclovir (500 mg three times daily for 7 days), valacyclovir (1 g three times daily for 7 days), or acyclovir (800 mg five times daily for 7 to 10 days) are minor, with headache and nausea being reported in about 8 to 20 percent of recipients. Patients with renal insufficiency require reduction in dosing.

Forty-five percent of patients over age 50 who develop shingles will experience pain persisting for more than 6 weeks after disappearance of the rash, i.e., *postherpetic neuralgia*. Postherpetic neuralgia is almost never seen in children who develop zoster and is rare (6 percent) in adults younger than 50. Patients with postherpetic neuralgia may benefit from topical therapy with capsaicin ointment as well as from systemic therapy with amitriptyline and carbamazepine.

Characteristic syndromes result from zoster eruptions involving the trigeminal and geniculate distribution. In 10 to 15 percent of cases, reactivation of virus in the trigeminal ganglia results in a rash in the distribution of the ophthalmic division of the trigeminal nerve (ophthalmic zoster). Vesicular eruption may be conjoined with conjunctivitis, keratitis, ocular muscle palsies, ptosis, and mydriasis. In rare cases, an attack is followed by the development of cerebral angiitis involving the ipsilateral carotid and/or middle cerebral arteries. Vascular compromise may lead to hemiplegia, aphasia, or other focal deficits contralateral to the side of the facial eruption. Reactivation of virus in the geniculate ganglion is reported to produce the Ramsay Hunt syndrome, consisting of facial palsy often associated with loss of taste in the anterior tongue, tinnitus, hearing loss, and vertigo. Zoster eruptions are found in the external auditory meatus.

HIV AND OTHER VIRAL NEUROPATHIES Isolated virus-induced peripheral or cranial neuropathies or plexopathies are unusual, with the exception of those associated with HIV infection (see below). CMV has been reported to produce both peripheral neuropathy and brachial plexus neuropathy. A similar syndrome may be seen with EBV. The incidence of CMV neuropathy is clearly increased in patients with AIDS. In some cases there has been evidence for direct viral infection, whereas in others the mechanism appears to be one of virus-induced segmental demyelination. CMV, HSV, EBV, VZV, mumps virus, and hepatitis B virus (HBV) also have been associated with Guillain-Barré syndrome. An almost identical syndrome can be seen in association with HIV infection, although these patients typically have a CSF pleocytosis rather than the classic albuminocytologic dissociation (elevated protein, no or few cells). Isolated cranial nerve palsies, especially of the facial nerve (Bell's palsy), have been attributed to VZV (Ramsay Hunt syndrome), HIV, EBV, enteroviruses, mumps virus, and HSV, although in many cases the etiologic relationship appears rather tenuous. Mumps, measles, and VZV may produce unilateral or bilateral nerve deafness. Seroepidemiologic studies also suggest a possible role for parainfluenza viruses, adenoviruses, and HSV in acute hearing loss.

CHRONIC AND PERSISTENT VIRAL CNS DISEASE

GENERAL CONSIDERATIONS From a practical point of view, chronic and persistent CNS viral diseases can be divided into those caused by conventional viruses and those caused by altered metabolism or accumulation of prions (Table 379-7).

HIV A complete discussion of the virologic aspects of HIV infection, of specific complications of HIV infection such as associated opportunistic infections, and of HIV therapy can be found in Chap. 308. We will focus here on the consequences for the central and peripheral nervous system of direct HIV infection.

Neurologic manifestations of HIV infection differ at different stages of illness (Fig. 379-3). Primary HIV infection can be associated with aseptic meningitis and more rarely with an acute encephalopathy. No clinical features clearly differentiate HIV aseptic meningitis from other viral meningitides, although the diagnosis should be strongly considered in patients with known risk factors for HIV infection. The syndrome is characterized by fever, headache, meningeal signs, and

Table 379-7

Chronic and Persistent CNS Diseases Caused by Viruses and Prions

Disease	Agent	Disease	Agent
Progressive multifocal leukoencephalopathy	JC virus	Creutzfeldt-Jakob disease	Prion
Subacute sclerosing panencephalitis	Measles virus	Gerstmann-Straussler-Scheinker disease	Prion
Progressive rubella panencephalitis	Rubella virus	Kuru	Prion
Tropical spastic paraparesis	HTLV-I	Fatal familial insomnia	Prion
AIDS	HIV	Alper's disease	Prion?

ABBREVIATIONS: HIV, human immunodeficiency virus; HTLV-I, human T cell leukemia virus, type I.

in some patients cranial nerve palsies (of nerves V, VII, VIII). The CSF shows a mononuclear pleocytosis, elevated protein level, and normal glucose level. HIV can be isolated from CSF, and p24 core protein may be present, which establishes the diagnosis. More commonly, the diagnosis is established by documenting HIV antibody seroconversion and intrathecal HIV antibody synthesis. In suspected cases, follow-up HIV serology should be obtained at 1, 2, and 3 months, because seroconversion may be delayed.

Persisting CSF pleocytosis also has been found in otherwise asymptomatic HIV-seropositive individuals. Seropositive individuals also may develop Guillain-Barré syndrome (GBS), chronic inflammatory demyelinating polyneuropathy (CIDP), or myopathy. HIV-associated GBS appears to be clinically indistinguishable from the syndrome that occurs in non-HIV-infected individuals. Patients present with acute onset of progressive extremity weakness, which may progress to respiratory failure. Bifacial weakness is common. Sensory symptoms may occur, but sensory signs are far less conspicuous than motor findings. All patients are areflexic or severely hyporeflexic. Findings in CIDP are similar but generally progress chronically rather than acutely and are not typically as severe. A diagnostic clue to HIV-associated GBS or CIDP may be the presence of a CSF pleocytosis in place of the typical albuminocytologic dissociation (no or few cells, elevated protein) seen in non-HIV cases. Electrophysiologic studies are consistent with demyelination (slowed conduction velocities, prolonged or absent F responses, and distal motor latencies, etc.). Extensive controlled trials of therapy in HIV-associated GBS and CIDP are not available. Plasmapheresis is the standard therapy for non-HIV-associated CIDP and GBS. Recent studies suggest that intravenous high-dose immunoglobulin may also be effective and associated with

FIGURE 379-3 The relative frequency and timing of major neurologic complications of direct HIV infection. Diseases that affect the CNS are shaded with diagonal lines; those that affect the peripheral nervous system are cross-hatched. The height of the boxes is a relative indicator of the frequency of each type of disease. (*From RT Johnson et al, FASEB J 2:2970, 1988, with permission.*)

few side effects, although some patients relapse following treatment. Both these treatments should be considered in HIV-positive individuals.

Progression of HIV infection from the asymptomatic state to more clinically advanced disease is associated with an increased incidence of neuropsychological abnormalities, including the development of HIV encephalopathy and dementia, also referred to as *AIDS-dementia complex* or *HIV-associated cognitive/motor complex*. Common early symptoms of cognitive impairment include difficulty concentrating, memory loss, slowness of thought, apathy, depression, social withdrawal, and personality changes. In distinction to "cortical" dementias such as Alzheimer's disease, aphasia, apraxia, and agnosia are uncommon, leading some investigators to classify HIV encephalopathy as a "subcortical dementia." At least 50 percent of patients will have associated signs or symptoms of motor dysfunction, including leg weakness, balance difficulty, ataxia, tremor, or pyramidal tract signs (hyperreflexia, extensor plantar responses). The illness progresses slowly over months, although mean survival time from the onset of severe dementia rarely exceeds 6 months. Laboratory studies are helpful in excluding or diminishing the possibility of other treatable processes. Twenty percent of patients will have CSF lymphocytic pleocytosis (<50 cells/μL), and 60 percent will have an elevated protein level. Hypoglycorrhachia is rare. CSF concentrations of β_2-microglobulin, neopterin, and quinolinate appear to correlate with the severity of HIV encephalopathy and may serve as useful markers of disease progression or response to antiviral therapy. CT and MRI typically show evidence of diffuse cerebral atrophy with widened sulci and ex vacuo ventricular enlargement. T2-weighted MRI spin-echo images show either patchy or diffuse white matter lesions. EEG findings are nonspecific, although some degree of generalized slowing is almost invariably present.

The neuropathologic hallmarks of AIDS encephalopathy are the presence of multinucleated giant cells seen throughout the cortex and white matter, microglial nodules, white matter pallor, and reactive gliosis. The multinucleated giant cells have been shown to contain HIV particles by electron microscopy and copious amounts of viral antigen and genome by immunocytochemistry and in situ hybridization. They appear to arise by syncytial fusion of infected monocyte-macrophage-microglial cells. These cells contain the bulk of HIV antigen and genome found in brain material. Endothelial cells and oligodendroglia may be found to contain HIV antigen or genome; neurons are rarely, if ever, positive. Neuronal dysfunction is not the result of productive infection with subsequent cell destruction. The mechanism by which HIV infection indirectly produces neuronal injury has not yet been established. Neurons may be injured as a result of cytokines, excitatory neurotoxins, or other soluble factors released by infected immune cells, macrophages, or glia. Alternatively, binding of gp120 or other viral proteins to neurons may result in alterations in ion channel conductance (e.g., of Ca^{2+}) or neurotransmitter levels, leading to cell injury (see also Chap. 308).

No definitive therapy for HIV dementia is available. Both zidovudine and didanosine have been reported to lead to improvement in some patients, although didanosine's limited CSF penetration may limit its usefulness. Some studies suggest that patients receiving higher doses of zidovudine (e.g., 1000 mg/d) do better than those receiving lower doses. Studies are under way to test the efficacy of calcium channel blockers, including nimodipine and memantine, in HIV dementia.

Symptomatic HIV-infected patients also may develop CIDP or mononeuropathy multiplex. Mononeuropathy multiplex typically presents with asymmetric multifocal peripheral and/or cranial nerve lesions. These may appear acutely as isolated regions of sensory loss or weakness in a peripheral nerve distribution. The pathogenesis appears to be ischemic injury to nerves resulting from arteritis of the vasa nervorum. In distinction to CIDP, the electrophysiologic studies suggest an axonal rather than a demyelinating lesion.

A distal symmetric painful sensory neuropathy is the most common form of neuropathy encountered in patients with clinically advanced AIDS and is present in at least one-third of patients. Most patients complain of painful distal paresthesia in the feet ("burning feet"),

which are often induced in causalgia-like fashion by pressure or contact. Walking may be difficult or impossible, and even minimal contact with blankets or sheets can produce severe discomfort. Findings on examination include a stocking-type sensory loss to pinprick, temperature, and touch sensation and loss of ankle reflexes. The knee jerks are usually intact. Motor changes (weakness, atrophy) are mild compared with the sensory signs and symptoms and are usually limited to weakness of the intrinsic foot muscles. Trophic changes, including atrophy of the skin, loss of hair, nail abnormalities, edema, and vasomotor disturbances, may be found. Patients with advanced HIV infection also may develop an autonomic neuropathy characterized by diarrhea, postural hypotension, and cardiac arrhythmias. Electrophysiologic studies are indicative of a distal sensorimotor axonopathy, which is consistent with findings on nerve biopsy. Conduction velocities and distal latencies are normal, but compound muscle action potentials in the legs and the sural sensory action potential are diminished in amplitude. HIV has been isolated from nerve biopsy specimens, although the source of virus (Schwann cells, axons, inflammatory cells) has not been established definitively.

Patients with advanced HIV infection may also develop CMV polyradiculopathy. This typically begins with involvement of the lumbosacral roots, resulting in pain and sensory loss in the feet and legs. Many patients have associated signs and symptoms of myelitis. The CSF shows a polymorphonuclear pleocytosis, and CMV DNA can be detected by CSF PCR. CMV antigen and genome can be detected in some biopsy specimens by immunocytochemistry, in situ hybridization, or PCR. Patients receiving either didanosine or dideoxycytidine also may develop neuropathic symptoms, and this possibility should be considered in the differential diagnosis. No adequate therapy exists. Patients with evidence of CMV infection should be treated with ganciclovir or foscarnet (see above). Analgesics, tricyclic antidepressants, anticonvulsants (including phenytoin and carbamazepine), and topical capsaicin ointment may be useful in the control of pain. Mineralocorticoids such as fludrocortisone may help control postural hypotension in patients with autonomic neuropathy.

A chronic progressive myelopathy affecting the posterior and lateral columns of the spinal cord is seen in 10 to 25 percent of AIDS patients. Patients develop a spastic ataxic paraparesis with diminished position and vibratory sense and urinary incontinence. Tibial somatosensory evoked responses are abnormal in virtually all patients. The clinical features resemble those seen in subacute combined degeneration secondary to vitamin B_{12} deficiency and those of nitrous oxide–induced myelopathy. Most patients (>90 percent) have associated HIV encephalopathy or dementia. Pathologic changes consist of vacuolar degeneration of the white matter of the lateral and posterior columns, typically maximal in the thoracic cord. The vacuolar areas result from severe edema within the myelin sheaths of nerve fibers and contain axonal spheroids and lipid-laden macrophages. HIV has been isolated from the spinal cord of affected individuals, and HIV genome has been found by in situ hybridization, although the role of direct viral infection versus indirect mechanism(s) of injury has not been established. No definitive therapy is available, and treatment with either zidovudine or didanosine is generally of little benefit.

In addition to vacuolar myelopathy, a variety of other myelopathic syndromes may occur in HIV-infected individuals. Ganglionitis of the lumbar and sacral dorsal root ganglia can result in secondary degeneration of the fasciculus gracilis within the posterior column of the spinal cord. The resulting clinical syndrome includes paresthesia and sensory loss (vibration, position sense) in the legs. Transverse myelitis also may result from infection with HSV, CMV, HSV plus CMV, or VZV, or from toxoplasmosis. Infection with HIV and HTLV-I together can occur, with the latter producing a spastic myelopathy (see next section).

Patients at any stage of HIV infection may develop myopathy. This is typically characterized by slowly progressive polymyositis-like proximal muscle weakness, myalgia, elevated muscle enzymes [creatine kinase, aldolase, lactate dehydrogenase, serum glutamic-oxaloacetic transaminase (SGOT)], and a myopathic pattern (brief low-amplitude motor unit potentials) on EMG testing. Muscle biopsy may show inflammation and/or myofiber degeneration and necrosis. Some patients have additional histologic changes, including nemaline rod and cytoplasmic bodies, mitochondrial abnormalities, and ragged red fibers. The pathogenesis of the syndrome has not been established. Direct HIV infection of muscle has not been detected, although HIV-infected monocytes, macrophages, and multinucleated giant cells may surround muscle fibers.

HIV-associated myopathy should be distinguished from myopathy as a complication of zidovudine therapy. Most patients with zidovudine myopathy have been receiving the drug for 6 months or more and often have higher enzyme levels and more pain than patients with non-zidovudine myopathy. Biopsy may help with the differential diagnosis, since zidovudine-related cases show more muscle fiber necrosis and less inflammation than patients with HIV myopathy. Discontinuation of zidovudine results in resolution of symptoms. Concurrent glucocorticoid therapy may allow continuation of zidovudine treatment.

TROPICAL SPASTIC PARAPARESIS AND HTLV-I–ASSOCIATED MYELOPATHY These two disorders are characterized by the development of slowly progressive spastic paraparesis, often associated with a neurogenic bladder (see Chap. 192). Symptoms typically appear during the third or fourth decades, and women are affected far more frequently than men. Most reported cases have been from Japan (HTLV-I–associated myelopathy), the Caribbean basin, parts of South America (Panama, Colombia, Peru, Brazil), the Seychelles Islands, and western Africa. Isolated cases have occurred in the southeastern United States and in many other locations. Neurologic examination shows a spastic paraparesis or paraplegia with hyperactive tendon reflexes, clonus, and extensor plantar responses. Although some patients have paresthesia, dyesthesia, or pain in the legs, sensory findings are usually mild (e.g., mild diminution in vibratory sense), and a true sensory level is only rarely found. Additional findings are seen in 5 to 20 percent of cases and can include brisk reflexes in the upper extremities, frontal release responses, cranial nerve abnormalities (optic neuropathy, deafness, nystagmus, diplopia, facial paresis), and cerebellar signs (tremor, dysmetria).

Tropical spastic myelopathies are multifactorial in nature and may be caused by a wide variety of toxic and nutritional factors. Several epidemiologic studies have unequivocally shown that infection with HTLV-I is the cause of an important subset of this disorder. Infection appears to be acquired through blood transfusion, sexual contact, intravenous drug use, and vertical transmission from mother to fetus. HTLV-I–associated cases are characterized by the presence of anti-HTLV-I antibodies in serum and CSF. The CSF/serum antibody index is elevated, indicative of intrathecal antibody synthesis. HTLV-I–specific CSF oligoclonal bands are often present. Between 25 and 60 percent of patients have a mild lymphocytic pleocytosis (<50 cells per microliter), and a higher percentage have a mild elevation in protein. HTLV-I genome can be found in CSF and peripheral blood lymphocytes using Southern blot hybridization or PCR amplification. Virus also can be isolated from the CSF and blood of affected individuals.

A number of abnormalities may be found on laboratory tests, although specific diagnosis requires viral isolation or positive serology. MRI of the spinal cord may show evidence of demyelination, and similar findings are occasionally found in the periventricular white matter in the cerebrum. Somatosensory evoked response studies may show evidence of posterior column dysfunction, even when clinical findings are mild or absent. Some patients have evidence of a demyelinating peripheral neuropathy with slowed conduction velocities, increased distal latencies, and slow or absent F waves. Pathologic examination of the spinal cord typically shows symmetric degeneration of the lateral columns encompassing the corticospinal tracts. Degenerative changes also may involve the posterior columns and spinocerebellar and spinothalamic tracts. There is an associated inflammatory infiltrate in the spinal leptomeninges, cord parenchyma, and surrounding vessels. Myelin destruction at times resembles the vacuolar myelopathy seen in association with AIDS.

The pathogenesis of the spinal cord disease has not been completely established. Both direct viral injury and immune-mediated processes may play a role. Recent evidence suggests that HTLV-I–specific cytotoxic T lymphocytes may be important in the production of immune-mediated spinal cord injury.

Currently there is no definitive therapy. Many patients benefit from oral prednisolone or equivalent glucocorticoid therapy. Zidovudine would be expected to be beneficial in limiting viral replication and associated direct cell injury.

PROGRESSIVE MULTIFOCAL LEUKOENCEPHALOPATHY As the name implies, progressive multifocal leukoencephalopathy (PML) is a progressive disorder characterized pathologically by multifocal areas of demyelination, which vary greatly in size and are scattered throughout the CNS. In addition to demyelination, there are characteristic cytologic alterations in both astrocytes and oligodendrocytes. Astrocytes are tremendously enlarged and contain hyperchromatic, deformed, and bizarre nuclei and frequent mitotic figures. Oligodendrocytes have enlarged, densely staining nuclei that contain viral inclusions formed by crystalline arrays of JC virus particles. Patients often present with visual deficits (45 percent), typically a homonymous hemianopia, and mental impairment (38 percent) (dementia, confusion, personality change). Motor weakness may not be present early but eventually occurs in 75 percent of cases.

CT and MRI remain the most valuable diagnostic studies in suggesting the diagnosis of PML. CT shows hypodense nonenhancing white matter lesions without associated edema or mass effect. Lesions are typically located periventricularly, in the centrum semiovale, in the parietal-occipital region, and in the cerebellum. MRI is more sensitive than CT and reveals hyperintense signal in the white matter on T2-weighted spin-echo images. MRI shows multifocal asymmetric, coalescing white matter lesions with a predilection for the occipital and parietal lobes. These lesions are generally nonenhancing on T1-weighted images following administration of Gd-DTPA or related contrast agents. EEG almost always shows focal or diffuse slowing, and abnormalities may occasionally precede those seen by CT. The CSF is typically normal, although mild elevation in protein and/or IgG may be found. Pleocytosis occurs in less than 25 percent of cases, is predominantly mononuclear, and rarely exceeds 25 cells per microliter. Recently, PCR amplification of JC virus DNA from CSF has shown promise as a diagnostic test for PML. The test has high specificity, but sensitivity has varied among studies. Rare cases of positive CSF PCR for JC virus DNA in the absence of clinical or radiographic evidence of PML have been described in HIV-infected patients. It remains to be established whether these results are false positive or are indicative of preclinical PML. The presence of oligoclonal bands, a substantial pleocytosis, or PMNs or red cells in the CSF should suggest such possibilities as acute multiple sclerosis, acute hemorrhagic leukoencephalitis, HIV-associated leukoencephalomyelopathy, multifocal VZV leukoencephalitis, or postinfectious or vaccinal immune-mediated encephalomyelitis.

Almost all patients (>95 percent) have an underlying immunosuppressive disorder. Prior to the HIV epidemic, common associated diseases included lymphoproliferative disorders, immune deficiency states, myeloproliferative disease, and chronic infectious or granulomatous diseases. Since 1984, the importance of these associated disorders has been dwarfed by that of AIDS. According to some recent estimates, more than 60 percent of currently diagnosed PML cases occur in patients with AIDS. Conversely, it has been estimated that nearly 1 percent of AIDS patients will develop PML. Early indications suggest that the basic clinicopathologic features of AIDS-associated PML do not differ significantly from those of non-AIDS-associated PML. Some patients with AIDS-associated PML have shown significant spontaneous improvement in the absence of therapy. Unfortunately, this appears to be the exception rather than the rule, and most cases pursue the same relentless downhill course to death that characterizes almost all reported cases of non-AIDS-associated PML.

CHAPTER 379
Aseptic Meningitis, Viral Encephalitis, and Prion Diseases

2449

Definitive diagnosis depends on identification of the characteristic neuropathologic abnormalities at biopsy or necropsy. The presence of JC virus antigen and genomic DNA can be confirmed by immunocytochemistry, in situ hybridization, and PCR amplification on brain tissue. However, detection of JC virus antigen or genomic material is not diagnostic of PML unless accompanied by characteristic pathologic changes, since both antigen and genomic material can be found in the brains of normal patients. Between 80 and 90 percent of the population is seropositive for JC virus by middle adult life. Virus may remain latent in brain or other tissues and be reactivated during immunosuppression. PML also may result from primary exposure to JC virus in an immunocompromised host, since 10 to 20 percent of individuals are seronegative at the time of disease diagnosis. As discussed above, PCR amplification of JC virus DNA from CSF appears to be a promising new diagnostic tool.

No effective therapy for PML is currently available. Anecdotal reports have described clinical and radiographic stabilization and in some cases improvement in sporadic patients treated with intravenous or intrathecal cytarabine alone or in combination with α-interferon. A multicenter trial supported by the National Institutes of Health that compared antiretroviral therapy alone to antiretroviral therapy plus either intravenous or intrathecal cytarabine in biopsy-documented HIV-associated PML failed to show any significant benefit from cytarabine treatment.

SUBACUTE SCLEROSING PANENCEPHALITIS This is a rare disease, with fewer than 10 cases per year reported in the United States. The incidence has declined substantially since the introduction of a measles vaccine. Most patients give a history of primary measles infection at an early age (≤2 years), which is followed after a latent interval of 6 to 8 years by the development of a progressive neurologic disorder. Eighty-five percent of patients are between 5 and 15 years old at diagnosis. Initial manifestations include poor school performance and mood and personality changes. As the disease develops, these nonspecific symptoms give way to progressive intellectual deterioration, focal and/or generalized seizures, myoclonus, ataxia, and visual disturbances. In the late stage of the illness, patients are unresponsive, quadriparetic, and spastic, with hyperactive tendon reflexes and extensor plantar responses. The EEG shows a characteristic periodic pattern with bursts every 3 to 8 s of high-voltage, sharp slow waves, followed by periods of attenuated ("flat") background. The CSF pattern may be diagnostic. The fluid is acellular with a normal or mildly elevated protein level and a markedly elevated gamma globulin level (>20 percent of total CSF protein). CSF antimeasles antibody levels are invariably elevated, and oligoclonal antimeasles antibodies are often present. CT and MRI show evidence of multifocal white matter lesions, cortical atrophy, and ex vacuo ventricular enlargement. Measles virus can be cultivated from brain tissue using special cocultivation techniques. Viral antigen can be identified immunocytochemically, and viral genome can be detected by in situ hybridization or PCR amplification. No definitive therapy is currently available. Treatment with Inosiplex (isoprinosine) (100 mg/kg per day) remains controversial but has been reported to prolong survival and produce clinical improvement in some patients.

PROGRESSIVE RUBELLA PANENCEPHALITIS This is an extremely rare disorder that affects mainly children with congenital rubella syndrome, although isolated cases have been reported following childhood rubella. All the approximately 20 cases reported to date have been in male children. After a latent period of 8 to 19 years, patients develop progressive neurologic deterioration. The initial manifestations are similar to those seen in SSPE and include decline in school performance, behavioral alterations, and seizures. These are followed by severe progressive dementia, prominent ataxia, pyramidal signs (spasticity, hyperreflexia, extensor plantar responses), and visual deterioration. Myoclonus may be present but is less prominent than in SSPE, whereas cerebellar signs are a great deal more prominent. In the terminal stages of the illness, patients are globally demented, mute, and quadriparetic, often with associated ophthalmoplegia. CSF shows a mild lymphocytic pleocytosis (<40 cells/μL), slightly elevated protein level [<1.5 g/L (<150 mg/dL)], markedly increased gamma globulin level (35 to 50 percent of total protein), and oligoclonal bands. The oligoclonal antibodies are specific for rubella virus antigens. The CSF/serum antirubella antibody index is markedly elevated, indicating high levels of intrathecal antirubella antibody synthesis. CT scans show ex vacuo ventricular enlargement with associated cortical atrophy. There may be hypodensity in the white matter, especially in the centrum semiovale. Cerebellar atrophy and associated fourth ventricle enlargement may be especially prominent. The EEG is nondiagnostic but is almost invariably abnormal with diffuse slowing. A few patients have a burst-suppression pattern similar to that encountered in SSPE. Biopsy or autopsy material shows perivascular lymphocytic and plasma cell cuffing in the white matter, leukomalacia of the centrum semiovale, and the atrophic and ex vacuo ventricular changes described above. Virus particles are not seen by electron microscopy, although rubella virus has been isolated from explant and cocultivation cultures of brain biopsy material in one reported case. The pathogenesis of the disease remains unclear. No therapy is currently available. Isoprinosine and amantadine are of no benefit. Universal prevention of both congenital and childhood rubella through the use of the available live attenuated rubella vaccine would be expected to eliminate the disease.

PRION DISEASES

Kuru, Creutzfeldt-Jakob disease (CJD), Gerstmann-Straussler-Scheinker (GSS) syndrome, and fatal familial insomnia, although traditionally included in discussions of viral CNS diseases, are due to the abnormal accumulation and/or metabolism of prion proteins. Prion proteins are encoded by a single-copy host gene (designated *PRNP*) present on the short arm of chromosome 20. The function of the normal cellular isoform of the *PRNP* gene (*PrP^c*) is unknown, although both membrane-associated and secreted forms exist. Neurons contain high concentrations of PrP^c, which is developmentally regulated.

A modified form, PrP^Sc, which is resistant to proteolytic digestion and spontaneously aggregates to produce rodlike or fibrillary particles (scrapie-associated fibrils, prion rods) can be identified by immunostaining in brains of animals and humans with prion diseases. The exact mechanism by which the normal cellular protein (PrP^c) is modified to its pathologic isoform (PrP^Sc), the method by which PrP^Sc replicates itself, and the way PrP^Sc accumulation leads to neuronal degeneration remain unknown.

Epidemiologic and clinical studies indicate that human prion diseases can be sporadic (CJD), infectious (kuru, rare cases of CJD), or genetic (GSS syndrome, familial CJD, fatal familial insomnia) in origin. The basic clinical features of each of these diseases are discussed below.

KURU This disease was previously endemic among members of the Fore linguistic tribal group of the Eastern Highlands area of Papua New Guinea. At its peak, the disease affected close to 1 percent of the population, although currently fewer than 10 cases per year are reported. The cardinal features of the illness were severe cerebellar ataxia with associated involuntary movements, including choreoathetosis, myoclonus, and tremor. These were associated with the subsequent development of mental impairment and frontal release signs. Brain material from affected individuals transmits the disease to primates. No new cases of the disease have been reported among individuals born since the cessation of ritual cannibalism in the affected areas. It has been suggested that ingestion of infected brain material during these rituals was responsible for disease transmission.

CREUTZFELDT-JAKOB DISEASE Most cases are sporadic, although 5 to 15 percent are familial with an autosomal dominant pattern of inheritance. Regions of high incidence and prevalence resulting from the presence of families with CJD, are scattered throughout the world, most prominently in parts of Libya and North Africa and in Slovakia. CJD is not contagious, but person-to-person spread of the disease has occurred following transplantation of corneas or dural grafts obtained from infected individuals. Isolated cases also have been attributed to improperly decontaminated neurosurgical instruments and stereotactic intracerebral depth electrodes. Approximately 50 cases have been reported in patients with panhypopituitarism who received supplemental cadaveric human growth hormone therapy and in patients who received cadaveric human gonadotropins for treatment of infertility.

CJD typically presents as a rapidly progressive dementia with prominent associated myoclonus. Clinical manifestations are protean and often include combinations of severe and progressive dementia, pyramidal and extrapyramidal motor disturbances, and signs and symptoms of cerebellar dysfunction. Clinical and pathologic subtypes with predominant involvement of specific regions of the brain have been described (e.g., occipital, thalamic, and cerebellar types). Early signs of mental impairment may be manifested as slowness in thinking, difficulty concentrating, impaired judgment, and memory loss. Mood changes and emotional lability may be combined with visual or other types of hallucinations. About a third of patients present initially with prominent cerebellar or visual disturbances, which may initially overshadow the mental impairment. Myoclonus occurs in more than 90 percent of patients and may be provoked or aggravated by startle. Additional motor signs and symptoms can include tremor, clumsiness, and choreoathetosis. As the disease progresses, about two-thirds of patients develop a parkinsonian extrapyramidal syndrome with hypokinesia and rigidity. Hyperreflexia, spasticity, and extensor plantar responses occur in about half of patients. The clinical presentation of CJD associated with use of cadaveric human pituitary hormone therapy differs from that of classic CJD. Patients are typically younger and often present with a kuru-like illness, in which cerebellar features may be more prominent initially than dementia.

Laboratory tests are helpful in excluding other causes of rapidly progressing dementia. The CSF is typically unremarkable, although the protein level may be mildly elevated. A pleocytosis is unusual and should prompt a thorough search for other processes. It has been suggested recently that two-dimensional isoelectric focusing of CSF proteins may show abnormal protein species, two of which (proteins designated 130 and 131) may be typical of Creutzfeldt-Jakob disease. These proteins appear to be identical to a brain protein designated 14-3-3. An immunoassay on CSF has been developed for this protein, which has been found in CSF from >90 percent of sporadic CJD cases. Approximately 4 percent of patients with other types of dementia, 50 percent of patients with viral encephalitis, and some patients with recent strokes may also have a positive CSF immunoassay for 14-3-3 protein. Further studies are needed to establish the utility of this test for noninvasive diagnosis of CJD. CT and MRI may show evidence of generalized cortical atrophy, but more typically the degree of clinical dementia appears disproportionate to the amount of tissue loss seen on CT and MRI. In some patients MRI has shown areas of high T2 signal intensity in the striatum. In some patients, sequential studies performed at biweekly or monthly intervals may show rapidly progressing loss of brain tissue and ex vacuo ventricular enlargement. The EEG may be quite useful in suggesting the diagnosis. The typical pattern of periodic sharp wave complexes consists of a generalized slow background interrupted by bilaterally synchronous sharp wave complexes occurring at intervals of 0.5 to 2.5 s and lasting for 200 to 600 ms. The classic EEG pattern is found in 75 to 95 percent of cases, although it may not be present very early or in the terminal stages of the disease. Sequential EEG studies may be useful if the initial recording fails to reveal the typical pattern.

The pathologic hallmarks of CJD are spongiform changes (small round vacuoles) within the neuropil, neuronal loss, hypertrophy and proliferation of glial cells, and absence of significant inflammation or white matter involvement. Pathologic changes are strongest in the cortex but are often prominent in the basal ganglia, cerebellum, and thalamus. The brainstem and spinal cord are usually spared. Recent studies indicate that the demonstration by immunostaining of protease-resistant prion proteins in brain material is a sensitive and specific marker for prion diseases. The finding of prion rods or scrapie-associated fibrils, which may be seen in electron micrographs of prepared brain material, also appears to be pathognomonic for prion diseases.

A recent summary of 300 cases of prion disease studied at the National Institutes of Health found that 79 percent of sporadic CJD cases were transmissible, 79 percent involved spongiform neuropathologic changes, and in 83 percent, protease-resistant prion proteins were detected in western immunoblots of brain tissue extracts. All iatrogenic CJD cases and all kuru cases were transmissible and had spongiform changes and positive immunoblots. Cases of familial CJD, GSS syndrome, and fatal familial insomnia showed more variable results. Taken together as a group, only 50 to 60 percent of these cases were transmissible or had positive immunoblots, although 71 percent involved spongiform changes.

CJD is invariably fatal, and no specific therapy is available. A number of drugs, including amantadine, have been reported to slow disease progression in isolated anecdotal case reports; however, the results have not been consistently reproducible.

Recent molecular genetic studies have established an unequivocal linkage between mutations in the *PRNP* gene and familial cases of CJD. Several mutations have been described, which may correlate with variations in the clinical phenotype of the disease in individual familial clusters. These include point mutations in codons 178, 200, and 210. Octarepeat inserts in the *PRNP* gene also occur in several families with CJD. No consistent *PRNP* gene mutation has been identified in cases of sporadic CJD. Some recent reports suggest that homozygosity at a polymorphic amino acid residue at codon 129 of the *PRNP* gene occurs more often than expected in patients with sporadic and iatrogenic CJD and kuru, although this possibility requires further confirmation.

Approximately a dozen cases of a variant form of CJD have been identified in the United Kingdom. It has been suggested that these cases are linked to bovine spongiform encephalopathy (BSE), perhaps as a result of human consumption or other exposure to BSE-infected bovine tissues. Patients have ranged in age from 19 to 41 years and developed a progressive illness leading to death within 7 to 23 months after onset. The clinical features included early and prominent behavioral disturbances and ataxia. Myoclonus and progressive dementia occurred in most patients as later features. The typical periodic EEG pattern usually associated with CJD did not occur. Neuropathologic features included spongiform change and prion protein (PrP) plaques. The PrP plaques resembled those seen in kuru and were often surrounded by a zone of spongiform change. PrP plaques were extensively distributed throughout the cerebrum and cerebellum.

GERSTMANN-STRAUSSLER-SCHEINKER SYNDROME This is a rare hereditary syndrome of spinocerebellar degeneration. Patients develop signs and symptoms of progressive cerebellar dysfunction in midlife, evidenced by unsteadiness, clumsiness, incoordination, and progressive gait difficulty. As the illness progresses, the cerebellar findings become increasingly severe and include ataxia, dysarthria, and nystagmus. Some patients have additional findings, which can include parkinsonian, pyramidal, and extrapyramidal findings; deafness; blindness; and gaze palsies. In distinction to their prominence in CJD, dementia and myoclonus are either absent or minor and are overshadowed by the cerebellar dysfunction.

Molecular genetic studies of GSS syndrome families have consistently demonstrated mutations in the PRNP gene, including point mutations at codons 102, 105, 117, 145, 180, 198, and 217. Although the clinical material is limited because of the rarity of the disease, it appears that ataxia is the dominant feature of the disease in families with the codon-102 mutation, whereas ataxia, dementia, and parkinsonism are seen in those with the codon-198 mutations.

FATAL FAMILIAL INSOMNIA Fatal familial insomnia (FFI) is a rapidly progressive autosomal dominant disease of middle or later life characterized by intractable insomnia, sympathetic hyperactivity and other autonomic and endocrine disturbances, dysarthria,

and motor system abnormalities, including myoclonus, tremor, ataxia,
hyperreflexia, and spasticity. Dementia is not prominent, although mild
CHAPTER 380
Nutritional and Metabolic Diseases of the Nervous System   **2451**

and motor system abnormalities, including myoclonus, tremor, ataxia,
hyperreflexia, and spasticity. Dementia is not prominent, although mild
memory and attention deficits are common. Patients often experience
complex hallucinations with the characteristics of "enacted dreams."
A variety of endocrine abnormalities also may occur, including loss
of the normal circadian fluctuations in melatonin, prolactin, and growth
hormone secretion; decreased secretion of adrenocorticotropic hormone; and elevated cortisol secretion. Pathologic changes include
atrophy and gliosis of specific thalamic nuclei and of the cerebellar
cortex and inferior olives. One patient has been described who had
spongiform changes in the involved areas and periodic sharp wave
complexes on EEG, but this appears exceptional rather than typical.
Sequencing of the *PRNP* gene from patients in two families with FFI
has shown an Asp→Asn mutation in codon 178, similar to that reported
in some cases of familial CJD. Brain material from patients in these
two families was found to contain the protease-resistant PrP^{Sc} isoform.
There have been no reports to date of successful transmission of the
disease from brain material of infected cases.

PUTATIVE PRION DISEASES There is one reported case of
transmission of a scrapie-like disease to rodents using brain material
from a 2½-year-old child diagnosed as having Alper's disease (progressive infantile poliodystrophy). This result has not been confirmed, and
no molecular genetic studies on the *PRNP* gene have been reported
from patients with Alper's disease.

BIBLIOGRAPHY

BALE JF: Viral encephalitis. Med Clin North Am 77:25, 1993
BERGER JR, CONCHA M: Progressive multifocal leukoencephalopathy: The
    evolution of a disease once considered rare. J Neurovirol 1:5, 1995
————, LEVY RM: *AIDS and the Nervous System*, 2d ed. New York, Lippincott-
    Raven, 1997
BOOSS J, ESIRI MM: *Viral Encephalitis*. Oxford, Blackwell Scientific, 1986
BROWN P et al: Human spongiform encephalopathy: The National Institutes
    of Health series of 300 cases of experimentally transmitted disease. Ann
    Neurol 35:513, 1995
CONNOLLY KJ, HAMMER SM: The acute aseptic meningitis syndrome. Infect
    Dis Clin North Am 4:599, 1990
FONG IW, TOMA E: The natural history of progressive multifocal leukoencepha-
    lopathy in patients with AIDS. Clin Infect Dis 20:1305, 1995
GESSAIN A, GOUT O: Chronic myelopathy associated with human T-lympho-
    tropic virus type 1 (HTLV-1). Ann Intern Med 117:933, 1992
GILLESPIE SM et al: Progressive multifocal leukoencephalopathy in persons
    infected with human immunodeficiency virus, San Francisco 1981–1989.
    Ann Neurol 30:597, 1991
HARRISON MJG, MCARTHUR JC: *AIDS and Neurology*. Edinburgh, Churchill
    Livingstone, 1995
JEFFERY DR et al: Transverse myelitis—retrospective analysis of 33 cases,
    with differentiation of cases associated with multiple sclerosis and parain-
    fectious events. Arch Neurol 50:532, 1993
JOHNSON RT: *Viral Infections of the Nervous System*. New York, Raven
    Press, 1982
LAKEMAN FD et al: Diagnosis of herpes simplex encephalitis: Application of
    polymerase chain reaction to cerebrospinal fluid from brain-biopsied pa-
    tients and correlation with disease. J Infect Dis 171:857, 1995
MCKENDALL RR (ed): *Handbook of Clinical Neurology*, vol 56/12: *Viral
    Disease*. Amsterdam, North-Holland, 1989
PRICE RW: Neurological complications of HIV infection. Lancet 348:445, 1996
PRUSINER SB: Inherited prion diseases. Proc Natl Acad Sci USA 91:4611, 1994
————, DEARMOND SJ: Prion diseases and neurodegeneration. Annu Rev
    Neurosci 17:311, 1994
————, HSIAO KK: Human prion diseases. Ann Neurol 35:385, 1994
ROOS KL (ed): Central nervous system infections. Semin Neurol 12:155, 1992
ROTBART HA: Enteroviral infections of the central nervous system. Clin Infect
    Dis 20:971, 1995
SIMPSON DA, TAGLIATI M: Neurologic manifestations of HIV infection. Ann
    Intern Med 121:769, 1994
SCHELD WM et al: *Infections of the Central Nervous System*, 2d ed. New
    York: Lippincott-Raven, 1997
TSAI TF: Arboviral infections in the United States. Infect Dis Clin North Am
    5:73, 1991
TYLER KL, MARTIN JB (eds): Contemporary Neurology Series, vol 41: *Infec-
    tious Diseases of the Central Nervous System*. Philadelphia, FA Davis, 1993
WEBER T et al: Clinical implications of nucleic acid amplification methods
    for the diagnosis of viral infections of the nervous system. J Neurovirol
    2:175, 1996

WHITLEY RJ: Viral encephalitis. N Engl J Med 323:242, 1990
WILL R et al: A new variant of Creutzfeldt-Jakob disease in the UK. Lancet
    347:921, 1996
WOOD M, ANDERSON M: *Major Problems in Neurology*, vol 16: *Neurological
    Infections*. London, Saunders, 1988

| 380 | *M. Flint Beal, Joseph B. Martin** |

NUTRITIONAL AND METABOLIC DISEASES OF THE NERVOUS SYSTEM

Nutritional and metabolic diseases of the central nervous system (CNS)
can be divided into two groups: acquired and inherited. Most metabolic
disturbances in adults, such as hypoxia, hypoglycemia, hepatic encephalopathy, uremia, and electrolyte abnormalities, are acquired disorders.
Nutritional diseases, many of which have prominent neurologic manifestations, remain prevalent, particularly those associated with chronic
alcoholism. Inherited metabolic diseases of late onset are relatively
infrequent, but some are important because they are prototypical and
have been explored at the genetic and biochemical levels. This is
particularly true of late-onset mitochondrial diseases. Other rare inherited metabolic disorders, such as lipid storage disease, may also present
in late life.

ACQUIRED METABOLIC DISORDERS OF THE NERVOUS SYSTEM

The acquired metabolic disorders of the nervous system include
anoxic-ischemic encephalopathy, hypoglycemia, hyperglycemic encephalopathy, hepatic encephalopathy, uremic encephalopathy, and
electrolyte or endocrine disturbances (see Chaps. 49 and 335).

EXCITOTOXIC CELL DEATH *Excitotoxicity* refers to neuronal death caused by activation of excitatory amino acid receptors.
Direct evidence for the role of excitatory amino acids in human neurologic disease arose from observations concerning the neurotoxicity of
domoic acid, a potent agonist of the kainic acid subtype of excitatory
amino acid receptors. Following consumption of mussels contaminated
with domoic acid, individuals can develop encephalopathy with complex partial seizures and memory disturbance. When death occurs, a
loss of neurons in the hippocampus can be demonstrated at necropsy.

Further compelling evidence for a role of excitotoxicity in hypoxia-
ischemia is derived from observations in experimental animals. Animal
models of stroke are associated with increased glutamate in the extracellular fluid, and neuronal damage is attenuated by glutamatergic
denervation or the administration of glutamate receptor antagonists.
The distribution of cells sensitive to ischemia corresponds closely with
that of *N*-methyl-D-aspartate (NMDA) receptors (except for cerebellar
Purkinje cells, which are vulnerable to hypoxia-ischemia but lack
NMDA receptors). Both competitive and noncompetitive NMDA antagonists are effective in preventing focal ischemia. In diffuse generalized hypoxia-ischemia, non-NMDA receptors (kainic acid and AMPA)
are activated. Antagonists to these receptors appear to be protective.
Hypoglycemia-induced brain damage is also attenuated by NMDA
antagonists.

Excitotoxicity causes an influx of calcium into the cell, and much of
the calcium is sequestered in mitochondria rather than in the cytoplasm.
Increased mitochondrial calcium causes metabolic dysfunction and
free radical generation. It also activates protein kinases, phospholipases, nitric oxide synthase, proteases, and endonucleases, and inhibits

* The authors acknowledge the contribution of Maurice Victor to this chapter
    in the 13th edition of this book.

protein synthesis. Activation of nitric oxide synthase generates nitric oxide (NO·), which can react with superoxide ($O_2\cdot$) to generate peroxynitrite ($ONOO^-$) (see Chap. 71), which may play a direct role in neuronal injury. Mice with knockout mutations of neuronal nitric oxide synthase and mice overexpressing superoxide dismutase are resistant to focal ischemia.

ANOXIA-ISCHEMIA Anoxic-ischemic encephalopathy is due to lack of delivery of oxygen to the brain because of hypotension or respiratory failure. The most common causes are myocardial infarction, cardiac arrest, shock, asphyxiation, paralysis of respiration, and carbon monoxide or cyanide poisoning. In some circumstances, hypoxia may predominate. Carbon monoxide and cyanide poisoning are termed *histotoxic hypoxia* since they cause a direct impairment of the respiratory chain.

Clinical Manifestations Mild degrees of hypoxia, such as occur at high altitudes, cause impaired judgment, inattentiveness, motor incoordination, and, at times, euphoria. With more severe hypoxia, such as occurs with circulatory arrest, consciousness is lost within seconds, but if circulation is restored within 3 to 5 min, a full recovery ensues. If anoxia persists beyond 3 to 5 min, cerebral damage is permanent. It is difficult to judge clinically the precise degree of hypoxia-ischemia. Some patients make a relatively full recovery after even 8 to 10 min of cerebral anoxia. A P_{O_2} as low as 2.7 kPa (20 mmHg) can be well tolerated if it develops gradually and normal blood pressure is maintained. The prognosis is better for patients with intact brainstem function, as indicated by normal pupillary light responses, intact doll's-head eye movements, and intact oculovestibular and corneal reflexes. Absence of these reflexes and the presence of persistently dilated pupils that do not react to light are grave prognostic signs. Long-term consequences of hypoxic-ischemic encephalopathy include persistent coma or stupor, dementia, visual agnosia, parkinsonism, choreoathetosis, cerebellar ataxia, myoclonus, and the Korsakoff amnestic state, which may be a consequence of selective damage to the hippocampus.

With severe hypoxia-ischemia, brain death is characterized by dilated, unresponsive pupils, absence of brainstem reflexes and respiration, and an isoelectric electroencephalogram (EEG). This diagnosis must be made with caution and in the absence of evidence of drug intoxication or hypothermia. Less severe anoxic damage can lead to the persistent vegetative state (see Chap. 24).

Pathologic Findings The principal histologic findings are extensive multifocal or diffuse laminar cortical necrosis, with almost invariable involvement of the hippocampus. The hippocampal CA1 neurons are the most vulnerable to even brief episodes of hypoxia-ischemia. Selective persistent memory deficits may occur after brief cardiac arrest. Scattered small areas of infarction or neuronal loss may be present in the deep forebrain nuclei, hypothalamus, or brainstem. In some cases, extensive bilateral thalamic scarring may affect thalamic and extrathalamic pathways that mediate arousal. The persistent vegetative state is thought to result from a complex interplay of discrete cortical and subcortical damage. A specific form of hypoxic-ischemic encephalopathy, so-called watershed infarcts (parieto-occipital), occur at the distal territories between the major cerebral arteries and can cause both cognitive deficits and weakness that is greater in proximal than in distal muscle groups.

DELAYED POSTANOXIC ENCEPHALOPATHY Delayed postanoxic encephalopathy is an uncommon phenomenon in which patients appear to make an initial recovery after a brief episode of cardiac arrest or strangulation, but then develop a relapse characterized by apathy, confusion, and agitation. Progressive neurologic deficits may include shuffling gait, diffuse rigidity and spasticity, persistent parkinsonism, and on occasion coma and death after 1 to 2 weeks. Widespread cerebral demyelination may be present. Carbon monoxide or cyanide intoxication causes delayed damage in both the putamen and the globus pallidus. Little clinical impairment is evident when the patient first regains consciousness, but a parkinsonian syndrome characterized by akinesia and rigidity with no tremor may develop. Symptoms can worsen over months, accompanied by increasing evidence of damage in the basal ganglia as shown by both computed tomography (CT) and magnetic resonance imaging (MRI).

Diagnosis Diagnosis depends on the history of a hypoxic-ischemic event such as cardiac arrest; blood pressures below 70 mm systolic and $Pa_{O_2} < 40$ mmHg are typical. Carbon monoxide intoxication can be confirmed by measurements of carboxyhemoglobin and is suggested by a cherry red color of the skin.

TREATMENT

Treatment is directed at restoration of normal cardiorespiratory function. Initial management is to secure a clear airway and institute artificial respiration. Cardiopulmonary resuscitation and the use of a cardiac defibrillator or pacemaker may be needed. Although neuroprotective agents are undergoing clinical investigation, none has demonstrated efficacy in improving neurologic outcome. Severe carbon monoxide intoxication is treated with hyperbaric oxygen. Seizures should be controlled by anticonvulsants. Posthypoxic myoclonus may respond to oral administration of clonazepam at doses of 1.5 to 10 mg daily.

HYPOGLYCEMIC ENCEPHALOPATHY (See Chaps. 334 and 335) Hypoglycemia typically causes confusion, seizures, stupor, coma, and occasionally hemiparesis or other focal neurologic findings. Blood glucose concentrations are typically <1.4 mmol/L (<25 mg/dL). Persistent hypoglycemia depletes cerebral energy supplies and can lead to irreversible neuronal damage. This process has been shown to involve excitotoxic mechanisms in animal studies.

Etiology Hypoglycemic encephalopathy is typically caused by accidental or deliberate overdoses of insulin or antidiabetic agents, insulin-secreting islet cell tumors or retroperitoneal sarcoma, protracted ethanol intoxication (in rare cases), or Reye's syndrome (in childhood).

Clinical Manifestations The symptoms of hypoglycemia may occur as three syndromes. In the acute syndrome, the initial symptoms are those of adrenergic activation and consist of nervousness, hunger, tachycardia and palpitations, anxiety, sweating, and tremor. These symptoms are frequently recognized by the patient and respond quickly to oral or parenteral glucose. If the syndrome progresses, patients develop increasing confusion, drowsiness, motor restlessness, myoclonic twitching, and seizures. Blood glucose levels of approximately 1 mM/L are associated with deep coma, dilated pupils, shallow respirations, and atonia. Subacute hypoglycemia is associated with an absence of adrenergic activation, and patients show slowing of thought processes and a gradual blunting of consciousness with retention of awareness. Hypothermia is commonly encountered in this form of the disorder. Chronic hypoglycemia, which typically occurs with islet cell tumors, is rare and is characterized by insidious changes in personality, memory, and behavior which may be construed as dementia. Some of these patients develop ataxia and, rarely, lower motor neuron involvement.

Pathology The neuropathologic effects of hypoglycemia are similar to those of anoxic injury. There is diffuse neuronal loss in the cerebral cortex and hippocampus, but Purkinje neurons are relatively spared.

TREATMENT

Rapid correction of hypoglycemia is critical to prevent neurologic damage. A 50% dextrose solution is administered initially. Blood glucose is then followed closely and maintained between 8 and 11 mM/L by constant infusion of a glucose-containing solution. Glucose levels must be monitored carefully to prevent the development of hypoglycemia in diabetics and to prevent recurrence of hypoglycemia in all subjects. Patients with acute or subacute hypoglycemia show rapid improvement. In patients with chronic hypoglycemia, glucose administration does not promptly relieve symptoms, suggesting the presence of neuronal injury. Clinical improvement after removal of the source of exogenous insulin is gradual and may extend over a period as long as a year.

Differential Diagnosis Episodes of hypoglycemia typically develop more slowly than those of hypoxia, and disturbances in cerebral function may not be apparent for 30 to 60 min, rather than within seconds or minutes. Large overdoses of insulin, however, can cause rapid onset of seizures and coma. Subacute and chronic hypoglycemia, as can occur with islet cell tumors, may masquerade as an episodic confusional state, dementia, or a seizure disorder. The diagnosis is established by demonstrating low blood glucose and elevated levels of insulin.

HYPERGLYCEMIC COMA Hyperglycemia is associated with two coma-producing syndromes in diabetics: hyperglycemia with ketoacidosis and hyperosmolar nonketotic hyperglycemia (see Chap. 334).

HYPERCARBIC ENCEPHALOPATHY Chronic emphysema, pulmonary fibrosis, and occasionally impaired central respiratory drive can lead to chronic respiratory acidosis with elevation of P_{CO_2} and a reduction in arterial P_{O_2}. Common sequelae are secondary polycythemia and "cor pulmonale."

Clinical Manifestations Manifestations include generalized or bilateral frontal headache, which is often intense and persistent, papilledema, mental dullness, drowsiness, confusion, stupor, and coma. At advanced stages a fast-frequency action tremor, as well as myoclonic twitching of the muscles, may be present. Interruption of voluntary movement characteristically causes brief lapses of sustained muscle contraction, known as asterixis. Patients frequently show indifference and inattention to the environment.

Pathogenesis The cerebral disorder is thought to be due to CO_2 narcosis, which causes cerebrovasodilation and leads to increased intracranial pressure. The P_{CO_2} may exceed 75 mmHg, and the oxygen saturation of blood ranges from 80 to 85 percent. The EEG frequently shows slowing in the theta and delta ranges.

℞ **TREATMENT**

Treatment consists of ventilation with an intermittent positive-pressure respirator. Cor pulmonale is treated with diuretics and agents to lower vascular resistance, as described in Chap. 233. It is imperative to avoid administering narcotics or other sedatives that can blunt the respiratory drive. Oxygen can also be dangerous, because it blunts the hypoxic respiratory drive. Oxygen should be administered only to raise the arterial oxygen level to the range of 50 to 55 mmHg. → *Respiratory failure is discussed in detail in Chap. 266.*

Differential Diagnosis Hypercapnia does not usually cause prolonged coma and does not result in irreversible brain damage. Asterixis is a feature of other metabolic encephalopathies as well, in particular of hepatic encephalopathy. Hypercapnia can be mistaken for a confusional psychosis or occasionally a chronic extrapyramidal syndrome that causes myoclonus or chorea.

HEPATIC ENCEPHALOPATHY (See Chap. 299) Chronic hepatic insufficiency, which is most frequently due to cirrhosis of the liver, results in portacaval shunting of blood and is often punctuated by episodes of stupor, coma, and other neurologic symptoms, termed *hepatic coma* or *portasystemic encephalopathy*. This condition is frequently triggered by gastrointestinal bleeding. In addition, hereditary hyperammonemic syndromes may cause episodic coma with or without seizures in infants (and rarely adults). Reye's syndrome is a hepatic encephalopathy that occurs in association with viral illnesses in children and involves acute brain swelling in conjunction with fatty infiltration of the liver and elevation of serum levels of liver enzymes and ammonia.

Clinical Features Chronic hepatic encephalopathy initially causes mental confusion and decreased motor activity, followed by progressive drowsiness, stupor, and coma. Brain edema, which can be visualized by MRI, may occur with acute hepatic encephalopathy. There are frequently lapses of sustained muscle contraction (asterixis).

Characteristic EEG abnormalities in the earliest stages of the confusional state consist of bilaterally synchronous delta waves, which are frequently triphasic and prominent in frontal regions. Fluctuating rigidity of the extremities, as well as grimacing, sucking, grasp reflexes, palmomental reflexes, Babinski's signs, and focal or generalized seizures, may be present.

The syndrome usually evolves slowly over days to weeks with drowsiness, confusion, and asterixis. In its mild form it needs to be distinguished from other confusional states. Recurrent hepatic encephalopathy can lead to persistent dementia and extrapyramidal syndromes, as described below.

Pathology and Pathogenesis The characteristic neuropathologic feature in patients who die in hepatic coma is an increase in the number and size of protoplasmic astrocytes (Alzheimer type II astrocytes) in the deep layers of the cerebral cortex and in the basal ganglia.

The pathogenesis of hepatic encephalopathy remains poorly understood. The disorder may be a consequence of elevated ammonia concentrations, which can cause a number of disturbances of intermediary metabolism. Elevated levels of glutamine in cerebrospinal fluid (CSF) levels are present in most patients with severe hepatic encephalopathy, possibly owing to the reaction of ammonia with α-ketoglutarate. This may impair the function of the Krebs cycle, leading to energy impairment. In animals, hepatic encephalopathy is accompanied by reductions in ATP concentrations. Much of the ammonia appears to arise from the action of urease-containing bacteria in the bowel, which can split urea. Ammonia is absorbed into the portal circulation, where it fails to serve as a substrate for nitrogen fixation because of either hepatocellular disease, portasystemic shunting of blood, or both.

℞ **TREATMENT**

The standard mode of treatment is to attempt to prevent elevated ammonia concentrations by dietary restriction of protein, mechanical cleansing of the colon, administration of antibiotics such as neomycin (1 g orally tid) to suppress or eliminate urease-producing organisms in the bowel, and administration of lactulose (30 to 50 mL orally tid), an osmotic laxative that acidifies the colonic contents. Liver transplantation has been successful in some patients and can reverse hepatic coma. → *See Chap. 298 for additional methods of treatment.*

CHRONIC ENCEPHALOPATHY (ACQUIRED HEPATO-CEREBRAL DEGENERATION) Clinical manifestations of this disorder are now less common owing to the widespread use of liver transplantation. Previously, patients would survive one or more episodes of hepatic coma and be left with residual neurologic abnormalities such as tremor of the head and arms, asterixis, grimacing, chorea, dysarthria, ataxia, and cognitive dysfunction. Some patients with chronic hepatic failure develop a slowly evolving syndrome of ataxia, choreoathetosis, and mild dementia characterized by slowness and indifference.

Pathology Chronic hepatocerebral degeneration is seen with all varieties of chronic liver disease. It is characterized neuropathologically by widespread hyperplasia of protoplasmic astrocytes in the cerebral and cerebellar cortices and in the thalamic and lenticular nuclei. Nerve cells often appear swollen and chromatolytic, accounting for the so-called Opalski cells. The protoplasmic astrocytes may contain periodic acid–Schiff (PAS)-positive glycogen granules.

CENTRAL PONTINE MYELINOLYSIS This disorder typically presents in a devastating fashion as quadriplegia and pseudobulbar palsy. Predisposing factors include severe underlying medical illness or nutritional deficiency; most cases are associated with hyponatremia, which is rapidly corrected by intravenous NaCl, or with other hyperosmolar states. The pathology consists of demyelination without inflammation in the base of the pons, with relative sparing of axons and nerve cells. Experimentally, central pontine myelinolysis can be reproduced by rapid correction of hyponatremia. MRI scans are useful in establishing the diagnosis (Fig. 380-1) and may also identify partial forms that present as confusion, dysarthria, and/or disturbances of conjugate gaze without quadriplegia. Therapeutic guidelines for the restoration of severe hyponatremia should aim for gradual correction, i.e., by no more than 10 mmol/L (10 meq/L) within 24 h and 20 mmol/L (20 meq/L) within 48 h.

HEREDITARY METABOLIC DISEASES OF LATE ONSET

MITOCHONDRIAL DISORDERS When glucose is used by the electron transport chain, it is converted into CO_2 and H_2O and produces 36 high-energy phosphates. In contrast, when glucose is converted to lactate by glycolysis, only 2 high-energy phosphates are produced. The brain has very high energy requirements and a limited capacity to use other substrates for ATP synthesis (see Chap. 335). The brain requires energy for basic housekeeping functions common to all cells and for specific functions such as maintaining ionic gradients. As much as 40 percent of all oxygen consumption in the brain is used to maintain the sodium-potassium gradient across the cell membrane. The energy reserves of the CNS are small, and irreversible cellular damage occurs after a brief deprivation of either glucose or oxygen.

The primary sites of oxidative phosphorylation are the mitochondria. Each mitochondrion has an outer membrane that is permeable to large molecules and an inner membrane that is relatively impermeable and contains the electron transport complexes. The electron transport complexes use both NADH and FADH, each of which is produced by the Krebs cycle and each of which donates electrons through transport enzymes on the inner mitochondrial membrane. The enzymes are designated complexes I through V. Complexes I and II collect electrons and transfer them to ubiquinone (coenzyme Q_{10}). The electrons then move sequentially to complex III, cytochrome c, complex IV, and finally to oxygen, the terminal electron acceptor. Concurrently, ejection of protons across the inner mitochondrial membrane results in an electrochemical proton gradient that stores potential energy. Complex V uses energy stored in the proton gradient to condense ADP with inorganic phosphate into ATP, which is then exchanged with ADP across the inner mitochondrial membrane by the adenine nucleotide translocase.

Kearns-Sayre Syndrome (See also Chap. 383) The first direct evidence that mitochondrial DNA is involved in human disease arose from the finding of large deletions in mitochondrial DNA from patients with myocardial myopathies and the detection of a missense mutation in mitochondrial DNA from patients with Leber's hereditary optic neuropathy. Subsequently, the molecular basis has been elucidated in other mitochondrial encephalomyopathies. Kearns-Sayre syndrome is characterized by progressive external opthalmoplegia, pigmentary reti-

FIGURE 380-1 Central pontine myelinolysis. Axial T2-weighted MR scan through the pons reveals a symmetric area of abnormal high signal intensity within the basis pantis (*arrows*).

nopathy, and one or more of the following: heart block, cerebellar ataxia, and cerebrospinal fluid protein concentration above 1.0 g/L (100 mg/dL). Onset is usually before age 20, and the prognosis is poor. CSF lactate and pyruvate levels are elevated. Muscle biopsy specimens typically show ragged red fibers. Large deletions of mitochondrial DNA are present. The course is progressively downhill, and most patients die in their third or fourth decade. Most cases appear to be sporadic mutations.

MERRF Myoclonic epilepsy with ragged red fibers (MERRF) is characterized by myoclonus, seizures, cerebellar ataxia, and mitochondrial myopathy. Onset is often in childhood or early adult life. Serum and CSF lactate and pyruvate levels are increased, and muscle biopsy specimens show ragged red fibers. The course of this illness is progressively downhill, and most patients die in the third or fourth decade with severe mental deterioration. Maternal relatives may be asymptomatic or have partial clinical syndromes. The pathogenic mutations have been demonstrated at nucleotide positions 8344 and 8356 in the lysine transfer RNA gene.

MELAS Mitochondrial encephalomyopathy, lactic acidosis, and strokelike episodes (MELAS) constitute another maternally inherited disorder characterized by recurrent strokelike episodes, migraine headaches, vomiting, seizures, and lactic acidosis. In most cases there is a point mutation at nucleotide position 3243 in the leucine transfer RNA gene.

Leigh Syndrome Maternally inherited Leigh syndrome is usually a disorder of infancy or childhood, rarely of early adulthood. These patients typically show psychomotor regression, seizures, dystonia, ataxia, optic atrophy, ophthalmoplegia, tremor, pyramidal signs, and respiratory abnormalities. CT or MRI scans show bilateral symmetric areas of signal abnormalities in the basal ganglia and brainstem. Lactic acidosis is common. These patients typically show a progressive downward course. In some families, mitochondrial point mutations have been described at position 8993 in the ATPase 6 gene.

Leber's Disease Leber's hereditary optic neuropathy was the first human disease linked to inherited point mutations in mitochondrial DNA. The phenotype is painless, subacute, bilateral visual loss with central scotomas and abnormal color vision. The mean age of onset is 23 years. Three to four times as many men as women are affected, for unclear reasons. Mitochondrial DNA mutations have been identified in at least eight genes, most encoding subunits of complex I but a few encoding subunits of complex IV. A small number of families with this disorder have degeneration in the basal ganglia with dystonia.

℞ TREATMENT

Many mitochondrial encephalomyopathies follow an episodic course. The most common therapy is to administer agents to stimulate residual electron transport enzyme activity, to supply precursors of coenzymes, or to administer artificial electron acceptors. Coenzyme Q_{10}, an essential component of the electron transport chain that may enhance ATP production and serve as an antioxidant, has been used in patients with mitochondrial disorders, but evidence for efficacy is limited. In a number of case reports, this treatment has been demonstrated to reduce lactate concentrations and to improve visual function. Other approaches have been to use vitamin K_3, nicotinamide, thiamine, riboflavin, and carnitine.

LIPID STORAGE DISORDERS (Inherited metabolic disorders of late life include the lipid storage disorders)

Metachromatic Leukodystrophy (See Chap. 346) Metachromatic leukodystrophy (MLD) may occur in adulthood (25 percent of cases) or in early childhood (75 percent). The mode of inheritance is autosomal recessive. Onset is insidious, and the disease course is progressive. The major clinical manifestation is cognitive deterioration, including forgetfulness, poor scholastic or job performance, and changes in personality. The possibility of psychiatric illness is frequently considered, but eventually mild cerebellar findings appear, with pyramidal signs, masked facies, and strange postures. The diagnosis is established by demonstrating diminished arylsulfatase A activity in white blood cells, serum, or urine; increased excretion of sulfatides in the urine; slowed nerve conduction velocity; and metachromatic material in nerve biopsy samples. No treatment is available, and deterioration progresses until the patient is demented, mute, and bedridden.

Adrenoleukodystrophy This inherited metabolic disorder is characterized by both a lipid storage abnormality and adrenal insufficiency and may present either with a progressive myelopathy or with cognitive findings, homonymous hemianopia, cortical blindness, hemiparesis, aphasia, or dementia. Typically, signs are asymmetric initially and progress intermittently, leading to diagnostic confusion. The diagnosis is usually made by finding low blood cortisol levels or deficient response to cosyntropin stimulation. Patients may develop either a progressive spastic paraparesis or a demyelinating polyneuropathy. There is increased urinary excretion of C22 to C26 fatty acids. The symptoms of adrenal insufficiency are treated by glucocorticoid replacement, but no effective treatment is available.

GM$_2$ Gangliosidosis GM$_2$ gangliosidosis (hexosaminidase A deficiency) can occur in young adults. The mode of inheritance is autosomal recessive, and both sexes are equally affected. Patients often develop progressive ataxia with mild signs of corticospinal disease and may have generalized seizures. The fundi are typically normal, but characteristic cherry red spots occur. In some cases the initial manifestations consist of motor neuron involvement with progressive weakness and muscle cramps, mimicking amyotrophic lateral sclerosis (see Chap. 370). The diagnosis is established by visualizing cytoplasmic bodies by electron microscopy or by detecting reduced hexosaminidase A activity in white blood cells. Gaucher's, Niemann-Pick, and Krabbe's diseases also occur rarely in adult life (see Chap. 346).

Ceroid Lipofuscinosis The Kufs type of ceroid lipofuscinosis is a lipid storage disease that can occur in either adolescence or early to mid-adult life. The disease is characterized by mental deterioration with seizures, ataxia, apoptosis, and spasticity. Diagnosis is made by skin or conjunctival biopsies that show lipofucsin storage material and characteristic abnormalities by electron microscopy.

NUTRITIONAL DISEASES

The vitamin deficiency diseases consist of the following neurologic diseases: (1) Wernicke's disease and Korsakoff's psychosis, (2) alcoholic cerebellar degeneration, (3) nutritional polyneuropathy, (4) pellagra, (5) deficiency amblyopia (nutritional optic neuropathy), (6) Strachan's syndrome, consisting of amblyopia, painful neuropathy, and orogenital dermatitis, (7) subacute combined degeneration of the spinal cord, (8) folic acid deficiency, and (9) vitamin E deficiency.

WERNICKE'S DISEASE OR ENCEPHALOPATHY Wernicke's encephalopathy is a common and preventable disorder due to a deficiency of thiamine (see Chap. 79). In the United States, alcoholics account for most cases, but patients are also at risk with malnutrition due to hyperemesis, starvation, renal dialysis, cancer, or acquired immunodeficiency syndrome. The characteristic clinical triad is that of ophthalmoplegia, ataxia, and global confusion. However, only one-third of patients with acute Wernicke's encephalopathy present with the classic clinical triad. Most patients are profoundly disoriented, indifferent, and inattentive, although rarely they have an agitated delirium related to ethanol withdrawal. If the disease is not treated, stupor, coma, and death may ensue. Ocular motor abnormalities include horizontal nystagmus on lateral gaze, lateral rectus palsy (usually bilateral), conjugate gaze palsies, and rarely ptosis. Gait ataxia probably results from a combination of polyneuropathy, cerebellar involvement, and vestibular paresis. The pupils are usually spared, but they may become miotic with advanced disease. Parenteral administration of thiamine in the early stages results in dramatic improvement in ocular motility, but horizontal nystagmus may persist.

Wernicke's disease is usually associated with other manifestations of nutritional disease, such as polyneuropathy, which is seen in 80 percent of patients (see Chap. 386). Rarely, amblyopia or spinal spastic ataxia occur. Tachycardia and postural hypotension may be related to impaired function of the autonomic nervous system or to the coexis-

tence of cardiovascular (wet) beriberi. Patients who recover show improvement in ocular palsies within hours after the administration of thiamine. Ataxia improves more slowly than the ocular motor abnormalities. Approximately half the patients recover incompletely and are left with a slow, shuffling, wide-based gait and an inability to walk tandem. Apathy, drowsiness, and confusion improve more gradually. As these symptoms recede, an amnestic state with impairment in recent memory and learning may become more apparent (Korsakoff's psychosis; see Chap. 386). Korsakoff's psychosis is a part of Wernicke's disease and may occur together with the other components of the illness (Wernicke-Korsakoff syndrome). Korsakoff's psychosis is frequently persistent; the residual mental state is characterized by gaps in memory, confabulation, and disordered temporal sequencing.

Pathology Lesions in the periventricular regions of the diencephalon, midbrain, and brainstem as well as the superior vermis of the cerebellum consist of symmetric discoloration of structures surrounding the third ventricle, aqueduct, and fourth ventricle, with petechial hemorrhages in occasional acute cases and atrophy of the mamillary bodies in most chronic cases. There is frequently endothelial proliferation, demyelination, a loss of neuropil, and some neuronal loss. These changes can be detected in some cases by MRI scanning (Fig. 380-2). The amnestic defect is related to lesions in the medial dorsal nuclei of the thalamus.

Etiology and Pathogenesis The specific factor responsible for the Wernicke-Korsakoff syndrome is a deficiency of thiamine. Thiamine is a cofactor of several enzymes, including transketolase, pyruvate dehydrogenase, and α-ketoglutarate dehydrogenase. Thiamine deficiency produces a diffuse decrease in cerebral glucose utilization and results in mitochondrial damage. Glutamate accumulates owing to impairment of α-ketoglutarate dehydrogenase activity and, in combination with the energy deficiency, may result in excitotoxic cell damage. Electron microscopy shows disintegrating mitochondria, chromatin clumping, and swelling of degenerating neurons in the diencephalic nuclei of thiamine-deficient rats, consistent with excitotoxicity. Cell degeneration can be blocked by an antagonist of the NMDA glutamate receptor.

℞ **TREATMENT**

Wernicke's disease is a medical emergency and requires immediate administration of thiamine, in a dose of 50 mg either intravenously or intramuscularly. The dose should be given daily until the patient resumes a normal diet and should be begun prior to treatment with

FIGURE 380-2 Wernicke's disease. Coronal T1-weighted postcontrast MR image reveals abnormal enhancement of the mammillary bodies (*arrows*), typical of acute Wernicke's encephalopathy.

intravenous glucose solutions. Glucose infusions may precipitate Wernicke's disease or acute cardiovascular beriberi in a previously unaffected patient or cause a rapid worsening of an early form of the disease. For this reason, thiamine should be administered to all alcoholic patients requiring parenteral glucose. The cardiovascular status of each patient should be carefully monitored.

NUTRITIONAL POLYNEUROPATHY (See also Chaps. 79 and 381)   Nutritional polyneuropathy is usually associated with alcoholism. It is present in most patients with Wernicke-Korsakoff syndrome. The neuropathy is identical to that seen with beriberi. The treatment is administration of B vitamins, including thiamine, pyridoxine, pantothenic acid, vitamin B_{12}, and folic acid.

ALCOHOLIC CEREBELLAR DEGENERATION   Cerebellar degeneration occurs frequently in chronic alcoholics. The symptoms usually evolve in a subacute fashion over several weeks to months. The cerebellar dysfunction predominantly affects the stance and the gait, which is wide-based. Legs are involved more severely than arms. Nystagmus and dysarthria occur infrequently. The pathologic changes consist of degeneration of neurons in the anterior and superior cerebellar vermis with loss of Purkinje cells. CT or MRI confirms cerebellar vermis atrophy. Abstinence, dietary replenishment, and supplemental B vitamins may produce moderate improvement in the gait ataxia as peripheral neuropathy resolves.

PELLAGRA (See Chap. 79)   Pellagra is a result of niacin deficiency. The neurologic symptoms consist of both an encephalopathy and a peripheral neuropathy. Early nonspecific symptoms consist of insomnia, fatigue, anxiety, nervousness, irritability, and depression. With advancing illness, there may be slowing of mental processes and impairment of memory. In some cases there is a spastic spinal syndrome consisting of spastic weakness of the legs, increased tendon reflexes, clonus, and extensor plantar responses.

Pathologic Features   The major neuropathologic changes in pellagra are swelling, chromatolysis, and loss of Nissl staining in neurons, particularly the large Betz cells of the motor cortex. The same changes are seen to a lesser extent in smaller pyramidal cells of cerebral cortex and in cells of the basal ganglia, cranial motor nuclei, dentate nuclei, and anterior horns of the spinal cord. The spinal cord lesions consist of symmetric degeneration of the dorsal columns and to a lesser extent the corticospinal tracts.

SUBACUTE COMBINED DEGENERATION OF THE SPINAL CORD (See Chap. 373)   This spinal cord disease due to vitamin B_{12} deficiency is typically associated with an acquired defect in intestinal absorption of vitamin B_{12} due to an intrinsic factor deficiency. Rarely, patients on highly restricted diets or with disease of the small intestine or gastric resection manifest the illness. Occasionally, the cause is an abnormal vitamin B_{12} binding protein.

Clinical Manifestations   Neurologic symptoms are present in most patients with B_{12} deficiency. The initial symptoms are generalized weakness and paresthesia consisting of tingling and "pins-and-needles" feelings. The paresthesia tends to persist and to cause distress. As the illness progresses, loss of vibration sense is more pronounced in the legs than the arms. Position sense is involved to a lesser extent. The motor defects are usually limited to the legs and include weakness, spasticity, increased deep tendon reflexes, clonus, and extensor plantar responses. At an early stage, the patellar and Achilles reflexes may be diminished, increased, or absent. The gait is initially ataxic but later becomes both spastic and ataxic.

Mental symptoms include irritability, apathy, somnolence, suspiciousness, confusional psychosis, and intellectual deterioration. Personality change and dementia may be the only manifestations. Optic neuropathy with impaired acuity and central scotomas often but not always improves with B_{12} replacement therapy. Neurologic symptoms may occur in the absence of anemia.

Pathology and Pathogenesis   The pathologic features consist of swelling of myelin sheaths followed by demyelination and astrocytic gliosis. The changes commence in the posterior columns of the lower cervical and upper thoracic region and spread up and down the spinal cord, followed by involvement of the lateral columns. In the optic nerves there is degeneration of myelinated fibers in the territory of the papillomacular bundles.

The pathogenesis is poorly understood. Vitamin B_{12} deficiency impairs the function of methionine synthetase and methylmalonyl CoA mutase. Impairment of the latter enzyme may lead to the production of abnormal fatty acids, which alters the production of myelin. The major defect, however, may result from impairment of methionine synthase activity, since hereditary cases of cobalamin deficiency have been described in which methylmalonyl CoA mutase activity was normal in the presence of neurologic abnormalities. Interestingly, dentists and others who have overexposure to nitrous oxide may develop neurologic symptoms identical to those in B_{12} deficiency. Prolonged exposure of rats to nitrous oxide inactivates methionine synthetase but has no effects on methylmalonyl CoA mutase. Methylation of myelin basic protein can stabilize its insertion in the myelin sheath, which could play a role in pathogenesis.

Diagnosis   Patients are typically screened by measurements of serum vitamin B_{12} levels. Rare patients become symptomatic with serum B_{12} concentrations in the low normal range. Intrinsic factor deficiency can be confirmed by a Shilling test (see Chap. 108). The presence of anti-intrinsic factor or anti-parietal cell antibodies confirms the diagnosis of pernicious anemia. In the rare instances in which these tests are inconclusive, documentation of elevated serum levels of methylmalonic acid and total serum homocysteine may substantiate the diagnosis, but these tests are expensive and are only performed in specialized laboratories. Their role in the screening of patients with nonspecific neuropsychiatric symptoms remains to be established.

℞ **TREATMENT**

Treatment consists of administration of cobalamin at a dosage of 1 mg (1000 μg) intramuscularly each day for 5 to 10 days, then weekly for a month, and then monthly for life. Folate administration may cause neurologic deterioration in vitamin B_{12}–deficient patients. Therefore, if folate therapy is indicated, it should not be given until cobalamin stores have been repleted for 1 to 2 weeks. The most important factor influencing the response to treatment is the duration of symptoms. Recovery is often complete if therapy is instituted within a few weeks of their onset. For this reason, treatment should be instituted on an emergent basis. If symptoms have been present for several months, the best that can be expected is arrest of progression of the disease.

FOLIC ACID DEFICIENCY   Folic acid deficiency occurs frequently, yet its role in the pathogenesis of nervous system disease is not firmly established. Neuropathies associated with some chronic malabsorption syndromes and accompanying chronic administration of phenytoin have been attributed to folate deficiency. Rare cases of subacute combined degeneration have been attributed to folic acid deficiency and have resolved after the institution of folate therapy.

VITAMIN E DEFICIENCY (See Chap. 79)   Vitamin E is a fat-soluble vitamin, and deficiency states occur with chronic malabsorption syndromes, such as in abetalipoproteinemia, following surgical resection of the intestine, and with hepatobiliary disease. Vitamin E deficiency also occurs in patients with mutations in the gene for the α-tocopherol transfer protein, which incorporates α-tocopherol into very low density lipoproteins in the liver. Three different mutations have been identified in families suffering from ataxia with vitamin E deficiency. The manifestations include peripheral neuropathy, ataxia, and proximal muscle weakness and resemble those of spinocerebellar degeneration. Pathologic features consist of degeneration of posterior columns, spinocerebellar tracts, posterior columns, dorsal root ganglia, and sensory roots. The pathogenesis of the lesions is of great interest, since vitamin E is known to be a major lipid-soluble antioxidant. It is therefore hypothesized that vitamin E deficiency leads to increased free radical generation and oxidative damage. Treatment consists of supplementation with 60 to 75 U of vitamin E. In patients with malabsorption, it may be necessary to administer other fat-soluble vitamins as well.

DEFICIENCY AMBLYOPIA Deficiency amblyopia (nutritional optic neuropathy, tobacco-alcohol amblyopia) is a form of visual impairment that complicates nutritional deficiency. The symptoms consist of dimness or blurring of vision and impairment of color vision, which then progresses insidiously over days to weeks. On examination, patients show reduced visual acuity and have bilateral and roughly symmetric central or centrocecal scotomas. Pallor of the temporal portion of the optic disc may be present.

Deficiency amblyopia, which was common among prisoners of war in the Far East, has also been associated with some cases of beriberi (due to thiamine deficiency) and pellagra (due to niacin deficiency). In the United States, most cases occur in heavy smokers who also consume alcohol. These cases of so-called tobacco-alcohol amblyopia are thought to be largely of nutritional origin. It has been hypothesized that smoking may contribute to optic nerve toxicity because of the cyanide in tobacco smoke. Cyanide may be detoxified by vitamin B_{12}–dependent mechanisms involving sulfated amino acids. Some cases of tobacco-alcohol amblyopia respond to vitamin B_{12} supplementation. Treatment otherwise consists of administration of a balanced diet, supplementation with vitamins, and restriction of alcohol when it is the cause of nutritional deficiency.

AMBLYOPIA, PAINFUL NEUROPATHY, AND OROGENITAL DERMATITIS (STRACHAN'S SYNDROME) The syndrome of amblyopia, painful neuropathy, and orogenital dermatitis (Strachan's syndrome), originally referred to as Jamaican neuritis, occurs among the undernourished populations of many tropical countries. The disorder occurred in the besieged population in Madrid during the Spanish Civil War and in prisoners of war during World War II in both the Middle and Far East, and an outbreak has occurred in Cuba. In the United States, this syndrome occurs occasionally in alcoholic patients.

The optic neuropathy is characterized by subacute onset of decreased visual acuity and color vision, central scotomas, pallor of the optic disc, and loss of papillomacular bundle fibers. The peripheral neuropathy consists of painful dysesthesia, areas of hyperesthesia, diminished ankle reflexes, decreased sensitivity to vibration, pinprick, and light touch, and rarely high-frequency hearing loss. A few patients have developed a myopathy with decreased posterior column sensation as well as mild spasticity with heightened reflexes, extensor plantar responses, and a spastic bladder.

An epidemic of optic and peripheral neuropathy affected more than 50,000 people in Cuba from 1991 to 1993. This outbreak was associated with tobacco use, particularly cigar smoking, and the risk was reduced with higher dietary intakes of thiamine, vitamin B_{12}, riboflavin, and niacin. In addition, higher serum concentrations of antioxidant carotenoids appear to be protective. Improved nutrition and supplementation with multivitamins have resulted in the disappearance of the syndrome.

BIBLIOGRAPHY

BEAL MF: Aging, energy and oxidative stress in neurodegenerative diseases. Ann Neurol 38:357, 1995

BECK WS: Neuropsychiatric consequences of cobalamin deficiency. Adv Intern Med 36:33, 1991

BUTTERWORTH RF: Pathophysiology of cerebellar dysfunction in the Wernicke-Korsakoff syndrome. Can J Neurol 20(Suppl 3):123, 1993

——— et al: Ammonia: Key factor in the pathogenesis of hepatic encephalopathy. Neurochem Pathol 6:1, 1987

CHARNESS MD et al: Ethanol and the nervous system. N Engl J Med 321:442, 1989

CHOI DW, ROTHMAN SM: The role of glutamate neurotoxicity in hypoxic-ischemic neuronal death. Annu Rev Neurosci 13:171, 1990

DININGER MN: Management of sodium abnormalities in patients with CNS disease. Clin Neuropharmacol 15:427, 1992

FRANCIS GS et al: Metachromatic leukodystrophy: Multiple nonfunctional and pseudodeficiency alleles in a pedigree: Problems with diagnosis and counseling. Ann Neurol 34:212, 1993

GOTODA T et al: Adult-onset spinocerebellar dysfunction caused by a mutation in the gene for the α-tocopherol-transfer protein. N Engl J Med 333:1313, 1995

JOHNS DR: Mitochondrial DNA and disease. N Engl J Med 333:638, 1995

KINNEY HC et al: Neuropathological findings in the brain of Karen Ann Quinlan. N Engl J Med 330:1469, 1994

LAURENO R: Central pontine myelinolysis following rapid correction of hyponatremia. Ann Neurol 13:232, 1983

LEE MS, MARSDEN CD: Neurological sequelae following carbon monoxide poisoning: Clinical course and outcome according to the clinical types and brain computed tomography scan findings. Movement Disord 9:550, 1994

LIEBER CS: Medical disorders of alcoholism. N Engl J Med 333:1058, 1995

OUHCHI K et al: Ataxia with isolated vitamin E deficiency is caused by mutations in the α-tocopherol transfer protein. Nat Genet 9:141, 1995

REYNOLDS EH et al: Subacute combined degeneration with high serum vitamin B_{12} level and abnormal vitamin B_{12} binding protein. Arch Neurol 50:739, 1993

ROMÁN GC: An epidemic in Cuba of optic neuropathy, sensorineural deafness, peripheral sensory neuropathy and dorsolateral myeloneuropathy. J Neurol Sci 127:11, 1994

RIZZO JF, LESSELL S: Tobacco amblyopia. Am J Ophthalmol 116:84, 1993

SERDARU M et al: The clinical spectrum of alcoholic pellagra encephalopathy. Brain 111:829, 1988

SHEVELL MI, ROSENBLATT DS: The neurology of cobalamin. Can J Neurol Sci 19:472, 1990

THE CUBA NEUROPATHY FIELD INVESTIGATION TEAM: Epidemic optic neuropathy in Cuba—clinical characterization and risk factors. N Engl J Med 333:1176, 1995

THE MULTI-SOCIETY TASK FORCE ON PVS: Medical aspects of the persistent vegetative state. N Engl J Med 330:1499, 1994

VICTOR M: Alcoholic dementia. Can J Neurol Sci 21:88, 1994

——— et al: *The Wernicke-Korsakoff Syndrome and Related Disorders Due to Alcoholism and Malnutrition.* Philadelphia, Davis, 1989

ZIEVE L: Pathogenesis of hepatic encephalopathy. Metab Brain Dis 2:147, 1987

SECTION 3
DISORDERS OF NERVE AND MUSCLE

381 | *Arthur K. Asbury*

DISEASES OF THE PERIPHERAL NERVOUS SYSTEM

Peripheral neuropathy is a general term indicating peripheral nerve disorders of any cause; the manifestations of such a disorder may be so bewildering and complex that it is difficult for the physician to know where to begin and how to proceed. Therefore, an assessment scheme is set forth to guide the examiner to correct diagnoses and management decisions (Fig. 381-1).

GENERAL DESCRIPTION Polyneuropathy is a common and important type of peripheral neuropathy. The prototypical picture of polyneuropathy occurs with acquired toxic or metabolic neuropathic states. The first symptoms tend to be sensory and consist of tingling, prickling, burning, or bandlike dysesthesias in the balls of the feet or tips of the toes, or in a general distribution over the soles (see Chap. 23). Symptoms and findings are usually symmetric and graded distally, but occasionally dysesthesias appear in one foot shortly before the other or are more pronounced in one foot. Some care and judgment is needed to avoid confusion with mononeuropathy multiplex. If the polyneuropathy remains mild, no objective motor or sensory signs may be detectable.

With progression, pansensory loss is usually found over both feet, ankle jerks are lost, and weakness of dorsiflexion of the toes, best demonstrated in the great toe, may be present. In some instances, the process begins with weakness in the feet, without sensory symptoms. As worsening occurs, sensory loss moves centripetally in a graded "stocking" fashion, and the patient may complain that the feet have a numb or "wooden" feeling or may say "I feel as though I'm walking on stumps." Patients have difficulty walking on their heels during examination and their feet may slap while walking. Later, the knee jerk reflex disappears, and foot drop becomes more apparent. By the time sensory disturbance has reached the upper shin, dysesthesias are usually noticed in the tips of the fingers. The degree of spontaneous pain varies but is often considerable. Light stimuli to hypesthetic areas, once perceived, may be experienced as extremely uncomfortable (hyperpathia). Unsteadiness of gait may be out of proportion to muscle weakness because of proprioceptive loss.

Worsening is more severe in the legs than in the arms and proceeds in a centripetal, symmetrically graded manner with pansensory loss, areflexia, and muscle atrophy; motor weakness is usually greater in the extensor muscles than in corresponding flexor groups. When the sensory disturbance reaches the elbows and mid-thighs, a tent-shaped area of hypesthesia often may be demonstrated on the lower abdomen. This area will grow broader, and its apex will extend rostrally toward the sternum as the neuropathy worsens. By this time, patients generally cannot stand or walk or hold objects in their hands.

In the most extreme cases, ventilatory capacity is impaired along with sphincteric function. Hypesthesia at the crown of the scalp may be present and may spread radially into both the trigeminal and the C2 distribution. Overall, nerve fibers are affected according to length of their axon, without regard to root or nerve trunk distribution—hence the aptness of the term *stocking-glove* to describe the pattern

of sensory deficit. In general, the motor deficit is also graded, distal, and symmetric.

Variations in disease manifestations are common and explain the diversity of clinical syndromes encountered. Variations occur in the rate of disease evolution, in whether progression is steady or fluctuating, in the eventual degree of severity, in the presence or absence of positive motor and sensory symptoms, in the symmetry of features and their distribution (proximal versus distal, arms versus legs, and motor versus sensory), in the relative proportions of dysfunction attributable to deficits in large and to small fibers, and in the relative importance of axonal and demyelinating processes (as assessed mainly by electrodiagnostic examination).

ASSESSMENT AND DIAGNOSIS OF NEUROPATHY
Clues to the diagnosis of specific peripheral neuropathies often lie in unnoticed or forgotten events occurring weeks or months prior to the onset of symptoms. Inquiry should be made about recent viral illnesses; other systemic symptoms; institution of new medications; exposures to solvents, pesticides, or heavy metals; the occurrence of similar symptoms in family members or coworkers; habits concerning alcohol; and the presence of known preexisting medical disorders. It is also useful to ask patients if they would feel well if free of their neuropathic symptoms, to obtain an idea of the presence or absence of an underlying systemic illness.

How did symptoms first appear? Even with distal polyneuropathies, symptoms may appear in the sole of one foot a few days or a week before the other, but usually the patient will describe a distal graded disturbance that moves evenly and symmetrically in centripetal fashion. Symptoms that first appear in the distribution of individual digital nerves, involving only half of a digit at a time, and then gradually spread and coalesce suggest a multifocal process (mononeuropathy multiplex), as might occur with a systemic vasculitis or cryoglobulinemia.

The evolution of neuropathy ranges from rapid worsening over a few days to an indolent process lasting many years. Polyneuropathies

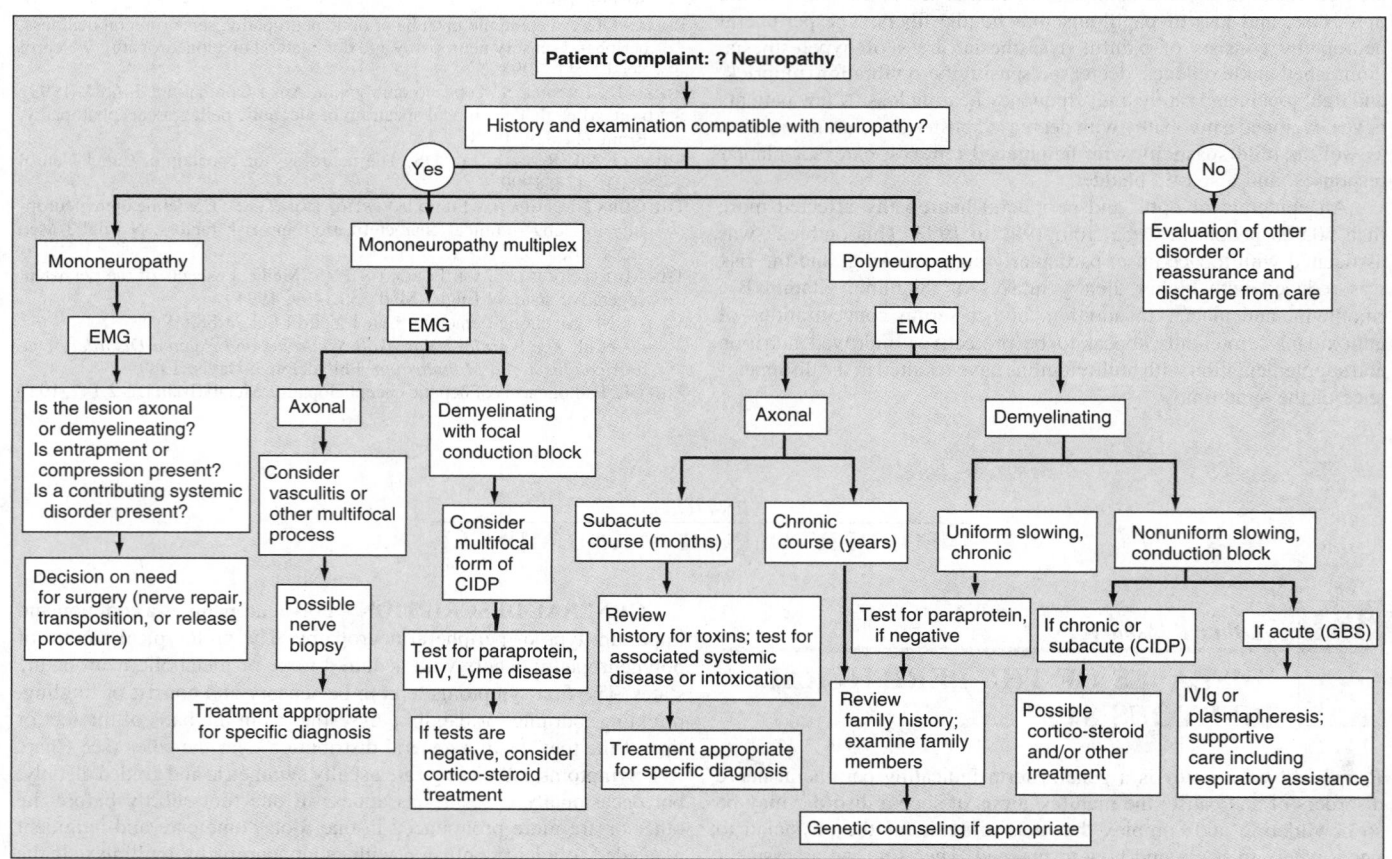

FIGURE 381-1 Approach to the evaluation of peripheral neuropathies. CIDP, chronic inflammatory demyelinating polyradiculoneuropathy; EMG, electro- myography; GBS, Guillain-Barré syndrome; HIV, human immunodeficiency virus; IVIg, intravenous immunoglobulin. *(After Asbury.)*

that progress slowly, over more than 5 years, are most likely to be genetically determined, particularly if the major manifestations are distal atrophy and weakness with few or no positive sensory symptoms. Diabetic polyneuropathy and paraproteinemic neuropathies also progress insidiously over 5 to 10 years. Axonal degeneration of toxic or metabolic origin tends to evolve over several weeks to a year or more, and the rate of progression of demyelinating neuropathies is highly variable, ranging from a few days in Guillain-Barré syndrome to many years in others.

Major fluctuations in the course of neuropathy raise two possibilities: (1) relapsing forms of neuropathy and (2) repeated toxic exposures. Slow fluctuation in symptoms taking place over weeks or months (reflecting changes in the activity of neuropathy) should not be confused with day-to-day variation or diurnal undulation of symptoms. The latter are common to all neuropathic disorders. An example is carpal tunnel syndrome, in which dysesthesia may be prominent at night but absent during the day.

Palpation of the nerve trunk to detect enlargement is a frequently forgotten part of the neurologic examination. In mononeuropathies, the entire course of the nerve trunk in question should be explored manually for focal thickening, for the presence of neurofibroma, point tenderness, or Tinel's phenomenon (generation of a tingling sensation in the sensory territory of the nerve by tapping along the course of the nerve trunk), and for pain elicited by stretching of the nerve trunk. In leprous neuritis, fusiform thickening of nerve trunks is frequent, and beading of nerve trunks may be encountered in amyloid polyneuropathy. In genetically determined hypertrophic neuropathies, uniform thickening of all nerve trunks may occur, often to the caliber of a clothesline or larger.

Most neuropathies involve nerve fibers of all sizes, but damage sometimes is restricted to either large or small fibers. In a polyneuropathy affecting mainly small fibers, diminished pinprick and temperature sensation, often with painful, burning dysesthesias, may predominate along with autonomic dysfunction, but with relative sparing of motor power, balance, and tendon jerks. Some cases of amyloid and distal diabetic polyneuropathies fall into this category. In contrast, large-fiber polyneuropathy is characterized by areflexia, sensory ataxia, relatively minor cutaneous sensory deficit, and variable but often severe motor dysfunction.

For patients with polyneuropathy or mononeuropathy multiplex, standard tests should include a complete blood count and measurement of erythrocyte sedimentation rate, urinalysis, chest x-ray, postprandial blood glucose determination, and serum protein electrophoresis. Further tests should be dictated by the combined results of the history and the physical and electrodiagnostic examination (see Fig. 381-1).

Electrodiagnosis Electrodiagnostic examination is a key procedure in all patients with suspected neuropathy (see Fig. 380-1). It is not generally possible to make the distinction between axonal and demyelinating disorders by clinical examination alone; here electrodiagnostic analysis is particularly useful. Electrodiagnostic features of demyelination are slowing of nerve conduction velocity (NCV), dispersion of evoked compound action potentials, conduction block (major decrease in amplitude of muscle compound action potentials on proximal stimulation of the nerve, as compared to distal stimulation), and marked prolongation of distal latencies (see Chap. 361). In contrast, axonal neuropathies are characterized by a reduction in amplitude of evoked compound action potentials with relative preservation of NCV. The distinction between a primarily demyelinating neuropathy and an axonal neuropathy is crucial because of the differing approaches to diagnosis and management.

Electrodiagnosis also helps to determine the presence or absence of a sensory involvement when that is not clear by clinical examination alone. It provides information about the distribution of subclinical findings, thus sharpening the diagnostic focus. The issues on which the clinician may ask the electrodiagnostician for clarification include the following:

1. The distinction between disorders primary to nerve and to muscle (neuropathy versus myopathy).

2. The distinction between root or plexus involvement and more distal nerve trunk involvement.
3. The distinction between generalized polyneuropathic processes and widespread multifocal nerve trunk involvement.
4. The distinction between upper and lower motor neuron weakness.
5. The distinction, in a given generalized polyneuropathic process, between primary demyelinating neuropathy and axonal degeneration.
6. The assessment, in both primary axonal and demyelinating neuropathies, of many factors bearing on the nature, activity, and likely prognosis of the neuropathy.
7. The assessment, in mononeuropathies, of the site of the lesion and its major effect on nerve fibers, especially the distinction between demyelinating conduction block and wallerian degeneration.
8. The characterization of disorders of the neuromuscular junction.
9. The identification, often in muscle of normal bulk and strength, of important features such as chronic partial denervation, fasciculations, and myotonia.
10. The analysis of cramp, and its distinction from physiologic contracture.

If in a particular instance of progressive polyneuropathy of subacute or chronic evolution the electrodiagnostic findings are those of an axonopathy, a long list of metabolic states and exogenous toxins comes under consideration (see Tables 381-1 and 381-2). If the course is protracted over several years, it raises the likelihood of the neuronal (axonal) form of peroneal muscular atrophy [hereditary motor and sensory neuropathy (HMSN) type II]; family members must be examined and additional attention given to the family history. If the electrodiagnostic findings indicate primary demyelination of nerve, on the other hand, the approach is entirely different. The possibilities then include acquired demyelinating neuropathy, thought to be immunologically mediated, and genetically determined neuropathies, some of which are marked by uniform and drastic slowing of nerve conduction velocities.

The flowchart in Fig. 381-1 summarizes the clinical and electrodiagnostic approach to evaluation and management of a neuropathic disorder. Using this scheme, the clinician determines for each patient the tempo, distribution, and severity of the disease, the functional impairment of the patient, and other features previously discussed, making a clinical judgment as to whether the problem represents a mononeuropathy, a mononeuropathy multiplex, or a polyneuropathy. Often this distinction is obvious. With the sum of clinical and electrodiagnostic information in hand, the differential diagnostic possibilities and management options will have been narrowed to only a few. The remainder of this chapter deals with the details of this formulation.

Nerve Biopsy The sural nerve at the ankle is the preferred site for cutaneous nerve biopsy. There are few indications to employ this invasive technique. The main one is in asymmetric and multifocal neuropathic disorders producing a clinical picture of mononeuropathy multiplex, the basis of which is still unclear after other laboratory investigations are complete. Diagnostic considerations include vasculitis, multifocal demyelinating neuropathies, amyloidosis, leprosy, and occasionally sarcoidosis. Nerve biopsy is also helpful when one or more cutaneous nerves are palpably enlarged. Another clinical application is in establishing the diagnosis in some genetically determined childhood disorders such as metachromatic leukodystrophy, Krabbe's disease, giant axonal neuropathy, and infantile neuroaxonal dystrophy. In all of these recessively inherited diseases, both the central nervous system (CNS) and the peripheral nervous system (PNS) are affected.

There is a tendency to carry out sural nerve biopsy in distal symmetric polyneuropathies of subacute or chronic evolution. This practice is discouraged because its yield is low. Nerve biopsy in this situation may be useful as part of an approved research protocol when the biopsy will provide crucial information not otherwise obtainable.

Table 381-1

Polyneuropathy Associated with Systemic Diseases

Systemic Disease (Occurrence)	Axonal*			Demyelinating*			Sensory vs. Motor†	Autonomic*	Comment
	Acute	Subacute	Chronic	Acute	Subacute	Chronic			
Diabetes mellitus (common)	−	±	+	−	±	+	S, SM, rarely M	± to +	See Table 381-4
Uremia (sometimes)	±	+	+	−	−	−	SM	±	Controllable with proper dialysis; curable with successful renal transplant
Porphyria (3 types) (rare)	+	±	−	−	−	−	M or SM	± to +	May be proximal > distal and may have atypical proximal sensory deficits
Hypoglycemia (rare)	±	+	±	−	−	−	M	−	Usually with insulinoma; arms often > legs
Vitamin deficiency, excluding B₁₂ (sometimes)	−	+	+	−	−	−	SM	±	Involves thiamine, pyridoxine, folate, pantothenic acid, and probably others
Vitamin B₁₂ deficiency (sometimes)	−	±	+	−	−	−	S	−	Neuropathy overshadowed by myelopathy
Critical illness (sepsis) (common)	−	+	±	−	−	−	M > S	−	Sepsis patients severely ill, often on ventilator
Chronic liver disease (sometimes)	−	−	−	−	−	+	S or SM	−	Usually mild or subclinical
Primary biliary cirrhosis (rare)	−	±	+	−	−	−	S	−	Intraneural xanthomas
Primary systemic amyloidosis (rare)	−	±	+	−	−	−	SM	+	Also in amyloidosis with myeloma or macroglobulinemia
Hypothyroidism (rare)	−	−	−	−	±	+	S	−	May respond to thyroid replacement
Chronic obstructive lung disease (rare)	−	±	+	−	−	−	S or SM	−	Severe pulmonary insufficiency
Acromegaly (rare)	−	−	+	−	−	−	S	−	Carpal tunnel syndrome also frequent
Malabsorption (sprue, celiac disease) (sometimes)	−	±	+	−	−	−	S or SM	±	Basis for neuropathy unclear; deficiency?
Carcinoma (sensory) (rare)	−	+	+	−	−	−	Pure S	−	Due to ganglionitic neuronopathy; mostly small cell lung or breast carcinoma; paraneoplastic
Carcinoma (sensorimotor) (sometimes)	−	+	+	−	−	−	SM	±	Sensorimotor axonal neuropathy; mostly with lung carcinoma
Carcinoma (late) (common)	−	+	+	−	−	−	S > M	±	Mild, probably related to weight loss and wasting
Carcinoma (demyelinating) (sometimes)	−	−	−	+	+	±	SM	−	Acute or relapsing demyelinating neuropathy
HIV infection (sometimes)	−	±	+	−	−	−	S >> M	−	Late stages of AIDS; other neuropathies occur; see text
Lyme disease (sometimes)	−	±	+	−	−	−	S > M	−	Variable picture; see text
Lymphoma, including Hodgkin's (sometimes)	−	+	+	+	+	±	See above	±	Same as with carcinomatous types
Polycythemia vera (rare)	−	±	+	−	−	−	S	−	Also many CNS manifestations; often shooting pains in limbs
Multiple myeloma, lytic type (sometimes)	−	±	+	−	−	−	S, M, or SM	±	Symptomatic neuropathy uncommon; subclinical neuropathy frequent
Multiple myeloma, osteosclerotic or solitary plasmacytoma type‡ (sometimes)	−	−	±	−	±	+	SM	−	May show severe slowing of nerve conduction velocity
Benign monoclonal gammopathy (sometimes):									
IgA	−	±	+	−	−	−	SM	−	IgM_κ (or occasionally
IgG	−	±	+	−	−	−	SM	−	IgM_λ) may bind to myelin-associated glycoprotein or glycolipids
IgM	−	−	−	−	±	+	SM or S	−	
Cryoglobulinemia (rare)	−	±	+	−	−	−	SM	−	May be mononeuropathy multiplex in presentation

* +, Usually; ±, sometimes; −, rare, if ever.
† S, sensory; M, motor; SM, sensorimotor.
‡ Some cases associated with POEMS syndrome (see text).

Table 381-2

Polyneuropathy Associated with Drugs and Environmental Toxins

	Axonal*			Demyelinating*			Sensory vs. Motor†	Autonomic*	CNS*	Comment
	Acute	Subacute	Chronic	Acute	Subacute	Chronic				
DRUGS‡										
Amiodarone (anti-arrhythmic)	−	−	+	−	−	+	SM	−	−	Dose-dependent neuropathy, reversible by decreasing dose
Aurothioglucose (antirheumatic)	±	±	−	+	+	−	SM	−	−	Idiosyncratic reaction; ? immune-mediated
Cisplatin (antineoplastic)	−	+	+	−	−	−	S	−	−	Severe sensory neuropathy, also ototoxicity; dose-related
Dapsone (dermatologic agent; used, e.g., for leprosy)	−	±	+	−	−	−	M	−	−	Dose-related pure motor neuropathy
Disulfiram (antialcoholism agent)	±	+	+	−	−	−	SM	−	±	Usually occurs after months of treatment
Hydralazine (antihypertensive)	−	±	+	−	−	−	S > M	−	−	A pyridoxine antagonist
Isoniazid	−	±	+	−	−	−	SM	±	−	A pyridoxine antagonist; neurotoxic in slow acetylators
Metronidazole (antiprotozoal)	−	−	±	−	−	−	S or SM	−	+	Dose-related central-peripheral distal axonopathy
Misonidazole (radiosensitizer)	−	±	+	−	−	−	S or SM	−	+	Neurotoxicity is the limiting factor
Nitrofurantoin (urinary antiseptic)	−	±	+	−	−	−	SM	−	−	Generally total dose-related; renal failure enhances toxicity
Nucleoside analogues (ddC, ddI, d4T) (antiretroviral agents)	±	+	+	−	−	−	S >> M	−	?	Dose-related; painful
Phenytoin (anticonvulsant)	−	−	+	−	−	−	S > M	−	−	After 20–30 years of phenytoin use
Pyridoxine (vitamin)	−	±	+	−	−	−	S	−	−	Occurs with large intake (>300 mg/d)
Suramin (antineoplastic)	+	+	−	+	+	−	M > S	−	−	Related to serum levels >350 mg/mL
Taxol (antineoplastic)	±	+	±	±	+	±	S > M	−	−	Dose-related
Vincristine (antineoplastic)	−	+	+	−	−	−	S > M	−	−	Sensory symptoms common, hands > feet; motor signs ominous; should stop treatment
TOXINS‡										
Acrylamide (flocculant; grouting agent)	−	±	+	−	−	−	S > M	±	+	Large-fiber neuropathy; sensory ataxia
Arsenic (herbicide; insecticide)	±	+	+	−	−	−	SM	±	±	Skin changes, Mees' lines in nails; painful; systemic effects
Diphtheria toxin	−	−	−	+	+	−	SM	−	−	Clinically very rare; can be confused with GBS
γ-Diketone hexacarbons (solvents)	−	±	+	−	−	+	SM	±	+	Neurofilamentous swelling of axons; these solvents now in restricted use
Inorganic lead	−	−	+	−	−	−	M > S or M	−	±	Selective motor neuropathy with prominent wrist drop
Organophosphates	−	±	+	−	−	−	SM	−	+	Brain and spinal cord also affected, the latter irreversibly
Thallium (rat poison)	−	+	+	−	−	−	SM	−	+	Also alopecia, Mees' lines in nails; painful

* +, Usually; ±, sometimes; −, rare, if ever.

† S, sensory; M, motor; SM, sensorimotor.

‡ The following drugs and environmental toxins are also neurotoxic, mainly to the peripheral nervous system:

Drugs: Amitriptyline, chloramphenicol, colchicine, ethambutol, nitrous oxide, perhexiline maleate, sodium cyanate, thalidomide, L-tryptophan

Environmental toxins: Allyl chloride, buckthorn berry, carbon disulfide, dimethylaminoproprionitrile, (DMAPN), ethylene oxide, metallic mercury, methyl bromide, polychlorinated biphenyls, styrene, trichlorethylene, vacor

POLYNEUROPATHY Although *polyneuropathy* connotes a widespread symmetric process, usually distal and graded, polyneuropathies are very diverse because of the extreme variability of tempo, severity, mix of sensory and motor features, and presence or absence of positive symptoms. The patient with a fulminant, severely dysesthetic sensory polyneuropathy and alopecia who is in the early phases of thallium intoxication bears little similarity to the patient with a 40-year history of insidiously progressive clumsiness of gait whose findings are foot drop, lower leg atrophy, pes cavus, and minimal asymptomatic distal sensory deficit (i.e., peroneal muscular atrophy, either type I or II; see Table 381-3). These two patients fall near opposite ends of the spectrum of polyneuropathy.

The classification of peripheral neuropathies has become increasingly complex as the capacity to discriminate new subgroups and identify new associations with toxins and systemic disorders improves. Further, our grasp of the pathophysiologic basis of the clinical phenomena observed in neuropathy has increased rapidly. But these advances are primarily descriptive; little progress has been made in understanding the fundamental pathogenic events in nervous tissue that eventuate in any of the polyneuropathies.

The important features of each major grouping of polyneuropathies are summarized below, and key aspects of specific polyneuropathies are given in Tables 381-1 to 381-5.

Acute Axonal Polyneuropathy In this setting, the term *acute* means evolution over days. Acute axonal polyneuropathies are relatively uncommon. Included are porphyric neuropathy and massive intoxications, often suicidal or homicidal in intent. For example, an individual receiving a large dose of arsenic (e.g., 100 mg of arsenous oxide) will become violently ill in a few hours with vomiting, diarrhea, and circulatory collapse. In 1 to 3 days, serious renal and liver failure will ensue, and between 14 and 21 days, painful polyneuropathy will appear, often as the systemic disorder abates. The polyneuropathy worsens over 2 to 3 weeks and then enters a plateau phase; recovery requires months.

Subacute Axonal Polyneuropathy Many instances of toxic and metabolic polyneuropathy are *subacute*, meaning they evolve over weeks, although even more of these may be chronic in evolution (months to years). Tables 381-1 and 381-2 offer many diagnostic possibilities. Management in almost all instances involves eliminating contact with the offending agent or treating the associated systemic order.

Chronic Axonal Polyneuropathy This category includes many more types of polyneuropathy, in part because the term *chronic* subsumes neuropathies that have progressed over periods from 6 months to 60 years. As a rough approximation, slow worsening for more than 5 years, absence of positive symptoms, deficits that are mainly motor, and absence of systemic disorder all favor a genetically determined neuropathy. Although these disorders are mostly autosomal dominant in inheritance, recessively inherited and X-linked varieties also occur (Table 381-3).

Acute Demyelinating Polyneuropathy For all practical purposes, this category is synonymous with Guillain-Barré syndrome (GBS). This acute, frequently severe, and fulminant polyneuropathy occurs at a rate of one case per million population per month, or approximately 3500 cases per year in the United States and Canada. Incidence patterns are similar worldwide. In over two-thirds of cases, an infection, either clinically overt or evidenced by serum titer rise, precedes the onset of neuropathy by 1 to 3 weeks. Herpesvirus infections (cytomegalovirus, Epstein-Barr virus) account for a large proportion of virus-triggered cases. Other cases appear to be triggered by *Campylobacter jejuni* gastroenteritis. A small proportion, less than 5 percent, occur within 1 to 4 weeks of a surgical procedure. GBS occurs on a background of lymphoma, including Hodgkin's disease, and in lupus erythematosus more frequently than can be attributed to chance alone.

Although the weight of evidence indicates that GBS is immune-mediated, the immunopathogenesis remains obscure. In 1976 to 1977, a flurry of some 500 cases followed the national swine flu vaccination program in the United States. This exceeded by severalfold the baseline incidence expected in this period in those vaccinated. The epidemiologic features of this outbreak resembled a point-source epidemic with an "incubation" period of 1 to 6 weeks. The reason why swine flu vaccine triggered GBS in 1976 to 1977 has never been discovered. In subsequent annual flu vaccine programs in the United States, no excess cases of GBS have been identified.

The clinical features of GBS include areflexic motor paralysis with or without sensory disturbance coupled with an acellular rise of total protein in the cerebrospinal fluid by the end of the first week of symptoms. Several subtypes of GBS are recognized. Approximately 80 percent of cases encountered in North America and Europe are demyelinating and inflammatory. An unusual variant, the Fisher syndrome, presents with ataxia, areflexia, and external ophthalmoplegia, but weakness often appears later in its course. Other variants are notable for an axonal pattern of electrodiagnostic findings and axonal pathology with little inflammation. Most patients with GBS are hospitalized, and about 30 percent require ventilatory assistance at some point during the illness. The prognosis is good; approximately 85 percent of patients make a complete or nearly complete recovery. The mortality rate is 3 to 4 percent. Management consists mostly of supportive care, but plasmapheresis also is important. Large, multicenter, controlled trials in North America and Europe have demonstrated a beneficial effect of plasmapheresis if initiated in the first 2 weeks of illness. Intravenous administration of high-dose immunoglobulin (2 g/kg body weight given over 5 days) is as effective as plasmapheresis, and is more easily administered. In contrast, glucocorticoid treatment has not been shown to be effective.

Other acute demyelinating polyneuropathies are rare and include buckthorn berry intoxication and diphtheritic polyneuritis (see Table 381-2).

Subacute Demyelinating Polyneuropathy Neuropathies in this category are heterogeneous in origin, although all are acquired. Most common is a relapsing and remitting neuropathy that has many clinical features in common with GBS but differs from GBS in tempo, course, and absence of discernible triggering events (see "Acquired Demyelinating Neuropathies," below). Previously mentioned toxins (buckthorn berry, diphtheria toxin, aurothioglucose) may also induce a picture of widespread subacute demyelination of peripheral nerves (see Table 381-2).

Chronic Demyelinating Polyneuropathy Although more common than the subacute neuropathies, chronic polyneuropathy with demyelinating features encompasses a wide diversity of disorders, including hereditary neuropathies, inflammatory neuropathies, and other acquired neuropathies associated with diabetes mellitus, dysproteinemias, other metabolic states, and some chronic intoxications. To complicate matters, many of these disorders present an electrodiagnostic picture of mixed axonal-demyelinative findings. Frequently it is difficult to determine which process—axonal degeneration or demyelination—is the primary event. Aspects of many of these neuropathies are included in Table 381-1 to 381-5 and in the sections below.

SPECIAL CATEGORIES OF NEUROPATHY Hereditary Neuropathies The major characteristics of this highly variegated group of disorders are summarized in Table 381-3. With the exception of the porphyric neuropathies, the onset of neuropathic dysfunction is insidious, and progression is indolent, occurring over years or decades. Most of these diseases are rare, with the striking exception of the dominantly inherited peroneal muscular atrophies (HMSN-I and HMSN-II; see Table 381-3). The prevalence of these disorders is roughly 1 case per 3000 to 6000 population. In peroneal muscular atrophy, phenotypic expression is often variable, so affected family members of a propositus may have no symptoms and minimal neurologic findings but (in HMSN-I) may still show severe reduction of nerve conduction velocity. Advances in molecular genetics have had a major impact on defining hereditary neuropathies. Two recent reviews are cited in the references, and Tables 362-1 and 380-3 outline what is known.

Table 381-3

Genetically Determined Neuropathies

Genetic Disorder	Inheritance/ Gene Location	Age of Onset	Basic Process	Other Features*	Other Systems Involved	Genetic Mutation	Comment
Charcot-Marie-Tooth (CMT) disease type 1A	AD 17p11.2-12	Decades 2–3	Demyelinating	Hypertropic change with onion bulbs; marked ↓ NCV	Rare; bony defects	Mutation in peripheral myelin protein gene (*PMP-22*)	Pes cavus, motor deficit predominates (see Chap. 363)
CMT disease type 1B	AD 1q22-23	Decades 2–3	Demyelinating	Hypertropic change with onion bulbs; marked ↓ NCV	—	Mutation in P_O gene	See Chap. 363
CMT disease type 2	AD 1p35-36 3q 7	Decades 3–5	Axonal	Marked ↓ NAP; slight ↓ NCV	—	Unknown	Genetic heterogeneity
Hereditary amyloid polyneuropathies	AD 18q11.2-12.1 9q33 11q23-24	Decades 3–6	Axonal	Small-fiber involvement; endoneurial amyloid deposition	In some families: cornea, kidneys, heart	Point mutations in transthyretin gene in most families	Dysautonomia often prominent
Hereditary sensory neuropathy type I (HSN-I)	AD Unknown	Decades 1–3	Neuronopathic	DRG neurons selectively involved	Sensorineural deafness (some families)	Unknown	Frequent distal mutilation—hands and feet
Porphyric neuropathy	AD 11q23-qter 14q	Adult life	Axonal	Neuropathy part of attacks; may be recurrent	Widespread cellular abnormality	Enzyme defects in porphyrin pathway	Acute intermittent porphyria, coproporphyria, and variegate porphyria
Hereditary liability to pressure palsy	AD 17p11.2-12	Decades 2–3	Demyelinating	Tomaculous changes in myelin	—	*PMP-22* gene deletions	Mostly ulnar, peroneal, and brachial plexus
Fabry's disease	X, R Xq21.33-22	Young males	Neuronopathic	Sensory neuronopathy, small DRG neurons	Kidney, skin, lung	Defect of α-galactosidase A	Neuropathy painful; often die of renal failure
CMT disease type 1, X-linked	D Xq13.1	Infancy to 2d decade	Demyelinating	Heterozygote females have symptoms	—	Defective gap junction protein (connexin 32)	—
Adrenomyeloneuropathy	X, R Xq28	Young males	? Axonal	Mild neuropathy, spastic paraparesis, baldness, hypogonadism	Adrenal cortex, cerebral white matter, spinal cord	Mutation in adrenoleukodystrophy (ALD) protein gene, a peroxisomal membrane transporter	See Chap. 363
Hereditary sensory neuropathy type II (HSN-II)	AR Unknown	Decades 1–3	Neuronopathic	DRG neurons selectively involved	—	Unknown	May be less severe than HSN-I
Déjerine-Sottas neuropathy, types A and B (HMSN-III)	Sporadic 1q22-23 17p11.2-12	1st decade	Demyelinating	Hypertrophic change with onion bulb formation	May be mentally retarded	*PMP-22* and P_O gene mutations	Marked nerve trunk enlargement (see Chap. 362)
CMT disease type 4A	AR 8q13-21.1	1st decade	Demyelinating	Hypomyelination; marked ↓ NCV	—	Unknown	—
Refsum's disease	AR Unknown	Decade 1 or 2	Demyelinating	Hypertropic change with onion bulb formation	Retinitis pigmentosa, ichthyosis, sensorineural deafness	Defect in α-oxidation of β-methylated fatty acids	Therapy consists of low-phytanate diet, plasmapheresis
Ataxia-telangiectasia	AR 11q22.1-22.3	Decade 1 or 2	Axonal	Neuropathy moderate	Cell nuclear aneuploidy, skin and scleral telangiectasia, cerebellar atrophy, immunopathy	Mutations in *ATM* gene	High incidence of early neoplasia (see Chap. 363)
Abetalipoproteinemia	AR Unknown	Decade 1 or 2	Neuronopathic	Large DRG neurons	Retinitis pigmentosa, acanthocytosis of red blood cells	Mutations in microsomal triglyceride transfer protein (*MTP*) gene	Proprioceptive disturbance marked; minimal small-fiber deficit (see Chap. 363)

(continued)

Table 381-3—*(continued)*

Genetically Determined Neuropathies

Genetic Disorder	Inheritance/ Gene Location	Age of Onset	Basic Process	Other Features*	Other Systems Involved	Genetic Mutation	Comment
Giant axonal neuropathy	AR Unknown	1st decade	Axonal	Massive segmented accumulation of neurofilaments in axons	Slowly progressive encephalopathy with Rosenthal fibers	Generalized disorder of 10-nm filaments	Intermediate filament masses in other cell types
Metachromatic leukodystrophy	AR 22q13.3-qter	1st decade	Demyelinating	Schwannopathy with cerebroside accumulation	Cerebral white matter disease predominates	Defect of arylsulfatase A	Infantile, juvenile, and adult-onset forms
Friedreich's ataxia	AR 9q13-21	1st decade	Axonal	Spinocerebellar and corticospinal tracts involved; also 1° sensory neuron	Cardiomyopathy (usual cause of death)	Controversial	Ataxia is both sensory and cerebellar

ABBREVIATIONS: A, autosomal; D, dominant; R, recessive; X, X chromosome; DRG, dorsal root ganglia; NAP, nerve action potential; NCV, nerve conduction velocity; CMT, Charcot-Marie-Tooth disease; HMSN, hereditary motor-sensory neuropathy; HSN, hereditary sensory neuropathy; PMP, peripheral myelin protein.

Table 381-4

Classification of Diabetic Neuropathies

Symmetric
1. Distal, primarily sensory polyneuropathy
   a. Mainly large fibers affected
   b. Mixed*
   c. Mainly small fibers affected*
2. Autonomic neuropathy
3. Chronically evolving proximal motor neuropathy*†

Asymmetric
1. Acute or subacute proximal motor neuropathy*†
2. Cranial mononeuropathy†
3. Truncal neuropathy*†
4. Entrapment neuropathy in the limbs

* Often painful.
† Recovery, partial or complete, is likely.

Acquired Demyelinating Neuropathies These disorders fall into two major groups, the acute form called Guillain-Barré syndrome and more chronic forms, usually referred to as *chronic inflammatory demyelinating polyradiculoneuropathy* (CIDP). The acquired demyelinating neuropathies account for a significant proportion of all cases of polyneuropathy and share a distinctive clinical, electrophysiologic, and pathologic pattern. The diagnosis rests on recognition of the clinical pattern and other features, including an elevated protein level in cerebrospinal fluid (CSF) not accompanied by pleocytosis, and electrophysiologic changes (marked slowing of conduction velocities, delayed late responses, prolonged distal latencies, dispersion of evoked responses, and evidence of conduction block). The course of GBS is acute and monophasic, whereas the more chronic forms pursue either a slowly progressive or a relapsing course. Cases with an intermediate course occur frequently enough to blur the distinction between GBS and CIDP.

This group of neuropathies is generally agreed to be immune-mediated, but the specific antigens involved, the crucial events of the immune response, and the reason it is activated are uncertain. Also unknown is whether GBS and CIDP share a common immunopathogenesis.

Management of CIDP involves a judicious mix of glucocorticoid therapy, plasmapheresis, administration of immunosuppressants such as azathioprine, cyclophosphamide, or cyclosporine, and administration of high-dose intravenous immunoglobulin. These powerful agents are used only if the disorder is severe enough to threaten walking.

Multifocal motor neuropathy is also a chronic acquired demyelinating neuropathy. It may mimic the lower-motor-neuron form of amyo-

Table 381-5

Sensory Neuropathies

Cause or Association	Course	Fiber Size Affected		Neuronopathy	Comment
		Small	Large		
TOXINS/DRUGS					
Cisplatin (antineoplastic)	Sub/Chr	+	+ +	+	Dose-related
Pyridoxine (vitamin, in megadose amounts)	Sub/Chr	+	+ +	+/−	Dose-related
Taxol (antineoplastic)	Acu/Sub	+ +	+	−	NGF may be protective
SYSTEMIC DISEASES					
Paraneoplastic	Sub	+	+ +	+ +	Most SCLC and breast
Sjögren's syndrome	Sub/Chr	+/−	+	+ +	Variable presentation
Dysproteinemia (mainly IgM$_\kappa$)	Chr	+	+ +	−	Demyelinating; may bind to MAG
IDIOPATHIC					
Acute sensory neuronopathy	Acu	+/−	+ +	+ +	Poor recovery; persistent deficit
Chronic ataxic neuropathy	Chr	+/−	+ +	Prob.	Gradual progression
HEREDITARY					
Many varieties (see Table 381-3)	Chr	Variable		Some	Progressive

ABBREVIATIONS: + +, most; +, some; ±, occasionally; Prob, probable; Acu, acute; Sub, subacute; Chr, chronic; NGF, nerve growth factor; MAG, myelin-associated glycoprotein; SCLC, small cell lung carcinoma.

tropic lateral sclerosis because of its features of weakness and atrophy without sensory disturbance. In many patients it is responsive to periodic high-dose intravenous immunoglobulin treatment.

Diabetic Neuropathies The neuropathies of diabetes mellitus are classified in Table 381-4. A limitation of this classification is that most patients do not fit neatly into any single category but instead have overlapping clinical features of several. For instance, many diabetics with distal, primarily sensory polyneuropathy also can be shown to have autonomic dysfunction, usually in the form of vasomotor disturbance in the limbs and abnormalities of sweating. Similarly, patients who develop a proximal motor syndrome may have dysautonomic features (including sexual impotence in males) and some degree of distal sensory polyneuropathy. To compound matters, such patients appear at risk of developing a cranial mononeuropathy. Pain is a frequent feature of diabetic neuropathies (see Table 381-4) but is variable in incidence and degree. The term *diabetic amyotrophy* should be avoided because of its ambiguity.

Diabetic neuropathies tend to occur in the setting of long-standing hyperglycemia (decades), whether the diabetes is insulin-dependent or not. By far the most common neuropathies related to diabetes mellitus are the diffuse sensory and autonomic types (categories 1 and 2 under "Symmetric" in Table 381-4). Sensory and autonomic polyneuropathy, chronic and indolent in evolution, may first be noticed in the third or fourth decade in patients with juvenile-onset diabetes but tends to occur after age 50 in patients with adult-onset diabetes. Focal and multifocal types of neuropathy are less common but quite dramatic (categories 1, 2, and 3 under "Asymmetric" in Table 381-4). They rarely occur before the age of 45 and are usually subacute or acute in onset. Cranial mononeuropathies are isolated sixth or third nerve palsies. The latter spares the pupil in three-fourths of cases, and some local pain or headache occurs in one-half. Truncal (thoracoabdominal) neuropathy is painful, involves one or more intercostal or lumbar nerves unilaterally, and frequently coexists with the asymmetric proximal motor neuropathy. The most evident features of asymmetric proximal motor neuropathy are weakened muscles innervated by the femoral and obturator nerves (quadriceps femoris, iliopsoas, adductor magnus) and ipsilateral loss of the knee jerk reflex. Sensory deficit is minor, but pain in the hip and anterior thigh may be prominent. In all these multifocal and focal neuropathies, the pain usually subsides within weeks to a year, and function is usually partly or completely recovered. The same is true for symmetric proximal motor neuropathy (category 3 under "Symmetric" in Table 381-4).

Focal and multifocal diabetic neuropathies are considered to be ischemic in origin, and ischemia may also underlie symmetric polyneuropathies, which are thought by some to involve abnormality of nerve metabolism.

Management of diabetic neuropathies is directed toward optimal control of hyperglycemia and symptomatic pain suppression. In the long-term Diabetes Control and Complications Trial completed recently in North America, patients who controlled their diabetes meticulously showed significantly less neuropathy. The role of aldose reductase inhibitors in preventing or reversing diabetic complications, including neuropathy, remains unclear. Entrapment neuropathies are frequently amenable to surgical decompression.

Neuropathies with Dysproteinemia An association between polyneuropathy and both multiple myeloma and macroglobulinemia has been recognized for many years. In the commonly encountered type of multiple myeloma, which has either lytic or diffuse osteoporotic bone lesions, clinically overt polyneuropathy is relatively infrequent, occurring in approximately 5 percent of patients. These neuropathies are sensorimotor, may be severe, and generally do not reverse with successful suppression of the myeloma. In most cases, electrodiagnostic and pathologic features are consistent with a process of axonal degeneration.

In contrast, myeloma with osteosclerotic features, although representing only 3 percent of all myelomas, is associated with polyneuropathy in almost one-half of cases. These neuropathies, which may also occur with solitary plasmacytoma, seem to be different from those linked to the lytic type of multiple myeloma in that they (1) often respond to radiation therapy or removal of the primary lesion, (2) are more frequently demyelinating in character, (3) are associated with different monoclonal proteins and light chains (almost all lambda as opposed to mostly kappa in the lytic type of multiple myeloma), and (4) frequently occur in association with other systemic findings. These include skin thickening, hyperpigmentation, hypertrichosis, organomegaly, endocrinopathy, anasarca, papilledema, and clubbing of fingers (POEMS syndrome: *p*olyneuropathy, *o*rganomegaly, *e*ndocrinopathy, *M* protein, and *s*kin changes). A great deal of attention has been paid to this curious syndrome in Japan, where it is more common, but the underlying mechanism remains unknown, other than the association with lambda light chains.

Benign monoclonal gammopathy with an IgM serum spike, and usually with kappa light chains, is described in association with demyelinating polyneuropathy, which often follows a protracted course and indolent progression. In about one-half of cases, the monoclonal serum protein binds to normal human peripheral myelin, specifically to myelin-associated glycoprotein. Treatment with high-dose intravenous immunoglobulin and potent immunosuppressants (chlorambucil, cyclophosphamide, or fludarabine) has been advocated.

Neuropathies with HIV Infection Neuropathies are common in infection with human immunodeficiency virus (HIV), but different types of neuropathy are seen according to the stage of the disease. GBS or CIDP are the neuropathies likely to occur following conversion to seropositivity and during the asymptomatic phase of HIV infection. Treatment is the same as for HIV-negative patients. In later, symptomatic stages, subacute to chronic mononeuritis multiplex, axonal in nature, can occur. In some cases, vasculitis of the vasa nervorum has been demonstrated.

The most common neuropathy is a distal, symmetric, mainly sensory polyneuropathy, which evolves slowly in the late symptomatic stages of HIV infection and frequently coexists with symptomatic encephalopathy and myelopathy (see Table 381-1 and Chap. 308). Improvement of this polyneuropathy with zidovudine treatment has been claimed. Also in the late stages, a severe, destructive, subacute, asymmetric polyradiculopathy involving the cauda equina may be seen; it is caused by an opportunistic infection of the nerve roots with cytomegalovirus. Ganciclovir, started early, can arrest the disorder.

Neuropathies with Lyme Disease A focal or multifocal radiculoneuropathy may occur weeks, months, or even years after primary infection by the tick-borne spirochete *Borrelia burgdorferi*. Although usually sensory and either dysesthetic or painful, the neuropathy is variable in distribution, affecting cranial nerves and spinal roots or nerves in a patchy, asymmetric fashion. Neuropathy is often chronic and persistent; CSF pleocytosis is the rule. In many, improvement occurs spontaneously, but the course is shortened by treatment with antibiotics, usually intravenous ceftriaxone (see Chap. 178).

Autonomic Neuropathy The autonomic nervous system regulates the visceral organs and vegetative functions (see Chap. 371). Many pharmacologic agents modify specific autonomic functions, but autonomic neuropathy (dysautonomia) with structural changes in pre- and postganglionic neurons can also occur. Usually autonomic neuropathy is a manifestation of a more generalized polyneuropathy also affecting somatic peripheral nervous function, as in diabetic neuropathy, GBS, and alcoholic polyneuropathy, but occasionally syndromes of pure pandysautonomia are encountered. Symptoms of dysautonomia are mainly negative (i.e., loss of function) and include postural hypotension with faintness or syncope, anhidrosis, hypothermia, bladder atony, obstipation, dry mouth and dry eyes from failure of salivary and lacrimal glands to secrete, blurring of vision from lack of pupillary and ciliary regulation, and sexual impotence in males. Positive phenomena (hyperfunction) may also occur and include episodic hypertension, diarrhea, hyperhidrosis, and either tachycardia or bradycardia. Autonomic neuropathies have many and diverse causes, and the classification is complex.

Pure Motor Neuropathy   Disorder affecting any level of the motor unit—anterior horn cell, motor axon, or neuromuscular junction—can result in a purely lower motor syndrome without sensory disturbance. Distinguishing anterior horn cell disorders (motor neuronopathies) from motor axonopathies may be difficult clinically because they share manifestations (weakness, muscle denervation atrophy, hypo- or areflexia, fasciculations). Electrodiagnostic examination may also fail to localize the primary site of the lesion (neuropathic versus neuronopathic) unless the lesion is demyelinating in nature, in which case it is by definition neuropathic.

Examples of motor neuronopathies include the lower-motor form of amyotrophic lateral sclerosis, poliomyelitis, hereditary spinal muscular atrophies, and adult variant of hexosaminidase A deficiency. Motor neuropathies may be seen with lead or dapsone intoxication, occasionally with porphyria, and also with multifocal motor neuropathy. The latter is a chronic asymmetric disorder of mid-life that may be associated with high titers of antiganglioside antibodies (particularly anti-GM$_1$), persistent conduction block on electrodiagnostic examination, or both. Neuromuscular junction disorders (e.g., Lambert-Eaton myasthenic syndrome, tick bite paralysis, other types of toxic neuromuscular blockade) can be recognized and localized electrodiagnostically. Some motor-sensory polyneuropathies have predominant motor symptoms and signs, such as hereditary motor-sensory neuropathies, GBS, and CIDP, but the subclinical sensory component is readily demonstrated electrodiagnostically or by quantitative sensory testing.

Pure Sensory Neuropathy   Clinical presentations involving primary sensation only (see Chap. 23) are not uncommon. Manifestations may (1) reflect mainly large afferent fiber involvement with deficits of vibratory and proprioceptive sense, areflexia, and sensory ataxia with or without tingling dysesthesias; (2) reflect mainly small afferent fiber involvement with numbness and cutaneous hypesthesia to pinprick and temperature stimuli, often with painful burning dysesthesias; or (3) be pansensory, with both large and small fiber manifestations. The pattern of distribution, although variable, is often distal and symmetric, particularly for large-fiber neuropathies.

The most severe and widespread of these pure sensory syndromes exhibit poor or no recovery, suggesting irreversible lesions of nerve cell bodies in dorsal root and trigeminal ganglia. These are frequently called *sensory neuronopathies*. With sensory neurotoxins, moderate doses lead to potentially reversible neuropathy, but high doses appear to cause neuronopathy (see Table 381-5).

Plexopathy   This term refers to disorders of either the brachial or the lumbosacral plexus. Lesions of the brachial plexus are characterized by motor and sensory signs different from those expected in either mononeuropathies of the upper limb or polyneuropathies. The usual causes are direct trauma to the plexus, idiopathic brachial neuritis (also called *neuralgic amyotrophy*), cervical rib or band, infiltration by malignant tumor, or prior radiation therapy. When the upper parts of the brachial plexus, arising from cervical roots 5 through 7, are affected, weakness and atrophy of shoulder girdle and upper arm muscles occur. Injuries to the lower brachial plexus, arising from the eighth cervical and first thoracic roots, produce distal arm weakness, atrophy, and focal sensory deficit in the forearm and hand. In general, idiopathic brachial neuritis, irradiation with greater than 60 Gy (6000 rad), and particular types of trauma (arm jerked downward) result in damage to the upper portions of the brachial plexus. In contrast, infiltration by malignant tumor, cervical rib or band, and certain other types of trauma (arm jerked upward) cause damage to the lower brachial plexus. Lumbosacral plexopathies are less common; they may be due to idiopathic lumbosacral plexitis, retroperitoneal hemorrhage, or malignant tumor infiltration or may occur in association with long-standing diabetes mellitus.

Miscellaneous Causes of Neuropathy   Ischemia of nerve severe enough to produce clinical symptoms has as its basis the widespread compromise of blood flow in the vasa nervorum. Typically, this is the result of small-vessel disease involving the vasa nervorum directly, as occurs with vasculitis, rather than large-vessel disease, such as atherosclerosis. Clinically, widespread disease of the vasa nervorum produces mononeuropathy multiplex, which electrodiagnostically has the features of a patchy axonal process.

Cold exerts direct deleterious effects on peripheral nerve, independent of ischemia. Cold injury to nerve occurs after prolonged exposure, usually of a limb, to moderately low temperatures, as with immersion of the feet in seawater; actual freezing of tissue is not required. Axonal degeneration of myelinated fibers is the pathologic expression of cold injury. Frequently, limbs affected by cold injury to nerve show sensory deficit and dysesthesias, cutaneous vasomotor instability, pain, and marked sensitivity to minimal cold exposure, which persist for many years. The pathophysiology of these phenomena is uncertain.

Trophic changes in severe neuropathy   The array of observable changes in completely denervated muscle, bone, and skin, including hair and nails, is well known, if incompletely understood. It is unclear what portion of the changes is due purely to denervation versus that caused by disuse, immobility, lack of weight bearing, and particularly recurrent, unnoticed, painless trauma. Considerable evidence favors the view that ulceration of skin, poor healing, tissue resorption, neurogenic arthropathy, and mutilation are the result of repeated heedless injury to insensitive parts. This sequence of events is avoidable with proper attention to and care of the insensitive parts by both patient and physician.

RECOVERY FROM NEUROPATHY   In contrast to axons in the CNS, peripheral nerve fibers have an excellent ability to regenerate under proper circumstances. The process of regeneration following axonal degeneration may take from 2 months to more than a year, depending on the severity of the neuropathy and the length of regeneration required. Whether regeneration takes place depends on whether the cause of the neuropathy has been eliminated, as by removal of a neurotoxic substance or correction of an abnormal metabolic state. A deficit secondary to demyelination may recover rapidly, since intact axons may remyelinate in just a few weeks. For example, a patient with GBS, in whom demyelination but no secondary axonal degeneration has occurred, may recover to normal strength from bedfastness and paralysis of arms and legs in as little as 3 to 4 weeks.

MONONEUROPATHY MULTIPLEX (MULTIFOCAL NEUROPATHY)   This term refers to simultaneous or sequential involvement of individual noncontiguous nerve trunks, either partially or completely, evolving over days to years. Since the disease process underlying mononeuropathy multiplex involves peripheral nerves in a multifocal and random fashion, progression of the disease involves a tendency for the neurologic deficit to become less patchy and multifocal and more confluent and symmetric. Some patients present with a distal symmetric neuropathy. Attention to the pattern of early symptoms is therefore important in making the judgment that a particular neuropathy is indeed a mononeuropathy multiplex.

Once that issue is settled, the next question is whether the process is primarily axonal or demyelinating. Almost one-third of all adults with the clinical syndrome of mononeuropathy multiplex have a clear-cut picture of a demyelinating disorder, often with multiple foci of persistent conduction block found by electrodiagnostic examination. Multifocal demyelinating neuropathy represents part of the spectrum of chronic acquired demyelinating neuropathy, that is, CIDP. Management of this multifocal subgroup is the same as for CIDP (see "Acquired Demyelinating Neuropathies," above).

The remaining two-thirds of patients with mononeuropathy multiplex have a picture by electrodiagnostic examination of axonal involvement that is heterogeneously distributed. Although ischemia should be suspected as the basis of neuropathy in these patients, only about one-half can be shown to have disease, usually vasculitis, affecting the vasa nervorum. Management of those with proven vasculitis of vasa nervorum is the same as treatment for systemic vasculitis (see Chap. 319). The cause of neuropathy remains undiagnosed in the remaining patients even on follow-up. Management in this group is conservative; in many patients the disease will stabilize or reverse, at least partially.

In individuals in whom vasculitic change in vasa nervorum can be demonstrated, any of a large number of underlying disorders may be responsible. The primary vasculitides of the polyarteritis nodosa group are the most frequent basis, followed closely by the vasculitis syndrome occurring in the course of other connective tissue disorders. In descending order of frequency, the latter are rheumatoid arthritis, systemic lupus erythematosus, and mixed connective tissue disease. Other rarer causes of mononeuropathy multiplex due to nerve ischemia from occlusion of vasa nervorum include mixed cryoglobulinemia, Sjögren's syndrome, Wegener's granulomatosis, progressive systemic sclerosis, Churg-Strauss allergic granulomatosis, and hypersensitivity angiitides (Chap. 319). Management of the neuropathy in each case depends on treatment of the responsible disease.

Mononeuropathy multiplex syndrome may also be seen as a manifestation of leprosy, sarcoidosis, certain types of amyloidosis, hypereosinophilia syndrome, cryoglobulinemia, and multifocal types of diabetic neuropathy.

MONONEUROPATHY *Mononeuropathy* refers to focal involvement of a single nerve trunk and therefore implies a local cause. Direct trauma, compression, and entrapment are the usual causes. Ulnar neuropathies, due to lesions either at the ulnar groove or in the cubital tunnel, and median neuropathy due to compression in the carpal tunnel constitute the great majority of mononeuropathies encountered in clinical practice. These are described below, and other common mononeuropathies are listed in Table 381-6.

In the absence of a history of trauma to the nerve trunk, factors favoring conservative management of a mononeuropathy include sudden onset, no motor deficit, few or no sensory findings (even though pain and sensory symptoms may be present), and no evidence of axonal degeneration by electrodiagnostic criteria. Factors favoring surgical intervention include chronicity and worsening neurologic deficit on examination, particularly if motor, and electrodiagnostic evidence that the lesion has produced a degree of wallerian degeneration.

Ulnar Neuropathy Complete ulnar paralysis results in a characteristic claw-hand deformity owing to wasting and weakness of many of the small hand muscles and hyperextension of the fingers at the metacarpophalangeal joints and flexion at the interphalangeal joints. The flexion deformity is most pronounced in the fourth and fifth fingers. Sensory loss occurs over the fifth finger, the ulnar aspect of the fourth finger, and the ulnar border of the palm. The superficial location of the nerve at the elbow makes it a common site of pressure palsy. The ulnar nerve may also become entrapped just distal to the elbow in the cubital tunnel formed by the aponeurotic arch linking the two heads of the flexor carpi ulnaris. Also, prolonged pressure on the base of the palm, as occurs with use of hand tools or bicycle riding, may result in damage to the deep palmar branch of the ulnar nerve, causing weakness of the small hand muscles but no sensory loss. See also Table 381-6.

Carpal Tunnel Syndrome The median nerve in the carpal tunnel lies in close quarters with nine tendons. Entrapment of the nerve at the wrist (*carpal tunnel syndrome*) may be secondary to excessive use of the wrist, tenosynovitis with arthritis, or local infiltration, for example, by a thickening of connective tissue as in acromegaly or by deposit of amyloid or by one of the mucopolysaccharidoses. Other systemic diseases associated with an increased incidence of carpal tunnel syndrome are hypothyroidism, rheumatoid arthritis, and diabetes mellitus, but underlying diseases account for only a small fraction of all cases. The main symptoms of carpal tunnel syndrome are nocturnal paresthesia of thumb, index, and middle fingers. With worsening, numbness demonstrable by pin examination occurs in that distribution, and eventually weakness and atrophy of the abductor pollicis brevis (thenar eminence) becomes evident. Treatment of carpal tunnel syndrome is surgical section of the carpal ligament to relieve entrapment. Incomplete lesions of the median nerve between the axilla and wrist may result in causalgia (a particularly severe type of burning pain; see Chap. 12). See also Table 381-6.

Tarsal Tunnel Syndrome The distal tibial nerve, along with several tendons and the posterior tibial artery, lies in the tarsal tunnel just posterior to the medial malleolus. Because of its superficial site, the distal tibial nerve is subject to compression or to direct trauma. Causes include sprain or fracture of the ankle, ill-fitting footwear, posttraumatic fibrosis, cysts, or ganglia adjacent to the nerve, arthritis, or tenosynovitis. Symptoms characteristically are pain in the ankle and the sole of the foot with paresthesia, particularly upon walking. On examination, the tibial nerve trunk in the tarsal tunnel is usually tender to palpation, sensory deficit should be demonstrable on the sole of the foot, and weakness of the toe plantar-flexor muscles may be noted. Electrodiagnostic examination and nerve block are useful in establishing the diagnosis. Definitive treatment is extensive surgical decompression of the tibial nerve in the tarsal tunnel. Tarsal tunnel syndrome, in terms of its pathophysiology and management, is similar to carpal tunnel syndrome, but it is much less common (see also Table 381-6).

OTHER FOCAL NEUROPATHIES **Peripheral Nerve Tumors** These tumors are mostly benign and can arise on any nerve trunk or twig. Although peripheral nerve tumors can occur anywhere in the body, including the spinal roots and cauda equina, many are subcutaneous in location and present as a soft swelling, sometimes with a purplish discoloration of the skin. Two major categories of peripheral nerve tumors are recognized: neurilemmoma (schwannoma) and neurofibroma. Neurilemmomas are usually solitary and grow in the nerve sheath, rendering the tumor relatively easy to dissect free. In contrast, neurofibromas tend to be multiple, grow in the endoneurial substance, which renders them difficult to dissect, may undergo malignant changes, and are the hallmark of von Recklinghausen's neurofibromatosis (NF1). This disease is characterized by an autosomal dominant inheritance pattern, any number of neurofibromas from one to thousands, five or more café au lait–pigmented skin lesions greater than 1.5 cm in diameter (80 percent of patients), axillary freckles (93 percent of patients), an increased incidence of seizure disorder and mental retardation, and an exceptionally high rate of spontaneous mutation. The gene for NF1 is on chromosome 17, and its protein product, neurofibromin, is a large, widely expressed protein that appears to regulate the proto-oncogene *ras*.

Herpes Zoster This is a sensory neuritis due to infection with varicella-zoster virus and is characterized by acute inflammation of one or more dorsal root ganglia. Lancinating pain and hyperalgesia over the skin surface supplied by the affected roots occur for 3 to 4 days, followed by the appearance in the same segment of a herpetic eruption characterized by painful raised blisters on reddened bases. Pain usually subsides in a few weeks. If the inflammatory process spreads to involve related motor roots, segmental motor weakness and wasting appear. Paralysis of the oculomotor nerves may occur in conjunction with involvement of the ophthalmic division of the trigeminal ganglion (ophthalmoplegic zoster). Facial paralysis may occur with involvement of the geniculate ganglion and herpetic eruption on the ipsilateral tympanic membrane or external ear canal (Ramsay Hunt syndrome).

In less than 5 percent of patients, neuropathic pain persists in the dermatomal distribution of the affected ganglia. This pain, known as *postherpetic neuralgia*, is intense, burning, hyperpathic, and unrelenting; it often dominates the lives of those affected. Advancing age is a risk factor for this outcome. In some patients, blunting of the pain to tolerable levels is achieved by use of carbamazepine or a tricyclic antidepressant such as desipramine (see also Chap. 12).

Leprous Neuritis This is a major worldwide cause of neuropathy. *Mycobacterium leprae* organisms readily invade Schwann cells in cutaneous nerve twigs, particularly those associated with unmyelinated nerve fibers. *M. leprae* thrives best in the coolest tissues in the body. Two major forms of leprous neuritis are recognized, tuberculoid and lepromatous, which actually represent the ends of a spectrum of disease, the middle of which is called dimorphous leprosy (patchy and multifocal involvement of skin and nerve). The treatment of a given case depends on where it falls in this spectrum (see Chap. 172). Tuberculoid (high-resistance) leprosy consists of a single patch of hypesthetic or anesthetic skin in any location. The skin patch is frequently thickened, reddened, or hypopigmented. If a superficially placed nerve trunk, typically a cutaneous nerve, courses just beneath the area of affected skin, it may be engulfed in the inflammatory reaction, resulting in an associated mononeuropathy. Such a nerve may be palpably enlarged and beaded. Lepromatous (low-resistance) leprosy is marked by immunologic tolerance and widespread skin thickening, cutaneous anesthesia, and anhidrosis, which spare only the warmest parts of the body, notably the axilla, the groin, and beneath the scalp hair. Motor signs (focal weakness and atrophy) result from damage to mixed nerves lying close to the skin, particularly the median, ulnar, peroneal, and facial nerves.

Bell's Palsy This seventh nerve palsy is due to inflammation of the facial nerve in the facial canal, the basis for which remains obscure. Edema may play a part in causing compression of nerve fibers, with resulting acute unilateral paralysis of facial muscles (see Chap. 372).

Sarcoidosis This may involve single or multiple peripheral nerves, producing asymmetric mononeuritis or polyneuritis. Unilateral or bilateral facial paralysis is described in association with parotitis and uveitis (Heerfordt's syndrome).

Table 381-6

Some Common Mononeuropathies

Nerve	Origin (Spinal Segments)	Muscles Innervated	Usual Site of Lesion	Clinical Features	Comments
UPPER EXTREMITY					
Suprascapular	C5, C6	Supraspinatus Infraspinatus	Suprascapular notch of scapula	Weakness of lateral rotation of the humerus	No sensory deficit
Long thoracic	C5–C7	Serratus anterior	Variable	Winging of scapula	No sensory deficit
Axillary	C5, C6	Deltoid, teres minor	Near shoulder joint	Weakness of shoulder abduction; atrophy of shoulder	Sensory deficit similar to C5 dorsal root lesion (see Figs. 23-2 and 23-3)
Radial	C5–T1	Triceps, brachioradialis, wrist, finger, and thumb extensors	Spiral groove of humerus	Wrist drop most obvious, also finger and thumb extensors paralyzed	Saturday night palsy (acute compression) is frequent cause
Posterior interosseous branch	C7, C8	Finger and thumb extensors	Edge of supinator muscle below elbow	Finger drop; wrist relatively spared	No sensory deficit
Ulnar	C8, T1	Ulnar flexor of the wrist, long flexors of 4th and 5th digits, and most intrinsic hand muscles	Ulnar groove at the elbow	Weakness of finger adduction and abduction and thumb adduction (see text); interosseous atrophy, claw-hand	May be acute or insidious; sensory symptoms/signs are distinctive (Figs. 23-2 and 23-3); see also text
			Cubital tunnel	Same as above	Often pain over medial proximal forearm (cubital tunnel)
			Medial base of palm	Intrinsic hand muscles only, interosseous atrophy	No sensory deficit
Median	C6–T1	Abductor pollicis brevis; more proximal muscles include forearm pronator, long finger and thumb flexors	Carpal tunnel	Characteristic sensory symptoms and deficit and inability to make a circle with thumb and index finger	Sensory deficit as per Figs. 23-2 and 23-3 (see text); known as carpal tunnel syndrome
Anterior interosseous branch	C7–T1	Long flexors of thumb and index and middle fingers	Anterior interosseus branch below the elbow	Weakness of pinch; pain in volar forearm	No sensory deficit
LOWER EXTREMITY					
Femoral	L2–L4	Iliopsoas (hip flexor) and quadriceps femoris (knee extensor)	Proximal to inguinal ligament	Knee buckling; absent knee jerk; weak anterior thigh muscles with atrophy	Association with diabetes mellitus; sensory disturbance as per Fig. 23-2
Lateral femoral cutaneous branch	L2, L3	None	Inguinal ligament	Dysesthetic hyperpathia of lateral thigh	Known as meralgia paresthetica
Obturator	L3, L4	Thigh adductors	Intrapelvic or at pubis	Weakness of hip adduction	Sensory deficit on medial thigh
Sciatic	L4–S3	Hamstring muscles, hip abductor, and all muscles below the knee	Near sciatic notch	Severe lower leg and hamstring weakness; flail foot; severe disability	Uncommon except from war wounds
Posterior tibial	L5–S2	Calf muscles (proximally), toe flexors and other intrinsic foot muscles	Tarsal tunnel, near medial malleolus	Pain and numbness of sole, weak toe flexors	Known as tarsal tunnel syndrome
Peroneal	L4–S1	Dorsiflexors of toes and foot, evertors of foot	At neck of fibula	Foot drop and weakness of foot eversion	Sensory deficit is similar in distribution to L5, S1 sensory roots

Polyneuritis Cranialis This is a relapsing and remitting mononeuropathy multiplex restricted to cranial nerves (see Chap. 372). It is usually associated with indolent tuberculous cervical adenitis (scrofula) or sarcoidosis. Treatment of the underlying condition will halt the cranial nerve palsies.

BIBLIOGRAPHY

ASBURY AK: New aspects of disease of the peripheral nervous system, in *Harrison's Textbook of Internal Medicine, Update IV.* New York, McGraw-Hill, 1983, pp 211–229

————, THOMAS PK: *Peripheral Nerve Disorders*, 2d ed. Oxford, Butterworth-Heinemann, 1995

BOLTON CF: The changing concepts of Guillain-Barré syndrome. N Engl J Med 333:1415, 1995

CHANCE PF, FISCHBECK KH: Molecular genetics of Charcot-Marie-Tooth disease and related neuropathies. Hum Mol Genet 3:1503, 1994

DAWSON DM et al: *Entrapment Neuropathies*, 2d ed. Boston, Little, Brown, 1991

DIABETES CONTROL AND COMPLICATIONS TRIAL RESEARCH GROUP: The effect of intensive treatment of diabetes on the development and progression of long-term complications in insulin-dependent diabetes mellitus. N Engl J Med 329:977, 1993

DYCK PJ et al (eds): *Diabetic Neuropathy.* Philadelphia, Saunders, 1987

————: *Peripheral Neuropathy*, 3d ed. Philadelphia, Saunders, 1992

GRIFFIN JW et al: Guillain-Barré syndrome in Northern China. The spectrum of neuropathological changes in clinically defined cases. Brain 118:577, 1995

LAYZER RB: *Neuromuscular Manifestations of Systemic Disease*, vol 25: *Contemporary Neurology Series.* Philadelphia, Davis, 1984

MAX MB et al: Effects of desipramine, amitriptyline, and fluoxetine on pain in diabetic neuropathy. N Engl J Med 326:1250, 1992

REES JH et al: *Campylobacter jejuni* infection and Guillain-Barré syndrome. N Engl J Med 333:1374, 1995

ROPPER AH et al: *Guillain Barré Syndrome.* Philadelphia, FA Davis, 1991

STEWART JD: *Focal Peripheral Neuropathies.* 2d ed. New York, Raven Press, 1993

SUTER U, SNIPES GJ: Biology and genetics of hereditary motor and sensory neuropathies. Annu Rev Neurosci 18:45, 1995

382 *Daniel B. Drachman*

MYASTHENIA GRAVIS AND OTHER DISEASES OF THE NEUROMUSCULAR JUNCTION

Myasthenia gravis (MG) is a neuromuscular disorder characterized by weakness and fatigability of skeletal muscles. The underlying defect is a decrease in the number of available acetylcholine receptors (AChRs) at neuromuscular junctions due to an antibody-mediated autoimmune attack. Treatment now available for MG is highly effective, although a specific cure has remained elusive.

PATHOPHYSIOLOGY In the neuromuscular junction (Fig. 382-1), acetylcholine (ACh) is synthesized in the motor nerve terminal and stored in vesicles (quanta). When an action potential travels down a motor nerve and reaches the nerve terminal, ACh from 150 to 200 vesicles is released and combines with AChRs that are densely packed at the peaks of postsynaptic folds. Channels in the AChRs open, permitting the rapid entry of cations, chiefly sodium, which produces depolarization at the end-plate region of the muscle fiber. If the depolarization is sufficiently large, it initiates an action potential that is propagated along the muscle fiber, triggering muscle contraction. This process is rapidly terminated by hydrolysis of ACh by acetylcholinesterase (AChE) and by diffusion of ACh away from the receptor.

In MG, the fundamental defect is a decrease in the number of available AChRs at the postsynaptic muscle membrane. In addition, the postsynaptic folds are flattened, or "simplified." These changes result in decreased efficiency of neuromuscular transmission. Therefore, although ACh is released normally, it produces small end-plate potentials which may fail to trigger muscle action potentials. Failure

of transmission at many neuromuscular junctions results in weakness of muscle contraction.

The amount of ACh released per impulse *normally* declines on repeated activity (termed *presynaptic rundown*). In the myasthenic patient, the decreased efficiency of neuromuscular transmission combined with the normal rundown results in the activation of fewer and fewer muscle fibers by successive nerve impulses and hence increasing weakness, or *myasthenic fatigue*. This mechanism also accounts for the decremental response to repetitive nerve stimulation seen on electrodiagnostic testing.

The neuromuscular abnormalities in MG are brought about by an autoimmune response mediated by specific anti-AChR antibodies. The anti-AChR antibodies reduce the number of available AChRs at neuromuscular junctions by three distinct mechanisms: (1) accelerated turnover of AChRs by a mechanism involving cross-linking and rapid endocytosis of the receptors; (2) blockade of the active site of the AChR, i.e., the site that normally binds ACh; and (3) damage to the postsynaptic muscle membrane by the antibody in collaboration with complement.

How the autoimmune response is initiated and maintained in MG is not completely understood. However, the thymus appears to play a role in this process. The thymus is abnormal in approximately 75 percent of patients with MG; in about 65 percent the thymus is "hyperplastic," with the presence of active germinal centers, while 10 percent of patients have thymic tumors (thymomas). Muscle-like cells within the thymus (myoid cells), which bear AChRs on their surface, may serve as a source of autoantigen and trigger the autoimmune reaction within the thymus gland.

CLINICAL FEATURES Myasthenia gravis is not rare, having a prevalence of at least 1 in 7500. It affects individuals in all age groups, but peaks of incidence occur in women in their twenties and thirties and in men in their fifties and sixties. Overall, women are affected more frequently than men, in a ratio of approximately 3:2. The cardinal features are *weakness* and *fatigability* of muscles. The weakness increases during repeated use (fatigue) and may improve following rest or sleep. The course of MG is often variable. Exacerbations and remissions may occur, particularly during the first few years after the onset of the disease. Remissions are rarely complete or permanent. Unrelated infections or systemic disorders often lead to increased myasthenic weakness and may precipitate "crisis" (see below).

The distribution of muscle weakness has a characteristic pattern. The cranial muscles, particularly the lids and extraocular muscles, are often involved early, and diplopia and ptosis are common initial complaints. Facial weakness produces a "snarling" expression when the patient attempts to smile. Weakness in chewing is most noticeable after prolonged effort, as in chewing meat. Speech may have a nasal timbre caused by weakness of the palate or a dysarthric "mushy" quality due to tongue weakness. Difficulty in swallowing may occur as a result of weakness of the palate, tongue, or pharynx, giving rise to nasal regurgitation or aspiration of liquids or food. In approximately 85 percent of patients, the weakness becomes generalized, affecting the limb muscles as well. The limb weakness in MG is often proximal and may be asymmetric. Despite the muscle weakness, deep tendon reflexes are preserved. If weakness of respiration becomes so severe as to require respiratory assistance, the patient is said to be in *crisis*.

DIAGNOSIS AND EVALUATION (Table 382-1) The diagnosis is suspected on the basis of weakness and fatigability in the typical distribution described above, without loss of reflexes or impairment of sensation or other neurologic function. The suspected diagnosis should always be confirmed definitively before treatment is undertaken; this is essential because (1) other treatable conditions may closely resemble MG and (2) the treatment of MG may involve surgery and the prolonged use of drugs with adverse side effects.

Anticholinesterase Test Drugs that inhibit the enzyme AChE allow ACh to interact repeatedly with the limited number of AChRs, producing improvement in the strength of myasthenic muscles. Edrophonium is used most commonly, because of the rapid onset (30 s) and short duration (about 5 min) of its effect. An objective end-point must be selected to evaluate the effect of edrophonium. The examiner should focus on one or more unequivocally weak muscle groups and evaluate their strength objectively. For example, weakness of extraocular muscles, impairment of speech, or the length of time that the patient can maintain the arms in forward abduction may be useful measures. An initial dose of 2 mg of edrophonium is given intravenously. If definite improvement occurs, the test is considered positive and is terminated. If there is no change, the patient is given an additional 8 mg intravenously. The dose is administered in two parts because some patients react to edrophonium with unpleasant side effects such as nausea, diarrhea, salivation, fasciculations, and rarely syncope. Atropine (0.6 mg) should be at hand for intravenous administration if these symptoms become troublesome.

False-positive tests occur in occasional patients with other neurologic disorders, such as amyotrophic lateral sclerosis, and in placebo-reactors. False-negative or equivocal tests also may occur. In some cases it is helpful to use a longer-acting drug such as neostigmine (15 mg given orally), since this permits more time for detailed evaluation of strength. In virtually all instances, it is desirable to carry out further testing to establish the diagnosis of MG definitively.

Electrodiagnostic Testing *Repetitive nerve stimulation* often provides helpful diagnostic evidence of MG. Anticholinesterase medication is stopped 6 to 24 h before testing. It is best to test weak muscles or proximal muscle groups. Electric shocks are delivered at a rate of two or three per second to the appropriate nerves, and action potentials are recorded from the muscles. In normal individuals, the amplitude of the evoked muscle action potentials does not change at these rates of stimulation. However, in myasthenic patients there is a rapid reduction in the amplitude of the evoked responses of more than 10 to 15 percent. As a further test, a single dose of edrophonium may be given to prevent or diminish this decremental reaction.

Antiacetylcholine Receptor Antibody As noted above, anti-AChR antibodies are detectable in the serum of approximately 80 percent of all myasthenic patients, but in only about 50 percent of patients with weakness confined to the ocular muscles. The presence of anti-AChR antibodies is virtually diagnostic of MG, but a negative test does not exclude the disease. The measured level of anti-AChR antibody does not correspond well with the severity of MG in different patients. However, in an individual patient, a treatment-induced fall in the antibody level often correlates with clinical improvement.

Table 382-1

Diagnosis of Myasthenia Gravis

History
  Diplopia, ptosis, weakness
  Weakness in characteristic distribution
  Fluctuation and fatigue: worse with repeated activity, improved by rest
  Effects of previous treatments
Physical examination
  Ptosis, diplopia
  Motor power survey: quantitative testing of muscle strength
  Forward arm abduction time (5 min)
  Vital capacity
  Absence of other neurologic signs
Laboratory testing
  Anti-AChR radioimmunoassay: ~90% positive in generalized MG; 50% in ocular MG; definite diagnosis if positive; negative result does not exclude MG
  Edrophonium chloride (Tensilon) 2 mg + 8 mg IV; highly probable diagnosis if *unequivocally* positive
  Repetitive nerve stimulation; decrement of >15% at 3 Hz: highly probable
  Single-fiber electromyography: blocking and jitter, with normal fiber density; confirmatory, but not specific
  For ocular or cranial MG: exclude intracranial lesions by CT or MRI

SOURCE: From Drachman.

Differential Diagnosis Other conditions that cause weakness of the cranial and/or somatic musculature include drug-induced myasthenia, Lambert-Eaton myasthenic syndrome (LEMS), neurasthenia, hyperthyroidism, botulism, intracranial mass lesions, and progressive external ophthalmoplegia. Treatment with *penicillamine* (used for scleroderma or rheumatoid arthritis) may result in true MG, but the weakness is usually mild, and recovery occurs within weeks or months after discontinuing its use. *Aminoglycoside antibiotics* in very large doses and *procainamide* can cause neuromuscular weakness in normal individuals or exacerbation of weakness in myasthenic patients.

The *Lambert-Eaton myasthenic syndrome* is a presynaptic disorder of the neuromuscular junction that can cause weakness similar to that of MG. The proximal muscles of the lower limbs are most commonly affected, but other muscles may be involved as well. Cranial nerve findings, including ptosis of the eyelids and diplopia, occur in up to 70 percent of patients and resemble features of MG. However, the two conditions are readily distinguished, since patients with Lambert-Eaton syndrome have depressed or absent reflexes, show autonomic changes such as dry mouth and impotence, and show incremental responses on repetitive nerve stimulation. It is now known that Lambert-Eaton syndrome is caused by autoantibodies directed against P/Q type calcium channels at the motor nerve terminals, resulting in impaired release of ACh, which can be detected in approximately 85 percent of LEMS patients. A majority of patients with this syndrome have an associated malignancy, most commonly small cell carcinoma of the lung, which is thought to trigger the autoimmune response. The diagnosis of Lambert-Eaton syndrome may signal the presence of the tumor long before it would otherwise be detected, permitting early removal. Treatment of the neuromuscular disorder involves plasmapheresis and immunosuppression, as for MG.

Neurasthenia may present with weakness and fatigue, but muscle testing usually reveals the "jerky release" characteristic of nonorganic disorders, and the complaint of fatigue in these patients means tiredness or apathy rather than decreasing muscle power on repeated effort. *Hyperthyroidism* is readily diagnosed or excluded by tests of thyroid function, which should be carried out routinely in patients with suspected MG. Abnormalities of thyroid function (hyper- or

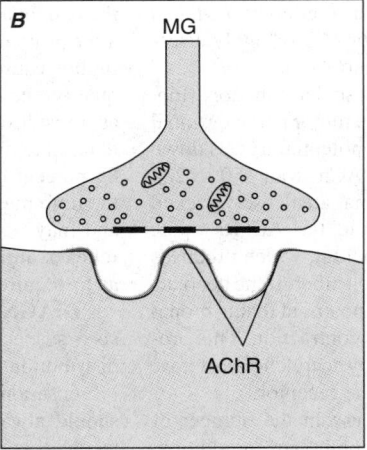

FIGURE 382-1 Diagrams of (*A*) normal and (*B*) myasthenic neuromuscular junctions. V, vesicles; M, mitochondria. See text for description of normal neuromuscular transmission. The MG junction shows reduced number of AChRs (stippling); flattened, simplified postsynaptic folds; a widened synaptic space; and a normal nerve terminal.

hypothyroidism) may increase myasthenic weakness. *Botulism* can cause myasthenic-like weakness, but the pupils are often dilated, and repetitive nerve stimulation gives an *incremental* rather than decremental response. Diplopia that mimics the symptoms of MG may occasionally be due to an *intracranial mass lesion* that compresses nerves to the extraocular muscles (e.g., sphenoid ridge meningioma), but magnetic resonance imaging (MRI) of the head and orbits usually reveals the lesion.

Progressive external ophthalmoplegia is a rare condition resulting in weakness of the extraocular muscles, which may be accompanied by weakness of the proximal muscles of the limbs, and a variety of other systemic features that are beyond the scope of this chapter. Most patients with this condition have mitochondrial disorders that can be detected on muscle biopsy (see Chap. 383).

Search for Associated Conditions (Table 382-2) Myasthenic patients have an increased incidence of several associated disorders. *Thymic abnormalities* occur in approximately 75 percent of patients, as noted above. Neoplastic change (thymoma) may produce enlargement of the thymus, which is detected by computed tomography (CT) or MRI scanning of the anterior mediastinum. Enlargement of the thymus in a patient over 40 years of age is highly suspicious of thymoma. *Hyperthyroidism* occurs in 3 to 8 percent of patients and may aggravate the myasthenic weakness. Tests of thyroid function should be obtained. Because of the *association of MG with other autoimmune disorders*, blood tests for rheumatoid factor and antinuclear antibodies should be carried out in all patients. Chronic infection of any kind can exacerbate MG and should be sought carefully. Finally, measurements of *ventilatory function* are valuable because of the frequency and seriousness of respiratory impairment in myasthenic patients.

Because of the side effects of glucocorticoids and other immunosuppressive agents used in the treatment of MG, a thorough medical investigation should be made, searching specifically for evidence of chronic or latent infection (such as tuberculosis or hepatitis), hypertension, diabetes, renal impairment, and glaucoma.

MEDICAL AND SURGICAL THERAPY (Fig. 382-2) The prognosis has improved strikingly as a result of advances in treatment; virtually all myasthenic patients can be returned to full productive lives with proper therapy. The most important methods used in the treatment of MG include anticholinesterase medications, immunosuppressive agents, thymectomy, and plasmapheresis or intravenous immunoglobulin.

Table 382-2

Disorders Associated with Myasthenia Gravis and Recommended Laboratory Tests

Associated disorders
 Disorders of the thymus: thymoma, hyperplasia
 Other autoimmune disorders: thyroiditis, Graves' disease, rheumatoid arthritis, lupus erythematosus, skin disorders, family history of autoimmune disorder
 Disorders or circumstances that may exacerbate myasthenia gravis: hyperthyroidism or hypothyroidism, occult infection, medical treatment for other conditions (aminoglycoside antibiotics, quinine, antiarrhythmic agents)
 Disorders that may interfere with therapy: tuberculosis, diabetes, peptic ulcer, gastrointestinal bleeding, renal disease, hypertension, asthma, osteoporosis

Recommended laboratory tests or procedures
 MRI or CT of mediastinum
 Tests for lupus erythematosus, antinuclear antibody, rheumatoid factor, antithyroid antibodies
 Thyroid-function tests
 Tuberculin test
 Chest radiography
 Fasting blood glucose measurement
 Pulmonary-function tests
 Bone densitometry in older patients

SOURCE: From RT Johnson, JW Griffin (eds): *Current Therapy in Neurologic Disease,* 4th ed. St. Louis, Mosby Year Book, 1993, p 379.

Anticholinesterase Medications   Anticholinesterase medication produces at least partial improvement in most myasthenic patients, although improvement is complete in only a few. There is no substantial difference in efficacy among the various anticholinesterase drugs; oral pyridostigmine is the one most widely used in the United States. As a rule, the beneficial action of oral pyridostigmine begins within 15 to 30 min and lasts for 3 to 4 h, but individual responses vary. Treatment is begun with a moderate dose, e.g., 60 mg three to five times daily. The frequency and amount of the dose should be tailored to the patient's individual requirements throughout the day. For example, patients with weakness in chewing and swallowing may benefit by taking the medication before meals so that peak strength coincides with mealtime. Long-acting pyridostigmine tablets may help to get the patient through the night but should never be used for daytime medication because of their variable absorption. The maximum useful dose of pyridostigmine rarely exceeds 120 mg every 3 h during daytime. Overdosage with anticholinesterase medication may cause increased weakness and other side effects. In some patients, muscarinic side effects of the anticholinesterase medication (diarrhea, abdominal cramps, salivation, nausea) may limit the dose tolerated. In these cases,

FIGURE 382-2   Algorithm for the management of myasthenia gravis. FVC, forced vital capacity.

propantheline bromide may be used to block the autonomic side effects without altering the beneficial effects on skeletal muscle. Loperamide is useful for the treatment of diarrhea.

Thymectomy Two separate issues should be distinguished: surgical removal of thymoma, and thymectomy as a treatment for myasthenia gravis. Surgical removal of a thymoma is necessary because of the possibility of local tumor spread, although most thymomas are benign. In the absence of a tumor, the available evidence suggests that up to 85 percent of patients experience improvement after thymectomy, and, of these, about 35 percent achieve drug-free remission. However, the improvement is typically delayed for months to years. The advantage of thymectomy is that it offers the possibility of long-term benefit, in some cases diminishing or eliminating the need for continuing medical treatment. In view of these potential benefits and of the negligible risk in skilled hands, thymectomy has gained widespread acceptance in the treatment of MG. It is the consensus that thymectomy should be carried out in all patients with generalized MG between the ages of puberty and at least 55 years. Whether thymectomy should be recommended in children, in adults over 55 years of age, and in patients with weakness limited to the ocular muscles is still a matter of debate. Thymectomy must be carried out in a hospital where it is performed regularly and where the staff is experienced in the pre- and postoperative management, anesthesia, and surgical techniques of total thymectomy.

Immunosuppression Immunosuppression using glucocorticoids, azathioprine, and other drugs is effective in nearly all patients with MG. The choice of which drugs to use should be guided by their relative benefits and risks for the individual patient. In general, clinical improvement begins somewhat more rapidly with steroid treatment than with the other immunosuppressive agents. The side effects of each drug may preclude its use in some patients, as indicated below.

Steroid therapy Glucocorticoids, when used properly, produce improvement in myasthenic weakness in the great majority of patients. The initial dose of prednisone should be relatively low (15 to 25 mg/d) to avoid the early weakening that occurs in about one-third of patients treated initially with a high-dose regimen. The dose is increased stepwise, as tolerated by the patient (usually by 5 mg/d at 2- to 3-day intervals), until there is marked clinical improvement or a dose of 50 mg/d is reached. This dose is maintained for 1 to 3 months and then is gradually modified to an alternate-day regimen over the course of an additional 1 to 2 months, until a dose of 100 mg on alternate days is reached. Generally, patients begin to improve within a few weeks after reaching the maximum dose, and improvement continues to progress for months or years. The prednisone dosage may gradually be reduced, but usually months or years may be needed to determine the minimum effective dose, and close monitoring is required by patient and doctor. *Few patients are able to do without prednisone entirely.* Patients on long-term glucocorticoid therapy must be followed carefully to prevent or treat adverse side effects. The most common errors in the steroid treatment of myasthenic patients include (1) insufficient persistence; improvement may be delayed and gradual; (2) too early, too rapid, or excessive tapering of steroid dosage; and (3) lack of attention to prevention and treatment of side effects. → *The management of patients treated with glucocorticoids is discussed in Chap. 332*

Other immunosuppressive drugs Azathioprine, cyclosporine, or occasionally cyclophosphamide is effective in many patients, either alone or in combination with glucocorticoid therapy. Azathioprine is the most widely used of these drugs because of its relative safety in most patients. Its therapeutic effect may add to that of glucocorticoids and/or allow the steroid dose to be reduced. However, up to 10 percent of patients are unable to tolerate azathioprine because of idiosyncratic reactions consisting of flulike symptoms of fever and malaise, bone marrow depression, or abnormalities of liver function. An initial dose of 50 mg/d should be used to test for adverse side effects. If this dose is tolerated, it is increased gradually until the white blood count falls to approxi-

mately 3000/μL. In patients who are receiving steroids concurrently, leukocytosis precludes the use of this measure. A reduction of the lymphocyte count below 1000/μL and/or an increase of the mean corpuscular volume may be used as indications of adequacy of azathioprine dosage. The typical dosage range is 2 to 3 mg/kg total body weight (including fat in obese patients). The beneficial effect of azathioprine takes at least 3 to 6 months to begin and even longer to peak.

Cyclosporine is approximately as effective as azathioprine and is being used increasingly in the management of MG. Its beneficial effect appears more rapidly than that of azathioprine. It may be used alone but usually is used as an adjunct to steroids, to permit reduction of the steroid dose. The usual dose of cyclosporine is 4 to 5 mg/kg per day, given in two divided doses (to minimize side effects). Side effects of cyclosporine include hypertension and nephrotoxicity, which must be closely monitored. "Trough" blood levels of cyclosporine are measured 12 h after the evening dose. The therapeutic range, as measured by radioimmunoassay, is 150 to 200 ng/L. Cyclophosphamide is reserved for patients refractory to the other drugs, because of its relatively high risk of adverse side effects, including late development of malignancies.

Plasmapheresis and Intravenous Immunoglobulin Administration In view of the antibody-mediated pathogenesis of MG, plasmapheresis has been used therapeutically. The plasma, which contains the pathogenic antibodies, is mechanically separated from the blood cells, which are returned to the patient. Plasmapheresis produces a short-term reduction in anti-AChR antibodies, with clinical improvement in many patients. It is useful as a temporary expedient in seriously affected patients or to improve the patient's condition prior to surgery (e.g., thymectomy).

The indications for the use of intravenous immunoglobulin are the same as those for plasma exchange: to produce rapid improvement to help the patient through a difficult period of myasthenic weakness, or prior to surgery. This treatment has the advantages of not requiring special equipment or large-bore venous access. The usual dose is 400 mg/kg per day for five successive days (total dose = 2 g/kg). Improvement occurs in about 70 percent of patients, beginning about 4 to 5 days after treatment and continuing for weeks to months. The mechanism of action of intravenous immunoglobulin is not known; the treatment has no consistent effect on the measurable amount of circulating AChR antibody. Adverse reactions are uncommon, but include headache, fluid overload, and rarely renal shutdown.

The long-term treatment of myasthenic patients requires other methods of therapy outlined earlier in this chapter.

Management of Myasthenic Crisis Myasthenic crisis is defined as an exacerbation of weakness sufficient to endanger life; usually it consists of respiratory failure caused by diaphragmatic and intercostal muscle weakness. Treatment should be carried out in an intensive care unit staffed with physicians experienced in the management of myasthenia gravis, respiratory insufficiency, infectious disease, and fluid and electrolyte therapy. The possibility that the deterioration could be due to excessive anticholinesterase medication ("cholinergic crisis") is best excluded by temporarily stopping anticholinesterase drugs. The most common cause of crisis is intercurrent infection. This should be treated *immediately*, because the mechanical and immunologic defenses of the patient can be assumed to be compromised. The myasthenic patient with fever and early infection should be treated like other immunocompromised patients. Early and effective antibiotic therapy, respiratory assistance, and pulmonary physiotherapy are essentials of the treatment program. As discussed above, plasmapheresis is frequently helpful in hastening recovery.

BIBLIOGRAPHY

DRACHMAN DB: Myasthenia gravis; medical progress. N Engl J Med 330:1797, 1994

GAJDOS P: Intravenous immune globulin in myasthenia gravis. Clin Exp Immunol 197:49, 1994

LENNON V: Serologic diagnosis of myasthenia gravis and the Lambert Eaton myasthenic syndrome, in *Handbook of Myasthenia Gravis and Myasthenic Syndromes*, RP Lisak (ed). New York, Marcel Dekker, 1994, p 149

SANDERS DB: *Myasthenia Gravis and Myasthenic Syndromes*. Philadelphia, Saunders, 1994

DISEASES OF MUSCLE

The muscle disorders discussed in this chapter include diseases that cause acute, subacute, or chronic muscle weakness. Some cause pain in addition to or instead of weakness. → *Dermatomyositis and polymyositis are discussed in Chap. 315.*

HEREDITARY MYOPATHIES

Muscular dystrophy refers to a group of hereditary progressive diseases. Each type of muscular dystrophy has unique phenotypic and genetic features (Table 383-1).

DUCHENNE MUSCULAR DYSTROPHY This X-linked recessive disorder, sometimes also called *pseudohypertrophic muscular dystrophy*, occurs with an incidence of about 30 per 100,000 liveborn males.

Clinical Features Duchenne dystrophy is present at birth, but the disorder usually becomes apparent between ages 3 and 5. The boys fall frequently and have difficulty keeping up with their friends when playing. Running, jumping, and hopping are invariably abnormal. By age 5, muscle weakness is obvious by muscle testing. On getting up from the floor, the patient uses his hands to climb up himself (Gowers' maneuver). In younger children, the calf muscles are usually enlarged from true muscle hypertrophy; later calf enlargement is appropriately called *pseudohypertrophy* since muscle is replaced by fat and connective tissue. Contractures of the heel cords and iliotibial bands become apparent by age 6, when toe walking is associated with a lordotic posture. Loss of muscle strength is progressive, with predilection for proximal limb muscles and the neck flexors; leg involvement is more severe than arm involvement. Between ages 8 and 10 walking may require the use of braces; joint contractures and limitations of hip flexion, knee, elbow, and wrist extension are made worse by prolonged sitting. By age 12, most patients are confined to a wheelchair. Contractures become fixed, and a progressive scoliosis often develops which may be associated with pain. The chest deformity associated with scoliosis impairs pulmonary function, which is already diminished by muscle weakness. By age 16 to 18, patients are predisposed to serious, sometimes fatal pulmonary infections. Other causes of death include aspiration of food and acute gastric dilation.

A cardiac cause of death is uncommon despite the presence of a cardiomyopathy in almost all patients. Congestive heart failure seldom occurs except with severe stress such as pneumonia. Cardiac arrhythmias are rare. The typical electrocardiogram (ECG) shows an increase net RS in lead V_1; deep, narrow Q waves in the precordial leads; and

RSR' or polyphyasic R waves in V_1. Intellectual impairment in Duchenne dystrophy is common; the average intelligence quotient (IQ) is approximately one standard deviation below the mean. Impairment of intellectual function appears to be nonprogressive and affects verbal ability more than performance. IQs of Duchenne patients are lower than those of children with comparably disabling and chronic disorders, indicating that the mental subnormality in Duchenne dystrophy is not solely a reflection of physical limitations. The basis for intellectual impairment in Duchenne dystrophy has not been established.

Laboratory Investigation Serum creatine phosphokinase (CK) levels are invariably elevated to between 20 and 100 times normal. The levels are abnormal at birth but decline late in the disease because of inactivity and loss of muscle mass. Electromyography (EMG) demonstrates features typical of myopathy. The muscle biopsy shows muscle fibers of varying size as well as small groups of necrotic and regenerating fibers. Connective tissue and fat replace lost muscle fibers.

Table 383-1

Progressive Muscular Dystrophies

Type of Muscular Dystrophy	Genetics	Clinical Features	Other Organ System Involvement
Duchenne	X-linked recessive; mutation of dystrophin gene	Onset before age 5 Progressive weakness of girdle muscles Inability to walk after age 12 Kyphoscoliosis Respiratory failure in 2d or 3d decade	Cardiomyopathy Mental impairment
Becker	X-linked recessive; mutation of dystrophin gene	Onset in early to late childhood Progressive weakness of girdle muscles Still able to walk at age 15 Respiratory failure after 4th decade	Cardiomyopathy
Limb-girdle (see Table 383-2)	Autosomal recessive; includes several disorders with linkage to chromosomes 2p, 4q, 5q, 13q, 17q, 15q; *also* Autosomal dominant; includes more than one disorder; one form maps to chromosome 5q	Onset in early childhood Slowly progressive weakness of shoulder and hip girdle muscles	Cardiomyopathy
Congenital	Autosomal recessive; includes disorders with linkage to chromosomes 6q and 9q	Onset at birth or in the first few months Hypotonia, contractures, delayed motor milestones Progression to respiratory failure in some; static course in others	Central nervous system abnormalities (hypomyelination and malformations) Eye abnormalities
Myotonic	Autosomal dominant; expansion of unstable triplet repeat at chromosome 19q13.3	Onset usually in 2d decade (but in infancy if born to affected mother) Slowly progressive weakness of eyelids, face, neck, distal limb muscles Myotonia	Cardiac conduction defects Mental impairment Cataracts Frontal baldness Gonadal atrophy Hypertension Deafness
Facioscapulohumeral	Autosomal dominant; maps to chromosome 14q	Onset before age 20 Slowly progressive weakness of face, shoulder girdle, foot dorsiflexion	Hypertension Deafness Coats' (eye) diseaes
Oculopharyngeal	Autosomal dominant; maps to chromosome 14q	Onset in 5th to 6th decade Slowly progressive weakness of extraocular, pharyngeal, and limb muscles	—

A definitive diagnosis of Duchenne dystrophy can be established on the basis of dystrophin deficiency in biopsied muscle tissue or mutation analysis on peripheral blood leukocytes as discussed below.

Genetics Duchenne dystrophy is caused by a mutation of the gene responsible for producing dystrophin. The latter is a 427-kDa protein localized to the inner surface of the sarcolemma of the muscle fiber. The dystrophin gene, estimated at 2000 kb in size, is one of the largest identified human genes. It is localized to the short arm of the X chromosome at Xp21. At present, mutations of the gene can be identified (in approximately two-thirds of Duchenne patients) using a battery of cDNA probes. Deletions are not uniformly distributed over the gene, but rather are most common near the beginning (5' end) and middle of the gene. Deletion size does not correlate with severity of disease. Less often, Duchenne dystrophy is caused by a gene duplication or point mutation. Identification of a specific mutation allows for an unequivocal diagnosis and makes possible accurate testing of potential carriers. Identification of such a mutation in amniotic fluid cells or chorionic villi permits prenatal diagnosis. In families without deletions or duplications, linkage analysis using probes recognizing restriction fragment length polymorphisms is also available.

Dystrophin determination of muscle tissue represents an accurate method of diagnosis of Duchenne dystrophy. The amount and alteration in the size of dystrophin can be determined by western blot analysis of muscle biopsy specimens. In addition, immunocytochemical staining of muscle with dystrophin antibodies can be used to demonstrate absence or deficiency of dystrophin localizing to the sarcolemmal membrane. Carriers of the disease may demonstrate a mosaic pattern, but dystrophin analysis of muscle biopsy specimens for carrier detection is not reliable.

Pathogenesis Dystrophin is part of a large complex of sarcolemmal proteins and glycoproteins (Fig. 383-1). In relation to human muscular dystrophies, it is useful to consider the constituents of the complex falling into three groups. *Group 1* includes dystrophin and the dystroglycans, α and β. Dystrophin binds to F-actin at its amino terminus and to β-dystroglycan at the carboxy terminus. β-dystroglycan in turn binds to α-dystroglycan, and extracellular glycoprotein. In the basal lamina, α-dystroglycan binds to laminin. *Group 2* is composed of the sarcoglycans, which have four transmembrane constituents: α-sarcoglycan (formerly called adhalin), β-sarcoglycan (previously called A3b), γ-sarcoglycan, and δ-sarcoglycan (the newest member to be identified). *Group 3* is composed of laminin, an integral component of the basal lamina, designated laminin 2 in skeletal muscle. It has a heterotrimeric molecular structure arranged in the shape of

a cross with one heavy α chain and two light chains, β1 and γ1. The laminin heavy α chain of skeletal muscle is designated lamina α2.

The function of each individual component of the dystrophin-glycoprotein complex is still under study. Nevertheless, important observations indicate that the dystrophin-glycoprotein complex confers stability to the sarcolemma. Furthermore, deficiency of one member of the complex causes loss of other components of the dystrophin-glycoprotein complex. For example, deficiency of dystrophin (Duchenne dystrophy) of α-sarcoglycan (limb-girdle dystrophy, see below) weakens the sarcolemma, causing membrane tears and a cascade of events leading to mucle fiber necrosis. This train of events happens repeatedly during the life of a muscular dystrophy patient.

℞ **TREATMENT**

Prednisone in a dose of 0.75 mg/kg per day has been shown to significantly alter the progression of Duchenne dystrophy for up to 3 years. Despite these favorable results, some patients clearly cannot tolerate glucocorticoid therapy. The weight gain represents a significant deterrent for some boys. Treatment must be tailored to the individual.

BECKER MUSCULAR DYSTROPHY This less severe form of X-linked recessive muscular dystrophy was described by Becker and Keiner in 1955. It is often called the benign form of pseudohypertrophic muscular dystrophy. Until recently, it was not known whether Duchenne and Becker muscular dystrophies were genetically distinct disorders. Molecular genetic studies now indicate that these dystrophies result from allelic defects of the same gene. Becker muscular dystrophy is approximately 10 times less frequent than Duchenne, with an incidence of about 3 per 100,000.

Clinical Features The pattern of muscle wasting in Becker muscular dystrophy closely resembles that seen in Duchenne. Proximal muscles, especially of the lower extremities, are prominently involved. As the disease progresses, weakness becomes more generalized. Significant facial muscle weakness is not a feature. Hypertrophy of muscles, particularly in the calves, is an early and prominent finding.

Most Becker patients first experience difficulties between ages 5 and 15 years, although onset in the third or fourth decade or even later can occur. By definition, Becker patients ambulate beyond age 15, allowing for a clinical distinction between Becker and Duchenne dystrophy. Becker dystrophy patients have a reduced life expectancy, but most survive into the fourth or fifth decade.

Mental retardation may be seen in Becker dystrophy, but it is not as common as in Duchenne. Cardiac involvement occurs in Becker dystrophy and may result in heart failure.

Laboratory Features The findings from serum CK measurement, EMG, and muscle biopsy closely resemble those in Duchenne dystrophy. The diagnosis of Becker muscular dystrophy requires western blot analysis of muscle biopsy samples demonstrating dystrophin of reduced amount or abnormal size. In addition, in Becker dystrophy, mutation analysis of DNA from peripheral blood leukocytes recognizes deletions and duplications of the dystrophin gene in approximately the same number of patients (65 percent) as in Duchenne. In both Becker and Duchenne dystrophies, the size of the DNA deletion does not predict clinical severity; however, in about 95 percent of Becker dystrophy patients, the DNA deletion does not alter the translational reading frame of messenger RNA. These "in-frame" mutations allow for production of some dystrophin, which accounts for the presence of altered rather than absent dystrophin on western blot analysis.

℞ **TREATMENT**

The use of prednisone has not been adequately studied in Becker dystrophy and other mild dystrophin-deficiency disorders.

LIMB-GIRDLE DYSTROPHY This term was introduced in 1954 in the Walton and Natrass revision of the classification of the muscular dystrophies. From the outset, it was apparent that limb-girdle dystrophy represented more than one disorder.

FIGURE 383-1 Dystrophin localizes to the cytoplasmic face of the membrane in a subsarcolemmal location. The syntrophin complex, composed of α, β1, and β2, is shown in its presumed place in relation to the dystrophin-glycoprotein complex. See text for further explanation.

Clinical Features Muscle weakness affects both males and females, with onset ranging from late in the first decade to the fourth decade. Most limb-girdle muscular dystrophies are progressive and affect the pelvic and shoulder girdle muscles. Respiratory insufficiency from diaphragm weakness may occur. The distribution of weakness and rate of progression vary from family to family. In some patients, cardiac involvement results in congestive heart failure or arrhythmias; occasional patients present with a cardiomyopathy. Intellectual function remains normal.

Laboratory Features An elevated serum CK level, myopathic EMG findings, and muscle biopsy features indicative of myopathy represent the characteristic changes in limb-girdle dystrophy. Careful attention to exclude phenotypically similar disorders, such as spinal muscular atrophy and metabolic and inflammatory myopathies, is required. The availability of western blot analysis for dystrophin sarcoglycans allows limb-girdle dystrophies to be distinguished unequivocally from Becker and Duchenne muscular dystrophies.

Genetics Limb-girdle dystrophy continues to refer to more than one disease transmitted by autosomal dominant and autosomal recessive inheritance. In a newly proposed genetic classification, *LGMD1* refers to the dominantly inherited cases, while *LGMD2* indicates recessive transmission. Presently, genetic linkage has established only a single, dominantly inherited disorder, LGMD1A. In contrast, the recessively inherited forms of LGMD now number six. In each case genetic linkage has been established, and the specific protein deficiency is known for most forms (Table 383-2 and Fig. 383-1). In LGMD2A the defect lies in a muscle-specific calcium-activated neutral protease, calpain 3. The sarcoglycans, α, β, γ, δ, are deficient in LGMDs 2C–F. In the latter deficiencies, the dystrophin-glycoprotein complex is affected, weakening the muscle membrane in a manner similar to Duchenne muscular dystrophy.

 TREATMENT

Supportive care, but not specific treatment, can be offered. Long leg braces are seldom helpful for adults. Wheelchairs may be essential or may be used to help preserve energy for work or recreational activities. Cardiac or respiratory muscle involvement may require individualized treatment.

CONGENITAL MUSCULAR DYSTROPHY This rare autosomal recessive disorder includes four subgroups with overlapping clinical features. Variable involvement of brain and eyes can help differentiate these conditions; two have been mapped to specific chromosomes, with a specific defect identified in one of these.

Clinical Features All the forms of congenital muscular dystrophy present at birth or in the first few months of life with hypotonia and proximal limb weakness. Varying degrees of joint contractures at the elbows, hips, knees, and ankles are seen in most patients. Contractures present at birth are referred to as *arthrogryposis*. Weakness of facial muscles may occur, but other cranial nerve musculature is spared. Severity varies greatly, but about half of affected individuals never achieve the ability to stand independently. Death may ensue because of respiratory insufficiency early in life. Some patients learn

to walk, although difficulty in motor activities (e.g., running) persists.

One variant of congenital muscular dystrophy has only the muscle features just described; three others have central nervous involvement. In patients with deficiency of laminin α2 (formerly called merosin) diffuse white matter changes typical of hypomyelination are seen by magnetic resonance imaging. There is no accompanying cerebral atrophy, ventricular dilation, or cerebellar hypoplasia. The clinical manifestation of the cerebral hypomyelination is mild, with learning disability as the most severe problem. In *Fukuyama congenital muscular dystrophy*, found mainly in Japan, patients are severely disabled and mentally retarded; most have seizures and die by age 20. Microcephaly and enlarged ventricles occur. Micropolygyria is common. In *cerebroocular-dysplasia muscular dystrophy*, the clinical features are like those of Fukuyama dystrophy, with the addition of eye abnormalities, including corneal defects, cataracts, retinal dysplasia, and hypoplasia of the optic nerve.

Laboratory Features Serum CK levels range from normal to 10 times normal. The EMG shows a myopathic pattern, and muscle biopsy samples demonstrate dystrophic features. In laminin α2 deficiency, the muscle lacks this protein.

Genetics The gene for laminin α2 maps to chromosome 6q22-23; specific mutations of the gene have been identified in some patients with this form of congenital muscular dystrophy. Deficiency of laminin α2 can adversely affect the dystrophin-glycoprotein complex (Fig. 383-1).

The gene for Fukuyama congenital muscular dystrophy has not been identified but has been mapped to the long arm of chromosome 9. The gene causing cerebroocular-dysplasia muscular dystrophy has not been mapped. In cases of congenital muscular dystrophy without brain or eye involvement, no candidate genes have been identified.

 TREATMENT

Supportive care and especially stretching to improve joint range of motion is important for congenital muscular dystrophies. Infants and very young children require special wheelchair modifications and adaptive seating to maximize functional capabilities.

MYOTONIC DYSTROPHY This disorder has an incidence of 13.5 per 100,000 live births and affects males and females equally. It is the most common adult muscular dystrophy.

Clinical Features The clinical expression of myotonic dystrophy varies widely and involves many systems other than muscle. Myotonic dystrophy patients have a typical "hatchet-faced" appearance due to temporalis, masseter, and facial muscle atrophy and weakness. Neck muscles, including the flexors and sternocleidomastoids, become involved early, as do distal limb muscles. Weakness of wrist extensors, finger extensors, and intrinsic hand muscles impairs function. Ankle dorsiflexor weakness may cause footdrop. Proximal muscles remain stronger throughout the course, although preferential atrophy and weakness of quadriceps muscles occur in many patients. Palatal, pharyngeal, and tongue involvement produce a dysarthric speech, nasal voice, and swallowing problems. Some patients have diaphragm and intercostal muscle weakness, resulting in respiratory insufficiency.

Myotonia, which usually appears by age 5, is demonstrable by percussion of the thenar eminence, the tongue, and wrist extensor muscles. Myotonia causes a slow relaxation of hand grip following a forced voluntary closure. Advanced muscle wasting makes myotonia more difficult to detect.

Congenital myotonic dystrophy is a more severe form of the disease and occurs in approximately 25 percent of infants of affected mothers. It is characterized by severe facial and bulbar weakness and neonatal respiratory insufficiency. Most patients will recover from respiratory distress. Congenital myotonic dystrophy patients usually have impaired intelligence.

Table 383-2

The Limb-Girdle Muscular Dystrophies Caused by Defects in Proteins Associated with the Muscle Membrane

Disease	Protein	Size	Chromosomal Localization
LGMD1A	Unknown	Unknown	5q31–33
LGMD2A	Calpain 3	95 kDa	15q15.1–15.3
LGMD2B	Unknown	Unknown	2p13.3
LGMD2C	γ-sarcoglycan	35 kDa	13q12
LGMD2D	α-sarcoglycan	50 kDa	17q12–21.33
LGMD2E	β-sarcoglycan	43 kDa	4q12
LGMD2F	δ-sarcoglycan	35 kDa	5q33–34

NOTE: LGMD, limb-girdle muscular dystrophy. Type 1A is autosomal dominant; types 2A–F are autosomal recessive.

Cardiac disturbances occur in most patients with myotonic dystrophy. Electrocardiographic abnormalities are common, including first-degree heart block and more extensive conduction system involvement. Complete heart block and sudden death can occur. Congestive heart failure occurs infrequently but may result from cor pulmonale secondary to respiratory failure. Mitral valve prolapse also occurs commonly in myotonic dystrophy patients.

Other features associated with myotonic dystrophy include intellectual impairment, hypersomnia, posterior subcapsular cataracts, frontal baldness, gonadal atrophy, insulin resistance, and decreased esophageal and colonic motility.

Laboratory Features The diagnosis of myotonic dystrophy can usually be made on the basis of clinical findings. Serum CK levels may be normal or mildly elevated. EMG evidence of myotonia will be found readily in most cases. Muscle biopsy shows muscle atrophy, which selectively involves type 1 fibers in 50 percent of cases. Typically, increased numbers of central nuclei can be seen. Necrosis of muscle fibers and increased connective tissue, common in other muscular dystrophies, do not usually occur in myotonic dystrophy.

Genetics Myotonic dystrophy is an autosomal dominant disorder. Evidence indicates that new mutations do not contribute to the pool of affected individuals. The disorder is transmitted by a mutation consisting of an unstable expansion of a CTG trinucleotide repeat sequence in a gene at 19q13.3. An increase in the severity of the disease phenotype in successive generations (genetic anticipation) is accompanied by an increase in the number of trinucleotide repeats. A similar type of mutation has been identified in fragile X syndrome (see Chap. 363). The unstable triplet repeat in myotonic dystrophy can be used for prenatal diagnosis. Congenital disease occurs almost exclusively in infants born to affected mothers; it is possible that sperm with greatly expanded triplet repeats do not function well.

The protein encoded by the region adjacent to the unstable repeat has a predicted amino acid composition homologous to a protein kinase (referred to as myotonin-protein kinase). Other genes may also be affected by the enlarged repeat.

A subset of patients with multisystemic disease features similar to myotonic dystrophy do not have the diagnostic expansion of trinucleotide repeats. Their weakness tends to be proximal rather than distal. This condition has been termed *pro*ximal *m*yotonic *m*yopathy (PROMM). At least a proportion of PROMM cases may be caused by a mutation at a different chromosome locus from that causing myotonic dystrophy.

℞ TREATMENT

The myotonia in myotonic dystrophy rarely warrants treatment. Phenytoin is the preferred agent for the occasional patient who requires an antimyotonia drug; other agents, particularly quinine and procainamide, may worsen cardiac conduction. Cardiac pacemaker insertion should be considered for patients with unexplained syncope or advanced conduction system abnormalities with evidence of second-degree heart block, or trifascicular conduction disturbances with marked prolongation of the PR interval. Molded ankle-foot orthoses will help prevent footdrop in patients with distal lower extremity weakness.

FACIOSCAPULOHUMERAL MUSCULAR DYSTROPHY This form of muscular dystrophy has an incidence of approximately 1 in 20,000. It is distinct from a somewhat similar disorder known as scapuloperoneal dystrophy.

Clinical Features The condition typically has an onset in childhood and young adulthood. In most cases, facial weakness is the initial manifestation, appearing as an inability to smile, whistle, or fully close the eyes. Weakness of the shoulder girdles, rather than the facial muscles, usually brings the patient to medical attention. Loss of scapular stabilizer muscles makes arm elevation difficult. Scapular winging becomes apparent with attempts at abduction and forward move-

ment of the arms. Biceps and triceps muscles may be severely affected, with relative sparing of the deltoid muscles. Weakness is invariably worse for wrist extension than for wrist flexion, and weakness of the anterior compartment muscles of the legs may lead to footdrop.

In most patients, the weakness remains restricted to facial, upper extremity, and distal lower extremity muscles. In 20 percent of cases, weakness progresses to involve the pelvic girdle muscles, and severe functional impairment and possible wheelchair confinement result.

Characteristically, patients with facioscapulohumeral dystrophy do not have involvement of other organ systems, although labile hypertension is common, and there is an increased incidence of nerve deafness. Coats' disease, a disorder consisting of telangiectasia, exudation, and retinal detachment, also occurs.

Laboratory Features The serum CK level may be normal or mildly elevated. EMG usually indicates a myopathic pattern. The muscle biopsy shows nonspecific features of a myopathy. A prominent inflammatory infiltrate, which is often multifocal in distribution, is present in some biopsy samples. The cause or significance of this finding is unknown.

Genetics An autosomal dominant inheritance pattern with almost complete penetrance has been established, but each family member should be examined for the presence of the disease, since approximately 30 percent of those affected are unaware of involvement. Facioscapulohumeral dystrophy has been linked to chromosome 4q35, but neither the gene nor the product is known. Nevertheless, deletions of telomeric heterochromatin at 4q35 are proved to be disease-causing with a great deal of certainty. In addition, there is a significant correlation between disease severity and the size of the 4q35-associated deletion. Carrier detection and prenatal diagnosis are possible. Most sporadic cases represent new mutations. Genetic heterogeneity has been documented for facioscapulohumeral dystrophy; in occasional families, the disease is linked to chromosome 4q.

℞ TREATMENT

No specific treatment is available; ankle-foot orthoses are helpful for patients with footdrop. Scapular stabilization procedures improve scapular winging but may not improve function.

OCULOPHARYNGEAL DYSTROPHY This form of muscular dystrophy represents one of several disorders characterized by *progressive external ophthalmoplegia*, which consists of slowly progressive ptosis and limitation of eye movements with sparing of pupillary reactions for light and accommodation. Patients usually do not complain of diplopia, in contrast to patients having conditions with a more acute onset of ocular muscle weakness (e.g., myasthenia gravis).

Clinical Features This is a late-onset form of muscular dystrophy. Oculopharyngeal muscular dystrophy usually presents with ptosis and/or dysphagia in the fourth to sixth decade. The extraocular muscle impairment is less prominent in the early phase but may be severe later. The swallowing problem may become debilitating and result in pooling of secretions and repeated episodes of aspiration. Mild neck and extremity weakness also occur.

Laboratory Features The serum CK level may be two to three times normal. Myopathic EMG findings are typical. On biopsy, muscle fibers are found to contain vacuoles, which by electron microscopy are shown to contain membranous whorls, accumulations of glycogen, and other nonspecific debris related to lysosomes. A distinct feature of oculopharyngeal dystrophy is the presence of tubular filaments, 8.5 nm in diameter, in muscle cell nuclei.

Genetics Oculopharyngeal dystrophy has an autosomal dominant inheritance pattern with complete penetrance. The incidence is high in French-Canadians and in Spanish-American families of the southwest United States. A large Jewish kindred of eastern European background has been reported. The gene for oculopharyngeal muscular dystrophy maps to the region on chromosome 14q containing the genes for the α and β heavy chains of cardiac myosin.

TREATMENT

Dysphagia can cause inanition and makes oculopharyngeal muscular dystrophy a potentially life-threatening disease. Cricopharyngeal myotomy may improve swallowing, although it does not prevent aspiration. Eyelid crutches can improve vision in patients in whom ptosis obstructs vision; candidates for ptosis surgery must be carefully selected; those with severe facial weakness are not suitable.

DISTAL MYOPATHIES Patients with predominantly distal weakness usually have a disease of peripheral nerve or anterior horn cells rather than of muscle. There is, however, a heterogeneous group of uncommon disorders of this type in which there is histopathologic and electrophysiologic evidence of myopathy. These distal myopathies can be separated into two types with onset in late adulthood and two types with onset in early adulthood.

The most familiar late adult–onset form was described by Welander. It is inherited as an autosomal dominant condition with onset in the fifth decade. Weakness begins in the hands, and distal anterior-compartment leg muscle involvement occurs later in the course. The serum CK level is either normal or mildly increased. Muscle biopsy shows vacuolated muscle fibers.

Another late adult–onset form of distal myopathy, also inherited as an autosomal dominant trait, was first recognized in non-Scandinavian patients and also occurs in Finland. Weakness begins in the anterior compartment of the distal lower extremities. The serum CK level is normal or mildly elevated. Muscle fibers often have vacuoles.

Both of the distal myopathies with onset in early adulthood have autosomal recessive inheritance. In one type, the weakness usually begins in the anterior compartment of the distal lower extremities, although in some cases it begins in the hands. The serum CK level is moderately elevated (less than 10 times normal), and muscle biopsies reveal a myopathy with many fibers showing vacuoles. The other form of early adult–onset distal myopathy (Miyoshi myopathy) is distinguished by weakness beginning in the posterior compartment, i.e., the gastrocnemius muscle. The serum CK level is markedly elevated (>10-fold), and biopsy shows a myopathy without vacuolated fibers. Miyoshi myopathy has been linked to chromosome 2p12-14.

CONGENITAL MYOPATHIES

These rare disorders are distinguished from muscular dystrophies by the presence of specific histochemical and structural abnormalities in muscle. Three major types are described: *central core disease, nemaline (rod) myopathy,* and *centronuclear (myotubular) myopathy.* Other rare types, such as multicore disease, fingerprint body myopathy, and sarcotubular myopathy, are not discussed here (see Griggs et al).

CENTRAL CORE DISEASE **Clinical Features** Patients with central core disease may have decreased fetal movements and breech presentation. Hypotonia and delay in motor milestones, particularly in walking, are common. Later in childhood, patients develop problems with stair climbing, running, and getting up from the floor. On examination, there is mild facial, neck-flexor, and proximal-extremity muscle weakness. Legs are more affected than arms. Skeletal abnormalities include congenital hip dislocation, scoliosis, and pes cavus; clubbed feet also occur. Most cases are nonprogressive, but exceptions are well documented.

Laboratory Features The serum CK level is usually normal. Needle EMG demonstrates a myopathic pattern. Muscle biopsy shows fibers with single or multiple central or eccentric discrete zones (cores) devoid of oxidative enzymes. Cores occur preferentially in type 1 fibers and represent poorly aligned sarcomeres associated with Z disk streaming.

Genetics Autosomal dominant inheritance is characteristic; sporadic cases also occur. The disease is caused by point mutations of the ryanodine receptor gene on chromosome 19q, encoding the calcium release channel of the sarcoplasmic reticulum of skeletal muscle; mutations of this gene also account for some cases of inherited malignant hyperthermia (see Chap. 363).

 TREATMENT

Specific treatment is not required, but establishing a diagnosis of central core disease is extremely important, because these patients have a known predisposition to *malignant hyperthermia* during anesthesia.

NEMALINE MYOPATHY The term *nemaline* refers to the distinctive presence in muscle fibers of rods or threadlike structures (Greek *nema,* "thread").

Clinical Features Nemaline myopathy is clinically heterogeneous. A severe neonatal form presents with hypotonia and feeding difficulties leading to early death. Most commonly, nemaline myopathy presents in infancy or childhood with delayed motor milestones. The course is nonprogressive or slowly progressive. The physical appearance may be striking because of the long, narrow facies, high-arched palate, and open-mouthed appearance due to a prognathous jaw. Other skeletal abnormalities include pectus excavatum, kyphoscoliosis, pes cavus, and clubfoot deformities. Facial and generalized muscle weakness are common. These two early childhood forms of nemaline myopathy are referred to as *congenital nemaline myopathy,* in contrast to an adult-onset disorder with progressive proximal weakness. Myocardial involvement is occasionally present in both the congenital and adult-onset forms of the disease.

Laboratory Features The serum CK level is usually normal or slightly elevated. The EMG in weak muscles demonstrates a myopathic pattern with occasional fibrillation potentials. Muscle biopsy demonstrates clusters of small rods (nemaline bodies), which occur preferentially, but not exclusively, in type 1 muscle fibers. The muscle often shows type 1 muscle fiber predominance. Rods originate from the Z disk material of the muscle fiber. In the severe neonatal variant, rods are commonly observed in the nucleus of muscle fibers.

Genetics Nemaline myopathy shows at least two patterns of inheritance: autosomal recessive and autosomal dominant with incomplete penetrance. Sporadic cases also occur. A gene for autosomal dominant nemaline myopathy maps to chromosome 1p, and a missense mutation in the α-tropomyosin gene (TPM3) has been found.

 TREATMENT

No specific treatment exists for this condition; some patients require bracing or surgery for the scoliosis as well as ankle-foot orthoses for distal lower extremity weakness.

CENTRONUCLEAR MYOPATHY **Clinical Features** Three distinct variants of the disease occur. A *neonatal form of centronuclear myopathy* presents with severe hypotonia and weakness at birth. Respiratory assistance may be required, and swallowing difficulties may necessitate a feeding tube. This form of the disease carries a poor prognosis and often results in death. The *late infancy–early childhood form of centronuclear myopathy* presents with delayed motor milestones. Later, difficulty with running and stair climbing becomes apparent. A marfanoid, slender body habitus, long narrow face, and high-arched palate are typical. Scoliosis and clubbed feet may be present. Most patients exhibit progressive weakness, some requiring wheelchairs. Progressive external ophthalmoplegia with ptosis and varying degrees of extraocular muscle impairment are characteristic of both the neonatal and the late-infantile forms.

A third variant, the *late childhood–adult type of centronuclear myopathy,* has an onset in the second or third decade. Patients have full extraocular muscle movements and rarely exhibit ptosis. There is mild, nonprogressive limb weakness and no associated skeletal abnormalities.

Laboratory Features Normal or slightly elevated CK levels occur in each of the forms of centronuclear myopathy. EMG studies often give distinctive results, showing positive sharp waves and fibrillation potentials, complex and repetitive discharges, and rarely myotonic discharges. Muscle biopsy specimens in longitudinal section demonstrate rows of central nuclei, often surrounded by a halo. In transverse sections, central nuclei are found in 25 to 80 percent of muscle fibers.

Genetics The gene for the neonatal form of centronuclear myopathy has been localized to Xq28, permitting identification of carriers and prenatal diagnosis. Inheritance pattern for the late infancy–early childhood disorder is probably autosomal recessive and for the late childhood–adult form, autosomal dominant.

℞ **TREATMENT**

Patients with the neonatal form of centronuclear myopathy require respiratory support and gastric feeding. For patients with the late infancy–early childhood disorder, ambulatory aids and orthotic devices and, less often, wheelchairs may be necessary. Occasional patients require scoliosis surgery.

DISORDERS OF MUSCLE ENERGY METABOLISM

Skeletal muscle uses two principal sources of energy—fatty acids and glucose. Abnormalities in either glucose or lipid utilization can be associated with distinct clinical presentations. The clinical presentation can range from an acute, painful syndrome with rhabdomyolysis and myoglobinuria to a chronic progressive muscle weakness simulating muscular dystrophy.

GLYCOGEN STORAGE AND GLYCOLYTIC DEFECTS

These disorders can be divided into those that cause exercise intolerance, particularly intermittent muscle pain and myoglobinuria, and those in which fixed muscle weakness is the predominant clinical feature. The latter can mimic limb-girdle muscular dystrophy or inflammatory myopathies.

Disorders of Glycogen Storage Causing Fixed Muscle Weakness Three clinical forms of acid maltase deficiency (*type II glycogenosis*) can be distinguished, all of which have autosomal recessive inheritance. The gene for acid maltase is found on the long arm of chromosome 17. *Infantile acid maltase deficiency* is the most common, with onset of symptoms in the first 3 months of life. Infants develop severe muscle weakness, cardiomegaly, hepatomegaly, and respiratory insufficiency. Glycogen accumulation in motor neurons of the spinal cord and brainstem contributes to muscle weakness. Death usually occurs by 1 year of age. In *childhood acid maltase deficiency*, the picture resembles muscular dystrophy. Delayed motor milestones result from proximal limb muscle weakness and involvement of respiratory muscles. The heart may be involved, but the liver and brain are unaffected. The *adult form of acid maltase deficiency* begins in the third or fourth decade. Respiratory failure and diaphragmatic weakness are often initial manifestations heralding progressive proximal muscle weakness. The heart and liver are not involved.

In all forms of acid maltase deficiency, the serum CK level is 2 to 10 times normal. EMG examination demonstrates a myopathic pattern, but other features are especially distinctive, including myotonic discharges, trains of fibrillation and positive waves, and complex repetitive discharges. EMG discharges are very prominent in the lumbosacral paraspinal muscles. The muscle biopsy shows vacuoles containing glycogen and the lysosomal enzyme acid phosphatase. Electron microscopy reveals membrane-bound and free tissue glycogen. Definitive diagnosis is established by enzyme determination in muscle.

No satisfactory treatment exists for acid maltase deficiency. A high-protein diet has been advocated, but efficacy has not been documented. Intravenous enzyme replacement has not shown benefit.

In *debranching enzyme deficiency (type III glycogenosis)*, a slowly progressive form of muscle weakness can develop after puberty. Rarely, myoglobinuria may be seen. Patients are usually diagnosed in infancy, however, because of hypotonia and delayed motor milestones, hepatomegaly, growth retardation, and hypoglycemia. *Branching enzyme deficiency (type IV glycogenosis)* is a rare and fatal glycogen storage disease characterized by failure to thrive and hepatomegaly. Hypotonia and muscle wasting may be present, but the skeletal muscle manifestations are minor compared to liver failure.

Disorders of Glycolysis Causing Exercise Intolerance Five glycolytic defects are associated with recurrent myoglobinuria: *myophosphorylase deficiency (type V glycogenosis), phosphofructokinase deficiency (type VII glycogenosis), phosphoglycerate kinase deficiency (type IX glycogenosis), phosphoglycerate mutase deficiency (type X glycogenosis)*, and *lactate dehydrogenase deficiency (glycogenosis type XI)*. The features of these conditions are summarized in Table 383-3. Myophosphorylase deficiency, also known as McArdle's disease, is by far the most common of the glycolytic defects associated with exercise intolerance. All are inherited as autosomal recessive traits, except for phosphoglycerate kinase deficiency, which is X-linked recessive. These five glycolytic defects result in a common failure to support energy production at the initiation of exercise, although the exact site of energy failure remains controversial.

Clinical manifestations in these five conditions usually begin in adolescence. Symptoms are precipitated by brief bursts of high-intensity exercise, such as running or lifting heavy objects. A history of myalgia and muscle stiffness usually precedes the intensely painful muscle contractures, which may be followed by myoglobinuria. Acute renal failure accompanies significant pigmenturia. Exercise tolerance can be enhanced by a slow induction phase (warm-up) or brief periods of rest allowing for the start of the "second-wind" phenomenon (switching to utilization of fatty acids).

Certain features help distinguish some enzyme defects. Varying degrees of hemolytic anemia accompany deficiencies of both phosphofructokinase (mild) and phosphoglycerate kinase (severe). In phosphoglycerate kinase deficiency, the usual clinical presentation is a seizure disorder associated with mental retardation; exercise intolerance is an infrequent manifestation.

In all of these conditions, the serum CK levels fluctuate widely and may be elevated even during symptom-free periods. CK levels over 200 times normal are expected accompanying myoglobinuria. All patients with suspected glycolytic defects leading to exercise intolerance should undergo a forearm exercise test (see Griggs et al. for details). Impaired rise in venous lactate is highly indicative of a glycolytic defect. In lactate dehydrogenase deficiency, venous levels of lactate will not increase, but pyruvate will rise to normal, after forearm exercise. In all glycolytic defects, a definitive diagnosis is made by analysis of muscle removed by biopsy.

Training may enhance the second-wind phenomenon, but attempts to raise blood glucose or to modify these disorders through diet have not been shown to be beneficial.

DISORDERS OF LIPID METABOLISM

Lipid is an important muscle energy source during rest and during prolonged, submaximal exercise. Fatty acids are derived from circulating very low density lipoprotein (VLDL) in the blood or from triglycerides stored in muscle fibers. Oxidation of fatty acids occurs in the mitochondria. To enter the mitochondria, a fatty acid must first be converted to an "activated fatty acid," acyl-CoA. The acyl-CoA must be linked with carnitine by the enzyme carnitine palmitoyltransferase (CPT) I for transport into the mitochondria. CPT 1 is present on the inner side of the outer mitochondrial membrane. Carnitine is removed by CPT II, an enzyme attached to the inside of the inner mitochondrial membrane, allowing transport of acyl-CoA into the mitochondrial matrix for β-oxidation.

CARNITINE DEFICIENCY Deficiency of this important substrate results in a myopathic and a systemic disorder.

Myopathic carnitine deficiency is associated with generalized muscle weakness, usually beginning in childhood. The clinical features overlap with those of muscular dystrophy and polymyositis. Patients develop progressive, painless proximal weakness. A severe cardiomyopathy may be present. Serum CK levels may be mildly to markedly (greater than 10-fold) elevated. The muscle biopsy shows striking lipid accumulation. Serum carnitine is normal. The cause for decreased muscle carnitine is not understood. Most cases are sporadic, but the inheritance pattern is thought to be autosomal recessive. Some patients respond to oral carnitine supplementation; this treatment should be tried in all cases. Other patients have responded to prednisone, riboflavin, or propranolol. A diet substituting medium-chain for long-chain triglycerides has been helpful in some cases.

Systemic carnitine deficiency usually presents in infancy and early childhood and is characterized by progressive weakness and episodes of hepatic encephalopathy with nausea, vomiting, confusion, coma, and early death. Carnitine levels are reduced in muscle, liver, kidney, and heart, but the low serum carnitine levels are especially useful in distinguishing this condition from the myopathic form. No single cause has been identified to explain the low serum carnitine levels. Decreased hepatic synthesis explains some cases, while increased urinary excretion is seen in others. Serum CK levels may be slightly elevated. The muscle biopsy may show lipid storage. In some cases, the liver, heart, and kidney show increased lipid. Treatment with oral carnitine supplementation or glucocorticoid administration has helped some, but not all, patients.

Secondary carnitine deficiency accompanies a variety of disorders in which carnitine deficiency is caused by decreased synthesis (cirrhosis), insufficient intake (parenteral nutrition), or excessive loss (renal dialysis, Fanconi's syndrome, or organic acidemia). Carnitine deficiency may also be seen in the muscular dystrophies, where it is thought to be a nonspecific result of loss of muscle tissue. Carnitine treatment has not been shown to clearly benefit patients with these secondary syndromes.

CARNITINE PALMITYOLTRANSFERASE DEFICIENCY
This disorder is the most common recognizable cause of recurrent myoglobinuria, more common than the glycolytic defects.

Clinical Features This disorder usually has its onset in the teenage years or early twenties. Muscle pain and myoglobinuria occur after prolonged exercise. Fasting predisposes to the development of symptoms. In contrast to disorders caused by defects in glycolysis, in which muscle cramps follow short, intense bursts of exercise, the muscle pain in CPT deficiency does not occur until the limits of utilization have been exceeded and muscle breakdown has already begun. Episodes of rhabdomyolysis may produce severe weakness. In contrast to carnitine deficiency, strength is normal between attacks.

Laboratory Findings Serum CK levels and EMG findings are both usually normal between episodes. A normal rise of venous lactate during forearm exercise distinguishes this condition from glycolytic defects, especially phosphorylase deficiency. Muscle biopsy does not show lipid accumulation and is usually normal between attacks. The diagnosis requires direct measurement of muscle CPT.

Genetics CPT deficiency is much more common in men than women (5:1); nevertheless, all evidence indicates autosomal recessive inheritance. A mutation in the gene for CPT II causes the disease in some individuals.

Rx TREATMENT
It has been suggested that frequent meals and a low-fat, high-carbohydrate diet can prolong exercise tolerance. Others suggest substituting medium-chain triglycerides in the diet. Neither approach has proven benefits.

Table 383-3

Glycolytic Defects Causing Exercise Intolerance

Enzyme Deficiency	Genetics	Clinical Features	Laboratory Features
Myophosphorylas deficiency (McArdle's disease)	Autosomal recessive; maps to chromosome 11	Exercise intolerance; myoglobinuria; male predominance	Elevated serum CK level No lactate rise on forearm exercise test Muscle weakness in 30%
Phosphofructokinase deficiency (Tarui's disease)	Autosomal recessive; maps to chromosome 1	Exercise intolerance; myoglobinuria; male predominance	Elevated serum CK level No lactate rise on forearm exercise test Mild hemolytic anemia
Phosphoglycerate kinase deficiency	X-linked recessive	*Most common presentation:* seizures, mental retardation, hemolytic anemia *Less commonly,* presentation includes exercise intolerance, myoglobinuria	Elevated serum CK level No lactate rise on forearm exercise test Hemolytic anemia
Phosphoglycerate mutase deficiency	Autosomal recessive	Exercise intolerance; myoglobinuria	Elevated serum CK level No lactate rise on forearm exercise test
Lactate dehydrogenase deficiency	Autosomal recessive, maps to chromosome 11	Exercise intolerance; myoglobinuria	Elevated serum CK level No lactate rise on forearm exercise test, *but* normal pyruvate rise

MYOADENYLATE DEAMINASE DEFICIENCY The muscle enzyme myoadenylate deaminase converts adenosine 5'-monophosphate (5'-AMP) to inosine monophosphate (IMP) with liberation of ammonia. Myoadenylate deaminase may play a role in regulating adenosine triphosphate (ATP) levels in muscles. Most subjects with myoadenylate deaminase deficiency have no symptoms. Many questions have been raised about the clinical effects of myoadenylate deaminase deficiency, and specifically its relationship to exertional myalgia and fatigability, but there is no consensus. There have been a few reports of patients with this disorder who have exercise-exacerbated myalgia and myoglobinuria. The full clinical significance of myoadenylate deaminase deficiency has not been established.

MITOCHONDRIAL MYOPATHIES

In 1972, Olson and colleagues recognized that muscle fibers with significant numbers of abnormal mitochondria could be highlighted using the modified trichrome stain; the term "ragged red fibers" was coined. By electron microscopy, the mitochondria in ragged red fibers are enlarged and often bizarrely shaped and have crystalline inclusions. Since that seminal observation, the understanding of these disorders of muscle (and other tissues, e.g., Leber's hereditary optic atrophy) has expanded (see also Chap. 380).

Mitochondria play a key role in energy production. Oxidation of the major nutrients derived from carbohydrate, fat, and protein leads to the generation of reducing equivalents (2H). The latter are transported through the respiratory chain in the process known as oxidative phosphorylation. The energy generated by the oxidation-reduction reactions of the respiratory chain is stored in an electrochemical gradient coupled to ATP synthesis.

A novel feature of mitochondria is their genetic composition. Each mitochondrion possesses a DNA genome that is distinct from that of the nuclear DNA. Human mitochondrial DNA (mtDNA) consists of a double-stranded, circular molecule comprising 16,569 base pairs. It codes for 22 transfer RNAs, 2 ribosomal RNAs, and 13 polypeptides of the respiratory chain enzymes. The genetics of mitochondrial diseases differs from those of chromosomal disorders. The DNA of mitochondria is directly inherited from the cytoplasm of the gametes, mainly from the oocyte. The sperm contributes very little of its mitochondria to the offspring at the time of fertilization. Thus, mitochondrial genes are derived almost exclusively from the mother, accounting for maternal inheritance of some mitochondrial disorders.

mtDNA DISORDERS OF MUSCLE Many different classifications of mitochondrial myopathies are possible. A convenient scheme allows for disorders to be grouped by the type of mtDNA mutation: deletions or point mutations (see also Chap. 380).

Disorders Associated with mtDNA Deletions The *Kearns-Sayre syndrome* (KSS) is a sporadic, noninherited disorder with onset before age 20. The characteristic findings include a triad of clinical features: progressive external ophthalmoplegia, pigmentary degeneration of the retina, and heart block. Some patients have only extraocular manifestations. KSS patients may also have short stature, ataxia, dementia, sensorineural hearing loss, diabetes, and hypothyroidism. In KSS, two populations of mtDNA, wild-type and mutant, are present in the same cell; the mutations in the latter consist of *single mtDNA deletions*. Heteroplasmy can be recognized on Southern blot analysis. The highest percentage of deleted mtDNA can be detected in postmitotic tissues, especially skeletal muscle. Other tissues can harbor the mutation (e.g., peripheral blood leukocytes, brain, liver, and fibroblasts). The absence of mutant mtDNA reflects both mitotic segregation early in embryogenesis and selection against a mutant cell line in a rapidly dividing tissue. KSS is not inherited, since mutations leading to an affected individual take place in the fertilized ovum.

Patients with *Pearson's marrow-pancreas syndrome*, a disorder of infancy characterized by refractory sideroblastic anemia and exocrine pancreatic dysfunction, may develop features of KSS in adolescence. Single mtDNA deletions account for Pearson's marrow-pancreas syndrome.

An *autosomal dominant disorder with progressive external ophthalmoplegia and proximal weakness* shares clinical features with KSS: hearing loss, ataxia, peripheral neuropathy, mental retardation, and hypoparathyroidism. Some of these patients also exhibit weakness of respiratory muscles, exercise intolerance, cataracts, and early death. The patients have ragged red fibers on muscle biopsy and *multiple mtDNA deletions*, rather than single deletions as in KSS. The mutation accounting for the autosomal dominant inheritance occurs in a *nuclear gene* that encodes a protein involved in the control of mtDNA replication. A failure or disruption of binding of this nuclear-encoded protein during mtDNA replication results in multiple deletions.

Disorders Associated with mtDNA Point Mutations *Myoclonic epilepsy and ragged red fibers*, called the *MERRF syndrome*, consists of mitochondrial myopathy, myoclonus, generalized seizures, intellectual deterioration, ataxia, and hearing loss. Extraocular movements are normal in MERRF. As with other mitochondrial disorders, individuals display varying manifestations of the disease. MERRF syndrome is maternally inherited. Most often, point mutations in the lysine transfer RNA gene of mtDNA can be found. This abnormality can be detected in mtDNA isolated from peripheral blood leukocytes or skeletal muscle and is useful for clinical diagnosis and genetic counseling. These mutations alter the normal conformation of the transfer RNA, impairing translation probably at the ribosomal level.

Mitochondrial myopathy, encephalopathy, lactic acidosis, and stroke-like episodes are referred to by the acronym *MELAS*. This disorder is a multisystem mitochondrial encephalomyopathy that begins in childhood after normal birth and early development. Patients have stunted growth and recurrent stroke-like episodes manifesting as hemiparesis, hemianopia, or cortical blindness. Episodic vomiting may occur, and some patients have hearing loss. Focal or generalized seizures and myoclonic epilepsy may be present. Full expression of the disease leads to dementia, a bedridden state, and death often before age 20. Lactic acidosis may be present. MELAS can be maternally inherited, but sporadic cases are common. No large pedigrees have been reported. In 80 to 90 percent of patients, a point mutation of the leucine transfer RNA gene of mtDNA has been identified at nucleotide 3243. Some patients with this same mutation have only diabetes mellitus and hearing loss. Rarely, an mtDNA mutation of subunit 4 of complex I (ND4) of the respiratory chain causes MELAS. Mutation analysis provides a specific diagnostic test that can be performed on peripheral blood leukocytes or skeletal muscle.

A clinical syndrome with combined features of *skeletal and cardiac myopathies associated with lactic acidosis* that is distinct from MELAS has been described with a point mutation at nucleotide 3260 of the leucine transfer RNA gene of mtDNA.

ENDOCRINE AND METABOLIC MYOPATHIES

Many endocrine disorders cause weakness. Muscle fatigue is more common than true weakness. The cause of weakness in these disorders is not well defined. It is not even clear that weakness results from disease of muscle as opposed to another part of the motor unit since the serum CK level is often normal (except in hypothyroidism), and the muscle histology is characterized by atrophy rather than destruction of muscle fibers. Nearly all endocrine myopathies respond to treatment.

THYROID DISORDERS (See Chap. 331) Abnormalities of thyroid function can cause a wide array of muscle disorders. These conditions relate to the important role of thyroid hormones in regulating the metabolism of carbohydrates and lipids as well as the rate of protein synthesis and enzyme production. Thyroid hormones also stimulate calorigenesis in muscle, increase muscle demand for vitamins, and enhance muscle sensitivity to circulating catecholamines.

Hypothyroidism Hypothyroid patients have frequent muscle complaints, and proximal muscle weakness occurs in about one-third of patients. Muscle cramps, pain, and stiffness occur commonly. Features of slow muscle contraction and relaxation occur in 25 percent of patients, and the relaxation phase of muscle stretch reflexes is characteristically prolonged. The serum CK level is often elevated (up to 10 times normal), even when there is minimal clinical evidence of muscle disease. In both children and adults, a distinct syndrome has been described. Severely hypothyroid children, especially boys, may have the Debré-Kocher-Sémélaigne syndrome, characterized by weakness, slowness of movement, and striking muscle hypertrophy, causing an "infant Hercules appearance." In adult hypothyroidism, Hoffman's syndrome results in prominent muscle enlargement and weakness with muscle stiffness. The cause of muscle enlargement in these two syndromes has not been determined. The muscle biopsy shows only muscle atrophy.

Hyperthyroidism Thyrotoxic patients commonly have proximal muscle weakness and atrophy on examination, but they rarely complain of the deficit. Muscle stretch reflexes are preserved and often brisk. Bulbar, respiratory, and even esophageal muscles may occasionally be affected, causing dysphagia, dysphonia, and aspiration. When bulbar involvement occurs, it is usually accompanied by chronic proximal limb weakness, but occasionally it presents in the absence of generalized thyrotoxic myopathy. Other neuromuscular disorders occur in association with hyperthyroidism, including periodic paralysis, myasthenia gravis, and a progressive ocular myopathy associated with proptosis (Graves' ophthalmopathy). Serum CK levels are low in thyrotoxic myopathy. The muscle histology usually shows only atrophy of muscle fibers.

PARATHYROID DISORDERS (See Chap. 354) **Hyperparathyroidism** Muscle weakness is an integral part of primary and secondary hyperparathyroidism. Proximal muscle weakness, muscle wasting, and brisk muscle stretch reflexes are the main features of this endocrinopathy. Serum CK levels are usually normal or slightly elevated. Serum calcium and phosphorus levels show no correlation with the clinical neuromuscular manifestations. Muscle biopsies show only varying degrees of atrophy without muscle fiber degeneration.

Hypoparathyroidism An overt myopathy due to hypocalcemia is rarely seen. Neuromuscular symptoms are usually related to localized or generalized tetany. Serum CK levels may be increased secondary to muscle damage following tetany. Hyporeflexia or areflexia is usually present and contrasts with the hyperreflexia seen in hyperparathyroidism.

ADRENAL DISORDERS (See Chap. 332)   Conditions associated with glucocorticoid excess cause a myopathy and, in fact, steroid myopathy is the most commonly diagnosed endocrine muscle disease. Steroid excess, either endogenous or exogenous (see "Toxic Myopathies," below), produces varying degrees of proximal limb weakness. Muscle wasting may be striking. A cushingoid appearance invariably precedes or accompanies clinical signs of myopathy. Histologic sections demonstrate muscle fiber atrophy rather than degeneration or necrosis of muscle fibers. Adrenal insufficiency commonly causes muscle fatigue. Objective weakness occurs less often and is typically mild.

In primary hyperaldosteronism, or Conn's syndrome, neuromuscular complications are due to potassium depletion. The clinical picture is one of persistent muscle weakness. Long-standing hyperaldosteronism may lead to proximal limb weakness and wasting. Serum CK levels may be elevated, and a muscle biopsy may demonstrate degenerating fibers, some with vacuoles. These changes relate to hypokalemia and are not a direct effect of aldosterone on skeletal muscle.

PITUITARY DISORDERS (See Chap. 328)   Patients with acromegaly usually show mild proximal weakness without muscle atrophy. Muscles often appear enlarged, but they have decreased forced generation. The duration of acromegaly, rather than the serum growth hormone levels, correlates with the degree of myopathy.

DIABETES MELLITUS (See Chap. 334)   Neuromuscular complications of diabetes mellitus are most often related to neuropathy with cranial and peripheral nerve palsies or distal sensorimotor polyneuropathy. "Diabetic amyotrophy" is now known to be a neuropathy affecting the proximal major nerve trunks and lumbosacral plexus. More appropriate terms for this disorder include *diabetic proximal neuropathy* and *lumbosacral plexopathy*.

The only notable myopathy of diabetes mellitus is ischemic infarction of thigh muscles. This condition occurs in patients with poorly controlled diabetes and presents with acute onset of pain, tenderness, and edema of one thigh with a palpable mass. The muscles most often affected include the vastus lateralis, thigh adductors, and biceps femoris. Computed tomography or magnetic resonance imaging can demonstrate focal abnormalities in the affected muscle. Imaging of the muscle may render muscle biopsy unnecessary.

VITAMIN DEFICIENCY   Vitamin D deficiency causes the only myopathy that occurs as an integral part of a vitamin deficiency. Vitamin D deficiency (see Chaps. 79 and 353) due to either decreased intake, decreased absorption, or impaired vitamin D metabolism (as occurs in renal disease) may lead to chronic muscle weakness. Pain reflects the underlying bone disease (osteomalacia). It has not been established that deficiency of other vitamins causes a myopathy.

MYOPATHIES OF SYSTEMIC ILLNESS   Systemic illnesses such as chronic respiratory, cardiac, or hepatic failure are frequently associated with severe muscle wasting and complaints of weakness. Strength testing often demonstrates mild weakness in such patients. Lack of endurance is a more significant problem.

Myopathy may be a manifestation of chronic renal failure, independent of the better known uremic polyneuropathy. Abnormalities of calcium and phosphorus homeostasis and bone metabolism in chronic renal failure result from a reduction in 1,25-dihydroxyvitamin D, leading to decreased intestinal absorption of calcium. Hypocalcemia, further accentuated by hyperphosphatemia due to decreased renal phosphate clearance, leads to secondary hyperparathyroidism. Renal osteodystrophy results from the compensatory hyperparathyroidism, which leads to osteomalacia from reduced calcium availability and to osteitis fibrosa from the parathyroid hormone excess. The clinical picture of the myopathy of chronic renal failure is identical to that of primary hyperparathyroidism and osteomalacia. There is proximal limb weakness with bone pain.

Gangrenous calcification represents a separate, rare, and sometimes fatal complication of chronic renal failure. In this condition, widespread arterial calcification occurs and results in ischemia. Extensive skin necrosis may occur along with painful myopathy and even myoglobinuria.

TOXIC MYOPATHIES

The classification of toxic myopathies is shown in Table 383-4. Drugs and chemicals may produce focal or generalized damage of skeletal muscle.

The most common cause of focal damage is the injection of narcotic analgesics. Three agents in particular—pentazocine, meperidine, and heroin—may cause a severe fibrotic reaction in muscle. Common injection sites include deltoid, triceps, gluteus maximus, and quadriceps muscles. The muscles become indurated and may have local abscess formation. Cutaneous ulcerations and depressions may occur. Severe joint contractures may develop.

Other drugs may induce generalized muscle weakness, particularly affecting the proximal muscles. In most cases the exact mechanism of drug toxicity is poorly understood. D-Penicillamine induces a condition simulating the clinical and pathologic picture of polymyositis. A similar condition has been reported with cimetidine. Procainamide may cause myositis as part of a systemic lupus–like reaction. Chloroquine administration may cause a vacuolar myopathy.

Zidovudine, used in the treatment of AIDS, produces proximal weakness and pain. On muscle biopsy, zidovudine myopathy demonstrates a distinctive pathologic alteration of skeletal muscle, affecting mitochondria and resembling ragged red fibers. In some patients, reintroduction of zidovudine in lower doses may be tolerated.

The cholesterol-lowering agents, including clofibrate, lovastatin, pravastatin, gemfibrozil, and niacin, have all been implicated as causes of myopathy. The hydroxymethylglutaryl-CoA (HMG-CoA) inhibitors, either alone or in combination with gemfibrozil, have caused rhabdomyolysis and myoglobinuria. Emetine hydrochloride (used for treatment of amebiasis), ε-aminocaproic acid (an antifibrinolytic agent), and perhexiline (used for angina pectoris) have all been observed to cause muscle weakness and muscle fiber necrosis following several weeks of therapy.

Drug-induced myopathy accompanied by proximal weakness occurs with glucocorticoid therapy. Glucocorticoid drugs fluorinated in the 9α-position, such as triamcinolone, dexamethasone, and betamethasone, are most likely to cause weakness, but chronic administration of any glucocorticoid, including prednisone, causes weakness. Divided-dose, as opposed to single-morning-dose, regimens produce more severe weakness. A single-dose, alternate-day regimen is yet less toxic. The clinical diagnosis of steroid-induced muscle weakness can be difficult if the medication is being used to treat an underlying inflammatory myopathy. The presence of a normal serum CK level, minimal or no changes of myopathy on EMG, and type 2 muscle fiber atrophy on biopsy are helpful in suggesting steroid-induced weakness.

Excess alcohol intake causes acute muscle weakness with rhabdomyolysis and myoglobinuria by several different mechanisms, including prolonged obtundation, seizures, hypokalemia, and hypophos-

---

Table 383-4

Toxic Myopathies

Causes of focal myopathies
  Pentazocine, meperdine, heroin
Causes of generalized myopathies
  Myotonia: propranolol, cyclosporine, iodides, clofibrate, penicillamine
  Elevated serum creatinine kinase without weakness: clofibrate, lovastatin
  Inflammatory: cimetidine, penicillamine, procainamide
  Muscle weakness and myalgias: chloroquine, clofibrate, colchicine, cyclosporine, emetine, ε-aminocaproic acid, glucocorticoids, labetalol, niacin, perhexilline, propranolol, vincristine, zidovudine
  Rhabdomyolysis and myoglobinuria: alcohol, amphetamine, barbiturates, clofibrate, cocaine, ε-aminocaproic acid, gemfibrozil, heroin, lovastatin, phencyclidine
  Malignant hyperthermia: ethyl chloride, ethylene, diethyl ether, gallamine, halothane, lidocaine, mepivacaine, methoxylflurane, trichloroethylene, succinylcholine

phatemia. The existence of a chronic myopathy causing slowly progressive weakness in this setting is controversial. Alcoholics often have chronic weakness resulting from neuropathy and poor nutrition.

A very serious drug-induced condition, *malignant hyperthermia*, occurs in susceptible individuals following exposure to certain general anesthetic and depolarizing muscle relaxants (Table 383-4). The local anesthetic amides, including lidocaine and mepivacaine, have also been implicated as precipitating agents.

PERIODIC PARALYSIS

Recent discoveries of the molecular defects in the primary periodic paralyses provide insight into their pathogenesis and form the basis for their classification. The major disorders constituting this group have some features in common (Table 383-5). Onset is usually early in life; episodic weakness *beginning* after age 25 is almost never due to periodic paralysis. Attacks typically occur after rest or sleep and almost never in the midst of vigorous activity, although antecedent exercise often provokes weakness. Patients remain alert during the attacks. Early in the course of these disorders, interattack strength is normal. After many years of attacks, interictal weakness develops and may be progressive. These disorders are amenable to treatment, and progressive weakness can be prevented and even reversed. Diagnosis is based on patient history and confirmed by appropriate evaluation of serum electrolytes during attacks, by evaluation of the response of strength to provocative testing with glucose, insulin, potassium, and cold, or by DNA analysis of the appropriate gene (Table 383-5).

CALCIUM CHANNEL DISORDERS OF MUSCLE **Hypokalemic Periodic Paralysis** Hypokalemic periodic paralysis (hypoKPP) causes episodic weakness, which usually affects proximal limb muscles more than distal ones; rarely, ocular, bulbar, or respiratory muscles are affected. Respiratory muscle weakness may prove fatal. Meals high in carbohydrate or sodium can provoke attacks. Reflexes become hypoactive, and cardiac arrhythmias may occur during attacks owing to low serum potassium. Men are more often affected because of decreased penetrance in women.

Diagnosis is established by demonstrating a low serum potassium level during a paralytic attack and by excluding secondary causes of hypokalemia. The molecular defect in the calcium channel can be defined in many patients. Muscle biopsy often shows the presence of single or multiple centrally placed vacuoles. Patients whose attacks are too infrequent for study of a spontaneous attack to be feasible

require provocative testing with glucose and insulin administration. Provocative tests are potentially hazardous and require careful monitoring.

The pathogenesis of paralytic attacks in hypoKPP is incompletely understood, even though mutations in the skeletal muscle calcium channel have been identified. The contractile apparatus is normal. The effects of insulin on potassium uptake in muscle suggest that an abnormality of the muscle membrane is involved. Weakness is often severe at levels of serum potassium that do not affect normal individuals. Moreover, attacks may occur when insulin levels are low.

The acute paralysis improves following the administration of potassium salts. Oral KCl (0.2 to 0.4 mmol/kg) should be given to patients with severe weakness and repeated at 15- to 30-min intervals depending on the response of the ECG, serum potassium, and muscle strength. Milder attacks usually resolve spontaneously. When patients are unable to swallow or are vomiting, intravenous therapy may be necessary. Small, repeated boluses of KCl (0.1 mmol/kg) may be administered over 5 to 10 min with careful monitoring of the ECG and serum potassium. If potassium is administered as a dilute solution (20 to 40 mmol/L) in 5% glucose or in physiologic saline solution, serum potassium may decline, and weakness may worsen. Mannitol is the preferred vehicle for administered intravenous potassium in such situations, since it facilitates rapid return of serum potassium to normal and will not cause the lowering of serum potassium that may occur when glucose or saline solutions are given.

The goal of therapy is to eliminate attacks, which also prevents interattack weakness. Before effective means of attack prevention became available, chronic progressive interattack weakness frequently caused serious disability. Prophylactic administration of potassium salts, even in large doses, does not prevent attacks, but acetazolamide (125 to 1000 mg/d in divided doses) abolishes attacks in most cases. The metabolic acidosis induced by acetazolamide may underlie the beneficial effect. Paradoxically, acetazolamide lowers the serum potassium level; to achieve an adequate response in some patients, it may be necessary to give supplementary potassium along with acetazolamide and to avoid high-carbohydrate meals. Chronic acetazolamide treatment may be associated with renal calculi, and patients should be monitored for this complication. In occasional patients, attacks may not respond to or may even be worsened by acetazolamide. In such patients, triamterene (25 to 100 mg/d) or spironolactone (25 to 100 mg/d) may prevent attacks.

SODIUM CHANNEL DISORDERS OF MUSCLE **Hyperkalemic Periodic Paralysis** Hyperkalemic periodic paralysis (hyperKPP) causes episodic weakness of limb muscles; cranial and respiratory muscles are rarely involved. The term "hyperkalemic" is misleading, since patients are often normokalemic during attacks. It is the fact that attacks are precipitated by potassium administration that best defines the disorder. Paresthesia and muscle pain are present during many attacks.

Diagnosis is suggested by a modest elevation of serum potassium during attacks in nearly half of patients; at times, however, the serum potassium is normal or even low. The so-called hyperkalemic and normokalemic forms of this disorder are not separate entities. Intravenous glucose-insulin loading does not precipitate weakness, but potassium-loading tests (0.05 to 0.15 g/kg) will induce weakness in such patients. Potassium-loading tests are potentially hazardous and are contraindicated in patients with renal disease and diabetes. Random serum potassium measurements may suggest the diagnosis, since potassium elevations are frequent during attack-free intervals. Electromyographic evidence

Table 383-5

Disorders Causing Periodic Paralysis

Feature	Hypokalemic Periodic Paralysis	Hyperkalemic Periodic Paralysis	Paramyotonia Congenita
Mode of inheritance	Autosomal dominant (67%) or sporadic (33%)	Autosomal dominant	Autosomal dominant
Myotonia	Eyelid only	Usually	Yes
Age of onset	Teens (invariably <30 years)	Infancy	Infancy
Attack frequency	Daily to yearly	Ranges from twice to thrice daily	With cold exposure; spontaneous attack rate <1/month
Attack duration	2–12 h (rarely longer)	1–2 h (occasionally longer)	2–24 h
Serum K⁺ level during attack	Decreased	Normal or increased (rarely low)	Normal or decreased (rarely elevated)
Effect of K⁺ loading	No change	Weakness	No change (occasionally weakness)
Effect of muscle cooling	No change	No change	Weakness
Fixed weakness occurs	Yes	Yes	Yes
Site of molecular defect	Calcium channel	Sodium channel	Sodium channel

of myotonia and the finding of vacuoles on muscle biopsy provide supporting data.

Paramyotonia Congenita Paramyotonia congenita (PC) causes attacks of paralysis either spontaneously or with cold provocation. PC with periodic paralysis is similar to hyperKPP except that it is characterized by paradoxical myotonia (i.e., myotonia worsening with activity) and objective cold sensitivity. Mutations in the skeletal muscle voltage-gated sodium channel SCN4A cause hyperKPP and PC (Fig. 383-2). In vitro study of these mutations demonstrates increased sodium conductance through the channels, which is consistent with findings in patient muscle samples.

In PC, attacks of weakness are seldom severe enough to require emergency treatment and are never fatal. Oral administration of glucose or other carbohydrate hastens recovery. Since interattack weakness may develop after repeated attacks, prophylactic treatment is usually indicated in PC. Thiazide diuretics (e.g., chlorothiazide, 250 to 1000 mg/d) are reported to be effective.

DISORDERS OF UNKNOWN PATHOGENETIC MECHANISM Thyrotoxic Periodic Paralysis This disorder is clinically indistinguishable from hypoKPP. It is common in young Latin American and Asian men, among whom up to 10 percent of thyrotoxic patients may have this condition. The thyrotoxicosis may be overlooked for many months. Occasionally, the only indication of thyrotoxicosis is a depressed level of thyroid-stimulating hormone. Acute attacks respond to potassium administration. Treatment of the underlying thyrotoxicosis abolishes attacks. Beta-adrenergic blocking agents are useful for reducing the frequency and severity of attacks while measures to control thyrotoxicosis are instituted. Acetazolamide is not helpful in preventing attacks. The pathogenesis of thyrotoxic periodic paralysis is uncertain, but there is evidence for a decrease in the activity of the calcium pump.

Andersen's Syndrome This is a rare disorder in which patients manifest periodic paralysis (hyperkalemic or hypokalemic), cardiac dysrhythmias (even when normokalemic), and dysmorphic features. Treatment of the episodic weakness is the same as for the other periodic paralyses, although cardiac status must be considered as well.

BIBLIOGRAPHY

BAROHN RJ: Distal myopathies and dystrophies. Semin Neurol 13:247, 1993

BRITTON CH et al: Human liver mitochondrial carnitine palmitoyltransferase I: Characterization of its cDNA and chromosomal localization and partial analysis of the gene. Proc Natl Acad Sci USA 92:1984, 1995

CAMPBELL KP: Adhalin gene mutations and autosomal recessive limb-girdle muscular dystrophy. Ann Neurol 38:353, 1995

CANNON SC: Ion-channel defects and aberrant excitability in myotonia and periodic paralysis. Trends Neurosci 19:3, 1996

DiMAURO S: Mitochondrial encephalomyopathies, in *The Molecular and Genetic Basis of Neurologic Disease*, RN Rosenberg et al (eds). Boston, Butterworth-Heinemann, 1993

DUBOWITZ V: The congenital myopathies, in *Muscle Disorders*, 2d ed, V Dubowitz (ed). London, Saunders, 1995

ELBAZ A et al: Hypokalemic periodic paralysis and the dihydropyridine receptor (CACNL1A3): Genotype/phenotype correlations for two predominant mutations and evidence for the absence of a founder effect in 16 Caucasian families. Am J Hum Genet 56:374, 1995

GRIGGS RC et al: The muscular dystrophies, in *Evaluation and Treatment of Myopathies*, RC Griggs et al (eds). Philadelphia, FA Davis, 1995

HELBLING-LECLERC A et al: Mutations in the laminin alpha$_2$-chain gene (LAMA2) cause merosin deficient congenital muscular dystrophy. Nat Genet 11:216, 1995

KISSEL JT et al: Endocrine myopathies, in *Handbook of Clinical Neurology*, vol 19, LP Rowland, S DiMauro (eds). New York, Elsevier, 1992

MENDELL JR et al: The childhood muscular dystrophies: Diseases sharing a common pathogenesis of membrane instability. J Child Neurol 10:150, 1995

PRIOR TW et al: Spectrum of small mutations in the dystrophin coding region. Am J Hum Genet 57:22, 1995

PTÁČEK LJ et al: Sodium channel mutations in acetazolamide-responsive myotonia congenita, paramyotonia congenita and hyperkalemic periodic paralysis. Neurology 44:1500, 1994

QUANE KA et al: Mutations in the ryanodine receptor gene in central core disease and malignant hyperthermia. Nat Genet 5:51, 1993

TAWIL R et al: Andersen's syndrome: Potassium-sensitive periodic paralysis, ventricular ectopy and dysmorphic features. Ann Neurol 35:326, 1994

VARDERIO E et al: Carnitine palmitoyltransferase II deficiency: Structure of the gene and characterization of two novel disease-causing mutations. Hum Mol Genet 4:19, 1995

FIGURE 383-2 The sodium channel is depicted here as a molecule containing four homologous domains. Each domain contains six putative membrane-spanning segments. The fourth segment of each domain is thought to act together as the "voltage sensor" for the channel and is cross-hatched in the figure. The tertiary structure of the protein in the membrane and the association of these segments is thought to form a pore through which ions could pass. Mutations that have been identified are shown along with the phenotype that they confer.

SECTION 4

CHRONIC FATIGUE SYNDROME

---

384 *Stephen E. Straus*

CHRONIC FATIGUE SYNDROME

DEFINITION *Chronic fatigue syndrome* is the current name for a disorder characterized by debilitating fatigue and a variety of associated physical, constitutional, and neuropsychological complaints (Table 384-1). The medical literature of the past three centuries informs us that this is not a new type of syndrome. Certain individuals, who were labeled in the past with diagnoses such as the vapors, neurasthe-

nia, effort syndrome, hyperventilation syndrome, chronic brucellosis, epidemic neuromyasthenia, myalgic encephalomyelitis, hypoglycemia, multiple chemical sensitivity syndrome, chronic candidiasis, chronic mononucleosis, chronic Epstein-Barr virus infection, and postviral fatigue syndrome, probably had what we now call chronic fatigue syndrome. The U.S. Centers for Disease Control and Prevention (CDC) developed in 1988 and revised recently a case definition based predominantly on symptoms and on the exclusion of other illnesses (Table 384-2).

EPIDEMIOLOGY Patients with chronic fatigue syndrome are twice as likely to be women as men and are generally 25 to 45

Table 384-1

Approximate Percentage of Patients with the Chronic Fatigue
Syndrome Reporting the Specific Symptoms

Symptom	Percentage
Fatigue	100
Difficulty concentrating	90
Headache	90
Sore throat	85
Tender lymph nodes	80
Muscle aches	80
Joint aches	75
Feverishness	75
Difficulty sleeping	70
Psychiatric problems	65
Allergies	55
Abdominal cramps	40
Weight loss	20
Rash	10
Rapid pulse	10
Weight gain	5
Chest pain	5
Night sweats	5

SOURCE: From SE Straus: The chronic mononucleosis syndrome. J Infect Diseases 157:405, 1988.

years old, although cases in childhood and in middle age have been described.

Cases are recognized in many developed countries. Most arise sporadically, but over 30 clusters of similar illness have been reported. The most famous of such "outbreaks" occurred in Los Angeles County Hospital in 1934; in Akureyri, Iceland, in 1948; in the Royal Free Hospital, London, in 1955; in Punta Gorda, Florida, in 1956; and in Incline Village, Nevada, and surrounding communities in 1985. While these clustered cases suggest a common environmental or infectious cause, none has been identified.

The prevalence of chronic fatigue syndrome is difficult to ascertain, since its estimate depends entirely on case definition. Chronic fatigue itself is a ubiquitous symptom, occurring in as many as 20 percent of patients attending a general medical clinic; the chronic fatigue syndrome is far less common. The CDC estimated that its original case definition for chronic fatigue syndrome is met by 2 to 7 individuals per 100,000 population. The revised case definition eliminated many of the ambiguities and some of the restrictions of the original definition. Although this definition will be easier for the clinician to apply, a slightly greater percentage of fatigued people will fulfill the revised criteria.

PATHOGENESIS The diverse names for the syndrome reflect the equally numerous and controversial hypotheses about its etiology.

Table 384-2

Revised CDC Criteria for Chronic Fatigue Syndrome

A case of chronic fatigue syndrome is defined by the presence of:
1. Clinically evaluated, unexplained, persistent or relapsing fatigue that is of new or definite onset; is not the result of ongoing exertion; is not alleviated by rest; and results in substantial reduction of previous levels of occupational, educational, social, or personal activities; and
2. Four or more of the following symptoms that persist or recur during six or more consecutive months of illness and that do not predate the fatigue:
   - Self-reported impairment in short-term memory or concentration
   - Sore throat
   - Tender cervical or axillary nodes
   - Muscle pain
   - Multijoint pain without redness or swelling
   - Headaches of a new pattern or severity
   - Unrefreshing sleep
   - Postexertional malaise lasting ≥24 h

SOURCE: Adapted from Fukuda et al.

Several common themes underlie attempts to understand the disorder: It is often postinfectious, it is associated with immunologic disturbances, and it is commonly accompanied by depression.

Some contemporary workers in the field espouse one or more of several viruses as potential etiologic agents. Among these are lymphotropic herpesviruses, retroviruses, and enteroviruses. The data on which these presumptions rest are as follows: First, chronic fatigue syndrome can be precipitated by a variety of acute infections. Some of the infecting organisms have the ability to persist in humans and cause chronic illness. Second, titers of antibodies to many infectious agents are elevated in patients with chronic fatigue. Included are antibodies to most herpesviruses, measles virus, rubella virus, and coxsackievirus B. Third, there are claims of increased levels of some viral antigens and nucleic acids in patients, although these assertions are not based on firm experimental evidence. While experience suggests that viruses can precipitate the syndrome, it is unlikely that they actually contribute to its long-term features. Common, persisting viruses may simply have a greater likelihood to reactivate because of inadequate immune restraints on them, while causing no symptoms.

Numerous subtle immunologic disturbances have been reported in patients with chronic fatigue syndrome. In addition to the elevated viral antibody titers mentioned above, there are also mild, nonspecific elevations in titers of antinuclear antibodies, modest immunoglobulin subclass reductions, mild deficiencies in mitogen-induced lymphocyte proliferation in vitro and in ensuing cytokine release, reduced natural killer cell activity, and shifts in lymphocyte phenotypes to greater than normal proportions of T cells expressing activation or differentiation markers. None of the immune findings appear in all patients, nor have any been correlated, as yet, with the severity of illness. None are specific for chronic fatigue syndrome; thus they remain nondiagnostic. An immune disturbance of some type, though, is in line with one favored theory that many of the symptoms of chronic fatigue syndrome derive from excessive cytokine release.

Recent controlled studies of patients with chronic fatigue syndrome documented abnormalities in endocrine function consistent with reduced production of corticotropin-releasing hormone in the hypothalamus. Mean serum cortisol concentrations were lower in patients than in controls; levels of adrenocorticotropic hormone (ACTH) were correspondingly high. Hypothetically, these neuroendocrine abnormalities could contribute to the impaired energy and mood of patients. Whatever their importance, these changes further indicate the complex and multifactorial nature of chronic fatigue syndrome.

Mild to moderate depression is evident in about two-thirds of patients. Much of this depression may be reactive, but the prevalence exceeds that seen in other chronic medical illnesses. Thus, some propose that chronic fatigue syndrome is fundamentally a psychiatric disorder and that the various neuroendocrine and immune disturbances arise secondarily.

MANIFESTATIONS The typical case of chronic fatigue syndrome arises suddenly in a previously active individual. An otherwise unremarkable flulike illness or some other acute stress is recalled with great clarity as the triggering event. Unbearable exhaustion is left in the wake of this incident. Other symptoms, such as headache, sore throat, tender lymph nodes, muscle and joint aches, and frequent feverishness, lead to the belief that an infection persists, and medical attention is sought. Over several weeks, the impact of reassurances proffered during that initial evaluation fades as other features of the syndrome become evident—disturbed sleep, difficulty in concentration, and depression (see Table 384-1).

Depending on the dominant symptoms and the beliefs of the patient, additional consultations may be sought from allergists, rheumatologists, infectious disease specialists, psychiatrists, ecologic therapists, homeopaths, or other professionals, frequently with unsatisfactory results. Once the pattern of illness is established, the symptoms may fluctuate somewhat. Many patients report that diverse complaints are linked—that during periods of greatest fatigue they perceive the most pain and difficulty with concentration. Patients also commonly assert that excessive physical or emotional stress may exacerbate their symptoms.

Most patients remain capable of balancing their limited resources to accommodate the obligations of family, work, or community. The discretionary activities are abandoned first. Some feel unable to engage in any gainful employment. A minority of individuals require help with the activities of daily living.

Ultimately, isolation, pathetic resignation, and frustration can mark the protracted course of illness. Patients may become angry at physicians for failing to acknowledge or resolve their plight. Fortunately, the chronic fatigue syndrome does not appear to progress. On the contrary, many patients experience gradual improvement, and a minority recover fully.

DIAGNOSIS Physical examination and routine laboratory tests are required to rule out other possible causes of the patient's symptoms. Prominent findings argue strongly in favor of other processes. No laboratory test, however esoteric or exotic, can diagnose this condition or measure its severity. Elaborate, expensive workups should therefore be avoided except in research settings. The great dilemma for patient and clinician alike is that chronic fatigue syndrome has no pathognomonic features and remains a constellation of symptoms and a diagnosis of exclusion.

TREATMENT

The primary responsibility of a physician confronted with a chronically fatigued patient is to address the cause by taking a thorough history, conducting a complete physical examination, judiciously using the laboratory, and, throughout this process, considering the differential diagnosis. If other illnesses are excluded, there are several points to address in the long-term care of a patient with chronic fatigue.

First, the patient should be informed about the illness and what is truly known of its pathogenesis; its potential impact on the physical, psychological, and social dimensions of life; and its prognosis. Patients are relieved when their complaints are taken seriously.

Second, periodic reassessment is appropriate to identify a possible underlying process that is late in declaring itself and to address intercurrent problems that must not be neglected as yet another subjective complaint.

Third, many symptoms of chronic fatigue syndrome respond to treatment. Nonsteroidal anti-inflammatory drugs alleviate headache, diffuse pain, and feverishness. Allergic rhinitis and sinusitis are common in patients with chronic fatigue syndrome; antihistamines or decongestants may be helpful. Although patients are often averse to psychiatric diagnoses, depression is a prominent symptom that should be confronted. Expert psychiatric assessment is sometimes advisable. Nonsedating antidepressants improve mood and disordered sleep and thereby attenuate the fatigue somewhat. Even modest improvements in symptoms can make an important difference in the patient's degree of self-sufficiency and ability to appreciate life's pleasures.

Fourth, practical advice should be given regarding lifestyle. The consumption of heavy meals with alcohol and caffeine at night can make it harder to sleep, compounding fatigue. Total rest is harmful. It leads to further deconditioning and the self-image of being an invalid. Exacerbation of exhaustion by strenuous exertion leads to total avoidance of exercise, so a moderate, carefully graded regimen needs to be encouraged.

Fifth, unproven treatments should be avoided. Controlled trials have established that acyclovir and intramuscular liver extract–folic acid–cyanocobalamin injections are of no value. Despite one encouraging study, other studies and clinical experience argue that high-dose intravenous immunoglobulin therapy is of no value. Countless anecdotes circulate regarding other traditional or nontraditional therapies. It is important to guide patients, flexibly, away from those therapeutic modalities which are most toxic, expensive, and unreasonable.

The physician should promote the patient's efforts toward improvement. A clinical trial in England showed behavioral therapy to be helpful. The therapy was aimed at dispelling cognitive distortions that lead to inactivity and despair. For chronic fatigue syndrome, as for many conditions, a comprehensive approach to physical, psychological, and social aspects is in order.

BIBLIOGRAPHY

ACHESON ED: The clinical syndrome variously called benign myalgic encephalomyelitis, Iceland disease and epidemic neuromyasthenia. Am J Med 26:569, 1959
BOCK GR, WHELAN J (eds): Ciba Found Symp 173, 1993
FUKUDA K et al: The chronic fatigue syndrome: A comprehensive approach to its definition and study. Ann Intern Med 121:953, 1994
HOLMES GP et al: Chronic fatigue syndrome: A working case definition. Ann Intern Med 108:387, 1988
STRAUS SE (ed): *Chronic Fatigue Syndrome*. New York, Marcel Dekker, 1994

SECTION 5
PSYCHIATRIC DISORDERS

---

385 | *Victor I. Reus*

MENTAL DISORDERS

The term "mental disorders," as defined in the 4th edition of the standard psychiatric Diagnostic and Statistical Manual (DSM-IV), encompasses a broad range of conditions characterized by patterns of abnormal behavioral and psychological signs and symptoms that result in dysfunction. The implication that mental disorders lack a physical cause is unfortunate and incorrect, and the term survives only for want of a better substitute. Mental disorders are highly prevalent in medical practice, although frequently unrecognized and untreated, and may present as either a primary disorder or as a comorbid condition. Physicians must be prepared to initiate prompt diagnosis and treatment planning of mental disorders to ensure that their patients receive appropriate medical services and that they have the best outcome possible.

The current nosologic system is multiaxial and assesses the presence or absence of a major mental disorder (axis I), any underlying personality disorder (axis II), general medical condition (axis III), psychosocial and environmental problems (axis IV), and overall rating of general psychosocial functioning (axis V). Given our current limited understanding of the etiology of most mental disorders, DSM-IV emphasizes phenomenology and is thus both empirical and atheoretical. The DSM-IV emphasis on strict operational criteria has resulted in high reliability for psychiatric diagnoses and in improved treatment and management.

Current changes in health care delivery underscore the need for primary care physicians to assume responsibility for the initial diagnosis and treatment of the most common mental disorders. Valid patient-based questionnaires have been developed that systematically probe for signs and symptoms associated with the most prevalent psychiatric diagnoses and guide the clinician into a more targeted historical assessment. Prime MD (from Roerig/Pfizer, New York) and the Symptom-Driven Diagnostic System for Primary Care (SDDS-PC) (from Pharmacia-Upjohn, Kalamazoo, MI) are inventories that require only 10 min to complete, in which patient responses can be linked to the formal diagnostic criteria of anxiety, mood, somatoform, and eating disorders, and alcohol abuse or dependence.

This chapter surveys the most commonly encountered conditions in general medical practice and focuses on illnesses whose treatment is likely to be the responsibility of the primary care practitioner rather than the specialist. A physician who refers patients to a psychiatrist must know not only when doing so is appropriate but also how to do it, since societal misconceptions and the stigma of mental illness impede the process. Primary care physicians should base referrals to a psychiatrist on the presence of the signs and symptoms of a mental disorder, and not simply on the absence of physical elements for a patient's complaint. Education of the patient and formation of an alliance are crucial to the success of treatment. Although some of the conditions and states discussed are outside the scope of primary care practice, their prompt recognition is often essential to avoid significant morbidity. When physicians encounter evidence of psychotic symptoms, mania, severe depression or anxiety, dissociative symptoms, suicidal or homicidal preoccupation, or a failure to respond to first-order treatment, consultation with a psychiatrist or transfer of care must be initiated. → *Eating disorders are discussed in Chap. 76.*

ANXIETY DISORDERS

Anxiety disorders, the most prevalent psychiatric illnesses in the general community, are present in 15 to 20 percent of medical clinic patients. Anxiety, defined as a subjective sense of unease, dread, or foreboding, can indicate a primary psychiatric condition, or it can be a component of, or reaction to, a primary medical disease. The primary anxiety disorders are classified according to their duration and course and the existence and nature of precipitants.

When evaluating the anxious patient, the clinician must first determine whether the anxiety antedates or postdates a medical illness or is due to a medication side effect. Approximately one-third of medical patients presenting with anxiety have an organic etiology for their psychiatric symptoms, but an anxiety disorder can also present with somatic symptoms in the absence of a diagnosable medical condition.

PANIC DISORDER   Clinical Manifestations   Panic disorder is defined by the presence of recurrent and unpredictable panic attacks, which are distinct episodes of intense fear and discomfort associated with a variety of physical symptoms, including palpitations, sweating, trembling, shortness of breath, chest pain, and dizziness, and a fear of impending doom or death (Table 385-1). Paresthesia, gastrointestinal distress, and feelings of unreality are also common. Panic attacks have a sudden onset, developing within 10 min and usually resolving over the course of an hour, and they occur in an unexpected fashion. The frequency and severity of panic attacks varies, ranging from once a week to clusters of attacks separated by months of well-being. The first attack is usually outside the home. Onset is usually in late adolescence to early adulthood. In some individuals, anticipatory anxiety develops over time and results in a generalized fear and a progressive avoidance of places or situations in which a panic attack might recur. *Agoraphobia*, which occurs commonly in patients with panic disorder, is an acquired irrational fear of being in places where one might feel trapped or unable to escape (Table 385-2). Typically it leads the patient into a progressive restriction in life-style and, in a literal sense, in geography. Because patients develop embarrassment about being housebound and dependent on the company of others to go out into the world, physicians may under-recognize the syndrome if they do not pursue direct questioning.

Differential Diagnosis   A diagnosis of panic disorder is made after an organic etiology for the panic attacks has been ruled out (Fig. 385-1). A variety of cardiovascular, respiratory, endocrine, and neurologic conditions can present with anxiety as the chief complaint, and patients with true panic disorder will often focus on one specific feature to the exclusion of others. Twenty percent of patients who present with syncope as a primary medical complaint, for example, have a primary mood, anxiety, or substance-abuse diagnosis, the most common being panic disorder. The differential diagnosis of panic disorder is complicated by a high rate of comorbidity with other psychiatric conditions, especially alcohol and benzodiazepine abuse, which patients initially use in an attempt at self-medication. Seventy-five percent of panic disorder patients will also satisfy criteria for major depression at some point in their illness.

When the history of present illness is nonspecific, physical examination and focused laboratory testing must be used to rule out organic anxiety states, such as those resulting from pheochromocytoma, thyrotoxicosis, or hypoglycemia. Electrocardiogram and echocardiogram may detect cardiovascular conditions associated with panic, such as paroxysmal atrial tachycardia and mitral valve prolapse, but in other conditions, such as hyperdynamic beta-adrenergic state, it is difficult to make a meaningful distinction between the independent psychiatric and cardiologic diagnoses. In two studies, panic disorder was the primary diagnosis in 43 percent of patients with chest pain who had normal coronary angiograms and was present in 9 percent of all outpatients referred for cardiac evaluation. Panic disorder has also been diagnosed in many patients referred for pulmonary function testing or having symptoms of irritable bowel syndrome.

Table 385-1

Diagnostic Criteria for Panic Attack

A discrete period of intense fear or discomfort, in which four (or more) of the following symptoms developed abruptly and reached a peak within 10 min:

1. Palpitations, pounding heart, or accelerated heart rate
2. Sweating
3. Trembling or shaking
4. Sensations of shortness of breath or smothering
5. Feeling of choking
6. Chest pain or discomfort
7. Nausea or abdominal distress
8. Feeling dizzy, unsteady, lightheaded, or faint
9. Derealization (feelings of unreality) or depersonalization (being detached from oneself)
10. Fear of losing control or going crazy
11. Fear of dying
12. Paresthesia (numbness or tingling sensations)
13. Chills or hot flushes

SOURCE: *Diagnostic and Statistical Manual of Mental Disorders,* 4th ed.

Table 385-2

Diagnostic Criteria for Agoraphobia

1. Anxiety about being in places or situations from which escape might be difficult (or embarrassing) or in which help may not be available in the event of having an unexpected or situationally predisposed panic attack or panic-like symptoms. Agoraphobic fears typically involve characteristic clusters of situations that include being outside the home alone; being in a crowd or standing in a line; being on a bridge; and traveling in a bus, train, or automobile.

   Note: Consider the diagnosis of specific phobia if the avoidance is limited to one or only a few specific situations, or social phobia if the avoidance is limited to social situations.

2. The situations are avoided (e.g., travel is restricted) or else are endured with marked distress or with anxiety about having a panic attack or panic-like symptoms, or require the presence of a companion.

3. The anxiety or phobic avoidance is not better accounted for by another mental disorder, such as social phobia (e.g., avoidance limited to social situations because of fear of embarrassment), specific phobia (e.g., avoidance limited to a single situation like elevators), obsessive-compulsive disorder (e.g., avoidance of dirt in someone with an obsession about contamination), posttraumatic stress disorder (e.g., avoidance of stimuli associated with a severe stressor), or separation anxiety disorder (e.g., avoidance of leaving home or relatives).

SOURCE: *Diagnostic and Statistical Manual of Mental Disorders,* 4th ed.

Etiology and Pathophysiology The etiology of panic disorder is unknown but appears to involve a genetic predisposition, altered autonomic responsivity, and social learning. Panic disorder shows familial aggregation, although the estimate of concordance in monozygotic twins is only 30 percent. Acute panic attacks appear to be associated with increased noradrenergic discharge in the locus ceruleus. Intravenous infusion of sodium lactate evokes an attack predictably in two-thirds of panic disorder patients, as do the alpha$_2$-adrenergic antagonist yohimbine and carbon dioxide inhalation. It is hypothesized that each of these stimuli activates a neural circuit involving noradrenergic neurons in the locus ceruleus and serotonergic neurons in the

dorsal raphe. Although the noradrenergic theory of panic attacks has proved empirically useful, a number of contradictory findings exist. For example, increases in noradrenergic metabolites are not consistently observed during provocative challenge testing. A serotonergic contribution is better established; infusion of the serotonin (5HT) agonist *m*-chlorophenylproperazine induces anxiety in panic-disorder patients but not in control subjects, and agents that block serotonin reuptake are therapeutic in preventing attacks. It is likely that panic-disorder

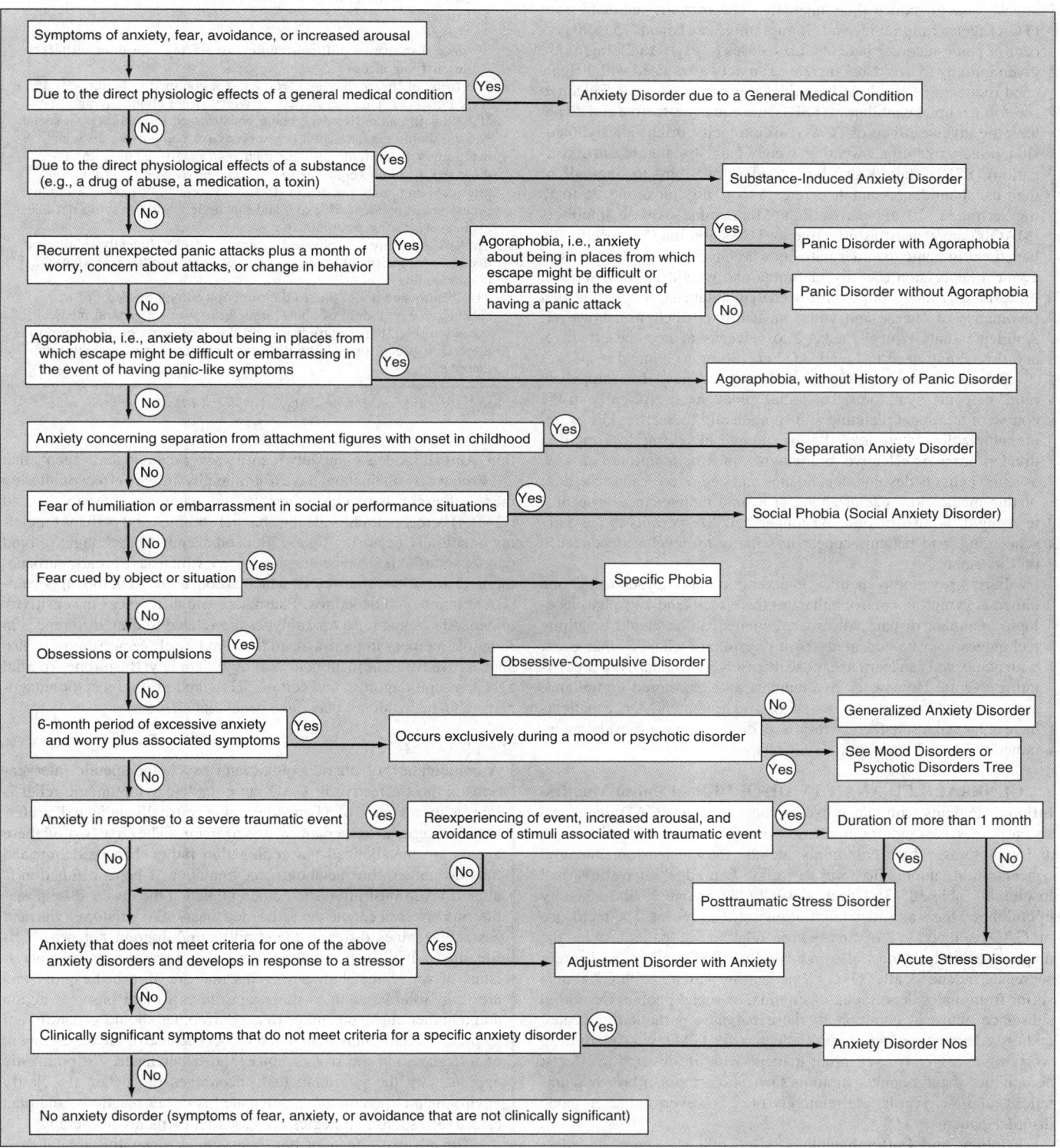

FIGURE 385-1 Differential diagnosis of anxiety disorders. NOS, not otherwise specified. (*From Diagnostic and Statistical Manual of Mental Disorders, 4th ed.*)

patients have a heightened sensitivity to somatic symptoms, which results in positive feedback to control autonomic systems and triggers increasing arousal, setting off the "panic attack" mechanism. Accordingly, successful therapeutic intervention involves altering the patient's cognitive interpretation of anxiety-producing experiences as well as preventing the attack itself.

℞ TREATMENT

Achievable goals of treatment are to decrease the frequency of panic attacks and to reduce their intensity. The tricyclic antidepressant (TCA) agents imipramine and clomipramine can benefit 75 to 90 percent of panic-disorder patients. Low doses (e.g., 10 to 25 mg/d) are given initially to avoid any increased anxiety associated with heightened monoamine levels in the initial stages of treatment. Selective serotonin reuptake inhibitors (SSRIs) are equally effective and do not have the adverse effects of TCAs (cardiotoxicity, orthostatic hypotension, urinary retention, sweating, weight gain, dry mouth, and constipation). SSRIs should also be started at one-third to one-half of their usual antidepressant dose (e.g., 5 to 10 mg fluoxetine, 25 to 50 mg sertraline, 10 mg paroxetine). Monoamine oxidase inhibitors (MAOIs) are at least as effective as TCAs and may be specifically beneficial in panic disorder patients who have comorbid features of atypical depression (i.e., hypersomnia and weight gain). Insomnia, orthostatic hypotension, and the need to maintain a low-tyramine diet (avoidance of cheese and wine) have limited their use, however. Antidepressants typically take 2 to 6 weeks to become effective, and doses may need to be adjusted according to clinical response.

Because of anticipatory anxiety and the need for immediate relief of panic symptoms, benzodiazepines are useful early in the course of treatment planning and sporadically thereafter. For example, alprazolam, starting at 0.5 mg qid and increasing to 4 mg/d in divided doses, is effective, but patients must be monitored closely, as some patients develop dependence and begin to escalate the dose of this medication. Clonazepam, at a final maintenance dose of 2 to 4 mg/d, is also helpful; its longer half life permits twice-daily scheduling, and patients appear less likely to develop dependence on this agent.

Early psychotherapeutic intervention and pyschoeducation aimed at symptom control enhances the effectiveness of pharmacologic treatment of panic disorder. Patients can be taught breathing techniques, can be educated about physiologic changes that occur with panic, and can learn to expose themselves voluntarily to precipitating events. Homework assignments and monitored compliance are important components of successful treatment. Once patients have achieved a satisfactory response, drug treatment must be maintained for 1 to 2 years to prevent relapse.

GENERALIZED ANXIETY DISORDER Clinical Manifestations Patients with generalized anxiety disorder (GAD) have persistent, excessive, and/or unrealistic worry associated with other signs and symptoms, which commonly include muscle tension, impaired concentration, autonomic arousal, feeling "on edge" or restless, and insomnia (Table 385-3). Onset is usually before age 20 and a history of childhood fears and social inhibition may be present. The incidence of GAD is increased in first-degree relatives of patients with the diagnosis; family studies also indicate that GAD and panic disorder segregate independently. Over 80 percent of patients with GAD also suffer from major depression, dysthymia, or social phobia. Comorbid substance abuse is common in these patients, particularly alcohol and/or sedative/hypnotic abuse. Patients with GAD readily admit to worrying excessively over minor matters, with life-disrupting effects; complaints of autonomic symptoms such as shortness of breath, palpitations, and tachycardia are relatively rare, however, unlike in panic disorder patients.

Etiology and Pathophysiology Generalized anxiety disorders are thought to result from aberrations in benzodiazepine receptor regula-

Table 385-3

Diagnostic Criteria for Generalized Anxiety Disorder

A. Excessive anxiety and worry (apprehensive expectation), occurring more days than not for at least 6 months, about a number of events or activities (such as work or school performance).
B. The person finds it difficult to control the worry.
C. The anxiety and worry are associated with three (or more) of the following six symptoms (with at least some symptoms present for more days than not for the past 6 months). **Note:** Only one item is required in children.
   1. Restlessness or feeling keyed up or on edge
   2. Being easily fatigued
   3. Difficulty concentrating or mind going blank
   4. Irritability
   5. Muscle tension
   6. Sleep disturbance (difficulty falling or staying asleep, or restless unsatisfying sleep)
D. The focus of the anxiety and worry is not confined to features of an Axis I disorder, e.g., the anxiety or worry is not about having a panic attack (as in panic disorder), being embarrassed in public (as in social phobia), being contaminated (as in obsessive-compulsive disorder), being away from home or close relatives (as in separation anxiety disorder), gaining weight (as in anorexia nervosa), having multiple physical complaints (as in somatization disorder), or having a serious illness (as in hypochondriasis), and the anxiety and worry do not occur exclusively during posttraumatic stress disorder.
E. The anxiety, worry, or physical symptoms cause clinically significant distress or impairment in social, occupational, or other important areas of functioning.
F. The disturbance is not due to the direct physiologic effects of a substance (e.g., a drug of abuse, a medication) or a general medical condition (e.g., hyperthyroidism) and does not occur exclusively during a mood disorder, a psychotic disorder, or a pervasive developmental disorder.

SOURCE: *Diagnostic and Statistical Manual of Mental Disorders*, 4th ed.

tion. Animal models of anxiety identify several anxiogenic agents that are structurally distinct but have a similar physiologic effect of altering the binding of benzodiazepines to the gamma-aminobutyric acid (GABA) A receptor/chloride ion channel complex and perhaps regulating a naturally occurring ligand. Benzodiazepines are thought to bind two separate GABA A receptor sites: type I, which has a broad neuroanatomic distribution, and type II, which is concentrated in the hippocampus, striatum, and neocortex. Pharmacologic differences in sensitivity to benzodiazepine receptor subtypes are related to drug differences in sedation, memory impairment, and antianxiety efficacy. Serotonin also appears to have a role in the neurobiology of anxiety. Buspirone, a partial $5HT_{1A}$ receptor agonist, and certain $5HT_{2A}$ and $5HT_{2C}$ receptor antagonists (e.g., nefazodone) may have beneficial effects.

℞ TREATMENT

A combination of pharmacologic and psychotherapeutic interventions is most effective in GAD but complete symptomatic relief is rare. A short course of a benzodiazepine is usually indicated, preferably lorazepam, oxazepam, or temazepam. (The first two of these agents are metabolized via conjugation rather than oxidation and thus do not exhibit metabolite accumulation if hepatic function is altered.) Administration should be initiated at the lowest dose possible and prescribed on an as-needed basis as symptoms warrant. Benzodiazepines differ in their milligram/kilogram potency, half-life, lipid solubility, metabolic pathways, and presence and characteristics of active metabolites. Agents that are absorbed rapidly and are lipid soluble, such as diazepam, have a rapid onset of action and a higher abuse potential. Benzodiazepines should generally not be prescribed for more than 4 to 6 weeks because of the development of tolerance and the risk of abuse and dependence. An optimistic approach by the physician that encourages the patient to clarify environmental precipitants, anticipate his or her reactions, and plan effective response strategies are essential elements of therapy.

The adverse effects of benzodiazepines generally parallel their relative half lives. Longer-acting agents, such as diazepam, chlordiazepoxide, flurazepam, clorazepate, halazepam, and prazepam, tend to show accumulation of active metabolites, with sedation, impairment of cognition, and psychomotor performance, while use of shorter-acting compounds, such as alprazolam and oxazepam, can result in daytime anxiety, early morning insomnia, and rebound anxiety and insomnia with discontinuation. Although patients develop tolerance to the sedative effects of benzodiazepines, they are less likely to habituate to the adverse psychomotor effects. It is generally easier to withdraw patients from the longer-half-life benzodiazepines. Withdrawal can be accomplished through gradual, step-wise dose reduction (by approximately 10 percent every 1 to 2 weeks) over a period of 6 to 12 weeks. It is usually much more difficult to taper patients off shorter-acting benzodiazepines. Physicians may need to switch the patient to a benzodiazepine with a longer half life or use an adjunctive medication, such as a beta blocker or carbamazepine, before attempting to discontinue the benzodiazepine. Withdrawal reactions vary in severity and duration; they can include depression, anxiety, delirium, lethargy, diaphoresis, tinnitus, autonomic arousal, unusual neuromuscular movements, and, rarely, seizures.

Buspirone, an azaspirone, is a nonbenzodiazepine anxiolytic agent. It is nonsedating, does not lead to tolerance or dependence, does not interact with benzodiazepine receptors or alcohol, and has no abuse or disinhibition potential. However, it requires several weeks to take effect and requires thrice-daily dosing (occasionally up to 20 mg tid). An extended release version of the drug has recently been introduced and may result in increased treatment adherence. Patients who were previously responsive to a benzodiazepine are unlikely to rate the drug as being equally effective. Patients with head injury or dementia who have symptoms of anxiety and/or agitation may do well with this agent.

Administration of benzodiazepines to geriatric patients requires special care. Such patients have increased drug absorption, decreased hepatic metabolism, protein binding, renal excretion, and an increased volume of distribution, which, together with the likely presence of comorbid medical illnesses and medication, dramatically increase the likelihood of toxicity. Iatrogenic psychomotor impairment can result in falls and fractures, confusional states, or motor vehicle accidents. If used, agents in this class should be started at the lowest possible dose, and results should be monitored closely. Benzodiazepines are contraindicated during pregnancy and lactation.

PHOBIC DISORDERS Clinical Manifestations The cardinal feature of phobic disorders is a marked and persistent fear of objects or situations, exposure to which results in an immediate anxiety reaction. The patient avoids the phobic stimulus, and this avoidance usually impairs occupational or social functioning. Panic attacks may be triggered by the phobic stimulus or may emerge spontaneously during the course of the illness. Unlike patients with other anxiety disorders, individuals with phobias experience anxiety only in specific and identifiable situations. Common phobias include fear of closed spaces (claustrophobia), fear of blood, and fear of flying. Social phobia is distinguished by a specific fear of social or performance situations in which the individual is exposed to unfamiliar individuals or to possible examination and evaluation by others. Examples include having to converse at a party, use public restrooms, and meet strangers. In each case, the affected individual is aware that the experienced fear is excessive and unreasonable given the circumstance. The specific content of a phobia may vary across gender, ethnic, and cultural boundaries.

Phobic disorders are common, with a 1-year prevalence rate of 9 percent and a lifetime rate of 10 to 11 percent. The onset is in childhood to early adulthood, and familial aggregation may occur. In female twins, concordance rates for agoraphobia, social phobia, and animal phobia of 23 percent for monozygotic twins and 15 percent for dizygotic twins are reported. Full criteria for diagnosis are usually evident first in adults, but behavioral avoidance in infancy of unfamiliar people, situations, or objects is common in the history of patients.

℞ TREATMENT

Recent controlled trials have documented the efficacy of several pharmacologic agents in the treatment of phobic disorders. Beta blockers are particularly effective in the treatment of "performance anxiety" (but not general social phobia) and appear to achieve their benefit by preventing the occurrence of peripheral manifestations of anxiety, such as perspiration, tachycardia, palpitations, and tremor. MAOIs alleviate social phobia independently of their antidepressant activity, and SSRIs appear to be effective also. Benzodiazepines can be helpful in reducing fearful avoidance, but the chronic nature of phobic disorders limits their usefulness.

Behaviorally focused psychotherapy is an important component of treatment, as relapse rates are high when medication is used as the sole treatment. Cognitive-behavioral strategies are the keystone of treatment and derive from the finding that patients' distorted perceptions and interpretations of fear-producing stimuli play a major role in perpetuation of phobias. Individual and group therapy sessions teach the patient to identify specific negative thoughts associated with the anxiety-producing situation, and help to reduce the patient's fear of loss of control. In desensitization therapy, hierarchies of feared situations are constructed and the patient is encouraged to pursue and master gradual exposure to the anxiety-producing stimuli.

Patients with social phobia, in particular, have a high rate of comorbid alcohol abuse, as well as of other psychiatric conditions (e.g., eating disorders), necessitating the need for parallel management of each disorder if anxiety reduction is to be achieved.

STRESS DISORDERS Clinical Manifestations Patients may develop significant anxiety after exposure to extreme trauma, defined as an event associated with either actual or threatened death or injury to oneself or another. The reaction may occur shortly after the traumatic exposure, (*acute stress disorder*) or be delayed in time and subject to recurrence (*posttraumatic stress disorder*, PTSD) (Table 385-4). In both syndromes, individuals experience associated symptoms of detachment and loss of emotional responsivity. The patient may feel depersonalized and unable to recall specific aspects of the trauma, though typically it is reexperienced through intrusions in thought, dreams, or flashbacks, particularly when cues of the original event are present. Accordingly, patients often actively avoid stimuli that precipitate recollections of the trauma and demonstrate a resulting increase in vigilance, arousal, and startle response. Patients with stress disorders are at increased risk for the development of other anxiety, mood, and substance-related disorders. Between 5 and 10 percent of Americans will at some time in their life satisfy the full criteria for PTSD with women more likely to be affected than men.

Risk factors for the development of PTSD include a past psychiatric history and personality characteristics of high neuroticism and extroversion. Studies of monozygotic and dizygotic twins showed a substantial influence of genetics on all symptoms associated with PTSD, with no evidence for an environment effect.

Etiology and Pathophysiology It is hypothesized that in PTSD there is impaired alpha$_2$-adrenergic receptor feedback inhibition to stress-induced release of norepinephrine from the locus ceruleus, with a progressive behavioral sensitization and generalization to stimulus cues associated with the original trauma. Increased noradrenergic activity at locus ceruleus projection sites in hippocampus and amygdala theoretically facilitates encoding of fear-based memories which persist and resist extinction. In clinical studies, diminished serotonergic effects, reduction in cortisol release, and increased sensitivity of cortisol to dexamethasone inhibition distinguish patients with PTSD from control subjects. Greater sympathetic responses to cues associated with trauma are shown by laboratory findings of increased release of norepinephrine in response to challenge. Altered alpha$_2$- and beta-adrenergic receptor binding and a lowered activity of platelet adenylate cyclase have also been reported.

Table 385-4

Diagnostic Criteria for Posttraumatic Stress Disorder

A. The person has been exposed to a traumatic event in which both of the following were present:
  1. The person experienced, witnessed, or was confronted with an event or events that involved actual or threatened death or serious injury, or a threat to the physical integrity of self or others.
  2. The person's response involved intense fear, helplessness, or horror. **Note:** In children, this may be expressed instead by disorganized or agitated behavior.
B. The traumatic event is persistently reexperienced in one (or more) of the following ways:
  1. Recurrent and intrusive distressing recollections of the event, including images, thoughts, or perceptions. **Note:** In young children, repetitive play may occur in which themes or aspects of the trauma are expressed.
  2. Recurrent distressing dreams of the event. **Note:** In children, there may be frightening dreams without recognizable content.
  3. Acting or feeling as if the traumatic event were recurring (includes a sense of reliving the experience, illusions, hallucinations, and dissociative flashback episodes, including those that occur on awakening or when intoxicated). **Note:** In young children, trauma-specific reenactment may occur.
  4. Intense psychological distress at exposure to internal or external cues that symbolize or resemble an aspect of the traumatic event.
  5. Physiologic reactivity on exposure to internal or external cues that symbolize or resemble an aspect of the traumatic event.
C. Persistent avoidance of stimuli associated with the trauma and numbing of general responsiveness (not present before the trauma), as indicated by three or more of the following:
  1. Efforts to avoid thoughts, feelings, or conversations associated with the trauma
  2. Efforts to avoid activities, places, or people that arouse recollections of the trauma
  3. Inability to recall an important aspect of the trauma
  4. Markedly diminished interest or participation in significant activities
  5. Feeling of detachment or estrangement from others
  6. Restricted range of affect (e.g., unable to have loving feelings)
  7. Sense of a foreshortened future (e.g., does not expect to have a career, marriage, children, or a normal life span)
D. Persistent symptoms of increased arousal (not present before the trauma), as indicated by two (or more) of the following:
  1. Difficulty falling or staying asleep
  2. Irritability or outbursts of anger
  3. Difficulty concentrating
  4. Hypervigilance
  5. Exaggerated startle response
E. Duration of the disturbance (symptoms in criteria B, C, and D) is more than 1 month
F. The disturbance causes clinically significant distress or impairment in social, occupational, or other important areas of functioning.

SOURCE: *Diagnostic and Statistical Manual of Mental Disorders*, 4th ed.

℞ TREATMENT

Acute stress reactions are usually self-limited, and treatment typically involves only the short-term use of benzodiazepines and supportive/expressive psychotherapy. The chronic and recurrent nature of PTSD, however, requires a more complex approach employing drug and behavioral treatments. TCAs such as imipramine and amitriptyline, the MAOI phenelzine, and the SSRIs (fluoxetine, sertraline, paroxetine) can all reduce anxiety, symptoms of intrusion, and avoidance behaviors. Trazodone, a sedating antidepressant, is frequently used at night to help with symptoms of insomnia (50 to 150 mg qid). Carbamazepine, valproic acid, or alprazolam have also independently produced symptomatic improvement in some patients in uncontrolled trials. There is frequent comorbidity with substance abuse, especially of alcohol.

Psychotherapeutic strategies are used in treatment of PTSD to help the patient overcome avoidance behaviors and demoralization and master fear of recurrence of the trauma; therapies that encourage the patient to dismantle avoidance behaviors through stepwise focusing on the experience of the traumatic event are the most effective.

OBSESSIVE-COMPULSIVE DISORDER   **Clinical Manifestations**   Obsessive-compulsive disorder (OCD) was previously considered a relatively rare condition, but recent epidemiologic data indicate a lifetime prevalence of 2 to 3 percent worldwide. OCD is characterized by obsessive thoughts and compulsive behaviors that impair everyday functioning. Fears of contamination and germs are common, as are handwashing, counting behaviors, and having to check and re-check such actions as whether a door is locked. The degree to which the disorder is disruptive for the individual varies, but in all cases obsessive-compulsive activities take up more than 1 h/d and are undertaken to relieve the anxiety triggered by the core fear. Patients often conceal their symptoms, usually because they are embarrassed by the content of their thoughts or the nature of their actions. Physicians must ask specific questions regarding recurrent thoughts and behaviors, particularly if physical clues such as chafed and reddened hands or patchy hair loss (from repetitive hair pulling, or *trichotillomania*) are present. Tics are sometimes associated with OCD. OCD usually has a gradual onset, beginning in early adulthood, but childhood onset is not rare. The disorder usually has a waxing and waning course, but some cases may show a steady deterioration in psychosocial functioning.

Etiology and Pathophysiology   A genetic contribution to OCD is suggested by a higher monozygotic than dizygotic concordance rate and the fact that familial studies show an aggregation with Tourette's disorder. OCD is more common in males and in first-born children.

The anatomic-physiologic disturbance in obsessive-compulsive behavior is thought to involve an alteration in a frontal-subcortical neural circuit involving the orbital frontal cortex, caudate nucleus, and globus pallidus. Neuroimaging studies have demonstrated a decrease in caudate nucleus volume, abnormalities in frontal lobe white matter, and increases in glucose metabolism in the orbital cortex of the frontal lobes and the head of the caudate nucleus. The caudate nucleus seems particularly involved in the acquisition and maintenance of habit and skill learning, and interventions that are successful in reducing obsessive-compulsive behaviors are paralleled by a comparable decrease in caudate glucose metabolic rate.

℞ TREATMENT

Clomipramine, fluoxetine, and fluvoxamine are approved for the treatment of OCD. Clomipramine is a TCA that is often tolerated poorly owing to significant anticholinergic and sedative side effects at the doses required to treat the illness (150 to 250 mg/d). Its efficacy in OCD is unrelated to its antidepressant activity. Fluoxetine (40 to 60 mg/d) and fluvoxamine (100 to 300 mg/d) are as effective as clomipramine and show a more benign side-effect profile. Fluvoxamine, a structurally unique SSRI, is metabolized through the hepatic P450 microsomal system (as is fluoxetine); it appears to inhibit the III A4 isoenzyme specifically and should not be given with other drugs that act on III A4, such as terfenadine and astemizole, because life-threatening cardiac arrhythmias may result. Only 50 to 60 percent of patients with OCD show an acceptable degree of improvement with pharmacotherapy alone. In treatment-resistant cases, augmentation with other serotonergic agents, such as buspirone, or with a neuroleptic or benzodiazepine may be beneficial. When a therapeutic response is achieved, long-duration maintenance therapy is usually indicated.

Drug treatment by itself is seldom sufficient. For many individuals, particularly those with time-consuming compulsions, behavior therapy will result in as much improvement as that afforded by medication. Effective techniques include having patients gradually increase their exposure to stressful situations, having them keep a diary to clarify stressors, and having them perform homework assignments where they substitute new activities for their compulsive behavior.

MOOD DISORDERS

Mood disorders are characterized by a disturbance in the regulation of mood, behavior, and affect. Mood disorders are subdivided into (1) depressive disorders, (2) bipolar disorders, and (3) depression in association with medical illness or alcohol and substance abuse (see Chaps. 386 through 388) (Fig. 385-2). Depressive disorders are differentiated from bipolar disorders by the absence of a manic or hypomanic episode. The etiopathogenic relationship between pure depressive syndromes and bipolar disorders is not well understood; depression occurs at increased frequency in families of bipolar individuals, but the reverse is not true, suggesting that depressive disorders are etiologically heterogeneous. Because of their common occurrence in general medical practice, mood disorders secondary to medical illness will be discussed first.

DEPRESSION IN ASSOCIATION WITH MEDICAL ILLNESS Depression occurring in the context of medical illness is difficult to evaluate. Depressive symptomatology may reflect the psychological stress of coping with the disease, may be caused by the disease process itself or by the medications used to treat it, or may simply coexist in time with the medical diagnosis.

Virtually every class of *medication* includes some agent that can induce depression. Antihypertensive drugs, anticholesterolemic agents, and antiarrhythmic agents are commonly-used classes of medications that can trigger depressive symptoms. Among the antihypertensive agents, beta-adrenergic blockers and, to a lesser extent, calcium channel blockers are the most likely to cause depressed mood. Iatrogenic depression should be considered in patients receiving, corticosteroids, antimicrobials, systemic analgesics, antiparkinsonian medications, and anticonvulsants. To decide whether a causal relationship exists between pharmacologic therapy and a patient's change in mood, it is necessary to examine the chronology of symptoms and sometimes ultimately to undertake an empirical trial of an alternative medication.

Twenty to thirty percent of *cardiac patients* manifest a depressive disorder; an even higher percentage endorse depressive symptomatology when self-reporting scales are used. Depressive symptoms following myocardial infarction have a negative effect on rehabilitation and predict a higher rate of mortality and medical morbidity. Depressed patients often show decreased variability in heart rate (an index of reduced parasympathetic nervous system activity), and this has been proposed as one mechanism by which depression may predispose individuals to ventricular arrhythmia and increased morbidity. Although TCAs have been used to treat depression in individuals with cardiac disease for a number of years, and although the quinidine-like effect of tricyclics may be useful in patients with preexisting arrhythmias, TCAs are contraindicated in patients with preexisting bundle branch block. They may also paradoxically precipitate arrhythmias in a subset of patients. Tricyclic-induced tachycardia is an additional concern in patients with congestive heart failure. Even though experience with the SSRIs is more limited, thus far they appear not to induce electrocardiographic changes or adverse cardiac events. SSRIs may interfere with hepatic metabolism of anticoagulants, however, resulting in an increase in the blood level of those drugs and in the bleeding time.

Epidemiologic surveys of depression in patients with *cancer* show a wide variability in prevalence, as might be predicted by differences in tumor site, severity of illness, and type of medical or surgical intervention. There is an overall mean prevalence of 25 percent, but depression occurs in 40 to 50 percent of patients with cancers of the pancreas or oropharynx. Assessment of the validity of prevalence rates is complicated by the fact that extreme cachexia may be misinterpreted as part of the symptom complex of the psychiatric diagnosis. The higher prevalence of depression in patients with pancreatic cancer nevertheless persists when patients are stratified and compared to others with advanced gastric cancer. Initiation of antidepressant medication in cancer patients has been shown to improve quality of life as well as mood. Psychotherapeutic approaches, particularly group therapy, may have some effect on short-term depression, anxiety, and pain symptoms and on recurrence rates and long-term survival. In a study of female patients with metastatic breast cancer, patients in group therapy had longer survival than control patients.

Depression occurs frequently in patients with *neurologic disorders*, particularly cerebrovascular disorders, Parkinson's disease, multiple sclerosis, and traumatic brain injury. Left-hemisphere strokes, particularly those involving the dorsal lateral frontal cortex, are most likely to cause depression. Both tricyclic and SSRI antidepressants are effective in the treatment of depression secondary to stroke, as are stimulant compounds and, in some patients, MAOIs.

The reported prevalence of depression in patients with *diabetes mellitus* varies from 8.5 to 27.3 percent, with the severity of the mood state correlating with the physical symptoms of illness and the degree of hyperglycemia. Pharmacologic treatment of depression is complicated by the fact that different antidepressants have different effects on blood glucose level. MAOIs can induce hypoglycemia and weight gain, while TCAs can lead to hyperglycemia and carbohydrate craving. SSRIs, like MAOIs, may cause a reduction in fasting plasma glucose, but they are easier to use. SSRIs result in better dietary and medication compliance.

Clinical hypothyroidism is frequently associated with features of depression, most commonly depressed mood and memory impairment. Hyperthyroid states may also present in a similar fashion, usually in geriatric populations. Improvement in mood usually follows normalization of thyroid function, but adjunctive antidepressant medication is sometimes required. Patients with more subtle thyroid dysfunction, such as subclinical hypothyroidism, can also experience symptoms of depression and cognitive difficulty that respond to thyroid replacement.

DEPRESSIVE DISORDERS **Clinical Manifestations** *Major depression* is defined as depressed mood on a daily basis for a minimum duration of 2 weeks (Table 385-5). An episode may be characterized by sadness, indifference or apathy, or irritability and is usually associated with change in a number of neurovegetative functions, including sleep patterns and appetite and weight, motor agitation or retardation, fatigue, impairment in concentration and decision making, feelings of shame or guilt, and thoughts of death or dying. Patients with endogenous depression have a profound loss of pleasure in all enjoyable activities, exhibit early morning awakening, feel that the dysphoric mood state is qualitatively different from sadness, and often notice a diurnal variation in mood (worse in morning hours). Paradoxically, these more severe features predict a good response to antidepressant treatment.

Approximately 15 percent of the general population experiences a major depressive episode at some point in life, and 6 to 8 percent of all outpatients in primary care settings satisfy diagnostic criteria for the disorder. Depression is often undiagnosed, however, and, even more frequently, it is treated inadequately. If a physician suspects the presence of a major depressive episode, the initial task is to determine whether it represents unipolar or bipolar depression or is one of the 10 to 15 percent of cases that are secondary to general medical illness or substance abuse. Physicians should also assess the risk of suicide by direct questioning, as patients are often reluctant to verbalize such thoughts without prompting. If specific plans are uncovered or if significant risk factors exist (e.g., a past history of suicide attempts, profound hopelessness, concurrent medical illness, substance abuse, or social isolation), the patient must be referred to a mental health specialist for immediate care. Nearly 15 percent of patients whose depressive illness goes untreated will commit suicide; most of these patients will have sought help from a physician within 1 month of their death.

In some depressed patients, the mood disorder does not appear to be episodic and is not as clearly associated with either psychosocial dysfunction or change from the individual's usual experience in life. *Dysthymic disorder* consists in a pattern of chronic (at least 2 years), ongoing, mild depressive symptoms that are less severe and less disabling than those found in major depression; the two conditions are sometimes difficult to separate, however, and can occur together ("double depression"). Interestingly, many patients who exhibit a profile of pessimism, disinterest, and low self-esteem respond to antidepressant treatment. Dysthymic disorder exists in approximately 5 percent of primary care patients.

Studies of various cultures have shown that external manifestations of depression differ but the core symptoms remain the same. The

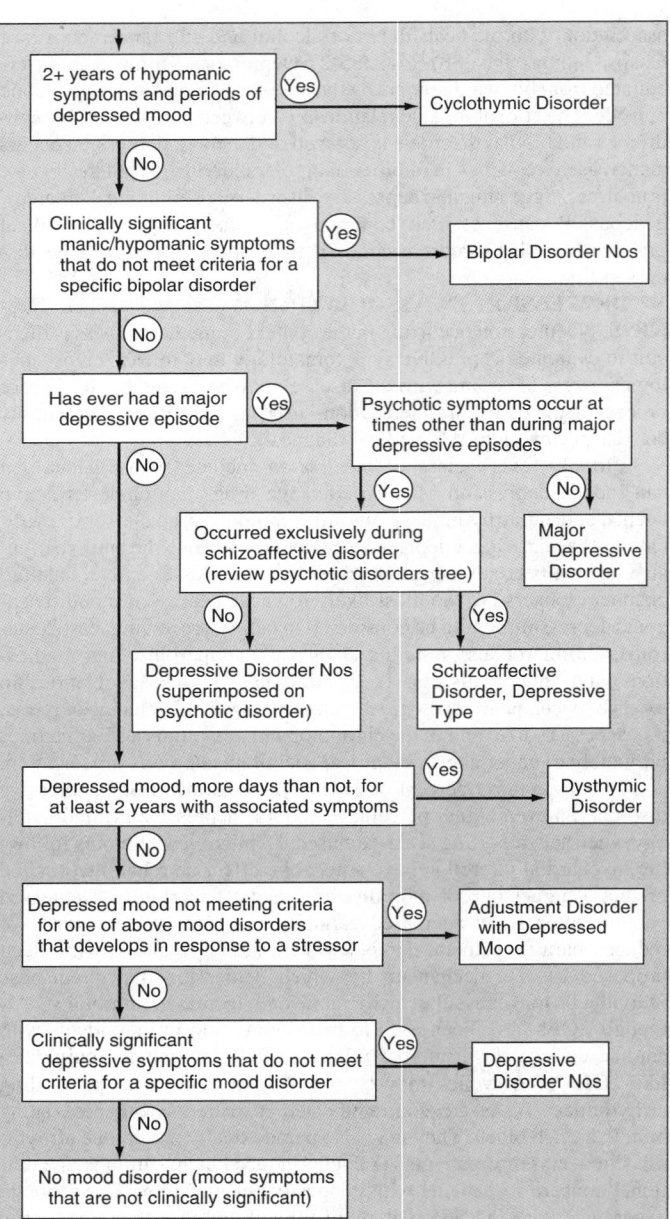

FIGURE 385-2 Differential diagnosis of mood disorders. NOS, not otherwise specified. *(From Diagnostic and Statistical Manual of Mental Disorders, 4th ed.)*

incidence of depression increases with age; the disorder is approximately twice as prevalent in women as in men, regardless of age. These gender differences were previously believed to reflect sociocultural factors, but recent longitudinal twin studies indicate that the liability to major depression in adult women is largely genetic in origin, and that the effect of environmental factors is transitory and does not affect lifetime prevalence. The relationship between psychological stress, negative life events, and the onset of depressive episodes remains unclear. Certainly, negative life events can precipitate and contribute to depression, but depression itself can be the source of stressful experiences as well.

Unipolar depressive disorders usually have their onset in early adulthood, and recurrences over the course of a lifetime are likely. The best predictor of future risk is the number of past episodes, making a prediction after a single episode unreliable; 50 to 60 percent of patients who have a first episode have at least one or two more episodes. Some patients experience multiple episodes that become more severe and frequent over time. The duration of an untreated episode varies greatly, ranging from a few months to 1 or more years. The pattern of

Table 385-5

CHAPTER 385
Mental Disorders   **2493**

Criteria for Major Depressive Episode

A. Five (or more) of the following symptoms have been present during the same 2-week period and represent a change from previous functioning; at least one of the symptoms is either (1) depressed mood or (2) loss of interest or pleasure.

Note: Do not include symptoms that are clearly due to a general medical condition, or mood-incongruent delusions or hallucinations.

1. Depressed mood most of the day, nearly every day, as indicated by either subjective report (e.g., feels sad or empty) or observation made by others (e.g., appears tearful). **Note:** In children and adolescents, can be irritable mood.
2. Markedly diminished interest or pleasure in all, or almost all, activities most of the day, nearly every day (as indicated by either subjective account or observation made by others).
3. Significant weight loss when not dieting or weight gain (e.g., a change of more than 5% of body weight in a month), or decrease or increase in appetite nearly every day. **Note:** In children, consider failure to make expected weight gains.
4. Insomnia or hypersomnia nearly every day.
5. Psychomotor agitation or retardation nearly every day (observable by others, not merely subjective feelings of restlessness or being slowed down).
6. Fatigue or loss of energy nearly every day.
7. Feelings of worthlessness or excessive or inappropriate guilt (which may be delusional) nearly every day (not merely self-reproach or guilt about being sick).
8. Diminished ability to think or concentrate, or indecisiveness, nearly every day (either by subjective account or as observed by others).
9. Recurrent thoughts of death (not just fear of dying), recurrent suicidal ideation without a specific plan, or a suicide attempt or a specific plan for committing suicide.

B. The symptoms do not meet criteria for a mixed episode.
C. The symptoms cause clinically significant distress or impairment in social, occupational, or other important areas of functioning.
D. The symptoms are not due to the direct physiologic effects of a substance (e.g., a drug of abuse, a medication) or a general medical condition (e.g., hypothyroidism).
E. The symptoms are not better accounted for by bereavement; i.e., after the loss of a loved one, the symptoms persist for longer than 2 months or are characterized by marked functional impairment, morbid preoccupation with worthlessness, suicidal ideation, psychotic symptoms, or psychomotor retardation.

SOURCE: *Diagnostic and Statistical Manual of Mental Disorders,* 4th ed.

recurrence and clinical progression in a developing episode is variable. Within an individual, there is often long-term stability in phenotype (presenting symptoms, and frequency and duration of episodes). In a minority of patients, the severity of the depressive episode may progress to psychotic symptomatology. A seasonal pattern of depression, called *seasonal affective disorder,* may manifest with onset and remission of episodes at predictable times of the year. This disorder is more common in women, whose symptoms are anergy, fatigue, weight gain, hypersomnia, and episodic carbohydrate craving. The prevalence increases with distance from the equator, and mood improvement can be accomplished with chronobiologic alteration of light exposure.

Etiology and Pathophysiology   The neurobiology of unipolar depression is poorly understood. Although evidence for genetic transmission is not as strong as in bipolar disorder, monozygotic twins have a higher concordance rate (46 percent) than dizygotic siblings (20 percent), with little evidence for effect of a shared family environment. Parallels between the affective, motor, and cognitive dysfunctions seen in unipolar depression and those observed in diseases of the basal ganglia have suggested that neural networks involving prefrontal cortex and the basal ganglia may be primary sites of deficit. This hypothesis is supported by positron emission tomography (PET) studies of brain glucose metabolism that show a decrease in metabolic rate in the caudate nuclei and frontal lobes in depressed patients that returns to normal with recovery. Single photon emission computed tomography (SPECT) studies show comparable changes in blood flow. Magnetic resonance imaging (MRI) findings include in some patients an increased frequency of subcortical white matter lesions. However, be-

cause these findings are more prevalent in patients with late onset of depressive illness, their significance remains unproven. A number of studies document increased ventricle-to-brain ratios in patients with recurrent depression, but whether this finding is state-dependent or represents true cerebral atrophy is controversial. Postmortem examination of brains of suicide victims suggest altered noradrenergic activity, including increased binding to alpha$_1$-, alpha$_2$-, and beta-adrenergic receptors in the cerebral cortex and a decreased total number and density of noradrenergic neurons in the locus ceruleus.

Involvement of the serotonin system is suggested by findings of lower plasma tryptophan levels, a decreased cerebrospinal fluid level of 5-hydroxyindolacetic acid (the principal metabolite of serotonin in brain), and decreased platelet serotonergic transporter binding. An increase in brain 5HT receptors in suicide victims is also reported, as are neuroendocrine changes consistent with either a pre- or postsynaptic dysfunction in the serotonin neuron. Depletion of blood tryptophan, the amino acid precursor of serotonin, rapidly reverses the antidepressant benefit in depressed patients who have been successfully treated. However, a decrement in mood after tryptophan reduction is considerably less robust in untreated patients, indicating that, if presynaptic serotonergic dysfunction occurs in depression, it likely plays a contributing rather than a directly causal role. Evidence suggests that reduced serotonergic activity in the central nervous system actually correlates with temperament, impulsivity, and aggression better than with mood state or diagnosis per se.

Neuroendocrine abnormalities that are consistent with the neurovegetative signs and symptoms of depression include (1) increased cortisol secretion, (2) an increase in adrenal size, (3) a decreased inhibitory response of glucocorticoids to dexamethasone, and (4) a blunted response of thyroid-stimulating hormone (TSH) level to infusion of thyroid releasing hormone (TRH). Less convincing evidence exists for (1) an alteration in the pituitary response to corticotropin-releasing hormone (CRH), (2) a decrease in growth hormone secretion and responsivity to growth hormone–releasing hormone (GHRH), and (3) a diminished gonadotropin response to gonadotropin-releasing hormone (GNRH). Changes in hypothalamic-pituitary-adrenal regulation suggest that depression may represent an adaptive dysregulation of the stress response that is either genetically mediated or secondary to exposure to significant stress during critical neuroendocrine encoding periods in early development. Rats stressed as pups by maternal separation have increased hypothalamic levels of CRH as adults and significantly greater release of adrenocorticotropic hormone (ACTH) and corticosterone in response to foot shock than do control animals. Interestingly, antidepressant treatment leads to normalization of pituitary-adrenal abnormalities in patients with depression, and amitriptyline and other antidepressants reduce CRH mRNA and increase glucocorticoid receptor mRNA in a time frame compatible with the onset of the clinical response.

Diurnal variations in symptom severity and alterations in circadian rhythmicity of a number of neurochemical and neurohumoral factors suggest that biologic differences may be secondary to a primary defect in regulation of biologic rhythms. Patients with major depression show consistent findings of a decrease in rapid eye movement (REM) sleep onset (REM latency), an increase in REM density, and in some subjects a decrease in stage IV delta slow wave sleep.

Although antidepressant drugs result in a blockade of neurotransmitter uptake within hours, their therapeutic effects typically emerge over several weeks, implicating neuroadaptive changes in second messenger systems, such as the G proteins, as a possible mechanism of action.

 TREATMENT

Treatment planning requires coordination of short-term symptom remission with longer term continuation and maintenance strategies designed to prevent relapse and recurrence. The most effective intervention for achieving remission and preventing relapse is medication, but combined treatment, incorporating psychotherapy to help the patient cope with decreased self-esteem and demoralization, demonstrably improves outcome (Fig. 385-3). Forty percent of primary care patients with depression drop out of treatment and discontinue medication if symptomatic improvement is not noted within a month, unless additional support is provided. Outcome improves with (1) increased intensity and frequency of visits during the first 4 to 6 weeks of treatment, (2) supplemental educational materials, and (3) psychiatric consultation as indicated. Despite the widespread acceptance and use of SSRIs, there is no convincing evidence that this class of antidepressant is more efficacious than TCAs. Sixty to seventy percent of all depressed patients respond to any drug chosen, if it is given in a sufficient dose for 6 to 8 weeks (Table 385-6). There is no ideal antidepressant; no current compound combines rapid onset of action, moderate half-life, a meaningful relationship between dose and blood level, a low side effect profile, minimal interaction with other drugs, and safety in overdose. A rational approach to selecting which antidepressant to use involves knowledge of differences in pharmacokinetic activity and matching of the patient's preference and medical history with the metabolic and side effect profile of the drug considered (Table 385-7). A previous response, or a family history of a positive response, to a specific antidepressant would suggest that that drug be tried first. Before initiating antidepressant therapy, the physician should evaluate the possible contribution of comorbid illnesses and consider their specific treatment. In individuals with suicidal ideation, particular atten

Table 385-6

Some Commonly Used Antidepressant Medications

Agent	Usual Daily Oral Therapeutic Dose Range, mg*
Imipramine	150–300
Amitriptyline	150–300
Desipramine	150–300
Nortriptyline	50–150
Doxepin	150–300
Protriptyline	15–60
Trimipramine	150–300
Maprotiline	150–200
Amoxapine	150–450
Trazodone	150–300
Bupropion	250–450
Chlomipramine	100–250
Fluoxetine	20–60
Sertraline	50–200
Paroxetine	20–60
Fluvoxamine	100–300
Nefazodone	300–500
Venlafaxine	125–375
Mirtazapine	15–45
Monoamine oxidase inhibitors	
Phenelzine	45–90
Tranylcypromine	30–50

* After titration; starting doses should be at or below the lowest dosage shown.

tion should be paid to choosing a drug with a low toxicity if taken in overdose. The SSRIs and other newer antidepressant drugs are distinctly safer in this regard; nevertheless, the advantages of TCAs have not been completely superseded. The existence of generic equivalents make them relatively cheap, and for several tricyclics, particularly nortriptyline, imipramine, and desipramine, relationships among dose, plasma level, and therapeutic response have been defined and make more specific individual treatment planning possible. The steady-state plasma level achieved for a given drug dose

FIGURE 385-3 A guideline for the medical management of major depressive disorder. SSRI, selective serotonin reuptake inhibitor; TCA, tricyclic antidepressant.

Table 385-7

Management of Antidepressant Side Effects

Symptoms	Comments and Management Strategies
Gastrointestinal	
Nausea, loss of appetite	Usually short-lived and dose-related; consider temporary dose reduction or administration with food and antacids
Diarrhea	Famotidine, 20–40 mg/d
Constipation	Wait for tolerance; try diet change, stool softener, exercise; avoid laxatives
Sexual dysfunction	Consider dose reduction; drug holiday
Anorgasmia/impotence; impaired ejaculation	Bethanechol, 10–20 mg, 2 h before activity, or cyproheptadine, 4–8 mg 2 h before activity, or bupropion, 100 mg bid or amantadine, 100 mg bid/tid
Orthostasis	Tolerance unlikely; increase fluid intake, use calf exercises/support hose; fludrocortisone, 0.025 mg/d
Anticholinergic	Wait for tolerance
Dry mouth, eyes	Maintain good oral hygiene; use artificial tears, sugar-free gum
Tremor/"jitteriness"	Antiparkinsonian drugs not effective; use dose reduction/slow increase; lorazepam, 0.5 mg bid, or propranolol, 10–20 mg bid
Insomnia	Schedule all doses for the morning; trazodone, 50–100 mg qhs
Sedation	Caffeine; schedule all dosing for bedtime; bupropion, 75–100 mg in afternoon
Headache	Evaluate diet, stress, other drugs; try dose reduction; amitriptyline, 50 mg/d
Weight gain	Decrease carbohydrates; exercise; consider fluoxetine
Loss of therapeutic benefit over time	Related to tolerance? Increase dose or drug holiday; Add amantadine, 100 mg bid, or buspirone, 10 mg tid

can vary more than tenfold between individuals. Plasma levels may help in understanding resistance to treatment and/or paradoxical drug toxicity. The principal disadvantages of TCAs are antihistamine side effects (sedation) and anticholinergic side effects (constipation, dry mouth, urinary hesitancy, and blurred vision). Severe cardiac toxicity due to conduction block or arrhythmias can also occur but is uncommon at therapeutic levels. Tricyclic agents are lethal in overdose, with desipramine carrying the greatest risk. Prescribing only a 10-day supply may be judicious. Most patients require a daily dose of 150 to 200 mg of imipramine or amitriptyline or its equivalent to achieve a therapeutic blood level of 150 to 300 ng/mL and a satisfactory remission; some patients show a partial effect at lower doses. Ethnic differences in drug metabolism are significant, with Hispanic, Asian, and African American patients generally requiring lower doses to achieve a comparable blood level than Caucasians.

Second-generation antidepressants include amoxapine, maprotiline, trazodone, and bupropion. Amoxapine is a dibenzoxazepine derivative that blocks norepinephrine and serotonin reuptake and has a metabolite that shows a degree of dopamine blockade. Long-term use of this drug carries a risk of tardive dyskinesia. Maprotiline is a potent noradrenergic reuptake blocker that has little anticholinergic effect but may produce seizures. Bupropion is a novel antidepressant whose mechanism of action is thought to involve enhancement of noradrenergic function. It has no specific anticholinergic, sedating, or orthostatic side effects and has a low incidence of impairment of sexual performance. It may, however, be associated with aversive stimulant-like side effects, may lower seizure threshold, and has an exceptionally short half-life, requiring multiple dosing.

SSRIs such as fluoxetine, sertraline, and paroxetine cause a lower frequency of anticholinergic, sedating, and cardiovascular side effects but a possibly greater incidence of gastrointestinal complaints, sleep impairment, and sexual dysfunction than do TCAs (Table 385-8). Akathisia, involving an inner sense of restlessness and anxiety, may also be more common, particularly during the first week of treatment. A serious concern, aside from drug interaction, is the risk of "serotonin syndrome," thought to result from hyperstimulation of brainstem $5HT_{1A}$ receptors and characterized by myoclonus, agitation, abdominal cramping, hyperpyrexia, hypertension, and potentially death. Combinations of serotonergic agonists should be monitored closely for this reason. Choice among the SSRIs relates principally to differences in half-life and issues of improved compliance versus increased risk of toxicity over time, and to variance in the risk of incurring adverse drug-drug interactions. Fluoxetine and its principal active metabolite, norfluoxetine, for example, have a combined half-life of almost 7 days, meaning that it takes 5 weeks to achieve steady-state levels and a similar period for the drug to leave the body once its use is discontinued. All the SSRIs may impair sexual function, resulting in diminished libido, impotence,

or difficulty in achieving orgasm. Sexual dysfunction frequently results in noncompliance, and should be asked about specifically in patients using SSRIs. Sexual dysfunction can sometimes be ameliorated by lowering the dose, by instituting drug holidays over the weekend (two or three times a month), or by treatment with amantadine (100 mg tid), bethanechol (25 mg tid), or buspirone (10 mg tid). Paroxetine appears to be more anticholinergic than either fluoxetine or sertraline, and sertraline carries a lower risk of producing an adverse drug interaction than the other two. Rare side effects of SSRIs include vasospastic angina and alterations of prothrombin time.

Venlafaxine, like imipramine, blocks the reuptake of both norepinephrine and serotonin, but it produces relatively little in the way of traditional tricyclic side effects. Unlike the SSRIs, it has a relatively linear dose-response curve. Patients should be monitored for a possible increase in diastolic blood pressure, and multiple daily dosing is required because of the drug's short half-life. Nefazadone is a selective $5HT_2$ receptor antagonist that also inhibits the presynaptic reuptake of serotonin and norepinephrine. Its side effects are similar to those of the SSRIs, and twice-daily dosing produces a steady state within 4 to 5 days. The drug is related structurally to trazodone, which is currently used more for its sedative than its antidepressant properties. Nefazadone appears to produce a lower incidence of sexual side effects than do the SSRIs. Mirtazapine is a recently introduced tetracyclic antidepressant that has a comparatively unique spectrum of activity. It increases noradrenergic and serotonergic neurotransmission through a blockade of central alpha$_2$-adrenergic auto- and heteroreceptors and postsynaptic $5HT_2$ and $5HT_3$ receptors. It is also strongly antihistaminic and, as such, may produce sedation at lower doses.

Each of the SSRIs, as well as nefazadone, may inhibit one or more cytochrome P450 enzymes (Table 385-8). Depending on the specific isoenzyme involved, the metabolism of a number of concomitantly administered medications can be dramatically affected. Fluoxetine and paroxetine, for example, by inhibiting 2D6, can cause dramatic increases in the blood level of type 1C antiarrhythmics, while sertraline and nefazadone, by acting on 3A4, may alter blood levels of terfenadine, carbamazepine, and astemizole. Because many of these compounds have a narrow therapeutic window and can cause iatrogenic ventricular arrhythmias when present at toxic levels, the possibility of an adverse drug interaction should be considered before initiation of therapy and at any time during the course of therapy when patient deterioration is noted.

Other treatment options include the MAOIs and electroconvulsive therapy. The MAOIs are highly effective, particularly in the treatment of atypical depression, but the risk of hypertensive crisis following intake of tyramine-containing food or sympathomimetic drugs makes them inappropriate as first-line agents. Common side effects include orthostatic hypotension, weight gain, insomnia, and sexual dysfunction. MAOIs should not be used in close temporal proximity with SSRIs because of the risk of serotonin syndrome. Electroconvulsive therapy is at least as effective as medication, but its use is reserved for treatment-resistant cases and delusional depressions.

Treatment response should be evaluated after approximately 2 months of therapy. Three-quarters of patients show an adequate response by this time, but if remission is inadequate, the patient should be questioned about medication compliance, and an increase in dose should be considered if side effects are not troublesome. Patients with an inadequate response to the higher dose should be offered an alternative medication. There are no data to guide predictably the choice of a second drug, although drugs of a significantly different class or structure may be recommended on theoretical grounds. However, individual patient responses vary even within a class of similar drugs. If the second medication trial fails, consultation with or referral to a mental health specialist is advised. Strategies for treatment then include combinations of antidepressants and/or adjunctive treatment with other classes of drugs, including lithium,

Table 385-8

Possible Drug Interactions with Selective Serotonin Reuptake Inhibitors

Agent	Effect
Monoamine oxidase inhibitors	Serotonin syndrome—absolute contraindication
Serotonergic agonists, e.g., tryptophan, fenfluramine	Potential serotonin syndrome
Drugs that are metabolized by P450 isoenzymes: tricyclics, other SSRIs, antipsychotics, beta blockers, codeine, terfenadine, astemizole, triazolobenzo-diazepines, calcium channel blockers	Delayed metabolism resulting in increased blood levels and potential toxicity—possible fatality secondary to QT prolongation with terfenadine or astemizole
Drugs that are bound tightly to plasma proteins, e.g., warfarin, coumadin	Increased bleeding secondary to displacement
Drugs that inhibit the metabolism of SSRIs by P450 isoenzymes, e.g., quinidine	Increased SSRI side effects

thyroid hormone, and dopamine agonists. Patients whose response to an SSRI disappears over time may benefit from the addition of buspirone (10 mg tid) or pindolol (2.5 mg tid) or small amounts of a tricyclic antidepressant such as desipramine (25 mg bid or tid). Once significant remission is achieved, drug treatment should be continued for at least 6 to 9 months to prevent relapse. In patients who have had two or more episodes of depression, indefinite maintenance treatment should be considered.

It is essential to counsel patients about depression and the medications they are receiving. An educational approach is best, describing what is known about the depressive syndrome and how the medications may help. Advice about side effects, and expected length of treatment and cautions about alcohol use are helpful. It is important that patients be given time to describe their experience and the impact it has had on them, their family, and their outlook. Occasional empathic silence may be as helpful for the treatment alliance as verbal reassurance.

BIPOLAR DISORDER **Clinical Manifestations** Bipolar disorder is common, affecting approximately 3 million persons in the United States, but often difficult to diagnose. It is characterized by unpredictable swings in mood from mania (or hypomania) to depression. Some patients suffer only from recurrent attacks of *mania*, which in its pure form is associated with increased psychomotor activity, excessive social extroversion, decreased need for sleep, impulsivity and impairment in judgment, and expansive, grandiose, and sometimes irritable mood (Table 385-9). In severe mania, patients may experience delusions and paranoid thinking indistinguishable from that associated with schizophrenia. About half of all patients with bipolar disorder present with a mixture of psychomotor agitation and activation with dysphoria, anxiety, and irritability. It may be difficult to distinguish *mixed mania* from *agitated depression*. In some bipolar patients (*bipolar II disorder*), the full criteria for mania are lacking, and recurrent depressions are separated by periods of mild activation and increased energy (hypomania). In *cyclothymic disorder*, there are numerous hypomanic periods, usually of relatively short duration, alternating with clusters of depressive symptoms that fail to meet the criteria of major depression, either in severity or duration. The mood fluctuations are chronic and should be present for at least 2 years before the diagnosis is made.

Manic episodes typically emerge over a period of days to weeks, but onset within hours is possible, usually in the early morning hours. An untreated episode of either depression or mania can last as short as several weeks or as long as 8 to 12 months, and rare patients have an unremitting chronic course. The term "rapid cycling" is used for patients who have four or more episodes of either depression or mania in a given year. This pattern occurs in 15 percent of all patients, almost all of whom are women. In some cases, rapid cycling is linked to an underlying thyroid dysfunction and, in others, iatrogenically triggered by prolonged antidepressant treatment.

Although bipolar illness is associated with frequent episodic recurrence, it was once thought to have a favorable prognosis and outcome. More recent data, however, show that approximately half of patients with the disorder have sustained difficulties in work performance and psychosocial functioning. The most frequent age of onset for bipolar disorder is between 20 and 30 years of age, but many individuals report premorbid symptoms in late childhood or early adolescence. The prevalence is similar for men and women, but there are gender differences in course, with women likely to have more depressive and men more manic episodes over a lifetime.

Differential Diagnosis The differential diagnosis of mania includes ruling out activation by stimulant and sympathomimetic compounds as well as secondary mania induced by hyperthyroidism, AIDS, or neurologic disorders, such as Huntington's or Wilson's disease, or cerebrovascular accidents. This distinction may be difficult to make, because comorbidity with alcohol and substance abuse is common,

either because of poor judgment and increased impulsivity or because of an attempt at self-medication.

Etiology and Pathophysiology Evidence for a genetic predisposition to bipolar disorder is significant. The concordance rate for monozygotic twin pairs approaches 80 percent, and segregation analyses are consistent with autosomal dominant transmission. Several chromosomal locations for the gene have been proposed in the last decade on the basis of linkage analysis in affected families. None has yet received independent confirmation. Two independent groups reported the results of complete genome scans. One reported weak evidence for linkage to loci on chromosomes 6, 13, and 15, while the other found a major gene locus and haplotype on 18q22-23 in two large Costa Rican pedigrees.

The pathophysiologic mechanisms underlying the profound and recurrent mood swings of bipolar disorder remain unknown. Cellular models of changes in membrane Na^+ and K^+ activated ATPase and proposals of disordered signal transduction mechanisms involving either the phosphoinositol system or guanine nucleotide binding proteins have received the most attention. Lithium reduces the supply of free inositol used to maintain the lipid precursors involved in intracellular signaling and blocks stimulation-induced increases in GTP binding capacity. Reduction of GTP and downstream effects on protein kinase C are being investigated as possible explanations for the therapeutic effects of the drug.

Neurophysiologic studies suggest that bipolar patients have altered circadian rhythmicity. A possible phase advance induced by desynchronization among controlling circadian oscillators is consistent with a finding that lithium increases period length and may exert its therapeutic benefit through a resynchronization of intrinsic rhythms keyed to the light/dark cycle (see Chap. 27). Neuroimaging techniques have also identified a higher rate of subcortical white matter abnormalities in bipolar patients than in age matched controls.

 TREATMENT

Lithium carbonate remains the mainstay of treatment in bipolar disorder, although sodium valproate is equally effective in acute mania. Carbamazepine is also efficacious (Table 385-10). The response rate to lithium carbonate is 70 to 80 percent in acute mania,

---

Table 385-9

Criteria for a Manic Episode

A. A distinct period of abnormally and persistently elevated, expansive, or irritable mood, lasting at least 1 week (or any duration if hospitalization is necessary).

B. During the period of mood disturbance, three (or more) of the following symptoms have persisted (four if the mood is only irritable) and have been present to a significant degree:
  1. Inflated self-esteem or grandiosity
  2. Decreased need for sleep (e.g., feels rested after only 3 hours of sleep)
  3. More talkative than usual or pressure to keep talking
  4. Flight of ideas or subjective experience that thoughts are racing
  5. Distractibility (i.e., attention too easily drawn to unimportant or irrelevant external stimuli)
  6. Increase in goal-directed activity (either socially, at work or school, or sexually) or psychomotor agitation
  7. Excessive involvement in pleasurable activities that have a high potential for painful consequences (e.g., engaging in unrestrained buying sprees, sexual indiscretions, or foolish business investments)

C. The symptoms do not meet criteria for a mixed episode.

D. The mood disturbance is sufficiently severe to cause marked impairment in occupational functioning or in usual social activities or relationships with others, or to necessitate hospitalization to prevent harm to self or others, or there are psychotic features.

E. The symptoms are not due to the direct physiologic effects of a substance (e.g., a drug of abuse, a medication, or other treatment) or a general medical condition (e.g., hyperthyroidism).

Note: Manic-like episodes that are clearly caused by somatic antidepressant treatment (e.g., medication, electroconvulsive therapy, light therapy) should not count toward a diagnosis of bipolar I disorder.

SOURCE: *Diagnostic and Statistical Manual of Mental Disorders,* 4th ed.

with beneficial effects appearing in 1 to 2 weeks. A prophylactic effect in prevention of recurrent mania, and, to a lesser extent, in the prevention of recurrent depression is documented. A simple cation, lithium is rapidly absorbed from the gastrointestinal tract and remains unbound to plasma or tissue proteins. Ninety-five percent of a given dose is excreted unchanged through the kidneys within 24 h.

Serious side effects from lithium administration are rare, but minor complaints such as gastrointestinal discomfort, nausea, diarrhea, polyuria, weight gain, skin eruptions, alopecia, and edema are common. Over time, urine concentrating ability may be decreased, but changes in function do not result in significant nephrotoxicity. In a small subset of patients in whom excessive polyuria occurs (>3000 mL per 24 h), dose or schedule adjustments or the adjunctive use of diuretics should be considered. Lithium exerts an antithyroid effect by interfering with the synthesis and release of thyroid hormones. Approximately 5 percent of patients taking lithium for 18 months or longer develop hypothyroidism, with women more likely to be affected than men. Iatrogenic hypothyroidism should be ruled out in any patient who experiences recurrence of depressive symptomatology during lithium treatment. More serious side effects include tremor, interference with concentration and memory, ataxia, dysarthria, and incoordination. Electrocardiographic (ECG) changes of T wave flattening and conduction delays may occur (see Table 385-2). There is suggestive but not conclusive, evidence that lithium is teratogenic, inducing cardiac malformations in the first trimester.

In the treatment of acute mania, lithium is initiated at 300 mg bid or tid, and the dose is then increased by 300 mg every 2 to 3 days to achieve blood levels of 0.8 to 1.2 mEq/L. Because the therapeutic effect of lithium may not appear until 7 to 10 days of treatment, adjunctive usage of lorazepam (1 to 2 mg every 4 h) or clonazepam (0.5 to 1 mg every 4 h), may be beneficial to control agitation. Antipsychotics are warranted in patients with severe agitation and who respond only partially to benzodiazepines. These agents should be discontinued in the transition to maintenance lithium therapy. Patients using lithium should be monitored closely, since the blood levels required to achieve a therapeutic benefit are close to those associated with neurotoxicity. Risk factors for neurotoxicity include concomitant medical illness, decrease in salt intake, or con-

current use of medications that may increase the serum level of lithium (neuroleptics, diuretics, and calcium channel blockers).

Valproic acid is an alternative in patients who cannot tolerate lithium or respond poorly to it. Valproic acid may be better than lithium for patients who have a rapid-cycling course (i.e., more than four episodes a year) or who present with a mixed or dysphoric mania. Valproic acid is usually started at 500 to 750 mg/d bid or tid. The dose is increased every several days to achieve blood levels in the range of 50 to 100 μg/mL, which typically are achieved at a dose of 1000 to 2500 mg/d. The most serious adverse effect of valproic acid is hepatoxicity, which may be fatal. Such cases are fortunately rare, but regular monitoring of liver enzymes, particularly during the first 90 days of treatment and periodically thereafter, is indicated.

Carbamazepine, although not formally approved by the Food and Drug Administration (FDA) for bipolar disorder, has clinical efficacy in the treatment of acute mania. Carbamazepine is initiated at 400 to 600 mg/d in divided doses, and the dose is increased to achieve a blood level of 4 to 12 mg/L. Carbamazepine may induce a benign leukopenia, but the risk of aplastic anemia is minimal. Nevertheless, it is wise to obtain a complete blood count (CBC) periodically.

The recurrent nature of bipolar mood disorder necessitates maintenance treatment. Maintenance of at least 0.8 mg/L blood lithium levels is important to achieve optimal prophylaxis. Antidepressant medications are sometimes required for the treatment of severe breakthrough depressions, but their use should generally be avoided during maintenance treatment because of the possible risk of precipitating mania or accelerating the cycle frequency. Loss of efficacy over time may be observed with any of the mood-stabilizing agents. In such situations, an alternative agent or combination therapy usually restores the therapeutic benefit.

SOMATOFORM DISORDERS

CLINICAL MANIFESTATIONS Patients with multiple somatic complaints that cannot be explained by a known medical condition or by the effects of alcohol or of recreational or prescription drugs are seen commonly in primary care practice; one survey indicates a prevalence of 5 percent. The somatoform disorders include a variety of conditions that differ in the symptoms present and in whether the symptoms are intentionally produced (Fig. 385-4). In *somatization disorder*, the patient presents with multiple physical complaints derived from different organ systems (Table 385-11). Onset is usually before age 30, and the disorder is persistent. Formal diagnostic criteria require the recording of at least four pain, two gastrointestinal, one sexual, and one pseudoneurologic symptom. Patients with somatization disorder often present with dramatic complaints, but the complaints are inconsistent. Symptoms of comorbid anxiety and mood are common and may be the result of drug interactions due to regimens initiated independently by different physicians. Patients with somatization disorder may be impulsive and demanding and frequently qualify for a formal comorbid psychiatric diagnosis. In *conversion disorder*, the symptoms focus on deficits that involve voluntary motor or sensory function and on psychological factors that initiate or exacerbate the medical presentation. Like somatization disorder, the deficit is not intentionally produced or simulated, as is the case in factitious disorder (malingering). In *hypochondriasis*, the essential feature is a belief of serious medical illness that persists despite reassurance and appropriate medical evaluation. As with somatization disorder, patients with hypochondriasis have a history of poor relationships with physicians stemming from their sense that they have been evaluated and treated inappropriately or inadequately. Hypochondriasis can be disabling in intensity and is persistent, with waxing and waning symptomatology.

In *factitious illnesses*, the patient consciously and voluntarily produces physical symptoms of illness. The term *Munchausen's syndrome* is reserved for individuals with particularly dramatic, chronic, or severe

Table 385-10

Clinical Pharmacology of Mood Stabilizers

Agent and Dosing	Side Effects and Other Effects
Lithium Starting dose: 300 mg bid or tid Therapeutic blood level: 0.8–1.2 mEq/L	*Common side effects:* nausea/anorexia/diarrhea, fine tremor, thirst, polyuria, fatigue, weight gain, acne, folliculitis, neutrophilia, hypothyroidism Blood level is increased by thiazides, tetracyclines, and NSAIDs Blood level is decreased by bronchodilators, verapamil, and carbonic anhydrase inhibitors *Rare side effects:* Neurotoxicity, renal toxicity, hypercalcemia
Carbamazepine Starting dose: 200 mg bid Therapeutic blood level: 4–12 μg/mL	*Common side effects:* Nausea/anorexia, sedation, rash, dizziness/ataxia Induces hepatic metabolism of other medications *Rare side effects:* Hyponatremia, agranulocytosis, Stevens-Johnson syndrome
Valproic acid Starting dose: 250 mg tid Therapeutic blood level: 50–125 μg/mL	*Common side effects:* Nausea/anorexia, weight gain, sedation, tremor, rash, alopecia Inhibits hepatic metabolism of other medications *Rare side effects:* Pancreatitis, hepatoxicity, Stevens-Johnson syndrome

ABBREVIATION: NSAID, nonsteroidal anti-inflammatory drug.

Table 385-11

Diagnostic Criteria for Somatization Disorder

A. A history of many physical complaints beginning before age 30 years that occur over a period of several years and result in treatment being sought or significant impairment in social, occupational, or other important areas of functioning.

B. Each of the following criteria must have been met, with individual symptoms occurring at any time during the course of the disturbance:
1. *Four pain symptoms:* a history of pain related to at least four different sites or functions (e.g., head, abdomen, back, joints, extremities, chest, rectum, during menstruation, during sexual intercourse, or during urination)
2. *Two gastrointestinal symptoms:* a history of at least two gastrointestinal symptoms other than pain (e.g., nausea, bloating, vomiting other than during pregnancy, diarrhea, or intolerance of several different foods)
3. *One sexual symptom:* a history of at least one sexual or reproductive symptom other than pain (e.g., sexual indifference, erectile or ejaculatory dysfunction, irregular menses, excessive menstrual bleeding, vomiting throughout pregnancy)
4. *One pseudoneurologic symptom:* a history of at least one symptom or deficit suggesting a neurologic condition not limited to pain (conversion symptoms such as impaired coordination or balance, paralysis or localized weakness, difficulty swallowing or lump in throat, aphonia, urinary retention, hallucinations, loss of touch or pain sensation, double vision, blindness, deafness, seizures; dissociative symptoms such as amnesia; or loss of consciousness other than fainting)

C. Either of the following:
1. After appropriate investigation, each of the symptoms in criterion B cannot be fully explained by a known general medical condition or the direct effects of a substance (e.g., a drug of abuse, a medication)
2. When there is a related general medical condition, the physical complaints or resulting social or occupational impairment are in excess of what would be expected from the history, physical examination, or laboratory findings

D. The symptoms are not intentionally produced or feigned (as in factitious disorder or malingering).

SOURCE: *Diagnostic and Statistical Manual of Mental Disorders,* 4th ed.

factitious illness. In true factitious illness, the sick role itself is gratifying. A variety of signs, symptoms, and diseases have been either simulated or caused by factitious behavior, the most common including chronic diarrhea, fever of unknown origin, intestinal bleeding or hematuria, seizures, and hypoglycemia. Factitious disorder is usually not diagnosed until 5 to 10 years after its onset, and it can produce significant social and medical costs. In *malingering,* the fabrication derives from a desire for some external reward, such as a narcotic medication or disability reimbursement.

℞ TREATMENT

Patients with somatization disorders are frequently subjected to multiple diagnostic testing and exploratory surgeries in an attempt to find their "real" illness. Such an approach is doomed to failure and does not address the core issue. Successful treatment is best achieved through behavior modification, in which access to the physician is tightly regulated and adjusted to provide a sustained and predictable level of support that is less clearly contingent on the patient's level of presenting distress. Visits can be brief and should not be associated with a need for a diagnostic or treatment action. Although the literature is limited, some patients with somatization disorder may benefit from antidepressant treatment. Fluoxetine and MAOIs have been found independently to be useful in reducing obsessive ruminations, dysphoria, and anxious preoccupation in patients with multiple somatic complaints.

The treatment of factitious disorder is complicated in that any attempt to confront the patient usually only creates a sense of humiliation and causes the patient to abandon treatment from that care giver. A better strategy is to introduce psychological causation as one of

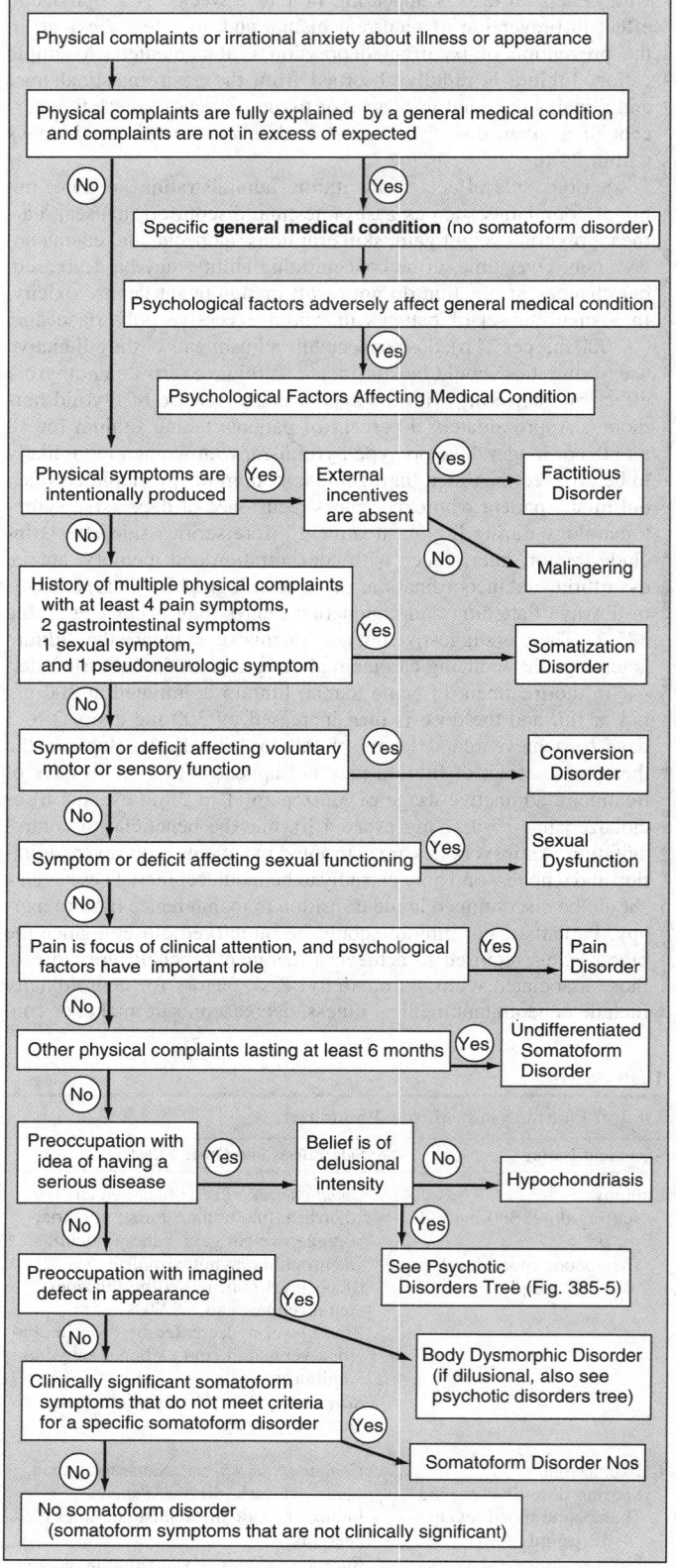

FIGURE 385-4 Differential diagnosis of somatoform disorders. NOS, not otherwise specified. (*From Diagnostic and Statistical Manual of Mental Disorders,* 4th ed.)

a number of possible explanations and to include factitious illness as an option in the differential diagnoses that are discussed. Without directly linking the treatment to the diagnosis, the patient can be offered a face-saving means by which the pathologic relationship with the health care system can be examined and alternative approaches to life stressors developed.

PERSONALITY DISORDERS

CLINICAL MANIFESTATIONS Personality disorders are characteristic patterns of thinking, feeling, and interpersonal behavior that are relatively inflexible and cause significant functional impairment or subjective distress for the individual. To qualify for the formal diagnosis, the observed behaviors should not be secondary to another mental disorder, nor should they be precipitated by substance abuse or a general medical condition. This distinction is often difficult to make in clinical practice, as personality change may be the first sign of serious neurologic, endocrine, or other medical illness. Patients with frontal lobe tumors, for example, can present with changes in motivation and personality while the results of the neurologic examination remain within normal limits. Personality traits are stable over time and environmental situation and are recognizable in adolescence or early adult life. Although DSM-IV portrays personality disorders as qualitatively distinct categories, there is an alternative perspective that personality characteristics vary as a continuum between normal functioning and formal mental disorder.

Personality disorders have been grouped into three clusters that share similar attributes. *Cluster A* includes paranoid, schizoid, and schizotypal personality disorders. It includes individuals who are odd and eccentric and who maintain an emotional distance from others. Individuals have a restricted emotional range and remain socially isolated. Patients with schizotypal personality disorder frequently have unusual perceptual experiences and express magical beliefs about the external world. The essential feature of paranoid personality disorder is a pervasive mistrust and suspiciousness of others to an extent that is unjustified by available evidence. *Cluster B* disorders include antisocial, borderline, histrionic, and narcissistic types and describe individuals whose behavior is impulsive, excessively emotional, and erratic. *Cluster C* incorporates avoidant, dependent, and obsessive-compulsive personality types, whose enduring traits are anxious or fearful in nature. These divisions have not been validated but are useful for understanding some patients whose psychological problems interfere with diagnosis and treatment. The boundaries between cluster types are to some extent artificial, and many patients who meet criteria for one personality disorder also meet criteria for aspects of another. In addition, the risk of a comorbid major mental disorder is increased in patients who qualify for a diagnosis of personality disorder.

℞ TREATMENT

Historically, recommended treatment for personality disorders was long-term psychotherapy, in which the pathologic patterns of interaction with the world at large could be relived and examined through the corrective emotional experience of the controlled therapeutic relationship. More recently, the recognition that personality derives in part from biologically determined components of temperament has given rise to the empirical use of drugs to treat specific symptom clusters as well as any coexisting major mental disorder. To this end, antidepressant medications and low-dose antipsychotic drugs have some efficacy in cluster A personality disorders, while anticonvulsant mood-stabilizing agents and MAOIs may be considered for patients with cluster B diagnoses who show marked mood reactivity, behavioral dyscontrol, and/or rejection hypersensitivity. Anxious or fearful cluster C patients often have a response to medication that parallels that for patients with axis I anxiety disorders. In all cases, it is important for both the physician and the patient to have reasonable expectations as to the possible effect of the medication and any associated side effects. Beneficial responses may be subtle and observable only over a span of time that affords an adequate sampling of life experience.

SCHIZOPHRENIA

CLINICAL MANIFESTATIONS Schizophrenia is no longer considered a single disease, but rather a group of illnesses that are phenomenologically and etiologically heterogeneous (Fig. 385-5). Schizophrenia is characterized by perturbations of language, percep-

tion, thinking, social activity, affect, and volition, but there are no pathognomonic features. The syndrome commonly begins in late adolescence, has an insidious onset, and, classically, a poor outcome, progressing from social withdrawal and perceptual distortions to a state of chronic delusions and hallucinations. Patients with schizophrenic syndrome may present with positive symptoms (such as conceptual

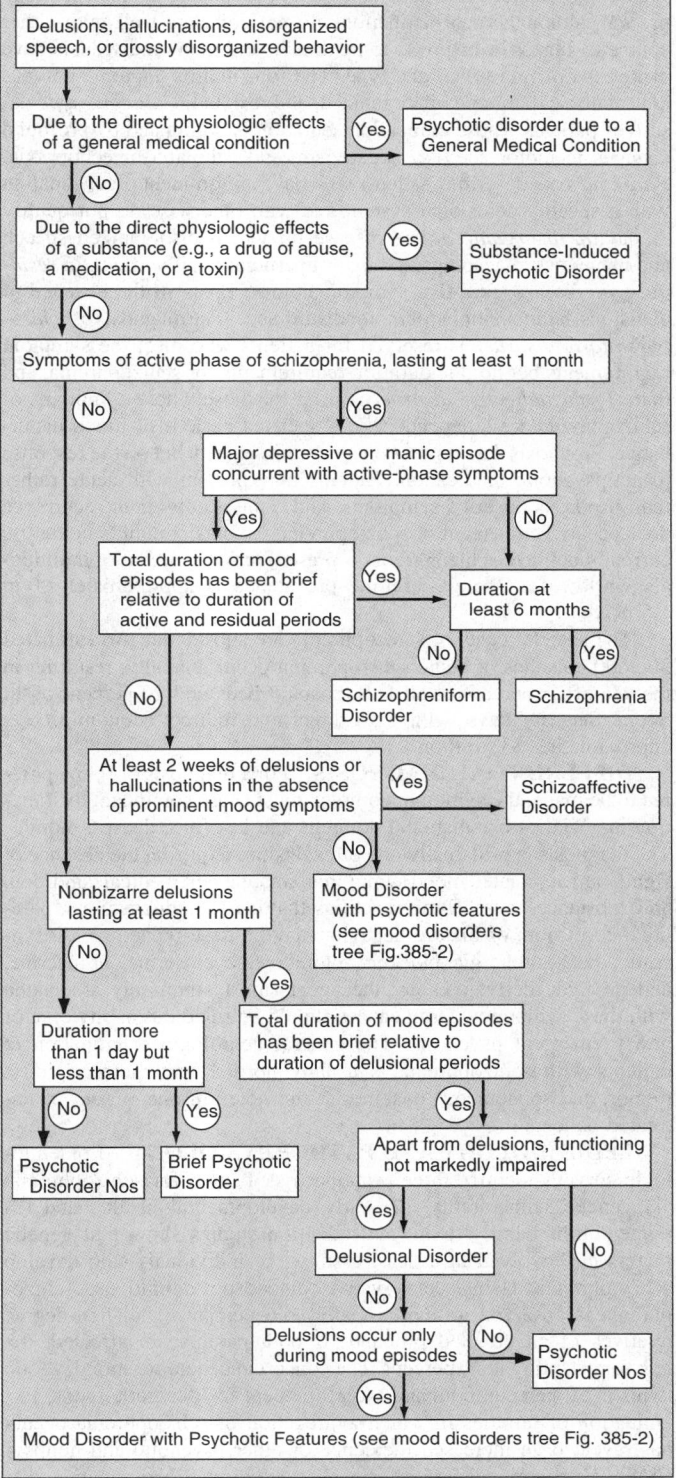

FIGURE 385-5 Differential diagnosis of psychotic disorders. NOS, not otherwise specified. *(From Diagnostic and Statistical Manual of Mental Disorders, 4th ed.)*

disorganization, delusions, or hallucinations) or negative symptoms (loss of function, anhedonia, decreased emotional expression, impaired concentration, and diminished social engagement). "Negative" symptoms predominate in one-third of the schizophrenic population and are associated with a poor long-term outcome and a poor response to drug treatment. However, marked variability in the course and individual character of symptoms is typical.

Schizophrenia can also be defined by the specific symptomatology present, although such distinctions do not correlate well with either course of illness or response to treatment, and many individuals have symptoms of more than one type. The four main symptom subtypes are catatonic, paranoid, disorganized, and residual. *Catatonic-type* describes patients whose clinical presentation is dominated by profound changes in motor activity, negativism, and echolalia or echopraxia. *Paranoid-type* describes patients who have a prominent preoccupation with a specific delusional system and who otherwise do not qualify as having *disorganized-type* disease, in which disorganized speech and behavior are accompanied by a superficial or silly affect. In *residual-type* disease, negative symptomatology exists in the absence of delusions, hallucinations, or motor disturbance. The diagnosis of *schizophreniform disorder* is reserved for patients who meet the symptom requirements but not the duration requirements for schizophrenia, and that of *schizoaffective disorder* is used for those whose symptoms of schizophrenia are independent of associated periods of mood disturbance. Prognosis depends not on symptom severity but on the response to antipsychotic medication. Patients may present with acute rather than insidious onset of symptoms, and remission without recurrence does occur. Ten percent of schizophrenic patients commit suicide. As currently defined, schizophrenia is present in 0.85 percent of individuals worldwide. Overall, lifetime prevalence is approximately 1 to 1.5 percent.

The societal costs of schizophrenia are substantial. An estimated 300,000 episodes of acute schizophrenia occur annually, resulting in the use of 25 percent of all U.S. hospital beds and 20 percent of all Social Security days, with total direct and indirect economic costs approximating $33 billion.

DIFFERENTIAL DIAGNOSIS   For a diagnosis of schizophrenia to be made, the symptom complex must cause significant dysfunction in social or occupational domains and last for at least 6 months. The diagnosis is principally one of exclusion, requiring the absence of significant associated mood symptoms, any relevant medical condition, and substance abuse. Drug reactions that cause hallucinations, paranoia, confusion, or bizarre behavior may be dose-related or idiosyncratic; beta-adrenergic blockers, clonidine, cycloserine, quinacrine, and procaine derivatives are the agents most commonly associated with these symptoms. Drug causes should be ruled out in any case of newly emergent psychosis. The general neurologic examination in patients with schizophrenia is usually normal, but motor rigidity, tremor, and spontaneous dyskinesias are noted in one-quarter of untreated patients.

EPIDEMIOLOGY AND PATHOPHYSIOLOGY   Epidemiologic surveys identify three principal risk factors for schizophrenia: (1) genetic vulnerability, (2) early developmental insults, and (3) winter birth. Family, twin, and adoption studies show that genetic factors are involved in at least a subset of individuals who develop schizophrenia. Using conservative diagnostic definitions, schizophrenia is observed in approximately 6.6 percent of all first-degree relatives of an affected proband. If both parents are affected, the risk for offspring is 40 percent. The concordance rate for monozygotic twins is 50 percent, compared to 10 percent for dizygotic twins. Examination of families in which aggregation of schizophrenia occurs has revealed an increased incidence of other psychotic and nonpsychotic psychiatric disorders as well, including schizoaffective disorder and *schizotypal* and *schizoid personality disorders*, the latter terms designating individuals who show a lifetime pattern of social and interpersonal deficits characterized by an inability to form close interpersonal relationships, eccentric behavior, and mild perceptual distortions.

There is increasing evidence that environmental influences modulate genetic factors in the expression of schizophrenia, and, in sporadic cases, may serve as a sufficient cause. Gestational and birth complications, including Rh factor incompatibility, prenatal exposure to influenza during the second trimester, and prenatal nutritional deficiency have been implicated. Studies of monozygotic twins discordant for schizophrenia have profiled neuroanatomic and morphologic differences between affected and unaffected siblings, supporting a "two-strike" etiology involving both genetic susceptibility and an environmental insult.

The proposed pathophysiology involves localized hypoxia during critical stages of neuronal migration and maturation. Neuroimaging and postmortem studies have identified a number of structural and functional abnormalities, including (1) enlargement of the lateral and third ventricles with associated cortical atrophy and sulcal enlargement, (2) volumetric reductions in the amygdala, hippocampus, right prefrontal cortex, and thalamus, (3) altered asymmetry of the planum temporale, and (4) decreases in neuronal metabolism in the thalamus and prefrontal cortex. Some, but not all, prospective studies record progressive reduction in hemispheric volume over years. Cytoarchitectural investigations reveal alterations in the size, orientation, and density of cells in the hippocampus and, in the prefrontal cerebral cortex, decreases in neuronal number and the density of interneurons in layer II as well as an increased density of pyramidal cells in layer V. These observations suggest that schizophrenia results from a disturbance in a cortical striatal–thalamic circuit resulting in deficits in sensory filtering and attentional behavior. Although the formal diagnostic requirements for schizophrenia are not usually met until early adult life, children who eventually develop the disorder may exhibit subtle deficits in motor function, cognition, and emotional expression from an early age.

The hypothesized alterations in cortical neuronal circuitry are paralleled clinically by impairments in attention and cortical information processing, autonomic nervous system activation, and habituation. Schizophrenic individuals are highly distractible and demonstrate a relative deficit in perceptual-motor speed, ability to shift attention, and filtering out of background stimuli. Event-related evoked potential studies of schizophrenia have defined a specific reduction in P300 amplitude to a novel stimulus, which implicates an impairment in cognitive processing, since earlier, more sensory-based components are unaffected. Impaired information processing aggregates in family members of schizophrenic probands.

Despite evidence for a genetic causation, the results of molecular genetic linkage studies in schizophrenia are inconclusive. Single reports of linkage of schizophrenia to loci on chromosomes 5, 11, and other regions have not been replicated. However, four separate groups, using 430 families from diverse populations worldwide, have identified an extended region on the short arm of chromosome 6 that appears to be linked to the disorder, while several others have reported a locus on chromosome 22.

The *dopamine hypothesis* of schizophrenia is based on the serendipitous discovery that agents that diminish dopaminergic activity have beneficial effects in reducing the acute symptoms and signs of psychosis, specifically agitation, anxiety, and hallucinations. Amelioration of delusions and social withdrawal is less dramatic. Thus far, however, evidence for increased dopaminergic activity is indirect. An increase in the activity of nigrostriatal and mesolimbic systems and a relative decrease in mesocortical tracts innervating the prefrontal cortex is hypothesized, although it is likely that other neurotransmitters, including serotonin, acetylcholine, glutamate, and GABA also contribute to the pathophysiology of the illness. Involvement of excitatory amino acids is postulated, based on the finding that NMDA receptor antagonists and channel blockers, such as phencyclidine (PCP) and ketamine, produce characteristic signs of schizophrenia in many normal individuals. These effects can be blocked by "atypical" neuroleptics like clozapine and olanzapine. NMDA receptors are located in high density in the frontal cortex, hippocampus, limbic system, and striatum regions suspected to be involved in schizophrenia. Levels of aspartate and glutamate are decreased in the brains of schizophrenics, while a co-localized neuropeptide antagonist compound, *N*-acetyl-aspartyl glutamate (NAAG), is increased. Evidence for reduced GABA transmission derives from decreased gene expression of glutamic acid decarboxylase in the dorsolateral prefrontal cortex of schizophrenic patients; such a deficit could be responsible for a loss of inhibition over dopaminergic activity in the basal ganglia.

℞ TREATMENT

Antipsychotic agents remain the cornerstone of acute and maintenance treatment of schizophrenia and are effective in the treatment of hallucinations, delusions, and thought disorders, regardless of etiology. The exact mechanism of action remains incompletely understood, but dopaminergic receptor blockade in the limbic system and basal ganglia appears to be an essential element, since the clinical potencies of traditional antipsychotic drugs parallel their affinities for the D_2 receptor, and even the newer "atypical" agents exert some degree of D_2 receptor blockade. All neuroleptics induce expression of the immediate-early gene c-*fos* in the nucleus accumbens, a dopaminergic site connecting prefrontal and limbic cortices. The clinical efficacy of newer atypical neuroleptics, however, may involve D_1, D_3, and D_4 receptor blockade, alpha$_1$ and alpha$_2$ noradrenergic activity, and/or the relationship between $5HT_2$ and D_2 receptor activity as well. In experimental investigations of a proposed glutaminergic deficiency model of schizophrenia, high-dose glycine therapy also shows encouraging evidence of efficacy.

Conventional neuroleptics differ in their potency and side-effect profile. Older agents, such as chlorpromazine and thioridazine, are more sedating and anticholinergic and more likely to cause orthostatic hypotension, while higher potency antipsychotics, such as haloperidol, perphenazine, and thiothixene, carry a higher risk of inducing extrapyramidal side effects. The model atypical antipsychotic agent is clozapine, a dibenzoazepine derivative that has a greater potency in blocking the $5HT_2$ than the D_2 receptor and a much higher affinity for the D_4 than the D_2 receptor. Its principal disadvantage is risk of blood dyscrasia, requiring regular monitoring of the CBC. Unlike other antipsychotics, clozapine does not cause a rise in prolactin level. Approximately 30 percent of patients have a better antipsychotic response to these agents than to traditional neuroleptics, suggesting that they will increasingly displace the older-generation drugs. *Clozapine* increases the activity of the immediate-early gene c-*fos* in the prefrontal cortex, the neuroanatomic region having the highest concentration of D_4 receptors and an area thought to mediate the specific executive functions that are prominently impaired in schizophrenia. *Risperidone*, a benzisoxazole derivative, is more potent at $5HT_2$ than D_2 receptor sites, like clozapine, but it also exerts significant alpha$_2$ antagonism, a property that may contribute to its perceived ability to improve mood and increase motor activity. Risperidone is not as effective as clozapine in treatment-resistant cases but does not carry a risk of blood dyscrasia.

Conventional antipsychotic agents are effective in approximately 70 percent of patients presenting with a first episode. Improvement may be observed within hours or days, but full remission usually requires 6 to 8 weeks. Since no antipsychotic drug is clearly superior to any other in efficacy (with the exception of clozapine in treatment-resistant groups), the choice of agent depends principally on the side-effect profile or on a past personal or family history of a favorable response to the drug in question. Equivalent treatment response can usually be achieved through relatively low doses of any drug selected, i.e., 4 to 6 mg/d of haloperidol, 400 mg/d of chlorpromazine, or 4 to 6 mg/d of risperidone. Doses in this range result in greater than 80 percent D_2 receptor blockade, and there is little evidence that higher doses increase either the rapidity or degree of response. Titration of the dose should proceed slowly, particularly with risperidone, for which 2 weeks to 1 month usually is required to arrive at an optimal level. Maintenance treatment requires careful attention to the possibility of relapse and monitoring for the development of a movement disorder. Intermittent drug treatment is less effective than regular dosing, but gradual dose reduction is likely to improve social functioning in many schizophrenic patients who have been maintained at high doses. If medications are completely discontinued, however, the relapse rate is about 60 percent within 6 months. Long-acting injectable preparations (haloperidol decanoate and fluphenazine decanoate) are considered when noncompliance with oral therapy leads to relapses. In treatment-resistant patients, a transition to clozapine usually results in rapid improvement, but a prolonged delay in response in some cases necessitates a 6- to 9-month trial for maximal benefit to occur.

Antipsychotic medications can cause a broad range of side effects, including lethargy, weight gain, postural hypotension, constipation, and dry mouth. Extrapyramidal symptoms such as dystonia, akathisia, and akinesia are also frequent with traditional agents and may contribute to poor compliance if not specifically addressed. Anticholinergic and Parkinsonian symptoms respond well to trihexyphenidyl, 2 mg bid, or benztropine mesylate, 1 to 2 mg bid. Akathisia may respond to beta blockers. In rare cases, more serious and occasionally life-threatening side effects may emerge, including ventricular arrhythmias, gastrointestinal obstruction, retinal pigmentation, obstructive jaundice, and neuroleptic malignant syndrome (characterized by hyperthermia, autonomic dysfunction, muscular rigidity, and elevated creatinine phosphokinase levels). The most serious adverse effects of clozapine are agranulocytosis, which has an incidence of 1 percent, and induction of seizures, which has an incidence of 10 percent. Weekly white blood cell counts are required, particularly during the first 3 months of treatment.

A severe side effect of long-term use of the classic antipsychotic agents is *tardive dyskinesia*, characterized by repetitive, involuntary, and potentially irreversible movements of the tongue and lips (buccolinguo-masticatory triad), and, in approximately half of cases, choreoathetoid movements of the limbs (see Chap. 21). Tardive dyskinesia occurs in one-quarter to one-half of all patients who are maintained on neuroleptics for longer than 6 months. The prevalence increases with age and with total dose and duration of drug administration, but as yet unknown individual factors play the greatest part in determining risk. The cause of tardive dyskinesia is unknown, but evidence suggests that chronic neuroleptic treatment increases the formation of free radicals and perhaps damages mitochondrial energy metabolism. Vitamin E may reduce abnormal involuntary movements if given early in the development of the syndrome. Other strategies for treatment include use of reserpine and anticholinergics, in addition to very gradual dose reduction. The higher efficacy of clozapine and risperidone in treating negative symptoms, together with their lower risk of tardive dyskinesia, has stimulated the development of additional atypical antipsychotic agents that are likely to revolutionize the treatment of schizophrenia. Quetiapine, olanzapine, ziprasidone, and sertindole promise to have a therapeutic efficacy comparable to that of clozapine without the latter's risk of causing agranulocytosis.

ASSESSMENT AND EVALUATION OF VIOLENCE

Primary care physicians may, in the course of routine medical practice, encounter situations in which familial, domestic, or societal violence is discovered or suspected. Depending on local laws, such an awareness can carry legal and moral obligations. Recent surveys document that child, spousal, and elder abuse is relatively common and that physicians are frequently the first point of contact for both victim and abuser. Between 1 and 2 million older Americans and 1.5 million U.S. children are thought to experience some form of physical maltreatment each year. Spousal abuse is thought to be even more prevalent. A recent broad-based survey of primary care internal medicine practices found that 5.5 percent of all female patients had experienced domestic violence in the previous year, and that these individuals were more likely to suffer from depression, anxiety, somatization disorder, and substance abuse and to have attempted suicide. When domestic violence is suspected, direct but nonjudgmental questioning should be pursued with each party separately—"Do you feel safe at home," and "If there's a disagreement or a conflict between the two of you, how is it worked out?" In addition to obvious and suggestive physical injury, individuals who are abused frequently express low self-esteem, vague somatic symptomatology, social isolation, and a passive feeling of loss of control. Although it is essential to treat these elements in the victim, the first obligation is to ensure that the perpetrator has taken responsibility for preventing any further violence. Substance abuse and/or dependence and serious mental illness in the abuser may contribute to the risk of harm and require direct intervention. Depending on the individual situation, law enforcement agencies, community resources such as support groups and shelters, and individual and family counseling can be appropriate components of a treatment plan. A safety plan should be formulated with the victim, in addition to the provision of information about abuse, its likelihood of recurrence, and its tendency to increase in severity and frequency. Antianxiety and antidepressant medications may sometimes be useful in treating the acute symptoms, but they should only be used if independent evidence for an appropriate psychiatric diagnosis exists. Antidepressants are generally not indicated when the diagnosis is linked to the social situation, such as an adjustment disorder with depressed mood. The most important element in treatment is the development of a supportive doctor-patient relationship that avoids further blame of the victim.

In certain circumstances, a significant potential for societal violence may be discovered. Sympathetic, but direct, questioning of potential violent impulses, access to weapons, recreational drug use, and specific homicidal ideation is necessary for appropriate evaluation and is sometimes therapeutic in its own right. The existence and possible contribution of such medical conditions as delirium and/or intoxication should be evaluated. Available disposition options for potentially violent patients include police custody, psychiatric hospitalization, and referral to home care, with involvement of family, friends, and care givers. In deciding which treatment option is most appropriate, clinicians should endeavor to establish an empathic interaction with the patient, while avoiding interventions or stimuli that might precipitate or increase the risk of violent behavior. Formal verbal limit setting may be necessary if the patient reveals the existence of a weapon or becomes increasingly agitated or verbally abusive. Use of the least restrictive intervention is generally the best approach during the initial evaluation.

MENTAL HEALTH PROBLEMS IN THE HOMELESS

There is increasing recognition of a high prevalence of mental disorders and substance abuse among homeless and impoverished populations. The total number of homeless individuals in the United States is estimated at 2 to 3 million, one-third of whom qualify as having a serious mental disorder. Poor hygiene and nutrition, substance abuse, psychiatric illness, physical trauma, and exposure to the elements combine to make the provision of medical care a challenging enterprise. Only a minority of individuals receive formal mental health care; the main points of contact are outpatient medical clinics and emergency departments. Primary care settings represent a critical site in which housing needs, treatment of substance dependence, and evaluation and treatment of psychiatric illness can most efficiently take place. Successful intervention is dependent on breaking down traditional administrative barriers to health care and recognizing the physical constraints and emotional costs imposed by homelessness. Simplifying health care instructions and follow-up, allowing frequent visits,

and dispensing medications in limited amounts that require ongoing contact are possible techniques for establishing a successful therapeutic relationship. Child neglect, resulting in developmental delay and emotional difficulty in addition to other health problems, is unfortunately common and necessitates an effort to independently evaluate the well being of any offspring.

BIBLIOGRAPHY

GENERAL

AMERICAN PSYCHIATRIC ASSOCIATION: Diagnostic and Statistical Manual of Mental Disorders, 4th ed. Washington DC, American Psychiatric Association, 1994

BROADHEAD WE et al: Development and validation of the SDDS-PC screen for multiple mental disorders in primary care. Arch Fam Med 4:211, 1995

HYMAN SE, NESTLER EJ: Initiation and adaptation: A paradigm for understanding psychotropic drug action. Am J Psychiatry 153:151, 1996

LACHS M, PILLEMER K: Abuse and neglect of elderly persons. N Engl J Med 332:437, 1995

McCAULEY J et al: The "battering syndrome": Prevalence and clinical characteristics of domestic violence in primary care internal medical practices. Ann Intern Med 123:737, 1995

OLDHAM JM et al: Comorbidity of axis I and axis II disorders. Am J Psychiatry 152:571, 1995

PSYCHOLOGICAL FACTORS IN MEDICAL ILLNESS

BUCKLEY RA: Differentiating medical and psychiatric illness. Psychiatr Ann 24:584, 1994

LINDEN W et al: Psychosocial interventions for patients with coronary artery disease. Arch Intern Med 156:745, 1996

McDANIEL JS et al: Depression in patients with cancer. Arch Gen Psychiatry 52:89, 1995

ANXIETY DISORDERS

BROWN C et al: Treatment outcomes for primary care patients with major depression and lifetime anxiety disorders. Arch Gen Psychiatry 153:1293, 1996

GOLDBERG RJ: Diagnostic dilemmas presented by patients with anxiety and depression. Am J Med 98:278, 1995

LYDIARD B et al: Panic disorder and gastrointestinal symptoms: Findings from the NIMH epidemiologic catchment area project. Am J Psychiatry 151:64, 1994

MAGEE WJ et al: Agoraphobia, simple phobia, and social phobia in the national comorbidity survey. Arch Gen Psychiatry 53:159, 1996

MARSHALL RD, KLEIN DF: Pharmacotherapy in the treatment of posttraumatic stress disorder. Psychiatr Ann 25:588, 1995

MOOD DISORDERS

BURVILL PW: Recent progress in the epidemiology of major depression. Epidemiol Rev 17:21, 1995

DEPRESSION GUIDELINE PANEL: Depression in Primary Care, vol 1: Detection and Diagnosis. Clinical Practice Guideline no 5. Rockville, MD, US Department of Health & Human Services, AHCPR Publication 93-0550, 1993

————: Depression in Primary Care, vol 2: Treatment of Major Depression. Clinical Practice Guideline no 5. Rockville, MD, US Department of Health & Human Services, AHCPR Publication 93-0551, 1993

HIRSCHFELD RMA: Algorithm for the evaluation and treatment of suicidal patients. Prim Psychiatry 3:26, 1996

KATON W et al: Collaborative management to achieve treatment guidelines. JAMA 13:1026, 1995

KUPFER DJ: Sleep research in depressive illness: Clinical implications—a tasting menu. Biol Psychiatry 38:391, 1995

PRICE LH, HENNINGER GR: Lithium in the treatment of mood disorders. N Engl J Med 331:591, 1994

SHERBOURNE CD et al: Subthreshold depression and depressive disorder: Clinical characteristics of general medical and mental health specialty outpatients. Am J Psychiatry 151:1777, 1994

SOLOMON DA et al: Course of illness and maintenance treatments for patients with bipolar disorder. J Clin Psychiatry 56:5, 1995

STURM R, WELLS KB: How can care for depression become more cost-effective? JAMA 273:51, 1995

SOMATOFORM DISORDERS, PERSONALITY AND BEHAVIORAL DISORDERS

DAVIS JM et al: Psychopharmacotherapy of the personality-disordered patient. Psychiatr Ann 25:614, 1995

Noyes R Jr et al: Somatization. Diagnosis and management. Arch Fam Med 4:790, 1995

SCHIZOPHRENIA

Andreasen NC et al: Symptoms of schizophrenia. Arch Gen Psychiatry 52:341, 1995

Carpenter WT Jr, Buchanan RW: Schizophrenia. N Engl J Med 330:681, 1994

———— et al: Patient response and resource management: Another view of clozapine treatment of schizophrenia. Am J Psychiatry 152:827, 1995

Kane JM: Schizophrenia. N Engl J Med 334:34, 1996

Kety SS et al: Mental illness in the biological and adoptive relatives of schizophrenic adoptees. Arch Gen Psychiatry 51:442, 1994

Wyatt RJ: Neurodevelopmental abnormalities and schizophrenia. Arch Gen Psychiatry 53:11, 1996

SECTION 6
ALCOHOLISM AND DRUG DEPENDENCY

386   *Marc A. Schuckit*

ALCOHOL AND ALCOHOLISM

Ninety percent of people drink alcohol, 40 to 50 percent of men have temporary alcohol-induced problems, and 10 to 20 percent of men and 3 to 10 percent of women develop pervasive and persistent alcohol-related problems (alcohol dependence or abuse—alcoholism). The usual alcoholic has a family and a job; only about 5 percent live on "skid row." Even light drinking may adversely interact with other medications; temporary heavier drinking can exacerbate most medical illnesses; and alcoholism can masquerade as many different medical disorders and psychiatric syndromes. The following sections describe the pharmacology and clinical effects of alcohol and identify circumstances in which drinking may cause a major medical or psychiatric problem or exacerbate a preexisting disorder.

PHARMACOLOGY OF ETHANOL: ABSORPTION AND METABOLISM   Ethanol is a weakly charged molecule that moves easily through cell membranes, rapidly equilibrating between blood and tissues. The effects of drinking depend in part on the amount of ethanol consumed per unit of body weight; the level of alcohol in the blood is expressed as milligrams or grams of ethanol per deciliter (e.g., 100 mg/dL or 0.1000 g/dL). In round figures, 340 mL (12 oz) of beer, 115 mL (4 oz) of nonfortified wine, and 43 mL (1.5 oz) (a shot) of 80-proof beverage each contain approximately 10 g of ethanol; 1 pint of 86-proof beverage contains approximately 160 g, and 1 L of wine contains approximately 80 g of ethanol. Congeners found in alcoholic beverages may contribute to body damage with heavy drinking; these include low-molecular-weight alcohols (e.g., methanol and butanol), aldehydes, esters, histamine, phenols, tannins, iron, lead, and cobalt.

Ethanol is a central nervous system (CNS) depressant that decreases activity of neurons, although some behavioral stimulation is observed at low blood levels. This drug has cross-tolerance and shares a similar pattern of behavioral problems with other brain depressants, including the benzodiazepines and barbiturates. Alcohol is absorbed from mucous membranes of the mouth and esophagus (in small amounts), from the stomach and large bowel (in modest amounts), and from the proximal portion of the small intestine (the major site). The rate of absorption is *increased* by rapid gastric emptying, by the absence of proteins, fats, or carbohydrates (which interfere with absorption), by the absence of congeners, by dilution to a modest percentage of ethanol (maximum absorption is seen at about 20 percent by volume), and by carbonation (e.g., champagne).

Between 2 percent (at low blood alcohol concentrations) and about 10 percent (at high blood alcohol concentrations) of ethanol is excreted directly through the lungs, urine, or sweat, but the greater part is metabolized to acetaldehyde in the liver. At least two metabolic routes, each with different optimal concentrations of ethanol (K_m), result in the metabolism of approximately one drink per hour. The *first* and clinically most important pathway occurs in the cell cytosol via alcohol dehydrogenase (ADH), with a K_m of about 2 mmol. This reaction produces acetaldehyde, which is then rapidly destroyed by aldehyde dehydrogenase (ALDH) in the cytosol and mitochondria. Each of these steps requires nicotinamide adenine dinucleotide (NAD) as a cofactor, and it is the increased ratio of the reduced cofactor (NADH) to NAD (NADH:NAD) that is responsible for many of the metabolic derangements observed after drinking. *Second*, microsomes of the smooth endoplasmic reticulum (the microsomal ethanol-oxidizing system, or MEOS), with a K_m of about 10 mmol, may be responsible for 10 percent or more of ethanol oxidation at high blood alcohol concentrations. Increased activity of this system can be induced by repeated exposure to ethanol.

The specific clinical significance of the first metabolite of alcohol, acetaldehyde, is not fully known, but low levels of this substance may cause stimulation and behavioral reinforcement. Accumulation of higher levels in liver, brain, or other body tissues may cause organ damage.

BEHAVIORAL EFFECTS, TOLERANCE, AND DEPENDENCE   The behavioral and physiologic effects of any drug depend on the dose, its rate of increase in plasma, the concomitant presence of other drugs or medical problems, and the past experience with the agent. With alcohol, an additional factor is whether blood alcohol levels are rising or falling; the effects of alcohol are more intense during the former period.

Even though "legal intoxication" requires a blood alcohol concentration of at least 80 to 100 mg/dL, behavioral, psychomotor, and cognitive changes are seen at levels as low as 20 to 30 mg/dL (i.e., after one to two drinks). Narcosis or deep sleep is induced in many people at twice the legal intoxication level, and even in the absence of concomitant medications, death can occur with levels between 300 and 400 mg/dL. Ethanol, either alone or in combination with agents such as benzodiazepines, is probably responsible for more toxic overdose deaths than any other agent.

Ethanol produces simultaneous changes in many neurotransmitters and also increases the fluidity of neuronal cell membranes. After repeated exposure to the drug, the body compensates in at least three ways to tolerate higher ethanol levels. *First*, after 1 to 2 weeks of daily drinking, the liver can increase the rate of ethanol metabolism by as much as 30 percent; i.e., there is *metabolic or pharmacokinetic tolerance*. This alteration disappears almost as rapidly as it develops. *Second, cellular or pharmacodynamic tolerance* probably occurs through complex neurochemical changes and alterations in cell membranes—adjustments that may contribute to physical dependence. *Third*, even at the same blood alcohol concentrations and level of neuronal adaptation, organisms can learn to adapt their behavior so as to function better than expected under drug influence *(behavioral tolerance)*.

Once the cells have adapted to chronic ethanol exposure, the structural or biochemical changes may not return to normal for several weeks or more. In the face of these adjustments, the neurons require ethanol to function optimally; i.e., the person is physically addicted. This physical condition is distinct from psychological dependence, a concept indicating that the person is psychologically uncomfortable without the drug.

NUTRITIONAL FACTORS One gram of ethanol has approximately 29.7 kJ (7.1 kcal) of energy, and a drink contains between 293.0 and 418.6 kJ (70 and 100 kcal) from ethanol and other carbohydrates. Therefore, 8 to 10 drinks can yield over 4186 kJ (1000 kcal) per day, but these are "empty" of nutrients such as minerals, proteins, and vitamins.

Any vitamin absorbed through the small intestine by active transport or stored in the liver may be deficient in even apparently well-nourished alcoholics. These include folate (folacin or folic acid), pyridoxine (B_6), thiamine (B_1), nicotinic acid (niacin, B_3), and vitamin A. Thiamine deficiency causes Wernicke's and Korsakoff's syndromes (see Chap. 380).

Low blood levels of potassium, magnesium, calcium, zinc, and phosphorus can occur as a consequence of dietary deficiency and acid-base imbalances during excess alcohol ingestion or withdrawal. Hypokalemia can lead to periodic muscle paralysis and areflexia. Deficiencies in magnesium can add to a clouded sensorium and other neurologic symptoms; hypocalcemia can cause tetany and weakness; low levels of zinc are speculated to contribute to gonadal dysfunction, anorexia, problems with wound healing, and immune deficiencies; and low phosphate levels can contribute to myocardial failure, brain dysfunction, weakness of muscles (including those of respiration), and white blood cell and platelet dysfunction.

An ethanol load in a fasting, healthy individual is likely to produce transient hypoglycemia within 6 to 36 h, secondary to the acute actions of ethanol on gluconeogenesis. This impairment is exacerbated by poor diet and by liver and pancreatic disease. As a result, glucose intolerance may be marked until the alcoholic has abstained for 2 to 4 weeks. Alcohol ketoacidosis, probably reflecting a decrease in fatty acid oxidation coupled with poor diet or recurrent vomiting, should not be misdiagnosed as diabetic ketosis. With the former, patients show an increase in serum ketones along with a mild increase in glucose but a large anion gap, a mild to moderate increase in serum lactate, and a β-hydroxybutyrate/lactate ratio of between 2:1 and 9:1 (with normal being 1:1).

THE EFFECTS OF ETHANOL ON BODY SYSTEMS

This overview of acute and chronic effects of alcohol on body systems outlines signs and symptoms that can aid in the recognition of the hidden alcoholic.

CENTRAL NERVOUS SYSTEM In addition to acute behavioral effects, an evening of heavy drinking can result in an alcoholic *blackout*, i.e., an episode of forgetting all or part of what occurred during drinking. This problem is experienced by 30 to 40 percent of men in their late teens and early 20s, most of whom do not go on to develop more serious and pervasive alcohol-related problems. Even after only a few drinks, alcohol acutely decreases *sleep* latency (helping people to fall asleep) and depresses rapid eye movement (REM) sleep early in the night, sometimes followed by later REM rebound associated with bad dreams. The consequence is to "fragment" sleep, causing a more rapid than normal alternation between sleep stages and a deficiency in deep sleep. The overall effect is likely to be repeated awakenings and a sense of restless sleep even in moderate drinkers.

Chronic intake of high doses of ethanol causes *peripheral neuropathy* in 5 to 15 percent of alcoholics (see Chap. 380), which is possibly related to thiamine deficiency. Patients complain of bilateral limb numbness, tingling, and paresthesia; symptoms are more pronounced distally than proximally. The treatment is abstinence and thiamine supplementation.

Wernicke's and Korsakoff's syndromes (alcohol-induced persisting amnestic disorder) are the result of thiamine deficiency in vulnerable individuals (possibly owing to interaction with a genetic

transketolase deficiency). Korsakoff's syndrome presents with profound anterograde amnesia (inability to learn new material) and a milder retrograde amnesia, along with possible impairment in visuospatial, abstract, and conceptual reasoning but with a normal intelligence quotient (IQ). While most patients demonstrate an acute onset of Korsakoff's syndrome in association with the neurologic stigmata seen with Wernicke's syndrome (e.g., sixth nerve palsy and ataxia), some individuals have a more gradual development of symptoms. Wernicke's syndrome responds rapidly to oral thiamine replacement (50 to 100 mg followed by 50 to 100 mg/d). However, only one-quarter of Korsakoff's patients achieve full recovery, one-half experience partial recovery, and one-quarter show no improvement with thiamine even after many months of supplementation.

About 1 percent of alcoholics with long histories of associated malnutrition develop *cerebellar degeneration*, a syndrome of progressive unsteady stance and gait often accompanied by mild nystagmus (see Chap. 380). Cerebellar atrophy is seen on computed tomography (CT) or magnetic resonance imaging (MRI), but the cerebrospinal fluid is usually normal. The major cause is probably nutritional, and identical symptoms can be seen with some forms of severe malnutrition alone. Treatment consists of abstinence and multiple vitamin supplementation, although improvement is often minimal.

Alcoholics can show severe *cognitive* problems and impairment in recent and remote memory for weeks to months after an alcoholic binge. Increased size of the brain ventricles and cerebral sulci are seen in up to 50 percent of chronic alcoholics, but these changes are often reversible, returning toward normal after a year or more of abstinence. Permanent CNS impairment (alcohol-induced persisting dementia) can develop and accounts for up to 20 percent of chronically demented patients. There is no single alcoholic dementia syndrome; rather, this label is used to describe patients who have apparently irreversible cognitive changes (possibly from diverse causes) in the midst of chronic alcoholism (see also Chap. 380).

Finally, almost every psychiatric syndrome can be seen during heavy drinking or subsequent withdrawal. These include intense *sadness* lasting for days to weeks in the midst of heavy drinking, which is classified as an alcohol-induced mood disorder in the Fourth Diagnostic and Statistical Manual of the American Psychiatric Association (DSM-IV); severe *anxiety* during alcohol withdrawal, often persisting for many months after cessation of drinking (alcohol-induced anxiety disorder); and auditory *hallucinations* and/or *paranoid delusions* in the absence of any obvious signs of withdrawal—a state now called alcohol-induced psychotic disorder. Whatever the cause, the treatment of alcohol-induced psychopathology includes abstinence and supportive care, with the likelihood of full recovery within several days to 6 weeks. Alcohol intake is an important part of the differential diagnosis of *any* patient with one of these psychological symptoms.

THE GASTROINTESTINAL SYSTEM Esophagus and **Stomach** Acute alcohol intake can result in inflammation of the esophagus (possibly secondary to reflux of gastric contents) and stomach (resulting from damage to the gastric mucosal barrier). Esophagitis can cause epigastric distress, and gastritis, the most frequent cause of gastrointestinal bleeding in heavy drinkers, can present with anorexia and abdominal pain. Chronic heavy drinking, if associated with violent vomiting, can produce a longitudinal tear in the mucosa at the gastroesophageal junction—a Mallory-Weiss lesion. Although many gastrointestinal problems are reversible, two complications of chronic alcoholism, esophageal varices secondary to cirrhosis-induced portal hypertension and atrophy of gastric cells, may be irreversible. → *See Chap. 283.*

Small Bowel Acutely, ethanol can cause hemorrhagic lesions of the duodenal villi and diarrhea secondary to increased small-bowel motility and decreased water and electrolyte absorption. Chronic alcoholism can contribute to diarrhea through its effects on the pancreas. → *See Chaps. 285 and 304.*

Pancreas Alcoholics commonly develop acute or chronic pancreatitis. → *See Chap. 304.*

Liver Ethanol absorbed from the small bowel is carried directly to the liver, where it becomes the preferred fuel; NADH accumulates and oxygen utilization escalates; gluconeogenesis is impaired (with a resulting fall in the amount of glucose produced from glycogen); lactate production increases; and there is a decreased oxidation of fatty acids in the citric cycle with an increase in fat accumulation within liver cells. In the healthy individual taking no medications, these changes are reversible, but with repeated exposure to ethanol, more severe changes in liver functioning are likely to occur. These include, in overlapping stages, fatty accumulation, alcohol-induced hepatitis, perivenular sclerosis, and cirrhosis. → *See Chap. 298.*

Increased Cancer Risk Cancer is the second leading cause of death in alcoholics (after cardiovascular disease); alcoholics have a rate of carcinoma 10 times higher than that in the general population. The sites with the greatest increase over expected rates include the head and neck, esophagus, cardia of the stomach, liver, pancreas, and, according to recent data, breast.

HEMATOPOIETIC SYSTEM Ethanol exerts multiple reversible acute and chronic effects on all blood cells. Alcohol alters acutely the production of red blood cells (RBC), and this effect reaches clinical significance after days to weeks of heavy drinking. The most common finding is an increase in RBC size (mean corpuscular volume, MCV), most often without anemia. This change appears to reflect the effect of alcohol on stem cells. If heavy drinking is accompanied by folic acid deficiency, there also can be hypersegmented neutrophils, reticulocytopenia, and hyperplastic bone marrow, and, if malnutrition is present, sideroblastic changes can be observed.

Chronic heavy drinking also can decrease production of most white blood cells (WBCs), decrease granulocyte mobility and adherence, and impair the delayed hypersensitivity response to new antigens (with a possible false-negative tuberculin skin test). While the changes in WBCs are usually temporary, they may contribute to the risk of infections and liver damage and perhaps to the increased risk of cancers in alcoholics. Alcohol also can cause toxic granulocytosis.

Many alcoholics present with mild thrombocytopenia (rarely associated with hemorrhage) due to a decrease in platelet survival and altered function; hypersplenism may occur as a complication of cirrhosis. Alcohol may decrease platelet aggregation and inhibit release of thromboxane A_2. These problems usually return toward normal within a week of abstinence.

CARDIOVASCULAR SYSTEM Modest doses of alcohol can have both deleterious and beneficial effects in individuals with normal cardiovascular status who take no medications. Ethanol acutely decreases myocardial contractility and causes peripheral vasodilation, resulting in a mild drop in blood pressure and a compensatory increased heart rate and cardiac output. Exercise-induced increases in cardiac oxygen consumption are higher after alcohol. A maximum of one to two drinks per day over long periods may decrease the risk of cardiovascular death, perhaps through an increase in high-density lipoprotein (HDL) cholesterol or changes in clotting mechanisms.

Although ethanol in low doses causes a mild acute drop in blood pressure, the consumption of three or more drinks per day results in a dose-dependent increase in blood pressure, which returns to normal within weeks of abstinence. As a result, heavy drinking is an important contributor to mild to moderate hypertension. Chronic heavy drinking can cause cardiomyopathy with symptoms ranging from unexplained arrhythmias in the presence of left ventricular impairment to heart failure with dilation of all four heart chambers and hypocontractility of heart muscle. Mural thrombi can form in the left atrium or ventricle, while heart enlargement exceeding 25 percent can cause mitral regurgitation. Finally, there is an association between cerebrovascular accidents and alcoholism, especially within 24 h of heavy drinking. Atrial or ventricular arrhythmias, especially paroxysmal tachycardia, also can occur after a binge in individuals showing no other evidence of heart disease—a syndrome known as the "holiday heart."

GENITOURINARY SYSTEM CHANGES, SEXUAL FUNCTIONING, AND FETAL DEVELOPMENT Acutely, modest ethanol doses (e.g., blood alcohol concentrations of 100 mg/dL or even less) can increase sexual drive in men. However, modest ethanol doses may simultaneously decrease erectile capacity. Even in the absence of liver impairment, a significant minority of chronic alcoholic men

may show irreversible testicular atrophy with concomitant shrinkage of the seminiferous tubules and loss of sperm cells (see Chap. 336).

The repeated ingestion of high doses of ethanol by women can result in amenorrhea, a decrease in ovarian size, absence of corpora lutea with associated infertility, and spontaneous abortions. Heavy drinking during pregnancy results in the rapid placental transfer of both ethanol and acetaldehyde, which may have serious consequences for fetal development. The *fetal alcohol syndrome* can include a mixture of any of the following: facial changes with epicanthal eye folds, poorly formed concha, and small teeth with faulty enamel; cardiac atrial or ventricular septal defects; an aberrant palmar crease and limitation in joint movement; and microcephaly with mental retardation. The specific amount of ethanol and/or specific time of vulnerability during pregnancy have not been defined, making it advisable for pregnant women to abstain completely.

OTHER EFFECTS OF ETHANOL Heavy drinking can produce an acute *alcoholic myopathy* characterized by painful and swollen muscles, high levels of serum creatine phosphokinase (CK), and, rarely, myoglobinemia and myoglobinuria. Effects on the *skeletal system* include alterations in calcium metabolism with an increased risk for fractures and osteonecrosis of the femoral head. *Hormonal* changes include an increase in cortisol levels, which can remain elevated during heavy drinking; inhibition of vasopressin secretion at rising blood alcohol concentrations and the opposite effect at falling blood alcohol concentrations (with the final result that most alcoholics are likely to be slightly overhydrated); a modest and reversible decrease in serum thyroxine (T_4); and a more marked decrease in serum triiodothyronine (T_3).

ALCOHOLISM (ALCOHOL ABUSE OR DEPENDENCE)

Because many drinkers occasionally imbibe to excess, temporary alcohol-related pathology is common in nonalcoholics. The time of heaviest drinking is usually the late teens to the late twenties, when between one-third and one-half of male drinkers experience some isolated (although potentially dangerous) alcohol-related social, occupational, or driving difficulty. These include alcohol-related blackouts, a single drunk driving arrest, and arguments with friends. This prevalent alcohol-related morbidity, however, is temporary and is a separate problem from alcohol dependence. The following sections describe diagnostic criteria for alcoholism, offer suggestions for identifying the usual (i.e., middle-class) alcoholic in everyday medical practice, review evidence that alcoholism is a biologic and genetically influenced disorder, and offer advice on intervention, detoxification, and rehabilitation of alcoholics.

DEFINITIONS AND EPIDEMIOLOGY DSM-IV defines alcohol dependence as repeated alcohol-related difficulties in at least three of seven areas of functioning. These include any combination of tolerance, withdrawal, taking larger amounts of alcohol over longer periods than intended, an inability to control use, spending a great deal of time associated with alcohol use, giving up important activities to drink, and continued use of alcohol despite physical or psychological consequences. This constellation of symptoms is likely to occur in both men and women, in individuals of all socioeconomic strata, and in people of all racial backgrounds. It also predicts a course of recurrent problems with the use of alcohol, and the consequent shortening of the life span by a decade or more. In the absence of alcohol dependence, an individual can be given a diagnosis of *alcohol abuse* if he or she demonstrates *repetitive* problems with alcohol in any one of four life areas, including an inability to fulfill major obligations, use in hazardous situations such as driving, legal problems, or use despite social or interpersonal difficulties.

Thus, the clinical diagnosis of alcohol abuse or dependence rests on the documentation of a pattern of *difficulties associated with alcohol use* and is *not* based on the quantity and frequency of alcohol consumption. This approach is used because an individual's pattern of drinking is difficult to establish and because the amount of alcohol associated with high blood levels differs with a person's age, sex, weight, percent body fat, and concomitant use of other medications. Thus, in screening for alcohol abuse or dependence in a clinical setting, it is important to probe for life problems and then attempt to tie in use of alcohol or another substance. A patient's pattern of life difficulties is important for a clinician to understand, and thus information regarding marital or job problems, legal difficulties, histories of accidents, medical problems, evidence of tolerance, etc., are important components of all evaluations and yield information that is of use even for nonalcoholic individuals.

The lifetime risk for alcohol dependence in most western countries is about 10 percent for men and 3 to 5 percent for women. When alcohol abuse is also considered, the rates double. The average alcoholic (just like the average person) is a blue-collar or white-collar worker or homemaker. Homeless or skid row alcoholics represent only 5 percent or less of the total.

GENETICS OF ALCOHOLISM Alcoholism is a multifactorial disorder in which biologic and genetic factors interact. The importance of genetic factors in alcoholism is supported by family, twin, and adoption studies. Close relatives of alcoholics who themselves have no other psychiatric disorder have an approximately fourfold increased risk for alcoholism but are not significantly more vulnerable to other psychiatric illnesses. The risk for the identical twin of an alcoholic is higher than for the fraternal twin of an alcohol-dependent person. Finally, adoption studies reveal that the fourfold increased risk for children of alcoholics is true even if they were adopted away at birth and raised without knowledge of the problems of their biologic parents.

The evidence supporting genetic influences in alcoholism has stimulated studies attempting to identify possible trait markers of a vulnerability toward the disorder before alcoholism appears. A 10-year followup of 453 men originally studied at age 20 has shown that subjects with alcoholic fathers demonstrated relatively lower levels of response to alcohol, including less intense subjective feelings of intoxication, less alcohol-related impairment in cognitive and psychomotor tests, and less intense alcohol-related changes in prolactin and cortisol secretion. This low level of response to alcohol at around age 20 was a powerful predictor of alcoholism a decade later. Taken as a whole, these data underscore the probability that alcoholism is biologically influenced and not related to a lack of "moral fiber." It is not surprising that the average alcoholic may continue to work, has a family, and may be difficult to identify if the physician persists with old stereotypes.

NATURAL HISTORY For the "average" alcoholic, the age of first drink and first minor problems (e.g., an argument with a friend while drunk or an alcoholic blackout) are similar to those in the general population. However, by the early to mid-twenties, most men and women moderate their drinking (perhaps learning from minor problems), whereas difficulties for alcoholics are likely to escalate, with the first major life problem from alcohol appearing in the mid-twenties to early forties. Once established, the course of alcoholism is likely to be one of exacerbations and remissions. As a rule there is remarkably little difficulty in stopping alcohol use when problems develop, and this step often is followed by days to months of carefully controlled drinking. Unfortunately, these periods are almost inevitably followed by escalations in alcohol intake and subsequent problems. The course is not hopeless, because a fifth or more of alcoholics achieve permanent abstinence without formal treatment or aid from self-help groups such as Alcoholics Anonymous (AA). However, should the alcoholic continue to drink, the life span is shortened by an average of 15 years, with the leading causes of death, in decreasing order, being heart disease, cancer, accidents, and suicide.

IDENTIFICATION OF THE ALCOHOLIC AND INTERVENTION Physicians even in affluent areas should recognize that 20 percent or so of patients have alcoholism. Therefore, it is important to pay attention to physical findings and laboratory tests that are likely to be abnormal in the alcoholic. These include a high-normal or slightly elevated MCV (e.g., 91 fL or higher), γ-glutamyl transferase (GGT) (30 or more units), serum uric acid [greater than 416 μmol/L (7 mg/dL)], carbohydrate-deficient transferrin (CDT) (20 g/L or more), and triglycerides [2.0 mmol/L (180 mg/dL) or more]. Mild and fluctuating levels of hypertension (e.g., 140/95), repeated infections such as pneumonia, and otherwise unexplained cardiac arrhythmias all suggest that the patient might be an alcoholic. Certain specific clinical findings also should raise suspicions, including cancer of the head and neck, esophagus, or cardia of the stomach as well as cirrhosis, unexplained hepatitis, pancreatitis, bilateral parotid gland swelling, and peripheral neuropathy.

Once the likelihood of alcoholism is established, only a few moments are needed to gather the history of alcohol-related life problems. The patient *and the spouse* or another close family member should be asked about patterns of accidents, marital difficulties, problems on the job, and driving-related difficulties, after which the role played by alcohol should be identified. All physicians should be able to take the time needed to gather such information. In addition, a simple 25-item form to be answered by the patient, the Michigan Alcohol Screening Test (MAST), is available to aid in identifying alcoholics. However, this is only a screening tool, and a careful face-to-face interview is still required for a meaningful diagnosis. The CAGE, which consists of asking about alcohol-related trouble *c*utting down, being *a*nnoyed by criticisms, *g*uilt, or use of an *e*ye-opener, can also be helpful as an initial screen.

After alcoholism is identified, the diagnosis must be shared with the patient. The presenting complaint can be used as an entrée to the alcohol problem. For instance, the patient complaining of insomnia or hypertension could be told that these are clinically important symptoms and that laboratory tests and physical findings indicate that alcohol appears to have contributed to the complaints and is increasing the risk for further medical and psychological problems. The physician should share information about the course of alcoholism and explore possible avenues of attacking the problem. Some patients and family members will benefit from the opportunity to read additional material, and several items are suggested in the reading list.

The process of intervention is rarely accomplished in one session. It is helpful to let patients know that they are responsible for their own actions and that the decision to quit drinking rests with them. For the person who refuses to stop drinking at the first intervention, a logical step is to "keep the door open," establishing future meetings so that help is available as problems escalate. In the meantime the family may benefit from counseling or referral to self-help groups such as Alanon (the Alcoholics Anonymous group for family members) and Alateen (for teenage children of alcoholics).

Those patients who refuse to stop but who want to "cut down" should be reminded that the average alcoholic successfully cuts back scores of times but that sooner or later drinking again escalates. The patient who refuses to stop might be offered a guideline of drinking no more than two drinks [115 mL (4 oz) of wine, 340 mL (12 oz) of beer, or 43 mL (1.5 oz) of 80-proof beverage amounts to one drink] in any 24-h period, but it is very unlikely that this measure will be effective for an extended period. This is another way of keeping the door open in the hope that the patient will return as drinking escalates.

TREATMENT OF THE ALCOHOL-RELATED WITHDRAWAL SYNDROME The Clinical Syndrome In the presence of ethanol-induced cellular tolerance, any sudden decrease in ethanol intake may lead to symptoms of withdrawal from the CNS-depressant effects. As with most syndromes, most patients do not develop every symptom, and the usual clinical picture is mild, resembling a mild to severe hangover that lasts several days. Features include a tremor of the hands (shakes or jitters); autonomic nervous system dysfunction such as increases in pulse, respiratory rate, and body temperature; insomnia, possibly accompanied by bad dreams; feelings of generalized anxiety or panic attacks; and gastrointestinal upset. Symptoms begin within 5 to 10 h of decreasing ethanol intake (addicted patients are likely to awaken in the morning with some signs of

CHAPTER 386
Alcohol and Alcoholism

2507

withdrawal), peak in intensity on day 2 or 3, and improve by day 4 or 5. Anxiety, insomnia, and mild levels of autonomic dysfunction may persist for 6 months or more as a protracted abstinence syndrome, which may contribute to the tendency to return to drinking.

Only 5 percent or fewer of alcoholics in withdrawal show severe symptoms such as delirium tremens (DTs), a state of confusion sometimes accompanied by visual, tactile, or auditory hallucinations. The likelihood of developing severe withdrawal symptoms increases with concomitant infections or medical problems, a prior history of withdrawal seizures or DTs, and higher quantity and frequency of drinking. These symptoms disappear as the mental state becomes clearer over a period of several days and are distinct from a temporary alcohol-induced psychotic disorder, which usually occurs with a clear sensorium as described earlier in this chapter.

A small percentage of alcoholics also demonstrate one or two generalized seizures ("rum fits"), usually within 48 h of stopping drinking. These are rarely focal in nature (unless there is underlying neuropathology), and electroencephalographic abnormalities are mild and usually return to normal within several days. There is no evidence that withdrawal seizures represent "latent" epilepsy.

℞ TREATMENT

The *first* and most important step is to perform a *thorough* physical examination in all alcoholics who are considering stopping drinking. It is necessary to evaluate organ systems likely to be impaired, including a search for evidence of liver failure, gastrointestinal bleeding, cardiac arrhythmia, and glucose or electrolyte imbalance.

The *second* step in treating withdrawal for even the typical well-nourished alcoholic is to give patients adequate nutrition and rest. All patients should be given oral multiple B vitamins, including 50 to 100 mg of thiamine daily for a week or more. Most patients enter withdrawal with normal levels of body water or mild overhydration, and intravenous fluids should be avoided unless there is evidence of hypotension or a history of recent excessive bleeding, vomiting, or diarrhea. Usually medications can be administered orally.

The *third* step in treatment is to recognize that the CNS symptoms were caused by rapid removal of the brain-depressant effects of ethanol. Symptoms can be alleviated by administering another CNS depressant and gradually decreasing the levels of the drug over a 3- to 5-day period. While many CNS depressants are effective, the *benzodiazepines* have the highest margin of safety and are, therefore, the preferred class of drugs in the treatment of alcohol withdrawal. Benzodiazepines with short half-lives (see Chap. 385) are especially useful for patients with serious liver impairment or evidence of preexisting encephalopathy or brain damage. On the other hand, short-half-life benzodiazepines, e.g., oxazepam or lorazepam, result in rapidly changing drug blood levels; administration every 4 h is required to avoid abrupt fluctuations in blood levels that may increase the risk for seizures. Therefore, most clinicians use drugs with longer half-lives, such as diazepam or chlordiazepoxide. The goal is to administer enough drug on day 1 to alleviate most of the symptoms of withdrawal (e.g., the tremor and elevated pulse), and then to decrease the dose by 20 percent on successive days over a period of 3 to 5 days. The approach is flexible; the dose is increased if signs of withdrawal escalate, and the medication is withheld if the patient is sleeping or shows signs of increasing orthostatic hypotension. The average patient requires 25 to 50 mg of chlordiazepoxide or 10 mg of diazepam given orally every 4 to 6 h on the first day.

The most effective treatment of delirium tremens remains controversial. Most clinicians use benzodiazepines, but despite as much as 300 mg or more per day of chlordiazepoxide, a patient might still remain awake and agitated. Since it is probable that the confused, agitated state will persist for 3 to 5 days regardless of the pharmacologic intervention used, drugs are given to control behavior rather than to change the course of the syndrome. Antipsychotic medications such as thioridazine or haloperidol are sometimes used, although they must be prescribed with care because they might lower the seizure threshold. The antipsychotic drugs have no place in the treatment of mild withdrawal symptoms.

The generalized seizures rarely require aggressive pharmacologic intervention beyond that given to the usual patient undergoing withdrawal, i.e., adequate doses of benzodiazepines. There is little evidence that phenytoin is effective in drug-withdrawal seizures, and the risk of seizures usually has passed by the time effective drug levels are reached. The rare patient with status epilepticus can be treated initially with intravenous diazepam. If anticonvulsants are used for alcohol-withdrawal seizures, they should be stopped within 5 to 7 days unless a cause for a persisting seizure disorder is documented.

While alcohol withdrawal is often treated in a hospital, efforts at reducing costs have resulted in experimentation with outpatient detoxification for alcoholics with mild abstinence syndromes. This outpatient approach is appropriate for patients in good physical condition who demonstrate mild signs of withdrawal despite low blood alcohol concentrations and for those without prior history of DTs or withdrawal seizures. Such individuals still require careful physical examination, evaluation of blood tests, and treatment with vitamin supplementation. Benzodiazepines can be given *in a 1- to 2-day supply* to be administered to the patient by a spouse or other family member four times a day. Patients are asked to *return daily* for evaluation of vital signs, and to come to the emergency room if signs and symptoms of withdrawal escalate.

REHABILITATION OF ALCOHOLICS After completing alcoholic rehabilitation, 60 percent or more of middle-class alcoholics maintain abstinence for at least a year, and many for a lifetime. There is no single best way to rehabilitate the alcoholic, and therapeutic approaches center on general supports that meet commonsense guidelines. Considering the lack of evidence for the superiority of any specific treatment type, it is best to keep interventions as simple, safe, and inexpensive as possible.

Maneuvers in rehabilitation fall into two general categories. *First* are attempts to help the alcoholic achieve and maintain a high level of motivation toward abstinence. These include educating the patient about alcoholism and teaching the family and/or friends to stop protecting the alcoholic from the problems caused by alcohol. The *second* series of maneuvers helps the patient to readjust to life without alcohol and to reestablish a functional lifestyle through personal counseling, vocational rehabilitation, family support, and sexual counseling.

There is no convincing evidence that inpatient rehabilitation is always more effective for the average alcoholic than is outpatient care. The decision to hospitalize can be made if (1) the patient has medical problems that are difficult to treat outside a hospital; (2) depression, confusion, or psychosis interferes with outpatient care; (3) the patient has such a severe life crisis that it is difficult to get his or her attention as an outpatient; (4) outpatient treatment has failed; or (5) the patient lives too far from the treatment center. If inpatient care is needed, free-standing treatment programs, units that are divisions of general hospitals, and those in psychiatric hospitals are all equally effective. The characteristics of the patient predict outcome more than any specific attribute of the program.

Whether the treatment begins in an inpatient or an outpatient setting, subsequent outpatient contact should be maintained for a minimum of 6 months and preferably a full year after abstinence is achieved. Counseling with an individual physician or through groups focuses on day-to-day living—emphasizing areas of improved functioning in the absence of alcohol (i.e., why it is a good idea to continue to abstain) and helping the patient to deal with free time without alcohol, develop a nondrinking peer group, and handle stresses on the job without alcohol.

The physician serves an important role in identifying the alcoholic, treating associated medical or psychiatric syndromes, overseeing detoxification, referring the patient to rehabilitation programs, and providing counseling. The physician also must regulate the use of medications during alcoholism rehabilitation. Once acute detoxification is complete (an average of 3 to 5 days), there is *no place* for hypnotics or antianxiety drugs in the treatment of most alcoholics. The patient has already demonstrated an inability to moderate the use of one brain depressant, alcohol, and is at considerable risk for abusing sleeping pills or antianxiety drugs. Anxiety and insomnia can be treated with behavior modification such as relaxation training, meditation, and exercise or through increased activity in hobbies or religion. For example, regarding insomnia, patients should be reassured that insomnia is normal after alcohol withdrawal and will improve over the subsequent weeks and months. They should then follow a rigid bedtime and awakening schedule and avoid any naps or the use of caffeine in the evenings. The sleep pattern will improve rapidly.

One medication that has been used in alcohol rehabilitation is disulfiram, usually given as 250 mg/d. This drug inhibits aldehyde dehydrogenase, causing very high levels of acetaldehyde to accumulate after alcohol is consumed. The disulfiram-ethanol reaction includes tremor, hypertension or hypotension, nausea and sometimes severe vomiting, and diarrhea. Disulfiram must not be given to persons for whom such a reaction could be dangerous, including patients with portal hypertension, diabetes mellitus, heart disease, or a history of stroke. Unfortunately, there is little convincing evidence from carefully controlled studies that disulfiram is significantly more effective than than placebo. As result, this drug should not be routinely prescribed.

Two medications, naltrexone and acamprosate, are reported to either decrease the amount of alcohol consumed or to shorten the period during which alcohol is used if a relapse occurs. While the mechanisms of action are not understood and the number of subjects on whom data are available is limited for naltrexone, both drugs may have a role in the future in alcohol rehabilitation. However, more data are required before routine clinical use can be justified.

Finally, an inexpensive, readily available, and dedicated additional support for all alcoholics is available in almost every community. Alcoholics Anonymous is a self-help group of recovering alcoholics (men and women who have stopped drinking, perhaps many years ago) that offers an effective model of abstinence, provides a sober peer group, and makes crisis intervention available when the urge to drink escalates. No matter what type of rehabilitation program is planned, the alcoholic should be offered the option of joining Alcoholics Anonymous.

BIBLIOGRAPHY

KENDLER KS et al: The structure of the genetic and environmental risk factors for six major psychiatric disorders in women. Arch Gen Psychiatry 52:374, 1995

LIEBER C: *Medical and Nutritional Complications of Alcoholism.* New York, Plenum, 1992

————: Medical disorders of alcoholism. N Engl J Med 333:1058, 1995

LITTEN RZ et al: Pharmacotherapies for alcoholism. Alcohol Clin Exp Res 15:620, 1991

PROJECT MATCH RESEARCH GROUP: Matching alcoholism treatments to client heterogeneity. J Stud Alcohol 58:7, 1997

SASS H et al: Relapse prevention by acamprosate. Arch Gen Psychiatry 53:673, 1996

SCHUCKIT MA: *Drug and Alcohol Abuse: A Clinical Guide to Diagnosis and Treatment,* 4th ed. New York, Plenum, 1995

————: *Educating Yourself About Alcohol and Drugs: A People's Primer.* New York, Plenum, 1995

————, SMITH TL: An 8-year follow-up of 450 sons of alcoholic and control subjects. Arch Gen Psychiatry 53:302, 1996

———— et al: The time course of development of alcohol-related problems in men and women. J Stud Alcohol 56:218, 1995

YERSIN B et al: Screening for excessive alcohol drinking. Comparative value of carbohydrate-deficient transferrin, gamma-glutamyltransferase, and mean corpuscular volume. Arch Intern Med 155:1907, 1995

OPIOID DRUG ABUSE AND DEPENDENCE

The principal effects of the opioids (opiate-like drugs) are a significant damping of pain perception along with modest levels of sedation and euphoria. Drugs in this category range from heroin, morphine, and codeine to many nonsteroidal prescription analgesics and many antitussive agents. Thus, the following comments have wide application in medicine and go far beyond the classical opiate-dependent person on the street.

Tolerance to any one opioid is likely to generalize to the others (i.e., cross-tolerance is likely), and all share a similar pattern of drug-related problems. Each of these substances is capable of producing dependence as defined in the *Fourth Diagnostic and Statistical Manual* of the American Psychiatric Association (DSM-IV), including evidence of physical addiction (and thus they all have some legal restrictions). The abstinence syndrome from any of the substances can be treated with administration of any of the others.

PHARMACOLOGY The prototypic opiates, morphine and codeine (3-methoxymorphine), are taken directly from the milky juice of the poppy *Papaver somniferum.* The semisynthetic drugs produced from the morphine or thebane molecules include hydromorphone, diacetylmorphine (heroin), and oxycodone. The purely synthetic opioids, sharing many of the basic properties of opium and morphine, include meperidine, propoxyphene, diphenoxylate, fentanyl, buprenorphine, methadone, and pentazocine. Despite claims to the contrary, all these substances (including almost all prescription analgesics) are capable of producing euphoria as well as psychological and physical dependence when taken in high enough doses over prolonged periods.

The opioids produce their effects by binding to different types of opioid receptors throughout the body, including the central nervous system. Endogenous opioid peptides (i.e., enkephalins, endorphins, dynorphin, and others) have been identified that appear to be natural ligands for opioid receptors. These peptides have a distinct distribution in the central nervous system (CNS). Recent evidence suggests that the receptors with which opioid peptides interact may be differentially engaged in production of the various opiate effects, such as analgesia, respiratory depression, constipation, and euphoria, but the data are not definitive. Substances capable of antagonizing one or more of these actions include nalorphine, levallorphan, cyclazocine, butorphanol, buprenorphine, and pentazocine, each of which has mixed agonist and antagonist properties, as well as naloxone and naltrexone, which are pure opiate antagonists. All antagonist drugs (including those with mixed agonist properties), if administered to a patient addicted to other narcotics, can precipitate opiate withdrawal symptoms. The availability of relatively specific antagonists has helped identify different receptor subtypes, including the μ_1 and μ_2 subtypes, which are thought to affect some of the more classical opioid actions such as pain control, constipation, and respiration; κ receptors, with possible similar functions along with sedation and effects on hormones; and δ receptors, thought to relate mostly to analgesia.

Opiate tolerance, dependence, and withdrawal are considered to be related phenomena and may share some common underlying mechanisms. Perhaps reflecting the actions of different classes of receptors, tolerance to various opiate actions may develop at different rates, and these same mechanisms may contribute to the diverse signs and symptoms characteristic of withdrawal. Biochemical systems that might contribute to the development of tolerance and dependence include alterations in neurotransmitters, including acetylcholine, serotonin, gamma-aminobutyric acid (GABA), and the catecholamines norepinephrine and dopamine. Behavioral conditioning also plays a role in maintaining dependence in at least some individuals.

All the opioid drugs are absorbed from the gastrointestinal system, the lungs, and/or the muscles. The most rapid and pronounced effects occur following intravenous administration, with only slightly less efficient absorption after smoking or inhaling the vapor ("chasing the dragon"), and the least intense actions are seen after absorption from the digestive tract. Most of the metabolism of opiates occurs in the liver, primarily through conjugation with glucuronic acid, and only small amounts are excreted directly in the urine or feces. The plasma half-lives of these drugs range from 2.5 to 3 h for morphine to more than 22 h for methadone and even longer for levomethadyl acetate (LAAM).

Street heroin typically contains only 5 to 10 percent of the opiate. The remainder consists of materials such as lactose and fruit sugars, quinine, powdered milk, phenacetin, caffeine, antipyrine, and strychnine, which are used to "cut" the drug and increase the profit margin. Any marked, unexpected increase in the purity of street drugs is likely to cause unintentional lethal overdoses in users expecting less effect from a "hit."

THE ACUTE AND CHRONIC EFFECTS OF OPIOID DRUGS ON BODY SYSTEMS

With the exception of overdose conditions and changes associated with physical addiction, most opiate actions are relatively benign and rapidly reversible. A major danger, however, comes through the use of contaminated needles by intravenous users. This practice is responsible for increased risks for hepatitis B and C, bacterial endocarditis, and infection with the human immunodeficiency virus (HIV), a major cause of mortality in injection drug users and their sexual partners (see Chap. 308).

Effects on Body Systems Acute changes in the *gastrointestinal (GI) system* are the result of decreased GI motility with resulting constipation and anorexia. Chronic GI problems in opiate-dependent people typically occur as a consequence of hepatitis in injection drug users.

The direct effects on opiate receptors in the CNS can result in intoxication-induced nausea and vomiting (medulla), decreased pain perception (spinal cord, thalamus, and periaqueductal gray region), euphoria (limbic system), and sedation (reticular activating system and striatum). The adulterants added to street drugs may contribute to some of the more permanent nervous system damage, including peripheral neuropathy, amblyopia, myelopathy, and leukoencephalopathy. Whether from the opiate, adulterants, or the consequences of dirty needles, at least one recent study revealed CNS defects in both computed tomographic and cognition evaluations of opiate-dependent people. Acute opiate administration results in decreases in luteinizing hormone (LH), with a subsequent decrease in testosterone, which might contribute to the decreased sex drive reported by most opiate-dependent people. Other hormonal changes include a decrease in the release of thyrotropin as well as increases in prolactin and possibly in growth hormone (see Chap. 328).

Acute changes in the *respiratory system* include respiratory depression, which results from a decreased response of the brainstem to carbon dioxide tension, a component of the drug overdose syndrome described below. At even low drug doses, this effect can be clinically significant in individuals with compromised lung activity. *Cardiovascular* changes tend to be relatively mild, with no direct opiate effect on heart rhythm or myocardial contractility, but there is a potential problem from orthostatic hypotension, probably secondary to dilation of peripheral vessels. Bacterial infections of both the lungs and heart valves can occur from contaminated needles; the latter can result in emboli and thus an increased risk for stroke.

The Toxic Reaction or Overdose Syndrome High doses of opiates taken intentionally (in a suicide attempt) or by a user who has misjudged the potency of the substance can result in a toxic reaction or overdose syndrome with a potentially lethal consequence. While toxic reactions are seen with all opiates, the more potent drugs such as fentanyl (80 to 100 times more powerful than morphine) are especially dangerous. The typical syndrome, which occurs immediately with intravenous overdose, includes shallow respirations at a rate of two to four per minute, pupillary miosis (with mydriasis once brain anoxia develops), bradycardia, a decrease in body temperature, and a general absence of responsiveness to external stimulation. If this medical emergency is not treated rapidly, symptoms can progress to cyanosis, and death can ensue from respiratory depression and cardiorespiratory arrest. Postmortem examination reveals few specific changes except for diffuse cerebral edema. An "allergic-like" reaction to intravenous heroin, apparently at least in part related to adulterants, also can occur and is characterized by decreased alertness, a frothy pulmonary edema, and an elevation in the blood eosinophil count.

The first step in treating any overdose is to support the vital signs through a respirator and other emergency procedures. The preferred, more definitive treatment for the typical opiate overdose is the intravenous or intramuscular administration of the narcotic antagonist naloxone in an initial dose of 0.2 mg (0.5 mL of the 10 mL vial) or more; this dose can be repeated in 3 to 10 min if no response occurs. It is important to titrate the dose relative to the patient's symptoms. Because the effects of this drug diminish within 2 to 3 h, the individual must be monitored for at least 24 h after a heroin overdose and 72 h after an overdose of a longer-acting drug such as methadone. If there is little response to naloxone alone, the possibility of a concomitant overdose with a benzodiazepine should be considered and a challenge with intravenous flumazenil, 0.2 to 0.5 mg/min up to a maximum of 3 mg, might be used. Patients who are physically addicted to an opioid are likely to experience a precipitous onset of an abstinence syndrome within 2 to 8 h after administration of the opioid antagonist, but aggressive treatment of this syndrome is not appropriate until all vital signs are relatively stable.

As with any drug overdose, treatment of either the typical or the "allergic" type of opiate toxic reaction often requires continued support of vital signs until the body detoxifies the substance. Patients may require a respirator (especially one using oxygen and positive-pressure breathing for the "allergic" type of overdose), intravenous fluids perhaps accompanied by pressor agents, to support blood pressure, and gastric lavage to remove any remaining drug, with care taken to use a cuffed endotracheal tube to prevent aspiration if the patient is not alert. It is important to evaluate and treat any possible anaphylactic reactions. Cardiac arrhythmias and/or convulsions, especially likely to be seen with codeine, propoxyphene, or meperidine, also need to be treated.

DIAGNOSIS AND NATURAL HISTORY OF OPIOID ABUSE AND DEPENDENCE

Repeated use of opiates to the point of developing multiple problems is a good indicator of the likelihood of future problems with the drug. The approach uses the same DSM-IV criteria for dependence as discussed for alcohol (see Chap. 386). Here, the patient develops repeated difficulties in any three of the criterion areas in any given year, showing a mixture of tolerance, withdrawal, use of greater amounts of opiates than intended, use despite consequences, and so on. Patients who do not have dependence but demonstrate repeated difficulties with the law, impaired ability to meet obligations, use in hazardous situations, or continued use despite problems can be labeled as having abuse.

Natural History Dependence on or abuse of opiates can be seen in at least three types of patients. First, evidence suggests that a minority of people with *chronic pain syndromes* (e.g., back, joint, and muscle disorders) misuse their prescribed drugs at various times. Of course, these comments deal with non-life-threatening chronic pain, not terminal illness, for which high doses of opiates can be important. If physical dependence is established, abstinence syndromes can then intensify the pain, promoting continued drug intake. A few precautions can help the physician to avoid contributing to physical dependence in chronic pain patients, particularly those who have demonstrated a history of misusing opioids. (1) The goal is to minimize the debilitating effects of pain with the understanding that discomfort may not be completely eliminated (see Chap. 12). (2) All possible efforts must be made to get the patient actively involved in and committed to improvement. (3) Analgesic medication should be only one component of treatment and limited to the oral administration of the least potent analgesic that is able to "take the edge off" the pain (e.g., ibuprofen or, if needed, propoxyphene). All such drugs should be coordinated through one physician. (4) Behavior modification techniques, such as muscle relaxation and meditation, and carefully selected exercises should be used as appropriate to help increase function and decrease pain. (5) Finally, nonmedicinal approaches, including electrical transcutaneous neurostimulation for muscle and joint disease, can be applied (see also Chap. 12).

The second group at high risk are *physicians, nurses,* and *pharmacists,* primarily because of their easy access to substances of abuse. Physicians may begin to use opiates to help them sleep or to reduce stress or physical aches and pains. These groups appear to be at especially high risk for developing dependence on the highly potent drugs such as fentanyl. Because of the growing awareness of these problems, impaired physician programs have been established in many hospitals and by most state medical societies. These groups attempt to identify and aid substance-impaired physicians, giving them peer support and education so as to help them achieve abstinence before problems escalate to the point of licensure revocation. In general, doctors are advised never to prescribe opiates for themselves or for members of their family—physicians deserve the same level of care and protection from future problems as their patients.

The third and most obvious group are those who buy their drugs on the street to get high. While some of these men and women have prior histories of severe antisocial problems, most have a relatively high level of premorbid functioning. The typical person begins using opiates occasionally, often after experimenting with tobacco, then alcohol, then marijuana, and then brain depressants or stimulants. Occasional opiate use, or "chipping," might continue for some time, and some individuals never escalate their intake to the point of developing dependence. Another pattern of temporary or intermittent abuse is represented by the experiences of Vietnam soldiers, most of whom had little or no prior experience with opiates and who found themselves in a situation of high stress and readily available drugs. Under these circumstances, as many as one-half tried opiates and, although many became physically addicted, those who had not misused drugs before Vietnam tended to return to drug-free status when back in their home communities.

Of course, opiate-dependent individuals are likely to continue to have experience with many other drugs. At least two of these often remain as problems during the course of opiate dependence. First, alcohol intake is classically used to moderate withdrawal problems, to enhance the opiate high, and as a substitute when the preferred drug is not readily available, including during methadone and other treatments. This pattern of problematic drinking, often meeting criteria for alcohol dependence, is seen in the course of opiate dependence in perhaps 50 percent of opiate-dependent persons. The second drug, cocaine, appears to be taken for many of the same reasons as alcohol and is often administered intravenously with the opiate in a mixture known as a "speedball." Dependence on these as well as other drugs must be addressed during opiate detoxification and rehabilitation.

Once persistent opiate use is established, the outcome is often extremely serious. At least 25 percent of such opiate abusers are likely to die within 10 to 20 years of active abuse, with death resulting from suicide, homicide, accidents, and infectious diseases such as tuberculosis, serum hepatitis, or AIDS. The mortality rate has escalated in recent years in response to the epidemic of AIDS among injection drug users, with an estimated 60 percent of these men and women carrying HIV (see Chap. 208). As many as 50 percent of male and 25 percent of female opiate-dependent persons turn to alcohol when their primary drug is not available, and many meet the criteria for secondary alcohol dependence. The prevalence of alcohol misuse is higher in drug treatment dropouts than in those who stay with therapy, and also in individuals who had alcohol problems before they developed opiate-related difficulties.

℞ **TREATMENT**

The key to diagnosis is to discard the erroneous stereotype that opiate-dependent men and women are always street people. Abuse or dependence is possible in any patient who demonstrates symptoms of what might be opiate withdrawal; anyone who has a chronic pain syndrome; physicians, nurses, and pharmacists or others with easy access to opiates; and all patients who repeatedly seek out prescription analgesics. The diagnosis is established by reviewing areas of life problems where opiates might be involved, beginning with the DSM-IV items for abuse and dependence.

Identification of the Patient, and Intervention The first step in treatment is identification of the opiate-dependent person—an especially difficult step with middle-class medical patients or physicians with an iatrogenic addiction. Therefore, it is important to take the time with *every* patient, especially those with complaints of pain, to gather a clinical history that includes the patterns of opiate use and the list of doctors and clinics from which they have received prescriptions. If the chronic use of opiates is suspected, gathering further data from an additional informant such as a spouse can be essential. Another indicator of an enhanced risk for opiate dependence is a history of pervasive antisocial problems beginning in the preteen years. Blood and urine screens can be used to identify opiates in patients in whom misuse is suspected, and clinicians should search for physical stigmata of misuse (e.g., needle marks).

After identifying opiate dependence, the next step is intervention. The need for active treatment of the abstinence syndrome can be presented, and the availability of help in establishing a drug-free life-style can be emphasized. The final decision, of course, rests with the patient. Much of this approach is presented in relation to alcoholism in Chap. 386.

The Symptoms of Withdrawal The withdrawal symptoms tend to be opposite to the acute effects of the drug and include nausea and diarrhea, coughing, lacrimation, mydriasis, rhinorrhea, profuse sweating, twitching muscles, and piloerection, or "goose bumps"; mild elevations in body temperature, respiratory rate, and blood pressure are also observed. In addition, sensations of diffuse body pain, insomnia, and yawning occur, along with intense drug craving. Drugs with a short half-life, such as morphine or heroin, cause symptoms typically within 8 to 16 h of the last dose (thus, many dependent individuals awake in mild withdrawal every morning); symptom intensity peaks within 36 to 72 h after discontinuation of the drug, and the acute syndrome disappears within 5 to 8 days. However, a protracted abstinence phase of mild symptoms (e.g., slight changes in pupillary size, autonomic dysfunction, changes in sleep pattern) may persist for 6 or more months. These lingering symptoms, which can be relieved by administering an opiate, probably contribute to relapse.

Treatment of the Withdrawal Syndrome Patients *must* receive a thorough physical examination, which includes an assessment of liver and neurologic function as well as identification of local and systemic infections, especially abscesses. Proper nutrition and rest must be initiated as soon as possible.

Effective treatment of withdrawal, however, also requires readministration of sufficient opiate medication on day 1 to decrease symptoms, followed by a more gradual withdrawal of the drug, usually over 5 to 10 days. Any opiate will work (they all have some level of cross-tolerance), but for ease of administration, many physicians prefer to use a long-acting drug such as methadone. In estimating the first day's dose from the patient's history, 1 mg of methadone is approximately equivalent to 3 mg of morphine, 1 mg of heroin, or 20 mg of meperidine. Most patients require between 10 and 25 mg of methadone orally given twice on day 1, with higher doses given if prominent symptoms of withdrawal are not dampened. After several days of a stabilized drug dose, the opiate is then decreased by 10 to 20 percent of the original day's dose each day.

Most states have restrictions on the prescription of opiates to dependent persons, and, in the absence of special permits, detoxification with opiates is often proscribed or limited to 1 month or less. Thus, pharmacologic treatments are often limited to symptomatic medication of diarrhea with kaopectate or a similar nonopiate, of "sniffles" with decongestants, and pain with nonopiate analgesics (e.g., ibuprofen). Another relatively successful nonopiate approach to the treatment of withdrawal is the use of the alpha$_2$-adrenergic agonist clonidine, used in part to decrease sympathetic nervous system overactivity. Given at doses of approximately 5 μg/kg (up to 0.3 mg given two to four times a day), clonidine decreases autonomic nervous system dysfunction in most patients undergoing opiate withdrawal. Opiates are more effective in relieving discomfort and pain, however, and clonidine is often not well tolerated because it produces high levels of sedation and orthostatic hypotension. Therefore, under most circumstances, opiates are the treatment of choice.

A special case of opiate withdrawal is seen in the newborn passively addicted by the mother's drug misuse during pregnancy. Some level of addiction develops in 50 to 90 percent of children of heroin-dependent mothers. As few as 25 percent of infants of methadone maintenance–addicted mothers show clinically relevant withdrawal symptoms, probably because of the longer half-life of this drug. The syndrome consists of irritability, crying, a tremor (in 80 percent), increased reflexes, increased respiratory rate, diarrhea, hyperactivity (in 60 percent), vomiting (40 percent), and sneezing/yawning/hiccuping (in 30 percent). The child usually has a low birth weight but may be otherwise unremarkable until the second day, when symptoms are likely to begin.

The treatment follows the same general steps used in the treatment of the physically addicted adult. The child must be carefully evaluated to rule out medical problems such as hypoglycemia, hypocalcemia, infections, and trauma; general support in a warm, quiet environment and regulation of electrolytes and glucose are also required. The infant with moderate to severe symptoms can be treated with any of the following: paregoric (0.2 mL orally every 3 to 4 h), methadone (0.1 to 0.5 mg/kg per day), phenobarbital (8 mg/kg per day), or diazepam (1 to 2 mg/kg every 8 h). Medication should be given in decreasing levels for 10 to 20 days. It is also possible to help treat the addicted infants of mothers on methadone maintenance by having the mother breast feed the infant while continuing to take methadone.

Rehabilitation of Opiate-Dependent Persons Despite some differences in demographics, the same general rules for rehabilitation apply to opiate-dependent persons as to alcoholics. The basic strategy includes beginning detoxification and general family support, and the process can benefit from the use of readings or referral to self-help groups. It is also important to establish realistic patient goals and a program of counseling and education to increase motivation toward abstinence. A long-term commitment to rebuilding a lifestyle without the substance is essential for preventing recidivism.

Most rehabilitation approaches have common elements, regardless of the drug involved. As described in several recent texts, patients are educated about their responsibility for improving their lives, and *motivation for abstinence* is increased by providing information about the medical and psychological problems that can be expected if addiction continues. Patients and families are helped to *establish an opiate-free life-style* by being educated about dealing with chronic pain and developing realistic vocational planning (e.g., for pharmacists, physicians, and nurses). The dependent person also should be encouraged to establish a drug-free peer group and to participate in self-help groups such as Narcotics Anonymous. Much of this advice and counseling can be given by the physician, but many clinicians refer patients to more formal drug programs, including methadone maintenance clinics, programs using narcotic antagonists, and therapeutic communities. Long-term follow-up of treated patients shows that approximately one-third of participants are completely drug free in the year before the follow-up interview and that a total of 60 percent are off opiates, although some are abusing other substances. Individuals who stay in methadone maintenance or in therapeutic communities show significant decreases in police and social problems and increases in job functioning. In general, the best prognosis is for those who are employed, who have higher levels of school completion, and who remain in treatment for at least 2 months. Dependence among health care deliverers, such as physicians, is treated with similar approaches. In addition, a closely supervised "diversion" procedure is usually instituted and carried out for 1 to 2 years or more.

METHADONE MAINTENANCE Maintenance programs with methadone and the even longer-acting agent LAAM should only be used along with education and counseling. It is important to note that drug maintenance is not aimed at "curing" opiate addiction; rather, it provides a substitute drug that is legally accessible, safer, can be taken orally, and has a long half-life so that it can be taken once a day. The goal is to help persons who have repeatedly failed in drug-free programs to improve functioning within the family and job, to decrease legal problems, and to improve health.

Methadone is a long-acting opiate that possesses almost all the physiologic properties of heroin. The recipient, who has been carefully screened to rule out prior psychiatric disorders, may be maintained on a relatively low dose (e.g., 30 to 40 mg/d); a better approach is to use a higher dose (100 to 120 mg/d), which may be more effective in blocking heroin-induced euphoria. There is some evidence that the higher methadone doses result in greater retention in treatment and consequently in lower levels of arrest and readdiction to street drugs. Three-quarters or more of patients, especially those receiving the higher doses, are likely to remain heroin-free for 6 months or longer. Methadone is administered in an oral liquid given once a day at the program center, with weekend portions taken by the patient at home. The longer-acting analogues, such as LAAM, can be given two or three times a week, with the dose of LAAM increased to as high as 80 mg three times a week if needed. After a period of maintenance (usually 6 months to 1 year or longer), the clinician should work closely with the patient to regulate the rate of drug decrease (by about 5 percent per week).

In the past, the British have used heroin maintenance with similar goals and following similar guidelines as those used for methadone. There is no evidence that heroin maintenance has any advantages over methadone maintenance, but the heroin approach does add the risk that the drug will be sold on the streets. These factors have contributed to the virtual abandonment of the heroin maintenance approach. Treatment with mixed agonists-antagonists such as buprenorphine has been proposed, especially to help the individual who is also using cocaine. However, at present these must be considered experimental.

OPIATE ANTAGONISTS The opiate antagonists (e.g., naloxone) compete with heroin and other opiates for opioid receptors, reducing the effects of the opiate agonists. Administered over long periods with the intention of blocking the "high" produced if the patient takes opiates, these drugs can be useful as part of an overall treatment approach that includes counseling and support. The most widely used antagonist in rehabilitation is naltrexone, which is effective for about 24 h and has few side effects. A dose of 50 mg of naltrexone per day will block 15 mg of heroin for 24 h, and higher doses (125 to 150 mg) are capable of blocking the effects of 25 mg of intravenous heroin for up to 3 days. Naltrexone is free of agonist properties and produces no known withdrawal symptoms when stopped, and its side effects tend to be mild. Patients should be free of opiates for a minimum of 5 days before beginning treatment with this medication, to avoid precipitating a withdrawal syndrome. In addition, they must be given a thorough physical examination and should be challenged with 0.4 or 0.8 mg of the shorter-acting agent naloxone to be certain they are able to tolerate the long-acting antagonist. Following this procedure, a test dose of 10 mg of naltrexone can be given, with the expectation that any withdrawal symptoms will be seen in 0.5 to 2 h. Several variations of this approach can be used with methadone maintenance, including a fairly rapid, medically supervised scheme. Over the next 10 days, the daily dose should be increased to about 100 mg on Mondays and Wednesdays and 150 mg on Fridays. Unfortunately, despite the apparent advantages of this treatment approach, patients demonstrate great resistance to continuing care. In one study, only about 60 percent of the patients completed 6 days of naltrexone induction, and only 10 percent remained in the program at the end of 6 months.

DRUG-FREE PROGRAMS Most existing halfway houses and recovery centers for opiate-dependent persons use some variant of the therapeutic community approach. This is an exception to the general preference for short-term inpatient rehabilitation, since care lasts up to a year while the person is taken out of the street culture and given a new life within the group. In this structure, members, including leaders who are themselves in the process of recovery, help participants gain insights into more successful life-styles for coping with problems.

As is true for treatments of all substance-use disorders, it is likely that counseling, behavioral treatments, and relatively simple approaches to psychotherapy add significantly to a positive outcome. Most approaches focus on teaching participants to handle stress better, enhancing their understanding of personality attributes, teaching better cognitive styles, and, through the process of relapse prevention, addressing issues that might contribute to increased craving, easy access to drugs, or periods of decreased motivation. A combination of these therapies with the approaches described above appears to give the best results.

Finally, it is important to briefly discuss prevention. Except for the terminally ill, physicians need to carefully monitor opiate drug use in their patients, keeping the doses as low as is practical and administering them over as short a period as the level of pain would warrant in the average person. Physicians must also be vigilant regarding their own risk for opiate abuse and dependence, *never* prescribing these drugs for themselves. For the nonmedical intravenous drug–dependent person, all possible efforts must be made to prevent AIDS, hepatitis, bacterial endocarditis, and other consequences of contaminated needles through methadone maintenance and by considering needle-exchange programs.

BIBLIOGRAPHY

AMERICAN PSYCHIATRIC ASSOCIATION: Practical guidelines for the treatment of substance use disorders. Am J Psychiatry 52(Suppl):1, 1995

BALL J, ROSS A: *The Effectiveness of Methadone Maintenance Treatments.* New York, Springer-Verlag, 1991

BONNER A, WATERHOUSE J: *Addictive Behaviour: Molecules to Mankind; Perspective on the Nature of Addiction.* New York, St. Martin's Press, 1996

COMMITTEE ON OPPORTUNITIES IN DRUG ABUSE RESEARCH: Pathways of Addiction. Washington DC, National Academy Press, 1995, pp 56–93

FINNEGAN LP: Neonatal abstinence syndrome: Assessment and pharmacotherapy, in *Neonatal Therapy: An Update*, FF Rubaltelli, B Granati (eds). New York, Elsevier, 1986

HUGHES PH et al: Prevalence of substance use among US physicians. JAMA 267:2333, 1992

KEENE J et al: Evaluation of syringe-exchange for HIV prevention among injecting drug users in rural and urban areas of Wales. Addiction 88:1063, 1993

MANFREDINI R et al: Emergency admissions of opioid drug abusers for overdose: A chronobiological study of enhanced risk. Ann Emerg Med 24:615, 1994

SCHUCKIT MA: *Drug and Alcohol Abuse: A Clinical Guide to Diagnosis and Treatment*, 4th ed. New York, Plenum, 1995

———: *Educating Yourself about Alcohol and Drugs: A People's Primer.* New York, Plenum, 1995

WEISS RD et al: The significance of a coexisting opioid use disorder in cocaine dependence: An empirical study. Am J Drug Alcohol Abuse 22:173, 1996

388 *Jack H. Mendelson, Nancy K. Mello*

COCAINE AND OTHER COMMONLY ABUSED DRUGS

Although there has been a decline in the occurrence of drug abuse–related problems, particularly among youths, the prevalence of drug abuse in the United States remained at epidemic levels during the mid-1990s and is believed to exceed that of other industrial nations. The primary data resources for assessing the scope and extent of drug abuse in the United States are the High School Senior Survey, the National Household Survey on Drug Abuse, and the Drug Abuse Warning Network (DAWN) supported by the National Institute on Drug Abuse (NIDA). During 1993, the National Household Survey on Drug Abuse revealed that 4.5 million persons in the United States used cocaine. Approximately 1.3 million persons (0.6 percent of the American population) stated that they self-administered cocaine on a frequent, monthly basis. The Drug Abuse Warning Network reported in 1993 that 30,900 cocaine-related emergency room visits occurred during the later part of 1992. Illnesses that prompted cocaine-related emergency room visits included cocaine-induced gastrointestinal, cardiovascular, and cerebrovascular disorders. Although there has been an encouraging trend of decreased cocaine abuse by young persons, the National Institute on Drug Abuse 1995 report *Epidemiologic Trends in Drug Abuse* noted that "the oldest age groups generally comprised the largest and fastest growing percentages of cocaine fatality." The report also highlighted that "cocaine (including crack) remains the nation's most serious drug problem." There is also increasing evidence that crack cocaine is frequently smoked with marijuana. A recent study indicated that a major cause of death of young adults in New York City was fatal injury associated with cocaine abuse.

Chronic drug abuse can be associated with a number of adverse health consequences, ranging from pulmonary disease to reproductive dysfunctions. Preexisting disorders such as hypertension and cardiac disease may be exacerbated by drug abuse, and the combined use of two or more drugs may accentuate medical complications associated with the abuse of one of them. The adverse health consequences of drug abuse are further complicated by AIDS, and drug abuse also increases the risk of exposure to the human immunodeficiency virus (HIV). Drug abuse contributes to the recent AIDS epidemic through HIV infection transmitted by needle-sharing by intravenous drug users and by adverse immunomodulatory effects of abused drugs. During 1993–1994, persons who self-administered drugs intravenously represented the largest single group with HIV infection in several major metropolitan areas in the United States, as well as urban areas in Scotland, Italy, Spain, Thailand, and China. Over 30 countries throughout Europe, North America, South America, Asia, Australia, and Africa have reported AIDS or HIV infection among intravenous drug users.

The initiation and continuation of drug abuse is determined by a complex interaction of the pharmacologic properties and relative availability of each drug, the personality and expectations of the user, and the environmental context in which the drug is used. Polydrug abuse—the concurrent use of several drugs with different pharmacologic effects—is increasingly common among individuals from all socioeconomic strata. There has been an alarming increase in a particularly dangerous form of polydrug abuse, the combined use of heroin and cocaine intravenously, called "speedballing." There is no simple explanation for this change in polydrug use patterns. Sometimes drug abusers attempt to attenuate one drug effect with another, as when heroin or alcohol is used to modulate the cocaine high. Sometimes one drug is used to enhance the effects of another, as with benzodiazepines and methadone, or cocaine plus heroin in methadone-maintained patients. Toxic drug interactions associated with polydrug abuse also contribute to adverse health consequences. This chapter discusses cocaine, marijuana, two hallucinogens [phencyclidine (PCP) and lysergic acid diethylamide (LSD)], and polydrug abuse. → *Alcohol and alcoholism are discussed in Chap. 386 and opioid drug abuse in Chap. 387.*

COCAINE Cocaine is a stimulant and local anesthetic with potent vasoconstrictor properties. The leaves of the coca plant (*Erythroxylon coca*) contain approximately 0.5 to 1 percent cocaine. The drug produces physiologic and behavioral effects when administered orally, intranasally, intravenously, or via inhalation following pyrolysis (smoking). It is now recognized that cocaine has potent pharmacologic effects on dopamine, norepinephrine, and serotonin neurons in the central nervous system. These effects include alteration and blockade of cellular membrane transport and prevention of the reuptake of biogenic amines. It has been postulated that cocaine-induced euphoria is due to cocaine-induced blockade of dopamine reuptake, but chronic cocaine use may cause dopamine depletion and impairment of dopaminergic function in the brain.

Prevalence of Cocaine Use Cocaine has become more widely available throughout the United States since its cost (relative to disposable income) has decreased considerably. Cocaine is no longer considered a "status" drug, since cocaine abuse occurs in virtually all social and economic strata of society. The prevalence of cocaine abuse in the general population has also been associated with an increase in cocaine abuse by heroin-dependent persons, including those in methadone maintenance programs. Intravenous cocaine is often used concurrently with intravenous heroin (the speedball)—a combination that purportedly attenuates the postcocaine "crash" and substitutes a cocaine "high" for the heroin "high" blocked by methadone. Intravenous use of cocaine plus heroin may further increase risk for HIV infection, both through needle sharing and through the combined immunosuppressive effects of the drugs.

Acute and Chronic Cocaine Intoxication Although cocaine is commonly self-administered by inhalation (snorting), there has been an increase in both intravenous administration and inhalation of pyrolyzed material via smoking. Following intranasal administration, changes in mood and feeling states are perceived within 3 to 5 min, and peak effects occur at 10 to 20 min. The effects rarely last more than 1 h following intranasal administration. Inhalation of pyrolyzed materials include smoking coca paste, a product produced by extracting cocaine preparations with flammable solvents, and cocaine free-base smoking. Coca paste is frequently contaminated with toxic solvents used in its preparation. Free-base cocaine, including the free base prepared with sodium bicarbonate (crack), is becoming increasingly popular because of the relative high potency of the compounds and their rapid onset of action (8 to 10 s following smoking).

Cocaine produces a brief, dose-related stimulation and enhancement of mood and dose-related increases in cardiac rate and blood pressure. Body temperature usually increases following cocaine administration, and high doses of cocaine may induce lethal pyrexia or hypertension. Because cocaine inhibits reuptake of catecholamines at adrenergic nerve endings, the drug potentiates sympathetic nervous system activity. Cocaine has a short plasma half-life of approximately 1 h. In humans, cocaine is primarily metabolized by plasma esterases, and cocaine metabolites are excreted in urine. The very short duration of euphorigenic effects of cocaine observed in chronic abusers is probably due to both acute and chronic tolerance. Frequent self-administration of the drug (two to three times per hour) is often reported by chronic cocaine abusers. Alcohol is used to modulate both the cocaine "high" and the dysphoria associated with the abrupt disappearance of cocaine's effects. A metabolite of cocaine, cocaethylene, has been detected in blood and urine of persons who concurrently abuse alcohol and cocaine. Cocaethylene induces changes in cardiovascular function similar to those of cocaine alone, and the pathophysiologic consequences of alcohol abuse plus cocaine abuse may be additive when both are used together.

The prevalent assumption that cocaine use is relatively safe is challenged by reports of death from respiratory depression, cardiac arrhythmias, and convulsions after cocaine snorting and intravenous administration. Disorders of cerebral blood flow and perfusion in cocaine-dependent persons have been detected with studies using single photon emission computed tomography (SPECT). Severe pulmonary disease may develop in individuals who smoke coca paste; this effect is attributed both to the direct effects of cocaine and to residual solvent contaminants in the smoked material. Hepatic necrosis has also been reported to occur in coca paste smokers. Although men and women who abuse cocaine may report that the drug enhances libidinal drive, chronic cocaine use causes significant loss of libido and adversely affects reproductive function. Impotence and gynecomastia have been observed in male cocaine abusers, and these abnormalities often persist for long periods following cessation of drug use. Women who abuse cocaine have reported major derangements in menstrual cycle function, including galactorrhea, amenorrhea, and infertility. Chronic cocaine abuse may cause persistent hyperprolactinemia as a consequence of cocaine-induced disorders of dopaminergic regulation of prolactin secretion by the pituitary. Cocaine abuse, particularly the smoking of crack by pregnant women, has been implicated as causing an increased risk of congenital malformations and of perinatal cardiovascular and cerebrovascular disease in the mother. However, cocaine abuse per se is probably not the sole cause of these perinatal disorders, since many problems associated with maternal cocaine abuse, including poor nutrition and health care status as well as polydrug abuse, also contribute to the risk for perinatal disease.

Numerous clinical reports, dating from the late nineteenth century, strongly suggest that protracted cocaine abuse may cause paranoid ideation and visual and auditory hallucinations, a state that resembles alcoholic hallucinosis. Psychological dependence on cocaine, as manifested by inability to abstain from frequent compulsive use, also has been reported. Although the existence of withdrawal syndromes involving psychomotor agitation and autonomic hyperactivity remains controversial, severe depression ("crashing") following cocaine intoxication may accompany drug withdrawal.

TREATMENT

Treatment of cocaine overdose is a medical emergency that involves resuscitation in an intensive care unit. Cocaine toxicity produces hypertension, tachycardia, tonic-clonic seizures, dyspnea, and ventricular arrhythmias. Intravenous diazepam in doses up to 0.5 mg/kg administered over an 8-h period has been shown to be effective for control of seizures. The systemic concomitants of a hypermetabolic state produced by cocaine toxicity with concurrent ventricular arrhythmias have been managed successfully by administration of 0.5 to 1.0 mg of propranolol intravenously. Since many instances of cocaine-related mortality have been associated with concurrent use of other illicit drugs (particularly heroin), the physician must be prepared to institute effective emergency treatment for multiple drug toxicity.

Treatment of chronic cocaine abuse requires combined efforts by family physicians, psychiatrists, and psychosocial care providers. Early abstinence from cocaine use is often complicated by symptoms of depression and guilt, insomnia, and anorexia, which may be as severe as those observed in major affective disorders. Individual and group psychotherapy, family therapy, and peer group assistance programs are often useful for inducing prolonged remission from drug use. A number of medications currently available for the treatment of various medical and psychiatric disorders have been administered to reduce the duration and severity of cocaine abuse and dependence. However, survey reports obtained from physicians specializing in the practice of addiction medicine indicate that no available medication is both safe and highly effective for either cocaine detoxification or maintenance of abstinence. A variety of psychotherapeutic and behavioral treatments for cocaine abuse have been attempted, and although some psychotherapeutic interventions are occasionally effective, no specific form of psychotherapy or behavioral modification has been determined to be uniquely beneficial for many persons who abuse or are dependent on cocaine.

MARIJUANA AND CANNABIS COMPOUNDS *Cannabis sativa* contains over 400 compounds in addition to the psychoactive substance, delta-9-tetrahydrocannabinol (THC). Marijuana cigarettes are prepared from the leaves and flowering tops of the plant, and a typical marijuana cigarette contains 0.5 to 1 g of plant material. Although the usual THC concentration varies between 5 and 20 mg, concentrations as high as 100 mg per cigarette have been detected. Hashish is prepared from concentrated resin of *Cannabis sativa* and contains a THC concentration of between 8 and 12 percent by weight. "Hash oil," a lipid-soluble plant extract, may contain a THC concentration of 25 to 60 percent, and it may be added to marijuana or hashish to enhance the THC concentration. Smoking is the most common mode of marijuana or hashish self-administration. During pyrolysis,

CHAPTER 388
Cocaine and Other Commonly Abused Drugs 2513

over 150 compounds in addition to the THC are released in the smoke. Although most of these compounds are not psychoactive, they do have potential physiologic effects.

THC is quickly absorbed from the lungs into blood and is then rapidly sequestered in tissues. It is metabolized primarily in the liver, where it is converted to 11-hydroxy-THC, a psychoactive compound, and more than 20 other metabolites. Most THC metabolites are excreted through the feces at a rate of clearance that is relatively slow in comparison to that of most other psychoactive drugs.

Prevalence of Marijuana Use   The National Institute on Drug Abuse 1995 report states that marijuana use, particularly by adolescents, is increasing significantly throughout the United States. Drug-related emergency department admissions increased greatly throughout the United States between 1992 and 1993. Most of these patients were males between the ages of 18 and 25. Marijuana-related emergency department admissions for males between the ages of 12 and 17 escalated by almost 100 percent during 1991 to 1993. Marijuana-filled cigars from which tobacco was removed ("blunts") were increasingly smoked by young adults in urban and some rural areas.

Acute and Chronic Marijuana Intoxication   Acute intoxication from marijuana and cannabis compounds is related to both the dose of THC and the route of administration. THC is absorbed more rapidly from marijuana smoking than from orally ingested cannabis compounds. Acute marijuana intoxication usually consists of a subjective perception of relaxation and mild euphoria resembling mild to moderate alcohol intoxication. This condition is usually accompanied by some impairment in thinking, concentration, and perceptual and psychomotor functions. Higher doses of cannabis may produce behavioral effects analogous to severe alcohol intoxication. Although the effects of acute marijuana intoxication are relatively benign in normal users, the drug can precipitate severe emotional disorders in individuals who have antecedent psychotic or neurotic problems. As with other psychoactive compounds, both set (user's expectations) and setting (environmental context) are important determinants of the type and severity of behavioral intoxication.

As is true of alcoholics, chronic marijuana abusers may lose interest in common socially desirable goals and devote steadily more time to drug acquisition and use. However, it should be emphasized that THC does not cause a specific and unique "amotivational syndrome." The range of symptoms sometimes attributed to marijuana use is difficult to distinguish from mild depression and the maturational dysfunctions often associated with protracted adolescence. Chronic use of marijuana has also been reported to increase the probability of exacerbation of psychotic symptoms in individuals with a past history of schizophrenia.

Physical Effects of Marijuana   Conjunctival injection and tachycardia are the most frequent immediate physical concomitants of smoking marijuana. Tolerance for marijuana-induced tachycardia develops rapidly among regular users; angina may be precipitated by marijuana smoking in persons with a history of coronary insufficiency. Exercise-induced angina may be increased after marijuana use to a greater extent than after tobacco cigarette smoking. Patients with cardiac disease should be strongly advised not to smoke marijuana or use cannabis compounds.

Significant decrements in pulmonary vital capacity have been found in regular daily marijuana smokers. Because marijuana smoking typically involves deep inhalation and prolonged retention of marijuana smoke, marijuana smokers may develop pulmonary disease such as chronic bronchial irritation. Impairment of single-breath carbon monoxide diffusion capacity (DL_{co}) is greater in persons who smoke both marijuana and tobacco than in tobacco smokers. Despite the well-documented association between tobacco smoking and lung cancer, at present there is no direct evidence that marijuana smoking induces lung cancer. However, heavy marijuana use among Americans may be too recent to permit detection of this problem.

Although marijuana has also been associated with adverse effects on a number of other systems, many of these studies await replication and confirmation. For example, the reported correlation between marijuana use and decreased testosterone levels in males has not been confirmed. Decreased sperm count and sperm motility and morphologic abnormalities of spermatozoa following marijuana use have also been reported. Administration of high doses of marijuana to female rhesus monkeys has revealed significant marijuana-induced suppression of pituitary gonadotropins and gonadal steroids. Carefully conducted prospective studies demonstrated a significant correlation between impaired fetal growth and development and heavy marijuana use during pregnancy. Marijuana also has been implicated in derangements of the immune response system, in chromosomal abnormalities, and in inhibition of DNA, RNA, and protein synthesis, but these findings have not been confirmed or related to any specific physiologic effect in humans. One report of cannabis-induced brain atrophy in young adults has not been confirmed in computed tomography studies of young men with histories of heavy marijuana smoking.

Tolerance and Physical Dependence   Habitual marijuana users rapidly develop tolerance to the psychoactive effects of marijuana and often smoke more frequently and try to secure more potent cannabis compounds. Tolerance for physiologic effects of marijuana develops at different rates; e.g., tolerance for marijuana-induced tachycardia develops rapidly, but tolerance for marijuana-induced conjunctival injection develops more slowly. Tolerance to both behavioral and physiologic effects of marijuana decreases rapidly upon cessation of marijuana use.

Withdrawal signs and symptoms have been reported in chronic cannabis users, with the severity of symptoms related to dosage and duration of use. These include tremor, nystagmus, sweating, nausea, vomiting, diarrhea, irritability, anorexia, and sleep disturbances. Withdrawal signs and symptoms observed in chronic marijuana users are usually relatively mild in comparison to those observed in heavy opiate or alcohol users and rarely require medical or pharmacologic intervention. Somewhat more severe and protracted abstinence syndromes may occur after sustained use of high-potency cannabis compounds for long periods.

LYSERGIC ACID DIETHYLAMIDE (LSD)   The serendipitous discovery of the psychedelic effects of LSD in 1947 culminated in an epidemic of LSD abuse during the 1960s. Imposition of stringent legal and regulatory constraints on the manufacture and distribution of LSD [classified as a Schedule I substance by the Food and Drug Administration (FDA)], as well as public recognition that the psychedelic experiences induced by LSD were a health hazard, has resulted in a significant reduction in LSD abuse. Although relatively few instances of LSD abuse have been reported, the drug still retains some popularity among adolescents and young adults. There are recent indications that the prevalence of LSD use among young persons has been accelerating in some communities in the United States.

LSD is a very potent drug; oral doses as low as 20 μg may induce profound psychological and physiologic effects. Tachycardia, hypertension, pupillary dilation, tremor, and hyperpyrexia occur within minutes following oral LSD ingestion in doses of 0.5 to 2 μg/kg. A variety of bizarre and often conflicting perceptual and mood changes, including visual illusions, synesthesias, and extreme lability of mood, usually occur within one-half hour after LSD intake. The action of LSD may persist for 12 to 18 h, even though the half-life of the drug is only 3 h.

Tolerance develops rapidly for LSD-induced changes in psychological function when the drug is used one or more times per day over a course of 4 days or more. Abrupt abstinence following continued use does not produce withdrawal signs or symptoms. To date there have been no clinical reports of death caused by the direct effects of LSD.

The most frequent acute medical emergency associated with LSD use is panic episodes, which may persist for up to 24 h (the "bad trip"). This problem is best managed by supportive reassurance ("talking down") and, if necessary, administration of small doses of anxiolytic drugs. Adverse consequences of chronic LSD use include enhanced risk for schizophreniform psychosis and derangements in memory function, problem solving, and abstract thinking. Treatment of these disorders is best carried out in specialized psychiatric facilities.

PHENCYCLIDINE (PCP) Phencyclidine, a cyclohexylamine derivative, is widely used in veterinary medicine to briefly immobilize large animals and is sometimes described as a dissociative anesthetic. PCP is easily synthesized, and its abusers are primarily young people and polydrug users. The true extent of PCP abuse is unknown, but recent national surveys indicate an increase in frequency of use.

Phencyclidine is taken orally, by smoking, or by intravenous injection. It is also used as an adulterant in illicitly sold THC, LSD, amphetamine, and cocaine. The most common street preparation, "angel dust," is a white granular powder which contains 50 to 100 percent of the drug. Low doses (5 mg) produce agitation, excitement, impaired motor coordination, dysarthria, and analgesia. Users may have horizontal or vertical nystagmus, flushing, diaphoresis, and hyperacusis. Behavioral changes include distortions of body image, disorganization of thinking, and feelings of estrangement. Higher doses of PCP (5 to 10 mg) may produce hypersalivation, vomiting, myoclonus, fever, stupor, or coma. PCP doses of 10 mg or more cause convulsions, opisthotonus, and decerebrate posturing which may be followed by prolonged coma.

The diagnosis of PCP overdose is difficult because the patient's initial symptoms may suggest an acute schizophrenic reaction. Confirmation of PCP use is possible by determination of PCP levels in serum or urine. PCP analysis is currently available at most toxicologic centers. Large quantities of PCP remain in urine for 1 to 5 days following high-dosage PCP intake.

PCP overdose requires prompt life-support measures, including treatment of coma, convulsions, and respiratory depression in a hospital intensive care unit. There is no specific antidote or antagonist for PCP. Excretion of PCP from the body can be enhanced by acidification of urine and gastric lavage. Death from PCP overdose may occur as a consequence of some combination of pharyngeal hypersecretion, hyperthermia, respiratory depression, severe hypertension, seizures, hypertensive encephalopathy, and intracerebral hemorrhage.

Acute psychosis associated with PCP use should be considered a psychiatric emergency, since patients may be at high risk for suicide or extreme violence toward others. Phenothiazines should not be used for treatment of acute PCP psychosis because they potentiate PCP's anticholinergic effects. Haloperidol (5 mg intramuscularly) has been administered on an hourly basis to suppress psychotic behavior. PCP, like LSD and mescaline, produces vasospasm of cerebral arteries at relatively low doses. Chronic PCP use has been shown to induce insomnia, anorexia, severe social and behavioral changes, and, in some cases, chronic schizophrenia.

POLYDRUG ABUSE Although drug abusers often report a preference for a particular drug, such as alcohol or opiates, the concurrent use of other drugs is common. Multiple drug use often involves substances having pharmacologic effects different from those of the preferred drug. Concurrent use of such dissimilar compounds as stimulants and opiates or stimulants and alcohol is not unusual. The diversity of reported drug use combinations suggests that achieving some perceptible change in state, rather than any particular direction of change (stimulation or sedation), may be the primary reinforcer in polydrug use and abuse. There is also evidence that intoxication with alcohol or opiates is associated with increased tobacco smoking, but marijuana smoking does not increase during alcohol intoxication. At present, there is relatively little systematic information available about drug interactions. However, it is known that the combined use of cocaine, heroin, and alcohol carries higher risks for toxic effects and adverse medical consequences than the use of a single drug.

A practical determinant of polydrug use patterns is the relative availability and cost of the drugs. There are many examples of situationally determined drug use patterns. For example, soldiers who became dependent on heroin in Vietnam seldom continued heroin use after leaving military service; but a significant proportion of them abused alcohol and became alcohol-dependent when they returned to the United States. Alcohol abuse, with its attendant medical complica-

tions, is one of the most serious problems encountered in former heroin addicts participating in methadone maintenance programs.

The physician must recognize that perpetuation of polydrug abuse and drug dependence is not necessarily a symptom of an underlying emotional disorder. Neither alleviation of anxiety nor reduction of depression accounts for the initiation and perpetuation of polydrug abuse. Severe depression and anxiety as frequently result from as precede polydrug abuse. There is also evidence that some of the most adverse consequences of drug use may reinforce continued polydrug abuse.

Adequate treatment of polydrug abuse, as well as other forms of drug abuse, requires innovative and eclectic programs of intervention. The first step in successful treatment is detoxification, a process which may be difficult because the patient has abused several drugs with different pharmacologic actions (e.g., alcohol, opiates, and cocaine). Since patients may not recall or may deny simultaneous multiple drug use, diagnostic evaluation should always include urinalysis for qualitative detection of psychoactive substances and their metabolites. Treatment of polydrug abuse requires hospitalization or inpatient residential care during detoxification and the initial phase of drug abstinence. When possible, specialized facilities for the care and treatment of chemically dependent persons should be used. Outpatient detoxification of polydrug abuse patients is likely to be ineffective and may be dangerous.

As in the treatment of alcohol abuse, no single therapeutic modality has been shown to be uniquely effective in inducing remission. Polydrug abuse is a chronic disorder with an unpredictable pattern of remission and recrudescence. Therapeutic management of chronic disorders such as cardiac or neoplastic disease should serve as a model for helping the person with polydrug abuse problems. Even temporary remissions with attendant physical, social, and psychological improvements are preferable to the continuation or progressive acceleration of polydrug abuse and its adverse medical and interpersonal consequences. In polydrug abuse, as in most chronic disorders, definitive "cures" are rare. The concerned physician should continue to assist polydrug abuse patients throughout the cyclic oscillations of this complex behavior disorder, recognizing that resumption of drug use may be the rule rather than the exception.

BIBLIOGRAPHY

CARROLL KM et al: Psychotherapy and pharmacotherapy for ambulatory cocaine abusers. Arch Gen Psychiatry 51:177, 1994

CREGLER LL, MARK H: Medical complications of cocaine abuse. N Engl J Med 315:1495, 1986

DAS G: Cocaine abuse in North America—A milestone in history. J Clin Pharmacol 33:296, 1993

FOLTIN RW, FISCHMAN MW: Smoked and intravenous cocaine in humans: Acute tolerance, cardiovascular and subjective effects. J Pharmacol Exp Ther 257:247, 1991

GAWIN FH: Cocaine addiction: Psychology and neurophysiology. Science 251:1580, 1991

———, ELLINWOOD EH JR: Cocaine and other stimulants. Actions, abuse, and treatment. N Engl J Med 318:1173, 1988

HALIKAS J et al: 1990–1991 Survey of pharmacotherapies used in the treatment of cocaine abuse. J Addict Dis 12:129, 1993

HOLLANDER JE: The management of cocaine-associated myocardial ischemia. N Engl J Med 333:1267, 1995

HOLMAN BL et al: Brain perfusion is abnormal in cocaine-dependent polydrug users: A study using technetium-99m-HMPAO and ASPECT. J Nucl Med 32:1206, 1991

JOHANSON CE, FISCHMAN MW: The pharmacology of cocaine related to its abuse. Pharmacol Rev 41:3, 1989

JONES RT: The pharmacology of cocaine smoking in humans, in *Research Findings on Smoking of Abused Substances*, NIDA Research Monograph vol. 99, CN Chiang, RL Hawks (eds). Washington, DC, U.S. Government Printing Office, 1990, pp 30–41

LEVIN JM et al: Gender differences in cerebral perfusion in cocaine abuse: Technetium-99m-HMPAO SPECT study of drug-abusing women. J Nucl Med 35:1902, 1994

MARZUK PM et al: Fatal injuries after cocaine use as a leading cause of death among young adults in New York City. N Engl J Med 332:1753, 1995

McCANCE EF et al: Cocaethylene: Pharmacology, physiology and behavioral effects in humans. J Pharmacol Exp Ther 274:215, 1995

MENDELSON JH, MELLO NK (eds): Medical Diagnosis and Treatment of Alcoholism. New York, McGraw-Hill, 1992

———: Management of cocaine abuse and dependence. N Engl J Med 334:965, 1996

——— et al: Acute effects of cocaine on plasma adrenocorticotropic hormone, luteinizing hormone and prolactin levels in cocaine-dependent men. J Pharmacol Exp Ther 263:505, 1992

MOLITERANO DJ et al: Coronary-artery vasoconstriction induced by cocaine, cigarette smoking, or both. N Engl J Med 330:454, 1994

NAJAVITS LM, WEISS RD: The role of psychotherapy in the treatment of substance-use disorders. Harvard Rev Psychiatry 2:84, 1994

NATIONAL INSTITUTE ON DRUG ABUSE: Epidemiologic Trends in Drug Abuse, vol 1: Highlights and Executive Summary. NIH Publication 95-3990, 1995

OM A et al: Management of cocaine-induced cardiovascular complications. Am Heart J 125:469, 1993

SUBSTANCE ABUSE AND MENTAL HEALTH SERVICES ADMINISTRATION OFFICE OF APPLIED STUDIES: The 1993 National Household Survey on Drug Abuse. US Department of Health and Human Services Public Health Service, 1993

SUBSTANCE ABUSE AND MENTAL HEALTH SERVICES ADMINISTRATION OFFICE OF APPLIED STUDIES: Preliminary Estimates from the Drug Abuse Warning Network (DAWN). Advance Report no. 2, 1993

WOODS JH, WINGER G: Phencyclidine and related substances, in Drug Abuse and Drug Abuse Research: The Third Triennial Report to Congress from the Secretary, Department of Health and Human Services. Washington, DC: U.S. Government Printing Office, 1991, p 145

389

John H. Holbrook

NICOTINE ADDICTION

Cigarette smoking is the principal cause of preventable disease, disability, and premature death in the United States. Nonetheless, each year more than one million American children and teenagers start smoking, and most established smokers have great difficulty in quitting. The addictive effects of nicotine account for most of this persistent personal and public health dilemma. Recognition of tobacco use as an addiction and of nicotine as the addictive drug is essential for effective patient management.

The primary criteria for defining drug addiction are compulsive use, psychoactive effects, and drug-reinforced behavior. Nicotine use fulfills these criteria because it produces a compelling urge to smoke, provides pleasurable alterations in mood, and motivates chronic tobacco-seeking and tobacco-using behavior. Tolerance and physical dependence, manifested by an abstinence-mediated withdrawal syndrome, contribute to the strong control exerted by nicotine on smoking behavior.

Smokers regulate their nicotine dose to obtain desired effects; these include both positive effects, such as pleasure and enhanced vigilance, and avoidance of the withdrawal syndrome. This syndrome is characterized by craving for tobacco products, depressed mood, insomnia, irritability, anxiety, difficulty concentrating, restlessness, and an increased appetite. Most of these symptoms peak in 1 to 2 days and return to baseline within 3 to 4 weeks of quitting; however, craving for tobacco products and hunger may persist for extended periods.

The use of tobacco products is a complex, learned behavior that is woven into the fiber of daily living and is linked to how the smoker deals with the world. Numerous daily activities, thoughts, and emotions serve as powerful cues to smoke. Such conditioned ties become paired with positive neuroregulatory effects of nicotine to reinforce the addictive process. Personal characteristics such as educational level, belief in one's ability to change, and coping skills are determinants of tobacco use. Similarly, environmental factors such as the level of acceptance of smoking in the home, peer group, workplace, and community norms influence smoking behavior.

PHYSICOCHEMICAL PROPERTIES OF CIGARETTE SMOKE Cigarette smoke is a heterogeneous aerosol produced by incomplete combustion of the tobacco leaf. It is composed of a gas phase in which particulate matter is dispersed. Mainstream smoke emerges from the mouthpiece during puffing. Sidestream smoke is emitted between puffs at the burning cone and from the mouthpiece. In the presence of the intense heat of combustion some tobacco constituents undergo thermic decomposition (pyrolysis). Volatile substances are distilled directly into the smoke. Unstable molecules recombine to generate new compounds (pyrosynthesis). Concentration of smoke constituents occurs as the smoke is filtered by unburnt tobacco and is redistilled by the burning cone. Some substances found in tobacco pass unchanged into cigarette smoke.

Approximately 92 to 95 percent of the total weight of mainstream smoke is present in the gas phase. Nitrogen, oxygen, and carbon dioxide account for 85 percent of the smoke's weight. The remaining gases and particulate matter are the substances of medical importance (Table 389-1) A variety of additives are used in the manufacturing of cigarettes; the influence of these substances on the composition and biologic activity of cigarette smoke is not known.

PHARMACOLOGY OF CIGARETTE SMOKE More than 4000 substances have been identified in cigarette smoke, including some that are pharmacologically active, antigenic, cytotoxic, mutagenic, and carcinogenic; these diverse biologic effects provide a framework for understanding the multiple adverse consequences of smoking. A pack-a-day cigarette smoker puffs more than 70,000 times a year, and, consequently, the membranes of the mouth, nose, pharynx, and tracheobronchial tree are exposed repetitively to tobacco smoke. Some constituents act directly on the membranes, while others are absorbed into the blood or are dissolved in saliva and swallowed.

Tissue and organ system responses to cigarette smoke inhalation are multiple and complex. Most studies in humans have dealt with exposure to whole smoke or to selected constituents thought to pose the greatest risk to health, such as nicotine and carbon monoxide.

Table 389-1

Selected Cigarette Smoke Constituents

Substance	Effect(s)
PARTICULATE PHASE	
"Tar"*	Carcinogen
Polynuclear aromatic hydrocarbons	Carcinogens
Nicotine	Neuroendocrine stimulant and depressant; addicting drug
Phenol	Cocarcinogen and irritant
Cresol	Cocarcinogen and irritant
β-Naphthylamine	Carcinogen
N-Nitrosonornicotine	Carcinogen
Benzo[a]pyrene	Carcinogen
Trace metals (e.g., nickel, arsenic, polonium 210)	Carcinogens
Indole	Tumor accelerator
Carbazole	Tumor accelerator
Catechol	Cocarcinogen
GAS PHASE	
Carbon monoxide	Impairs oxygen transport and utilization
Hydrocyanic acid	Ciliotoxin and irritant
Acetaldehyde	Ciliotoxin and irritant
Acrolein	Ciliotoxin and irritant
Ammonia	Ciliotoxin and irritant
Formaldehyde	Ciliotoxin and irritant
Oxides of nitrogen	Ciliotoxin and irritant
Nitrosamines	Carcinogen
Hydrazine	Carcinogen
Vinyl chloride	Carcinogen

* The aggregate of particulate matter in cigarette smoke after subtracting nicotine and moisture.

Relatively little is known about the individual effects and interactions of other potentially toxic smoke constituents that are present in low concentrations.

Nicotine is a highly toxic alkaloid that is both a ganglionic stimulant and depressant. Many of its complex effects are mediated by catecholamine release. Nicotine also increases serum concentrations of glucose, cortisol, free fatty acids, vasopressin, and β-endorphin.

Carbon monoxide interferes with oxygen transport and utilization. Because cigarette smoke contains 2 to 6 percent carbon monoxide, smokers inhale concentrations as high as 400 parts per million (ppm) and develop elevated carboxyhemoglobin (COHb) levels. The range of COHb found in smokers is 2 to 15 percent, while levels for nonsmokers are near 1 percent. The average COHb level of moderate cigarette smokers is 5 percent. Chronic, mild elevations of COHb due to smoking are a common cause of mild polycythemia and may produce subtle impairment of central nervous system function.

Cigarette smoke and its condensate are carcinogenic in several species of animals. The major identified carcinogens in cigarette smoke are polynuclear aromatic hydrocarbons, aromatic amines, and nitrosamines (Table 389-1). Cocarcinogens present in cigarette smoke, such as catechol, greatly enhance its carcinogenicity.

Potent pulmonary irritants and ciliotoxins are found in cigarette smoke (Table 389-1). These substances increase bronchial mucus secretion and mediate acute and chronic decreases in pulmonary and mucociliary function.

EPIDEMIOLOGY   Data from large prospective studies of populations in several countries have shown that cigarette-smoking men have 70 percent higher overall death rates than nonsmokers. About half of all regular cigarette smokers will eventually die because of smoking. The effect on mortality is proportionately greatest in younger age groups. The excess mortality of female smokers has been somewhat less than that of male smokers, but it has increased. Cigarette smoking is the largest single health risk in the United States and is responsible for an estimated 430,000 premature deaths each year; this is equivalent to approximately one out of every five deaths. Coronary heart disease (CHD) and lung cancer are the chief contributors to smoking-related excess mortality. In the United States, cigarette smokers also experience more disability due to chronic illness and report significantly more days absent from work than do nonsmokers. Cigarette smoking causes immeasurable personal loss and suffering.

A strong dose-response relationship exists between cigarette smoking and excess mortality, as measured by the age at onset of smoking, the number of cigarettes smoked, the number of years of smoking, and the depth of inhalation. Cessation of smoking is associated with a decrease in the excess mortality. These observations together with clinical, experimental, and pathologic studies indicate that smoking, per se, causes the excess mortality.

CHARACTERISTICS OF SMOKERS   Demographic, anthropometric, physiologic, and laboratory features that distinguish cigarette smokers from nonsmokers are due both to baseline differences between these groups and to the effects of smoking. Smokers drink more alcohol, coffee, and tea than do nonsmokers. Their weight and blood pressure are slightly less and their heart rate is slightly faster than those of nonsmokers. In women, the menopause comes earlier in smokers than in nonsmokers. Smokers have impaired maximum exercise performance and impaired immune systems compared to nonsmokers. A markedly increased number of pulmonary alveolar macrophages is present in smokers, and the function and metabolism of these cells are abnormal. When compared with nonsmokers, smokers show small increases in hematocrit, total white blood cell count, and platelet count, as well as small decreases in leukocyte vitamin C levels, serum uric acid, and albumin. In smokers, the ratio of high-density lipoprotein cholesterol to low-density lipoprotein cholesterol is reduced.

CLINICAL CORRELATIONS   Large population studies have shown a strong association between cigarette smoking and several diseases. Atherosclerotic cardiovascular disease, cancer, and chronic obstructive pulmonary disease account for most of the excess mortality and morbidity due to smoking.

Individual patient risks due to cigarette smoking vary widely. Factors that influence these risks include the duration, intensity, and type of smoke exposure; genetically mediated susceptibility; occupational and environmental exposures; use of medication; and coexisting risk factors and diseases.

Cardiovascular Disease   Cigarette smoking is a major cause of coronary heart disease, and premature CHD is one of its most important medical consequences (see Chap. 244). Approximately 20 percent of the 500,000 CHD deaths occurring each year in the United States is attributable to smoking. Cigarette smoking, hypertension, and hypercholesterolemia are the three major CHD risk factors. Smoking acts both independently of and synergistically with these other CHD risk factors. There is a dose-response relationship between CHD risk and cigarette smoking. CHD death rates are 60 to 70 percent greater in male smokers than nonsmokers. Sudden death may be the first manifestation of CHD, and it is two to four times more likely to occur in younger male cigarette smokers than in nonsmokers. Women cigarette smokers are also at greater risk of developing CHD than nonsmokers, and the use of both cigarettes and oral contraceptives increases this risk approximately tenfold. Those who continue to smoke after an acute myocardial infarction are more likely to die from CHD than are those who quit smoking. Smokers who undergo coronary artery bypass surgery have increased perioperative mortality compared to nonsmokers. Cigarette smoking contributes to both coronary atherosclerosis and acute ischemic, thrombotic, and arrhythmic coronary events. Cigarette smoking may interfere with the efficacy of medications used to treat CHD, such as propranolol.

Cigarette smoking is an important cause of cerebrovascular disease and accounts for an estimated 15 percent of the 150,000 stroke deaths that occur each year in the United States. Large epidemiologic studies in men and women have shown an increased risk of stroke among smokers compared to nonsmokers, a dose-response relationship between smoking and stroke risk, and a decrease in stroke risk with smoking cessation. Among women, subarachnoid hemorrhage is more likely to occur in smokers than nonsmokers, and the use of both cigarettes and oral contraceptives greatly increases this risk.

Cigarette smoking is the most powerful risk factor for arteriosclerosis obliterans and thromboangiitis obliterans. It also aggravates peripheral ischemia and may adversely affect peripheral bypass grafts. The mortality rate for atherosclerotic aortic aneurysm is greater in male smokers than nonsmokers.

Cigarette smoking is not a risk factor for the development of hypertension; however, hypertensives who smoke are at a greater risk of developing malignant hypertension and of dying from hypertension. Because of the association with chronic obstructive pulmonary disease, cigarette smoking is an important factor leading to chronic pulmonary heart disease.

Cancer   Cigarette smoking is the single most important cause of cancer mortality in the United States, accounting for 30 percent of all cancer deaths. In spite of the well-documented cause-and-effect relationship between cigarette smoking and lung cancer, more Americans continue to die from this cancer than from any other tumor (see Chap. 90). In 1991, an estimated 143,000 lung cancer deaths occurred in the United States; 85 percent of these deaths were attributable to cigarette smoking. The risk of developing lung cancer is quantitatively related to cigarette smoke exposure. Men who smoke one pack a day increase their risk tenfold compared with nonsmokers; men who smoke two packs a day may increase their risk more than 25 times compared with nonsmokers. Asbestos workers who smoke cigarettes are at especially high risk for developing lung cancer. Cigarette consumption by women increased rapidly in the United States during the past 50 years, and lung cancer mortality among smokers is currently increasing faster in women than in men. Lung cancer has become the leading cause of cancer death among American women.

Cigarette smoking is a cause of laryngeal, oral, pharyngeal, esophageal, and bladder cancer in men and women. Cigarette smoking is an important contributory factor for the development of kidney and pancreatic cancer; it is associated with cancer of the stomach and uterine cervix. Cigarette smoking may also be associated with leukemia, hepatoma, nonmelanoma skin cancer, and cancer of the anus and vulva.

Respiratory Disease Cigarette smoking is the major cause of chronic obstructive pulmonary disease (COPD), that is, chronic bronchitis and emphysema (see Chap. 258). Of the estimated 80,000 deaths from COPD in the United States in 1991, 82 percent were attributable to smoking, and many of these deaths were preceded by prolonged respiratory disability. There is a dose-response relationship between COPD death rates and cigarette smoking. Depending upon the extent of smoke exposure, the mortality rate due to COPD is 4 to 25 times higher in male cigarette smokers than in nonsmokers. Although the death rate from COPD among female smokers is somewhat lower than among male smokers, it is increasing much more rapidly in female than in male smokers. Chronic cough, sputum production, and breathlessness are much more common in smokers. Smokers are more likely than nonsmokers to show abnormalities in a number of pulmonary function tests, including measurements of elastic recoil, airflow in large and small airways, and diffusing capacity. Mild airflow obstruction in small airways may be present even in teenage smokers.

Cigarette smoking has been associated with an increased incidence of respiratory infections and deaths from pneumonia and influenza. Postoperative respiratory complications and spontaneous pneumothorax are also more common in smokers. Because tobacco smoke may increase airway obstruction, asthmatics should be urged not to smoke. Chronic stomatitis and chronic laryngitis occur more frequently in smokers than in nonsmokers.

Pregnancy Smoking may delay conception, and smoking during pregnancy may affect the fetus adversely. Infants whose mothers smoked during pregnancy weigh, on average, 170 g less than infants whose mothers did not smoke. This effect probably results from impaired uteroplacental circulation. Maternal smoking during pregnancy increases the risk of spontaneous abortion, fetal death, neonatal death, and the sudden infant death syndrome. This increased risk may be much greater in pregnancies already at high risk owing to other factors. Smoking during pregnancy may also adversely affect the long-term physical growth and intellectual development of the child.

Gastrointestinal Disorders Gastric and duodenal ulcer disease is more prevalent in male and female cigarette smokers than in nonsmokers and causes more deaths in male smokers than in nonsmokers. Smoking impairs spontaneous and drug-induced healing of peptic ulcers, increases the likelihood of duodenal ulcer recurrence, inhibits pancreactic bicarbonate secretion, and decreases the pressure of esophageal and pyloric sphincters. Smoking also prevents the inhibition of nocturnal gastric secretion by histamine H_2-receptor antagonists.

Other Conditions Cigarette smoking is a risk factor for premature facial wrinkling, osteoporosis in women, and sexual dysfunction in men. It may also be associated with Graves' disease, cataracts, macular degeneration, degenerative disk disease, and sleep disturbances.

Depression Recent studies indicate that the prevalence of cigarette smoking is increased among those who have had a major depressive disorder. Furthermore, smoking cessation rates are lower among depressed smokers compared to nondepressed smokers. What role antidepressants could play in such individuals who are attempting to quit smoking remains to be determined.

Involuntary Smoke Inhalation Indoor atmospheres and other confined spaces are often contaminated by tobacco smoke, which is inhaled involuntarily by both smokers and nonsmokers. Most of the atmospheric pollutants arise from sidestream smoke. It contains greater concentrations of many smoke constituents than does mainstream smoke, but since sidestream smoke is diluted in a large volume of air, the smoke exposure from involuntary inhalation is less than that associated with smoking.

Initially, involuntary or passive smoking was thought to cause primarily an irritant effect such as ocular burning. It is now recognized as a cause of lung cancer in nonsmokers. Parental smoking in the home is associated with an increased risk of acute respiratory illnesses, middle-ear effusions, chronic respiratory symptoms, and slightly impaired lung function in children. Involuntary smoke inhalation may also cause CHD.

Drug Effects Tobacco smoke constituents induce hepatic microsomal enzyme systems that are important in the metabolism of several drugs. For example, cigarette smoking increases the metabolism of propranolol, propoxyphene, and theophylline. Hence, changes in smoking behavior may cause significant alterations of serum drug levels that may result in either drug toxicity or failure of drug treatment.

TYPES OF SMOKING Filter-tipped cigarettes and lower-tar and -nicotine cigarettes now account for more than 95 and 55 percent of sales, respectively. Lung cancer and laryngeal cancer are the only tobacco-related diseases for which the use of lower-tar and -nicotine cigarettes has been shown to result in risk reduction, compared with the use of higher-tar and -nicotine cigarettes; however, compared with not smoking or quitting, the benefits are minimal. Consumers who choose lower-tar and -nicotine cigarettes and then smoke a larger number of cigarettes or inhale more frequently or deeply may actually increase their exposure to harmful substances.

Cigar and pipe smokers usually inhale less smoke than cigarette smokers, presumably because the alkaline pH of cigar and pipe tobacco makes it more irritating to the respiratory tract. The smoke exposure and overall mortality rates of pipe and cigar smokers in the United States are substantially less than those of cigarette smokers; however, death rates of cigarette, cigar, and pipe smokers are approximately equal for carcinoma of the oral cavity, larynx, and esophagus, sites where exposures to cigarette, cigar, and pipe smoke are similar. The mortality rates of most cigar and pipe smokers for cancer at other sites, CHD, and COPD are not greatly elevated above the rates of nonsmokers, but cigar and pipe smokers who inhale consistently may experience adverse health effects comparable with those of cigarette smokers.

The use of chewing tobacco and snuff may produce plasma nicotine levels comparable to those of cigarette smokers and lead to nicotine dependence or addiction. The use of such smokeless tobacco products also increases the risk for oral cancer.

CESSATION OF SMOKING In the United States between 1965 and 1991, the prevalence of smoking in adults declined from 52 to 28 percent of men and 34 to 23 percent of women. Each year in the United States, approximately 1.3 million smokers stop smoking. In 1991 there were an estimated 46.3 million current adult smokers and 43.5 million former smokers. In recent years, the smoking prevalence among senior high school students has leveled off at about 20 percent. The rate of decline in smoking prevalence among the least educated Americans lags behind other groups.

Benefits Smoking cessation produces immediate and long-term physical, psychological, and economic benefits. Within days of quitting the sense of smell and taste may improve. One year after quitting there is a substantial decrease in risk for a myocardial infarction. Total mortality among former smokers decreases almost to that of nonsmokers 15 years after quitting. When chronic smoking produces permanent damage, as it does in the case of emphysema, the benefits of cessation are more modest, such as a slowing in the rate of decline of pulmonary function. The U.S. Surgeon General summarized the major and immediate health benefits of cessation that are valid for men and women of all ages and for those with and without smoking-related disease. Former smokers live, on the average, longer than continuing smokers. Cessation reduces the risk for tobacco-related cancers, myocardial infarction, cerebrovascular disease, and chronic obstructive pulmonary disease. Women who quit smoking prior to pregnancy, or during the first trimester, eliminate the risk of delivering a low-birth-weight baby. The health benefits of quitting smoking far exceed the risks of the average 2.3- to 6.8-kg (5- to 15-lb) weight gain or any adverse psychological effects that may occur after quitting.

Cessation Process Most American smokers would like to quit. Eighty percent have attempted to stop smoking during their lifetime, and 30 percent have stopped for at least one day during the previous year. Most of these attempts to quit are only temporarily successful. Smoking cessation is a dynamic, cyclic process that leads to overcoming an addictive behavior. Smokers move through a series of stages in their attempts to quit, including thinking about quitting, deciding to quit, attempting to quit, and maintaining the ex-smoker status. Most successful quitters relapse and recycle through these stages three or four times before attaining long-term abstinence. Fewer than 5 percent of smokers move directly to the confirmed ex-smoker status without experiencing relapses. Factors encouraging long-term cessation include decreased social acceptability of smoking, increased concern about the health consequences of active and passive smoking, and increased costs of tobacco products. Factors contributing to relapse include craving for nicotine, weight gain, social pressures, and attempts to cope with negative feelings and interpersonal conflicts.

Cessation Methods More than 90 percent of confirmed ex-smokers quit without formal assistance. Quitting "cold turkey" is the method used by more than 80 percent of successful ex-smokers. However, heavy smokers and those most addicted to nicotine may benefit from participation in a cessation program. Organized programs employ a variety of approaches, including self-help, physician advice and counseling, use of medication, group therapy, and behavioral training. With such methods 20 to 30 percent 1-year abstinence rates are commonly reported.

Recent meta-analyses of approximately 300 controlled clinical trials document the effectiveness of smoking cessation treatments. The three modalities that are especially effective are nicotine replacement therapy, social support through clinician-provided encouragement and assistance, and skills training on techniques to achieve and maintain smoking cessation. The most effective programs offer multiple treatment modalities, involvement of physician and nonphysician health personnel, and a clear nonsmoking message presented in a variety of formats over time.

Physician Guidelines Physicians have unique opportunities and effective tools to promote smoking cessation. Seventy percent of American smokers visit a physician at least once a year. Some of these visits occur when the patient is experiencing symptomatic illness. In such settings, patients may be especially responsive to cessation messages, and quit rates may be substantially enhanced. Even brief, physician-delivered stop-smoking messages may double the spontaneous smoking cessation rate. Treatment of nicotine addiction is at least as cost-effective as treating other common medical problems such as hypertension and hypercholesterolemia.

Nicotine addiction should be viewed as a chronic medical problem requiring long-term commitment and management skills. Each patient's smoking status should be noted on the problem list. The primary goal for each clinic visit should be to assist the smoker to move one step closer to quitting. The three essential phases for physician management are assessment, intervention, and follow-up (Table 389-2). During the assessment phase, data are collected on health status, nicotine addiction, quitting experience, and interest in quitting. If the patient doesn't want to stop smoking, the clinician should review the risks of smoking, recommend quitting, and defer further action until the next clinic visit. Most patients are interested in quitting and progress to the intervention phase. Smokers are taught about the benefits of quitting and the cyclical cessation process. The smoker is advised to choose a quit date and to go "cold turkey." When possible, the recommendation to stop smoking is related to the patient's unique needs and risk factors. A cessation method(s) is chosen and implemented. Physicians often provide educational material, counseling, and nicotine replacement therapy. Both nicotine chewing gum and transdermal patches improve cessation rates. Transdermal nicotine doubles smoking cessation rates and should be the pharmacotherapy of choice for most smokers; this effect is independent of the intensity of psychosocial interventions. The proper uses, contraindications, and side effects of these products should be understood. For example,

Table 389-2

Physician Guidelines for Managing Nicotine Addiction

Assessment
1. Smoking history
2. Level of nicotine addiction
3. Health status
4. Quitting experience
5. Interest in quitting

Intervention
1. Education
   a. Benefits of cessation
   b. Cessation process
   c. Withdrawal syndrome
2. Giving advice to quit
   a. Personalized message
   b. Quit date
   c. "Cold turkey"
3. Selection of cessation method(s)
   a. Self-help
   b. Physician-assisted
   c. Nicotine replacement
   d. Behavioral training
   e. Group therapy
4. Implementation of method
5. Meeting of special needs

Follow-up
1. Measurement of progress
2. Provision of support
3. Dealing with relapse
4. Consideration of alternative methods
5. Consideration of referral

nicotine replacement therapy should not be used when the patient is still smoking. The likelihood of success with any cessation method is enhanced when the clinician responds to individual concerns such as weight gain and helps the smoker to develop practical strategies to avoid relapse. The final phase, follow-up, involves assessing progress, providing support, and dealing with relapse. The last should not be viewed as failure but as part of the cyclic process leading to cessation. Follow-up discussions may focus on alternative cessation methods or referral to a smoking cessation specialist.

Political, social, and cultural forces play a critical role in the individual decision to start or stop smoking. For this reason, physicians should lead and support efforts to increase tobacco excise taxes, to eliminate all tobacco advertisements and promotional activities, and to ban smoking in public places.

PREVENTION In the United States, more than 90 percent of cases of first tobacco use occurs before high school graduation. The average age of first smoking a cigarette is 14.5 years and of becoming a daily smoker is 17.7 years. Approximately 40 percent of teenage smokers who experiment with a few cigarettes become regular smokers. Even though most adolescent smokers want to quit, they are unable to do so because of nicotine addiction. Because few people start to smoke after the age of 18 years, primary smoking prevention in the pediatric and adolescent age groups is an essential step to reduce the toll of tobacco use. Young people who have been trained to resist social pressures, who appreciate the difficulty of quitting, and who understand the health consequences of smoking are less likely to start smoking.

BIBLIOGRAPHY

AMERICAN PSYCHIATRIC ASSOCIATION: Practice guideline for the treatment of patients with nicotine dependence. Am J Psychiatry 153:1, 1996

DOLL R et al: Mortality in relation to smoking: 40 years' observations on male British doctors. BMJ 309:901, 1994

GRIES JM et al: Chronopharmacokinetics of nicotine. Clin Pharmacol Ther 60:385, 1996

HENNINGFIELD JE: Nicotine medications for smoking cessation. N Engl J Med 333:1196, 1995

KESSLER DA: Nicotine addiction in young people. N Engl J Med 333:186, 1995

US DEPARTMENT OF HEALTH AND HUMAN SERVICES: *The Health Consequences of Smoking: Nicotine Addiction. A Report of the Surgeon General.* DHHS (CDC) Publication 88-8406, 1988

————: *Preventing Tobacco Use Among Young People. A Report of the Surgeon General.* DHHS (CDC), National Center for Chronic Disease Prevention and Health Promotion, Office on Smoking and Health, 1994

————: *Smoking Cessation and Prevention.* Clinical Practice Guideline Number 18, Agency for Health Care Policy and Research Publication No. 96-0692, Public Health Service, DHHS, 1996

390

Howard Hu, Frank E. Speizer

SPECIFIC ENVIRONMENTAL AND OCCUPATIONAL HAZARDS

It cannot be overemphasized that an appropriate environmental/occupational history is an essential part of the medical workup of many chronic diseases. The general approach to the patient whose illness may have been caused or exacerbated by environmental or occupational hazards is detailed in Chap. 5.

As stated in Chap. 5, the term *hazards* in this context is generally synonymous with *toxins* and *toxic exposures* and encompasses chemical factors as well as other risks posed by the physical environment and by selected natural phenomena. These hazards may exist in the general environment or in the workplace. Strictly speaking, smoking, alcohol ingestion, nutritional factors, and infectious agents can also be considered chemical or environmental hazards.

Once a specific hazard has been identified as a factor in the pathogenesis of an illness or as an imminent threat, the clinical approach must include the development of a strategy for preventing further exposure and for treating the specific manifestations of the illness, using antidotes and supportive measures. In the following chapters, specific hazards are considered, including acute poisoning and drug overdose; heavy metal poisoning; disorders caused by venoms, bites, and stings; drowning and near-drowning; electrical injuries; and radiation injury. The health effects of ambient air pollution, occupational respiratory exposures, passive smoking, and assorted toxic air pollutants are discussed briefly in Chap. 254. Space does not allow specific discussion in this text of many other important categories of hazards, such as organic solvents; chemicals used in the plastics, synthetic textiles, and rubber industries; and pesticides. The reader should consult other detailed texts or electronic information sources for clinical data on these topics. In this volume, however, brief attention is focused on several selected issues in light of recent developments in research that have enhanced our understanding of the way these hazards may interact with human behavior and consequently pose increased risks to both individuals and society.

HAZARDOUS WASTE AND GROUNDWATER CONTAMINATION The term *hazardous waste* embodies toxic chemicals, radioactive materials, and biologic or infectious wastes. In many communities, hazardous waste has emerged as a major public health concern. In the United States, some 50,000 sites (defined by specific criteria) have been estimated to contain hazardous chemicals; 1000 or so of these have been included as "Superfund sites" on a National Priority List drawn up by the Environmental Protection Agency (EPA). New or unrecognized sites are likely to exist as well. These sites may require long-term remedial action. The spectrum of substances contained at the sites is wide and theoretically may include any of some 30,000 chemicals that are commonly used in commerce. However, the EPA keeps fewer than 200 chemicals on a special hazardous substance list in light of their toxicity, the frequency with which they are encountered, and other factors. One difficulty in anticipating risks associated with hazardous waste sites is that the substances are usually present in mixtures whose composition is seldom fully known. In addition, with respect to toxicity, chemicals may interact with one another in an additive, protective, or synergistic fashion, and little knowledge exists on which to base predictions regarding the interactions of these complex mixtures.

Waste-site employees and the surrounding community can incur hazardous exposures through the inhalation of toxic vapors or dusts emanating directly from a waste site or an on-site incinerator; the ingestion of water contaminated by surface runoff or by material leaching through soil into surface water or groundwater; the ingestion of contaminated plants, fish, or other wildlife; or direct contact. This last risk is particularly likely for children, who may enter a poorly secured site. Perhaps the exposure of greatest concern to community residents has been the contamination of groundwater by volatile organic compounds or solvents (VOCs); together, the widespread detection of low levels of VOCs in groundwater and the several studies suggesting an association between heavy VOC contamination of drinking water and cancer probably account for the high priority given in public opinion polls to avoiding cancer risks. A 1983 study found that 11 of the 20 chemicals most commonly detected at National Priority List waste sites were VOCs (Table 390-1).

Current regulatory policy rests on the assumption that there is no threshold below which a carcinogen exerts no effect or risk. Thus, once a substance is identified as a probable carcinogen (see below), it is regulated to a concentration that is believed to be accompanied by an acceptable level of risk. Clearly, great uncertainty exists regarding methods used to classify drinking-water carcinogens and to extrapolate the risks related to exposure to these substances. Regardless, VOC contamination in groundwater is likely to continue to be a high-priority issue in the public arena.

ENVIRONMENTAL CARCINOGENS Based on studies and reviews of the literature by the International Agency for Research on Cancer, enough evidence exists to classify around 50 substances and processes as probably or definitely carcinogenic in humans (Table 390-2). Some processes are deemed carcinogenic on the basis of epidemiologic evidence, even though the specific causative agent cannot always be clearly identified. Tumor promoters are not distinguished from tumor initiators in this listing, and the chemical structures and modes of action are diverse. Around 150 additional agents and processes have been designated as possibly carcinogenic on the basis of studies of bacteria and animals as well as human epidemiologic studies. The extent to which inferences can be made from nonhuman studies is controversial but certainly depends on minimal standards in the execution of such studies. For example, the Interagency Regulatory Liaison Group recommends that for a carcinogen assay to be considered positive, the test must have been performed on at least 50 animals of each sex in two different species with at least three dose groups (control and two dose levels) over the lifetime of the animals.

BUILDING-RELATED ILLNESSES Reports of discomfort and symptoms in relation to office environments began in the United

Table 390-1

Volatile Organic Compounds Most Frequently Detected in 1983 at National Priority List Hazardous Waste Sites (in Order of Frequency and Detection) and (When Known) Associated Cancer Risks

Chemical	Risk Level*
Trichloroethylene	3.0
Toluene	
Benzene	1.0
Chloroform	0.43
Tetrachloroethylene	0.7
1,1,1-Trichloroethane	
Ethylbenzene	
Trans-1,2-dichloroethane	0.4
Xylene	
Dichloromethane	
Vinyl chloride	0.02

* Concentration in water (μg/L) equivalent to a lifetime cancer risk of 1×10^{-6}. Risk estimates used in these calculations were derived from the U.S. Environmental Protection Agency (1990).

States in the 1970s. Research has led to the recognition that some building-related illnesses have a clear etiology; these illnesses include hypersensitivity diseases, infections, and exacerbations of asthma due to airborne irritants. However, the majority of such complaints, particularly those of mucous membrane irritation, fatigue, and headache, have no clear etiology. Terms such as *sick-building syndrome* (SBS; also called *tight-building syndrome*) have been used to designate this constellation of symptoms, which have been found in most investigations to occur most often in sealed buildings with centrally controlled mechanical ventilation. Early characterizations of SBS as mass psychogenic illness have not been borne out in the majority of cases by subsequent epidemiologic investigations. Since indoor air-exchange rates were sharply reduced in the 1970s to conserve energy, current hypotheses focus on inadequate dilution of irritants arising from building materials (such as formaldehyde-containing particle board), office supplies (such as carbonless copy paper and photocopy developer solution), and personal care products used by occupants as risk factors for SBS. Confirmation of these hypotheses and further characterization of SBS await additional research.

MULTIPLE-CHEMICAL SENSITIVITY The multiple-chemical sensitivity (MCS) syndrome is a diagnosis that has increasingly been given to patients with a wide variety of symptoms that they attribute to exposure at very low levels to a number of commonly encountered chemicals. The syndrome usually begins after a well-defined environmental event, such as a reaction to a more clearly toxic dose of an organic solvent, pesticide, or respiratory irritant. Some cases of MCS begin as SBS. Affected persons commonly report symptoms such as fatigue, malaise, headache, dizziness, lack of concentration, memory loss, and "spaciness"—symptoms that overlap somewhat with those of other diagnoses of uncertain etiology, such as chronic fatigue syndrome. The pathogenesis of MCS is obscure, and no proven methods exist for its diagnosis, evaluation, and treatment. Case series suggesting a high prevalence of affective disorders indicate that psychological factors may play a role in causing MCS and/or in determining its severity; however, evidence does not support MCS as a purely psychogenic illness. Some patients have debilitating symptoms that are precipitated by incidental exposures to substances as common as perfumes, motor vehicle exhaust, and paint vapors. Other than the ruling out of other treatable conditions and the avoidance of exacerbating exposures, no specific recommendations for the management of MCS patients can yet be made. A recent panel of European scientists convened by the World Health Organization recommended that the designation MCS be replaced by the term *idiopathic environmental illness* (IEI).

GLOBAL CLIMATIC CHANGES An increasing body of evidence indicates that human activities are responsible for global climatic changes, which, in turn, may be directly or indirectly increasing human exposure to environmental hazards. The depletion of stratospheric ozone by chlorinated fluorocarbons, with a consequent increase in ultraviolet radiation exposure, has been firmly established. Increased risks of skin cancers and cataracts are accepted as results of this phenomenon. Less clear is whether the immunosuppressive effects of ultraviolet radiation detected in animals and in vitro have significant clinical impacts on human resistance to infection. Although uncertainties in climate modeling persist, an increasing if not overwhelming amount of evidence indicates that anthropogenic greenhouse gases are fostering global warming. A prominent concern is that global warming can abet the introduction and dissemination of serious infectious diseases, such as mosquito-borne infections (malaria, dengue, and viral encephalitis) and waterborne infectious and toxin-related illnesses (cholera, shellfish poisoning). The World Health Organization has identified global warming as one of the largest public health challenges facing the twenty-first century.

Table 390-2

Substances and Processes Classified as Definitely or Probably Carcinogenic by the International Agency for Research on Cancer

Aflatoxins	Estrogen, nonsteroidal
Aluminum production	Estrogen, steroidal
4-Aminobiphenyl	Furniture and cabinet working
Analgesic mixtures containing phenacetin	Hematite mining, underground, with exposure to radon
Arsenic and arsenic compounds	Iron and steel founding
Asbestos	Isopropyl alcohol manufacture, strong-acid process
Auramine manufacture	Magenta manufacture
Azathioprine	Melphalan
Benzene	8-Methoxypsoralen (Methoxsalen) plus ultraviolet radiation
Benzidine	
Betel quid with tobacco	Mineral oils, untreated and mildly treated
N,N-bis(2-chloroethyl)-2-naphthylamine (Chlornaphazine)	
	MOPP (combined therapy with nitrogen mustard, vincristine, procarbazine, and prednisone) and other combined chemotherapy including alkylating agents
Bis(chloromethyl)ether and chloromethyl methyl ether (technical-grade)	
Boot and shoe manufacture and repair	
1,4-Butanediol dimethanesulfonate (Myleran)	
Chlorambucil	Mustard gas (sulfur mustard)
1-(2-Chloroethyl)-3-(4-methylcyclohexyl)-1-nitrosourea (methyl-CCNU)	2-Naphthylamine
	Nickel and nickel compounds
	Oral contraceptives, combined
Chromium compounds, hexavalent	Oral contraceptives, sequential
Coal gasification	Rubber industry
Coal-tar pitches	Shale oils
Coal tars	Soots
Coke production	Talc-containing asbestiform fibers
Cyclophosphamide	Tobacco products, smokeless
Diethylstilbestrol	Tobacco smoke
Erionite	Treosulfan
Estrogen replacement therapy	Vinyl chloride

BIBLIOGRAPHY

BOURBEAU J et al: Prevalence of sick building syndrome symptoms in office workers before and after being exposed to a building with an improved ventilation system. Occup Environ Med 53:204, 1996

GOLDBERG MS et al: Incidence of cancer among persons living near a municipal solid waste landfill site in Montreal, Quebec. Arch Environ Health 50:416, 1995

JEEVAN A, KRIPKE ML: Ozone depletion and the immune system. Lancet 342:1159, 1993

PATZ JA et al: Global climate change and emerging infectious diseases. JAMA 275:217, 1996

SPARKS PJ et al: Multiple chemical sensitivity syndrome: A clinical perspective. I. Case definition, theories of pathogenesis, and research needs. II. Evaluation, diagnostic testing, treatment, and social considerations. J Occup Med 36:718, 1994

US ENVIRONMENTAL PROTECTION AGENCY: *Health Effects Assessment Summary Tables*, first/second quarters, FY-1990. Washington, DC, Office of Solid Waste and Emergency Response, 1990

WORLD HEALTH ORGANIZATION: *Climate Change and Human Health*. Geneva, World Health Organization, 1996

391

391

Christopher H. Linden, Frederick H. Lovejoy, Jr.

POISONING AND DRUG OVERDOSAGE

Poisoning refers to the development of harmful effects following exposure to chemicals. In a sufficient dose, substances that are usually innocuous, such as oxygen and water, can cause poisoning. Conversely, in small amounts, poisons such as arsenic and cyanide can be consumed without ill effect. Hence, a given substance may or may not be harmful depending on the conditions of exposure. *Overdosage* is exposure to excessive amounts of a substance normally intended for consumption and does not necessarily imply poisoning

Poisoning may be local (limited to the eyes, skin, lungs, or gastrointestinal tract), systemic, or both, depending on dose, absorption, distribution, potency, and host susceptibility. Absorption and distribution are influenced by properties of the substance (molecular size, degree of ionization, lipid and water solubility, protein binding) and of the biologic barriers (membrane composition, pore size, chemical transport systems) through which it penetrates.

Local poisoning results from nonspecific chemical reactions such as oxidation, protein denaturation, desiccation, and solvent activity. Its severity and reversibility depend on the dose (concentration), contact time, potency of the chemical, and type and condition of the exposed surface. The nature, extent, severity, and reversibility of systemic poisoning depend on the dose, potency, and metabolic disposition of the chemical, the functional reserve of the individual, and the presence of secondary complications (shock, hypoxia). Other variables that influence toxicity include coexisting illnesses, previous chemical exposure (e.g., enzyme induction or inhibition, tolerance), and individual differences in biologic response, tissue concentration (pharmacodynamics), and/or absorption, distribution, metabolism, and elimination (pharmacokinetics). *The effects of an overdose begin sooner, peak later, and last longer than those of therapeutic doses.*

EPIDEMIOLOGY

In the United States, chemical exposures result in over 5 million requests for medical advice or treatment each year. The common routes of exposure are ingestion (74 percent), dermal exposure (87 percent), inhalation (5 percent), ophthalmic exposure (6 percent), bites and stings (3 percent), and parenteral injections (0.3 percent). Exposures most frequently involve cleaning agents, analgesics, cosmetics, plants, cough and cold preparations, and hydrocarbons. Most exposures are acute, accidental, occur in the home, result in minor or no toxicity, and involve children under 6 years of age. Pharmaceuticals are involved in 41 percent of exposures and 75 percent of serious or fatal poisonings.

Accidental exposures can result from the improper use of chemicals at work or play, product mislabeling, label misreading, mistaken identification of unlabeled chemicals, uninformed self-medication, and dosing errors by nurses, parents, pharmacists, physicians, and the elderly. Excluding the recreational use of ethanol, attempted suicide is the most common reason for intentional exposure. Unintended poisonings may result from the intentional use of drugs for psychotropic effects (abuse) or excessive self-dosing (misuse).

About 5 percent of victims of chemical exposure require hospitalization. They account for 5 to 10 percent of all ambulance transports, emergency room visits, and intensive care unit admissions, and up to 30 percent of psychiatric admissions are prompted by attempted suicide via overdosage. Suicide attempts also account for most serious or fatal poisonings. Most deaths are due to carbon monoxide poisoning and occur before arrival at a hospital. Most drug-related fatalities are due to analgesics, antidepressants, sedative-hypnotics, stimulants and street drugs, cardiovascular drugs, asthma medications, and antihistamines.

Nonpharmaceutical agents implicated in fatal poisoning include alcohols and glycols, automotive products, inorganic chemicals, hydrocarbons, and cleaning agents.

DIAGNOSIS

Although poisoning can mimic other illnesses, the correct diagnosis usually can be established by the history, physical examination, routine and toxicologic laboratory evaluations, and clinical course. The *history* should include the time, route, duration, and circumstances (location, surrounding events, and intent) of exposure; the name and amount of each drug, chemical, or ingredient involved; the time of onset, nature, and severity of symptoms; the time and type of first aid measures provided; and the medical and psychiatric history.

In many cases the victim is confused, comatose, unaware of an exposure, or unable or unwilling to admit to one. Suspicious circumstances include unexplained illness in a previously healthy person; a history of psychiatric problems (particularly depression); recent changes in health, economic status, or social relationships; and onset of illness while working with chemicals or after ingesting food, drink (especially ethanol), or medications. Patients who become ill soon after arriving from a foreign country or after arrest for criminal activity should be suspected of having illicit drugs concealed in body cavities (the gastrointestinal tract). Family, friends, paramedics, police, pharmacists, physicians, and employers should be questioned regarding habits, hobbies, behavior changes, available medications, and antecedent events. A search of the clothes, belongings, and place of discovery may reveal a suicide note or a container of drugs or chemicals. The imprint code on pills and the label on chemical products may be used to identify the ingredients and potential toxicity of a suspected poison by consulting a reference text, a computerized chemical database, the manufacturer, or a regional poison information center.

The *physical examination* should focus initially on the vital signs and cardiopulmonary and neurologic status. The physiologic state can be characterized as excited, depressed, discordant, or normal on the basis of the pulse, blood pressure, respiratory rate, temperature, and mental status. A differential diagnosis can then be formulated (Table 391-1). Examination of the eyes (for nystagmus, pupil size, and pupil reactivity), abdomen (for bowel activity and bladder size), and skin (for burns, bullae, color, warmth, moisture, pressure sores, and puncture marks) may narrow the diagnosis to a particular disorder. Grading the severity of poisoning (Table 391-2) is useful for assessing the clinical course and response to treatment.

The patient also should be examined for evidence of trauma and underlying illnesses. Except in the case of carbon monoxide, theophylline, and drugs that cause hypoglycemia or hypoxia, seizures and neurologic dysfunction due to poisoning are nonfocal. Hence, focal findings should prompt evaluation for a structural central nervous system (CNS) lesion. When the history is unclear, all orifices should be examined for the presence of chemical burns and drug packets. The odor of breath or vomitus and the color of nails, skin, or urine may provide diagnostic clues.

Laboratory assessment may be helpful in the differential diagnosis of poisoning (Fig. 391-1). An anion-gap metabolic acidosis can be caused by a number of substances (Table 391-1); it is characteristic of methanol, ethylene glycol, and salicylate intoxication but can occur in any poisoning that results in hypoxia, hypotension, or seizures. The serum lactate concentration is low (less than the anion gap) in the former and high (nearly equal to the anion gap) in the latter. An abnormally low anion gap can be due to poisoning with bromide, iodine, lithium, or nitrate or to hypercalcemia or hypermagnesemia. An osmolal gap—the difference between the measured serum osmolality and the calculated osmolality [from the serum sodium, glucose, and blood urea nitrogen (BUN)]—of more than 10 mmol/L indicates the presence of a low-molecular-weight solute such as an alcohol, glycol, or ketone or an unmeasured electrolyte or sugar. Such a gap can also be due to diabetic ketoacidosis or lactic acidosis. The osmolal gap provides an estimate of the amount of anion present (Table 391-3). Ketosis can be due to acetone, isopropyl alcohol, and salicylate. Hypoglycemia may be due to poisoning with beta-adrenergic blocking agents, quinine, ethanol, oral hypoglycemic agents, and salicylates, whereas hyperglycemia suggests poisoning with acetone, a beta-adrenergic agonist, a calcium channel–blocking agent, iron, or theophylline. Hypokalemia can be caused by barium, a beta-adrenergic agonist, a diuretic, theophylline, or toluene; hyperkalemia suggests poisoning with an alpha-adrenergic agonist, a beta-adrenergic blocker, digitalis, or fluoride. Poisons that cause specific signs, symptoms, and other laboratory abnormalities are listed in the bibliography.

Pulmonary edema (adult respiratory distress syndrome, or ARDS) can be caused by poisoning with carbon monoxide, cyanide, an opioid, paraquat, phencyclidine, a sedative-hypnotic, or salicylate; by inhalation of irritant gases, fumes, or vapors (ammonia, metal oxides, mercury); or by prolonged anoxia, hyperthermia, or shock. Aspiration pneumonia is common in patients with coma, seizures, and petroleum distillate ingestion. Radiopaque densities may be visible on abdominal x-rays following the ingestion of calcium salts, chloral hydrate, chlorinated hydrocarbons, heavy metals, illicit drug packets, iodinated compounds, potassium salts, psychotherapeutic agents, lithium, phenothiazines, enteric-coated tablets, or salicylates.

Table 391-2

Severity of Stimulant and Depressant Poisoning and Drug Withdrawal

Severity	Signs and Symptoms
STIMULANT POISONING	
Grade 1	Diaphoresis, flushing, hyperreflexia, irritability, mydriasis, tremors
Grade 2	Confusion, fever, hyperactivity, hypertension, tachycardia, tachypnea
Grade 3	Delirium, mania, hyperpyrexia, tachyarrhythmias
Grade 4	Coma, convulsions, cardiovascular collapse
DEPRESSANT POISONING	
Grade 1	Lethargic but arousable; able to answer questions and follow commands
Grade 2	Comatose; withdraws from pain; brainstem and deep tendon reflexes intact
Grade 3	Comatose; no response to pain; most reflexes absent; respiratory depression
Grade 4	Comatose; no response to pain; reflexes absent; respiratory and cardiovascular depression

Bradycardia and atrioventricular (AV) block may occur in patients poisoned by antiarrhythmic agents, beta blockers, calcium channel blockers, cholinergic agents (carbamate and organophosphate insecticides), digitalis, lithium, phenylpropanolamine, or tricyclic antidepressants. QRS- and QT-interval prolongation may be caused by hyperkalemia and by membrane-active drugs (Table 391-1). Ventricular

Table 391-1

Differential Diagnosis of Poisoning Based on Physiologic Status as Determined by Vital Signs and CNS Activity

Excited	Depressed	Discordant	Normal
Sympathomimetic syndrome	**Sympatholytic syndrome**	**Asphyxiants**	**Agents with slow absorption**
Amphetamines	Alpha-adrenergic blockers	Carbon monoxide	Carbamazepine
Bronchodilators (beta₂-adrenergic agonists)	Angiotensin converting enzyme inhibitors	Cyanide	Digitalis preparations
Caffeine	Antiarrhythmics	Hydrogen sulfide	Dilantin Kapseals
Cocaine	Antidepressants (tricyclic)	Inert gases	Enteric-coated pills
Decongestants (alpha-adrenergic agonists)	Beta-adrenergic blockers	Irritant fumes, gases, vapors	Lomotil
Ergot alkaloids	Calcium channel blockers	Methemoglobinemia	Salicylates
MAO inhibitors	Clonidine	Nitrophenol herbicides	Sustained-release preparations
Theophylline	Decongestants (imidazolines)	**Central nervous system syndromes**	**Agents with slow distribution**
Thyroid hormones	Digitalis	Disulfiram	Digitalis preparations
Anticholinergic syndrome	**Cholinergic syndrome**	Dystonic/extrapyramidal reactions	Heavy metals
Antidepressants (tricyclic)	Bethanechol	Isoniazid	Lithium
Antihistamines	Carbamate insecticides	Neuroleptic malignant syndrome	Salicylates
Antiparkinsonian agents	Echothiophate	Serotonin syndrome	**Agents that are activated metabolically**
Antispasmodics (GI, GU)	Myasthenia gravis drugs (e.g., pyridostigmine)	Strychnine	Acetaminophen
Belladonna alkaloids	Organophosphate insecticides	Volatile hydrocarbon inhalation	Chloramphenicol
Cyclobenzaprine	Physostigmine	**Membrane-active agents**	Chlorinated hydrocarbons
Mydriatics (topical)	Pilocarpine	Amantadine	Ethylene glycol
Orphenadrine	Urecholine	Antiarrhythmic agents	L-thyroxine
Plants/mushrooms	**Opioid syndrome**	Antidepressants (cyclic)	Methanol
Phenothiazines	Analgesics	Beta-adrenergic blockers	Paraquat
Hallucinogenic syndrome	Antidiarrheal agents	Fluorides	Certain methemoglobin inducers
LSD and its analogues	Antispasmodics (GI)	Heavy metals	**Inhibitors of metabolic pathways**
Marijuana	Heroin	Lithium	Disulfiram
Mescaline and its analogues	Opium	Local anesthetics	Inhibitors of thyroid hormone synthesis
Phencyclidine	**Sedative-hypnotic syndrome**	Meperidine	Monoamine oxidase inhibitors
Withdrawal syndrome	Alcohols	Neuroleptic agents	Salicylates
Antidepressants	Anticonvulsants	Propoxyphene	**Inhibitors of nucleic acid synthesis**
Beta-adrenergic blockers	Barbiturates	Quinine and related antimalarial agents	Anticancer agents
Clonidine	Benzodiazepines	**Metabolic acidosis (low lactate; high anion gap)**	Antiviral agents
Ethanol	Bromide	Alcoholic ketoacidosis	Immunosuppressive drugs
Opioids	Ethchlorvynol	Ethylene glycol	Mushrooms (amatoxins)
Sedative-hypnotics	γ-Hydroxybutyrate	Methanol	Podophylline
	Hydrocarbons	Metformin/phenformin	**Nontoxic exposure**
	Glutethimide	Paraldehyde	**Psychogenic illness**
	Methyprylon	Salicylate	
	Muscle relaxants	Sulfur/sulfate	
		Toluene	

FIGURE 391-1 Differential diagnosis of poisoning based on the results of routine laboratory tests. Dashed lines indicate possible pathways.

tachyarrhythmias may be seen in poisoning with digitalis, membrane-active drugs, sympathomimetics, or agents that potentiate the effects of endogenous catecholamines such as chloral hydrate and aliphatic or halogenated hydrocarbons.

Analysis of urine and blood (and occasionally of gastric contents and chemical samples) may be useful to confirm or rule out suspected poisoning. Interpretation of laboratory data requires knowledge of the tests used for screening and confirmation (thin-layer, gas-liquid, or high-performance liquid chromatography; colorimetric and fluorometric assays; enzyme-multiplied and radioimmunoassays; gas chromatography; mass spectrometry), their sensitivity (limit of detection) and specificity, the best type of biologic specimens for analysis, and the best time to obtain such specimens. Personal communication with the laboratory is essential. A negative result on a screen may mean the poison is not detectable by the test used or that its concentration is too low for detection at the time of sampling. In the latter case, repeating the test at a later time may yield a positive result.

Table 391-3

Solute Effects on Serum Osmolality

Agent	Approximate Serum Concentrations (mg/dL) of Solute That Will Increase the Serum Osmolality by 1 mmol/kg
Alcohols	
Ethanol	4.6
Isopropanol	6.0
Methanol	2.6
Glycols	
Ethylene glycol	5.2
Propylene glycol	7.6
Ketones	
Acetone	5.8
Electrolytes	
Calcium	4 (2 mmol/L)
Magnesium	2.4 (2 mmol/L)
Sugars	
Mannitol	18
Sorbitol	18

Although some rapid screening tests are available, comprehensive screening tests require 2 to 6 h for completion, and immediate management must be based on the history, physical examination, and routine ancillary tests. In addition, when the patient is asymptomatic or when the clinical picture is consistent with the reported history, qualitative screening is neither clinically useful nor cost-effective. It is of greatest value in patients with severe or unexplained toxicity such as coma, seizures, cardiovascular instability, metabolic or respiratory acidosis, and nonsinus cardiac rhythms. Quantitative analysis is useful for poisoning with acetaminophen, acetone, alcohol (including ethylene glycol), antiarrhythmics, antiepileptics, barbiturates, digoxin, heavy metals, lithium, salicylate, and theophylline and for carboxyhemoglobinemia and methemoglobinemia. Results can often be available within an hour.

The *response to antidotes* may be assessed for diagnostic purposes. Resolution of altered mental status and abnormal vital signs within minutes of intravenous administration of dextrose, naloxone, or flumazenil is virtually diagnostic of hypoglycemia, narcotic poisoning, and benzodiazepine intoxication, respectively. The prompt reversal of acute dystonic (extrapyramidal) reactions following an intravenous dose of benztropine or diphenhydramine confirms the diagnosis of a drug etiology. Vin rosé urine color following a diagnostic dose of deferoxamine can be used to confirm iron poisoning when measurements of serum iron and total iron-binding capacity are not immediately available. Although reversal of both central and peripheral manifestations of anticholinergic poisoning by physostigmine is diagnostic, physostigmine may cause arousal in patients with CNS depression of any etiology.

In the absence of a history of chemical exposure the *clinical course* may suggest a diagnosis of poisoning. Poisoning typically evolves and resolves more rapidly than other disorders. Signs and symptoms characteristically develop within an hour of acute exposure, peak within several hours, and resolve over hours to days. However, the absence of signs and symptoms soon after an overdose does not rule out a poisoning.

℞ **TREATMENT**

General Principles Treatment goals include support of vital signs, prevention of further poison absorption, enhancement of poison elimination, administration of specific antidotes, and prevention of reexposure (Table 391-4). The treatment depends on the identity of the poison, the route and amount of exposure, the time of presentation relative to the time of exposure, and the severity of poisoning. Knowledge of toxin pharmacokinetics and pharmacodynamics is essential.

During the *pretoxic phase*, prior to the onset of manifestations, decontamination is the highest priority, and treatment is based solely on the history. The maximum potential toxicity based on the greatest possible exposure should be assumed. When appropriate, gastrointestinal decontamination to minimize absorption and decrease the severity of toxicity is the first priority. Since decontamination is more effective the sooner performed, the initial history should be focused, and the physical examination should be brief. It is also advisable to establish intravenous access and initiate cardiac monitoring, particularly in patients with potentially serious ingestions or unclear histories. The choice of decontamination procedure depends on the predicted toxicity; the availability, efficacy, and contraindications of the procedure; and the nature, severity, and risk of complications. For the home management of patients with accidental ingestions, reliable histories, and mild predicted toxicity, emesis can be induced with ipecac syrup. For patients treated in medical facilities, activated charcoal has comparable or greater efficacy, has fewer contraindications and complications, and is less invasive than ipecac or gastric lavage. Alternative methods should be used if the ingested agent is not well adsorbed by activated charcoal. Unless there has been a witnessed ingestion of a potentially severe overdose and the patient is comatose, the use of a large-bore gastric lavage tube is inappropriate, since serious complications (aspiration or esophageal perforation) may result from the forcible use of a lavage tube in an uncooperative patient.

When an accurate history is not obtainable and a poison causing delayed toxicity or irreversible damage is suspected, blood and urine should be sent for toxicologic screening and, if indicated, for quantitative analysis. During absorption and distribution, blood levels may be greater than those in tissue and may not correlate with toxicity. However, high blood levels of agents whose metabolites are more toxic than the parent compound (acetaminophen, ethylene glycol, or methanol) may indicate the need for additional interventions (antidotes, dialysis).

After evaluation and decontamination, some patients may be sent home because the predicted toxicity is minimal or the time of expected maximal toxicity has passed without incident. Observation for at least 4 to 6 h after gastrointestinal tract decontamination ensures that most patients who remain asymptomatic can be discharged safely. However, longer observation may be necessary for patients who have ingested agents that slow gastric emptying and intestinal motility and thus will have slowed dissolution, absorption,

and distribution characteristics, or agents that have to be converted in the body to active metabolites (Table 391-1). In such patients, documentation of a charcoal stool prior to discharge should prevent delayed absorption and subsequent toxicity.

The *toxic phase* is the time between the onset of poisoning and the peak effects. Management is based primarily on clinical and laboratory findings. Resuscitation and stabilization are the first priority. All symptomatic patients should have an intravenous line, supplemental oxygen, cardiac monitoring, continuous observation, and baseline laboratory, electrocardiographic (ECG), and x-ray evaluation. Patients with altered mental status, particularly those with coma or seizures, should be given an intravenous bolus of glucose, naloxone, and thiamine and additional antidotes as indicated. Decontamination measures should be initiated as soon as possible. Further absorption of ingested agents should be limited by administering activated charcoal. Gastric evacuation by the use of ipecac syrup or lavage is appropriate for agents not adsorbed by charcoal. Since aspiration is a hazard, ipecac syrup should be used with extreme caution in the presence of actual or potential CNS dysfunction. Charcoal may be given by mouth or by a stomach tube. The rare patient who deteriorates after this regimen should be lavaged and given additional charcoal. Administration of charcoal both before and after gastric lavage may be more effective than giving it only after lavage. In critically ill patients, an initial dose of charcoal can be given by a small-bore nasogastric tube (no. 18 French or smaller) while monitoring and supportive measures are being initiated. Once the patient is stable, lavage through a large-bore orogastric tube can be followed with a second dose of charcoal.

Measures that enhance poison elimination may shorten the duration of toxicity and lessen its severity. However, the risks must be weighed against the benefits. Diagnostic certainty (usually via laboratory confirmation) is generally a prerequisite. Intestinal dialysis with repetitive doses of activated charcoal is generally safe and can enhance the elimination of many poisons. Diuresis and chelation therapy are effective in enhancing the elimination of a relatively small number of poisons, and their use is associated with potential complications. Extracorporeal methods are effective in removing many poisons, but the expense and risk make their use reasonable only in patients who would otherwise not have a favorable outcome.

Patients with severe poisoning (coma, respiratory depression, hypotension, cardiac conduction abnormalities, cardiac arrhythmias, hypothermia or hyperthermia, seizures), those needing close monitoring or antidotes or enhanced elimination therapy, those showing progressive clinical deterioration, and those with significant underlying medical problems should be admitted to an intensive care unit. Patients with mild to moderate toxicity can be managed on a general medical service, intermediate care unit, or emergency department observation area, depending on the anticipated duration and level of monitoring needed (intermittent clinical observation versus continuous clinical, cardiac, and respiratory monitoring). Patients who have attempted suicide require continuous observation until they are thought unlikely to make further attempts.

During the *resolution phase* of poisoning, supportive care should continue until the patient is alert and laboratory and ECG abnormalities are resolved. Repeat charcoal dosing may prevent rebound toxicity when depressed gastrointestinal function improves and the substances still in the gut are absorbed or when active metabolites are formed. Since chemicals are eliminated from the blood before tissues, blood levels are generally lower than tissue levels during this phase and once again may not correlate with toxicity. This is particularly true when extracorporeal elimination procedures are used. Because of redistribution, a rebound increase in blood level and clinical relapse may occur after the termination of such procedures. When a metabolite is responsible for toxic effects, continued treatment of an asymptomatic patient may be necessary because of a blood level predictive of subsequent toxicity (acetaminophen, ethylene glycol, and methanol).

Supportive Care The goal of supportive therapy is to maintain physiologic homeostasis until detoxification is accomplished and

Table 391-4

Fundamentals of Poisoning Management

SUPPORTIVE CARE

Airway protection	Treatment of seizures
Oxygenation/ventilation	Correction of temperature abnormalities
Treatment of arrhythmias	Correction of metabolic derangements
Hemodynamic support	Prevention of secondary complications

PREVENTION OF FURTHER POISON ABSORPTION

Gastrointestinal decontamination	Decontamination of other sites
Syrup of ipecac-induced emesis	Eye decontamination
Gastric lavage	Skin decontamination
Activated charcoal	Body cavity evacuation
Whole bowel irrigation	
Catharsis	
Dilution	
Endoscopic/surgical removal	

ENHANCEMENT OF POISON ELIMINATION

Multiple-dose activated charcoal	Extracorporeal removal
Forced diuresis	Peritoneal dialysis
Alteration of urinary pH	Hemodialysis
Chelation (see Chap. 397)	Hemoperfusion
	Hemofiltration
	Plasmapheresis
	Exchange transfusion
	Hyperbaric oxygenation

ADMINISTRATION OF ANTIDOTES

Neutralization by antibodies	Metabolic antagonism
Neutralization by chemical	Physiologic antagonism
binding	

PREVENTION OF REEXPOSURE

Adult education	Notification of regulatory agencies
Child-proofing	Psychiatric referral

to prevent and treat secondary complications such as aspiration, bedsores, cerebral and pulmonary edema, pneumonia, rhabdomyolysis, renal failure, sepsis, thromboembolic disease, and generalized organ dysfunction due to prolonged hypoxia or shock.

Respiratory care is an important component of supportive care. In addition to those needing endotracheal intubation for mechanical ventilation, many patients require semielective endotracheal intubation for protection against aspiration of gastrointestinal contents and of the poison itself. The gag reflex alone is not a reliable indicator of the need for intubation. Since patients may maintain airway patency while being stimulated but not if left unattended, those who cannot respond to voice or who are unable to sit and drink fluids without assistance are best managed by prophylactic intubation. Patients with severe excitation also may require intubation for airway protection (due to the risk or existence of seizures) and sedation or paralysis for control of agitation and prevention of hyperthermia, acidosis, and rhabdomyolysis. Since clinical assessment of respiratory function is often inaccurate, the need for oxygenation and ventilation is best determined by oximetry or analysis of arterial blood gases.

Drug-induced pulmonary edema is usually noncardiac rather than cardiac in nature. Profound CNS depression and cardiac conduction abnormalities suggest the latter etiology. Measurement of pulmonary artery pressure may be necessary to establish etiology and direct appropriate therapy. Extracorporeal membrane oxygenation may be appropriate for severe but reversible respiratory failure.

Cardiovascular manifestations include arrhythmias caused by direct cardiotoxicity, abnormal cardiovascular reflexes, or metabolic derangements. Supraventricular tachycardia associated with hypertension and CNS excitation is almost always due to agents that cause general excitation (see Table 391-1). Most cases are mild or moderate in severity and require only observation or nonspecific sedation with a benzodiazepine. For cases that are severe or associated with hemodynamic instability, with chest pain, or with ECG evidence of ischemia, specific therapy is indicated. Hypoxia, hypoglycemia, and other metabolic causes of sympathetic stimulation also should be ruled out. For patients with sympathetic hyperactivity, treatment with a combined alpha and beta blocker (labetalol), a calcium channel blocker (verapamil or diltiazem), or a combination of a beta blocker and a vasodilator (esmolol and nitroprusside) is preferred. For those with anticholinergic poisoning, physostigmine is the treatment of choice. Supraventricular tachycardia without hypertension is generally secondary to vasodilation or hypovolemia and responds to fluid administration.

Lidocaine and phenytoin are generally safe for ventricular tachyarrhythmias, but beta blockers can be hazardous unless the arrhythmia is clearly due to sympathetic hyperactivity. In poisoning with tricyclic antidepressants (and probably in poisoning with all membrane-active agents (Table 391-1) quinine and procainamide are contraindicated (because of similar electrophysiologic effects), but sodium bicarbonate may be therapeutic. Magnesium sulfate and overdrive pacing (by isoproterenol or a pacemaker) may be useful in patients with torsade de pointes and prolonged QT intervals. Magnesium and antidigoxin antibodies are used in patients with severe digitalis poisoning. Invasive (esophageal or intracardiac) ECG recording may sometimes be necessary to determine the origin (ventricular or supraventricular) of wide-complex tachycardias (see Chap. 231). If the patient is hemodynamically stable, however, it may be prudent to observe rather than to treat with another potentially harmful cardioactive agent. Arrhythmias may be resistant to drug therapy until underlying acid-base and electrolyte derangements, hypoxia, and hypothermia are corrected.

Bradyarrhythmias associated with hypotension generally should be treated as described in Chap. 230. In beta-blocker and calcium channel–blocker poisoning, the administration of glucagon and calcium, respectively, may be effective. Antibody therapy may be indicated for digitalis poisoning. The management of hypotension is described in Chap. 38. If hypotension is unresponsive to volume expansion, norepinephrine or high-dose dopamine may be necessary.

Intraaortic balloon pump counterpulsation or full cardiopulmonary bypass pump circulatory support should be considered for severe but reversible cardiac failure.

Central nervous system manifestations are an important component of poisoning. Drug-induced seizures may be due to direct or indirect CNS neuroreceptor stimulation (or inhibition), neuronal membrane destabilization, ischemia, edema, or metabolic abnormalities. Seizures due to excessive stimulation of catecholamine receptors (sympathomimetic or hallucinogen poisoning and drug withdrawal) or decreased activity of gamma-aminobutyric acid (GABA) (isoniazid poisoning) or glycine (strychnine poisoning) are best treated with enhancers of GABA effects such as benzodiazepines or barbiturates. Since benzodiazepines and barbiturates act by slightly different mechanisms (the former increases the frequency and the latter increases the duration of chloride channel opening in response to GABA), therapy with both may be effective when neither is effective alone. Seizures caused by isoniazid, which inhibits the synthesis of GABA, may not respond to GABA-enhancer therapy until GABA synthesis is restored, because enhancers cannot work in the absence of GABA. High doses of pyridoxine, which facilitates the synthesis of GABA, are often necessary to terminate such seizures. For poisons with central dopaminergic effects (phencyclidine), an agent with opposing activity, such as haloperidol, may be useful. Seizures resulting from membrane destabilization (beta-blocker or cyclic antidepressant poisoning) may require a membrane-active agent such as phenytoin as well as a GABA agonist. In rare cases (anticholinergic or cyanide poisoning), specific antidotal therapy may be necessary.

The treatment of seizures secondary to ischemia, edema, or metabolic abnormalities should include correction of the underlying cause. Since prolonged convulsions can lead to rhabdomyolysis and severe acidosis, neuromuscular paralysis is indicated in refractory cases. Electroencephalographic (EEG) monitoring and continuing treatment of seizures are necessary to prevent permanent neurologic damage.

Temperature extremes; metabolic, hepatic, and renal abnormalities; and secondary complications should be treated by standard measures.

Prevention of Poison Absorption GASTROINTESTINAL DECONTAMINATION *Activated charcoal*, as a suspension in water either alone or with a cathartic, is given orally via a nippled bottle (for infants), or via a cup, straw, or small-bore nasogastric tube. The recommended dose is 1 to 2 g/kg body weight, using 8 mL of diluent per gram of charcoal if a premixed formulation is not available. Palatability may be increased by adding a sweetener (sorbitol) or a flavoring agent (cherry, chocolate, or cola syrup) to the suspension. Charcoal adsorbs ingested poisons within the gut lumen, allowing the charcoal-toxin complex to be evacuated with stool. The complex also can be removed from the stomach by induced emesis or lavage. In vitro, charcoal adsorbs 90 percent or more of most poisons when given in a tenfold ratio to the toxin. Charged (ionized) chemicals such as mineral acids, alkalis, and highly dissociated salts of cyanide, fluoride, iron, lithium, and other inorganic compounds are not well adsorbed by charcoal. Experimentally, charcoal decreases the absorption of other chemicals by an average of 73 percent when given within 5 min of administration, 51 percent when given at 30 min, and 36 percent at 60 min. Charcoal is as or more effective as ipecac syrup or gastric lavage. Lavage followed by charcoal is more effective than charcoal alone, and charcoal before and after lavage is more effective than charcoal alone or charcoal after lavage. In general, treatment with charcoal alone gives a better clinical outcome than treatment with ipecac followed by charcoal or lavage followed by charcoal. Side effects of charcoal include nausea, vomiting, and diarrhea or constipation. Charcoal also may prevent the absorption of orally administered therapeutic agents. Complications include mechanical obstruction of the airway, aspiration, vomiting, and bowel obstruction and infection caused by inspissated charcoal.

Charcoal is contraindicated in patients who have ingested corrosives because it obscures endoscopy.

Gastric lavage is performed using a no. 28 French orogastric tube in children and a no. 40 French tube in adults with volumes of about 5 mL fluid per kilogram of body weight. Except for infants, tap water is acceptable. The patient should be placed in Trendelenburg and left lateral decubitus positions to prevent aspiration (even if an endotracheal tube is in place). Experimentally, lavage decreases chemical absorption by an average of 52 percent if performed within 5 min of ingestion, 26 percent if performed at 30 min, and 16 percent if performed at 60 min. Its efficacy is similar to that of ipecac. Significant amounts of ingested drug are recovered in one-tenth of patients. As with ipecac, its effect on the clinical outcome of poisoned patients is not known. Aspiration is a common complication (occurring in up to 10 percent of patients), especially when lavage is improperly performed. Serious complications (tracheal lavage, esophageal and gastric perforation) occur in approximately 1 percent of patients. For this reason, only a physician should insert the lavage tube, and the patient must be restrained (with pharmacologic sedation if necessary) during the procedure. Gastric lavage is contraindicated in patients who have ingested corrosives or petroleum distillate hydrocarbons because of the risk of aspiration-induced hydrocarbon pneumonitis and gastroesophageal perforation.

Syrup of ipecac is administered orally in a dose of 30 mL for adults, 15 mL for children, and 10 mL for small infants. Clear liquids also should be given. Ipecac irritates the stomach and stimulates the central chemoreceptor trigger zone. Vomiting usually occurs approximately 22 min after administration. The dose may be repeated if vomiting does not occur. Experimentally, ipecac decreases chemical absorption by an average of 60 percent if given within 5 min of ingestion, 32 percent if given at 30 min, and 30 percent if given at 60 min. Because there are no suitable control groups, its efficacy in overdose patients is not established. Side effects include lethargy in children (12 percent) and protracted vomiting (8 to 17 percent). Chronic ipecac use (by patients with anorexia nervosa or bulimia) may cause electrolyte and fluid abnormalities, cardiac toxicity, and myopathy. Except for aspiration, serious complications are rare. Isolated cases of gastric and esophageal tears and perforations and stroke have been reported. Ipecac is contraindicated in patients with recent gastrointestinal surgery, CNS depression, or seizures, and in those who have ingested corrosives or rapidly acting CNS poisons (camphor, cyanide, tricyclic antidepressants, propoxyphene, strychnine).

Whole-bowel irrigation is performed by administering a bowel-cleansing solution containing electrolytes and polyethylene glycol (Golytely, Colyte) orally or by gastric tube at a rate of up to 0.5 L/h in children and 2.0 L/h in adults until rectal effluent is clear. The patient must be in a sitting position. Although data are limited, whole-bowel irrigation may be as or more effective than the previously discussed procedures and may be particularly useful in patients who have ingested foreign bodies, drug packets, slow-release medications, and agents that are poorly adsorbed by charcoal.

Cathartic salts (disodium phosphate, magnesium citrate and sulfate, sodium sulfate) or *saccharides* (mannitol, sorbitol) promote the rectal evacuation of gastrointestinal contents. The most effective cathartic is sorbitol in a dose of 1 to 2 g/kg of body weight. Alone, cathartics do not prevent poison absorption. Their primary use is to prevent constipation following charcoal administration. Abdominal cramps, nausea, and occasional vomiting are side effects. Complications of repeated dosing include hypermagnesemia and excessive diarrhea. The agents are contraindicated in patients who have ingested corrosives and in those with preexisting diarrhea. Magnesium-containing cathartics should not be used in patients with renal failure.

Dilution is accomplished by having the patient drink 5 mL/kg of body weight of water or another clear liquid as soon as possible after the ingestion of a corrosive (acids, alkali). Dilution also may be used as an adjunct to ipecac syrup administration. Otherwise, it is not indicated because it may increase the dissolution rate (and hence absorption) of capsules, tablets, and other solids.

Endoscopic or surgical removal of poisons may be useful in rare situations, such as ingestion of a potentially toxic foreign body that fails to transit the gastrointestinal tract, a potentially lethal amount of a heavy metal (arsenic, iron, mercury, thallium), or agents that have coalesced into gastric concretions or bezoars (barbiturates, gluthethimide, heavy metals, lithium, meprobamate, sustained-release preparations). Patients who ingest multiple packets of cocaine and then become toxic owing to packet leakage or rupture require immediate surgical intervention.

DECONTAMINATION OF OTHER SITES Immediate, copious flushing with water, saline, or another available clear, drinkable liquid is the initial treatment for topical exposures (particularly with corrosives and solvents). Saline is preferred for eye irrigation. A triple wash (water, then soap, then more water) may be best for dermal decontamination. Inhalational exposures should be treated initially with fresh air or oxygen. The removal of liquids from body cavities such as the vagina or rectum is best accomplished by irrigation. Solids (drug packets, pills) should be removed manually with visual guidance.

Enhancement of Poison Elimination Although the elimination of most poisons can be accelerated by therapeutic interventions, pharmacokinetic efficacy (removal of drug at a rate greater than that accomplished by intrinsic elimination) and the resulting clinical benefits (in terms of a shortened duration of toxicity or improved outcome) are often more theoretical than proven. Hence the decision to use such a procedure should be based on the actual or predicted toxicity and the potential efficacy, cost, and risks of therapy.

MULTIPLE-DOSE ACTIVATED CHARCOAL Repeated oral dosing with charcoal (with sorbitol as needed to enhance gastrointestinal motility) can enhance the elimination of some chemicals. A dose of 1 g/kg body weight every 2 to 4 h, adjusted downward to avoid regurgitation in patients with decreased gastrointestinal motility, is generally recommended. Experimentally, this treatment enhances the elimination of most drugs and chemicals tested (carbamazepine, dapsone, diazepam, digoxin, glutethimide, meprobamate, methotrexate, phenobarbital, phenytoin, salicylate, theophylline, valproic acid). The efficacy approaches that of hemodialysis for some agents (theophylline). Multiple-dose therapy is not effective in accelerating elimination of chlorpropamide, imipramine, or agents that adsorb poorly to charcoal.

FORCED DIURESIS AND ALTERATION OF URINARY pH Diuresis and ion trapping via alteration of urine pH may prevent the renal reabsorption of poisons that undergo excretion by glomerular filtration and active tubular secretion. Since membranes are more permeable to nonionized molecules than to their ionized counterparts, acidic (low-pK_a) poisons are ionized and trapped in an alkaline urine, and basic poisons are ionized and trapped in an acid urine. Saline diuresis can enhance the renal excretion of alcohols, bromide, calcium, fluoride, lithium, meprobamate, potassium, and isoniazid. Alkaline diuresis (a urine pH of 7.5 or greater and a urine output of 3 to 6 mL/kg body weight per hour) enhances the elimination of chlorphenoxyacetic acid herbicides, chlorpropamide, diflunisal, fluoride, methotrexate, phenobarbital (and probably other long-acting barbiturates), sulfonamides, and salicylates. Contraindications include congestive heart failure, renal failure, and cerebral edema. Acid-base, fluid, and electrolyte parameters should be monitored carefully. Saline diuresis may enhance the excretion of bromide, calcium, fluoride, lithium, meprobamate, potassium, and isoniazid. Acid diuresis enhances the renal elimination of amphetamines, chloroquine, cocaine, local anesthetics, phencyclidine, quinidine, quinine, strychnine, sympathomimetics, tricyclic antidepressants, and tocainide. Its use, however, has been largely abandoned because risks are significant and clinical efficacy has not been established.

EXTRACORPOREAL REMOVAL Peritoneal dialysis, hemodialysis, charcoal or resin hemoperfusion, hemofiltration, plasmapheresis, and exchange transfusion are capable of removing any toxin from the bloodstream. The toxins most amenable to enhanced elimination by dialysis have low molecular mass (<500 Da), high water solubility, low protein binding, small volumes of distribution (<1 L/kg body weight), prolonged elimination (long half-life), and high dialysis clearance relative to total-body clearance. The efficacy of the other forms of extracorporeal removal is not limited by molecular weight, water solubility, or protein binding.

Dialysis should be considered in cases of severe poisoning due to barbiturates, bromide, chloral hydrate, ethanol, ethylene glycol, isopropyl alcohol, lithium, methanol, procainamide, theophylline, salicylate, and possibly heavy metals. Although hemoperfusion may be more effective in removing some of these poisons, it does not correct associated acid-base and electrolyte abnormalities. Hemoperfusion should be considered in cases of severe poisoning due to chloramphenicol, disopyramide, and hypnotic-sedatives (barbiturates, ethchlorvynol, glutethimide, meprobamate, methaqualone), phenytoin, procainamide, and theophylline. Both techniques require central venous access and systemic anticoagulation and often result in transient hypotension. Hemoperfusion also may cause hemolysis, hypocalcemia, and thrombocytopenia. Peritoneal dialysis and exchange transfusion are less effective but may be used when other procedures either are not available, are contraindicated, or are technically difficult (e.g., in infants). Exchange transfusion removes poisons affecting red blood cells (as in methemoglobinemia or arsine-induced hemolysis). The efficacy of other extracorporeal elimination procedures has not been defined.

Candidates for these invasive treatments include patients with severe toxicity who deteriorate despite aggressive supportive therapy; those with potentially prolonged, irreversible, or fatal toxicity; those with dangerous blood levels of toxins; those who lack the capacity for self-detoxification because of liver or renal failure; and those with a serious underlying illness or complication that will adversely affect recovery.

OTHER TECHNIQUES The elimination of heavy metals can be enhanced by chelation and urinary excretion of the metal-chelator complex, and the elimination of carbon monoxide can be increased by hyperbaric oxygenation, as discussed in the sections on the specific poisons.

Administration of Antidotes Antidotes counteract the effects of poisons by neutralizing them (e.g., antibody-antigen reactions, chelation, chemical binding) or by antagonizing their physiologic effects (e.g., activation of opposing nervous system activity, provision of competitive metabolic or receptor substrate). Antidotes can significantly reduce morbidity and mortality, but most antidotes are potentially toxic. Poisons or conditions with specific antidotes include acetaminophen, anticholinergic agents, anticoagulants, benzodiazepines, beta blockers, calcium channel blockers, carbon monoxide, cholinergic agents, cyanide, digitalis, drugs that cause dystonic reactions, ethylene glycol, fluoride, heavy metals, hydrogen sulfide, hypoglycemic agents, isoniazid, methemoglobinemia, narcotics, sympatomimetics, and Vacor. Since the safe use of antidotes requires correct identification of a specific poisoning or syndrome, antidotal therapy is discussed with the conditions for which they are indicated.

Prevention of Reexposure Poisoning is a preventable illness. Unfortunately, some adults and children are poison-prone, and recurrences are common. Adults with accidental exposures should be instructed regarding the safe use of medications and chemicals (according to labeling instructions). Confused patients may need assistance with the administration of medications. Errors in dosing by health care providers require special educational efforts. Patients should be advised to avoid circumstances that result in chemical exposure or poisoning. Appropriate agencies and health departments should be notified in cases of environmental or workplace exposure. The best approach with young children and patients with intentional overdose is to limit access to poisons. In households where children live or visit, alcoholic beverages, medications, household products (automotive, cleaning, fuel, pet-care, toiletry products), nonedible plants, and vitamins should be kept out of reach or in locked or

child-proof cabinets. Depressed or psychotic patients should receive psychiatric assessment, disposition, and follow-up. They should be given prescriptions for a limited supply of drugs and with a limited number of refills and be monitored for compliance and response to therapy.

SPECIFIC POISONS

The poisons discussed in this section are common, produce life-threatening toxicity, or require unique therapeutic interventions. Poisons not mentioned here are described in the referenced texts. → *Alcohol, cocaine, hallucinogens, and opioids are discussed in Chaps. 386 to 388, and heavy metal poisoning is discussed in Chap. 397.*

ACETAMINOPHEN At therapeutic doses, acetaminophen is metabolized to sulfate and glucuronide conjugates that are excreted in the urine. Minor amounts are excreted unchanged or as mercapturic acid after conjugation with hepatic glutathione. Following an acute overdose of ≥140 mg/kg body weight, the sulfate and glucuronide pathways become saturated, resulting in an increased fraction of acetaminophen metabolized to mercapturic acid. Once hepatic glutathione is depleted, reactive metabolites are formed that bind covalently to hepatocytes and cause cell lysis. Acetaminophen is absorbed rapidly from the stomach and small bowel and has a volume of distribution of 1 L/kg body weight. Plasma concentrations range from 160 to 660 μmol/L (0.5 to 2.0 mg/dL) following therapeutic doses. The plasma half-life is usually 2 to 4 h but may be prolonged if hepatotoxicity develops.

Clinical Toxicity Early manifestations of poisoning are nonspecific and not predictive of subsequent hepatotoxicity. Within 2 to 4 h of ingestion, nausea, vomiting, diaphoresis, and pallor develop. CNS depression is absent unless depressant drugs are coingested. Within 24 to 48 h, hepatotoxicity is evidenced by right upper quadrant tenderness and mild hepatomegaly. Renal function also may be impaired. Laboratory evidence of hepatic toxicity includes prolongation of the prothrombin time and elevation of serum bilirubin and transaminase activity (aspartate transaminase, alanine transaminase). Severe poisoning may cause hepatic failure. A twofold prolongation of prothrombin time and/or a serum bilirubin level greater than 68 μmol/L (4 mg/dL) on the third to fifth day after ingestion indicate hepatotoxicity. Histologic evidence of liver damage varies from cytolysis to centrilobular necrosis. In patients who recover, liver function returns to normal within 1 week, and liver histology returns to normal within 3 months.

Diagnosis A serum acetaminophen level above the lower line on the Rumack Matthew nomogram (Fig. 391-2) between 4 and 24 h after ingestion indicates possible hepatotoxicity and the need for antidote therapy.

℞ **TREATMENT**

In patients who present within 4 h of ingestion, initial treatment involves gastrointestinal decontamination. Activated charcoal should be administered. (Charcoal does not interfere significantly with acetylcysteine therapy.) In patients with a potentially toxic acetaminophen level, acetylcysteine is given at a loading dose of 140 mg/kg body weight, followed by a maintenance dose of 70 mg/kg body weight every 4 h for 17 additional doses. Treatment is most effective if started within 8 to 10 h of an overdose. Side effects include nausea, vomiting, and epigastric discomfort. If treatment is started before the serum level is known and if the level is subsequently shown to be below the toxic level, therapy may be discontinued.

ACIDS AND ALKALI Common alkaline products include industrial-strength bleach, drain cleaners (sodium hydroxide), surface cleaners (ammonia, phosphates), laundry and dishwasher detergents (phosphates, carbonates), disk batteries, denture cleaners (borates, phosphates, carbonates), and Clinitest tablets (sodium hydroxides). Acids are used in toilet bowl cleaners (hydrofluoric, phosphoric, and

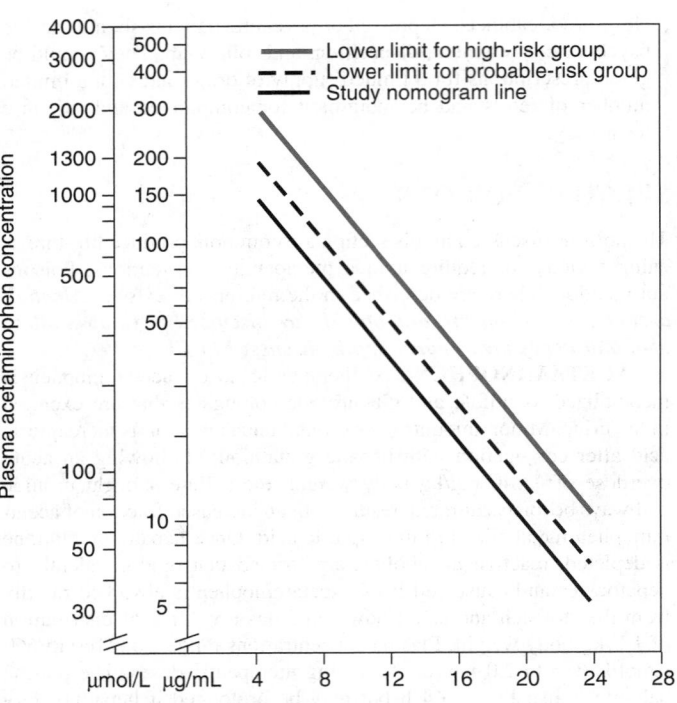

FIGURE 391-2 Nomogram to define risk according to initial plasma aceta-minophen concentration. (*After BH Rumack, H Matthew, Pediatrics 55:871, 1975.*)

sulfuric acids), soldering fluxes (hydrochloric acid), antirust compounds (hydrofluoric and oxalic acids), automobile battery fluid (sulfuric acid), and stone cleaners (hydrofluoric and nitric acids).

Alkalis produce liquefactive necrosis with rapidly penetrating tissue burns and a higher risk of perforation of the esophagus and stomach than do acids. Acids produce coagulative necrosis. Both may burn the mouth, esophagus, and stomach. The lack of oral involvement does not rule out esophageal or gastric injury. Liquids tend to produce superficial, often circumferential burns over a larger surface area, while solids and tablets cause localized but deeper burns. The severity of the burn relates to the contact time, the amount ingested, and the pH (especially if <2 or >12) of the ingested product. Corrosives other than acids and bases that cause similar toxicity include household bleach (sodium hypochlorite), hydrogen peroxide, hydrazine, and phenol.

Clinical Toxicity Burns of the mouth result in excess salivation, pain, dysphonia, and dysphagia and are manifested by erythema, edema, ulceration, and necrosis. Deep burns may destroy mucosal nerve endings and produce anesthesia. Esophageal symptoms and signs include drooling, painful swallowing, retrosternal pain, and neck tenderness. Vomiting of blood and mucus may occur. Esophageal perforation following alkali ingestion is suggested by increased severity of chest pain, often with respiratory distress. Epigastric pain, vomiting, and tenderness may occur with burns to the stomach. Aspiration of acids and alkalis may cause fulminant tracheitis and bronchial pneumonia. In severe cases, hypotension, shock, metabolic acidosis, liver and renal dysfunction, hemolysis, and disseminated intravascular coagulation may be seen. Deep burns, particularly if extensive or circumferential, may be followed by fibrosis with stricture formation and obstruction of the esophagus (alkalis) or of the gastric outlet (acids).

Diagnosis Symptoms, history, and physical findings usually suggest the diagnosis. Endoscopy, best performed 12 to 24 h after ingestion in all symptomatic patients, documents the anatomic site and often the severity of the injury. Chest and abdominal x-rays and routine laboratory values should be obtained to evaluate for aspiration, perforation, and organ dysfunction. Residual effects of the ingestion can be assessed by barium swallow.

℞ **TREATMENT**

Treatment consists of immediate dilution with milk or water. Weak acid or basic solutions should not be used because the heat of neutralization may cause thermal burns and increase tissue injury. Glucocorticoids and Silastic esophageal stents have traditionally been used for alkali burns to prevent esophageal stricture formation. Their efficacy is not proven. Animal studies suggest that glucocorticoids should be begun immediately on presentation. If used, a dose of 1 to 2 mg of prednisone per kilogram every 4 to 6 h for at least 2 weeks is suggested. Prophylactic broad-spectrum antibiotic use is also recommended. Glucocorticoids are not useful for acid burns. Antacids should be used for burns of the stomach. Esophageal stricture or gastric outlet obstruction may require subsequent dilatation and bouginage or surgical reconstruction.

ANTIARRHYTHMIC DRUGS Only drugs that act by blocking myocardial cell-membrane sodium channels are discussed here. These agents can be divided into three subclasses: class IA (disopyramide, procainamide, and quinidine), class IB (lidocaine, mexiletine, phenytoin, and tocainide), and class IC (encainide, moricizine, propafenone, and flecainide). The pharmacology is presented in Chap. 231. Because of toxicity, some agents have been withdrawn from the market but are still available for compassionate use. Antiarrhythmic drugs are rapidly absorbed (except for disopyramide and sustained-release formulations), have volumes of distribution ranging from 1 to 10 L/kg, have half-lives of 3 to 16 h, and are eliminated mainly by hepatic metabolism.

Clinical Toxicity The acute ingestion of more than twice the usual daily dose is potentially toxic. Onset of toxicity occurs within 1 h, and the effects peak within several hours. Toxicity also may develop during chronic therapeutic use. Manifestations include nausea, vomiting, and diarrhea, followed by lethargy, confusion, ataxia, bradycardia, hypotension, and cardiovascular collapse. Anticholinergic effects (blurred vision, dry mucosae) may be seen in disopyramide poisoning. Quinidine and class IB agents may cause agitation, dysphoria, and seizures. Nonspecific ECG findings include bradycardia with AV block and QRS-interval prolongation. Ventricular tachycardia, ventricular fibrillation (including the polymorphous form, torsade de pointes), and QT-interval prolongation are characteristics of poisoning due to class IA and IC drugs. Depressed myocardial contractility and arrhythmias may lead to decreased cardiac output and pulmonary edema. Hypoglycemia and mild hypokalemia may be seen with disopyramide and quinidine intoxication, respectively.

Diagnosis Toxicology screening will detect most of these agents. Measurement of serum levels may confirm an overdose and indicate the need for monitoring.

℞ **TREATMENT**

Treatment consists of gastrointestinal decontamination and supportive therapy. Hypotension, bradyarrhythmias, and seizures are treated with standard measures. Patients with persistent hypotension and bradycardia require monitoring of pulmonary arterial pressure. Cardiac pacing, intraaortic balloon pump counterpulsation, and cardiopulmonary bypass may be necessary. Ventricular tachyarrhythmias that cause hemodynamic instability should be treated with lidocaine and bretylium. Sodium bicarbonate or sodium lactate (1 mmol/kg by intravenous bolus) may be effective for tachyarrhythmias due to class IA or IC agents. Mild hypokalemia may be protective, and potassium levels that do not fall below 3.0 mmol/L may be best treated by close monitoring. For torsade de pointes (polymorphous or atypical ventricular tachycardia), magnesium sulfate (4 g or 40 mL of a 10% solution given intravenously as an initial dose) and overdrive pacing (with isoproterenol or electricity) may be effective. Hemodialysis and hemoperfusion may enhance the elimination of disopyramide, the active procainamide metabolite *N*-acetylprocainamide, and possibly other agents.

ANTICHOLINERGIC AGENTS   Agents with anticholinergic properties include antihistamines (H₁ receptor blockers and over-the-counter hypnotics), belladonna alkaloids and related agents (atropine, glycopyrrolate, homatropine, hyoscine, ipratropium, scopolamine), drugs for Parkinson's disease (benztropine, biperiden, trihexyphenidyl), mydriatics (cyclopentolate, tropicamide), phenothiazines, skeletal muscle relaxants (cyclobenzaprine, orphenadrine), smooth muscle relaxants (clidinium, dicyclomine, isometheptene, oxybutynin), tricyclic antidepressants, and a variety of plants (such as *Datura stramonium* and jimson weed) and mushrooms. More properly called *antimuscarinics*, these agents are competitive inhibitors of acetylcholine only at CNS and parasympathetic postganglionic muscarinic neuroreceptors. They are absorbed efficiently, but absorption can be delayed following an overdose. The antihistamines, belladonna agents, Parkinson's drugs, and smooth muscle relaxants are weak bases (pK_a 8–9), exhibit variable binding to plasma proteins (18 to 98 percent), and have moderate volumes of distribution (2 to 6 L/kg). They are eliminated primarily by hepatic metabolism and have half-lives of 2 to 12 h.

Clinical Toxicity   Manifestations usually begin within an hour of acute overdosage and 1 to 3 days after beginning treatment in the case of chronic poisoning. Toxic doses are only slightly greater than therapeutic doses. CNS manifestation include agitation, ataxia, confusion, delirium, hallucinations, and movement disorders (choreoathetoid and picking movements). Lethargy, respiratory depression, and coma may occur. Peripheral nervous system findings include decreased or absent bowel sounds, dilated pupils, dry skin and mucosal surfaces, urinary retention, and increases in pulse rate, blood pressure, respiratory rate, and temperature. The first-generation H₁ blockers (diphenhydramine and probably others) can also cause tricyclic antidepressant–like cardiotoxicity and seizures, and the second-generation H₁ blockers (astemizole, terfenadine) can cause QT-interval prolongation with subsequent ventricular tachyarrhythmias, especially torsade de pointes.

Diagnosis   The diagnosis is suggested by the characteristic manifestations and supported by demonstrating the presence of the agents in the urine. Serum assays are not generally available. The diagnosis can be confirmed by demonstrating resolution of anticholinergic toxicity in response to physostigmine.

℞ **TREATMENT**

Treatment involves gastrointestinal decontamination, supportive measures, and, in severe cases, therapy with physostigmine. Activated charcoal adsorbs these agents effectively. Agitation may respond to benzodiazepines, and comatose patients may require intubation and mechanical ventilation. Cardiovascular toxicity and arrhythmias should be treated as described for antiarrhythmics, phenothiazines, or tricyclic antidepressants. Physostigmine, an acetylcholinesterase inhibitor, reverses anticholinergic toxicity. It is indicated primarily for uncontrolled agitation and hallucinations. The dose is 1 to 2 mg given intravenously over 2 min; the dose can be repeated if there is an incomplete response or recurrent toxicity. If signs of cholinergic poisoning occur (see "Organophosphate and Carbamate Insecticides," below), they can be reversed by atropine in half the amount of physostigmine given. Physostigmine should not be given for seizures or for coma; its arousal effects are nonspecific and cannot be used for diagnostic purposes. Physostigmine is contraindicated in the presence of cardiac conduction defects or ventricular arrhythmias because it can cause asystole in such patients.

BARBITURATES   Barbiturates bind to the GABA receptor and prolong the opening of the chloride channels in response to GABA, thereby inhibiting excitable cells of the CNS and other tissues. Long-acting barbiturates are effective for 6 to 12 h and include mephobarbital, barbital, phenobarbital, and primidone. Agents with intermediate (3 to 6 h), short (1 to 3 h), and ultrashort (<30 min) durations of action include amobarbital, aprobarbital, butabarbital, butalbital; hexobarbital, pentobarbital, and secobarbital; and methohexital, thiamylal, and thiopental, respectively.

Barbiturates are well absorbed from the stomach and the small bowel. With therapeutic doses, plasma concentrations generally peak in 1 to 4 h (earlier for short-acting agents than for long-acting ones). Barbiturates are weak acids with pK_a values ranging from 7.2 to 8.5, volumes of distribution of 0.8 to 1.5 L/kg of body weight, and 45 to 70 percent protein binding in the plasma. Most barbiturates are primarily metabolized by the liver. Some long-acting agents are converted to active metabolites: mephobarbital to barbital, and primidone to phenobarbital and phenylethylmalonamide (PEMA). In contrast to short-acting agents, long-acting ones also undergo significant renal excretion: 95 percent for barbital, 25 to 33 percent for phenobarbital, 15 to 42 percent for primidone, and 95 percent for PEMA. Half-lives range from 1 h for ultrashort-acting agents to 6 d for long-acting ones.

Clinical Toxicity   Barbiturates cause CNS depression ranging from confusion and lethargy to deep coma. Hypothermia, hypotension, pulmonary edema, and cardiac arrest may occur in severe cases. Pupils are generally constricted but may dilate in terminal phases. Pressure sores and bullous skin lesions can develop with prolonged coma. Maximal toxicity usually occurs within 4 to 6 h but may be delayed to 10 h or more after overdosage with long-acting barbiturates.

Diagnosis   Signs of toxicity usually appear when serum concentrations of long-acting barbiturates exceed 170 μmol/L (4 mg/dL) and those of short-acting barbiturates exceed 88 μmol/L (2 mg/dL). Because of tolerance, the degree of CNS depression relative to ingested dose is dependent on prior exposure to the drug.

℞ **TREATMENT**

Initial management involves gastrointestinal decontamination. Barbiturates are well adsorbed by activated charcoal. Hemodynamic and respiratory support and correction of temperature and electrolyte derangements may be necessary. Since short-acting barbiturates are predominantly metabolized by the liver, diuresis is ineffective. Renal elimination of phenobarbital (and probably other long-acting agents) is enhanced by alkalinization of urine to a pH of 8 (by giving intravenous sodium bicarbonate) and by saline diuresis. Elimination can also be enhanced by repeated doses of activated charcoal. Hemodialysis and hemoperfusion are effective in removing both long- and short-acting barbiturates, but their use is seldom necessary.

BENZODIAZEPINES   Benzodiazepines potentiate the inhibitory effect of GABA on CNS neurons by binding to GABA receptors and increasing the frequency of opening of chloride channels in response to GABA stimulation.

Long-acting benzodiazepines include chlordiazepoxide, clonazepam, clorazepate, diazepam, flurazepam, prazepam, and quazepam. Short-acting agents include alprazolam, lorazepam, and oxazepam; ultrashort-acting agents include estazolam, midazolam, temazepam, and triazolam. All benzodiazepines are well absorbed from the gastrointestinal tract, exhibit 85 to 99 percent protein binding in the plasma, are lipid soluble, and have an apparent volume of distribution of 0.3 to 2 L/kg body weight. They are weak acids with pK_a values ranging from 1.3 to 6.2. Benzodiazepines are eliminated mainly by hepatic metabolism, and some have pharmacologically active metabolites. Metabolites are generally excreted in the urine, whereas only a small amount of the parent compound is excreted unchanged by the kidneys. Half-lives range from as little as 2 h for short-acting agents to up to 8 days for long-acting ones.

Clinical Toxicity   Effects are evident within 30 min of an overdose and include weakness, ataxia, and drowsiness. Coma and respiratory depression are rare but can occur with ultrashort-acting agents and when benzodiazepines are combined with other CNS depressants. Paradoxical excitation may occur early in the course of poisoning.

Diagnosis   The diagnosis can sometimes be confirmed by identification of metabolites in urine. However, routine screening tests do not detect many benzodiazepines so that a negative result does not exclude the diagnosis. A response to flumazenil is a more sensitive diagnostic test.

℞ TREATMENT

Initial management includes gastrointestinal decontamination with single-dose as well as repeated-dose activated charcoal. Respiratory support should be provided as necessary. Flumazenil, a competitive benzodiazepine receptor antagonist, can reverse CNS and respiratory depression and obviate the need for endotracheal intubation. It is administered intravenously in incremental doses of 0.2, 0.3, and 0.5 mg at 1-min intervals until the desired effect is achieved or a cumulative dose of 3 to 5 mg has been given. Since flumazenil has a relatively short duration of action, patients must be monitored carefully for relapse. Should relapse occur, treatment can be repeated (at intervals of 20 min with a maximum dose of 3 mg/h). Failure to respond to flumazenil suggests that benzodiazepines are not the cause of poisoning. Flumazenil can cause seizures in patients who have coingested stimulants and tricyclic antidepressants and in patients who are physically dependent on benzodiazepines as a result of chronic high-dose use. A starting dose of 0.1 mg should be used in patients at risk for withdrawal. Extracorporeal drug removal is not of clinical benefit.

BETA-ADRENERGIC BLOCKING AGENTS Beta-adrenergic blocking agents include acebutolol, atenolol, betaxolol, bisoprolol, carteolol, esmolol, labetalol, metoprolol, nadolol, penbutolol, pindolol, propranolol, sotalol, and timolol. These drugs act by competitively blocking beta-adrenergic neurohumoral receptors. At therapeutic doses, some beta blockers act predominantly on $beta_1$ receptors and are "cardioselective" (acebutolol, atenolol, betaxolol, metoprolol), some have partial agonist or sympathomimetic activity (acebutolol, carteolol, pindolol, timolol, and possibly penbutolol), and some have quinidine-like antiarrhythmic effects (acebutolol, metoprolol, pindolol, propranolol, sotalol, and possibly betaxolol). Antiarrhythmic effects are due to a reduction of sodium and calcium influx during membrane depolarization (phase 0) as a consequence of decreased production of cyclic AMP by adenylate cyclase. This activity defines beta blockers as class II antiarrhythmics. Beta blockers decrease cardiac contractility by directly inhibiting the release of calcium from sarcoplasmic reticulum.

Beta blockers are absorbed rapidly and well, exhibit variable protein binding (5 to 93 percent), and have low water solubility and variable volumes of distribution (0.23 to 10.0 L/kg body weight). Most beta blockers are eliminated predominantly by hepatic metabolism. Atenolol, carteolol, nadolol, and sotalol are eliminated primarily by renal excretion, and esmolol is metabolized by serum esterases.

Clinical Toxicity Effects usually begin within 1/2 h following an overdose and peak within 2 h. Common findings include nausea, vomiting, and diarrhea, followed by bradycardia, hypotension, and CNS depression. However, agents with sympathomimetic activity can cause hypertension and tachycardia. CNS effects vary from lethargy and confusion to coma and seizures and tend to be more pronounced with highly lipophilic agents (acebutolol, metoprolol, pindolol, propranolol, and timolol). The skin is often pale and cool. Bronchospasm and pulmonary edema are uncommon unless there is a history of asthma, chronic obstructive pulmonary disease, or congestive heart failure. Metabolic abnormalities include hyperkalemia and hypoglycemia (as a direct result of beta-adrenergic receptor blockade) and metabolic acidosis (due to seizures, shock, or respiratory depression). ECG manifestations include all degrees of AV block, bundle branch block, prolonged QRS duration, and asystole. Sotalol may cause QT-interval prolongation with ventricular tachycardia, ventricular fibrillation, and torsade de pointes. Patients with mild poisoning usually recover within 6 to 12 h, whereas those with severe poisoning may be symptomatic for 24 to 48 h.

Diagnosis The diagnosis is made on the basis of the history and clinical presentation. A toxicology screen may identify the presence of beta blockers, but blood levels are not generally available nor helpful in guiding therapy.

℞ TREATMENT

Treatment includes gastrointestinal decontamination, nonspecific supportive measures, and the administration of glucagon and calcium. Because gastric emptying procedures may produce vagal stimulation and exacerbate bradyarrhythmias, monitoring should be instituted first. Treatment of bradycardia and hypotension should begin with atropine, isoproterenol, and vasopressors (dopamine, dobutamine, epinephrine, and norepinephrine have been used with variable success, alone or in combination). With severe poisoning, these agents may be ineffective, and glucagon, calcium, cardiac pacing (external or internal), and intraaortic balloon pump support may be necessary. Glucagon, which stimulates adenylate cyclase by a nonadrenergic mechanism, should be given at an initial dose of 5 to 10 mg. Patients who respond favorably should then be given an infusion of 1 to 5 mg/h. Calcium, which may reverse nonadrenergic negative inotropic effects, should be given in the same initial dose as described for calcium channel blocker poisoning. Patients with altered mental status also should have a bedside glucose determination or be given an intravenous bolus of glucose. Bronchospasm may be treated with an inhaled beta agonist, subcutaneous epinephrine, and intravenous aminophylline. Lidocaine, magnesium (as for antiarrhythmic poisoning), or overdrive pacing may be used for sotalol-induced ventricular tachyarrhythmias. Extracorporeal elimination procedures are probably not of benefit, with the possible exceptions of atenolol, carteolol, metoprolol, nadolol, and sotalol.

CALCIUM CHANNEL BLOCKERS Calcium channel blockers include amlodipine, bepridil, diltiazem, felodipine, flunarizine, isradipine, lacidipine, nicardipine, nifedipine, nimodipine, nisoldipine, nitrendipine, and verapamil. These agents act by decreasing the influx of calcium across slow calcium channels in the membranes of myocardial and vascular smooth-muscle cells during phases 2 (plateau) and 4 (spontaneous depolarization) of the action potential. Electrophysiologic effects include decreases in cardiac contractility, heart rate [sinoatrial (SA) node rate], and AV nodal conduction. These actions define calcium channel blockers as class IV antiarrhythmics. At therapeutic doses, diltiazem and verapamil have significant effects on cardiac conduction and contractility. Bepridil also has class I antiarrhythmic activity. All calcium channel blockers cause vasodilation.

Calcium channel blockers are absorbed rapidly and exhibit high (80 to 99 percent) protein binding in the plasma. Most have distribution volumes ranging from 1 to 8 L/kg body weight. They are eliminated mainly by hepatic metabolism, and the half-lives typically range from 1 to 24 h.

Clinical Toxicity Effects begin within 1/2 to 1 h of ingestion of amounts 5 to 10 times the usual therapeutic dose. Toxicity may be delayed for many hours following overdoses of sustained-release preparations. Clinical manifestations include bradycardia, hypotension, and CNS depression. Invasive monitoring almost invariably reveals a low peripheral vascular resistance and normal or increased cardiac output. Mental status changes range from confusion and drowsiness to coma and seizures and are due both to direct membrane effects and to cerebral hypoperfusion. Hypotension may precipitate myocardial ischemia, and depression of cardiac function may lead to pulmonary edema. ECG findings include all degrees of AV block, prolonged QRS and QT intervals (mainly with verapamil), evidence of ischemia or infarction, and asystole. Metabolic acidosis (secondary to shock) and hyperglycemia (resulting from the inhibition of insulin release) may be present. Serum calcium levels, however, remain normal.

Diagnosis The diagnosis is based primarily on the clinical presentation. These agents can be detected by appropriate screening tests. Serum levels are not generally available but can be useful in confirming overdosage when the history is inconclusive.

℞ TREATMENT

Gastrointestinal tract decontamination should be accomplished as soon as possible. Symptomatic bradycardia should be treated with atropine, calcium, isoproterenol, glucagon, and electrical (external or internal) pacing. Calcium, as a 10% chloride or gluconate salt solution, is given in a dose of 0.2 mL/kg body weight (up to 10 mL) intravenously over 5 min. This dose may be repeated up to four times in patients with a partial, transient, or absent response, provided that serum calcium levels are monitored. A continuous calcium infusion (0.2 mL/kg body weight per hour up to a maximum of 10 mL/h) may be appropriate when relapse occurs after an initial bolus. Although electrical pacing is often required, glucagon, in the same dose as for beta-blocker poisoning, should be tried first. Hypotension that persists despite resolution of bradycardia should be treated with fluids and vasopressors. Amrinone, dopamine, dobutamine, glucagon, and norepinephrine, alone or in combination, have been used. Restoring perfusion is particularly important in patients with organ ischemia. Intraaortic balloon pump support should be used in patients unresponsive to the preceding measures. Patients with mild toxicity usually recover within a few hours, whereas those with severe toxicity or overdose with sustained-release preparations may remain symptomatic for 24 h or longer. Extracorporeal removal techniques are unlikely to be of benefit.

CARBON MONOXIDE Carbon monoxide is produced in large amounts in industrial processes as well as by gasoline engines, home appliances, and the incomplete combustion of wood, natural gas, and tobacco products. In addition, methylene chloride, a solvent in paint removers, is metabolized to carbon monoxide.

Carbon monoxide is absorbed rapidly through the lungs and binds to hemoglobin (forming carboxyhemoglobin) with an affinity 210 times that of oxygen. This binding reduces oxygen transportation by hemoglobin and also decreases the release of oxygen to tissues (the oxygen dissociation curve shifts to the left). Carbon monoxide also binds to myoglobin, decreasing its oxygen-carrying capacity, and to mitochondrial cytochrome oxidase, inhibiting cellular respiration. The net effect is profound tissue hypoxia, anaerobic metabolism, and lactic acidosis. Once carbon monoxide exposure is discontinued, dissociation of the hemoglobin–carbon monoxide complex occurs, and carbon monoxide is excreted through the lungs. In room air, the carboxyhemoglobin half-life is 4 to 6 h; the half-life decreases to 40 to 80 min when breathing 100% oxygen and to 15 to 30 min with hyperbaric oxygen therapy. The apparent half-life after methylene chloride exposure is considerably longer.

Clinical Toxicity Manifestations of carbon monoxide poisoning include shortness of breath, dyspnea, tachypnea, headache, emotional lability, confusion, impaired judgment, clumsiness, and syncope. Nausea, vomiting, and diarrhea also may occur. Cerebral edema, coma, respiratory depression, and pulmonary edema occur with severe poisoning. Cardiovascular manifestations include ischemic chest pain, arrhythmias, heart failure, and hypotension. In comatose patients, blisters and bullae may develop over pressure points. Myoglobinuria secondary to muscle necrosis may result in renal failure. A cherry red color of skin and mucous membranes is rare, and cyanosis is usual. Visual field defects, blindness, and venous engorgement with papilledema or optic atrophy may be noted. Measurement of arterial blood gases reveal metabolic acidosis, a normal P_{O_2}, decreased oxygen saturation (by co-oximetry but not when calculated or measured by pulse oximetry), and a variable P_{CO_2}.

After brief exposure, carboxyhemoglobin fractions of 15 to 20 percent are associated with mild symptoms, of 20 to 40 percent with moderate symptoms, and of 40 to 50 percent with severe symptoms. Fractions above 60 percent are often fatal. With prolonged exposure, toxicity occurs at lower percentages. Serum creatine phosphokinase (CK) and lactate dehydrogenase (LHD) levels may be elevated.

Patients with loss of consciousness are at risk for developing neuropsychiatric sequelae 1 to 3 weeks after exposure. Manifestations vary from subtle personality changes and intellectual impairment to gross neurologic deficits such as blindness, deafness, incoordination, and parkinsonism.

Diagnosis The diagnosis is confirmed by determining the carboxyhemoglobin fraction. If this cannot be measured, the difference between the oxygen saturation calculated from the P_{O_2} and that measured by co-oximetry can be used to estimate the carboxyhemoglobin fraction.

℞ TREATMENT

The patient should be removed from the site of exposure. In conscious patients, oxygen should be administered by a non-rebreather mask at 10 L/min until carbon monoxide levels are less than 10 percent and all symptoms have resolved. Infants and pregnant women require treatment for several more hours, because fetal hemoglobin has a high affinity for carbon monoxide. Endotracheal intubation and mechanical ventilation with 100% oxygen are indicated in patients with coma, significant CNS dysfunction, or cardiovascular instability. Arrhythmias and hypotension are treated by usual measures. Patients with coma, syncope, or seizures and those with less severe signs or symptoms of neurologic or cardiovascular dysfunction that do not resolve with oxygen and supportive therapy are candidates for hyperbaric oxygen therapy. Hyperbaric oxygenation shortens the duration of toxicity and may prevent delayed sequelae.

CYANIDE Hydrogen cyanide is used as a fumigant rodenticide and in chemical syntheses. Cyanide salts are used in photography, metallurgy, electroplating, metal cleaning, and ore refining. Organic cyanide compounds (nitriles) are used in the synthetic rubber industry, artificial nail removers, and rodenticides. Cyanogenic glycosides are present in the seeds of the chokeberry, cherry, plum, peach, apricot, pear, bean, apple, and crabapple.

Cyanide inhibits mitochondrial cytochrome oxidase and hence blocks electron transport, resulting in decreased oxidative metabolism and oxygen utilization. Lactic acidosis occurs as a consequence of anaerobic metabolism. Cyanide is rapidly absorbed from the stomach, lungs, mucosal surfaces, and unbroken skin. In the stomach it reacts with hydrochloric acid, liberating hydrocyanic acid, which is absorbed as cyanide ion. Cyanide is 60 percent protein-bound, is concentrated in red cells, and has a volume of distribution of 1.5 L/kg body weight. Cyanide is metabolized by the mitochondrial enzyme rhodanase, which mediates the transfer of sulfur from thiosulfate to the cyanide ion, producing thiocyanate, which in turn is excreted in the urine.

Clinical Toxicity The potentially lethal dose of potassium or sodium cyanide is 200 to 300 mg and of hydrocyanic acid is 50 mg. Effects begin within seconds of inhalation and within 30 min of ingestion. Initial manifestations of cyanide poisoning include headache, faintness, vertigo, excitement, anxiety, a burning sensation in the mouth and throat, dyspnea, tachycardia, and hypertension. Nausea, vomiting, and diaphoresis are common. A bitter almond odor may be detected on the breath. Later effects include coma, convulsions, opisthotonus, trismus, paralysis, respiratory depression, pulmonary edema, arrhythmias, bradycardia, and hypotension. A rough correlation exists between blood cyanide levels and symptoms: Levels less than 8 μmol/L (0.02 mg/L) are associated with no symptoms; 20 to 40 μmol/L (0.05 to 0.1 mg/dL) with flushing and tachycardia; 40 to 100 μmol/L (0.1 to 0.25 mg/dL) with obtundation; 100 to 200 μmol/L (0.25 to 0.3 mg/dL) with coma and respiratory depression; and levels greater than 120 μmol/L (0.3 mg/dL) with death. With significant poisoning, lactic acidosis and narrowing of the arteriovenous oxygen saturation difference may be present. ECG abnormalities include both tachyarrhythmias and bradyarrhythmias, such as nodal or idioventricular rhythm, AV dissociation, and progressive slowing of heart rate.

Diagnosis Although measurement of the whole-blood cyanide level will confirm the diagnosis, cyanide assays are not routinely available. The diagnosis and treatment decisions must therefore be based on clinical findings.

℞ TREATMENT

Initial management involves general supportive measures and gastrointestinal decontamination. Antidotal therapy using amyl nitrite, sodium nitrite, and sodium thiosulfate (the Lilly cyanide antidote kit) coupled with high-dose oxygen should be administered as soon as possible to patients with altered mental status, abnormal vital signs, or metabolic acidosis. The rationale for antidotal therapy is as follows. Nitrites induce methemoglobinemia. Methemoglobin has a higher affinity for cyanide than does cytochrome oxidase and thus promotes its dissociation from this enzyme. Thiosulfate reacts with the cyanide as the latter is slowly released from cyanomethemoglobin, forming the relatively nontoxic thiocyanate, which is excreted in the urine. Oxygen reverses the binding of cyanide to cytochrome oxidase sites and enhances the efficacy of sodium nitrite and sodium thiosulfate, in addition to acting as a substrate for metabolism.

Amyl nitrite is administered for 30 s of each minute. The ampule is broken between two pads of gauze and placed over the airway while the patient breathes spontaneously or is ventilated by a bag-mask unit. A new ampule should be used every 3 min. This process is continued while sodium nitrite is being prepared, but it may be omitted if endotracheal intubation has been performed. Sodium nitrite is administered intravenously as a 3% solution at a rate of 2.5 to 5.0 mL/min up to a total dose of 10 to 15 mL (300 to 450 mg). Sodium thiosulfate is then administered intravenously as a 25% solution at a dose of 50 mL (12.5 g) given over 1 to 2 min. With recurrent or persistent symptoms, half or full doses of both sodium nitrite and sodium thiosulfate are administered. Hyperbaric oxygen therapy should be considered in patients who fail to respond to antidotal therapy.

DIGOXIN Poisoning with digitalis (cardiac glycoside) occurs most often during therapeutic or suicidal use of digoxin and on occasion with plant (oleander) ingestion. Cardiac glycosides act by inhibiting the enzyme sodium-potassium ATPase, leading to increased intracellular levels of Na^+ and Ca^{2+} and decreased intracellular K^+ levels. Digoxin is slowly absorbed and slowly distributed. Serum levels may not correlate with pharmacologic effects for up to 8 h following a therapeutic oral dose. Digoxin is 25 to 30 percent protein-bound in the plasma, has a large volume of distribution of 5 to 6 L/kg body weight, and is localized in skeletal muscle, liver, and heart. Elimination is primarily by renal excretion. The half-life ranges between 36 and 45 h, is prolonged in hepatic failure and in renal failure, and may be shortened in overdose. Approximately 60 percent of a dose is excreted unchanged by the kidneys, and the remainder is metabolized by the liver to inactive metabolites. Therapeutic serum concentrations range from 0.6 to 2.5 nmol/L (0.5 to 2.0 ng/mL).

Clinical Toxicity Symptoms of toxicity include vomiting, confusion, delirium, and occasionally hallucinations, blurred vision, photophobia, scotomata, and disturbed color perception. Cardiac manifestations include sinus arrhythmia, sinus bradycardia, and all degrees of atrioventricular block. Premature ventricular contractions, bigeminy, ventricular tachycardia, and fibrillation also occur. The combination of supraventricular tachyarrhythmia and AV block is highly suggestive of digitalis toxicity. While bradyarrhythmias and hypokalemia are common with chronic intoxication, tachyarrhythmias and hyperkalemia are generally seen with acute poisoning. Similarly, serum digoxin levels may be minimally elevated or even therapeutic in chronic toxicity, whereas they are usually markedly elevated following acute overdose. Clinical toxicity occurs with digoxin levels in excess of 3.8 to 6.4 nmol/L (3 to 5 ng/mL), and levels as high as 64 to 77 nmol/L (50 to 60 ng/mL) have been seen following acute overdose.

Diagnosis The diagnosis is confirmed by finding an elevated serum digoxin level. Since toxicology screening tests do not detect cardiac glycosides, a quantitative drug level must be ordered specifically.

℞ TREATMENT

Gastrointestinal decontamination should be accomplished as soon as possible. Since emesis and gastric intubation may cause vagal stimulation and worsen existing conduction block, activated charcoal is preferred. Repeated doses should be administered because this therapy also can enhance elimination of digoxin. Diuresis, hemodialysis, and hemoperfusion are ineffective, however. Potassium, magnesium, and calcium abnormalities should be corrected. Electrical pacing may be necessary when sinus bradycardia and second- and third-degree heart block result in hypotension and fail to respond to atropine, isoproterenol, or antibody therapy. Magnesium sulfate (as for antiarrhythmic poisoning), phenytoin, and lidocaine may be useful in the treatment of ventricular tachyarrhythmias. Digoxin-specific Fab-fragment antibodies should be administered to patients with potentially life-threatening toxicity not immediately responsive to the above. Following antibody administration, cardiac arrhythmias and hyperkalemia are generally corrected within an hour; the antibodies are given intravenously over 30 min, unless cardiac arrest has occurred, in which case the solution is given as a bolus. The drug-antibody complex is excreted in the urine with a half-life of 16 to 20 h. In patients with renal failure, the drug-antibody complex is metabolized over a period of days to weeks. Although free digoxin levels decrease rapidly to zero following antibody administration, routine methods used to measure digoxin do not differentiate between bound and unbound drug, so that drug levels do not correlate with toxicity after antibody therapy. Antibodies cross-react with other cardiac glycosides, but larger doses may be needed for toxicity not involving digoxin.

Each 40 mg vial of antibody can neutralize 0.6 mg of digoxin. Formulas and tables for calculating the dose of antibody based on body weight and post-distribution serum digoxin level or the amount of drug acutely ingested are available in the package insert. Unfortunately, toxicity may occur before distribution is complete or before levels are available. In addition, the amount of an acute overdose may be unknown, and calculated doses often exceed the effective dose (leading to costly overtreatment). The following doses are therefore suggested. With chronic digoxin intoxication, when total-body drug load only slightly exceeds the therapeutic amount and when patients may be dependent on digoxin for its inotropic effects, an antibody dose of 1 to 2 vials is usually sufficient. In acute poisoning drug levels are generally higher, and 5 to 10 vials are usually required. These doses can be repeated as necessary.

ETHYLENE GLYCOL Ethylene glycol is a colorless, odorless, sweet-tasting, water-soluble liquid that is used as a solvent for paints, plastics, and pharmaceuticals and in the manufacture of explosives, fire extinguishers, foams, hydraulic fluids, windshield cleaners, radiator antifreeze, and de-icer preparations.

Ethylene glycol is absorbed rapidly, and levels peak approximately 2 h after ingestion. Ethylene glycol has a volume of distribution of 0.6 to 0.8 L/kg body weight. It is oxidized by alcohol dehydrogenase to glycoaldehyde, which is metabolized successively to glycolic acid, glyoxylic acid, and oxalic acid. As much as 20 percent is excreted unchanged in the urine. The half-life ranges from 3 to 8 h. Since alcohol dehydrogenase has a higher affinity for ethanol than for ethylene glycol, ethanol is metabolized preferentially when both alcohols are present, and the half-life of ethylene glycol is then prolonged to about 17 h.

Ethylene glycol and its metabolites produce CNS depression. Ethylene glycol is more potent than ethanol in this respect. The glycolic acid metabolite is even more toxic than ethylene glycol. It causes a metabolic acidosis with an increased anion gap and interstitial and tubular damage to the kidney. Glyoxylic acid is more toxic still, but it is metabolized rapidly to oxalic acid and contributes little to the organ toxicity. Oxalic acid may precipitate as calcium oxalate crystals in the brain, heart, kidney, lung, pancreas, and urine and cause hypocalcemia.

Clinical Toxicity As little as 120 mg/kg body weight or 0.1 mL/kg body weight (one swallow) of pure ethylene glycol can result in a potentially toxic blood concentration of 3 mmol/L (20 mg/dL). Effects of the parent compound begin 30 min after ingestion and include nausea, vomiting, slurred speech, ataxia, nystagmus, and lethargy. A faint, sweet aromatic odor may be detected on the breath. Coma, seizures, respiratory depression, cardiovascular collapse, and death may occur. Effects caused by metabolites begin 4 to 12 h after ingestion. At this stage, the patient appears more ill than intoxicated. Manifestations include tachypnea, hypotension, agitation, confusion, lethargy, coma, and seizures. Hypocalcemia occurs in one-third of patients. Leukocytosis is present in most. In severe cases, adult respiratory distress syndrome, cyanosis, pulmonary edema, and cardiomegaly may be seen. Laboratory findings include metabolic acidosis, an increased anion gap (low bicarbonate and chloride), and abnormal urinalysis (crystalluria). Acute tubular necrosis manifested by proteinuria, oliguria, and anuria typically becomes evident 12 to 24 h following ingestion. Renal failure may be permanent but typically lasts days to weeks.

Diagnosis The diagnosis is established by measuring ethylene glycol and glycolic acid levels. In the absence of a history of exposure, the diagnosis is suggested by the finding of an ethanol-like intoxication with an elevated serum osmolality early in the course and with an increased-anion-gap metabolic acidosis and oxalate crystals in the urine later in the course. In the absence of ethanol, signs of intoxication occurs with ethylene glycol levels >8 mmol/L (50 mg/dL).

℞ **TREATMENT**

Gastrointestinal lavage and activated charcoal should be administered. Supportive measures include protection of the airway, ventilatory and circulatory support, and anticonvulsants for seizures. Hypocalcemia is treated with intravenous calcium salts. Metabolic acidosis should be corrected with sodium bicarbonate; large doses may be required. Alkalinization of the urine enhances the excretion of acid metabolites. Fluids and diuretics may reverse oliguria but do not increase the rate of elimination of ethylene glycol. Indications for ethanol therapy include an elevated osmolal gap or an increased anion gap in a symptomatic patient, a history or strong suspicion of ethylene glycol ingestion and a low or undetectable ethanol level, or an ethylene glycol concentration greater than 3 mmol/L (20 mg/dL). A serum ethanol level of at least 20 mmol/L (100 mg/dL) is required to inhibit the metabolism of ethylene glycol (higher levels may be needed with very high ethylene glycol concentrations). The loading dose of ethanol is 10 mL/kg of 10 percent ethanol intravenously or 1 mL/kg of 95 percent ethanol by mouth; the maintenance dose is 1.5 ml/kg per hour of 10 percent ethanol intravenously or 3 mL/kg per hour of 10 percent ethanol intravenously during hemodialysis. Serum ethanol and ethylene glycol concentrations should be monitored frequently. Therapy should be continued until the ethylene glycol level in blood falls below 1.5 mmol/L (10 mg/dL). Because they are cofactors in the pathway of ethylene glycol metabolism, supplemental folate (50 mg qid), pyridoxine (50 mg qid), and thiamine (100 mg qid) may be beneficial. Hemodialysis enhances the elimination of ethylene glycol and its toxic metabolites. Indications for hemodialysis include metabolic acidosis not readily correctable with bicarbonate and ethanol therapy, lack of clinical improvement despite treatment, ethylene glycol concentrations greater than 8 mmol/L (50 mg/dL), or any detectable level of blood ethylene glycol in the presence of renal failure.

HYDROCARBONS Hydrocarbons exist in a number of forms, including aromatic hydrocarbons, such as xylene and toluene, halogenated hydrocarbons, such as carbon tetrachloride and trichlorethane, and petroleum distillate hydrocarbons, such as gasoline, lacquer thinner, mineral seal oil, kerosene, and lighter fluid.

All hydrocarbons are CNS depressants and irritants of the gastrointestinal and pulmonary systems. They are absorbed rapidly following inhalation or pulmonary aspiration. Aromatic and halogenated hydrocarbons are also absorbed following ingestion and are toxic to the heart, liver, and kidneys. Aromatic hydrocarbons also can cause bone marrow suppression and skeletal muscle damage. Petroleum distillate hydrocarbons are poorly absorbed following ingestion.

Clinical Toxicity Hydrocarbons produce CNS excitation in low doses and depression in high doses. Rarely, coma and seizures occur. Psychosis, cerebral and cerebellar atrophy, encephalopathy, and peripheral neuropathy can result from chronic inhalation. Other effects include nausea, vomiting, abdominal pain, hepatitis, renal tubular acidosis, acute hepatic or renal failure, and rhabdomyolysis. Sudden death due to myocardial irritability and ventricular fibrillation may occur following hydrocarbon sniffing. After ingestion, hydrocarbons cause burning of the mouth and throat with subsequent nausea, vomiting, and diarrhea. Aspiration into the lungs may occur with ingestion or as a result of vomiting and cause pneumonia. Following aspiration, chest x-ray abnormalities include infiltrates, atelectasis, effusions, pneumothorax, and pneumatoceles. Renal tubular acidosis with decreased serum bicarbonate, calcium, phosphate, and potassium and increased serum chloride may result from chronic aromatic hydrocarbon inhalation.

Diagnosis The diagnosis is based on the clinical presentation. Assays for assessing hydrocarbons in blood are not routinely available.

℞ **TREATMENT**

The ingestion of aromatic and halogenated hydrocarbons requires prompt gastric lavage. More than one episode of ipecac-induced emesis is contraindicated, and the role of activated charcoal is controversial. Since the ingestion of other types of hydrocarbons is unlikely to result in systemic toxicity and since the risk of aspiration during gastric decontamination is greater than the potential benefit, decontamination is contraindicated for these ingestions. Supportive therapy includes oxygen, respiratory support, and monitoring of liver, renal, and myocardial function. Metabolic abnormalities should be corrected, and patients with aspiration paneumonitis should be monitored for superimposed bacterial infection. Glucocorticoids are ineffective.

HYDROGEN SULFIDE Hydrogen sulfide is a rapidly acting, malodorous ("rotten eggs"), colorless, irritating gas. It is encountered in the petroleum and mining industries, tanning of leather, vulcanization of rubber, the production of synthetic fabrics, metal refining, the production of heavy water for atomic reactors, and glue and felt manufacturing. It is also found in sewers, sulfur springs, and the holds of fishing vessels, and as a byproduct of manure storage.

The hydrogen sulfide anion inhibits electron transport in the cytochrome oxidase system, thereby inhibiting aerobic metabolism with resultant cellular anoxia and lactic acidosis. Hydrogen sulfide is detoxified to sulfate products, which are excreted principally by the kidneys.

Clinical Toxicity Exposure to low concentrations of hydrogen sulfide results in rhinitis, conjunctivitis, and pharyngitis. Inhalation of large amounts causes headache, vertigo, nausea, vomiting, confusion, seizures, and coma. Hypoventilation, hypoxia, cyanosis, metabolic acidosis, pneumonia, and pulmonary edema can occur.

Diagnosis The diagnosis is based on the characteristic clinical features, including the breath odor, the setting, and the rapidity of onset.

℞ **TREATMENT**

Treatment begins with prompt removal of the victim from the site of exposure. The airway should be cleared, ventilation should be assisted when indicated, and 100% oxygen should be administered. The use of amyl and sodium nitrite should be considered when patients fail to respond rapidly to oxygen. Nitrites promote the dissociation of sulfide ions from cytochrome oxidase by providing an alternative binding site (methemoglobin). They also enhance detoxification by acting as a catalyst for sulfide oxidation. Except for cardiac arrest, no clear-cut indications for nitrite administration exist. For optimal effectiveness, they must be used immediately in symptomatic patients (sulfide oxidation is so rapid that the amount of sulfide bound to cytochrome is minimal by the time the patient presents for treatment). The dose schedule is the same as for cyanide poisoning (thiosulfate is not necessary). Hyperbaric oxygen should be considered in patients who do not respond to the preceding measures.

IRON   Iron preparations contain ferrous salts that vary in elemental iron content (20 percent in the sulfate salt, 33 percent in the fumarate, 12 percent in the gluconate, and 35 percent in the succinate). Ingestion of 20 mg/kg body weight of elemental iron typically produces gastrointestinal symptoms, and 60 mg/kg body weight may cause systemic toxicity.

Ferrous iron is absorbed into mucosal cells of the duodenum and jejunum and is oxidized to ferric iron and bound to ferritin. It is then slowly released into the plasma, where it is bound to transferrin, an iron-specific binding globulin, and transported to tissues. Iron levels in serum usually peak 4 to 6 h after overdosage (later for delayed-release formulations). Iron bound to transferrin is nontoxic. With overdosage, free iron that exceeds the iron-binding capacity of transferrin and high ferritin levels cause tissue damage and lead to the release of vasoactive substances such as serotonin and histamine. Increased capillary permeability, vasodilation, and fluid loss result in hypotension and metabolic acidosis. Free iron also injures mitochondria, causes lipid peroxidation, and may result in renal, hepatic, myocardial, and pulmonary injury.

Clinical Toxicity   Initial manifestations include vomiting and diarrhea (often bloody). X-rays may reveal iron tablets in the stomach or small bowel. A positive x-ray, fever above 38.5°C, hyperglycemia greater than 8.5 mmol/L (150 mg/dL), and leukocytosis (white blood cell count greater than 15,000/μL) are associated with serum iron levels above 50 μmol/L (300 μg/dL) and the potential for systemic toxicity. Systemic effects occur later and include lethargy, hypotension, and metabolic acidosis and, with severe poisoning, seizures, coma, pulmonary edema, and vascular collapse. Jaundice, elevated hepatic enzyme levels, prolongation of prothrombin time, and hyperammonemia are indicative of liver injury. Proteinuria and cells in the urine indicate renal injury. Pulmonary edema and hemorrhage are seen with severe overdose. In the recovering patient, gastric ulcerations and scars may cause outlet obstruction. Overgrowth of *Yersinia enterocolitica* with sepsis is a rare complication of iron overload.

Diagnosis   A serum iron concentration above 50 μmol/L (300 μg/dL) is potentially toxic. Serious poisoning is generally associated with levels above 80 μmol/L (500 μg/dL). A positive urine deferoxamine provocative challenge test (see below) is also diagnostic.

℞ TREATMENT
Ingested iron is best removed by either ipecac-induced emesis or a large orogastric tube. An x-ray film following gastric lavage will show the success of the decontamination procedure. Whole-bowel irrigation, endoscopic removal, or gastrostomy may be necessary for large quantities of iron tablets or when concretions form. Activated charcoal is ineffective. Although bicarbonate lavage may cause the formation and removal of the insoluble ferrous carbonate salt, its effectiveness is not proven. Oral deferoxamine may bind the iron remaining in the stomach and form the less toxic ferrioxamine. Since the amount of the deferoxamine that would be required for the typical overdosage is prohibitively large, this therapy is rarely useful. Intravenous sodium bicarbonate should be used to correct metabolic acidosis. Hypotension may respond to volume expansion. Coagulation abnormalities should be treated with vitamin K or blood products.

When the serum iron level or the clinical findings indicate potential systemic toxicity, parenteral deferoxamine should be administered. If levels are not immediately available, or if the patient has mild clinical toxicity, deferoxamine can be given intramuscularly in a challenge dose of 50 mg/kg up to 2 g. A vin rosé urine color indicates the presence of ferrioxamine and means that free iron is present in the circulation. In those with a positive challenge test or with significant clinical toxicity, deferoxamine should be given intravenously at a rate of 10 to 15 mg/kg per hour. When iron levels exceed 180 μmol/L (1000 μg/dL), larger deferoxamine doses (up to 30 mg/kg per hour) can be given initially. Once the patient is asymptomatic or improved, deferoxamine therapy should be discontinued. Exchange transfusion or plasmapheresis to remove the iron-desferal (ferrioxamine) complex should be reserved for patients with renal failure or for those who fail to respond to the preceding therapy.

ISONIAZID   Toxic doses of isoniazid decrease the synthesis of the inhibitory CNS neurotransmitter GABA by competing with pyridoxal-5-phosphate, a cofactor for the enzyme glutamic acid decarboxylase. Decreased GABA can result in seizures and consequently in increased lactate production by muscle. Since isoniazid also inhibits the metabolism of lactate to pyruvate, intractable lactic acid acidosis may occur. Isoniazid is rapidly absorbed, mainly from the small intestine. Serum concentrations peak within 1 to 2 h. The volume of distribution is approximately 0.6 L/kg body weight. Serum protein binding is slight. Isoniazid is eliminated primarily by acetylation to acetylisoniazid followed by hydrolysis to isonicotinic acid. Approximately 15 percent of an ingested dose of isoniazid is excreted unchanged by the kidneys. The serum half-life of isoniazid in overdose is approximately 1 to 4 h.

Clinical Toxicity   Effects begin within 30 min of ingestion of doses greater than 20 mg/kg body weight. Symptoms include nausea, vomiting, dizziness, slurred speech, lethargy, and confusion. The major manifestations include coma, respiratory depression, generalized seizures, and lactic acid acidosis. Seizures are protracted and relatively unresponsive to standard anticonvulsant therapy. Acidosis does not occur when seizures are prevented.

Diagnosis   The diagnosis is confirmed by measuring isoniazid in blood; the assay must be ordered specifically, since routine screening tests do not detect the drug. Toxicity occurs with concentrations as low as 15 μmol/L (2 mg/L). Significant symptoms are seen with serum concentrations greater than 30 to 35 μmol/L (4 to 5 mg/L).

℞ TREATMENT
Initial therapy consists of prompt gastrointestinal decontamination and supportive measures. Ipecac-induced vomiting should be avoided, because of the high incidence of seizures. Isoniazid is well adsorbed by activated charcoal. Seizures can sometimes be treated with benzodiazepines and barbiturates. Administration of pyridoxine (vitamin B$_6$), which reverses isoniazid-induced enzyme inhibition, is usually necessary for treating seizures. Diazepam is synergistic with pyridoxine. Bicarbonate may be necessary to correct acidosis. Pyridoxine should be given intravenously in an amount equal to the ingested dose of isoniazid. When the ingested dose is not known, 5 g of pyridoxine should be administered. Pyridoxine should be given over 5 min to patients with seizures but over 30 min in the absence of seizures. Cessation of seizures and correction of metabolic acidosis are prompt, but the patient may not awake for several hours. The dose may be repeated if the response is partial or if symptoms recur. Saline diuresis enhances the excretion of isoniazid, and the drug is efficiently removed by hemodialysis. These therapies are rarely necessary because of the efficacy of pyridoxine.

ISOPROPYL ALCOHOL   Isopropyl alcohol is a component of rubbing alcohol, solvents, aftershave lotions, antifreeze, and window cleaners. Its metabolite, acetone, is found in cleaners, solvents, and nail polish removers. It is absorbed rapidly from the stomach and the lungs but only minimally through skin. It is distributed in body water and has a volume of distribution of 0.6 L/kg body weight. Its half-life ranges from 3 to 6 h. Isopropyl alcohol is metabolized to acetone in the liver by the enzyme alcohol dehydrogenase, and the acetone is excreted by the kidneys and lungs with a half-life of 20 to 30 h. Up to 20 percent of isopropyl alcohol is excreted unchanged through the kidneys. Isopropyl alcohol and acetone are about twice as potent as ethanol as CNS depressants.

Clinical Toxicity Effects begin within 30 min of ingestion and include vomiting, abdominal discomfort, and sometimes hematemesis. A characteristic smell of rubbing alcohol may be noted. CNS manifestations include headache, dizziness, confusion, and excitation. With severe ingestion, obtundation, coma, respiratory depression, hypothermia, and hypotension may occur. Hypoglycemia may be seen. Isopropyl alcohol can cause a falsely elevated serum creatinine level. A mild anion-gap acidosis, ketonemia, and increased serum osmolality may be present.

Diagnosis Measurement of the serum level must be ordered specifically, since routine screening tests do not detect isopropyl alcohol or acetone. Isopropyl alcohol levels of 8 to 17 mmol/L (50 to 100 mg/dL) produce lethargy; concentrations greater than 25 to 33 mmol/L (150 to 200 mg/dL) are associated with coma; and concentrations greater than 66 to 84 mmol/L (400 to 500 mg/dL) are potentially fatal.

 TREATMENT

Gastrointestinal decontamination must be instituted soon after ingestion. Gastric lavage will suffice. Activated charcoal is ineffective. Supportive measures should include intravenous fluids and bicarbonate to correct dehydration, shock, and acidosis. Isopropyl alcohol and acetone are removed efficiently by hemodialysis, which should be considered in patients who have high serum levels and do not respond to conservative therapy.

LITHIUM Lithium is most commonly available as the carbonate or the citrate salt. Lithium may substitute for cellular cations (K^+ and Na^+), thereby interfering with adenylate cyclase activation, inhibiting neurotransmitter (norepinephrine) release, and reducing the activity of Na^+, K^+-ATPase.

The drug is absorbed rapidly from the gastrointestinal tract and reaches peak levels within 2 to 4 h of ingestion (later with overdosage and with sustained-release preparations). It has negligible plasma protein binding and a volume of distribution of approximately 0.6 L/kg body weight. Removal from the body is primarily (95 percent) by glomerular filtration, with significant reabsorption (80 percent) by the proximal tubules. Lithium clearance is increased by alkalinization of the urine and decreased by hypovolemia and hyponatremia. The serum half-life ranges from 18 to 36 h; therapeutic levels range from 0.6 to 1.2 mmol/L.

Clinical Toxicity Effects begin 1 to 4 h after acute overdosage, but the onset can be insidious with chronic poisoning. Gastrointestinal effects include nausea, vomiting, and diarrhea; neuromuscular effects include weakness, fasciculations, and twitching; CNS effects include ataxia, tremor, myoclonus, choreoathetosis, seizures, confusion, and coma; and cardiovascular effects include arrhythmias and hypotension. Hyperthermia may occur. Laboratory abnormalities include leukocytosis, hyperglycemia, albuminuria, glycosuria, and nephrogenic diabetes insipidus. ECG changes include sinus tachycardia or bradycardia, flattened or inverted T waves, atrioventricular block, and a prolonged QT interval. In chronic intoxication signs and symptoms occur at lower serum levels than with acute intoxication.

Diagnosis Lithium is not detected by routine screening tests, so measurement of the serum level must be requested specifically. In chronic poisoning, serum levels between 3 and 4 mmol/L may be associated with severe toxicity. In acute poisoning, serum levels may exceed 8 mmol/L despite minimal symptoms. Serum levels should be measured serially because absorption may be prolonged following overdosage.

 TREATMENT

Within 2 to 4 h following ingestion, gastrointestinal decontamination is indicated. Lithium is poorly adsorbed by activated charcoal. Since most patients vomit spontaneously, lavage and bowel irrigation are the treatments of choice, particularly for sustained-release formulations. Supportive therapy includes standard treatments for seizures, CNS depression, hypotension, and arrhythmias. Symptomatic pa-

tients with serum concentrations greater than 2 mmol/L require intravenous saline to correct dehydration and achieve a normal urine output. Diuresis and alkalinization of the urine are recommended to enhance renal excretion of lithium. Hemodialysis is indicated for severe intoxication when the serum lithium level is >3 mmol/L. It may need to be repeated or prolonged to prevent serum levels from rebounding when it is stopped.

METHANOL Methanol is a component of shellacs, varnishes, paint removers, Sterno, windshield-washer solutions, and copy machine fluid. It is also a denaturant used to make ethanol unfit for consumption. Methanol, a slightly less potent CNS depressant than ethanol, is metabolized to formaldehyde and formic acid, which in turn causes metabolic acidosis and injury to the retina.

Methanol is absorbed rapidly and completely from the gastrointestinal tract, and levels peak within 1 to 2 h of ingestion. It is distributed throughout body water, with a volume of distribution of 0.7 L/kg body weight. Its protein binding is negligible. Elimination occurs mainly by hepatic metabolism, with up to 10 percent excreted unchanged by the lungs and kidneys. Elimination follows first-order kinetics with a half-life of about 3 h at low serum levels (less than about 15 mmol/L or 50 mg/dL) and converts to zero-order kinetics with an elimination rate of 3 mmol/L per hour (10.5 mg/dL per hour) at higher levels. The half-life of elimination at low serum levels is approximately 14 to 20 h, and at high serum levels it is 24 to 30 h. Ethanol competes with methanol for metabolism by alcohol dehydrogenase and increases the elimination half-life of methanol to 30 to 35 h.

Clinical Toxicity Onset is variable and may be delayed. Absence of signs and symptoms soon after ingestion should not be equated with absence of subsequent toxicity. Early manifestations are caused by methanol itself, and late manifestations are due to the metabolite formic acid. Initially, nausea, vomiting, abdominal pain, headache, vertigo, and an ethanol-like intoxication occur. An increased osmolal gap may be present. Late manifestations include coma, seizures, an increased anion gap, metabolic acidosis, and retinal injury. Ophthalmologic manifestations occur 15 to 19 h or later after ingestion and include clouding and diminished vision, dancing and flashing spots, dilated or fixed pupils, hyperemia of the disk, retinal edema, and blindness. These changes are potentially reversible with prompt institution of therapy. With severe poisoning, myocardial depression, bradycardia, and shock may occur.

Diagnosis Early in the course, the diagnosis is suggested by ethanol-like intoxication and an elevated serum osmolality and is confirmed by measurement of the serum methanol level [usually greater than 6 mmol/L (20 mg/dL)]. Later, the diagnosis is suggested by an increased-anion-gap metabolic acidosis and elevated serum methanol or formate levels.

 TREATMENT

Gastrointestinal decontamination is indicated soon after ingestion. Gastric aspiration is the treatment of choice. Supportive measures should include volume replacement, respiratory care, and treatment of seizures. Acidosis should be corrected with sodium bicarbonate; large amounts may be required. Alkalinization of the urine enhances the elimination of formic acid. Supplemental thiamine and folate, which enhance the metabolism of formic acid, are recommended in the same doses as for ethylene glycol toxicity. Ethanol therapy is indicated in patients who are symptomatic or who have an increased osmolar gap, increased-anion-gap metabolic acidosis, or a methanol level exceeding 6 mmol/L (20 mg/dL) and a low or undetectable ethanol level. The loading and maintenance doses of ethanol are the same as for ethylene glycol. Ethanol levels must be monitored frequently to document that they are in the therapeutic range of 20 to 30 mmol/L (100 to 150 mg/dL). Therapy should be continued until the serum methanol level falls below 3 mmol/L (10 mg/dL) and all signs of toxicity are resolved. Hemodialysis enhances the elimination of methanol and formic acid and is indicated when methanol levels exceed 15 mmol/L (50 mg/dL), for patients with visual signs or elevated formic acid levels, and when clinical or metabolic abnormalities are unresponsive to the preceding therapy.

METHEMOGLOBINEMIA Methemoglobinemia results from exposure to chemicals that oxidize the iron in hemoglobin from its ferrous (Fe^{2+}) to its ferric (Fe^{3+}) state. Concomitant oxidation of hemoglobin protein may cause its precipitation (as Heinz bodies) and a hemolytic anemia (with bite cells seen on peripheral blood smear). Oxidizing agents include aniline and its derivates, aminophenols, aminophenones, chlorates, dapsone, local anesthetics such as benzocaine, nitrites, nitrates, naphthalene, nitrobenzene and related chemicals, oxides of nitrogen, phenazopyridine, primaquine and related antimalarials, and sulfonamides.

Methemoglobin (ferric hemoglobin) cannot carry oxygen and, when present in excess, results in a functional anemia. It also shifts the oxygen-dissociation curve to the left, limiting the release of oxygen to tissues. Symptoms are due to hypoxia and anaerobic metabolism.

Various systems normally operate to keep methemoglobin at physiologic levels (1 percent of the total hemoglobin concentration). Oxidant inactivation systems utilize ascorbic acid and sulfhydryl agents such as glutathione. Mechanisms for converting methemoglobin back to oxyhemoglobin include NADH-methemoglobin reductase (responsible for 95 percent of baseline reducing capacity), NADPH-methemoglobin reductase, and the ascorbic acid and glutathione systems. When supplied with the cofactor methylene blue, the capacity of the NADPH-methemoglobin reductase is greatly increased. Because this enzyme is dependent on NADPH, individuals with glucose-6-phosphate dehydrogenase deficiency have profound impairment in the ability to reduce methemoglobin after oxidant exposure.

Clinical Toxicity Cyanosis that is unresponsive to oxygen and may have a gray-brown hue occurs with methemoglobin levels greater than 15 percent (15 g/L or 1.5 g/dL absolute methemoglobin). Patients are otherwise asymptomatic, however, until methemoglobin levels exceed 20 to 30 percent, at which point fatigue, headache, tachycardia, dizziness, and weakness develop. At levels greater than 45 percent, dyspnea, bradycardia, hypoxia, acidosis, seizures, coma, and cardiac arrhythmias may occur. Levels greater than 70 percent are rapidly fatal. Hemolytic anemia may cause hyperkalemia and renal failure.

Diagnosis The diagnosis is confirmed by measuring the methemoglobin level by co-oximetry, a feature of some arterial blood gas analyzers. If co-oximetry is not available, methemoglobin levels can be estimated as the difference between the oxygen saturation calculated from the P_{O_2} and that measured directly. Oxygen saturation measured by pulse oximetry may be falsely normal. Blood with high levels of methemoglobin is chocolate colored when placed on filter paper and compared with normal blood. The chocolate color does not revert to pink when oxygen is bubbled through a tube of blood but does return to normal when 10% potassium cyanide is added. Finally, the toxic screen on blood or urine may identify the drug or chemical that served as the oxidizing agent.

℞ TREATMENT
The toxin, if recently ingested, should be removed by gastrointestinal decontamination. Most oxidizing agents are eliminated by metabolism, making diuresis ineffective. Supplemental oxygen should be administered. Dialysis may be useful, depending on the specific compound. Methylene blue is indicated for methemoglobin levels above 30 percent (cyanosis alone is not an indication for methylene blue therapy). In patients with anemia or cardiovascular disease, methylene blue may be indicated at lower levels when manifestations of hypoxia are present. Methylene blue is given at a dose of 1 to 2 mg/kg body weight as a 1% solution over 5 min. If a clinical response is not observed within 1 h, the dose may be repeated. A methemoglobin level of 40 g/L can be expected to decrease by half

in 1 to 2 h. As long as the oxidizing agent remains in the body, methemoglobin will be generated, and additional doses may be necessary. Side effects of methylene blue include precordial pain, dyspnea, restlessness, apprehension, and tremor; a transient blue color to the skin and urine; and the induction of methemoglobinemia at doses greater than 7 mg/kg of body weight. Methylene blue is contraindicated in patients with glucose-6-phosphate dehydrogenase deficiency because it can cause hemolysis. If the methemoglobin level is very high, if the patient is refractory to methylene blue, or if the patient is deficient in glucose-6-phosphate dehydrogenase, exchange transfusion may be indicated.

MONOAMINE OXIDASE INHIBITORS Monoamine oxidase (MAO) inhibitors include furazolidone, isocarboxazid, nialamide, pargyline, phenelzine, procarbazine, and tranylcypromine. These agents block monoamine oxidase, thus inhibiting a major pathway for catabolism of neurotransmitters such as dopamine, norepinephrine, and serotonin. Toxicity results from accumulation of neurotransmitters and hence potentiation of their actions.

MAO inhibitors are absorbed efficiently from the gastrointestinal tract. The volume of distribution is not known but is probably large. These drugs are eliminated mainly by hepatic metabolism, and less than 5 percent is excreted unchanged in the urine. The plasma half-life of phenelzine and tranylcypromine at therapeutic doses is 24 h.

Clinical Toxicity Effects may not begin until 6 to 12 h after ingestion and may not peak until 24 h after ingestion. Initial effects include dilated pupils, hyperpyrexia, tachycardia, hypertension, and tachypnea. Nausea and vomiting also may occur. Agitation, hyperactivity, and confusion may be coupled with fasciculations, twitching, tremor, and rigidity. Cardiovascular collapse and CNS depression are late effects in severe poisoning.

Diagnosis The diagnosis is made on the basis of the clinical presentation. Toxic levels of MAO inhibitors have not been established, and no assay methods are commonly available.

℞ TREATMENT
Gastrointestinal decontamination should be performed as soon as possible. Benzodiazepines should be given for neuromuscular hyperactivity. Hyperthermia should be treated with external cooling and sedation and in severe cases with neuromuscular paralysis. Severe hypertension and tachycardia should be treated with nitroprusside and propranolol, respectively. Hypotension should be treated with volume expanders, and pressor therapy should begin at lower than normal initial doses because of the possibility of an exaggerated response. In fact, before any drug is given, potential adverse interactions with MAO inhibitors should be researched. Arrhythmias can be treated by usual measures. Diuresis, hemodialysis, and hemoperfusion are not effective. No specific antidote exists. Because of persistence of MAO inhibition, drug therapy and diet should be carefully controlled for 7 to 10 days after stopping the agents.

MUSCLE RELAXANTS Muscle relaxants include orphenadrine, methocarbamol, baclofen, chlorphenesin, cyclobenzaprine, chlorzoxazone, and carisoprodol. Muscle relaxants have some direct effects on muscle but act mainly as CNS depressants. They also depress spinal synaptic reflexes, prolong synaptic recovery time, and reduce repetitive discharges. Baclofen enhances the effects of GABA, and cyclobenzaprine and orphenadrine have anticholinergic activity. Muscle relaxants are absorbed rapidly and completely, and blood levels peak 1 to 2 h after ingestion. The half-lives of these drugs vary; most have half-lives between 2 and 6 h. Most muscle relaxants are metabolized by the liver to derivatives that are generally inactive and are excreted by the kidneys. Baclofen, an exception, is largely excreted unchanged in the urine.

Clinical Toxicity Effects of carisoprodol, chlorphenesin, chlorzoxazone, and methocarbamol include nausea, vomiting, dizziness, headache, nystagmus, hypotonia, and central nervous system depression. Cyclobenzaprine and orphenadrine may cause agitation, hallucinations, tachycardia, mydriasis, hyperthermia, and dry skin and mucosa. Orphenadrine can also cause ventricular tachyarrhythmias. Baclofen causes CNS depression, hypothermia, excitability, delirium, myoclonus, seizures, cardiac conduction abnormalities, tachycardia, bradycardia, and hypotension.

Diagnosis The diagnosis is supported by detecting the drugs on comprehensive urine screening. Quantitative measurements of serum levels are not routinely available.

 TREATMENT
Initial management includes prompt gastrointestinal decontamination. Muscle relaxants are well adsorbed by a single dose of activated charcoal. Repetitive charcoal administration may be used for baclofen. Diuresis is ineffective. The efficacy of hemodialysis or hemoperfusion is not established. Physostigmine (1 to 2 mg intravenously over 2 to 5 min) will reverse the anticholinergic effects of orphenadrine and cyclobenzaprine but should be reserved for patients with severe hallucinations and hyperactivity.

NONSTEROIDAL ANTI-INFLAMMATORY DRUGS
Nonsteroidal anti-inflammatory drugs (NSAIDs) include diclofenac, diflunisal, etodolac, fenoprofen, flurbiprofen, ibuprofen, indomethacin, ketoprofen, ketorolac, meclofenamate, mefenamic acid, naproxen, oxaprozin, piroxicam, phenylbutazone, sulindac, and tolmetin. NSAIDs inhibit prostaglandin synthesis by blocking cyclooxygenase. They are absorbed rapidly, and blood concentrations peak 1 to 2 h after ingestion. They are highly bound (greater than 90 percent) to plasma protein and have volumes of distribution of less than 1.0 L/kg body weight. The pK_a ranges from 3.5 to 6.3. They are metabolized mainly by conjugation, oxidation, and hydroxylation. A small portion (1 to 15 percent) is eliminated unchanged by the kidneys. Half-lives vary from 1 to 16 h except in the case of phenylbutazone, which has a half-life of 2 to 4 days.

Clinical Toxicity Effects are usually mild and include nausea, vomiting, abdominal pain, drowsiness, headache, glycosuria, hematuria, and proteinuria. Acute renal failure and hepatitis are rare. Diflunisal may produce hyperventilation, tachycardia, and sweating. Ibuprofen sometimes causes metabolic acidosis, coma, and seizures. Seizures are relatively common in mefenamic acid and phenylbutazone poisoning and occur rarely with ketoprofen and naproxen. Coma, respiratory depression, and cardiovascular collapse or arrest can occur with mefenamic acid and phenylbutazone. Metabolic acidosis is relatively common in phenylbutazone poisoning and occurs rarely with naproxen.

Diagnosis Comprehensive toxicology screening will identify these drugs in the urine, but quantitative analysis is not useful.

 TREATMENT
Therapy for NSAID poisoning includes gastrointestinal decontamination and supportive care. Repeated doses of activated charcoal may be of benefit for indomethacin, phenylbutazone, and piroxicam. Renal excretion is not increased by diuresis, and protein binding limits the efficacy of hemodialysis. Although experience with hemoperfusion is limited, this method might be useful in patients with hepatic or renal failure and severe clinical toxicity.

ORGANOPHOSPHATE AND CARBAMATE INSECTICIDES Organophosphorus insecticides include chlorpyrifos, phosphorothioic acid (Diazinon), dichlorvos, fenthion, malathion, and parathion, and carbamate insecticides include aldicarb, propoxur (Baygon), carbaryl, and bendiocarb (Ficam). (Numerous others are available.) The nerve gas sarin is an organophosphate, and therapeutic carbamates include ambenonium, neostigmine, physostigmine, and pyridostigmine. Organophosphorus insecticides irreversibly inhibit acetylcholinesterase and cause accumulation of acetylcholine at muscarinic and nicotinic synapses and in the CNS. Carbamates reversibly inhibit this enzyme. Organophosphates are absorbed through the skin, lungs, and gastrointestinal tract, are distributed widely in tissues, and are slowly eliminated by hepatic metabolism. The oxidative metabolites of parathion and malathion (paraoxon, malaoxon) are the active forms of the

agents. Subsequent hydrolysis produces inactive metabolites. Carbamates are eliminated rapidly by serum and liver enzymes.

Clinical Toxicity The time from exposure to the onset of toxicity varies from minutes to hours but usually is between 30 min and 2 h. Muscarinic effects include nausea, vomiting, abdominal cramps, urinary and fecal incontinence, increased bronchial secretions, cough, wheezing, dyspnea, sweating, salivation, miosis, blurred vision, lacrimation, and urinary frequency and incontinence. In severe poisoning, bradycardia, conduction block, hypotension, and pulmonary edema may occur. Nicotinic signs include twitching, fasciculations, weakness, hypertension, tachycardia, and in severe cases paralysis and respiratory failure. CNS effects include anxiety, restlessness, tremor, convulsions, confusion, weakness, and coma. Toxicity due to carbamates is shorter in duration and usually less severe than that due to organophosphates. Most patients recover within 24 to 48 h, but fat-soluble organophosphates may cause effects for weeks to months. Death is most often due to pulmonary toxicity.

Diagnosis A reduction of cholinesterase activity in plasma and in red blood cells to less than 50 percent of normal confirms the diagnosis. A reduction in red blood cell cholinesterase activity is more specific; however, this test is less readily available, and some organophosphates inhibit only one type of cholinesterase. With carbamate insecticides, depression in plasma or red blood cell cholinesterase levels is transient because of the rapid reversibility of the inhibition. Since cholinesterase assays are not routinely or rapidly available, the initial diagnosis is clinical. Insecticides may be identified in urine by specific testing.

 TREATMENT
Contaminated clothing should be removed, and the skin should be washed with soap and water. The patient should be removed from the site of inhalation exposure, and in the case of ingestion, gastrointestinal decontamination should include use of activated charcoal. Supportive measures include oxygen administration, ventilatory assistance, and treatment of seizures. Atropine, a muscarinic receptor antagonist, should be administered for muscarinic effects. A dose of 0.5 to 2 mg of atropine is given intravenously every 15 min until bronchial and other secretions have dried. Pupil size and heart rate cannot be used as end-points. Repeated doses or a constant atropine drip may be necessary for several days. Pralidoxime (2-PAM), an oxime that reactivates cholinesterases, is indicated for nicotinic symptoms due to organophosphate poisoning. The dose is 1 to 2 g intravenously over 5 to 20 min. The dose may be repeated every 4 to 6 h. Neither atropine nor pralidoxime is particularly effective at reversing CNS effects. The use of pralidoxime in carbamate poisoning is controversial. It is usually unnecessary, but its use is safe, particularly if it is administered in conjunction with atropine.

PHENOTHIAZINES Phenothiazines include chlorpromazine, fluphenazine, mesoridazine, perphenazine, prochlorperazine, promazine, promethazine, thioridazine, and trifluoperazine derivatives. Haloperidol, loxapine, pimozide, and thiothixene differ structurally but have similar pharmacologic activity. The principal mechanism of action of these agents is related to inhibition of dopaminergic neurotransmission in the CNS, but they also block some alpha-adrenergic, histaminergic, muscarinic, and serotonergic actions. Some phenothiazines have a quinidine-like effect on the heart. These agents are absorbed efficiently from the gastrointestinal tract, exhibit 90 to 95 percent protein binding in plasma, and have large apparent volumes of distribution (10 to 40 L/kg body weight). They are eliminated slowly by hepatic metabolism with half-lives of 20 to 40 h. Only 1 percent is excreted unchanged in the urine. Most metabolites are inactive.

Clinical Toxicity Effects begin within 30 to 60 min of ingestion and include lethargy, obtundation, respiratory depression, hypotension, hypothermia, and coma. Pupils are often constricted, and the skin is usually warm and dry. Other anticholinergic effects may be evident (see "Anticholinergic Agents," above). Cardiac effects include supraventricular tachycardia, atrioventricular block, and atrial and ventricular arrhythmias. Torsade de pointes, prolonged PR, QRS, and QT intervals, and U- and T-wave abnormalities may be seen with thioridazine and its metabolite mesoridazine. The neuroleptic malignant syndrome (see Chap. 18) rarely, if ever, occurs following acute overdose. In acute dystonic reactions, sustained muscle contractions may result in abnormal posturing of the eyes, face, tongue, jaw, neck, back, abdomen, and pelvis, but the patient remains alert. These reactions are idiosyncratic rather than dose-related.

Diagnosis The diagnosis is supported by detecting the presence of these agents on toxicologic screening of the urine. Quantitative measurement is not helpful.

℞ TREATMENT

Gastrointestinal decontamination should be accomplished as soon as possible. Treatment is supportive. Diuresis and dialysis are ineffective. Seizures should be treated with anticonvulsants, and hypotension should be managed with volume expanders and pressor agents. Arrhythmias are treated by standard agents. Quinidine and procainamide, however, should be avoided. Sodium bicarbonate and magnesium may be useful for ventricular tachyarrhythmias associated with intraventricular conduction delays and prolonged QT intervals, respectively. Physostigmine is sometimes useful for anticholinergic toxicity (see "Anticholinergic agents," above).

Acute dystonic reactions respond rapidly to intravenous diphenhydramine (1 mg/kg body weight given over 2 min) or benztropine (1 to 2 mg). Doses may be repeated in 20 min if the response is incomplete. Treatment is generally continued with an oral formulation for 2 to 3 days to prevent recurrence of symptoms.

SALICYLATES All salicylates have pharmacologic activity similar to that of the NSAIDs, and aspirin also inhibits platelet aggregation. Following overdosage, salicylates increase the sensitivity of respiratory centers in the brain to changes in P_{O_2} and P_{CO_2}, resulting in an increased rate and depth of respiration. Later, salicylates uncouple oxidative phosphorylation and increase the metabolic rate, oxygen consumption, glucose utilization, and heat production. They also inhibit the Krebs cycle and block carbohydrate and lipid metabolism, resulting in ketoacidosis. Salicylates inhibit the synthesis of clotting factors in the liver and cause prolongation of the prothrombin time.

Salicylates are well absorbed both from the stomach and the small bowel, but absorption may continue for 24 h or longer following an overdose. Therapeutic blood levels range from 0.7 to 1.4 mmol/L (10 to 20 mg/dL). In the plasma, 50 to 80 percent of drug is bound to albumin. These drugs have a small volume of distribution (0.2 L/kg body weight), which increases with the dose and duration of poisoning. Because salicylate is a weak acid with a pK_a of 3, the unbound portion in the serum exists mainly in an ionized state. Acidosis increases the un-ionized fraction and promotes the distribution of salicylate into brain, liver, and other tissues. Salicylates are eliminated by both hepatic metabolism and renal excretion. The half-life is 2 to 3 h after a single therapeutic dose. Saturation of hepatic metabolic pathways results in a prolonged half-life (20 to 36 h) following overdose. Alkalinization of the urine to a pH of 8 enhances renal excretion by causing the un-ionized drug in the lumen of the renal tubules to ionize; the ionized drug cannot be reabsorbed.

Clinical Toxicity Manifestations begin 3 to 6 h after overdosage and include vomiting, sweating, tachycardia, hyperpnea, fever, tinnitus, lethargy, confusion, respiratory alkalosis, and an alkaline urine (pH >6). Vomiting, diaphoresis, and hyperventilation may lead to dehydration and acute renal failure. An increased-anion-gap metabolic acidosis with an acidic urine (pH <6) may develop. In cases of severe poisoning, convulsions, coma, respiratory depression, and cardiovascular collapse may ensue. Other complications include cerebral and pulmonary edema and myocardial failure. Elevation of the hematocrit, white blood cell count, and platelet count; hypernatremia; hyperkalemia; hypoglycemia; and prolongation of the prothrombin time may be seen. Acid-base disturbances include respiratory alkalosis coupled with metabolic acidosis (40 to 50 percent), respiratory alkalosis (20 percent), metabolic acidosis (20 percent), and mixed respiratory and metabolic acidosis (5 to 10 percent). Lactic and other organic acids are responsible for an increased anion gap.

Diagnosis Salicylates are identified by a positive ferric chloride test in urine. This test is usually included in routine screening procedures. If not, specific serum measurement must be ordered. In the case of an acute single ingestion, a peak level of less than 3 mmol/L (40 mg/dL) is associated with no symptoms, one of 3 to 7 mmol/L (40 to 100 mg/dL) with mild to moderate manifestations, and one of greater than 7 mmol/L (100 mg/dL) with severe toxicity. Because of delayed and prolonged absorption, levels should be assayed serially. In chronic poisoning, symptoms may occur at levels only slightly above the therapeutic range.

℞ TREATMENT

Gastrointestinal decontamination is indicated if an ingested dose is greater than 150 mg/kg body weight. Because of delayed absorption, decontamination may be helpful 12 to 24 h after ingestion. If serum salicylate levels rise, whole-bowel irrigation and/or endoscopic removal of bezoars should be considered. Elimination may be increased by repeated administration of activated charcoal. Parenteral fluids should be given to replace fluid losses and to produce a brisk urine flow. Supplemental glucose and oxygen should be given. Electrolyte and metabolic abnormalities should be corrected. Prolongation of prothrombin time should be corrected with intravenous vitamin K. Seizures should be controlled with benzodiazepines or barbiturates. Myocardial failure should be treated with standard therapy. In symptomatic patients treatment should include saline diuresis and alkalinization of the urine to a pH of 8 to enhance urinary excretion. Depending on severity, one to three ampules (44 to 131 mmol) of bicarbonate and 20 to 60 mmol of potassium should be added to a liter of intravenous fluid containing dextrose and administered at a rate of 2 to 6 mL/kg per hour. Electrolytes, calcium, acid-base status, urine pH, and fluid balance must be monitored carefully during such therapy. When acidosis is present, bicarbonate increases the serum pH and limits the tissue uptake of salicylates. If cerebral or pulmonary edema is present, alkalinization is contraindicated. Salicylates are effectively removed by hemodialysis, which should be considered with severe overdose, cerebral edema, failure of conventional therapy, or compromised renal or hepatic function.

STIMULANTS Amphetamines, bronchodilators such as albuterol and metaproterenol, and decongestants such as ephedrine, pseudoephedrine, phenylephrine, and phenylpropanolamine stimulate alpha- and beta-, beta-, and alpha-adrenergic receptors, respectively. These agents are absorbed rapidly from the gastrointestinal tract, reaching peak plasma levels 1 to 2 h after ingestion. They are weak bases with pK_a values ranging from 8 to 10 and a volume of distribution of 2 to 6 L/kg body weight. These agents are eliminated by a combination of hepatic metabolism and renal excretion of unchanged drug. Excretion is enhanced in an acid urine and slowed in an alkaline urine. Half-lives range from 2 to 8 h to 6 to 34 h, depending on urine flow and pH.

Clinical Toxicity Effects are seen within 30 to 60 min after ingestion and include nausea, vomiting, diarrhea, and abdominal cramps. Talkativeness, irritability, confusion, delirium, headache, combativeness, auditory and visual hallucinations, tremors, tachycardia, palpitations, hypertension, and hyperreflexia are common. Other findings may include dilated pupils, dry mouth, pallor, and tachypnea. Hyperpyrexia, seizures, rhabdomyolysis, hypertensive crisis, intracranial hemorrhage, cardiac arrhythmias, and cardiovascular collapse may occur in cases of severe overdose. Bronchodilators may cause hypotension as a result of beta-adrenergic-mediated vasodilation, and decongestants may cause reflex bradycardia secondary to alpha-adrenergic-mediated hypertension.

Diagnosis This diagnosis is supported by finding these agents in the urine by toxicology screening. Quantitative measurement is not useful.

 TREATMENT

Gastrointestinal decontamination should be accomplished as soon as possible. Supportive care includes treatment of agitation and seizures with benzodiazepines or barbiturates; of hypertension with labetalol, nifedipine, or phentolamine; of hyperpyrexia with cooling blankets; and of agitation with sedatives and, if necessary, with paralyzing agents. Lidocaine and propranolol are preferred for the treatment of ventricular tachyarrhythmias. Although theoretically effective for enhancing drug elimination, acid diuresis is not recommended, owing to lack of documented clinical efficacy and risks of side effects such as worsening of acidosis and triggering of myoglobinuric renal failure.

THEOPHYLLINE Theophylline causes the release of endogenous catecholamines and prolongs their effects by inhibiting the degradation of cyclic AMP by phosphodiesterase. Theophylline is absorbed rapidly from the stomach and upper small bowel. Following overdose, serum levels peak 1 to 2 h after ingestion of liquid preparations, 2 to 4 h after ingestion of tablets, and 6 to 24 h after ingestion of sustained-release preparations. Theophylline is approximately 60 percent bound to albumin and has a low volume of distribution (0.6 L/kg body weight). Therapeutic serum levels are 55 to 110 μmol/L (10 to 20 mg/L). Theophylline is eliminated primarily by hepatic metabolism, which is saturable at levels in the high therapeutic range. The serum half-life, normally 4 to 6 h, is therefore prolonged in overdoses. Only 5 percent of the theophylline is excreted unchanged by the kidneys. Theophylline elimination is also decreased with impaired liver function, congestive heart failure, viral infections, and concomitantly administered drugs such as cimetidine, erythromycin, and quinolone antibiotics.

Clinical Toxicity Effects begin 30 min to 2 h following overdose and include nausea, vomiting, restlessness, irritability, agitation, tachypnea, tachycardia, and muscle tremors. Coma, hypotension, respiratory depression, generalized tonic-clonic and focal convulsions, and rhabdomyolysis may occur in cases of severe poisoning. Convulsions are often protracted, repetitive, and resistant to therapy. Cardiovascular effects include atrial arrhythmias, multifocal premature ventricular contractions, idioventricular rhythms, ventricular tachycardia, and ventricular fibrillation. Metabolic abnormalities include ketosis, metabolic acidosis, increased serum amylase levels, hyperglycemia, and decreased serum levels of potassium, calcium, and phosphorus. Toxicity occurs at lower theophylline levels with chronic than with acute poisoning, and mortality rates are higher after chronic ingestion.

Diagnosis Theophylline is not detected by routine urine screening; measurement of its level in serum must be requested specifically. Cardiac arrhythmias and seizures occur following chronic ingestion at serum levels of 200 to 300 μmol/L (40 to 60 mg/L). Similar toxicity, along with hypotension, hypokalemia, and metabolic abnormalities, generally occurs at levels above 400 to 500 μmol/L (80 to 100 mg/L) following acute overdose. Because of prolonged and delayed absorption after overdosage, levels should be measured serially to determine the peak concentration.

 TREATMENT

Initial therapy involves prompt gastrointestinal decontamination. Theophylline is well adsorbed by activated charcoal. With sustained-release forms, decontamination should be considered up to 12 to 24 h following ingestion. Repeated doses of charcoal shorten the serum half-life by approximately 50 percent. Metoclopramide and ondansetron may be necessary for controlling theophylline-induced vomiting. Extreme tachycardia should be treated with propranolol or esmolol. Hypotension is treated with volume expansion or propranolol. Benzodiazepines and barbiturates are useful for convulsions and hyperactivity. Phenytoin is ineffective. Treatment of ventricular tachyarrhythmias should include propranolol as well as

standard antiarrhythmics. Diuresis is ineffective for enhancing removal of theophylline. Hemodialysis and hemoperfusion are effective in removing theophylline and are indicated in patients with severe toxicity or with a serum level greater than 500 μmol/L (100 mg/L) after acute overdosage and greater than 300 μmol/L (60 mg/L) with chronic poisoning.

TRICYCLIC ANTIDEPRESSANTS Commonly available tricyclic compounds include amitriptyline, imipramine, chlomipramine, desipramine, doxepin, nortriptyline, protriptyline, and trimipramine. Related agents include amoxapine, bupropion, maprotiline, and trazodone. These agents block reuptake of synaptic transmitters such as norepinephrine, dopamine, and serotonin in the CNS. In addition, they have anticholinergic activity, alpha-adrenergic blocking activity, and quinidine-like effects on the heart. Antidepressants that selectively inhibit the reuptake of serotonin (fluoxetine, paroxetin, sertraline) or norepinephrine and serotonin (venlafaxine) do not cause a toxicity similar to that produced by the tricyclics; CNS depression is mild, and cardiotoxicity is virtually nonexistent.

Tricyclics are well absorbed from the gastrointestinal tract, and serum levels peak within 2 to 6 h of an overdose. In rare cases, anticholinergic effects result in prolonged absorption and delayed peak levels (6 to 12 h following ingestion). Tricyclics exhibit high protein binding in the plasma. They have large volumes of distribution, in the range of 20 to 40 L/kg body weight. Elimination is mainly by hepatic metabolism, with an initial demethylation sometimes generating pharmacologically active metabolites. Subsequent steps of metabolism result in metabolites of increasing polarity, which are then excreted by the kidneys. Less than 5 percent of the parent compound is excreted unchanged in urine. The half-lives of tricyclics and their metabolites range from 25 to 30 h but may be longer in the overdose setting.

Clinical Toxicity Effects generally develop within 30 min of overdose and peak in 2 to 6 h. In cases of low overdose, anticholinergic effects predominate (see "Anticholinergic Agents," above). In cases of high overdose, marked CNS depression is coupled with cardiotoxicity, seizures, and hypotension. Ventricular tachyarrhythmias, atrioventricular and intraventricular conduction delays, terminal bradycardia, and decreased cardiac output may occur. Aspiration pneumonia and pulmonary edema also may develop. In fatal cases death usually occurs either within 6 h of ingestion or much later from multiple organ failure or pulmonary complications. Prolongation of the QRS complex (greater than 100 ms) is a characteristic feature. Increasing duration of the QRS complex correlates with an increased risk of cardiac arrhythmias and seizures. A terminal QRS right-axis deviation and a R wave greater than the S wave in lead AVR of the ECG are sensitive indicators of cardiotoxicity.

Diagnosis The diagnosis is supported by the presence of these drugs in the urine on routine screening tests. Serum levels are diagnostic and generally correlate with severity. Serum levels of active metabolites should be summed with that of the parent compound when estimating the serum concentration. Levels less than about 1000 nmol/L (300 ng/mL) are therapeutic. Levels over 3300 nmol/L (1000 ng/mL) indicate serious poisoning.

 TREATMENT

Ipecac-induced emesis is contraindicated with tricyclic ingestions. Gastric lavage is indicated for comatose patients with recent ingestion. Activated charcoal in single and repeated doses should be administered. Treatment includes support of respiration and volume expansion and norepinephrine or high-dose dopamine for hypotension. Seizures should be treated with benzodiazepines and barbiturates. Phenytoin is of uncertain benefit. Acidosis worsens the likelihood of arrhythmias and should be corrected. Sodium bicarbonate should be given as a bolus following a seizure and as an infusion to maintain a serum pH of 7.40 to 7.50 in patients with QRS prolongation. Treatment of ventricular tachyarrhythmias should include sodium bicarbonate (0.5 to 1 mmol/kg of body weight), lidocaine, and bretyllium. Phenytoin is often recommended, but its efficacy is not established. Beta-adrenergic blockers and class 1A antiarrhythmics (quinidine, procainamide, and disopyramide) should be avoided. Cardiac pacing and invasive hemodynamic support may be necessary for severe cardiovascular depression. Physostigmine (see "Anticholinergic Agents," above) will reverse low-dose anticholinergic effects and may be administered in cases of mild poisoning if the ECG is normal and deterioration has been excluded by a suitable period of observation.

BIBLIOGRAPHY

GENERAL ASPECTS

AMDUR MO et al (eds): *Casarett and Doull's Toxicology: The Basic Science of Poisons*, 5th ed. New York, McGraw-Hill, 1996

EPIDEMIOLOGY

LITOVITZ TL et al: 1994 annual report of the American Association of Poison Control Centers Toxic Exposure Surveillance System. Am J Emerg Med 13:551, 1995

DIAGNOSIS

AABAKKEN et al: Osmollal and anion gaps in patients admitted to an emergency medical department. Hum Exp Toxicol 13:131, 1994

BRADBERRY SM, VALE JA: Disturbances of potassium homeostasis in poisoning. Clin Toxicol 33:295, 1995

BRETT AS: Implication of discordance between clinical impression and toxicology analysis in drug overdose. Arch Intern Med 148:437, 1988

COUNCIL OF SCIENTIFIC AFFAIRS, AMERICAN MEDICAL ASSOCIATION: Scientific issues in drug testing. JAMA 257:3110, 1987

HEPLER BR et al: Role of the toxicology lab in the treatment of acute poisoning. Med Toxicol 1:61, 1986

HOFFMAN RS, GOLDFRANK LR: The poisoned patient with altered consciousness. Controversies in the use of the "coma cocktail." JAMA 274:562, 1995

KELLERMANN AL et al: Impact of drug screening in suspected overdose. Ann Emerg Med 16:1206, 1987

OLSON KR et al: Physical assessment and differential diagnosis of the poisoned patient. Med Toxicol 2:52, 1987

OSTER JR et al: Use of the anion gap in clinical medicine. South Med J 81:229, 1988

TREATMENT

ALBERTSON TE et al: Superiority of activated charcoal alone compared with ipecac and activated charcoal in the treatment of acute toxic ingestions. Ann Emerg Med 18:56, 1989

BRETT AS et al: Predicting the clinical course of intentional drug overdose: Implications for utilization of the intensive care unit. Arch Intern Med 147:133, 1987

COOMEY DO: *Activated Charcoal in Medical Applications*. New York, Marcel Dekker, 1995

CURTIS RA et al: Efficacy of ipecac and activated charcoal/cathartic: Prevention of salicylate absorption in a simulated overdose. Arch Intern Med 144:48, 1984

GARRETTSON LK, GELLER RJ: Acid and alkaline diuresis: When are they of value in the treatment of poisoning? Drug Safety 5:220, 1990

GOLDBERG MJ et al: An approach to the management of the poisoned patient. Arch Intern Med 146:1381, 1986

KING WD: Syrup of ipecac: A drug review. Clin Toxicol 17:353, 1980

KORNBERG AE, DOLGIN J: Pediatric ingestions: Charcoal alone versus ipecac and charcoal. Ann Emerg Med 20:648, 1991

KRENZELOK EP et al: Gastrointestinal transit times of cathartics combined with charcoal. Ann Emerg Med 14:1152, 1985

KULIG K et al: Management of acutely poisoned patients without gastric emptying. Ann Emerg Med 14:562, 1985

LITOVITZ TL: The anecdotal antidotes. Emerg Med Clin North Am 2:145, 1984

MANNO BR, MANNO JE: Toxicology of ipecac: A review. Clin Toxicol 10:221, 1977

McCARRON MM, WOOD JD: The cocaine "body packer" syndrome: Diagnosis and treatment. JAMA 250:1417, 1983

MERRIGIAN KS et al: Prospective evaluation of gastric emptying in the self-poisoned patient. Am J Emerg Med 8:479, 1990

MINOCHA A, SPYKER DA: Acute overdose with sustained-release drug formulations: Perspectives in treatment. Med Toxicol 1:300, 1986

NEUVONEN PJ: Clinical pharmacokinetics of oral activated charcoal in acute intoxications. Clin Pharmacokinet 7:465, 1982

————, OLKKOLA KT: Oral activated charcoal in the treatment of intoxications: Role of single and repeated doses. Med Toxicol 3:33, 1988

PARK GD et al: Expanded role of charcoal in the poisoned and overdosed patient. Arch Intern Med 146:969, 1986

PETERSON RG, PETERSON LN: Cleansing the blood: Hemodialysis, peritoneal dialysis, exchange transfusion, charcoal hemoperfusion, forced diuresis. Pediatr Clin North Am 33:675, 1986

POND SM: Diuresis, dialysis and hemoperfusion: Indications and benefits. Emerg Med Clin North Am 2:29, 1984

ROSENBERG J et al: Pharmacokinetics of drug overdose. Clin Pharmacokinet 6:161, 1981

SHANNON M et al: Carthartics and laxatives: Do they still have a place in management of the poisoned patient? Med Toxicol 1:247, 1986

SPYKER DA, MINOCHA A: Toxicodynamic approach to the management of the poisoned patient. J Emerg Med 6:117, 1988

STEAD AH, MOFFAT AC: A collection of therapeutic, toxic and fatal blood drug concentrations in man. Hum Toxicol 3:437, 1983

STEWART JJ: Effects of emetic and cathartic agents on the gastrointestinal tract and the treatment of toxic ingestion. Clin Toxicol 20:199, 1983

TENEBEIN M: Whole bowel irrigation as a gastrointestinal decontamination procedure after acute poisoning. Med Toxicol 3:77, 1988

———— et al: Efficacy of ipecac-induced emesis, orogastric lavage, and activated charcoal for acute drug overdose. Ann Emerg Med 16:838, 1987

WHEELER-USHER DH et al: Gastric emptying: Risk versus benefit in the treatment of acute poisoning. Med Toxicol 1:142, 1986

ZACCARA G et al: Clinical features, pathogenesis, and management of drug-induced seizures. Drug Safety 5:109, 1990

REFERENCE TEXTS

BASENT RC, CRAVEY RH: *Disposition of Toxic Drugs and Chemicals in Man*, 4th ed. Foster City, CA, Chemical Toxicity Institute, 1995

BLOCK JB: *The Signs and Symptoms of Chemical Exposure*. Springfield, IL, Charles C Thomas, 1980

CLAYTON GD, CLAYTON FE (eds): *Patty's Industrial Hygiene and Toxicology*, 4th ed. New York, Wiley, 1993

DANGAARD J: *Symptoms and Signs in Occupational Disease: A Practical Guide*, Copenhagen, Year Book Medical Publishers, 1978

ELLENHORN MJ, BARCELOUX DG: *Medical Toxicology: Diagnosis and Treatment of Human Poisoning*. New York, Elsevier, 1988

GOLDFRANK LR et al (eds): *Goldfrank's Toxicologic Emergencies*, 5th ed. Norwalk, CT, Appleton and Lange, 1994

GOSSELIN RE: *Clinical Toxicology of Commercial Products: Acute Poisoning*, 5th ed. Baltimore, Williams & Wilkins, 1984

HADDAD LM, WINCHESTER JF: *Clinical Management of Poisoning and Drug Overdose* 2d ed. Philadelphia, Saunders, 1990

HAYES WJ, LAW ER: *Handbook of Pesticide Toxicology*. San Diego, Academic Press, 1991

LAMPE KF, McCANN MA (eds): *AMA Handbook of Poisonous and Injurious Plants*. Chicago, American Medical Association, 1985

RUMACK BH (eds): *Poisindex Information System* (updated quarterly). Denver, Micromedex

SULLIVAN JB, KRIEGER GR: *Hazardous Materials Toxicology: Clinical Principles of Environmental Health*. Baltimore, Williams & Wilkins, 1992

SPECIFIC POISONS

ACETAMINOPHEN

FLANAGAN RJ: The role of acetylcysteine in clinical toxicology. Med Toxicol 2:93, 1987

PRESCOTT LF: Paracetamol overdose. Drugs 25:290, 1983

SMILKSTEIN MJ et al: Efficacy of oral *N*-acetylcysteine in the treatment of acetaminophen overdose. N Engl J Med 319:1558, 1988

ACIDS AND ALKALIS

ANDERSON KD et al: Controlled trial of corticosteroids in children with corrosive injury of the esophagus. N Engl J Med 323:637, 1990

FRIEDMAN EM, LOVEJOY FH JR: The emergency management of caustic ingestions. Emerg Med Clin North Am 2:77, 1984

HOWELL JM et al: Steroids for the treatment of corrosive esophageal injury: A statistical analysis of past studies. Am J Emerg Med 10:421, 1992

WASON S: The emergency management of caustic ingestions. J Emerg Med 2:175, 1984

ANTIARRHYTHMIC DRUGS

DUNBAR DN, PENTEL PR: Antiarrhythmic drug toxicity, in *Intensive Care Medicine*, 3d ed, JM Rippe et al (eds). Boston, Little, Brown, 1995

FREEDMAN MD et al: Extracorporeal pump assistance—a novel treatment for acute lidocaine poisoning. Eur J Clin Pharmacol 22:129, 1982

HRUBY K, MISSLIVETZ J: Poisoning with oral antiarrhythmic drugs. Int J Clin Pharmacol 23:253, 1985

STRATMAN HG, KENNEDY HL: Torsade de pointes associated with drugs and toxins: Recognition and management. Am Heart J 113:1470, 1987

BARBITURATES

BOLDY DAR et al: Treatment of phenobarbitone poisoning with repeat oral administration of activated charcoal. Q J Med 235:997, 1986

MATTHEW H: Barbiturates. Clin Toxicol 8(5):495, 1975

MCCARRON MM et al: Short-acting barbiturate overdosage: Correlation of intoxication score with serum barbiturate concentration. JAMA 248:55, 1982

BENZODIAZEPINES

HOJER J et al: Diagnostic utility of flumazenil in coma with suspected poisoning: A double-blind, randomized controlled study. BMJ 301:1308, 1990

KULKA PJ, LAUVEN PM: Benzodiazepine antagonists: An update of their role in the emergency care of overdose patients. Drug Safety 7:381, 1992

THE FLUMAZENIL IN BENZODIAZEPINE INTOXICATION STUDY GROUP (Bayer MJ et al): Treatment of benzodiazepine overdose with flumazenil. Clin Ther 14:978, 1992

BETA BLOCKERS

CRITCHLEY JA, UNGAR A: The management of acute poisoning due to beta-adrenoreceptor antagonists. Med Tox Adverse Drug Exp 4:32, 1989

HEATH A: β-Adrenoceptor blocker toxicity: Clinical features and therapy. Am J Emerg Med 2:518, 1984

WEINSTEIN RS: Recognition and management of poisoning with beta-adrenergic blocking agents. Ann Emerg Med 13:1123, 1984

CALCIUM CHANNEL BLOCKERS

HERRINGTON DM et al: Nifedipine overdose. Am J Cardiol 81:344, 1986

MCMILLAN R: Management of acute severe verapamil intoxication. J Emerg Med 6:193, 1988

SNOVER SW, BOCCHINO V: Massive diltiazem overdose. Ann Emerg Med 15:1221, 1986

CARBON MONOXIDE

DOLAN MC: Carbon monoxide poisoning. Can Med Assoc J 133:392, 1985; Symposium—carbon monoxide poisoning—mechanism of damage, late sequelae and therapy. Clin Toxicol 23:247, 1985

MOFENSON HC et al: Carbon monoxide poisoning. Am J Emerg Med 2:254, 1984

TIBBLES PM, PERROTTA PL: Treatment of carbon monoxide poisoning: A critical review of human outcome studies comparing normobaric oxygen with hyperbaric oxygen. Ann Emerg Med 24:269, 1994

CYANIDE

CARAVETI M, LITOVITZ T: Pediatric cyanide intoxication and death from acetonitrile-containing cosmetic. JAMA 260:3740, 1988

GRAHAM DL et al: Acute cyanide poisoning complicated by lactic acidosis and pulmonary edema. Arch Intern Med 137:1051, 1977

HALL AH et al: Clinical toxicology of cyanide: North American clinical experiences, in *Clinical and Experimental Toxicology of Cyanides*, B Ballantyne, TC Marrs (eds). Bristol, Wright, 1987, p 312

DIGOXIN

SMITH TW et al: Digitalis glycosides: Mechanisms and manifestations of toxicity. Prog Cardiovasc Dis 26:413, 1984 (part I); 26:495, 1984 (part II); 27:26, 1984 (part III)

TABOULET P et al: Clinical features and management of digitalis poisoning—rationale for immunotherapy. Clin Toxicol 31:247, 1993

WENGER TL et al: Treatment of 63 severely digitalis-toxic patients with digoxin-specific antibody fragments. J Am Coll Cardiol 5:118A, 1985

ETHYLENE GLYCOL

GABOW PA et al: Organic acids in ethylene glycol intoxication. Ann Intern Med 105:16, 1986

JACOBSEN D, MCMARTIN KE: Methanol and ethylene glycol poisonings: Mechanism of toxicity, clinical course, diagnosis and treatment. Med Toxicol 1:309, 1986

PARRY MF, WALLACH R: Ethylene glycol poisoning. Am J Med 57:143, 1974

HYDROCARBONS

ANAS N et al: Criteria for hospitalizing children who have ingested products containing hydrocarbons. JAMA 246:840, 1981

STREICHEN M et al: Syndromes of solvent sniffing in adults. Ann Intern Med 94:785, 1981

TRUEMPIER E et al: Clinical characteristics, pathophysiology and management of hydrocarbon ingestion: Case report and review of the literature. Pediatr Emerg Care 3:187, 1987

HYDROGEN SULFIDE

HOIDAL CR et al: Hydrogen sulfide poisoning from toxic inhalations of roofing fumes. Ann Emerg Med 15:826, 1986

SMITH RP: Management of acute sulfide poisoning. Arch Environ Health 31:166, 1976

WHITECRAFT DD et al: Hydrogen sulfide poisoning treated with hyperbaric oxygen. J Emerg Med 3:23, 1985

IRON

BANNER W et al: Iron poisoning. Pediatr Clin North Am 33:393, 1986

PROUDFOOT AT et al: Management of acute iron poisoning. Med Toxicol 1:83, 1986

TENEBEIN M et al: Myocardial failure and shock in iron poisoning. Hum Toxicol 7:281, 1988

ISONIAZID

ORLOWSKI JP et al: Treatment of potentially lethal dose isoniazid ingestion. Ann Emerg Med 17:73, 1988

WASON S et al: Single high-dose pyridoxine treatment for isoniazid overdose. JAMA 246:1102, 1981

YARBROUGH B, WOOD J: Isoniazid overdose treated with high-dose pyridoxine. Ann Emerg Med 12:303, 1983

ISOPROPYL ALCOHOL

LACOUTURE PG et al: A review of acute isopropyl alcohol intoxication: Diagnosis and management. Am J Med 75:680, 1983

NATOWICZ M et al: Pharmacokinetic analysis of a case of isopropyl intoxication. Clin Chem 31:326, 1985

LITHIUM

AMDISEN A: Clinical features and management of lithium poisoning. Med Toxicol 3:18, 1988

DYSON EH et al: Self-poisoning and therapeutic intoxication with lithium. Human Toxicol 6:326, 1987

MAO INHIBITORS

KAPLAN RF et al: Phenelzine overdose treated with dantrolene sodium. JAMA 255:642, 1986

LINDEN CH: Monoamine oxidase inhibitor overdose. Ann Emerg Med 13:1137, 1984

METHANOL

JACOBSEN D, MCMARTIN KE: Methanol and ethylene glycol poisoning: Mechanism of toxicity, clinical course, diagnosis and treatment. Med Toxicol 1:309, 1986

OSTERLOH JD et al: Serum formate concentrations in methanol intoxication as a criterion for hemodialysis. Ann Intern Med 104:200, 1986

SWARTZ RD et al: Epidemic methanol poisoning: Clinical and biochemical analysis of a recent episode. Medicine 60:373, 1981

METHEMOGLOBINEMIA

CURRY S: Methemoglobinemia. Ann Emerg Med 11:214, 1982

HALL AH et al: Drug and chemical-induced methaemoglobinaemia. Med Toxicol 1:253, 1986

HARVEY JW, KEITT AS: Studies of the efficacy and potential hazards of methylene blue therapy in aniline-induced methaemoglobinaemia. Br J Haematol 53:29, 1983

MUSCLE RELAXANTS

BAILEY DN: Meprobamate ingestion: A five-year review of cases with serum concentrations and clinical findings. Am J Clin Pathol 75:102, 1981

COHEN MD et al: Atropine in the treatment of baclofen overdose. Am J Emerg Med 4:552, 1986

NONSTEROIDAL ANTI-INFLAMMATORY DRUGS

COURT H, VOLANS GN: Poisoning after overdose with nonsteroidal anti-inflammatory drugs. Adverse Drug React Acute Poisoning Rev 3:1, 1984

HALL AH et al: Ibuprofen overdose: 126 cases. Ann Emerg Med 15:1308, 1986

VALE JA, MEREDITH TJ: Acute poisoning due to nonsteroidal anti-inflammatory drugs: Clinical features and management. Med Toxicol 1:11, 1986

ORGANOPHOSPHATE AND CARBAMATE INSECTICIDES

MINTON NA, MURRAY VSG: A review of organophosphate poisoning. Med Toxicol 3:350, 1988

NAMBA T et al: Poisoning due to organophosphate insecticides. Am J Med 50:475, 1971

SENANAYAKE N, KARALLIEDDE L: Neurotoxic effects of organophosphorus insecticides: An intermediate syndrome. N Engl J Med 316:761, 1987

PHENOTHIAZINES

BARRY D et al: Phenothiazine poisoning: A review of 48 cases. Calif Med 118:1, 1983

BENOWITZ NL et al: Cardiopulmonary catastrophes in drug-overdosed patients. Med Clin North Am 63:267, 1979

BORYS DJ et al: Acute fluoxetine overdose: A report of 234 cases. Am J Emerg Med 10:115, 1992

LEE A: Treatment of drug-induced dystonic reactions. J Am Coll Emerg Phys 8:453, 1979

SALICYLATES

BRENNER BE, SIMON RR: Management of salicylate intoxication. Drugs 24:335, 1987

GAUDREAULT P et al: The relative severity of acute vs chronic salicylate poisoning in children: A clinical comparison. Pediatrics 70:566, 1982

TEMPLE AR: Acute and chronic effects of aspirin toxicity and their treatment. Arch Intern Med 141:364, 1981

THISTED B et al: Acute salicylate poisoning in 177 consecutive patients treated in an ICU. Acta Anaesthesiol Scand 31:312, 1987

STIMULANTS

AARON CK: Sympathomimetics. Emerg Med Clin North Am 8:513, 1990

LINDEN CH et al: Amphetamines. Top Emerg Med 7:18, 1985

PENTEL P: Toxicity of over-the-counter stimulants. JAMA 252:1898, 1984

THEOPHYLLINE

GAUDREAULT P, GUAY J: Theophylline poisoning. Med Toxicol 1:169, 1986

OLSON KR et al: Theophylline overdose: Acute single ingestion versus chronic repeated overmedication. Am J Emerg Med 3:386, 1985

PARK GD et al: Use of hemoperfusion for treatment of theophylline intoxication. Am J Med 74:961, 1983

SHANNON MW, LOVEJOY FH JR: The influence of age versus peak concentration on life-threatening events after chronic theophylline intoxication. Arch Intern Med 150:2045, 1990

TRICYCLIC ANTIDEPRESSANTS

BOEHNERT MT, LOVEJOY FH JR: Value of QRS duration versus the serum drug level in predicting seizures and ventricular arrhythmias after an acute overdose of tricyclic antidepressants. N Engl J Med 313:474, 1985

CROME P: Poisoning due to tricyclic antidepressant overdose. Med Toxicol 1:261, 1986

FROMMER DA et al: Tricyclic antidepressant overdose: A review. JAMA 257:521, 1987

LIEBELT EL et al: ECG lead a VR versus QRS in predicting seizures and arrhythmias in acute tricyclic antidepressant toxicity. Ann Emerg Med 26:195, 1995

392

Robert L. Norris, Scott Oslund, Paul S. Auerbach

DISORDERS CAUSED BY REPTILE BITES AND MARINE ANIMAL ENVENOMATIONS

Few topics in medicine are as controversial or as influenced by tradition as the management of bites and stings from venomous creatures. Because the incidence of serious bites and stings is relatively low in developed nations, there is a paucity of relevant clinical research and literature, and therapeutic decision-making is often based on anecdotal information. Furthermore, the different responses of different species to various toxins make it difficult to extrapolate data from animal studies to clinical application. This chapter outlines general principles for the evaluation and management of victims of venom poisoning by certain reptiles and marine creatures and presents a clinical approach to these emergencies.

VENOMOUS SNAKEBITE

EPIDEMIOLOGY The venomous snakes of the world are classified in Table 392-1. A number of snakes in the family Colubridae (traditionally thought of as harmless snakes) can be dangerous to humans because of toxic salivary secretions. The incidence of venomous snakebites is low in most developed countries, but in regions of the world where people are engaged in manual agriculture, often with exposed lower extremities, attack rates are higher. About 30,000 to 40,000 persons die each year from venomous snakebite; incomplete reporting in disadvantaged regions probably makes this range an underestimate.

ANATOMY The typical snake-venom apparatus consists of paired venom glands—one on each side of the head, below and behind the eye—connected by ducts to hollow, anterior maxillary teeth. In viperids, these teeth are large, mobile fangs that retract against the roof of the mouth when the animal is at rest. In elapids and sea snakes, the fangs are only slightly enlarged and are fixed in an erect position. For reasons that are unclear but may be related to the venom apparatus itself, venomous snakes can bite without injecting any venom. Approximately 20 percent of pit viper bites and an even higher percentage of bites inflicted by some other snake families (up to 75 percent for sea snakes) are "dry."

Differentiation of venomous from nonvenomous snake species can be difficult unless one is familiar with local fauna. Viperids are characterized by somewhat triangular heads (a feature shared with many harmless snakes); elliptical pupils (also seen in the nonvenomous boas and pythons as well as some colubrids); enlarged maxillary fangs; subcaudal scalation that involves a single scale running the full width of the ventral surface of the tail for several rows just distal to the anal plate (as opposed to the two scales in each subcaudal row in most nonvenomous snakes); and, in the case of the pit vipers, the heat-sensing pits (foveal organs) for which they are named, located slightly inferior and anterior to the eyes on each side. Color pattern is notoriously unhelpful in identifying most venomous snakes except for the coral snakes, whose other body characteristics are similar to those of harmless colubrids. The American coral snakes can be identified by red, yellow (or white), and black bands completely encircling the body; a few species have red and black bands only. North of Mexico City, the immediate contiguity of red and yellow bands is fairly reliable for distinguishing a coral snake from one of its harmless colubrid mimics. Further south, differentiation by color pattern is less reliable.

Immunodiagnostic techniques have been developed for species identification of the snakes involved in bites. An enzyme-linked immunoassay (ELISA) can be used to identify a specific type of snake venom in a victim's blood, wound aspirate, or urine, and this method is finding clinical application around the world. However, no commercial ELISA kit is currently available in the United States.

VENOMS AND CLINICAL MANIFESTATIONS Snake venoms are complex mixtures of enzymes, low-molecular-weight polypeptides, glycoproteins, and metal ions. The enzymes and polypeptides affect the human body in a multisystem fashion. Among the deleterious components are hemorrhagins that render the vasculature leaky and thus cause both local and systemic bleeding; various proteolytic enzymes that cause local tissue necrosis, affect the coagulation pathway at various steps, or impair organ function; myocardial depressant factors that reduce cardiac output; and neurotoxins that act either pre- or postsynaptically to inhibit peripheral nerve impulses. Most snake venoms can adversely affect multiple organs.

Contact with either of the venom apparatuses produces immediate and intensely painful stings. The affected part should be immersed immediately in hot water (see below). Accessible embedded spines should be removed but may break off and remain lodged in the victim. Residual dye from the surface of a spine remaining after the spine's removal may mimic retained spines but is otherwise of no consequence. Soft tissue radiography or magnetic resonance imaging can confirm the presence of retained spines; this finding may warrant referral for attempted surgical removal if the spines are located near vital structures (e.g., joints, neurovascular bundles). Retained spines may cause the formation of granulomas that are amenable to excision or to intra-lesional injection with triamcinolone hexacetonide (5 mg/mL).

Cone shells are predatory, carnivorous mollusks. The most danger-ous of these creatures are found in the Indian and Pacific oceans. A neurotoxic venom comprising multiple peptides is delivered through harpoon-like darts propelled from an extensible proboscis. Clinically, the sting is like that of a bee. The victim may report wound, perioral, and generalized paresthesia. Bulbar dysfunction and systemic muscular paralysis indicate severe envenomation. The sting of the geographer cone (*Conus geographus*) can cause cerebral edema, coma, and death due to respiratory or cardiac failure. Immediately after envenomation, a circumferential pressure-immobilization dressing 15 cm wide should be applied over a gauze pad measuring approximately 7 cm by 7 cm by 2 cm that has been placed directly over the sting. The dressing should be applied at venous-lymphatic pressure with the preservation of distal arterial pulses. Once the victim has been transported to the nearest medical facility, the bandage can be released. Provision should be made for cardiovascular and respiratory support.

Serious envenomations and deaths have followed bites of the Australian blue-ringed octopuses (*Octopus maculosus* and *Octopus lunulata*). Although these animals rarely exceed 20 cm in length, their venom contains a potent neurotoxin (maculotoxin) that inhibits peripheral nerve transmission by blocking sodium conductance. Within several minutes of a serious envenomation, oral and facial numbness develops and rapidly progresses to total flaccid paralysis, including failure of respiratory muscles. If respirations are assisted, the victim may remain awake although completely paralyzed. Since there is no antidote, treatment is supportive. Immediately after envenomation, attempts should be made to limit the dispersion of venom by application of a pressure-immobilization or a venous-lymphatic pressure dressing. Hot-water immersion and cryotherapy are ineffective. Artificial respi-ration should be provided. Even with serious envenomations, signifi-cant recovery often takes place within 4 to 10 h. Sequelae are uncom-mon unless related to hypoxia.

VERTEBRATES A number of marine vertebrates, including stingrays, scorpionfish, catfish, surgeonfish, and weeverfish, are capa-ble of envenoming humans. The management of most of these stings is similar.

A stingray injury is both an envenomation and a traumatic wound. The venom, which contains serotonin, 5'-nucleotidase, and phospho-diesterase, causes immediate and intense pain that may last up to 48 h. Systemic effects include weakness, diaphoresis, nausea, vom-iting, diarrhea, dysrhythmias, syncope, hypotension, muscle cramps, fasciculations, paralysis, and (in rare cases) death.

The designation *scorpionfish* encompasses members of the family Scorpaenidae and in fact includes not only scorpionfish but also lionfish and stonefish. A complex venom with neuromuscular toxicity is deliv-ered through 12 or 13 dorsal, two pelvic, and three anal spines. Pectoral spines do not contain venom. The severity of envenomation depends on the species of fish, the number of stings, and the amount of venom released. In general, the sting of a stonefish is regarded as the most serious (severe to life-threatening); that of the scorpionfish is of inter-mediate seriousness; and that of the lionfish is the least serious. Like that of a stingray, the sting of a scorpionfish is immediately and intensely painful. Pain from a stonefish envenomation may last for days. The systemic manifestations are similar to those of stingray envenomations but may be more pronounced, particularly in the case of a stonefish sting. The rare deaths following stonefish envenomation usually occur within 6 to 8 h.

Two species of marine catfish, *Plotosus lineatus* (the oriental catfish) and *Galeichthys felis* (the common sea catfish), as well as several species of freshwater catfish are capable of stinging humans. Venom is delivered through a single dorsal spine and two pectoral spines. Clinically, a catfish sting is comparable to that of a stingray, although marine catfish envenomations are generally more severe than those of their freshwater counterparts. Surgeonfish (doctorfish, tang), weeverfish, and horned venomous sharks have also been implicated in human envenomations.

The stings of stingrays, scorpionfish (lionfish, scorpionfish, stone-fish), catfish, weeverfish, venomous horned sharks, and surgeonfish are treated in a similar fashion. Except for stonefish and serious scorpi-onfish envenomations (see below), no antivenin is available. The af-fected part should be immersed immediately in nonscalding hot water (113°F/45°C) for 30 to 90 min or until there is significant relief of pain. This measure also helps to inactivate the heat-labile components of the venoms. Recurrent pain may respond to repeated hot-water treatment. Cryotherapy is contraindicated. Opiates will help alleviate the pain, as will local wound infiltration or regional nerve block with 1% lidocaine, 0.5% bupivacaine, and sodium bicarbonate mixed in a 5:5:1 ratio. After soaking and anesthetic administration, the wound must be explored and debrided. Radiography may be helpful in the identification and location of foreign bodies. After exploration and debridement, the wound should be vigorously irrigated with warm sterile water, saline, or 1% povidone-iodine in solution. Unless imme-diate wound closure is necessary for hemostasis, wounds should be left open to heal by secondary intention or to undergo delayed primary closure. Tetanus immunization should be updated. Antibiotic treatment should be considered for serious wounds and for envenomation in immunocompromised hosts. The initially administered antibiotics should cover *Staphylococcus* and *Streptococcus* species. If the victim is immunocompromised or an infection develops, antibiotic coverage should be broadened to include *Vibrio* species.

SOURCES OF ANTIVENINS AND OTHER ASSISTANCE
An antivenin for stonefish (and severe scorpionfish) envenomation made in Australia by the Commonwealth Serum Laboratories (CSL; 45 Poplar Road, Parkville, Victoria, Australia 3052; 61-3-389-1911; fax: 61-3-389-1434) is available in the United States through the pharmacies of Sharp Cabrillo Hospital Emergency Department, San Diego, CA, at (619) 221-3429, and Community Hospital of Monterey Peninsula (CHOMP) Emergency Department, Monterey, CA, at (408) 625-4900.

Polyvalent sea snake antivenin is available from CSL or CHOMP. If sea snake antivenin is unavailable, tiger snake (*N. scutatus*) antivenin should be used.

Divers Alert Network, a nonprofit organization designed to assist in the care of injured divers, may also help with the treatment of marine injuries. The network can be reached 24 h a day at (919) 684-8111 or on the Internet at http://www.dan.ycg.org.

BIBLIOGRAPHY

SNAKES AND LIZARDS

DART RC et al: Validation of a severity score for the assessment of crotalid snakebite. Ann Emerg Med 27:321, 1996
KUNKEL DB et al: Reptile envenomations. J Toxicol Clin Toxicol 21:503, 1983–1984
MINTON SA, NORRIS RL: Non-North American venomous reptile bites, in *Wilderness Medicine: Management of Wilderness and Environmental Emergencies,* 3d ed, PS Auerbach (ed). St. Louis, Mosby, 1995, pp 710–730
RUSSELL FE: *Snake Venom Poisoning.* New York, Scholium International, 1983
SULLIVAN JB et al: North American venomous reptile bites, in *Wilderness Medicine: Management of Wilderness and Environmental Emergencies,* 3d ed, PS Auerbach (ed). St. Louis, Mosby, 1995, pp 680–709
SWAROOP S, GRAB B: Snakebite mortality in the world. Bull World Health Org 10:35, 1954

MARINE CREATURES

AUERBACH PS: Marine envenomation, in *Wilderness Medicine: Management of Wilderness and Environmental Emergencies,* 3d ed, PS Auerbach (ed). St. Louis, Mosby, 1995, pp 1327–1374
————: Marine envenomations. N Engl J Med 325:486, 1991
BROWN CK, SHEPHERD SM: Marine trauma, envenomations, and intoxications. Emerg Med Clin North Am 10:385, 1992
HALSTEAD BW, AUERBACH PS: *Dangerous Aquatic Animals of the World: A Color Atlas: With Prevention, First Aid, and Emergency Treatment Procedures.* Princeton, Darwin Press, 1992, 29–124, 241–252
MEIER J, WHITE J (eds): *Handbook of Clinical Toxicology of Animal Venoms and Poisons.* Boca Raton, FL, CRC Press, 1996, pp 89–176

393 | *James H. Maguire, Andrew Spielman*

ECTOPARASITE INFESTATIONS AND ARTHROPOD BITES AND STINGS

Ectoparasites are arthropods or helminths that *infest* the skin of other animals from which they derive sustenance. They may penetrate beneath the surface of the host or attach superficially by their mouthparts. These organisms damage their hosts by inflicting direct injury, by eliciting a hypersensitivity reaction, or by inoculating toxins or pathogens. The main medically important ectoparasites are arachnids (including mites and ticks), insects (including lice, fleas, and flies), pentastomes (tongue worms), and leeches. Arthropods may also harm humans through brief encounters in which they take a blood meal or attempt to defend themselves by biting, stinging, or inoculating venoms. Various arachnids (spiders, scorpions), insects (including bees, hornets, wasps, ants, flies, bugs, caterpillars, and beetles), millipedes, and centipedes produce ill effects in this manner. More people in the United States die each year as a consequence of arthropod stings than from poisonous snake bites.

ECTOPARASITE INFESTATIONS

SCABIES The human itch mite, *Sarcoptes scabiei,* which infests some 300 million persons each year, is one of the most common causes of itching dermatoses throughout the world. Gravid female mites measuring 0.3 to 0.4 mm in length burrow superficially beneath the stratum corneum for a month, depositing two or three eggs a day. Nymphs that hatch from these eggs mature in about 2 weeks through a series of molts and then emerge as adults to the surface of the skin, where they mate and subsequently reinvade the skin of the same or another host. Transfer of newly fertilized female mites from person to person occurs by intimate personal contact and is facilitated by crowding, uncleanliness, and sexual promiscuity. Medical practitioners are at particular risk of infestation. Transmission via sharing of contaminated bedding or clothing is infrequent because these mites cannot survive much more than a day without host contact. In the United States, scabies may account for 2 to 5 percent of visits to dermatologists; involved particularly often are children, immigrants from developing countries, and close household contacts. Outbreaks occur in nursing homes, mental institutions, and hospitals.

The itching and rash associated with scabies derive from a sensitization reaction directed against the excreta that the mite deposits in its burrow. For this reason, an initial infestation remains asymptomatic for 4 to 6 weeks, and a reinfestation produces a hypersensitivity reaction without delay. Scratching generally destroys the burrowing mite, but symptoms remain even in its absence. Burrows become surrounded by infiltrates of eosinophils, lymphocytes, and histiocytes, and a generalized hypersensitivity rash later develops in remote sites.

By destroying these pathogens, immunity and associated scratching limit most infestations to fewer than 15 mites per person. Hyperinfestation with thousands or millions of mites, a condition known as *crusted* (or *Norwegian*) *scabies,* may result from glucocorticoid use, immunodeficiency diseases (including AIDS), and neurologic and psychiatric illnesses that interfere with itching and scratching.

Patients with scabies report intense itching that worsens at night and after a hot shower. Typical burrows may be difficult to find because they are few in number and may be obscured by excoriations. Burrows appear as dark wavy lines in the epidermis that measure 3 to 15 mm and end in a small pearly bleb that contains the female mite. Such lesions generally develop on the volar wrists, between the fingers, on the elbows, and on the penis. Small papules and vesicles, often accompanied by eczematous plaques, pustules, or nodules, are symmetrically distributed in these sites and in skin folds under the breasts and around the navel, axillae, belt line, buttocks, upper thighs, and scrotum. Except in infants, the face, scalp, neck, palms, and soles are spared. Burrows and other typical lesions may be sparse in persons who wash frequently, and topical glucocorticoid treatment and bacterial superinfection may alter the appearance of the rash. Superinfection with nephritogenic strains of streptococci has led to acute glomerulonephritis. Crusted scabies resembles psoriasis in its typical widespread erythema, thick keratotic crusts, scaling, and dystrophic nails. Characteristic burrows are not seen in crusted scabies, and patients usually do not itch, although their infestations are highly contagious and have been responsible for outbreaks of classic scabies in hospitals. Bacteremia occurs frequently in AIDS patients with crusted scabies and prominent fissures. Persons with massive infestations occasionally present with diffuse pruritus and generalized papules or with minimal or no cutaneous signs.

A diagnosis of scabies should be considered in patients with pruritus and symmetric polymorphic skin lesions in characteristic locations, particularly if there is a history of household contact with a case. Burrows should be sought and unroofed with a sterile needle or scalpel blade, and the scrapings should be examined microscopically for the mite, its eggs, and its fecal pellets. A drop of mineral oil facilitates removal of the sample. Biopsies or scrapings of papulovesicular lesions also may be diagnostic. In the absence of identifiable mites or mite products, the diagnosis is based on clinical presentation and history. The possibility of other sexually transmitted diseases should be excluded in adults with scabies.

For the treatment of scabies, 5% permethrin cream is less toxic than the once commonly used 1% lindane preparations and is effective against lindane-tolerant infestations. Both scabicides are applied thinly but thoroughly behind the ears and from the neck down after bathing and are removed 8 h later with soap and water. Lindane is absorbed through the skin, and its overuse has led to seizures and aplastic anemia. It should not be applied to pregnant women or infants. Alternatives include topical crotamiton cream, benzyl benzoate, and sulfur ointments. Successful treatment of crusted scabies requires the application first of a keratolytic agent such as 6% salicylic acid (to improve the penetration of scabicides) and then of scabicides to the scalp, face, and ears (with care to avoid the eyes). Repeated treatments or the sequential use of several agents may be necessary. A single oral dose of ivermectin (200 µg/kg) effectively treats scabies in otherwise healthy persons. Patients with crusted scabies may require two or more doses of ivermectin.

Although effectively treated scabies infestations become noninfectious within a day, itching and rash due to hypersensitivity frequently persist for weeks or months. Unnecessary retreatment of the affected patients may provoke contact dermatitis. Antihistamines, salicylates, and calamine lotion relieve itching during treatment, and topical glucocorticoids are useful for the pruritus that lingers after effective treatment. An oral antibiotic may be necessary for bacterial superinfections that fail to resolve with antiscabietic therapy. To prevent reinfestations, bedding and clothing should be washed in hot water, and close contacts, even if asymptomatic, should be treated simultaneously.

SARCOPTIC MANGE (ANIMAL SCABIES) Persons who have close contact with dogs may become transiently infested by the

℞ TREATMENT

Field Management   First-aid or "field" measures to be used in the management of venomous snakebite should focus on delivery of the victim to definitive medical care as quickly as possible; the victim should be as inactive as is feasible to limit systemic spread of the venom. Beyond this, any measure employed should at least do no further harm.

After viperid bites, local mechanical suction may be beneficial if applied to the puncture wounds within 3 to 5 min. A useful device is the Extractor (Sawyer Products, Safety Harbor, FL), which delivers one atmosphere of negative pressure to the wound. Suction should be continued for at least 30 min. Mouth suction should be avoided as it inoculates the wound with oral flora and theoretically can also result in the absorption of venom by the rescuer through lesions of the upper digestive tract. A proximal lymphatic-occlusive constriction band may limit the spread of venom if applied within 30 min. To avoid compounding of tissue necrosis, however, the band should not be allowed to interrupt arterial flow. A bitten extremity should be splinted if possible and kept at approximately heart level. Incisions into the bite site should never be made, and no form of cooling or electric shock is advantageous.

For elapid or sea snake bites, the Australian pressure-immobilization technique, in which the entire bitten extremity is wrapped with an elastic or crepe bandage and then splinted, is highly beneficial. The bandage is applied as tightly as it would be to treat a sprained ankle. This technique greatly restricts the absorption and circulation of venom from the bite site. However, an assessment of the potential utility of this method in viperid poisoning requires further research, as it may compound local tissue damage following these bites.

Hospital Management   Once in the hospital, the victim should be closely monitored (vital signs, cardiac rhythm, and oxygen saturation) while a history is quickly obtained and a brief but thorough physical examination is performed. The level of erythema/swelling in a bitten extremity should be marked and the circumferences measured in several locations every 15 min until swelling has stabilized. Large-bore intravenous access in unaffected extremities should be obtained in the event that hypotension develops. Early hypotension is due to pooling of blood in the pulmonary and splanchnic vascular beds; hours later, hemolysis and loss of intravascular volume into soft tissues may play important roles. Fluid resuscitation with normal saline or Ringer's lactate should be initiated for clinical shock. If the blood pressure response is inadequate after the administration of 20 to 40 mL/kg body weight, then a trial of 5% albumin (10 to 20 mL/kg) is in order. If volume resuscitation fails to improve tissue perfusion, vasopressors (e.g., dopamine) should be administered. Invasive hemodynamic monitoring (central venous and/or pulmonary arterial pressures) can be helpful in such cases. Central access must be obtained with extra caution if coagulopathy is evident.

Blood should be drawn for laboratory evaluation (including determination of blood type and cross-matching) as soon as possible, before the effects of circulating venom interfere with typing. Also important are a complete blood count to evaluate the degree of hemorrhage or hemolysis, studies of renal and hepatic function, coagulation studies to identify signs of consumptive coagulopathy, and testing of urine for blood or myoglobin. In severe cases or in the face of significant comorbidity, arterial blood gas studies, electrocardiography, and chest radiography may be necessary.

Attempts to locate a source of appropriate antivenin should begin early in all cases of known venomous snake-

bite, regardless of symptoms. If signs or symptoms develop, they may progress rapidly, making any delay in the administration of antivenin dangerous for the victim. Antivenins rarely offer cross-protection against snake species other than those used in their production unless the species are closely related. An example of good cross-protection is in the use of Australian tiger snake (*Notechis scutatus*) antivenin for sea snake bites (see below). The package insert accompanying a particular antivenin should be consulted for information regarding the spectrum of coverage. In the United States, assistance in finding antivenin can be obtained 24 hours a day from the University of Arizona Poison and Drug Information Center (520-626-6016).

Rapidly progressive and severe local findings (soft tissue swelling, ecchymosis, petechiae, etc.) or manifestations of systemic toxicity (signs and symptoms or laboratory abnormalities) are indications for the administration of intravenous antivenin. The package insert outlines techniques for reconstitution of antivenin (when necessary), skin-testing procedures (for potential allergy), and appropriate starting doses. Most antivenins are of equine origin and carry a risk of anaphylactic, anaphylactoid, and delayed-hypersensitivity reactions. Skin testing does not always reliably predict which patients will have an allergic reaction to equine antivenin; a skin test can be either false negative or false positive. Before antivenin infusion, the patient should receive appropriate loading doses of intravenous antihistamines (e.g., diphenhydramine, 1 mg/kg to a maximum of 100 mg; and cimetidine, 5 to 10 mg/kg to a maximum of 300 mg) in an effort to limit acute reactions. Expanding the patient's intravascular volume with crystalloids may also be beneficial in this regard (unless contraindicated by the patient's cardiac status). Epinephrine should be immediately available, and the antivenin dose to be administered should be diluted (e.g., in 1000 mL of normal saline, Ringer's lactate, or 5% dextrose in water for adults or in 20 mL/kg for children). This volume can be decreased if necessary for the treatment of patients with compromised cardiovascular reserve. The antivenin infusion should be started slowly, with the physician at the bedside to intervene in the event of an acute reaction. The rate of infusion can be increased gradually in the absence of allergic phenomena until the total starting dose has been administered (over a period of 1 to 4 h). Further antivenin may be necessary if clinical abnormalities worsen. Laboratory values should be rechecked hourly, particularly if abnormal, until stability is ensured.

The management of a life-threatening envenomation in a victim with an apparent allergy to antivenin requires significant expertise. Consultation with a poison specialist, an intensive care specialist, or an allergist is recommended. Often, antivenin can still be adminis-

Table 392-1

Venomous Snakes of the World

Family	Subfamily	Representative Species	Remarks
Viperidae	Crotalinae	Rattlesnakes (*Crotalus* and *Sistrurus* species), water moccasins and copperheads (*Agkistrodon* species), lancehead vipers (*Bothrops* species)	New World and Asian pit vipers
	Viperinae	Russell's viper (*Vipera russelli*), saw-scaled viper (*Echis carinatus*), puff adder (*Bitis arietans*)	European, Asian, African vipers
Elapidae		Cobras (*Naja* species), mambas (*Dendroaspis* species), taipan (*Oxyuranus scutellatus*)	Temperate and tropical New and Old World; all venomous terrestrial snakes of Australia
Hydrophiidae		Pelagic sea snake (*Pelamis platurus*)	Pacific and Indian oceans
Atractaspididae		Burrowing asps (*Atractaspis* species)	Africa, Middle East
Colubridae		Boomslang (*Dispholidus typus*), twig snake (*Thelotornis kirtlandii*)	Rear-fanged snakes with toxic salivary secretions

tered in these situations under closely controlled conditions and with intensive premedication (e.g., with epinephrine, antihistamines, and steroids).

Care of the bite wound should include application of a dry sterile dressing and splinting of the extremity with padding between the digits. Because of the risk of central spread of venom, an extremity should be elevated only when antivenin is available. Tetanus immunization should be updated as appropriate. The use of prophylactic antibiotics is controversial, as the incidence of secondary infection following venomous snakebite appears to be low. Many authorities, however, prescribe a broad-spectrum antibiotic (such as ampicillin or a cephalosporin) for the first few days.

If swelling in the bitten extremity raises concern that subfascial muscle edema may be impeding tissue perfusion (muscle-compartment syndrome), intracompartmental pressures should be checked by any minimally invasive technique (e.g., the wick catheter). If pressures are elevated, prompt surgical consultation for possible fasciotomy should be obtained while antivenin administration continues. Compartment syndromes, however, are quite rare after snakebites.

Whether or not antivenin is given, any patient with signs of venom poisoning should be admitted to the hospital for observation for at least 24 h. A patient with an apparently "dry" bite should be watched for at least 6 to 8 h before discharge. An occasional viperid "dry" bite progresses to significant toxicity after a delay of several hours, and the onset of systemic symptoms is commonly delayed for a number of hours after bites by several of the elapids (especially the coral snakes) and sea snakes. Patients bitten by these reptiles should be observed in the hospital for 24 h.

MORBIDITY AND MORTALITY The overall mortality rates for venomous snakebite are low in areas of the world with rapid access to medical care and appropriate antivenin. In the United States, for example, the mortality rate is <1 percent for victims who receive antivenin. Eastern and western diamondback rattlesnakes (*Crotalus adamanteus* and *Crotalus atrox*, respectively) are responsible for most snakebite deaths in the United States. Snakes responsible for large numbers of deaths in other regions of the world include the cobras (*Naja* species) of Asia and Africa, the carpet and saw-scaled vipers of the Middle East and Africa (*Echis* species), Russell's viper (*Vipera russelli*) of the Middle East and Asia, the large African vipers (*Bitis* species), and the lancehead pit vipers of Central and South America (*Bothrops* species).

The incidence of morbidity in terms of permanent functional loss in a bitten extremity is difficult to estimate but is probably substantial. Such loss may be due to muscle, nerve, or vascular injury or to scar contracture. In the United States, such loss due to snakebite tends to be much more common and severe after rattlesnake bites than after bites by copperheads or water moccasins.

LIZARD BITES

Bites from the two species of venomous lizards (the gila monster, *Heloderma suspectum*, of the southwestern United States and the Mexican beaded lizard, *Heloderma horridum*) are infrequent and usually follow attempts to capture or handle these creatures. The wounds are characterized by soft tissue trauma with surrounding local edema and occasionally local cyanosis and ecchymosis. Broken teeth may be embedded in the wounds. The venom contains proteases and phospholipases, and systemic effects may include hypotension, weakness, dizziness, and diaphoresis.

First-aid measures for these bites best follow the guidelines listed above for viperid bites. If the biting lizard is still attached to the victim, mechanical opening of its jaws may be required for its removal.

The sparseness of the data on the pathophysiologic effects of helodermatid venom precludes specific recommendations regarding laboratory evaluation, but routine studies (complete blood count, coag-

ulation studies, electrolyte analysis, blood typing and cross-matching, urinalysis, and electrocardiography) are prudent in anything other than a trivial envenomation. Wounds should be cleansed thoroughly and irrigated when possible. Tetanus immunization should be updated as indicated. Soft tissue radiography of the bite site and sterile probing under local anesthesia may identify retained teeth. An extremity should be splinted and elevated, but antibiotic treatment is not usually required. Systemic care is supportive (e.g., use of intravenous normal saline or Ringer's lactate for hypotension). No commercial antivenin exists. Pain due to local venom effects and mechanical trauma can be treated with opiates and regional nerve blocks. The mortality rate is extremely low.

MARINE ENVENOMATIONS

Management of venom poisoning by marine creatures is similar to that of venomous snakebite in that much of the treatment administered is supportive in nature. A few specific marine antivenins can be used when appropriate.

INVERTEBRATES Hydroids, fire coral, jellyfish, Portuguese man-of-war, and sea anemones possess specialized stinging cells called nematocysts. The venoms from these organisms are mixtures of proteins, carbohydrates, and other components. The clinical syndrome following envenomation by any of these species is similar but of variable severity. Victims usually report immediate prickling or burning, pruritus, paresthesia, and painful throbbing with radiation. A legion of neurologic, cardiovascular, respiratory, rheumatologic, gastrointestinal, renal, and ocular symptoms have been described. Victims in unstable condition with hypotension or respiratory distress should be treated supportively. During stabilization, the skin should be immediately decontaminated with a forceful jet of vinegar (5% acetic acid) or rubbing alcohol (40% to 70% isopropyl alcohol), which inactivates nematocysts. For the venomous box-jellyfish (*Chironex fleckeri*), vinegar should be used. Perfume, aftershave lotion, and high-proof ethanol are less efficacious and may in fact be detrimental. Shaving the skin helps remove remaining nematocysts. Freshwater irrigation and rubbing lead to further stinging by adherent nematocysts and should be avoided. After decontamination, application of anesthetic ointments (lidocaine, benzocaine), antihistamine creams (diphenhydramine), or steroid lotions (hydrocortisone) may be helpful. Persistent pain following decontamination may be treated with morphine or meperidine. Muscle spasms may respond to 10% calcium gluconate (5 to 10 mL) or diazepam (5 to 10 mg) given intravenously. An antivenin is available from Commonwealth Serum Laboratories (see last section of this chapter) for stings from the venomous box-jellyfish found in Australian waters.

Touching of a sea sponge may result in dermatitis. If contact occurs, the skin should be gently dried and adhesive tape used to remove embedded spicules. Vinegar should be applied immediately and then for 10 to 30 min three or four times a day. Rubbing alcohol may be used if vinegar is unavailable. After spicule removal and skin decontamination, a steroid or antihistamine cream may be applied to the skin. Severe vesiculation should be treated with a 2-week course of systemic glucocorticoids.

Annelid worms (bristleworms) possess rows of soft, cactus-like spines capable of inflicting painful stings. Contact results in symptoms similar to those of nematocyst envenomation. Without treatment, pain usually subsides over several hours, but inflammation may persist for up to a week. Victims should resist the urge to scratch, since scratching may fracture retrievable spines. Visible bristles should be removed with forceps and adhesive tape, a commercial facial peel, or a thin layer of rubber cement. Use of vinegar, rubbing alcohol, or dilute ammonia or a brief application of unseasoned meat tenderizer (papain) may provide additional relief. Local inflammation should be treated with topical or systemic glucocorticoids.

Sea urchins possess either hollow, venom-filled, calcified spines or triple-jawed, globiferous pedicellariae with venom glands. Their venom contains several toxic components, including steroid glycosides, hemolysins, proteases, serotonin, and cholinergic substances.

mites responsible for zoonotic scabies; such infestation less often follows contact with cats and horses. Zoonotic mites are unable to propagate on the human host or to produce their elongate burrows, and the characteristic pruritic papulovesicular rash is self-limited.

CHIGGER AND OTHER MITE INFESTATIONS Chiggers are the larvae of trombiculid (harvest) mites that normally feed on mice in grassy or brush-covered sites in the tropics, subtropics, and (less frequently) in temperate areas during warm months. They wait for hosts on low vegetation and attach themselves to passing animals or to people. The larva then pierces the skin of its host and deposits a tubelike structure in the dermis through which it imbibes lymph and tissue juices. This highly antigenic "stylostome" serves as the focus of an exceptionally pruritic papule that may be 2 cm in diameter and that develops within hours of attachment in persons previously sensitized to mite antigen. Scratching invariably destroys the body of a mite attached to a person. These lesions generally vesiculate and develop a hemorrhagic base. Itching and burning last for weeks. The rash is most common on the ankles or near tight-fitting clothes that obstruct the mites' movements. Chiggers are the vectors of scrub typhus in tropical and subtropical parts of Asia. Repellents are useful for preventing chigger bites.

Certain mesostigmatid mites that infest the nests of mice or birds feed on human beings when their usual hosts have been displaced. For example, intense episodes of itching dermatitis in humans may follow the removal of trash from a human residence or the departure of pigeons that have been nesting on a window air-conditioner. Other mites that infest grain, straw, cheese, or other animal products occasionally produce similar episodes. Mouse mites are the vectors of rickettsialpox in cities of the northeastern United States. Although sanitary measures effectively prevent rickettsialpox, removal of accumulated refuse may result in a transient period of elevated risk.

Diagnosis of mite-induced dermatitides (including those caused by chiggers) relies heavily on a history of exposure to the source of the mite, since the tiny mite may escape notice or may already have fallen off or been scratched off the lesions. Antihistamines or topical steroids effectively reduce mite-induced pruritus.

Species of *Demodex*, the follicle mite, live in hair follicles and sebaceous glands of the face and ears. The worm-like mites measure up to 0.4 mm in length and, if carefully sought, can be found on almost all persons. They appear not to cause disease, although their density is high in persons with rosacea. House dust mites of the genus *Dermatophagoides* infest houses throughout the world, living on furniture and rugs and feeding on shed human dander. Exposure to their allergens causes asthma, rhinitis, conjunctivitis, and eczema in persons with house dust allergies. Management includes immunotherapy with mite extracts and environmental interventions such as frequent vacuuming and removal of rugs from bedrooms to reduce mite density.

TICK INFESTATIONS AND TICK PARALYSIS In the United States, hard ticks (Ixodidae) have increased in abundance since the mid-1900s to become the most common carriers of vector-borne diseases. Deer ticks of the genus *Ixodes* transmit the pathogens of Lyme disease, babesiosis, and human granulocytic ehrlichiosis. Other ticks, such as *Dermacentor variabilis* (the dog tick), *Dermacentor andersoni* (the wood tick), and *Amblyomma americanum* (the Lone Star tick), are vectors of tularemia, Rocky Mountain spotted fever, Colorado tick fever, and human monocytic ehrlichiosis. Outside the United States, hard ticks transmit pathogenic rickettsiae and arboviruses as well. Soft ticks (Argasidae) of the genus *Ornithodoros* transmit tick-borne relapsing fever (see Chap. 177). Except in parts of Africa, soft ticks rarely attack human beings, and relapsing fever occurs only sporadically in the United States.

Ticks attach and feed painlessly; blood is their only food. Their secretions, however, produce local reactions, a febrile illness, or paralysis. Local reactions to tick bites vary from small pruritic papules to chronic nodules, or "tick granulomas," that reach several centimeters in diameter and may require surgical excision. Tick-induced fever, associated with headache, nausea, and malaise, usually resolves within 24 to 36 h after the tick is removed. Tick paralysis is an ascending flaccid paralysis believed to be caused by a toxin in tick saliva that causes neuromuscular block and decreased nerve conduction. Throughout the world, this rare complication has followed the bites of more than 40 kinds of tick—most commonly, dog and wood ticks in the United States. Children, especially girls with long hair, are most often affected. Weakness begins in the lower extremities 5 to 6 days after the tick's attachment and ascends symmetrically over several days to result in complete paralysis of the extremities and cranial nerves. Deep tendon reflexes are diminished or lacking altogether, but sensory examination and findings on lumbar puncture are typically normal. Removal of the tick results in improvement within a few hours and usually in complete recovery after several days. Failure to remove the tick may lead to death from aspiration or respiratory paralysis. Diagnosis depends on finding the tick, which often is hidden beneath hair. An antiserum to the saliva of *Ixodes holocyclus*, the usual cause of tick paralysis in Australia, effectively reverses paralysis caused by these ticks. Ticks should be removed by firm traction with a forceps placed near their point of attachment. The site of attachment should be disinfected (e.g., with tincture of iodine). Removal of ticks during the first 48 h of attachment prevents transmission of the agents of Lyme disease and babesiosis. Gentle handling to avoid rupture of ticks and use of gloves may avert accidental contamination with tick fluids containing pathogens. Protective measures against ticks include avoidance of brushy vegetation, use of protective clothing sprayed with 0.5% permethrin, and application of a repellent containing *N,N*-diethyl-*m*-toluamide (DEET). The cuffs of trousers should be tucked inside the socks.

PEDICULOSIS (LOUSE INFESTATIONS) All three species of human louse feed at least once a day on human blood. *Pediculus humanus* var. *capitis* infests the head, *P. humanus* var. *corporis* the clothing, and *Pthirus pubis* mainly the hair of the pubis. Females cement their eggs (nits) firmly to hair or clothing. The saliva of lice produces an intensely irritating maculopapular or urticarial rash in sensitized persons.

Head lice are transmitted directly from person to person and occasionally by shared headgear and grooming implements. The prevalence is highest among school-aged girls who wear long hair; black children are less frequently infested than other children. Excoriations of pruritic lesions on the scalp, neck, and shoulders lead to oozing, crusting, matting of hair, bacterial infections, and regional lymphadenopathy.

Body lice remain in clothing except when feeding and cannot survive more than a few hours away from the human host. It follows, therefore, that *P. humanus* var. *corporis* mainly infests disaster victims or indigent persons who do not change their clothes. Transmission by direct contact or by sharing of clothing and beds is enhanced under crowded conditions. The fact that the body louse leaves febrile persons or corpses as they become cold facilitates the transmission of typhus, louse-borne relapsing fever, and trench fever (see Chap. 179). Pruritic lesions are particularly common around the neckline. Chronic infestations result in the postinflammatory hyperpigmentation and thickening of skin known as *vagabonds' disease*.

The cosmopolitan crab or pubic louse is transmitted mainly by sexual contact but can infest eyelashes, axillary hair, and hair in other sites as well as pubic hair. Intensely pruritic lesions and 2- to 3-mm blue macules (maculae ceruleae) develop at the site of bites. Blepharitis commonly accompanies infestations of the eyelashes.

A suspected diagnosis of pediculosis is confirmed by the finding of nits or adult lice on hairs or in clothing. The preferred treatment is 1% permethrin creme rinse, which kills both lice and eggs and is available without prescription. An alternative, 0.5% malathion, requires a prescription and may not be as effective. Other agents, such as the more toxic 1% lindane and pyrethrins with piperonyl butoxide, are not ovicidal and require a second application 1 week after the first to kill hatching nymphs. Dead or hatched nits, which remain attached to hair sheaths, may falsely suggest an active infection. Lindane-resistant head lice have been reported. After louse infestations have been treated with insecticide, the hair should be combed with a fine-toothed nit comb to remove nits. Combs and brushes should be disinfected in hot water at 65°C for 5 min or soaked in insecticide for 1 h. Body lice can be eliminated by bathing and application of topical pediculicides from head to foot. Clothes and bedding are deloused by heat sterilization in a dryer at 65°C for 30 min or by fumigation. Infestations with pubic lice are treated with topical pediculicides except for eyelid infestations (*phthiriasis palpebrum*), which respond to a coating of petroleum applied for 3 to 4 days or 1% yellow oxide of mercury ointment applied four times daily for 2 weeks.

FLEA INFESTATIONS AND TUNGIASIS Fleas are wingless insects 2 to 4 mm long that feed on the blood of human beings and other warm-bodied animals. Common human-biting fleas include the dog and cat fleas (*Ctenocephalides* species) and the rat flea (*Xenopsylla cheopis*), which inhabit the nests and resting sites of their hosts. Larval fleas feed on pellets of dried host blood that the adult fleas eject from their rectums while feeding. The high-jumping adults attack human beings or other available warm-bodied animals when the usual host abandons or is driven from its nest. The human flea (*Pulex irritans*) infests human bedding and furniture but mainly in relatively humid buildings that lack central heating. Sensitized persons develop erythematous pruritic papules, urticaria, and occasionally vesicles and bacterial superinfection at the site of the bite. Treatment consists of antihistamines and antipruritics.

Fleas transmit plague, murine typhus, the rat and dog tapeworms, and possibly *Bartonella henselae*. Flea infestations are eliminated by frequent cleaning of the nesting sites and bedding of the host or judicious dusting or spraying of insecticides such as pyrethrin, DDT, or malathion.

Human infestations with *Tunga penetrans* (the chigoe flea, sand flea, or jigger) occur in tropical regions of Africa and the Americas. Adults live in sandy soil and burrow under the skin between toes, under nails, or on the soles of bare feet. The fleas engorge on blood and grow from pinpoint to pea size over a 2-week period. The lesions resemble a white pustule with a central black depression and may be pruritic or painful. Occasional complications include tetanus, bacterial infections, and autoamputation of toes. Tungiasis is treated by removal of the intact flea with a sterile needle or scalpel.

MYIASIS Myiasis refers to infestations by maggots, mainly due to the larvae of metallic-colored screw-worm flies or botflies. Maggots invade living or necrotic tissue or body cavities and produce different clinical syndromes depending on the species of fly.

Furuncular Myiasis In forested parts of Central and South America, larvae of *Dermatobia hominis* (the human botfly) produce boil-like subcutaneous nodules 2 to 3 cm in diameter. The adult female captures a mosquito or other bloodsucking insect and deposits her eggs beneath its abdomen. When the carrier insect attacks a human or bovine host several days later, the warmth and moisture of the host's surface stimulate the larvae to hatch and penetrate the skin. After 6 to 12 weeks, the larvae mature and drop to the ground, where they pupate. The African tumbu fly, *Cordylobia anthropophaga*, produces similar lesions. Dozens of eggs are deposited on sand or drying laundry that is contaminated with urine or sweat. Larvae hatch on contact with the body, penetrate the skin, and produce boils from which they emerge 8 or 9 days later. A diagnosis of furuncular myiasis is suggested by uncomfortable lesions with a central breathing pore that emits bubbles when submerged in water. Tumbu fly larvae can be removed by manual expression after the air pore is coated with petroleum to suffocate the larvae and induce them to emerge. *Dermatobia* larvae often require surgical excision.

Creeping Dermal Myiasis Maggots of the horse botfly, *Gasterophilus intestinalis*, do not mature after penetrating human skin but migrate for weeks in the epidermis. The resulting pruritic and serpiginous eruption resembles cutaneous larva migrans caused by *Ancylostoma braziliense*. Horseback riders become infested when eggs deposited on the flank of the horse hatch against their bare legs. The

black spines of the larvae can be identified after mineral oil is smeared over the lesion. Larva are removed with a needle. The larvae of the cattle botfly (*Hypoderma* species) invade more deeply and produce boil-like swellings.

Wound and Body Cavity Myiasis Certain flies are attracted to blood and pus, and their newly hatched larvae enter wounds or diseased skin. Larvae of species such as *Phaenicia sericata*, the green-bottle fly, remain superficial and confined to necrotic tissue and were used in the past to debride purulent wounds. Other species, including the screw-worms (*Chrysomyia bezziana* in Asia and Africa and *Cochliomyia hominivorax* in Latin America) and the flesh fly (*Wohlfahrtia vigil* in northern North America), invade more deeply into viable tissue and produce large suppurating lesions. Larvae that infest wounds also may infest body cavities such as the mouth, nose, ears, sinuses, anus, vagina, and lower urinary tract, particularly in unconscious or otherwise debilitated patients. The consequences range from harmless colonization to destruction of the nose, meningitis, and deafness. Treatment involves removal of maggots and debridement of tissue.

Other Forms of Myiasis The maggots responsible for furuncular and wound myiasis also may cause ophthalmomyiasis. Sequelae include nodules in the eyelid, retinal detachment, and destruction of the globe. In addition, the adult sheep botfly, *Oestrus ovis*, may deposit larvae in the eyes of persons tending sheep and goats, and the larvae may produce a conjunctival infestation and acute conjunctivitis. True intestinal myiasis occurs when eggs or larvae of the drone fly (*Eristalis tenax*) are ingested with contaminated food, mature in the gut, and cause enteritis. Most instances in which maggots are found in human feces are the result of larviposition by flesh flies on recently passed stools.

PENTASTOMIASIS Pentastomids, or tongue worms, are parasites with characteristics of both helminths and arthropods and are classified in a separate phylum. The wormlike adults inhabit the respiratory passages of reptiles and carnivorous mammals. Human infestation with *Linguatula serrata* is common in the Middle East and occurs in the Sudan following ingestion of encysted larval stages in raw liver or lymph nodes of sheep and goats, the intermediate hosts. The larvae migrate to the nasopharynx and produce an acute self-limiting syndrome known as *halzoun* (*Marrara* in the Sudan), which is characterized by pain and itching of the throat and ears, coughing, hoarseness, dysphagia, and dyspnea. Severe edema may cause obstruction and necessitate tracheostomy, and ocular invasion has been described. Diagnostic larvae measuring 5 to 10 mm in length are found in the copious nasal discharge or vomitus. Human beings become infected with *Armillifer armillatus* by ingesting eggs in contaminated food or drink or after handling the definitive host, the African python. Larvae encyst in various organs but rarely cause symptoms unless they compress vital structures or perforate an organ during migration. Cysts occasionally require surgical removal as they enlarge during molting, but they are usually encountered as an incidental finding at autopsy. There are reports of the cutaneous larva migrans syndrome due to other pentastomes (*Reighardia* and *Sebekia* species) in Southeast Asia and Central America.

LEECH INFESTATIONS Medically important leeches are annelid worms that attach to their hosts with chitinous cutting jaws and draw blood with muscular suckers. The medicinal leech, *Hirudo medicinalis*, is still used occasionally to reduce venous congestion in surgical flaps or replanted body parts. This practice has been complicated by wound infections, myonecrosis, and sepsis due to *Aeromonas hydrophila*, which colonizes the gullets of commercially available leeches.

Ubiquitous aquatic leeches that parasitize fish, frogs, and turtles readily attach to the skin of human beings and avidly suck blood. More notorious are the land leeches (*Haemadipsa*) that live in moist vegetation of tropical rain forests. Attachment is usually painless. Hirudinin, a powerful anticoagulant secreted by the leech, causes continued bleeding after the leech has detached. Healing of the wound is slow, and bacterial infections are not uncommon. Several species of aquatic leeches in Africa, Asia, and southern Europe can enter through the mouth, nose, and genitourinary tract and attach to mucosal surfaces at sites as deep as the esophagus and trachea. Bleeding may be intense. Externally attached leeches are removed by steady gentle traction. Removal is hastened by application of alcohol, salt, vinegar, or a flame to the leech. Internally attached leeches may detach on exposure to gargled saline or may be removed by forceps.

DELUSIONAL INFESTATIONS The groundless conviction that one is infested with arthropods or other parasites is an extremely difficult disorder to treat and unfortunately is not rare. Patients report infestations of their skin, clothing, or homes and describe sensations of something moving in or on their skin. Excoriations often accompany complaints of pruritus or insect bites. Patients bring in as evidence of infestation specimens that are identified microscopically as plant-feeding or peridomestic arthropods, pieces of skin, vegetable matter, or inanimate objects. In suspected cases, it is imperative to rule out true infestations and neuropathies, environmental irritants such as fragments of fiberglass, and other causes of tingling or prickling sensations. Pharmacotherapy with pimozide, which blocks dopamine receptors, has been more helpful than psychotherapy in treating this disorder.

ARTHROPOD BITES AND STINGS

SPIDER BITES Of the more than 30,000 recognized species of spider, only about 100 defend themselves aggressively and have fangs sufficiently long to penetrate human skin. The venom that spiders use to immobilize and digest their prey can cause necrosis of skin and systemic toxicity. While the bites of most spiders are painful but not harmful, envenomations of the brown or fiddle spiders (*Loxosceles* species), widow spiders (*Latrodectus* species), and other species may be life-threatening. Identification of the offending spider should be attempted, since specific treatments exist for bites of widow and brown recluse spiders and since injuries attributed to spiders are frequently due to other causes.

Recluse Spider Bites and Necrotic Arachnidism Severe necrosis of skin and subcutaneous tissue follows envenomation by *Loxosceles reclusa*, the brown recluse spider, and by at least four other species of *Loxosceles* in the southern and midwestern United States. Other spiders that produce necrotic ulceration include the hobo spider (*Tegenaria agrestis*) in the Pacific Northwest, the sac spiders (*Chiracanthium* species) throughout the United States and abroad, the South American brown spider *Loxosceles laeta* in Central and South America, and other *Loxosceles* species in Africa and the Middle East. All these spiders measure 7 to 15 mm in body length and 2 to 4 cm in leg span. Recluse spiders are brown and have a dark violin-shaped spot on their dorsal surface; hobo spiders are brown with gray markings; and sac spiders may be pale yellow, green, or brown.

These spiders are not aggressive toward human beings and bite only if threatened or pressed against the skin. They hide under rocks and logs or in caves and animal burrows, and they emerge at night to hunt other spiders and insects. They invade homes, particularly in the fall, and seek dark and undisturbed hiding spots in closets, in folds of clothing, or under furniture and rubbish in storage rooms, garages, and attics. Bites often occur while the victim is dressing and are sustained primarily to the arms, neck, and lower abdomen.

The clear viscous venoms of these spiders contain an esterase, alkaline phosphatase, protease, and other enzymes that produce tissue necrosis and hemolysis. Sphingomyelinase B, the most important dermonecrotic factor, binds cell membranes and promotes chemotaxis of neutrophils, leading to vascular thrombosis and an Arthus-like reaction. Initially, the bite is painless or produces a stinging sensation. Within the next few hours, the site becomes painful and pruritic, with central induration surrounded by a pale zone of ischemia and a zone of erythema. In most cases, the lesion resolves without treatment over 2 to 3 days. In severe cases, the erythema spreads, and the center of the lesion becomes hemorrhagic and necrotic with an overlying bulla. A black eschar forms and sloughs several weeks later, leaving an ulcer that may be ≥25 cm in diameter and eventually a depressed scar. Healing usually takes place within 3 to 6 months but may take as long as 3 years if adipose tissue is involved. Local complications include injury to nerves and secondary infection. Fever, chills, weak-

ness, headache, nausea, vomiting, myalgia, arthralgia, maculopapular rash, and leukocytosis may develop within 72 h of the bite. In rare instances, acute complications such as hemolytic anemia, hemoglobinuria, and renal failure are fatal.

Initial management includes local cleansing, application of sterile dressings and cold compresses, and elevation and loose immobilization of the affected limb. Analgesics, antihistamines, antibiotics, and tetanus prophylaxis should be administered if indicated. Within the first 48 to 72 h, the administration of dapsone, a leukocyte inhibitor, may halt the progression of lesions that are becoming necrotic. Dapsone is given in oral doses of 50 to 100 mg twice daily after glucose-6-phosphate dehydrogenase deficiency has been ruled out. The efficacy of locally or systemically administered glucocorticoids has not been demonstrated, and a potentially useful *Loxosceles*-specific antivenin has not been approved for use in the United States. Debridement and later skin grafting may be necessary after signs of acute inflammation have subsided, but immediate surgical excision of the wound is detrimental. Patients should be monitored closely for signs of hemolysis, renal failure, and other systemic complications.

Widow Spider Bites The bite of the female widow spider is notorious for the effect of its potent neurotoxin. *Latrodectus mactans*, the black widow, has been found in every state of the United States except Alaska and is most abundant in the southeast. It measures up to 1 cm in body length and 5 cm in leg span, is shiny black, and has a red hourglass marking on the ventral abdomen. Other dangerous North American *Latrodectus* species include *L. geometricus* (the brown widow), *L. bishopi* (the red widow), *L. variolus*, and *L. hesperus*, and there are related species in other temperate and subtropical parts of the world.

Widow spiders spin their webs under stones, logs, plants, or rock piles or in dark spaces in barns, garages, and outhouses. Bites are most common in the summer and early autumn and occur when the web is disturbed or when the spider is trapped or provoked. The buttocks or genitals are sites of bites incurred by humans while sitting in an outdoor privy.

The initial bite goes unnoticed or is perceived as a sharp pinprick. Two small red marks, mild erythema, and edema develop at the fang entrance site. The oily yellow venom that is injected does not produce local necrosis, and some persons experience no other symptoms. However, alpha-latrotoxin, the most active component of the venom, binds irreversibly to nerves and causes release and eventual depletion of acetylcholine, norepinephrine, and other neurotransmitters from presynaptic terminals. Within 30 to 60 min, painful cramps spread from the bite site to large muscles of the extremities and the trunk. Extreme rigidity of the abdominal muscles and excruciating pain may suggest peritonitis, but the abdomen is not tender on palpation. Other features include salivation, diaphoresis, vomiting, hypertension, tachycardia, labored breathing, anxiety, headache, weakness, fasciculations, paresthesia, hyperreflexia, urinary retention, uterine contractions, and premature labor. Rhabdomyolysis and renal failure have been reported, and respiratory arrest, cerebral hemorrhage, or cardiac failure may end fatally, especially in very young, elderly, or debilitated persons. The pain begins to subside during the first 12 h but may recur during several days or weeks before resolving spontaneously.

Treatment consists of local cleansing, application of ice packs, and tetanus prophylaxis. Hypertension that does not respond to analgesics and antispasmodics, such as benzodiazepines or methocarbamol, requires specific antihypertensive medication. Intravenous administration of one or two vials of a widely available equine antivenin rapidly relieves pain and can be life-saving. Because of the risk of anaphylaxis and serum sickness, antivenin should be reserved for severe cases involving respiratory arrest, uncontrollable hypertension, seizures, or pregnancy.

Envenomations by Tarantulas and Other Spiders Tarantulas are long-lived, hairy spiders of which 30 species are found in the United States, primarily in the southwest. The tarantulas that have become popular household pets are usually imported species with bright colors and a leg span of up to 25 cm. Tarantulas bite only when threatened and cause no more harm than a bee sting, but the venom occasionally provokes deep pain and swelling. Several species are covered with urticating hairs that are launched in the thousands when a threatened spider rubs its hind legs across the dorsal abdomen. These hairs penetrate human skin and produce pruritic papules that last for weeks. Treatment of bites includes local washing and elevation of the bitten area, tetanus prophylaxis, and analgesic administration. Antihistamines and topical or systemic glucocorticoids are given for exposure to urticating hairs.

Atrax robustus, the Sydney funnel-web spider of Australia, and *Phoneutria* species, the South American banana spiders, are among the most dangerous spiders in the world because of their aggressive behavior and potent neurotoxins. Envenomation by *A. robustus* causes a rapidly progressive neuromotor syndrome that can be fatal within 2 h. The bite of the banana spiders causes severe local pain followed by profound systemic symptoms and respiratory paralysis that can lead to death within 2 to 6 h. Specific antivenins for envenomation by each of these spiders are available. *Lycosa* species (wolf spiders) are found throughout the world and may produce painful bites and transient local inflammation.

SCORPION STINGS Scorpions are crablike arachnids that feed on ground-dwelling arthropods and small lizards, which they grasp with a pair of frontal pinchers and paralyze by injecting venom from a stinger on the tip of the tail. Painful but relatively harmless scorpion stings need to be distinguished from the potentially lethal envenomations that are produced by about 30 of the approximately 1000 known species and cause more than 5000 deaths worldwide each year. Scorpions feed at night and remain hidden during the day in crevices or burrows or under wood, loose bark, or rocks on the ground. They seek cool spots under buildings and often enter houses, where they get into shoes, clothing, or bedding or enter bathtubs and sinks in search of water. Scorpions sting human beings only when disturbed.

Scorpions of the United States Of the 40 or so scorpion species in the United States, only the bark scorpion (*Centruroides sculpturatus* or *Centruroides exilicauda*) produces a venom that can be lethal. Stings of the other species, such as the common striped scorpion *Centruroides vittatus* and the large *Hadrurus arizonensis*, cause immediate sharp local pain followed by edema, ecchymosis, and a burning sensation. Symptoms typically resolve within a few hours, and skin does not slough. Allergic reactions to the venom sometimes develop.

The deadly *C. sculpturatus* of the southwestern United States and northern Mexico measures about 7 cm in length and is yellow-brown in color. Its venom contains neurotoxins that cause sodium channels to remain open and neurons to fire repetitively. In contrast to the stings of nonlethal species, *C. sculpturatus* envenomations are usually associated with little swelling, but prominent pain, paresthesia, and hyperesthesia can be accentuated by tapping on the affected area (the tap test). These symptoms soon spread to other locations; dysfunction of cranial nerves and hyperexcitability of skeletal muscles develop within hours. Patients present with restlessness, blurred vision, abnormal eye movements, profuse salivation, lacrimation, rhinorrhea, slurred speech, difficulty in handling secretions, diaphoresis, nausea, and vomiting. Muscle twitching, jerking, and shaking may be mistaken for a seizure. Complications include tachycardia, arrhythmias, hypertension, hyperthermia, rhabdomyolysis, and acidosis. Symptoms progress to maximal severity in about 5 h and subside within a day or two, although pain and paresthesia can last for weeks. Fatal respiratory arrest is most common among young children and the elderly.

Other Dangerous Scorpions Envenomations by *Leiurus quinquestriatus* in the Middle East and North Africa, by *Mesobuthus tamulus* in India, by *Androctonus* species along the Mediterranean littoral and in North Africa and the Middle East, and by *Tityus serrulatus* in Brazil cause massive release of endogenous catecholamines with hypertensive crises, arrhythmias, pulmonary edema, and myocardial damage. Acute pancreatitis occurs with stings of *Tityus trinitatis* in Trinidad, and central nervous toxicity complicates stings of *Parabuthus* and *Buthotus* scorpions of South Africa. Tissue necrosis and hemolysis may follow stings of the Iranian *Hemiscorpius lepturus*.

TREATMENT

Identification of the offending scorpion aids in planning therapy. Stings of nonlethal species require at most ice packs, analgesics, or antihistamines. Because most victims of dangerous envenomations (such as those produced by *C. sculpturatus*) experience only local discomfort, they can be managed at home with instructions to return to the emergency department if signs of cranial-nerve or neuromuscular dysfunction develop. Aggressive supportive care and judicious use of antivenin can reduce or eliminate mortality from more severe envenomations. Keeping the patient calm and applying pressure dressings and cold packs to the sting site decrease the absorption of venom. Although narcotics and sedatives can control restlessness and hypertension, these agents interfere with protective airway reflexes and should not be given to patients with neuromuscular symptoms unless endotracheal intubation is planned. Hypertension and pulmonary edema respond to nifedipine, nitroprusside, hydralazine, or prazosin, and bradyarrhythmias can be controlled with atropine.

Commercially prepared antivenins are available in several countries for some of the most dangerous species. A caprine *C. sculpturatus* antivenin[1] is available as an investigational drug only in Arizona. Because of the risk of anaphylaxis or serum sickness following administration of goat serum, use of the antivenin is controversial. Intravenous administration of antivenin rapidly reverses cranial-nerve dysfunction and muscular symptoms but does not affect pain and paresthesia.

Prevention In scorpion-infested areas, shoes, clothing, bedding, and towels should be shaken and inspected before being used. Removal of wood, stones, and debris from yards and campsites eliminates hiding places for scorpions, and household spraying of insecticides can deplete their source of food.

HYMENOPTERA STINGS Insects that sting to defend their colonies or subdue their prey belong to the order Hymenoptera, which includes apids (bees and bumblebees), vespids (wasps, hornets, and yellow jackets), and ants. Their venoms contain a wide array of amines, peptides, and enzymes that are responsible for local and systemic reactions. Although the toxic effect of multiple stings can be fatal, nearly all of the 50 or more deaths due to hymenopteran stings in the United States each year are the result of allergic reactions.

Bee and Wasp Stings Bees lose their venom apparatus in the act of stinging and subsequently die, while vespids can sting numerous times in succession. The familiar honeybees (*Apis mellifera*) and bumblebees (*Bombus* and other genera) attack when a colony is disturbed, but the extremely aggressive Africanized honeybees respond to minimal intrusions rapidly and in large numbers. Since their introduction into Brazil in 1957, these "killer bees" have spread through South and Central America to the southern United States.

The common vespids in the United States include the yellow jacket, notable for the yellow and black bands on its abdomen; the bald-faced hornet, with a black body and a white face; the brown hornet, measuring 2.5 to 3.5 cm in length; and the paper wasps, which have variously colored elongate bodies. Vespids sting in defense of their nests, which they often build near human dwellings and suspend from eaves or shubbery, plaster onto walls, or burrow into wood or soil. Yellow jackets feed on sugary substances and decaying meat and are annoyingly abundant at recreation sites and around garbage, particularly in the late summer and fall.

Venom is produced in glands at the posterior end of the abdomen and is expelled rapidly by contraction of muscles of the venom sac, which has a capacity of up to 0.1 mL in large insects. The venoms

---

[1] This agent had not been approved by the Food and Drug Administration for this purpose at the time of publication.

of different species of hymenopterans are biochemically and immunologically distinct. Direct toxic effects are mediated by mixtures of low-molecular-weight compounds such as serotonin, histamine, and acetylcholine and several kinins. Polypeptide toxins in honeybee venom include mellitin, which damages cell membranes; mast cell–degranulating protein, which causes histamine release; apamin, a neurotoxin; and adolapin, which has anti-inflammatory action. Enzymes in venom include hyaluronidase, which allows the spread of other venom components, and phospholipases, which may be among the major venom allergens. There appears to be little cross-sensitization between honeybee and wasp venoms.

Uncomplicated stings cause immediate pain, a wheal-and-flare reaction, and local edema and swelling that subside in a few hours. Stings from accidentally swallowed insects may induce life-threatening edema of the upper airways. Multiple stings can lead to vomiting, diarrhea, generalized edema, dyspnea, hypotension, and collapse. Rhabdomyolysis and intravascular hemolysis may cause renal failure. Death from the direct effects of venom has followed 300 to 500 honeybee stings.

Large local reactions that spread ≥10 cm around the sting site over 24 to 48 h are not uncommon. These reactions may resemble cellulitis but are caused by hypersensitivity rather than secondary infection. Such reactions tend to recur on subsequent exposure but seldom are accompanied by anaphylaxis and are not prevented by venom immunotherapy.

An estimated 0.4 to 4.0 percent of the U.S. population exhibits clinical immediate-type hypersensitivity to insect stings, and 15 percent may have asymptomatic sensitization manifested by positive skin tests. Persons who experience severe allergic reactions are likely to have similar reactions after subsequent stings; occasionally, adults who have had mild reactions later experience serious reactions. Mild anaphylactic reactions from insect stings, as from other causes, consist of nausea, abdominal cramping, generalized urticaria, flushing, and angioedema. Serious reactions, including upper airway edema, bronchospasm, hypotension, and shock, may be rapidly fatal. Severe reactions usually begin within 10 min of the sting and only rarely develop after 5 h. Unusual complications, including serum sickness, vasculitis, neuritis, and encephalitis, develop several days or weeks after a sting.

℞ TREATMENT

Stingers embedded in the skin should be scraped or brushed off with a blade or a fingernail but not removed with forceps, which may squeeze more venom out of the venom sac. The site should be cleansed and disinfected and ice packs used to slow the spread of venom. Elevation of the affected site and administration of analgesics, oral antihistamines, and topical calamine lotion relieve symptoms; application of meat tenderizer containing papain is of no proven value. Large local reactions may require a short course of oral therapy with glucocorticoids. Patients with numerous stings should be monitored for 24 h for evidence of renal failure or coagulopathy.

Anaphylaxis is treated with subcutaneous injection of 0.3 to 0.5 mL of epinephrine hydrochloride in a 1:1000 dilution; treatment is repeated every 20 to 30 min if necessary. Intravenous epinephrine (2 to 5 mL of a 1:10,000 solution administered by slow push) is indicated for profound shock. A tourniquet may slow the spread of venom. Parenteral antihistamines, fluid resuscitation, bronchodilators, oxygen, intubation, and vasopressors may be required. Patients should be observed for 24 h for recurrent anaphylaxis.

Prevention Persons with a history of allergy to insect stings should carry a sting kit with a preloaded syringe containing epinephrine for self-administration in case of a sting. These patients should seek medical attention immediately after using the kit. To avoid stings when outdoors, individuals can wear shoes and protective clothing and avoid attracting insects with sweet foods, bright-colored clothes, perfumes, or cosmetics.

Venom Immunotherapy Repeated injections of purified venom produce a blocking IgG antibody response to venom and reduce the

incidence of recurrent anaphylaxis from between 50 and 60 percent to less than 5 percent. Honeybee, wasp, yellow jacket, and mixed vespid venoms are commercially available for desensitization and for skin testing. Adults with a history of anaphylaxis should undergo desensitization. Results of skin tests and venom-specific radioallergosorbent tests aid in the selection of patients for immunotherapy and guide the design of such treatment. A 3- to 5-year course of immunotherapy usually eliminates the risk of anaphylaxis.

Stings of Fire Ants and Other Ants All ants that are large enough can bite human beings, and some can secrete repugnant substances when handled. Stinging fire ants are an important medical problem in the United States. The imported fire ants *Solenopsis richteri* and *Solenopsis invicta* were introduced from South America into Alabama in 1918 and now infest urban and rural areas of southern states from Texas to North Carolina, where each year they sting up to 60 percent of the inhabitants of some cities. They excavate open fields and yards to build tall mounds that can harbor 200,000 worker ants. Slight disturbances of the mounds have provoked massive outpourings of ants and as many as 10,000 stings on a single person. Waterborne ants bite on contact during times of flooding.

Red-brown or brown-black fire ants attach to human skin with powerful mandibles and rotate their bodies around their heads while repeatedly injecting venom with posteriorly situated stingers. The alkaloid venom consists of cytotoxic and hemolytic piperidines and several proteins with enzymatic activity. The initial wheal-and-flare reaction, burning, and itching resolve in about 30 min, and a sterile pustule develops within 24 h. The pustule ulcerates over the next 48 h and then heals a week or 10 days later unless it becomes secondarily infected. Large areas of erythema and edema lasting several days are not uncommon and in extreme cases may compress nerves and blood vessels. Anaphylaxis occurs in about 1 to 2 percent of persons, and seizures and mononeuritis have been reported. Stings are treated with ice packs, topical glucocorticoids, and oral antihistamines. Covering pustules with bandages and antibiotic ointment may prevent bacterial infection. Epinephrine and supportive measures are indicated for anaphylactic reactions. Whole-body extracts are available for skin testing and immunotherapy, which appears to lower the rate of anaphylactic reactions.

The western United States is home to harvester ants (*Pogonomyrmex* species) as well as to less aggressive fire ants not yet displaced by the introduced species. The painful local reaction following harvester ant stings often extends to lymph nodes and may be accompanied by anaphylaxis. Large Australian bulldog ants and the aggressive South American *Paranopera* ants deliver extremely painful stings and may cause systemic symptoms. Velvet ants that inhabit sandy beaches in the United States and sting the bare feet of bathers are actually wingless female wasps of the genus *Dasymutilla*.

OTHER ARTHROPOD BITES AND ENVENOMATIONS
Dipteran (Fly) Bites In the process of feeding on vertebrate blood, adults of certain fly species inflict painful bites, produce local allergic reactions, or transmit infectious diseases. Unlike insect stings, insect bites rarely cause anaphylaxis. Mosquitoes are ubiquitous pests and are the vectors of malaria, filariasis, yellow fever, dengue, and viral encephalitides. Their bite typically produces a wheal and later a pruritic papule. In the United States, a similar reaction follows the bite of tiny but aggressive midges known as "no-see-ums," which attack in swarms during warm months, or of other *Culicoides* species that transmit "nonpathogenic" filariae in tropical climates. The bite of the small humpbacked blackfly of the genus *Simulium* leaves a large bleeding puncture and painful and pruritic sores that are slow to heal; regional lymphadenopathy, fever, or anaphylaxis occasionally ensues. Blackflies are common summertime nuisances in the United States and Canada and are vectors of onchocerciasis in Africa and Latin America. The widely distributed tabanids, including deerflies (*Chrysops* species) and horseflies (*Tabanus* species), are stout flies measuring 10 to 25 mm in length that attack during the day and produce large and painful

bleeding punctures. Deerflies transmit loiasis in African equatorial rain forests and tularemia in the United States and elsewhere. Tsetse flies of the genus *Glossina* transmit African trypanosomiasis in sub-Saharan Africa. Tiny phlebotomine sand flies are the vectors of leishmaniasis, bartonellosis (Carrión's disease), sand-fly fever, and other arboviral infections in warm climates. *Stomoxys calcitrans*, the stable fly, which resembles a large housefly, is a fierce biter of human beings and domestic animals and a major pest in seacoast areas.

Treatment of fly bites is symptom-based. Topical application of antipruritic agents, glucocorticoids, or antiseptic lotions may relieve the itching and pain. Allergic reactions may require oral antihistamines. Antibiotics may be necessary for large bite wounds that become secondarily infected. Personal protection measures against biting flies include avoidance of infested areas, application of a DEET-containing repellent to exposed skin, and use of protective clothing and bed nets treated with permethrin.

Hemipteran (True Bug) Bites Several true bugs of the family Reduviidae inflict bites that produce allergic reactions and are sometimes painful. The cosmopolitan bedbug (*Cimex* species) hides in mattresses, behind bedboards, and under loose wallpaper during the day and takes its blood meal at night. The bite is painless, but sensitized persons develop erythema, itching, and wheals around a central hemorrhagic punctum. The cone-nose bugs, so called because of their elongated heads, include the assassin and wheel bugs, which feed on other insects and bite human beings only in self-defense, and the kissing bugs, which routinely feed on vertebrate blood. Assassin and wheel bugs inhabit many parts of the world, including the southwestern and southern United States, where they are notorious for their painful bites. The bites of the nocturnally feeding kissing bugs are painless and occur commonly in groups on the face and other exposed parts of the body. Reactions to such bites depend on prior sensitization and include tender and pruritic papules, vesicular or bullous lesions, giant urticaria, fever, lymphadenopathy, and anaphylaxis. *Triatoma infestans* and other species of kissing bug are the vectors of *Trypanosoma cruzi* in South and Central America and Mexico, but transmission of *T. cruzi* to human beings by species indigenous to the United States is exceedingly rare. Bug bites are treated with topical antipruritics or oral antihistamines. Persons with anaphylactic reactions to reduviid bites should keep an epinephrine kit available.

Centipede Bites and Millipede Dermatitis The fangs of centipedes of the genus *Scolopendra* can penetrate human skin and deliver a venom that produces intense burning pain, swelling, erythema, and lymphangitis. Dizziness, nausea, and anxiety are occasionally described, and rhabdomyolysis and renal failure have been reported. Treatment includes washing of the site, application of cold dressings, oral analgesic administration or local lidocaine infiltration, and tetanus prophylaxis. Species of *Scolopendra*, measuring up to 25 cm, occur widely in the southern United States and other areas with warm climates worldwide. The smaller house centipede *Scutigera coleoptrata*, which is common throughout the United States, is harmless.

Millipedes, unlike centipedes, do not bite but rather secrete and in some cases eject defensive fluids that burn and discolor human skin. Affected skin turns brown overnight and may blister and exfoliate. Secretions in the eye cause intense pain and inflammation that may lead to corneal ulceration and blindness. Management includes irrigation with copious amounts of water or saline, use of analgesics, and local care of denuded skin. Millipedes are found throughout the world in leaf litter and under rocks.

Caterpillar Stings and Dermatitis The surface of caterpillars of several moth species is covered with hairs or spines that produce mechanical irritation and may contain or be coated with venom. Contact with these caterpillars causes an immediate burning sensation followed by local swelling and erythema and occasionally by regional lymphadenopathy, nausea, vomiting, and headache; shock, seizures, and coagulopathy are rare complications. In the United States, stings are most often caused by io moth larvae and puss as well as saddleback and brown-tail moth caterpillars as they cling to leaves and branches. Contact with even detached hairs of other caterpillars, such as gypsy moth larvae (*Lymantria dispar*) in the northeastern United States, can produce a pruritic urticarial or papular rash hours later. Spines may be deposited on tree trunks and drying laundry or may be airborne and cause irritation of the eyes and upper airways. Treatment of caterpillar stings consists of repeated application of adhesive or cellophane tape to remove the hairs, which can then be identified microscopically. Local ice packs, topical steroids, and oral antihistamines relieve symptoms.

Beetle Vesication When disturbed, blister beetles extrude cantharidin, a low-molecular-weight toxin that produces thin-walled blisters measuring up to 5 cm in diameter 2 to 5 h after contact with the beetle. The blisters are not painful or pruritic unless broken, and they resolve without treatment in a week to 10 days. Nephritis may follow unusually heavy cantharidin exposure. In the southern United States, blister beetles of several *Epicauta* species are abundant in the summer months. Contact occurs when people sit on the ground, work in the garden, or deliberately handle the beetles. In other countries, different species of beetle produce different vesicants. No treatment is necessary, although ruptured blisters should be kept clean and bandaged until healing is complete.

BIBLIOGRAPHY

Auerbach PS (ed): *Wilderness Medicine*, 3d ed. St. Louis, Mosby, 1995

Beaucher WN, Farnham JE: Gypsy-moth-caterpillar dermatitis. N Engl J Med 306:1301, 1982

Burgess I: *Sarcoptes scabiei* and scabies. Adv Parasitol 33:235, 1994

Centers for Disease Control and Prevention: Necrotic arachnidism—Pacific Northwest, 1988–1996. Morb Mort Week Rep 45:433, 1996

Clark RF et al: Clinical presentation and treatment of black widow spider envenomation: A review of 163 cases. Ann Emerg Med 21:782, 1992

deShazo RD et al: Reactions to the stings of the imported fire ant. N Engl J Med 323:462, 1990

Drabick JJ: Pentastomiasis. Rev Infect Dis 9:1087, 1987

Goddard J: *Physician's Guide to Arthropods of Medical Importance*. Boca Raton, FL, CRC Press, 1993

Hall M, Wall R: Myiasis of humans and domestic animals. Adv Parasitol 35:257, 1995

Meinking TL et al: The treatment of scabies with ivermectin. N Engl J Med 333:26, 1995

Millikan LE: Mite infestations other than scabies. Semin Dermatol 12:22, 1993

Peters W: *A Colour Atlas of Arthropods in Clinical Medicine*. London, Wolfe, 1992

Reisman RE: Insect stings. N Engl J Med 331:523, 1994

Tan BB et al: Double-blind controlled trial of effect of house dust-mite allergen avoidance on atopic dermatitis. Lancet 347:15, 1996

Williams ST et al: Severe intravascular hemolysis associated with brown recluse spider envenomation. A report of two cases and review of the literature. Am J Clin Pathol 104:463, 1995

394 *Jerome H. Modell*

DROWNING AND NEAR-DROWNING

It is an unexpected tragedy when a previously healthy person dies or is exposed to severe cerebral hypoxia and suffers permanent brain damage. For many years, drowning was considered a "fight for survival": Arms flailing and screaming for help, a person who could not swim struggled to remain on the surface of the water to reach safety. This situation, however, is rarely reported by persons at the scene of aquatic emergencies. Furthermore, no single set of circumstances comprises drowning or near-drowning. It may be a secondary event following such precursors as head or spinal trauma, hypoxia-induced unconsciousness, or unconsciousness due to preexisting cardiovascular disease, sudden cardiac death, or myocardial infarction. The initiating event is usually unknown, so the drowned or near-drowned victim must be treated based on probable physiologic effects of the near-drowning itself. If survival with normal brain function is to occur, a thorough understanding of the pathophysiology of drowning and an organized approach to therapy are imperative.

PATHOPHYSIOLOGY OF DROWNING Approximately 90 percent of drowning victims aspirate fluid into their lungs. In those who do not aspirate fluid, hypoxemia results simply from apnea. In those who do aspirate, the volume and the composition of the fluid determine the physiologic basis of the hypoxemia. Freshwater aspiration alters the surface tension properties of pulmonary surfactant and makes alveoli unstable, which causes a decreased ventilation/perfusion ratio. Some alveoli collapse and become atelectatic, which produces a true or absolute intrapulmonary shunt, while others are poorly ventilated and produce a relative shunt; in either case, significant pulmonary venous admixture occurs. Fresh water in the alveoli is hypotonic and is rapidly absorbed and redistributed throughout the body. While some have proposed that water continues to enter the lungs after death, at autopsy, the lungs of victims who died in the water frequently contain little water. These findings support the premise that active respiration determines the volume of water aspirated.

Hypertonic seawater pulls additional fluid from the plasma into the lungs, and thus the alveoli are fluid-filled but perfused, which causes substantial pulmonary venous admixture. With both types of water, pulmonary edema may occur secondary to events such as fluid shifts, a change in capillary permeability, or cerebral hypoxia, which causes neurogenic pulmonary edema. Regardless of the cause, pulmonary edema adds to the ventilation/perfusion abnormality.

Water that is grossly contaminated with bacteria or that contains particulate matter may complicate the picture. Particulate matter can obstruct the smaller bronchi and respiratory bronchioles. Grossly contaminated water increases the risk of severe pulmonary infection. Neither problem is sufficiently common, however, to justify recommending specific therapy routinely for all victims.

At least 85 percent of near-drowned victims are thought to aspirate 22 mL/kg of water or less, which does not significantly affect blood volume or serum electrolyte concentrations. After resuscitation, by the time blood is analyzed, serum electrolyte concentrations usually are normal or close to normal. Significant changes are documented in only approximately 15 percent of those who cannot be resuscitated and only rarely in those who are resuscitated. These findings suggest that either a small amount of water was aspirated, fluid was rapidly redistributed, or both. Therefore, electrolyte disturbance rarely needs treatment. When a large quantity of water is aspirated, seawater causes hypovolemia, which concentrates extracellular electrolytes, and fresh water causes acute hypervolemia. If enough water is aspirated that plasma becomes severely hypotonic and the patient is hypoxemic,

red cell membranes can rupture, and plasma hemoglobin and serum potassium concentrations increase significantly. However, this development has been reported only rarely. With rapid redistribution of fluid and development of pulmonary edema, even freshwater victims frequently demonstrate hypovolemia by the time they reach the hospital.

Hypercarbia, which is associated with apnea and/or hypoventilation, is less often documented by blood gas analysis than is hypoxemia. While hypoxemia due to pulmonary venous admixture persists in all near-drowned victims who aspirate water, hypercarbia is usually corrected sooner with artificial mechanical ventilation and improved minute ventilation and, thus, is reported in only a small percentage of victims evaluated at the hospital. Besides hypoxemia, metabolic acidosis also persists in most patients. Abnormal cardiovascular function, usually ascribed to hypoxemia, is brief with effective, timely therapy. Abnormality in renal function is uncommon, but when it does occur, it too is secondary to hypoxemia, altered renal perfusion, or, in extremely rare circumstances, significant hemoglobinuria.

TREATMENT OF NEAR-DROWNING The first step is retrieving the victim from the water, and, if necessary, performing artificial ventilation and circulation. The American Heart Association recommends that an abdominal thrust not be used routinely in victims of submersion. This recommendation was upheld by a special committee of the Institute of Medicine convened in 1994 specifically to evaluate the efficacy of an abdominal thrust in the treatment of near-drowned victims. In these patients, an abdominal thrust may lead to regurgitation of gastric contents and, thus, to aspiration of the vomitus. Further, an abdominal thrust may delay ventilatory or circulatory resuscitation. Therefore, an abdominal thrust should only be used when the airway is obstructed with a foreign body or when the victim fails to respond to mouth-to-mouth ventilation.

Because emergency services and intensive pulmonary and cardiovascular care have improved during the past two decades, central nervous system depression now presents the major therapeutic challenge in near-drowning. The rate of survival with normal cerebral function varies considerably in retrospective studies. Some factors that adversely influence survival are prolonged submersion, delay in initiation of effective cardiopulmonary resuscitation, severe metabolic acidosis (pH < 7.1), asystole upon arrival to a medical facility, fixed dilated pupils, and a low Glasgow coma score (<5). None of these predictors is absolute, however, and normal survivors have been reported in all of the above categories. Absence of cortical evoked potentials does indicate irreversibility of the cerebral hypoxic lesion; this test, however, cannot be done in the field to guide rescuers. A comparison of outcomes between one institution that added brain preservation techniques to intensive pulmonary and circulatory treatment and another institution that did not found no significant differences.

Hypothermia appears to be protective, but only if it occurs early, at the time of the accident, in which case it increases the victim's chance of cerebral salvage after relatively long periods of acute hypoxia and cardiac arrest. While hypothermia prolongs tolerance to hypoxia, it also can precipitate fatal cardiac arrhythmia; thus, its occurrence can be helpful on the one hand and harmful on the other. The diving reflex produces bradycardia, breath-holding, and circulatory redistribution when the face is submerged in cold water. However, the effect of the diving reflex in explaining cerebral recovery after prolonged immersion has not been specifically documented.

Significant pulmonary venous admixture usually persists even after successful resuscitation; therefore, supplemental oxygen should be administered until arterial blood gas analysis confirms that oxygen is no longer needed. Intravenous access should be established as soon as possible. The trachea should be intubated if necessary for airway maintenance or to facilitate mechanical ventilatory support. Electrocardiographic monitoring will facilitate prompt treatment of cardiac arrhythmia.

Victims should be transported to a hospital for definitive testing of the adequacy of ventilation and blood gas exchange, cardiac activity, and effective circulating blood volume. Other variables, such as serum electrolyte concentrations, renal function, and cerebral status, should be analyzed as indicated.

The single most effective treatment for hypoxemia, regardless of cause, is mechanical ventilatory support including continuous positive airway pressure (CPAP). After freshwater aspiration, improvement in ventilation/perfusion matching is more consistent when CPAP is combined with mechanical inflation of the lung than with spontaneous respiration. The question of whether CPAP should be combined with spontaneous respiration or with mechanical ventilation should be decided by whether the specific patient can perform the necessary work of breathing, adequately eliminate carbon dioxide, and adequately match ventilation/perfusion ratios. Positive airway pressure should be withdrawn gradually as the lungs stabilize and ventilation/perfusion ratio returns toward normal.

The pH in near-drowned victims is commonly significantly acidotic, which, in turn, can depress cardiac function. The metabolic component of the acidosis, if it results in a pH < 7.20, should be corrected pharmacologically, although there is some disagreement on this point. With cardiovascular instability, cannulation of the pulmonary artery with a Swan-Ganz catheter or evaluation by transesophageal echocardiography is indicated. Many patients will be hypovolemic from loss of fluid into the lung as pulmonary edema or from decreased venous return secondary to increased intrathoracic pressure during mechanical ventilatory support.

Because recovery after long periods of submersion under frigid conditions has been reported, body temperature should be taken into account before a decision is made to terminate therapy. The body temperature of victims depends not only on the temperature of the water from which they are retrieved but also on how well they were insulated by clothing. The volume of water actually aspirated is also important, because a large volume, if distributed before cardiac arrest occurs, can produce rapid central cooling. Thus, cold water can be protective when it produces total-body hypothermia, which decreases metabolic oxygen requirement. On the other hand, cold water may also contribute to the accident if hypothermia occurs before total submersion, and severe, or even fatal, cardiac arrhythmia results. Several methods of rewarming hypothermic victims have been advocated, but any technique that increases oxygen utilization, such as shivering, should be avoided.

Regardless of the conditions surrounding a drowning or near-drowning, treatment should adhere to the following sequence of priorities (Fig. 394-1):

1. Remove the victim from the water as soon as possible and stabilize the patient's head and neck if trauma is suspected.

2. Immediately follow the ABCs of cardiopulmonary resuscitation—even in the water if this does not endanger the rescuer.

3. If the patient is unconscious, protect the airway as needed with endotracheal intubation.

4. Establish venous access as soon as possible.

5. Provide supplemental oxygen and ventilatory support until each is no longer needed. This can be judged from analysis of arterial blood for oxygen tension, carbon dioxide tension, and pH.

6. Monitor cardiac rhythm with an electrocardioscope as soon as possible.

7. Monitor body temperature and restore it to normal.

8. If the patient has persistent respiratory insufficiency, provide intensive pulmonary support with CPAP and mechanical ventilation therapy as necessary.

9. If the patient has cardiovascular instability, evaluate cardiac output and effective circulatory volume by invasive monitoring, and measure serum electrolyte concentrations.

10. Evaluate and treat renal function and cerebral status as indicated.

FIGURE 394-1 Treatment of a near-drowned victim should follow a sequence of priorities. *Guidelines only; assumes victim had normal arterial blood gas values (ABGs) before near-drowning. Abbreviations/definitions: CPAP, continuous positive airway pressure; CPR, cardiopulmonary resuscitation; $F_{I_{O_2}}$, fraction of inspired oxygen; intubate: endotracheal intubation; ICU, intensive care unit; NaHCO₃, bicarbonate; Pa_{O_2}/Pa_{CO_2}, arterial oxygen/carbon dioxide tension; pHa, arterial pH. (*Modified from Graves and Layon.*)

Glucocorticoid therapy, prophylactic antibiotic therapy, and monitoring of intracranial pressure are no longer recommended.

ACCIDENT PREVENTION Because drowning begins as an accident that results in a medical problem, the definitive strategy is to prevent the accident. For those victims in whom the accident is secondary to a medical condition, as in persons susceptible to syncope or seizure, the only way to prevent the accident is to identify those who ought to avoid the water or to encourage them to use the buddy system. For young children, early swimming lessons, vigilant caretakers, and stringent laws governing pool enclosures are needed. Those who teach parenting classes should routinely warn parents about the risk of toddlers' drowning in such household fixtures as toilets, buckets of water, and even washing machines. Preventing accidents during boating, athletics, and other water-related recreational activities requires public education. Rules associated with these activities to maximize safety and judicious, responsible behavior should be portrayed as life-saving measures. Similarly, drinking alcohol, a "ubiquitous catalyst" to drowning, should be portrayed as life-threatening whenever water is nearby.

BIBLIOGRAPHY

AMERICAN HEART ASSOCIATION: Guidelines for cardiopulmonary resuscitation and emergency cardiac care. JAMA 268:2171, 1992

BOHN DJ et al: Influence of hypothermia, barbiturate therapy, and intracranial pressure monitoring on morbidity and mortality after near-drowning. Crit Care Med 14:529, 1986

FULLER RH: The 1962 Welcome Prize Essay. Drowning and the postimmersion syndrome. A clinicopathologic study. Milit Med 128:22, 1963

GRAVES SA, LAYON AJ: Drowning and near-drowning, in *Emergency Medicine: A Comprehensive Review*, 3d ed, TC Kravis et al (eds). New York, Raven, 1993, pp 689–700

MODELL JH: Drowning. N Engl J Med 328:253, 1993

————: *Pathophysiology and Treatment of Drowning and Near-Drowning*. Springfield, IL, Charles C Thomas, 1971

———— et al: Clinical course of 91 consecutive near-drowning victims. Chest 70:231, 1976

ORNATO JP: The resuscitation of near-drowning victims. JAMA 256:75, 1986

ROSEN P et al (eds): *The Use of the Heimlich Maneuver in Near-Drowning*. Committee on the Treatment of Near-Drowning Victims, Institute of Medicine, Washington, DC, 1994

395 *Alan R. Dimick*

ELECTRICAL INJURIES

EPIDEMIOLOGY The exact incidence of electrical injury is unknown. Each year in the United States, approximately 1000 deaths, constituting roughly 1 percent of all accidental deaths, are attributed to electric current. The prevalence of electrical technology in modern society has resulted in more people experiencing electrical injury. The current treatment of electrical injury has resulted in a low mortality, ranging from 3 to 15 percent, but the amputation rate remains high, and disfigurement due to extensive soft tissue destruction is frequent. More than 60 percent of the electricity-related fatalities occur in males, with the highest incidence among those 20 to 34 years of age. Approximately one-third of *high-voltage* injuries occur in electrical workers, one-third in construction workers, and the remainder from non-work-related events. One-half of *low-voltage* injuries occur at home, most of them to young children. Burn center referral is usually necessary for electrical burns.

PATHOPHYSIOLOGY Electrical burns result from the conversion of electrical energy into heat. Factors that determine the severity and distribution of injury include the type of current (direct or alternating), the quantity of the current (amperage), the potential of the current (voltage), the resistance offered by the body, the pathway of the current, and the duration of contact. These variables are interrelated, and their interactions produce the varied spectrum of injury seen clinically.

Direct and alternating current have different effects. At low voltages (<1000 V), the low-frequency (40 to 150 Hz) alternating current range, which is used almost exclusively for incandescent lighting and appliances, is three times more dangerous than direct current. Immediate death can result from ventricular fibrillation, central respiratory arrest, or asphyxia due to tetanic respiratory muscle contractions. Tetanic muscle spasms, which freeze the contact point to the power source, tend to increase the flow of current and the severity of injury. Cutaneous burns may be entirely absent or minimal. In contrast, at high voltages, high-frequency alternating current and direct current are equally lethal.

Survivals from electric shocks of greater than 100,000 V and deaths from as little as 50 V have occurred, which underscores the interplay of the variables already noted. Clinically, the severity of injury relates primarily to the voltage. Low-voltage contact, while potentially lethal, does not result in the magnitude of tissue necrosis seen with high-voltage injury. Tissue resistance is an important factor in determining both the initiation of current flow and its subsequent path. A person completing a circuit between two contact points has a resistance that is the sum of the skin resistances at both contact points plus the internal body resistance. If skin resistance is high, there will be considerable local tissue destruction. Conversely, if skin resistance is low, systemic effects, such as those on the heart and brain, predominate. Skin resistance varies widely according to the thickness, cleanliness, and wetness of the skin. The resistance of skin in water is only about 0.1 percent of the resistance of dry skin. The extent of tissue damage can be explained by the differing resistances of various tissues. Listed in the order of increasing magnitude of resistance are nerves, blood vessels, muscle, skin, tendon, fat, and bone.

All tissues and organs can be affected by electrical injury. The cutaneous burns are often limited, with variable deep tissue damage. Appreciation of this special property of electrical wounds is critical in their management. Skin wounds are typically leathery or charred areas of full-thickness skin loss. The entry and exit sites are usually depressed, giving the appearance that current exploded the tissues. The arc burn is produced by current coursing external to the body from contact to ground, favoring a path of least resistance. The flexor surfaces of the wrist, elbow, and axilla are most often involved, because the hand is the most commonly involved body part. After several days, the demarcation between viable and nonviable tissue becomes more obvious. Flame burns of the skin may result from ignition of clothing by electrical arcing and may be full-thickness burns because of the prolonged exposure of the dazed victim to the flame.

The most severe cardiopulmonary manifestations occur at the time of the injury. These include anoxia and ventricular fibrillation, which may cause immediate death due to respiratory or cardiac arrest. Major electrical injury is accompanied by a 3 to 15 percent incidence of acute renal failure, which is greater than the incidence after thermal burns.

Nervous tissue is highly susceptible to electrical injury because of its low resistance. Neurologic deficits can be seen initially or up to 3 years later, and neurologic aberrations are the most frequent nonfatal sequelae of electrical injury. An important diagnostic point is to ask the patient if the details of the accident are remembered. An inability to recall recent events indicates that electricity entered the body, erasing recent memory. This loss of recent memory is used by psychiatrists treating severely depressed people by means of electroshock therapy. Lesions of the central nervous system may cause varying levels of consciousness and respiratory and motor paralysis, which are usually transient; recovery is the rule. If the effects are permanent, they often assume the character of cortical encephalopathy or hemiplegia with or without aphasia. Spinal cord damage is the most common permanent sequela of electrical injury and is seldom complete. Many deficits seen initially resolve spontaneously; others may not develop until 6 to 9 months after the electrical injury. Permanent deficits may not be seen for days to months, are of gradual onset, and progress slowly. Often these disturbances are not noted until the rehabilitative phase of recovery, when gait abnormalities become evident. Peripheral nerves may be burned directly or may be compressed by surrounding edema or scar tissue. Neuropathies also can develop in unburned limbs. Autonomic nervous system dysfunction may be seen in both the acute and recovery phases. Reflex sympathetic dystrophy or causalgia can occur. Late onset of burning pain, frequently associated with vasomotor, trophic, and dermal changes, is characteristic.

Cataracts characteristically occur following high-voltage injuries. The incidence of these lesions, which are usually bilateral, may be as great as 30 percent when electrical contact is made above the clavicles, particularly when the entry wound is on the head. The latent period between the accident and the onset of blurred vision averages 6 months but ranges from a few weeks to 3 years.

Direct vascular injury is more common after electrical injury than after any other type of burn. The blood flow in large arteries and veins is usually sufficient to dissipate the heat generated by the electric current. However, smaller vessels may experience significant heat-related damage, resulting in thrombosis. Direct vascular injury probably contributes to the high amputation rate after high-voltage electrical injury. Delayed hemorrhage from mural necrosis of large blood vessels also may occur.

Associated injury in electrical accidents can be due to falls of considerable distance or to the explosive effects of the current. Fractures of the vertebrae and long bones and dislocations also may result from the violent tetanic muscle contractions.

℞ TREATMENT

At the scene of the accident, the patient must be separated immediately from the electric current, but rescuers must not touch or approach the patient until the current has been shut off to avoid injury to themselves. Flames should then be extinguished.

Cardiopulmonary support must be initiated if necessary and maintained during transport. Aggressive life support is essential, because victims of high-voltage electrical injury may be resuscitated successfully without permanent neurologic damage even after a prolonged cessation of vital functions. Because blunt trauma and skeletal injury may both coexist, a thorough history and careful physical examination are essential. Accurate assessment of the extent and nature of the burns is essential to the determination of subsequent therapy. Neurologic status must be evaluated repeatedly during convalescence because it changes frequently.

Fluid replacement is essential in the initial management. Hypovolemia results from the rapid loss of fluid into damaged tissues. Small entry and exit wounds may lead to underestimation of the underlying injury, so fluid requirements may be grossly underestimated. Ringer's lactate should be infused rapidly (0.5 to 1 mL/kg per hour) as necessary to correct hypovolemia and to maintain urinary output. Large volumes of fluid are necessary in high-voltage injury because the fluid and electrolyte needs are much greater than in patients with thermal burns of equivalent surface area. The adequacy of resuscitation is monitored, with urinary output being the single most reliable indicator of circulatory status. The presence of urinary hemoglobin and myoglobin necessitates treatment with mannitol, and the urine should be made alkaline to prevent precipitation of these pigments in the kidney. When hemoglobinuria and/or myoglobinuria is present, the rate and volume of the crystalloid infusion must be sufficient to maintain a minimum urine output of 100 mL/h. This infusion is continued until the urine is grossly clear of pigment. Acute renal failure, if it occurs, is treated as described in Chap. 270. Red blood cell transfusion, plasma, dextran, or other plasma expanders are unnecessary during the acute resuscitative phase.

Low-Voltage Injury Injuries resulting from low-voltage current, such as those related to household appliances, are usually small and limited to the area of contact. These burns frequently involve the hands, feet, or, in children, the corners of the mouth, lips, and tongue. The evolution of tissue injury and vascular necrosis from the current itself are complete within 7 to 10 days. During this time, the wounds are allowed to slough and heal by contracture. Small but deep contact injuries on the trunk and extremities may be excised and grafted as necessary when the extent of the slough is evident. Early excision and local flap repair are rarely indicated. Delayed bleeding from the lip, seen in one-quarter of these injuries, is usually readily controlled by direct pressure.

High-Voltage Injury High-voltage injuries with devitalized skin, fat, and muscle are fundamentally surgical problems. They usually involve a limited amount of the total body surface, have upper-extremity contact points, and require amputation or other surgical procedures. They may affect any organ system. The ultimate treatment goals are stabilization of the patient, salvage of the limb, debridement of devitalized tissue, wound coverage, and rehabilitation. Prolonged expectant nonsurgical therapy only increases the risk of invasive infection.

The timing of surgical debridement and its aggressiveness are controversial issues. Opinions range from early total excision with primary wound closure to the now outmoded expectant nonsurgical approach. Most surgeons favor an intermediate approach, individualizing according to the amount of tissue destruction and the location and type of the injury. Major amputations and surgical debridement are usually performed 2 to 4 days following injury, when the extent of necrosis is reasonably well defined but the risk of significant infection is small. High-voltage electrical burns frequently produce muscle compartment syndromes requiring fasciotomy. Circumferential deep limb burns due to associated flame or arc burns also may require escharotomy or fasciotomy. Indications for surgical decompression include loss of distal pulses, impaired capillary filling, paresthesia, and rigid muscle compartments. Decompression of the carpal tunnel is especially important owing to the high incidence of electrical injury to hands. If done expeditiously, this procedure may save a hand.

Debridement When possible, formal amputation and major debridement are delayed for 2 to 4 days following injury. During this interval, neurologic and cardiopulmonary abnormalities usually stabilize or resolve, and the demarcation between viable and nonviable tissues becomes more evident. Because these wounds are prone to anaerobic infection, particularly myonecrosis with clostridia, aqueous penicillin is given prophylactically from the time of admission until debridement is complete. Antibiotic administration should be further guided by identification of infecting organisms. Local wound care is started immediately and includes mechanical cleansing followed by the application of topical antibacterial agents and cotton gauze dressings. Silver sulfadiazine cream has excellent antibacterial activity but penetrates only a few millimeters into the tissues. Sulfamylon, a burn cream containing mafenide (a carbonic anhydrase inhibitor that readily penetrates soft tissue), may be advantageous in deep injuries and, therefore, is the topical agent of choice in the prevention and/or treatment of deep-seated infections. However, when absorbed, this drug causes a bicarbonate diuresis resulting in systemic acidosis.

Coverage of open wounds usually requires skin grafting. Deep electrical injuries frequently result in complex soft tissue wounds, which may require skin flaps for coverage. Nutritional support is essential and should be instituted early. As with other types of burns, appropriate splints should be fashioned and applied, and an aggressive program of physical therapy should be formulated and instituted. Psychological counseling is usually beneficial for patients who require a major amputation or other mutilating surgical procedure.

LIGHTNING INJURY

When the difference in potential between the undersurface of a cloud that becomes progressively more negative and the surface of the earth, which is positive, exceeds the insulator strength of air, electrical energy discharges as lightning. There are four mechanisms of lightning strike:

direct strike, flashover phenomenon, side flash, and stride potential. A direct strike consists of a major current flow directly through the victim. It is the most serious type of strike and is facilitated by metal objects such as golf clubs, umbrellas, or tools carried during a thunderstorm. In flashover, the lightning travels on the outside of the body; this type of strike is facilitated by wet garments and sweat. Side flash occurs when the current splashes from a building, tree, or other person and then travels to the victim. Stride potential occurs when the lightning strikes the ground close to a victim with one foot touching the ground closer to the point of the lightning strike than the other foot. In this position, there will be a potential electrical difference between the legs called *stride potential*. The lightning current may enter one leg, pass up and through the victim's body, and exit through the other leg. Stride potential and side-flash strikes can involve several individuals at once and may contribute to the multiple casualties often associated with lightning strike.

The pathophysiology of lightning injury is similar to that described for other electrical injuries. Lightning is direct current. The voltage of lightning may range from 3 million to 200 million volts and may carry a current of between 2000 and 3000 A. Lightning victims have a very short exposure to current because of the brief duration of lightning strike, which usually lasts only 1 to 100 ms. Most of the current may flash over the outside of the body. In contrast, contact with current from high-voltage electrical injuries may be prolonged, since the victim may become frozen to the current source. The injuries resulting from lightning strikes are similar to those from direct current and alternating current, as described above. Thus, treatment is essentially the same as for other types of electrical injury. The best form of treatment is prevention, consisting of avoidance of dangerous situations during rainstorms and electrical storms, such as standing near tall structures and metal poles or beneath metal shelters. It is erroneous to assume that once lightning strikes it is safe to venture into the open; another strike may occur in the same location. Many towers and churches have sustained multiple strikes.

BIBLIOGRAPHY

GROSSMAN AR et al: Auditory and neuropsychiatric behavior patterns after electrical injury. J Burn Care Rehab 14:169, 1993

GRUBE BJ et al: Neurologic consequences of electrical burns. J Trauma 30:254, 1990

HANUMADASS ML et al: Acute electrical burns: A 10-year clinical experience. Burns 12:427, 1986

JORDAN MH et al: Lightning strike to the head. J Trauma 36:113, 1994

LICHTENBERG R et al: Cardiovascular effects of lightning strikes. J Am Coll Cardiol 21:531, 1993

LIFSCHULTZ BD, DONOGHUE ER: Deaths caused by lightning. J Forensic Sci 38:353, 1993

PATTEN BM: Lightning and electrical injuries: A review. Neurol Clin 10:1047, 1992

SAFFLE JR et al: Recent outcomes in the treatment of burn injury in the U.S. J Burn Care Rehab 16:219, 1995

396 *L. Chinsoo Cho, Eli Glatstein*

RADIATION INJURY

All human beings are constantly exposed to ionizing radiation. The sources of radiation include both the natural environment and man-made products. The natural sources include the cosmic radiation from space and radiation from the ground and from inhaled and ingested materials. Airline travel and mining both increase exposure to the background radiation. For example, air travel at 30,000 ft exposes individuals to a dose equivalent of 0.5 mrem/h. Radiation originating in the body comes mainly from radioactive potassium, which emits beta and gamma rays. Lungs are exposed to irradiation from inhaled air, which contains small amounts of radioactive radon. The cosmic exposure contributes approximately 28 mrem per year. The ground and internal sources contribute approximately 26 and 27 mrem per year, respec-

tively. The most prominent man-made sources of radiation include x-ray equipment, nuclear weapons, and radioactive medications.

TERMINOLOGY AND DEFINITIONS

The first major unit of radiation exposure was the roentgen (R), defined as an amount of x-rays or gamma rays that produces a specific amount of ionization in a unit of air under standard temperature and pressure (Table 396-1); this quantity can be measured directly in an ionization chamber. The rad, or *r*adiation *a*bsorbed *d*ose, is defined as 100 ergs/g of tissue. Thus, the rad represents a net deposition of energy in a three-dimensional volume, because x-rays attenuate as they traverse tissue. The rad has been replaced by the Système Internationale (SI) unit of the gray (Gy), which represents 100 rad. Roentgens and rads can be converted by means of various tables; the relation between them depends on photon energy.

The above definitions reflect physical variables. The unit that reflects the biologic response and that can be used to compare the effects of various types of radiation is the unit of *dose equivalence*, the rem (*r*oentgen *e*quivalent in *m*an). The rem has been replaced by the SI unit, the sievert (Sv). These units reflect the exposure or absorption dose multiplied by a biologic factor that represents the biologic effectiveness of the specific type of radiation (see below).

TYPES OF IONIZING RADIATION

The absorption of energy from radiation in tissue often leads to excitation or ionization. Excitation involves elevation of an electron in an atom or molecule to a higher energy state without actual ejection of the electron. Ionization involves actual ejection of one or more electrons from the atom. Ionizing radiation is subclassified as electromagnetic (photon) or particulate radiation (Table 396-2). X-rays and gamma rays are examples of electromagnetic photon radiation. They differ only in their source: X-rays are produced mechanically, by making electrons strike a target, which causes the electrons to give up their kinetic energy as x-rays, while gamma rays are produced by nuclear disintegration of radioactive isotopes. The wavelength λ of the electromagnetic radiation is related to the frequency v by the formula $\lambda v = c$, where c is the speed of light. Thus, wavelength is inversely proportional to frequency. The wavelength for x-rays is on the order of 10^{-10} m (1 Å).

X-rays can be thought of as packets of energy, or photons. X-rays have no mass or charge, travel in straight lines, and attenuate continuously as they traverse tissue. Gamma rays have similar properties. Each photon contains an amount of energy equal to hv, where h is Planck's constant. The critical difference between nonionizing and ionizing radiation is the energy of individual photons, not the energy of the total dose. The energy in keV of a particular x-ray or gamma ray can be calculated to be equal to 12.4 divided by the wavelength in angstroms.

Table 396-1

Units and Definitions

Unit	Quantity Measured	Definition
Roentgen (R)	Exposure	Amount of x-rays or gamma rays that produces a specific amount of ionization in a given volume of air
Rad	Dose	100 ergs deposited per gram of tissue
Gray (Gy)	Dose	SI unit of dose; equals 100 rad
Rem	Dose equivalence	Unit that reflects the biologic response. It is used to compare various types of radiation
Sievert (Sv)	Dose equivalence	SI unit of dose equivalence; equals 100 rem

Table 396-2

Common Types of Ionizing Radiation

Type	Mass	Charge	Comment
Electromagnetic			
X-ray	0	0	X-rays and gamma rays
Gamma ray	0	0	do not differ except in the source. Gamma rays are produced intranuclearly, and x-rays are produced extranuclearly (i.e., mechanically).
Particulate			
Electron (e)	9.1×10^{-31} kg	-1	—
Proton (p)	$2000 \times e$	$+1$	Exhibits a Bragg peak
Neutron (n)	$2000 \times e$	0	Cannot be accelerated by an electrical field
Alpha particle	$2p + 2n$ $\sim 8000 \times e$	$+2$	Helium nucleus

Types of *particulate radiation* include electrons, protons, alpha particles, neutrons, negative pi-mesons, and heavy charged ions; these have discrete mass and charge (except for neutrons, which lack charge) (see Table 396-2). *Electrons*, or *beta particles*, are small and negatively charged, and can be accelerated to close to the speed of light. They decelerate fairly rapidly in tissue and penetrate it to only a limited depth. Thus, electron beams are often used to treat superficial problems. *Protons* are positively charged and have a mass about 2000 times that of an electron. Protons stop abruptly, depending on their energy; in the process of sudden deceleration, most of their energy is given up, which tends to cause ionization just before the proton stops. This region of enhanced ionization, sometimes called the Bragg peak, means that proton beams exert their effects in a relatively compact region. *Alpha particles* are helium nuclei, consisting of two protons and two neutrons. The mass and charge are great enough that these particles do not penetrate far through matter unless they have tremendous energy; even a piece of paper is enough to protect against most alpha particles. Because these particles are charged, they can be accelerated in electrical fields.

Neutrons are similar in mass to protons (having an atomic mass of 1), but they are not charged and therefore cannot be accelerated in an electrical field. Neutron beams are produced by colliding charged particles into a suitable target or are emitted as a fission product of heavy radioactive atoms. *Heavy charged ions* are nuclei of heavier elements that have a positive charge owing to the stripping away of some or all of the orbiting electrons.

Equal doses of different types of radiation do not necessarily produce equal biologic effects. One gray of neutrons produces a greater biologic effect than 1 Gy of x-rays. The biologic effects produced by a given dose of radiation can be quantified by the relative biologic effectiveness (RBE) value, which relates them to the effects produced by 250 kV photon radiation as a standard. The RBE value will be greater for more densely ionizing radiation, such as neutrons. In general, the RBE value depends on the linear energy transfer (see below), the dose, the dose rate, and the nature of the biologic system. Gamma rays and x-rays generally have an RBE of approximately 1. Beta radiation (electrons) also has an RBE of approximately 1. The exact RBE value depends on the specific energy. Higher-energy x-rays are associated with a slightly lower RBE value. Neutrons and alpha particles have RBEs of about 3 for most biologic systems.

The linear energy transfer (LET) is the amount of ionization occurring per unit length of the radiation track. It is usually expressed as kilovolts per micron, and it increases with the square of the charge of the incident particle. High-LET radiation is biologically different from low-LET (i.e., conventional) radiation: Hypoxic and oxygenated cells respond similarly to high-LET irradiation, whereas it takes about three times as much low-LET radiation to produce a given killing effect in hypoxic cells as in oxygenated cells. It is thought that low-LET radiation must produce multiple hits on DNA to destroy a cell, whereas high-LET radiation need produce only a single hit on DNA to kill a cell. Representative values of LET and RBE are given in Table 396-3.

There are three major ways in which radiation, especially x-rays, is absorbed and results in ionization: the *photoelectric effect*, the *Compton effect*, and *pair production*. At low energies (30 to 100 keV), as in diagnostic radiology, the photoelectric effect is important. In this process, the incident photon interacts with an electron in one of the outer shells of an atom (typically K, L, or M). If the energy of the photon is greater than the binding energy of the electron, then the electron is expelled from the orbit with a kinetic energy that is equal to the energy of the incident photon minus the binding energy of the electron. The photoelectric effect varies as a function of the cube of the atomic number of the material exposed (Z^3); this fact explains why bone is visualized much better than soft tissue on radiographs.

At higher energies, as used in therapeutic radiology, the Compton effect dominates. In this process, the incident photon interacts with an electron in an orbital shell. Part of the incident photon energy appears as kinetic energy of electrons, and the residual energy continues as a less energetic deflected photon.

At energy levels above 1.02 MeV, the photons may be absorbed through pair production. In this process, both a positron and an electron are produced in the absorbing material. A positron has the same mass as an electron but has a positive instead of a negative charge. The positron travels a very short distance in the absorbing medium before it interacts with another electron. When that happens, the entire mass of both particles is converted to energy, with the emission of two photons in exactly opposite directions.

BIOLOGIC EFFECTS OF RADIATION

Radiation must generally produce double-strand breaks in DNA to kill a cell, owing partly to the high capacity of mammalian cells for repairing single-strand damage. Radiation can also produce effects indirectly by interacting with water (which makes up approximately 80 percent of a cell's volume) to generate free radicals, which can damage the cell. Free radicals are highly reactive chemical entities that lack a stable number of outer-shell electrons. A free radical is not stable and has a life span of a fraction of a second. It is estimated that most x-ray–induced cell damage is due to the formation of hydroxyl radicals, as follows:

$$\text{Ionizing radiation} + H_2O \rightarrow H_2O^+ + e^-$$
$$H_2O^+ + H_2O \rightarrow H_3O^+ + OH\cdot$$
$$OH\cdot \rightarrow \text{Cell damage}$$

Cell killing is the result of radiation damage. The biologic effects on epithelial cell reproduction are typically expressed only when the damaged cells attempt to divide. Another biologic effect is the induction of cancerous growth by mutation many years after radiation exposure. It is clear that patients who receive low doses of radiation in childhood have a significant risk of neoplasm two to three decades after their exposure; this risk is significantly higher than that of the population as a whole.

Table 396-3

LET and RBE Values

Type of Radiation	LET Values, keV/μm
Cobalt-60 gamma rays	0.2
250-keV x-rays	2.0
10 MeV protons	4.7

Type of Radiation	RBE Values (Quality Factors)
X-rays, gamma rays, and electrons	1
Neutrons	3–20
Heavy particles	1–20

Chromosome breaks can occur when cells are irradiated. The broken ends of chromosomes can combine with broken ends of different chromosomes. These abnormal combinations are most readily seen during mitosis. Chromosome abnormalities typically occur in cells irradiated in the G1 phase of the cell cycle, before the doubling of genetic material. If cells are irradiated in the G2 phase, chromatid aberrations may result. The frequency of chromosomal aberrations in peripheral circulating lymphocytes correlates with dose received. The dose can be estimated by comparing the chromosomal changes to in vitro cultures exposed to controlled doses of irradiation. The minimum dose that can be detected by peripheral lymphocyte analysis is about 10 to 20 rem. Lymphocyte analysis may provide evidence of recent total-body exposure.

CELL SURVIVAL CURVE The dose-response curve for all mammalian cells appears to have a linear-quadratic relationship. In simple terms, the mathematical model that explains the relationship between the dose and the fraction of surviving cells has both linear and exponential components. The linear component results from double-stranded chromosomal breaks produced by single hits. The exponential component represents breaks produced by multiple hits. Figure 396-1 shows the shape of a typical survival curve for mammalian cells exposed to radiation. The fraction of cells surviving is plotted on a semilogarithmic scale. For alpha particles or low-energy neutrons, the dose-response curve is a straight line from the origin. There appears to be no shoulder, which is thought to represent the accumulation of sublethal events within the cells beyond which one additional hit will cause cell death, and which also reflects the cell's ability to repair sublethal injury. Thus, the survival rate is an exponential function of the dose. In the case of x-rays or gamma rays, the dose-response curve has a shoulder, which is followed by a straight-line curve as the dose is increased.

D_0 represents the straight-line portion of the curve; it is the dose required to reduce the fraction of surviving cells to 37 percent of its previous value. D_0 represents the dose at which each cell receives an average of one lethal hit. The number N is defined by extrapolating the D_0 line directly back to the Y axis and is a measure of the width of the shoulder; presumably it represents the cell's repair capability. D_q is the dose at which the straight portion of the curve intersects a horizontal line drawn through unity; it represents a quasi-threshold dose.

In all mammalian cell lines studied, increases in the radiation dose decrease the survival rate of cells; i.e., there is no absolute radioresistance for mammalian cells, although relative resistance is common. Membrane-based resistance mechanisms, commonly responsible for resistance to chemotherapy, have not been identified with radiation.

Four important processes that occur after radiation exposure can be summarized as the "four R's" of radiobiology. The first is *repair*. Repair is temperature dependent and is thought to represent the enzymatic mechanisms for healing intracellular injury. The second R is *reoxygenation*. Reoxygenation represents a process whereby oxygen (and other nutrients) actually are better distributed to viable cells following radiation injury and cell killing. The third R is *repopulation*, the ability of the cell population to continue to divide and to replace dying and dead cells. The fourth R is *redistribution*, which reflects the variability of a cell's radiosensitivity over the cell cycle. Radiosensitivity can vary through cell

cycle by as much as a factor of 3. The G1 phase has the most variable length of all the phases of the cell cycle. For most cell lines, cells that have a short G1 period are most sensitive at the G2/mitosis interface, less sensitive in G1, and most resistant toward the end of the synthesis (S) period.

When radiation works as an anticancer treatment, it works because of differences in the four Rs between tumor cells and normal tissues. Those differences are best exploited by radiotherapy regimens that employ dose fractionation.

CLINICAL FINDINGS RELATED TO FRACTIONATION The clinical radiation response may be related to the interactions of various growth factors and cytokines. For example, radiation can induce growth factors and cytokines such as tumor necrosis factor (TNF), interleukin (IL) 1, and others to be released by irradiated cells. TNF can induce proliferation of fibroblasts and enhance the inflammatory response. TNF and IL-1 have been shown to radioprotect hematopoietic cells in vitro by increasing the D_0 of the cell survival curve. TNF also has been shown to enhance killing of a human tumor cell line when added before irradiation. TNF may produce radioprotection or radiosensitization depending on the cell type, and it remains unclear what degree of sensitization or protection can be derived from TNF. Other factors implicated in the radiation response are basic fibroblast growth factor and platelet-derived growth factor-β, which may be associated with late effects of radiation on vessels. Cytokines are induced by transcriptional activation after exposure to ionizing radiation. Interactions of these factors may modify the clinical response to radiation exposure.

The rate and the length of functional recovery of normal tissues are related to the number of stem cells surviving after irradiation. The volume of the irradiated tissue will also influence the rate of recovery from the radiation as well as the severity of the side effects. If the stem cells are destroyed in the irradiated volume and there is inadequate

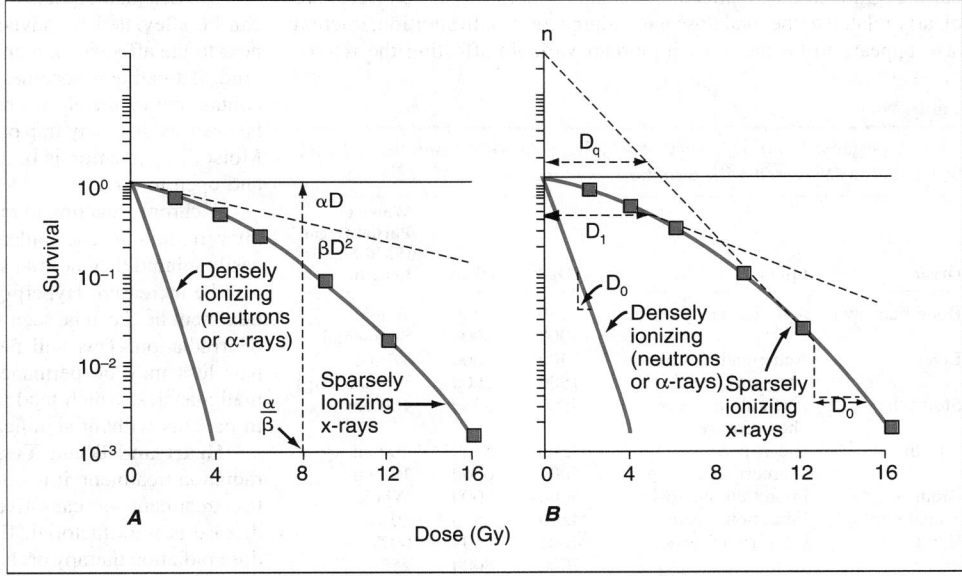

FIGURE 396-1 Shape of survival curve for mammalian cells exposed to radiation. The fraction of cells surviving is plotted on a logarithmic scale against dose on a linear scale. For alpha particles or low-energy neutrons (said to be densely ionizing) the dose-response curve is a straight line from the origin (i.e., survival is an exponential function of dose). The survival curve can be described by just one parameter, the slope. For x-rays or gamma rays (said to be sparsely ionizing), the dose-response curve has an initial linear slope, followed by a shoulder; at higher doses the curve tends to become straight again. *A*. The experimental data are fitted to a linear-quadratic function. There are two components of cell killing: one is proportional to dose (αD), while the other is proportional to the square of the dose (βD^2). The dose at which the linear and quadratic components are equal is the ratio α/β. The linear-quadratic curve bends continuously but is a good fit to experimental data for the first few decades of survival. *B*. The curve is described by the initial slope (D_1), the final slope (D_0), and a parameter that represents the width of the shoulder, either n or D_q. (From Hall, with permission.)

replacement from adjacent tissues, radiation injury will persist. True late effects develop independent of early reactions; they occur despite recovery from acute radiation injury.

Table 396-4 shows the frequency of radiation tolerance seen with fractionated radiotherapy at 5 years of follow-up. These numbers are rough estimates at best. The clinical manifestations of irradiation will depend on the volume of the organ irradiated, the total dose, the dose per fraction, and the length of time taken to deliver the dose. In addition, the cellular consequences of treatment can be progressive over time. Thus, length of follow-up is also crucial in judging clinical sequelae.

Central Nervous System   Traditionally, the central nervous system (CNS) has been described as relatively resistant to radiation-induced changes. When the human brain is treated with standard fractionation (1.8 to 2.0 Gy/d), acute reactions are seldom observed.

Subacute CNS reactions to radiation treatment are more common. The clinical manifestations may include Lhermitte's sign, which is a self-limited paresthesia occurring with flexion of the neck. It is believed to be due to transient demyelination of the spinal cord following significant radiation exposure. It can be seen 1 to 3 months after completion of radiation treatment to the spinal cord. The frequency of Lhermitte's sign varies according to the type of radiation therapy and can be as high as 15 percent after the mantle radiation treatments commonly employed to treat Hodgkin's disease. Mild encephalopathy and focal neurologic changes can occur after irradiation limited to the cranium. If radiation treatments to the brain are given at the same time that chemotherapeutic agents are administered, the effects can be more severe, presumably reflecting altered permeability to the drugs. The effect of cranial irradiation is believed to be secondary to radiation effects on the replicating oligodendrocytes and possibly on the microvasculature. Both clinical and radiologic changes may simulate tumor progression and can often pose diagnostic and treatment dilemmas.

Post-irradiation pathology and associated clinical symptoms typically begin 6 to 36 months after radiation therapy. These effects are clearly related to the total dose and volume treated. In addition, fraction size appears to be the most important variable affecting the rate of

Table 396-4

Class 1 Organs: Fatal or Severe Morbidity Following Cumulative Doses of Radiation Delivered with Standard Fractionation

Organ	Injury	TD$_{5/5}$*	TD$_{50/5}$†	Whole or Partial Organ (Field Size or Length)
Bone marrow	Aplasia, pancytopenia	250	450	Whole
		3000	4000	Segmental
Liver	Acute and chronic hepatitis	2500	4000	Whole
		1500	2000	Whole (strip)
Stomach	Perforation, ulcer, hemorrhage	4500	5500	100 cm
Intestine	Ulcer, perforation, hemorrhage	4500	5500	400 cm
		5000	6500	100 cm
Brain	Infarction, necrosis	5000	6000	Whole
Spinal cord	Infarction, necrosis	4500	5500	10 cm
Heart	Pericarditis, pancarditis	4500	5500	60%
		7000	8000	25%
Lung	Acute and chronic pneumonitis	3000	3500	100 cm
		1500	2500	Whole
Kidney	Acute and chronic nephrosclerosis	1500	2000	Whole (strip)
		2000	2500	Whole
Fetus	Death	200	400	Whole

* TD$_{5/5}$ is the minimal tolerance dose—the dose that, when administered to a given patient population under a standard set of treatment conditions, results in a rate of severe complications of 5 percent or less within 5 years of treatment.
† TD$_{50/5}$ is the maximal tolerance dose—the dose that, when administered to a given population of patients under a standard set of treatment conditions, results in a rate of severe complications of 50 percent within 5 years of treatment.
SOURCE: From Rubin et al, 1975.

post-irradiation brain necrosis. Neurocognitive changes can also be seen in children after cranial irradiation. The important pretreatment factors that predict the degree of late CNS effects include the age at which cranial irradiation was given and neurocognitive functional level at the time of treatment.

A unique late effect of cranial irradiation combined with chemotherapy, known as leukoencephalopathy, has been described in some patients. Leukoencephalopathy is a necrotizing reaction usually noted 4 to 12 months after combined treatment with methotrexate and cranial irradiation. Dementia and dysarthria may progress to seizures, ataxia, or death.

Transverse myelitis after radiation treatment is a spinal cord reaction similar to cerebral necrosis. This syndrome consists of progressive and irreversible leg weakness, and loss of bladder function and sensation referrable to a single spinal cord level. Flaccid paralysis eventually occurs. Symptoms can occur as early as 6 months after radiation treatment, but the usual time to onset is 12 to 24 months. There is no known correlation between Lhermitte's sign and transverse myelitis.

Skin   Skin reaction can be seen within 2 weeks of fractionated radiotherapy, a delay that correlates with the time required for cells to move from the basal to the keratinized layer of skin. The severity of the reaction depends on the amount of skin dose per fraction and the total dose delivered to an area of skin. Erythema is observed, soon followed by dry desquamation. The skin at this time can be erythematous, warm, and sometimes edematous. There is dilation of the vessels in the upper dermis and an associated inflammatory infiltration with granulocytes, macrophages, eosinophils, plasma cells, and lymphocytes.

Modern high-energy radiotherapy machines often do not produce significant skin reactions. When a severe skin reaction occurs, it is usually located where the beam strikes the skin tangentially. *Moist desquamation* consists of eruption of the epidermal layer. Healing is through re-epithelialization from cells of less affected basal layers. When skin reactions are severe, treatment interruptions are needed to permit healing.

Dry desquamation is treated conservatively. Symptoms of dryness can be alleviated by advising the patient to wear only cotton fabric next to the affected skin and to refrain from the use of irritants of any kind. If treatment becomes necessary, hydrophilic agents that do not contain heavy metals are recommended. Petroleum jellies should not be used, as they may trap bacteria and increase the chance of infection. Moist desquamation is best managed by leaving the affected area dry and open to air.

A chronic reaction to radiation can be seen starting 6 to 12 months after irradiation. The epidermis is usually atrophic, and it may be more easily injured than normal skin. The amount of interstitial fibrosis may also be increased. Hyperpigmentation of irradiated skin outlining the treatment field can be seen within a couple of months after completion of irradiation. This will fade gradually. The skin becomes thin, and hair loss may be permanent. Radiation therapy can induce second malignancies, which tend to be more aggressive than cancers arising in patients without significant radiation exposure.

Heart and Blood Vessels   When cardiac disease appears after radiation treatment, it is often difficult to tell to what extent the radiation treatment was causative. The pathogenesis of atherosclerotic heart disease is multifactorial. Exposure of a large heart volume to high-dose radiation therapy probably enhances the development of coronary artery disease. Acute "pericarditis" may result from cardiac irradiation. The symptoms may include chest pain and fever, with or without pericardial effusion. This syndrome is usually self-limited and typically manifests itself a few months after treatment. Asymptomatic pericardial effusion may be the most common manifestation of radiation-induced heart disease. It is usually detected by chest x-ray and confirmed by an echocardiogram.

Most patients with symptomatic radiation-induced constrictive pericarditis will have received more than 40 Gy to a large portion of the heart. The risk increases significantly with cardiac doses greater than 50 Gy.

Chronic cardiac changes may have their onset from 6 months to several years after irradiation. The clinical symptoms may indicate chronic constrictive disease due to pericardial, myocardial, and endocardial fibrosis—a pancarditis. The clinical signs may include dyspnea, chest pain, venous distention, pleural effusion, and paradoxical pulse.

Lung The clinical symptoms of radiation pneumonitis can be separated into early and late phases. During the early phase, clinical manifestations may include dyspnea, cough, and fever. Shortness of breath is relatively infrequent. It is more common to observe only the radiologic changes on a chest x-ray, without clinical symptoms. The clinical signs and symptoms of radiation pneumonitis may appear in 3 to 6 weeks if a large region of lung is irradiated to a dose above 25 Gy. An infiltrate outlining the treatment field may become evident on the chest x-ray. Radiation changes should not occur outside the treated field. Computed tomography can often help in distinguishing radiation pneumonitis from other causes of the infiltrate. The incidence of radiation pneumonitis can be reduced with careful treatment planning designed to lower the total dose given to the treated lung volume. Permanent scarring that results in respiratory compromise may develop if the dose and the volume of lung irradiated are excessive. Dyspnea and cough may be severe and debilitating.

There may be a role for glucocorticoids, especially in patients with hypoxemia. Patients with symptoms of radiation pneumonitis may respond rapidly to glucocorticoids, but the medication has little effect on fibrotic changes. Steroid treatment must be tapered very slowly to avoid rebound exacerbation of symptoms, which can prove lethal for some patients. Prophylactic administration of steroids is of questionable merit. Unless the symptoms are severe, it is preferable to provide supportive care, including bronchodilators and oxygen at the lowest possible $F_{I_{O_2}}$.

Digestive Tract The limited available human data show that pathologic changes of the epithelial layer occur early during radiation treatments. The underlying submucosa may become edematous, with dilation of capillaries. Recovery from radiation damage can be expected within a few weeks after completion of radiation therapy, provided that sufficient numbers of stem cells are left. The radioresponsiveness of the aerodigestive tract, like that of other strctures, is not uniform but varies according to the location.

Patients often have symptoms from radiation exposure that are similar to other forms of acute gastritis. The clinical signs include epigastric pain, loss of appetite, nausea, and vomiting. Decreased gastric acidity is observed after 15 to 20 Gy of fractionated radiation therapy. The tolerance of the stomach to radiation is also aggravated by addition of systemic chemotherapy, such as therapy with 5-fluorouracil.

The germinal centers of the bowel mucosa are in the crypts of Lieberkühn. Newly formed cells move upward along the walls of the crypts as transitional cells, undergoing maturation. The epithelial lining of the small bowel is the most rapidly renewed system in the human body and it is completely renewed in 3 to 6 days. Within 12 to 24 h after the first dose of radiation therapy, pathologic evidence of dead cells are seen in the mucosal lining. Complete denudation of the mucosal surface rarely occurs during a regular course of radiation treatment because of the high capacity of the mucosa for regeneration. However, a focal area of erosion may be seen. The histologic appearance may be nearly normal within 2 to 3 weeks after radiation therapy.

Clinical manifestations of acute radiation enteropathy are nausea and vomiting, diarrhea, and cramping pain. Relevant factors contributing to the pathogenesis of diarrhea include malabsorption and alterations in the intestinal bacterial flora. The severity of symptoms, as in other anatomic areas, is proportional to the irradiated volume and the total dose.

The symptoms of chronic radiation enteropathy include diarrhea, abdominal cramping, nausea, malabsorption, vomiting, and obstruction. Progressive fibrosis, perforation, fistula formation, and stenosis of the irradiated portion of the bowel can also occur during the chronic phase of radiation enteropathy. Most clinical manifestations of chronic changes occur between 6 months and 5 years after radiation therapy.

Conservative noninvasive treatment can frequently control gastrointestinal symptoms. A low-residue or elemental diet may be beneficial.

When nonsurgical treatment fails to relieve severe symptoms, surgical intervention is often indicated.

Bladder Radiation injury to the bladder generally becomes symptomatic 3 to 6 weeks after the start of treatment, and symptoms usually subside 3 to 4 weeks after completion of radiation therapy. Patients often complain of increased frequency and dysuria. Cystoscopy often shows diffuse mucosal changes similar to those of acute cystitis. Sometimes desquamation and ulceration can be seen. Without infection, urinary symptoms are managed symptomatically. Concurrent chemotherapy with cytotoxic agents such as cyclophosphamide increases the severity of the acute bladder reaction.

The late effects of high radiation doses to the bladder may include interstitial fibrosis, telangiectasia, and ulceration. The blood vessels may be dilated and prone to rupture, resulting in painless hematuria. These changes are often difficult to distinguish from tumor recurrence and progression. A contracted bladder may result from doses in excess of 60 Gy.

Testis and Ovaries In general, type B spermatogonia are exquisitely sensitive to the effects of radiation. The type A spermatogonia are thought to be more resistant because their longer cell cycle time allows considerable variation in radiosensitivity among different phases of the cell cycle. Sertoli cells and Leydig cells are less radiosensitive than the spermatogonia. FSH and LH elevation have been observed after as little as 75 cGy. Doses as low as 10 cGy to the testicles may result in injury to the type B spermatogonia. The single dose required for permanent sterilization on normal human males is not clearly established but it is believed to be between 6 and 10 Gy. In normal human males, sperm count recovery requires 9 to 18 months after a fractionated dose of 8 to 100 cGy.

The radiation dose necessary to induce ovarian failure is age dependent. A single dose of 3 to 4 Gy can induce amenorrhea in almost all women over 40 years of age. In young women, oogenesis is much less sensitive to radiation than spermatogenesis in men.

ACUTE TOTAL-BODY IRRADIATION The data regarding the acute effects of total-body irradiation on humans come primarily from Japanese survivors of the atomic bomb, Marshallese exposed to radioactive fall-out in 1954, and persons exposed to radiation from the recent Chernobyl accident. Early symptoms of acute total-body irradiation last for a limited time. This is known as the *prodromal radiation syndrome*. Clinical manifestations depend on the total-body dose. At doses in excess of 100 Gy to the total body, death usually occurs 24 to 48 h later from neurologic and cardiovascular failure. This is known as the *cerebrovascular syndrome*. Because cerebrovascular damage causes death very quickly, the failures of other systems do not have time to develop.

At doses between 5 and 12 Gy, death may occur in a matter of days as a result of the *gastrointestinal syndrome*. The symptoms during this period may include nausea, vomiting, and prolonged diarrhea for several days leading to dehydration, sepsis, and death. A total-body dose of greater than 1000 cGy is uniformly fatal unless supportive therapy (fluid, electrolytes, blood products, and antibiotics) is given. The process of intestinal denudation depends on the dose and may take between 3 and 120 days. Death from intestinal denudation usually occurs before the full effects of radiation on the blood-forming elements are seen.

At total-body doses between 2 and 8 Gy, death may occur several weeks after exposure and is due to effects on the bone marrow, which results in the *hematopoietic syndrome*. The full effect of radiation is not apparent until the mature hematopoietic cells are depleted. Death from the hematologic damage occurs at about 20 to 30 days after exposure, and the risk of death continues over the next 30 days. Clinical symptoms during this period may include chills, fatigue, and petechial hemorrhage. Peripheral blood lymphopenia develops during the first 12 to 48 h after any significant exposure. Beyond 5 to 6 Gy, the rate and magnitude of the drop are not well correlated to radiation exposure. Some stem cells may survive acute exposure to 10 Gy or more. Anemia from red cell depression usually does not occur because of the long half-life of erythrocytes.

It is estimated that the $LD_{50/60}$ (the dose at which 50 percent of the population is dead by 60 days) is around 325 cGy if support is not given. There is considerable variability in the total-body dose tolerated. The very young and the old are more radiosensitive than middle-aged and young adult individuals. Females in general appear to be more tolerant of radiation than males. Persons exposed to less than 2 Gy will require little or no therapy, but they should probably be observed closely with daily blood counts for a few days.

There is a considerable controversy regarding the utility of bone marrow transplantation for patients exposed to acute total body irradiation. At doses less than 800 cGy, the patient is likely to survive with supportive care. Most people exposed to doses higher than 1000 cGy will die from the gastrointestinal syndrome. Therefore, 800 to 1000 cGy may be the dose range in which bone marrow transplantation could have a role, although the Chernobyl experience did not confirm that. It is difficult to estimate the dose received by a given patient after radiation exposure. This is an important point, because bone marrow transplantation is most effective if it is performed within the first 3 to 5 days after exposure. It is, therefore, extremely important to estimate the received dose quickly.

RADIATION AND CANCER INDUCTION Some nonlethal changes in DNA sequences caused by irradiation may cause malignant transformations. Thus, it is not surprising that second neoplasms can be caused by exposure to ionizing radiation. However, paradoxically, this risk is actually less with doses above a certain level. It is unclear whether there is a "safe" dose that will not have any adverse biologic effect. It should be emphasized that the estimates of the risk of developing cancer after low-level exposure to ionizing radiation are often derived by extrapolation from the risks for higher doses and acute exposures. Predicted risks of cancer are, therefore, prone to modification depending on the assumptions made about the data available for analysis.

Throughout the history of human exposure to ionizing radiation, there have been documented cases of increased rates of cancer after exposure to radiation. The populations studied include survivors of the atomic bomb during World War II, radium watch dial painters who shaped their brush tips with their tongue, patients who have undergone multiple fluoroscopic examinations for tuberculosis, patients who received spinal irradiation for ankylosing spondylitis, patients who received breast irradiation for postpartum mastitis, and others. Exposure to ionizing radiation at an earlier age appears to increase the chance of developing radiation-induced carcinomas. However, the radiation-induced cancers have an age of onset similar to that of the native cancers, and the available data argue against radiation as the only cause of the increased incidence of cancers seen after exposure to radiation. Table 396-5 shows examples of cancer observed in specific situations.

Table 396-5

Examples of Radiation-Induced Cancers

Types of Exposure	Types of Cancer Observed
Neck irradiation during infancy for benign conditions	Thyroid carcinoma
Radiation therapy for other malignant tumors	Thyroid carcinoma
	Breast cancer
	Gastric cancer
	Melanoma
	Lung cancer
	Sarcomas in the field
Cranial irradiation	Central nervous system tumors
Breast irradiation for postpartum mastitis	Breast cancer
Brush-licking by radium dial painters	Bone sarcomas
Uranium mining	Lung cancer
In utero exposure	Leukemia

Because a safe dose of radiation is unknown at present, it is prudent to avoid routine exposures to ionizing irradiation.

BIBLIOGRAPHY

Cox JD: Moss' *Radiation Oncology: Rationale, Technique, Results*, 7th ed. St. Louis, Mosby, 1994

Glatstein E, Carter SK: The chronic toxicity of cancer treatment, in *Principles of Cancer Treatment*, SK Carter et al (eds). New York, McGraw-Hill, 1982, pp 221–236

Hall EJ: *Radiobiology for the Radiologist*, 4th ed. Philadelphia, Lippincott, 1994

Hallahan D et al: The role of cytokines in radiation oncology, in *Important Advances in Oncology 1993*, VT DeVita Jr et al (eds). Philadelphia, Lippincott, 1993

Karas JS, Stanbury JB: Fatal radiation syndrome from an accidental nuclear excursion. N Engl J Med 272:755, 1965

Khan FM: *The Physics of Radiation Therapy*, 2d ed. Baltimore, Williams & Wilkins, 1993

Littlefield LG, Lushbaugh CC: Cytogenetic dosimetry for radiation accidents: "The good, the bad, and the ugly," in *The Medical Basis for Radiation Accident Preparedness*, vol 2: *Clinical Experience and Follow-up Since 1979*, RC Ricks, SA Fry (eds). New York, Elsevier, 1990, pp 461–478

Mettler FA Jr, Upton AC: *Medical Effects of Ionizing Radiation*, 2d ed, Philadelphia, Saunders, 1995

Perez CP, Brady LW: *Principles and Practice of Radiation Oncology*, 2d ed, Philadelphia, Lippincott, 1992

Rubin P et al (eds): *Radiation Biology and Radiation Pathology Syllabus*, set RT 1: *Radiation Oncology*. Chicago, American College of Radiology, 1975
——— et al: Late effects of normal tissues consensus conference. Int J Radiat Oncol Biol Phys 31:5, 1995

Schwade JG, Lichter AS: Management of acute effects of radiation therapy, in *Principles of Cancer Treatment*, SK Carter et al (eds). New York, McGraw-Hill, 1982, pp 212–220

Tepper JE (ed): Normal tissue effects of radiation therapy. Semin Radiat Oncol 4:2, 1994

397 *Howard Hu*

HEAVY METAL POISONING

Metals constitute a major category of toxins that pose a significant threat to health through occupational as well as environmental exposures. One indication of their importance relative to other potential hazards is their ranking by the U.S. Agency for Toxic Substances and Disease Registry, which lists all hazards present in toxic waste sites according to their prevalence and the severity of their toxicity. The first, second, third, and sixth hazards on the list are heavy metals: lead, mercury, arsenic, and cadmium, respectively. This chapter offers specific information on the sources and metabolism of each of these metals as well as on the toxic effects produced by each and the appropriate treatment for poisoning by each.

The intrinsic atomic stability of metals allows their relatively easy tracing and measurement in biologic material, although the clinical significance of the levels measured is not always clear. Metals are inhaled primarily as dusts and fumes (the latter defined as tiny particles generated by combustion). Metal poisoning can also result from exposure to vapors (e.g., mercury vapor in the manufacture of fluorescent lamps). When metals are ingested in contaminated food or drink or through hand-to-mouth activity (implicated especially often in children), their gastrointestinal absorption varies greatly with the specific chemical form of the metal and the nutritional status of the host. Once a metal is absorbed, blood is the main medium for its transport, with the precise kinetics dependent on diffusibility, binding forms, rates of biotransformation, availability of intracellular ligands, and other factors. Some organs (such as bone, liver, and kidney) sequester metals in relatively high concentrations for years. Most metals are excreted through renal clearance and gastrointestinal excretion; some proportion is also excreted through salivation, perspiration, exhalation, lactation, skin exfoliation, and loss of hair and nails.

Some metals, such as copper and selenium, are essential to normal metabolic function as trace elements (see Chap. 80) but are toxic at high levels of exposure. Others, such as lead and mercury, are xenobiotic and theoretically are capable of exerting toxic effects at any level of exposure. Indeed, much research is currently focused on the contribution of low-level xenobiotic metal exposure to chronic diseases and to subtle changes in health that may have significant public health consequences.

The most important component of treatment for metal toxicity is the termination of exposure. Another component is the use of *chelating agents*, which are used to bind metals into stable cyclic compounds with relatively low toxicity and to enhance their excretion. The principal chelating agents are dimercaprol (British Anti-Lewisite, BAL), edetate (EDTA), succimer (DMSA, dimercaptosuccinic acid), and penicillamine; their specific use depends on the metal involved and the clinical picture. Activated charcoal does not bind metals and thus is of limited usefulness in cases of acute metal ingestion.

Besides the four metals discussed in detail in this chapter, several others deserve mention. *Aluminum* contributes to the encephalopathy seen in patients with severe renal disease who are undergoing dialysis (see Chap. 354). High levels of aluminum are found in the neurofibrillary tangles in the cerebral cortex and hippocampus of patients with Alzheimer's disease as well as in the drinking water and soil of areas with an unusually high incidence of Alzheimer's disease. The experimental and epidemiologic evidence for the aluminum–Alzheimer's disease link is so far relatively weak, however, and it cannot be concluded that aluminum is a causal agent or a contributing factor in neurodegenerative disease. Hexavalent *chromium* is corrosive and sensitizing. Workers in the chromate and chrome pigment production industries have consistently had an excess risk of lung cancer. The introduction of *cobalt* chloride as a fortifier in beer led to outbreaks of fatal cardiomyopathy among heavy consumers. Occupational exposure (e.g., of some miners, dry-battery manufacturers, and arc welders) to *manganese* can cause a Parkinsonian syndrome within 1 to 2 years, including gait disorders; postural instability; a masked, expressionless face; tremor; and psychiatric symptoms. *Nickel* exposure induces an allergic response, and inhalation of nickel compounds with low aqueous solubility (such as nickel subsulfide and nickel oxide) in occupational settings is associated with an increased risk of cancer of the lung. Overexposure to *selenium* may cause local irritation of the respiratory system and eyes, gastrointestinal irritation, liver inflammation, loss of hair, depigmentation, and peripheral nerve damage. Workers exposed to certain organic forms of *tin* (particularly trimethyl and triethyl derivatives) have developed psychomotor disturbances including tremor, convulsions, hallucinations, and psychotic behavior.

Finally, *thallium*, which is a component of some insecticides, metal alloys, and fireworks, is absorbed through the skin as well as through ingestion and inhalation. Severe poisoning follows a single ingested dose of >1 g or >8 mg/kg. Nausea and vomiting, abdominal pain, and hematemesis precede confusion, psychosis, organic brain syndrome, and coma. Thallium is radiopaque. Induced emesis or gastric lavage is indicated within 4 to 6 h of acute ingestion; Prussian blue prevents absorption and is given orally at 250 mg/kg in divided doses. Unlike other types of metal poisoning, thallium poisoning may be less severe when activated charcoal is used to interrupt its enterohepatic circulation. Other measures include forced diuresis, treatment with potassium chloride (which promotes renal excretion of thallium), and peritoneal dialysis.

LEAD

SOURCE Lead has been mined and used in industry and in household products for centuries. The dangers of lead toxicity, the clinical manifestations of which are known as *plumbism*, have been known since ancient times. The twentieth century has seen both the greatest-ever exposure of the general population to lead and an extraordinary amount of new research on lead toxicity.

Populations are exposed to lead chiefly via paints, cans, plumbing fixtures, and leaded gasoline. The intensity of these exposures, while recently decreased by regulatory actions, remains high in some segments of the population because of the deterioration of lead paint used in the past and the entrainment of lead from paint and vehicle exhaust into soil and house dust. Many other environmental sources of exposure exist, such as leafy vegetables grown in lead-contaminated soil, improperly glazed ceramics, lead crystal, and certain herbal folk remedies. Many industries, such as battery manufacturing, demolition, painting and paint removal, and ceramics, continue to pose a significant risk of lead exposure to workers and surrounding communities.

New research on lead toxicity has been stimulated by advances in toxicology and epidemiology as well as by a shift of emphasis in toxicology away from binary outcomes (life/death; 50 percent lethal dose) to grades of function, such as neuropsychological performance, indices of behavior, blood pressure, and kidney function.

Tests for levels of lead in blood have facilitated both research on lead and surveillance of individuals at risk. Blood lead is now measured with stringent quality controls in commercial laboratories throughout the United States. Measurement of the blood lead levels of children 6 months to 5 years of age is currently mandated by some states, and the U.S. Occupational Safety and Health Administration (OSHA) requires the testing of workers who may be exposed to lead in the course of their jobs.

METABOLISM Elemental lead and inorganic lead compounds are absorbed through ingestion or inhalation. Organic lead (e.g., tetraethyl lead, the lead additive to gasoline) is absorbed to a significant degree through the skin as well. Pulmonary absorption is efficient, particularly if particle diameters are <1 μm (as in fumes from burning lead paint). Children absorb up to 50 percent of the amount of lead ingested, whereas adults absorb only about 10 to 20 percent. Gastrointestinal absorption of lead is enhanced by fasting and by dietary deficiencies in calcium, iron, and zinc; such absorption is minimal, however, for lead in the form of lead sulfide, a common constituent of mining waste. Lead is absorbed into blood plasma, where it equilibrates rapidly with extracellular fluid, crosses membranes (such as the blood-brain barrier and the placenta), and accumulates in soft and hard tissues. In the blood, around 95 to 99 percent of lead is sequestered in red cells, where it is bound to hemoglobin and other components. As a consequence, lead is usually measured in whole blood rather than in serum. The largest proportion of absorbed lead is incorporated into the skeleton, which contains more than 90 percent of the body's total lead burden. Lead is excreted mainly in the urine (in a process that depends on glomerular filtration and tubular secretion) and in the feces. Lead also appears in hair, nails, sweat, saliva, and breast milk. The half-life of lead in blood is approximately 25 days; in soft tissue, about 40 days; and in the nonlabile portion of bone, more than 25 years. Thus, blood lead levels may decline significantly while the body's total burden of lead remains heavy.

The toxicity of lead is probably related to its affinity for cell membranes and mitochondria, as a result of which it interferes with mitochondrial oxidative phosphorylation and sodium, potassium, and calcium ATPases. Lead impairs the activity of calcium-dependent intracellular messengers and of brain protein kinase C. In addition, lead stimulates the formation of inclusion bodies that may translocate the metal into cell nuclei and alter gene expression.

CLINICAL TOXICOLOGY Symptomatic lead poisoning in childhood generally develops at blood lead levels exceeding 3.9 μmol/L (80 μg/dL) and is characterized by abdominal pain and irritability followed by lethargy, anorexia, pallor (resulting from anemia), ataxia, and slurred speech. Convulsions, coma, and death due to generalized cerebral edema and renal failure occur in the most severe cases. Subclinical lead poisoning [blood lead level >1.4 μmol/L (>30 μg/dL)] can cause mental retardation and selective deficits in language, cognitive function, balance, behavior, and school performance despite the lack of discernible symptoms. Epidemiologic studies and meta-analyses of studies regarding lead's effect on the intellectual function of children indicate that cognition is probably impaired in a dose-related fashion at blood lead levels well below 1.4 μmol/L (30 μg/dL) and that no threshold for this effect is likely to exist above the lowest measurable blood lead level of 0.05 μmol/L (1 μg/dL). The impact is greatest when the exposure is of long duration and when it takes place around the age of 2 years.

In adults, symptomatic lead poisoning usually develops when blood lead levels exceed 3.9 μmol/L (80 μg/dL) for a period of weeks and is characterized by abdominal pain, headache, irritability, joint pain, fatigue, anemia, peripheral motor neuropathy, and deficits in short-term memory and the ability to concentrate. Encephalopathy is rare. A "lead line" sometimes appears at the gingiva-tooth border after prolonged high-level exposure. Some individuals develop these symptoms and signs at lower blood lead levels [1.9 to 3.9 μmol/L (40 to 80 μg/dL)] and/or with briefer periods of exposure. Chronic subclinical lead exposure is associated with interstitial nephritis, tubular damage (with tubular inclusion bodies), hyperuricemia (with an increased risk of gout), and a decline in glomerular filtration rate and chronic renal failure. Epidemiologic evidence also suggests that blood lead levels in the range of 0.34 to 1.7 μmol/L (7 to 35 μg/dL) are associated with increases in blood pressure, decreases in creatinine clearance, and decrements in cognitive performance that are too small to be detected as a lead effect in individual cases but nevertheless may contribute significantly to the causation of chronic disease.

An additional issue for both children and adults is whether lead that has accumulated in bone and lain dormant for years can pose a threat later in life, particularly at times of increased bone resorption such as pregnancy, lactation, and senile osteoporosis. Elevation of the bone lead level appears to be a risk factor for anemia and hypertension. Hyperthyroidism has been reported to cause lead toxicity in adults by mobilizing stores of bone lead acquired during childhood.

Genetic polymorphisms of the gene that codes for aminolevulinic acid dehydratase, a critical enzyme in the production of heme, may confer differences in susceptibility to lead retention and toxicity; 15 percent of Caucasians have a variant form of this gene. This issue is the focus of continued research.

LABORATORY FINDINGS In 1991, the Centers for Disease Control and Prevention designated 0.48 μmol/L (10 μg/dL) as the blood lead level of concern in children. A specific set of interventions is recommended when the level exceeds this value. OSHA requires the regular measurement of blood lead in lead-exposed workers and the maintenance of blood lead levels below 1.9 μmol/L (40 μg/dL). Concentrations of heme precursors (such as δ-aminolevulinic acid) in plasma and urine are sometimes increased at blood lead levels as low as 0.73 μmol/L (15 μg/dL). Levels of protoporphyrin (free erythrocyte or zinc) rise—although not consistently—once blood lead levels have exceeded 1.2 μmol/L (25 μg/dL) for several months. Lead-associated anemia is usually normocytic and normochromic and may be accompanied by basophilic stippling. Lead-induced peripheral demyelination is reflected by prolonged nerve conduction time and subsequent paralysis, usually of the extensor muscles of the hands and feet ("wrist and foot drop"). An increased density at the metaphyseal plate of growing long bones ("lead lines") can develop in children and resemble those seen in rickets. Children with high-level lead exposure sometimes develop Fanconi's syndrome, pyuria, and azotemia. Adults chronically exposed to lead can develop elevated serum creatinine levels, decreased creatinine clearance rates, and chronic changes and intranuclear inclusion bodies (detected at renal biopsy). Deficits may be apparent in neuropsychometric tests of both children and adults; these abnormalities by themselves are not pathognomonic. X-ray fluorescence is being investigated as a method for estimating long-term accumulation of lead in bone.

℞ **TREATMENT**

It is absolutely essential to prevent further exposure of affected individuals to lead. Cases of lead poisoning should be reported to OSHA (if the exposure is occupational) and to local boards of health

so that home evaluations can be performed. Pharmacologic treatment for lead toxicity entails the use of chelating agents, principally edetate calcium disodium (CaEDTA), dimercaprol, penicillamine, and succimer, which is given orally and has relatively few side effects. Chelation is recommended for the treatment of all children whose blood lead levels are greater than 2.7 μmol/L (55 μg/dL), with the addition of dimercaprol if lead encephalopathy is found. Chelation is also recommended for children if blood lead levels are between 1.2 and 2.7 μmol/L (25 and 55 μg/dL) and the total amount of lead excreted in urine during the 8 h after a single dose of edetate calcium disodium exceeds 9.7 μmol/L (200 μg/dL). Chelation is recommended for adults if blood lead levels exceed 3.9 μmol/L (80 μg/dL) or if blood lead levels exceed 2.9 μmol/L (60 μg/dL) and symptoms have developed. The ability of chelation to improve subclinical outcomes (such as performance on psychometric testing) at lower levels of blood lead in both children and adults is the subject of current research.

MERCURY

SOURCE Metallic mercury (Hg^0) is used in thermometers, dental amalgams, and some batteries. Mercurous mercury (Hg^+) and mercuric mercury (Hg^{2+}) can be combined with other chemicals, such as carbon, chlorine, or oxygen, to form inorganic or organic mercury compounds. All three forms of mercury are toxic to various degrees. Organic mercury compounds are slowly broken down into inorganic compounds; conversely, inorganic mercury can be converted by microorganisms in soil and water into the organic compound methyl mercury. Fish, particularly tuna and swordfish, can concentrate methyl mercury at high levels; such contamination of fish by industrial runoff and their subsequent ingestion was responsible for the Minamata Bay epidemic of mercury poisoning in Japan in 1955. Occupational exposure to inorganic mercury compounds continues in some chemical, metal-processing, electrical-equipment, automotive, and building industries and in medical and dental services. Environmental exposure probably takes place most commonly through ingestion of contaminated fish and through inhalation of the vapor generated by ordinary dental amalgam, which typically contains about 50 percent metallic mercury. There is also concern about exposure to drinking water contaminated by toxic waste sites included on the National Priority List, almost half of which contain mercury, and about the inhalation of fumes from incinerators burning mercury-contaminated waste products. Whether the latter types of exposure confer a significant risk of toxicity is controversial.

METABOLISM Elemental mercury is not well absorbed by the gastrointestinal tract and is excreted almost entirely in the feces after being ingested; however, when left standing, mercury is volatilized at room temperature into a vapor that is well absorbed by the lungs. Once absorbed, mercury in this form is lipid soluble, crosses the blood-brain barrier and the placenta, and can be oxidized by catalase and hydrogen peroxide into mercuric chloride, which is retained by the kidney and brain for years. Elemental mercury in blood has a half-life of approximately 60 days and is excreted mainly in the urine and feces.

The gastrointestinal and dermal absorption of inorganic mercury is significant. Large overdoses disrupt gastrointestinal barriers, further enhancing absorption. Once absorbed, inorganic mercury breaks down into metallic and mercuric mercury. Relatively little of this mercury crosses the blood-brain barrier; most is excreted in the urine or feces, with a half-life of 40 days, or is retained by the kidneys as mercuric mercury.

Organic mercury, particularly methyl mercury, can evaporate and undergo pulmonary absorption. Forms that are ingested (e.g., in contaminated fish) are well absorbed. Only small amounts are absorbed through the skin. Absorbed organic mercury is lipid soluble, readily crosses the blood-brain barrier and the placenta, appears in breast milk, and concentrates in the kidneys and central nervous system. Methyl mercury is acetylated in the liver, excreted in bile, reabsorbed, and then excreted in urine. Methyl mercury can also be conjugated

Exposure to mercury in any form stimulates the kidney to produce metallothionein, a metal-binding protein that affords partial protection against mercury toxicity.

CLINICAL TOXICOLOGY Inhalation of metallic mercury vapor is the form of mercury exposure that has been best studied in terms of toxicity. High levels of exposure are most likely in an occupational setting in which mercury vapors are generated by heat-induced volatilization of metallic mercury. Cough, dyspnea, and tightness or burning pain in the chest are common symptoms that may be accompanied by diffuse infiltrates or a pneumonitis-like appearance on chest x-ray. Respiratory distress, pulmonary edema, lobar pneumonia, fibrosis, and desquamation of the bronchiolar epithelium can occur in relatively severe cases and have sometimes led to death. Acute inhalation of mercury vapor can also cause neurologic toxicity manifested by tremors (beginning in the hands), emotional lability, headaches, and polyneuropathy. Chronic exposure to metallic mercury produces a characteristic intention tremor and mercurial *erethism*, a constellation of findings including excitability, memory loss, insomnia, timidity, and sometimes delirium that was described in workers with occupational exposure in the felt-hat industry—hence the expression "mad as a hatter." Dentists with occupational exposure to mercury score below normal on neurobehavioral tests of motor speed, visual scanning, verbal and visual memory, and visuomotor coordination. Low-level exposure from dental amalgams may also be associated with adverse immunologic reactions in individuals with certain major human leukocyte antigen genotypes; further research is needed in this area.

Acute high-dose ingestion of inorganic mercury causes severe gastrointestinal corrosion with nausea, vomiting, hematemesis, and abdominal pain; acute renal failure, cardiovascular collapse, and shock may ensue. The lethal dose of inorganic mercury is estimated to be in the range of 10 to 42 mg/kg. Lower levels of exposure cause milder forms of gastrointestinal inflammation, gingivitis and loosening of the teeth, increased blood pressure and tachycardia, and the nephrotic syndrome. Symptoms similar to erethism may develop. Skin exposure to mercuric salts can cause exfoliative dermatitis.

Ingestion of organic mercury compounds is followed by diarrhea, tenesmus, and blisters of the upper gastrointestinal tract. The fatal dose of organic mercury is estimated at 10 to 60 mg/kg. People who ingested flour contaminated with N-(ethylmercuri)-p-toluenesulfonanilide developed bradycardia, QT prolongation, ST-segment depression, and T-wave inversions. The neurotoxicity resulting from organic mercury exposure is characterized by paresthesia; impaired peripheral vision, hearing, taste, and smell; slurred speech; unsteadiness of gait and limbs; muscle weakness; irritability; memory loss; and depression. In general, such symptoms begin at doses above 1.7 mg/kg. Autopsy findings suggest that lesions in the basal ganglia and gray matter of the cortex and cerebellum are chiefly responsible for these symptoms. Organic mercury exposure, primarily through the ingestion of grain treated with mercuric fungicides or of contaminated fish, is also associated with an increased risk of fetal toxicity. After the 1955 mercury poisoning outbreak in Minamata, Japan, exposed mothers gave birth to infants with mental retardation; retention of primitive reflexes; cerebellar symptoms; dysarthria; hyperkinesia; hypersalivation; atrophy of the cerebral cortex, corpus callosum, and cerebellum; and abnormal neuronal cytoarchitecture. This last change may reflect derangement of neuronal migration during fetal development.

Exposure of children to mercury in any of its forms can cause a particular syndrome known as *acrodynia*, or pink disease. This condition is characterized by flushing, itching, swelling, tachycardia, elevated blood pressure, excessive salivation or perspiration, irritability, weakness, morbilliform rashes, and desquamation of the palms and soles.

LABORATORY FINDINGS Levels of mercury in blood and urine should not exceed 180 nmol/L (3.6 μg/dL) and 0.7 μmol/L (15 μg/L), respectively. Symptoms may develop when blood and urine mercury levels exceed 1 μmol/L (20 μg/dL) and 3 μmol/L (60 μg/L),

respectively. If a baseline 24-h urinary mercury value is low, repetition of the measurement after a single 2-g oral dose of succimer may be useful in documenting elevated renal mercury burdens in retired mercury-exposed workers; an increase of more than 20 μg in a 24-h urine sample suggests previous exposure. Levels in hair may be used as a dosimeter for chronic organic mercury exposure; neurobehavioral dysfunction in children may occur if the maternal mercury concentration in hair exceeds 30 nmol/g (6 μg/g).

℞ **TREATMENT**

Acute ingestion of mercuric salts can be treated by induced emesis or gastric lavage. Polythiol resins can be administered orally to bind mercury in the gastrointestinal tract. The most effective chelating agents are dimercaprol, succimer, and penicillamine, which have active mono- or dithiol groups. Acute inorganic mercury poisoning can be treated with dimercaprol at a dose not exceeding 24 mg/kg per day and given intramuscularly in divided doses. Therapy is usually given in 5-day courses separated by several days of rest. The N-acetyl form of penicillamine is also useful at a dose of 30 mg/kg per day in divided doses. Peritoneal dialysis, hemodialysis, and extracorporeal regional complexing hemodialysis with succimer have all been used with some success in the treatment of patients with renal failure.

Chronic inorganic mercury poisoning is best treated with N-acetyl penicillamine.

ARSENIC

SOURCE Significant exposure to arsenic occurs through both anthropogenic and natural sources. Arsenic is released into the air by volcanoes and is a natural contaminant of some deep-water wells. Occupational exposure to arsenic is common in the smelting industry (in which arsenic is a byproduct of ores containing lead, gold, zinc, cobalt, and nickel) and is increasing in the microelectronics industry (in which gallium arsenide is responsible). Low-level arsenic exposure continues to take place in the general population (as do some cases of high-dose poisoning) through the commercial use of inorganic arsenic compounds in common products such as wood preservatives, pesticides, herbicides, fungicides, and paints; through the consumption of foods and the smoking of tobacco treated with arsenic-containing pesticides; and through the burning of fossil fuels in which arsenic is a contaminant. Arsenic was also a major ingredient of Fowler's solution and continues to be found in some folk remedies.

METABOLISM The toxicity of an arsenic-containing compound depends on its valence state (zero-valent, trivalent, or pentavalent), its form (inorganic or organic), and the physical aspects governing its absorption and elimination. In general, inorganic arsenic is more toxic than organic arsenic, and trivalent arsenite is more toxic than pentavalent and zero-valent arsenic. The normal intake of arsenic by adults occurs primarily through ingestion and averages around 50 μg/d (range, 8 to 104 μg/d). Most (around 64 percent) of this amount is accounted for by organic arsenic from fish, seafood, and algae; the specific arsenic compounds obtained from these sources are arsenobentaine and arsenocholine, which are relatively nontoxic and are rapidly excreted in unchanged form in the urine. After absorption, inorganic arsenic accumulates in the liver, spleen, kidneys, lungs, and gastrointestinal tract. It is then rapidly cleared from these sites but leaves a residue in keratin-rich tissues such as skin, hair, and nails. Arsenite (+5) undergoes biomethylation in the liver to the less toxic metabolites methylarsenic acid and dimethylarsenic acid; biomethylation can quickly become saturated, however, and the result is the deposition of increasing doses of inorganic arsenic in soft tissues. Arsenic, particularly in its trivalent form, inhibits critical sulfhydryl-containing enzymes. In the pentavalent form, the competitive substitution of arsenic for phosphate can lead to rapid hydrolysis of the high-energy bonds in compounds such as ATP.

CLINICAL TOXICOLOGY Acute arsenic poisoning from ingestion results in increased permeability of small blood vessels and inflammation and necrosis of the intestinal mucosa; these changes manifest as hemorrhagic gastroenteritis, fluid loss, and hypotension. Delayed cardiomyopathy accompanied by electrocardiographic abnormalities may develop. Symptoms include nausea, vomiting, diarrhea, abdominal pain, delirium, coma, and seizures. A garlicky odor may be detectable on the breath. Acute tubular necrosis and hemolysis may develop. The reported lethal dose of arsenic ranges from 120 to 200 mg in adults and is 2 mg/kg in children. Arsine gas causes severe hemolysis within 3 to 4 h of exposure and can lead to acute tubular necrosis and renal failure.

In chronic arsenic poisoning, the onset of symptoms comes at 2 to 8 weeks. Typical findings are skin and nail changes, such as hyperkeratosis, hyperpigmentation, exfoliative dermatitis, and Mees' lines (transverse white striae of the fingernails); sensory and motor polyneuritis manifesting as numbness and tingling in a "stocking-glove" distribution, distal weakness, and quadriplegia; and inflammation of the respiratory mucosa. Epidemiologic evidence has linked chronic consumption of water containing arsenic at concentrations in the range of 10 to 1820 ppb with vasospasm and peripheral vascular insufficiency culminating in "blackfoot disease," a gangrenous condition affecting the extremities. Chronic arsenic exposure has also been associated with a greatly elevated risk of skin cancer and possibly of cancers of the lung, liver (angiosarcoma), bladder, kidney, and colon.

LABORATORY FINDINGS When acute arsenic poisoning is suspected, an x-ray of the abdomen may reveal ingested arsenic, which is radiopaque. The serum arsenic level may exceed 0.9 μmol/L (7 μg/dL); however, arsenic is rapidly cleared from the blood. Electrocardiographic findings may include QRS complex broadening, QT prolongation, ST-segment depression, T-wave flattening, and multifocal ventricular tachycardia. Urinary arsenic should be measured in 24-h specimens collected after 48 h of abstinence from seafood ingestion; normally, levels of total urinary arsenic excretion are less than 0.67 μmol/d (50 μg/d). Arsenic may be detected in the hair and nails for months after exposure. Abnormal liver function, anemia, leukocytosis or leukopenia, proteinuria, and hematuria may be detected. Electromyography may reveal features similar to those of Guillain-Barré syndrome.

℞ **TREATMENT**

Vomiting should be induced with ipecac in the alert patient with acute arsenic ingestion. Gastric lavage may be useful; activated charcoal with a cathartic (such as sorbitol) may be tried, although its efficacy is not clear. Aggressive therapy with intravenous fluid and electrolyte replacement in an intensive-care setting may be lifesaving. Dimercaprol is the chelating agent of choice and is administered intramuscularly at an initial dose of 3 to 5 mg/kg on the following schedule: every 4 h for 2 days, every 6 h on the third day, and every 12 h thereafter for 10 days. (An oral chelating agent may be substituted.) Succimer is sometimes an effective alternative, particularly if adverse reactions to dimercaprol develop (such as nausea, vomiting, headache, increased blood pressure, and convulsions). In cases of renal failure, doses should be adjusted carefully, and hemodialysis may be needed to remove the chelating agent–arsenic complex. Arsine gas poisoning should be treated supportively with the goals of maintaining renal function and circulating red-cell mass. Other than the avoidance of additional exposure, specific treatment is not of proven benefit in chronic arsenic toxicity. Recovery, particularly from the resulting peripheral neuropathy, may take months and may never be complete.

CADMIUM

SOURCE Environmental exposure to cadmium can result from the ingestion of basic foodstuffs, especially grains, cereals, and leafy vegetables, which readily absorb cadmium occurring naturally or in soil contaminated by sewage sludge, fertilizers, and polluted groundwater. Serious cadmium poisoning can follow the contamination of food and water by mining effluents, as took place in the 1946 outbreak of *itai-itai* ("ouch-ouch") disease (so named because cadmium-induced bone toxicity caused painful bone fractures) in the Jintzu River basin in Japan. Airborne cadmium can be released during smelting or during the incineration of municipal waste containing plastics and nickel-cadmium batteries. Cigarette smoke contains cadmium. Occupational exposure takes place in the metal-plating, pigment, battery, and plastics industries.

METABOLISM The normal daily intake of cadmium through ingestion or inhalation is from 20 to 40 μg, although only 5 to 10 percent of this amount is absorbed. Most absorbed cadmium is concentrated in the liver and kidneys. In erythrocytes and soft tissues, cadmium is bound to metallothionein, a low-molecular-weight protein that mitigates the toxicity of the unbound ion. This complex is filtered at the glomerulus but is then reabsorbed by the proximal tubules. The lack of an effective elimination pathway is responsible for cadmium's biologic half-life of 10 to 30 years. The toxicity of cadmium may involve its binding to key cellular sulfhydryl groups, its competition with other metals (zinc and selenium) for inclusion in metalloenzymes, and its competition with calcium for binding sites on regulatory proteins such as calmodulin.

CLINICAL TOXICOLOGY Acute high-dose cadmium inhalation can cause severe respiratory irritation with pleuritic chest pain, dyspnea, cyanosis, fever, tachycardia, nausea, and life-threatening noncardiogenic pulmonary edema. The onset of symptoms may be delayed from 4 to 24 h. Acute exposure through ingestion can cause severe nausea, vomiting, salivation, abdominal cramps, and diarrhea. Single lethal oral doses have reportedly ranged from 350 to 8900 mg. Chronic effects of cadmium exposure are dose-dependent and include anosmia, yellowing of the teeth, emphysema, minor changes in liver function, microcytic hypochromic anemia unresponsive to iron therapy, renal tubular dysfunction characterized by proteinuria and increased urinary excretion of β_2-microglobulin, and (with prolonged poisoning) osteomalacia leading to bone lesions and pseudofractures. In follow-up studies of occupationally exposed workers, β_2-microglobulinuria was found to be irreversible. Associations with hypertension, prostate cancer, and lung cancer have been suggested by some studies but await confirmation.

LABORATORY FINDINGS The daily level of excretion of cadmium by persons without known cadmium exposures is usually below 10 nmol/L (1 μg/L or 1 μg/g of creatinine). This level increases somewhat with age and smoking. Toxicity, including renal dysfunction, is considered unlikely until the urinary cadmium level exceeds 100 nmol/L (10 μg/g of creatinine). Serum cadmium levels reflect recent rather than chronic exposure and generally are below 30 nmol/L (0.3 μg/dL) in unexposed persons. A blood level exceeding 500 nmol/L (5 μg/dL) is considered toxic. An increased urinary concentration of β_2-microglobulin is the most sensitive indicator of an elevated cadmium dose and of nephropathy but may also be detected in other renal diseases, such as chronic pyelonephritis.

℞ **TREATMENT**

There is no proven effective treatment for cadmium poisoning. Succimer has been used as an antagonist for cadmium intoxication in animals. Although there is no published experience in humans, this drug might be considered for therapy. Chelation therapy is not useful, and use of dimercaprol is contraindicated as this agent may exacerbate nephrotoxicity. Avoidance of further exposure and supportive therapy (including vitamin D if osteomalacia exists) are the mainstays of management.

BIBLIOGRAPHY

GENERAL

APOSHIAN HV et al: Mobilization of heavy metals by newer, therapeutically useful chelating agents. Toxicology 97:23, 1995

CHRISTENSEN J: Human exposure to toxic metals: Factors influencing interpretation of biomonitoring results. Sci Total Environ 166:89, 1995

FRIBERG L, ELINDER CG: Biological monitoring of toxic metals. Scand J Work Environ Health 1:7, 1993

GOYER RA: Nutrition and metal toxicity. Am J Clin Nutr 61:646S, 1995

WENNBERG A: Neurotoxic effects of selected metals. Scand J Work Environ Health 20:65, 1994

LEAD

BALBUS-KORNFELD JM et al: Cumulative exposure to inorganic lead and neurobehavioural test performance in adults: An epidemiological review. Occup Environ Med 52:2, 1995

GOLDMAN R et al: Lead poisoning from mobilization of bone stores during thyrotoxicosis. Am J Ind Med 25:417, 1994

HU H et al: The relationship between bone lead and hemoglobin. JAMA 272:1512, 1994

———— et al: The relationship of blood and bone lead to hypertension among middle-aged to elderly men. JAMA 275:1171, 1996

KIM R et al: A longitudinal study of low-level lead exposure and renal function in men from the Normative Aging Study. JAMA 275:1177, 1996

LOCKITCH G: Perspectives on lead toxicity. Clin Biochem 26:371, 1993

SMITH MC et al: A polymorphism in the delta-aminolevulinic acid dehydratase gene is a possible modifier of the pharmacokinetics of lead. Environ Health Perspect 103:248, 1995

MERCURY

CLARKSON TW: Mercury: Major issues in environmental health. Environ Health Perspect 100:31, 1993

CORBIN SB, KOHN WG: The benefits and risks of dental amalgam: Current findings reviewed. J Am Dent Assoc 125:381, 1994

ENESTROM S, HULTMAN P: Does amalgam affect the immune system? A controversial issue. Int Arch Allergy Immunol 106:180, 1995

HARADA M: Minamata disease: Methylmercury poisoning in Japan caused by environmental pollution. Crit Rev Toxicol 25:1, 1995

NGIM CH et al: Chronic neurobehavioural effects of elemental mercury in dentists. Br J Ind Med 49:782, 1992

ROELS HA et al: Urinary excretion of mercury after occupational exposure to mercury vapour and influence of the chelating agent meso-w,e-dimercaptosuccinic acid (DMSA). Br J Ind Med 48:247, 1991

ARSENIC

BATES MN et al: Arsenic ingestion and internal cancers: A review. Am J Epidemiol 135:462, 1992

HEAVEN R et al: Arsenic intoxication presenting with macrocytosis and peripheral neuropathy, without anaemia. Acta Haematol 92:142, 1994

KELAFANT GA et al: Arsenic poisoning in central Kentucky: A case report. Am J Ind Med 24:723, 1993

CADMIUM

BASINGER MA et al: Antagonists for acute oral cadmium chloride intoxication. J Toxicol Environ Health 23:77, 1988.

LAUWERYS RR et al: Cadmium: Exposure markers as predictors of nephrotoxic effects. Clin Chem 40:1391, 1994

STAESSEN J, LAUWERYS R: Health effects of environmental exposure to cadmium in a population study. J Hum Hypertens 7:195, 1993

WAALKES MP, REHM S: Cadmium and prostate cancer. J Toxicol Environ Health 43:251, 1994

A

LABORATORY VALUES OF CLINICAL IMPORTANCE

INTRODUCTORY COMMENTS

All laboratory appendices should be interpreted with caution since normal values differ widely among clinical laboratories. The values given in this Appendix are meant primarily for use with this text. In preparing the Appendix, the editors have taken into account the fact that the system of international units (SI, système international d'unités) is now used in most countries and in most medical and scientific journals.[1] However, clinical laboratories in many countries continue to report values in traditional units. Therefore, both systems are used in the Appendix. Values in SI units appear first, and traditional units appear in parentheses after the SI units. The dual system is also used in the text except for (1) those instances in which the numbers remain the same but only the terminology is changed (mmol/L for meq/L or IU/L for mIU/mL), when only the SI units are given; and (2) most pressure measurements (e.g., blood and cerebrospinal fluid pressures), when the traditional units (mmHg, mmH$_2$O) are used. In all other instances in the text the SI unit is followed by the traditional unit in parentheses. The SI base units, SI derived units, other units of measure referred to in Appendix A, and SI prefixes are listed in Tables A-1 to A-3 at the end of Appendix A. Conversions from one system to another can be made as follows:

$$mmol/L = \frac{mg/dL \times 10}{atomic\ weight}$$

$$mg/dL = \frac{mmol/L \times atomic\ weight}{10}$$

ASCITIC FLUID

See Chapter 46

BODY FLUIDS AND OTHER MASS DATA

Body fluid, total volume: 50 percent (in obese) to 70 percent (lean) of body weight
    Intracellular: 0.3–0.4 of body weight
    Extracellular: 0.2–0.3 of body weight
Blood
    Total volume:
        Males: 69 mL per kg body weight
        Females: 65 mL per kg body weight
    Plasma volume:
        Males: 39 mL per kg body weight
        Females: 40 mL per kg body weight
    Red blood cell volume:
        Males: 30 mL per kg body weight (1.15–1.21 L/m^2 of body surface area)
        Females: 25 mL per kg body weight (0.95–1.00 L/m^2 of body surface area)

[1] Young DS: Implementation of SI units for clinical laboratory data. Ann Intern Med 106:114, 1987

CEREBROSPINAL FLUID[2]

		Conversion Factor (CF) C × CF = SI
Osmolarity	292–297 mmol/kg water (292–297 mOsm/L)	—
Electrolytes:		
Sodium	137–145 mmol/L (137–145 meq/L)	—
Potassium	2.7–3.9 mmol/L (2.7–3.9 meq/L)	—
Calcium	1.0–1.5 mmol/L (2.1–3.0 meq/L)	0.5
Magnesium	1.0–1.2 mmol/L (2.0–2.5 meq/L)	0.5
Chloride	116–122 mmol/L (116–122 meq/L)	—
CO$_2$ content	20–24 mmol/L (20–24 meq/L)	—
P$_{CO_2}$	6–7 kPa (45–49 mmHg)	0.1333
pH	7.31–7.34	—
Glucose	2.2–3.9 mmol/L (40–70 mg/dL)	0.05551
Lactate	1–2 mmol/L (10–20 mg/dL)	0.1110
Total protein:	0.2–0.5 g/L (20–50 mg/dL)	0.01
Albumin	0.066–0.442 g/L (6.6–44.2 mg/dL)	0.01
IgG	0.009–0.057 g/L (0.9–5.7 mg/dL)	0.01
IgG index[3]	0.29–0.59	
Oligoclonal bands (OGB)	<2 bands not present in matched serum sample	
Ammonia	15–47 μmol/L (25–80 μg/dL)	0.5872
Creatinine	44–168 μmol/L (0.5–1.9 mg/dL)	88.40
Myelin basic protein	<4 μg/L	—
CSF pressure	50–180 mmH$_2$O	—
CSF volume (adult)	~150 mL	—
Leukocytes		
Total	<5 per mL	—
Differential:		
Lymphocytes	60–70 percent	
Monocytes	30–50 percent	
Neutrophils	None	—

[2] Since cerebrospinal fluid concentrations are equilibrium values, measurements of the same parameters in blood plasma obtained at the same time are recommended. However, there is a time lag in attainment of equilibrium, and cerebrospinal levels of plasma constituents that can fluctuate rapidly (such as plasma glucose) may not achieve stable values until after a significant lag phase.

[3] $IgG\ index = \dfrac{CSF\ IgG(mg/dL) \times serum\ albumin(g/dL)}{Serum\ IgG(g/dL) \times CSF\ albumin(mg/dL)}$

CHEMICAL CONSTITUENTS OF BLOOD

See also function tests, especially "Metabolic and Endocrine Tests."

	Conversion Factor (CF) $C \times CF = SI$
Acetoacetate, plasma: <100 μmol/L (<1 mg/dL)	97.95
Albumin, serum: 35–55 g/L (3.5–5.5 g/dL)	10.00
Aldolase: 0–100 nkat/L (0–6 U/L)	16.67
Alpha$_1$ antitrypsin, serum: 0.8–2.1 g/L (85–213 mg/dL)	0.01
Alpha fetoprotein (adult), serum: <30 μg/L (<30 ng/mL)	—
Aminotransferases, serum:	
Aspartate (AST, SGOT): 0–0.58 μkat/L (0–35 U/L)	0.01667
Alanine (ALT, SGPT): 0–0.58 μkat/L (0–35 U/L)	0.01667
Ammonia, as NH$_3$, plasma: 6–47 μmol/L (10–80 μg/dL)	0.5872
Amylase, serum: 0.8–3.2 μkat/L; 60–180 U/L	0.01667
Angiotensin-converting enzyme (ACE): <670 nkat/L (<40 U/L)	16.67
Anticonvulsant drug levels: see Fig. 365-8	
Arterial blood gases:	
[HCO$_3^-$]: 21–28 mmol/L (21–30 meq/L)	—
P$_{CO_2}$: 4.7–5.9 kPa (35–45 mmHg)	0.1333
pH: 7.38–7.44	—
P$_{O_2}$: 11–13 kPa (80–100 mmHg)	0.1333
Ascorbic acid (vitamin C), serum: 23–57 μmol/L (0.4–1.0 mg/dL)	56.78
Barbiturates, serum: normal, nondetectable	
Phenobarbital, "potentially fatal" level: approximately 390 μmol/L (9 mg/dL)	43.06
Most short-acting barbiturates, "potentially fatal" levels: approximately 150 μmol/L (35 mg/L)	4.419
β-Hydroxybutyrate, plasma: <300 μmol/L (<3 mg/dL)	96.05
Bilirubin, total, serum (Malloy-Evelyn): 5.1–17 μmol/L (0.3–1.0 mg/dL)	17.10
Direct, serum: 1.7–5.1 μmol/L (0.1–0.3 mg/dL)	17.10
Indirect, serum: 3.4–12 μmol/L (0.2–0.7 mg/dL)	17.10
Calciferols (vitamin D), plasma:	
1,25-dihydroxyvitamin D [1,25(OH)$_2$D]: 40–160 pmol/L (16 to 65 pg/mL)	2.4
25-hydroxyvitamin D [25(OH)D]: 20–200 nmol/L (8–80 ng/mL)	2.496
Calcium, ionized: 1.1–1.4 mmol/L (4.5–5.6 mg/dL)	0.2495
Calcium, plasma: 2.2–2.6 mmol/L (9–10.5 mg/dL)	0.2495
Carbon dioxide content, plasma (sea level): 21–30 mmol/L (21–30 meq/L)	—
Carbon dioxide tension (P$_{CO_2}$), arterial blood (sea level): 4.7–5.9 kPa (35–45 mmHg)	0.1333
Carbon monoxide content, blood: symptoms with over 20 percent saturation of hemoglobin	
Carotenoids, serum: 0.9–5.6 μmol/L (50–300 μg/dL)	0.01863
Ceruloplasmin, serum: 270–370 mg/L (27–37 mg/dL)	10.00
Chloride, serum (as Cl$^-$): 98–106 mmol/L (98–106 meq/L)	—
Cholesterol: see Table A-4	
Complement, serum:	
C3: 0.55–1.20 g/L (55–120 mg/dL)	0.01
C4: 0.20–0.50 g/L (20–50 mg/dL)	0.01
Copper, serum: 11–22 μmol/L (70–140 μg/dL)	0.1574

	Conversion Factor (CF) $C \times CF = SI$
Creatine kinase, serum (total):	
Females: 0.17–1.17 μkat/L (10–70 U/L)	0.01667
Males: 0.42–1.50 μkat/L (25–90 U/L)	0.01667
Creatine kinase-MB: 0–7 μg/L	—
Creatinine, serum: <133 μmol/L (<1.5 mg/dL)	88.40
Digoxin serum:	
Therapeutic level: 0.6–2.8 nmol/L (0.5–2.2 ng/mL)	1.281
Toxic level: >3.1 nmol/L (>2.4 ng/mL)	1.281
Ethanol, blood:	
Behavioral changes: >4.3 mmol/L (>20 mg/dL)	0.2171
Legal intoxication: >17 mmol/L (>80 mg/dL)	0.2171
Coma and death: >65 mmol/L (>300 mg/dL)	0.2171
Fatty acids, free (nonesterified), plasma: 180 mg/L (<18 mg/dL)	10.00
Ferritin, serum:	
Women: 10–200 μg/L (10–200 ng/ml)	
Men: 15–400 μg/L (15–400 ng/ml)	
Fibrinogen, plasma: see "Hematologic Evaluations: Platelets and Coagulation"	—
Fibrinogen split products: see "Hematologic Evaluations: Platelets and Coagulation"	—
Folic acid, red cell: 340–1020 nmol/L cells (150–450 ng/mL cells)	2.266
Folic acid, serum: 7–36 nmol/L cells (3–16 ng/mL cells)	—
Gastrin, serum: 40–200 ng/L (40–200 pg/mL)	—
Glucose (fasting), plasma:	
Normal: 4.2–6.4 mmol/L (75–115 mg/dL)	0.05551
Diabetes mellitus: >7.8 mmol/L [>140 mg/dL (on more than one occasion)]	0.05551
Glucose, 2 h postprandial, plasma:	
Normal: <7.8 mmol/L (<140 mg/dL)	0.05551
Impaired glucose tolerance: 7.8–11.1 mmol/L (140–200 mg/dL)	0.05551
Diabetes mellitus: >11.1 mmol/L on more than one occasion (>200 mg/dL)	0.05551
Hemoglobin, blood (sea level):	
Male: 140–180 g/L (14–18 g/dL)	10.00
Female: 120–160 g/L (12–16 g/dL)	10.00
Hemoglobin A$_{1c}$: up to 6 percent of total hemoglobin	—
Immunoglobulins, serum:	
IgA: 0.9–3.2 g/L (90–325 mg/dL)	0.01
IgD: 0–0.08 g/L (0–8 mg/dL)	0.01
IgE: <0.00025 g/L (<0.025 mg/dL)	0.01
IgG: 8.0–15.0 g/L (800–1500 mg/dL)	0.01
IgM: 0.45–1.5 g/L (45–150 mg/dL)	0.01
Iron, serum: 9–27 μmol/L (50–150 μg/dL)	0.1791
Iron-binding capacity, serum: 45–66 μmol/L (250–370 μg/dL)	0.1791
Saturation: 0.2–0.45 (20–45 percent)	
Lactate dehydrogenase, serum: 1.7–3.2 μkat/L (100–190 U/L)	0.01667
Lactate dehydrogenase isoenzymes, serum (agarose):	
Fraction 1 (of total): 0.14–0.25 (14–26 percent)	0.01
Fraction 2: 0.29–0.39 (29–39 percent)	0.01
Fraction 3: 0.20–0.25 (20–26 percent)	0.01
Fraction 4: 0.08–0.16 (8–16 percent)	0.01
Fraction 5: 0.06–0.16 (6–16 percent)	0.01
Lactate, venous plasma: 0.6–1.7 mmol/L (5–15 mg/dL)	0.1110
Lead, serum: <1.0 μmol/L (<20 μg/dL)	0.04826
Lipase, serum: 0–2.66 μkat/L (0–160 U/L)	0.01667
Lipids: see Table A-4	

	Conversion Factor (CF) C × CF = SI
Lipids, triglyceride, serum: see "Triglycerides"	—
Lipoprotein: see Table A-4	—
Lithium, serum:	
Therapeutic level: 0.6–1.2 mmol/L (0.6–1.2 meq/L)	—
Toxic level: >2 mmol/L (2 meq/L)	—
Magnesium, serum: 0.8–1.2 mmol/L (1.8–3 mg/dL)	0.4114
Osmolality, plasma: 285–295 mmol/kg serum water (285–295 mosmol/kg serum water)	
Oxygen content:	
Arterial blood (sea level): 17–21 volume percent	—
Venous blood, arm (sea level): 10 to 16 volume percent	—
Oxygen percent saturation (sea level):	
Arterial blood: 0.97 mol/mol (97 percent)	0.01
Venous blood, arm: 0.60–0.85 mol/mol (60–85 percent)	0.01
Oxygen tension (P_{O_2}) blood: 11–13 kPa (80–100 mmHg)	0.1333
pH, blood: 7.38–7.44	—
Phenytoin, plasma: See Fig. 365-8	
Phosphatase, acid, serum: 0.90 nkat/L (0–5.5 U/L)	—
Phosphatase, alkaline, serum: 0.5–2.0 nkat/L (30–120 U/L)	—
Phosphorus, inorganic, serum: 1.0–1.4 mmol/L (3–4.5 mg/dL)	0.3229
Potassium, serum: 3.5–5.0 mmol/L (3.5–5.0 meq/L)	—
Protein, total, serum: 55–80 g/L (5.5–8.0 g/dL)	10.00
Protein fractions, serum:	
Albumin: 35–55 g/L [3.5–5.5 g/dL (50–60 percent)]	10.00
Globulin: 20–35 g/L [2.0–3.5 g/dL (40–50 percent)]	10.00
Alpha$_1$: 2–4 g/L [0.2–0.4 g/dL (4.2–7.2 percent)]	10.00
Alpha$_2$: 5–9 g/L [0.5–0.9 g/dL (6.8–12 percent)]	10.00
Beta: 6–11 g/L [0.6–1.1 g/dL (9.3–15 percent)]	10.00
Gamma: 7–17 g/L [0.7–1.7 g/dL (13–23 percent)]	10.00
Pyruvate, venous, plasma: 60–170 μmol/L (0.5–1.5 mg/dL)	113.6
Quinidine, serum:	
Therapeutic range: 4.6–9.2 μmol/L (1.5–3 mg/L)	3.082
Toxic range: 15.4–18.5 μmol/L (5–6 mg/L)	3.082
Salicylate, plasma: 0 mmol/L	—
Therapeutic range: 1.4–1.8 mmol/L (20–25 mg/dL)	0.07240
Toxic range: >2.2 mmol/L (>30 mg/dL)	0.07240
Sodium, serum: 136–145 mmol/L (136–145 meq/L)	—
Steroids: see "Metabolic and Endocrine Tests"	—
Transferrin, serum: 2.3–3.9 mg/L (230–390 μg/dL)	10.00
Triglycerides: <1.8 mmol/L (<160 mg/dL)	0.01129
Troponin I, serum: 0–0.4 μg/L (0–0.4 ng/mL)	—
Troponin T, serum: 0–0.1 μg/L (0–0.1 ng/mL)	—
Urea nitrogen, serum: 3.6–7.1 mmol/L (10–20 mg/dL)	0.3570
Uric acid, serum:	
Men: 150–480 μmol/L (2.5–8.0 mg/dL)	59.48
Women: 90–360 μmol/L (1.5–6.0 mg/dL)	59.48
Vitamin A, serum: 0.7–3.5 μmol/L (20–100 μg/dL)	0.03491
Vitamin B$_{12}$, serum: 148–443 pmol/L (200–600 pg/mL)	0.7378
Zinc, serum: 11.5–18.5 μmol/L (75–120 μg/dL)	0.1530

CIRCULATORY FUNCTION TESTS

Arteriovenous oxygen difference: 30–50 mL/L
Cardiac output (Fick): 2.5–3.6 L/m^2 of body surface area per minute
Contractility indexes:
    Maximum left ventricular dp/dt: 1650 mmHg/s (range, 1320–1880, mmHg/s)
    (dp/dt)/DP when DP = 40 mmHg: 37.6 ±12.2 s^{-1} (DP, diastolic pressure)
    Mean normalized systolic ejection rate (angiography): 3.32 ± 0.84 end-diastolic volumes per second
    Mean velocity of circumferential fiber shortening (angiography) 1.66 ± 0.42 circumferences per second
Ejection fraction, stroke volume/end-diastolic volume (SV/EDV): normal range: 0.55–0.78; average: 0.67
End-diastolic volume: 75 mL/m^2 (range, 60–88 mL/m^2)
End-systolic volume: 25 mL/m^2 (range, 20–33 mL/m^2)
Left ventricular work:
    Stroke work index: 30–110 (g·m)/m^2
    Left ventricular minute work index: 1.8–6.6 [(kg·m)/m^2]/min
    Oxygen consumption index: 110–150 mL
Maximum oxygen uptake: normal range 20–60 mL/min; average: 35 mL/min
Pulmonary vascular resistance: 20–120 (dyn·s)/cm^5 (2–12 kPa·s/L)
Systemic vascular resistance: 770–1500 (dyn·s)/cm^5 (77–150 kPa·s/L)

GASTROINTESTINAL TESTS

See also "Stool Analysis."

Absorption tests:
    D-Xylose absorption test: After an overnight fast, 25 g xylose is given in aqueous solution by mouth. Urine collected for the following 5 h should contain 33–53 mmol (5–8 g) (or >20 percent of ingested dose). Serum xylose should be 1.7–2.7 mmol (25–40 mg/dL) 1 h after the oral dose.
    Vitamin A absorption test: A fasting blood specimen is obtained and 200,000 units of vitamin A in oil is given by mouth. Serum vitamin A levels should rise to twice fasting level in 3–5 h.
Bentiromide test (pancreatic function): 500 mg bentiromide (chymex) orally; p-aminobenzoic acid (PABA) measured in plasma and/or urine
    Plasma: >3.6 (±1.1) μg/mL at 90 min
    Urine: >50 percent recovered as PABA in 6 h
Gastric juice:
    Volume:

	Conversion Factor (CF) C × CF = SI
24 h: 2–3 L	
Nocturnal: 600–700 mL	
Basal, fasting: 30–70 mL/h	
Reaction:	
pH: 1.6–1.8	
Titratable acidity of fasting juice: 4–9 μmol/s (15–35 meq/h)	0.261
Acid output:	
Basal:	
Females (mean ± 1 SD): 0.6 ± 0.5 ρmol/s (2.0 ± 1.8 meq/h)	0.2778
Males (mean ± 1 SD): 0.8 ± 0.6 μmol/s (3.0 ± 2.0 meq/h)	0.2778
Maximal (after subcutaneous histamine acid phosphate 0.004 mg/kg body weight and preceded by 50 mg promethazine or after betazole 1.7 mg/kg body wt or pentagastrin 6 μg/kg body wt):	
Females (mean ± 1 SD): 4.4 ± 1.4 μmol/s (16 ± 5 meq/h)	0.2778
Males (mean ± 1 SD): 6.4 ± 1.4 μmol/s (23 ± 5 meq/h)	0.2778

Conversion
Factor (CF)
C × CF = SI

Basal acid output/maximal acid output ratio: 0.6 or less

Gastrin, serum: 40–200 ng/L (40–200 pg/mL) —

Secretin test (pancreatic exocrine function): 1 unit per kg body wt, intravenously

Volume (pancreatic juice): >2.0 mL/kg in 80 min —

Bicarbonate concentration: >80 mmol/L (>80 meq/L) —

Bicarbonate output: >10 mmol in 30 min (>10 meq in 30 min) —

METABOLIC AND ENDOCRINE TESTS

Conversion
Factor (CF)
C × CF = SI

Adrenocorticotropin (ACTH) plasma, 8 A.M.: 2–11 pmol/L (9–52 pg/mL) | 0.2202

Adrenal cortex function tests: see Chap. 332 —

Adrenal medulla function tests: see Chap. 333 —

Adrenal steroids, plasma:

Aldosterone, 8 A.M.: <220 pmol/L (patient supine, 100 meq Na and 60–100 meq K intake) (<8 ng/dL) | 27.74

Cortisol:

8 A.M.: 140–690 nmol/L (5–25 μg/dL) | 27.59

4 P.M.: 80–330 nmol/L (3–12 μg/dL) | 27.59

Dehydroepiandrosterone (DHEA): 7–31 nmol/L (2–9 μg/L) | 3.467

Dehydroepiandrosterone sulfate (DHEA sulfate): 1.3–6.8 μmol/L (500–2500 μg/L) | 0.002714

11-Deoxycortisol (compound S): <30 nmol/L (<1 μg/dL) | 28.86

17-Hydroxyprogesterone:

Women: follicular phase, 0.6–3 nmol/L (0.20–1 μg/L); luteal phase 1.5–10.6 nmol/L (0.5–3.5 μg/L) | 3.026 / 3.026

Men: 0.2–9 nmol/L (0.06–3 μg/L) | 3.026

Adrenal steroids, urinary excretion

Aldosterone: 14–53 nmol/d (5–19 μg/d) | 2.774

Cortisol, free: 55–275 nmol/d (20–100 μg/d) | 2.759

17-Hydroxycorticosteroids: 5.5–28 μmol/d (2–10 mg/d) | 2.759

17-Ketosteroids:

Men: 20–69 ρmol/d (6–20 mg/d) | 3.467

Women: 20–59 μmol/d (6–17 mg/d) | 3.467

Angiotensin II, plasma, 8 A.M.: 10–30 nmol/L (10–30 pg/mL) —

Arginine vasopressin (AVP), plasma:

Random fluid intake: 1.5–5.6 pmol/L (1.5–6 ng/L) | 0.92

Calcitonin, plasma: <50 ng/L (<50 pg/mL) —

Catecholamines, urinary excretion:

Free catecholamines: <590 nmol/d (<100 μg/d) | 5.911

Epinephrine: <275 nmol/d (<50 μg/d) | 5.458

Metanephrines: <7 μmol/d (<1.3 mg/d) | 5.458

Norepinephrine: 89–473 nmol/d (15–80 μg/d) | 5.91

Vanillylmandelic acid (VMA): <40 μmol/d (<8 mg/d) | 5.046

Glucagon, plasma: 50–100 ng/L (50–100 pg/mL) —

Gonadal function tests: see Chaps. 336 and 337 —

Gonadal steroids, plasma:

Androstenedione:

Women: 3.5–7.0 nmol/L (1–2 ng/mL) | 3.492

Men: 3.0–5.0 nmol/L (0.8–1.3 ng/mL) | 3.492

Conversion
Factor (CF)
C × CF = SI

Estradiol:

Women: 70–220 pmol/L (20–60 pg/mL), higher at ovulation | 3.671

Men: <180 pmol/L (<50 pg/mL) | 3.671

Progesterone:

Men, prepubertal girls, preovulatory women, and postmenopausal women: <6 nmol/L (<2 ng/mL) | 3.180

Women, luteal, peak: 6–60 nmol/L (2–20 ng/mL) | 3.180

Testosterone:

Women: <3.5 nmol/L (<1 ng/mL) | 3.467

Men: 10–35 nmol/L (3–10 ng/mL) | 3.467

Prepubertal boys and girls: 0.17–0.7 nmol/L (0.05–0.2 ng/mL) | 3.467

Gonadotropins, plasma:

Women, mature, premenopausal, except at ovulation:

FSH: 1.4–9.6 IU/L (1.4–9.6 mIU/mL) —

LH: 0.8–26 IU/L (0.8–26 mIU/mL) —

Ovulatory surge:

FSH: 2.3–21 IU/L (2.3–21 mIU/mL) —

LH: 25–57 IU/L (25–57 mIU/mL) —

Postmenopausal women:

FSH: 34–96 IU/L (34–96 mIU/mL) —

LH: 40–104 IU/L (40–104 mIU/mL) —

Men, mature:

FSH: 0.9–15 IU/L (0.9–15 mIU/mL) —

LH: 1.3–13 IU/L (1.3–13 mIU/mL) —

Children of both sexes, prepubertal:

LH: 1.0–5.9 IU/L (1.0–5.9 mIU/mL) —

Growth hormone, after 100 g glucose by mouth: <2 μg/L (<2 ng/ml) —

Human chorionic gonadotropin, β subunit (β-hCG), plasma:

Men and nonpregnant women: <3 IU/L (<3 mIU/mL) —

Insulin, serum or plasma, fasting: 43–186 pmol/L (6–26 μU/mL) | 7.175

Insulin-like growth factor I (somatomedin C, IGF-1/SM C): see Chap. 329 —

Oxytocin: random 1–4 pmol/L (1.25–5 ng/L) | 0.80

Ovulatory peak in women 4–8 pmol/L (5–10 ng/L) —

Pancreatic islet function tests: see Chap. 334 —

Parathyroid function tests: see Chap. 354 —

Pituitary function tests: see Chaps. 328 to 330 —

Pregnancy tests: see Chap. 337 —

Prolactin, serum: 2–15 μg/L (2–15 ng/mL) —

Renin-angiotensin function tests: see Chap. 332 —

Semen analysis: see Chap. 336 —

Thyroid function tests:

Dynamic tests of thyroid function: see Chap. 331 —

Radioactive iodine uptake, 24 h: 5–30 percent (range varies in different areas due to variations in iodine intake) —

Resin T_3 uptake: 0.25–0.35 (25–35 percent) (varies among laboratories; for calculation of free T4 estimate, see Chap. 331) | 0.01

Reverse triiodothyronine (rT_3), plasma: 0.15–0.61 nmol/L (10–40 ng/dL) | 0.01536

Thyroid-stimulating hormone (TSH): 0.4–5 mU/L (0.4–5 μU/mL) —

Thyroxine (T_4), serum radioimmunoassay: 64–154 nmol/L (5–12 μg/dL) | 12.86

Triiodothyronine (T_3), plasma: 1.1–2.9 nmol/L (70–190 ng/dL) | 0.01536

PULMONARY FUNCTION TESTS

See Table A-9

RENAL FUNCTION TESTS

	Conversion Factor (CF) $C \times CF = SI$
Clearances (corrected to 1.72 m² body surface area):	
Measures of glomerular filtration rate:	
Insulin clearance (Cl):	
Males (mean ± 1 SD): 2.1 ± 0.4 mL/s (124 ± 25.8 mL/min)	0.01667
Females (mean ± 1 SD): 2.0 ± 0.2 mL/s (119 ± 12.8 mL/min)	0.01667
Endogenous creatinine clearance: 1.5–2.2 mL/s (91–130 mL/min)	0.01667
Urea: 1.0–1.7 mL/s (60–100 mL/min)	0.01667
Measures of effective renal plasma flow and tubular function:	
p-Aminohippuric acid clearance (Cl_{PAH}):	
Males (mean ± 1 SD): 10.9 ± 2.7 mL/s (654 ± 163 mL/min)	0.01667
Females (mean ± 1 SD): 9.9 ± 1.7 mL/s (594 ± 102 mL/min)	0.01667
Concentration and dilution test:	
Specific gravity of urine:	
After 12-h fluid restriction: 1.025 or more	—
After 12-h deliberate water intake: 1.003 or less	—
Protein excretion, urine: <0.15 g/d (<150 mg/d)	0.01
Males: 0–0.06 g/d (0–60 mg/d)	0.01
Females: 0–0.09 g/d (0–90 mg/d)	0.01
Specific gravity, maximal range: 1.002–1.028	—
Tubular reabsorption, phosphorus: 79–94 percent of filtered load	—

HEMATOLOGIC EVALUATIONS

See also "Chemical Constituents of Blood."

	Conversion Factor (CF) $C \times CF = SI$
Bone marrow: see Table A-6	—
Carboxyhemoglobin:	
Nonsmoker: 0–0.023 (0–2.3 percent)	0.01
Smoker: 0.021–0.042 (2.1–4.2 percent)	0.01
Erythrocyte:	
Count: 4.15–4.90 × 10¹²/L (4.15–4.90 × 10⁶/mm³)	—
Distribution width: 0.13–0.15 (13–15 percent)	—
Glucose-6-phosphate dehydrogenase: 12.1 ± 2 IU/gHb (WHO)	—
Life span:	
Normal survival: 120 days	—
Chromium-labeled, half-life ($t_{1/2}$): 28 days	—
Mean corpuscular hemoglobin (MCH): 28–33 pg/cell (28–33 pg/cell)	—
Mean corpuscular hemoglobin concentration (MCHC): 320–360 g/L (32–36 g/dL)	10.00
Mean corpuscular volume (MCV): 86–98 fl (86–98 μm³)	—
Ham's test (acid serum): negative	—
Haptoglobin, serum 0.5–2.2 g/L (50–220 mg/dL)	0.01
Hematocrit	
Males: 0.42–0.52 (42–52%)	—
Females: 0.37–0.48 (37–48%)	—

	Conversion Factor (CF) $C \times CF = SI$
Hemoglobin:	
Plasma: 0.01–0.05 g/L (1–5 mg/dL)	0.01
Whole blood:	
Males: 8.1–11.2 mmol/L (13–18 g/dL)	—
Females: 7.4–9.9 mmol/L (12–16 g/dL)	—
Hemoglobin A₂ (HbA₂): 0.015–0.035 (1.5–3.5 percent)	0.01
Hemoglobin, fetal (HbF): <0.02 (<2 percent)	0.01
Leukocytes:	
Alkaline phosphatase (LAP): 0.2–1.6 μkat/L (13–100 μ/L)	—
Count: 4.3–10.8 × 10⁹/L (4.3–10.8 × 10³/mm³)	
Differential:	
Neutrophils: 0.45–0.74 (45–74 percent)	
Bands: 0–0.04 (0–4 percent)	
Lymphocytes: 0.16–0.45 (16–45 percent)	
Monocytes: 0.04–0.10 (4–10 percent)	
Eosinophils: 0–0.07 (0–7 percent)	
Basophils: 0–0.02 (0–2 percent)	
Methemoglobin: <2 mg/L (<2 μg/mL)	—
Osmotic fragility:	
Slight hemolysis: 0.45–0.39 percent	—
Complete hemolysis: 0.33–0.30 percent	—
Platelets and coagulation parameters:	
Alpha₂ antiplasmin: 70–130 percent	
Antithrombin III: 80–120 percent	
Bleeding time:	
Simplate: <7 min	
Euglobulin lysis time: >2 h	
Factor II: 60–100 percent	
Factor V: 60–100 percent	
Factor VII: 60–100 percent	
Factor IX: 60–100 percent	
Factor X: 60–100 percent	
Factor XI: 60–100 percent	
Factor XII: 60–100 percent	
Factor XIII: 60–100 percent	
Fibrinogen: 200–400 mg/dL	
Plasminogen: 2.4–4.4 CTA U/mL	
Protein C (antigenic assay): 58–148 percent	
Protein S (antigenic assay): 58–148 percent	
Partial thromboplastin time (activated PTT): comparable to control	
Prothrombin time (quick one-stage): control ± 1 s	
Platelets: 130–400 × 10⁹/L (130,000–400,000/mm³)	
Thrombin time: control ± 3 s	
von Willebrand's antigen: 60–150 percent	
Protoporphyrin, free erythrocyte (FEP): 0.28–0.64 μmol/L of red blood cells (16–36 μg/dL of red blood cells)	0.0177
Red cells: (see "Erythrocytes")	
Schilling test: 7–40 percent of orally administered vitamin B₁₂ excreted in urine	
Sedimentation rate:	
Westergren, <50 years of age:	
Males: 0–15 mm/h	
Females: 0–20 mm/h	
Westergren, >50 years of age:	
Males: 0–20 mm/h	
Females: 0–30 mm/h	
Sucrose hemolysis: negative	
Viscosity	
Plasma: 1.7–2.1	
Serum: 1.4–1.8	
White blood cells: (see "Leukocytes")	

STOOL ANALYSIS

Conversion
Factor (CF)
$C \times CF = SI$

Bulk:
    Wet weight: <197.5 (115 ± 41) g/d — —
    Dry weight: <66.4 (34 ± 15) g/d — —
Alpha$_1$ antitrypsin: 0.98 (±0.17) mg/g dry weight stool — —
Coproporphyrin: 600–1500 nmol/d (400–1000 μg/d)   1.527
Fat (on diet containing at least 50 g fat): <6.0 (4.0 ± 1.5) g/d when measured on a 3-day (or longer) collection
    Percent of dry weight: 0.30 (<30.4 percent)   0.01
    Coefficient of fat absorption: >0.95 (>95 percent)   0.01
Fatty acid:
    Free: 0.01–0.10 (1–10 percent of dry matter)   0.01
    Combined as soap: 0.005–0.12 (0.5–12 percent of dry matter)   0.01
Nitrogen: <1.7 (1.4 ± 0.2) g/d — —
Protein content: minimal — —
Urobilinogen: 68–470 μmol/d (40–280 mg/d)   1.693
Water: 0.65 (approximately 65 percent)   0.01

URINE ANALYSIS

See also "Metabolic and Endocrine Tests"

Conversion
Factor (CF)
$C \times CF = SI$

Acidity, titratable: 20–40 mmol/d (20–40 meq/d) — —
Ammonia: 30–50 mmol/d (30–50 meq/d) — —
Amylase: 35–260 Somogyi units/h — —
Amylase/creatinine clearance ratio [(Cl$_{am}$/Cl$_{cr}$) × 100]: 1–5 — —
Bentiromide (pancreatic function): 50 percent excreted in 6 h as p-amino benzoic acid (PABA) after 500 mg oral bentiromide — —
Calcium (10 meq/d or 200-mg/d calcium diet): <3.8 mmol/d (<7.5 meq/d)   0.5
Catecholamines: see under "Metabolic and Endocrine Tests"
Copper: 0–0.4 μmol/d (0–25 μg/d)   0.01574
Coproporphyrins (types I and III): 150–460 nmol/d (100–300 μg/d)   1.527
Creatine, as creatinine:
    Adult males: <380 μmol/d (<50 mg/d)   7.625
    Adult females: <760 μmol/d (<100 mg/d)   7.625
Creatinine: 8.8–14 mmol/d (1.0–1.6 g/d)   8.840
Glucose, true (oxidase method): 0.3–1.7 mmol/d (50–300 mg/d)   0.5551
5-Hydroxyindoleacetic acid (5-HIAA): 10–47 μmol/d (2–9 mg/d)   5.230
Lead: <0.4 μmol/d (<80 μg/d)   0.004826
Protein: <0.15 g/d (<150 mg/d)   0.1
Porphobilinogen: none — —
Potassium: 25–100 mmol/d [25–100 meq/d (varies with intake)] — —
Sodium: 100–260 mmol/d [100–260 meq/d (varies with intake)] — —
Urobilinogen: 1.7–5.9 μmol/d (1–3.5 mg/d)   1.693
D-Xylose excretion: 5 to 8 g within 5 h after oral dose of 25 g — —

Table A-1

SI and Other Units

Quantity	Name of Unit	Symbol for Unit	Derivation of Units
SI BASE UNITS			
Length	meter	m	
Mass	kilogram	kg	
Time	second	s	
Thermodynamic temperature	Kelvin	K	
Amount of substance	mole	mol	
SI DERIVED UNITS			
Area	square meter	m²	
Force	newton	N	$(m \cdot kg)/s^2$
Pressure	pascal	Pa	$N \cdot m^2$
Work, energy	joule	J	$N \cdot m$
Celsius temperature	degree Celsius	°C	K
OTHER UNITS RETAINED FOR USE			
Time	minute	min	
	hour	h	
	day	d	
Volume	liter	L	

Table A-2

Radiation Derived Units

Quantity	Old Unit	SI Unit	Name for SI Unit (and Abbreviation)	Conversion
Activity	curie (Ci)	Disintegrations per second (dps)	becquerel (Bq)	1 Ci = 3.7 × 10¹⁰ Bq 1 mCi = 37 mBq 1 μCi = 0.037 MBq or 37 GBq 1 Bq = 2.703 × 10⁻¹¹ Ci
Absorbed dose	rad	joule per kilogram (J/kg)	gray (Gy)	1 Gy = 100 rad 1 rad = 0.01 Gy 1 mrad = 10⁻³ cGy
Exposure	roentgen (R)	coulomb per kilogram (C/kg)	—	1 C/kg = 3876 R 1 R = 2.58 × 10⁻⁴ C/kg 1 mR = 258 pC/kg
Dose equivalent	rem	joule per kilogram (J/kg)	sievert (Sv)	1 Sv = 100 rem 1 rem = 0.01 Sv 1 mrem = 10 μSv

Table A-3

SI Prefixes and Their Symbols

Factor	Prefix	Symbol for Prefix
10⁹	giga	G
10⁶	mega	M
10³	kilo	k
10²	hecto	h
10¹	deka	da
10⁻¹	deci	d
10⁻²	centi	c
10⁻³	milli	m
10⁻⁶	micro	μ
10⁻⁹	nano	n
10⁻¹²	pico	p
10⁻¹⁵	femto	f
10⁻¹⁸	alto	a

Table A-4

Classification of Total Cholesterol, LDL-Cholesterol, and HDL-Cholesterol Values

	Total Plasma Cholesterol	LDL-Cholesterol	HDL-Cholesterol	Conversion Factor (C to SI)
Desirable	<5.20 mmol/L (<200 mg/dL)	<3.36 mmol/L (<130 mg/dL)	>1.55 mmol/L (>60 mg/dL)	0.02586
Borderline	5.20–6.18 mmol/L (200–239 mg/dL)	3.36–4.11 mmol/L (130–159 mg/dL)	0.9–1.55 mmol/L (35–60 mg/dL)	0.02586
Undesirable	≥6.21 mmol/L (≥240 mg/dL)	≥4.14 mmol/L (≥ 160 mg/dL)	<0.9 mmol/L (<35 mg/dL)	0.02586

SOURCE: Modified from the report of the Expert Panel on Detection, Evaluation, and Treatment of High Blood Cholesterol in Adults: Second Report of the National Cholesterol Education Program (NCEP) expert panel on detection, evaluation, and treatment of high blood cholesterol (Adult Treatment Panel II). Circulation 89:1329, 1994.

Table A-5

Normal Values of Doppler Echocardiographic Measurements in Adults

	Range	Mean
RVD (cm)	0.9 to 2.6	1.7
LVID (cm)	3.5 to 5.7	4.7
Posterior LV wall thickness (cm)	0.6 to 1.1	0.9
IVS wall thickness (cm)	0.6 to 1.1	0.9
Left atrial dimension (cm)	1.9 to 4.0	2.9
Aortic root dimension (cm)	2.0 to 3.7	2.7
Aortic cusps separation (cm)	1.5 to 2.6	1.9
Percentage of fractional shortening	34 to 44%	36%
Mitral flow (m/sec)	0.6 to 1.3	0.9
Tricuspid flow (m/sec)	0.3 to 0.7	0.5
Pulmonary artery (m/sec)	0.6 to 0.9	0.75
Aorta (m/sec)	1.0 to 1.7	1.35

NOTE: RVD, right ventricular dimension; LVID, left ventricular internal dimension; LV, left ventricle; IVS, interventricular septum.
SOURCE: From H Feigenbaum, *Echocardiography,* 5th ed, Philadelphia. Lea & Febiger, 1994

Table A-6

Differential Nucleated Cell Counts of Bone Marrow

	Normal, Mean%*	Range, %†		Normal, Mean%*	Range, %†
Myeloid	56.7		Erythroid	25.6	
Neutrophilic series	53.6		Pronormoblasts	0.6	0.2–1.3
Myeloblast	0.9	0.2–1.5	Basophilic normoblasts	1.4	0.5–2.4
Promyelocyte	3.3	2.1–4.1	Polychromatophilic normoblasts	21.6	17.9–29.2
Myelocyte	12.7	8.2–15.7			
Metamyelocyte	15.9	9.6–24.6	Orthochromatic normoblasts	2.0	0.4–4.6
Band	12.4	9.5–15.3	Megakaryocytes	<0.1	
Segmented			Lymphoreticular	17.8	
Eosinophilic series	3.1	1.2–5.3	Lymphocytes	16.2	11.1–23.2
Basophilic series	<0.1	0–0.2	Plasma cells	2.3	0.4–3.9
			Reticulum cells	0.3	0–0.9

* From MM Wintrobe et al, *Clinical Hematology,* 8th ed. Philadelphia, Lea & Febiger, 1981.
† Range observed in 12 healthy men.

Table A-7

Erythrocytes and Hemoglobin: Normal Values at Various Ages

Age	Red Blood Cell Count,* 10¹²/L	Hemoglobin,* g/L (g/dL)	Vol. Packed RBCs,* mL/dL	Corpuscular Values			
				MCV, fL	MCH, pg	MCHC, g/L (g/dL)	MCD, μm
Days 1–13	5.1 ± 1.0	195 ± 50 (19.5 ± 5)	54.0 ± 10.0	106–98	38–33	340–360 (36–34)	8.6
Days 14–60	4.7 ± 0.9	140 ± 33 (14 ± 3.3)	42.0 ± 7.0	90	30	330 (33)	8.1
3 months to 10 years	4.5 ± 0.7	122 ± 23 (12.2 ± 2.3)	36.0 ± 5.0	80	27	340 (34)	7.7
11–15 years	4.8	131 (13.14)	39.0	82	28	340 (34)	
Adults:							
Females	4.8 ± 0.6	140 ± 20 (14 ± 2)	42.0 ± 5.0	90 ± 7	29 ± 2	340 ± 20 (34 ± 2)	7.5 ± 0.3
Males	5.4 ± 0.9	160 ± 20 (16 ± 2)	47.0 ± 5.0	90 ± 7	29 ± 2	340 ± 20 (34 ± 2)	7.5 ± 0.3

* The range of values represents almost the extremes of observed variations (93 percent or more) at sea level. The blood values of healthy persons should fall well within these mean ± SD figures.
NOTE: MCV, mean corpuscular volume; MCH, mean corpuscular hemoglobin; MCHC, mean corpuscular hemoglobin concentration; MCD, mean corpuscular diameter.
SOURCE: MM Wintrobe et al, *Clinical Hematology,* 8th ed, Philadelphia, Lea & Febiger, 1981.

Table A-8

Normal Leukocyte Count, Differential Count, and Hemoglobin Concentration at Various Ages

Age	Leukocytes, Total	Neutrophils Total	Band	Segmented	Eosinophils	Basophils	Lymphocytes	Monocytes
12 mo	11.4(6.0–17.5)	3.5(1.5–8.5)	0.35	3.2	0.3(0.05–0.7)	0.05(0–0.20)	7.0(4.0–10.5)	0.55(0.05–1.1)
		31	*3.1*	*28*	*0.4*	*0.4*	*61*	*4.8*
4 yr	9.1(5.5–15.5)	3.8(1.5–8.5)	0.27(0–1.0)	3.5(1.5–7.5)	0.25(0.02–0.65)	0.05(0–0.20)	4.5(2.0–8.0)	0.45(0–0.8)
		42	*3.0*	*39*	*2.8*	*0.6*	*50*	*5.0*
6 yr	4.3(1.5–8.0)	0.25(0–1.0)	4.0(1.5–7.0)	4.0(1.5–7.0)	0.23(0–0.65)	0.05(0–0.20)	3.5(1.5–7.0)	0.40(0–0.8)
		51	*3.0*	*48*	*2.7*	*0.6*	*42*	*4.7*
10 yr	8.1(4.5–13.5)	4.4(1.8–8.0)	0.24(0–1.0)	4.2(1.8–7.0)	0.20(0–0.60)	0.04(0–0.20)	3.1(1.5–6.5)	0.35(0–0.8)
		54	*3.0*	*51*	*2.4*	*0.5*	*38*	*4.3*
21 yr	7.4(4.5–11.0)	4.4(1.8–7.7)	0.22(0–0.7)	4.2(1.8–7.0)	0.20(0–0.45)	0.04(0–0.20)	2.5(1.0–4.8)	0.30(0–0.8)
		59	*3.0*	*56*	*2.7*	*0.5*	*34*	*4.0*

NOTE: Values are expressed as "cells $\times 10^9$/L." The numbers in italic are percentages.

SOURCE: E Beutler et al (eds), *Williams Hematology*, 5th ed, New York, McGraw-Hill, 1995. By permission.

Table A-9

Summary of Values Useful in Pulmonary Physiology

	Symbol	Typical Values Man Aged 40, 75 kg, 175 cm Tall	Woman Aged 40, 60 kg, 160 cm Tall
PULMONARY MECHANICS			
Spirometry—volume-time curves:			
Forced vital capacity	FVC	4.8 L	3.3 L
Forced expiratory volume in 1 s	FEV_1	3.8 L	2.8 L
FEV_1/FVC	$FEV_1\%$	76%	77%
Maximal midexpiratory flow	MMF (FEF 25–27)	4.8 L/s	3.6 L/s
Maximal expiratory flow rate	MEFR (FEF 200–1200)	9.4 L/s	6.1 L/s
Spirometry—flow-volume curves:			
Maximal expiratory flow at 50% of expired vital capacity	V_{max} 50 (FEF 50%)	6.1 L/s	4.6 L/s
Maximal expiratory flow at 75% of expired vital capacity	V_{max} 75 (FEF 75%)	3.1 L/s	2.5 L/s
Resistance to airflow:			
Pulmonary resistance	RL (R_L)	<3.0 (cmH$_2$O/s)/L	
Airway resistance	Raw	<2.5 (cmH$_2$O/s)/L	
Specific conductance	SGaw	>0.13 cmH$_2$O/s	
Pulmonary compliance:			
Static recoil pressure at total lung capacity	Pst TLC	25 ± 5 cmH$_2$O	
Compliance of lungs (static)	CL	0.2 L cmH$_2$O	
Compliance of lungs and thorax	C(L + T)	0.1 L cmH$_2$O	
Dynamic compliance of 20 breaths per minute	C dyn 20	0.25 ± 0.05 L/cmH$_2$O	
Maximal static respiratory pressures:			
Maximal inspiratory pressure	MIP	>90 cmH$_2$O	>50 cmH$_2$O
Maximal expiratory pressure	MEP	>150 cmH$_2$O	>120 cmH$_2$O
LUNG VOLUMES			
Total lung capacity	TLC	6.4 L	4.9 L
Functional residual capacity	FRC	2.2 L	2.6 L
Residual volume	RV	1.5 L	1.2 L
Inspiratory capacity	IC	4.8 L	3.7 L
Expiratory reserve volume	ERV	3.2 L	2.3 L
Vital capacity	VC	1.7 L	1.4 L
GAS EXCHANGE (SEA LEVEL)			
Arterial O$_2$ tension	Pa$_{O_2}$	12.7 ± 0.7 kPa (95 ± 5 mmHg)	
Arterial CO$_2$ tension	Pa$_{CO_2}$	5.3 ± 0.3 kPa (40 ± 2 mmHg)	
Arterial O$_2$ saturation	Sa$_{O_2}$	0.97 ± 0.02 (97 ± 2%)	
Arterial blood pH	pH	7.40 ± 0.02	
Arterial bicarbonate	HCO$_3^-$	24 + 2 meq/L	
Base excess	BE	0 ± 2 meq/L	
Diffusing capacity for carbon monoxide (single breath)	DL$_{CO}$	0.42 mLCO/s/mmHg (25 mL CO/min/mmHg)	
Dead space volume	V$_D$	2 ml/kg body wt	
Physiologic dead space; dead space-tidal volume ratio	V$_D$/V$_T$		
Rest		≤35% V$_T$	
Exercise		≤20% V$_T$	
Alveolar-arterial difference for O$_2$	P(A − a)$_{O_2}$	≤2.7 kPa ≤20 kPa (≤20 mmHg)	

INSTRUCTIONS FOR COLLECTION AND TRANSPORT OF SPECIMENS FOR CULTURE

It is absolutely essential that the microbiology laboratory be informed of the site of origin of the sample to be cultured and of the infections that are suspected. This information determines the selection of culture media and the length of culture time.

Type of Culture (Synonyms)	Specimen	Minimum Volume	Container	Other Considerations
BLOOD				
Blood, routine (blood culture for aerobes, anaerobes, and yeasts)	Whole blood	10 mL in each of 2 bottles for adults and children; 5 mL, if possible, in each of 2 bottles for infants; less for neonates	See below.[a]	See below.[b]
Blood for fungi/ *Mycobacterium* spp.	Whole blood	10 mL in each of 2 bottles, as for routine blood cultures, or in Isolator tube requested from laboratory	Same as for routine blood culture	Specify "hold for extended incubation," since fungal agents may require 4 weeks or more to grow.
Blood, Isolator (lysis centrifugation)	Whole blood	10 mL	Isolator tubes	Use mainly for isolation of fungi, *Mycobacterium,* or other fastidious aerobes and for elimination of antibiotics from cultured blood in which organisms are concentrated by centrifugation.
RESPIRATORY TRACT				
Nose	Swab from nares	1 swab	Sterile culturette or similar transport system containing holding medium	Swabs made of calcium alginate may be used.
Throat	Swab of posterior pharynx, ulcerations, or areas of suspected purulence	1 swab	Sterile culturette or similar swab specimen collection system containing holding medium	See below.[c]
Sputum	Fresh sputum (not saliva)	2 mL	Commercially available sputum collection system or similar sterile container with screw cap	*Cause for rejection:* Care must be taken to ensure that the specimen is sputum and not saliva. Examination of Gram's stain, with number of epithelial cells and PMNs noted, can be an important part of the evaluation process. Induced sputum specimens should not be rejected.
Bronchial aspirates	Transtracheal aspirate, bronchoscopy specimen, or bronchial aspirate	1 mL of aspirate or brush in transport medium	Sterile aspirate or bronchoscopy tube, bronchoscopy brush in a separate sterile container	Special precautions may be required, depending on diagnostic considerations (e.g., *Pneumocystis*).
STOOL				
Stool for routine culture; stool for *Salmonella, Shigella,* and *Campylobacter*	Rectal swab or (preferably) fresh, randomly collected stool	1 g of stool or 2 rectal swabs	Plastic-coated cardboard cup or plastic cup with tight-fitting lid. Other leak-proof containers are also acceptable.	If *Vibrio* spp. are suspected, the laboratory must be notified, and appropriate collection/transport methods should be used.
Stool for *Yersinia, E. coli* O157	Fresh, randomly collected stool	1 g	Plastic-coated cardboard cup or plastic cup with tight-fitting lid	*Limitations:* Procedure requires enrichment techniques.
Stool for *Aeromonas* and *Plesiomonas*	Fresh, randomly collected stool	1 g	Plastic-coated cardboard cup or plastic cup with tight-fitting lid	*Limitations:* Stool should not be cultured for these organisms unless also cultured for other enteric pathogens.

(continued)

Type of Culture (Synonyms)	Specimen	Minimum Volume	Container	Other Considerations
UROGENITAL TRACT				
Urine	Clean-voided urine specimen or urine collected by catheter	0.5 mL	Sterile, leak-proof container with screw cap or special urine transfer tube	See below.[d]
Urogenital secretions	Vaginal or urethral secretions, cervical swabs, uterine fluid, prostatic fluid, etc.	1 swab or 0.5 mL of fluid	Transwab containing Amies transport medium or similar system containing holding medium for *Neisseria gonorrhoeae;* modified Todd-Hewitt broth for group B *Streptococcus* surveillance cultures	Vaginal swab samples for "routine culture" should be discouraged whenever possible unless a particular pathogen is suspected. For detection of multiple organisms (e.g., group B *Streptococcus, Trichomonas, Chlamydia,* or *Candida* spp.), 1 swab per test should be obtained.
BODY FLUIDS, ASPIRATES, AND TISSUES				
Cerebrospinal fluid (lumbar puncture)	Spinal fluid	1 mL for routine cultures; ≥5 mL for *Mycobacterium*	Sterile tube with tight-fitting cap	Do not refrigerate; transfer to laboratory as soon as possible.
Body fluids	Aseptically aspirated body fluids	1 mL for routine cultures	Sterile tube with tight-fitting cap. Specimen may be left in syringe used for collection if the syringe is capped before transport.	For some body fluids (e.g., peritoneal lavage samples), increased volumes are helpful for isolation of small numbers of bacteria.
Biopsy and aspirated materials	Tissue removed at surgery, bone, anticoagulated bone marrow, biopsy samples, or other specimens from normally sterile areas	1 mL of fluid or a 1-g piece of tissue	Sterile "culturette"-type swab or similar transport system containing holding medium. Sterile bottle or jar should be used for tissue specimens.	Accurate identification of specimen and source is critical. Enough tissue should be collected for both microbiologic and histopathologic evaluations.
Wounds	Purulent material or abscess contents obtained from wound or abscess without contamination by normal microflora	2 swabs or 0.5 mL of aspirated pus	Culturette swab or similar transport system or sterile tube with tight-fitting screw cap. For simultaneous anaerobic cultures, send specimen in anaerobic transport device or closed syringe.	*Collection:* Abscess contents or other fluids should be collected in a syringe (see above) when possible to provide an adequate sample volume and an anaerobic environment.
SPECIAL RECOMMENDATIONS				
Fungi	Specimen types listed above may be used. When urine or sputum is cultured for fungi, a first morning specimen is usually preferred.	1 mL or as specified above for individual listing of specimens. Large volumes may be useful for urinary fungi.	Sterile, leak-proof container with tight-fitting cap	*Collection:* Specimen should be transported to microbiology laboratory within 1 h of collection. Contamination with normal flora from skin, rectum, vaginal tract, or other body surfaces should be avoided.
Mycobacterium (acid-fast bacilli)	Sputum, tissue, urine, body fluids	10 mL of fluid or small piece of tissue. Swabs should not be used.	Sterile container with tight-fitting cap	Detection of *Mycobacterium* spp. is improved by use of concentration techniques. Smears and cultures of pleural, peritoneal, and pericardial fluids often have low yields. Multiple cultures from the same patient are encouraged. Culturing in liquid media shortens the time to detection.
Legionella	Pleural fluid, lung biopsy, bronchoalveolar lavage fluid, bronchial/transbronchial biopsy. Rapid transport to laboratory is critical.	1 mL of fluid; any size tissue sample, although a 0.5-g sample should be obtained when possible	—	—
Anaerobic organisms	Aspirated specimens from abscesses or body fluids	1 mL of aspirated fluid or 2 swabs	An appropriate anaerobic transport device is required.[e]	Specimens cultured for obligate anaerobes should be cultured for facultative bacteria as well.

(continued)

Type of Culture (Synonyms)	Specimen	Minimum Volume	Container	Other Considerations
SPECIAL RECOMMENDATIONS (*Continued*)				
Viruses[f]	Respiratory secretions, wash aspirates from respiratory tract, nasal swabs, blood samples (including buffy coats), vaginal and rectal swabs, swab specimens from suspicious skin lesions, stool samples (in some cases)	1 mL of fluid, 1 swab, or 1 g of stool in each appropriate transport medium	Fluid or stool samples in sterile containers or swab samples in viral culturette devices (kept on ice but not frozen) are generally suitable. Plasma samples and buffy coats in sterile collection tubes should be kept at 4 to 8°C. If specimens are to be shipped or kept for a long time, freezing at −80°C is usually adequate.	Most samples for culture are transported in holding medium containing antibiotics to prevent bacterial overgrowth and viral inactivation. Many specimens should be kept cool but not frozen, provided they are transported promptly to the laboratory. Procedures and transport media vary with the agent to be cultured and the duration of transport.

[a] For samples from adults and children, two bottles (smaller for pediatric samples) should be used: one with dextrose phosphate, tryptic soy, or another appropriate broth and the other with thioglycollate or another broth containing reducing agents appropriate for isolation of obligate anaerobes. For special situations (e.g., suspected fungal infection, culture-negative endocarditis, or mycobacteremia), different blood collection systems may be used (Isolator systems; see table).

[b] *Collection:* An appropriate disinfecting technique should be used on both the bottle septum and the patient. Do not allow air bubbles to get into anaerobic broth bottles. *Special considerations:* There is no more important clinical microbiology test than the detection of blood-borne pathogens. The rapid identification of bacterial and fungal agents is a major determinant of patients' survival. Bacteria may be present in blood either continuously (as in endocarditis, overwhelming sepsis, and the early stages of salmonellosis and brucellosis) or intermittently (as in most other bacterial infections, in which bacteria are shed into the blood on a sporadic basis). Most blood culture systems employ two separate bottles containing broth medium: one that is vented in the laboratory for the growth of facultative and aerobic organisms and a second that is maintained under anaerobic conditions. In cases of suspected continuous bacteremia/fungemia, two or three samples should be drawn before the start of therapy, with additional sets obtained if fastidious organisms are thought to be involved. For intermittent bacteremia, two or three samples should be obtained at least 1 h apart during the first 24 h.

[c] Normal microflora includes alpha-hemolytic streptococci, saprophytic *Neisseria* spp., diphtheroids, and *Staphylococcus* spp. Aerobic culture of the throat ("routine") includes screening for and identification of beta-hemolytic *Streptococcus* spp. and other potentially pathogenic organisms. Although considered components of the normal microflora, organisms such as *Staphylococcus aureus, Haemophilus influenzae,* and *Streptococcus pneumoniae* will be identified by most laboratories, if requested. When *Neisseria gonorrhoeae* or *Corynebacterium diphtheriae* is suspected, a special culture request is recommended.

[d] (1) Clean-voided specimens, midvoid specimens, and Foley or indwelling catheter specimens that yield ≥50,000 organisms/mL and from which no more than three species are isolated should have organisms identified. (2) Straight-catheterized, bladder-tap, and similar urine specimens should undergo a complete workup (identification and susceptibility testing) for all potentially pathogenic organisms, regardless of colony count. (3) Certain clinical problems (e.g., acute dysuria in women) may warrant identification and susceptibility testing of isolates present at concentrations of <50,000 organisms/mL.

[e] Aspirated specimens in capped syringes or other transport devices designed to limit oxygen exposure are suitable for the cultivation of obligate anaerobes. A variety of commercially available transport devices may be used. Contamination of specimens with normal microflora from the skin, rectum, vaginal vault, or another body site should be avoided. Collection containers for aerobic culture (such as dry swabs) and inappropriate specimens (such as refrigerated samples; expectorated sputum; stool; gastric aspirates; and vaginal, throat, nose, and rectal swabs) should be rejected as unsuitable.

[f] Laboratories generally use diverse methods to detect viral agents, and the specific requirements for each specimen should be checked before a sample is sent.

Bold number indicates the start of the chapter that contains the main discussion of the topic; numbers with "f" and "t" refer to figure and table pages and are listed at the end of the entries.

Verruga
clin
d

ISBN 0-07-020291-5

90000

9 780070 202917

TOPICAL CONTENTS